HURST'S THE HEART

NOTICE

HURST'S THE HEART

TENTH EDITION

Editors

VALENTIN FUSTER M.D., Ph.D.
Director, The Zena and Michael A. Wiener Cardiovascular Institute
Richard Gorlin, M.D./Heart Research Foundation, Professor of Cardiology, Vice Chairman, Department of Medicine, The Mount Sinai School of Medicine
New York, New York

R. WAYNE ALEXANDER, M.D., PhD.
R. Bruce Logue Professor and Chair
Department of Medicine
Emory University School of Medicine
Atlanta, Georgia

ROBERT A. O'ROURKE, M.D.
Charles Conrad Brown Distinguished Professor in Cardiovascular Disease
University of Texas Health Science Center at San Antonio
San Antonio, Texas

Associate Editors

ROBERT ROBERTS, M.D.
Don W. Chapman Professor of Medicine and Chief of Cardiology
Professor of Cell Biology, Molecular Physiology and Biophysics, Director, Bugher Foundation Center for Molecular Biology in the Cardiovascular System
Baylor College of Medicine
Director, Specialized Center for Research in Heart Failure
Houston, Texas

SPENCER B. KING III, M.D.
J.B. and Dottie Fuqua Chair of Cardiology, The Fuqua Heart Center
Co-Director, Atlanta Cardiovascular Research Institute, Clinical Professor of Medicine
Atlanta, Georgia

HEIN J. J. WELLENS, M.D.
Professor and Chairman of the Department of Cardiology
Academic Hospital Maastricht
Maastricht, The Netherlands

McGRAW-HILL
Medical Publishing Division

New York St. Louis San Francisco Auckland Bogotá Caracas Lisbon London Madrid Mexico City Milan Montreal New Delhi San Juan Singapore Sydney Tokyo Toronto

McGraw-Hill

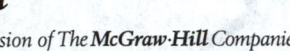

A Division of The **McGraw·Hill** *Companies*

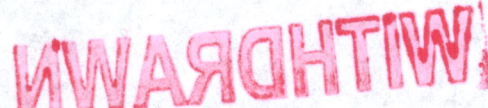

Hurst's
THE HEART
Tenth Edition

1234567890 DOWDOW 09876543210

ISBN 0-07-135694-0 (Single vol. ed.)
0-07-135693-2 (2-vol. set ed.)
0-07-135695-9 (Vol. 1)
0-07-135696-7 (Vol. 2)

This book was set in Times Roman by The PRD Group, Inc.
The editors were Darlene B. Cooke, Susan R. Noujaim, and Lester A. Sheinis.
The production supervisor was Richard C. Ruzycka.
The text designer was Marsha Cohen / Parallelogram Graphics.
The cover designer was Aimee Nordin.
The indexer was Irving Condé Tullar.
R. R. Donnelley and Sons Company was printer and binder.

This book is printed on acid-free paper.

Library of Congress Cataloging-in-Publication Data

Hurst's the heart / editors, Valentin Fuster ... [et al.].—10th ed.
p. ; cm.
Rev. ed. of: Hurst's the heart, arteries and veins. 9th ed. © 1998.
Includes bibliographical references and index.
ISBN 0-07-135694-0 (single vol.)—ISBN 0-07-135693-2 (2 vol. set)
1. Cardiovascular system—Diseases. 2. Heart—Diseases. I. Fuster, Valentin. II. Hurst's the heart, arteries and veins
[DNLM: 1. Cardiovascular Diseases. WG 100 H9662 2001]
RC667.H88 2001
616.1—dc21

00-061611

CONTENTS

Part 3

HEART FAILURE

Part 4

RHYTHM AND CONDUCTION DISORDERS

Part 5

SYNCOPE, SUDDEN DEATH, AND CARDIOPULMONARY RESUSCITATION

Part 6

CORONARY HEART DISEASE

Part 13

THE HEART, ANESTHESIA, AND SURGERY

Part 14

MISCELLANEOUS DISEASES AND CONDITIONS

Part 15

DISEASES OF THE GREAT VESSELS AND PERIPHERAL VESSELS

Part 16

COST-EFFECTIVE STRATEGIES, INSURANCE, AND LEGAL PROBLEMS

CONTRIBUTORS

Masood Akhtar, M.D.
Clinical Professor of Medicine
University of Wisconsin Medical School
Milwaukee Clinical Campus
Sinai Samaritan Medical Center
and St. Luke's Medical Center
Milwaukee Heart Institute
Milwaukee, Wisconsin
Chapter 26

R. Wayne Alexander, M.D., Ph.D.
R. Bruce Logue Professor and Chair
Department of Medicine
Emory University School of Medicine
Atlanta, Georgia
Chapters 6 and 42

Jeffrey L. Anderson, M.D.
Professor of Internal Medicine
Chief
Division of Cardiology
University of Utah School of Medicine
University of Utah Medical Center
Salt Lake City, Utah
Chapter 73

David S. Bach, M.D.
Associate Professor of Medicine
University of Michigan School of Medicine
University of Michigan
Ann Arbor, Michigan
Chapter 74

George L. Bakris, M.D.
Professor of Preventive Medicine and Internal Medicine
Vice-Chairman
Department of Preventive Medicine
Director
Hypertension Clinical Research Center
Rush-Presbyterian-St. Luke's Medical Center
Chicago, Illinois
Chapter 51

Ainat Beniaminovitz, M.D.
Assistant Professor of Medicine
Attending Physician
Columbia Presbyterian Medical Center
New York, New York
Chapter 69

Daniel S. Berman, M.D.
Professor of Medicine
University of California School of Medicine
Director, Nuclear Cardiology
Cedars Sinai Medical Center
Cedars-Sinai Medical Center
Los Angeles, California
Chapter 16

Gerald J. Berry, M.D.
Associate Professor of Pathology
Director of Cardiac Pathology
Stanford University School of Medicine
Stanford University Medical Center
Stanford, California
Chapter 22

Alan L. Bisno, M.D.
Professor and Vice-Chairman
Department of Medicine
University of Miami School of Medicine
Chief, Medical Service
VA Medical Center
Miami, Florida
Chapter 55

Henry R. Black, M.D.
Charles J. and Margaret Roberts Professor
Associate Dean for Research
Rush Medical College
Chair
Department of Preventive Medicine
Rush-Presbyterian-St. Luke's Medical Center
Chicago, Illinois
Chapter 51

Daniel G. Blanchard, M.D.
Associate Professor of Medicine
Director
Non-Invasive Cardiac Laboratories
University of California
San Diego Medical Center
UCSD Medical Center
San Diego, California
Chapter 13

Teresa J. Bohlmeyer, M.D.
Assistant Professor of Medicine
University of Colorado
Health Sciences Center
Division of Cardiology
UCHSC
Denver, Colorado
Chapter 66

Wendy M. Book, M.D.
Assistant Professor
Division of Cardiology
Emory University School of Medicine
Atlanta, Georgia
Chapter 71

Harisios Boudoulas, M.D., Ph.D.
Professor of Medicine and Pharmacy
Academician
Division of Cardiology
Ohio State University Medical Center
Director
Overstreet Teaching and Research Laboratory
Division of Cardiology
Ohio State University Medical Center
Columbus, Ohio
Chapter 32

Michael R. Bristow, M.D., Ph.D.
Professor of Medicine
Head
Division of Cardiology
Director
Temple Hoyne Buell Laboratories
Director
Heart Failure Program
Associate Director
Heart Transplant Program
University of Colorado Health Sciences Center
Denver, Colorado
Chapter 66

Bruce R. Brodie, M.D.
Clinical Professor of Medicine
Director
LeBauer Cardiovascular Research Foundation
University of North Carolina Teaching Service
The Moses H. Cone Memorial Hospital
Greensboro, North Carolina
Chapter 46

Christopher P. Cannon, M.D.
Assistant Professor of Medicine
Harvard Medical School
Associate Physician
Cardiovascular Division
Brigham and Women's Hospital
Associate Physical Cardiovascular Division
Brigham and Women's Hospital
Boston, Massachusetts
Chapter 44

Louis R. Caplan, M.D.
Professor of Neurology
Harvard Medical School
Chief
Cerebrovascular Disease
Beth Israel Deaconess Medical Center
Boston, Massachusetts
Chapter 89

Agustin Castellanos, M.D.
Director
Clinical Electrophysiology
Professor of Medicine
University of Miami—Jackson Memorial Hospital
Miami, Florida
Chapters 11, 24, 31

Simon Chakko, M.D.
Professor of Medicine
Department of Medicine
University of Miami School of Medicine
Chief
Cardiology Section
Veterans Affairs Medical Center
Chief
Cardiology Section
VA Medical Center
Miami, Florida
Chapter 55

Nisha Chandra-Strobos, M.D.
Professor and Director
Coronary Intensive Care Unit
Johns Hopkins Hospital
Division of Cardiology
Bayview Medical Center
Baltimore, Maryland
Chapter 34

Pamela Charney, M.D.
Professor of Clinical Medicine
Associate Professor of Clinical Obstetrics
& Gynecology and Women's Health
Director
General Internal Medicine
Women's Health Residency Track
Jacobi Medical Center—Adult Primary Care Pavilion
Bronx, New York
Chapter 87

Melvin D. Cheitlin, M.D.
Emeritus Professor of Medicine–UCSF
San Francisco General Hospital
San Francisco, California
Chapter 70

James T. T. Chen, M.D.
Professor of Radiology
Duke University Medical Center
Durham, North Carolina
Chapter 12

Michael B. Clark, M.D., F.A.C.C.
Chief Medical Director
Senior Vice President
Swiss RE Life & Health
Life Reassurance Corporation
Stamford, Connecticut
Chapter 95

Stephen D. Clements, Jr., M.D.
Professor of Medicine (Cardiology)
Emory University School of Medicine
Atlanta, Georgia
Chapter 49

Denton A. Cooley, M.D.
President and Surgeon-in-Chief
Texas Heart Institute
Surgeon-in-Chief
Texas Heart Institute
Houston, Texas
Chapter 77

Ralph B. D'Agostino, Sr., Ph.D.
Department of Mathematics
Boston University College of Arts and Sciences
Boston, Massachusetts
Chapter 1

Karina W. Davidson, Ph.D.
Assistant Research Professor
Mount Sinai School of Medicine
Integrative Behavioral Cardiology Program
The Zena and Michael A. Wiener Cardiovascular Institute
Mount Sinai Medical Center
New York, New York
Chapter 98

Michael J. Davies, M.D.
Professor of Cardiovascular Pathology
St. George's Hospital Medical Center
London, England
Chapter 36

John E. Deanfield, M.D.
Professor of Cardiology
Institute of Child Health
University College London
Consultant Cardiologist
Great Ormond Street Hospital for Children
London, United Kingdom
Chapter 64

Anthony N. DeMaria, M.D.
Professor and Chief of Cardiology
University of California San Diego School of Medicine
UCSD Medical Center
San Diego, California
Chapter 13

Regis DeSilva, M.D.
Associate Professor of Medicine
Harvard Medical School
Director of Medical Education
Cardiovascular Division
Beth Israel Deaconess Medical Center
Boston, Massachusetts
Chapter 29A

Thomas F. Dodson, M.D.
Associate Professor of Surgery
Vice Chairman of Education
Program Director of General Surgery Residency Program
Emory University School of Medicine
Section of Vascular Surgery
The Emory Clinic
Atlanta, Georgia
Chapter 91

Gerald W. Dorn III, M.D.
Professor of Medicine
Staff Cardiologist
University of Cincinnati Medical Center
Cincinnati, Ohio
Chapter 5

John S. Douglas, Jr., M.D.
Professor of Medicine
Cardiology
Emory University School of Medicine
Director
Interventional Cardiology and Cardiac Catheterization Laboratories
Cardiac Cath Lab
Emory University Hospital
Atlanta, Georgia
Chapters 15, 40, 45

Mark Doyle, M.D.
Associate Professor of Medicine
University of Alabama at Birmingham
Birmingham, Alabama
Chapter 18A

Victor J. Dzau, M.D.
Hersey Professor of the Theory and Practice of Physic (Medicine) and Chairman of Department of Medicine
Brigham and Women's Hospital
Boston, Massachusetts
Chapter 8

Kim A. Eagle, M.D.
Albion Walter Henleh Professor of Internal Medicine
Chief
Division of Cardiology and Chief of Clinical Cardiology
Division of Cardiology
University of Michigan Medical Center
Ann Arbor, Michigan
Chapter 74

Robert H. Eckel, M.D.
Professor of Medicine and of Physiology and Biophysics
University of Colorado Health Sciences Center
University of Colorado Health Sciences Center
Denver, Colorado
Chapter 83

William D. Edwards, M.D.
Professor of Pathology
Mayo Graduate School of Medicine
Consultant in Pathology
Division of Anatomic Pathology
Mayo Clinic
Rochester, Minnesota
Chapter 2

William J. Elliott, M.D., Ph.D.
Professor of Preventive Medicine
Internal Medicine, and Pharmacology
Attending Physician
Rush University School of Medicine
Rush-Presbyterian-St. Luke's Medical Center
Chicago, Illinois
Chapter 51

Domien Engelen, M.D.
Department of Cardiology
Academic Hospital Maastricht
Maastricht, The Netherlands
Chapter 43

Maurice Enriquez-Sarano, M.D., F.A.C.C.
Associate Professor of Medicine
Consultant
Cardiovascular Diseases and Internal Medicine
Mayo Clinic
Rochester, Minnesota
Chapter 57

Erling Falk, M.D., Ph.D.
Professor
Department of Cardiology Research
AARHUS University Hospital (Skejby)
Aarhus N, Denmark
Chapter 35

Michael E. Farkouh, M.D., F.R.C.P., M.Sc.
Assistant Professor of Medicine
Mount Sinai School of Medicine
Director
Telemetry Unit
Consultant
Mount Sinai Diabetes
Mount Sinai Medical Center
New York, New York
Chapter 78

ZAHI A. FAYAD, Ph.D.
Assistant Professor
Mount Sinai Medical School
Director
Cardiovascular MRI Research
Mount Sinai Medical Center
New York, New York
Chapter 18B

GERALD F. FLETCHER, M.D.
Professor of Medicine
Mayo Medical School
Jacksonville, Florida
Chapter 85

THOMAS R. FLIPSE, M.D.
Consultant
Cardiovascular Diseases
Mayo Clinic Jacksonville
Jacksonville, Florida
Chapter 85

THOMAS K. F. FOO, Ph.D.
Chief Scientist
Cardiovascular MRI
Development
Applied Science Laboratory
GE Medical Systems
Baltimore, Maryland
Chapter 18B

ROBERT H. FRANCH, M.D.
Professor of Medicine
Emory University School of Medicine
Atlanta, Georgia
Chapter 15

GARY S. FRANCIS, M.D.
Professor of Medicine
Director
Coronary Intensive Care Unit
George M. and Linda H. Kaufman
Center for Heart Failure
The Cleveland Clinic Foundation
Cleveland, Ohio
Chapter 20

O. HOWARD FRAZIER, M.D.
Chief
Cardiopulmonary Transplantation
Director
Surgery Research
Cullen Cardiovascular Research
Laboratories
Texas Heart Institute
Texas Medical Center
Houston, Texas
Chapter 77

MICHAEL D. FREED, M.D.
Associate Professor of Pediatrics
Harvard Medical School
Senior Associate in Cardiology
Children's Hospital
Boston, Massachusetts
Chapter 63

WILLIAM T. FRIEDEWALD, M.D.
Clinical Professor of Medicine and
Public Health
Columbia University School of
Medicine
Public Health Division of Epidemiology
Columbia-Presbyterian Medical Center
New York, New York
Chapter 95

WILLIAM H. FRISHMAN, M.D.
Professor of Medicine and
Pharmacology
Chairman
Department of Medicine
Director of Medicine
Westchester Medical Center
New York Medical College
Valhalla, New York
Department of Medicine
New York Medical College
Valhalla, New York
Chapters 21 and 81

VICTOR F. FROELICHER, M.D.
Professor of Medicine
Stanford University School of Medicine
Division of Cardiovascular Medicine
Director
ECG Exercise Lab
VA Medical Center
Palo Alto, California
Chapter 14

ROBERT L. FRYE, M.D.
Rose M. and Morris Eisenberg
Professor of Medicine
Mayo Clinic
Rochester, Minnesota
Chapter 57

VALENTIN FUSTER, M.D., Ph.D.
Director
The Zena and Michael A. Wiener
Cardiovascular Institute
Richard Gorlin, M.D./Heart Research
Foundation
Professor of Cardiology
Vice Chairman
Department of Medicine
The Mount Sinai School of Medicine
New York, New York
Chapters 18B, 35, 44, 78, 93

JOHN P. GASSLER, M.D.
Fellow
Cardiovascular Diseases
Cleveland Clinic Foundation
Cleveland, Ohio
Chapter 20

WILLIAM GERIN, M.D.
Associate Professor
The Zena and Michael A. Wiener
Cardiovascular Institute
The Mount Sinai School of Medicine
New York, New York
Chapter 98

GUIDO GERMANO, Ph.D.
Director
Nuclear Medicine Physics
Cedars-Sinai Medical Center
Associate Professor of Radiological
Science
University of California Los Angeles
School of Medicine
Los Angeles, California
Chapter 16

GARY GERSTENBLITH, M.D.
Professor of Medicine
The Johns Hopkins School of Medicine
Attending Physician
The Johns Hopkins Hospital
Director
Clinical Trials Cardiology Division
The John Hopkins Hospital
Baltimore, Maryland
Chapter 86

Edward M. Gilbert, M.D.
Associate Professor of Medicine
Director
Heart Failure Treatment Program
Division of Cardiology
University of Utah Health Sciences Center
Salt Lake City, Utah
Chapter 66

Anton P. M. Gorgels, M.D., Ph.D.
Department of Cardiology
Academic Hospital Maastricht
Maastricht, The Netherlands
Chapter 43

Kathy K. Griendling, M.D.
Professor of Medicine
Emory University School of Medicine
Emory University, Cardiology
Atlanta, Georgia
Chapter 6

Scott M. Grundy, M.D., Ph.D.
Professor of Internal Medicine
University of Texas
Southwestern Medical Center at Dallas
Director
Center for Human Nutrition
University of Texas, Southwestern Medical Center at Dallas
Dallas, Texas
Chapter 38

Gary L. Grunkemeier, M.D.
Director
Medical Data Research Center
Providence Health System
Portland, Oregon
Chapter 60

Robert J. Hall, M.D.
Director
Cardiac Education
St. Luke's Episcopal Hospital and Texas Heart Institute
Clinical Professor of Medicine
Baylor College of Medicine and University of Texas Medical School at Houston
St. Luke's Episcopal Hospital
Houston, Texas
Chapter 77

David G. Harrison, M.D.
Professor of Medicine
Emory University
Cardiology
Atlanta, Georgia
Chapter 6

Gerard Helft, M.D., Ph.D., A.C.C.A.
Research Fellow
Mount Sinai School of Medicine
The Zena and Michael A. Wiener Cardiovascular Institute
New York, New York
Chapter 18B

Brian D. Hoit, M.D.
Professor of Medicine
Case Western Reserve University
Co-director of Echocardiography
Attending Physician
University Hospitals of Cleveland
Cleveland, Ohio
Chapters 68 and 72

Larry H. Hollier, M.D., F.A.C.S., F.A.C.C., F.R.C.S. (Eng)
Julius Jacobson II, M.D.
Professor of Surgery
Chairman
Department of Surgery
Mount Sinai School of Medicine
Julius H, Jacobson II, M.D.
Professor of Vascular Surgery
Chairman
Department of Surgery
Mount Sinai Medical Center
New York, New York
Chapter 93

Carl C. Hug, Jr., M.D., Ph.D.
Attending Physician in Cardiothoracic Anesthesiology and Intensive Care
Emory University Hospital
Professor of Anesthesiology and Pharmacology
Emory University Hospital
Atlanta, Georgia
Chapter 49

Sharon A. Hunt, M.D.
Professor, Cardiovascular Medicine
Stanford University
Department of Cardiothoracic Surgery
Stanford, California
Chapter 22

Alberto Interian, Jr., M.D.
Professor of Medicine
Director
Electrophysiology Laboratory
Director
Electropathophysiology Laboratory
University of Miami School of Medicine
Division of Cardiology
Miami, Florida
Chapter 11

Mark E. Josephson, M.D.
Professor of Medicine
Harvard Medical School
Director
Harvard-Thorndike Electrophy
Beth Israel Deaconess Medical Center
Boston, Massachusetts
Chapter 33

William B. Kannel, M.D., M.P.H., F.A.C.C.
Professor of Medicine and Public Health
Boston University School of Medicine
Professor of Medicine and Public Health
Framingham Heart Study
Framingham, Massachusetts
Chapter 1

Samir R. Kapadia, M.D.
Acting Assistant Professor
University of Washington
Interventional Cardiologist
Puget Sound Health Care System
Seattle, Washington
Chapter 92

Joel A. Kaplan, M.D.
Dean
School of Medicine
Vice President for Health Affairs
University of Louisville School of Medicine
University of Louisville School of Medicine
Abell Administration Center
Louisville, Kentucky
Chapter 75

Marinka Kartalija, M.D.
Resident
Department of Internal Medicine
University of Utah School of Medicine
Salt Lake City, Utah
Chapter 73

Bradley B. Keller, M.D.
Chief
Division of Pediatric Cardiology
Director
Pediatric Cardiovascular Research Program
Jennifer Gill, Associate Professor of Pediatrics
Division of Pediatric Cardiology
University of Kentucky College of Medicine
Lexington, Kentucky
Chapter 9

Morton J. Kern, M.D.
Professor of Medicine
Director of Cardiac Catheterization Laboratory
St. Louis University Medical Center
St. Louis, Missouri
Chapter 15

Spencer B. King III, M.D.
Clinical Professor of Medicine
Emory University School of Medicine
J. B. and Dottie Fuqua Chair of Cardiology
The Fuqua Heart Center
Co-director
Atlanta Cardiovascular Research Institute
Atlanta, Georgia
Chapters 15 and 45

E. Martin Kloosterman, M.D.
Servicio de Electrofisiologia
Hospital Naval Pedro Mallo
Hospital Militar Cosme Argerich
Buenos Aires, Argentina
Chapter 24

Harlan Krumholz, M.D., M.Sc.
Associate Professor of Medicine
Cardiology
Yale University of Medicine
New Haven, Connecticut
Chapter 94

Edward G. Lakatta, M.D.
Adjunct Professor of Physiology
University of Maryland School of Medicine
Professor of Medicine
The Johns Hopkins School of Medicine
National Institute on Aging
Gerontology Research Center
Laboratory of Cardiovascular Science
Baltimore, Maryland
Chapter 86

Gaetano Antonio Lanza, M.D.
Assistant Professor
Catholic University of the Sacred Heart
Institute of Cardiology
Catholic University of the Sacred Heart
Rome, Italy
Chapter 37

Thierry H. LeJemtel, M.D.
Professor of Medicine
Albert Einstein College of Medicine
Bronx, New York
Chapter 21

Martin M. LeWinter, M.D.
Professor of Medicine
University of Vermont
Director
Cardiology Unit
University of Vermont
Fletcher Allen Health Care
MCHV Campus
Burlington, Vermont
Chapter 3

Richard P. Lewis, M.D.
Professor of Internal Medicine
Ohio State College of Medicine and Public Health
Columbus, Ohio
Chapter 32

Richard P. Lifton, M.D.
Chairman
Department of Genetics
Professor of Genetics
Internal Medicine and Molecular Biophysics and Biochemistry
Yale University School of Medicine
Associate Investigator
Howard Hughes Medical Institute
Yale University
New Haven, Connecticut
Chapter 7

Joseph Lindsay, Jr., M.D.
Director
Section of Cardiology
Washington Hospital Center
Professor of Medicine
The George Washington University School of Health Care Sciences
Washington Hospital Center
Washington, District of Columbia
Chapter 88

Bernard Lown, M.D.
Professor of Cardiology (Emeritus)
Harvard School of Public Health
Senior Physician
Brigham and Women's Hospital
Brookline, Massachusetts
Chapter 29A

Bruce W. Lytle, M.D.
Surgeon
Department of Thoracic and Cardiovascular Surgery
The Cleveland Clinic Foundation
Cleveland, Ohio
Chapter 48

JOHN J. MAHMARIAN, M.D.

Associate Professor of Medicine
Baylor College of Medicine
Assistant Director
Nuclear Cardiology Laboratory
The Methodist Hospital
Section of Cardiology
Baylor College of Medicine
Houston, Texas
Chapter 17

JOSEPH F. MALOUF, M.D.

Associate Professor of Medicine
Cardiovascular Consultant
Mayo Clinic
Rochester, Minnesota
Chapter 2

DONNA M. MANCINI, M.D.

Associate Professor of Medicine
Medical Director
Cardiac Transplant
New York Presbyterian Hospital
New York, New York
Chapter 69

MICHAEL L. MARIN, M.D.

Henry Kaufmann Professor of Vascular Surgery
Director of Endovascular Surgery
Mount Sinai Medical Center
New York, New York
Chapter 93

ROGER R. MARKWALD, Ph.D.

Professor and Chairman
Department of Cell and Biology and Anatomy
Medical University of South Carolina
Department of Cell Biology and Anatomy
Charleston, South Carolina
Chapter 9

BARRY J. MARON, M.D.

Director
Cardiovascular Research
Division, Minneapolis Heart Institute Foundation
Minneapolis, Minnesota
Chapter 67

DAVID J. MARON, M.D.

Assistant Professor of Medicine
Division of Cardiovascular Medicine
Director
Preventive Cardiology
Vanderbilt University Medical Center
Division of Cardiovascular Medicine
Nashville, Tennessee
Chapter 38

ATTILIO MASERI, M.D.

Professor of Cardiology
Director
Institute of Cardiology
Catholic University of the Sacred Heart
Institute of Cardiology
Rome, Italy
Chapter 37

JAY W. MASON, M.D.

Jack M. Gill Professor and Chairman
Department of Medicine
University of Kentucky
Lexington, Kentucky
Chapter 65

HUGH A. MCALLISTER, JR., M.D.

Chief
Department of Pathology
St. Luke's Episcopal Hospital and Texas Heart Institute (Emeritus)
Clinical Professor of Pathology
Baylor College of Medicine
Adjunct Professor of Pathology
University of Texas Medical School
Houston, Texas
Chapter 77

JOHN H. MCANULTY, M.D.

Professor and Head of Cardiology
Oregon Health Sciences University
Portland, Oregon
Chapters 61 and 82

WILLIAM M. MCDONALD, M.D.

Associate Professor
Department of Psychiatry and Behavioral Sciences
Emory University School of Medicine
Fuqua Center for Late-Life Depression
Atlanta, Georgia
Chapter 80

JAMES METCALFE, M.D.

Professor of Medicine (Emeritus)
Oregon Health Sciences University
School of Medicine
Portland, Oregon
Chapter 82

LUISA MESTRONI, M.D.

Associate Professor of Medicine
Director
Molecular Genetics
University of Colorado Cardiovascular Institute
Director
Molecular Genetics
University of Colorado Cardiovascular Institute
Fitzsimons Hospital
Aurora, Colorado
Chapter 66

WILLIAM E. MITCH, M.D.

Director
Renal Division
Garland Herndon Professor of Medicine
Emory University School of Medicine
Emory University, Cardiology
Atlanta, Georgia
Chapter 84

RAUL D. MITRANI, M.D.

Associate Professor of Medicine
Director
Arrhythmia and Pacemaker Center
University of Miami Medical Center–Jackson Memorial Hospital
Miami, Florida
Chapter 31

DOUGLAS C. MORRIS, M.D.

J. Willis Hurst, Professor and Vice Chair
Department of Medicine
Emory University
Director
Emory Heart Center
Atlanta, Georgia
Chapter 49

Dominique L. Musselman, M.D.
Assistant Professor of Psychiatry
Psychiatry and Behavioral Sciences
Emory University School of Medicine
Atlanta, Georgia
Chapter 80

Robert J. Myerburg, M.D.
Director
Division of Cardiology
Professor of Medicine and Physiology
University of Miami School of Medicine
Division of Cardiology
Miami, Florida
Chapters 11, 24, 31

Elizabeth G. Nabel, M.D.
Scientific Director
Clinical Research Program
National Heart, Lung, and Blood Institute
National Institutes of Health
Bethesda, Maryland
Chapter 8

Ira S. Nash, M.D.
Associate Director
The Zena and Michael A. Wiener Cardiovascular Institute
Assistant Professor of Medicine
Mount Sinai School of Medicine
Mount Sinai Medical Center
New York, New York
Chapters 96 and 97

Steven D. Nelson, M.D.
Associate Professor of Medicine
Director
Cardiac Electrophysiology
Ohio State University Hospitals
Columbus, Ohio
Chapter 32

Charles B. Nemeroff, M.D., Ph.D.
Chair
Reunette W. Harris Professor and Chairman
Department of Psychiatry and Behavioral Sciences
Emory University School of Medicine
Atlanta, Georgia
Chapter 80

John H. Newman, M.D.
Chief of Medical Services
Elsa S. Harrigan Professor of Pulmonary Medicine
VAMC Nashville
Nashville, Tennessee
Chapter 54

Steve E. Nissen, M.D.
Professor of Medicine
Ohio State University
Vice-Chairman
Department of Cardiology
Cleveland Clinic Foundation
Cleveland, Ohio
Chapter 47

R. Joe Noble, M.D., F.A.C.C.
Clinical Professor of Medicine
Indiana University School of Medicine
Consulting Cardiologist
The Care Group
and St. Vincent's Hospital and Health Care Center
Northside Cardiology
Indianapolis, Indiana
Chapter 25

Peter A. O'Callaghan, M.D.
Clinical and Research Fellow in Cardiology
Department of Cardiological Sciences
St. Georges Hospital Medical School
London, England
Chapter 30

William W. O'Neill, M.D., F.A.C.C.
Director
Division of Cardiology
Co-Director
Beaumont Heart Center
William Beaumont Hospital
Royal Oak, Michigan
Chapter 46

Lionel H. Opie, M.D., D.Phil, F.R.C.P.
Professor of Medicine
Co-Director
Cape Heart Centre
University of Cape Town Medical School
Cape Town, South Africa
Chapter 81

Robert A. O'Rourke, M.D.
Charles Conrad Brown, Distinguished Professor in Cardiovascular Disease
University of Texas Health Science Center
San Antonio, Texas
Chapters 10, 40, 58

George Osol, Ph.D.
Professor and Director of Research
Department of Obstetrics and Gynecology
University of Vermont College of Medicine
Burlington, Vermont
Chapter 3

Eegen C. Palma, M.D., F.A.C.C.
Assistant Professor of Medicine
Albert Einstein College of Medicine
Electrophysiologist
Montefiore Medical Center
Division of Cardiology
Bronx, New York
Chapter 28

Stephen O. Pastan, M.D.
Associate Professor of Medicine
Emory University School of Medicine
Atlanta, Georgia
Chapter 84

THOMAS A. PEARSON, M.D., M.P.H., Ph.D.
Albert D. Kaiser Professor and Chair
Community and Preventive Medicine
Professor of Medicine
University of Rochester School of Medicine and Dentistry Attending Physician
Department of Medicine
Director
Preventive Cardiology Clinic
Co-Director
Stony Heart Program
University of Rochester Medical Center
Rochester, New York
Chapter 38

THOMAS G. PICKERING, M.D., D.Phil
Professor of Medicine
Director
Integrative and Behavioral Cardiology Program
The Zena and Michael Wiener Cardiovascular Institute
Mount Sinai Medical Center
New York, New York
Chapter 98

DUANE S. PINTO, M.D.
Cardiology Fellow
Clinical Instructor in Medicine
Beth Israel Deaconess Medical Center
Divison of Cardiology
Boston, Massachusetts
Chapter 33

GERALD M. POHOST, M.D.
Mary Gertrude Waters Professor of Cardiovascular Medicine
Professor of Medicine and Radiology
University of Alabama
Birmingham, Alabama
Chapter 18A

PAUL POIRIER, M.D., F.R.C.P.C.
Associate Professor of Medicine
Laval University School of Medicine
Director
Cardiac Rehabilitation Program
Quebec Heart Institute
Laval Hospital
Quebec, Canada
Chapter 83

MICHAEL POON, M.D.
Assistant Professor of Medicine (Cardiology)
Director of the Mount Sinai Pulmonary Hypertension Program
Medical Director of the Joseph H. Hazen Ambulatory Cardiac Care Center
Mount Sinai Medical Center
New York, New York
Chapter 93

CRAIG M. PRATT, M.D.
Director
Coronary Care Unit
Professor of Medicine
Baylor College of Medicine
The Methodist Hospital
Houston, Texas
Chapter 42

ERIC N. PRYSTOWSKY, M.D.
Director
Clinical Electrophysiology Laboratory
St. Vincent Hospital
Indianapolis, Indiana
Consulting Professor of Medicine
Duke University Medical Center
Durham, North Carolina
Northside Cardiology, PC
Indianapolis, Indiana
Chapter 25

SHAHBUDIN H. RAHIMTOOLA, M.D.
George C. Griffith Professor of Cardiology
Division of Cardiology
LAC + USC Medical Center
Los Angeles, California
Chapters 56, 57, 60, 61

ELLIOT J. RAYFIELD, M.D.
Clinical Professor of Medicine
Mount Sinai School of Medicine
Attending Physician
Mount Sinai Hospital
New York, New York
Chapter 78

DAVID L. REICH, M.D.
Vice Chair for Academic Affairs
Co-Director of Cardiothoracic Anesthesia
Professor of Anesthesiology
Mount Sinai Medical School
Department of Anesthesiology
New York, New York
Chapter 75

PAUL M. RIDKER, M.D., M.P.H.
Associate Professor of Medicine
Harvard Medical School
Director
Center for Cardiovascular Disease Prevention
Birgham and Women's Hospital
Harvard Medical School
Boston, Massachusetts
Chapter 38

STEFANO RIGATTIERI, M.D.
Resident in Cardiology
Catholic University of the Sacred Heart
Institute of Cardiology
Rome, Italy
Chapter 37

WILLIAM C. ROBERTS, M.D.
Medical Director
Baylor Cardiovascular Institute
Clinical Professor of Medicine
Hahnemann Medical School
Philadelphia, Pennsylvania
Baylor Cardiovascular Institute
Baylor University Medical Center
Dallas, Texas
Chapter 76

ROBERT ROBERTS, M.D.
Don W. Chapman Professor of Medicine
Chief of Cardiology
Professor of Cell Biology
Director of Bugher Foundation Center for Molecular Biology
Baylor College of Medicine
Houston, Texas
Chapters 4, 7, 9, 42, 62

Luz-Maria Rodriguez, M.D.

Associate Professor of Cardiology
University of Maastricht
Staff Physician
Cardiology
University Hospital Maastricht
The Netherlands
Maastricht, The Netherlands
Chapter 29

Thom W. Rooke, M.D.

Professor of Medicine
Mayo Clinic
Rochester, Minnesota
Chapter 90

Lewis J. Rubin, M.D.

Professor of Medicine
Director of Pulmonary Critical
Care Medicine
University of California San Diego
Director
Division of Pulmonary/Critical Care
Medicine
UCSD Medical Center
La Jolla, California
Chapter 52

Jeremy N. Ruskin, M.D.

Director
Cardiac Arrhythmia Service
Massachusetts General Hospital
Associate Professor of Medicine
Harvard Medical School
Boston, Massachusetts
Chapter 30

Thomas J. Ryan, M.D.

Professor of Medicine
Boston University School of Medicine
Senior Consultant
and Emeritus Chief of Cardiology
Boston, Massachusetts
Chapter 42

Merle A. Sande, M.D.

Professor and Chairman
Department of Medicine
Clarence M. and Ruth N. Birrer
Presidential Endowed Chair in Internal
Medicine
University of Utah School of Medicine
Salt Lake City, Utah
Chapter 73

Tommaso Sanna, M.D.

Consultant
Catholic University of the Sacred Heart
Institute of Cardiology
Rome, Italy
Chapter 37

Stephen F. Schaal, M.D.

Professor of Medicine
Ohio State University
College of Medicine and Public Health
Columbus, Ohio
Chapter 32

Hartzell V. Schaff, M.D.

Stuart W. Harrington
Professor of Surgery
Division of Cardiology
Mayo Clinic
Rochester, Minnesota
Chapter 57

Melvin M. Scheinman, M.D.

Professor of Medicine
University of California San Francisco
Medical Center
San Francisco, California
Chapter 28

Heinrich R. Schelbert, M.D., Ph.D.

Professor of Pharmacology and
Radiological Sciences
Chief
Nuclear Medicine Services
Department of Molecular and Medical
Pharmacology
UCLA School of Medicine
Los Angeles, California
Chapter 19

Robert C. Schlant, M.D.

Professor of Medicine (Cardiology)
Emory University School of Medicine
Atlanta, Georgia
Chapter 40

John S. Schroeder, M.D.

Professor of Medicine
Stanford University School of Medicine
Stanford, California
Chapter 22

Steven P. Schulman, M.D.

Associate Professor of Medicine
Director of CCU
The Johns Hopkins University School
of Medicine
Baltimore, Maryland
Chapter 86

Robert J. Schwartz, Ph.D.

Professor of Cell Biology
Baylor College of Medicine
Houston, Texas
Chapter 9

James B. Seward, M.D.

Professor of Medicine & Pediatrics
Director
Echocardiography Laboratory
Consultant in Cardiovascular Diseases
Mayo Clinic
Rochester, Minnesota
Chapter 2

James Shaver, M.D.

Professor of Cardiovascular Disease
University of Texas Health Science
Center
San Antonio, Texas
Chapter 10

Leslee J. Shaw, M.D.

Associate Professor of Medicine and
Health Policy and Management
Director
Technology Evaluation Center
Emory University
Rowland School of Public Health
Atlanta, Georgia
Chapter 16

Halit Silbershatz, Ph.D.

Associate Director of Biometrics
Pfizer Pharmaceuticals, Inc.
New York, New York
Chapter 1

Mark Silverman, M.D.

Professor of Cardiovascular Disease
University of Texas Health Service
Center
San Antonio, Texas
Chapter 10

Robert B. Smith III, M.D.
John E. Skandalakis, Professor of Surgery
Emory University School of Medicine
Medical Director
Emory University Hospital
Chief
Vascular Surgery
Atlanta, Georgia
Chapter 91

Andrew L. Smith, M.D.
Assistant Professor
Division of Cardiology
Emory University School of Medicine
Medical Director
Heart Failure and Transplant Programs
Emory Health Care
Atlanta, Georgia
Chapter 71

Edmund H. Sonnenblick, M.D.
Professor of Medicine
Albert Einstein College of Medicine
Bronx, New York
Chapters 20 and 21

Albert Starr, M.D.
Professor of Surgery
Oregon Health Sciences University
Director
Heart Institute
Providence St. Vincent Medical Center
Starr Wood Cardiac Group
Portland, Oregon
Chapter 60

Panagiotis N. Symbas, M.D.
Professor of Cardiothoracic Surgery
Emory University
Director of Cardiothoracic Surgery
Grady Hospital
Atlanta, Georgia
Chapter 79

A. Jamil Tajik, M.D.
Thomas J. Watson, Jr., Professor of Medicine and Pediatrics
Chair
Division of Cardiovascular Diseases
Consultant
Division of Cardiovascular Diseases
Mayo Clinic
Rochester, Minnesota
Chapter 2

Victor F. Tapson, M.D., F.C.C.P.
Associate Professor
Division of Pulmonary and Critical Care
Director
Lung Transplant Program
Duke University Medical Center
Durham, North Carolina
Chapter 53

Thomas J. Thom, B.A.
Epidemiology and Biometry Program
Division of Heart and Vascular Diseases
National Heart, Lung, and Blood Institutes
Bethesda, Maryland
Chapter 1

Carl Timmermans, M.D.
Associate Professor of Cardiology
University of Maastricht
Staff Physician
Cardiology
University Hospital Maastricht
Maastricht, The Netherlands
Chapter 29

Jeffrey A. Towbin, M.D.
Professor of Pediatrics (Cardiology) and Molecular and Human Genetics
Associate Chief
Pediatrics Director
Heart Failure and Transplant Program
Texas Children's Hospital Foundation
Chair
Pediatric Molecular Cardiac Research
Molecular and Human Genetics
Baylor College of Medicine
Houston, Texas
Chapter 62

Kent Veland, M.D.
Professor Emeritus
Department of OB/GYN
Stanford University School of Medicine
Stanford, California
Chapter 82

Albert L. Waldo, M.D.
The Walter H. Pritchard Professor of Cardiology and Professor of Medicine
Case Western Reserve University
Cleveland, Ohio
Director
Cardiac Electrophysiology Program
Division of Cardiology
University Hospitals of Cleveland
Cleveland, Ohio
Chapter 23

Bruce F. Waller, M.D.
Clinical Professor of Medicine and Pathology
Indiana University School of Medicine
Director
Cardiovascular Pathology Registry
St. Vincent Hospital
Cardiologist
The Care Group
Medical Director
The Care Group Laboratory
Indianapolis, Indiana
Chapter 39

Richard A. Walsh, M.D.
John H. Hord Professor and Chairman of the Department of Medicine
Case Western Reserve University
Physician-in-Chief
University Hospitals of Cleveland
Cleveland, Ohio
Chapter 5

Carole A. Warnes, M.D., M.R.C.P., F.A.C.C.
Professor of Medicine
Mayo Medical School
Consultant Division of Cardiovascular Diseases
Internal Medicine
Pediatric Cardiology
and Adult Congenital Heart Disease Clinic
Mayo Clinic
Rochester, Minnesota
Chapter 64

David D. Waters, M.D.
Professor of Medicine
University of California, San Francisco
Division of Cardiology
San Francisco General Hospital
San Francisco, California
Chapter 41

William S. Weintraub, M.D.
Professor of Medicine
Cardiology
Director
Emory Center for Outcomes Research (ECOR)
Emory University
Division of Cardiology
Atlanta, Georgia
Chapter 94

Myron L. Weisfeldt, M.D.
Chairman
Department of Medicine
Samuel Bard Professor of Medicine
Columbia University College of Physicians and Surgeons
Columbia Presbyterian Medical Center
New York, New York
Chapter 34

Hein J. J. Wellens, M.D.
Professor of Cardiology
University of Maastricht
Chairman
Department of Cardiology
University Hospital Maastricht
Maastricht, The Netherlands
Chapters 29 and 43

Nanette K. Wenger, M.D.
Professor of Medicine (Cardiology)
Emory University School of Medicine
Consultant
Emory Heart and Vascular Center
Chief of Cardiology
Grady Memorial Hospital
Emory University School of Medicine
Atlanta, Georgia
Chapter 50

Paul Wennberg, M.D.
Instructo of Medicine
Senior Associate Consultant
Cardiovascular Division
Mayo Clinic
Rochester, Minnesota
Chapter 90

Andy Wessels, Ph.D.
Professor
Medical University of South Carolina
Medical University of South Carolina
Chapter 9

Susan Wilansky, M.D.
Medical Director
Non-Invasive Cardiac Imaging
St. Luke's Episcopal Hospital/Texas Heart Institute
St. Luke's Episcopal Hospital
Houston, Texas
Chapter 77

Andrew L. Witt, Ph.D.
Professor and Associate Chairman
Department of Pharmacology
College of Physicians and Surgeons
Columbia University
New York, New York
Chapter 23

Raymond L. Woosley, M.D., Ph.D.
Professor and Chairman
Department of Pharmacology
Georgetown University Medical Center
Washington, District of Columbia
Chapter 27

Stephen G. Worthley, M.B.B.S., F.R.A.C.P.
Research Fellow
Mount Sinai School of Medicine
The Zena and Michael A. Wiener Cardiovascular Institute
New York, New York
Chapter 18B

Sanjay S. Yadav, M.D.
Director, Carotid Intervention
Staff Cardiologist
Vascular Medicine
The Cleveland Clinic Foundation
Cleveland, Ohio
Chapter 92

PREFACE

In 1966 the first edition of Hurst's *The Heart* was published after more than five years of planning by Dr. J. Willis Hurst and his colleagues at Emory University. This was the first textbook on cardiovascular disease to be multiauthored and comprehensive with expert discussions on the basic science of cardiovascular diseases and the diagnosis and treatment of specific disorders involving the heart arteries, and veins.

Contributing authors were carefully chosen and the various chapters of the textbook were meticulously reviewed by the editors to provide completeness without overlap. This 1966 text was extensively referenced and the index of the book was written by the contributing authors and editors themselves. The first edition of *The Heart* was designed as a reference source for its readers as well as providing clinically relevant material for use in the diagnosis and treatment of cardiovascular disease in the 1960s.

The tenth edition of *The Heart* is considerably different from the previous nine editions. It approaches the entire discipline of cardiovascular disease, from basic science through clinical disease states, with all chapters written by most prominent experts in the field. Thus, from the description of the latest advances in molecular cardiology, including the promising cardiovascular applications of the human genome project, the book approaches in depth all the recent major advances in clinical cardiology, including the description of the most up-to-date practice guidelines.

Sixteen new chapters have been added and about 60 percent of the chapters have been radically modified. Specifically new, and we believe unique, aspects of this tenth edition of *The Heart* are the following:

1. Within the basic section of the book there are three new chapters devoted to molecular, cellular, and vessel wall biology;
2. also, in the basic section there are three new chapters devoted to the human genome, molecular development and embriology, and genetic therapy;
3. as a practical new understanding of the anatomy of *The Heart*, the group at the Mayo Clinic has written an outstanding chapter based on clinical imaging;
4. in the section devoted to diagnostic modalities, there are four new superb chapters on computed tomography of the heart, magnetic resonance imaging of the heart, magnetic resonance imaging of the vascular systsem, and cardiac positron emission tomography;
5. two timely new clinincal chapters; diabetes in cardiovascular disease and cardiac disease in women;
6. a new aspect of this tenth edition is a chapter on practice guidelines in cardiovascular disease, which we expect will be very practical for the daily approach to the patient and as a teaching tool for residents and fellows;
7. finally, there is a new and unique chapter on extended cardiovascular medicine, which, we predict, outlines a strong trend toward the future.

From the moment that the outstanding group of authors accepted to participate in this tenth edition of *The Heart* to the moment of the book appearing on the shelves has only taken fifteen months. This is an absolute record for a textbook of this size and complexity. Such an approach represents the highest tribute and acknowledgment to our authors for their extraordinary and timely contribution.

We thank J. Willis Hurst, M.D., editor of the first seven editions, for his constant and enthusiastic encouragement, as well as Robert C. Schlant, M.D., who contributions to the first nine editions of *The Heart* have been responsible for the foundation of this tenth edition. Importantly, this edition would not have been possible without the many extensive contributions and personal sacrifices of two individuals at McGraw-Hill, Darlene B. Cooke and Susan R. Noujaim. We would also like to thank Lester A. Sheinis and Richard C. Ruzycka for their efforts in getting the book produced on time.

Finally we wish to acknowledge the support of our families and the many sacrifices they have made to make this volume possible. Our wives remain our greatest support and strength; Maria Fuster, Jane W. Alexander, Suzann O'Rourke, Donna Roberts, Gail King, and Inez Wellens.

HURST'S
THE HEART

PART ONE

BASIC FOUNDATIONS OF CARDIOLOGY

CHAPTER 1

CARDIOVASCULAR DISEASES IN THE UNITED STATES AND PREVENTION APPROACHES

Thomas J. Thom / William B. Kannel* / Halit Silbershatz / Ralph B. D'Agostino, Sr.

The large and long-term decline in mortality from the cardiovascular diseases accounted for almost 4 of the 5.6-year increase in life expectancy in the United States attained between 1965 and 1995.[1] The 55 percent decline in the age-corrected death rate for total cardiovascular disease between 1950 and 1996 indicates the extent to which these leading causes of death are subject to preventive and therapeutic measures. These diseases, however, still account for 41 percent of all deaths and are leading causes of morbidity and health care utilization. Control of these diseases should focus on prevention because of its inherent benefits, its apparent role in the mortality reductions, and its potential given the presence of modifiable risk factors in millions of Americans.

CARDIOVASCULAR DISEASES

Major Cause of Morbidity and Mortality

The most common cardiovascular diseases are hypertension and heart disease, but the basis for most cardiovascular diseases is atherosclerosis, which is almost universally present in U.S. adults and is manifest clinically as coronary heart disease (CHD), cerebrovascular disease (stroke), or peripheral arterial disease. The likelihood of developing one of these diseases is high, and they affect the health of nearly 59 million Americans.[2] In 1999, these diseases were projected to account for $178 billion in health care expenditures in the United States—2 percent of the gross domestic product (Fig. 1-1). These diseases also account for an estimated $108 billion in lost productivity due to illness and premature mortality. These expenditures and indirect costs are by far the largest for any diagnostic group.

During the past 30 years, there have been major reductions in mortality rates for the various forms of cardiovascular disease (Fig. 1-2). Cardiovascular diseases, however, continue to be the most common threat to life and health. The lifetime risk of developing CHD after age 40 is 49 percent in men and 32 percent in women.[3] Even at age 70, the risk is 35 percent for men and 24 percent for women. CHD is the leading or second leading cause of death beginning at age 45 in men and in women.[4] An estimated 8 percent of the U.S. population, 20 million persons, have some form of heart disease.[5] About 50 million, 20 percent of the total population and one-fourth of the adult population, have hypertension, defined as a systolic blood pressure of 140 mmHg or greater, a diastolic blood pressure of 90 mmHg or greater, or normal blood pressure levels maintained by use of antihypertensive medication.[1,2] Thirty-two percent of persons with heart disease and 36 percent of those with stroke are limited in their usual activity by the condition.[6]

* Department of Preventive Medicine and Epidemiology, Evans Department of Clinical Research, Boston University School of Medicine, Boston, Massachusetts, and the Framingham Heart Study. Framingham Study research is supported by NIH/NHLBI Contract N01-HC-38038 and the Visiting Scientist Program that is supported by Servier Amérique.

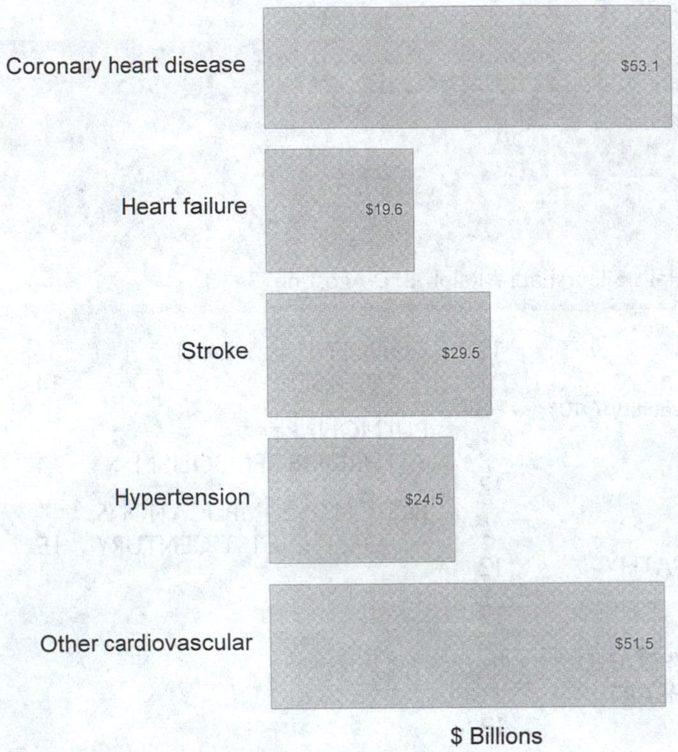

FIGURE 1-1 Health expenditures for cardiovascular diseases, United States, 1999 (includes expenditures for hospital, home, and nursing home care; physician and other professionals; and drugs). (From the American Heart Association and National Heart, Lung, and Blood Insitute.[2])

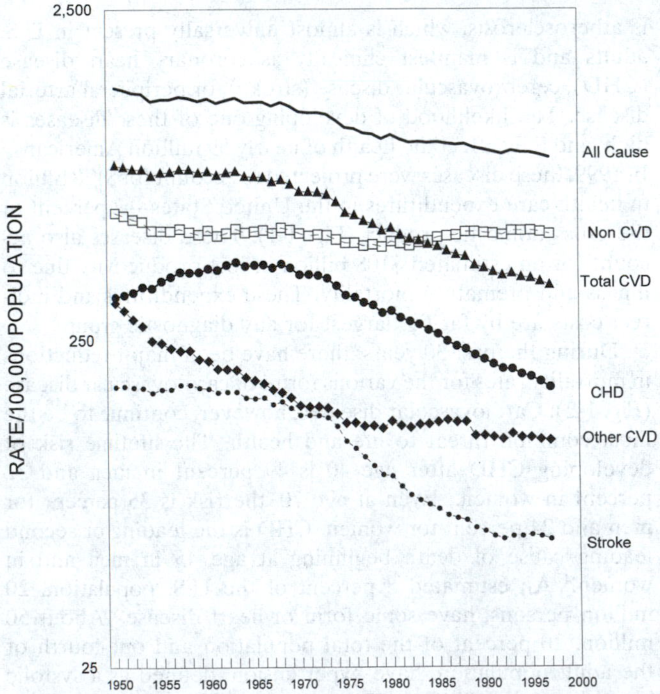

FIGURE 1-2 Age-adjusted death rates for selected causes of death; United States, 1950–1997 (adjusted to U.S. population 2000) CVD, cardiovascular disease; CHD, coronary heart disease. (From *Vital Statistics of the United States*, National Center for Health Statistics.)

Heart disease and hypertension, respectively, are the third and fourth most common chronic conditions causing limitation of activity.[1] Almost 60 percent of those with hypertension are under 65 years of age, and about 50 percent of persons with heart disease are under that age.[5] The prevalence and mortality from the cardiovascular diseases increase with decreasing levels of family income and education.[5,7] Between 1990 and 1992 in the United States, heart disease and hypertension accounted for an estimated 542 million days of restricted activity and 206 million bed days.[6] In 1997, there were an estimated 33 million days in short-stay hospitals, 60 million visits to physicians' offices, 5 million outpatient visits, and 616,000 patients receiving home health care (in 1996) for the cardiovascular diseases.[8–11]

In 1997, cardiovascular diseases accounted for 41 percent of all deaths in the United States, a total of 952,000.[1] Largely because there are many more older women than older men in the U.S. population, the analogous percentage is higher in women (42 percent) than in men (39 percent), and the number of deaths from cardiovascular diseases is greater in women than in men.[4] Of all cardiovascular disease deaths, 36 percent occurred "prematurely," i.e., before 75 years of age. Atherosclerosis, when manifested as CHD, cerebrovascular disease, or peripheral arterial disease, accounted for 71 percent of all deaths from the cardiovascular diseases in 1997.[1] Heart disease is the leading cause of death in all racial groups.[4] Stroke ranks third highest in whites, blacks, and Asians in the U.S. population; fourth in Hispanics; and fifth in Native Americans.[12] Age-adjusted death rates for cardiovascular disease in 1997 were highest in black males, next highest in white males, and then followed by black females and white females.[2] Rates are not quite as high in Native Americans, Asian Americans, and Hispanic Americans.

Unfortunately, national incidence and case fatality data for the cardiovascular diseases do not exist. Data from the Framingham (Massachusetts) Heart Study, which began in 1948, and the Framingham Offspring Study provide reliable estimates for 44 years of follow-up of a defined population sample of men and women aged 35 to 94, the original cohort, and for 20 years of follow-up of their offspring. The average annual rates of first major cardiovascular events rose from 7 per 1000 men at ages 35 to 44 years to 68 per 1000 at ages 85 to 94 (Table 1-1). For women, comparable rates are achieved 10 years later in life, with the gap narrowing with advancing age. CHD is the predominant cardiovascular event, comprising more than one-half of all such events in men and in women under age 75 (Table 1-2). The proportions of cardiovascular events due to CHD decline with age, as the proportions due to stroke and congestive heart failure (CHF) increase with age. Under age 75, there is a higher proportion of cardiovascular events due to CHD in men than in women and a higher proportion due to CHF in women than in men (see Tables 1-1 and 1-2).

Secular Trends

The trend in mortality from total cardiovascular disease has been downward since about 1940, with long-term declines for the three subgroups—rheumatic, cerebrovascular, and hypertensive diseases—and a decline for CHD since the mid-1960s.[1] The coronary decline antedates effective antithrombolytic and antihypertensive treatment. Prior to 1940, cardiovascular mor-

TABLE 1-1 Incidence of Major Cardiovascular Events: Framingham Study, 44-Year Follow-Up of Cohort and 20-Year Follow-Up of Offspring[a]

	Cardiovascular Disease, All Types		Coronary Heart Disease		Stroke and Transient Ischemic Attack		Congestive Heart Failure		Peripheral Arterial Disease	
Age	Men	Women	Men	Women	Men	Women	Men	Women	Men	Women
35–44	7	3	4	1	[b]	[b]	[b]	[b]	[b]	[b]
45–54	15	7	10	4	2	1	2	1	2	1
55–64	26	15	21	10	4	3	4	2	5	3
65–74	39	24	24	14	11	8	9	6	8	5
75–84	59	40	33	18	20	15	18	12	7	5
85–94	68	63	35	28	12	25	39	31	7	1
35–64[c]	17	9	12	5	2	2	2	1	3	2
65–94[c]	44	30	27	16	13	11	12	9	8	5

[a]Average annual incidence per 1000 persons free of specified disease.
[b]Results are omitted when fewer than five individuals experience an event.
[c]Age-adjusted rates.
SOURCE: The Framingham Study.

tality increased and became the predominant cause of death because of control of infectious and parasitic diseases and an epidemic increase in fatal coronary attacks. Cardiovascular mortality declined just less than 1 percent per year in the 1950s and 1960s. The decline became more precipitous in the 1970s, with the rate falling 3 percent per year since then. For CHD, there has been more than a 58 percent decline in the age-adjusted death rate between the peak of mortality in 1963 and 1997; the current decline is 2 to 3 percent per year. For stroke, the rate of decline was 4 to 6 percent per year in the 1970s and early 1980s, but the decline slowed and has been less than 1 percent per year between 1990 and 1996.

The decline in cardiovascular mortality, including the steep rise and fall in CHD mortality, indicates that the major cause of mortality is controllable. Whether attributable more to beneficial changes in disease-promoting lifestyle or to better medical care of those already afflicted, it is clear that cardiovascular disease in most patients is not an inevitable burden of aging or genetic makeup. Although the causes of the decline in cardiovascular mortality are uncertain, the decline has been substantial, sustained, and real. The decline has coincided with increased efforts to achieve healthier living habits and with improvements in the ambient burden of cardiovascular risk factors.

Unfortunately, there are very few statistics on trends in morbidity, particularly incidence. Some, but not all, studies suggest that there have been declines in incidence and case fatality of CHD and stroke.[13,14] For myocardial infarction (MI), declines have been reported from most international sites in the MONICA (Monitoring Trends in Cardiovascular Diseases) studies.[15] This is important because reduction in mortality without a decline in the incidence rate would indicate that better medical care were responsible, whereas a reduction in both incidence and mortality would suggest that environmental influences and/or preventive measures have improved. If reduction in mortality continues, the size of the elderly population will continue to increase over and above increases due to demographic effects.

TABLE 1-2 Percentage of First Cardiovascular Events by Type of Event: Framingham Study, 44-Year Follow-Up of Cohort and 20-Year Follow-Up of Offspring

	Cardiovascular Disease, All Types (N)		Coronary Heart Disease (%)		Stroke and Transient Ischemic Attack (%)		Congestive Heart Failure (%)		Peripheral Arterial Disease (%)	
Age	Men	Women	Men	Women	Men	Women	Men	Women	Men	Women
35–54	352	200	76.1	60.9	9.6	13.8	5.0	10.6	9.3	14.8
55–64	437	329	69.9	62.2	11.1	14.6.	5.2	8.7	13.9	14.6
65–74	358	364	57.9	53.6	20.8	24.5	7.2	8.4	14.1	13.5
75–94	199	312	51.0	39.3	26.0	35.0	13.5	16.8	9.4	8.9

SOURCE: The Framingham Study.

Risk Factors and Subclinical Disease

Observational studies in populations such as the Framingham Study have documented factors that increase the risk of cardiovascular diseases.[16,17] These include atherogenic attributes such as dyslipidemia, hypertension, glucose intolerance, and elevated fibrinogen; living habits that promote them; indicators of unstable lesions; and signs of compromised circulation, e.g., measures of subclinical arterial disease. Risk factors can be classified into the lipids, metabolic factors, hemostatic factors, blood pressure, and lifestyle factors. Some are modifiable. They promote cardiovascular disease in both sexes at all ages but with different strengths. Diabetes and high-density lipoprotein (HDL) cholesterol operate with greater power in women. Cigarette smoking is particularly influential in men, is noncumulative, and loses some of its adverse impact shortly after quitting. Some risk factors, such as blood lipids, impaired glucose tolerance, uric acid, and fibrinogen, have smaller risk ratios in advanced age, but this lower relative risk is offset by a high absolute risk. In fact, most of the major risk factors remain relevant in the elderly. Obesity or weight gain promotes or aggravates all the atherogenic risk factors, and physical indolence worsens some of them and predisposes to cardiovascular events at all ages. Systolic blood pressure and isolated systolic hypertension are major risk factors at all ages in both sexes. The ratio of total to HDL cholesterol is used by many as a convenient lipid risk factor profile (see also Chap. 53).

Beyond age 65, women become nearly as vulnerable to cardiovascular mortality as men.[4] The predisposing modifiable risk factors for CHD, stroke, peripheral arterial disease, and cardiac failure are similar in the young and old in men and women.[16] An attenuated risk ratio for some risk factors at advanced age is offset by a greater incidence of cardiovascular disease. Consequently, the attributable risk and the potential benefit of treatment rise with age. In old age, average atherogenic total and low-density lipoprotein (LDL) cholesterol levels are considerably higher in women than in men. Cardiovascular risk profiles comprising the major risk factors predict CHD as efficiently in the elderly as in the young. This, and the fact that the decline in cardiovascular mortality has included the elderly, suggests the potential for intervention.

Evidence from the Framingham Study suggests that the presence of certain risk factors in women can attenuate their advantage in cardiovascular risk over that in men. The male-female gap in incidence closes with advancing age. After menopause, risk escalates two- to threefold, with more infarction and sudden death. A high total to HDL cholesterol ratio of 7.5 or greater virtually eliminates the female advantage. Diabetes has twice the relative impact on risk in women, almost canceling the female advantage. Electrocardiographic evidence of left ventricular hypertrophy has a greater relative impact on risk in women. The residual effect of triglycerides after consideration of HDL cholesterol appears to be greater in women than in men.

The major modifiable risk factors that contribute powerfully to cardiovascular disease are highly prevalent in the population. Trends in their prevalence and differences in their impact on the various atherosclerotic sequelae are noteworthy. Despite 30 years of appreciable decline in the percentage of persons who smoke cigarettes, one-fourth of adults, 49 million, still smoke.[2] Despite declining trends in mean total serum cholesterol level, more than 50 percent of American adults, 98 million, have blood cholesterol levels of 200 mg/dL or greater, and of these, 39 million have levels of 240 mg/dL or greater. Fifty million have hypertension, but fortunately, treatment and control of this condition improved considerably since the early 1970s.[1,2] Not improving is obesity. One-third of adults, 106 million, are overweight, defined as a body mass index greater than 25 kg/m2. An estimated 10 million persons are at increased risk of cardiovascular disease because they have diabetes.[2] Another highly prevalent risk factor is sedentary lifestyle. It plays a role in the prevalence of overweight, dyslipidemia, and hypertension and, thus, cardiovascular disease. There also are persons under 18 years of age who have one or more modifiable risk factors.[1,12]

More recent additions to the list of risk factors include homocystinemia. In the general population, 29 percent have deficient enough vitamin B intake to elevate homocystine to more than 14 μmol/L.[18] Inadequate intake of vitamins B_{12} and B_6 and folate account for 67 percent of the elevated homocystine encountered in the general population. An estimated 25 percent of the population have Lp(a) lipoprotein cholesterol values greater than 20 mg/dL.[19] Small, dense LDL (pattern B) occurs in 11.1 percent of the population and in 50 percent of patients with CHD.[20] Fibrinogen greater than 300 mg/dL occurs in 30 percent of the population. Other novel risk factors are leukocyte count, estrogen deficiency, factor VII, endogenous tissue plasminogen activator, plasminogen activator inhibitor type 1, D-dimer, C-reactive protein, and possibly *Chlamydia pneumoniae*.[16,17]

Very early asymptomatic cdiovascular disease can be diagnosed by noninvasive testing, such as magnetic resonance imaging (MRI) and computed tomographic (CT) scanning. Well-established clinical indicators include left ventricular hypertrophy, audible vascular bruits, a positive exercise electrocardiogram (ECG), absent arterial pulses in the limbs and neck, regional wall motion abnormality on the echocardiogram, reduced ankle-arm blood pressure ratio, sonographic evidence of carotid wall thickness, reduced left ventricular ejection fraction, and presence of coronary calcium.

No individual risk factor is essential or sufficient in the causation of cardiovascular disease; causation is multifactorial. Indeed, the risk posed by one factor is generally enhanced in the presence of another. Thus multivariate risk factor assessment gives the most useful measure of the joint effect of the risk factors.[16] Multivariate analyses help provide a better understanding of the pathogenesis of the disease and guidelines for prevention. Based on the absolute, relative, and attributable risks imposed by the various risk factors, the older concepts of *normal* have evolved to optimal values associated with long-term freedom from disease. As a consequence, acceptable blood pressures, blood glucose levels, and lipid values have been revised downward.[16] Multifactorial risk functions based on the Framingham Study data, composed of the major identified risk factors, have been shown to predict the rate of occurrence of coronary disease in a variety of U.S. population samples, suggesting that much of the cardiovascular disease in the population is attributable to these factors[21] (see also Chap. 41).

CORONARY HEART DISEASE

CHD kills and disables people in their most productive years and in 1999 was estimated to account for $53 billion in medical care costs and $47 billion in indirect economic costs.[2] Each year

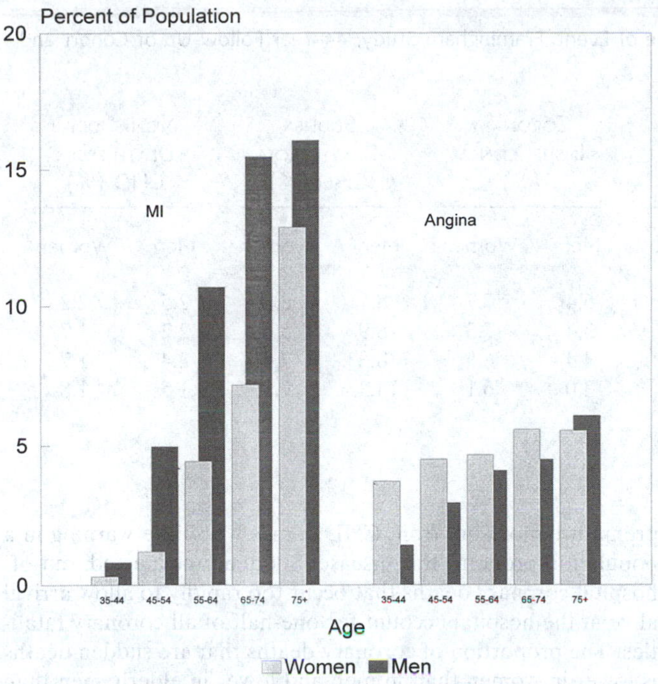

FIGURE 1-3 Prevalence of MI and angina pectoris by age and sex, United States, 1988–1994 (self-reported myocardial infarction and Rose angina from health interviews). MI, myocardial infarction. (From the National Health and Nutrition Examination Survey, 1988–1994, National Center for Health Statistics.)

there are more hospitalizations for CHD than for any broad diagnostic group, with the exceptions of births, all respiratory diseases, all digestive diseases, and all injuries.[8]

Prevalence

In the United States, an estimated 12 million people have CHD, about one-half of whom have acute MI and half have angina pectoris.[2] For men, prevalence of MI is 1 percent at ages 35 to 44 years and 16 percent at age 75 and over (Fig. 1-3). In women, the prevalence is less than 1 percent at ages 35 to 44 years and 13 percent at age 75 and over.

Incidence

In the United States, CHD causes about 650,000 new heart attacks each year and 450,000 recurrent attacks.[2] The incidence in women lags behind that in men by 10 years for total CHD and by 20 years for more serious clinical manifestations such as MI and sudden death (Tables 1-1 and 1-3). Male predominance is least striking for uncomplicated angina pectoris. The first coronary presentation for women is more likely to be angina, whereas in men it is more likely to be MI (Table 1-4). In men, more angina occurs after MI than before. Only 20 percent of coronary attacks are preceded by long-standing angina; the percentage is lower if the infarction is silent or unrecognized. In premenopausal women, serious manifestations of CHD such as infarction or sudden death are relatively rare. The incidence and severity of CHD increase with age in both sexes (see Table 1-3 and Table 1-4). There seems to be a more precipitous increase for women after menopause, with CHD rates in postmenopausal women two to three times those of women the same age who remain premenopausal.[21] This applies whether the menopause is natural or surgical and, in the latter case, whether or not the ovaries are removed. The sex ratio in incidence narrows progressively with advancing age.

Unrecognized MIs are common in the Framingham Study, numbering at least one in three infarctions (Fig. 1-4). Half the unrecognized infarctions are silent, and the rest are atypical so that neither the patient nor the physician entertains the possibility.[22] More than half these persons eventually develop some overt clinical manifestations of CHD and hence come under medical care. Angina is less frequent in individuals with unrecognized MI than in those with recognized symptomatic MI, either before or after the infarction occurs. Despite the apparent mild nature of unrecognized MI, t risk of subsequent mortality is nearly the same as in patients with recognized infarction. Diabetic men and hypertensive persons of both sexes are particularly susceptible to silent or unrecognized MIs.

Prognosis

In patients who survive the acute stage of an MI, the morbidity and mortality range from 1.5 to 15 times that of the general population, depending on the person's sex and clinical outcome (Table 1-5). The rates of occurrence of reinfarction, sudden death, angina pectoris, cardiac failure, and stroke are all substantial. The relative and absolute risks of these events are as great in women as in men after MI. Within 6 years following a recognized MI, 18 percent of men and 35 percent of women have a recurrent infarction, and 27 percent of men and 14 percent of women develop angina. About 22 percent of men and 46 percent of women are disabled with cardiac failure; 8 percent of men and 11 percent of women will have a stroke. Sudden death will be experienced by 7 percent of men and 6

TABLE 1-3 Incidence of Specified Clinical Manifestations of Coronary Heart Disease: Framingham Study, 44-Year Follow-Up of Cohort and 20-Year Follow-Up of Offspring[a]

	Angina Pectoris		Myocardial Infarction		Sudden Death	
Age	Men	Women	Men	Women	Men	Women
35–44	4	1	2	[b]	[b]	[b]
45–54	8	3	5	1	1	[b]
55–64	12	7	10	3	3	1
65–74	11	8	14	5	3	1
75–84	8	7	19	10	6	1
85–94	[b]	5	26	17	[b]	5
35–64[c]	8	4	6	2	2	1
65–94[c]	10	8	16	7	3	1

[a]Average annual incidence rate per 1000 persons free of coronary heart disease.
[b]Results are omitted when fewer than five individuals experienced event.
[c]Age-adjusted rates.
SOURCE: The Framingham Study.

TABLE 1-4 Percentage of First Events of Coronary Heart Disease by Type of Event: Framingham Study, 44-Year Follow-Up of Cohort and 20-Year Follow-Up of Offspring

	Coronary Heart Disease, All Types (*N*)		Myocardial Infarction[a] (%)		Angina Pectoris (%)		Coronary Insufficiency (%)		Sudden Death from CHD (%)		Non-sudden Death from CHD (%)	
Age	Men	Women	Men	Women	Men	Women	Men	Women	Men	Women	Men	Women
35–54	236	91	45.3	29.7	37.7	58.2	6.4	7.7	8.1	2.2	2.5	2.2
55–64	358	233	42.2	26.2	43.3	59.2	3.4	7.3	8.9	5.6	2.2	1.7
65–74	253	231	51.0	33.3	34.0	51.1	4.4	6.5	8.3	7.4	2.4	1.7
75–94	133	165	59.4	54.6	21.8	30.3	3.0	6.1	14.3	7.3	1.5	1.8

[a]Recognized or unrecognized.
SOURCE: The Framingham Study.

percent of women. The prognosis is nearly as bad, sometimes worse, following an unrecognized MI (see Table 1-5).

Mortality

CHD is the leading single cause of death in adults in the United States, accounting for 1 in 5 deaths.[4] In 1997, there were 466,000 coronary deaths. Mortality from this disease increases with age, but CHD is also a prominent cause of death in adults at the peak of their productive lives. Heart disease is the leading cause of death in men and women in every racial or ethnic group except Asian-American females.[2] The CHD death rate is almost three times higher in men than in women at ages 25 to 34, but this ratio declines to 1.6 by ages 75 to 84. The coronary death rate is more than 50 percent higher in blacks than in whites at ages 25 to 34, and this difference disappears by age 75. CHD mortality is not as high among the Hispanic population as it is among blacks and whites.

In a substantial number of CHD deaths, the progression from inapparent clinical disease to death is swift. Much of the premature mortality from CHD comes with little warning in a population prone to this disease. Sudden, unexpected, out-of-hospital coronary deaths that occur too rapidly to allow arrival alive at the hospital account for one-half of all coronary fatalities. The proportion of coronary deaths that are sudden deaths is lower in women than in men and lower in elderly men than in the young (Fig. 1-5). The percentage of sudden coronary deaths that occur without prior CHD, however, is much greater in women than in men (Fig. 1-6). In 50 percent of men and 63 percent of women who died suddenly, there was no prior overt evidence of coronary disease (see also Chap. 36).

There is a higher risk of death in patients with a prior coronary attack, yet most CHD deaths arise from the population who are still free of symptomatic CHD.[23] Hence primary prevention ultimately appears to offer more to society than secondary prevention. After MI, sudden death occurs at four to six times the rate in the general population. The first year following a recognized MI is especially dangerous, with 25 percent of men and 38 percent of women succumbing (Fig. 1-7). Long-term survival following unrecognized MI is only slightly better than for recognized MIs, and survival is better for women than for men (Table 1-6). In men under age 65 with uncomplicated angina pectoris, the survival picture is nearly the same as it is for recognized MI and is much worse than the survival in women (see also Chap. 38).

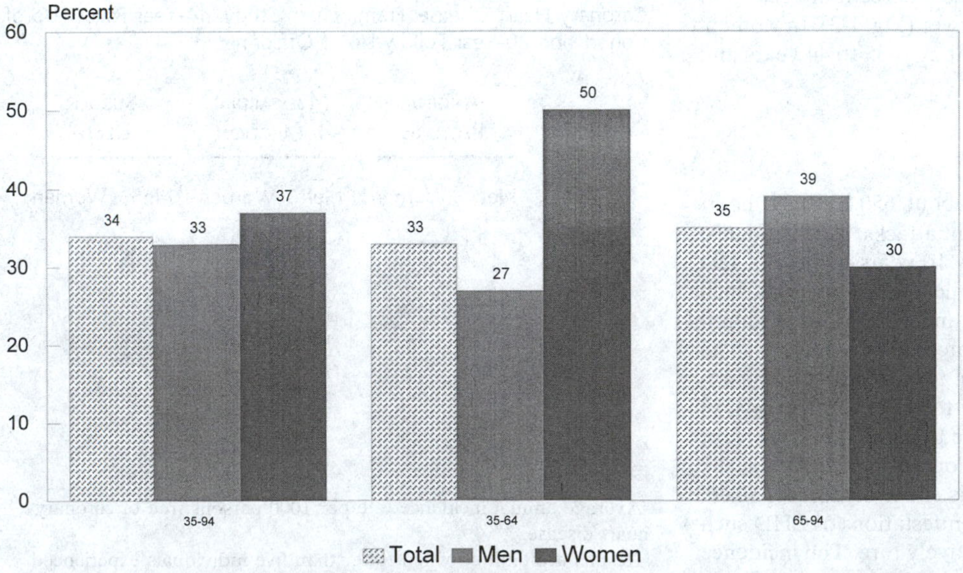

FIGURE 1-4 Percentage of MIs that are unrecognized (Framingham Study 44-year follow-up of cohort and 20-year follow-up of offspring).

HYPERTENSION

Hypertension, present in 50 million Americans, is one of the most powerful contributors to cardiovascular morbidity and mortality: the 600,000 annual cases of stroke, 1.1 million annual heart attacks, 400,000 annual new cases of CHF, and most of the nearly 1 million annual deaths from cardiovascular and kidney diseases.[2,4]

TABLE 1-5 Six-Year Prognosis Following Myocardial Infarction: Framingham Study, 44-Year Follow-Up of Cohort and 20-Year Follow-Up of Offspring[a]

	Men		Women	
	Percent	Risk Ratio[b]	Percent	Risk Ratio[b]
Recognized				
Death	37	2.5	60	5.1
Sudden death	7	2.2	6	4.4
Myocardial infarction	18	2.2	35	9.6
Angina pectoris	27	4.1	14	2.3
Cardiac failure	22	5.4	46	15.4
Stroke/TIA	8	2.4	11	3.1
Unrecognized				
Death	46	2.5	34	2.4
Sudden death	5	1.7	2	2.1
Myocardial infarction	19	2.0	18	3.6
Angina pectoris	11	1.6	17	3.2
Cardiac failure	27	5.8	21	6.2
Stroke/TIA	13	3.5	7	1.5

[a]Surviving 30 days.
[b]Standardized morbidity and mortality ratios (times 0.01).
SOURCE: The Framingham Study.

Prevalence

In a 1988–1994 national survey of persons aged 20 to 74 years, the prevalence of hypertension, i.e., systolic blood pressure of 140 mmHg or greater or diastolic blood pressure of 90 mmHg or greater or on antihypertensive medication, was 24 percent in white men, 19 percent in white women, 35 percent in black men, and 34 percent in black women.[24] Prevalence increases with age and is highest among blacks and the elderly (Fig. 1-8). Isolated systolic hypertension is a common and distinctly hazardous condition in the elderly. There is evidence from the Systemic Hypertension in the Elderly Program (SHEP) and the Syst-Eur trial that treatment of this form of hypertension in the elderly is distinctly efficacious not only against stroke but also against coronary disease.[25,26] Persons with hypertension face serious excess risks of cardiovascular sequelae, and since much of this excess risk is attributable to mild hypertension, there is need for intervention through preventive lifestyle modification, if not through drug treatment. Because of the higher prevalence of milder hypertension, almost 60 percent of the excess mortality attributable to hypertension comes from this blood pressure range. The risks of cardiovascular sequelae are proportional to the blood pressure level at any age and in both sexes and are increased whether the elevation is systolic or diastolic. Approximately one-half of persons who suffer a first heart attack and two-thirds who suffer a first stroke have blood pressures greater than 160/95 mmHg.

Although there is a rise in blood pressure with age in both sexes, in most affluent populations this is not universal, and it does not imply that blood pressure inevitably must rise with age or that in those whose pressures do rise it reflects a normal aging process. In the United States, there is about a 20 mmHg systolic and 10 mmHg diastolic rise in mean pressures from age 30 to age 64. Systolic pressures continue to rise in women into their eighties and in men into their seventies. Diastolic pressures level off earlier and in men decline beyond age 55. The pressures start lower in young-adult women and rise more steeply in middle age (50 and over), and they equal those of men in their fifties and then progressively exceed those of men in later life; this crossover is observed for both systolic and diastolic pressures. In some populations in the world, blood pressure does not rise with age.

For the following discussion, *hypertension* means that a patient has blood pressure of 160/95 mmHg or greater or is on antihypertensive medication; *under control* means that a patient is on antihypertensive medication and has blood pressure of less than 160/95 mmHg. Between the periods 1971–1972 and 1988–1994, there have been large improvements in the percentage of hypertensive patients who (1) are aware of their hypertension (from 51–88 percent), (2) are on antihypertensive medication (from 36–79 percent), and (3) are under control (from 16–65 percent).[1] Although an improving trend is also seen at the 140/90 mmHg and greater level of control, using this definition, 46 percent still do not have medication prescribed for their hypertension.[2]

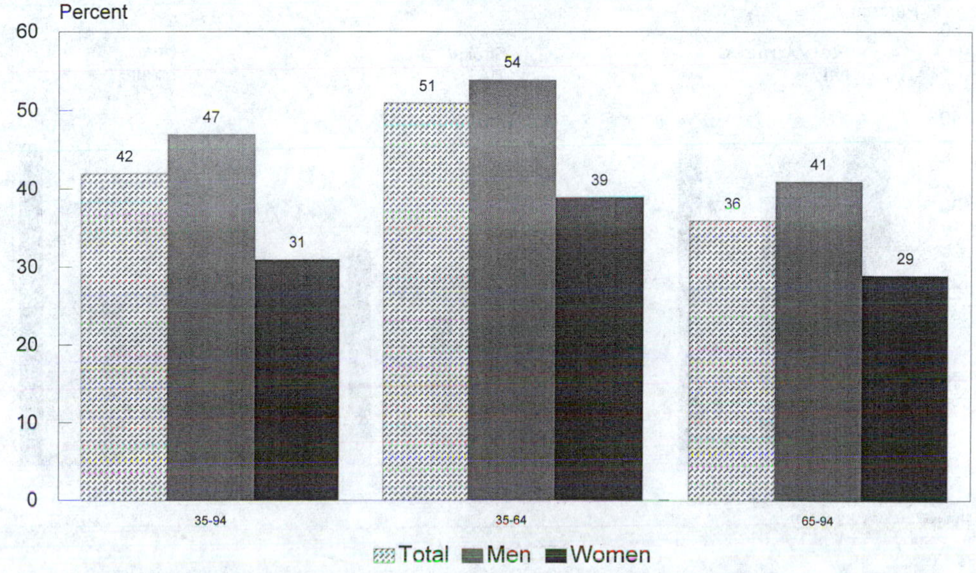

FIGURE 1-5 Percentage of CHD deaths as sudden deaths (Framingham Study 44-year follow-up of cohort and 20-year follow-up of offspring).

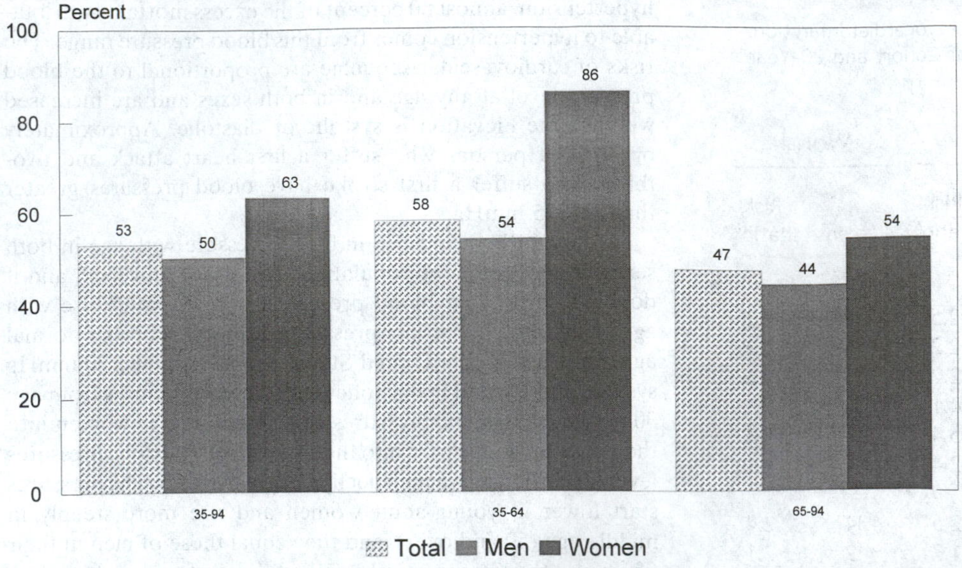

FIGURE 1-6 Percentage of sudden deaths without prior CHD (Framingham Study 44-year follow-up of cohort and 20-year follow-up of offspring).

Determinants

While genetic susceptibility plays a large role in hypertension, this may be only permissive, requiring one or more environmental cofactors such as salt intake, alcohol, or weight gain to bring on hypertension. Of all the identifiable determinants of hypertension, weight gain and adiposity, particularly abdominal in distribution, seem to be predominant. New underlying causes of hypertension are discovered every decade, but the causes of the vast majority of cases remain undetermined. Of the identifiable causes, chronic renal diseases, renovascular disease, and oral contraceptives head the list. Routine search for underlying causes not suggested by signs or symptoms is usually unrewarding and often counterproductive. Recent research suggests that insulin resistance occurring in association with obesity may play a fundamental role[27] (see also Chaps. 41 and 56).

Incidence

Longitudinal observation of blood pressures as people age reveals a different pattern than cross-sectional prevalence data. The reason for this difference is obscure. Diastolic pressures are essentially parallel in both sexes, with women's pressures consistently below those of men at all ages. In women, systolic pressures are initially lower than in men but subsequently rise more steeply with age. They converge at age0 with those of men but never exceed them. With advancing age in both genders, a progressive and disproportionate rise in systolic pressure occurs that is presumed to result from loss of arterial elasticity. Blacks have higher blood pressures than whites in most Western cultures.

STROKE

Prevalence

Two percent of the U.S. adult population, 4.4 million people, have cerebrovascular disease (stroke).[2] More than 1 million of these individuals are limited in their usual activity.[6] Prevalence rises from 2 percent in men at 45 to 54 years to 12.5 percent for men aged 75 and over and from 1 to 10.7 percent in the respective age groups in women (Fig. 1-9). In the Framingham Study, the most common variety of complete stroke is atherothrombotic brain infarction, which accounts for 61 percent of all strokes (excluding transient ischemic attacks).[28] Next most common are cerebral embolus (24 percent), intracerebral hemorrhage, and subarachnoid hemorrhage. Intracerebral hemorrhage apparently has declined most in recent years (see also Chap. 99).

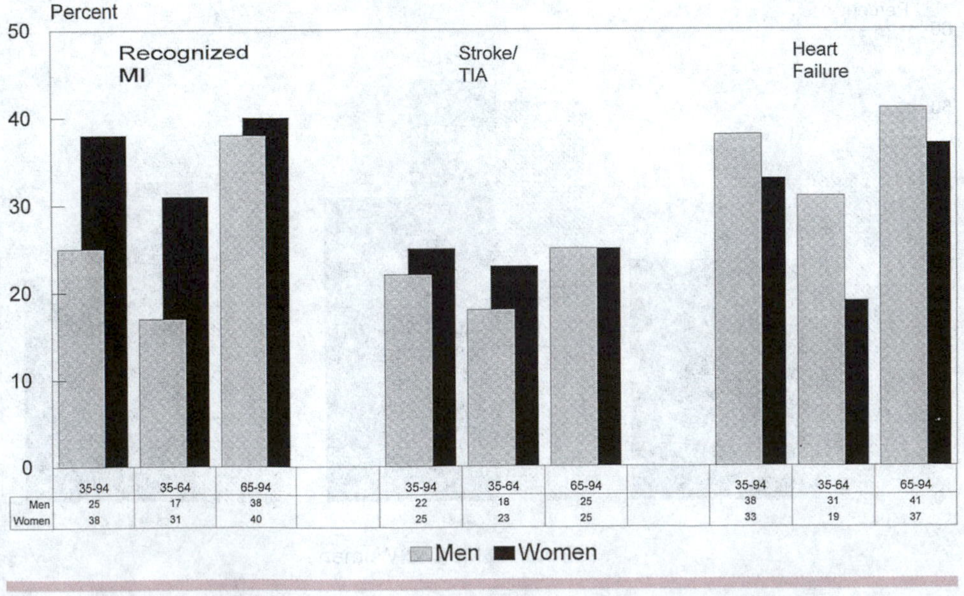

FIGURE 1-7 Percentage dead within 1 year following initial cardiovascular event (Framingham Study 44-year follow-up of cohort and 20-year follow-up of offspring).

Incidence and Disability

In the Framingham Study, the chance of having a stroke before age 70 was 5 percent for both sexes.[28] Annual incidence in the Atherosclerosis Risk in Communities Study was 5.3 per 1000 persons at risk in black men aged 45 to 64 years, 4.0 in black women,

TABLE 1-6 Deaths Per 100 Persons at Risk by Time Interval Following Initial Cardiovascular Event and Survival for 30 Days: Framingham Study, 44-Year Follow-Up of Cohort and 20-Year Follow-Up of Offspring

Interval Length (years)	Angina Pectoris Uncomplicated		Recognized Myocardial Infarction		Unrecognized Myocardial Infarction		Stroke/Transient Ischemic Attacks		Intermittent Claudication		Congestive Heart Failure	
	Men	Women	Men	Women	Men	Women	Men	Women	Men	Women	Men	Women
Ages 35–64 Years												
1–2	2	1	11	12	8	9	12	14	1	1	29	22
2–4	7	4	18	16	14	13	19	22	2	1	46	30
4–8	15	12	27	28	30	29	30	30	13	9	61	44
8–12	32	25	45	47	52	41	51	53	35	23	80	70
12–16	51	37	56	71	74	52	69	68	57	41	90	81
16–20	66	52	69	84	85	60	80	77	72	67	93	87
Ages 65–94 Years												
1–2	2	4	24	17	12	10	20	18	1	1	35	30
2–4	9	9	35	23	23	24	32	28	2	1	56	42
4–8	23	26	50	46	40	52	46	42	16	12	73	57
8–12	51	41	69	69	69	70	74	69	51	38	91	85
12–16	75	60	85	89	90	84	89	83	71	69	98	94
16–20	92	79	91	95	97	89	95	92	93	88	100	97

SOURCE: The Framingham Study.

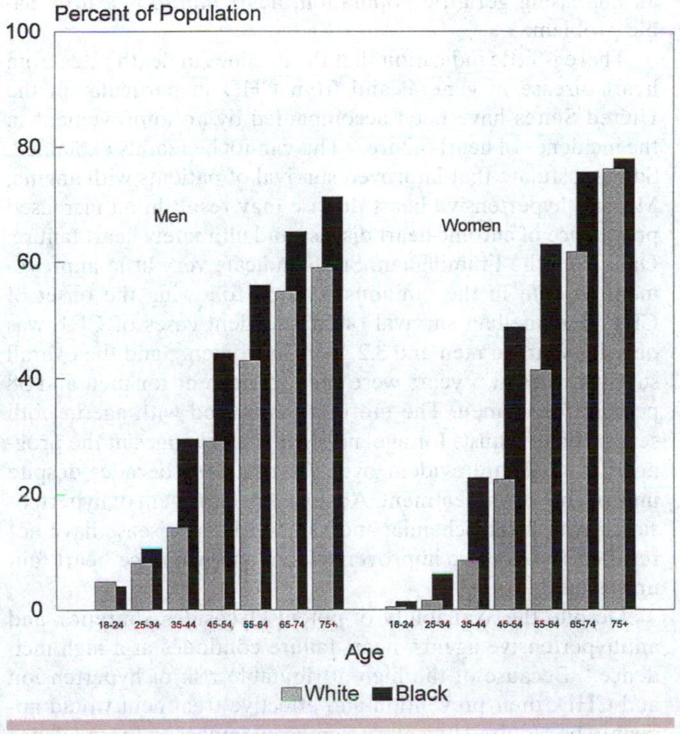

FIGURE 1-8 Prevalence of hypertension by age, race, and sex; United States, 1988–1994 (hypertension: 140/90 mmHg or greater or on antihypertensive medication). (From the National Health and Nutrition Examination Survey, National Center for Health Statistics.)

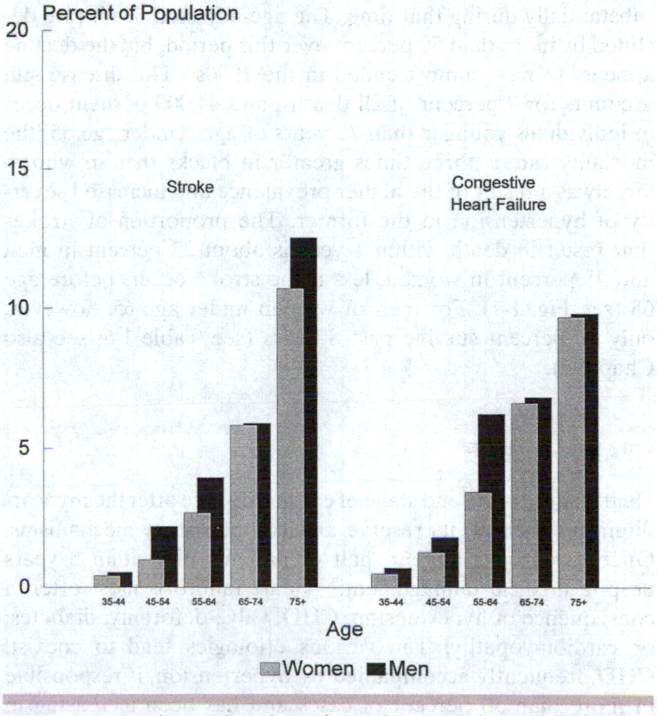

FIGURE 1-9 Prevalence of stroke and CHF by age and sex, United States, 1988–1994 (self-reported stroke and congestive heart failure from health interviews). (From the National Health and Nutrition Examination Survey, National Center for Health Statistics.)

2.0 in white men, and 1.5 in white women.[29] Of the incident events, 83 percent were ischemic strokes, 10 percent were hemorrhagic, and 7 percent were subarachnoid hemorrhage. Among the 54 percent classified as definite thrombotic brain infarctions, 38 percent were classified as lacunar, more than twice as many in blacks as in whites. The time course of functional recovery is strongly related to initial stoke severity.[30] Of survivors of an initial event, 50 to 70 percent return to functional independence, but 15 to 30 percent become permanently dependent. Institutional care is required by 20 percent at 3 months after onset.[31]

Stroke attacks have become less severe in recent years, but prevention is essential for dealing effectively with the problem of stroke because of the irreversibility of established ischemic brain damage and the neurologic deficit it induces. The underlying cerebrovascular disease is not a necessary consequence of aging. Modifiable contributing factors offer the possibility of prevention in identified stroke candidates. Stroke prevention requires early and sustained treatment of persons with hypertension, cardiac disorders (especially atrial fibrillation), and transient cerebral ischemic attacks.

Mortality

Cerebrovascular disease, the third leading cause of death, was responsible for 207,000 deaths in the United States in 1974, but by 1997, the number had declined to 160,000.[4,12] This decline is remarkable because the population of older persons increased substantially during that time. The age-adjusted death rate declined by more than 50 percent over this period, but the decline appears to have almost ended in the 1990s.[1] This disease still accounts for 7 percent of all deaths, and 44,000 of them occur in individuals younger than 75 years of age. Under age 65, the mortality rate is three times greater in blacks than in whites, largely as a result of the higher prevalence and increased severity of hypertension in the former. The proportion of strokes that result in death within 1 year is about 22 percent in men and 25 percent in women, less if the stroke occurs before age 65 (see Fig. 1-7). For men or women under age 65, however, only 50 percent survive past 8 years (see Table 1-6; see also Chap. 99).

HEART FAILURE

Heart failure is the end stage of cardiac disease after the myocardium has used all its reserve and compensatory mechanisms. Once overt signs appear, half of patients die within 5 years despite medical management.[32] Heart failure is most often a consequence of hypertension, CHD, valve deformity, diabetes, or cardiomyopathy. The various etiologies tend to coexist. CHD, frequently accompanied by hypertension, is responsible in more than 50 percent of cases and has been increasing in prevalence among new cases of heart failure. Left ventricular hypertrophy, hypertension, and valvular diseases are diminishing determinants. The risk of cardiac failure is increased two- to sixfold with CHD, angina conferring half the risk compared with MI. The dominant cause continues to be hypertension, which precedes failure in 75 percent of patients.

An estimated 4.8 million Americans have CHF.[2] The prevalence increases with age to exceed 10 percent after age 60 (see Fig. 1-9). Each year there are an estimated 400,000 new cases.[2] In 1997, there were 43,000 deaths nominally classified to heart failure as the underlying cause and about another 200,000 where heart failure was listed on the death certificates as a secondary cause. The death rate increased in most years between 1968 and 1997. The rate of hospitalizations for heart failure increased between three and four times between 1970 and 1997 in patients aged 45 to 64 and 65 and over.[2,8] In 1997, heart failure was the first-listed discharge diagnosis in 957,000 hospital discharges and a secondary diagnosis in another 2.1 million discharges.[8] Twenty percent of all hospital discharges of patients aged 65 and over had heart failure as a primary or secondary diagnosis. The percentage of CHF patients who died in hospitals, however, decreased from 11.3 percent in 1981 to 5.0 percent in 1996.[1] Visits to physicians' offices for CHF increased from 1.7 million in 1980 to 3.2 million in 1995. The prevalence is similar in men and women, but it is higher in blacks than whites. It increased substantially as measured in national surveys in 1976–1980 and 1988–1994 (see also Chaps. 23 and 41).

Based on the Framingham Study, heart failure is equally frequent in men and women, and the annual occurrence approaches 10 per 1000 population after 65 years of age (see Table 1-1). Survival following the diagnosis of heart failure is worse in men than in women, but even in women fewer than 15 percent survive much longer than 8 to 12 years (see Table 1-6). The prognosis is not much better than for most forms of cancer. The 1-year fatality rate for heart failure is high, with one in five patients dying. Sudden death is a common mode of exitus, occurring at six to nine times the general population rate. With an increasing geriatric population, heart failure is a formidable problem.

There is little indication that the declines in death rates from heart disease in general and from CHD in particular in the United States have been accompanied by an improvement in the incidence of heart failure.[33] This cannot be readily explained. Some postulate that improved survival of patients with angina, MI, and hypertensive heart disease may result in an increased prevalence of chronic heart disease and ultimately heart failure. Data from the Framingham Study indicate very little improvement to date in the ominous outlook following the onset of CHF. The median survival of 652 incident cases of CHF was only 1.7 years in men and 3.2 years in women,[33] and the overall survival rates at 5 years were only 25 percent for men and 38 percent for women. The mortality increased with age in both sexes. If one adjusts for age, no significant changes in the prognosis of CHF are evident over the past four decades despite improvements in treatment. Advances in treatment of hypertension, myocardial ischemia, and valvular heart disease have not resulted in dramatic improvements in survival once heart failure ensues.

Despite the availability of potent glycosides, diuretics, and antihypertensive agents, heart failure continues at a high incidence.[34] Because of the high attributable risk of hypertension and CHD, their prevention and effective treatment would appear to be required to make a significant impact on the incidence of congestive heart failure.

IDIOPATHIC CARDIOMYOPATHY

Reliable estimates of the prevalence and incidence of idiopathic dilated (congestive) and hypertrophic cardiomyopathies are unavailable because of their comparatively uncommon occurrence in the general population. The National Center for Health Statistics data from 1996 assigned 27,501 deaths to cardiomyopathy, hypertrophic cardiomyopathy accounting for only 1 percent.[4,35] Alcoholic heart muscle disease (cardiomyopathy) appears to account for 8 percent of deaths due to cardiomyopathy. This condition appears to be 2.5 times as frequent in blacks as in whites. Mortality from cardiomyopathy was highest in older persons, men, and blacks. Death rates rose sharply in the 1970s and 1980s but for reasons that are unclear. This apparent increase could be an artifact of changes in diagnostic criteria and death certification practices. In 1997, cardiomyopathy was the primary diagnosis for 39,000 hospitalizations and 261,000 days of hospital care, but 443,000 hospitalizations had cardiomyopathy listed as a secondary diagnosis[8] (see also Chaps. 72 and 73).

ARRHYTHMIAS

Arrhythmias are a major cause of morbidity in heart failure and rheumatic heart disease and are a contributor to half the mortality from CHD. Many such victims die suddenly, without warning. Together with heart failure, arrhythmias are often the final common pathways of terminal heart disease. Estimates of morbidity and mortality are difficult to obtain. There is good evidence, however, that atrial fibrillation is the most common of the serious arrhythmias and is responsible for substantial morbidity and mortality in the general population.[36] Although the true frequency of arrhythmias is not known, in 1997 there were an estimated 3.5 million hospital discharges with arrhythmias as the primary (635,000) or secondary diagnosis, with two-thirds being due to atrial fibrillation.[8] Between 1982 and 1995, the rate of hospitalization for atrial fibrillation about doubled.[1] In 1995, there were an estimated 3.3 million visits to physicians' offices for arrhythmias, more than due to the cerebrovascular diseases.

The Framingham Study reported estimates for atrial fibrillation. In that population, prevalence rose from 0.5 percent at ages 50 to 59 years to almost 9 percent at ages 80 to 89 years.[36] Between 1968 and 1989, age-adjusted prevalence tripled in men but did not change appreciably in women. These trends are unexplained. Incidence also doubles with each successive age decade, to reach almost 5 percent per year at ages 85 to 94 years.

Most cases of atrial fibrillation evolved following development of overt cardiovascular disease. Heart failure, MI, and valvular heart disease were the most powerful precursors, with the relative risks as much as sixfold. Hypertensive cardiovascular disease was the most common prior cardiovascular disease, largely because of its great frequency in the general population. Impaired glucose tolerance was the other major risk factor predisposing substantially to atrial fibrillation.

Atrial fibrillation is associated with increased risks of cardiovascular morbidity and mortality. After adjusting for various factors, there was a three- to fivefold increased risk of stroke, the chief hazard of atrial fibrillation. Atrial fibrillation decreases survival and is associated with a near doubling of the risk of mortality, after adjusting for associated cardiovascular conditions (see Chap. 27).

RHEUMATIC FEVER AND RHEUMATIC HEART DISEASE

Rheumatic fever is a prominent cause of serious valvular heart disease. Acute rheumatic fever and subsequent rheumatic heart disease remain important cardiovascular problems in the tropical and subtropical developing countries of South America, Africa, the Middle East, and Asia, and there have been outbreaks in the United States in recent years.[37] Although preventable, rheumatic fever occurs more frequently because of overcrowding, the deceptive self-limited nature of symptoms in streptococcal pharyngitis, and the mild and often clinically inapparent nature of streptococcal infections. The availability of penicillin to treat these infections, living conditions that are less crowded than formerly, and evolution of different strains of *Streptococcus* have made rheumatic fever uncommon in the United States, although the incidence remains high in subgroups such as blacks, Puerto Ricans, Mexican Americans, and Native Americans (see Chap. 62). Because this disease has not been eradicated in this country, there is a need to define its incidence and prevalence more accurately as well as those of the infective endocarditis that may follow in order to pinpoint those at risk (see also Chap. 82).

An estimated 1.8 million persons have rheumatic heart disease in the United States, more than 6 per 1000 persons.[2] About 15 percent of these persons are limited in activity because of the resulting chronic carditis.[6] There is no national estimate of annual incidence. A study in Tennessee reported a range from 0.5 to 1.88 new cases per 100,000 school-aged children in 1977–1981, with the lowest rates in the affluent suburbs.[37] Occurrence tends to be concentrated in the lower socioeconomic subgroups, perhaps due to factors of nutrition, hygiene, and access to medical care. Rheumatic fever is rare before age 3, occurring most frequently between 5 and 15 years of age, when streptococcal infections are most frequent. During epidemics of streptococcal pharyngitis, the rheumatic fever attack rate may be 3 percent, whereas in endemic situations it is usually only 0.3 percent (see also Chap. 62).

With the decline in rheumatic fever in the United States, its clinical manifestations also have moderated so that carditis is detected in fewer than 20 percent of acutely affected patients.[38] The annual mortality has declined to about 5000 deaths per year. Because the cardiac sequelae of rheumatic fever are still seen in adults and adequate treatment can reduce attacks by 90 percent, rheumatic fever and rheumatic heart disease remain the two most preventable serious cardiovascular disorders. It seems clear that at least part of the decline in rheumatic fever was due to prompt antistreptococcal treatment by physicians. The decline in rheumatic fever, however, appears to have antedated the advent of antistreptococcal agents. We are currently unable to explain the reasons for the decline in rheumatic fever definitely, possibly because we do not fully understand its etiologic factors (see Chap. 62).

OTHER VALVULAR DISEASE

In the two decades since mitral valve prolapse was described, the syndrome was thought to be a frequently diagnosed valvular deformity, more common in women. This assessment was based on studies that had patient selection bias and diagnostic criteria that were less specific than those used today. In a community population study, with false-positive results, false-negative results, and selection bias greatly minimized, the picture looks quite different.[39] The Framingham Study reports that prevalence is no more than 1 to 2 percent, no more common in women than in men, and diagnosis of associated cardiovascular sequelae is low. This assessment also has its limitations. Study results are based on a white population only, confidence limits around the prevalence estimates are large, results are subject to a survival bias, and patients with mitral valve prolapse that resulted in sudden death may not have been included in the cohort. The major importance of mitral valve prolapse may be the threat of endocarditis, which must be rare, and arrhythmias, which may be common (see Chap. 65).

Little information is available on the prevalence of valvular heart disease in the general population. Most prevalence estimates come from surgical studies and small numbers of patients referred for diagnosis. The Framingham Study has estimated prevalence of mitral, tricuspid, and aortic regurgitation in their population sample using color Doppler echocardiography routinely obtained on all participants.[40] Some degree of mitral and tricuspid regurgitation was seen in 19 and 15 percent of men and 19 and 18 percent of women, respectively. Aortic regurgitation was found in 13 percent of men and 8.5 percent of women.

Rheumatic heart disease is no longer the most frequent cause of valve disease. Mitral valve prolapse and degeneration of congenital aortic valve lesions are now the most common causes.[41] Aortic stenosis also may result from atherosclerotic degeneration of the valve in diabetes with dyslipidemia. It is the most common valve lesion in the elderly having valve replacement.[42] Aortic root or annular dilatation is responsible for most aortic regurgitation, of which 40 to 60 percent is of unknown cause.

CONGENITAL HEART DISEASE

About one million persons in the United States have congenital cardiovascular disease, and each year an estimated 32,000 babies, about 8 per 1000 live births, are born with this disease.[2,43] Of the new cases, 8 to 13 percent have atrial sepal defects, 6 to 11 percent have patent ductus arteriosus, and 20 to 25 percent have ventricular sepal defects. The prevalence of congenital heart disease at birth as determined during the infant's brief stay in the hospital is likely to be underestimated, and recognition of specific lesions may be inaccurate.[44] Most data are deficient for a diagnosis after the first week of life. Prevalence data based on autopsy findings are unreliable because they reflect a fraction of the deaths and relate only to fatal lesions. Most information comes from retrospective studies based extensively on referral practices.

Structural abnormalities of the heart or intrathoracic great vessels seem to affect 8 to 10 of every 1000 infants born alive in the United States. If bicuspid aortic valves and mitral valve prolapse manifested later in life are included, the rate may well exceed 1 percent of live births. About 1 newborn per 1000 live births has a cardiac birth defect that cannot be managed medically or surgically. Most infants who previously would have died now survive to adult life because of improved treatment, but 5 to 6 of these infants per 1000 live births require frequent medical or surgical attention shortly after birth or later in childhood.

Except for the recent unexplained twofold increase in ventricular sepal defects and the threefold increase in patent ductus arteriosus, the incidence of most congenital heart diseases has remained stable. Rubella vaccine has reduced rubella-caused congenital heart disease, and congenital heart defects associated with Down's syndrome are less common because older women are having fewer babies. Pregnancies may be terminated if prenatal screening reveals Down's syndrome. Preventive strategies are impeded by lack of knowledge of the cause of most congenital heart disease, although it is known that alcohol, trimethadione, and lithium can cause cardiac defects. The majority of congenital heart disease may involve complex genetic-environmental interactions that remain to be elucidated (see Chaps. 69 and 70).

About 75 of each 1000 live births in the United States are premature, with the infants weighing less than 2500 g.[12] Almost half of premature infants weighing less than 1750 g will maintain patency of their ductus arteriosus, possibly because their immature lungs do not properly metabolize prostaglandins that cause the ductus to remain open.[45] The growing number of teratogens identified appears to account for only 5 percent of all human malformations, and single mutant genes are said to be responsible for only 3 percent of cases.

In 1997, deaths in infancy from congenital cardiovascular disease occurred at the rate of 0.5 per 1000 live births, about one-half the rate that occurred in 1980.[8] The 1-year fatality rate among the estimated 32,000 new cases at birth each year was about 6.5 percent in 1997. About 25 percent of infants with congenital heart disease have a malformation incompatible with life beyond the first year; possibly half of these can be treated surgically to improve the quality of life, if not to produce a cure. About 2.5 per 1000 live-born infants require specialized services for diagnosis and treatment of congenital heart disease shortly after birth, and another 2.5 per 1000 will need these resources later in childhood.

With the exception of bicuspid aortic valve in older patients, ventricular septal defect is the most common variety, accounting for 30 percent of congenital heart disease. Some 75 percent of congenital heart disease in infants and children is encompassed by seven defects: ventricular sepal defect, pulmonary stenosis, patent ductus arteriosus, tetralogy of Fallot, aortic stenosis, coarctation of the aorta, and transposition of the great arteries. There is an excess of birth defects in blacks. The rate among siblings is 17 per 1000 compared with 2.6 per 1000 in the general population (see Chap. 70).

PULMONARY THROMBOEMBOLISM

More than 95 percent of pulmonary emboli arise from deep venous thrombi in the legs (above the knee); the remainder arise from the right cardiac chambers or other veins. The majority of deaths occur suddenly and can be avoided only by prophylaxis. Patients who survive to reach the hospital for medical treatment generally have a good outlook, with little morbidity and resolution of the emboli.

Estimates of mortality from pulmonary embolism vary depending on the source and accuracy of data. Pulmonary emboli are probably directly responsible for 50,000 deaths annually in the United States. If untreated, recurrent episodes are frequent, and more than 25 percent will be fatal. More than 60 percent of fatalities occur within 1 hour of onset; hence pulmonary embolism is likely to be confused with sudden coronary death. It is estimated that pulmonary embolism is grossly underdiagnosed, since only 10 to 30 percent of autopsied cases with evidence of embolism had an antemortem diagnosis.[46]

Among the U.S. population, the age-adjusted death rate for pulmonary embolism decreased 33 percent between 1979 and 1997.[4] The decline was greater in whites than in blacks and greater in men than in women. The rate of hospital discharges with a primary or secondary diagnosis of pulmonary embolism declined 38 percent from 7 per 10,000 population in 1979 to 4.3 in 1997.[8] Death rates and hospital rates for pulmonary embolism increase with age and are higher in men than in women and in blacks than in whites.[4] It was listed on 115,000 hospital records in 1997.[8] The incidence is even more uncertain. Only 10 percent of cases occur in normal persons without predisposing factors such as chronic cardiopulmonary and malignant disease, estrogen therapy, orthopedic trauma, immobilization, operative procedures, obesity, pregnancy, or blood dyscrasias. The elderly are more vulnerable.

Postoperative pulmonary emboli alone produce 4000 to 8000 deaths annually.[47] It is a major cause of death postpartum and in patients hospitalized for orthopedic conditions. Evidence from Britain suggests that the annual mortality from pulmonary embolism has been increasing for several decades despite anticoagulant drugs. More than 5 million persons over age 45 undergo major surgery each year in the United States; 1 or 2 of each 1000 will die postoperatively from pulmonary embolism. The recent advent of low-dose heparin prophylaxis may reduce this risk substantially (see Chap. 60).

PREVENTIVE IMPLICATIONS FOR THE 21ST CENTURY

Examination of the incidence, prevalence, mortality, natural history, and risk factors of cardiovascular disease suggests the greatest benefits will be from a preventive approach. Further innovations in diagnosis and treatment for cardiovascular disease undoubtedly will improve the outlook of patients surviving the initial attack, but this can have only a limited impact because of the high initial mortality. When the heart or brain is infarcted, no therapy can be expected to restore full function. If the initial presentation is sudden death, therapy is unavailing. A preventive approach involving correction of predisposing factors in advance of the overt clinical expression of the disease can be expected to have a greater impact. To date, application of preventive measures of proven efficacy has been suboptimal.[48] Their application in the next century, even for the growing elderly population, has immense potential for primary and secondary prevention. Evidence is accumulating that medical therapy (vigorous risk-factor control) may be at least as effective as surgical or invasive revascularization in preventing recurrence of MI, progression of angina to MI, and premature CHD mortality. The potential benefits for primary prevention of MI by modification of risk factors has been demonstrated by a meta-analysis and reviews of the larger and more rigorous epidemiologic studies.[49] A multifactorial approach to risk reduction offers the best opportunity for saving patients at high risk and preventing the development of high-risk status in the first place.[50]

CHD often strikes without warning: One in five coronary attacks presents as sudden death, and two-thirds of the deaths occur in the community too precipitously to be brought under medical attention. While some strokes may give warning by transient ischemic attacks, most do not. Even when they do, intervention at that stage does not necessarily avoid a permanently damaging stroke or prolong life. Heart valves damaged by degenerative and rheumatic heart disease and infective endocarditis can be repaired surgically or replaced by prosthetic appliances; this approach often requires potentially dangerous anticoagulants to prevent emboli, and valve failure and hemolysis are distressingly common. Although such patients live longer, more comfortable lives than formerly, their survival does not approach that of patients with rheumatic fever who have been kept from progressing to severe valve damage by antibiotic prophylaxis against recurrent disease. Hypertension that progresses to target-organ involvement is less manageable than if vigorously treated prior to such manifestations. The first sign of target-organ involvement is often a stroke, MI, or sudden death. Half of such events occur before evidence of organ involvement is discovered on routine biennial examination. In some respects, the occurrence of symptoms more properly may be regarded as a medical failure rather than as the initial indication for treatment (see Chap. 58).

A major impact on cardiovascular morbidity and mortality in the 21st century should derive from the practice of preventive medicine, from public health measures to alter lifestyle to one more favorable to cardiovascular health, and from health education to inform people of what they must do to protect their cardiovascular health. Recent expansion and improvements in these measures have occurred, conceivably contributing significantly to the 36 percent decline in cardiovascular mortality during the past two decades, which is responsible for most of the decline in overall mortality.[2]

The epidemiologic and clinical trial evidence of the cardiovascular diseases in the 20th century has set the stage for opportunities in the next century to direct research and public health activities that can substantially reduce the risk and impact of cardiovascular disease. Foremost among those opportunities is implementation of comprehensive preventive programs of government regulation, health education, and preventive medicine designed to control the major identified cardiovascular risk factors. This includes exploring further the underlying basis for clustering of atherogenic risk factors and the prevalence and impact of insulin resistance, promoting cardiovascular risk profiles to more efficiently target high-risk cardiovascular disease candidates for preventive measures, and finding better ways to implement preventive measures against obesity, insulin resistance, and cigarette smoking. The potential is large if physicians can be induced to more aggressively implement the proven measures recommended to prevent cardiovascular disease.

References

1. National Heart, Lung, and Blood Institute. *Morbidity and Mortality Chartbook on Cardiovascular, Lung, and Blood Diseases*, 1998. US Dept of Health and Human Services; 1998. *http://www nhlbi.nih.gov/index.htm.*
2. American Heart Association. *1999 Heart and Stroke: Statistical Update.* Dallas: American Heart Association, 1999. *http://www.am hrt.org.*
3. Lloyd-Jones DM, Larson MG, Beiser A, Levy D. Lifetime risk of developing coronary heart disease. *Lancet* 1999; 353:89–92.
4. National Center for Health Statistics. Detailed statistical tables: General mortality: GMWK1 Total deaths for each cause by 5-year age group, United States 1993, 1994, 1995, 1996, and 1997. *http://www.cdc.gov/nchswww..*

5. National Center for Health Statistics, Benson V, Marano MA. Current estimates from the National Health Interview Survey, United States, 1995. *Vital and Health Statistics, Series 10(199)* DHHS pub no (PHS) 98-1527. US Government Printing Office; 1998. *http://www.cdc.gov/nchswww/.*
6. National Center for Health Statistics, Collins JG. Prevalence of selected chronic conditions, United States, 1990-1992. *Vital and Health Statistics* 10(194), DHHS pub no (PHS) 97-1522. US Government Printing Office; 1997. *http://www.cdc.gov/nchswww/.*
7. Rogot E, Sorlie PD, Johnson NJ, et al. Second data book: A study of 1.3 million persons: By demographic, social, and economic factors: 1979-1985 follow-up: US National Longitudinal Mortality Study. US Dept of Health and Human Services, National Institutes of Health, pub no 92-3297; 1992.
8. National Center for Health Statistics, Lawrence L, Hall MJ. 1997 Summary: National Hospital Discharge Survey. *Advance Data from Vital and Health Statistics* 308, DHHS pub no (PHS) 99-1250. US Government Printing Office; 1999. *http://www.cdc.gov/nchswww/.*
9. National Center for Health Statistics, Woodwell DA. National ambulatory medical care survey: 1997 summary. *Advance Data from Vital and Health Statistics* 305, DHHS pub no (PHS) 99-1250. US Government Printing Office; 1999. *http://www.cdc.gov/nchswww/.*
10. National Center for Health Statistics, McCraig LF. National hospital ambulatory medical care survey: 1997 outpatient department summary. Advance Data from Vital and Health Statistics 307, DHHS pub no (PHS) 96-1250. US Government Printing Office; 1999. *http://www.cdc.gov/nchswww/.*
11. National Center for Health Statistics, Haupt BJ. An overview of home health and hospice care patients: 1996 National Home and Hospice Care Survey. *Advance Data from Vital and Health Statistics* 297, DHHS pub no (PHS) 98-1250. US Government Printing Office; 1998. *http://www.cdc.gov/nchswww/.*
12. National Center for Health Statistics. *Health, United States, 1998.* DHHS pub no (PHS) 98-1232. US Government Printing Office; 1998. *http://www.cdc.gov/nchswww/.*
13. Hunink MG, Goldman L, Tosteson, et al. The recent decline in mortality from coronary heart disease, 1980-1990: The effect of secular trends in risk factors and treatment. *JAMA* 1997; 277: 535–542.
14. Rosamond WD, Chambless LE, Folsom AR, et al. Trends in the incidence of myocardial infarction and in mortality due to coronary heart disease, 1987-1994. *New Engl J Med* 1998; 339:861–867.
15. Tunstall-Pedoe H, Kuulasmaa K, Mahonen M, et al. Contributions of trends in survival and coronary-event rates to changes in coronary heart disease mortality: 10-year results from 37 WHO MONICA project populations. *Lancet* 1999; 353:1547–1557.
16. Kannel WB, Wilson PWF. An update on coronary risk factors. *Med Clin North Am* 1995; 79:951–971.
17. Braunwald E. Shattuck lecture: Cardiovascular medicine at the turn of the millennium: Triumphs, concerns, and opportunities. *New Engl J Med* 1997; 337:1360–1369.
18. Selhub J, Jacques PF, Wilson PWF, et al. Vitamin status and intake as primary determinants of homocystinemia in an elderly population. *JAMA* 1993; 270:2693–2698.
19. Dammerman M, Breslow JL. Genetic basis of lipoprotein disorders. *Circulation* 1995; 92:505–512.
20. Superko HR. Small-dense LDL: The new coronary artery disease risk factor and how it is changing the treatment of coronary artery disease. *Prev Cardiol* 1998; 1:16–24.
21. Levy D, Wilson PWF. Atherosclerotic cardiovascular disease: An epidemiologic perspective. In: Topol EJ, ed. *Textbook of Cardiovascular Medicine.* Philadelphia: Lippincott-Raven; 1998:13–29.
22. Kannel WB. Clinical misconceptions dispelled by epidemiologic research. *Circulation* 1995; 92:3350–3360.
23. Kannel WB, Wilson PWF, D'Agostino RB, Cobb J. Sudden coronary death in women. *Am Heart J* 1998; 136:205–212.
24. Thom TJ, Roccella EJ. Trends in blood pressure control and mortality. In: Izzo JL, Black HR, eds. *Hypertension Primer: The Essentials of High Blood Pressure: Basic Science,* 2d ed. Dallas: American Heart Association; 1999:268–270.
25. SHEP Cooperative Research Group. Prevention of stroke by antihypertensive drug treatment in older persons with isolated systolic hypertension. Final results of the Systolic Hypertension in the Elderly Program. *JAMA* 1991; 265:3255–3264.
26. Staessen JA, Fagard R, Thijs L, et al. Randomized double-blind comparison of placebo and active treatment for older patients with isolated systolic hypertension. The Systolic Hypertension in Europe (Syst-Eur) Trial investigators. *Lancet* 1997; 350:757–764.
27. Reaven GM, Lithell H, Landsberg L. Hypertension and associated metabolic abnormalities: The role of insulin resistance and the sympathoadrenal system. *New Engl J Med* 1996; 334:374–381.
28. Wolf PA, D'Agostino RB. Epidemiology of stroke. In: Barnett HJM, Mohr JP, Stein BM, eds. *Stroke: Pathophysiology, Diagnosis, and Management,* Chap 1. New York: Churchill-Livingstone; 1998:3–28.
29. Rosamond WD, Folsom AR, Chambless LE, et al. Stroke incidence and survival among middle-aged adults: 9-year follow-up of the Atherosclerosis in Communities (ARIC) cohort. *Stroke* 1999; 30:736.
30. Jorgensen HS, Nakayama H, Raaschou H, et al. Outcome and time course of recovery in stroke: II. Time course of recovery. The Copenhagen Stroke Study. *Arch Phys Med Rehabil* 1995; 76:406–412.
31. Asplund K, Stegmayr B, Peltonen M. From the twentieth to the twenty-first century: A public health perspective on stroke. In: Ginsberg MD, Bogousslavsky J, eds. *Cerebrovascular Disease: Pathophysiology, Diagnosis, and Management,* Vol 2, Chap 64. Boston: Blackwell Science; 1998.
32. Kannel WB, Ho K, Thom T. Changing epidemiological features of cardiac failure. *Br Heart J* 1994; 72:S3–S9.
33. Gillum RF. Epidemiology of heart failure in the United States. *Am Heart J* 1993; 126:1042–1047.
34. Ho KKL, Pinsky JL, Kannel WB, et al. The epidemiology of heart failure: The Framingham Study. *J Am Coll Cardiol* 1993; 22: 6A–13A.
35. Gillum RF. The epidemiology of cardiomyopathy in the United States. In: Zipes P, Rowlands DJ, eds. *Progress in Cardiology.* Philadelphia: Lea and Febiger; 1989:11–21.
36. Kannel WB, Wolf PA, Benjamin EJ, Levy D. Prevalence, incidence, prognosis, and predisposing conditions for atrial fibrillation: Population-based estimates. *Am J Cardiol* 1998; 82:2N–9N.
37. Bisno AL. The resurgence of acute rheumatic fever in the United States. *Annu Rev Med* 1990; 41:319–329.
38. Persellin RH. Acute rheumatic fever. Changing manifestations. *Ann Intern Med* 1978; 89:1002–1003.
39. Freed LA, Levy D, Levine RA, et al. Prevalence and clinical outcome of mitral valve prolapse. *New Engl J Med* 1999; 341:1–2.
40. Singh JP, Evans JC, Levy D, et al. Prevalence and clinical determinants of mitral, tricuspid, and aortic regurgitation (The Framingham Study). *Am J Cardiol* 1999; 83:897–902.
41. Moller JH, Nakib A, Elliott RS, Edwards LE. Symptomatic aortic stenosis in first year of life. *J Pediatr* 1966; 69:728–734.
42. Rahimtoola SH. Valvular heart disease. In: Stein J, ed. *Internal Medicine,* 3d ed. St Louis: Mosby-Year Book; 1994:202–234.
43. Engle MA. Congenital heart disease. *J Am Coll Cardiol* 1999; 33:905–908.
44. Gillum RF. Epidemiology of congenital heart disease in the United States. *Am Heart J* 1994; 127:919–927.
45. Michaelson M. *Report on a Study of Congenital Cardiovascular Malformations: Etiology, Incidence, Natural History and Organiza-*

tion of Diagnostic and Therapeutic Service. Geneva: World Health Organization, Regional Office for Europe, 1979.

46. Moser KM. Pulmonary thromboembolism. In: Isselbacher KJ, Braunwald E, Wilson JD, et al, eds. *Harrison's Principles of Internal Medicine*, 13th ed. New York: McGraw-Hill; 1994:1214–1220.
47. Clagett GP, Anderson FA Jr, Levine MN, et al. Prevention of venous thromboembolism. *Chest* 1995; 108(suppl):3125–3345.
48. Rogers WJ, Bowlby LJ, Chandra NC, et al. Treatment of myocardial infarctions in the United States (1990 to 1993): Observations from the National Registry of Myocardial Infarction. *Circulation* 1994; 90:2103–2113.
49. Manson JE, Tosteson H, Ridker PM, et al. The primary prevention of myocardial infarction. *New Engl J Med* 1992; 326:1406–1416.
50. Grundy SM, Pasternak R, Greenland P. Assessment of cardiovascular risk by use of multiple risk-factor assessment equations: A statement for healthcare professionals from the American Heart Association and the American College of Cardiology, *Circulation* 1999; 34:1348–1349.

C H A P T E R 2

FUNCTIONAL ANATOMY OF THE HEART

Joseph F. Malouf / William D. Edwards / A. Jamil Tajik / James B. Seward

BACKGROUND

The study of the heart and great vessels has come a long way since the days of Andreas Vesalius, the great 16th-century anatomist who recognized the impact of anatomy on the practice of medicine.[1] During the European Renaissance, the tomographic approach to the study of cardiac anatomy became popular because of its artistic-based correlations. This is vividly depicted in the drawings of Leonardo da Vinci[2] (Fig. 2-1), who was called the first comparative anatomist since Aristotle. During the ensuing nearly four hundred years, however, interest in cardiac anatomy was very sporadic and limited to a few zealous and pioneering physicians, anatomists, and artists.

The 19th century ushered in the era of anatomic dissection for the study of physiologic and pathophysiologic processes. Virchow in 1885 described the *inflow-outflow method of cardiac dissection* that followed the direction of blood flow.[3] It was quick and simple and became the dissection method of choice. The works of Virchow and Osler paved the way to understanding the pathophysiologic basis of such diseases as pulmonary embolism, endocarditis, and heart failure.[4] Renewed interest in the study of cardiac anatomy and pathology was facilitated by the rise in autopsy rates in Europe and North America during the first half of the 20th century.[5] Herrick described the clinical features of coronary thrombosis.[5] Later, Blumgart, Schlesinger, and Zoll advanced our understanding of coronary artery disease through elegant clinicopathologic correlations.[5]

These achievements notwithstanding, however, they were limited to postmortem examinations. The advent of cardiac surgery in the 1950s, followed by coronary angiography, was a major impetus for promoting the study of in vivo clinicopathologic anatomic correlations. While cardiac surgeons were quick to appreciate the importance of having a detailed understanding of cardiac anatomy, clinical cardiologists were more interested in pathophysiology. However, with the introduction of noninvasive imaging techniques [echocardiography, computed tomography (CT), magnetic resonance imaging (MRI), and single-photon-emission computed tomography (SPECT)] over the past two decades, the perception of cardiac anatomy and pathophysiology radically changed for all of medicine in general and cardiology in particular.

With increasing use of tomographic techniques in the diagnosis and management of cardiovascular diseases, there has been a corresponding decrease in the use of autopsy for anatomic correlations. The reasons for this decrease are complex and controversial and include an increased confidence in technology, lack of reimbursement for the cost of autopsy, and rescinding the mandate for autopsies for hospital accreditation.[4] Nonetheless, autopsy still uncovers unexpected processes in about 15 percent of cases and is an invaluable tool for quality assurance programs.

Today, at the beginning of the 21st century, there is a resurgence in the clinicopathologic correlative approach to cardiovascular morphology. In particular, the tomographic presentation of cardiac structure, which had remained dormant for over a century, has become relevant because the diagnostic techniques used today are tomographic in nature.[6] The specialties associated with cardiovascular diseases have been quick to embrace these newer anatomic presentations. Echocardiography was brought into the operating room, and with the advent of transesophageal echocardiography, the cardiologist became an indispensable member of the surgical team.[7,8] Because of increasingly more sophisticated cardiac surgical techniques, coupled with closer interaction between the cardiac surgeon and the noninvasive cardiologist, there has been a growing demand for precise diagnostic tools with greater spatial and temporal resolution to guide the planning of surgical procedures and, therefore, to ensure their success.[7,8]

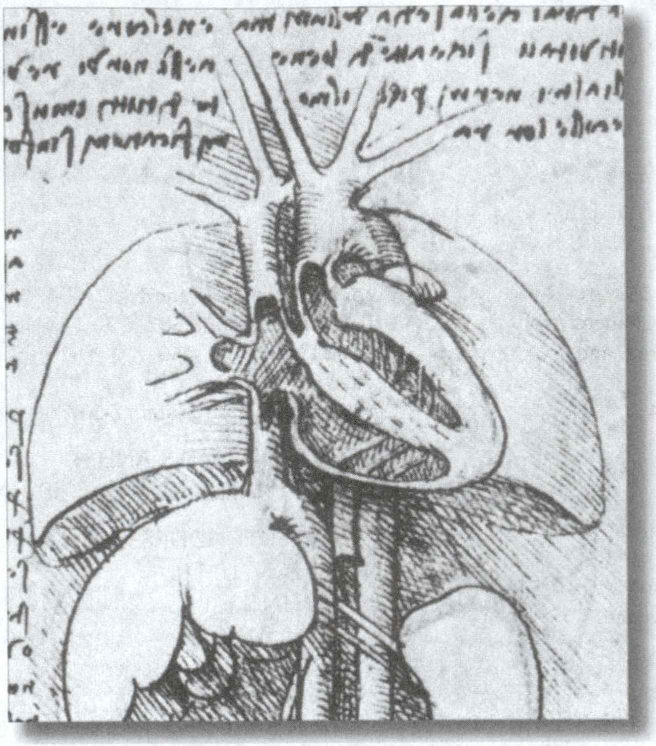

FIGURE 2-1 Four-chamber tomographic section of the heart as illustrated by Leonardo da Vinci. Note the thin-walled right ventricle and thick-walled left ventricle and detailed anatomic connections. (From O'Malley and Saunders,[2] with permission.)

The interest in cardiac anatomy among cardiologists is by no means limited to those involved in imaging the heart. Over the past few years, there has been an explosion of interest in anatomically guided electrophysiologic mapping and ablation techniques, which are increasingly guided by intracardiac ultrasound.[9–13] It has thus become feasible to accurately pinpoint the anatomic location of the source of many arrhythmias[9–13] (Figs.

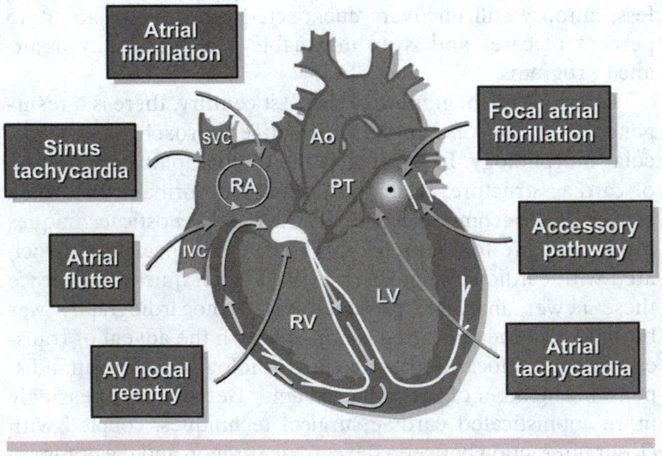

FIGURE 2-2 Anatomic considerations in the treatment of supraventricular arrhythmias. AV, atrioventricular; Ao, ascending aorta; IVC, inferior vena cava; LV, left ventricle; PT, pulmonary trunk; RA, right atrium; RV, right ventricle; SVC, superior vena cava. (Courtesy of Dr. Douglas L Packer, Mayo Clinic, Rochester, Minnesota.)

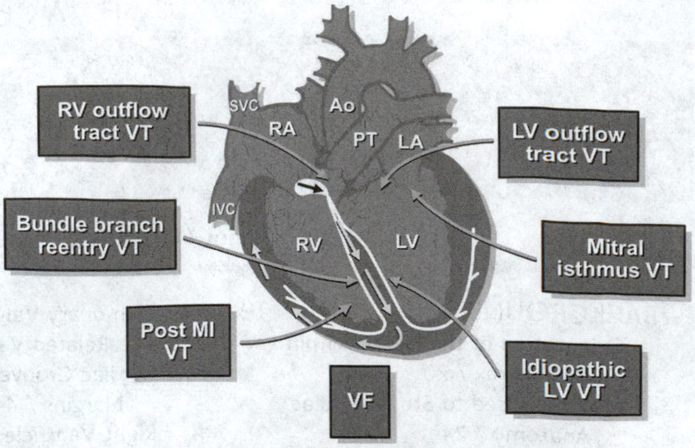

FIGURE 2-3 Anatomic considerations in the treatment of ventricular arrhythmias. LV, left ventricle; LA, left atrium; MI, myocardial infarction; VT, ventricular tachycardia; VF, ventricular fibrillation; other abbreviations as in Fig 2-2. (Courtesy of Dr. Douglas L Packer, Mayo Clinic, Rochester, Minnesota.)

2-2 and 2-3). By providing the electrophysiologist with a real-time visual "road map," the "search and destroy" mission during an ablation procedure will be made much easier and results, as well as complications, recognized immediately.[9–13] By providing a new window to the heart, real-time anatomic-electrophysiologic correlations also may help to enhance our understanding of the mechanisms of propagation of various arrhythmias.

In this technologically driven era, a *new* appreciation of cardiac anatomy has emerged as the cornerstone for clinical cardiology. The purpose of this chapter is to describe the anatomy of the heart by principally using the tomographic format prevalent in current CT, MRI, and echocardiography, with special emphasis and focus on clinically relevant anatomic details. We will make only a passing note of the next generation of imaging techniques. The intent is to emphasize the important anatomic features of various cardiovascular disease processes relative to diagnosis and management.

Orientation of the Heart Within the Thorax

The body may be viewed in three standard anatomic planes: (1) frontal (coronal), (2) horizontal (transverse), and (3) sagittal that are orthogonal to one another.[6,7] However, the three primary planes of the heart [short axis (transverse), four-chamber (frontal), and long-axis (sagittal)] do not correspond to the standard anatomic planes of the body[6,7] (Fig. 2-4, Plate 1). *Incorrect photographic or artistic orientation of surgical or autopsy specimens of the heart, presented out of context, can result in the display of two-dimensional images in nonanatomic positions and actually contribute to misconceptions regarding the position of the heart within the thorax*[6] (Fig. 2-5, Plate 2).

Thus, first, when describing the orientation of a specific organ such as the heart, one must take into account both the position of the heart and the position of adjacent structures such as the thoracic aorta and esophagus. When interpreting two-dimensional images, clinicians must avoid making correlations that yield impossible anatomy[6] (Fig. 2-6). Accurate anatomic diagnoses require close interdisciplinary interactions between cardiovascular pathologists, clinicians, radiologists, anesthesiologists,

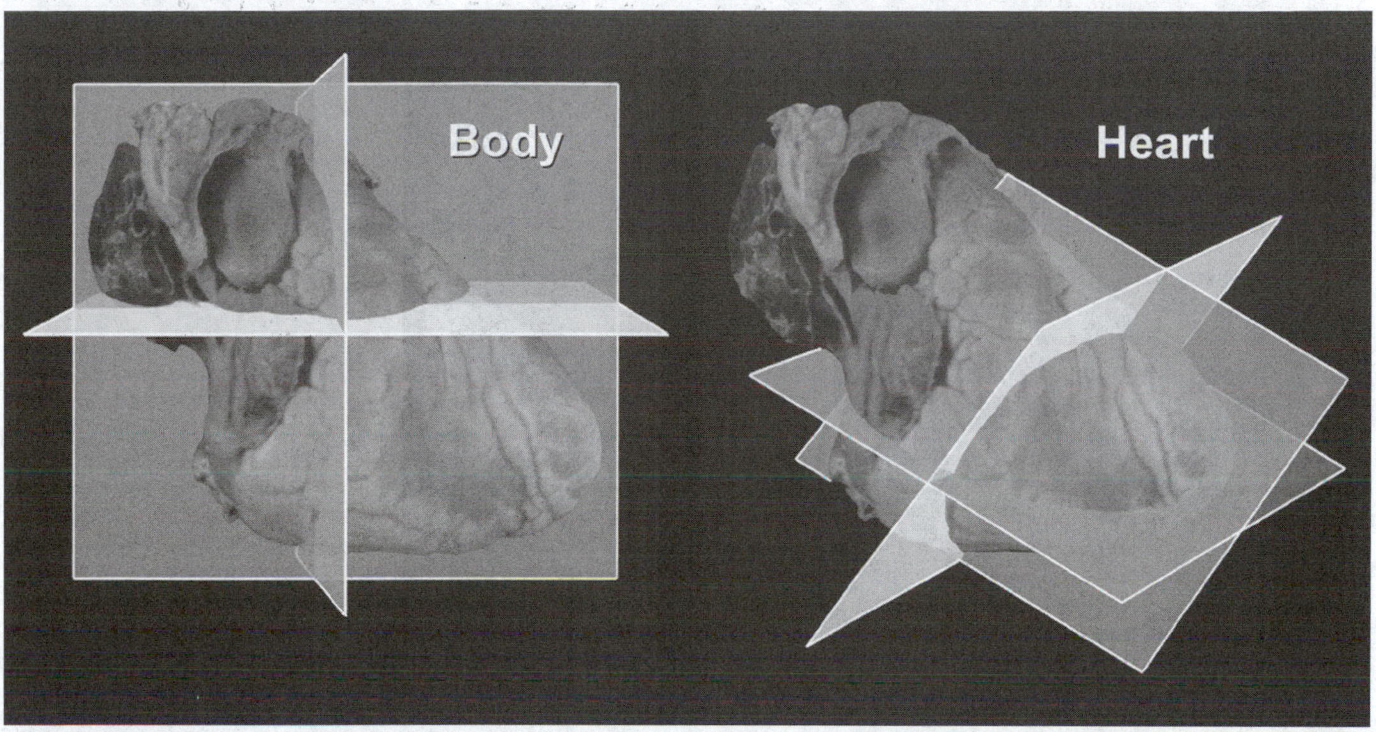

FIGURE 2-4 (Plate 1) The three primary planes of the body (*left*) and heart (*right*). Note that the planes of the body are aligned with vertical midline structures, such as the esophagus. In contrast, the major axis of the heart is oriented obliquely. Thus the heart's long and short axes do not lie in the same plane as the body's long and short axes. The body planes cut the heart obliquely and not in its primary planes. Conversely, the heart's primary planes cut the body obliquely.

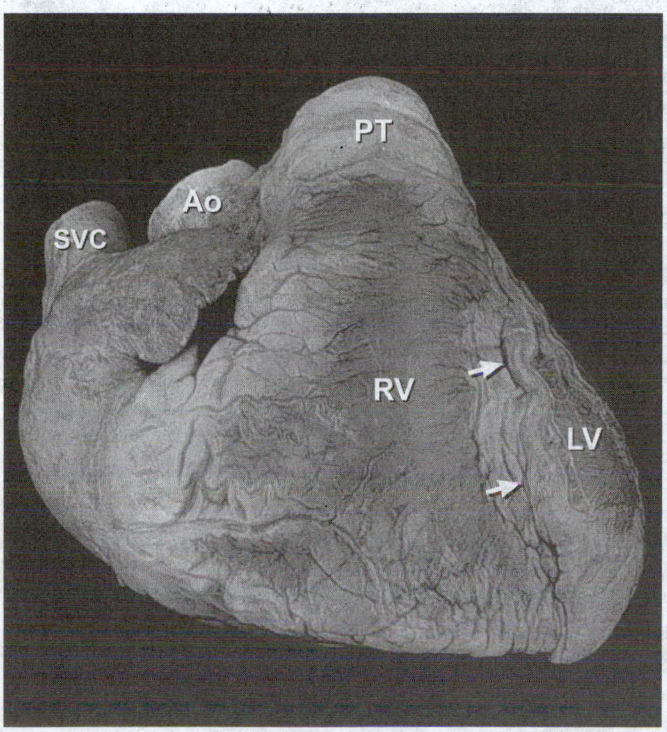

A

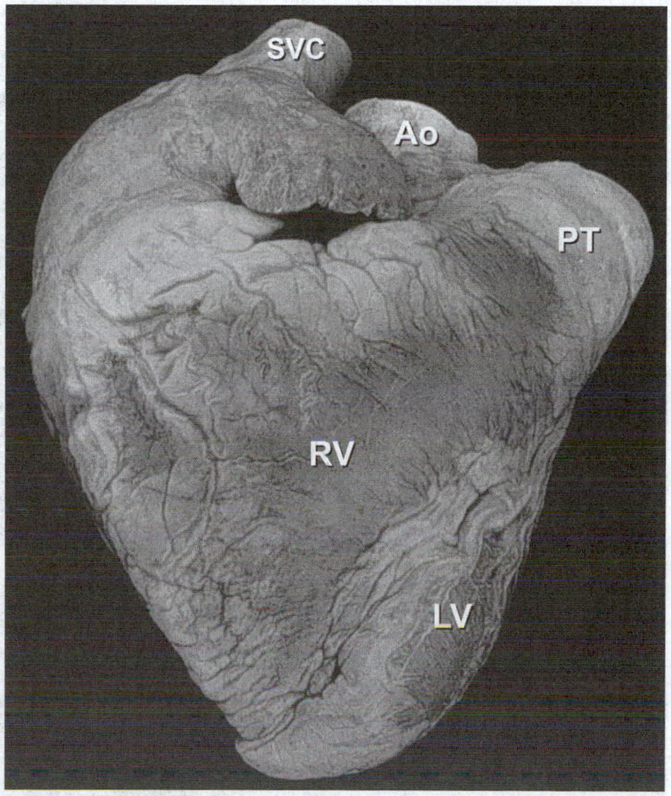

B

FIGURE 2-5 (Plate 2) *A.* Anterior view of the heart in its usual anatomic position with its apex directed from right to left. Arrows point to the anterior interventricular groove. *B.* Nonanatomic positioning of the normal heart with its apex directed downward, thereby resembling a "valentine." The position of the cardiac apex is normally leftward (levocardia) but may anomalously be rightward (dextrocardia) or midline and inferiorly (mesocardia). Ao, ascending aorta; LV, left ventricle; PT, pulmonary trunk; RV, right ventricle; SVC, superior vena cava.

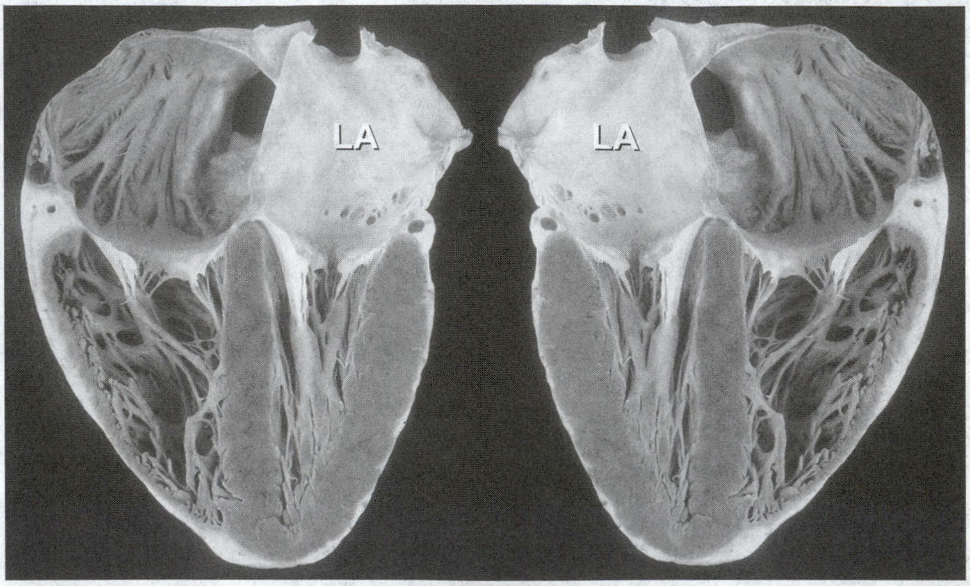

FIGURE 2-6 Apex-down four-chamber view of the heart (*left*) and an anatomically impossible mirror-image photograph (*right*). Mirror-image depiction (though unfortunately commonly used in publications) does not correspond to normal anatomic reality. Obviously, three-dimensional anatomic correctness is essential for accurate clinicopathologic correlations. LA, left atrium.

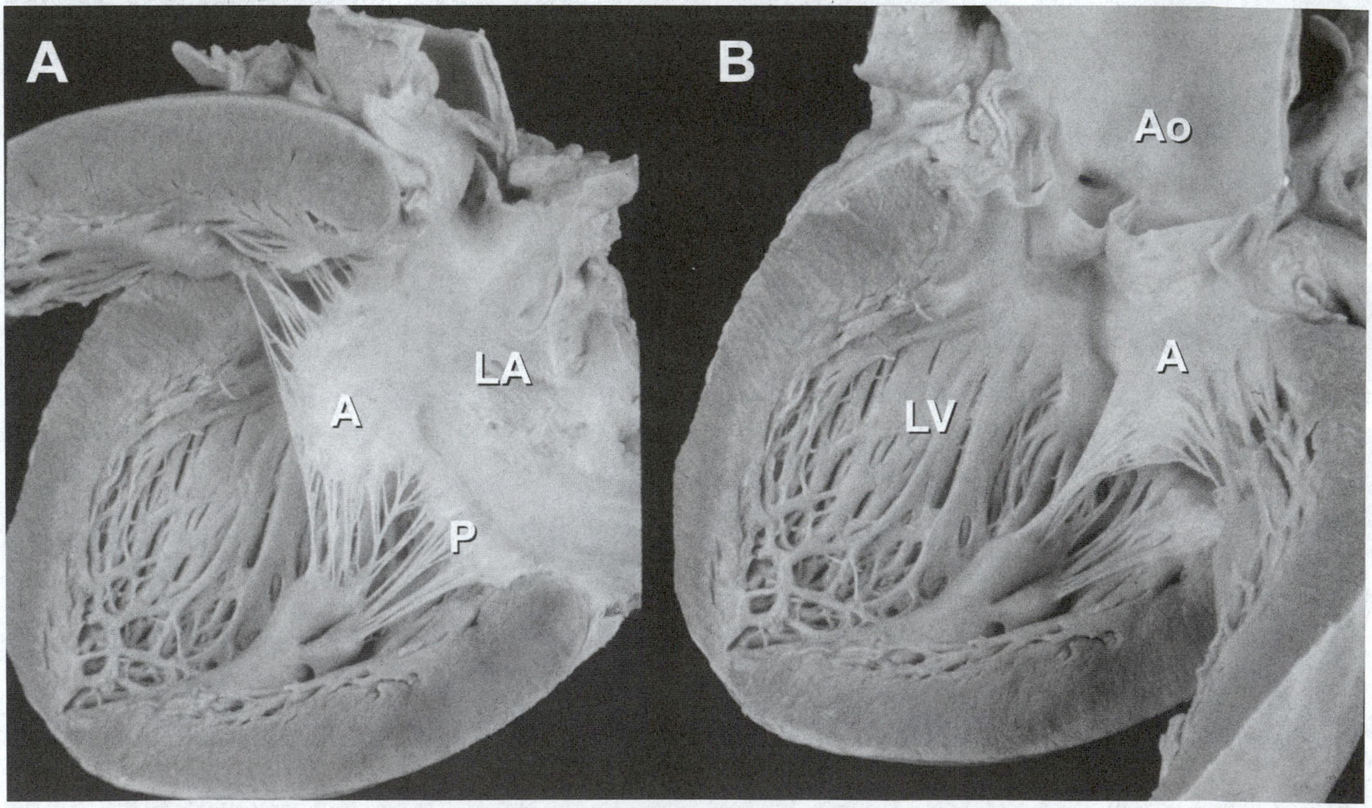

FIGURE 2-7 Inflow-outflow method of cardiac dissection. *A.* Left ventricular inflow view. *B.* Left ventricular outflow view. A, anterior mitral leaflet; Ao, ascending aorta; LA, left atrium; LV, left ventricle; P, posterior mitral leaflet.

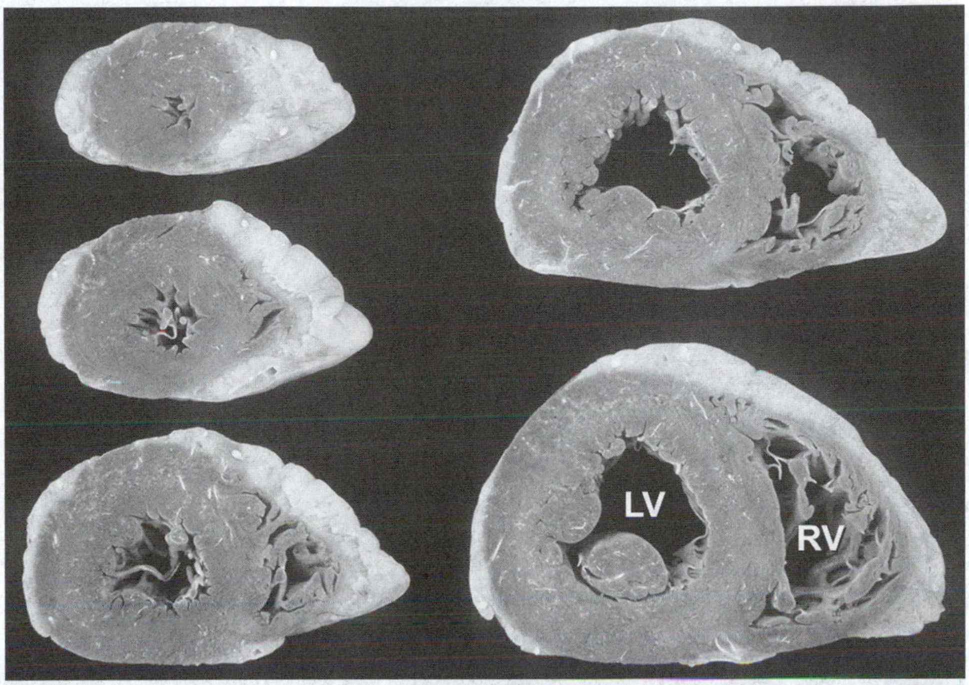

FIGURE 2-8 (Plate 3) Ventricular slice method of cardiac dissection. Display of five slices (LV, left ventricle; RV, right ventricle) viewed as though looking from the base of the heart toward the apex.

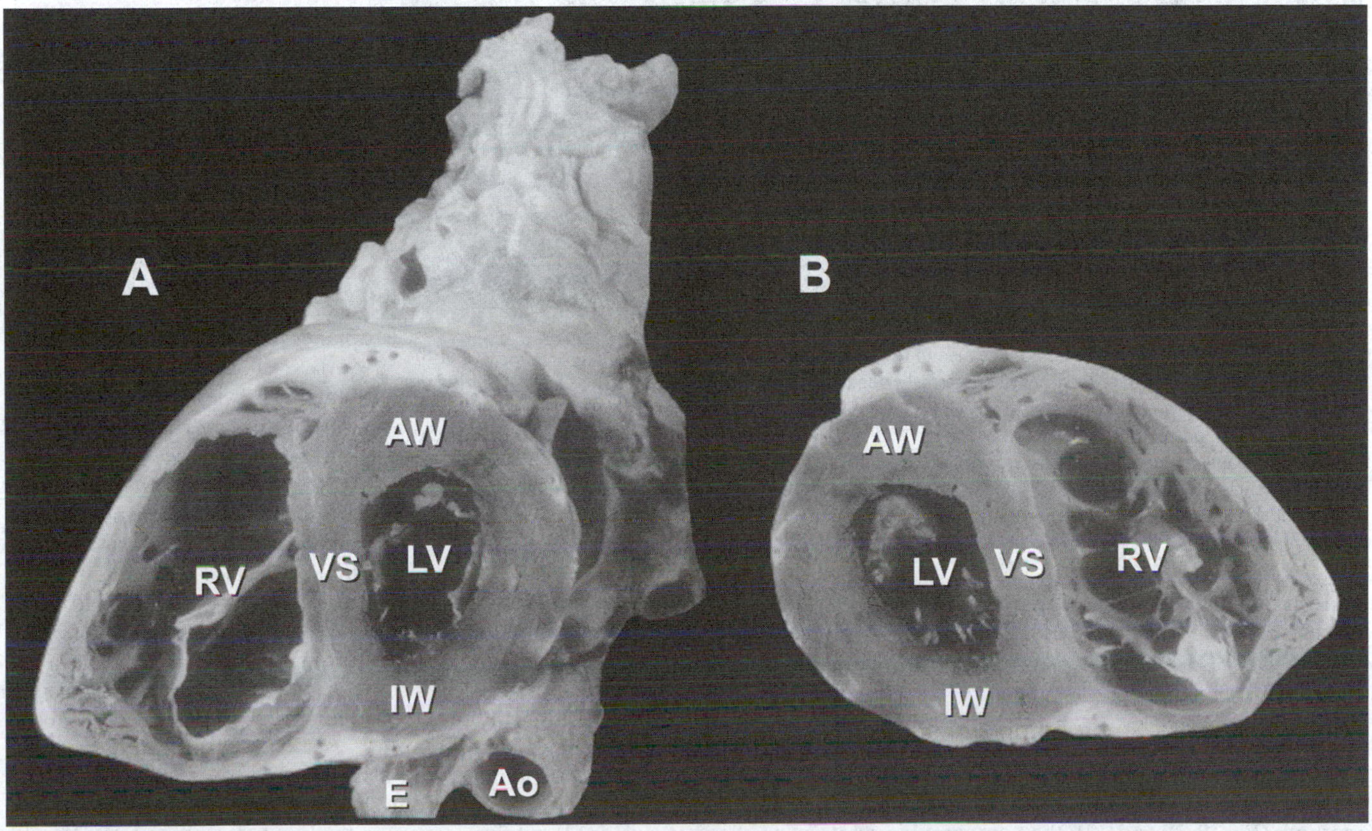

FIGURE 2-9 (Plate 4) Bisected cardiac specimen, viewed in the short axis. *A.* The specimen is viewed from the apex toward the base. The esophagus (E) is posterior and adjacent to the both the thoracic aorta (Ao) and the inferior wall of the left ventricle (LV). The right ventricular (RV) cavity is to the left. *B.* The other half of the bisected specimen is viewed as though looking from the base toward the apex (comparable with Fig. 2-8). AW, anterior wall; IW, inferior wall; VS, ventricular septum.

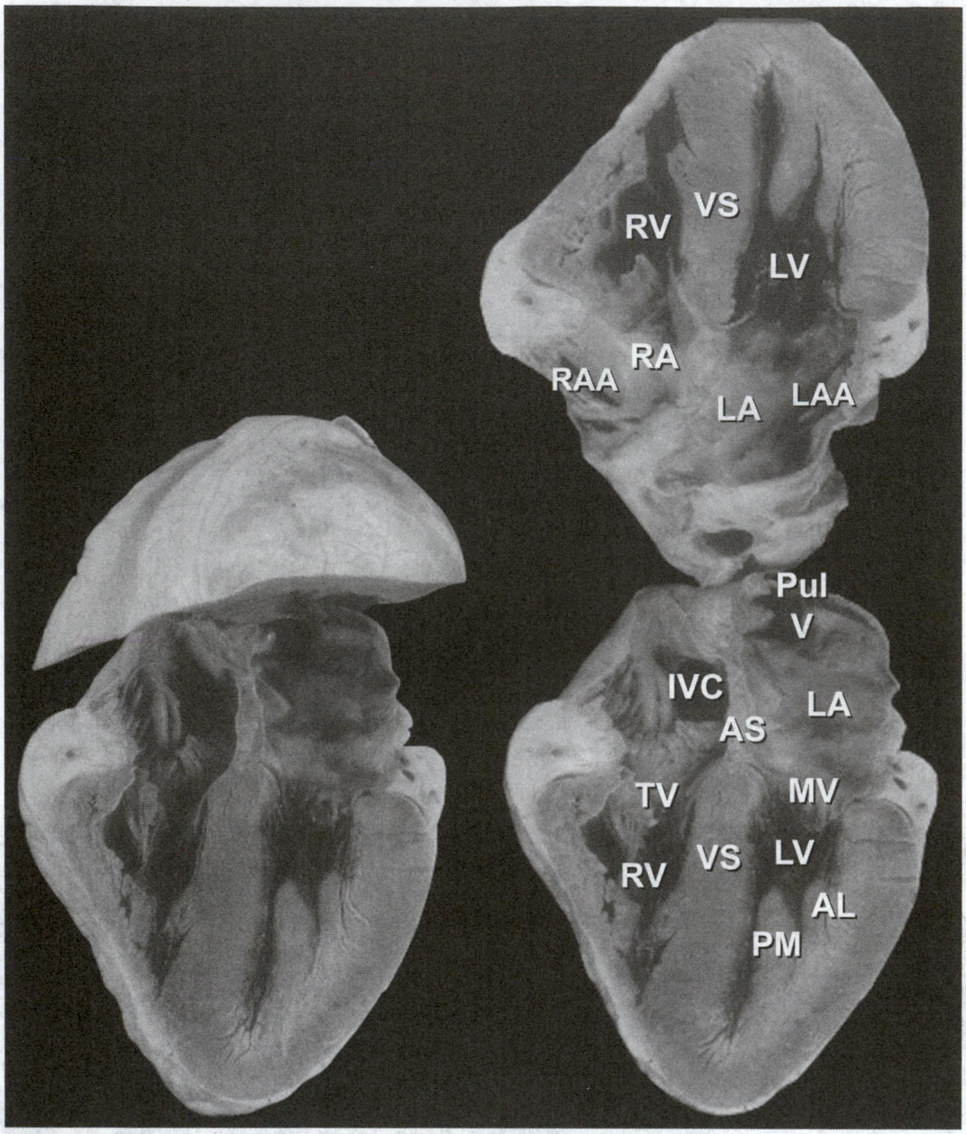

FIGURE 2-10 (Plate 5) Bisected cardiac specimen in the four-chamber view parallel to the base-apex axis of the heart. (*Left*) The bisected specimen has been partially opened to show the relative relationship of the bisected halves. (*Right*) The two components of the bisected specimen are opened completely. Note the positions of the pulmonary veins posteriorly and the positions of the atrial appendages at the atrioventricular groove. AL, anterolateral papillary muscle; AS, atrial septum; IVC, inferior vena cava; LA, left atrium; LAA, left atrial appendage; LV, left ventricle; MV, mitral valve; PM, posteromedial papillary muscle; PulV, pulmonary vein; RA, right atrium; RAA, right atrial appendage; RV, right ventricle; TV, tricuspid valve; VS, ventricular septum.

and surgeons and emphasize a critical need for teamwork and a "common language" when describing cardiac anatomy and pathology.

Methods Used to Study Cardiac Anatomy

The two conventional approaches to the study of cardiac anatomy that have stood the test of time are (1) the inflow-outflow method (Fig. 2-7) and (2) the tomographic ventricular slice method[3,6] (Fig. 2-8, Plate 3). Although the inflow-outflow method readily demonstrates disease processes in a given cardiac chamber or valve, it does not allow simultaneous visualization of the effects of that process on contiguous structures.[6] Furthermore, the inflow-outflow method does not correspond well to clinical tomographic imaging modalities except possibly cavitary angiography.[6] With the ventricular slice technique (see Fig. 2-8), the ventricles are "bread sliced" perpendicular to the plane of the ventricular septum. This technique is ideal for the evaluation of ischemic heart disease but may need to be carried basally, well beyond the papillary muscle tips.[6]

TOMOGRAPHIC METHOD

Renaissance anatomists such as da Vinci used the *tomographic approach* principally because of its *artistic correlations*.[2] Modern anatomists and pathologists have resorted to this method because it correlates with conventional diagnostic tomographic-anatomic techniques. With this method, cardiac dissection involves bisecting the heart into two pieces using a single plane of section.[6] Anatomy contained within the depth of each section fosters a perception of three-dimensional anatomy. Commonly used planes bisect the heart perpendicular to the base-apex axis (*short-axis "transverse" views*) (Fig. 2-9, Plate 4) or parallel to it (*long-axis and four-chamber "frontal" views*)[6] (Fig. 2-10, Plate 5). Planes that bisect the heart parallel to the conventional body planes (frontal "coronal", transverse "short-axis", and sagittal "long-axis" views) (Fig. 2-11, Plate 6) replicate *body tomography*.[6,14]

The *short-axis tomographic planes*[6,7] of the heart (Fig. 2-12) are similar to the ventricular slice method but differ in two important respects. The "bread slicing" of the heart is continued to the base of the heart and great vessels, and the slices are oriented as though the heart were being viewed from the apex toward the base rather than in the opposite direction, as has been the case with the ventricular slice technique. Photographs should correspond with diagnostic tomographic scans.

The *long-axis and four-chamber planes* are orthogonal to the short-axis planes. The four-chamber planes of cardiac dissection (Fig. 2-13) involve sectioning the heart along both lateral walls, from apex to base, such that both ventricles and both atria are included in the plane of section.[6,7] The long-axis two-chamber method (Fig. 2-14) involves bisecting the heart from the left ventricular apex through the mitral orifice and into the left

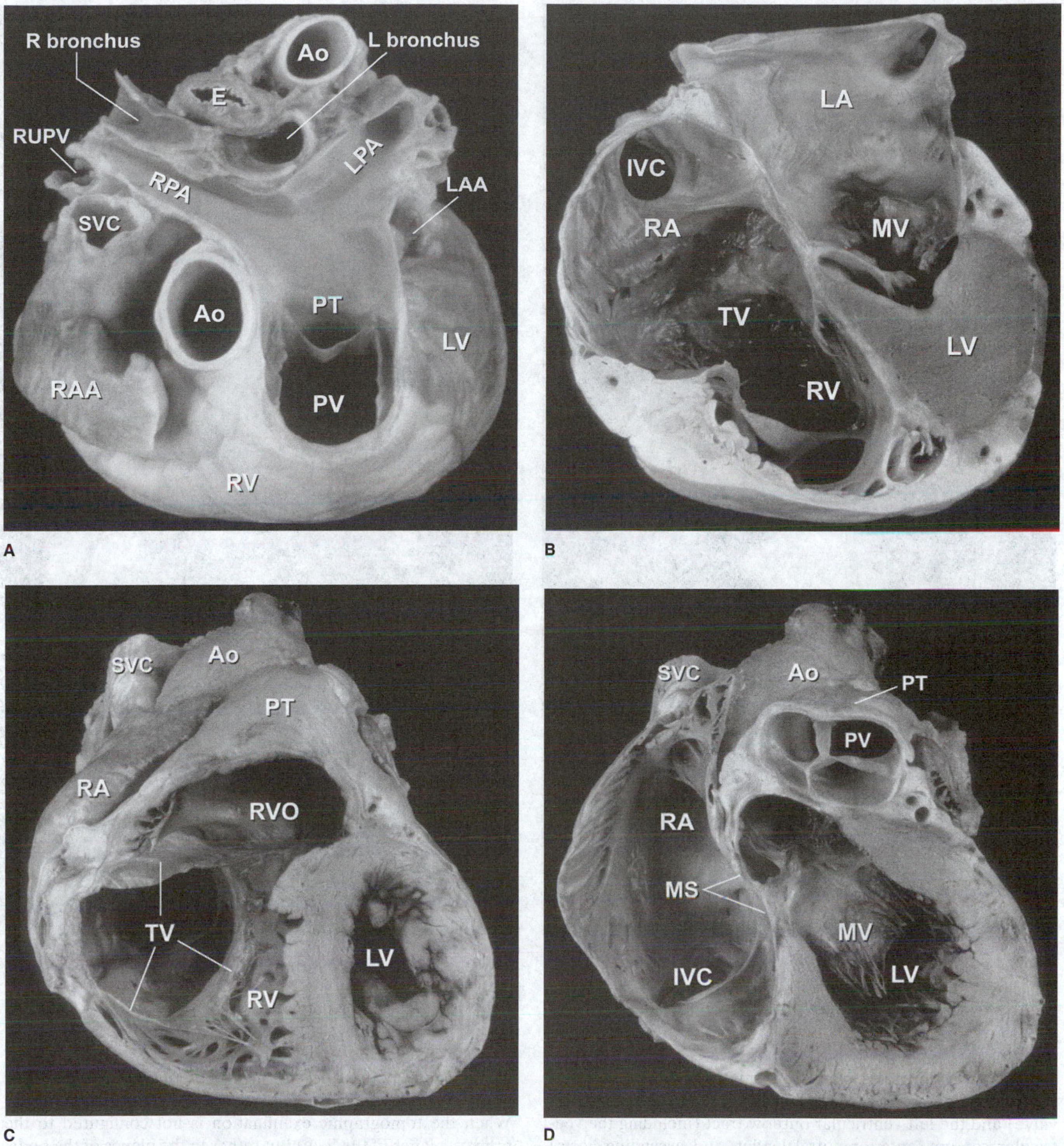

FIGURE 2-11 (Plate 6) Tomographic cardiac dissection along the body primary planes. *A,B*. Transverse sections (looking from head toward feet) at the level of the great vessels (*A*) or the cardiac chambers (*B*). The aortic arch travels over the left bronchus and the right pulmonary artery. *C,D*. Frontal sections (looking from anterior to posterior) through both ventricles (*C*) or left ventricle and right atrium (*D*). *E,F*. Parasagittal sections looking from right (*E*) to left (*F*). Ao, ascending aorta; CS, coronary sinus; E, esophagus; IA, innominate artery; IVC, inferior vena cava; LA, left atrium; LAA, left atrial appendage; LB, left bronchus; LCX, left circumflex coronary artery; LIV, left innominate vein; LLPV, left lower pulmonary vein; LPA, left pulmonary artery; LUPV, left upper pulmonary vein; LSA, left subclavian artery; LV, left ventricle; MS, membranous ventricular septum; MV, mitral valve; PS, pericardial sac; PT, pulmonary trunk; PV, pulmonary valve; RA, right atrium; RAA, right atrial appendage; RPA, right pulmonary artery; RUPV, right upper pulmonary vein; RV, right ventricle; RVO, right ventricular outflow; SVC, superior vena cava; TV, tricuspid valve.

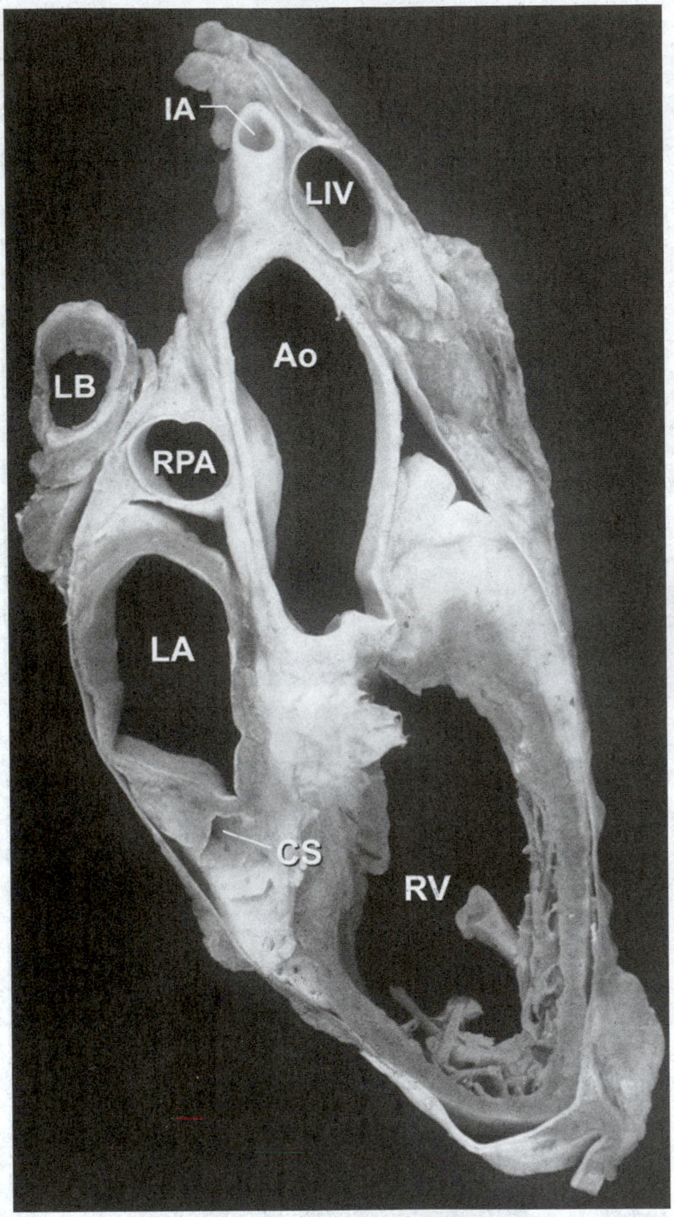

E

FIGURE 2-11 (*Continued*)

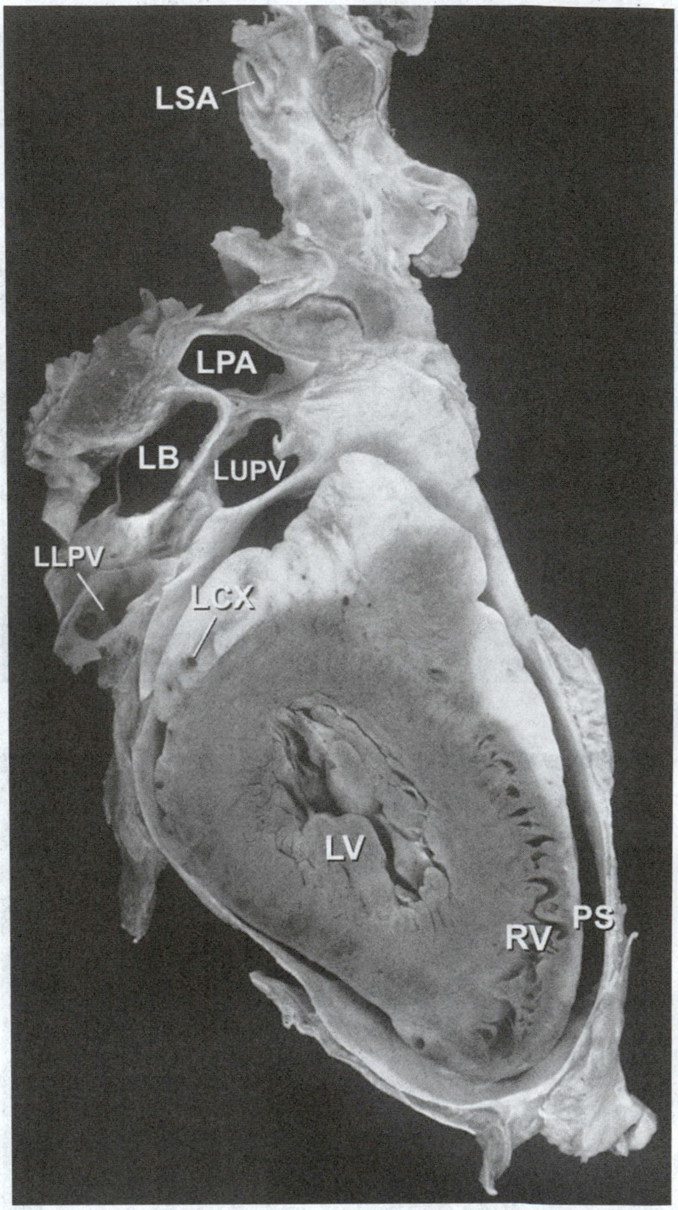

F

FIGURE 2-11 (*Continued*)

atrium.[6,7] The long-axis plane can cut through both the left ventricular inflow tract (including the left atrium and mitral valve) and the left ventricular outflow tract (including the ventricular septum, anterior mitral leaflet, and ascending aorta) (Fig. 2-15). This plane also cuts obliquely through the right ventricular outflow tract.[6,7]

These three tomographic planes of the heart have been particularly useful in echocardiography. Serial sections within each plane produce a collage of anatomic slices (Fig. 2-16, Plate 7) that can be used for three-dimensional reconstruction, which is beyond the scope of this chapter. The tomographic planes of section can be tailored to the different imaging modalities. *Thus echocardiography and* SPECT *generally employ the primary planes of the* heart. *In contrast, CT and MRI use the primary planes of the* body. *The parasagittal or oblique planes of the body serve radionuclide angiography and left ventriculography.*[6] When the tomographic examination is not configured to the primary planes of the heart but rather to the planes of the body, the terms *short, long,* and *frontal* can be misleading (Figs. 2-17 and 2-18).

Pathologic lesions in both congenital and acquired heart diseases often involve contiguous chambers, valves, or vessels. The tomographic method is the optimal technique for demonstrating intracardiac relationships and is ideal for any disease that involves several cardiac chambers. The proliferation of noninvasive tomographic imaging techniques makes this method particularly ideal for clinicopathologic correlations.

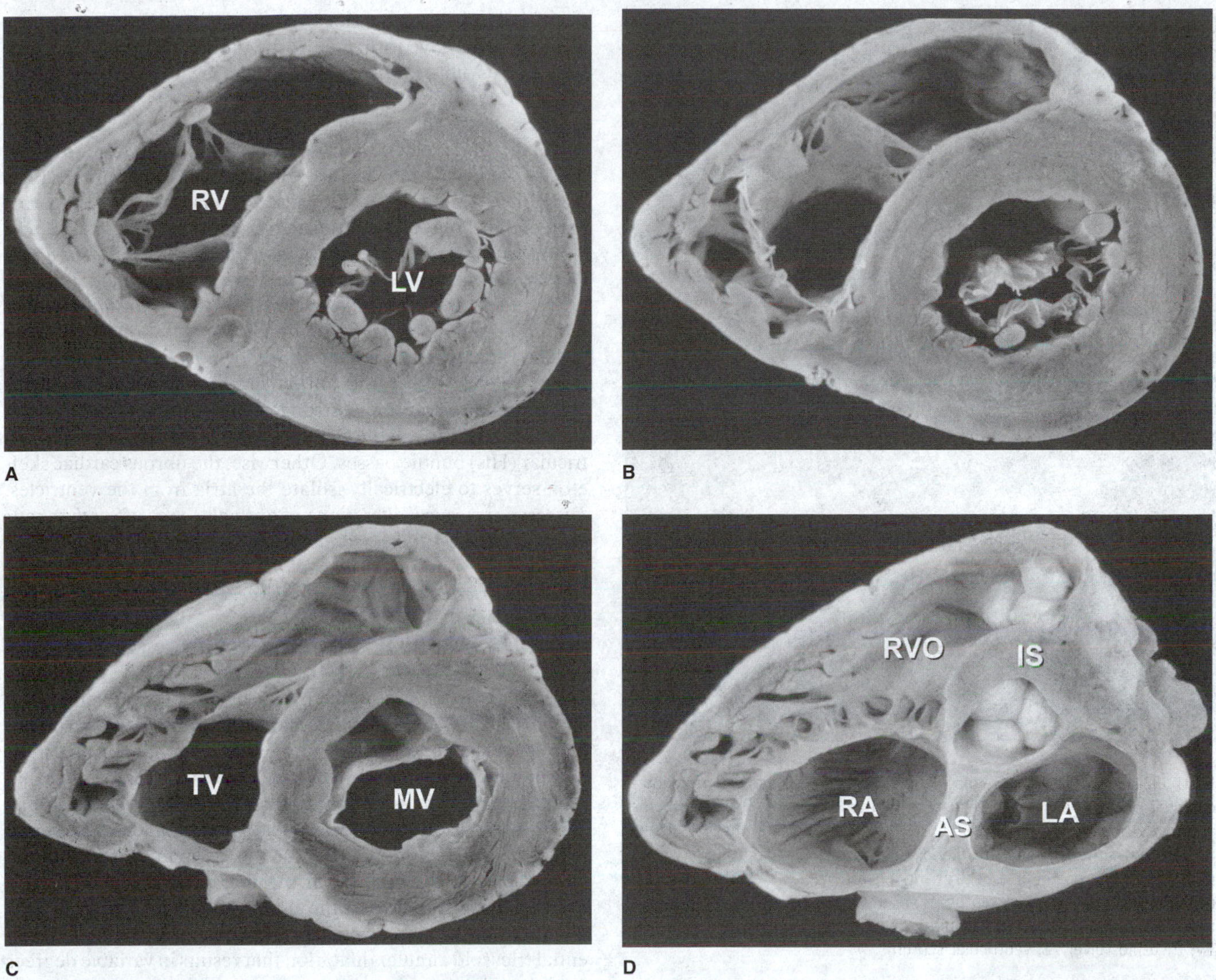

FIGURE 2-12 *A–D*. Tomographic cardiac dissections along the heart's primary short-axis plane. This method of tomographic dissection shows the crescentic right ventricle (RV) and circular left ventricle (LV). The atrioventricular valves are sectioned at the level of their papillary muscles (in *A*), chordae tendineae (in *B*), atrioventricular valve leaflets (in *C*), and their annuli and the semilunar valves (in *D*). The infundibulum septum (IS) separates the pulmonary and aortic valves. The atrial septum (AS) separates the tricuspid and mitral valves and abuts the posterior (noncoronary) cusp of the aortic valve. LA, left atrium; MV, mitral valve; RA, right atrium; RVO, right ventricular outflow; TV, tricuspid valve.

Limitations of tomographic dissection can be overcome by photography, computer imagery, and interestingly, the use of glue. After each tomographic section has been produced and photographed, the bisected specimens can be glued back together using any cyanoacrylate glue such as Krazy Glue or Superglue and resectioned along a different tomographic plane.[6] A step-by-step photographic documentation is necessary, since once the specimen has been glued and recut, the preceding tomographic plane of section will be available only in the photograph and not in the actual specimen.

CORRELATIVE ANATOMY

This section in this chapter is an illustrated review of applied cardiac anatomy. The clinical significance of the anatomy described is highlighted in italics.

Pericardium

The fibrous (parietal) pericardium is a resilient sac that envelops the heart and attaches onto the great vessels.[15] Almost the entire ascending aorta and main pulmonary artery and portions of both venae cavae and all four pulmonary veins are intrapericardial (Fig. 2-19). *These are important anatomic landmarks to remember when evaluating diseases of the pericardium. Given the intrapericardial location of the ascending aorta, diseases such as localized aortic wall hematoma, aortic dissection, or aortic rupture can produce a rapidly fatal hemopericardium. Because the sac is collagenous, with little elastic tissue, it cannot stretch acutely. In patients with total anomalous pulmonary venous connection, the confluence of pulmonary veins is intrapericardial. In contrast, the right and left pulmonary arteries and ductal artery (ductus arteriosus) are extrapericardial structures.*[16]

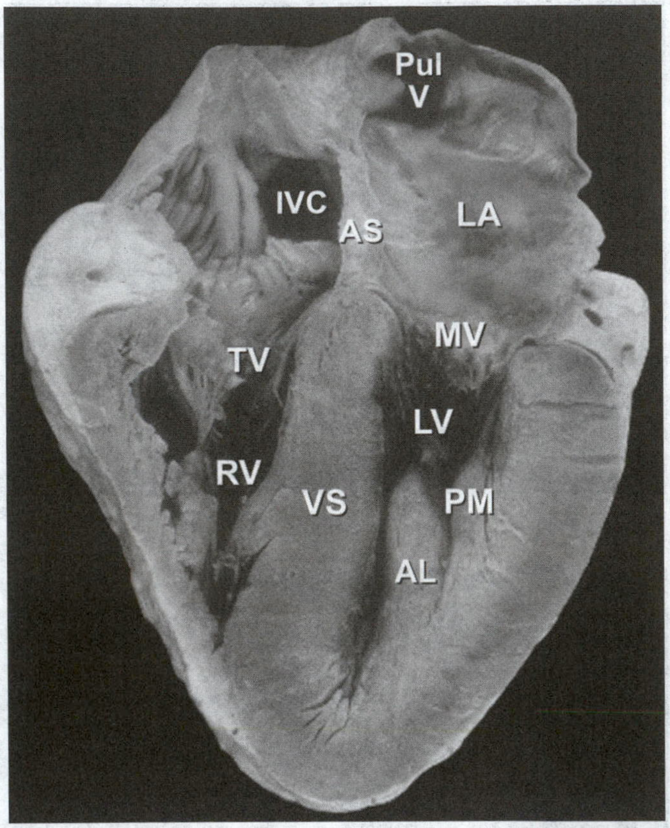

FIGURE 2-13 Tomographic cardiac dissection along the heart's primary four-chamber plane. The heart is viewed as though one were looking from the anterosuperior surface toward the posteroinferior surface. In the floor of the right atrium is the orifice of the inferior vena cava (IVC). The pulmonary veins (PulV) enter the posterior aspect of the left atrium. AL, anterolateral mitral papillary muscle; AS, atrial septum; LA, left atrium; LV, left ventricle; MV, mitral valve; PM, posteromedial mitral papillary muscle; RV, right ventricle; TV, tricuspid valve; VS, ventricular septum.

The serous pericardium forms the delicate inner lining of the fibrous pericardium as well as the outer lining of the heart and great vessels (visceral pericardium). Over the heart, it is referred to as the epicardium, and it contains the epicardial coronary arteries and veins, autonomic nerves, lymphatics, and a variable amount of adipose tissue. The junctions between the visceral and parietal pericardium lie along the great vessels and form the pericardial reflections. The reflections along the pulmonary veins and vena cavae are continuous and form a posterior midline cul-de-sac known as the *oblique sinus*. Behind the great arteries, the *transverse sinus* forms a tunnel-like passageway (Fig. 2-20). *After open-heart surgery, localized accumulation of blood within the oblique sinus can produce isolated left atrial tamponade.*[16] *Similarly, a hematoma adjacent to the low-pressure right atrium can cause isolated right atrial tamponade.* With increasing age and with obesity, fat can accumulate within the parietal pericardium and epicardium.[16] *When imaging the heart, it is important not to misinterpret fat as an abnormal structure or a tumor.*

Cardiac Skeleton

The four cardiac valves are anchored to their annuli, or valve rings. These fibrous rings, at the base of the heart, join to form the fibrous skeleton of the heart[16] (Fig. 2-21). The centrally located aortic valve forms the cornerstone of the cardiac skeleton, and its fibrous extensions abut each of the other three valves. The cardiac skeleton contains not only the four valve annuli but also the membranous septum and the aortic intervalvular, right, and left fibrous trines. The fibrous trigones form the anatomic substrate for direct mitral-aortic continuity[16] (Figs. 2-21, Plate 8, and 2-22). The intervalvular fibrosa also forms part of the floor of the transverse sinus (see Figs. 2-22 and 2-33). *In patients with infective endocarditis of the mitral or aortic valves, the infection may burrow through the intervalvular fibrosa and produce fistulas betwn the left ventricle and the adjacent left atrium, ascending aorta, or transverse sinus.*[17]

The right fibrous trigone, also known as the *central fibrous body*, welds together the aortic, mitral, and tricuspid valves and forms the largest and strongest component of the cardiac skeleton. It is through the right fibrous trigone that the atrioventricular (His) bundle passes. Otherwise, the fibrous cardiac skeleton serves to electrically isolate the atria from the ventricles. *Diseases or surgical alterations of one valve may affect the shape or angulation of adjacent valves (e.g., aortic valve replacement causing severe mitral regurgitation) and may affect the nearby coronary arteries or conduction tissue.*[17]

Tricuspid Valve

The tricuspid valve is comprised of five components (i.e., annulus, leaflets, commissures, chordae tendineae, and papillary muscles). The anterior tricuspid leaflet is the largest and most mobile and forms an intracavitary curtain that partially separates the inflow and outflow tracts of the right ventricle (Fig. 2-23). The posterior leaflet is usually the smallest. The septal leaflet is the least mobile because of its many direct chordal attachments to the ventricular septum. A distensible fibroadipose annulus is unique to the tricuspid valve.[17] Consequently, dilatation of the right ventricle commonly produces circumferential tricuspid annular dilatation that results in variable degrees of tricuspid valve regurgitation.[16]

Mitral Valve

The mitral apparatus is comprised of the same five components as the tricuspid valve. Competent mitral valve function is a complex process that requires the proper interaction of all components, as well as adequate left atrial and left ventricular function. *Abnormalities of the mitral valve apparatus may involve any of these components or combinations thereof. The pattern of pathologic involvement often determines the feasibility of mitral valve repair (surgical or percutaneous).*[18] The mitral valve annulus forms a complete fibrous ring that is firmly anchored along the circumference of the anterior leaflet by the tough fibrous skeleton of the heart[17] (see Fig. 2-21). Therefore, dilatation of the mitral valve annulus primarily affects the posterior leaflet. *All current operative mitral repair techniques are based on this principle of asymmetric annular dilatation. Mitral valve annuloplasty reduces the mitral valve inlet area by reducing the circumference of the posterior leaflet.*[17] *This is the rationale for using a partial posterior annuloplasty ring.*

Unlike the other cardiac valves, the mitral valve has only two leaflets. The anterior leaflet is large and semicircular, and it partially separates the ventricular inflow and outflow tracts

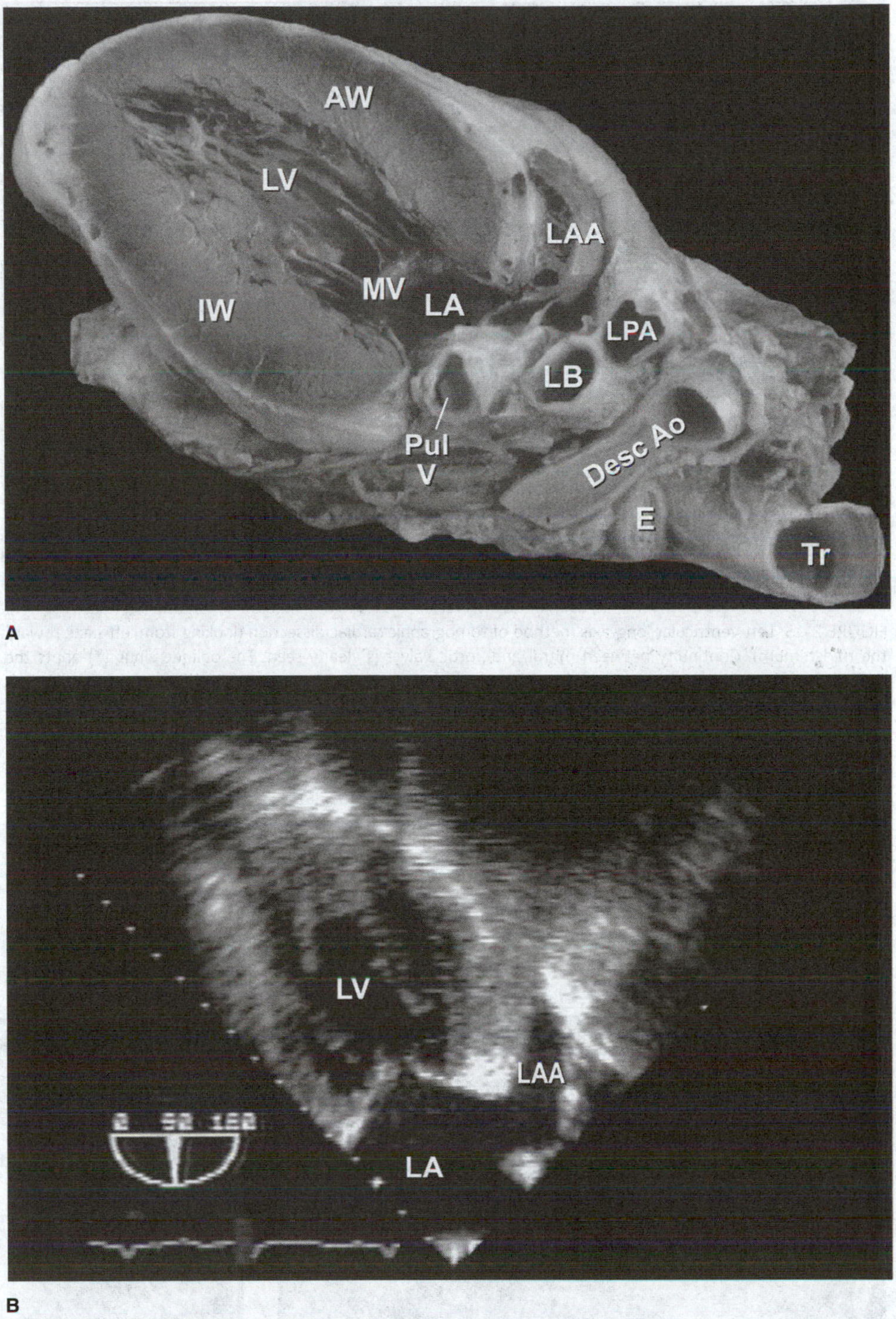

FIGURE 2-14 Tomographic cardiac dissection along the heart's primary long-axis plane. *A*. Tomographic section showing the left ventricle and left atrium. The mitral valve is also well demonstrated. The left atrial appendage is located anteriorly. The specimen is viewed as though one were looking from the tip of the left scapula toward the right nipple. *B*. Analogous two-chamber transesophageal view. AW, anterior wall; Desc Ao, descending thoracic aorta; E, esophagus; IW, inferior wall; LA, left atrium; LAA, left atrial appendage; LB, left bronchus; LPA, left pulmonary artery; LV, left ventricle; MV, mitral valve; PulV, pulmonary vein; Tr, trachea.

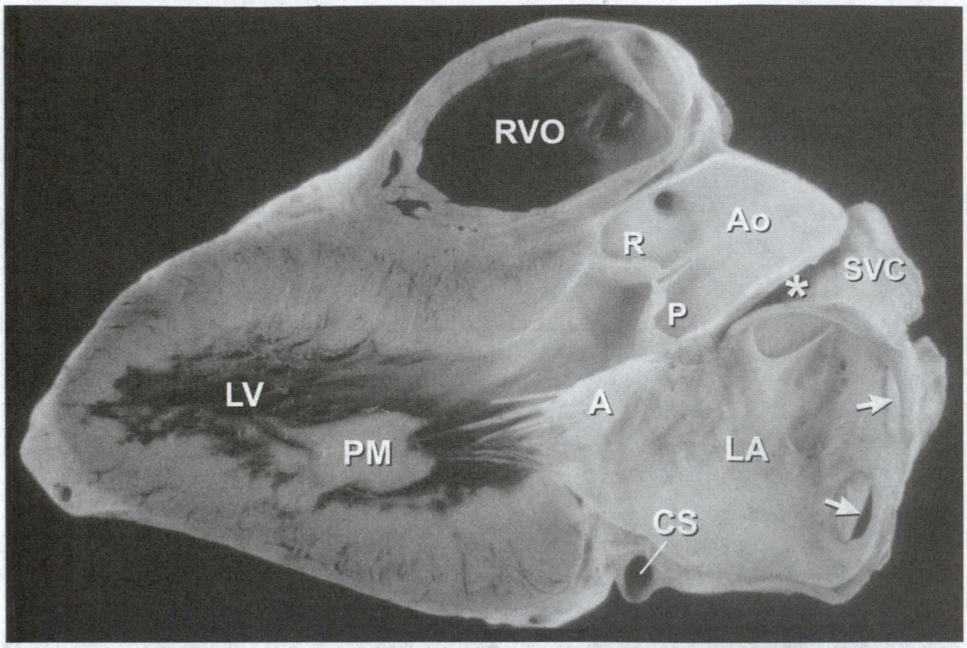

FIGURE 2-15 Left ventricular long-axis method of tomographic cardiac dissection (looking from left flank toward the midsternum). Continuity between mitral and aortic valves is clearly seen. The oblique sinus (*) abuts the wall of the left atrium. A, anterior mitral leaflet; Ao, ascending aorta; CS, coronary sinus; LA, left atrium; LV, left ventricle; P, posterior aortic cusp; PM, posteromedial mitral papillary muscle; R, right aortic cusp; RVO , right ventricular outflow; SVC, superior vena cava; arrows point to the right upper and lower pulmonary veins.

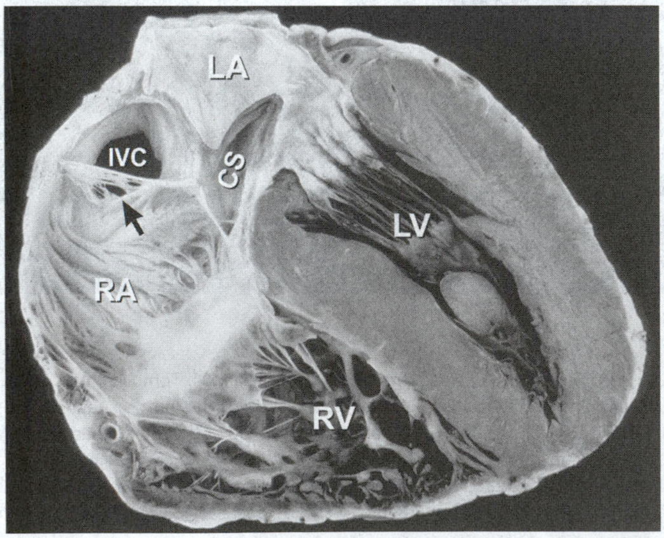

A

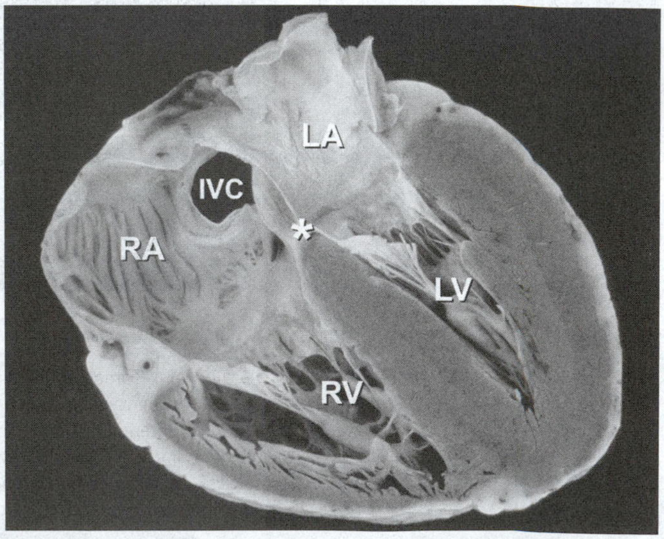

B

FIGURE 2-16 (Plate 7) Collage of four-chamber tomographic sections cutting from inferior wall to anterosuperior wall showing coronary sinus (*A*), internal cardiac crux (*) (*B*), and aortic valve (*C*). Ao, ascending aorta; CS, coronary sinus; IVC, inferior vena cava; LA, left atrium; LV, left ventricle; RA, right atrium; RV, right ventricle; arrow in *A* points to a fenestrated eustachian valve.

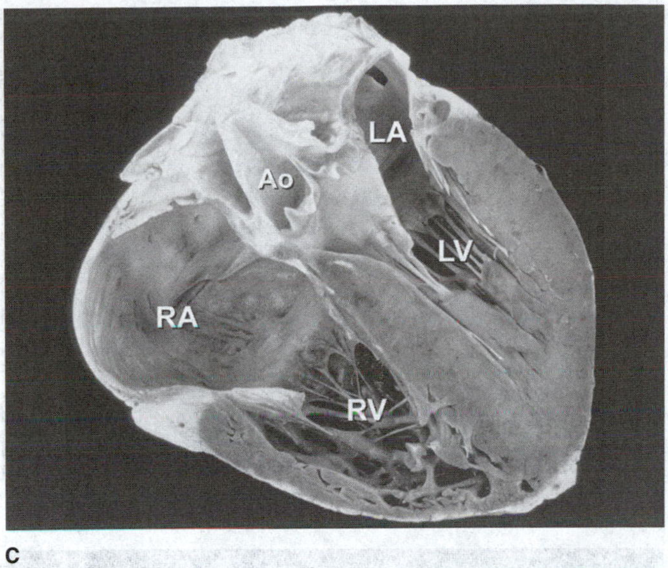

FIGURE 2-16 (*Continued*)

(see Fig. 2-23). However, unlike its right-sided counterpart, it also forms part of the outflow tract. *In patients with hypertrophic obstructive cardiomyopathy, the anterior mitral leaflet may be drawn toward the basal anterior septum because of the Venturi effect, resulting in midsystolic outflow obstruction and mitral regurgitation.*[16] The posterior mitral leaflet is rectangular and usually is divided into three scallops. The middle scallop is the largest of the three in more than 90 percent of normal hearts. Occasionally, however, either the anterolateral or the posteromedial scallop is larger, and rarely there are accessory scallops[15,17] (Fig. 2-24, Plate 9). *Posterior mitral leaflet prolapse usually involves the middle scallop and may be associated with chordal rupture.* Both mitral leaflets are normally similar in area. The anterior leaflet is twice the height of the posterior leaflet but has half its annular length.[17] With advanced age, the mitral leaflets thicken somewhat, particularly along their closing edges.[15]

The commissures are cleftlike splits in the leaflet tissue that represent the sites of separation of the leaflets (Figs. 2-25 and 2-26*A*). Beneath the two mitral commissures lie the anterolateral and posteromedial papillary muscles, which arise from the left ventricular free wall (see Figs. 2-18*B* and 2-25). Commissural chords arise from each papillary muscle and extend in a fanlike array to insert into the free edge of both leaflets adjacent to the commissures (major commissures)[17] (see Figs. 2-24 and 2-26*A*, Plate 10) or into two adjacent scallops of the posterior leaflet (minor commissures) (see Figs. 2-24 and 2-25). *In contrast*

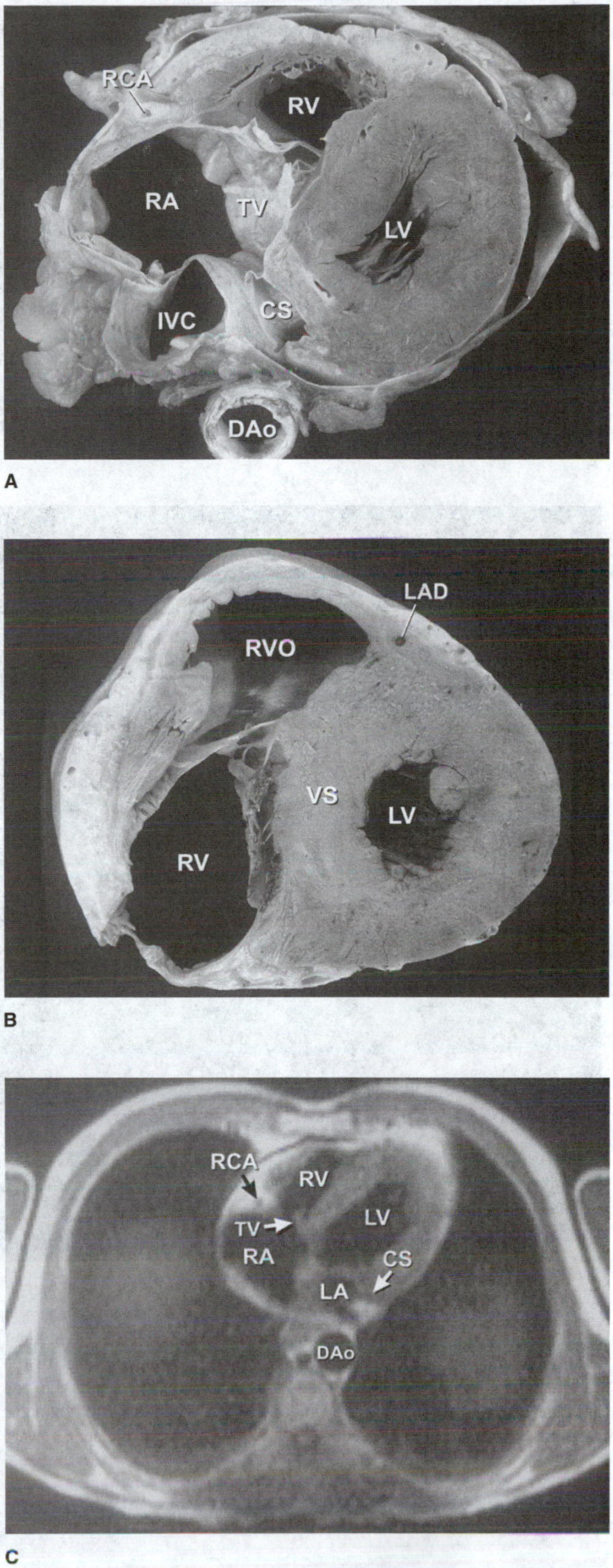

FIGURE 2-17 Tomographic sections of the heart in the transverse (*A*) and frontal (*B*) planes of the body. A tomographic section in the transverse plane of the body (*A*) results in a four-chamber view of the heart. A tomographic section along the frontal plane of the body (*B*) results in an oblique short-axis view of the heart. *C*. MRI image corresponding to *A*. CS, coronary sinus; DAo, descending thoracic aorta; IVC, inferior vena cava; LA, left atrium; LAD, left anterior descending coronary artery; LV, left ventricle; RA, right atrium; RCA, right coronary artery; RV, right ventricle; RVO, right ventricular outflow; TV, tricuspid valve; VS, ventricular septum.

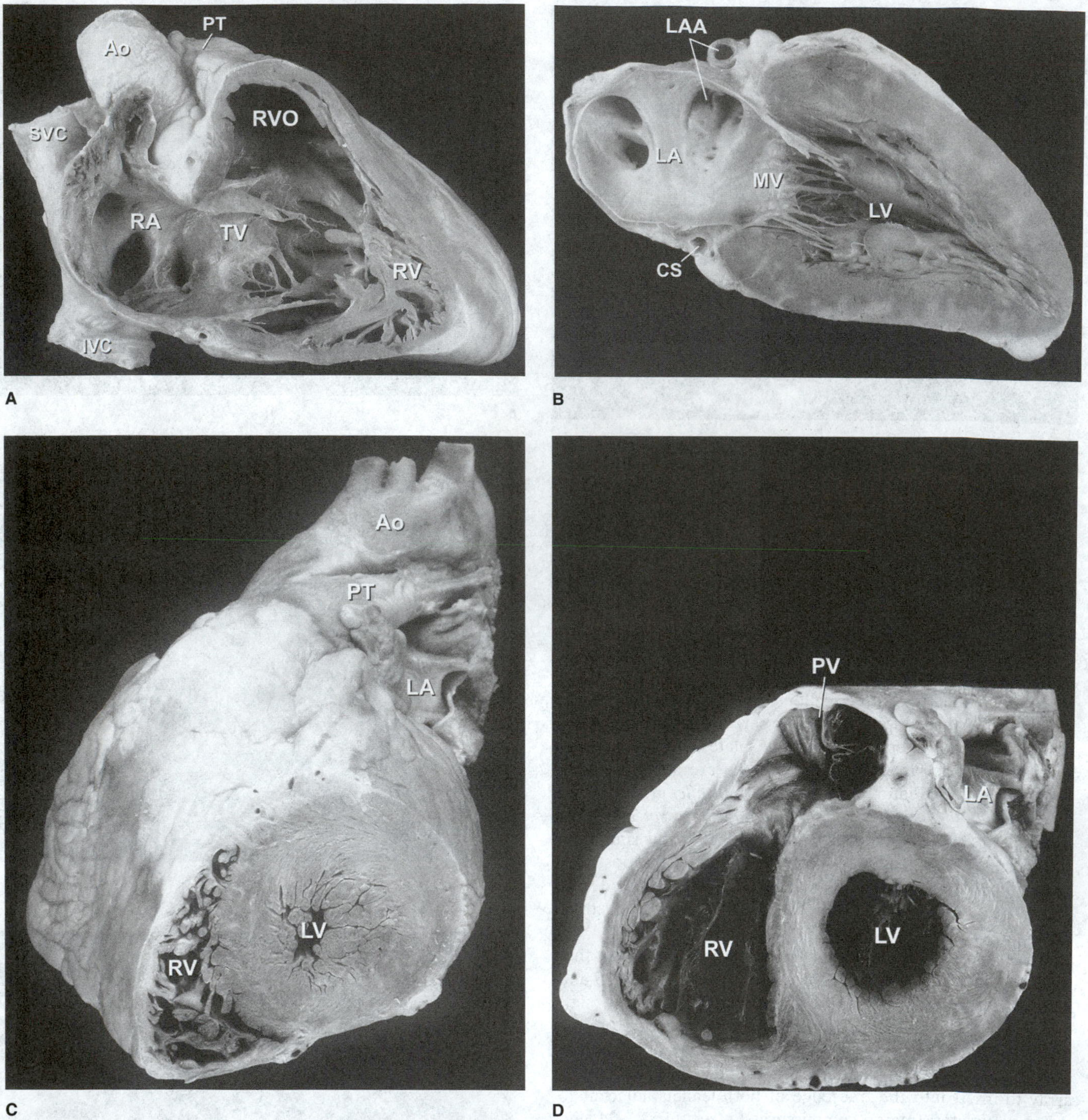

FIGURE 2-18 Oblique methods of tomographic cardiac dissection. *A, B.* Right anterior oblique sections, viewed from the right, are taken parallel to the ventricular and atrial septa, may include the right side of the heart (*A*) or the left side of the heart (*B*), and are similar to the two-chamber tomographic sections. *C,D.* Left anterior oblique sections, viewed from the apex toward the base, may be taken at various levels and are similar to the short-axis tomographic sections. Ao, aorta; CS, coronary sinus; IVC, inferior vena cava; LA, left atrium; LAA, left atrial appendage; LV, left ventricle; MV, mitral valve; PT, pulmonary trunk; PV, pulmonary valve; RA, right atrium; RV, right ventricle; RVO, right ventricular outflow; SVC, superior vena cava; TV, tricuspid valve.

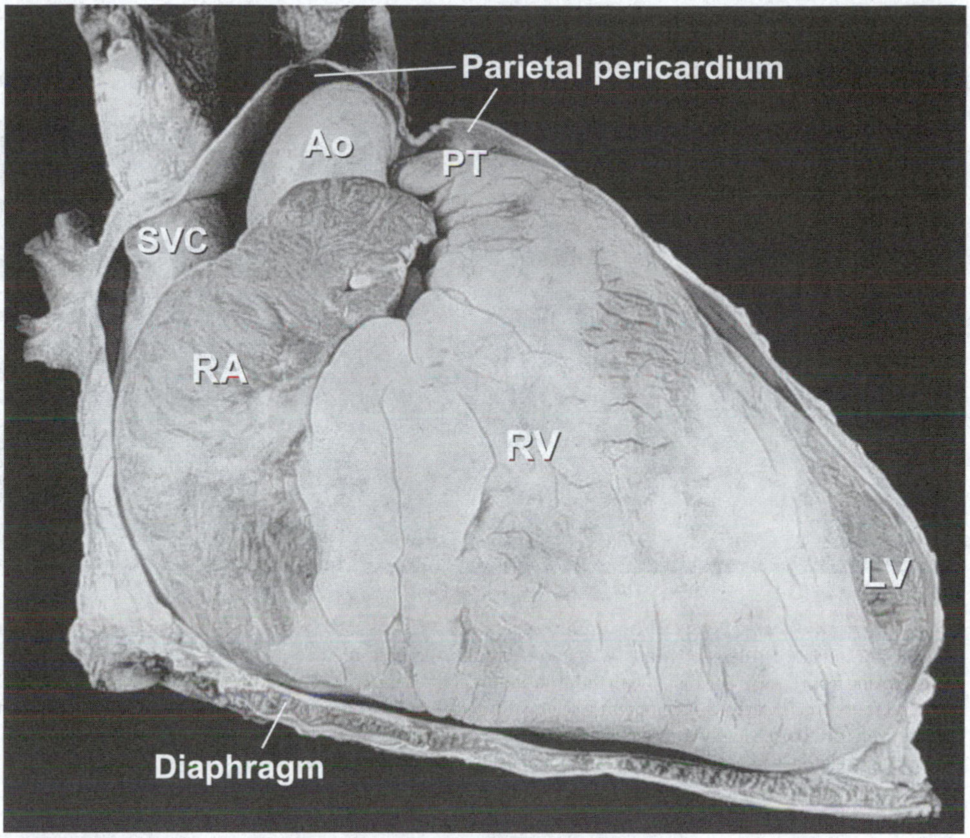

FIGURE 2-19 Anterior view of the heart. The anterior portion of the parietal pericardium has been removed, exposing the intrapericardial portions of the superior vena cava (SVC), ascending aorta (Ao), and pulmonary trunk (PT). LV, left ventricle; RA, right atrium; RV, right ventricle.

to congenital clefts, a true commissure is always associated with an underlying papillary muscle and an intervening array of chordae tendineae.[17] The attachments of commissural chords precisely demarcate the commissure. *Because the commissural chords are seldom elongated, they serve as accurate reference points for determining the proper closing plane for the leaflets during surgical repair.*

The anterolateral papillary muscle is commonly single and usually has a dual blood supply from the left coronary circulation.[16] In contrast, the posteromedial papillary muscle usually has multiple heads and is most commonly supplied only by the right coronary artery.[16] Small left atrial branches supply the most basal aspects of the mitral leaflets.[17]

Papillary muscle contraction pulls the two leaflets toward one another and thereby promotes valve closure. The line of closure for either mitral leaflet is not its free edge but an ill-defined junction between a thin, clear zone and a thicker, rough zone[17] (see Fig. 2-26, Plate 10). The major chordae supporting a leaflet insert into its free edge and rough zone. The chordae tendineae anchor and support the leaflets and, by doing so, prevent leaflet prolapse during ventricular systole. Two particularly prominent rough zone chords, referred to as *strut chordae*, insert along each half of the ventricular surface of the anterior mitral leaflet and provide additional leaflet support.[17] They may contain cardiac muscle and tend to calcify with age. Unlike the tricuspid valve, the normal mitral leaflets have no chordal insertions into the ventricular septum.[16]

The functional orifice of the mitral valve is defined by its narrowest diastolic cross-sectional area. This may be at the annulus when there is extensive annular calcification or close to the papillary muscle tips in patients with rheumatic mitral stenosis.

Mitral valve prolapse is characterized by thickened and redundant leaflets, annular dilatation (with or without calcium), and thickened and elongated chordae tendineae (with or without rupture). Prolapse of the posterior leaflet occurs more frequently than that of the anterior leaflet. Rheumatic involvement of the mitral valve causes chordal shortening and thickening without annular dilatation. Rheumatic mitral stenosis is produced by chordal and commissural fusion, often with calcification, whereas rheumatic mitral insufficiency results from scar retraction of leaflets and chords.[15] *Chronic postinfarction mitral regurgitation is associated with left ventricular dilatation and scarring of a papillary muscle and its subjacent ventricular free wall. Acute postinfarction mitral regurgitation may be associated with partial*

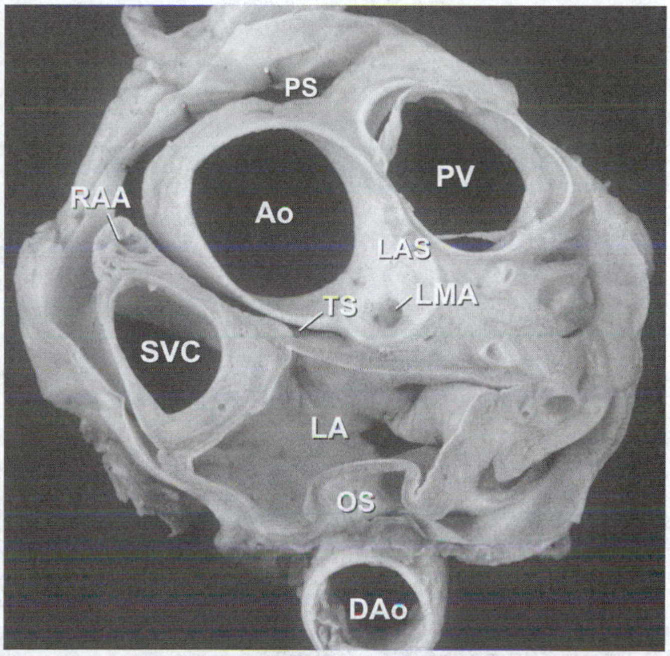

FIGURE 2-20 Tomographic section in the short-axis plane of the body, looking from apex toward the base, showing the oblique (OS) and transverse (TS) pericardial sinuses. Ao, ascending aorta; DAo, descending thoracic aorta; LA, left atrium; LAS, left aortic sinus; LMA, left main coronary artery: PS, pericardial sac; PV, pulmonary valve; RAA, right atrial appendage; SVC, superior vena cava.

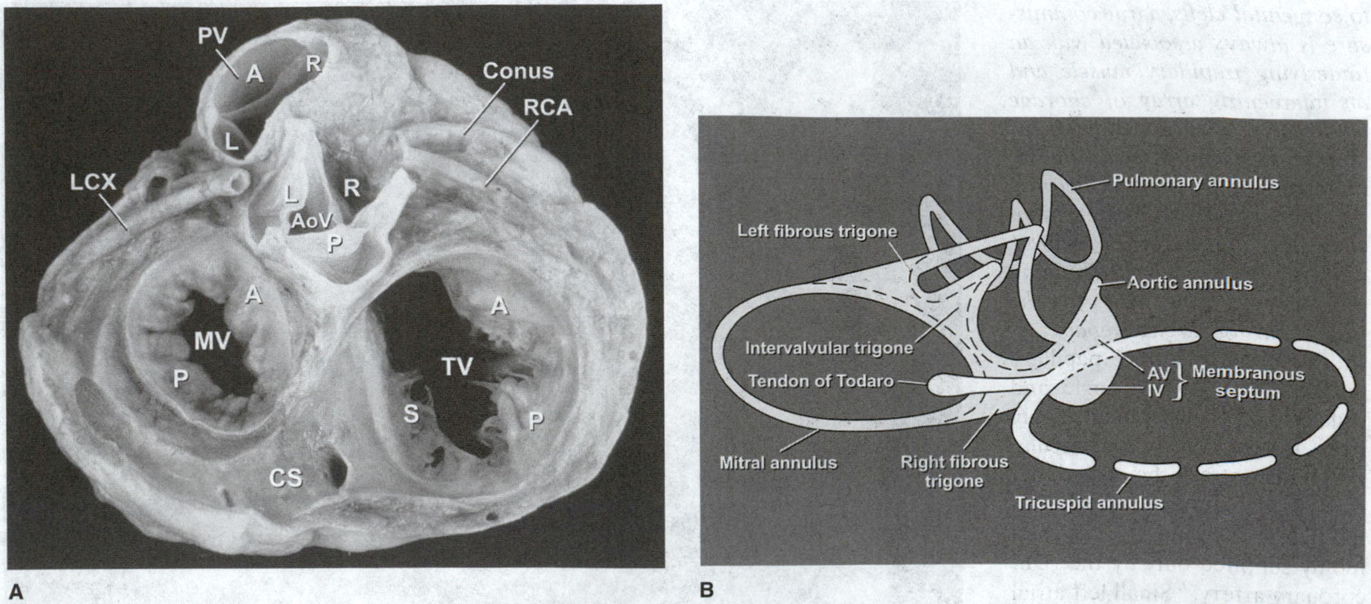

FIGURE 2-21 (Plate 8) Base of heart. *A*. Section through the base of the heart, looking from base toward apex, with the atria and great arteries removed, shows all four cardiac valves. *B*. A comparable schematic diagram of the fibrous cardiac skeleton. The centrally located aortic valve forms the cornerstone of the cardiac skeleton. Its fibrous extensions anchor and support the other three valves. *A*, anterior; AoV, aortic valve; AV, atrioventricular; CS, coronary sinus; IV, interventricular; L, left; LCX, left circumflex coronary artery; MV, mitral valve; P, posterior; PV, pulmonary valve; R, right; RCA, right coronary artery; S, septal; TV, tricuspid valve.

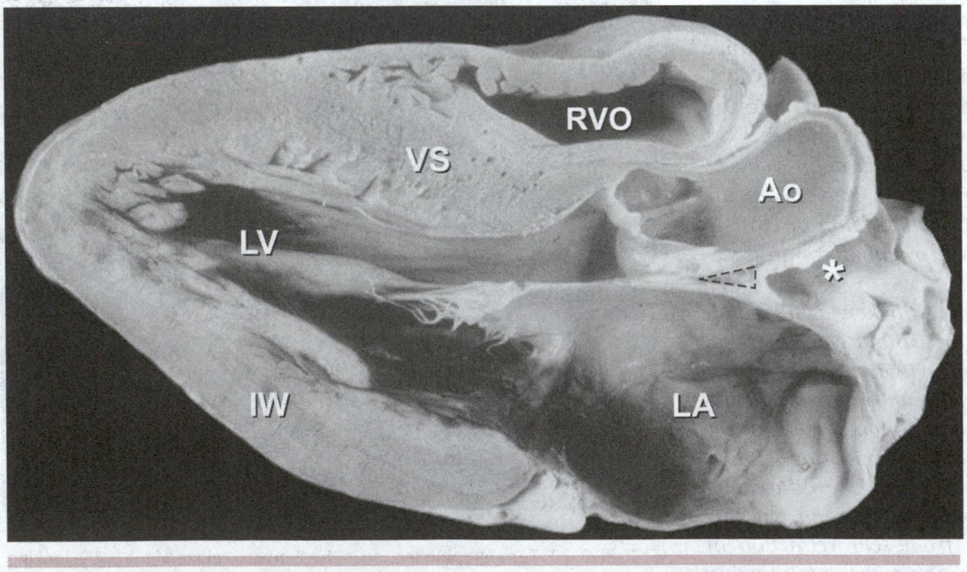

FIGURE 2-22 Long-axis section of the left ventricle. The intervalvular fibrosa (dashed triangle) lies between the anterior mitral leaflet and the posterior cusp of the aortic valve and abuts the floor of the transverse pericardial sinus (*). Ao, ascending aorta; IW, inferior wall; LA, left atrium; LV, left ventricle; RVO, right ventricular outflow; VS, ventricular septum.

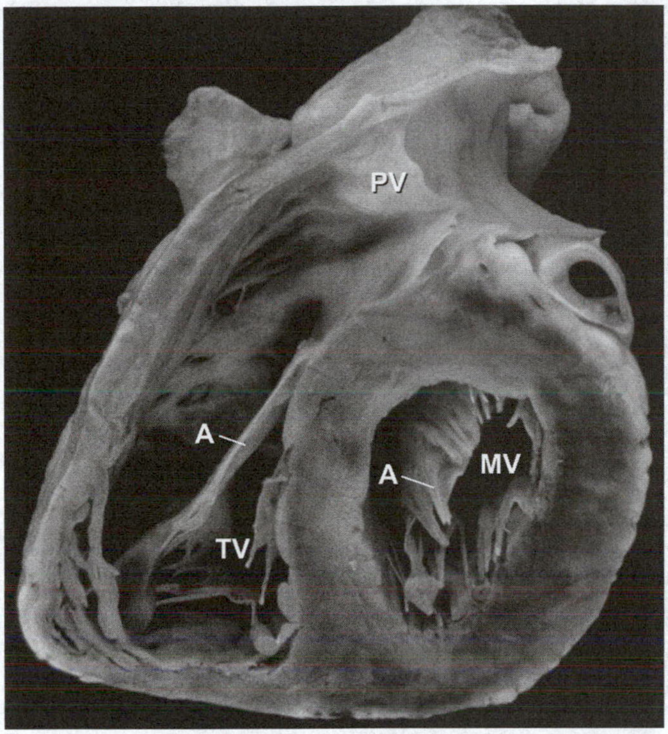

FIGURE 2-23 This oblique short-axis view of the heart shows the triangular-shaped tricuspid orifice (TV) and the elliptical mitral orifice (MV) at midleaflet level. The anterior tricuspid and anterior mitral leaflets (A) separate the inflow and outflow tracts of the right and left ventricles, respectively, and are parallel to one another. PV, pulmonary valve.

or complete rupture of a papillary muscle, usually the posteromedial one.

Anatomically important structures during mitral valve surgery include the left circumflex coronary artery, which courses within the left atrioventricular groove near the anterolateral commissure, and the coronary sinus, which courses within the left atrioventricular groove adjacent to the annulus of the posterior mitral leaflet[17] (see Fig. 2-21*A*).

Aortic Valve

The aortic valve, like the pulmonary valve, is comprised of three components (i.e., annulus, cusps, and commissures). In contrast to the mitral and tricuspid valves, the two semilunar valves have no tensor apparatus (i.e., chordae tendineae or papillary muscles). The commissures form tall, peaked spaces between the attachments of adjacent cusps (Figs. 2-27 and 2-28) and attain the level of the aortic sinotubular junction, the ridge that separates the sinus and tubular portions of the ascending aorta (originally described by Leonardo da Vinci as the "suprortic ridge")[15] (see Fig. 2-28). The functional aortic valve orifice may be at the sinotubular junction or proximal to it.[17]

The three half-moon-shaped (semilunar) aortic cusps form pocket-like tissue flaps that are avascular. In only about 10 percent of hearts are they truly equal in size. In two-thirds of hearts, either the right or posterior cusp is larger than the other two.[17] Just below the free edge of each cusp is a ridgelike closing edge (see Fig. 2-28). At the center of each cusp the closing edge meets the free edge and forms a small fibrous mound, the *nodule of Arantius*[15] (see Fig. 2-28). Between the free and closing edges, to each side of the nodule, are two crescent-shaped areas known as the *lunulas* that represent the sites of cusp apposition during valve closure.[15] Lunular fenestrations, near the commissures, are common and increase in size and incidence with age[15] (Fig. 2-29). However, owing to their position distal to the closing edge, they rarely produce valvular incompetence.[17] When viewed from above, the linear distance along the closing edge of a cusp is much greater than the straight-line distance between its two commissures[15] (see Fig. 2-27). This extra length of cusp tissue is necessary for nonstenotic opening and nonregurgitant closure of the valve.[15] Normally, the diameter of the aortic annulus at the hinge points of the aortic valve is about equal to the diameter of the ascending aorta at the sinotubular junction.[8]

These are important anatomic details in patients undergoing aortic valve repair. In hearts from adults with bicuspid valves and other congenital aortic valve disease, the annular diameter is usually enlarged. In contrast, patients with normal aortic cusps and central aortic regurgitation show enlargement at the level of the sinotubular junction.[7]

A prebypass intraoperative transesophageal long-axis view of the left ventricular outflow tract is used to measure the aortic valve annular diameter prior to replacement by a homograft. By doing so, precious bypass time is saved while the homograft is being prepared.[8] *Disease processes that produce commissural fusion such as rheumatic valvulitis or which decrease cusp mobility such as fibrosis or calcification may lead to aortic stenosis.*[15] *In contrast, those disorders which decrease cusp size such as rheumatic valvulitis or which cause aortic root dilatation may lead to aortic regurgitation.*[15] *Combinations of these processes may produce combined stenosis and regurgitation.*

The commissure between the right and posterior aortic cusps overlies the membranous septum (Fig. 2-30) and contacts the commissure between the anterior and septal leaflets of the tricuspid valve (see Fig. 2-40). The commissure between the right and left aortic cusps contacts its corresponding pulmonary commissure and overlies the infundibular septum (see Fig. 2-12*D*). The intervalvular fibrosa, at the commissure between the left and posterior aortic cusps, fuses the aortic valve to the anterior mitral leaflet.[15,17]

During aortic valve replacement, the anterior mitral leaflet, left bundle branch, or coronary ostia may be injured inadvertently.[17] *Annular abscesses due to infective endocarditis involving the aortic valve may burrow into adjacent structures and thereby produce endocarditis of the other valves, conduction disturbances with septal involvement, aortoatrial, aortopulmonary artery, or aortoventricular fistulas, pericarditis, or fatal hemopericardium.*[15]

Pulmonary Valve

The pulmonary valve is virtually identical in design to the aortic valve.[17] The pulmonary artery sinuses are partially embedded within the muscle bundles of the right ventricular infundibulum, particularly adjacent to the right and left sinuses.[16,19] *In pulmonary valve atresia with an intact ventricular septum, hypertrophy of the muscle bundles and the narrow right ventricular outflow tract accentuate this relationship.*[19] Also, unlike the aortic valve,

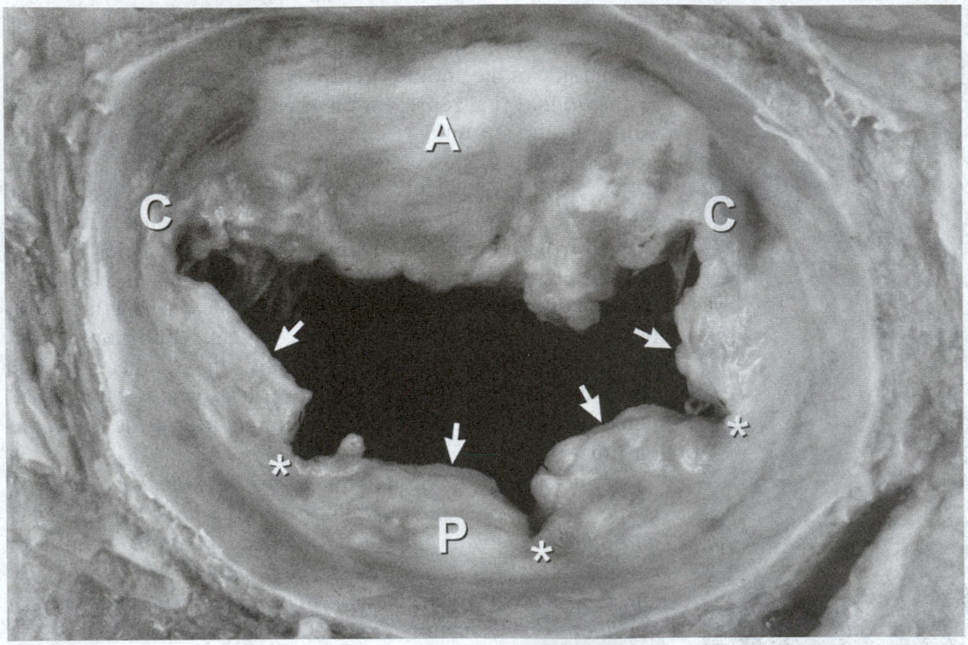

FIGURE 2-24 (Plate 9) Mitral valve, viewed from left atrial aspect. Minor commissures (*) divide the posterior leaflet into four scallops (arrows). A, anterior; C, major commissures; P, posterior.

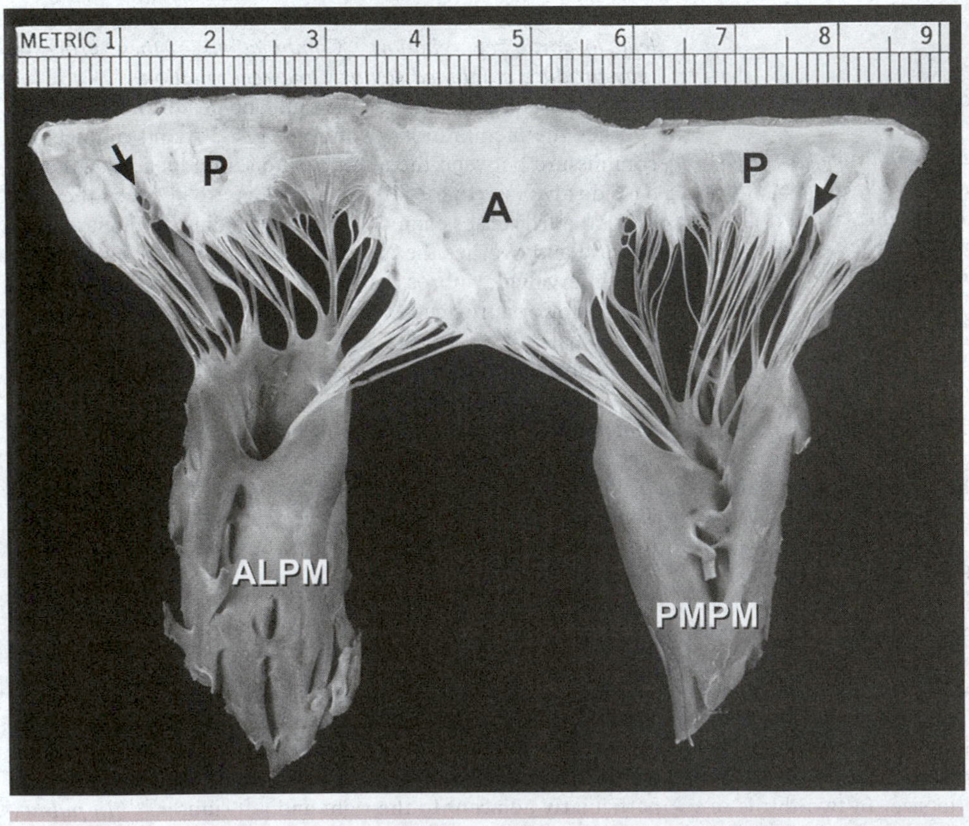

FIGURE 2-25 Gross anatomy of the mitral valve and papillary muscle–chordal apparatus, as demonstrated in an excised and unfolded valve. Each commissure overlies a papillary muscle. Arrows point to minor commissures. A, anterior leaflet; ALPM, anterolateral papillary muscle; P, posterior leaflet; PMPM, posteromedial papillary muscle.

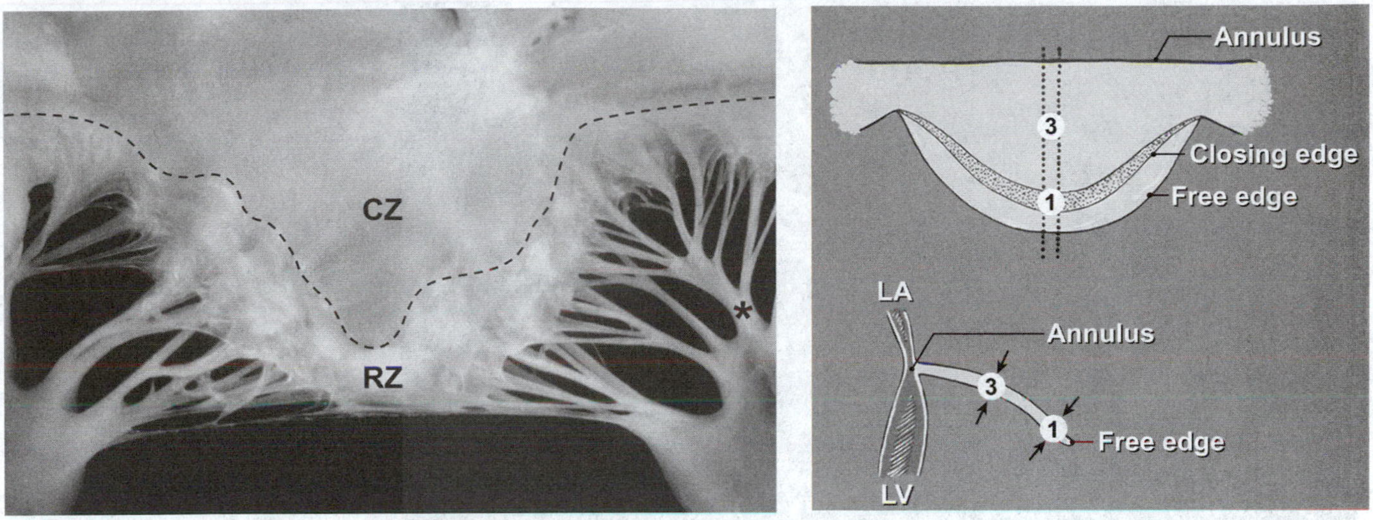

A B

FIGURE 2-26 (Plate 10) Components of the mitral valve. *A*. Each leaflet has a large clear zone (CZ) and a smaller rough zone (RZ) between its free edge and closing edge (dotted line). A fanlike commissural chorda tendinea (*) connects the tip of the papillary muscle to the commissure. *B*. Schematic diagram of an open anterior mitral leaflet comparable to *A*. Section obtained along the dotted lines shows the relationship of the mitral annulus and free edge to the closing edge.

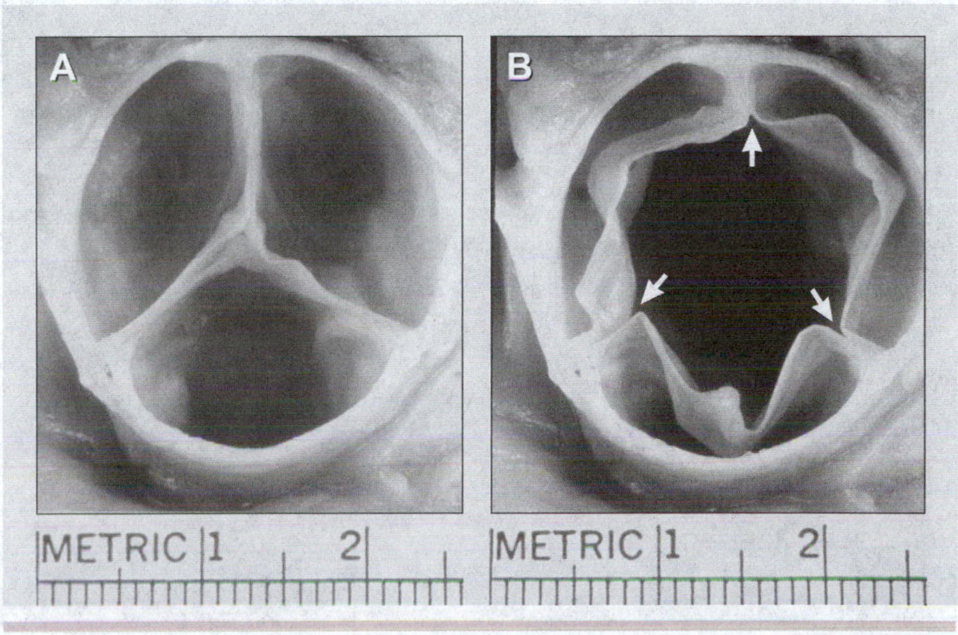

FIGURE 2-27 Each cusp of a semilunar valve is pocket-shaped. The aortic valve is viewed from above in simulated closed (*A*) and open (*B*) positions, showing the three commissures (arrows). Note that the length of the closing edge exceeds the straight-line distance between the commissures.

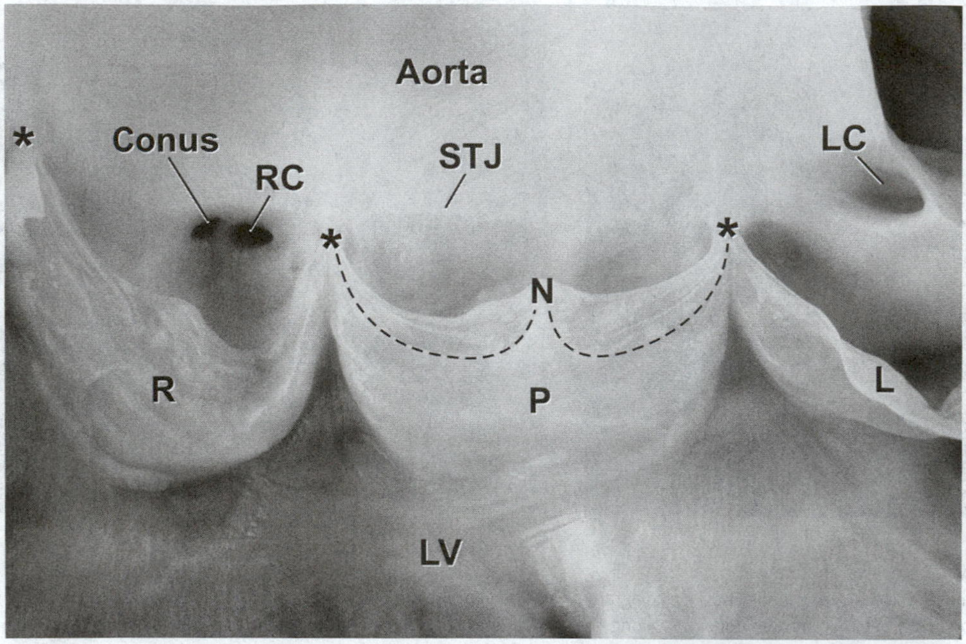

FIGURE 2-28 An opened aortic valve shows the right (R), left (L), and posterior (P) cusps. The dashed line marks the closing edge. Between the free and closing edges of each cusp are two lunular areas, representing the surfaces of apposition between adjacent cusps during valve closure. The commissures (*) attain the level of the aortic sinotubular junction (STJ). Conus, conus coronary ostium; LC, left coronary ostium; LV, left ventricle; N, nodule of Arantius; RC, right coronary ostium.

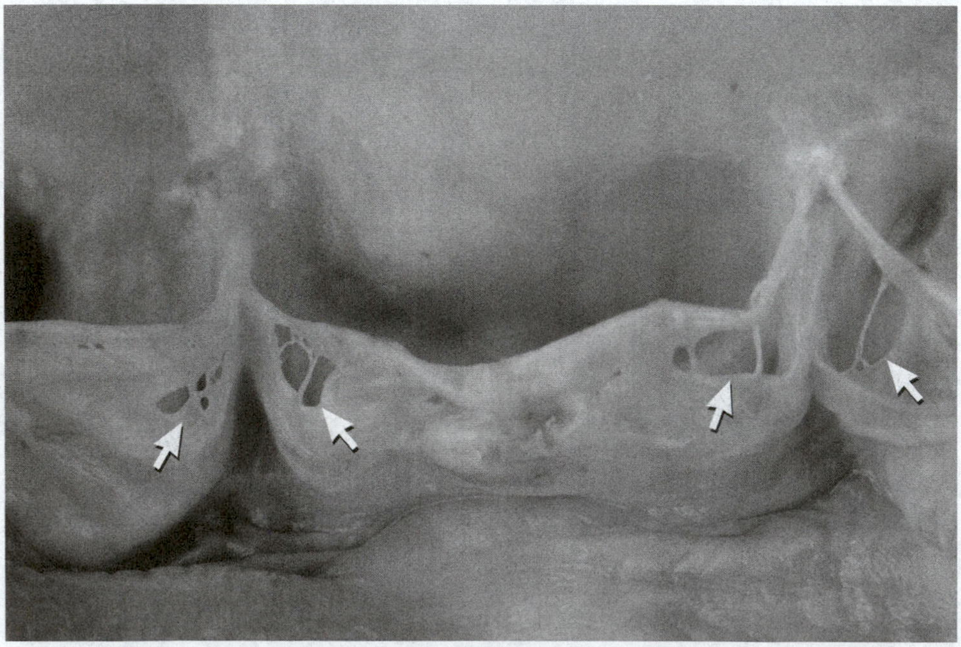

FIGURE 2-29 Aortic cusp fenestrations (arrows) occurring in the lunular regions near the commissures. This is a common age-related degenerative finding and normally accounts for little or no aortic valve regurgitation.

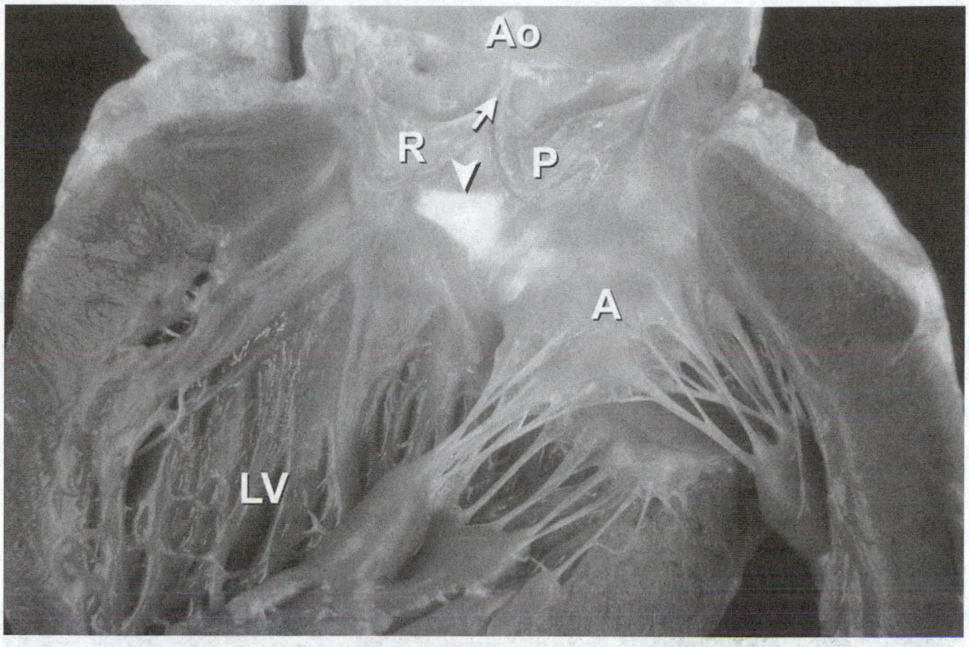

FIGURE 2-30 The commissure between the right and posterior aortic cusps (arrow) overlies the transilluminated membranous septum (arrowhead). A, anterior mitral leaflet; Ao, ascending aorta; LV, left ventricle; P, posterior aortic cusp; R, right aortic cusp.

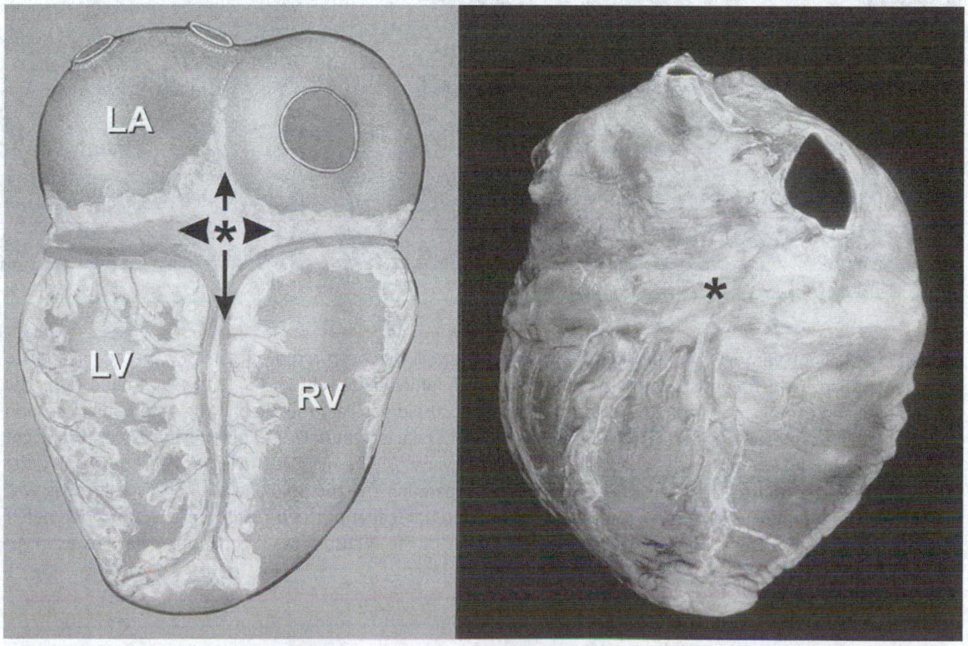

FIGURE 2-31 View of the diaphragmatic aspect of the heart shows the intersection of the atrioventricular (arrowheads), posterior interventricular (long arrow), and interatrial (small arrow) grooves at the external cardiac crux (*). (*Left*) Diagram. (*Right*) Cardiac specimen. LA, left atrium; LV, left ventricle; RV, right ventricle.

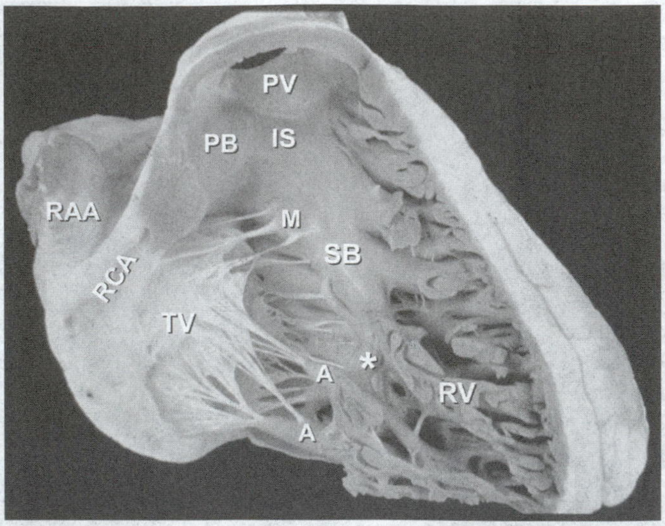

A

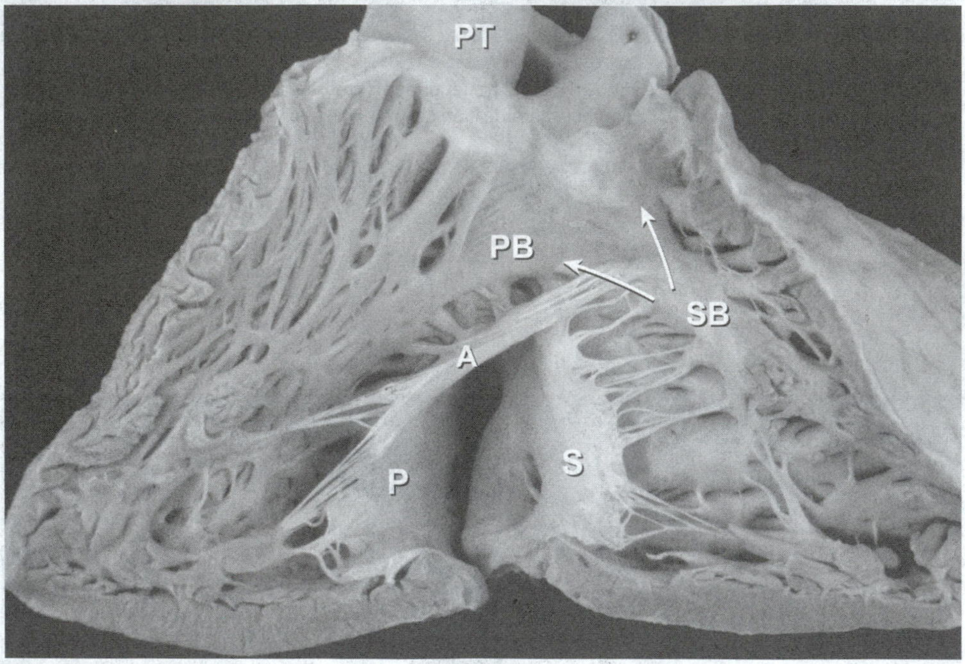

B

FIGURE 2-32 Right ventricle. *A*. The right ventricular free wall has been removed to show the archlike crista supraventricularis, which consists of the parietal band (PB), infundibular septum (IS), and septal band (SB). The moderator band (*) joins the septal band to the anterior tricuspid papillary muscle (*A*). The anteroapical portion of the chamber is heavily trabeculated. M, medial tricuspid papillary muscle; PV, pulmonary valve; RAA, right atrial appendage; RCA, right coronary artery; TV, tricuspid valve. *B*. The right ventricle has been opened by the inflow-outflow method to show the parietal band (PB) separating the tricuspid and pulmonary valves, as well as the two upper limbs (arrows) of e septal band (SB). *A*, anterior leaflet of the tricuspid valve; P, posterior leaflet of the tricuspid valve; PT, pulmonary trunk; S, septal leaflet of the tricuspid valve; other abbreviations as in *A*.

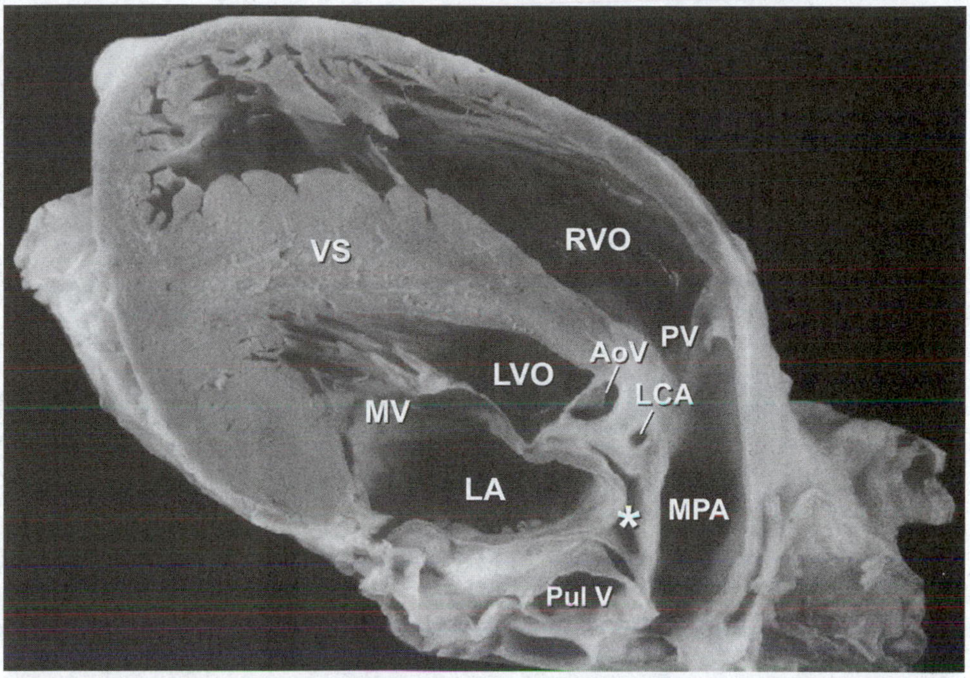

FIGURE 2-33 Long-axis view of the right ventricular outflow (RVO) tract showing the pulmonary valve (PV) and main pulmonary artery (MPA). AoV, aortic valve; LA, left atrium; LCA, left coronary artery; LVO, left ventricular outflow; MV, mitral valve; PulV, pulmonary vein; VS, ventricular septum; *, transverse sinus.

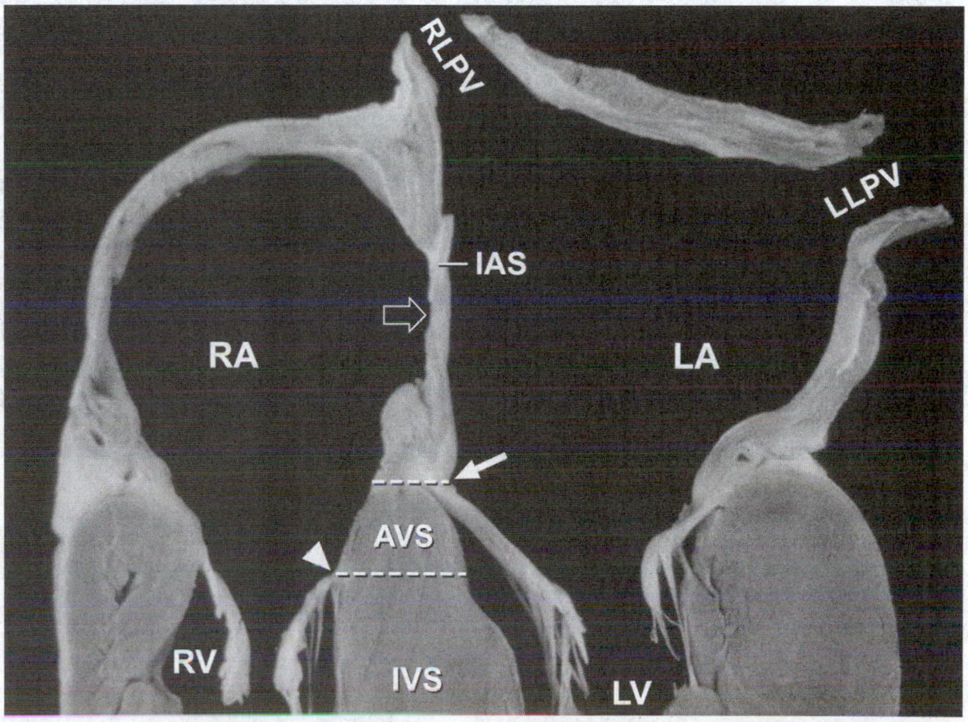

FIGURE 2-34 (Plate 11) Four-chamber slice of the heart shows the characteristic normal apical displacement of the tricuspid valve septal leaflet insertion (arrowhead) when compared with septal insertion of the mitral valve (solid arrow). This tomographic section also shows the interatrial septum (IAS), atrioventricular septum (AVS), and interventricular septum (IVS). Open arrow points to fossa ovalis. LA, left atrium; LLPV, left lower pulmonary vein; LV, left ventricle; RA, right atrium; RLPV, right lower pulmonary vein; RV, right ventricle.

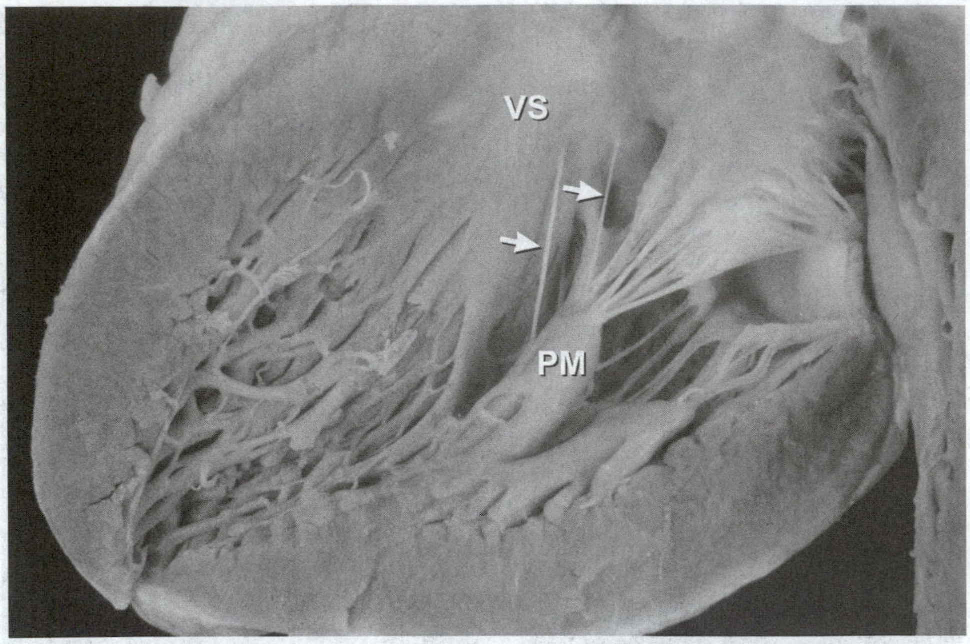

A

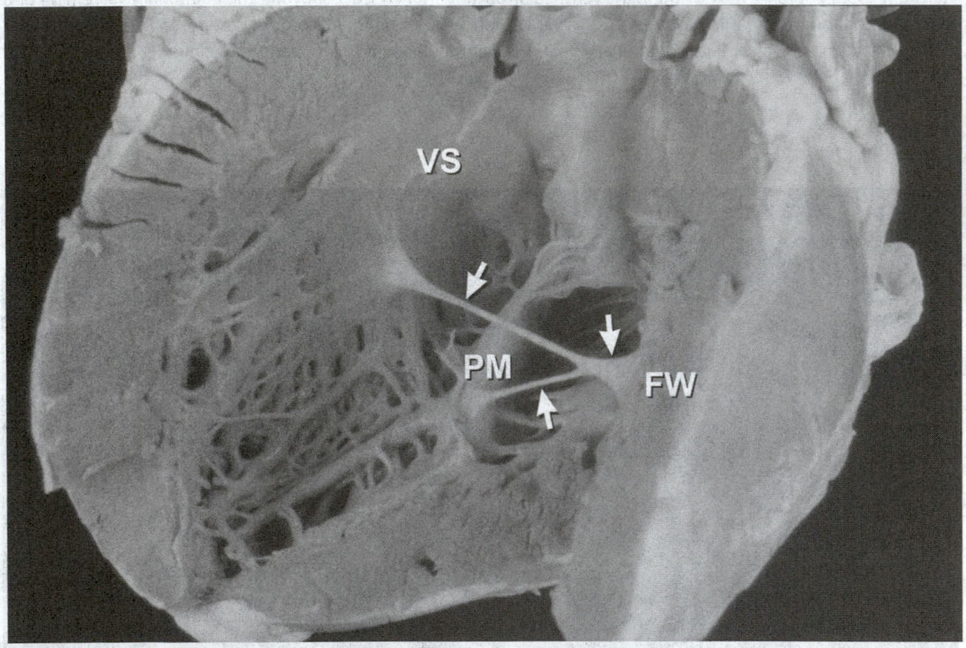

B

FIGURE 2-35 Various locations of left ventricular false tendons. *A*. Two false tendons (arrows) from posteromedial mitral papillary muscle (PM) to ventricular septum (VS), representing the most common location. *B*. Complex branching false tendon (arrows) with origin from the left ventricular free wall (FW) and insertions into the ventricular septum (VS) and base of posteromedial mitral papillary muscle (PM).

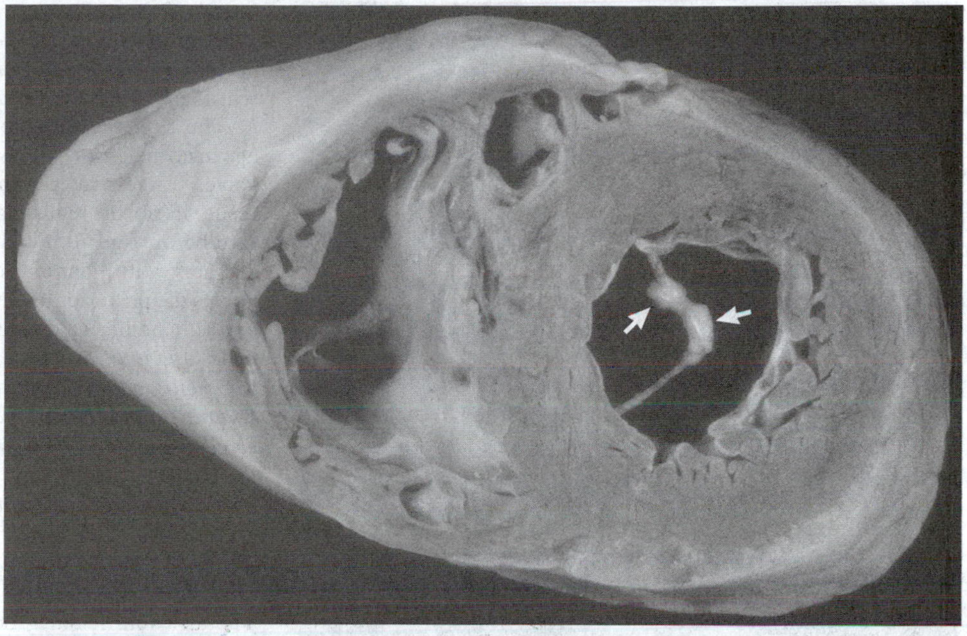

FIGURE 2-36 (Plate 12) Calcified left ventricular false tendon (arrows) seen in short-axis view.

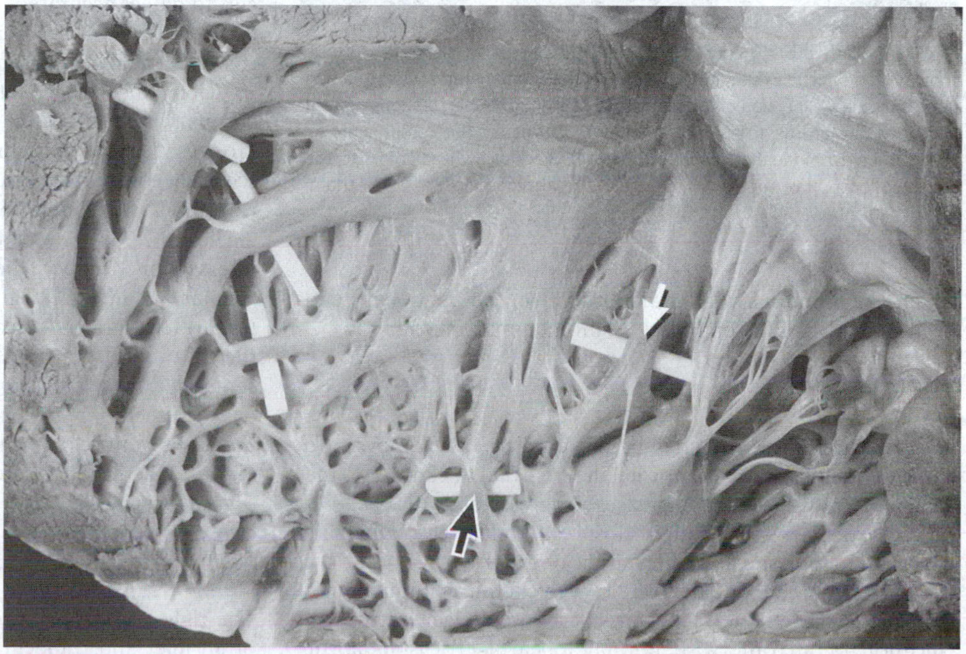

FIGURE 2-37 Prominent left ventricular trabeculations. Multiple large muscle bundles extend from the anterior free wall to the septum (probes). A single muscle bundle extends from the posteromedial mitral papillary muscle to the posterior septum (probe with white arrow), and one bundle extends from one portion of the posterior septum to another (probe with black arrow). Such trabeculations become even more prominent in noncompaction of the left ventricular myocardium.

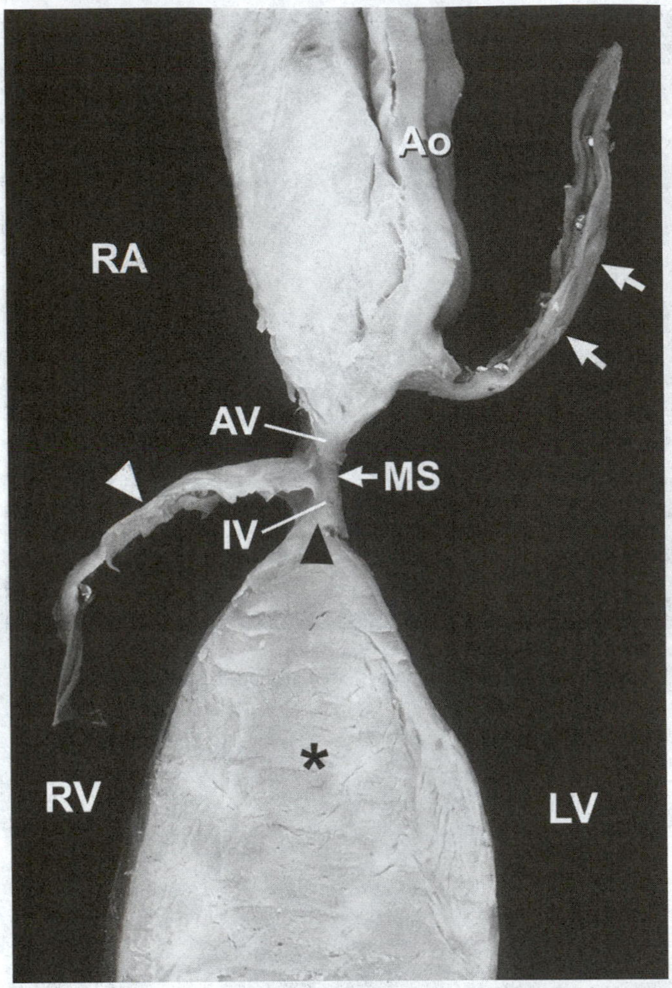

FIGURE 2-38 (Plate 13) Four-chamber tomographic slice through the aortic root (Ao) and aortic valve (arrows) showing the small membranous (MS) and large muscular (*) portion of the ventricular septum. The membranous septum is divided into atrioventricular (AV) and interventricular (IV) components by the septal tricuspid leaflet (white arrowhead). Black arrowhead points to the expected location of the AV (His) bundle. LV, left ventricle; RA, right atrium; RV, right ventricle.

which is continuous with the mitral valve, the pulmonary and tricuspid valves are separated by infundibular muscle.[17]

Age-Related Valve Changes

Several age-related changes in the cardiac valves may have clinical significance.[20] In normal hearts, the thickness of the aortic and mitral leaflets increases progressively with each decade, particularly along their closure margins.[20] Probably the most common clinical manifestation of these changes is aortic valve sclerosis, characterized by valve thickening without hemodynamic dysfunction.[20] However, age-related degenerative calcification of an otherwise normal-appearing tricuspid aortic valve may result in progressive aortic stenosis.[20]

Age-related thickening along the nodule of Arantius and closing edges may be associated with the formation of whisker-like projections called *Lambl's excrescences*. These fine fibrous-like strands also can develop on the mitral valve.[17] *They are readily detected by echocardiography and have been associated with cardioembolic stroke.*[21] *Larger clusters, having the appearance of a sea anemone, are considered to be either neoplastic or reactive and are known as* papillary fibroelastomas.[22]

The circumferences of all four cardiac valves increase with age in normal hearts. This is particularly evident in the semilunar valves.[20] Age-related annular dilatation of the aortic valve can result in aortic regurgitation.[20] Mitral annular calcification is rare before age 70 but is present in 40 percent of women over age 90.[20] Mitral annular calcification almost invariably only involves the posterior leaflet and forms a C-shaped ring of annular and subannular calcium.[17] *Mitral annular calcification may impede subannular ventricular contraction, thereby resulting in mitral regurgitation. Because of the proximity of the posteromedial commissure to the atrioventricular (His) bundle, mitral annular calcification may be associated with atrioventricular block.*[20] *With the increasing size of the aging population, degenerative calcific aortic disease is increasing in frequency.*[20]

Cardiac Grooves, Crux, and Margins

The atrioventricular groove encircles the heart and defines its base. It separates the atria from the ventricles (Fig. 2-31). The two ventricles are separated by the anterior and posterior (inferior) interventricular grooves, which define the plane of the ventricular septum (see Figs. 2-5*A* and 2-31).

With age, fat tends to accumulate in increasing amounts in the epicardium, particularly in the atrioventricular grooves.[20,23] *Increased epicardial fat deposits may be associated with increased risk of cardiac rupture after acute transmural myocardial infarction.*[23] Excess fat in the atrial septum is called *lipomatous hypertrophy* and may result in a thickness that exceeds that of the ventricular septum. Fat in the right ventricular free wall is difficult to detect accurately clinically; its excess accumulation may be associated with increasing age, obesity, or arrhythmogenic right ventricular cardiomyopathy.[24]

Along the surface of the heart, the right and circumflex coronary arteries travel in the right and left atrioventricular grooves, respectively, and the left anterior and posterior descending coronary arteries course along the anterior and posterior (or inferior) interventricular grooves, respectively (see Figs. 2-5*A* and 2-31). The external cardiac crux is the cross-shaped intersection between the atrioventricular, posterior interventricular, and interatrial grooves (see Fig. 2-31). Its internal counterpart (the internal crux) is the posterior intersection between the mitral and tricuspid annuli and the atrial and ventricular septa (see Figs. 2-16*B* and 2-34, Plate 11).

The junction between the anterior and inferior free walls of the right ventricle forms a sharp angle known as the *acute margin*. The rounded lateral wall of the left ventricle forms the *obtuse margin*.[15]

Right Ventricle

The right ventricle is a right-anterior structure. It is comprised of an inlet and trabecular and outflow segments[15] (Fig. 2-32). The inlet component extends from the tricuspid annulus to the insertions of the papillary muscles. An apical trabecular zone extends inferiorly beyond the attachments of the papillary muscles toward the ventricular apex and about halfway along the anterior wall.[15] *This muscular meshwork is the site of insertion of transvenous ventricular pacemaker electrodes. During right ventricular endomyocardial biopsy, tissue generally is obtained from the trabeculated apex. Disruption of a portion of the tricuspid support apparatus is a potential complication of right-sided heart instrumentation (e.g., right ventricular endomyocardial biopsy).*[17] The outflow portion, also known as the conus (meaning "cone") or *infundibulum* (meaning "funnel"), is a smooth-walled muscular subpulmonary channel[15,17] (see Fig. 2-32).

A prominent arch-shaped muscular ridge known as the *crista supraventricularis* separates the tricuspid and pulmonary valves. It is made up of three components (i.e., parietal band, infundibular septum, and septal band) that may appear as distinct structures or may merge together[15,17] (see Fig. 2-32). The parietal band is a free-wall structure, whereas the adjacent infundibular septum is intracardiac and separates the two ventricular outflow tracts beneath the right and left cusps of both semilunar valves[15,17] (Figs. 2-12D and 2-33). The septal band forms a Y-shaped muscle, the two upper limbs of which cradle the infundibular septum. From this branching point of the septal band emanates the medial tricuspid papillary muscle[15,17] (see Fig. 2-32). The moderator band forms an intracavitary muscle that connects the septal band with the anterior tricuspid papillary muscle (see Fig. 2-32*A*).

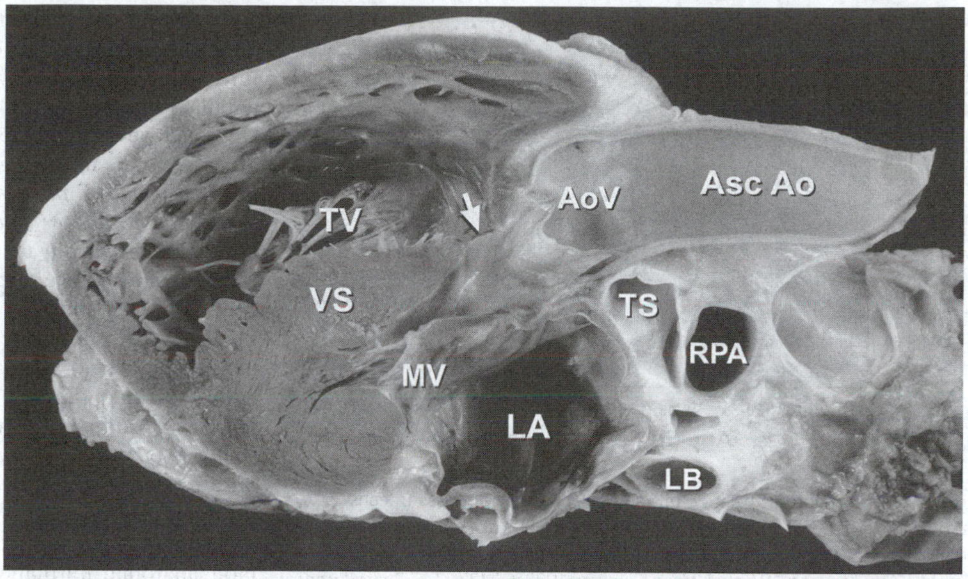

FIGURE 2-39 Tomographic section of the heart along a long-axis plane of the body. The aortic root lies in this plane. The left ventricle and aortic valve are cut obliquely. The membranous ventricular septum (arrow) lies beneath the right and posterior aortic cusps. AoV, aortic valve; Asc Ao, ascending aorta; LA, left atrium; LB, left bronchus; MV, mitral valve; RPA, right pulmonary artery; TS, transverse sinus; TV, tricuspid valve; VS, muscular ventricular septum.

Left Ventricle

The left ventricle, like the right ventricle, is made of an inlet portion comprised of the mitral valve apparatus, a subaortic outflow portion, and a finely trabeculated apical zone.[17] The left ventricular free wall is normally thickest toward the base and thinnest toward the apex, where it averages only 1 to 2 mm in thickness, even in hypertrophied hearts.[17] Structurally, the left and right ventricles differ considerably.[15,17] Normally, the left ventricular free-wall and septal thicknesses are three times the thickness of the right ventricular free wall. The mitral and aortic valves share fibrous continuity, whereas the parietal band separates the tricuspid and pulmonary valves. Whereas the mitral valve has an elliptical orifice and no septal attachments, the tricuspid valve has a triangular orifice and numerous direct septal attachments (see Fig. 2-23). The right ventricular apex is much more trabeculated than its counterpart on the left (see Figs. 2-9*B* and 2-18*C*). *The distinctive differences in apical trabeculations persist even in markedly hypertrophied or dilated hearts.*[17]

The annular attachment of the septal leaflet of the tricuspid valve inserts more apically than that of the anterior mitral leaflet, allowing distinction between the right and left ventricles by four-chamber imaging (Fig. 2-34). *Exceptions include partial atrioventricular septal defects and double-inlet ventricles in which the two valve annuli are at the same level. Ebstein's anomaly is characterized by exaggeration of apical displacement of the septal and posterior tricuspid leaflets resulting in an atrialized portion of the right ventricular chamber.*[16,17] *Morphologic differentiation of the right and left ventricles is particularly important in congeni-*

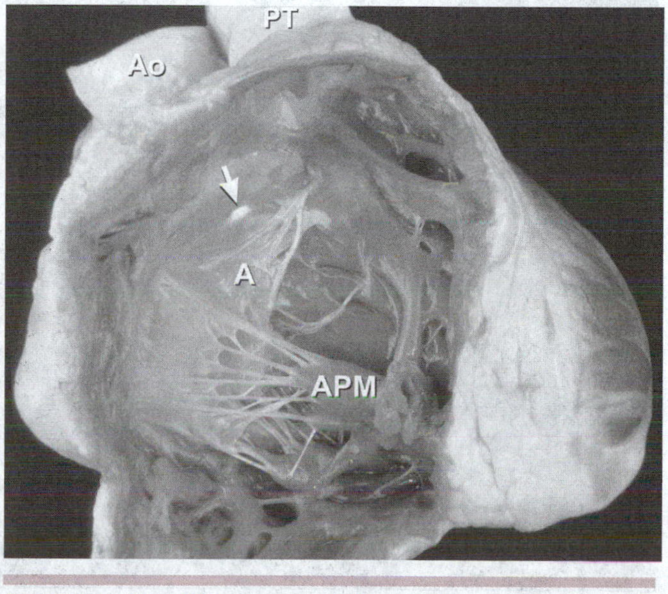

FIGURE 2-40 (Plate 14) A view of the right ventricle. Transilluminated membranous ventricular septum (arrow) in contact with the commissure between the anterior and septal leaflets of the tricuspid valve. A, anterior tricuspid leaflet; Ao, ascending aorta; APM, anterior tricuspid papillary muscle; PT, pulmonary trunk.

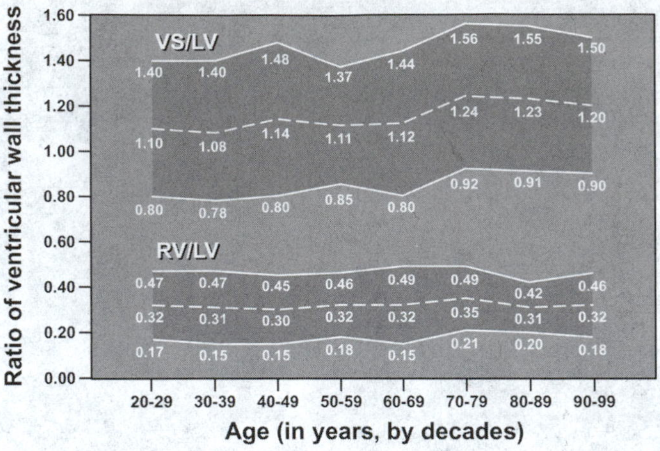

FIGURE 2-41 (Plate 15) Ratios of ventricular wall thicknesses (means ± 2 standard deviations) versus age. RV/LV, ratio of right to left ventricular wall thickness; VS/LV, ratio of ventricular septal to left ventricular free wall thickness. (From Kitzman DW, et al. *Mayo Clin Proc* 1988; 63:137–146. Reproduced with permission of Mayo Foundation.)

tal heart disease. The morphologic tricuspid valve virtually always connects to a morphologic right ventricle, whereas the morphologic mitral valve connects to a morphologic left ventricle.[15,16] Because of the rightward bulging of the ventricular septum, the left ventricular chamber appears circular in cross section, whereas the right ventricular chamber has a crescentic appearance (see Fig. 2-23). Tomographic segmental left ventricular anatomy will be reviewed in the section on coronary arteries.

Left ventricular false tendons, also referred to as *pseudotendons* or *bands*,[25] are discrete, thin, cordlike fibromuscular structures that connect two walls, the two papillary muscles, or a papillary muscle to a wall, usually the ventricular septum (Fig. 2-35). However, false tendons, as the name implies, are not attached to the mitral leaflets. *Chordal attachments between the mitral leaflets and the ventricular septum are abnormal and are usually associated with atrioventricular septal defects or straddling atrioventricular valves*.[16] False tendons are common anatomic variants of the normal left ventricle, occurring in 50 percent of hearts, and may become calcified with age (Fig. 2-36, Plate 12). They are more frequently observed in men, but their incidence does not appear to be age-related.[25] *It has been suggested that they may be the cause of innocent systolic musical murmurs*.[25] *Although they are readily detectable by echocardiography, they may be misinterpreted by the inexperienced sonographer as pathologic structures such as ruptured chords, mural thrombi, or vegetations*.[17,25]

Prominent left ventricular trabeculations[26] are another common anatomic normal variant that may be an even greater source of misinterpretation by two-dimensional echocardiography in patients with suspected mural thrombus. They are defined as discrete, thick muscle bundles that generally connect the free wall to the septum (Fig. 2-37). Less common attachments include papillary muscle to the septum, septum to septum, or free wall to free wall. *In noncompaction of the left ventricular myocardium*,[27,28] *also known as* spongy myocardium, *there is persistence of multiple prominent ventricular trabeculations and deep intertrabecular recesses caused by arrest in the normal in utero process of myocardial compaction. The associated clinical manifestations and age at onset of symptoms (i.e., typically a dilated cardiomyopathy) are highly variable.*

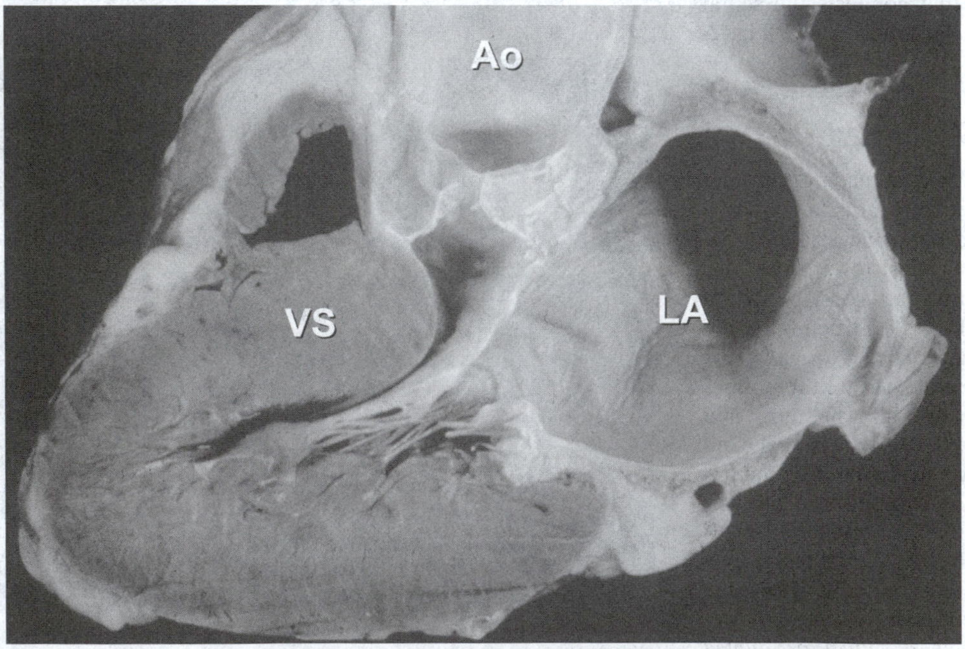

FIGURE 2-42 Age-related changes in the left-sided cardiac structures. Normal heart from an 84-year-old man demonstrates shortening of the base-to-apex (long-axis) dimension, decreased internal left ventricular dimension, aortic root dilatation, left atrial enlargement, and sigmoid-shaped septum. (Compare with Fig. 2-15 from an 18-year-old man.) Ao, ascending aorta; LA, left atrium; VS, ventricular septum.

Ventricular Septum

The ventricular septum is a complex intracardiac partition that can be considered to comprise four parts: inlet, trabecular, membranous, and infundibular. The plane of the infundibular portion (see Figs. 2-12*D* and 2-33) is different from that of the three other portions. *This anatomic relationship is important in many forms of congenital heart disease in which the infundibular septum is dissociated from the remainder of the ventricular septum (e.g., malalignment forms of ventricular septal defects in tetralogy of Fallot and in double-outlet right ventricle)*.[15–17]

The ventricular septum also may be divided into muscular and membranous portions[15–17] (Figs. 2-38, Plate 13, and 2-39). The membranous septum lies beneath the right and posterior (noncoronary) aortic cusps (see Fig. 2-30) and contacts the mitral and tricuspid annuli (Fig. 2-40, Plate 14). The

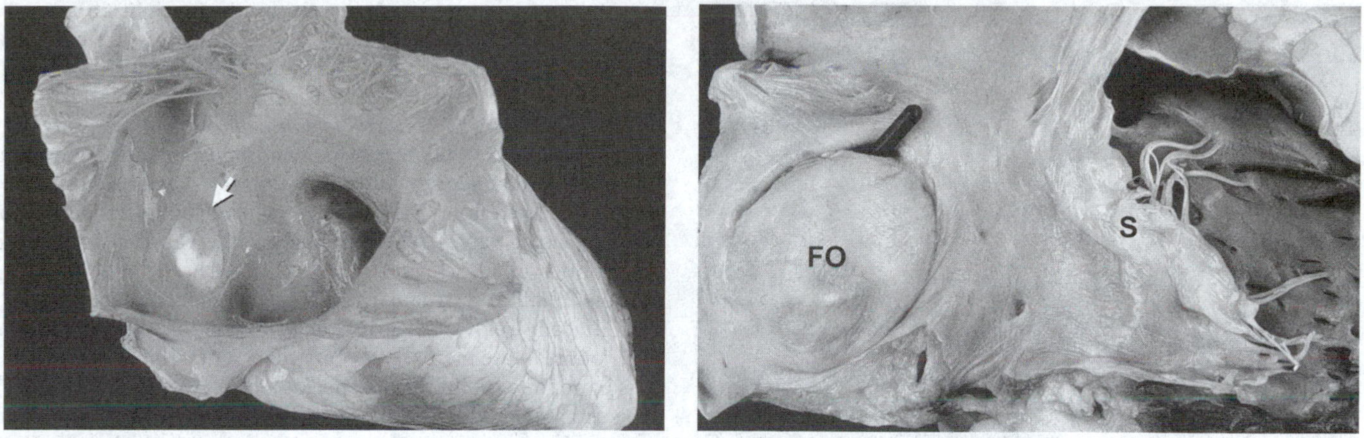

A B

FIGURE 2-43 *A*. Fossa ovalis. Opened right atrium shows the thick muscular limbus of the atrial septum (arrow), in contrast to the thin valve of the fossa ovalis (transilluminated). *B*. Patent foramen ovale (black probe) as seen from the right atrium. There is also an aneurysm of the valve of the fossa ovalis (FO). S, septal leaflet of the tricuspid valve.

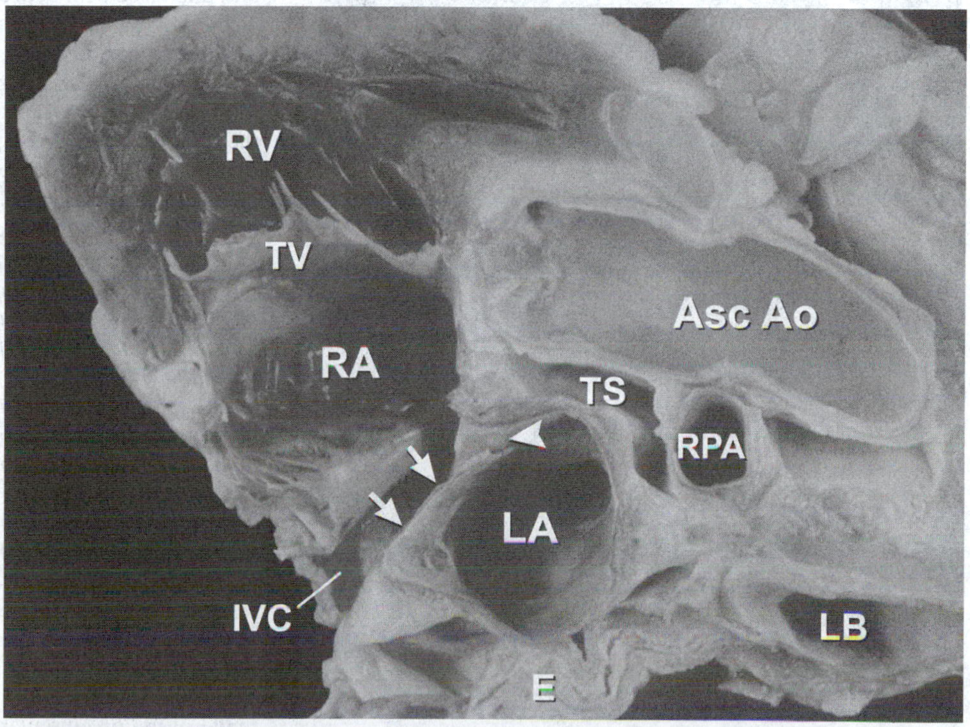

FIGURE 2-44 Tomographic section of the heart along a long-axis of the body. The valve of the fossa ovalis (arrows) and a patent foramen ovale (arrowhead) are seen in this view. Asc Ao, ascending aorta; E, esophagus; IVC, inferior vena cava; LA, left atrium; LB, left bronchus; RA, right atrium; RPA, right pulmonary artery; RV, right ventricle; TS, transverse sinus; TV, tricuspid valve.

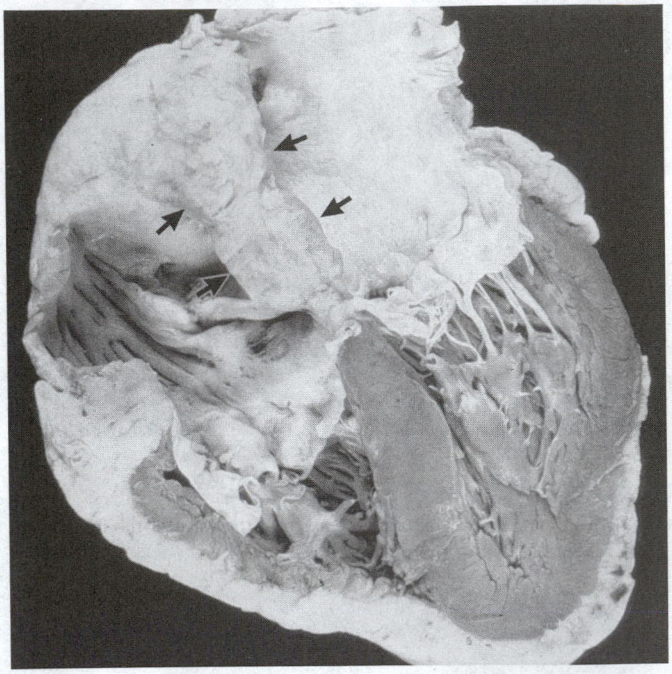

FIGURE 2-45 (Plate 16) Four-chamber slice through the heart showing lipomatous hypertrophy of the atrial septum (arrows).

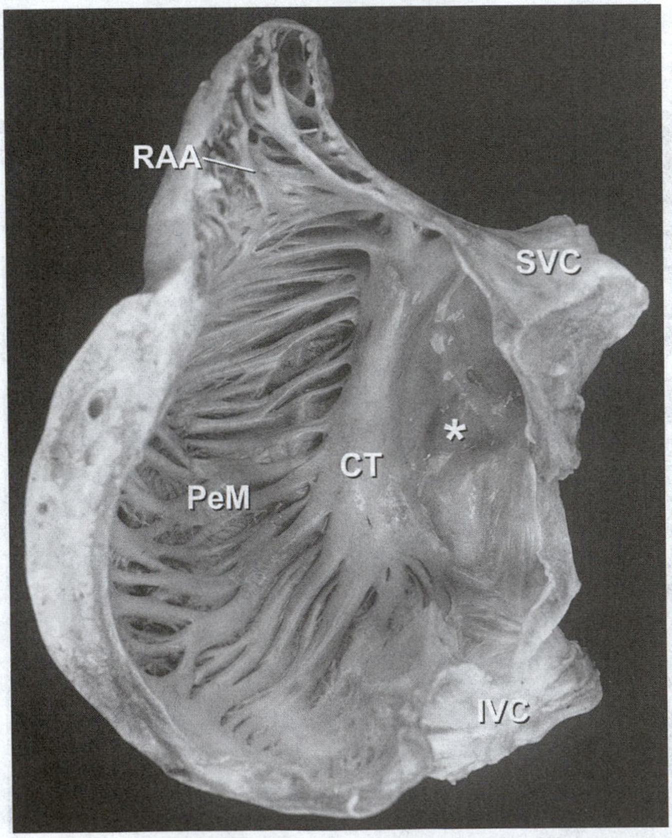

FIGURE 2-46 Right atrial free wall showing separation of the posterior smooth-walled (*) portion from the anterior muscular portion with its pectinate muscles (PeM) and right atrial appendage (RAA) by the crista terminalis (CT). IVC, inferior vena cava; SVC, superior vena cava.

membranous septum in conjunction with the right fibrous trigone with which it is continuous fuses the commissure between the right and posterior aortic cusps to the commissure between the anterior and septal tricuspid leaflets (see Fig. 2-21*B*). *The majority of clinically significant ventricular septal defects involve the membranous septum.*[17] Owing to normal angulation between the infundibular septum and remaining ventricular septum, the septal surface follows the course of an inverted S (moving from apex to aortic valve). The basal half of the ventricular septum is smooth-walled, while the apical half is characterized by numerous small and irregularly arranged trabeculations.[15–17]

Clinically relevant age-related anatomic changes include a disproportionate increase in ventricular septal thickness regardless of gender and in the absence of a history of hypertension.[20] This is associated with an appreciable increase in the ratio of ventricular septal to left ventricular free-wall thickness often exceeding 1.3 in patients older than age 60[20] (Fig. 2-41, Plate 15). This may be due in part to accentuation of the sigmoid shape of the basal septum[15,20] (Fig. 2-42). *Age-related ventricular septal angulation may have clinical importance because it may mimic certain features of hypertrophic cardiomyopathy,*[15,20] *particularly if complicated by the indiscriminate use of diuretics or afterload-reducing agents.*

Atrial Septum

When viewed from its right aspect, the atrial septum is comprised of interatrial and atrioventricular regions[16,17] (see Fig. 2-34). The interatrial portion is characterized by the fossa ovalis, which is the anatomic hallmark of a morphologic right atrium (Fig. 2-43*A*). Its outer muscular rim is a horseshoe-shaped limbus, and its central depression is the valve of the fossa ovalis[16,17] (see Fig. 2-43*A*). The potential interatrial passageway between the limbus and the valve (which is patent throughout fetal life) is the foramen ovale (Figs. 2-43*B* and 2-44). When viewed from the left atrium, the atrial septum is entirely interatrial, since the atrioventricular component lies below the mitral annulus, between the left ventricle and right atrium. Likewise, the limbus of the fossa ovalis is completely covered by its opaque valve and is not directly visible from the left atrium.[15]

The foramen ovale is anatomically closed in about two-thirds of adults, but in the remaining one-third it remains patent and, therefore, a potential source for shunts and paradoxical embolism. Stretching of the atrial septum, when the atria are markedly dilated, can transform a patent foramen ovale into an acquired atrial septal defect. The posterior aortic sinus abuts against the interatrial septum (see Fig. 2-12*D*). *During transseptal procedures, care must be taken to stay within the confines of the valve of the fossa ovalis in order to avoid perforation of an aortic sinus.*[16] *Echocardiography may help guide transseptal puncture during balloon mitral valvuloplasty or closure of an atrial septal defect with an occluder device.*[13] *Fenestrations of the valve of the fossa ovalis are the most common cause of congenital atrial septal defects. Redundant valve tissue may form an aneurysm of the valve of the fossa ovalis.*

The atrioventricular (AV) portion of the atrial septum is made of major muscular and minor membranous components and separates the right atrium from the left ventricle[16,17] (see Figs. 2-34 and 2-38). *This explains why there is a potential for left-ventricular-to-right-atrial shunts.*[16,17] *The AV septum corresponds roughly to the triangle of Koch, an important anatomic surgical*

THE COLOR PLATES

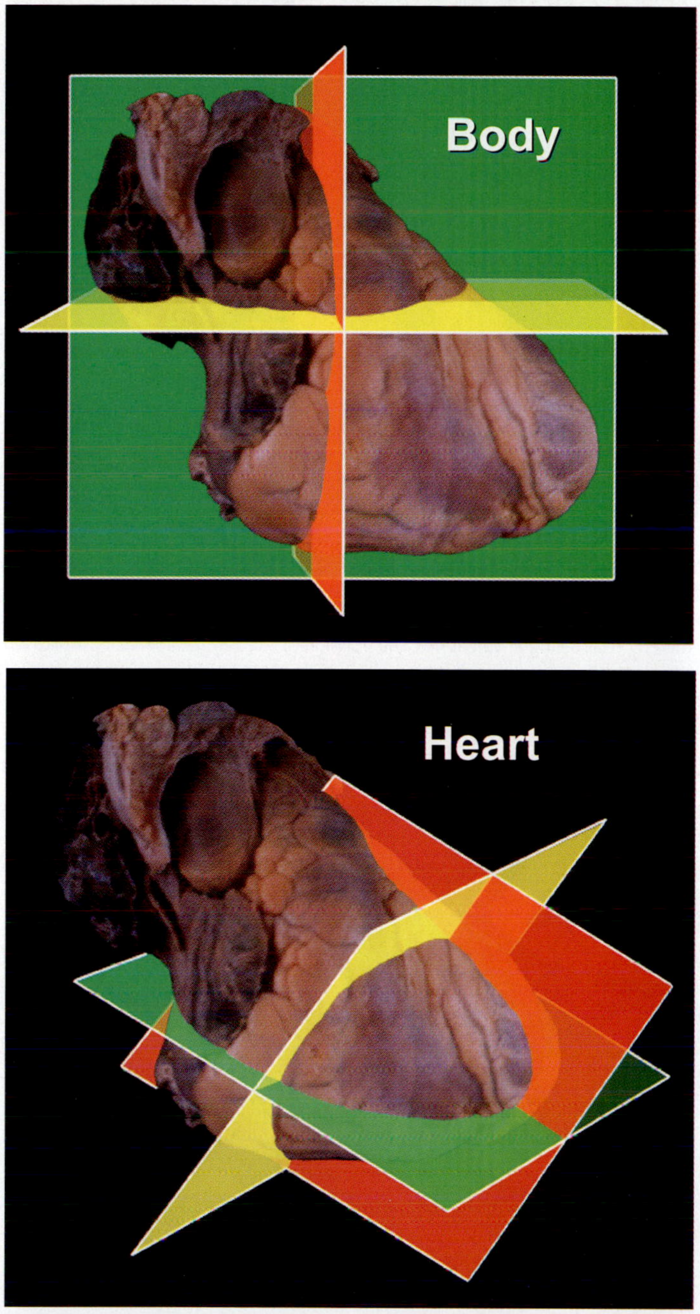

Plate 1 (FIGURE 2-4) The three primary planes of the body (*top*) and heart (*bottom*). Note that the planes of the body are aligned with vertical midline structures, such as the esophagus. In contrast, the major axis of the heart is oriented obliquely. Thus the heart's long and short axes do not lie in the same plane as the body's long and short axes. The body planes cut the heart obliquely and not in its primary planes. Conversely, the heart's primary planes cut the body obliquely.

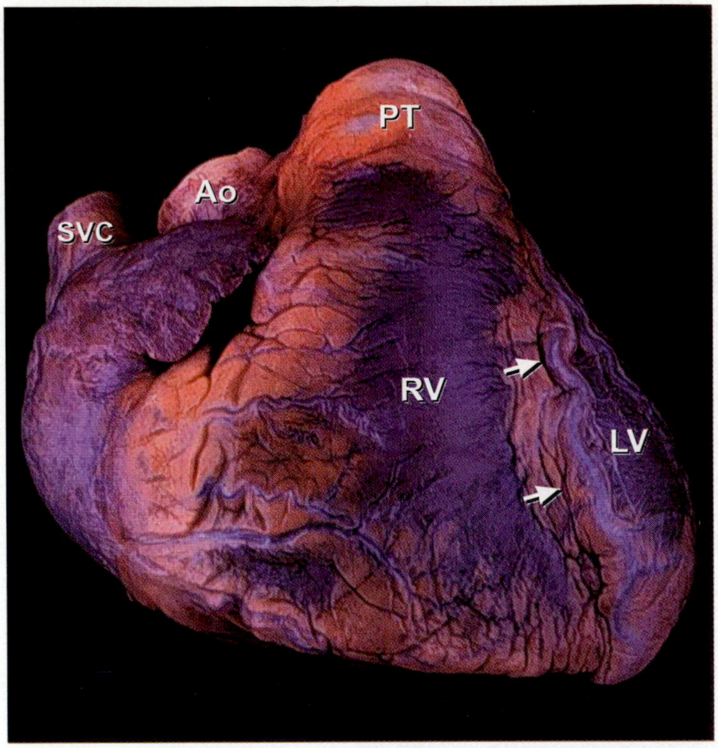

A

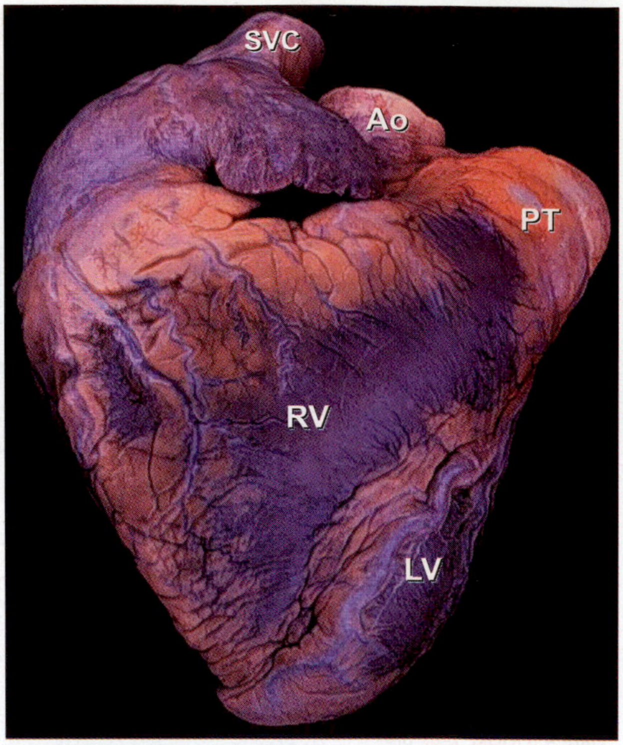

B

Plate 2 (FIGURE 2-5) *A.* Anterior view of the heart in its usual anatomic position with its apex directed from right to left. Arrows point to the anterior interventricular groove. *B.* Nonanatomic positioning of the normal heart with its apex directed downward, thereby resembling a "valentine." The position of the cardiac apex is normally leftward (levocardia) but may anomalously be rightward (dextrocardia) or midline and inferiorly (mesocardia). Ao, ascending aorta; LV, left ventricle; PT, pulmonary trunk; RV, right ventricle; SVC, superior vena cava.

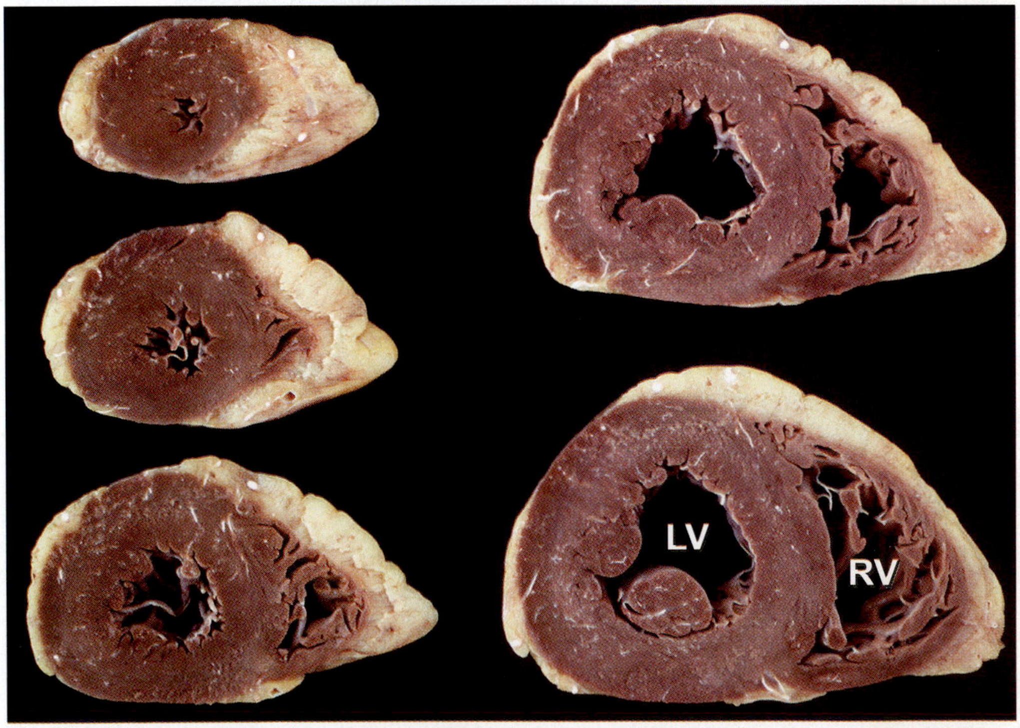

Plate 3 (FIGURE 2-8) Ventricular slice method of cardiac dissection. Display of five slices (LV, left ventricle; RV, right ventricle) viewed as though looking from the base of the heart toward the apex.

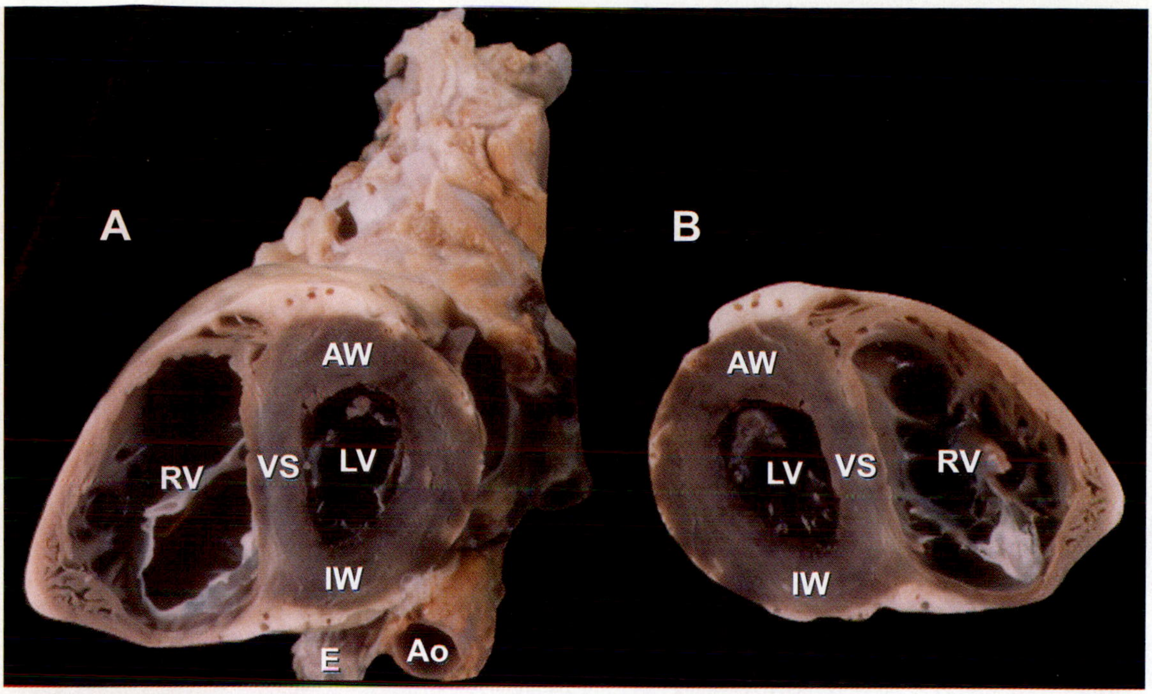

Plate 4 (FIGURE 2-9) Bisected cardiac specimen, viewed in the short axis. *A*. The specimen is viewed from the apex toward the base. The esophagus (E) is posterior and adjacent to both the thoracic aorta (Ao) and the inferior wall of the left ventricle (LV). The right ventricular (RV) cavity is to the left. *B*. The other half of the bisected specimen is viewed as though looking from the base toward the apex (comparable with FIGURE 2-8). AW, anterior wall; IW, inferior wall; VS, ventricular septum.

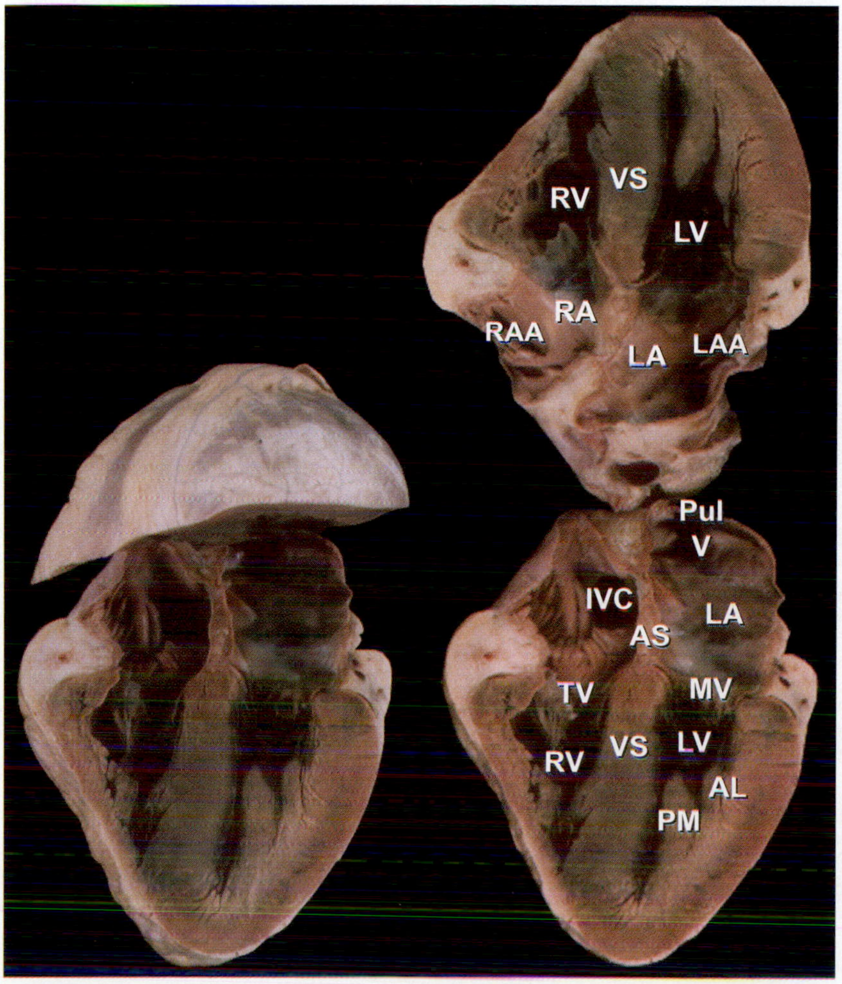

Plate 5 (FIGURE 2-10) Bisected cardiac specimen in the four-chamber view parallel to the base-apex axis of the heart. (*Left*) The bisected specimen has been partially opened to show the relative relationship of the bisected halves. (*Right*) The two components of the bisected specimen are opened completely. Note the positions of the pulmonary veins posteriorly and the positions of the atrial appendages at the atrioventricular groove. AL, anterolateral papillary muscle; AS, atrial septum; IVC, inferior vena cava; LA, left atrium; LAA, left atrial appendage; LV, left ventricle; MV, mitral valve; PM, posteromedial papillary muscle; PulV, pulmonary vein; RA, right atrium; RAA, right atrial appendage; RV, right ventricle; TV, tricuspid valve; VS, ventricular septum.

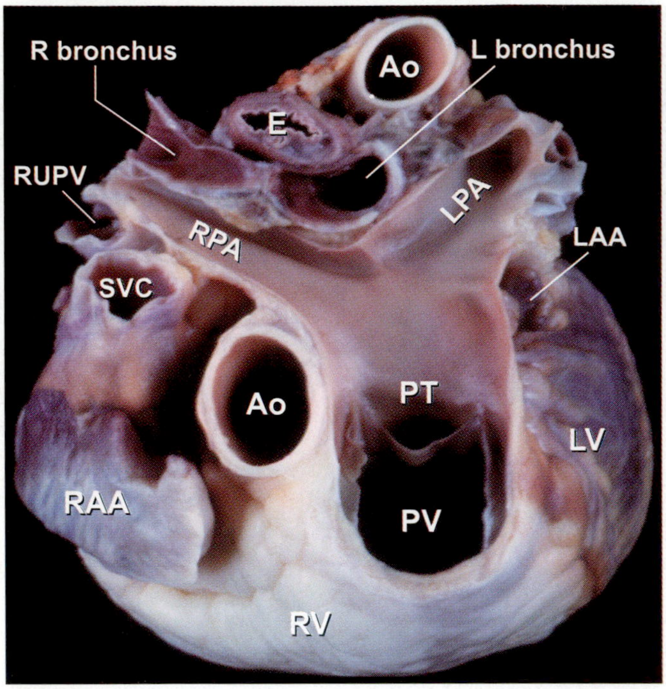
R bronchus
Ao
L bronchus
E
RUPV
LPA
RPA
LAA
SVC
Ao
PT
LV
RAA
PV
RV

A

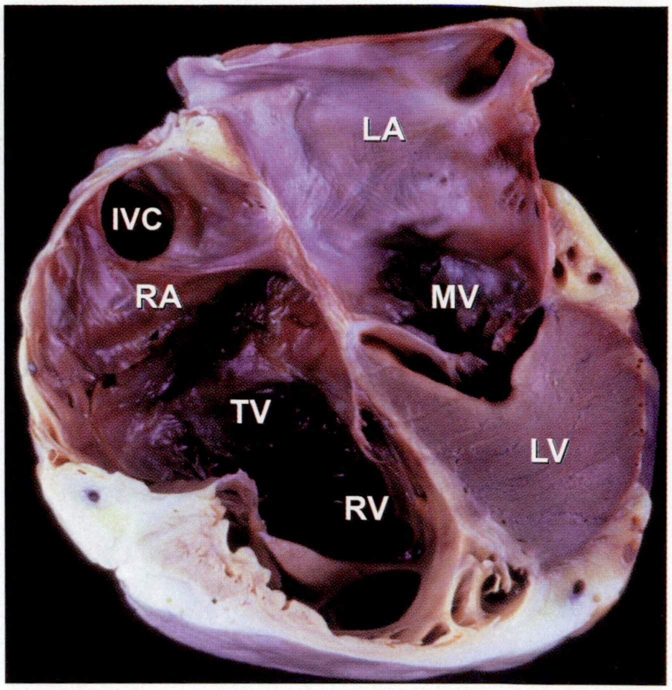
LA
IVC
RA
MV
TV
LV
RV

B

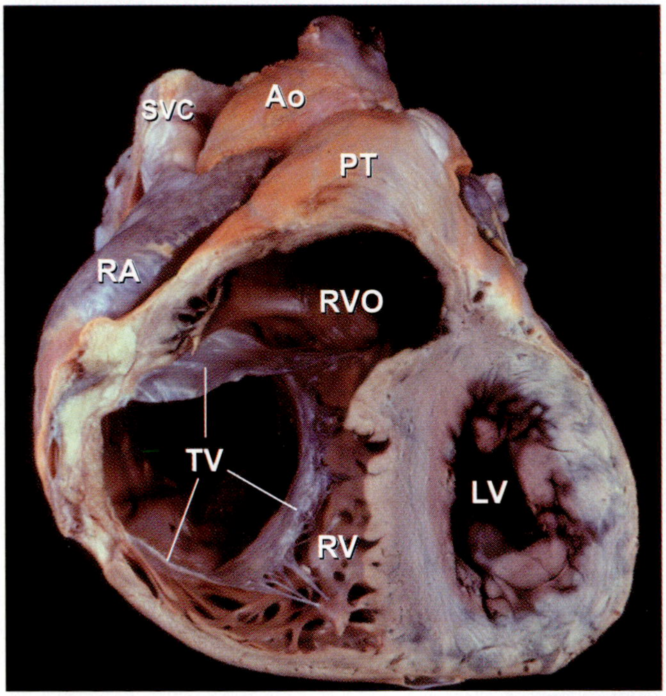
SVC
Ao
PT
RA
RVO
TV
LV
RV

C

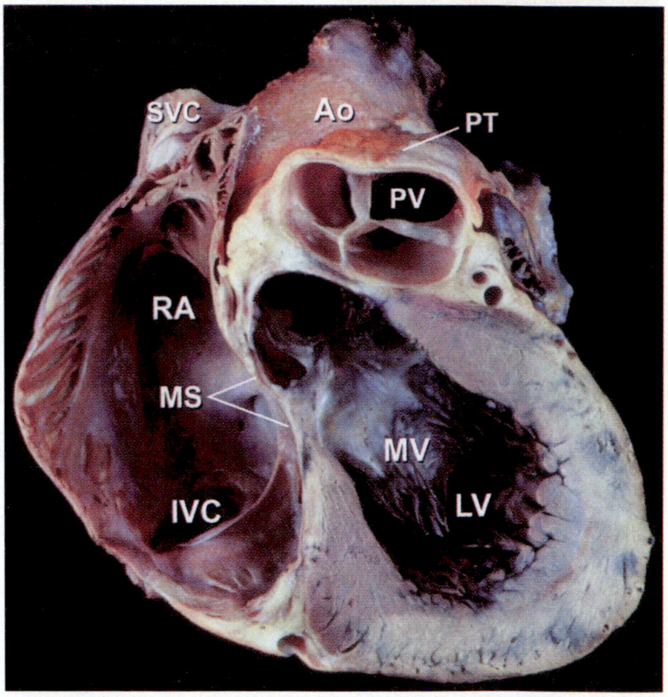
SVC
Ao
PT
PV
RA
MS
MV
IVC
LV

D

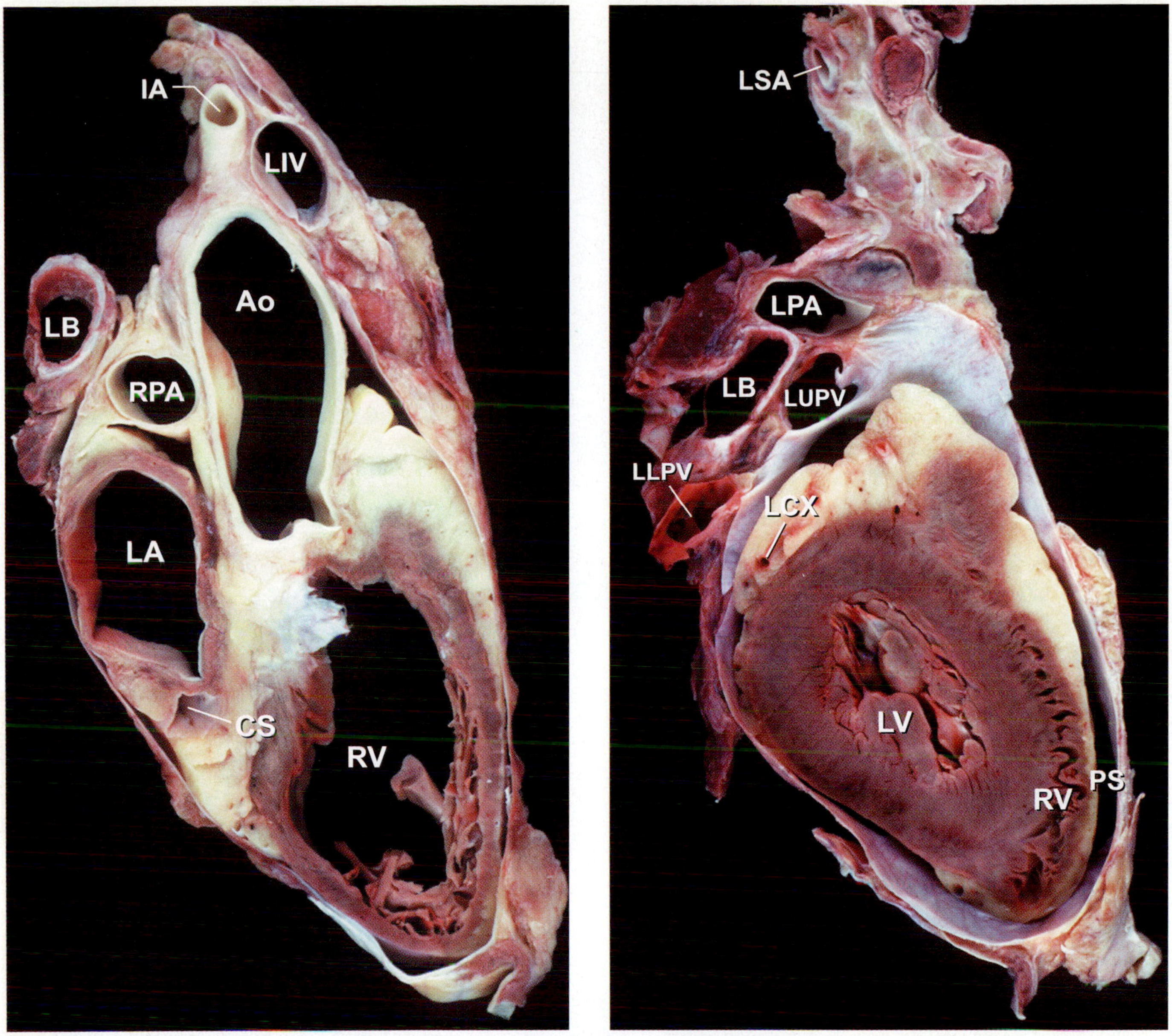

Plate 6 (FIGURE 2-11) Tomographic cardiac dissection along the body primary planes. *A*,*B*. Transverse sections (looking from head toward feet) at the level of the great vessels (*A*) or the cardiac chambers (*B*). The aortic arch travels over the left bronchus and the right pulmonary artery. *C*,*D*. Frontal sections (looking from anterior to posterior) through both ventricles (*C*) or left ventricle and right atrium (*D*). *E*,*F*. Parasagittal sections looking from right (*E*) to left (*F*). Ao, ascending aorta; CS, coronary sinus; E, esophagus; IA, innominate artery; IVC, inferior vena cava; LA, left atrium; LAA, left atrial appendage; LB, left bronchus; LCX, left circumflex coronary artery; LIV, left innominate vein; LLPV, left lower pulmonary vein; LPA, left pulmonary artery; LUPV, left upper pulmonary vein; LSA, left subclavian artery; LV, left ventricle; MS, membranous ventricular septum; MV, mitral valve; PS, pericardial sac; PT, pulmonary trunk; PV, pulmonary valve; RA, right atrium; RAA, right atrial appendage; RPA, right pulmonary artery; RUPV, right upper pulmonary vein; RV, right ventricle; RVO, right ventricular outflow; SVC, superior vena cava; TV, tricuspid valve.

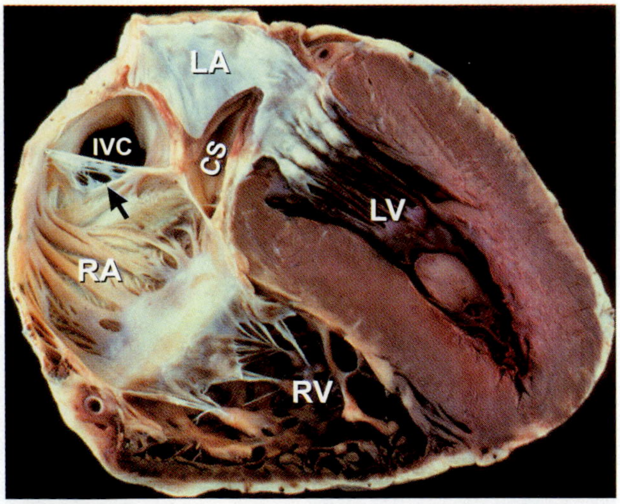

A

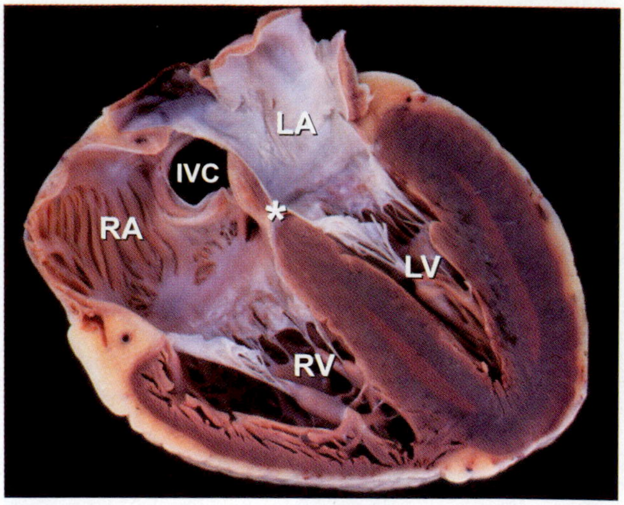

B

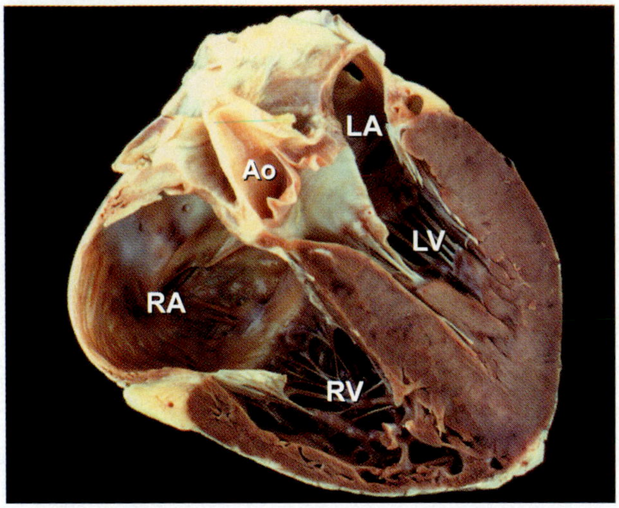

C

Plate 7 (FIGURE 2-16) Collage of four-chamber tomographic sections cutting from inferior wall to anterosuperior wall showing coronary sinus (*A*), internal cardiac crux (*) (*B*), and aortic valve (*C*). Ao, ascending aorta; CS, coronary sinus; IVC, inferior vena cava; LA, left atrium; LV, left ventricle; RA, right atrium; RV, right ventricle; arrow in *A* points to a fenestrated eustachian valve.

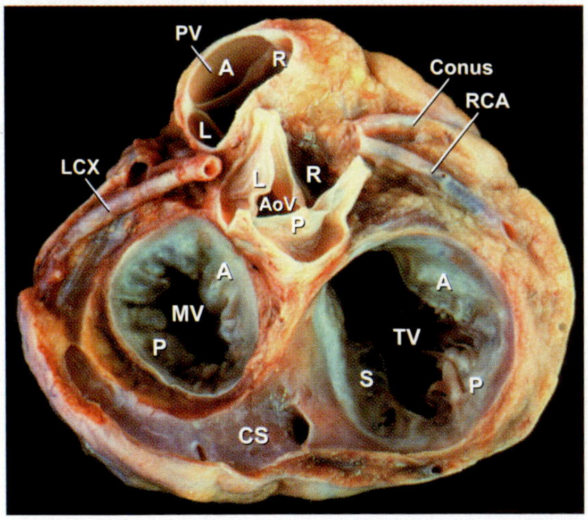

A

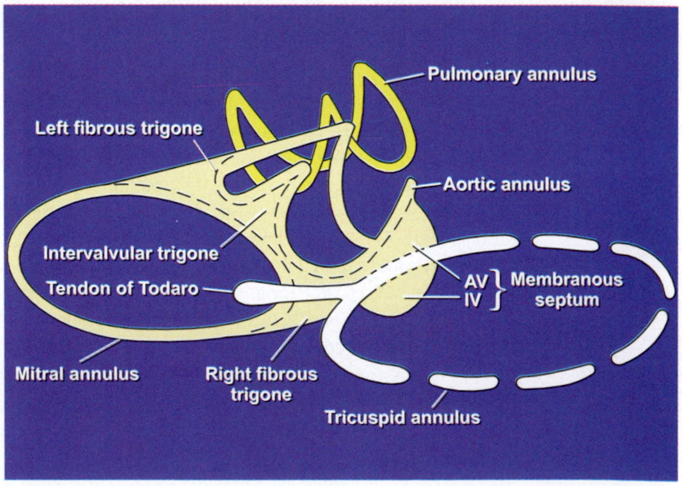

B

Plate 8 (FIGURE 2-21) Base of heart. *A*. Section through the base of the heart, looking from base toward apex, with the atria and great arteries removed, shows all four cardiac valves. *B*. A comparable schematic diagram of the fibrous cardiac skeleton. The centrally located aortic valve forms the cornerstone of the cardiac skeleton. Its fibrous extensions anchor and support the other three valves. *A*, anterior; AoV, aortic valve; AV, atrioventricular; CS, coronary sinus; IV, interventricular; L, left; LCX, left circumflex coronary artery; MV, mitral valve; P, posterior; PV, pulmonary valve; R, right; RCA, right coronary artery; S, septal; TV, tricuspid valve.

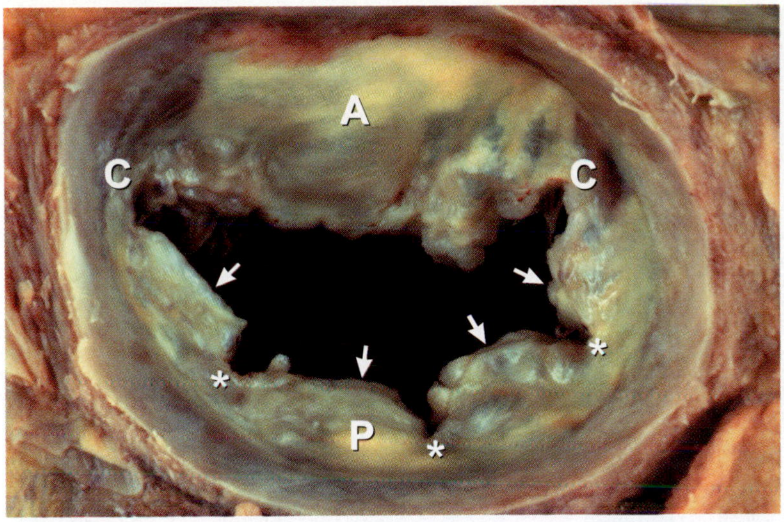

Plate 9 (FIGURE 2-24) Mitral valve, viewed from left atrial aspect. Minor commissures (*) divide the posterior leaflet into four scallops (arrows). A, anterior; C, major commissures; P, posterior.

Plate 10 (FIGURE 2-26) Components of the mitral valve. *A*. Each leaflet has a large clear zone (CZ) and a smaller rough zone (RZ) between its free edge and closing edge (dotted line). A fanlike commissural chorda tendinea (*) connects the tip of the papillary muscle to the commissure. *B*. Schematic diagram of an open anterior mitral leaflet comparable to *A*. Section obtained along the dotted lines shows the relationship of the mitral annulus and free edge to the closing edge.

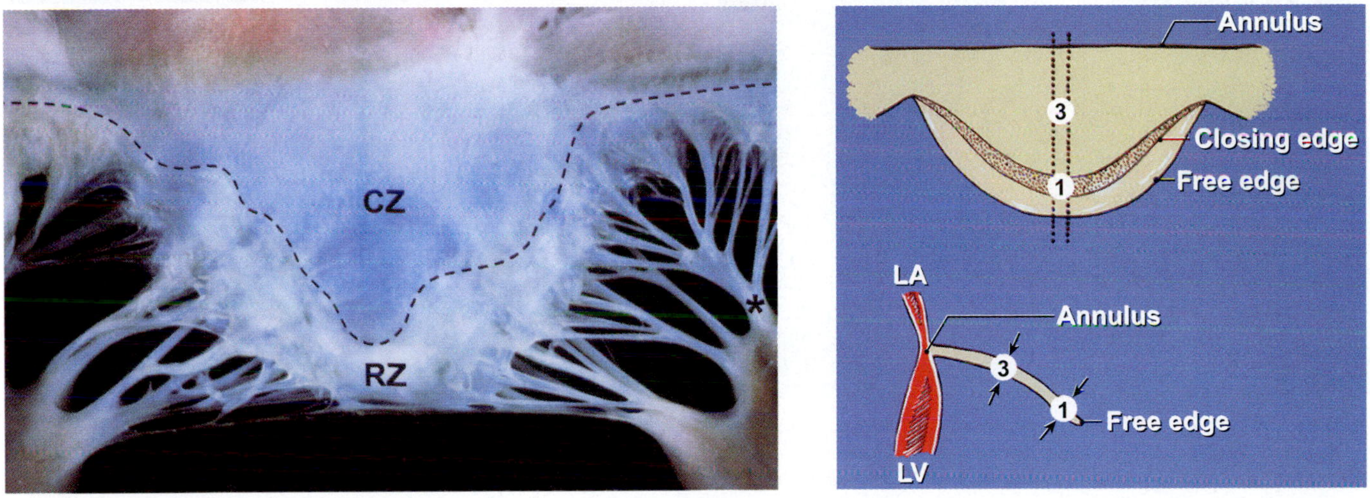

A

B

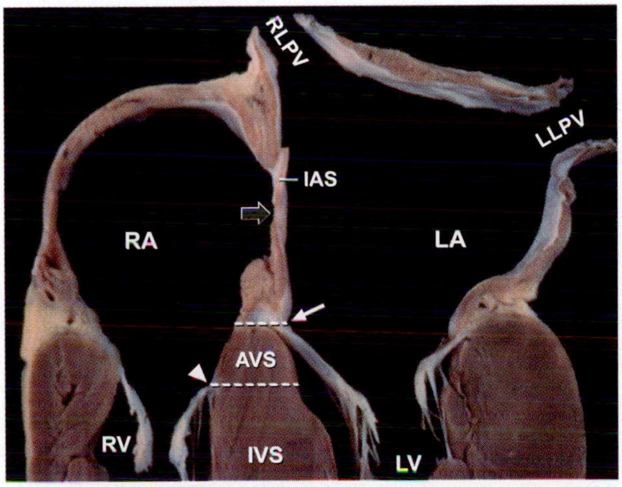

Plate 11 (FIGURE 2-34) Four-chamber slice of the heart shows the characteristic normal apical displacement of the tricuspid valve septal leaflet insertion (arrowhead) when compared with septal insertion of the mitral valve (solid arrow). This tomographic section also shows the interatrial septum (IAS), atrioventricular septum (AVS), and interventricular septum (IVS). Open arrow points to fossa ovalis. LA, left atrium; LLPV, left lower pulmonary vein; LV, left ventricle; RA, right atrium; RLPV, right lower pulmonary vein; RV, right ventricle.

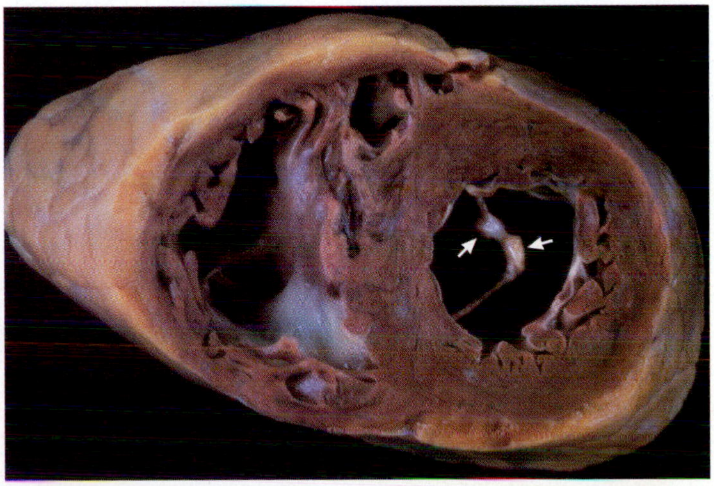

Plate 12 (FIGURE 2-36) Calcified left ventricular false tendon (arrows) seen in short-axis view.

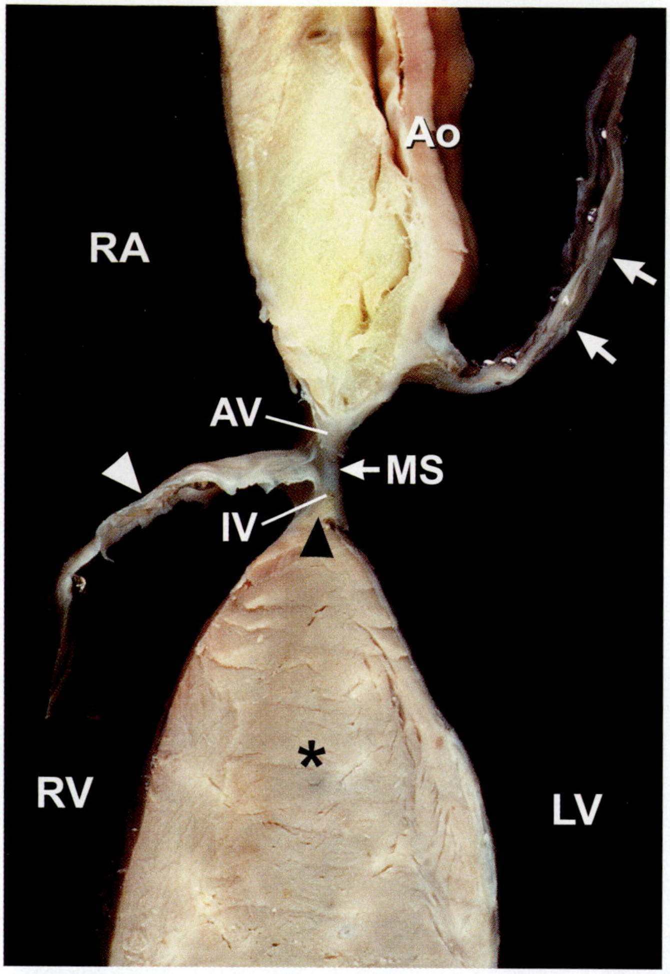

Plate 13 (FIGURE 2-38) Four-chamber tomographic slice through the aortic root (Ao) and aortic valve (arrows) showing the small membranous (MS) and large muscular (*) portion of the ventricular septum. The membranous septum is divided into atrioventricular (AV) and interventricular (IV) components by the septal tricuspid leaflet (white arrowhead). Black arrowhead points to the expected location of the AV (His) bundle. LV, left ventricle; RA, right atrium; RV, right ventricle.

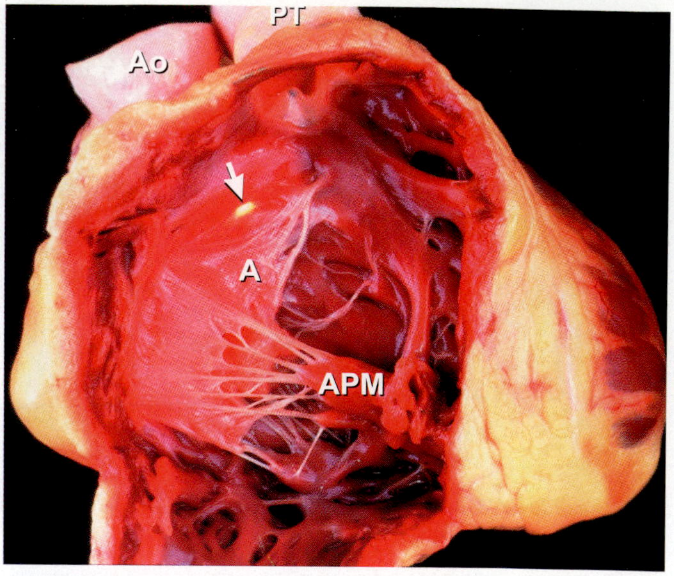

Plate 14 (FIGURE 2-40) A view of the right ventricle. Transilluminated membranous ventricular septum (arrow) in contact with the commissure between the anterior and septal leaflets of the tricuspid valve. A, anterior tricuspid leaflet; Ao, ascending aorta; APM, anterior tricuspid papillary muscle; PT, pulmonary trunk.

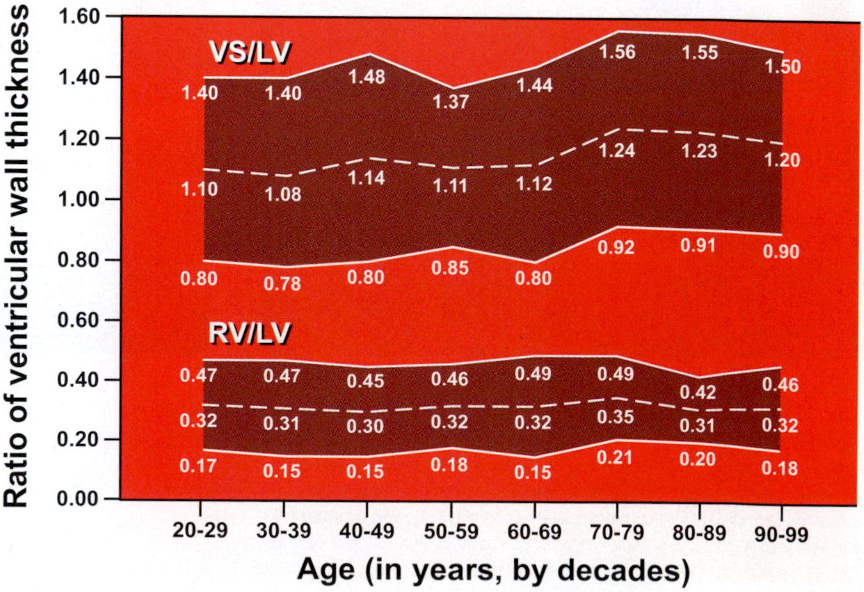

Plate 15 (FIGURE 2-41) Ratios of ventricular wall thicknesses (means |||pm 2 standard deviations) versus age. RV/LV, ratio of right to left ventricular wall thickness; VS/LV, ratio of ventricular septal to left ventricular free wall thickness. (From Kitzman DW, et al. *Mayo Clin Proc* 1988; 63:137–146. Reproduced with permission of Mayo Foundation.)

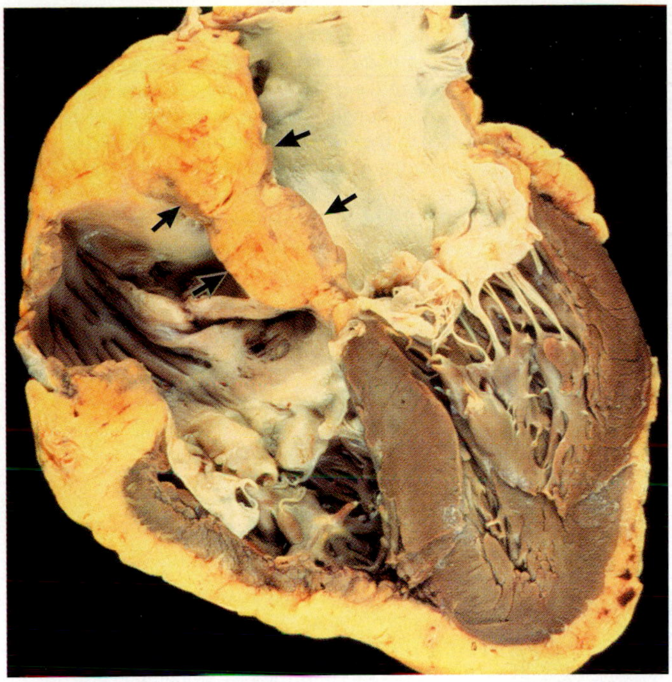

Plate 16 (FIGURE 2-45) Four-chamber slice through the heart showing lipomatous hypertrophy of the atrial septum (arrows).

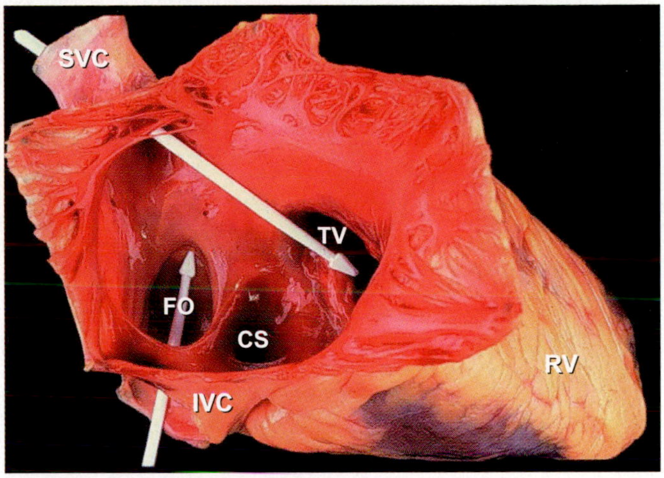

Plate 17 (FIGURE 2-47) Opened right atrium. Two arrow-shaped probes show that superior vena caval flow is directed toward the tricuspid orifice and inferior vena caval flow is directed toward the fossa ovalis (FO). CS, coronary sinus; IVC, inferior vena cava; RV, right ventricle; SVC, superior vena cava ; TV, tricuspid valve.

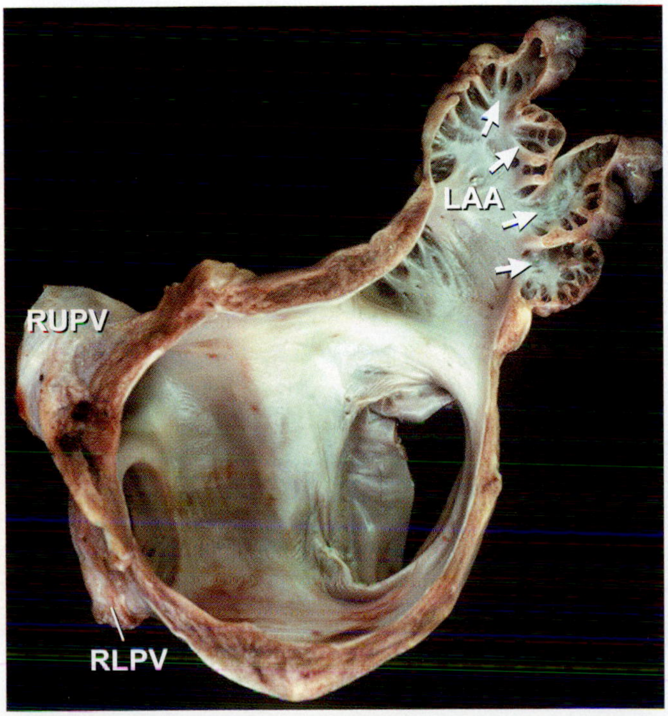

A

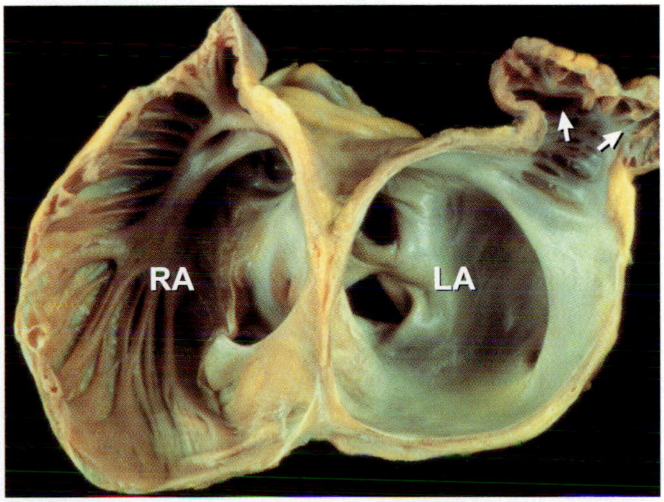

B

Plate 18 (FIGURE 2-49) Left atrial appendages (LAA). *A.* Left atrial free wall showing appendage with four lobes (arrows). *B.* Biatrial specimen demonstrating left atrial appendage with two lobes (arrows). LA, left atrium; RA, right atrium; RLPV, right lower pulmonary vein; RUPV, right upper pulmonary vein.

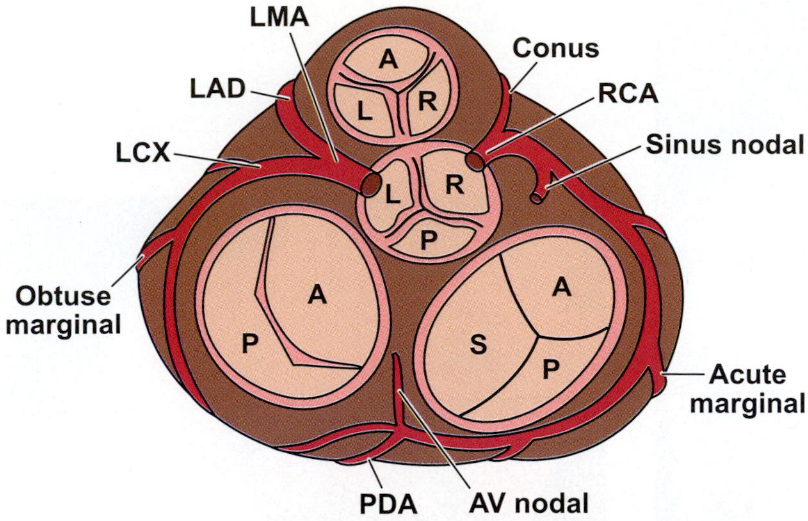

Plate 19 (FIGURE 2-50) Schematic diagram of coronary artery distribution viewed at the base of the heart. In this right-dominant system, the right coronary artery (RCA) gives rise to the posterior descending artery (PDA), and the left main coronary artery (LMA) gives rise to the left anterior descending (LAD) and left circumflex (LCX) branches. A, anterior; AV, atrioventricular; L, left; P, posterior; R, right; S, septal.

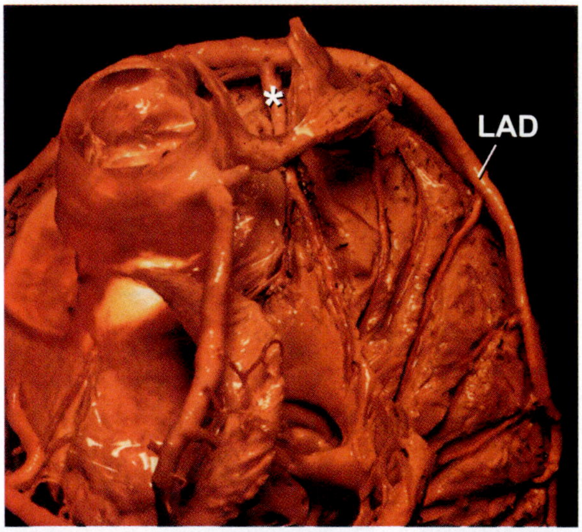

Plate 20 (FIGURE 2-53) Septal branches of the left anterior descending coronary artery (LAD); * points to the first septal perforator. (From McAlpine,30 with permission.)

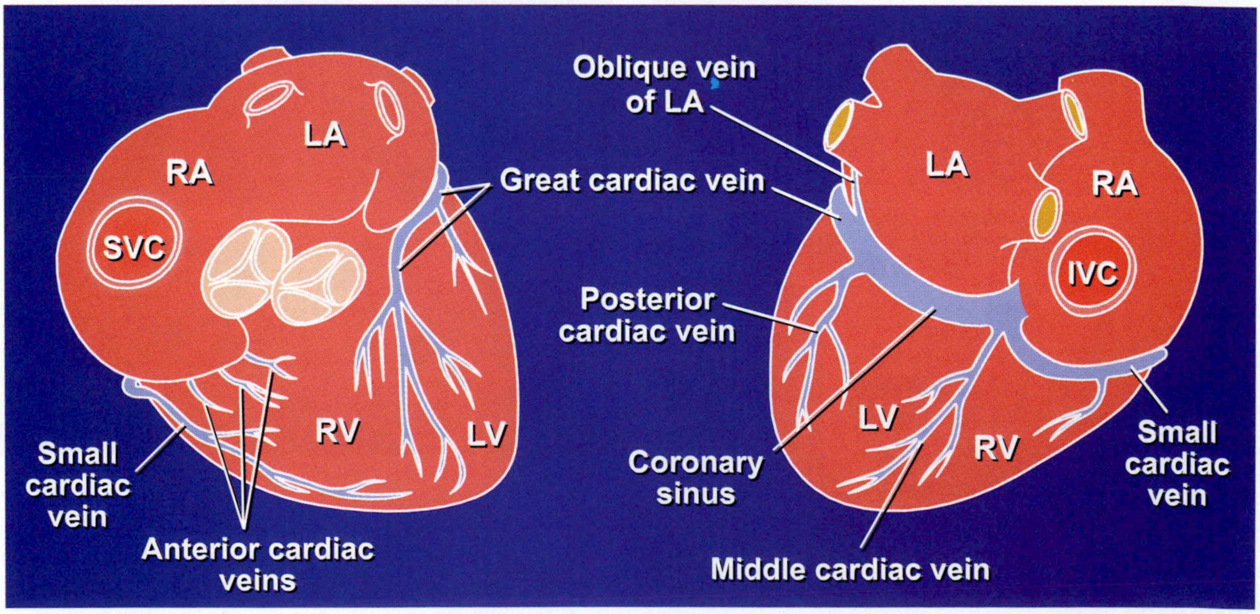

Plate 21 (FIGURE 2-55) Schematic diagram of the coronary venous circulation. IVC, inferior vena cava; LA, left atrium; LV, left ventricle; RA, right atrium; RV, right ventricle; SVC, superior vena cava.

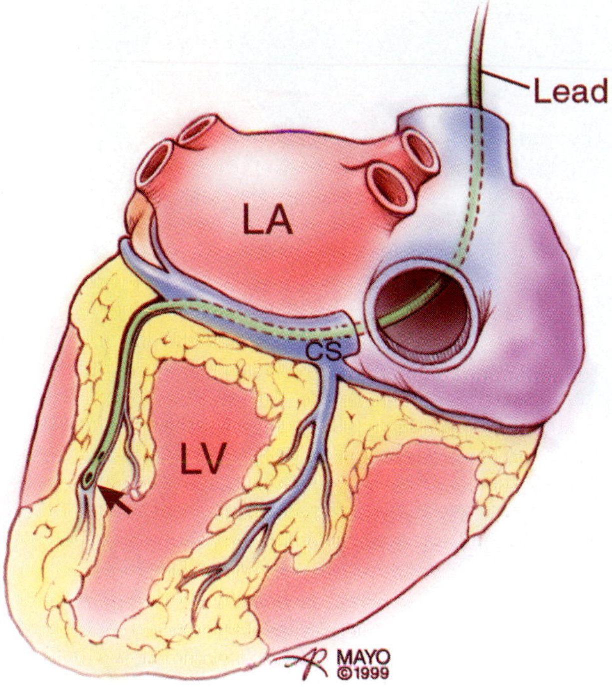

Plate 22 (FIGURE 2-56) Schematic diagram shows placement of the tip of a pacing/mapping catheter within a coronary vein (arrow) via the coronary sinus (CS). LA, left atrium; LV, left ventricle.

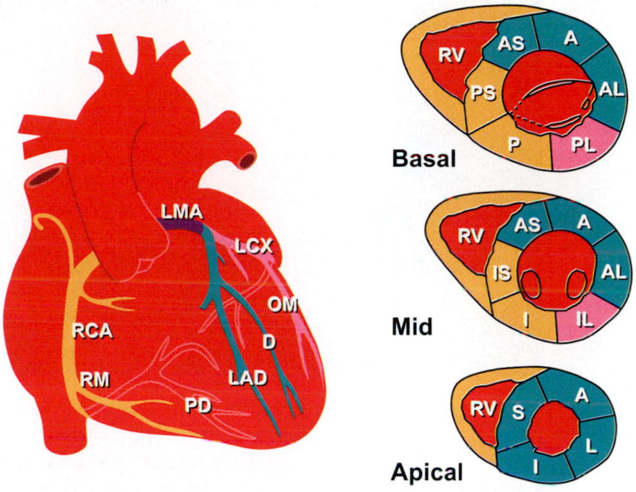

Plate 23 (FIGURE 2-60) Coronary distribution using a 16-segment model. D, diagonal branch of the left anterior descending coronary artery; LAD, left anterior descending coronary artery; LCX, left circumflex coronary artery; LMA, left main coronary artery; OM, obtuse marginal branch of the circumflex coronary artery; PD, posterior descending coronary artery; RCA, right coronary artery; RM, right marginal branch; other abbreviations as in Fig. 2-58.

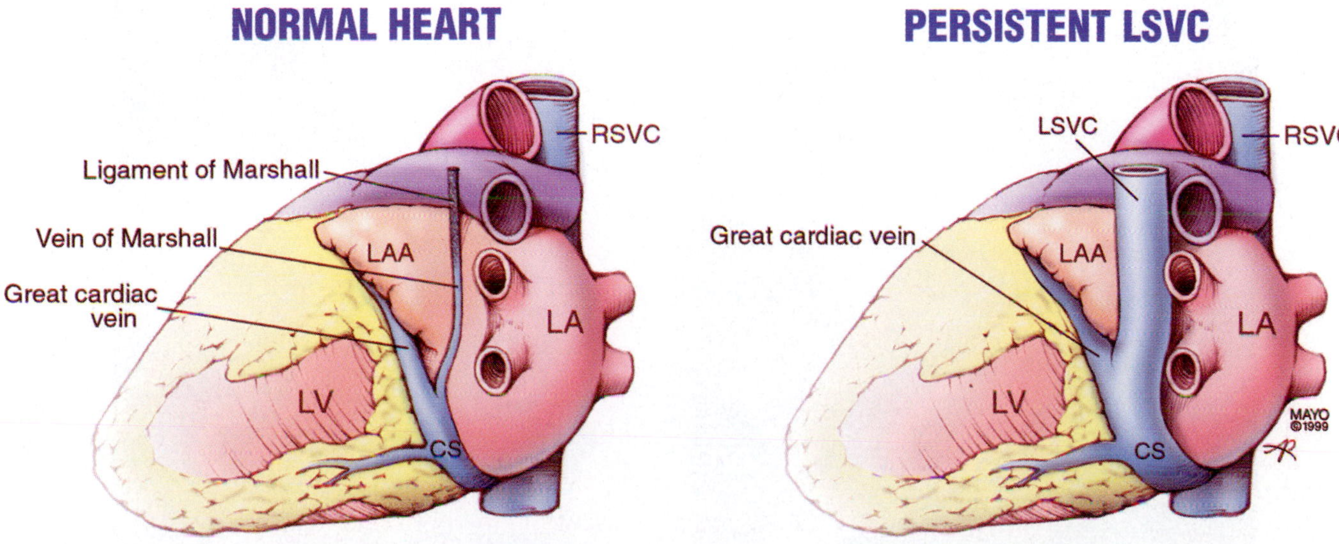

Plate 24 (FIGURE 2-64) Schematic diagrams showing the ligament/vein of Marshall in normal hearts (*left*) and persistent left superior vena cava (LSVC) (*right*). CS, coronary sinus; LA, left atrium; LAA, left atrial appendage; LV, left ventricle; RA, right atrium; RSVC, right superior vena cava.

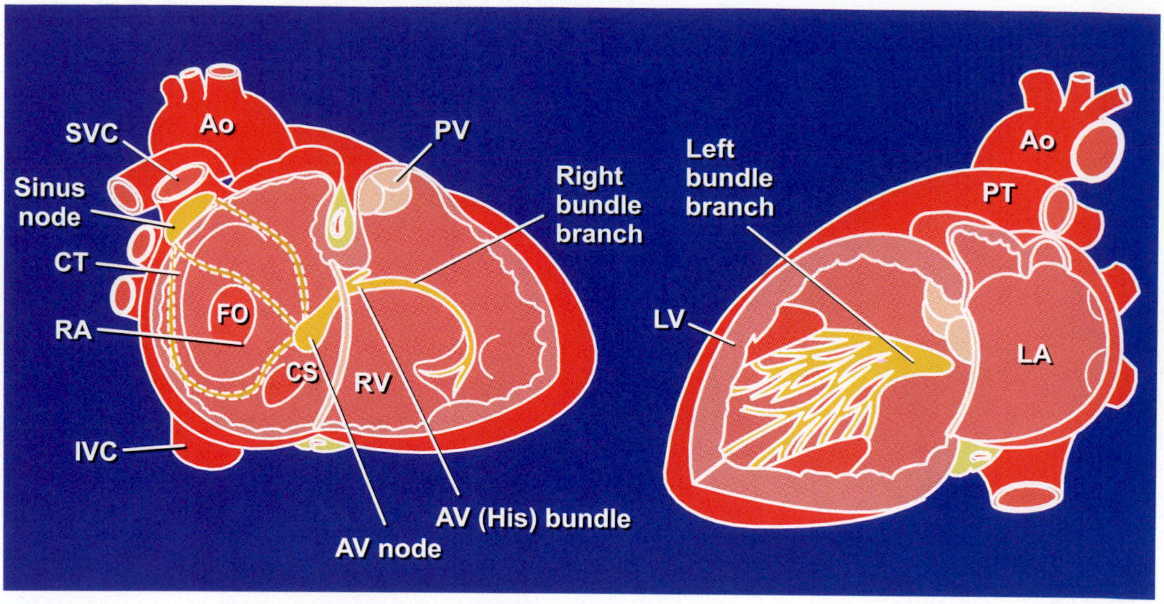

Plate 25 (FIGURE 2-67) Schematic diagram of the cardiac conduction system. (*Left*) The right side of the heart showing the sinus node, atrioventricular (AV) node, AV (His) bundle, and right bundle branch. (*Right*) The left side of the heart showing incomplete anatomic separation of the left bundle into antero and posterior fascicles. Ao, ascending aorta; AV, atrioventricular; CS, coronary sinus; CT, crista terminalis; FO, fossa ovalis; IVC, inferior vena cava; LA, left atrium; LV, left ventricle; PT, pulmonary trunk; PV, pulmonary valve; RA, right atrium; RV, right ventricle; SVC, superior vena cava.

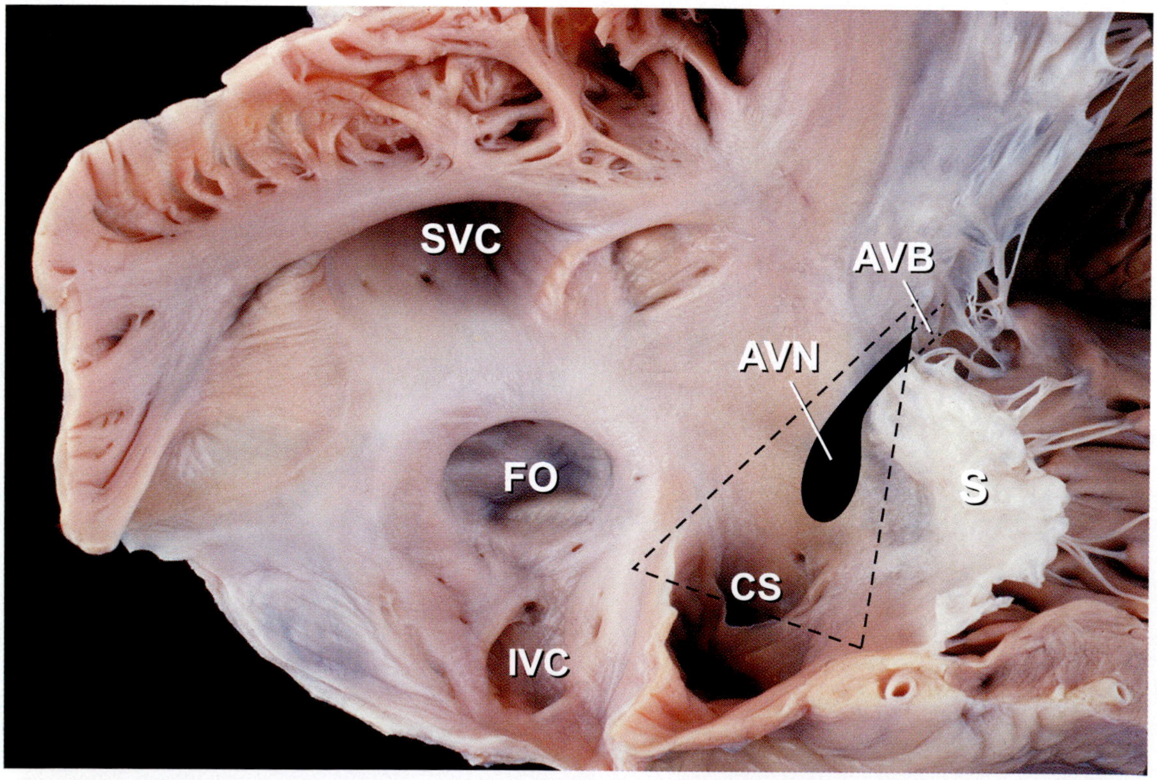

Plate 26 (FIGURE 2-68) The atrioventricular node (AVN) lies within the triangle of Koch (dashed triangle), and the AV (His) bundle (AVB) travels through the tricuspid annulus to rest along the summit of the ventricular septum. CS, coronary sinus; FO, fossa ovalis; IVC, inferior vena cava; S, septal leaflet of the tricuspid valve; SVC, superior vena cava.

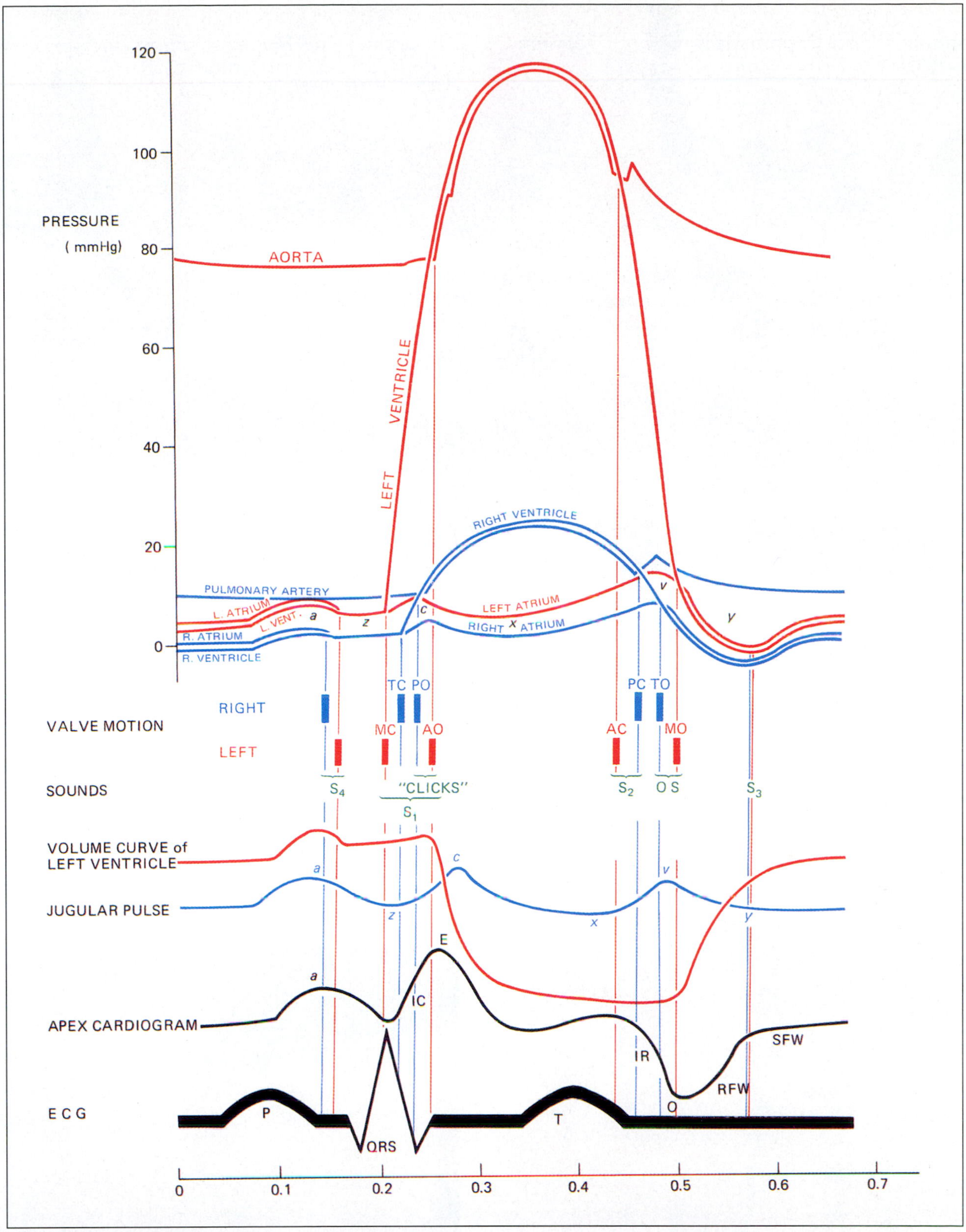

Plate 27 (FIGURE 3-1) Electrical and mechanical events during the cardiac cycle. Shown are pressure curves of great vessels and cardiac chambers, valvular events, timing of heart sounds, LV volume curve, jugular venous pulse wave, and electrocardiogram (ECG). MC and TC, mitral and tricuspid valve closure; PO and AO, pulmonic and aortic valve opening; AC and PC, aortic and pulmonic valve closure; TO and MO, tricuspid and mitral valve opening.

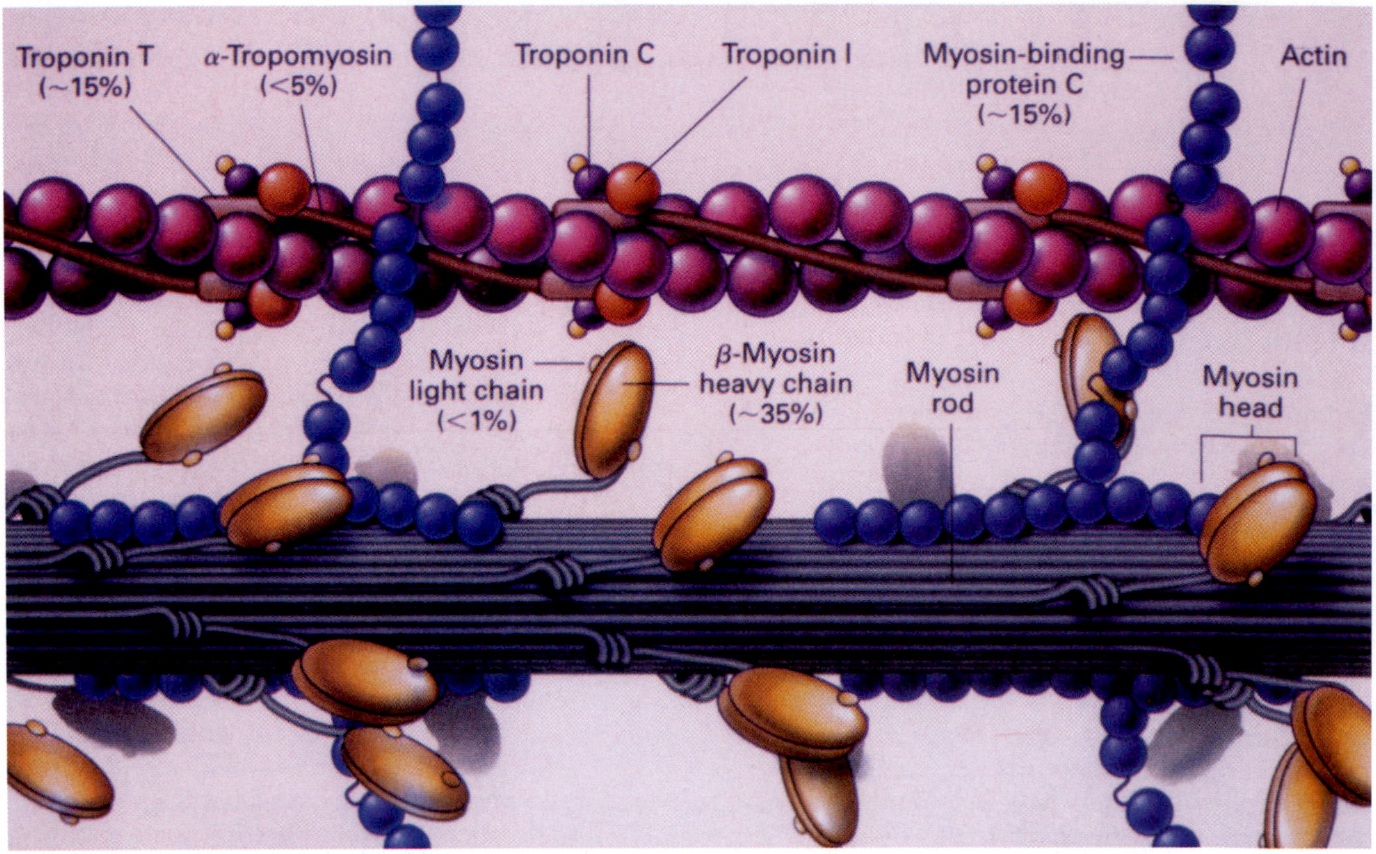

Plate 28 (FIGURE 3-8) Cartoon of sarcomeric proteins (titin not shown). (From Spirito P, Seidman CE, McKenna WJ, Maron BJ. The management of hypertrophic cardiomyopathy. *New Eng J Med* 1997; 336:775. Reprinted with permission of the publisher.)

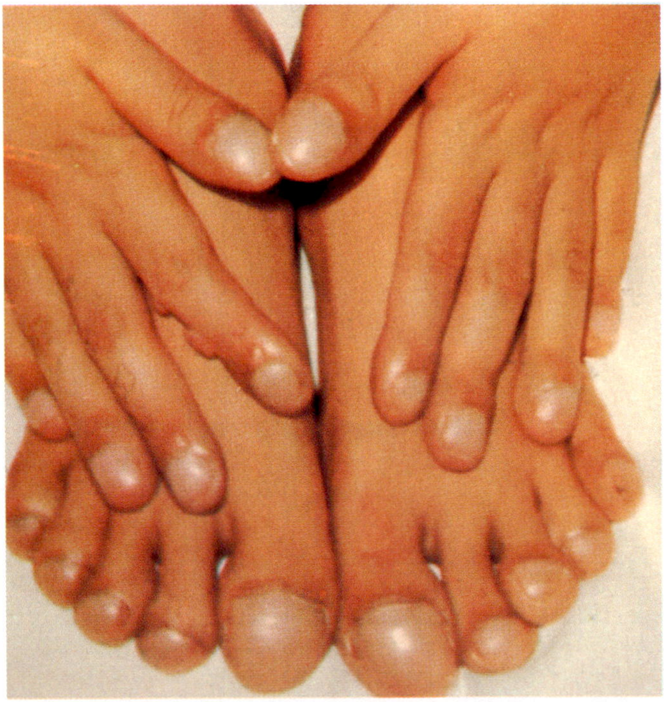

Plate 29 (FIGURE 10-12) *Symmetric cyanosis*. Equal cyanosis and clubbing of hands and feet due to transposition of great vessels and a ventricular septal defect without patent ductus arteriosus.

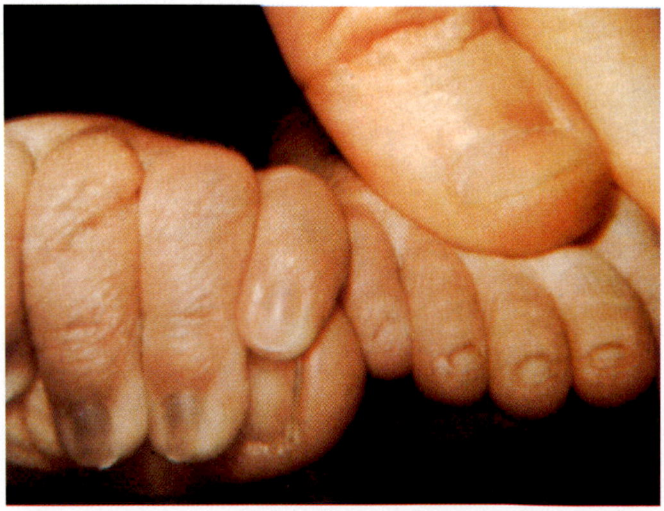

Plate 30 (FIGURE 10-13) *Differential cyanosis*. Cyanosis of fingers (*left*) greater than that of toes due to transposition of great vessels with patent ductus arteriosus.

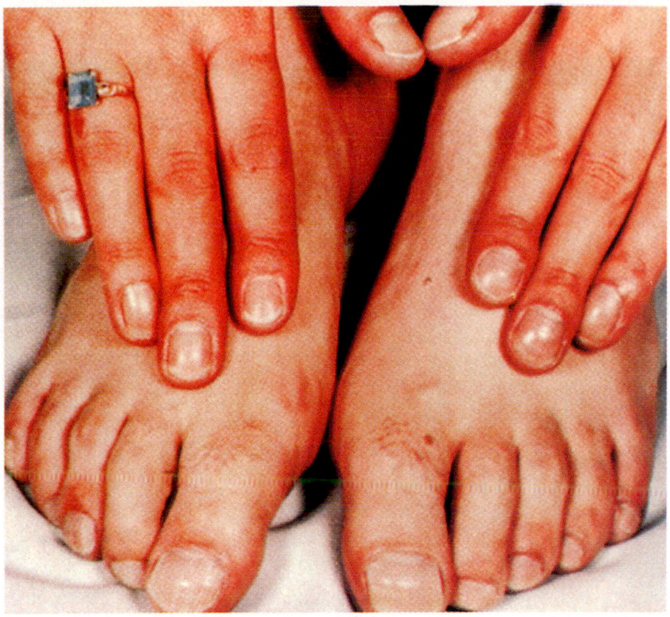

Plate 31 (FIGURE 10-14) *Differential cyanosis*. Clubbing of left hand (compare thumbs) and cyanosis of left hand and all toes due to patent ductus arteriosus with pulmonary hypertension and normally related great vessels. (Courtesy of Dr. Joseph K. Perloff, University of California, Los Angeles.)

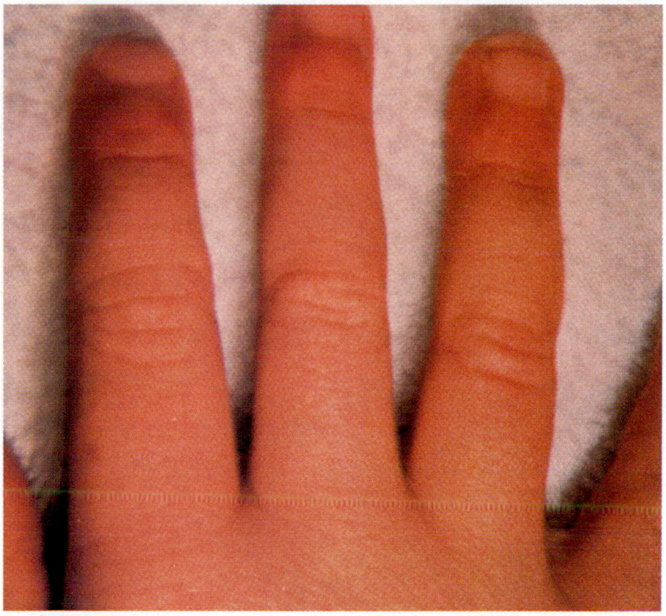

Plate 32 (FIGURE 10-15) *Tuft erythema*. Erythema of fingertips due to small right-to-left shunt from AV canal defect.

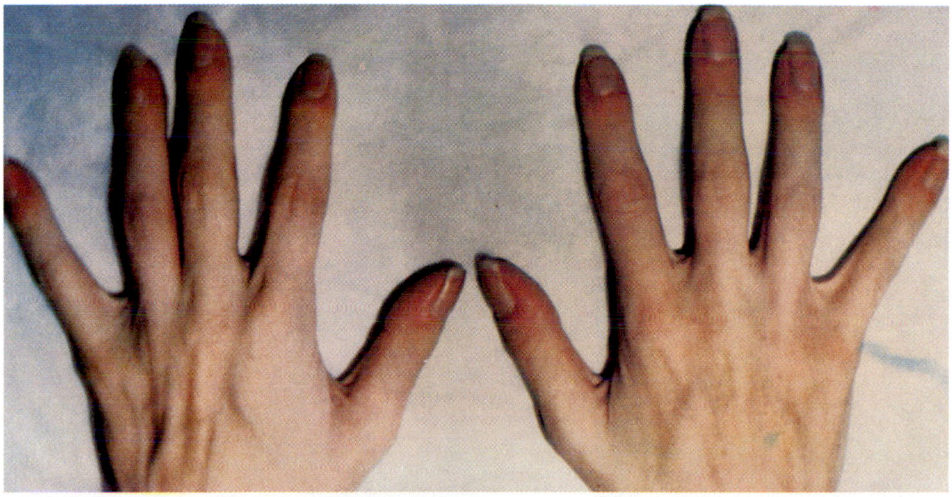

Plate 33 (FIGURE 10-16) Clubbing due to bacterial endocarditis.

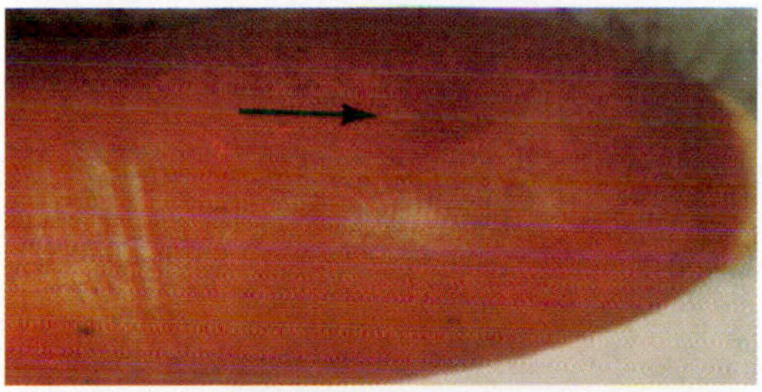

A

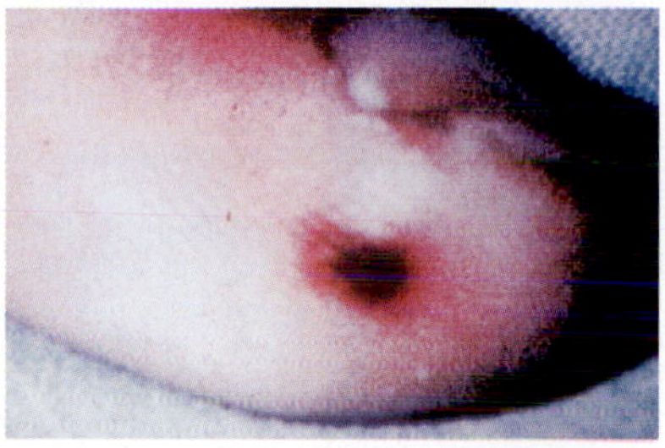

B

Plate 34 (FIGURE 10-17) *Bacterial endocarditis: A.* Valvular infection associated with a tender, purplish nodule (Osler's node) in the finger pad (arrow). *B. Osler's node.*

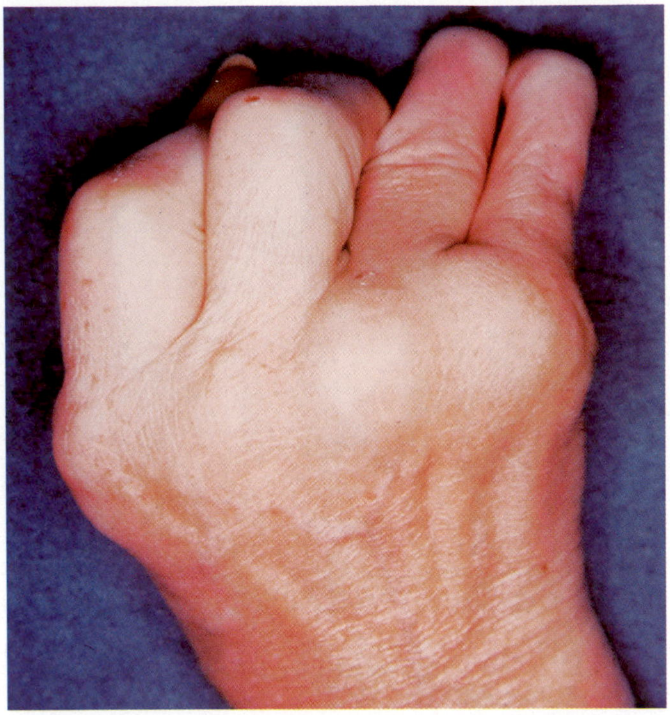

Plate 35 (FIGURE 10-24) *Rheumatoid arthritis:* with ulnar deviation of the fingers, flexion of the distal interphalangeal joints with hyperextension of the proximal interphalangeal joints.

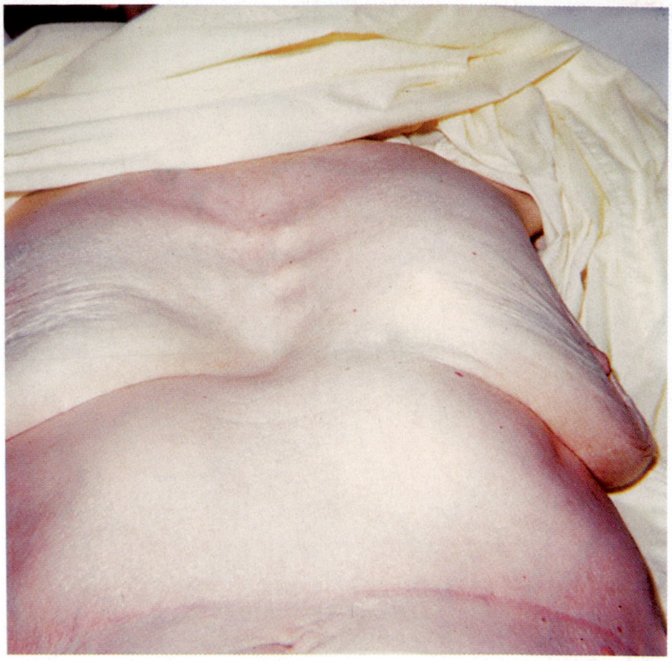

Plate 36 (FIGURE 10-27) Marked pectus excavatum.

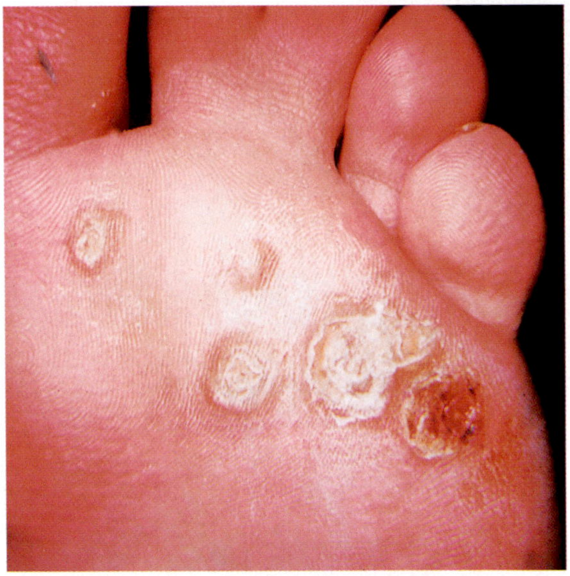

Plate 37 (FIGURE 10-30) *Hyperkeratotic lesions* encrusted on the soles of the feet in Reiter's syndrome.

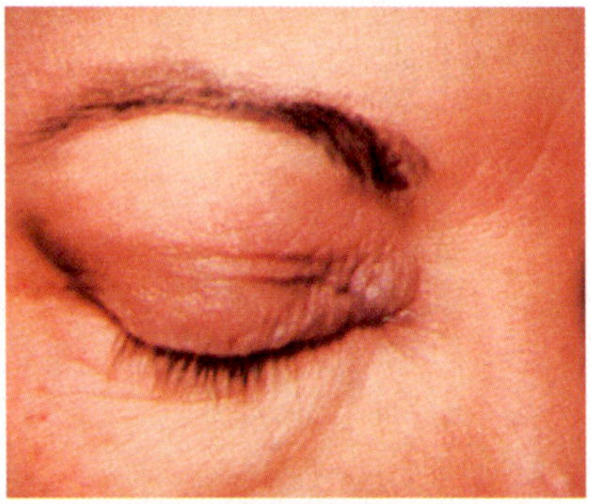

Plate 38 (FIGURE 10-32) *Dermatomyositis*. A violaceous hue and edema of upper eyelid may be associated with myocardial disease.

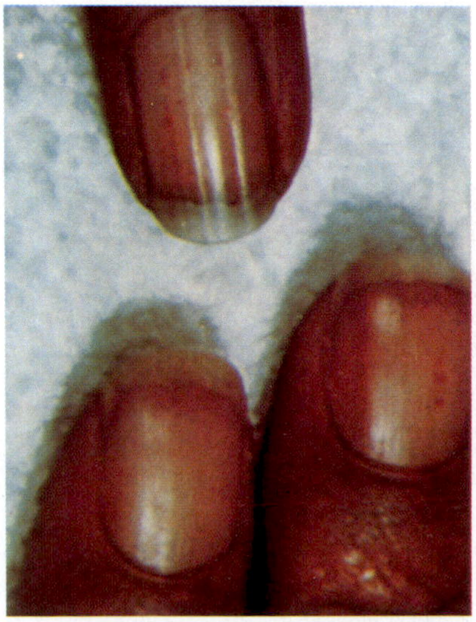

Plate 39 (FIGURE 10-37) Hereditary hemorrhagic telangiectasia. Telangiectasia under nails. (From Silverman ME, Hurst JW. The hand and the heart. *Am J Cardiol* 1968; 22:609. Used with permission from the publisher.)

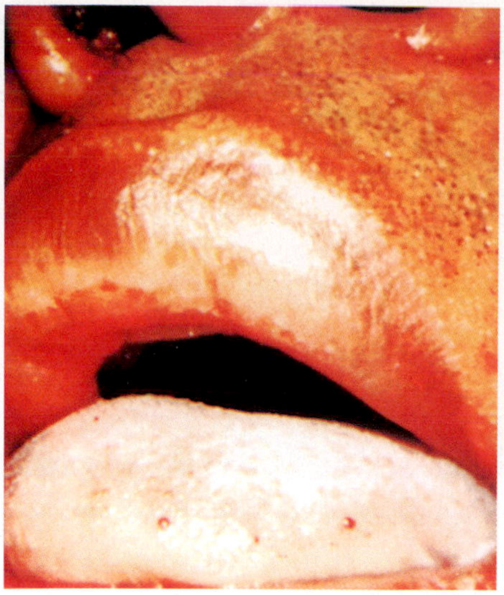

Plate 40 (FIGURE 10-38) Hereditary hemorrhagic telangiectasia. Telangiectasia of tongue and lips may be associated with a pulmonary arteriovenous fistula.

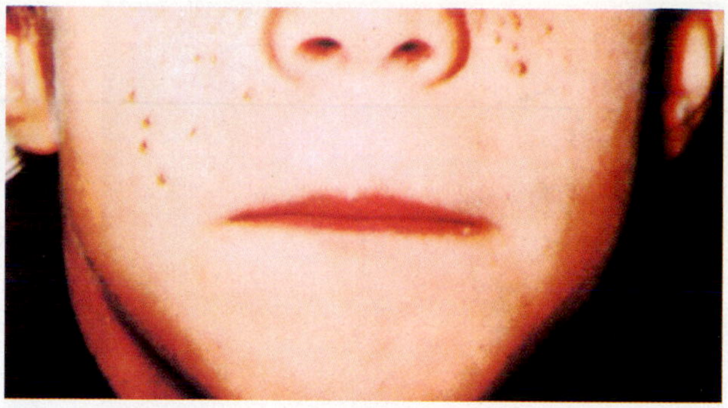

Plate 41 (FIGURE 10-39) Tuberous sclerosis. Adenoma sebaceum may be associated with rhabdomyomas of the myocardium.

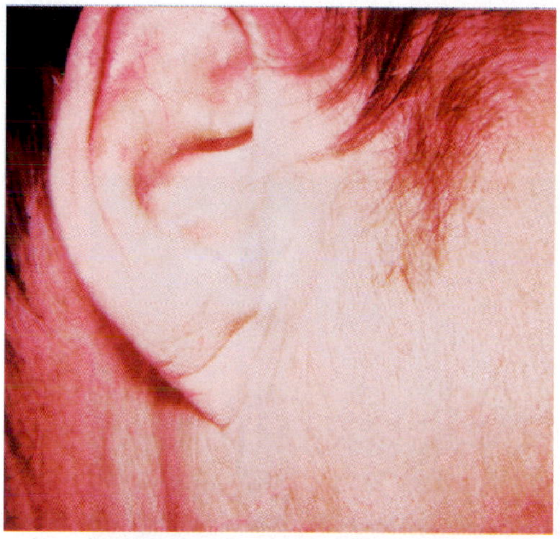

Plate 42 (FIGURE 10-40) Horizontal ear creases often are associated with the presence of extensive CAD.

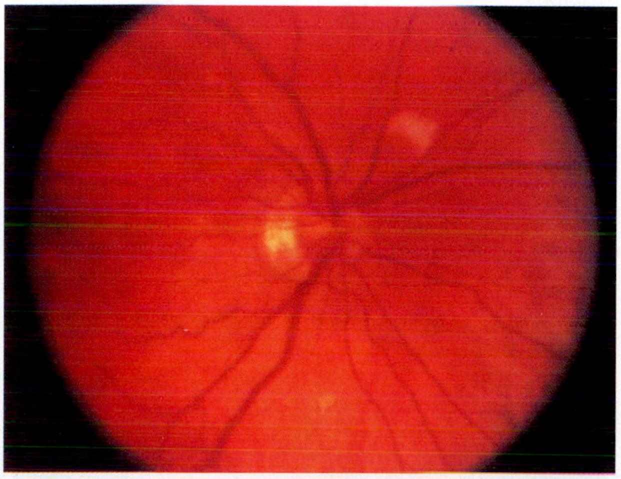

Plate 43 (FIGURE 10-47) Retinal cotton-wool spot. Cotton-wool spots are most frequently found close to the optic disk. Although they occur in acute uncontrolled systemic hypertension, the more common cause now, in younger patients, is infection with the human immunodeficiency virus (HIV). This normotensive 37-year-old man had no visual symptoms and no other retinopathy. There is a myopic crescent at the temporal disk edge, which is not abnormal. He died of complications related to the acquired immunodeficiency syndrome (AIDS) 2 years later.

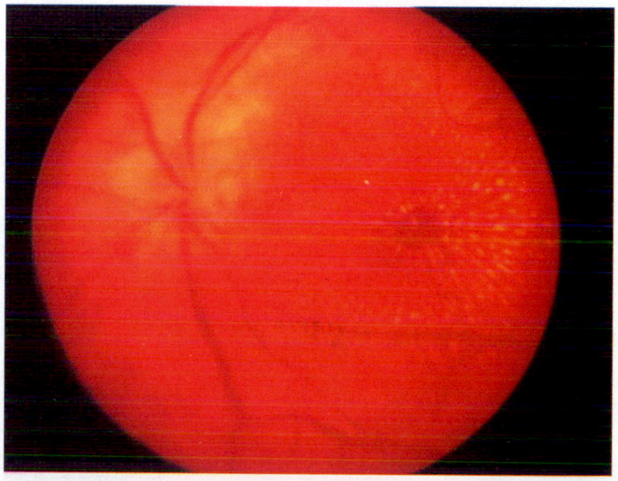

Plate 44 (FIGURE 10-48) Disk swelling and hard exudate in a macular "star" pattern. In this hypertensive patient with periarteritis nodosa, vascular leakage has led to the deposit of hard exudates around the fovea. Radial perifoveal connective tissue results in the star pattern of the exudate. Note also that the optic disk is edematous, with blurred margins, secondary to hypertension.

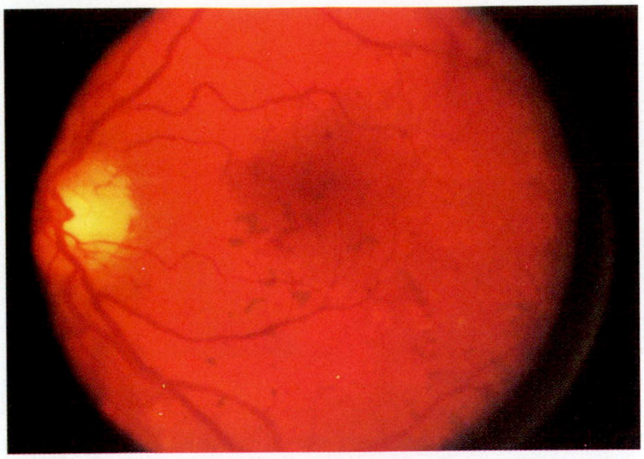

Plate 45 (FIGURE 10-49) Background diabetic retinopathy. Retinal microaneurysms, dot-and-blot hemorrhages, and a few fine upper temporal hard exudates are diagnostic of early diabetic retinopathy. The patient had no visual symptoms, but retinopathy of this magnitude can often be seen in patients with insulin-requiring diabetes of 15 or more years' duration.

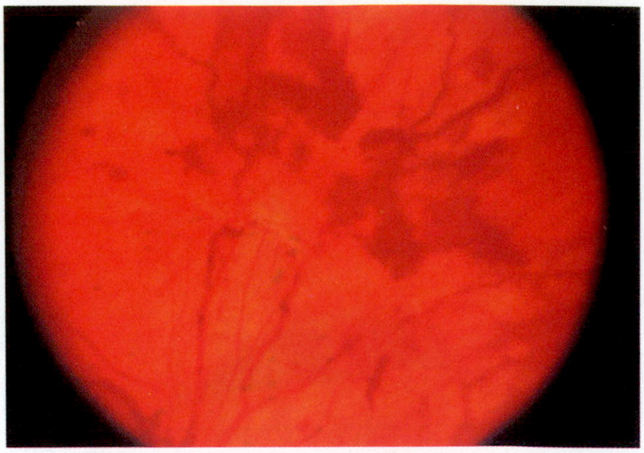

Plate 46 (FIGURE 10-50) Proliferative diabetic retinopathy with preretinal hemorrhage. When neovascularization develops, preretinal and vitreous hemorrhages are much more likely to occur. Easily visible neovascularization either in the periphery of the retina, as in this diabetic patient, or at the disk is an indication for immediate panretinal laser photocoagulation.

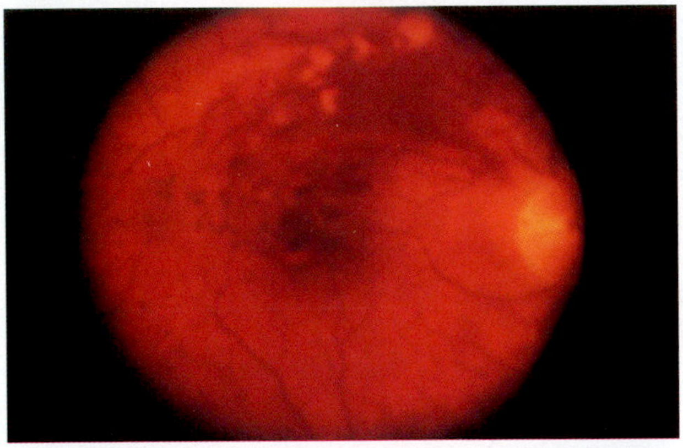

Plate 47 (FIGURE 10-52) Branch retinal vein obstruction. Thickening of the retinal arterial wall in diabetes and hypertension may compromise the lumen of the vein, where they share a common adventitial sheath at an arteriovenous crossing. The resulting obstruction produces hemorrhage retinopathy in the drainage area of the affected vein. Note here how the flame-shaped pattern of blood outlines the arcuate pattern of the nerve fibers as they run toward the optic disk.

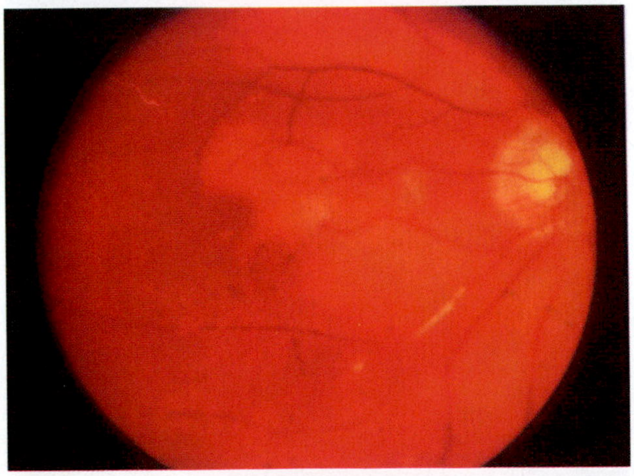

A

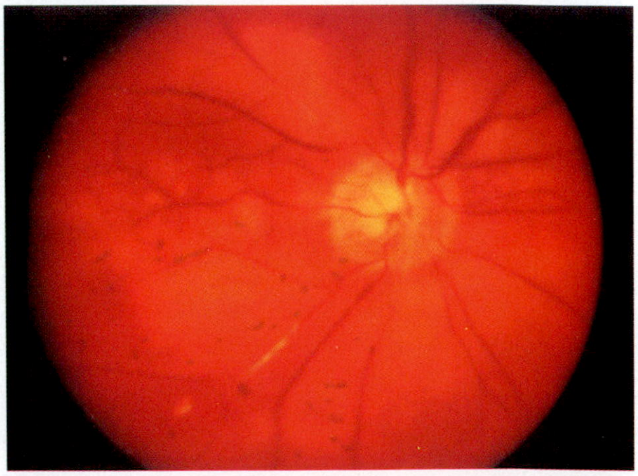

B

Plate 48 (FIGURE 10-53) Embolic retinal arterial obstruction (*A* and *B*). Cholesterol crystals may dislodge from the walls of the heart, aortic arch, or carotids. Carried into the retinal circulation as Hollenhorst plaques, they seldom obstruct the arterioles completely. Although amaurosis fugax is more common, the embolic burden may occasionally be so large as to produce retinal infarction. Note in the photograph of the macular area (*A*) that this patient's fovea remains red, while there is a pale, cloudy swelling nasal to it. This has produced a half "cherry-red" spot. With complete central retinal artery occlusion, the red foveal area is completely surrounded by pale swollen retina. Hollenhorst cholesterol plaques can be seen in both the upper and lower temporal retinal arteries. In *A*, the inferior temporal arteriole demonstrates "boxcar" segmentation of the blood column, indicative of very slow flow.

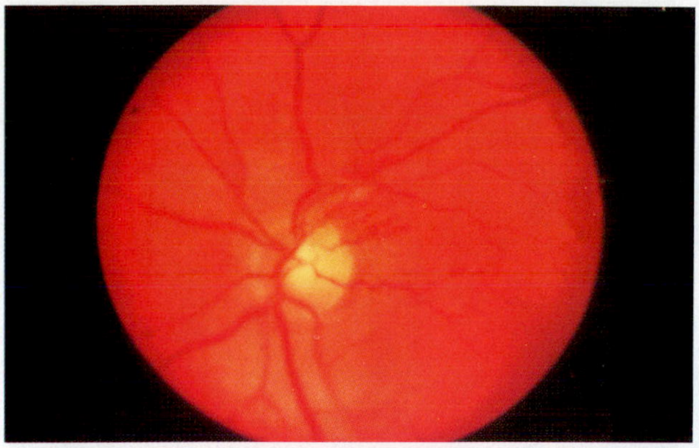

Plate 49 (FIGURE 10-54) Neovascularization after branch retinal vein obstruction. New vessels may develop late after obstruction of a branch of the central retinal vein. These most often serve to shunt flow around the obstructed vessel site and are thus not as exuberantly proliferative as those seen in diabetic retinopathy.

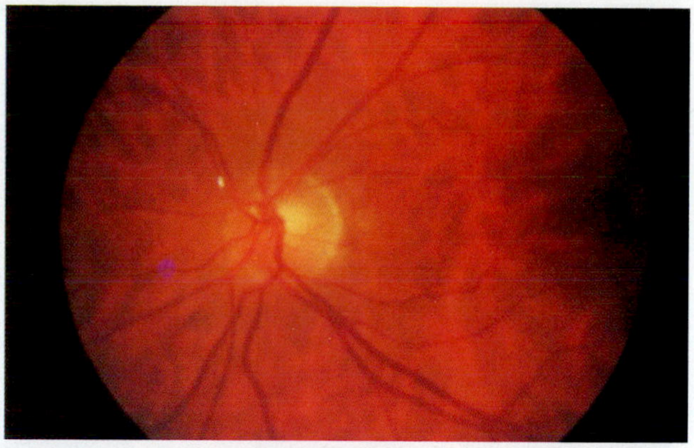

Plate 50 (Fig. 10-56) Calcific retinal embolus associated with aortic valvular disease. Calcific aortic valvular disease and valve replacement surgery may result in retinal emboli. Like cholesterol emboli, these calcific flecks lodge at arterial bifurcations but seldom obstruct flow completely. They are white and glitter in the ophthalmoscope beam. Somewhat similar emboli may be seen after the intravenous injection of illicit drugs expanded with talc.

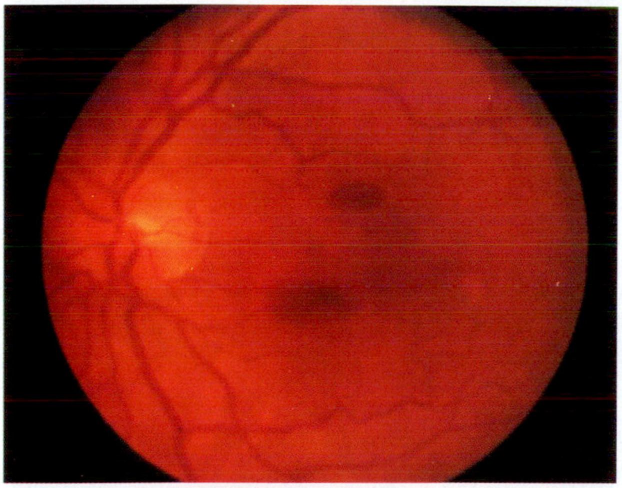

Plate 51 (FIGURE 10-57) Retinal hemorrhages after cardiac catheterization. Following cardiac catheterization, symptomatic and asymptomatic retinal hemorrhages may occur. The latter are more common. Presumably, these are the result of embolic events. Note, in this recently catheterized patient, the two oval hemorrhages and a small area of cloudy swelling just inferior and temporal to the fovea.

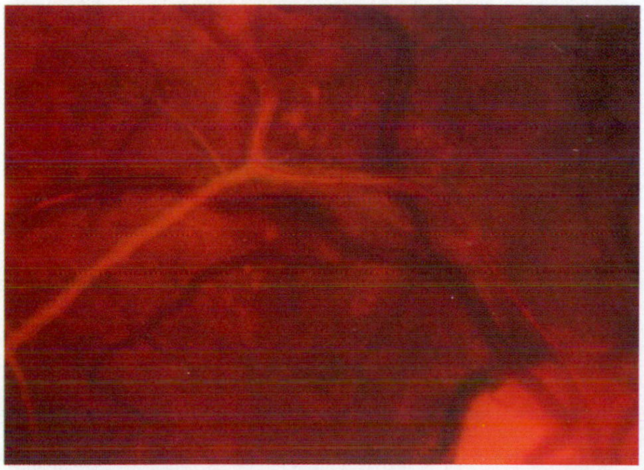

A

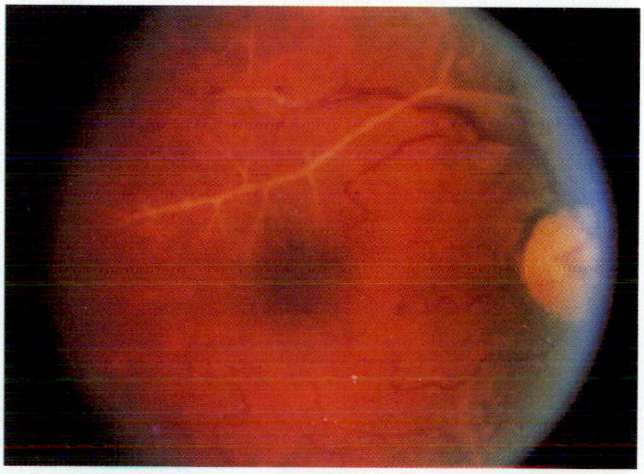

B

Plate 52 (FIGURE 10-59) *A.* Retinal arteriosclerosis. This 75-year-old hypertensive woman has marked arteriosclerosis of the upper temporal retinal arteriole and its branches. When the narrowed blood column can no longer be seen, the thickened wall produces the "silver-wire" appearance seen here. Where the arteriole crosses its associated vein, the course of the vein is altered, and its blood column cannot be seen. This venous "nicking" and "banking" is associated with impairment of outflow, and the affected veins become darker, larger, and more tortuous. *B.* Low-power view showing the silver-wire arteriole.

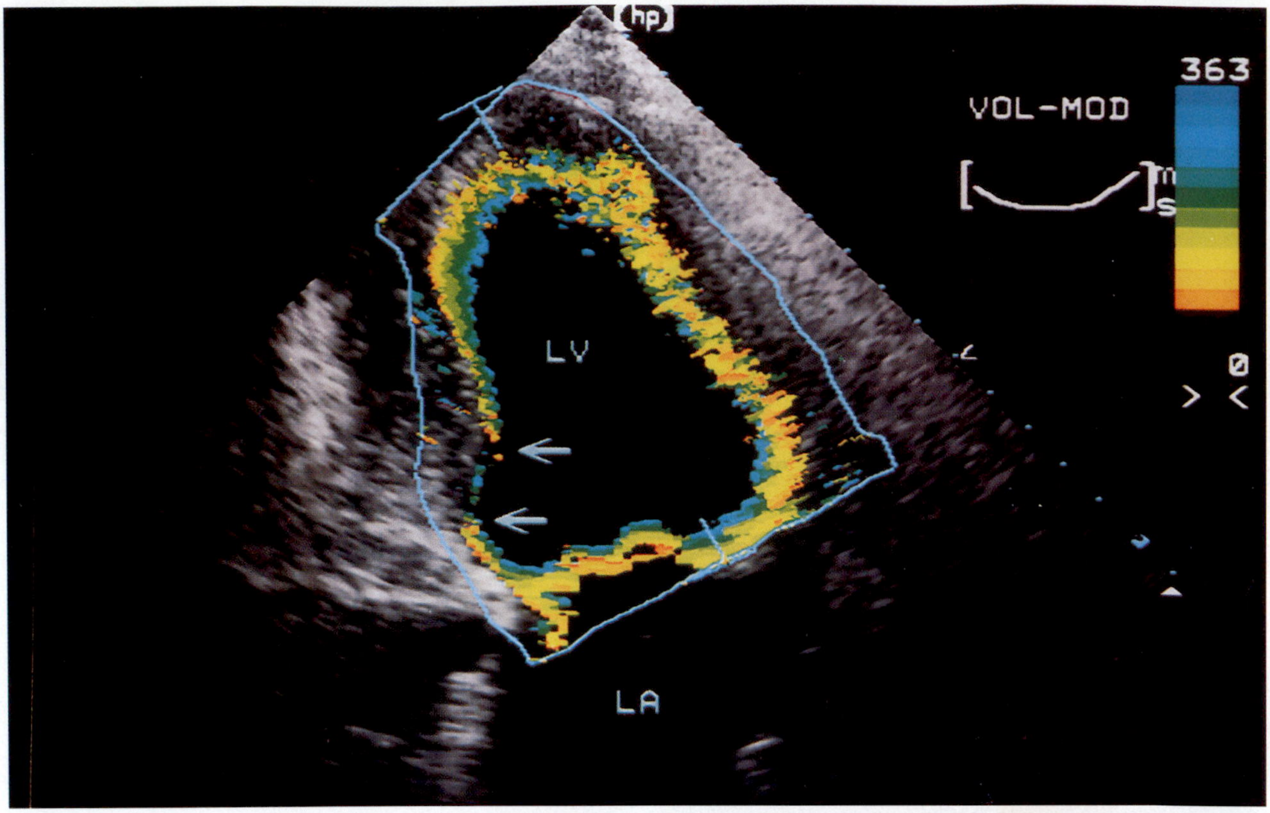

Plate 53 (FIGURE 13-23) Color kinesis image (apical two-chamber view) from a patient with an inferobasal infarction. Systolic motion in this area (*arrows*) is markedly diminished.

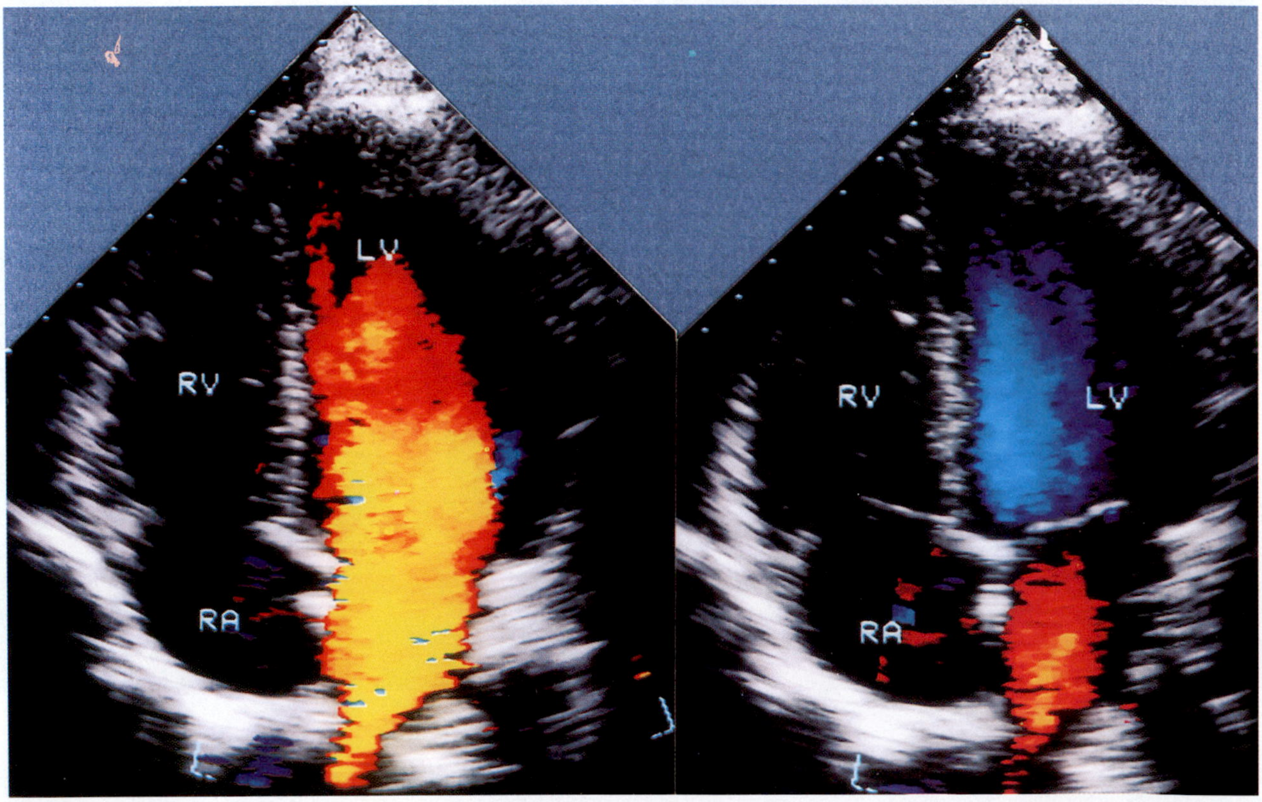

Plate 54 (FIGURE 13-30) Apical four-chamber images with color-flow Doppler during diastole and systole. Red flow indicates movement toward the transducer (diastolic filling); blue flow indicates movement away from the transducer (systolic ejection).

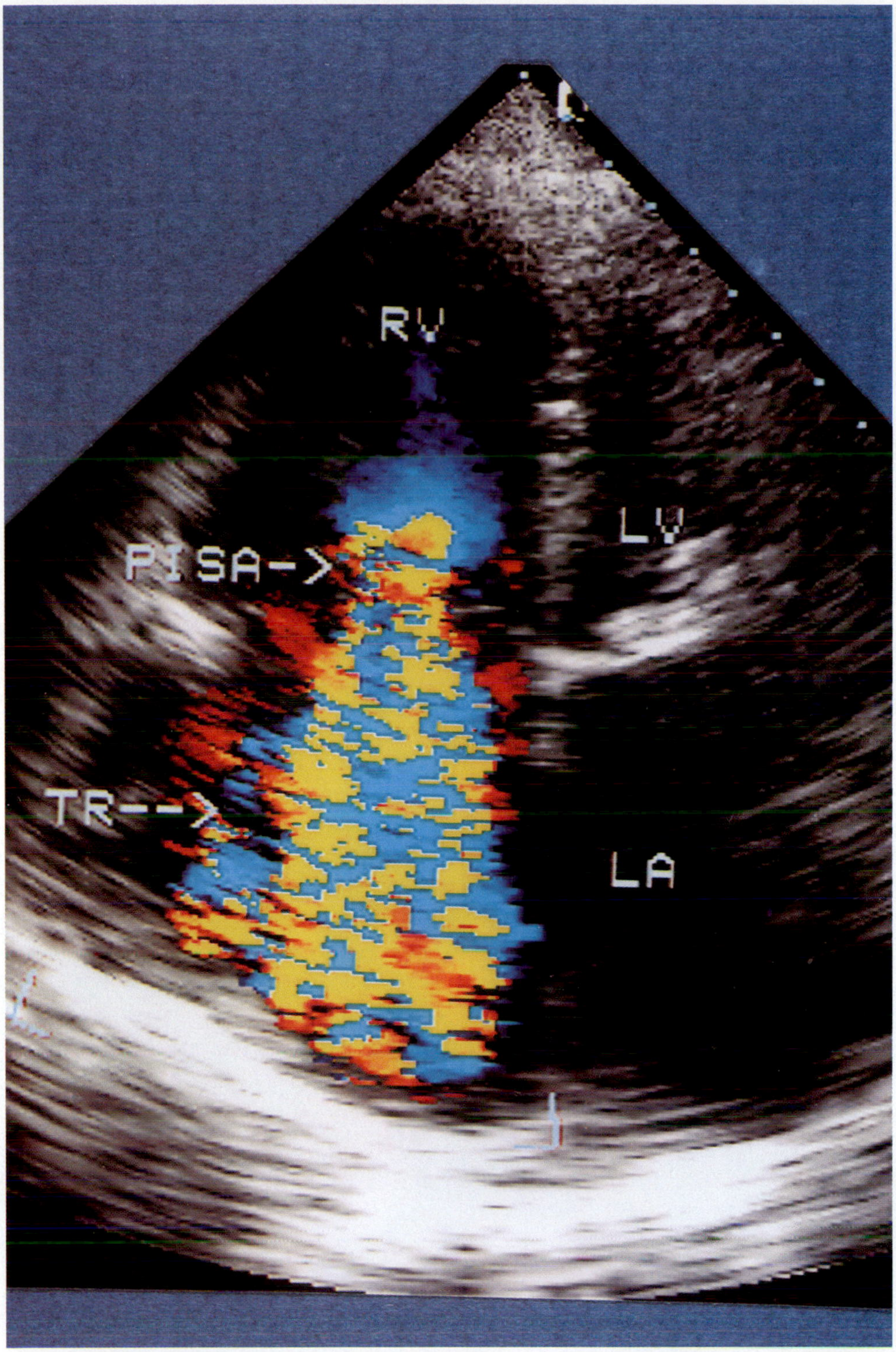

Plate 55 (FIGURE 13-31) Apical four-chamber view of severe tricuspid regurgitation. The Doppler color jet fills the RA. PISA = proximal isovelocity surface area; LV = left ventricle; LA = left atrium; RV = right ventricle.

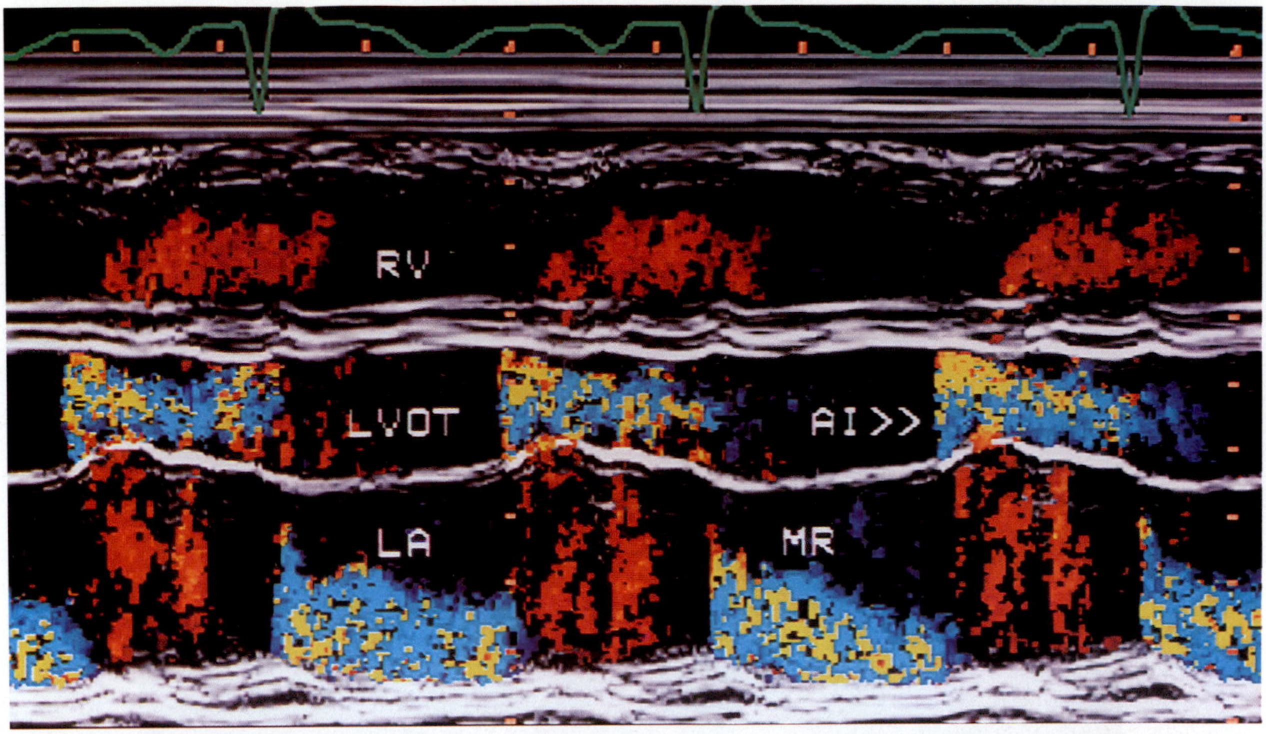

Plate 56 (FIGURE 13-32) Color-flow Doppler superimposed on an M-mode image. The transducer is in parasternal position, and the cursor is directed through the left ventricular outflow tract (LVOT) and left atrium (LA). The patient under study has both aortic insufficiency (AI) and mitral regurgitation (MR). RV = right ventricle.

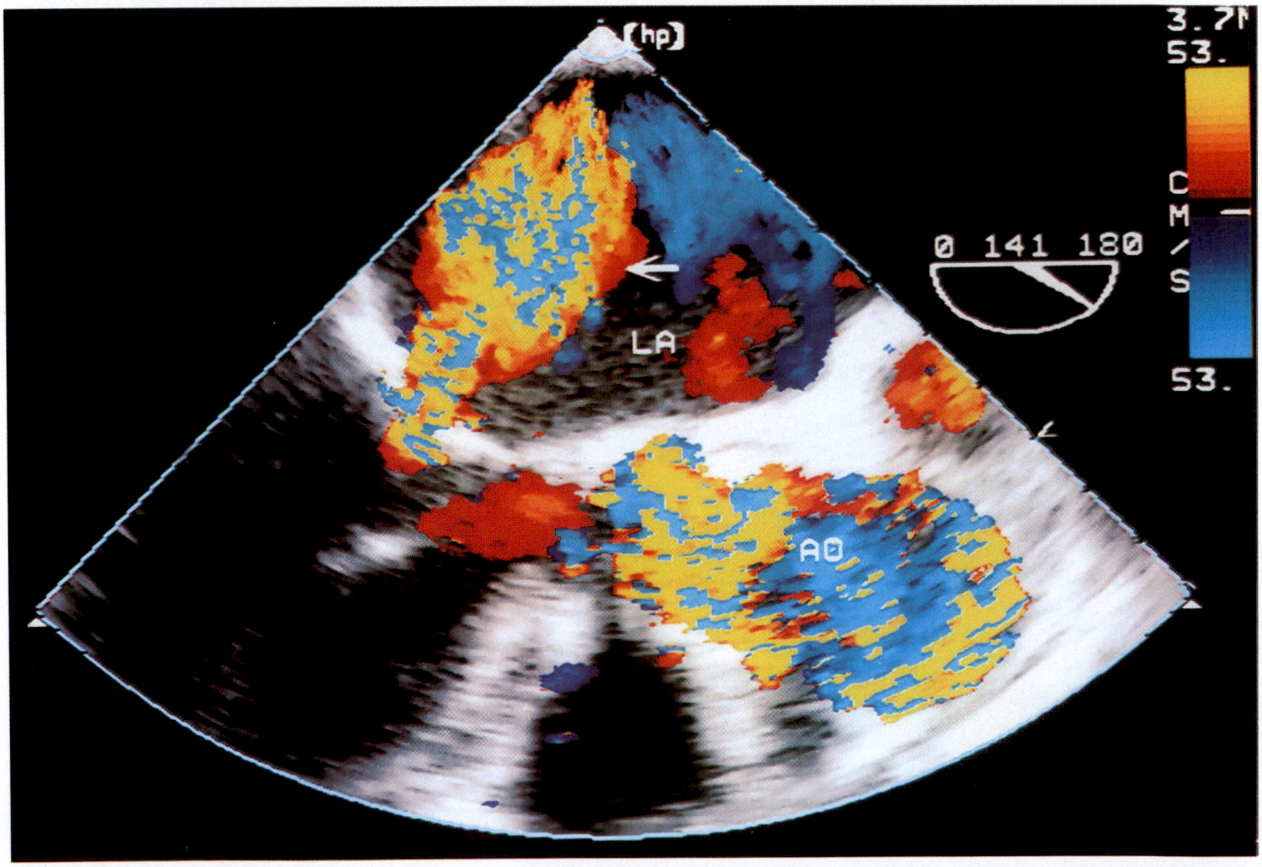

Plate 57 (FIGURE 13-49) Transesophageal echocardiography image (three-chamber plane) demonstrating a jet of mitral regurgitation (*arrow*) in the left atrium (LA). AO = aorta; LV = left ventricle.

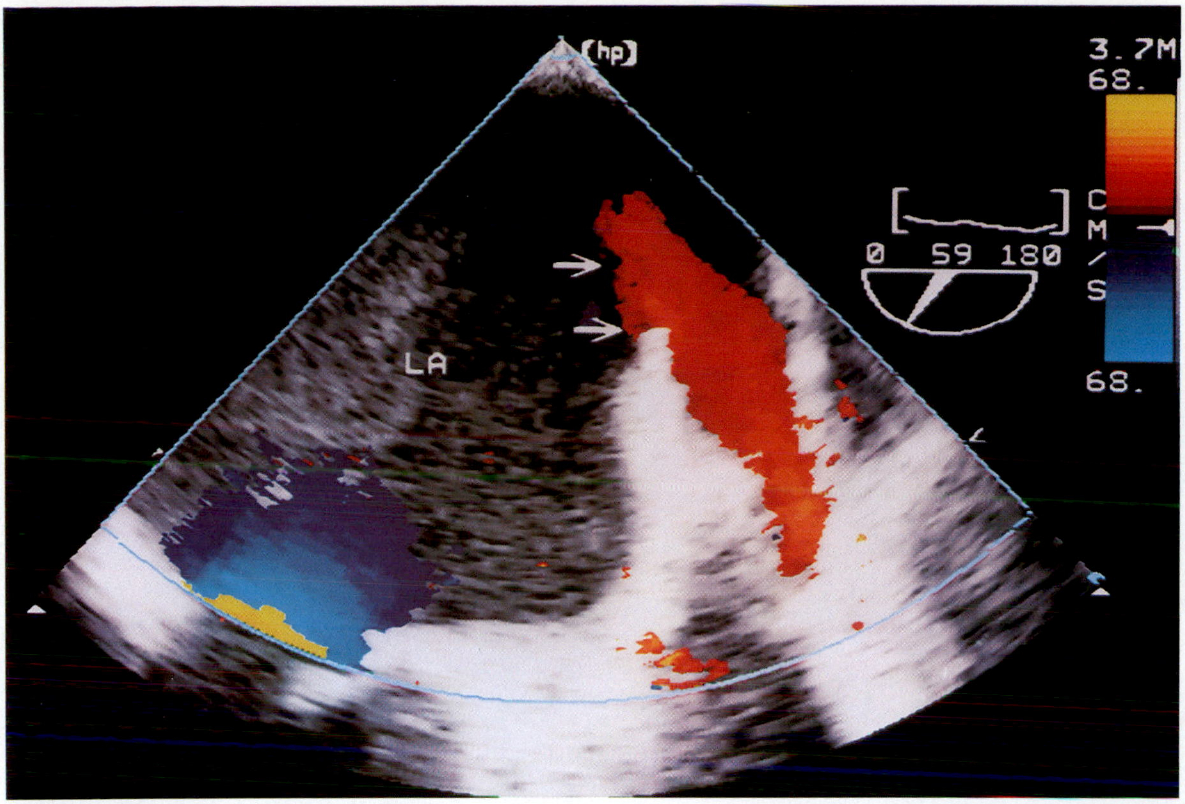

Plate 58 (FIGURE 13-50) Transesophageal echocardiography image of pulmonary venous flow (*arrows*) entering the left atrium (LA) during diastole.

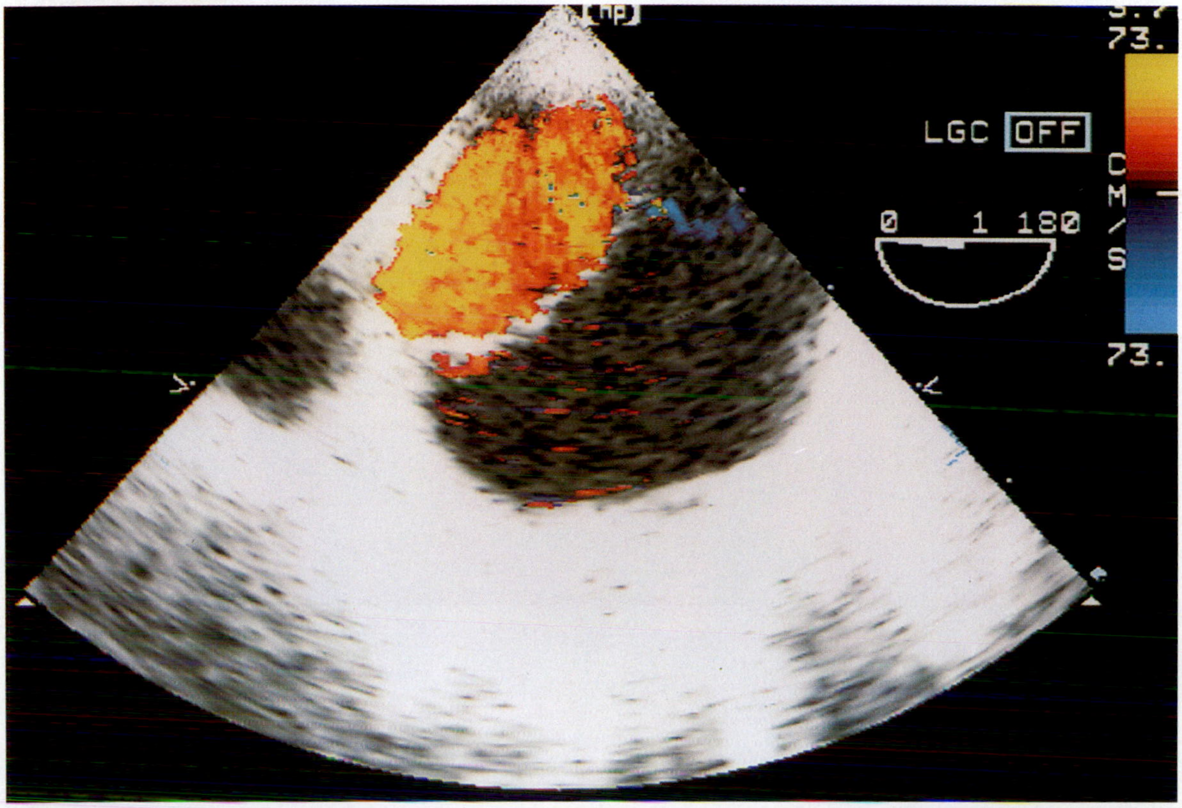

Plate 59 (FIGURE 13-51) Transverse TEE image of a descending aortic dissection. The true lumen is color-coded orange. The false lumen is mostly devoid of flow, but a small blue jet of communication between the two channels is present.

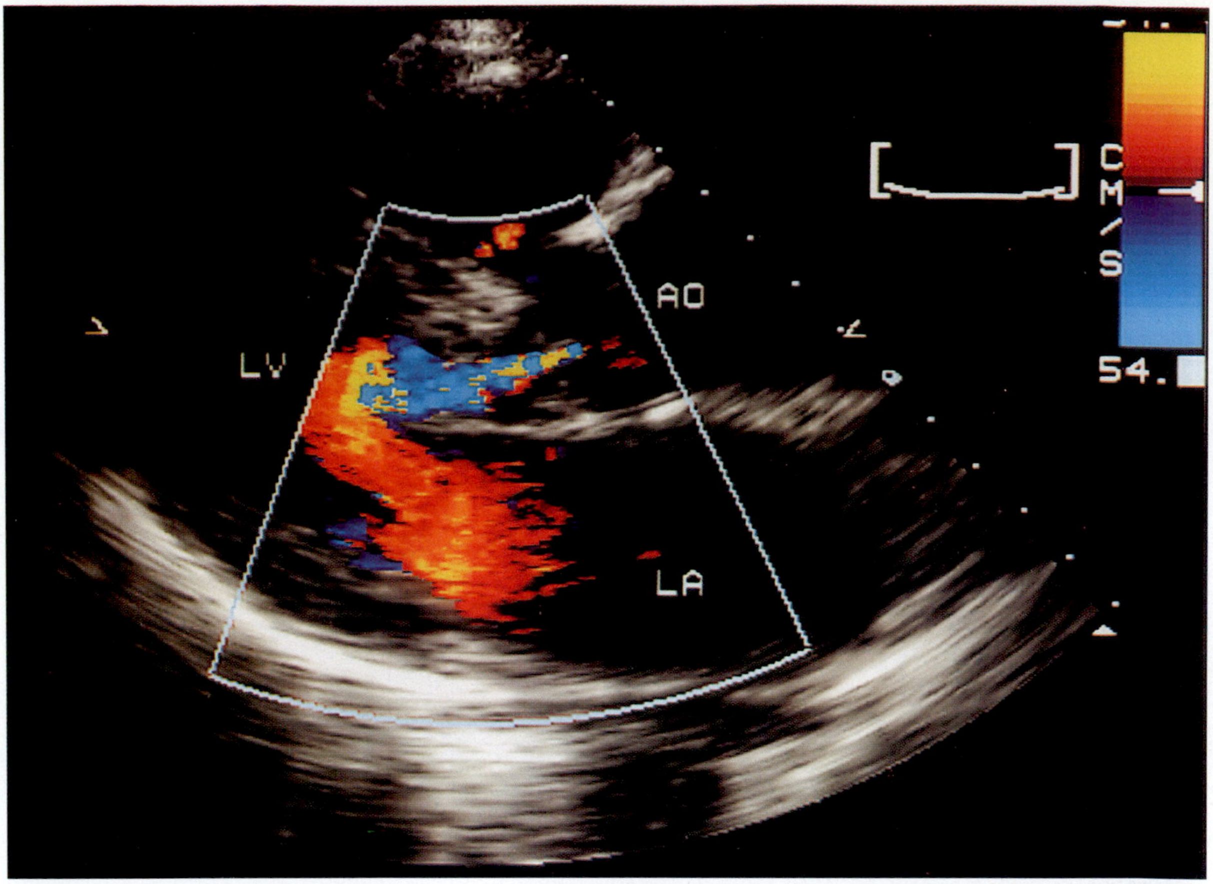

A

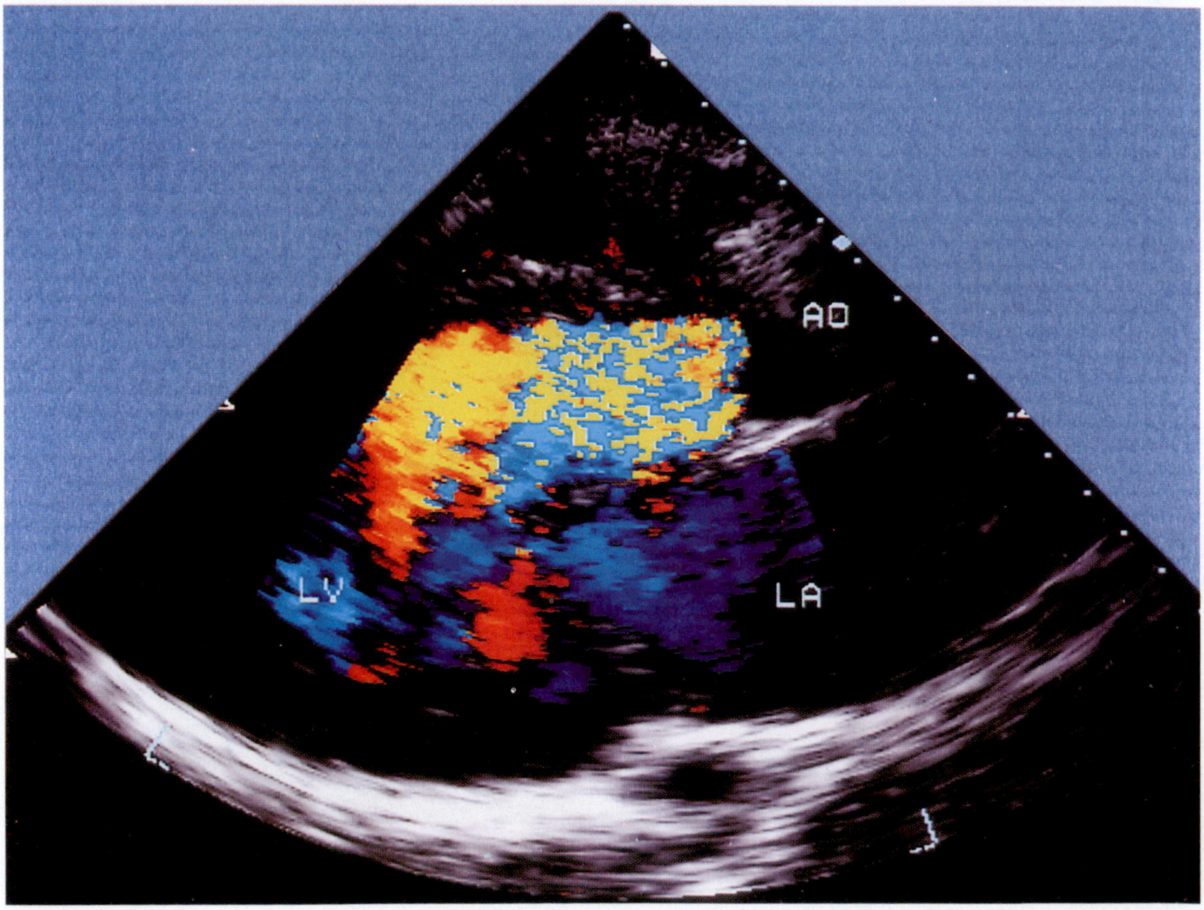

B

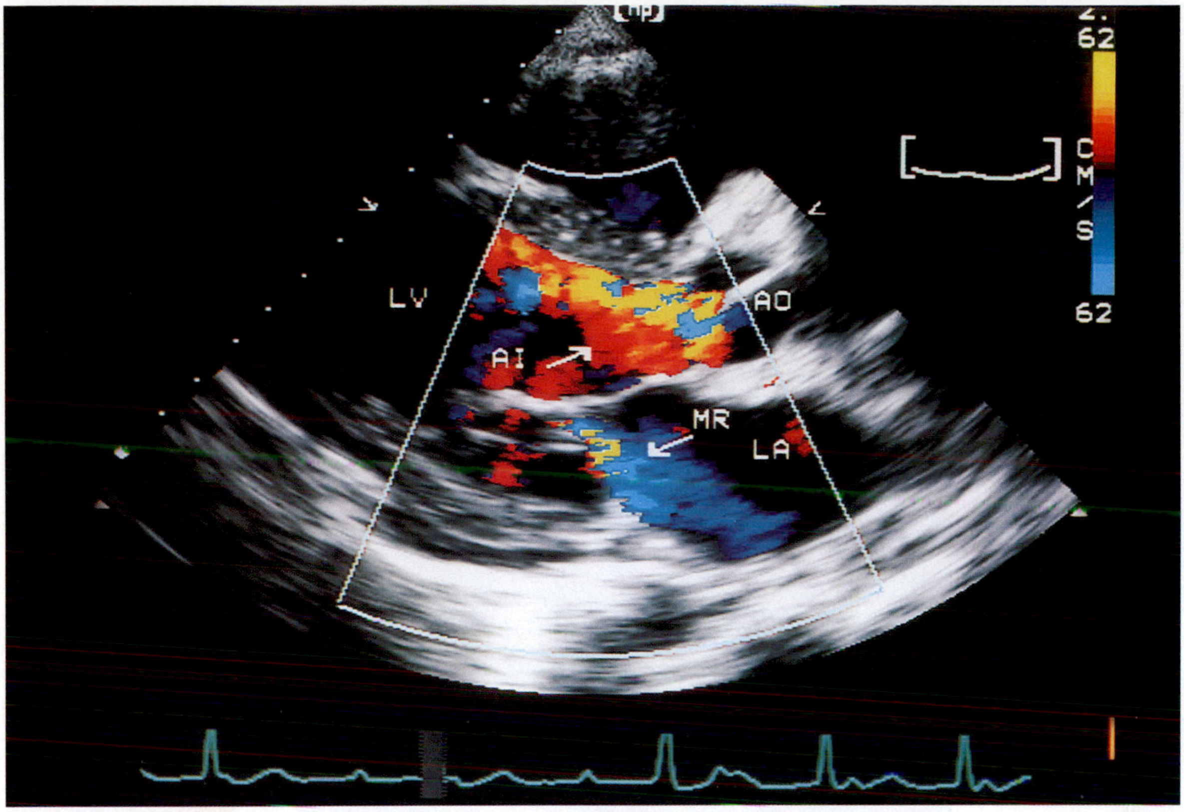

C

Plate 60 (FIGURE 13-64) *A.* Parasternal long-axis plane showing a multicolor jet (indicating turbulent flow) of aortic regurgitation in the left ventricular outflow tract. The jet is narrow in width, suggesting mild regurgitation. AO = aorta; LA = left atrium; LV = left ventricle. *B.* Parasternal long-axis plane with color-flow Doppler imaging. The aortic regurgitant (AR) color jet is as wide as the left ventricular outflow tract, suggesting severe AR. AO = aorta; LA = left atrium; LV = left ventricle. *C.* Parasternal long-axis image of acute severe aortic insufficiency (AI). The accompanying marked elevation of left ventricular (LV) diastolic pressure causes diastolic mitral regurgitation (MR). AO = aorta; LA = left atrium.

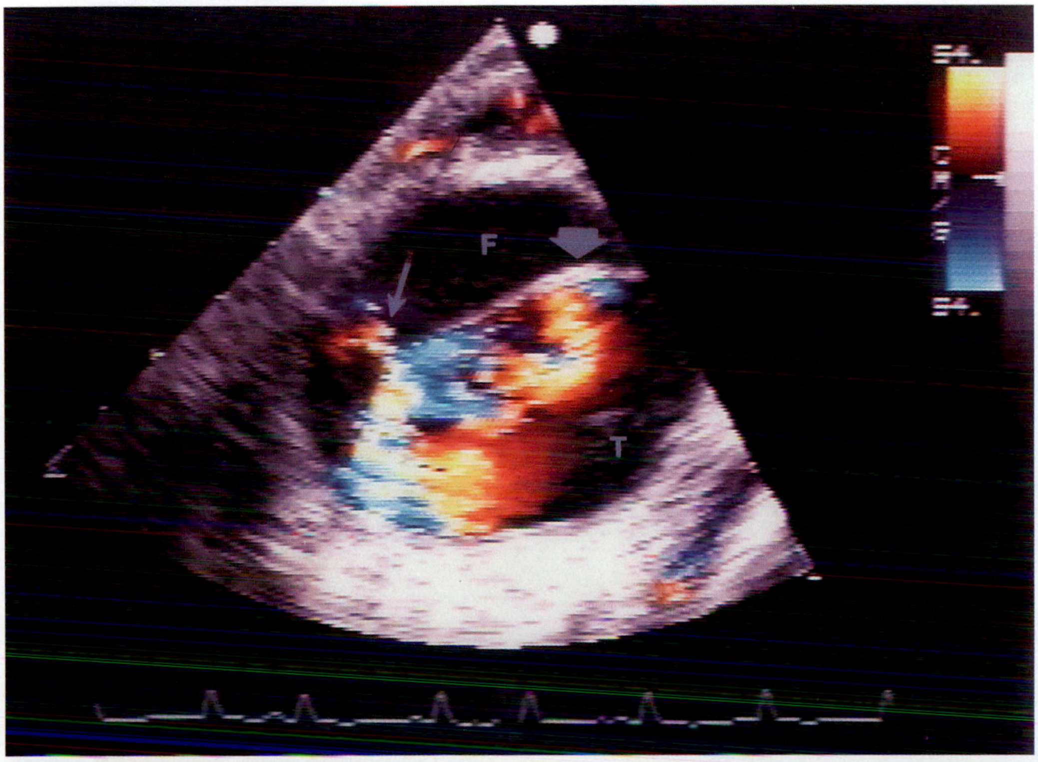

Plate 61 (FIGURE 13-69) Transverse TEE view of an aortic dissection. The false (F) and true (T) lumens are separated by an intimal flap (*large arrow*). The communication between the two channels is visible (*small arrow*).

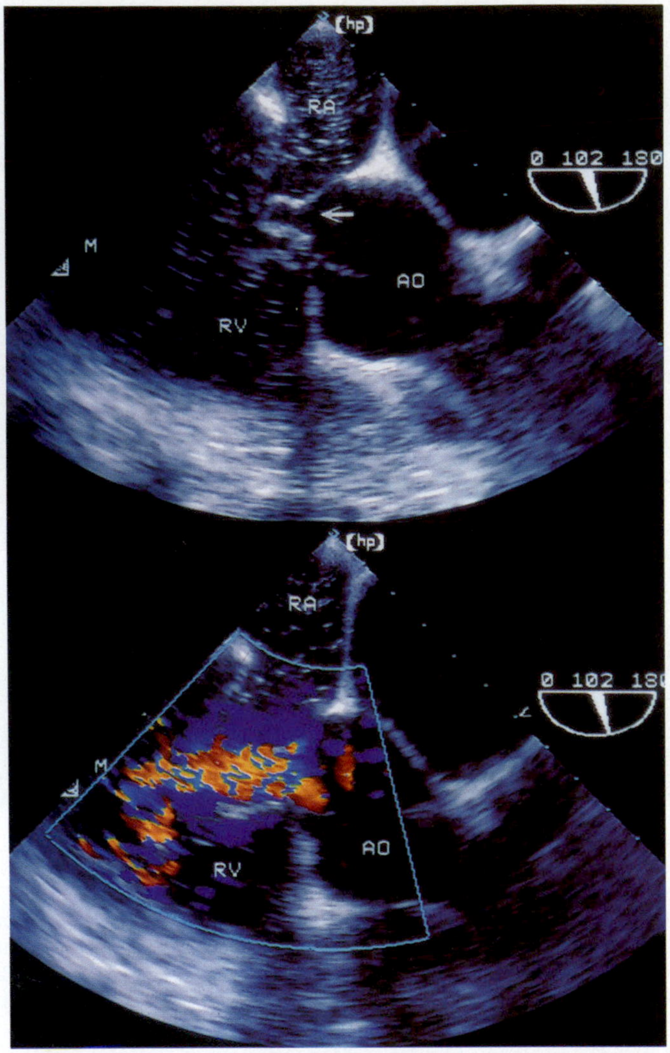

Plate 62 (FIGURE 13-70B) TEE image of a ruptured sinus of Valsalva aneurysm. The upper image shows focal aneurysmal dilatation of the right coronary sinus with the appearance of a "windsock." Color Doppler (*lower image*) reveals a high-velocity flow jet from the aorta into the right ventricle. Agitated saline was injected intravenously to highlight right heart structures.

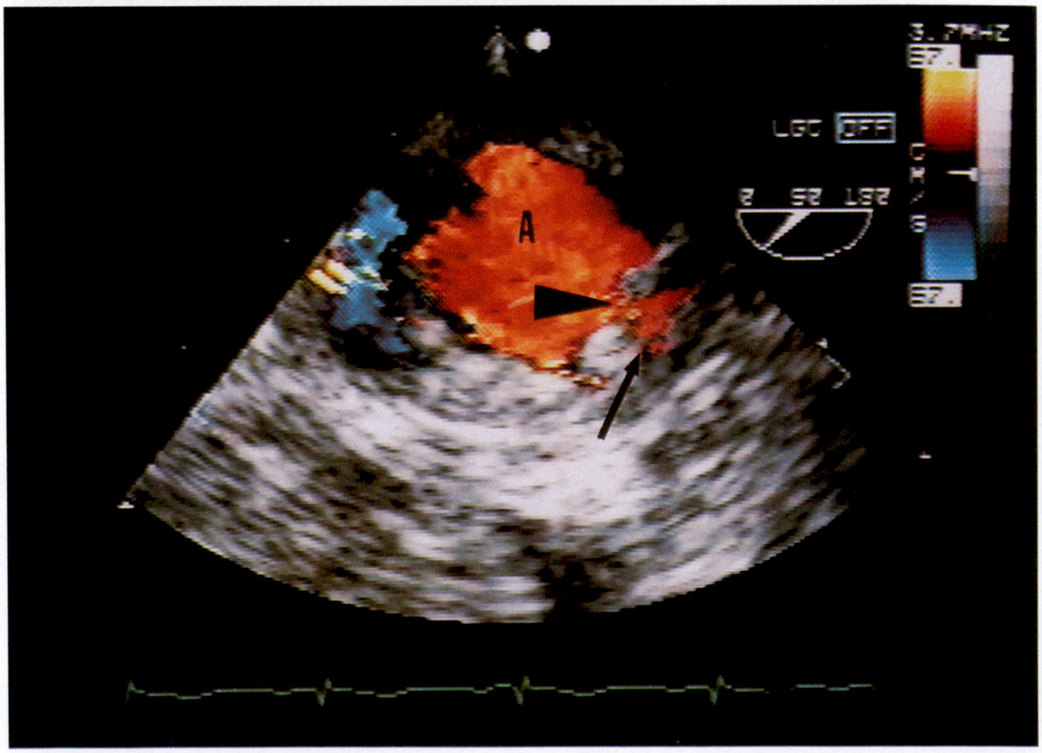

Plate 63 (FIGURE 13-71) Transverse TEE view of penetrating ulceration in the proximal portion of the descending aorta (A). The mouth of the ulcer crater is visible (*large arrowhead*), as is blood flow within the atheroma (*arrow*).

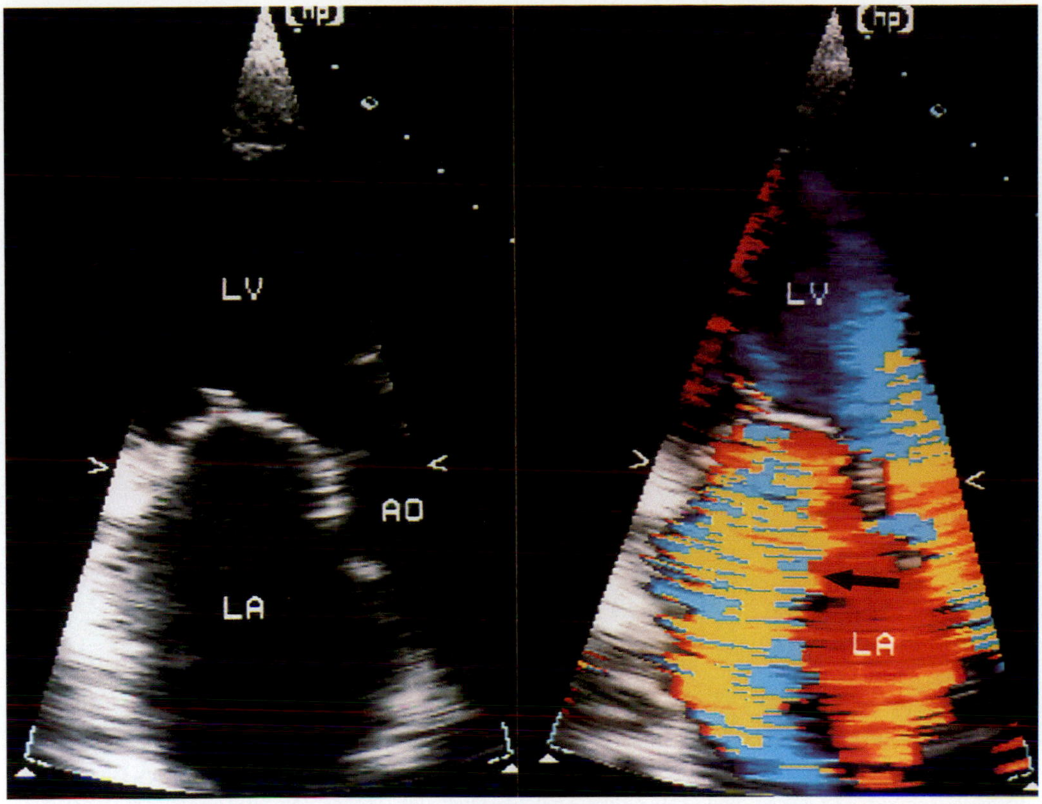

A

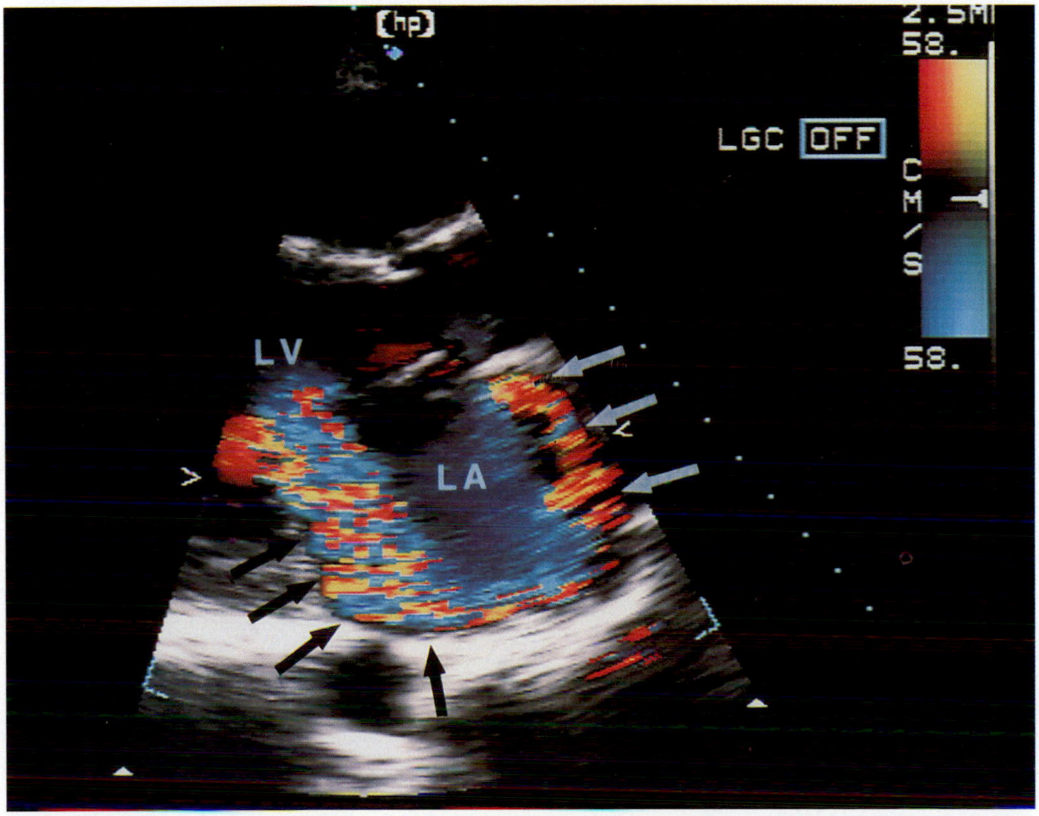

B

Plate 64 (FIGURE 13-77) *A.* Mitral regurgitation. *Left:* apical three-chamber plane. Right: same plane with color Doppler imaging. A large jet of mitral regurgitation (*arrow*) is present. AO = aorta; LA = left atrium; LV = left ventricle. *B.* Parasternal long-axis view from a patient with angiographically proved severe mitral regurgitation. The color Doppler jet in this case is directed posteriorly and eccentric (*black arrows*). The jet hugs the wall of the left atrium (LA) and wraps around all the way to the aortic root (*white arrows*). LV = left ventricle.

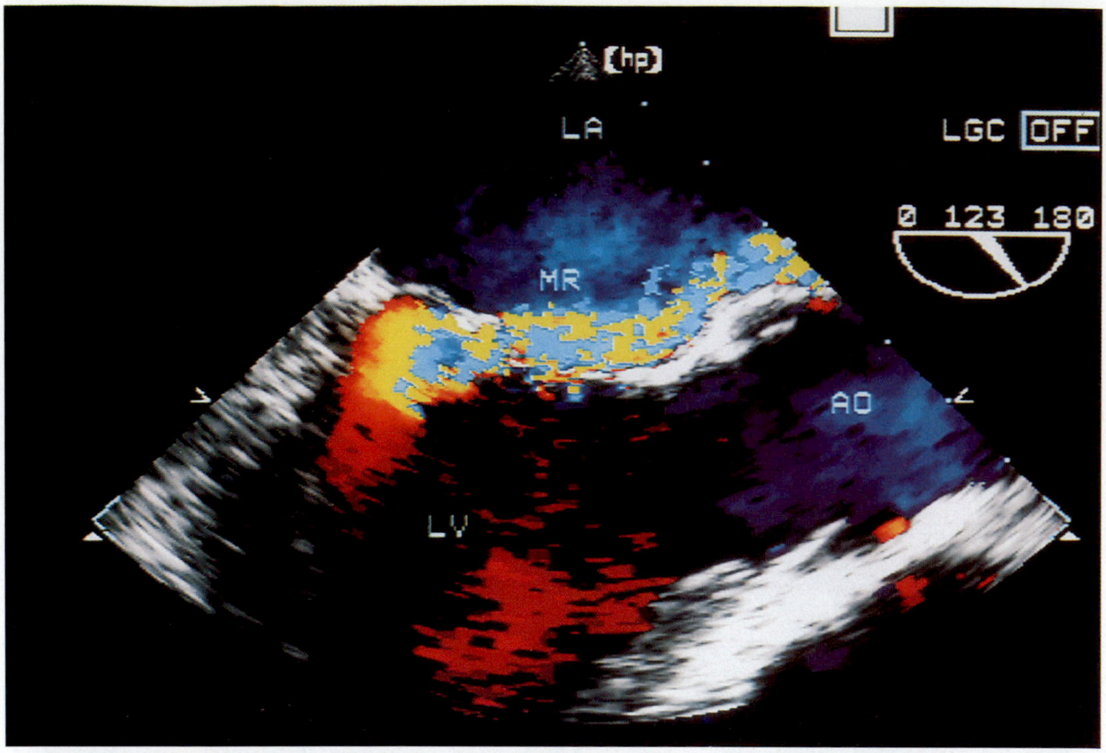

Plate 65 (FIGURE 13-78) TEE images from a case of severe mitral regurgitation secondary to a flail posterior mitral valve leaflet. *A.* abnormal coaptation and prolapse of the posterior leaflet is apparent. *B.* Color Doppler imaging demonstrates an eccentric jet of MR directed anteriorly toward the aortic root (AO). LA = left atrium; LV = left ventricle.

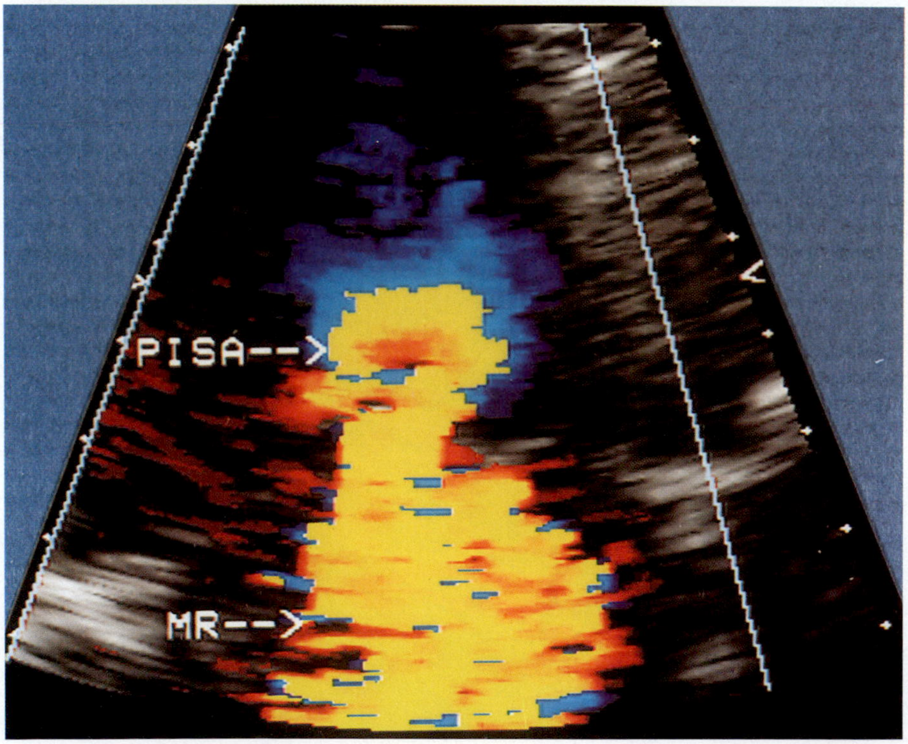

Plate 66 (FIGURE 13-80) *A.* Proximal isovelocity surface area (PISA). See text for details. Q = flow; FCR = flow convergence region; r = radius of isovelocity hemisphere; Vr = velocity of flow at distance r from the orifice. (From Bargiggia GS, Tronconi L, Sahn DJ, et al. A new method for quantitation of mitral regurgitation based on color flow Doppler imaging of flow convergence proximal to regurgitant orifice. *Circulation* 1991; 84:1481–1489, with permission.) *B.* Magnified view (from the apical four-chamber plane) of mitral regurgitation (MR) demonstrating color Doppler flow convergence proximal to the mitral valve (PISA).

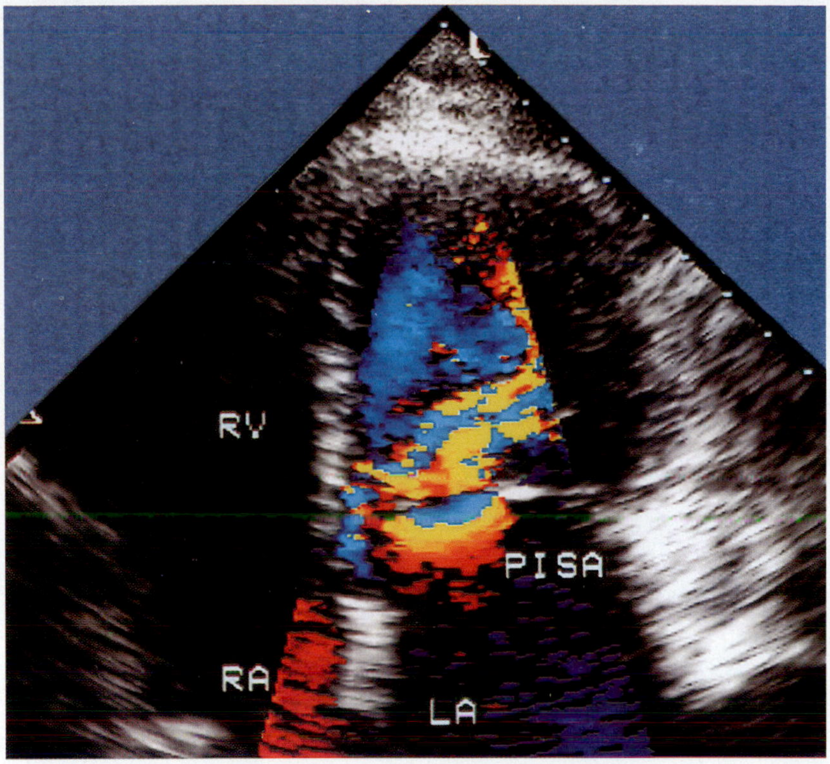

Plate 67 (FIGURE 13-81) Apical four-chamber plane in mitral stenosis. Color flow imaging in the mitral valve region shows flow convergence (PISA) proximal to the valve during diastole. LA = left atrium; RA = right atrium; RV = right ventricle.

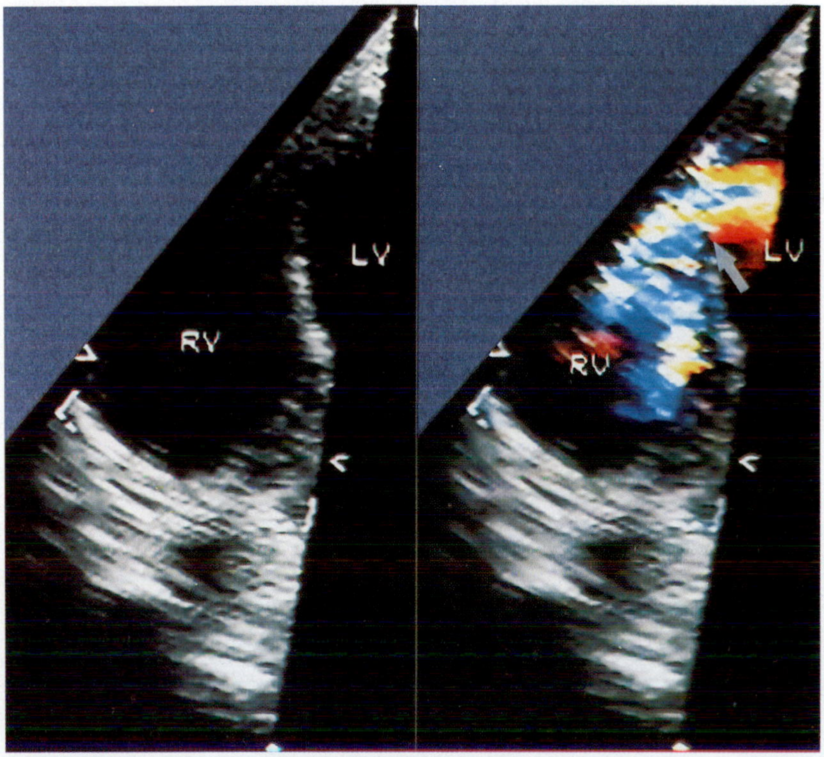

Plate 68 (FIGURE 13-102) Modified apical four-chamber image of a distal septal ventricular septal rupture. With 2D imaging (*left*), the distal septum is incompletely visualized. With color Doppler imaging, however, a high-velocity aliased color jet is seen in the right ventricle (RV). In addition, an area of flow convergence is seen on the left ventricular (LV) side of the rupture (*arrow*).

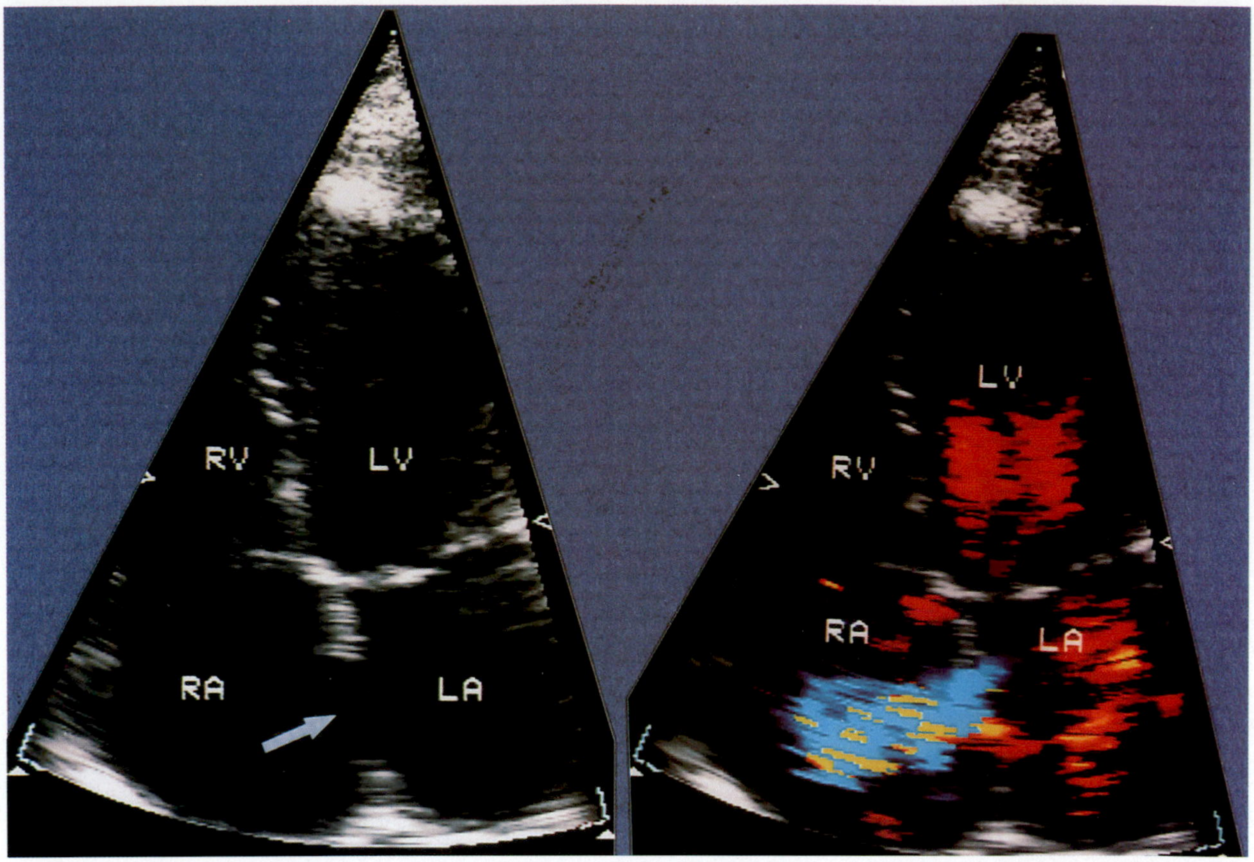

Plate 69 (FIGURE 13-110) Apical four-chamber view of an ostium secundum atrial septal defect (ASD). On the left, a defect in the mid atrial septum is apparent (*arrow*). On the right, there is color flow through the shunt. RV = right ventricle; RA = right atrium; LA = left atrium; LV = left ventricle.

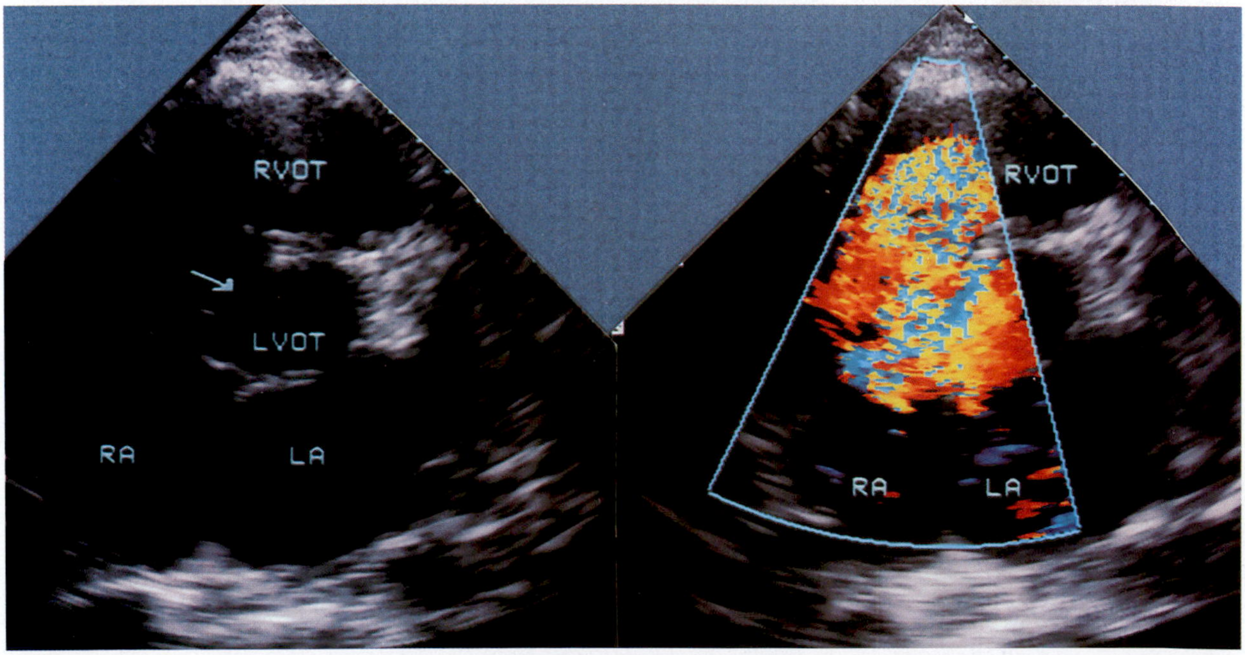

Plate 70 (FIGURE 13-114) Parasternal short-axis images of a large perimembranous ventricular septal defect (VSD) (*arrow*) without (*left*) and with (*right*) superimposed color flow Doppler. A large, turbulent color jet crosses the VSD during systole (*right*). RVOT = right ventricular outflow tract; RA = right atrium; LA = left atrium; LVOT = left ventricular outflow tract.

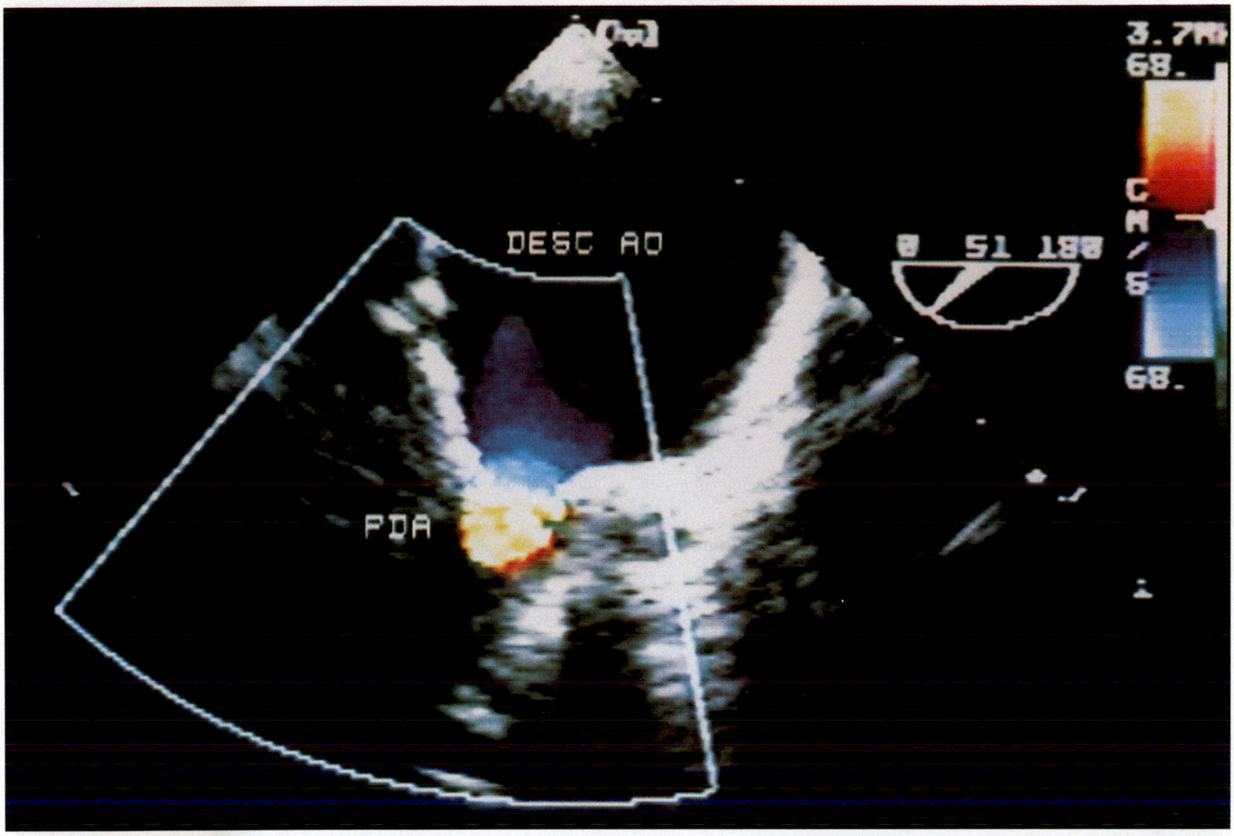

A

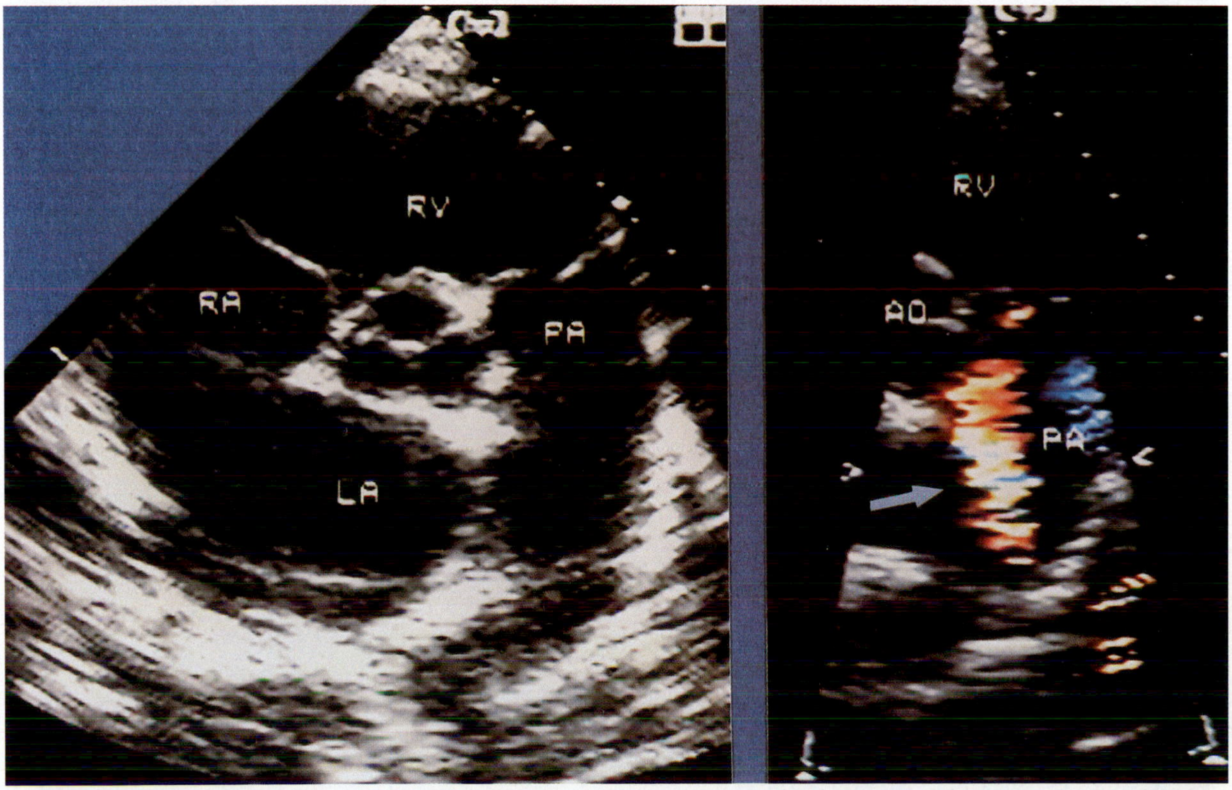

B

Plate 71 (FIGURE 13-115) *A*. Transesophageal image of a patent ductus arteriosus (PDA). Color Doppler imaging shows flow from the descending aorta (DESC AO) into the PDA. (Courtesy of Bruce J. Kimura, M.D.) *B*. Parasternal short-axis images at the aortic valve level. On the left, the pulmonary artery (PA) is somewhat enlarged. On the right, color imaging reveals diastolic flow within the PA, consistent with a patent ductus arteriosus. RV = right ventricle; RA = right atrium; LA = left atrium; AO = aorta.

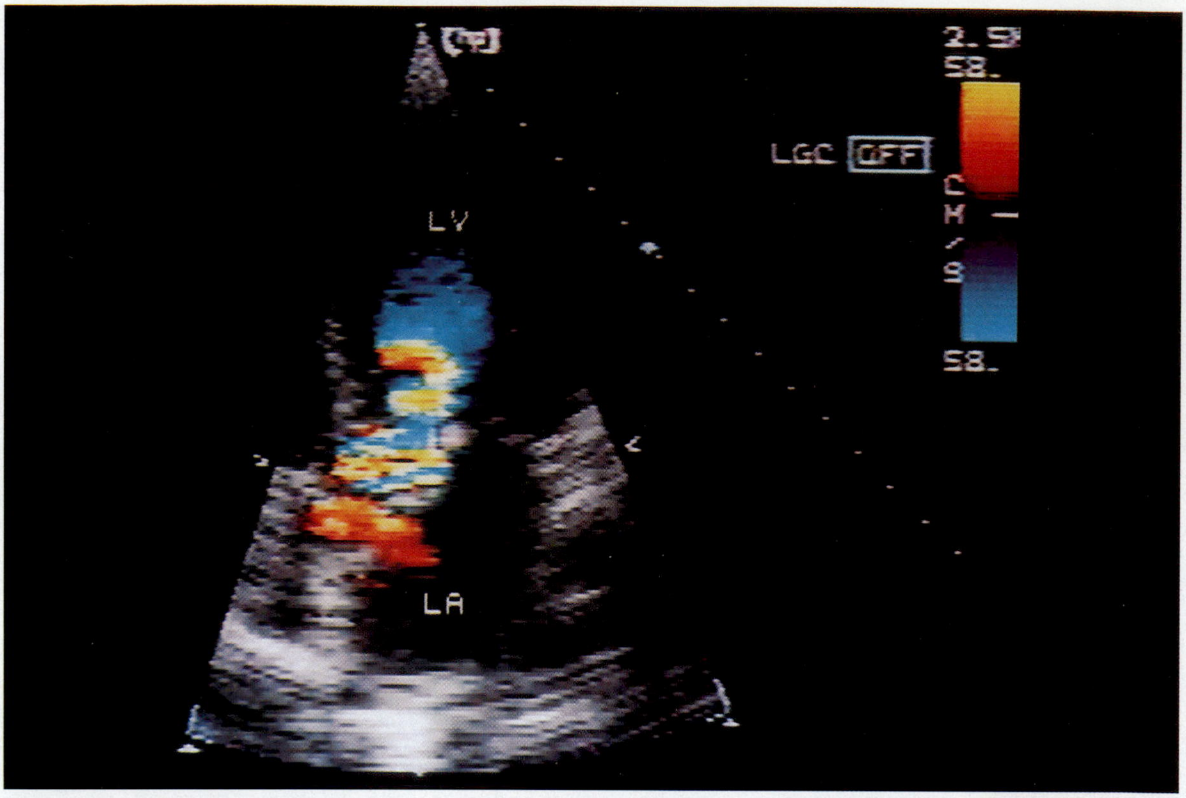

Plate 72 (FIGURE 13-122) Apical five-chamber view of discrete subaortic stenosis with color-flow Doppler, demonstrating aliasing and proximal flow convergence in the left ventricular outflow tract. LV = left ventricle; LA = left atrium.

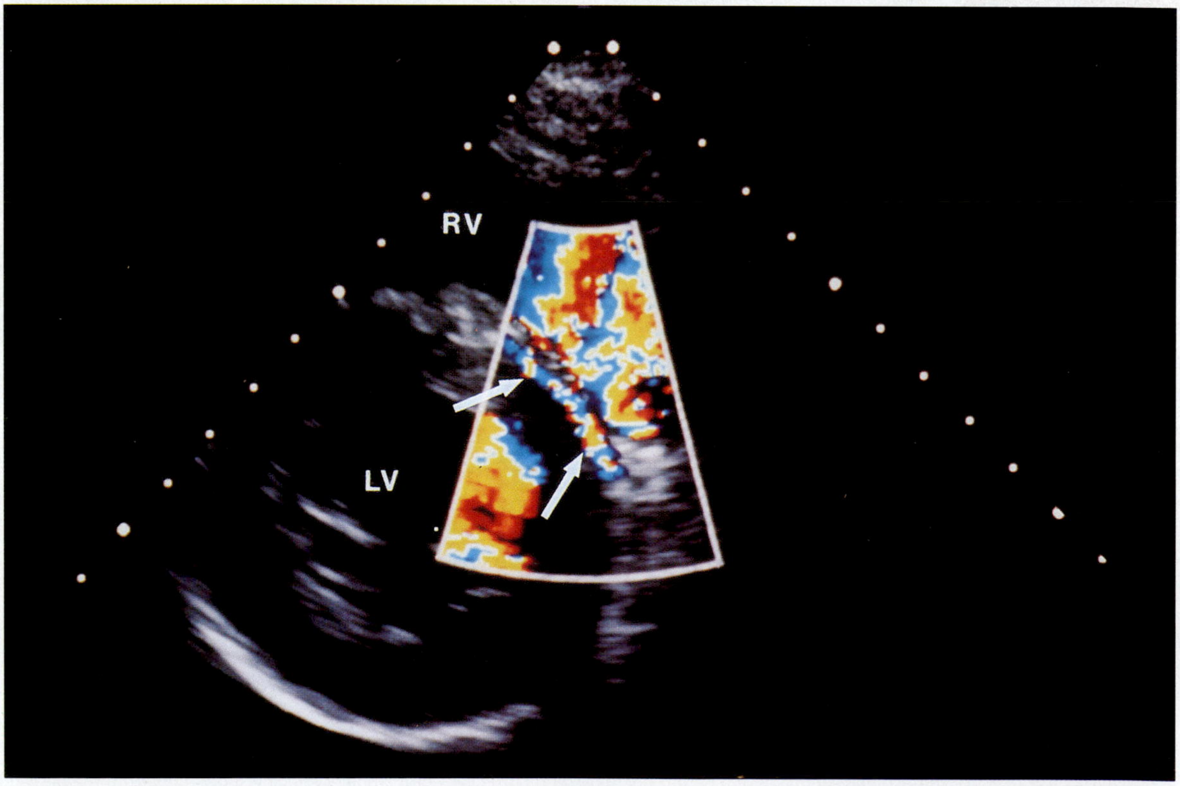

Plate 73 (FIGURE 13-141) Transthoracic short-axis image of a coronary artery within the interventricular septum (*arrows*). LV= left ventricle; RV = right ventricle.

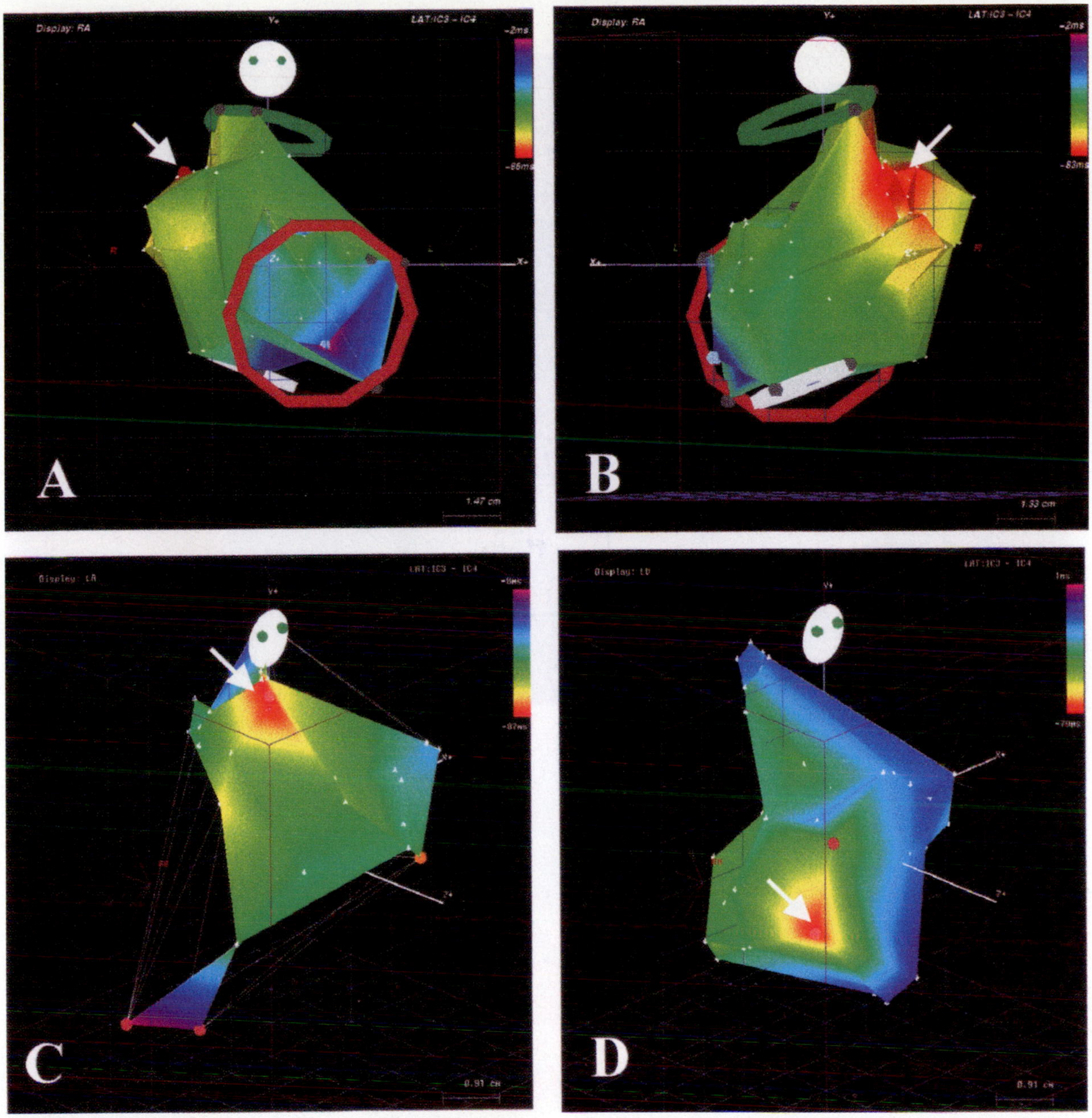

Plate 74 (FIGURE 24-5) Catheter-based mapping of the right atrium using a nonfluoroscopic electroanatomic mapping system that allows computer storage and recall of multisite activation patterns. Panels A and B demonstrate the activation sequence during normal sinus rhythm, with the earliest activation in the region of the sinus node (*arrows*) shown from (*A*) anterior and (*B*) posterior perspectives. The sequence of activation is indicated by the gradation of the color scale, based upon the reference times shown in the spectral bar. *C* and *D* were recorded from another patient who had episodic ectopic atrial tachycardia. In this oblique view, the sequence of activation during sinus rhythm is shown in *C*, with the earliest site of activation in red (*arrow*) representing the region of the sinus node. *D* was recorded during a low right atrial ectopic tachycardia. The earliest site of activation is indicated by the arrow.

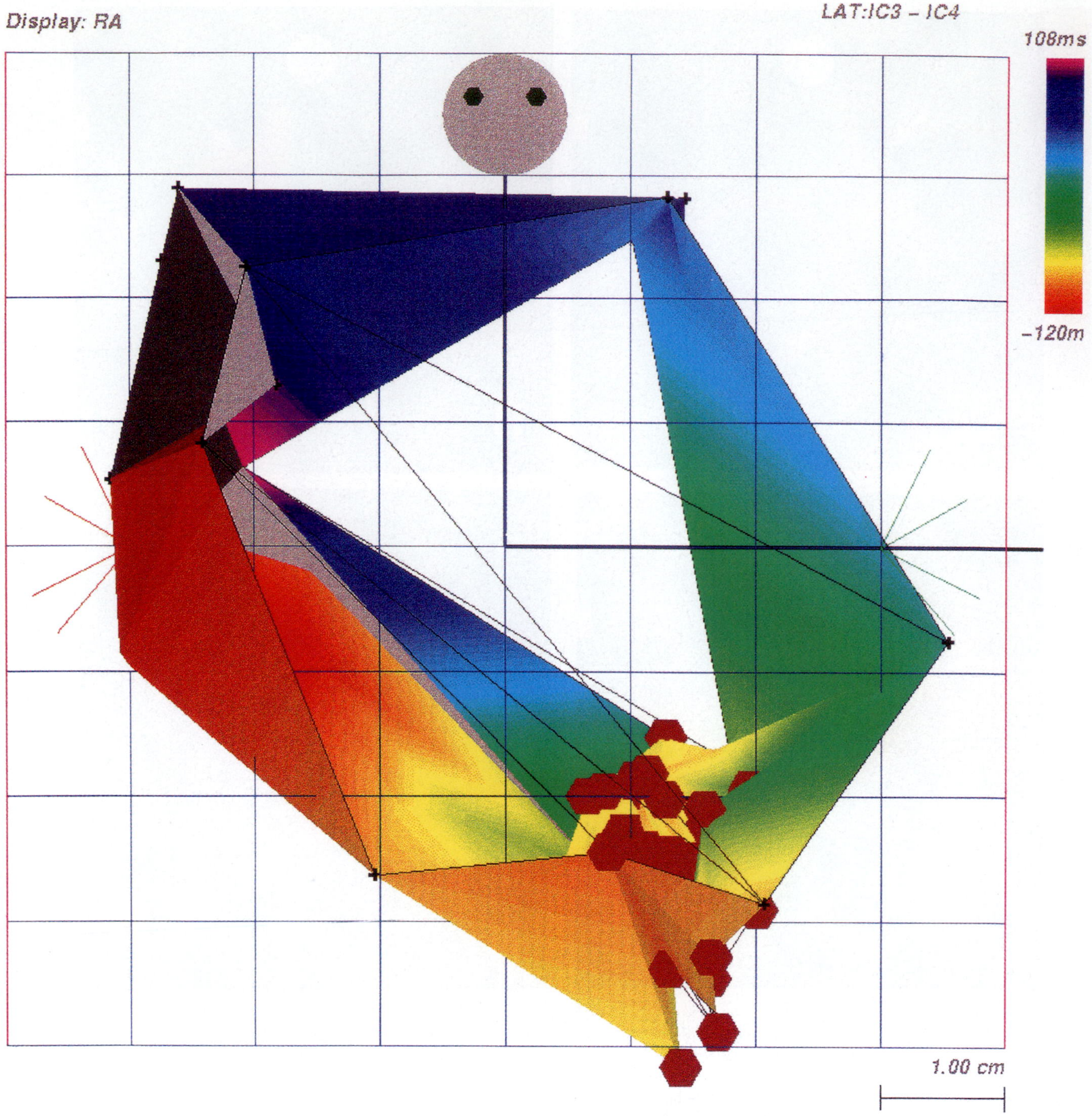

Plate 75 (FIGURE 26-3) Anterior-posterior view of the right atrium during typical, inferior vena cava (IVC)-tricuspid valve annulus isthmus-dependent atrial flutter using the Biosense CARTO system. The *red* shows the earliest activation with respect to the timing reference (typically the proximal coronary sinus recording), and the *blue* and the *violet* represent areas of late activation. The *gray* areas are where early activation meets late activation, a characteristic of reentrant tachycardias. The *brown* hexagons mark the location of radiofrequency lesions positioned on the isthmus to ablate the atrial flutter. RA = right atria.

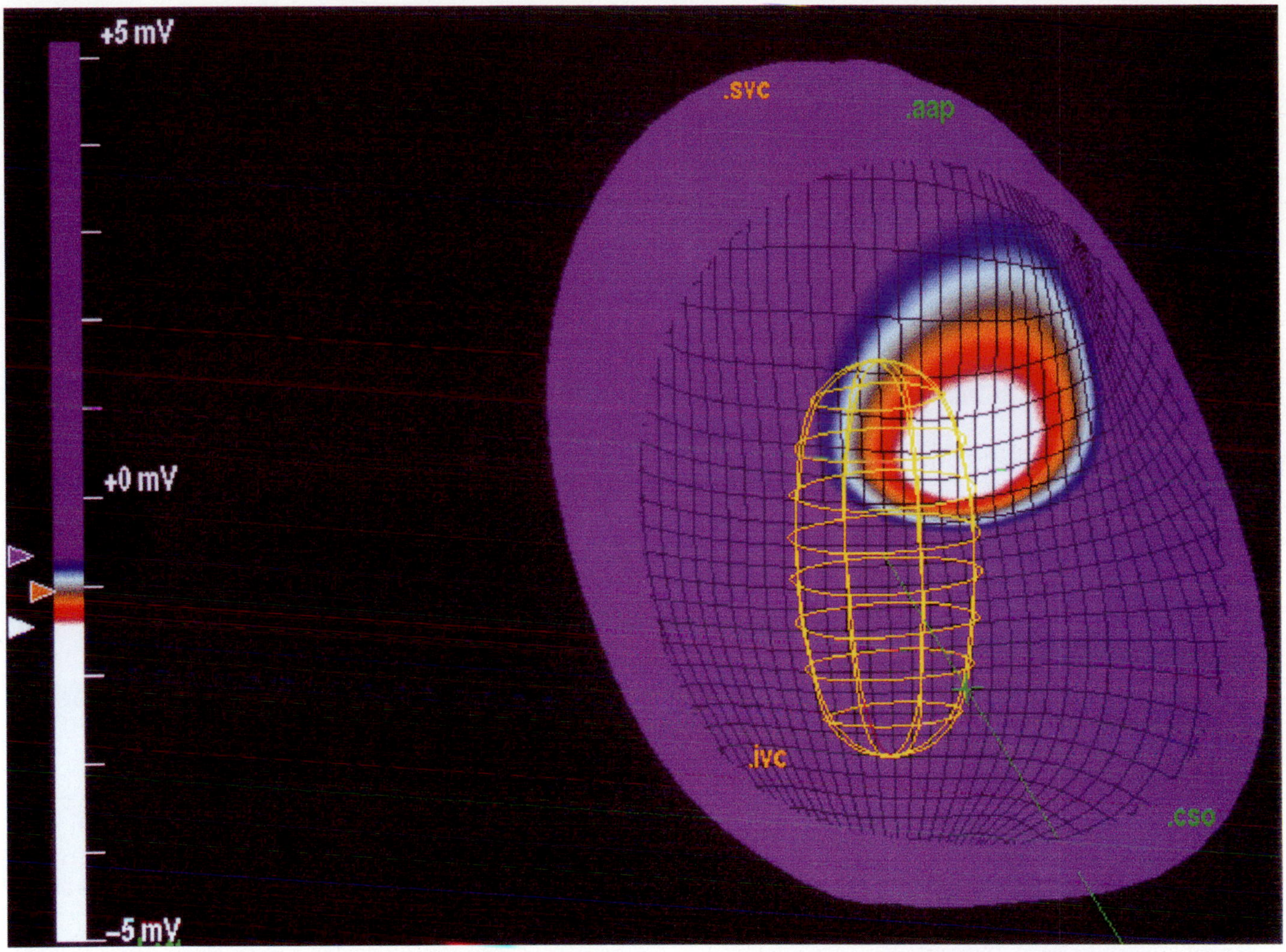

Plate 76 (FIGURE 26-4) Activation of the right atrium during focal atrial tachycardia, mapped with the Endocardial Solutions EnSite 3000 system. The *white* represents tissue that is fully activated, and *purple* is tissue that is not yet activated. SVC = superior vena cava; IVC = inferior vena cava.

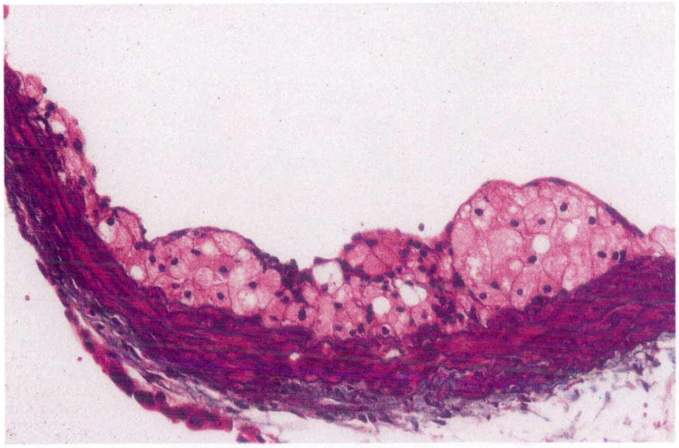

Plate 77 (FIGURE 35-1) An early atherosclerotic lesion (fatty streak) in the aortic root of a 3-month-old apolipoprotein $E^{-/-}$ mouse fed a high-fat Western-type diet for 6 weeks. The lesion consists of lipid-laden monocyte-derived macrophage foam cells and a few lymphocytes (T cells) beneath an intact endothelium. Elastin trichrome stain.

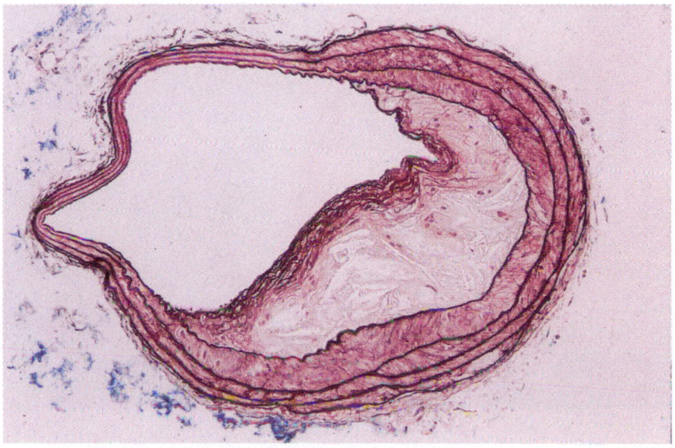

Plate 78 (FIGURE 35-2) An advanced atherosclerotic plaque in the brachiocephalic trunk of a 6-month-old apolipoprotein $E^{-/-}$ mouse fed normal chow. The plaque appears vulnerable morphologically, consisting of a lipid-rich core with cholesterol crystals covered by a thin fibrous cap. Orcein, staining elastic tissue black.

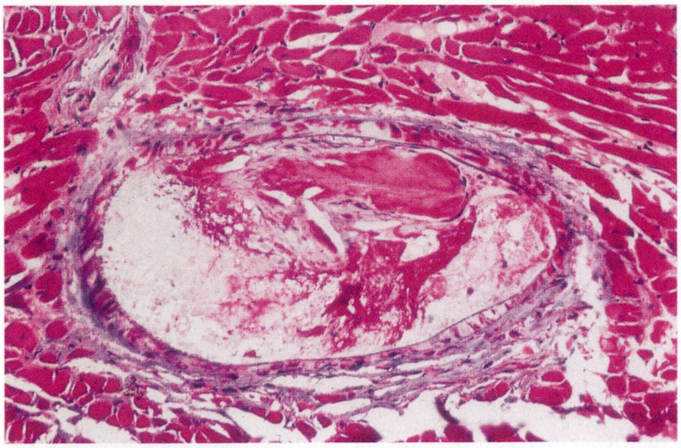

Plate 79 (FIGURE 35-3) Ruptured coronary plaque with occlusive thrombosis superimposed (natural death of a 21-month-old apolipoprotein $E^{-/-}$ mouse). Spontaneous plaque rupture and/or luminal thrombosis are extremely rare in animal models of atherosclerosis. Elastin trichrome stain.

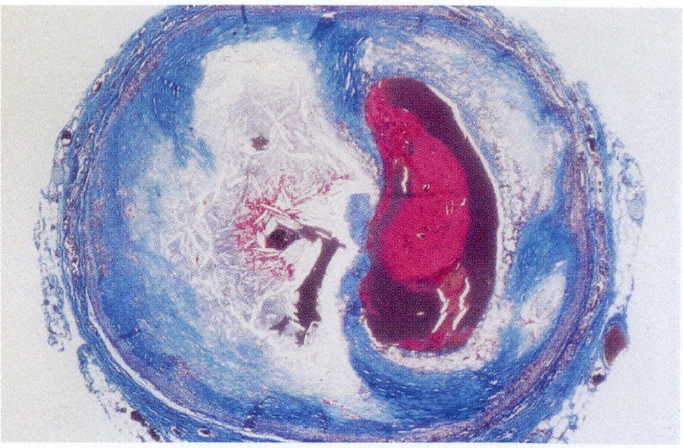

Plate 80 (FIGURE 35-5) Cross-sectioned coronary artery, containing a vulnerable plaque (large lipid-rich core covered by a thin fibrous cap) with ruptured surface and a nonocclusive luminal thrombosis superimposed. Trichrome stain.

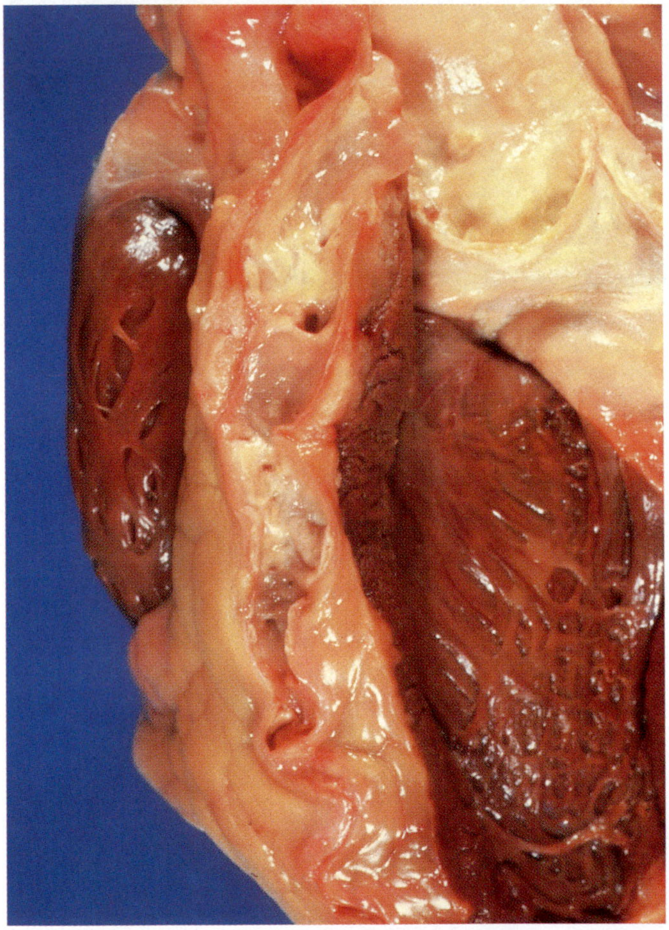

A

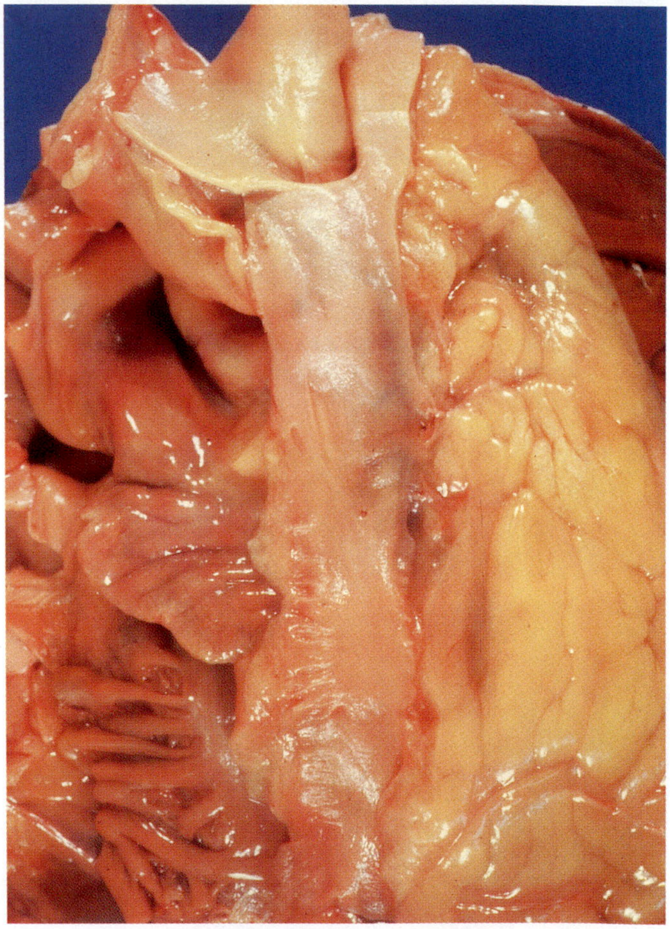

B

Plate 81 (FIGURE 35-8) Experiment of nature, illustrating the pathogenetic role of blood pressure in atherogenesis. The left anterior descending coronary artery (LAD) is departing normally and thus exposed to systemic blood pressure; the LAD is severely atherosclerotic, stiff, and calcified (*A*). In contrast, the right coronary artery (RC) is originating anomalously from the lower-pressure pulmonary trunk; the RC is elastic and compliant without atherosclerosis (*B*).

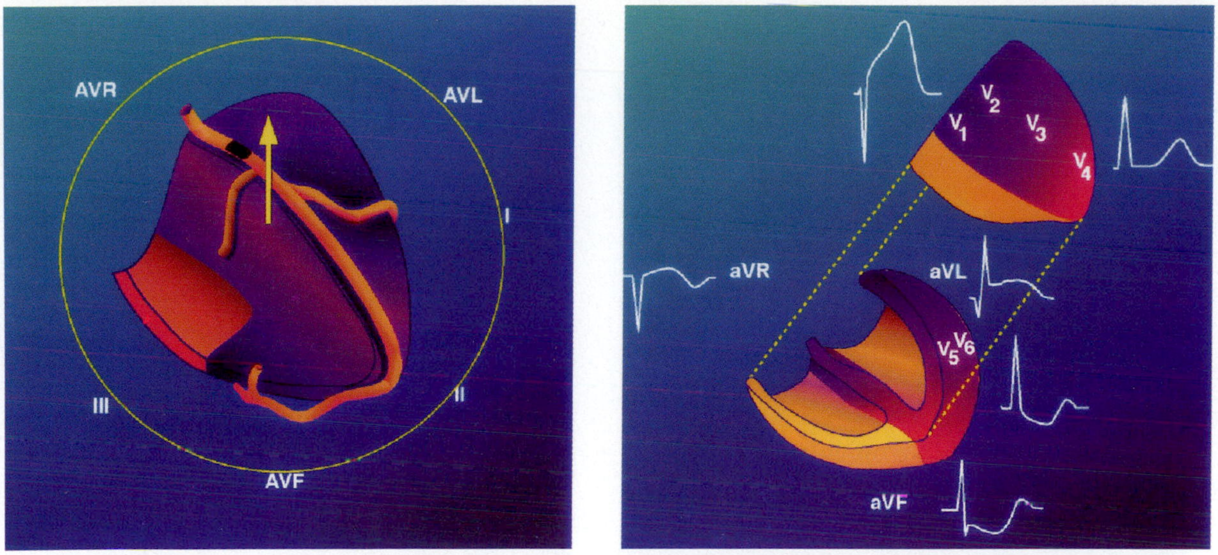

Plate 82 (FIGURE 43-2) Areas of left ventricular ischemia in LAD occlusion proximal to the first septal and first diagonal branch. *Left panel:* There is ischemia of the left ventricle. The ST-segment vector points in a superior direction because ischemia predominates in the basal areas. *Right panel:* The superiorly oriented ST vector leads to ST-segment elevation in lead aVR and lead V1 and ST-segment depression in the inferior leads and in V5 and V6.

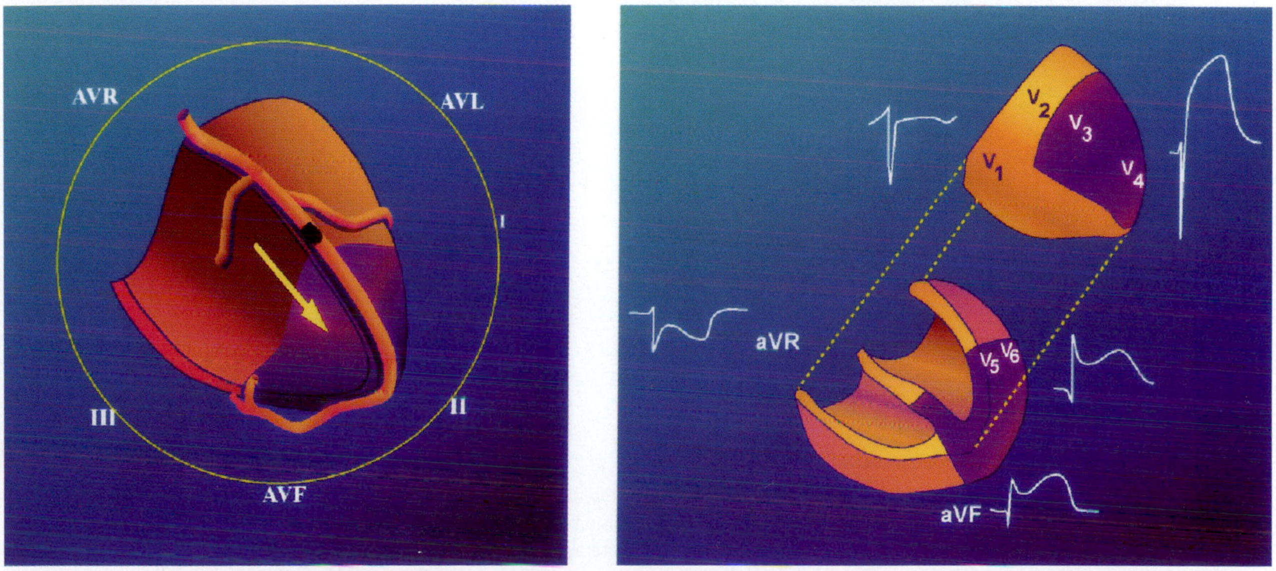

Plate 83 (FIGURE 43-4) Ischemic areas in distal LAD occlusion. *Left panel:* The ST vector points inferiorly due to ischemia of the inferoapical area. *Right panel:* The inferiorly directed ST vector leads to ST-segment depression in lead aVR and ST-segment elevation in the inferior leads.

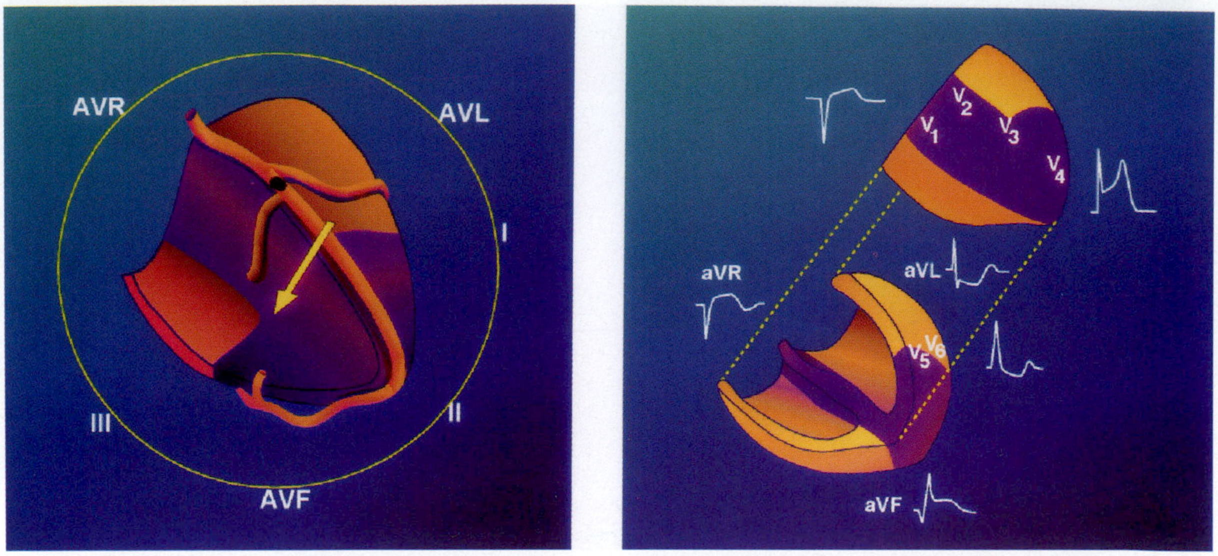

Plate 84 (FIGURE 43-6) Ischemic areas in LAD occlusion between the first diagonal (or intermediate) and first septal branch. *Left panel:* Predominance of ischemia in the septal-apical area leads to an ST-segment vector pointing in a rightward direction. *Right panel:* Apart from ST-segment elevation in the precordial leads, ST-segment elevation is also seen in leads III and aVR. Negativity of the ST segment is seen in lead aVL.

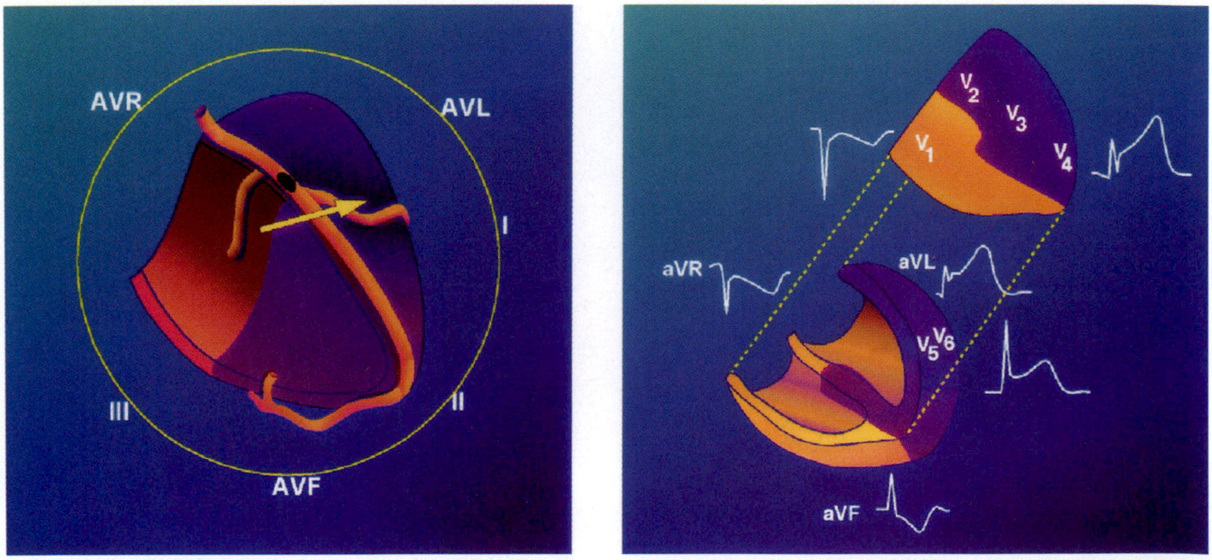

Plate 85 (FIGURE 43-8) Ischemic areas in LAD occlusion distal to the septal and proximal to the first diagonal branch. *Left panel:* Predominance of ischemia in the lateral area leading to an ST vector pointing in that direction. *Right panel:* The lateral orientation of the ST vector leads to ST-segment negativity of leads III and aVR. Lead II is isoelectric due to the perpendicular orientation of the ST vector in that lead. The lateral leads I and aVL show ST-segment elevation.

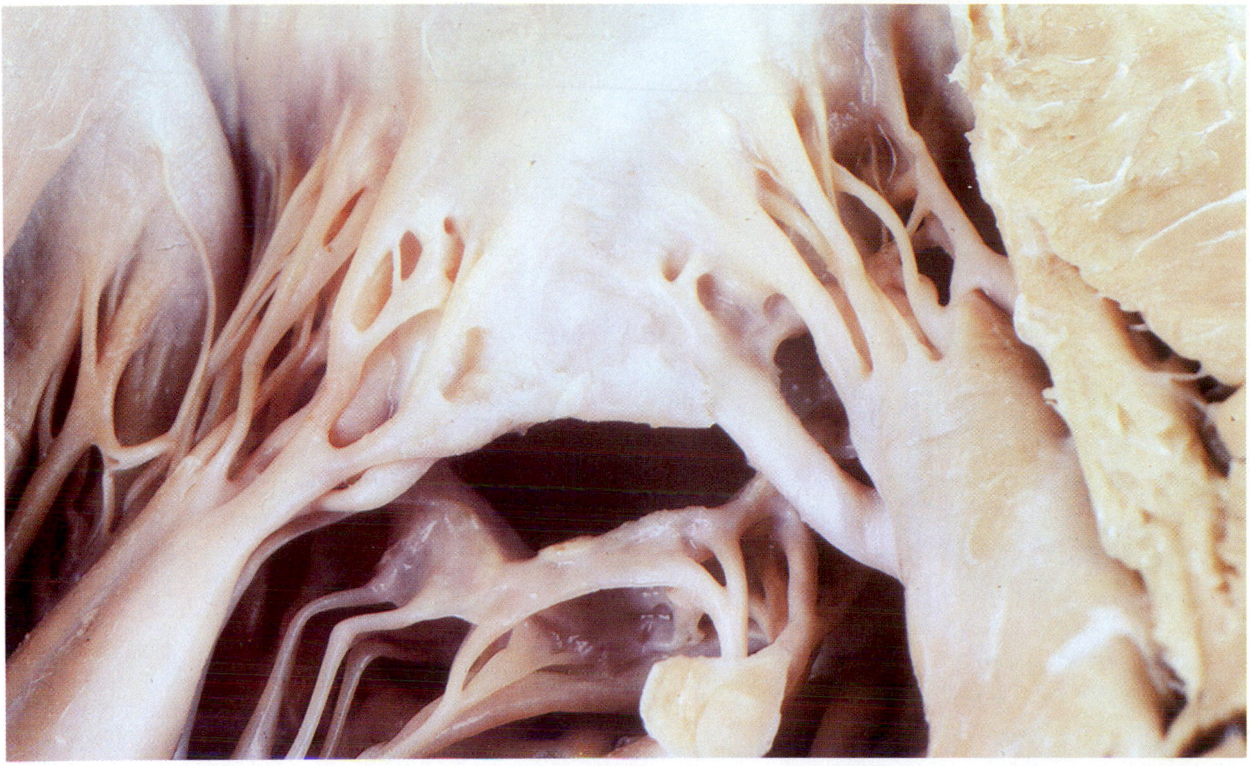

Plate 86 (FIGURE 57-7) Anatomic example of rheumatic MR. Note the thickening of the leaflet and chordae and the retraction of the mitral tissue. (Courtesy of Dr. W. D. Edwards.)

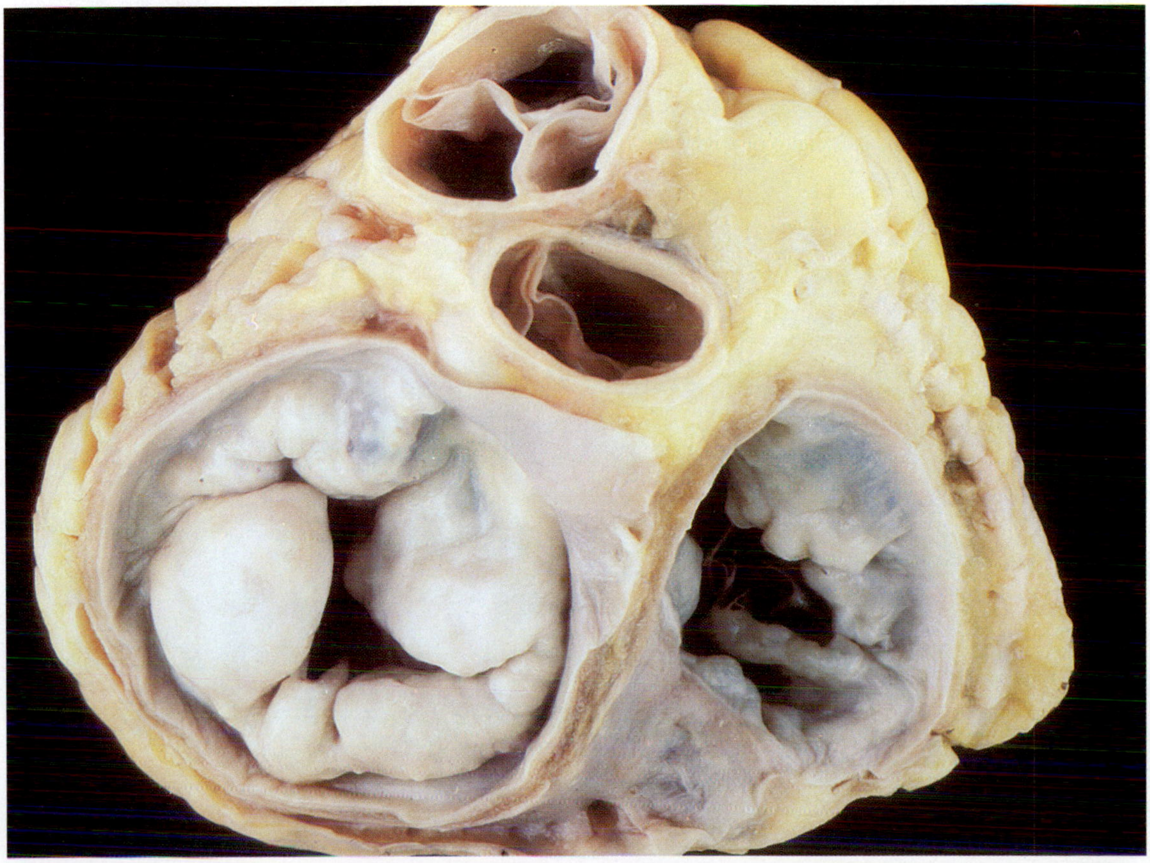

Plate 87 (FIGURE 57-8) Anatomic example of MR due to mitral valve prolapse seen from the atrial view (the mitral orifice is on the left of picture). Note the redundancy of the leaflets with excess tissue. (Courtesy of Dr. W. D. Edwards.)

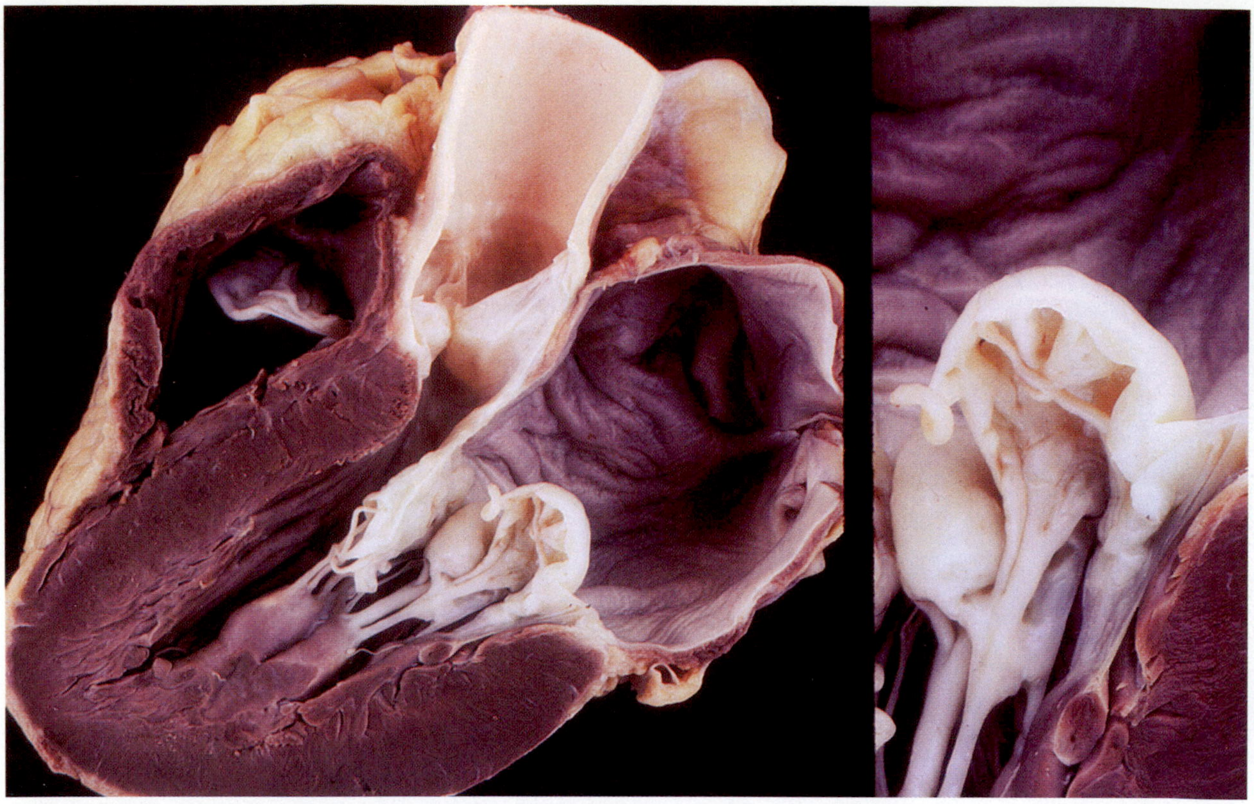

Plate 88 (FIGURE 57-9) Anatomic example of a flail posterior leaflet with ruptured chord. On the right of the picture, closeup view of the ruptured chord. Otherwise the left atrium is enlarged and the valvular tissue normal. (Courtesy of Dr. W. D. Edwards.)

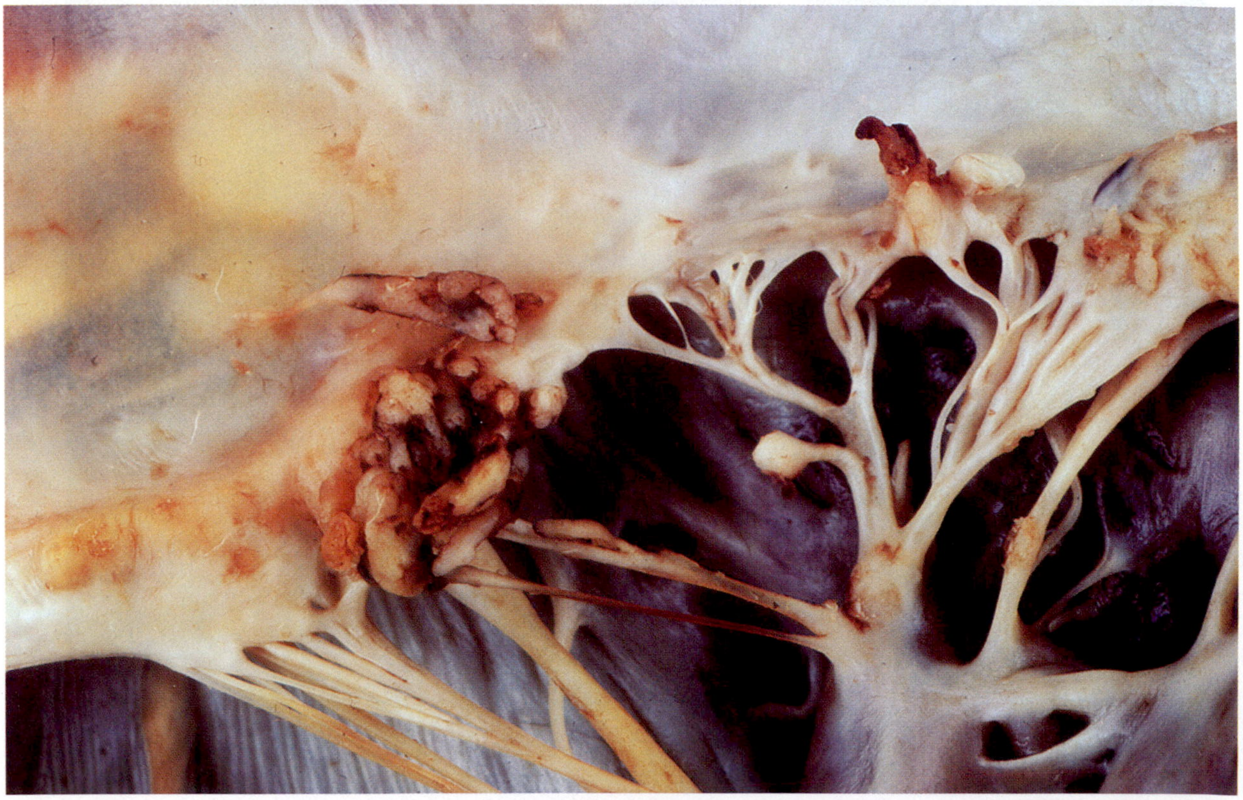

Plate 89 (FIGURE 57-10) Anatomic example of MR due to endocarditis. Note the vegetations of the anterior leaflet and the ruptured chords. (Courtesy of Dr. W. D. Edwards.)

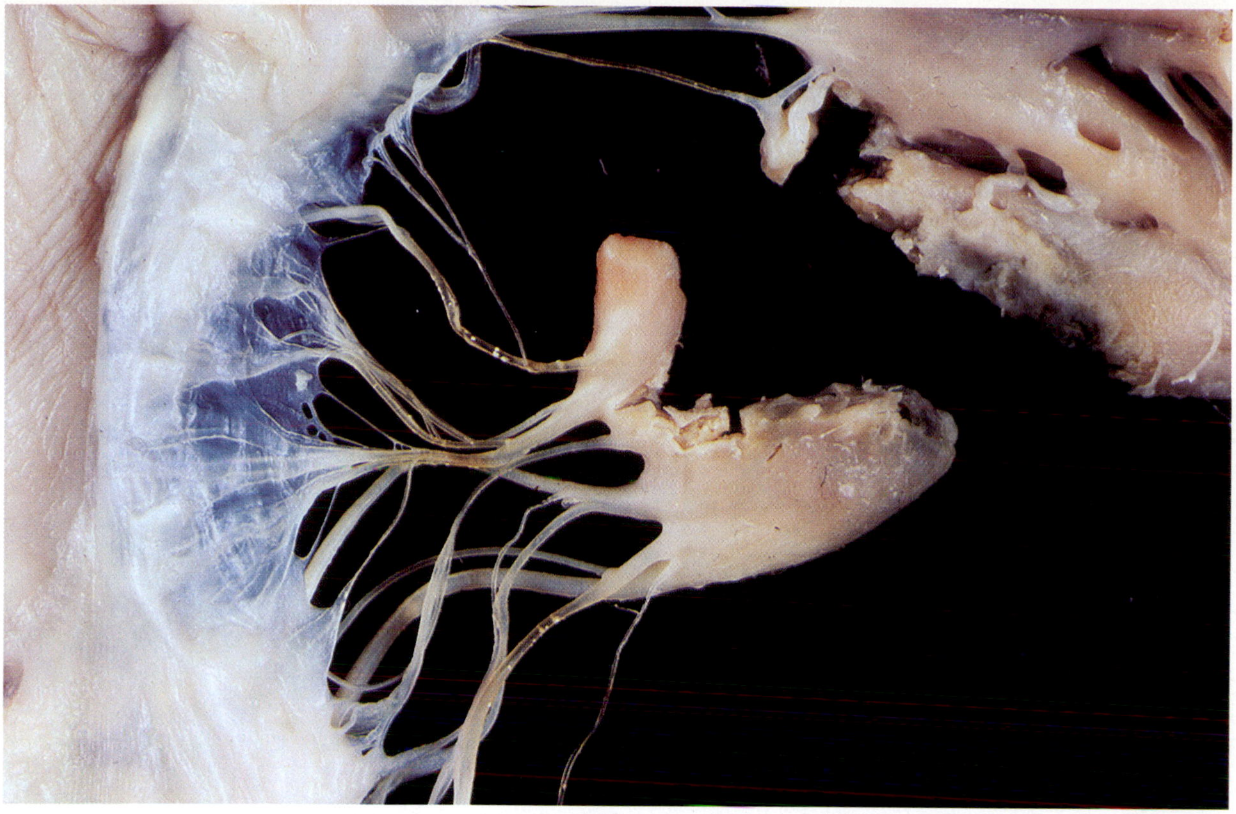

Plate 90 (FIGURE 57-11) Anatomic example of a ruptured posterior papillary muscle. Note the normal valvular tissue otherwise. (Courtesy of Dr. W. D. Edwards.)

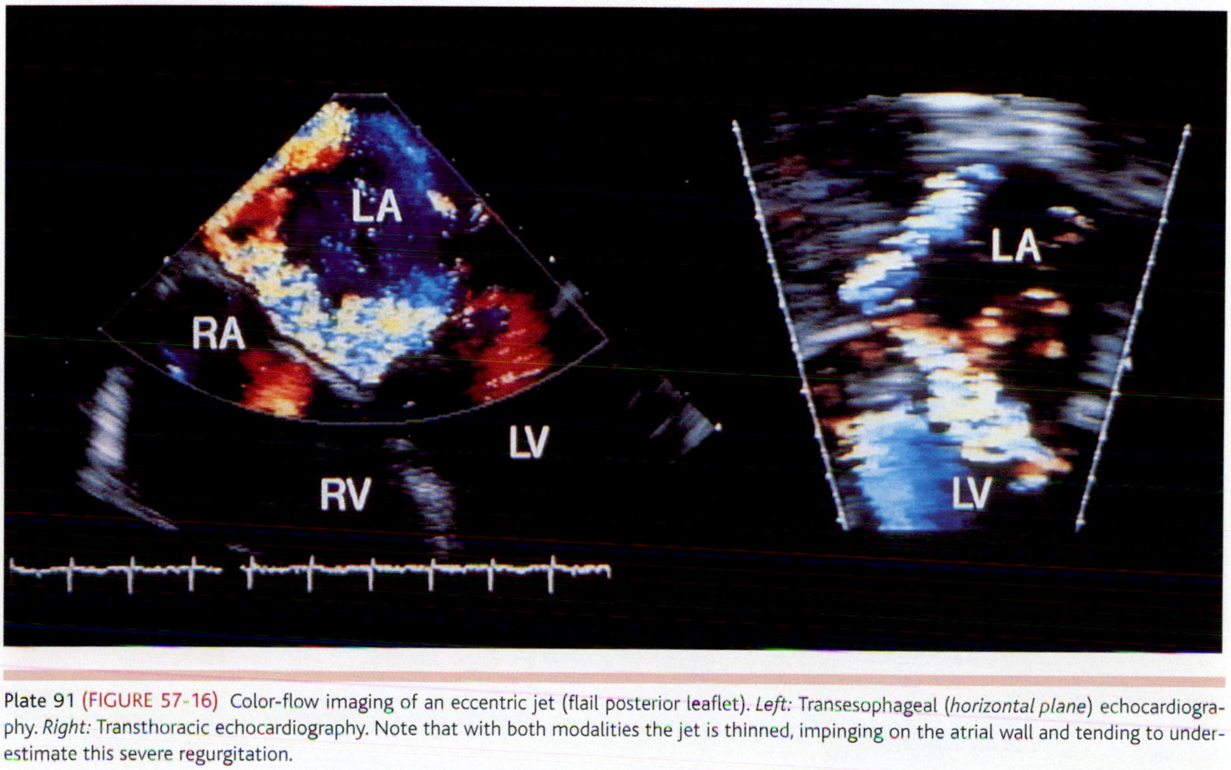

Plate 91 (FIGURE 57-16) Color-flow imaging of an eccentric jet (flail posterior leaflet). *Left:* Transesophageal (*horizontal plane*) echocardiography. *Right:* Transthoracic echocardiography. Note that with both modalities the jet is thinned, impinging on the atrial wall and tending to underestimate this severe regurgitation.

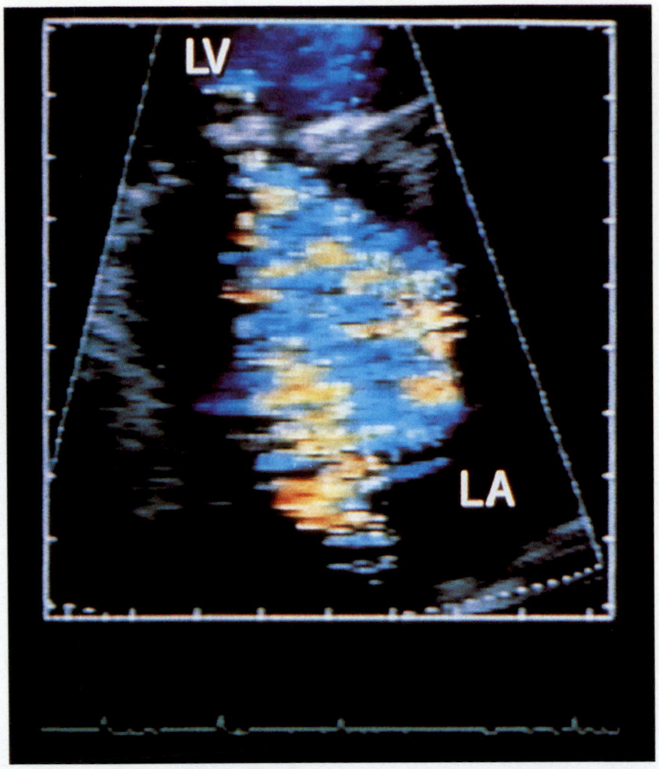

Plate 92 (FIGURE 57-17) Color flow imaging of a central jet of a functional mitral regurgitation by transthoracic echocardiography. Note that the jet is free, expands in the left atrium, and tends to overestimate this moderate regurgitation.

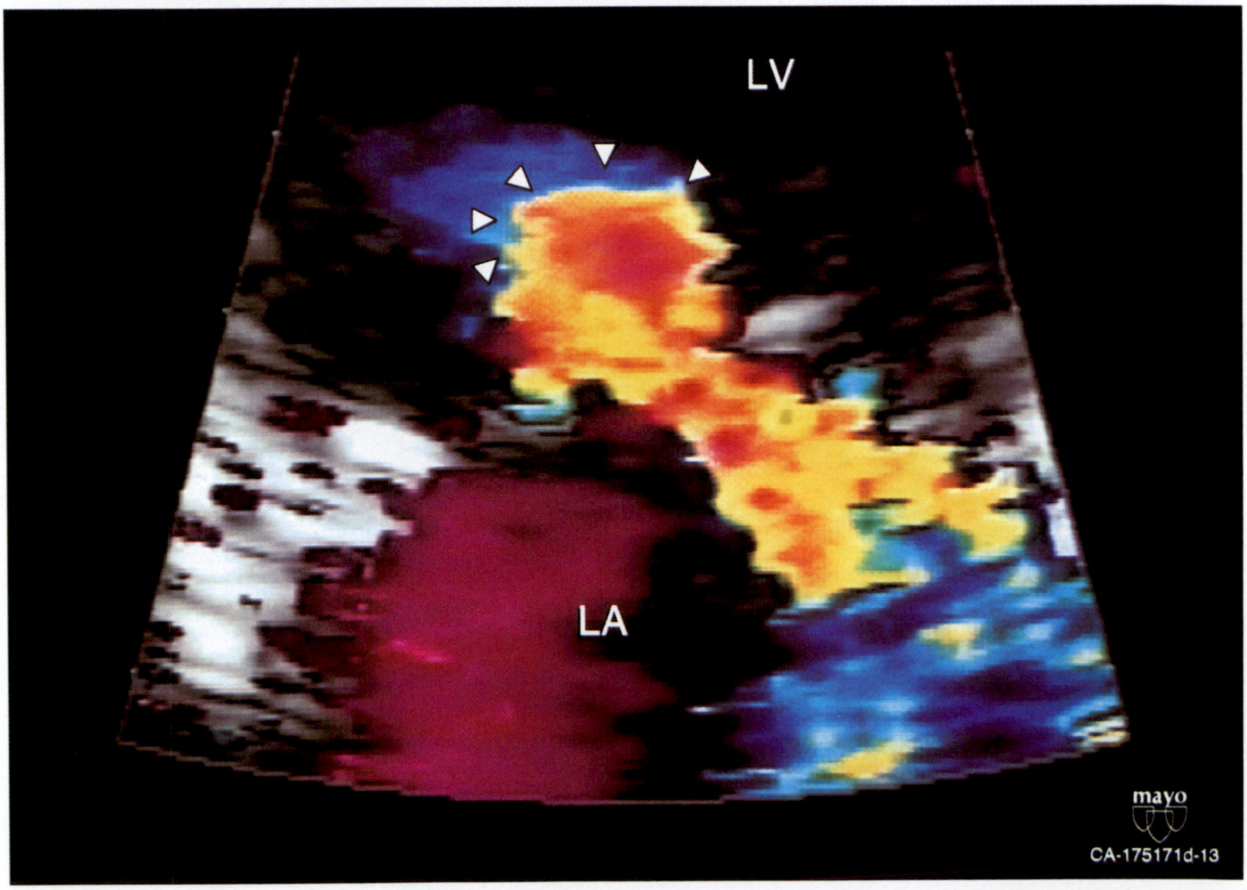

Plate 93 (FIGURE 57-19) Color flow imaging of the proximal flow convergence of a mitral regurgitation due to a flail posterior leaflet (by transthoracic echocardiography). The downward baseline shift of the color-flow scale enlarges the size of the flow convergence, which is easily measurable.

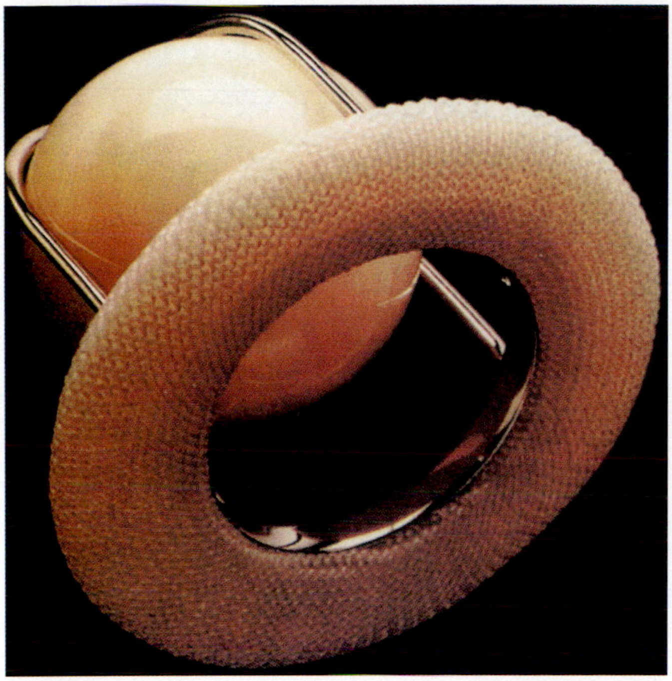

Plate 94 (FIGURE 60-1) Starr-Edwards caged ball valve. The ball is a silicone rubber polymer, impregnated with barium sulfate for radiopacity, which oscillates in a cage of cobalt-chromium alloy. When the valve opens, blood flows through the circular primary orifice and a secondary orifice between the ball and the housing. In the aortic position, there is a tertiary orifice between the ball and the aortic wall.

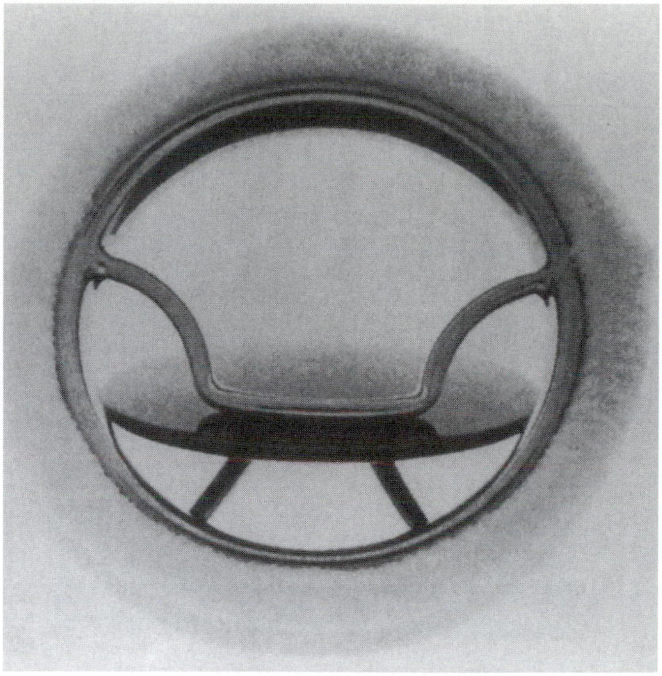

A

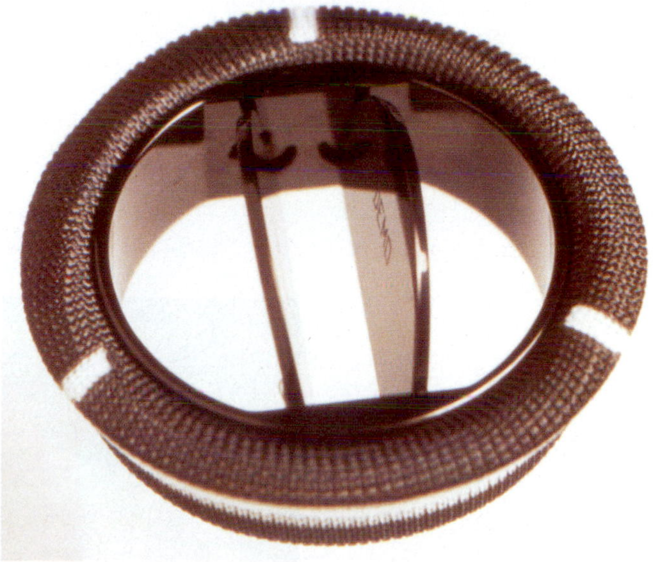

B

Plate 95 (FIGURE 60-2) Bileaflet valves. The St. Jude Medical valve (*A*) has leaflets that open to an angle of 85 degrees from the plane of the orifice and travel from 55 to 60 degrees to the fully closed position, depending on valve size. The original version, whose housing did not rotate within the sewing ring, has been supplemented by a model that does rotate for intraoperative adjustment. The Carbomedics valve (*B*) has flat leaflets that open to 78 to 80 degrees and close at an angle of 25 degrees with the horizontal and has a carbon-coated surface on the sewing ring to inhibit thrombus formation.

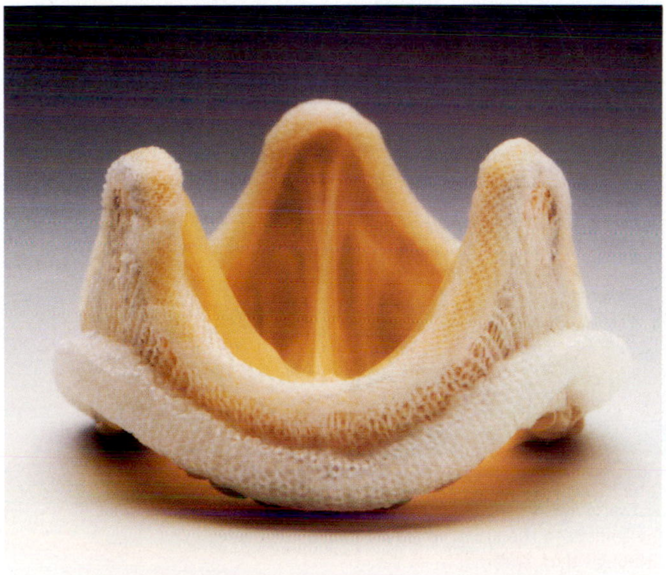

Plate 96 (FIGURE 60-3) Stented porcine valves. The Carpentier-Edwards SupraAnnular Valve is designed to be implanted above rather than within the aortic annulus. It has low-pressure fixation and a cone-shaped stent which flares out at the top to improve leaflet durability.

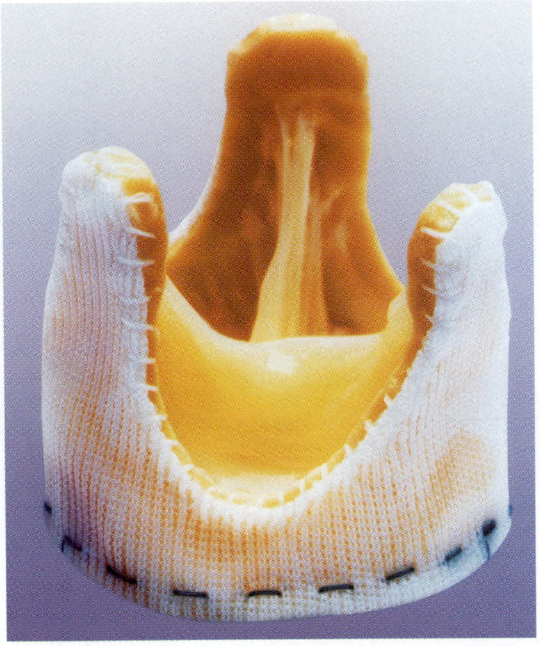

A

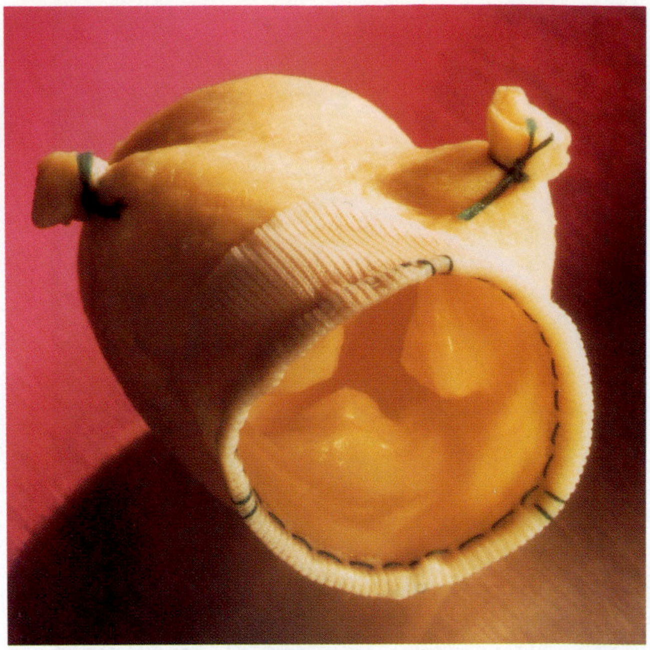

B

Plate 97 (FIGURE 60-4) St. Jude Toronto SPV (*A*) and Medtronic Freestyle (*B*) stentless porcine valves. The Toronto SPV is designed to be used as a subcoronary valve replacement. The Freestyle can be implanted using any of the methods of implantation used for homografts: subcoronary implantation of the valve alone, aortic root replacement, or cylinder (root) inclusion.

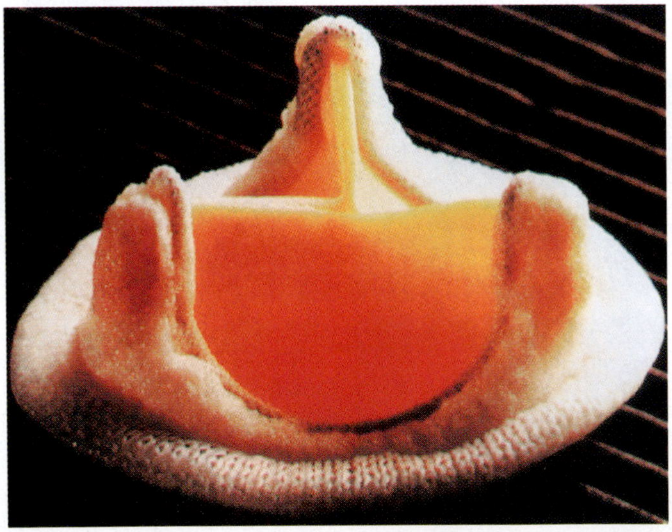

Plate 98 (FIGURE 60-5) The Carpentier-Edwards Perimount pericardial bioprosthesis uses a method of mounting the leaflets to the stent, which does not depend on retaining stitches passed through the pericardium—a design weakness of previous pericardial valves. Instead, the leaflets are anchored behind the stent pillars.

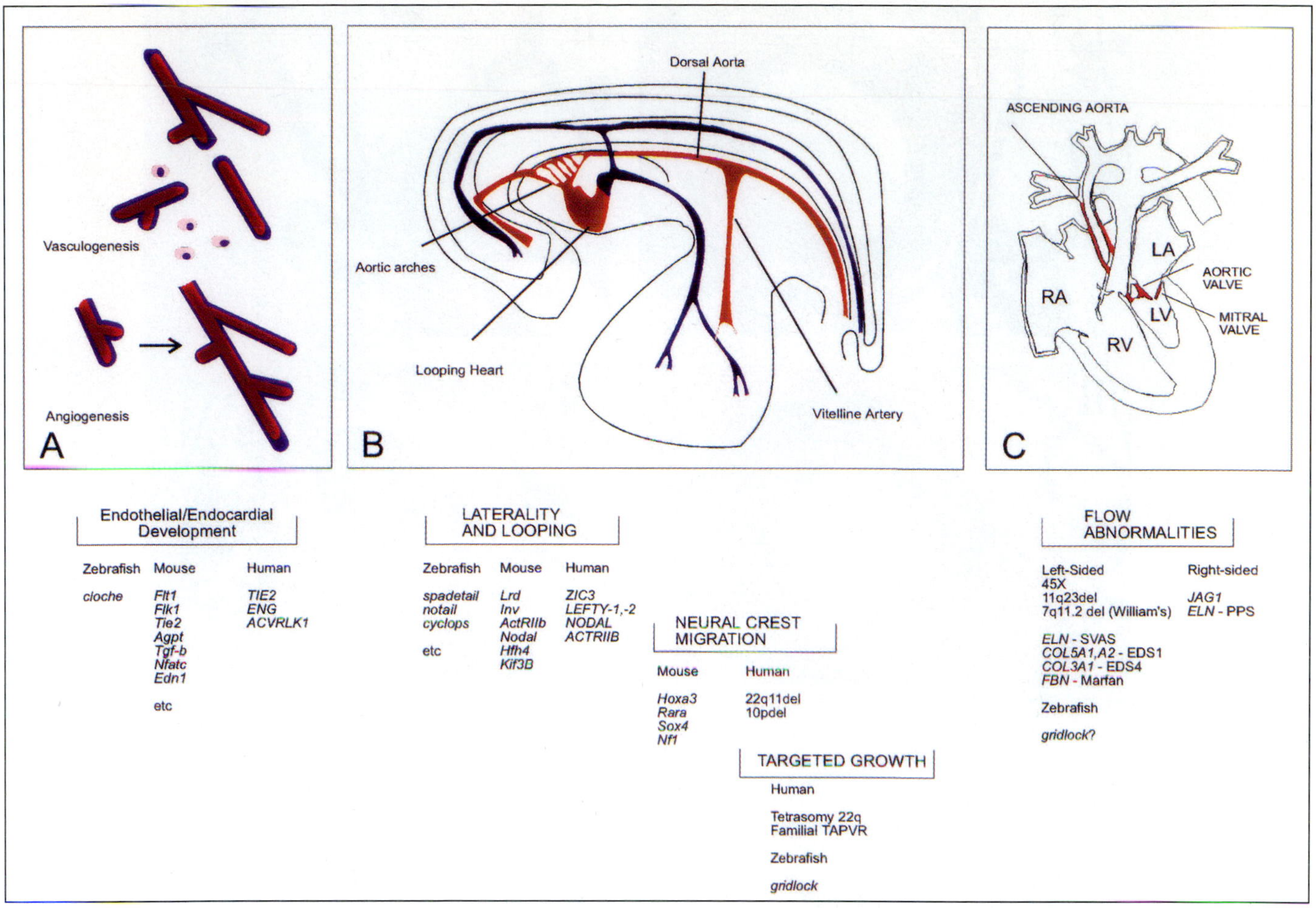

Plate 99 (FIGURE 62-16) Genetic defects causing congenital heart disease with or without genetic syndromes. Mutants from zebrafish, mouse, and human relating to primary developmental processes or maintenance of the vascular system are illustrated, including those of vasculogenesis and angiogenesis (*A*), embryonic development of the vascular system (*B*), and LV outflow tract obstruction (*C*).

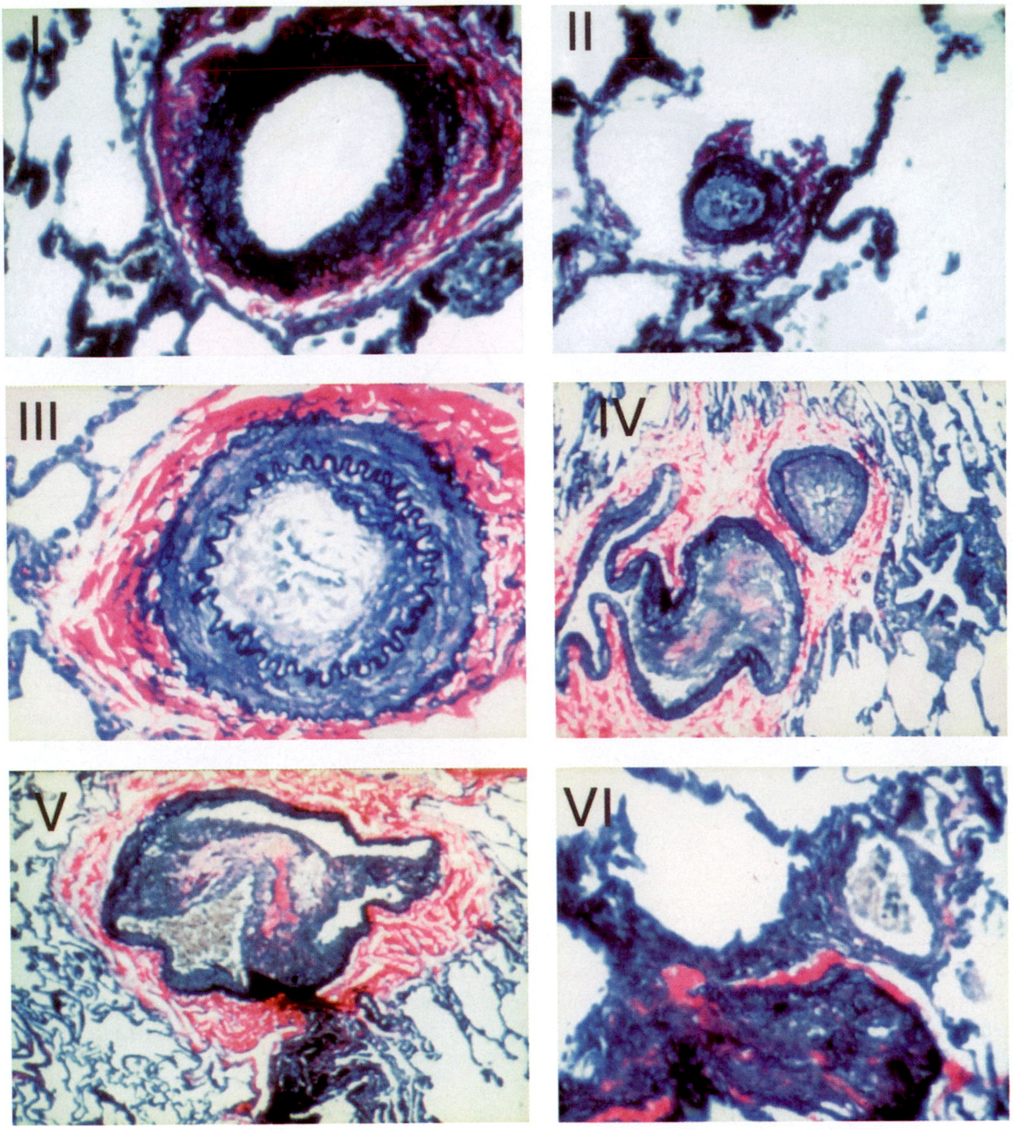

Plate 100 (FIGURE 63-4) Pulmonary vascular changes by the Heath and Edwards criteria (see text). Grades 1–6 are represented by panels I–VI, respectively.

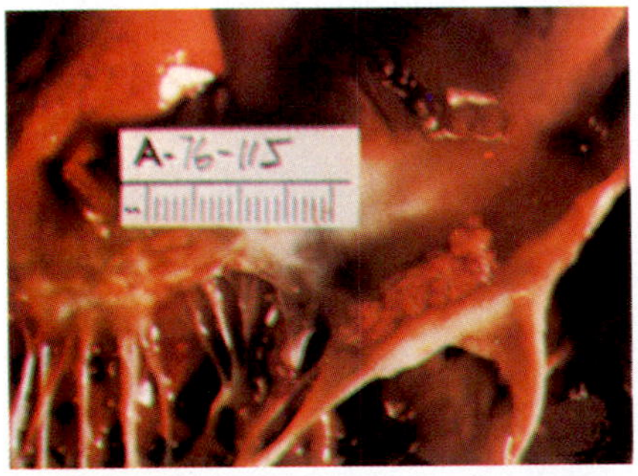

Plate 101 (FIGURE 73-3) Typical vegetation of nonbacterial thrombotic endocarditis found at necropsy in a cachectic patient who died with disseminated lung cancer.

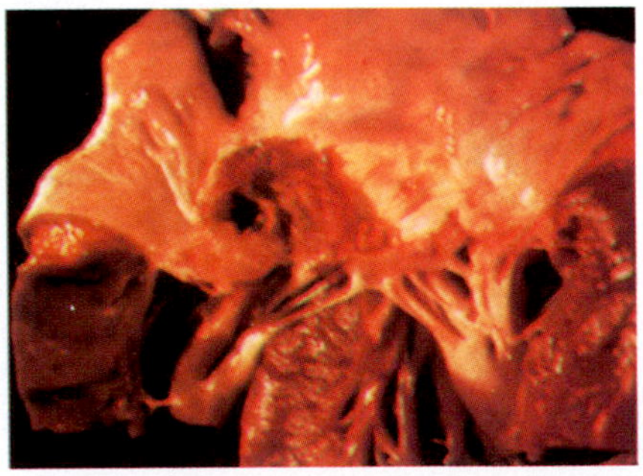

Plate 102 (FIGURE 73-5) Typical vegetation of bacterial endocarditis, complicated by perforation of the anterior mitral valve leaflet. Note that the valve shows preexisting chronic rheumatic disease, with thickening, deformity, and fusion of chordae tendineae.

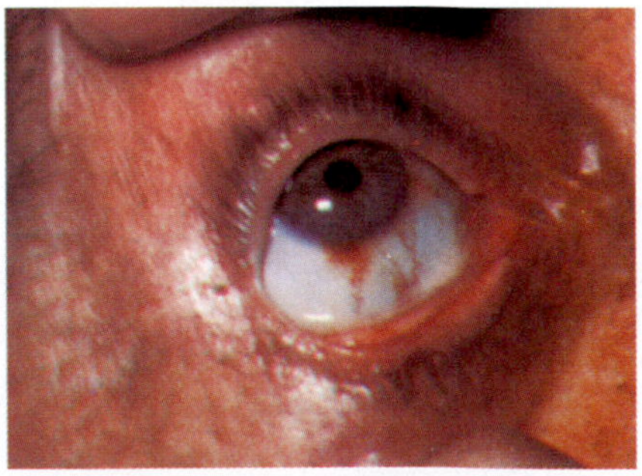

Plate 103 (FIGURE 73-7) Typical conjunctival petechiae in a patient with subacute bacterial endocarditis due to *Streptococcus sanguis*.

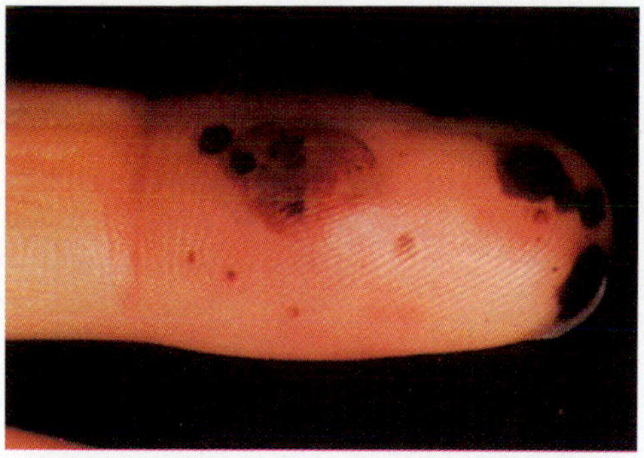

Plate 104 (FIGURE 73-8) Ischemic, hemorrhagic, and pustular lesions on the extremities in acute *Staphylococcus aureus* endocarditis.

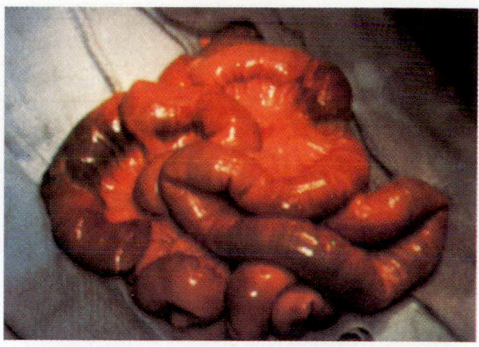

Plate 105 (FIGURE 73-9) Segmental ischemia and necrosis in the gut, presenting as acute abdomen.

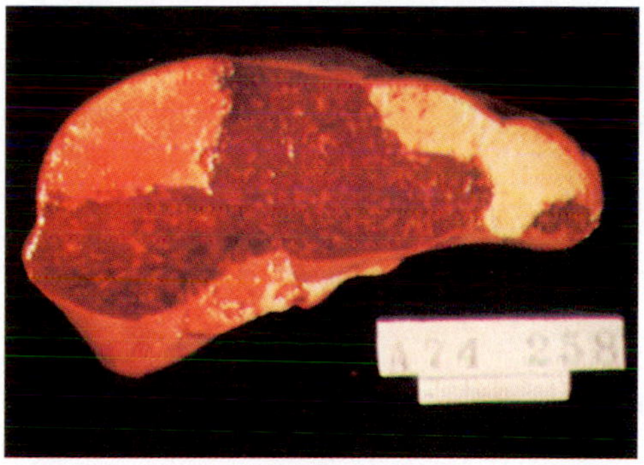

Plate 106 (FIGURE 73-10) Infarctions in the spleen.

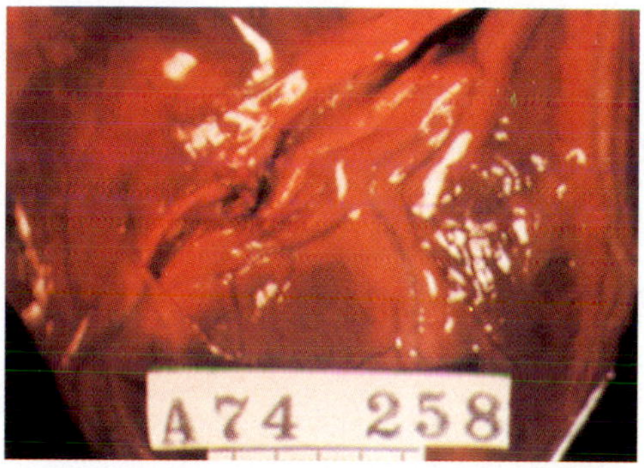

Plate 107 (FIGURE 73-11) An infected embolus in a coronary artery.

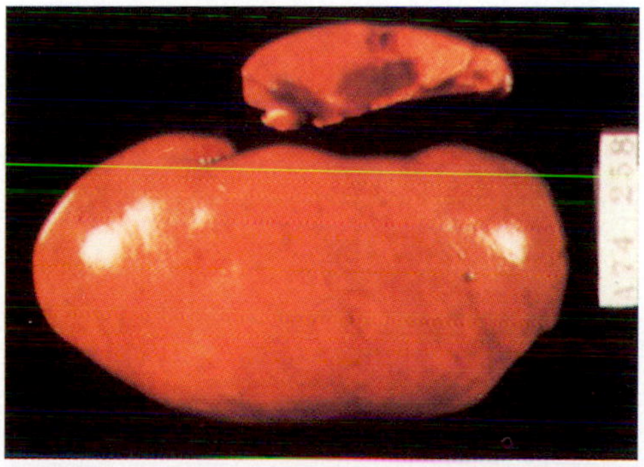

Plate 108 (FIGURE 73-12) Kidney from a patient with subacute bacterial endocarditis, showing two abnormalities: (1) typical ischemic infarctions due to emboli and (2) swelling and petechiae (flea-bitten kidney) due to immune-complex glomerulonephritis.

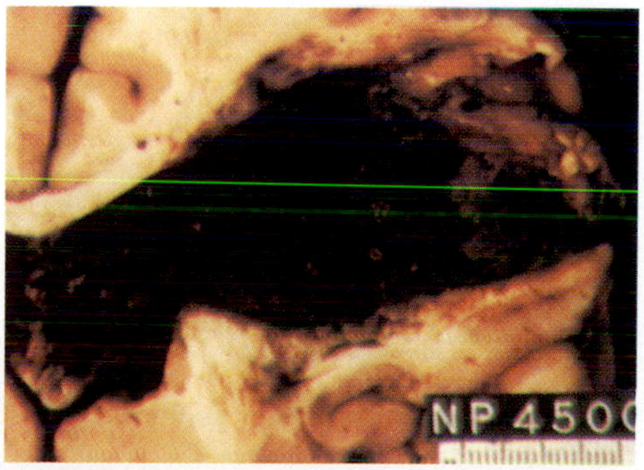

Plate 109 (FIGURE 73-13) Massive cerebral hemorrhage with intraventricular extension due to rupture of a small, peripheral mycotic aneurysm. The patient had been bacteriologically cured of *Staphylococcus epidermidis* endocarditis several weeks previously. Cultures of the blood, valve, and aneurysm taken at necropsy were negative.

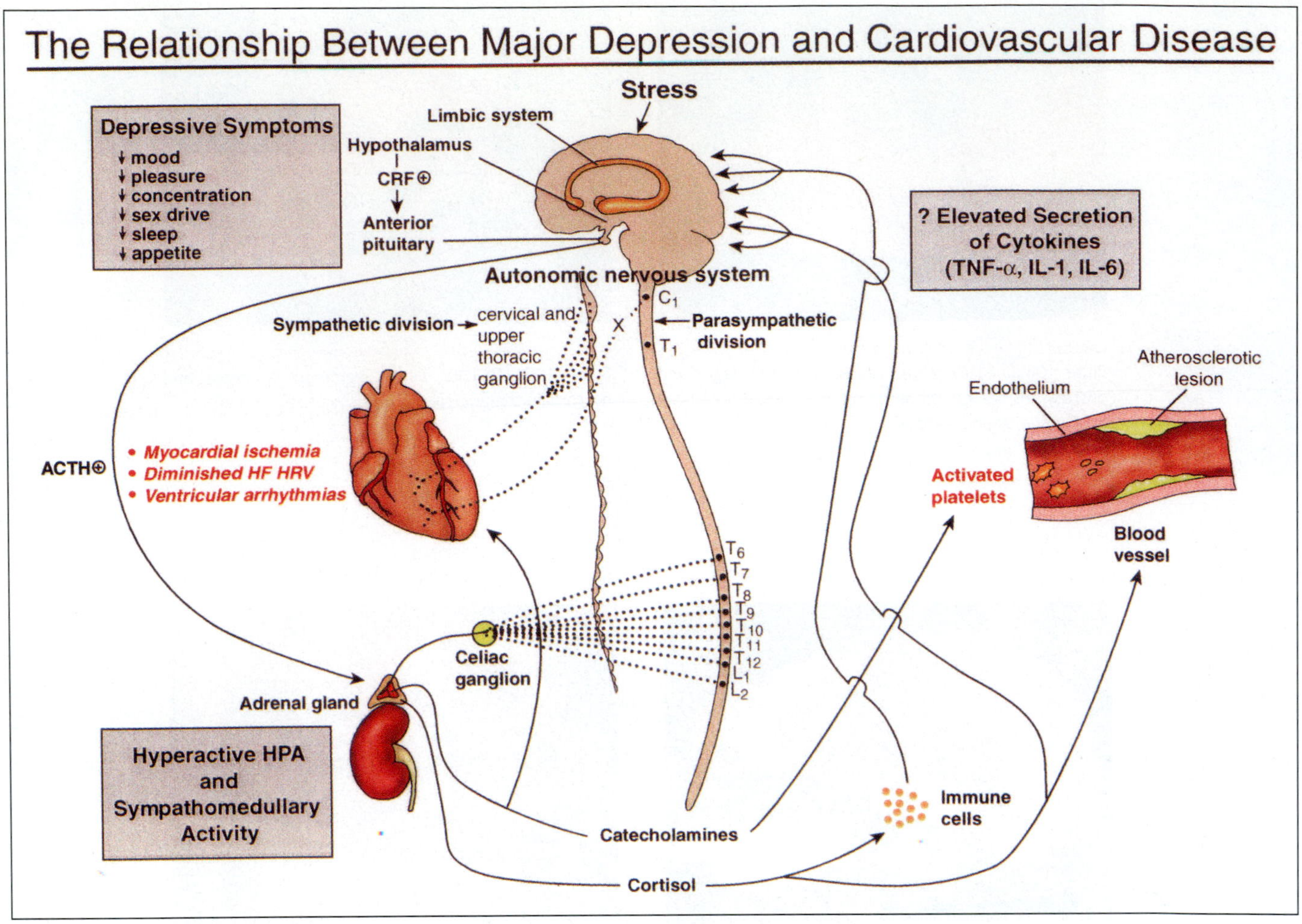

Plate 110 (FIGURE 80-1) Hypothetical schema of pathophysiologic findings associated with depression that probably contribute to increased susceptibility to cardiovascular disease. Autonomic nervous system innervation of the heart via the parasympathetic vagus (X) nerve and sympathetic (postganglionic efferents from the cervical and upper thoracic paravertebral ganglia) nerves is shown. CRF = corticotropin-releasing factor; ACTH = corticotropin; TNF-α = tumor necrosis factor α IL-1 = interleukin-1; IL-6 = interleukin-6; HRV = heart rate variability; HPA = hypothalamic-pituitary-adrenocortical axis.

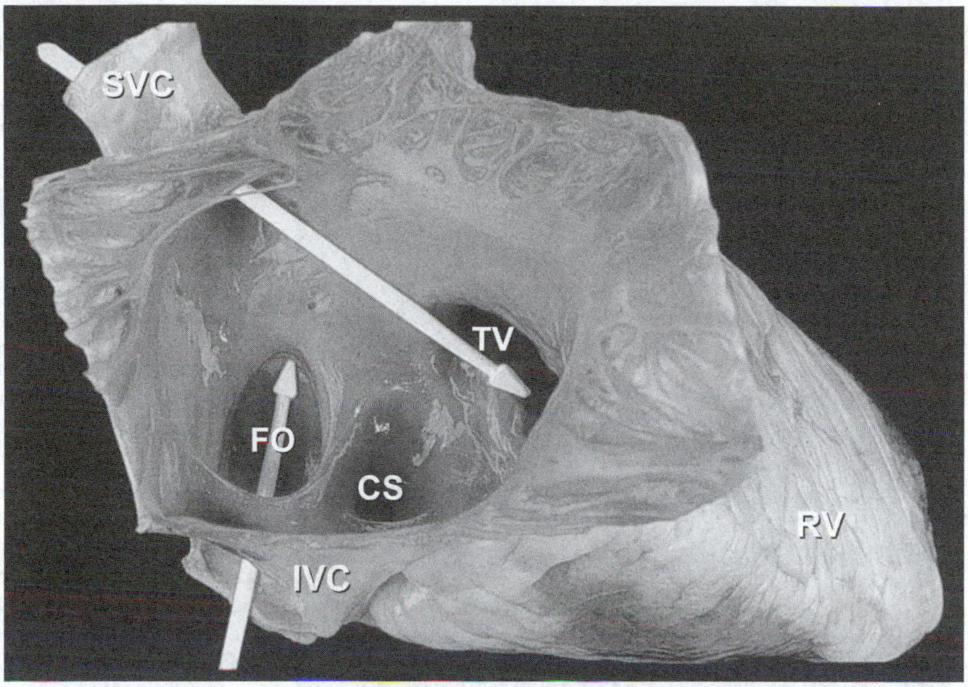

FIGURE 2-47 (Plate 17) Opened right atrium. Two arrow-shaped probes show that superior vena caval flow is directed toward the tricuspid orifice and inferior vena caval flow is directed toward the fossa ovalis (FO). CS, coronary sinus; IVC, inferior vena cava; RV, right ventricle; SVC, superior vena cava ; TV, tricuspid valve.

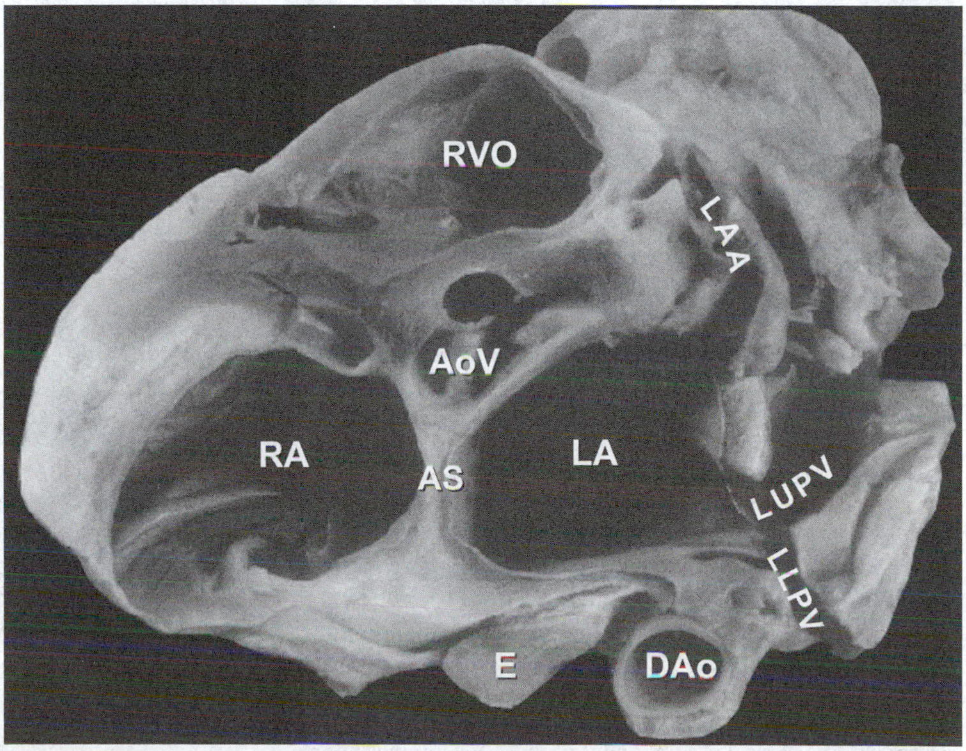

FIGURE 2-48 Oblique, short-axis cut at the base of the heart. The esophagus (E) is posterior and adjacent to the left atrium (LA) and adjacent to the descending thoracic aorta (DAo). The left upper pulmonary (LUPV) and left lower pulmonary vein (LLPV) are clearly seen. The right ventricular outflow tract (RVO) is anterior. AS, atrial septum; AoV, aortic valve; LA, left atrium; LAA, left atrial appendage; RA, right atrium.

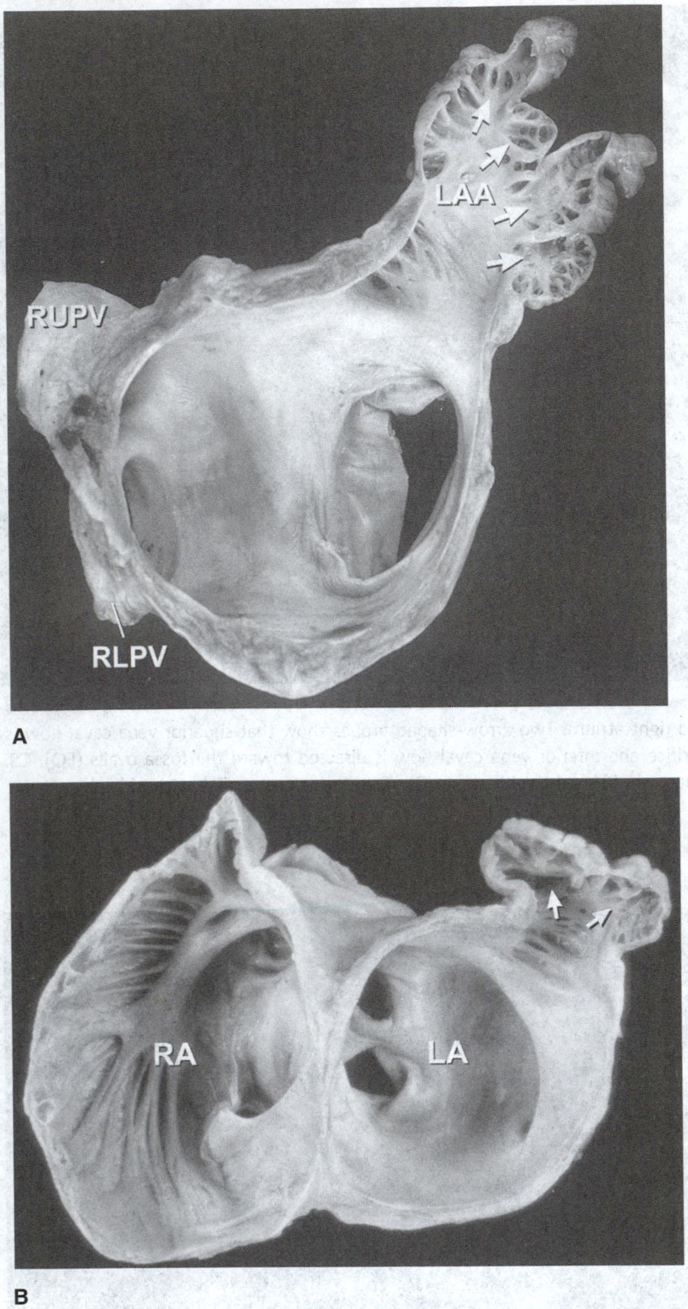

FIGURE 2-49 (Plate 18) Left atrial appendages (LAA). A. Left atrial free wall showing appendage with four lobes (arrows). B. Biatrial specimen demonstrating left atrial appendage with two lobes (arrows). LA, left atrium; RA, right atrium; RLPV, right lower pulmonary vein; RUPV, right upper pulmonary vein.

landmark because it contains the AV *node and proximal portion of the* AV *(His) bundle. Thus, during tricuspid annuloplasty procedures and patch closures of membranous ventricular septal defects, care must be taken to avoid injury to the conduction system.*[16,17] The muscular component of the AV septum is interposed between the membranous septum anteriorly and the internal cardiac crux posteriorly.

When defects occur in the muscular atrioventricular septum, the mitral annulus usually drops to the same level as the tricuspid annulus, so the defect becomes primarily interatrial (primum atrial septal defect), and the AV *conduction tissues are displaced inferiorly*. Lipomatous hypertrophy of the atrial septum is characterized by excessive accumulation of adipose tissue within the limbus of the fossa ovalis but always sparing the valve of the fossa[7,15–17] (Fig. 2-45, Plate 16). Lipomatous hypertrophy of the atrial septum occurs commonly but not exclusively in older and obese persons.[15–17] *Although readily detected by echocardiography, it may be misinterpreted as a thrombus or tumor.*[7]

Right Atrium

A prominent internal muscle ridge, the crista terminalis (Fig. 2-46), separates the right atrial free wall into a smooth-walled posterior region that receives the venae cavae and coronary sinus and a muscular anterior region that is lined by parallel pectinate muscles and from which the right atrial appendage emanates.[15–17] *Pectinatus* is Latin for "comb," and the pectinate muscles and crista terminalis resemble the teeth and backbone of a comb, respectively.[17] The right atrial appendage abuts the right aortic sinus and overlies the proximal right coronary artery (see Fig. 2-52). *The right atrial free wall is paper thin between pectinate muscles and therefore can be perforated easily by stiff catheters.*[15–17]

Inferior vena caval blood flow is directed by the eustachian valve toward the foramen ovale, and superior vena caval blood is directed toward the tricuspid valve[15] (Fig. 2-47, Plate 17). *Thus transseptal cardiac catheterization is more easily accomplished via the inferior vena cava, whereas instrumentation of the right ventricular apex (e.g., endomyocardial biopsy, placement of ventricular pacemaker lead) is more easily accomplished via the superior vena cava.*[15]

Left Atrium

The pulmonary vein orifices lie on the posterolateral (left pulmonary veins) and posteromedial (right pulmonary veins) as-

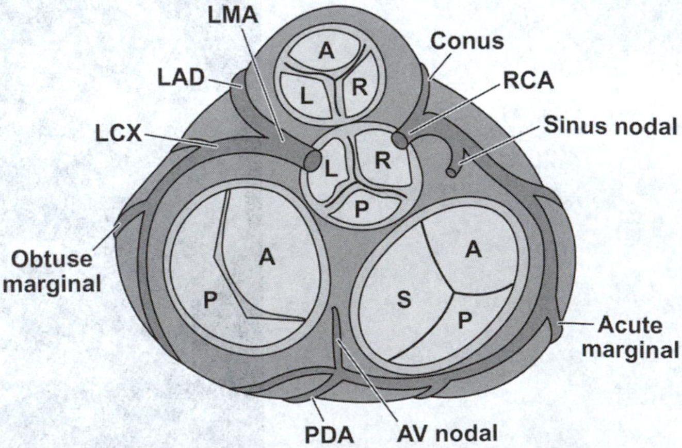

FIGURE 2-50 (Plate 19) Schematic diagram of coronary artery distribution viewed at the base of the heart. In this right-dominant system, the right coronary artery (RCA) gives rise to the posterior descending artery (PDA), and the left main coronary artery (LMA) gives rise to the left anterior descending (LAD) and left circumflex (LCX) branches. A, anterior; AV, atrioventricular; L, left; P, posterior; R, right; S, septal.

pects of the left atrial cavity. The left and right upper pulmonary veins are directed anterosuperiorly, whereas the lower veins enter the left atrium nearly perpendicular to the posterior atrial wall[15–17] (Figs. 2-15 and 2-48). *Left atrial muscle extends some distance within the pulmonary veins. The resultant cuff of muscle acts as a sphincter during atrial systole and may be the source of focal atrial fibrillation that is amenable to catheter ablation*[9–13] (see Fig. 2-2).

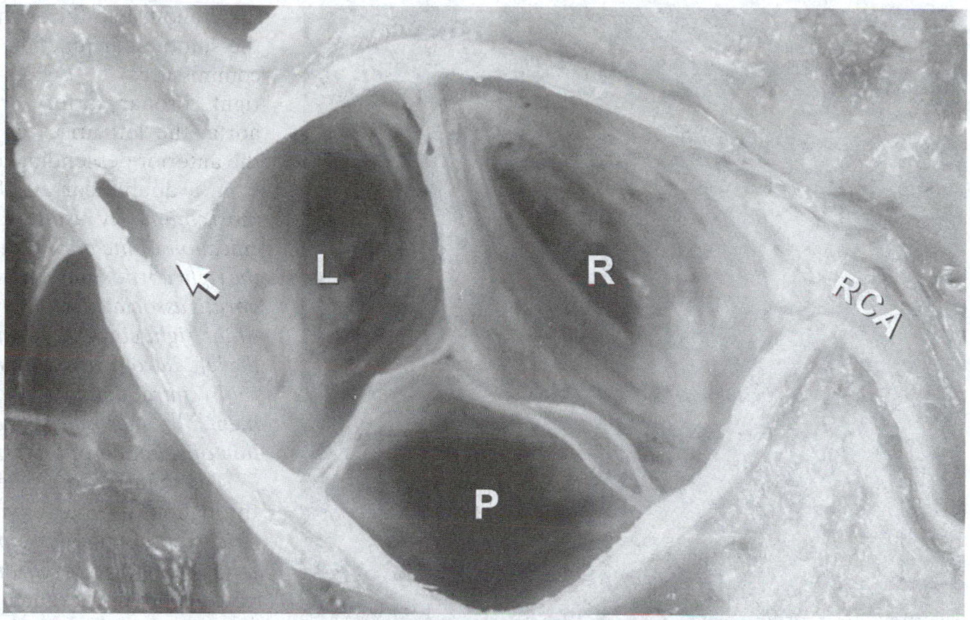

FIGURE 2-51 Differences in angulation at the origins of the right (RCA) and left main (arrow) coronary arteries. L, left aortic cusp; P, posterior aortic cusp; R, right aortic cusp.

The atrial appendage arises anterolaterally and lies in the left atrioventricular groove atop the proximal portion of the left circumflex coronary artery and, in some individuals, the left main coronary artery[16] (see Figs. 2-21*A* and 2-48). The left atrial appendage is smaller, more tortuous, and less pyramidal than its right atrial counterpart.[15–17] At least 80 percent are multilobed (up to four lobes, but the most frequent finding is two lobes)[29] (Fig. 2-49, Plate 18). There are also age- and sex-related differences in the dimensions of the appendage.[20] *With increasing use of transesophageal echocardiography to search for a cardiac source of embolism and to guide cardioversion and percutanous balloon valvuloplasty procedures, a thorough appreciation of the variations in normal left atrial appendage morphology has become important because a thrombus may be missed if all lobes in the appendage are not visualized.* In contrast to the right atrial free wall, the left has no crista terminalis and no pectinate muscles outside its appendage.[15–17]

The coronary sinus travels along the posterior wall of the left atrium within the left atrioventricular groove (see Fig. 2-21*A*). *In patients with persistent left superior vena cava, which most commonly drains into a dilated coronary sinus, the left-sided cava courses between the left atrial appendage and the left upper pulmonary vein.*[17] *The venous structure can be misinterpreted as the descending thoracic aorta, a mass, or a pathologic cavity.*

The esophagus and descending thoracic aorta are in contact with the posterior left atrial wall (see Figs. 2-20 and 2-48). *Accordingly, esophageal carcinomas may compress, infiltrate, or perforate the left atrium, and descending thoracic aortic aneurysms may compress this chamber.*[15] *A large hiatal hernia also can abut against the left atrium and resemble a mass.*

The marked increase in the incidence of atrial fibrillation from the fourth to the ninth decades of life may be due in part to the age-associated dilatation of the left atrium.[20]

Coronary Arteries and Veins

A detailed description of the spectrum of coronary artery anatomy including the many variations in the number and size of branches and course of the different arteries is beyond the scope of this chapter. The interested reader is referred to the elegant

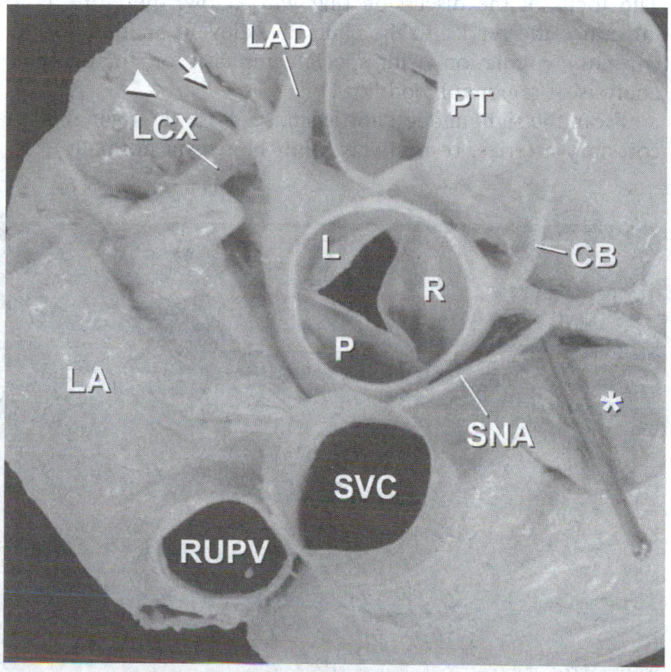

FIGURE 2-52 The right coronary artery gives rise to the conus branch (CB). A rod retracts the right atrial appendage (*) to disclose the sinus node artery (SNA). Arrow points to an intermediate left coronary artery; arrowhead points to a circumflex marginal branch. L, left aortic cusp; LA, left atrium; LAD, left anterior descending coronary artery; LCX, left circumflex coronary artery; P, posterior aortic cusp; PT, pulmonary trunk; R, right aortic cusp; RUPV, right upper pulmonary vein; SVC, superior vena cava. (From McAlpine,[30] with permission.)

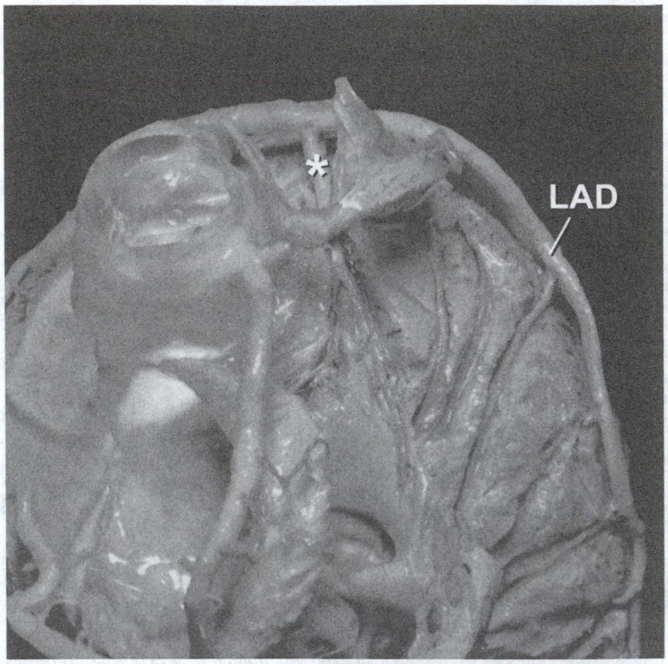

FIGURE 2-53 (Plate 20) Septal branches of the left anterior descending coronary artery (LAD); * points to the first septal perforator. (From McAlpine,[30] with permission.)

anatomic work by McAlpine published almost 25 years ago.[30] The focus of the discussion that will follow, therefore, is to introduce the reader to the clinically relevant anatomy of the coronary circulation, with special emphasis on tomographic analysis of regional blood flow.

From the right and left aortic sinuses arise the right and left coronary arteries, respectively, and their ostia normally originate about two-thirds the distance from the aortic annulus to the sinotubular junction and about midway between theaortic commissures[15–17] (Figs. 2-28 and 2-50, Plate 19). Whereas the right coronary artery arises nearly perpendicularly from the aorta, the left arises at an acute angle[15] (Fig. 2-51). Rarely, the anterior descending and circumflex arteries arise separately from a double-barrel left coronary ostium.[15–17] *Ostial stenosis most commonly results from atherosclerosis and degenerative calcification of the aortic sinotubular junction, which often overlies the right aortic sinus.*[17] *Less often it is due to aortic dissection or to aortitis associated with syphilis or ankylosing spondylitis. Stenosis of the right coronary ostium is much more frequent than that of the left. Iatrogenic ostial injury may complicate coronary angiography, intraoperative coronary perfusion, or aortic valve replacement.*[15–17] *Atherosclerosis or thrombosis of the most proximal portion of either coronary artery may mimic true ostial stenosis.*

The right coronary artery is embedded in adipose tissue throughout its course within the right atrioventricular groove. *Tricuspid annuloplasty or replacement may be complicated by injury to the right coronary artery.*[17] In 50 to 60 percent of persons, its first branch is the conus artery (Fig. 2-52), which supplies the right ventricular outflow tract and forms an important collateral anastomosis (circle of Vieussens), just below the pulmonary valve, with an analogous branch from the left anterior descending coronary artery.[15–17] In about a third of patients, the conus artery arises independently from the aorta[17] (see Fig. 2-28). The infundibular septum is supplied by the descending septal artery, which usually originates from the proximal right or conus coronary artery.[15–17] Among the numerous marginal branches of the right coronary artery that supply the remainder of the right ventricular free wall, the largest branch travels along the acute margin from base to apex[15–17] (see Fig. 2-50). In at least 70 percent of human hearts, the posterior descending artery arises from the distal right coronary artery (see Fig. 2-50). The posterior descending and distal posterolateral branches of a dominant right coronary artery supply the basal and middle inferior wall, basal (inlet) inferior septum, right bundle branch, AV node, AV (His) bundle, posterior portion of the left bundle branch, and posteromedial mitral papillary muscle.[17]

The left main coronary artery travels for a very short distance along the epicardium between the pulmonary trunk and left atrium (see Figs 2-50 and 2-52). It then divides into anterior descending and circumflex arteries (see Figs. 2-50 and 2-52). An intermediate artery also may arise at this division, thus forming a trifurcation rather than a bifurcation, and follows the course of a circumflex marginal branch[15–17] (see Fig. 2-52).

The left anterior descending coronary artery (LAD) courses within the epicardial fat of the anterior interventricular groove, wraps around the cardiac apex, and travels a variable distance along the inferior interventricular groove toward the cardiac base. Its septal perforating branches supply the anterior septum and apical septum. The first septal perforating branch supplies the AV (His) bundle and proximal left bundle branch[17] (Fig. 2-53, Plate 20). *In patients with symptomatic hypertrophic obstructive cardiomyopathy, nonsurgical septal reduction by percutaneous transluminal occlusion of septal branches of the* LAD *is a new therapeutic approach aimed at reducing the outflow gradient.*[31] *The long-term effects of this procedure are currently unknown.* The epicardial diagonal branches of the LAD supply the anterior left ventricular free wall, part of the anterolateral mitral papillary muscle, and the medial one-third of the anterior

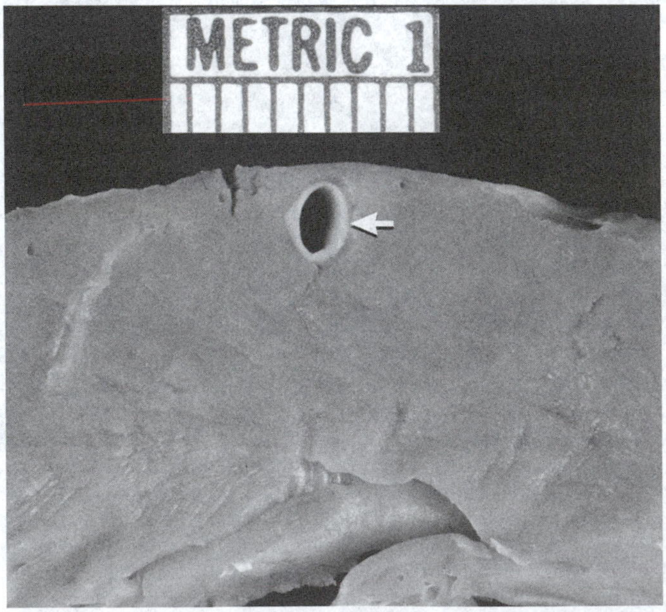

FIGURE 2-54 Intramyocardial course of the left anterior descending coronary artery (arrow).

right ventricular free wall.[15–17] Although short segments of the LAD may travel within the myocardium (covered by a so-called myocardial bridge) (Fig. 2-54), the resulting systolic luminal narrowing is probably benign in the vast majority of people.[17] *However, whereas the prevalence of myocardial bridging is only 0.5 to 1.6 percent in the general population, it is reported to be 28 percent in children and 30 to 50 percent in adults with hypertrophic cardiomyopathy.*[32] *More important, myocardial bridging appears to be associated with a poor prognosis (higher incidence of myocardial ischemia and sudden death) in patients with hypertrophic cardiomyopathy regardless of age.*[32]

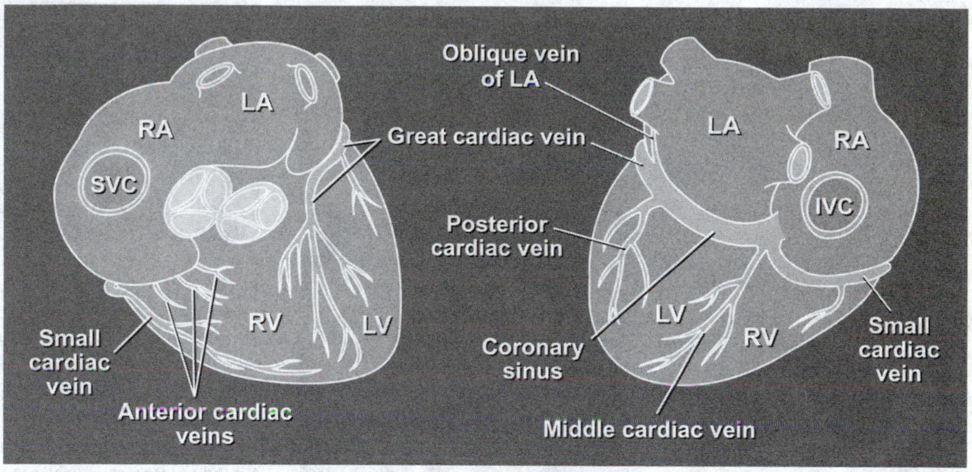

FIGURE 2-55 (Plate 21) Schematic diagram of the coronary venous circulation. IVC, inferior vena cava; LA, left atrium; LV, left ventricle; RA, right atrium; RV, right ventricle; SVC, superior vena cava.

The left circumflex coronary artery courses within the adipose tissue of the left atrioventricular groove (see Fig. 2-21*A*) and commonly terminates just beyond its large obtuse marginal branch (see Fig. 2-50). It supplies the lateral left ventricular free wall and a portion of the anterolateral mitral papillary muscle.[15–17]

Along the inferior surface of the heart, the length of the right coronary artery varies inversely with that of the circumflex artery. The artery that crosses the cardiac crux and gives rise to the posterior descending branch represents the dominant coronary artery. Dominance is right in 70 percent of human hearts, left in 10 percent, and shared in 20 percent.[15–17] *In patients with a congenitally bicuspid aortic valve, the incidence of left coronary dominance is 25 to 30 percent.*[17]

The coronary venous circulation is comprised of coronary sinus, cardiac veins, and thebesian venous systems[15–17] (Fig. 2-55, Plate 21). The great cardiac vein travels in the anterior interventricular groove beside the left anterior descending coronary artery and in the left atrioventricular groove beside the left circumflex artery.[15–17] The great cardiac vein and other cardiac veins, such as the left posterior and middle cardiac veins, drain into the coronary sinus, which courses along the posteroinferior aspect of the left atrioventricular groove and empties into the right atrium[15–17] (see Fig. 2-21*A*). The ostium of the coronary sinus is guarded by a crescent-shaped valvular remnant, the thebesian valve. Rarely, the coronary sinus drains directly into the left atrium.[17]

During cardiac operations, cardioplegic solution may be administered retrogradely into the coronary sinus. In patients with the Wolff-Parkinson-White preexitation syndrome and left-sided bypass tracts, the ablation catheter during electrophysiologic studies can be positioned within the coronary sinus and great cardiac vein adjacent to the mitral valve ring in order to localize the aberrant conduction pathway.[17] *The coronary veins, via the coronary sinus, provide access to percutaneous epicardial mapping and pacing of the ventricles and ablation of subepicardial arrhythmogenic foci*[33] (Fig. 2-56, Plate 22). *Some patients with ischemic cardiomyopathy may be poor candidates for conventional revascularization procedures (e.g., coronary artery bypass graft surgery or angioplasty) because their epicardial coronary arteries are diffusely diseased. Since in virtually all people the coronary veins run parallel to the entire course of coronary arteries, alternative percutaneous revascularization methods that use the coronary veins as a bypass conduit for coronary arterial flow are being explored.*[34–36] *Myocardial revascularization is achieved by either connecting the coronary artery proximal and distal to a stenosis to its companion coronary vein (similar to a conventional bypass graft) or by retroperfusion through the ve-*

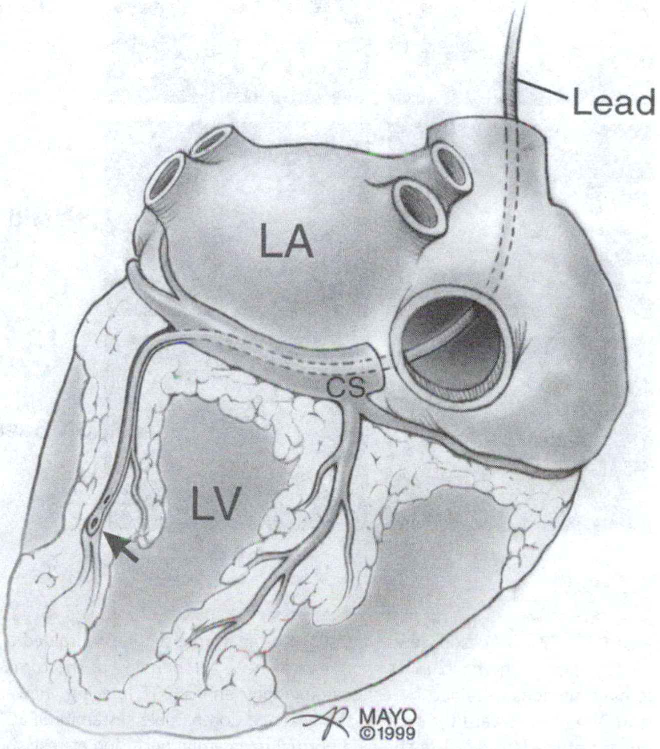

FIGURE 2-56 (Plate 22) Schematic diagram shows placement of the tip of a pacing/mapping catheter within a coronary vein (arrow) via the coronary sinus (CS). LA, left atrium; LV, left ventricle.

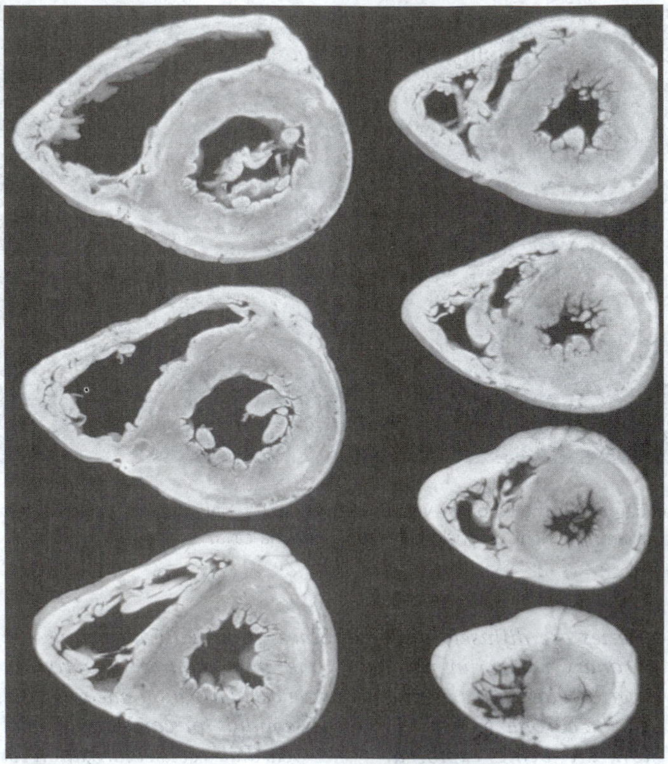
A

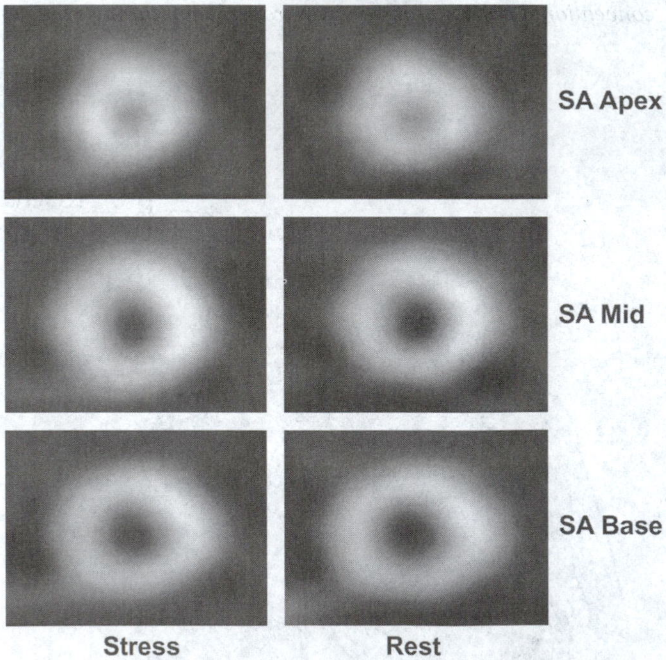

B

FIGURE 2-57 Short-axis views. A. Collage of anatomic sections obtained by "bread slicing" the heart in its short-axis plane, corresponding to the tomographic sections obtained by echocardiography and SPECT imaging, viewed from the apex toward the base of the heart. B. Comparable sestamibi SPECT images of the left ventricle showing normal myocardial perfusion at rest and with exercise. SA, short axis.

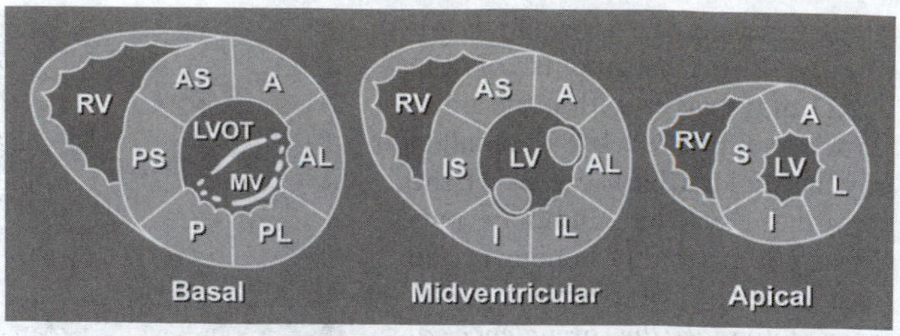

FIGURE 2-58 Schematic diagram of the three levels of short-axis tomographic views used in echocardiography for 16-segment wall motion analysis. A, anterior; AL, anterolateral; AS, anterior ventricular septum; I, inferior; IL, inferolateral; IS, inferior ventricular septum; L, lateral; LV, left ventricle; LVOT, left ventricular outflow tract; P, posterior; PL, posterolateral; PS, posterior ventricular septum; RV, right ventricle; S, septum. The most basal segment of the inferior wall is the anatomically true posterior segment. At this level, the adjacent ventricular septum is commonly referred to as either the *basal posterior septum* or the *basal inferior septum* and the adjacent lateral wall as either the *basal posterolateral wall* or the *basal inferolateral wall.*

nous microvasculature if the artery and vein are only connected proximal to the stenosis. Coronary veins, unlike saphenous veins, are not removed, thus preserving their adventitia and blood supply.[34-36]

Coronary artery disease is associated with regional abnormalities in ventricular structure and function. Because analysis of segmental myocardial perfusion or contractility is the cornerstone of tomographic imaging techniques [stress echocardiography, SPECT imaging, positron emission tomography

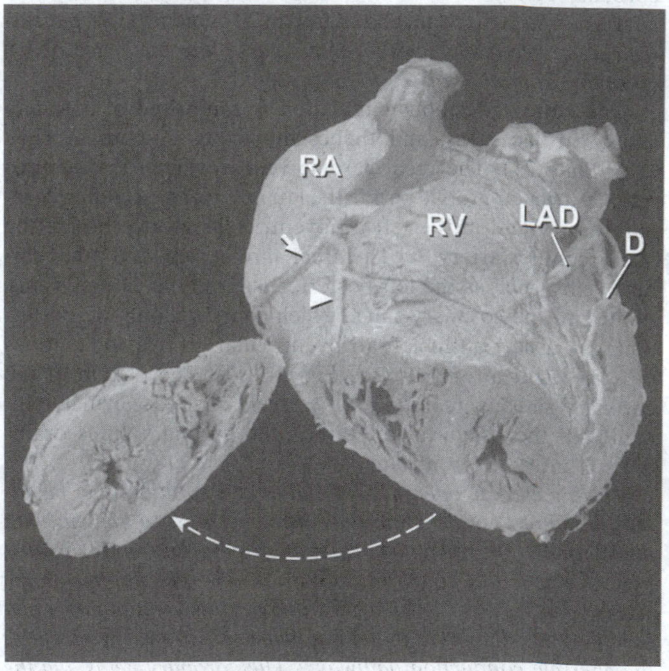

FIGURE 2-59 Regional coronary flow, with a short-axis slice of the heart. A large diagonal branch (D) of the left anterior descending coronary artery (LAD) supplies the lateral wall, and an acute marginal branch (arrowhead) of the right coronary artery (arrow) supplies the anterior right ventricular free wall. The distal segment of the LAD is intramural. RA, right atrium; RV, right ventricle. (From McAlpine,[30] with permission.)

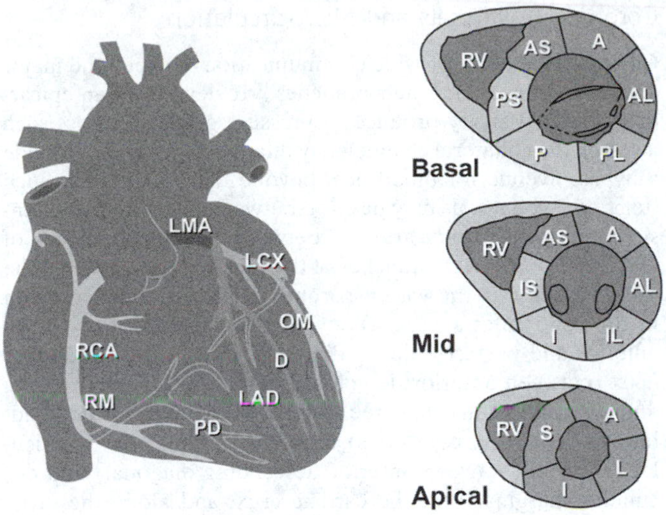

FIGURE 2-60 (Plate 23) Coronary distribution using a 16-segment model. D, diagonal branch of the left anterior descending coronary artery; LAD, left anterior descending coronary artery; LCX, left circumflex coronary artery; LMA, left main coronary artery; OM, obtuse marginal branch of the circumflex coronary artery; PD, posterior descending coronary artery; RCA, right coronary artery; RM, right marginal branch; other abbreviations as in Fig 2-58.

(PET), and MRI], for clinicopathologic correlations (Fig. 2-57), a combination tomographic and segmental approach to coronary artery anatomy is recommended.[17,37,38] Ventricular mass is made of the left and right ventricular free walls and the partitioning ventricular septum. Three levels (i.e., basal, midventricular, and apical) are used to divide the base-apex length of the left ventricle into thirds (Fig. 2-58). The basal third includes that portion between the mitral annulus and the tips of the papillary muscles. The midventricular third is from the papillary muscle to the most apical insertion point of these muscles into the left ventricular free wall. The apical third includes the remainder of the ventricle, from the insertion of the papillary muscles to the left ventricular apex. A similar approach can be applied to the right ventricle.[15–17,37] The ventricular septum can be divided into anteroseptal, septal, and inferoseptal segments, and the left ventricular free wall is divided into anterior, lateral, and inferior segments at the basal and midventricular levels (see Fig. 2-58). The left ventricular apical level consists of four segments (i.e., septum, inferior, lateral, and anterior) (see Fig. 2-58).

This regional approach is not arbitrary and has been verified by studies of normal, dilated, and hypertrophied hearts. According to this system, there are 16 left ventricular segments that can be evaluated for regional abnormalities. This regional approach also can be used to assess transmural infarct size, because the percentage of left ventricular mass contributed by any particular region is not altered in any significant manner by symmetric hypertrophy or dilatation.[17]

Regional Coronary Artery Supply

The ventricular regions described tend to correlate well with common patterns of coronary arterial distribution[15–17] (Figs. 2-59 and 2-60, Plate 23). Any specific epicardial coronary artery generally will supply a certain cluster of regions. For example, in a typical right-dominant system, the left anterior descending coronary artery would supply the midventricular and basal segments of the anterior and anterolateral walls and anterior septum and all apical segments. The left circumflex artery would supply the midventricular and basal inferolateral segments, and the right coronary artery would supply the midventricular and basal inferior wall and inferior septum (see Fig. 2-60). However, because the patterns of coronary distribution are so highly variable, these correlations between coronary blood flow and regional anatomy are not precise. For example, a hyperdominant right coronary artery may supply the apex, and a large, obtuse marginal branch of the circumflex artery may supply the anterolateral or inferior wall. Also, any given myocardial region may, in some people, receive its blood supply from the branches of two independent major epicardial arteries.[15–17] In old age, the coronary arteries become dilated and tortuous (Fig. 2-61).

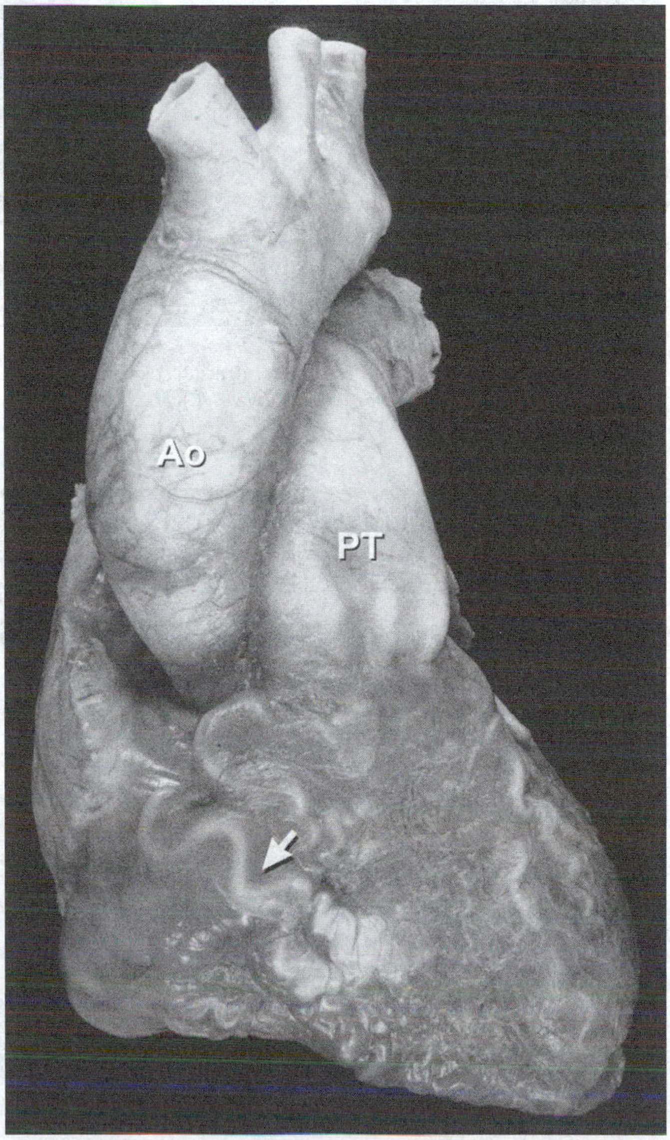

FIGURE 2-61 Tortuous coronary arteries (arrow) typically seen in the elderly with nondilated hearts. Ao, ascending aorta; PT, pulmonary trunk.

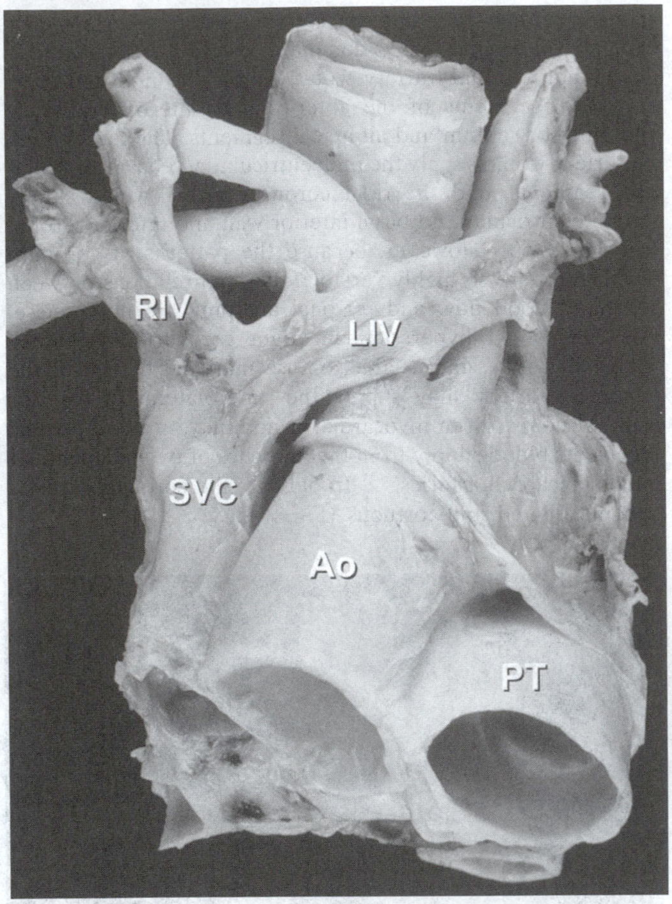

FIGURE 2-62 The longer left (LIV) and shorter right (RIV) innominate veins normally join to form the right superior vena cava (SVC). Ao, ascending aorta; PT, pulmonary trunk.

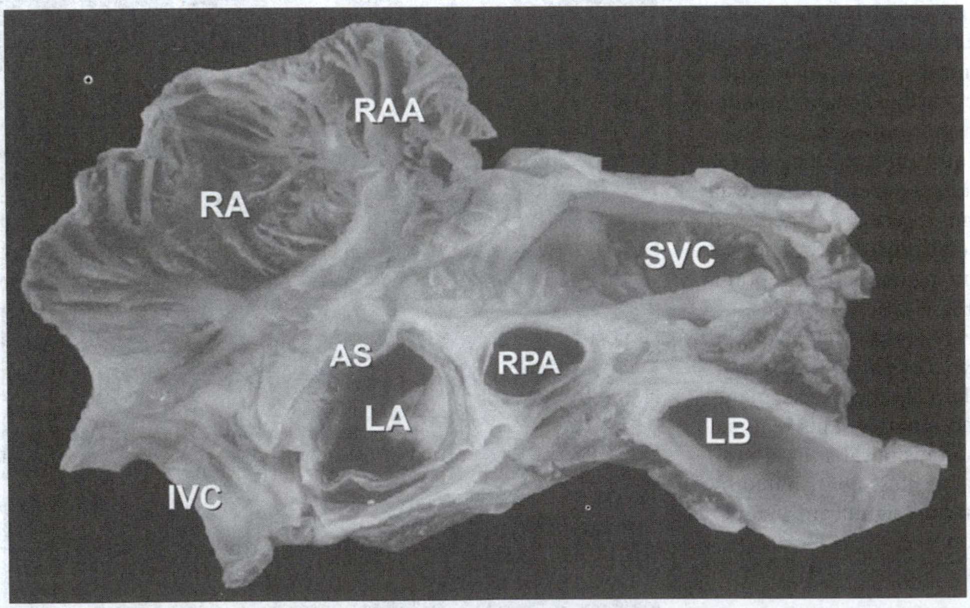

FIGURE 2-63 Long-axis view of the superior vena cava (SVC) and inferior vena cava (IVC). The specimen is viewed from the left looking toward the free wall of the right atrium. The right atrium (RA) and its appendage (RAA) are anterior. This is a commonly used tomographic plane in transesophageal echocardiography. AS, atrial septum; LA, left atrium; LB, left bronchus; RPA, right pulmonary artery.

Coronary Collaterals and Microcirculation

Collateral channels provide communication between the major coronary arteries and their branches.[17] If stenosis of an epicardial coronary artery produces a pressure gradient across such a vessel, the collateral channel may dilate with time and provide a bypass avenue for blood flow beyond the obstruction. Such functional collaterals may develop between the terminal extensions of two coronary arteries, between the side branches of two arteries, between branches of the same artery, or within the same branch (via the vasa vasorum). These are most common in the ventricular septum (between septal perforators of the anterior and posterior descending arteries), in the ventricular apex (between anterior descending septal perforators), in the anterior right ventricular free wall (between anterior descending and right or conus arteries), in the anterolateral left ventricular free wall (between anterior descending diagonals and circumflex marginals), at the cardiac crux, and along the atrial surfaces (between the right and left circumflex arteries).[17]

The intramural coronary vessels form the microcirculation. There are age-related variations in the pattern of distribution of the coronary microcirculation.[39] *Angina-like chest pain in some patients with angiographically normal epicardial coronary arteries (i.e., syndrome X, or microvascular angina) may be secondary to abnormal vasodilator reserve or vasoconstriction of the coronary microcirculation.*[40] *Abnormal flow reserve of the coronary microcirculation is seen in both dilated and hypertrophied hearts. In the latter, structural changes in the coronary arterioles can be found on histologic examination of the myocardium.*[41–43] *In patients with symptomatic hypertrophic cardiomyopathy without angiographic evidence of epicardial coronary artery disease, myocardial tissue obtained during surgical myectomy may show smaller than normal coronary arteriolar lumina.*[43] *Postmortem analysis of hearts with hypertrophic cardiomyopathy also has revealed coronary arterioles with abnormally thick walls.*[43] *With contrast echocardiography, it may be possible to noninvasively visualize intramyocardial arterioles and study coronary flow reserve.*[44] *Demonstration of an intact microvascular circulation in akinetic myocardium following acute myocardial infarction, using PET or SPECT imaging or contrast echocardiography, is evidence of viability of the affected segment.*[44] *The creation of intramyocardial channels with* CO_2 *laser transmyocardial revascularization has been associated with augmentation of collateral flow to ischemic myocardium through angiogenesis.*[45]

Cardiac Lymphatics

The myocardial lymphatics drain toward the epicardial surface, where they merge to form the right and left lymphatic channels,

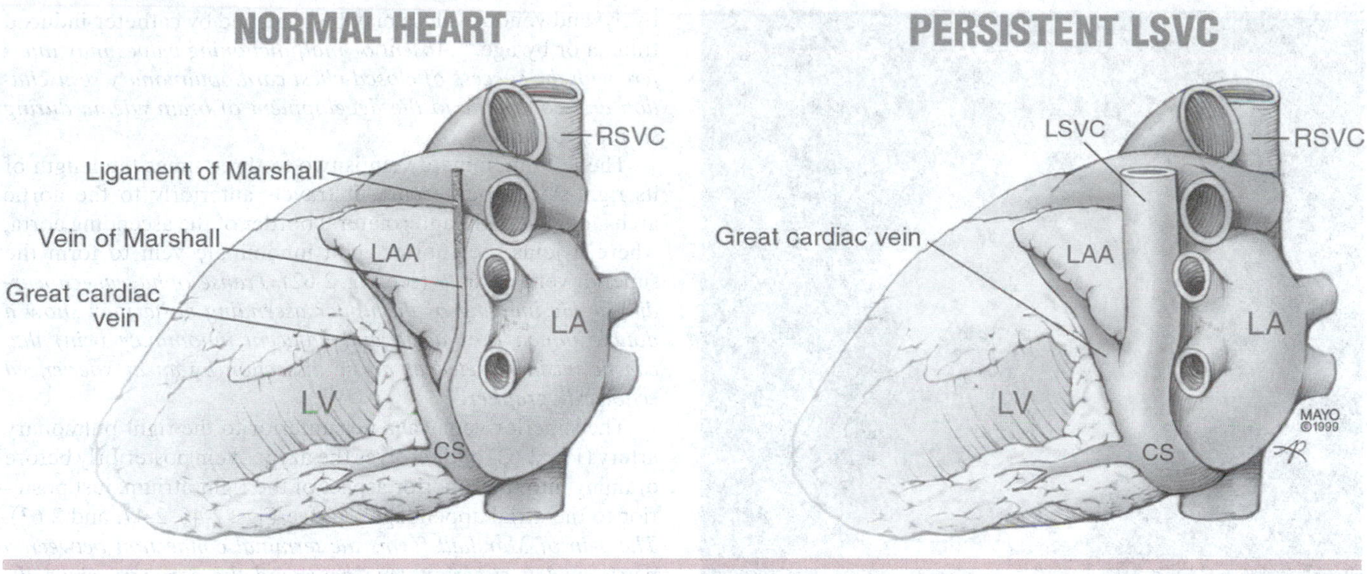

FIGURE 2-64 (Plate 24) Schematic diagrams showing the ligament/vein of Marshall in normal hearts (*left*) and persistent left superior vena cava (LSVC) (*right*). CS, coronary sinus; LA, left atrium; LAA, left atrial appendage; LV, left ventricle; RA, right atrium; RSVC, right superior vena cava.

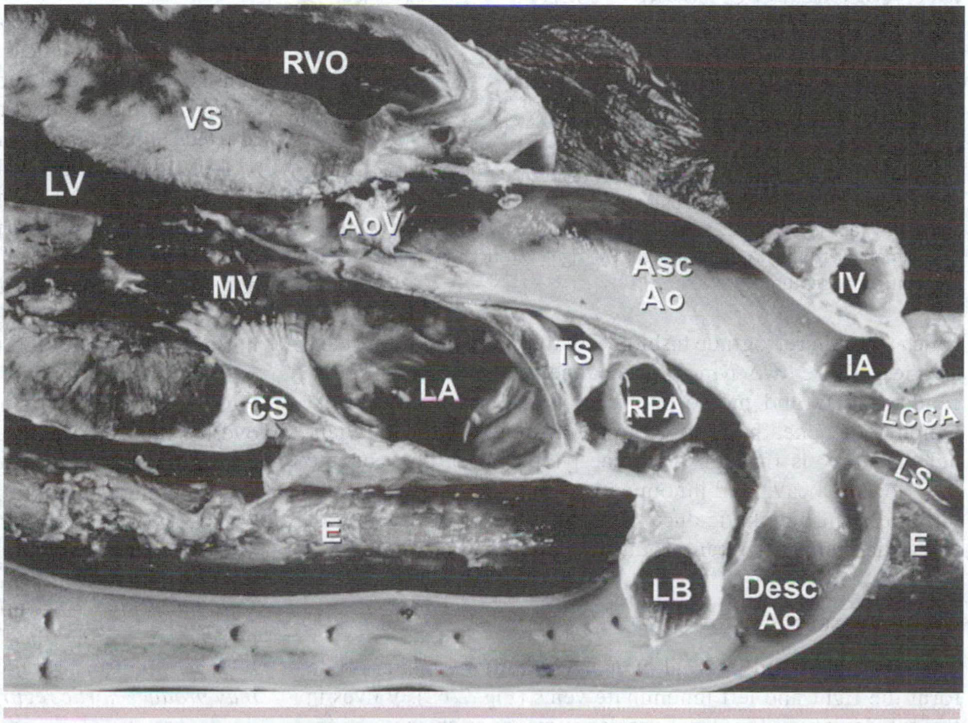

FIGURE 2-65 Thoracic aorta. The entire thoracic aorta has been cut in a tomographic manner. The aortic arch travels over the left bronchus and the right pulmonary artery. Asc Ao, ascending aorta; AoV, aortic valve; CS, coronary sinus; Desc Ao, descending thoracic aorta; E, esophagus; IA, innominate artery; IV, innominate vein; LA, left atrium; LB, left bronchus; LCCA, left common carotid artery; LS, left subclavian artery; LV, left ventricle; MV, mitral valve; RPA, right pulmonary artery; RVO, right ventricular outflow; TS, transverse sinus; VS, ventricular septum.

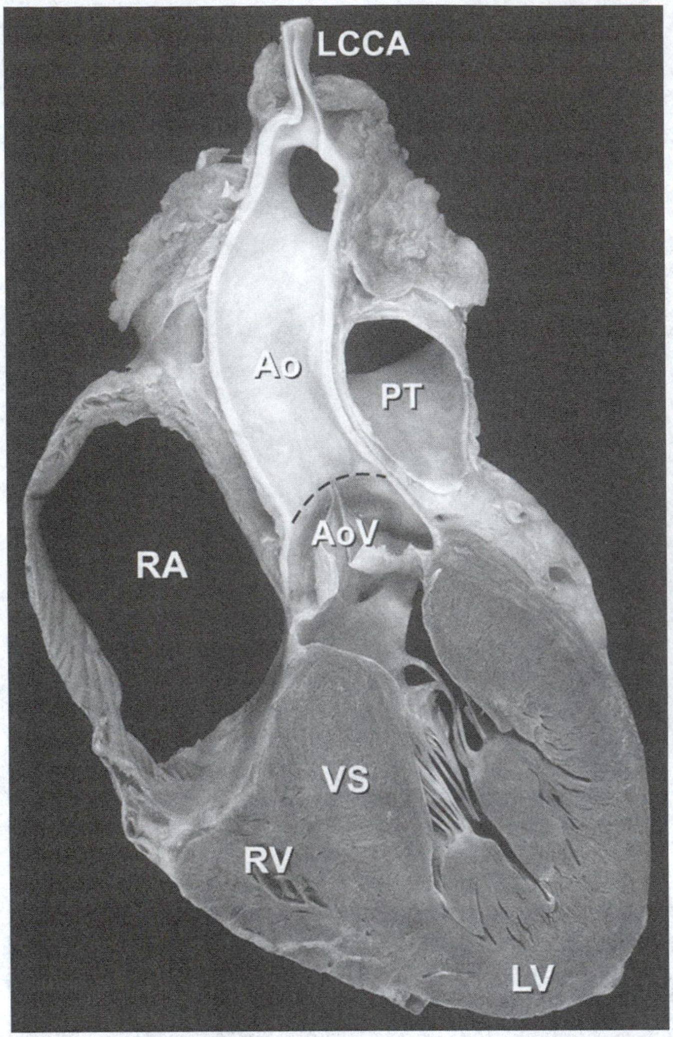

FIGURE 2-66 Tomographic section of the heart in the frontal plane of the body showing the aortic sinotubular junction (dashed line). Ao, ascending aorta; AoV, aortic valve; LCCA, left common carotid artery; LV, left ventricle; PT, pulmonary trunk; RA, right atrium; RV, right ventricle; LV, left ventricle; VS, ventricular septum.

which travel in retrograde fashion with their respective coronary arteries. These two lymphatic channels travel along the ascending aorta and merge before draining into a pretracheal lymph node beneath the aortic arch. This single lymphatic channel then travels through a cardiac lymph node, between the superior vena cava and innominate artery, and finally empties into the right lymphatic duct. Metastatic tumor obstruction of epicardial lymphatics can produce a pericardial effusion.[15–17]

Great Vessels

The subclavian and internal jugular veins merge bilaterally to form the right and left innominate veins (Fig. 2-62). Valves in the subclavian and internal jugular veins, near their junctions with the innominate veins, are important anatomic structures that help maintain unidirectional antegrade blood flow not only in the normal state but also in the setting of elevated right-sided heart filling pressures.[46] Subclavian and internal jugular venous valves are absent in 2 and 6 percent of people, respectively, and venous valves may be damaged by catheter-induced trauma or by age.[46] *Absent or malfunctioning valves may interfere with the success of closed-chest cardiopulmonary resuscitation and contribute to the development of brain edema during such a procedure.*[46]

The left innominate vein is two to three times the length of its right-sided counterpart. It travels anteriorly to the aortic arch along the right anterolateral border of the ascending aorta, where it joins the shorter right innominate vein to form the superior vena cava[15–17] (see Fig. 2-62). *Transesophageal echocardiographic imaging of the upper ascending aorta may show a double lumen (i.e., aorta and adjacent innominate vein) that can be misinterpreted as aortic dissection by an inexperienced echocardiographer.*[7]

The superior vena cava lies anterior to the right pulmonary artery (Fig. 2-63) and receives the azygos vein posteriorly before draining into the superior aspect of the right atrium, just posterior to the atrial appendage[15–17] (see Figs. 2-46, 2-47, and 2-63). *The vein of Marshall forms the terminal connection between a persistent left superior vena cava and the coronary sinus. Its vestigial remnant in normal adults is the ligament of Marshall* (Fig 2-64, Plate 24). *Both vein and ligament are a potential source of arrhythmias.* The ostium of the inferior vena cava is guarded by a crescent-shaped, often fenestrated flap of tissue, the eustachian valve[15–17] (see Fig. 2-16*A*), that is readily seen by echocardiography. Although generally small, the eustachian valve may become so large that it can produce a double-chambered right atrium.[16] Also, when either the eustachian or thebesian valve is large and fenestrated, it is referred to as a *Chiari net*.[15–17] *By echocardiography, a Chiari net may be misinterpreted as a mass.*

The thoracic aorta arises at the level of the aortic valve and is divided into three segments: ascending aorta, aortic arch, and descending thoracic aorta (Fig. 2-65). The ascending aorta consists of sinus and tubular portions, which are demarcated by the sinotubular junction (Figs. 2-28 and 2-66). *This is the site at which supravalvular aortic stenosis is often most severe.*[15–17]

Behind the aortic valve cusps are three outpouchings, or sinuses (of Valsalva). The right aortic sinus abuts against the ventricular septum and right ventricular parietal band and is covered in part by the right atrial appendage (see Figs. 2-30 and 2-52). In contrast, the left aortic sinus rests against the anterior left ventricular free wall and a portion of the anterior mitral leaflet, abuts the left atrial free wall, and is covered in part by the pulmonary trunk and left atrial appendage (see Figs. 2-20 and 2-21*A*). The posterior (noncoronary) aortic sinus overlies the ventricular septum and a part of the anterior mitral leaflet, forms part of the transverse sinus, abuts the atrial septum, and indents both atrial free walls[15–17] (see Figs. 2-12*D* and 2-22). *Rupture of the right and posterior aortic sinuses of Valsalva may result in a communication with the right ventricular outflow tract or right atrium, whereas rupture of the left aortic sinus of Valsalva leads to a communication with the left atrium or left ventricular outflow tract. Annuloaortic ectasia is associated with hypertension, aortic medial degeneration, and advanced age and may produce aortic regurgitation, ascending aortic aneurysm, or aortic dissection.*[15–17]

The aortic arch gives rise to the innominate, left common carotid, and left subclavian arteries in that order (see Fig. 2-65). In about 10 percent of people, the innominate and left common carotid arteries share a common ostium, and in 5 percent of people, the left vertebral artery arises directly from

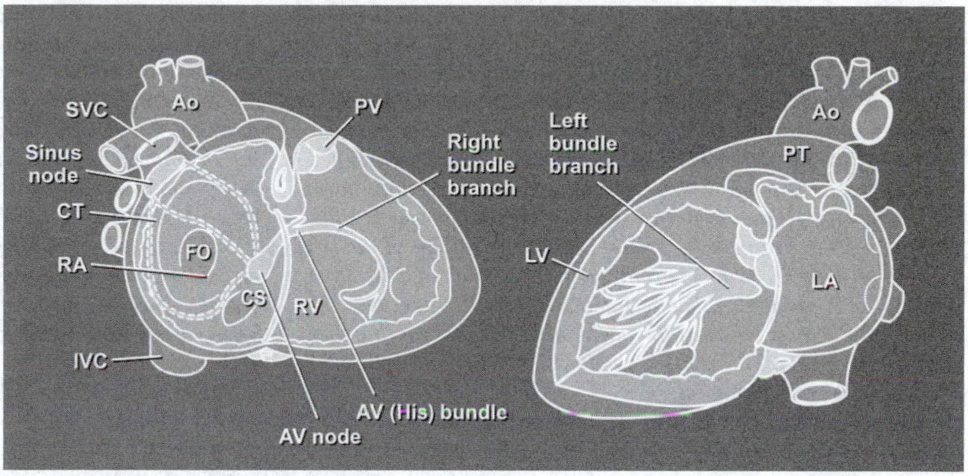

FIGURE 2-67 (Plate 25) Schematic diagram of the cardiac conduction system. (*Left*) The right side of the heart showing the sinus node, atrioventricular (AV) node, AV (His) bundle, and right bundle branch. (*Right*) The left side of the heart showing incomplete anatomic separation of the left bundle into antero and posterior fascicles. Ao, ascending aorta; AV, atrioventricular; CS, coronary sinus; CT, crista terminalis; FO, fossa ovalis; IVC, inferior vena cava; LA, left atrium; LV, left ventricle; PT, pulmonary trunk; PV, pulmonary valve; RA, right atrium; RV, right ventricle; SVC, superior vena cava.

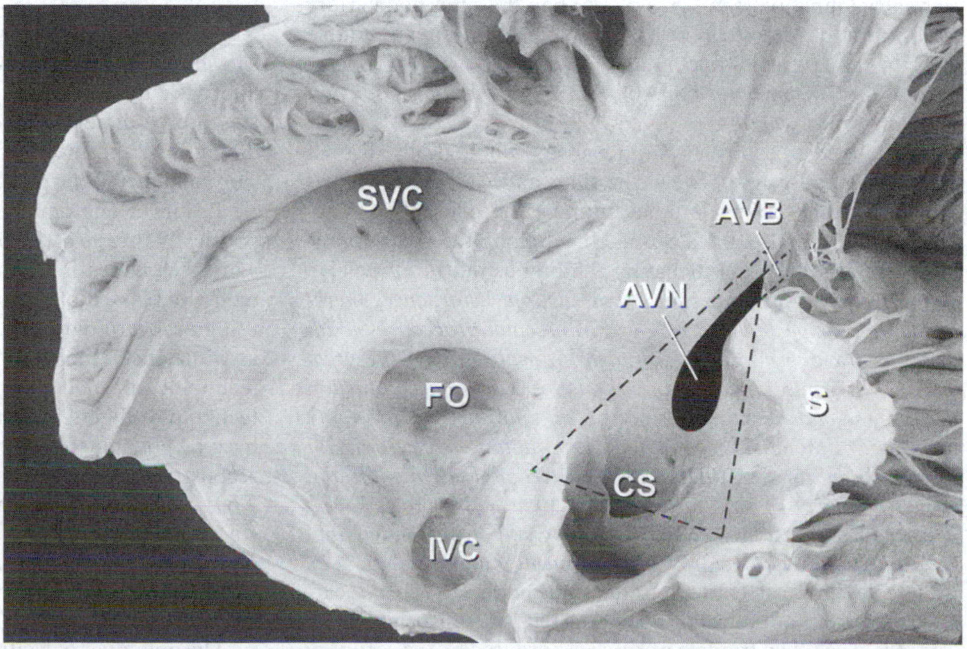

FIGURE 2-68 (Plate 26) The atrioventricular node (AVN) lies within the triangle of Koch (dashed triangle), and the AV (His) bundle (AVB) travels through the tricuspid annulus to rest along the summit of the ventricular septum. CS, coronary sinus; FO, fossa ovalis; IVC, inferior vena cava; S, septal leaflet of the tricuspid valve; SVC, superior vena cava.

the aortic arch, between the left common carotid and left subclavian arteries.[17] The ligamentum arteriosum (ductal artery ligament) represents the vestigial remnant of the fetal ductal artery, which when patent connects the proximal left pulmonary artery to the undersurface of the aortic arch.[17] *Most coarctations occur just distal to the left subclavian artery* (see Fig. 2-69). *When thoracic aortic dissection does not involve the ascending aorta (Debakey type III and Stanford type B), the intimal tear is commonly near the ligamentum arteriosum or the ostium of the left subclavian artery.*[17] *Nonpenetrating deceleration chest trauma, as may occur in motor vehicle accidents, commonly involves the aorta in the region between the aortic arch and descending thoracic aorta and may be associated with aortic transection or pseudoaneurysm formation.*[17]

The descending thoracic aorta lies adjacent to the left atrium, esophagus, and vertebral column. The pulmonary trunk (or main pulmonary artery) emanates from the right ventricle and travels to the left of the ascending aorta. As it bifurcates, the left pulmonary artery courses over the left bronchus, whereas the right pulmonary artery travels beneath the aortic arch and behind the superior vena cava (see Figs. 2-11*A* and 2-63). Thus the *left* bronchus and the *right* pulmonary artery normally travel beneath the aortic arch.

Cardiac Conduction System

The cardiac conduction system consists of the sinus node, internodal tracts, AV node, AV (His) bundle, and right and left bundle branches[15–17] (Fig. 2-67, Plate 25). The sinus node is located sub-epicardially in the terminal groove, close to the junction between the superior vena cava and right atrium. The sinus node artery arises from the right coronary artery in 55 percent of people. Its course may place it in contact with the base of the right atrial appendage and the superior vena cava–right atrial junction (see Fig. 2-52). When the sinus node artery arises from the left circumflex artery (45 percent), it may course close to the left atrial appendage. *During such surgical operations as the Mustard and Fontan procedures, the sinus node and its artery are susceptible to injury.*[16,17]

By light microscopy, there are no morphologically distinct conduction pathways between the sinus and AV nodes.[17] However, electrophysiologic studies support the concept of functional preferential pathways that travel along the crista terminalis and atrial septum including the limbus but not the valve of the fossa ovalis.[17] *Internodal conduction disturbances therefore are not expected as a result of transseptal procedures. With the Mustard operation for complete transposition of the great arteries, there may be severe disturbance of internodal conduction because the entire septum is resected, and the surgical atriotomy may disrupt the crista terminalis.*[17] *Lipomatous hypertrophy of the atrial septum may interfere with internodal conduction and induce a variety of atrial arrhythmias. Ventricular preexcitation is most commonly associated with aberrant bypass tracts that span the annulus of the tricuspid or mitral valve* (see Fig. 2-2).

The AV node, in contrast to the sinus node, is a sub*endo*cardial structure that is located within the triangle of Koch[15–17] (Fig. 2-68, Plate 26). The triangle of Koch is bordered by the coronary sinus ostium posteroinferiorly and the septal tricuspid annulus anteriorly. *Because of its right atrial location near the tricuspid annulus, the AV node is susceptible to injury during tricuspid annuloplasty and during plication procedures for Ebstein's anomaly.*[15–17]

The AV (His) bundle arises from the distal portion of the AV node and travels along the ventricular septum adjacent to the membranous septum[15–17] (see Fig. 2-68). *The AV conduction tissue is generally remote from the defect in the outlet, inlet, and muscular forms of ventricular septal defect but travels along the inferior margin of a membranous ventricular septal defect.* The AV bundle travels through the central fibrous body (right fibrous trigone) and therefore is closely related to the annuli of the aortic, mitral, and tricuspid valves. *Thus, during operative procedures involving these valves or a membranous ventricular septal defect, care must be taken to avoid injury to the His bundle. Whereas in normal hearts the AV bundle courses along the posteroinferior rim of the membranous septum, it courses along the anterosuperior rim of the membranous septum in hearts with AV discordance.* The AV bundle receives a dual blood supply from the AV nodal artery and the first septal perforator of the left anterior descending coronary artery.[17]

The right bundle branch emanates from the distal portion of the AV bundle and forms a cordlike structure that travels along the septal and moderator bands toward the anterior tricuspid papillary muscle (see Fig. 2-67). In contrast, the left bundle branch represents a broad fenestrated sheet of subendocardial conduction fibers that spread along the septal surface of the left ventricle[15–17] (see Fig. 2-67). The right and left bundle branches receive dual blood supply from the septal perforators of the left anterior descending coronary artery and posterior descending coronary arteries.[17] Left ventricular pseudotendons may contain conduction tissue from the left bundle branch.[17] *Following right ventriculotomy for reconstruction of the right ventricular outflow tract, the ECG shows a pattern of right bundle-branch block even though the right bundle is not disrupted.*[16]

NEW DEVELOPMENTS AND FUTURE CHALLENGES

The future holds promise for an integrated multidimensional approach to the study of cardiac anatomy that incorporates static three-dimensional data, the elements of time (the fourth dimension) and motion, and physiologic (pressure and perfusion) and metabolic parameters.[47–49] Until recently, the geometric fusion of anatomy and function was not possible without physically invading the body. With the currently available imaging techniques, multidimensional anatomy and physiology are mentally reassembled from the sequential tomographic images using echocardiography, MRI or CT, or multiple scintigraphy, as with SPECT imaging.[47] With the advances made in medical technology propelled by the rapid developments in computer technology, digital imaging, and data-storage techniques, it has become possible to electronically perform virtual dissection and reconstruction of the heart and cardiovascular system[47–49] (Fig. 2-69). Furthermore, multidimensional imaging allows continued study of any human organ of interest because of the ability to permanently store anatomic images and physiologic features for retrieval, comparison for change, and ultimately, physical replication.[47–49]

The potential realization of virtual anatomy notwithstanding, standardization of the various tomographic approaches to image acquisition in a manner that conforms with anatomic correctness remains a major challenge that has to be overcome if multidimensional cardiac imaging is to become a clinical reality. There is current progress in this direction. Real-time three-

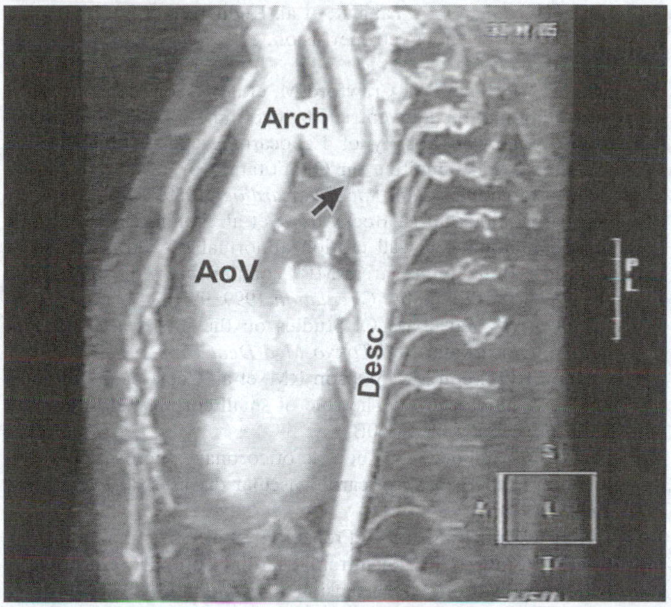

FIGURE 2-69 Real-time three-dimensional CT reconstruction of the thoracic aorta in a patient with coarctation (arrow) distal to the left subclavian artery. AoV, aortic valve. Desc, descending thoracic aorta.

dimensional reconstruction of the heart using identical CT and two-dimensional tomographic sectioning of the heart is now possible. Virtual vivisection may soon become reality. It will allow virtual surgery (dry runs prior to the actual operation) and dissection of the heart into its various functional components, be it anatomic, physiologic, or metabolic, either separately or in various combinations. Because of these advances in multimedia technology, the centuries-old great divide between physiologists and anatomists has been relegated to the history books.

ANATOMY NOT ADDRESSED AND QUANTUM COMPUTING

Fine-detailed anatomy such as that of the conduction system and microvasculature is not available to the usual anatomic dissection. Additionally, tissue histology or molecular biologic assessment is not obtained routinely by the dissectionist. At the other end of the spectrum, three-dimensional gross anatomic dissection of contiguous structures is also normally not available. How does metastatic cancer throughout the system relate to a primary tumor in the gut?

These and other desirable anatomic and histologic dissections await the future of increasing computer technology. Both pathologic and living tissues someday will be dissected and analyzed not by destructive cutting but by digital imagery. Today's computers have introduced the information era. Information has become a commodity expanding our ability to access useful data. Within the next two decades, however, we will have evolved to the quantum era where all that has been discussed in this chapter plus gross and microscopic anatomy will be possible within an electronic environment. Reality will be broken down into its base parts or characteristics and then reformatted relative to the desired information. Gross anatomy, physiology, tissue characteristics, and even histopathology can be dissected and presented as a quantifiable geometric image.

References

1. Callahan JA, Key JD. Foundations of cardiology. In: Giuliani ER, Fuster V, Gersh BJ, et al, eds. *Cardiology Fundamentals and Practice*, 2d ed: Vol 1. St Louis: Mosby-Year Book; 1991:3–25.
2. O'Malley CD, Saunders JB. *Leonardo da Vinci on the Human Body*. New York: Greenwich House; 1982:223.
3. Ackermann DM, Edwards WD. Anatomic basis for tomographic analysis of the pediatric heart at autopsy. *Perspect Pediatr Pathol* 1988; 12:44–68.
4. Landefeld CS, Goldman L. The autopsy in clinical medicine. *Mayo Clinic Proc* 1989; 64:1185–1189.
5. Hurst JW, King SB, Friesinger GC, et al. Atherosclerotic coronary heart disease: Angina pectoris, myocardial infarction, and other manifestations of myocardial ischemia. In: *Hurst's the Heart,* 6th, ed. New York: McGraw-Hill; 1986:882–1008.
6. Edwards WD. Anatomic basis for tomographic analysis of the heart at autopsy. *Cardiol Clin* 1984; 2:485–506.
7. Seward J. Transesophageal echocardiographic anatomy. In: Freeman W, Seward J, Khandheria B, Tajik AJ, eds. *Transesophageal Echocardiography*. Boston: Little, Brown; 1994:55–101.
8. Stewart W. Intraoperative echocardiography. In: Topol EJ, ed. *Textbook of Cardiovascular Medicine*. Philadelphia: Lippincott-Raven; 1998:1497–1525.
9. Packer DL, Johnson SB. Intracardiac ultrasound guidance of linear lesion creation for ablation of atrial fibrillation. *J Am Coll Cardiol* 1998; 31:333A.
10. Chu E, Fitzpatrick AP, Chin MC, et al. Radio-frequency catheter ablation guided by intracardiac echocardiography. *Circulation* 1994; 89:1301–1305.
11. DeLurgio DB, Frohwein SC, Walter PF, et al. Anatomy of atrioventricular nodal reentry investigated by intracardiac echocardiography. *Am J Cardiol* 1997; 80:231–234.
12. Bruce CJ, Packer DL, Seward J. Transvascular imaging: Feasibility study using a vector phased array ultrasound catheter. *Echocardiography* 1999; 16:425–430.
13. Fu M, Hung JS, Lo PH, et al. Intracardiac echocardiography via the transvenous approach with use of 8F 10-MHz ultrasound catheters. *Mayo Clin Proc* 1999; 74:775–783.
14. Nazarian GK, Julsrud PR, Ehman RL, et al. Correlation between magnetic resonance imaging of the heart and cardiac anatomy. *Mayo Clinic Proc* 1987; 62:573–583.
15. Edwards WD. *Anatomy of the Cardiovascular System: Clinical Medicine*, Vol 6. Philadelphia: Harper & Row; 1984:1–24.
16. Edwards WD. Cardiac anatomy and examination of cardiac specimens. In: Emmanouilides G, Reimenschneider T, Allen H, Gutgesell H, eds. *Moss & Adams' Heart Disease in Infants, Children, and Adolescents*, 5th ed. Baltimore: Williams & Wilkins; 1995:70–105.
17. Edwards WD. Applied anatomy of the heart. In: Giuliani ER, Fuster V, Gersh BJ, et al, eds. *Cardiology Fundamentals and Practice*, 2d ed: Vol 1. St Louis: Mosby-Year Book; 1991:47–112.
18. McAfee MK, Schaff HV. Valve repair for mitral insufficiency. *Cardiology* 1990; 20:35–43.
19. Arom KV, Edwards JD. Relationship between right ventricular muscle bundles and pulmonary valve: Significance in pulmonary atresia with intact ventricular septum. *Circulation* 1976; 54:79–83.
20. Kitzman D, Edwards WD. Minireview: Age-related changes in the anatomy of the normal human heart. *J Gerontol Med Sci* 1990; 45:M33–39.
21. Freedberg RS, Goodkin GM, Perez JL. Valve strands are strongly associated with systemic embolization: A transesophageal echocardiographic study. *J Am Coll Cardiol* 1995; 26:1709–1712.

22. Burke A, Virmani R. *Atlas of Tumor Pathology: Tumors of the Heart and Great Vessels in Papillary Fibroelastoma.* Washington DC: Armed Forces Institute of Pathology; 1996:47–54.
23. Roberts WC, Roberts JD. The floating heart too fat to sink: Analysis of 55 necropsy patients. *Am J Cardiol* 1983; 52:1286–1289.
24. Cristina B, Gaetano T, Domenico C, et al. Arrhythmogenic right ventricular cardiomyopathy: Dysplasia, dystrophy, or myocarditis. *Circulation* 1996; 94:983–991.
25. Luetmer PH, Edwards WD, Seward JB, et al. Incidence and distribution of left ventricular false tendons: An autopsy study of 483 normal human hearts. *J Am Coll Cardiol* 1986; 8:179–183.
26. Boyd MT, Seward JB, Tajik AJ, et al. Frequency and location of prominent left ventricular trabeculations at autopsy in 474 normal human hearts: Implications for evaluation of mural thrombi by two-dimensional echocardiography. *J Am Coll Cardiol* 1987; 9:323–326.
27. Ritter M, Oechslin E, Sutsch G. Isolated noncompaction of the myocardium in adults. *Mayo Clin Proc* 1997; 72:26–31.
28. Agmon Y, Connolly H, Olson L, et al. Noncompaction of the ventricular myocardium. *J Am Soc Echocardiogr* 1999; 20:859–863.
29. Veinot JP, Harrity PJ, Gentile F, et al. Anatomy of the normal left atrial appendage: A quantitative study of age-related changes in 500 autopsy hearts: Implications for echocardiographic examination. *Circulation* 1997; 96:3112–3115.
30. McAlpine W. *Heart and Coronary Arteries: An Anatomic Atlas for Radiologic Diagnosis and Surgical Treatment.* New York: Springer-Verlag; 1975.
31. Naqueh SF, Lakkis NM, He ZX, et al. Role of myocardial contrast echocardiogrhy during nonsurgical septal reduction therapy for hypertrophic obstructive cardiomyopathy. *J Am Coll Cardiol* 1988; 32:225–229.
32. Yetman AT, McCrindle BW, MacDonald C, et al. Myocardial bridging in children with hypertrophic cardiomyopathy: A risk factor for sudden death. *New Engl J Med* 1998; 339:1201–1209.
33. Gras D, Mabo P, Tang T, et al. Multisite pacing as a supplemental treatment of congestive heart failure: Preliminary results of the Medtronic Inc in Sync Study. *PACE* 1998; 21:2249–2255.
34. Kar S, Nordlander R. Coronary veins: An alternate route to ischemic myocardium. *Heart Lung* 1992; 21:148–157.
35. Kar S, Drury JK, Hajduczki I, et al. Synchronized coronary venous retroperfusion for support and salvage of ischemic myocardium during elective and failed angioplasty. *J Am Coll Cardiol* 1991; 18:271–282.
36. Lazar HL, Haan CK, Yang X, et al: Reduction of infarction size with coronary venous retroperfusion. *Circulation* 1992; 86:11351–11352.
37. Schiller NB, Shah PM, Crawford M, et al. Recommendations for quantitation of the left ventricle by two-dimensional echocardiography: American Society of Echocardiography Committee on Standards, Subcommittee on Quantitation of Two-Dimensional Echocardiograms. *J Am Soc Echocardiogr* 1989; 2:358–367.
38. Nagel E, Lehmkuhl H, Bocksch W, et al. Noninvasive diagnosis of ischemia-induced wall motion abnormalities with the use of high-dose dobutamine stress MRI comparison with dobutamine stress echocardiography. *Circulation* 1999; 99:763–770.
39. Ichikawa H, Matsubara O. Studies on the microvasculature of human myocardium *Bull Tokyo Med Dent Univ* 1977; 24:53–65.
40. Cannon RO, Leon MB, Watson RM, et al. Chest pain and "normal" coronary arteries: The role of small coronary arteries. *Am J Cardiol* 1985; 55:50B–60B.
41. Parodi O, Sambuceti G. The role of coronary microvascular dysfunction in the genesis of cardiovascular diseases. *Q J Nucl Med* 1996; 40:9–16.
42. Schwartzkopff B, Motz W, Frenzel H, et al. Structural and functional alterations of the intramyocardial coronary arterioles in patients with arterial hypertension. *Circulation* 1993; 88:993–1002.
43. Krams R, Kofflard MJM, Duncker DJ, et al. Decreased coronary flow reserve in hypertrophic cardiomyopathy is related to remodeling of the coronary microcirculation. *Circulation* 1998; 97:23–233.
44. Oh JK, Seward JB, Tajik AJ. Contrast echocardiography. In: Weinberg RW, Simmons LA, Madrigal R, eds. *The Echo Manual*, 2d . Philadelphia: Lippincott-Raven; 1999:245–249.
45. Kantor B, McKenna CJ, Caccitolo JA, et al. Transmyocardial and percutaneous myocardial revascularization: Current and future roles in the treatment of coronary artery disease. *Mayo Clin Proc* 1999; 74:585–592.
46. Harmon J Jr, Edwards WD. Venous valves in subclavian and internal jugular veins. *Am J Cardiovasc Pathol* 1987; 1:51–54.
47. Maclellan-Tobert SG, Buithieu J, Belohlavek M, et al: Three-dimensional imaging used for virtual dissection, image banking and physical replications of anatomy and physiology. *Echocardiography* 1998; 15:89–98.
48. Bruining N, Roelandt J, Grunst G, et al. Three-dimensional echocardiography: The gateway to virtual reality. *Echocardiography* 1999; 16:417–423.
49. Seward JB, Belohlavek M, Kinter T, et al. Evolving era of multidimensional medical imaging. *Mayo Clin Proc* 1999; 74:399–414.

CHAPTER 3

NORMAL PHYSIOLOGY OF THE CARDIOVASCULAR SYSTEM

Martin M. LeWinter / George Osol

The cardiovascular system functions to deliver oxygen, nutrients, and other essential molecules to the tissues and carry waste products (e.g., carbon dioxide, metabolic end products) to the organs responsible for their elimination (i.e., lungs, liver, kidney). To accomplish these functions, a system with two separate circulations in series has evolved. The pulmonary circulation is a low-resistance, high-capacitance vascular bed specialized for bidirectional gas exchange with the environment. The systemic circulation consists of multiple, relatively high resistance vascular beds specialized for the delivery of oxygen and nutrients to tissues and extraction of carbon dioxide and metabolic waste products. Blood is a solvent that dissolves and transports the substances required for and produced by metabolic processes. It travels sequentially through the two circulations and is pumped by two highly adapted pumps in series. The latter are combined in one organ, the heart, that is under coordinated local and neurohumoral control. Each side of the heart is composed of two chambers, a thin-walled atrium that accepts venous blood from its respective circulation and also has a booster pump function and a thicker-walled ventricle that pumps the blood to its respective circulation.

A key aspect of the cardiovascular system is that it must function under a wide variety of demands. Thus, during the stress of exercise, the amount of blood pumped, the *cardiac output* (CO), must increase fourfold or more.[1,2] Extremes of temperature (e.g., during exercise) require that the cardiovascular system function to maximize heat loss or conservation. Beat-to-beat variations in loading of the heart related to normal functions such as respiration require exquisitely fine tuning of the stroke volume (SV) produced by each side of the heart. Moreover, the system has little or no room for error; even a slight, sustained mismatch of left- and right-sided SV would result in a catastrophe. This chapter reviews the cellular and organ-level cardiac and vascular mechanisms nature has devised to accomplish these tasks.

CARDIAC FUNCTION

The Cardiac Cycle

As a departure point, we begin this section by considering the sequence of events that occur at the organ level during the course of a single heartbeat, or cardiac cycle (Fig. 3-1, Plate 27). Before mechanical activity begins, an electric signal is delivered to the myocardium (see Chaps. 11 and 23). Electrical signaling is accomplished by specialized conduction system tissue that controls heart rate (HR) by responding to a variety of influences (especially sympathetic and parasympathetic stimulation), provides a normal sequence of activation of the heart chambers that in turn maximizes efficient contraction and filling, and at the cellular level, initiates the biochemical processes that underlie contraction. With respect to HR, conduction system cells have the general property of undergoing spontaneous electrical depolarization and thereby functioning as pacemakers that control the rate of beating. The sinus node, located in the right atrium (RA) near the superior vena caval junction, is the component of the conduction system that has the fastest rate of spontaneous depolarization and therefore provides normal control of HR. It is under the direct influence of the autonomic nervous and neuroendocrine systems, which modulate beat-to-beat and longer-term variations in HR.

At the body surface, activity of the specialized conduction system and spread of the electric impulse is represented by the electrocardiogram (ECG), which is caused by electrical potential differences generated by the heart (see Chap. 11). At the cellular level, electrical excitation consists of transmission of a membrane-based depolarizing and then repolarizing current called the *action potential* (AP) that is propagated through the cardiac chambers via the specialized conduction system, ultimately reaching individual atrial and ventricular myocytes.

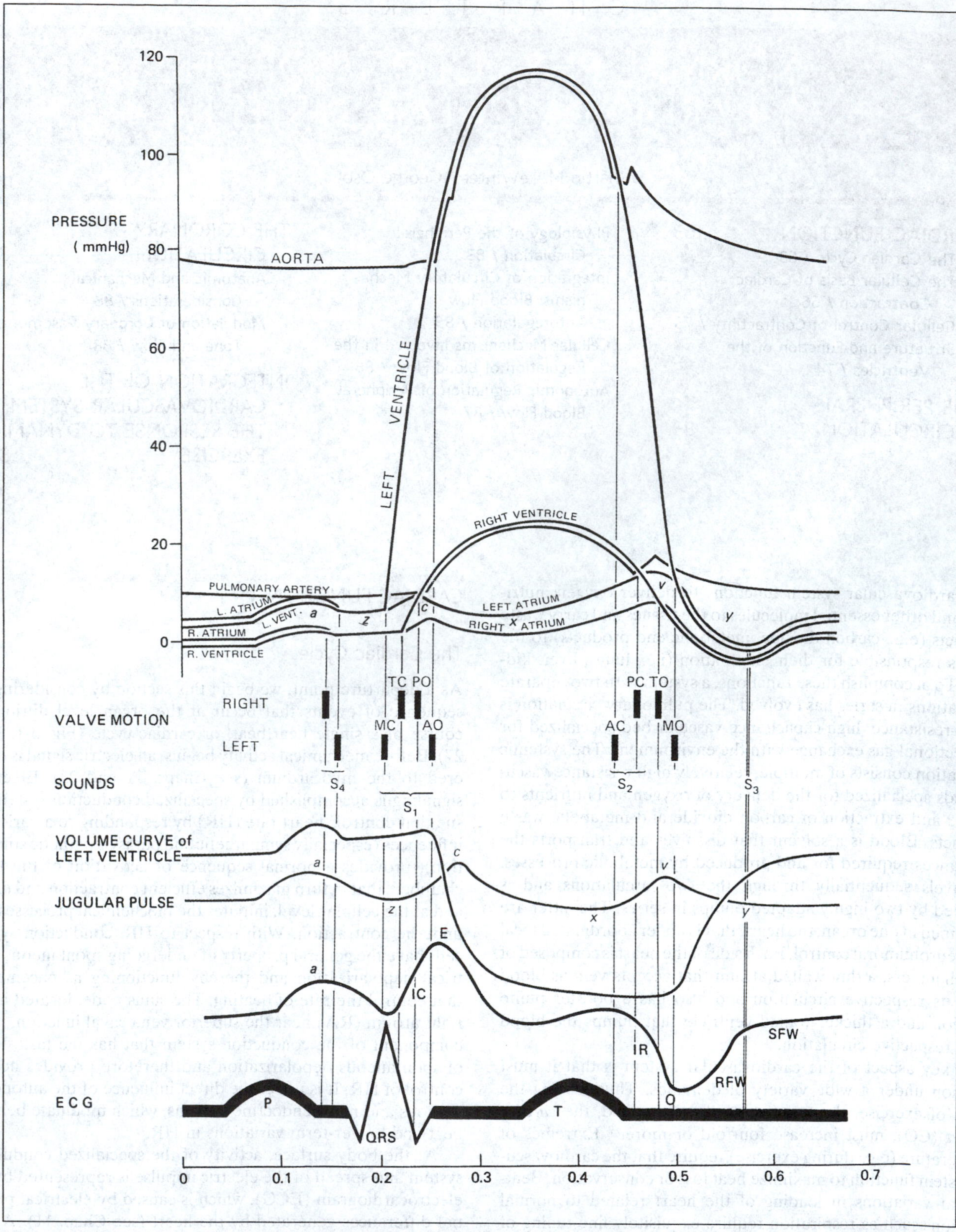

FIGURE 3-1 (Plate 27) Electrical and mechanical events during the cardiac cycle. Shown are pressure curves of great vessels and cardiac chambers, valvular events, timing of heart sounds, LV volume curve, jugular venous pulse wave, and electrocardiogram (ECG). MC and TC, mitral and tricuspid valve closure; PO and AO, pulmonic and aortic valve opening; AC and PC, aortic and pulmonic valve closure; TO and MO, tricuspid and mitral valve opening.

The electric signal (AP) begins in the sinoatrial node and then traverses specialized conduction tissue in both atria, spreading to atrial myocytes and causing atrial contraction (the P wave of the ECG). The atrial conduction system tissue then converges at the atrioventricular node region, consisting of the atrioventricular node itself and the more distal His bundle. These structures are located in the junctional tissue where interatrial and interventricular septa meet. The atrioventricular node is an area of relatively slow conduction that is responsible for most of the normal delay between atrial and ventricular contraction (the PR interval of the ECG). A properly timed delay maximizes the booster pump function of the atria and also protects the ventricles from excessively rapid stimulation. From the His bundle, electrical excitation spreads through large, intraventricular fascicles, the left and right bundles. The left bundle branches into two smaller branches, the left anterior and posterior fascicles. Both bundle-branch systems then ramify within the ventricular myocardium. The smallest branches of the specialized conduction tissue are Purkinje system fibers. The electric signal is transmitted from the Purkinje fibers to individual ventricular myocytes, which contract following a series of cellular events described below. Depolarization of ventricular myocardium accounts for the QRS complex of the ECG. Within the myocardium, the AP spreads from myocyte to myocyte through specialized structures called *intercalated disks,* which contain low-resistance gap junctions across which current flows preferentially. The left ventricle (LV), most massive of the cardiac chambers, is the largest source of electrical potential differences. Electrical activation of the LV begins in the interventricular septum, spreads toward the anteroapical region, and reaches the posterobasal portion last. Activation of the right ventricle (RV) begins slightly after the LV.

This pattern of normal electrical activation causes a coordinated sequence of contraction and relaxation of the cardiac chambers, resulting in ejection of blood by the ventricles into the aorta and pulmonary artery (PA), followed by relaxation and filling. The fact that interference with the normal electrical activation sequence almost always adversely affects cardiac function is strong evidence that normal activation is also the most efficient.

By convention, the mechanical cycle (see Fig. 3-1) is considered to begin at ventricular end diastole (ED), the instant just before systole, when the ventricles begin to actively generate tension as signaled by a sudden, rapid rise in intraventricular pressure. Soon after ventricular systolic pressure begins to rise, it exceeds atrial pressure, at which time the mitral and tricuspid valves close. Ventricular pressures then continue to rise rapidly until aortic (Ao) and PA pressures are exceeded, resulting in opening of the Ao and pulmonic valves and onset of the period of *ejection* of blood into the systemic and pulmonary circulations. Between mitral/tricuspid valve closure and Ao/pulmonic valve opening, ventricular volume is constant. This phase of the cycle is termed *isovolumic* or *isovolumetric contraction*. As ejection proceeds, ventricular and Ao/PA pressures rise and then fall together. The Ao and pulmonic valves close, and ejection ends when ventricular pressure falls below Ao and PA pressure. This event is signaled by the *dicrotic notch* of the respective arterial pressures. In the LV, a period then ensues during which pressure continues to fall rapidly until it drops below left atrial (LA) pressure, when the mitral valve opens. Since Ao and mitral valves are closed during this period, volume is constant, and it is termed *isovolumic* or *isovolumetric relaxation*. Although pulmonic valve closure and tricuspid valve opening are shown as separated significantly in time in Fig. 3-1, the point at which RV pressure falls below PA pressure is actually so low (slightly above the point at which it falls below RA pressure) that the RV isovolumic relaxation period is almost nonexistent.[3]

The time when ventricular pressure falls below atrial pressure signals the onset of the *ventricular filling period*. (There is disagreement as to the best conceptual definition of the *onset of diastole*. One is that contraction and relaxation should be viewed as linked events. Diastole therefore does not begin until relaxation is complete. As will be seen, ventricular filling begins *before* relaxation ends. A second is that diastole begins when ventricular filling commences. A third is that diastole begins when the ventricular myocardium begins to relax, i.e., at about the time ventricular systolic pressure begins to fall. Each definition has merit, and there is no need to take sides in the debate.) Immediately after the atrioventricular (AV) valves open, there is rapid inflow of blood into the ventricles. The latter is caused by an AV pressure gradient (typically several millimeters of mercury) that develops immediately after the AV pressure crossover (Fig. 3-2). Ventricular pressure normally declines by

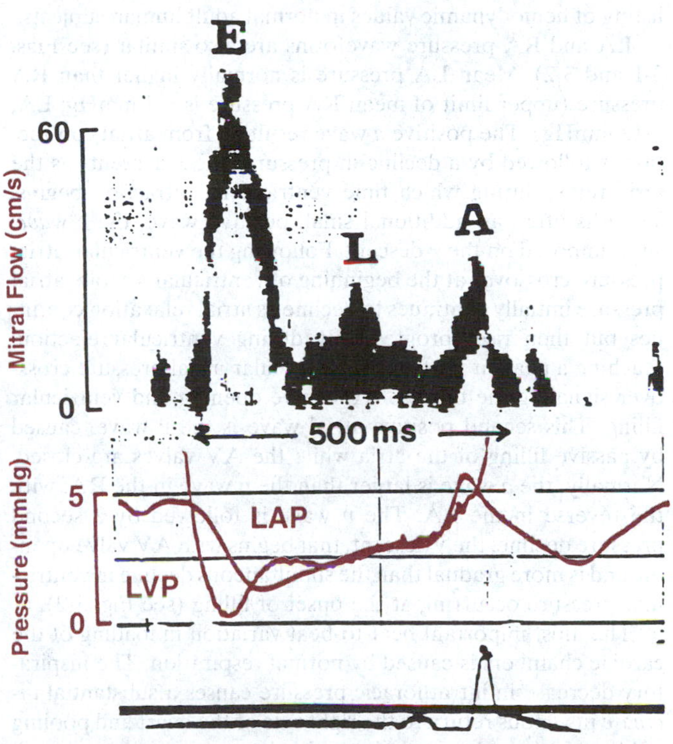

FIGURE 3-2 Mitral flow recorded with a Doppler probe in the mitral annulus and simultaneous LA (LAP) and LV (LVP) pressures in a dog. Note initial gradient immediately after LV pressure crosses LA pressure. As shown here, when recorded with high-fidelity manometers, this is typically followed by a brief reversal of the gradient and then, following the slow-filling phase, by atrial contraction and a second increase in the gradient. Note rapid, early transmitral mitral flow (E wave) and smaller contribution of atrial contraction (A wave). The record also reveals a middiastolic increase in flow (L wave) that is occasionally observed. (From Yellin EL, Nikolic SD. Diastolic suction and the dynamics of LV filling. In: Gaasch WH, LeWinter MM, eds. *LV Diastolic Dysfunction and Heart Failure*. Philadelphia: Lea & Febiger, 1994:92. Reproduced with permission of the publisher.)

at least several millimeters of mercury immediately after the onset of filling and then rises rapidly after reaching its minimum value. Following this initial *rapid filling phase,* ventricular pressure plateaus, the AV gradient diminishes markedly, and filling slows and actually may come to a complete halt (*diastasis*). Slow filling is immediately succeeded by the final filling event, contraction of the atria, which results in a second increase in the AV gradient and injection of an additional bolus of blood into the ventricle. The increase in pressure caused by atrial contraction is the *a wave*. Because of its brief duration, it has relatively little effect on *mean* atrial pressure. Thus normal atrial pump function augments ventricular filling with little risk of an excessive increase in atrial pressure and attendant circulatory congestion. With a normal PR interval, ventricular contraction begins during atrial relaxation.

Ventricular volume changes as a function of time are similar on the right and the left sides, except for the virtual absence of isovolumic relaxation on the right (see Fig. 3-1). Systolic pressure waveforms, of course, differ. The thick-walled LV generates a much higher pressure than the RV, reflecting the high-resistance systemic vascular bed. Pressure waveforms during filling are qualitatively similar in both ventricles but normally on the order of a few to as many as 7 to 8 mmHg higher in the left, reflecting the less distensible, thicker-walled LV chamber. Table 3-1 is a listing of hemodynamic values in normal adult human subjects.

LA and RA pressure waveforms are also similar (see Figs. 3-1 and 3-2). Mean LA pressure is normally higher than RA pressure (upper limit of mean RA pressure is ~7 mmHg; LA, ~12 mmHg). The positive *a* wave resulting from atrial contraction is followed by a decline in pressure (the *x* descent) as the atria relax, during which time ventricular contraction begins. There is often an additional small positive wave, the *c wave,* superimposed on the *x* descent. Following the ventricular-atrial pressure crossover at the beginning of ventricular systole, atrial pressure initially continues to decline as atrial relaxation continues but then rises progressively during ventricular ejection, reaching a peak at time of the ventricular-atrial pressure crossover signaling the onset of AV valve opening and ventricular filling. This second positive atrial wave is the *v* wave, caused by passive filling of the atria while the AV valves are closed. Normally, the *a* wave is larger than the *v* wave in the RA, with the reverse in the LA. The *v* wave is followed by a second pressure decline, the *y* descent, that begins with AV valve opening and is more gradual than the simultaneous decline in ventricular pressure occurring at the onset of filling (see Fig. 3-2).

The most important beat-to-beat variation in loading of the cardiac chambers is caused by normal respiration. The inspiratory decrease in intrathoracic pressure causes a substantial *increase* in venous return to the right side of the heart and pooling of blood in the pulmonary circulation in association with a small decrease in venous return to the left side of the heart. As a result of the relative changes in left- and right-side heart filling during inspiration, RV SV increases in relation to LV SV. This prolongs RV ejection time and delays pulmonic valve closure, accounting for the inspiratory increase in splitting of the second heart sound (see Chap. 10).

TABLE 3-1 Hemodynamic Values in Normal Recumbent Adults

Measurement	Range	Mean
Cardiac index, liters/min per m^2	2.8–4.2	3.4
SV, mL/beat	30–65	47
Arteriovenous oxygen difference, mL per liter of blood	30–48	38
Intravascular pressure,[a] mmHg		
Brachial artery		
Systolic	90–140	—
Diastolic	60–90	—
Mean	70–105	85
LV		
Systolic	90–140	—
ED	5–12	—
LA or PA wedge		
Mean	5–12	—
PA		
Systolic	15–28	—
Diastolic	5–16	—
Mean	10–22	16
RV		
Systolic	15–28	—
ED	0–8	—
RA		
Mean	0–8	—
LV volume index (mL/m^2)		
ED	50–90	—
ES	15–25	—
Resistance, dyn·s/cm^5		
Total systemic	900–1400	1150
Systemic arteriolar	600–900	850
Total pulmonary	150–250	200
Pulmonary arteriolar	45–120	70

[a]Baseline for pressure measurements one-half of anteroposterior chest diameter. 1 mmHg = 133.332; Pa = 0.133 kPa.

The Cellular Basis of Cardiac Contraction

Cardiomyocytes may be considered to consist of three systems: (1) a sarcolemmal excitation system that participates in spread of the AP and functions as a switch initiating the intracellular events giving rise to contraction, (2) an intracellular excitation-contraction coupling (ECC) system that amplifies and converts the electric excitation signal to a chemical signal that, in turn, activates the (3) contractile system, a molecular motor based on formation of chemical crossbridges between two proteins, actin and myosin (Fig. 3-3).

EXCITATION SYSTEM

This system is also discussed in Chap. 23. The cellular AP consists of a transient, local transsarcolemmal depolarizing current that raises the transmembrane potential from its normal resting value of negative 80 to 90 mV to slightly positive values, followed by a depolarizing current that returns the potential to its resting value[4–6] (Fig. 3-4). The AP is initiated within the specialized conduction tissue and is propagated to individual myocytes. It results from a series of coordinated changes in the conductance of specific ionic species through variably gated sarcolemmal channels. The earliest and largest component of membrane depolarization is caused by a rapid, inward Na current. The resting potential is established and maintained by the transsarcolemmal Na-K-ATPase, which uses energy from ATP hydrolysis to pump Na ions out of the cytoplasm.

With respect to initiation of contraction, the most important component of the AP is a relatively *slow, inward Ca current* through voltage-sensitive, L-type (for long-lasting) Ca channels[5,7,8] (Ca^{2+} influx in Fig. 3-4). These channels open, and the current begins when transmembrane potential reaches −35 to −20 mV and, because of its slow kinetics, continues well after the Na current has ceased. The Ca current is mainly responsible for the AP plateau phase. It ceases when L-type channels become inactivated, and regenerative currents (mainly K efflux) begin the repolarization process. L-type channels, also termed *dihydropyridine (DHP) receptors,* are concentrated in invaginations of the sarcolemma called the *transverse-tubule system,* in close proximity to sarcoplasmic reticulum membrane–associated *ryanodine receptor* (RyR) Ca release channels (discussed below).

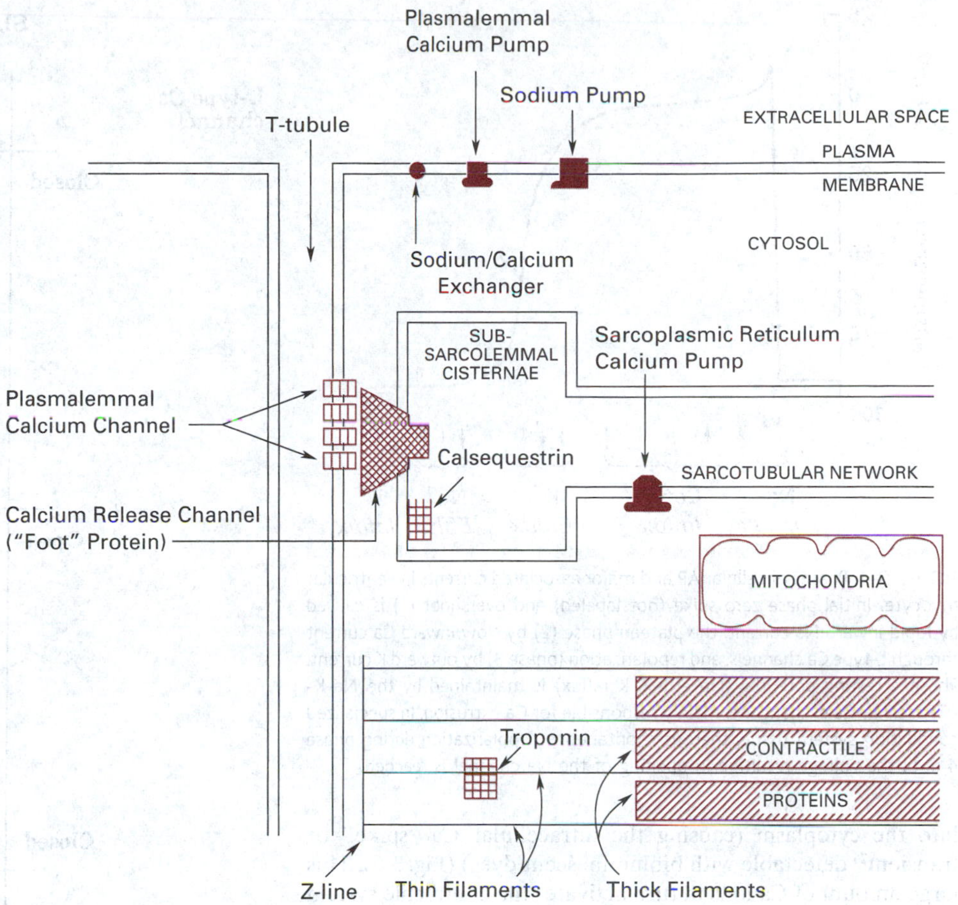

FIGURE 3-3 Schematic diagram of the major cellular components involved in contraction of the myocyte (see text). (Modified from Katz AM. *Physiology of the Heart*, 2d ed. New York: Raven, 1992. Reprinted with permission of the publisher.)

The AP results in a net movement of Ca ions into and a net movement of Na ions out of the cytoplasm. Ionic balance is restored mainly by another sarcolemmal ion-transport mechanism, the *Na-Ca exchanger.*[7,9–11] The exchanger is a shuttle that moves one Ca ion out of the cell against its concentration gradient while using energy from the Na gradient to move one Na ion into the cell. The exchanger also can function in so-called reverse mode, moving a Ca ion into the cytoplasm and a Na ion out.[9–11] Normally, the reverse mode does not contribute significantly to inward movement of Ca ions.

EXCITATION-CONTRACTION COUPLING SYSTEM

ECC is accomplished by the *sarcotubular system,* an arrangement of specialized sarcolemmal and intracellular membranes that functions to control and amplify the ability of the AP to switch the activity of the contractile system on and off. It does so by creating electrochemical signals between the sarcolemma and intracellular organelles; these signals occur much more rapidly than would be possible by simple diffusion of the signaling molecule (in this case, Ca ions).

The sarcotubular system consists of two main components, transverse or T-tubules and the sacroplasmic reticulum (SR)[7,12,13] (see Fig. 3-3). T-tubules are transverse invaginations of the sarcolemma that are concentrated at the Z line of the sarcomere (see below). The SR is a longitudinally oriented system of intracellular membranous sacs and tubules consisting of collar-like structures encircling the contractile filaments at 1- to 2-μm spacings and forming repeating closed compartments that extend along the length of each myofibril from cross striation to cross striation. At the end of each collar is a bulge (*cistern*) that closely abuts a T-tubule, creating a *dyad* or sometimes a *triad* structure. The gap between the cistern and nearby T-tubule is bridged by structures called *feet.*

The SR contains a large store of Ca ions that are released into the cytoplasm as a result of a process termed *Ca-induced Ca release* (CICR)[7,8,14–21] that takes place within or near the dyad. At any point in time, the bulk of Ca ions within the SR is associated with binding proteins, for example, calsequestrin. The details of CICR have been illuminated by Ca "spark" studies employing Ca concentration–sensitive bioluminescent intracellular dyes in conjunction with confocal microscopy[17–21] (Fig. 3-5). As indicated earlier, DHP receptor Ca channels are concentrated in the T-tubule region forming the dyad. The adjacent SR membranes in the dyad contain Ca release channels (RyRs)[7,8,16,22–25] that bridge the cisternal membrane near the foot proteins of the dyad. When the AP depolarizes the cell membrane in the dyad region, the voltage-sensitive DHP receptor channel gate opens, allowing movement of Ca from the extracellular space across the sarcolemma into the gap region of the dyad. Nearby RyR channels are activated (opened) by the local rise in Ca concentration in the dyad,[7,22–25] resulting in very rapid release of much larger amounts of Ca ions from the SR cisternae

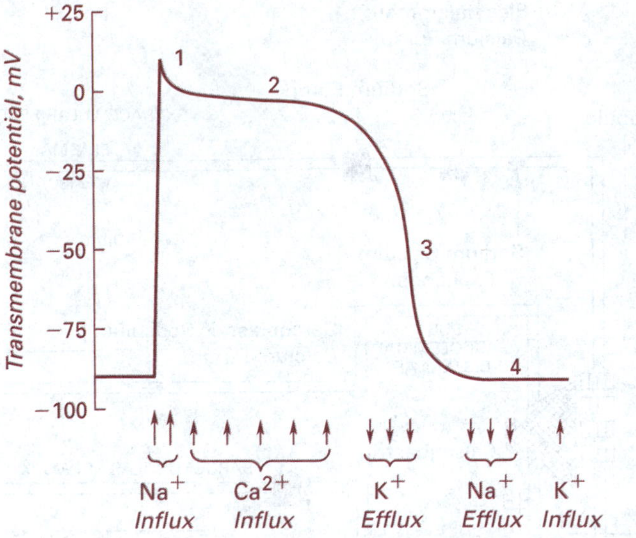

FIGURE 3-4 Phases of cellular AP and major associated currents in ventricular myocyte. Initial phase zero spike (not labeled) and overshoot (1) is caused by rapid inward Na current, the plateau phase (2) by slow inward Ca current through L-type Ca channels, and repolarization (phase 3) by outward K current. Phase 4 resting potential (Na efflux, K influx) is maintained by the Na-K-ATPase. Na-Ca exchanger is mainly responsible for Ca extrusion. In specialized conduction system tissue, there is spontaneous depolarization during phase 4 until the voltage resulting in opening of the Na channel is reached.

into the cytoplasm (causing the intracellular Ca "spike" or transient[26] detectable with bioluminescent dyes) (Fig. 3-6). This large amount of Ca ions in turn activates the contractile system (see below).

The amplification of Ca release inherent in CICR occurs because each DHP release channel induces release of Ca from more than one RyR channel (the exact number is unknown) and because of the very large Ca concentration gradient between the SR and the cytoplasm.[7,8,16,22–25] CICR results in an increase in the intracellular Ca concentration from a diastolic value of approximately 0.1 μM to 1 to 10 μM at the peak of the Ca transient. However, the actual amount of Ca released per beat constitutes only a small amount of the total stored (due to the binding proteins). The increase in intracellular Ca concentration is very transient because free Ca ions rapidly bind to the contractile proteins and are also removed from the cytoplasm by the Na-Ca exchanger and a specialized pump, the SR Ca ATPase (SERCA2).

In order for contraction to be turned off (i.e., for relaxation to occur), Ca ions bound to the contractile proteins must be returned to their storage sites in the SR, and the relatively small number that enter during the AP must be transported back to the extracellular space. As indicated earlier, the Na-Ca exchanger is primarily responsible for extrusion of Ca out of the cytoplasm. There is also a sarcolemmal Ca pump that uses energy from ATP hydrolysis, but this does not appear to be an important means of Ca extrusion. The most important mechanism of reuptake of Ca ions by the SR is pumping by SERCA2, a SR membrane–spanning protein[7,13,27] (see Fig. 3-3). SERCA2 uses energy from ATP hydrolysis to rapidly pump the bulk of Ca ions released during CICR back into the SR. It competes with the contractile proteins and other potential uptake sites (Na-Ca exchanger, sarcolemmal ATPase, mitochondria) for Ca

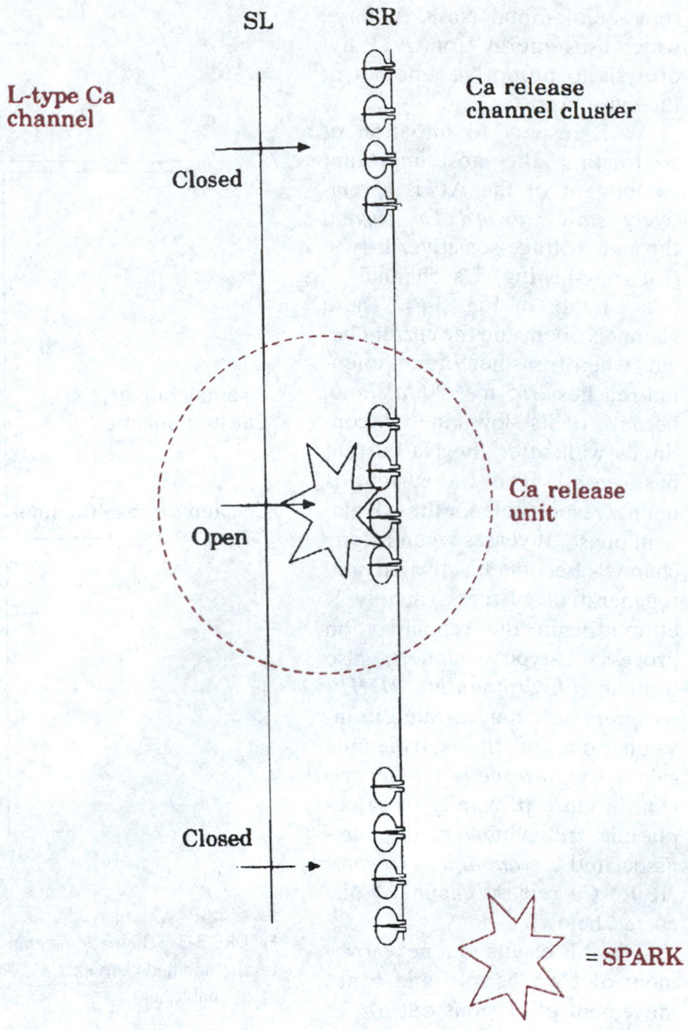

FIGURE 3-5 Schematic of Ca-induced Ca release from SR resulting in a Ca "spark." Opening of sarcolemmal (SL) L-type Ca channel results in movement of a relatively small amount of Ca ions into the cell. The latter causes opening of a number of nearby RyR channels (Ca release unit) with local release of a large amount of Ca ions from the SR and appearance of a "spark," as bioluminescent dye responds to change in local Ca concentration. (From Williams.[8] Reproduced with permission of the publisher.)

ions. Pump stoichiometry is two Ca ions for each ATP hydrolyzed. Functionally, Ca ions pumped back into the SR initially enter a "reuptake pool" and then move to a "release" pool.

The SERCA2 pump is partially self-regulating, since its speed increases in proportion to free Ca concentration (see below). It is also regulated by a closely associated SR protein, phospholamban (PLB), a key modulator of cardiac responses to adrenergic signaling.[28–33] PLB is a 52-amino-acid protein with a hydrophobic domain anchored in the SR membrane and a hydrophilic domain containing three phosphorylation sites. PLB inhibits SERCA2 activity, as exemplified by transgenic PLB knockout mice with increased basal cardiac contractility due to increased Ca cycling per beat but blunted adrenergic responses.[30,31] β-Adrenergic stimulation results in phosphorylation of PLB by activation of cyclic AMP-dependent protein kinase A (PKA). This reduces the inhibitory effect of PLB on SERCA2,

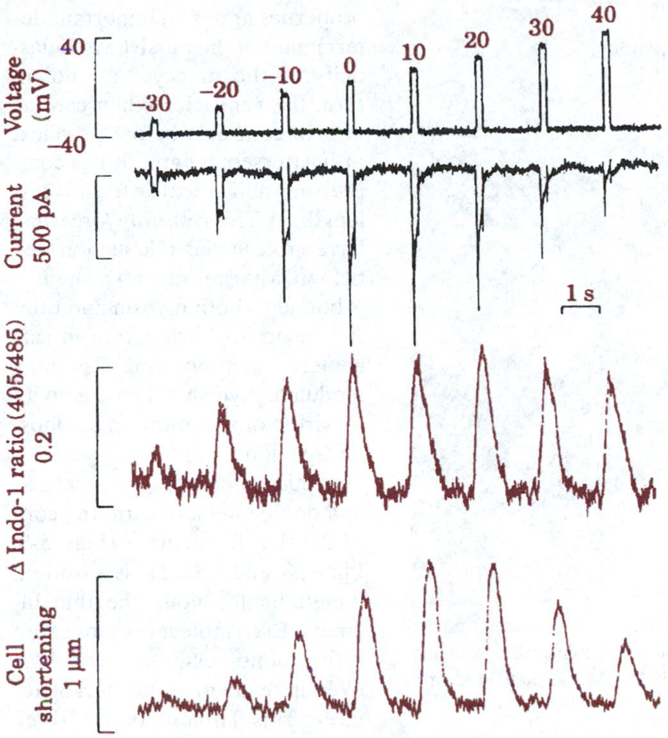

FIGURE 3-6 Intracellular Ca transient obtained with the bioluminescent dye Indo-1 is shown in the middle of this figure. It reflects the average instantaneous intracellular Ca ion concentration. The L-type Ca channel current modified by voltage clamping is shown in the top panel, and myocyte shortening is shown in the bottom panel. Note the voltage dependence of the Ca current and the parallel changes in both the Ca transient and shortening. (From Williams.[8] Reproduced with permission of the publisher.)

resulting in increased Ca cycled per beat and an increased reuptake rate. These effects increase the rate and force of contraction as well as relaxation rate. (In addition to PLB phosphorylation, adrenergic stimulation of PKA also causes phosphorylation of L-type Ca channels,[8,15,34] resulting in increased transsarcolemmal Ca current and increased CICR via RyR channels.)

CONTRACTILE SYSTEM

The basic building block of the contractile system is the sarcomere[12] (Fig. 3-7), a recurring arrangement of the proteins responsible for mechanical activity. Adult myocytes are capable of increasing the numbers and changing the arrangement of sarcomeres in response to physiologic or pathologic changes in demands. An increase in sarcomeres in parallel increases force-producing capacity; an increase in series increases shortening capacity. Each sarcomere is composed of two bundles of longitudinally oriented filaments.[12] *Thick filaments,* approximately 1.6 μm long, are composed of myosin molecules in a trigonal array at the center of the sarcomere's length. Cardiac myosin is a member of a large family of myosins that function in various molecular motors. In addition to myosin, two other proteins are associated with the thick filament, titin and myosin-binding protein C. At each end of this array, a set of approximately 1-μm-long *thin filaments* composed of actin and the proteins tropomyosin (Tm) and troponin (Tn) interdigitates with the thick filaments. The other ends of the thin filaments extend to the ends of the sarcomere, where they attach to a transverse

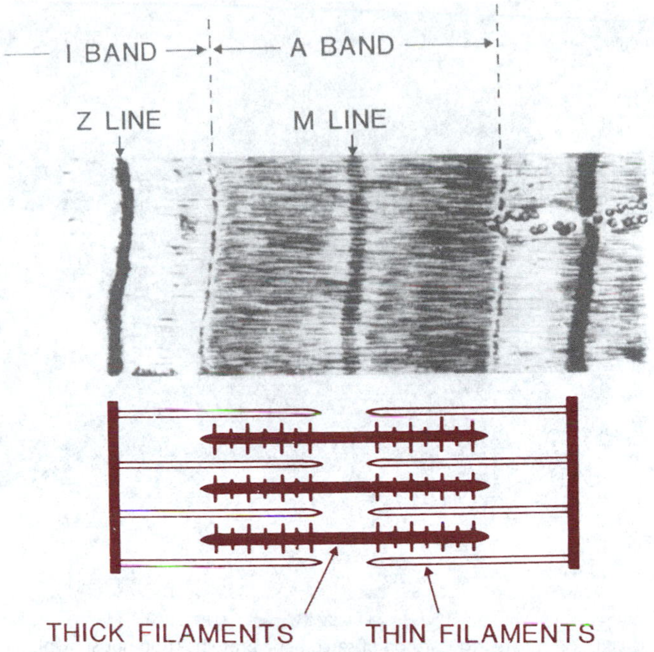

FIGURE 3-7 (*Top*) Electronmicrograph of sarcomere. (*Bottom*) Schematic (see text). (From Woledge et al.[58] Reproduced with permission of the publisher.)

structure, the *Z-line*. The distance between sequential Z-lines is the sarcomere length. At a length of 2.2 μm (length at which maximal force is produced), the central end of each thin filament overlaps 0.7 μm of the distal ends of the thick filaments (the *overlap zone*). The 0.3-μm length of nonoverlapped thin filaments extending to the Z-line and the corresponding 0.3 μm of nonoverlapped thin filaments in the adjacent sarcomere constitute the *I-band*. The centrally positioned thick filaments constitute the *A-band*. Alternating A- and I-bands are responsible for the *striated* appearance of cardiac muscle. Thick filaments are joined at the *M-line* in the middle of the sarcomere.

As just indicated, a portion of each myosin molecule is oriented longitudinally to form the thick filament. In addition, a portion of the molecule protrudes from the thick filament surface and can move freely in the space between the thick and thin filaments (Fig. 3-8, Plate 28). This protruding portion includes the myosin *heavy chain* that forms the crossbridge, the molecular structure that interacts with actin and is responsible for conversion of chemical energy (high-energy phosphate bonds) to mechanical energy (force and motion).[35,36] The crossbridge head (myosin heavy chain) is a complex protein containing a domain that binds with actin and a site of ATPase activity.[37,38] Two auxiliary proteins (*light chains*) that have a role in maintaining the structural requirements for force generation (*essential light chain*) and providing fine control of force and motion (*regulatory light chain*) are adsorbed to the surface of the heavy chain. In mammalian cardiac muscle, myosin heavy chain exists primarily as two isoforms, alpha and beta.[37] The alpha isoform has higher ATPase activity and more rapid rates of crossbridge formation and velocity than beta and is dominant in adult small mammals.[38–42] The beta isoform is dominant in adult large mammals, including humans. Titin is a giant protein anchored in the Z-line on one end and closely associated with myosin on its other end.[43] A segment of titin has springlike

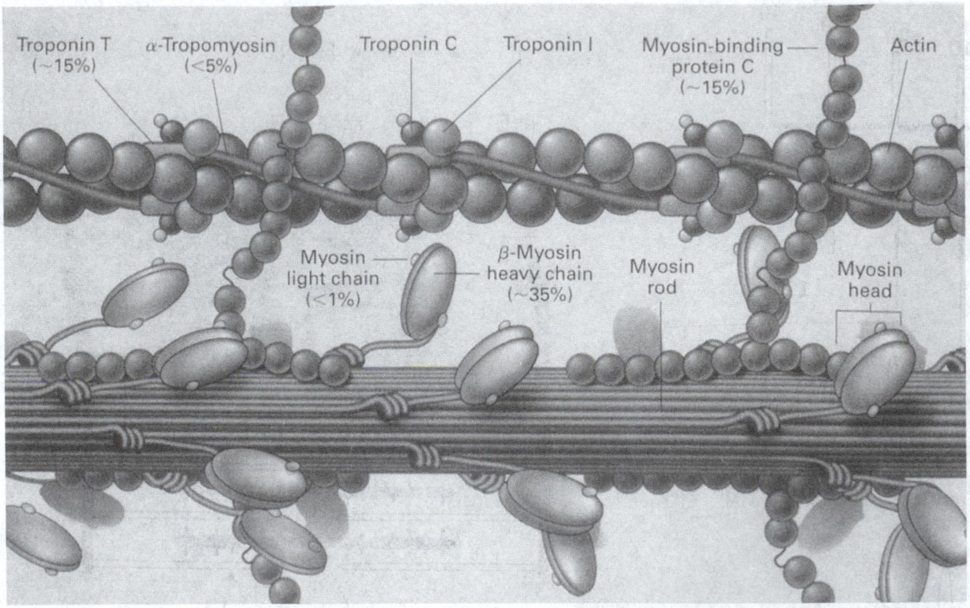

FIGURE 3-8 (Plate 28) Cartoon of sarcomeric proteins (titin not shown). (From Spirito P, Seidman CE, McKenna WJ, Maron BJ. The management of hypertrophic cardiomyopathy. *New Eng J Med* 1997; 336:775. Reprinted with permission of the publisher.)

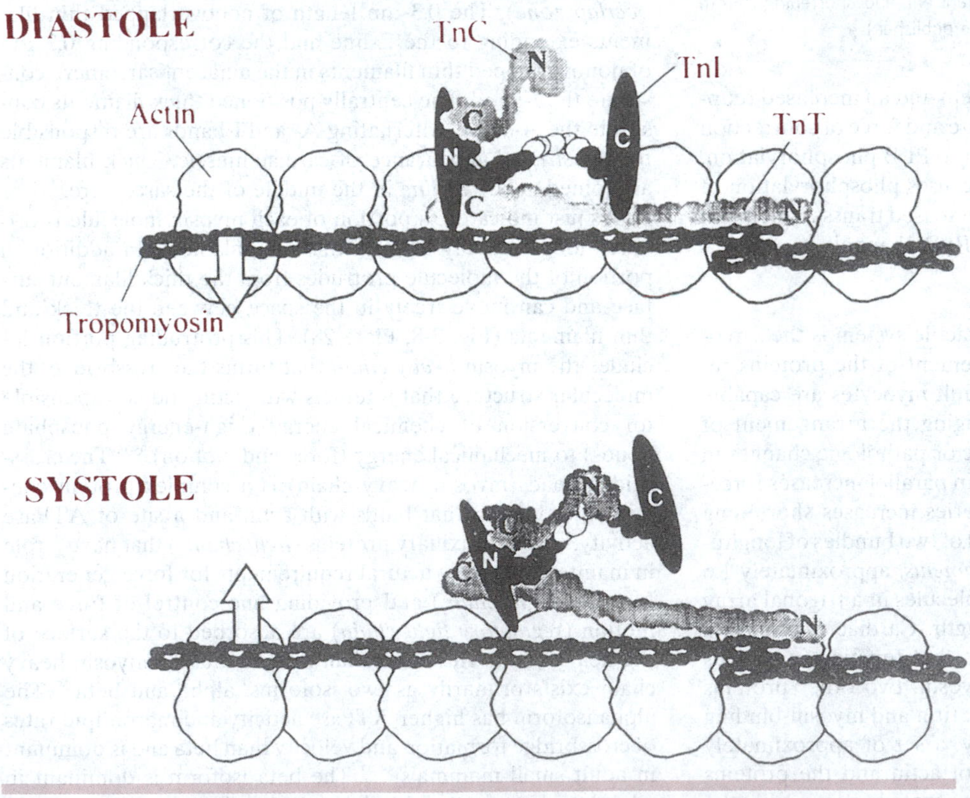

FIGURE 3-9 Cartoon of the thin filament with actin and regulatory proteins, Tm and Tn complex, showing conformational differences between inactive state (diastole) and activation (systole). C, COOH terminus; N, NH_2 terminus. (From Solaro and Rarick.[48] Reproduced with permission from the publisher.)

properties and is an important determinant of the passive viscoelasticity of the myocyte[43,44] and, in turn, the ventricle. When cardiac muscle contracts below its slack, or unstressed, length, titin is compressed and recoils to its rest length.[43,44] This *restoring force* may have a role in diastolic suction (see below). Myosin-binding protein C is bound to both myosin and titin. It appears to have a role in sarcomere assembly and also may modulate myosin ATPase activity by virtue of variations in its phosphorylation.[45]

Actin monomers are arranged in a double helix to form the core of the thin filament[46–48] (Figs. 3-8, Plate 28, and 3-9). Tm is adsorbed longitudinally along the thin filament. Each molecule spans seven actin monomers, with a short overlap segment at the ends of adjacent Tms. Tn, composed of three subunit proteins, TnC, TnI, and TnT, is adsorbed on Tm, also in a ratio of 1 per 7 actin monomers. TnC contains a Ca-binding site, TnI variably binds to Tm and TnC (depending on activation), and TnT links Tn to Tm at the overlap zone. The combined Tm-Tn complex is responsible for the ability of Ca ions, binding to TnC, to act as a switch initiating crossbridge formation. TnI and TnT, the myosin regulatory light chain, and myosin-binding protein C all have phosphorylatable sites (mainly serines and threonines).[48,49] Phosphorylation of these contractile proteins, especially TnI and TnT, modulates the activity of myosin ATPase, as described below.

The sequence of events that ensues when the contractile system is activated by Ca ions entering the cytoplasm as a result of CICR may be summarized as follows[46–48] (see Fig. 3-9): In diastole, with low Ca concentration, Tm occupies a position on actin that inhibits interaction between actin and myosin. Strong binding between TnI and Tm appears to be responsible for maintaining this position. In the *steric blocking* model of Huxley,[50] it was hypothesized that in diastole Tm physically blocks any actin-myosin interaction; i.e., crossbridges are detached. It now appears that the situation is more complex.[48,51,52] At diastolic Ca concentrations, crossbridges exist in both a truly detached or *blocked* state and a weakly attached, non-force-producing state. Moreover, it is proposed that weakly attached crossbridges exist in two states, *closed* and *open*, depending on variations in the position of Tm on actin. With activation, Ca ions bind to TnC and cause a complex rearrangement of the Tn complex, with the most important element probably being a switch to strong binding of TnI to TnC rather than to Tm. The latter, in turn, causes a change in the position of Tm on actin that releases inhibition of actin-myosin interaction and, in addition, probably directly influences the kinetics of crossbridge formation by increasing the rate of transitions from the various non-force-producing to force-producing states.

Two other factors appear to be important in this process of *thin filament activation*. One is *nearest-neighbor interactions*[47,48] along the actin monomers, such that binding of Ca to Tn causes the process of crossbridge formation to spread down the thin filament (perhaps to as many as 12 to 14 adjacent monomers). This property appears to be related to activation-induced structural changes in TnT and Tm. The second is strong binding of actin to myosin,[48,53,54] which begins to occur once inhibition of the actin-myosin reaction is relieved. In and of itself, strong binding seems to encourage additional thin filament activation. Under most physiologic conditions, systolic Ca concentration does not achieve a level resulting in maximum force and/or shortening; i.e., the muscle is *submaximally* activated. Cardiac muscle is also highly cooperative; i.e., the relation between Ca concentration and force/shortening between diastolic and maximally activated levels is very steep (Fig. 3-10). This property is thought to be due to both nearest-neighbor interactions and strong actin-myosin binding. Functionally, this means that contractile reserve can be recruited with modest changes in Ca concentration.

Regardless of the details of thin filament activation, when Ca binds to TnC, the crossbridge cycle is switched on, and actin and myosin undergo a chemical reaction powered by ATP hydrolysis in which a series of transitions are made from detached/weakly bound states to force-producing states and back.[35,36,38,55–59] ATP hydrolysis actually occurs in conjunction with the transition from force production back to detached/weakly bound states. Energy released from hydrolysis of one high-energy phosphate bond is stored in the form of a molecular conformational change in the head of the crossbridge. While the myosin head is strongly bound to actin on the activated thin filament, conformational energy is released, causing the myosin head to rotate slightly as would the oar of a rower seated on the actin filament (Fig. 3-11). This motion generates a force propelling the thin filament along the thick filament toward

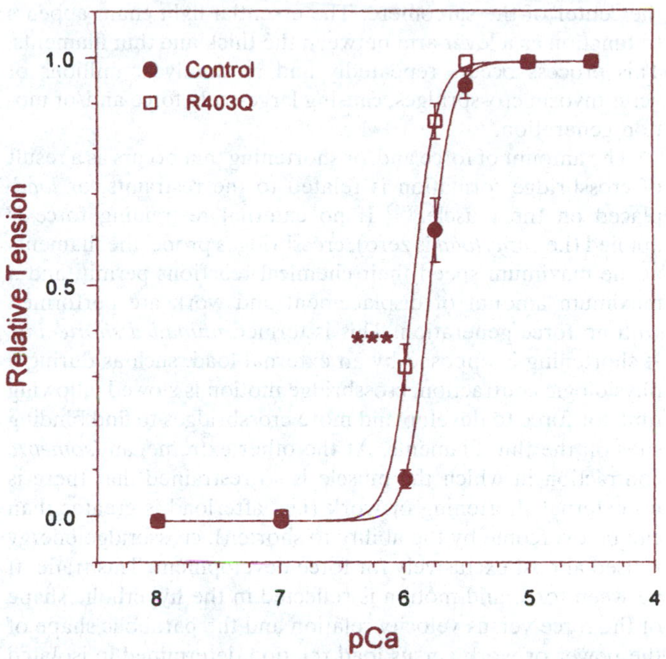

FIGURE 3-10 Relation between log Ca concentration (pCa) and isometric tension in detergent-treated ("skinned") strips of mouse cardiac muscle. R403Q indicates a transgenic animal with a mutation causing hypertrophic cardiomyopathy; control is wild type. Skinning results in loss of integrity of the sarcolemma and all intracellular membranes, leaving sarcomeric proteins intact. In skinned strip, the ionic milieu of the contractile proteins can be manipulated and their behavior studied in isolation from the excitation and ECC systems. Note very steep relation between isometric tension and pCa between relaxing (pCa >7) and fully activating Ca concentrations (pCa 5) in both strips. The relation is shifted to the left in R403Q mice. (From Blanchard E, Seidman C, Seidman JG, et al. Altered crossbridge kinetics in the αMHC[403/+] mouse model of familial hypertrophic cardiomyopathy. *Circ Res* 1999; 84:475. Reprinted with permission of the publisher.)

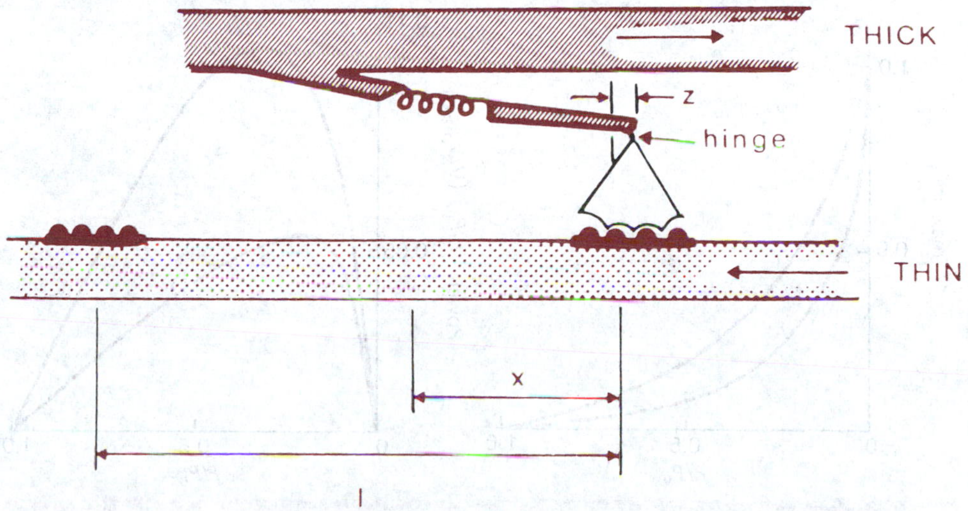

FIGURE 3-11 Schematic of the mechanical interaction between the myosin head (triangular structure) and actin located on the thin filament. Letter *z* denotes the distance moved by the thick filament as a result of rotation of the head region (see text). (From Woledge et al.[58] Reproduced with permission of the publisher.)

the center of the sarcomere. The essential light chain appears to function as a lever arm between the thick and thin filaments. This process occurs repeatedly and randomly at millions of actin-myosin crossbridges, causing large-scale force and/or motion generation.

The amount of force and/or shortening that occurs as a result of crossbridge formation is related to the restraints, or *load,* placed on the muscle.[58-60] If no external restraining force is applied (i.e., *afterload* is zero), crossbridges propel the filaments at the maximum speed their chemical reactions permit, and a maximum amount of displacement and work are performed with no force generation. This is termed *unloaded shortening.* If shortening is opposed by an external load, such as during a physiologic contraction, crossbridge motion is slowed, allowing time for force to develop and more crossbridges to find binding sites on the thin filaments. At the other extreme, an *isometric* contraction in which the muscle is so restrained that there is no external shortening or work (i.e., afterload is greater than can be overcome by the ability to shorten), crossbridge energy is used almost exclusively for force development. This tradeoff between force and motion is reflected in the hyperbolic shape of the force versus velocity relation and the parabolic shape of the power or work versus load relation determined in isolated cardiac muscle (Fig. 3-12). There is also a reciprocal relation between load on the muscle and crossbridge cycling rate.[58-60] That is, the speed of the chemical reactions driving crossbridge attachment and detachment is sensitive to load and/or the resulting strains or displacements within the sarcomere. The mechanism of this relationship is uncertain, but it is a fundamental property of cardiac muscle that is required for normal function.

Another key determinant of mechanical performance of an activated sarcomere is its initial length, as reflected by the initial length of the muscle (its *preload*)[48-50,61,62] (Fig. 3-13). Force (or shortening) is maximal at an initial sarcomere length of approximately 2.2 μm and falls off very rapidly below approximately 2 μm. The ascending length–active tension/force relation is mainly caused by changes in activation of crossbridges as a function of sarcomere length.[61,62] This is most likely related to the fact that because the sarcomere maintains a constant volume, thick and thin filaments move farther apart at shorter sarcomere lengths.[63] The resulting change in geometry causes a decrease in the effective activation at any concentration of Ca; i.e., fewer crossbridges are formed. This *length-dependent activation* is the primary mechanism at the sarcomere level of the Frank-Starling law of the heart, i.e., the increase in contractile performance as ventricular preload increases. Previously it was thought that the Frank-Starling relation was best explained by changes in thick and thin filament overlap,[35,55] but the latter is probably a modest contributor at best. Although a *descending limb* of the length-tension relation is evident in isolated muscle, it does not appear to be present in the intact ventricle.

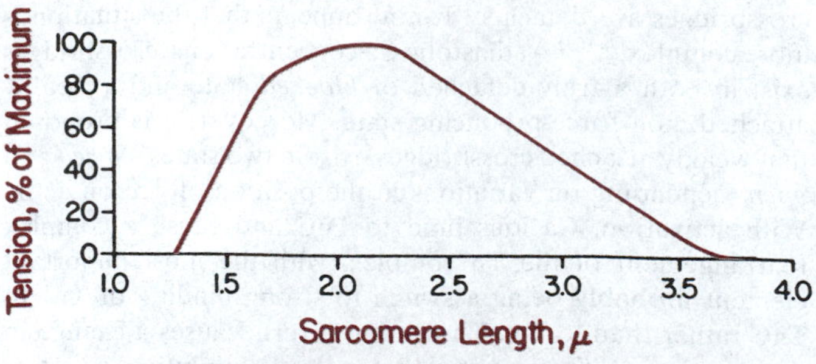

FIGURE 3-13 Schematic of relation between sarcomere length and developed tension (or force). Note fall in tension at lengths below approximately 2.2 μm. At very long sarcomere lengths, thick-thin filament overlap is reduced, resulting in descending limb of relation (not observed in ventricle). (Modified from Braunwald E, Ross J Jr, Sonnenblick EH, eds. *Mechanisms of Contraction of the Normal and Failing Heart.* Boston, Little, Brown, 1976:77.)

MYOCYTE RELAXATION

Myocyte relaxation is a complex process whose rate is determined by three main factors: the kinetics of crossbridge cycling (particularly the rate at which the crossbridges transition from a force-producing to a non-force-producing state), the affinity of Ca ions for TnC, and the activity and affinity of the main Ca reuptake and extrusion mechanisms.[64,65] All else being equal, slower kinetics of crossbridge cycling, increased Ca affinity for TnC, and reduced activity of SERCA2 and/or the Na-Ca exchanger slow relaxation. Relaxation is also modulated by the load on the myocyte, at least in part because of the aforementioned dependence of crossbridge cycling kinetics on load. As noted previously, relaxation also may be influenced by restoring forces generated by compression of titin.

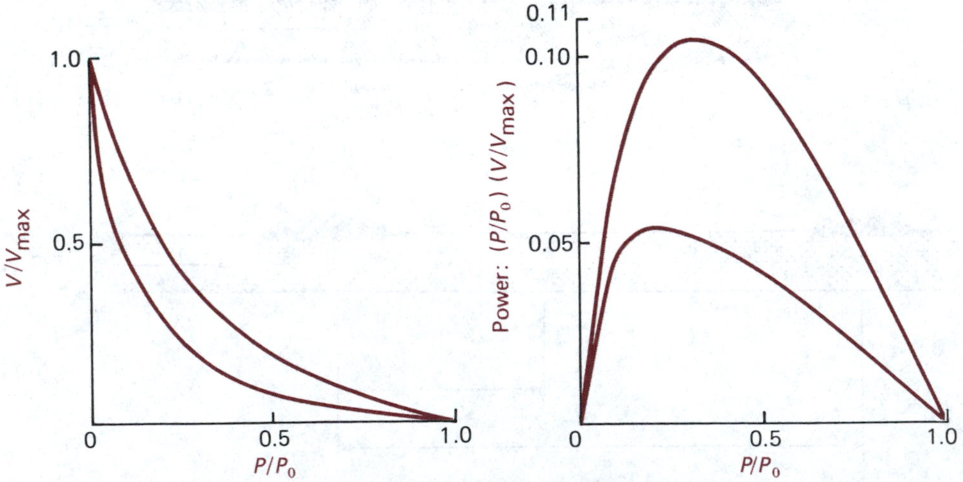

FIGURE 3-12 (*Left*) Force (*P*) versus velocity (*V*) relation for two muscles with differing contractile performance. Velocity normalized to maximum unloaded value (V_{max}) and force to maximum isometric value (P_0). (*Right*) Normalized force versus power (force × velocity) for same muscles. Power is maximal at midrange force values. (Modified from Woledge et al.[58] Reproduced with permission of the publisher.)

ENERGY METABOLISM AND MECHANOENERGETICS

Myocytes are heavily dependent on oxidative metabolism and endowed with large numbers of mitochondria. Under basal conditions, myocytes preferentially take up and oxidize fatty acids to generate ATP.[66–68] During stress, however, glucose uptake, glycogenolysis, and glycolysis become increasingly important. Certain ion pumps, e.g., SERCA2, may be especially dependent on glycolytic ATP.[69] Nitric oxide (NO) generated by vascular endothelium decreases myocardial oxygen consumption (VO_2) due to a direct effect on mitochondrial respiration, and may have a significant role in normal control of energy production and utilization.[70–72]

The processes that account for the great majority of myocardial energy consumption are crossbridge cycling (myosin ATPase), Ca reuptake by the SR (SERCA2), and basal metabolism.[59] Each crossbridge cycle consumes one high-energy phosphate bond, although at very rapid cycling rates it may be possible for one ATP to fuel more than one cycle. SERCA2 uses one high-energy phosphate bond for every two Ca ions pumped. As indicated earlier, the rate of energy consumption is heavily dependent on loading conditions and resulting work and power generation.[58,59] The thermodynamic efficiency of heart muscle, its total mechanical energy output divided by its total chemical energy input, is uncertain, in large measure because of difficulties in quantifying *total* energy output. A more conventional approach is estimation of efficiency of external work production.[58] External work efficiency is heavily dependent on loading conditions, ranging from a maximum under unloaded conditions to zero for an isometric contraction. Additional mechanoenergetic concepts are discussed below under ventricular function.

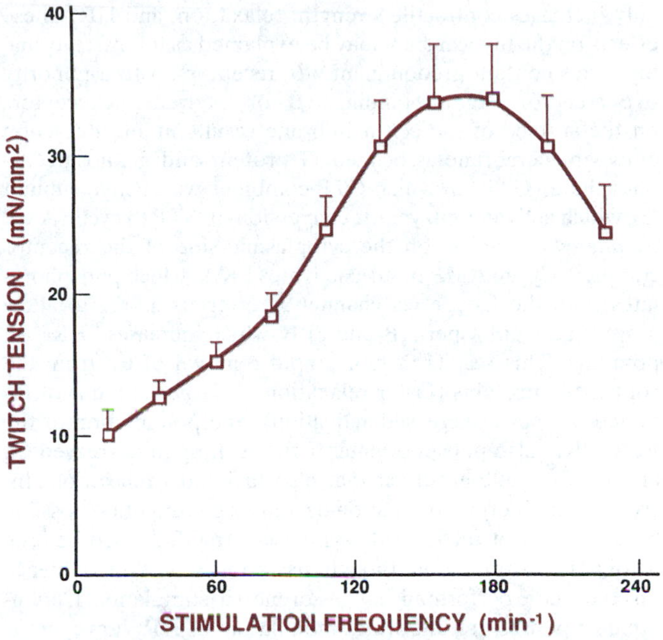

FIGURE 3-14 Example of average relation between developed force and stimulation frequency in strips of human myocardium obtained by epicardial biopsy from a group of patients undergoing coronary bypass surgery, all with normal LV contraction patterns. Note the marked increase in force as contraction frequency increases from typical basal level of 60 per minute to a value of 170 to 180 per minute, at which force is maximal (see text).

Cellular Control of Contractility

This section is divided into intrinsic and extrinsic control systems. *Intrinsic control* includes adaptive mechanisms that are components of the normal mechanical behavior of cardiac muscle. *Extrinsic control* includes both adaptive mechanisms that require the elaboration/secretion of a cardioactive substance by the myocyte or some other cell type and classic neurohumoral modulation of myocyte function.

INTRINSIC CONTROL SYSTEMS

The most obvious is the *length-dependent activation* underlying the Frank-Starling relation. This allows heart muscle to adjust its performance on a beat-to-beat basis, e.g., with respiration and changes in body position, and is discussed further under ventricular function.

Another important intrinsic control mechanism is the *force-frequency relation* (FFR)[73–75] (Fig. 3-14). At a basal rate of 60 per minute, the duration of the myocardial twitch contraction is such that relaxation would be incomplete at rates achieved during exercise and cause impaired diastolic filling. Therefore, the myocardium must have mechanisms that automatically speed contraction and relaxation at rapid rates. In conjunction with this abbreviation of contraction, the strength of contraction is markedly enhanced, allowing maintenance of SV even though less time is available for filling and emptying. The mechanism of the positive FFR involves increased and more rapid Ca cycling per beat as frequency increases.[8,59,76–79] Factors contributing to this include the direct effect of a greater number of APs per unit time, causing intracellular accumulation of Ca ions, as well as increases in SR Ca pumping. Thus Ca entry increases directly with more frequent opening of L-type Ca channels and indirectly when the Na-Ca exchanger extrudes excess Na ions arising from the increased frequency of sarcolemmal Na channel opening. Operating in isolation, these factors would risk elevation of diastolic Ca concentration. However, SR Ca pump speed increases concomitantly, increasing relaxation rate and abbreviating the contraction. In addition to PLB, SERCA2 activity is under the control of another protein, *Ca-activated calmodulin kinase,* which increases SERCA2 activity in response to increased Ca concentration and has built-in frequency sensitivity. Slight, transient increases in Ca ions, even if insufficient to directly activate the kinase, are held in binding sites long enough so that repeated increases are summated. This averaging process results in increased speed of the SERCA2 pump in response to increased average and instantaneous Ca concentration.

The FFR appears to depend on the intactness of multiple elements of Ca handling, as evidenced by the fact that it is depressed in a number of conditions in which the myocardium is diseased and/or subjected to chronic stress.[73,74,76,80] The ratio of SERCA2 pumps to PLB protein has been proposed as an important determinant of its magnitude.[77] Moreover, the FFR is markedly amplified by increased β-adrenergic stimulation.[75] Thus, during stress, increased adrenergic stimulation not only increases HR but also increases the magnitude of FFR occurring in response to the increase. This amplification appears to be related to cyclic AMP-mediated phosphorylation of PLB.[30]

EXTRINSIC CONTROL SYSTEMS

The best understood, most extensively characterized and important extrinsic control mechanism is modulation of contractility by adrenergic and cholinergic neural discharge and circulating catecholamines.[75,81–85] Increased adrenergic stimulation markedly increases contractile strength, relaxation, and HR. These effects on the myocardium may be explained as follows: Normal myocytes contain predominantly β_1 receptors, with a minority of β_2 receptors. Agonist binding to β_1- or β_2-adrenergic receptors on the surface of the cell membrane results in an interaction between membrane-associated G protein and guanosine triphosphate (GTP) in which GTP combines with active subunit G_s, which activates enzymatic conversion of ATP to cyclic AMP by *adenylate cyclase* on the cytoplasmic side of the receptor complex. Cyclic AMP in turn activates PKA, which phosphorylates both the L-type Ca channel, altering its gating to allow more Ca ion entry per AP, and PLB, which increases SERCA2 pumping. This results in more rapid removal of Ca from the contractile proteins (faster relaxation), a larger amount of Ca cycled per beat (increased activation), and potentiation of the FFR. PKA also phosphorylates TnI, resulting in decreased Ca affinity for TnC, an effect that also facilitates relaxation. Increased cholinergic stimulation decreases contractility, possibly by activation of nitric oxide synthase-3 (NOS-3) (see below). Cholinergic stimulation, though, has a much weaker influence on contractile performance than adrenergic stimulation. Cholinergic responses are important modulators of HR, however.

A number of other naturally occurring substances modulate myocyte function. These include circulating neurohormones as well as molecules produced by myocytes themselves and vascular endothelium. Alterations in these substances and their effects on myocardial function may be critically important in disease. The normal physiologic roles of these substances have been variably and in no case fully delineated, but they are almost certainly less important than the intrinsic and extrinsic control systems already discussed. Accordingly, some but not all will be discussed briefly. These substances and their complex signaling pathways are also discussed in Chaps. 5 and 6.

NO is produced in endothelial cells in proximity to cardiac myocytes and in myocytes themselves.[70-72,86,87] NOS-3 is the predominant form of nitric oxide synthase in the myocyte. NOS-3 is Ca-sensitive and is activated by levels of intracellular Ca achieved during normal beating and by muscarinic cholinergic agonists. NO produced in the myocyte or in adjacent endothelium has a negative inotropic effect, mediated via cyclic GMP.[72,86,88] The mechanism appears to involve myofilament desensitization to Ca, possibly via protein kinase G phosphorylation of TnI. NOS-3 activation also blunts catecholamine responses. Inflammatory cytokines also activate NOS-3,[88] an observation that may be important in disease. Endothelial-derived NO may have somewhat different effects than myocyte-derived NO. Thus endothelial-selective, NO-dependent vasodilators cause early and somewhat accelerated relaxation with only a modest negative inotropic effect. Although effects of NO on contractile performance have been observed in normal humans, their physiologic significance is uncertain. *Atrial natriuretic peptide* (ANP) and *brain natriuretic peptide* (BNP) produced in atria and ventricles, respectively, are naturally occurring vasodilators and diuretics. These substances appear to have effects on myocyte function similar to endothelial-derived NO. While increased secretion of these hormones has great significance in heart failure, their role in normal physiologic control of myocyte function also has not been defined.

A number of agonists, including α_1*-adrenergic agonists*,[89] *endothelin-1* (ET-1),[90-92] and *angiotensin II* (ATII),[93-95] influence myocyte function through activation of phospholipase with resulting production of inositol triphosphate (IP_3) and diacylglycerol (DAG).[96-98] (It is now well established that the heart has its own ATII-generating system.[93-95]) IP_3 increases the release of intracellular Ca during contraction through as yet poorly understood mechanisms. DAG appears to be more importantly involved in myocyte functional responses. Its effects are mediated through activation of protein kinase C (PKC).[96-100] The effects of DAG and PKC activation have been somewhat controversial. This may be related to the fact that the effects of DAG or its analogs administered intracellularly (the normal "route") differ from those when they are administered extracellularly.[98] On balance, activation of PKC by the preceding agonists appears to result in a complex, slowly appearing, sustained positive inotropic effect. Mechanisms that may account for this effect are increased intracellular Ca due to phosporylation of L-type Ca channels and PLB. In addition, phosphorylation of the sarcolemmal Na-H exchanger may increase contractility by increasing intracellular pH. However, activation of PKC also has distinctive and contrasting effects on the contractile proteins via phosphorylation of both TnT and TnI.[47,48,101] The result is a reduction in myofibrillar ATPase activity with attendant decreases in crossbridge cycling rate, an effect that by itself would reduce measures of contractility such as rate of tension development or shortening, as well as relaxation rate. The integrated response to agents such as ET-1 is a net positive inotropic effect that may be relatively economical with respect to energy consumption because of the concomitant effects on crossbridge cycling.

Structure and Function of the Ventricles

ARCHITECTURE

The human LV is a thick-walled chamber (average approximately 1.0 cm at ED) with a truncated ellipsoid shape composed of spiraling, sheetlike layers of myocyte bundles (Fig. 3-15). The orientation of the bundles changes from subepicardium to subendocardium, progressing from relatively longitudinal (in relation to the long axis of the ellipsoid) to roughly circumferential fibers occupying about the middle two-thirds of the wall to longitudinal fibers once again in the subendocardium.[102] Regional wall thickness parallels the local radius of curvature. Near the apex, where the radius is small, thickness is relatively small. Variations in thickness may function to equalize regional wall stress.

Contraction of the LV is associated with a wringing motion, or torsion, characterized by a counterclockwise rotation that progressively increases from base to apex.[103] Torsion is important for normal ejection and is an inherent feature of the normal spread of excitation and the connections between the fiber bundles.[104] It also is likely a storage mechanism for potential energy generated during systole that is converted to kinetic energy during diastole, assisting filling by suction.[105] This complex architecture results in efficient conversion of the shortening of individual myocytes and fibers to wall thickening, which is ultimately responsible for ejection of blood. Thus, even though individual fibers shorten only about 10 percent, the normal LV ejects about two-thirds of its ED volume. Interventricular septal fibers have a similar orientation and are continuous with those of the LV free wall. As a result, the septum normally functions as a part of the LV; i.e., during contraction, its endocardial surface under-

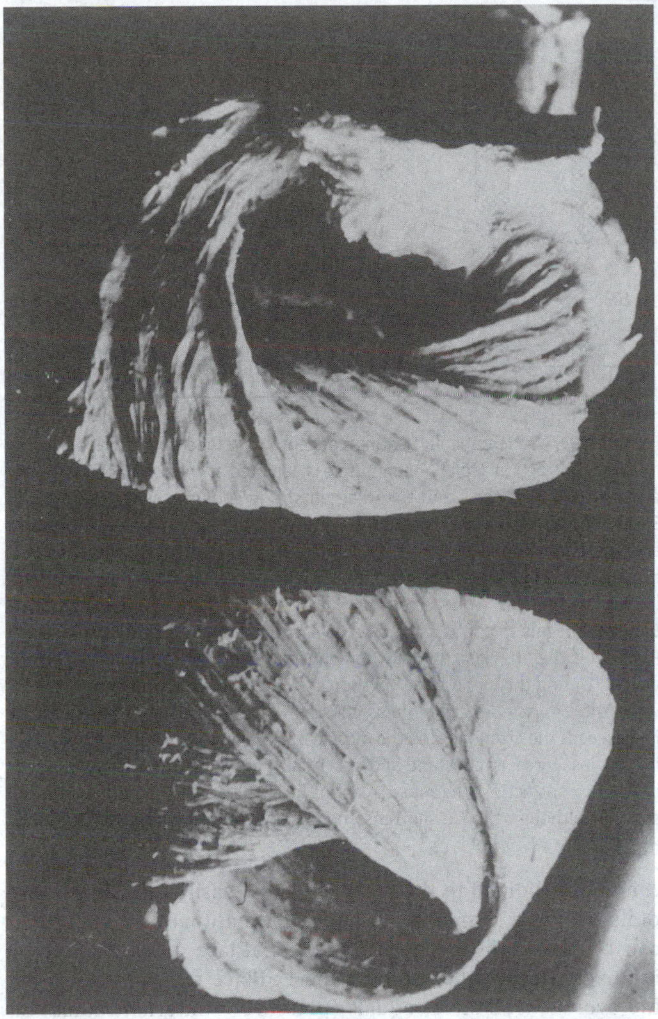

FIGURE 3-15 Three-dimensional architecture of LV, illustrating spiraling bundles of myofibers (see text). (From Streeter.[102] Reprinted with permission of the publisher.)

goes more or less symmetric inward movement toward the center of the LV.

In line with the high-capacitance/low-resistance nature of the pulmonary vascular bed, the RV is much thinner-walled than the LV (3 to 4 mm in an adult human) and appears crescentic in cross section.[102] Its contraction has been likened to that of a bellows. The RV inflow and outflow portions are functionally distinct, with inflow contraction preceding outflow contraction.[106] A significant fraction of the mechanical output of the RV appears to be related to energy transfer from the LV through the interventricular septum (systolic ventricular interaction).[107] This is supported by the observation that destruction of much of the free wall of the RV is remarkably well tolerated.

Ventricular myocardium also has a well-developed connective tissue matrix.[108–110] Cardiac collagen is organized into a weave of fibers that forms a netlike structure around the myofibers (groups of six or more myocytes), as well as connections that link adjacent myofibers and strutlike projections connecting to adjacent blood vessels. The latter may function to help maintain vessel patency during contraction. The collagen network of the ventricles is an important determinant of their passive filling properties (see discussion below). The last major component of the ventricles is the vascular bed, described below.

THE VENTRICLE AS A PUMP

Normal pumping of the ventricles requires that they deliver appropriate amounts of blood to the tissues at acceptably low filling pressures (FPs). Thus the most physiologically relevant means of characterizing the pump is to construct a *function curve* relating FP to a measure of mechanical output (SV, minute volume, work, power). Ventricular function curves display a prominent *Frank-Starling effect,* manifest as a curvilinear relationship between FP and output (once again, there is no descending limb in the normal ventricle) (Fig. 3-16). As discussed earlier, at the myocyte level, the Frank-Starling effect is mainly caused by increased myofilament Ca sensitivity at longer sarcomere lengths. Thus a function curve relating ED *volume* (ventricular *preload*) to mechanical output is a more accurate representation of the ventricular Frank-Starling effect. However, in the clinical setting, FP (pulmonary capillary wedge or RA pressure) is usually more readily available than volume. Whether FP or volume is employed, changes in intrinsic contractile performance result in upward or downward shifts of the ventricular function curve. However, characterization of ventricular performance in terms of function curves relating FP to output is a "black box" approach; alterations in diastolic compliance (see below) produce effects that are indistinguishable from alterations in contractile performance.

The normal heart can pump adequate amounts of blood to meet the needs of the body under the most stressful conditions. Indeed, maximal CO normally is not limited by pumping capacity but by the ability of the systemic circulation, via venoconstriction and the systemic venous system of valves and muscular

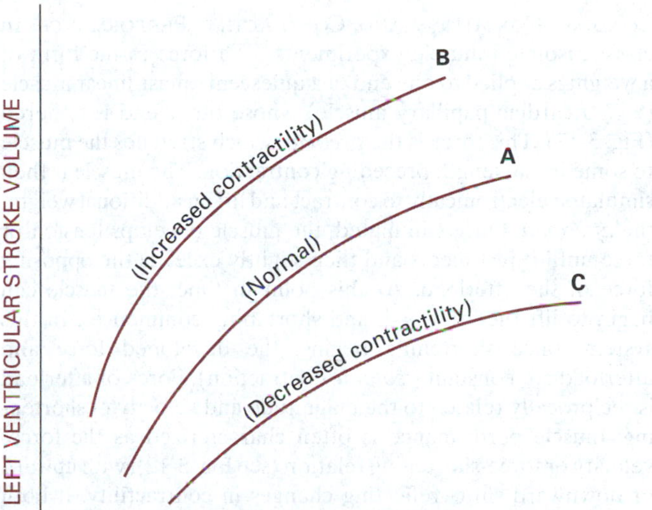

FIGURE 3-16 LV function curves relating SV to ED pressure (see text). *A.* Normal function. *B,C.* Augmented and depressed contractility, respectively, as occur with increases or decreases in adrenergic stimulation. Because ED pressure is plotted, identical shifts could be observed with altered diastolic compliance.

pumps, to return blood to the heart.[111] Under pathologic conditions, pumping capacity may limit CO.

THE VENTRICLE AS A MUSCLE

For convenience, it is useful to consider contraction (systolic performance) as distinct from relaxation and filling (diastolic performance). This distinction is arbitrary, however. The two aspects of function overlap and interact.

Systolic Function Systolic performance of the ventricle traditionally is characterized in terms of loading conditions (preload, afterload) and contractility.[112] Although *contractility* is a term that is employed frequently and often perfectly reasonably, it is difficult to define. We use it here as a *comparative concept* to connote differences in the intrinsic level of contractile performance either before or after some intervention *in the same heart* or *between different hearts* that cannot be accounted for by differences in loading conditions. Thus one way to define a change or difference in contractility is as a change or difference in contractile performance when loading conditions are unchanged or can be accounted for, e.g., increased shortening despite increased afterload. Unfortunately, this is often impossible in the intact heart, especially in the clinical setting. Further, any definition of contractility that attempts to neatly separate it from loading conditions inevitably encounters the fundamental problem that the two are not really separable. A good example of this problem is the Frank-Starling relation, in which *preload* influences *intrinsic* contractile performance by modulating myofilament Ca sensitivity. Similarly, afterload, by influencing shortening, determines instantaneous length and myofilament Ca sensitivity during the course of contraction. Thus, while contractility is a useful concept, the notion that it is possible to define *load-independent* contractility indices is not entirely realistic.

Loading Conditions and Contractile Performance In classic, isolated muscle experiments,[58,60] a force in the form of a weight is applied to one end of a quiescent, quasi-linear muscle (e.g., a cardiac papillary muscle) whose other end is tethered (Fig. 3-17). This force is the *preload,* which stretches the muscle to some initial length preceding contraction. The muscle is then simulated electronically to contract and lift an additional weight, the *afterload.* Once stimulated, the muscle develops tension or force until it just meets and then slightly exceeds the opposing force of the afterload. At this point in time, the muscle can begin to lift the afterload, and shortening commences. In this system, once shortening begins, the developed force and afterload are constant (*isotonic* contraction). Force or afterload is reciprocally related to the magnitude and velocity of shortening; muscle performance is often characterized as the force-velocity or force-shortening relation (see Fig. 3-12), with upward or downward shifts reflecting changes in contractility. If both ends of the muscle are tethered, or if the afterload simply exceeds the force-generating capacity of the muscle, an *isometric* contraction ensues, in which tension is generated, but no shortening occurs. By varying the preload, the Frank-Starling effect (see Fig. 3-13) can be delineated by relating the initial length to shortening (isotonic contraction) or developed tension or force (isometric contraction).

In isolated muscle, load also can be expressed as *stress* (force normalized to cross-sectional area). Normalization allows comparison of muscles of different size. Normalization for stress

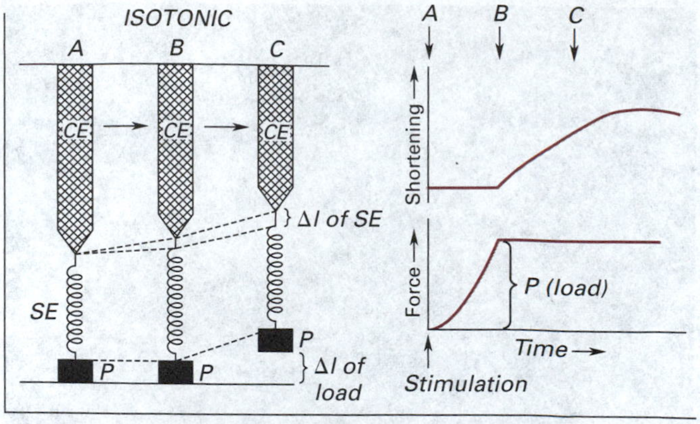

FIGURE 3-17 Schematic illustrating concept of preload and afterload during isotonic contraction. (*Left*) Linear muscle is depicted as consisting of contractile element (CE) (i.e., thick and thin filaments) and spring in series (SE). (*Right*) Shortening and force are depicted. *A*. Muscle is at rest, with one end tethered and the other connected to a weight (P). P is supported, however, so that muscle is only subjected to a fraction of weight (or load). This relatively small load is the preload, which stretches the muscle to the initial, resting length. *B*. Muscle begins to contract. In order to shorten, it must lift the entire weight P, which is the afterload. Initially, force increases but is insufficient to lift the weight. During this period, the CE shortens and reciprocally lengthens the SE, while total muscle length remains constant. Eventually, the developed force just exceeds the afterload, and the muscle begins to shorten (*C*). Once shortening begins, force is constant and essentially equal to the afterload. In an isometric contraction, the muscle cannot lift the load and therefore does not shorten (although the CE shortens and SE lengthens by the same amount).

can be transferred to the ventricle, most easily the LV because of its relatively symmetrical shape. Estimation of LV wall stress can be accomplished by using the LaPlace relation.[113] For a relatively thick-walled sphere, the LaPlace relation states that the average wall stress equals (pressure × internal radius) divided by twice the wall thickness. Variants of this equation can be employed to account for the actual shape of the LV, fiber orientation, and other geometric and structural features. Thus, for an ellipsoid, the ratio of the long to short axis (a measure of how ellipsoidal the shape is) modifies the stress; as shape changes from less to more spherical, wall stress increases.

Use of the LaPlace relation allows an estimate of the stress "seen" by the myofibers as the ventricle fills and then contracts against its afterload. In diastole, the stress applied to the myofibers constitutes their preload and determines initial length at the beginning of the next contraction. During contraction, the stress resulting from both the preload and the afterload (or systolic load) determines the velocity and extent of ejection. Total systolic load presented to the LV by the vascular system has two components, a resistive load determined at the level of small systemic arteries and arterioles by microvascular tone and a smaller capacitive load determined by the properties of the large arteries, which absorb a certain amount of blood pumped via expansion of their walls.[114] As mentioned earlier, a component of vascular load is caused by reflection of pressure waves back to the heart from the periphery. In contrast to classic, isolated muscle experiments, during ventricular contraction, both afterload and developed wall stress vary.

Estimates of *systolic* stress using the LaPlace relation are helpful clinically in assessing and comparing contractile performance.[115] This can accomplished by relating some measure of shortening [e.g., ejection fraction (EF), defined as SV/ED volume] or shortening velocity [e.g., mean velocity of circumferential fiber shortening (V_{cf}); see discussion below] to a measure of systolic stress [e.g., peak, end-systolic (ES), or mean]. The ventricle behaves in a qualitatively similar fashion as isolated muscle; i.e., afterload (wall stress) is reciprocally related to shortening. As shown in Fig. 3-18, the stress-shortening relation can be characterized in a normal population with single data points obtained invasively or using noninvasive techniques such as echocardiography and cuff sphygmomanometry. If the value in a given patient falls above or below the normal range, this may indicate an alteration in intrinsic contractile performance.

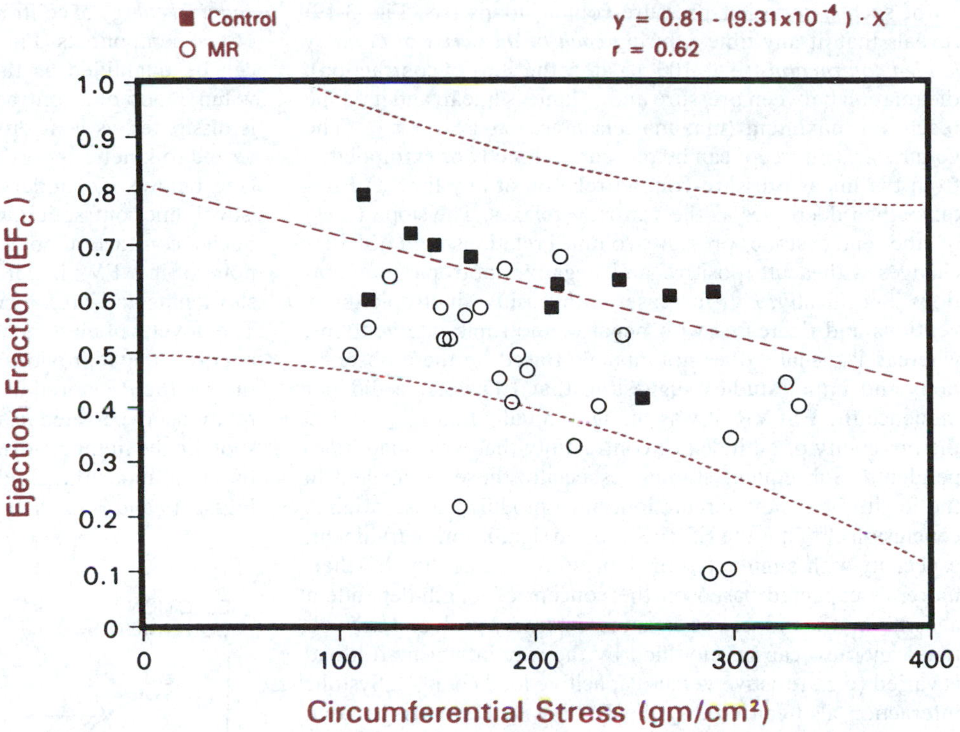

FIGURE 3-18 Relation between EF and circumferential stress (with 95 percent confidence intervals) in human subjects with normal ventricular function (control, filled squares) and mitral regurgitation (MR, open circles) (see text). Some MR patients fall below confidence intervals. (From Starling et al.[115] Reproduced with permission of publisher.)

Clinically, the most commonly employed index of ventricular contractile function is the EF (from angiography, echocardiography, or radionuclide ventriculography). Fractional shortening (minor axis diameter shortening/ED minor axis diameter) is calculated routinely from the echocardiogram and is interchangeable with EF, provided there are no regional wall motion abnormalities. Both these shortening measurements are sensitive to alterations in preload and afterload.[112] Thus normal values are indicative of normal intrinsic contractile function only if loading conditions are also normal.

Elastance Concepts in the Assessment of Ventricular Contractile Function As an alternative to characterization of systolic function in terms of stress and shortening, Suga and Sagawa proposed an elastance approach.[116–118] This is based on the empirical observation that during systole the ventricle behaves like a spring with a time-varying elastance (or stiffness) that increases from a minimum at ED to a maximum at ES (Fig. 3-19). The elastance of a spring is the slope of the linear relation between the stress or force applied to stretch it and its length normalized to its unstressed or rest length. A "stiffer" spring requires a larger stress to extend it by a given length. By analogy, ventricular elastance is the relation between pressure and volume at any time during systole normalized to a volume at which the pressure is zero (*dead volume,* V_0 or V_d).

At any time during contraction, elastance can be estimated by varying loading conditions and generating a series of pressure-volume loops with varying ES volumes. In their original studies, Suga and Sagawa used isolated, perfused canine ventricles with controlled loading conditions and volumes.[116,117] Analy-

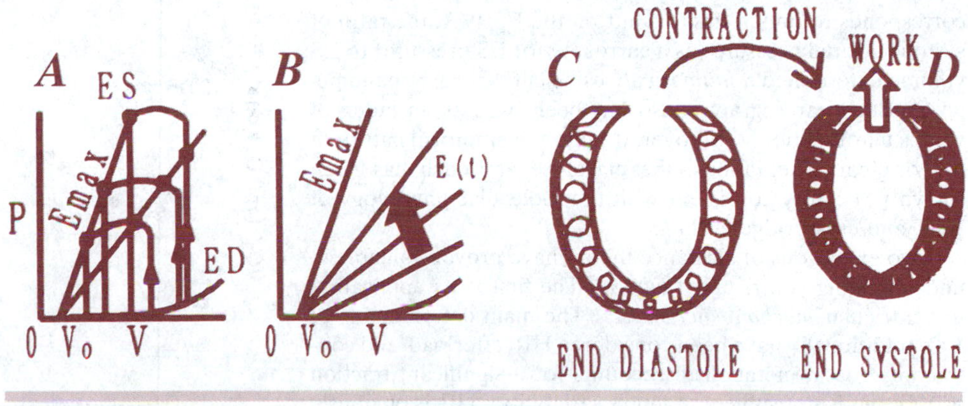

FIGURE 3-19 Schematic of elastance concept (see text). *A.* Series of variably loaded pressure-volume loops. Filled circles connected by straight lines occur at same time *t* during contraction. E_{max} is line connecting points at ES. *B.* Elastance *E(t)* increases at each time *t* during contraction until it reaches maximal value at ES. Increased contractility increases slope at any time *t*, including ES (E_{max}); vice versa for decreased contractility. *C,D.* The concept that the ventricle behaves like a spring of increasing stiffness (increased slope of elastance relations) during contraction. (From Suga H, Takaki M, Matsubara H, Goto Y. Energy costs of PVA and E_{max}: Constancy and variability. In: LeWinter MM, Suga H, Watkins MW, eds. *Cardiac Energetics: From E_{max} to Pressure-Volume Area.* Boston, Kluwer, 1996:2. Reprinted with permission of publisher.)

sis of such a series of pressure-volume loops (see Fig. 3-19) reveals that at any time t during *each of the series of variably loaded contractions* (e.g., 100 ms after the start of contraction), the relation between pressure and volume is linear, and its slope reaches a maximum (maximal elastance) at ES, or t_{max}. (The volume axis intercept can be measured directly or extrapolated from the linear pressure-volume relation at any time t.) Elastance then decreases as the ventricle relaxes. The slope (E_{max}) of the end-systolic pressure-volume relationship (ESPVR) changes with acute positive and negative inotropic interventions. Specifically, E_{max} increases with positive inotropic interventions and decreases with negative inotropic interventions, whereas V_0 usually does not change. Based on these observations and initial studies suggesting that ED volume did not influence the ESPVR, it was thought initially that E_{max} offered the possibility of an index of contractility that was "load independent." Subsequent studies, especially those performed in the in situ heart and circulation, have modified these original conclusions.[118] Thus the ESPVR is often significantly curvilinear, especially with augmented or depressed contractility. Furthermore, as expected based on the concept of length-dependent activation, it is influenced to some extent by preload (ED volume) and also can be modified by the way in which afterload is varied (e.g., resistive versus capacitive load change). Systolic interaction also can modify the ESPVR.[119] E_{max} must be used with caution in comparing different hearts because of difficulties in normalizing ES relationships for size and variable curvilinearity. To overcome these problems, the ESPVR has been modified by calculating ES myocardial stiffness based on wall stress estimates, and comparative analyses have been devised that take curvilinearity into account.[115,120–123] Last, the pressure-volume approach does not include rate of change of these parameters and therefore does not capture power output,[58,112] an important aspect of performance.

Despite the aforementioned cautions, the ESPVR has proven to be a useful conceptual approach to assessment of contractile function in the experimental laboratory and the clinic. Measurements have been made in hearts as small as that of the mouse,[124] whereas estimation of ES pressure and/or stress-volume relations can be obtained in patients.[115,125] Although it corresponds to only a single point on the ESPVR, the ratio of systolic arterial pressure (as a surrogate for ES pressure) to ES volume determined *noninvasively* using cuff sphygmomanometry and echocardiography also has been used as an index of ventricular function. Moreover, despite the empirical nature of the original observations, the elastance approach has been shown to be very consistent with the molecular physiology of ECC and crossbridge cycling.[126]

Two extensions of elastance theory have proven valuable in understanding ventricular function. The first is its application to ventricular *mechanoenergetics*.[127] The main determinants of VO_2 traditionally have been considered HR, afterload, and contractility (basal metabolism accounts for a significant fraction of VO_2 but is not subject to much variability). HR is obviously a critical determinant of energy consumption per unit time. However, the difficulty in even defining contractility was discussed earlier. Moreover, it is not obvious how contractility or afterload is related *quantitatively* to the two major energy-consuming processes in heart, ECC and crossbridge cycling.

As proposed by Suga,[127] use of elastance theory to quantify mechanoenergetics is based on quantification of the *total mechanical energy* of contraction. Total mechanical energy consists of two components (Fig. 3-20, top), *external work* (EW), which can be quantified as the area enclosed within the pressure-volume loop of a contraction, and *potential energy* (PE), which is dissipated as heat during relaxation and possibly also converted to kinetic energy used for filling the ventricle by suction (see below). To understand PE in this context, consider an isovolumic contraction, which can be produced experimentally. Such a contraction obviously generates mechanical energy, but none of it is EW; i.e., it is all PE. As afterload is reduced and shortening and work increase, the ratio of EW to PE increases. The novelty of elastance theory in quantifying total mechanical energy is that it provides a basis for quantifying PE. In elastance theory, the PE stored in a spring is the area under its elastance relationship between its rest length and its actual length. Correspondingly, in the ventricle, PE for any beat can be considered the area under the ESPVR between its ES point and V_0 (see Figs. 3-19 and 3-20). The sum of EW and PE is total mechanical

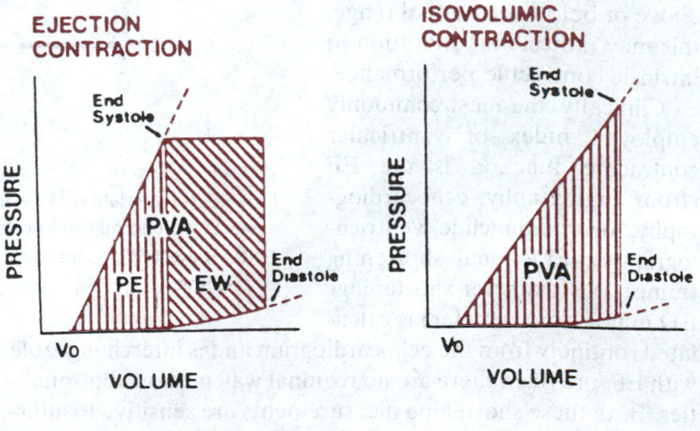

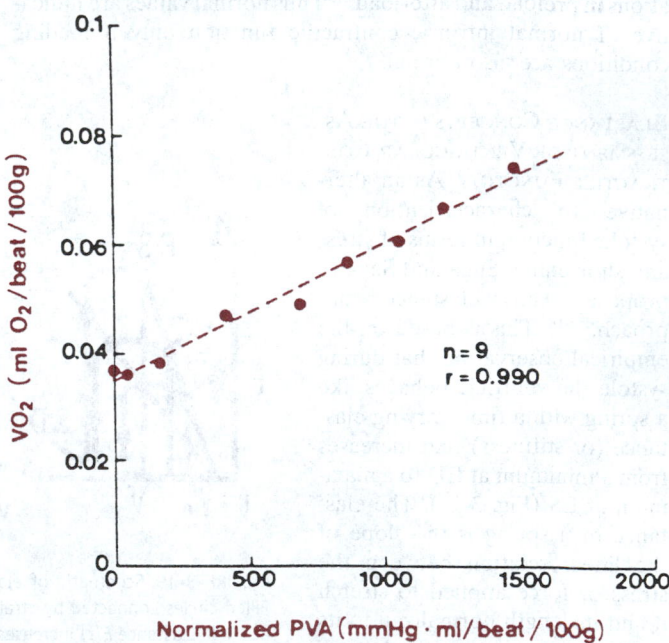

FIGURE 3-20 (*Top*) Schematic of VO_2-PVA concept (see text). In ejecting contraction, PVA = EW + PE; in isovolumic contraction, PVA = PE only. (*Bottom*) Correlation of PVA with VO_2. (From Goto et al.[128] Reproduced with permission of publisher.)

energy and is termed *pressure-volume area* (PVA). The relation between PVA and VO_2 requires knowledge of the ESPVR and can be delineated by widely varying loading conditions while measuring LV VO_2. This is done most easily in isolated, perfused heart preparations.[123,127,128] PVA has a remarkably high linear correlation with VO_2 in several species, under a variety of loading conditions, and in both normal and abnormal hearts[123,124,127,128] (see Fig. 3-20, bottom).

The linear VO_2-PVA relation has a positive VO_2 axis intercept (see Fig. 3-20), unloaded VO_2, or O_2 consumption at zero PVA, when virtually no mechanical energy is produced. Unloaded VO_2 is largely accounted for by basal metabolism and Ca pumping by SERCA2, which continue under unloaded conditions. Subtraction of unloaded VO_2 from total VO_2 provides an estimate of VO_2 used by the contractile machinery, or PVA-dependent VO_2. Since VO_2 can be converted to units of energy, the ratio of PVA to PVA-dependent VO_2 (total mechanical energy output divided by total chemical energy input), or simply the inverse slope of the linear VO_2-PVA relation, is an estimate of the *efficiency* of conversion of O_2 to mechanical energy by the contractile machinery. Variations in myosin ATPase activity modulate efficiency assessed in this fashion.[124,129]

Based on the preceding analyses, it can be understood how changes in afterload and contractility as well as preload can alter myocardial energy demands and consumption (see Fig. 3-20). Assuming no change in ED volume or afterload, increased contractility increases E_{max}, resulting in a smaller ES volume and increased EW at any preload. Even though ES volume is smaller, which in and of itself decreases PE, this is at least partially compensated by increased E_{max}, which serves to increase the area under the ESPVR. The net result is increased PVA in association with more energy used for crossbridge cycling by the contractile machinery. Most positive inotropic interventions increase the amount of Ca cycled per beat and, in turn, energy consumption by SERCA2, resulting in increased unloaded VO_2. Increased afterload increases the level of pressure at which the pressure-volume loop intersects the ESPVR, increasing PE with variable effects on EW but a net increase in PVA. In the whole LV, increases in preload have not been considered to markedly alter myocardial energy demands. Assuming constant contractility (ESPVR) and afterload, it is evident that changes in ED volume (preload) should modify EW and therefore PVA and VO_2 in direct proportion to the magnitude of the change. However, it is likely that under basal conditions the LV operates at an ED volume not too far from the point at which the diastolic pressure-volume relation becomes relatively steep. Thus there is not a great deal of room for the LV to acutely increase its preload (although its FP certainly may increase considerably). This may explain the modest effect of preload on VO_2.

A second application of elastance theory is ventricular-vascular coupling.[130,131] Just as the ventricle can be considered in terms of an elastance relationship, systemic arteries also can be characterized by an elastance relationship. Arterial elastance is largely a function of the properties of the large arteries. There exists an optimal relationship between ventricular and arterial elastance at ES such that energy transfer from the heart to the periphery is most efficient; i.e., the largest possible proportion of total mechanical VO_2 is converted to EW. In essence, this merely states that arterial loading influences the point at which the pressure-volume loop intersects the ESPVR and therefore the proportion of PVA converted to EW. The normal heart and vascular system operate at nearly optimal ventricular-vascular coupling. Vasoactive drugs can influence ventricular-vascular coupling. Moreover, in heart failure, coupling is adversely affected, resulting in less efficient transfer of energy from the heart to the vascular system.[132]

OTHER APPROACHES TO ASSESSMENT OF SYSTOLIC VENTRICULAR PERFORMANCE Following is a sampling of a number of indexes that have been proposed to assess systolic function. Maximal rate of pressure rise (max *dP/dt*) is very sensitive to changes in intrinsic contractile performance but also varies somewhat with preload.[133,134] It is not markedly influenced by changes in afterload. Max *dP/dt* is especially useful in quantifying acute changes in contractility. Its use for comparisons between different patients is limited by large interindividual variations. *Mean circumferential fiber shortening* velocity (V_{cf})[135,136] is LV internal minor axis shortening ÷ (ejection time × ED minor axis dimension). It is readily calculated from echocardiograms. Although quite sensitive to changes in afterload (as is any shortening measurement), it is a useful measure of intrinsic contractile performance if afterload is normal or can be accounted for. *Maximal ventricular power index*[137] is attractive because of its physiologic importance; i.e., it takes into account both the work done by the ventricle and the time over which it is generated. This index has been normalized to minimize effects of loading and has the potential for noninvasive determination. Two empirical indexes have been devised that appear to be relatively afterload-insensitive. One of these is preload recruitable stroke work,[138] the relationship between ED volume (or strain) and stroke work. The other is the relationship between ED volume and max *dP/dt*.[139,140] Both are linear and in essence representations of the Frank-Starling relation; by incorporating ED volume, length-dependent activation is an intrinsic component of these indexes.

Diastolic Function In addition to meeting widely varying physiologic demands for blood flow, the heart must do so at levels of FP that do not result in circulatory congestion. This requires a normal sequence of relaxation and filling. Ventricular relaxation begins at about ES (defined as the time of maximal elastance, slightly before Ao valve closure), continues through isovolumic relaxation, and does not reach completion until after AV valve opening. Before filling commences, several factors combine to determine relaxation rate, represented by isovolumic pressure decline (Fig. 3-21). After filling begins, but before relaxation is complete, other factors related to the level of ventricular volume and/or the rate of ventricular volume change also influence ventricular diastolic pressure. Once relaxation is complete, the so-called passive properties of the ventricle dominate the relation between pressure and volume as filling continues through ED.

During isovolumic relaxation, pressure falls exponentially. The rate of isovolumic pressure fall (a measure of relaxation rate) therefore has been quantified as a time constant (τ)[141,142] or simply the time to reach one-half of some starting value ($T_{1/2}$, typically measured beginning at peak negative *dP/dt*).[143] Peak negative *dP/dt*, maximal rate of pressure fall, also has been used but is less accurate. The determinants of the rate of isovolumic pressure fall are as follows:[65,141,142,144] First, as discussed earlier, myocyte relaxation rate is determined by the

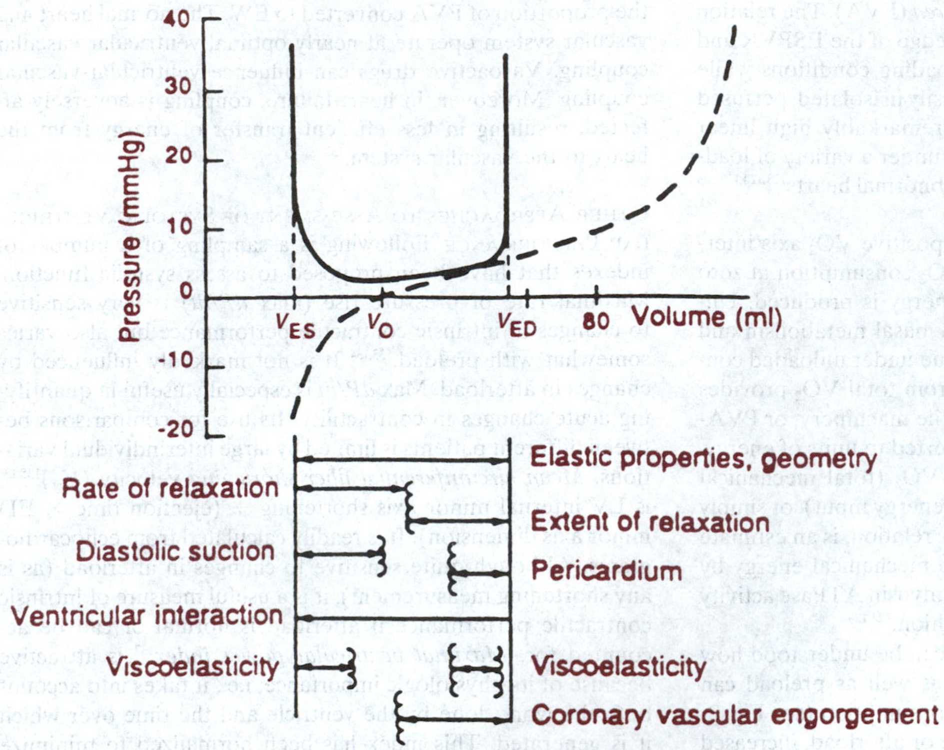

FIGURE 3-21 Determinants of relation between LV diastolic pressure and volume during filling. Solid line, LV pressure during isovolumic relaxation, filling, and isovolumic contraction; dashed line, positive and negative portions of passive pressure-volume relation. V_{ES}, ES volume; V_o, equilibrium volume or zero pressure intercept of passive pressure-volume relation (which is not same as dead volume of ESPVR); V_{ED}, ED volume. (From Gilbert JC, Glantz SA. Determinants of LV filling and of the diastolic pressure-volume relation. *Circ Res* 1989; 64:828. Reproduced with permission of publisher.)

balance between the avidity of the contractile proteins for Ca and the rate at which SERCA2 and other uptake and extrusion mechanisms remove Ca from the contractile proteins and restore the cytoplasmic concentration to normal diastolic levels. In some pathologic conditions, e.g., certain types of ischemia, diastolic Ca may not be restored to normal.[145] Relaxation is therefore incomplete, and crossbridge cycling continues during diastole, resulting in increased diastolic tension. Isovolumic relaxation is also modulated by the load on the myocardium.[141,142,144,146–150] Increased afterload through all of systole or beginning early in systole (*a contraction load*) results in delayed relaxation. Changes in load occurring late during systole (*a relaxation load*) cause opposite effects. Although changes in relaxation load may be considered to be of theoretical interest only, this may not be the case. Normal arterial waves reflected from the periphery return to the ventricle at about ES and may function to accelerate relaxation. When arteries become noncompliant, e.g., with aging, reflected waves return earlier and therefore may be converted to a contraction load, with delay of relaxation. Last, a normal temporal and spatial activation sequence results in the most rapid relaxation rate.[151]

As soon as ventricular pressure falls below atrial pressure, filling commences. As noted earlier, the magnitude and rate of ventricular filling are determined by the instantaneous AV pressure gradient (see Fig. 3-2). It is self-evident that the gradient is determined by properties of both ventricle and atrium. Immediately after AV valve opening, the rapid period of filling begins in association with a gradient of several millimeters of mercury (see Fig. 3-2). This corresponds to the E wave of mitral inflow measured with echocardiographic-Doppler techniques. During rapid filling, both ventricular and atrial pressures initially fall, but ventricular pressure falls faster than atrial pressure. Ventricular pressure soon reaches a minimum and then increases throughout the rest of diastole. The peak AV gradient occurs at or near the time of minimum ventricular pressure. (As noted earlier, it is common to observe a brief period of gradient reversal during the latter portion of rapid filling. Due to inertial effects, there is no retrograde mitral flow.) Rapid filling is succeeded by the variable slow filling phase during which the AV gradient is small to negligible. During this phase, a small, secondary increase in inflow (the L wave) is observed occasionally. The length of the slow filling phase is markedly dependent on HR, being maximal at slow rates and disappearing at rapid rates. Atrial contraction increases the AV gradient once again and injects an additional volume of blood into the ventricle.

The ventricular properties that determine pressure and the AV gradient during filling are as follows: As indicated earlier, relaxation continues past the time of AV valve opening. Therefore, the same factors (Ca reuptake, load) that modulate *isovolumic* pressure fall also influence pressure *after filling begins*. However, effects of load on relaxation rate may differ somewhat once filling begins.[144,148,150]

In addition to the ongoing process of relaxation, *restoring forces* generated during contraction also influence ventricular pressure during the early, rapid filling phase.[152–154] By a restoring force, we mean PE generated during contraction in the form of a deformation(s) of the myocyte and/or the ventricle that can be converted into kinetic energy during diastole, accelerating flow of blood from atrium to ventricle. Restoring forces are caused by functional springs whose compression during contraction is converted to elastic recoil during diastole and filling by *suction*. When present, this active, energy-requiring driving force for filling results in lowering of ventricular pressure relative to atrial pressure and a larger AV gradient. Restoring forces are probably generated by two interrelated mechanisms. One is contraction of the ventricle to an ES volume below equilibrium volume (V_{eq}), the volume at which, in the *fully relaxed* state, the pressure inside and outside the chamber is equal (transmural pressure = 0). With contraction below V_{eq}, the fully relaxed intracavitary pressure is negative with respect to the outside, and the chamber may be considered to be under compression. If allowed to fill, the PE stored in the walls results

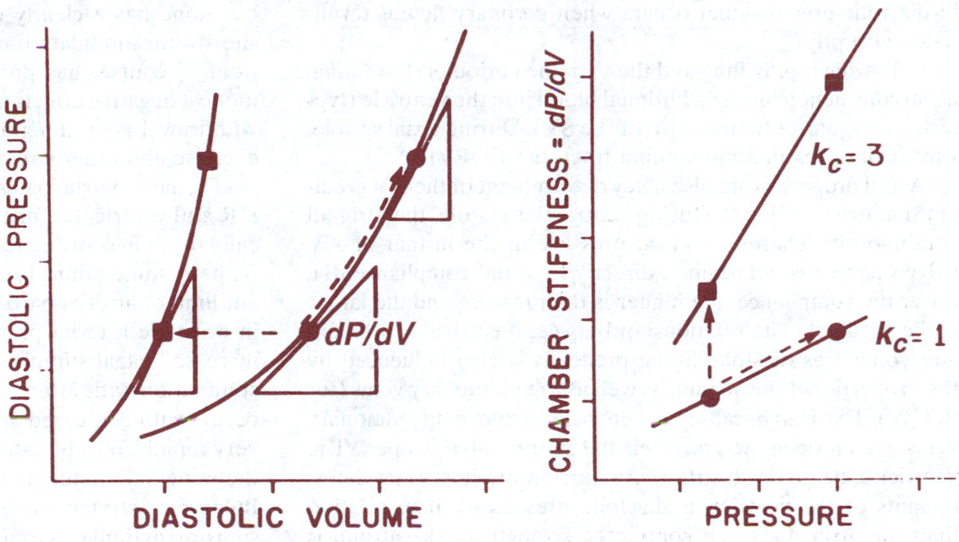

FIGURE 3-22 (*Left*) EDPVR in two ventricles with differing passive diastolic properties. Chamber stiffness is *dP/dV* at any point on the EDPVR. Chamber compliance is its inverse. Stiffer chamber (left) has steeper overall slope. (*Right*) Same data plotted as pressure versus chamber stiffness. Because of exponential nature of EDPVR, result is a straight line. Its slope (k_c) is a chamber-stiffness constant that characterizes the overall slope of the EDPVR. (From Gaasch.[157] Reprinted with the permission of the publisher.)

in elastic recoil and filling until V_{eq} is reached. As noted earlier, titin appears to be the site of a restoring force in the myocyte. The second mechanism involves complex, contraction-dependent three-dimensional deformations that are normally dissipated (by elastic recoil) during isovolumic relaxation and the early phase of ventricular filling. One of these is torsional rotation. The magnitude of these deformations increases as ES volume decreases;[103–105,155] hence they parallel compressive forces related simply to contraction below V_{eq}. As a corollary, whether and how much of a restoring force is present are critically dependent on the ES volume in relation to V_{eq}. The *sine qua non* of suction is a negative transmural pressure early during diastole, but this is rarely observed because filling is occurring rapidly and is driven simultaneously by the atrial pressure. Thus the presence of suction is ordinarily obscured. However, suction appears to be important at diastolic volumes within the physiologic range and especially during the stress of exercise, when ES volume decreases.[103,104] A second myocardial property that theoretically influences ventricular pressure during rapid filling is *viscous resistance to stretch,* i.e., intrinsically greater stiffness at high lengthening rates due to elements that behave like dashpots.[156] This property does not appear to be significant under normal physiologic conditions, however.

Relaxation and the generation of restoring forces are dynamic aspects of filling whose influence varies with time. Underlying these time varying properties is the passive ventricular pressure-volume relationship, the exponential relation between pressure and volume in the fully relaxed state.[157] We will refer to this as the *end-diastolic pressure-volume relationship* (EDPVR) (Fig. 3-22). (Although usually considered only at positive transmural pressures, as discussed earlier and as shown in Fig. 3-21, the EDPVR has a negative-pressure portion. The volume at zero transmural pressure is once again V_{eq}.) Passive *chamber compliance* is the ratio of change in volume to change in pressure at any point on the EDPVR. Because the EDPVR is exponential, passive compliance is inversely related to volume. The inverse of chamber compliance is *passive chamber stiffness*. The EDPVR is determined mainly by the geometry of the ventricular chamber, especially the chamber volume to wall thickness ratio, and the intrinsic stiffness of the myocardial tissue itself. Thus, all else being equal, increases in wall thickness or myocardial stiffness increase its slope. Intrinsic stiffness is the change in stress (force normalized to cross-sectional area) occurring in association with a given change in strain (extension of the tissue above some initial length or area). Passive myocardial stiffness is largely accounted for by the properties of titin[43,44] at relatively low volumes and by connective tissue at larger volumes. Throughout all of relaxation and filling, a portion of the pressure in the ventricle is dictated by its position on its EDPVR. Early during filling, the relation between ventricular pressure and volume is determined by relaxation and elastic recoil (when present), superimposed on the EDPVR; the EDPVR alone is the prime determinant of ventricular pressure once relaxation is complete.

The EDPVR is modified by external restraints. The most important is the parietal pericardium.[158] The pericardial sac has a relatively small reserve volume; at total heart volumes in the physiologic range, the pressure in the sac is very low in relation to left-side FPs. However, with relatively modest increments in volume above the physiologic range, the *pericardial* pressure-volume relation becomes quite steep (noncompliant), and the pressure rises rapidly. This external pressure acting on the surface of the heart is transmitted to the chambers and serves to restrain further filling; i.e., it decreases chamber compliance. Even under physiologic conditions, however, pericardial pressure is significant in relation to right-side FPs, which are normally lower than left-side FPs. Thus effective pericardial pressure is normally responsible for a significant fraction of right-side FP. Restraint to filling by the pericardium becomes quite important when the heart dilates rapidly, e.g., after RV myocardial infarction. The interventricular septum constitutes about one-third of the LV wall; diastolic pressure in the RV is therefore also an external restraint to filling of the LV (and vice versa). That is, a component of LV diastolic pressure is transmitted from the RV, an effect termed *diastolic interaction*.[158] Diastolic interaction is normally modest but can become important when RV diastolic pressure is elevated, often in conjunction with augmented pericardial restraint.

An additional factor that influences the EDPVR is the volume of blood in the myocardial vascular bed, or myocardial *turgor*.[159] A significant component of pressure in the fully relaxed ventricle is accounted for by turgor. This component is almost certainly reasonably constant under normal physiologic conditions because coronary blood volume is more or less constant. The significance of turgor is evident from the substantial drop in diastolic pressure that occurs when coronary flow is terminated abruptly.[159]

Following rapid filling and the variable period of slow filling, atrial contraction injects additional blood into the ventricle (typically one-quarter to one-third of the SV). During atrial systole, ventricular pressure and volume track the EDPVR.[157]

Atrial properties are also a key determinant of the AV gradient that drives filling.[160] During ventricular systole, the atria fill continuously. Therefore, atrial pressure at the instant of AV valve opening is determined directly by atrial compliance; the lower the compliance, the higher is the pressure and the larger is the gradient. The relationship between ventricular pressure and volume as diastolic filling proceeds is also influenced by the properties of the atrium, as well as the pulmonary veins (for the LV). This is so because the ventricle, atrium, and pulmonary veins are an open system when the mitral valve is open. The ventricles, being much stiffer, are much more important determinants of the ventricular diastolic pressure-volume relation than the atria. Last, the contractile strength of the atrium is obviously a determinant of the gradient during atrial systole.

SHORT-TERM MODULATION OF VENTRICULAR FUNCTION

Heart Rate The ventricle has a positive FFR with an optimal frequency that parallels the myocardial FFR.[74,75] As indicated earlier, this is an important means of modulating ventricular function that is intimately connected with changes in adrenergic stimulation. Changes in contraction frequency also influence relaxation and filling. There is some shortening of relaxation in conjunction with the positive FFR even without concurrent increases in adrenergic stimulation.[73] Moreover, with increased HR, diastole is shortened much more than systole, especially the slow-filling phase.

Paracrine Modulation of Ventricular Function This has been discussed previously in the section on cellular control of contractility. It is important to emphasize that the significance of these factors with respect to *normal* ventricular function is not established. In the ventricle, these factors tend to have more prominent effects on relaxation than on contraction.[161] NO and endothelial-dependent vasodilators cause very modest depression of systolic function and an earlier onset of ventricular relaxation. Substances whose effects are mediated by the IP_3 second-messenger system (ET-1, α-adrenergic agonists) have more or less opposite effects.

Neurohumoral Responses The most important short-term neurohumoral modulation occurs as a result of variations in sympathetic and parasympathetic stimulation caused by both cardiac neural activity and circulating catecholamines. Stimulation of β-adrenergic receptors results in increased HR and contractility and more rapid relaxation. These effects are due to the influence of adrenergic stimulation on the sinus node and specialized conduction system and, within the myocyte, activation of adenyl cyclase with increases in cyclic AMP. Increases in HR also allow the heart to use the FFR. Adrenergic stimulation interacts with the FFR not only by increasing HR but also by increasing the gain of the relationship.[75] There are many other myocyte cell surface receptors (e.g., α-adrenergic, dopaminergic, histaminergic, angiotensin II, and endothelin receptors), but none has a clearly delineated, significant role in normal, short-term modulation of ventricular function. Vagal stimulation, of course, has profound HR slowing effects as well as modest negative effects on contractility. Correspondingly, vagal withdrawal is an integral component of HR responses during exercise and other stresses.

The heart participates in a number of reflexes that modulate HR and ventricular function in the short term.[162–165] These typically result in coordinated changes in parasympathetic and sympathetic stimulation. Thus the heart is a component of the efferent limb of arterial baro- and chemoreceptors. Acute increases in systemic arterial pressure result in slowing of HR due to increased vagal stimulation and decreased sympathetic neural stimulation with attendant effects on contractility; the reverse occurs with decreased arterial pressure. Vagal responses occur very rapidly, on a beat-to-beat basis, whereas changes in sympathetic neural stimulation take somewhat longer to take effect. Pulmonary stretch receptors are largely responsible for normal sinus arrhythmia. Atrial stretch receptors also may modulate HR via the Bainbridge reflex, resulting in tachycardia with increased intravascular volume. Ventricular mechanoreceptors that discharge with deformation are activated when volume decreases. Discharge results in vagally mediated bradycardia and hypotension and appears to be involved in vasovagal syncope. Chemoreceptors on the ventricular epicardium also connect to vagal efferents and may discharge in response to prostaglandins secreted into the pericardial sac.

Ventricular Interaction Diastolic ventricular interaction has been discussed previously. The ventricles also interact during systole. Left-to-right systolic interaction was mentioned earlier. There is also a modest amount of right-to-left interaction.[119] As a result, an abrupt increase in PA pressure results in a small increase in LV contractile performance. Both diastolic and systolic ventricular interaction function as internal feedback mechanisms that modulate SV on a beat-to-beat basis to ensure that left- and right-side heart outputs remain equal over time. Obviously, even tiny differences in output summated over time would have disastrous consequences.

Coronary Perfusion Changes in coronary perfusion pressure and/or flow per se can influence ventricular function.[166,167] Increases augment systolic performance and may cause some decrease in passive compliance. Modest decreases insufficient to cause myocardial ischemia likely have opposite effects. A component of the influence of coronary perfusion on ventricular function is related to turgor. In addition to modulation of diastolic compliance, stretching of myocardial tissue due to increased turgor appears to augment the Frank-Starling effect. It is also possible that stretch-activated Ca channels[168] open as turgor increases with resulting increased activation of the myocardium. Because of *coronary autoregulation,* these effects of coronary perfusion are probably of minor importance under normal physiologic conditions.

LONG-TERM MODULATION OF VENTRICULAR FUNCTION

Chronic nonphysiologic stresses modulate ventricular function by causing pathologic hypertrophy. Chronic alterations in the demands placed on the cardiovascular system within the physiologic range can cause modest changes in cardiac mass.[169,170] However, measurable changes require very substantial changes in demand. Thus endurance athletes develop modest, physiologic hypertrophy characterized by increased ventricular chamber volume with little or no increase in wall thickness. This adaptation allows for a greater SV.

THE PERIPHERAL CIRCULATION

The essence of normal *vascular* function lies in adjusting total and regional peripheral resistance, as needed, to accommodate the metabolic demands of various organs and in ensuring adequate venous return to the heart. The goal of this section is to first provide an understanding of transcapillary exchange, the process by which tissues are nourished and normal fluid balance maintained, and to then consider the underlying physiologic mechanisms responsible for changes in regional and total peripheral resistance.

Physiology of the Peripheral Circulation

PRINCIPLES OF CAPILLARY EXCHANGE

The exchange of gases, nutrients, water, and waste material occurs at the capillary level and is governed by the interplay of two opposing but balanced forces. At the proximal end of a capillary, intravascular pressure slightly exceeds tissue pressure. The gradient in hydrostatic pressure results in hydraulic *ultrafiltration,* a process characterized by the movement of fluid through the capillary wall and into the extracellular compartment. Composed of a single layer of endothelial cells, the capillary acts as a selective filter. The degree of selectivity varies with the physical properties of the endothelium in different tissues. Passage of relatively large molecules (e.g., proteins) is largely impeded, although some leakage occurs with subsequent reabsorption into lymphatic vessels and a return to the circulation. As a result of ultrafiltration, the concentration of solute (plasma osmolarity) increases along the length of a capillary, and the associated force (termed *oncotic pressure*) acts to pull extracellular fluid back into the capillary lumen through a process of *reabsorption*. This fundamental concept was first described by Ernest Starling in 1896 and is therefore known as the *Starling hypothesis,* mathematically expressed as follows:

$$Q_f = k[(P_c + \pi_i) - (P_i + \pi_p)]$$

where Q_f is fluid movement across the capillary wall, P_c is capillary hydrostatic pressure, π_i is interstitial fluid oncotic pressure, P_i is interstitial fluid hydrostatic pressure, π_p is plasma oncotic pressure, and k is a filtration constant for capillary membrane.

A positive Q_f value indicates net filtration, whereas a negative value connotes net reabsorption. In general, if filtration exceeds reabsorption, an edematous state develops; conversely, if reabsorption exceeds filtration, plasma volume expands (primarily on the venous side), and cellular/extracellular volume decreases. It should be noted, however, that not every capillary behaves in the idealized fashion predicted by the Starling hypothesis. For example, in the renal glomerulus, hydrostatic pressures are elevated along the entire length of the capillary; hence filtration predominates. In the intestinal mucosa, the elevated oncotic forces result primarily in reabsorption, with little or no filtration.

Transcapillary exchange is modulated by a series of integrated mechanisms ranging from central neural control of CO and total peripheral resistance (the primary determinants of blood pressure) to local mechanisms within the microcirculation that modulate capillary pressure and regional blood flow. During the last decade, our appreciation of the latter has increased substantially, and it is now clear that metabolic and myogenic factors within the microcirculation play a major role in determining upstream resistance and, hence, pressure within a capillary bed.

The presence of actin and myosin in some endothelial cells, particularly those of postcapillary venules (also a site of fluid exchange), argues for the existence of a cytoskeletal mechanism for governing the geometry of interendothelial pores or clefts.[171] The state of the cytoskeleton is, in turn, regulated by physical and chemical signals that impinge on the capillary. A number of molecules, such as histamine, adenosine, and NO, are able to alter the permeability characteristics of the endothelium and lead to rapid and significant changes in permeability. For example, *vascular endothelial growth factor* (VEGF) is a peptide that binds to receptors on the endothelium and initiates a series of intracellular signal-transduction events that result in greatly augmented permeability. Recent observations suggest that this pathway involves a receptor tyrosine kinase that is coupled to phospholipase C, an enzyme whose activation leads to the generation of second messengers that modulate both enzymatic and ionic events within the endothelial cell, including activation of protein kinase C, generation of NO, and changes in the endothelial cytoskeleton.[172] Finally, in some organs such as the brain or kidney, transcapillary exchange may be subject to modulation by pericytes, specialized cells that encircle the capillary endothelium and contribute to permeability/barrier functions by mechanisms that are as yet poorly defined. Under normal conditions, it is essential that the vascular resistance upstream of the capillary bed be regulated in such a way so as to maintain capillary pressure at levels at which normal fluid exchange may occur. The remainder of this section therefore is devoted to reviewing the principal mechanisms by which the cells of the arterial and arteriolar wall regulate arterial tone and hence vascular resistance and capillary pressure.

PERIPHERAL RESISTANCE AND ITS DETERMINANTS

Pressure, flow, and resistance are related most often through Poiseuille's equation, which was first formulated in 1842. Based on a series of careful observations of water flowing through rigid tubes, Poiseuille demonstrated that the resistance to flow R through a tube is proportional to tube length L and fluid viscosity η and inversely proportional to the tube radius to the fourth power (r^4). These variables can be related to each other in the following way:

$$R = 8\eta L/\pi r^4$$

Poiseuille's equation applies to the behavior of Newtonian fluids flowing in a nonpulsatile, nonturbulent (laminar) manner through rigid tubes. Although the vascular system satisfies none of these parameters, the equation is useful because it predicts that flow Q is proportional to r^4 (and inversely proportional to resistance: $Q \alpha r^4$, or $Q \alpha 1/R^4$, where r is radius and R is resistance), i.e., given the same initial pressure, doubling the inner radius of a tube will result in a sixteenfold (2^4) increase in flow. Estimates from intact vascular networks suggest that this may be an overestimation and that a third-power equation ($Q \propto r^3$) may be more accurate.[173] Nevertheless, it is clear that relatively minor changes in arterial caliber can produce large changes in resistance and flow.

The relationship between vascular resistance and blood flow may be defined by an equation that is analogous to Ohm's law for the flow of electrons, where flow = perfusion pressure/resistance. The complete formulation includes the main determinants of resistance (labeled as above in Poiseuille's equation) and is called *Poiseuille's law:*

$$Q = PP\pi r^4/8\eta L$$

where Q is flow, PP is perfusion pressure, and the determinants of resistance (inverted during the simplification of the quotient) are signified as above. Although flow resistance also can be affected by the viscosity of the blood (η) and the length of the vessel (L), as predicted by the Poiseuille formula, these parameters are normally relatively invariant within the adult cardiovascular system. For this reason, lumen diameter is the single most powerful determinant of vascular resistance (and blood flow) under physiologic conditions. Its control is the primary end point for a variety of physiologic mechanisms.

Most of the pressure drop between large conduit arteries and capillaries occurs in vessels having lumen diameters of a few hundred microns or less. For this reason, small arteries and arterioles are considered to be of primary importance in regulating and determining peripheral resistance. These muscular vessels have a high wall-thickness to lumen diameter ratio and usually contain one to three layers of circumferentially oriented vascular smooth muscle cells. They also normally possess some degree of basal tone and are capable of diameter changes that range from fully open to virtually closed. Hence their potential to affect resistance is considerable. In contrast, large conduit arteries such as the aorta only constrict by 10 to 20 percent. Unless they become diseased, they are of minor importance to peripheral resistance and blood flow control. The relationship between blood pressure, blood flow velocity, and total cross-sectional area in various blood vessels of the systemic circulation is summarized in Fig. 3-23.

Larger vessels do contribute significantly to resistance in some organs, such as the brain,[174] primarily due the more linear geometry of the arterial vasculature. In a *serial arrangement* of tubes, total resistance R_t is the sum of individual resistance elements ($R_t = R_1 + R_2 + R_3$, etc.). Conversely, in regional circulations in which vessels are highly and sequentially branched, resistance tends to be localized to smaller (<50 μm) arteries. This occurs because a greater number of *parallel elements* lowers the overall resistance of the array. This makes sense because, given the same driving pressure, there are more tubes to conduct flow, and in this case, total resistance is defined by a reciprocal relationship ($1/R_t = 1/R_1 + 1/R_2 + 1/R_3$, etc.). These concepts are shown in Fig. 3-24.

SYSTEMIC HEMODYNAMICS

In healthy adults, 15 percent of the blood is contained within the systemic arterial system. The remainder is distributed between

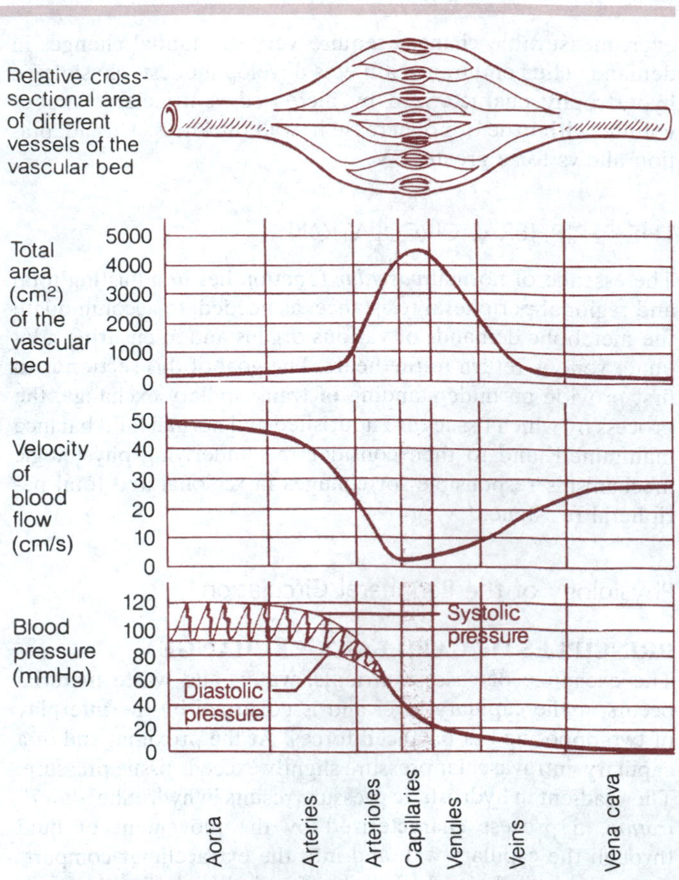

FIGURE 3-23 Relations between total cross-sectional area of the vascular bed (cm²), velocity of blood flow (cm/s), and blood pressure (mmHg) in various vessels in systemic circulation. (From Marieb EN. *Human Anatomy and Physiology*. Redwood City, CA: Benjamin/Cummings; 1989:629. Reproduced with permission of the publisher.)

capillaries (5 percent), veins (66 percent), heart (6 percent), and pulmonary circulation (8 percent). The peripheral circulation distributes CO throughout the various tissues and organs of the body. The elasticity of large conduit arteries such as the aorta serves to absorb and dampen the highly pulsatile and discontinuous flow from the heart (the Windkessel effect). As a result, the amplitude of pressure pulsations is diminished in smaller vessels and capillaries and is virtually absent in the venous circulation. Mean pressure also decreases from a value of 90 to 95 mmHg in large arteries to about 30 mmHg in capillaries and less than 20 mmHg in veins. The peripheral circulation must adapt rapidly to changes in arterial pressure and variations in end-organ metabolic demands. Even actions we take for granted, such as getting out of bed, challenge the cardiovascular system. Thus, owing to gravitational forces, cerebral perfusion pressure and venous return are suddenly reduced, leading to transient feelings of dizziness in some individuals (orthostatic hypotension). At the same time, capillary pressures in the ankles may rise to exceed 90 or 100 mmHg. As another example, the metabolic demands of exercise require major redistribution of CO to increase perfusion of coronary, pulmonary, and skeletal muscle circulations, diminish splanchnic flow, and still maintain cerebral blood flow (Table 3-2). Regulatory mechanisms therefore must be bidirectional, i.e., allow blood flow to either increase or decrease on demand. For this to occur, the venous circulation must be able to adjust its capacitance and modulate venous return, and the arterial vasculature must operate at a point from which it can either dilate or constrict to increase or decrease flow. Because it is impossible to dilate a vessel that is already fully relaxed, some portion of the arterial circulation must operate in a state of partial constriction or tone. This theoretical supposition is supported by experimental studies in which the infusion of vasodilators into the afferent vasculature results in substantial increases in blood flow, demonstrating a dilator "reserve" (Fig. 3-25) that can only be accounted for by the presence of basal tone.

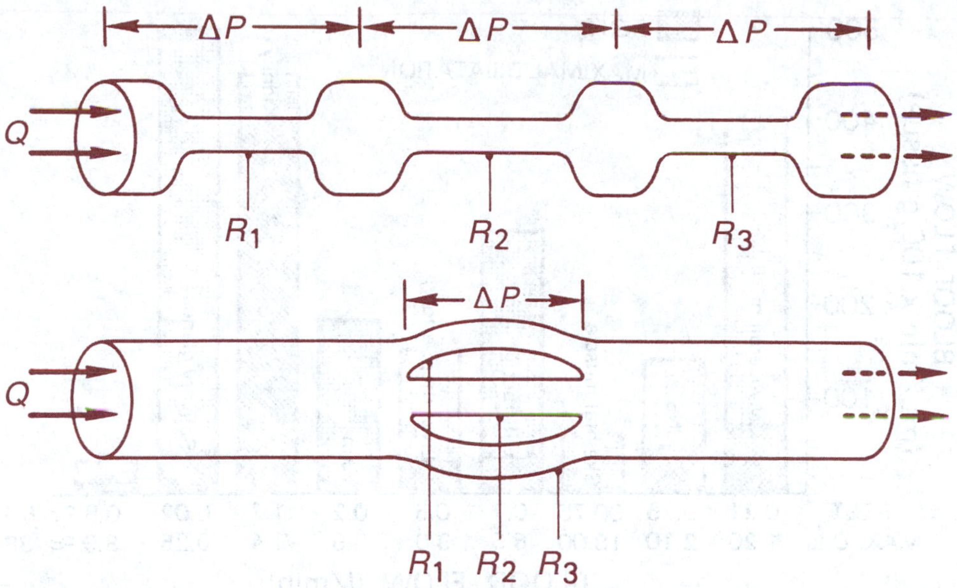

FIGURE 3-24 Illustration of principle of resistance elements arranged in series versus parallel. (*Top*) If the driving pressurer (ΔP) across each series resistance is 3 mmHg, and flow (Q) is 1 mL/min, each resistance (R) would be ΔP/Q, or 3 mmHg/mL per minute, and total resistance (R_t) would be 9 mmHg/mL per minute. (*Bottom*) In parallel resistances, if driving pressure (ΔP) is 3 mmHg, and flow (Q) is 1 mL/min, total resistance is $1/R_1 + 1/R_2 + 1/R_3$, or 1 mmHg/mL per minute. When three resistances are in parallel, total resistance is only one-ninth that with resistances in series, so it would take a ΔP of only 1 mmHg to produce a 1 mL/min flow. (From Smith JJ, Kampine JP. *Circulatory Physiology: The Essentials*. Baltimore: Williams & Wilkins, 1990:20. Reprinted with permission of the publisher.)

Integration of Circulatory Mechanisms: Blood Flow Autoregulation

Minute-to-minute control of the peripheral circulation involves a complex interplay between several physiologic mechanisms, mainly neural, myogenic, and endothelial. Metabolites released from adjacent tissues also impinge on the vascular wall (metabolic regulation). The importance of each varies with ambient conditions. Under resting conditions, skeletal muscle arteries and arterioles operate in a highly constricted state, and perfusion is relatively low. Physical activities such as running or swimming result in manyfold increases in skeletal muscle blood flow due to a combination of increased CO and arterial dilation. The proportion of CO directed to skeletal muscles increases from 20 to more than 70 percent, and total blood flow is increased by as much as tenfold (see Table 3-2).

During exercise, dilation of skeletal muscle arteries and arterioles occurs due to metabolic factors such as adenosine and potassium and hydrogen ions that diffuse from adjacent myocytes into the vascular wall and induce hyperpolarization and relaxation of vascular smooth muscle either directly or indirectly by stimulating the release of endothelial factors such as NO and prostacyclin.[175] Increased flow itself serves as a stimulus for further vasodilation, presumably through shear stress-induced release of vasoactive substances from the endothelium.[176] The degree of local circulatory control can be quite remarkable. This is perhaps best illustrated by studies of cerebral blood flow using inhaled isotopes such as xenon in combination with scanning devices that produce a topographic map of cortical flow.[177] These studies show that when an individual begins to play the piano with his or her right hand, cerebral blood flow increases markedly, but only in the opposite hemisphere in the area of the motor cortex that controls finger and hand movements. Similarly, the act of speaking increases blood flow to the speech areas, solving mathematical equations augments flow to the frontal lobe, visual stimuli to the occipital cortex, and so on. At the same time, global cerebral flow is unaltered in the face of changing blood pressure, a phenomenon called *autoregulation*.

Autoregulation is the ability of an organ to maintain a constant blood flow despite changes in systemic arterial pressure. Although most organs can autoregulate blood flow, this phenomenon is particularly well developed in the cerebral, coronary, and renal circulations and is principally effected by adjustments in the caliber of smaller arteries and arterioles. Autoregulatory effectiveness is determined by the ability of the

TABLE 3-2 Distribution of Tissue Blood Flow during Exercise

	Tissue Blood Flow (mL/min)		
Organ	Rest	Light Exercise	Strenuous Exercise
Skeletal muscle	1200	4500	12,500
Heart	250	350	750
Brain	750	750	750
Skin	500	1500	1,900
Kidney	1100	900	600
Abdominal viscera	1400	1100	600
Miscellaneous	600	400	400
TOTAL CO	5800	9500	17,500

SOURCE: Modified from Martini FH. *Fundamentals of Anatomy and Physiology*. Upper Saddle River, NJ: Prentice-Hall; 1998:735.

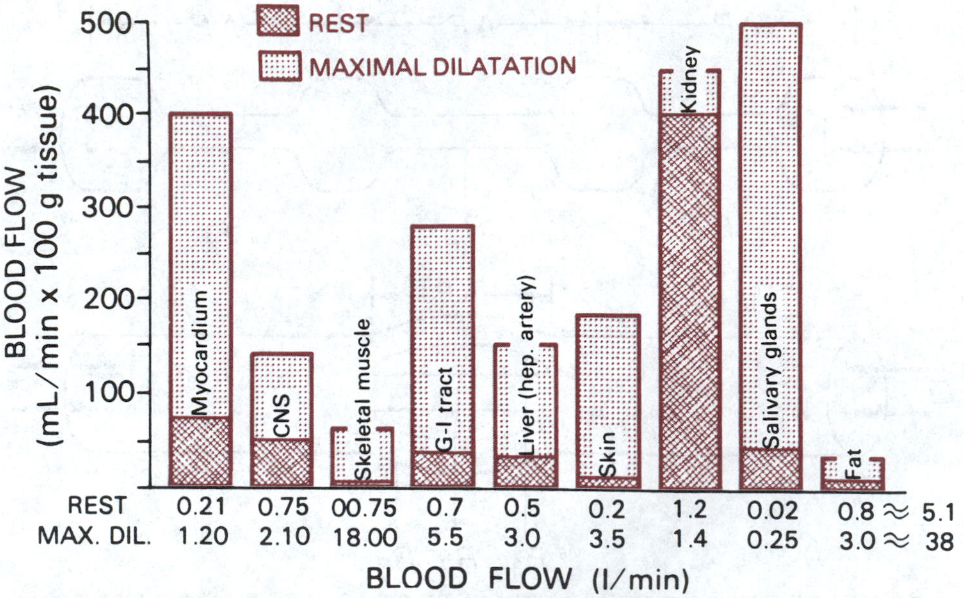

FIGURE 3-25 Regional blood flow at rest (shaded areas) and at maximal dilatation (stippled areas) per organ and per 100 g tissue, illustrating the concept of arterial/arteriolar vasodilator reserve. (From Mellander S, Johansson B. Control of resistance, exchange and capacitance functions in the peripheral circulation. *Pharmacol Rev* 1968; 20:117. Reprinted with permission of the publisher.)

arteries to constrict to increased and dilate to decreased pressure so as to keep total flow relatively constant. This involves an interaction between several mechanisms, myogenic, endothelial, neural, and metabolic; others, such as tissue pressure or tubuloglomerular feedback, may occur within the cranium and kidneys, respectively.

Autoregulation occurs over a range of pressures with both upper and lower limits. If perfusion pressure falls below a certain point, tissue hypoperfusion will ensue. Transmural pressures above the upper limit of autoregulation, on the other hand, result in a "breakthrough" phenomenon in which forced dilatation of arteries occurs, leading to loss of vasomotor tone. Large increases in organ blood flow, transmission of high intravascular pressures to capillaries and veins, and vessel leakage and rupture potentially may result. Forced dilatation is thought to be important in the development of hypertensive encephalopathy, a condition characterized by increases in cerebral blood flow and extravasation of fluid and protein from the microcirculation. Experimental studies have shown that leakage occurs initially in postcapillary venules, although arteriolar damage and changes in permeability have been documented as well.[178] The ability to autoregulate flow must be reserved for some organs (e.g., brain, heart, and kidney) but not all; if increased blood pressure stimulated arterial constriction throughout the body, total peripheral resistance would increase, raising pressure further via a positive-feedback mechanism that could have dire consequences. An equally dangerous situation would occur with a fall in blood pressure and potentially lead to vascular collapse. Thus simultaneous and opposite changes in arterial and arteriolar tone and/or adjustments in venous capacitance and plasma volume (driven by nervous and endocrine systems) must occur to prevent the development of either hyper- or hypotension.

Cellular Mechanisms Involved in the Regulation of Blood Flow

VASCULAR TONE AND ITS DETERMINANTS

Vascular tone generally increases with decreasing arterial size and is greatest in the smaller arteries and arterioles that play a primary role in determining peripheral resistance and regulating regional blood flow.[179] The level of tone at any time reflects an integration of multiple excitatory and inhibitory pathways that converge on the ultimate effector, vascular smooth muscle (VSM), to "set" the level of tone. Changes in the physical forces impinging on the vascular wall (shear stress, transmural pressure), neurotransmitter release from nerves (most often located at the medial-adventitial junction), or the concentration of metabolites released from surrounding tissues all modulate the set point to either increase or decrease arterial tone, lumen diameter, and resistance. VSM itself is capable of constricting in response to pressure or stretch. Because this occurs in isolated arterial segments that have been denuded of endothelium and in the absence of metabolic or neural factors, it appears to be a pure response of VSM to pressure or stretch and therefore is termed *myogenic tone* (see ref. 179 for review).

The endothelium, situated at the interface between blood and VSM, is also an important modulator of tone via release of a number of vasoactive factors having both inhibitory (e.g., NO, prostacyclin) and excitatory (e.g., ET-1, thromboxane) effects on VSM.[180] Moreover, in many arteries the endothelium is coupled to VSM through numerous myoendothelial junctions—areas where membranes of endothelium and VSM are in close contact.[181] The nature of the contact varies but may occur through low-resistance gap junctions that allow bidirectional transfer of information and propagation of dilatation or constriction. Spontaneous vasomotion and, in some cases, upstream ("ascending") vasodilatation have been observed in vivo in several circulatory beds and may involve cooperativity between endothelium and VSM in determining network resistance.[182]

MYOGENIC PROPERTIES OF VASCULAR SMOOTH MUSCLE

Arterial constriction to increased perfusion pressure was first described by Bayliss in 1902. Since then, myogenic responses have been documented in arteries, arterioles, and veins. The fundamental question of how a vessel is able to sense intravascular pressure and/or flow has proven difficult to answer. The identity of the myogenic sensor—the structure(s) that convert physical force into VSM contraction—has thus far eluded investigators. Some putative candidates are integrins (molecules embedded in the membrane that link the extracellular matrix with the cytoskeleton) and stretch-activated cation channels.[183] Recent studies have elucidated many of the intracellular signal-transduction pathways involved in myogenic tone. Myogenicity appears to involve a cooperativity between ionic and enzymatic mechanisms, with Ca entry and activation of the phospholipase C/protein kinase C cascade being central among them. Transmural pressure leads to depolarization of the VSM membrane and activation of L-type Ca channels that allow extracellular Ca to enter the VSM cell. Ca entry activates a variety of enzymes and promotes contraction through calmodulin-mediated myosin light chain phosphorylation that initiates actomyosin ATPase activity and crossbridge (actin and myosin) cycling. At the same time, membrane enzymes such as phospholipase C and protein kinase C become activated; many of these enzymes are Ca-dependent. Enzyme activation leads to kinase-induced phosphorylation of a number of other intracellular enzymes and ion channels (e.g., K channels) located in the membrane, as well as modulation of intracellular Ca stores through phosphoinositides such as IP_3.[179,183] Although Ca is required for constriction (inhibition of entry with channel blockers eliminates myogenic tone), enzymatic activity may "sensitize" the contractile proteins to the effects of Ca. Tone is thus controlled by a combination of mechanisms that (1) regulate VSM Ca levels (Ca entry and extrusion) and (2) modulate the effect of Ca on the contractile proteins (Ca sensitivity).

The feedback mechanisms for myogenic behavior are poorly understood but may involve Ca-induced activation of K channels whose opening facilitates K efflux and membrane hyperpolarization, opposing the depolarizing effect of transmural pressure and stabilizing membrane potential at the appropriate level.[184] An intriguing concept, first reported in cardiomyocytes,[185] invokes control of a subset of K channels that have been implicated in basal tone (KCa, or Ca-activated K channels) by highly localized intracellular "hot spots" of Ca, i.e., Ca sparks.[186] In this scenario, Ca is released from the SR in a discrete fashion that leads to localized concentrations of Ca within the cytoplasm. The proximity of the SR release site to the KCa channels, which are proteins embedded in the plasma membrane, leads to their activation. The resulting outward K current produces membrane hyperpolarization that, in turn, inhibits voltage-sensitive Ca channels, decreasing Ca entry and leading to vascular relaxation. Hence Ca sparks produce vasodilation indirectly by activating KCa channels but have little direct effect on spatially averaged intracellular Ca concentration, which regulates contraction.

ENDOTHELIAL INFLUENCES ON VASCULAR SMOOTH MUSCLE CONTRACTILITY

Although the importance of the endothelium as a nonthrombogenic surface has been known for some time, its role in modulating arterial tone was unrecognized until the early 1980s, when Furchgott and Zawadski[187] observed that this cell type was obligatory for the relaxation response to acetylcholine. Although cholinergic vasodilation in vivo had been recognized, its mechanism was difficult to study because the event rarely could be reproduced in vitro. In their landmark paper, Furchgott and Zawadski[187] reported that endothelial denudation abolished relaxation to acetylcholine and hypothesized that cholinergic stimulation led to the release of a substance that relaxed VSM. This compound, initially called *endothelium-derived relaxing factor* (EDRF), was subsequently shown to be NO. NO is a gas produced during the conversion of the amino acid L-arginine into L-citrulline by the enzyme NO synthase.[188] In addition to its vasodilatory actions, NO is now known to be an important cytotoxic molecule used by the immune system, a neurotransmitter, a modulator of cell division,[189] and, as discussed earlier, a modulator of myocardial function and energy metabolism.

It is now clear that the endothelium performs a variety of chemo- and mechanotransduction functions and releases a host of vasoactive molecules in response to physical and chemical stimulation.[180] In addition to NO, the latter include ET-1[190] and dilator and constrictor prostaglandins (e.g., prostacyclin and thromboxane, respectively). There is also experimental evidence for a non-NO factor that hyperpolarizes VSM. This substance has been termed *endothelium-derived hyperpolarizing factor* (EDHF).[191] Endothelial secretions diffuse to adjacent VSM to activate a variety of signal-transduction mechanisms that alter intracellular concentrations of cyclic AMP (induced by prostaglandins), cyclic GMP (via NO), phospholipase C (ET-1), and membrane potential (EDHF). Release of endothelium-derived vasoactive molecules is controlled by a variety of factors, both chemical and physical. The endothelium is exposed to much higher levels of shear stress than most other tissues. Shear is thought to be an important stimulus for a number of endothelial events, including hyperpolarization (opening of K channels), Ca influx, up- and down-regulation of mRNA for many proteins (e.g., adhesion molecules, tissue plasminogen activator, heat shock proteins), induction of G proteins and a number of kinases (protein kinase C, mitogen activated protein kinase), cytoskeletal rearrangement, and release of cytokines and growth factors.[176] There is also evidence that shear stress modulates arterial growth and remodeling through an endothelium-dependent mechanism.[192] Altered small artery endothelial function (most often characterized by diminished release of vasodilator substances) has been reported in vascular diseases such as hypertension and diabetes.[193,194] In larger arteries, abnormal flow patterns (turbulence, eddy currents) associated with reduced shear stress may lead to metabolic derangements in endothelial function and accelerate the development of atherosclerotic lesions.

Autonomic Regulation of Peripheral Blood Flow

Most arteries and veins receive direct sympathetic innervation. Sympathetic tone contributes to maintenance of arterial and venous pressure under normal and stressful conditions. Sympathetic efferent activity is determined by a complex interaction of neurons in the spinal cord, medulla, pons, hypothalamus, limbic system, and portions of the forebrain and, as discussed earlier, by feedback signals arising from cardiovascular mechano- and chemoreceptors localized in discrete baroreceptor centers in the carotid sinuses, aortic arch, and the heart. The two central nervous system (CNS) areas that appear to be of principal importance in regulating sympathetic outflow are the nucleus tractus solitarius (NTS) and the rostral ventral lateral medulla (RVLM). The influence of the NTS on the RVLM is inhibitory: In animals, bilateral lesions lead to malignant hypertension. Sympathetic denervation produces widely varying effects on organ blood flow. Cerebral and coronary circulations are virtually unaffected, most likely as a result of the dominance of intrinsic autoregulatory mechanisms, whereas denervation of the skin or skeletal muscle produces substantial increases in blood flow. During intense sympathetic activation, large amounts of epinephrine (and, to a lesser extent, norepinephrine) are released from the adrenal medulla in response to activation of sympathetic preganglionic afferents. Blood pressure increases markedly, and significant redistribution of CO occurs (e.g., simultaneous increased perfusion of skeletal muscle and decreased splanchnic flow). Moreover, stimulation of the venous circulation increases venous return, thereby augmenting CO.

The efferent fibers of the cranial division of the parasympathetic system innervate the blood vessels of the head and viscera; those of the sacral division supply the vasculature of the large bowel, bladder, and genitalia. Resistance vessels are not thought to receive parasympathetic innervation, and the effect of the parasympathetic system on total resistance is minor. The parasympathetic system generally produces effects opposite those of the sympathetic division, i.e., decreased cardiac rate and output and vascular relaxation, but is thought to be of secondary importance in peripheral vascular regulation.

THE CORONARY CIRCULATION

Anatomic and Mechanical Considerations

The right and left main coronary arteries (CAs) arise at the root of the aorta and provide the blood supply to the myocardium. The right CA normally supplies the inferior surface of the LV, the RV and RA, whereas the left CA divides into circumflex and anterior descending branches that perfuse the rest of the LV and the LA. In about 10 percent of cases the left circumflex branch rather than the right CA supplies the inferior LV. Branches from the main CAs ramify and penetrate the myocardium, forming dense capillary beds. Most venous blood returns to the RA via the coronary sinus; there is also communication between the cardiac chambers and myocardium via arteriosinusoidal channels. Delivery of blood to the myocardium is complicated by compression of intramyocardial vessels during systole, which induces retrograde flow in epicardial CAs.[195–201] As a consequence, the bulk of coronary flow occurs during diastole, and the upstream perfusion pressure is the Ao *diastolic* pressure. The subendocardial layer of the myocardium is more susceptible to hypoperfusion because ventricular diastolic pressure opposes the driving pressure for flow. Moreover, compression of microvessels during systole is more prominent in the subendocardium. There has been some uncertainty about the actual driving pressure for nutrient flow, in particular whether the downstream pressure should be considered RA/coronary sinus pressure or a higher value related to tissue forces that cause collapse of the microcirculation (i.e., a critical closing pressure).

Modulation of Coronary Vasomotor Tone and Flow

The distribution of coronary vascular resistance is complex and dependent on type of vessel, region, and specific vasomotor stimuli.[198,200] Arterioles clearly comprise the main component of resistance, but small arteries and venules also contribute in a coordinated fashion to control flow to specific regions. Some vasodilators and contrictors preferentially dilate small arteries rather than arterioles. Resistance in subendocardial microvessels appears to be significantly lower than in the subepicardium. Modulation of coronary vascular resistance is exceedingly complex, and only a brief discussion will be undertaken here (see ref. 200 and Chap. 37 for additional details). As the heart varies its mechanical performance over a wide range of physiologic demands, the coronary circulation must keep pace. For example, nutritive coronary flow increases by as much as 400 percent during exercise. Since upstream Ao diastolic pressure does not change markedly during exercise (or even decreases), this requires an ability to markedly dilate coronary resistance vessels. The most potent mechanism of modulation of coronary resistance and flow is endogenous autoregulation. As discussed earlier, this is the ability of the coronary circulation to maintain flow constant over a wide range of perfusion pressures and/or alter flow in response to increased metabolic demands by changing its resistance.[198,200] Autoregulation occurs at the level of small arteries, arterioles, and venules and appears to be due to both *myogenic* and *metabolically mediated* responses.[198,200,201] As discussed earlier, a myogenic response is the ability of vessels to alter tone as a direct response to changes in pressure and/or flow. This is most prominent in arterioles and results in constriction when perfusion pressure is increased and dilatation when pressure is reduced. Although myogenic responses play a role in autoregulation, the most important factors are those related to changes in the washout of metabolites. (Of course, changes in perfusion pressure and flow themselves alter metabolite concentration.) The actual metabolites and effector mechanisms responsible for autoregulation are incompletely defined, but the effects are most prominent in small arterioles. There is much evidence that local release of adenosine (a potent coronary dilator) under conditions of increased metabolic demand is a key mediator of autoregulation.[198,200,202,203] However, other endogenous vasoactive mechanisms also contribute. For example, local release of K and activation of ATP-sensitive K channels in small arteries and arterioles also may have a role.[204] Moreover, adenosine release itself may activate ATP-sensitive K channels. NO appears to have a significant role in autoregulation as well (see below).

Neurohumorally mediated responses also play a role in modulation of coronary vascular resistance.[198,200] Their importance under *normal physiologic conditions* is uncertain. α-Adrenergic responses are well documented in the coronary circulation. α-Adrenergic agonists constrict large epicardial and small coronary arteries/arterioles (>100 μm in diameter) and dilate smaller arterioles. At physiologic perfusion pressure, the main effect appears to be constriction of small arteries. While there is evidence of α-adrenergic activity under physiologic conditions, endogenous mechanisms mask and/or counteract this vasoconstrictive influence. Thus endothelial release of NO occurs concomitant with α-adrenergic activity. β-Adrenergic receptors are present in coronary vessels and cause dilation of large arteries and resistance vessels. However, this influence is difficult to distinguish from and likely of minor importance compared with autoregulation.

Constrictive and dilatory substances produced by the endothelium play a key role in many, if not all, of the changes in coronary tone occurring in response to a variety of physiologic stimuli, including autoregulation in general and adenosine, serotonin, acetylcholine, and adrenergic stimulation.[198,200,205,206] These endothelial-derived substances include prostaglandins, ET-1, endothelium-derived hyperpolarizing factor,[207] and

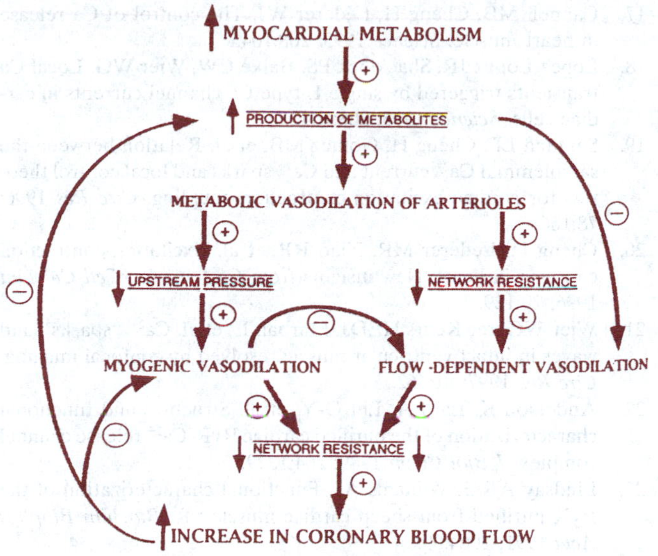

FIGURE 3-26 Schematic diagram of integrated response of metabolic, myogenic and flow-mediated regulation of coronary vascular resistance and flow during increase in metabolic demand. Plus sign indicates vasodilatory feedforward steps in response to initial increase in demand. Minus sign indicates negative-feedback processes that limit vasodilation. Events marked by lines ("Production of Metabolites") occur as a reaction to metabolic or vascular changes. Bolded items are metabolic or vasoactive adjustments. (From Muller et al.[200] Reprinted with permission of the publisher.)

NO.[198,200,204–209] At present, there is considerable information about the physiologic role of NO, but relatively little is known about the others. Although NO is a coronary vasodilator, it produces somewhat heterogeneous effects and may have quantitatively different influences on large arteries versus resistance vessels. NO appears to be the key effector of autoregulatory responses to normal physiologic stimuli, including tachycardia and vasodilation during exercise,[208–210] and is intimately connected to responses to the endothelial-derived substances mentioned earlier, as well as a variety of vasoactive drugs.

The response of the coronary circulation to changes in demand requires the coordination of the multiple modulatory mechanisms discussed earlier. The integrated response consists of heterogeneous effects that depend on the type of vessel and the region of the myocardium, which together increase nutritive flow. A scheme illustrating the complex interactions involved in the response to an increase in demand is shown in Fig. 3-26.

INTEGRATION OF THE CARDIOVASCULAR SYSTEM: THE RESPONSE TO DYNAMIC EXERCISE

Integrated functioning of the heart and peripheral and coronary circulations is exemplified by responses to dynamic exercise, especially isotonic activities such as walking, running, and swimming that entail repetitive shortening of skeletal muscle against relatively low loads. The coordinated response maximizes flow to working skeletal muscle and the heart; minimizes flow to nonworking muscle, visceral organs, and the kidneys; and ensures that flow to the brain is not compromised (see Table 3-2). In the periphery, local vasodilatory influences reduce resistance in vascular beds of working muscle. Cutaneous beds also dilate in order to facilitate heat transfer. In contrast, neurohumorally mediated responses cause vasoconstriction in nonworking skeletal muscle, abdominal viscera, and the kidneys. With isotonic exercise involving large muscle groups, there is usually a decrease in total systemic vascular resistance.

O_2 delivery to the myocardium is augmented by increased coronary flow caused by autoregulatory vasodilatation in response to increased metabolic demands. In addition to increased O_2 delivery, O_2 consumption is augmented by increased extraction, with lowering of coronary sinus O_2 saturation. Myocardial use of glycolytic metabolism increases, and NO produced in the coronary endothelium may facilitate shifts in mitochondrial respiration that tend to minimize increases in energy demands.

As noted earlier, in the normal circulation the ability to return blood to the heart is the limiting factor for increases in CO during exercise. In order to increase venous return, systemic venoconstriction decreases the volume of blood in venous reservoirs, resulting in a shift of blood volume to the arterial circulation and the heart. Working skeletal muscles in conjunction with venous valves themselves function as pumps to return blood to the heart, and increased respiratory rate causes the intrathoracic pressure to be negative a larger proportion of the time, which directly assists venous return to the right side of the heart.

In the heart itself, increased adrenergic stimulation caused by the coordinated effects of increased central nervous outflow and circulating catecholamines, along with parasympathetic withdrawal, results in increased HR (as much as three- to fivefold at maximum exercise), accelerated AV conduction, and enhanced contractility. Increased force and velocity of contraction are achieved through the effects of adrenergic stimulation (via cyclic AMP) and the FFR on Ca delivery to the myofilaments. Their effects on Ca reuptake and myofilament Ca sensitivity speed myocardial relaxation so that increased HR does not occur at the expense of incomplete relaxation. During upright exercise, ED volume remains relatively constant; during supine exercise, it increases somewhat.[211] Reflecting increased contractility, the ESPVR shifts leftward, and ES volume decreases. The combination of relatively constant or modestly increased ED volume and reduced ES volume results in a variable increase in SV and EF. With respect to augmenting CO, however, the increase in HR is considerably more important than the increase in SV.

The combination of increased HR and SV with resulting marked shortening of diastole means that ventricular filling must occur much more rapidly than under resting conditions. This is partly accomplished by the aforementioned increase in relaxation rate. However, it is likely that an increase in the generation of restoring forces due to the smaller ES volume as well as increased deformations such as torsion result in increased suction. Thus the same mechanisms causing increased force of contraction (adrenergic stimulation, FFR) also result in more rapid diastolic filling at lower ventricular pressures.

Systolic systemic arterial pressure increases substantially during dynamic exercise as a result of increased contractility and SV, while diastolic arterial pressure decreases because systemic resistance decreases. Obviously, pulse pressure increases. Minimum ventricular diastolic pressure decreases (more rapid relaxation, increased suction) with little or no change in ED pressure. Finally, coordinated changes in arterial elastance may function to optimize ventricular-vascular coupling and efficiency of conversion of chemical energy to EW by the contractile machinery.

Predominantly isometric exercise involving relatively brief bursts of skeletal muscle shortening against a heavy load (e.g., weight lifting, handgrip) evoke different responses. This type of exercise does not require a marked and/or sustained increase in CO with selective distribution to working muscles and heart. Thus many of the complex, integrated responses present during sustained isotonic exercise are unnecessary. However, isometric exercise does elicit reflex-mediated increases in sympathetic stimulation causing increased systemic vascular resistance and arterial pressure, HR, and cardiac contractility. The increases in systolic blood pressure are comparable with those during isotonic exercise, whereas the increases in HR are much smaller in magnitude.

References

1. Smith EE, Guyton AC, Manning RD, White RJ. Integrated mechanisms of cardiovascular response and control during exercise in the normal human. *Prog Cardiovasc Dis* 1976; 18:421.
2. Brengelmann GL. Circulatory adjustments to exercise and heat stress. *Annu Rev Physiol* 1983; 45:191.
3. Myhre ESP, Slinker BK, LeWinter MM. Absence of RV isovolumic relaxation in open-chest anesthetized dogs. *Am J Physiol* 1992; 263:H1587.
4. Fozzard HA, Arnsdorf MF. Cardiac electrophysiology. In: Fozzard HA, Haber E, Jennings RB, Katz AM, Morgan HE, eds. *The Heart and Cardiovascular System*, 2d ed. New York: Raven Press; 1991:63.
5. Pelzer D, Pelzer S, McDonald TF. Ca channels in heart. In: Fozzard HA, Haber E, Jennings RB, Katz AM, Morgan HE, eds. *The Heart and Cardiovascular System*, 2d ed. New York: Raven Press; 1991:1049.
6. Fozzard HA, Hanck DA: Na channels. In: Fozzard HA, Haber E, Jennings RB, Katz AM, Morgan HE, eds. *The Heart and Cardiovascular System*, 2d ed. New York, Raven Press; 1991:1091.
7. Gibbons WR, Zygmunt AC. ECC in the heart. In: Fozzard HA, Haber E, Jennings RB, Katz AM, Morgan HE, eds. *The Heart and Cardiovascular System*, 2d ed. New York: Raven Press; 1991:1249.
8. Williams AJ. The functions of two species of Ca channel in cardiac muscle ECC. *Eur Heart J* 1997; 18(suppl A):A27.
9. Yao A, Su Z, Nonaka A, et al. Effects of overexpression of the Na^+-Ca^{2+} exchanger on $[Ca^{2+}]_i$ transients in murine ventricular myocytes. *Circ Res* 1998; 82:657.
10. Grantham CJ, Cannell MB. Ca^{2+} influx during the cardiac AP in guinea pig ventricular myocytes. *Circ Res* 1996; 79:194.
11. Sipido KR, Maes M, Van de Werf F. Low efficiency of Ca^{2+} entry through the Na^+-Ca^{2+} exchanger as trigger for Ca^{2+} release from the SR. *Circ Res* 1997; 81:1034.
12. Sommer JR, Jennings RB. Ultrastructure of cardiac muscle. In: Fozzard HA, Haber E, Jennings RB, Katz AM, Morgan HE, eds. *The Heart and Cardiovascular System*, 2d ed. New York: Raven Press; 1991:3.
13. Lytton J, MacLennan DH Sr. In: Fozzard HA, Haber E, Jennings RB, Katz AM, Morgan HE, eds. *The Heart and Cardiovascular System*, 2d ed. New York: Raven Press; 1991:1203.
14. Stern MD. Theory of ECC in cardiac muscle. *Biophys J* 1992; 63:497.
15. McDonald TF, Pelzer S, Trautwein W, Pelzaer DJ. Regulation and modulation of Ca channels in cardiac, skeletal, and smooth muscle cells. *Physiol Rev* 1994; 74:365.
16. Carl SL, Felix K, Caswell AH, et al. Immunolocalization of sarcolemmal dihydropyridine receptor and SR triadin and RyR in rabbit ventricle and atrium. *J Cell Biol* 1995; 129:673.
17. Cannell MB, Cheng H, Lederer WJ. The control of Ca release in heart muscle. *Science* 1995; 268:1045.
18. Lopez-Lopez JR, Shacklock PS, Balke CW, Wier WG. Local Ca transients triggered by single L-type Ca channel currents in cardiac cells. *Science* 1995; 268:1042.
19. Santana LF, Cheng H, Gomez MB, et al. Relation between the sarcolemmal Ca^{2+} current and Ca^{2+} sparks and local control theories for cardiac excitation-contraction coupling. *Circ Res* 1996; 78:166.
20. Cheng H, Lederer MR, Xiao RP, et al. Excitation-contraction coupling in heart: New insights from Ca^{2+} sparks. *Cell Calcium* 1996; 20:129.
21. Wier WG, ter Keurs HEDJ, Marban E, et al. Ca^{2+} "sparks" and waves in intact ventricular muscle resolved by confocal imaging. *Circ Res* 1997; 81:462.
22. Anderson K, Lai FA, Liu Q-Y, et al. Structure and functional characterization of the purified cardiac RyR-Ca^{2+} release channel complex. *J Biol Chem* 1989; 264:1329.
23. Lindsay ARG, Williams AJ. Functional characterization of the RyR purified from sheep cardiac muscle SR. *Biochim Biophys Acta* 1991; 1064:89.
24. Sitsapesan R, Williams AJ. Gating of the native and purified cardiac SR Ca^{2+}-release channel with monovalent cations as permeant species. *Biophys J* 1994; 67:1484.
25. Sitsapesan R, Williams AJ. Regulation of the gating of the sheep cardiac SR Ca^{2+}-release channel by luminal Ca^{2+}. *J Membr Biol* 1994; 266:11144.
26. Kao JPY, Harootunian AT, Tsien RY. Photochemically generated cytosolic Ca pulses and their detection by fluo-3. *J Biol Chem* 1989; 264:8171.
27. Schatzmann HJ. The Ca pump at the surface membrane and at the SR. *Annu Rev Physiol* 1989; 51:473.
28. Tada M, Kirchberger MA, Repke DI, Katz AM. The stimulation of Ca transport in cardiac SR by adenosine 3′:5′-monophosphate-dependent protein kinase. *J Biol Chem* 1974; 249:6174.
29. Fujii J, Zarain-Herzberg A, Willard HF, et al. Structure of the rabbit phospholamban gene, cloning of the human cDNA, and assignment of the gene to chromosome 6. *J Biol Chem* 1991; 266:11669.
30. Luo W, Grupp IL, Harrer J, et al. Targeted ablation of the phospholamban gene is associated with markedly enhanced myocardial contractility and loss of β-agonist stimulation. *Circ Res* 1994; 75:401.
31. Luo W, Wolska BM, Grupp IL, et al. Phospholamban gene dosage effects in the mammalian heart. *Circ Res* 1996; 78:839.
32. Kadambi VJ, Ponniah S, Harrer J, et al. Cardiac-specific overexpression of phospholamban alters Ca kinetics and resultant cardiomyocyte mechanics in transgenic mice. *J Clin Invest* 1996; 97:533.
33. Koss KL, Kranias EG. Phospholamban: A prominent regulator of myocardial contractility. *Circ Res* 1996; 79:1059.
34. Katz AM. Cardiac ion channels. *New Eng J Med* 1993; 328:1244.
35. Huxley AF. Muscle structure and theories of contraction. *Prog Biophys Biophys Chem* 1957; 7:255.
36. Spudich JA. How molecular motors work. *Nature* 1994; 372:515.
37. McNally EM, Kraft R, Bravo-Zehnder M, et al. Full-length rat alpha and beta cardiac myosin HC sequences. *J Mol Biol* 1989; 210:665.
38. Rayment L, Holden H, Whittaker M, et al. Structure of the actin-myosin complex and its implications for muscle contraction. *Science* 1993; 261:58.
39. Pagani ED, Julian FJ. Rabbit papillary muscle myosin isozymes and the velocity of muscle shortening. *Circ Res* 1984; 54:586.
40. VanBuren P, Harris DE, Alpert NR, Warshaw DM. Cardiac V_1 and V_3 myosins differ in their mechanical activities in vitro. *Circ Res* 1995; 77:439.
41. Cuda G, Cooke R, Sellers JR. In vitro actin filament sliding

velocities produced by mixtures of different types of myosin. *Biophys J* 1997; 72:1767.
42. Winegrad S. How actin-myosin interactions differ with different isoforms of myosin. *Circ Res* 1998; 82:1109.
43. Labeit S, Kolmer B. Titins: Giant proteins in charge of muscle ultrastructure and elasticity. *Science* 1995; 270:293.
44. Helmes M, Trombitas K, Granzier H. Titin develops restoring force in rat cardiac myocytes. *Circ Res* 1996; 79:619.
45. Winegrad S. Cardiac myosin binding protein C. *Circ Res* 1999; 84:1117.
46. Holmes KC, Popp D, Gebhard W, Kabsch W. Atomic model of the actin filament. *Nature* 1995; 347:44.
47. Tobacman LS. Thin filament-mediated regulation of cardiac contraction. *Annu Rev Physiol* 1996; 58:447.
48. Solaro RJ, Rarick HM. Tn and Tm: Proteins that switch on and tune in the activity of cardiac myofilaments. *Circ Res* 1998; 83:471.
49. Weisberg A, Windegrad S. Relation between crossbridge structure and actomyosin ATPase activity in rat heart. *Circ Res* 1998; 83:60.
50. Kress M, Huxley HE, Faruqi R, Hendrix J. Structural changes during activation of frog muscle studied by time resolved x-ray diffraction. *J Mol Biol* 1986; 188:325.
51. McKillop DFA, Geeves MA. Regulation of the interaction between actin and myosin subfragment 1: Evidence for three states of the thin filament. *Biophys J* 1993; 65:693.
52. Geeves MA, Lehrer SS. Dynamics of the muscle thin filament regulatory switch: The size of the cooperative unit. *Biophys J* 1994; 67:273.
53. Swartz DR, Moss RL. Influence of a strong binding myosin analog on Ca sensitive mechanical properties of skinned skeletal muscle fibers. *J Biol Chem* 1992; 267:20497.
54. Moss RL. Ca^{2+} regulation of mechanical properties of striated muscle: Mechanistic studies using extraction and replacement of regulatory proteins. *Circ Res* 1992; 70:865.
55. Huxley AF. Muscular contraction. *J Physiol* 1974; 243:1.
56. Eisenberg E, Hill TL, Chen Y. Cross-bridge model of muscle contraction. *Biophys J* 1980; 29:195.
57. Kawai M, Brandt PW. Sinusoidal analysis: A high resolution method for correlating biochemical reactions with physiologic processes in activated skeletal muscle of rabbit, frog and crayfish. *J Muscle Res Cell Motil* 1980; 1:279.
58. Woledge RC, Curtin NA, Homsher E. *Energetic Aspects of Muscle Contraction*. London: Academic Press; 1985.
59. Alpert NA, Mulieri LA, Hasenfuss G. Myocardial chemo-mechanical energy transduction. In: Fozzard HA, Haber E, Jennings RB, Katz AM, Morgan HE, eds. *The Heart and Cardiovascular System*, 2d ed. New York: Raven Press; 1991:111.
60. McMahon TA. *Muscles, Reflexes, and Locomotion*. Princeton, NJ: Princeton University Press; 1984.
61. Lakatta EG. Starling's law of the heart is explained by an intimate interaction of muscle length and myofilament Ca activation. *J Am Coll Cardiol* 1987; 10:1157.
62. Lakatta EG. Length modulation of cardiac performance: Frank-Starling law of the heart. In: Fozzard HA, Haber E, Jennings RB, Katz AM, Morgan HE, eds. *The Heart and Cardiovascular System*, 2d ed. New York: Raven Press; 1991:1325.
63. McDonald KS, Moss RL. Osmotic compression of single cardiac myocytes eliminates the reduction in Ca^{2+} sensitivity of tension at short sarcomere length. *Circ Res* 1995; 77:199.
64. Apstein CS, Morgan JP. Cellular mechanisms underlying LV diastolic dysfunction. In: Gaasch WH, LeWinter MM, eds. *LV Diastolic Dysfunction and Heart Failure*. Philadelphia: Lea & Febiger; 1994:3.
65. Gillebert TC, Sys SU. Physiologic control of relaxation in isolated cardiac muscle and intact LV. In: Gaasch WH, LeWinter MM, eds. *LV Diastolic Dysfunction and Heart Failure*. Philadelphia: Lea & Febiger; 1994:25.
66. Gordon EE, Morgan HE. Principles of metabolic regulation. In: Fozzard HA, Haber E, Jennings RB, Katz AM, Morgan HE, eds. *The Heart and Cardiovascular System*, 2d ed. New York: Raven Press; 1991:151.
67. Tahiliani AG. Myocardial fatty acid metabolism. In: Fozzard HA, Haber E, Jennings RB, Katz AM, Morgan HE, eds. *The Heart and Cardiovascular System*, 2d ed. New York: Raven Press; 1991:1599.
68. Stanley WC, Lopaschuk GD, Hall JL, McCormack JG. Regulation of myocardial carbohydrate metabolism under normal and ischaemic conditions: Potential for pharmacological interventions. *Cardiovasc Res* 1997; 33:243.
69. Eberli FR, Weinberg EO, Grice WN, et al. Protective effect of increased glycolytic substrate against systolic and diastolic dysfunction and increased coronary resistance from prolonged global underperfusion and reperfusion in isolated rabbit hearts perfused with erythrocyte suspensions. *Circ Res* 1991; 68:466.
70. Bernstein RD, Ochoa FY, Xu X, et al. Function and production of NO in the coronary circulation of the conscious dog during exercise. *Circ Res* 1996; 79:840.
71. Xie Y-W, Shen W, Zhao G, et al. Role of endothelium-derived NO in the modulation of canine myocardial mitochondrial respiration in vivo. *Circ Res* 1996; 79:381.
72. Kelly RA, Balligand J-L, Smith TW. NO and cardiac function. *Circ Res* 1996; 79:363.
73. Mulieri LA, Hasenfuss G, Leavitt B, et al. Altered myocardial force-frequency relation in human heart failure. *Circulation* 1992; 85:1743.
74. Liu CP, Ting CT, Lawrence W, et al. Diminished contractile response to increased HR in intact human LV hypertrophy: Systolic versus diastolic determinants. *Circulation* 1993; 88:1893.
75. Ross J Jr, Miura T, Kambayashi M, et al. Adrenergic control of the force-frequency relation. *Circulation* 1995; 92:2327.
76. Hasenfuss G, Schillinger W, Lehnart SE, et al. Relationship between Na^{+}-Ca^{2+} exchanger protein levels and diastolic function of failing human myocardium. *Circulation* 1999; 99:641.
77. Meyer M, Bluhm WF, He H, et al. Phospholamban-to-SERCA2 ratio controls the force-frequency relationship. *Am J Physiol* 1999; 276:H779.
78. Hasenfuss G, Mulieri LA, Holubarsch C, et al. Energetics of Ca cycling in nonfailing and failing human myocardium. *Basic Res Cardiol* 1992; 87(suppl 2):81.
79. Blanchard EL, Leavitt BJ, Mulieri LA, Alpert NR. Dynamic Ca requirements for activation of human ventricular muscle calculated from tension independent heat. *Basic Res Cardiol* 1992; 87(suppl 1):245.
80. Mulieri LA, Leavitt BJ, Martin BJ, et al. Myocardial force-frequency defect in mitral regurgitation heart failure is reversed by forskolin. *Circulation* 1993; 88:2700.
81. Susanni EE, Vatner DE, Homcy CJ. The beta-adrenergic receptor/adenyl cyclase system. In: Fozzard HA, Haber E, Jennings RB, Katz AM, Morgan HE, eds. *The Heart and Cardiovascular System*, 2d ed. New York: Raven Press; 1991:1685.
82. Vatner SF. Sympathetic mechanisms regulating myocardial contractility in conscious animals. In: Fozzard HA, Haber E, Jennings RB, Katz AM, Morgan HE, eds. *The Heart and Cardiovascular System*, 2d ed. New York: Raven Press; 1991:1709.
83. Koch WJ, Milano CA, Lefkowitz RJ. Transgenic manipulation of myocardial G protein-coupled receptors and receptor kinases. *Circ Res* 1996; 78:511.
84. Ishikawa Y, Homcy CJ. The adenyl cyclases as integrators of transmembrane signal transduction. *Circ Res* 1997; 80:297.
85. Xiao R-P, Avdonin P, Zhou Y-Y, et al. Coupling of β_2-adrenoceptor to G_i proteins and its physiological relevance in murine cardiac myocytes. *Circ Res* 1999; 84:43.
86. Kaye DM, Wiviott SD, Balligand J-L, et al. Frequency-dependent activation of a constitutive NO synthase and regulation of con-

tractile function in adult rat ventricular myocytes. *Circ Res* 1996; 78:217.
87. Andries LJ, Brutsaert DL, Sys SU. Nonuniformity of endothelial constitutive NO synthase distribution in cardiac endothelium. *Circ Res* 1998; 82:195.
88. Haque R, Kan H, Finkel MS. Effects of cytokines and NO on myocardial E-C coupling. *Basic Res Cardiol* 1998; 93(suppl 1):86.
89. Graham RM, Perez DM, Hwa J, Piascik MY. α_1-Adrenergic receptor subtypes: Molecular structure, function, and signaling. *Circ Res* 1996; 78:737.
90. Jiang T, Pak E, Zhang H, et al. Endothelin-dependent actions in cultured AT-1 cardiac myocytes. *Circ Res* 1996; 78:724.
91. McClellan G, Weisberg A, Winegrad S. Effect of endothelin-1 on actomyosin ATPase activity. *Circ Res* 1996; 78:1044.
92. Endoh M, Fujita S, Yang H-T, et al. Endothelin: Receptor subtypes, signal transduction, regulation of Ca^{2+} transients and contractility in rabbit ventricular myocardium. *Life Sci* 1998; 62:1485.
93. Hoit BD, Shao Y, Kinoshita A, et al. Effects of angiotensin II generated by an angiotensin converting enzyme-independent pathway on LV performance in the conscious baboon. *J Clin Invest* 1985; 95:1519.
94. Wilny A, Clozel J-P, Rein J, et al. Functional and biochemical analysis of angiotensin II-forming pathways in the human heart. *Circ Res* 1997; 80:219.
95. Sadoshima J. Versatility of the angiotensin II type 1 receptor. *Circ Res* 1998; 82:1352.
96. Kaku T, Lakata E, Filburn C. α-Adrenergic regulation of phosphoinositide metabolism and protein kinase C in isolated cardiac myocytes. *Am J Physiol* 1991; 260:C635.
97. Heller-Brown J, Martinson AE. Phosphoinositide-generated second messengers in cardiac signal transduction. *Trans Cardiovasc Med* 1992; 2:209.
98. Pi Y, Sreekumar R, Xupei H, Walker JW. Positive inotropy mediated by diacylglycerol in rat ventricular myocytes. *Circ Res* 1997; 81:92.
99. Rouet-Benzineb P, Mohammadi K, Perennec J, et al. Protein kinase C isoform expression in normal and failing hearts. *Circ Res* 1996; 79:153.
100. Puceat M, Vassort G. Signalling by protein kinase C isoforms in the heart. *Mol Cell Biochem* 1996; 157:65.
101. Solaro RJ, Van Eyk J. Altered interactions among thin filament proteins modulate cardiac function. *J Mol Cell Cardiol* 1996; 28:217.
102. Streeter DD Jr. Gross morphology and fiber geometry of the heart. In: Berne RM, Sperelakis N, eds. *Handbook of Physiology*, Sec 2: *The Cardiovascular System*, Vol 1: *The Heart*. Bethesda, MD: American Physiological Society; 1979:61.
103. Buchalter MB, Weiss JL, Rogers WJ, et al. Noninvasive quantification of left ventricular rotational deformation in normal humans using magnetic resonance myocardial tagging. *Circulation* 1990; 81:1236.
104. Arts T, Veenstra PC, Reneman RS. Epicardial deformation and LV wall mechanics during ejection in the dog. *Am J Physiol* 1982; 243:H379.
105. Rademakers FE, Buchalter MB, Rogers WL, et al. Dissociation between LV untwisting and filling. *Circulation* 1992; 85:1572.
106. Raines RA, LeWinter MM, Covell JW. Regional shortening patterns of canine right ventricle. *Am J Physiol* 1976; 231:1395.
107. Yaku H, Slinker BK, Bell SP, LeWinter MM. Effects of free wall ischemia and bundle branch on systolic ventricular interaction in dog hearts. *Am J Physiol* 1994; 266:H1087–H1094.
108. Robinson TF, Cohen-Gould L, Factor SM. Skeletal framework of mammalian heart muscle: Arrangements of inter- and pericellular connective tissue structures. *Lab Invest* 1983; 49:482.
109. Robinson RF, Cohen-Gould L, Remily R, et al. Extracellular structures in heart muscle. In: Harris P, Poole-Wilson PA, eds. *Advances in Myocardiology*, Vol 5. New York: Plenum Press; 1985:243.
110. Weber KT. Cardiac interstitium: Extracellular space of the myocardium. In: Fozzard HA, Haber E, Jennings RB, Katz AM, Morgan HE, eds. *The Heart and Cardiovascular System*, 2d ed. New York: Raven Press; 1991:1465.
111. Guyton AC. The circulation. In: Guyton AC, Nall JE, eds. *Textbook of Medical Physiology*, 9th ed. Philadelphia: WB Saunders; 1996:239.
112. Shroff SG, Janicki J, Weber KT. Mechanical and energetic behavior of the intact left ventricle. In: Fozzard HA, Haber E, Jennings RB, Katz AM, Morgan HE, eds. *The Heart and Cardiovascular System*, 2d ed. New York: Raven Press; 1991:129.
113. Mirsky I. Review of various theories for the evaluation of left ventricular wall stresses. In: Mirsky I, Ghista DN, Sandler H, eds. *Cardiac Mechanics*. New York: Wiley; 1974:381.
114. Cohn JN. Cardiac consequences of vasomotor changes in the periphery: Impedance and preload. In: Fozzard HA, Haber E, Jennings RB, Katz AM, Morgan HE, eds. *The Heart and Cardiovascular System*, 2d ed. New York: Raven Press; 1991:1369.
115. Starling MR, Kirsh MM, Montgomery DG, Gross MD. Impaired left ventricular contractile function in patients with long-term mitral regurgitation and normal EF. *J Am Coll Cardiol* 1993; 22:239.
116. Suga H, Sagawa K, Shoukas AA. Load independence of the instantaneous pressure-volume ratio of the canine left ventricle and effects of epinephrine and HR on the ratio. *Circ Res* 1973; 32:314.
117. Sagawa K. The ES pressure-volume relation of the ventricle: Definition, modifications and clinical use. *Circulation* 1981; 63:1223.
118. Kass DA, Maughan WL. From "E_{max}" to pressure-volume relations: A broader view. *Circulation* 1991; 77:1203.
119. Slinker BK, Goto Y, LeWinter MM. Systolic direct ventricular interaction affects left ventricular contraction and relaxation in the intact dog circulation. *Circ Res* 1989; 65:307.
120. Suga H, Hisano R, Goto Y, Yamada O. Normalization of ES pressure-volume relation and E_{max} of different sized hearts. *Jpn Circ J* 1984; 48:136.
121. Mirsky I, Tajimi T, Peterson KL. The development of the entire ES pressure-volume and EF-afterload relations: A new concept of systolic myocardial stiffness. *Circulation* 1987; 76:343.
122. Mirsky I, Corin WJ, Murakami T, et al. Correction for preload in the assessment of myocardial contractility in aortic and mitral valve disease: Application of the concept of systolic myocardial stiffness. *Circulation* 1988; 78:68.
123. Kameyama T, Chen Z, Bell SP, Maughan D, et al. Mechanoenergetic alterations during the transition from cardiac hypertrophy to failure in Dahl salt sensitive rats. *Circulation* 1998; 98:2911.
124. Kameyama T, Chen Z, Bell SP, et al. Mechanoenergetic studies in isolated mouse hearts. *Am J Physiol* 1998; 274:H366.
125. Takeuchi M, Igarashi Y, Tomimoto S, et al. Single beat estimation of the slope of the ES pressure-volume relation in the human ventricle. *Circulation* 1991; 83:202.
126. Burkhoff D, Schnellbacher M, Stennett RA, et al. Explaining load-dependent ventricular performance and energetics based on a model of E-C coupling. In: LeWinter MM, Suga H, Watkins MW, eds. *Cardiac Energetics: From E_{max} to Pressure-Volume Area*. Boston: Kluwer; 1995:41.
127. Suga H. Ventricular energetics. *Physiol Rev* 1990; 70:247.
128. Goto Y, Slinker BK, LeWinter MM. Similar normalized E_{max} and O_2 consumption-pressure volume area relation in rabbit and dog. *Am J Physiol* 1988; 255:H366.
129. Goto Y, Slinker BK, LeWinter MM. Decreased contractile efficiency and increased nonmechanical energy cost in hyperthyroid rabbit heart. *Circ Res* 1990; 66:999.
130. Sunagawa K, Maughan WL, Sagawa K: Optimal arterial resis-

tance for the maximal stroke work studied in isolated canine left ventricle. *Circ Res* 1985; 56:586.
131. Hayashida K, Sunagawa K, Noma M, et al. Mechanical matching of the left ventricle with the arterial system in exercising dogs. *Circ Res* 1992; 71:481.
132. Asanoi H, Sasayama S, Kameyama T. Ventriculoarterial coupling in normal and failing heart in humans. *Circ Res* 1989; 65:483.
133. Furnival CM, Linden RJ, Snow HM. Inotropic changes in the left ventricle: The effect of changes in heart rate, aortic pressure, and end-diastolic pressure. *J Physiol* (*Lond*) 1970; 211:359.
134. Peterson KL, Sklovan D, Ludbrook P, et al. Comparison of isovolumic and ejection phase indices of myocardial performance in man. *Circulation* 1974; 49:1088.
135. Karliner JS, Gault JH, Eckberg D, et al. Mean velocity of fibre shortening: A simplified measure of left ventricular myocardial contractility. *Circulation* 1971; 44:323.
136. Ross J Jr. Afterload mismatch and preload reserve: A conceptual framework for the analysis of ventricular function. *Prog Cardiovasc Dis* 1976; 18:255.
137. Nakayama M, Chen CH, Nevo E, et al. Optimal preload adjustment of maximal ventricular power index varies with cardiac chamber size. *Am Heart J* 1998; 136:281.
138. Glower DD, Spratt JA, Snow ND, et al. Linearity of the Frank-Starling relationship in the intact heart: The concept of preload recruitable stroke work. *Circulation* 1985; 71:994.
139. Little WC. The left ventricular dP/dt_{max}-end-diastolic volume relation in closed chest dogs. *Circ Res* 1985; 56:808.
140. Little WC, Park RC, Freeman GL. Effects of regional ischemia and ventricular pacing on left ventricular dP/dt_{max}-end-diastolic volume relation. *Am J Physiol* 1987; 252:H993.
141. Weiss JL, Frederiksen JW, Weisfeldt ML. Hemodynamic determinants of the time-course of fall in canine left ventricular pressure. *J Clin Invest* 1976; 58:751.
142. Karliner JS, LeWinter MM, Mahler F, et al. Pharmacologic and hemodynamic influences on the rate of isovolumic left ventricular relaxation in conscious dogs. *J Clin Invest* 1977; 60:511.
143. Mirsky I. Assessment of diastolic function: Suggested methods and future considerations. *Circulation* 1984; 69:836.
144. Brutsaert DL, Sys SU. Relaxation and diastole of the heart. *Physiol Rev* 1989; 69:1228.
145. Wexler LF, Weinberg EO, Ingwall JS, Apstein CS. Acute alterations in diastolic left ventricular chamber distensibility: Mechanistic differences between hypoxemia and ischemia in isolated perfused rabbit and rat hearts. *Circ Res* 1989; 59:515.
146. Gaasch WH, Blaustein AS, Andrias CW, et al. Myocardial relaxation: II. Hemodynamic determinants of rate of left ventricular isovolumic pressure decline. *Am J Physiol* 1980; 239:H1.
147. Yellin EL, Hori M, Yoram C, et al. Left ventricular relaxation in the filling and nonfilling intact canine heart. *Am J Physiol* 1986; 250:H620.
148. Gillebert TC, Sys SU, Brutsaert DL. Influence of loading patterns on peak length-tension relation and on relaxation in cardiac muscle. *J Am Coll Cardiol* 1989; 13:483.
149. Zile MR, Gaasch WH. Load-dependent left ventricular relaxation in conscious dogs. *Am J Physiol* 1991; 261:H691.
150. Leite-Moreira AF, Gillebert TC. Non-uniform course of left ventricular pressure fall and its regulation by load and contractile state. *Circulation* 1994; 90:2481.
151. Gillebert TC, Lew WYW. Nonuniformity and volume loading independently influence isovolumic relaxation rates. *Am J Physiol* 1989; 257:H1927.
152. Nikolic S, Yellin EL, Tamura K, et al. Passive properties of the left ventricle: diastolic stiffness and restoring forces. *Circ Res* 1988; 62:1210.
153. Ingels NB Jr, Daughters GT II, Nikolic SD, et al. Left atrial pressure-clamp servomechanism demonstrates left ventricular suction in canine hearts with normal mitral valves. *Am J Physiol* 1994; 267:H354.
154. Bell SP, Fabian J, Higashiyama A, et al. Restoring forces assessed with left atrial pressure clamps. *Am J Physiol* 1996; 270:H1015.
155. Hansen DE, Daughters GT II, Alderman EL, et al. Torsional deformation of the left ventricular midwall in human hearts with intramyocardial markers: Regional heterogeneity and sensitivity to the inotropic effects of abrupt rate changes. *Circ Res* 1988; 62:941.
156. Pouleur H, Karliner JS, LeWinter MM, Covell W. Diastolic viscous properties of the intact left ventricle. *Circ Res* 1979; 45:410.
157. Gaasch WH. Passive elastic properties of the left ventricle. In: Gaasch WH, LeWinter MM, eds. *Left Ventricular Diastolic Dysfunction and Heart Failure*. Philadelphia: Lea & Febiger; 1994:143.
158. LeWinter MM, Myhre ESP, Slinker BK. Influence of the pericardium and ventricular interaction on diastolic function. In: Gaasch WH, LeWinter MM, eds. *Left Ventricular Diastolic Dysfunction and Heart Failure*. Philadelphia: Lea & Febiger; 1994:103.
159. Apstein CS, Grossman W. Opposite initial effects of supply and demand ischemia on left ventricular diastolic compliance: The ischemia-diastolic paradox. *J Mol Cell Cardiol* 1987; 19:119.
160. Yellin EL, Nikolic S, Frater RWM. Left ventricular filling dynamics and diastolic function. *Prog Cardiovasc Dis* 1990; 32:247.
161. Shah AM, Grocott-Mason RM, Pepper CB, et al. The cardiac endothelium: Cardioactive mediators. *Prog Cardiovasc Dis* 1996; 39:239.
162. Mark AL, Mancia G. Cardiopulmonary baroreflexes in humans. In: Shepherd JT, Abboud FM, eds. *Handbook of Physiology*, Sec 2: *The Cardiovascular System*, Vol 3. Bethesda, MD: American Physiological Society; 1983:795.
163. Shepherd JT. Cardiac mechanoreceptors. In: Fozzard HA, Haber E, Jennings RB, Katz AM, Morgan HE, eds. *The Heart and Cardiovascular System*, 2d ed. New York: Raven Press; 1991:1481.
164. Waldrop TG, Eldridge FL, Iwamoto GA, et al. Central neural control of respiration and circulation during exercise. In: Rowell LB, Shepherd JT, eds. *Handbook of Physiology*, Sec 12: *Exercise Regulation and Integration of Multiple Systems*. New York: American Physiological Society; 1996:333.
165. Mitchell JH, Victor RG. Neural control of the cardiovascular system: Insights from muscle sympathetic nerve recordings in humans. *Med Sci Sports Exerc* 1996; 28(suppl S):S60.
166. Goto Y, Slinker BK, LeWinter MM. Effect of coronary hyperemia on E_{max} and oxygen consumption in blood-perfused rabbit hearts: Energetic consequences of Gregg's phenomenon. *Circ Res* 1991; 68:482.
167. Schulz R, Heusch G. The relationship between regional blood flow and contractile function in normal, ischemic, and reperfused myocardium. *Basic Res Cardiol* 1998; 93:455.
168. Ruknudin A, Sachs F, Bustamente JO. Stretch-activated ion channels in tissue-cultured chick heart. *Am J Physiol* 1993; 264:H960.
169. Maron BJ, Pelliccia A, Spataro A, Granata M. Reduction in LV wall thickness after deconditioning in highly trained Olympic athletes. *Br Heart J* 1993; 69:125.
170. Maron BJ, Pelliccia A, Spirito P. Cardiac disease in young trained athletes: Insights into methods for distinguishing athlete's heart from structural heart disease, with particular emphasis on hypertrophic cardiomyopathy. *Circulation* 1995; 91:1596.
171. Lum H, Malik AB. Regulation of vascular endothelial barrier function. *Am J Physiol* 1994; 267:L223.
172. Wu HM, Yuam Y, Zawieja DC, et al. Role of phospholipase C, protein kinase C, and Ca in VEGF-induced venular hyperpermeability. *Am J Physiol* 1999; 276:H535.
173. Mayrovitz HN, Roy J. Microvascular blood flow: Evidence indicating a cubic dependence on arteriolar diameter. *Am J Physiol* 1983; 245:H1031.
174. Heistad DD, Kontos HA. Cerebral circulation. In: Shepard JT, Abboud FM, eds. *Handbook of Physiology*, Sec 2: *The Cardiovas-*

cular System. Bethesda, MD: American Physiological Society; 1983:137.
175. Koller A, Dornyei G, Kaley G. Flow-induced responses in skeletal muscle venules: Modulation by NO and prostaglandins. *Am J Physiol* 1998; 275:H831.
176. Burnstock G. Release of vasoactive substances from endothelial cells by shear: Stress and purinergic mechanosensory transduction. *J Anat* 1999; 194:335.
177. Lassen NA, Ingvar DH, Skinhoj E. Brain function and blood flow. *Sci Am* 1978; 239:62.
178. Mayhan WG. Disruption of blood brain barrier during acute hypertension in adult and aged rats. *Am Physiol* 1990; 258:H173.
179. Davis MJ, Hill MA. Signaling mechanisms underlying the vascular myogenic response. *Physiol Rev* 1999; 79:387.
180. Davies PF. Flow-mediated endothelial mechanotransduction. *Physiol Rev* 1995; 75:519.
181. Little TL, Xia J, Duling BR. Dye tracers define differential endothelial and smooth muscle coupling patterns within the arteriolar wall. *Circ Res* 1995; 76:498.
182. Segal SS, Welsh DG, Kurjiaka DT. Spread of vasodilation and vasoconstriction along feed arteries and arterioles of hamster skeletal muscle. *J Physiol* 1999; 516:283.
183. Meininger GA, Davis MJ. Cellular mechanisms involved in the vascular myogenic response. *Am J Physiol* 1992; 263:H657.
184. Brayden JE, Nelson MT. Regulation of arterial tone by activation of Ca-dependent K channels. *Science* 1992; 256:532.
185. Cheng HH, Lederer WJ, Cannell MB. Ca sparks: Elementary events underlying excitation-contraction coupling in heart muscle. *Science* 1992; 256:532.
186. Nelson MT, Cheng H, Rubart M, et al. Relaxation of arterial smooth muscle by Ca sparks. *Science* 1995; 270:633.
187. Furchgott RF, Zawadski JV. The obligatory role of endothelial cells in the relaxation of arterial smooth muscle by acetylcholine. *Nature* 1980; 288:373.
188. Ignarro LJ, Buga GM, Wood K, et al. Endothelium-derived relaxing factor produced and released from artery and vein is NO. *Proc Natl Acad Sci USA* 1987; 84:2965.
189. Ignarro LJ. Physiology and pathophysiology of NO. *Kidney Int* 1996; 55:S2.
190. Highsmith RF, Blackburn K, Schmidt DJ. Endothelin and Ca dynamics in vascular smooth muscle. *Annu Rev Physiol* 1992; 54:257.
191. Feletou M, Vanhoutte PM. The alternative: EDHF. *J Mol Cell Cardiol* 1999; 31:15.
192. Driss AB, Benessiano JP, Levy BI, et al. Arterial expansive remodeling induced by high flow rates. *Am J Physiol* 1997; 272:H851.
193. De Artinano AA, Gonzalez VL. Endothelial dysfunction and hypertensive vasoconstriction. *Pharmacol Res* 1999; 40:113.
194. Arnal JF, Dinh-Xaun AT, Pueyo M, et al. Endothelium-derived NO and vascular physiology and pathology. *Cell Mol Life Sci* 1999; 55:1078.
195. Chilian WM, Marcus ML. Effects of coronary and extravascular pressure on intramyocardial and epicardial blood velocity. *Am J Physiol* 1985; 248:H170.
196. Hoffman JI, Spaan JA. Pressure-flow relations in coronary circulation. *Physiol Rev* 1990; 70:331.
197. Farhi ER, Klocke FJ, Mates RE, et al. Tone-dependent waterfall behavior during venous pressure elevation in isolated canine hearts. *Circ Res* 1991; 68:392.
198. Olsson RA, Bunger R, Spaan JAE. Coronary circulation. In: Fozzard HA, Haber E, Jennings RB, Katz AM, Morgan HE, eds. *The Heart and Cardiovascular System*, 2d ed. New York: Raven Press; 1991:1393.
199. Austin RE Jr, Smedira NG, Squiers TM, Hoffman JI. Influence of cardiac contraction and coronary vasomotor tone on regional myocardial blood flow. *Am J Physiol* 1994; 266:H2542.
200. Muller JM, Davis MJ, Chilian WM. Integrated regulation of pressure and flow in the coronary microcirculation. *Cardiovasc Res* 1996; 32:668.
201. Dube GP, Bemis KG, Greenfield JC Jr. Distinction between metabolic and myogenic mechanisms of coronary hyperemic response to brief diastolic occlusion. *Circ Res* 1991; 68:1313.
202. Ely SW, Matherne GP, Coleman SD, Berne RM. Inhibition of adenosine metabolism increases myocardial interstitial adenosine concentration and coronary flow. *J Mol Cell Cardiol* 1992; 24:1321.
203. Stepp DW, Van Bibber R, Kroll K, Feigl EO. Quantitative relation between interstitial adenosine concentration and coronary blood flow. *Circ Res* 1996; 79:601.
204. Ishibashi Y, Duncker DJ, Zhang J, Bache RJ. ATP-sensitive K^+ channels, adenosine, and NO-mediated mechanisms account for coronary vasodilatation during exercise. *Circ Res* 1998; 82:346.
205. Furchgott RF. The 1989 Ulv von Euler Lecture: Studies on endothelium-dependent vasodilatation and the endothelium-derived relaxing factor. *Acta Physiol Scand* 1990; 139:257.
206. DiCarlo PE, Gimbrone MA Jr. Vascular endothelium. In: Fuster V, Ross R, Topol EJ, eds. *Atherosclerosis and Coronary Artery Disease*. Philadelphia: Lippincott-Raven; 1996:387.
207. Popp R, Fleming I, Busse R. Pulsatile stretch in coronary arteries elicits release of endothelium-derived hyperpolarizing factor: A modulator of arterial compliance. *Circ Res* 1998; 82:696.
208. Egashira K, Katsuda Y, Mohri M, et al. Role of endothelium-derived NO in coronary vasodilatation induced by pacing tachycardia in humans. *Circ Res* 1996; 79:331.
209. Recchia FA, Senzaki H, Saeki A, et al. Pulse pressure-related changes in coronary flow in vivo are modulated by NO and adenosine. *Circ Res* 1996; 79:849.
210. Zhao G, Zhang X, Xu X, et al. Short-term exercise training enhances reflex cholinergic NO-dependent coronary vasodilatation in conscious dogs. *Circ Res* 1997; 80:868.
211. Bar-Shlomo B-Z, Druck MN, Morch JE, et al. Left ventricular function in trained and untrained healthy subjects. *Circulation* 1982; 65:484.

CHAPTER 4

PRINCIPLES OF MOLECULAR CARDIOLOGY

Robert Roberts

Application of the techniques of recombinant DNA to cardiovascular disorders appears to be essential and appropriate to overcome several of the major obstacles to immediate and future progress.[1-3] The heart exhibits three characteristic adaptive responses to changes in its environment: the constitutive adaptive mechanism—namely, myofibril stretch that regulates cardiac output on a beat-to-beat basis (Starling's law)[4]; modulation of excitation contraction coupling through intramyofibril calcium leading to increased heart rate and force of contraction; and the long-term adaptation of compensatory growth (see Chap. 5). The first two adaptations were characterized extensively in the 20th century through the development, refinement, and application of hemodynamic techniques. In the 21st century, the molecular basis for the growth response will be elucidated and will include deciphering the basis for cardiac differentiation and development. This will be necessary if one desires to therapeutically modulate growth. Similarly, elimination of restenosis after angioplasty probably will require disruption of smooth muscle migration and proliferative response.[5] Unraveling the molecular basis of hereditary cardiac disorders is well underway, and with completion of the Human Genome Project within the next couple of years, this will be accelerated considerably[6,7] (see Chap. 62).

We have already entered the era of genetically engineered drugs such as recombinant tissue plasminogen activator (rt-PA),[8] which initiated a paradigmatic shift in the therapy of myocardial infarction, resulting in an acute mortality of only 6 percent.[9] The era referred to as *pharmacogenomics* is rapidly approaching, in which therapy will be individualized on the basis of a patient's genotype.[10]

HISTORICAL PERSPECTIVE OF MOLECULAR BIOLOGY

In 1953, Watson and Crick[11,12] proposed the double-helix model for DNA structure based on the results of x-ray defraction studies by Franklin and Wilkins.[13,14] The implications of DNA being a double helix, in which each strand is a mirror image of the other, were evident, namely, that one strand could serve as a template for the synthesis of a daughter strand, thus providing the means whereby genetic information could be perpetuated from parent to offspring. In 1957, Kornberg[15] described DNA polymerase, the enzyme necessary for the synthesis of DNA that was essential to recombinant DNA technology. Marmor and colleagues showed that the double helix of DNA, when subjected to high temperatures,[16,17] could be separated into its separate strands (denatured), and decreasing the temperature resulted in the reannealing, or hybridizing, of the strands, thus returning them to their previous double-stranded nature. This specific hybridization, or "base pairing" of complementary nucleotide strands, provides both the rationale and the practical basis for much of recombinant DNA technology. Crick had suggested correctly that the genetic code would be written in codons of three nucleotides for each amino acid.[12] The specific combination of three nucleotides that code for each amino acid was unraveled by Leder and Nirenberg[18] and Nishimura et al.[19] Several other necessary components were discovered subsequently, including the enzyme DNA ligase, which joins DNA fragments together.[20] All this information was known in the 1960s, as was the complete DNA code, as well as messenger RNA and the cytoplasmic ribosomal RNA for protein synthesis, but recombinant technology was not yet born and, in fact, for the next few years did not appear promising.

Many important discoveries, including those from the 1950s, played a role in recombinant technology, but four that really brought it to fruition and made possible modern molecular biology occurred between the years of 1970 and 1977. A major obstacle to the manipulation of DNA was its large size with no means to cut it into smaller pieces of known specific size. This obstacle was overcome by the discovery of restriction endonucleases that made it possible to cut DNA into smaller pieces in a predictable fashion.[21,22] These endonucleases, more commonly referred to as *restriction enzymes,* recognize specific sequences of DNA consisting of anywhere from four to eight nucleotides and specifically cut the DNA molecules at their recognition sites, making it possible to use and manipulate DNA fragments in a variety of procedures and reactions. In 1972, the enzyme reverse transcriptase was discovered by Baltimore[23] and Temin and Mizutani[24] simultaneously, making it possible to translate messenger RNA (mRNA) into its complementary DNA (cDNA). Shortly after the first molecule was cloned,[25] recombinant DNA techniques were born, as was modern molecular biology. In 1975, Sanger and Coulson[26] and Maxim and Gilbert[27] developed techniques for the rapid sequencing of DNA. In addition to these four developments, polymerase chain reaction (PCR), a more recently developed technique to rapidly amplify small amounts of DNA or RNA several million-fold, is also having a revolutionary effect on medicine and other fields.

NUCLEIC ACIDS

The Essentials of Nucleic Acids

The human genome is known to contain about three billion base pairs, which contain information that would more than fill a 500,000-page textbook. The DNA is contained in 46 chromosomes consisting of 44 autosomal and 2 sex chromosomes, but each chromosome is one continuous DNA molecule around which is wrapped several proteins. The smallest chromosome, 21, has more than 50 million base pairs, whereas chromosome 1, the largest, has over 250 million base pairs. There is enough DNA to form several hundred thousand genes; however, it is estimated that only about 67,000 genes encode for a human being. This would indicate that less than 5 percent of DNA is used to code for protein. The remainder of the DNA is used to provide spacing, structure, regulatory information, and other as yet unknown functions.

DNA consists of four building blocks referred to as *nucleotides* or merely as *bases*. A nucleotide consists of a nitrogenous base, a 5-carbon sugar (deoxyribose), and a phosphate group (Fig. 4-1). There are two purine bases (adenine and guanine) and two pyrimidine bases (cytosine and thymine) (Fig. 4-2). The triphosphate molecule is bonded to the 5′ carbon of the sugar, and the base is bonded to the 1′ carbon of the sugar. Each DNA molecule consists of millions of nucleotides joined together in a linear fashion through the phosphate group, which forms a bond with the hydroxyl group of the 3′ carbon of the next sugar. The phosphate groups form the backbone of the molecule, but because they are water-soluble, they face outward. Attached to the inner side of the sugar is the hydrophobic base, which faces inward to shield it from the aqueous environment. The molecule forms a right-sided spiral coil with a turn every 10 nucleotides (3.4 nm), referred to as a *right-sided α-helix,* and pairs with its complementary strand to form the so-called double helix (Fig. 4-3). The center of the molecule consists of the bases that face inward and are opposite to each other. This arrangement provides for the hydrogen bonding between the bases that keeps the two strands together. The hydrogen bonds are perpendicular to the helical axis. The directionality of the strands is referred to as *5′ to 3′* or *3′ to 5′*, which is based on the position of the carbons in the sugar. The end of the molecule with a phosphate or hydroxyl group on the 5′ carbon is termed the *5′ end,* whereas the end with a free terminal 3′ carbon is referred to as the *3′ end*. It is important to distinguish the two ends because the enzyme DNA polymerase always initiates replication of DNA from the 5′ end and proceeds to the 3′ end. There seems to be no constraints on which bases can be adjacent to each other; however, the hydrogen binding between the bases of the two chains is highly specific, since adenine (A) always pairs with thymine (T), and guanine (G) always pairs with cytosine (C). The sugars and the phosphate groups are always the same, whereas the sequence of the bases varies and determines the nature of the hereditary information to be passed onto the progeny. The specificity of this "base pairing" is the basis of the ability of DNA to replicate itself and pass on the genotype characteristics and also forms the basis for the specificity of essentially all the procedures used in recombinant DNA technology. During the process of DNA replication, the strands separate, and new strands form complementary to the original strands, resulting in two additional identical molecules.

Transcription (from DNA to RNA)

The central dogma of molecular biology is that DNA produces RNA, which in turn produces a polypeptide, the latter being the molecules that make up proteins that provide the cell structure and perform the functions of the cell (Fig. 4-4). The genetic information inherited by each individual is encoded by the sequence of the bases of the DNA (the genotype), which is translated into proteins and provides the observable characteristics of the individual (the phenotype). This overall process from DNA to protein, however, must first go through the intermediary step of RNA. The process whereby mRNA is synthesized using DNA as the template is referred to as *transcription* (Fig. 4-5). Transcription and the processing of mRNA occur in the nucleus of the cell, separated by the nuclear membrane from the cytoplasm of the cell. The process of transcription is initiated by attachment of the enzyme RNA polymerase II to specific recognition sites where the DNA is double-stranded, but on activation by the enzyme, the strands now selectively unwind and separate (Fig. 4-6). The binding site of RNA polymerase II is always located on the 5′ end of the gene, and the enzyme remains attached to a single strand of DNA as it travels in the 3′ direction. The DNA immediately in front of it separates into two strands with just one strand of DNA (antisense) acting as a template for the synthesis of mRNA. Thus, in contrast to DNA, mRNA is a single-stranded polynucleotide. Messenger RNA also differs from DNA in that deoxyribose, the sugar found in DNA, is replaced by ribose. Moreover, uracil (U) replaces thymine (T), and like thymine, uracil pairs exclusively

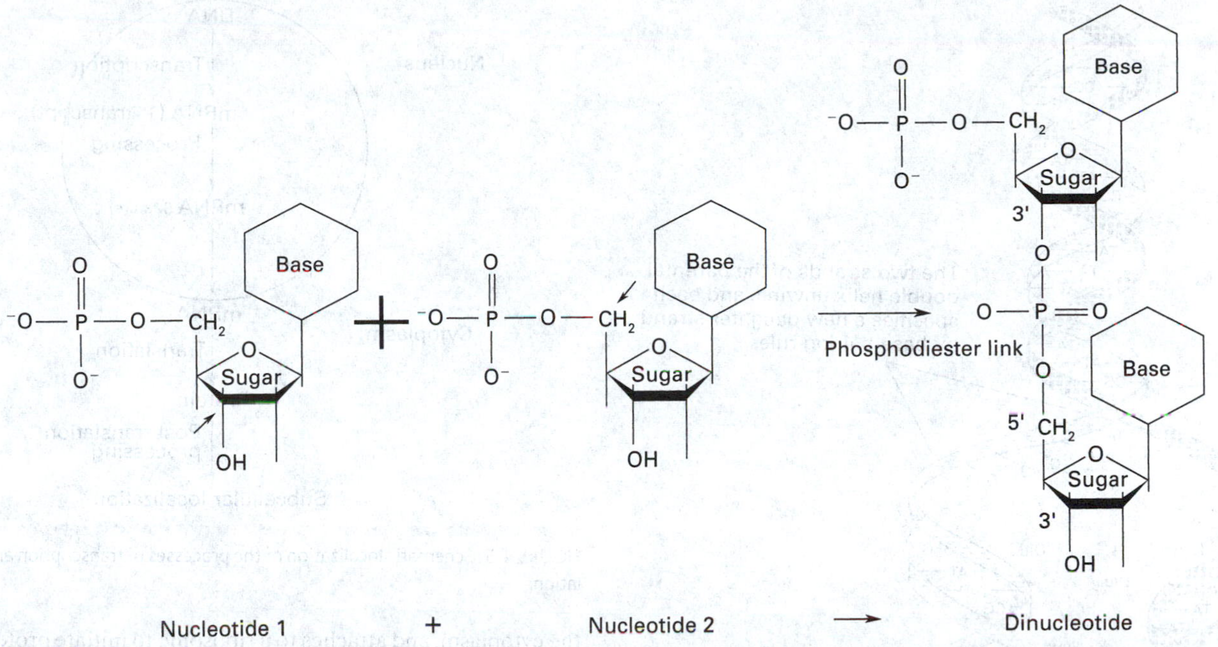

FIGURE 4-1 Formation of polynucleotides from nucleotide precursors. Nucleotides are joined together by a phosphodiester linkage to form a nucleic acid. Arrows indicate the carbon atoms of deoxyribose that are joined by phosphodiester bonds to form polynucleotides. Note that the bases are attached to 1′ carbon position of the sugar molecule and face the interior of the molecule. The backbone is formed by the sugar linked by phosphate groups binding to 5′ and 3′ carbons of the sugar. (From Mares A Jr, Towbin J, Bies RG, Roberts R. Molecular biology for the cardiologist. *Curr Probl Cardiol* 1992; 17:9–72. Reproduced with permission from the publisher and authors.)

with adenine (A). Thus, by this mechanism, each adenine (A) of DNA pairs with uracil (U) of RNA, each cytosine (C) of DNA pairs with guanine (G) of RNA, each thymine (T) of DNA pairs with adenine (A) of RNA, and each guanine (G) of DNA pairs with cytosine (C) of RNA.

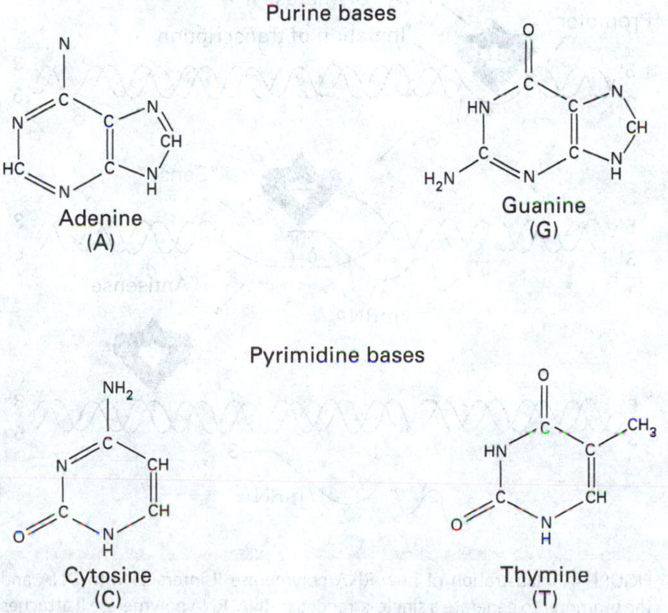

FIGURE 4-2 The common purine and pyrimidine bases found in DNA. Uracil is substituted for thymine in RNA. (From Mares A Jr, Towbin J, Bies RG, Roberts R. Molecular biology for the cardiologist. *Curr Probl Cardiol* 1992; 17:9–72. Reproduced with permission from the publisher and authors.)

The mRNA, as transcribed from the DNA, is referred to as the *primary transcript,* or sometimes as *immature mRNA,* and is a complementary copy of the DNA (Fig. 4-7). Since protein synthesis occurs in the cytoplasm, the mRNA must exit the nucleus, but prior to transport, it undergoes extensive posttranscriptional processing primarily through three main events: (1) addition of a methylated guanosine (4-methylguanosine residue) to the 5′ end, referred to as a *cap,* which is important for the initiation of translation; (2) addition of a long tail of repeated adenine nucleotides, called the *poly(A) tail,* to the 3′ region of the mRNA, which is essential for stability of the message in the cytoplasm; and (3) the primary transcript, which contains introns and exons, undergoes a specific splicing process whereby the introns are removed and the exons are properly respliced together prior to exit from the nucleus as mature mRNA. The process of splicing is, in part, performed by molecules referred to as *small nuclear ribonucleoproteins* (snRNPs), which consist of RNA molecules tightly associated with a group of about 10 different proteins. Exons survive the mRNA processing and exit the nucleus (hence the name) as part of the mature mRNA. The mRNA consists of three distinct regions. The exons of the 5′ end are not translated into protein but signal the beginning of mRNA translation and contain sequences that direct the mRNA to the ribosome in the cytoplasm for protein synthesis. The exons in the second region, referred to as the *coding region,* contain the information that determines the amino acid sequence of the protein. The exons of the 3′ end do not code for protein but for signals that terminate translation and direct the addition of the poly(A) tail. Introns are portions of the gene included in the primary mRNA transcript but which are spliced out of the mature mRNA. The process of splicing out introns and rejoining exons is an important means of introducing ge-

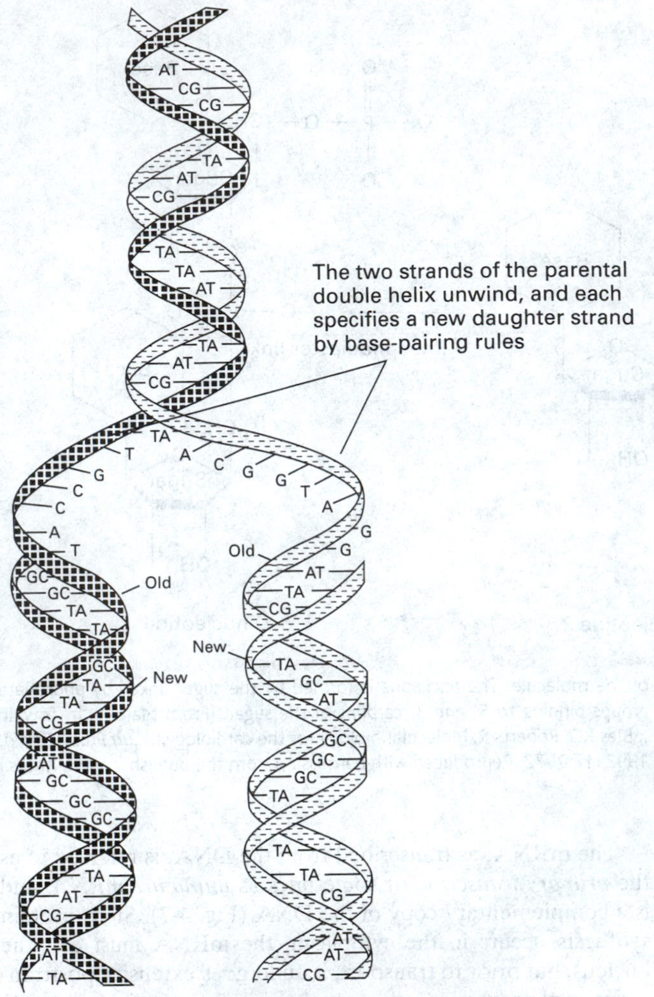

FIGURE 4-3 DNA replication conserves the nucleotide sequence. DNA is a double-stranded helical molecule bound together by the nucleotide bases contained on each individual strand. During cell division, two identical copies of the original parental strand are made by unwinding the DNA and then synthesis of a complementary second strand to make two identical new daughter strands.

netic diversity, since one mRNA may provide several different mRNAs that code for different polypeptides (this will be discussed further under gene regulation). The primary transcript undergoes extensive shortening such that the mature mRNA often represents only 10 percent of the primary transcript. The mature mRNA exits the nucleus through nuclear pores, enters

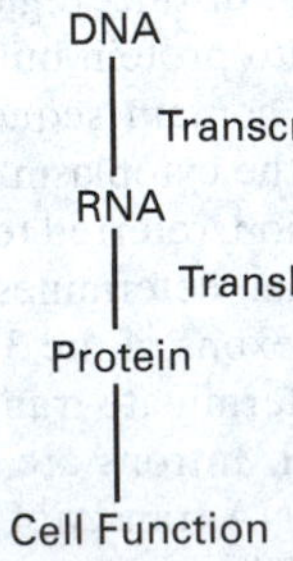

FIGURE 4-4 Central dogma of molecular biology.

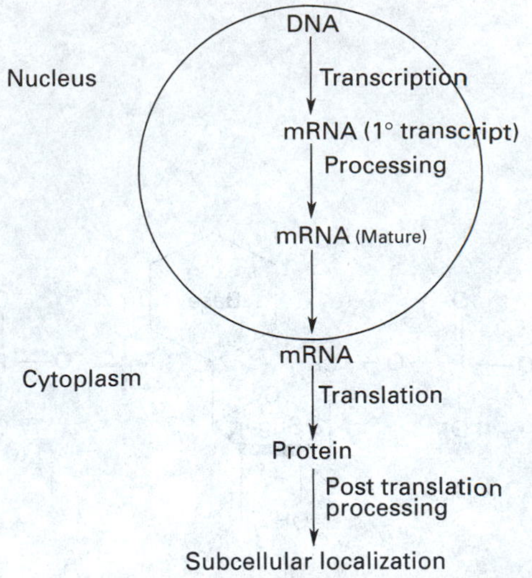

FIGURE 4-5 Schematic localization of the processes of transcription and translation.

the cytoplasm, and attaches to a ribosome to initiate protein synthesis.

Translation

The final process whereby the nucleic acids of the mRNA code for a specific polypeptide is referred to as *translation*. This process is the most complex of the various processes that occur in the flow from genomic DNA (gene) to mature protein. The alphabet of the DNA or its single-stranded complementary mRNA is that of the four nucleotides (bases), whereas that of the protein is the 20 amino acids. Crick in 1961,[11] while trying

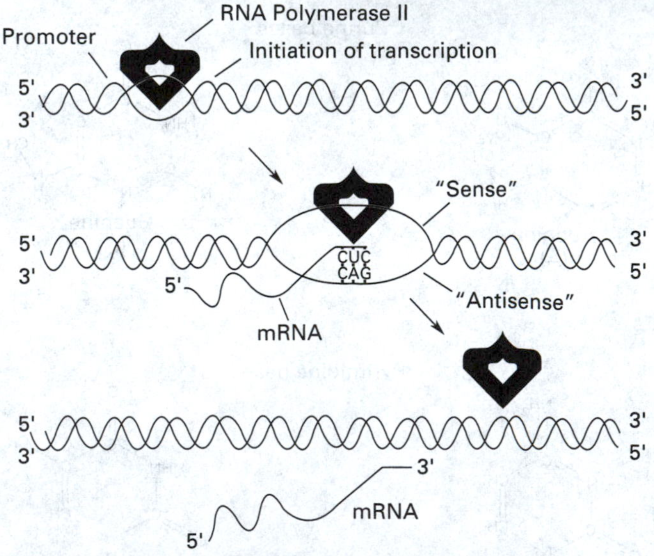

FIGURE 4-6 Illustration of how RNA polymerase II interacts with DNA and the promoter to generate a single-stranded mRNA. RNA polymerase II attaches to the initiation site promoted by the 5′ promoter sequence. mRNA is synthesized in the 5′ to 3′ direction from just one strand, the antisense strand. The specificity of base pairing between mRNA and the antisense strand provides for an mRNA with sequences complementary to that of the antisense strand and identical to that of the sense strand.

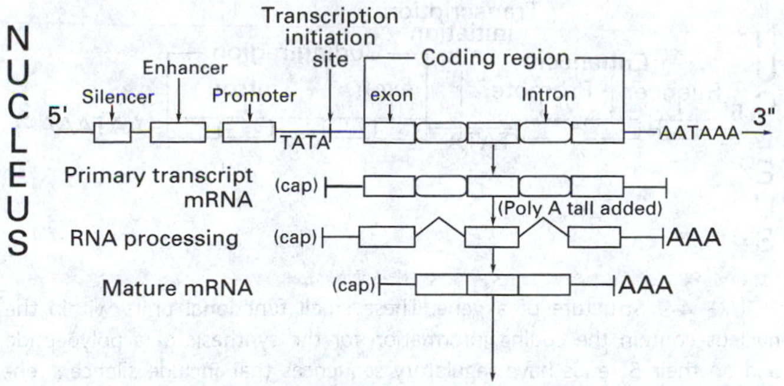

FIGURE 4-7 Transcription. Transcription occurs in the nucleus, producing mRNA that is processed into mature mRNA and transported to the cytoplasm. In the cytoplasm, translation occurs, with the mRNA coding for specific amino acids that are linked together to form a polypeptide and ultimately to form a mature protein. (From Mares A Jr, Towbin J, Bies RG, Roberts R. Molecular biology for the cardiologist. *Curr Probl Cardiol* 1992; 17:9–72. Reproduced with permission from the publisher and authors.)

to determine the code for translation from DNA to protein, showed that the genetic code was written in triplets of bases, with each amino acid being encoded by three base pairs referred to as a *codon* and specific amino acids determined by the sequence of the codon. The mRNA codons dictate which amino acids are to be selected, and the order of the codons dictates the sequence of the amino acids in the protein. Determination of the codons for each amino acid was completed in 1966. There are four different nucleotides to form the triplets; thus the number of combinations (4^3) is 64, but there are only 20 amino acids. There is considerable redundancy, referred to as *degeneracy,* and this results in most of the amino acids having more than one codon. In addition to codons for each amino acid, there is also the codon AUG, which is the start codon that initiates protein synthesis and also codes for methionine. To stop translation, there are three codons, UAA, UAG, and UGA, that signal the end of a particular polypeptide. Translation into protein requires two other RNA species, ribosomal RNA (rRNA) and transfer RNA (tRNA). The mRNA, after exiting the nucleus, recognizes the ribosome, which is the site of protein synthesis. The ribosome moves along an mRNA molecule, translating each of its codons in a 5′ to 3′ direction to assemble the polypeptide from its amino (N-terminal) to its carboxy (C-terminal) ends (Fig. 4-8).

The mRNA does not interact directly with amino acids but rather through adaptor molecules—referred to as transfer RNA (tRNA)—to which amino acids are covalently joined by a highly specific enzyme (aminoacyl tRNA synthetase) using ATP. There is at least one tRNA species corresponding to each of the 20 naturally occurring amino acids. The aminoacyl tRNA synthetase performs a special function of activating the amino acids and ensuring that each amino acid is joined to its tRNA and to no other. The structure of tRNA is now known in great detail, and its specificity is attributed to the sequence of three nucleotides complementary to the codon exposed at one end of the folded tRNA molecule, which, on the tRNA, is referred to as the *anticodon*. The amino acid receptor site is exposed at the other end. Amino acids thus are specified at two recognition steps: one in which a specific enzyme joins the amino acid to a specific tRNA and the other in which the tRNA serving as an adaptor molecule joins the amino acid to the ribosomal-mRNA complex through a codon-anticodon specific-base-pairing interaction between the mRNA and the tRNA. Once the process of protein synthesis is initiated, the ribosome moves along the mRNA joining the amino acids via peptide bonds in the sequence specified by the mRNA to form the mature polypeptide. The process of protein synthesis from this complex of mRNA and ribosome involves over 100 enzymes. The steps involved consist of initiation, elongation, and termination of the polypeptide, with each process having its own enzymes.

The mature polypeptide consists of amino acids joined together by peptide bonds; the mature protein, however, often consists of multiple covalently bound polypeptides, and many undergo other modifications referred to as *posttranslational changes*. A more detailed analysis of protein synthesis is given in Chap. 5. Encoded in the polypeptide are other features that have been determined by the mRNA, namely, leader sequences

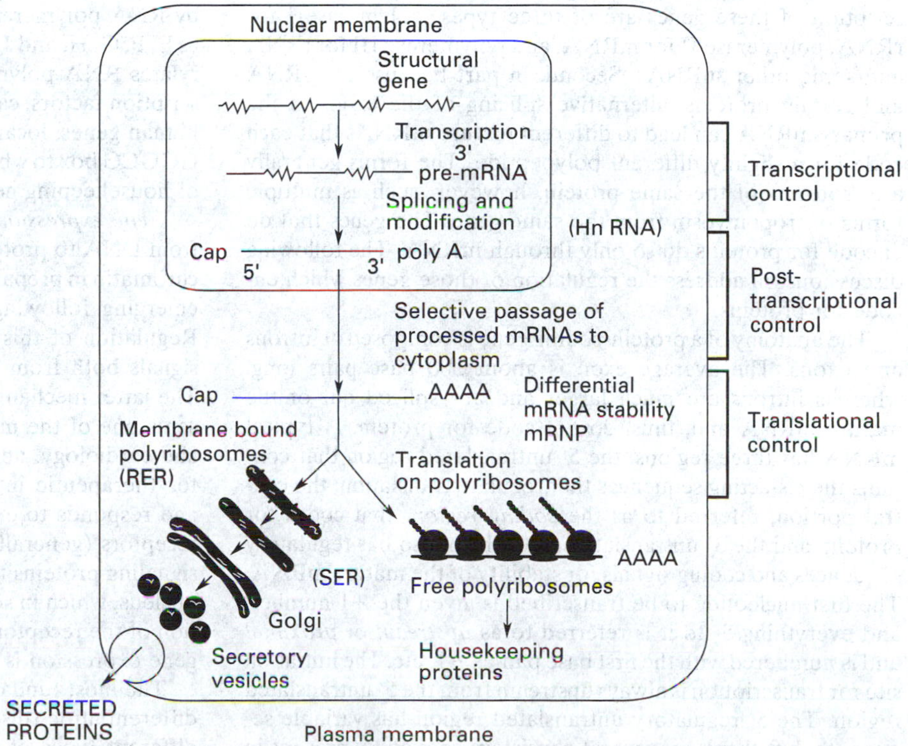

FIGURE 4-8 A summary of the multiple steps involved in gene expression from the genomic DNA to the protein showing how the protein destined for secretion follows a systematic path different from proteins destined to remain in the cytoplasm. (From Campbell PN, Smith AD. Nucleic acids and protein biosynthesis. In: Campbell PN, Smith AD, eds. *Biochemistry Illustrated*, 2d ed. New York: Churchill Livingstone; 1988:111. Reproduced with permission from the publisher.)

that will direct the protein to either intracellular membranes, the plasma membrane, or organelles such as the mitochondria. There is also considerable proteolytic activity following entry of the molecule into its organelle, or membrane, as the leader sequences are removed. There are also the processes whereby disulfhydryl bonds are formed or glycosylation occurs (in the Golgi apparatus) (see Fig. 4-8). The mRNAs generally are not long-lived due to their rapid degradation by RNAses and so may last from only a few minutes to many hours. A single mRNA may code for only a few copies of the polypeptide or several thousand. The average estimate is 1400. In contrast, rRNAs and tRNAs are much less rapidly degraded and therefore have acquired the name *stable RNAs*. Their relative concentration in the cell, in large part, reflects their stability, with more than 80 percent being rRNAs, 15 percent being tRNAs, and less than 5 percent being mRNAs.

Gene Structure, Expression, and Regulation

The concept that one gene leads to one protein remains basic to the central dogma of molecular biology but does, in some cases, need to be modified slightly in view of recent observations. In the classic sense, a gene consists of a discrete unit of DNA that encodes for a specific polypeptide. Two observations must be noted: First, transcription produces two end points—ribonucleic acid (RNA) and protein. The products, or rRNA, tRNA, and small nuclear RNA (snRNA), do not get translated into protein but rather perform functions during posttranscription and translation that are pivotal to expression of the mRNA that does code for protein. The polymerases necessary for transcription of these genes are of three types, polymerase I for rRNA, polymerase II for mRNA, and polymerase III for tRNA and some other snRNAs. Second, in part because of snRNA and certain proteins, alternative splicing of the exons in the primary mRNA can lead to different mature mRNAs that each code for a slightly different polypeptide. The forms generally are isoforms of the same protein, however, such as multiple forms of tropomyosin from the same gene. The genes that do encode for proteins do so only through mRNA. The following discussion will address the regulation of those genes which encode for proteins.

The anatomy of a protein-coding gene is composed of introns and exons. The average exon is about 300 base pairs long, whereas introns are much larger and are spliced out of the mature mRNA and, thus, do not code for protein. A typical mRNA has three regions: the 5′ untranslated region that contains the cis-acting sequences that regulate translation; the central portion, referred to as the *coding region,* that codes for protein; and the 3′ untranslated end, which also has regulatory sequences and coding signals for stability of the mature mRNA. The first nucleotide to be transcribed is given the +1 number, and everything 5′ to it is referred to as *upstream* or *proximal* and is numbered with the first base pair as −1, etc. The initiation site for transcription is always upstream from the 5′ untranslated region. The 5′ regulatory untranslated region has variable sequences, but there are several consistent sequences present in the same position in most human genes. Polymerase II has no affinity for DNA and can only bind after several transcription factors have bound. The site of transcription and its direction are determined by a TATA box, which has a consensus sequence of TATAA(T)AA(T) and is found at base pairs −25 to −30

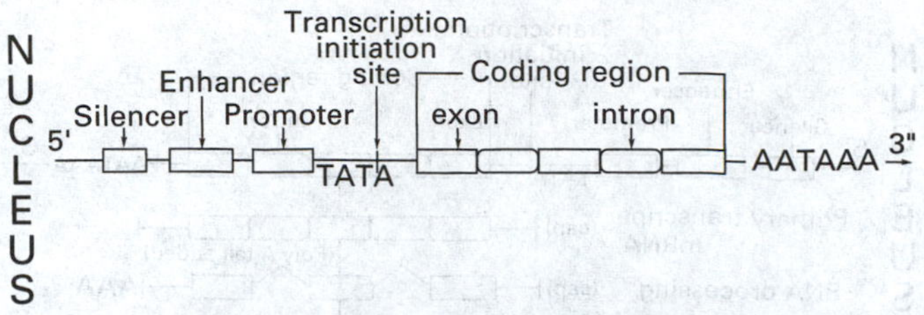

FIGURE 4-9 Structure of a gene. These small functional units within the nucleus contain the coding information for the synthesis of a polypeptide and on their 5′ ends have regulatory sequences that include silencers, enhancers, and promoters. The coding region consisting of exons (code for protein) as well as intervening noncoding sequences (introns) is followed by a 3′ noncoding region that is translated into the mRNA. The 3′ end appears important for exit of the mRNA from the nucleus and its stability in the cytoplasm but does not code for protein. The TATA is the initiation site for polymerase and is present in most eukaryotes at about 10 to 30 base pairs 5′ from the start codon (TAC) of the coding region. The AATAA will become the recognition site on the mRNA to which attaches an enzyme that cleaves the 3′ region and replaces the distal portion with a poly(A) tail. (From Mares A Jr, Towbin J, Bies RG, Roberts R. Molecular biology for the cardiologist. *Curr Probl Cardiol* 1992; 17:9–72. Reproduced with permission from the publisher and authors.)

upstream from the start site. A large complex of transcription factors (more than 25 proteins) binds to the TATA box in preparation for RNA polymerase II binding and transcription. Collectively, these transcription factors are referred to as *transcription factors for polymerase II* (TFII), with letters designating the different factors. TFIID binds first, then TFIIB, followed by RNA polymerase II, followed by several TFII factors such as E, F, G, H, and J, etc. TFIIH has kinase activity and phosphorylates RNA polymerase II, which now, independent of transcription factors, can initiate transcription. In addition, in many human genes, located at about base pair −200 upstream is the GGGCG box to which SP1 binds, and this is felt to be a regulator of housekeeping genes (Fig. 4-9).

Gene expression refers to all the processes required to go from DNA to protein, from the initial unfolding of the nuclear chromatin in preparation for transcription to the mature protein emerging following completion of posttranslational changes. Regulation of this process occurs at all levels in response to signals both from within the cell and from the environment. The latter mechanism is of particular interest because it represents one of the major areas of research in molecular biology and cardiology, and it is also an area that has great potential for therapeutic intervention. The cell maintains its integrity and responds to external stimuli through signals that activate receptors (generally in the cell membrane). These in turn use signaling proteins to transfer their message to the cytoplasm or nucleus, which in some way modifies gene expression. Delineation of the receptor, the signaling proteins, and where and how gene expression is altered are of prime importance.

The most fundamental level of gene regulation involves cell differentiation (discussed later). The body contains at least 200 different types of cells that have been programmed by their genes to perform highly specialized functions. All cells have the same DNA and the same genes, but only those genes which are expressed determine the cell's phenotype. Cardiac myocytes, for example, are characterized by a set of proteins that specialize in contractile activity, whereas hepatocytes specialize in the synthesis and catabolism of proteins. Selective gene expression is the basis of cell differentiation. Cell growth and replication occur in what is termed the *undifferentiated cell* but, through complex mechanisms, give rise to cells that cease to replicate and are programmed to take on specialized functions (cell differentiation). In the process of cell differentiation, genes—particularly those concerned with cell proliferation and undifferentiated functions—are down-regulated, whereas those genes coding for the proteins that perform the specialized functions are up-regulated. Once cells are differentiated, protein synthesis, however, remains a dynamic process to maintain cell integrity. Most of gene regulation is concerned with the maintenance of cellular integrity, and the genes responsible for this basal function are referred to as *housekeeping genes*. Housekeeping genes are constitutively regulated, as opposed to genes responsible for cell differentiation and growth, which are developmentally regulated. It is estimated that organs use about 10,000 genes (constitutive) to maintain their integrity, with one exception—the brain, which is estimated to use around 20,000 genes. Gene regulation may be classified under the following headings: pretranscription, transcription, posttranscription, translation, and posttranslation.[28]

Pretranscriptional regulation refers to the decompaction of the DNA and exposure of the region about to undergo transcription. The total DNA of a single cell would measure about 1 m in length, yet in the nucleus it is markedly compacted and is folded around specific proteins, the dominant class being histone. The coiling of the DNA appears to be in domains that can be exposed when transcription is activated. It is also at this level that methylation plays a part. Heavily methylated genes, made insensitive to digestion by the enzyme DNAse, tend not to be transcribed, whereas other areas sensitive to digestion appear to be very active in transcription. The precise mechanisms involved with chromatin conformational changes or exposure of the gene for transcription are, at present, relatively unknown. There is evidence, however, that methylation is involved in regulating cell differentiation.

The role of transcriptional control is a major rate-limiting step to gene expression. While transcription is catalyzed by the enzyme RNA polymerase II, the enzyme by itself cannot initiate transcription and acts only with the help of additional transcriptional factors. In addition to the promoter sequences previously described (TATA box and CG box), several DNA sequences in conjunction with their DNA-binding proteins act as either promoters, enhancers, or silencers of transcription and will be defined subsequently (see Fig. 4-9). The 5′ upstream region, immediately adjacent to the transcription initiation site and including the area that binds RNA polymerase II, is referred to as the *promoter region*. This region contains sequences that are specific binding sites for proteins referred to as *transacting factors,* or *transcriptional factors*. The protein-binding sites are often referred to as *cis-acting sequences* because they are on the same DNA molecule on which they act. The transcription factors (also referred to as *DNA-binding proteins*) are referred to as *transacting factors* (acting at a distance) because they are encoded by genes that may even be on another chromosome. The average promoter binding site consists of several hundred base pairs grouped into motifs of 4 to 10 base pairs.[29] It is hypothesized that all the motifs have to be bound by transcription factors of the appropriate nature and in the appropriate sequence for transcription to occur.

The promoter sequences and their corresponding DNA-binding proteins may act ubiquitously or may be tissue-specific. Promoters often increase transcription of a class of genes rather than a single gene. Another type of DNA sequence that increases transcription is referred to as an *enhancer* (see Fig. 4-9). Enhancers differ from promoter sequences in that they may be upstream or downstream from the coding region and be separated by as many as hundreds of thousand base pairs and are effective in either the 5′ to 3′ or 3′ to 5′ direction. An extreme example is the DNA sequence that enhances expression of the gene for hemoglobin, which is located more than 1 million base pairs from the transcription initiation site. These enhancers, like promoters, consist of several small motifs of 4 to 10 base pairs, and when bound by their corresponding DNA-binding proteins (transcription factors), they have a positive influence on gene transcription. Another regulatory DNA sequence that is similar to enhancers in size and location but exerts a negative influence on transcription is referred to as a *silencer* or *repressor*. It is believed that enhancer and silencer sequences, when bound by transcription factors, communicate with promoters by DNA looping that is induced by the binding. This DNA binding that brings the enhancer, silencer, and promoter in close proximity is the mechanism responsible for the action-at-a-distance phenomenon seen in human gene regulation.

The genes that encode proteins regulating cardiac growth are many: growth factors, growth factor receptors, intracellular signaling proteins that relay growth signals from the extracellular milieu, and ultimately, transcription factors that regulate RNA polymerase and selectively induce or down-regulate gene expression.[30] Several DNA-binding proteins are recognized (transcription factors) (Fig. 4-10), including the zinc-finger, leucine-zipper, helix-loop-helix, MADS domain, and helix-turn-helix proteins. The zinc-finger type of protein is used by developmental genes called *GATA factors* and the receptors for circulating hormones, including the glucocorticoids, progesterones, androgens, mineralocorticoids, estrogen, thyroxine, vitamin D_3, and retinoic acid. These hormones, which are lipophilic, penetrate the cell membrane and activate an intracellular receptor or nuclear receptor, which, in turn, activates gene expression through the zinc-finger transcription proteins. Many of the growth-related signaling proteins, such as c-fos, jun-B, and c-jun, dimerize through leucine-zipper proteins prior to binding to DNA. For example, c-fos dimerizes with c-jun and subsequently binds to DNA.[31] Transcription factors such as the *myo-D* family genes, which are the master genes for inducing differentiation of skeletal muscle, contain a helix-loop-helix motif. The MADS domain proteins include myocyte enhancer factor 2 (MEF2) and the serum response factor (SRF). The helix-turn-helix proteins include homeodomain-containing proteins that are important in the development of prokaryotes and eukaryotes.

Another level at which gene expression may be regulated is that of mRNA processing, whereby the introns are removed and the exons spliced together to provide the mature mRNA. In the majority of instances, each exon present in the gene is incorporated into a mature mRNA via ligation of consecutive pairs of exons and removal of all introns. This constitutive splicing process produces a single gene product from each transcriptional unit, even when the coding sequence is split into many separated exons. In other instances, however, nonconsec-

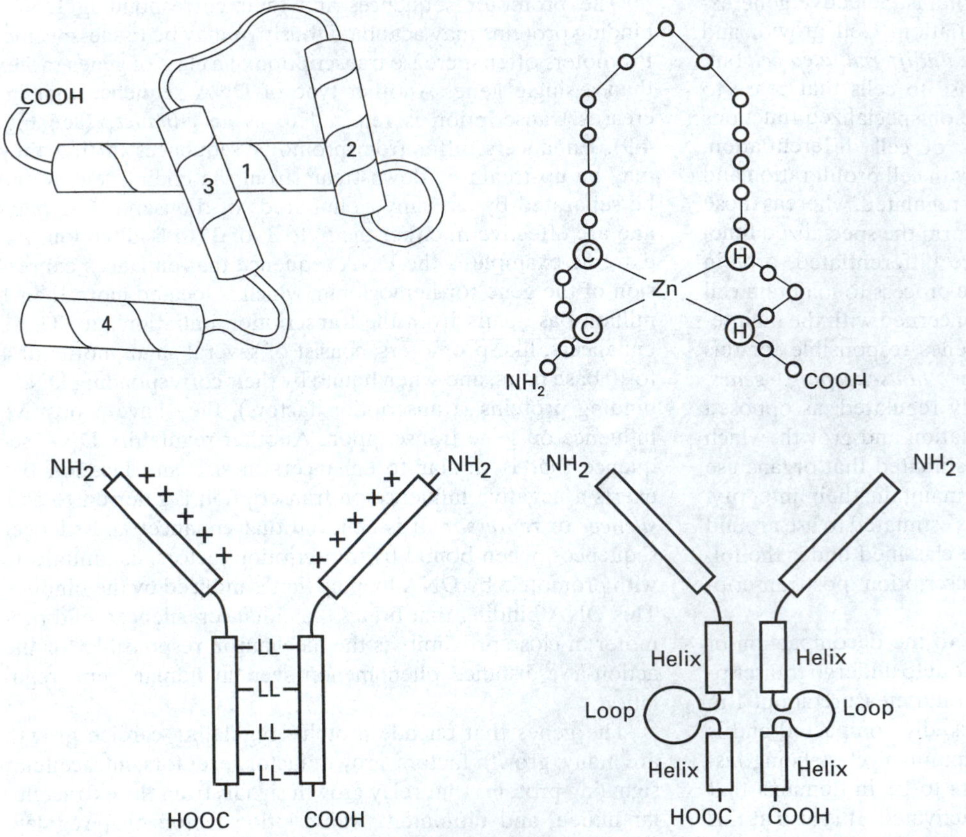

FIGURE 4-10 Types of transcription factors that affect gene activation. Schematic representation of the shapes of four types of protein transcription factors that bond to DNA and influence gene activation. Helix-turn-helix is a protein with two α-helices separated by a β-turn. Leucine zippers are protein dimers with entering leucine amino acids. Zinc fingers have a peptide loop connected at the base by a zinc ion tetrahedran between cysteine and/or histidine in amino acids. The helix-loop-helix consists of α-helix but uses leucine zippers and has a loop between the α-helices. The darkened areas are believed to be the regions of the protein that interact with the DNA to modulate transcription.

utive exons are joined in the processing of some gene transcripts, and this alternative pattern of primary mRNA splicing can exclude individual exons from mature mRNA in some transcripts and include them in others. The use of such differential splicing patterns creates mRNAs that generate a variety of proteins from a single gene. Differential splicing is particularly prevalent in genes of muscles and has been shown to occur in three of the eight major sarcomeric proteins studied thus far—myosin heavy chains, tropomyosin, and troponin T (skeletal and cardiac).

The 3′ non-protein-coding region of the mature mRNA contains the poly(A) tail, which is essential for message stability. It is believed that protein synthesis is, in part, regulated on the basis of alterations in message stability. The precise mechanism whereby an mRNA is induced to remain stable and encode several thousand polypeptides as opposed to being extremely unstable and encoding only a few molecules is not well understood. Nevertheless, it is likely to be an important step in regulating the response to cytoplasmic signals that require rapid synthesis of a particular polypeptide. Synthesis of a polypeptide initiated via transcription is estimated to take several minutes, whereas synthesis of a protein initiated through translation requires only seconds. Regulation of gene expression also occurs at the translational and posttranslational levels. Proteins are often translated as precursors that must undergo proteolytic cleavage. Others must undergo cleavage of leader sequences that are attached to direct them to their particular subcellular compartment. Other posttranslational modifications include protein glycosylation, the addition of polysaccharides and lipids, and the formation of disulfide bonds. Finally, polypeptides often polymerize with similar or different polypeptides to form complex tertiary structures that make up the mature proteins. The folding of polypeptides into mature proteins is guided by a group of genes that encode for so-called chaperone genes. Regulation of gene expression at the protein synthesis level is more fully discussed in Chap. 5.

Molecular Biology and the Basis for Recombinant DNA Technology

Modern molecular biology, initiated in the 1970s,[27,32] was in part due to four pivotal discoveries or inventions: restriction enzymes, reverse transcription, cloning, and DNA sequencing. Since DNA consists simply of four nucleotides joined together, it is a monotonous, repetitive molecule that, at first glance, offers no landmarks to recognize that a particular segment of DNA codes for a particular mRNA. The discovery of the restriction endonucleases provided the genetic scalpel to cut DNA into smaller pieces of predictable size that could be used in a variety of procedures. The unique feature of these enzymes is that each recognizes a specific sequence of DNA of 4 to 8 base pairs and cleaves the molecule at that particular site. Thus one knows precisely where the enzyme cuts, and using a number of different enzymes, one can identify the site and number of recognition sites for each enzyme in a fragment of DNA of interest and develop what is referred to as a *restriction map*. These enzymes also made it possible to cut DNA from different sources in a predictable manner in preparation for ligating them together into a recombinant molecule. Restriction endonucleases are obtained from bacteria, and enzymes have been purified that recognize more than 100 different cleavage sites. A restriction endonuclease is named after the bacterium from which it was isolated, taking the first letter of the genus of the bacterium, the first two letters of the species, and the first letter of the strain. An example of this would be an enzyme from *Haemophilus influenzae* referred to as *Hind-III*. The III simply refers to the third restriction endonuclease enzyme isolated

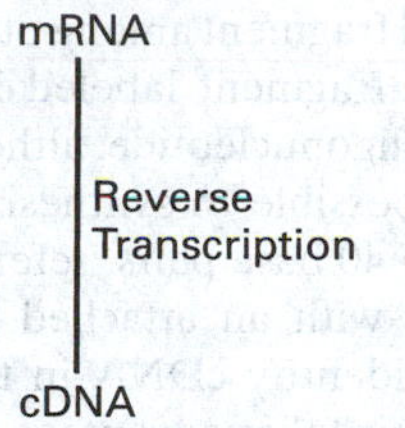

FIGURE 4-11 Generation of a complementary DNA (cDNA). Taking advantage of the enzyme reverse transcriptase, mRNA is converted to DNA, referred to as *complementary DNA* (cDNA). The DNA is single-stranded and complementary to the sequence of RNA, except thymine now replaces uracil. Using DNA polymerase, one can then make the single-stranded DNA into double-stranded cDNA. The cDNA can be used as a probe to identify specific sequences or genes of the genomic DNA, or it can be inserted into vectors to be cloned or expressed in a variety of hosts.

from that particular species of bacteria. Thus the availability of restriction endonucleases made it possible to digest DNA into smaller molecules that could be manipulated and used in a variety of reactions and to develop a restriction map as well as develop chimeric DNA molecules, the latter being the essence of recombinant DNA technology.

The discovery that retroviruses contain an enzyme that catalyzes the formation of DNA from RNA, referred to as *reverse transcriptase,* revolutionized molecular biology. The resulting so-called complementary DNA (cDNA) (represented by the appropriate complementary bases for the mRNA, except, of course, with thymine replacing uracil) binds to the nucleotide sequences from which the particular mRNA was originally derived (Fig. 4-11). Messenger RNA, as discussed previously, codes for a specific polypeptide and is derived from a discrete, specific unit of DNA referred to as a *gene*. Reverse transcriptase reverses this process so that a cDNA is generated from an mRNA (coding part of the gene) and can be used as a gene to express the protein. The cDNA is reinserted into the genome of a vector (virus or plasmid) and subsequently replicated in an appropriate host, such as a bacterium, which made possible the first cloning of the gene. Radioactive labeling of a cDNA provides an extraordinarily powerful tool to develop known chromosomal landmarks and to isolate and identify particular genes. The labeled cDNA, referred to as a *probe,* or *indicator molecule,* is a routine, essential tool used to identify and isolate DNA or RNA fragments of interest. Development of rapid-sequencing techniques made it possible to sequence several thousand of bases per day. It is expected that a by-product of the Human Genome Project will be technology to sequence millions of bases per day.

Two features essential to all techniques of recombinant DNA technology need to be highlighted: The first is the ability of DNA to denature and anneal, or hybridize. The double-stranded DNA, held together by hydrogen bonding of the corresponding complementary bases, will, on exposure to high temperatures (95°C), separate into two strands, but under appropriate conditions (55°C), the complementary strands will again anneal precisely as originally and return to their normal double-stranded state. The process of separating into separate strands is referred to as *denaturation,* and the recombining process is known as *annealment,* or *hybridization,* with the latter term preferred if the two DNA fragments are from different sources. Second, the strands come together identically to the parent molecule because of complementary base pairing, whereby A must bind to T and C to G.

Unique Features of Recombinant DNA Technology

The techniques of recombinant DNA are unique and are not limited by some of the restrictions imposed on other scientific techniques.[3] Some of these are the abilities (1) to perform the structure-function analysis of a selected molecule or a portion thereof in the intact living cell or organism, (2) to isolate and identify genes responsible for hereditary diseases, (3) to unravel the molecular basis for the regulation of growth (including the heart), and (4) to generate large quantities of protein present only in trace amounts that otherwise would not be available, as well as the opportunity to genetically engineer proteins for maximum benefit with the least side effects. The techniques routinely used in molecular biology consist of electrophoresis, Southern and Northern blotting, DNA cloning, polymerase chain reaction (PCR), electrophoretic mobility shift assay, and the development of gene libraries. Techniques related to vessel wall biology and gene transfer are discussed in Chap. 8.

Isolation of DNA

Since the DNA of all human tissues is the same, practically any tissue can be used to obtain a DNA sample. It requires only a microgram for most procedures. In humans, lymphocytes are commonly used because they are very accessible and the DNA can be extracted easily. Lymphocytes are also used because they can be transformed by Epstein-Barr virus into an immortal cell line that can provide a continuous, renewable source of DNA. The cells can be grown in culture, frozen for years (from which samples can be obtained), thawed, and regrown, providing a renewable source of DNA for several decades. A sample of 10 to 15 mL of whole blood typically would yield about 50 to 100 μg of genomic DNA. If one's interest is restricted to the DNA sequences that are expressed, one would isolate mRNA and, using it as a template, employ reverse transcriptase to derive its cDNA. cDNA molecules represent the expressed form of a gene and thus can be used as probes to select the specific genomic DNA segments from which the mRNA was transcribed. Myocardial biopsies obtained under appropriate conditions provide adequate tissue for most DNA or RNA analyses.

Digestion and Electrophoretic Separation of DNA

One of the important physical properties of the DNA molecule is that each individual nucleotide possesses a net negative charge resulting from the phosphate group. Thus fragments of different sizes exposed to an electric field tend to migrate toward the positive electrode at differential rates depending on their size, with small fragments migrating faster than larger ones. This process of separation based on electric charge is called *electrophoresis.*[33] The DNA sample, after being digested into fragments of different size by a restriction endonuclease, is added to a gel matrix such as agarose or acrylamide. After separation by electrophoresis, the pattern of the DNA can be visualized under an ultraviolet lamp with a fluorescent dye such as ethidium bromide (Fig. 4-12). Agarose gel electrophoresis will separate fragments from 1000 to 60,000 base pairs (60 kb) in size, and polyacrylamide gels effectively separate fragments smaller than

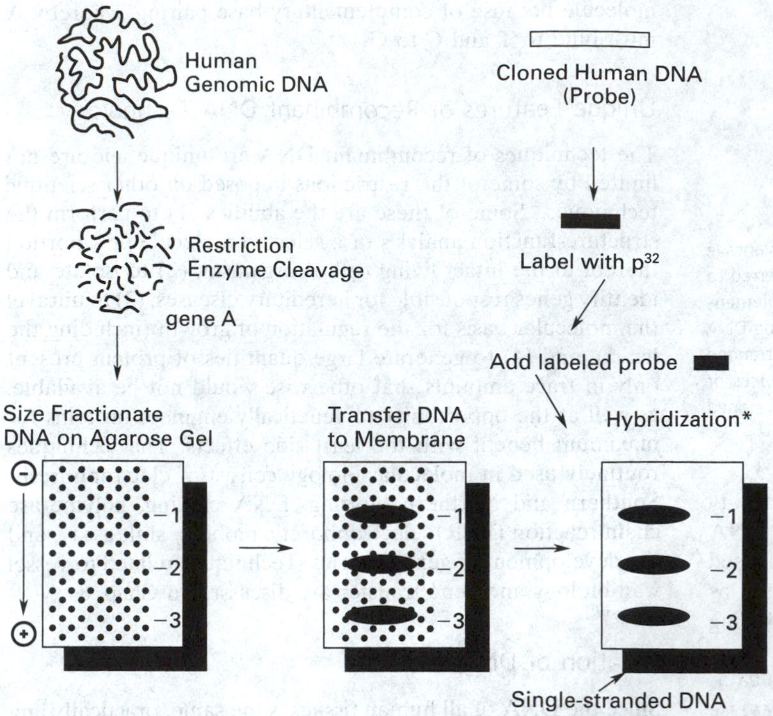

FIGURE 4-12 Southern blotting technique. The DNA is cleaved with an appropriately selected restriction endonuclease. The digested fragments are separated by electrophoresis on agarose gel, and the fragments of gene A are located at positions 1, 2, and 3 but cannot be seen against the background of many other randomly occurring DNA fragments. The DNA is denatured and transferred to a membrane in an identical pattern to what it was on the agarose gel. It is difficult to manipulate anything on a soft gel or to remove it. Once transferred to the membrane (filter), a solid support system, the DNA is much easier to handle. A DNA probe (cDNA) that has been labeled with ^{32}P is hybridized to its cDNA and visualized after exposure of the nylon membrane to an autoradiograph. The transfer of the DNA from the gel to the membrane developed by Southern was a major innovation illustrated in the next figure. (From Mares A Jr, Towbin J, Bies RG, Roberts R. Molecular biology for the cardiologist. *Curr Probl Cardiol* 1992; 17:9–72. Reproduced with permission from the publisher and authors.)

1000 base pairs (1 kb). The recent development of pulse-field gel electrophoresis (PFGE) made possible the separation of DNA fragments even up to 2000 kb in size. In this technique, the electric field is alternated in different directions, forcing the molecules of DNA to reorient between each pulse of electric current. Thus this technique is particularly suitable for isolating and characterizing large segments of DNA, such as to identify a known gene.

As noted previously, prior to electrophoresis, the DNA must be digested with one of the restriction endonucleases. The size of the fragments resulting from digestion will depend on the type of restriction endonuclease used, i.e., whether they recognize sequences of 4, 5, 6, or 8 base pairs. Enzymes recognizing a 4-base-pair sequence will cut the DNA into much smaller fragments than one that recognizes an 8-base-pair sequence.

Development of a DNA Probe

A nucleic acid probe is a fragment of nucleic acid to which has been attached a label such as a radioisotope or a fluorescent compound, making it possible to easily detect and recognize the desired fragment among other native DNA molecules. The fragment labeled is usually cDNA or a synthetic oligonucleotide, although it could be RNA. It is now possible to synthesize DNA fragments of up to 30 to 40 base pairs, referred to as *oligonucleotides,* that, with an attached label, can be used as probes to identify cDNA in the human genome or mRNA. This takes advantage of the fact that at high temperatures, the double-stranded DNA probe and the native DNA will break into separate strands. On recombining at random, the labeled DNA probe can bind with either its original complementary strand or the native DNA that is complementary to the probe and thus provide a means of isolating a fragment of native genomic DNA. A probe is necessary in most recombinant DNA procedures to detect the molecule of interest following electrophoresis.

Southern, Northern, and Western Blotting

A procedure to separate and detect specific DNA fragments, referred to as *Southern blotting,* is named after E. M. Southern, who developed it in 1975.[34] Genomic DNA is isolated and digested into small fragments with restriction enzymes, and the fragments are separated by gel electrophoresis as described previously. Following separation, DNA fragments are denatured chemically into single-strand fragments. It is very difficult to handle gels and even more impractical to store them. Southern developed a technique whereby these separated single-strand fragments in the gel could be transferred by capillary action to a solid support medium (nylon or nitrocellulose membrane) and fixed permanently by heating. The pattern on the membrane reflects identically the pattern induced by electrophoresis on the gel. The process used to produce a Southern blot is illustrated schematically in Fig. 4-12. The nylon membrane and its attached single-strand DNA fragments are then incubated with a radioactively labeled complementary probe. The hybridized, radioactive double-strand product, on exposure to x-ray film (autoradiography), will exhibit the pattern of the radiolabeled DNA fragments (Fig. 4-13). In summary, the electrophoretic separation of DNA followed by its transfer to a nylon membrane for subsequent identification by radioactive hybridization is referred to as *Southern blotting,* and the autoradiogram as a *Southern blot*. The same approach to detect mRNA is referred to as *Northern blotting*. This procedure also can be used for detection of proteins, in which case it is referred to as *Western blotting* (Table 4-1). The only significant difference in detecting protein versus nucleic acid by this procedure is the probe, which is an antibody rather than an oligonucleotide, or cDNA. However, as in Southern and Northern blotting, the probe may be labeled with a radioactive isotope, a fluorescent tag, or some visual colorimetric substance.

Cloning of a Gene

DNA cloning is a technique used to produce large quantities of a specific DNA fragment of interest.[35] It generally is quite feasible to produce a billion copies of a DNA fragment by routine bacterial cloning techniques. The DNA fragment of interest (insert) is inserted into the DNA of a vector, and the vector is amplified in an appropriate host cell. The host provides amplification of the DNA of both the vector and the foreign insert. The prerequisites for cloning are (1) isolation of the DNA fragment of interest, (2) a vector, which is often an extrachromosomal segment of DNA with the ability to propagate independently of the host DNA, (3) a restriction endonuclease to digest both the insert and the vector so the DNA ends will be compatible for ligation (as illustrated in Fig. 4-14), (4) a DNA ligase to ligate the insert into the vector, (5) a means to introduce the vector into the host cell, and (6) a means to differentiate the host cells that have incorporated the vector from those which have not. Standard vectors used in cloning have circular DNA and fall into three classes: (1) plasmids harvested from bacterial cells (a *plasmid* is an extrachromosomal segment of DNA present in bacteria that is self-replicating and on which are located certain genes that express resistance to ampicillin or other antibiotics), (2) bacteriophages (commonly referred to merely as *phages,* they are viruses that invade and multiply in bacterial cells), and (3) an artificially developed vector (referred to as a *cosmid*). The insert and vector are enzymatically ligated together by DNA ligase into circular DNA, and the recombinant product (hence the name *recombinant*) is incorporated into a host such as a bacterium or a mammalian cell for amplification (Fig. 4-15). In order to identify whether or not the particular DNA of interest has been replicated in the host, a so-called selection gene, such as one responsible for ampicillin resistance, is incorporated into the vector. The bacteria are grown in media containing ampicillin so that only those with the resistance gene will survive. Since the resistance gene is attached to the DNA fragment of interest, it indicates that colonies (bacteria) or plaques (phage) that survive must contain the gene of interest. The size of the insert is a limitation in cloning. Plasmids can only accommodate inserts up to approximately 15,000 base pairs, phages up to 25,000 base pairs, and cosmids up to 45,000 base pairs. Recently, a new vector has been developed, namely, bacterial artificial chromosomes (BACs), that accommodates DNA fragments of up to 200,000 base pairs. The yeast artificial chromosome (YAC),[36] developed several years ago, accommodates DNA inserts of up to 2 million base pairs but is extremely difficult to work with on a routine basis; in contrast, the BACs are as convenient as plasmids or phages. This has markedly accelerated the cloning of large fragments of DNA. Cloning, as discussed, is performed to obtain multiple copies of DNA, and unless specifically designed, the DNA is neither transcribed into mRNA nor translated into protein. If one desires to express a particular DNA fragment or gene, one must then use what is referred to as an *expression vector.* It is imperative to provide a promoter element that is appropriate for the host, and the gene must contain the appropriate 5′ untranslated region for binding to the ribosome as well as the appropriate 3′ region for stability of the message. An example would be the expression of rt-PA in mammalian cells, whereby the protein is expressed and secreted to be harvested and processed commercially for use as a thrombolytic agent.

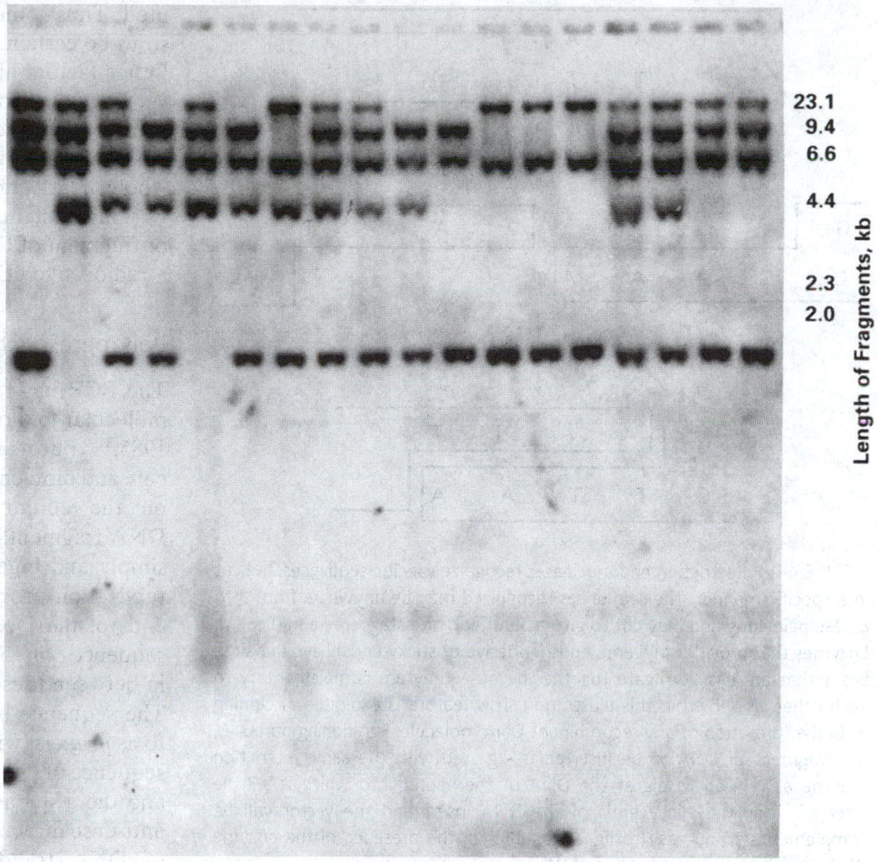

FIGURE 4-13 A typical Southern blot with distinct bands. Each vertical lane consists of DNA from a separate individual. All the individual DNAs were digested with the same restriction endonuclease. Following separation on electrophoresis and transfer to a nylon membrane, hybridization was performed with the selected radioactive probe, and thus only those fragments complementary to the probe are visualized. This is an analysis of a family with hypertrophic cardiomyopathy, and the different patterns reflect restriction fragment length polymorphisms (RFLPs) characteristic of the marker locus, which is linked to the disease locus. (From Mares A Jr, Towbin J, Bies RG, Roberts R. Molecular biology for the cardiologist. *Curr Probl Cardiol* 1992; 17:9–72. Reproduced with permission from the publisher and authors.)

TABLE 4-1 Separation and Identification oF Molecular Species

Procedures	Molecule	Labeled Probe
Southern blotting	DNA	DNA or cDNA
Northern blotting	RNA	DNA or cDNA
Western blotting	Protein	Antibody

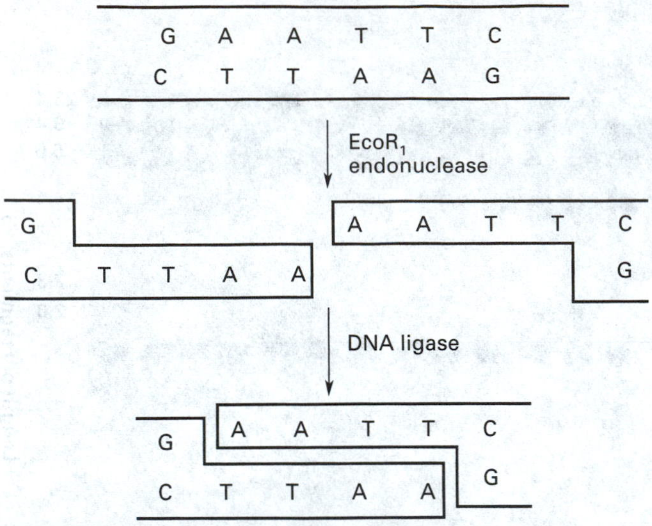

FIGURE 4-14 Restriction endonucleases recognize specific sequences and cut in a specific manner. The sequences recognized may be anywhere from 3 to 8 base pairs long and may cut to give a blunt end or a staggered end (EcoR1). Enzymes that provide staggered ends (cohesive or sticky ends) have unpaired bases that are easy to ligate together because they are complementary to each other, as shown in this illustration. This feature is exploited in cloning or in the formation of any recombinant DNA molecule. For cloning purposes, the fragment of DNA to be inserted is digested with the same restriction enzyme as is used to digest the DNA of the vector into which it will be inserted. Thus the sticky ends of the DNA insert and the vector will be complementary and easy to ligate together in the presence of the enzyme DNA ligase, as illustrated in Fig. 4-15.

Development of Gene Libraries

Gene libraries are usually called either genomic or cDNA libraries. A *genomic library* refers to one made from genomic DNA. A library is a collection of DNA fragments that have been cloned in an appropriate vector and grown in a particular host, usually bacteria. A major difference between a genomic and a cDNA library is that a genomic library contains DNA fragments composed of introns and exons, whereas a cDNA library is made from mRNA that represents genes expressed in a particular organ and does not have introns. The cDNA library contains genes specifically expressed in a particular tissue only. In contrast, a genomic library, whether derived from the heart or another tissue, will have the same genes. To make a human genomic library, one must first isolate the whole genome of a cell, cut it into fragments with a restriction enzyme, and insert the fragments into a vector replicated in an appropriate host, usually bacteria.[37] To increase the odds that enough fragments are cloned to represent the whole genome, certain calculations are necessary. It is assumed that the recognition site for a particular restriction enzyme occurs at random. For the restriction enzyme EcoR1, with a 6-base-pair recognition site, the average size of each fragment will be $4^6 = 4096$ base pairs. In contrast, if the recognition site involves 4 base pairs, each fragment would be $4^4 = 256$ base pairs long. If the 6-base-pair cutter were used for the human genome, the result would be the 3 billion base pairs of the human genome divided by 4096 to produce roughly 750,000 fragments requiring 750,000 colonies or clones. However, the recognition sites are not evenly or randomly distributed. Thus some fragments are larger and others are smaller, so to be certain, at least 1 million colonies would be required. Other factors also must be considered, such as the choice of vector with respect to insert size. Any part of the library that is used can be replaced by regrowing it, and thus the library is a permanent, renewable source of DNA. cDNA libraries of the whole heart and specific structures of the heart such as the Purkinje system are now available. To isolate a particular gene or fragment of DNA or cDNA from a library generally requires a radioactive cDNA probe.

Polymerase Chain Reaction

The PCR has revolutionized application of the techniques of molecular biology. This technique was not developed until 1985,[38,39] but its impact already has been felt throughout medicine and biotechnology. This procedure, conveniently and without the tedium of cloning, can provide 1 million copies of a DNA fragment in 3 to 4 h and 1 billion copies within 24 h. PCR simply and ingeniously takes advantage of the natural DNA replication process. One must know the sequence of the two ends of the DNA fragment that is to be amplified, but short sequences of 15 to 30 base pairs are adequate, and fragments in between these sequences as large as 20 kb can be amplified. The sequence is used to make two oligonucleotides, referred to as *primers,* with one for each end of the DNA fragment. The sequence of one primer is complementary to the sense direction, and the sequence of the other is made complementary to the antisense direction. The primers are used to prime the synthesis of cDNA strands and are designed such that the DNA between the primers is the fragment of interest to be amplified. If mRNA is to be amplified, it is first converted to a cDNA using the enzyme reverse transcriptase. The primers (oligonucleotides) and the necessary bases are added in excess, together with the enzyme Taq DNA polymerase (which catalyzes DNA synthesis) and a sample containing the DNA to be amplified. There are three steps to each cycle. Initially, one must denature the DNA (separate the primers and the native DNA) into separate strands, which is done by increasing the temperature to 95°C. The temperature is then decreased to 50°C so that the primers and native DNA will reanneal to their complementary base sequences. The native DNA strands will bind not only to each other but also to the primers. The temperature is now increased to 65°C for synthesis of the new DNA fragments. Synthesis in the presence of Taq1 polymerase is initiated at the 5′ end, and further nucleotides are added in the 5′ to 3′ direction to provide the desired double-stranded DNA fragment. Taq1 DNA polymerase, isolated from *Thermus aquaticus,* is thermostable, which is of tremendous advantage in performing the PCR reaction. Since the high temperatures of up to 95°C do not destroy this polymerase, it negates the need to add DNA polymerase between each cycle. Furthermore, since Taq polymerase has an optimal activity at around 70°C, one can significantly accelerate DNA synthesis. The cycle is then repeated, and after about 30 cycles over 3 h, one should have about 1 million copies. There are many clinical applications for PCR. To make a diagnosis of viral myocarditis, for example, one can use PCR to amplify from a myocardial biopsy any specific viral RNA or DNA for which primers can be made. The sensitivity of most conventional techniques is inadequate to detect molecules unless present in 50,000 to 100,000 copies per cell. In contrast, only one copy of

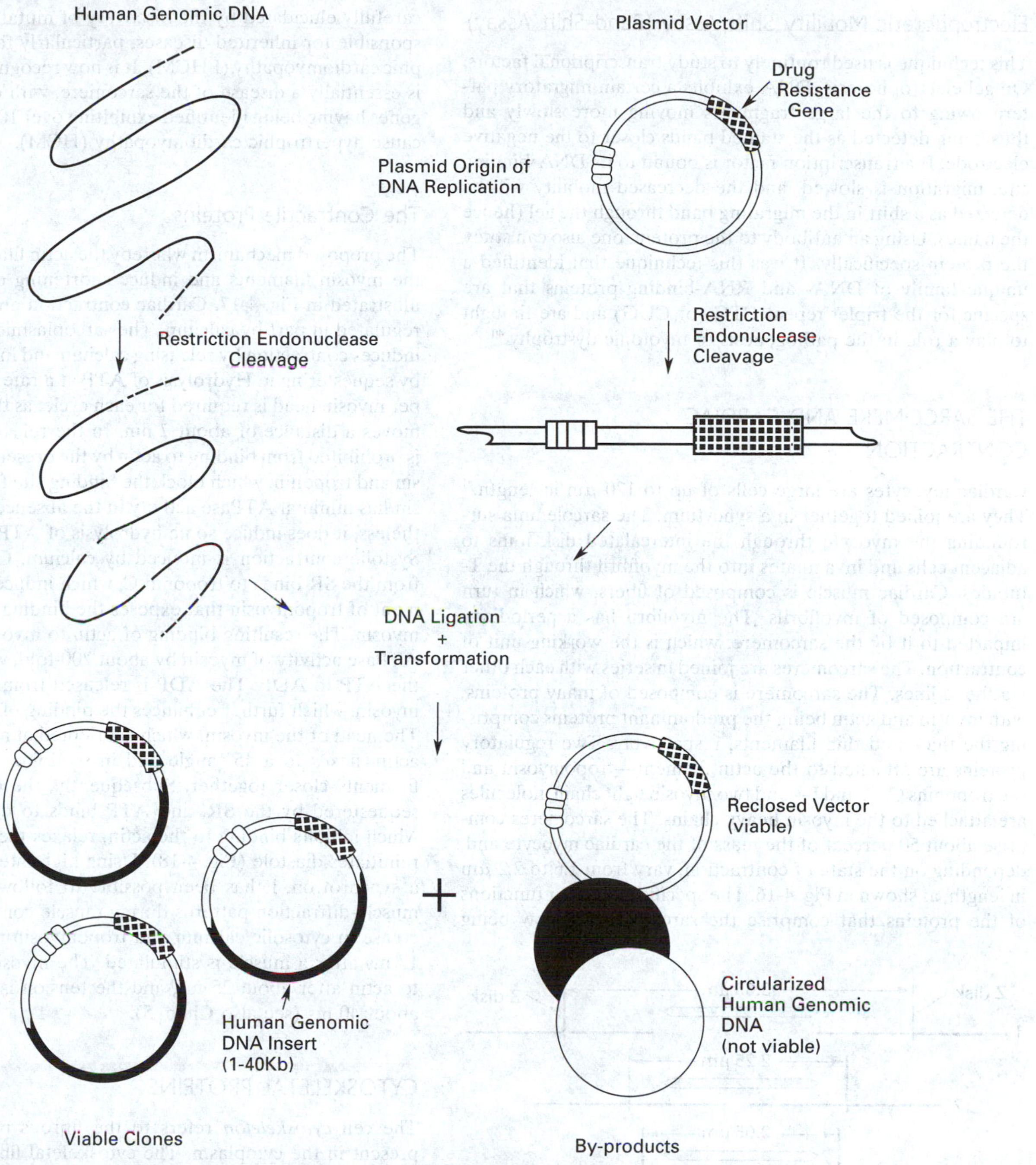

FIGURE 4-15 DNA cloning. The basic objective of cloning is to provide multiple copies of a DNA fragment of interest. The fundamental principles for in vitro cloning of specific DNA fragments are as follows: (1) The human genome DNA of interest is isolated after digested by a restriction endonuclease, which is often referred to as the *DNA insert.* (2) A DNA vector is selected (shown on the right); the vector is a plasmid that has circular DNA and contains the necessary replication site and the reporter gene (drug resistance gene) to subsequently recognize which host has the insert. The vector and the DNA fragment to be inserted are digested with the same restriction endonuclease so that the ends are complementary for ligation. (3) DNA ligase ligates compatible insert and vector ends together. (4) Finally, host cells are transformed by incorporating vectors containing insert fragments and are identified by characteristics encoded by resident genes on the vector. Some of the clones will be viable and others not. (From Mares A Jr, Towbin J, Bies RG, Roberts R. Molecular biology for the cardiologist. *Curr Probl Cardiol* 1992; 17:9–72. Reproduced with permission from the publisher and authors.)

RNA or DNA is needed for detection by PCR, and in 3 to 4 h, up to 1 million copies can be generated, which is adequate abundance for detection by most conventional techniques. PCR offers exquisite diagnostic sensitivity and specificity for determining the etiology of cardiac disorders such as myocarditis, and in patients undergoing cardiac transplantation, it is used for detecting infection or immunologic rejection. Another application of PCR is to detect and amplify mutations associated with hereditary disorders. One also can sequence DNA directly from PCR without the need for cloning.

Electrophoretic Mobility Shift Assay (Band-Shift Assay)

This technique is used routinely to study transcriptional factors. On gel electrophoresis, DNA exhibits a certain migratory pattern owing to the large fragments moving more slowly and thus being detected as the stained bands closer to the negative electrode. If a transcription factor is bound to its DNA-binding site, migration is slowed, and the decreased mobility will be detected as a shift in the migrating band through the gel (hence the name). Using an antibody to the protein, one also can study the protein specifically. It was this technique that identified a unique family of DNA- and RNA-binding proteins that are specific for the triplet repeat CTG (or CUG) and are thought to play a role in the pathogenesis of myotonic dystrophy.[40]

THE SARCOMERE AND CARDIAC CONTRACTION

Cardiac myocytes are large cells of up to 120 μm in length.[41] They are joined together in a syncytium. The sarcolemma surrounding the myocyte through the intercalated disk joins to adjacent cells and invaginates into the myofibril through the T-tubules. Cardiac muscle is composed of fibers, which in turn are composed of myofibrils. The myofibril has a periodicity imparted to it by the sarcomere, which is the working unit of contraction. The sarcomeres are joined in series with each other via the Z-lines. The sarcomere is composed of many proteins, with myosin and actin being the predominant proteins comprising the thick and thin filaments, respectively. Two regulatory proteins are attached to the actin filament—tropomyosin and the troponins C, T, and I—and two myosin light chain molecules are attached to the myosin heavy chains. The sarcomeres comprise about 50 percent of the mass of the cardiac myocyte and, depending on the state of contraction, vary from 1.6 to 2.2 μm in length, as shown in Fig. 4-16. The specific molecular functions of the proteins that comprise the sarcomere are now being carefully elucidated by the discovery of mutations that are responsible for inherited diseases, particularly familial hypertrophic cardiomyopathy (FHCM). It is now recognized that FHCM is essentially a disease of the sarcomere, with eight sarcomeric genes having being identified exhibiting over 100 mutations that cause hypertrophic cardiomyopathy (HCM).

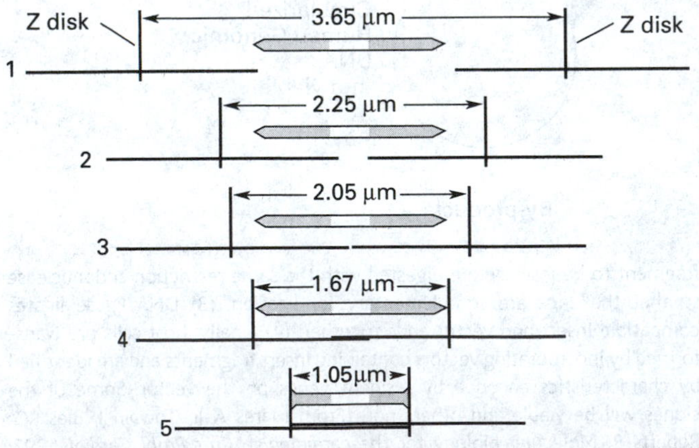

FIGURE 4-16 Relationship of sarcomere length and tension generated during isometric contraction of striated muscle. Maximum tension is generated at sarcomere lengths that allow maximum interaction of myosin heads and actin filaments (positions 2 and 3). If the sarcomere length is too short (positions 4 and 5), actin filaments overlap one another and prevent optimal interaction with myosin heads. (From Darnell J, Lodish H, Baltimore D, eds. *Molecular Cell Biology*. New York: Scientific American Books, W. H. Freeman; 1990. Reproduced with permission from the publisher.)

The Contractile Proteins

The proposed mechanism whereby the actin filaments slide over the myosin filaments and induce shortening or contraction is illustrated in Fig. 4-17. Cardiac contraction and relaxation are regulated in part by calcium. The sarcoplasmic reticulum (SR) induces contraction by releasing calcium and induces relaxation by sequestering it. Hydrolysis of ATP at a rate of one molecule per myosin head is required for each cycle, as the actin filament moves a distance of about 7 nm. In the relaxed state, myosin is prohibited from binding to actin by the presence of tropomyosin and troponin, which block the binding site for myosin. Myosin has minimal ATPase activity in the absence of actin; nevertheless, it does induce some hydrolysis of ATP to ADP and P_i. Systolic contraction is induced by calcium. Calcium released from the SR binds to troponin C, which induces a slight movement of tropomyosin that exposes the binding site on actin for myosin. The resulting binding of actin to myosin increases the ATPase activity of myosin by about 200-fold, which hydrolyzes the ATP to ADP. The ADP is released from the head of the myosin, which further enhances the binding of myosin to actin. The head of the myosin, which is oriented at a 90° angle to the actin, flexes to a 45° angle and in so doing moves the actin filaments closer together. Subsequently, the calcium is again sequestered by the SR, and ATP binds to the myosin head, which inhibits binding to the actin, relaxes the sarcomere, and reinitiates diastole (Fig. 4-18). Using high-intensity x-ray from a synchrotron, it has been possible to follow the changes in muscle-diffraction patterns during muscle contraction. The increase in cytosolic calcium and tropomyosin movement occur 17 ms after a muscle is stimulated. The myosin head attaches to actin after about 25 ms, and the tension is generated after about 40 ms (see also Chap. 5).

CYTOSKELETAL PROTEINS

The cell *cytoskeleton* refers to the fibrous proteins that are present in the cytoplasm. The cytoskeletal fibers give the cell strength and rigidity and control movement within the cell. For example, the microtubules provide the tracks along which vesicles are transported by tubulin-binding molecules. These cytoskeletal proteins form three major classes subdivided according to size into microfilaments,[42] microtubules, and intermediate filaments.[43] The microfilaments are polymers of the protein subunit actin; the microtubules are polymers of the subunits of α- and β-tubulin, and the intermediate filaments are polymers of five different rod-shaped protein subunits. The polymerization and depolymerization of these fibers are closely regulated by the cell. Just as FHCM is essentially a sarcomeric disease, it appears that familial dilated cardiomyopathy (FDCM) is a disease of cytoskeletal proteins. Mutations in dystrophin,[44] α-dystroglycan,[44] α-sarcoglycan,[45] metavinculin,[46] actin,[47] and desmin[48] have all been shown to be associated with FDCM.

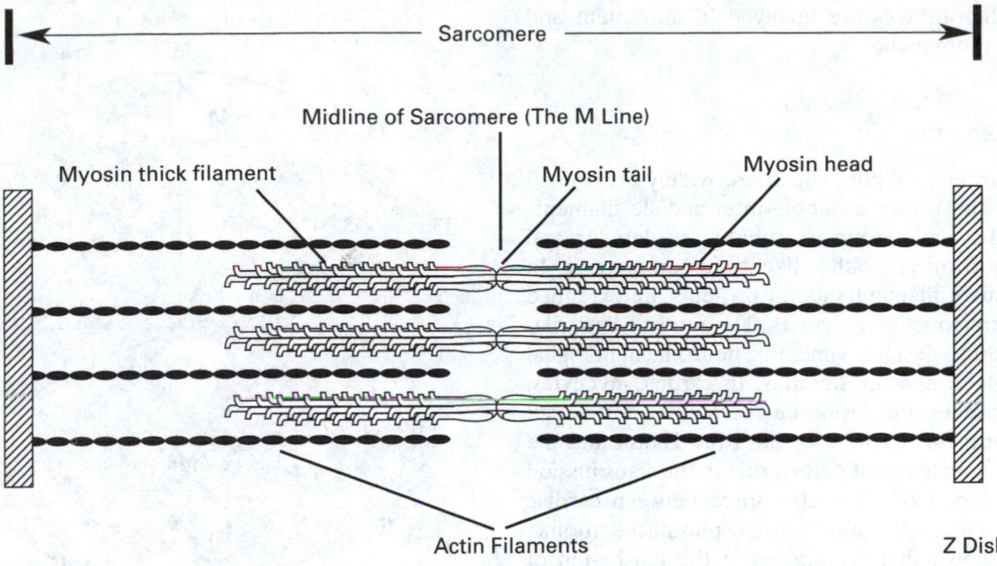

FIGURE 4-17 Sarcomere ultrastructure.

Microfilaments

In addition to the actin thin filaments of the sarcomere, which help to generate the force of contraction, actin filaments are distributed throughout the cytoplasm of essentially all cells and serve to transmit force. To serve its role as a transmitter of force, actin is linked to several other proteins. The dual function of actin is exemplified in the thin sarcomere filaments that generate force by mutations that induce FDCM,[47] whereas other mutations in the portion of the molecule that transmits force induce FHCM.[49] Titan, which binds myosin to the Z-line, is essential to the velocity and force developed by myosin-actin interaction, as is nebulin, which attaches actin to the Z-line. Dystrophin is the protein encoded by the gene responsible for Duchenne muscular dystrophy and is known to be a subsarcolemmal protein with the function of anchoring actin to the plasma membrane. Spectrin, which binds actin to the plasma membrane, has several isoforms, one of which is specific to the heart.[50]

Microtubules

Microtubules are about 24 nm in diameter, varying widely in length from a fraction of a micrometer to tens of micrometers. The microtubule wall is made up of globular subunits about 4 to 5 nm in diameter, and these subunits are arranged in 13 longitudinal rows encircling the hollow-appearing center. This basic design is present in practically all microtubules. Colchicine, which inhibits microtubule assembly, does so by binding

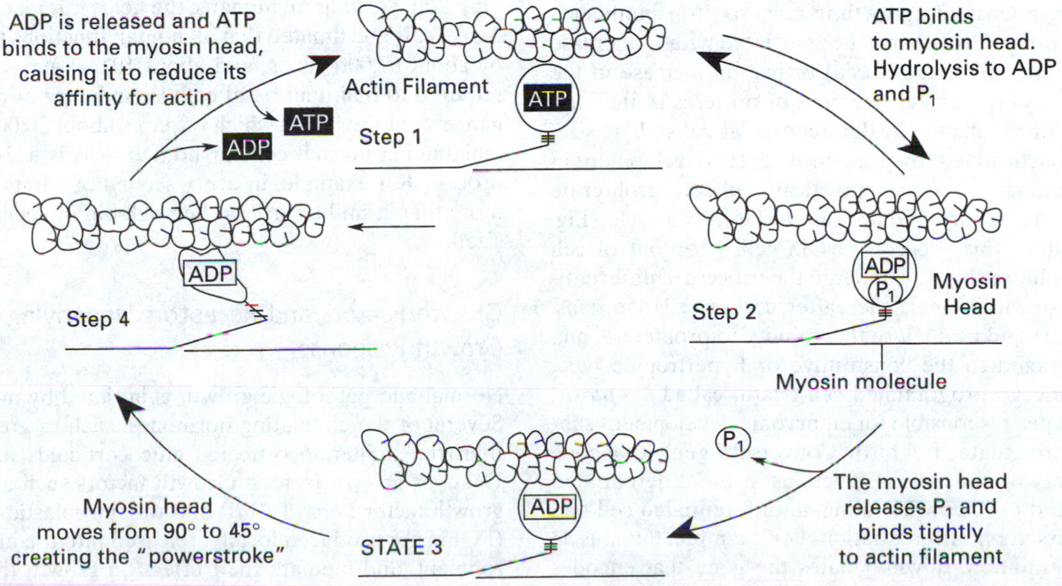

FIGURE 4-18 Molecular basis of myocardial contraction. (Adapted with permission from Alberts B, Bray A, Lewis J, et al, eds. *Molecular Biology of the Cell*, 2d ed. New York: Garland; 1991:621.)

to the tubulin. Microtubules are involved in movement and organization of cell organelles.

Intermediate Filaments

In contrast to actin and tubulin, which are widely distributed among cell types, the rather insoluble intermediate filaments are tissue- and cell-specific. Actin and tubulin are globular, and the polymers they form are rather like beads on a string. In contrast, intermediate filament subunit proteins are extended molecules that form ropelike polymers. The intermediate filament proteins include desmin, vimentin, neurofilaments, glial fibrillary acid protein, and the keratins. In cardiac myocytes, desmin filaments connect the desmosomes from one muscle cell to another and form the scaffold for both the Z-disk and the myofibrils. The desmin filament plays a role in the transmission of the stress and strain of contractile force between cardiac myocytes. It also connects the nucleus to the plasma membrane. Recently, it was shown that a mutation in the tail region of desmin causes FDCM.[48] Mutations in the rod region induce a phenotype exhibiting skeletal and cardiac manifestations, whereas mutations in the tail region exhibit only a cardiac phenotype.[48] The restriction of the phenotype to cardiac tissue suggests a specific cardic function for the tail domain.

MOLECULAR BASIS FOR CELLULAR GROWTH

Patterns of Growth (Hyperplasia, Hypertrophy, and Constitutive)

The molecular genetic basis for growth is somewhat distinct,[51,52] depending on when in the life of the organism it occurs, and may be divided into four phases: the embryonic phase of development and cellular differentiation (to be discussed later) occurring in utero, the rapidly growing phase prior to and during puberty, the normal constitutive maintenance growth throughout life, and compensatory growth in response to stimuli such as exercise or injury. Growth may be associated with an increase in the number of cells (hyperplasia) or just an increase in the size (hypertrophy) or just replacement of proteins as they are catabolized with no change in the number of cells, their size, or function (constitutive growth). During early development in the fetal and embryonic stages, practically all cells proliferate as well as increase in size and are said to be in cell cycle (Fig. 4-19). Throughout this process, certain cells drop out of cell cycle, cease proliferating, and undergo the process of differentiation. At birth or within weeks thereafter, certain cells of organs, such as the heart and brain, lose their ability to proliferate, and growth is restricted to the constitutive or hypertrophic type. Some cells undergo programmed cell death, called *apoptosis*. Many of the genes responsible for embryonic development subsequently downregulate after birth. Conversely, genes that code for proteins serving specialized functions in the differentiated cell are inhibited in the proliferating, undifferentiated cell and are only expressed on differentiation. For example, the muscle cell, on differentiation, downregulates the gene that encodes for BB creatine kinase and upregulates the gene that encodes for MM creatine kinase. Similarly, upregulation occurs for the genes that encode for myosin, actin, and other sarcomeric proteins essential to the contractile performance of the cell. It is estimated that the human body has a total of 10^{14} cells but only about 200 different types defined by their specific function. The specialized functions of a cell are determined by the repertoire of genes expressed in that particular cell.

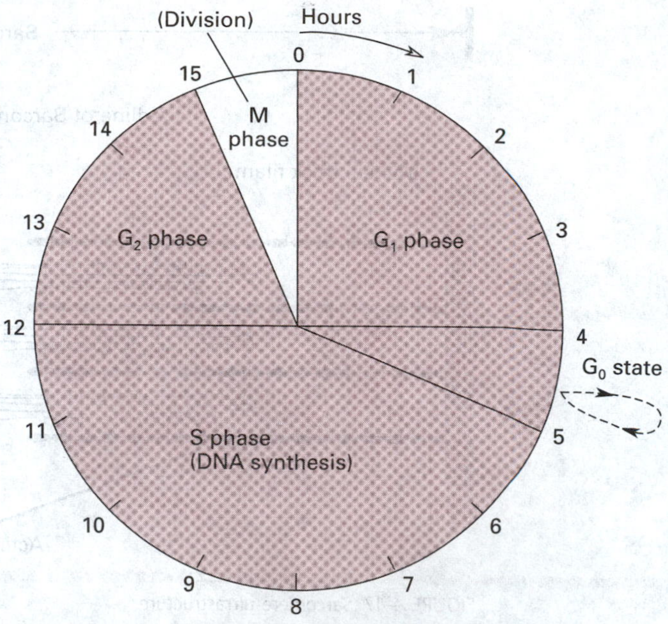

FIGURE 4-19 The cell cycle in a mammalian cell having a generation time of 16 h. The three phases spanning the first 15 h or so—the G1 (first gap) phase, and S (synthetic) phase, and the G2 (second gap) phase—make up the interphase, during which DNA and other cellular macromolecules are synthesized. The remaining hour is the M (mitotic) phase, during which the cell actually divides.

In the adult heart, most of normal growth is constitutive. It is estimated that most of the proteins of the heart are replaced every 5 days, except collagen, which replaces itself every 120 days; with hypertrophy, however, the half-life of collagen is only 17 days. Thus, in humans, the heart is replaced about every 3 weeks. It is estimated that all human functions are determined by about 67,000 genes, and about 10,000 genes (proteins) are required to maintain basal cellular integrity of a particular organ, except the brain, which requires about 20,000 genes. Thus, maintaining normal cellular homeostasis is a dynamic growth process. For example, in every second of a human being's life, more than a million trillion hemoglobin molecules are synthesized.

Growth Factors and Receptors Underlying the Growth Response

Normal and pathologic growth is initiated by multiple factors. Several of the circulating hormones, such as growth hormone, thyroxine, mineralocorticoids, glucocorticoids, and angiotensin II, act as growth factors. Growth factors such as transforming growth factor beta (TGFβ) and the fibroblastic growth factors (FGFs) are produced locally, released into the immediate environment, and mediate their effect on growth through what is termed *paracrine* or *autocrine mechanisms. Paracrine* refers to a growth factor that is secreted and affects the growth of adjacent cells. *Autocrine* refers to a growth factor that binds to the

TABLE 4-2 Cascade for Relaying Growth Signals

Receptor
↓
Coupling protein
↓
Signaling molecule
↓
Effector protein (transcription factor)

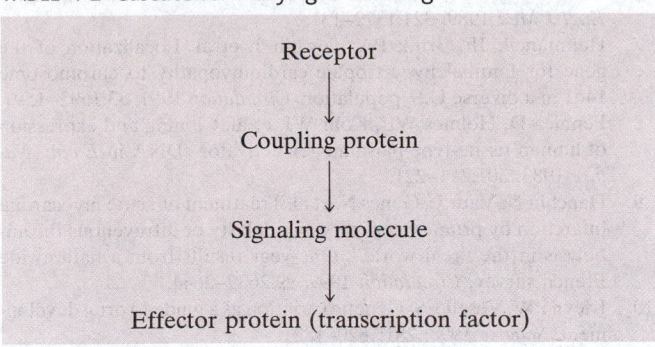

receptors of the same cell from which it was produced and secreted. *Intracrine* refers to a growth factor that induces growth in the same cell from which it was produced without being secreted. An external stimulus that influences growth is detected by a receptor that usually sits on the cell's surface as an intramembrane receptor and is relayed through several signaling or transducing proteins to the nucleus of the cell, where the ultimate effector molecule is a transcription factor (Table 4-2). The effector molecule also may affect growth through regulation of translation. The latter, however, is usually more transient, whereas a sustained change in growth almost always is mediated through transcription. The signaling proteins usually involve kinases and phosphatases, which through phosphorylation transfer ATP to amplify the signal and by dephosphorylation decrease it or in some way alter it (Fig. 4-20). Regulation of protein synthesis also may result from altered stability of mRNA. The growth response to circulating hormones or locally produced growth factors occurs several hours after the initial stimulation and is more likely to occur if two or more growth factors have been activated (see Chap. 5). In the case of the heart, a common signal is increased intraventricular pressure, which results in compensatory hypertrophy (see Chap. 5).

THE CARDIAC GROWTH RESPONSE

The growth response of the myocardium to injury, whether it be myocardial infarction, hypertension, or valvular disease, is a major determinant of morbidity and mortality. Growth is the major long-term adaptive mechanism of the heart (see Chap. 5). In hypertrophy, the sarcomeres are added in parallel, which gives rise to thickened walls of the cardiac chambers.[53] In contrast, in cardiac dilatation, the growth is achieved by adding sarcomeres in sequence.[54] It remains to be determined whether dilated cardiomyopathy occurring as a pathologic entity is a normal compensatory response or represents abnormal growth or an inadequate growth response.

Developmental growth in utero or during prepuberty and puberty is associated with orchestrated stimuli from a variety of hormones such as growth hormone. This is in sharp contrast to the restricted cardiac growth observed in the adult in response to injury. For example, in aortic constriction, the left ventricle responds with increased mass, while the right ventricle is not affected. Hammond et al.[55] in 1979 demonstrated that the growth stimulus was indeed localized to the affected organ. Left

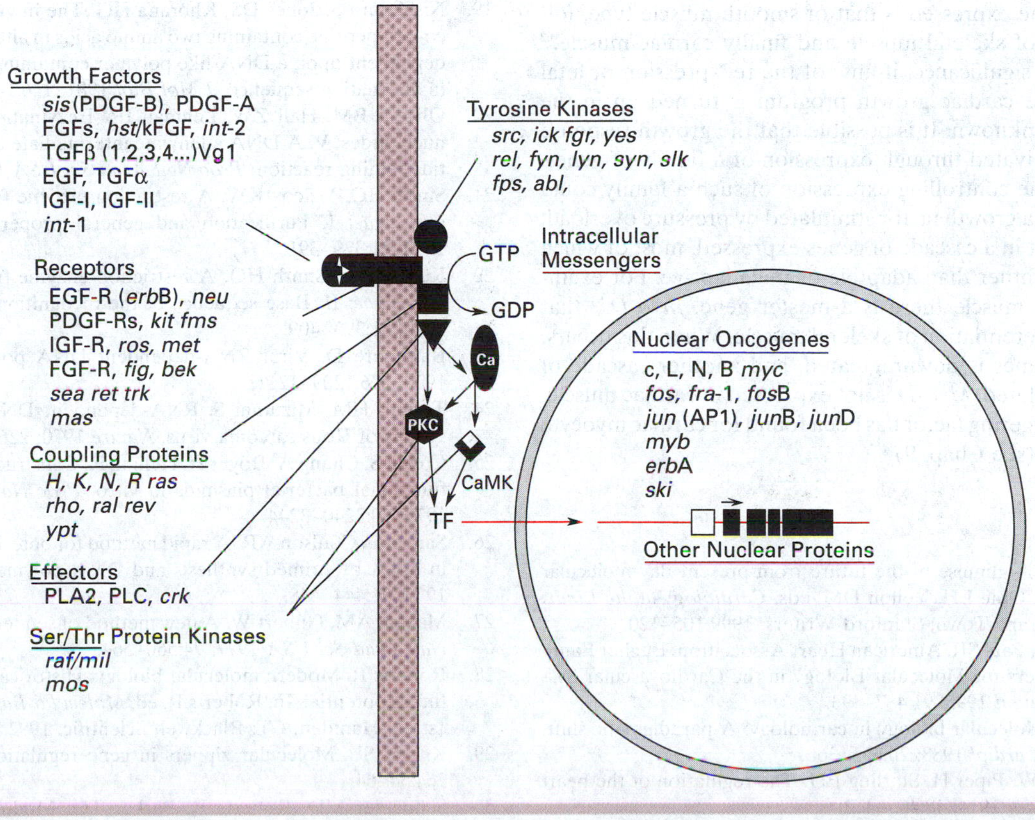

FIGURE 4-20 Illustration of many proteins with varied functions for which oncogenes are known to encode. It is clear from this diagram that oncogenes encode proteins that function as growth factors, receptors, coupling proteins, signaling proteins, and transcription factors.

ventricular hypertrophy was induced by aortic coarctation in the dog. Supernatants of the homogenized, hypertrophied left ventricle from dogs with aortic coarctation and normal dogs were used to perfuse a normal canine heart. Messenger RNA of the perfused heart was increased by extracts from the hypertrophied left ventricle but not from the normal myocardium, indicating the presence of a growth factor in the hypertrophied ventricle. This established the presence of a localized cellular stimulus acting through autocrine, paracrine, or intracrine mechanisms to induce cardiac hypertrophy. This was confirmed by Imamura et al.[56] in 1990; they showed that hypertrophy occurs in the left ventricle in response to aortic coarctation without growth in other chambers of the heart, while banding the pulmonary artery induced hypertrophy of the right ventricle without involvement of the left ventricle. Similarly, hypertrophy induced by volume overload, myocardial infarction,[57] or other forms of injury is restricted to the cardiac chamber involved. Despite the myocyte not increasing in number in the adult heart during hypertrophy, certain other features are interesting and unique. Cardiac myocytes, during their normal growth response, exhibit DNA synthesis (multiple nuclei)[58] and the reexpression of several fetal proteins otherwise expressed only in embryonic cells.[59] The rational basis for the reexpression of fetal protein is not obvious. The response has been referred to as *adaptive, maladaptive,* or part of a *triggered program response.*[28] The atrial natriuretic factor gene is expressed in the atria and ventricles in the embryonic state but not in the normal adult ventricle. It is reexpressed in the ventricle during hypertrophy.[60] Calcium ATPase, an enzyme essential to cardiac contractility, is decreased in the hypertrophied human ventricle.[61] It is well documented in the developing mammalian heart in utero that the initial actin gene expressed is that of smooth muscle type, followed by that of skeletal muscle and finally cardiac muscle.[62] The functional significance, if any, of the reexpression of fetal genes when the cardiac growth program is turned on in the adult heart is unknown. It is possible that the growth response can only be activated through expression of a family of genes. The master gene controlling expression of such a family could be triggered by a growth factor stimulated by pressure overload; this could result in a cascade of genes expressed, most of which are incidental rather than adaptive or maladaptive. For example, in skeletal muscle there is a master gene, *myo-D,*[63] that triggers the differentiation of skeletal muscle. When this occurs, a cascade of genes is downregulated, and another cascade of genes is upregulated. *Myo-D* is not expressed in cardiac muscle, and no such triggering factor has been found for cardiac myocyte differentiation (see Chap. 9).

References

1. Roberts R. A glimpse of the future from present day molecular genetics. In: Opie LH, Yellon DM, eds. *Cardiology at the Limits III*, 3d ed. Cape Town: Stanford Writers; 1999:105–120.
2. Morgan HE, Paul SR. American Heart Association: Bugher Foundation Centers for Molecular Biology in the Cardiovascular System. *Circulation* 1995; 91:487–493.
3. Katz AM. Molecular biology in cardiology: A paradigmatic shift. *J Mol Cell Cardiol* 1988; 20:355–366.
4. Patterson SW, Piper H, Starling EH. The regulation of the heart beat. *J Physiol* 1914; 48:465–472.
5. Baek S, March KL. Gene therapy for restenosis: Getting nearer the heart of the matter. *Circ Res* 1999; 82:295–305.
6. Jarcho JA, McKenna W, Pare JAP, et al. Mapping a gene for familial hypertrophic cardiomyopathy to chromosome 14q1. *New Engl J Med* 1989; 321:1372–1378.
7. Hejtmancik JF, Brink PA, Towbin J, et al. Localization of the gene for familial hypertrophic cardiomyopathy to chromosome 14q1 in a diverse U.S. population. *Circulation* 1991; 83:1592–1597.
8. Pennica D, Holmes WE, Kohr WJ, et al. Cloning and expression of human tissue-type plasminogen activator cDNA in *E coli. Nature* 1983; 301:214–221.
9. Danchin N, Vaur L, Genes N, et al. Treatment of acute myocardial infarction by primary coronary angioplasty or intravenous thrombolysis in the "real world": One-year results from a nationwide French survey. *Circulation* 1999; 99:2639–2644.
10. Kleyn PW, Vesell ES. Genetic variation as a guide to drug development. *Science* 1998; 281:1820–1821.
11. Watson JD, Crick FHC. Molecular structure of nucleic acids: A structure for deoxyribose nucleic acid. *Nature* 1953; 171:737–738.
12. Watson JD, Crick FHC. Genetic implications of the structure of deoxyribonucleic acid. *Nature* 1953; 171:964–967.
13. Franklin RE, Gosling RG. Molecular configuration in sodium thymonucleate. *Nature* 1953; 171:740–741.
14. Wilkins MHF, Stokes AR, Wilson HR. Molecular structure of deoxypentose nucleic acids. *Nature* 1953; 171:738–740.
15. Schekman R, Weiner A, Kornberg A. Multienzyme systems of DNA replication. *Science* 1956; 186:987–993.
16. Marmor J, Lane L. Strand separation and specific recombination of deoxyribonucleic acids: Biological studies. *Proc Natl Acad Sci USA* 1960; 46:453–461.
17. Doty P, Marmor J, Eigner J, Schildkraut C. Strand separation and specific recombination in deoxyribonucleic acids: Physical chemical studies. *Proc Natl Acad Sci USA* 1960; 46:461–476.
18. Leder P, Nirenberg M. RNA codewords and protein synthesis: II. Nucleotide sequence of a valine RNA codeword. *Proc Natl Acad Sci USA* 1964; 52:420–427.
19. Nishimura S, Jones DS, Khorana HG. The in vitro synthesis of a co-polypeptide containing two amino acids in alternative sequence dependent upon a DNA-like polymer containing two nucleotides in alternating sequence. *J Mol Biol* 1981; 146:1–21.
20. Olivera BM, Hall ZW, Lehman IR. Enzymatic joining of polynucleotides: V. A DNA adenylate intermediate in the polynucleotide joining reaction. *Proc Natl Acad Sci USA* 1968; 61:237–244.
21. Smith HO, Wilcox KW. A restriction enzyme from *Hemophilias influenzae*: I. Purification and general properties. *J Mol Biol* 1970; 51:379–391.
22. Kelly TJ Jr, Smith HO. A restriction enzyme from *Hemophilias influenzae*: II. Base sequence of the recognition site. *J Mol Biol* 1970; 51:393–409.
23. Baltimore D. Viral RNA-dependent DNA polymerase. *Nature* 1970; 226:1209–1211.
24. Termin HM, Mizutani S. RNA-dependent DNA polymerase in virions of Rous sarcoma virus. *Nature* 1970; 226:1211–1213.
25. Cohen S, Chang A, Boyer H, Helling R. Construction of biological functional bacterial plasmids in vitro. *Proc Natl Acad Sci USA* 1973; 70:3240–3244.
26. Sanger F, Coulson AR. A rapid method for determining sequences in DNA by primed synthesis and DNA polymerase. *J Mol Biol* 1975; 94:444–448.
27. Maxam AM, Gilbert W. A new method of sequencing DNA. *Proc Natl Acad Sci USA* 1977; 74:560–564.
28. Roberts R. Modern molecular biology: Historical perspective and future potential. In: Roberts R, ed. *Molecular Basis of Cardiology,* 1st ed. Hamden, CT: Blackwell Scientific; 1992:1–15.
29. Knight SL. Molecular zippers in gene regulation. *Sci Am* 1991; 264:54–64.
30. Schneider MD, Roberts R, Parker TG. Modulation of cardiac genes by mechanical stress: The oncogene signalling hypothesis. *Mol Biol Med* 1991; 8:167–183.

31. Falvey E, Schibler U. How are the genes regulators regulated? *FASEB J* 1991; 5:309–314.
32. Brenner S. *Molecular Biology: A Selection of Papers*. San Diego: Academic Press; 1989.
33. Aaij C, Borst P. The gel electrophoresis of DNA. *Biochim Biophys Acta* 1972; 269:192–200.
34. Southern EM. Detection of specific sequences among DNA fragments separated by gel electrophoresis. *J Mol Biol* 1975; 98:503–517.
35. Sambrook J, Fritsch EF, Maniatis T. Analysis and cloning of eucaryltic genomic DNA. In: *Molecular Cloning: A Laboratory Manual*. Cold Spring Harbor, NY: Cold Spring Harbor Laboratory Press; 1989:9.14–9.23.
36. Schwarz DC, Cantro CR. Separation of yeast chromosome-sized DNAs by pulsed field gradient gel electrophoresis. *Nucl Acids Res* 1984; 37:67–76.
37. Hunt T, Kozak M, Lindahl T, Varmus HE. The molecular organization of cells. In: Alberts B, Bray D, Lewis, J, et al., eds. *Molecular Biology of the Cell*, 2d ed. New York: Garland Publishing; 1989:201–274.
38. Saiki RK, Scharf S, Faloona F, et al. Enzymatic amplification of beta-globin genomic sequences and restriction site analysis for diagnosis of sickle cell anemia. *Science* 1985; 230:1350–1354.
39. Saiki RK, Gelfand DH, Stoffel S, et al. Primer-directed enzymatic amplification of DNA with a thermostable DNA polymerase. *Science* 1988; 239:487–491.
40. Timchenko LT, Timchenko NA, Caskey T, Roberts R. Novel proteins with binding specificity for DNA CTG repeats and RNA CUG repeats: Implications for myotonic dystrophy. *Hum Mol Genet* 1996; 5:115–121.
41. Alberts B, Bray D, Lewis J, et al. *Molelcular Biology of the Cell*, 3d ed. New York: Garland Publishing; 1994.
42. Mitsui T. Induced potential model of muscular contraction mechanism and myosin molecular structure. *Adv Biophys* 1999; 36:107–158.
43. Honda H, Nakamoto T, Sakai R, Hirai H. p130(Cas), an assembling molecule of actin filaments, promotes cell movement, cell migration, and cell spreading in fibroblasts. *Biochem Biophys Res Commun* 1999; 262:25–30.
44. Bies RD, Maeda M, Roberds SL, et al. A 5′ dystrophin duplication mutation causes membrane deficiency of α-dystroglycan in a family with X-linked cardiomyopathy. *Am J Hum Genet* 1997; 29:3175–3188.
45. Nigro V, Okazaki Y, Belsito A, et al. Identification of the Syrian hamster cardiomyopathy gene. *Hum Mol Genet* 1997; 6(601): 607–607.
46. Maeda M, Holder E, Lowes B, et al.. Dilated cardiomyopathy associated with deficiency of the cytoskeletal protein metavinculin. *Circulation* 1997; 95:17–20.
47. Olson TM, Michels VV, Thibodeau SN, et al. Actin mutations in dilated cardiomyopathy, a heritable form of heart failure. *Science* 1998; 280:750–752.
48. Li D, Tapscott T, Gonzalez O, et al. Desmin mutation responsible for idiopathic dilated cardiomyopathy. *Circulation* 1999; 100:461–464.
49. Mogensen J, Klausen IC, Pedersen AK, et al. α-Cardiac actin is a novel disease gene in familial hypertrophic cardiomyopathy. *J Clin Invest* 1999; 103:R39–R42.
50. Vybiral T, Williams JK, Winkelman JC, et al. Human cardiac and skeletal muscle spectrins: Differential expression and localization. *Cell Motil Cytoskel* 1992; 21:291–304.
51. Black BL, Olson EN. Transcriptional control of muscle development by myocyte enhancer factor-2 (MEF2) proteins. *Annu Rev Cell Dev Biol* 1998; 14:167–196.
52. Borg TK, Nakagawa M, Carver W, Terracio L. Overview: Extracellular matrix, receptors, and heart development. In: Clark EB, Markwald RR, Takao A, eds. *Developmental Mechanisms of Heart Disease*, 1st ed. Armonk, NY: Futura; 1995:175–184.
53. Tamura T, Onodera T, Said S, Gerdes AM. Correlation of myocyte lengthening to chamber dilation in the spontaneously hypertensive heart failure (SHHF) rat. *J Mol Cell Cardiol* 1998; 30:2175–2181.
54. Gerdes AM, Capasso JM. Structural remodeling and mechanical dysfunction of cardiac myocytes in heart failure. *J Mol Cell Cardiol* 1995; 27:849–856.
55. Hammond GL, Wieben E, Markert CL. Molecular signals for initiating protein synthesis in organ hypertrophy. *Proc Natl Acad Sci USA* 1979; 76:2455–2459.
56. Imamura SI, Matsuoka R, Hiratsuka E, et al. Local response to cardiac overload on myosin heavy chain gene expression and isozyme transition. *Circ Res* 1990; 66:1067–1073.
57. Rubin SA, Correa M, Rabines A, Fishbein MC. Beta blockade alters myosin heavy chain gene expression after rat infarction. *Circulation* 1989; 80:II-458.
58. Clubb JR, Bishop FJ, Bishop SP. Formation of binucleated myocardial cells in the neonatal rat: An index for growth hypertrophy. *Lab Invest* 1984; 40:571–577.
59. Parker TG, Packer SE, Schneider MD. Peptide growth factors can provoke "fetal" contractile protein gene expression in rat cardiac myocytes. *J Clin Invest* 1990; 85:507–514.
60. Seidman CE, Wong DW, Jarcho JA, et al. Cis-acting sequences that modulate atrial natriuretic factor gene expression. *Proc Natl Acad Sci USA* 1988; 85:4104–4108.
61. Mercadier JJ, Lompre AM, Duc P, et al. Altered sarcoplasmic reticulum Ca^{2+}-ATPase gene expression in the human ventricle during end-stage heart failure. *J Clin Invest* 1990; 8:305–309.
62. Ruzicka DL, Schwartz RJ. Sequential activation of a α-actin gene transcripts mark the onset of cardiomyocyte differentiation. *J Cell Biol* 1988; 107:2575–2586.
63. Davis RL, Weintraub H, Lassar AB. Expression of a single transfected cDNA converts fibroblasts to myoblasts. *Cell* 1987; 51:987–1000.

CHAPTER 5

MOLECULAR AND CELLULAR BIOLOGY OF THE NORMAL, HYPERTROPHIED, AND FAILING HEART

Richard A. Walsh

INTRODUCTION

Growth of the heart is a dynamic process that occurs during embryogenesis, postnatal development, maturity, and senescence and in response to changing environmental and pathologic conditions. Cardiac growth occurs at the cellular level as a consequence of the interplay between *hyperplasia* (increase in cell number) and *hypertrophy* (increase in cell size) or a combination of both processes. The relative importance of each of these two mechanisms depends upon the cell type, developmental stage, and the nature of the growth stimulus. These two forms of cell growth are variably modulated by *apoptosis,* or programmed cell death.[1,2] This phenomenon is of importance in the determination of heart shape and chamber formation during cardiogenesis and may contribute to altered cardiac chamber geometry in response to pathologic stimuli. Physiologic and pathologic cardiovascular growth are generally mediated by developmental programs, mechanical deformation, and injury in various combinations. These processes stimulate a repertoire of biochemical signals that alter the cardiovascular phenotype. The application of molecular and cell biological approaches to this problem is rapidly defining the precise factors responsible for normal and pathologic growth of the heart and the mechanisms responsible for altered cardiac function.

CARDIAC GROWTH AND HYPERTROPHY

Cardiac hypertrophy is a process wherein there is an increase in chamber mass produced largely by an increase in the size of terminally differentiated cardiomyocytes. Although cardiomyocytes make up only one-third of the total cell number, they are responsible in aggregate for over 70 percent of cardiac volume. Cardiac hypertrophy may be reasonably categorized as either physiologic or pathologic (Fig. 5-1).

Physiologic Hypertrophy

Physiologic hypertrophy includes cardiogenesis during embryonic development, postnatal cardiac growth, a modest additional increase in heart size that evolves during senescence, and the increase in heart size that occurs in response to athletic conditioning. The earliest stage of cardiac growth in utero depends on a genetically determined developmental program, since it can occur in the absence of contractile activity. Subsequently, mechanical forces become increasingly important in the development of the normal cardiac phenotype. Throughout the embryonic period and for a few weeks after birth, cardiac growth occurs as a consequence of hyperplasia and hypertrophy of myocytes (see Chap. 9). Classically, adult myocytes have been described as terminally differentiated—that is, incapable of reentering the cell cycle. This issue is currently undergoing reexamination. It is critical to make a distinction between DNA synthesis and cell division. In the adult cardiomyocyte, DNA synthesis may clearly result in either multinucleation or polyploidy (an increase in the DNA content of a single nucleus). By contrast, there is little evidence that cardiomyocytes are capable of division under normal conditions after the early postnatal period.[3,4] The capacity to reactivate hyperplasia in the terminally differentiated cardiomyocyte is an area of intense research interest, with potentially important therapeutic implications in the hypertrophied and failing heart.[5]

From birth to maturation, the mammalian heart undergoes a sixfold increase in mass. The normal heart/body weight ratio is species-specific. The largest hearts relative to body size occur in animals with survival requirements that depend on sustained exercise rather than on burst activity.[6] In humans, intense, prolonged exercise training can produce an increase in cardiac mass. Isotonic exercise, such as running, produces *eccentric hypertrophy,* characterized by a normal ratio of wall thickness to

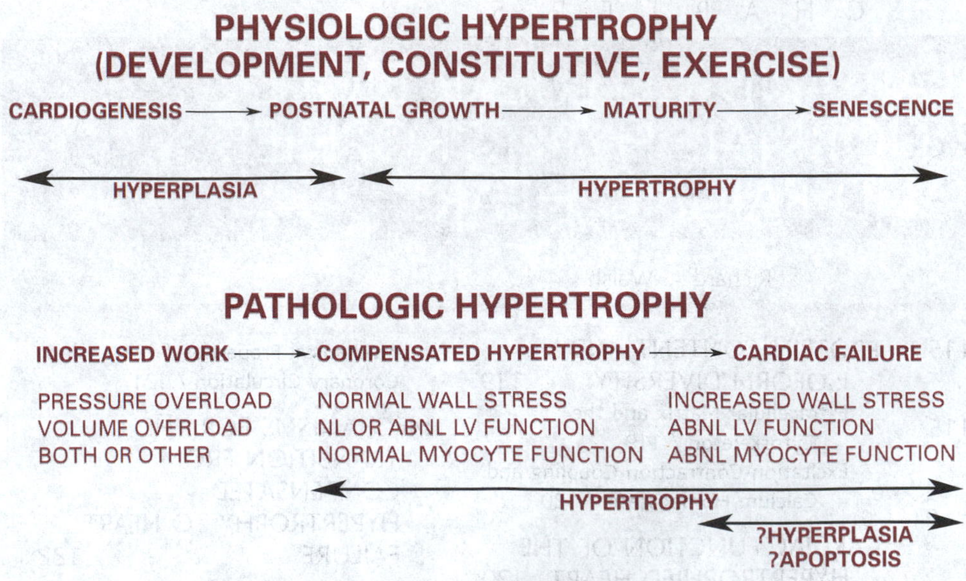

FIGURE 5-1 Relative roles of cardiomyocyte hypertrophy, hyperplasia, and apoptosis in physiologic and pathologic cardiac hypertrophy, along with the functional differences between compensated hypertrophy and heart failure.

dimension, whereas isometric exercise, such as weight lifting, stimulated *concentric hypertrophy,* associated with an increased ratio of wall thickness to dimension.[7] Senescent animals and humans free of organic heart disease develop mild concentric left ventricular hypertrophy as a consequence of age-related decreases in the distensibility of the peripheral vasculature.[8] The molecular, biochemical, and physiologic changes associated with physiologic hypertrophy differ both qualitatively and quantitatively from those that occur during pathologic hypertrophy. Physiologic studies in animal models and humans have demonstrated no substantial alterations in isolated muscle or intact heart function. There is also little evidence of alterations in the molecular determinants of excitation-contraction coupling. Most importantly, epidemiologic data fail to demonstrate adverse risk associated with the modest hypertrophy that occurs as a consequence of athletic conditioning. It is, therefore, important clinically to distinguish physiologic hypertrophy from hypertrophic cardiomyopathy in athletes (see Chap. 67).

Pathologic Hypertrophy

Pathologic hypertrophy is an important adaptive response to abnormal global or regional increase in cardiac work. Initially, the increase in cardiac mass serves to normalize wall stress and permit normal cardiovascular function at rest and during exercise in *compensated hypertrophy*. If the stimulus for pathologic hypertrophy is sufficiently intense or prolonged, *decompensated hypertrophy* and heart failure ensue. Pathologic hypertrophy may be caused by pressure overloading, as in systemic or pulmonary arterial hypertension, left ventricular outflow obstruction, or aortic coarctation. Pressure overloading produces an increase in systolic wall stress and results in concentric ventricular hypertrophy. Volume overloading, as occurs in mitral or aortic regurgitation or as a result of arteriovenous fistulas, also produces pathologic hypertrophy. These latter conditions induce an increase in either diastolic wall stress (mitral regurgitation) or both systolic and diastolic wall stress (aortic regurgitation and arteriovenous fistulas) and result in eccentric left ventricular hypertrophy. Regional hypertrophy that occurs in viable myocardium adjacent to and remote from an area of infarction has the characteristics of eccentric hypertrophy.

There are exceptions to the principle that pathologic hypertrophy occurs as a result of excessive increases in external work. For example, hypertrophic cardiomyopathy is produced by point mutations of the sarcomeric proteins, in particular the β-myosin heavy chain. These mutations result in massive asymmetric or concentric hypertrophy in the absence of augmented peripheral hemodynamic requirements (see Chap. 62). It is possible that the massive myofibrillar disarray that characterizes this genetic form of hypertrophy increases internal cardiac work, which, in turn, increased cardiac mass.[9,10] Genetically engineered mice with cardiac-specific postnatal overexpression of the β_2 adrenergic receptor[11] or targeted ablation of the phospholamban gene[12] have enhanced cardiac function throughout life but no significant increase in cardiac mass. By contrast, similar cardiac overexpression of the sarcoplasmic reticulum–binding protein calsequestrin in mice results in hypofunction of the heart, with decreased external work and substantial cardiac hypertrophy.[13] Finally, tachycardia-induced heart failure in animal models and humans is associated with increased external cardiac work, decreased cardiac function, and no alteration in cardiac mass. These recent observations suggest a critical reexamination of the primary role of mechanotransduction in the etiology of pathologic hypertrophy.

Mechanisms for the Development of Cardiac Hypertrophy

STIMULI AND SIGNAL TRANSDUCTION PATHWAYS

Stretch-Induced Growth Factors Dynamic or static stretch of neonatal or adult cardiomyocytes, papillary muscle, isolated heart, or intact heart produces increased cardiac protein synthesis and resultant cellular hypertrophy.[14] The process by which stimuli in the physical domain activate intracellular growth-signaling pathways is known as *mechanotransduction.*[15] There is evidence that this process may be accomplished in the cardiomyocyte by stretch-activated sarcolemmal ion channels, G protein–coupled receptors, NA^+/H^+ antiporters, tyrosine kinase–containing receptors, and/or an extracellular matrix–integrin linked pathway. These cell-surface mechanotransducers then activate cytosolic signal transduction pathways that initiate gene transcription and translation of increased quantities of protein (Fig. 5-2). Important signal transduction pathways that are clearly activated by mechanical deformation include protein kinase C (PKC), mitogen activated protein (MAP) kinases,

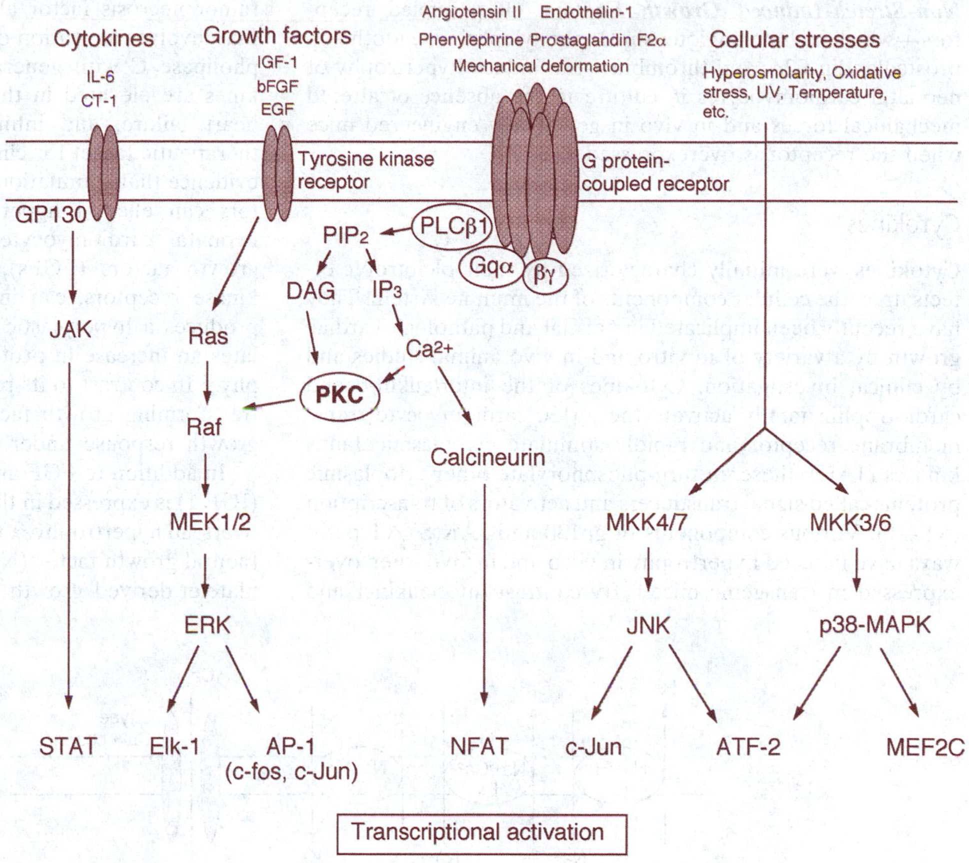

FIGURE 5-2 A schema for signal-transduction pathways that activate transcriptional regulation and induce hypertrophic genes. G protein–coupled receptor agonists binding to their receptors activate phospholipase C (PLC) β_1 via the dissociated α subunit of a GTP-binding protein of the Gq class (Gqα). PLCβ_1 catalyzes the hydrolysis of phosphatidyl-inositol bisphosphate (PIP_2) into diacylglycerol (DAG), which activates protein kinase C (PKC) and inositol trisphosphate (IP_3), which stimulates calcium release from intracellular stores. PKC activated by DAG and ± calcium initiates cascades of phosphorylation. One of the downstream targets of PKC is the ras-raf mitogen-activated protein kinase (MAPK) cascade. Insulin-like growth factor (IGF)-1, basic fibroblast growth factor (bFGF), or epidermal growth factor (EGF) interacts with cognate membrane tyrosine kinase receptors, which activate ras by the growth factor receptor–bound protein. Ras activates raf, MAPK/ERK-activating kinase (MEK), and extracellular signal regulated kinase (ERK). Cellular stresses activate other members of the MAPK family, c-Jun N-terminal kinase (JNK) and p38-MAPK, but precise signaling elements are not as well defined as in the ERK cascade. The MAPK kinase (MKK) and small G proteins are likely to be involved. Ras, either directly or indirectly, may activate JNK and p38-MAPK. Signaling through interleukin-1 (IL-1) and cardiotrophin-1 (CT-1) receptors involves gp130, which acts as a signal-transducing receptor component. The binding of ligands to their cognate receptors results in receptor dimerization, autophosphorylation, and activation of the associated Janus kinase (JAK). In turn, JAK activates members of the STAT (signal transducer and activator of transcription) family. PKC activation increases calcium concentration through phosphorylation of L-type calcium channel and IP_3 mediated calcium release from intracellular stores. This leads to stimulation of the calcium-dependent phosphatase calcineurin. Activated calcineurin dephosphorylates nuclear factor of activated T lymphocytes (NFAT), which translocates into the nucleus to interact with multiple transcription factors.

stress-activated protein kinase, and possibly cyclic adenosine monophosphate (cAMP)–dependent protein kinase.[16] In particular, stretch of neonatal cultured cardiomyocytes produces G protein–mediated activation of membrane-bound phospholipase C, which, in turn, hydrolyzes phosphatidylinositol bisphosphate (PIP_2) to inositol trisphosphate (IP_3) and diacylglycerol (DAG). Diacylglycerol then activates PKC.[17,18] Phosphorylation of downstream cytosolic and nuclear proteins and transcription factors by PKC is known to be of critical importance for growth in a number of cell types, while inositol triphosphate is an important modulator of cytosolic calcium homeostasis by the interaction with its receptor on the sarcoplasmic reticulum. Angiotensin II receptor coupling appears to play a critical role in the activation of phospholipase C;[19,20] however, α_1-adrenergic and endothelin receptor stimulation can also activate this pathway, with resultant hypertrophy in the neonatal cardiomyocytes and in transgenic mice.[21–23]

Current information suggests that mechanotransduction and a number of interrelated autocrine, paracrine, and endocrine effects of hormones and growth factors mediate cardiac hypertrophy[24] (Fig. 5-2). The resultant activation of multiple signal transduction pathways, which have demonstrable cross talk and considerable redundancy, provides a powerful mechanism by which the heart can respond to changing chronic hemodynamic requirements. A point of downstream convergence of multiple signal transduction pathways in the heart and noncardiac systems appears to be the phosphorylation of mitogen-activated protein kinase [MAPK, also known as extracellular signal regulated kinase (ERK)].[25] Mammalian MAPKs are serine-threonine protein kinases that are activated by signal transduction pathways coupled to both phosphatidylinositol hydrolysis/PKC activation and receptor protein tyrosine kinases (Fig. 5-2). Of particular importance to cardiac hypertrophy is the observation that important transcription factors (c-*jun*, c-*myc*, p62[TCF]) are known substrates of MAPK phosphorylation. Recently, transfection of an antisense nucleotide to MAPK was shown to prevent hypertrophy in cardiomyocytes. Information from noncardiomyocyte cell systems, neonatal and adult myocytes, and genetically engineered mice has demonstrated considerable complexity, redundancy, and cross talk among these and other intracellular signaling pathways in the development of the cardiac hypertrophy phenotype in response to stretch and other stimuli.[26] In particular, ischemia, hypoxia, oxidative stress, neurohormones, and cytokines can activate downstream signaling and resultant nuclear transcriptional events, including cardiomyocyte hypertrophy and fibroblast hyperplasia.

Non-Stretch-Induced Growth Factors Gαq-coupled receptors—which include angiotensin II, phenylephrine, endothelin, prostaglandin F2α, and thrombin—can induce hypertrophy of neonatal cardiomyocytes in culture in the absence of altered mechanical forces and in vivo in genetically engineered mice when the receptor is overexpressed.[27]

Cytokines

Cytokines were initially characterized by their pleiotropic effects upon the cellular components of the immune system. They have recently been implicated in normal and pathologic cardiac growth by a variety of in vitro and in vivo animal studies and by clinical investigation. Cytokines of the interleukin-6 and cardiotrophin family activate the gp130 cardiomyocyte transmembrane receptor and rapidly stimulate cytoplasmic Janus kinases (JAK); these, in turn phosphorylate other cytoplasmic proteins called signal transducers and activators of transcription (STAT). Various components of gp130 and JAK-STAT pathways have induced hypertrophy in vitro and in vivo when overexpressed in transgenic mice.[28] By contrast interleukin-1 and tumor necrosis factor alpha (TNF-α) use a distinct pathway that involves activation of a phosphatidylcholine-specific phospholipase C with generation of diacylglycerol.[29] These cytokines are elevated in the plasma of patients with congestive heart failure, and inhibition of their effects is a current therapeutic target for clinical heart failure. There is increasing evidence that stimulation of cell-surface tyrosine-kinase receptors can elicit a hyperplastic or hypertrophic response in neonatal cardiomyocytes. Both acidic and basic fibroblast growth factors (FGFs), which act as ligands for tyrosine-kinase receptors, can induce myocyte growth.[30] Acidic FGF produces a hyperplastic response, whereas basic FGF stimulates an increase in protein synthesis with resultant hypertrophy.[31] In contrast to its role in vascular smooth muscle growth, transforming growth factor beta (TGF-β) does not induce a growth response under these conditions.[32]

In addition to FGF and TGF-β, insulin-like growth factor 1 (IGF-1) is expressed in the myocardium in response to pressure overload hypertrophy.[33] These and other peptide growth factors [neural growth factor (NGF), epidermal growth factor (EGF), platelet-derived growth factor (PDGF), and insulin] bind to receptor tyrosine kinases (RTK). These receptors undergo ligand-mediated homodimerization with resultant autophosphorylation of tyrosine residues on the cytoplasmic domain. These tyrosine complexes recruit signaling molecules such as the monomeric GTP-binding protein P21 ras to the membrane, where transient complexes stimulate downstream signaling to the nucleus. Increasing evidence using loss of function and gain of function in in vitro studies of neonatal myocytes implicates this signaling molecule and its downstream effector raf-1 as potential mediators of cardiac growth.[34]

Hormones

Thyroid hormone is generally considered the classic hormonal mediator of cardiac hypertrophy. Administration of excess thyroid hormone to experimental animals produces increased heart weight that is associated with transcriptionally mediated alterations in the myosin heavy chains (MHCs), calcium-cycling proteins, and other functional constituents of the cardiomyocyte in small animals and primates.[35] Thyroid hormone–induced hypertrophy appears to be an indirect effect of the T_3-mediated increased oxygen consumption and resultant augmentation of cardiac work. For ex-

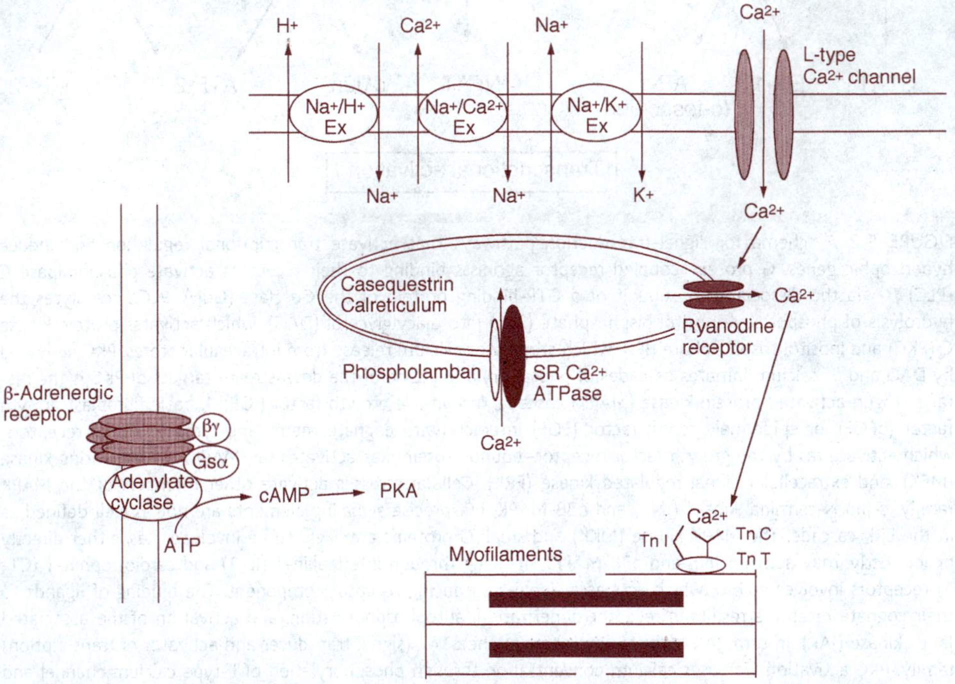

FIGURE 5-3 Schematic diagram of cardiomyocyte signaling pathways that regulate calcium levels and excitation-contraction coupling. Calcium enters into the cytosol via the voltage-sensitive L-type channel. Calcium then interacts with the ryanodine receptor, which triggers augmented calcium release from the sarcoplasmic reticulum (SR). Calcium is bound to troponin (Tn) C, which activates actin myosin cross-bridge development and shortening. Hydrolysis of ATP to ADP mediated by the ATPase at the head of myosin molecules in the thick filament provides energy for the process. Tn I inhibits cross-bridge formation when calcium is not bound to Tn C. Tn T anchors the Tn complex to the thin filament actin. Calcium is then released and resequestered into the SR by an ATPase where it is bound to the SR storage proteins calsequestrin and calreticulum. Phospholamban in its dephosphorylated state inhibits SR ATPase activity and phosphorylation relieves this inhibition. Binding of agonist to the β-adrenergic receptor activates adenylate cyclase via dissociation of the Gsα subunit. Adenylate cyclase generates cyclic AMP from ATP, which, in turn, activates cyclic AMP–dependent protein kinase A (PKA). PKA regulates myocardial contractility by phosphorylation of the L-type calcium channel, leading to increased calcium entry, by phosphorylating phospholamban and resultant enhanced SR ATPase activity, and by phosphorylating regulatory proteins of the myofilament leading to decreased calcium sensitivity. The net enhancement of intracellular calcium concentration is restored by the coordinated activity of the Na^+-H^+ and Na^+-Ca^{2+} exchangers (Ex).

ample, heterotopic transplantation of a nonworking rat heart into the abdominal aorta of the hyperthyroid animal is unassociated with hypertrophy, despite the presence of the transcriptionally mediated effects of the hormone in the transplanted organ and hypertrophy and typical transcriptional events in the native working heart.[36,37]

In addition to the indirect effects of thyroid hormone on cardiac growth, other endocrine mediators of hypertrophy have been examined. Growth hormone, which mediates its effects in large part though IGF-1, may be a mediator of physiologic hypertrophy. By contrast, there is preliminary evidence that retinoic acid and vitamin D may inhibit cardiac growth.[38,39]

Calcium Signaling

Increases in intracellular calcium have been associated with hypertrophic cardiomyocyte growth in vitro (see Figs. 5-2 and 5-3).[40,41] For example, use of the calcium ionophore BAYK8644 enhances while application of a membrane-permeable calcium chelator inhibits the cellular hypertrophic response by affecting calcium-calmodulin–dependent protein kinase. In addition, calcineurin, a phosphatase activated by intracellular calcium, dephosphorylates nuclear factor for activation of transcription (NFAT), which translocates to the nucleus, where it activates numerous transcription factors such as GATA-4. In vitro and in vivo studies using genetically engineered mice have demonstrated that augmented levels of activity of calcineurin, NFAT, or both can initiate a hypertrophic response. However, the relative role of this pathway in normal and pathologic growth of the heart is unclear at this time.[42,43]

PROTEIN CONTENT AND ISOFORM DIVERSITY

The hallmark of cardiac hypertrophy is a net increase in protein synthesis above protein degradation. Under normal circumstances, these two processes are matched and result in nitrogen balance. Since the average half-life of cardiac proteins is 5 days, the composition of the adult heart is regenerated approximately every 3 weeks. The more rapid rate of cardiac growth in response to increased hemodynamic load could result from an augmentation in either the efficiency or the capacity of protein synthesis or a combination of the two.[44,45] Efficiency of protein synthesis is usually measured as moles of amino acid incorporated per milligram of cellular RNA per hour; capacity is assessed by determining the number of milligrams of RNA per gram of tissue. Experiments in a variety of systems indicate that the critical determinant for cardiac hypertrophy is an increased capacity for protein synthesis, which is mediated by augmented ribosomal content. Protein degradation appears to be modestly increased in cardiac hypertrophy and may play a critical role in the distinctive geometry of the ventricles in response to pressure or volume overloading, regression of hypertrophy, and cardiac atrophy.[46,47] The mechanisms for protein degradation in the heart involve the activation of both lysosomal and cytosolic proteases. Posttranslational processes are increasingly being recognized as important factors in the production of the cardiac phenotype in cardiac hypertrophy and failure.[35,48]

In addition to increased total protein content, cardiac hypertrophy is characterized by alterations in the relative abundance and isoform composition of the cardiomyocyte contractile, regulatory, and calcium-cycling proteins and other subcellular constituents. These processes provide an additional degree of plasticity for the heart to adapt to changing functional requirements. It is clear that there is considerable species specificity in the capacity for isoform switching. In small mammals with rapid heart rates, such as mice and rats, imposition of a pressure overload produces a transcriptionally mediated shift from the α- to the β-MHC and from cardiac to skeletal α-actin.[49–51] α-Myosin has a three- to sevenfold greater ATPase activity than β-myosin. The greater abundance of β-MHC in response to pressure overload in small animals increases the efficiency of force development by producing the same absolute muscle tension at a slower rate.[52] Despite identical cardiac muscle mechanics in response to hypertrophy, large animals with slower heart rates, including humans, possess β-MHC almost exclusively throughout embryogenesis and postnatal development.[53] It is possible that, in higher mammalian species, altered myosin ATPase in response to pressure-overload hypertrophy may be mediated in part by a posttranslationally produced low-molecular-weight variant of the β-MHC or isoform shifts in other myofibrillar proteins. For example, cardiac isoforms exist for essential and regulatory light chains, troponin (I, C, and T), tropomyosin, and the sarcolemmal Na^+, K^+-ATPase. Isoform switching of each of the components of the cardiomyocyte has been reported in hypertrophy and failure, but the functional significance of this has been unclear. The ability to ablate or overexpress these isoforms in genetically engineered mice will more clearly elucidate their role in the normal and hypertrophied heart.

Extracellular Matrix and the Cytoskeleton

Although cardiomyocytes make up the bulk of cardiac mass by volume, they are tethered in an extensive extracellular network of collagen and other structural proteins, including fibronectins and proteoglycans. The extracellular and intracellular myofibrillar scaffolding is a critical determinant of cardiac shape during normal and pathologic cardiac growth.[54–56] Collagen is synthesized principally by fibroblasts but also by vascular smooth muscle cells in response to a variety of pathologic stimuli, including increased oxidative and mechanical stress, ischemia, and inflammation. Most of the molecules and signal transduction pathways operant in cardiomyocyte growth play a role in hyperplasia of fibroblasts and in the elaboration of collagen. The resultant fibrosis produces altered myocardial stiffness and arrhythmogenesis in ischemic heart disease, cardiac hypertrophy, and congestive heart failure. Collagen synthesis is continuously and variably offset by extracellular matrix resorption mediated by matrix metalloproteinases (MMPs). The activity of these enzymes is increased in dilated cardiomyopathy. Conversely, the activity of a class of enzymes known as tissue inhibitors of matrix metalloproteinases (TIMPs) is reduced in this setting. The resultant excessive collagenolyses may induce myofibrillar slippage and contribute to the dilated thin-walled chamber geometry that characterizes acute and chronic heart failure. This process has been termed *chamber remodeling* by clinicians.[57]

Cardiomyocytes are tethered to the extracellular matrix by membrane-spanning proteins called *integrins*. The extracellular portion of these molecules binds to fibronectins in the extracellular matrix while the cytoplasmic domain is associated with a nonreceptor tyrosine kinase called focal adhesion kinase

(FAK).[58] Downstream targets for FAK phosphorylation are the SRC kinases src and fyn. This pathway is differentially activated by mechanical stretch ischemia and oxidative stress in the myocardium and provides an additional mechanism for altered growth during pathologic conditions.[59] Perimyocyte extracellular proteins such as dystrophin and dystrophin-related proteins contribute to normal cardiogenesis; when altered in abundance, they can produce a cardiomyopathy in Duchenne's muscular dystrophy and some familial cardiomyopathies, respectively (see Chap. 62).

The cardiomyocyte cytoskeleton is the intracellular scaffolding that provides a framework for the orderly arrangement of sarcomeres in striated cardiac and skeletal muscle. Titin—the third most abundant protein in the heart—desmin, and vinculin have differing intracellular spatial distributions that contribute to resting tension of cardiac muscle. The amount and polymerization status of the proteins that make up the microtubular network of the cardiomyocyte cytoplasm (tubulin and β actin) are important determinants of the viscous properties of heart muscle and contribute to altered cardiac function in pathologic states.[60,61]

Cardiac hypertrophy and failure are associated with changes in the relative abundance of the various intra- and extracellular structural proteins. All forms of cardiac hypertrophy are associated with increased collagen deposition in the extracellular matrix, which contributes to the observed alterations in passive chamber and muscle properties. Pressure overload (but not volume overload) hypertrophy has been associated with changes in the levels of the cytoskeletal proteins titin, desmin, and tubulin. Depolymerization of tubulin with colchicine reversed abnormalities in cardiac function in feline right ventricular hypertrophy but not in guinea pig left ventricular hypertrophy.[60,61]

Excitation-Contraction Coupling and Calcium Homeostasis (see Fig. 5-3)

Cardiomyocyte membrane depolarization is initiated by the intracellular movement of sodium through its ion channel, while repolarization is achieved by the extracellular movement of potassium via a family of sarcolemal K^+ channels. Membrane depolarization enhances the transmembrane conductance of calcium through a dihydropyridine-sensitive *l*-channel. The resultant increase in cytosolic calcium concentration permits binding of this cation to the ryanodine receptor on the surface of the sarcoplasmic reticulum. This process results in release of calcium from sarcoplasmic reticulum stores and further elevation of cytosolic calcium concentrations. The resultant hundredfold elevation of calcium permits binding to the myofilament regulatory protein troponin C. Calcium binding to troponin C promotes a steric movement of troponin I away from the actin binding site on the myosin molecule. This permits actin-myosin cross-bridge formation and resultant tension development. The activity of troponin I can be modulated via phosphorylation by protein kinase A and C, while the affinity of troponin C for calcium is altered by intracellular pH. These processes may result in substantial alteration of myofilament calcium. Energy for cross-bridge cycling is produced by hydrolysis of ATP via myosin ATPase. Calcium is released from troponin C and resequestered into the sarcoplasmic reticulum by a specific SR-ATPase. The activity of this enzyme is inhibited by the phosphoprotein phospholamban. Phosphorylation of phospholamban by cAMP (PKA)-dependent protein kinases, protein kinase C, or calcium-calmodulin–dependent protein kinase results in disinhibition and resultant enhancement of calcium uptake in the SR. Steady-state sarcoplasmic reticulum calcium content is determined by the abundance of the anionic storage proteins calsequestrin and calreticulum. Reequilibration of cytosolic sodium and potassium levels produced by the depolarization and repolarization cycle is facilitated by the activity of the sarcolemmal Na^+,K^+-ATPase. Extrusion of transarcolemmal mediated calcium influx is mediated by the coordinated interplay between the membrane situated Na^+-H^+ and Na^+-Ca^{2+} exchangers. Isolated changes in the stoichiometry between the sarcoplasmic reticulum ATPase and its inhibitor, phospholamban, have been demonstrated to have functional significance in genetically engineered mice. Targeted ablation of phospholamban enhanced cardiac inotropic and lusitropic function, whereas cardiac-specific overexpression produced the opposite result.[62,63]

CARDIAC FUNCTION OF THE HYPERTROPHIED HEART

The phenotypic consequences of the increased cardiac mass and altered protein abundance and composition of the hypertrophied heart are considerable and depend upon the model utilized; the animal species; and the nature, intensity, and duration of the hypertrophic stimulus. Taken together, available clinical and animal studies suggest that functional alterations evolve along a continuum from normal chamber and myocyte function to abnormal chamber and normal myocyte function to abnormalities of both chamber and myocyte function (Fig. 5-1).

Electrical Properties

The most typical electrical abnormality of the hypertrophied heart is prolongation of the duration of the action potential.[64] Recent studies using the single-cell voltage-clamp technique have begun to elucidate the ionic mechanisms responsible for this phenomenon. In mild hypertrophy, increases in calcium and calcium-activated currents (including the NA^+/Ca^{2+} exchanger) appear to be important. In severe hypertrophy, prolongation of the action potential is also determined importantly by a reduction in the potassium currents Ik*l* and Ito. The relations between these changes in membrane current properties of hypertrophied hearts and altered mechanical behavior at the myocyte and whole-heart level are not clearly understood at present. Hypertrophied myocardium is more likely than normal tissue to precipitate arrhythmias. The mechanisms for arrhythmogenesis are multifactorial and are operant at the tissue and cardiomyocyte levels. Increased dispersion of refractoriness and slowed conduction results from myocyte loss and fibrosis. Prolongation of the duration of the action potential increases the likelihood of early afterdepolarizations, which may result in triggered arrhythmias. Reduced coronary artery flow reserve and accelerated atherosclerosis of epicardial coronary vessels predispose toward ischemia-induced arrhythmias.[65] In concert, these mechanisms contribute to the finding of cardiac hypertrophy as the most powerful predictor of cardiovascular mortality in the Framingham Study (see Chap. 1).

The application of molecular biological and molecular genetic approaches is providing increasing insight into the cellular mechanisms of arrhythmogenesis. Normal cardiomyocyte excitation and arrhythmogenesis involve voltage-dependent ion channels, mechanosensitive channels, sarcolemmal electrogenic transporters, and gap junctions. The latter are two channels or connexins that enable ion current flow between and among cardiomyocytes. Connexons are composed of a class of molecules called *connexins*. Isoform diversity of the connexins are determinants of ion conductance and sensitivity.[66,67] The genes for each of the cardiomyocyte ion channels, transporters, and connexins have been cloned. Structure–function relations are being defined in vitro using site-directed mutagenesis and in vivo using loss of function or gain of function mutations in genetically engineered mice. In parallel, the abundance and/or function of the molecular determinants of excitability and arrhythmogenesis are beginning to be elucidated in animal models and human cardiovascular disease (see Chap. 23).

Genetic linkage analysis of familial arrhythmias and resultant identification of culprit gene defects of cardiomyocyte ion channels or channel modulators has provided complementary insight into the cellular mechanisms of arrhythmogenesis. The long-QT syndrome is now known to result from mutations in genes responsible for various outwardly rectifying potassium channels and the cardiomyocyte sodium channel.[68–70] Analyses of other inherited arrhythmias are under way.

Mechanical Properties

Mechanical function of the hypertrophied heart has been studied at the isolated myocyte, muscle, and chamber levels and in the intact circulation.[71–73] The results of these studies have revealed variable alterations in the rate and extent of contraction and relaxation, in the amount of force development, and in resting muscle and chamber properties. In the intact circulation, altered systolic and diastolic function is a composite result of subcellular changes in the myocyte, changes in the extracellular matrix, altered chamber geometry and mass, altered ventricular-vascular coupling, and the modulatory effects of neural and hormonal influences.

The earliest changes in mechanical performance observed in isometrically contracting papillary muscles extracted from hypertrophied hearts consist of a prolongation of time to peak tension and relaxation, despite normal peak twitch tension normalized for cross-sectional area of the muscle.[74] Afterloaded isotonically shortening papillary muscle preparations from hypertrophied hearts of a variety of animal species typically reveal a decrease in the force-velocity relationship and a depression of V_{max} (the extrapolated maximal unloaded shortening velocity).[75] V_{max} has been directly related to the calcium-activated myosin ATPase activity. Both myosin and myofibrillar ATPase activity are typically depressed in hypertrophied myocardium. In small rodents, this is due to the transcriptionally mediated switch from α- to β-MHC. In higher mammals including humans, the decreased myosin ATPase activity of the hypertrophied heart may be due to alterations in the troponin isoform composition[76] or the posttranslational generation of a lower molecular variant of the β-MHC.[48]

The dissociation between depressed rate-dependent indices of contraction and relaxation and normal maximal force development and extent of shortening in early cardiac hypertrophy has also been demonstrated in isolated cardiomyocytes and in the intact circulation of the nonhuman primate.[71,73] *These results suggest the rate of cross-bridge cycling is reduced but that the effective number of active cross bridges per unit of myocardium is preserved in compensated cardiac hypertrophy.* In decompensated hypertrophy, reduced absolute levels of force development and diminished contractility ultimately ensue.

In addition to alteration in excitation-contraction coupling and relaxation, the increased cardiac mass and changes in geometry significantly affect passive muscle and chamber properties of the hypertrophied heart. Concentric hypertrophy is characterized by an increased resting muscle and chamber stiffness, which results in an increase in pulmonary venous pressure for any given left ventricular volume. The resultant pulmonary congestion at rest or with exercise is an important determinant of symptoms in patients with hypertensive left ventricular hypertrophy or hypertrophic cardiomyopathy and normal or elevated ejection fraction. Pure volume overload hypertrophy, as occurs with mitral regurgitation, is typically associated with no change or a decrease in passive muscle or chamber stiffness. As a result, patients with chronic volume overload may remain asymptomatic for long periods despite appreciable increase in regurgitant fraction (see also Chaps. 56 and 57).

Coronary Circulation

Clinicians have long recognized that myocardial blood flow may be abnormal in the hypertrophied heart, since such patients may have exertional angina, resting or exercise-induced electrocardiographic or perfusion abnormalities, or pathologic evidence of subendocardial fibrosis, despite the presence of angiographically normal epicardial coronary arteries.

Morphologic studies of hypertrophied hearts from experimental animals and patients with pressure-overload hypertrophy demonstrate that the ratio of capillaries to myocytes remains unchanged.[77] Since myocyte cross-sectional area is increased, there is a resultant increase in nutrient diffusion distance in the hypertrophied heart. This anatomic change results in a reduced vasodilatory reserve in response to various stimuli in experimental and clinical studies.[78] Myocardial blood flow and oxygen consumption per unit of myocardium are normal in compensated pressure overload–left ventricular hypertrophy, where wall stress has been normalized by an increase in wall thickness. The impairment in vasodilatory reserve produces evidence of ischemia during increased myocardial oxygen demand. In right ventricular pressure-overload hypertrophy, differences in perfusion between the ventricles result in increased right ventricular blood flow per unit of myocardial mass at rest and no increase in minimum coronary resistance of hypertrophied right ventricular myocardium.[79]

Few data are available regarding changes in the coronary circulation in experimental or clinical volume-overload hypertrophy. Most studies have reported normal resting flow values per unit of myocardial mass. In contrast to pressure overload, volume-overload hypertrophy has been associated with normal or mildly increased minimum coronary resistance and normal or mildly decreased coronary reserve.[80] The coronary circulatory abnormalities associated with cardiac hypertrophy appear to be reversible with removal of the hypertrophic stimulus and resultant decreased chamber mass.[81]

Important recent studies have begun to elucidate the molecular and cellular mechanisms responsible for reversible functional consequences of ischemia and ischemia reperfusion. The syndrome of *myocardial stunning,* which refers to the variable period of regional or global myocardial hypofunction consequent to ischemia and reperfusion, is believed to involve two mechanisms. Either hydroxy-free radical generation, calcium overload, or both may be involved.[82] Downstream effects of these two pathologic processes include activation of protein kinase C, tyrosine kinases, and stress-activated kinases. In addition, proteolytic degradation of troponin I has been observed and is associated with uncoupling of excitation from contraction due to reduced myofilament calcium sensitivity. Transgenic overexpression either of a PKC isoform or the proteolytic degradation product of troponin I in mice produces both myocardial dysfunction and reduced myofilament calcium sensitivity responsiveness.[83]

Brief repetitive periods of ischemia and reperfusion also produce a powerful cardioprotective effect against myocardial necrosis. This process, called *ischemic preconditioning,* is also associated with activation of similar signal transduction pathways. The precise mechanism(s) for reduced myocyte cell death from necrosis, apoptosis, or both are presently unclear. *Hibernation* or myocardial hypofunction associated with reduced steady-state coronary blood flow may, in fact, result from repetitive periods of stunning.

MECHANISMS FOR THE TRANSITION FROM COMPENSATED HYPERTROPHY TO HEART FAILURE

In contrast to hypertrophied skeletal muscle, chronically increased work eventually results in depressed contractility and relaxation of the hypertrophied heart. Compensated hypertrophy, which is characterized by abnormal chamber function but preserved muscle and myocyte function, evolves into a decompensated phase characterized by abnormal chamber, muscle, and myocyte function (Fig. 5-1). Attempts to elucidate the underlying mechanisms for this transition have involved multidisciplinary studies of clinical end-stage heart failure, longitudinal studies in experimental animals, and characterization of cardiovascular function in genetically engineered mice, where attempts are made to mimic human disease (Fig. 5-4).[84]

Current information suggests that decompensated hypertrophy may result from a number of mechanisms that are both intrinsic and extrinsic to the cardiomyocyte. These include necrosis; apoptosis;[85,86] altered growth secondary to altered signal transduction pathways; alterations in cardiomyocyte contractile, regulatory, calcium-cycling, and structural proteins; alterations in the extracellular matrix, and remodeling (Fig. 5-4). Because of the complex combinatorial alterations that occur in human heart failure and conventional animal models of hypertrophy, studies in genetically engineered mice in which a protein of interest is either overexpressed or ablated using homologous recombination hold particular promise in determining the relative importance of various candidate genes. For example, mice bearing the mutation in the β-MHC that occurs in familial cardiomyopathy have many features of the human disease.[87] Overexpression of the α subunit of the G protein that couples to the β-adrenergic receptor has produced dilated fibrotic hearts with altered cardiovascular function.[88] Overexpression or ablation of genes involved in cardiomyocyte calcium-cycling proteins has been associated with altered heart function and abnormal calcium kinetics. It is of interest that, with few exceptions,[89] the resultant cardiac phenotype has failed to reproduce completely human decompensated hypertrophy and failure. This observation further supports the multifactorial nature of the condition and the importance of genetic background on the phenotype observed after loss-of-function or gain-of-function genetic engineering.

A common prominent feature of many experimental and clinical studies of decompensated hypertrophy and failure is a derangement of cardiomyocyte calcium homeostasis (Fig. 5-3). Studies of human cardiomyocytes extracted from the hearts of patients with end-stage heart failure have revealed elevated diastolic calcium levels with either no change or a reduction in the amplitude of the calcium transient.[90–93] Longitudinal studies of hypertrophy in experimental animals have revealed depression of steady-state mRNA levels[94] and sarcoplasmic reticulum ATPase and phospholamban proteins in decompensated, but not compensated, pressure-overload hypertrophy.[72] These changes were associated with distinctive contractile depression of isovolumically contracting heart func-

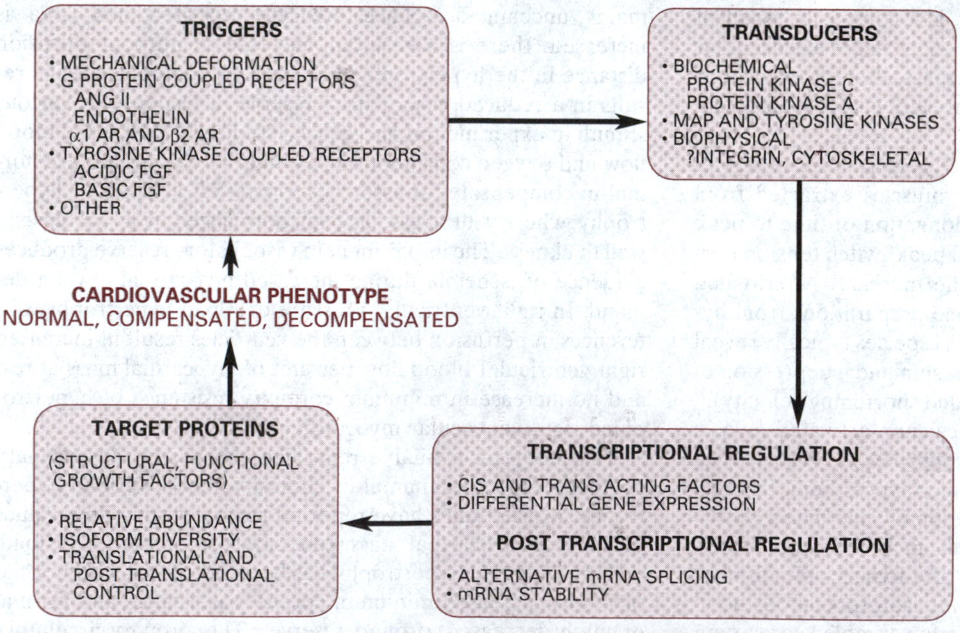

FIGURE 5-4 Schematic diagram of the mechanisms responsible for the development of the anatomic and functional cardiac phenotypes in physiologic and pathologic hypertrophy. Abnormalities at one or multiple levels in this putative closed-loop system may be responsible for the transition between compensated and decompensated hypertrophy.

tion, increases in the EC_{50}, and decreases in the V_{max} for sarcoplasmic reticular membrane uptake of calcium. Transgenic overexpression of the sarcoplasmic reticulum ATPase inhibitor phospholamban depressed cardiomyocyte function and calcium kinetics, whereas targeted ablation of the phosphoprotein produced the opposite result. Whether altered levels of the calcium-cycling proteins occur by transcriptional, translational, or posttranslational levels is currently unknown. In addition to altered levels of the various calcium-cycling proteins in hypertrophy and heart failure, there is evidence that abnormal spatial organization of the *l*-channel and SR may be contributory. Specifically, increased distance between the *l*-channel and the ryanodine receptor may contribute to abnormal calcium cycling.[95]

In addition to altered calcium homeostasis, there is increasing evidence that abnormal signal transduction plays a critical role in the development of cardiac hypertrophy and failure. In vitro studies with neonatal myocytes have demonstrated that phenylephrine, endothelin, and angiotensin II cause cardiomyocyte hypertrophy. These vasoactive peptides have cognate receptors that signal via the α subunit of the Gq protein (see Fig. 5-2). Cardiac-specific overexpression of Gαq produced cardiac hypertrophy, apoptosis, and contractile depression in transgenic mice.[96,97] By contrast, overexpression of a protein inhibitor of Gαq in a similar manner prevented cardiac hypertrophy due to pressure overload.[98] Transgenic overexpression of receptors that couple through Gαq, such as α_1 and angiotensin II, produces a similar phenotype: cardiac-specific postnatal overexpression of the calcium-sensitive PKC isoform B produced cardiac hypertrophy and failure. Pretreatment of mice overexpressing PKC B with a highly specific inhibitor prevented or reversed this hypertrophy–heart failure phenotype.[99] Part of the contractile depression observed with excess PKC B activity was due to phosphorylation of troponin I and resultant reduced myofilament calcium sensitivity.[100] Augmented PKC activity and elevated levels of the calcium-sensitive PKC α and β isoforms, but not Gαq, were found in human end-stage cardiomyopathic heart failure.[101,102] It is also known that PKC may be stimulated by pathophysiologic levels of stretch[103] and ischemia-reperfusion and directly by oxidative stress.[33] Taken together, these lines of evidence suggest that *PKC mediated signal transduction plays a critical role in the development of cardiac hypertrophy and failure.*[104]

A variety of studies with end-stage human cardiomyopathic heart tissue, conventional animal models, and genetically engineered mice suggest that apoptosis may contribute to the heart failure phenotype.[105] The key issue that remains unclear is the quantitative importance of the phenomenon. This problem is further complicated by the fact that a number of signaling molecules (e.g., Gαq and TNF-α) produce both hypertrophy and apoptosis. By contrast, gp130 heterodimerizes with LIF (leukemia inhibitory factor) receptor to permit binding of the interleukin-6 family of cytokines, such as cardiotrophin 1. Receptor binding stimulates the hypertrophic response while inhibiting apoptosis. Elimination of the gp130 by loss of function mutations of the gene results in mice that have structurally normal hearts. However, when a pressure overload is imposed, a rapidly progressive dilated cardiomyopathy ensues, which is associated with massive apoptosis.[106] The application of molecular genetic and biological approaches to elucidate mechanisms responsible for myocardial hypertrophy, cardiac failure, arrhythmogenesis, and ischemic dysfunction will permit improved diagnostic and therapeutic approaches to congenital and acquired heart diseases.[107]

References

1. Thompson CB. Apoptosis in the pathogenesis and treatment of disease. *Science* 1995; 267:1456–1462.
2. Vaux DL, Strasser A. The molecular biology of apoptosis. *Proc Natl Acad Sci USA* 1996; 93:2239–2244.
3. Dorée M, Galas S. The cyclin-dependent protein kinases and the control of cell division. *FASEB J* 1994; 8:1114–1121.
4. Peter M, Herskowitz I. Joining the complex: Cyclin dependent kinase inhibitory proteins and the cell cycle. *Cell* 1994; 79: 181–184.
5. Field LJ. Atrial natriuretic factor-SV40 T antigen transgenes produce tumors and cardiac arrhythmias in mice. *Science* 1988; 239:1029–1033.
6. Clark AJ. General physiology of hearts of cold-blooded vertebrates. In: Barcroft JSJ, ed. *Comparative Physiology of the Heart.* New York: Macmillan; 1927:151.
7. Ford LE. Heart size. *Circ Res* 1976; 39:297–303.
8. Walsh RA. Cardiovascular effects of the aging process. *Am J Med* 1987; 82:34–40.
9. Marian AJ, Roberts R. Recent advances in the molecular genetics of hypertrophic cardiomyopathy. *Circulation* 1995; 92:1336–1347.
10. Watkins H, Rosenzweig A, Hwang DS, et al. Characteristics and prognostic implications of myosin missense mutations in familial hypertrophic cardiomyopathy. *N Engl J Med* 1992; 326:1108–1114.
11. Milano CA, Allen LF, Rockman HA, et al. Enhanced myocardial function in transgenic mice overexpressing the β_2-adrenergic receptor. *Science* 1994; 264:582–586.
12. Hoit BD, Khoury SF, Kranias EG, et al. In vivo echocardiograph detection of enhanced left ventricular function in gene-targeted mice with phospholamban deficiency. *Circ Res* 1995; 77:632–637.
13. Sato Y, Ferguson DG, Sako H, et al. Cardiac-specific overexpression of mouse cardiac calsequestrin is associated with depressed cardiovascular function and hypertrophy in transgenic mice. *J Biol Chem* 1998; 273:28470–28477.
14. Cooper G IV. Cardiocyte adaptation to chronically altered load. *Annu Rev Physiol* 1987; 49:501–518.
15. Watson PA. Mechanical activation of signaling pathways in the cardiovascular system. *Trends Cardiovasc Med* 1996; 6:73–79.
16. Sugden PH, Bogoyevitch MA. Intracellular signalling through protein kinases in the heart. *Cardiovas Res* 1995; 30:478–492.
17. Komuro I, Katoh Y, Kaida T, et al. Mechanical loading stimulates cell hypertrophy and specific gene expression in cultured rat cardiac myocytes. *J Biol Chem* 1991; 266:1265–1268.
18. Sadoshima J, Jahn L, Takahashi T, et al. Molecular characterization of the stretch-induced adaptation of cultured cardiac cells. *J Biol Chem* 1992; 267:10551–10560.
19. Sadoshima J, Xu Y, Slayter HS, et al. Autocrine release of angiotensin II mediates stretch-induced hypertrophy of cardiac myocytes in vitro. *Cell* 1993; 75:977–984.
20. Yamazaki T, Komuro I, Kudoh S, et al. Angiotensin II partly mediates mechanical stress-induced cardiac hypertrophy. *Circ Res* 1995; 77:258–265.
21. Knowlton KU, Michel MC, Itani M, et al. The α_{1A}-adrenergic receptor subtype mediates biochemical, molecular, and morphologic features of cultured myocardial cell hypertrophy. *J Biol Chem* 1993; 268:15374–15380.
22. Bogoyevitch MA, Glennon PE, Andersson MB, et al. Endothelin 1 and fibroblast growth factors stimulate the mitogen-activated protein kinase signaling cascade in cardiac myocytes. *J Biol Chem* 1994; 269:1110–1119.
23. Milano CA, Dolber PC, Rockman HA, et al. Myocardial expres-

sion of a constitutively active α_{B1}-adrenergic receptor in transgenic mice induces cardiac hypertrophy. *Proc Natl Acad Sci USA* 1994; 91:10109–10113.

24. Sadoshima J, Izumo S. Mechanical stretch rapidly activates multiple signal transduction pathways in cardiac myocytes: Potential involvement of an autocrine/paracrine mechanism. *EMBO J* 1993; 12:1681–1692.
25. Sugden PH, Clerk A. Regulation of mitogen-activated protein kinase cascades in the heart. *Adv Enzyme Regul* 1998; 38:87–98.
26. Hunter JJ, Chien KR. Signaling pathways for cardiac hypertrophy and failure. *N Engl J Med* 1999; 341:1276–1283.
27. Paradis P, Dali-Youcef N, Paradis FW, et al. Overexpression of angiotensin II type I receptor in cardiomyocytes induces cardiac hypertrophy and remodeling. *Proc Natl Acad Sci USA* 2000; 97:931–936.
28. Hirota H, Yoshida K, Kishimoto T, et al. Continuous activation of gp130, a signal-transducing receptor component for interleukin 6–related cytokines, causes myocardial hypertrophy in mice. *Proc Natl Acad Sci USA* 1995; 92:4862–4866.
29. Muller G, Ayoub M, Storz P, et al. PKC zeta is a molecular switch in signal transduction of TNF-alpha, bifunctionally regulated by ceramide and arachidonic acid. *EMBO J* 1995; 14:1961–1969.
30. Cummins P. Fibroblast and transforming growth factor expression in the cardiac myocyte. *Cardiovasc Res* 1993; 27:1150–1154.
31. Parker TG, Packer SE, Schneider MD. Peptide growth factors can provoke "fetal" contractile protein gene expression in rat cardiac myocytes. *J Clin Invest* 1990; 85:507–514.
32. Roberts AB, Roche NS, Winokur TS, et al. Role of transforming growth factor-β in maintenance of function of cultured neonatal cardiac myocytes. *J Clin Invest* 1992; 90:2056–2062.
33. Sacca L, Fazio S. Cardiac performance: Growth hormone enters the race. *Nat Med* 1996; 1:29–31.
34. Glennon PE, Kaddoura S, Sale EM, et al. Depletion of mitogen-activated protein kinase using an antisense oligodeoxynucleotide approach downregulates the phenylephrine induced hypertrophic response in rat cardiac myocytes. *Circ Res* 1996; 78:954–961.
35. Khoury SF, Hoit BD, Dave V, et al. Effects of thyroid hormone on left ventricular performance and regulation of contractile and Ca^{2+} cycling proteins in the baboon: Implications for the force-frequency and relaxation-frequency relationships. *Circ Res* 1996; 79:727–735.
36. Klemperer JD, Ojamaa K, Klein I. Thyroid hormone therapy in cardiovascular disease. *Prog Cardiovasc Dis* 1996; 38:329–336.
37. Klein I, Hong C. Effects of thyroid hormone on cardiac size and myosin content of the heterotopically transplanted rat heart. *J Clin Invest* 1986; 77:1694–1698.
38. Zhou MD, Sucov HM, Evans RM, et al. Retinoid-dependent pathways suppress myocardial cell hypertrophy. *Proc Natl Acad Sci USA* 1995; 92:7391–7395.
39. Wu J, Garami M, Cheng T, et al. 1,25(OH)$_2$ vitamin D$_3$ and retinoic acid antagonize endothelin-stimulated hypertrophy of neonatal rat cardiac myocytes. *J Clin Invest* 1996; 97:1577–1588.
40. Sei CA, Irons CE, Sprenkle AB, et al. The alpha-adrenergic stimulation of atrial natriuretic factor expression in cardiac myocytes requires calcium influx, protein kinase C, and calmodulin-regulated pathways. *J Biol Chem* 1991; 266:15910–15916.
41. Sadoshima J, Qiu Z, Morgan JP, et al. Angiotensin II and other hypertrophic stimuli mediated by G protein-coupled receptors activate tyrosine kinase, mitogen-activated protein kinase, and 90-kD S6 kinase in cardiac myocytes: The critical role of Ca^{2+}-dependent signaling. *Circ Res* 1995; 76:1–15.
42. Sugden PH. Signaling in myocardial hypertrophy: Life after calcineurin? *Circ Res* 1999; 84:633–646.
43. Walsh RA. Calcineurin inhibition as therapy for cardiac hypertrophy and heart failure: Requiescat in pace? *Circ Res* 1999; 84: 741–743.
44. Morgan HE, Gordon EE, Kira Y, et al. Biochemical mechanisms of cardiac hypertrophy. *Annu Rev Physiol* 1987; 49:533–543.
45. Hannan R, Luyken J, Rothblum LI. Regulation of ribosomal DNA transcription during contraction-induced hypertrophy of neonatal cardiomyocytes. *J Biol Chem* 1996; 271:3213–3220.
46. Samarel AM. Hemodynamic overload and the regulation of myofibrillar protein degradation. *Circulation* 1993; 87:1418–1420.
47. Samarel AM, Parmacek MS, Magid NM, et al. Protein synthesis and degradation during starvation-induced cardiac atrophy in rabbits. *Circ Res* 1987; 60:933–941.
48. Henkel RD, VandeBerg JL, Shade RE, et al. Cardiac beta myosin heavy chain diversity in normal and chronically hypertensive baboons. *J Clin Invest* 1989; 83:1487–1493.
49. Morkin E. Regulation of myosin heavy chain genes in the heart. *Circulation* 1993; 87:1451–1460.
50. Walsh RA, Henkel R, Robbins J. Cardiac myosin heavy- and light-chain gene expression in hypertrophy and heart failure. *Heart Failure* 1990; 6:238–243.
51. Boheler KR, Chassagne C, Martin X, et al. Cardiac expression of α- and β-myosin heavy chains and sarcomeric α-actins are regulated through transcriptional mechanisms. *J Biol Chem* 1992; 267:12979–12985.
52. Cooper G IV. Load and length regulation of cardiac energetics. *Annu Rev Physiol* 1990; 52:505–522.
53. Hixson JE, Henkel RD, Britten ML, et al. α-Myosin heavy chain cDNA structure and gene expression in adult, fetal, and premature baboon myocardium. *J Mol Cell Cardiol* 1989; 21:1073–1086.
54. Weber KT, Brilla CG. Pathological hypertrophy and cardiac interstitium. *Circulation* 1991; 83:1849–1865.
55. Borg T, Rubin K, Carver W, et al. The cell biology of the cardiac interstitium. *Trends Cardiovasc Med* 1991; 6:65–70.
56. Prockop DJ, Kivirikko KI. Collagens: Molecular biology, diseases, and potentials for therapy. *Annu Rev Biochem* 1995; 64:403–434.
57. Swynghedauw B. Molecular mechanisms of myocardial remodeling. *Physiol Rev* 1999; 79:215–262.
58. Schlaepfer DD, Hanks SK, Hunter T, et al. Integrin-mediated signal transduction linked to Ras pathway by GRB2 binding to focal adhesion kinase. *Nature* 1994; 372:786–791.
59. Takeishi Y, Abe J, Lee JD, et al. Differential regulation of p90 ribosomal S6 kinase and big mitogen-activated protein kinase 1 by ischemia/reperfusion and oxidative stress in perfused guinea pig hearts. *Circ Res* 1999; 85:1164–1172.
60. Collins JF, Pawloski-Dahm C, Davis MG, et al. The role of the cytoskeleton in left ventricular pressure overload hypertrophy and failure. *J Mol Cell Cardiol* 1996; 28:1435–1443.
61. Tsutsui H, Kshihara K, Cooper G. Cytoskeletal role in the contractile dysfunction of hypertrophied myocardium. *Science* 1993; 260:682–687.
62. Kadambi VJ, Ponniah S, Harrer JM, et al. Cardiac-specific overexpression of phospholamban alters calcium kinetics and resultant cardiomyocyte mechanics in transgenic mice. *J Clin Invest* 1996; 97:533–539.
63. Luo W, Grupp IL, Harrer J, et al. Targeted ablation of the phospholamban gene is associated with markedly enhanced myocardial contractility and loss of agonist stimulation. *Circ Res* 1994; 75:401–409.
64. Hart G. Cellular electrophysiology in cardiac hypertrophy and failure. *Cardiovasc Res* 1994; 28:933–946.
65. Pye MP, Cobbe SM. Mechanisms of ventricular arrhythmias in cardiac failure and hypertrophy. *Cardiovasc Res* 1992; 26: 740–750.
66. Severs NJ. Pathophysiology of gap junctions in heart disease. *J Cardiovasc Electrophysiol* 1994; 5:462–475.
67. Saffitz JE, Davis LM, Darrow BJ. The molecular basis of anisotropy: Role of gap junctions. *J Cardiovasc Electrophysiol* 1995; 6:498–510.

68. Curran ME, Splawski I, Timothy KW, et al. A molecular basis for cardiac arrhythmia: *HERG* mutations cause long QT syndrome. *Cell* 1995; 80:795–803.
69. Wang Q, Shen J, Splawski I, et al. *SCN5A* mutations associated with an inherited cardiac arrhythmia, long QT syndrome. *Cell* 1995; 80:805–811.
70. Sanguinetti MC, Jiang C, Curran ME, et al. A mechanistic link between an inherited and an acquired cardiac arrhythmia: *HERG* encodes the I_{kr} potassium channel. *Cell* 1995; 81:299–307.
71. Dorn GW II, Robbins J, Ball N, et al. Myosin heavy chain regulation and myocyte contractile depression after LV hypertrophy in aortic banded mice. *Am J Physiol* 1994; 267:H400–H405.
72. Kiss E, Ball N, Kranias EG, et al. Differential changes in cardiac phospholamban and sarcoplasmic reticular Ca^{2+}-ATPase protein levels: Effects on Ca^{2+} transport and mechanics in compensated pressure-overload hypertrophy and congestive heart failure. *Circ Res* 1995; 77:759–764.
73. Hoit BD, Shao Y, Gabel M, et al. Disparate effects of early pressure overload hypertrophy on velocity-dependent and force-dependent indices of ventricular performance in the conscious baboon. *Circulation* 1995; 91:1213–1220.
74. Cooper G IV, Tomanek RJ, Ehrhardt JC, et al. Chronic progressive pressure overload of the rat right ventricle. *Circ Res* 1981; 48:488–497.
75. Bing OHL, Matsushita S, Fanburg BL, et al. Mechanical properties of rat cardiac muscle during experimental hypertrophy. *Circ Res* 1971; 28:234–245.
76. Anderson PAW, Greig A, Mark TM, et al. Molecular basis of human cardiac troponin T isoforms expressed in the developing, adult, and failing heart. *Circ Res* 1995; 76:681–686.
77. Bache RJ. Effects of hypertrophy on the coronary circulation. *Prog Cardiovasc Dis* 1988; 31:403–440.
78. Breisch EA, White FC, Bloor CM. Myocardial characteristics of pressure overload hypertrophy: A structural and functional study. *Lab Invest* 1984; 51:333–342.
79. Murray PA, Vatner SF. Reduction of maximal coronary vasodilator capacity in conscious dogs with severe right ventricular hypertrophy. *Circ Res* 1981; 48:25–33.
80. Hultgren PB, Bove AA. Myocardial blood flow and mechanics in volume overload-induced left ventricular hypertrophy in dogs. *Cardiovas Res* 1981; 15:522–528.
81. Isoyama S, Ito N, Kuroha M, et al. Complete reversibility of physiological coronary vascular abnormalities in hypertrophied hearts produced by pressure overload in the rat. *J Clin Invest* 1989; 84:288–294.
82. Bolli R, Marbán E. Molecular and cellular mechanisms of myocardial stunning. *Physiol Rev* 1999; 79:609–634.
83. Murphy AM, Kogler H, Georgakopoulos D, et al. Transgenic mouse model of stunned myocardium. *Science* 2000; 287:488–491.
84. Anonymous. *Cardiovascular Physiology in the Genetically Engineered Mouse.* Norwell, MA: Kluwer Academic Publishers, 1998.
85. Teiger E, Dam TV, Richard L, et al. Apoptosis in pressure overload induced heart hypertrophy in the rat. *J Clin Invest* 1996; 97:2891–2897.
86. Cheng W, Li B, Kajstura J, et al. Stretch-induced programmed myocyte cell death. *J Clin Invest* 1995; 96:2247–2259.
87. Geisterfer-Lowrance AAT, Christe M, Conner DA, et al. A mouse model of familial hypertrophic cardiomyopathy. *Science* 1996; 272:731–734.
88. Iwase M, Bishop SP, Uechi M, et al. Adverse effects of chronic endogenous sympathetic drive induced by cardiac Gs α overexpression. *Circ Res* 1996; 78:517–524.
89. Edwards JG, Lyons GE, Micales BK, et al. Cardiomyopathy in transgenic *myf5* mice. *Circ Res* 1996; 78:379–387.
90. D'Agnolo A, Luciani GB, Mazzucco A, et al. Contractile properties and Ca^{2+} release activity of the sarcoplasmic reticulum in dilated cardiomyopathy. *Circulation* 1992; 85:518–525.
91. Schwinger RHG, Böhm M, Schmidt U, et al. Unchanged protein levels of SERCA II and phospholamban but reduced Ca^{2+} uptake and Ca^{2+}-ATPase activity of cardiac sarcoplasmic reticulum from dilated cardiomyopathy patients compared with patients with nonfailing hearts. *Circulation* 1995; 92:3220–3228.
92. Meyer M, Schillinger W, Pieske B, et al. Alterations of sarcoplasmic reticulum proteins in failing human dilated cardiomyopathy. *Circulation* 1995; 92:778–784.
93. Hasenfuss G, Reinecke H, Studer R, et al. Relation between myocardial function and expression of sarcoplasmic reticulum Ca^{2+}-ATPase in failing and nonfailing human myocardium. *Circ Res* 1994; 75:434–442.
94. Feldman AM, Weinberg EO, Ray PE, et al. Selective changes in cardiac gene expression during compensated hypertrophy and the transition to cardiac decompensation in rats with chronic aortic banding. *Circ Res* 1993; 73:184–192.
95. Gomez AM, Valdivia HH, Cheng H, et al. Defective excitation-contraction coupling in experimental cardiac hypertrophy and heart failure. *Science* 1997; 276:800–806.
96. D'Angelo DD, Sakata Y, Lorenz NJ, et al. Transgenic G alpha q overexpression induces cardiac contractile failure in mice. *Proc Natl Acad Sci USA* 1997; 94:8121–8126.
97. Sakata Y, Hoit BD, Liggett SB, et al. Decompensation of pressure-overload hypertrophy in G alpha q–overexpressing mice. *Circulation* 1998; 97:1488–1495.
98. Akhter SA, Luttrell LM, Rockman HA, et al. Targeting the receptor-Gq interface to inhibit in vivo pressure overload myocardial hypertrophy. *Science* 1998; 280:574–577.
99. Wakasaki H, Koya D, Schoen FJ, et al. Targeted overexpression of protein kinase C $beta_2$ isoform in myocardium causes cardiomyopathy. *Proc Natl Acad Sci USA* 1997; 94:9320–9325.
100. Takeishi Y, Chu G, Kirkpatrick DM, et al. In vivo phosphorylation of cardiac troponin I by protein kinase C $beta_2$ decreased cardiomyocyte calcium responsiveness and contractility in transgenic mouse hearts. *J Clin Invest* 1998; 102:72–78.
101. Bowling N, Walsh RA, Song G, et al. Increased protein kinase C activity and expression of Ca^{2+}-sensitive isoforms in the failing human heart. *Circulation* 1999; 99:384–391.
102. Jalili T, Takeishi Y, Song G, et al. PKC translocation without changes in G alpha q and PLC-beta protein abundance in cardiac hypertrophy and failure. *Am J Physiol* 1999; 277:H2298–H2304.
103. Paul K, Ball N, Dorn GW II, et al. Left ventricular stretch stimulates angiotensin II–mediated phosphatidylinositol hydrolysis and protein kinase C epsilon isoform translocation in adult guinea pig hearts. *Circ Res* 1997; 81:643–650.
104. Jalili T, Takeishi Y, Walsh RA. Signal transduction during cardiac hypertrophy: The role of G alpha q, PLC beta I, and PKC. *Cardiovasc Res* 1999; 44:5–9.
105. Guerra S, Leri A, Wang X, et al. Myocyte death in the failing human heart is gender dependent. *Circ Res* 1999; 85:856–866.
106. Hirota H, Chen J, Betz UA, et al. Loss of a gp130 cardiac muscle cell survival pathway is a critical event in the onset of heart failure during biomechanical stress. *Cell* 1999; 97:189–198.
107. Cohn JN, Bristow MR, Chien KR, et al. Report of the National Heart, Lung, and Blood Institute Special Emphasis Panel on Heart Failure Research. *Circulation* 1997; 95:766–770.

C H A P T E R 6

MOLECULAR AND CELLULAR BIOLOGY OF BLOOD VESSELS

Kathy K. Griendling / David G. Harrison / R. Wayne Alexander

It has become apparent that a diverse number of pathologic processes all contribute to common vascular diseases such as atherosclerosis and hypertension. During the past several years, these pathologic events have been defined with increasing clarity at a cellular and molecular level, and strategies are emerging to treat these primary processes rather than simply treating the secondary manifestations of vascular disease. Because of this, understanding normal function of vascular cells and how these are altered by various vascular insults has become essential for both basic investigators and clinicians caring for patients with peripheral vascular disease, coronary artery disease, and hypertension. This chapter is designed to introduce important concepts in vascular biology and to emphasize how fundamental aspects of vascular control are altered by common disease conditions.

STRUCTURE OF THE VESSEL WALL

Arteries consist of three layers: the innermost intima, the media, and the outermost adventitia. The intima is comprised of a single layer of endothelial cells embedded in an extracellular matrix. The internal elastic lamina separates the intima from the media. The media consists of smooth muscle cells, elastic laminae, bundles of collagen fibers, and elastic fibrils, all embedded in an extracellular matrix. The adventitia is the most variable layer, containing dense fibroelastic tissue, nutrient vessels, and nerves.

The actual composition of each of these layers varies with the type of blood vessel. Large, conduit arteries are typically referred to as *elastic arteries,* because of their high ratio of elastic laminae to smooth muscle cells. Muscular arteries are generally smaller and have a prevalence of smooth muscle cells, whereas arterioles consist of only one to two layers of smooth muscle cells. Capillaries are the smallest vessels, made up of a single layer of endothelial cells that are occasionally apposed to pericytes—smooth muscle-like cells that serve a contractile and synergistic nutritive function. The venous system has a similar architecture to that of the arterial system, the main difference being the orientation and mass of the smooth muscle cells within the wall.

Physiologically, the two best understood cell types in the vascular system are the endothelial and vascular smooth muscle cells (VSMCs). The endothelial cell is generally oriented with the direction of blood flow parallel to the main axis of the vessel. Endothelial cells are held together by junctional complexes that regulate permeability and control cell-to-cell communication. The smooth muscle cell is a spindle-shaped cell whose orientation varies with the type of artery, but is generally helical in large, elastic arteries and concentric in muscular arteries. Vascular smooth muscle cells contain three types of filaments: thick (myosin), thin (actin), and intermediate. The proteins that form these filaments undergo phosphorylation upon exposure to certain vasoactive agonists, thus altering their orientation and interactions and supporting force development (see below). In normal arteries, the smooth muscle cells are primarily in the aforementioned *contractile* phenotype. In contrast, in response to vascular insults such as hyperlipidemia or angioplasty, smooth muscle cells lose their contractile phenotype and acquire a so-called *synthetic* phenotype. This is characterized by a loss of contractile proteins, a rounded shape, and a dramatic change in biochemical properties. This change in phenotype and function is thought to be important in the genesis of the myointimal cell that populates the atherosclerotic subintimal space.

PHYSIOLOGY OF THE ENDOTHELIAL CELL

Normal endothelial cell function is crucial to homeostasis in the vascular system. During the past decade, it has become apparent that diseases such as atherosclerosis are ultimately manifestations of endothelial dysfunction. The endothelium has three major functions: (1) it is a metabolically active secretory tissue; (2) it serves as an anticoagulant, antithrombotic surface; and (3) it provides a barrier to the indiscriminant passage of blood constituents into the arterial wall. The implications of these physiologic properties for vascular biology will be considered separately.

Endothelial Cell Metabolism and Secretion of Vasoactive Factors

As discussed in more detail below, endothelial cells secrete vasoactive substances that play a major role in the control of vascular tone. These molecules include vasodilators such as prostacyclin, endothelial-derived relaxing factor (EDRF), and endothelial-derived hyperpolarizing factor (EDHF).[1-3] In addition, the endothelium produces vasoconstrictor substances, including endothelin[4] and vasoconstrictor prostanoids.[5]

Endothelial cells also manufacture and secrete substances such as factor VIII antigen, von Willebrand's factor, tissue factor, thrombomodulin, and tissue plasminogen activator, which are all involved in coagulation/fibrinolytic pathways. Structural components of the extracellular matrix synthesized by these cells include collagen, elastin, glycosaminoglycans, and fibronectin.[6,7] The composition of the extracellular matrix is dynamically modulated by matrix metalloproteinases, enzymes that degrade matrix protein and participate in its remodeling. These enzymes are secreted by both endothelial and smooth muscle cells.[8,9] In addition, endothelial cells synthesize and secrete heparans and growth factors that regulate smooth muscle cell proliferation.[10-13] Finally, endothelial cells are able to clear and metabolically alter bloodborne and locally produced substances, including plasma lipids and lipoproteins,[14] adenine nucleotides and nucleosides,[15] serotonin, catecholamines, bradykinin, and angiotensin I.[16]

Endothelial cells are involved in the metabolism of plasma lipids in several ways. Lipoprotein lipase, an enzyme that hydrolyzes triglycerides into constituent fatty acids, is bound to the endothelial cell surface by heparan sulfates.[17] The interaction of this enzyme with chylomicrons or very low density lipoprotein (VLDL) particles results in the release of free fatty acids, which can then cross the subendothelial space to the underlying smooth muscle or inflammatory cells in atherosclerosis. In addition, endothelial cells possess receptors for low-density lipoprotein (LDL),[18] which regulate the transport and modification of LDL. Normally, LDL receptors are downregulated because receptor processing is inhibited in the nonproliferating monolayer.[18] There are, however, two other pathways for uptake of LDL. First, LDL can be transported across the endothelium by an unknown, active, receptor-independent mechanism.[19] Second, modified, or oxidized LDL can be taken up by "scavenger" LDL receptors,[20] the expression of which is unaffected by the growth state of the endothelial cells. These cells also have the capacity to modify LDL,[21] thus enhancing its uptake and ultimately leading to an increase in cholesterol esters in the vessel wall and, importantly, facilitating LDL uptake by inflammatory cells in disease.

The Endothelial Cell and Thrombosis

Quiescent endothelial cells normally present an antithrombotic surface that resists platelet adhesion and does not activate coagulation. (For a more detailed discussion of thrombosis, see Chap. 44.) The continuity of the endothelium is essential to this function, and nonthrombogenicity has been attributed in part to the negative charge on the surface of these cells.[22] Endothelial cells are, however, capable of synthesizing and secreting prothrombotic factors, especially when stimulated with cytokines or other inflammatory agents. The endothelium thus represents a functional antithrombotic-thrombolytic/thrombotic balance. Potent anticoagulants elaborated by the endothelium include prostacyclin, which inhibits platelet aggregation,[23] heparin-like molecules,[24] and thrombomodulin, which activates protein C.[25] In addition, antithrombin III binds to the surface-bound heparin-like molecules and serves as a clearance (via internalization) molecule for thrombin, as well as a thrombin inhibitor.[26] These cells also produce tissue plasminogen activator (tPA) and plasminogen activator inhibitor I (PAI-I), and can bind plasminogen on their surface via fibronectin and thrombospondin.[27] The relative amounts of tPA and PAI-I can be upregulated or downregulated, respectively, by thrombin, angiotensin II, and other vasoactive substances to control clot lysis.[28]

As alluded to earlier, the endothelium, under conditions of injury or inflammation, may become prothrombotic (Fig. 6-1). On stimulation with inflammatory cytokines, endothelial cells increase the surface expression of tissue factor[29] and leukocyte adhesion molecules,[30] and decrease the expression of thrombomodulin.[29] Thrombin itself stimulates further production of von Willebrand's factor,[31] which, along with thrombospondin and fibronectin, participates in the thrombotic response. Furthermore, endothelial cells can bind factor IX,[32] which, when tissue factor is expressed, can be activated by tissue factor VIIa complex, leading to activation of factor X in the presence of factor VIII. Activated factor X (Xa) can then promote assembly of the prothrombinase complex. Thus, under inflammatory conditions, endothelial cells can amplify the prothrombotic response. Not all of the factors controlling the expression of pro- and antithrombotic/fibrinolytic molecules are known, but it is clear that the endothelium functions as a major regulator of hemostasis.

Barrier Function and Endothelial Cell Permeability

There are three ways that the endothelium regulates influx of macromolecules into the arterial wall: intercellular tight junctions, vesicles and/or transendothelial channels, and the lipid phase of the endothelial membrane. These pathways enable the intact endothelium to serve as a barrier, preventing or impeding highly mitogenic, thrombotic, or vasoactive substances from

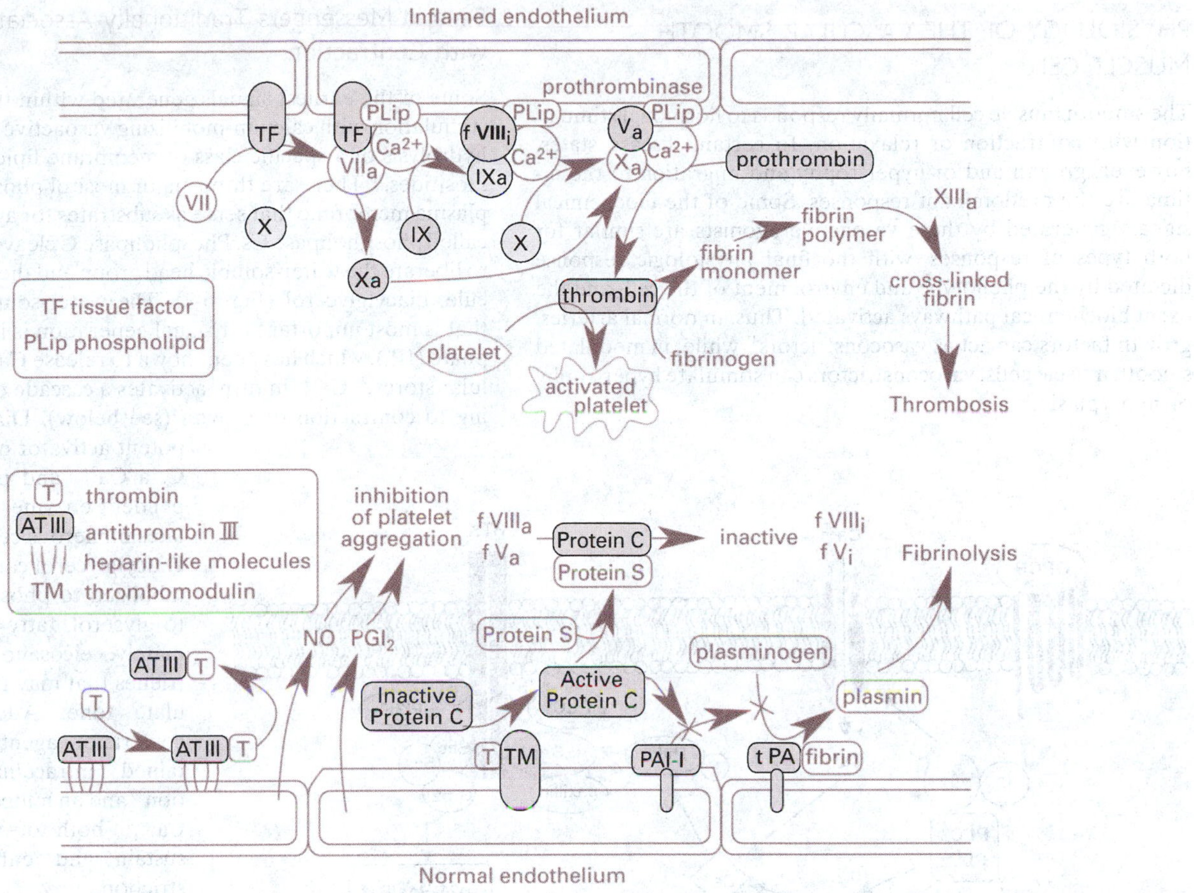

FIGURE 6-1 Pathways of thrombosis and thrombolysis. Under normal conditions, the endothelium is antithrombotic. Antithrombin III (ATIII) binds thrombin and serves to clear thrombin from the circulation. Prostacyclin (prostaglandin I_2, PGI_2) inhibits platelet aggregation, and thrombomodulin (TM) activates protein C, which inhibits plasminogen activator inhibitor I (PAI-I) and interacts with protein S to inactivate activated factors V and VIII, thus limiting thrombosis. Since PAI-I inhibits the tissue plasminogen activator (tPA)-catalyzed conversion of plasminogen to plasmin, PAI-I inhibition leads to accumulation of plasmin and fibrinolysis. Upon stimulation with inflammatory cytokines, there is increased expression of tissue factor on the endothelial cell surface. Tissue factor participates in the activation of factor X, which, in turn, promotes assembly of the prothrombinase complex, producing thrombin. Under these conditions, endothelial cells thus amplify the thrombotic response. (Courtesy of Bernard Lassègue, Ph.D.)

coming into direct contact with the underlying vascular smooth muscle. Each route has both active and passive components, and the extent to which they are utilized depends to a certain degree on the location of the endothelial cells. Thus, capillaries and postcapillary venules respond to vasoactive agents, some of which (histamine, prostaglandins) are secreted by the endothelial cell itself, with increased flux through tight junctions.[33] The tight junctions found in arteries tend to be more occlusive, but may also be influenced by hypertension[34] and various agonists. Vesicular transport is mainly utilized by the cell to transfer water-soluble macromolecules from the luminal surface to the abluminal surface, but the permanence of such structures and whether they form transendothelial channels is a matter of debate. It has recently been shown that caveolae, vesicles containing the structural protein caveolin that are pinched off from the plasma membrane, are involved in transendothelial transport of macromolecules. Multiple such vesicles may link together to form functional pores from the luminal to abluminal surface.[35,36] Lipid-phase transport has been proposed as a mechanism whereby lipid-soluble molecules (e.g., free fatty acids) could be transferred to the abluminal surface of the endothelial cell.[37] These molecules could enter the outer leaflet of the membrane from the circulation and diffuse along the lipid bilayer to be released or bind to extracellular matrix components in the subintimal area.

Another major mechanism modulating endothelial barrier formation occurs via contraction of these cells in a fashion analogous to smooth muscle contraction. This occurs in response to a variety of agonists, including thrombin, histamine, and ionomycin, and results in cell shape change that opens gap junctions between cells. It is likely that this contractile response is a major mechanism for edema formation in response to histamine and bradykinin and is also involved in solute transport. This phenomenon is mediated by a series of intracellular signaling events, including activation of protein kinase C, myosin light chain phosphorylation, activation of tyrosine kinases, and stimulation of the small G-protein Rho.[38–40]

Thus, the endothelium has both passive and active roles in the control of vascular permeability by acting as a physical permeability barrier and by modulating the expression of cell surface and secreted agonists and molecules that are capable of altering permeability.

PHYSIOLOGY OF THE VASCULAR SMOOTH MUSCLE CELL

The smooth muscle cell normally responds to hormonal stimulation with contraction or relaxation. In certain disease states, however, growth and/or hypertrophy and migration to the intima are the predominant responses. Some of the biochemical signals generated by these vasoactive agonists are similar for both types of responses, with the final physiologic response dictated by the phenotype and environment of the cell, and the exact biochemical pathways activated. Thus, in normal arteries, growth factors can act as vasoconstrictors[41] while, in modulated smooth muscle cells, vasoconstrictors can stimulate hypertrophy or hyperplasia.[42]

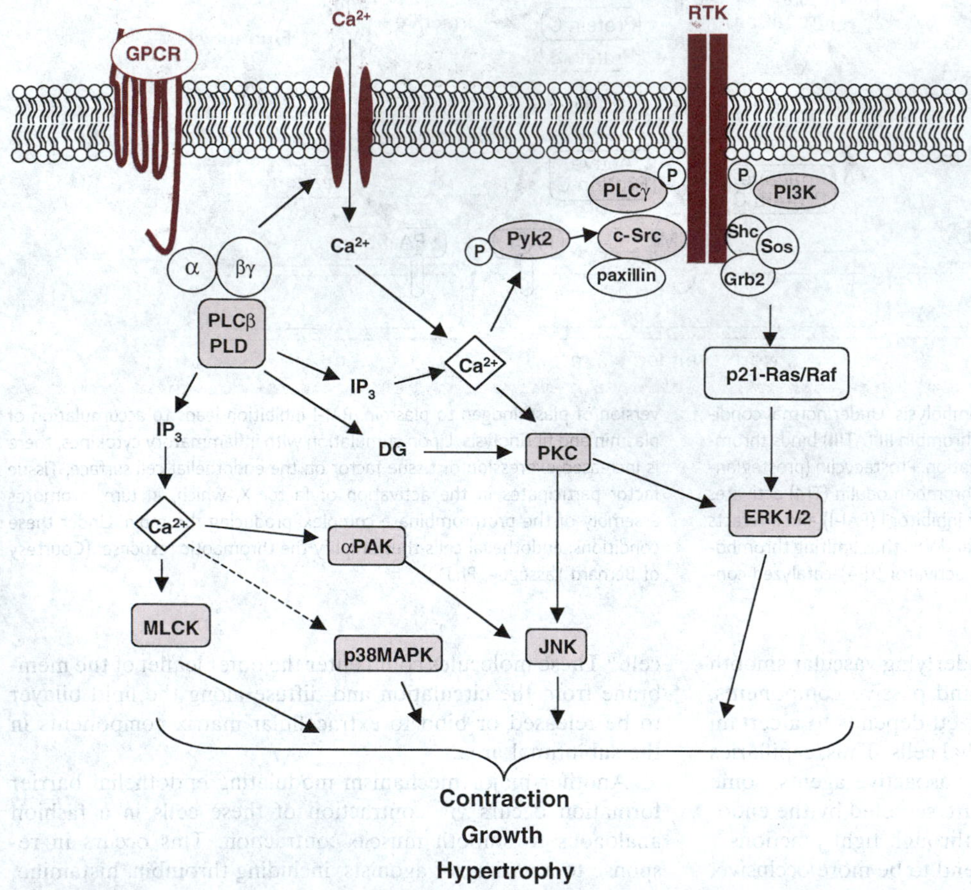

FIGURE 6-2 Signaling pathways in vascular smooth muscle. Vasoconstrictor agonists interact with specific G protein-coupled receptors (GPCRs) on vascular smooth muscle. These receptors are linked to a heterotrimeric G protein ($\alpha\beta\gamma$), which then couples to one or more phospholipase Cs (PLCs) or phospholipase D (PLD). PLC cleaves the inositol phospholipids to yield diacylglycerol (DG) and inositol phosphates, in particular, inositol trisphosphate (IP_3). IP_3 releases calcium from intracellular stores, and, along with DG, activates the Ca^{2+}- and phospholipid-dependent enzyme protein kinase C (PKC). Ca^{2+} activates numerous other kinases, including p21-activated kinase (αPAK), Pyk2, and myosin light chain kinase (MLCK). PLD cleaves phosphatidylcholine to release phosphatidic acid, which is converted to DG. PKC is involved in activation of the mitogen-activated protein kinase (MAPK) cascade, including extracellular signal-regulated kinases (ERK1/2) and Jun kinase (JNK). Growth factors activate receptor tyrosine kinases (RTKs), Src, PLC-γ, and phosphatidylinositol 3-kinase (PI3K). RTKs also phosphorylate and form a signaling complex with paxillin and adapter proteins such as Shc, which binds Grb-2 and Sos and ultimately mediates the conversion of Ras to its active form. Ras phosphorylates Raf1, which in turn leads to activation of the MAP Kinase cascade.

Second Messengers Traditionally Associated with Contraction

Some of the earliest signals generated within the cell following stimulation with calcium-mobilizing vasoactive agonists involve hydrolysis of a specific class of membrane lipids: the phosphoinositides.[43] There are three major inositol phospholipids in the plasma membrane that serve as substrates for a class of enzymes called phospholipase Cs. Phospholipase C cleaves phospholipids to liberate the water-soluble head group and the lipophilic molecule, diacylglycerol (Fig. 6-2). The water-soluble head group that is most important for signal generation is inositol trisphosphate (IP_3), which has been shown to release Ca^{2+} from intracellular stores.[44] Ca^{2+}, in turn, activates a cascade of enzymes leading to contraction or growth (see below). Diacylglycerol is a potent activator of protein kinase C, a Ca^{2+}- and phospholipid-dependent enzyme that phosphorylates numerous cellular proteins.[45] Diacylglycerol can be further metabolized to phosphatidic acid or to glycerol, fatty acids, and, ultimately, eicosanoids and leukotrienes that may themselves modulate tone. Additionally vasoconstrictor agents cause a sustained intracellular alkalinization[46] and an influx of extracellular Ca^{2+},[47] both of which serve to sustain and enhance vasoconstriction.

Contraction Cascade

Contractions induced by various vasoactive hormones differ not only in magnitude and time course, but also differ between vessels. In general, there is an initial, rapid component of force generation and a more sustained phase of contraction. Some agonists, such as angiotensin II, induce only a transient constriction of many vessels, whereas others, including norepinephrine and vasopressin, nearly always cause a sustained contraction. The initial phase of force development has been shown to depend on the formation of actin-myosin cross-bridges, but the mechanisms underlying the sustained phase of contraction are less clear.

A sliding-filament mechanism similar to that found in skeletal muscle is thought to regulate phasic contraction of smooth muscle. Force generation is accomplished by attachment of the myosin heads (or cross-bridges) to actin fila-

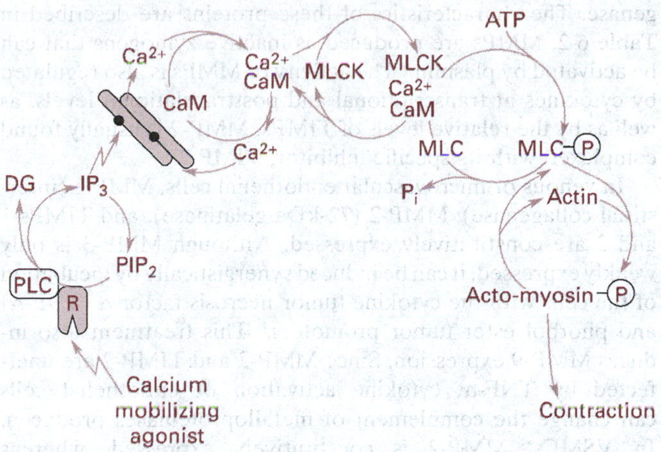

FIGURE 6-3 Contraction cascade. Activation of smooth muscle by a vasoconstrictor hormone leads to a cascade of biochemical signals, ultimately resulting in phosphorylation of actomyosin, cross-bridge formation, and force generation. The release of Ca^{2+} from intracellular stores is one of the major initiating events, since Ca^{2+} combines with calmodulin to activate myosin light chain kinase. This enzyme phosphorylates the myosin light chain, which is then able to interact with actin. ABBREVIATIONS: R = receptor; PLC = phospholipase C; DG = diacylglycerol; PIP_2 = phosphatidylinositol 4,5-bisphosphate; IP_3 = inositol trisphosphate; CaM = calmodulin; MLCK = myosin light chain kinase; MLC = myosin light chain; P = phosphate. (Courtesy of Bernard Lassègue, Ph.D.)

ments. This attachment catalyzes ATP hydrolysis to generate tension and occurs in a cyclic manner for the duration of the stimulus. Smooth muscle has a relatively greater content of actin and a lower content of myosin than does skeletal muscle and, in contrast to skeletal muscle, the major site of calcium regulation of smooth muscle actomyosin is on the myosin molecule. Smooth muscle myosin consists of two large subunits, each with a molecular weight of 200 kDa, and two small subunits of 20 and 16 to 17 kDa, known as the *myosin light chains*. Force generation in smooth muscle is regulated by the phosphorylation/dephosphorylation of the 20-kDa protein (Fig. 6-3). Once phosphorylation occurs, actin-activated Mg^{2+}-ATPase activity is stimulated, resulting in cross-bridge cycling. Myosin light chain phosphorylation is mediated by an enzyme known as myosin light chain kinase (MLCK). This protein associates with calmodulin, a calcium-binding protein required for activation of numerous cytoplasmic enzymes. Thus, when Ca^{2+} increases within the cell in response to hormonal stimulation, it binds to calmodulin, which, in turn, associates with MLCK, converting it from an inactive to an active form. MLCK then phosphorylates the myosin light chain, enabling actin activation of the Mg^{2+}-ATPase ultimately resulting in cross-bridge formation. When the intracellular Ca^{2+} concentration drops below about 100 nM, Ca^{2+} dissociates from calmodulin, calmodulin detaches from MLCK, and MLCK becomes inactive. Myosin light chain phosphatase activity then predominates, myosin is dephosphorylated, and cross-bridge cycling ceases. During sustained contraction, however, the intracellular Ca^{2+} concentration is low, and energy consumption is reduced, suggesting the development of a latch-bridge, or of a low cycling state.[48] Alternatively, the sensitivity of the contractile apparatus to Ca^{2+} may be increased, a response posited to be regulated by protein kinase C.[49]

Biochemical Signals Traditionally Associated with Proliferation

Classic growth factors, such as platelet-derived growth factor (PDGF), activate many of the same signaling pathways as do vasoconstrictors: phosphoinositide hydrolysis, Ca^{2+} mobilization and influx, Na^+/H^+ exchange and intracellular alkalinization. Receptors for these growth factors are intrinsic tyrosine kinases, leading to the tyrosine phosphorylation of numerous proteins that are essential for growth. The importance of tyrosine phosphorylation in mediating the growth response is shown by the observation that mutant PDGF receptors, which lack the normal, intrinsic tyrosine kinase domain, are incapable of mediating proliferation in response to PDGF.[50] In addition, tyrosine kinase inhibitors have been shown to inhibit growth.[51] There is also increasing evidence that tyrosine phosphatases can counteract the mitogenic effects of growth factors by inhibiting tyrosine phosphorylation of specific substrates.[52]

A complex of substrates becomes associated with activated growth factor receptors and subsequently activates multiple signaling cascades leading to the final cellular response.[53] Some proteins, such as phospholipase C-γ, the tyrosine kinase c-Src, and phosphatidylinositol-3-kinase, bind directly to receptor tyrosine kinases, whereas others, including the tyrosine kinase Pyk-2 and the cytoskeletal protein paxillin, associate with the receptor via linker proteins such as Grb and Shc. Upon addition of growth factors, the receptors dimerize and auto-tyrosine phosphorylate, and each of the aforementioned proteins is phosphorylated on tyrosine, presumably leading, either directly or indirectly via association with the activated receptor, to their activation. In addition, Shc and Grb2 link these receptors to Ras, a ubiquitous GTPase that initiates a kinase cascade that includes mitogen-activated protein kinase (MAP kinase) and ultimately leads to growth. Recent evidence suggests that many of these proteins are also activated by seven-transmembrane-spanning G-protein-coupled receptors,[54] an observation that may partially explain the growth-promoting properties of some vasoconstrictor hormones.

An additional pathway that is activated under some conditions by growth factors and vasoactive agonists is phospholipase D-mediated hydrolysis of plasma membrane phosphatidylcholine.[55] In this reaction, phosphatidic acid and choline are released. This pathway is receiving increasing attention because phosphatidic acid may have a role in mediating the growth response[56] and because phospholipase D activation seems to be required for the proliferative response.[57]

Growth

Vascular smooth muscle cell growth occurs via two processes: hypertrophy and hyperplasia. In general, hypertrophy occurs in response to long-term stimulation with vasoconstrictor-type agents, whereas hyperplasia occurs in response to the classic growth factors. Hypertrophy is characterized by an increase in smooth muscle cell mass due to increased protein synthesis and has been shown to occur in response to angiotensin II[58] and thrombin[59] and in large vessels during hypertension. Hyperplasia is characterized by cell replication and is stimulated by growth factors such as PDGF and fibroblast growth factor (FGF)[60-62] following vascular injury. The biochemical processes leading to hypertrophy and hyperplasia are currently under investigation. It is clear that the aforementioned tyrosine kinase pathways are important in both types of growth.[53,54] In addition, generation of reactive oxygen species, including superoxide and hydrogen peroxide, serves to transduce the growth signal by activating specific proteins such as p38 mitogen-activated protein kinase and Akt/protein kinase B.[63,64]

THE EXTRACELLULAR MATRIX

The extracellular matrix is a major component of the vessel wall. It is the medium through which nutrients are transported, a repository for products secreted by the cells of the vascular wall, the site of accumulation of cell debris, and a substrate for migration and proliferation of endothelial cells, monocytes, and vascular smooth muscle cells. The matrix consists of several proteins that have distinct functions in maintaining the integrity of the wall (Table 6-1).

Extracellular matrix degradation and reformation is an extremely important biological process with profound clinical implications. It is impossible for vascular cells to hypertrophy, proliferate, or migrate without an initial degradation of the matrix. One of the earliest events in angiogenesis is the degradation of the extracellular matrix to enable tube (capillary) formation. Vascular cells, including endothelial cells, VSMCs, resident macrophages and fibroblasts, may secrete matrix metalloproteinases (MMPs), enzymes that selectively digest the individual components of the matrix. In addition, these cells elaborate tissue inhibitors of metalloproteinases (TIMPs).[8]

MMPs belong to three main groups: the type IV collagenases (also called gelatinases), the stromelysins, and interstitial collagenase. The characteristics of these proteins are described in Table 6-2. MMPs are produced as inactive zymogens that can be activated by plasmin.[9] The activity of MMPs is also regulated by cytokines at transcriptional and posttranslational levels, as well as by the relative levels of TIMPs. MMP-2 is usually found complexed with its specific inhibitor, TIMP-2.

In venous or microvascular endothelial cells, MMP-1 (interstitial collagenase), MMP-2 (72-kDa gelatinase), and TIMPs-1 and 2 are constitutively expressed. Although MMP-3 is only weakly expressed, it can be induced synergistically by incubation of the cells with the cytokine tumor necrosis factor α (TNF-α) and phorbol ester tumor promoters.[8] This treatment also induces MMP-9 expression. Since MMP-2 and TIMP-2 are unaffected by TNF-α, cytokine activation of endothelial cells can change the complement of metalloproteinases produced. In VSMCs, MMP-2 is constitutively expressed, whereas MMP-1, MMP-9 (92-kDa gelatinase), and MMP-3 (stromelysin) are induced by cytokines such as interleukin 1 and TNF-α.[9] Cytokines can also activate MMP-2 zymogen.[65] Thus, cytokine stimulation increases the range of active metalloproteinases secreted by smooth muscle cells to encompass proteases capable of degrading all the major matrix components. In contrast, although TIMP-1 and TIMP-2 are constitutively expressed by vascular smooth muscle, their expression is unaffected by cytokines.[9] The net effect of cytokines on the vascular wall may be to tip the balance between the production of MMPs and TIMPs in favor of extracellular matrix degradation and remodeling.

Of particular importance, several reactive oxygen species have been shown to stimulate both activation and expression of MMPs, in particular MMP-9.[66,67] This is likely to be very important in diseases like atherosclerosis and hypertension, where vascular oxidant stress is increased. Activated macrophages accumulate at shoulder regions of the atherosclerotic plaque and secrete both MMPs and reactive oxygen species,[66,68] contributing to plaque rupture in this region.

TABLE 6-1 Components of the Extracellular Matrix

Matrix Component	Function
Proteoglycans	Resistance to deformation Arterial permeability, filtration, ion exchange Transport and deposition of plasma elements Regulation of cellular metabolism
Collagens (types I and III)	Mechanical strength
Collagens (types IV, V, and VI)	Attachment of vascular cells to the matrix Components of the basal lamina Linking collagens to noncollagenous structures
Elastin	Regulation of vascular elasticity
Fibronectin	Cell-cell adhesion Cell-substrate adhesion Cell motility Specific binding of collagen, heparin
Laminin	Attachment of endothelial cells to type IV collagen

ENDOTHELIAL CELL-VASCULAR SMOOTH MUSCLE INTERACTIONS

Endothelial Control of Vascular Tone

The endothelium serves a dual function in the control of vascular tone (Fig. 6-4). It secretes relaxing factors such as nitric oxide and adenosine, and constricting factors such as the endothelins. Vessel tone thus depends on the balance between these factors, as well as on the ability of the smooth muscle cell to respond to them. The most important regulatory molecules are discussed separately.

ENDOTHELIUM-DERIVED RELAXING FACTOR/NITRIC OXIDE

An EDRF was first described by Furchgott and Zawadzki,[2] who observed that aortic rings dilated in response to acetylcholine only when the rings maintained an intact endothelium. The predominant form of EDRF, derived from L-arginine by the action of the enzyme nitric oxide synthase (NOS), is nitric oxide (NO), or a closely related nitroso compound.[62]

Many factors have been shown to regulate the release of EDRF/NO[69] by increasing intracellular Ca^{2+}. These include hormones such as acetylcholine, norepinephrine, bradykinin,

TABLE 6-2 Matrix Metalloproteinases and Inhibitors

Class	Nomenclature	Molecular Weight[a]	Vascular Cell Type	Expression
Interstitial collagenase	MMP-1	~45	VSMC, EC, microvascular EC	Inducible by PDGF, PMA, IL-1, VEGF
Type IV collagenase	MMP-9, gelatinase B, type V gelatinase	92	VSMC, EC	Inducible by IL-1α, PMA; inhibited by retinoic acid
	MMP-2, gelatinase A, type IV gelatinase	72	VSMC, wounded EC, microvascular EC	Constitutive, ↑ by TNF-α, IL-1α (VSMC); ⇅ by retinoic acid (EC)
Stromelysin	MMP-3	50	VSMC, EC, microvascular EC	Inducible by IL-1 (VSMC); TNF-α, PMA (EC)
TIMP-1	Inhibits MMPs	30	VSMC, EC, microvascular EC	Constitutive
TIMP-2	Inhibits MMP-2	~20	VSMC, EC, microvascular EC	Constitutive, ↑ by retinoic acid (EC)

[a]The molecular weight of MMP-1 and MMP-3 depends on the species.
ABBREVIATIONS: EC = endothelial cell; IL = interleukin; MMP = matrix metalloproteinase; PDGF = platelet-derived growth factor; PMA = phorbol 12,13-myrisate acetate; TIMP = tissue inhibitor of metalloproteinase; TNF = tumor necrosis factor; VEGF = vascular endothelial growth factor;
VSMC = vascular smooth muscle cell.

thrombin, ATP, and vasopressin; the platelet-derived factors, serotonin and histamine; fatty acids; ionophores; and physical forces. NO easily crosses the smooth muscle cell membrane and binds to the heme moiety of the soluble guanylate cyclase, thereby enhancing the formation of cyclic GMP. Cyclic GMP, in turn, reduces intracellular Ca^{2+} concentrations leading todephosphorylation of the myosin light chain and relaxation.[70] It should be noted that the drug nitroglycerin exerts its vasodilator effects by being converted to NO, thus substituting for a natural product. Deficiency in release of active NO is an important contributing factor leading to vasospasm.

NO is produced by the action of the enzyme NOS, which oxidizes the guanidino nitrogens of L-arginine to form citrulline and NO. This enzyme has been cloned from brain (nNOS, for neuronal NOS, type I),[71] macrophages (iNOS, for inducible NOS, type II),[72] and endothelial cells (eNOS, for endothelial NOS, type III).[73] The three isoforms of NOS share important consensus sequences for NADPH, flavin adenine dinucleotide, and flavin mononucleotide cofactor-binding sites, as well

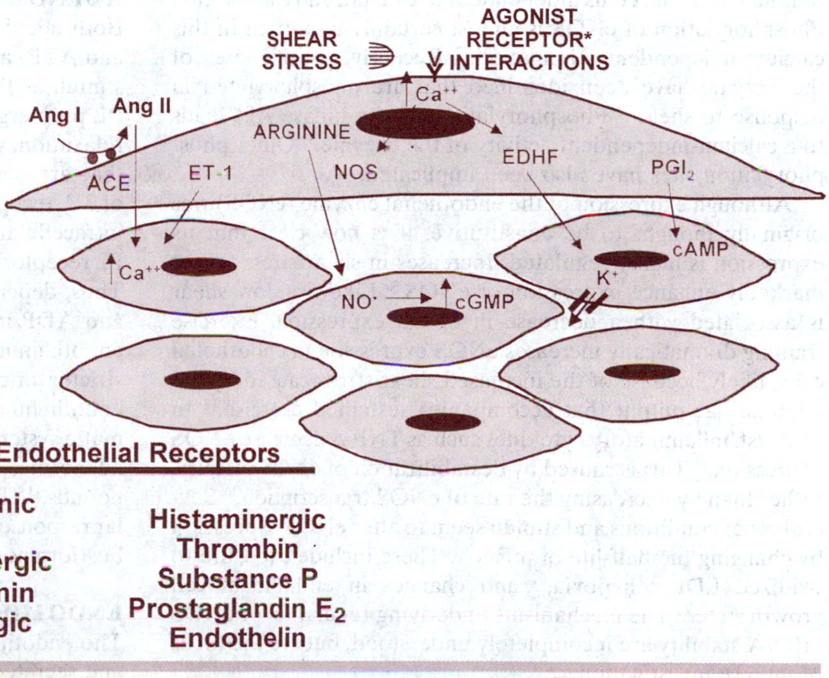

FIGURE 6-4 Endothelial control of vascular tone. Endothelial cells synthesize and secrete both vasodilator substances (NO, EDHF, and PGI_2) and vasoconstrictor compounds (Ang II and ET-1). Secretion of these factors occurs in response to receptor stimulation and hemodynamic forces such as shear stress. Vessel tone depends on the balance between these factors, as well as on the ability of the smooth muscle cells to respond to them. ABBREVIATIONS: NO· = nitric oxide; NOS = nitric oxide synthase; EDHF = endothelial-derived hyperpolarizing factor; PGI_2 = prostaglandin I_2; ACE = angiotensin-converting enzyme; Ang = angiotensin; ET-1 = endothelin-1; cGMP = cyclic guanosine monophosphate; cAMP = cyclic adenosine monophosphate; 5-HT-5-hydroxytryptamine.

as a Ca^{2+}-calmodulin-binding site. During the past several years, a great deal has been learned about how these enzymes function.[74] All NO synthases function as homodimers, and each subunit consists of a carboxy-terminal reductase domain and an amino-terminal oxygenase domain, connected by a calmodulin-binding region. The NADPH- and flavin-binding sites reside in the reductase domain, where electrons derived from NADPH are stored by the flavins. For both the neuronal and endothelial isoforms of the enzymes, increases in intracellular calcium lead to calmodulin binding to the calmodulin-binding site, which in turn enables electrons to flow from the reductase domain to the amino-terminal oxygenase domain. This region contains binding sites for heme, tetrahydrobiopterin, and L-arginine. Electrons transferred from the reductase domain are initially bound by the ferrous iron in the prosthetic heme group. The precise role of tetrahydrobiopterin remains unknown, although it appears critical in allowing electrons to be transferred from the heme to the guanidino nitrogens of L-arginine, resulting in the formation of NO. Interestingly, when tetrahydrobiopterin or L-arginine is absent, the electron flows to molecular oxygen, resulting in the formation of the superoxide anion.[75] This phenomenon has been termed *uncoupling* of NOS, and there are substantial data that this may occur in a variety of disease states, perhaps because of oxidation of tetrahydrobiopterin.

Although increases in intracellular calcium clearly activate eNOS via stimulation of calmodulin, there are additional ways that the enzyme is activated that seem independent of calmodulin or calcium. For example, shear stress acutely stimulates the release of NO from the endothelium, and this depends only on calcium during the first few seconds of the response.[76] The continued activation of eNOS in response to several minutes or hours of shear seems independent of calcium and calmodulin. Phosphorylation of eNOS is almost certainly important in this calcium-independent stimulation.[77] Recently, specific sites of the enzyme have been identified that are phosphorylated in response to shear.[78] Phosphorylation by the kinase Akt leads to a calcium-independent activity of the enzyme.[79] Other phosphorylation sites have also been implicated.

Although expression of the endothelial enzyme (eNOS) was originally thought to be constitutive, it is now clear that its expression is highly regulated. Increases in shear stress rather markedly enhance expression of eNOS.[80] Likewise, low shear is associated with a decrease in eNOS expression. Exercise training dramatically increases eNOS expression in endothelial cells, likely because of the increased shear stress caused by the high cardiac output that accompanies sustained exercise.[81] In contrast, inflammatory cytokines such as TNF-α decrease eNOS expression.[73] This is caused by destabilization of eNOS mRNA, rather than by decreasing the rate of eNOS transcription.[82] Several other conditions and stimuli seem to alter eNOS expression by changing the half-life of mRNA. These include exposure to oxidized LDL,[83] hypoxia,[84] and changes in endothelial cell growth state.[85] The mechanisms underlying regulation of eNOS mRNA stability are incompletely understood, but are the focus of intense investigation.

ENDOTHELIUM-DERIVED HYPERPOLARIZING FACTOR

Shortly after the identification of the EDRF, it was suspected that the endothelium could release more than one relaxing factor, depending on the vessel size, the stimulus, and the species studied. Initial studies showed that some vasodilators produce hyperpolarization of the vascular smooth muscle membrane in an endothelium-dependent manner. It is now clear that this is due to the release of a hyperpolarizing factor from the endothelium that is almost certainly different than NO.[86] Its production is stimulated by many of the same stimuli that evoke the release of NO and depends on intracellular calcium. Although there is some debate regarding the nature of this factor, increasing evidence suggests that it is a cytochrome P450 metabolite of arachidonic acid and perhaps other fatty acids.[87] This epoxide, when released from the endothelium, opens calcium-activated potassium channels in the adjacent vascular smooth muscle, resulting in vasodilation.[88] It has also been shown that these epoxides have important anti-inflammatory effects.[89]

PROSTACYCLIN

Prostacyclin, or prostaglandin I_2 (PGI_2), which is a prostanoid derived from the action of cyclooxygenase on arachidonic acid, is released by the endothelium and relaxes vascular smooth muscle by increasing its intracellular content of cyclic AMP.[90] Prostacyclin is also platelet suppressant and antithrombotic, and reduces the release of growth factors from endothelial cells and macrophages.[23] Among the agonists that stimulate prostacyclin synthesis are bradykinin (one of the most potent), substance P, platelet-derived growth factor and epidermal growth factor, and adenine nucleotides,[23] whereas aspirin has been shown to inhibit it transiently. Therapeutically, the debate about the appropriate dose of aspirin in ischemic coronary syndromes revolves around finding a dose that will inhibit platelet function without inhibiting endothelial PGI_2 synthesis.

ADENOSINE AND RELATED COMPOUNDS

Both adenine nucleosides (adenosine) and nucleotides (ADP and ATP) are released by the endothelium in response to such stimuli as thrombin[91] and flow.[92] Adenine nucleosides bind to P1 purinergic receptors that activate cyclic AMP leading to relaxation, whereas adenine nucleotides stimulate P2 receptors that are coupled to phosphoinositide hydrolysis. Stimulation of P2 receptors in endothelial cells results in an increase in intracellular Ca^{2+} and release of EDRF/prostacyclin,[93] whereas P2 receptors on vascular smooth muscle mediate contraction.[94] Thus, depending on the relative amounts of adenosine, ATP, and ADP in the vessel wall, and the presence of a functional endothelium, these compounds can have a net dilatory or constrictor effect on vascular smooth muscle. Additionally, the endothelium possesses an extracellular ectonucleotidase enzymatic system that mediates the conversion of ATP or ADP to adenosine, thereby regulating the local levels of these compounds.[15] These systems are important in determining the vascular response to ADP released from platelets at the site of thrombus formation.

ENDOTHELIN

The endothelins are a family of closely related peptides made and secreted by endothelial cells in some, but not all, vascular beds. There are three endothelins (ET-1, 2, and 3), all of which are 18 amino acid peptides. Endothelins are initially synthesized as preproendothelin, which undergoes preprocessing to big-endothelin. Big-endothelin is released and is converted to active endothelin by the endothelin-converting enzyme. The vascular effects of endothelin are mediated by endothelin receptors, of which three subtypes have been identified (ET-A, B, and C). The receptors have differing specificity for the individual endothelin peptides and activate somewhat different signaling pathways. In the vessel, the ET-A receptor is predominantly found on vascular smooth muscle, whereas the ET-B receptor resides on endothelial cells. Activation of the former stimulates potent vasoconstriction, whereas activation of the latter stimulates release of NO and thus favors vasodilation.[95]

The slow, intense, and sustained contraction caused by ET-1 appears to be the result of activation of the phosphoinositide/protein kinase C signaling pathway, as well as of opening voltage-dependent L-type calcium channels.[96] Importantly, even low, subthreshhold concentrations of ET-1 enhance vasoconstriction to a variety of other vasoconstrictor agents, including serotonin, angiotensin II, and α-adrenergic agonists, seemingly via activation of protein kinase C. This has been suggested to contribute to the *rebound phenomenon* that occurs after nitroglycerin has been administered for several days and suddenly discontinued.[97]

ET-1 is also a potent growth factor for smooth muscle,[98] is a chemoattractant for monocytes,[99] and plays a role in nitroglycerin tolerance.[97] Importantly, angiotensin II has been shown to stimulate the production of ET-1 by VSMCs in culture[100] and, in vivo, some of the hypertensive effect of angiotensin II is mediated by endothelin.[101]

ANGIOTENSIN-CONVERTING ENZYME

Endothelial cells synthesize and express on their surface angiotensin-converting enzyme (ACE),[102] the protein that converts angiotensin I to the potent vasoconstrictor angiotensin II and degrades and inactivates bradykinin. Of note, vascular cells contain almost all components of the renin/angiotensin system, and thus local production of angiotensin II can contribute importantly to vascular function. This local production of angiotensin II can explain why ACE inhibitors and angiotensin receptor antagonists are often effective even when the circulating levels of renin or angiotensin II are not elevated.

Endothelial Control of Vascular Growth

As with vascular tone, the endothelium also exerts a dual effect on vascular growth (Fig. 6-5). Both growth-promoting and growth-inhibitory factors are made and secreted by endothelial cells, making them pivotal in the control of smooth muscle responsiveness. Endothelial cells are involved in two types of vascular growth: angiogenesis and abnormal growth of smooth muscle during disease.

ANGIOGENESIS

Angiogenesis in vivo occurs during normal wound healing and during the vascularization of solid tumors. It is a complex process involving degradation of the basement membrane, the migration and proliferation of endothelial cells, and tube formation. Several factors have been shown to stimulate angiogenesis, including FGF, vascular endothelial growth factor (VEGF), transforming growth factor α (TGF-α), angiogenin, transforming growth factor-β (TGF-β), TNF-α,[103] and insulin-like growth factor 1 (IGF-1).[104] Their properties are summarized in Table 6-3. Some of these factors stimulate angiogenesis by inducing endothelial cell migration and proliferation (FGF and VEGF); others appear to do so by stimulating endothelial cell

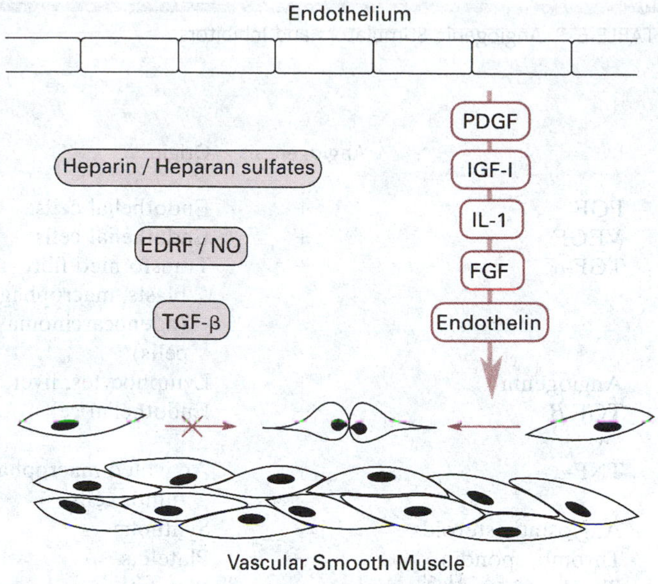

FIGURE 6-5 Endothelial control of vascular growth. As with vasoactive substances, endothelial cells make and secrete both growth-promoting (*white boxes*) and growth-inhibitory (*colored boxes*) compounds. Under normal conditions, the net effect of the endothelium is growth inhibitory. ABBREVIATIONS: EDRF = endothelial-derived relaxing factor; NO = nitric oxide; TGF-β = transforming growth factor-β; PDGF = platelet-derived growth factor; IGF-I = insulin-like growth factor-I; IL-1 = interleukin-1; FGF = fibroblast growth factor. (Courtesy of Bernard Lassègue, Ph.D.)

differentiation (TGF-β and TNF-α) or by activating a secondary cell type to produce angiogenic factors (angiogenin, TGF-β, and TNF-α). Angiogenesis may be negatively regulated by both naturally occurring and synthetic compounds. It can be inhibited by the combination of heparin and cortisone,[105] thrombospondin, platelet factor IV, and γ-interferon. Many of these agents bind to heparin, suggesting that they exert their growth-inhibitory effects by blocking the action of heparin-binding growth factors, such as FGF. It is likely that the control of angiogenesis rests on the maintenance of a balance between the stimulatory and inhibitory factors, the regulation of which is not yet fully understood.

ENDOTHELIAL-DERIVED INHIBITORS OF SMOOTH MUSCLE CELL GROWTH

Normally, smooth muscle cells are relatively refractory to growth stimuli and are maintained in a quiescent, differentiated state. It has been proposed, based on at least two lines of evidence, that the endothelium is important in maintaining this smooth muscle phenotype. First, removal of the endothelium experimentally allows initiation of the mitogenic response and, second, regrowth of normal endothelium inhibits further proliferation.[106] One mechanism by which such a tonic inhibitory influence on smooth muscle cell growth could be effected is the secretion by endothelial cells of specific inhibitors of cell proliferation. Alternatively, the endothelium could be an effective barrier limiting access of bloodborne growth factors to vascular smooth muscle. Attention so far has focused on heparin and other glycosaminoglycans (including heparan sulfate) as possible candidates for endothelial-derived growth-inhibitory factors. Heparin inhibits VSMC mitogenesis and migration in

TABLE 6-3 Angiogenic Stimulators and Inhibitors

	Angiogenesis	Origin	Release	Endothelial Cell Proliferation	Endothelial Cell Chemotaxis	Tubule Formation
FGF	+	Endothelial cells	Cell lysis	+ +	+ (EC)	+
VEGF	+	Endothelial cells	Secreted	+ +	+	+
TGF-α	+	Transformed fibroblasts, macrophages (adenocarcinoma cells)	Secreted	+ +		
Angiogenin	+	Lymphocytes, liver	Secreted	0	−	
TGF-β	+	Endothelial cells	Secreted	−	−(EC) + (Monocytes)	+
TNF-α	+	Activated macrophages, tumor cells	Secreted	−	+	+
Angiostatic steroids	−	Synthetic	−	−		
Thrombospondin	−	Platelets	Secreted	−		
Platelet factor IV	−	Platelets	Secreted	−		
γ-Interferon	−	Activated T cells, macrophages	Secreted	−		

ABBREVIATIONS: EC = endothelial cell; FGF = fibroblast growth factor; TGF = Transforming growth factor; TNF = tumor necrosis factor; VEGF = vascular endothelial growth factor.

vivo and in vitro, and reduces neointimal proliferation if administered during the first 3 days after vascular injury.[107] However, the inhibition is not complete, and it seems likely that other endothelial cell factors may be involved. Another possibility is NO, which is usually associated with vascular relaxation. NO is released tonically from the endothelium of large arteries, which have a relatively minor role in the control of vascular tone, suggesting that it may have an additional function in these vessels. Studies on cultured VSMC have shown that pharmacologic agents such as sodium nitroprusside and 8-bromo-cyclic GMP, which mimic the effect of NO on vascular smooth muscle G kinase, can inhibit mitogenesis.[108] This raises the possibility that NO may have an important role in maintaining the normal artery in a state refractory to mitogens. It is of interest that the myointimal proliferation in response to balloon injury can be inhibited by overexpression of NO synthase using gene transfer techniques.[109,110] Finally, endothelial cells have been shown to make and secrete TGF-β,[12] which is subsequently activated by smooth muscle cells. This growth factor inhibits smooth muscle growth directly[111] and alters PDGF secretion,[112] as well as extracellular matrix composition. The extracellular matrix may itself have a very important influence on smooth muscle proliferation.

The response of VSMCs to growth factors depends on the balance of the hormonal and environmental influences to which the cells are subjected. For example, intact arteries are relatively unresponsive to FGF, only showing a proliferative response when the endothelium has been damaged or removed.[61] This raises the possibility that the cellular mechanism of action of factors secreted by the endothelial cells is to induce a protein or factor in smooth muscle cells that makes them refractory to mitogenic stimulation. One candidate for such a protein is a tyrosine phosphatase. As already noted, most growth factors activate a cascade of tyrosine kinases as an initial step in the mitogenic stimulus. The level of tyrosine in cellular proteins is also controlled by tyrosine phosphatases, enzymes that remove phosphates from tyrosine residues. Thus, in cells with very active tyrosine phosphatases, tyrosine kinases may be unable to induce a sustained phosphorylation of proteins on tyrosine, theoretically inhibiting the growth response. Evidence for such a mechanism of growth control is only now becoming available, with the discovery that somatostatins act as growth inhibitors in neoplastic cells through activation of a tyrosine phosphatase.[52] Angiopeptin, a somatostatin analog, has been shown to inhibit neointimal proliferation after balloon injury,[113] suggesting that activators of tyrosine phosphatases may be important in growth control in the vasculature. These observations raise the possibility that one of the mechanisms by which endothelial cells help to maintain smooth muscle quiescence is by the induction of tyrosine phosphatase activity in the smooth muscle cells.

ENDOTHELIAL-DERIVED STIMULATORS OF SMOOTH MUSCLE CELL GROWTH

Endothelial cells have the capacity to secrete several factors that are thought to be involved in the abnormal smooth muscle cell growth seen during atherogenesis and hypertension. As noted previously, the most well studied of these factors is PDGF, so named because it was originally isolated from platelets. PDGF is a dimer, composed of two distinct peptide chains (designated A and B chains), and can be produced as an AB heterodimer or as an AA or BB homodimer. Endothelial cells contain the mRNA for both peptides,[112] although the precise form in which PDGF is secreted is unclear. Release of PDGF from the endothelium is regulated by second messengers such as cAMP and activators of protein kinase C; other growth factors including TGF-β, FGF, and TNF; circulating factors; and locally produced factors such as thrombin.[112] A second growth factor made and secreted by endothelial cells is IGF-1,[13] which is a progression factor that facilitates movement of cells through the cell cycle but, by itself, is not a particularly strong mitogen. In vitro, it enhances the mitogenic effect of PDGF on smooth muscle.[114] IGF-1 production by endothelium has been shown to be regulated by PDGF and has been shown to be a major player in vascular hypertrophy and hyperplasia.[115]

Other factors made by the endothelium that are able to alter smooth muscle proliferation include interleukin 1 (IL-1), FGF, and endothelin. IL-1 is an inflammatory cytokine that has numerous vascular effects in addition to mitogenesis, including the stimulation of procoagulant activity,[116] induction of leukocyte adhesiveness (see below), and inhibition of contraction.[117] IL-1 regulates its own expression,[118] and, in addition, its production is regulated by TNF-α,[103] lipopolysaccharide, and γ-interferon.[118] As already noted, basic FGF has been detected in endothelial cells[17] and acts as a potent smooth muscle mitogen, particularly after denuding injury.[61] FGF does not contain the signal peptide that usually provides a mechanism for transporting proteins out of cells and thus may not be secreted by endothelial cells. It is, however, present and stored in the subendothelial matrix and may be released on cell lysis or death.[119] FGF released from VSMCs may be particularly important in the growth response induced by injury to the arterial wall after balloon angioplasty. FGF bound to the matrix can be released by heparin and proteinases,[120] suggesting that the matrix may serve as a store for rapidly mobilizing this growth factor. Finally, the vasoconstrictor endothelin has also been shown under certain circumstances to act as a smooth muscle mitogen,[121] possibly by increasing PDGF-A chain secretion in the smooth muscle cells themselves.

ENDOTHELIAL CELL-LEUKOCYTE INTERACTIONS

Endothelial cells participate actively in the development of inflammatory reactions. They are central to the recruitment of leukocytes to sites of inflammation by secreting chemotactic molecules and expressing adhesion molecules that interact with surface proteins on leukocytes.

Inflammatory cytokines increase synthesis of vasodilators by the endothelium, which causes increased blood flow to the injured area. Histamine, which is released at the site of vascular inflammation, also contracts endothelial cells in certain areas, thus increasing permeability.[122] Cytokines stimulate endothelial secretion of leukocyte chemoattractant proteins (interleukin 8) and monocyte chemotactic protein 1 (MCP-1), and expression of adhesion molecules such as intercellular adhesion molecules 1 and 2 (ICAM-1 and ICAM-2), endothelial leukocyte adhesion molecule 1 (E-selectin), vascular cell adhesion molecule 1 (VCAM-1), and GMP-140, which are important regulators of leukocyte accumulation on the vascular surface.[123] E-selectin and GMP-140 bind resting, but not activated, neutrophils; VCAM-1 binds to the VLA-4 antigen on monocytes and T lymphocytes; and ICAM-1 and 2 bind to the LFA-1 integrin receptor on B lymphocytes.[123] The expression of these molecules appears to be differentially regulated by cytokines, thrombin, and histamine,[123] so that their surface expression determines the type of leukocytes attached to the endothelial monolayer. It has been suggested that the sequential accumulation of different leukocyte classes at sites of inflammation can be explained by the differential induction of these endothelial cell adhesion molecules.[124] Leukocyte adhesion molecules and chemoattractant proteins are also likely to be important in atherogenesis (see below).

ENDOTHELIAL RESPONSES TO HEMODYNAMIC INFLUENCES

In addition to being influenced by the interaction of circulating blood cells, VSMCs, and matrix, the endothelium responds to the physical forces of pressure, stretch, and shear stress imposed by the hemodynamics of the circulation. Flow-mediated, endothelium-dependent vasodilation has been described in many vascular beds,[125] and shear stress has been proposed to play a role in controlling endothelial cell proliferation.[126] Elevated pressure, stretch of the vessel wall, and shear stress have all been shown independently to affect endothelial cell morphology and/or function. Pressure alone appears to have a role in the generalized hypertrophy of the vessel wall that occurs during hypertension. Studies in cultured cells have shown that stretching endothelial cells leads to changes in cell shape, intracellular signal generation with an increase in calcium concentration, and proliferation.[126] Shear stress has numerous effects on endothelial cells. Initially, it was found that exposure of endothelial cell monolayers to elevated shear stresses in vitro caused them to align in the direction of flow. This reorientation was accompanied by changes in the cytoskeleton of the cells, including reorganization and alignment of the actin filaments and microtubules (Fig. 6-6). Similar mechanisms presumably also account for the orientation of endothelial cells parallel to the longitudinal axis in areas of laminar flow in the arterial system. The function of endothelial cells is also altered by shear stress: a K^+ current is activated; secretion of vasoactive and growth factors, including NO, endothelin, prostacyclin, and basic FGF (bFGF) is increased; tissue factor expression is increased; uptake of LDL is elevated; and tPA secretion is increased.[126]

The importance of these observations lies in the variation in hemodynamic forces throughout the circulation. High pressure, such as that which occurs in hypertension, causes changes in the morphology and function of the vessel wall.[127] In addition, the areas of the vasculature exposed to low shear stress (branch points and curvatures) exhibit a predilection to the formation of atherosclerotic lesions.[128] It is thus clear that the hemodynamic environment of the endothelium and underlying smooth muscle is a potentially powerful regulator of vascular function.

The mechanism(s) by which the endothelial cell can sense and transduce mechanical signals has not been defined definitively. Possibilities include signaling through focal adhesion complexes, a surface mechanoreceptor, a flow-sensitive ion channel, changes in cytoskeletal stress due to deformation, and flow-dependent gradients of bioactive substances along the surface of the cell. Recent data have implicated heterotrimeric G-protein activation.[129] Furthermore, caveolae, which are budding, membrane vesicular structures as described previously, are rich in signaling molecules such as G proteins and may be involved in signal generation in response to shear stress.[130]

ENDOTHELIAL DYSFUNCTION AND VASCULAR SMOOTH MUSCLE ABNORMALITIES

In general, the normal endothelium is in an inhibitory mode–inhibiting contraction, thrombosis, white cell adhesion, and vas-

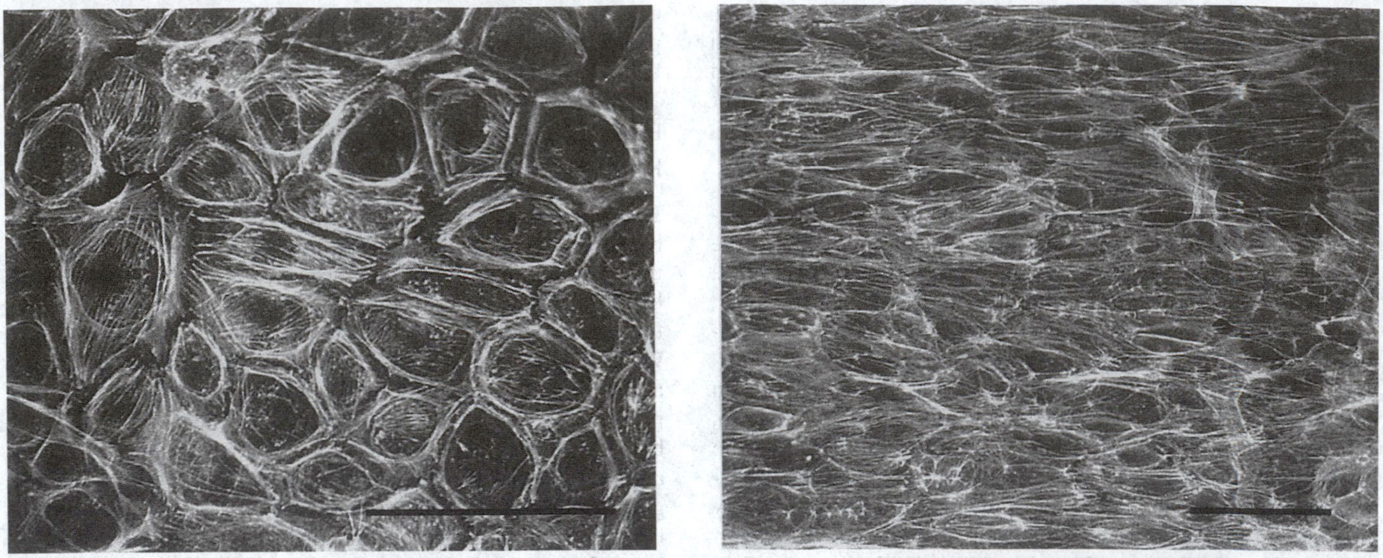

FIGURE 6-6 Effect of shear stress on endothelial cells. In bovine aortic endothelial cells grown in static conditions, F-actin filaments assume a random orientation as visualized by rhodamine-labeled phalloidin staining (*left*). Upon exposure to shear stress (30 dynes/cm^2, 24 h), these filaments align (*right*). Bars = 100 μm. (Courtesy of Lula Hilenski, Ph.D.)

cular smooth muscle growth (Figs. 6-4 and 6-5). *Endothelial dysfunction* is one of the important concepts that has developed in vascular biology over the last decade. Implicit in the term is the recognition that the fundamental or normal functions of the endothelium are not fixed, but are mutable. Thus, the endothelium in a given area may lose its vasodilator predominance, become prothrombotic or less thrombolytic, begin to support leukocyte adherence (which may be a normal response in the inflammatory process), or stimulate rather than inhibit smooth muscle migration and proliferation. *It is likely that endothelial dysfunction accounts ultimately for a large portion of cardiovascular diseases.*

Oxidative Stress and Vascular Disease

In the past several years, it has become clear that vascular cells, including endothelial, vascular smooth muscle, and adventitial cells, can produce reactive oxygen species (ROS). These include superoxide anion, hydrogen peroxide, NO, and peroxynitrite. In numerous pathophysiologic conditions, the production of ROS in the vascular wall is increased, resulting in a situation commonly referred to as *oxidant or oxidative stress*. Several enzyme systems have been implicated in production of ROS.

Recent studies suggest that an NADH/NADPH-driven oxidase is a major source of ROS in endothelial and vascular smooth muscle cells. This oxidase is a multisubunit enzyme that has only partial similarity to the neutrophil respiratory burst oxidase. For example, in VSMCs, the subunit p22phox has been shown to be critical for its function, whereas the gp91phox subunit appears to be absent.[131] In endothelial cells, the existence of all of the neutrophil subunits has been demonstrated, although it is not clear that they function together to produce ROS as they do in the neutrophil.[132] The adventitia also contains fibroblasts and macrophages that express multiple oxidase subunits.[133] Importantly, the NADH/NADPH vascular oxidase is activated by several pathophysiologic stimuli, including angiotensin II, mechanical stretch, cytokines, and thrombin.[134–137]

A second source of ROS is eNOS. As discussed previously, in the absence of tetrahydrobiopterin or L-arginine, this enzyme becomes "uncoupled" so that it produces hydrogen peroxide and superoxide, rather than NO.[75,138] Importantly, this uncoupling process seems to occur in several common disease states, including hypercholesterolemia,[139] hypertension,[140] and diabetes, although the mechanisms responsible for this process are poorly understood.

An important source of radicals in the vasculature is the lipoxygenases and in particular 12,15-lipoxygenase. These do not form superoxide, but react directly with unsaturated fatty acids (e.g., linoleic or arachidonic acid) to form a lipid radical (L$^\cdot$), which in turn can react with molecular oxygen to produce alkoxy radicals (LO$^\cdot$) and lipid peroxy radicals (LOO$^\cdot$). These lipid radicals are biologically very active and can stimulate gene expression, consume NO, oxidize NADH, and serve as a source of other radicals.[141]

Other sources of ROS in vascular cells are xanthine oxidase, cytochrome P450, cyclooxygenase, and mitochondrial electron transport.[141] There is now substantial interest in the role of these various sources of ROS and how they contribute to vascular oxidant stress.

In the next several paragraphs, we consider how endothelial dysfunction and vascular smooth muscle abnormalities contribute to several vascular diseases. A recurring theme in these conditions is that ROS play a central role. For example, superoxide rapidly reacts with NO, forming the strong oxidant peroxynitrite. The latter can oxidize lipids, damage lipid membranes, deplete cellular thiols, and alter function of several enzymes.[142] This inactivation of NO alters vasomotion and can predispose one to or even cause hypertension.[143] A substantial component of VSMC hypertrophy caused by angiotensin II is mediated by hydrogen peroxide.[144] ROS also contribute to vascular inflammation by stimulating expression of adhesion molecules in endothelial cells.[145] These issues discussed in the context of several vascular diseases.

Atherosclerosis

Atherosclerosis is the prototypical disease characterized by endothelial dysfunction, which may explain many of its cardinal features. Thus, mononuclear and lymphocytic infiltration, hypercontractility, LDL modification, smooth muscle cell growth, and intimal migration are likely related to abnormalities of the endothelium induced by hyperlipidemia, hypertension, smoking, and unknown hereditary factors. The pathogenesis of atherosclerosis viewed as a disease of endothelial dysfunction is depicted in Fig. 6-7. (For a more detailed discussion, see Chap. 41.)

Clinically, endothelial dysfunction in atherosclerosis has primarily been defined by impairment of endothelial-dependent relaxation.[146] This defect, which likely accounts for the vasospastic tendency of diseased arteries, appears to be attributable to defective generation or delivery of active EDRF/NO.[147] Coronary endothelial-dependent vasodilator function is impaired in patients with risk factors such as hypercholesterolemia, prior to angiographically demonstrable coronary disease.[148] As previously discussed, increased inactivation of NO by the superoxide anion is likely one cause of this abnormality.[147,149] Other causes may include "uncoupling" of the eNOS enzyme, altered calcium signaling of eNOS, and diminished expression of the eNOS enzyme, which clearly occurs late in the atherosclerotic process.[150] Of note, LDL and cytokines have been shown to downregulate eNOS by destabilizing the eNOS mRNA. This is prevented by HMG-CoA reductase inhibitors even without lowering of cholesterol. New evidence suggests that this process involves the lipid modification of the small GTPase Rho by the attachment of a geranylgeranyl and lipid moiety, which facilitates its localization to the cell membrane, suggesting a new target for the HMG-CoA reductase inhibitors.[151]

A second manifestation of a dysfunctional endothelium that is apparent very early after initiation of cholesterol feeding in animals is the recruitment of monocytes and macrophages into the vessel wall.[152] This recruitment is likely the result of induction of VCAM-1 expression,[153] as well as secretion of MCP-1.[154] The molecular linkage between hyperlipidemia and MCP-1/adhesion molecule expression is unknown, but may reflect in part the oxidative stress imposed by this change in milieu. Inflammatory cytokines are also important mediators of adhesion molecule expression,[155] and their production by the endothelium and inflammatory cells in the vessel wall may also contribute to adhesion molecule expression in both the early and the late stages of the disease.

The intimal proliferation observed in atherosclerotic lesion formation results from migration and hyperplasia of VSMCs[156] and accumulation of extracellular matrix.[157] Proliferation has been attributed to growth factors such as PDGF, FGF, and IGF-1. Since these growth factors can be produced by the endothelium in vitro, it is very likely that the dysfunctional endothelium in atherosclerosis also produces growth factors while shifting from a growth-inhibitory to a growth-promoting mode. Furthermore, there is evidence that products of oxidative metabolism may also release growth factors and activate matrix metalloproteinases,[67] thus contributing to intimal lesion formation on multiple levels.

The recent advances in our understanding of vessel wall biology provide insight into the biological mechanisms responsible for the pathogenesis of atherosclerosis. A unifying concept of the disease has arisen that revolves around endothelial dysfunction mediated by changes in oxidative metabolism. Oxidative stress and oxidatively modified LDL thus assume central roles in atherogenesis (Fig. 6-7). As discussed previously, a major source of lipid oxidation is lipoxygenase. Recently, the 12,15-lipoxygenase gene has been deleted in mice. When these animals were crossed with apolipoprotein E–deficient mice (which spontaneously develop atherosclerosis), atherosclerotic lesion development was strikingly reduced.[158] These data indicate that 12- and 15-lipoxygenases are almost certainly involved in the atherosclerotic process. The role of oxidized LDL is discussed more completely in Chap. 35, and the relationship of the cell biology of atherosclerosis to coronary ischemic syndrome is discussed in Chap. 41.

Hypertension

Hypertension is characterized by dysfunction of both endothelium and vascular smooth muscle. In chronic hypertension, endothelium-dependent relaxations are impaired in both conduit and resistance arteries.[159–162] Relaxations to some platelet factors are also altered, but have been found to be augmented or diminished, depending on the hypertensive model studied.[163] Furthermore, the endothelium-dependent constrictor activity is increased in some models of hypertension.[163] These alterations in endothelial function would tend to increase the tone of hypertensive vessels. The mechanism responsible for this effect is not entirely clear. Data from experimental animals make it seem likely that the alterations in endothelium-dependent responses in hypertension result from a combination of altered endothelial and VSMC function.

Hypertension is also characterized by an increase in vessel wall mass. In the aortas of spontaneously hypertensive and Goldblatt hypertensive rats, this increase can be attributed to an increase in the size of the existing smooth muscle cells.[164,165] Hypertrophy is accompanied by an increase in ploidy; that is, an increased DNA content per cell.[164,165] In contrast, resistance vessels from these same animals appear to increase their mass by hyperplasia of the smooth muscle cells.[166] The stimuli responsible for these changes in the hypertensive vascular wall are unknown. Vascular remodeling appears to have two stages: (1) an initial, reversible intense vasoconstriction mediated by neural or endogenous signals, followed by (2) a remodeling of the vessel wall characterized by increased smooth muscle mass and narrowing of the vessel lumen. There is some evidence that this response is dependent on the presence of the endothelium.[127]

Vasospasm

When the endothelium becomes dysfunctional as in atherosclerosis, the underlying smooth muscle cells often become hyperreactive to certain vasoconstrictor stimuli, including serotonin and ergonovine.[167] Coronary spasm leading to myocardial infarction is one of the most clinically relevant problems arising from this phenomenon. Proposed mechanisms underlying this vasoconstrictor abnormality that can result in total occlusion include

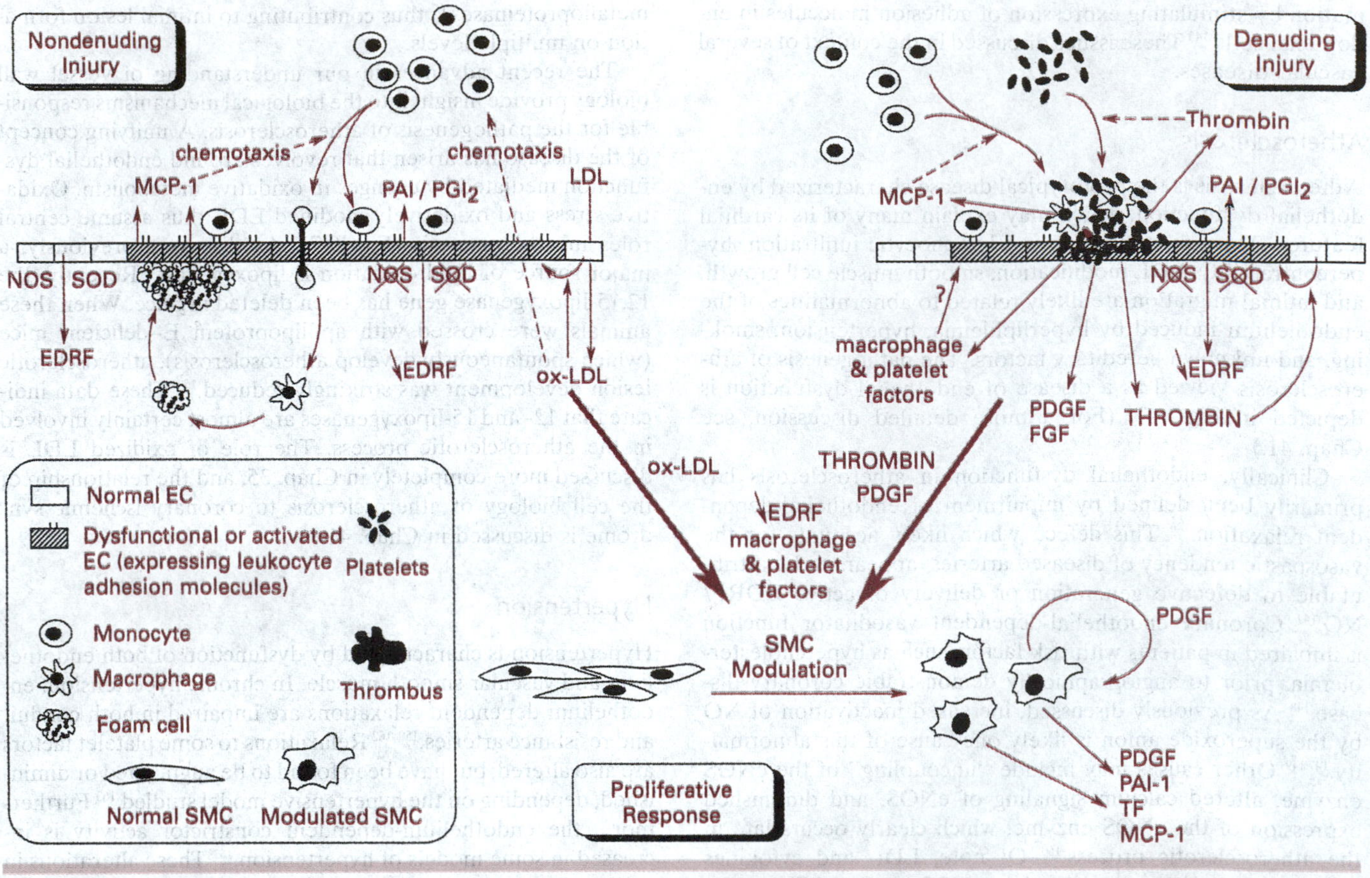

FIGURE 6-7 Theoretical initiating events in vascular lesion formation. *Nondenuding injury:* Low-density lipoprotein (LDL) enters the subendothelial space where it is converted to oxidized LDL (ox-LDL), which induces monocyte chemoattraction and endothelial dysfunction. Dysfunctional endothelial cells (ECs) express cell adhesion molecules (ICAM, ELAM, and VCAM), leading to increased monocyte adhesion and movement into the vessel wall. Monocytes in the vessel wall differentiate into macrophages, take up lipids, and remain locally as foam cells, subsequently evolving into fatty streaks. The foam cells in the fatty streak and the overlying endothelium express monocyte chemotactic protein 1 (MCP-1), resulting in further enhanced monocyte chemoattraction and adhesion. Dysfunctional ECs may synthesize less nitric oxide synthase (NOS) or superoxide dismutase (SOD, an enzyme that metabolizes oxygen radicals that have been shown to inactivate NO). This decreases endothelial-derived relaxing factor (EDRF) release/activity. The loss of EDRF together with the direct effects of ox-LDL, or growth factors secreted by the foam cells or endothelium, act on the quiescent contractile smooth muscle cells in the vessel wall, giving rise to the proliferative phenotype, with division and migration into the intima. *Denuding injury:* Loss of endothelium leads to platelet deposition, tissue factor-mediated activation of extrinsic coagulation to generate thrombin, cleavage of fibrinogen to fibrin, and the formation of thrombus. Thrombin gives rise to endothelial expression of adhesion molecules and consequent monocyte attachment, together with secretion of platelet granular constituents. Monocytes enter the thrombus and differentiate into phagocytic macrophages expressing tissue factor and MCP-1. This leads to further monocyte chemoattraction into the vessel wall. Smooth muscle cell proliferation is produced by (1) thrombin generation at the site of denuding injury, (2) platelet-derived growth factor (PDGF) or other growth factors released from platelets in the thrombus, (3) factors secreted by the macrophages ingesting the thrombus, and (4) the loss of EDRF activity caused by endothelial dysfunction. *Proliferative response:* Modulated smooth muscle cells (SMCs) proliferate and synthesize factors that promote plaque development. SMCs synthesize (1) PDGF and other growth factors that cause self-perpetuating autocrine or paracrine stimulation of SMC proliferation, (2) tissue factor (TF) and plasminogen activator inhibitor 1 (PAI-1) that act locally to produce thrombin or inhibit fibrinolysis of the fibrin network used to facilitate cell migration, and (3) MCP-1, which increases monocyte chemoattraction into the lesion, thereby leading to lesion development. (We thank Drs. Laurence Harker, Josiah Wilcox, and Bernard Lassègue for their creative and intellectual development of this figure.)

supersensitivity of the smooth muscle cells to constrictor stimuli and loss of endothelial-dependent relaxing mechanisms. The increased tendency toward thrombus formation in dysfunctional endothelium, due to a loss of the normal anticoagulant properties, also promotes the release of thrombus-related factors (serotonin, thromboxane A_2, ADP, thrombin, and PDGF) in the vicinity of the smooth muscle cells, which can promote vasoconstriction.[168]

Restenosis

Restenosis is the development of a neointima that occurs following angioplasty, often leading to reocclusion of the initial lesion. The response of the arterial wall to the injury induced by angioplasty (removal of the endothelium and stretching of the vessel wall) involves several distinct events (Fig. 6-7). Removal of the endothelium not only alters the paracrine hormonal environment in which VSMCs exist, but it also exposes a thrombogenic surface to which platelets and other circulating factors can adhere, resulting in the formation of a thrombus. In addition, injury to the underlying smooth muscle may release factors such as FGF, which have mitogenic effects on the remaining smooth muscle cells. Finally, infiltration and subsequent activation of macrophages into the denuded vessel wall bring an additional set of hormonal influences to bear on the vascular smooth muscle. The pathophysiologic consequences of these complex events include migration and proliferation of smooth muscle cells into the intimal area, resulting in the formation of a neointima over a period of weeks to months.

Balloon injury has been extensively studied in several animal models, including pigs, rabbits, rats, and baboons. In the rat carotid artery, the events following injury can be divided into three stages: initial (injury to 48 h), migratory (3 to 7 days), and proliferative (7 days to 3 to 4 weeks). During the initial response to injury, growth-related genes in the smooth muscle cells are induced, including c-fos, PDGF-A, PDGF-β receptor,[169] and MCP-1.[170] It also appears that deep injury to smooth muscle cells results in an outpouring of FGF, a potent smooth muscle mitogen.[119] This initial response does not appear to depend on platelet factors, but does appear to be directly related to the removal of the endothelium.[106] During the migratory phase, a large increase of thymidine incorporation in the vessel wall occurs, accompanied by further increases in the mRNA encoding IGF-I[171] and the PDGF-β receptor.[169] This phase of the response can be modulated by platelet factors and inhibited by the endothelium.[106] Finally, the proliferative phase is characterized by marked intimal thickening, with a decreased percentage of thymidine-labeled cells. Some of the increased area is due to deposition of extracellular matrix, and the majority of the proliferative activity occurs at the luminal surface of the vessel. This proliferative phase seems ultimately to be inhibited by regrowth of normal-functioning endothelium.

Thus, during the process of restenosis after angioplasty, both the loss of endothelium and the transformation of smooth muscle cells appear to contribute to neointimal formation. At least two lines of evidence implicate the endothelium as having a crucial role in the response of the vessel wall to injury. First, removal of the endothelium allows initiation of the mitogenic response and, second, regrowth of normal endothelium inhibits further proliferation. Furthermore, gentle denudation with a nylon loop, accompanied by rapid regeneration of endothelium, results in significantly less neointimal proliferation.[172] In addition, proliferating smooth muscle cells have characteristics distinct from the differentiated smooth muscle cells in the medial layer. Their cytoskeleton is similar to that found in cultured cells. It seems likely, therefore, that two of the most important causes of restenosis are the loss of endothelium-derived growth-inhibitory factors and the transformation of smooth muscle cells into a phenotype able to respond to platelet- and endothelial-derived factors with proliferation.

ROS are not only thought to be centrally involved in the pathogenesis of atherosclerosis, but very likely are major mediators of the proliferative, hypertrophic, and fibrotic responses that frequently occur in arteries after percutaneous transluminal coronary angioplasty (PTCA) resulting in renarrowing or restenosis of the lumen (see Chap. 45). Migration and growth of VSMCs into the intima contribute significantly to restenosis, and intracellular signaling pathways mediating growth, hypertrophy, and migration are stimulated by ROS.[173,174] As discussed previously, both proinflammatory pathways and matrix metalloproteinases, which facilitate vascular remodeling, involve redox-sensitive controlling mechanisms. The apparent broad role for oxidative signaling mechanisms in the vascular wall led to testing of the concept that antioxidants might inhibit restenosis. The production of superoxide is increased in vessels following balloon injury and, in the porcine model of restenosis, vitamins E and C have been shown to reduce neointimal development.[175,176] Further, several clinical studies have shown that the potent antioxidant probucol reduces late lumen loss after balloon angioplasty.[177–179] Larger clinical trials are under way to test the hypothesis that antioxidants are effective in inhibiting the vascular remodeling processes leading to post-PTCA restenosis.

FUTURE DIRECTIONS

Defining the molecular and cellular basis for dysfunction of the arterial wall in vascular diseases provides information critical to developing clinical strategies for patient management, as well as new therapeutic targets. It is now clear that both endothelial function and smooth muscle function are compromised by a variety of risk factors for vascular disease, due in part to oxidative stress. Further research is required to determine at a more basic level the molecular events that link these risk factors to these diseases. In the near future, the human genome will be fully sequenced, and via the use of bioinformatics, it will be possible to identify genetic profiles that predispose people to the development of vascular pathologies. Clinical trials in the future will be targeted to these populations in new and powerful ways, and basic research will address the roles of these newly identified genes in vascular physiology and pathophysiology.

References

1. Moncada S, Vane JR. Arachidonic acid metabolites and the interaction between platelets and blood vessel walls. *N Engl J Med* 1979; 300:1142.
2. Furchgott RF, Zawadski JV. The obligatory role of endothelial cells in the relaxation of arterial smooth muscle by acetylcholine. *Nature* 1980; 228:373.
3. Taylor SG, Weston AH. Endothelium-derived hyperpolarizing factor: A new endogenous inhibitor from the vascular endothelium. *Trends Pharmacol Sci* 1988; 9:272.
4. Yanagisawa Y, Kurihara H, Kimura S, et al. A novel potent vasoconstrictor peptide produced by vascular endothelial cells. *Nature* 1988; 332:411.
5. Lin L, Balazy M, Pagano PJ, et al. Expression of prostaglandin H_2-mediated mechanism of vascular contraction in hypertensive rats: Relation to lipoxygenase and prostacyclin synthase activities. *Circ Res* 1994; 74:197.
6. Stenmark KR, Orton EC, Reeves JT, et al. Vascular remodeling in neonatal pulmonary hypertension. *Chest* 1988; 93:127S.
7. Sato T, Arai K, Ishiharajima S, et al. Role of glycosaminoglycan and fibronectin in endothelial cell growth. *Exp Mol Pathol* 1987; 47:202.
8. Hanemaaijer R, Koolwijk P, le Clercq L, et al. Regulation of matrix metalloproteinase expression in human vein and microvascular endothelial cells: Effects of tumor necrosis factor alpha, interleukin 1 and phorbol ester. *Biochem J* 1993; 296:803.
9. Galis ZS, Muszynski M, Sukhova GK, et al. Cytokine-stimulated

human vascular smooth muscle cells synthesize a complement of enzymes required for extracellular matrix digestion. *Circ Res* 1994; 75:181.

10. Castellot JJ Jr, Addonizio ML, Rosenberg R, et al. Cultured endothelial cells produce a heparin-like inhibitor of smooth muscle cell growth. *J Cell Biol* 1981; 90:372.
11. Zerwes HG, Risau W. Polarized secretion of a platelet-derived growth factor-like chemotactic factor by endothelial cells in vitro. *J Cell Biol* 1987; 105:2037.
12. Hannan RL, Kourembanas S, Flanders KC, et al. Endothelial cells synthesize basic fibroblast growth factor and transforming growth factor beta. *Growth Factors* 1988; 1:7.
13. Delafontaine P, Bernstein KE, Alexander RW. Insulin-like growth factor I gene expression in vascular cells. *Hypertension* 1991; 17:693.
14. Wang-Iverson P, DeRosa PM, Brown WV. Plasma lipoprotein interaction with endothelial cells. In: Ryan U, ed. *Endothelial Cells*. Boca Raton, FL: CRC; 1988:179.
15. Gordon EL, Pearson JD, Slakey LL. The hydrolysis of extracellular adenine nucleotides by cultured endothelial cells from pig aorta. *J Biol Chem* 1986; 33:15,496.
16. Cary DA, Mendelsohn FA. Effect of forskolin, isoproterenol and IBMX on angiotensin converting enzyme and cyclic AMP production by cultured bovine endothelial cells. *Mol Cell Endocrinol* 1987; 53:103.
17. Shimada K, Gill PJ, Silbert JE, et al. Involvement of cell surface heparan sulfate in the binding of LPL to cultured bovine endothelial cells. *J Clin Invest* 1981; 68:995.
18. Vlodavsky I, Fielding PE, Johnson LK, et al. Inhibition of low density lipoprotein uptake in confluent endothelial cell monolayers correlates with a restricted surface receptor redistribution. *J Cell Physiol* 1979; 100:481.
19. Hashida R, Anamizu C, Kimura J, et al. Transcellular transport of lipoprotein through arterial endothelial cells in monolayer culture. *Cell Struct Funct* 1986; 11:31.
20. Baker DP, Van Lenten BJ, Fogelman AM, et al. LDL, scavenger and beta-VLDL receptors on aortic endothelial cells. *Arteriosclerosis* 1984; 4:357.
21. Morel DW, DiCorleto PE, Chisolm GM. Endothelial and smooth muscle cells alter low density lipoprotein in vitro by free radical oxidation. *Arteriosclerosis* 1984; 4:357.
22. Danon D, Skutelsky E. Endothelial surface charge and its possible relationship to thrombogenesis. *Ann NY Acad Sci* 1976; 275:47.
23. Gryglewski RJ, Botting RM, Vane JR. Mediators produced by the endothelial cell. *Hypertension* 1988; 12:530.
24. Rosenberg RD, Rosenberg JS. Natural anticoagulant mechanisms. *J Clin Invest* 1984; 74:1.
25. Esmon CT, Owen WG. Identification of an endothelial cofactor for thrombin-catalyzed activation of protein C. *Proc Natl Acad Sci USA* 1981; 78:2249.
26. Van Iwaarden F, Acton DS, Sixma JJ, et al. Internalization of antithrombin III by cultured human endothelial cells and its subcellular localization. *J Lab Clin Med* 1989; 113:717.
27. Podor TJ, Curriden SA, Loskutoff DJ. The fibrinolytic system of endothelial cells. In: Ryan US, ed. *Endothelial Cells*. Boca Raton, FL: CRC; 1988:127.
28. Vaughan DE. Fibrinolytic balance, the renin-angiotensin system and atherosclerotic disease. *Eur Heart J* 1998; 19(suppl G):G9.
29. Schorer AE, Moldow CF. Production of tissue factor. In: Ryan US, ed. *Endothelial Cells*. Boca Raton, FL: CRC; 1988:85.
30. Whelan J, Ghersa P, Hooft-an-Huijsduijnen R, et al. An NF kappa B-like factor is essential but not sufficient for cytokine induction of endothelial leukocyte adhesion molecule 1 (ELAM-1) gene transcription. *Nucleic Acids Res* 1991; 19:2645.
31. Sporn LA, Marder VJ, Wagner DD. Von Willebrand factor released from Weibel-Palade bodies binds more avidly to extracellular matrix than that secreted constitutively. *Blood* 1987; 69:1531.
32. Stern DM, Nawroth PP. Modulation of endothelial cell coagulant properties. In: Ryan US, ed. *Endothelial Cells*. Boca Raton, FL: CRC; 1988:149.
33. Svensjo E, Grega GJ. Evidence for endothelial cell-mediated regulation of macromolecular permeability by post-capillary venules. *Fed Proc* 1986; 45:89.
34. Huttner I, Boutet M, Rona G, et al. Studies on protein passage through arterial endothelium: III. Effect of blood pressure levels on the passage of fine structural protein tracers through rat arterial endothelium. *Lab Invest* 1973; 29:536.
35. Feng D, Nagy JA, Pyne K, et al. Pathways of macromolecular extravasation across microvascular endothelium in response to VPF/VEGF and other vasoactive mediators. *Microcirculation* 1999; 6:23.
36. Feng Y, Venema VJ, Venema RC, et al. VEGF-induced permeability increase is mediated by caveolae. *Invest Ophthalmol Vis Sci* 1999; 40:157.
37. Scow RO, Blanchette-Mackie EJ, Smith LC. Role of capillary endothelium in the clearance of chylomicrons: A model for lipid transport from blood by lateral diffusion in cell membranes. *Circ Res* 1976; 39:149.
38. Garcia JG, Davis HW, Patterson CE. Regulation of endothelial cell gap formation and barrier dysfunction: Role of myosin light chain phosphorylation. *J Cell Physiol* 1995; 163:510.
39. Garcia JG, Schaphorst KL, Shi S, et al. Mechanisms of ionomycin-induced endothelial cell barrier dysfunction. *Am J Physiol* 1997; 273:L172.
40. Garcia JG, Verin AD, Schaphorst K, et al. Regulation of endothelial cell myosin light chain kinase by rho, cortactin, and p60. *Am J Physiol* 1999; 276:L989.
41. Berk BC, Alexander RW, Brock TA, et al. Vasoconstriction: A new activity for platelet-derived growth factor. *Science* 1986; 232:87.
42. Owens GK. Control of hypertrophic vs. hyperplastic growth of vascular smooth muscle cells. *Am J Physiol* 1989; 257:H1755.
43. Berridge MJ, Irvine RF. Inositol trisphosphate, a novel second messenger in cellular signal transduction. *Nature* 1984; 312:315.
44. Yamamoto H, van Breeman C. Inositol 1,4,5-trisphosphate releases calcium from skinned cultured smooth muscle cells. *Biochem Biophys Res Commun* 1985; 130:270.
45. Nishizuka Y. The role of protein kinase C in cell surface signal transduction and tumour promotion. *Nature* 1984; 308:693.
46. Berk BC, Aronow MS, Brock TA, et al. Angiotensin II-stimulated Na^+/H^+ exchange in cultured vascular smooth muscle cells: Evidence for protein kinase C-dependent and -independent pathways. *J Biol Chem* 1987; 262:5057.
47. Brock TA, Alexander RW, Ekstein LS, et al. Angiotensin increases cytosolic free calcium in cultured vascular smooth muscle cells. *Hypertension* 1985; 7:I-105.
48. Dillon PF, Aksoy MO, Driska SP, et al. Myosin phosphorylation and the cross-bridge cycle in arterial smooth muscle. *Science* 1981; 211:495.
49. Morgan KG. Role of calcium ion in maintenance of vascular smooth muscle tone. *Am J Cardiol* 1987; 59:24A.
50. Williams LT. Signal transduction by the platelet-derived growth factor receptor. *Science* 1989; 243:1564.
51. Clegg KB, Sambhi MP. Inhibition of epidermal growth factor-mediated DNA synthesis by a specific tyrosine kinase inhibitor in vascular smooth muscle cells of the spontaneously hypertensive rat. *J Hypertens* 1989; 7:S144.
52. Liebow C, Reilly C, Serrano M, et al. Somatostatin analogues inhibit growth of pancreatic cancer by stimulating tyrosine phosphatase. *Proc Natl Acad Sci USA* 1989; 86:2003.
53. Ullrich A, Schlessinger J. Signal transduction by receptors with tyrosine kinase activity. *Cell* 1990; 81:203.
54. Luttrell LM, Daaka Y, Lefkowitz RJ. Regulation of tyrosine

kinase cascades by G-protein-coupled receptors. *Curr Opin Cell Biol* 1999; 11:177.

55. Lassègue B, Alexander RW, Clark M, et al. Angiotensin II-induced phosphatidylcholine hydrolysis in cultured vascular smooth-muscle cells: Regulation and localization. *Biochem J* 1991; 276:19.
56. Moolenaar WH, Kruijer W, Tilly BC, et al. Growth factor-like action of phosphatidic acid. *Nature* 1986; 323:171.
57. Kondo T, Inui H, Konishi F, et al. Phospholipase D mimics platelet-derived growth factor as a competence factor in vascular smooth muscle cells. *J Biol Chem* 1992; 267:23,609.
58. Berk BC, Vekshtein V, Gordon HM, et al. Angiotensin II-stimulated protein synthesis in cultured vascular smooth muscle cells. *Hypertension* 1989; 13:305.
59. Berk BC, Taubman MB, Griendling KK, et al. Thrombin-stimulated events in cultured vascular smooth muscle cells. *Biochem J* 1991; 274:799.
60. Golden MA, Au YPT, Kirkman TR, et al. Platelet-derived growth factor activity and mRNA expression in healing vascular grafts in baboons. *J Clin Invest* 1991; 87:406.
61. Lindner V, Lappi DA, Baird A, et al. Role of basic fibroblast growth factor in vascular lesion formation. *Circ Res* 1991; 68:106.
62. Myers PR, Minor RL, Guerra R Jr, et al. The vasorelaxant properties of the endothelium derived relaxing factor more closely resemble S-nitrosocysteine than nitric oxide. *Nature* 1990; 345:161.
63. Ushio-Fukai M, Alexander RW, Akers M, et al. p38MAP kinase is a critical component of the redox-sensitive signaling pathways by angiotensin II: Role in vascular smooth muscle cell hypertrophy. *J Biol Chem* 1998; 273:15,022.
64. Ushio-Fukai M, Alexander RW, Akers M, et al. Reactive oxygen species mediate the activation of Akt/protein kinase B by angiotensin II in vascular smooth muscle cells. *J Biol Chem* 1999; 274:22,699.
65. Sato H, Takino T, Okada Y, et al. A matrix metalloproteinase expressed on the surface of invasive tumor cells. *Nature* 1994; 370:61.
66. Galis ZS, Asanuma K, Godin D, et al. *N*-Acetyl-cysteine decreases the matrix-degrading capacity of macrophage-derived foam cells: New target for antioxidant therapy? *Circulation* 1998; 97:2445.
67. Rajagopalan S, Meng XP, Ramasamy S, et al. Reactive oxygen species produced by macrophage-derived foam cells regulate the activity of vascular matrix metalloproteinases in vitro. *J Clin Invest* 1996; 98:2572.
68. Galis ZS, Sukhova GK, Lark MW, et al. Increased expression of matrix metalloproteinases and matrix degrading activity in vulnerable regions of human atherosclerotic plaques. *J Clin Invest* 1994; 94:2493.
69. Furchgott RF, Vanhoutte PM. Endothelium-derived relaxing and contracting factors. *FASEB J* 1989; 3:2007.
70. Rapoport RM, Draznin MB, Murad F. Endothelium-dependent relaxation in rat aorta may be mediated through cyclic GMP-dependent protein phosphorylation. *Nature* 1983; 306:174.
71. Bredt DS, Hwang PM, Glatt CE, et al. Cloned and expressed nitric oxide synthase structurally resembles cytochrome P-450 reductase. *Nature* 1991; 351:714.
72. Lyons CR, Orloff GJ, Cunningham JM. Molecular cloning and functional expression of an inducible nitric oxide synthase from a murine macrophage cell line. *J Biol Chem* 1992; 267:6370.
73. Nishida K, Harrison DG, Navas JP, et al. Molecular cloning and characterization of the constitutive bovine aortic endothelial nitric oxide synthase. *J Clin Invest* 1992; 90:2092.
74. Stuehr DJ. Mammalian nitric oxide synthases. *Biochim Biophys Acta* 1999; 1411:217.
75. Vasquez-Vivar J, Kalyanaraman B, Martasek P, et al. Superoxide generation by endothelial nitric oxide synthase: The influence of cofactors. *Proc Natl Acad Sci USA* 1998; 95:9220.
76. Kuchan MJ, Frangos JA. Role of calcium and calmodulin in flow-induced nitric oxide production in endothelial cells. *Am J Physiol* 1994; 266:C628.
77. Corson MA, James NL, Latta SE, et al. Phosphorylation of endothelial nitric oxide synthase in response to fluid shear stress. *Circ Res* 1996; 79:984.
78. Gallis B, Corthals GL, Goodlett DR, et al. Identification of flow-dependent endothelial nitric-oxide synthase phosphorylation sites by mass spectrometry and regulation of phosphorylation and nitric oxide production by the phosphatidylinositol 3-kinase inhibitor LY294002. *J Biol Chem* 1999; 274:30,101.
79. Dimmeler S, Fleming I, Fisslthaler B, et al. Activation of nitric oxide synthase in endothelial cells by Akt-dependent phosphorylation. *Nature* 1999; 399:601.
80. Uematsu M, Ohara Y, Navas JP, et al. Regulation of endothelial cell nitric oxide synthase mRNA expression by shear stress. *Am J Physiol* 1995; 269:C1371.
81. Sessa WC, Pritchard K, Seyedi N, et al. Chronic exercise in dogs increases coronary vascular nitric oxide production and endothelial cell nitric oxide synthase gene expression. *Circ Res* 1994; 74:349.
82. Yoshizumi M, Perrella MA, Burnett JC Jr, et al. Tumor necrosis factor downregulates an endothelial nitric oxide synthase mRNA by shortening its half-life. *Circ Res* 1993; 73:205.
83. Liao JK, Shin WS, Lee WY, et al. Oxidized low-density lipoprotein decreases the expression of endothelial nitric oxide synthase. *J Biol Chem* 1995; 270:319.
84. Liao JK, Zulueta JJ, Yu FS, et al. Regulation of bovine endothelial constitutive nitric oxide synthase by oxygen. *J Clin Invest* 1995; 96:2661.
85. Searles CD, Miwa Y, Harrison DG, et al. Posttranscriptional regulation of endothelial nitric oxide synthase during cell growth. *Circ Res* 1999; 85:588.
86. Feletou M, Vanhoutte PM. The alternative: EDHF. *J Mol Cell Cardiol* 1999; 31:15.
87. Fisslthaler B, Popp R, Kiss L, et al. Cytochrome P450 2C is an EDHF synthase in coronary arteries. *Nature* 1999; 401:493
88. Hayabuchi Y, Nakaya Y, Matsuoka S, et al.: Endothelium-derived hyperpolarizing factor activates Ca^{2+}-activated K^+ channels in porcine coronary artery smooth muscle cells. *J Cardiovasc Pharmacol* 1998; 32:642.
89. Node K, Huo Y, Ruan X, et al. Anti-inflammatory properties of cytochrome P450 epoxygenase-derived eicosanoids. *Science* 1999; 285:1276.
90. Ito T, Ogawa K, Enomoto I, et al. Comparison of the effects of PGI_2 and PGE_1 on coronary and systemic hemodynamics and coronary arterial cyclic nucleotide level in dogs. *Adv Prostaglandin Thromboxane Leukotriene Res* 1980; 7:641.
91. Carwile LE, Ager A, Gordon JL. Effects of neutrophil elastase and other proteases on porcine aortic endothelial prostaglandin I_2 production, adenine nucleotide release, and responses to vasoactive agents. *J Clin Invest* 1984; 74:1003.
92. Milner P, Bodin P, Loesch A, et al. Rapid release of endothelin and ATP from isolated aortic endothelial cells exposed to increased flow. *Biochem Biophys Res Commun* 1990; 170:649.
93. Pearson JD, Slakey LL, Gordon JL. Stimulation of prostaglandin production through purinoceptors on cultured porcine endothelial cells. *Biochem J* 1983; 214:273.
94. O'Connor SE, Wood BE, Leff P. Characterization of P2x-receptors in rabbit isolated ear artery. *Br J Pharmacol* 1990; 101:640.
95. Luscher TF, Wenzel RR. Endothelin and endothelin antagonists: Pharmacology and clinical implications. *Agents Actions Suppl* 1995; 45:237.
96. Simonson MS, Dunn MJ. Cellular signaling by peptides of the endothelin gene family. *FASEB J* 1990; 4:2989.
97. Münzel T, Giaid A, Kurz S, et al. Evidence for a role of endothelin

1 and protein kinase C in nitroglycerin tolerance. *Proc Natl Acad Sci USA* 1995; 92:5244.
98. Hafizi S, Allen SP, Goodwin AT, et al. Endothelin-1 stimulates proliferation of human coronary smooth muscle cells via the ET(A) receptor and is co-mitogenic with growth factors. *Atherosclerosis* 1999; 146:351.
99. Achmad TH, Rao GS. Chemotaxis of human blood monocytes toward endothelin-1 and the influence of calcium channel blockers. *Biochem Biophys Res Commun* 1992; 189:994.
100. Sung CP, Arleth AJ, Storer BL, et al. Angiotensin type 1 receptors mediate smooth muscle proliferation and endothelin biosynthesis in rat vascular smooth muscle. *J Pharmacol Exp Ther* 1994; 271:429.
101. Rajagopalan S, Bech-Laursen J, Borthayre A, et al. A role for endothelin-1 in angiotensin II mediated hypertension. *Hypertension* 1997; 30:29.
102. Gumkowski F, Kaminska F, Kaminiski M, et al. Heterogeneity of mouse vascular endothelium: In vitro studies of lymphatic, large blood vessel and microvascular endothelial cells. *Blood Vessels* 1987; 24:11.
103. Klagsbrun M, D'Amore PA. Regulators of angiogenesis. *Ann Rev Physiol* 1991; 53:217.
104. Hansson HA, Brandsten C, Lossing C, et al. Transient expression of insulin-like growth factor I immunoreactivity by vascular cells during angiogenesis. *Exp Mol Pathol* 1989; 50:125.
105. Folkman J, Langer R, Linhardt RJ, et al. Angiogenesis inhibition and tumor regression caused by heparin or a heparin fragment in the presence of cortisone. *Science* 1983; 221:719.
106. Clowes AW, Clowes MM, Fingerle J, et al. Regulation of smooth muscle cell growth in injured artery. *J Cardiovasc Pharmacol* 1989; 14:S12.
107. Clowes AW, Clowes MM. Kinetics of cellular proliferation after arterial injury. IV. Heparin inhibits rat smooth muscle mitogenesis and migration. *Circ Res* 1986; 58:839.
108. Garg UC, Hassid A. Nitric oxide generating vasodilators and 8-bromo cyclic GMP inhibit mitogenesis and proliferation of cultured rat vascular smooth muscle cells. *J Clin Invest* 1989; 83:1774.
109. Von der Leyen HE, Gibbons GH, Morishita R, et al. Gene therapy inhibiting neointimal vascular lesion: In vivo transfer of endothelial cell nitric oxide synthase gene. *Proc Natl Acad Sci USA* 1995; 92:1137.
110. Janssens S, Flaherty D, Nong Z, et al. Human endothelial nitric oxide synthase gene transfer inhibits vascular smooth muscle cell proliferation and neointima formation after balloon injury in rats. *Circulation* 1998; 97:1274.
111. Owens GK, Geisterfer AA, Yang YW, et al. Transforming growth factor-beta-induced growth inhibition and cellular hypertrophy in cultured vascular smooth muscle cells. *J Cell Biol* 1988; 107:771.
112. Kavanaugh WM, Harsh GR IV, Starksen NF, et al. Transcriptional regulation of the A and B chain genes of PDGF in microvascular endothelial cells. *J Biol Chem* 1988; 263:8470.
113. Conte JV, Foegh ML, Calcagno D, et al. Peptide inhibition of myointimal proliferation following angioplasty in rabbits. *Transplant Proc* 1989; 21:3686.
114. Clemmons DR. Exposure to platelet-derived growth factors modulate the porcine aortic smooth muscle cell response to somatomedin-C. *Endocrinology* 1985; 117:77.
115. Delafontaine P. Insulin-like growth factor I and its binding proteins in the cardiovascular system. *Cardiovasc Res* 1995; 30:825.
116. Bevilaqua MP, Gimbrone MA Jr. Modulation of endothelial cell procoagulant and fibrinolytic activities by inflammatory mediators. In: Ryan US, ed. *Endothelial Cells.* Boca Raton, FL: CRC; 1988:107.
117. Beasley D, Cohen RA, Levinsky NG. Interleukin 1 inhibits contraction of vascular smooth muscle. *J Clin Invest* 1989; 83:331.
118. Schindler R, Ghezzi P, Dinarello CA. IL-1 induces IL-1 IV. IFN-gamma suppresses IL-1 but not lipopolysaccharide-induced transcription of IL-1. *J Immunol* 1990; 144:2216.
119. Lindner V, Reidy MA. Proliferation of smooth muscle cells after vascular injury is inhibited by an antibody against basic fibroblast growth factor. *Proc Natl Acad Sci USA* 1991; 88:3739.
120. Bashkin P, Doctrow S, Klagsbrun M, et al. Basic fibroblast growth factor binds to subendothelial extracellular matrix and is released by heparinase and heparin-like molecules. *Biochemistry* 1989; 28:1737.
121. Hirata Y, Takagi Y, Fukuda Y, et al. Endothelin is a potent mitogen for rat vascular smooth muscle cells. *Atherosclerosis* 1989; 78:225.
122. Majno G, Shea SM, Leventhal M. Endothelial contraction induced by histamine-type mediators: An electron microscopic study. *J Cell Biol* 1969; 42:647.
123. Pober JS, Cotran RS. What can be learned from the expression of endothelial adhesion molecules in tissues? *Lab Invest* 1991; 64:301.
124. Pober JS, Cotran RS. The role of endothelial cells in inflammation. *Transplantation* 1990; 50:537.
125. Marshall JJ, Kontos HA. Endothelium-derived relaxing factors: A perspective from in vivo data. *Hypertension* 1990; 16:371.
126. Nerem RM, Girard PR. Hemodynamic influences on vascular endothelial biology. *Toxicol Pathol* 1990; 18:572.
127. Schwartz SM, Majesky MW, Dilley RJ. Vascular remodeling in hypertension and atherosclerosis. In: Laragh JH, Brenner BM, eds. *Hypertension: Pathophysiology, Diagnosis and Management*, New York: Raven; 1990:521.
128. Asakura T, Karino T. Flow patterns and spatial distribution of atherosclerotic lesions in human coronary arteries. *Circ Res* 1990; 66:1045.
129. Traub O, Berk BC. Laminar shear stress: Mechanisms by which endothelial cells transduce an atheroprotective force. *Arterioscler Thromb Vasc Biol* 1998; 18:677.
130. Rizzo V, McIntosh DP, Oh P, et al. In situ flow activates endothelial nitric oxide synthase in luminal caveolae of endothelium with rapid caveolin dissociation and calmodulin association. *J Biol Chem* 1998; 273:34,724.
131. Ushio-Fukai M, Zafari AM, Fukui T, et al. p22phox is a critical component of the superoxide-generating NADH/NADPH oxidase system and regulates angiotensin II-induced hypertrophy in vascular smooth muscle cells. *J Biol Chem* 1996; 271:23,317.
132. Jones SA, O'Donnell VB, Wood JD, et al. Expression of phagocyte NADPH oxidase components in human endothelial cells. *Am J Physiol* 1996; 271:H1626.
133. Pagano PJ, Clark JK, Cifuentes-Pagano ME, et al. Localization of a constitutively active, phagocyte-like NADPH oxidase in rabbit aortic adventitia: Enhancement by angiotensin II. *Proc Natl Acad Sci USA* 1997; 94:14,438.
134. Griendling KK, Minieri CA, Ollerenshaw JD, et al. Angiotensin II stimulates NADH and NADPH oxidase activity in cultured vascular smooth muscle cells. *Circ Res* 1994; 74:1141.
135. Howard AB, Alexander RW, Nerem RM, et al. Cyclic strain induces an oxidative stress in endothelial cells. *Am J Physiol* 1997; 272:C421.
136. De Keulenaer GW, Alexander RW, Ushio-Fukai M, et al. Tumor necrosis factor-α activates a p22phox-based NADH oxidase in vascular smooth muscle cells. *Biochem J* 1998; 329:653.
137. Patterson C, Ruef J, Madamanchi NR, et al. Stimulation of a vascular smooth muscle cell NAD(P)H oxidase by thrombin: Evidence that p47(phox) may participate in forming this oxidase in vitro and in vivo. *J Biol Chem* 1999; 274:19,814.
138. Xia Y, Tsai AL, Berka V, et al. Superoxide generation from endothelial nitric-oxide synthase: A Ca^{2+}/calmodulin-dependent and tetrahydrobiopterin regulatory process. *J Biol Chem* 1998; 273:25,804.
139. Verhaar MC, Wever RM, Kastelein JJ, et al. 5-Methyltetrahy-

drofolate, the active form of folic acid, restores endothelial function in familial hypercholesterolemia. *Circulation* 1998; 97:237.
140. Cosentino F, Patton S, d'Uscio LV, et al. Tetrahydrobiopterin alters superoxide and nitric oxide release in prehypertensive rats. *J Clin Invest* 1998; 101:1530.
141. Harrison DG, Galis Z, Parthasarathy S, et al. Oxidative stress and hypertension. In: Izzo JL, Black HR, eds. *Hypertension Primer*. Baltimore: Lippincott, Williams and Wilkins; 1999:163.
142. Beckman JS, Koppenol WH. Nitric oxide, superoxide, and peroxynitrite: The good, the bad, and ugly. *Am J Physiol* 1996; 271:C1424.
143. Bech-Laursen J, Rajagopalan S, Galis Z, et al. Role of superoxide in angiotensin II-induced but not catecholamine-induced hypertension. *Circulation* 1997; 95:588.
144. Zafari AM, Ushio-Fukai M, Akers M, et al. Novel role of NADH/NADPH oxidase-derived hydrogen peroxide in angiotensin II-induced hypertrophy of rat vascular smooth muscle cells. *Hypertension* 1998; 32:488.
145. Marui N, Offerman M, Swerlick R, et al. Vascular cell-adhesion molecule-1 (VCAM-1) gene transcription and expression are regulated through an antioxidant sensitive mechanism in human vascular endothelial cells. *J Clin Invest* 1993; 92:1866.
146. Treasure CB, Klein JL, Weintraub WS, et al. Beneficial effects of cholesterol-lowering therapy on the coronary endothelium in patients with coronary artery disease. *N Engl J Med* 1995; 332:481.
147. Minor RL, Myers PR, Guerra R, et al. Diet-induced atherosclerosis increases the release of nitrogen oxides from rabbit aorta. *J Clin Invest* 1990; 86:2109.
148. McLenachan JM, Williams JK, Fish RD, et al. Loss of flow-mediated endothelium-dependent dilation occurs early in the development of atherosclerosis. *Circulation* 1991; 84:1273.
149. Mügge A, Elwell JH, Peterson TE, et al. Chronic treatment with polyethylene-glycolated superoxide dismutase partially restores endothelium-dependent vascular relaxations in cholesterol-fed rabbits. *Circ Res* 1991; 69:1293.
150. Harrison DG. Cellular and molecular mechanisms of endothelial cell dysfunction. *J Clin Invest* 1997; 100:2153.
151. Laufs U, Liao JK. Post-transcriptional regulation of endothelial nitric oxide synthase mRNA stability by Rho GTPase. *J Biol Chem* 1998; 273:24,266.
152. Hansson GK, Seifert PS, Olsson G, et al. Immunohistochemical detection of macrophages and T lymphocytes in atherosclerotic lesions of cholesterol-fed rabbits. *Arterioscler Thromb* 1991; 1:745.
153. Cybulsky MI, Gimbrone MA Jr. Endothelial expression of a mononuclear leukocyte adhesion molecule during atherogenesis. *Science* 1991; 251:788.
154. Wang JM, Sica A, Peri G, et al. Expression of monocyte chemotactic protein and interleukin-8 by cytokine-activated human vascular smooth muscle cells. *Arterioscler Thromb* 1991; 11:1166.
155. Meager A. Cytokine regulation of cellular adhesion molecule expression in inflammation. *Cytokine Growth Factor Rev* 1999; 10:27.
156. Ross R. The pathogenesis of atherosclerosis: An update. *N Engl J Med* 1986; 314:488.
157. Stary HC. Changes in components and structure of atherosclerotic lesions developing from childhood to middle age in coronary arteries. *Basic Res Cardiol* 1994; 89:17.
158. Cyrus T, Witztum JL, Rader DJ, et al. Disruption of the 12/15-lipoxygenase gene diminishes atherosclerosis in apo E-deficient mice. *J Clin Invest* 1999; 103:1597.
159. Alexander RW. Hypertension and the pathogenesis of atherosclerosis: Oxidative stress and the mediation of arterial inflammatory response—A new perspective. *Hypertension* 1995; 25:155.
160. Li J, Zhao SP, Li XP, et al. Non-invasive detection of endothelial dysfunction in patients with essential hypertension. *Int J Cardiol* 1997; 61:165.
161. Panza JA, Quyyumi AA, Brush JE Jr, et al. Abnormal endothelium-dependent vascular relaxation in patients with essential hypertension. *N Engl J Med* 1990; 323:22.
162. Panza JA, Quyyumi AA, Callahan TS, et al. Effect of antihypertensive treatment on endothelium-dependent vascular relaxation in patients with essential hypertension. *J Am Coll Cardiol* 1993; 21:1145.
163. Luscher TF, Vanhoutte PM. Endothelium-dependent contractions to acetylcholine in the aorta of the spontaneously hypertensive rat. *Hypertension* 1986; 8:344.
164. Owens GK, Schwartz SM. Alterations in vascular smooth muscle mass in the spontaneously hypertensive rat: Role in cellular hypertrophy, hyperploidy and hyperplasia. *Circ Res* 1982; 51:280.
165. Owens GK, Schwartz SM. Vascular smooth muscle cell hypertrophy and hyperploidy in the Goldblatt hypertensive rat. *Circ Res* 1983; 53:491.
166. Halpern W, Warshaw DM, Mulvany MJ. Mechanical and morphological properties of arterial resistance vessels in young and old spontaneously hypertensive rats. *Circ Res* 1979; 45:250.
167. Vita JA, Treasure CB, Nabel EG, et al. Coronary vasomotor response to acetylcholine relates to risk factors for coronary artery disease. *Circulation* 1990; 81:491.
168. Rubanyi GM. Endothelium-derived relaxing and contracting factors. *J Cell Biochem* 1991; 46:27.
169. Majesky MW, Reidy MA, Bowen-Pope DF, et al. PDGF ligand and receptor gene expression during repair of arterial injury. *J Cell Biol* 1990; 111:2149.
170. Taubman MB, Rollins BJ, Poon M, et al. JE mRNA accumulates rapidly in aortic injury and in platelet-derived growth factor-stimulated vascular smooth muscle cells. *Circ Res* 1992; 70:314.
171. Cercek B, Fishbein MC, Forrester JS, et al. Induction of insulin-like growth factor I messenger RNA in rat aorta after balloon denudation. *Circ Res* 1990; 66:1755.
172. Fingerle J, Au YP, Clowes AW, et al. Intimal lesion formation in rat carotid arteries after endothelial denudation in absence of medial injury. *Atherosclerosis* 1990; 10:1082.
173. Berk BC. Redox signals that regulate the vascular response to injury. *Thromb Haemost* 1999; 82:810.
174. Griendling KK, Ushio-Fukai M. Redox control of vascular smooth muscle proliferation. *J Lab Clin Med* 1998; 132:9.
175. Nunes GL, Robinson K, Kalynych A, et al. Vitamins C and E inhibit O_2^- production in the pig coronary artery. *Circulation* 1997; 96:3593.
176. Nunes GL, Sgoutas DS, Redden RA, et al. Combination of vitamins C and E alters the response to coronary balloon injury in the pig. *Arterioscler Thromb Vasc Biol* 1995; 15:156.
177. Cote G, Tardif JC, Lesperance J, et al. Effects of probucol on vascular remodeling after coronary angioplasty: Multivitamins and Probucol Study Group. *Circulation* 1999; 99:30.
178. Rodes J, Cote G, Lesperance J, et al. Prevention of restenosis after angioplasty in small coronary arteries with probucol. *Circulation* 1998; 97:429.
179. Tardiff J-C, Cote G, Lesperance J, et al. Prevention of restenosis by pre- and post-PTCA probucol therapy: A randomized clinical trial. *Circulation* 1996; 94:I-91.

CHAPTER 7

UNRAVELING THE HUMAN GENOME AND ITS FUTURE IMPLICATIONS FOR CARDIOLOGY

Robert Roberts / Richard Lifton

THE HUMAN GENOME

The term *genome* refers to all of the DNA, including the genes, responsible for an organism. The term *proteome* refers to all of the proteins responsible for an organism. The genes exert all of their influence through the proteins they produce. In general, the dogma is still true that each gene produces a unique protein, although it is preferable to refer to the end product as a polypeptide, since some proteins are made of two or more polypeptides and occasionally certain genes, through alternative splicing, may produce more than one polypeptide. The human genome is contained in 23 pairs of chromosomes. Twenty-two of these pairs are homologous chromosomes (one from the father and one from the mother), referred to as autosomes, and the remaining pair contain the sex chromosomes, which in the male consists of an X and a Y chromosome and in the female of two X chromosomes. Only a small portion of the X and Y chromosomes are homologous which is referred to as the pseudoautosomal region. Each pair of autosomal homologous chromosomes carries the same set of genes, with one inherited from each parent. Despite their homology and potentially identical function, some of the genes have a slightly different DNA sequence from that of the corresponding gene on their homologous partner, which may slightly or markedly alter their function. For example, the gene encoding for angiotensin-converting enzyme (ACE) has three forms (alleles): D, DI, and II. Thus, the chromosome from the mother may have the D form and the homologous chromosome from the father the I form; nevertheless, both genes encode for ACE and convert angiotensinogen to angiotensin II. However, there is increased plasma enzyme activity associated with the D form, leading to an exaggeration of ACE function. Studies suggest that individuals who are homozygous for the DD gene are predisposed to develop cardiac hypertrophy.[1,2] These minor differences give rise to individual's genetic distinguishing features and in some instances predispose to the disease.

It is estimated that the difference in the DNA sequence among all humans is about 0.1 percent, which means that 99.9 percent of the DNA sequence is identical. However, there is a difference in over 3 million bases of the DNA sequence. Each chromosome is a long molecule made of DNA. DNA is made up of only four bases: adenine (A), guanine (G), cytosine (C), and thymidine (T). If one visualizes a chromosome, it consists of repetitions of these four bases and is extremely monotonous. Nevertheless, the sequence of these four bases determines all of one's inherited characteristics. The average length of a chromosome is about 135,000,000 base pairs. The longest chromosome, chromosome 1, has over 250,000,000 base pairs. The smallest, chromosome 21, has only 50,000,000 base pairs. The 23 chromosomes together contain a total of 3 billion base pairs (Table 7-1). Genes themselves are discrete units with a start and stop point and vary in size from 10,000 to 2,000,000 base pairs. The estimated average is about 20,000 base pairs. Despite the fact that the whole of the human genome has 3 billion base pairs, it is estimated that only about 3 percent is used to make genes.[3] Genes themselves do not participate in specific functions, but function through an intermediary, their single-stranded templates, referred to as messenger RNA (mRNA). The mRNA leaves the nucleus and goes to the ribosome in the cytoplasm, where it provides the template for protein synthesis. It is estimated there are between 50,000 and 100,000 genes.[3]

The intervening DNA sequences between the genes that do not exit the nucleus are referred to as introns, and the DNA sequences transcribed into mRNA that exits the nucleus to form the template for protein synthesis are referred to as exons. The function of the introns is largely unknown. A small proportion of the introns has the important regulatory function of determining when and how often the gene make, mRNA. Another function of the introns is, presumably, maintaining the structure and integrity of the DNA molecule. On a simple mathematical basis, the introns also offer some protection of the genes from mutations. The natural mutation rate is 1 every 200,000 years per

TABLE 7-1 The Human Genome

Base pairs	3 billion
Genes estimated	50,000–100,000
Percent of DNA contained in genes	<3%

gene. The mutation rate is higher in the introns, but, since the intron is not expressed in the protein, they are benign and nondisease producing. The DNA used to make genes consists of just one copy of each gene per chromosome. However, the introns not infrequently have many repeating units of the same sequence throughout the genome. The most frequent example of this is the ALU repeats, which consists of a 300-base pair repeat with over 500,000 copies scattered throughout the human genome. The role of these repeat sequences is also not known, but they may play a role as replication or initiation sites for duplication of DNA. While foreign DNA is usually destroyed, some, such as the genomes of retroviruses, does get incorporated into the human genome. It is estimated that 35 percent of the human genome is composed of DNA from evolutionary relics of mobile DNA elements transposed into the human genome with no known function.[4] Mutations that induce single-gene diseases inherited as Mendelian disorders occur at a frequency of less than 1 percent. In contrast, mutations that induce more subtle changes (genes that predispose to polygenic diseases; e.g., DD versus II) or none at all may be located in exons or introns and occur more frequently, in the range of 10 to 20 percent. One form of these polymorphisms, single-nucleotide polymorphisms,[5,6] which occur every 1000 base pairs, is discussed subsequently as the most promising marker for identifying genes responsible for polygenic diseases.

THE HUMAN GENOME PROJECT

The Human Genome Project is the first large international effort in the history of biological research.[7] The overall objective of the Human Genome Project was to determine the sequence of the bases throughout each chromosome of the human genome, which is a total of 3 billion bases. The Human Genome Project was initiated on October 1, 1990, to be completed in the year 2005.[8] The National Institutes of Health and the Department of Energy in the United States are expected to produce 60 to 70 percent of the sequences, with the remainder from the Sanger Institute, at Cambridge, England, and other international partners.[7] However, with improvements in technology and increasing demands, the timetable has been accelerated. Initially, the Human Genome Project announced that it would have all of the genes sequenced by the year 2003, and most recently it was announced that a rough draft of 90 percent of the human sequences will be available by the spring of 2000.[7] At least two commercial enterprises involved in sequencing human genes have claimed they will have all of the human genes sequenced by the year 2001.[9] Regardless of the precise timetable and whether every gene is to be identified as indicated, it is now evident there will be an avalanche of genes available to the cardiologist within the next 2 to 3 years. At the end of 1999, only one-third of the human genome was sequenced, and there were less than 1000 human genes available in GenBank. There will be at least 20,000 to 30,000 genes, if not more, available within the first couple of years of the new millenium. It is part of the policy of the Human Genome Project that all of these genes will be available to the public. As it is sequenced, each gene is entered into a publicly accessible database and available at no cost. In the United States, GenBank (accessible at http://www.ncvi.nlm.nih.gov) run by the National Center for Biotechnology Information, serves as the public repository of sequence information. The results of the efforts of the publicly funded Human Genome Project consist not only of DNA sequences of the various genes but also of the intervening sequences. In addition, each sequence is anchored to one of the known genetic markers, integrating the physical and genetic maps. The first chromosome to be sequenced was chromosome 22, which was announced in November 1999. Investigators from Great Britain, the United States, and Japan teamed up to sequence 32,000,000 bases. While there remain some gaps, there is general agreement that essentially all of the genes of chromosome 22, together with most of the intervening sequences, have been sequenced.[10]

Charles Delisi, of the Department of Energy, in commenting on the initiation of the Human Genome Project, stated that the goal was to decipher the blueprint for the development of a single fertilized egg into a complex organism of more than 10^{13} cells. The blueprint is written in a coded message given by the sequence of nucleotide bases—the As, Cs, Gs, and Ts—that are strung along the DNA molecules in the human genome. The goal was to sequence from one end to the other and then to try to decipher all of the instructions included in this massive coding sequence. In 1990, the best of the laboratories were probably sequencing only a few hundred bases per day; at that rate, it would have required centuries to complete the human genome. However, technological improvements have enabled some laboratories engaged in the Human Genome Project to sequence more than 1 million bases per day. While the overall objective was to sequence the human genome, other goals completed along the way markedly accelerated the efforts of all investigators involved in biological or medical research. The first goal was to develop a genetic map. This meant developing markers along each chromosome that would be readily identifiable and highly informative signposts for the identification of nearby genes. This goal has now been achieved. Investigators in France and the United States published 6000 markers spaced less than 1 million base pairs apart throughout the entire human genome.[11] Thus, a complete set of genetic markers is now available for each chromosome. This provided the necessary tool for widespread application of genetic linkage analysis, a technique that has led to the mapping of numerous genes responsible for disease of the cardiovascular system (Chap. 62) and other organs.

The next goal was to develop a genomic physical map. This map would involve sequence tagged sites (STSs) throughout the genome that has been completed.[12] Over 50,000 STSs were given their approximate chromosomal location which made it possible to relate them to the location of a locus genetically linked to a disease of interest.[13] The next goal was to develop a physical map of that part of the DNA that is expressed as genes. These markers are referred to as expressed sequence tags (ESTs) and contain short sequences of 200 to 300 base pairs. These sequences are unique and believed to represent a specific gene. If, indeed, each one of these ESTs represents a gene, we are at present in the position of having available 60,000 genes to be identified.[14] One may wonder how it is possible to obtain such ESTs and be certain that they represent only sequences that are expressed in genes. As indicated previously, all genes are first synthesized as single-stranded mRNA that leaves the nucleus to travel to the ribosome in the cytoplasm, where it serves as a template for its unique protein product. Thus, if one extracted all of the RNA in the cell, it would include all of the mRNAs and, thus, at that moment in time, all of the genes expressed in that cell. This is, in fact, the approach for obtaining ESTs: mRNA is isolated from cells of all organs in the body, and collectively they represent all of the body's expressed genes. The mRNA is then converted to complementary deoxyribonucleic acid (cDNA) with the enzyme reverse transcriptase, and sequences from these cDNAs are amplified by polymerase chain reaction. From these amplified sequences, unique sequences are selected and entered into GenBank as ESTs. These ESTs are cloned in vehicles such as bacteria and, thus, provide a library of human ESTs. Many of these ESTs are now being mapped to their chromosomal location to be used as markers to find genes responsible for disease. The ultimate aim is to have an EST every 100,000 base pairs evenly distributed throughout the 23 chromosomes. The development of the genetic map and that of the physical map, which followed, were great contributions that have tremendously accelerated the efforts of all investigators throughout the world in identifying genes responsible for disease.

FUNCTIONAL GENOMICS (PROTEOMICS)

One of the great accomplishments—and perhaps the greatest of the twenty-first century or even the new millenium—will be the identification of all the genes responsible for humankind. This development is often compared to another great landmark in physics, namely, the identification of the table of physical elements. This analogy emphasizes a very important point for the future. The table of physical elements (periodic table) provided the physicists with the tools to determine the composition of the earth, to understand many natural phenomena, and also to create artificial constructs, many that were essential to modern civilization and others that were destructive, such as the atomic bomb. Identification of the genes will be to the biologist or physician what discovering the physical elements was to the physicist. Leroy Hood refers to the human genetic map as the "periodic table of life." The identification of all human genes provides the tools for the first step: determining gene function and how to manipulate genes to benefit humankind. Determining the function of known and unknown genes was addressed at a recent workshop in Cold Spring Harbor, New York.[15] At present, we know of only about 2000 proteins. Thus, we do not know the protein composition of most genes and so would not be expected to know their function. It was estimated that determining the function of 100,000 genes by conventional techniques—namely, eliminating the gene from the mouse by homologous recombination or overexpressing the gene (transgenic mouse)—would take a century. The theme of Human Genome Project II will undoubtedly be determining functions of the proteins, and the project has been referred to by several names emphasizing function, such as The Proteome, Gene Health and Disease, or Functional Genome II. It is imperative that the efforts to determine the functions of human genes receive a boost from improved technology and increased awareness. New approaches are already emerging from the Human Genome Project to address this issue.

In parallel with the progress for sequencing the human genome has been the success of efforts to sequence simpler genomes of single-cell organisms. The first organism for which the genome was sequenced and the genes identified was *Haemophilus influenzae,* in 1995, consisting of 1.4 million base pairs and 1740 genes. Within 3 years of this initial effort, the genomes of over 40 single-cell organisms were completely sequenced and all of the genes identified. Several notable organisms were sequenced: *Saccharomyces cerevisiae,*[16] which is the cause of vaginitis, and spirochete *Treponema pallidum,*[17] which causes syphilis. These organisms, many of which are bacterial, offer the potential for the diagnosis and treatment of human infectious diseases, whether they affect the heart or other organs. Identification of the genes responsible for these various organisms has ushered in a new era for antibiotics based on a variety of molecular mechanisms made possible through the identification of genes and the various pathways they regulate. A significant step forward in our understanding of the function of human genes came with the sequencing of the genome responsible for *Caenorhabditis elegans* (*C. elegans*).[18] This was the first multicellular organism for which the genome and all of its genes have been sequenced. *C. elegans,* although a tiny worm that is not visible to the naked eye, has 959 cells, all of which have been identified and characterized. Its genome consists of over 97,000,000 base pairs, with a total of over 19,000 genes. This represents one-fifth of the number of genes present in the human genome. The more important features are, however, that 36 percent of the genes in *C. elegans* are virtually identical to human genes, with many others having homologous consensus. The *C. elegans* is a transparent worm, and, thus, it is possible under the microscope to observe development from a single cell to a multicellular organism and now to do so with the armamentarium of knowing all the genes. Thus, it should be possible, by determining the function of many genes in *C. elegans* homologous to human genes, to learn of their approximate function in humans. Several other multicellular organisms are being sequenced, including the fruit fly (*Drosophila*)[19] and the mouse, which will provide an immense opportunity for determining the function of human genes with similar functions.[20] This will considerably accelerate our efforts to determine the function of human genes and how to utilize them to diagnose, prevent, and cure disease.

COMPUTERIZED GENE BANK NETWORKS AND BIOINFORMATICS

It became evident to investigators and physicians involved with genetics that the amount of information to be derived from unraveling the genome would be exhaustive. It was thus necessary to develop a computerized network of gene databases in which information would be rapidly entered worldwide and available worldwide at no cost. GenBank, a computerized network of gene banks, was established in the United States, Britain, and Japan, and all investigators have agreed to input their data daily. This database resource has been invaluable to medical scientists throughout the world. Information on DNA and genes from all species is entered into this network and cataloged for readily accessible use. Over 2 billion DNA bases have been collected from over 39,000 species, and that number is rapidly expanding on a daily basis. There are over 500,000 queries per day for information from GenBank alone. The information in GenBank provides available access to all investigators identifying genes.

The storage of gene sequences is likely to directly contribute to the determination of gene function. The functions of certain genes are often first determined in simple organisms, such as single-cell bacteria or viruses. It is also well recognized that certain genes, because of their function, have been conserved through evolution. Thus, when a DNA sequence is identified in the human genome with consensus sequence to one of the genes of known function in simpler organisms, one immediately has an important clue to the function of that sequence in humans. Such comparative genomic techniques are expected to significantly accelerate our search for the function of genes. A DNA sequence from the human genome with unknown function can be entered into a gene bank network such as GenBank (http://www.ncvi.nlm.nih.gov) and a consensus sequence sought. It is possible with GenBank to travel back in time over 1 billion years to very simple organisms of which much more is known of the function of their genes. Although the human genome may contain 100,000 genes, it is highly likely that many of these genes can be grouped into families that have a common function, such as the genes that encode for kinases. These proteins all have a common function: the transfer of high-energy phosphate from one compound to another. Therefore, genes encoding for kinases will share this common functional motif. This common motif can be used to group unknown genes that have the motif in their sequences to encode for kinases. It is estimated there are over 3000 genes encoding for various kinases. Thus, in addition to computerized comparative genomics, another function of bioinformatics is to cluster based on common functional motifs. Another emerging contribution from bioinformatics is the grouping of genes that have in common a functioning pathway, whether it be that of metabolism or message signaling. Several such signaling pathways have been identified, including the map kinases, the inositol phosphatases, and the tyrosine kinases. It is expected that several metabolic pathways, such as glycolysis, the Kreb's cycle, the hexosmonophosphate shuttle, and others, will have a common group of genes. The cascade of signaling proteins responsible for growth and development of the heart is likely to be very similar across the invertebrate, vertebrate, and mammalian cardiac genetic systems. It is of note that all mammals have a similarly sized genome of 3 billion bases with an estimated 100,000 genes. Similarly, the network of molecules that process the electrical activity to decipher and analyze messages in the brain is likely to have common genetic pathways. It is anticipated that information on human disease-causing genes available from GenBank will be transmitted to nursing stations and made available to all personnel, including physicians, nurses, genetic counselors, and others. Determining the function of genes through such bioinformatics techniques as comparative genomics and gene clustering is likely to contribute greatly to our understanding of the role of genes in human physiology and disease.

THE DNA CHIP TECHNOLOGY

A major obstacle in applying the progress made in molecular genetics to the practice of medicine is inability to detect mutations rapidly and accurately. At the turn of the millenium, there were already 1000 genes in GenBank known to cause disease, with over 25,000 mutations. To perform genetic screening for known mutations and determine individuals at risk for disease is still a formidable task at an unacceptable cost. The various techniques for detecting mutations are time consuming, expensive, and, ideally, require confirmation by DNA sequencing. Technologies to perform these tasks on a daily basis with results available within a reasonable time from hours to days are essential. Several technologies are evolving, the most promising being the DNA microarray chip.[21] Several thousand genes are attached to glass or plastic, and each base is color coded to detect mismatches in hybridization (mismatch mutations; Fig. 7-1). This technique has the potential for robust high-throughput detection of thousands of mutations within hours. Other techniques include high-pressure liquid chromotography and mass spectrometry, both of which also have the potential for high-throughput analysis. Genetic testing of individuals, for example, with familial hypertrophic cardiomyopathy (FHCM) or arrhythmogenic right ventricular dysphasia could prevent the death of thousands of individuals each year in competitive sports. Another use of the DNA chip technology is in the field of pharmacogenomics, or genoptying to individualize therapy. This technique could also provide screening for multiple genes that are up- or down-regulated during the response of a particular organ to various physiologic or pathologic stimuli.

RESTORATIVE BIOLOGY

It is highly likely that, within the first decade of the new millenium, significant progress will be made in our ability to generate organs. While the average human has over 200 trillion cells, it is estimated there are only about 206 distinct cells as defined by a unique function. These cells are derived from stem cells that are pluripotent, which means that with appropriate stimulation they can develop into any kind of cell. There are two types of stem cells: embryonic and adult.[22,23] Embryonic stem cells have not yet specialized into any type of cell and are obtained from two sources: (1) fetal tissues from miscarriages or abortions, and (2) in vitro embryos discarded by fertility clinics that cannot be implanted. Adult stem cells are committed to develop into a specific cell but have some limited capacity to be directed to develop into some other cell. At present, investigators have been relatively unsuccessful in obtaining stem cells from most organs in adults. Stem cells in limited numbers have been obtained from bone marrow, liver, and skeletal muscle. These stem cells, exposed to the appropriate cardiac growth factor, would be expected to develop into cardiac myocytes.[24] There are already considerable preliminary data to show that fibroblasts can be transformed into skeletal muscle.[25,26] The key gene that commits a cell to become a skeletal muscle cell has been identified, namely, MyoD. Transfection with MyoD has been shown to induce the phenotype of skeletal muscle in fibroblasts and several other cells.[26] Myocardial infarction may be thought of as a myocyte deficiency disease in which a part of the myocardium is replaced by fibrous scar tissue. Myoblast, an adult skeletal muscle stem cell, has been transplanted with some success into the heart of a rat that had undergone a previous myocardial infarction.[27] Bone marrow stem cells are being used with some degree of success in regenerating bone marrow in the treatment of leukemias. The National Institutes of Health has already

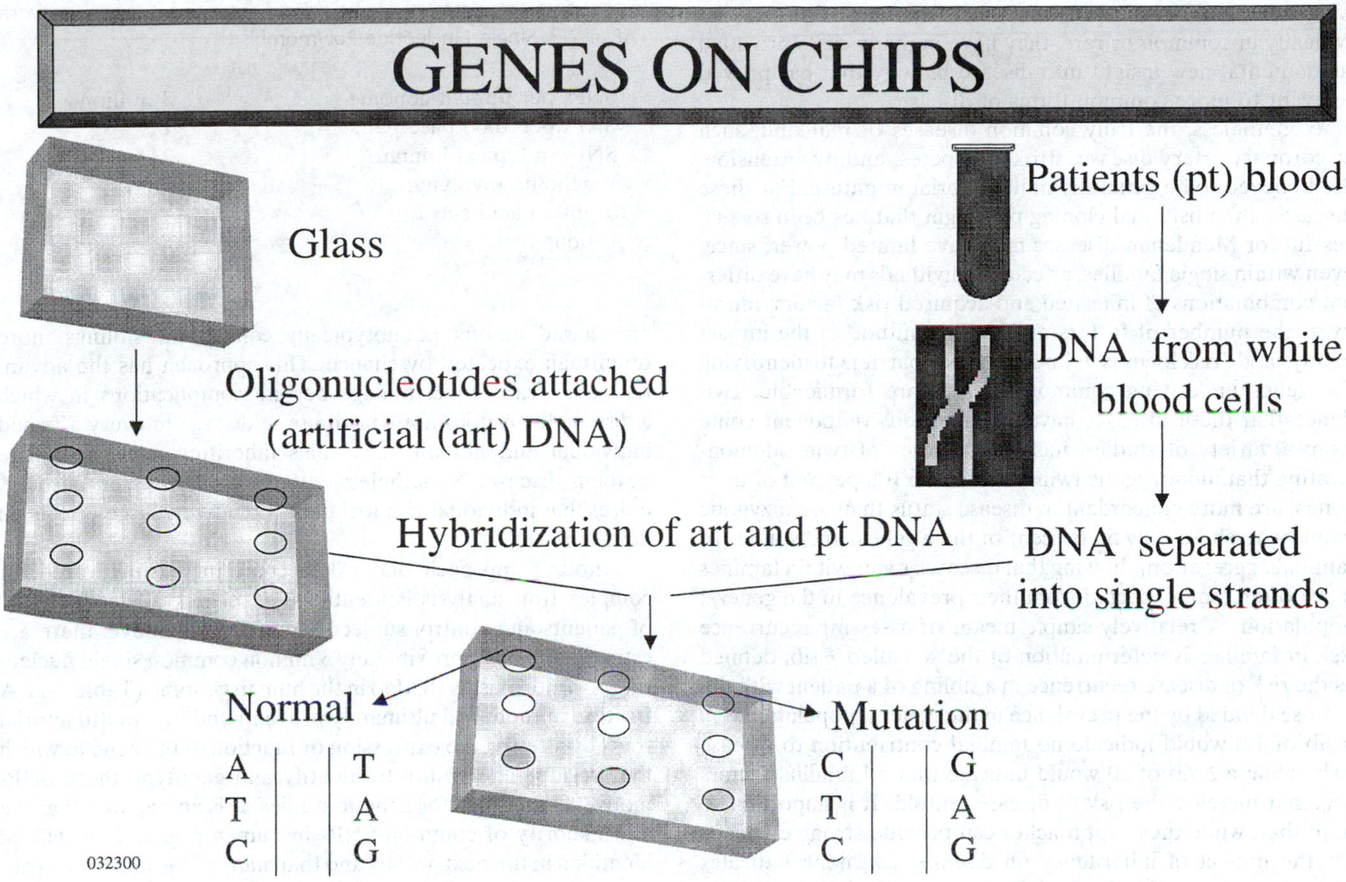

FIGURE 7-1 Illustrated here is the means of detecting genes or their mutations. Oligonucleotides are single short strands of DNA of about 15 to 30 bases artificial synthesized to have the sequence of the desired gene. These oligonucleotides are bound to glass with each of the four bases labeled with a distinct fluorescent color. The DNA extracted from the patient's white blood cells is denatured into separate strands and brought in contact with the artificial oligonucleotides DNA. If the sequence in the patients DNA is complementary to the oligonucleotide, hybridization will occur and the laser beam will detect the appropriate colors. If there is a mutation present, there will be a mismatch and a different color will be exhibited by the laser indicating where the mutation is.

developed goals to begin the pursuit of research to repair or regenerate human organs (www.bioethics.gov). Extensive research will be required to understand the molecular factors necessary to convert stems cells into a pretargeted, specific cell. Nevertheless, this research has great potential for diseases such as myocardial infarction.

A NEW ERA FOR UNRAVELING POLYGENIC DISORDERS

The extraordinary similarities in the height, weight, body habitus, and facial features of identical twins underscore the extremely limited variation in physical features of individuals who share complete genetic identity. The wide variation that is seen in these features among unrelated individuals in the general population strongly implies that much of this variation is attributable to variation in DNA sequence. Therefore, it comes as no surprise that this same principle applies to variation in disease susceptibility and that virtually all human diseases have an inherited component. In some cases, referred to as Mendelian diseases, mutation in a single gene is sufficient to produce disease in a high proportion of individuals inheriting that mutation. For other diseases, the inherited contribution is more subtle, requiring inheritance of variants in a number of genes, with disease development also being influenced by environmental factors. In this setting, inheritance of a particular genetic variant may be neither necessary nor sufficient for disease development. These genetically complex diseases thus have multifactorial determination.

With the development of complete genetic maps of the human genome, a new approach to identifying genes contributing to Mendelian diseases, called positional cloning, became available.[28] Positional cloning proceeds in several stages: (1) the collection of families' segregating traits of interest; (2) determination of the chromosomal location of disease genes by comparing the inheritance of chromosome segments to the inheritance of disease in families; (3) refinement of the interval containing the disease gene and identification of genes in the disease interval; and (4) screening genes in the interval for mutations that alter the structure or expression of the encoded protein. In the Mendelian paradigm, independent mutations that alter the encoded protein and segregate specifically with the disease in families constitute proof that the disease gene has been identified. This approach has to date resulted in identification of nearly 1000 human disease genes, of which over 100 are associated with cardiac diseases, and almost all have been identified within the last decade. While these Mendelian disorders are typically uncommon or rare, they have in many cases provided fundamental new insight into disease biology that has proved relevant to more common forms of disease.

Nonetheless, the truly common diseases of mankind, such as coronary artery disease, stroke, diabetes, and hypertension, are believed to be generally multifactorial in nature. For these diseases, the positional cloning paradigm that has been so successful for Mendelian diseases may have limited power, since, even within single families, affected individuals may have different combinations of inherited and acquired risk factors; moreover, the number of factors and the magnitude of the impact of any single risk locus is unknown. These barriers to identifying the genes underlying common diseases are formidable. Evidence that these diseases have an inherited component come from a variety of studies, including studies of twins, demonstrating that monozygotic twins, who share 100 percent of their genes, are more concordant in disease status than are dizygotic twins, who share only 50 percent of their genes, and studies of familial aggregation, showing that diseases recur within families more often than expected from their prevalence in the general population. A relatively simple means of assessing recurrence risk in families is determination of the so-called δ sib, defined as the risk of disease recurrence in a sibling of a patient with the disease divided by the prevalence in the general population.[29] A δ sib of 1.0 would indicate no familial contribution to disease risk, while a δ sib of 10 would indicate that all familial factors together increase the risk of disease tenfold. It is important to note that, while these approaches can provide strong evidence for the impact of inheritance on disease risk, none indicates how many genes underlie the inherited disease risk, their mode of transmission, or the magnitude of the effect imparted by any single locus. For example, the same tenfold familial increase in disease risk could be determined by the effects of two genes, each imparting fivefold increased risk, or, alternatively, 50 genes, each imparting 1.2-fold increased risk. The best study design for identifying underlying disease genes is considerably confounded by this imprecise knowledge.

There are a number of potential approaches to unraveling the inherited contribution to these complex disorders. One is to simplify the analysis by identifying sub- or intermediate phenotypes in which the genetic contribution is more homogeneous or contributes to a larger fraction of disease risk. For example, the considerable etiologic heterogeneity of coronary artery disease can be reduced by focusing on cases sharing diabetes, hypertension, or hypercholesterolemia as contributing factors. Similarly, further refinement of these subgroups might define physiologic subsets with more homogeneous genetic contribution, potentially defining Mendelian subsets to which the power of Mendelian genetics can be applied.[30]

Despite this potential, few useful intermediate phenotypes have been defined for common diseases, often requiring investigation of non-Mendelian traits. In this setting, linkage approaches like those used for Mendelian diseases might be successful if any single locus imparts a relatively large effect on disease risk, and collecting large extended kindreds may be worthwhile. In the absence of evidence of a substantial Mendelian component, a modification of the linkage approach analyzing large numbers of sibling or relative pairs concordant or discordant for disease has potential advantages. In this approach, one scans the genome for chromosome segments that are shared among phenotypically concordant siblings more often than expected by chance. This approach has the advantage that can detect linkage despite complications in which a disease locus does not contribute to disease in every affected individual and not all individuals inheriting a disease allele develop disease. Nonetheless, success with this approach requires that individual risk loci impart relatively large effects on disease risk.[31]

TABLE 7-2 Single Nucleotide Polymorphisms

SNPs per human genome	3 million
SNPs per 1000 base pairs	1
SNPs in typical human genome involving amino acid substitutions	24,000–40,000

Another approach that will become increasingly used for complex trait analysis is identification of risk alleles by study of patients and control subjects. As indicated above, there are estimated to be approximately 3 million common single nucleotide polymorphisms (SNPs) in the human genome (Table 7-2). A fraction of them will ultimately prove to underlie multifactorial traits by altering the expression or function of the gene in which they reside. The ability to identify and genotype these SNPs motivates their use for genetic studies. It is anticipated that the vast majority of common SNPs in human populations will be identified in the next 5 years and that many of the alleles contributing to common diseases will be found among them. If one tested a SNP whose variation contributes to, for example, coronary artery disease, comparison of SNPs allele frequencies in patients with the disease and in a matched cohort of control subjects free of disease would demonstrate a significantly different distribution of allele frequencies. This approach has substantially higher power than does linkage to detect variants with small effects on disease risk.[31] This case-control approach is associated with a number of important caveats, however. First, patients and control subjects must be well matched for genetic background. If they are not, many SNPs will show a false-positive association with disease. This is a current and serious problem with case-control studies. Unless disease associations are highly reproducible using the same SNP alleles and the same clinical phenotype, their significance should be regarded with caution. One means of eliminating this vexing problem is to collect the parents of affected individuals to permit use of transmission disequilibrium.[32] If a SNP allele contributes to disease risk, it ought to be transmitted from a heterozygous parent to an affected offspring more often than the expected Mendelian proportion of 0.5. This test thus eliminates the problem of poorly matched cases and control subjects and holds considerable promise for the investigation of complex genetic traits. Proof that a disease-associated SNP is itself a functional variant contributing to disease may be problematic, since some of these SNPs may well be common alleles in the population. Proof can be pursued by clinical studies of the physiology of individuals with and without the disease allele, biochemical studies of the wild-type and variant gene and gene product in vitro, and construction and investigation of animal models based on the variant gene.

A second caveat regarding this SNP approach is that at present we have a limited number of SNPs for examination and also a limited capacity for SNP genotyping. As a result, we cannot readily perform comprehensive genome-wide searches for disease variants with this approach, instead being limited to investigation of candidate genes. While this approach may prove successful, we are currently largely limited to implicating genes in pathways we can already associate with disease. There are two approaches to extending this case-control approach to a genome-wide analysis. One is to investigate populations that have been established from a small number of founders in relatively recent times. In such cases, one expects relatively long ancestral chromosome segments to be preserved in the present-day population such that genetic markers at considerable distance from one another remain in *linkage disequilibrium*. Thus, one may be able to screen for the chromosome location of disease susceptibility loci using a relatively modest number of SNPs distributed across the genome; proceeding from initial map location would be analogous to the positional cloning paradigm for Mendelian traits. Alternatively, with identification of complete SNP maps of the human genome, we will have many or all of the common SNPs in hand; one can contemplate performing extremely high-density SNP genotyping in outbred populations to identify disease susceptibility alleles. In order to retain analytic power, this approach may require performance of 10^9 to 10^{10} genotypes; such a study is clearly beyond the capacity of present implemented technology but is not inconceivable in the future.[31]

Ultimately, one can envision that alleles that contribute to susceptibility to common disease will be identified. These findings will have important consequences for clinical medicine. First, these findings will permit identification of individuals with specific inherited disease susceptibility before disease has become manifest, affording new opportunity for targeted lifestyle or pharmacologic intervention in individual patients. Second, identification of these susceptibility alleles will define the physiologic pathways that contribute to disease, providing "validated targets" whose altered activity can be predicted with high likelihood to alter disease development; these will highlight opportunities for development of new therapies. Third, we currently treat multifactorial diseases as though they are of homogeneous causation, with largely empiric therapies. The ability to identify specific risk alleles in individual patients may afford the opportunity to tailor treatment in individual patients to the specific inherited abnormalities underlying their disease susceptibility.

BIOETHICAL IMPLICATIONS AND GENETIC COUNSELING

Molecular genetics will soon be part of routine clinical practice. While most genetic screening currently performed for cardiovascular disease is done as part of a research protocol, many diseases, such as the familiar cardiomyopathies or those associated with the long Q-T syndrome, will soon enter the realm of routine genetic screening and diagnosis. It is estimated that less than 5 to 10 percent of cardiologists have any understanding of genetic testing and that even fewer are capable of interpreting the results of genetic testing. It is well recognized that there are too few genetic counselors and medical geneticists to meet present demands, let alone the demands within a few years, following the exposition of the human genome.[33] It was realized from the very beginning of the Human Genome Project that, in parallel with the scientific effort, there had to be a formal initiative to plan for the ethical, legal, and societal implications (ELSI) of this new paradigm. The National Institutes of Health have allocated 5 percent of the budget of the Human Genome Project for ELSI and the U.S. Department of Energy has allocated 3 percent of the HGP budget. A detailed review of the Human Genome Project and the ELSI have been prepared by the U.S. Department of Energy and the Human Genome Project and made available on the internet (http://www.ornl.gov/hgmis/tko/).

The working group for ELSI developed an agenda with the following main goals: (1) stimulate research on issues through grant making; (2) refine the research agenda through workshops, commissioned papers, and invited lectures; (3) solicit public input; (4) provide massive education through multiple media, including the internet; and (5) encourage international collaboration. A major objective would be to develop policies regarding professional, institutional, governmental, and societal levels to ensure that genetic information would be used to maximize benefit to individuals and society. Three issues were identified as particularly important: privacy of genetic information, safety and efficacy of new testing options, and fairness in the use of genetic information.

The Hereditary Susceptibility Working Group of the National Action Plan on Breast Cancer (NAPBC), coordinated by the Public Health Service Office on Women's Health, recently joined with the National Institutes of Health/Department of Energy ELSI group to address the issue of genetic information in the workplace. The working group recommendations are as follows:

1. Employment organizations should be prohibited from using genetic information to affect the hiring of an individual or to affect the terms, conditions, privileges, benefits, or termination of employment unless the employment organization can prove that this information is job related and consistent with business necessity.
2. Employment organizations should be prohibited from using genetic information or requiring collection or disclosure of genetic information prior to a conditional offer of employment, and, under all other circumstances, employment organizations should be prohibited from requesting or requiring collection or disclosure of genetic information unless the employment organization can prove that this information is job related and consistent with business necessity, or otherwise mandated by law. Written and informed consent should be required for each request, collection, or disclosure.
3. Employment organizations should be restricted from access to genetic information contained in medical records released by individuals as a condition of employment, in claims filed for reimbursement of health care costs, and other sources.
4. Employment organizations should be prohibited from releasing genetic information without prior written authorization of the individual. Written authorization should be required for each disclosure and include to whom the disclosure will be made.
5. Violators of these provisions should be subject to strong

enforcement mechanisms, including a private right of action.

6. The task force recommends genetic testing be made available to individuals in the context of clinical investigation and research; however, the information obtained must remain available only to the patient, physician, and investigator. Information must not be made available to any other party or individual.

In regard to genetic diagnosis and screening, there is as yet no consensus on who should undergo genetic testing, how to protect the privacy of the results, or how this information should be applied in the routine practice of medicine. Most genetic testing in cardiology at present is performed as part of research and as such is regulated by RRC (Recombinant Regulatory Committee) and the local institutional review board. In a recent Bethesda, Maryland, conference of the American College of Cardiology on Bioethics and Molecular Genetics,[33] there was a consensus that certain rules must be followed in the routine use of genetic testing: (1) informed written consent must be obtained prior to obtaining the sample; (2) every effort should be made to provide the necessary education in terms understandable to the concerned individual, and (3) genetic testing must not be performed unless accompanied with counseling. The Bethesda conference offered the following guidelines, recognizing that they will continue to evolve and are as yet not definitive:[34]

1. The use of genetic testing and diagnosis as a research tool should continue along the guidelines outlined for research.
2. Genetic testing (usually prenatal) for devastating fetal disease or early-onset disease, such as Down's syndrome, is performed routinely and should be continued. It has been shown that, if the results are positive, whether the parents seek an abortion or not, the information provided is considered beneficial.
3. Use of genetic testing in someone with a phenotype to confirm or exclude a genetic cause should be permitted. An example would be FHCM with concomitant hypertension.
4. In families with a known history of a familial disease, genetic testing when sought by a family member should be performed. Testing of other members of the family should be performed only at their request.
5. Testing at birth or during childhood for asymptomatic disorders that develop later in life remains investigational until more data are available.

It has been customary not to perform genetic screening in high school students unless there is an immediate medical benefit. However, recent studies[35] from Montreal and Hong Kong show that genetic screening during high school has successfully decreased the incidence of Tay-Sachs disease and β-thalassemia. A major issue associated with the cardiovascular disorder FHCM, the most common cause of sudden death in the young, particularly in the athlete, is whether athletes at the high school and college level with a family history or suspected HCM phenotype should be screened prior to participating in competitive sports.[36]

A NEW PARADIGM FOR MEDICINE

The genetic revolution that has already begun will usher in the beginning of a new paradigm in the diagnosis and treatment of cardiac disorders. Physicians traditionally have been taught to diagnose and treat disease. Cardiology in the past 50 years has advanced more than perhaps in the previous 2000 years.[37] Nevertheless, despite our ability to diagnose, we seldom know the precise molecular defect or pathogenesis of a particular phenotype. In the near future, a single blood sample will make available to the physician 100,000 etiologies with their multiple mutations. This represents a new era in which specific etiologies will be looking for their respective diseases. This will further challenge the physician to attempt to associate genes with physiological functions and mutations with disease. The physician will be well positioned to advance functional genomics through translational research at the bedside. In fact, until recently, physicians who saw individuals without complaints were often questioned as to the appropriateness of their practice. We are now entering an era of prevention, and thousands of genetic risk factors will soon be available on which to base comprehensive and effective preventive therapies. In the near future, physicians will yearn to assess individuals early in life in the hope of aborting major disease, such as atherosclerosis, hypertension, cancer, and osteoporosis. This, too, will represent a new paradigm for all physicians. It will stimulate changes in health care delivery as well as means to finance such programs. The developent of an electronic medical record will be essential, and protection of the individual's rights and privacy will be paramount.[34]

References

1. Marian AJ. Genetic risk factors for myocardial infarction. *Curr Opin Cardiol* 1999; 13:171–178.
2. Schunkert H, Dzau VJ, Tank SS, et al. Increased rat cardiac angiotensin converting enzyme activity and mRNA levels in pressure overload left ventricular hypertrophy: Effects on coronary resistance, contractility and relaxation. *J Clin Invest* 1990; 86:1913–1920.
3. Fields C, Adams MD, White O, Venter JC. How many genes in the human genome? *Nature Genet* 1994; 7:345–346.
4. Bestor TH, Bycko B. Creation of genomic methylation patterns. *Nature Genet* 1996; 12:363–367.
5. Halushka MK, Fan J-B, Bentley K, et al. Patterns of single-nucleotide polymorphisms in candidate genes for blood-pressure homeostasis. *Nature Genet* 1999; 22:239–247.
6. Cargill M, Altshuler D, Ireland J, et al. Characterization of single-nucleotide polymorphisms in coding regions of human genes. *Nature Genet* 1999; 22:231–238.
7. Collins FS. Shattuck Lecture: Medical and societal consequences of the human genome project. *N Engl J Med* 1999; 341:28–37.
8. Cooper NG, ed. *The Human Genome Project: Deciphering the Blueprint of Heredity.* Mill Valley, CA: University Science Books; 1994:359.
9. Marshall E. A high-stakes gamble on genome sequencing. *Science* 1999; 284:1906–1909.
10. Normile D, Pennisi E. Team wrapping up sequence of first human chromosome. *Science* 1999; 285:2038.
11. Murray JC, Buetow KH, Weber JL, et al. A comprehensive human linkage map with centimorgan density. Cooperative Human Linkage Center (CHLC). *Science* 1994; 265:2049–2054.
12. Olson M, Hood L, Cantor C, Botstein D. A common language for physcial mapping of the human genome. *Science* 1989; 245:1434–1435.
13. Ward T, Davies KE. The leading role of STSs in genome mapping. *Hum Mol Genet* 1993; 8:1097–1098.

14. Deloukas P, Schuler GD, Gyapay G, et al: A physical map of 30,000 human genes. *Science* 1998; 282:744–746.
15. Abboud FM, Bassingthwaighte JB, Bond EC, et al: The Banbury Conference: Genomics to physiology and beyond: How do we get there? *Physiologist* 1997; 40:205–211.
16. Holstege FC, Jennings EG, Wyrick JJ, et al. Dissecting the regulatory circuitry of a eukaryotic genome. *Cell* 1998; 95:717–728.
17. Fraser C, Norris S, Weinstock G, et al. Complete genome sequence of *Treponema pallidum,* the syphilis spirochete. *Science* 1999; 281:375–388.
18. Hodgkin J, Horowitz RS, Jasny BR, Kimble J. *C. elegans:* Sequence to biology. *Science* 1998; 282:2011–2017.
19. Garza DAJ, Burke D, Hartl D. Mapping the *Drosophila* genome with yeast artificial chromosomes. *Science* 1989; 246:641–646.
20. Li J, Hampton T, Morgan JP, Simons M. Stretch-induced VEGF expression in the heart. *J Clin Invest* 1997; 100:18–24.
21. Kononen J, Bubendorf L, Kallioniemi A, et al. Tissue microarrays for high-throughput molecular profiling of tumor specimens. *Nature Med* 1998; 4:844–847.
22. Thomson JA, Itskovitz-Eldor J, Shapiro SS, et al. Embryonic stem cell lines derived from human blastocyst. *Science* 1998; 282:1145–1147.
23. Gearhart J. New potential for human embryonic stem cells. *Science* 1998; 282:1061–1062.
24. Solter D, Gearhart J. Putting stem cells to work [see comments]. *Science* 1999; 283:1468–1470.
25. Weintraub H, Davis R, Tapscott S, et al. The myoD gene family: Nodal point during specification of the muscle cell lineage. *Science* 1991; 251:761–766.
26. Sartorelli V, Kurabayashi M, Kedes L. Muscle-specific gene expression: A comparison of cardiac and skeletal muscle transcription strategies. *Circ Res* 1993; 72:925–931.
27. Murray CE, Wiseman RW, Schwartz SM, Hauschka SD. Skeletal myoblast transplantation of repair of myocardial necrosis. *J Clin Invest* 1996; 98:2512–2523.
28. Botstein D, White RL, Skolnick M, Davis RW. Construction of a genetic linkage map in man using restriction fragment length polymorphisms. *Am J Hum Genet* 1980; 32:314–331.
29. Risch N. Linkage strategies for genetically complex traits: II. The power of affected relative pairs. *J Genet Hum* 1990; 46:229–241.
30. Lipton RP. Molecular genetics of human blood pressure variation. *Science* 1996; 272:676–680.
31. Risch N, Merikangas K. The future of genetic studies of complex human diseases. *Science* 1996; 273:1516–1517.
32. Spielman RS, McGinnis RE, Ewens WJ. Transmission test for linkage disequilibrium: The insulin gene region and insulin-dependent diabetes mellitus (IDDM). *Am J Hum Genet* 1993; 52:506–516.
33. Collins FS. Preparing health professionals for the genetic revolution. *JAMA* 1997; 278:1285–1286.
34. Roberts R, Ryan TJ. 29th Bethesda Conference, Task Force 3: Clinical research in a molecular era and the need to expand its ethical imperatives. *J Am Coll Cardiol* 1998; 31:917–949.
35. Kronn D, Jansen V, Ostrer H. Carrier screening for cystic fibrosis, Gaucher disease, and Tay-Sachs disease in the Ashkenazi Jewish population: The first 1000 cases at New York University Medical Center, New York, NY. *Arch Intern Med* 1998; 158:777–781.
36. Corrado D, Basso C, Schiavon M, Thiene G. Screening for hypertrophic cardiomyopathy in young athletes. *N Engl J Med* 1998; 339:364–369.
37. Roberts R. A glimpse of the future from present day molecular genetics. In: Opie LH, Yellon DM, eds. *Cardiology at the Limits III.* Cape Town: Stanford Writers; 1999:105.

C H A P T E R 8

CARDIOVASCULAR TISSUE MODIFICATION BY GENETIC APPROACHES

Elizabeth G. Nabel / Victor J. Dzau

The field of cardiovascular gene therapy had its origins in the mid-1980s as a result of rapid advances in the molecular genetics of the cardiovascular system. The cloning of genes important for the development and function of the cardiovascular system increased our understanding of the normal biology and pathology of cardiac diseases. In turn, this genetic information provided new opportunities for novel therapeutics using gene-transfer approaches.

Somatic gene transfer is the introduction of recombinant genetic material (DNA or RNA) into host cells such that gene expression within the host cell is altered to achieve a therapeutic effect. The genetic material includes eukaryotic genes (often with transcriptional regulatory elements) and RNA that encodes intracellular or secreted gene products. *Vectors* are used commonly to introduce the genetic material into cells (Table 8-1). These vectors include replication-incompetent viruses and biochemical substances. The genetic material can be delivered directly into vascular or myocardial cells in vivo, referred to as *direct gene transfer,* or into tissues, such as a venous bypass graft ex vivo that in turn is returned to the host. This latter approach is termed *indirect gene transfer.* Local delivery catheters are required for the introduction of vectors and cells (Fig. 8-1).

This chapter reviews our current understanding of genetic therapies, including stem cell biology, for cardiovascular diseases. This discussion will examine vector systems for delivering genes, disease targets and preclinical animal models, recent results of clinical trials, and new, emerging opportunities for cell transplantation with pluripotent stem cells.

VECTORS FOR GENE TRANSFER

Viral Vectors

RETROVIRAL VECTORS

Retroviruses were the first viruses adapted for use as vectors owing to the simplicity of their genomes and their capacity to stably integrate their genome into the host chromosome. A retroviral vector is constructed in several steps.[1,2] First, the structural genes required for viral replication are deleted to render the vector nonreplicating. After insertion of the exogenous gene of interest into the viral backbone, the recombinant retrovirus contains the exogenous gene, regulatory sequences, and packaging signals but lacks the actual structural genes required to produce a complete virion. It requires a helper cell to produce infectious viral particles. Nabel et al. demonstrated the feasibility of transfecting blood vessels with foreign DNA in vivo by transfecting pig iliofemoral arteries with a recombinant amphotropic retroviral vector containing a β-galactosidase gene.[3,4] Several cell types in the vessel wall were transduced, including endothelial and vascular smooth muscle cells. Using a β-galactosidase retroviral vector to modify endothelial cells, Wilson et al.[5] demonstrated β-galactosidase expression up to 5 weeks after transfection in prosthetic vascular grafts seeded with the genetically transformed cells. Retroviral vectors have not been effective vectors for cardiovascular applications because they require actively dividing cells for integration and expression of the viral genome. Since most myocardial and vascular cells are not dividing, transfection efficiency with retroviral vectors in these cells has been low.

ADENOVIRAL VECTORS

Adenoviral vectors are widely used for cardiovascular gene transfer because adenoviruses infect nondividing cells and do not integrate into the host genome. Adenoviruses are double-stranded linear DNA viruses that in their wild type cause a self-limited respiratory tract infection in humans.[6] The wild-type adenovirus genome is a 36-kDa DNA molecule that is divided into 100 map units. The majority of adenoviral vectors are derived from adenovirus serotypes 2 and 5. These vectors are constructed by deletion of the E1 region (map units 1–9) of the genome that normally encodes E1A and E1B motifs that are required for the expression of late viral genes and for the induction of the lytic phase of the virus. Without the E1 region, the virus cannot replicate. This region is replaced with the

TABLE 8-1 Gene Transfer Vectors

Viral vectors	Nonviral vectors
Retrovirus	Cationic liposomes
Adenovirus	Fusigenic liposomes
Adeno-associated virus	DNA plasmid vectors

transgene of interest, up to 7.5 kb in size. Because the E1 deletion renders them replication-incompetent, adenoviral vectors are propagated in a helper cell line that expresses E1 protein in transfection. These vectors can be produced in high titers for in vivo delivery.[7] Adenoviral vectors enter mammalian cells by receptor-mediated endocytosis and $\alpha 2\beta 3$ integrins.[8] Aortic smooth muscle cells[9] and cardiac myocytes[10] were transfected successfully using replication-defective adenovirus carrying the β-galactosidase or chloramphenicol acetyltransferase reporter gene, respectively. In vivo transfection by adenoviral vectors was demonstrated in vascular tissue by direct infusion into vessels,[9,11,12] in myocardial tissue by direct injection into the myocardium,[10,13] and in the circulation after adenoviral infection of skeletal muscle.[14] Limitations of the first-generation adenoviral vectors include transient gene expression and host inflammatory and immune responses against the transgene[15] and viral antigens.[16,17] These limitations are being overcome by the development of "gutted" adenoviral vectors.[18] These vectors retain viral

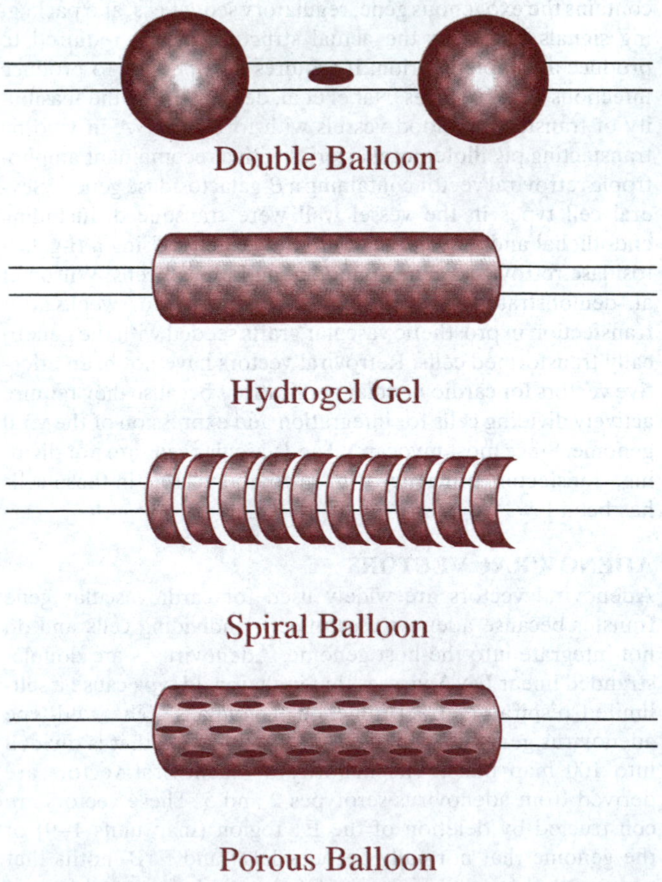

FIGURE 8-1 Catheters for cardiovascular gene therapy. (From Nabel,[95] with permission.)

coat proteins for receptor attachment and internalization but lack other viral proteins that are immunogenic.

ADENO-ASSOCIATED VIRAL VECTORS

Adeno-associated virus (AAV) is a defective human parvovirus that is not able to replicate unless a helper virus, such as adenovirus, is also present.[19] There are several features that make AAV an attractive vector. The virus can be prepared at high titer, is not pathogenic in humans, and infects a broad range of cell lines.[20] Wild-type AAV integrates in a site-specific manner in a 7-kb region of human chromosomes.[20,21] The AAV genome is a single-stranded, linear, 5-kb DNA molecule. The genome is flanked by two 145-bp inverted terminal repeats (ITRs) that contain the sequences required for packing, integration, and DNA replication. The coding region contains two open reading frames (ORFs). Either of these ORFs can be replaced with the transgene and regulatory elements to construct an AAV vector. The ORF can only accept a transgene of 4 to 5 kb, thus limiting the size of the transgene insert. Propagation of AAV vectors requires AAV Rep and Cap proteins and five adenoviral proteins: E1A, E1B, E2A, E4, and VA. These are complex packaging requirements, and thus it has been difficult to construct a packaging cell line. Instead, AAV vectors are propagated by cotransfection of the AAV vector with a plasmid wild-type or mutant helper adenovirus. AAV vectors have been used very successfully when injected into skeletal muscle to produce proteins secreted into the circulation, such as factor IX for hemophilia B.[22] Cardiovascular applications include cardiac myocytes, where Svensson et al. have demonstrated stable expression.[23] Whether AAV vectors can be adapted to efficiently transduce vascular endothelial cells and smooth muscle cells is not known.

Nonviral Vectors

CATIONIC LIPOSOMES

The encapsulation of DNA in artificial lipid membranes (i.e., liposomes) can facilitate its uptake and cellular transport. Cationic liposomes have been used for cellular delivery of DNA[24] and antisense oligonucleotides.[25] The activity of cationic liposomes is postulated to be mediated by (1) spontaneous capture of the negatively charged polynucleotides with cationic lipids by a condensation reaction, (2) increased cellular uptake due to interaction of positively charged complexes with negatively charged biologic membranes, and (3) membrane fusion (or transient membrane destabilization) with the plasmalemma or the endosome to achieve delivery into the cytoplasm while avoiding degradation in the lysosomal compartment. Recent data indicate that movement of DNA from the cytoplasm to the nucleus and successful dissociation of DNA from the lipid complex appear to be important variables for lipid-mediated gene transfer.[26] Expression of recombinant genes after cationic lipid-mediated gene transfer has been demonstrated in vivo in several animal models.[27-29] Gene expression after liposome-mediated arterial gene transfer may be augmented in the presence of ongoing proliferation (e.g., intimal proliferation after balloon injury).[30]

FUSIGENIC LIPOSOMES

This method uses a combination of fusigenic proteins of the Sendai virus (hemagglutinating virus of Japan) and neutral liposomes. Hemagglutinating virus of Japan (HVJ) is an RNA virus that belongs to the paramyxovirus family, which has HN and F glycoproteins on its envelope. HN binds with glycol-type sialic acid and degrades the receptor by its own neuraminidase activity. F glycoprotein is cleaved to generate a hydrophobic fusion peptide by proteases, and the activated F protein can interact directly with the cellular lipid bilayer and induces fusion. A nuclear protein, namely, high-mobility group 1 (HMG-1), that binds DNA enhances the integration of transfected DNA into the nucleus.[31] HVJ liposomes consist of neutral liposomes complexed with ultraviolet (UV) light-inactivated HVJ virus. It is postulated that after fusion of the liposome complex with the cell membrane, the DNA is released directly into the cytosol without undergoing endocytosis, thereby reducing lysosomal destruction of the DNA construct and facilitating the nuclear uptake.[32] HVJ liposome methods have been employed successfully for gene transfer in vivo to liver,[31] kidney,[33] and vasculature.[34,35]

PLASMID DNA

Direct injection of plasmid DNA in cardiac or skeletal muscle results in stable transfection of a small percentage of cells.[36] Following direct injection to the heart muscle, expression of a reporter gene was demonstrated for up to 4 weeks.[37] Expression of injected genes can be targeted to specific cell types in vivo (e.g., cardiac muscle cells) and can be modulated by the hormonal status of the animal.[38]

SYNTHETIC OLIGONUCLEOTIDES

Antisense oligonucleotides (ASOs) are short, 10- to 30-bp, chemically synthesized DNA molecules that are designed to be complementary to the coding sequence of a target RNA. ASOs can be introduced into cells simply by diffusion or complexed with liposomes, such as HVJ.[32] Inside the cell, ASOs form double-stranded complexes with their complementary RNA and decrease translation of RNA. Mechanisms of antisense inhibition include interference with ribosome binding and processing of mRNA, interference with mRNA conformation or mRNA splicing, and RNase-H activation of mRNA digestion.[39,40]

ASOs are attractive agents for in vivo gene therapy. They can be chemically synthesized in large quantities, and they do not require a viral component for in vivo delivery. However, there are several limitations to their use in vivo. ASOs have a short half-life in vivo due to nuclease degradation. Chemical modifications, such as substitution of sulfur for one of the nonbridging oxygens of a phosphate group (phosphorothiorates), renders ASOs more stable to degradation in serum.[41] Several nonspecific effects of ASOs have been noted that account in part for their biologic effect.[39,42] ASOs can have nonspecific cytotoxic effects due to binding to intracellular and cell surface proteins. Some ASOs affect the expression of multiple genes in addition to the gene of interest. This effect is sequence-specific and cannot be controlled for by scrambled oligonucleotides. ASOs containing C_pG dinucleotides have been shown to have nonantigen activation of the humoral immune system.[43] Despite these relative limitations, ASOs are well suited to the treatment of diseases where transient

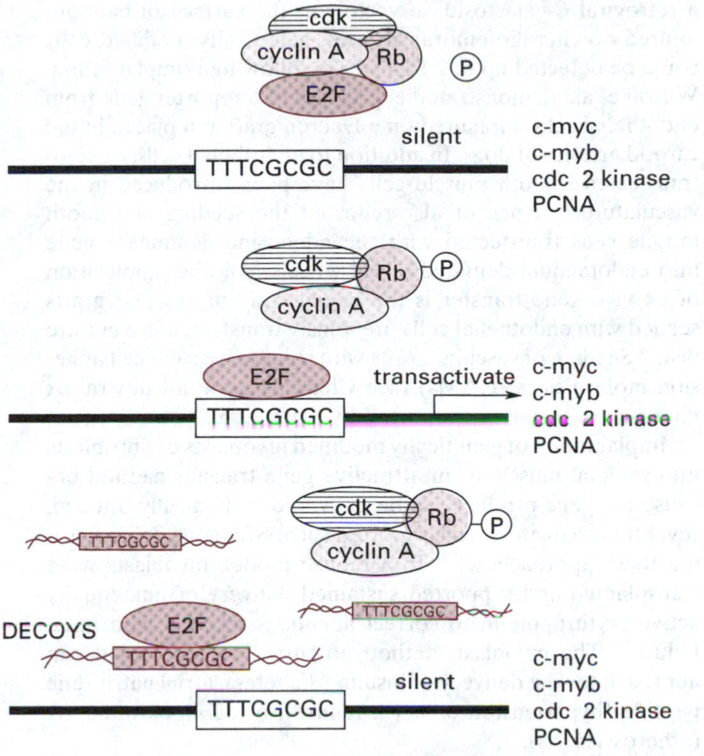

FIGURE 8-2 Principal of E2F "decoy" strategy. TTTCGCGC is the consensus sequence for the E2F binding site. In the quiescent cell state, the transcription factor E2F is complexed with Rb (retinoblastoma gene product), cyclin A, and the cyclin-dependent kinase cdk2 (*top*). Phosphorylation of Rb releases free E2F, which binds to cis elements of the cell cycle regulatory genes, resulting in the transactivation of these genes (*middle*). The E2F decoy cis-element double-stranded oligonucleotide binds to free E2F, preventing E2F-mediated transactivation of cell cycle regulatory genes (*bottom*). (From Morishita et al.,[45] with permission.)

reductions in gene expression are required. ASOs theoretically can be used to specifically reduce the expression of one or more genes. The uptake of ASOs can be enhanced by complexing the oligonucleotide with cationic liposomes[25] or HVJ liposomes.[34,35]

Synthetic double-stranded oligonucleotides containing binding sites for transcription factors serve as "decoys" to block the binding of nuclear factors to promoter regions of targeted genes, resulting in the inhibition of gene transactivation.[41,44] Morishita et al.[45] have shown that a single administration of an E2F decoy (containing the E2F cis element) that binds the transcription factor E2F inhibits smooth muscle cell hyperplasia in a rat carotid balloon injury model[45] (Fig. 8-2). The binding of E2F prevents it from transactivating the gene expression of cell cycle regulatory proteins such as PCNA, c-myc, and cdk2, thereby inhibiting vascular smooth muscle cell proliferation and subsequent neointimal formation in vivo.

CELLULAR TRANSPLANTATION

The implantation of cells expressing recombinant genes into the heart or vasculature is termed *ex vivo gene transfer*. Nabel et al.[3] demonstrated a cell-based vascular gene-transfer technique. By reimplanting endothelial cells transfected ex vivo with a retroviral β-galactosidase vector on the surface of balloon-injured porcine iliofemoral arteries, genetically modified cells could be detected up to 2 to 4 weeks following reimplantation. Wilson et al.[5] demonstrated expression of a reporter gene from endothelial cells implanted on a Dacron graft and placed in the carotid arteries of dogs. In addition to endothelial cells, ex vivo-transfected smooth muscle cells have been introduced in the vasculature.[46] Lynch et al.[47] reported the seeding of smooth muscle cells transfected with the adenosine deaminase gene into endothelium-denuded blood vessels. Another application of ex vivo gene transfer is the engineering of vascular grafts seeded with endothelial cells previously transfected in a culture dish.[48] Seeding of vascular grafts with soluble vascular cell adhesion molecules (sVCAMs) (see Chap. 5) using adenoviral ex vivo gene transfer was reported by Chen et al.[49]

Implantation of genetically modified myoblasts or fibroblasts into skeletal muscle is an attractive gene-transfer method because the gene product can be delivered systemically. Indeed, several investigators have reported successful gene delivery using these approaches.[50–52] In a mouse model, myoblasts were transplanted and supported sustained delivery of functionally active erythropoietin to correct anemia associated with renal failure.[53] The myoblast method potentially could provide an approach for the delivery of insulin (diabetes), atrial natriuretic peptide (hypertension or heart failure), or apolipoprotein AI (atherosclerosis).

GENE TRANSFER AND VASCULAR DISEASE

Gene transfer into the vasculature has been used to investigate the pathophysiology of vascular diseases and to develop novel therapies for these diseases. This field has expanded rapidly in the past decade. A number of models in the mouse, rat, rabbit, dog, and pig have been created to dissect vascular pathophysiology in peripheral, coronary, renal, pulmonary, and cerebral blood vessels. A full discussion of these animal models is beyond the scope of this chapter, and the reader is guided to pertinent reviews.[54–58]

Experimental Applications of ASOs

INTIMAL HYPERPLASIA

Simons et al.[59] reported that the administration of ASOs against c-myb applied by pluronic gel to the adventitial layer of rat carotid arteries inhibited neointimal hyperplasia in response to balloon injury. Data from Morishita et al.[34] demonstrated that a single HVJ liposome-mediated administration of ASOs against proliferating cell nuclear antigen (PCNA) and cdc2 kinase inhibited neointimal lesion formation after balloon injury for at least 8 weeks after transfection. The combination of antisense cdc2 kinase and cdk2 kinase oligonucleotides also resulted in almost complete inhibition of neointima formation.[35] Bennett et al.[60] showed an inhibition of vascular smooth muscle cell proliferation by administration of c-myc ASOs to the adventitial surface of injured carotid arteries in a pluronic gel solution. Two other studies reported inhibition of neointima formation after application of ASOs. Delivery of antisense PCNA oligonucleotides by pluronic gel (in a rat carotid model) and of antisense c-myc oligonucleotides by direct application through a porous balloon (in a porcine coronary artery model) resulted in significant inhibition of neointimal hyperplasia.[61,62]

VEIN GRAFT DISEASE

Autologous vein grafts remain the most commonly used conduits for surgical revascularization of the heart and lower extremities. Given the failure of traditional therapies at improving long-term vein graft function, gene therapy offers a new opportunity for reducing the morbidity and increased costs associated with the current limitations on functional graft survival. The vein graft offers an unusual opportunity for combining intact tissue in vivo gene-transfer techniques with the increased safety of an ex vivo application of the transfection medium. Manipulation of transfection conditions, including increased exposure time and controlling components of the transfection medium, also can be more easily achieved. Some researchers have begun to explore the possibility of ex vivo virus-mediated gene transfer in autologous vein grafts. Chen et al.[49] demonstrated the expression of the marker gene β-galactosidase along the luminal surface and in the adventitia of porcine vein grafts infected with a replication-deficient adenoviral vector at the time of surgery. In this same study, short-term expression of soluble VCAM-1 was documented after transfection of vein grafts.

The Dzau laboratory hypothesized that genetic engineering could alter the ability of the grafts to mount a hyperplastic response to acute injury while leaving intact their ability to respond to chronic hemodynamic stress via a hypertrophic response, such as that seen in arteries exposed to hypertension. This group used HVJ liposomes to deliver a combination of ASOs to cdc2/PCNA to rabbit veins at the time of grafting into the carotid artery and observed a greater than 90 percent inhibition of smooth muscle cell (SMC) proliferation during the first postoperative week[63] (Fig. 8-3). This blockade of cell cycle progression resulted in a near-complete inhibition of neointimal hyperplasia. Instead, the vein graft wall was shifted to an adaptive process of medial hypertrophy. Having redirected the genetically engineered grafts away from neointimal hyperplasia and toward medial hypertrophy as an adaptation to the arterial environment, the susceptibility of these ASO-treated grafts to accelerated atherogenesis was tested. Control ASO-treated and untreated grafts placed in cholesterol-fed rabbits developed significant foam cell lesions and plaque within 6 weeks after surgery. ASO-treated grafts that had remained free of neointima formation, however, resisted macrophage invasion and the development of macroscopic plaque. This inhibition of cell cycle progression is likely to have effects on the phenotypes of the vascular cells undergoing remodeling after vein grafting, and these changes are likely to affect the proatherogenic environment of the normal graft wall. For example, the endothelium of ASO-treated grafts retained more of its capacity to produce nitric oxide and resist monocyte adhesion in comparison with untreated or control ASO-treated grafts.[64]

Gene Transfer and Vascular Remodeling

Molecular cardiovascular research has resulted in significant gains in the knowledge of disease processes at cellular and molecular levels and has led to the characterization of expressed genes in diseased blood vessels. These gene products play autocrine and/or paracrine roles in vascular pathophysiology.

Nabel et al.[65] overexpressed an expression vector encoding a secreted form of fibroblast growth factor 1 (FGF-1) in porcine arteries. FGF-1 expression was associated with intimal thickening of the transfected vessels together with neocapillary formation in the expanded intima. These findings suggest that FGF-1 induces intimal hyperplasia in the arterial wall in vivo, and through its ability to stimulate angiogenesis in the neointima, FGF-1 could stimulate neovascularization of atherosclerotic plaques. In the same porcine model, the overexpression of transforming growth factor β1 (TGF-β1) in normal arteries resulted in substantial production of extracellular matrix accompanied by intimal and medial hyperplasia.[65] These findings demonstrated that TGF-β1 differentially modulates extracellular matrix production and cellular proliferation in the arterial wall and plays a reparative role in response to arterial injury. The increased production of extracellular matrix that accompanied the intimal and medial hyperplasia was not observed following expression of other growth factor genes in the vessel wall, including genes for platelet-derived growth factor (PDGF-BB)[27,66] or the secreted form of FGF-1.[62] Porcine arteries transfected with human PDGF-BB demonstrated intimal hyperplasia with increased numbers of intimal smooth muscle cells. An increased deposition of procollagen, however, as seen in TGF-β1-transfected vessels, was not observed. By stimulating the formation of extracellular matrix, it is possible that TGF-β1 could promote healing following vascular injury, limiting the extensive cellular intimal hyperplasia observed with PDGF-BB.[66]

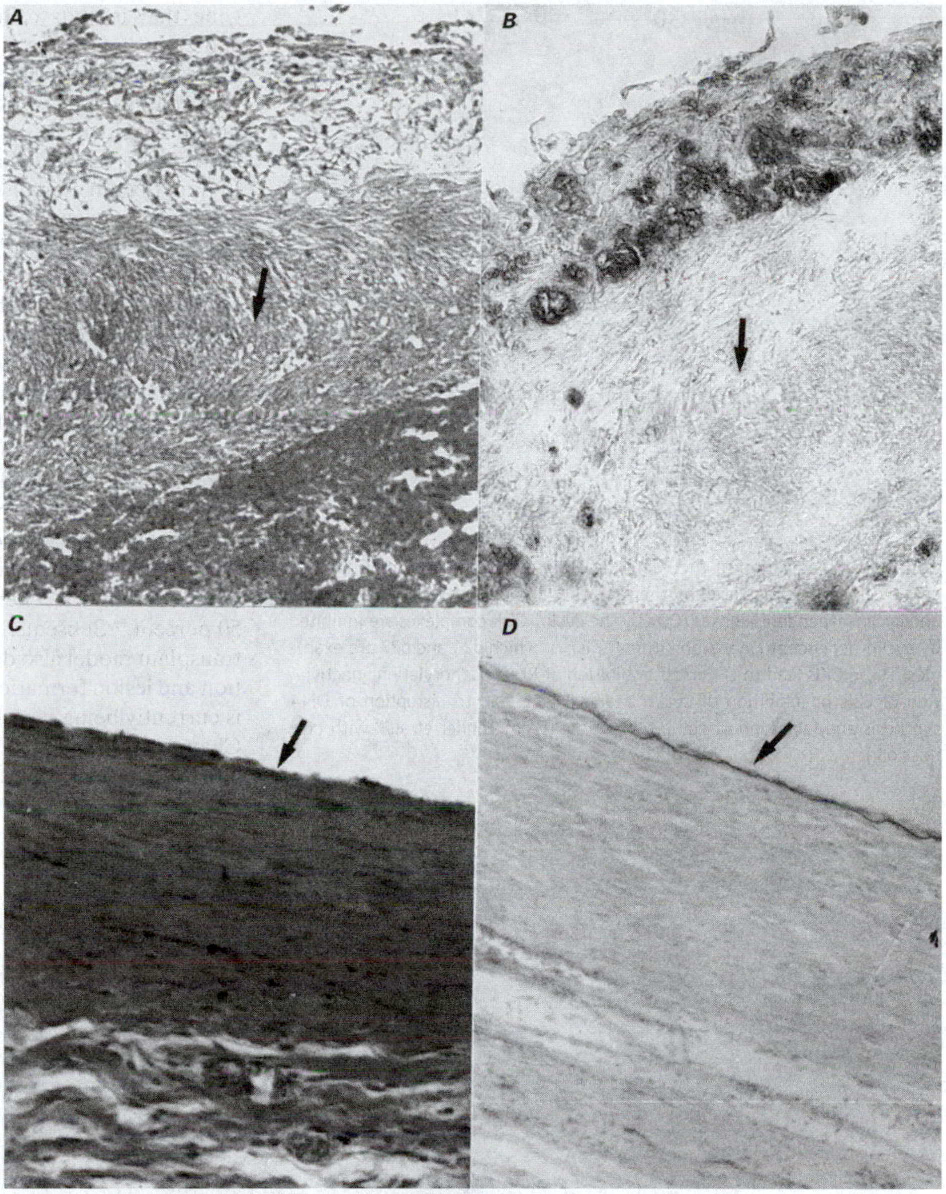

FIGURE 8-3 Control oligonucleotide-treated (*A* and *B*) and ASO (against cdc2 kinase/PCNA)-treated vein grafts (*C* and *D*) in hypercholesterolemic rabbits 6 weeks after surgery (×70). Sections of 5 mm were stained with hematoxylin/van Gieson (*A* and *C*) and a monoclonal antibody against rabbit macrophages (*B* and *D*). Arrows indicate the location of the internal elastic lamina. (From Mann et al.,[63] with permission.)

The pathogenesis of vascular diseases such as hypertension involves a process of vascular remodeling associated with increased vascular hypertrophy and activation of the local angiotensin system. Angiotensin II has been shown to stimulate the growth and proliferation of vascular smooth muscle as well as collagen biosynthesis in vitro. Its in vivo role has been inferred from experiments using angiotensin converting enzyme (ACE) inhibitors. Since these drugs produce hemodynamic effects, a direct role of local angiotensin in vascular remodeling was not clear. To study the local effects of angiotensin, Morishita et al.[67] overexpressed ACE within the vascular wall. Immunoreactive ACE activity was noted in medial vascular smooth muscle cells as well as in intimal endothelial cells. Vascular ACE activity was associated with increased DNA synthesis and vascular protein content via the local production and action of vascular angiotensin II without changes in systemic blood pressure. Parallel to these biochemical changes, medial thickening of ACE-transfected vessel segments was noted, without changes in luminal diameters, implying medial wall hypertrophy by local production of angiotensin II. In a subsequent study, Nakajima et al.[68] demonstrated that overexpression of the type 2 angiotensin II (AT2) receptor in balloon-injured rat carotid arteries exerts an antiproliferative effect, counteracting the growth action of AT1 receptors.

One approach to the treatment of vascular diseases that are characterized by excessive cell proliferation is to overexpress a

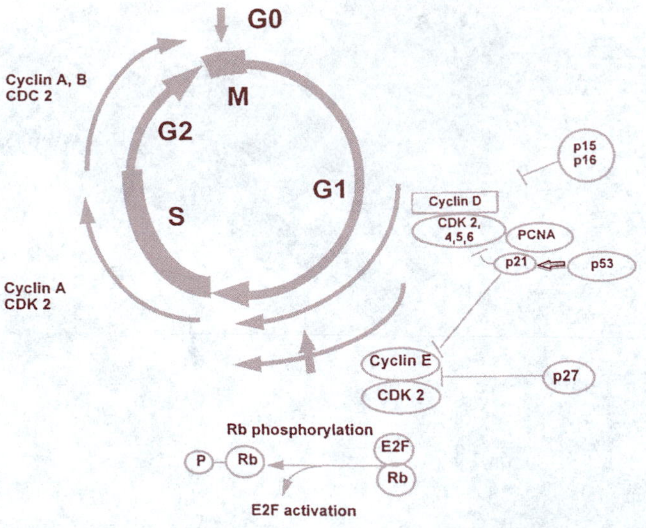

FIGURE 8-4 Regulation of the cell cycle. Progression through the G1 phase of the cell cycle is regulated by the assembly and phosphorylation of cyclins and cyclin-dependent kinases (CDKs). The cyclin-CDK complexes are inhibited by cyclin-dependent kinase inhibitors (CKIs), of which p21 and p27 are examples. These CKIs lead to G1 arrest. Inhibition of Rb phosphorylation, inactiviation of E2F, or inhibition of cyclin A and B also lead to disruption of DNA synthesis and inhibition of cell proliferation. (From Tanner et al.,[96] with permission.)

gene that inhibits cellular proliferation. It is important that expression of the gene proceed during the time period when intimal cells undergo proliferation following vascular injury. This may vary between animal models, and it is likely that in humans, cell proliferation following angioplasty, stent placement, or bypass graft surgery may proceed over a longer period of time than in animal models. Nonetheless, several gene products have proven efficacious in appropriate animal models of vascular injury. Most of these approaches are based on arresting vascular cells in G1 or S phase of the cell cycle (Fig. 8-4). One approach is to express the herpes simplex virus thymidine kinase gene (*HSVtk*). *HSVtk* encodes for the enzyme thymidine kinase that phosphorylates the nucleoside analog ganciclovir or acyclovir into a metabolite that disrupts replication of DNA during S phase of the cell cycle. A by-product of this biochemical reaction is diffusible to adjacent cells, where it is incorporated in replicating cells, leading to inhibition of cell replication. This property is termed a *bystander effect* and allows for inhibition of replication in a greater number of cells than transfected. This model was established initially in a pig peripheral artery model of vascular injury, where intimal hyperplasia was decreased by 50 percent.[69] Subsequent investigations in the rat, rabbit, and a transplant model also demonstrated reductions in cell proliferation and lesion formation by about 50 percent.[70–73] This approach is currently being investigated in a model of in-stent restenosis. Chang et al.[74] demonstrated that localized arterial infection with a replication-defective adenovirus encoding a nonphosphorylatable, constitutively active form of the retinoblastoma gene product at the time of angioplasty significantly reduced SMC proliferation and neointima formation in both the rat carotid and porcine femoral artery models of restenosis. The cyclin-dependent kinase inhibitors p21 and p27 that arrest smooth muscle cells in G1 phase of the cell cycle are also potent negative regulators of lesion formation after vascular injury.[75–78] Ras proteins are key transducers of mitogenic signals from the cell membrane to the nucleus. The local delivery of vectors expressing *ras* transdominant negative mutants, which interfere with ras function, reduced neointimal lesion formation in a rat carotid artery balloon-injury model.[79]

To assess the effect of endothelial cell nitric oxide synthase (ecNOS) on vessel lesion formation, a DNA vector encoding ecNOS was expressed in a rat model of arterial injury[80] (Fig. 8-5). Four methods were used to verify ecNOS expression: transgene protein expression by Western blot, localization of enzyme expression by in situ histochemical staining, enzymatic activity of the transgene product, and vascular reactivity in

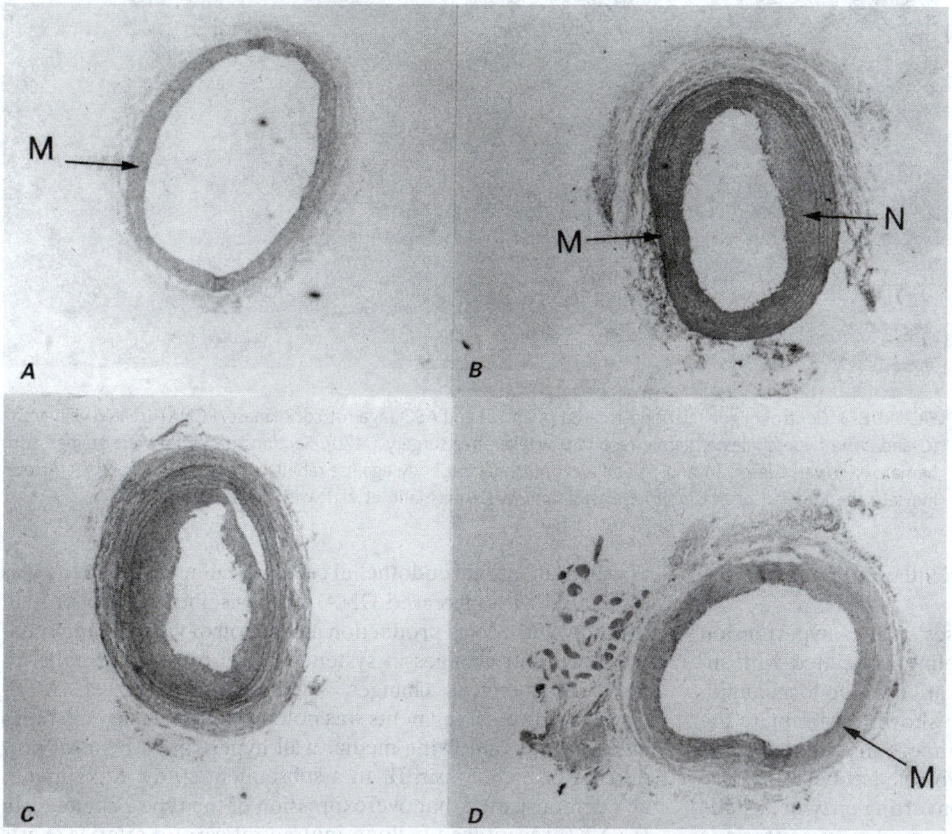

FIGURE 8-5 Inhibition of neointimal hyperplasia by in vivo gene transfer of endothelial cell nitric oxide synthase (ecNOS) in balloon-injured rat carotid arteries. *A.* Normal artery. *B.* Injured, untransfected artery. *C.* Injured, control vector-transfected artery. *D.* Injured, ecNOS-transfected artery. M, media; N, neointima. (From von der Leyen et al.,[80] with permission.)

response to the transgene. Overexpression of ecNOS led to vasorelaxation and 70 percent inhibition of neointima formation after balloon injury. This same approach has been investigated in a pig coronary model.[81] The loss of ecNOS may play a fundamental role in the pathogenesis of vascular diseases, including atherosclerosis. The overexpression of ecNOS may be useful for gene therapy of neointimal hyperplasia and associated local vasospasm after vascular injury.

Angiogenesis

Angiogenic growth factors may be useful to augment collateral artery development in animal models of myocardial and hind limb ischemia. Initial studies using intramuscular injections of angiogenic proteins, including basic fibroblast growth factor (bFGF) and acidic fibroblast growth factor (aFGF) into the hind limbs of rabbits with surgically induced ischemia lead to increased capillary densities and augmented blood flow.[82,83] These findings have been extended to gene-transfer approaches using vascular endothelial growth factor (VEGF). Following gene transfer of VEGF via a hydrogel balloon, increased numbers of capillary vessels also were observed in a rabbit model of hind limb ischemia, and improvement of resting and maximum flow was achieved that was comparable with that of a single administration of VEGF protein.[84] Intracoronary delivery of a recombinant adenovirus that encodes FGF-5 has been shown to induce collateral blood flow and restore myocardial function in a pig model of myocardial ischemia.[85] While the studies are encouraging, our understanding of the process by which VEGF, angiopoietin, and other angiogenic proteins lead to blood vessel formation and maturation is still incomplete.

MYOCARDIAL GENE TRANSFER

Direct injection of DNA into myocardial tissue has been shown to be effective in local delivery of a transgene to the heart. Lin et al.[37] reported in vivo expression of β-galactosidase in cardiac myocytes for at least 4 weeks after direct injection into the left ventricle. Direct injections of a major histocompatibility complex (*MHC*) gene and the reporter gene *luciferase* under the control of an MHC promoter also resulted in the regulated expression of these genes.[38] Subsequent studies also showed increased gene expression after myocardial injection of adenoviral vectors.[10,13]

Healing and remodeling of the ventricle after myocardial infarction remain as important clinical problems. Some candidate genes (e.g., those for TGF-β1 and myogenin) may enhance the healing and recovery of myocytes after injury associated with infarction. The induction of neovascularization or angiogenesis in ischemic myocardium after coronary artery occlusion using gene transfer may salvage myocardium at risk by enhancing blood supply to the ischemic areas. Indeed, intracardiac myoblast grafts stably transfected with an inducible TGF-β1 construct were associated with increased DNA synthesis in vascular endothelial cells, consistent with a sustained angiogenic response.[86] The success of intracardiac grafting with genetically modified cardiomyocytes depends on the ability of grafts to couple with host myocytes. Soonpaa et al.[87] demonstrated that fetal cardiomyocytes isolated from transgenic mice carrying a fusion protein of the cardiac α-MHC promoter with a β-galactosidase reporter gene were connected to the host myocardium by nascent intercalated disks formed after grafting. Chronic heart failure is accompanied by a reduction in the number of myocardial β-adrenergic receptors and inotropic responsiveness. Cardiac-specific overexpression of a β_2-adrenergic receptor in a transgenic animal model with subsequent increased myocardial function suggests a potential gene-therapy approach to heart failure.[88]

CLINICAL TRIALS

Clinical trials in cardiovascular gene therapy have gone forward in two areas: vascular proliferative diseases and angiogenesis. The results of a Phase I/II randomized study of a cell cycle inhibitor have been reported recently.[89] In this study, cell cycle blockade by ex vivo gene therapy of experimental vein grafts was accomplished with a dominant negative transcription decoy, E2F, that leads to G1 arrest and inhibition of cell proliferation. The investigators hypothesized that this transcription decoy would inhibit the neointimal hyperplasia and subsequent accelerated atherosclerosis that lead to human bypass graft failure. This hypothesis was tested in a prospective, randomized, controlled trial to investigate the safety and biologic efficacy of intraoperative gene therapy in patients receiving bypass vein grafts. Patients undergoing infrainguinal bypass grafting were randomized to decoy oligodeoxynucleotide (which binds and inactivates E2F), scrambled oligodeoxynucleotides, or no treatment. Oligonucleotide was delivered to grafts intraoperatively by ex vivo pressure-mediated transfection. Since this was a Phase I/II study, the primary end points were safety and inhibition of target cell cycle regulatory genes and of DNA synthesis in the grafts. The investigators found that the E2F decoy treatment reduced proliferating-cell nuclear antigen and c-myc mRNA concentrations as well as cell proliferation indices. Twelve months later, there were fewer clinical complications in the E2F treatment group, defined as fewer graft occlusions, revisions, or severe lesions. The investigators concluded that the intraoperative transfection of human bypass vein grafts with E2F decoy oligodeoxynucleotide was not only safe and feasible but also achieved inhibition of cell cycle genes and cell replication.[89]

Several protocols have now been initiated to promote angiogenesis for myocardial and peripheral ischemia. These studies have administered recombinant protein, plasmid DNA, or adenoviral vectors encoding bFGF, VEGF, aFGF, or FGF-4 by direct injection into the heart or limb muscle or by direct intracoronary infusion. Thus different genes, vectors, routes of delivery, and tissues are being examined. These studies to date have been Phase I (i.e., safety and toxicity) studies in which clinical efficacy is not an end point due to the small number of patients. Some of these Phase I protocols have been completed and reported. In a study to treat myocardial ischemia, recombinant aFGF was injected directly into the anatomosis site of the left internal mammary artery (LIMA) and into the left anterior descending artery (LAD) of patients undergoing coronary bypass surgery.[90] Patients with peripheral ischemia have been treated with direct injections of plasmid DNA encoding VEGF.[91] These Phase I studies are promising. The treatments to date have been safe, with no substantial toxicities. Progression to Phase II/III studies in which dose escalation, double-blind randomization, and measurements of clinical efficacy are performed is warranted.

STEM CELL BIOLOGY

Recently, pluripotent human stem cells have been discovered or derived from human embryos.[92] These stem cells have the potential to differentiate into any kind of cell and thus may be used to treat or cure many diseases, including heart disease, diabetes, Parkinson's disease, Alzheimer's disease, and others.[93] There are two types of stem cells: embryonic and adult stem cells. Embryonic stem (ES) cells have not become differentiated and hence are pluripotent. Adult stem cells have undergone differentiation, and their potential to regenerate damaged tissue is limited. There is controversy surrounding stem cell research with regard to funding for the derivation of human embryonic stem cells and for research on ES cells once derived.

The following scenario could be envisioned. ES cells are derived by culturing a several-day-old human embryo or blastocyst. The trophoblast will form the placenta, while the inner cell mass will form the embryo. The inner cell mass is isolated. This tissue contains ES cells that have the potential to differentiate into any kind of tissue. The ES cells are cultured in media to grow colonies of cells. Special factors can be applied to encourage differentiation. Subpopulations of cells can be separated, i.e., bone marrow cells, cardiac myocytes, neurons, etc. The differentiated cells are then engineered to be an immunologic match with the patient and then can be administered. For example, ES cells that have differentiated into cardiac myocytes can be injected into a patient having sustained a myocardial infarction or heart failure.

SUMMARY AND FUTURE DIRECTIONS

Since the 1980s, there has been remarkable progress in the design of vectors, the enhancement of gene expression by optimizing regulatory units, the development of animal models, and the translation of basic science studies into clinical applications. Despite this progress, there are significant hurdles and challenges that must be met if the promise of gene therapy is to be fulfilled. There is a persistent need for improved vectors that increase transgene expression and program expression specifically to cardiovascular tissues. Cell-specific promoters are being studied. Improved catheters are needed to deliver vectors and transgenes to vascular and myocardial tissues.[94] A better understanding of the pathways leading to cardiovascular diseases will permit more careful delineation of candidate target genes. There is no doubt, however, that enthusiasm and optimism remain high that this technology can lead to successful cardiovascular therapies.

References

1. Boris-Lawrie K, Temin HM. The retroviral vector: Replication cycle and safety considerations for retrovirus-mediated gene therapy. *Ann NY Acad Sci* 1994; 716:59–70.
2. Danos O, Mulligan RC. Expression of retroviral trans-acting functions from complementary crippled genomes: A system for helper free packaging of retroviral vectors. *J Cell Biochem* 1988; 12:172–178.
3. Nabel EG, Plautz G, Boyce FM, et al. Recombinant gene expression in vivo within endothelial cells of the arterial wall. *Science* 1989; 244:1342–1344.
4. Nabel EG, Plautz G, Nabel GJ. Site-specific gene expression in vivo by direct gene transfer into the arterial wall. *Science* 1990; 249:1285–1288.
5. Wilson JM, Birinyi LK, Salomon RN, et al. Implantation of vascular grafts lined with genetically modified endothelial cells. *Science* 1989; 244:1344–1346.
6. Horwitz M. The adenoviruses. In: Fields B, Knipe D, eds. *Virology*. New York: Raven Press; 1990:1723–1742.
7. Wilson JM. Adenoviruses as gene-delivery vehicles. *New Engl J Med* 1996; 334:1185–1187.
8. Wickman TJ, Mathias P, Cheresh DA, et al. Integrins $\alpha v\beta 3$ and $\alpha v\beta 5$ promote adenovirus internalization but not virus attachment. *Cell* 1983; 73:309–319.
9. Guzman RJ, Lemarchand P, Crystal RG, et al. Efficient and selective adenovirus-mediated gene transfer into vascular neointima. *Circulation* 1993; 88:2838–2848.
10. Kass-Eisler A, Falck-Pedersen E, Alvira M, et al. Quantitative determination of adenovirus-mediated gene delivery to rat cardiac myocytes in vitro and in vivo. *Proc Natl Acad Sci USA* 1993; 90:11,498–11,502.
11. Barr J, Kalynych AM, Tripathy SK, et al. Efficient catheter-mediated gene transfer into the heart using replication-defective adenovirus. *Gene Ther* 1994; 1:51–58.
12. Lemarchand P, Jones M, Yamada I, et al. In vivo gene transfer and expression in normal uninjured blood vessels using replication-deficient recombinant adenovirus vectors. *Circ Res* 1993; 72:1132–1138.
13. Guzman RJ, Lemarchand P, Crystal RG, et al. Efficient gene transfer into myocardium by direct injection of adenovirus vectors. *Circ Res* 1993; 73:1202–1207.
14. Tripathy SK, Goldwasser E, Lu MM, et al. Stable delivery of physiological levels of recombinant erythropoietin to the systemic circulation by intramuscular injection of replication-defective adenovirus. *Proc Natl Acad Sci USA* 1994; 91:11,557–11,561.
15. Tripathy SK, Black HB, Goldwasser E, et al. Immune responses to transgene-encoded proteins limit the stability of gene expression after injection of replication-defective adenovirus vectors. *Nature Med* 1996; 2:545–550.
16. Yang Y, Ertl J, Wilson JM. MHC class 1-restricted cytotoxic T lymphocytes to viral antigens destroy hepatocytes in mice infected with E1-deleted recombinant adenoviruses. *Immunity* 1994; 1:433–442.
17. Yang Y, Li Q, Ertl HC, Wilson JM, et al. Cellular immunity to viral antigens limits E1-deleted adenoviruses for gene therapy. *Proc Natl Acad Sci USA* 1994; 91:4407–4411.
18. Hartigan-O'Connor D, Amalfitano A, Chamberlain JS. Improved production of gutted adenovirus in cells expressing adenovirus preterminal protein and DNA polymerase. *J Virol* 1999; 73:7835–7841.
19. Muzyczka N. Use of adeno-associated virus as a general transduction vector for mammalian cells. *Curr Top Microbiol Immunol* 1992; 158:97–129.
20. Rolling F, Samulski RJ. AAV as a viral vector for human gene therapy: Generation of recombinant virus. *Mol Biotechnol* 1995; 3:9–15.
21. Kotin R, Linden R, Berns K. Characterization of a preferred site on human chromosome 19q for integration of adeno-associated virus DNA by nonhomologous recombination. *EMBO J* 1992; 11:5071–5078.
22. Herzog RW, Yang EY, Couto LB, et al. Long-term correction of canine hemophilia B by gene transfer of blood coagulation factor IX mediated by adeno-associated viral vector. *Nature Med* 1999; 5(1):56–63.
23. Svensson EC, Marshall DJ, Woodard K, et al. Efficient and stable

transduction of cardiomyocytes after intramyocardial injection or intracoronary perfusion with recombinant adeno-associated virus vectors. *Circulation* 1999; 99:201–205.
24. Felgner PL, Gader TR, Holm M, et al. Lipofectin: A highly efficient, lipid mediated DNA-transfection procedure. *Proc Natl Acad Sci USA* 1987; 84:7413–7417.
25. Bennett CF, Chiang MY, Chan H, et al. Cationic lipids improve antisense oligonucleotide uptake and prevent degradation in cultured cells and in human serum. *Mol Pharmacol* 1992; 41:1023–1033.
26. Zabner J, Fasbender AJ, Moninger T, et al. Cellular and molecular barriers to gene transfer by a cationic lipid. *J Biol Chem* 1995; 270:18,997–19,007.
27. Nabel EG, Yang Z, Liptay S, et al. Recombinant platelet-derived growth factor B gene expression in porcine arteries induces intimal hyperplasia in vivo. *J Clin Invest* 1993; 91:1822–1829.
28. Nabel EG, Yang Z, Plautz G, et al. Recombinant fibroblast growth factor-1 promotes intimal hyperplasia and angiogenesis in arteries in vivo. *Nature* 1993; 362:844–846.
29. Leclerc G, Gal D, Takeshita S, et al. Percutaneous arterial gene transfer in a rabbit model: Efficiency in normal and balloon-dilated atherosclerotic arteries. *J Clin Invest* 1992; 90:936–944.
30. Takeshita S, Gal D, Leclerc G, et al. Increased gene expression after liposome-mediated arterial gene transfer associated with intimal smooth muscle cell proliferation. *J Clin Invest* 1994; 93:652–661.
31. Kaneda Y, Iwai K, Uchida T. Increased expression of DNA cointroduced with nuclear protein in adult rat liver. *Science* 1989; 243:375–378.
32. Okada Y, Koseki I, Kim J, et al. Modification of cell membranes with viral envelopes during fusion of cells with HVJ (Sendai virus). *Exp Cell Res* 1975; 93:368–378.
33. Isaka Y, Fujiwara Y, Ueda N, et al. Glomerulosclerosis induced by in vivo transfection of transforming growth factor-β or platelet-derived growth factor gene into the rat kidney. *J Clin Invest* 1993; 92:2597–2601.
34. Morishita R, Gibbons GH, Ellison KE, et al. Single intraluminal delivery of antisense cdc2 kinase and proliferating-cell nuclear antigen oligonucleotides results in chronic inhibition of neointimal hyperplasia. *Proc Natl Acad Sci USA* 1993; 90:8474–8478.
35. Morishita R, Gibbons GH, Ellison KE, et al. Intimal hyperplasia after vascular injury is inhibited by antisense cdk2 kinase oligonucleotides. *J Clin Invest* 1994; 93:1458–1464.
36. Wolff J, Malone R, Williams P, et al. Direct gene transfer into mouse muscle in vivo. *Science* 1990; 247:1465–1468.
37. Lin H, Parmacek MS, Morle G, et al. Expression of recombinant gene in myocardium in vivo after direct injection of DNA. *Circulation* 1990; 82:2217–2221.
38. Kitsis RN, Buttrick PM, McNally EM, et al. Hormonal modulation of a gene injected into rat heart in vivo. *Proc Natl Acad Sci USA* 1991; 88:4138–4142.
39. Stein CA, Cheng YC. Antisense oligonucleotides as therapeutic agents: Is the bullet really magical? *Science* 1993; 261:1004–1012.
40. Cohen JS. Oligonucleotide therapeutics. *Trends Biotechnol* 1992; 10:87–91.
41. Bielinska A, Schivdasani RA, Zhang L, et al. Regulation of gene expression with double-stranded phosphothiolate oligonucleotides. *Science* 1990; 250:997–1000.
42. Epstein SE, Speir E, Finkel T. Do antisense approaches to the problem of restenosis make sense? *Circulation* 1993; 88:1351–1353.
43. Krieg AM, Yi A, Matson S, et al. CpG motifs in bacterial DNA trigger direct B-cell activation. *Nature* 1995; 374:546–549.
44. Sullenger BA, Gallardo HF, Ungers GE, et al. Overexpression of TAR sequences renders cells resistant to human immunodeficiency virus replication. *Cell* 1990; 63:601–608.
45. Morishita R, Gibbons GH, Horiuchi M, et al. A novel molecular strategy using cis element "decoy" of E2F binding site inhibits smooth muscle proliferation in vivo. *Proc Natl Acad Sci USA* 1995; 92:5855–5859.
46. Plautz G, Nabel EG, Nabel GJ. Introduction of vascular smooth muscle cells expressing recombinant genes in vivo. *Circulation* 1991; 83:578–583.
47. Lynch CM, Clowes MM, Osborne RA, et al. Long-term expression of human adenosine deaminase in vascular smooth muscle cells of rats: A model for gene therapy. *Proc Natl Acad Sci USA* 1992; 89:1138–1142.
48. Dichek DA, Neville RF, Zwiebel JA, et al. Seeding of intravascular stents with genetically engineered endothelial cells. *Circulation* 1989; 80:1347–1353.
49. Chen S, Wilson JM, Muller DWM. Adenovirus-mediated gene transfer of soluble vascular cell adhesion molecule to porcine interposition vein grafts. *Circulation* 1994; 89:1922–1928.
50. Yao SN, Smith KJ, Kurachi K. Primary myoblast-mediated gene transfer: Persistent expression of human factor IX in mice. *Gene Ther* 1994; 1:99–107.
51. Barr E, Leiden JM. Systemic delivery of recombinant proteins by genetically modified myoblasts. *Science* 1991; 254:1507–1509.
52. Dhawan J, Pan LC, Pavlath GK, et al. Systemic delivery of human growth hormone by injection of genetically engineered myoblasts. *Science* 1991; 254:1509–1512.
53. Hamamori Y, Samal B, Tian J, et al. Myoblast transfer of human erythropoietin gene in a mouse model of renal failure. *J Clin Invest* 1995; 95:1808–1813.
54. Barr E, Leiden JM. Somatic gene therapy for cardiovascular diseases: Recent advances. *Trends Cardiovasc Med* 1994; 4:57–63.
55. Nabel EG. Gene therapy for cardiovascular disease. *Circulation* 1995; 91:541–548.
56. Ooboshi H, Welsh MJ, Rios CD, et al. Adenovirus-mediated gene transfer in vivo to cerebral blood vessels and perivascular tissue. *Circ Res* 1995; 77:7–13.
57. Muller DW, Gordon D, San H, et al. Catheter-mediated pulmonary vascular gene transfer and expression. *Circ Res* 1994; 75:1039–1049.
58. Crystal RG. Transfer of genes to humans: Early lessons and obstacles to success. *Science* 1995; 270:404–410.
59. Simons M, Edelman ER, DeKeyser JL, et al. Antisense c-*myb* oligonucleotides inhibit intimal arterial smooth muscle cell accumulation in vivo. *Nature* 1992; 359:67–70.
60. Bennett MR, Anglin S, McEwan JR, et al. Inhibition of vascular smooth muscle cell proliferation in vitro and in vivo by c-*myc* antisense oligonucleotides. *J Clin Invest* 1994; 93:820–828.
61. Shi Y, Fard A, Galeo A, et al. Transcatheter delivery of c-*myc* antisense oligomers reduces neointimal formation in a porcine model of coronary artery balloon injury. *Circulation* 1994; 90:944–951.
62. Simons M, Edelman ER, Rosenberg RD. Antisense proliferating cell nuclear antigen oligonucleotides inhibit intimal hyperplasia in a rat carotid artery injury model. *J Clin Invest* 1994; 93:2351–2356.
63. Mann MJ, Gibbons GH, Kernoff RS, et al. Genetic engineering of vein grafts resistant to atherosclerosis. *Proc Natl Acad Sci USA* 1995; 92:4502–4506.
64. Mann MJ, Gibbons GH, Tsao PS, et al. Cell cycle inhibition leads to preservation of endothelial function in genetically engineered vein grafts. *J Clin Invest* 1997; 99:1295–1301.
65. Nabel EG, Shum L, Pompili VJ, et al. Direct transfer of transforming growth factor β1 gene into arteries stimulates fibrocellular hyperplasia. *Proc Natl Acad Sci USA* 1993; 90:10,579–10,763.
66. Pompili VJ, Gordon D, San H, et al. Expression and function of a recombinant PDGF B gene in porcine arteries. *Arterioscl Thromb Vasc Biol* 1995; 15:2254–2264.
67. Morishita R, Gibbons GH, Ellison KE, et al. Evidence for direct local effect of angiotensin in vascular hypertrophy: In vivo gene transfer of angiotensin converting enzyme. *J Clin Invest* 1994; 94:978–984.

68. Nakajima M, Hutchinson HG, Fujinaga M, et al. The angiotensin II type 2 (AT2) receptor antagonizes the growth effects of the AT1 receptor: Gain-of-function study using gene transfer. *Proc Natl Acad Sci USA* 1995; 92:10,663–10,667.
69. Ohno T, Gordon D, San H, et al. Gene therapy for vascular smooth muscle cell proliferation after arterial injury. *Science* 1994; 265:781–784.
70. Chang MW, Ohno T, Gordon D, et al. Adenovirus-mediated transfer of the herpes simplex virus thymidine kinase gene inhibits vascular smooth muscle cell proliferation and neointima formation following balloon angioplasty. *Mol Med* 1995; 1:172–181.
71. Guzman RJ, Hirschowitz EA, Brody SL, et al. In vivo suppression of injury-induced vascular smooth muscle cell accumulation using adenovirus-mediated transfer of the herpes simplex virus thymidine kinase gene. *Proc Natl Acad Sci USA* 1994; 91:10,732–10,736.
72. Simari R, San H, Rekhter M, et al. Regulation of cellular proliferation and intimal formation following balloon injury in atherosclerotic rabbit arteries. *J Clin Invest* 1996; 98:225–235.
73. Rekhter MD, Shah N, Simari RD, et al. Graft permeabilization facilitates gene therapy of transplant atherosclerosis in a rabbit model. *Circulation* 1998; 98:1335–1341.
74. Chang MW, Barr E, Seltzer J, et al. Cytostatic gene therapy for vascular proliferative disorders with a constitutively active form of the retinoblastoma gene product. *Science* 1995; 267:518–522.
75. Chang MW, Barr E, Lu MM, et al. Adenovirus-mediated overexpression of the cyclin/cyclin-dependent kinase inhibitor, p21 inhibits vascular smooth muscle cell proliferation and neointima formation in the rat carotid artery model of balloon angioplasty. *J Clin Invest* 1995; 96:2260–2268.
76. Yang Z, Simari R, Perkins N, et al. Role of the p21 cyclin-dependent kinase inhibitor in limiting intimal cell proliferation in response to arterial injury. *Proc Natl Acad Sci USA* 1996; 93:1905–1910.
77. Chen D, Krasinski K, Sylvester A, et al. Down regulation of cyclin-dependent kinase 2 activity and cyclin A promoter activity in vascular smooth muscle cells by p27(KIP1), an inhibitor of neointima formation in the rat carotid artery. *J Clin Invest* 1997; 99:2334–2341.
78. Tanner FC, Boehm M, Akyurek LM, et al. Differential effects of the cyclin-dependent kinase inhibitors p27(Kip1), p21(Cip1), and p16(Ink4) on vascular smooth muscle cell proliferation. *Circulation* 2000; 101:2022–2025.
79. Indolfi C, Avvedimento EV, Rapacciuolo A, et al. Inhibition of cellular *ras* prevents smooth muscle cell proliferation after vascular injury in vivo. *Nature Med* 1995; 1:541–545.
80. von der Leyen HE, Gibbons GH, Morishita R, et al. Gene therapy inhibiting neointimal vascular lesion: In vivo gene transfer of endothelial-cell nitric oxide synthase gene. *Proc Natl Acad Sci USA* 1995; 92:1137–1141.
81. Varenne O, Pislaru S, Gillijns H, et al. Local adenovirus-mediated transfer of human endothelial nitric oxide synthase reduces luminal narrowing after coronary angioplasty in pigs. *Circulation* 1998; 98:919–926.
82. Pu LQ, Sniderman AD, Brassard R, et al. Enhanced revascularization of the ischemic limb by means of angiogenic therapy. *Circulation* 1993; 88:208–215.
83. Unger EF, Banai S, Shou M, et al. Basic fibroblast growth factor enhances myocardial collateral flow in a canine model. *Am J Physiol* 1994; 266:H1588–H1595.
84. Takeshita S, Weir L, Chen D, et al. Therapeutic antiogenesis following arterial gene transfer of vascular endothelial growth factor in a rabbit model of hindlinb ischemia. *Biochem Biophys Res Commun* 1996; 227:628–635.
85. Giordano FJ, Ping P, McKirnan MD, et al. Intracoronary gene transfer of fibroblast growth factor-5 increases blood flow and contractile function in an ischemic region of the heart. *Nature Med* 1996; 2:534–539.
86. Koh GY, Kim S, Klug MG, et al. Targeted expression of transforming growth factor-β1 in intracardiac grafts promotes vascular endothelial cell DNA synthesis. *J Clin Invest* 1995; 95:114–121.
87. Soonpaa MH, Koh GY, Klug MG, et al. Formation of nascent intercalated disks between grafted fetal cardiomyocytes and host myocardium. *Science* 1994; 264:98–101.
88. Milano CA, Allen LF, Rockman HA, et al. Enhanced myocardial function in transgenic mice overexpressing the β_2-adrenergic receptor. *Science* 1994; 264:582–586.
89. Mann MJ, Whittemore AD, Donaldson MC, et al. Ex-vivo gene therapy of human vascular bypass grafts with E2F decoy: The PREVENT single-centre, randomised, controlled trial. *Lancet* 1999; 354:1493–1498.
90. Isner JM, Pieczek A, Schainfeld R, et al. Clinical evidence of angiogenesis after arterial gene transfer of phVEGF165 in patient with ischaemic limb. *Lancet* 1996; 348:370–374.
91. Tsurumi Y, Takeshita S, Chen D, et al. Direct intramuscular gene transfer of naked DNA encoding vascular endothelial growth factor augments collateral development and tissue perfusion. *Circulation* 1996; 94:3281–3290.
92. Makino S, Mayazi K, Fuji M, et al. Cardiomyocytes can be generated from marrow stromal cells in vitro. *J Clin Invest* 1999; 103:697–705.
93. Leiden JM. Beating the odds: A cardiomyocyte cell line at last. *J Clin Invest* 1999; 103:591–592.
94. Riessen R, Isner JM. Prospects for site-specific delivery of pharmacologic and molecular therapies. *J Am Coll Cardiol* 1994; 23:1234–1244.
95. Nabel EG. Gene therapy for cardiovascular diseases. *J Nucl Cardiol* 1999; 6:69–75.
96. Tanner FC, Yang ZY, Simari RD, et al. Gene transfer and vascular remodeling. In: LaFont A, Topol E, eds. *Arterial Remodeling.* Boston: Kluwer Academic Publishers; 1997:549–556.

CHAPTER 9

MOLECULAR DEVELOPMENT OF THE HEART

Bradley B. Keller / Andy Wessels / Robert J. Schwartz / Robert Roberts / Roger R. Markwald

The wide spectrum of congential cardiovascular anomalies that present from the prenatal period into adulthood has challenged clinicians and scientists for centuries.[1,2] Equally daunting historically have been the complex and varied descriptions of cardiac embryology and the pathogenesis of congenital cardiovascular malformations.[3-6] Fortunately, scientific advances, including the availability of cell-specific immunohistochemistry, rapid advances in molecular biological techniques, expansion of investigations into integrated embryonic cardiovascular physiology, and dramatic improvements in the three-dimensional imaging of the embryonic cardiovascular anatomy, make the specific determination of pathogenesis for most cardiovascular anomalies a realistic goal in the next decade (Fig. 9-1).[7-11]

This chapter will discuss current ideas about normal development of the heart and vasculature and illustrate how this knowledge can help one understand the pathogenesis of congenital cardiovascular malformations. As with all complex developmental events, cardiovascular morphogenesis must be defined in a stepwise fashion, and this chapter details some of these pivotal developmental events. Although many of the mechanisms that lead to the development of the fully septated, four-chambered vertebrate heart are interdependent (e.g., the formation of the muscular ventricular septum and the membranous portion of the atrioventricular septum), many of these events are discussed in separate sections for clarity. It needs to be emphasized, however, that none of these remodeling events are isolated processes (e.g., formation of the outflow tract and closure of the interventricular foramen). The information presented in this chapter focuses on human development. However, a rapidly growing number of animal models generated by using sophisticated molecular biological techniques are becoming available and will accelerate the investigation of a wide variety of aspects related to normal and aberrant cardiovascular morphogenesis.

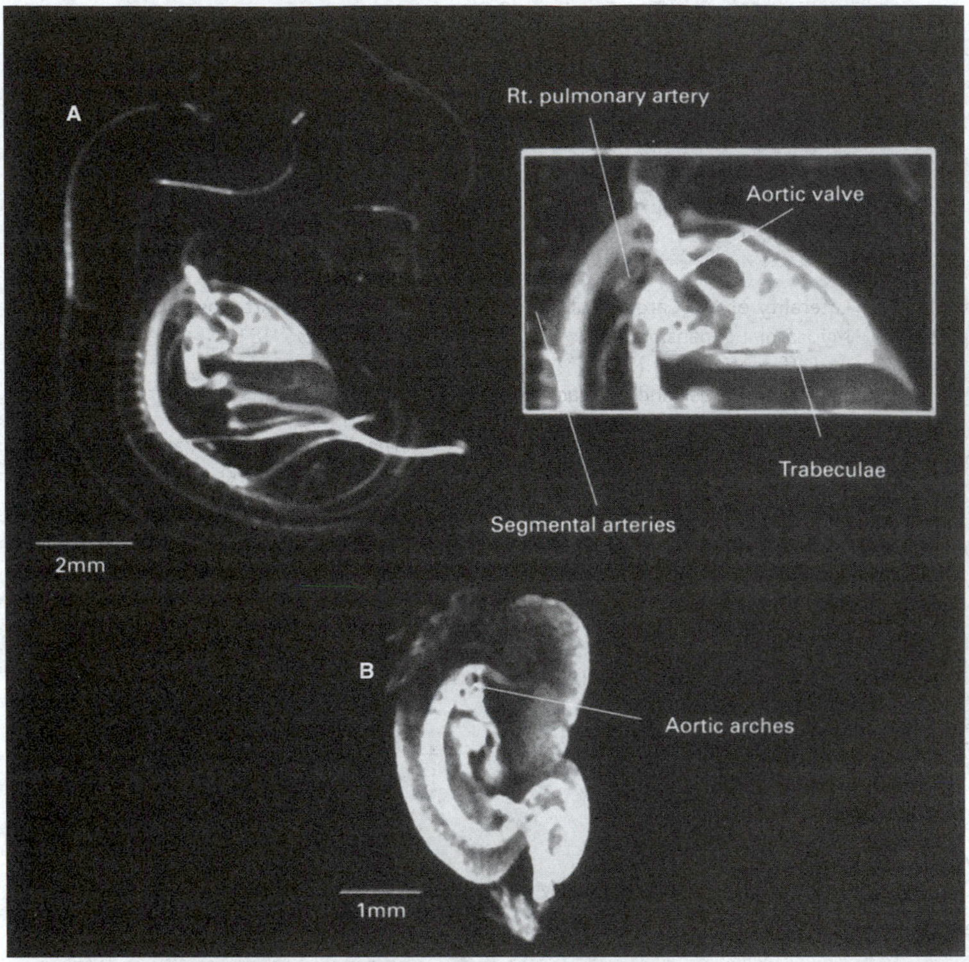

FIGURE 9-1 Magnetic resonance (MR) microscopy of mouse embryos at embryonic days 12.5 (*A*) and 9.5 (*B*). These embryos were perfused with BSA-DTPA-Gd, an MR contrast agent, to enhance the signal from cardiovascular structures. These volume-rendered images, based on three-dimensional T1-weighed scans, demonstrate the cardiac chambers, cardiac valves, aortic arches, intersegmental vessels, cranial vasculature, and hepatic vasculature. Scale bars are marked as 2 mm or 1 mm. Rt = right. (Data courtesy of Brad Smith, University of Michigan.)

MOLECULAR DEVELOPMENT OF THE HEART TUBE

Embryo Patterning

Morphogenesis of the heart begins with the initial patterning of the embryo that determines the three axes of the embryo: anterior-posterior, dorsal-ventral, and left-right. These axes are imprinted onto the cellular program as cell populations expand to form the embryo and extraembryonic tissues. Specific genes have been identified that alter axis determination in a range of species, including the mouse.[12,13] After determination of the embryo axes, subpopulations of cells are programmed in a segmental body plan. Much of the current understanding of the body plan comes from developmental studies of *Drosophila*, an insect with a head, thorax, and abdomen.[14] In mammals, maternal gene products control the cell through the first two cell cycles and then control switches to the embryonic genome. These patterning (homeobox) genes are arranged along the anterior-posterior axis of the embryo.[15] Structural asymmetry is apparent at the blastodisc stage, when the primitive streak defines the anterior-posterior axis and the dorsal-ventral axis is defined by the position of the yolk sac. Myocyte commitment in the chick embryo occurs in the early blastula stage, followed by clonal expansion in the bilateral heart-forming regions located in the lateral splanchnic folds after gastrulation. Molecular studies also have confirmed the segmental patterning of the cardiac tube, linking gene products with morphologic boundaries between segments that eventually integrate to form the future atria, ventricles, and outflow tract in chick, mouse, and human hearts.[16]

The process of mesoderm formation is integral to the organization of the primary axis of the embryo and the differentiation of the right and left sides. At the blastodisc stage of development, there are two primitive germ layers—endoderm and ectoderm—and then the endoderm layer splits into splanchnic and visceral layers with interposed mesodermal cells (Fig. 9-2). Mesoderm is formed as ectodermal cells migrate through the primitive streak coursing adjacent to Hensen's node (organizer). Hensen's node contains retinoic acid and serves as an embryonic organizer that may confer positional information on the mesodermal cells.[17] At this critical phase in cell determination, exogenous retinoic acid is extremely teratogenic. Interestingly, retinoic acid has a gradient-like effect on the determination of the heart tube, with the greatest effect at the arterial pole and the smallest effect at the venous pole.[18] After migration, this crescent of mesodermal cells forms the precardiac region from which the heart and the precursor cells of the great vessels originate.

Molecular Factors Involved in Cardiogenesis

Defining the molecular basis that underlies the establishment and maintenance of cardiac muscle differentiation has presented a fundamental challenge in developmental biology and molecular genetics. Despite the shared expression of numerous contractile protein genes by both cardiac and skeletal striated muscles, the molecular mechanisms for cell determination, differentiation, and tissue patterning are quite distinct. The following section presents some of the current, relevant information on molecular cardiogenesis, as defects in these molecular mechanisms have been shown to be associated with structural and/or functional heart diseases in children and adults (Fig. 9-3).

Basic Helix-Loop-Helix Factors and Muscle Development

One of the initial, critical discoveries related to muscle development was the observation that a specific transcription factor, Myo-D, expressed in myoblasts[19] is sufficient to convert a variety of mesodermal and nonmesodermal cell types to stable myoblasts with active muscle-specific gene expression. Using Myo-D as a probe, several additional regulatory factors that specify skeletal muscle cell lineage in fibroblasts have been identified: myogenin,[20,21] Myf5,[22] MRF4-herculin, and Myf6.[23–25] These factors share extensive homology within a basic region and an HLH motif that mediate DNA binding and dimerization, respectively.[26] HLH proteins share the ability to recognize the DNA consensus sequence CANNTG, known as an *E-box,* which first was identified with the immunoglobulin enhancer[26] and subsequently was found in regulatory regions of most muscle-specific genes. Thus, the regulatory paradigm for skeletal muscle differentiation is centered on the bHLH myogenic regulatory factors, but Myo-D, myogenin, Myf5, MRF-4, and Myf6 are not expressed in the heart.[27]

In the heart, there are other basic HLH factors. dHAND and eHAND are two bHLH transcription factors that share high homology in their bHLH regions and show segment-specific expression patterns.[28] In the mouse, HAND expression coincides with that of other cardiac transcription factors. dHAND expressed in the endocardium is maintained throughout the straight heart tube but is restricted to the conotruncus and the future right ventricle as the heart tube forms a loop. eHAND expressed in the myocardium rapidly becomes restricted to the conotruncus and the left ventricle.[29] Expression of dHAND and eHAND precedes separation of the two ventricles, representing early chamber specification. In addition to cardiac expression, dHAND (HAND1) is expressed in early trophoblast tissue and is required for the nutritional support of the developing mouse embryo.[30] It is of interest that *Nkx-2.8* has an expression pattern that overlaps eHAND, being restricted to the rostral and caudal regions of the heart tube after looping and being expressed in the endoderm of the pharyngeal arches. The deletion of dHAND by gene targeting showed that dHAND expression is necessary for the formation of the right ventricle.[29,31] Thus, it appears that dHAND may specify the right ventricle, and eHAND the left ventricle. In addition, dHAND and eHAND specify right ven-

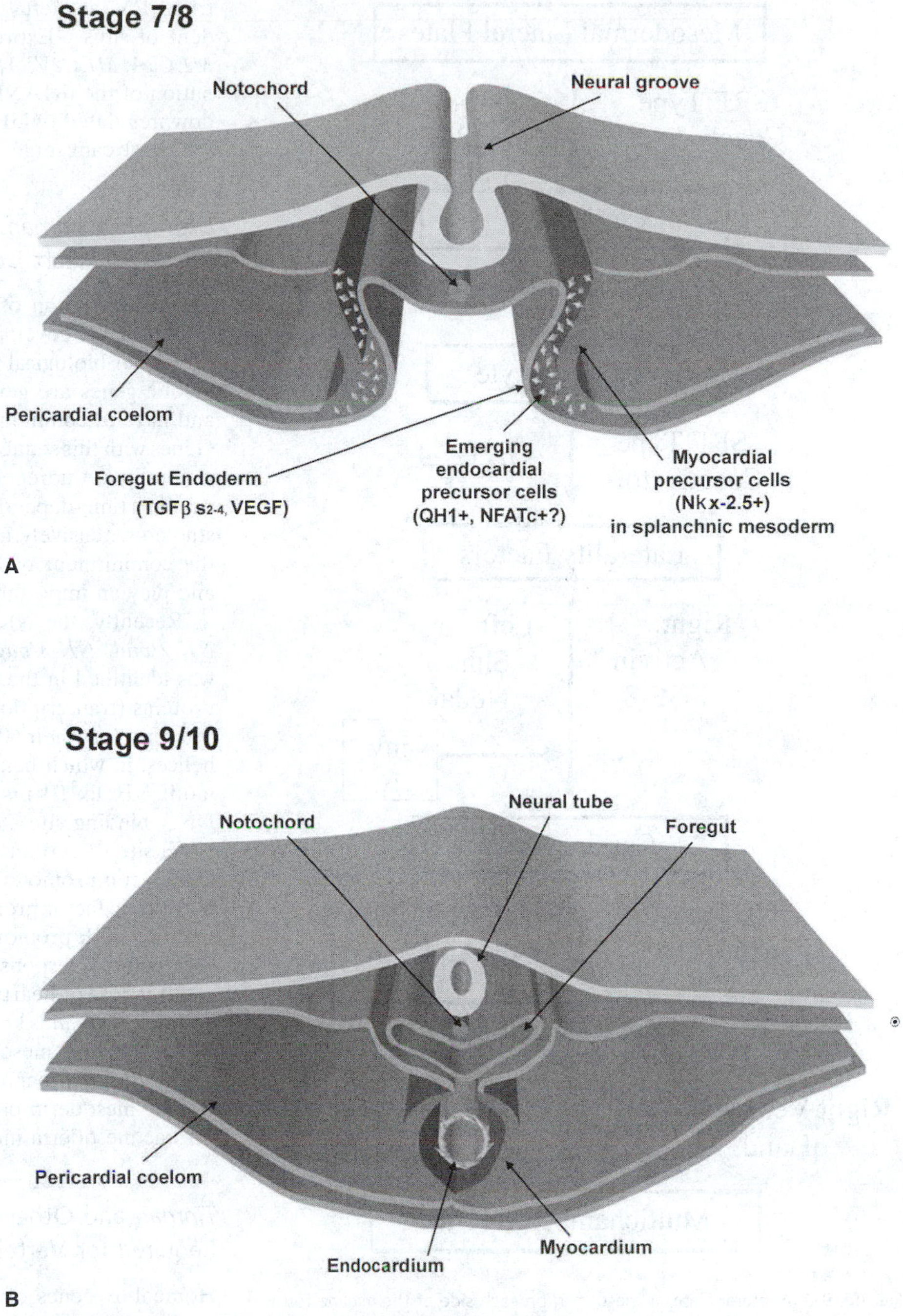

FIGURE 9-2 The postgastrulation morphogenetic events involved in the formation of the tubular heart. The upper panel represents a chick embryo at stage 7/8 H/H, demonstrating the emergence of endocardial precursor mesenchymal cells from the splanchnic mesoderm, which gives rise to the future myocardium. It is proposed that the formation of both endocardium and myocardium is induced by adjacent endoderm. The lower panel shows that subsequent to the migration and assembly of endocardial precursor mesenchymal cells during stages 7–8 H/H, the cellular plexus coalesces to form the definitive endocardial tube enveloped by the myocardial tube. Note that the endocardium is still in close proximity to the ventral side of the foregut. (Courtesy of Yukiko Sugi, Cardiovascular Developmental Biology Center, Medical University of South Carolina.)

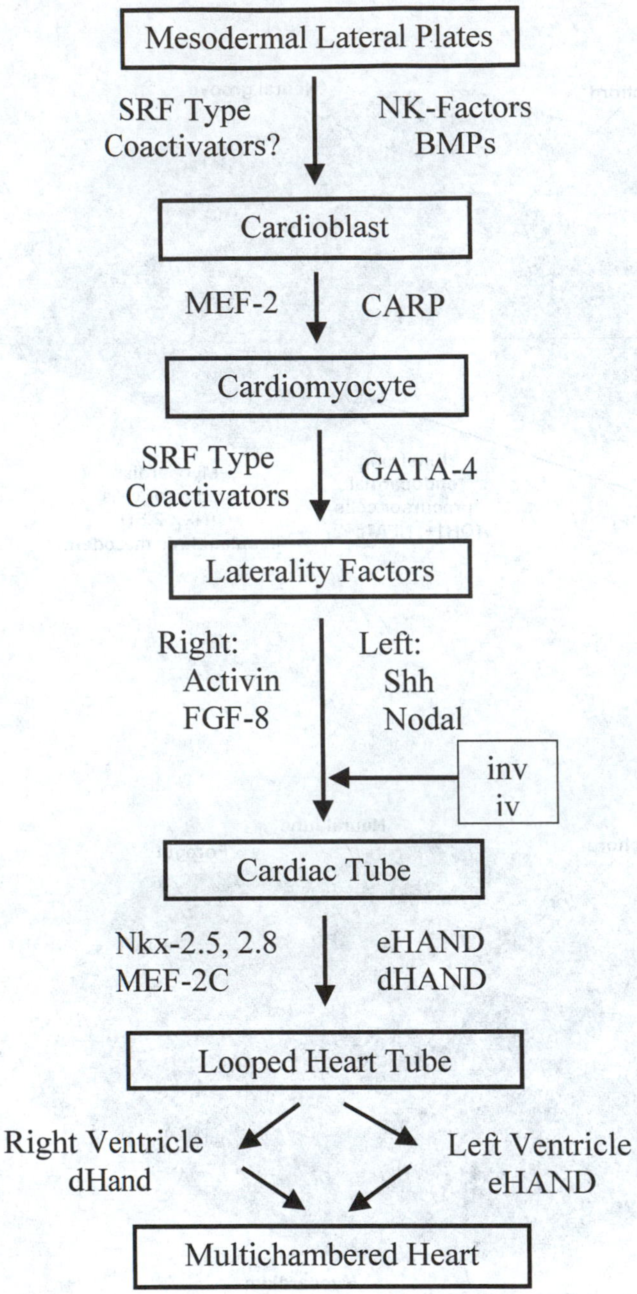

FIGURE 9-3 A lateral plate of mesoderm on each side of the midline forms the progenitor for the development of the heart and portions of the great vessels. The NK-Factor homeobox genes, such as *Nkx2.5*, in combination with multiple other genes, such as the serum response factor (SRF), are responsible for activating commitment of these undifferentiated cells to cardioblasts. Myocyte enhancer factor (MEF) has a binding site in practically all muscle genes and is essential to the development of cardiac myocytes. The CARP gene is downstream of *Nkx2.5* in the cardiac lineage. The genes responsible for the fusion of the two lateral mesodermal plates into a single tube are unknown, but experiments show that GATA-4 is necessary, along with SRF and many other genes yet to be identified. Genes involved in laterality include *Activin, FGF-9, Shh*, and *nodal*. The cardiac tube that forms a loop to the right requires *Nkx* genes and the *eHAND* and *dHAND* as well as *inv* (inversion of embryonic turning) and *iv* genes. The *dHAND* gene is responsible for the formation of the right ventricle, and the *eHAND* for that of the left ventricle.

tricle (RV) and left ventricle (LV) specific morphology independent of situs.[32] Expression of cardiac-specified genes *αMHC, MLC2A, MLC2V, ANE,* and *Nkx-2.5* was not affected by elimination of the dHAND gene. GATA-4 in the myocardium was downregulated by dHAND-deficient hearts and appears to be a downstream target of dHAND.

Drosophila tinman Is Required for Insect Heart Development

The identification of molecular mechanisms involved specifically in heart development has depended on the investigation of simpler biological models, including the fly *Drosophila*. Homeotic genes are genes that determine a change in structure and have in common a domain that codes for 60 amino acids. Genes with this sequence, referred to as homeobox (*Hox*) genes, generally are upregulated during early differentiation and appear in a time-dependent sequence. Homeobox genes have been studied extensively in *Drosophila,* where they are involved in the commitment of cells to specific developmental pathways and play an important role in pattern formation.[33]

Recently, the NK homeobox family of genes (*NK-1/S59, NK-2/vnd, NK-3/bagpipe,* and *NK-4/msh-2/tinman* and *H6*) was identified in the mouse.[34] Nkx-2 factors are DNA-binding proteins (transcriptional factors) that are capable of activating transcription; their 60-amino-acid homeodomain includes three helices, in which helix II and helix III form a helix-turn-helix motif.[35] Helix III fits across the AT-rich major groove of the DNA binding site. *Nkx-2.5* has been shown to bind to novel NKE sites,[36] certain serum response elements of the cardiac alpha-actin promoter,[37] and the NKE sites in the cardiac atrial natriuretic factor promoter.[38] Gajewski and associates[39] showed that two NKE promoter sites direct *Drosophila* MEF2(dMEF2) expression in response to *tinman*. Mutations in the *tinman* gene result in loss of heart formation in the *Drosophila* embryo.[40] In addition, *tinman* is known to regulate NK-3/bagpipe expression in the visceral mesoderm[41] and the expression of dMEF2.[39] These observations suggest that *tinman* may be involved in cardiac mesoderm patterning and make it a likely marker for cardiac mesoderm induction.

Tinman and Other Related NK-2 Genes Are Required for Vertebrate Heart Morphogenesis

Homeobox genes of the NK class also may function in early cardiac development in vertebrates. The murine NK-2 homeobox gene *Nkx-2.5/Csx* is expressed in early cardiac progenitor cells before cardiogenic differentiation and continues through adulthood.[42,43] Superimposed on the appearance of *Nkx-2.5* in cardiac progenitor cells is the sequential expression of the cell type–restricted cardiac alpha-actin and MHC genes.[42] The *Nkx-2.5* factors identified in other vertebrates, such as zebrafish,[44] *Xenopus,*[45] and chickens,[46] were highly related in sequence and expression pattern to the mouse gene and to cardiac development.

The similarity in expression patterns between *Nkx-2.5, XNkx-2.5, ceh-22, tinman,* and *bagpipe* suggested that the function of these genes might be conserved. Another member of the Nkx-2 family, *Nkx-2.8,* which was recently isolated from avian species, is closely related to *Xenopus*, chicken, and zebrafish *Nkx-2.5* homeoboxes and is expressed in the developing embryo in the lateral plate mesoderm and underlying pharyngeal endoderm.[47] An attractive hypothesis is that these homeodomain factors function in phylogenetically conserved myogenic pathways occurring in muscle types that do not utilize the Myo-D family. Whether the vertebrate *Nkx-2.5* or other Nkx-2-related genes expressed in the early heart play a role in heart specification or whether they are downstream regulators of cardiac gene expression remains to be determined. In this respect, it is interesting to note that although it does not inhibit formation of the cardiac tube, homologous recombination knockouts of the endogenous murine *Nkx-2.5* gene do result in cardiac dysmorphogenesis at the looping stages of development and embryonic lethality.[48]

The partially overlapping expression pattern of *Hox* genes in embryos has led to the concept of a "*Hox* code."[49] The term *Hox code* means that a particular combination of *Hox* genes is functionally active in a region and thus specifies the developmental fate of this region. The existence of eight Nkx-2 family members, their overlapping DNA-binding specificities, and, most important, their partially overlapping patterns of expression raise the possibility of an "Nkx code."[47] Overexpression of *Nkx-2.5* in a zebrafish embryo results in an enlarged heart.[44] Thus, inactivation of the Nkx genes by homologous recombination and their overexpression as transgenes offer promise in addressing the functional significance of the expression domains and thus also of the Nkx code. As is mentioned below, patients with secundum atrial septal defect have been identified to have specific mutations in the human homolog to the *Nkx2.5* gene.[49]

Cardiac-Restricted Ankyrin Repeat Protein Gene

The cardiac-restricted ankyrin repeat protein (*CARP*) gene encodes a nuclear coregulator for cardiac gene expression which lies downstream of the cardiac homeobox gene *Nkx 2.5* and is an early marker of the cardiac muscle cell lineage.[50] The expression of the *CARP* gene is developmentally downregulated and dramatically induced as part of the embryonic gene program during cardiac hypertrophy. A distinct 5′ cis regulatory element directs heart segment–specific expression, such as atrial versus ventricular and left versus right. In addition, a 213-base-pair sequence element of the gene confers conotruncal segment–specific expression.[50] In addition, an essential GATA-4-binding site is present in the proximal upstream regulatory region of the gene and cooperative transcriptional regulation is mediated by *Nkx2.5* and GATA-4. This cooperative regulation is dependent on the binding of GATA-4 to its cognate DNA sequence in the promoter, which suggests that *Nkx2.5* controls CARP expression, at least in part, through GATA-4.[50]

SRF and MEF2, MADS Box Factors Involved with Cardiogenesis

Serum response factor generally was presumed to be a ubiquitous and constitutive trophic factor[51] but was later shown to be highly expressed in the embryonic heart.[52] Serum response factor (SRF) represents an ancient DNA-binding protein whose relatives shared a highly conserved DNA-binding/dimerization domain of 90 amino acids, termed the *MADS box*. SRF-related proteins that are capable of binding to sites found in the regulatory regions of both nonmuscle- and muscle-specific genes also belong to the MADS box family of trophic factors.[53] SRF-related proteins are capable of binding MEF2 sites, CTA(A/T)4TAG, which can be found in the regulatory regions of both nonmuscle- and muscle-specific genes.[54,55] Like SRF, MEF2 factors contain a MADS box and an adjacent MEF2 box. Expression and mutagenesis studies in *Drosophila* have shown that MEF2 proteins are necessary for myogenic differentiation during development[56,57] and are activated by *tinman*.[39]

In the mouse embryo, MEF2 genes are highly expressed in the early heart and skeletal muscle progenitor cells before the induction of cardiac and skeletal muscle structural genes, implicating MEF2 as key regulator of cardiac and skeletal muscle differentiation programs.[58–60] Four MEF2 genes have been isolated in vertebrate species and are referred to as MEF2A-MEF2D.[60,61] The four MEF2 gene products are highly homologous in the MADS box domain but are divergent in the carboxy termini, arising from alternative splicing mechanisms. MEF2C shows a tissue-restricted expression pattern, being expressed exclusively in skeletal muscle, brain, and spleen, and is induced by myogenin in fibroblasts during myogenic differentiation in tissue cultures.[62]

Transactivation of the Cardiac Alpha-Actin Gene by Nkx-2.5 and SRF

Gilman and coworkers[63,64] showed that human SRF interacts with a novel human homeodomain protein, Phox, which shows similarity to the homeodomains of two murine Pax genes. The highest similarity is to a partial murine cDNA termed S8[65] and to MHox, a novel homeodomain protein expressed in mesoderm.[66] Phox interacts with SRF to enhance the exchange of SRF with its binding site in the *c-fos* gene. It has been shown that *Nkx-2.5* transactivates the cardiac alpha-actin gene by binding to SRF, but only after SRF has bound to DNA.[67]

The Role of the GATA Family in Cardiogenesis

The GATA family of proteins has been subdivided, with GATA-1/2/3 being linked to hematopoiesis and GATA-4/5/6 thought to be involved with cardiac, gut, and blood vessel formation. Each of the six GATA proteins contains a highly specific DNA-binding domain consisting of two C4 zinc fingers that bind to the DNA sequence element (A/T)GATA(A/G) and that may be able to interchange with each other. GATA-4 and 6 have been found to be expressed in a developmentally and lineage-specific pattern within cardiac mesoderm and gut epithelium.[68–70] GATA-5 expression is restricted to the endocardium. Experiments have shown that GATA-4 regulates the expression of cardiac-specific genes such as cardiac troponin C[71] and alpha-MHC.[72] Mice without the GATA-4 gene display a severe defect in the formation of the cardiac tube. Several studies have demonstrated that the GATA-4 transcription factor plays an important role in regulating cardiac-specified genes and appears to be downstream to the *Nkx-2.5* gene.

Cardiogenesis, an Nkx-2-Dependent Paradigm

An attractive hypothesis from the analysis of these NK-2 homologues is that these homeodomain factors function in phylogenetically conserved pathways in muscle cell types that do not utilize the Myo-D family. Expression of *Nkx-2.5* in fibroblasts demonstrated that downstream targets such as the cardiac alpha-actin gene are not directly activated by *Nkx-2.5* alone but require the collaboration of additional factors, such as SRF.[37,67] Whether the vertebrate *Nkx-2.5* or other Nkx-2-related genes with SRF are sufficient to play the primary role in heart specification and serve as regulators of other downstream cardiac genes remains to be determined. It is reasonable to postulate that the vertebrate MEF2C genes and the GATA-4 factor are high in the hierarchical order of regulatory factors that, in combination with *Nkx-2.5* and SRF, specify the cardiac cell lineage.

Role for Bone Morphogenic Proteins in Initiating Early Myocardial Cell Differentiation

One type of signaling molecule responsible for cardiogenic commitment was identified to be composed of the bone morphogenic proteins (BMPs), which are members of the transforming growth factor-beta family of signaling molecules. BMP-2 and -4 appear to be capable of inducing the cardiac regulatory factors *Nkx-2.5* and GATA-4 when ectopically applied to regions of chick embryos that usually are not specified to become heart tissue.[46] In mice with the BMP-4 gene eliminated (knockout mice), there was little or no mesoderm differentiation. Some of the mice deficient for BMP-2 gene that lacked *Nkx-2.5* expression also failed to develop beyond the early stages of looping.[73] Thus, BMPs appear to have an early influence on cardiogenesis and *Nkx-2.5* expression.

Laterality of the Cardiac Tube

Correct laterality is fundamental to the developing embryo, and situs solitus has the lowest risk of congenital cardiovascular malformations.[74] The first grossly asymmetric feature to develop is the heart tube, which forms from the fusion of cardiac primordia at the midline (see Fig. 9-2). Subsequently, the initially symmetric heart acquires a dextral loop. The tubular heart initiates rhythmic contractions at about day 23 in humans and then undergoes rightward looping. This pattern of left-right asymmetry occurs in all vertebrate internal organs as a result of a signaling cascade present before gastrulation. On the right side of Hensen's node, the secreted morphogen activin represses Sonic hedgehog (Shh) expression and induces expression of the genes for the activin receptor and fibroblast growth factor 8. On the left side, Shh induces Nodal expression in lateral plate mesoderm and subsequent left-sided expression of the bicoid-like homeobox gene *Pitx2*. The homeobox gene *Nkx3.2* is asymmetrically expressed in the anterior left lateral plate mesoderm (LPM) and head mesoderm in the chick embryo.[75] Misexpression of the normally left-sided signals Nodal, Lefty2, and Shh on the right side or ectopic application of retinoic acid results in upregulation of *Nkx3.2* contralateral to its normal expression on the left. FGF8 is an important negative determinant of asymmetric *Nkx3.2,* and ectopic application of FGF8 on the left side blocks *Nkx3.2* expression, whereas an FGF receptor-1 antagonist implanted on the right side results in bilateral *Nkx3.2* expression in the LPM.[75]

There is a genetic basis for left-right asymmetry, as several types of unlinked mutations affecting left-right laterality exist in mice and humans. For example, in the offspring of *iv* mice (lacking the *iv* gene), 50 percent have situs inversus.[76] The *iv* gene has been mapped to mouse chromosome 12 and has been identified to code for the structural protein dynein. The *inv* (inversion of embryonic turning) gene mapped to chromosome 4 causes complete reversal of left-right symmetry and cardiac looping.[77,78] *Nkx3.2* expression also was found to be asymmetric in the mouse LPM, but unlike in the chick, it was expressed in the right LPM. In the inversion of embryonic turning (inv) mouse mutant, which has aberrant left-right (L-R) development, *Nkx3.2* was expressed predominantly on the left side. Thus, *Nkx3.2* transcripts accumulate on opposite sides of mouse and chick embryos, although in both the mouse and the chick, *Nkx3.2* expression is controlled by the L-R signaling pathways.

Myocardial Expansion and Differentiation

Retrovirus labeling studies have demonstrated that the ventricular myocardium expands by a process of clonal expansion of the epitheliod myocytes of the cardiac tube (see Figure 9-7).[79,80] The regulation of myocyte specification and differentiation is complex and probably involves cell adhesion molecules, including N-cadherin, extracellular proteases, and morphogenetic signals from the transforming growth factor-beta (TGF-beta) and FGF families of growth and differentiation factors.[80–84]

The Neural Crest and Cardiac Development

The cardiac neural crest is an important migratory cell population that contributes to cardiovascular morphogenesis. The cardiac neural crest arises from the dorsal margin of the neural tube before fusion and migrates ventrally to form the autonomic ganglia, melanocytes, and Schwann cells. The crest cells move in waves through the branchial arches during the first 4 weeks of human development. The eventual fate of the neural crest cells likely is determined long before the initial phenotypic expression of a heart tube by activation of the cellular gradients of *Hox* genes and other morphoregulating factors.[85,86] The cranial neural crest region defines a developmental field that includes the heart, hindbrain, face, and branchial arch derivatives.

Experimental disruption of cranial neural crest produces a spectrum of abnormalities. In a series of elegant ablation and chick quail chimera studies, Kirby and Waldo defined the range of cardiac neural crest that is integral to the septation of the conotruncal region of the heart and branchial arch derivatives, including facial abnormalities, thymus, parathyroid, and autonomic derivatives.[85] These neural crest cells are site-specific and carry information for the formation of structures appropriate to their origin rather than being defined at the destination of migration.

Several genes have been identified as important in the proper migration and differentiation of the cardiac neural crest. The Splotch mutant mouse is characterized by a mutation in the *Pax-3* gene.[87] Homozygote Splotch mutants have a complete neural crest ablation phenotype, including persistent truncus arteriosus and aortic arch anomalies,[88] similar to the CV phenotype of neural crest ablation in the chick embryo.[86,89] *Hox* gene abnormalities also are associated with defects in the derivatives of cranial neural crest. A transgenic murine model of *Hox* 1.1 overexpression has neural crest ectomesenchymal tissue abnormalities, including cleft palate, nonfused pinnae, and open eyes. *Hox* 1.5-deficient mice have features of DiGeorge's syndrome.[86] In humans, DiGeorge's syndrome, velo-cardio-facial syndrome, and conotruncal anomaly face syndrome are associated with chromosomal deletions in the 22q11 region on the long arm of chromosome 22.[90–93] Recent studies have indicated a number of candidate factors in the pathogenesis of these syndromes (referred to as catch22 syndrome). In addition, retinoic acid is a potent teratogen in humans and produces a syndrome involving all the derivatives of the cranial neural crest.[94]

Myocyte Differentiation

In the human embryo, the heart begins to contract at day 17 as the machinery of contraction and relaxation becomes functional. These functional units include the sarcomere, composed of the contractile elements; the mitochondria, containing the enzymes for energy production and modulation; and the sarcolemma, the cell envelope with specialized components of the t tubular system linked to the sarcoplasmic reticulum. In the mature myocardium, sarcomeres are organized parallel to the lines of peak systolic stress. In the embryonic myocyte, myofibrils initially appear disarrayed and become aligned as development proceeds.[95] Despite this disordered appearance, the contraction pattern of the early embryonic heart is isotropic.[96]

The temporal and spatial expression of contractile proteins in the developing heart is under intense investigation. At the precardiac tube stage, smooth muscle alpha-actin is the only isoform present. With formation of the cardiac tube, there is progressive expression of the cardiac form of sarcomeric actin with the onset of cardiac pumping. The alpha smooth muscle actin may act as a scaffolding during assembly of the sarcomere.[97,98]

Mitochondria multiply concurrently with the myofibrils in the differentiating myocyte. In the mature heart, mitochondrial enzymes are the major source of high-energy phosphate necessary for contraction and probably begin this function during embryonic development. In the chick, the mitochondria account for about 10 percent of myocyte volume.[95] In the rat embryo, total volume increases from 22 to 34 percent between days 6 and 10, and the mitochondria also change morphologically with development, becoming larger with more cristae and a denser matrix.[99] The myocyte mitochondrial volume fraction correlates directly with heart rate and oxygen consumption among animals.[100]

Maturation of the sarcoplasmic reticulum and the apparatus for excitation-contraction coupling occurs coincident with the structural morphogenesis of the embryonic heart. The sarcolemma contains ion pumps, channels, and exchangers that maintain chemical and charge differences between extracellular and intracellular spaces.[101] During maturation of the heart, the resting potential increases (becomes more negative) in both birds and mammals [102,103] Ca^{2+} influx through Ca^{2+} channels may play a relatively important role in transsarcolemmal Ca^{2+} influx in the immature heart. However, peak Ca^{2+} current density is actually decreased compared with that measured in mature cells.[104,105] Although Ca^{2+} influx by way of the Na^+–Ca^{2+} exchanger is less important for excitation-contraction coupling in mature myocardium, Na^+–Ca^{2+} exchange may play an important role in myocytes from relatively immature rabbit hearts.

Relaxation, an active process by which the myocardium returns to steady state after contraction, depends on rapid removal of Ca^{2+} from troponin C. This is mediated primarily by active transport of Ca^{2+} back into the sarcoplasmic reticulum (SR). The SR Ca^{2+} pump ATPase (SERCA2a) usually couples hydrolysis of adenosine triphosphate (ATP) to active Ca^{2+} transport. The rate of SR Ca^{2+} uptake correlates well with the observed rate of myocardial relaxation. Regulation of SR Ca^{2+} pump activity is mediated by the intrinsic SR protein phospholamban. Ca^{2+} also is removed from the myofilaments by extrusion across the cell membrane. In the steady state, the amount of Ca^{2+} removed from the myocyte equals the amount entering through the Ca^{2+} channels.[106]

Segmental Basis of Heart Tube Formation

Formation of the cardiac tube is a complex morphogenetic event. The primitive, bilateral heart tubes each contain an inner layer of endocardium, a middle layer of cardiac jelly, and an outer layer of myocardium. At the cephalic end of the embryo (on each side of the midsagittal plane), myocytes within a section of each heart tube acquire contractile elements, and the position of the heart tubes shifts first to be parallel and close to each other within the cephalic part of the developing body cavity (intraembryonic coelom), ventral to the foregut, followed by fusion of the heart tubes in the ventral midline to form the linear or straight heart tube.[4,5,107–109]

It is important to note that the primitive linear heart tube does not contain all the segments present in the mature heart. During morphogenesis, the proximal portion of the aortic sac is incorporated into the outflow tract of the right ventricle (along with migrating neural crest cells) and the sinus venosus is incorporated into developing atria. Thus, each "segment" of the mature heart arises at a unique time during embryogenesis.[110] One critical aspect of this segmental assembly and maturation of the heart is that there likely are both temporal and spatial "windows" that are developmentally regulated, and this may explain why similar morphogens such as retinoic acid produce a wide spectrum of teratogenic effects depending on the time in gestation of exposure. Another aspect of this segmental paradigm is the concept that cardiac morphogenesis depends on molecular and cellular as well as mechanical interactions between the respective segments in the developing heart.[110]

Cardiac Jelly

Prior to looping, the acellular space between the myocardium and the endocardium in the heart is filled with a deformable extracellular matrix. This "cardiac jelly" forms before cardiac tube fusion and is closely associated with the primordial myocytes.[111] At the pretubular heart stages, the extracellular matrix contains collagen types I and IV, fibronectin, and laminin. The primordial endothelial cells destined to form the endocardium interact and migrate through this matrix during the establishment of the primitive, bilateral heart tubes. Radioactive labeling has demonstrated that proteins produced in the myocardium flow toward the endocardium and are incorporated into the basal lamina.[112] The cardiac jelly has a variety of functions related to hemodynamic performance, cardiac looping and cell migration in cardiac septation, and the formation of the endocardial cushion valves at the atrioventricular (AV) junction and outflow tract of the heart.

The protein composition of the cardiac jelly modulates differentiation of the endothelium. Recent information explains the role of genes from the TGF-beta family of peptide growth

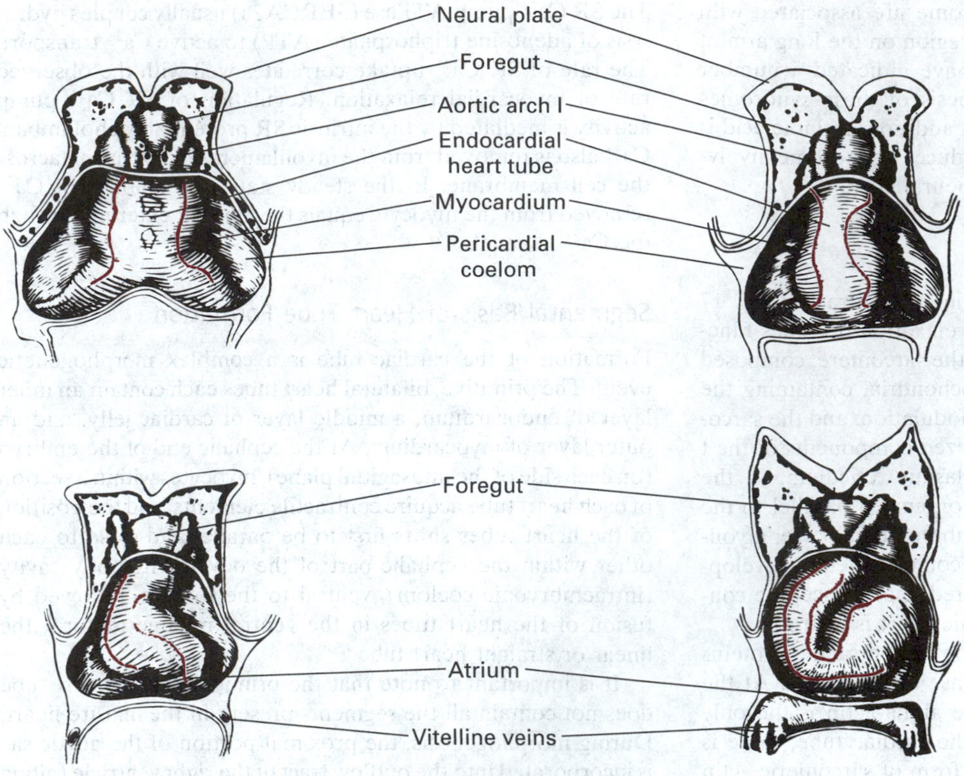

FIGURE 9-4 Schematic ventral dissections of human embryos of different ages, showing formation of the heart loop. (Adapted from Davis CL. Development of the human heart from its first appearance to the state found in embryos of 20 paired somites. *Contrib Embryol* 1927; 19:245. Reproduced with permission from the Carnegie Institution of Washington.)

factors as regulators of morphogenesis.[113] TGF-beta2 proteins are in the extracellular matrix and are an integral component of the morphogenetic changes at the AV cushion level, acting through second messengers such as protein kinase C.[114] In addition, fibronectin probably serves to set up migratory pathways in the cardiac jelly. These protein strands are arranged radially in the cushion, presumably along the lines of stress. The fibronectin strands also may serve as a template for the fibrous skeleton of the AV valve leaflets.[115–117] The extracellular matrix proteins stimulate transdifferentiation of the endocardium in these regions, prompting endothelial cells to transform to mesenchymal cells which migrate into the cushion matrix. Laminin and type IV collagen are stabilizing signals or markers, since these compounds are absent in the cushion regions but are present adjacent to the endocardial cells that maintain a typical epithelial integrity.

Endocardial Maturation

The endothelial cells that make up the lining of the embryonic heart initially are arranged as a single sheet. This squamous-like sheet has the morphologic features of an active tissue, including microvilli, ruffles, and intercellular openings.[118] The endocardium participates in the formation of endocardial cushions at the AV junction and in the outflow tract.[119] Transdifferentiation of the endocardium occurs in the endocardial cushions, where cells round up, produce pseudopodia, and migrate into the cardiac jelly.[120] These cells eventually make up a portion of the fibrous skeleton of the cardiac valves. Inductive chemical signals from the myocardium contribute to the endocardial transdifferentiation and regulate the migration of the mesenchymal cells.[120] In addition, hemodynamic alterations can influence the orientation of endocardial cells on the endocardial cushions[121] and the loci of dead and dying cells in the chick embryo heart.[122] This interaction likely is similar to the relation between the endothelium and smooth muscle of the mature vascular bed.[123] Finally, expansion of the endocardium is critical to the process of ventricular trabeculation, as is discussed below.

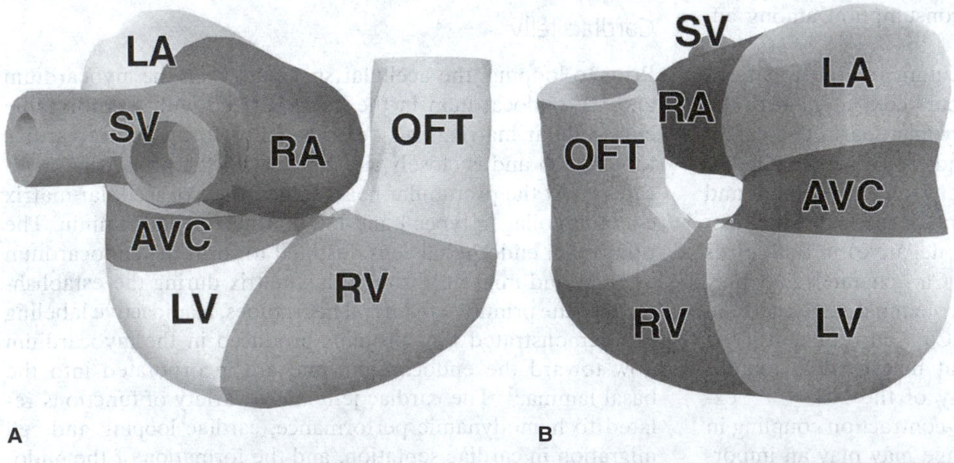

FIGURE 9-5 Schematic representation of the tubular heart during looping. Panel *A* depicts an inferior view of the heart, while panel *B* represents a superior view. Note that at this stage (approximately 4 weeks of development in the human), all the segments are more or less arranged in series. From inflow to outflow: V = sinus venosus; RA = right atrium; LA = left atrium; AVC = atrioventricular canal; LV = left ventricle; RV = right ventricle; OFT = outflow tract.

Looping

Following the formation of the straight heart tube, the human embryo is about 2 mm long and 23 days old. At the cephalic (or cranial) end of the myocardial heart tube, the nonmyocardial aortic sac can be recognized. The aortic sac is connected to the first pair of aortic arches and later also to the second, third, fourth, and sixth arches (the fifth pair of aortic arches does not normally develop in mammals or is very rudimentary). The extreme caudal part of the myocardial tube receives the paired confluence of veins that lie extrapericardially and are embedded in mesenchyme. In the early tubular stage, the heart hangs suspended from the ventral foregut by the so-called dorsal mesocardium. This structure disintegrates in the midportion of the tube, leaving the heart connected at the anterior pole at the level of the aortic sac and at the posteriorly located venous pole (atria and sinus venosus). At least three different biomechanical mechanisms may act in combination to generate the characteristic bend to the right of the cardiac tube: locally constrained growth, active cell deformation, and prestressed dorsal mesocardium.[124]

As the tubular heart continues to grow, it bends to the right and anteriorly (Fig. 9-4). This results in a compound sigmoid structure with a so-called d-loop (rightward) configuration. At this stage, it is easy to distinguish the sinus venosus, the common atrium, the atrioventricular canal, the future left and right ventricles, and the outflow segment. Internally, the developing muscular interventricular septum is recognizable, its crest characteristically expressing the molecular marker GLN2/HNK-1.[125,126] It is important to note that at this stage, all the future segments of the heart are still basically connected in series and that the common atrium connects, via the atrioventricular canal, completely to the left ventricle [i.e., double-inlet left ventricle (DILV)], while the outflow tract is connected exclusively to the right ventricle [i.e., double-outlet right ventricle (DORV)]. This is schematically depicted in Fig. 9-5.

The transition from a tubular heart in which the future segments are arranged in series (atrium to LV to RV to outflow tract) into a four-chambered heart in which the definitive chambers are arranged in parallel, separated by septa and valves, raises two important questions. The first is how the right atrium becomes connected to the right ventricle, and the second is how the left ventricle gains access to the aortic portion of the outflow tract. The remodeling of the so-called inner curvature of the looping heart tube plays an important role in this process and involves a rightward expansion of the AV canal and a concomitant leftward shift of the aorta. Immunohistochemical studies have demonstrated that this remodeling is intimately related to the development of the so-called primary ring (Fig. 9-6).[125,126] In the postnatal human heart, derivatives of the primary ring are found in the AV conduction system, in the right AV junction (the right AV ring), and behind the aorta (the retroaortic root branch) (Fig. 9-7).[126]

ANOMALIES

Ventricular Inversion with Transposition of the Great Arteries If the cardiac tube loops to the left and anterior (L-loop) rather than to the right and anterior, most of the structures

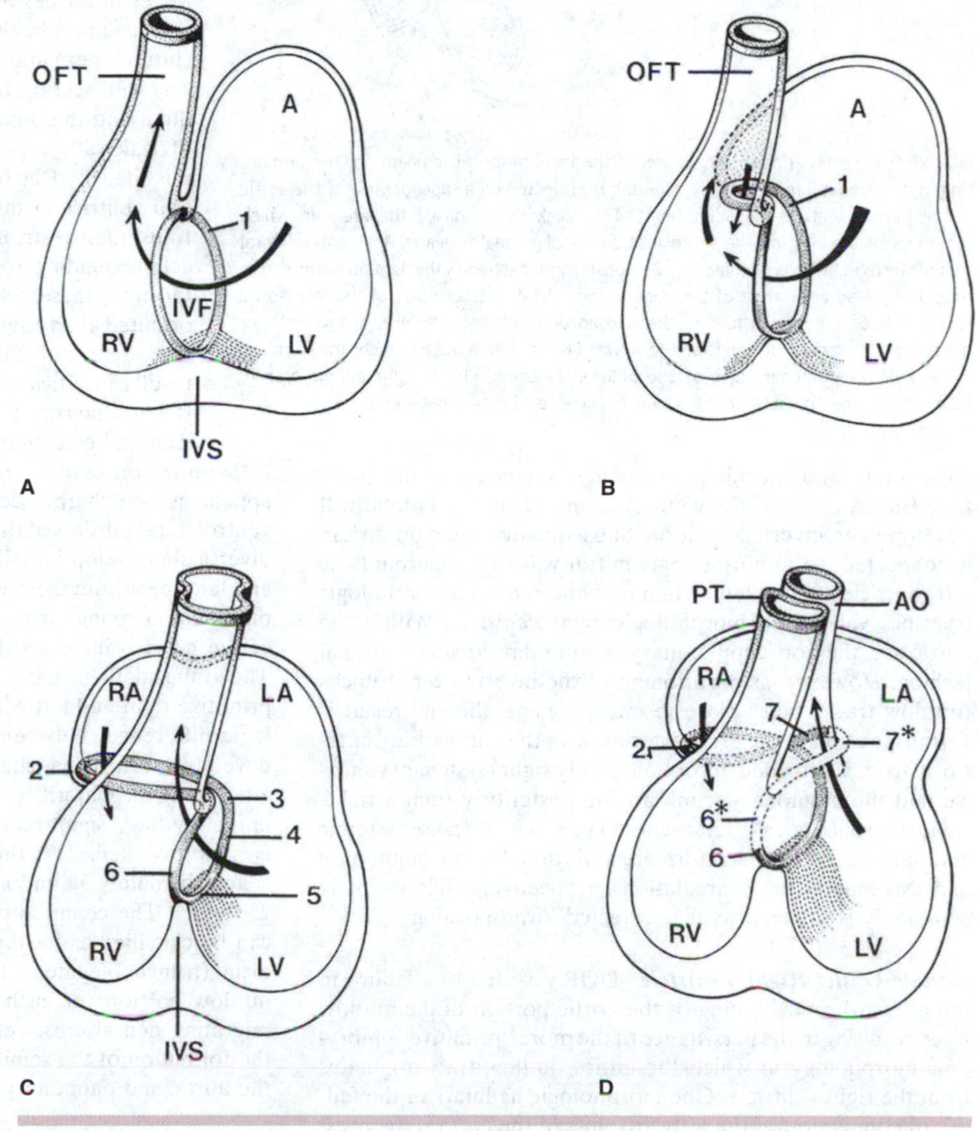

FIGURE 9-6 Schematic representation of the location of the so-called primary ring (characterized by the expression of the antigen GIN2) in different stages of human development. The drawings illustrate the development of the conduction system as a derivative of the primary ring but also show that the changes in the topography of the ring tissue reflects (1) the rightward expansion of the atrioventricular canal and (2) the leftward shift ("wedging") of the developing aorta. 1 = "primary ring"; 2 = right atrioventricular ring; 3 = atrioventricular nodal area; 4 = penetrating His bundle; 5 = crest of interventricular septum; 6 = septal branch; 7 = retroaortic branch. Areas indicated with an asterisk have lost their expression. The Carnegie stages of development presented in the drawings a to d are a = stage 14; b = stage 15; c = stage 17; d = stage 18–19. (Adapted from Wessels et al.[125])

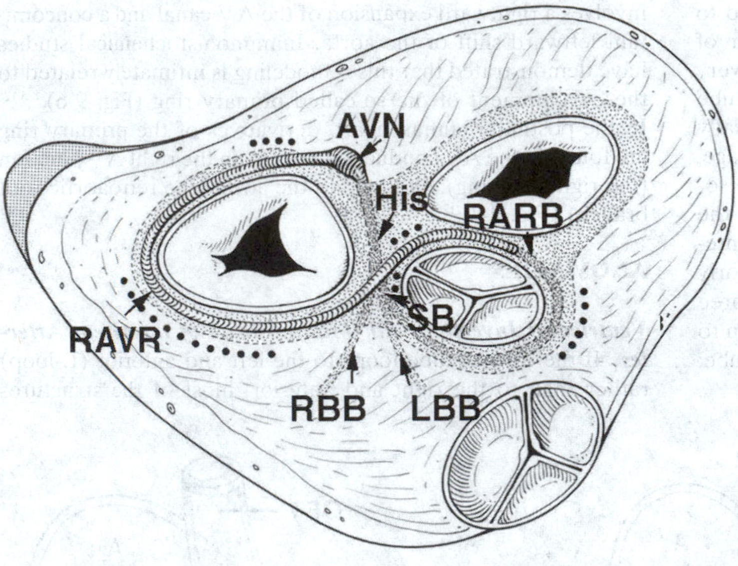

FIGURE 9-7 Schematic representation of the localization of remnants of the primary ring in the neonatal human heart. The ring is projected on a superior view of the aortic mitral fibrous unit of the adult heart. The black dots indicate the areas in which remnants of the ring are detected in a series of neonatal hearts. 1 = anterolateral part of the right atrioventricular ring; 2 = posteromedial part of the right atrioventricular ring; 3 = "dead-end" tract of the conduction axis; 4 = lateral part of the retroaortic rootbranch; 5 = posterior part of the retroaortic rootbranch. AVN = atrioventricular node; AoV = semilunar valve of the aorta; LBB = left bundle branch; mi = mitral valve; PuV = semilunar valve of the pulmonary trunk; Rbb = right bundle branch; SB = septal branch; tri = tricuspid valve. (Adapted from Wessels et al.[126])

adjacent to and including ventricular segments of the heart tube (the AV valves, the ventricles, and the arterial roots) will develop in an inverted position. Subsequently, the right atrium is connected via a morphologic mitral valve to a morphologic left ventricle and the left atrium is connected via a morphologic tricuspid valve to a morphologic right ventricle. Within the aortic sac, the aorticopulmonary septum develops in a normal fashion. However, as partitioning of the inverted conotruncus (outflow track) takes place in mirror image, the end result is L-transposition of the great arteries, with the aorta arising anteriorly from a left-sided, morphologically right (systemic) ventricle and the pulmonary trunk arising posteriorly from a right-sided, morphologically left (venous) ventricle. Because systemic and pulmonary venous return are still routed to the pulmonary and systemic arterial circulations, respectively, this anomaly commonly is referred to as "corrected" transposition.

Double-Outlet Right Ventricle DORV is due to a failure in the leftward repositioning of the aortic portion of the outflow tract, resulting in the persistence of the more "primitive" embryonic morphology in which the entire outflow tract originates from the right ventricle. One morphologic hallmark of the failure of completion of the leftward shift of the aorta is the presence of myocardial tissue between the left AV valve and the aorta (mitral-aortic separation). This anomaly is found after a wide range of hemodynamic, metabolic, and genetic insults to the embryo, suggesting that the phenotype of the DORV may be a final common expression of a range of primary abnormalities that result in the persistence of the embryonic configuration.[127]

Myocardial Trabeculation

The processes of primary myocardial trabeculation, expansion of secondary and tertiary myocardial trabeculae, and myocardial compaction are critical to the structural maturation of the ventricular chambers. This process results in the transformation of the smooth-walled endocardial lining into complex three-dimensional structure of the right and left ventricular myocardium. Rapid cell division and interposition of endothelial cells along the right and left ventrolateral borders of the endocardial tube is associated with a rapid resorption of cardiac jelly, resulting in myocardial ridges and trabeculae lined with single layers of endocardial cells.[128] The initial number and orientation of the myocardial ridges differ between species.[129] In general, myocardial trabeculation begins at the ventricular outer curvature (future apex) and then extends proximally and distally. The intersection between the outer, compact myocardium and the base of the trabeculae probably is a site of peak wall stress, and myocyte division is most active at this site.[130,131] Retroviral marker studies also have shown that ventricular myocardial growth is associated with a transmural distribution of clonally related myocardial cells extending from the epi- to the endocardium.[79,80] Of note, these cells reside in muscle bundles that are oriented at an angle to the longitudinal axis of the heart, consistent with the adult myocardial architecture that results in efficient twist and contraction.[79,80] However, the mechanisms that regulate clonal myocardial expansion and compaction have not been defined.

With the onset of myocardial trabeculation, diverticula first appear as two sharply defined areas along the right and left ventrolateral borders of the endocardial tube (Fig. 9-8).[132] These diverticula develop initially at the expense of the cardiac jelly and later penetrate the myocardium as it increases in thickness, producing a spongy mass of trabeculae.[128] The filling capacity of the heart is increased by the added intertrabecular spaces. The trabeculating embryonic heart now can be divided into primitive right and left ventricles as there are distinct morphologic differences between the trabecular architectures of the developing ventricular chambers. The developing LV is trabeculated along the majority of its greater curvature, while the developing RV has a significant portion of the greater curvature that is smooth-walled.[133] At this stage of development, the embryo is approximately 3 mm long and has an ovulation age of about 25 days.[107] The common outflow tract of the developing heart can be classified as having a proximal (conus) segment and a distal (truncus) segment. The conus eventually septates into the outflow portions of each ventricle with the incorporation of migrating neural crest cells, while the truncus contributes to the formation of the semilunar valves and the development of the aortic and pulmonary roots.

ANOMALIES

Noncompaction of the Ventricular Myocardium Noncompaction of the ventricular myocardium is a rare, familial congenital cardiomyopathy that results from incomplete compaction of the trabecular embryonic myocardium.[134,135] The characteristic echocardiographic findings consist of multiple, prominent myo-

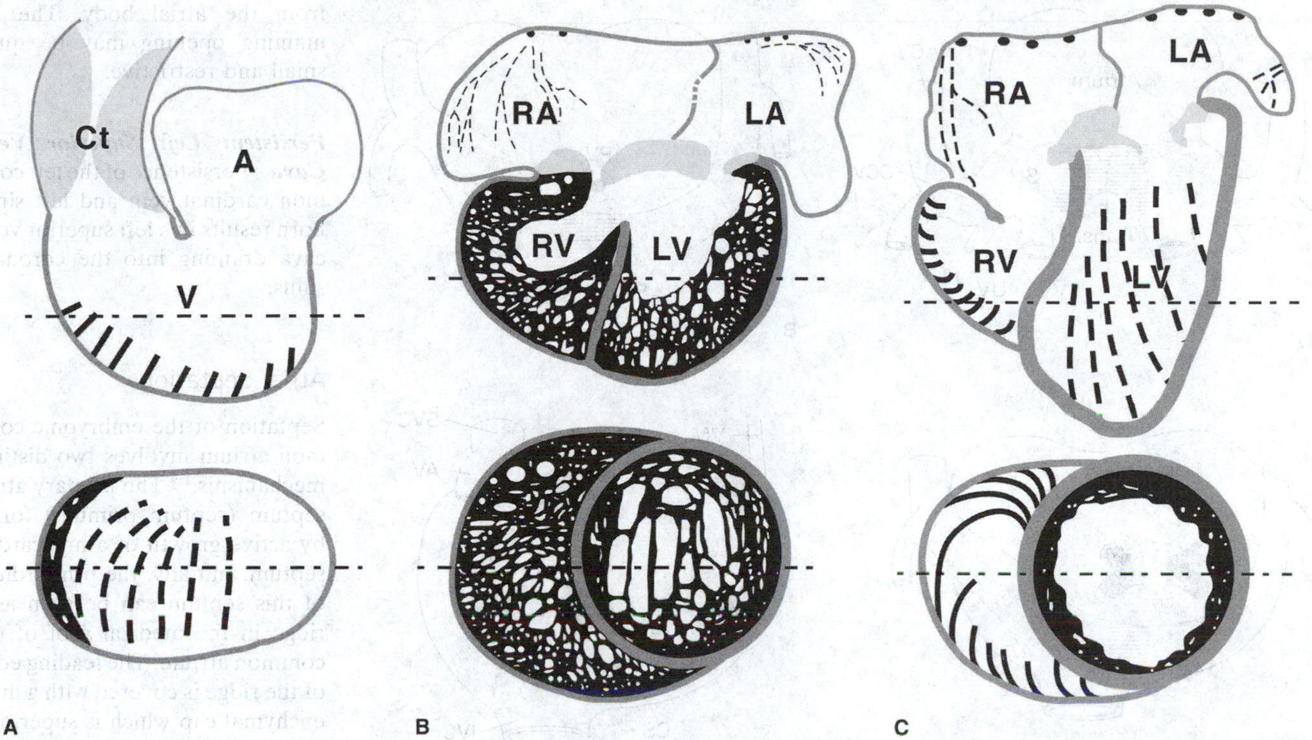

FIGURE 9-8 Schematic representation of myocardial trabecular development in the chick embryo. *A.* At the onset of ventricular trabeculation [around Hamburger-Hamilton (HH) stage 17], the process is limited to the primitive ventricle (V), while the inner curvature of the cardiac loop remains smooth. *B.* Transverse and frontal sections that show the distribution of secondary trabeculae (around HH stage 28). *C.* Mature tertiary trabecular pattern (HH stage 45). Only two of the principal bundles are shown in the left ventricle for clarity. In both ventricles, the trabeculae are arranged in a counterclockwise apicobasal spiral (viewed from base to apex). Differences between the right and left ventricles relate primarily to geometric differences (cone/crescent versus cylinder/prolate ellipsoid). Ct = conotruncus; At = primitive atrium. (Adapted from Sedmera et al.[144])

cardial trabeculations and deep intertrabecular recesses communicating with the left ventricular cavity. The disease uniformly affects the left ventricle with or without concomitant RV involvement and results in systolic and diastolic ventricular dysfunction and clinical heart failure. Recent studies have characterized this disease in both children and adults. A higher incidence of Wolff-Parkinson-White syndrome was found in children, whereas left bundle branch block was more rare than reported in adults. Familial recurrence is high.[136] Recently, a case of ventricular noncompaction was identified in a patient who also had a haplotype deletion on the long arm of chromosome 5.[137] The affected region included the locus for the cardiac-specific homeobox gene *Nkx2.5,* suggesting an association between ventricular myocardial noncompaction and haploinsufficiency of *Nkx2.5.*

MECHANISMS OF CARDIAC SEPTATION

Cardiac and Extracardiac Orientation

Because of rapid growth and the progressive curvature of the longitudinal axis of the embryo during organogenesis, it is critical to define cardiac morphogenesis, including septation, with reference to extracardiac morphologic landmarks that relate to the longitudinal axis of the embryo.[138] In the following discussion of cardiac septation, therefore, the diaphragm (septum transversum) is assumed to maintain an approximately horizontal position, as it does in the mature heart. The terms *anterior, posterior, superior,* and *inferior* are employed accordingly. Although the formation of the various cardiac septa occurs almost simultaneously, for clarity it is necessary to consider their development separately.

Cardiac Septation

Cardiac septation involves the formation of several septal (myocardial and mesenchymal/fibrous) and valvar structures. All the original tissues of the tubular heart (myocardium, endocardium, endocardial cushion tissues) as well as the so-called extracardiac cell populations, which arrive in the heart at relatively late stages of development (neural crest, epicardium, ventral neural tube cells), appear to play a role during valvuloseptal morphogenesis.

The Sinus Venosus

In the 3-mm human embryo, the sinus venosus consists of a central, transverse portion of the sinus venosus and the right and left sinus horns (Fig. 9-9). The sinus venosus receives three pairs of veins: the omphalomesenteric (vitelline) veins, the umbilical (allantoic) veins, and the common cardinal veins. The proximal portions of the umbilical veins soon disappear. As a result of the increased blood flow associated with the right and left systemic veins, the right sinus horn and the proximal cardinal

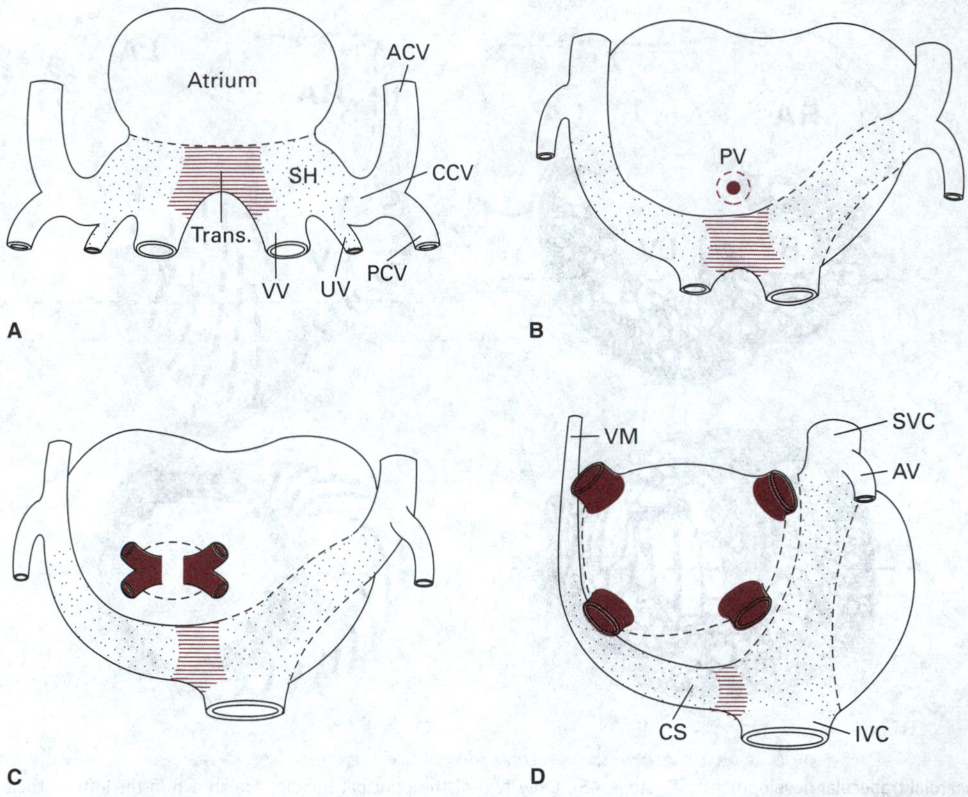

FIGURE 9-9 Posterior view of the atria and sinus venosus in embryos. *A.* 3-mm CR length; *B.* 5-mm CR length; *C.* 12-mm CR length. *D.* Newborn. Diagrammatic. A(C)CV = anterior (common) cardinal vein; AV = azygos vein; CS = coronary sinus; IVC = inferior vena cava; PCV = posterior cardinal vein; PV = pulmonary vein; SH = sinus horn; UV = umbilical vein; VM = vein of Marshall; VV = vitelline vein. (From Van Mierop LHS, Wiglesworth FW. Isomerism of the cardiac atria in the asplenia syndrome. *Lab Invest* 1962; 11:1303. Copyright by U.S. and Canadian Academy of Pathology.)

and vitelline veins attain a vertical position, increase in size, and form the smooth-walled, intercaval part of the atrium. The transverse portion and the proximal left sinus horn become the coronary sinus. Infolding of the sinoatrial junctional tissue at the right border of the sinoatrial foramen results in the formation of the right venous valve.[139,140] The left valve develops as a result of active growth, similar to that of the primary atrial septum (i.e., the left valve does not develop as a fold) (Fig. 9-10). Thus, the vertical sinoatrial orifice is flanked on each side by a valvelike structure in the 4- to 6-mm human embryo. Superiorly, the venous valves join to form the septum spurium. The venous valves, particularly the right venous valve, are relatively large in the 16-mm embryo. The superior aspect of the right venous valve eventually develops into the crista terminalis, or terminal crest. The left sinus valve fuses partly with the atrial septum. Inferiorly, the left venous valve intersects with the inferior part of the right venous valve. As a result, the right venous valve becomes divided into the relatively large inferior vena caval (or eustachian) valve and a smaller coronary sinus (or thebesian) valve.

ANOMALIES

Cor Triatriatum Dexter Complete persistence of the right venous valve of the embryonic heart produces a septum in the right atrium, separating the intercaval part of the right atrium from the atrial body. The remaining opening may be quite small and restrictive.

Persistent Left Superior Vena Cava Persistence of the left common cardinal vein and left sinus horn results in a left superior vena cava draining into the coronary sinus.

Atrial Septation

Septation of the embryonic common atrium involves two distinct mechanisms.[139] The primary atrial septum (septum primum) forms by active growth of a myocardial septum. Initially, the primordium of this septum can be seen as a ridge in the medical roof of the common atrium. The leading edge of the ridge is covered with a mesenchymal cap which is superiorly continuous with the superior AV cushion and inferiorly with the inferior AV cushion. As the primary septum descends from the roof of the atrium toward the atrioventricular canal, thus decreasing the size of the primary interatrial foramen, the mesenchymal leading edge continues to fuse with the AV cushions, which are also in the process of fusing. These events result in closure of the primary interatrial foramen (or ostium primum) and the formation of the central fibrous body (see Figure 9-12). Concomitantly, perforations appear in the superior aspect of the primary. The perforations coalesce, resulting in the secondary atrial foramen (ostium secundum). Next, the secondary atrial septum develops as an infolding of the atrial roof located between the primary septum and the left venous valve. The foramen ovale is the opening bordered by the free edge of the septum secundum. After fusion of the septum primum with the septum secundum, the foramen ovale becomes the fossa ovalis.

Development of the Pulmonary Veins

The so-called pulmonary pit, the future portal of entry for the main pulmonary vein, is recognizable at around 28 days of gestation and is situated in the midline of the inferior portion of the common atrium before atrial septation is initiated. The pulmonary pit is flanked by two myocardial reflections that are referred to as the left and right pulmonary ridges, respectively.[141] This pulmonary pit, actually an invagination of the endocardium into the dorsal mesocardium, can be traced toward the pulmonary mesenchyme as an endothelial strand. Remodeling of the tissues surrounding the pulmonary pit results in incorporation of the ostium of the pulmonary vein in the wall of the left ventricle.

ANOMALIES

Atrial Septal Defect at the Fossa Ovalis This defect, which often is referred to as a secundum-type atrial septal defect, is due to malformation of the primary atrial septum, resulting in an oversized ostium secundum. Frequently, the atrial defect is further enlarged by a hypoplastic septum secundum. Total absence of both the septum primum and the septum secundum (common atrium) is rare and almost always is associated with a form of persistent AV canal.

Anomalous Pulmonary Venous Connection The total form of anomalous pulmonary venous connection presumably is due either to lack of development or to a premature involution of the common pulmonary vein. A number of types of pulmonary venous to systemic venous connections occur, depending on which of the early embryonic channels connecting the pulmonary venous bed to the systemic venous circulation remains patent.

Cor Triatriatum Sinister If incorporation of the common pulmonary vein into the left atrium does not take place and the common pulmonary venous ostium remains narrow, the result is a septum-like structure that may derive from the left pulmonary ridge and divides the left atrium into two components: One receives the pulmonary veins, and the other gives access to the mitral valve and the left atrial appendage.

The Atrioventricular Canal

Division of the AV canal into left-sided and right-sided orifices occurs as a result of fusion of the superior and inferior AV cushions, which are first evident in the 6-mm crown-rump (CR)-length human embryo. At this stage, the common AV canal is located exclusively over the left ventricle. The superior aspect of the developing interventricular septum is continous with the right aspect of the AV junctional myocardium.

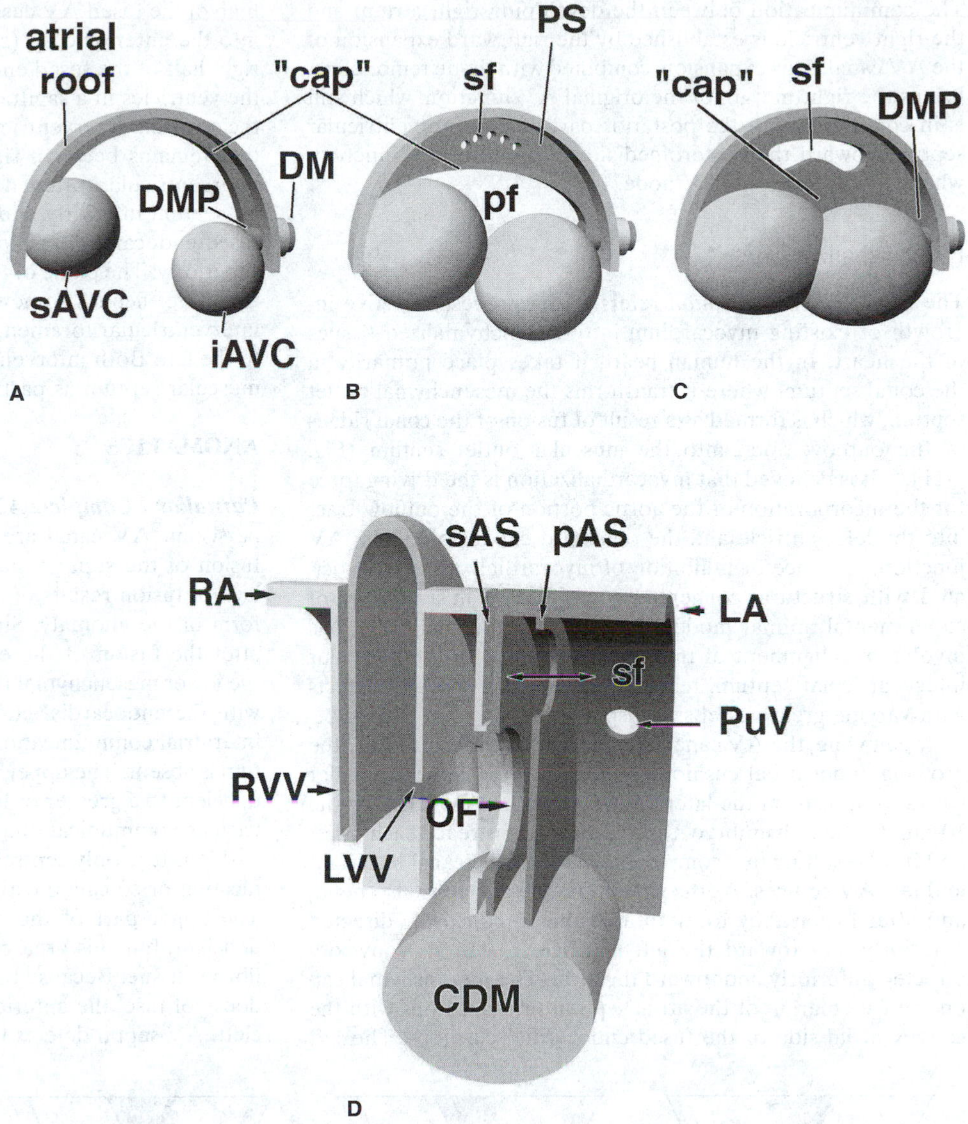

FIGURE 9-10 A model for the development of the atrial septal complex in the human heart. Panels *A–C* of this cartoon illustrate the key events in the formation of the primary atrial septum (*A–C*). Panel *D* schematically depicts the formation of the atrial septum and venous valves. Panel *A* represents a heart at approximately $4\frac{1}{2}$ weeks of development. The AV cushions can be distinguished but have not yet fused. The leading edge of the primary septum is covered by a mesenchymal cap which is in continuity with the dorsal mesenchymal protrusion of the dorsal mesocardium. Panel *B* represents the situation at approximately 6 weeks of development. The leading edge of the primary atrial septum, covered with a mesenchymal cap, is now approaching the AV cushions, which are in the process of fusing. Within the myocardial portion of the primary septum, multiple fenestrations represent the developing secondary foramen. Completion of fusion of the mesenchymal tissues at 6 to 7 weeks of development (panel *C*) results in the closure of the primary interatrial foramen. At this time, a prominent secondary foramen can be found within the superior portion of the primary septum. The cartoon in panel *D* shows how the secondary atrial septum is formed as a result of infolding of the atrial roof. This occurs at the margin between the myocardium and the left and right atrial expression domain. The myocardium of the primary atrial septum is part of the left atrial expression domain; the orifice of the pulmonary vein also is surrounded by myocardium with a left atrial molecular phenotype. This panel also illustrates that based on the gene expression patterns, the left venous valve develops as a myocardial structure with a right atrial molecular phenotype, whereas the right venous valve (just like the secondary atrial septum) develops by infolding, in this case of the junctional tissue between the right atrium and the sinus venosus. iAVC = inferior atrioventricular cushion; sAVC = superior atrioventricular cushion; DM = dorsal mesocardium; DMP = dorsal mesenchymal protrusion; pf = primary foramen; PS = primary atrial septum; sf = secondary foramen; LA = left atrium; RA = right atrium; OF = oval fossa; pAS = primary atrial septum; sAS = secondary atrial septum; PuV = pulmonary vein; LVV = left venous valve; RVV = right venous valve (From Wessels et al.[139])

The communication between the developing right atrium and the right ventricle is established by the rightward expansion of the AV canal. This expansion, combined with tissue remodeling, brings the right margin of the original AV junction, which still is in continuity with the posterior part of the interventricular septum, toward the posteromedial aspect of the AV junction, where it will form the AV node.[16,125]

Myocardialization

The term *myocardialization* refers to the process of active ingrowth of existing myocardium into mesenchymalized tissues of the heart. In the human heart, it takes place primarily in the conal septum, where it transforms the mesenchymal outlet septum, which is formed as a result of fusion of the conal ridges of the outflow tract, into the muscular outlet septum (Fig. 9-11).[142] It is believed that myocardialization is the driving force for the incorporation of the aortic portion of the outflow tract into the left ventricle and the rightward expansion of the AV junction. Absence or inhibition of myocardialization is associated with structural congenital heart disease in a number of experimental animal models.[143] Most of these malformations involve malalignment of the outlet septum with the muscular interventricular septum, resulting in ventricular septal defects with varying great vessel size disparity.[110]

Meanwhile, the AV canal has enlarged to the right, while the growing endocardial cushions project into the lumen. Smaller cushions appear on the lateral borders of the AV canal. In the 10-mm CR-length embryo, the major cushions reach each other and fuse, resulting in a complete division of the canal into right and left AV orifices. At the same time the cushions also bend, and after fusion they form an arch that is concavely directed anteriorly and toward the left ventricle[143] with its convexity directed anteriorly and toward the atria. The mesenchymal cap on the free margin of the atrial septum primum fuses with the convex atrial side of the fused endocardial cushions. The left limb of the fused AV cushion eventually becomes incorporated into the anterior cusp (aortic leaflet) of the mitral valve. The right half of the fused endocardial cushions comes to lie within the ventricles in a sagittal orientation somewhat to the right of the muscular interventricular septum. Thus, the communication that remains between right and left ventricles, the secondary interventricular foramen, is bordered by the muscular ventricular septum inferiorly and anteriorly, the right extremity of the fused endocardial cushions posteriorly, and the conal septum superiorly. The plane of the secondary interventricular foramen therefore inclines somewhat to the right; that of the primary interventricular foramen, as we have seen, has come to deviate to the left. Both interventricular foramens share the top of the muscular septum as part of their inferior borders.

ANOMALIES

Partial and Complete AV Canal Defect The several forms of persistent AV canal are due to various degrees of failure of fusion of the superior and inferior AV canal cushions. Total lack of fusion results in a single AV ostium, i.e., the complete form of the anomaly. Since the arch or bay normally formed after the fusion of the endocardial cushions fails to develop, the lower mesenchymal border of the atrial septum cannot fuse with the endocardial cushions. The result is a low-lying large interatrial communication, and the AV part of the cardiac septum is absent. The upper part of the ventricular septum remains deficient to a greater or lesser degree, and there is an interventricular communication. In the partial forms, the endocardial cushions fuse only centrally. The result is an interatrial communication or so-called ostium primum–type atrial septal defect. The upper part of the muscular ventricular septum remains deficient, but this area of the ventricular septum is closed by fibrous tissue. Because the left side of the endocardial cushions does not fuse, the anterior or aortic cusp of the mitral valve is cleft. AV septal defects frequently are associated with trisomy 21 in humans and trisomy 16 in mice.[127] Genetic markers in patients without trisomy 21 also are under investigation.

Ventricular Septal Defect Some forms of perimembranous ventricular septal defect may be due to failure of fusion of the right extremity of the fused endocardial cushions, the upper border of the muscular ventricular septum, and the conal septum. Since the endocardial cushions fuse normally, there is no cleft in the anterior mitral valve cusp, and there also is no interatrial communication.

Single Ventricle, Left Ventricular Type with Rudimentary Outflow Chamber, or Double-Inlet Left Ventricle. If the AV canal becomes divided into two separate ostia (by the fusing AV cushions) but fails to expand to the right,

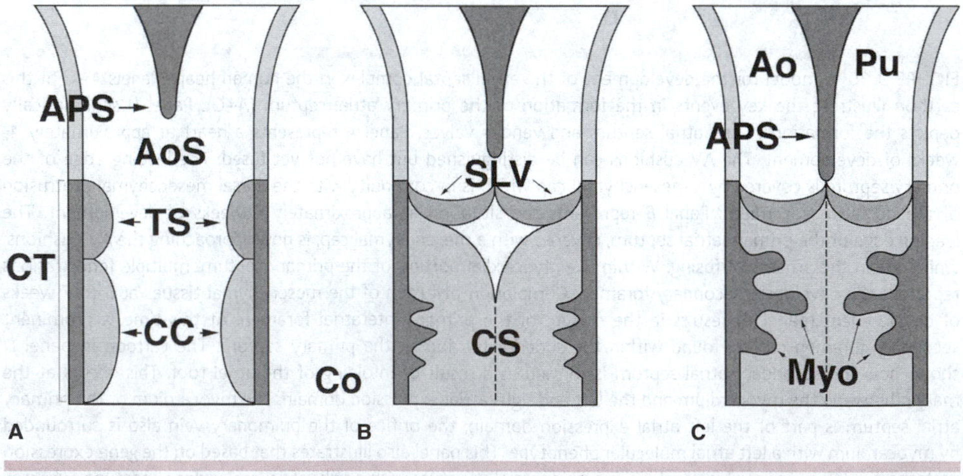

FIGURE 9-11 Schematic drawing of some of the developmental events involved in the septation of the outflow tract. Panel *A* depicts the stage in which the endocardial cushion tissues in the outflow tract (conal cushions and truncal swellings) and the aorticopulmonary septum have not yet fused. Panel *B* illustrates that the truncal swellings contribute to the formation of the semilunar valves of the aorta and the pulmonary trunk, whereas the fusing conal cushions are forming the mesenchymal outlet septum. At this stage, the conal myocardium starts to myocardialize the outlet septum. Panel *C* shows one of the final stages. The aorticopulmonary septum has now completely separated the aorta and pulmonary trunk above the level of the semilunar valves, while below the valves the outlet septum divides the outlet segment of the heart in a subaortic and subpulmonary outlet.

thus retaining its far leftward position, both ostia connect only to the primitive left ventricle. As a result, a communication between the right atrium and the right ventricle does not develop. The communication between the large ventricular chamber (i.e., left ventricle) and the rudimentary outflow chamber (i.e., right ventricle) represents the persistence of the primary interventricular foramen.

The Ventricles

As was mentioned above, the AV canal communicates exclusively with the primitive (or embryonic) left ventricle in the 5-mm CR-length human embryo and blood from the left ventricle reaches the primitive (or embryonic) right ventricle only by way of the primary interventricular foramen. In the developing human heart, the myocardium surrounding the interventricular foramen is characterized by the expression of the GFlN2/HNK antigen and is termed the "primary interventricular ring."[125]

The ventricles enlarge through centrifugal growth of the myocardium. The trabecular myocardium progresses from primary to secondary to tertiary trabeculations, while the compact outer myocardial layer remains relatively thin.[144] Coalescence of the secondary trabeculations into larger tertiary trabeculations occurs after septation, coincident with the formation of the AV valve leaflets.[145] The trabeculae positioned at the border between the developing left and right ventricle coalesce to form the major portion of the muscular ventricular septum.[115] On the right side, a large trabecula, the trabecula septomarginalis,[146] appears early (in embryos about 9 mm in CR length) and runs from the anteroinferior border of the primary interventricular foramen toward the apex.

ANOMALIES

Muscular Ventricular Septal Defect Failure of compaction and fusion of the trabecular portion of the ventricular septum results in the most common congenital cardiovascular anomaly, the isolated muscular ventricular septal defect.

The Truncus Arteriosus

The embryonic "outflow tract" consists of the conus, truncus, and aortic sac and functions as the conduit between the primitive right ventricle and the aortic arches. Septation of the conotruncal area of the outflow tract begins in embryos about 6 mm in CR length with the appearance of two opposing truncal cushions. One of these cushions is located along the dextrosuperior truncal endocardium (dextrosuperior truncal cushion), and the other on the sinistroinferior wall (sinistroinferior truncal cushion). Coincident with the expansion of the conotruncus, the cushions rapidly enlarge and fuse to form the truncal septum, thus dividing the truncus into aortic and pulmonary channels. The truncus is the first part of the heart to septate (at the 7-mm CR-length stage). Proximally, the truncal cushions merge with the superior aspects of the conal cushions, which are the comparable mesenchymal masses within the conus. Distally, the undivided portion of the truncus and the aortic sac enlarge to form the truncoaortic sac. Simultaneously, the origin and course of the sixth arches shift leftward, aligning with right ventricular outflow, and the origin and course of the fourth aortic arches shift rightward, aligning with left ventricular outflow. At the same time, a population of cells derived from the cardiac neural crest contributes to the formation of a vertical septum, the aorticopulmonary septum (APS), in the aortic sac.[89] The APS fuses with the truncal septum to complete septation of the aorta and the pulmonary trunk.[127,133,143,146,147]

ANOMALIES

Persistent Truncus Arteriosus If the truncal cushions remain hypoplastic and fail to fuse, partitioning of the truncus arteriosus does not take place. If, in addition to the hypoplastic truncal cushions, both intercalated valve cushions persist, the result is a quadricuspid truncal valve. Usually, fusion occurs between adjacent valve anlagen, resulting in an apparently tricuspid truncal valve with one larger cusp containing a fused raphe. In the great majority of cases, the aorticopulmonary septum does develop, and a short common pulmonary trunk arises from the persistent trunk. The ductus arteriosus is almost always absent, except when it is associated with interruption of the aortic arch. In experimental models, persistent truncus arteriosus can be produced after selected ablation of neural crest tissue, as was mentioned above.[85]

Aorticopulmonary Septal Defect This anomaly may be due to malalignment and/or failure of fusion between the distal truncal septum and the aorticopulmonary septum. Both arterial valves are present, but there is a communication of varying size (aorticopulmonary window) between the ascending aorta and the pulmonary trunk.

The Conus

The conal cushions make their appearance at about the same time as the truncal cushions. One is located on the dextrodorsal wall, and the other on the sinistroventral wall of the conus. On the right side, the dorsal conal cushion becomes contiguous with the superior truncal cushion, and on the left, the ventral conal cushion becomes contiguous with the inferior truncal cushion. Fusion of the conal cushion begins proximally and then progresses rapidly, completing the partition of the conal septum by the 14- to 15-mm CR-length stage in the human embryo. Conal septation reduces and then closes the small secondary interventricular foramen, which was bordered by the conal septum, the top of the muscular ventricular septum, and the right extremities of the fused endocardial cushions. The mesenchymal conal septum eventually becomes muscularized by myocardialization, resulting in the muscular outlet septum.[142]

ANOMALIES

Ventricular Septal Defect, Eisenmenger Type A large basilar septal defect, dextroposition of the aortic valve, and a hypoplastic or absent infundibular septum probably are due to hypoplasia or absence of the conal cushions.

Ventricular Septal Defect, Supracristal Type The supracristal type of ventricular septal defect probably is due to either simple failure of truncal and conal septal fusion or septal malalignment, which prevents fusion.

Tetralogy of Fallot The primary anomaly in tetralogy of Fallot probably is an anterior displacement to a varying degree of the conal septum, leading to unequal partitioning of the conus and reduction of the right ventricular infundibulum. A large basilar ventricular septal defect and dextroposition of the aortic valve result from failure of the displaced conal septum to participate in closure of the interventricular foramen. Pulmonary vascular hypoplasia probably is a secondary result of diminished forward blood flow. As was mentioned above, tetralogy of Fallot frequently is associated with 22q11 deletion, particularly in the setting of severe pulmonary atresia or when associated with extracardiac anomalies.

DEVELOPMENT OF THE HEART VALVES

The Atrioventricular Valves

Initially, the tubular embryonic heart functions as a peristaltoid pump, relying on endocardial cushions to function as valves and regional variations in conduction velocity to facilitate forward flow. The endocardial cushions develop in the areas characterized by slow contraction and relaxation and, in combination with the specialized myocardium with which they are associated, serve to promote antegrade blood flow. Initially, it is possible to distinguish only two AV cushions: the inferior (iAVC) and the superior (sAVC) cushions. Fusion of these two cushions results in the formation of the two AV orifices. At later stages, the so-called lateral AV cushions appear. Over time, the cushion-derived tissues develop into the thin mature AV valve cusps.[148] The sAVC contributes to the aortic leaflet of the mitral valve, and the iAVC to the septal and posteroinferior leaflet of the tricuspid valve. The right lateral AVC contributes to the formation of the anterosuperior leaflet of the tricuspid valves, and the left lateral AVC is involved in the formation of the parietal leaflet of the mitral valve. Although the cushion-derived tissues form the main component of the leaflets (Fig. 9-12), it is important to note that an essential step in the morphogenesis of the valves is the delamination of the developing leaflets from the underlying ventricular myocardium.[149,150]

ANOMALIES

Tricuspid Valve Atresia and Mitral Valve Atresia Tricuspid and mitral valve atresias are anomalies that probably are due to abnormal formation and/or premature fusion of the endocardial cushion tissue that borders the AV canal during or shortly after partitioning of the AV canal.

Ebstein's Anomaly of the Tricuspid Valve Ebstein's anomaly of the tricuspid valve probably is due to an abnormality in the process of myocardial delamination required for AV valve and chordal formation.

The Arterial Valves

The primordia of the semilunar valves become visible as small tubercles on the distal extensions of each truncal cushion after truncal partitioning in the 9-mm embryo. One of each pair is assigned to the pulmonary and aortic channels, respectively. On the walls of both aortic and pulmonary channels, opposite the fused truncus cushions, a third small cushion appears.[146] These two intercalated valve cushions form the third member of each arterial valve primordium. Both the aortic and pulmonary roots, consisting of the sinuses of Valsalva and the semilunar valves, probably are derived from the truncus arteriosus and the truncal and intercalated valve cushions.

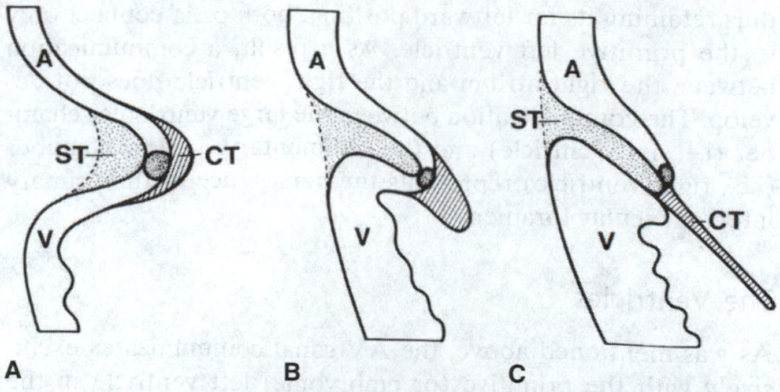

FIGURE 9-12 Schematic drawings of the formation of the atrioventricular junction in the human heart. *A*. The situation at the atrioventricular junction at 4 to 5 weeks of development. Myocardial continuity between atrium and ventricle occurs through the myocardium of the atrioventricular canal. The AV junction is sandwiched between the tissues of the AV sulcus at the epicardial side and the AV cushion at the endocardial side. *B*. With progressive remodeling of the AV junction, the sulcus tissues expand toward the midline of the AV canal as the cushion tissue remodels. *C*. With completion of this process, continuity is lost between atrial and ventricular myocardium. A = atrium; V = ventricle; ST = sulcus tissue; AV = myocardium of the atrioventricular canal; CT = cushion tissue. (Adapted from Wessels et al.[148])

ANOMALIES

Bicuspid Arterial Valves A bicuspid aortic or pulmonary valve is due to a failure of development of an intercalated valve cushion, resulting in a valve with two equal-size cusps, neither containing a raphe, or to fusion of adjacent valve anlagen, in which case the cusps are generally unequal in size, with the larger containing a raphe of varying length.

Arterial Valve Stenosis or Atresia Fusion of two or all three of the arterial valve anlagen probably results in stenosis or atresia of the valve.

Absent Arterial Valves Failure of the arterial valve anlagen to develop may explain the rare occurrence of absence of the pulmonary or aortic valve.

AORTIC ARCH DEVELOPMENT

Aortic arch development involves the sequential development and then the involution of six arch pairs. The first pair of arches in the 3-mm CR-length embryo is large when the second pair is just forming (Fig. 9-13*A*). Caudally, the dorsal aortas fuse to 0form a single vessel, and then vessel fusion progresses cranially. In a 4-mm embryo, the first and second arches have largely disappeared (Fig. 9-13*B*). The third aortic arch is well developed, and the fourth and sixth arches are being formed as ventral and dorsal sprouts of the aortic sac and dorsal aorta, respectively. The ventral portion of the sixth arch already has as its major branch the primitive pulmonary artery even though

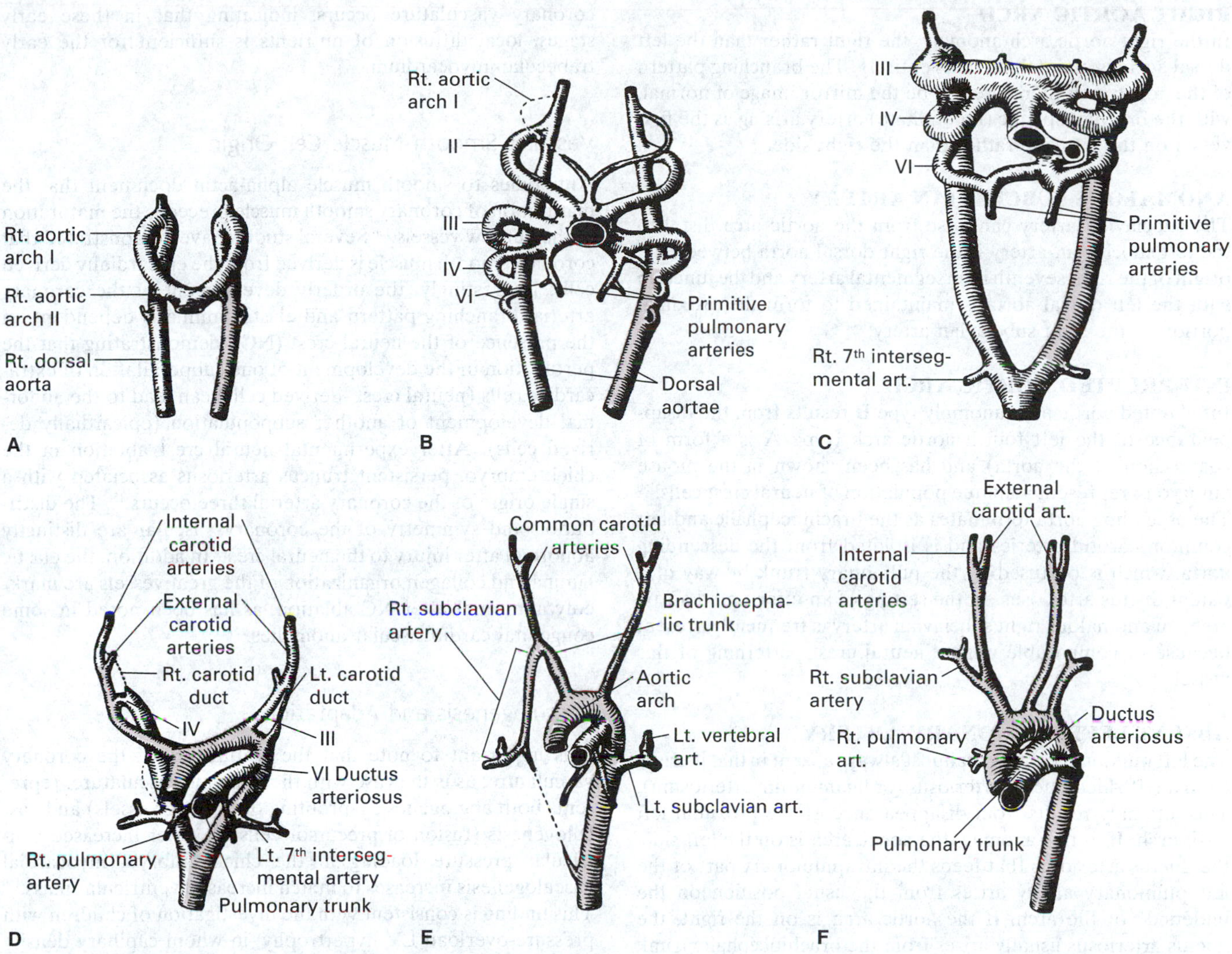

FIGURE 9-13 Development of the aortic arch system. Embryos of (*A*) 3 mm, (*B*) 4 mm, (*C*) 10 mm, (*D*) 14 mm, (*E*) 17 mm, (*F*) neonate. (Adapted from Congdon ED. Transformation of the aortic arch system during the development of the human embryo. *Contrib Embryol* 1922; 14:47.)

the arch itself has not yet been completed. Of note, in mammals the fifth aortic arch is rudimentary. By the 10-mm embryo stage, the first two aortic arches have regressed; the third, fourth, and sixth are present; and the truncoaortic sac has been divided by the formation of the aorticopulmonary septum so that the six arches are now continuous with the pulmonary trunk (Fig. 9-13*C*). Of note, the seventh cervical intersegmental arteries arise from the dorsal aorta near the midline and form the subclavian arteries. In a 14-mm embryo, the dorsal aortas between the third and fourth arches have disappeared and the third arches begin to elongate (Fig. 9-13*D*). At this point, the dorsal portion of the right sixth arch has disappeared, though the left sixth arch persists as the ductus arteriosus. The aortic sac has been broadened to contribute to the brachiocephalic trunk on the right and part of the definitive aortic arch up to the origin of the left third arch (common carotid artery). Finally, by the 17-mm embryo stage, the right dorsal aorta has become atrophic between its junction with the left dorsal aorta and the origin of the right seventh intersegmental artery has become attenuated and later disappears (Fig. 9-13*E*). The remaining components of the right dorsal aorta and right fourth aortic arch form the proximal subclavian artery. After birth, the distal part of the left sixth aortic arch, the ductus arteriosus, normally also involutes to form the ligamentum arteriosum. Thus, most aortic arch anomalies are secondary to abnormal retention or disappearance of various embryonic segments.

Anomalies

PATENT DUCTUS ARTERIOSUS

Persistence of the ductus arteriosus postnatally frequently occurs in permature infants as a result of delayed ductal involution. However, persistence of a large ductus arteriosus also occurs in isolation and in association with a variety of congenital cardiovascular malformations.

DOUBLE AORTIC ARCH

Double aortic arch is a result of persistence and continued patency of the segment of the right dorsal aorta between the origin of the right seventh intersegmental artery and its junction with the left dorsal aorta.

RIGHT AORTIC ARCH

In the right aortic arch anomaly, the right rather than the left dorsal aorta is maintained in its entirety. The branching pattern of the aortic arch therefore will be the mirror image of normal, with the brachiocephalic (innominate) artery arising as the first vessel on the left side rather than the right side.

ANOMALOUS SUBCLAVIAN ARTERY

The subclavian artery can arise from the aortic arch distal to the left subclavian artery if the right dorsal aorta between the origin of the right seventh intersegmental artery and the junction with the left dorsal aorta is maintained to form the proximal portion of the right subclavian artery.[150]

INTERRUPTED AORTIC ARCH

Interrupted aortic arch anomaly type B results from the disappearance of the left fourth aortic arch (type A is a form of coarctation of the aorta) and has been shown in the mouse embryo to represent a unique population of neural crest cells.[150] The ascending aorta terminates as the brachiocephalic and left common carotid arteries and is isolated from the descending aorta, which is perfused by the pulmonary trunk by way of a patent ductus arteriosus. In the setting of an interrupted aortic arch, an anomalous right subclavian artery is frequently present because of comparable unique neural crest patterning of this vessel.[150]

ABSENT LEFT PULMONARY ARTERY

The left pulmonary artery is almost always absent in that it arises from a left-sided ductus arteriosus (or ligamentum arteriosum). This anomaly results from disappearance of the proximal left sixth arch. If in this anomaly the aortic arch is on the left side, the ductus arteriosus that feeds the intrapulmonary part of the left pulmonary artery arises from the usual position on the underside of the arch. If the aortic arch is on the right, the ductus arteriosus usually arises from the brachiocephalic trunk with the left common carotid and left subclavian arteries as a trifurcation or, rarely, from a diverticulum of the descending aorta. Usually the left subclavian artery in such cases also arises from the diverticulum.

CORONARY ARTERY DEVELOPMENT

Endothelial Cell Origin

Coronary vascular endothelial maturation closely parallels the development of the embryonic epicardium.[151] A series of cell-fate studies has revealed that the coronary endothelial cells as well as coronary smooth muscle cells derive from the so-called proepicardium, a cluster of cells attached to the ventral wall of the sinus venosus. As cells from the proepicardium spread out and cover the surface of the heart, a subpopulation of epicardially derived cells (EPDCs) transdifferentiate and migrate into the myocardial cell layers,[152–155] where they contribute to the formation of the coronary network. A part of this network reaches the mesenchymal border of the aortic annulus.[151] Initially, multiple connections between the coronary vascular plexus and the aortic root are present; however, only two connections persist. It is interesting to note that the heart begins to pump blood before perfusion by the coronary vasculature occurs, indicating that in these early stages, local diffusion of nutrients is sufficient for the early trabecular myocardium.

Vascular Smooth Muscle Cell Origin

Antibodies to smooth muscle alpha-actin document that the maturation of coronary smooth muscle precedes the maturation of the outflow vessels.[156] Several studies have demonstrated that coronary smooth muscle is derived from the epicardially derived cells. Interestingly, the orderly development of the coronary arterial branching pattern and elastic lamina is dependent on the presence of the neural crest (NC), demonstrating that the pertubation in the development of one subpopulation of extracardiac cells (neural crest–derived cells) can lead to the abnormal development of another subpopulation (epicardially derived cells). After experimental neural crest ablation in the chick embryo, persistent truncus arteriosus associated with a single origin of the coronary arterial three occurs.[156] The distribution and symmetry of the coronary vascular are distinctly abnormal after injury to the neural crest. In addition, the elastic lamina and collagen organization of the great vessels are markedly abnormal after NC ablation, as has been noted in some congenital cardiovascular anomalies.[157]

Vasculogenesis and Adaptation

It is important to note that the maturation of the coronary vasculature, as is the case with the systemic vasculature, represents both angiogenesis (sprouting of existing vessels) and vasculogenesis (fusion of precursor cells).[158] After increased ventricular pressure loading in the chick embryo, myocardial vasculogenesis increases to match increased ventricular mass.[159] This finding is consistent with the investigation of children with pressure-overload LV hypertrophy, in whom capillary density remains unchanged.[160]

ANOMALIES

Anomalous Origin of the Left Coronary Artery Occasionally, the left coronary artery is found to arise from the pulmonary artery, and rarely from other aortic arch vessels. The developing coronary vessels perforate the aortic annulus in association with specific immunohistochemical markers, and so it is likely that when this patterning event is altered, anomalies occur.

Abnormal Origin and Course of Coronary Arteries Numerous variations in the architecture and course of the coronary arteries occur in association with structural cardiovascular malformations. For example, an anomalous origin of the left anterior descending coronary artery from the right coronary artery occurs in association with tetralogy of Fallot. Unfortunately, the mechanisms for these associations have not been defined.

Coronary Arterial Fistulas Coronary arterial fistulas occasionally occur in isolation and also occur in association with pulmonary valve atresia with an intact ventricular septum. The mechanics responsible for these anomalies are unknown.

CONDUCTION SYSTEM DEVELOPMENT

The development of the conduction system has fascinated cardiovascular embryologists from the moment it became clear that a subpopulation of specialized myocytes is responsible for the regulation of the cardiac impulse in the heart.[161] During the last decade, several studies have revealed new aspects regarding the development of the conduction system. Immunohistochemical studies have shown that the developing conduction system in humans and other vertebrates is characterized by the expression of a unique set of antigens and genes, some of which also are expressed in the nervous system, sometimes referred to as neuromuscular markers (Fig. 9-14).[125,162,163] Retroviral cell-targeting and -tracing methods have defined subpopulations of cardiomyocytes that differentiate into Purkinje's cells within the trabecular myocardium.[125,164,165] Altered patterns of ventricular depolarization have been recognized in association with structural heart defects, such as the pattern of depolarization noted with endocardial cushion defects, and conduction abnormalities associated with atrial septum defects, as has been observed in patients with mutations in the *Nkx2.5* and *TBX5* (Holt Oram syndrome) genes.[166]

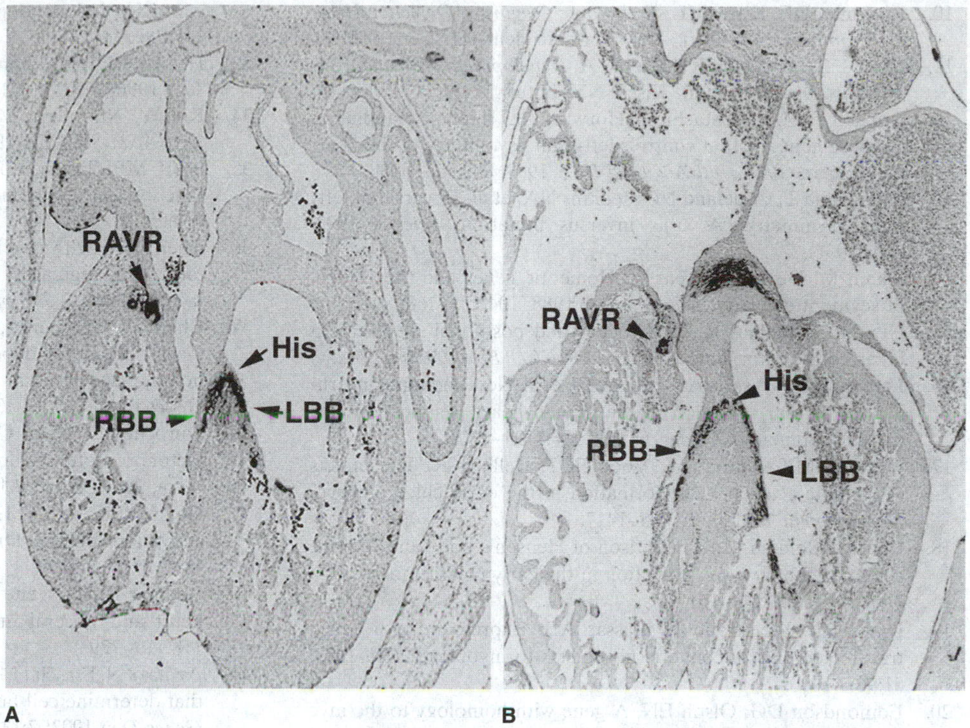

FIGURE 9-14 Expression of neuromuscular markers in the developing vertebrate heart. Panel *A* shows a transverse section of a human heart at 6 weeks of development immunohistochemically stained for the presence of a carbohydrate moiety recognized by the monoclonal antibody GIN2 (see also Wessels et al.[125]). The section shown in panel *B* is from a rabbit embryo at 15 days of development and is immunohistochemically stained for the presence of neurofilaments (Wessels et al.[139]). RAVR = right atrioventricular ring bundle; His = bundle of His; LBB = left bundle branch; RBB = right bundle branch.

CARDIOVASCULAR INNERVATION

Despite numerous descriptive studies regarding the location of cardiac ganglia, little is known regarding the immunohistochemical cues required for the patterning of myocardial innervation. NC cell migration is critical for this process, as NC cells serve as precursors for the cardiac nerves and ganglia.[85] Cardiac ganglia and nerves are present in the 7-week gestation human embryo.[167] The density of cardiac innervation exhibits a gradient of decreasing density from the atrium to the ventricle. It is interesting to note that functional adrenergic receptors are present on the embryonic heart before histologic evidence of autonomic nerves.[168] The differential appearance and distribution of peptide-containing nerves indicate that there is a maturational order to the autonomic and sensory components of the developing human heart.[167]

FUNCTIONAL MATURATION OF THE EMBRYONIC HEART

Obviously, cardiovascular morphogenesis is influenced directly by the dynamic mechanical environment of the pulsatile embryonic heart. An overview of functional maturation, while critical, is beyond the scope of this chapter. The reader is referred to reviews of embryonic functional maturation in vertebrate and invertebrate species.[167,170]

References

1. Von Haller A. *Sur la formation du coeur dans le poulet.* Lausanne, 1758.
2. Neill CA, Clark EB. Tetralogy of Fallot: The first 300 years. *Tex Heart Inst J* 1994; 21:272–279.
3. Anderson RH. Simplifying the understanding of congenital malformations of the heart. *Int J Cardiol* 1991; 32:131–142.
4. Van Mierop LHS. Morphological development of the heart. In: Berne RM, ed. *Handbook of Physiology*, section 2, vol. I. Bethesda, MD: American Physiological Society; 1979:1.
5. Clark EB, Van Mierop LHS. Cardiac development. In: Adams FH, Emmanoulides GC, Riemenschneider TA, eds. *Heart Disease in Infants, Children, and Adolescents*, 4th ed. Baltimore: Williams & Wilkins; 1989:1.
6. Wenick ACG. Embryology of the heart. In: Anderson RH, Macartney FJ, Shinebourne EA, Tynan M, eds. *Pediatric Cardiology*, vol. 1. New York: Churchill Livingstone; 1987:83.
7. Ferrens VJ, Rosenquist GC, Weinstein C. *Cardiac Morphogenesis.* New York: Elsevier; 1985.
8. Nora JJ, Takao A. *Congenital Heart Disease: Causes and Processes.* Mount Kisco, NY: Futura; 1984.
9. Clark EB, Takao A. *Developmental Cardiology: Morphogenesis and Function.* Mount Kisco, NY: Futura; 1990.

10. Bockman DE, Kirby ML. *Embryonic Origins of Defective Heart Development.* New York: New York Academy of Sciences; 1990.
11. Clark EB, Markwald RR, Takao A. *Developmental Mechanisms of Heart Disease.* Mount Kisco, NY: Futura; 1995.
12. Brueckner M, D'Eustachio P, Horwich AL. Linkage mapping of a mouse gene, iv, that controls left-right asymmetry of the heart and viscera. *Proc Natl Acad Sci USA* 1989; 86:5035–5038.
13. Yokoyama T, Copeland NG, Jenkins NA, et al. Reversal of left-right asymmetry: A situs inversus mutation. *Science* 1993; 260:679–682.
14. Akam M, Dawson I, Tear G. Homeotic genes and the control of segment diversity. *Development* 1988; 104:123–168.
15. Hunt P. Krumlauf R. HOX codes and positional specification invertebrate embryonic axes. *Annu Rev Cell Biol* 1992; 8:227–256.
16. Lamers WH, Wessels A, Verbeek FJ, et al. New findings concerning ventricular septation in the human heart: Implications for maldevelopment. *Circulation* 1992; 86:1194–1205.
17. Osmond MK, Butler AJ, Voon FCT, Bellairs R. The effects of retinoic acid on heart formation in the early chick embryo. *Development* 1991; 113:1405–1417.
18. Chen Y, Solursh M. Comparison of Hensen's node and retinoic acid in secondary axis induction in the early chick embryo. *Dev Dyn* 1992; 195:142–151.
19. Davis RL, Weintraub H, Lassar AB. Expression of a single transfected cDNA converts fibroblasts to myoblasts. *Cell* 1987; 51:987–1000.
20. Edmondson DG, Olson EN. A gene with homology to the myc similarity region of MyoD1 is expressed during myogenesis and is sufficient to activate the muscle differentiation program. *Genes Dev* 1989; 3:628–640.
21. Wright WE, Sassoon DA, Lin VK. Myogenin, a factor regulating myogenesis, has a domain homologous to Myo D. *Cell* 1989; 56:607–617.
22. Braun T, Buschhausen-Denker G, Bober E, et al. A novel human muscle factor related to but distinct from MyoD1 induces myogenic conversion in 10T1/2 fibroblasts. *EMBO* J 1989; 8:701–709.
23. Rhodes SJ, Konieczny SF. Identification of MRF4: A new member of the muscle regulatory factor gene family. *Genes Dev* 1989; 3:2050–2061.
24. Miner JH, Wold B. Herculin, a fourth member of the MyoD family of myogenic regulatory genes. *Proc Natl Acad Sci USA* 1990; 87:1089–1093.
25. Braun T, Bober E. Winter B, et al. Myf-6, a new member of the human gene family of myogenic determination factors: Evidence for a gene cluster on chromosome 12. *EMBO J* 1990; 9:821–831.
26. Murre C, McCaw PS, Baltimore D. A new DNA binding and dimerization motif in immunoglobulin enhancer binding, daughterless, MyoD, and myc proteins. *Cell* 1989; 56:777–783.
27. Sasson D, Lyons G, Wright WE, et al. Expression of two myogenic regulatory factors myogenin and MyoD1 during mouse embryogenesis. *Nature* 1989; 41:303–307.
28. Srivastava D. Segmental regulation of cardiac development by the basic Helix-Loop-Helix transcription factors dHAND and eHAND. In: Harvey RP, Rosenthal N, eds. *Heart Development.* San Diego: Academic Press; 1999:143.
29. Srivastava D, Thomas T, Lin Q, et al. Regulation of cardiac mesodermal and neural crest development by the bHLH transcription factor, dHAND. *Nat Genet* 1997; 16:154–160.
30. Riley P, Anson-Cartwright L, Cross JC. The Hand1 bHLH transcription factor is essential for placentation and cardiac morphogenesis. *Nat Genet* 1998; 18:271–275.
31. Lin Q, Schwarz J, Bucana C, Olson EN. Control of mouse cardiac morphogenesis and myogenesis by transcription factor MEF2C. *Science* 1997; 276:1404–1407.
32. Thomas T, Yamagishi H, Overbeek PA, et al. The bHLH factors, dHAND and eHAND, specify pulmonary and systemic cardiac ventricles independent of left-right sidedness. *Dev Biol* 1998; 15; 196:228–236.
33. Harvey RP. NK-2 homeobox genes and heart development. *Dev Biol* 1996; 178:203–216.
34. Kim Y, Nirenberg M. Drosophila NK-homeobox genes. *Proc Natl Acad Sci USA* 1989; 86:7716–7720.
35. Scott MP, Tamkun JW, Hertzell GW III. The structure and function of the homeodomain. *Biochem Biophys Acta* 1989; 989:25–48.
36. Chen CY, Schwartz RJ. Identification of novel DNA binding targets and regulatory domains of a murine tinman homeodomain factor, Nkx-2.5. *J Biol Chem* 1995; 270:15,628–15,633.
37. Chen CY, Croissant J, Majesky M, et al. Activation of the cardiac a-actin promoter depends upon serum response factor, tinman homologue, Nkx-2.5, and intact serum response elements. *Dev Genet* 1996; 19:119–130.
38. Durocher D, Chen CY, Ardati A, et al. The atrial natriuretic factor promoter is a downstream target for Nkx-2.5 in the myocardium. *Mol Cell Biol* 1996; 16:4648–4655.
39. Gajewski K, Kim Y, Lee YM, et al. D-mef2 is a target for tinman activation during Drosophila heart development. *EMBO J* 1997; 16:515–522.
40. Bodmer R. The gene tinman is required for specification of the heart and visceral muscles in Drosophila. *Development* 1993; 118:719–729.
41. Azpiazu N, Frasch H. Tinman and bagpipe: Two homeobox genes that determine cell fates in the dorsal mesoderm of Drosophila. *Genes Dev* 1993; 7:1325–1340.
42. Lints TJ, Parsons LM, Hartley L, et al. Nkx-2.5: A novel murine homeobox gene expressed in early heart progenitor cells and their myogenic descendants. *Development* 1993; 119:419–431.
43. Komuro I, Izumo S. Csx: A murine homeobox-containing gene specifically expressed in the developing heart. *Proc Natl Acad Sci USA* 1993; 90:8145–8149.
44. Chen JN, Fishman MC. Zebrafish tinman homolog demarcates the heart field and initiates myocardial differentiation. *Development* 1996; 122:3809–3816.
45. Tonissen KF, Drysdale TA, Lints TJ, et al. XNkx-2.5, a Xenopus gene related to Nkx-2.5 and tinman: Evidence for a conserved role in cardiac development. *Dev Biol* 1994; 162:325–328.
46. Schwartz RJ, Olson EN. Building the heart piece by piece: Modularity of cis-elements regulating Nkx2-5 transcription. *Development* 1999; 126:4187–4192.
47. Reecy JM, Yamada M, Cummings K, et al. Chicken Nkx-2.8: A novel homeobox gene expressed in early heart progenitor cells and pharyngeal pouch-2 and -3 endoderm. *Dev Biol* 1997; 188:295–311.
48. Lyons I, Parsons LM, Hartley L, et al. Myogenic and morphogenetic defects in the heart tubes of murine embryos lacking the homeobox gene Nkx2-5. *Genes Dev* 1995; 9:1654–1666.
49. Schott JJ, Benson DW, Basson CT, et al. Congenital heart disease caused by mutations in the transcription factor NKX2-5. *Science* 1998; 281:108–111.
50. Kuo H, Chen J, Ruiz-Lozano P, et al. Control of segmental expression of the cardiac-restricted ankyrin repeat protein gene by distinct regulatory pathways in murine cardiogenesis. *Development* 1999; 126:4223–4234.
51. Teisman R. Identification of a protein-binding site that mediates transcription response of the c-fos gene to serum factors. *Cell* 1986; 46:567–574.
52. Croissant JD, Kim JH, Eichele G, et al. Avian serum response factor expression restricted primarily to muscle cell lineages is required for a-actin gene transcription. *Dev Biol* 1996; 177: 250–264.
53. Dalton S, Treisman R. Characterization of SAP-1, a protein recruited by serum response factor to the c-fos serum response element. *Cell* 1992; 68:597–612.

54. Pollock R, Treisman R. Human SRF-related proteins: DNA-binding properties and potential regulatory targets. *Genes Dev* 1991; 5:2327–2341.
55. Gossett LA, Kelvin DJ, Sternberg EA, Olson EN. A new myocyte-specific enhancer-binding factor that recognizes a conserved element associated with multiple muscle-specific genes. *Mol Cell Biol* 1989; 9:5022–5033.
56. Bour BA, O'Brien MA, Lockwood ML, et al. Drosophila MEF2, a transcription factor, is essential for myogenesis. *Genes Dev* 1995; 9:730–741.
57. Lilly B, Zhao B, Ranganayakulu G, et al. Requirement of MADS domain transcription factor D-MEF2 for muscle formation in Drosophila. *Science* 1995; 267:688–693.
58. Edmondson DG, Lyons GE, Martin JF, Olson EN. Mef-2 gene expression marks the cardiac and skeletal muscle lineages during mouse myogenesis. *Genes Dev* 1994; 120:1251–1263.
59. Yu Y-T, Breitbart RE, Smoot LB, et al. Human myocyte-specific enhancer factor 2 comprises a group of tissue restricted MADS box transcription factors. *Genes Dev* 1992; 6:1783–1798.
60. Chien KR, Zhu H, Knowlton KU, et al. Transcriptional regulation during cardiac growth and development. *Annu Rev Physiol* 1993; 55:77–95.
61. Breitbart RE, Liang C, Smott LB, et al. A fourth human MEF-2 transcription factor, hMEF-2d, is an early marker of the myogenic lineage. *Development* 1993; 118:1095–1106.
62. Martin JF, Miano JM, Hustad CM, et al. A Mef2 gene that generates a muscle-specific isoform via alternative mRNA splicing. *Mol Cell Biol* 1994; 14:1647–1656.
63. Grueneberg DA, Natesan S, Alexandre C, Gilman MZ. Human and Drosophila homeodomain proteins that enhance the DNA-binding activity of serum response factor. *Science* 1992; 257:1089–1095.
64. Grueneberg DA, Simon KJ, Brennan K, Gilman M. Sequence-specific targeting of nuclear signal transduction pathways by homeodomain proteins. *Mol Cell Biol* 1995; 15:3318–3326.
65. Opsltsein D, Vogels JE, Robert B, et al. The mouse homeobox gene, S8, is expressed during embryogenesis predominantly in mesenchyme. *Mech Dev* 1991; 34:29–42.
66. Cserjesi P, Lilly B, Bryson L, et al. MHox: A mesodermally-restricted homeodomain protein that binds an essential site in the muscle creatine kinase enhancer. *Development* 1992; 115: 1087–1101.
67. Chen CY, Schwartz RJ. Recruitment of the tinman homolog Nkx-2.5 by serum response factor activates cardiac a-actin gene transcription. *Mol Cell Biol* 1996; 16:6372–6384.
68. Charron F, Nemer M. GATA transcription factors and cardiac development. *Semin Cell Dev Biol* 1999; 10:85–91.
69. Laverriere AC, MacNeill C, Mueller C, et al. GATA4/5/6, a subfamily of three transcription factors transcribed in developing heart and gut. *J Biol Chem* 1994; 269:23,177–23,184.
70. Morrisey EE, Ip HH, Lu MM, Parmacek MS. GATA-6: A zinc finger transcription factor that is expressed in multiple cell lineages derived from lateral mesoderm. *Dev Biol* 1996; 177: 309–322.
71. Ip HS, Wilson DB, Heikinheimo M, et al. The GATA-4 transcription factor transactivates the cardiac muscle specific troponin C promoter-enhancer in nonmuscle cells. *Mol Cell Biol* 1994; 14:7515–7526.
72. Mokentin JD, Lin Q, Duncan S, Olson EN. Requirement of the transcription factor GATA4 for heart tube formation and ventral morphogenesis. *Genes Dev* 1997; 11:1061–1072.
73. Zhang HB, Bradley A. Mice deficient for BMP2 are nonviable and have defects in amnion/chorion and cardiac development. *Development* 1996; 122:2977–2986.
74. Morgan MJ. The asymmetrical genetic determination of laterality: Flatfish, frogs and human handedness. In: *Biological Asymmetry and Handedness*. Wiley Chichester Ciba Foundation Symposium 162, 1991:234.
75. Schneider A, Mijalski T, Schlange T, et al. The homeobox gene NKX3.2 is a target of left-right signaling and is expressed on opposite sides in chick and mouse embryos. *Curr Biol* 1999; 9:911–914.
76. Layton WM. Random determination of developmental process: Reversal of normal visceral asymmetry in the mouse. *J Hered* 1976; 67:336–338.
77. Yokoyama T, Copeland NG, Jenkins NA, et al. Reversal of left-right asymmetry: A situs inversus mutation. *Science* 1993; 260:679–682.
78. Morgan D, Turnpenny L, Goodship J, et al. Inversin, a novel gene in the vertebrate left-right axis pathway, is partially deleted in the inv mouse. *Nat Genet* 1998; 20:149–156.
79. Mikawa T, Borisov A, Brown AM, Fischman DA. Clonal analysis of cardiac morphogenesis in the chicken embryo using a replication-defective retrovirus: I. Formation of the ventricular myocardium. *Dev Dyn* 1992; 193:11–23.
80. Mikawa T, Cohen-Gould L, Fischman DA. Clonal analysis of cardiac morphogenesis in the chicken embryo using a replication-defective retrovirus: III. Polyclonal origin of adjacent ventricular myocytes. *Dev Dyn* 1992; 195:133–141.
81. Linask KK. N-Cadherin localization in early heart development and polar expression of Na^+, K^+-ATPase, and integrin during pericardial coelom formation and epithelialization of the differentiating myocardium. *Dev Biol* 1992; 151:213–224.
82. Parlow MH, Bolender DL, Kokan-Moore NP, Lough J. Localization of bFGF-like proteins as punctate inclusions in the preseptation myocardium of the chicken embryo. *Dev Biol* 1991; 146:139–147.
83. Lyons KM, Jones CM, Hogan BL. The TGF-beta-related DVR gene family in mammalian development. *Ciba Found Symp* 1992; 165:219–230.
84. Sugi Y, Sasse J, Lough J. Inhibition of precardiac mesoderm cell proliferation by antisense oligodeoxynucleotide complementary to fibroblast growth factor-2 (FGF-2). *Dev Biol* 1993; 157:28–37.
85. Kirby ML, Waldo KL. Role of neural crest in congenital heart disease. *Circulation* 1990; 82:332–340.
86. Chisaka O, Capecchi MR. Regionally restricted developmental defects resulting from targeted disruption of the mouse homeobox gene Hox-1.5. *Nature* 1991; 350:473–474.
87. Conway SJ, Godt RE, Hatcher CJ, et al. Neural crest is involved in development of abnormal myocardial function. *J Mol Cell Cardiol* 1997; 29:2675–2685.
88. Epstein JA. PAX3, neural crest and cardiovascular development. *Trends Cardiovasc Med* 1996; 6:255–261.
89. Kirby ML. Contribution of neural crest to heart and vessel morphology. In: Harvey RP, Rosenthal N, eds. *Heart Development.* San Diego: Academic Press; 1999:179.
90. Lammer EJ, Opitz JM. The DiGeorge anomaly as a developmental field defect. *Am J Med Genet Suppl* 1986; 2:113–127.
91. Wilson DI, Cross IE, Goodship JA, et al. DiGeorge syndrome with isolated aortic coarctation and isolated ventricular septal defect in three sibs with a 22q11 deletion of maternal origin. *Br Heart J* 1991; 66:308–312.
92. Scambler PJ, Kelly D, Lindsay E, et al. Velo-cardio-facial syndrome associated with chromosome 22 deletions encompassing the DiGeorge locus. *Lancet* 1992; 339:1138–1139.
93. Driscoll DA, Budarf ML, Emanuel BS. A genetic etiology for DiGeorge syndrome: Consistent deletions and microdeletions of 22q11. *Am J Hum Genet* 1992; 50:924–933.
94. Lammer EJ, Chen DT, Hoar R, et al. Retinoic acid embryopathy *N Engl J Med* 1985; 313:837–841.
95. Clark EB, Hu N, Dummett JL, et al. Ventricular function and morphology in the chick embryo stage 18 to 29. *Am J Physiol* 1986; 250:H407–H413.

96. Taber LA, Keller BB, Clark EB. Cardiac mechanics in the stage 16 chick embryo. *J Biomech Eng* 1992; 114:427–434.
97. Ruzicka DL, Schwartz RJ. Sequential activation of alpha actin genes during avian cardiogenesis: Vascular smooth muscle alpha actin gene transcripts mark the onset of cardiomyocyte differentiation. *J Cell Biol* 1988; 107:2575–2586.
98. Sugi Y, Lough J. Onset of expression and regional deposition of alpha-smooth and sarcomeric actin during avian heart development. *Dev Dyn* 1992; 193:116–124.
99. Sordahl LA, Crow CA, Draft GH, Schwartz A. Some ultrastructural and biochemical aspects of heart mitochondria associated with development. *J Mol Cell Cardiol* 1972; 4:1–10.
100. Barth E, Stammler G, Speiser B, Schaper J. Ultrastructural quantitation of mitochondria and myofilaments in cardiac muscle from 10 different animal species including man. *J Mol Cell Cardiol* 1992; 24:669–681.
101. Mahony L. Cardiac membrane structure and function. In: Burggren WW, Keller BB, eds. *Development of Cardiovascular Systems: Molecules to Organisms*. New York: Cambridge University Press; 1997:18.
102. Bernard C. Establishment of ionic permeabilities of the myocardial membrane during embryonic development of the rat. In: Lieberman M, Sano T, eds. *Development and Physiological Correlates of Cardiac Muscle*. New York: Raven Press; 1975:169.
103. Rosen MR, Danilo PJ. Developmental electrophysiology of the heart. In: Polin RA, Fox WW, eds. *Fetal and Neonatal Physiology*. Philadelphia: Saunders; 1992:656.
104. Osaka T, Joyner RW. Developmental changes in calcium currents of rabbit ventricular cells. *Circ Res* 1991; 68:788–796.
105. Wetzel GT, Chen F, Klitzner TS. Ca^{2+} channel kinetics in acute isolated fetal, neonatal and adult rabbit cardiac myocytes. *Circ Res* 1993; 72:1065–1074.
106. Bridge JHB, Smolley JR, Spitzer KW. The relationship between charge movements associated with I_{ca} and $I_{Na\text{-}Ca}$ in cardiac myocytes. *Science* 1990; 248:376–378.
107. Davis CL. Description of a human embryo having 20 paired somites. *Contrib Embryol* 1923; 15:1–52.
108. Davis CL. The cardiac jelly of the chick embryo. *Anat Rec* 1924; 27:201–202.
109. Van Mierop LHS. Embryology of the heart. In: Netter FH, ed. *The CIBA Collection of Medical Illustrations*, vol 5, part 1. Summit, NJ: CIBA; 1969:112.
110. Markwald RR, Trusk T, Gittenberger-de Groot AC, Poelman R. Cardiac morphogenesis: Formation and septation of the primary heart tube. In: Kavlock R, Datson G, eds. *Handbook of Experimental Pharmacology*. Vol 124. Berlin: Springer Verlag; 1998:11.
111. Drake CJ, Davis LA, Walters L, Little CD. Avian vasculogenesis and the distribution of collagens I, IV, laminin and fibronectin in the heart primordia. *J Exp Zool* 1990; 255:309–322.
112. Markwald RR, Mjaatvedt CH, Krug EL. Induction of endocardial cushion tissue formation by adheron-like molecular complexes derived from the myocardial basement membrane. In: Clark EB, Takao A, eds. *Developmental Cardiology: Morphogenesis and Function*. Mount Kisco, NY: Futura; 1990:191.
113. Lyons KM, Jones CM, Hogan BLM. The TGF-β-related DVR gene family in mammalian development. In: *Postimplantation Development in The mouse*. Ciba Foundation Symposium 165. Chichester, UK: Wiley; 1992:219.
114. Runyan RB, Potts JD, Sharma RV, et al. Signal transduction of a tissue interaction during embryonic heart development. *Cell Regul* 1990; 1:301–313.
115. Chin C, Gandour-Edwards R, Oltjen S, Choy M. Fate of the atrioventricular endocardial cushions in the developing chick heart. *Pediatr Res* 1992; 32:390–393.
116. Garcia-Martinez V, Sanchez-Quintana D, Hurle JM. Histogenesis of the semilunar valves: An immunohistochemical analysis of tenascin and type-I collagen distribution in developing chick heart valves. *Cell Tissue Res* 1990; 259:299–304.
117. Potts JD, Vincent EB, Runyan RB, Weeks DL. Sense and antisense TGF beta 3 mRNA levels correlate with cardiac valve induction. *Dev Dyn* 1992; 193:340–345.
118. Pexieder T. Prenatal development of the endocardium: A review. *SEM* 1981; 2:223–253.
119. Noden DM. Origins and patterning of avian outflow tract endocardium. *Development* 1991; 111:867–876.
120. Markwald RR, Mjaatvedt CH, Krug EL, Sinning AR. Inductive interaction in heart development: Role of cardiac adherons in cushion tissue formation. In: Bockman DE, Kirby ML, eds. *Embryonic Origins of Defective Heart Development. Ann NY Acad Sci* 1990; 588:13–25.
121. Icardo JM, Hurle JM, Ojeda JL. Endocardial cell polarity during the looping of the heart in the chick embryo. *Dev Biol* 1982; 90:203–209.
122. Pexieder T. Cell death in the morphogenesis and teratogenesis of the heart. *Adv Anat Embryol Cell Biol* 1975; 51:1–100.
123. Dzau VJ, Krieger JE. Molecular biology of hypertension. In: Roberts R, ed. *Molecular Basis of Cardiology*. Boston: Blackwell; 1993:325.
124. Taber LA, Lin IE, Clark EB. Mechanics of cardiac looping. *Dev Dyn* 1995; 203:42–50.
125. Wessels A, Vermeulen JLM, Verbeek FJ, et al. Spatial distribution of "tissue-specific" antigens in the developing human heart and skeletal muscle: III. An immunohistochemical analysis of the distribution of the neural tissue antigen GIN2 in the embryonic heart: Implications for the development of the atrioventricular conduction system. *Anat Rec* 1992; 232:97–111.
126. Wessels A, Mijnders TA, de Gier-de Vries C, et al. Expression of myosin heavy chain in neonatal human hearts. *Cardiol Young* 1992; 2:318–334.
127. Gittenberger-de Groot A. Principles of abnormal cardiac development. In. Burggren WW, Keller BB, eds. *Development of Cardiovascular Systems: Molecules to Organisms*. New York: Cambridge University Press; 1996:259.
128. Icardo JM, Fernandez-Teran A. Morphologic study of ventricular trabeculation in the embryonic chick heart. *Acta Anat* (*Basel*) 1987; 130:264–274.
129. Pexieder T, Christen Y, Vuillemin M, Patterson DR. Comparative morphometric analysis of cardiac organogenesis in chick, mouse, and dog embryos. In: Nora JJ, Takao A, eds. *Congenital Heart Disease: Causes and Processes*. Mount Kisco, NY: Futura; 1984:423.
130. Taber LA, Hu N, Pexieder T, et al. Residual strain in the ventricle of the stage 16-24 chick embryo. *Circ Res* 1993; 72:455–462.
131. Thompson RP, Lindroth JR, Wong YMM. Regional differences in DNA-synthetic activity in the preseptation myocardium of the chick. In: Clark EB, Takao A, eds. *Developmental Cardiology: Morphogenesis and Function*. Mount Kisco, NY: Futura; 1990:219.
132. Streeter GL. Developmental horizons in human embryos: Description of age groups XI, 13-20 somites, and age group XII, 21-29 somites. *Contrib Embryol* 1942; 30:211–246.
133. Van Mierop LHS, Alley RD, Kausel HW, Stranahan A. The anatomy and embryology of endocardial cushion defects. *J Thorac Cardiovasc Surg* 1962; 43:71–83.
134. Chin TK, Perloff JK, Williams RG, et al. Isolated noncompaction of left ventricular myocardium: A study of eight cases. *Circulation* 1990; 82:507–513.
135. Agmon Y, Connolly HM, Olson LJ, et al. Noncompaction of the ventricular myocardium. *J Am Soc Echocardiogr* 1999; 12:859–863.
136. Ichida F, Hamamichi Y, Miyawaki T, et al. Clinical features of isolated noncompaction of the ventricular myocardium: Long-

term clinical course, hemodynamic properties, and genetic background. *J Am Coll Cardiol* 1999; 34:233–240.

137. Pauli RM, Scheib-Wixted S, Cripe L, et al. Ventricular noncompaction and distal chromosome 5q deletion. *Am J Med Genet* 1999; 85:419–423.
138. Pexieder T, Christen Y. Quantitative analysis of the shape development in the chick embryo heart. In: Pexieder T, ed. *Mechanisms of Cardiac Morphogenesis and Teratogenesis*. New York: Raven Press; 1981:49.
139. Wessels A, Anderson RH, Markwald RR, et al. Atrial development in the human heart: An immunohistochemical study with emphasis on the role of mesenchymal tissues. *Anat Rec*, in press.
140. Seo JW, Kim AEK, Brown NA, Wessels A. Section directed cryosectioning of specimens for scanning electron microscopy: A new method to study cardiac development. *Micr Res Techn* 1995; 30:491–495.
141. Neill CA: Development of the pulmonary veins. *Pediatrics* 1956; 18:880–887.
142. Van den Hoff MJB, Bennington RW, Moorman AFM, et al. Myocardialization in the developing heart. *Dev Biol* 1999; 212:477–490.
143. Van Mierop LHS, Alley RD, Kausel HW, Stranahan A. Pathogenesis of transposition complexes: I. Embryology of the ventricles and great arteries. *Am J Cardiol* 1963; 12:216–225.
144. Sedmera D, Pexieder T, Hu N, Clark EB. Developmental changes in the myocardial architecture of the chick. *Anat Rec* 1997; 248:421–432.
145. Streeter GL. Developmental horizons in human embryos: Description of age groups XV, XVI, XVII, XVIII, being the third issue of a survey of the Carnegie Collection. *Contrib Embryol* 1948; 32:133–204.
146. Pexieder T. Conotruncus and its septation at the advent of the molecular biology era. In: Clark EB, Markwald RR, Takao A, eds. *Developmental Mechanisms of Heart Disease*. Mount Kisco, NY: Futura; 1995:227.
147. Dor X, Corone P. Embryologie cardiaque: Malformations (I). In: *Embryologie Cardiaque—Editions Techniques—Encyclopedie Medico-Chirurgicale*. Paris: 11001 C[30], 1992:1–20.
148. Wessels A, Markman MWM, Vermeulen JLM, et al. The development of the atrioventricular junction in the human heart: An immunohistochemical study. *Circ Res* 1996; 78:110–117.
149. Lamers WH, Wessels A, Moorman AFM, et al. Formation of the tricuspid valve in the human heart. *Circulation* 1995; 91:111–121.
150. Bergwerff M, Verberne ME, DeRuiter MC, et al. Neural crest cell contribution to the developing circulatory system: Implications for vascular morphology? *Circ Res* 1998; 82:221–231.
151. Poelman RE, Gittenberger-de Groot AC, Metlink MMT, et al. Development of the cardiac/coronary vascular endothelium, studied with antiendothelial antibodies, in chicken-quail chimeras. *Circ Res* 1993; 73:559–568.
152. Perez-Pomares JM, Macias D, Garcia-Garrido L, Munoz-Chapuli R. Contribution of the primitive epicardium to the subepicardial mesenchyme. *Dev Dyn* 1997; 210:96–105.
153. Perez-Pomares JM, Macias D, Garcia-Garrido L, Munoz-Chapuli R. The origin of the subepicardial mesenchyme in the avian embryo: An immunohistochemical and quail-chick chimera study. *Dev Biol* 1998; 200:57–68.
154. Dettman RW, Denetclaw W Jr, Ordahl CP, Bristow J. Common epicardial origin of coronary vascular smooth muscle, perivascular. *Dev Bio* 1998; 193:169–181.
155. Gittenberger-de Groot AC, Vrancken Peeters MP, Mentink MM, et al. Epicardium-derived cells contribute a novel population to the myocardial. *Circ Res* 1998; 82:43–52.
156. Hood LC, Rosenquist TH. Coronary artery development in the chick: Origin and deployment of smooth muscle cells, and the effects of neural crest ablation. *Anat Rec* 1992; 234:291–300.
157. Rosenquist TH, Modis L. Spatial disorder of collagens in the great vessels, associated with congenital heart defects. *Anat Rec* 1991; 229:116–124.
158. Risau W. Vasculogenesis, angiogenesis and endothelial cell differentiation during embryonic development. In: Feinberg RN, Sherer GK, Auerbach R, eds. *The Development of the Vascular System*, Vol 14. Basel: Karger; 1991:1:58.
159. Rakusan K, Flanagan MF, Geva T, et al. Morphometry of human coronary capillaries during normal growth and the effect of age in left ventricular pressure-overload hypertrophy. *Circulation* 1992; 86:38–46.
160. Tomanek RJ, Phan BP, Hu N, Clark EB. Myocardial vascularization is accelerated in chick embryos with increased afterload and ventricular mass (abstract). *FASEB J* 1996; 10:A579.
161. Anderson RH, Becker AE, Wenink ACG. The development of the conducting tissues. In: Roberts EA, ed. *Cardiac Arrhythmias in the Neonate, Infant and Child*. New York: Appleton-Century-Crofts; 1978.
162. Gorza L, Vitadello M. Distribution of conduction system fibers in the developing and adult rabbit heart revealed by an antineurofilament antibody. *Circ Res* 1989; 65:360–369.
163. Ikeda T, Iwasaki K, Shimokawa I, et al. Leu-7 immunoreactivity in human and rat embryonic hearts, with special reference to the development of the conduction tissue. *Anat Embryol* 1990; 182:553–562.
164. Wessels A, Vermeulen JLM, Verbeek FJ, et al. Spatial distribution of "tissue-specific" antigens in the developing human heart and skeletal muscle: III. An immunohistochemical analysis of the distribution of the neural tissue antigen GlN2 in the embryonic heart: Implications for the development of the atrioventricular conduction system. *Anat Rec* 1992; 231:97–111.
165. Gourdie RG, Mima T, Thompson RP, Mikawa T. Terminal diversification of the myocyte lineage generates Purkinje fibers of the cardiac conduction system. *Development* 1995; 121:1423–1431.
166. Li QY, Newbury-Ecob RA, Terrett JA, et al. Holt-Oram syndrome is caused by mutations in TBX5, a member of the Brachyury (T) gene family. *Nat Genet* 1997; 15:21–29.
167. Gordon L, Polak JM, Moscoso GJ, et al. Development of the peptidergic innervation of human heart. *J Anat* 1993; 183: 131–140.
168. St Petery LB, Van Mierop LHS. Evidence for the presence of adrenergic receptors in 3-day-old chick embryo. *Am J Physiol* 1977; 232:H250–H254.
169. Keller BB. Functional maturation and coupling of the embryonic cardiovascular system. In: Clark EB, Markwald PR, and Takao A, eds. *Developmental Mechanisms of Heart Disease*. Mount Kisco, NY: Futura; 1995:367.
170. Keller BB. Embryonic cardiovascular function, coupling, and maturation: A species view. In: Burggren W, Keller BB, eds. *Development of Cardiovascular Systems: Molecules to Organisms*. New York; Cambridge University Press; 1996:65.

PART TWO

GENERAL EVALUATION OF THE PATIENT

CHAPTER 10

THE HISTORY, PHYSICAL EXAMINATION, AND CARDIAC AUSCULTATION

Robert A. O'Rourke / James A. Shaver / Mark E. Silverman

In the assessment of patients with definite or suspected heart disease, relevant information can be acquired from the history, physical examination, chest roentgenogram, electrocardiogram, and other routine laboratory tests. These data, when integrated properly, result in an accurate diagnosis and appropriate decisions regarding therapy in many patients. In other patients, more information is necessary, and additional, more technical, and usually more expensive noninvasive cardiac tests such as echocardiography or radionuclide studies are needed. In some patients, the general assessment indicates the need for cardiac catheterization and contrast angiography, with or without additional noninvasive cardiac testing. For example, the proper approach to certain patients with symptomatic coronary artery disease may include both coronary arteriography and cardiac catheterization (anatomy and hemodynamics), as well as myocardial perfusion imaging with thallium or technetium sestamibi (extent of inducible ischemia).

Not all patients need every test, and the skillful use of low-technology approaches, including the history and general examination, may preclude the need for additional studies or may determine which of a wide variety of available sophisticated tests should be chosen for a particular patient. This chapter is divided into three sections. The first section concerns the proper application of the history and its use to delineate the differential diagnosis in patients who present with certain common cardiovascular symptoms. The second section details the essential components of the *physical examination* and their usefulness in establishing a likely diagnosis when specific abnormal findings are detected. Finally, the third section focuses on cardiac auscultation.

THE HISTORY

Elements of Accurate History Taking

A carefully obtained history is the cornerstone in the evaluation of a patient with known or suspected cardiac disease.[1,2] A deliberate, compassionate interview forms the basis for a patient-physician relationship that may continue for days, months, or years. Unfortunately, the interview may result in adversary roles for physician and patient if the interviewer appears hurried, demands exact answers, shows impatience, insists on exploring areas that are uncomfortable to the patient, fails to establish eye contact, accepts multiple interruptions during the discussion, seems to treat dreaded diseases casually, gives nonverbal signs of personal unhappiness, or appears to be unsympathetic.[2] When the medical interview is unsatisfactory due to poor communication and lack of rapport, inaccurate information often will be obtained.[2] Also, important facts not revealed during a meticulous initial history usually are not detected later as workup progresses and the patient and physician become focused on high-technology studies and more aggressive therapeutic interventions.[1]

The patient's chief complaint, which requires further elaboration and investigation, may not identify the patient's most serious problem. Symptoms other than the patient's chief complaint must be defined.[2] Rather than focusing entirely on the patient's present illness, the interviewer should note all existing symptoms and establish a present illness for each of these.[2]

A medical questionnaire given to the patient well in advance of the interview is useful. The patient can then record important data more accurately because of the time available for reflection and the checking of details.[2] Any abnormalities indicated on the questionnaire must be defined more completely during the interview, and related areas should be discussed.[2]

A proper interpretation of the past history is important, and the physician should not accept a past event as a fact when the evidence is not well established. Knowledge obtained from family members about the patient's symptoms and his or her response to the illness is extremely important.[2]

Importantly, serious heart disease can occur in patients with mild or no symptoms. Also, knowing the sensitivity, specificity, and predictive value of an answer to a question and of the presence or absence of a physical sign provides the physician with a better perspective. The physician must determine whether or not the history obtained is sufficient to support a decision-making process about the patient.[2] While many patients with severe heart disease have no symptoms, others have many symptoms associated with minor or no disease.

Some patients deny the presence of symptoms because they cannot accept the reality of the situation, whereas others may purposefully withhold information because they may lose their jobs if the truth were revealed.[2] Still other patients may overstate their symptoms for personal gain. Elderly patients, sedentary patients, and patients whose physical activity is limited by another illness may have no symptoms because they do not perform adequate physical effort to produce them.[2]

Past and Family History

The past history may provide important clues to the presence of cardiovascular disease. A definite history of rheumatic fever may be useful in defining the cause of a heart murmur, whereas a negative history of rheumatic fever does not exclude it.[2] A history of hypertension in a family member increases the likelihood that the patient has essential hypertension.[2] Previous trauma may be the cause of constrictive pericarditis, a thoracic aortic aneurysm, an arteriovenous fistula, and other types of cardiac lesions. A detailed history of the use of medications, addicting drugs, and alcohol, each of which may cause heart disease, is essential. A past history of pulmonary embolism, thrombophlebitis, or systemic embolism should be ascertained.

A history of dental work, some other diagnostic or therapeutic procedure, or recent infection suggests the possibility of infective endocarditis in a patient with valvular heart disease. Patients often give a history of having had a "heart attack," which, in fact, may have been an episode of unstable angina, heart failure, or arrhythmia. The "heart attack" history often becomes "myocardial infarction" in the patient's medical record unless more information about the episode is obtained or documentation of the event is reviewed.[1]

Many patients are referred who have had several catheterizations, percutaneous coronary interventions, angioplasties, and one or more coronary bypass operations in addition to multiple noninvasive tests. A thorough and often time-consuming review of records from other institutions, operative notes, cineangiographic films, and noninvasive studies often will provide an accurate assessment of the patient's current status without the unnecessary repetition of expensive and potentially risky procedures.[1]

Past and present therapeutic regimens must be reviewed carefully. Various treatment programs may have been inappropriate or suboptimal. The drugs currently used for the treatment of cardiovascular diseases have a larger number of potential side effects that can result in both cardiovascular and noncardiovascular symptoms (see Chap. 81).

Multiple risk factors for developing coronary artery disease (CAD) have been identified, including age, male sex, hypertension, hypercholesterolemia, low high-density lipoprotein (HDL) cholesterol, cigarette smoking, diabetes, and a family history of premature atherosclerosis (see Chap. 38). The presence or absence of risk factors can increase or decrease the statistical likelihood that an individual patient has CHD.

Patients should be questioned about previous health evaluations. In addition to being examined at the time of routine physicals or in association with other medical treatment, patients often have been examined for the military service, for athletics, or for insurance, and they may have been told of a heart murmur or hypertension on those occasions.[2] Rejection by the military or an insurance company is often due to a cardiovascular abnormality. Many patients have not seen a physician in the recent past or ever had a careful examination of the cardiovascular system.

The increasing hemodynamic burden of pregnancy may cause an otherwise marginally compensated cardiac patient to become symptomatic. Specific inquiry should be made about heart failure, edema, dyspnea, or prescribed prolonged periods of bed rest during pregnancy.[1] Many normal women have had a murmur detected during pregnancy (see Chap. 82). A history of illicit parenteral drug use should raise the suspicion of infective endocarditis, especially in a febrile patient (see Chap. 73). Cocaine can cause coronary artery vasospasm and also raise myocardial oxygen demand by increasing heart rate and blood pressure. Angina, myocardial infarction, and sudden cardiac death have been well documented after cocaine use (see Chap. 71).

A history of moderate to excessive alcohol consumption, an enlarged heart on prior chest roentgenogram, periods of rapid weight gain or loss, and other illnesses may provide important information, as may questions concerning prior diagnoses made by the patient or by medical personnel.[1]

A family history of congenital heart disease indicates a higher risk of a congenital heart lesion (see Chap. 63). The patient's mother may give a history of rubella during the first few months of pregnancy; this increases the likelihood that the patient has patent ductus arteriosus, pulmonic valve stenosis, coarctation of the pulmonary arteries, or atrial septal defect.

Although most of the common cardiovascular diseases are sporadic, there are several examples in which genetic transmission can occur (see Chap. 62). These include mitral valve prolapse and the hypertrophic or dilated cardiomyopathies. Other genetically determined disorders include some of the inborn errors of metabolism, muscular dystrophies, Ehlers-Danlos syndrome, Marfan's syndrome, and the long Q-T syndromes with or without deafness (see Chaps. 62 and 63).

Symptoms Associated with Cardiovascular Disease

CHEST PAIN

Chest pain or chest discomfort is the foremost manifestation of myocardial ischemia and results from a disparity between myocardial oxygen demand and coronary blood flow in patients with CAD.[3] The most common causes of myocardial ischemia are coronary atherosclerosis, coronary vasoconstriction, and coronary artery thrombosis, the latter occurring particularly in patients with acute coronary syndromes such as acute myocardial infarction and unstable angina (see Chaps. 41 and 42). An increase in myocardial oxygen demand ($M\dot{V}O_2$) or demand ischemia, a decrease in or inadequate blood flow (supply ischemia), or their combination may be responsible for anginal chest pain (see Chap. 40).

The mechanism responsible for cardiac pain is not clearly understood. Nonmedullated small sympathetic nerve fibers that parallel the coronary arteries are thought to provide the afferent sensory pathway for angina; these enter the spinal cord in the C8-T4 segments.[4] Impulses are transmitted to corresponding spinal ganglia and then through the spinal cord to the thalamus and cerebral cortex. Angina pectoris, like other pain of visceral origin, is often poorly localized and is commonly referred to the corresponding segmental dermatomes.

The differential diagnosis of chest pain is extensive.[5] In addition to angina pectoris and myocardial infarction, other cardiovascular diseases, gastrointestinal diseases, psychogenic diseases, neuromuscular diseases, and diseases of the pulmonary system must be considered (Table 10-1; see also Table 40-6). An accurate interpretation of the etiology and significance of chest discomfort is critically dependent on a carefully taken history. Important clinically relevant information may be missed if the *overenthusiastic use of noninvasive or invasive diagnostic methods* replaces rather than augments direct physician-patient communication (see Chap. 40).

The original subjective description of angina pectoris by

TABLE 10-1 Differential Diagnosis of Chest Pain

1. Angina pectoris/myocardial infarction
2. Other cardiovascular causes
   a. Likely ischemic in origin
      (1) Aortic stenosis
      (2) Hypertrophic cardiomyopathy
      (3) Severe systemic hypertension
      (4) Severe right ventricular hypertension
      (5) Aortic regurgitation
      (6) Severe anemia/hypoxia
   b. Nonischemic in origin
      (1) Aortic dissection
      (2) Pericarditis
      (3) Mitral valve prolapse
3. Gastrointestinal
   a. Esophageal spasm
   b. Esophageal reflux
   c. Esophageal rupture
   d. Peptic ulcer disease
4. Psychogenic
   a. Anxiety
   b. Depression
   c. Cardiac psychosis
   d. Self-gain
5. Neuromusculoskeletal
   a. Thoracic outlet syndrome
   b. Degenerative joint disease of cervical/thoracic spine
   c. Costochondritis (Tietze's syndrome)
   d. Herpes zoster
   e. Chest wall pain and tenderness
6. Pulmonary
   a. Pulmonary embolus with or without pulmonary infarction
   b. Pneumothorax
   c. Pneumonia with pleural involvement
7. Pleurisy

William Heberden[6] in the late eighteenth century has not been surpassed. It is quoted in Chap. 40.

Angina pectoris is defined as chest pain or discomfort of cardiac origin that usually results from a temporary imbalance between myocardial oxygen supply and demand. It may occur only with exertion or spontaneously at rest; various subtypes are defined in Chap. 40. The quality of the chest discomfort is usually described as "tightness," "pressure," "burning," "heaviness," "aching," "strangling," or "compression." Usually the patient is able to describe a deep rather than a superficial origin of the pain. Since the qualitative description of the pain is greatly influenced by the patient's intelligence, education, and social/cultural background, a definition of other characteristics of the chest discomfort is often extremely important in evaluating the symptoms appropriately. The most important of these characteristics are the *precipitating factors* for the onset of pain, its *mode of onset and duration,* its *pattern of disappearance,* and its *location.* Classically, the discomfort is induced by exercise, emotion, eating, or cold weather.

A recognizable pattern of reproducibility of chest pain by certain activities is an important characteristic of angina. Often, patients develop pain with exertion after meals, and there is a greater tendency for arm work, which involves a greater element of isometric exercise than isotonic leg exercise, to produce distress.[7–9] Occasionally, angina will dissipate despite continued exercise (the walk-through phenomenon) or will not occur when a second exercise effort is undertaken that previously produced chest discomfort (warm-up phenomenon).

Both circumstances may be attributed to the opening of functioning coronary arterial collaterals during the initial myocardial ischemia. Angina commonly occurs after the patient has eaten a heavy meal or when the patient is excited, angry, or tense. Cold showers increase blood pressure and heart rate, whereas hot showers cause an augmented cardiac output in response to vasodilation. Either may precipitate angina after exercise. The chest pain during any type of activity is often made worse by the use of tobacco. All the hemodynamic changes resulting from the use of nicotine increase the myocardial oxygen demand.

Angina pectoris characteristically has a crescendo pattern at onset and "builds up." Pains, often described as "shooting" or "stabbing," that reach their maximum intensity virtually instantaneously are often not angina but are of musculoskeletal or neural origin. Angina is usually relieved within 5 to 20 min by rest, with or without the use of vasodilator drugs such as nitroglycerin, although nitroglycerin characteristically hastens relief. Failure to obtain relief with rest or nitroglycerin suggests another cause of pain or actual impending myocardial infarction. The reproducible relief of chest pain in an appropriate time frame (within 10 min) can be strong evidence favoring ischemia. A trial of nitroglycerin can be a useful diagnostic strategy. Patients with angina pectoris usually are classified functionally from class I to class IV (Table 10-2), depending on the amount of activity necessary to induce chest pain.[10]

Localizing the site of chest discomfort provides additional information in determining its cause. Anginal pain is ordinarily retrosternal or felt slightly to left of the midline, beside or partly under the sternum. It is rarely isolated to the cardiac apex in the inframammary region. The chest pain of myocardial ischemia tends to radiate bilaterally across the chest into the arms (left more than right) and into the neck and lower jaw. Occasionally, radiation to the back or occiput is noted. In the arms, the pain passes down the ulnar and volar surface to the wrist and then only into the ulnar fingers, rarely into the thumb or down the outer (extensor) surface of the arm, which has a different dermatome pattern. Pain occasionally may be felt only in the arm or may start in the arm and radiate to the chest. Attention to the gestures that the patient uses in characterizing and localizing the site of pain may be useful in determining its etiology. One or two clenched fists held by the patient over the sternal area (Levine's sign) is much more indicative of ischemic pain than is a finger pointed to a small, circumscribed area in the left inframammary region. The latter more likely represents chest pain of psychogenic origin.

As indicated earlier, the *duration* of chest pain also may be a useful differentiating feature. Angina pectoris rarely lasts less than 1 min or more than 20 min in the absence of myocardial infarction or persistent arrhythmias. Most patients with angina report prompt relief in less than 5 min after cessation of activity or with the use of sublingual nitroglycerin. Delayed relief of chest pain by sublingual nitroglycerin may be ascribed to a placebo effect. Since nitrates are generalized smooth muscle relaxants, pain due to diffuse esophageal spasm or biliary colic also may be relieved by these same agents. Carotid sinus massage by the physician frequently will relieve anginal chest pain because of the resulting reflex bradycardia and the decrease in systolic blood pressure, thus reducing myocardial oxygen demand.[11] Carotid sinus massage should be performed only in the absence of extracranial occlusive cerebrovascular disease as manifest by carotid bruits or decreased carotid arterial pulsations and with careful auscultatory monitoring of the heart rate. The Valsalva maneuver also may relieve anginal pain by decreasing myocardial wall tension as a result of the reduced

TABLE 10-2 Canadian Cardiovascular Society Functional Classification of Angina Pectoris

I.	Ordinary physical activity, such as walking and climbing stairs, does not cause angina. Angina results from strenuous or rapid or prolonged exertion at work or recreation.
II.	Slight limitation of ordinary activity. Walking or climbing stairs rapidly, walking uphill, walking or stair climbing after meals, in cold, in wind, or when under emotional stress, or only during the few hours after awakening. Walking more than two blocks on the level and climbing more than one flight of ordinary stairs at a normal pace and under normal conditions.
III.	Marked limitations of ordinary physical activity. Walking one to two blocks on the level and climbing more than one flight under normal conditions.
IV.	Inability to carry on any physical activity without discomfort—anginal syndrome may be present at rest.

SOURCE: Modified from Campeau L. Letter to the editor. *Circulation* 1976; 54:522. Reproduced with permission from the American Heart Association, Inc., and the author.

venous return and left ventricular volume accompanying the increase in intrathoracic pressure. *Associated symptoms*—such as nausea, vomiting, faintness, fatigue, or diaphoresis—often accompany severe episodes of myocardial ischemia in both men and women.[12] Severe myocardial ischemia often produces marked dyspnea due to a large increase in left ventricular (LV) diastolic filling pressure, sometimes producing an "angina equivalent" in the absence of chest discomfort.

Linked angina is a term applied to definite episodes of angina in patients with established CAD caused by gastrointestinal factors not related to an increase in cardiac work.[13] Episodes typically are induced by stooping or occur after eating; they can be mimicked by esophageal acid stimulation, which can reduce coronary blood flow (CBF).[13]

No consideration of myocardial ischemia as a likely cause of chest discomfort is complete without carefully considering the chest pain in the context of known risk factors for CAD (see above).

Angina pectoris should be considered a symptom and not a specific disease. Coronary arteriographic studies have demonstrated that more than 90 percent of patients with chest pain precipitated by exercise and relieved by rest have angiographic evidence of significant CAD. However, other diseases may be associated with classic angina pectoris (see below).

Several reports have described certain patients with typical exertional chest discomfort and arteriographically normal coronary arteries.[14,15] These patients are more likely to be females, have fewer coronary risk factors, have variable responses to various antianginal agents, and less commonly, have more relief of pain by sublingual nitroglycerin than patients with occlusive CAD. Although the underlying cause of this condition remains unsettled, the life expectancy of these patients appears no different from that of an age- and sex-matched population without chest discomfort (see Chap. 40).

There is some evidence that abnormal function of small coronary arteries may cause limited CBF responses to stress or pharmacologic vasodilators in a subset of patients with anginal chest pain despite angiographically normal coronary arteries (*microvascular angina*).[16–22] In the past, investigators arguing for or against the existence of this syndrome often have used the term *syndrome X* to describe their patient cohort.[23] Syndrome X appears to include a heterogeneous group of patients with a wide spectrum of chest pain and a variety of vascular and smooth muscle hypersensitive constrictor responses. Multiple research studies continue in an effort to explain syndrome X.[24–30] It should be distinguished from the *metabolic syndrome X* of insulin resistance (glucose intolerance), hypertension, hyperlipidemia, and upper body obesity (see Chaps. 40 and 78).

Some patients with CAD experience angina at rest as a complication or an isolated clinical manifestation of ischemic heart disease.[11] Myocardial ischemic pain at rest more likely results from an acute reduction in CBF than from an increase in $M\dot{V}O_2$. Possible causative factors include isolated coronary artery spasm or embolism, coronary artery spasm superimposed on coronary atherosclerosis, and coronary thrombosis with spontaneous thrombolysis.[31–34] In patients with progressive coronary atherosclerosis, however, ischemic rest pain also may result from intermittent arrhythmias that increase $M\dot{V}O_2$ or decrease CBF or from labile hypertension with its increased wall stress. Chest pain at rest may occur only as nocturnal angina. In addition to the preceding mechanisms, nocturnal angina, also known as *angina decubitus*, may be produced by the increase in wall stress and thus $M\dot{V}O_2$ secondary to redistribution of the intravascular blood volume in the recumbent position.

The relative hypercapnia and acidosis that occur during sleep also may contribute to nocturnal angina. This condition also has been accompanied by concomitant rapid eye movement sleep patterns on the electroencephalogram, which may be associated with augmented sympathetic discharge increasing $M\dot{V}O_2$ or causing coronary constriction[8–11] (see Chap. 40).

Despite the more malignant natural history observed in many patients with rest angina, particularly associated with ST-T—wave changes, the predictive value of the history alone is not as accurate as with exertional angina. The quality of pain is usually similar to that of exertional angina, but the discomfort may be more severe and its duration longer. In addition, angina at rest is commonly associated with nausea, vomiting, and diaphoresis. The onset of shortness of breath during or after the beginning of chest discomfort suggests that the pain is due to extensive myocardial ischemia and usually results from an acute elevation of LV filling pressure secondary to the development of a large, transiently ischemic myocardial segment. Such patients are commonly found to have multivessel occlusive CAD on arteriography.

Chest pain or discomfort resulting from *myocardial infarction* (MI) is qualitatively similar to angina at rest. Differentiation between the pain resulting from ischemia and that due to MI is usually impossible based on the history alone.[7–9] Pain associated with transmural Q-wave MI is usually more severe and longer lasting than anginal pain and is often associated with nausea, vomiting, and diaphoresis. In addition, MI is frequently accompanied by symptoms of sustained LV dysfunction (dyspnea, orthopnea) and evidence of autonomic nervous system hyperactivity (tachycardia, diaphoresis, bradycardia).[7–9] Painless or atypical presentations of MI, however, occur in up to 30 percent of patients, particularly in diabetic patients and the elderly. Thus determination of serial serum enzymes, isoenzymes, and other serum markers (e.g., troponin I), providing evidence of myocardial necrosis, and serial electrocardiograms (ECGs), indicating myocardial injury, are necessary to establish the diagnosis in most patients (see Chaps. 42 and 43).

There are two groups of *cardiovascular diseases causing chest pain that is not due to coronary atherosclerosis* (see Table 10-1). The first group consists of cardiac diseases causing myocardial ischemia-related angina in the absence of CAD; ischemia is due to hemodynamic changes associated with an inadequate CBF in relation to a normal or increased myocardial oxygen demand. Among these are *aortic valve stenosis* (see Chap. 56), *hypertrophic cardiomyopathy* (see Chap. 67), and *systemic arterial hypertension* (see Chap. 51), in which LV systolic pressure and LV wall tension are greatly increased or LV hypertrophy is present.[7–9] Chest pain due to myocardial ischemia also can occur with severe aortic regurgitation (see Chap. 56). The large ventricular volume load and increased ventricular dimensions result in increased $M\dot{V}O_2$, and the reduced diastolic perfusion pressure of the coronary arteries results in a relatively inadequate CBF. Occasionally, very severe anemia or hypoxia also may produce myocardial ischemia by an inadequate oxygen blood supply even in the absence of associated CAD as well as increases in angina in the presence of obstructive coronary artery disease.[7–9] In addition, severe right ventricular (RV) systolic hypertension, as often occurs with pulmonic stenosis or pulmonary hypertension, may cause exertional angina, presumably on the basis of RV subendocardial ischemia.[35]

A second group of cardiac diseases causing chest pain that is not usually due to myocardial ischemia includes *pericarditis* (see Chap. 72), aortic dissection (see Chap. 88), and mitral valve prolapse (see Chap. 58). Pericarditis is a relatively common cause of chest pain.[36] The chest pain of pericarditis is most often sharp and penetrating in quality, and patients often obtain relief by sitting up and bending forward (see Chap. 72). The cardinal diagnostic feature of pericardial pain is its frequent worsening by changes in body position, during deep inspiration, and occasionally, on swallowing. The chest discomfort may radiate to the shoulders, upper back, and neck because of irritation of the diaphragmatic pleura, which is innervated through the phrenic nerve by fibers originating in cervical sympathetic ganglia C3–C5. Therefore, the chest discomfort associated with pericarditis is due predominantly to parietal pleural irritation. Occasionally, the pain of acute benign, presumptive viral pericarditis may mimic that observed in acute MI. Importantly, the most common cause of pericarditis in middle-aged or older people is acute MI. The pericarditis usually occurs several days after the myocardial necrosis and must be distinguished from recurrent infarction or ischemia. Pericarditis also may be a cause of chest pain after cardiac surgery and may be a complication of aortic dissection, with leakage into the pericardium.

Aortic dissection (see Chap. 88) may be misdiagnosed on initial presentation as an acute MI; indeed, MI is a recognized complication of aortic dissection. The pain with dissection, however, is usually of sudden onset as compared with the pain of myocardial ischemia, which builds in intensity with time.[37] Patients frequently characterize the pain as excruciating, the most severe discomfort that they have ever experienced, and as having a tearing quality, commonly localized to the interscapular area. The discomfort may radiate widely into the neck, back, abdomen, flanks, and legs and may migrate, depending on the location and progression of the aortic dissection and the amount of arterial luminal compression. Neurologic symptoms and signs may occur when dissection involves the cerebral arteries. With the exception of patients with Marfan's syndrome (see Chaps. 66 and 76) or idiopathic cystic medial necrosis, most patients with aortic dissection have a history of long-standing systemic arterial hypertension or evidence of it on physical examination.

Psychogenic chest discomfort is a common type of recurrent chest pain that may be difficult to separate from angina pectoris, particularly when it occurs in patients with multiple risk factors for CAD or in otherwise asymptomatic patients with well-documented CAD. The most common psychogenic cause of chest discomfort is anxiety[38] (see Chap. 80). Psychogenic chest pain is often described as sharp or stabbing, is commonly localized to the left inframammary area, and is usually sharply circumscribed. Descriptors such as "stabbing" or "lightning-like" may be used to describe extremely short (<1 min) episodes of pain. At times, the pain may persist for many hours or several days. Patients often note psychogenic pain at rest. Also, nonvocal communication, such as a flat or worried facial expression, retarded motor activity, and hand wringing, may indicate underlying depression. Observation of the patient during pain that occurs spontaneously or during exercise testing often provides insight into a potential psychogenic etiology. Patients with anxiety often have multiple complaints such as breathlessness, giddiness, and palpitations. Associated symptoms, such as air hunger, circumoral paresthesias, globus hystericus, and multiple somatic complaints, may suggest a neurasthenic personality or hyperventilation syndrome.

Pain originating in the gastrointestinal tract, particularly that of esophageal origin, is commonly confused with ischemic chest pain.[39] Diffuse esophageal spasm, a neuromuscular motor disorder of the esophagus characterized by chest pain, is the extracardiac condition most frequently confused with angina pectoris. Esophageal spasm may occur at any age but is more common in individuals in the fifth decade. The pain is usually retrosternal; may be burning, squeezing, or aching in quality; and often radiates to the back, arms, and jaw. It usually begins during or after a meal and can last minutes or hours. In some patients, the pain may be precipitated or exacerbated by exercise, and relief may be obtained with nitroglycerin, which also relaxes esophageal smooth muscle. A useful feature in the differentiation of diffuse esophageal spasm from ischemic chest discomfort is its frequent association with pain as a result of swallowing, dysphagia, and the regurgitation of gastric contents. Episodes of pain frequently are precipitated either by extremely hot or cold drinks or by an emotional upset. The diagnosis of diffuse esophageal spasm is based on the history, the exclusion of cardiac and musculoskeletal causes of chest pain, and the demonstration of abnormal esophageal motility on cineesophagograms or by esophageal manometry.

Reflux esophagitis results from mucosal irritation produced by failure of the lower esophageal sphincter to prevent regurgitation of highly acidic gastric contents into the distal esophagus.[40–42] The pain is usually epigastric or retrosternal, burning in quality, and frequently precipitated by the recumbent position or by bending over. "Heartburn" and regurgitation often occur after meals or ingestion of coffee or after postural changes. Patients are often awakened by chest discomfort due to acid reflux occurring in the recumbent position. Many of these patients are obese and report relief of discomfort from food, antacids, or elevation of the head of the bed. Dysphagia may result from stricture formation secondary to long-standing esophageal reflux. An upper gastrointestinal series may demonstrate hiatal hernia, but this does not establish the diagnosis of esophagitis or esophageal reflux. Esophagoscopy and esophageal biopsy may demonstrate mucosal lesions and are useful for assessing the severity of inflammation and for excluding malignancy. Sphincter incompetence may be documented by the use of esophageal manometry. Esophageal acid perfusion testing (Bernstein test) often will provoke the patient's characteristic symptoms, and distal esophageal pH monitoring will detect gastroesophageal reflux.[41]

Acute esophageal rupture, a serious and often rapidly lethal event, causes severe retrosternal pain secondary to the chemical mediastinitis produced by acidic gastric contents.[7–9] Spontaneous rupture usually results from a prolonged bout of vomiting or retching after a heavy meal. Rupture is a recognized iatrogenic complication of esophageal instrumentation. The pain varies in location depending on the rupture's site and position. The diagnosis is based on symptoms and signs of mediastinal air following vomiting or esophageal instrumentation.

Although peptic ulcer disease and biliary colic are less commonly confused with chest pain of cardiac origin, myocardial ischemic pain occasionally may be described as burning in character and located near the epigastrium.

Diseases involving the neuromuscular-skeletal systems may cause pain affecting dermatome patterns similar to those occurring with angina pectoris.[7–9] The thoracic outlet syndromes, in which various neural and vascular structures are compressed, may produce symptoms that are sometimes confused with cardiac chest pain. Although compression of the neurovascular bundle by a cervical rib or the scalenus anterior muscle may cause discomfort radiating to the head and neck, the shoulder region, or the axilla, most patients experience pain in the upper extremity resulting from somatic nerve compression, usually in the distribution of the ulnar nerve.[8–11] The presence of associated paresthesias, the presence of pain unrelated to physical exercise, the worsening of discomfort, and its aggravation by certain body positions are useful differentiating characteristics. The diagnosis of thoracic outlet syndrome can be confirmed in many patients by careful physical and neurologic examination.

Tietze's syndrome, or idiopathic costochondritis, is an occasional cause of anterior chest wall pain that is aggravated by movement and deep breathing. The reproduction of the chest pain syndrome by direct pressure over the involved costochondral junction or the relief of pain after local infiltration with lidocaine is a helpful diagnostic maneuver.[43] Degenerative arthritis of the cervical and thoracic vertebrae may cause bandlike pain confined to the chest, neck, or back that often radiates to the arms.[7–9] Radiologic evidence of degenerative changes involving the cervical and thoracic vertebrae is often found in asymptomatic elderly patients. The production or exacerbation of pain by various postures, movement, sneezing, or coughing is more useful in the diagnosis of chest discomfort due to vertebral disease.[7–9]

The *preeruptive stage of herpes zoster* may be characterized by bandlike chest pain over one or more dermatomes. The advanced age of the patient, additional symptoms of malaise, headache and fever, the presence of hyperesthesia of the involved area on physical examination, and the eventual eruption of typical lesions 4 or 5 days after the onset of symptoms will result in the correct diagnosis. Chest wall pain and tenderness may occur for unknown reasons.[44] The discomfort may be reproduced by pressure over the painful area and by movements of the thorax such as bending, twisting, or turning. The variable duration of the pain and the absence of relief by nitroglycerin distinguish it from angina.

The syndrome of acute massive *pulmonary embolism* with its associated acute pulmonary hypertension and low cardiac output occasionally may simulate acute MI, since myocardial ischemia may be present in both conditions. The quality of chest pain may be identical to that observed in patients with nonradiating ischemic chest pain or may be pleuritic, as described below. The associated signs of severe dyspnea, tachypnea, and intense cyanosis, accompanied by profound anxiety and agitation, however, favor the diagnosis of pulmonary embolism[8–11] (see Chap. 54). The clinical setting may suggest the diagnosis because of the known increased likelihood of pulmonary embolism in the postpartum or postoperative state, during long trips, in patients with congestive heart failure and peripheral edema, and in those with deep-vein thrombophlebitis. Measurements of arterial blood gases, abnormal pulmonary perfusion-ventilation scans, and if needed, pulmonary arteriography will establish the correct diagnosis.[7–9]

Other pulmonary conditions associated with chest discomfort, such as pneumothorax, are rarely confused with ischemic chest pain because of additional characteristic clinical features. Spontaneous pneumothorax usually occurs in otherwise healthy males in the third and fourth decades. The clinical presentation is usually characterized by the abrupt onset of agonizing unilateral pleuritic chest pain associated with severe shortness of breath. The plain or expiratory chest film provides the definitive diagnosis. Chest pain associated with pneumonias of various etiologies, as well as pulmonary infarctions as a consequence of pulmonary embolus, may result from pleural irritation. The discomfort is sharp, varies acutely with breathing, and frequently is accompanied by a reduced inspiratory effort. Associated signs of pulmonary parenchymal infection or infarction usually indicate the underlying diagnosis.

EXTRATHORACIC PAIN

Intermittent claudication of the lower extremities due to peripheral atherosclerosis (see Chap. 90) may present as discomfort during exercise in the arch of the foot, calf of the leg, thighs, hips, or gluteal region.[7–9] Acute arterial occlusion in the lower extremities due to systemic embolism may cause the sensation of hypesthesia.[2] Intermittent claudication of the upper extremities or masseter muscles is usually due to nonatherosclerotic causes of arterial disease, such as arteritis.[2] The pain of Raynaud's disease may be noted in the fingers after exposure to cold, with pallor of the fingers prior to the sensation of pain. Pain and swelling of lower extremities may be caused by thrombophlebitis (see Chap. 90).

Head pain secondary to myocardial ischemia may be felt in the jaw, hard palate, cheek, and sometimes deep in the ear canals. The pain of temporal arteritis, commonly localized to the temporal area, often is associated with abnormal vision and polymyalgia rheumatica.[76] Migraine headache, frequently accompanied by nausea, scotoma, and intolerance to light, is vascular in origin and may be incapacitating.[2] A severe headache may be present in patients with uncontrolled hypertension (see Chap. 51).

Pain in the abdomen, often localized to the midabdomen and lower portion of the back, may be produced by an expanding or rupturing atherosclerotic abdominal aneurysm. Abdominal angina due to vascular disease of the mesenteric arteries is discussed in Chap. 88. The liver is often painful and tender in severe right-sided heart failure, with worsening of the pain during activity.[2]

Various types of *joint pain* may be associated with heart disease. Rheumatic fever, rheumatoid arthritis, lupus erythematosus, psoriatic arthritis, ankylosing spondylitis, gonococcal arthritis, Reiter's syndrome, and Lyme disease may be associated with valvular, myocardial, or pericardial disease.[2]

RESPIRATORY SYMPTOMS

Dyspnea is defined as difficult or labored respiration or the unpleasant awareness of one's respiration. It has many causes. A clue to the etiology is obtained from the factors that precipitate or relieve it.[1] Chronic dyspnea can be caused by heart failure, pulmonary disease, anxiety, obesity, poor physical fitness, pleural effusions, and asthma.[2] Acute dyspnea may occur with acute pulmonary edema, hyperventilation, pneumothorax, pulmonary embolism, pneumonia, and airway obstruction.[2]

Dyspnea on effort, a frequent symptom, is usually due to congestive heart failure, chronic pulmonary disease, or physical deconditioning (see Chap. 20). The amount of activity necessary to produce dyspnea needs definition. A recent or dramatic increase in the dyspnea is more likely to be due to the development of heart failure than to lung disease. When heart and lung disease coexist, however, the determination of the relative contribution of pulmonary and cardiac dysfunction to dyspnea can be very difficult.

Cheyne-Stokes respiration is a form of periodic breathing characterized by cycles beginning with shallow respirations that increase in rate and depth to significant hyperpnea, followed by decreasing rate and depth of respiration, and then a period of apnea that may last 15 s or longer.[1] This form of respiration occurs in advanced congestive heart failure and in some forms of central nervous system disease. Cheyne-Stokes respiration often occurs during sleep without the patient's awareness and is often reported by others.

Orthopnea results from an increase in hydrostatic pressure in the lungs that occurs with assumption of the supine position. It consists of cough and dyspnea in some patients with LV failure or mitral valve disease and necessitates the use of two or more pillows on lying down. The patient with severe obstructive lung disease, especially acute asthma, also cannot lie flat comfortably.

Paroxysmal nocturnal dyspnea (PND) is the occurrence of dyspnea during sleep, commonly 2 to 3 h after going to bed, that is relieved by assuming the upright position. Dyspnea usually does not recur after the patient goes back to sleep. Episodes can be mild, or they can be severe with wheezing, coughing, gasping, and apprehension.[1] Some episodes will progress to pulmonary edema. The probable mechanism for this *relatively specific symptom* of left-sided heart failure is the increase in central blood volume in the supine position.

A dry, nonproductive cough, occurring with effort or at rest, may be related to the pulmonary congestion associated with heart failure (see Chap. 20). Although dyspnea is usually present, cough may dominate the clinical picture. The cough that accompanies acute pulmonary edema is often associated with frothy, pink-tinged sputum, whereas the sputum associated with chronic bronchitis is usually white and mucoid.[2] The sputum associated with pneumonia is often thick and yellow, and that due to pulmonary infarction may be bloody, as may the sputum associated with cancer of the lung or bronchiolectasis. Cough also may be caused by angiotensin-converting enzyme inhibitors, which are often prescribed for heart failure or hypertension.

Recurrent coughing due to heart failure is often thought to be due to bronchitis, and patients with chronic bronchitis may cough more when heart failure ensues.[2] Patients with a high pulmonary blood flow due to congenital left-to-right shunts are subject to pulmonary infection. Patients with a high pulmonary venous pressure are more vulnerable to the development of pulmonary edema when they have viral pneumonitis than are patients with normal pulmonary venous pressure. This particularly applies to patients with mitral stenosis.

Hemoptysis occurs in many cardiac disorders. Posterior epistaxis due to systemic hypertension may cause blood-streaked sputum; patients on anticoagulants may have epistaxis that mimics hemoptysis. Epistaxis, however, is usually easily differentiated from bloody sputum. Bright red pulmonary venous blood from rupture of submucosal pulmonary venules may be expectorated by patients with pulmonary venous hypertension due to mitral stenosis or severe LV failure.[2] Darker blood or clots often occur with pulmonary emboli.

Pink, frothy sputum may be produced during acute pulmonary edema. Blood-streaked sputum is a feature of the "winter bronchitis" of mitral stenosis.[2] Massive hemoptysis with exsanguination or death from asphyxiation can follow rupture of an aortic aneurysm or one of the cardiac chambers into the bronchial tree.[2] Rupture of a pulmonary artery by the balloon of an indwelling pulmonary artery catheter can cause abrupt, severe hemoptysis in hospitalized patients.

Wheezing associated with dyspnea may be due to lung or heart disease. If the symptoms have developed recently in an adult over age 40, other clues indicating heart disease should be sought. Wheezing due to heart disease is termed *cardiac asthma.*

EDEMA AND ASCITES

Edema is a common symptom or finding in patients with right- or left-sided heart failure. Fluid retention in heart failure results from increased venous pressure and abnormal activity of salt-retaining hormones (see Chap. 20). In an average-sized person, 5 to 10 lb of excess fluid is required for edema to become apparent; a history of recent weight gain often will correlate with a deterioration in clinical status. The amount of weight loss in response to treatment for heart failure in the past will relate to the severity of the problem. Minor degrees of edema are evident only after a period of dependency of the legs and will decrease after rest. Presacral edema may be most obvious when the patient has been at bed rest. Although edema of cardiac origin may progress to anasarca, cardiac edema rarely involves the face or upper extremities. Edema mainly affecting the face and arms is more likely to be due to venous or lymphatic obstruction by clot or neoplasm. Facial edema is a feature of the nephrotic syndrome, angioneurotic edema, and glomerulonephritis. Swelling or "puffiness" of the hands and fingers is not usually a symptom of cardiac disease. Persistent edema in the legs from which veins were harvested at the time of bypass surgery is common. Other causes of edema—such as varicosities, obesity, tight girdle, renal insufficiency, or cirrhosis with hypoproteinemia—must be considered.[1] A patient with chronic congestive heart failure may detect edema of the ankles and lower legs during the day and note that it diminishes during the night. It is important to ascertain whether edema of the extremities preceded or followed dyspnea on effort. The calcium antagonists may produce bilateral edema of the lower legs. Edema may occur in one or both legs following the harvesting of veins for conduits in patients undergoing coronary artery bypass graft (CABG) surgery.

Patients will be aware of ascites because of increased abdominal girth. Previously comfortable trousers or skirts may no longer fit. Bending at the waist is uncomfortable, with ill-defined abdominal fullness. Patients with severe edema due to congestive heart failure may develop ascites; however, ascites is particularly common in patients with constrictive pericardial disease, sometimes occurring before peripheral edema becomes obvious (see Chap. 72). Ascitic fluid is formed when elevated venous pressure leads to transudation of fluids from the serosal surfaces. Other causes of ascites—such as cirrhosis, nephrosis, and tumor—must be excluded.

FATIGUE AND WEAKNESS

Fatigue and *weakness* may be due to many causes and therefore are not specific symptoms for heart disease. The most common cause of these symptoms is anxiety and depression. Anemia, thyrotoxicosis, and other chronic disease states may be associated with fatigue and weakness.

When a patient with heart disease is volume overloaded, or when there is pulmonary congestion due to heart disease, the patient is likely to complain of dyspnea. With vigorous diuretic therapy, this complaint may be replaced by symptoms of fatigue and weakness,[2] probably related to inadequate cardiac output (see Chap. 21). The heart fails in its prime objective of nourishing all the tissues and organs of the body, including the skeletal muscles. As congestive heart failure worsens, fatigue may replace dyspnea as the major symptom. Beta blockers used to treat angina or hypertension often cause fatigue and lethargy. Hypotension or hypokalemia caused by diuretics can result in fatigue and weakness, as can relative hypovolemia due to the use of angiotensin-converting enzyme inhibitors.

Severe fatigue related to effort may result from transient global myocardial ischemia in patients with extensive CAD. Dyspnea and hypotension also may occur at the same time as the severe fatigue as *angina equivalents*.[2]

PALPITATION

Most normal individuals are intermittently aware of their heart action, particularly at the time of physical and emotional stress. When the heart action is more vigorous than usual or its perception is unpleasant, the term *palpitation* is appropriate.[1] The patient may complain of a "pounding," "stopping," "jumping," or "racing" in the chest. Palpitation is frequently a benign symptom without any serious cardiac disease present; at other times it may indicate a potentially life-threatening condition. Simple premature beats may be perceived as a "floating" or "flopping" sensation in the chest due to the more forceful beat that occurs after the pause following the premature beat. Sometimes a transient feeling of fullness in the neck (due to cannon a waves) is perceived with premature beats. Certain patients perceive almost every premature beat, whereas others are totally unaware of frequent or advanced arrhythmias. A report of skips or irregularity during uninterrupted sinus rhythm is not uncommon. Generally, thin, tense individuals are likely to be more aware of their cardiac activity than others. Individuals with and without arrhythmias often are aware of their cardiac activity when they first lie down on their side to sleep, especially if they lie on their left side.[1]

Rapid heart action of a paroxysmal tachycardia usually begins and terminates abruptly and causes a pounding sensation in the chest.[1] Patients often will indicate whether the tachycardia is regular or irregular and may be able to tap out the rate and rhythm of the episode (see Chap. 24). Chest pressure suggesting angina may occur with an episode of tachycardia even in young, healthy patients without CAD. Patients with CAD, however, often develop severe angina with a sustained arrhythmia because of increased $M\dot{V}O_2$. Depending on the rate and mechanism of the arrhythmia, faintness and syncope may be described during questioning. Nevertheless, sustained ventricular tachycardia can occur in the setting of serious underlying cardiac disease without a significant compromise in hemodynamics (see Chap. 24). Syncope due to tachyarrhythmias may occur without the patient being aware of palpitations.

SYNCOPE

Cardiac *syncope* (fainting) is defined as the transient loss of consciousness due to inadequate cerebral blood flow secondary to an abrupt decrease in cardiac output (see Chap. 32). *Near syncope* refers to the clinical situation in which the patient feels dizzy and weak and tends to lose postural tone but does not lose consciousness. In assessing the patient with syncope, one determines if there were precipitating factors, premonitory symptoms, injury with the episode, seizure activity or incontinence, or a postictal state.[1] Injury during an episode suggests a sudden profound loss of body tone and increases the likelihood of more serious causes. Brief, unsustained seizure activity can occur with syncope due to a cardiac arrhythmia.

The patient may be incontinent during cardiogenic syncope, but an aura, sustained tonic-chronic movements, tongue biting, and confusion or drowsiness after the event are more characteristic of syncope due to central nervous system disease. In contrast, return of consciousness to the alert state is prompt after reversal of the arrhythmia causing cardiac syncope.[1] The common faint (*vasovagal syncope*) results from bradycardia and hypotension caused by excessive vagal discharge. It is often associated with some precipitating event such as a "heavy" meal in a warm room and has brief premonitory signs and symptoms such as nausea, yawning, diaphoresis, and sometimes the feeling of decreased hearing or vision.[1] There is frequently sufficient warning that the patient does not fall abruptly. The results of head-up tilt-table testing indicate a vasovagal mechanism in some patients with syncope who do not have premonitory symptoms (see Chap. 32). Following a fainting episode, the patient may be pale and diaphoretic and have a slow heart rate. Syncope occurring in the setting of any gastrointestinal symptoms is likely to be vagal in origin. A history of similar episodes during the preceding several years is common in patients with vagal syncope.

A hypersensitive carotid sinus can cause syncope. A history of episodes during an activity such as shaving, wearing of a tight collar, or extreme turning of the head may occur but is unusual even when a sensitive carotid sinus is shown to be the cause of syncope. Syncope following urination (micturition syncope) may occur at the time of rapid decompression of a distended bladder, which typically occurs after a period of sleep. Paroxysms of coughing, usually in patients with underlying pulmonary disease, can result in syncope. Very fast or slow arrhythmias may decrease the cardiac output enough to cause alterations in consciousness, ranging from abrupt profound syncope to mild light-headedness. Stokes-Adams syncope is caused by intermittent complete heart block, sinus arrest, or ventricular tachyarrhythmias[77] (see Chap. 32). It is characterized by abrupt loss of consciousness without warning, a variable period of unconsciousness (seconds to minutes), and then a rapid return of normal mental status without amnesia or a postictal state.

In the presence of several LV outflow obstruction (aortic stenosis or hypertrophic cardiomyopathy), loss of consciousness with effort may occur. Syncope can be due either to the heart's inability to increase its output in response to the peripheral vasodilatation that occurs during exercise or to a tachyarrhythmia. Intermittent obstruction of a cardiac valve by an intracavitary tumor or thrombus is a rare cause of syncope that occasionally may be precipitated when the patient changes position (see Chap. 77).

Many normal subjects experience transient light-headedness with rapid changes in position. This is more common in older patients, since the ability of the peripheral vasculature to respond is attenuated with aging (see Chap. 86). Postural hypotension is a well-defined cause of fainting or dizziness that usually occurs when the individual is upright and often just after rising from a supine or sitting position. Possible causes include peripheral neuropathy, autonomic dysfunction, volume depletion, or drug side effects.

OTHER CEREBRAL SYMPTOMS

Patients with decreased cardiac output secondary to heart failure may become mentally confused and disoriented. Such symptoms also may be due to hypoxia, to drugs that are invariably prescribed for such patients, and to renal or hepatic failure.[2] A completed stroke may be caused by a lacunar infarct, cerebral hemorrhage, cerebral arterial thrombosis, or a cerebral embolus (see Chap. 89). A transient cerebral ischemic attack is commonly due to an embolus. The embolus may originate in an atheromatous ulcer in the carotid artery system or the aortic arch; be related to infective endocarditis, a recent MI, atrial fibrillation, or clots on a prosthetic valve; or originate in the leg veins and pass through a patent foramen ovale to the brain (see Chap. 89).

The patient with cardiogenic shock or with a severe tachyarrhythmia who also has considerable intracranial or extracranial vascular disease may develop such severe cerebral hypoxia that coma occurs. Hypoxic encephalopathy may follow cardiac resuscitation and occasionally occurs after cardiopulmonary bypass for cardiac surgery. A cerebral abscess may occur in patients with congenital heart disease and a right-to-left shunt.[2]

FEVER, CHILLS, AND SWEATS

Patients with rheumatic fever usually do not have chills. Chills are common in patients with bacterial endocarditis. Symptoms of fever, chills, or sweats in any patient with a heart murmur should lead one to suspect infective endocarditis (see Chap. 73). A history of valvular heart disease is not a prerequisite for a diagnosis of endocarditis, since previously normal valves become infected. A history of recent dental work, genitourinary surgery, or illicit drug use increases the suspicion of infective endocarditis. Fever may accompany pericarditis. Myalgia, chills, and fever on rare occasions may be related to MI, presumably because of some form of immunologic response to the necrotic myocardial tissue. An intracardiac tumor (myxoma) may produce systemic symptoms in the absence of infection. Low-grade fever in a patient with heart failure may be a sign of pulmonary emboli.[2] A profuse "cold sweat" mediated by sympathetic discharge often accompanies early stages of acute MI. Excessive sweating may occur in patients with severe aortic regurgitation. Diaphoresis is often a sign of congestive heart failure in infants.

HOARSENESS

Although usually unrelated to cardiovascular disease, *hoarseness* can occur in patients with an aortic aneurysm that involves the left recurrent laryngeal nerve. Mitral stenosis occasionally may produce hoarseness due to the pressure of a large pulmonary artery on the recurrent laryngeal nerve. Pericardial effusion may be related to myxedema, which may be associated with a coarse, low-pitched voice. Hoarseness and loss of voice may occur following the use of an endotracheal tube during cardiac surgery.

INDIGESTION, HICCUPS, AND DYSPHAGIA

Many patients with angina pectoris due to CAD erroneously attribute their symptoms to *indigestion* or heartburn. Also, patients with heartburn, esophageal reflux, and esophageal spasm may believe they have angina pectoris. *Hiccups* occasionally may occur in patients with MI and are common during the postoperative period after cardiac surgery. *Dysphagia* may occur in patients with progressive systemic sclerosis, an aortic arch anomaly, or an extremely large left atrium.

GASTROINTESTINAL SYMPTOMS

Anorexia, nausea, and vomiting may occur as a result of digitalis excess. Hepatomegaly associated with tricuspid valve disease or severe right-sided heart failure may cause right-upper-quadrant epigastric pain and fullness as well as anorexia. Abdominal pain due to visceral ischemia or infarction may occur in a patient who has had a period of very low cardiac output. The pain of some gastrointestinal diseases may be referred or extend to the chest or back and lead to confusion with myocardial ischemia.

ABNORMAL SKIN COLOR

Although *cyanosis* is a sign rather than a symptom, patients or family members may describe cyanosis during the history. *Cyanosis* is a bluish color of the skin or mucous membranes caused by excess amounts of reduced hemoglobin. About 4 g of reduced hemoglobin is required for cyanosis to be apparent (see Chap. 63). Severely anemic patients will not exhibit cyanosis. A distribution of cyanosis involving the mucous membranes as well as the periphery (central cyanosis) is caused by the admixture of venous blood at the level of the heart or great vessels. A patient or a family member may detect that the cyanosis is more intense in the feet than in the hands. This differential cyanosis suggests a right-to-left shunt through a patent ductus arteriosus in a patient with Eisenmenger physiology (see Chap. 63). Peripheral cyanosis does not involve the mucous membranes but is the result of slow peripheral flow with accumulation of excess reduced hemoglobin in the setting of circulatory failure, shock, or peripheral vasospasm.

Jaundice may be detected by a patient or by a member of the family. As a rule, hepatic congestion due to heart failure will not produce jaundice. When jaundice does occur in a patient with heart failure, it is appropriate to consider pulmonary infarction in addition to hepatic congestion or cirrhosis of the liver. Hemolysis of red blood cells may occur in patients with prosthetic valves and can produce jaundice.[2]

A history of flush of face and trunk, sometimes accentuated by alcohol, should lead one to search for the other signs and symptoms of carcinoid heart disease[2] (see Chap. 77). Cardiomyopathies due to hemochromatosis should be considered in the patient with diabetes whose skin color has changed from normal to bronze.[2] A slatelike color of the skin, hands, and nose may develop in patients who take amiodarone.

EMBOLIZATION

The entry of a blood clot, vegetation, or tumor fragment from the heart into the systemic circulation results in arterial embolus. Clots may occur in the left atrium behind a stenotic mitral valve, within a ventricular aneurysm, or in the left ventricle of a patient with cardiomyopathy. While many emboli originate in the heart, arteriosclerotic material in the ascending and descending aorta often embolizes to the periphery.[1] Many emboli are asymptomatic. Symptoms of a stroke occur with emboli to the cerebral vessels. MI can result from an embolus to a coronary artery. Hematuria, flank pain, and hypertension can result from embolization to a renal artery. The abrupt development of a cold, painful extremity follows embolic obstruction of an arm or leg

TABLE 10-3 The Old New York Heart Association Functional Classification

Class 1	No symptoms with ordinary physical activity.
Class 2	Symptoms with ordinary activity. Slight limitation of activity.
Class 3	Symptoms with less than ordinary activity. Marked limitation of activity.
Class 4	Symptoms with any physical activity or even at rest.

SOURCE: The Criteria Committee of the New York Heart Association. *Diseases of the Heart and Blood Vessels: Nomenclature and Criteria for Diagnosis of the Heart and Great Vessels.* 6th ed. New York: New York Heart Association/Little, Brown; 1964. Reproduced with permission from the New York Heart Association, Inc., and the publisher.

artery.[1] Emboli from the vegetations of acute endocarditis may produce characteristic areas of vascular necrosis in the fingers or toes (see Chap. 77). Severe atherosclerosis in the abdominal aorta and iliac vessels can be responsible for showers of peripheral emboli with multiple small, reddish blue lesions on the lower extremities sometimes causing small areas of gangrene. An embolic event may be the presenting manifestation of previously unrecognized cardiac disease.

INSOMNIA

The most common causes of insomnia are mental conflict, emotional disturbances, and depression. Heart failure, however, also may cause insomnia. The patient with Cheyne-Stokes respirations (see above) may sleep during the apneic phase and wake during the hyperpneic phase of the condition. Occasionally, patients with pulmonary congestion due to heart failure have insomnia before they develop nocturnal dyspnea.

Classification of Cardiac Disability

Several classifications have been proposed and used for many years for the systematic and reproducible grading of disability due to cardiac disease. Although the complete New York Heart Association method of classifying cardiac diagnoses, originally proposed many years ago, is not widely used now, the portion of the classification that concerns functional capacities[45] is still commonly used (Table 10-3). Although the Canadian Cardiovascular Society's grading system for angina (see Table 10-2) is more widely used for patients with chest pain, both classifications continue to be used in the medical literature and in clinical practice, particularly as criteria for the inclusion of heart patients in multicenter clinical trials.

THE PHYSICAL EXAMINATION

Important information concerning the patient with definite or suspected heart disease is often obtained by a careful and deliberate physical examination, which includes a general inspection of the patient, an indirect measurement of the arterial blood pressure in both arms and one or both lower extremities, an examination of central and peripheral arterial pulses, an evaluation of the jugular venous pressure and pulsations, palpation of the precordium, and cardiac auscultation. Based on the results of this rather inexpensive evaluation, a definite diagnosis often is made, and selected noninvasive and invasive testing is ordered only when appropriate.

General Inspection of the Patient

The art of bedside medicine begins with a careful overall appraisal of the patient. This visual approach is of great advantage in seeking clues to the etiology of cardiovascular disease. Since this discussion is organized according to the specific type of heart involvement, diseases that cause several problems are mentioned more than once. Each disorder is italicized, and its major manifestations are described the first time it is named.

Syndromes Associated with Congenital Heart Disease

Congenital heart disease syndromes may be classified into heritable disorders, connective tissue disorders, inborn areas of metabolism, chromosomal abnormalities, sporadic disorders, and teratogenic disorders (see also Chaps. 62–64 and 76). Occasionally, a particular syndrome falls into more than one category. In the first category, the *Ellis-van Creveld syndrome,* a common disorder in the Amish population, is a heritable form of dwarfism characterized by short extremities, polydactyly, dysplastic teeth and nails, and multiple frenula binding the upper eyelid to the alveolar ridge (Fig. 10-1). Over half the patients have heart disease, usually a large atrial septal defect or a single atrium.[46]

The *thrombocytopenia–absent radius* (TAR) *syndrome* includes bilateral radial aplasia with a persistent thumb and thrombocytopenia and may be associated with an ostium secundum atrial septal defect (ASD) and/or tetralogy of Fallot. The Holt-Oram syndrome, an autosomal dominant trait, combines an ASD or other congenital heart disease with a thumb[47] (Fig. 10-2) that may be absent, hypoplastic, bifid, triphalangeal, or unusually long. *Tabatznik's syndrome* (heart-hand syndrome type II) is characterized by hypoplastic deltoids, skeletal anomalies of the forearm, bradydactyly, and atrial fibrillation. In the *Laurence-Moon-Bardet-Biedl syndrome,* mental retardation, polydactyly, obesity, retinitis pigmentosa, and hypogonadism occur with a variety of congenital heart diseases.[48]

Arteriovenous fistulas involving the lung, liver, and mucous membranes are associated with multiple telangiectasias in patients with the hereditary hemorrhagic telangiectasis (*Osler-Weber-Rendu syndrome*).[49] *Cornelia de Lange's syndrome* is characterized by bushy, confluent eyebrows, downward-slanting eyes, a small mandible, low-set ears, hirsutism, long eyelashes, a broad, flat, upturned nose, severe growth and mental retardation, and a peculiar "chicken wing" extremity with a single thumblike digit (Fig. 10-3). A ventricular septal defect (VSD), patent ductus arteriosus, pulmonic stenosis, anomalous venous return, or ASD may be present.

There appears to be an increased incidence of congenital heart disease in children with a cleft palate or lip.[50] In the *Pierre Robin syndrome,* the cleft palate is associated with a hypoplastic mandible causing a "shrewlike" face (Fig. 10-4). A cleft palate, micrognathia, low-set ears, and truncus arteriosus may be present in the familial *third and fourth pharyngeal pouch syndromes.*

Cutis laxis is a generalized disruption of elastic fibers with diminished skin resilience, frequent hernias, and pulmonary

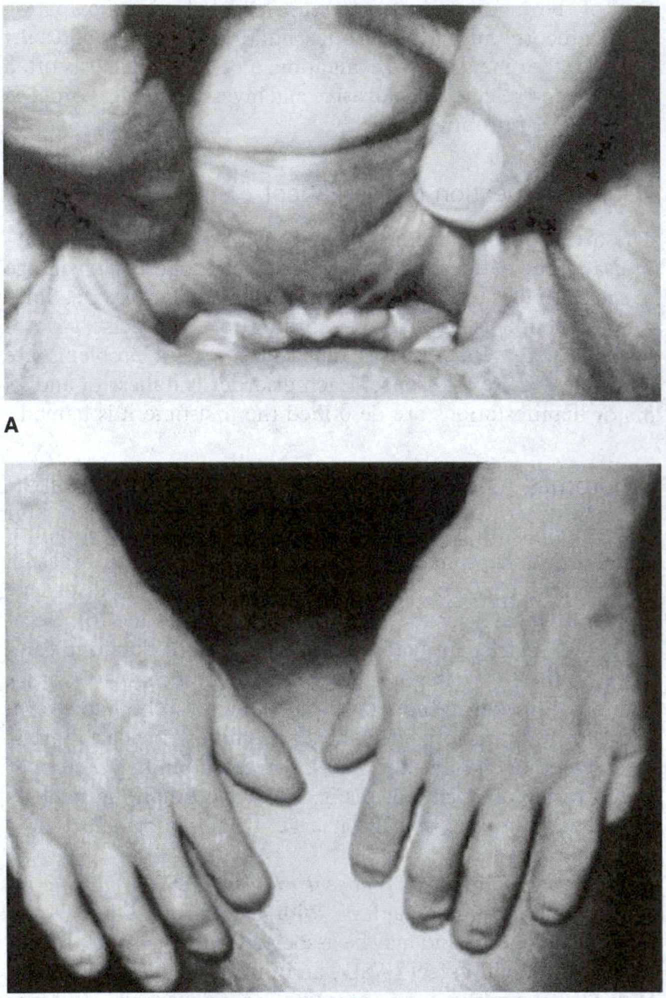

A

B

FIGURE 10-1 *Ellis-van Creveld syndrome. A.* Typical "lip tie" due to multiple frenulum. *B.* Polydactyly. This patient has a large septal defect.

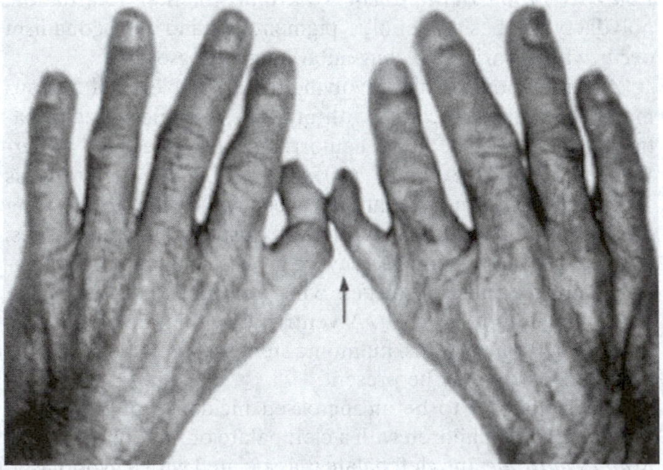

FIGURE 10-2 *Holt-Oram syndrome:* fingerized thumb (arrow) associated with an atrial septal defect.

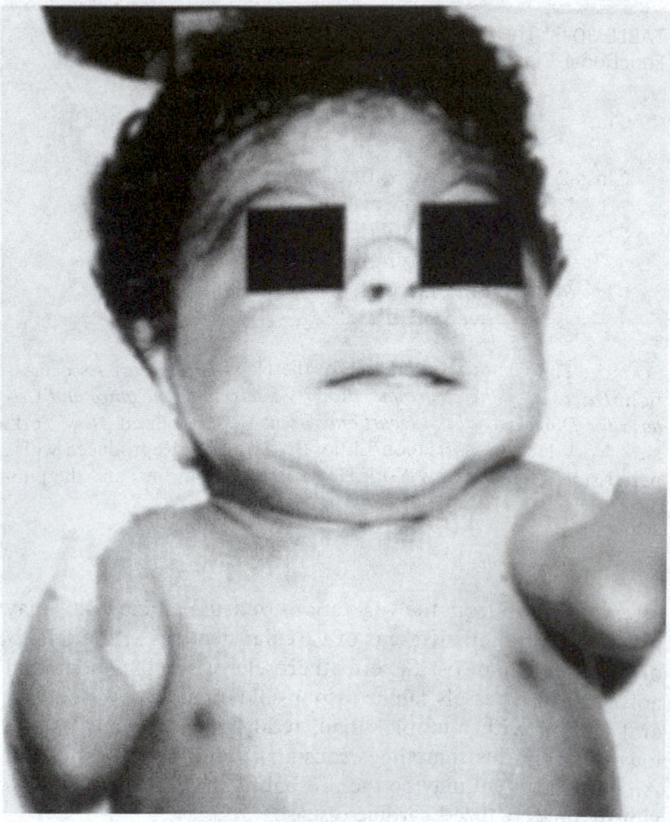

FIGURE 10-3 *Cornelia de Lange's syndrome:* low hairline, hirsutism, bushy brows, phocomelia, and a single thumblike digit. May be associated with ventricular septal defect.

artery branch stenosis.[51] Patients with the *Ehlers-Danlos syndrome* (Fig. 10-5*A*, *B*) have hyperextensible joints and hyperelastic and friable skin that is often associated with arterial dilatation and rupture, aortic regurgitation, or mitral valve prolapse.[52] Patients with osteogenesis imperfecta have brittle bones, blue sclera, and short legs and have an increased incidence of aortic and mitral regurgitation.[53] Patients with pseudoxanthoma elasticum (see Chap. 76), who have degeneration of dermal elastic fibers and retinal angioid streaks, can develop aortic regurgitation and CAD (Fig. 10-6).

Marfan's syndrome, an autosomal dominant trait, is suggested by skeletal features such as increased height, long fingers, narrow palms, lax joints, kyphoscoliosis, pectus excavatum or carinatum, an elongated face, high-arched palate, and flat feet[54] (Fig. 10-7*A-C*). The legs are disproportionately long, resulting in an abnormal ratio of the upper-to-lower segments of at most 0.85. The arm span many exceed the height. When a patient with Marfan's syndrome clenches the hand around a flexed thumb, the thumb protrudes past the ulnar side of the hand. Such a patient also can easily encircle the wrist by grasping it with the fifth finger and thumb of the other hand (see Fig. 10-7*B*). Other signs include bilateral subluxation of the lens, severe myopia, and blue sclera (see Fig. 10-7*D*). Subcutaneous tissue is sparse. Valvular disease is common; patients with Marfan's syndrome usually have mitral valve prolapse (see Chap. 58), minimal to severe mitral regurgitation, a dilated and often calcified mitral annulus, and eventual chordal rupture. Aortic

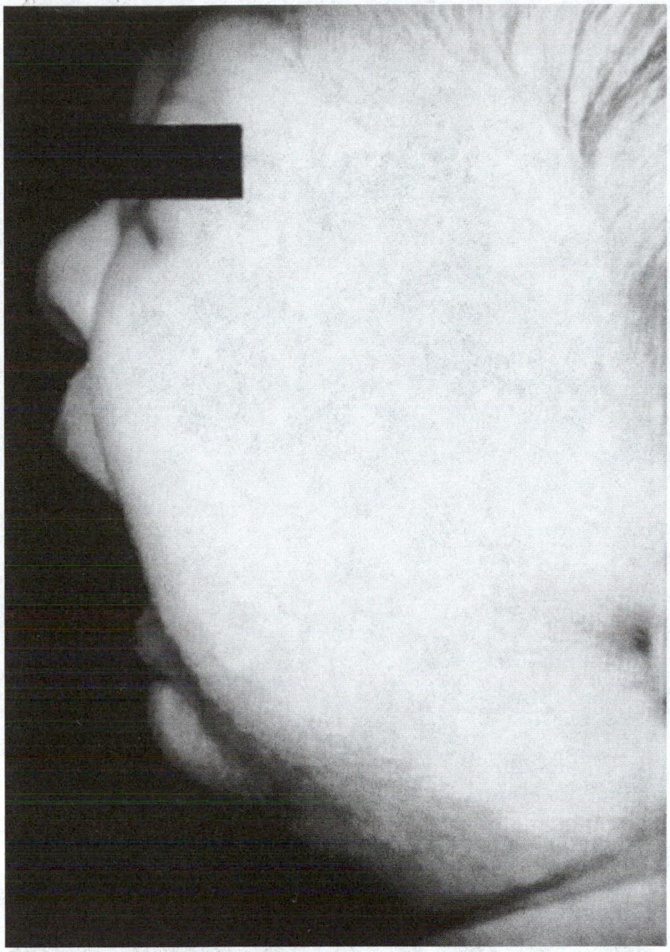

FIGURE 10-4 *Pierre Robin syndrome*: hypoplastic mandible associated with a ventricular septal defect.

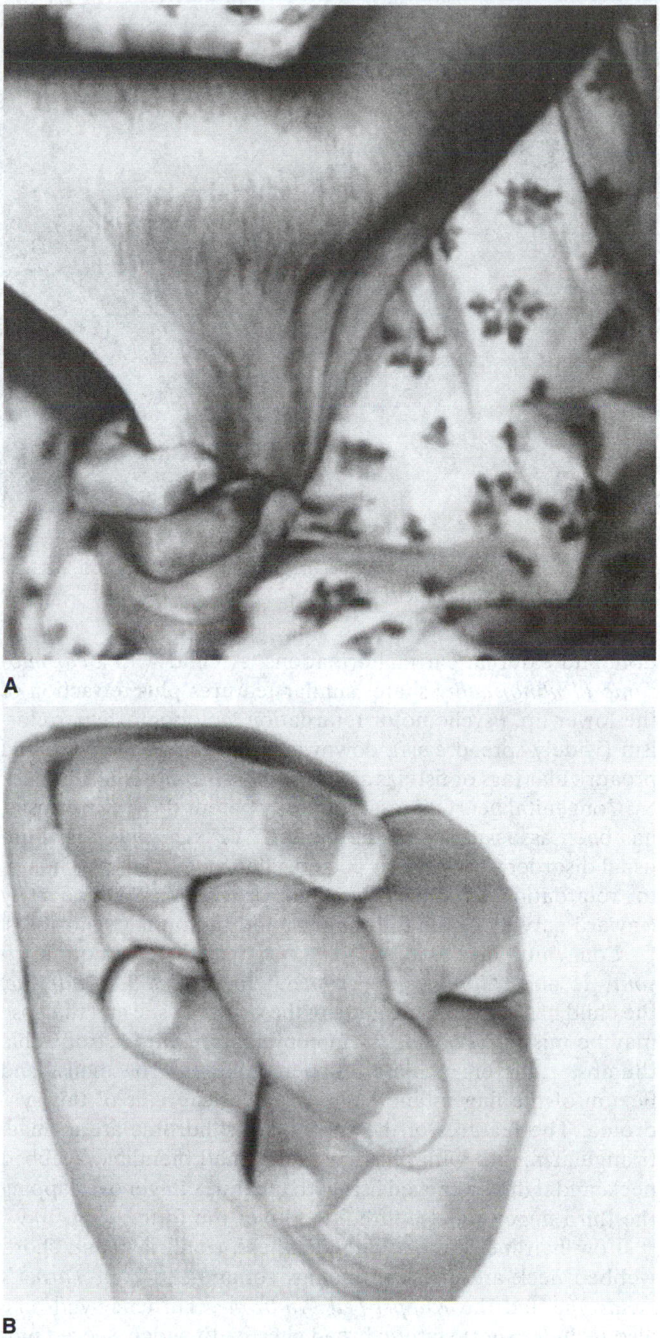

FIGURE 10-5 *Ehlers-Danlos syndrome. A.* Hyperextensible skin. *B.* Lax joints. Redundant chordae tendineae and arterial rupture may occur.

regurgitation is a consequence of a dilated aortic root, prolapse of the aortic cusps, or aortic dissection (see Chap. 76).

Aortic regurgitation also has been described in patients with inborn errors of metabolism including *Morquio's syndrome* (mucopolysaccharidosis IV) and *Scheie's syndrome* (mucopolysaccharidosis V).[55] Patients with Morquio's syndrome are identified by their short stature, short neck, barrel chest, broad mouth, short nose, widely spaced teeth, and cloudy cornea. In Scheie's syndrome, growth retardation, sternal protrusion, facial abnormalities, and cloudy cornea are present. In *Fabry's disease*, angiokeratomas identified as purplish pinpoint skin lesions occur on the lips, underarm, buttocks, scrotum, and penis (Fig. 10-8). Cardiomyopathy, ischemic heart disease, and conduction defects beginning in the third decade are associated with this sex-linked recessive disorder, in which there is a genetic deficiency of the enzyme α-galactosidase A.[56]

Many chromosomal abnormalities have been associated with congenital heart disease. The well-recognized characteristics of *Down's syndrome* (trisomy 21) include a small head, shallow orbits, epicanthal folds, low-set ears, widely spaced eyes (hypertelorism), Brushfield's white spots of the iris, protruding tongue, transverse palmar creases, and mental retardation (see Chap. 64). Congenital heart disease occurs in 40 to 60 percent of patients; a VSD or endocardial cushion defect is the most frequent.[57] Less commonly, tetralogy of Fallot, secundum ASD, patent ductus arteriosus, and other abnormalities are present.[58,59]

Klinefelter's syndrome is characterized by gynecomastia, small testicles, a eunuchoid appearance, tall stature, and long extremities. Associated ASD's have been described.[58]

Patients with abnormalities involving chromosomes 1, 9, 11, and 22 often have congenital heart disease.[59] The findings with *chromosome 1 abnormalities* include a peaked nose, micrognathia, and long, tapering fingers. Children with *chromosome 9 abnormalities* have a prominent forehead, hypertension, anteverted nostrils, a long upper lip, a short neck, mental retarda-

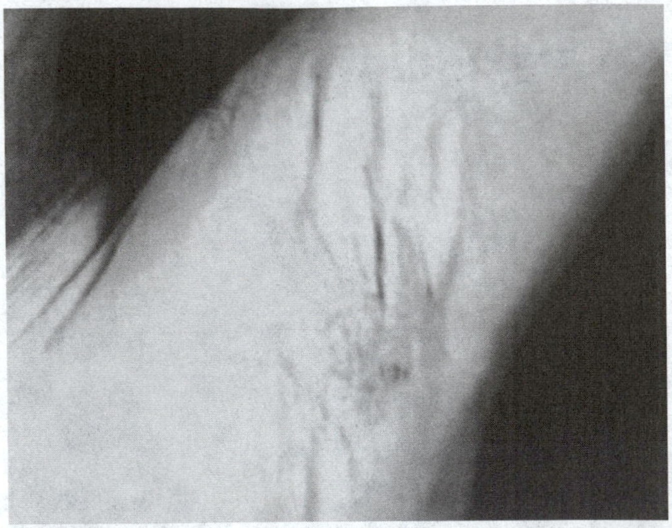

FIGURE 10-6 *Pseudoxanthoma elasticum*: grooved skin in a typical location. Arterial calcification may occur.

tion, and external ear malformations. A child with a *chromosome 11 abnormality* shares similar features plus retraction of the lower lip. Psychomotor retardation, coloboma, hypertelorism (widely spread eyes), downward slanting of the eyes, and preauricular tags or fistulas are clues to a *chromosome 22 defect*.

Congenital heart disease, primarily patent ductus arteriosus, has been associated with the *49 XXXXY syndrome*. This unusual disorder should be suspected when a child has psychomotor retardation, hypoplastic genitals, prognathism, clinodactyly (inward curving of the fifth finger), and radioulnar synostoses.

Congenital heart disease of varied types is common in *trisomy 13* and *trisomy 18 syndromes*.[60] In *trisomy 13 syndrome*, the child has a cleft palate and lip; the ocular tissue and the nose may be missing. Polydactyly in combination with retroflexible thumbs, transverse creases, hyperconvex narrow nails, and flexion of the fingers and hands are characteristic of this syndrome. The features of the trisomy 18 syndrome are a small, triangular mouth with receding chin, small mandible, webbed neck, and tightly clenched fists with the index finger overlapping the third finger and the fifth finger over the fourth (Fig. 10-9).

Low hairline, low-set ears, deafness, small jaw, and short, webbed neck are physical findings common to both *Turner's syndrome* and the *Klippel-Feil syndrome*. Turner's syndrome also includes short stature, broad chest with widely spaced nipples, epicanthal folds, widely spaced eyes, pigmented moles, ptosis, clinodactyly, and a shortened fifth finger[61] (Fig. 10-10). Coarctation of the aorta, aortic stenosis, and hypertrophic cardiomyopathy are the usual cardiovascular considerations. The Klippel-Feil syndrome may cause facial asymmetry, cleft palate, torticollis, scoliosis, deafness, strabismus, and hydrocephaly. VSD is the most common associated cardiac disorder.[62]

There are many sporadic disorders associated with congenital heart disease. An imperforate anus may be associated with a cardiovascular malformation.[63] This may occur as an isolated

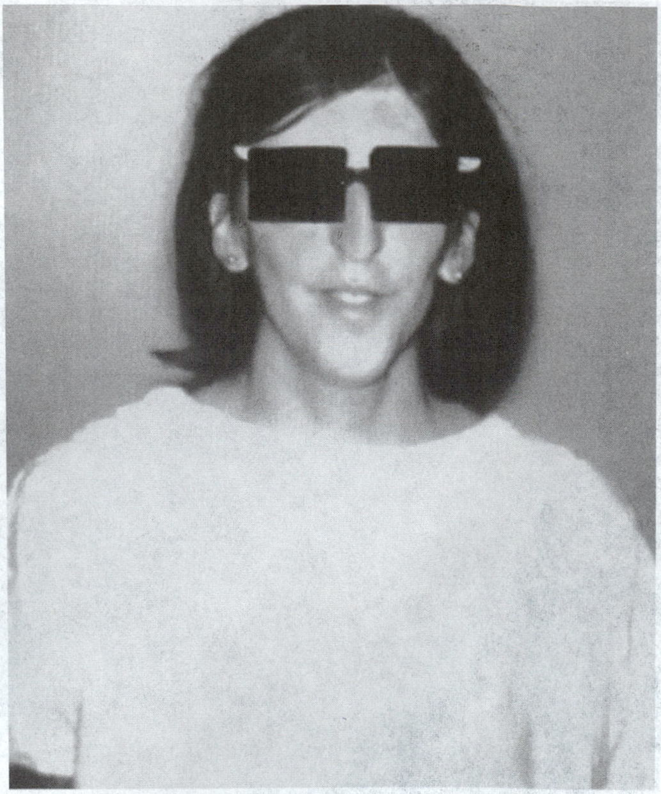

A

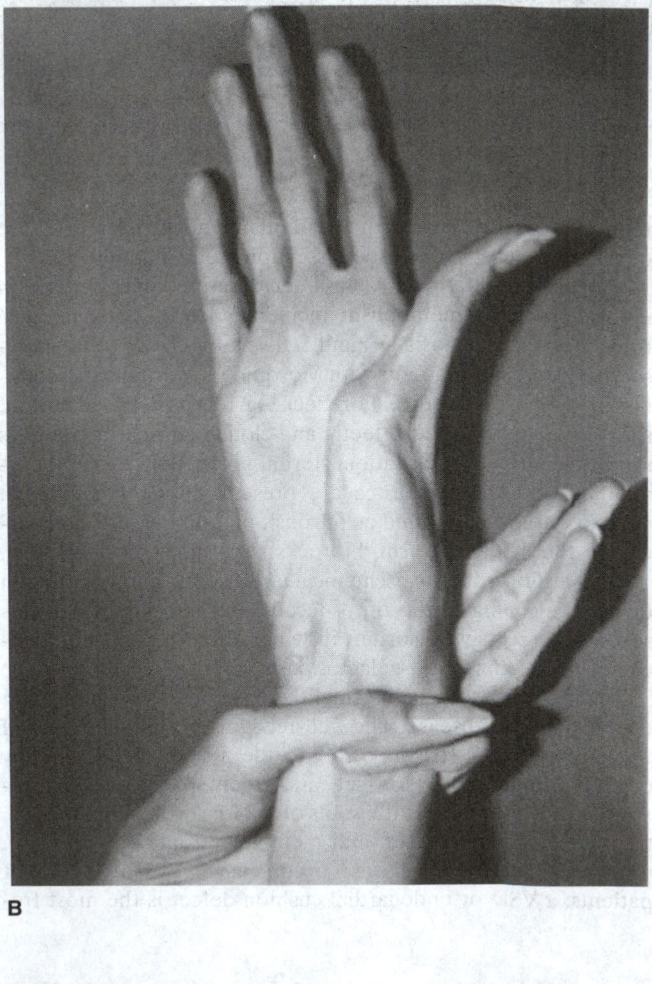

B

FIGURE 10-7 *Marfan's syndrome. A.* Long, narrow face. *B.* Arachnodactyly and positive wrist sign. *C.* High-arched palate. *D.* Ectopia lentis associated with aortic aneurysm and severe aortic regurgitation in a teenage girl.

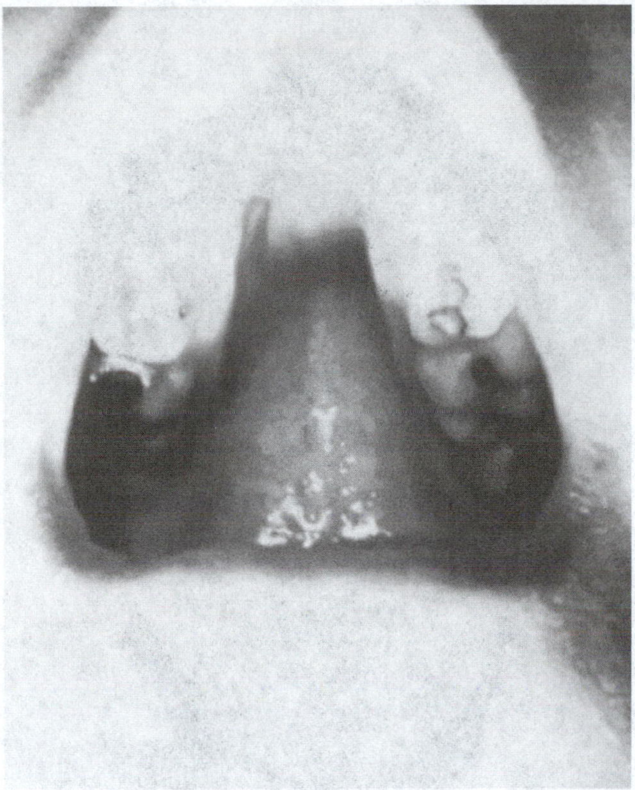

C

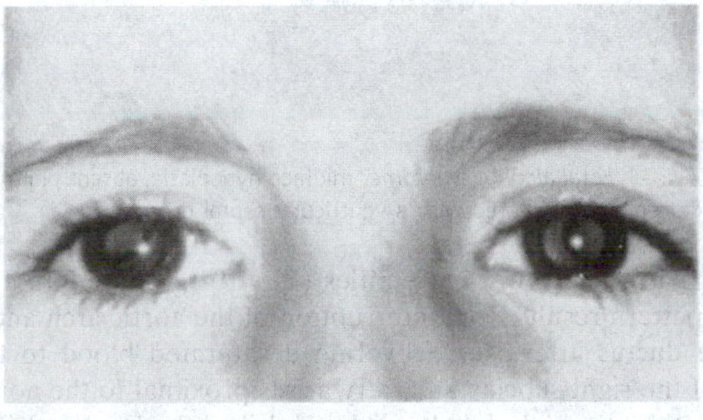

D

FIGURE 10-7 (*Continued*)

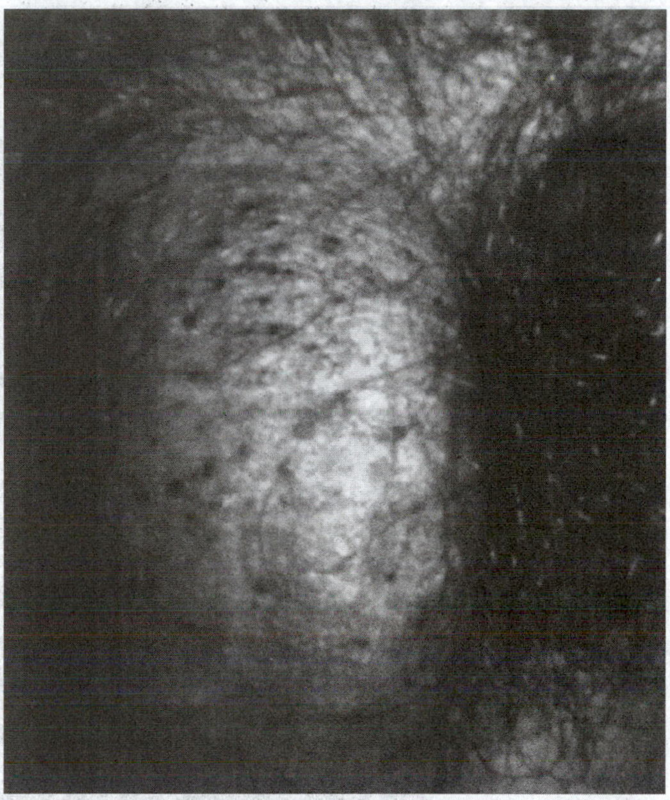

FIGURE 10-8 *Fabry's disease*: dark-red angiokeratomas on the penis may be linked with coronary artery disease.

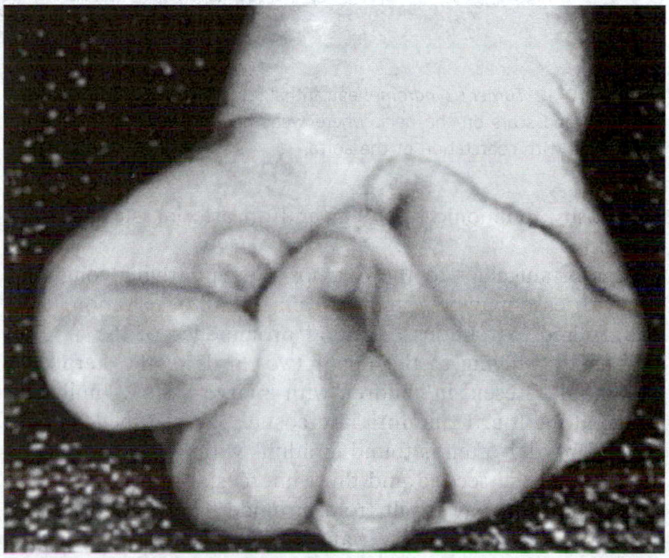

FIGURE 10-9 *Trisomy 18 syndrome*: tightly clenched fist with overlapping index and fifth fingers. A ventricular septal defect was present.

finding or as a component of the *VATER association*,[64] the *asplenia syndrome*,[65] the *CHARGE syndrome*[66] (*coloboma, heart disease, atresia choanae, retarded growth, genital hypoplasia, ear anomalies*), or *cat's-eye pupil*[67] (a fissure of the iris and choroid associated with a cardiac defect). The VATER association includes vertebral defect, tracheoesophageal fistula, and radial and renal dysplasia. A ventricular defect occurs in 80 percent of these patients. The asplenia syndrome is associated with a high incidence of complex congenital heart disease. Cardiovascular malformations are found in 15 to 25 percent of newborns with omphalocele.[68]

Teratogenic effects resulting in congenital heart disease may be alcohol-induced, the result of rubella during pregnancy, or induced by phenytoin, thalidomide, or lithium.[69] From 30 to 40 percent of children born to alcoholic mothers are affected with the *fetal alcohol syndrome*.[70] These children have an undeveloped-appearing central face because of maxillary hypoplasia, a small and upturned nose, an indistinct or smooth philtrum, micrognathia, and a thin upper lip and vermilion (Fig. 10-11). ASDs and VSDs are most common, but many other cardiac defects also can be found. The teratogenic effects of the rubella syndrome include cataracts, deafness, and microcephaly. The most frequent congenital cardiac disorders are patent ductus

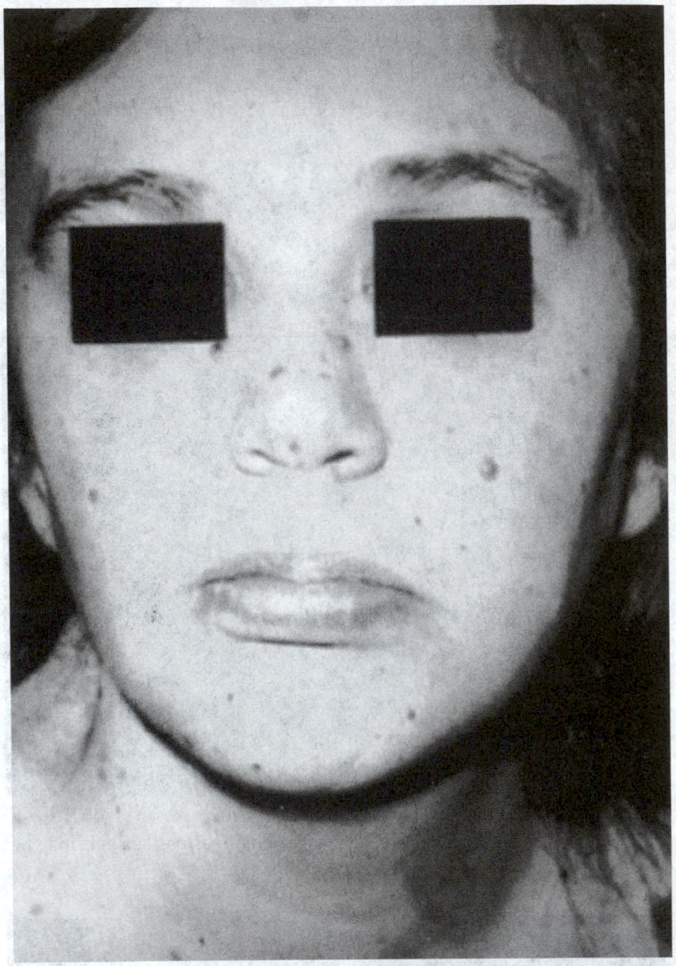

FIGURE 10-10 *Turner's syndrome:* epicanthal folds, pigmented moles, hypertelorism, and scars on the neck where webs have been removed. May be associated with coarctation of the aorta.

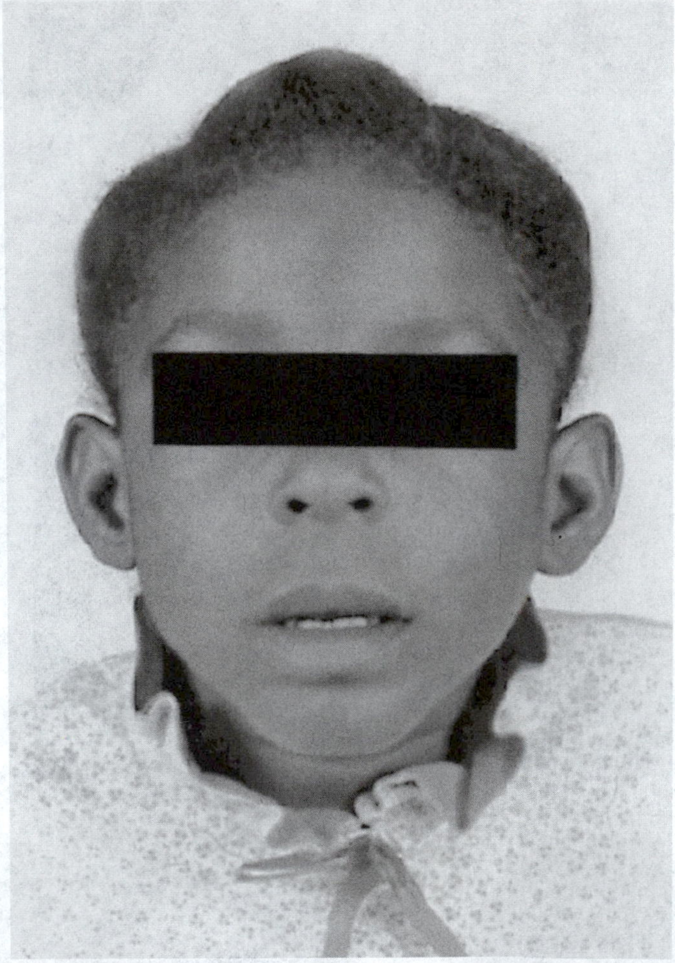

FIGURE 10-11 *Fetal alcohol syndrome:* midface hypoplasia, absent philtrum, and microcephaly associated with a ventricular septal defect.

arteriosus, pulmonic valvular and/or arterial stenosis, and ASD.[71]

Important clues to the diagnosis of underlying congenital heart disease may be obtained from careful observation of the thorax and extremities. Bilateral prominence of the anterior chest with bulging of the upper two-thirds of the sternum is commonly present in children with a large VSD. A unilateral bulge at the fourth and fifth intercostal spaces at the lower left sternal border often is found in adults with VSDs. A bulge in the area of the second and third intercostal spaces at the left sternal border may result from an underlying ASD. Scoliosis is commonly present in cyanotic congenital heart disease. Underdeveloped musculature of the lower extremities compared with the upper extremities occurs with coarctation of the aorta. Clubbing of the digits and cyanosis of the skin or nails suggest congenital heart disease with right-to-left shunting of blood (Fig. 10-12, Plate 29).

Differential cyanosis often provides a clue to exact pathologic anatomy.[72] Cyanosis and clubbing of the toes associated with pink fingernails of the right hand and minimal cyanosis and clubbing of the left hand are due to pulmonary hypertension with normally related great vessels and a reversed shunt, with the patent ductus arteriosus bringing unoxygenated blood to the left arm and lower extremities (Fig. 10-13, Plate 30). The same pattern results from interruption of the aortic arch and a patent ductus arteriosus delivering desaturated blood to the legs. If the right subclavian artery arises proximal to the aortic obstruction, the right hand may be pink and the left hand cyanotic. When an anomalous right subclavian artery originates from the descending aorta, however, both hands are cyanotic. Cyanosis of the fingers greater than that in the toes suggests complete transposition of the great vessels with preductal coarctation or complete interruption of the aortic arch, pulmonary hypertension, and a reverse shunt through a patent ductus arteriosus delivering oxygenated blood to the lower extremities (Fig. 10-14, Plate 31). In this anomaly, the presence of aortic coarctation can be distinguished from complete interruption of the aortic arch. Slightly less cyanosis of the left arm when compared with the right arm favors aortic coarctation, whereas intense symmetric cyanosis of both arms is seen with complete aortic interruption. Red fingertips ("tuft erythema") may signify a small, intermittent right-to-left shunt with only slight reduction in arterial oxygen saturation (Fig. 10-15, Plate 32).

Anotia (congenital absence of the pinna) and facial paralysis may be signs of an underlying VSD and pulmonic stenosis.[73] The presence of any congenital somatic abnormality always should prompt a search for congenital heart disease. Extracar-

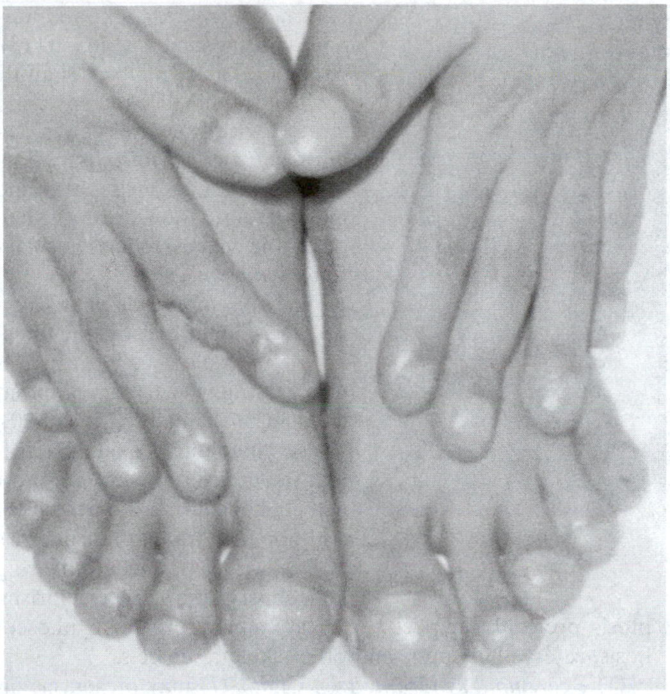

FIGURE 10-12 (Plate 29) *Symmetric cyanosis*. Equal cyanosis and clubbing of hands and feet due to transposition of great vessels and a ventricular septal defect without patent ductus arteriosus.

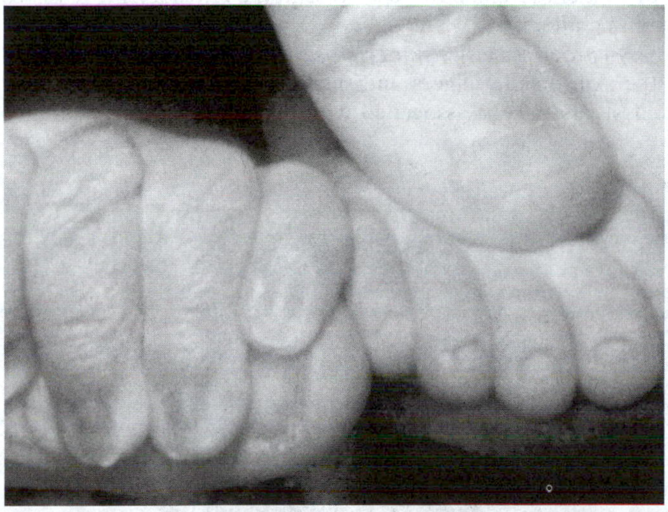

FIGURE 10-13 (Plate 30) *Differential cyanosis*. Cyanosis of fingers (*left*) greater than that of toes due to transposition of great vessels with patent ductus arteriosus.

diac anomalies were found in 25 percent of infants seen during the first year for significant cardiac disease in one study.[74] The defects were commonly found in the musculoskeletal system and were associated with specific syndromes.

Disorders Affecting the Valves

The cutaneous lesions of *infective endocarditis* (see Chap. 73) include Osler's nodes, Janeway lesions, clubbing of the fingers (Fig. 10-16, Plate 33), splinter hemorrhages of the nails, and

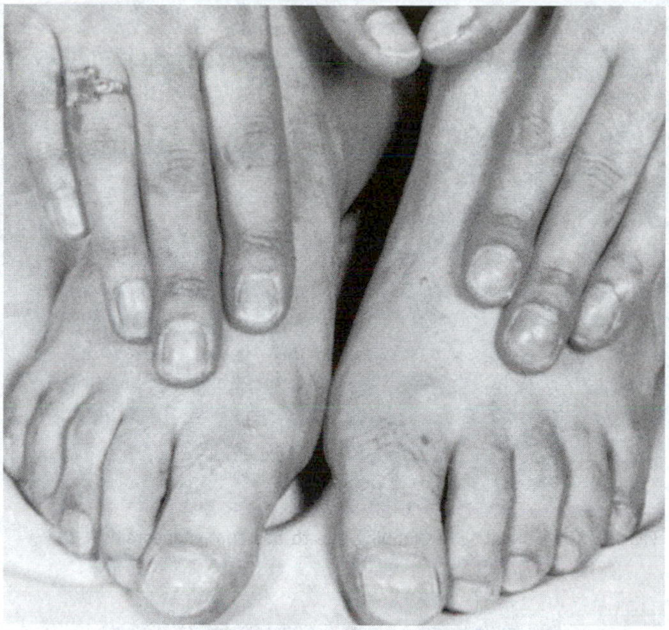

FIGURE 10-14 (Plate 31) *Differential cyanosis*. Clubbing of left hand (compare thumbs) and cyanosis of left hand and all toes due to patent ductus arteriosus with pulmonary hypertension and normally related great vessels. (Courtesy of Dr. Joseph K. Perloff, University of California, Los Angeles.)

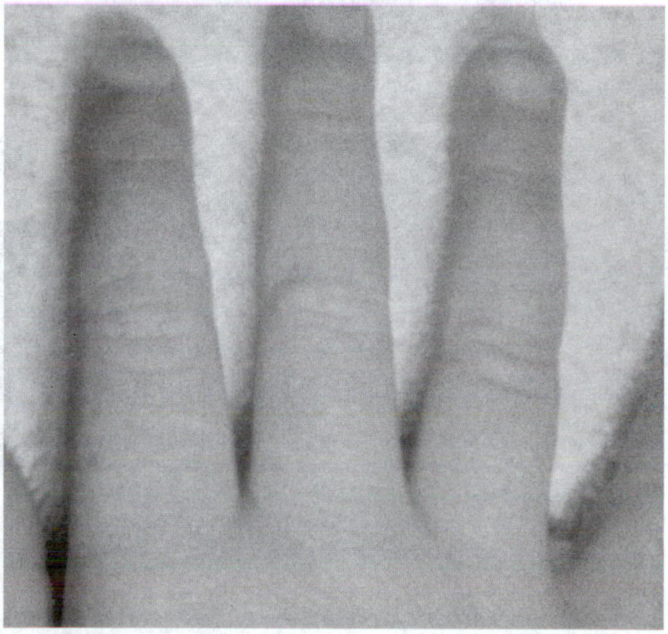

FIGURE 10-15 (Plate 32) *Tuft erythema*. Erythema of fingertips due to small right-to-left shunt from AV canal defect.

petechiae.[75,76] *Osler's nodes* are reddish purple, tender nodules typically found in the distal pad of the finger or toe (Fig. 10-17, Plate 34). By contrast, *Janeway lesions* are hemorrhagic but nontender and involve the palms or soles. Splinter hemorrhages are linear and black and affect the distal third of the fingernail. They are also present in many unrelated diseases and may result from trauma in otherwise healthy people.

Certain features suggest primary valvular heart disease (see

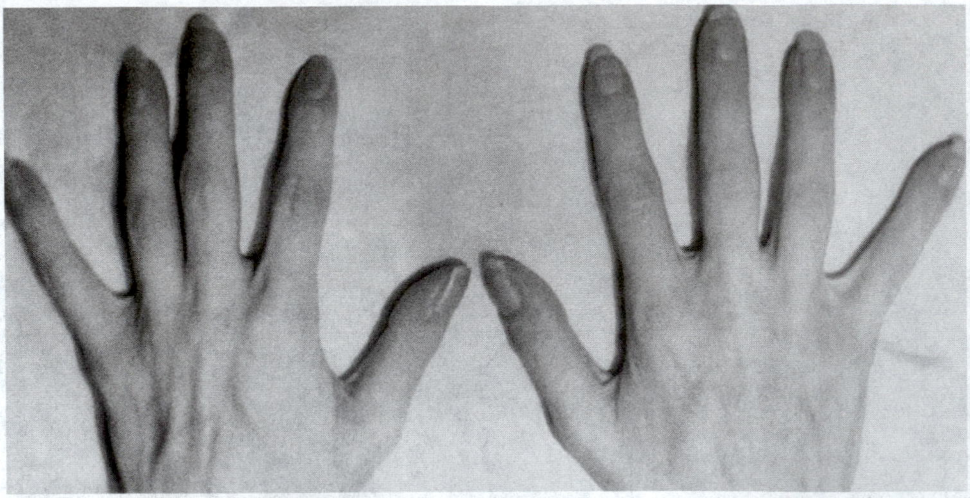

FIGURE 10-16 (Plate 33) Clubbing due to bacterial endocarditis.

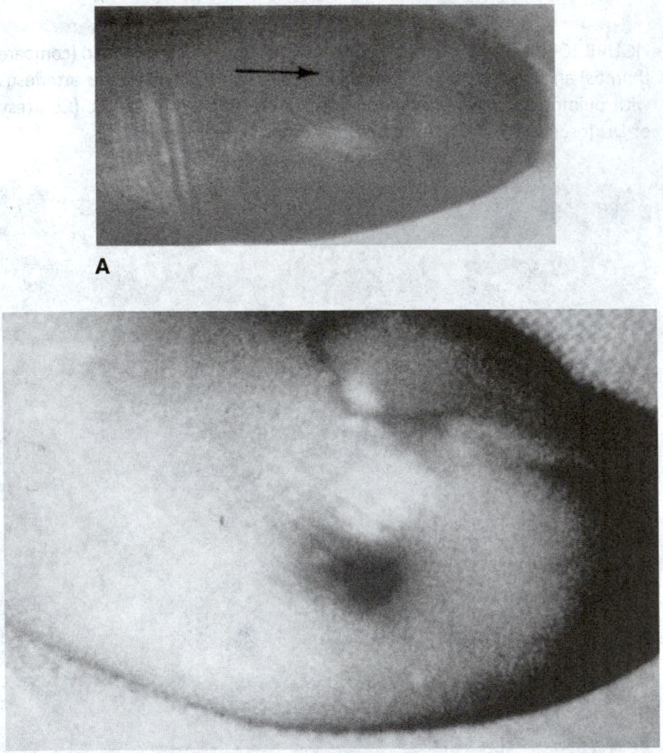

A

B

FIGURE 10-17 (PLATE 34) *Bacterial endocarditis: A.* Valvular infection associated with a tender, purplish nodule (Osler's node) in the finger pad (arrow). *B. Osler's node* from another patient.

Chaps. 56, 57, and 59). Pulmonic stenosis may be part of Noonan's syndrome, Turner's syndrome (previously discussed), Rubinstein-Taybi syndrome, rubella syndrome (see above), the multiple-lentigines syndrome, pulmonary valve dysplasia, or Watson's syndrome. In *Noonan's syndrome,*[77] the characteristic findings include ptosis, low-set ears, downward-slanting eyes, webbed neck, hypertelorism, low posterior hairline, short stature, mental retardation, and normal chromosomes (Fig. 10-18). Broad toes and thumbs, a slanting forehead, a thin, beaked nose, and large, low-set ears are seen in *Rubinstein-Taybi syndrome*[78] (Fig. 10-19). Café-au-lait spots and mental retardation are linked to pulmonic valve stenosis in *Watson's syndrome.*

The *multiple-lentigines syndrome* is identified by the presence of multiple tan to brown macules varying in size from pinpoint to 5 cm in diameter (Fig. 10-20). These cutaneous lesions may affect the entire body but are most heavily concentrated on the neck and upper thorax. Other findings in this syndrome include hearing loss, short stature, hypertelorism, ptosis, prognathism, pectus excavatum or carinatum, kyphoscoliosis, café-au-lait spots, and other skeletal defects.[79]

The *carcinoid syndrome* (see Chap. 77) may present as intense flushing of the face; a chronic cyanotic hue and telangiectasia may be present. Stenosis and/or regurgitation of the tricuspid and/or pulmonic valves often results when hepatic metastases are present.[80] When a patent ductus arteriosus, lung metastases, or a patent foramen ovale is present, the left-sided heart valves can be affected.

In *progressive systemic sclerosis* (scleroderma), tightening of the skin on the fingers and then the hands, forearms, upper chest, and face is associated with hair loss and disappearance

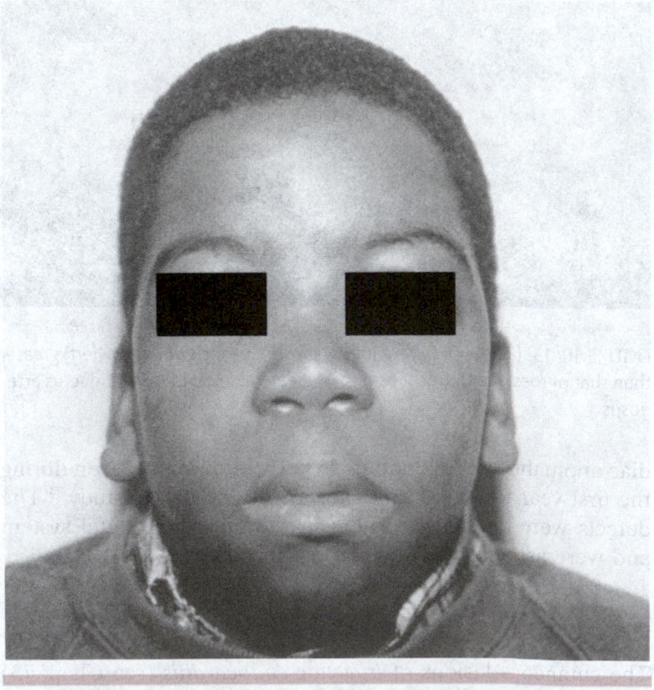

FIGURE 10-18 *Noonan's syndrome:* ptosis, hypertelorism, and low-set ears associated with valvular pulmonic stenosis.

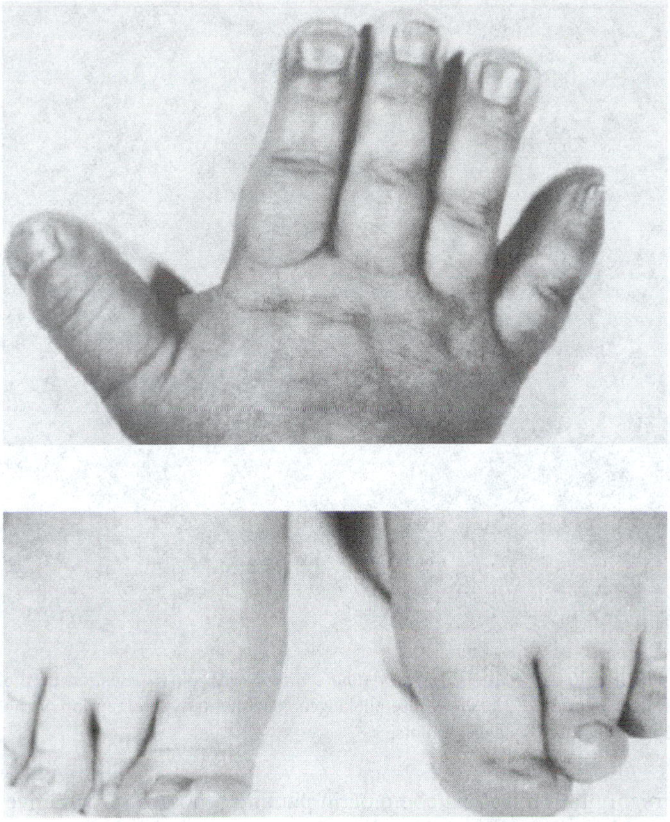

FIGURE 10-19 *Rubinstein-Taybi syndrome* may be associated with a variety of congenital heart defects. (From Silverman ME, Hurst JW. The hand and heart. *Am J Cardiol* 1968; 22:718. Reproduced with permission from the publisher and authors.)

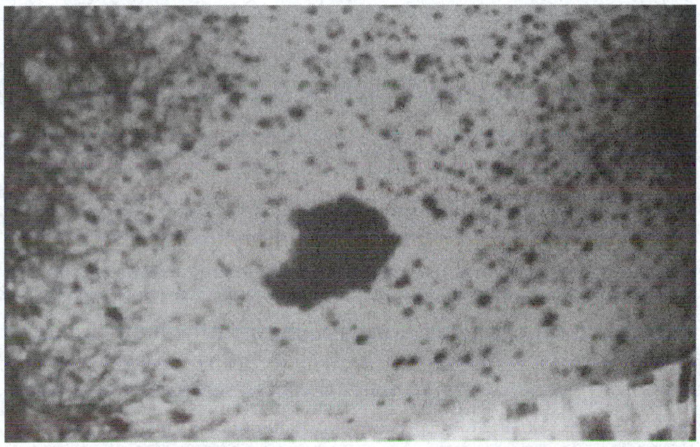

FIGURE 10-20 *Multiple lentigines syndrome:* dark-brown macular lesions of the abdomen associated with hypertrophic subaortic stenosis. (From Silverman ME. Visual clues to diagnosis. *Primary Cardiology*, October 1986. Reproduced with permission from the publisher and author.)

of subcutaneous tissue and skin creases (Fig. 10-21). Flexion contractures on the fingers may cause a clawlike hand deformity. Raynaud's phenomenon is an early manifestation. The *CREST syndrome* (*calcinosis, Raynaud's esophageal involvement, sclerodactyly,* and *telangiectasia*) is a variant of scleroderma (Fig. 10-22). Although valvular changes include thickening of the edges of the mitral, aortic, and tricuspid valves, as well as thick-

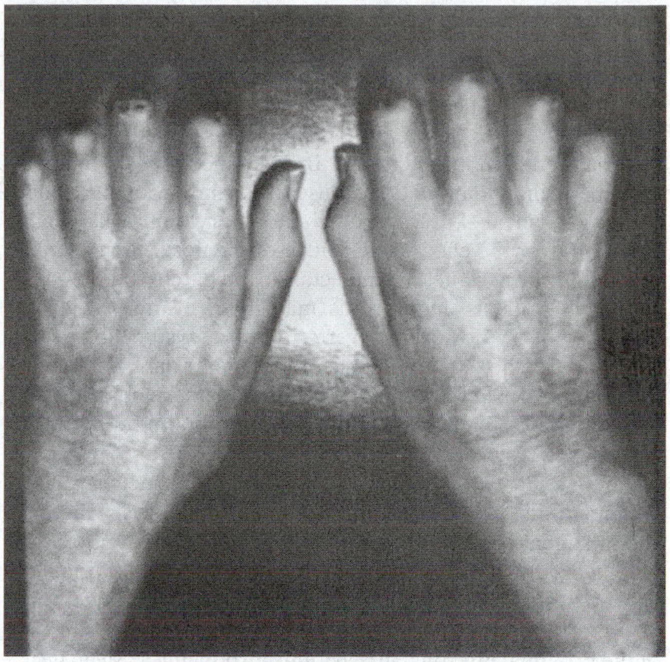

FIGURE 10-21 *Scleroderma:* clawlike hand deformity and shiny, tight skin. May be linked with myocardial fibrosis.

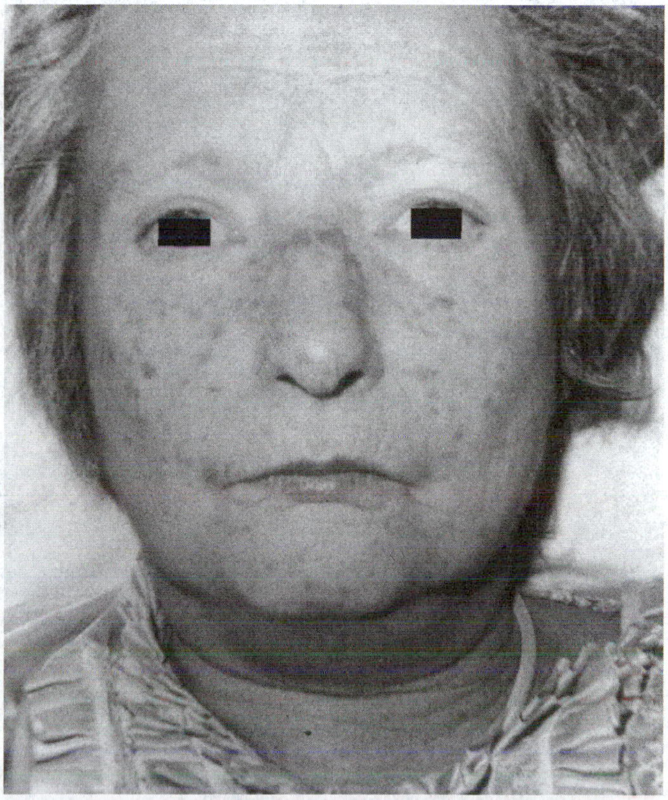

FIGURE 10-22 *CREST syndrome*. Telangiectasia of the face in a patient with Raynaud's phenomenon and sclerodactyly.

ening and shortening of the mitral chordae, the resulting valve disease is rarely significant.[81]

Joint disease associated with cardiac valvular disease is frequent with systemic lupus erythematosus, rheumatoid arthritis, rheumatic fever, polychondritis, ankylosing spondylitis, alkaptonuria, and Whipple's disease. In systemic lupus erythematosus, the joint inflammation is usually symmetric and nondeforming. Typical skin lesions include an erythematous, scaling eruption over the cheeks and bridge of the nose, circumscribed reddish purple plaques, telangiectasia, and patchy hair loss (Fig. 10-23). Verrucous endocarditis may involve any of the four cardiac valves; however, severe valvular dysfunction is unusual.[82,83] Sessile, small, nonbacterial vegetations and valvular thickening causing regurgitation rather than stenosis may be more common in patients with antiphospholipid antibodies[84] (see Chap. 76).

In patients with *rheumatoid arthritis,* the metacarpophalangeal joints, proximal interphalangeal joints, wrists, metatarsophalangeal joints, shoulders, knees, ankles, and elbows are involved with inflammation and subsequent destruction. Advanced disease results in ulnar deviation of the fingers and flexion of the distal interphalangeal joints with hyperextension of the proximal interphalangeal joints, producing a "swan neck" deformity and a Z-shaped configuration of the thumb (Fig. 10-24, Plate 35). Subluxation of the metacarpophalangeal joints with interosseal muscle wasting and thickening of the wrists are common. Granulomatous aortic or mitral valve disease with regurgitation is most common in patients who are seropositive and have subcutaneous nodules or classic rheumatoid deformities.[85] Rheumatic fever, often with cardiac involvement, should be suspected in patients with erythema marginatum, urticaria, and migratory polyarthritis involving the large joints (see Chap. 55). Subcutaneous nodules are found less frequently. Marked ulnar deviation at the metacarpophalangeal joints, suggesting rheumatoid arthritis, can be due to repeated attacks of rheumatic fever and is known as *Jaccoud's* or *post-rheumatic fever arthritis*. In contrast to rheumatoid arthritis, the fingers can be moved freely into a correct alignment, and x-rays of the hands are normal. It also occurs in systemic lupus erythematosus (SLE).

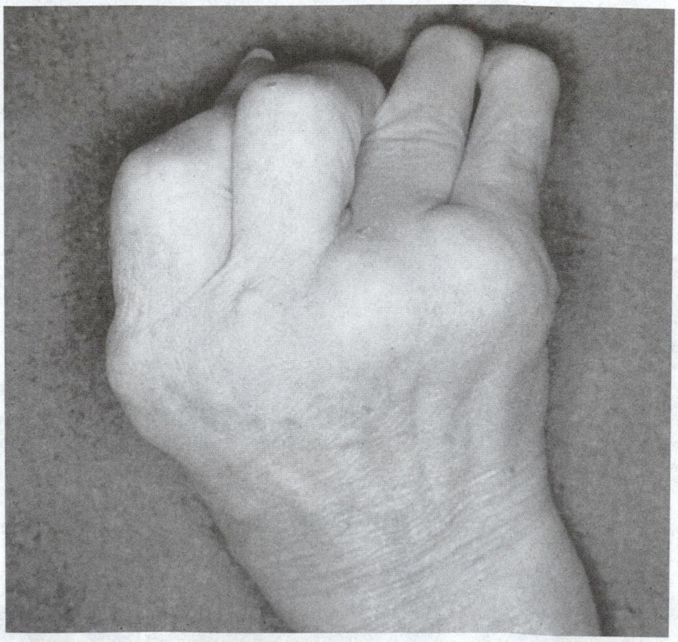

FIGURE 10-24 (Plate 35) *Rheumatoid arthritis:* with ulnar deviation of the fingers, flexion of the distal interphalangeal joints with hyperextension of the proximal interphalangeal joints.

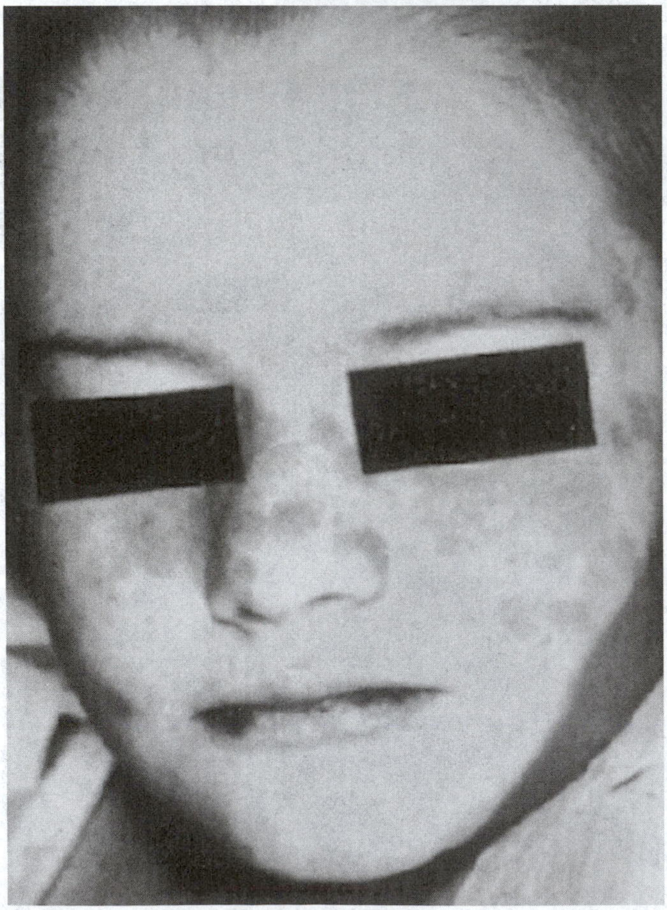

FIGURE 10-23 *Systemic lupus erythematosus:* butterfly rash associated with pericardial, myocardial, and endocardial disease.

Polychondritis causes an inflammatory destruction of the cartilage of the face, resulting in a saddle-shaped collapse of the nose or a cauliflower ear. Aortic regurgitation, aortic aneurysm, and rarely aortic root dissection are associated[86] (Fig. 10-25).

Chronic synovitis involving the fibrocartilaginous joints of the spine occurs in patients with ankylosing spondylitis. The disease may be confined to a sacroiliac area or spread slowly upward. The patient with advanced disease is bent forward, is unable to stand upright, and must walk with a stiff and halting gait (Fig. 10-26). Aortic regurgitation due to thickening and shortening of the aortic cusps from perivascular inflammation and fibrosis occurs in up to 10 percent of patients.[87] Mitral regurgitation and complete heart block also may occur. Cogan's syndrome, consisting of ophthalmic inflammation and audiovestibular symptoms, is another cause of vasculitis involving the aortic root and leading to aortic regurgitation and coronary disease.[88]

Whipple's disease is suggested by the combination of polyarthritis, abdominal pain, and diarrhea. Aortic and mitral regurgitation and endocarditis are known complications.[89] Aortic or mitral valvular disease also may be due to an accumulation of homogentisic acid in *alkaptonuria*. Blue-black, stiff pinnae and

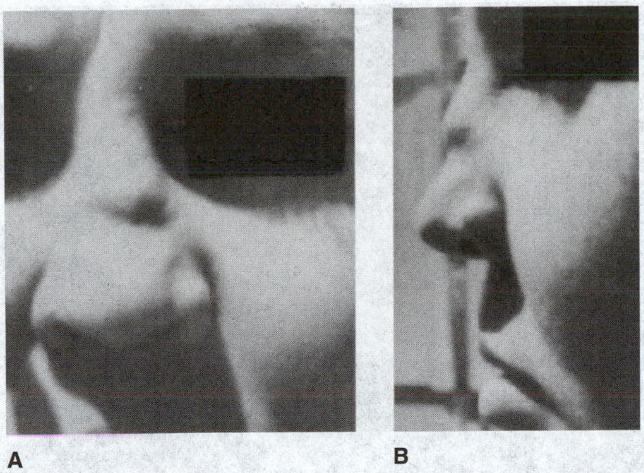

FIGURE 10-25 *Polychondritis. A,B.* Destruction of cartilage of the nose, producing a "saddle nose" in association with aortic regurgitation. (Courtesy of Dr. Warren Sarrell, Anniston, AL.)

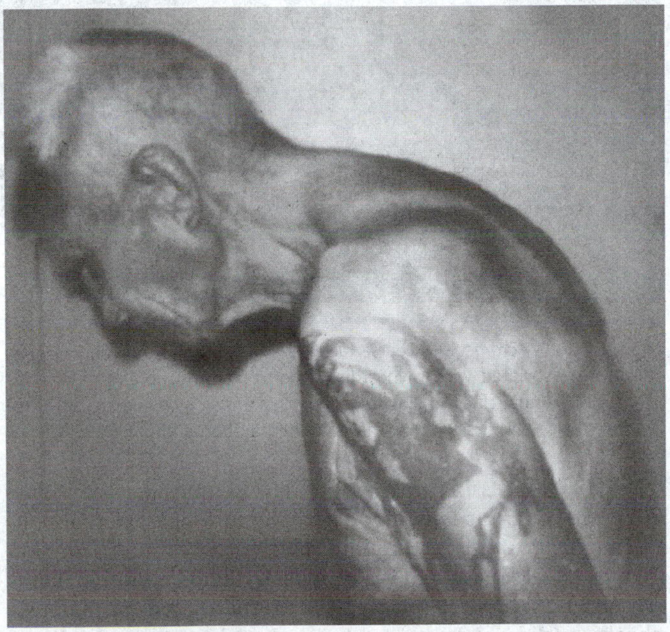

FIGURE 10-26 *Ankylosing spondylitis:* immobile, curved spine with forward jutting of head. May be seen with AV block or aortic regurgitation. (From Silverman ME. Visual clues to diagnosis. *Primary Cardiology*, June 1987. Reproduced with permission from the publisher, author, and patient.)

joints are important clues to this inherited disorder of tyrosine metabolism.

External signs of mitral valve prolapse (see Chap. 58) include a straight thoracic spine, pectus excavatum, scoliosis, hypomastia, joint laxity, and various neuromuscular disorders. Systolic and rarely diastolic murmurs have been described with chest wall deformities due to *straight-back syndrome* and *pectus excavatum* (Fig. 10-27, Plate 36) that may impinge on or displace the heart.

Disorders Associated with Cardiomyopathy

Hypertrophic cardiomyopathy (see Chap. 67) has been associated with *Friedreich's ataxia*, Turner's syndrome, Noonan's syndrome, Fabry's disease, neurofibromatosis, and the multiple-

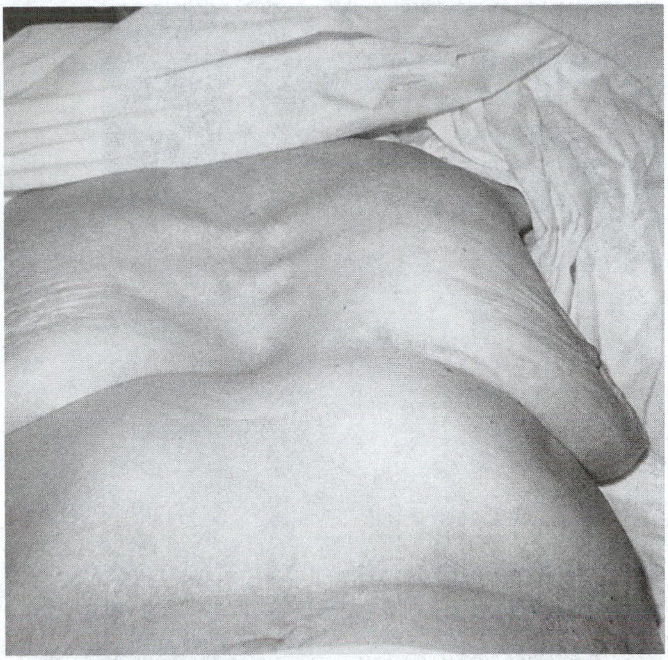

FIGURE 10-27 (Plate 36) Marked pectus excavatum.

lentigines syndrome. Friedreich's ataxia is a spinocerebellar degenerative disorder that results in a broad-based, lurching gait, impaired vibration, position, and joint sense, and incoordination. Kyphoscoliosis and pes cavus (high instep, retraction of the toes at the metatarsophalangeal joints, and hammer toes) are two important physical signs (Fig. 10-28). Concentric and asymmetric LV hypertrophy that may evolve into a dilated cardiomyopathy have each been described.[90]

Myocardial hypertrophy may be secondary to extreme obesity or acromegaly. With acromegaly, the broad forehead, thickened skin, and enlarged nose, lip, and tongue produce coarsened facial features (Fig. 10-29), whereas elongation of the mandible leads to prognathism and overbite. The large, sausage-shaped fingers and spadelike configuration of the hands are typical.[91]

Cor pulmonale and RV hypertrophy may be secondary to pulmonary hypertension caused by *kyphoscoliosis, restrictive lung disease, progressive systemic sclerosis, upper airway blockade* by enlarged tonsils[126] and adenoids, or the *sleep apnea syndrome* associated with extreme obesity.[92,93]

Myocarditis (see Chap. 69) occurs with SLE, rheumatic fever, Reiter's syndrome,[94] Kawasaki's disease,[95] Lyme arthritis,[96] and occasionally, Whipple's disease. Reiter's syndrome is characterized by conjunctivitis and hyperkeratotic coalescing lesions encrusted on the soles and palms, associated with arthritis and urethritis (Fig. 10-30, Plate 37). Kawasaki's disease begins with fever, nonexudative conjunctivitis, dry, fissured lips, cervical adenopathy, and a strawberry tongue. Later, the palms and soles become indurated and purplish red and then peel. A widespread erythematous rash may appear and then desquamate. *Lyme arthritis*, caused by the spirochete *Borrelia burgdorferi*, begins with a red macule or papule and then develops into an expanding erythematous rash with a bright red border known as *erythema migrans* (Fig. 10-31). The center of the rash may clear, indurate, blister, or become necrotic. Multiple annular lesions may develop.

Diseases that cause myocardial fibrosis include dermatomyositis, Duchenne's and Becker's muscular dystrophy, myotonic

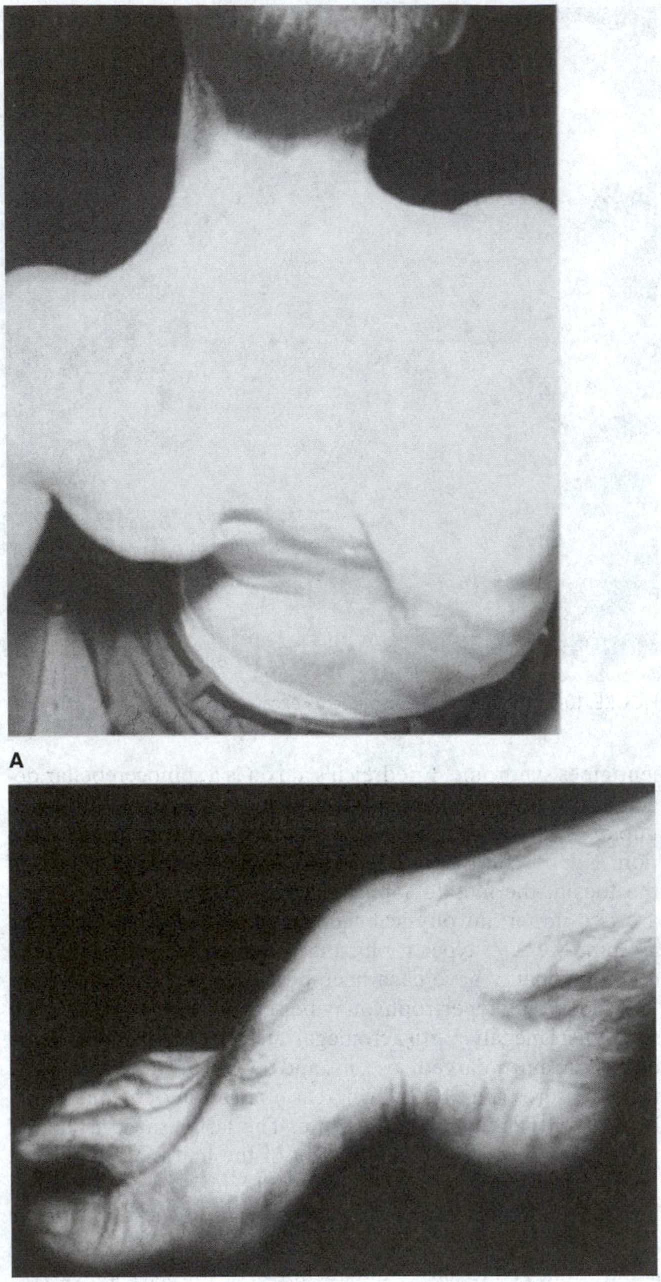

FIGURE 10-28 *Friedreich's ataxia* (photographs from different patients). *A.* Kyphoscoliosis. *B.* Pes cavus. Myocardial fibrosis and hypertrophy are often present. (From Silverman ME. Visual clues to diagnosis. *Primary Cardiology*, June 1987. Reproduced with permission from the publisher and authors.)

muscular dystrophy, Kearns-Sayres syndrome, Friedreich's ataxia, sarcoidosis, and progressive systemic sclerosis (see Chaps. 62 and 76). With dermatomyositis, an erythematous eruption and periorbital heliotropic discoloration affects the face (Fig. 10-32, Plate 38), and a scaly, erythematous rash may cover the knuckles, sparing the interphalangeal region.[97] A waddling gait and pseudohypertrophic calves are characteristic of Duchenne's muscular dystrophy. The ECG is commonly consistent with fibrosis of the posterior left ventricle.[98] In *myotonic dystrophy,* drooping eyelids, cataracts, a receding hairline, and

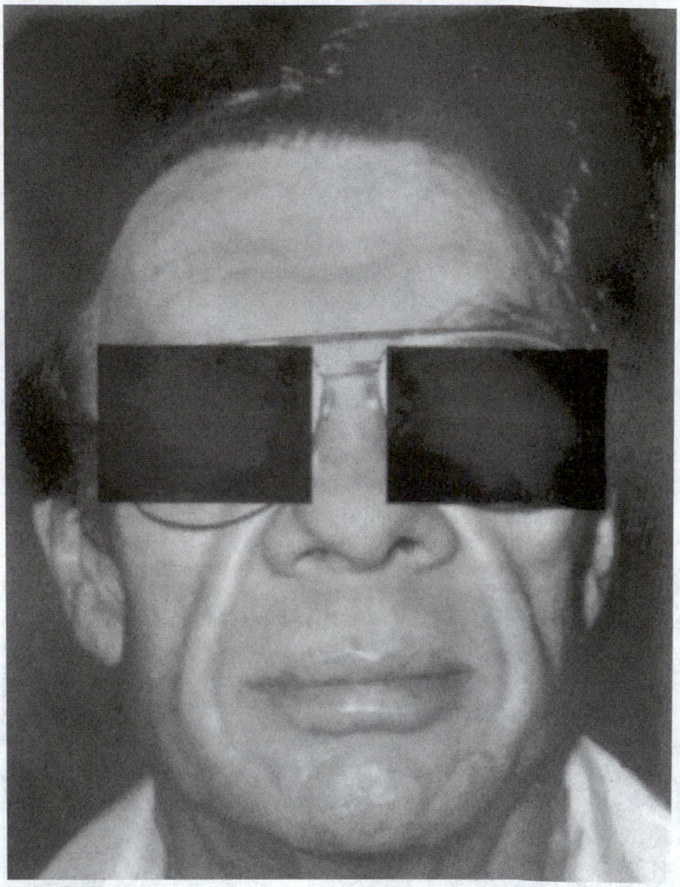

FIGURE 10-29 *Acromegaly.* Coarse facial features, folds of skin, and prognathism are associated with myocardial hypertrophy and fibrosis. (From Silverman ME. Visual clues to diagnosis. *Primary Cardiology*, February1987. Reproduced with permission from the publisher, author, and patient.)

a masklike expression are present.[99] The *Kearns-Sayre syndrome* is a form of ocular muscular dystrophy in which external ophthalmoplegia, ptosis, and retinitis pigmentosa occur.[100] The skin manifestations of sarcoidosis include erythema nodosum, lupus pernio (a red or violet plaque with a predilection for the nose, cheeks, eyelids, and ears), and waxy translucent papules found on the cheeks, periorbital area, ears, nasolabial folds, and elsewhere.[101] Uveitis, bilateral parotid and lacrymal gland enlargement, and arthritis are other signs (see Chap. 68).

Isolated noncompaction of the LV myocardium is characterized by numerous, prominent ventricular trabeculations, deep intertrabecular recesses, arrhythmias, and a distinctive facial dysmorphism.

Infiltrative diseases of the myocardium include Wilson's disease, Cori's disease, Fabry's disease, hemochromatosis, amyloidosis, glycogen storage disease, and sarcoidosis (see Chap. 68). *Wilson's disease* is an autosomal recessive disorder in which copper accumulates in tissues, including the myocardium.[102] Arrhythmias, autonomic dysfunction, and cardiomyopathy have been reported. Kayser-Fleischer rings, usually golden-brown in color and circling the edge of the cornea, provide a major clue to the correct diagnosis.

Cori's disease (type III glycogenosis) is suspected when a patient has xanthomas and a yellowish skin. In *hemochromatosis,* the skin has a bronze or slate-gray coloration; myocar-

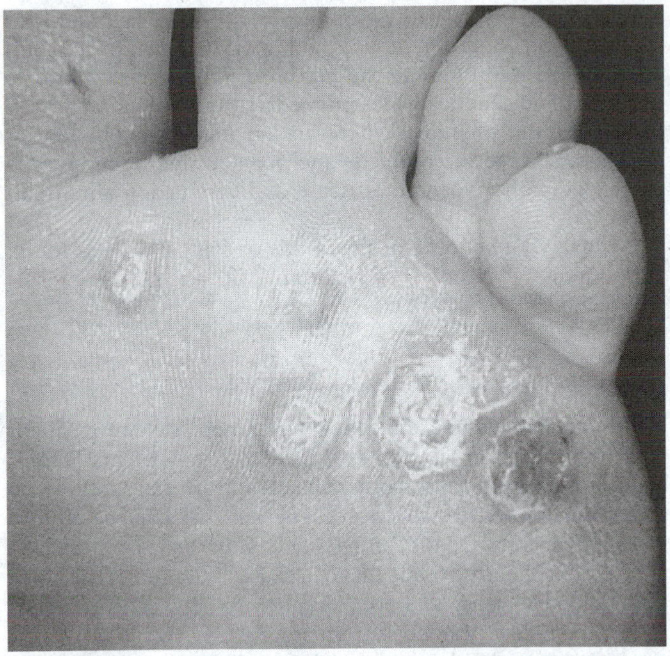

FIGURE 10-30 (Plate 37) *Hyperkeratotic lesions* encrusted on the soles of the feet in Reiter's syndrome.

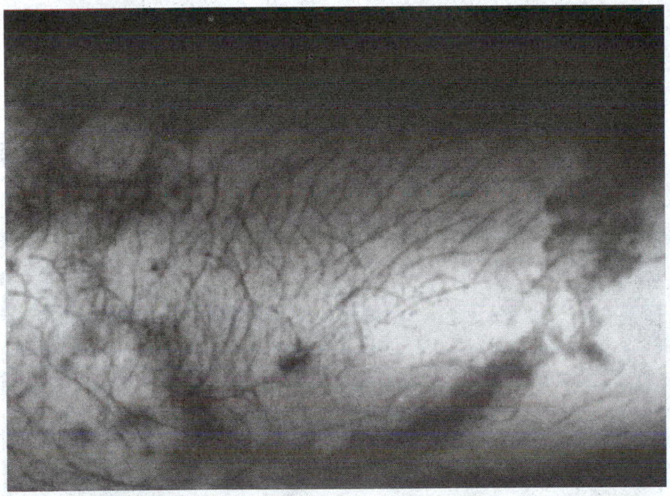

FIGURE 10-31 *Lyme arthritis:* annular expanding rash with a clear central area. May be associated with pericarditis and AV block. (From Silverman ME. Visual clues to diagnosis. *Primary Cardiology*, December 1986. Reproduced with permission from the publisher and author.)

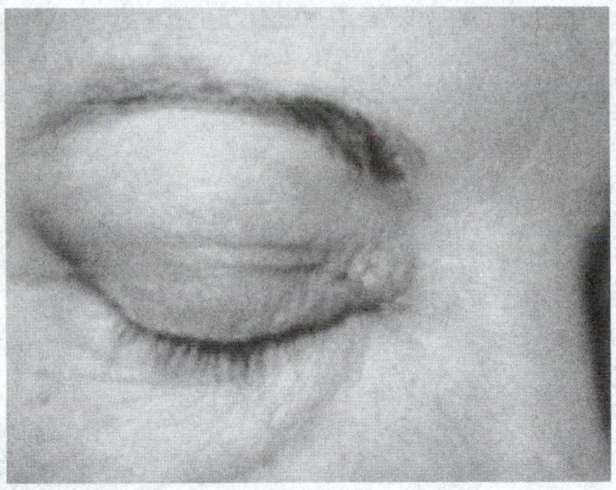

FIGURE 10-32 (Plate 38) *Dermatomyositis*. A violaceous hue and edema of upper eyelid may be associated with myocardial disease.

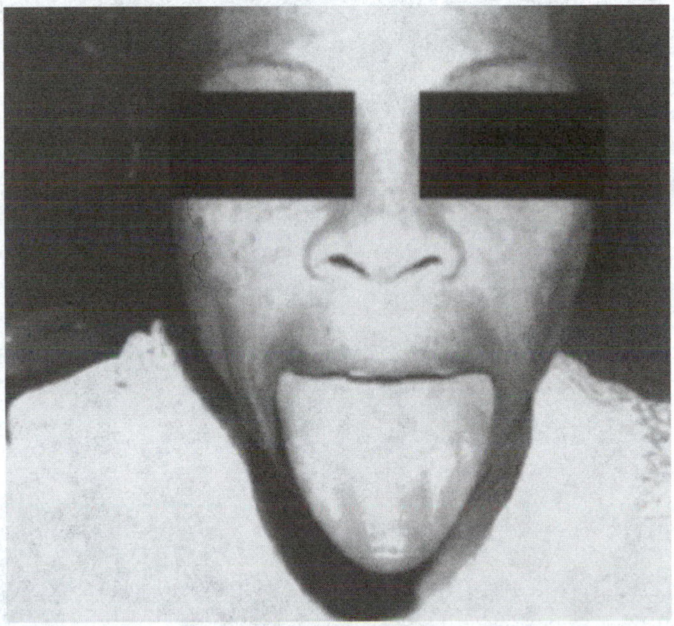

FIGURE 10-33 *Amyloidosis*. Enlarged tongue may be a sign of an infiltrative cardiomyopathy. (From Silverman ME. Visual clues to diagnosis. *Primary Cardiology*, November1987. Reproduced with permission from the publisher, author, and patient.)

dial infiltration with iron deposits often causes a dilated or rarely a restrictive cardiomyopathy associated with arrhythmias and heart failure.[103] Macroglossia and waxy nodules of the skin and eyelids, which may hemorrhage when pinched, are clues to the diagnosis of *amyloidosis*[104] (Fig. 10-33) (see Chap. 68). Glycogen storage disease and myxedema also can enlarge the tongue.

Disorders Associated with Pericardial Disease

Pericarditis may be a result of Reiter's syndrome, Whipple's disease, Kawasaki's disease, SLE, rheumatoid arthritis,[105] rheumatic fever, sarcoidosis, scleroderma, dermatomyositis, hemochromatosis, Behçet's disease, Degos' disease, uremia, mulibrey nanism, polychondritis, hypothyroidism, or metastatic disease among others (see Chap. 72). The components of *Behçet's disease* include erythema nodosum, superficial phlebitis, oral and genital ulcers, and iritis.[106] Patients with *Degos' disease* (malignant atrophic papulosis) present with painless, oval cutaneous lesions that have a white center and surrounding erythema. In this rapidly fatal disease, occlusive fibrosis of small and medium-sized arteries produces pleuritis and pericarditis. In far-advanced renal disease, urochrome pigmentation of the skin and uremic frost are cutaneous manifestations. The term *mulibrey nanism* describes a syndrome involving muscle, liver, brain, and eyes.[107] These patients have a triangular face, bulging forehead, low nasal bridge, growth retardation, pigmentary changes in the fundus, hemangiomas, and constrictive pericarditis. Hypothyroidism, a cause of often massive pericardial effusions, thickens the face and causes dry hair, puffy eyelids, and an enlarged tongue.

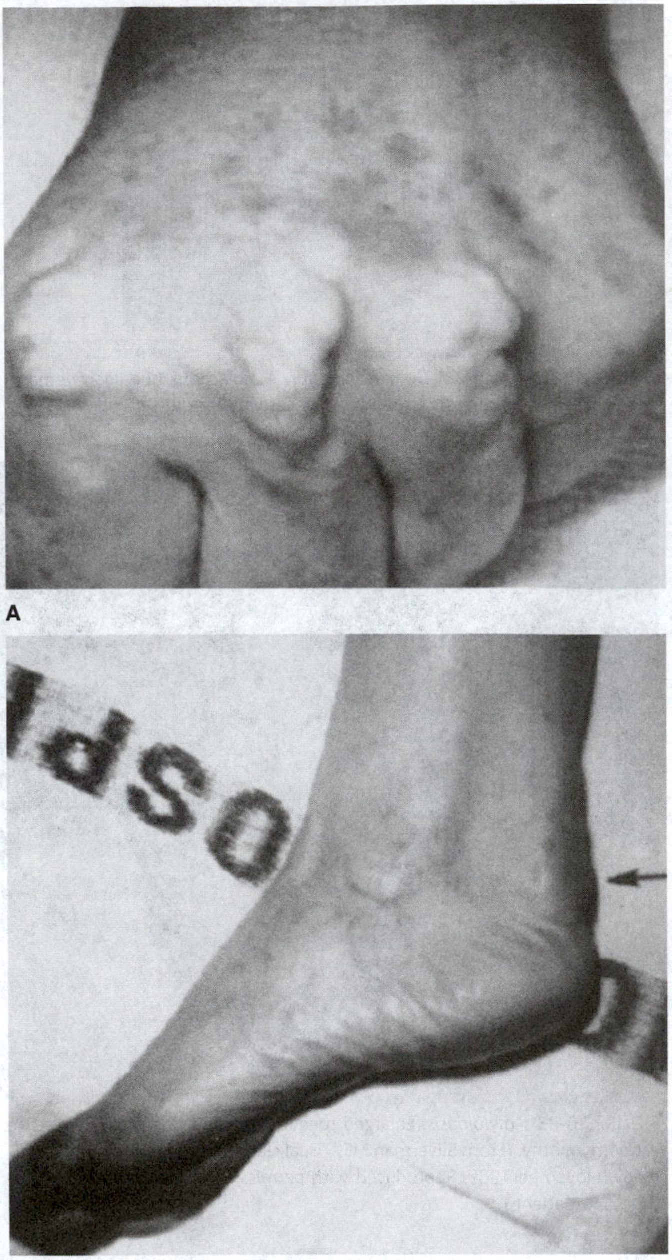

A

B

FIGURE 10-34 *Hyperlipidemia:* xanthomata associated with coronary artery disease. *A.* On the extensor tendons of the hand. *B.* On the Achilles tendon (arrow).

Disorders Causing Conduction System Disease

Acquired causes of atrioventricular (AV) block or bundle-branch block include sarcoidosis,[101] rheumatic fever, gout, Reiter's syndrome,[108] dermatomyositis, amyloidosis, Kawasaki's disease,[95] ankylosing spondylitis,[109] SLE,[83] and Lyme arthritis.[96] In gout, uric acid crystals may form nodules affecting the conduction system. AV block may be an early cardiac manifestation of ankylosing spondylitis.

Inherited or congenital disorders associated with conduction defects include SLE, Fabry's disease, Friedreich's ataxia, Kearns-Sayre syndrome, multiple-lentigines syndrome, muscular dystrophy, myotonic dystrophy, tuberous sclerosis, and Refsum's disease. Maternal lupus is an important cause of congenital complete AV block in the newborn.[82] In *Refsum's disease,* a lipidosis and genetically determined neuropathy characterized by high levels of phytanic acid, cerebellar ataxia, night blindness, deafness, ichthyosis, cataracts, and polyneuropathy have been associated with myocardial disease and conduction abnormalities.

Syndactyly (webbing of the hands or feet) has been found with a long QT interval—a syndrome with a high risk of sudden death.[110]

Disorders Affecting the Vascular System

Aortic aneurysms and dissection (see Chap. 88) are frequent cardiovascular complications of Marfan's and Ehlers-Danlos syndromes. Aneurysms of other vessels and arterial rupture also may occur. A progressive looseness of skin producing pendulous folds and droopy eyelids can be due to cutis laxa, a generalized destruction of elastic tissue that can cause dilatation of the aorta or pulmonary artery and aortic rupture.[51]

Coronary artery stenosis from atherosclerosis can be associated with hyperlipidemia,[111] cerebrotendinous xanthomatoses, Werner's syndrome, uremia, progeria, acromegaly, and diabetes mellitus. *Hyperlipidemia* may be suspected when xanthomas or arcus senilis are present. Xanthelasma usually involve the upper eyelid. When they occur before age 50, there is a strong association with familial hypercholesterolemia and premature CAD. Eruptive xanthomata are recognized as papules with yellow

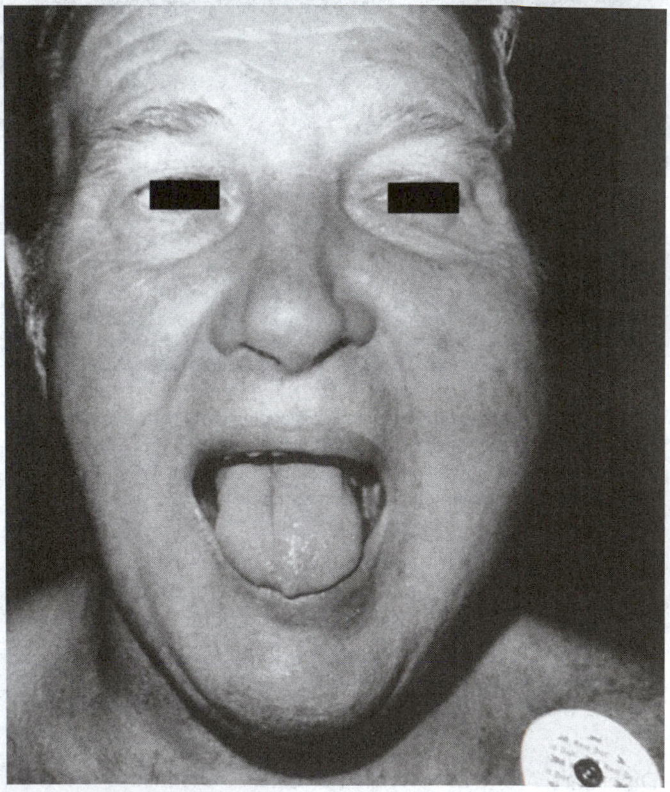

FIGURE 10-35 *Klippel-Trenaunay syndrome:* hypertrophy of left side of face and tongue in a patient with port-wine stains, gigantism of digits, and varicose veins.

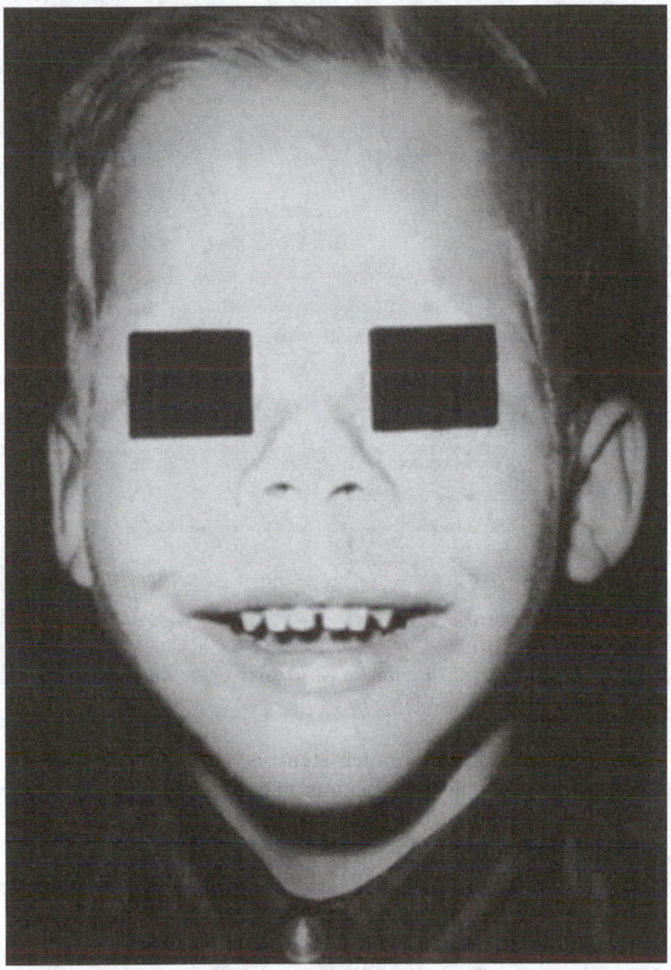

FIGURE 10-36 *Supravalvular aortic stenosis:* turned-up nose, broad cheeks, large mouth with peg-shaped teeth, and large ears.

centers surrounded by an erythematous halo. They often appear with a sudden outbreak of discrete 1- to 4-cm lesions on the buttocks, back, thighs, and exterior surfaces of the knees and elbows. They indicate a very high level of triglycerides and are associated with hyperlipidemia, diabetes mellitus, pancreatitis, myxedema, and the nephrotic syndrome. Tendon xanthomata are firm, painless nodules that thicken the exterior tendons of the hand, the Achilles tendons, and sometimes the tendons of the knees and elbows (Fig. 10-34). *Cerebrotendinous xanthomatosis* is a rare disorder in which tendon xanthomata, cataracts, dementia, ataxia, neuropathy, and accelerated atherosclerosis are present. Tuberous xanthomata are yellow to deep-orange papules erupting over the elbows, knees, buttocks, and heels. They may coalesce or be pedunculated and are a manifestation of hyperlipidemia, myxedema, and liver disease. Large, orange, lobulated tonsils are a finding in *Tangier disease,* in which there is deficiency of high-density lipoprotein.

In *Werner's syndrome,* the skin is tightly stretched over the underlying bones.[112] There is marked loss of subcutaneous tissue, and ulcerations occur over the legs. Severe coronary atherosclerosis often results in MI at an early age. Physical findings in diabetes mellitus may include tight skin and necrobiosis diabeticorum, an atrophy of the skin of the lower extremities characterized by ovoid plaques with central telangectasia and a violet, undurated perimeter. *Progeria* is a rare disorder in which the face is small and prematurely aged, the eyes bulge, and the nose is beaked. Severe atherosclerosis with early MI is a common cause of death in early life.[113] A diagonal earlobe crease and short tufts of ear-canal hair curiously have been associated with coronary artherosclerosis.[114] There is a modest correlation between male-pattern baldness involving the vertex of the scalp in men under 55 years of age and an increased risk of MI.[115] Patients resemble those with Marfan's syndrome because they have long extremities, pectus carinatum, and kyphoscoliosis. Pseudoxanthoma elasticum has been associated with fibrosis of the coronary artery and calcification of peripheral arteries[116] (see Chap. 76). A glycosphingolipid is deposited in the arterial endothelium of patients with Fabry's disease and may result in angina pectoris or MI. Patients with Hurler's syndrome have mental retardation, a large, boat-shaped head, a broad nose, large lips, small, widely spaced teeth, and a large, protuberant tongue. Glycosaminoglycan deposition in the coronary arteries is present.[117] Myocardial fibrosis due to repeated coronary small-vessel spasm has been postulated to be a result of progressive systemic sclerosis.[81]

Vasculitis may be due to SLE, rheumatoid arthritis, Behçet's disease,[108] Kawasaki's disease, and polyarteritis. Cutaneous infarction, nodules, petechiae, livedo reticularis, gangrenous digits, MI, heart failure, and hypertension may be due to polyarteritis[118] (see Chap. 76).

Arteriovenous shunts may be found in extensive skin disease, hereditary *hemorrhagic telangiectasia,* and the Klippel-Trenaunay-Weber syndrome. *Kaposi's sarcoma* or exfoliative dermatitis due to psoriasis may divert the blood supply through shunts in the skin to produce high-output cardiac failure. Clues to underlying arteriovenous fistula as a cause of high-output failure include a barely discernible scar from a knife wound or a surgical incision. Telangiectasias of the fingertips, face, palate, lips, and tongue, as well as pulmonary and hepatic arteriovenous fistulas, are components of *hereditary hemorrhagic telangiectasia.*[44] The triad of anomalies that Klippel-Trenaunay-Weber syndrome

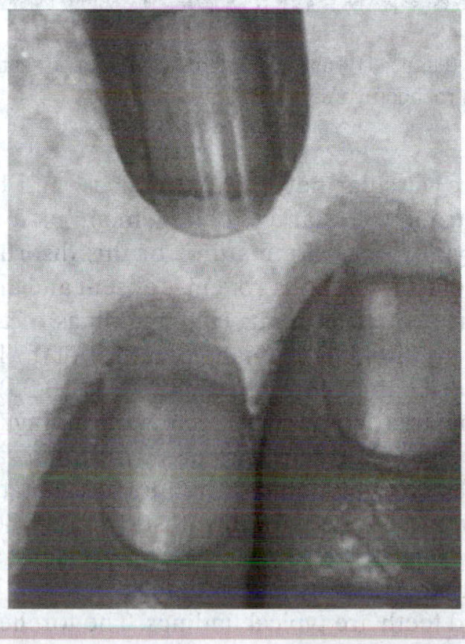

FIGURE 10-37 (Plate 39) Hereditary hemorrhagic telangiectasia. Telangiectasia under nails. (From Silverman ME, Hurst JW. The hand and the heart. *Am J Cardiol* 1968; 22:609. Used with permission from the publisher.)

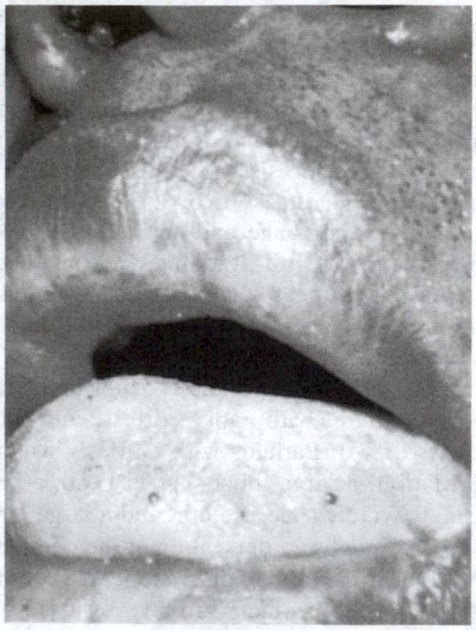

FIGURE 10-38 (Plate 40) Hereditary hemorrhagic telangiectasia. Telangiectasia of tongue and lips may be associated with a pulmonary arteriovenous fistula.

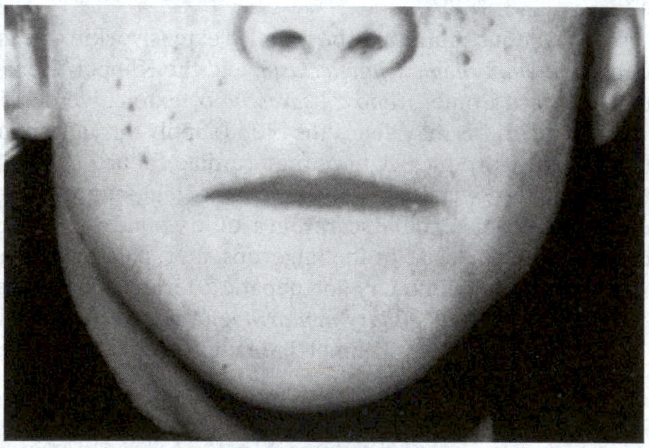

FIGURE 10-39 (Plate 41) Tuberous sclerosis. Adenoma sebaceum may be associated with rhabdomyomas of the myocardium.

comprises are vascular nevus, large varices, and bony or soft tissue hypertrophy.[119] Marked enlargement of a limb(s) and facial hemihypertrophy are features of this disorder, in which part or all of the deep venous system is absent and arteriovenous malformation is often present. Hemangiomas of the skin also may indicate multinodular hemangiomatosis of the liver, a cause of high-output heart failure in infancy (Fig. 10-35).

Stenosis of large arteries may occur with supravalvular aortic stenosis, rubella syndrome, Turner's syndrome, and neurofibromatosis. The face of a child with supravalvular aortic stenosis (Williams syndrome) is almost diagnostic (Fig. 10-36). The head is small, with an elflike appearance; the cheeks are full and baggy; and the mouth is large.[120] Thick lips and peg-shaped, widely spaced teeth are typical findings. The forehead is prominent and broad. Mental retardation is often present. The supravalvular aortic stenosis may be a localized ridge or a diffuse narrowing of the aorta beginning just above the sinuses of Valsalva. Pulmonic artery branch stenosis is frequently present. Coarctation of the aorta is a common cardiac lesion in Turner's syndrome,[61] and neurofibromatosis has been associated with renal artery stenosis.

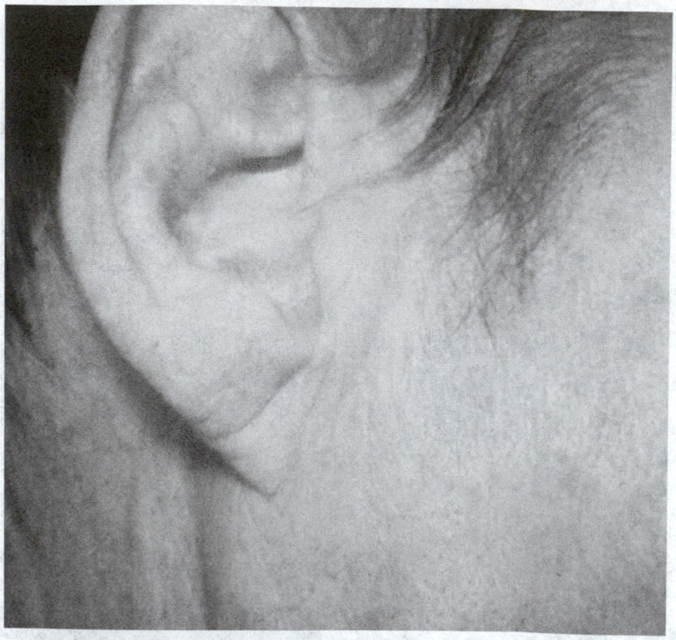

FIGURE 10-40 (Plate 42) Horizontal ear creases often are associated with the presence of extensive CAD.

Facial swelling and jugular venous distention may be early signs of *superior vena caval obstruction* from clot or tumor.

Miscellaneous Disorders

Multiple lentigines, cutaneous myxomas, myxoid fibroadenomas of the breast, and various endocrine abnormalities are features of a recently described inherited disorder in which single or multiple cardiac myxomas occur.[121] Telangiectasia of the tongue and lips or under the fingernails may be associated with a pulmonary arteriovenous fistula (Figs. 10-37 and 10-38, Plates 39 and 40). A susceptibility to atrial fibrillation and atrial flutter has been documented in patients who have facioscapulohumeral muscular dystrophy.[122] Sinus node dysfunction, elbow contractures, and humeroperoneal weakness are manifestations of Emery-Dreifuss muscular dystrophy.[123]

Single or multiple rhabdomyomas may develop within the myocardium and cause heart failure, valvular obstruction, or arrhythmias in patients with tuberous sclerosis[124] (Fig. 10-39, Plate 41). The diagnosis is suggested by the presence of yellow-brown angiofibromas (adenoma sebaceum) on the face, subungual fibromas around the fingernail, café-au-lait spots, and subcutaneous nodules. Finally, horizontal ear creases often are associated with the presence of extensive CAD (Fig. 10-40, Plate 42).

MEASUREMENT OF ARTERIAL BLOOD PRESSURE

A pneumatic cuff with a mercury or aneroid manometer for the noninvasive assessment of arterial blood pressure is the most commonly used method for determining the status of the circulation and the interaction between the heart and arterial system. Blood pressure deviations from normal often provide important diagnostic information in patients with a variety of cardiac and noncardiac diseases. Accordingly, the blood pressure is best recorded by the physician during his or her *initial* physical examination.

Physical Determinants of the Arterial Pressure

The arterial blood pressure, a measure of lateral force per unit area of vascular wall, is quantitated as millimeters of mercury or dynes per square centimeter. The factors responsible for the peak systolic blood pressure include the volume and velocity of LV ejection, the peripheral arteriolar resistance, the distensibility of the arterial wall, the viscosity of the blood, and the end-diastolic volume in the arterial system.[125] The subsequent diminution in pressure during diastole is, in turn, determined by blood viscosity, arterial distensibility, peripheral resistance to flow, and length of the cardiac cycle.[125] Important physical factors affecting arterial distensibility include (1) the elastic modulus of the arterial wall, the ratio of stress (force acting to deform the wall) to strain (the proportional deformation produced), and (2) the geometry of the arterial wall, i.e., the internal radius (r) and wall thickness (h), which govern wall tension (T) according to the modified Laplace equation $T = Pr/h$, where P is intravascular pressure. A decrease in elasticity or an increase in radius results in diminished distensibility and a greater rise in pressure per unit volume of blood.[126]

The mean arterial pressure is the product of the cardiac output and the total peripheral resistance, the latter often being increased by many mechanisms, including α-adrenergic stimulation, the renin-angiotensin system, or other circulating hormonal or humoral factors.[127]

Methods for Measuring the Arterial Pressure

DIRECT METHODS

In 1733, Stephen Hales recorded the arterial pressures in animals by cannulation and use of a blood-filled glass column.[128] Current techniques for the direct and continuous measurement of arterial pressure use the electromanometer, a transducer that converts mechanical energy into an electric signal suitable for amplification, display, and recording. The artery is cannulated with a saline-filled catheter or needle that mechanically couples the circulation to the arterial manometer. Pressures are recorded using atmospheric pressure as the "zero" reference level, and intravascular pressures are further referenced to the level of the heart by addition or subtraction of a gravitation factor. The gravitation factor is expressed by the formula pgh, where p is the density of blood (in grams per milliliter), g is the acceleration due to gravity (980 cm/s), and h is the transducer height (centimeters) above or below the horizontal plane of the heart.

The strain-gauge manometer is commonly used for the precise and accurate measurement of the arterial pressure. However, error may originate in the catheter or coupling system, in which the properties of inertia, friction, and elasticity interact to produce damping of the frequency response. Systems may be overdamped or underdamped, both of which can result in signal distortion. Nevertheless, the appropriate combination of an inelastic cardiac catheter and connecting tube filled with bubble-free fluid produces "critical" damping in which the system response is constant to some desirable frequency level and adequate for the clinical recording of intravascular pressures.[125]

Measurement errors also occur when an end-hole catheter is positioned axial to flow in a vessel and may become especially important during high arterial flow, when kinetic energy may exceed 10 percent of the total fluid energy. Also, pressure transients due to catheter whip can falsely elevate the measured arterial pressure.[125]

Miniature, self-flushing strain-gauge manometers attached directly to an intravascular catheter or needle eliminate many of the problems related to transducer mounting and flushing and overdamping by connective tubing. The most satisfactory method for reducing measurement errors, however, is the use of intravascular electromanometers mounted on cardiac catheters or surgically implanted in the vascular wall.

INDIRECT METHODS

The invention of the pneumatic cuff manometer (Riva-Rocci, 1896) and the subsequent discovery and use of the arterial sounds (Korotkoff, 1905) permitted indirect measurement of the arterial pressure. The mercury manometer is the "gold standard," and the more fragile aneroid manometer should be calibrated against the mercury manometer at least every 6 months. Semiautomatic electronic devices, if used, should be validated according to Association for the Advancement of Medical Instrumentation (AAMI) guidelines.[129] The most commonly used noninvasive method is based on the auscultatory detection of low-pitched Korotkoff sounds over a peripheral artery at a point distal to cuff compression of the artery. McCutcheon and Rushmer[130] described two major components of these sounds: the initial transient (k_{-i}) and the compression murmur (k_c), which coincide with the opening tap and rumble sounds of Rodbard.[131] The initial sound k_{-i} occurs when cuff pressure reaches arterial pressure and likely results from abrupt arterial opening and vascular distention. The intensity of this initial sound depends on the slope of the pressure pulse and the level of the distal arterial pressure at the time of arterial opening, the sound being louder with vasodilatation and high-velocity flow and softer with arterial constriction or circulatory collapse. The initial transient is probably caused by oscillation of the arterial walls as the occluded segment is suddenly opened by systolic pressure, and the compression murmur is caused by a turbulent jet of flow distal to the partially compressed segment.

The Korotkoff sounds have been divided into five phases occurring in sequence as the occluding pressure declines (Table 10-4). To avoid error, the observer must be prepared to recognize two normal Korotkoff sound variations associated with blood pressure (BP) reading. (1) The *ausculatory gap* is a period of silence occurring during Korotkoff phases I and II. This disappearance of sound is temporary and is usually short, but the gap can occur over a period of 40 mmHg. It seems to be associated with higher BP readings. (2) An absent Korotkoff phase V occurs when sounds are heard to "0." When this is the case, phase IV should be recorded along with phase V. In this case, phase IV is the best reference for diastolic pressure.

Proper technique is important for obtaining accurate measurements. The inflatable rubber bag within the compression cuff should have a width that is 20 percent greater than the limb diameter and a length adequate to encompass two-thirds the limb. The cuff should be applied snugly, with the inflatable

TABLE 10-4 Phases of the Korotkoff Sounds

Phase I
The pressure level at which the first faint, consistent tapping sounds are heard. The sounds gradually increase in intensity as the cuff is deflated. The first of at least two of these sounds is defined as the systolic pressure.
Phase II
The time during cuff deflation when a murmur of swishing sounds are heard.
Phase III
The period during which sounds are crisper and increase in intensity.
Phase IV
The time when a distinct, abrupt, muffling of sound (usually of a soft blowing quality) is heard. This is defined as the diastolic pressure in anyone in whom sounds continue to zero.
Phase V
The pressure level when the last regular blood pressure sound is heard and after which all sound disappears. This is defined as the diastolic pressure unless sounds are heard to zero.

bag positioned over the artery, at the level of the heart. Before auscultation, the cuff is quickly inflated to a pressure 20 mmHg above the systolic, as indicated by obliteration of the radial pulse. The stethoscope is then applied lightly but firmly over the artery, and auscultatory pressure is determined by noting the onset (peak systole) and behavior of the Korotkoff sounds as the cuff is deflated at a rate of about 3 mmHg per second. When the sounds disappear, the bag should be rapidly decompressed and 1 or 2 min allowed to pass before repeat determinations are made. When possible, the blood pressure should be taken with the subject upright as well as supine. Determination of the blood pressure in both arms is recommended, especially in the elderly. An American Heart Association hypertension primer recommends that the systolic pressure be recorded as the point at which the first tapping sounds occur for two consecutive beats (phase I) and that the diastolic pressure in adults be recorded as the point at which sounds become inaudible. In children and in adults with a hyperkinetic circulation, the diastolic pressure should be recorded as the point at which muffling of the sounds occurs (onset of phase IV). The arterial pressures at both the onset of muffling (phase IV) and the disappearance of sound (phase V) should be recorded. The mean blood pressure can be estimated by the addition of one-third the pulse pressure (systolic pressure minus diastolic pressure) to the diastolic pressure.

Patients with atrial fibrillation may have a significant beat-to-beat variation in their arterial pressure. Accordingly, the indirect blood pressure should be measured several times and the average noted.

This indirect method provides several potential sources of error due to improper equipment, inaccurate detection of the Korotkoff sounds, and observer techniques.[125] The standard pneumatic cuff often may be unsatisfactory for pressure measurement in the arms or in the legs of very obese subjects.[132] The arterial pressure may be underestimated if the cuff is deflated too rapidly, particularly when bradycardia or an irregular rhythm is present or if inadequate inflation does not result in complete arterial occlusion. When the cuff is deflated too slowly or is immediately reinflated for multiple pressure determinations, the resulting venous congestion may elevate the diastolic pressure artificially and falsely decrease the systolic pressure by decreasing the intensity of phase I or phase II sounds to an inaudible level.

Studies correlating direct and indirect blood pressure measurements have been characterized by considerable variability between individual subjects but in general have shown a good correlation between indirect and direct measurements of blood pressure in the arm. The observed trend has been for the indirect method to underestimate systolic pressure by several millimeters of mercury, to overestimate diastolic pressure by several millimeters of mercury when phase IV is used as an end point, and to slightly underestimate diastolic pressure in normal individuals when phase V is taken as the end point.

Home blood pressure recordings using manual or automatic inflation and deflation of the cuff and detection of Korotkoff sounds by a microphone, stethoscope, or ultrasonic transducer are being used with increasing frequency for the ambulatory assessment of patients with hypertension. In general, ambulatory blood pressure devices do not meet the standards for automated devices of the Association for the Advancement of Medical Instrumentation.[129,133–135]

More recently, arterial tonometry has been used as a completely noninvasive method for monitoring the arterial pressure. This probe, with a micromanometer in its tip, operates on the principle of a piezo-resistive transducer of cantilever construction.[136–141]

Normal Arterial Pressure

Normal pressures have been defined on the basis of values included within two standard deviations of the mean of pressures obtained in a large population of apparently healthy individuals. The normal blood pressure range varies with age, sex, and socioracial grouping.[142] In the United States, the pressure increases rapidly during the first few days of life and then increases gradually, with a slightly greater increment in systolic than in diastolic values, throughout life. The pressure tends to be higher in Western, industrialized societies than in Asian, African, and technically undeveloped societies.

With increasing age and into senescence, the aorta undergoes progressive dilatation and elongation, with increasing stiffness of its walls.[143] As a result of this diminished vascular distensibility, there is an increase in systolic arterial pressure with less change in diastolic pressure.[144]

The normal blood pressure limits for adults (below 40 years of age and of mixed sex and race) living in the United States are approximately 100 to 140 mmHg systolic and 60 to 90 mmHg diastolic. In an individual subject, however, baseline pressures above or below these levels do not define a pathologic state, since the physiologic range of normal for an individual may overlap with the statistical range of abnormality.[125] The systolic arterial pressure rises slowly and progressively in most Americans between the ages of 20 and 60 and more rapidly later, increasing by about 20 mmHg between the ages of 60 and 80.[145] Diastolic pressure usually rises very little after age 45.[153] Data from the Framingham Study and then from more recent studies (e.g., MRFIT, SHEP, Syst-Eur) have shown a clear correlation between systolic pressure and cardiovascular events, a reduction in events with reduction of systolic blood pressure,[146–151] or even a negative association between diastolic blood pressure and events.[152]

In mildly to moderately hypertensive persons, the blood pressure "casually" recorded by a physician is significantly higher than the average value of a series of intermittent, indirect determinations or continuous direct recordings made during normal activity.[153] To estimate basal blood pressure, measurements have been obtained during sleep, when the subject first awakens in the morning while still recumbent, or after several hours of reclining.

Factors contributing to variations in an individual's blood pressure during daily activities include (1) body posture, (2) state of muscular, cerebral, or gastrointestinal activity, (3) emotional or painful stimuli, (4) environmental factors such as temperature and noise level, and (5) the use of tobacco, coffee, alcohol, and other drugs with direct or neurally mediated vasomotor properties.[125,154] Twenty-four-hour pressures, obtained from normal and hypertensive subjects with an automatic recorder, have shown considerable variability with activity and emotional stimuli.[155–156] The average diurnal pattern of blood pressure consists of an increase throughout the day and early evening and a significant, rapid decline to a low point during the early, deep stage of sleep.

With normal respiration, the peak systolic blood pressure is greater during expiration than during inspiration by as much as 10 mmHg. An augmentation of this difference occurs in patients with pericardial tamponade (pulsus paradoxus; see Chap. 72) and during hyperventilation.

Isotonic exercise in both the supine and upright positions produces a moderate increase in blood pressure (systolic pressure greater than mean greater than diastolic pressure). Sustained isometric muscular contractions produce an abrupt increase in systolic, mean, and diastolic blood pressure that depends on the strength of the contraction.[157]

Abnormal Arterial Pressure

INCREASED PULSE PRESSURE

An increase in arterial pulse pressure is commonly observed during routine blood pressure recordings. This usually is due to an increase in stroke volume and ejection velocity, often with a decrease in peripheral resistance. Fever, anemia, hot weather, exercise, pregnancy, hyperthyroidism, or arteriovenous fistulas may produce this change. Several cardiac diseases, such as aortic regurgitation, patent ductus arteriosus, and truncus arteriosus, also can result in a widened pulse pressure. An increased pulse pressure due to a large stroke volume may occur with complete heart block or marked sinus bradycardia.[125]

Atherosclerosis of the large arteries often reduces arterial compliance and results in an elevated systolic pressure with a normal or even decreased stroke volume. The systolic hypertension of the elderly does not necessarily represent a change in arteriolar resistance. Efforts to lower this type of systolic pressure elevation are often appropriate but can result in diminished peripheral perfusion (see Chap. 51). The increased pulse pressure associated with systemic arteriovenous fistulas is less common; a relative tachycardia may be the only clinical clue. Compression of a systemic arteriovenous fistula can produce a prompt slowing of the heart rate (Branham's sign).

REDUCED PULSE PRESSURE

A narrow pulse pressure is uncommon in normal subjects but may result from an increased peripheral resistance (increased circulating catecholamines in heart failure), decreased stroke volume (severe aortic stenosis), and/or markedly decreased intravascular volume (diabetic ketoacidosis).[125]

UNEQUAL PULSE PRESSURES

The diagnostic importance of blood pressure differences between right and left arms has been enhanced in recent years by the recognition of supravalvular aortic stenosis and this "choana effect" in children and of the subclavian steal syndrome in adults.[158] Most patients with the former have greater than 20 mmHg higher blood pressure in the right arm. The subclavian steal syndrome, often accompanied by symptoms of cerebrovascular insufficiency, usually results in a pronounced lowering or absence of brachial artery pressure in the ipsilateral extremity.[125]

A progressive increase in systolic pressure normally occurs as the point of measurement is moved peripherally from the central aorta (Fig. 10-41), and the increment in systolic pressure is equivalent in the large arteries of the upper arm and the thigh. Direct recordings of femoral and brachial arterial pressures (systolic, diastolic, and mean) in adults[159] and children[160] and indirect measurement of popliteal and brachial artery pressures using appropriate pressure cuffs[161] have demonstrated that mean pressures are equal at these sites. A difference in arm and leg pressures may occur because of coarctation of the aorta or acquired disease such as aortic dissection, aortic arch syndrome, or the subclavian steal syndrome.[125]

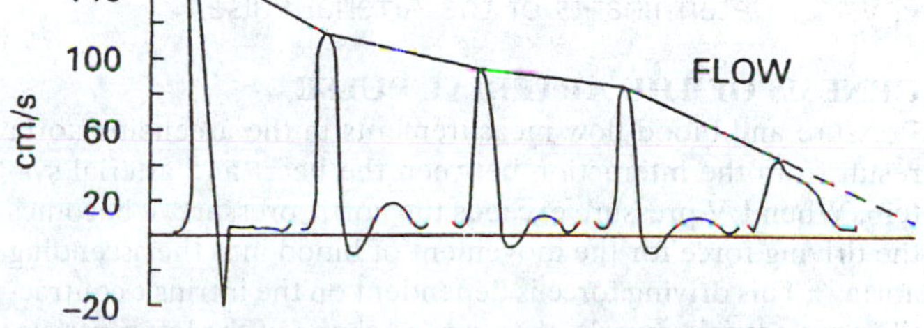

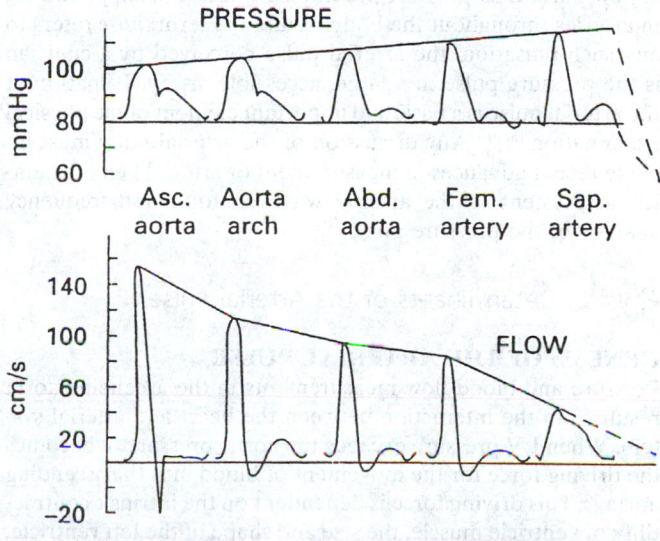

FIGURE 10-41 Micromanometer and catheter tip flow velocity as change in contour of pressure waves (above) and flow waves (below) between the ascending aorta and the saphenous artery. (From Vlachopoulos C, O'Rourke MF. The arterial pulse. *Curr Probl Cardiol* 2000; 25:296–346.)

Pulsus Alternans

Pulsus alternans may be detected by palpating a peripheral artery. The femoral artery is probably best for this purpose. One must, of course, be certain the heart rhythm is normal. The sphygmomanometer can be used to measure accurately the beat-to-beat variation in pressure that characterizes pulsus alternans.

Pulsus alternans, which is discussed at greater length later in this chapter, occurs in patients with severe heart disease who exhibit impaired LV contraction. It also can occur for a few beats following supraventricular tachycardia in normal persons or when the respiratory rate is half the pulse rate. This may be apparent when pulsus paradoxus is present in patients with cardiac tamponade.

Pulsus Paradoxus

A normal person may exhibit a 10- to 12-mmHg drop in systolic pressure during normal inspiration. A fall in pressure greater than this amount may be identified in patients with acute cardiac tamponade, constrictive pericarditis, severe obstructive lung disease, and restrictive cardiomyopathy.

Pulsus paradoxus is best detected by inflating the blood pressure cuff above systolic pressure and then slowly releasing it. As the cuff pressure is gradually reduced, the blood pressure sounds become audible during expiration. The difference in pressure between the first audible sound heard on expiration and the pressure level at which the sounds are heard during all phases of respiration gives a measurement of magnitude of pulsus paradoxus. The mechanism of pulsus paradoxus is discussed in Chap. 72.

THE ARTERIAL PULSE

The arterial pulse is as any periodic fluctuation that is caused by the heart and occurs at the same frequency as the heartbeat. Ejection of blood with every cardiac contraction is converted to *flow* pulsations, *pressure* pulsations, and *dimension* pulsations in arteries throughout the body. While the term *pulse* refers to any such pulsation, the arterial pulse perceived by a clinician is the pressure pulse in a large, accessible artery. Palpation of the arterial pulse is a basic and important element of the physical examination.[162–166] Any discussion of the arterial pulse must include recent advances in measurement of arterial hemodynamics, assessment of the arterial wave contour, and frequency analysis of the pressure pulse.[162–170]

Physical Determinants of the Arterial Pulse

GENESIS OF THE ARTERIAL PULSE

Pressure and blood flow measurements in the ascending aorta result from the interaction between the heart and arterial system. When LV pressure exceeds the aortic pressure, it becomes the driving force for the movement of blood into the ascending aorta.[162] This driving force is dependent on the intrinsic contractility of ventricle muscle, the size and shape of the left ventricle, and the heart rate. It is opposed by several forces that impede the development of flow and are interrelated in a complex manner. Three major determinants of arterial impedance include (1) resistance, (2) inertia, and (3) compliance.

Resistance is related to blood viscosity and the geometry of the vasculature; it opposes flow and is unaffected by changes in heart rate. Inertia, which is related to the mass of the column of blood, opposes the rate of change of arterial blood flow (i.e., acceleration) and depends on the heart rate. Compliance is related to the distensibility of the vascular walls, opposes changes in arterial blood volume, and also depends on the heart rate. The heart rate dependency of inertia and compliance introduces phase shifts between instantaneous pressure and flow in a pulsatile system.[167] Inertia and compliance are important determinants of the character of ventricular ejection, especially in early systole, when flows and pressures are changing rapidly.

The arterial pulse wave begins with aortic valve opening and the onset of LV ejection. Aortic pressure rises rapidly in early systole because the LV stroke volume enters the aorta faster than it flows to distal sites. The rapid-rising portion of the arterial pressure curve is often termed the *anacrotic limb* (from the Greek, meaning "upbeat"). In experimental animals and in humans, peak proximal aortic flow velocity occurs slightly earlier than peak pressure.[167] After its peak, aortic pressure declines as ventricular ejection slows and peripheral blood flow continues. During isovolumic relaxation, a transient reversal of flow from the central arteries toward the ventricle just prior to aortic valve closure is associated with an incisura on the descending limb of the aortic pressure pulse. The subsequent smaller, secondary positive wave has been attributed to the elastic recoil of the aorta and aortic valve but is partially due to reflected waves from more distal arteries. Subsequently, aortic pressure decreases again as further "runoff" in the peripheral circulation occurs in diastole.

The proximal aortic pulse pressure is directly proportional to the ratio of stroke volume to arterial distensibility, but multiple factors influence this complex relationship.[171] Arterial distensibility diminishes as the distending arterial pressure increases. Accordingly, the pulse pressure for a constant stroke volume will be larger if the mean blood pressure is elevated. In addition, arterial distensibility varies inversely with the rate of rise of intraluminal pressure. When the systolic ejection rate increases, the stiffer arterial wall results in a greater pulse pressure. Finally, the arterial pulse pressure is modified by reflected pressure waves and by the rate of blood flow from arterioles to veins.

CONTOUR OF THE ARTERIAL PULSE

Pulsatile changes in arterial diameter are virtually identical to the pressure pulse, with minor differences explained in terms of nonlinear elasticity and viscosity of the arterial wall. In 1939, Hamilton and Dow defined the pressure wave contour in different arteries in terms of wave reflection between the aortic valve and peripheral sites.[172] The pulse waveform recorded at any site of the arterial tree is the sum of a forward waveform and a backward-traveling one that is the "echo" of the incident wave reflected at peripheral sites. *Wave reflection is an important determinant of LV load and CBF.* A reflected wave occurring at systole increases systolic pressure and thereby increases ventricular afterload. In contrast, occurrence of the reflected wave at diastole is highly desirable because augmentation of pressure during diastole aids coronary perfusion.

Conventionally, the pulse is described in the *time domain,* where it is considered as a change in arterial pressure with time. An alternative approach that has the advantage of being quantitative is to analyze the pulse in the *frequency domain.*

Pulse is conceived as a composite wave that can be resolved into component harmonics like a musical wave. Impedance is the measure of the opposition to flow presented by a system and can be approached quantitatively when harmonic analysis is used to relate frequency components of pressure and flow pulses.[173-178] Study of impedance provides valuable insights for several issues of vascular mechanics.

Usually, there is a linear relation between pressure and flow at the same point in an artery and between pressures at different points in the arterial system. From impedance curves, it is possible to identify the factors responsible for the relation between the pulsatile pressure and flow. Furthermore, the coefficient of reflection in peripheral vessels can be calculated from the relation of resistance to the minimal and subsequent values of impedance modulus. The peripheral arterial pressure wave recorded is the summation of the incident (initial) and reflected waves. The systemic circulation has been represented by a simple asymmetric T-tube model that emphasizes the importance of wave reflection at two arteriolar reflecting sites in the upper and lower parts of the body.[169] An important patient study indicates major reflection sites at the aortic level of the renal arteries and at a point distal to the terminal abdominal aorta bifurcation.[170]

PERIPHERAL TRANSMISSION OF THE ARTERIAL PULSE

As the normal aortic pulse wave is transmitted peripherally, significant changes in its contour occur due to (1) distortion and damping of pulse wave components, (2) different rates of transmission of various components, (3) distortion or exaggeration by reflected, resonant, or standing waves, (4) conversion of kinetic energy into hydrostatic or potential energy, (5) differences in distensibility and caliber of the arteries, and (6) changes in the vessel wall due to age and/or disease.[176]

The arterial pressure pulse enters the proximal aorta and travels distally at a velocity many times faster than maximum blood flow. The pressure wave is accompanied by a traveling wave distending the arterial wall, the pulse wave velocity increasing as arterial wall distensibility diminishes.[171] This normally occurs distally, as the arteries branch into smaller channels and their walls become stiffer. With increasing age or with systemic hypertension, however, arterial wall distensibility diminishes, and pulse wave velocity is correspondingly greater.

The pulse wave arrives progressively later at more peripheral sites when timed from the QRS complex on the ECG. Representative time delays from the central aorta are as follows: carotid, 30 ms; brachial, 60 ms; radial, 80 ms; and femoral, 75 ms.

The arterial pulse wave undergoes a progressive change in shape during its transmission distally (Fig. 10-41). The pulse pressure and systolic amplitude increase, and the ascending limb of the pulse wave becomes steeper. The incisura of the central aorta pulse is gradually replaced by a smoother, somewhat later dicrotic notch that occurs at lower pressure levels. The dicrotic notch and the following positive secondary or dicrotic wave probably result from the summation of the forward pulse wave and reflected waves from the peripheral vessels.[162]

EXAMINATION OF THE ARTERIAL PULSE

All major arterial pulses should be examined bilaterally for both patency and waveform characteristics. The thickness and hardness of the arterial walls often can be assessed by "rolling" the vessel against underlying tissue. A pulse in the foot should not be considered absent unless examined with the foot in a dependent position. Otherwise, the arterial pulses usually are examined with the patient supine and with the trunk of the body slightly elevated.

The examiner uses tactile receptors in the tips of the fingers to sense movement of the arterial wall associated with the pressure pulse as it passes the site of palpation. Measurements in the proximal aorta show cyclic movement in both diameter and length proportional to the pulse pressure. In more peripheral arteries with connective tissue attachments, however, the detectable movement is small and variable, with radial expansion by only about 2 percent of the end-diastolic cross-sectional area.[162]

The usual technique for palpating the arterial pulse is to press with the examining fingers until the maximum pulse is sensed. The pulse is felt as changing displacement superimposed on the "baseline" displacement produced by compressing the artery. The examiner should apply varying degrees of pressure while concentrating on the separate phases of the pulse wave. This method, referred to as *trisection,* is useful for assessing the upstroke, systolic peak, and diastolic slope of the arterial pulse.[176] Controversy exists as to how many fingers should be used to palpate the pulse; the examiner should use whichever method he or she prefers.

Palpation of the carotid artery is preferred for assessing cardiac performance, since the carotid pulse corresponds more closely to the central aortic pressure. In certain cardiac diseases (e.g., aortic regurgitation), however, the abnormalities detected in the carotid pulse are accentuated in the more peripheral pulses. For determining the cardiac rate and rhythm, the radial pulse most often is used, but if it is irregular, cardiac auscultation often provides more reliable information. To evaluate the integrity of the peripheral arterial blood supply and to localize any lesions that exist, the arterial pulses in all four extremities should be examined and compared (see also Chap. 90).

Inspection of the carotid arterial and jugular venous pulsations should be performed at the same time. The carotid pulse is usually best examined with the sternocleidomastoid muscles relaxed and with the head rotated slightly toward the examiner. The carotid pulse may be timed from the first heart sound, which is heard slightly before the pulsation. The carotid pulse should be palpated in the lower half of the patient's neck in order to avoid carotid sinus compression. Occasionally, it is useful to palpate two arteries simultaneously (e.g., radial and femoral) to detect an apparent pulse wave delay, such as occurs in patients with coarctation of the aorta.

The examination of arterial pulses in the abdomen and upper and lower extremities should be performed carefully in all patients and compared using a scale such as the following: 0 = complete absence of pulsation; 1+ = small or reduced pulsation; 2+ = normal or average pulsation; and 3+ = large or bounding pulsation. Furthermore, auscultation over the major arteries should be performed, since an audible bruit may be a clue to partial occlusion or may indicate transmission (e.g., carotid) of a cardiac murmur.

NORMAL ARTERIAL PULSE

The normal carotid pulse has a smooth, rapid upstroke or ascending limb to a smooth, dome-shaped summit (see Fig. 10-42). Then a downstroke occurs that is somewhat less rapid than the upstroke. The dicrotic notch and secondary diastolic wave

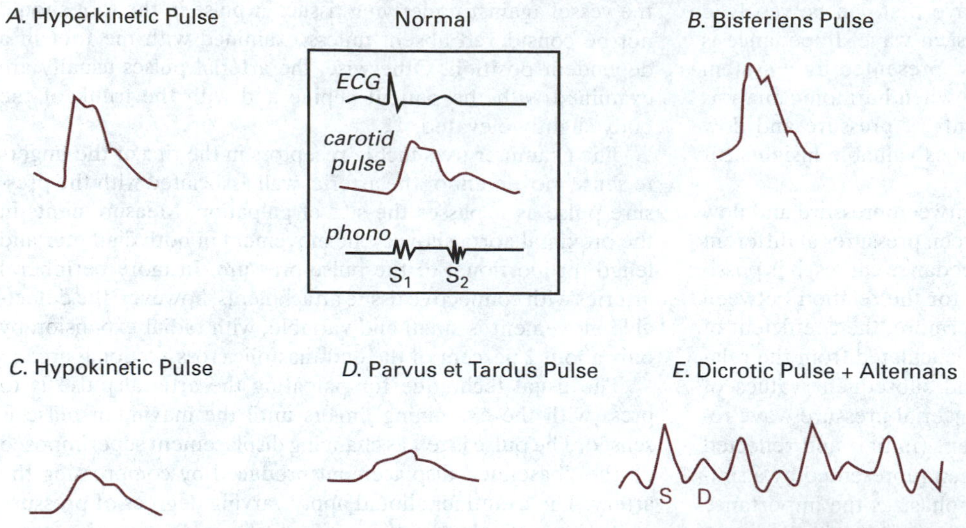

FIGURE 10-42 Schematic representation of the normal carotid arterial pulse, five types of abnormal pulses, and pulsus alternans. ECG, electrocardiogram; phono, phonocardiogram; S_1, S_2, first and second heart sounds; S, systole; D, diastole.

pulse wave velocity is decreased, and the later tidal and diastolic waves are further displaced from the percussion wave.

Impairment of the pulse of one or both carotid arteries is usually produced by atherosclerosis, but multiple other causes include thrombosis, embolus, arteritis, and diseases of the aortic arch. Kinking of the carotid or brachiocephalic artery is relatively frequent, particularly in hypertensive patients, and may simulate aneurysmal dilatation. Femoral pulses may be diminished in the child or young adult as a result of coarctation of the aorta. In most adults, however, the diminution of the femoral pulsation is caused by atherosclerosis of the abdominal aorta, aortic bifurcation, or ileofemoral arteries (see also Chap. 90).

usually are not felt but may be palpable in some normal individuals, particularly during fever, exercise, or excitement. The dicrotic notch usually occurs about 300 ms after the onset of the pulse wave when corrected for heart rate.

In arteries distal to the carotid, the pulse wave arrives later and has a steep initial wave that rises to a high peak pressure, whereas the diastolic pressure and the mean pressure are slightly lower. The systolic upstroke time (onset of pulse wave to its peak) tends to be shorter, but the apparent LV ejection time (onset of pulse wave to incisura) is longer in more peripheral arterial pulses. In the brachial artery, the heart rate-corrected systolic upstroke time averages 120 ms (range, 90–160 ms), and the systolic ejection time averages about 320 ms (range, 280–360 ms).

Graphic recordings of the arterial pulses frequently show two positive deflections during systole, the first shoulder being referred to as the *percussion wave* and the second as the *tidal wave*. In the normal proximal aortic pulse, the percussion wave is due to arrival of the impulse generated by LV ejection, the tidal wave may represent its echo from the upper part of the body, and the dicrotic or diastolic wave is a reflection from the lower part of the body.[166] The contour of the distal pulses can be explained in similar terms, with altered time relations between incident and reflected waves at different distances from peripheral reflecting sites.

With aging, there is a relative increase in the second (tidal) systolic wave and the height of the incisura relative to the first systolic wave.[162,177,179,180] The systolic upstroke time is longer, and the amplitude and duration of the diastolic wave tend to be less prominent.

ABNORMAL ARTERIAL PULSES

In hypertension and arteriosclerosis, the pressure pulse amplitude is increased, the tidal wave is prominent, and the diastolic wave is absent. All features of the pulse can be explained by increased wave velocity.[162,177] Reflected waves return to the proximal aorta during late systole, augmenting the tidal wave and increasing systolic pressure. With systemic hypotension, the

HYPERKINETIC ARTERIAL PULSE

Large, bounding arterial pulses usually indicate the rapid ejection of an increased volume of blood from the left ventricle (see Fig. 10-42*A*). Commonly, the arterial pulse pressure is increased, and the peripheral arterial resistance diminished. The hyperdynamic arterial pulse is sometimes referred to in terms that describe a particular component of the pulse wave. Thus the *water-hammer pulse,* named after a Victorian toy, refers to an extremely rapid, forceful ascending limb of the arterial pulse wave.[181] By contrast, *collapsing pulse* refers to a quick, marked decrease in the arterial pulse wave following its peak. Hyperkinetic pulses often are more prominent in the brachial, radial, and femoral arteries than in the carotid artery. The term *Quincke pulse* refers to visible small pulsations in the nail bed of patients with hyperdynamic arterial pulses from any cause, including aortic regurgitation.

Hyperkinetic arterial pulses occur in normal subjects with a hyperkinetic circulation (e.g., exercise, fever), patients with cardiovascular diseases associated with increased stroke volume, and subjects with marked bradycardia and an extremely large stroke volume (e.g., athletes). A hyperdynamic arterial pulse also occurs in patients with an abnormally rapid runoff of blood from the arterial system (e.g., patent ductus arteriosus, arteriovenous fistulas). Patients on chronic hemodialysis often have hyperdynamic pulses produced by the combination of a surgical arteriovenous fistula, anemia, and hypertension.

In aortic regurgitation, the rapid-rising, bounding arterial pulse results from increases in both stroke volume and the rate of LV ejection. The early systolic flow often produces palpable vibrations manifest as a thrill on the steep ascending limb. Later in systole, the rate of ventricular ejection and the arterial pulse wave decrease sharply, often resulting in systolic collapse.

BISFERIENS ARTERIAL PULSE

The bisferiens (from the Latin, meaning "twice beating") pulse has a waveform characterized by two positive waves during systole (see Fig. 10-42*B*). The pulse wave upstroke rises rapidly and forcefully, producing the first systolic peak (percussion wave). A brief decline in pressure is followed by a smaller and somewhat slower-rising positive pulse wave (tidal wave). Abnormalities of LV ejection and reflected waves from peripheral arteries contribute to the prominence of the second systolic wave in the bisferiens pulse. The bisferiens pulse, usually felt in the carotid artery, is sometimes more easily palpable in a brachial or radial artery. A bisferiens pulse often occurs in patients with pure aortic regurgitation and in patients with combined aortic stenosis and severe aortic regurgitation.[182] It also can occur in other conditions associated with the rapid ejection of an increased stroke volume from the left ventricle (e.g., exercise, fever, patent ductus arteriosus).

The bisferiens pulse often is present in patients with hypertrophic cardiomyopathy, many of whom have a pressure gradient in the LV outflow tract.[183] In this syndrome, the midsystolic negative wave usually coincides with a marked decrease in the rate of LV ejection. The second systolic wave, or tidal wave, most likely is produced by reflected waves from the periphery. The bisferiens pulse may be elicited by maneuvers that decrease the LV size or increase its contractility. The most characteristic aspect of the arterial pulse in hypertrophic cardiomyopathy is its rapid rate of rise. A physical finding nearly specific for hypertrophic cardiomyopathy is a much smaller arterial pressure pulse in the cardiac cycle following a premature ventricular beat (see Chap. 67).

HYPOKINETIC ARTERIAL PULSE

A small, weak arterial pulse is frequently present in patients with a diminished stroke volume (see Fig. 10-42*C*). Usually, the decreased stroke output is associated with decreased rate and duration of LV ejection, and there is a narrow arterial pulse pressure despite an increased arterial resistance. Common causes include hypovolemia, LV failure, and mitral or aortic valve stenosis.

PARVUS ET TARDUS PULSE

Patients with moderate or severe valvular aortic stenosis often have an arterial pulse that is small and has a delayed systolic peak.[184–186] Occasionally, there may be a detectable shoulder on the upstroke of the carotid pulse, referred to as *anacrotic*[184] (see Fig. 10-42*D*). Palpable coarse vibrations often are present as a systolic thrill over the slowly rising carotid pulse. The parvus et tardus pulse is much easier to detect in the carotid arteries than in more distal arteries.

Most middle-aged patients with uncomplicated severe aortic stenosis have a parvus et tardus pulse, but this pulse also may occur in relatively mild stenosis. Conversely, an apparently normal arterial pulse is not unusual in elderly patients with severe aortic stenosis who have decreased distensibility of the large arteries, which also alters the character of the arterial pulse.[162,164] Severe LV failure often results in a small, weak pulse that may be difficult to distinguish from that of aortic stenosis.

DICROTIC ARTERIAL PULSE

The dicrotic (from the Greek *dikrotos,* meaning "double beating") pulse is a twice-peaked pulse with one peak in systole and the second in diastole, the latter due to an accentuated and palpable dicrotic wave that follows the second heart sound[187] (see Fig. 10-42*E*). It is usually felt best in the carotids, although it also may be palpated over more peripheral arteries. Major abnormalities include a short systolic ejection phase, a low dicrotic notch, a large diastolic wave, a narrow pulse pressure, a diminished rate of rise of the pulse, and the lack of distinct percussion and tidal waves. The dicrotic pulse is most common in young or middle-aged patients with impaired LV performance. It is usually associated with a low cardiac output, markedly diminished stroke volume, elevated LV end-diastolic pressure, and high systemic arterial resistance. In general, the dicrotic wave becomes less prominent with age, hypertension, generalized atherosclerosis, and diabetes. Rarely, the dicrotic wave can be palpated in young, febrile patients in whom none of the other abnormal features of the dicrotic pulse are present.

PULSUS ALTERNANS

In pulsus alternans, beats occur at regular intervals with a regular alternation of the systolic height of the pressure pulses[188,189] (see Fig. 10-42*E*). Rarely, pulsus alternans is so marked that the weaker pulses are not felt at all. When pulsus alternans is noticed first after a premature beat, the extent of the difference in systolic pressure in alternating beats may decline for several cycles until the pulse amplitude is again constant. The initiation of post-premature ventricular beat pulsus alternans is probably related to the increased duration of LV filling after the premature beat, resulting in a greater end-diastolic volume and hence increased contractile force due to the Frank-Starling mechanism.

Sustained pulsus alternans (see Chap. 20) is seen in severe depression of LV performance with an alteration in aortic flow, systolic LV pressure, aortic systolic pressure, LV *dP/dt*, and LV end-diastolic pressure. Sustained pulsus alternans likely is due to alteration of the contractile state of at least part of the myocardium, which may be caused by the failure of electromechanical coupling in some cells during the weaker contraction.[189] A subsequent stronger contraction would then represent contraction of all cells, some of which were potentiated.[190]

Pulsus alternans may be better appreciated when palpating a distal artery, which normally has a slightly wider pulse pressure than the carotid artery. The patient's respiration should be held, since the small changes in arterial pressure caused by normal respiration may obscure the recognition of pulsus alternans. Pulsus alternans can be confirmed by using a sphygmomanometer and is usually associated with a LV third heart sound.

PULSUS PARADOXUS

A *paradoxical pulse* is defined as a marked decrease in the pulse amplitude during normal quiet inspiration or a decrease in the systolic arterial pressure by more than 10 mmHg. The normal small decline in systolic blood pressure probably is produced predominantly by relative pooling of blood in the pulmonary vessels during inspiration and also may reflect the delayed transmission through the lungs of the preceding expiratory fall in venous pressure and RV cardiac output.[176]

In patients with cardiac tamponade, fluid accumulation in the pericardium increases intrapericardial pressure, and the heart's filling capacity is reduced. During inspiration, the expected augmentation of venous return to the right side of the heart occurs despite the elevated intrapericardial pressure.[191] The diminished thoracic pressure also causes a pooling of blood in the pulmonary veins and capillaries and diminishes pulmonary venous return to the left atrium. Since the high intrapericardial pressure limits flow to the heart and the total cardiac filling capacity is limited, the increase in right-sided heart volume with inspiration causes an obligatory decrease in left-sided heart filling. This, along with the pooling of blood in the pulmonary bed, produces a decline in LV stroke volume and systolic blood pressure during inspiration.[192]

Pulsus paradoxus is common with cardiac tamponade but infrequent with constrictive pericarditis (see Chap. 72). Different hemodynamic mechanisms contribute to the production of a paradoxical pulse in certain patients with superior vena cava obstruction, asthma, or obstructive airways disease; in some patients with pulmonary embolism or shock; and in some patients after thoracotomy.[176]

The extent of pulsus paradoxicus can be quantitated by cuff sphygmomanometry as the pressure difference between the first discernible Korotkoff sound on expiration and the pressure level at which Korotkoff sounds are audible during all phases of respiration.

EFFECTS OF ARRHYTHMIAS ON THE ARTERIAL PULSE

Premature Ventricular Depolarizations A premature ventricular depolarization may be associated with no pulse, a small-amplitude pulse, or a normal arterial pulse depending on timing and whether or not the LV pressure generated is able to open the aortic valve.[193] The arterial pulse following a premature beat usually is greatly enhanced because of decreased aortic impedance, increased LV filling, and augmented LV contractility. At times, premature ventricular beats are so common as to produce an irregularly irregular pulse. Then the presence of cannon *a* waves in the jugular venous pulse should alert one to the correct diagnosis.

Tachyarrhythmias The ECG is usually needed for the definitive diagnosis of any abnormality of heart rate or rhythm. On the other hand, careful observation of the arterial and jugular venous pulses frequently leads to the correct diagnosis. Simultaneous cardiac auscultation is also frequently helpful.

Most tachycardias associated with a regular pulse are of supraventricular origin. In sinus tachycardia, the arterial pulse will slow gradually with carotid sinus pressure and then again increase gradually. Paroxysmal atrial tachycardia has an "all or none" response. In patients with atrial flutter, carotid sinus pressure will increase the block at the AV junction, the pulse rate slowing and subsequently returning to its original rate in a "jerky" fashion.

In patients with ventricular tachycardia and AV dissociation, the variation in the atrial ventricular sequence of contraction and resulting variation in pulse amplitude often may be detected by palpation.[194]

An irregularly irregular pulse with a varying pulse pressure is usually the result of atrial fibrillation; however, multifocal atrial tachycardia is also a common cause of this finding in patients with severe chronic obstructive lung disease.

Bradyarrhythmias An unusually slow heart rate frequently is associated with a decrease in the rate of rise and amplitude of the arterial pressure pulse. Complete heart block often is readily diagnosed by the variability in the arterial pulse amplitude, the changing intensity of the first heart sound, and intermittent cannon *a* waves in the jugular venous pulse, all due to the time-dependent variable contribution of atrial contraction to ventricular filling.

EFFECTS OF DRUG THERAPY ON THE ARTERIAL PULSE

Pulse wave analysis provides important information about the actions of drugs that, most importantly, may not be apparent with conventional methods.[162] *Nitrates* decrease central systolic pressure substantially while they have no or minimal effect on peripheral systolic pressure (Fig. 10-43).[162a] *Beta-blocking* agents have variable effect depending on their intrinsic properties. Nonselective agents tend to increase late systolic pressure augmentation; in contrast, those agents with vasodilating properties have the opposite effect. Both angiotensin-converting enzyme (ACE) inhibitors and calcium-channel blockers have significant effects on the arterial pulse by reducing late systolic pressure augmentation. These actions can be explained on the basis of wave reflection. Reduction of wave reflection is an important advantage in the logical treatment of hypertension and heart failure.

THE VENOUS PULSE

An accurate assessment of the venous pulse is an integral part of the physical examination because it provides information concerning both the mean right atrial pressure and the hemodynamic events in the right atrium.[165] Factors influencing the right atrial and central venous pressure (CVP) include the total blood volume, thedistribution of blood volume, and the strength of right atrial contraction.

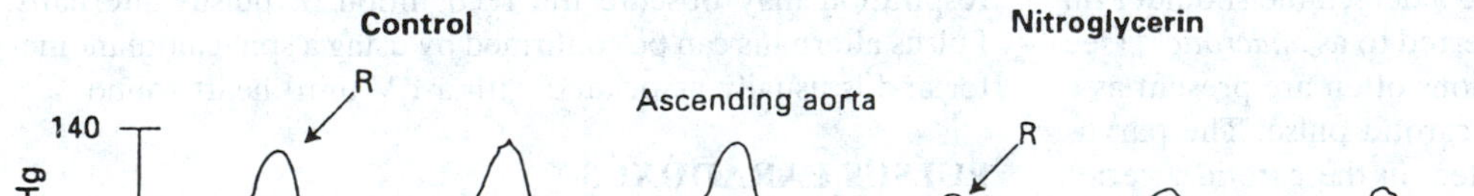

FIGURE 10-43 Pressure waves recorded directly in the ascending aorta (*top*) and brachial artery (*bottom*) under control conditions (*left*) and after 0.3 mg sublingual nitroglycerin (*right*) in a human adult. X, height the pressure would have without reflection (R). (From Kelly et al.,[162a] with permission.)

Venous blood returning from the systemic capillaries is nonpulsatile. Changes in volume flow created by skeletal muscles and the respiratory pump are nonsynchronous with the pulsatile activity of the heart. Changes in flow and pressure caused by right atrial and ventricular filling, however, produce pulsations in the central veins that are transmitted toward the peripheral veins, opposite to the direction of blood flow. With the possible exception of the *c* wave, which is the combined result of carotid arterial impact and an upward movement of the tricuspid valve, the pulsations observed in the neck are produced by right atrial and ventricular activity.[195]

Examination of the Jugular Venous Pulse

The two main objectives of the bedside examination of the neck veins are estimation of the CVP and inspection of the waveform.[197] Usually, the right internal jugular vein is superior for both purposes. In most normal subjects, the maximum pulsation of the internal jugular vein is observed when the trunk is inclined by less than 30°. In patients with an elevated venous pressure, it may be necessary to elevate the trunk further, sometimes to as much as 90°. When the neck muscles are relaxed, shining a beam of light tangentially across the skin overlying the internal jugular vein often exposes its pulsations. Simultaneous palpation of the left carotid artery aids the examiner in deciding which pulsations are venous.

Measurements of Venous Pressure

The difference between venous distention and venous pressure elevation must be considered. Veins may be markedly dilated with minimal increase in pressure or may not be visibly distended despite a very high venous pressure.[196] Venous pressure may be estimated by examining the veins on the dorsum of the hand. With the patient sitting or lying at a 30° elevation or greater, the arm is slowly and passively raised from a dependent position. When the venous pressure is normal, the veins collapse when the dorsum of the hand reaches the level of the sternal angle of Louis. Unfortunately, local venous obstruction or augmented peripheral venous constriction may diminish the accuracy of estimating CVP by this method.

The external or internal jugular veins also may be used to estimate venous pressure.[196] Because of its more direct route to the right atrium, the internal jugular vein is superior for the estimation of venous pressure and assessment of the venous waveform. The patient is examined at the optimal degree of trunk elevation for visualization of venous pulsations. The vertical distance from the top of the oscillating venous column to the level of the sternal angle is generally less than 3 cm. Greatly elevated venous pressure may be missed by failing to elevate the patient's head adequately. It may be necessary to actually have the patient sit upright. If the "pulsating meniscus" is very high, pulsations may not be apparent in the lower neck. When venous engorgement is marked, the patient's earlobe may pulsate, and even the veins on the top of the head may be distended.

In patients suspected of RV failure but having a normal resting venous pressure, the abdominojugular test is useful.[196] With the patient breathing normally, firm pressure is applied with the palm of the hand to the upper right quadrant of the abdomen for 10 s or more. The patient should be instructed to continue to breathe normally during the test. In most subjects, the jugular venous pressure is not altered significantly. In some normal patients there is a transient increase in jugular venous pressure with a rapid return to or near baseline in less than 10 s. The dysfunctioning right ventricle, however, is unable to accept the increment in blood volume due to enhanced venous return without a marked increase in its filling pressure, which is transmitted to the neck veins. In patients with RV failure, which often results from left-sided heart failure, the venous pressure either rises rapidly and then partially declines slowly during continued abdominal compression or remains elevated by 4 cm of blood or more until the abdominal pressure is released (Fig. 10-44). Ducas et al.[198] also studied the abdominojugular test and confirmed its clinical value.

Analysis of Venous Waveforms

Again, the patient's trunk should be inclined to whatever elevation is necessary to reveal the top of the oscillating venous

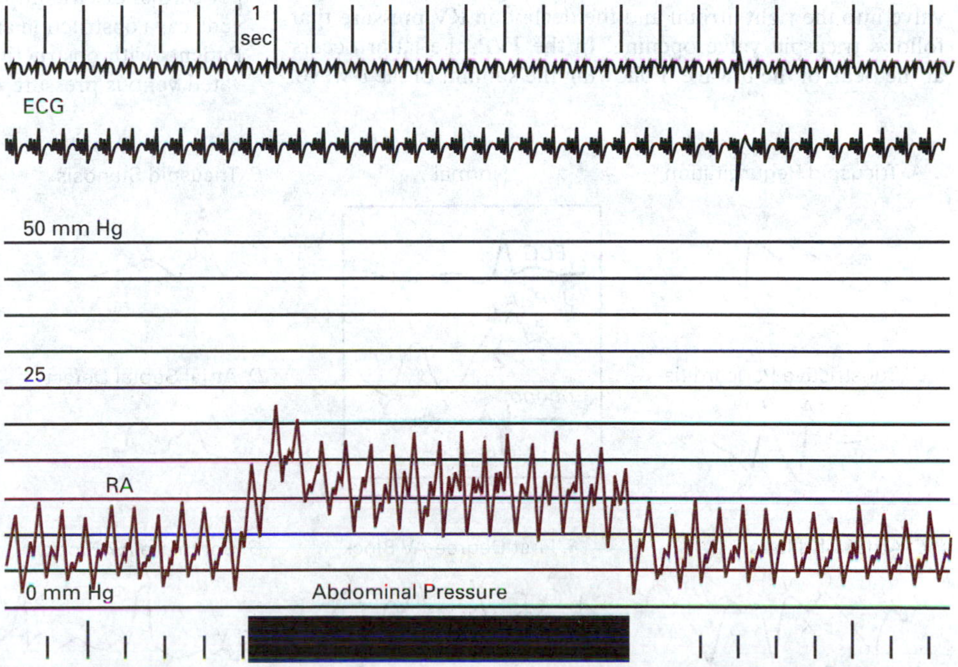

FIGURE 10-44 Elevation in RA pressure observed during abdominal pressure in patient with mild congestive heart failure. (From Ewy GA. The abdominojugular test: Technique and hemodynamic correlates. *Ann Intern Med* 1989; 109:456. Used with permission from the publisher and author.)

column.[199] Slow, deep inspiration will increase the amplitude of the presystolic *a* wave while decreasing the mean right atrial pressure. This is a useful technique for identifying the site at which the pulsations will be best visualized. Simultaneous palpation of the left carotid artery and cardiac auscultation aid the examiner in relating the venous pulsations to the timing of the cardiac cycle.

Normal Venous Pulse

The normal *jugular venous pulse* (JVP) reflects phasic pressure changes in the right atrium and consists of three positive waves and two negatives troughs (Fig. 10-45). It is useful to refer to the events of the cardiac cycle (Plate 2). The positive presystolic *a* wave is produced by right atrial (RA) contraction and is the dominant wave in the JVP, particularly during inspiration. During atrial relaxation, the venous pulse descends from the summit of the *a* wave. Depending on the PR interval, this descent may continue until a plateau (*z* point) is reached just prior to RV systole. More often, the descent is interrupted by a second positive venous wave, the *c* wave, that is produced by bulging of the tricuspid valve into the right atrium during RV isovolumic systole and by the impact of the carotid artery adjacent to the jugular vein.[200] Following the summit of the *c* wave, the JVP contour declines, forming the normal negative systolic wave, the *x* wave. The *x* descent is due to a combination of atrial relaxation, the downward displacement of the tricuspid valve during RV systole, and the ejection of blood from both ventricles (see Chap. 3).

The positive, later systolic *v* wave in the JVP results from the increase in blood volume in the venae cavae and right atrium during ventricular systole when the tricuspid valve is closed. After the peak of the *v* wave is reached, the RA pressure decreases because of the diminished bulging of the tricuspid valve into the right atrium and the decline in RV pressure that follows tricuspid valve opening. In the JVP, the latter occurs at the peak of the *v* wave. Following the summit of the *v* wave, there is a negative descending limb, referred to as the *y* descent or diastolic collapse, which is due to the tricuspid valve opening and the rapid inflow of blood into the right ventricle. The initial *y* descent corresponds to the RV rapid-filling phase. The trough of the *y* wave occurs in early diastole and is followed by the ascending limb of the *y* wave, which is produced by the continued diastolic inflow of blood into the right side of the heart. The velocity of this ascending pressure curve depends on the rate of venous return and the distensibility of the chambers of the right side of the heart. When diastole is long, the ascending limb of the *y* wave is often followed by a small, brief, positive wave, the *h* wave, that occurs just prior to the next *a* wave. At times, there is a plateau phase rather than a distinct *h* wave. With increasing heart rate, the *y* trough and *y* ascent are followed immediately by the next *a* wave.

Usually, there are three visible major positive waves (*a*, *c*, and *v*) and two negative waves (*x* and *y*) when the pulse rate is below 90 beats per minute and the PR interval is normal. With faster heart rates, there is often fusion of some of the pulse waves, and an accurate analysis of the waveform is more difficult.

Abnormal Venous Pulse

ELEVATED VENOUS PRESSURE

The most common cause of an elevated jugular venous pressure is an increased RV pressure such as occurs in patients with pulmonic stenosis, pulmonary hypertension, or RV failure secondary to left-sided heart failure or RV infarction. The venous pressure also is elevated when obstruction to RV inflow occurs, as with tricuspid stenosis or RA myxoma, or when constrictive pericardial disease impedes RV inflow. It also may result from vena cava obstruction and, at times, an increased blood volume. Patients with obstructive pulmonary disease may have an elevated venous pressure only during expiration.

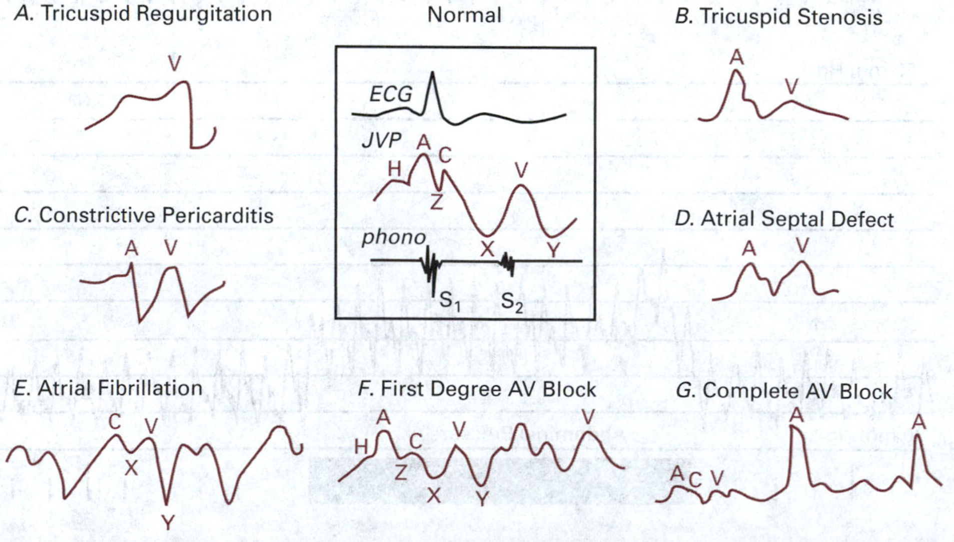

FIGURE 10-45 Schematic representation of the normal JVP, four types of abnormal JVPs, and the JVPs in three arrhythmias. See text under "Normal Venous Pulse" for definition of H, A, Z, C, X, V, and Y.

KUSSMAUL'S SIGN

Normally, during inspiration, there is an increase in the *a* wave of the JVP but a decrease in the mean jugular venous pressure as a result of the increased filling of the right-sided chambers associated with the decrease in intrathoracic pressure. *Kussmaul's sign* denotes an inspiratory increase in the venous pressure, which may occur in patients with severe constrictive pericarditis when the heart is unable to accept the increase in RV volume without a marked increase in the filling pressure. Although Kussmaul's sign was first described in patients with constrictive pericarditis, its most common cause is severe right-sided heart failure, regardless of etiology. The presence of Kussmaul's sign is also useful in the diagnosis of RV infarction[201] (see Chap. 72).

ABNORMALITIES OF THE *a* WAVE

The *a* wave in the JVP is absent when there is no effective atrial contraction, such as in atrial fibrillation (see Fig. 10-45*E*). In certain other conditions, the *a* wave may not be apparent. In sinus tachycardia, the *a* wave may fuse with the preceding *v* wave, particularly if the PR interval is prolonged. In some patients with sinus tachycardia, the jugular *a* wave may occur during the *v* or *y* descent and may be small or absent. In the presence of first-degree AV block, a discrete *a* wave with ascending and descending limbs is often completed prior to the first heart sound, and the *ac* interval is prolonged (see Fig. 10-45*F*).

Large *a* waves are of considerable diagnostic value (see Fig. 10-45*B*). When giant *a* waves are present with each beat, the right atrium is contracting against an increased resistance. This may result from obstruction at the tricuspid valve (tricuspid stenosis or atresia, right atrial myxoma) or conditions associated with increased resistance to RV filling.[200] A giant *a* wave is more likely to occur in patients with pulmonic stenosis or pulmonary hypertension in whom both the atrial and ventricular septa are intact.

Cannon *a* waves occur when the right atrium contracts while the tricuspid valve is closed during RV systole.[200] Cannon *a* waves may occur either regularly or irregularly and are most common in the presence of arrhythmias (see Fig. 10-45*G*).

ABNORMALITIES OF THE *x* WAVE

The most important alteration of the normally negative systolic collapse (*x* wave) of the JVP is its obliteration or even replacement by a positive wave. This is usually due to tricuspid regurgitation. Although atrial relaxation may contribute to the normal *x* descent, the development of atrial fibrillation does not obliterate the *x* wave except in the presence of tricuspid regurgitation. Accordingly, the occurrence of a positive wave in the JVP during ventricular systole is strong evidence of tricuspid regurgitation (Fig. 10-46*A*). Mild tricuspid regurgitation lessens and shortens the downward *x* wave as the regurgitation of blood into the right atrium produces a positive wave that diminishes the usual systolic fall in venous pressure. In some patients with moderate tricuspid regurgitation, there is a fairly distinct positive wave during ventricular systole between the *c* and *v* waves. This abnormal systolic waveform is usually referred to as a *v* or *cv* wave, although it has also been referred to as an *r* (regurgitant) or an *s* (systolic) wave. In patients with constrictive pericarditis, the *x* descent wave during systole is often more prominent than the early diastolic *y* wave (see Fig. 10-45*C* and Chap. 72).

ABNORMALITIES OF THE *v* WAVE

The positive, late systolic *v* wave results from the increasing RA blood volume during ventricular systole when the tricuspid valve normally is closed. With mild tricuspid regurgitation, the *v* wave and the obliteration of the *x* descent result in a single, large positive systolic wave (ventricularization) (see Figs. 10-45*A* and 10-46).

Normally in the JVP the *v* wave is lower in amplitude than the *a* wave. In patients with an ASD, however, the *a* and *v* waves are often equal in the right atrium and the JVP (see Fig. 10-46*D*). In patients with constrictive pericarditis and sinus

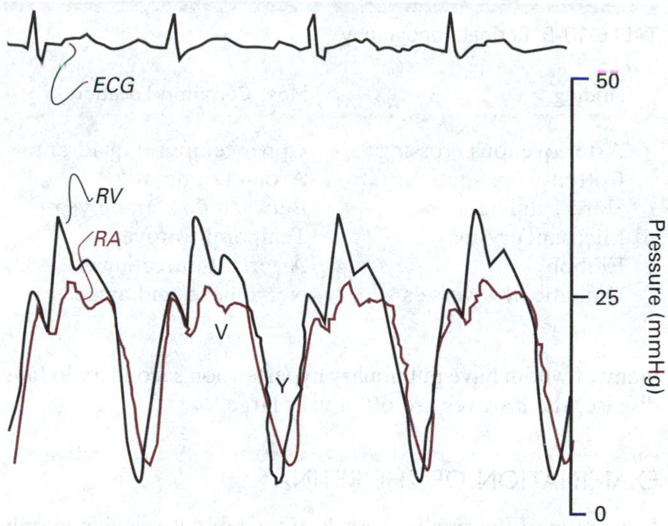

FIGURE 10-46 Right ventricular (RV) and right atrial (RA) pressure curves and simultaneous ECG from a patient with severe tricuspid regurgitation. Note ventricularization of the RA pressure curve.

rhythm, the RA *a* and *v* waves also may be equal, but the venous pressure is increased, which is unusual with isolated ASD. In patients with constrictive pericarditis who are in atrial fibrillation, the *cv* wave is prominent and the *y* descent rapid.

ABNORMALITIES OF THE *y* TROUGH

The *y* descent, or diastolic collapse, is produced mainly by the tricuspid valve opening and the rapid inflow of blood into the right ventricle. A rapid, deep *y* descent in early diastole occurs with severe tricuspid regurgitation (see Fig. 10-45*A*). A venous pulse characterized by a sharp *y* descent, a deep *y* trough, and a rapid ascent to the baseline is seen in patients with constrictive pericarditis or with severe right-sided heart failure. A slow *y* descent in the JVP suggests an obstruction to RV filling and may be the only abnormal finding in patients with tricuspid stenosis or right atrial myxoma (see Fig. 10-45*B*). In both constrictive pericarditis and severe right-sided heart failure, the venous pressure is elevated with a sharp *y* dip in the JVP (see Chap. 72). The presence of a large positive systolic venous wave favors the diagnosis of severe heart failure.

Effects of Arrhythmias on the Venous Pulse

Large *a* waves in the JVP during arrhythmias are present when the *P* wave (atrial contraction) occurs between the onset of the QRS complex and the termination of the T wave (see Fig. 10-46*G*). Such cannon *a* waves may occur regularly in junctional rhythm. More commonly, they occur irregularly when AV dissociation accompanies premature ventricular beats, ventricular tachycardia, or complete heart block. The *a* wave is absent in patients with atrial fibrillation, and flutter *a* waves at a regular rate of 250 to 300 per minute occasionally are observed in patients with atrial flutter and varying degrees of AV block. Patients with multifocal atrial tachycardia often have prominent and somewhat variable *a* waves in the JVP. In these patients,

TABLE 10-5 Retinal Topography

Finding	Most Common Location
Arteriovenous crossings	Upper temporal quadrant
Cotton-wool spots	Around optic disk
Hard exudates	Between disk and fovea
Microaneurysms	Temporal to fovea
Emboli	Arterial bifurcations
Diabetic new vessels	Nerve head and arcades

many of whom have pulmonary hypertension secondary to lung disease, the *a* waves are often very large.

EXAMINATION OF THE RETINA*

Inspection of the smaller vessels of the body is possible in only three areas: the retina, the conjunctiva, and the nail beds. The ophthalmoscope has made the retina by far the easiest and most rewarding site.[201] Viewing this two-dimensional vascular display is generally much easier if the pupils are dilated. Pulse and blood pressure determinations should be made prior to the instillation of rapidly acting mydriatics, since both may increase after absorption of the drops. The pupils are left undilated in patients in whom the iris seems closely apposed to the cornea and in those with a history of closed-angle glaucoma. Examination of the retina should proceed methodically. Best pupillary dilatation is maintained if the optic disk is observed first. Assess for evidence of edema and blurred margins and for cupping with sharp contours. Rule out neovascularization or the pallor of optic atrophy. Next, scan along the superior temporal arcade, inspecting the arteries carefully for embolic plaques at each bifurcation. Observe the arteriovenous crossing for obscuration of the vein and for pronounced nicking and banking of the vessels. The lower arcade and the nasal vessels may be inspected next. Avoid the macular area until all else has been viewed because the pupil constricts most intensely when this area is illuminated. To discover diabetic microaneurysms early, look just temporal to the fovea, along the horizontal raphe. To find cotton-wool infarcts, look circularly around the disk two disk diameters out. Using this method, the retina can be efficiently searched for evidence of cardiovascular disease[201] (Table 10-5).

Alterations in retinal caliber along the course of a single artery or vein are more important than estimates of arteriovenous ratios or absolute vascular diameter. Determining the degree of tortuosity of straightening are of little value where the veins are large, dark, and tortuous.

Variations in the caliber of a single vessel are more important than determinations of arteriovenous ratios. These changes may take the form of focal narrowing, sometimes called *beading* or *spasm*.

Thickening of the Vascular Wall

Normally, only the blood column is visible when the retinal vessels are viewed. When changes in the walls do occur, they

* This text is modified from Chap. 11 by N. Banks Anderson, Jr., in the ninth edition of *The Heart.*

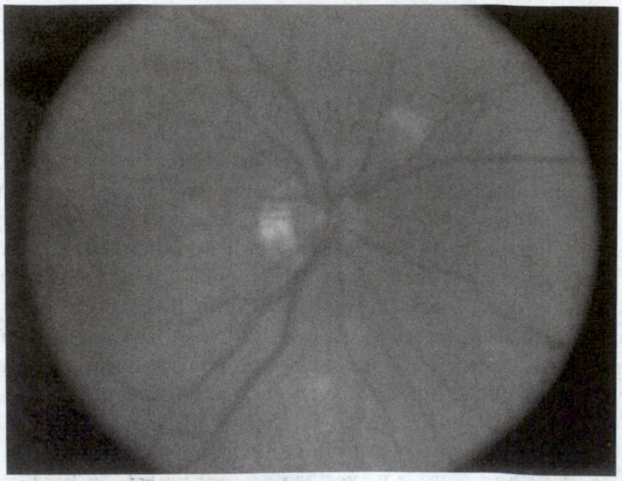

FIGURE 10-47 (Plate 43) Retinal cotton-wool spot. Cotton-wool spots are most frequently found close to the optic disk. Although they occur in acute uncontrolled systemic hypertension, the more common cause now, in younger patients, is infection with the human immunodeficiency virus (HIV). This normotensive 37-year-old man had no visual symptoms and no other retinopathy. There is a myopic crescent at the temporal disk edge, which is not abnormal. He died of complications related to the acquired immunodeficiency syndrome (AIDS) 2 years later.

are most visible along the sides of the vessels, since the location of the tangential line of sight presents a greater thickness to the viewer. Fatty exudate (hard exudate) may collect along venous walls (never arteries), particularly in diabetic exudative retinopathy.

Arteriosclerosis

In arteriosclerosis, medial smooth muscle (which may hypertrophy in chronic hypertension) becomes hyalinized with the deposition of collagen. As the wall thickens, the vessel takes on a burnished coppery luster; with further thickening, this may transmute to silver.

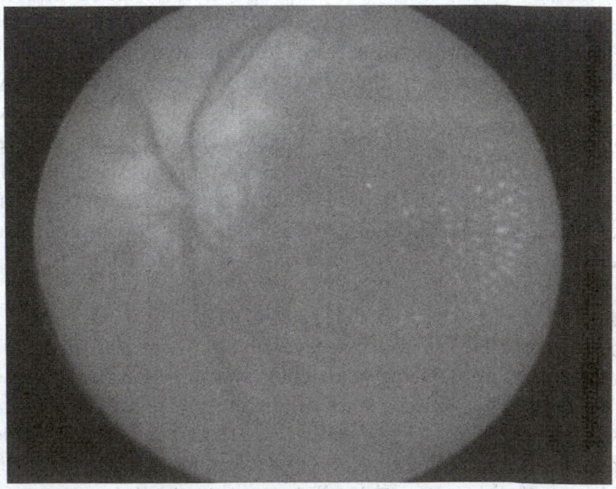

FIGURE 10-48 (Plate 44) Disk swelling and hard exudate in a macular "star" pattern. In this hypertensive patient with periarteritis nodosa, vascular leakage has led to the deposit of hard exudates around the fovea. Radial perifoveal connective tissue results in the star pattern of the exudate. Note also that the optic disk is edematous, with blurred margins, secondary to hypertension.

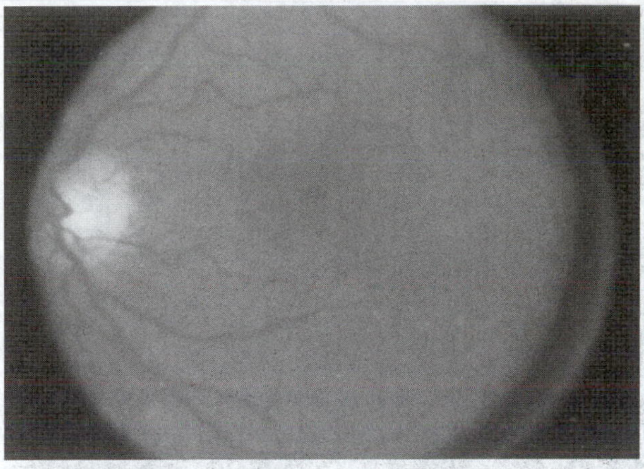

FIGURE 10-49 (Plate 45) Background diabetic retinopathy. Retinal microaneurysms, dot-and-blot hemorrhages, and a few fine upper temporal hard exudates are diagnostic of early diabetic retinopathy. The patient had no visual symptoms, but retinopathy of this magnitude can often be seen in patients with insulin-requiring diabetes of 15 or more years' duration.

Arteriovenous Compressions

Arteriovenous compressions or "nicking" results from the sharing by the artery and vein of a common adventitial sheath at their crossings. Arteriosclerotic thickening impedes venous outflow at these locations, with venous tortuosity, engorgement, and darkening of the flood column distal to the compression.[201]

Atherosclerosis

Retinal atheromata have a predilection for the bifurcation and bends within the first two branches of the central retinal artery, appearing as segments of irregular yellowish sheathing and having the crystalline knobbiness of a salted pretzel stick.[210]

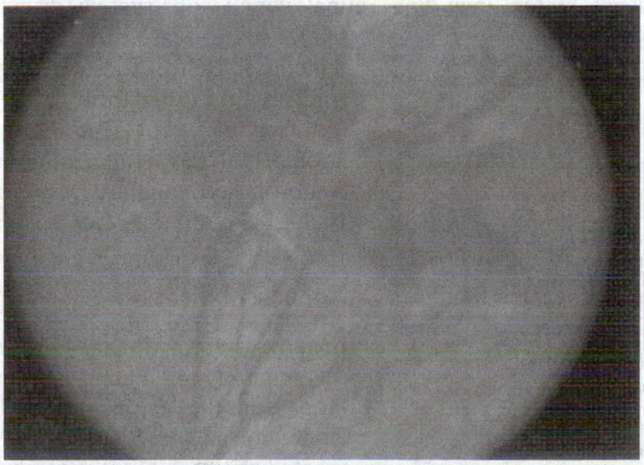

FIGURE 10-50 (Plate 46) Proliferative diabetic retinopathy with preretinal hemorrhage. When neovascularization develops, preretinal and vitreous hemorrhages are much more likely to occur. Easily visible neovascularization either in the periphery of the retina, as in this diabetic patient, or at the disk is an indication for immediate panretinal laser photocoagulation.

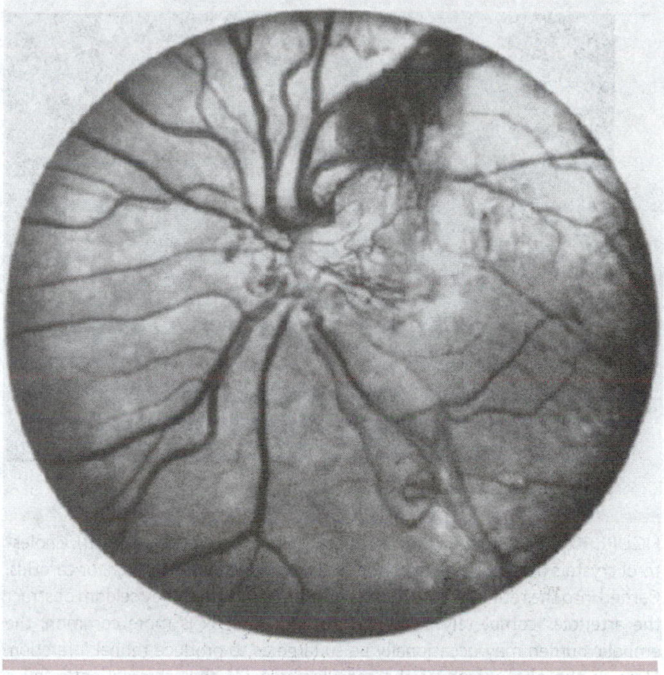

FIGURE 10-51 Proliferative diabetic retinopathy, left eye. There is extensive neovascularization of the disk with an associated small intravitreal hemorrhage that obscures the upper temporal vessels. Along the inferior temporal arcade is another area of neovascularization. These new vessels are incorporated in fibrous membranes that may tent up the vessels and cause traction detachments of the retina, as at the lower right edge of the photograph.

Cotton-Wool Spots

Cotton-wool spots are generally a sign of serious systemic disease. They may be seen in patients with severe hypertension, blood dyscrasias, collagen diseases, or hemorrhagic shock. Cotton-wool spots also are seen frequently in patients with acquired immunodeficiency syndrome (AIDS) (Fig. 10-47, Plate 43). Cotton-wool "exudates" are not exudates but consist of a cluster

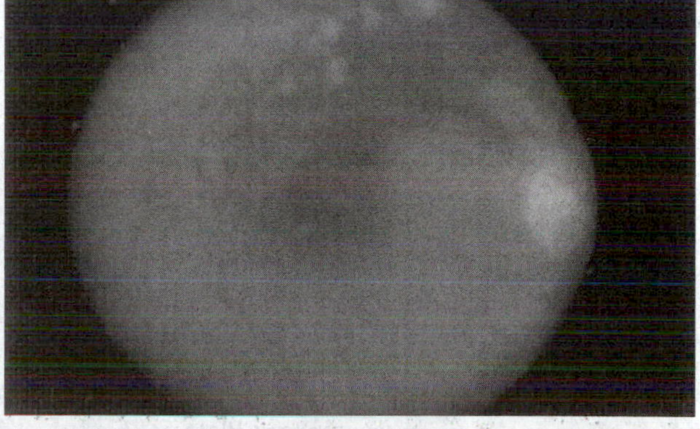

FIGURE 10-52 (Plate 47) Branch retinal vein obstruction. Thickening of the retinal arterial wall in diabetes and hypertension may compromise the lumen of the vein, where they share a common adventitial sheath at an arteriovenous crossing. The resulting obstruction produces hemorrhage retinopathy in the drainage area of the affected vein. Note here how the flame-shaped pattern of blood outlines the arcuate pattern of the nerve fibers as they run toward the optic disk.

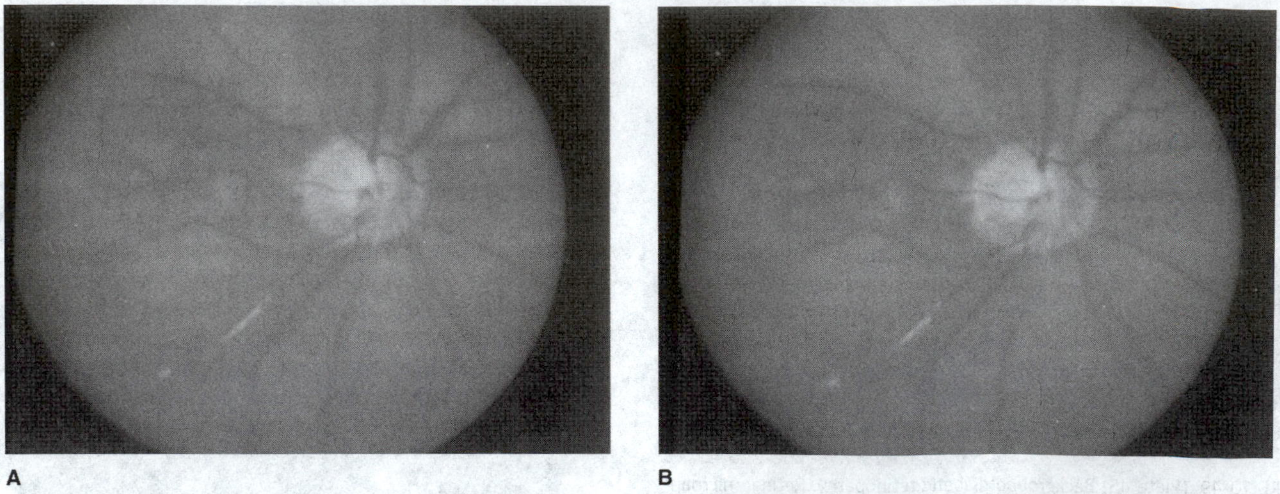

FIGURE 10-53 (Plate 48) Embolic retinal arterial obstruction (*A* and *B*). Cholesterol crystals may dislodge from the walls of the heart, aortic arch, or carotids. Carried into the retinal circulation as Hollenhorst plaques, they seldom obstruct the arterioles completely. Although amaurosis fugax is more common, the embolic burden may occasionally be so large as to produce retinal infarction. Note in the photograph of the macular area (*A*) that this patient's fovea remains red, while there is a pale, cloudy swelling nasal to it. This has produced a half "cherry-red" spot. With complete central retinal artery occlusion, the red foveal area is completely surrounded by pale swollen retina. Hollenhorst cholesterol plaques can be seen in both the upper and lower temporal retinal arteries. In *A*, the inferior temporal arteriole demonstrates "boxcar" segmentation of the blood column, indicative of very slow flow.

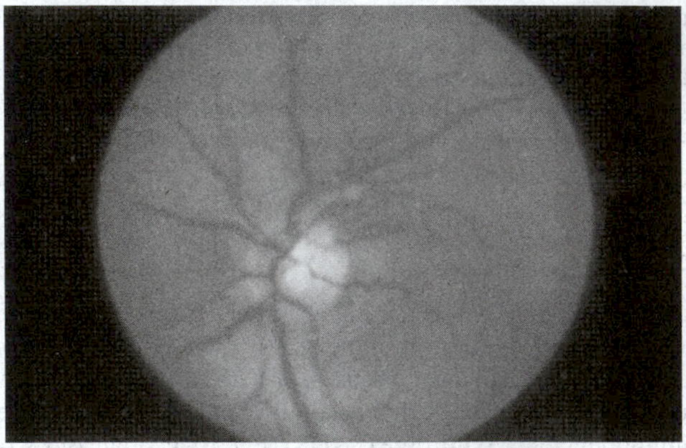

FIGURE 10-54 (Plate 49) Neovascularization after branch retinal vein obstruction. New vessels may develop late after obstruction of a branch of the central retinal vein. These most often serve to shunt flow around the obstructed vessel site and are thus not as exuberantly proliferative as those seen in diabetic retinopathy.

of cell-like swollen ends of fragmented axons (cytoid bodies) in an area of edematous retina.[201]

Hard Exudates

Hard exudates are most likely residues of edema. They occur in situations where the vessels become leaky, and as the more watery component of the extravasation is resorbed, the lipid residue forms a hard, yellow, waxy deposit. These deposits may surround the leaking vessel in a circinate ring or may accumulate in the macula, radiating from the fovea in the spokes of a macular "star" (Fig. 10-48, Plate 44).

Microaneurysms

Microaneurysms are not unique to diabetes but occur in many disease states, including retinal venous obstructive disease, sickle cell disease, the dysproteinemias, Behçet's disease, sarcoidosis, and other forms of uveitis. They may represent abortive attempts at revascularization of compromised capillary bed (Fig. 10-49, Plate 45).

TABLE 10-6 Emboli of Cardiovascular Significance

Type	Appearance	Significance
Platelet	Dull pink to gray often with associated fibrin	Downstream vegetations, mural thrombi
Hollenhorst plaque	Glistening yellow-orange plaques at bifurcations	Downstream atheroma (containing cholesterol)
Calcium plaque	Glistening white plaques	Calcific aortic stenosis
Roth spot	Hemorrhage with gray-white center (see Plate 51, Fig. 10-57)	Blood dyscrasia or septic embolus as in subacute bacterial endocarditis
Fat embolus	Fuzzy-bordered gray-white spot without hemorrhage	Severe trauma with long bone fractures
Myxoma	Disk edema, retinal edema in arterial supply zone	Life-threatening atrial myxoma

Neovascularization

In neovascularization the new vessels generally originate from capillaries from the venous side of the circulation and are associated with greater or lesser degrees of fibrosis. In all cases, however, the new vessels are incorporated in an associated fibrous membrane (Fig. 10-50, Plate 46; Fig. 10-51).

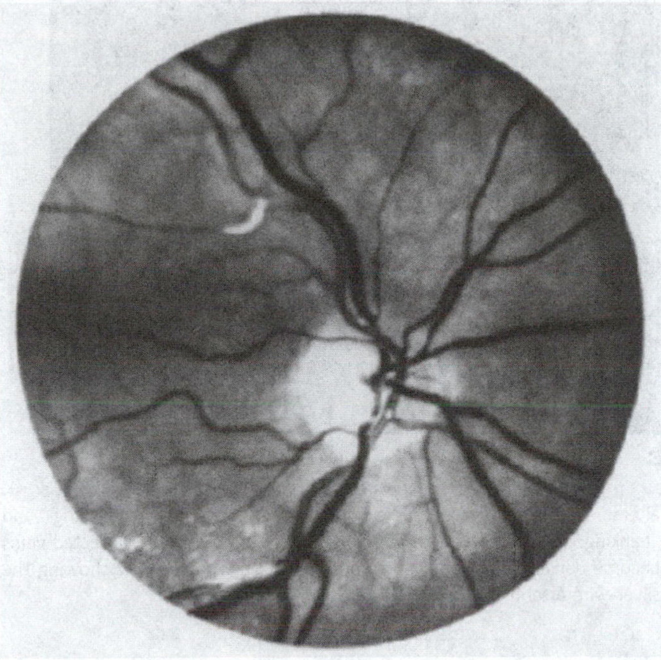

FIGURE 10-55 Retinal emboli often lodge at bifurcations, as in this patient with carotid atherosclerosis. Note that the embolic material often seems larger than the containing vessel, as in the embolus at the lower left edge of the photograph. Emboli may damage the vessel wall and cause leakage, as can be seen by the exudate deposited about the inferior embolus. Hollenhorst cholesterol plaques rarely obstruct arterial flow completely, and this patient maintained vision.

Retinal Hemorrhage

Hemorrhage into the retina indicates further breakdown in the integrity of the vascular wall. When the hemorrhage occurs in the inner retina, as in hypertension, it assumes a feathery flame shape as it is molded and dispersed by the nerve fibers coursing toward the disk. In obstruction of the central retinal vein, the fundus may be splattered with blood (Fig. 10-52, Plate 47).

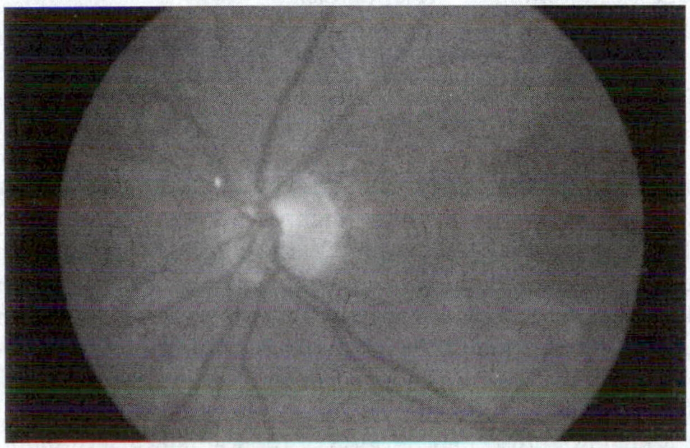

FIGURE 10-56 (Plate 50) Calcific retinal embolus associated with aortic valvular disease. Calcific aortic valvular disease and valve replacement surgery may result in retinal emboli. Like cholesterol emboli, these calcific flecks lodge at arterial bifurcations but seldom obstruct flow completely. They are white and glitter in the ophthalmoscope beam. Somewhat similar emboli may be seen after the intravenous injection of illicit drugs expanded with talc.

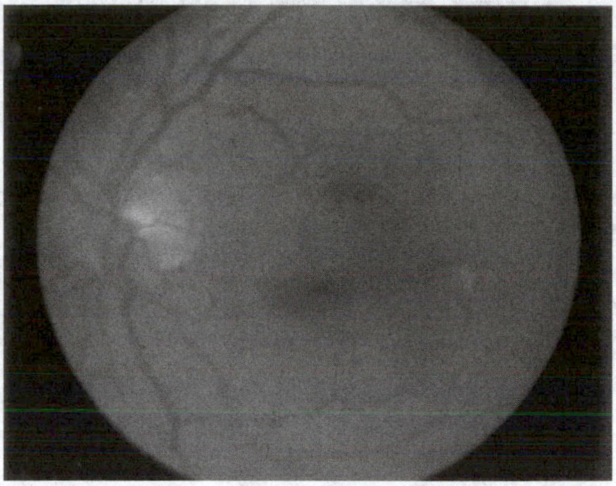

FIGURE 10-57 (Plate 51) Retinal hemorrhages after cardiac catheterization. Following cardiac catheterization, symptomatic and asymptomatic retinal hemorrhages may occur. The latter are more common. Presumably, these are the result of embolic events. Note, in this recently catheterized patient, the two oval hemorrhages and a small area of cloudy swelling just inferior and temporal to the fovea.

Vascular Occlusion

When the central artery or one of its branches is occluded, the nonperfused retinal area becomes cloudy in a matter of minutes. At the fovea, where the retina is one cell layer thick and nourished by the choroid, the normal color and transparency persist. By contrast with the surrounding pallor, the fovea then has a cherry-red appearance (Fig. 10-53, Plate 48). Occlusions of branches of the central vein produce edema and hemorrhage in the drained area. As collateral drainage channels develop (see

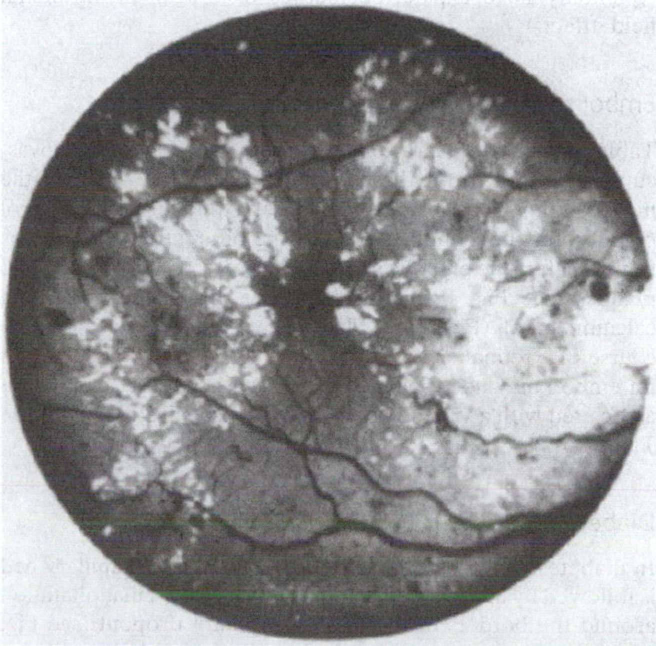

FIGURE 10-58 Exudative diabetic retinopathy, right eye, illustrating microaneurysms, dot-and-blot hemorrhages, and venous engorgement with extensive deposits of hard, yellow exudate.

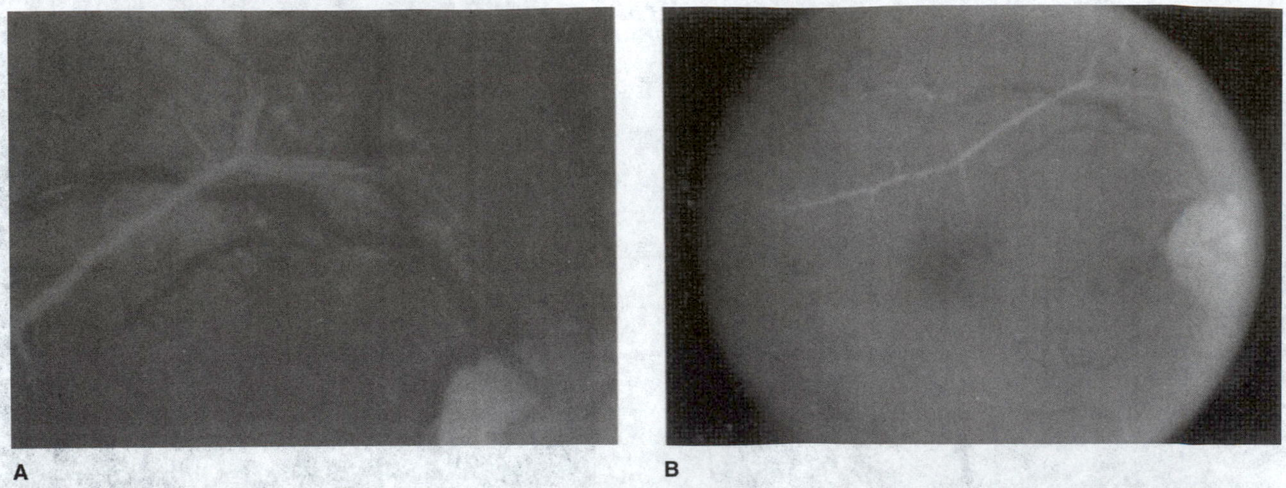

FIGURE 10-59 (Plate 52) *A.* Retinal arteriosclerosis. This 75-year-old hypertensive woman has marked arteriosclerosis of the upper temporal retinal arteriole and its branches. When the narrowed blood column can no longer be seen, the thickened wall produces the "silver-wire" appearance seen here. Where the arteriole crosses its associated vein, the course of the vein is altered, and its blood column cannot be seen. This venous "nicking" and "banking" is associated with impairment of outflow, and the affected veins become darker, larger, and more tortuous. *B.* Low-power view showing the silver-wire arteriole.

Fig 10-52 and Plate 47), the edema and hemorrhagic retinopathy subside, leaving white-walled veins, neovascularization, and microaneurysms in the affected area (Fig. 10-54, Plate 49).

Optic Disk Edema

The term *papilledema* is reserved for the form of disk edema that is the result of increased intracranial pressure. It therefore has an etiologic connotation and is not used generally to mean optic disk edema. *Papillitis* is the term applied to inflammatory disk edema. Patients with anterior ischemic optic neuropathy commonly have a pale, edematous disk with an altitudinal field effect.

Embolism

Table 10-6 lists the characteristics of retinal emboli of cardiovascular significance. Of these, platelet emboli are at once the most common and the most evanescent. Hollenhorst cholesterol plaques may be identified at the same bifurcations for months to years after the embolic shower. Platelet emboli, Hollenhorst plaques (see Fig. 10-53, Plate 48; Fig. 10-55, Plate 49), and calcium emboli (Fig. 10-56, Plate 50) are usually seen along the course of a retinal artery. Roth spots (Fig. 10-57, Plate 51) and fat emboli may not appear to be intravascular and may not be associated with a vessel that is ophthalmoscopically visible (see Table 10-6).[201]

Diabetes Mellitus

In diabetes mellitus, focal loss of a portion of the capillary bed is followed by microaneurysm formation and vascular dilatation around the borders of the area of capillary dropout (see Fig. 10-49 and Plate 45). Vascular leakage occurs with dot and blot hemorrhages and deposits of hard exudate (Fig 10-58). New blood vessels develop along the vascular arcades and at the optic nerve head (see Figs. 10-50 and 10-51 and Plate 50).

Vasoconstriction of the arterial tree and thickening of the arterial vessel walls with consequent reduction in lumen diameter are homeostatic responses to hypertension. Arteriosclerotic narrowing of the vessels acts to insulate the capillary bed from the elevated pressure of the arterial supply. These arteriosclerotic changes are visible as narrowing, increases in central light reflexes, and copper and silver "wiring" of the arteries (Fig. 10-59, Plate 52). Radial arrangement of such exudate deposits in the macula produces a "star" (see Fig 10-48 and Plate 48). Hemorrhage may occur in the retinal layers in a characteristic flame pattern, and focal ischemia in the nerve fiber may result in cotton-wool microinfarcts. In severe hypertensive decompensation, the optic nerve head becomes swollen and edematous (see Fig. 10-48 and Plate 48).

Hypertensive patients should be classified as to whether or not their retinal circulation is compensated or has decompensated with observable edema, cotton-wool spots, flame hemorrhages, or swelling of the optic disk.[201]

PHYSICAL EXAMINATION OF THE CHEST, ABDOMEN, AND EXTREMITIES

Physical examination of the lungs is an important noninvasive technique requiring only a stethoscope.[202] Wheezing and a pleural friction rub are detected only by the clinical evaluation. The pleural friction rub may be a clue to the diagnosis of pulmonary infarction. Pleural fluid due to heart failure is usually located in the right pleural space. When pleural fluid is localized predominately to the left, a cause other than or in addition to heart failure, such as pulmonary infarction, should be considered.

A pneumothorax may develop as a consequence of spontaneous mediastinal emphysema or may be iatrogenic, due to procedures.[202] Hyperresonance and diminished breath sounds may be due to pulmonary emphysema. Signs of pulmonary consolidation may be due to pneumonia or pulmonary infarction. Wheezing and rales may be due to bronchial disease. Heart failure may be associated with rales in the lung bases, wheezing, and pleural fluid. Importantly, heart failure frequently is not associated with rales, since interstitial pulmonary edema usually does not produce rales.[202]

The diameter of the *abdominal* aorta should be determined in every patient[202] (see Chap. 88). An abdominal aortic aneurysm may be missed if the examiner fails to assess the area above the umbilicus.

Specific abnormalities of the abdomen may be secondary to heart disease. A large, tender liver is common in patients with heart failure or constrictive pericarditis. Systolic hepatic pulsations are frequent in patients with tricuspid regurgitation. A palpable spleen is a common but late sign in patients with severe heart failure and is also often present in patients with infective endocarditis.

Although hepatic cirrhosis is the most common cause of ascites, the latter may occur with heart failure alone, although it is less common with the use of diuretic therapy. Severe tricuspid regurgitation, as caused by infective endocarditis in drug addicts, may produce prominent systolic pulsation of the internal jugular veins in the neck, a large, moving, and pulsating liver, and ascites. Constrictive pericarditis should be considered when the ascites is out of proportion to peripheral edema. In many such patients, the heart is normal in size or only slightly enlarged, a pericardial "knock" is heard, and there is a rapid x and/or y descent in the internal jugular vein pulsation.[202] Restrictive cardiomyopathy can mimic constrictive pericarditis, but the heart is usually moderately large in patients with restrictive cardiomyopathy. When there is an arteriovenous fistula in the abdomen, a continuous murmur may be heard over the abdomen. Fistulas due to trauma and surgery may occur.

A systolic bruit may be heard over the kidney areas and may signify renal artery stenosis, particularly in patients with systemic hypertension. A systolic bruit often is auscultated over the abdominal aorta, but its presence does not indicate the severity of disease of the aorta.[202]

Examination of the upper and lower extremities may provide important diagnostic information (see Chap. 90). The clinical detection of arterial disease and thrombophlebitis is important. Atherosclerosis of the peripheral arteries may produce intermittent claudication of the buttock, calf, thigh, or foot, with severe disease resulting in tissue damage of the toes. Peripheral atherosclerosis is an important risk factor for ischemic heart disease, and its presence increases the likelihood of coronary atherosclerosis. Thrombophlebitis often causes pain in the calf or thigh or edema, and its presence should raise the consideration of pulmonary emboli as well. Edema is a late sign of heart failure, and its predictive value as a diagnostic sign is poor. It frequently involves the right leg prior to the left. Considerable heart failure and a resulting weight gain may be present without edema being present. Edema of the lower extremities may be secondary to local factors such as varicose veins or thrombophlebitis or the removal of veins at CABG surgery. Under such circumstances, the edema often occurs in only one leg.

Edema may result from restrictive garments, and venous stasis often is secondary to a long trip in a car or airplane.[202] Edema may be due to salt and water retention in patients with primary renal disease. In the differential diagnosis of edema, local factors should be considered first. If local factors can be excluded, the cause of the salt and water retention should be determined with an assessment for evidence of primary renal disease. Rarely, peripheral edema can be an early sign of lymphatic obstruction produced by metastatic disease in the pelvis or abdomen.

Since the invention of the stethoscope by Laennec in 1826, cardiac auscultation has played a key role in the evaluation of patients with cardiovascular disease. New diagnostic techniques developed in recent years have led to a better understanding of the relationship between intracardiac pressure, flow, and valve motion and the resulting sound phenomena on the other. The analysis of heart sounds and murmurs by phonocardiography, together with information obtained by cardiac catheterization, angiography, echocardiography, and cardiac surgery, has made cardiac auscultation a precise discipline based on firm physiologic principles.[203]

INSPECTION AND PALPATION OF THE PRECORDIUM

Inspection and palpation of the cardiac pulsations of the anterior chest have been practiced by physicians since ancient times and have a solid scientific basis. The results of precordial inspection and palpation have been correlated with noninvasive studies, hemodynamic data, and surgical and autopsy studies[202,203] and remain an important part of the cardiovascular examination. Their usefulness depends on an understanding of cardiovascular physiology, the proficiency of the examiner, and his or her ability to integrate findings with history, the information obtained by other portions of the physical examination, the ECG, the chest roentgenogram, and other diagnostic tests.

Precordial Pulsations Due to the Heartbeat

Precordial pulsations, reflecting underlying movement of the heart and great vessels, occur principally in seven areas of the anterior chest[204,205] (Fig. 10-60):

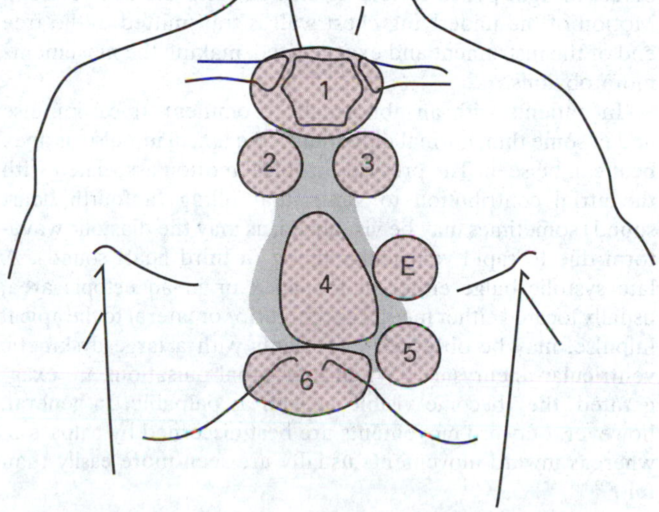

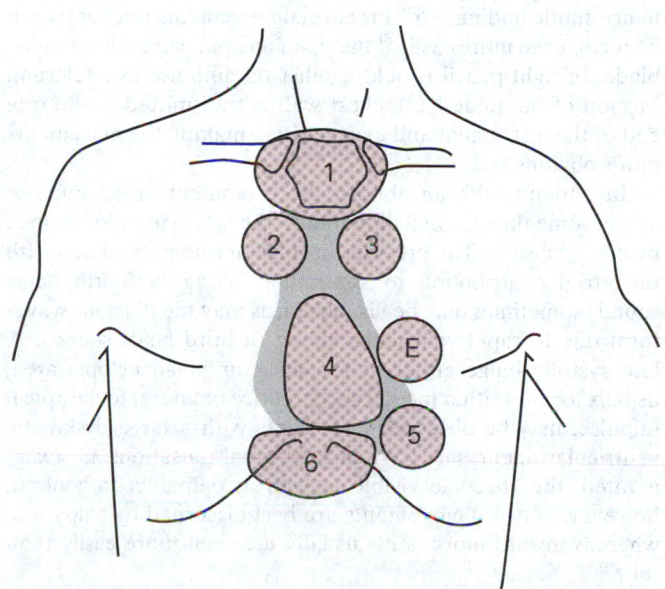

FIGURE 10-60 Seven areas to be examined for abnormal cardiovascular pulsations by inspection and palpation. (From Schlant RC, Hurst JW. *Examination of the Precordium: Inspection and Palpation*. New York: American Heart Association; 1990:1–28. Used with permission from the publisher and authors.)

1. The sternoclavicular area
2. The aortic area
3. The pulmonic area
4. The RV (left parasternal) area
5. The LV (apical) area
6. The epigastric area
7. Ectopic (variable-location) areas

While the cardiac apex is usually produced by the left ventricle, it is sometimes produced by an enlarged right ventricle that displaces the left ventricle laterally and posteriorly. Occasionally, the cardiac position is abnormal due to dextroposition, dextroversion, dextrocardia, or other changes in intrathoracic structures. Although the cardiac apex impulse is commonly referred to as the *point of maximal impulse* (PMI), the two terms are not necessarily synonymous, since the maximal precordial pulsation may be produced by an enlarged or hypertrophied right ventricle, a dilated aorta or pulmonary artery, or a LV wall-motion abnormality. Therefore, precordial pulsations should be described by their location, timing, contour, and duration.

Inspection of the Precordium

The examiner should first inspect the thorax from the foot of the bed with the subject supine, the legs horizontal, and the head and trunk elevated to approximately 30°.[205] The patient may have a barrel-shaped chest with an increased anteroposterior diameter, a straight-back syndrome, pectus excavatum, pectus carinatum, kyphoscoliosis, or ankylosing spondylitis. Each may produce or be associated with cardiac abnormalities. Asymmetry of the thorax due to convex bulging of the precordium suggests the presence of heart disease since childhood. Exaggerated movements of the cardiac apex often can be detected from this observation point.

Next, the examiner should move to the patient's right side and observe the patient's chest tangentially rather than from above. A light beam directed across the precordium may enhance subtle findings.[205,206] Precordial movements frequently can be recognized more easily if the tip of an applicator stick, tongue blade, or light pencil is held against the impulse as a fulcrum. Motion of the underlying chest wall is transmitted to the free end of the instrument and exaggerated, making the movements more obvious.

In patients with an abnormally prominent apical impulse and in some thin, normal individuals, the apical impulse or apex beat can be seen. The presystolic apical motion associated with the atrial contribution to ventricular filling (a fourth heart sound) sometimes may be visualized, as may the diastolic waveform due to rapid ventricular filling (a third heart sound). A late systolic bulge either at the apex or in an ectopic area, usually located either medial and superior or lateral to the apical impulse, may be observed in patients with a large dyskinetic ventricular aneurysm.[203] When precordial pulsations are exaggerated, they become visible as well as palpable. In general, however, outward movements are best discerned by palpation, whereas inward movements usually are seen more easily than felt.[202,203]

Palpation of the Precordium

With Tietze's syndrome, pain, sometimes with swelling and tenderness, may affect the costochondral, chondrosternal, or xiphosternal joints and may be reproduced by touching. Palpation also may reveal tender superficial veins on the anterior chest (Mondor's disease), a rare etiology of chest discomfort.[206] Collateral vessels in the posterior intercostal spaces may be palpable in patients with aortic coarctation.[206]

Palpation of the precordium is also best performed from the right side, with the patient supine and the upper trunk elevated 30°. Palpation with the right hand usually provides more information. Patients with suspected cardiovascular disease also should be examined in the left lateral decubitus position, rotated 45 to 90°.[207] In this position, the normal LV impulse may be displaced several centimeters leftward and may appear more prominent and sustained. The size of the apex impulse rather than its distance from the midsternal or midclavicular line determines its normality.[207] Often, the apex impulse and other palpable events such as a LV rapid filling wave (S_3) or presystolic *a* wave (S_4) may be felt only in this position.

The location and size of the cardiac apex impulse should be defined, its contour characterized, and any abnormal precordial pulsations identified. The palm of the hand, ventral surface of the proximal metacarpals, and fingers should all be used for optimal appreciation of specific movements. The fingers appear to be particularly insensitive to movements of relatively large amplitude and very low frequency. This is consistent with the clinical observation that an examiner's hand occasionally can be seen to move up and down with precordial motion, although the same movements are imperceptible by palpation alone. By contrast, higher-frequency events, such as the vibrations associated with abnormally loud aortic or pulmonic components of the second heart sound, are easily palpable, even though the amplitude of their movement is not readily visible.[204]

The pads of the fingers are most useful for detecting LV and normal RV motion, whereas the palm and proximal metacarpals are usually best used for palpating larger, low-frequency movements such as the parasternal systolic lift of RV hypertrophy.[204] Varying pressure with the hand is often quite useful. High-frequency movements such as ejection sounds, valve closure sounds, and mitral opening snaps are detected more easily with the hand held firmly against the chest, whereas low-frequency movements such as ventricular diastolic filling events are best recognized with light pressure with the fingertips.

Thrills are palpable vibrations from murmurs or bruits ordinarily associated with grade 4/6 murmurs or louder. The location of a thrill often helps identify its origin. Thrills are palpated most easily with the fingertips or with firm pressure, using either the palm of the hand or the proximal metacarpals. Sometimes thrills are felt better during a held end-expiration with moderate pressure applied from the right hand on top of the left hand, which is placed on the chest. Occasionally, palpable murmurs are more readily detected with the right palm placed over the anterior chest and the left hand supporting the posterior thorax with equal force.[205]

To detect abnormal RV motion, the heel of the hand should be placed over the lower half of the sternum with the patient's breath held at end-expiration. The parasternal lift due to RV hypertrophy is often better visualized than actually felt. In patients with chronic obstructive pulmonary disease, subxiphoid and epigastric palpation with the patient's breath held at end-inspiration is useful for assessing RV motion.

Proper patient positioning is important. The location of the apex impulse is usually described in terms of its distance from the midsternal or midclavicular line and the intercostal space in which it is located. Although heart size is commonly estimated based on the size and location of the apex impulse with the patient supine, this is not always a reliable indicator of LV end-diastolic volume. The apex impulse is often faint or not palpable with the patient supine because of the distance of the ventricular apex from the chest wall. Palpation of the cardiac apex with the patient in the left lateral position, however, permits optimal assessment of the size (diameter) and contour of the systolic outward movement at the apex; diastolic movements are also best appreciated with the patient in this position. Since the apex impulse may shift several centimeters laterally when the patient rotates to the left lateral position, however, the location of the apex impulse may be incorrect in this position. Palpation with simultaneous cardiac auscultation often is useful for identifying the systolic or diastolic timing of precordial pulsations. Simultaneous palpation of the apical impulse and carotid pulse may be helpful in assessing the severity of aortic stenosis. An appreciable lag time between the onset of the apex impulse and carotid pulse usually indicates severe aortic stenosis.

Physiology of Precordial Motion

Although only the apical impulse is palpable normally, a brief RV systolic motion can be felt at the left sternal edge in asthenic individuals. With the onset of isovolumic LV contraction, there is anterior movement of the left ventricle toward the chest walls (see Fig. 10-61). Counterclockwise rotation of the left ventricle along its longitudinal axis occurs as the cardiac apex moves anteriorly and makes contact with the chest wall in early systole.[208] The maximal outward movement occurs coincident with or just after aortic valve opening. After rapid early ejection, the left ventricle moves away from the chest wall, and the apex retracts during latter systole and returns to baseline well before the second heart sound.[204] The outward apex movement in early systole normally is palpable, but the later systolic inward movement is only visible (Fig. 10-61). Palpable movements of the apex in diastole result from LV filling. The early diastolic outward movement due to rapid ventricular filling (F wave), which corresponds to the normal S_3, is occasionally palpable in normal children and young adults (see Fig. 10-61). Later diastolic filling due to left atrial contraction (*a* wave) is not normally palpable. Precordial motion is modified by age, chest wall thickness, lung disease, and pleural or pericardial effusion.

AREA 1: STERNOCLAVICULAR AREA PULSATIONS

The sternoclavicular area (see Fig. 10-60) includes the right and left sternoclavicular joints, the ma-

Type of movement and associated clinical condition	Graphic Representation (palpable features in heavy line)	Location and accompanying features
NORMAL ADULT APEX IMPULSE	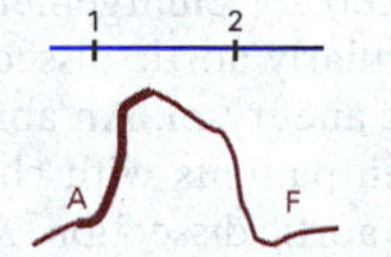	Cardiac apex; moderate systolic thrust; A and F waves usually imperceptible
HYPERKINETIC APEX IMPULSE Normal Child Hyperdynamic states Ventricular septal defect Patent ductus arteriosus Mitral regurgitation Aortic regurgitation	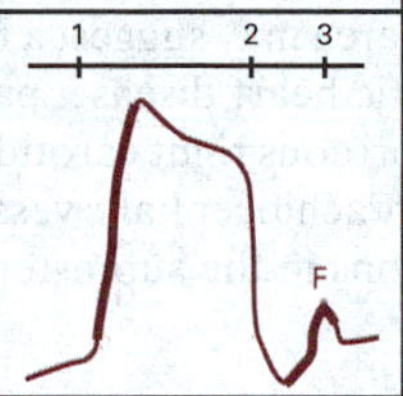	Exaggerated thrust at cardiac apex; F wave may be palpable, coincident with third heart sound
HYPERKINETIC RIGHT VENTRICULAR IMPULSE Atrial septal defect Pulmonary regurgitation	Same as above	Maximal at left sternal edge in third and fourth intercostal spaces
SUSTAINED APEX IMPULSE Left ventricular hypertrophy, as in: Aortic stenosis Hypertension Insert: a variation that may occur in hypertrophic cardiomyopathy	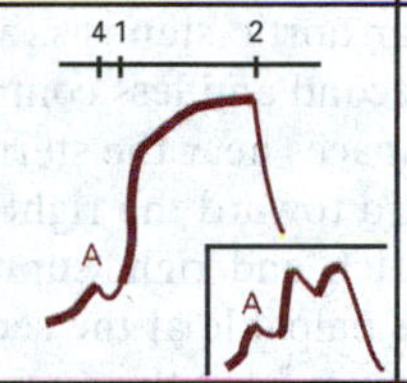	Maximal at cardiac apex; A wave may be visible and palpable coincident with fourth heart sound
SUSTAINED RIGHT VENTRICULAR IMPULSE Right ventricular hypertrophy, as in: Pulmonary hypertension Pulmonary stenosis	Same impulse as in Sustained above	Maximal at left sternal edge in third and fourth intercostal spaces
ECTOPIC LEFT VENTRICULAR IMPULSE Ventricular aneurysm	Same impulse as in Sustained above	Maximal over mid-precordium rather than at apex
LEFT ATRIAL EXPANSION Severe mitral regurgitation	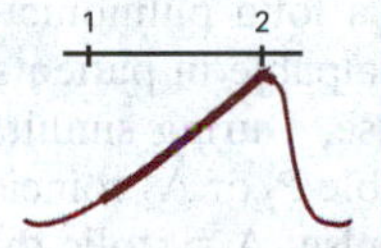	Left sternal edge or entire precordium; hyperkinetic apex impulse due to left ventricular volume overload
PULMONARY ARTERY PULSATION Pulmonary hypertension	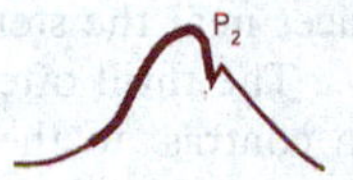	Second left intercostal space; palpable P_2
INWARD MOVEMENT DURING SYSTOLE Constrictive pericarditis Tricuspid regurgitation; primary	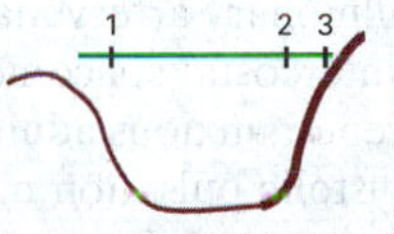	Cardiac apex or entire precordium; reversal of direction during systole as compared with preceding examples
DIASTOLIC MOVEMENTS Cardiomyopathy	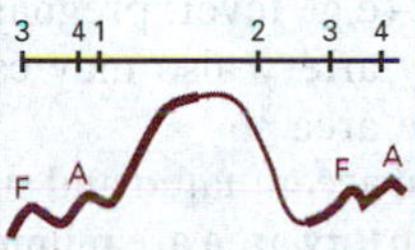	Cardiac apex; systolic movement may be inconspicuous; diastolic movements F and A correspond to 3rd and 4th heart sounds which may merge in tachycardia to form a summation gallop

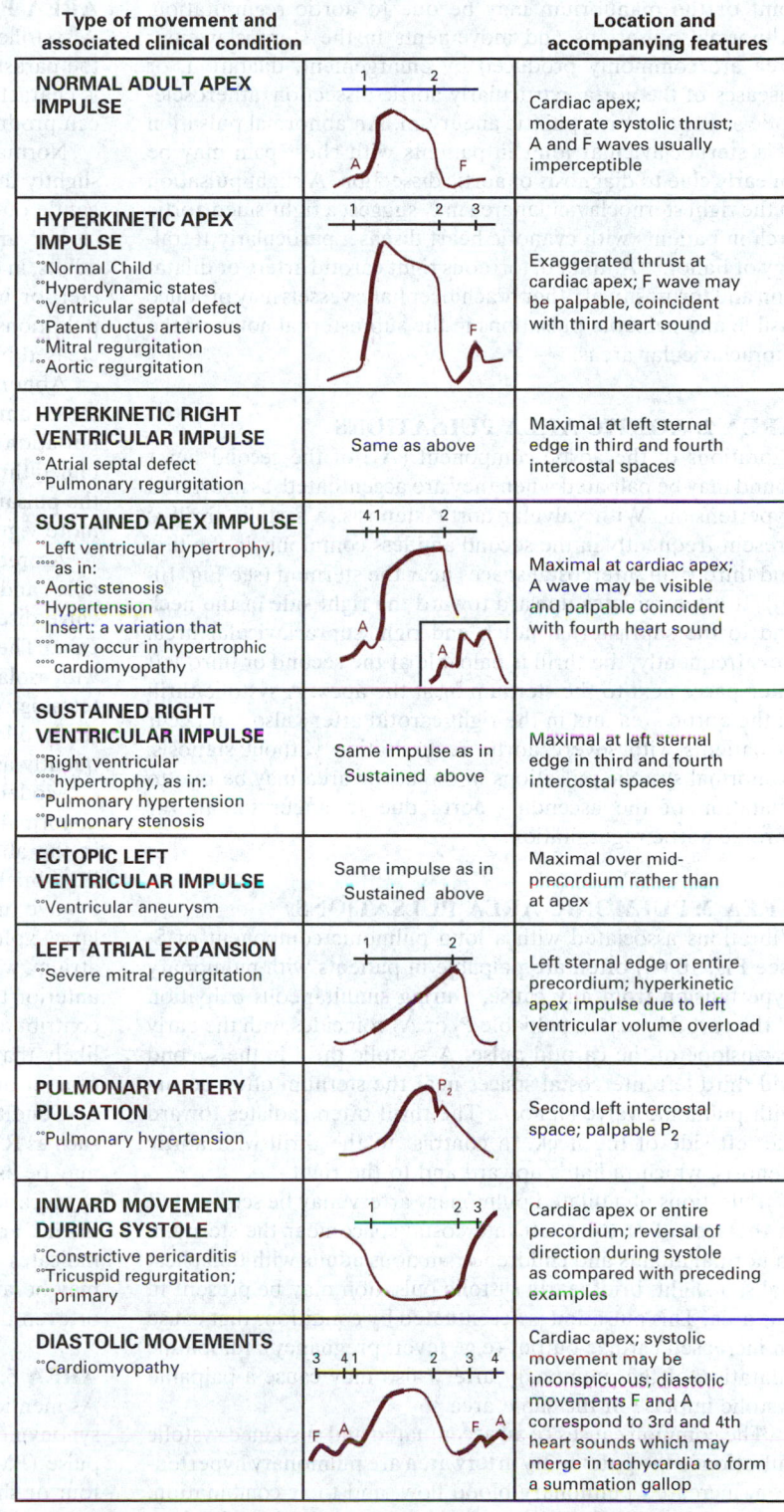

FIGURE 10-61 Graphic representation of apical movements in health and disease. Heavy line indicates palpable features. P_2, pulmonary component of second heart sound; A, atrial wave, corresponding to a fourth heart sound (S_4) or atrial gallop; F, filling wave, corresponding to third heart sound (S_3) or ventricular gallop. (From Willis P IV. Inspection and palpation of the precordium. In: Hurst JW, ed. *The Heart*, 7th ed. New York: McGraw-Hill; 1990:164. Reproduced with permission from the publisher and author.)

nubrium, and the upper sternum. Usually, no pulsation is noted in this area. A slight, brief systolic pulsation of a sternoclavicular joint or the manubrium may be due to aortic regurgitation. Abnormal pulsations and movements in the sternoclavicular area are commonly produced by enlargement, dilatation, or diseases of the aorta, particularly aortic dissection, atherosclerotic aneurysm, or syphilitic aneurysm. An abnormal pulsation of a sternoclavicular joint in patients with chest pain may be an early clue to diagnosis of aortic dissection. A slight pulsation in the right sternoclavicular area may suggest a right-sided aortic arch in patients with cyanotic heart disease, particularly tetralogy of Fallot.[204] A kinked, tortuous right carotid artery or dilatation and tortuosity of other brachiocephalic vessels may produce visible and palpable pulsations in the suprasternal notch or the supraclavicular areas.

AREA 2: AORTIC AREA PULSATIONS

Vibrations of the aortic component (A_2) of the second heart sound may be palpated when they are accentuated, as in arterial hypertension. With valvular aortic stenosis, a systolic thrill is present frequently in the second and less commonly in the first and third right intercostal spaces near the sternum (see Fig. 10-60). It often radiates upward toward the right side of the neck and to the suprasternal notch and right supraclavicular area. Less frequently, the thrill is palpable at the second or third left interspaces next to the sternum or at the apex. A systolic thrill in the aortic area and in the right carotid artery also can occur in patients with severe aortic regurgitation without stenosis. Abnormal systolic pulsations in the aortic area may be due to dilatation of the ascending aorta due to aneurysm and/or chronic aortic regurgitation.

AREA 3: PULMONIC AREA PULSATIONS

Vibrations associated with a loud pulmonic component of S_2 (see Fig. 10-60) often are palpable in patients with pulmonary hypertension from any cause. During simultaneous palpation of the carotid pulse, a palpable P_2 or A_2 coincides with the early downslope of the carotid pulse. A systolic thrill in the second and third left intercostal spaces near the sternum often occurs with pulmonic valve stenosis. The thrill often radiates toward the left side of the neck, in contrast to the thrill with aortic stenosis, which radiates upward and to the right.

Pulsations of a dilated pulmonary artery may be seen or felt in the second or third left intercostal space near the sternum. In normal infants and children or anxious adults with thin chest walls, a slight, brief, early systolic pulsation may be present in this area. This pulsation is accentuated by conditions that cause an increased cardiac output (e.g., fever, pregnancy). Idiopathic dilatation of the pulmonary artery also may cause a palpable systolic impulse in the same area.[205]

The common causes of an accentuated and sustained systolic pulsation in the pulmonary artery area are pulmonary hypertension, increased pulmonary blood flow, and their combination. In general, pulmonary hypertension causes a relatively slow, sustained, and forceful pulmonary artery pulsation, whereas a large pulmonary blood flow (e.g., ASD) produces an extremely active, more vigorous, but less sustained pulsation. Valvular pulmonary stenosis with poststenotic dilatation of the pulmonary artery may be associated with a palpable, sustained pulsation in this area, often with a slow rise of the initial phase.

AREA 4: LEFT PARASTERNAL—RIGHT VENTRICULAR OR TRICUSPID AREA PULSATIONS

A systolic thrill in the third, fourth, or fifth intercostal space in the parasternal area to the left of the sternum (see Fig. 10-60) is characteristic of VSD, although tricuspid regurgitation also can produce a thrill here.

Normally, the lower left parasternal region retracts very slightly during systole, and RV activity is not palpable. Slight, gentle outward pulsations of the lower sternum and left parasternal area may be recorded in normal children and young adults, in thin adults with a small anteroposterior thoracic diameter, or in patients with pectus excavatum. Sometimes, these pulsations can be palpated in the subxiphoid area and are increased by hyperdynamic cardiac function.

Abnormal pulsations of the sternal and left parasternal areas most commonly are due to RV hypertrophy or dilatation. The pulsation associated with RV hypertension is usually more sustained throughout systole and tends to rise more gradually than the pulsation produced by a RV volume load, which usually is more vigorous but often briefer.[203,208]

A predominant RV pressure load occurs with pulmonic stenosis and pulmonary hypertension due to LV failure, mitral valve disease, a left-to-right shunt, or pulmonary vascular disease. The sustained anterior precordial pulsation associated with isolated valvular pulmonic stenosis may not occur with tetralogy of Fallot because the thick right ventricle is not excessively dilated. ASD and VSD are two congenital lesions frequently associated with a RV volume load.

Moderate or severe mitral regurgitation may produce an abnormal late systolic anterior left parasternal pulsation even in the absence of pulmonary hypertension.[209] This precordial lift is brisk, and its greatest force coincides with the accentuated *v* wave in the left atrial pressure wave. It likely is due to the large volume of blood regurgitated into the expanding left atrium, which is located centrally behind the right ventricle and anterior to the spine. While expansion of the left atrium may contribute somewhat to the anterior motion of the heart, it is likely that most of the anterior motion and force is the result of a jet or squid effect.

Conditions associated with a decrease in RV compliance, such as RV hypertrophy secondary to pulmonary hypertension, may be associated with a palpable "right sided" S_4 in this area or, occasionally, in the epigastric area. Although a palpable S_3 in this area may reflect a large RV volume load, it usually indicates RV dysfunction or failure. RV S_3 and S_4 vibrations may be augmented during inspiration and may be attenuated or even disappear during expiration (see below).

AREA 5: APICAL AREA PULSATIONS

As mentioned earlier, the apex impulse (see Fig. 10-60) is not synonymous with maximum impulse or point of maximum impulse (PMI). The location, size, and character (duration, contour or shape, amplitude, and apparent force) of the apex impulse should be determined.[207] The examiner should focus on one phase of the cardiac cycle at a time and correlate the findings with other cardiovascular events.

The normal apex (apical) impulse usually is located within 10 cm of the sternal midline, at or within the left midclavicular line in the fifth intercostal space, when the patient is supine. It may be located lateral to the midclavicular line when associated with a high diaphragm, pregnancy, marked pectus excavatum, or other conditions that displace a normal heart to the left. The normal apex impulse is less than 3 cm in diameter and in most instances is considerably smaller. The early systolic outward movement of the apical area (Fig. 10-61) begins at about the same time as that of the S_1, just before the upstroke of the carotid pulse. Peak outward motion normally occurs with or just after blood is ejected into the aorta; then the apex normally moves inward. The outward movement of the apical impulse is normally not excessively forceful and is felt only during the first third of systole.

The apex impulse may be hyperkinetic or hyperdynamic with increased amplitude in normal individuals who have a thin chest wall, a flat chest, or a depressed sternum. Lying on the left side may cause a normal apical impulse to move laterally and to have increased amplitude and duration[207]; however, it still should not exceed a diameter of greater than 3 cm. A hyperdynamic apex impulse also may be found in anxious children, in patients with high cardiac output states, and in patients with a mild to moderate LV volume load from mitral or aortic regurgitation. The apex impulse is more sustained when mitral or aortic regurgitation is more severe or when LV systolic function is decreased.[204] In general, a greatly sustained apex impulse indicates either marked LV hypertrophy or depressed LV systolic function, whereas LV dilatation displaces the apex impulse laterally and inferiorly[207,210] (see Fig. 10-61).

Concentric LV hypertrophy without an increase in LV cavity size may occur in systemic hypertension, valvular aortic stenosis, and hypertrophic cardiomyopathy. Characteristically, the apex impulse is not displaced but is both abnormally forceful and sustained.[204,205] An S_4 vibration may be palpable or visible or both.

Severe LV dilatation—whether due to volume load or ventricular failure—may displace the apex impulse laterally and inferiorly and cause a marked increase in size. The duration of the apex impulse is more sustained in patients with LV systolic dysfunction, particularly when associated with marked LV dilatation.

Important information about relative amounts of ventricular hypertrophy and dilatation often can be obtained from the apex impulse. Thus, in valvular aortic stenosis, with marked concentric LV hypertrophy but little or no dilatation, the apex impulse characteristically is small, forceful, and sustained but not displaced. A presystolic S_4 often is palpable at the apex. By contrast, in severe aortic regurgitation with marked dilatation of the left ventricle plus considerable eccentric hypertrophy, there is a diffuse apex impulse with increased force, duration, and amplitude, and it is displaced laterally and inferiorly.[205]

In some patients with acute MI, a sustained apex impulse may simulate that due to LV hypertrophy.[201] Those developing mitral regurgitation secondary to MI (papillary muscle dysfunction) may manifest LV dilatation and hypertrophy by a displaced and sustained, forceful, large apex impulse.[211] A late systolic bulge at the cardiac apex may be due to a functional LV aneurysm, occasionally resulting in a bifid apex impulse. In other patients, a late systolic bulge may be palpable in an ectopic area between the apex impulse and the left parasternal area.

A bifid apex impulse during systole also may be due to marked LV dilatation and hypertrophy in patients with both aortic stenosis and regurgitation or in patients with hypertrophic cardiomyopathy.[212] Infrequently, a faint systolic notch or vibration is palpable in the apex impulse of patients with mitral valve prolapse at the moment of a nonejection midsystolic click. Systolic retraction of the apical impulse usually indicates either constrictive pericarditis or severe tricuspid regurgitation with marked RV dilatation (see Fig. 10-61). An apical systolic thrill most commonly is produced by mitral regurgitation and often is diffuse, whereas a diastolic thrill is usually produced by mitral stenosis and is localized to a small, discrete periapical area.

Diastolic Events: Palpable Third and Fourth Heart Sounds

During early diastole, brief outward chest wall movement corresponding to a LV filling or a third heart sound (S_3) occasionally may be seen or felt, even if it is not audible with a stethoscope (see Fig. 10-61). In children and young adults, the presence of an early diastolic ventricular filling sound (S_3) and movement is usually normal. On the other hand, the presence of such a movement or sound in a sedentary adult or a patient with heart disease usually indicates an elevated LV diastolic pressure and volume and likely ventricular decompensation, often with a decreased ejection fraction. Patients with acute MI or transient myocardial ischemia during angina pectoris frequently develop a transient palpable and audible ventricular filling S_3, which reflects the acutely decreased ventricular compliance. A palpable ventricular rapid filling wave (S_3) may be present in patients with LV failure from any cause; however, hemodynamic systolic ventricular failure is often not always present when a ventricular filling wave or sound occurs in the presence of volume loading and dilatation of the left ventricle, as with mitral regurgitation or aortic regurgitation.

The presystolic left atrial contribution to the apical impulse (referred to as the *atrial impulse* or *a* wave) may be detected during late diastole, just prior to S_1 (see Fig. 10-61). Usually, a palpable atrial impulse coincides with an audible fourth heart sound and is associated with an increased LV end-diastolic pressure and decreased compliance. In general, an S_4 is not normally palpable but may be felt at the apex with its associated S_4 in some normal adults if the PR interval is long and circulation is hyperdynamic.[202] In some patients with ischemic heart disease, a palpable apical S_4 may develop or become more prominent during an episode of angina pectoris or even during exertion without chest pain. A palpable presystolic impulse, S_4, or both occur frequently in patients with acute MI, and these are also frequently present in other conditions producing a decrease in LV compliance and increased end-diastolic pressure.

In a patient with mitral valve disease, the presence of a palpable left-sided atrial impulse or S_4, a palpable left-sided ventricular filling sound or S_3, or an abnormally sustained apical impulse is evidence against the diagnosis of isolated important mitral stenosis and suggests the presence of coincident LV disease.

A double, or bifid, apical impulse may be present in various circumstances, most commonly in the combination of an outward movement during ventricular systole and a second outward pulsation during diastole.[205] The diastolic impulse may occur either in early diastole (S_3) or in late diastole or presystole (S_4).

A bifid apical impulse with two systolic impulses may be present in patients with hypertrophic obstructive cardiomyopathy, complete left bundle branch block (LBBB), or MI. If these patients also develop a palpable impulse during either early

(S_3) or late (S_4) diastole, a triple or trifid apical impulse may occur. When such patients develop both a palpable S_3 and a palpable S_4, it is occasionally possible to see and feel a quadruple apical impulse.

AREA 6: EPIGASTRIC AREA PULSATIONS

Some normal and many hyperkinetic individuals have visible or palpable pulsations of the aorta in the epigastric area (see Fig. 10-61). Abnormally large pulsations of the aorta may be due to an aortic aneurysm or aortic regurgitation. Hepatic movements may be identified in the epigastric area, particularly in patients with tricuspid regurgitation, tricuspid stenosis, or marked RV dilatation, hypertrophy, and hyperactivity.

In some patients with pulmonary hypertension due to chronic lung disease, the detection of RV hypertrophy by precordial palpation is difficult because the shape of the chest often conceals the enlarged right ventricle. To detect abnormal RV pulsations in patients with emphysema, the palm of the right hand should be placed on the epigastric area and moved cephalad while gently sliding the fingers under the rib cage. Aortic pulsations can be detected by the palmar surface of the fingers, and pulsations due to RV hypertrophy can be felt in the fingertips.

AREA 7: ECTOPIC AREA PULSATIONS

Occasionally, cardiac pulsations are encountered in areas other than those described previously, i.e., between the pulmonary and apical areas (see Fig. 10-61). Ischemic heart disease is the most common cause of an ectopic systolic pulsation, which may occur transiently during an episode of angina pectoris. A similar paradoxical systolic outward movement may be detected after acute MI and may persist; more commonly, it disappears within a few weeks. A persistent paradoxical ectopic pulsation also may be found in patients who develop a ventricular aneurysm after MI. Ectopic pulsations on the anterior chest wall also can be found in patients with cardiomyopathies of varying etiologies. In patients with severe mitral regurgitation and a giant left atrium that extends to the right, an ectopic systolic pulsation of the atrium occasionally may be felt in the right anterior or lateral chest or in the left axilla.[205]

Percussion versus Inspection and Palpation of the Precordium

When performed by a skilled examiner, percussion of the heart can provide an estimate of cardiac size and shape. Percussion of the heart only gives information about the location of the borders of cardiac dullness, whereas precordial inspection and palpation provide both information about the location of the outer limits of cardiac pulsations and a determination of the size and character of the pulsations. Although percussion has been used in the diagnosis of pericardial effusion, it has limited value when the results are objectively correlated with the diagnosis as determined by more sensitive and specific noninvasive and invasive testing.

CARDIAC AUSCULTATION

The Stethoscope

The physician must choose a stethoscope that fits the ears comfortably with the right angulation, has as short a segment of flexible tubing as possible, and is equipped with a diaphragm and a bell. Selection of the proper earpieces for comfort and the best transmission of sound is based on individual preference and is best evaluated by trial and error. A snug, comfortable fit depends on the size of the earpieces as well as the angle at which they enter the ear canal; the angulation of the rigid metal tubing therefore must be chosen to suit the comfort of the individual. The rubber tubing should be as short as feasible; experience indicates that tubing about 12 in (30 cm) long is the best compromise. Rapaport and Sprague[213] have shown that thick-walled tubing about 3 mm in diameter is best suited to transmit sounds and murmurs.

The human ear is most sensitive to auditory vibrations that occur in the frequency range between 1000 and 4000 to 5000 Hz; the sensitivity falls off sharply when the frequency of vibration is below 1000 Hz. This is particularly true of low-frequency sounds, which must be of considerably greater amplitude to reach the threshold of audibility than sounds of higher frequency. Most cardiovascular sounds and murmurs of diagnostic importance are between 30 and 1000 Hz, thereby placing the auscultator at considerable disadvantage.[214] Therefore, a stethoscope requires *both a diaphragm and a bell,* and each must be applied to the chest wall with optimal pressure. The diaphragm, which is fairly rigid, brings out the high frequencies and attenuates the lows. When the diaphragm is used to accentuate high-pitched sounds, it should be pressed very firmly against the skin. This technique will make a high-frequency murmur, such as the faint diastolic blowing murmur of aortic valve regurgitation, audible along the left sternal border when it would otherwise be missed. The bell tends to accentuate the low-frequency sounds and to filter out the high-pitched tones. Often, low-frequency sounds are more easily appreciated by palpation than by auscultation; in these situations, the stethoscope should be placed very lightly on the skin, with just enough pressure to seal the edge at the point of maximal impulse. With very light pressure of the bell, the low-pitched sounds are accentuated; however, with firm pressure of the bell against the skin, the skin itself becomes a relatively tight diaphragm, and the low-frequency sounds are suppressed. Although this technique can be very helpful, the stethoscope always should be equipped with a valve system that permits one to switch from the diaphragm to the bell with ease.

Examination of the Patient

The examination should take place in a quiet room that is well lighted and comfortably heated. The patient should be properly gowned, with adequate exposure to the waist. The examining table should be large enough that the patient can be instructed to lie flat, sit up, or roll to one side with complete ease. Usually, the physician will examine from the right side, and it is equally important that the physician be comfortable.

Prior to auscultation, the clinician should take advantage of the information obtained from the history as well as from the examination of the arterial, venous, and cardiac pulsations. When abnormalities are found, their auscultatory counterparts should be pursued diligently. For example, prominent *a* waves in the jugular venous pulse should alert the clinician to search carefully for a low-pitched, right-sided fourth heart sound (S_4) or the subtle presystolic murmur of tricuspid stenosis, whereas large *v* waves that augment with inspiration should suggest tricuspid regurgitation. The presence of pulsus alternans always should demand a careful search for third and fourth heart sounds (S_3, S_4), as well as for the presence of functional mitral or tricuspid regurgitation, often present in severe cardiac decompensation. A rapid, jerky rise of the carotid pulse may be the clue to the diagnosis of hypertrophic cardiomyopathy, which can be confirmed by manipulating the systolic murmur with maneuvers that change the pre- and afterloading conditions of the heart.

There are four primary areas of cardiac auscultation: (1) the primary and secondary aortic areas in the second right interspace and the third left interspace adjacent to the sternum, respectively, (2) the pulmonary area in the second left interspace, (3) the tricuspid area in the fourth and fifth interspaces adjacent to the left sternal border, and (4) the mitral area at the cardiac apex. This does not mean to imply that auscultatory events arising from each valve are heard only in their respective areas. The murmur of aortic stenosis in the elderly is often heard best (and at times only) at the apex, whereas the murmur of a flail posterior mitral leaflet may radiate to the base and simulate the murmur of aortic stenosis. Ejection sounds arising from the stenotic aortic valve are usually most prominent at the apex, whereas the opening snap of mitral stenosis is heard best midway between the tricuspid and mitral areas. The murmur of tricuspid regurgitation may be appreciated best at the classic mitral area if the right ventricle occupies the apex. Furthermore, cardiac auscultation should not be restricted to just these four areas. For example, the murmur of aortic regurgitation secondary to abnormalities of the aortic root may be heard best to the right of the sternum, whereas the murmur of tricuspid regurgitation in the emphysematous patient with pulmonary hypertension may be heard best in the epigastrium. The continuous murmur of a patent ductus arteriosus is heard just below the left clavicle, whereas the murmur of large bronchial collaterals may be most prominent in the posterior thorax. Again, the overall clinical presentation will guide one to the appropriate area to auscultate.

During auscultation, one listens both specifically and selectively for heart sounds and then for murmurs, first during systole and then during diastole. As described by Levine and Harvey,[215] the physician should adopt a systematic approach to listening. The patient should be lying on his or her back, and each area should be surveyed with both chest pieces. In each area examined, the physician listens specifically for the first heart sound (S_1), noting its intensity, constancy, presence of splitting, and variation with respiration. This is followed by selective listening for the second heart sound (S_2), noting the same characteristics. Then extra sounds are searched for and carefully listened to, first in systole and then in diastole, with mental notations as to their time of appearance, pitch, and other characteristics that may identify them as gallop sounds, ejection sounds, or valve-opening sounds. Whether the examination is initiated at the base by listening to S_2 or at the apex by listening to S_1 depends on the physician's preference. Of greater importance is that the examination be performed in a methodical, systematic way, with the physician listening intently for one event at a time. Attention is then first turned to systole and then to diastole for the presence of murmurs. After this general survey, the physician listens selectively for certain sounds and murmurs. With the bell applied lightly to the skin at the apex, the patient is instructed to roll onto the left side, and the clinician selectively "tunes in" to diastole and the low-frequency range. This allows the physician to determine the presence or absence of diastolic filling sounds or diastolic rumbles arising from the AV valves. The examination is continued with the patient in the sitting position. While the patient leans slightly forward during quiet respiration, the clinician can optimally appreciate splitting of S_2. With the patient's breath held in deep expiration, the physician examines the aortic and pulmonic areas with the diaphragm firmly pressed against the chest wall, selectively "tuning in" to the high-frequency range in an effort to hear the faint blowing diastolic murmur of aortic regurgitation or, if the clinical situation warrants, the presence of a pericardial friction rub. Sounds and murmurs such as these are discovered only when they are searched out carefully with intent listening and concentration.

Auscultation of the heart should be considered a dynamic exercise. In addition to being auscultated in the left lateral ducubitus position, the patient should, when possible, also be examined while standing, squatting, and during the Valsalva maneuver and following its release. This type of dynamic examination changes the pre- and afterloading conditions of the heart and may yield diagnostic information because of the typical response of heart sounds and murmurs to these maneuvers.

HEART SOUNDS

Heart sounds are of two types: high-frequency transients associated with the abrupt terminal checking of valves that are closing or opening and low-frequency sounds related to early and late diastolic filling events of the ventricles. Sounds related to closing and opening of the AV valves include mitral and tricuspid closing sounds (M_1, T_1), nonejection sounds, and the opening snaps; sounds related to closing and opening of the semilunar valves include aortic and pulmonic closure sounds (A_2, P_2) and early valvular ejection sounds or clicks. Low-frequency sounds include the physiologic heart sound (S_3) and the pathologic S_3 gallop associated with early ventricular filling events and the presystolic atrial S_4 gallop associated with late diastolic events resulting from the atrial contribution to ventricular filling. With tachycardia, these sounds may fuse, producing a summation gallop.[216,217]

The First Heart Sound

The first heart sound (S_1) as recorded by high-resolution phonocardiography consists of four sequential components: (1) small, low-frequency vibrations, usually inaudible, that coincide with the beginning of LV contraction and felt to be muscular in origin, (2) a large, high-frequency vibration, easily audible, related to mitral valve closure (M_1), (3) a second high-frequency component, following closely, related to tricuspid valve closure (T_1), and (4) small, low-frequency vibrations that coincide with accelerated flow of blood into the great vessel. The two major components normally audible at the left lower sternal border are the louder M_1 followed by T_1. They are separated by only 20 to 30 ms, and at the apex in the normal subject, and only a single sound (M_1) is usually appreciated. Splitting of the first heart sound is less evident with the tachycardia following coughing or with sustained handgrip exercises

ECHOCARDIOGRAPHIC CORRELATES AND SPLITTING OF S_1

The first high-frequency component of S_1 coincides with the complete coaptation of the anterior and posterior leaflets of the mitral valve. This sound is due to the sudden deceleration of blood setting the entire cardiohemic system into vibration when the elastic limits of the closed, tensed valves are met. It is unlikely that complete coaptation of the complex valve leaflets and final tensing are simultaneous; presumably it is the latter event that is associated with vibrations perceived as M_1. When T_1 is more widely separated from M_1, however, identical echocardiographic correlates have been demonstrated in patients with wide splitting of S_1 due to Ebstein's anomaly of the tricuspid valve.[216] This exaggerated T_1, or "sail sound," and its wide separation from M_1 have been a helpful sign in the diagnosis of this entity.[217] Wide splitting of S_1 with normal sequencing (M_1, T_1) is also present in right bundle branch block of the proximal type as well as in LV pacing, ectopic beats, and idioventricular rhythms originating from the left ventricle due to a delayed contraction of the right ventricle. In a similar manner, pacing from the right ventricle and ectopic beats and idioventricular rhythms originating from the right ventricle will produce reversed splitting of S_1 (T_1, M_1) due to delay in LV contraction. Reversed splitting of S_1 also may be present in patients with hemodynamically significant obstruction of the mitral valve, since mitral valve closure is delayed due to the increased left atrial pressure, which must be overcome by the rising LV pressure before closure can occur. Similar delay in M_1 also may be found in mitral obstruction secondary to left atrial myxoma.

HEMODYNAMIC CORRELATES OF S_1

Figure 10-62 illustrates the sound and pressure correlates of M_1. The first high-frequency component of M_1 coincides with the downstroke of the left atrial *c* wave and is delayed from the left ventricular–left atrial pressure crossover by 30 ms. In the past, these findings have caused considerable confusion regarding the origin of both M_1 and T_1, since it was assumed that these sounds occurred at AV pressure crossover. However, the elegant studies of Laniado et al.[218] established that forward flow continued for a short period following left ventricular–left atrial pressure crossover due to the inertia of mitral flow, with M_1 occurring 20 to 40 ms later, coincidentally with cessation of mitral flow and closure of the valve. An even greater delay between the occurrence of T_1 and right ventricular–right atrial pressure crossover has been shown,[219] and O'Toole et al.[220] have shown that T_1 also coincides with the downstroke of the right atrial *c* wave. These hemodynamic data, together with the echocardiographic correlates of M_1 and T_1, confirm the prime role played by the AV valves in the genesis of S_1.

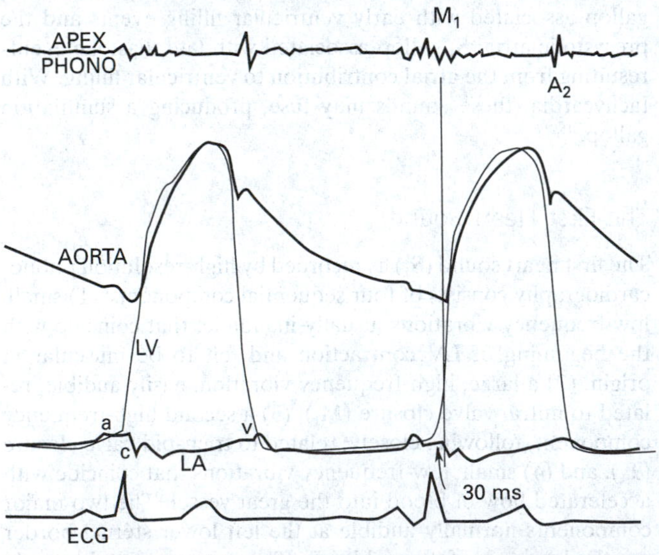

FIGURE 10-62 The apex phonocardiogram is displayed simultaneously with the cardiac cycle, as recorded by high-fidelity catheter-tipped micromanometers in the central aorta, left ventricle (LV), and left atrium (LA). The first high-frequency component of M_1 is coincident with the downstroke of the left atrial *c* wave and is separated from left ventricular–left atrial pressure crossover by an interval of 30 ms. (From Shaver JA, Saderni R, Reddy PS, et al. Normal and abnormal heart sounds in cardiac diagnosis: I. Systolic sounds. *Curr Probl Cardiol* 1985; 10:10–53. Reproduced with permission from the publisher and authors.)

INTENSITY OF S_1

The primary factors determining intensity of S_1 are (1) integrity of valve closure, (2) mobility of the valve, (3) velocity of valve closure, (4) status of ventricular contraction, (5) transmission characteristics of the thoracic cavity and thorax, and (6) physical characteristics of the vibrating structures.

Integrity of Valve Closure In rare situations, usually in the setting of severe mitral regurgitation, there is inadequate coaptation of the mitral leaflets to a degree that valve closure is not effective. As a result, abrupt halting of the retrograde blood column during early ventricular contraction does not occur, and S_1 may be markedly attenuated or absent. Such may be the case in severe mitral regurgitation due to a flail mitral leaflet, as shown in Fig. 10-63.

Mobility of the Valve Severe calcific fixation of the mitral valve with complete immobilization will cause a markedly attenuated M_1. This is seen most commonly in the setting of long-standing mitral stenosis.

Velocity of Valve Closure The velocity of valve closure is the most important factor affecting the intensity of S_1 and is determined by the timing of mitral valve closure in relation to the LV pressure rise in early systole.[221] The relative timing of left atrial and LV systole may vary this relationship. As the PR interval progressively decreases from 130 to 30 ms, there is a progressive increase in the intensity of M_1 and progressive delay in M_1 relative to the onset of LV contraction. When left atrial and LV systole occur almost simultaneously at a PR interval of 10 ms, however, S_1 again becomes soft. At short PR intervals (30–70 ms), the mitral valve leaflets are maximally separated by atrial contraction at the onset of LV systole. With LV contraction, the mitral valve closes at a high velocity with a large excursion. This results in a loud, late M_1 occurring on a steeper part of the LV pressure curve when the retrograde blood column is suddenly decelerated at the moment the elastic limits of the mitral valve are met. At longer PR intervals, there is less separation of the mitral valve leaflets, which have already begun to close with atrial relaxation. When LV systole begins, there is less excursion of the mitral valve until tensing occurs, and S_1 occurs earlier relative to the onset of LV contraction at a lower LV pressure. Thus less force is applied to the mitral valve, its closing velocity is decreased, and less energy is generated when a column of retrograde blood is abruptly halted, resulting in a softer M_1.

The clinical finding of marked variation in the intensity of S_1 in a patient with a slow heart rate often will alert the clinician at the bedside to the diagnosis of complete heart block with AV dissociation. Other conditions in which there are beat-to-beat variations in the intensity of S_1 include Mobitz type I heart block and ventricular tachycardia with AV dissociation. Variations in the intensity of S_1 also occur with atrial fibrillation with both normal and stenotic AV valves. The loud S_1 occurs at short RR intervals, whereas a softer S_1 occurs at longer RR intervals when the valve leaflets have closed partially.[222]

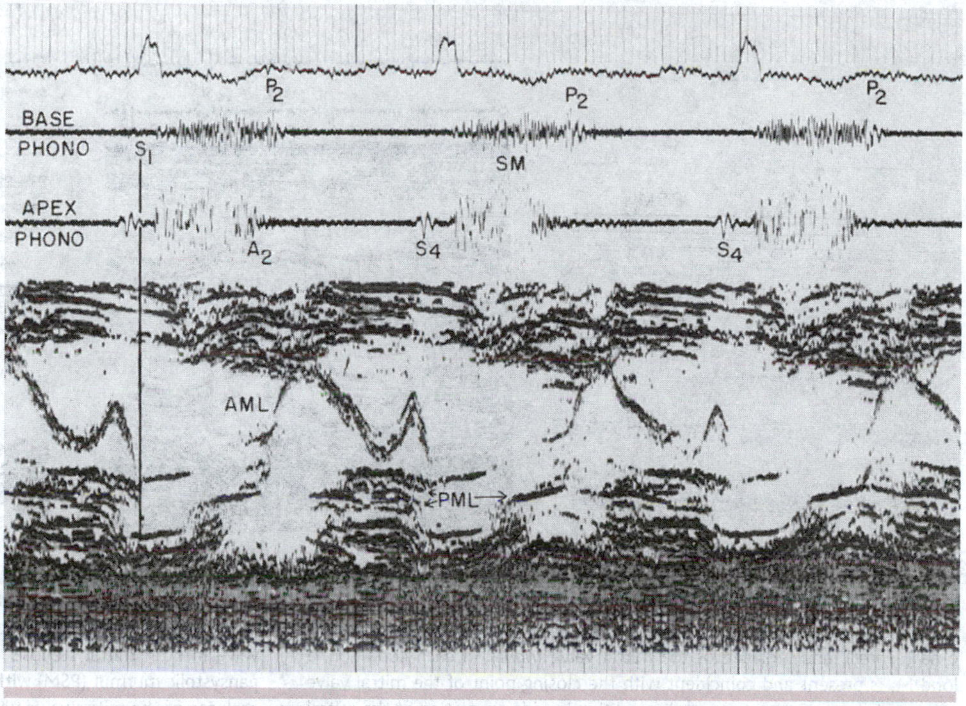

FIGURE 10-63 Base and apex phonocardiograms are recorded simultaneously with the mitral valve echocardiogram in a 62-year-old man who developed acute mitral regurgitation secondary to rupture of the chordae tendinae of a myxomatous valve. During diastole, multiple echoes arise from the flail posterior mitral leaflet (PML), and during early ventricular systole, effective mitral valve closure does not occur, resulting in an inaudible low-frequency vibration on the apex phonocardiogram. During systole, there is separation of the anterior (AML) and posterior mitral leaflets, resulting in severe mitral regurgitation. The murmur has a crescendo-decrescendo contour simulating the murmur of aortic stenosis ending prior to A_1. Wide physiologic splitting of S_1 is present. The prominent S_4 present on the apex phonocardiogram was associated with an apical presystolic impulse. (From Shaver JA. The physical examination in cardiac diagnosis. *Cardiol Consult* 1985; 6:3. Reproduced with permission from the publisher and author.)

The position of the mitral valve at the onset of ventricular systole may be altered not only by the relative timing of atrial and ventricular systole but also by altering the rate of LV filling during atrial systole. Leonard et al.[221] have shown that the timing and intensity of both S_1 and S_4 in hypertensive patients can be influenced by variations in venous return. It is suggested that the mitral leaflets have a greater separation when venous return is decreased to the noncompliant hypertensive left ventricle because there is more effective atrial volume transport into a relatively underfilled ventricle. This results in a softer S_4 that migrates toward an increased S_1. When venous return is increased, the atrial contribution of ventricular filling is now operating on the steeper portion of the LV pressure volume curve. The S_4 becomes louder and earlier, and S_1 is decreased in amplitude due to partial atriogenic closure of the mitral valve. This is the most likely explanation of a soft S_1 frequently noted in hypertensive patients with normal PR intervals.

Status of Ventricular Contraction The status of ventricular contractility is also an independent factor determining the amplitude of S_1.[221,222] In normal subjects, both exercise and catecholamine infusion have been shown to increase the amplitude of S_1, whereas administration of β-blocking agents decreases it.[221] In both situations, the prime factor in altering the intensity of S_1 is the rate of pressure development in the ventricle. This increased rate of pressure development partially explains why S_1 is increased in patients with anemia, arteriovenous fistulas, pregnancy, anxiety, and fever. It is also likely that these high-output states, often associated with tachycardia, result in wider separation of the AV valves at the onset of ventricular systole due to high flow through a shortened diastolic period. Similarly, the loud T_1 in an ASD is due to high flow through the tricuspid valve, secondary to the left-to-right shunt at the atrial level. A decrease in the intensity of S_1 associated with a decrease in the rate of LV pressure development may be found in myxedema, cardiomyopathy, and acute MI.[223,224] Beat-to-beat variation in the intensity of S_1 (auscultatory alternans) also has been found in patients with pulsus alternans, in whom beat-to-beat alteration in the rate of LV pressure development occurs.

Transmission Characteristics of the Thoracic Cavity and Chest Wall The degree of attenuation of heart sounds generated by the vibrating cardiohemic system is a function of both sound frequency and the distance of the heart from the chest wall. The higher-frequency heart sounds are attenuated to a greater extent than are lower-frequency sounds. Conditions such as obesity, emphysema, and large pleural or pericardial effusions will decrease the intensity of all auscultatory events, whereas a thin body habitus would tend to increase the intensity.

Physical Characteristics of the Vibrating Structures Alterations in the physical characteristics of the vibrating structures also may vary the intensity of S_1. Both MI and ischemia induced by pacing have been shown to decrease the intensity of S_1 secondary to these alterations.[224]

S_1 IN PATHOLOGIC CONDITIONS

Careful attention to the intensity of S_1 is an extremely important aspect of cardiac auscultation, often giving clues to the proper diagnosis and degree of abnormality of the involved structures. The following conditions are examples where alterations in the intensity of S_1 play a key role in the correct diagnosis.

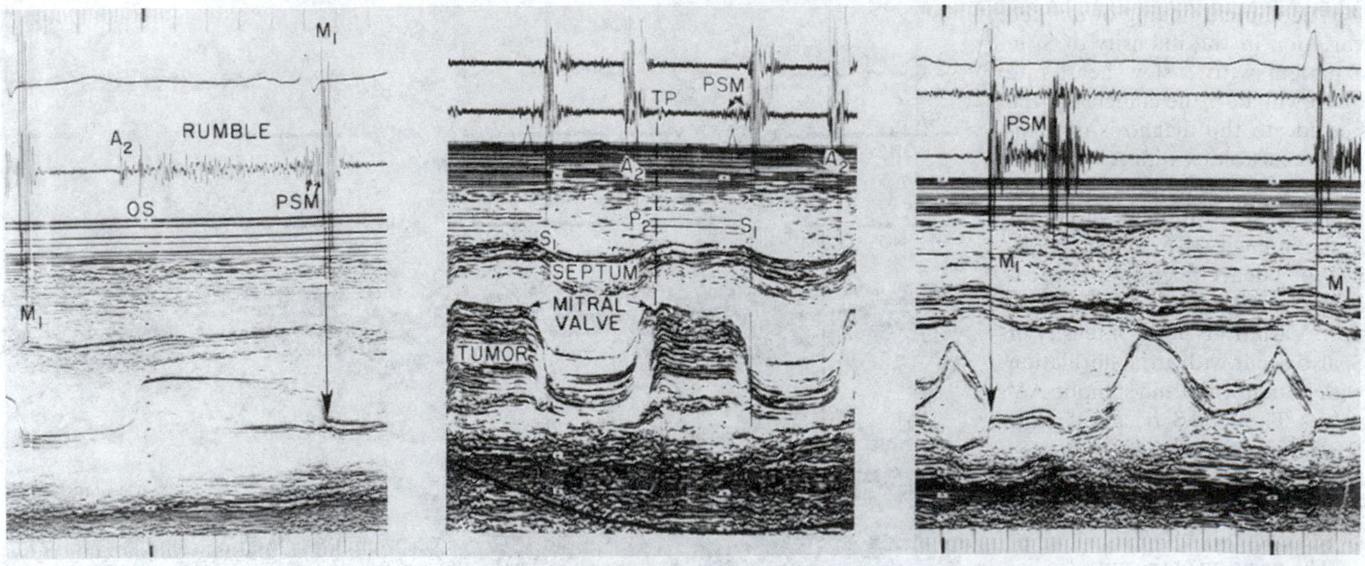

FIGURE 10-64 Simultaneous phonocardiograms are recorded with the mitral valve echocardiograms in three patients: mitral stenosis (*left*), left atrial myxoma (*center*), and prolapse of the mitral valve (*right*). In each condition, a loud M_1 is present and coincident with the closing point of the mitral valve echocardiogram. Common to each condition is wide separation of the mitral leaflets at the onset of LV systole, with high-velocity closure occurring over a large excursion. In the left panel, a mobile stenotic valve is demonstrated, and a loud opening snap is coincident with the E point. In the center panel, an early diastolic tumor plop (TP) is coincident with the maximal excursion of the tumor during its rapid descent into the ventricle. Note the presystolic crescendo murmur (PSM) occurring during the rapid closure of the mitral valve in both mitral stenosis and left atrial myxoma. In the right panel, a pansystolic murmur (PSM) with late systolic accentuation is secondary to the prolapse of the mitral valve with late systolic hammocking. (From Shaver JA. Current uses of phonocardiography in clinical practice. In: Rapaport E, ed. *Cardiology Update: Reviews for Physicians. New York*: Elsevier; 1981:370. Reproduced in part (center panel) with permission from the publisher and author. Copyright 1981 by Elsevier Science Publishing Co, Inc.)

S1 in Mitral Stenosis A loud, late M_1 is the hallmark of hemodynamically significant mitral stenosis.[225] When M_1 is loud, it is associated with a loud opening snap, and the intensity of both M_1 and the opening snap correlates with valve motility (Fig. 10-64, *left*). When calcific fixation of the stenotic mitral valve occurs, M_1 is soft, and the opening snap is absent. The relationship between sound and pressure and echocardiographic mitral valve motion is shown in Fig. 10-65. Significant scarring of the mitral valve is evident as a result of the rheumatic process. The increased left atrial pressure delays the time of pressure crossover between the left atrium and the left ventricle. As a result, M_1 occurs later and at a much higher than normal LV pressure, at a time when there is a more rapid rate of development of LV pressure. The presystolic gradient between the left atrium and the left ventricle prevents preclosure of the mitral valve leaflets. As a result, the closure of the leaflet begins from a domed position within the LV cavity and takes place over a much greater distance than normal following the onset of LV contraction. Both these factors increase the velocity of mitral valve closure and the momentum of blood directed toward the mitral valve leaflets, resulting in a loud M_1 when the elastic limits of the stenotic mitral valve are met. A similar mechanism is responsible for the booming S_1 with after vibrations in left atrial myxoma (see Fig. 10-65, *center*).

S1 in Mitral Valve Prolapse Tei et al.[226] have reported a loud M_1 heard over the apex in patients with nonrheumatic mitral regurgitation; this is indicative of holosystolic mitral valve prolapse (see Fig. 10-64, *right*). Patients with the more common middle to late systolic prolapse have a normal S_1, whereas a soft or absent S_1 may indicate a flail mitral leaflet (see Fig. 10-65). The increased amplitude of leaflet excursion with prolapse beyond the line of closure explains the loud M_1 associated with holosystolic prolapse. An alternate explanation may be a summation of a normal M_1 and an early nonejection click of valvular prolapse.

S1 and LBBB In LBBB, M_1 is decreased in intensity and is frequently delayed, at times resulting in reversal of sequence of S_1.[227] The reason for the delay and the decreased intensity of M_1 in this condition is multifactional, with different mechanisms operative in different patients, depending on the degree of completeness of the LBBB, the site of block (proximal versus peripheral), and especially the status of LV function.[228] The primary factors involved are (1) delay in onset of LV contraction, (2) degree of LV dysfunction, (3) presence of concomitant first-degree heart block, and (4) presence of a noncompliant left ventricle facilitating atriogenic preclosure of the mitral valve. It is likely that more than one factor is operative in most patients with LBBB, with one or two factors predominating.

S1 in Acute Aortic Regurgitation One of the important auscultatory findings in acute aortic regurgitation is attenuation or absence of M_1.[222] Severe regurgitation into a left ventricle that has not had time to adapt to the acute volume overload causes a marked increase in the LV end-diastolic pressure, resulting in premature closure of the normal mitral valve in middiastole. With the onset of LV systole, minimal mitral valve excursion occurs, causing a marked reduction in the intensity of M_1.

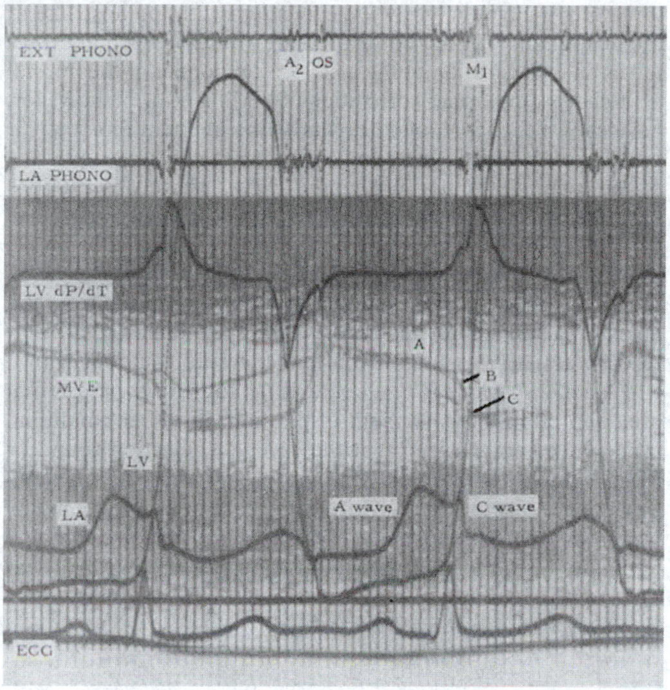

FIGURE 10-65 External sound, equisensitive LV and left atrial pressures (catheter-tipped micromanometer), LV *dP/dt*, and left atrial sound are recorded simultaneously with the mitral valve echocardiogram in a patient with hemodynamically significant mitral stenosis. A significant presystolic gradient is present due to atrial contraction, and the onset of the rapid closure of the mitral valve (*B*) is delayed until the LV pressure exceeds left atrial pressure. This occurs 40 ms after the beginning of the LV pressure rise at a time when LV *dP/dt* is much higher than normal. Following left atrial–left ventricular pressure crossover, there is rapid ventriculogenic closure of the mitral valve (*BC*), resulting in a very loud M_1 coincident with the *C* point of the mitral valve echocardiogram. Its separation from A_2 is determined by both the level of the left atrial pressure and the rate of LV pressure decline. (From Shaver JA, et al. Normal and abnormal heart sounds in cardiac diagnosis: I. Systolic sounds. *Curr Probl Cardiol* 1985; 10:10–53. Reproduced with permission from the publisher and the authors.)

Systolic Ejection Sounds

Ejection sounds are early systolic ejection events that can originate from either the left or the right side of the heart. These sounds may be classified as valvular, arising from deformed aortic or pulmonic valves, or as vascular, or root events caused by the rapid, forceful ejection of blood into the great vessels. The presence or absence of valvular ejection sounds is of great benefit in defining the level of RV or LV outflow tract obstruction, whereas root ejection sounds give insight into abnormalities of the great vessels with or without systemic or pulmonary hypertension.

AORTIC VALVULAR EJECTION SOUNDS

Aortic valvular ejection sounds are found in nonstenotic congenital bicuspid valves and in the entire spectrum of mild to severe stenosis of the aortic valve. This sound introduces the typical ejection murmur of aortic stenosis, is widely transmitted, and is often heard best at the apex. The aortic valvular ejection sound is delayed 20 to 40 ms after the onset of pressure rise in the central aorta and is coincident with the sharp anacrotic notch on the upstroke of the aortic pressure curve. The sound is coincident with the maximal excursion of the domed valve when its elastic limits are met.[229] The abrupt deceleration of the oncoming column of blood sets the entire cardiohemic system into vibration, the lower-frequency components being recorded as the anacrotic notch and the high-frequency components representing the valvular ejection sound. Inherent in this mechanism of sound production is the ability of the deformed valve to move. With severe calcific fixation of the valve, no excursion or piston-like ascent of the deformed valve is possible; therefore, no sudden tensing of the valve leaflets or abrupt deceleration of the column of blood occurs. Sound and motion correlates identical to those demonstrated by cineangiography have been found with phonoechocardiography, clearly showing the onset of the ejection sound to be coincident with the maximal opening of the valve[230] (Fig. 10-66). The intensity of the ejection sound correlates directly with the mobility of the valve, but there is no correlation between intensity and the severity of the obstruction. In mobile, nonstenotic bicuspid valves, the ejection sound is not only loud but also widely separated from S_1 due to the prolonged excursion of the mobile valve. The presence of an

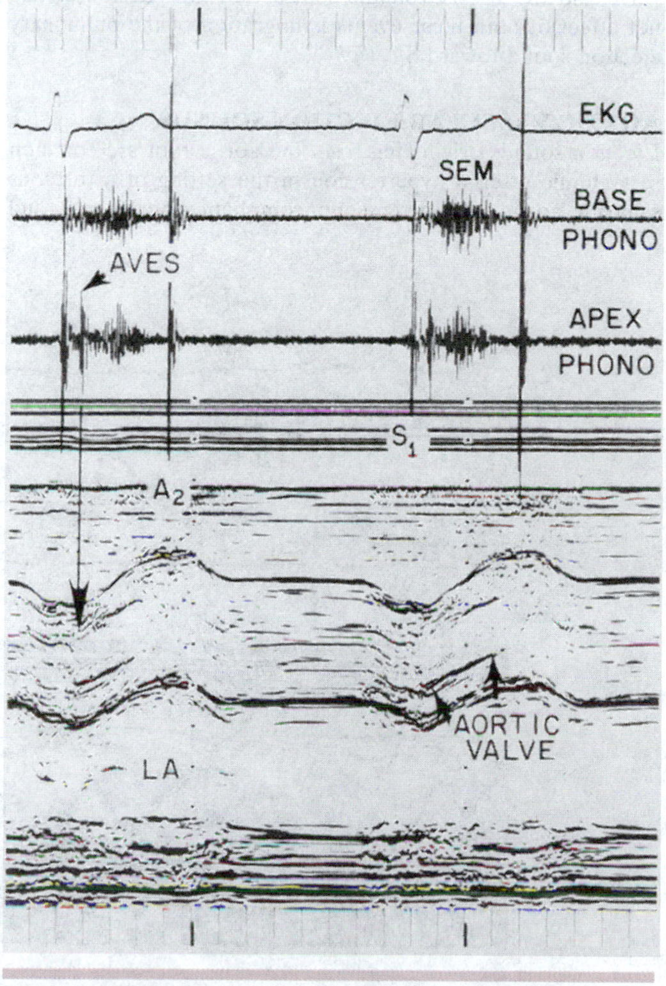

FIGURE 10-66 Base and apex phonocardiograms are recorded simultaneously with the aortic valve echocardiogram in a young man with valvular aortic stenosis. A prominent aortic valvular ejection sound (AVES) is recorded at the apex and is coincident with the maximal excursion of the aortic valve in early systole. It is followed by a crescendo-decrescendo systolic ejection murmur (SEM) that ends well before a loud A_2.

aortic valvular ejection sound is a valuable physical finding at the bedside; it not only defines the LV outflow obstruction at the valvular level but also gives insight into the mobility of the valve (see Fig. 10-66).

PULMONIC VALVULAR EJECTION SOUNDS

Pulmonic valvular ejection sounds have identical sound and pressure correlates as aortic valvular ejection sounds.[231] Echocardiographic correlations also have shown that the onset of the pulmonary ejection sound occurs at the maximal excursion of the stenotic pulmonary valve. In contrast to the aortic valvular ejection sounds and to most right-sided auscultatory events, the pulmonic sound or ejection click decreases in intensity or disappears with inspiration in mild to moderate pulmonic stenosis. In very mild valvular pulmonic stenosis, respiratory variation may be absent.[231] In very severe valvular obstruction, a vigorous atrial contraction can completely preopen the pulmonic valve in diastole, causing a crisp preejection sound. In this situation, RV pressure at the time of the atrial kick actually can exceed pulmonary artery end-diastolic pressure.[231] As the severity of the pulmonic stenosis increases, both the excursion of the deformed valve and the RV isovolumic contraction time decrease. The net effect of both these events is migration of the pulmonary ejection sound toward S_1.

AORTIC VASCULAR EJECTION SOUNDS

Ejection sounds originating from the aortic root are common in systemic arterial hypertension in the setting of a tortuous sclerotic aortic root, a tight, noncompliant arterial tree, and forceful LV ejection. They are coincident with the upstroke of the high-fidelity central aortic pressure and have been interpreted as an exaggeration of the ejection component of the normal S_1. Echocardiographic correlations by Mills et al.,[230] however, have shown that this sound occurs at the moment of complete opening of the aortic valve and always on the pressure upstroke of the high-fidelity aortic pressure curve. These observations have led them to conclude that this sound probably originates from the valve leaflets.

In contrast to the ejection sound of the stenotic aortic valve, these aortic root sounds tend to be poorly transmitted from the aortic area and are not heard well at the apex. It may be difficult to differentiate this sound from the tricuspid component of a widely split S_1, which is best heard at the fourth left parasternal area and often increases with inspiration. In either condition, it should be emphasized that the benign S_1 ejection sound or M_1-T_1 complex is frequently misinterpreted as a pathologic S_4-S_1 sequence. Factors that favor the presence of an S_4-S_1 complex are an associated palpable presystolic apical impulse, optimal audibility of the S_4 with the stethoscope bell applied lightly at the apex, and a change in the intensity of the S_4 with maneuvers that vary venous return.

PULMONARY VASCULAR EJECTION SOUNDS

Vascular or root ejection sounds also may arise from the pulmonary artery, and the common denominator is dilatation of the pulmonary artery.[231] This dilatation can be idiopathic or secondary to severe pulmonary hypertension. Although it has been stated that this sound is louder during expiration, there is no

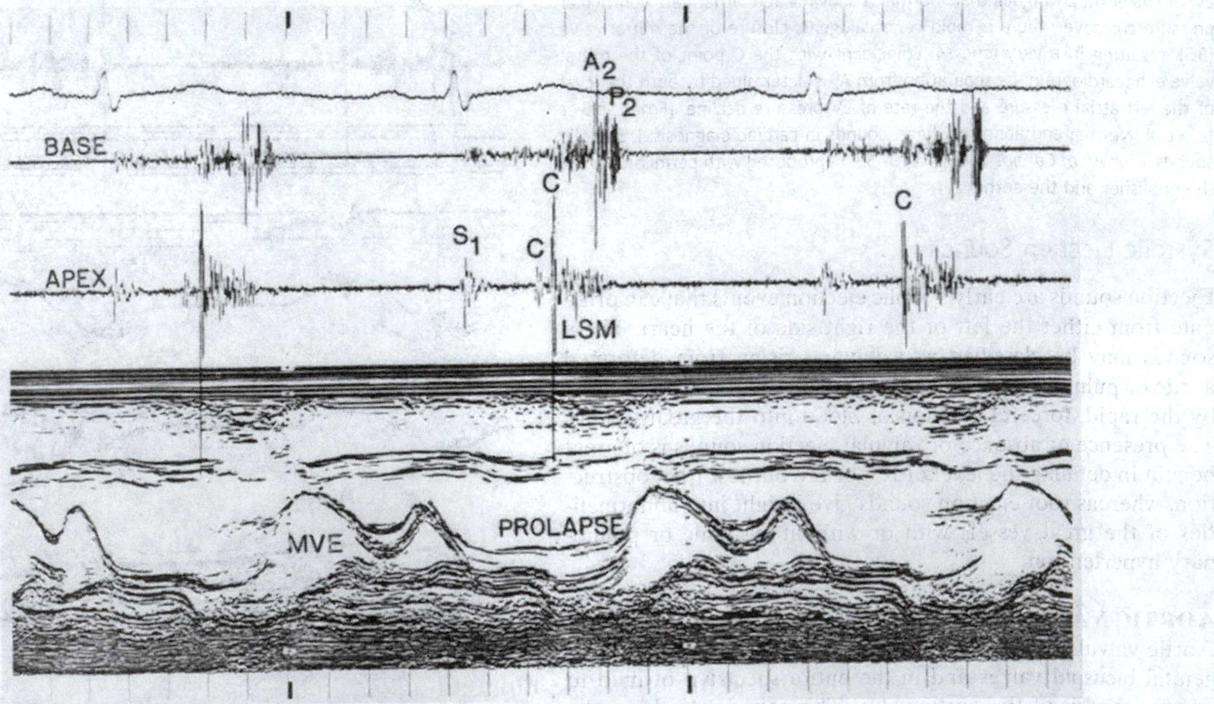

FIGURE 10-67 Simultaneously recorded base and apex phonocardiograms and mitral valve echocardiogram (MVE) demonstrating the frequent association of a late systolic murmur with a prominent late systolic click. Although the murmur is well transmitted to the base, the click transmits poorly. In the first two complexes, an additional softer click precedes the click murmur complex. The last complex shows only a single click, demonstrating the variability of the auscultatory findings even at rest. The large click occurs at maximal prolapse, and the smaller click occurs near the onset of echocardiographic prolapse.

consensus on this point. Unlike splitting of S_1, which is heard best at the mitral or tricuspid area, this sound is louder in the second and third left intercostal spaces.

Echocardiographic correlates of the pulmonary root ejection sound show it to be coincident with complete opening of the pulmonary valve, occurring during the upstroke of the high-fidelity pulmonary artery pressure recording. This has led to the conclusion that these vascular ejection sounds may originate from semilunar valve cusps that have undergone changes in structure in response to increased pressure. Other investigators have found that the pulmonary root ejection sounds in the setting of pulmonary hypertension coincide with the upstroke of the high-fidelity pulmonary artery pressure tracing, whereas in both idiopathic dilatation of the pulmonary artery and ASD, this sound occurs during the upstroke of the pulmonary pressure tracing.[231] In each of these conditions, it has been suggested that this sound is related to sudden checking of the rapidly accelerating blood column by the "tight" or "loose" pulmonary artery when its elastic limits are met.

Nonejection Sounds

The midsystolic click due to prolapse of the mitral or tricuspid valve is the most frequent cause of systolic nonejection sounds and is often associated with a systolic regurgitant murmur. Although originally thought to be extracardiac in origin, confirmation of their valvular origin has been shown by angiographic,[232,233] intracardiac phonocardiographic,[234,235] and echocardiographic studies.[236,237] As originally proposed by Reid,[238] the cause of this sound is due to tensing of the AV valves during systole. As with other high-frequency cardiac sounds, it is produced by vibrations of the entire cardiohemic system when the elastic limits of the prolapsed valve are suddenly reached.

The presence of a nonejection click on physical examination is sufficient to make the diagnosis of mitral valve prolapse (MVP). The sound has a sharp, high-frequency clicking quality and, although often confined to the apex, can be transmitted widely on the precordium. It may be an isolated finding, occurring most often in middle to late systole, or there may be multiple clicks, presumably as a result of different areas of the large, redundant, scalloped mitral leaflets prolapsing at different times. Numerous echocardiographic studies have shown the presence of the characteristic mid- to late-systolic prolapse as well as holosystolic prolapse in patients with clicks. All these patterns may be seen in the presence of an isolated systolic click, click and late systolic murmur, or a late systolic murmur alone. The click usually occurs at the time of maximal prolapse.

A feature of MVP is the variability of the auscultatory findings from examination to examination and even from beat to beat (Fig. 10-67). The timing of the click or the click and late systolic murmur varies considerably with changes in posture[239] (Fig. 10-68). In the upright posture, the heart becomes smaller due to decreased venous return, and the click moves earlier in systole. Angiographic studies have confirmed an earlier and greater degree of prolapse in the upright posture compared with the supine position. Squatting, which causes an immediate increase in venous return and afterload, increases LV volume, resulting in later prolapse and movement of the click toward S_2. At the bedside, these simple maneuvers are helpful in differentiating the nonejection click from early ejection sounds, a split S_2, or an S_3 (see Chap. 58).

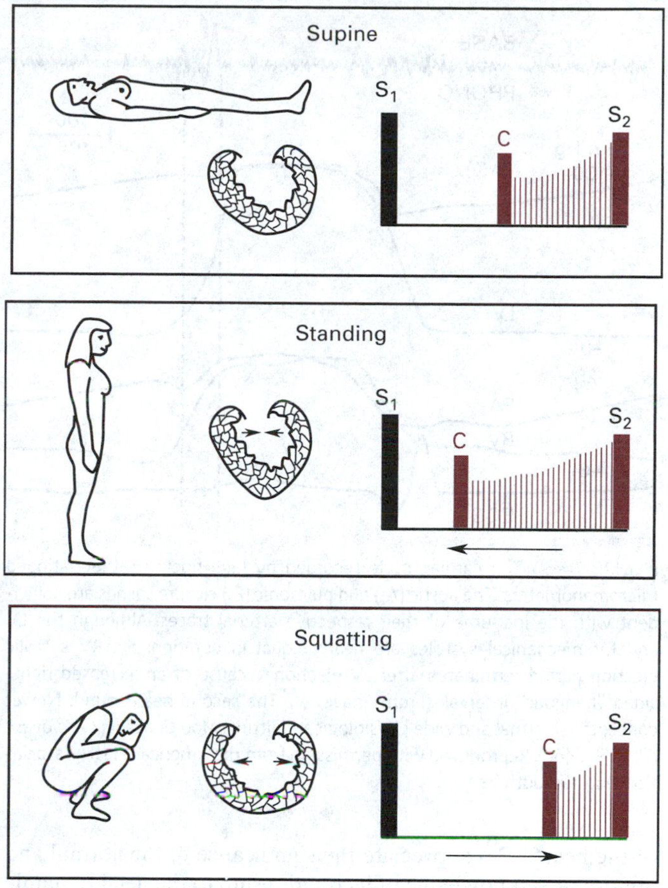

FIGURE 10-68 A midsystolic nonejection sound (*C*) occurs in mitral valve prolapse and is followed by a late systolic murmur that crescendos to S_1. With assumption of the upright posture, venous return decreases, the heart becomes smaller, the *C* moves closer to S_1, and the mitral regurgitant murmur has an earlier onset. With prompt squatting, both venous return and afterload increase, the heart becomes larger, the *C* moves toward S_2, and the duration of the murmur shortens. (From Shaver JA. *Examination of the Heart*, Part IV: Auscultation. Dallas: American Heart Association; 1990:13. Reproduced with permission from the publisher and the authors.)

In general, maneuvers that decrease LV volume—such as sitting, standing, or strain of the Valsalva maneuver—cause the click to move closer to S_1. Maneuvers that increase LV volume move the click toward S_2 (see Chap. 58).

Although the most common cause of nonejection clicks is prolapse of the AV valves, systolic sounds have been reported in patients with left-sided pneumothorax, adhesive pericarditis, atrial myxomas, LV aneurysm, aneurysm of the membranous ventricular septum associated with a VSD, and incompetent heterograft valves. The presence of these conditions usually can be recognized by the clinical setting and by the absence of the typical changes in the timing of the click associated with physiologic and pharmacologic maneuvers.

The Second Heart Sound

Leatham[240] has emphasized the importance of the S_2 in the cardiac examination by labeling it as the "key to auscultation

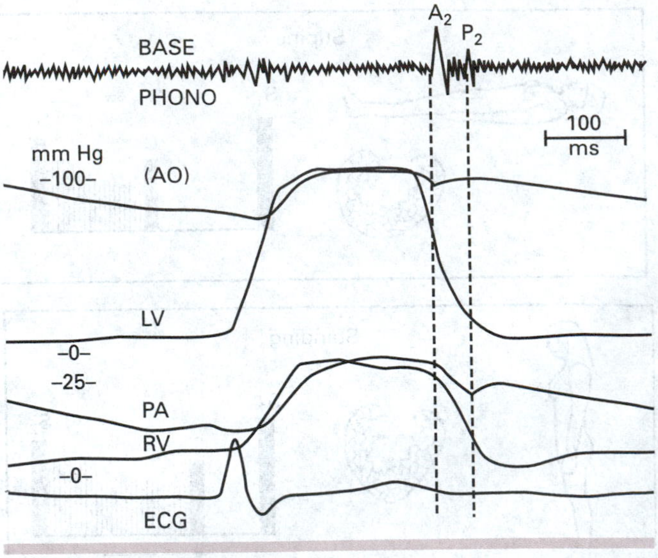

FIGURE 10-69 The cardiac cycle recorded by high-fidelity catheter-tipped micromanometers. The aortic (A_2) and pulmonic (P_2) closure sounds are coincident with the incisurae of their respective arterial traces. Although the LV and RV mechanical systoles are nearly equal in duration, the RV systolic ejection period terminates after LV ejection because of an increased right-sided "hangout" interval. (From Shaver JA. The second heart sound: Newer concepts: I. Normal and wide physiological splitting. *Mod Concepts Cardiovasc Dis* 1997; 46:7. Reproduced with permission from the American Heart Association and the authors.)

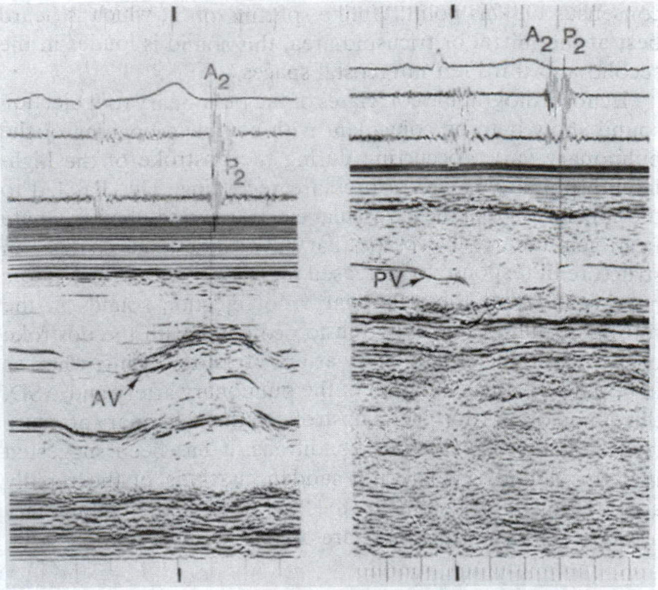

FIGURE 10-70 (*Left*) The base and apex phonocardiograms are recorded simultaneously with the aortic valve echocardiogram. The first high-frequency component of A_2 is coincident with the completion of closure of the aortic valve. (*Right*) Base and apex phonocardiograms are recorded with the pulmonary valve echocardiogram. The first high-frequency component of P_1 is coincident with the completion of closure of the pulmonic valve. (From Shaver JA, et al. Normal and abnormal heart sounds in cardiac diagnosis: I. Systolic sounds. *Curr Probl Cardiol* 1985: 10:43. Reproduced with permission from the publisher and the authors.)

of the heart." To appreciate the significance of the normal and abnormal S_2, knowledge of its relationship to the hemodynamic events of the cardiac cycle is essential.[241–242] Figure 10-69 records the two components of S_2 simultaneously with the cardiac cycle by high-fidelity catheter-tipped micromanometers. The A_2 and P_2 are coincident with the incisura of the aorta and pulmonary artery pressure trace, respectively, and terminate the LV and RV ejection periods. RV ejection begins prior to LV ejection, has a longer duration, and terminates after LV ejection, resulting in P_2 normally occurring after A_2. RV and LV systole are nearly equal in duration, and the pulmonary artery incisura is delayed relative to the aortic incisura, primarily due to a larger interval separating the pulmonary artery incisura from the RV pressure compared with the same left-sided event. This interval has been called the "hangout" interval, a purely descriptive term coined in our laboratory over 15 years ago. Its duration is felt to be a reflection of the impedance of the vascular bed into which the blood is being received.[243] Normally, it is less than 15 ms in the systemic circulation and only slightly prolongs the LV ejection time. In the low-resistance, high-capacitance pulmonary bed, however, this interval is normally much greater than on the left, varying between 43 and 86 ms, and therefore contributes significantly to the duration of RV ejection. Awareness of this interval is essential for proper understanding of normal physiologic splitting and for the abnormal splitting seen in conditions where significant alterations in pulmonary vascular impedance have occurred.

ECHOCARDIOGRAPHIC CORRELATIONS AND MECHANISMS OF SOUND PRODUCTION

Figure 10-70 illustrates the relationship between the aortic and pulmonary valve echocardiogram and A_2 and P_2. The first high-frequency component of both A_2 and P_2 is coincident with completion of closure of the aortic and pulmonic valve leaflets. A_2 and P_2 are not due to the clapping together of the valve leaflets but are produced by the sudden deceleration of retrograde flow of the blood column in the aorta and pulmonary artery when the elastic limits of the tensed leaflets are met. This abrupt deceleration of flow sets the cardiohemic system into vibration; the lower-frequency vibrations are recorded as in the incisura of the great vessels, whereas the higher-frequency components result in A_2 and P_2. This pressure gradient across the valves is the result of both the level of the diastolic pressure in the great vessel and the rate of pressure decline in the ventricle and is consistent with the well-known clinical observation of increased intensity of A_2 and P_2 in systemic and pulmonary hypertension.

NORMAL PHYSIOLOGIC SPLITTING

Normally during expiration, A_2 and P_2 are separated by an interval of less than 30 ms and are heard by the clinician as a single sound.[244] During inspiration, both components become distinctly audible as the splitting interval widens, primarily due to a delayed P_2, although an earlier A_2 contributes to a lesser degree[245] (Fig. 10-71). The traditional explanation of normal splitting was that the delayed P_2 during inspiration was secondary to increased venous return, prolonging the duration of RV systole, whereas a concomitant decrease in venous return to the left side of the heart shortened LV systole. More recent studies have shown that the delayed P_2 and early A_2 associated with inspiration are due to a complex interplay between dynamic changes in pulmonary vascular impedance and changes in systemic and pulmonary venous return.[245]

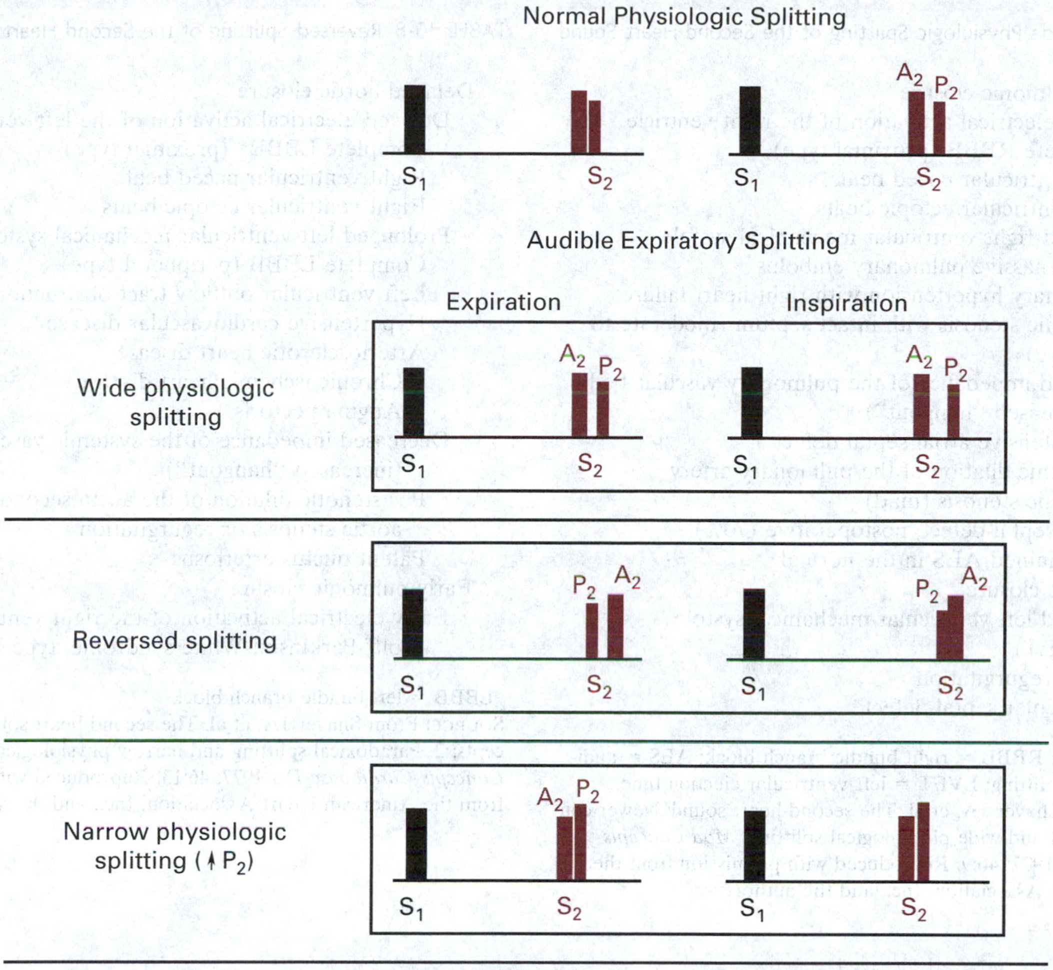

FIGURE 10-71 (*Top*) Normal physiologic splitting. During expiration, A_2 and P_2 are separated by less than 30 ms and are appreciated as a single sound. During inspiration, the splitting interval widens, and A_2 and P_2 are clearly separated into two distinctly audible sounds. (*Bottom*) Audible expiratory splitting. In contrast to normal physiologic splitting, two distinct sounds are easily heard during expiration. Wide physiologic splitting is due to delay in P_2. Reversed splitting is due to delay in A_2, resulting in paradoxical movement; i.e., with inspiration, P_2 moves toward A_2, and the splitting interval narrows. Narrow physiologic splitting is seen in pulmonary hypertension, and both A_2 and P_2 are heard during expiration at a narrow splitting interval due to an increased intensity and high-frequency composition of P_2. (From Shaver JA. *Examination of the Heart*, Part IV: Auscultation. Dallas: American Heart Association; 1990:17. Reproduced with permission from the publisher and the authors.)

On auscultation, splitting of S_2 is usually best heard at the second or third left intercostal space; the normal P_2 is softer than A_2 and is rarely audible at the apex. When P_2 is heard at the apex, either significant pulmonary hypertension is present or the apex is occupied by the right ventricle—a situation seen commonly in normotensive ASD. The absolute value of inspiratory splitting varies with age and depth of respiration. In younger subjects, maximal splitting during inspiration averages 40 to 50 ms; with age, this value decreases such that a single S_2 during both phases of respiration may be normal in subjects older than age 40.[246]

ABNORMAL SPLITTING

All conditions in which abnormal splitting of S_2 exists can be identified at the bedside by the presence of audible expiratory splitting (>30 ms)—i.e., the ability to hear two distinct sounds during expiration[246] (see Fig. 10-71). This finding must be present when the patient is auscultated in both the supine and upright positions. There are three causes of audible expiratory splitting: (1) wide physiologic splitting primarily due to delayed P_2, (2) reversed splitting primarily due to delayed A_2, and (3) narrow physiologic splitting as seen in pulmonary hypertension, where A_2 and P_2 are heard as two distinct sounds during expiration at a narrow splitting interval. Tables 10-7 and 10-8 classify the common causes of wide physiologic splitting and reversed splitting of S_2 according to the abnormality of the cardiac cycle responsible for the altered timing of A_2 and P_2. In each table, the cardiac cycle has been divided into three phases (see Fig. 10-69): (1) the electromechanical couple interval, the time from the onset of the Q wave to the rise of ventricular pressure, (2) ventricular mechanical systole, the sum of the isovolumic contraction time plus the ejection period minus the "hangout" interval (abnormalities of this interval exclude those conditions in which prolongation of the "hangout" interval is primarily responsible for the increased ejection time), and (3) "hangout" or impedance interval, the time between the incisura of the arterial trace and the ventricular pressure at the same level

TABLE 10-7 Wide Physiologic Splitting of the Second Heart Sound

Delayed pulmonic closure
- Delayed electrical activation of the right ventricle
  - Complete RBBB (proximal type)
  - Left ventricular paced beats
  - Left ventricular ectopic beats
- Prolonged right ventricular mechanical systole
  - Acute massive pulmonary embolus
  - Pulmonary hypertension with right heart failure
  - Pulmonic stenosis with intact septum (moderate to severe)
- Decreased impedance of the pulmonary vascular bed (increased "hangout")
  - Normotensive atrial septal defect
  - Idiopathic dilation of the pulmonary artery
  - Pulmonic stenosis (mild)
  - Atrial septal defect, postoperative (70%)
  - Unexplained AES in the normal

Early aortic closure
- Shortened left ventricular mechanical systole (LVET)
  - Mitral regurgitation
  - Ventricular septal defect

ABBREVIATIONS: RBBB = right bundle branch block; AES = audible expiratory splitting; LVET = left ventricular ejection time.
SOURCE: From Shaver JA, et al. The second heart sound: Newer concepts: 1. Normal and wide physiological splitting. *Mod Concepts Cardiovasc Dis* 1977; 46:9. Reproduced with permission from the American Heart Association, Inc., and the authors.

TABLE 10-8 Reversed Splitting of the Second Heart Sound

Delayed aortic closure
- Delayed electrical activation of the left ventricle
  - Complete LBBB* (proximal type)
  - Right ventricular paced beat
  - Right ventricular ectopic beats
- Prolonged left ventricular mechanical systole
  - Complete LBBB (peripheral type)
  - Left ventricular outflow tract obstruction
  - Hypertensive cardiovascular disease
  - Arteriosclerotic heart disease
    - Chronic ischemic heart disease
    - Angina pectoris
- Decreased impedance of the systemic vascular bed (increased "hangout")
  - Poststenotic dilation of the aorta secondary to aortic stenosis or regurgitation
  - Patent ductus arteriosus

Early pulmonic closure
- Early electrical activation of the right ventricle
  - Wolff-Parkinson-White syndrome, type B

*LBBB = left bundle branch block.
SOURCE: From Shaver JA, et al. The second heart sound: Newer concepts: 2. Paradoxical splitting and narrow physiological splitting. *Mod Concepts Cardiovasc Dis* 1977; 46:13. Reproduced with permission from the American Heart Association, Inc., and the authors.

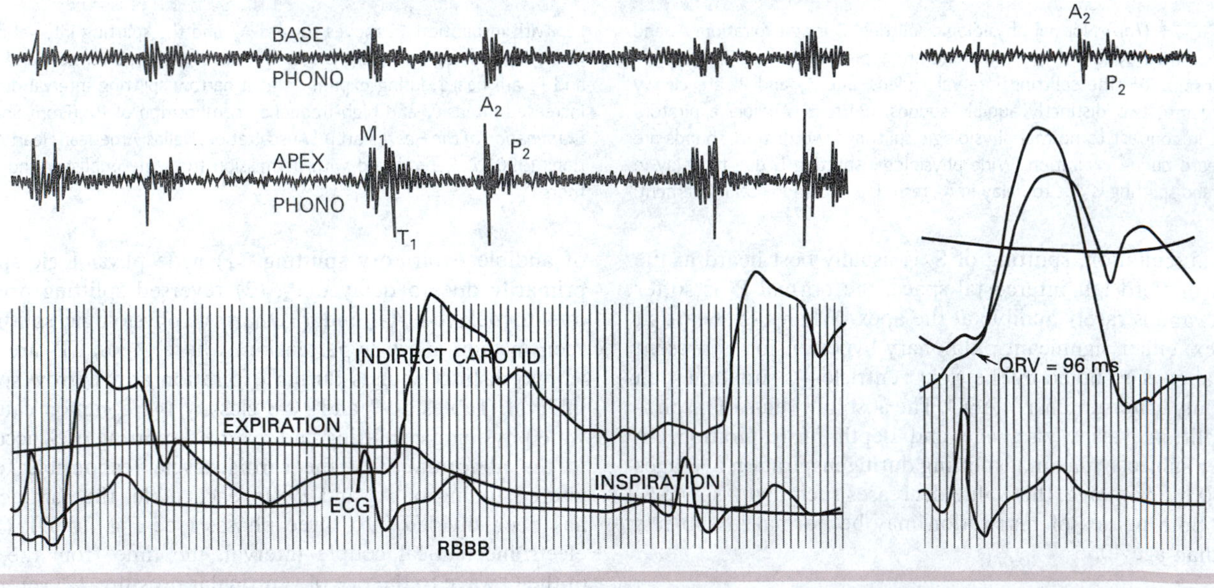

FIGURE 10-72 (*Left*) Wide physiologic splitting of S_2 is seen in a patient with complete right bundle branch block. Audible expiratory splitting that widens normally with inspiration is present. Note also the wide splitting of the first heart sound into its mitral (M_1) and tricuspid (T_1) components, as recorded at the apex. (*Right*) The base phonocardiogram is recorded simultaneously with high-fidelity catheters in the right ventricle and pulmonary artery during cardiac catheterization. There is marked prolongation of the Q to the onset of the RV pressure rise of 96 ms, resulting in wide physiologic splitting of S_2. The delayed P_2 is secondary to delayed activation of the right ventricle. (From Shaver JA. Current uses of phonocardiography in clinical practice. In: Rapaport E, ed. *Cardiology Update: Reviews for Physicians*. New York: Elsevier; 1981:337. Reproduced originally in part (left panel) with permission from the publisher and author, and from Shaver JA, et al. Normal and abnormal heart sounds in cardiac diagnosis: I. Systolic sounds. *Curr Probl Cardiol* 1985; 10:48. Reproduced in total with permission from the publisher and authors.)

as the incisura (includes all conditions in which prolongation of this interval is primarily responsible for the increased ejection time).

Wide Physiologic Splitting of S2 An example of wide physiologic splitting of S_2 due to delayed electrical activation of the right ventricle secondary to right bundle branch block is shown in Fig. 10-72. Prolongation of RV mechanical systole secondary to severe pulmonary hypertension and pulmonic stenosis are also responsible for a delayed P_2. Classic wide, fixed splitting of S_2 is found in patients with ASD. A composite in Fig. 10-73 documents the role played by decreased impedance of the pulmonary vascular bed in the audible expiratory splitting found in ASD, idiopathic dilatation of the pulmonary artery, and mild pulmonic stenosis with aneurysmal dilatation of the pulmonary artery. In each case, there is a marked increase in the "hangout" interval, as measured by high-fidelity pressure tracings. Wide physiologic splitting secondary to a decreased LV ejection time occurs in patients with acute mitral regurgitation.

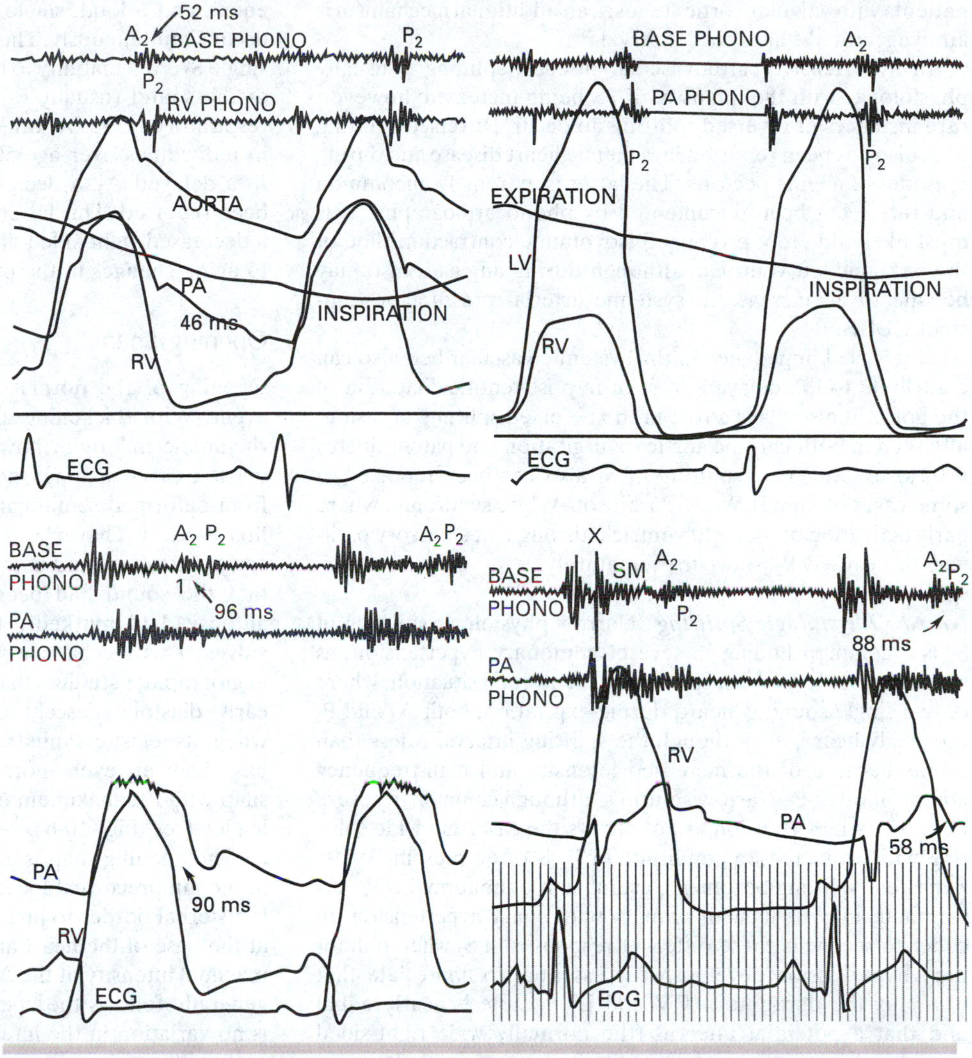

FIGURE 10-73 (*Upper left*) Sound and pressure correlates of S_2 in a 45-year-old woman with a normotensive atrial septal defect (shunt 2:1). Wide, fixed splitting of S_2 is demonstrated; P_2 and A_2 are coincident with their respective incisurae, and the duration of the "hangout" interval is nearly equal to the A_2-P_2 interval. (*Upper right*) Simultaneous RV and LV pressures clearly show that the duration of RV and LV systole is equal. (*Lower left*) Sound and pressure correlates of a patient with idiopathic dilatation of the pulmonary artery. P_2 is coincident with the incisura of the pulmonary artery and separated from the RV pressure tracing by a "hangout" interval of 90 ms (almost identical to the splitting interval). (*Lower right*) Similar sound and pressure correlates in a patient with mild valvular pulmonic stenosis and aneurysmal dilatation of the pulmonary artery. Most of the delay in P_2 is due to a wide "hangout" interval of 56 ms. In each patient all pressures are recorded by catheter-tipped micromanometers. (From Shaver JA, et al. Second heart sound: The role of altered greater and lesser circulation. In: Leon DF, Shaver JA, eds. *Physiologic Principles of Heart Sounds and Murmurs*. Monograph 46. New York: American Heart Association;1975:63. Reproduced originally in part (top panel) with permission from the publisher and the authors, and from Shaver JA. The second heart sound: Hemodynamic determinants. *Acta Cardiol* 1985; 40:12. Reproduced in total with permission from the publisher and authors.)

Reversed Splitting of S2 Almost all cases of reversed splitting of S_2 are due to a delay in A_2. As a result, the sequence of closure sounds is reversed, with P_2 preceding A_2. At the bedside, this abnormality is recognized by paradoxical movement of A_2 and P_2 with respiration.[247] During inspiration, P_2 moves toward A_2, and the splitting interval narrows, whereas during expiration, the two components separate, and audible expiratory splitting is present (see Fig. 10-71). The presence of reversed splitting of S_2 almost always indicates significant underlying cardiovascular disease.

Both RV ectopic and paced beats produce a delay in the onset of LV contraction, resulting in reversed splitting of S_2. The mechanism responsible is a delayed activation of the left ventricle, prolonging the Q to LV pressure rise interval. The most common cause of reversed splitting is complete LBBB, which can be due either to delayed activation of the left ventricle, as seen in isolated proximal block, or to prolonged mechanical systole (primarily isovolumic contraction time), as seen in proximal or peripheral block invariably associated with significant LV dysfunction. Delay often exists in the onset of LV pressure rise when isovolumic contraction time is markedly prolonged, since in most cases of LBBB varying degrees of both mechanisms are present, with one predominating.

Reversed splitting of S_2 may occur in a patient with hypertrophic cardiomyopathy and is due to the large systolic pressure gradient and prolonged LV relaxation.[248] Although both these mechanisms may contribute to the reversed splitting observed in patients with valvular aortic stenosis, an additional mechanism is an exaggerated "hangout" interval.[249]

In hypertensive cardiovascular disease, splitting is usually physiologic, with the intensity of A_2 being increased; however, rare instances of reversed splitting do occur. Reversed splitting of S_2 also has been reported in ischemic heart disease and during episodes of angina pectoris. The latter is extremely uncommon and rarely has been documented by phonocardiography. It is most likely due to a prolonged isovolumic contraction time of the ischemic left ventricle, although during angina it also may be due to an increase in systemic arterial pressure or transient LBBB.[250]

Decreased impedance in the systemic vascular bed also can contribute to the delayed A_2 seen in poststenotic dilatation of the aorta. It also plays a role in the reversed splitting occasionally seen in both chronic aortic regurgitation and patent ductus arteriosus. Reversed splitting of S_2 also has been reported in some cases of type B Wolff-Parkinson-White syndrome, where early activation of the right ventricle through an accessory pathway has caused P_2 to occur prematurely.

Narrow Physiologic Splitting Narrow physiologic splitting of S_2 is a common finding in severe pulmonary hypertension, as shown in Fig. 10-71.[251] In contrast to the normal situation, where only a single sound is heard during expiration, both A_2 and P_2 are easily heard, even though the splitting interval is less than 30 ms because of the increased intensity and high-frequency composition of P_2. Narrow splitting, although common in severe pulmonary hypertension, is not always the case, and wide splitting with an increased amplitude of P_2 is often present. Wide, persistent splitting becomes a useful sign of abnormal RV performance in patients with primary pulmonary hypertension. In order to reconcile these different responses in S_2 when pulmonary hypertension develops, it is essential to appreciate that normally the duration of RV and LV systole is nearly equal and that a potential interval (the normally wide right-sided "hangout" interval) can be encroached on as the pulmonary hypertension progressively decreases the capacitance and increases the resistance of the pulmonary vascular bed[252] (see Fig. 10-69). Thus a spectrum of the width of splitting may be seen in pulmonary hypertension, depending on the degree of selective prolongation of RV systole, always in the setting of a narrow "hangout" interval. Furthermore, it is clear that varying degrees of splitting may be seen in the same patient during different stages of the disease process producing the pulmonary hypertension. Similar hemodynamic correlates have been found in patients having hyperkinetic pulmonary hypertension secondary to large ASDs. Fixed splitting of S_2 occasionally has been documented in severe RV failure secondary to pulmonary hypertension. This usually has been attributed to the inability of the compromised right ventricle to accept the augmented venous return associated with inspiration.

SINGLE S_2

All conditions listed in Table 10-8 that delay A_2 may produce a single S_2 when the splitting interval becomes less than 30 ms. Also, conditions in which one component of S_2 is either absent or inaudible will produce a single S_2 (e.g., truncus arteriosus, severe tetralogy of Fallot, severe semilunar valve stenosis, pulmonary atresia, and most cases of tricuspid atresia). In Eisenmenger's VSD, the duration of RV and LV systole is necessarily equal, and a loud, single S_2 is appreciated because A_2 and P_2 occur simultaneously. The most common cause of an apparently single S_2 is the inability to hear the fainter of the two components of the sound (usually P_2) because of emphysema, obesity, or respiratory noise. Another common cause of single S_2 is seen in individuals over age 50. Although this has been attributed to a delayed A_2, a decreased inspiratory delay in P_2 also has been reported. This latter finding has been shown to be due to a decreased right-sided "hangout" interval, most likely related to aging changes in the pulmonary vascular bed.

Opening Snaps

Opening of the normal AV valve is almost always a silent event. With thickening and deformity of the leaflets, usually rheumatic in origin, however, a sound is generated in early diastole in a manner analogous to ejection sounds arising from deformed semilunar valves. The term *opening snap* was first used by Thayer[253] in 1908 to describe the high-frequency early diastolic sound in mitral stenosis. Thayer also recognized that the sound had been absent in those patients who, on autopsy, had markedly thickened and essentially immobile valves. This mechanism was confirmed by hemodynamic and angiographic studies that showed sudden checking of the early diastolic descent of the funnel-shaped stenotic valve when its elastic limits were met.[254] Phonoechocardiography has given an even more precise correlation of the opening snap with the maximum opening motion of the anterior mitral leaflet (see Fig. 10-64, *left*).

The opening snap is a crisp, sharp sound that can be heard in the midprecordial location, usually best in the area from the left sternal border to just inside the apex. Often it is heard well at the base of the heart and frequently is not well heard at the maximal intensity of the diastolic murmur. The diastolic rumble generally follows the opening snap by a short interval. There is no variation in the intensity or timing of the mitral opening snap with respiration.

As with ejection sounds of valvular origin, the intensity of the mitral opening snap correlates well with the mobility of the valve. A loud opening snap is found in mobile stenotic valves with good excursions (see Fig. 10-64, *left*), whereas the opening snap is absent with severe calcific fixation of the valve. The intensity of M_1 parallels the intensity of the opening snap; mobile valves having a loud opening snap have an accentuated M_1, and immobile valves having a decreased or absent opening snap have marked attenuation of M_1. Although the presence of valvular calcification decreases valve mobility and the audibility of the opening snap, the sound is actually found in 50 to 60 percent of patients with calcific valves.

The opening snap follows A_2 by an interval of 0.03 to 0.15 s. In patients with mild mitral stenosis, the interval is usually long, whereas in patients with more severe stenosis, the A_2-opening snap interval is shorter. The A_2-opening snap interval in atrial fibrillation can vary with cycle length. With a short preceding RR interval, the left atrium has not had time to empty, the left atrial pressure remains high, and the A_2-opening snap interval is short. With a longer preceding RR interval, the left atrial pressure falls, and the A_2-opening snap interval widens.

There have been a number of attempts to use the A_2-opening snap interval to predict the level of left atrial pressure and the severity of mitral stenosis.[255] The opening snap occurs at the maximal mitral valve opening shortly after left ventricular–left atrial pressure crossovers. Factors that influence the timing of the opening snap relative to A_2 are (1) the rate of LV pressure decline, (2) the level of the LV pressure at the time of A_2, and (3) the level of the left atrial pressure. Increasing severity of mitral stenosis is usually accompanied by an increasing left atrial pressure and therefore a shortening of the A_2-opening snap interval. Because this interval is multifactorially determined, there is an imperfect correlation between the A_2-opening snap interval and the mitral valve area.[256] Tricuspid valve stenosis also can produce an opening snap.[258] This sound is frequently not detected because the findings of coexisting mitral stenosis, which is almost invariably present, overshadow those of tricuspid stenosis. The maximum intensity of the tricuspid opening snap tends to be found closer to the left sternal border, and unlike the mitral snap, the intensity of the tricuspid snap increases with inspiration. When present, it generally follows the mitral opening snap.[257] An early diastolic sound also can be caused by a right or left atrial myxoma. Although the clinical findings of a left atrial myxoma may be similar to those of mitral stenosis, the echocardiographic picture is classic (see Fig. 10-64, *center*). The tumor "plop" occurs at the maximal diastolic descent of the myxoma.

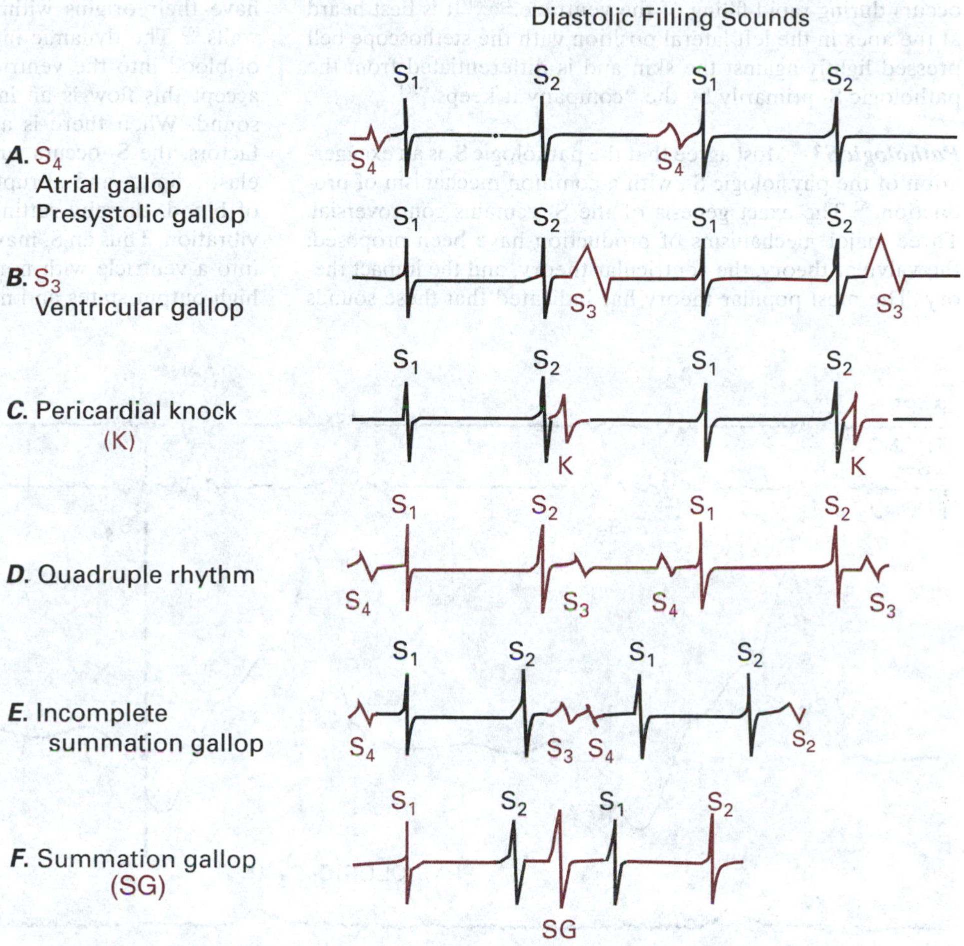

FIGURE 10-74 A. The S_4 occurs in presystole and is frequently called an atrial, or presystolic, gallop. *B.* The S_3 occurs during the rapid phase of ventricular filling. It is a normal finding and is commonly heard in children and young adults, disappearing with increasing age. When it is heard in a patient with cardiac disease, it is called a pathologic S_3, or ventricular gallop, and usually indicates ventricular dysfunction or AV valvular incompetence. *C.* In constrictive pericarditis, a sound in early diastole, the pericardial knock (K), is heard earlier and is louder and higher-pitched than the usual pathologic S_3. *D.* A quadruple rhythm results if both S_4 and S_3 are present. *E.* At faster heart rates, the S_3 and S_4 occur in rapid succession and may give the illusion of a middiastolic rumble. *F.* When the heart rate is sufficiently fast, the two rapid phases of ventricular filling reinforce each other, and a loud summation gallop (SG) may appear; this sound may be louder than either the S_3 or S_4 alone. (From Shaver JA. *Examination of the Heart*, Part IV: Auscultation. Dallas: American Heart Association; 1990:27. Reproduced with permission from the publisher and the authors.)

Although an opening snap is rarely heard with normal valves, it may be heard in situations where high flow exists across the AV valves.[258] An early diastolic sound is frequently present in large ASDs coincident with maximal opening of the tricuspid valve. Other conditions in which functional opening snaps have been found include large VSDs, thyrotoxicosis, and tricuspid atresia with a large ASD. The opening snap must be differentiated from other early diastolic sounds such as the S_3, the pulmonary component of a widely split S_2, and a pericardial knock. At the bedside, differentiation of an opening snap from P_2 is made by noting that the maximal intensity is near the apex rather than at the pulmonary area and that there is lack of movement with respiration. During continuous respiration, it is often possible to appreciate three sounds on inspiration, occurring in rapid sequence in the pulmonary area, and only two components on expiration.

The Third and Fourth Heart Sounds

The third and fourth heart sounds (S_3, S_4) are low-frequency events related to early and late diastolic filling of the ventricles (Fig. 10-74). When they are heard in disease states, they are called *gallop sounds,* and their presence gives valuable information to the clinician regarding the status of ventricular function and compliance.

THE THIRD HEART SOUND

Physiologic S3 The physiologic S_3 is a benign finding commonly heard in children, adolescents, and young adults, but it is rarely present in adults after age 40 and, when present, is often associated with a thin, asthenic body habitus. This is a low-frequency sound that follows A_2 by 120 to 200 ms and occurs during rapid filling of the ventricle.[259,260] It is best heard at the apex in the left lateral position with the stethoscope bell pressed lightly against the skin and is differentiated from the pathologic S_3 primarily by the "company it keeps."[261]

Pathologic S3 Most agree that the pathologic S_3 is an exaggeration of the physiologic S_3, with a common mechanism of production.[262] The exact genesis of the S_3 remains controversial. Three major mechanisms of production have been proposed: the valvular theory, the ventricular theory, and the impact theory. The most popular theory has indicated that these sounds have their origins within the left or right ventricle or their walls.[263] The dynamic interplay between the force of delivery of blood into the ventricle and the ability of the ventricle to accept this flow is an important factor in the genesis of this sound. When there is appropriate interaction between these factors, the S_3 occurs when the ventricle suddenly reaches its elastic limits and abruptly decelerates the onrushing column of blood, thereby setting the entire cardiohemic system into vibration. Thus an S_3 may be produced by excessive rapid filling into a ventricle with normal or increased compliance, as with high-output states and mitral regurgitation, or by a normal or less than normal rate of filling into a ventricle with decreased compliance, as in patients with hypertrophic cardiomyopathy. Likewise, decreased rates of filling into overfilled ventricles with large end-systolic volumes, as seen in patients with poor LV function and congestive heart failure, will produce this sound.[264]

Although this mechanism is likely responsible for the sound recorded within the ventricular cavity and on its epicardial surface, Reddy et al.[217,265] have reported convincing data that the sound heard with the stethoscope can be due to the dynamic impact of the heart with the chest wall. The force of the impact and resulting intensity of S_3 depend primarily on the size of the heart, the motion of the heart within the thorax, and the chest wall configuration. This theory explains the S_3 present in hyperdynamic states as well as those with an increased end-systolic volume secondary to LV dysfunction. In the latter, the space between the enlarged heart and the lateral chest wall is diminished, thereby facilitating a more forceful impact in early diastole. This results in an exaggerated rapid filling wave on the apex cardiogram and the prominent S_3 pathognomonic of congestive failure (Fig. 10-75, *lower panel*). Table 10-9 tabulates the major factors responsible for the production of the S_3 as recorded within the left ventricle and on the chest wall.

A convenient classification of physiologic and pathologic states with an S_3 is presented in Table 10-10. Both the intensity and timing of the pathologic S_3 associated with LV dysfunction are related to the patient's volume status. With diuresis, the S_3 may decrease in intensity or disappear, and it tends

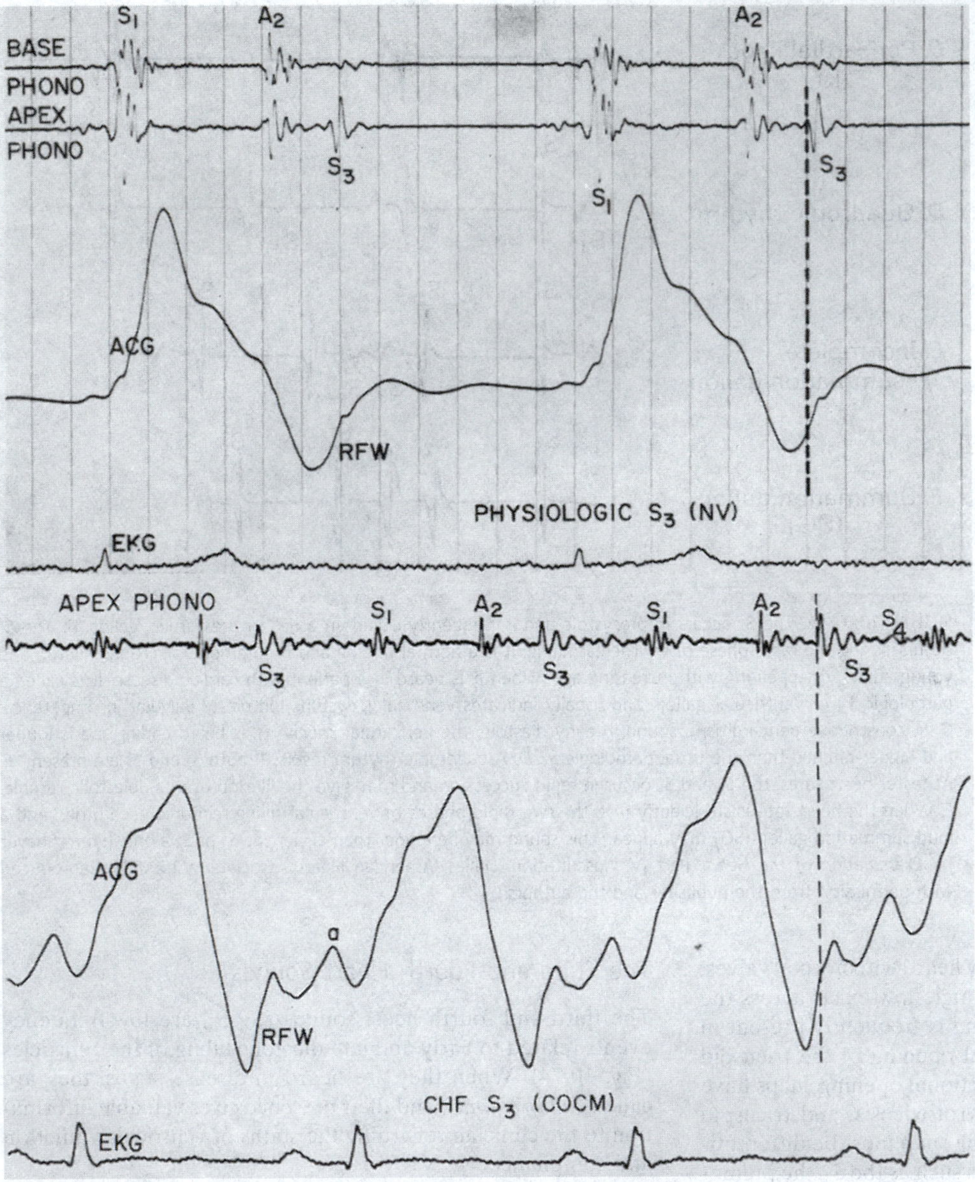

FIGURE 10-75 (*Top*) A physiologic S_3 (normal variant) recorded in a 24-year-old woman without evidence of cardiovascular disease. The onset of the S_3 occurs during the rapid filling wave (RFW) of the ACG between the *O* and *F* points. The remainder of the cardiovascular examination was entirely within normal limits. (*Bottom*) A very prominent S_3 gallop is recorded in a patient with severe congestive cardiomyopathy (COCM). On physical examination, there was a small-volume carotid pulse and marked engorgement of the neck veins with elevated venous pressure. The ACG shows a very prominent presystolic pulsation (a), and an extremely rapid filling wave is present. The onset of the S_3 occurs during the RFW of the ACG. The first heart sound is soft. (From Shaver JA. Early diastolic events associated with the physiologic and pathologic S_3. *J Cardiogr.* 1984; 14(suppl 5):30. Reproduced with permission from the publisher and the authors.)

TABLE 10-9 Hemodynamic Determinants of the S_3

Ability of the ventricle to accept flow during the rapid phase of diastolic filling
Rate of relaxation of the ventricle
End-systolic or residual volume of the ventricle
Compliance of the relaxed ventricle
Nonobstructed atrioventricular valve
Atrial pressure head
Atrial blood volume
Atrial compliance
Dynamic impact of the heart with the chest wall
Architecture of the thorax
Cardiac size
Cardiac motion within the thorax
Phase of respiration
Position of the patient

SOURCE: From Shaver JA, et al. Early diastolic events associated with the physiologic and pathologic S_3. *Am J Cardiol* 1984; 14(suppl 5):45. Reproduced with permission from the publisher and authors.

to move away from A_2. A loud, persistent S_3 with cardiomyopathy or acute MI is an ominous sign associated with high mortality, whereas prompt subsidence with therapy suggests a more favorable outlook. LV third heart sounds are heard best at the apex, whereas RV third heart sounds are heard at the lower left sternal edge and may increase in intensity with inspiration.

In chronic aortic regurgitation, even though end-diastolic volume is increased, end-systolic volume may not be increased until LV dysfunction develops. As LV dysfunction develops, the ejection fraction decreases, resulting in an increased end-systolic volume, and a pathologic S_3 appears in these patients.[266]

TABLE 10-10 Third Heart Sound (S_3), Ventricular Diastolic Gallop, Protodiastolic Gallop, and Pericardial Knock

Physiologic S_3—children and young adults
Decreased prevalence with increasing age
Pathologic S_3
Ventricular dysfunction—poor systolic function, increased end-diastolic and end-systolic volume, decreased ejection fraction, and high filling pressures
Idiopathic dilated cardiomyopathy
Ischemic heart disease
Valvular heart disease
Congenital heart disease
Systemic and pulmonary hypertension
Excessively rapid early diastolic ventricular filling
Hyperkinetic states
Anemia
Thyrotoxicosis
Arteriovenous fistula
Atrioventricular valve incompetence
Left-to-right shunts
Restrictive myocardial or pericardial disease
Constrictive pericarditis (pericardial knock)
Restrictive cardiomyopathy
Hypertrophic cardiomyopathy?

An S_3 is very common in acute aortic regurgitation and is usually followed by the middiastolic component of the Austin Flint rumble.

A pathologic S_3 resulting from excessive early diastolic filling is common in hyperkinetic states and AV valve regurgitation and often initiates a short flow rumble. It is often present in large left-to-right shunts due to high flow across the mitral valve with VSD or patent ductus arteriosus and with high flow across the tricuspid valve with ASD. The presence of this sound in these conditions does not imply congestive heart failure, and such patients may maintain normal myocardial contractility for years after the S_3 is detected.[267] Pathologic third heart sounds are heard in both restrictive and hypertrophic cardiomyopathy. In constrictive pericarditis, an early prominent sound of a somewhat higher frequency is heard—the *pericardial knock*. The evidence to date points to the simultaneous occurrence of the pericardial knock and the termination of rapid filling of the ventricles. Whether this relationship is causal or coincidental is unclear. The apex cardiac pulsation may show systolic retraction followed by an exaggerated diastolic impulse. The pericardial knock usually increases in intensity with inspiration and occurs near the nadir of the *y* descent of the jugular venous pulse. Atrial fibrillation is commonly present in severe constrictive pericarditis, and at times the loud early knock may be confused with the opening snap of mitral stenosis.

THE FOURTH HEART SOUND

Precordial vibrations resulting from atrial contraction are normally neither palpable nor audible. Under pathologic conditions, forceful atrial contraction generates a low-frequency sound (S_4) just prior to S_1 (also termed the *atrial diastolic gallop* or the *presystolic gallop*). Atrial contraction must be present for production of an S_4. It is absent in atrial fibrillation and in other rhythms in which atrial contraction does not precede ventricular contraction. The S_4 follows the onset of the P wave of the ECG by approximately 70 ms. Audibility of the S_4 depends not only on its intensity and frequency but also on its separation from S_1. The degree of this separation is determined primarily by the PR interval, but it is also somewhat influenced by the PS_4 and the QS_1 intervals. A loud S_1 also may mask the audibility of a preceding softer S_4. The S_4 is best heard at the apex impulse with the patient turned in the left lateral position. It varies considerably with respiration, usually being heard best during expiration. A left-sided S_4 may radiate to the brachiocephalic and carotid vessel and be best heard in the areas in patients with severe lung disease or who are very obese. A left-sided S_3 may do likewise. A left-sided S_4 and S_3 may also be augmented post-tussively and with sustained handgrip exercise. Both the intensity and timing of the S_4 are closely related to the end-diastolic volume of the ventricle. Maneuvers that increase venous return increase the audibility by increasing the intensity of the sound and by causing it to occur earlier, thereby separating it further from S_1. Decreased venous return does the opposite. Audible fourth heart sounds are usually accompanied by a palpable presystolic apical impulse in the absence of obesity, emphysema, etc., but occasionally, palpable presystolic impulses are not audible. The S_4 generated by a forceful right atrial contraction is usually heard best at the lower left sternal border. Unlike the left-sided S_4, it tends to be accentuated with inspiration. It is also accompanied by prominent *a* waves in the JVP and is occasionally audible over the right jugular vein.[268]

TABLE 10-11 Fourth Heart Sound (S_4), Atrial Diastolic Gallop, and Presystolic Gallop

- Physiologic—recordable rarely audible
- Pathologic
  - Decreased ventricular compliance
    - Ventricular hypertrophy
      - Left or right ventricular outflow obstruction
      - Systemic or pulmonary hypertension
      - Hypertrophic cardiomyopathy
    - Ischemic heart disease
      - Angina pectoris
      - Acute myocardial infarction
      - Old myocardial infarction
      - Ventricular aneurysm
    - Idiopathic dilated cardiomyopathy
  - Excessively rapid late diastolic filling secondary to
    - Vigorous atrial systole
    - Hyperkinetic states
      - Anemia
      - Thyrotoxicosis
    - Arteriovenous fistula
    - Acute atrioventricular valve incompetence
  - Arrhythmias
    - Heart block

As with the S_3, both the ventricular origin of the S_4 sound due to the abrupt deceleration of the atrial contribution to late diastolic filling and the impact theory have been proposed.[270] It is likely that the former is responsible for the sounds recorded within the ventricular cavities or on their epicardial surfaces, whereas the latter mechanism is responsible for the S_4 auscultated at the chest wall.

The presence of an S_4, particularly when associated with a palpable presystolic apical impulse, is an abnormal finding. Although it is considered to be a normal finding in older subjects by some investigators,[269] others feel strongly that a definite S_4 in a middle-aged or older person is unlikely to be a normal event.[268] Conditions such as obesity, emphysema, or barrel-chest deformity may hinder the clinical detection of both an S_4 and an apical presystolic impulse.

The common pathologic conditions in which S_4 is heard are listed in Table 10-11. A forceful atrial contraction into a hypertrophied, noncompliant ventricle almost always produces an early and easily audible and recordable S_4. The severe LV hypertrophy present in systemic hypertension, severe valvular aortic stenosis, and hypertrophic cardiomyopathy often is responsible for a loud S_4 (Fig. 10-76). In each case, the S_4 is associated with a prominent apical presystolic impulse and is widely separated from S_1.

An audible S_4 with a palpable presystolic impulse is common in patients with ischemic heart disease during an acute episode of angina and in the early phases of transmural MI. Its prevalence is also increased with prior MI; however, audible fourth

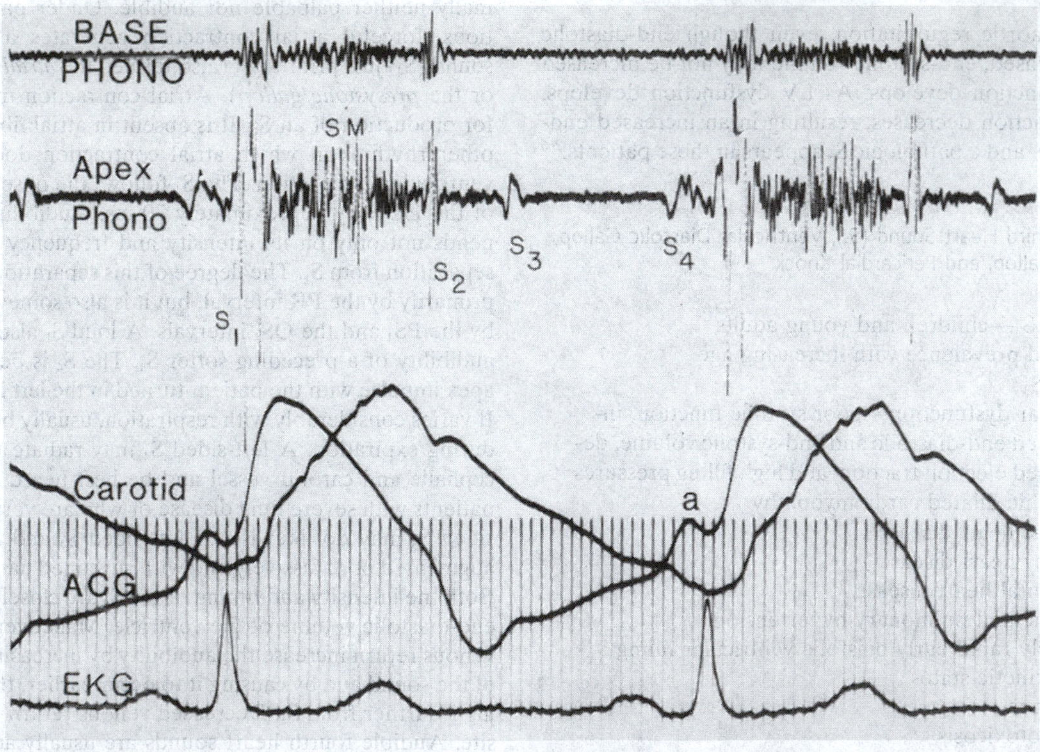

FIGURE 10-76 Atrial diastolic (ADG) and ventricular diastolic gallops (VDG) are recorded in an adult with severe calcific aortic stenosis. The ADG is associated with a prominent presystolic apical impulse (a), and the VDG occurs during the rapid filling wave of the ACG. The carotid pulse has a very slow rate of rise and a markedly prolonged LV ejection time. The classic diamond-shaped systolic ejection murmur (SM) is present at the base and apex. Note the higher-frequency composition of the SM at the apex but preservation of the crescendo-decrescendo pattern. (From Shaver JA. Current uses of phonocardiography in clinical practice. In: Rapaport E, ed. *Cardiology Update: Reviews for Physicians*. New York: Elsevier; 1981:356. Reproduced with permission from the publisher and author. Copyright 1981 by Elsevier Publishing Co., Inc.)

heart sounds in patients with ischemic heart disease without prior infarction or hypertension are uncommon.[217] In patients with LV aneurysm or idiopathic or ischemic cardiomyopathy, abnormal fourth heart sounds are commonly present and often associated with an S_3, producing a quadruple rhythm. If tachycardia is present, or if the PR interval is prolonged, S_3 and S_4 may fuse, giving rise to a loud summation gallop (see Fig. 10-74).

Quadruple rhythms are common in hyperkinetic states where the S_3 is due to excessively rapid early diastolic filling and the S_4 results from a forceful atrial contraction into a volume-loaded ventricle. With varying degrees of tachycardia, incomplete summation may occur, simulating a diastolic rumble, or complete fusion may occur, generating a loud summation gallop (see Fig. 10-74). In acute AV valve regurgitation, vigorous atrial contraction into an acutely volume-loaded ventricle can produce an S_4 associated with a presystolic apical impulse. At times it may be difficult to appreciate because of the masking effect of the loud systolic murmur. This contrasts with most patients with chronic mitral regurgitation, who do not have an S_4 but frequently have an S_3.

Presystolic and isolated diastolic fourth heart sounds as well as summation gallops may be heard with varying degrees of heart block. First-degree heart block facilitates audibility of the S_4 because it further separates S_4 from S_1. In 2:1 heart block, an isolated S_4 may be heard in diastole, and a presystolic S_4 may be audible because of the increase in diastolic volume. In complete heart block, S_4 may be heard randomly throughout diastole, and when it occurs simultaneously with rapid early ventricular filling, a loud summation gallop may occur. Fourth heart sounds also have been reported in ventricular systole when atrial contraction occurred during systole in a patient with heart block. The occurrence of an S_4 when the mitral valve is closed excludes its ventricular origin due to either a pressure or volume change and is in keeping with the impact theory of S_4 sound production.[217]

Prosthetic Valve Sounds

The sounds produced by prosthetic valves are varied, depending on the type of valve, its position, and whether or not it is functioning normally. Mechanical valves produce opening and closing clicks that are easily audible and in many patients can be heard even without a stethoscope. Ball-in-cage valves such as the Starr-Edwards produce the loudest and most distinctive opening and closing clicks in any position as long as there is normal valve and ventricular function. In the aortic position, a crisp opening click occurs 0.06 to 0.07 s after S_1 and is coincident with maximal ball excursion, as demonstrated by echocardiography. The metallic ball of the Starr-Edwards valve also produces multiple early systolic clicks when the freely moving ball bounces against the cage during early systolic ejection. These clicks occur during the harsh systolic ejection murmur. Absence or decrease in intensity of these clicks can occur with valve obstruction or LV dysfunction. A decrease in the intensity of the opening and closing clicks, which normally have an intensity ratio of more than 0.5, and the absence of the opening click are also indications of valve malfunction.

In the mitral position, a prominent opening click occurs 0.05 to 0.15 s after A_2. Narrowing of this interval indicates an elevation of left atrial pressure, which may be due to either valvular obstruction or regurgitation. Interference with ball motion also can produce prolongation or significant beat-to-beat variation of this interval. A closing click is also prominent. Just as is seen with the normal S_1, there is variability in the intensity of the closing click, with the changing RR intervals of atrial fibrillation being louder with short RR intervals and softer with long intervals. A decreased intensity with first-degree AV block also occurs due to partial atriogenic closure of the valve, thus reducing the ball excursion and therefore the click intensity. Although a decreased intensity of the valve clicks occurs with valve malfunction, the presence of normal ball motion on an echocardiogram suggests that a nonvalvular cause such as severe LV dysfunction is responsible for the decreased intensity.

The auscultatory findings of disk valve prostheses vary, depending on the type of disk valve. Central occluder valves such as the Beall valve, which was used predominantly in the mitral and tricuspid positions, produce distinct, audible opening and closing sounds. The more commonly used tilting-disk valves do not ordinarily produce audible opening sounds in either the aortic or mitral position.[205] The closing sounds of disk valves are distinct and easily heard in both aortic and mitral positions. LV dysfunction, first-degree AV block, or another arrhythmia that causes the disk to move to a partially closed position prior to the onset of ventricular contraction will result in a softer sound. This finding must be distinguished from malfunction caused by either fibrosis or thrombus disturbing the disk motion. Auscultation of the bileaflet St. Jude valve is similar to that of the tilting-disk valve.

The sounds produced by tissue prosthetic valves are more like normal heart sounds than the sounds from a mechanical valve.[205] In the aortic position, an opening sound is usually not audible. In the mitral position, an opening sound is audible in about 50 percent of patients at an interval of 0.07 to 0.11 s after A_2.

EXTRACARDIAC SOUNDS

Pacemaker Sounds

High-frequency sounds of brief duration are occasionally present in patients with transvenous pacemakers located in the RV apex. They are extracardiac in origin, occurring nearly synchronously (within 6–10 ms) with the pacemaker spike, and are due to stimulation of intercostal nerves adjacent to endocardial electrodes.[270] This stimulus results in contraction of the intercostal muscles, and frequently twitching of the muscle can be observed. The presence of these sounds always should suggest possible myocardial perforation by the endocardial lead, although this is not always present. Stimulation of the pectoral muscles, as well as diaphragmatic stimulation, also has been reported to produce these extracardiac sounds. They also have been observed in patients having transthoracically placed epicardial leads.

Pericardial Friction Rub

Inflammation of the pericardial sac with or without fluid may cause a pericardial friction rub. These friction sounds are very high-pitched, leathery, and scratchy in nature. They seem close to the ear and are auscultated best with the patient leaning forward or in the knee-chest position, holding his or her breath after forced expiration. The pericardial rub may have three components during the intervals of the cardiac cycle when the heart has the greatest excursions within the pericardial sac—at the time of atrial systole, at the time of ventricular contraction, and during rapid early diastolic filling. The usual friction rub occurs during the first two intervals, although three-component rubs may be heard. Triple-component friction rubs are common in uremic pericarditis, particularly when the underlying cardiac disease is hypertension. In this situation, the heart is hyperkinetic due to both pressure and volume overload as well as to the anemia associated with renal failure. Pericardial friction rubs are very common in the acute phase of transmural MI, although they often last for only a few hours. There is a common misconception that friction rubs are not heard when there is a large amount of fluid in the pericardial sac; this is not the case, because usually some portions of the visceral and parietal pericardial surfaces are in contact despite the large amount of fluid (see Chap. 72).

Occasionally, certain midsystolic (ejection) murmurs have a scratchy character and may be misinterpreted as friction rubs. This is particularly true of the short, scratchy pulmonic ejection murmur heard in hyperthyroidism (Means-Lerman sign).[271] Such scratchy sounds should not be considered to be a friction rub unless both systolic and diastolic components are heard.

Mediastinal Crunch: Hamman's Sign

When air is present in the mediastinum, a series of scratchy sounds (Hamman's sign[272]) may occur, related indirectly to both heartbeat and respiratory excursion. These sounds occur most frequently during ventricular systole and in a random fashion. The diagnosis of mediastinal emphysema may be confirmed by crepitation in the neck secondary to subcutaneous air. These crunching sounds due to air in the mediastinum are common following cardiac surgery.

HEART MURMURS

A *cardiac murmur* is defined as a relatively prolonged series of auditory vibrations of varying intensity (loudness), frequency (pitch), quality, configuration, and duration.[273] Although the exact physical principles that govern the production of murmurs have been debated for years, most authorities now agree that turbulence is the prime factor responsible for most murmurs. Turbulence arises when blood velocity becomes critically high due to high flow, flow through an irregular or narrow area, or a combination of both. Leatham has attributed the production of murmurs to three main factors: (1) high flow rate through normal or abnormal orifices, (2) forward flow through a constricted or irregular orifice or into a dilated vessel or chamber, and (3) backward or regurgitant flow through an incompetent valve, septal defect, or patent ductus arteriosus. Frequently, a combination of these factors is operative.

While the intensity of a systolic murmur is not always proportional to the hemodynamic disturbance, grading the loudness of a murmur from 1 to 6 as described by Freeman and Levine[274] is generally used. A *grade 1 murmur* is so faint that it can be heard only with special effort. A *grade 2 murmur* is faint but can be heard easily. A *grade 3 murmur* is moderately loud, a *grade 4 murmur* is very loud, and a *grade 5 murmur* is extremely loud and can be heard if only the edge of the stethoscope is in contact with the skin but cannot be heard if the stethoscope is removed from the skin. A *grade 6 murmur* is exceptionally loud and can be heard with the stethoscope just removed from contact with the chest. Experience has shown that systolic murmurs of grade 3 or more in intensity are usually hemodynamically significant.[275] Systolic thrills usually are associated with murmurs of grade 4 or louder. The intensity of the murmur varies directly with the velocity of blood flow across the area of murmur production. The velocity, in turn, is directly related to the pressure head that drives the blood across the murmur-producing area. For example, high velocity of flow through a small VSD produces a loud murmur, whereas a large flow at low velocity through an ASD produces no murmur. The *intensity* of a murmur as auscultated at the chest wall is also determined by the transmission characteristics of the tissues intervening between the source of the murmur and the stethoscope. Obesity, emphysema, and the presence of significant pericardial or pleural effusion will decrease the intensity of a murmur, whereas a thin, asthenic body habitus often will accentuate it.

The frequency of a murmur bears a direct relationship to the velocity of blood flow, as does the intensity of the murmur. The low-velocity flow resulting from a small pressure head across a stenotic mitral valve produces a low-pitched rumbling murmur, whereas the large diastolic pressure gradient across a regurgitant aortic valve causes a high-pitched murmur. A recent study has further demonstrated that the dominant frequencies contained in heart murmurs due to stenotic lesions are directly related to the instantaneous jet velocities distal to the associated obstruction. Occasionally, the frequency composition of the same systolic murmur may vary, depending on the area auscultated. For example, the systolic murmur of aortic stenosis frequently sounds higher-pitched at the apex than at the base.[276] Some murmurs such as the "cooing dove" regurgitant murmur of a ruptured or retroverted aortic cusp, the systolic "whoop" or "honk" of mitral valve prolapse, or the high-pitched systolic murmur of a degenerated bioprosthetic valve—have a very distinctive musical quality.

In addition to the intensity and frequency of murmurs, their *timing* also should be described. There is seldom any difficulty distinguishing between systole and diastole, since systole is considerably shorter at normal heart rates. At rapid heart rates, however, the durations of these two intervals approach each other. Under such circumstances, the examiner usually can time the murmur by simultaneous palpation of the lower right carotid artery or can rely on the fact that the second heart sound (S_2) is usually the louder sound at the base. Once S_2 is identified, murmurs can be located properly in the cardiac cycle as systolic or diastolic. If the murmur in question is at the apex, the proper timing can be ensured by the "inching" technique popularized by Harvey and Levine.[215] This consists of slowly moving the stethoscope down from the base to the apex while repeatedly fixing the cardiac cycle in mind, using S_2 as a reference point. With sinus tachycardia, carotid sinus pressure may temporarily slow the rate and make it possible to differentiate systole from diastole. Continuous murmurs are heard throughout the cardiac cycle in systole and diastole and usually have their peak intensity around S_2.

The *location* and *radiation* of a murmur are determined multifactorially by the site of origin, intensity, and direction of blood flow, as well as by the physical characteristics of the chest. The duration and time intensity contour (murmur *envelope*) of a specific murmur are intimately related to the instantaneous pattern of blood flow velocity causing the murmur.

Systolic Murmurs

Systolic murmurs may be classified into two basic categories—ejection (midsystolic) murmurs and regurgitant murmurs. This simple classification is attractive because it has a physiologic as well as a descriptive basis. Systolic *ejection* murmurs are due to forward flow across the LV or RV outflow tract, whereas systolic *regurgitant* murmurs are due to retrograde flow from a high-pressure cardiac chamber to a low-pressure chamber.[277]

SYSTOLIC EJECTION (MIDSYSTOLIC) MURMURS

The systolic *ejection* murmur begins shortly after the pressure in the left or right ventricle exceeds the aortic or pulmonic diastolic pressure sufficiently to open the aortic or pulmonic valve. As a result, there is a delay between the S_1, which occurs shortly after AV pressure crossover, and the beginning of the murmur (Fig. 10-77). The murmur then waxes and wanes in a crescendo-decrescendo fashion often described as "diamond shaped" or "spindle shaped" in configuration. The

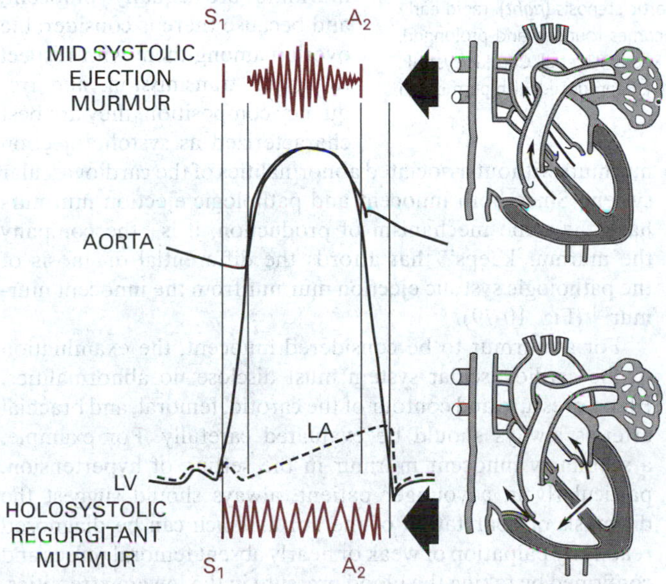

FIGURE 10-77 Midsystolic ejection murmurs are caused by forward flow across the LV or RV outflow tract, whereas pansystolic regurgitant murmurs are caused by retrograde flow from a high-pressure cardiac chamber to a low-pressure one. (*Left*) Diagrammatic representation of the midsystolic ejection murmur and the pansystolic regurgitant murmur, as related to LV, aortic, and left atrial (LA) pressures. The systolic ejection murmur occurs during the period of LV ejection; the onset of the murmur is separated from S_1 by the period of isovolumic contraction and the crescendo-decrescendo murmur terminates before A_2. The pansystolic regurgitant murmur begins with, or may replace, S_1, and the murmur continues up to and through A_2 as LV pressure exceeds left atrial pressure during the period of isovolumic relaxation. The murmur has a plateau configuration and varies little with respiration. (*Right*) Flow diagram. (Left panel reproduced from Reddy PS, Shaver JA, Leonard JJ. Cardiac systolic murmurs: Pathophysiology and differential diagnosis. *Prog Cardiovasc Dis* 1971; 14:19. Entire figure reproduced with permission from Shaver JA. Systolic murmurs. *Heart Dis Stroke* 1993; 2:10.)

murmur ends before the semilunar valve closure on the side from which it originates. The contour of the time-intensity pattern or envelope of the murmur corresponds to the contour of the flow velocity, and the murmur is heard when the sound produced during the peak turbulence exceeds the audible threshold. Thus not only is the overall intensity of the murmur proportional to the rate of ventricular ejection, but also its shape depends on the instantaneous flow velocity during the period of ejection. As can be seen in Fig. 10-78, during normal LV ejection, a disproportionately large volume flow occurs in early systole. If velocity of flow exceeds the murmur threshold, a short midsystolic or ejection murmur results, and its envelope corresponds to the flow velocity pattern. If the stroke volume of the ventricle is increased, this pattern of ejection persists in an exaggerated fashion; the resulting murmur has a tendency to peak early in systole and fade out about halfway through the ejection phase. Such murmurs have been referred to as "kite shaped" and are common in high-output states or conditions such as aortic regurgitation or heart block, where stroke volume is high.

The flow characteristics of normal RV ejection are somewhat different. Early ejection rates are not nearly as high, and the flow curve peaks somewhat later, having a more rounded contour. This flow pattern may well explain some of the long systolic ejection murmurs heard in ASDs and the straight-back syndrome, where only minimal gradients are found across the RV outflow tract.[278] With true valvular obstruction, rapid early ejection is no longer possible; the aortic flow velocity patterns become rounded, resulting in the more symmetric murmur of aortic stenosis. In such cases, the instantaneous flow pattern is determined by the instantaneous pressure head with the resulting high correlation between the contour of the pressure gradient and the murmur envelope. If LV or RV obstruction is severe, systole is prolonged, and closure sound of the semilunar valve is delayed. The murmur, however, always stops before the closure sound on the side from which it originates, although it may envelop the closure sound of the opposite side of the circulation. Because of the high correlation between the shape of the murmur and its underlying flow velocity characteristics, careful attention must be given during auscultation to the shape and duration of the murmur as well as to its intensity.

The intensity of ejection murmurs closely parallels changes in cardiac output. Any condition that increases forward flow—such as exercise, anxiety, fever, or increased stroke volume associated with the long diastolic filling period after a premature beat—increases the intensity of the murmur. Likewise, conditions that decrease cardiac output—congestive heart failure, beta blockade, or other negative inotropic agents—will decrease the intensity of the ejection murmur. This intimate relationship to flow, particularly with beat-to-beat variations, usually will allow the clinician to differentiate a systolic ejection murmur from a systolic regurgitant murmur. Furthermore, definitive diagnosis of the systolic murmur often can be made during auscultation by careful attention to the response of the murmur to various bedside maneuvers that alter the flow and loading conditions of the heart.[279] These maneuvers include respiration, the strain and release phases of the Valsalva maneuver, standing, squatting, passive leg elevation, isometric handgrip exercise, inhalation of amyl nitrite, and transient arterial occlusion.

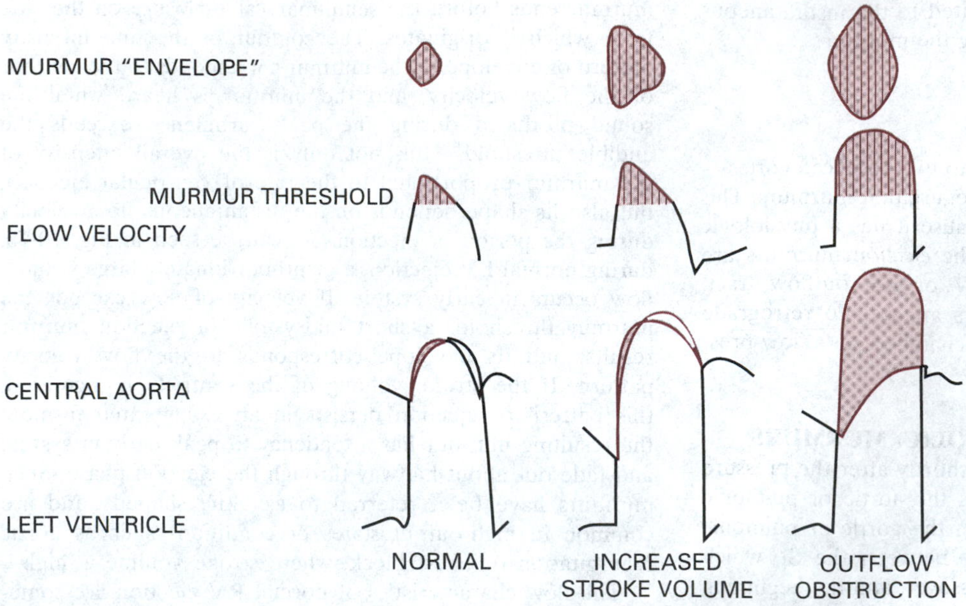

FIGURE 10-78 The simultaneous time-intensity course of the murmur "envelope," aortic flow velocity, and LV and central aortic pressure. During normal LV ejection (*left*), peak flow velocity is early, with two-thirds of the ventricular volume ejected during the first half of systole. The murmur threshold may be exceeded during the early peak flow and the corresponding murmur envelope inscribed. (*Center*) Exaggeration of the normal pattern of LV ejection with a high stroke volume, as in high-output states. With critical aortic stenosis (*right*), rapid early ejection is no longer possible; the flow velocity is increased, and the contour becomes rounded and prolonged, producing the typical diamond-shaped murmur of aortic stenosis. (Modified from Reddy PS, et al. Cardiac systolic murmurs: Pathophysiology and differential diagnosis. *Prog Cardiovasc Dis* 1971; 14:4. Reproduced with permission from the publisher and the authors.)

Innocent Murmurs

Innocent murmurs are always systolic ejection in nature and occur without evidence of physiologic or structural abnormalities in the cardiovascular system when peak flow velocity in early systole exceeds the murmur threshold.[275] These murmurs are almost always less than grade 3 in intensity and vary considerably from examination to examination and with body position and level of physical activity. They are not associated with a thrill or with radiation to the carotid arteries or axillae. They may arise from flow across either the normal LV or RV outflow tract and always end well before semilunar valve closure.

Innocent murmurs are found in approximately 30 to 50 percent of all children. In young children, especially children aged 3 to 8 years, the vibratory systolic (Still's) murmur is common. It has a very distinctive quality described as "groaning," "croaking," "buzzing," or "twanging." It is heard best along the left sternal border at the third or fourth interspace and disappears by puberty. Considerable controversy exists as to the origin of the vibratory systolic murmur. Regardless of the exact cause, most authorities agree that this murmur originates from flow in the LV outflow tract.

Innocent systolic ejection murmurs also have been attributed to flow in the normal RV outflow tract and have been termed *innocent pulmonic systolic murmurs* because the site of their maximal intensity is auscultated best in the pulmonic area at the second left interspace with radiation along the left sternal border. These are low to medium in pitch, with a blowing quality, and are common in children, adolescents, and young adults. Stein et al.,[280] who used high-fidelity catheter-tipped micromanometers to record intracardiac sound and pressure in the aorta and pulmonary artery in adults with normal valves, invariably recorded the ejection murmur in the region of the aortic valve. They concluded that these murmurs, despite their precordial location, were aortic in origin.

In adults over age 50, innocent murmurs due to flow in the LV outflow tract are often heard and may be of a higher frequency, with a musical quality, and frequently loudest at the apex. They may be associated with a tortuous, dilated sclerotic aortic root, often in the setting of systolic hypertension. Mild sclerosis of the aortic valve also may be present.

The preceding descriptive breakdown of innocent murmurs is based primarily on age, precordial location, and distinctive acoustic qualities. Since all these murmurs are equally innocent, and because there is considerable overlap among them with respect to origin, transmission, and frequency composition, they are best characterized as systolic ejection murmurs without associated abnormalities of the cardiovascular system. Since both innocent and pathologic ejection murmurs have the same mechanism of production, it is "the company the murmur keeps" that affords the differential diagnosis of the pathologic systolic ejection murmur from the innocent murmur[281] (Fig. 10-79).

For a murmur to be considered innocent, the examination of the cardiovascular system must disclose no abnormalities. Blood pressure and contour of the carotid, femoral, and brachial arteries always should be evaluated carefully. For example, a seemingly innocent murmur in the setting of hypertension, particularly in a younger patient, always should suggest the diagnosis of coarctation of the aorta, which can be diagnosed readily by palpation of weak or nearly absent femoral pulses and confirmed by taking the blood pressure in the lower extremities. There should be no elevation of the jugular venous pulse, and the contour of the jugular pulse should be normal, without exaggeration of either the *a* or *v* wave. Evidence of cardiac enlargement on physical examination should be absent, and palpation of the apex in the left lateral position should show no evidence of a presystolic impulse, sustained systolic motion, or hyperdynamic circulation. On auscultation, normal physiologic splitting should be present. A physiologic S_3 is often present in association with an innocent murmur in children and young adults but should not be heard after age 30. An S_4 is rarely heard in normal children and adults (younger than 50 years) and always should be considered to be abnormal when associated with a presystolic impulse. Systolic ejection sounds of valvular origin as well as midsystolic nonejection sounds should be absent because their presence points to minor abnormalities of the semilunar and AV valves, respectively (see Fig. 10-79). The remainder of the physical examination should show no evidence of a cardiac cause of pulmonary or systemic congestion. In almost all patients with innocent murmurs, the ECG and the cardiac silhouette on chest x-ray should be normal.

The supraclavicular arterial murmur or bruit is a common finding in normal individuals, particularly children and adolescents. These murmurs are maximal in intensity above the clavicles and tend to be louder on the right, although they are often heard bilaterally. The bruit begins shortly after S_1, is diamond-shaped, and is of brief duration, usually occupying less than half of systole. Although the exact mechanism is unknown, it is related to peak flow velocity near the origin of the normal subclavian, innominate, or carotid artery. When particularly prominent, this murmur may transmit to the basal region of the heart and simulate a systolic ejection murmur. However, unlike the cardiac ejection murmur, the supraclavicular murmur is always louder above the clavicles than below them. Complete compression of the subclavian artery may cause the murmur to disappear completely, whereas partial compression occasionally may intensify it. Hyperextension of the shoulders is a simple bedside maneuver that may decrease the intensity of the murmur and cause it to disappear completely. In the adult, the supraclavicular murmur must be distinguished from the murmur of true organic carotid obstruction, this latter murmur being longer, often extending through S_2, and frequently associated with a history suggestive of transient ischemic attacks.

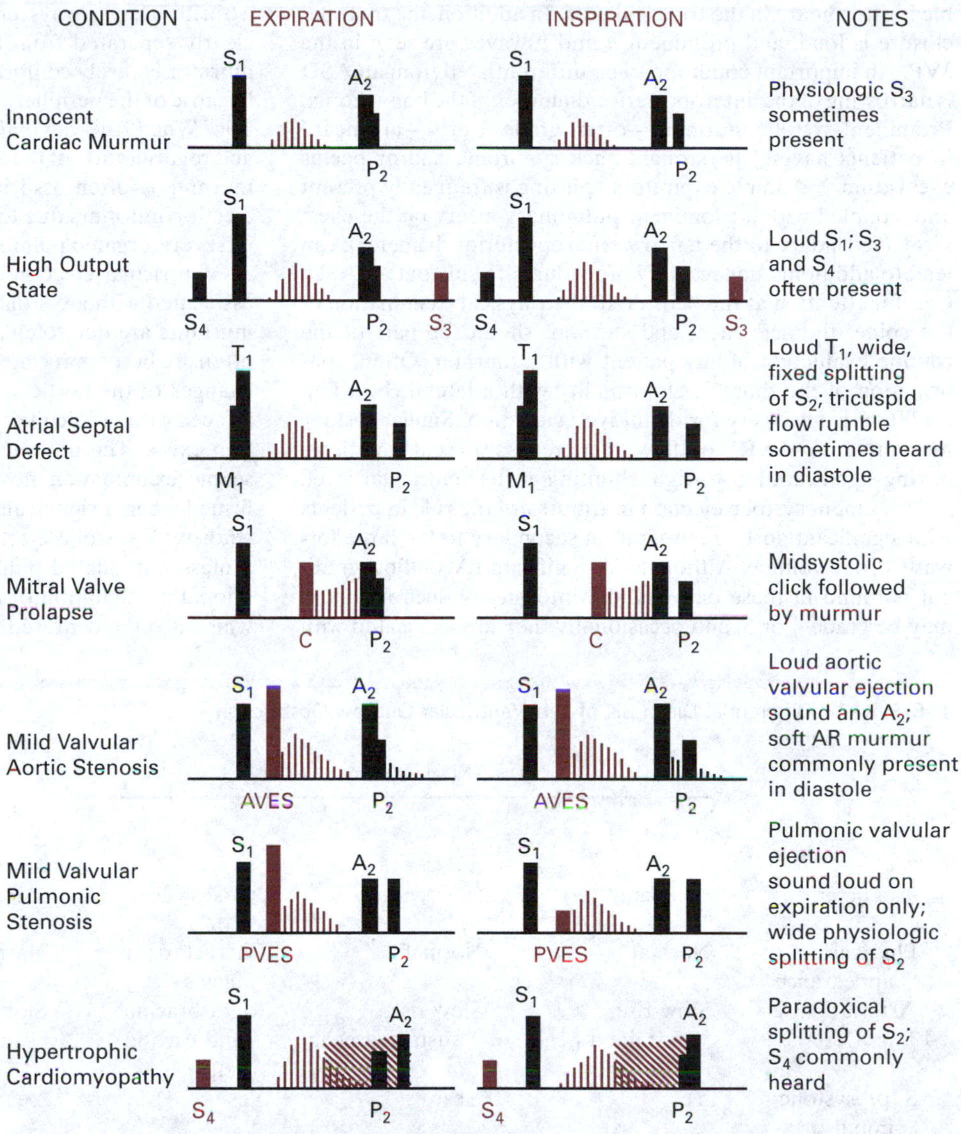

FIGURE 10-79 The differential diagnosis of the innocent murmur versus the pathologic systolic murmur is made by the "company the murmur keeps." The innocent murmur must be found in the setting of an otherwise normal cardiovascular examination. C, midsystolic nonejection sound; AVES, aortic valvular ejection sound; PVES, pulmonic valvular ejection sound; AR, aortic regurgitation. (From Shaver JA, et al. *Examination of the Heart*, Part IV. Auscultation. Dallas: American Heart Association; 1990:40. Reproduced with permission from the publisher and the authors.)

Functional Systolic Ejection Murmurs

Systolic ejection murmurs produced by high cardiac output states are functional and flow-related but are excluded from the category of innocent murmurs because of their associated altered physiologic state. These include the cardiac murmurs of thyrotoxicosis, pregnancy, anemia, fever, exercise, and peripheral arteriovenous fistula, which are best interpreted in light of the total presentation of the patient (see Fig. 10-77). Although these murmurs are often grade 3 and occasionally grade 4 in intensity, they always end well before S_2 and are only rarely confused with obstruction of the LV or RV outflow tract. The large stroke volume associated with high-degree heart block often produces a functional systolic murmur; when found in the setting of complete heart block, beat-to-beat variations in the intensity of the murmur are present due to the random contribution of atrial systole to LV filling.

The functional systolic murmur in patients with a hemodynamically significant ASD is due to the increased flow in the RV outflow tract secondary to the left-to-right shunt at the atrial level. It is easily diagnosed at the bedside "by the company it keeps." The hallmark of this condition is wide, fixed splitting of S_2. When the shunt is large (more than 2.5:1), a hyperdynamic parasternal impulse is usually present, and a diastolic flow rumble is often heard in the tricuspid area. In addition, the tricuspid closure is loud, and prominent *a* and *v* waves are seen in the JVP. An important condition to be differentiated from an ASD is narrowing of the anteroposterior diameter of the bony thorax. Prominent systolic murmurs—often grade 3 or 4—are heard in patients having the straight-back syndrome and/or pectus excavatum.[282] Audible expiratory splitting is frequently present and, coupled with a prominent pulmonary artery on the chest x-ray (secondary to the narrow anteroposterior diameter), can lead to additional unnecessary procedures to rule out an ASD. Careful attention at the bedside to the physical examination of the spine, thoracic cage, and sternum should be part of the routine evaluation of any patient with a murmur. Often, confirmation of the thoracic abnormality with a lateral chest film is all that is necessary for definitive evaluation. Similar systolic murmurs from the RV outflow tract are also present in patients having significant left-to-right shunting at the ventricular level.

Prominent systolic ejection murmurs are the rule in patients with significant aortic regurgitation secondary to the large forward stroke volume. Although no significant LV outflow gradient is found in these patients, the intensity of such murmurs may be grade 4 or 5, and occasionally they are associated with a thrill. They always end well before aortic closure and are clearly separated from the early regurgitant murmur. Such a murmur is rarely confused with significant valvular obstruction because of the peripheral findings of wide-open aortic regurgitation. When true valvular obstruction is present (mixed stenosis and regurgitation of the aortic valve), the longer systolic ejection murmur is often associated with a prominent thrill. Systolic ejection murmurs due to large RV stroke volume are also seen in severe organic pulmonic valvular regurgitation.

Ventricular ejection into a dilated great vessel is commonly associated with a systolic ejection murmur. In the elderly, such murmurs are due to ejection into a dilated, sclerotic aorta and often are best appreciated at the apex. Frequently, degenerative changes of the aortic valve are also present, and the clinician is faced with a difficult decision as to whether or not true obstruction exists. The presence of significant calcification on fluoroscopic examination favors true obstruction and can be confirmed when a significant gradient is demonstrated by Doppler studies. A systolic ejection murmur due to RV ejection into a massively dilated pulmonary artery is frequently present in idiopathic dilatation of the pulmonary artery (see Fig. 10-73), which is often confused with an ASD due to the wide auditory

TABLE 10-12 Differential Diagnosis of Left Ventricular Outflow Obstruction

	Congenital Aortic Stenosis				
Parameter	Valvular	Subvalvular	Supravalvular	Acquired Aortic Stenosis	Hypertrophic "Obstructive" Cardiomyopathy
Physical appearance	Normal	Normal	Characteristic facies	Normal	Normal
Arterial pulse	Slow rise, sustained peak	Slow rise, sustained peak	Right brachial and carotid > left	Slow rise, sustained peak	Brisk rise, unsustained double peak
S_4 presystolic impulse	Yes	Yes	Yes	Yes	Yes
Left ventricular systolic impulse	Sustained, single	Sustained, single	Sustained, single	Sustained, single	Sustained, may be double
Aortic ejection sound	Typical ↓ with calcif.	Rare	Rare	Common ↓ with calcif.*	Rare exception
Midsystolic ejection murmur; maximal site	First or second right interspace	First or second right interspace	First right interspace and over right carotid	First or second right interspace; apex in elderly	Apex, lower left sternal edge
Second sound splitting	Usually normal or single	Usually normal or single	Usually normal or single	Usually single or reversed	Usually reversed or single
Intensity of aortic closure	Normal or increased or ↓ with calcif.*	Normal or decreased	Normal or decreased	Decreased or absent with calcif*	Normal
Murmur of aortic regurgitation	Common	Common	Uncommon	Common	Rare exception

*Calcif. = calcification.

Source: Modified from Reddy PS, et al. Cardiac systolic murmurs: Pathophysiology and differential diagnosis. *Prog Cardiovasc Dis* 1971; 14:6. Reproduced with permission from the publisher and authors.

expiratory splitting present in this condition. The prominent pulmonary ejection sound also may be confused with a loud tricuspid closure sound of a patient with an ASD. Short systolic ejection murmurs, frequently associated with a prominent late pulmonary ejection sound, are also seen in dilated pulmonic arteries secondary to severe pulmonary hypertension of any cause. Physical findings of severe pulmonary hypertension are always present, including a prominent parasternal impulse and increased intensity of the pulmonic component of S_2, which is well heard at the apex. Prominent *a* waves in the neck and a right-sided S_4 that increases with inspiration are present if the ventricular septum is intact. If the pulmonary hypertension is associated with intracardiac shunting, cyanosis frequently is present. A high-pitched, early diastolic murmur of pulmonic regurgitation secondary to severe pulmonary hypertension often is present.

LV Outflow Tract Murmurs

Obstruction to LV outflow may be congenital or acquired and may be located at the valvular, supravalvular, or subvalvular level. Stenosis is occasionally present at more than one level. In the clinical evaluation, one should attempt to define the severity and the level of obstruction. A summary of this differential diagnosis can be found in Table 10-12 (see Chap. 56).

The murmur of fixed stenosis of the LV outflow tract, regardless of the site, is crescendo-decrescendo, and its contour closely parallels the instantaneous pressure gradient. As long as cardiac output is maintained, there is an excellent correlation between the intensity and length of the murmur with severity of obstruction. Although there is a tendency toward late peaking of the murmur with increasing severity of the obstruction, this delayed peaking has not been found to correlate as well with the severity of valvular obstruction in aortic stenosis as it has in pulmonic stenosis.[283] The murmur of significant fixed LV outflow tract obstruction usually is best heard in the second right and second and third left interspaces near the sternum. It radiates widely into the neck and along the great vessels. With radiation to the apex, particularly in the elderly patient, the high-frequency components of the murmur predominate, and the apical murmur has a high pitch and often a musical quality. This characteristic change in the pitch between the proximal and distal radiation of the murmur is a repeated source of confusion on auscultation. There is an almost overpowering urge to call it a separate murmur of mitral regurgitation; however, observations repeatedly demonstrate that this murmur, regardless of its timbre or harmonics, retains a spindle-shaped configuration whenever it is heard or recorded. The murmur of aortic stenosis varies directly with the length of the preceding diastole; the longer the preceding ventricular filling period, the louder is the systolic murmur (Fig. 10-80). In contrast, the apical murmur of mitral regurgitation is associated with little or no variation in intensity with varying cycle lengths. This observation is useful in patients with atrial fibrillation or frequent premature contrac-

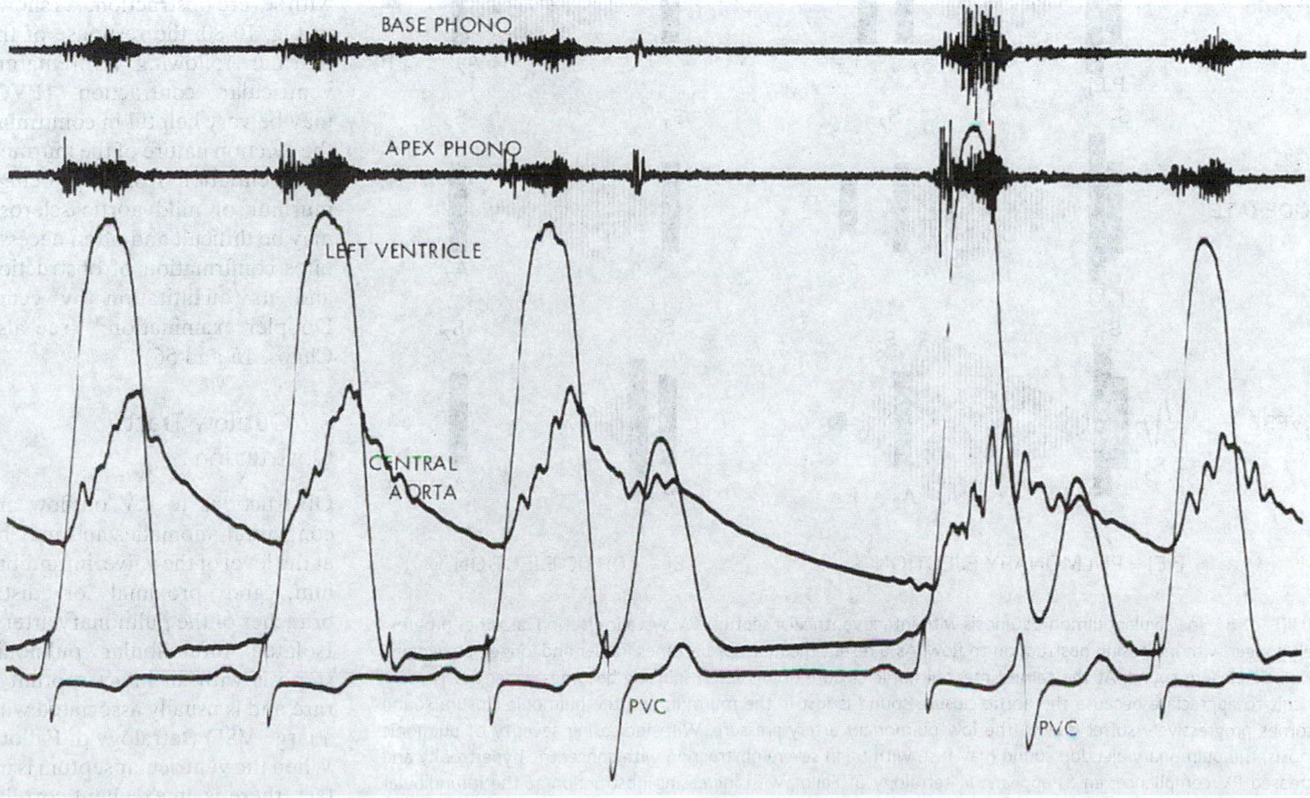

FIGURE 10-80 Effect of the long diastolic filling period following a premature ventricular contraction (PVC) on the intensity of a systolic ejection murmur (SEM). There is a marked increase in the intensity of the aortic stenosis murmur recorded at the base and at the apex. Despite the higher-frequency content of the apical murmur, this response clearly identifies this murmur as ejection in nature. (From Paley H. Left ventricular outflow tract obstruction: Heart sounds and murmurs. In: Leon DF, Shaver JA, eds. *Physiologic Principles of Heart Sounds and Murmurs*. Monograph 46. Dallas: American Heart Association; 1975:112. Reproduced with permission from the publisher and the author.)

tions and helps to identify whether an apical murmur is due to radiation of an ejection murmur or is an additional regurgitant murmur of mitral regurgitation. Beat-to-beat variations in the intensity of the murmur of aortic stenosis have been noted in both pulsus alternans and AV dissociation.

A loud early systolic valvular ejection sound or click is the hallmark of congenital valvular aortic stenosis, and its presence defines the obstruction at the valvular level (see Fig. 10-66). As discussed earlier in this chapter, its intensity correlates well with the motility of the valve, and there is little correlation with the severity of the obstruction. It disappears when the valve becomes immobile due to calcific fixation and is absent in fixed subaortic stenosis. With progressive increase in the severity of the outflow obstruction, the duration of LV ejection is prolonged, resulting in narrow, single, or reversed splitting of S_2. Reversed splitting of S_2 in aortic stenosis in the absence of LBBB is always associated with severe obstruction (see Chap. 56).

Regardless of the site of obstruction, significant stenosis always results in LV hypertrophy, with a decreased diastolic compliance. Clinically, this is manifest as a presystolic apical pulsation on palpation and as an S_4 on auscultation (see Fig. 10-76). In patients older than age 12, the S_4 is generally associated with a LV diastolic pressure above 11 mmHg and a left atrial *a*-wave peak of about 13 mmHg. The relationship between the severity of obstruction and the presence of S_4 gallops is indirect, reflecting hypertrophy and decreased compliance of the left ventricle rather than obstruction per se.

Because of the frequent coexistence of hypertensive or arteriosclerotic heart disease in elderly patients with calcific aortic stenosis, the presence of an S_4 is nonspecific and correlates poorly with the severity of obstruction. The S_3 gallops also may be heard in LV outflow tract obstruction, particularly when decompensation occurs (see Fig. 10-76).

The diagnosis of hemodynamically significant aortic stenosis in the elderly presents a particularly difficult problem. The murmur is often of low intensity due to the decreased cardiac output and poor LV function. An ejection sound or click is rarely present, due to calcific fixation of the valve leaflets, and S_2 is of low amplitude. The murmur is often loudest at the apex, has a high-frequency content, and may be difficult to define as ejection in nature because S_1 and A_2 may be poorly heard and therefore lost as landmarks defining the onset and end of mechanical systole.[283] In most patients with severe aortic stenosis, no A_2 is heard, and the systolic murmur obliterates P_2. In the elderly, the rate of rise of the carotid pulse may be nearly normal due to the hard, sclerotic vessels even with severe obstruction. As shown in Fig. 10-80, the response of the murmur following a premature ventricular contraction (PVC) may be very helpful in confirming the ejection nature of the murmur. Differentiation from the benign murmur of mild aortic sclerosis may be difficult and often necessitates confirmation of obstruction and its quantitation by echo-Doppler examination[284] (see also Chaps. 15 and 56).

RV Outflow Tract Obstruction

Obstructions to RV outflow are congenital anomalies and may be at the level of the valve, infundibulum, and proximal or distal branches of the pulmonary artery. Isolated infundibular pulmonic stenosis with an intact septum is rare and is usually associated with a large VSD (tetralogy of Fallot). When the ventricular septum is intact, there is an excellent correlation between both the intensity and duration of the murmur and the severity of obstruction.[285] Figure 10-81 contrasts the auscultatory findings of progressively

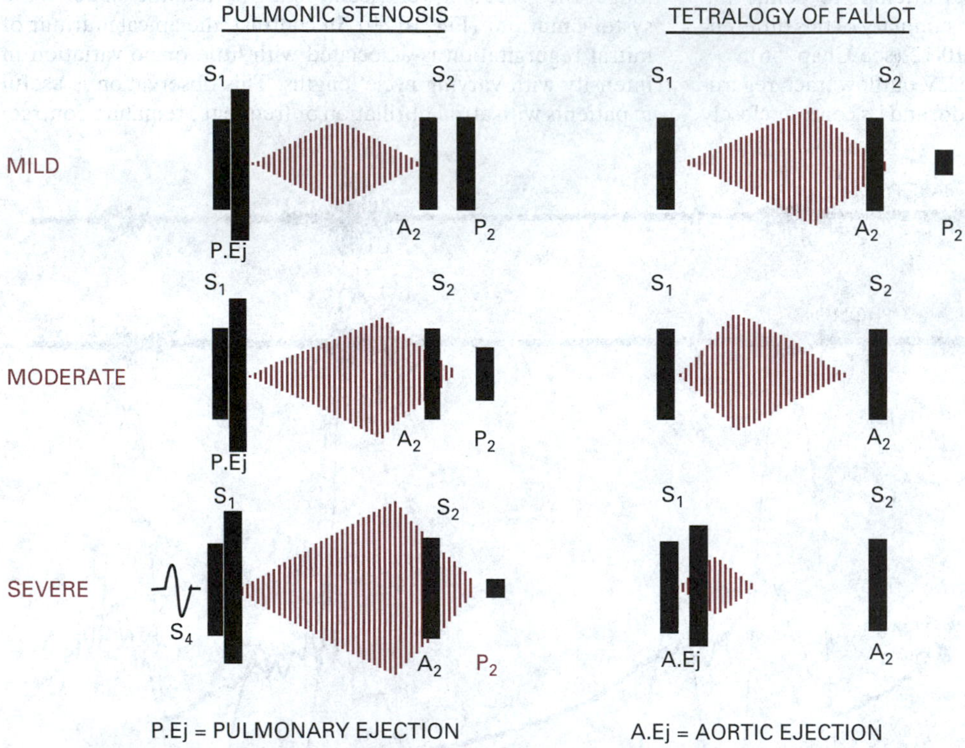

FIGURE 10-81 In valvular pulmonic stenosis with intact ventricular septum, RV systolic ejection becomes progressively longer with increasing obstruction to flow. As a result, the murmur becomes louder and longer, enveloping the aortic closure sound. At the same time, pulmonic closure occurs later; splitting becomes wider but is more difficult to appreciate because the aortic closure sound is lost in the murmur; and the pulmonic closure sound becomes progressively softer due to the low pulmonary artery pressure. With increasing severity of pulmonic stenosis, the pulmonary ejection sound may fuse with S_1. In severe obstruction with concentric hypertrophy and decreased RV compliance, an S_4 appears. In tetralogy of Fallot, with increasing obstruction at the infundibular area, more and more RV blood is shunted across a silent VSD with less flow across the obstructed RV outflow tract. With increasing obstruction, the murmur becomes shorter, earlier, and fainter. The pulmonic closure sound is absent in severe tetralogy of Fallot. The dilated aorta receives almost all the cardiac output from both ventricular chambers, and there is an aortic ejection sound (Aej). (From Leonard J, et al: *Examination of the Heart*, Part 4: Auscultation. Dallas: American Heart Association; 1974:45. Reproduced with permission from the publisher and authors.)

more severe valvular pulmonic stenosis with an intact ventricular septum with those in tetralogy of Fallot with progressively more severe RV outflow obstruction.[286] As with valvular aortic stenosis, an early systolic ejection sound defines the level of obstruction at the valve. In mild to moderate valvular obstruction, the intensity of this sound is markedly attenuated or may disappear with inspiration. In more severe valvular obstruction, this sound may fuse with S_1 or actually may present as a presystolic click when the pressure generated by a forceful right atrial contraction exceeds RV end-diastolic pressure, causing doming of the stenotic valve in late diastole. Although obstruction to RV outflow in tetralogy of Fallot is usually at the infundibular level, valvular stenosis also may be present. In this setting, a pulmonary valvular ejection sound introduces a systolic murmur, and little variation in the intensity of the ejection sound is found with respiration.

The classic late peaking of the systolic ejection murmur of severe pulmonic stenosis with an intact ventricular septum is demonstrated in Fig. 10-82. Note that the late vibrations of the murmur completely envelop A_2, whereas P_2 is markedly delayed and decreases in intensity secondary to the low pulmonary artery closing pressure. In moderate to severe valvular pulmonic stenosis, an excellent correlation has been found between the A_2-P_2 interval and the RV peak pressure. When the ventricular septum is intact in severe RV outflow obstruction, prominent *a* waves are present in the JVP in association with a right-sided S_4 that may increase with inspiration. Neither of these is present in uncomplicated tetralogy of Fallot. Occasionally, in very severe pulmonic stenosis, a low-pitched presystolic murmur may be present due to forward flow across the stenotic valve that has been opened prematurely by forceful right atrial contraction in late diastole. Such patients are often cyanotic due to right-to-left shunting through a patent foramen ovale.

In isolated infundibular obstruction, a pulmonic ejection sound is usually not encountered, and the pulmonic closure (P_2) is usually not audible except in the mildest cases. Both valvular pulmonic stenosis and isolated infundibular pulmonic stenosis with an intact septum can be differentiated from tetralogy of Fallot by noting the marked intensification of the ejection murmur after the inhalation of amyl nitrite. In contrast, the murmur of tetralogy of Fallot shortens and decreases in intensity.

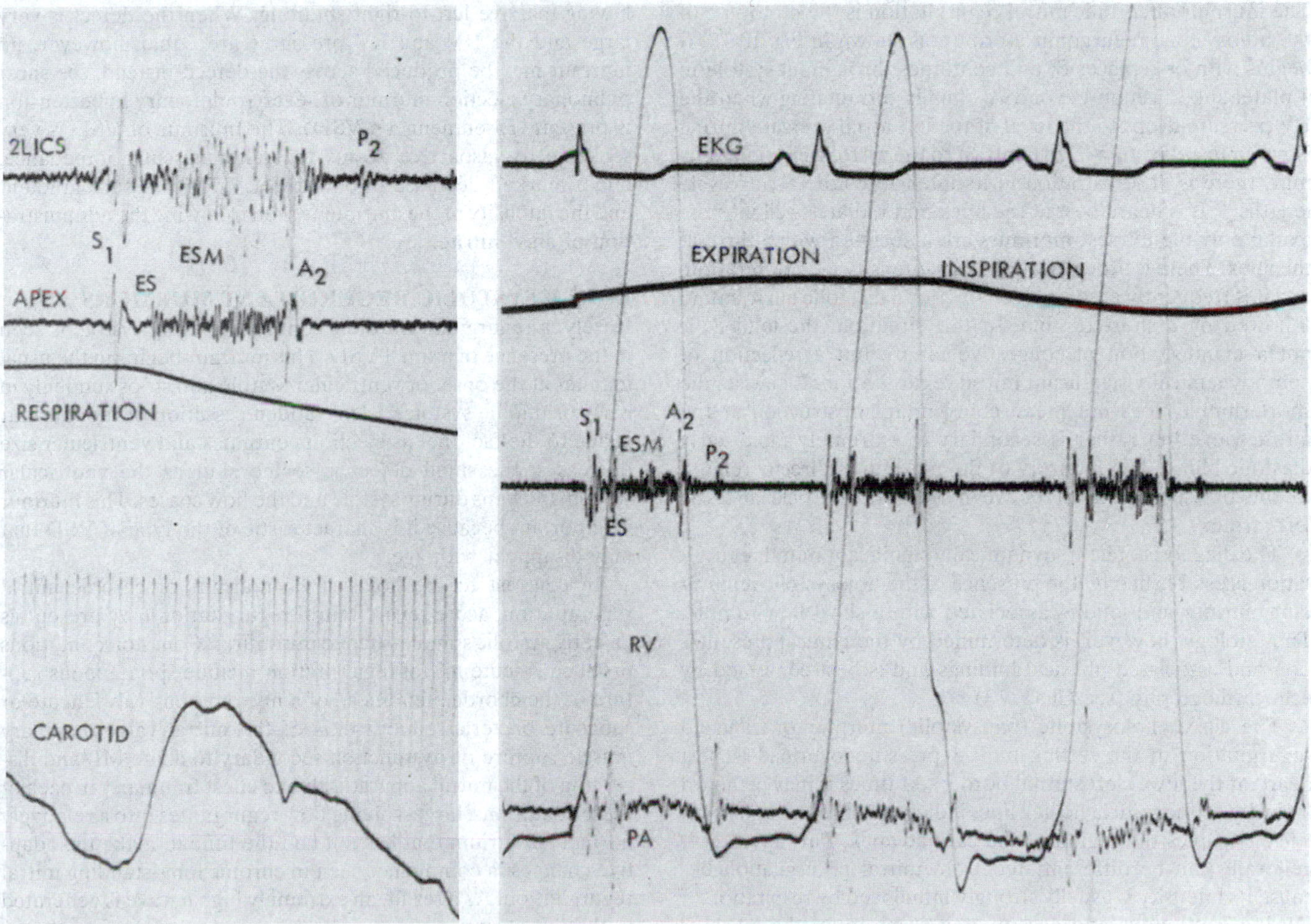

FIGURE 10-82 (*Left*) The phonocardiogram of a patient with severe valvular pulmonic stenosis as recorded at the second left intercostal space (2LICS) and the apex. The long ejection murmur (ESM) has late systolic peaking and spills through A_2. There is a marked delay in P_2, which is very small in amplitude. (*Right*) At cardiac catheterization, the markedly delayed P_2 is shown to be secondary to a very large systolic pressure gradient, and its decreased intensity is due to the low pulmonary artery pressure at the time of valve closure. The late peaking of the ejection murmur correlates with the maximal pressure gradient between the right ventricle and the pulmonary artery. (From Curtiss EI, et al. First and second heart sound. In: Horwitz LD, ed. *Signs and Symptoms in Cardiology*. Philadelphia: Lippincott; 1985:200. Reproduced with permission from the publisher and authors.)

In branch stenosis of the pulmonary artery, there is a systolic murmur of varying intensity at the upper left sternal border that is widely transmitted to the right side of the chest, back, and both axillae. The murmur is usually less harsh and of higher pitch than the murmur of valvular stenosis. With more peripheral branch stenosis, systolic ejection murmurs or even continuous murmurs may be heard over the lung fields. The wide radiation of this murmur is particularly helpful in alerting the clinician to this type of right-sided obstruction.

Systolic Regurgitant Murmurs

Systolic regurgitant murmurs are produced by retrograde flow from a chamber of high pressure to a chamber of lower pressure. The classic examples of such murmurs are the holosystolic (pansystolic) murmur of mitral regurgitation, tricuspid regurgitation, and VSD. Since there is usually a high-pressure differential between the two chambers throughout systole, the murmurs are holosystolic in duration, high-pitched and blowing in quality, and plateaulike in configuration.

HOLOSYSTOLIC REGURGITANT MURMURS

The murmur of chronic mitral regurgitation is the prototype of the holosystolic regurgitant murmur, as shown in Fig. 10-77. It begins with or replaces S_1 and continues throughout systole in a plateaulike fashion beyond A_2, finally terminating when the LV pressure drops to the level of the left atrial pressure during isovolumic relaxation.[287] In contrast to the systolic ejection murmur, there is little variation in its intensity with varying cycle lengths.[288] It is heard best at the apex and radiates well into the axilla; only the loudest murmurs are associated with a thrill at the apex. There is little variation in its intensity with respiration, and it is frequently accompanied by a loud diastolic filling sound followed by a short rumble. In this situation, the loud S_3 is not a manifestation of congestive failure but a reflection of hemodynamically significant mitral regurgitation. Likewise, the short rumble does not mean concomitant obstruction at the mitral valve but rather is secondary to extremely rapid early diastolic filling. The intensity of the murmur is directly related to the pressure gradient between the left ventricle and the left atrium.

The diagnosis of hemodynamically significant mitral regurgitation is established by the presence of the holosystolic regurgitant murmur and loud S_3 associated with a short flow rumble. The etiology, however, is determined by the clinical presentation and associated physical findings and is best confirmed by echocardiography (see Chap. 13).

The classic holosystolic (pansystolic) murmur of tricuspid regurgitation in the setting of RV pressure overload is best heard at the lower left sternal border. At times it may be heard laterally to the midclavicular line, indicating that the right ventricle occupies the region of the cardiac apex. Furthermore, it generally can be differentiated from mitral regurgitation because its intensity is usually strongly influenced by respiration.[289] During continuous and accentuated respiration, the murmur increases in intensity with inspiration due to the increased venous return and RV filling associated with inspiration. The inspiratory increase in loudness of right-sided auscultatory events is known as *Carvallo's sign*. Careful inspection of the JVP while auscultating the murmur will be of further help in defining its tricuspid origin, showing a prominent v wave with a rapid y descent that augments during inspiration. In severe RV failure, this respiratory variation may be absent, but it may reappear as the state of compensation improves. With severe tricuspid regurgitation, a short flow rumble introduced by an S_3 can be present, just as with mitral regurgitation, and both will increase with inspiration.[290]

The holosystolic murmur of VSD is heard best just off the sternal border in the fourth, fifth, and sixth intercostal spaces and is usually accompanied by a forceful thrill.[291] The murmur does not radiate to the axilla as with mitral regurgitation and does not have the respiratory variation characteristic of tricuspid regurgitation. Wide physiologic splitting with an easily heard P_2 is usually present when the left-to-right shunt is hemodynamically significant. When the shunt is large, there is a left ventricular S_4 followed by a short flow rumble. The regurgitant murmur is due to high-velocity flow from the high-pressure left ventricle to the lower-pressure right ventricle, and its intensity correlates poorly with the degree of left-to-right shunting. For example, a grade 5 murmur may be associated with a very high velocity flow through a small hemodynamically insignificant muscular VSD (Roger). On the other hand, an equally loud murmur associated with a thrill may be present with a larger defect having massive left-to-right shunting. When the defect is very large and the RV and LV pressures are equal, however, no murmur may be produced across the defect; instead, the short pulmonary ejection murmur of severe pulmonary hypertension is present (Eisenmenger's VSD). The murmur of VSD is very sensitive to vasoactive agents that alter vascular impedance, and a marked decrease in both the LV-RV pressure gradient and the intensity of the murmur is seen following the administration of amyl nitrite.

EARLY SYSTOLIC REGURGITANT MURMURS

Rarely, a regurgitant murmur confined to early systole is seen in the presence of a small VSD. This murmur begins in the usual manner at the onset of ventricular systole and stops suddenly in early or middle systole.[292] The sudden cessation of the murmur is due to the fact that as ejection continues and ventricular size decreases, the small defect is sealed shut as the ventricular septum thickens during systole and the flow ceases. This murmur is important because it is characteristic of the type of VSD that may disappear with age.

In contrast to the holosystolic murmur of chronic mitral regurgitation, acute severe mitral regurgitation may present as an early systolic spindle-shaped murmur.[293] Common conditions producing acute mitral regurgitation include spontaneous rupture of the chordae tendineae of a myxomatous valve, acute or subacute bacterial endocarditis of the mitral valve, papillary muscle rupture or dysfunction secondary to acute MI, and disruption of the mitral apparatus due to chest trauma.[294] In each of these conditions, large-volume flow regurgitates into a relatively normal left atrium that has not had the time to make the adaptive changes in compliance seen in chronic long-standing mitral regurgitation. As a result, an extremely high v wave is generated in the left atrium.

This high v wave abolishes the left ventricular–left atrial gradient during the latter part of systole, resulting in termination of retrograde flow and abbreviation of the systolic murmur. As shown in a patient with acute mitral regurgitation secondary to spontaneous rupture of the chordae tendineae of a myxomatous valve, the murmur ends before A_2. Audible expiratory splitting with an accentuated P_2 is present at the base, and a loud S_4 is recorded at the apex. The presence of the S_4 associated with a prominent presystolic impulse on palpation is an important clue that indicates the acute nature of the mitral regurgitation and is rarely present in mitral regurgitation of a chronic nature. The systolic murmur of acute mitral regurgitation, which can mimic ejection murmurs, may have classic radiation to the axilla and back, especially if it is due to prolapse of the anterior leaflet of the valve with flow directed over the posterior leaflet. When the murmur is loud, it may be conducted to the top of the head and to the sacrum along the spinal column. Occasionally, the murmur is conducted to the base of the heart and great vessels, simulating aortic stenosis. The quick-rising carotid pulse with rapid falloff, as well as the wide physiologic splitting of the second heart sound, helps differentiation from aortic stenosis.[295]

The systolic murmur of organic tricuspid regurgitation is often unimpressive and presents as an early systolic murmur ending well before A_2, even in the presence of severe regurgitation.[296] In this condition, the RV pressure is nearly normal, and massive regurgitation may be present with only a small pressure differential between the right ventricle and the right atrium. The small pressure head results in a low-velocity flow, minimal turbulence, and a soft, abbreviated murmur. Occasionally, only minimal early systolic vibrations are heard. In most patients, large *v* waves are readily apparent in the JVP. The murmur retains the characteristic inspiratory augmentation seen in right-sided regurgitant murmurs and is frequently associated with an S_4 that increases in intensity with inspiration. A right-sided S_4 and a prominent diastolic tricuspid flow rumble are the rule when the tricuspid regurgitation is acute, as in endocarditis of the tricuspid valve. After total excision of the tricuspid valve for infective endocarditis related to intravenous drug abuse, the systolic murmur is often very unimpressive or may be completely absent. Giant *v* waves in the neck are easily visible, however, and palpable venous thrills and a murmur at the base of the neck may be present secondary to rapid retrograde flow in the jugular system.[297] Other causes of organic tricuspid regurgitation include carcinoid heart disease, RV infarction, chest trauma, and damage of the tricuspid valve during open heart surgery.

MID- AND LATE-SYSTOLIC REGURGITANT MURMURS

Midsystolic murmurs can occur with mitral regurgitation due to papillary muscle dysfunction.[298] The timing of the murmur of papillary muscle dysfunction also may be late systolic, and the murmur may be either intermittent or constant. It occurs with ischemia or infarction of either the posteromedial or anterolateral papillary muscle. Often these murmurs are transient, being provoked by episodes of ischemia.

Varying degrees of mitral valve prolapse are the most frequent cause of a late-systolic murmur, and this entity is one of the most common causes of systolic murmurs seen in clinical practice[299] (see Chap. 58). The murmur is best heard at the apex and often has a tendency to a late systolic crescendo. It is frequently introduced or accompanied by nonejection clicks. These clicks may be single or multiple, and they can occur independently without an accompanying systolic murmur. As shown in Fig. 10-67, the click occurs near the time of maximal prolapse in midsystole, and the late-systolic murmur continues up to and through A_2 due to prolapse of the posterior leaflet during the remainder of systole.

The timing and intensity of these murmurs vary with physiologic and pharmacologic maneuvers that alter the end-diastolic volume of the heart (see Fig. 10-68). These murmurs are also sensitive to conditions that alter the peripheral vascular impedance as well as the inotropic state of the heart. These variations in the timing and duration of the murmur can be understood most easily by considering mitral valve prolapse as a condition in which the valve is too big for the ventricle (see Chap. 58). This valvuloventricular disproportion manifests itself at a given geometric size and configuration during LV contraction. These dynamic changes can best be appreciated at the bedside by examining the patient in the supine, left lateral, sitting, and standing positions as well as during prompt squatting. Late-systolic murmurs also may originate from prolapse of the tricuspid valve (see Chap. 59).

Levine and Harvey[215] described a musical, apical systolic murmur that they called a "whoop" because it simulated the "whoop" of whooping cough. These murmurs are loud, high-pitched, musical, sonorous, and vibratory, are best heard at the apex in late systole, and are frequently intermittent. They may vary strikingly with respiration, from beat to beat, and from examination to examination. They are often preceded by clicks and originate in the mitral valve. They are associated with ballooning of the mitral valve or mitral regurgitation (or both), and their unusual quality is secondary to the high-frequency vibrations of the mitral apparatus. The systolic "whoop" or "honk," together with late systolic murmurs, with or without associated clicks, is part of a continuum representing abnormalities of the mitral valve apparatus of varying etiologies. Similar honking noises, with or without clicks, may arise from the tricuspid valve and also have been produced by transvenous pacemaker catheters situated across the valve. These murmurs are best auscultated at the fourth left intercostal space and have the typical inspiratory augmentation of tricuspid murmurs (see Chap. 59).

MURMUR OF HYPERTROPHIC "OBSTRUCTIVE" CARDIOMYOPATHY

The classic cardiac findings of hypertrophic cardiomyopathy (HCM) with a LV outflow gradient are demonstrated in Fig. 10-83, and the echocardiogram on the right gives insight into the mechanism of production of the systolic murmur. Systolic anterior motion of the mitral apparatus impinges on the massively thickened septum, producing high-velocity flow in middle and late systole, resulting in a midsystolic ejection murmur usually with its maximal intensity at the left sternal edge.[300] Varying degrees of mitral regurgitation also may be present during systole due to the distorted mitral apparatus. Frequently, on auscultation, the skilled clinician has difficulty deciding whether the systolic murmur found in HCM is ejection or regurgitant in nature.[301] Usually, the murmur recorded by the precordial phonocardiogram is actually the summation of the murmurs of LV outflow obstruction and mitral regurgitation as transmitted to the chest wall.[302]

In patients with dynamic LV outflow gradients, the intensity of both the systolic ejection murmur and the mitral regurgitant murmur varies directly with the magnitude of the pressure gradient. Thus physiologic maneuvers and pharmacologic interventions that increase the pressure gradient will increase the inten-

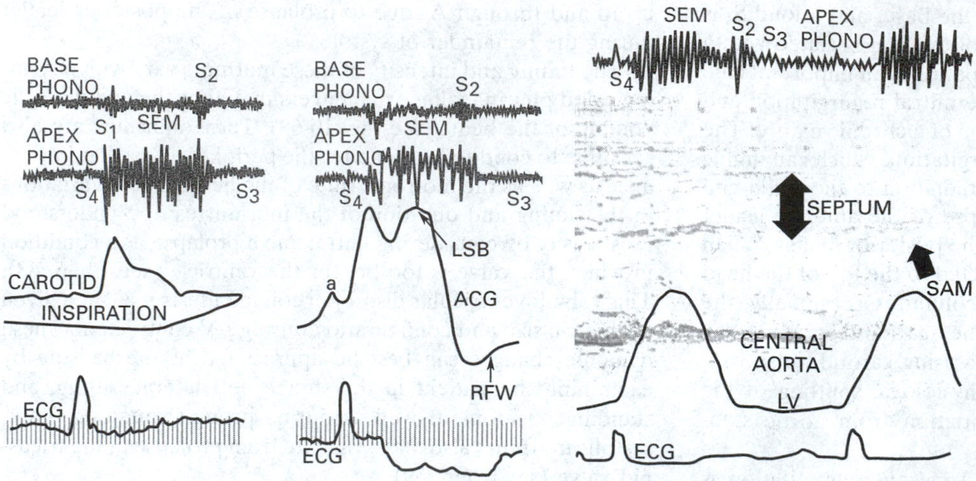

FIGURE 10-83 Simultaneous base and apex phonocardiograms are recorded with the carotid pulse and ACG in the left and center panels, respectively, in a 54-year-old man with hypertrophic cardiomyopathy. The carotid pulse rises rapidly and has a late systolic plateau and a prolonged ejection period. Prominent S_4 and S_1 are demonstrated and are associated with the a wave and the rapid filling wave (RFW), respectively, of the ACG. Note the late systolic bulge (LSB) on the ACG. S_2 is single. A loud, grade 5 systolic ejection murmur is present and is of greatest intensity at the apex. In the right panel, the apical systolic murmur is recorded together with the M-mode echocardiogram. Simultaneous high-fidelity LV and central aortic pressures are recorded by catheter-tipped micromanometers. Marked thickening of the interventricular septum and SAM of the mitral valve are present on the echocardiogram. A large systolic pressure gradient is demonstrated beginning shortly after the onset of the SAM. (From Shaver JA, et al. Phonoechocardiography and intracardiac phonocardiography in hypertrophic cardiomyopathy. *Postgrad Med J*. 1986; 62:538. Reproduced with permission from the publisher and the authors.)

sity of the precordial murmur, and vice versa. Decreases in LV preload and afterload or increases in LV contractility are associated with increases in the pressure gradient and the intensity of the murmur, whereas increases in LV preload and afterload or decreases in LV contractility will decrease the pressure gradient and the intensity of the murmur.[303,304] For example, the upright posture and the strain phase of the Valsalva maneuver decrease venous return and LV preload, and the murmur increases in intensity. On reclining or with prompt squatting, augmented venous return increases LV preload, and the murmur decreases in intensity. Vasoactive drugs such as amyl nitrite decrease blood pressure, and a marked increase in the intensity of the murmur occurs, whereas vasoconstrictive drugs such as phenylephrine increase the afterload, and the murmur is decreased or abolished (see Chap. 67).

These responses to vasoactive drugs should be compared with the diametrically opposite responses shown in a patient with a holosystolic murmur of chronic mitral regurgitation.

In the absence of a LV outflow gradient at rest or with provocation, the murmur of HCM is less impressive. Although a short ejection murmur is usually recorded due to rapid early LV ejection, it is often softer and extends through less of systole than when a gradient is present. There is also little variation in the intensity with changes in preload, afterload, or contractility.

In HCM with and without a gradient across the LV outflow tract, massive LV hypertrophy is present, and a prominent presystolic impulse associated with a LV S_4 is the rule when normal sinus rhythm is present. An S_3 is also a common finding in patients with HCM, and occasionally there is an early diastolic rumble that may mimic the diastolic murmur of mitral stenosis. Such rumbles are felt to be due to the increased impedance to LV filling secondary to the decreased diastolic compliance of the left ventricle.

Diastolic Murmurs

Diastolic murmurs have two basic mechanisms of production. Diastolic filling murmurs or rumbles are due to forward flow across an AV valve, whereas diastolic regurgitant murmurs are due to retrograde flow across an incompetent semilunar valve[305] (Fig. 10-84).

DIASTOLIC FILLING MURMURS (RUMBLES)

Diastolic rumbles are caused by forward flow across the AV valves and are delayed from their respective semilunar closure sound by the isovolumic relaxation period. Only following this period, when the atrial pressure exceeds the declining ventricular pressure, do the AV valves open and filling begins. Since there are two phases of rapid ventricular filling—early diastole and presystole—these murmurs have a tendency to be most prominent during these two filling periods. Because the velocity of flow is relatively low, these murmurs have a low-frequency content and are rumbling in character.

Diastolic Rumbles due to Obstruction of the AV Valve The murmur of mitral stenosis is heard best at the apex in the left lateral position, and its duration correlates well with the duration of the mitral diastolic gradient. Its intensity is related to the severity of the obstruction and to the flow across the valve.[306] As a result, there is poor correlation between the intensity of the murmur and the severity of the obstruction; e.g., high flow across a mild obstruction may produce a loud rumble, whereas low flow across a severely stenotic valve may produce a very soft murmur or may be silent. When the stenotic mitral valve is mobile, the murmur is introduced by a prominent opening snap (see Fig. 10-64, *left*). The duration of the interval between A_2 and the opening snap correlates well with the level of left atrial pressure; the shorter the A_2–opening snap interval, the higher is the left atrial pressure, and vice versa. The S_1 is also loud when the stenotic valve is mobile and is usually preceded by a crescendo murmur. Although originally attributed to increased flow secondary to left atrial systole, phonoechocardiographic studies have suggested that this short "presystolic" murmur is actually due to high-velocity antegrade flow through a progressively narrowing mitral orifice during very early (isovolumic) ventricular systole (see Fig. 10-64, *left*). This mechanism also may be responsible for the brief crescendo presystolic murmur observed in patients with mitral stenosis in atrial fibrillation following a short cycle length. The exact physical principles causing the production of this crescendo murmur are still in question.

Although the intensity of the diastolic rumble in mitral stenosis correlates poorly with the severity of obstruction, there is an excellent correlation of severity with the duration of the murmur. When sinus tachycardia or rapid atrial fibrillation is present, a rumble starting with an opening snap and continuing to S_1 may not be meaningful because of the short diastolic time. Carotid sinus pressure may be very helpful in temporarily slowing the heart rate, thereby allowing the clinician to uncover the potential length of the rumble.

Obstruction of the mitral orifice also can be produced by a left atrial tumor. The diastolic murmur may be very similar to that produced by mitral stenosis (as shown in Fig. 10-64, *center*). A loud tumor "plop" is present instead of the opening snap, and the presystolic crescendo murmur occurs as the protruding tumor mass returns rapidly through the mitral orifice into the left atrium during early ventricular systole. A systolic murmur of mitral regurgitation also may be present, and both murmurs may vary from examination to examination and with changes in body position.

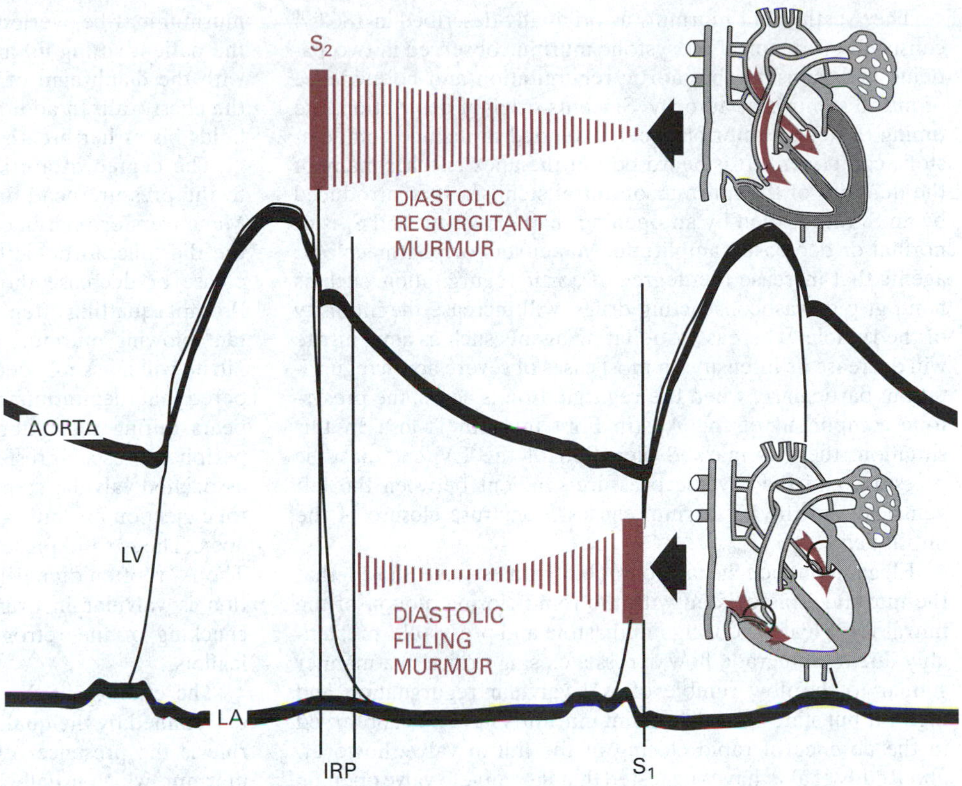

FIGURE 10-84 Diastolic filling murmurs or rumbles are caused by forward flow across the AV valves, whereas diastolic regurgitant murmurs are caused by retrograde flow across incompetent semilunar valves. (*Left*) Diagrammatic representation of the diastolic filling murmur and the diastolic regurgitant murmur as related to LV, aortic, and left atrial (LA) pressures. The diastolic filling murmur occurs during the diastolic filling period and is separated from S_2 by the isovolumic relaxation period. The rumbling murmur is most prominent during rapid, early ventricular filling and presystole, terminating with S_1. The diastolic regurgitant murmur begins immediately after S_2 and continues in a decrescendo fashion up to S_1, closely paralleling the aortic LV diastolic pressure gradient. (*Right*) Flow diagram. (From Shaver JA. Diastolic murmurs. *Heart Dis Stroke* 1993; 1:98–103. Reproduced with permission from the American Heart Association.)

The murmur of tricuspid stenosis is usually heard in the xiphoid area just off the sternal border. Since right atrial systole occurs earlier than left, the diastolic murmur of tricuspid stenosis may have a crescendo-decrescendo configuration. Even when the PR interval is normal, the presystolic accentuation of the diastolic rumble may terminate before S_1. Since tricuspid stenosis almost always occurs in the presence of mitral stenosis, this diastolic diamond-shaped murmur, which augments during inspiration, and the presence of large *a* waves in the JVP are clues to this additional diagnosis. When atrial fibrillation is present, the murmur is in middiastole and has the typical inspiratory augmentation. A tricuspid opening snap, which usually follows the mitral opening snap, also may be present and may initiate the murmur.

Diastolic Rumbles due to High Flow Across the AV Valves High-velocity flow across the normal or insufficient AV valve may result in short middiastolic rumbles often accompanied by an S_3 and should not be confused with murmurs produced by true obstruction of the AV valves. Such rumbles are common in both VSD and patent ductus arteriosus due to the large flow across the mitral valve secondary to the left-to-right shunt.[307] Likewise, the left-to-right shunt in a large ASD often produces a tricuspid rumble. Similar low-pitched rumbling murmurs also may be present in hyperkinetic states and occasionally are heard in patients with complete heart block and increased diastolic blood flow in each cardiac cycle. Common to all these conditions is high-volume flow during the latter phase of the rapid filling period. Phonoechocardiography has shown that these murmurs occur during the rapid closing motion of the mitral valve, suggesting a functional "obstruction" during the period of rapid early diastolic filling.[308] Identical phonoechocardiographic correlates also have been shown with mitral and tricuspid regurgitation, where early diastolic filling is also extremely rapid. With tricuspid regurgitation, the early rumble will increase with inspiration, typical of right-sided murmurs across the tricuspid valve. During rapid atrial fibrillation, ventriculogenic closure of the normal mitral valve during the rapid filling phase of a short cardiac cycle may cause a "presystolic" murmur by a similar mechanism.

Mitral valvulitis during an episode of acute rheumatic fever may cause a short diastolic rumble, the *Carey Coombs murmur*.[309] This rumble, especially in children or in the presence of fever and anemia, may be introduced by an S_3 rather than by an opening snap. This combination of an S_3 with a short rumble indicates that there is not enough obstruction to the valve to alter the characteristics of rapid early ventricular filling.

The Austin Flint murmur, as originally described in 1862,[310] consisted of an apical presystolic murmur observed in two patients with considerable aortic regurgitation and no evidence of mitral stenosis at autopsy. Since its original description, the timing of this murmur has been extended to include a middiastolic component. It is heard best at the apex and has many of the qualities of the murmur of mitral stenosis. It is introduced by an S_3 rather than by an opening snap, however, and S_1 is of normal or decreased amplitude. Maneuvers or pharmacologic agents that increase the degree of aortic regurgitation, such as hand grip or vasoconstricting drugs, will increase the intensity of the rumble, whereas vasodilating agents such as amyl nitrite will decrease its intensity. In most cases of severe aortic regurgitation, particularly when the regurgitation is acute, the presystolic component of the Austin Flint murmur is lost. In this situation, there is marked elevation of the LV end-diastolic pressure, and the reverse pressure gradient between the left ventricle and the left atrium causes premature closure of the mitral valve.

Elegant phonoechocardiographic studies have shown that the murmur is associated with the rapid closing motion of the mitral valve leaflets during middiastole and presystole, presumably due to antegrade flow across a closing orifice in a manner similar to the flow rumble of AV valvular regurgitation and high-output states.[311] Austin Flint murmurs have been observed in the absence of rapid closing of the mitral valve, however, and Reddy et al.[312] have suggested that incomplete valve opening rather than excessively rapid closure rates may be the essential requirement for producing the increased mitral flow velocity. One echo-Doppler study has suggested that patients with an Austin Flint murmur usually have an aortic regurgitant jet aimed directly at the mitral valve, causing deformity and shuddering of the valve, in contrast to patients with equally severe regurgitation, in whom the murmur is absent.[313] Right-sided Austin Flint murmurs of similar quality have been reported in association with severe pulmonic regurgitation associated with pulmonary hypertension.[314]

DIASTOLIC REGURGITANT MURMURS

Holodiastolic Aortic Regurgitant Murmurs The early diastolic murmur of aortic regurgitation is blowing and high-pitched in character and is often more difficult to record than to hear because of its high-frequency content. Since isovolumic relaxation of the left ventricle is very rapid, a large gradient quickly develops between the aortic and LV diastolic pressures, and the murmur builds up to maximum intensity almost immediately after A_2. As diastole progresses, the gradient between the two chambers falls slowly, and the murmur envelope closely parallels the pressure drop in a decrescendo fashion up to S_1. When the aortic regurgitation is valvular in origin, the murmur is usually best heard at the third and fourth left parasternal areas. The finding that the murmur is heard best to the right of the sternum should alert the clinician to an aortic root etiology of the regurgitation.[315] It should be pointed out that this finding is helpful only if present, since most patients with aortic regurgitation secondary to dilatation of the aortic root have the usual radiation with peak intensity to the left of the sternum. Although the frequency content of the murmur is in a range advantageous to the human ear, the amplitude of the vibrations may be quite small and the murmur quite faint. Therefore, the murmur may be overlooked if the examiner does not listen with the patient sitting up and leaning forward and does not listen with the diaphragm of the stethoscope pressed firmly against the chest wall. In addition, one should listen while the patient holds his or her breath after deep expiration.

The degree of aortic regurgitation is directly proportional to the pressure head driving the flow in a retrograde fashion. Maneuvers or pharmacologic agents that increase or decrease the diastolic aortic–left ventricular pressure gradient will increase or decrease the intensity of the regurgitant murmur. Prompt squatting often will bring out a very faint aortic regurgitant blowing murmur at the bedside, and inhalation of amyl nitrite will markedly decrease its intensity. It should be remembered that the murmur of mild aortic regurgitation often disappears during the latter stages of pregnancy due to the low peripheral vascular resistance. Pure aortic regurgitation without associated valvular stenosis may present with a prominent systolic ejection murmur as well as an Austin Flint rumble at the apex. The carotid pulse is rapid-rising and has a large volume. The A_2 is often diminished or even absent when the regurgitation is valvular in origin due to inadequate coaptation and checking of the retrograde blood column by the deformed leaflets.

The etiology of the aortic regurgitation usually cannot be determined by the quality of the murmur. An exception to this rule is the presence of a "cooing dove" or musical diastolic murmur, which usually denotes a rupture or retroversion of an aortic cusp. Such ruptures occur secondary to trauma, bacterial endocarditis, and occasionally in the presence of arteriosclerotic involvement of the aortic valve. Retroversion and subsequent rupture of the aortic valve with a musical murmur are also a complication of syphilitic aortic regurgitation (see Chap. 56).

Abbreviated Aortic Diastolic Regurgitant Murmur The murmur of very mild aortic regurgitation may be abbreviated and may end by middiastole. This is particularly true of the functional aortic regurgitant murmur of systemic arterial hypertension. As the volume of blood in the aorta decreases during diastole, the aortic annulus becomes smaller, and coupled with the decreasing aortic–left ventricular diastolic gradient, retrograde flow ceases, and the murmur disappears.

The murmur of aortic regurgitation also may be abbreviated if the aortic regurgitation is acute. Acute regurgitation of blood into a ventricle that has not had time to adapt to a large-volume load results in marked elevation of the LV end-diastolic pressure and equilibration of the aortic and LV diastolic pressures. With this, retrograde flow ceases, and the murmur disappears in the latter part of diastole. In the syndrome of acute aortic regurgitation, there may be preclosure of the mitral valve, resulting in a soft or absent S_1 as well as absence of the presystolic component of the Austin Flint murmur. The auscultatory findings of acute versus chronic aortic regurgitation are contrasted in Fig. 10-85. Common causes of acute aortic regurgitation include aortic valve endocarditis, trauma, acute aortic dissection, and dehiscence of an aortic valve prosthesis (see Chap. 56).

Holodiastolic Pulmonic Regurgitant Murmur Pulmonic regurgitation is found most commonly in the setting of severe pulmonary hypertension and dilatation of the pulmonary artery with inadequate coaptation of the leaflets of the pulmonic valve.

The functional murmur of pulmonic regurgitation (Graham Steell murmur)[316] is similar in both frequency and contour to that of aortic regurgitation because the hemodynamics responsible for their production are identical. The differential diagnosis is made by the "company the murmur keeps," and when it is associated with the peripheral signs of hemodynamically significant aortic regurgitation or with the findings of severe pulmonary hypertension, there is rarely a problem. However, when rheumatic mitral stenosis is the primary lesion, the semilunar regurgitant murmur may be secondary either to associated rheumatic aortic regurgitation or to the Graham Steell murmur if the pulmonary hypertension is severe. Careful investigation of the semilunar blowing murmur in the setting of mitral stenosis has shown that it is almost always due to aortic regurgitation, even when significant pulmonary hypertension is present.[317] More common causes of the Graham Steell murmur of functional pulmonary regurgitation are primary pulmonary hypertension and Eisenmenger's syndrome.

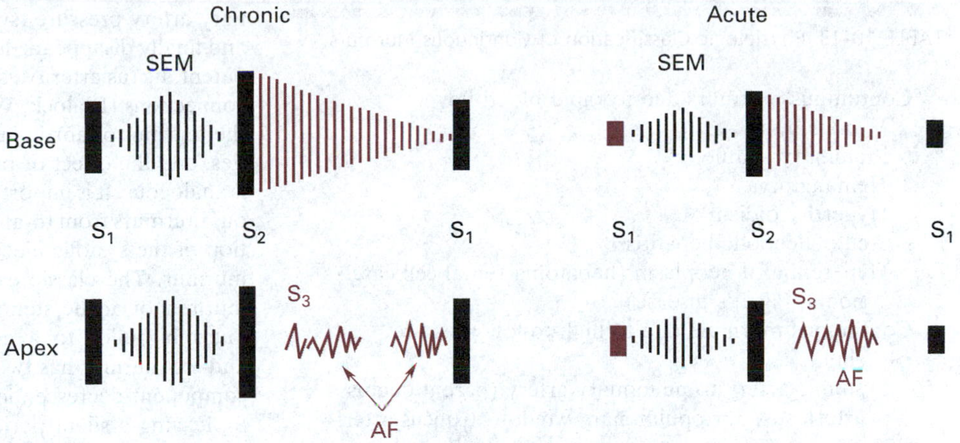

FIGURE 10-85 Diagram contrasting the auscultatory findings in chronic and acute aortic regurgitation. In chronic aortic regurgitation, a prominent systolic ejection murmur (SEM), resulting from the large forward stroke volume, is heard at the base and apex and ends well before S_2. The aortic diastolic regurgitant murmur begins with S_2 and continues in a decrescendo fashion, terminating before S_1. At the apex, the early diastolic component of the Austin Flint (AF) murmur is introduced by a prominent S_3. A presystolic component of the AF is also heard. In acute aortic regurgitation, there is a significant decrease in the intensity of the SEM compared with chronic aortic regurgitation because of the decreased forward stroke volume. S_1 is markedly decreased in intensity because of preclosure of the mitral valve, and at the apex the presystolic component of the AF murmur is absent. The early diastolic murmur at the base ends well before S_1 because of the equilibration of the LV and aortic end-diastolic pressure. Significant tachycardia is usually present. (From Shaver JA. Diastolic murmurs. *Heart Dis Stroke* 1993; 1:98-103. Reproduced with permission from the American Heart Association.)

Early diastolic murmurs occasionally are heard in end-stage renal failure, particularly when there is concurrent anemia, hypertension, and fluid overload. Doppler echocardiography demonstrated that these murmurs are usually pulmonic in origin.[318] They are often transient in nature and are related to fluid overload. Such murmurs are diminished by extracellular fluid removal and reflect correctable pulmonary hypertension.[318]

Delayed Pulmonic Regurgitant Murmur The murmur of organic (non-pulmonary hypertensive) pulmonary regurgitation is quite different in quality and duration as compared with either aortic regurgitation or the Graham Steell murmur of pulmonary hypertension.[319] The murmur is delayed from P_2 by a short interval and then builds up quickly to a crescendo followed by a decrescendo that ends well before S_1. In organic pulmonic regurgitation, the pulmonary artery pressure may be normal, and the diastolic gradient between the pulmonary artery and right ventricle may be very small, resulting in low-velocity retrograde flow and a lower-pitched murmur. The murmur is heard only during the period of maximal gradient in early and middle diastole, as the pulmonary artery pressure begins to equilibrate with the RV end-diastolic pressure in the latter part of diastole. This type of murmur may be congenital or acquired, as with pulmonary valve endocarditis, carcinoid syndrome, or surgical procedures on the pulmonic valve. It is often associated with a prominent systolic ejection murmur secondary to the large RV stroke volume.

CONTINUOUS MURMURS

A *continuous murmur* is defined as one that begins in systole and extends through S_2 into part or all of diastole. It need not occupy the entire cardiac cycle; therefore, a systolic murmur that extends into diastole without stopping at S_2 is considered to be continuous even if it fades completely before the subsequent S_1. A physiologic classification of continuous murmurs as described by Myers[320] is detailed in Table 10-13.

Continuous Murmurs due to Rapid Blood Flow High-velocity blood flow through veins and arteries may cause a continuous murmur. The cervical venous hum is a continuous murmur with diastolic accentuation and is easily heard in almost all children. This murmur also can be heard in healthy adults and is present in nearly all women in the later stages of pregnancy. High cardiac output states such as thyrotoxicosis and anemia are also associated with easily heard venous hums. This murmur is usually poorly heard in the supine position, and its presence in this position in an adult strongly suggests a hyperdynamic circulatory state. Peak intensity is in the supraclavicular fossa just lateral to the sternocleidomastoid muscle, and it is usually more prominent on the right side. When the murmur is loud, it may radiate below the clavicles and occasionally can be confused with the continuous murmur of patent ductus arteriosus. This error should never be made, however, because the cervical venous hum can be terminated easily by digital compression of the JVP.

The mammary souffle is another example of a continuous murmur occurring in 10 to 15 percent of pregnant women during the second and third trimesters and in the early postpartum period, particularly in lactating women, and is heard between the second and sixth anterior intercostal spaces. This murmur may be obliterated by firm pressure on the stethoscope or by digital pressure applied just lateral to the site of auscultation and therefore should not be confused with the continuous murmur of patent ductus arteriosus or with arteriovenous

TABLE 10-13 Physiologic Classification of Continuous Murmurs

Continuous murmurs due to rapid blood flow
Venous hum
Mammary souffle
Hemangioma
Hyperthyroidism
Acute alcoholic hepatitis
Hyperemia of neoplasm (hepatoma rental cell carcinoma, Paget's disease)
Continuous murmurs due to high-to-low pressure shunts
Systemic artery to pulmonary artery (parent ductus arteriosus, aortopulmonary window, truncus arteriosus, pulmonary atresia, anomalous left coronary, bronchiectasis, sequestration of the lung)
Systemic artery to right heart (ruptured sinus of Valsalva, coronary artery fistula)
Left-to-right atrial shunting (Lutembacher's syndrome, mitral atresia plus atrial septal defect)
Venovenous shunts (anomalous pulmonary veins, portosystemic shunts)
Arteriovenous fistula (systemic or pulmonic)
Continuous murmurs secondary to localized arterial obstruction
Coarctation of the aorta
Branch pulmonary stenosis
Carotid occlusion
Celiac mesenteric occlusion
Renal occlusion
Femoral occlusion
Coronary occlusion

SOURCE: From Myers JD. The mechanisms and significances of continuous murmurs. In: Leon DF, Shaver JA, eds. *Physiologic Principles of Heart Sounds and Murmurs*. Monograph 46. New York: American Heart Association; 1975:202. Reproduced with permission from the American Heart Association, Inc., and author.

fistula. The mammary souffle disappears after termination of lactation. Other causes of continuous murmurs due to rapid blood flow through arterial or venous channels are outlined in Table 10-13.

Continuous Murmurs due to High-to-Low-Pressure Shunts A group of congenital cardiovascular anomalies has shunting from the high-pressure systemic (aortic) circulation to the low-pressure pulmonary arterial circulation, resulting in a large gradient between the two systems throughout the cardiac cycle. The murmur of patent ductus arteriosus is the classic example of this type of anomaly. It is heard best in the left infraclavicular area and the second left intercostal space. The peak intensity of the murmur is at the time of S_2, after which it gradually wanes until it terminates before S_1.[221] The length of the murmur is determined by the difference in the vascular resistance between the greater and lesser circulation. As the pulmonary vascular resistance increases, the diastolic pressure in the pulmonary artery approaches and finally reaches systemic levels, diminishing and finally abolishing diastolic flow and the diastolic portion of the murmur. With equilibration of aortic and pulmonary artery pressure, systolic flow across the shunt diminishes and finally disappears, leaving the ductus silent (Eisenmenger's patent ductus arteriosus). Surgically produced aortopulmonary connections (Blalock, Waterston, and Pott's shunts), as well as the murmur of aortic pulmonary window, have identical qualities, and the effect of pulmonary hypertension on their length is analogous. It is important to distinguish these types of continuous murmurs from to-and-fro murmurs. The latter is a combination of the systolic ejection murmur and a semilunar diastolic murmur. The classic example of a to-and-fro murmur is the murmur of aortic stenosis and regurgitation. The continuous murmur builds to a crescendo around S_2, whereas the to-and-fro murmur has two components. The midsystolic ejection component decrescendos and may disappear as it approaches S_2, leaving a silent period before the onset of the regurgitant murmur. Truncus arteriosus is a rare congenital anomaly and probably produces a continuous murmur only if there is coexisting pulmonary artery stenosis (see Chap. 63). In the presence of severe RV outflow obstruction, bronchial collateral arteries can enlarge their normal precapillary anastomoses with pulmonary arteries, and the resulting aortic pulmonary fistula can produce a continuous murmur. This murmur can be heard in the same location as the patent ductus but radiates widely, especially over the posterior thorax. Large bronchial collateral arteries producing such continuous murmurs are more common with pulmonary atresia but also occur with tetralogy of Fallot. Bronchial artery–pulmonary artery collaterals sufficient to produce continuous murmurs are also found in far-advanced bronchiectasis and sequestration of the lung (see Chap. 63).

An anomalous left coronary artery arising from the pulmonary artery may cause a continuous murmur when the left-to-right shunt flow is large; it is usually best heard at the left sternal border. In this condition, the origin of the right coronary artery is from the aorta, and the left-to-right shunt is from the high-pressure right coronary arterial bed through large arterial collaterals to the left coronary system, which empties into the low-pressure pulmonary artery.

Sinus of Valsalva aneurysms may cause continuous murmurs when they rupture into the right side of the heart. In almost all cases, rupture occurs from the right and noncoronary sinuses into the right atrium or the right ventricle.[321] The murmur is heard maximally at the lower sternal border or xiphoid over the area corresponding to the fistulous tract. Diastolic accentuation of this murmur is an important sign to differentiate ruptured sinus from patent ductus arteriosus or arteriovenous fistula. Systolic suppression of the murmur is due to both mechanical narrowing of the fistulous tract during systole as well as the probable Venturi effect created by the rapid ejection of blood past the aortic origin of the fistula.

Coronary artery fistulas usually empty into the right atrium or ventricle and cause a continuous murmur that is best heard to either the left or the right of the lower sternal area. Since the majority of coronary flow occurs during diastole, the diastolic component of the murmur is louder. When the coronary artery fistula empties into a high-pressure right ventricle, only a diastolic murmur may be heard because the pressure gradient across the shunt is reduced during systole. Left-to-right shunting through an uncomplicated ASD produces no murmur audible on the chest wall because of the minimal pressure gradient and absence of turbulence. When mitral valve obstruction is present, as with Lutembacher's syndrome or mitral atresia, however, there can be a high-pressure gradient between the left and right atria across a small defect, and a continuous murmur may be present.[322] This murmur increases in intensity with inspiration and decreases with the Valsalva maneuver. Occasionally, a small ASD is produced following transseptal catheterization or balloon valvuloplasty for mitral stenosis, and a continuous murmur is produced due to high-velocity flow resulting from the large pressure gradient from the left to the right atrium.

Total anomalous pulmonary venous drainage into a systemic vein may produce a continuous venous hum usually heard in the pulmonary area or the left infraclavicular area. Frequently, a constriction at the junction of the anomalous venous conduit and the innominate vein or superior vena cava may cause augmentation of the murmur (see Chap. 63).

Arteriovenous fistulas between peripheral vessels produce a classic continuous murmur with systolic accentuation caused by shunting of a large volume of blood at rapid flow rates from a high-pressure artery into a low-pressure vein. These murmurs are best heard at the site of the fistula. Local compression of the veins may decrease the intensity of the murmur by raising venous pressure and reducing the arteriovenous pressure gradient. Complete obliteration of the fistula will terminate the murmur, and if the shunt is of considerable magnitude, a baroreceptor-mediated reflex bradycardia may occur (Branham's sign). Likewise, a reflex tachycardia will occur on release of the obstruction. Pulmonary arteriovenous fistulas usually produce only a systolic murmur because the peripheral vascular resistance of the normal lung is very low, and the normally small diastolic pressure gradient from pulmonary artery to pulmonary vein is not significantly increased by the presence of the fistula.

Continuous Murmur Secondary to Localized Arterial Obstruction Localized stenosis of systemic or pulmonary arteries may produce a continuous murmur or bruit if the obstruction is critical and adequate collateral flow is not available.[323] Most partially obstructed arteries have only systolic murmurs that are delayed relative to cardiac systole, depending on the transit time of pulsatile flow from the heart to the site of obstruction. This lack of diastolic gradient is explained by the fact that the collateral arteries around the obstruction deliver adequate flow such that the diastolic pressure on either side of the localized obstruction is essentially equal. Thus a localized, partial arterial obstruction characteristically produces only a systolic murmur or bruit. If adequate collateral flow is not present, however, a diastolic and a systolic pressure gradient can be produced, together with a continuous murmur with systolic accentuation. Depending on the degree of inadequacy of collaterals, the murmur is truly continuous when collateral circulation is essentially nonexistent, or it extends only partially through diastole when collateral flow is somewhat compromised. Such is the case in severe coarctation of the aorta, where, in addition to the systolic and/or continuous murmurs heard over the thorax and produced by rapid blood flow through the tortuous intercostal collaterals, a continuous murmur may be produced at the site of the coarctation. This latter murmur is best heard over the back midline between the scapulae.

Continuous murmurs also may arise from branch pulmonary stenosis or partial obstruction of a major pulmonary artery occluded by a massive pulmonary embolus. Other common locations of continuous murmurs secondary to localized arterial obstructions are listed in Table 10-13. Common to all these murmurs is critical narrowing of the vessel with inadequate collateral flow such that a continuous pressure gradient is produced throughout the cardiac cycle. Murmurs produced by obstruction of major coronary arteries are rarely loud enough to be transmitted to the chest wall. When audible, they produce only diastolic murmurs, even with inadequate collateral circulation.

References

1. Vanden Belt RJ. The history. In: Chizner M, ed. *Classic Teachings in Clinical Cardiology: A Tribute to W. Proctor Harvey.* Cedar Grove, NJ: Laennec; 1996:41–54.
2. Hurst JW, Morris DC. The history: Symptoms and past events related to cardiovascular disease. In: Schlant RC, Alexander RW, O'Rourke RA, et al., eds. *The Heart*, 8th ed. New York: McGraw-Hill; 1994:205–216.
3. O'Rourke RA. Chest pain. In: Schlant RC, Alexander RW, O'Rourke RA, et al., eds. *The Heart*, 8th ed. New York: McGraw-Hill; 1994:459–467.
4. Sampson JJ, Cheitlin M. Pathophysiology and differential diagnosis of cardiac pain. *Prog Cardiovasc Dis* 1971; 13:507–531.
5. O'Rourke RA. Diagnostic approach to the patient with chest pain compatible with definite or suspected angina pectoris. In: Sobel BE, ed. *Medical Management of Heart Disease.* New York: Marcel Dekker; 1996:4–22.
6. Heberden W. Some accounts of a disorder of the breast. *Med Trans* 1772; 2:59.
7. Murray DR, O'Rourke RA, Walling AD, Walsh RA: History and physical examination in myocardial ischemia and acute myocardial infarction. In: Francis G, Alpert J, eds. *Coronary Care*, 2d ed. Boston: Little, Brown; 1995:73–95.
8. Dell'Italia LJ. Chest pain. In: Stein JH, ed. *Internal Medicine*, 5th ed. Boston: Little, Brown; 1998:125–129.
9. Christie LG Jr, Conti CR. Systemic approach to evaluation of angina-like chest pain: Pathophysiology and clinical testing with emphasis on objective documentation of myocardial ischemia. *Am Heart J* 1981; 102:897–912.
10. Campeau L. Letter to the editor. *Circulation* 1976; 54:522.
11. Levine SA. Carotid sinus massage: A new diagnostic test for angina pectoris. *JAMA* 1962; 182:1332–1356.
12. Douglas PS, Ginsberg GS. The evaluation of chest pain in women. *New Engl J Med* 1996; 334:1311–1315.
13. Chauhan A, Mullins PA, Taylor G, et al. Cardioesophageal reflex: A mechanism for "linked angina" in patients with angiographically proven coronary artery disease. *J Am Coll Cardiol* 1996; 27:1621–1628.
14. Epstein SE, Talbot TL. Dynamic coronary tone in precipitation, exacerbation and relief of angina pectoris. *Am J Cardiol* 1981; 48:797–803.
15. Proudfit WL, Shrey ED, Sones FM Jr. Selective cine coronary arteriography: Correlation with clinical findings in 1000 patients. *Circulation* 1996; 33:901–910.
16. Cannon RO III: Microvascular angina: Cardiovascular investigations regarding pathophysiology and management. *Med Clin North Am* 1991; 75:1097–1118.
17. Cannon RO III, Cattau EL Jr, Yakshe PN, et al. Coronary flow reserve, esophageal motility, and chest pain in patients with angiographically normal coronary arteries. *Am J Med* 1990; 88:217–222.
18. Panza JA, Epstein S, Quyyumi AA. Circadian variation in vascular tone and its relation to α-sympathetic vasoconstrictor activity. *New Engl J Med* 1991; 325:986–990.
19. Crake T, Canepa-Anson R, Shapiro L, Poole-Wilson PA. Con-

tinuous recording of coronary sinus oxygen saturation during atrial pacing in patients with coronary artery disease or with syndrome X. *Br Heart J* 1988; 59:31–38.
20. Cannon RO III, Schenk WH, Quyyumi A, et al. Comparison of exercise testing with studies of coronary flow reserve in patients with microvascular angina. *Circulation* 1991; 83(suppl III):III-77–III-81.
21. Kaski JC, Tousoulis D, Galassi AR, et al. Epicardial coronary artery tone and reactivity in patients with normal coronary arteriograms and reduced coronary flow reserve (syndrome X). *J Am Coll Cardiol* 1991; 18:50–54.
22. Cannon RO III, Peden DB, Berkebile C, et al. Airway hyperresponsiveness in patients with microvascular angina: Evidence for a diffuse disorder of smooth muscle responsiveness. *Circulation* 1990; 82:2011–2017.
23. Kemp HG. Left ventricular function in patients with the anginal syndrome and normal coronary arteries. *Am J Cardiol* 1973; 32:375–376.
24. Attilio M. Syndrome X: Still an appropriate name. *J Am Coll Cardiol* 1991; 17:1471–1472.
25. Levy RD, Cunningham D, Shapiro LM, et al. Diurnal variation in left ventricular function: A study of patients with myocardial ischaemia, syndrome X, and of normal controls. *Br Heart J* 1987; 57:148–153.
26. Spinelli L, Ferro G, Genovese A, et al. Exercise-induced impairment of diastolic time in patients with X syndrome. *Am Heart J* 1990; 119:829–833.
27. Kern MJ. Extracting the coronary artery from syndrome X: Is epicardial vasomotion physiologic in patients with normal coronary arteriograms and reduced coronary flow reserve? *J Am Coll Cardiol* 1991; 18:55–56.
28. Galassi AR, Kaski JC, Pupita G, et al. Lack of evidence for alpha-adrenergic receptor-mediated mechanisms in the genesis of ischemia in syndrome X. *Am J Cardiol* 1989; 64:264–269.
29. Epstein SE, Cannon RO III, Bonow RO. Exercise testing in patients with microvascular angina. *Circulation* 1991; 83(suppl III):III-73–III-76.
30. Cannon RO III, Quyyumi AA, Schenke WH, et al. Abnormal cardiac sensitivity in patients with chest pain and normal coronary arteries. *J Am Coll Cardiol* 1990; 16:1359–1366.
31. Maseri A, ed. *Ischemic Heart Disease.* New York: Churchill-Livingstone; 1995:1–713.
32. Hillis DL, Braunwald E. Medical progress: Coronary-artery spasm. *New Engl J Med* 1978; 229:695–702.
33. Prinzmetal M, Kennamer R, Merliss R, et al. Angina pectoris: 1. A variant form of angina pectoris. *Am J Med* 1959; 26:375–388.
34. Herrick JB. Clinical features of sudden obstruction of the coronary arteries. *JAMA* 1912; 59:2015–2020.
35. Ross RS, Babe BM. Right ventricular hypertension as a cause of angina. *Circulation* 1960; 22:801–802.
36. Spodick DH. Pitfalls in the recognition of pericarditis. In: Hurst JW, ed. *Clinical Essays on the Heart*, Vol V. New York: McGraw-Hill; 1985:95–111.
37. Eagle KA, DeSanctis RW. Dissecting aortic aneurysm. *Curr Probl Cardiol* 1989; 14:227–228.
38. Katon W, Hall ML, Russo J, et al. Chest pain: Relationship of psychiatric illness to coronary arteriographic results. *Am J Med* 1988; 84:1–9.
39. Mellow MH. A gastroenterologist's view of chest pain. *Curr Probl Cardiol* 1983; 9:1–36.
40. Rose S, Achkar E, Easley KA. Follow-up of patients with noncardiac chest pain: Value of esophageal testing. *Dig Dis Sci* 1994; 39:2063–2068.
41. Bernstein LM, Grain RC, Pacini R. Differentiation of esophageal pain from angina pectoris: Role of esophageal acid perfusion test. *Medicine* 1962; 41:145–162.
42. Atkinson M. Monitoring esophageal pH. *Gut* 1987; 28:509–514.
43. Wolf E, Stern S. Costosternal syndrome: Its frequency and importance in differential diagnosis of coronary heart disease. *Arch Intern Med* 1976; 136:1289–1291.
44. Epstein SE, Gerber LN, Boren JS. Chest wall syndrome: A common cause of unexpected pain. *JAMA* 1979; 241:2793–2797.
45. The Criteria Committee of the New York Heart Association. *Diseases of the Heart and Blood Vessels: Nomenclature and Criteria for Diagnosis of the Heart and Great Vessels*, 6th ed. New York: New York Heart Association/Little, Brown; 1964.
46. McKusick VA, Egeland JA, Eldridge R, Krusem DE. Dwarfism in the Amish: I. The Ellis-van Creveld syndrome. *Bull Johns Hopkins Hosp* 1964; 115:306–330.
47. Basson CT, Solomon SD, Weissman B, et al. Genetic heterogeneity of heart-hand syndromes. *Circulation* 1995; 91:1326–1329.
48. Green JS, Parfrey PS, Harnett JD, et al. The cardinal manifestations of Bardet-Biedl syndrome, a form of Laurence-Moon-Biedl syndrome. *New Engl J Med* 1989; 321:1002–1009.
49. Guttmacher AE, Marchuk DA, White RI Jr. Hereditary hemorrhagic telangiectasia. *New Engl J Med* 1995; 333:918–926.
50. Shah CV, Pruyansky S, Harris WS. Cardiac malformations with facial clefts. *Am J Dis Child* 1970; 119:238–244.
51. Beighton P. The dominant and recessive forms of cutis laxa. *J Med Genet* 1972; 9:916–925.
52. Takahashi T, Koide T, Yamaguchi H, et al. Ehlers-Danlos syndrome with aortic regurgitation, dilation of the sinuses of Valsalva, and abnormal dermal collagen fibrils. *Am Heart J* 1992; 123:1709–1712.
53. Hortop J, Tsipouras P, Hanley JA, et al. Cardiovascular involvement in osteogenesis imperfecta. *Circulation* 1986; 73:54–61.
54. Marsalese DL, Moodie DS, Vacante M, et al. Marfan's syndrome: Natural history and long-term follow-up of cardiovascular involvement. *J Am Coll Cardiol* 1989; 14:422–428.
55. Schieken RM, Kerber RE, Iowasecu VV, Zellinger H. Cardiac manifestations of the mucopolysaccharidoses. *Circulation* 1975; 52:700–705.
56. Fisher EA, Desnick RJ, Gordon RE, et al. Fabry disease: An unusual cause of severe coronary disease in a young man. *Ann Intern Med* 1992; 117:221–223.
57. Tandon R, Edwards JE. Cardiac malformations associated with Down's syndrome. *Circulation* 1973; 47:1349–1355.
58. Rosenthal A. Cardiovascular malformations in Klinefelter's syndrome: Report of three cases. *J Pediatr* 1972; 80:471–473.
59. Lewandowski RC Jr, Yunis J. New chromosomal syndromes. *Am J Dis Child* 1975; 129:515–529.
60. Musewe NN, Alexander DJ, Teshima I, et al. Echocardiographic evaluation of the spectrum of cardiac anomalies associated with trisomy 13 and trisomy 18. *J Am Coll Cardiol* 1990; 15:673–677.
61. Subramaniam PN. Turner's syndrome and cardiovascular anomalies. *Am J Med Sci* 1989; 297:260–262.
62. Helmi C, Pruzansky S. Craniofacial and extracranial malformations in the Klippel-Feil syndrome. *Cleft Palate J* 1980; 17:65–88.
63. Greenwood RD, Rosenthal A, Nadas AS. Cardiovascular malformations associated with imperforate anus. *J Pediatr* 1975; 86: 576–579.
64. Quan L, Smith DW. The VATER association. *J Pediatr* 1973; 82:104–107.
65. Freedom RM. The asplenia syndrome: A review of significant extracardiac structural abnormalities in 29 necropsied patients. *J Pediatr* 1972; 81:1130–1133.
66. Cyran SE, Martinez R, Daniels S, et al. Spectrum of congenital heart disease in CHARGE association. *J Pediatr* 1987; 110: 576–578.
67. Ho CK, Kaufman RL, Podos SM. Ocular colobomata, cardiac defect, and other anomalies. *J Med Genet* 1975; 12:289–293.
68. Greenwood RD, Rosenthal A, Nadas AS. Cardiovascular malformations associated with omphalocele. *J Pediatr* 1974; 85:818–821.

69. Nora JI, Nora AH. Maternal transmission of congenital heart diseases: New recurrence risk figures and the questions of cytoplasmic inheritance and vulnerability to teratogens. *Am J Cardiol* 1987; 59:459–463.
70. Sandor GGS, Smith DF, McLeod PM. Cardiac malformations in the fetal alcohol syndrome. *J Pediatr* 1981; 98:771–773.
71. Rowe RD. Maternal rubella and pulmonary artery stenosis. *J Pediatr* 1963; 32:180–185.
72. Aziz K, Sanyal SK, Goldblatt E. Reversed differential cyanosis. *Br Heart J* 1968; 30:288–290.
73. Pearl W. Syndrome of anotia, facial paralysis, and congenital heart disease. *J Pediatr* 1984; 105:441–442.
74. Jaigesimi P, Antia AV. Extracardiac defects in children with congenital heart disease. *Br Heart J* 1979; 42:475–479.
75. Naidu R, O'Rourke RA. Infective endocarditis In: Cohn JN, Rakel RE, Bupc ET, eds. *Current Therapy*, 53 ed. Philadelphia: Saunders; 2000 (in press).
76. Proudfit WL. Skin signs of infective endocarditis. *Am Heart J* 1983; 106:1451–1453.
77. Burch M, Sharland M, Shinebourne E, et al. Cardiologic abnormalities in Noonan syndrome: Phenotypic diagnosis and echocardiographic assessment of 118 patients. *J Am Coll Cardiol* 1993; 22:1189–1192.
78. Gellis SS, Feingold M. Rubinstein-Taybi syndrome. *Am J Dis Child* 1971; 121:327–328.
79. St. John Sutton MG, Tajik AJ, Giuliana ER, et al. Hypertrophic obstruction cardiomyopathy and lentiginosis: A little known neural ectodermal syndrome. *Am J Cardiol* 1981; 47:214–217.
80. Pellikka PA, Tajik AJ, Khandheria BK, et al. Carcinoid heart disease: Clinical and echocardiographic spectrum in 74 patients. *Circulation* 1993; 87:1188–1196.
81. Goldman AP, Kotler MN. Heart disease in scleroderma. *Am Heart J* 1985; 110:1043–1046.
82. Waltuck J, Buyon JP. Autoantibody-associated congenital heart block: Outcome in mothers and children. *Ann Intern Med* 1994; 120:544–551.
83. Boumpas DT, Austin HA III, Fessler BJ, et al. Systemic lupus erythematosus: Emerging concepts: I. Renal, neuropsychiatric, cardiovascular, pulmonary and hematologic disease. *Ann Intern Med* 1995; 122:940–950.
84. Hojnik M, George J, Ziporen L, Shoenfeld Y. Heart valve involvement (Libman-Sacks endocarditis) in the antiphospholipid syndrome. *Circulation* 1996; 93:1579–1587.
85. Nomier AM, Turner RA, Watts LE. Cardiac involvement in rheumatoid arthritis. *Arthritis Rheum* 1979; 22:561–564.
86. Bowness P, Hawley JC, Morris T, et al. Complete heart block and severe aortic incompetence in relapsing polychondritis. *Arthritis Rheum* 1991; 34:97–100.
87. Bergfeldt L, Edhag O, Rajs J. HLA-B27–associated heart disease. *Am J Med* 1984; 77:961–967.
88. Livingston JZ, Casale AS, Hutchins GM, Shapiro EP. Coronary involvement in Cogan's syndrome. *Am Heart J* 1992; 123: 528–530.
89. McAllister HA, Fenogho JJ. Cardiac involvement in Whipple's disease. *Circulation* 1975; 52:152–156.
90. Casazza F, Morpurgo M. The varying evolution of Friedreich's ataxia cardiomyopathy. *Am J Cardiol* 1996; 77:895–898.
91. Lie JT, Grossman SJ. Pathology of the heart in acromegaly: Anatomic findings in 27 autopsied patients. *Am Heart J* 1980; 100:41–52.
92. Sofer S, Weinhouse E, Tal A, et al. Cor pulmonale due to adenoidal or tonsillar hypertrophy or both in children. *Chest* 1988; 93:119–127.
93. Parish JM, Shepard JW. Cardiovascular effects of sleep disorders. *Chest* 1990; 97:1220–1225.
94. Collins P. Aortic incompetence and active myocarditis in Reiter's disease. *Br J Vener Dis* 1972; 48:300–303.
95. Dajani AS, Taubert KA, Gerber MA, et al. Diagnosis and therapy of Kawasaki disease in children. *Circulation* 1993; 87:1776–1780.
96. Cox J, Krajden M. Cardiovascular manifestations of Lyme disease. *Am Heart J* 1991; 122:1449–1455.
97. Stern R, Goldbold JH, Chess O, Kagen LJ. ECG abnormalities in polymyositis. *Arch Intern Med* 1984; 144:2185–2189.
98. Perloff JK. Cardiac rhythm and conduction in Duchenne's muscular dystrophy: A prospective study of 20 patients. *J Am Coll Cardiol* 1984; 3:1263–1268.
99. Badano L, Autore C, Fragola PV, et al. Left ventricular myocardial function in myotonic dystrophy. *Am J Cardiol* 1993; 71:987–991.
100. Kenny D, Wetherbee J. Kearns-Sayre syndrome in the elderly: Mitochondrial myopathy with advanced heart block. *Am Heart J* 1990; 120:440–443.
101. Shammas RL, Movahed A. Sarcoidosis of the heart. *Clin Cardiol* 1993; 16:462–472.
102. Kuan P. Cardiac Wilson's disease. *Chest* 1987; 91:579–583.
103. Olson LJ, Edwards WD, McCall JT, et al. Cardiac iron deposition in idiopathic hemochromatosis: Histologic and analytic assessment of 14 hearts from autopsy. *J Am Coll Cardiol* 1987; 10:1239–1243.
104. Kyle RA. Amyloidosis. *Circulation* 1995; 91:1269–1271.
105. Hara KS, Ballard DJ, Ilstrup DM, et al. Rheumatoid pericarditis: Clinical features and survival. *Medicine* 1990; 69:81–91.
106. Di Eusanio G, Mazzola A, Gregorini R, et al. Left ventricular aneurysm secondary to Behçet's disease. *Ann Thorac Surg* 1991; 51:131–135.
107. Turiteri L, Perheentupa J, Rapola J. The cardiopathy of mulibreynanism: A new inherited syndrome. *Chest* 1974; 65:628–631.
108. Deer T, Rosencrance JG, Chillag SA. Cardiac conduction manifestations of Reiter's syndrome. *South Med J* 1991; 84:799–800.
109. Bergfeldt L, Edhag O, Vedin L, Vallin H. Ankylosing spondylitis: An important cause of severe disturbances of the cardiac conduction system. *Am J Med* 1982; 73:187–191.
110. Marks ML, Trippel DL, Keating MT. Long QT syndrome associated with syndactyly identified in females. *Am J Cardiol* 1995; 76:744–745.
111. Sprecher DL, Schaefer EJ, Kent KM, et al. Cardiovascular features of homozygous familial hypercholesterolemia: Analysis of 16 patients. *Am J Cardiol* 1984; 54:20–30.
112. Cohen JI, Arnett EN, Kolodny AL, Roberts WC. Cardiovascular features of the Werner syndrome. *Am J Cardiol* 1987; 59:493–495.
113. Dyck JD, David TE, Burke B, et al. Management of coronary artery disease in Hutchinson-Gilford syndrome. *J Pediatr* 1987; 111:407–410.
114. Elliott WJ, Powell LH. Diagonal earlobe creases and prognosis in patients with suspected coronary artery disease. *Am J Med* 1996; 100:205–211.
115. Lesko SM, Rosenberg L, Shapiro S. A case-control study of baldness in relation to myocardial infarction in men. *JAMA* 1993; 269:998–1003.
116. Bowen J, Boudoulas H, Wooley CF. Cardiovascular disease of connective tissue origin. *Am J Med* 1987; 82:481–488.
117. Braunlin EA, Hunter DW, Krivit W, et al. Evaluation of coronary artery disease in the Hurler syndrome by angiography. *Am J Cardiol* 1992; 69:1487–1489.
118. Przybojewski JZ. Polyarteritis nodosa in the adult: Report of a case with repeated myocardial infarction and a review of cardiac involvement. *S Afr Med J* 1981; 60:512–518.
119. You CK, Rees J, Gillis DA, Steeves J. Klippel-Trenaunay syndrome: A review. *Can J Surg* 1983; 26:399–403.
120. Pagon RA, Bennett FC, LaVeek B, et al. Williams syndrome. *J Pediatr* 1987; 80:85–91.
121. Carney JA, Kruska LS, Beauchamp CD, Gordon H. Dominant

inheritance of the complex of myxomas, spotty pigmentation, and endocrine overactivity. *Mayo Clin Proc* 1986; 61:165–172.
122. Stevenson WG, Perloff JK, Weiss JN, Anderson TL. Facioscapulohumeral muscular dystrophy: Evidence for selective, genetic electrophysiologic cardiac involvement. *J Am Coll Cardiol* 1990; 15:292–299.
123. Hopkins LC, Jackson JA, Elsas LJ. Emery-Dreifuss humeroperoneal muscular dystrophy: An X-linked myopathy with unusual contractures and bradycardia. *Ann Neurol* 1981; 10: 230–237.
124. Gibbs JL. The heart and tuberous sclerosis. *Br Heart J* 1985; 54:596–599.
125. Nutter DO. Measurements of the systolic blood pressure. In: Hurst JW, ed. *The Heart*, 5th ed. New York: McGraw-Hill; 1982.
126. Asmar R, Benetos A, London G, et al. Aortic distensibility in normotensive, untreated and treated hypertensive patients. *Blood Pressure* 1995; 4:48–54.
127. Frohlich ED. Hypertension in the elderly. *Curr Probl Cardiol* 1988; 13:313–367.
128. Hales S. *Statistical Essays: Containing Haema-staticks; or, an Account of Some Hydraulick and Hydrostatical Experiments Made on the Blood and Blood-Vessels of Animals.* London: Innys W, Manby R; 1733.
129. Grim NC, Grim CE. Blood pressure measurements. In: Izzo JL, Black HE, eds. *AHA Hypertension Primer*, 2d ed. New York: American Heart Association; 1998:295–298.
130. McCutcheon EP, Rushmer RF. Korotkov sounds: An experimental critique. *Circ Res* 1967; 20:149–161.
131. Rodbard S. The components of the Korotkov sounds. *Am Heart J* 1967; 74:278–282.
132. Neilsen PR, Janniche H. The accuracy of auscultatory measurement of arm blood pressure in very obese subjects. *Acta Med Scand* 1974; 196:403–409.
133. Littler WA, Komsuoglar B. Which is the most accurate method of measuring blood pressure? *Am Heart J* 1989; 117:723–728.
134. Evans CE, Haynes RB, Goldsmith CH, Hewson SA. Home blood pressure-measuring devices: A comparative study of accuracy. *J Hypertens* 1989; 7:133–142.
135. White SB, Berson AS, Robbins C, et al. National standard for measurement of resting and ambulatory blood pressure with automated sphygmomanometers. *Hypertension* 1993; 21: 504–509.
136. Kelly RP, Haywood C, Ganis J, et al. Noninvasive registration of the arterial pressure waveform using high-fidelity applanation tonometry. *J Vasc Med Biol* 1989; 1:142–149.
137. Nichols WW, O'Rourke MF, eds. *McDonald's Blood Flow in Arteries*, 4th ed. London: Edward Arnold; 1998.
138. Chen CH, Ting CT, Nussbacher A, et al. Validation of carotid artery tonometry as a means of estimating augmentation index of ascending aortic pressure. *Hypertension* 1996; 27:168–175.
139. Liang YL, Teede H, Kotsopoulos D, et al. Non-invasive measurements of arterial structure and function: Repeatability, interrelationships and trial sample size. *Clin Sci* 1998; 95:669–679.
140. Wilkinson IB, Fuchs SA, Jansen IM, et al. Reproducibility of pulse wave velocity and augmentation index measure by pulse wave analysis. *J Hypertens* 1998; 16:2079–2084.
141. Siebenhofer A, Kemp C, Sutton A, Williams B. The reproducibility of central aortic blood pressure measurements in healthy subjects using applanation tonometry and sphygmocardiography. *J Hum Hypertens* 1999; 13:625–629.
142. Frohlich ED, Gifford RW, Hall WD. Hypertensive cardiovascular disease. In: 18th Bethesda Conference Report: Cardiovascular Disease in the Elderly. *J Am Coll Cardiol* 1987; 10(suppl A):57A–59A.
143. Cohn JN, Finkelstein SM. Abnormalities of vascular compliance in hypertension, aging and heart failure. *J Hypertens* 1992; 10:S61–S64.
144. O'Rourke MF. *Arterial Function in Health and Disease.* New York: Churchill-Livingstone; 1982.
145. Wei Y, Gersh BJ. Heart disease in the elderly. *Curr Probl Cardiol* 1987; 12:1–65.
146. Kannel WB. Historic perspectives on the relative contributions of diastolic and systolic blood pressure elevation to cardiovascular risk profile. *Am Heart J* 1999; 138:205–210.
147. Kannel WB, Wolf PA, McGee DL. Systolic blood pressure, arterial rigidity, and risk of stroke: The Framingham Study. *JAMA* 1998; 245:1225–1229.
148. Rutan GH, Kuller LH, Neaton JD, et al. Mortality associated with diastolic hypertension among men screened for Multiple Risk Factors Intervention Trial (MRFIT). *Circulation* 1988; 77:504–514.
149. SHEP Cooperative Research Group. Prevention of stroke by antihypertensive drug treatment in older persons with isolated hypertension: Final results of the Systolic Hypertension in the Elderly Program (SHEP). *JAMA* 1991; 265:3255–3264.
150. Staessen JA, Fagard R, Thijs L, et al. Randomised double-bond comparison of placebo and active treatment for older patients with isolated systolic hypertension. The Systolic Hypertension in Europe (syst-Eur) trail investigators. *Lancet* 1997; 350;757–764.
151. O'Rourke MF. Isolated systolic hypertension, pulse pressure, and arterial stiffness as risk factors for cardiovascular disease. *Curr Hypertens Reps* 1999; 3:204–211.
152. Franklin SS, Khan SA, Wong ND, et al. The importance of pulse pressure and systolic blood pressure in predicting coronary heart disease in older adults: The Framingham Heart Study. *Circulation* 1999; 100:354–360.
153. Kaplan NM. *Clinical Hypertension*, 5th ed. Baltimore: Williams & Wilkins; 1990.
154. Safar ME, Frohlich ED. The arterial system in hypertension: A prospective view. *Hypertension* 1995; 26:10–14.
155. Littler WA, Honour AJ, Pugsley DJ, Sleight PL. Continuous recording of direct arterial pressure in unrestricted patients. *Circulation* 1975; 51:1101–1106.
156. Richardson DW, Honour AJ, Fenton DW, et al. Variation in arterial pressure throughout the day and night. *Clin Sci* 1964; 26:445–460.
157. Donald KW, Lind AR, McNicol GW, et al. Cardiovascular response to sustained contractions. *Circ Res* 1967; 20(suppl 1): 15–30.
158. Wooley CF, Hosier DM, Booth RW, et al. Supravalvular aortic stenosis. *Am J Med* 1961; 31:717–725.
159. Pascarelli EF, Bertrand CA. Comparison of blood pressure in the arms and legs. *New Engl J Med* 1964; 270:693–698.
160. Park MK, Guntheroth WG. Direct blood pressure measurements in brachial and femoral arteries in children. *Circulation* 1979; 42:231–237.
161. Felix WR, Hochbert HM, George MED, et al. Ultrasound measurement of arm and leg blood pressure. *JAMA* 1973; 226:1096–1099.
162. Vlachopoulos C, O'Rourke M. Genesis of the normal and abnormal arterial pulse. *Curr Probl Cardiol* 2000; 296–346 (in press).
162a. Kelly RP, Gibbs HH, O'Rourke MF, et al. Nitroglycerin has a favorable effect on left ventricular afterload than apparent from measurement of pressure in a peripheral artery. *Eur Heart J* 1990; 11:138–144.
163. Crawford MH. Inspection and palpation of venous and arterial pulses: In: *Examination of the Heart*, Part 2. New York: American Heart Association; 1990.
164. O'Rourke MF, Kelly R, Avolio A. *The Arterial Pulse.* Philadelphia: Lea & Febiger; 1992.
165. Ewy GA. Venous and arterial pulsations: Bedside insights into hemodynamics. In: Chizner M, ed. *Classic Teachings in Clinical Cardiology: A Tribute to W. Proctor Harvey.* Cedar Grove, NJ: Laennec; 1996:65–84.

166. O'Rourke MF. The arterial pulse in health and disease. *Am Heart J* 1971; 82:687–702.
167. Murgo JP, Westerhof N, Giolma JP, Altobelli SA. Aortic input impedance in normal man: Relationship to pressure wave shapes. *Circulation* 1980; 62:105–116.
168. O'Rourke MF. Pressure and flow waves in systemic arteries and the anatomic design of the arterial system. *J Appl Physiol* 1967; 23:139–149.
169. O'Rourke MF, Auido AP. Pulsatile flow and pressures in human systemic arteries: Studies in man and in a multibranched model of the human systemic arterial tree. *Circ Res* 1980; 46:363–372.
170. Murgo JP, Westerhof N, Giolma JO, Altobelli SA. Effects of exercise on aortic impedance and pressure wave shapes in normal man. *Circ Res* 1981; 48:334–343.
171. Marx HJ, Yu PN. Clinical examination of the arterial pulse. *Prog Cardiovasc Dis* 1967; 10:207–235.
172. Hamilton WF, Dow P. An experimental study of the standing waves in the pulse propagated through the aorta. *Am J Physiol* 1939; 125:48.
173. O'Rourke MF. Vascular impedance in studies of arterial and cardiac function. *Physiol Rev* 1982; 62:570–623.
174. O'Rourke MF, Mancia G. Arterial stiffness. *J Hypertens* 1999; 17:1–4.
175. O'Rourke MF, Taylor MG. Input impedance of the systemic circulation. *Circ Res* 1967; 20:365–380.
176. Schlant RC, Felner MJ. The arterial pulse: Clinical manifestations. *Curr Prob Cardiol* 1977; 2:1–50.
177. Franklin SS, Gustin W IV, Wong ND, et al. Hemodynamic patterns of age-related changes in blood pressure: The Framingham Heart Study. *Circulation* 1997; 96:308–315.
178. Benetos A, Laurent S, Hoeks AP, et al. Arterial alterations with aging and high blood pressure: A noninvasive study of carotid and femoral arteries. *Arterioscler Thromb* 1993; 13:90–97.
179. Armentano R, Megnien JL, Simon A, et al. Effects of hypertension on viscoelasticity of carotid and femoral arteries in humans. *Hypertension* 1995; 26:48–54.
180. Safar ME, Frohlich ED. The arterial system in hypertension: A prospective view. *Hypertension* 1995; 26:10–14.
181. Corrigan DJ. On permanent patency of the mouth of the aorta, or inadequacy of the aorta valves. *Edinburgh Med Surg* 1832; 37:225–245.
182. Ikram H, Nixon PGF, Fox JA. The hemodynamic implications of the bisferiens pulse. *Br Heart J* 1964; 26:452–459.
183. Wigle ED. The arterial pressure pulse in muscular subaortic stenosis. *Br Heart J* 1963; 25:97–105.
184. Deane CR, Needleman L. The cause of pulsus tardus in arterial stenosis. *Radiology* 1995; 194:28–30.
185. Bude RO, Rubin JM, Platt JF, et al. Pulsus tardus: Its cause and potential limitations in detection of aortic stenosis. *Radiology* 1994; 190:779–784.
186. Dow P. The development of the anacrotic and tardus pulse of aortic stenosis. *Am J Physiol* 1940; 131:432.
187. Ewy GA, Rios JC, Marcus FI. The dicrotic arterial pulse. *Circulation* 1969; 39:655–661.
188. White PD. Alternation of the pulse: A common clinical condition. *Am J Med Sci* 1915; 150:82–96.
189. Mitchell JH, Sarnoff SJ, Sonnenblock EH. The dynamics of pulsus alternans: Alternating end-diastolic fiber length as a causative factor. *J Clin Invest* 1963; 42:55–63.
190. Freeman GL, Widman LE, Campbell JM, Colston JT. An evaluation of the onset of pulsus alternans in closed-chest dogs. *Am J Physiol* 1992; 262:H278–H284.
191. Shabetai R, Fowler NO, Fenton JC, Masangkay M. Pulsus paradoxus. *J Clin Invest* 1965; 44:1882–1898.
192. Shabetai R, Fowler NO, Guntheroth WG. The hemodynamics of cardiac tamponade and constrictive pericarditis. *Am J Cardiol* 1970; 26:480–498.
193. Otsuji Y, Toda H, Kisanuki A, et al. Influence of left ventricular filling profile during preceding control beats on pulse pressure during ventricular premature contractions. *Eur Heart J* 1994; 15:462–467.
194. Garratt CJ, Griffith MJ, Young G, et al. Value of physical signs in the diagnosis of ventricular tachycardia. *Circulation* 1994; 90:3103–3107.
195. Hurst JW, Schlant RC. Examination of the veins and their pulsation. In: Hurst JW, ed. *The Heart*, 4th ed. New York: McGraw-Hill; 1978:193–201.
196. Ewy GA, Marcus FI. Bedside estimation of the venous pressure. *Heart Bull* 1968; 17:41.
197. Ewy GA. The abdominojugular test: Technique and hemodynamic correlates. *Ann Intern Med* 1989; 108:456–460.
198. Ducas J, Magder S, McGregor M. Validity of the hepatojugular reflux as a clinical test for congestive heart failure. *Am J Cardiol* 1983; 52:1299–1303.
199. Dell'Italia L, Starling MR, O'Rourke RA. Physical examination for exclusion of hemodynamically important right ventricular infarction. *Ann Intern Med* 1983; 99:608–612.
200. Stonjic BB, Brecker SJ, Xiao HB, Gibson DG. Jugular venous *a* wave in pulmonary hypertension: New insights from a Doppler echocardiographic study. *Br Heart J* 1992; 68:187–191.
201. Anderson WB. Examination of the retina: In: Alexander AW, Schlant RC, Fuster W, eds. *Hurst's The Heart*, 9th ed. New York: McGraw-Hill; 1998:343–349.
202. Hurst JW, Robinson PH. Physical examination of the chest, abdomen and extremities. In: Hurst JW, et al., eds. *The Heart*, 7th ed. New York: McGraw-Hill; 1990:242–243.
203. Shaver JA. Cardiac auscultation: A cost-effective diagnostic skill. *Curr Probl Cardiol* 1995; 20:443–530.
204. Willis PW IV. Inspection and palpation of the precordium. In: Hurst JW, ed. *The Heart*, 7th ed. New York: McGraw-Hill; 1990:163–169.
205. Schlant RC, Hurst JW. *Examination of the Precordium: Inspection and Palpation.* New York: American Heart Association; 1990:1–28.
206. Abrams J. Precordial palpation: Let your fingers do the walking. In: Chizner M, ed. *Classic Teachings in Clinical Cardiology: A Tribute to W. Proctor Harvey.* Cedar Grove, NJ: Laennec; 1996:85–103.
207. Eilen SD, Crawford MH, O'Rourke RA. Accuracy of precordial palpation for detecting increased left ventricular volume. *Ann Intern Med* 1983; 99:628–630.
208. Abrams J. *Essentials of Cardiac Physical Diagnosis.* Philadelphia: Lea & Febiger; 1987.
209. Ronon JA Jr, Steelman RB, DeLeon AC Jr, et al. The clinical diagnosis of acute severe mitral insufficiency. *Am J Cardiol* 1971; 27:284–290.
210. Abrams J. Precordal palpation. In: Horwitz LD, Graves BM, eds. *Signs and Symptoms in Cardiology.* Philadelphia: Lippincott; 1985:156–177.
211. Harvey WP. Some pertinent physical findings in the clinical evaluation of acute myocardial infarction. *Circulation* 1969; 39/40(suppl IV):IV-175–IV-181.
212. Shah PM. Newer concepts in hypertrophic obstruction cardiomyopathy, part II. *JAMA* 1979; 242:1771–1776.
213. Rapaport MB, Sprague HB. The effects of tubing bore on stethoscope efficiency. *Am Heart J* 1951; 42:605–609.
214. Butterworth JS, Chassin MR, McGrath R, et al. *Cardiac Auscultation.* New York: Grune & Stratton; 1960.
215. Levine SA, Harvey SP. *Clinical Auscultation of the Heart*, 2d ed. Philadelphia: Saunders; 1959.
216. Shaver JA, Salerni R, Reddy PS. Normal and abnormal heart

sounds in cardiac diagnosis: I. Systolic sounds. *Curr Probl Cardiol* 1985; 10:1–68.

217. Reddy PS, Salerni R, Shaver JA. Normal and abnormal heart sounds in cardiac diagnosis: II. Diastolic sounds. *Curr Probl Cardiol* 1985; 10:1–55.
218. Laniado S, Yellin EL, Miller H, Frater WM. Temporal relation of the first heart sound to closure of the mitral valve. *Circulation* 1973; 47:1006–1014.
219. Mills P, Craige E. Echophonocardiography. *Prog Cardiovasc Dis* 1978; 20:337.
220. O'Toole JD, Reddy PS, Curtiss EI, et al. The contribution of tricuspid valve closure to the first heart sound: An intracardiac micromanometer study. *Circulation* 1976; 53:752–758.
221. Thompson ME, Shaver JA, Leon DF, et al. Pathodynamics of first heart sound. In: Leon DF, Shaver JA, eds. *Physiologic Principles of Heart Sounds and Murmurs* (Monograph 46). New York: American Heart Association; 1975:8–18.
222. Shah PM. Hemodynamic determinants of the first heart sound. In: Leon DF, Shaver JA, eds. *Physiologic Principles of Heart Sounds and Murmurs* (Monograph 46). New York: American Heart Association; 1975:2–7.
223. Delman AJ. Hemodynamic correlates of cardiovascular sounds. *Annu Rev Med* 1967; 18:139–158.
224. Adolph RJ, Stephens JF, Tanaka K. The clinical value of frequency analysis of the first heart sound in myocardial infarction. *Circulation* 1970; 41:1003–1014.
225. Thompson ME, Shaver JA, Heidenreich FP, et al. Sound, pressure and motion correlates in mitral stenosis. *Am J Med* 1970; 49:436–450.
226. Tei C, Shah PM, Cherian G, et al. The correlates of an abnormal first heart sound in mitral valve prolapse syndromes. *New Engl J Med* 1982; 307:334–339.
227. Burggraf GW. The first heart sound in left bundle branch block: An echophonocardiographic study. *Circulation* 1981; 63:429–435.
228. Shaver JA, Rahko PS, Grines CL, et al. Effect of left bundle branch block on the events of the cardiac cycle. *Acta Cardiol* 1988; 4:459–467.
229. Shaver JA, Griff FW, Leonard JJ. Ejection sounds of left-sided origin. In: Leon DF, Shaver JA, eds. *Physiologic Principles of Heart Sounds and Murmurs* (Monograph 46). New York: American Heart Association; 1975:27–34.
230. Mills PG, Brodie B, McLaurin L, et al. Echocardiographic and hemodynamic relationships of ejection sounds. *Circulation* 1977; 56:430–436.
231. Martin CE, Shaver JA, O'Toole JD, et al. Ejection sounds of right-sided origin. In: Leon DF, Shaver JA, eds. *Physiologic Principles of Heart Sounds and Murmurs* (Monograph 46). New York: American Heart Association; 1975:35–44.
232. Barlow JB, Pocock WA, Marchand P, Denny M. The significance of late systolic murmurs. *Am Heart J* 1963; 66:443–452.
233. Criley JM, Lewis KB, Humphries JO, Ross RS. Prolapse of the mitral valve: Clinical and cine-angiocardiographic findings. *Br Heart J* 1966; 28:488–496.
234. Ronan JA, Perloff JK, Harvey WP. Systolic clicks and the late systolic murmur. *Am Heart J* 1965; 70:319–325.
235. Leon DF, Leonard JJ, Kroetz FW, et al. Late systolic murmurs, clicks, and whoops arising from the mitral valve. *Am Heart J* 1966; 72:325–336.
236. Kerber RE, Isaeff DM, Hancock EW. Echocardiographic patterns in patients with the syndrome of systolic click and late systolic murmur. *New Engl J Med* 1971; 284:691–693.
237. Popp RL, Brown OR, Silverman JF, Harrison D. Echocardiographic abnormalities in the mitral valve prolapse syndrome. *Circulation* 1974; 49:428–433.
238. Reid JVO. Mid-systolic clicks. *S Afr Med J* 1961; 35:353–355.
239. Fontana ME, Pence HL, Leighton RF, Wooley CF. The varying clinical spectrum of the systolic click-late systolic murmur syndrome: A postural auscultatory phenomenon. *Circulation* 1970; 41:807–816.
240. Leatham A. The second heart sound, key to auscultation of the heart. *Acta Cardiol* 1964; 19:395–416.
241. Shaver JA, O'Toole JD. The second heart sound: Newer concepts: I. Normal and wide physiologic splitting. *Mod Concepts Cardiovasc Dis* 1977; 46:7–12.
242. Shaver JA. Clinical implications of the hangout interval. *Int J Cardiol* 1984; 5:391–398.
243. Shaver JA, Nadolny RA, O'Toole JD, et al. Sound pressure correlates of the second heart sound: An intracardiac sound study. *Circulation* 1974; 49:316–325.
244. Adolph RJ. Second heart sound: Role of altered electromechanical events. In: Leon DF, Shaver JA, eds. *Physiologic Principles of Heart Sounds and Murmurs* (Monograph 46). New York: American Heart Association; 1975:45–57.
245. Leatham A, Towers M. Splitting of the second heart sound in health. In: Proceedings of the Thirtieth Annual General Meeting of the British Cardiac Society, Glasgow, May 10, 1951. *Br Heart J* 1951; 13:575.
246. Adolph RJ, Fowler NO. The second heart sound: A screening test for heart disease. *Mod Concepts Cardiovasc Dis* 1970; 39: 91–96.
247. Shaver JA, O'Toole JD. The second heart sound: Newer concepts: 2. Paradoxical splitting and narrow physiological splitting. *Mod Concepts Cardiovasc Dis* 1977; 46:13–16.
248. Alvares RF, Shaver JA, Gamble WH, Goodwin JF. The isovolumic relaxation period in hypertrophic cardiomyopathy. *J Am Coll Cardiol* 1984; 3:71–81.
249. Gamble WH, Shaver JA, Alvares RF, et al. A critical appraisal of diastolic time intervals as a measure of relaxation in left ventricular hypertrophy. *Circulation* 1983; 68:76–87.
250. Martin CE, Shaver JA, Leonard JJ. Physical signs, apex cardiography, phonocardiography, and systolic time intervals in angina pectoris. *Circulation* 1972; 46:1098–1114.
251. Wood P. Pulmonary hypertension. *Br Med Bull* 1952; 8:348–353.
252. Dell'Italia LJ, Walsh RA. Acute determinants of the hangout interval in the pulmonary circulation. *Am Heart J* 1988; 16:1289–1297.
253. Thayer WS. The early diastolic heart sound. *Trans Assoc Am Phys* 1908; 13:326–357.
254. Ross RS, Criley JM, Morgan RH. Cineangiography in mitral valve disease. *Trans Assoc Am Phys* 1961; 74:271–279.
255. Oriol A, Palmer WH, Nakhjavan F, McGregor M. Prediction of left atrial pressure from the second sound-opening snap interval. *Am J Cardiol* 1965; 16:184–188.
256. Rahko PS, Shaver JA, Salerni R, et al. Echophonocardiographic estimates of pulmonary artery wedge pressure in mitral stenosis. *Am J Cardiol* 1985; 55:462–469.
257. Tavel ME. Opening snaps: Mitral and tricuspid. In: Leon DF, Shaver JA, eds. *Physiologic Principles of Heart Sounds and Murmurs* (Monograph 46). New York: American Heart Association; 1975:85–91.
258. Millward DK, McLaurin LP, Craige E. Echocardiographic studies to explain opening snaps in the presence of nonstenotic mitral valves. *Am J Cardiol* 1973; 31:64–70.
259. Sloan AW, Campbell FW, Henderson AS. Incidence of the physiological third heart sound. *Br Med J* 1952; 2:853–855.
260. Harvey WP, Stapleton J. Clinical aspects of gallop rhythm with particular reference to diastolic gallops. *Circulation* 1958; 18: 1017–1024.
261. Craige E. Gallop rhythm. *Prog Cardiovasc Dis* 1967; 10:246–260.
262. Shaver JA, Reddy PS, Alvares FR. Early diastolic events associated with the physiologic and pathologic S_3. *J Cardiol* 1984; 14(suppl V):30–46.
263. Shah PM, Jackson D. Third heart sound and summation gallop.

In: Leon DF, Shaver JA, eds. *Physiologic Principles of Heart Sounds and Murmurs* (Monograph 46). New York: American Heart Association; 1975:79–84.

264. Reddy PS, Meno F, Curtiss EI, O'Toole JD. The genesis of gallop sounds: Investigation by quantitative phono- and apex cardiography. *Circulation* 1981; 63:922–933.

265. Shaver JA, Reddy PS, Alvares RF, Salerni R. Genesis of the physiologic third heart sound. *Am J Noninvas Cardiol* 1987; 1:39–55.

266. Abdulla AM, Frank MJ, Erdin RA Jr, Canedo M. Clinical significance and hemodynamic correlates of the third heart sound gallop in aortic regurgitation. *Circulation* 1981; 64:464–471.

267. Stapleton JF. Third and fourth heart sounds. In: Horwitz LD, Groves BM, eds. *Signs and Symptoms in Cardiology*. Philadelphia: Lippincott; 1985:214–226.

268. Fowler NO, Adolph RJ. Fourth sound gallop or split first sound? *Am J Cardiol* 1972; 30:441–444.

269. Spodick DH, Quary-Pigotti VM. Fourth heart sound as a normal finding in older persons. *New Engl J Med* 1973; 288: 140–141.

270. Harris A. Pacemaker "heart sound." *Br Heart J* 1967; 29: 608–615.

271. Lerman J, Means JH. Cardiovascular symptomatology in exophthalmic goiter. *Am Heart J* 1932; 8:55–65.

272. Hamman L. Spontaneous mediastinal emphysema. *Bull Johns Hopkins Hosp* 1939; 64:1–21.

273. Soffer A, Feinstein A, Luisada AA, et al. Glossary of cardiologic terms related to physical diagnosis and history. *Am J Cardiol* 1967; 20:285–286.

274. Freeman AR, Levine SA. Clinical significance of systolic murmurs: Study of 1000 consecutive "non-cardiac" cases. *Ann Intern Med* 1933; 6:1371–1385.

275. O'Rourke RA. Cardiac murmurs. In: Goldman L, Braunwald E, eds. *Cardiology for the Primary Physician*. Philadelphia: Saunders; 1998:155–173.

276. Gallavardin L, Ravault P. Le souffle du retrecissement aortique puet changer de timbre et devenir musical dans sa propagation apexienne. *Lyon Med* 1925; 135:523–529.

277. Shaver JA. Systolic murmurs. *Heart Dis Stroke* 1993; 2:9–17.

278. Murgo JP, Altobelli SA, Dorethy JF, et al. Normal ventricular ejection dynamics in man during rest and exercise. In: Leon DF, Shaver JA, eds. *Physiologic Principles of Heart Sounds and Murmurs* (Monograph 46). New York: American Heart Association; 1975:92–101.

279. Lembo NJ, Dell'Italia LJ, Crawford MH, O'Rourke RA. Bed side diagnosis of systolic murmurs. *New Engl J Med* 1988; 318:1572–1578.

280. Stein PD, Sabbah HN. Aortic origin of innocent murmurs. *Am J Cardiol* 1977; 39:665–671.

281. Shaver JA. Innocent murmurs. *Hosp Med* 1978; 8–35.

282. deLeon AC Jr. "Straight back" syndrome. In: Leon DF, Shaver JA, eds. *Physiologic Principles of Heart Sounds and Murmurs* (Monograph 46). NewYork: American Heart Association; 1975:197–208.

283. Gamboa R, Hugenholtz PG, Nadas AS. Accuracy of the phonocardiogram in assessing severity of aortic and pulmonic stenosis. *Circulation* 1964; 30:35–46.

284. Aronow WS, Kronzon I. Correlation of prevalence and severity of valvular aortic stenosis determined by continuous-wave Doppler echocardiography with physical signs of aortic stenosis in patients aged 62 to 100 years with aortic systolic ejection murmurs. *Am J Cardiol* 1987; 60:399–401.

285. Vogelpoel L, Schrire V. Auscultatory and phonocardiographic assessment of pulmonary stenosis with intact ventricular septum. *Circulation* 1960; 22:55–72.

286. Zuberbuhler JR, Lenox CC, Neches WH, et al. Auscultatory spectrum of the tetralogy of Fallot. In: Leon DF, Shaver JA, eds. *Physiologic Principles of Heart Sounds and Murmurs* (Monograph 46). New York: American Heart Association; 1975: 187–192.

287. O'Rourke RA, Crawford MH. Mitral valve regurgitation. *Curr Probl Cardiol* 1984; 9:1–52.

288. Karliner JS, O'Rourke RA, Kearney DJ, Shabetai R. Hemodynamic explanation of why the murmur of mitral regurgitation is independent of cycle length. *Br Heart J* 1973; 35: 397–401.

289. Rivero Carvallo JM. Signo para el diagnostico de las insufficiencias tricuspideas. *Arch Inst Cardiol Mex* 1946; 16:531–540.

290. Wooley CF. The spectrum of tricuspid regurgitation. In: Leon DF, Shaver JA, eds. *Physiologic Principles of Heart Sounds and Murmurs* (Monograph 46). New York: American Heart Association; 1975:139–148.

291. Leatham A, Segal BL. Auscultatory and phonocardiographic findings in ventricular septal defect with left-to-right shunt. *Circulation* 1962; 25:318–327.

292. Leatham A. The spectrum of ventricular septal defect. In: Leon DF, Shaver JA, eds. *Physiologic Principles of Heart Sounds and Murmurs* (Monograph 46). New York: American Heart Association; 1975:135–138.

293. Ronan JA Jr, Steelman RB, DeLeon AC, et al. The clinical diagnosis of acute severe mitral insufficiency. *Am J Cardiol* 1971; 27:284–290.

294. Perloff JW, Roberts WC. The mitral apparatus: Functional anatomy of mitral regurgitation. *Circulation* 1972; 46:227–239.

295. Braunwald E. Mitral regurgitation. *New Engl J Med* 1969; 281:425–433.

296. Rios JC, Massumi RA, Breesmen WT, Sarin RK. Auscultatory features of acute tricuspid regurgitation. *Am J Cardiol* 1969; 23:4–11.

297. Amidi M, Irwin JM, Salerni R, et al. Venous systolic thrill and murmur in the neck: A consequence of severe tricuspid insufficiency. *J Am Coll Cardiol* 1986; 7:942–945.

298. Burch GE, DePasquale NP, Phillips HJ. Clinical manifestations of papillary muscle dysfunction. *Arch Intern Med* 1963; 112: 158–163.

299. Barlow JB, Bosman CK, Pocock WA, Marchand P. Late systolic murmurs and nonejection ("mid-late") systolic clicks. *Br Heart J* 1968; 30:203–217.

300. Wigle ED, Sasson Z, Henderson MA, et al. Hypertrophic cardiomyopathy: The importance of the site and the extent of hypertrophy. A review. *Prog Cardiovasc Dis* 1985; 28:1–83.

301. Shaver JA, Alvares RF, Reddy PS, Salerni R. Phonoechocardiography and intracardiac phonocardiography in hypertrophic cardiomyopathy. *Postgrad Med J* 1986; 62:537–543.

302. Murgo JP, Miller JW. Hemodynamic, angiographic and echocardiographic evidence against impeded ejection in hypertrophic cardiomyopathy. In: Goodwin JF, ed. *Heart Muscle Disease*. Lancaster, England: MTP Press; 1985:187–211.

303. Shah PM. Controversies in hypertrophic cardiomyopathy. *Curr Probl Cardiol* 1986; 11:563–613.

304. Shaver JA, Salerni R, Curtiss EI, Follansbee WP. A clinical presentation and noninvasive evaluation of the patient with hypertrophic cardiomyopathy. In: Shaver JA, Brest AN, eds. *Cardiomyopathies: Clinical Presentation, Differential Diagnosis, and Management* (Cardiovascular Clinics). Philadelphia: Davis, 1988:149–192.

305. Shaver JA. Diastolic murmurs. *Heart Dis Stroke* 1993; 2:98–103.

306. Wood P. An appreciation of mitral stenosis. *Br Med J* 1954; 1:1051–1063.

307. Craige E. Phonocardiography in interventricular septal defects. *Am Heart J* 1960; 60:51–60.

308. Fortuin NJ, Craige E. Echocardiographic studies of genesis of mitral diastolic murmurs. *Br Heart J* 1973; 35:75–81.
309. Coombs CF. *Rheumatic Heart Disease.* New York: William Wood; 1924:190.
310. Flint A. On cardiac murmurs. *Am J Med Sci* 1862; 44:29–54.
311. Craige E. The Austin Flint murmur. In: Leon DF, Shaver JA, eds. *Physiologic Principles of Heart Sounds and Murmurs* (Monograph 46). NewYork: American Heart Association; 1970: 160–165.
312. Reddy PS, Curtiss EI, Salerni R, et al. Sound pressure correlates of the Austin Flint murmur: An intracardiac sound study. *Circulation* 1976; 53:210–217.
313. Rahko PS. Doppler and echocardiographic characteristics of patients having an Austin Flint murmur. *Circulation* 1991; 83:1940–1950.
314. Green EW, Agruss NS, Adolph RJ. Right-sided Austin Flint murmur. *Am J Cardiol* 1973; 32:370–374.
315. Harvey WP, Corrado MA, Perloff JK. "Right-sided" murmurs of aortic insufficiency. *Am J Med Sci* 1963; 245:533–543.
316. Steell G. The murmur of high pressure in the pulmonary artery. *Med Chron* 1888; 9:182–188.
317. Runco V, Molnar W, Meckstroth CV, Ryan JM. The Graham Steell murmur versus aortic regurgitation in rheumatic heart disease. *Am J Med* 1961; 31:71–80.
318. Perez JE, Smith CA, Meltzer VN. Pulmonic valve insufficiency: A common cause of transient diastolic murmurs in renal failure. *Ann Intern Med* 1985; 103:497–502.
319. Runco V, Levin HS. The spectrum of pulmonic regurgitation. In: Leon DF, Shaver JA, eds. *Physiologic Principles of Heart Sounds and Murmurs* (Monograph 46). New York: American Heart Association; 1975:175–182.
320. Myers JD. The mechanisms and significances of continuous murmurs. In: Leon DF, Shaver JA, eds. *Physiologic Principles of Heart Sounds and Murmurs* (Monograph 46). New York: American Heart Association; 1975:201–208.
321. Minkoff SM, Fort ML, Sharp JT. Rupture of an aneurysm of the sinus of Valsalva into the right atrium. *Am J Cardiol* 1967; 19:278–284.
322. Ross J Jr, Braunwald E, Mason DT, et al. Interatrial communication and left atrial hypertension: A cause of continuous murmur. *Circulation* 1963; 28:853–860.
323. Myers JD, Murdaugh HV Jr, McIntosh HD, Blaisdell RK. Observations on continuous murmurs over partially obstructed arteries. *Arch Intern Med* 1956; 97:726–737.

CHAPTER 11

THE RESTING ELECTROCARDIOGRAM

Agustin Castellanos / Alberto Interian, Jr. / Robert J. Myerburg

What is commonly called an *electrocardiogram* (ECG) is the graph obtained when the electrical potentials of an electrical field originating in the heart are recorded at the body surface.[1-4] Although the ECG gives very useful clinical information, it only provides an approximation of the voltage produced by the source. The ECG has not been able to achieve interesting new insights into its own *basic* theoretic limitations, which some have considered as the solutions of the "forward" problem and the "inverse" problem of electrocardiography.[1,2] Whereas the former seeks the description of a specific electrocardiographic pattern in response to a specific local or regional intracardiac change in electrical activity, the latter seeks to predict the behavior of the cardiac generator from potentials recorded at the body surface.[1,2] Nevertheless, recent experimental studies have provided new information capable of expanding the clinical usefulness of the ECG, as will be discussed throughout this chapter. The ECG has many uses: It may serve as an independent marker of myocardial disease; it may reflect anatomic, hemodynamic, molecular, ionic, and drug-induced abnormalities of the heart; and it may provide information that is essential for the proper diagnosis and therapy of many cardiac[1] problems[4] (see also Chap. 24). In fact, it is the most commonly used laboratory procedure for the diagnosis of heart disease. Underreading or misreading due to insufficient knowledge of pathologic conditions, overreading due to an inability to recognize technical errors, and most important, failure to correlate ECG findings with the clinical findings may result in iatrogenic heart disease. Every physician interpreting ECGs as well as those learning electrocardiographic interpretation should read the *Guidelines for Electrocardiography of the American College of Cardiology, American Heart Association Task Force.*[4]

VENTRICULAR DEPOLARIZATION AND REPOLARIZATION

Fluxes of ions across the cell membranes cause the differences in voltage between resting and activated myocardial cells. To understand the electrical forces produced by the heart as a whole at the body surface, it has been conventional to first discuss the electrical properties of a hypothetical muscle strip from the free wall of the left ventricle extending from endocardium to epicardium.[5–7] In the resting or polarized state, the charges are at rest. A unipolar electrode facing the epicardial side of the strip, such as V_6, registers an isoelectric line.[5–13] If activation of this relatively large muscle strip starts in the endocardial side, it initiates the process called *depolarization*.[5–13] The *sequence* of this process is thus from endocardium to epicardium. Depolarization has been described as a moving wave *with the positive charges in front of the negative charges*. The previously mentioned lead V_6 overlying the epicardium of the left ventricle will record a positivity because it consistently faces positive charges throughout the entire depolarization sequence.[5–13] On the other hand, the *sequence* of ventricular repolarization is from epicardium to endocardium.[5–13] The *negative charges,* however, travel *in front* because repolarization tends to reestablish the resting, polarized state of the previously depolarized cells. As a consequence of the latter, V_6 will record a positive deflection (T wave) because it constantly faces positive charges throughout the entire repolarization sequence. The earlier epicardial end of repolarization has been attributed to the shorter duration of repolarization that epicardial cells have in comparison with endocardial cells. Thus repolarization finishes at the epicardium while it still has not been completed at the endocardium. Hence the *sequence* of repolarization is, as noted previously, from epicardium to endocardium. This simplistic view is of didactic value only because it fails to take into consideration the role played by the M cells described by Antzelevitch et al.[14] since the beginning of this decade. According to these authors, M cells play a determining role in the inscription of the T wave because currents flowing down voltage gradients on either side of the usual (but not necessarily) mid-myocardial cells determine both the height and width of the T wave, as well as the degree to which the ascending or descending limbs of the T wave are interrupted.

ELECTROCARDIOGRAPHIC LEADS

To record an ECG, an electric circuit between the heart and the electrocardiograph must be completed.[11] For this purpose, electrodes are placed on different parts of the body surface and are connected to the instrument by means of cables.[11] Thus the whole system consists of an instrument, electrodes, cables, and leads.

Bipolar Standard Leads

An ECG lead can be defined as a pair of terminals with designated polarity, each of which is connected either directly or via a passive-active network to recording electrodes. In 1913, Einthoven et al.[3] developed a method of studying the electrical activity of the heart by representing it graphically in a *two-dimensional* geometric figure, namely, an equilateral triangle. There are several simplifying assumptions on which Einthoven's hypothesis is founded[3–13]: (1) The body is a homogeneous volume conductor. Although the conductivity of the various tissues is not the same, the differences are not great enough to invalidate that the body can be considered as a homogeneous volume conductor. (2) The sum of all the electric forces, or the mean of all the forces generated during the cardiac cycle, can be considered as originating in a dipole located in the electrical center of the heart. (3) Electrodes placed on the right arm (RA), left arm (LA), and left leg (LL) are used to pick up the potential variations on these extremities. Standard (bipolar) leads (I, II, and III) are obtained by recording, respectively, the potential differences between LA and RA, LL and RA, and LL and LA. These leads record potential variations in a single frontal plane only. (4) Attachment between these limb electrodes, on the forearms and limbs, corresponds to a position in the root of the corresponding limb. For example, an electrode in the right forearm records the electrical activity that reaches the right shoulder. It should be pointed out that when the electrodes are placed proximally to the roots of the extremities, they lose their relatively "far" distance from the heart. Hence Einthoven's equilateral theory does not hold. The latter is of importance to understand why leads placed proximally to the roots of the extremities, such as those used for exercise testing and coronary care unit and Holter monitoring, by being only "equivalent" to the corresponding bipolar leads, are in some cases markedly different from the "true" standard bipolar leads.

Wilson Central Terminal

The sum of the potentials from the right arm (RA), left arm (LA), and left leg (LL) is equal to zero throughout the cardiac cycle with respect to any point at the body surface.[3,5,6,13] Lead wires attached to electrodes on each limb are connected together, through 5000-Ω resistors, at a point. When this common point—*Wilson's central terminal*—is attached to the negative pole of the ECG machine and an "exploring" electrode is connected to the positive pole, the potential variations recorded will be those of the latter only. A lead taken by this method is called a *unipolar lead.* Actually, the central terminal is not zero because the RA, LA, and LL are not equidistant from each other and from the heart, the body tissues vary in resistance, and the heart and extremities do not lie in exactly the same plane in the body. The potential of the central terminal has been said to average around 0.3 mV.[9]

Unipolar Extremity Leads

At present, unipolar extremity leads are obtained by disconnecting the input to the central terminal of Wilson from the extremity being explored. This results in a one-and-a-half increase in their voltage. These *augmented* (a) extremity leads are the ones usually used for clinical electrocardiography and are labeled aV_R, aV_L, and aV_F.[5,9,13]

Unipolar Precordial Leads

The unipolar precordial ECG is obtained by placing the exploring electrode (connected to the positive pole of the ECG machine) on the classic six locations of the anterior and left portions of the chest.[5,6,13] The central terminal is used as the indifferent electrode. Precordial (V) leads yield a positive deflection when facing positive charges and negative deflections when facing negative charges.[5,6,12,13,15–17] They do this according to what Wilson called the *solid-angle concept*.[5,13] A solid angle is merely an imaginary cone extending from the site in the chest throughout the heart. The precordial electrode is at its apex, and its base is at the opposite epicardial surface.[13] This concept is most important to understand precordial lead morphologies. According to Wilson's scalar concept of electrocardiography, this occurs because the solid angle subtended by the corresponding lead records the electrical activity from the regions of the heart over which the lead is placed as well as from distant regions.[5,13] Thus, if V_2 is placed over (thereby facing) the right ventricle, part of the initial positive ventricular deflection reflects right ventricular activation, with the corresponding electrical forces moving toward the electrode.[13] Most portions of the terminal S wave represent activation of muscle other than the right ventricle (septum and free left ventricular wall), reflecting electrical forces moving away from the electrode.[13] Acceptance that the amount of muscle activity recorded by various unipolar leads is not the same implies different "real" duration of depolarization and repolarization, irrespective of that supposedly resulting from the projections of a vector on an idealized horizontal lead axis (see sections on QT dispersion and vectorcardiography). For practical purposes, the peak of the r (or R) wave in precordial leads gives a rough estimate of the moment of arrival of excitation (*intrinsicoid* deflection) at the muscle underneath the electrode.[13] This encompasses a considerable number of muscle fibers (given by the solid-angle concept), however—in fact, a greater number than if the electrode is placed directly on the epicardial surface.[13] In the latter case, the moment of arrival of excitation at the electrode affects a lesser number of fibers and is thus given by the *intrinsic* deflection.[13]

NORMAL ACTIVATION OF THE HEART: VENTRICULAR DEPOLARIZATION

After emerging from the sinus node, the cardiac impulse propagates throughout the atria in its journey toward the atrioventricular (AV) node. The *normal* P wave (resulting from activation of the myocardium of both atria) is a consequence of, but does not directly represent, sinus node activity. During sinus rhythm, the right atrium is activated before the left atrium.[6] This explains why high-fidelity recordings of the P waves of some normal persons show a small notch at the top. The latter simply reflects the normal asynchrony existing between the atria.[6] Because of the anatomic position of the sinus node, the sequence of atrial depolarization occurs in an inferior, leftward, and somewhat posterior direction. The normal P waves are always positive in leads I, II, aV_F, and V_3 to V_6 and negative in lead aV_R. According to the anatomic position of the heart, the P wave may be diphasic in V_1 and aV_L or negative in the latter lead. Atrial repolarization, also called T_a, is directly opposite in polarity to the P wave.[6,11] It is usually not seen because it coincides with the PR segment (not to be confused with the PR interval) and QRS complex. The PR interval (used to estimate AV conduction time) includes conduction through the "true" AV structures (AV node, His bundle, bundle branches, and main divisions of the left bundle branch), as well as through those parts of the atria located between sinus and AV nodes.[8] The onset of ventricular depolarization (given by the beginning of the normal q wave) reflects activation of the left side of the interventricular septum. This has been attributed to the fact that the left bundle system is shorter than the right bundle branch.[8,15] In addition, the large fanlike distribution of the ramifications of the fascicles of the left bundle branch on the left septal surface produces activation of a greater number of ordinary muscle cells per unit of time.[6,8,15] For this reason, the normal initial depolarization is oriented from left to right, therefore explaining the small q wave in lead V_6 and the small r wave in lead V_1. After the cardiac impulse descending through the right bundle branch reaches the right septal surface, the interventricular septum is activated in both directions. Septal activation is thereafter encompassed within or neutralized by free-wall activation. The most distal ramifications of both bundle branches (Purkinje fibers) form networks within the subendocardial regions of both ventricular walls. The latter are activated as soon as the multiple ramifications emerge from the Purkinje fibers.[6,15] The greater mass of the left ventricular (LV) free wall explains why LV free-wall events overpower those of the interventricular septum and right ventricular free wall.

ELECTRICAL AXIS

The *electrical axis* (EA) may be defined as a vector originating in the center of Einthoven's equilateral triangle.[3,13] A *vector* is a mathematical value expressed as an arrow that has magnitude, sense, and direction. On the other hand, *scalar* values only have magnitude. When applied to the EA of the QRS complexes, the vector that represents it also gives the direction of the activation process as projected in the plane of the limb leads. Its length represents the manifest potential of the dipole in the center of the triangle. These general considerations apply either to the instantaneous EA (the vector indicating the direction of the impulse at the instant at which it is determined) or to the mean EA (which is the resultant of all instantaneous electrical axes). Although the term *EA* can be used in reference to any of the major components of the ECG (P, T, or QRS), it is generally applied to the QRS. There are many methods for

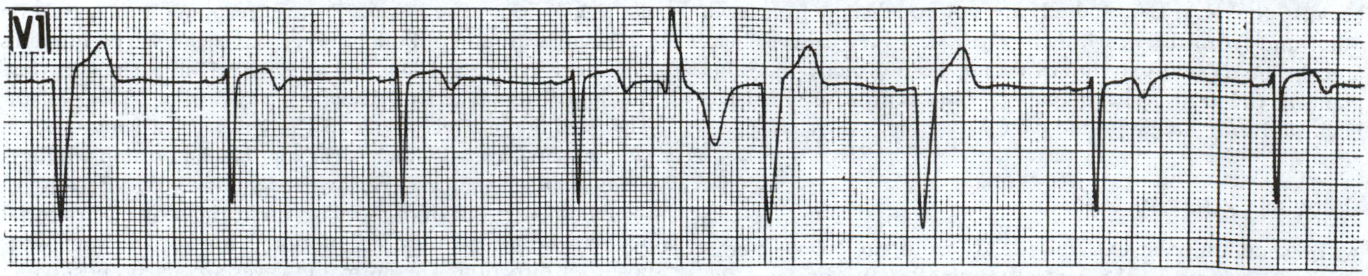

FIGURE 11-1 Tachycardia-dependent complete left bundle branch block. Negative, T waves become manifest (when the left bundle branch block disappears) in leads showing a predominant negative (S wave) deflection. The patient had "primary" conduction system disease with no other evidence of organic heart disease. These changes have been attributed to the type of long-term memory effects that become manifest after disappearance of an abnormal sequence of depolarization.

determining the mean EA. The one recommended by electrocardiographers of the classical school consists of calculating the net areas enclosed by the QRS complex in leads I, II, and III.[3,6,7,12,13] The net area is the absolute sum of the positive and negative areas of the QRS complex in the corresponding lead. One of the drawbacks of this method is that the absolute values of the net area cannot be determined *accurately* by inspection. Since the absolute magnitude of the EA is not of fundamental clinical importance, it has been recommended that arbitrary units be used. When this is done, the results can be counterchecked by using Einthoven's law. For example, if in a given case lead I is +4 units, lead II is +2 units, and lead III is −2 units, the calculation is accurate because the sum of leads I and III (+4 plus −2) must always equal lead II (+2). After having determined the net area, the results are plotted on the sides of the triangle, and perpendiculars are dropped from two or all three leads. The perpendiculars will meet at a point away from the center of the triangle. A line drawn from the latter to the former defines the mean EA. A simpler, though less precise, method of calculating the quadrant (or parts of a quadrant) in which the EA is located consists of using the maximal QRS deflection in leads I and aV_F and, when necessary, lead II. This method is inexact from the mathematical viewpoint but has the value of simplicity.[15,16]

VENTRICULAR GRADIENT

The relationship between the EA of the QRS complex and the T wave was referred to by Wilson as the *ventricular gradient*.[17] In contrast to what occurs in an epicardial-to-endocardial muscle strip (as mentioned previously), in the isolated muscle strip, the *sequence* of ventricular depolarization occurs in the same direction as that of repolarization.[12] Although the QRS and T deflections have opposite polarity, the algebraic sum of QRS and T *areas* is zero. In the human heart, however, not only is the sequence different, but the pathways of ventricular depolarization and repolarization are not exactly the same.[12] Thus the algebraic sum of QRS and T *areas* is no longer zero. Therefore, a *gradient* is said to exist. The ventricular gradient can be calculated by determining the electrical axis of the QRS and T (using *areas*) and then obtaining the resultant by the parallelogram method. Wilson considered that the ventricular gradient could be of help in differentiating between T-wave inversion of various causes (primary changes) and the obligatory secondary T-wave changes resulting from abnormalities in depolarization, such as bundle branch block, ventricular hypertrophy, ventricular pacing, and preexcitation syndromes.[12,13,17] In practice, calculation of the ventricular gradient is difficult and time consuming because it has to be determined by areas and not maximal amplitude.

Apparent Challenges to the Concept of the Ventricular Gradient

Rosenbaum et al.[18] studied the prolonged depolarization occurring during long periods of ventricular stimulation and found two types of altered ventricular repolarization. One, corresponding to Wilson's classic theory, was transient and proportional in magnitude to the QRS complex but of opposite polarity. The other, concealed by (and during) the former, required a longer time (even days) to reach maximal effect as well as to disappear, becoming apparent *only when* normal activation recurred (Fig. 11-1). The latter type was attributed to modulated electrotonic interactions occurring during cardiac activation in such a way that repolarization was accelerated at ventricular sites where depolarization begins and delayed in areas where depolarization terminates. T-wave changes appearing after pro-

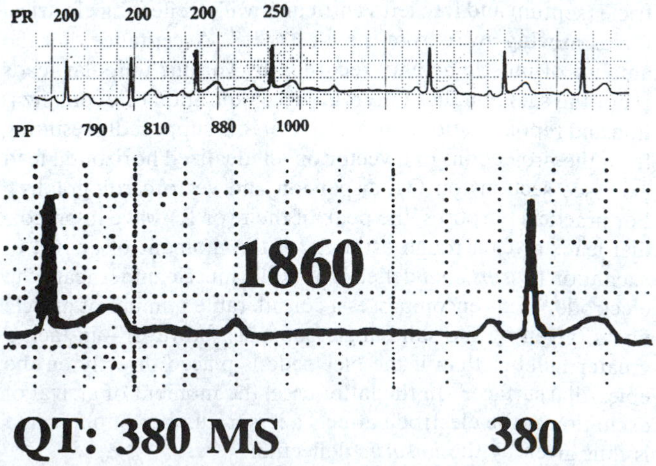

FIGURE 11-2 Vagal-induced AV nodal block in a young person without structural heart disease. All values are expressed in milliseconds. The uncorrected QT interval does not increase at the end of an 1860-ms (RR) pause. This can be due to the form of short-term cardiac memory whereby the QT interval "remembers" its prepause values because of the slow adjustment to abrupt changes in cycle length in otherwise *normal* subjects.

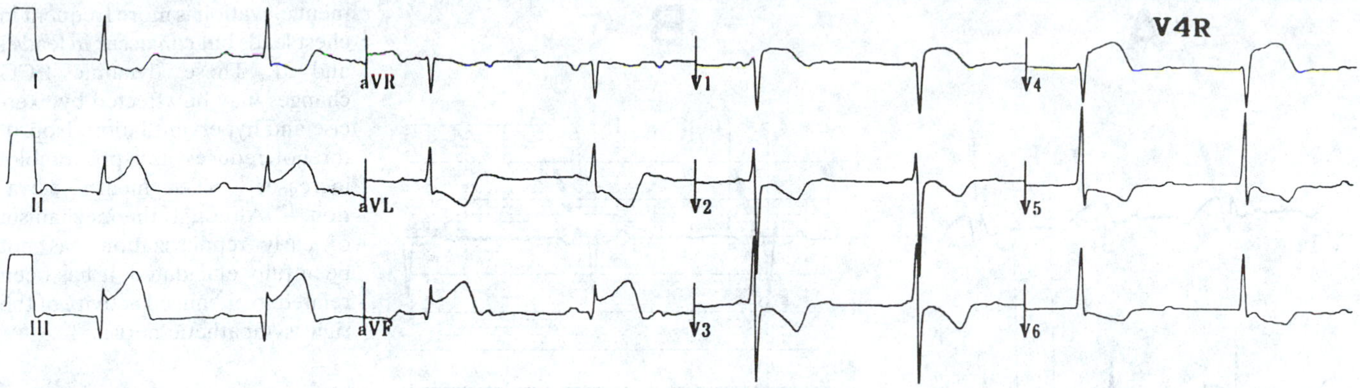

FIGURE 11-3 Acute inferior (diaphragmatic) MI showing "indicative" ST-segment elevation in leads reflecting the inferior wall (II, III, and aV_F). Reciprocal changes are seen in the diametrically opposed leads (I and aV_L) located in the same (frontal) plane. V_{4R} showed evidence of right ventricular MI. There was complete AV block with an AV junctional rhythm.

longed depolarization was no longer present showed accumulation and (fading) *long-term* memory for variable time (see "Secondary ST-T-Wave Changes," below).[18] Recently, Goyal et al.[19] reported the occurrence of *short-term* memory after periods of altered ventricular repolarization as short as 1 min in duration. In addition, according to Surawicz,[20] the term *memory* also has been applied to gradual adjustments of action potential duration (corresponding to QT intervals) after abrupt changes in cycle lengths (events influenced by past history) without necessarily requiring abnormal ventricular repolarization (Fig. 11-2). The cellular mechanism responsible for any form of cardiac memory is beyond the scope of this chapter.

ABNORMAL ST-SEGMENT CHANGES

In orthodox ECG language, *injury* implies *abnormal* ST-segment changes, *necrosis* implies *abnormal* Q waves, and *ischemia* implies *symmetric* T-wave inversion (or elevation).[5–7,9–13,16] Following conventional ECG theory, several authors consider that ECG "injury" occurs because the affected cells are unable to maintain their normal polarization during diastole.[5–7,12,16,21] Various hypotheses have been postulated to explain how this diastolic hypopolarization or generalized diastolic depolarization is manifested as abnormal ST-segment shifts in the surface ECG[21–24] (Fig. 11-3). One hypothesis is based on the existence of a diastolic current of "injury." During the control (diastolic) period, both membrane resting potential and surface ECG baseline are at their normal level. At the onset of injury, the resting intracellular potential decreases (e.g., from 90 to 70 mV), and the ECG baseline shifts below its preinjury level. Because the injured cells leak negative ions, their *exterior* becomes relatively negative (or less positive) than that of the normal cells. Thus a "current of injury" flows between the negative ("injured") zone and the positive ("normal") region.[10] This produces a negative displacement of the surface ECG *baseline* in the leads facing the injured region. In the surface ECG, depolarization (by virtue of the electrical negativization of the nonaffected area) practically reduces the potential difference between noninjured and injured regions. Therefore, the ST segment remains at the preinjury level, which is relatively *elevated* in reference to the injury baseline.[21–24] Consequently, the ST segment appears to be abnormally displaced above the latter. Note that the apparent presence of a systolic current of injury actually reflects disappearance of the diastolic current of injury. Finally, after the end of repolarization, the current of injury between injured and noninjured regions is reestablished, and the ECG baseline is again depressed (as it was immediately before depolarization).

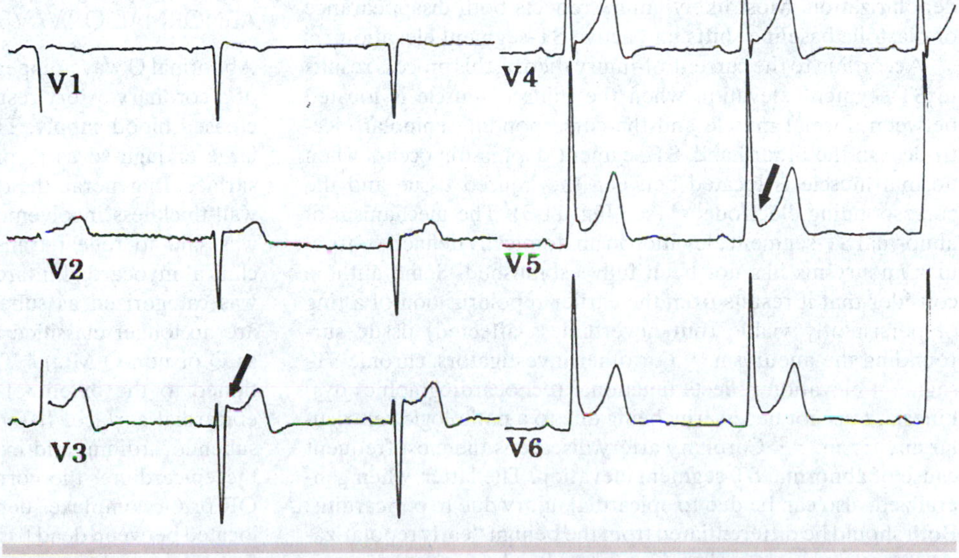

FIGURE 11-4 Early repolarization. This normal variant is characterized by narrow QRS complexes with J-point and ST-segment elevation in the chest leads. Left chest leads often show tall R waves with a distinct notch or slur in their downstroke (*arrow* in V_5), while the right chest leads may display ST segments having a "saddleback" or "humpback" shape (*arrow* in V_3).

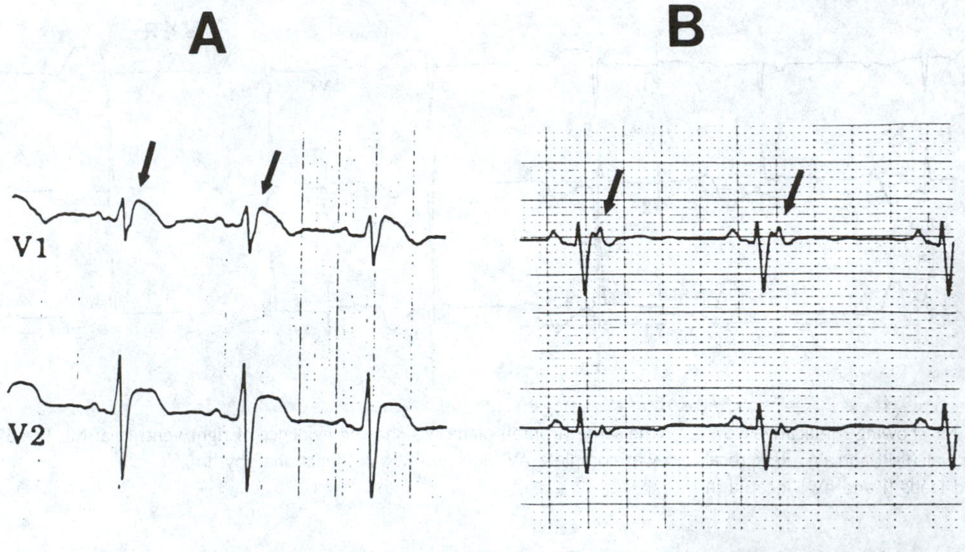

FIGURE 11-5 *A.* Nonischemic ST-segment elevation in the right precordial leads in a young patient with the Brugrada syndrome. *B.* Epsilon wave of a patient with arrhythmogenic right ventricular dysplasia.

Since the precise moment at which injury starts is not recorded in the usual alternating-current (ac) electrocardiographic recordings, the baseline that is almost invariably recorded is the postinjury baseline.[10] It also has been shown that the abnormal ST-segment elevation in leads facing the affected zone does not merely represent the (passive) return of the baseline to its preinjury level but reflects a true, active, positive displacement.[10,21–24] Thus, when depolarization of both normal and injured regions has occurred, the surface of the normal cells will (on account of their greater initial polarization) be able to accumulate more negative ions. Hence the normal regions become more negative than the injured regions, which are relatively more positive. In consequence, the ST segment becomes actively elevated above and beyond the preinjury baseline because of the relative potential difference existing at the end of depolarization. Most likely, injury reflects both disappearance of diastolic baseline shifts and active ST-segment elevation.[10,24]

According to the current-of-injury theory, this process results in ST-segment elevation when the injured muscle is located between normal muscle and the corresponding unipolar electrode. On the other hand, ST-segment depression occurs when normal muscle is located between the injured tissue and the corresponding electrode[10,12] (see Fig. 11-3). The mechanism of abnormal ST-segment elevation in anatomically defined ventricular aneurysms has not been fully established. Some authors consider that it results from the earlier repolarization of a ring of persistently viable (but nevertheless affected) tissue surrounding the aneurysm.[8,10] For other investigators, chronic ST-segment elevation reflects functional (echocardiographic) dyskinesia, thus not necessarily being due to a pathologic ventricular aneurysm.[8,25–27] Coronary artery disease is the most frequent cause of abnormal ST-segment elevation. The latter, when generalized, also can be due to epicardial injury due to pericarditis. Both should be differentiated from the benign "early repolarization" pattern, a normal variant.[28,29] In its classic form, there is J-point elevation (of no more than 3 mm) with an upwardly concave ST segment. R waves may be tall and at times have a distinct notch and slur on the downstroke (Fig. 11-4). ST-segment elevation is more frequent in chest leads but can occur in leads I and II. These dynamic ECG changes may be affected by exercise and hyperventilation. Isoproterenol reduces and propranolol increases ST-segment elevation.[30,31] Although the mechanism of early repolarization has not been fully elucidated, it has been related to enhanced activity of the right sympathetic nerves.[30]

SELECTIVE NONISCHEMIC ST-SEGMENT ELEVATION IN THE RIGHT PRECORDIAL LEADS

High-takeoff ST segments of either the caved or saddleback type localized to the right chest leads associated with different degrees of right bundle block with or without T-wave inversion and sudden death due to ventricular fibrillation are seen in the *Brugada syndrome*[32] (Fig. 11-5, *left*). This is a familial entity ascribed to a "primary" electrophysiologic abnormality. Similar findings were reported in the familial cardiomyopathy and sudden cardiac death syndrome described by Corrado et al.[33] Strong Na channel blocking drugs can produce ST-segment elevations even in patients without any evidence of syncope or ventricular fibrillation.[34] The changes produced by potassium are discussed in the section of hyperkalemia (below). Slight ST-segment elevation with an incomplete right bundle branch block pattern showing an epsilon wave has been described in arrhythmogenic right ventricular dysplasia[35] (see Fig. 11-5, *right*).

ABNORMAL Q WAVES

Abnormal Q waves appearing several hours after total occlusion of a coronary artery result from necrosis secondary to the decreased blood supply. The number of affected cells has to be large enough so as to produce changes reflected at the body surface. In general, the depth of the Q wave is proportional to wall-thickness involvement.[7] Thus, in lead aV_F a QS complex was said to reflect transmural necrosis. On the other hand, clinical myocardial infarction (MI) without abnormal Q waves was categorized as subendocardial infarction. Presently, MIs are no longer classified as transmural or subendocardial (but as Q or non-Q MIs).[36] The duration of the Q wave is proportioned to the extent of the area of necrosis parallel to the epicardial surface. If the latter is large enough, starts in the subendocardium, and extends toward (but not quitereaching) the epicardium, the corresponding unipolar leads will record QR or Qr complexes depending on the amount of living tissue located between dead tissue and the recording electrode. Therefore, abnormal Q waves may occur in MIs that are not completely transmural.[7,36] The following changes have been said to be equivalent to Q waves in non-Q-wave MI: R/S ratio changes, acute frontal plane right-axis deviation, new left-axis deviation or left bundle branch block, initial and terminal QRS notching, and some types of "poor r-wave progression."[36] Although the concept of non-Q-wave MI as a discrete clinicopathologic entity, different from Q-wave MI, has gained almost universal acceptance, it was challenged recently by a group of respectable electrocardiographers.[36]

In the course of the clinical entity known as *acute myocardial infarction* (MI), persisting Q waves are usually (but not invariably, as will be discussed subsequently) due to anatomic (lack of blood flow-related) necrosis. Abnormal Q waves also can occur transiently in unstable angina, Prinzmetal's angina, coronary artery spasm (without chest pain), and exercise-induced ischemia. This has been attributed to an intensity of cellular affectation ("injury") severe enough to produce a significant degree of hypopolarization (to, let us say, around 60 mV). Because the cells become electrically unexcitable (even though they are not anatomically, irreversibly necrotic),[7,8,15,16] abnormal Q waves occur. Spontaneous recanalization of an occluded vessel, spontaneous reversion of the ischemia, or spasm and interventions (pharmacologic or mechanical) that improve cellular metabolism and oxygenation can restore the normal polarization. If these cells become again excitable, the abnormal Q waves may disappear or vanish.[16,37] Ischemic necrosis usually takes longer to appear than the accelerated abnormal Q waves seen in the majority of patients with Q-wave MI after successful thrombolysis or effective coronary artery angioplasty performed early in the course of the process.[5] The genesis of these Q waves is not well understood.[37] Some authors consider them an expression of the acceleration of necrosis secondary to explosive cell swelling in already irreversibly injured tissue.[31] Because some of these Q waves also tend to disappear quickly, other authors consider that they reflect factors other than myocardial necrosis, such as reversal of regional dysmetabolism or the occurrence of transient interstitial ischemia or hemorrhage.[38] Profound and prolonged ischemia can cause myocardial stunning with reversible functional, metabolic, ultrastructural, and electrophysiologic abnormalities.[39] Thus transient Q waves may be the ECG counterpart (electrical stunning) of the corresponding mechanical stunning.[37–40] It is possible for myocardial stunning to lag behind electrical recovery.[37] *Myocardial stunning* should be differentiated from *myocardial hibernation*. The latter is a term used in reference to mechanical dysfunction of an ischemic area that is not transient but chronic.[41,42] Although the ECG counterpart of this type of mechanical dysfunction requires further study, it is conceivable that (in some cases) the disappearance of chronic Q waves after coronary artery bypass surgery with improvement of wall motion abnormalities indicates that these Q waves were due not to cellular death but to cellular hibernation[41,42] (see also Chaps. 37 and 40). Finally, abnormal Q waves need not be the end result of coronary artery disease because they may be seen after primary (due to infections or drugs) cellular necrosis and in other pathologic processes such as myocardial infiltration and certain types of interventricular septal (and LV) hypertrophy, Wolff-Parkinson-White syndrome, and muscular dystrophies.[43]

ISCHEMIC T-WAVE CHANGES

Symmetric T waves, inverted or upright (as in "hyperacute" T waves), characteristic of ECG "ischemia," have been considered to reflect a type, or degree, of cellular affection resulting only in action potentials of increased duration.[7,10,16] Because the QT interval recorded at the body surface can be considered as the sum of all action potentials (i.e., of the QT intervals of individual cells), any process (such as ECG ischemia) that increases action potential duration will cause prolongation of ventricular depolarization and QT interval. T-wave inversions[7,10] do not always reflect "physiologic" ischemia (due to decreased blood supply) because they also can be seen in evolving pericarditis, myocardial contusion, and increased intracranial pressure, as well as in the right chest leads of young patients (persistent juvenile pattern).[43]

SECONDARY ST-T-WAVE CHANGES

Alterations in the sequence of (and sometimes delay in) ventricular depolarization (such as those produced by bundle branch blocks, ventricular pacing, ectopic ventricular impulse formation, preexcitation syndromes, and ventricular hypertrophy) result in a change in the sequence of ventricular repolarization. The latter causes nonischemic T-wave inversions (secondary T-wave changes) in leads showing a predominantly positive QRS deflection.[6,10,12,17] As mentioned earlier in the discussion of ventricular gradient and cardiac memory, disappearance of these alterations in ventricular depolarization may be followed by narrow QRS complexes with negative T waves[18] (see Fig. 11-1). After disappearance of "complete" left bundle branch block

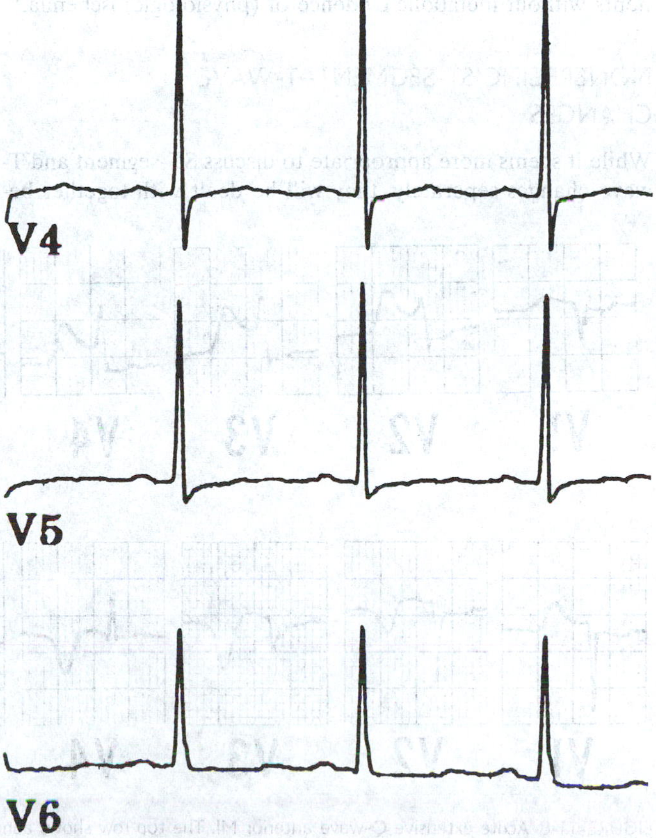

FIGURE 11-6 Nonspecific (nondiagnostic) ST-segment–T-wave changes, the most common abnormalities in ECG interpretation.

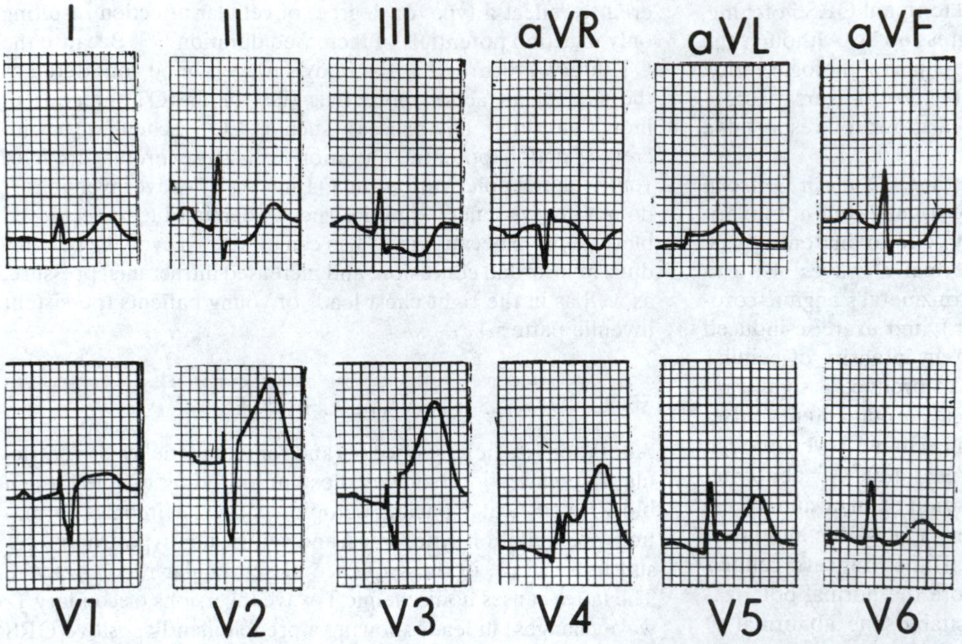

FIGURE 11-7 Acute extensive anterior wall MI showing abnormal ST-segment changes and hyperacute T waves.

(LBBB) and in right ventricular pacing, inverted T waves appear in leads (such as V_1 and V_2) where the S wave predominates (see Fig. 11-1). Finally, marked ST-segment changes may occur *during* rapid supraventricular tachycardias, even in young patients without metabolic evidence of (physiologic) ischemia.[44]

NONSPECIFIC ST-SEGMENT–T-WAVE CHANGES

While it seems more appropriate to discuss ST-segment and T-wave changes separately, they will be dealt with together because of their often coexistence. While nonspecific (or rather, nondiagnostic) ST-segment–T-wave changes are the most commonly diagnosed ECG abnormalities, they have not been categorized adequately and represent different findings for various interpreters.[45] In the classic paper, Friedberg and Zager[46] considered depth of ST-segment depression and T-wave inversion as well as their contour (Fig. 11-6).[46] When analyzed without clinical information, this diagnosis was made in 40 percent of 410 abnormal ECGs. The number was reduced to 10 percent, however, when clinical data became available. In the absence of structural heart disease, these changes can be due to a variety of physiologic (i.e., hyperventilation, anxiety, body position, food, neurogenic influences, and temperature), pharmacologic (i.e., antiarrhythmic and psychotropic drugs, digoxin), and extracardiac (i.e., electrolyte abnormalities, upper gastrointestinal processes, allergic reactions, etc.) factors.[45]

U WAVE

A number of hypotheses have been advanced to explain the genesis of the U wave. Foremost among them is the relationship to late repolarization of the Purkinje system. A criticism of this hypothesis is that the conducting system does not have sufficient mass to generate a large deflection at the body surface. The recent identification of another population of (M) cells between epicardium and endocardium may provide the necessary mass to produce not only U waves but also the J (or Osborn) wave characteristic of hypothermia.[14] What sometimes appears to be a U wave merging with a T wave simple may be a notched T wave whose ascending or descending limbs are interrupted by differences in the end of the composite action potential of epicardial and M cells.[14] The normal U wave, most prominent in leads V_2 and V_3, has the same polarity as the T wave and is approximately 10 percent of its amplitude. A large positive U wave may be due to hypokalemia and multiple antiarrhythmic drugs. In orthodox ECG interpretation, merging of T and U is still considered a stage in hypokalemia but

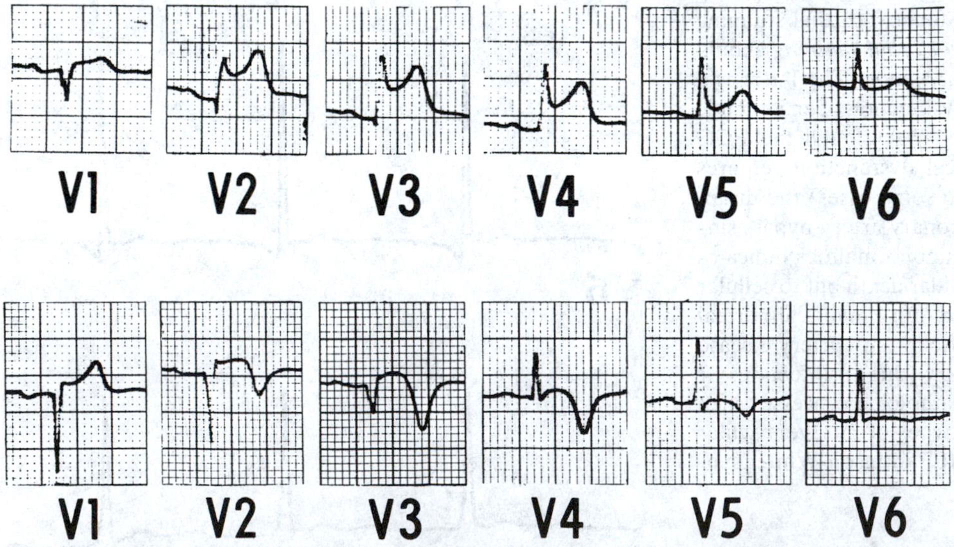

FIGURE 11-8 Acute extensive Q-wave anterior MI. The top row shows abnormal ST-segment elevation at the moment of appearance of (small) q waves in V_1, V_2, and V_3. Note that R waves are taller than q waves in leads (V_2 and V_3), where the reverse is expected. In the bottom row, Q waves are deeper, ST segments are less elevated, and ischemic T waves can be seen clearly.

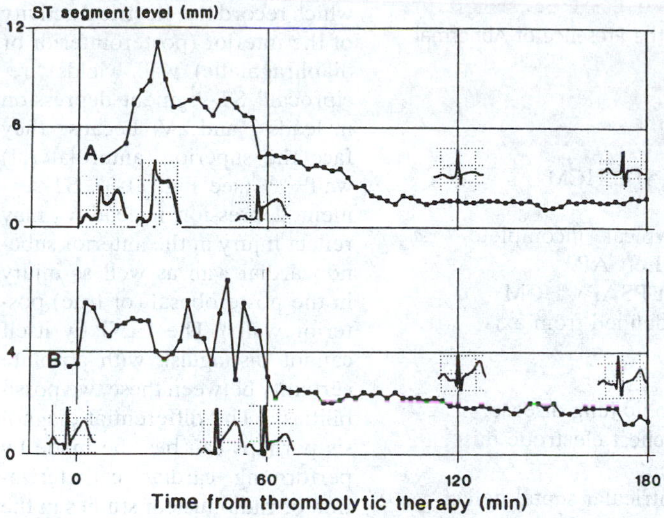

FIGURE 11-9 Plots of ST-segment levels versus time from therapy in two selected patients with patency of the infarct-related vessel at 60 min. Note that a 50 percent decrease in ST-segment levels within 60 min occurred only when measurements were made from the peak ST-segment level (highest ST-segment level measurement within the first 60 min).

can result from such drugs as quinidine and sotalol.[14] According to Antzelevitch, repolarization of the His-Purkinje system was first suggested by Watanabe as the most likely cause of the "real" U wave.[14] Causes of negative U waves are ischemia, hypertension, and occasionally, right ventricular enlargement.[45]

ACUTE MI

Although a recent article challenged this distinction,[36] MIs are no longer classified as transmural and subendocardial but as Q-wave and non-Q-wave.[36,47–50] In the thrombolytic era, the prevalence of the latter seems to be greater than that of the former (see Chap. 42), presumably due to a reduction in infarct size.[42–44] The prethrombolytic "classic" evolution of acute MI has been transformed by pharmacologic therapy and interventional techniques.[49,50] The succession of events in the course of a Q-wave MI is from hyperacute positive T waves (on occasion) to ST-segment elevation to abnormal Q waves to T-wave inversion[49,50] (Figs. 11-7 and 11-8). Commonly, two or more of these findings appear together, depending on the timing of the first recorded static ECG. Acceleration of these phases can occur with effective reperfusion. The time course of ST-segment elevation is a good predictor of reperfusion. Because prethrombolytic 12-lead ECG studies on ST-segment evolutions were based on static recordings obtained at fixed time intervals, it became clear that continuous monitoring in the coronary care unit (which falls outside the realm of this chapter) was essential to adequately record the dynamics of ST-segment trends (Figs. 11-9 and 11-10). Sensitivity increases as frequency of monitoring increases.[51–53] Continuous monitoring is thus essential to evaluate occurrence of reperfusion. Resolution of ST-segment elevation has been defined as a progressive decrease within 40 to 60 min to less than 50 percent of its maximally elevated value.[51,52] It has been suggested that in patients treated with thrombolytics, the dichotomization for Q-wave and non-Q-wave MI should be made by the predischarge, rather than the 24-h, ECG due to possible crossover from one group to another.[54]

Aspects of the ECG other than ST-segment changes may be altered particularly during acute, anterior-wall MI. In fact, the same degree of ST-segment elevation in V_2 and V_3 with disappearance of the S waves indicates a greater degree of affectation than with preservation of this negative wave[55] (see Fig. 11-8, *top*).

LOCATION OF THE SITE OF Q-WAVE MI

Table 11-1 shows an acceptable classification for the ECG location of MI according to leads showing abnormal Q waves. In addition, it depicts other processes that may result in false patterns of Q-wave MI. During the acute phase, ST-segment changes give a clue to the area at risk, but because of the normal variability in coronary anatomy and the presence of previous

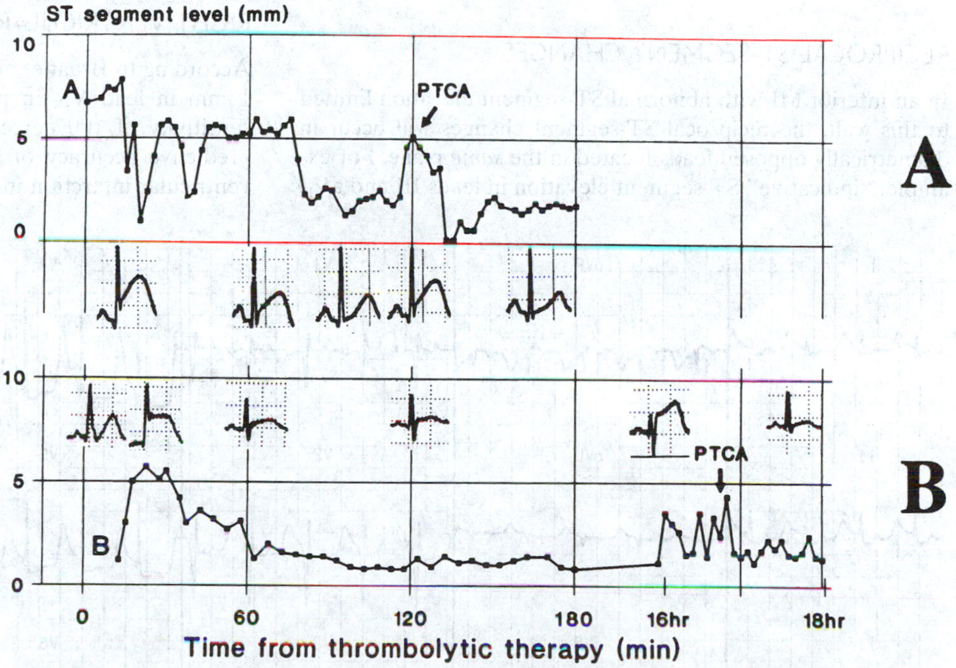

FIGURE 11-10 Assessment of thrombolytic therapy in patients with acute MI by ST-segment monitoring. Plots of ST-segment levels versus time from initiation of therapy in two selected patients with angiographic reocclusion. Patient A showed wide ST-segment shifts in the first 40 min, angiographic and electrocardiographic reperfusion at 90 min, and reocclusion at 120 min that required coronary angioplasty (PTCA). Patient B had successful thrombolysis within 60 min of initiation of therapy. At 16 h, ST-segment elevation recurred, and PTCA was performed.

TABLE 11-1 Electrocardiographic Location of Infarction Sites Based on the Presence of Abnormal Q Waves

Site	Leads	False Patterns
Inferior (diaphragmatic)	II, III, aV_F	WPW (PSAP), HCM
Inferolateral	II, III, aV_F, V_4–V_6	
"True" posterior (posterobasal)	V_1*	RVH, "atypical" incomplete RBBB, Left AP
Inferoposterior	II, III, aV_F, V_1*	WPW (left PSAP), HCM
Inferior-right ventricular	II, III, aV_F plus V_{4R}–V_{6R} or V_1–V_3	ASMI as defined from axis
Anteroseptal	V_1, V_2, V_3	LVH, chronic lung disease, LBBB, chest electrode misplacement
Anterolateral	I, II, V_4–V_6	HCM, ventricular septal defect
Extensive anterior	I, aV_L, V_1–V_6	
High lateral	I, aV_L	
Anterior (apical)	V_3–V_4	
Posterolateral	V_4–V_6, V_1*	WPW (LFWAP)
Right ventricular	V_{4R} with V_{4R}–V_{6R} or V_1–V_3	ASMI

*Tall R wave, "reciprocal" to changes in "indicative" back lead.

NOTE: ASMI = anteroseptal myocardial infarction; HCM = hypertrophic cardiomyopathy; LBBB = left bundle branch block; LFWAP = left free-wall accessory pathway; PSAP = posteroseptal accessory pathway; WPW = Wolff-Parkinson-White syndrome; RVH = right ventricular hypertrophy.

occlusions, there is sometimes more than one possible explanation for a specific ECG pattern.[55]

RECIPROCAL ST-SEGMENT CHANGES

In an inferior MI with abnormal ST-segment elevation limited to this wall, the reciprocal ST-segment changes will occur in diametrically opposed leads located in the *same* plane. For example, "indicative" ST-segment elevation in leads III and aV_F, which record the electrical activity of the inferior (posteroinferior or diaphragmatic) wall, yields "reciprocal" ST-segment depression in leads I and aV_L because they face the superior (anterolateral) wall[11,56,57] (see Fig. 11-3). ST-segment depression in lead V_2 may reflect injury in the anterior subendocardial wall as well as injury in the posterobasal (or true) posterior wall.[10] The ECG by itself cannot distinguish with absolute certainty between these two possibilities.[10] The differential diagnosis perhaps can best be made by performing cardiac catheterization or radionuclear studies in the acute phase of the MI, when the ST-segment changes are still present. Another way is by analyzing ST-segment changes occurring during percutaneous transluminal coronary angioplasty in patients with proven single-vessel disease.[58,59] This has shown that reciprocal ST-segment depression in leads V_2 and V_3 can occur during balloon occlusions of dominant right, as well as of dominant left, coronary arteries.[59]

RIGHT VENTRICULAR MI

According to Braat et al.,[60] an ST-segment elevation of at least 1 mm in lead V_{4R} in patients with *acute inferior MI* had a sensitivity of 100 percent, a specificity of 87 percent, and a predictive accuracy of 92 percent for the diagnosis of right ventricular infarction in patients with ST-segment elevation in leads II, III, and aV_F (see Fig. 11-3). These changes disappeared within 10 to 18 h after the onset of chest pain in 50 percent of their patients and after 72 h in the remaining patients.[60] In addition to V_{4R}, ST-segment elevation can be seen in leads V_5 and V_{6R} and in some cases (with decreasing amplitude) in V_1, V_2, and even V_3. It is possible for ST-segment depression in V_5 and V_6 to be reciprocal to right ventricular involvement (see Fig. 11-3).

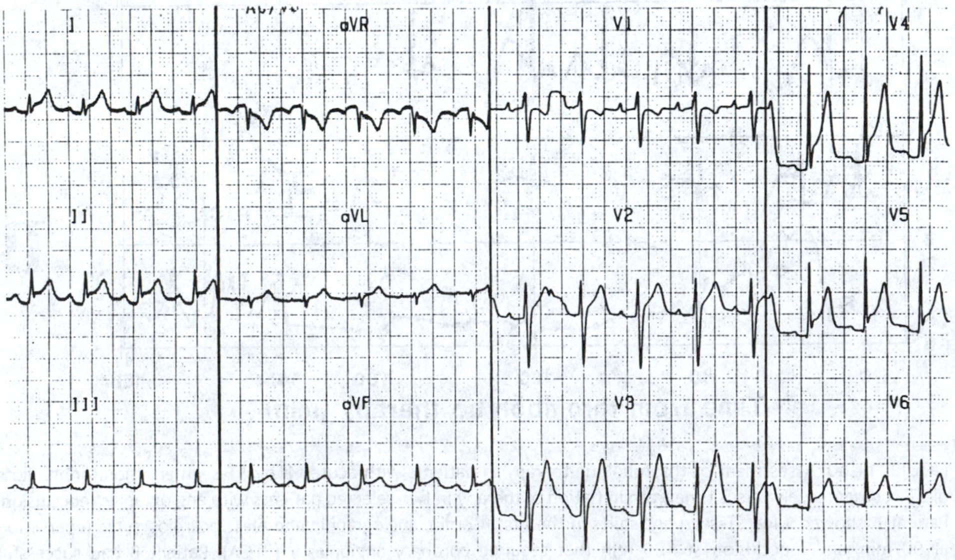

FIGURE 11-11 Acute nonspecific pericarditis showing ST-segment elevation in all leads except aV_R and V_1.

PERICARDITIS

The ECG pattern of acute (generalized) pericarditis not due to MI is produced by the associated epimyocarditis, which in turn results in diffuse epicardial "injury."[6] The

ST segments can be elevated in all leads except aV_R and, rarely, in V_1 (Fig. 11-11). Symmetric T-wave inversion (due to epicardial "ischemia") usually develops after the ST segments have returned to the baseline (but can appear during the injury stage).[6] Neither reciprocal ST-segment changes nor abnormal Q waves are seen. In most cases of acute pericarditis, the PR segment is depressed (see Fig. 11-11). Average ECG resolution occurs in close to 2 weeks.[11] The ECG pattern of acute pericarditis has to be differentiated from the normal variant referred to as *early repolarization* (see Fig. 11-4).

FASCICULAR BLOCKS

Generalities

There are several ways of proving that a given QRS pattern is due to a specific type of conduction abnormality.[15,57,61] First is extrapolation from animal experiments.[15,61] Second is ECG-pathologic correlation.[15,61] Third is an analysis of QRS changes produced by the inadvertent section of the conduction fascicles during open heart surgery or catheter-induced trauma.[62] Fourth is a comparison of tracings obtained before, during, and after the appearance or disappearance of conduction disturbances that are either persistent or (spontaneously or iatrogenically) intermittent. Under such circumstances, the QRS changes produced by fascicular block occur side by side with the control morphologies.[8,15,61,62,63] The various criteria proposed for diagnosis of fascicular blocks, though empirical, have been accepted for a very pragmatic reason: the need to interpret clinical ECGs. In reality, the sensitivity and specificity of these criteria require independent confirmation.[61,64] One can speculate that the latter may be provided by newer methods of intraoperative and body surface mapping and refinements in the technique of phase imaging or even perhaps Carto mapping, since few centers in the United States are currently performing histopathologic studies of the distal intraventricular conduction system.

Left Anterior Fascicular Block

In left anterior fascicular block (LAFB), the posteroinferior regions of the LV endocardium are activated abnormally before the anterosuperior LV area.[8,15] After emerging from the posteroinferior division of the left bundle branch, the impulse first propagates in an inferior, rightward, and usually anterior direction for a short period of time, producing q waves in leads I and aV_L and r waves in leads II, III, and aV_F (see Fig. 11-12). Thereafter, the general direction of the activation process (which determines the direction of the EA) occurs in a superior and leftward direction. Consequently, from the ECG viewpoint, the fascicles of the left branch behave more as if they were "superior" and "inferior" rather than "anterior" and "posterior" (Figs. 11-12 and 11-13). For this reason, the most significant abnormalities produced by LAFB, in the absence of complete right bundle branch block (RBBB), occur in the standard and unipolar extremity leads rather than in the precordial leads[8,15] (see Figs. 11-12 and 11-13). S waves frequently are recorded V_5 and V_6 because the depolarization wave first moves towards

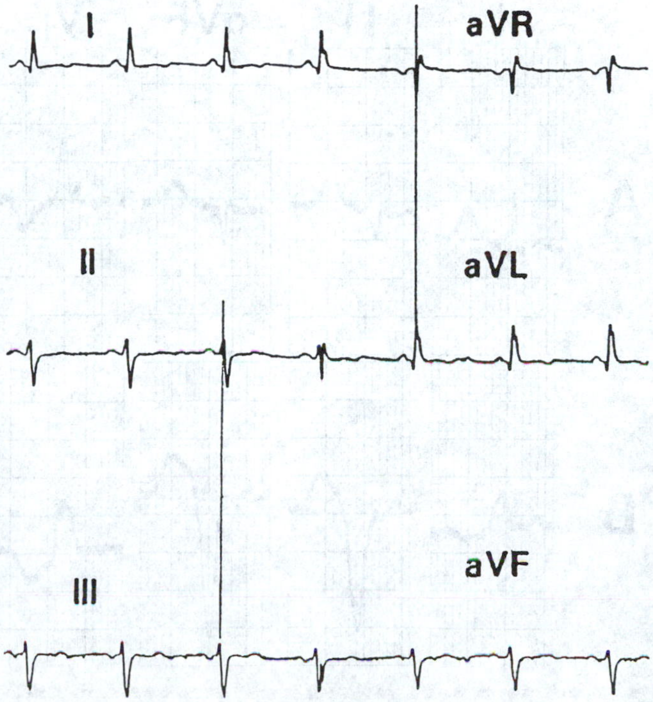

FIGURE 11-12 LAFB in a patient with primary conduction system disease. QRS duration: 0.10 s. At normal paper speeds (25 mm/s), the relationship between the peaks of the R waves (*vertical lines*) in simultaneously recorded leads II and III and aV_L and aV_R cannot be determined with the desired accuracy (see Fig. 11-13).

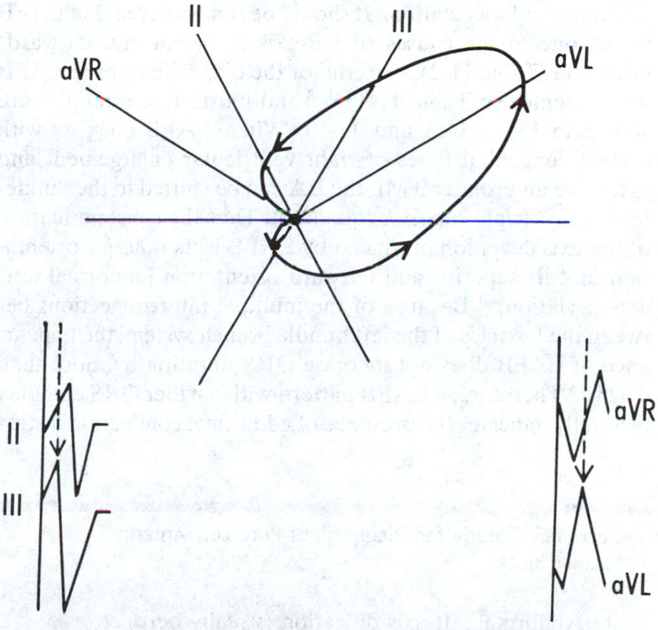

FIGURE 11-13 Derivation of electrocardiographic leads from a frontal plane QRS loop showing LAFB. Due to the counterclockwise rotation of the left superior loop, the peak of the R in aV_L preceded the peak of this deflection in aV_R (lower right). Furthermore, because the initial portion of the loop was inscribed on the positive half of the axis of lead III before it was inscribed on the positive half of the axis of lead II, the peak of the R in the former lead occurred before that in the latter lead. (From Castellanos A, Pina L, Zaman L, et al. Recent advances in the diagnosis of fascicular blocks. *Cardiol Clin* 1987; 5:469–488. Reproduced with permission from the publisher and authors.)

TABLE 11-2 Causes of Abnormal (−30° to −90°) Left-Axis Deviation

Cause	Characteristic Features
1. Left anterior fascicular block	1. rS complexes in lead II with positive T waves
2. Extensive inferior wall (AC5)MI	2. Qr complexes in lead II with ST-segment elevation and/or T-wave inversion
3. Extensive inferior wall MI with possible (AC7)LAFB	3. QS pattern in leads II, III, and aV_F with ST-segment elevation and/or T-wave inversion
4. Wolff-Parkinson-White syndrome (posteroseptal accessory pathway)	4. Short PR interval; delta wave
5. Hyperkalemia	5. Wide QRS complexes; peaked T waves
6. Pulmonary emphysema	6. Low voltage; peaked P waves, S waves in standard and precordial leads
7. Right ventricular apical pacing	7. Pacemaker spikes; predominantly negative ventricular deflections in V_1
8. Middle cardiac vein pacing	8. Pacemaker spikes; predominantly positive QRS deflections in V_1
9. Left coronary arteriography	9. Knowledge that dye was injected in left coronary artery

SOURCE: Used with permission from Castellanos and Myerburg.[15]

them and later, because of their relatively low position, away, in a more superior direction. The degree of left-axis deviation required for the diagnosis of complete LAFB has been a subject of debate and speculation.[8] It should be remembered that LAFB is but one of the causes of left-axis (superior and leftward) deviation (Table 11-2). Criteria for the diagnosis of pure LAFB are presented in Table 11-3,[8,64–68] and illustrative examples are shown in Figs. 11-12 and 11-13. When LAFB coexists with certain congenital types of right ventricular enlargement and extensive anterolateral MI, the EA can be shifted to the "undeterminate" (right superior) quadrant. Thus the constant feature of the axis deviation produced by LAFB is its *superior* orientation, not its superior and leftward orientation (abnormal left-axis deviation).[61] Because of the multiple interconnections between the fascicles of the left bundle branch system, the appearance of LAFB does not increase QRS duration by more than 0.025 s.[8] Therefore, a LAFB pattern with a wider QRS complex generally indicates the presence of additional conduction disturbances such as RBBB (Fig. 11-14, *top*), MI, or intraventricular conduction delays due to free wall fibrosis. Masquerading RBBB is said to be present when (with the classic findings in lead V_1) lead I shows what seems to be a left bundle branch block (LBBB) due to the absence of q and S waves (see Fig. 11-14, *bottom*). This pattern has been attributed to a terminal delay perpendicular to lead I associated with diffuse intramyocardial fibrosis.[15]

TABLE 11-3 Criteria for Diagnosis of Pure Left Anterior Fascicular Block

1. Abnormal left-axis deviation (usually between −45 and −60°)
2. rS complexes in leads II, III, and aV_F and qR complexes in leads I and aV_L
3. Delayed intrinsicoid deflection in leads I and aV_L
4. Peak of r wave in lead III occurring earlier than peak of r wave in lead II
5. Peak of R wave in lead aV_L occurring earlier than peak of R wave in aV_R

SOURCE: From Castellanos et al.[61] and Milliken,[64] with permission.

Left Anterior Fascicular Block Coexisting with MI

The ECG changes imposed by MIs of different locations on the LAFB are shown in Fig. 11-15. An inferior wall MI can be masked by a LAFB if the infarction does not involve the areas first depolarized by the impulse emergency from the unaffected fascicle.[8] In these cases, an r (slurred or not) can be seen in leads III and aV_F. It also has been stated that the change in left septal activation produced by the fascicular block may produce small r waves in V_1, V_2, and V_3 capable of modifying

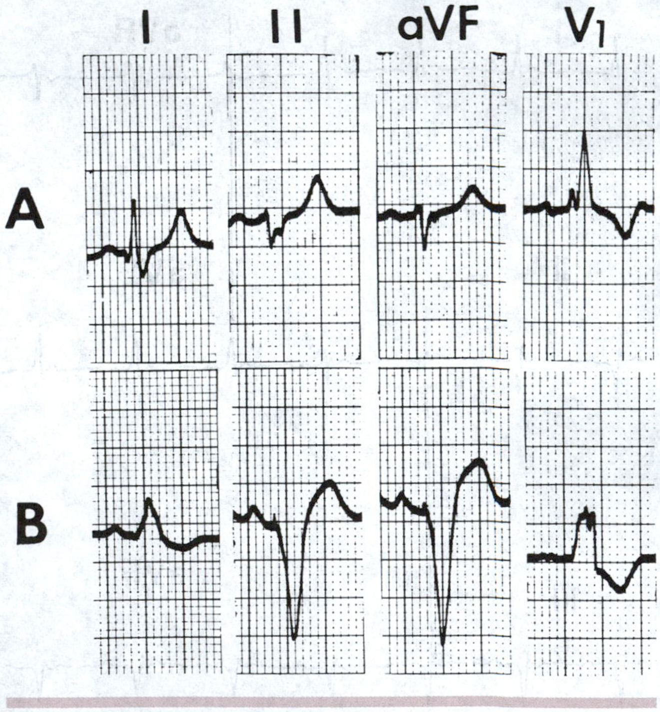

FIGURE 11-14 LAFB with wide QRS complexes. Whereas panel *A* shows LAFB with RBBB, these conduction disturbances coexist with diffuse septal and inferoposterior fibrosis in panel *B*. Consequently, the expected small q wave and the wide S wave in lead I are not present. This pattern has been called "masquerading" bundle branch block because the standard leads suggest LBBB, while the chest leads are diagnostic of RBBB.

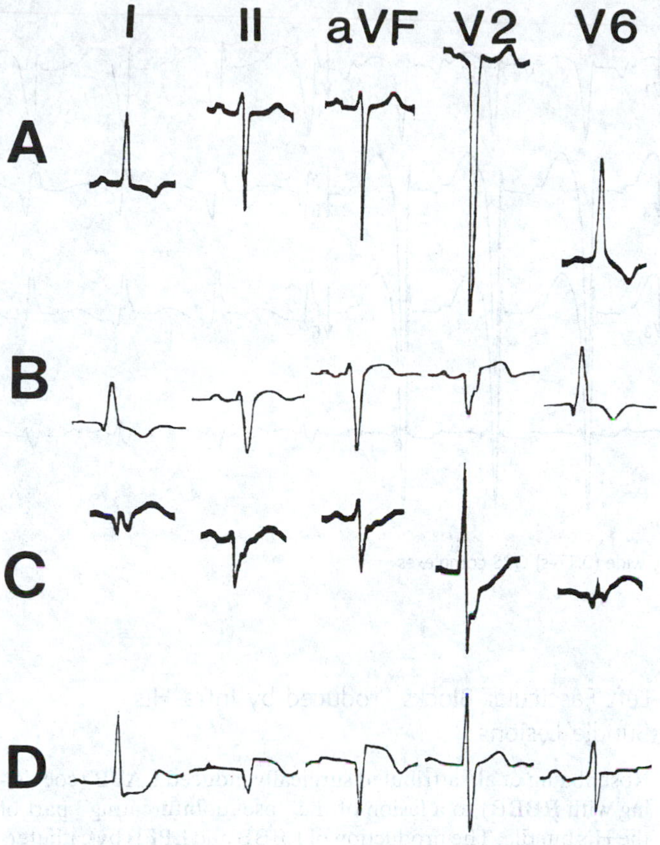

FIGURE 11-15 Diagnosis of LAFB associated with MI. Diagnostic feature given in parentheses. *A.* LAFB and anteroseptal MI (QR or QS complex in right chest leads). *B.* LAFB and anterolateral MI (abnormal Q wave in leads I and V_6). *C.* LAFB and anterolateral MI with electrical axis in the right superior quadrant (Q wave in leads I and V_6). *D.* LAFB and inferior wall MI (QR or QS complexes and elevation of J point and ST segments in leads II and III).

the characteristics QS complexes produced by anteroseptal MI in these leads.[8]

Nonspecific Intraventricular Conduction Delays

Several names have been applied to the conduction disturbances occurring in the left-sided Purkinje-myocardial junctions, left septal surface, or free wall of the left ventricle: *arborization block, diffuse (nonspecific) intraventricular block, peri-infarction block, parietal block, focal block,* etc.[8,66–75] These conduction disturbances have different electrogenetic mechanisms. Thus the cellular "affectation" due to acute injury resulting from coronary artery disease, hyperkalemia, drugs, and intracoronary injections of contrast material occurs within (inside) the affected regions.[5,15,75] Blocks occurring in subacute or chronic MI after the appearance of abnormal Q waves (peri-infarction block) (Fig. 11-16), as well as those occurring in the presence of diffuse myocardial fibrosis (Fig. 11-17), are due to the circuitous and irregular activation of living cells surrounding areas of fibrotic tissue.[68–75]

Left Posterior Fascicular Block

In pure left posterior fascicular block (LPFB), the impulse emerges from the unblocked anterosuperior division, thus producing small q waves in leads II, III, and aV_F.[8,15] Thereafter, the impulse moves through the electrically predominant left ventricle in an inferior and rightward direction, thus explaining the S waves in leads I and aV_L as well as the R waves in leads II, III, and aV_F.[8,15] Radiologic studies of the human heart in situ have shown that the paraseptal regions of the posteroinferior (diaphragmatic) surface of the anatomic *left* ventricle are spatially located more to the *right* than certain (anterior) portions of the anatomic right ventricle.[15] Since the portions of the left ventricle that are spatially located to the right are less than those located superiorly, the degree of right-axis deviation produced by pure LPFB is of lesser magnitude than that of left-

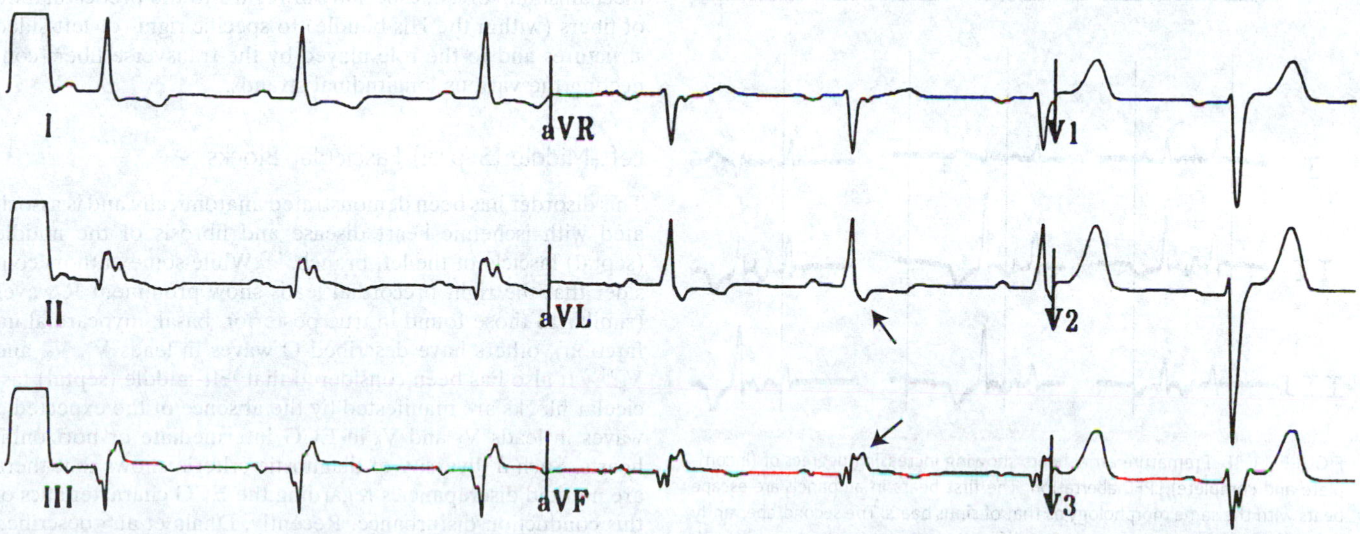

FIGURE 11-16 Type of nonspecific intraventricular conduction delay known as *peri-infarction block*. The patient had an evolving inferior wall MI. The wide (0.14-s) ventricular complexes show a predominantly terminal delay (*arrows*) and notching (more evident in the inferior leads) without a typical LBBB or RBBB morphology.

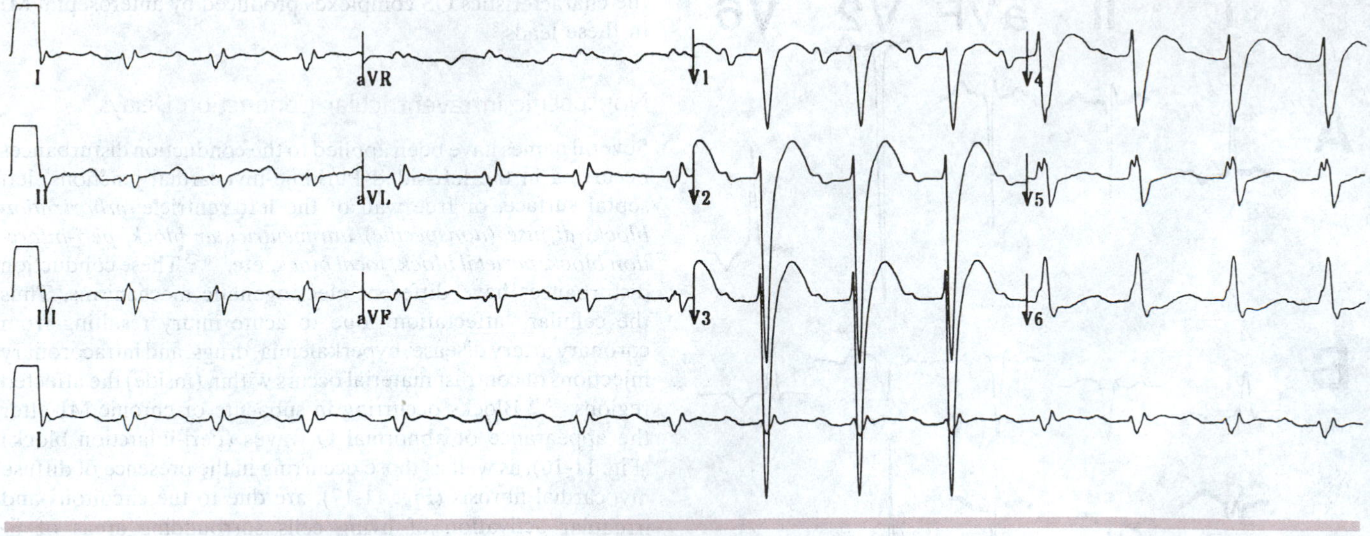

FIGURE 11-17 Nonspecific intraventricular conduction delay characterized by very wide (0.17-s) QRS complexes not showing a typical RBBB or LBBB pattern.

axis deviation produced by LAFB.[15] The hallmark of LPFB, therefore, is an "inferior" axis shift as much as "right" axis deviation (Figs. 11-18 to 11-20). Because a similar sequence of ventricular activation also can occur in right ventricular hypertrophy, pleuropulmonary disease (acute or chronic), and extremely vertical anatomic heart positions due to a slender body build or chest wall deformities, it is evident that the diagnosis of "pure" LPFB cannot be made from the ECG alone. Additional clinical, radiologic, or pathologic information is required for this purpose.[8,15,61,66] The changes imposed in LPFB by MIs of different locations are depicted in Figs. 11-18 to 11-20.

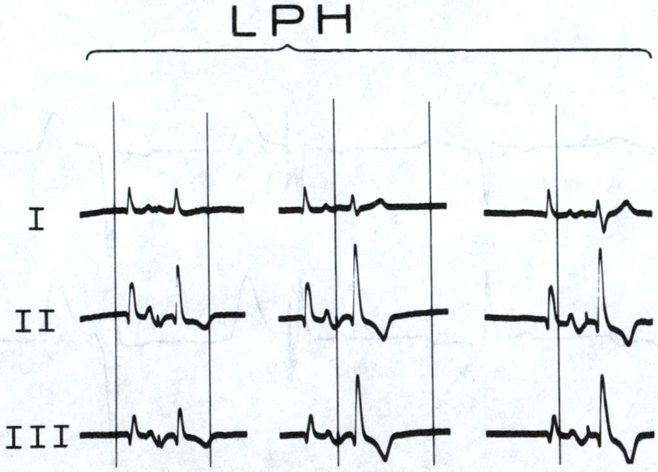

FIGURE 11-18 Premature atrial beats showing increasing degrees of (incomplete and complete) LPFB aberration. The first beats in all panels are escape beats with the same morphology as that of sinus beats. The second, aberrantly induced ventricular complexes show different degrees of right-axis shift with an increase in size of the R waves in leads II and III. Note that the fundamental characteristic of LPFB was not right-axis deviation (beyond +90°) but an inferior-axis shift. (From Castellanos A, Myerburg RJ. *The Hemiblocks in Myocardial Infarction*. New York: Appleton-Century-Crofts; 1976. Reproduced with permission from the publisher and authors.)

Left Fascicular Blocks Produced by Intra-His Bundle Lesions

Rosenbaum et al.[8] attributed surgically induced LAFB (coexisting with RBBB) to a lesion of the "pseudobifurcating" part of the His bundle. The production of LBBB and LPFB by catheters located in the right-sided cavities, however, cannot be explained by assuming direct affectation of these left-sided structures.[76,77] Nevertheless, they have been reported and attributed to the His bundle trauma produced by Swan-Ganz catheters.[76,77] In fact, certain clinical and experimental studies have shown that some bundle branch block patterns could be normalized by distal His bundle pacing.[78] Longitudinal dissociation of conduction within a usually diseased His bundle should be present for this to occur. There is, however, disagreement as to the mechanism involved, especially in regard to the predestination of fibers (within the His bundle) to specific right- or left-sided structures and to the role played by the transverse fibers connecting the various longitudinal strands.[77–80]

Left-Middle (Septal) Fascicular Blocks

This disorder has been demonstrated anatomically and is associated with ischemic heart disease and fibrosis of the middle (septal) fascicle of the left branch.[81,82] While some authors consider that the right precordial leads show prominent R waves (similar to those found in true posterior, basal, myocardial infarction), others have described Q waves in leads V_1, V_2, and V_3.[81,82] It also has been considered that left-middle (septal) fascicular blocks are manifested by the absence of the expected q waves in leads V_5 and V_6 in ECG intermediate or horizontal hearts. Such a diversity of diagnostic criteria shows that there are marked discrepancies regarding the ECG characteristics of this conduction disturbance. Recently, Dhala et al.[83] described what they considered as the unmasking of the trifascicular conduction system by catheter ablation of the right bundle branch with a diseased left intraventricular conduction system. In these cases, ablation-induced damage to "predestined" fibers in a diseased His bundle cannot be totally excluded.

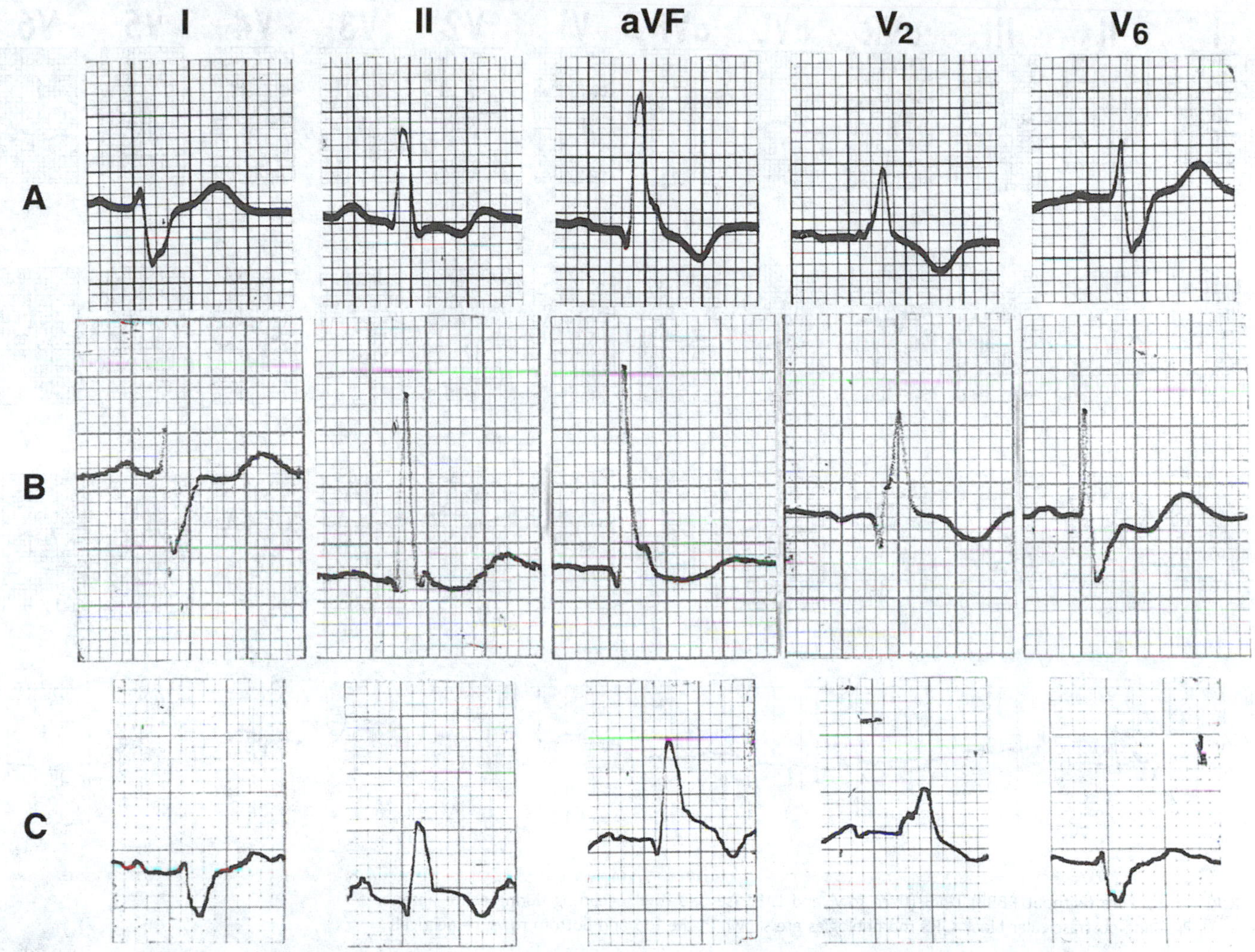

FIGURE 11-19 LPFB with RBBB. *A.* No MI. *B.* Anteroseptal MI (note q wave in V_2). *C.* Inferior MI (note ST-segment elevation and T-wave inversion in leads II and aV_F with slight ST-segment depression in lead I). The differences in QRS complexes between *A* and *C* are not very marked because pure LPFB may produce an almost abnormal Q wave in the inferior leads.

Complete RBBB

A "complete" RBBB pattern (with QRS duration of ≥0.12 s) does not necessarily reflect the existence of a total conduction block in the right branch. This pattern only indicates that the entire or major parts of both ventricles are activated by the impulse emerging from the left branch.[15,84,85] Thus a significant degree of conduction delay ("high grade" or "incomplete" RBBB) can produce a similar pattern. In pure complete RBBB, the EA should not be deviated *abnormally* either to the left or to the right. These axis deviations reflect coexisting fascicular block (see Figs. 11-14 and 11-19) or right ventricular hypertrophy.

Incomplete RBBB Pattern

For many years what has been proven with endocardial (catheter) and epicardial mapping has been recognized—namely, that incomplete RBBB "patterns" can be produced by various mechanisms[84–90]: (1) different degrees of conduction delays through the main trunk of the right bundle branch, (2) an increased conduction time through an elongated right bundle branch that is stretched because of a concomitant enlargement of the right septal surface, (3) a diffused Purkinje-myocardial delay due to right ventricular (RV) stretch or dilatation, (4) surgical trauma or disease-related interruption of the major ramifications of the right branch ("distal" RBBB), or (5) congenital variations of the distribution of the major distal ramifications resulting in a slight delay in activation of the crista supraventricularis.[6] In arrhythmogenic RV dysplasia, the S wave in V_1 is followed by a sharp, wide, positive deflection (epsilon wave; Fig. 11-5*B*) attributed to delayed ventricular activation (postexcitation) in some RV myocardial fibers.[39] Wide QRS complexes in this lead (wider than in other precordial leads) were attributed to a "parietal" block superimposed on a RBBB.[35]

Concealed RBBB

A minor conduction delay in the main trunk of the right bundle branch or in its major ramifications may be "concealed" (not

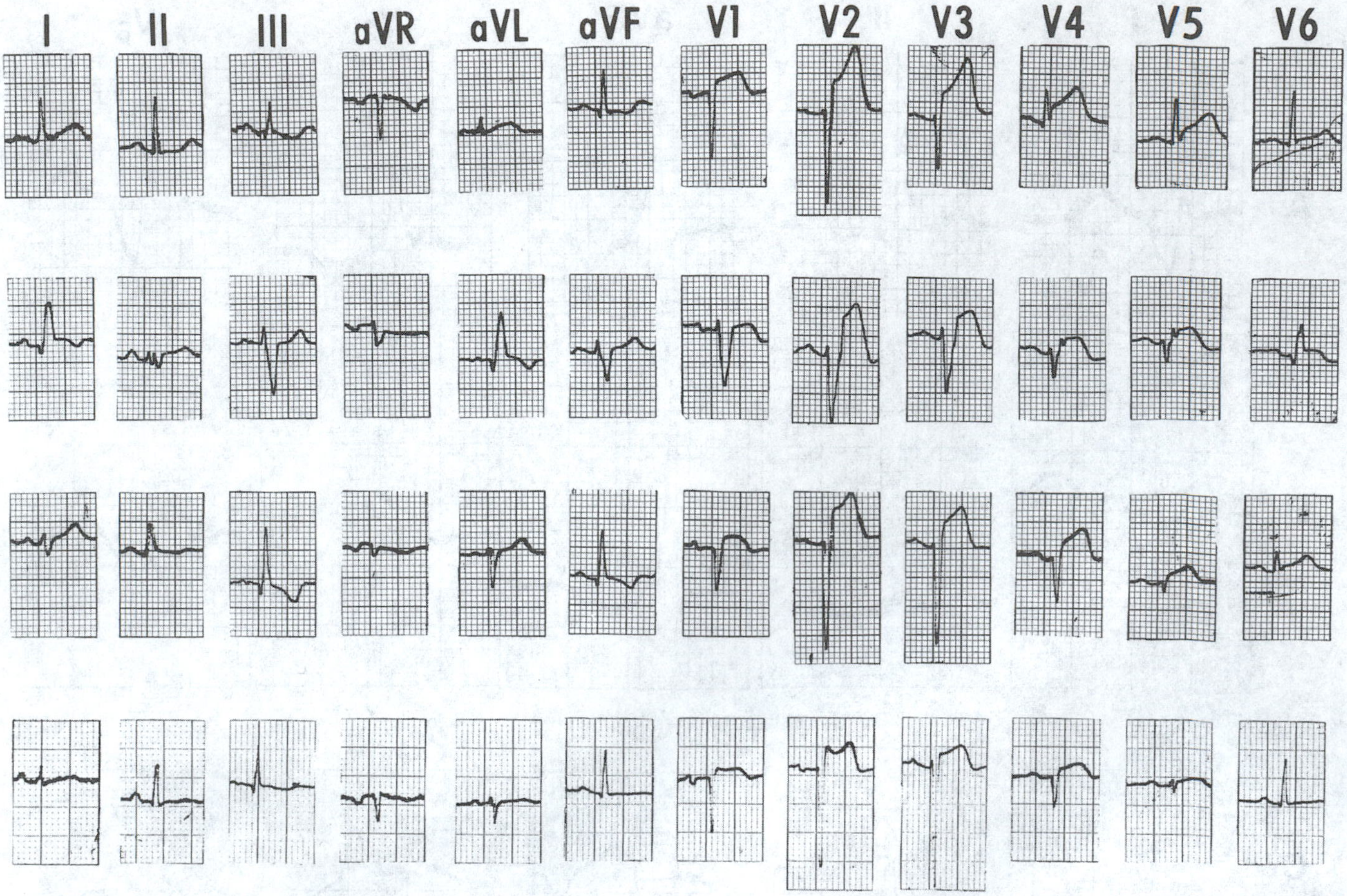

FIGURE 11-20 Pure (without RBBB) LPFB (third row) and LAFB (second row) occurring during acute anterior wall MI. Pre- and postfascicular block QRS morphologies are shown in the top and bottom rows, respectively.

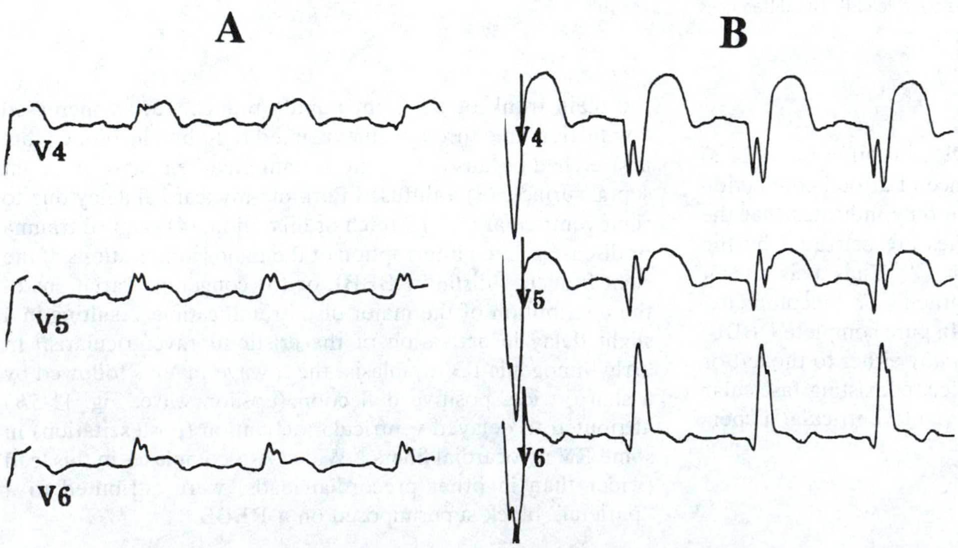

FIGURE 11-21 Morphologic characteristics of complete LBBB complicated by acute anterior MI. *A.* Abnormal ST-segment elevation without q waves (QRS duration: 0.14 s). *B.* Abnormal ST-segment elevation, obtained from another patient, persisted after the appearance of abnormal Q waves (QRS duration: 0.13 s).

manifested in the surface ECG) when there are coexisting (and of greater degree) conduction disturbances in the main left bundle branch, the anterosuperior division of the left bundle branch, and/or the free LV wall.[8,15] An RBBB also can be concealed in some patients with Wolff-Parkinson-White syndrome if the ventricular insertion of the accessory pathway causes preexcitation of the RV regions that would be activated late because of the RBBB.[91]

Complete LBBB

This conduction disturbance is characterized by wide (>0.11 s) QRS complexes. The diagnostic criteria consist of prolongation of the QRS complexes (>0.11 s) with neither a q nor an S wave in leads

I, aV_L, and a *properly placed* V_6. A wide R wave with a notch on its top ("plateau") is seen in these leads. Apparently, the EAs of most *uncomplicated* complete LBBBs usually are not located beyond 30°.[8,15,16] Complete LBBB with abnormal left-axis deviation indicates a great degree of left Purkinje and myocardial disease.

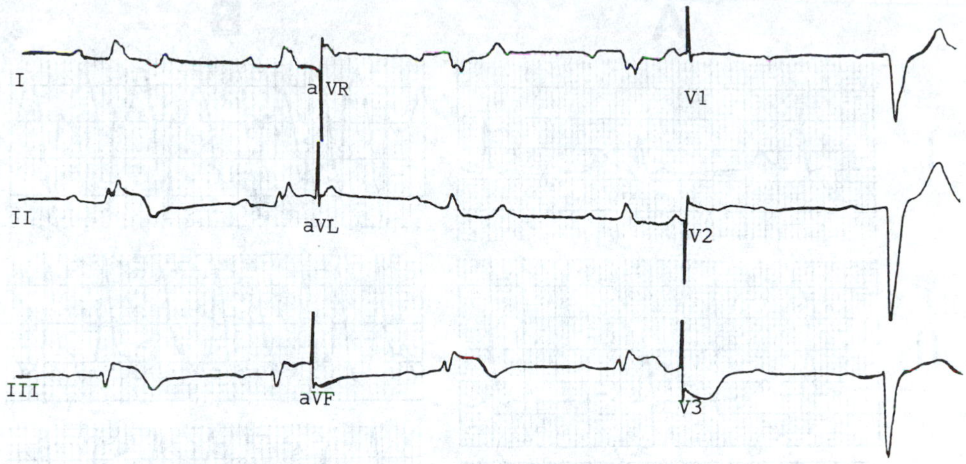

FIGURE 11-22 Morphologic features of complete LBBB complicated by acute inferior MI. There is abnormal ST-segment elevation in leads II, III, and aV_F (QRS duration: 0.14 s). AV block is also present.

Complete LBBB with Acute MI

The classic pattern of LBBB may not be modified by a small area of myocardial necrosis. This explains why thrombolytics may be given if clinical findings characteristic of MI occur in patients with a LBBB pattern. Recent studies, however, have shown that occlusions of a coronary artery by either an angioplasty balloon or (a presumably large) MI can produce ST-segment changes as in the absence of a conduction disturbance.[112] Recently, Sgarbossa[92] has suggested that ST-segment elevation of 1 mm or more concordant with QRS polarity has a high specificity and sensitivity. ST-segment elevation of 5 mm or more discordant with QRS polarity, ST-segment depression of 1 mm or more in V_1, V_2, and V_3, and (sudden) positive T waves in V_4 and V_5 have a high specificity but a low sensitivity. The latter can occur transiently during acute ischemia (pseudonormalization) without myocardial necrosis or be persistently present in cases where its significance is unclear. Examples of LBBB complicated by acute anterior and inferior MI are shown in Figs. 11-21 and 11-22. The above-mentioned criteria also can be applied to diagnose acute MI in patients with pacemakers.[92,93]

Complete LBBB with Old MI

Normally, in complete LBBB, the impulse emerges from the right bundle branch and propagates inferiorly, to the left, and slightly anteriorly. This orientation of the initial forces tends to abolish previously present inferiorly and laterally located abnormal Q waves characteristic of inferior and lateral wall MIs.[15,93,94] If the infarction is anteroseptal, however, the impulse cannot propagate toward the left. Instead, the initial vectors point toward the free wall of the right ventricle because now the RV free-wall forces are not neutralized by the normally preponderant septal and/or initial LV free-wall forces.[15] Thus a small q wave will be recorded in leads I, V_5, and V_6, where it is not normally present in complete LBBB (Fig. 11-23*A*). For a recent review of this subject, see Ref. 92. Similar findings can be seen in paced beats when in lead I the spike is followed by a well-defined q wave (see Fig. 11-23*B*). Several studies reported that Q waves in lead I or in two or more lateral leads (I, aV_L or V_5 and V_6) have high specificity but moderate sensitivity.[92] The sign of Cabrera and Friedland (late notching of S waves in V_3 through V_5) has been found to have higher to moderate specificity and moderate to low sensitivity.[94] Notching of the upstroke of the R wave in leads I, aV_L, V_5, and V_6 (sign of Chapman) has a sensitivity of 21 percent and a specificity of 82 percent.[94]

Complete LBBB with LV Hypertrophy

This is discussed under "LV Hypertrophy," below.

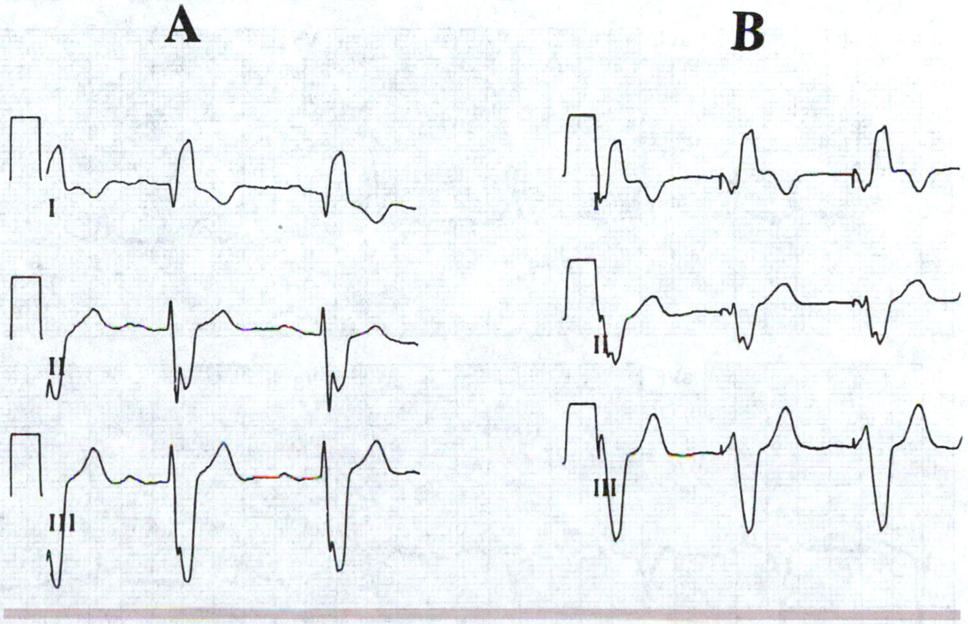

FIGURE 11-23 *A*. Complete LBBB with old anterior MI. Abnormal Q waves are present in lead I (QRS duration: 0.18 s). *B*. Pacing-induced complete LBBB pattern in a patient with old anterior MI. There are abnormal Q waves in lead I after spikes (QRS duration: 0.20 s). Note resemblance between natural and artificial (electrically induced) QRS patterns.

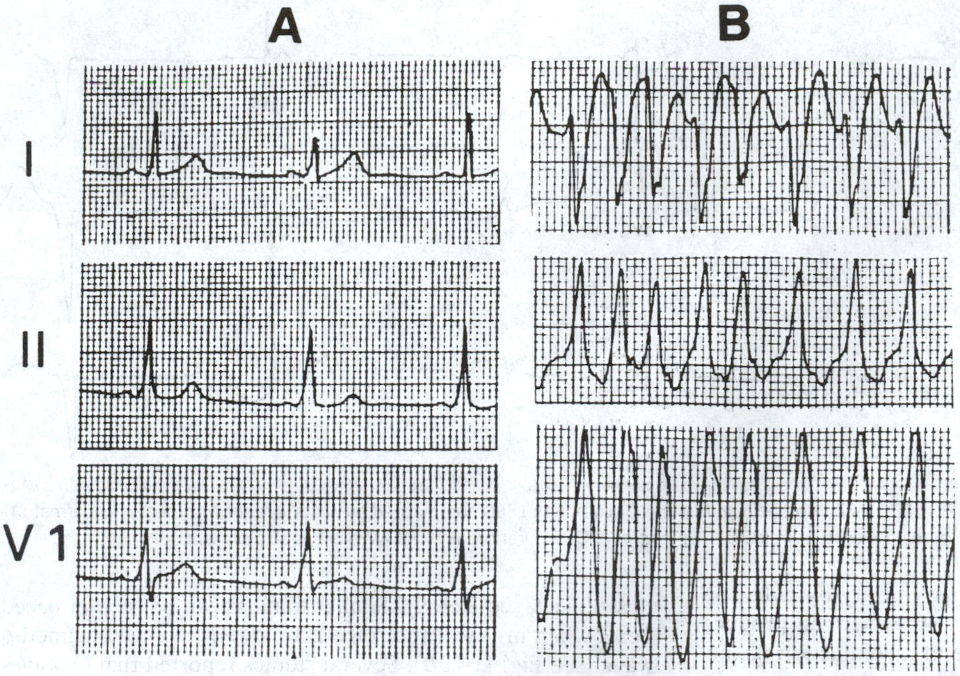

FIGURE 11-24 Wolff-Parkinson-White syndrome in a patient with a left free-wall accessory pathway. *A.* Sinus rhythm with fusion beats showing different degrees of preexcitation. *B.* Maximal preexcitation during atrial fibrillation. Note marked change in QRS duration and electrical axis.

Incomplete LBBB Pattern

An incomplete LBBB pattern can be diagnosed if leads I and an *appropriately placed* V_6 show an R wave not preceded by a q wave.[6] Lead V_1 shows rS or QS complexes, and lead V_2 shows rS complexes. Although QRS duration usualy ranges between 0.08 and 0.11 s, this *pattern* can be observed with QRS durations of 0.12 and 0.13 s.

Wide QRS Complexes in Patients with Manifest Preexcitation Syndromes

The characteristic pattern of manifest Wolff-Parkinson-White syndrome during sinus rhythm is well known.[95–103] The ventricular complex is a fusion beat resulting from ventricular activation by two wave fronts.[116–126] The degree of preexcitation (amount of muscle activated through the accessory path-

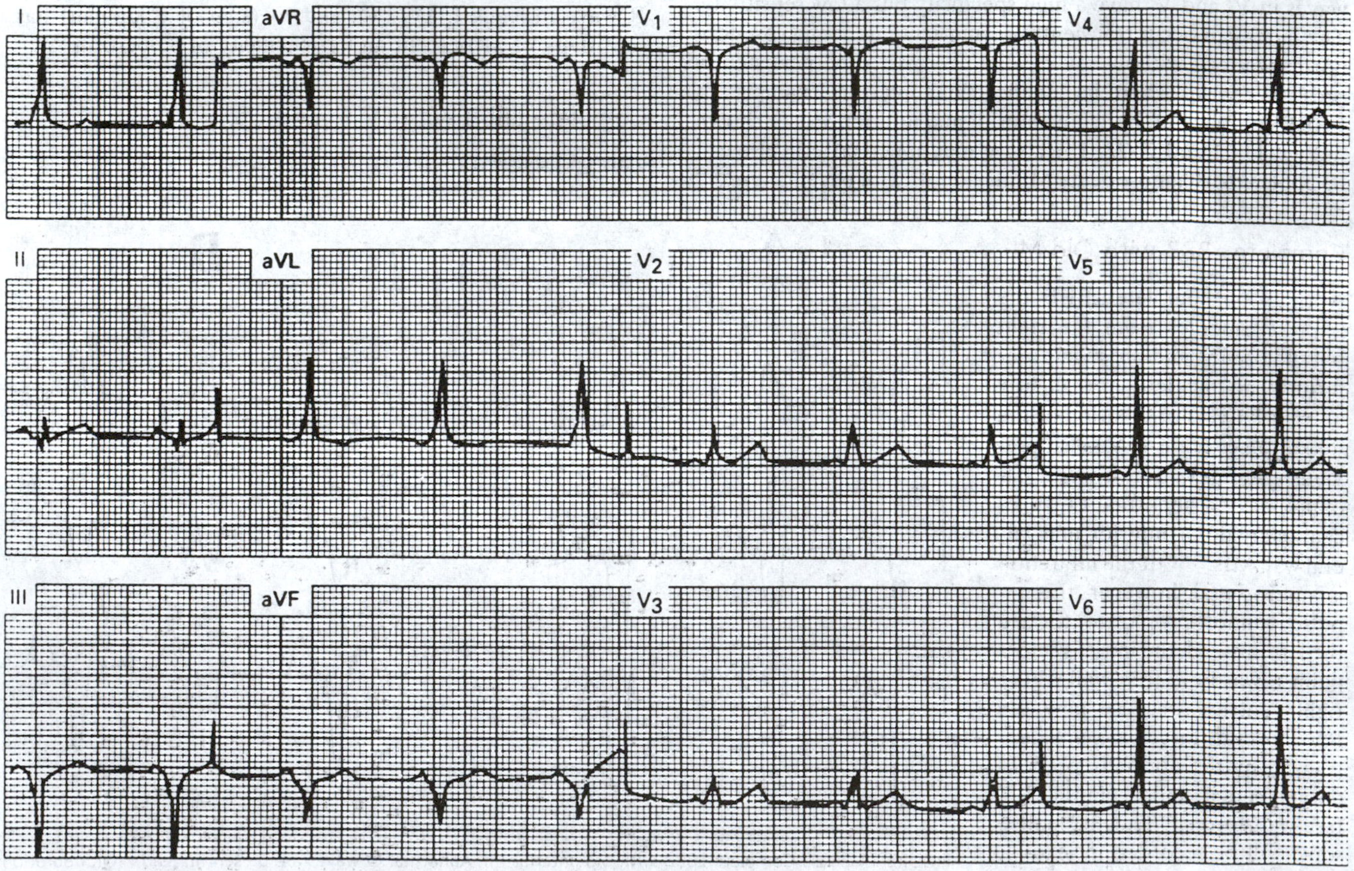

FIGURE 11-25 Wolff-Parkinson-White syndrome in a patient having a posteroseptal accessory pathway. Note short PR intervals with negative delta waves in leads III and aV_F (false pattern of inferior MI). Lead V_2 shows all-positive QRS complexes.

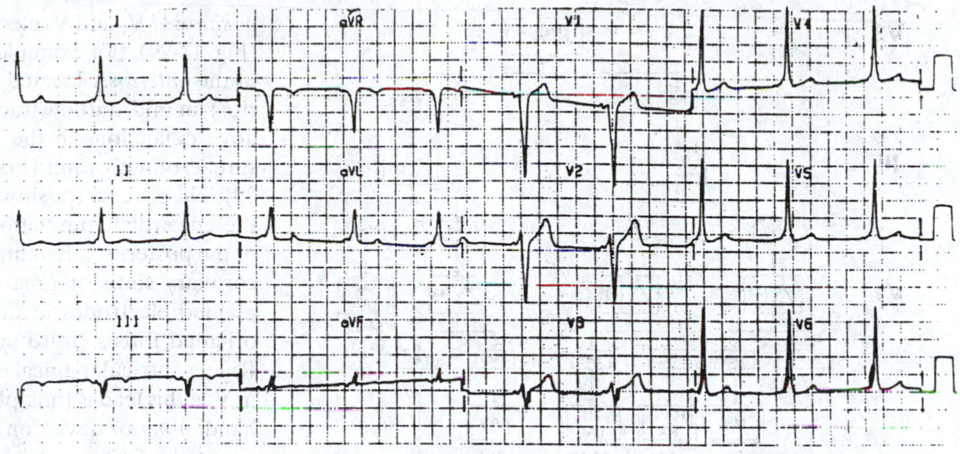

FIGURE 11-26 Wolff-Parkinson-White syndrome in a patient with a right free-wall accessory pathway. Note LBBB "pattern" characterized for diagnostic (of accessory pathway location) purposes by a QRS duration greater than 0.09 s in lead I with rS complexes in leads V_1 and V_2. The electrical axis is approximately +15°.

way) is variable and depends on many factors. Foremost among these are the distance between the sinus node and atrial insertion of the accessory pathway and, more important, the differences in refractory period duration and in conduction time through the normal pathway and the accessory pathway. Other things being equal, a patient with rapid (enhanced) AV nodal conduction will have a smaller delta wave than a patient with slow conduction through the AV node. Moreover, if there is total block at the AV node or His-Purkinje system, the impulse will be conducted exclusively via the accessory pathway bundle.[96,99–101] Consequently, the QRS complexes are different from fusion beats, although the direction of the delta wave remains the same. Moreover, the QRS complexes are as wide as (and really simulating) those produced by artificial or spontaneous beats arising in the vicinity of the ventricular end of the accessory pathway.[96,99–101] The original ECG classification of manifest Wolff-Parkinson-White syndrome proposed by Rosenbaum et al.[97] is now of historical interest only. Nevertheless, initial noninvasive determination of the anatomic position of the accessory pathway is of great clinical importance because of the introduction of surgical and catheter ablative techniques for symptomatic cases of preexcitation.

Toward the end of the millennium, Basiouny et al.[104] reported that there were 41 publications dealing with methods for localizing the accessory pathways of patients with preexcitation syndrome. Of these, they analyzed what they considered the most important algorithms available for this purpose. The interested reader can consult this article.[104] For the purposes of this chapter and due to space limitations, we will refer to the pioneer study of Milstein et al.,[102] who analyzed the direction of the delta wave and divided the mitral and tricuspid ring areas where the pathways are located into various segments. These investigators considered that only four segments were necessary. This appeared logical, for at the time that this method was proposed, most ablations were performed surgically.[102,103] Left free-wall accessory pathways are characterized by isoelectric and even positive delta waves in leads I, aV_L, V_5, or V_6. Lead V_1 shows R or Rs complexes (Fig. 11-24). During sinus rhythm, the electrical axis may be normal, but when atrial fibrillation develops and exclusive accessory pathway conduction occurs, the EA is deviated to the right and inferiorly (see Fig. 11-24). Posteroseptal accessory pathways show negative delta waves in leads III and aV_F and R waves in V_2. An Rs (or RS) wave in V_1 suggests a left posteroseptal pathway; a QS complex in the same lead may correspond to a right posteroseptal pathway (Fig. 11-25). Right free-wall accessory pathways display an LBBB pattern defined, for purposes of accessory pathway localization, by an R wave greater than 0.09 s in lead I and rS complexes in leads V_1 and V_2 with an electrical axis ranging between +30 and −60° (Fig. 11-26).

Right anteroseptal accessory pathways show an LBBB pattern (as defined) with an electrical axis ranging between +30

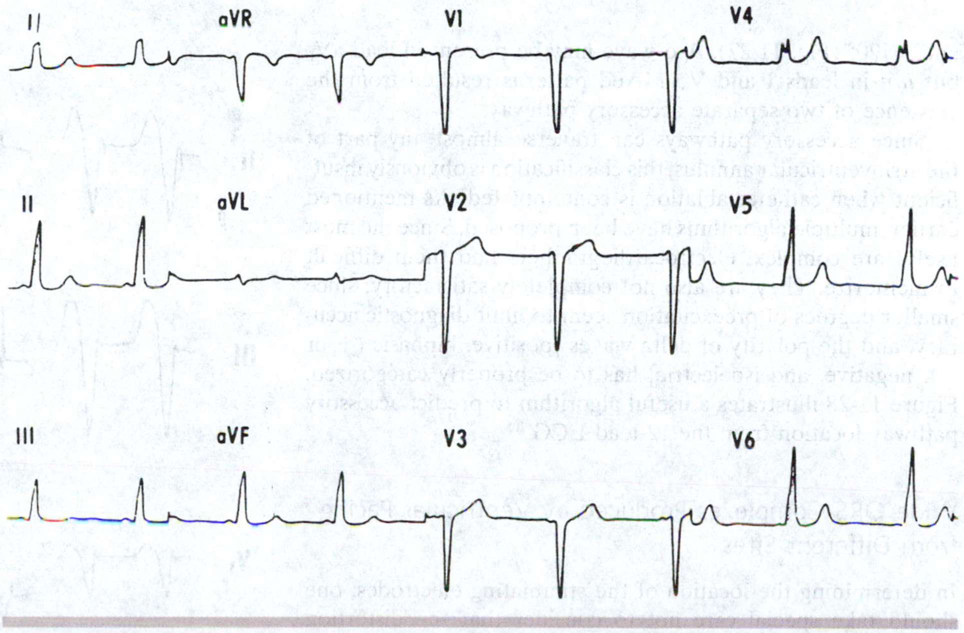

FIGURE 11-27 Wolff-Parkinson-White syndrome in a patient with a right anteroseptal accessory pathway. Note LBBB pattern (as defined in Fig. 11-26). The most important difference with the latter is that the electrical axis points more vertically, toward +60°, thereby being located within the range of the axis (+30 to +120°) reported for right anteroseptal accessory pathways.

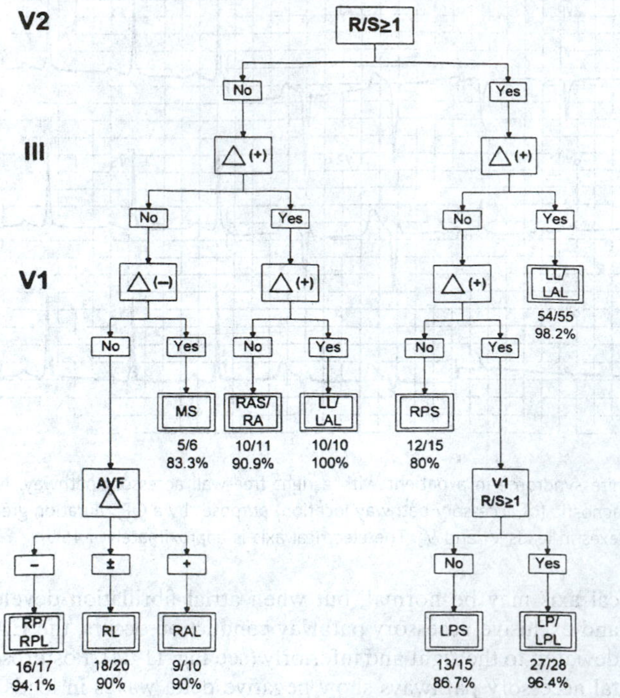

FIGURE 11-28 Useful algorithm to predict accessory pathway location from the 12-lead ECG. Step 1: Analysis of R/S ratio in V_2. Step 2: Existence of positive (+) delta wave in lead III (initial 40 ms). Step 3: Existence of positive or negative (−) delta wave in V_1 (initial 60 ms). Step 4: Delta-wave polarity in aV_F (initial 40 ms) or analysis of R/S ratio in V_1 (± = biphasic or isoelectric). The accuracy of the algorithm for each location in 187 prospective patients is also shown at the bottom. LAL, left anterolateral; LL, left lateral; LP, left posterior; LPL, left posterolateral; LPS, left posteroseptal; MS, midseptal; RA, right anterior; RAL, right anterolateral; RAS, right anteroseptal; RL, right lateral; RP, right posterior; RPL, right posterolateral; RPS, right posteroseptal. (From Chiang et al.[105] Reproduced with permission from the publisher and authors.)

and +120° (Fig. 11-27). A q wave may be present in lead aV_L but *not* in leads I and V_6. Mixed patterns resulted from the existence of two separate accessory pathways.

Since accessory pathways can traverse almost any part of the atrioventricular annulus, this classification is obviously insufficient when catheter ablation is contemplated. As mentioned earlier, multiple algorithms have been proposed. Since the most useful are complex, electrocardiographers find them difficult to memorize. They are also not completely satisfactory, since smaller degrees of preexcitation seem to limit diagnostic accuracy, and the polarity of delta waves [positive, biphasic (+ or −), negative, and isoelectric] has to be properly categorized. Figure 11-28 illustrates a useful algorithm to predict accessory pathway location from the 12-lead ECG.[105]

Wide QRS Complexes Produced by Ventricular Pacing from Different Sites

In determining the location of the stimulating electrodes, one should take special care not to consider that the distortion produced by large unipolar spikes constitutes parts of the pacing-induced QRS complexes. It is best *not* to describe the electrically produced ventricular beats as having an RBBB or LBBB morphology, since what is relevant is the polarity of the *properly positioned* V_1 and V_2 electrodes and the direction of the EA[106,107] (Fig. 11-29). For example, endocardial or epicardial stimulation of the *anteriorly* located right ventricle at any site [apical (inferior), or mid/outflow tract (superior)] yields predominantly negative deflections in the right chest leads due to the *posterior* spread of activation (first and second vertical rows in Fig. 11-29). The reverse (positive deflections in V_1 and V_2) occurs when the epicardial stimulation of the superior and lateral portions of the posterior left ventricle by catheter electrodes in the distal coronary sinus or great and middle cardiac veins (or by implanted electrodes in the nearby muscle) results in *anteriorly* oriented forces (third and fourth vertical rows in Fig. 11-29). Right ventricular apical pacing may produce positive deflections in V_1 if this lead is (mis)placed above its usual level. On the other hand, *superior* deviation of the electrical axis only indicates that a spatial *inferior* ventricular site has been stimulated, regardless of whether this site is the apical portion of the right ventricle or the inferior part of the left ventricle, the latter being paced through the middle cardiac vein (first and fourth vertical rows in Fig. 11-29). Conversely, an *inferior* vertical axis is simply a consequence of pacing from a *superior* site, which can be the endocardium of the RV outflow tract or the epicardium of the posterosuperior and lateral portions of the left ventricle (second and third vertical rows in Fig. 11-29). The changes produced on the basic ECG patterns of paced beats produced by MI were briefly discussed in the section of LBBB and MI. The method discussed above to locate the site of impulse initiation during pacing is simpler than the more complicated ones used to determine the ventricular sites of exit from accessory pathways (cross-

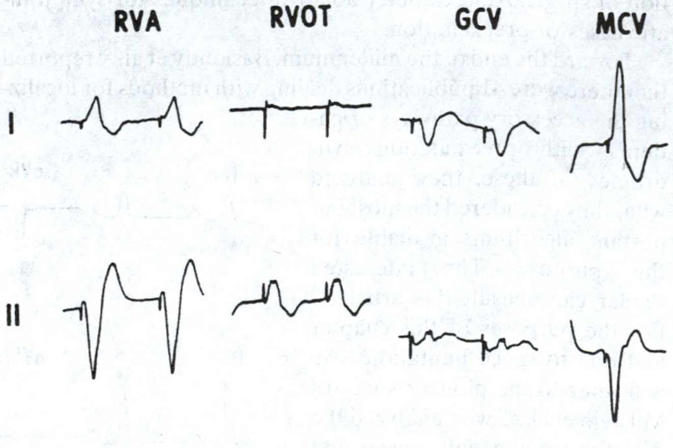

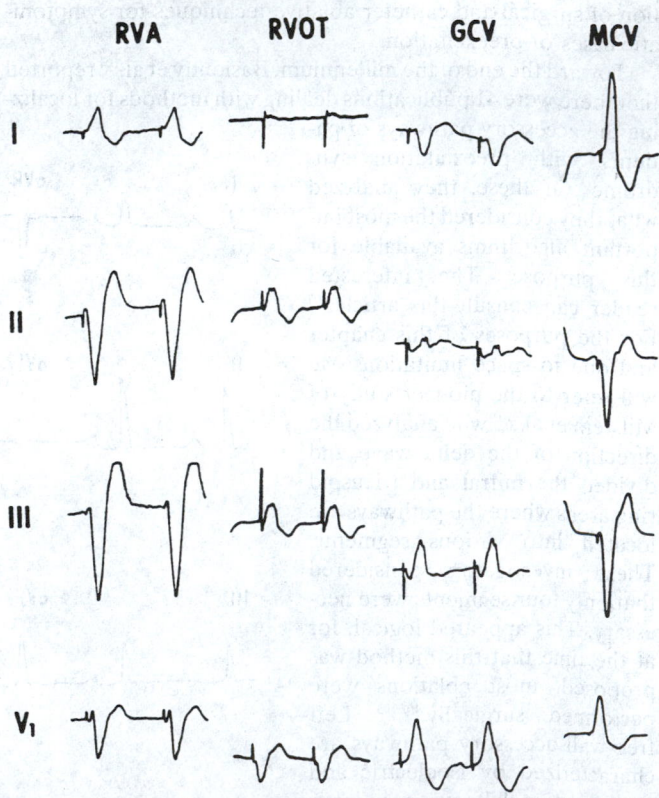

FIGURE 11-29 QRS changes (location of the electrical axis and polarity of lead V_1) produced by pacing from right ventricular apex (RVA), right ventricular outflow tract (RVOT), great cardiac vein (GCV), and middle cardiac vein (MCV).

ing the AV junction), which require the use of right anterior oblique and, specially, left anterior oblique projections. The currently used nomenclature for accessory pathway location was discussed recently and challenged by a group of notable experts in the field of preexcitation.[108]

Left Atrial Hypertrophy

Munuswamy et al.,[109] using M-mode echocardiography as the "gold standard," evaluated the specificity and sensitivity of the most important clues for determining left atrial hypertrophy. These included (1) P wave duration greater than 0.11 s and notched P wave with an interpeak interval in excess of 0.04 s and (2) negative phase of P in V_1 longer than 0.04 s and greater than 1 mm in lead V_1. There are, however, problems when applying these criteria in a given ECG. For example, according to Josephson,[110] prolonged duration of the P wave and of (posteriorly directed) terminal forces reflected delayed left atrial activation, not left atrial enlargement. In fact, most criteria mentioned above also apply for intraatrial block. Moreover, a negative P wave in lead V_1[110] may reflect improper (high) placement of this lead, a common error made by ECG technicians. Generally, if the previously mentioned findings are found in patients with LV enlargement or mitral stenosis, left atrial hypertrophy is most likely present, but in their absence, such findings usually indicate an intraatrial conduction defect. In any case, the ECG pattern of left atrial hypertrophy results from a hypertrophy-induced (stretching) intraatrial conduction delay.

LV HYPERTROPHY

As emphasized by Surawicz,[111] since the advent of other noninvasive techniques, there has been a changing role for the ECG in the diagnosis of ventricular hypertrophy. Necropsy studies have exposed the superiority of echocardiography (see Chap. 13) with respect to electrocardiography to detect LV hypertrophy.[111] Echocardiography is also a better method for the serial follow-up of changes during progression or regression of LV hypertrophy. Multiple criteria have been proposed to diagnose LV hypertrophy using necropsy or echocardiographic information[49,112–115] (Tables 11-4 and 11-5). Of these, the Sokolow-Lyon criterion (SV_1 + RV_{5-6} ≥35 mm) is the most specific (>95 percent) but is not very sensitive (≈45 percent) (see Table 11-4). The Romhilt-Estes score has a specificity of 90 percent and a sensitivity of 60 percent in studies correlated with echocardiography. The following are some of the other criteria[49]: The Casale (modified Cornell) criterion (Ra_{VL} + SV_3 >28 mm in men and >20 in women) is somewhat more sensitive but less specific than the Sokolow-Lyon criterion.[116] The Talbot criterion[117] (R ≥16 mm in a_{VL}) is very specific (>90 percent), even in the presence of MI and ventricular block, but not very sensitive. The Koito and Spodick criterion[118] (RV_6 > RV_5) claims a specificity of 100 percent and a sensitivity of more than 50 percent. According to Hernandez Padial,[119] a total 12-lead QRS voltage of greater than 120 mm is a good ECG criterion of LV hypertrophy in systemic hypertension and is better than those most frequently used. With echocardiography as the "gold standard," several authors postulated ECG criteria for diagnosis of LV hypertrophy in the presence of complete LBBB and LAFB[120,121] (Tables 11-6 and 11-7). The high sensitivity and specificity re-

TABLE 11-4 Electrocardiographic Criteria for Left Ventricular Enlargement

	Sensitivity		
Specificity Accuracy Voltage Criteria	(%)	(%)	(%)
RI + S_{III} > 25 mm	10.6	100	55
RVL > 7.5 mm	22.5	96.5	59.5
RVL > 11 mm	10.6	100	55
RVF > 20 mm	1.3	99.5	50
SV_1 + RV_{5-6} > 35 mm (Sokolow-Lyon)	55.6	89.5	73
In V_1–V_6, the tallest S + the tallest R > 45 mm	45	93	69
RV_{5-6} > 26 mm	25	98	62
Romhilt-Estes score	See Table 11-5		

SOURCE: Used with permission from Bayes de Luna.[49]

TABLE 11-5 Point Score System of Romhilt and Estes for Diagnosis of Left Ventricular Hypertrophy

1. Amplitude, 3 points
   Any of the following:
   a. Largest R or S wave in the limb leads ≥ 20 mm
   b. S wave in V_1 or V_2 ≥ 30 mm
   c. R wave in V_5 or V_6 ≥ 30 mm
2. ST-T-segment changes (typical pattern of left ventricular strain with the ST-T-segment vector shifted in direction opposite to the mean QRS vector)
   Without digitalis, 3 points
   With digitalis, 1 point
3. Left atrial involvement, 3 points
   Terminal negativity of the P wave in V_1 is 1 mm or more in depth with a duration of 0.04 s or more
4. Left-axis deviation: −30° or more, 2 points
5. QRS duration ≥ 0.09 s, 1 point
6. Intrinsicoid deflection in V_5, V_6 = 0.05 s, 1 point

Note: sensitivity, 54%; specificity, 97%.
SOURCES: From Bayes de Luna[49] and Romhilt and Estes,[115] with permission.

TABLE 11-6 Criteria for Diagnosis of Left Ventricular Hypertrophy in Presence of Complete Left Bundle Branch Block

1. RaV_L ≥ 11 mm
2. Electrical axis ≥ 40° (or S_2 ≥ R_1)
3. SV_1 + RV_5 or RV_6 ≥ 40 mm
4. SV_2 ≥ 30 and SV_3 ≥ 25 mm

Sensitivity (%)	Specificity (%)
24	100
39	100
58	97
75	90

Note: Left ventricular hypertrophy diagnosed by echocardiography when left ventricular mass is 115 g/m² or more.
SOURCE: Used with permission from Kafka et al.[120]

TABLE 11-7 Criteria for Diagnosis of Left Ventricular Hypertrophy in Presence of Left Anterior Fascicular Block*

Study	ECG Criteria	Sensitivity (%)	Specificity (%)	Positive Predictive Value (%)	Negative Predictive Value (%)
Bozzi and Figini	$SV_1 + (RV_5 + SV_5) \geq 25$ mm	69	92	90	73
Milliken	$RaV_L \geq 13$ mm	35	92	82	56
Milliken	SIII ≥ 15 mm	38	87	77	57
Gerstch et al.[143]	SIII + maximal sum of R+S in any single precordial lead	96	87	89	95
Reevaluated Gerstch criteria†		80	55	78	58

*Left ventricular hypertrophy diagnosed by echocardiography when left ventricular mass is ≥ 124 g/m².
†Unpublished observations performed in our department.
SOURCE: Used with permission from Gerstch et al.[121]
SOURCE: See text.

ported by Gertsch et al.[121] for diagnosis of LV hypertrophy with LAFB have not been corroborated in preliminary studies performed in our department (unpublished observations; nevertheless indicated in Table 11-7).

PROCESSES PRODUCING OR LEADING TO RV HYPERTROPHY AND ENLARGEMENT

RV hypertrophy is manifest in the ECG only when the RV forces predominate over those of the left ventricle. Since the latter has, roughly, three times more mass than the former, the right ventricle may double in size (when the left ventricle is normal) or triple its weight (when there is significant LV hypertrophy) and still not result in the necessary requirements to pull the electrical forces anteriorly and to the right. For these reasons, RV hypertrophy cannot be recognized easily in adult patients. Despite these limitations, the ECG manifestations of RV hypertrophy or enlargement can be subdivided into the following main types[1] (see Figs. 11-11, 11-12, and 11-16): (1) the posterior and rightward displacement of the QRS forces associated with low voltage, as seen in patients with pulmonary emphysema (Fig. 11-30), (2) the incomplete RBBB pattern *with right-axis deviation* occurring in patients with chronic lung disease and some congenital cardiac malformations resulting in volume overloading of the right ventricle (Fig. 11-31), (3) the true posterior wall MI pattern with normal to low voltage of the R wave in V_1 of mitral stenosis (Fig. 11-32), and (4) and the classic RV hypertrophy and strain pattern seen in young patients with congenital heart disease (producing pressure overload) or in adult patients with high-pressure ("primary" pulmonary) hypertension (Fig. 11-33). False patterns of RV hypertrophy may occur in patients with true posterior (basal) MI, complete RBBB with LPFB, and Wolff-Parkinson-White syndrome resulting from AV conduction through left free wall or posteroseptal accessory pathways.

ELECTROLYTE IMBALANCES

Because multiple factors can affect ventricular repolarization in diseased hearts, the finding characteristic of a specific electrolyte abnormality may be modified, and even mimicked, by various pathologic processes and the effects of certain drugs. In practice, the major problem with the ECG diagnosis of electrolyte imbalance is not the negative ECG with abnormal serum values but the production of similar changes by other conditions in patients with normal serum values.[122]

Hyperkalemia

The initial effect of acute hyperkalemia is the appearance of peaked T waves with a narrow base (Fig. 11-34, *left*). The diagnosis of hyperkalemia is almost certain when the duration of the base is 0.20 s or less (with rates between 60 and 110 beats per minute).[122] As the degree of hyperkalemia increases, the QRS complex widens (Fig. 11-35), with the electrical axis usually being deviated abnormally to the left and only rarely to the right. In addition, the PR interval prolongs, and the P wave

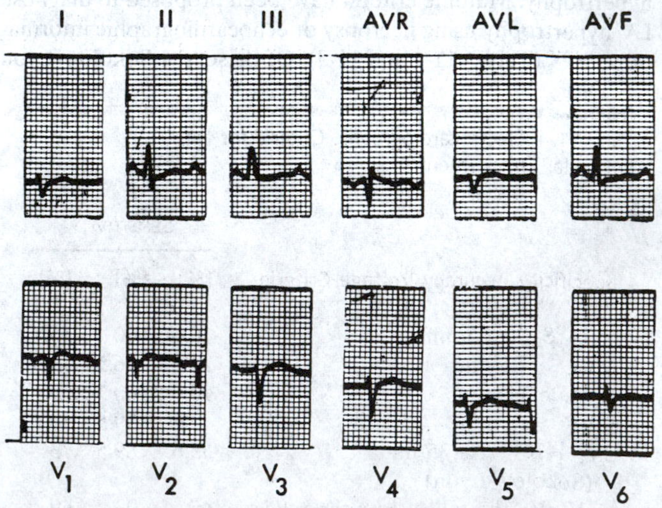

FIGURE 11-30 ECG taken on a patient with pulmonary emphysema showing slight right-axis deviation with small rS complexes in lead I, an electrically vertical heart position, overall tendency to low voltage, and rS complexes in all chest leads. (From Lemberg and Castellanos.[151] Reproduced with permission from the publisher and authors.)

flattens until it disappears.[45,122] If untreated, death ensues either due to ventricular standstill or coarse, slow ventricular fibrillation. Death also can result if wide QRS complexes occurring at fast rates are diagnosed as ventricular tachycardia and the patient is treated with antiarrhythmic drugs. On the other hand, class IA, IC, and III drugs as well as large doses of tricyclic antidepressants (especially when ingested for suicidal purposes) also can produce marked QRS widening. These processes, however, do not coexist with narrow-based, peaked T waves. Rarely, hyperkalemia produces (in the absence of coronary artery disease) a degree of ST-segment elevation in the right chest leads capable of suggesting anteroseptal myocardial injury (see Fig. 11-35). These constitute the "dialyzable currents of injury in potassium intoxication" reported by Levine et al.[123]

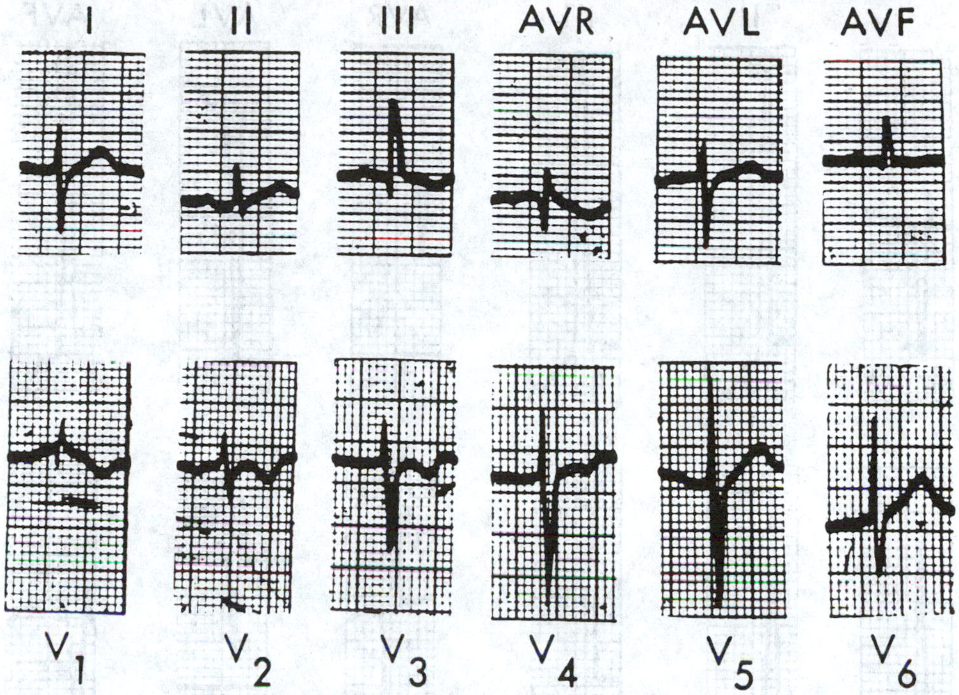

FIGURE 11-31 ECG from a patient with RV enlargement (volume overload in type) due to a small atrial septal defect (ostium secundum). Right-axis deviation was associated with an incomplete RBBB pattern (rsR' complexes in lead V_1). (From Lemberg and Castellanos.[151] Reproduced with permission from the publisher and authors.)

Hypokalemia

The abnormal and delayed repolarization that occurs in hypokalemia is best expressed as QU, rather than QT, prolongation, since at times it can be difficult to differentiate between notching of the T wave and T- and U-wave fusion.[122] On the basis of the previously mentioned M cells, these U waves are part of notched T waves, suggesting that that term be used in place of U. As the serum potassium level falls, the ST segment becomes progressively more depressed, and there is a gradual blending of the T wave into what appears to be a tall U wave (Fig. 11-36, *top*). An ECG pattern similar to that of hypokalemia can be produced by some antiarrhythmic drugs, especially quinidine and, experimentally, DL-sotalol. In any case, when repolarization is greatly prolonged, ventricular arrhythmias, including the so-called torsades de pointes, can occur.

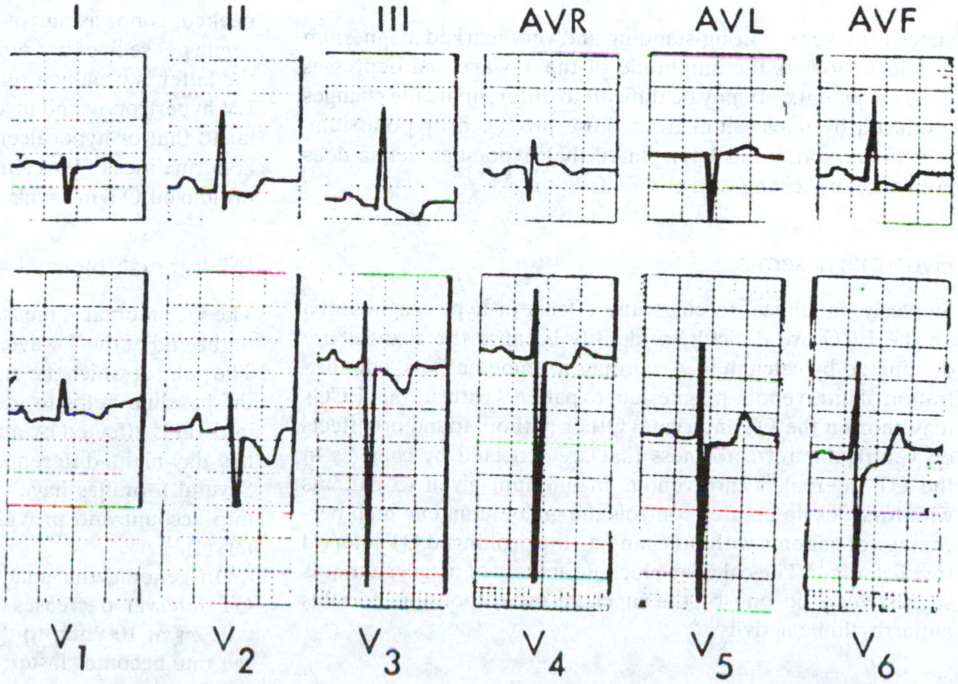

FIGURE 11-32 ECG from a patient with RV hypertrophy due to pure mitral stenosis showing P "mitrale," right-axis deviation, an all-positive deflection (R wave of only approximately 5 mm) in V_1, and rS complexes from V_2 to V_6. (From Lemberg and Castellanos.[151] Reproduced with permission from the publisher and authors.)

Hypomagnesemia

Hypomagnesemia does not produce QU prolongation unless the coexisting hypokalemia (with which it is almost invariably asso-

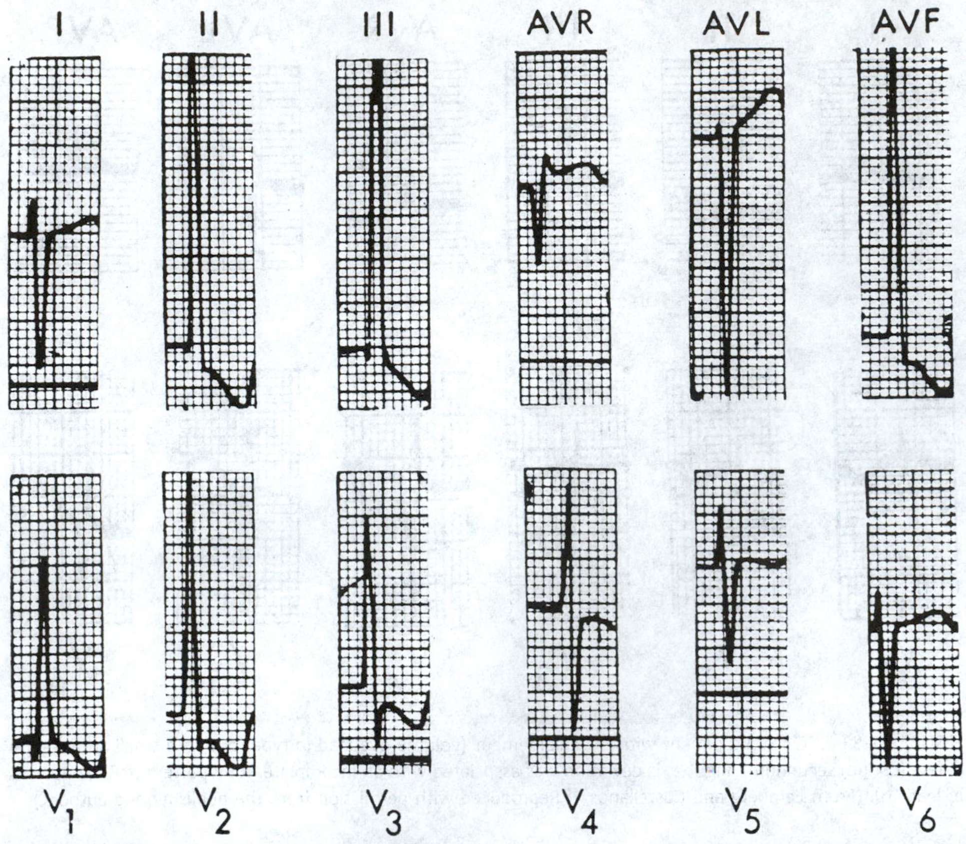

FIGURE 11-33 ECG from a 17-year-old patient who had RV enlargement (pressure overloading in type) due to severe pulmonic stenosis. Note extreme right-axis deviation, overall high voltage, and qR complexes in lead V_1 without an incomplete RBBB pattern. (From Lemberg and Castellanos.[151] Reproduced with permission from the publisher and authors.)

ciated) is severe.[122] Long-standing and very marked magnesium deficiency lowers the amplitude of the T wave and depresses the ST segment.[122] It may be difficult to differentiate the changes produced by magnesium from those produced by potassium. For this reason, it has been stated that hypomagnesemia does not cause any changes in the ECG.[45]

Hypermagnesemia

Similarly, in clinical tracings, the effects of hypermagnesemia on the ECG are difficult to identify because the changes are dominated by calcium.[124] According to some authors, administration of intravenous magnesium to patients with normal ECGs may shorten the QT interval.[45] Other authors found no effects on ventricular refractoriness that are reflected by changes in the QT interval.[125] Intravenous magnesium given to patients with torsades de pointes controls the arrhythmia in a high percentage of patients without changing the prolonged QT interval significantly.[126] The calcium-blocking activity of magnesium was suggested to be one of the mechanisms responsible for this antiarrhythmic activity.[146]

Hypercalcemia

During sinus rhythm with normal rates, the QT interval is short (see Fig. 11-36, *bottom*). In some cases, the Q-to-apex of T intervals is also short. If factors known to modify the QT interval are not present, it has been said that a reasonably accepted correlation exists between the duration of the interval and serum calcium levels.[122] Occasionally, the ST segment disappears, and the T waves may become inverted in left and right chest leads. Digitalis also shortens the QT interval but produces its characteristic "effects" in leads where the R waves predominate. The classic upward concavity of the ST segment is seen in the left chest leads in patients with LV hypertrophy and in leads V_1 and V_2 when there is RV hypertrophy (with predominantly positive deflections in these leads).

Hypocalcemia

The typical ECG pattern of hypocalcemia consists of QT prolongation at the expense of the ST segment.[45,122] The T wave is usually of normal width but can be narrow if there is coexisting (moderate) hyperkalemia (see Fig. 11-34*B*). A very marked injury (with the so-called hyperacute ST-T changes) can produce a similar pattern, but in such cases the T wave, though peaked, is not as narrow based. It has been said that hypocalcemia per se does not produce T-wave inversion. When present, the latter is usually a reflection of coexisting processes such as LV hypertrophy and incomplete LBBB. An ECG pattern similar to that of hypocalcemia can be produced by some organic abnormalities of the central nervous system and by congenitally prolonged QT intervals (see below).

QT Interval: Normal and Prolonged

The QT interval is measured from the beginning of the q wave to the end of the T wave.[1,11] The latter may be difficult to define. The point at which the maximal downslope of the T wave crosses the baseline helps to identify the end of this wave.[45] The QT interval is affected by autonomic tone and cathecolamines and has day-night differences. It varies with heart rate and sex. Several formulas have been proposed to take these variables into account and provide a corrected measurement (QTc interval).[127]

In general, the unadjusted (noncorrected), usually resting QT interval decreases from ±0.42 s at rates of 50/min to ±0.32 s at 100/min to ±0.26 s at 150/min.[9,11] During exercise, the rate becomes faster; the QTc first increases until reaching, approximately, a rate of 120/min, thereafter again decreasing.[128] Although the value of the normal QTc is open to question, it is still used in routine computer interpretations. Because the 12-lead ECG shows a normal degree of QT and QTc dispersion, indexes have been used to quantify the extent of heterogeneity in ventricular repolarization. The difference between the longest and shortest QT interval is referred to as *QT dispersion*.[129–134] Since 1990 it has been used as a prognostic marker not only in patients with prolonged QT intervals but also in those with acute MI.[130–132] The upper limits of normal vary with different investigators; a value of 65 may be an acceptable compromise according to Antzelevitch.[14] Others may disagree. Coumel et al.[133] emphasized that QT dispersion could be an illusion or a reality.[133] Inferred from the oncoming section on spatial vectorcardiography, the fact is that a truly *spatial* QRS-T loop cannot yield *abnormal* QT dispersion, for in planar projections of this spatial loop (as well as in the standard and unipolar extremity leads of the ECG) the shortest interval occurs because the terminal forces are perpendicular to the plane or derived lead. On the other hand, if precordial leads are considered scalar leads capable of recording (as stated in a previous section) local potentials with different durations, then QT dispersion is a reality.

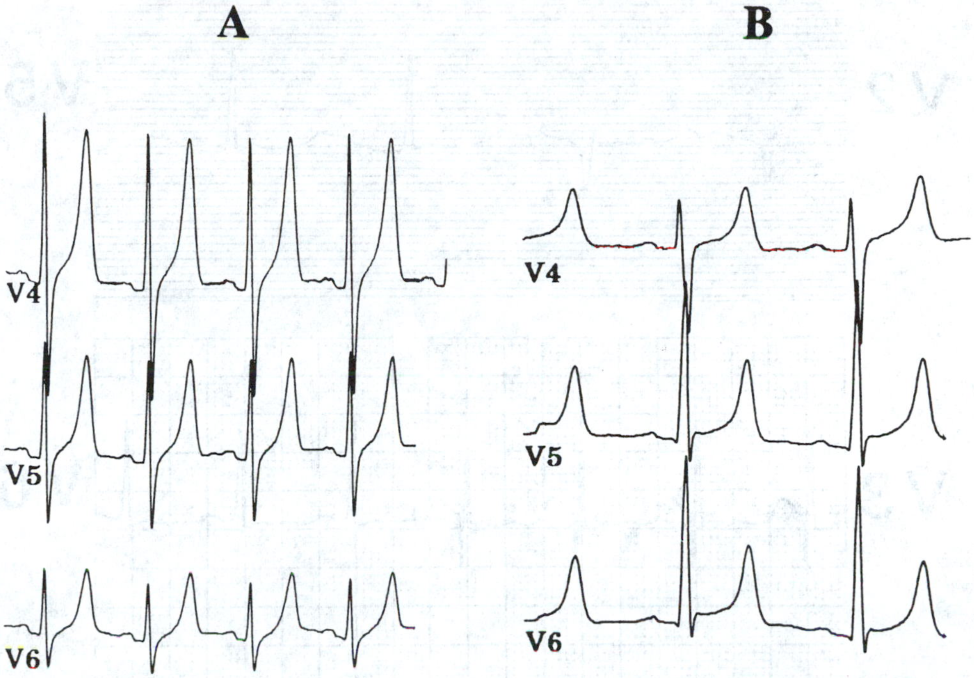

FIGURE 11-34 Electrocardiographic manifestations of early hyperkalemia. The nonprolonged QRS complex is followed by a peaked T wave having a very narrow base. Uncorrected and corrected QT intervals of 0.32 and 0.44 s, respectively (*A*). Hyperkalemia with hypocalcemia characterized by prolongation of the QT interval at the expense of the ST segment preceding the narrow-based T wave. Uncorrected and corrected QT intervals of 0.52 and 0.53 s, respectively (*B*).

The M-cell studies of Antzelevitch allow for the differentiation of this global "dispersion" (derived from *multiple* leads) from "local" transmural dispersion in *single* leads reflecting the time elapsing between the peak of the T wave (given by the end of the composite epicardial action potentials) and the end of the T wave (given by the end of the composite M-cell action potentials).[14]

The QT intervals are shortened with hypercalcemia, pure hyperkalemia, digoxin, and acidosis.[45] Prolongation of the QT interval may be congenital or acquired and is an important marker for malignant ventricular arrhythmias (see Chap. 24). A partial list of conditions causing a prolonged QT or, in some instances, prolonged QU intervals (delayed repolarization) is given in Table 11-8.[45]

Hypothermia

Characteristic ECG changes develop when the body temperature drops to approximately 30°C.[11] The QT interval becomes prolonged. In addition, a deflection, called an *Osborn wave*, appears in a place said to be located between the end of the QRS complex and the beginning of the ST segment[135] (Fig. 11-37). This deflection has been attributed to delayed depolarization, to a current of injury, or to "early" repolarization.[153] In leads facing the left ventricle, the deflection is positive, and its size is inversely related to body temperature.

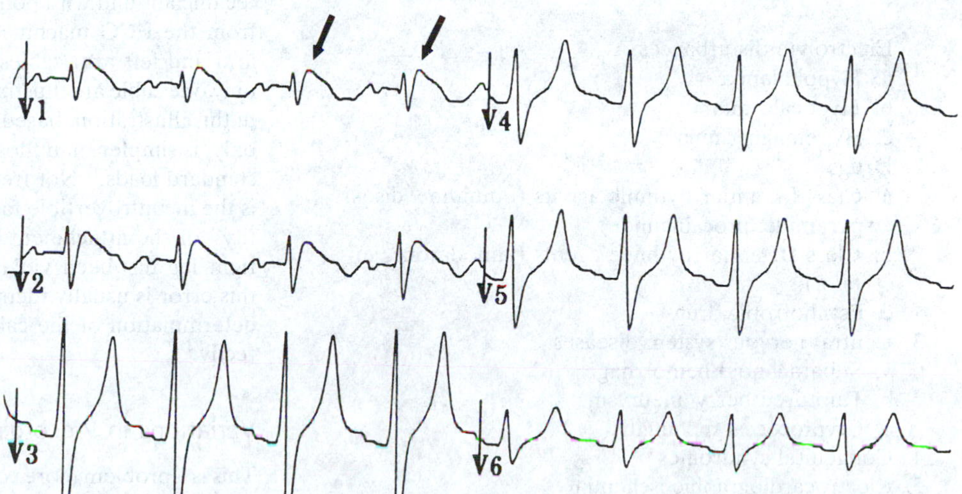

FIGURE 11-35 Advanced hyperkalemia. The wide (0.14-s) QRS complexes are followed by peaked T waves (best seen in lead V_3). The hyperkalemia-induced ST-segment elevation in lead V_1 (*arrows*), known as the *dialyzable currents of injury*, disappeared after appropriate treatment.

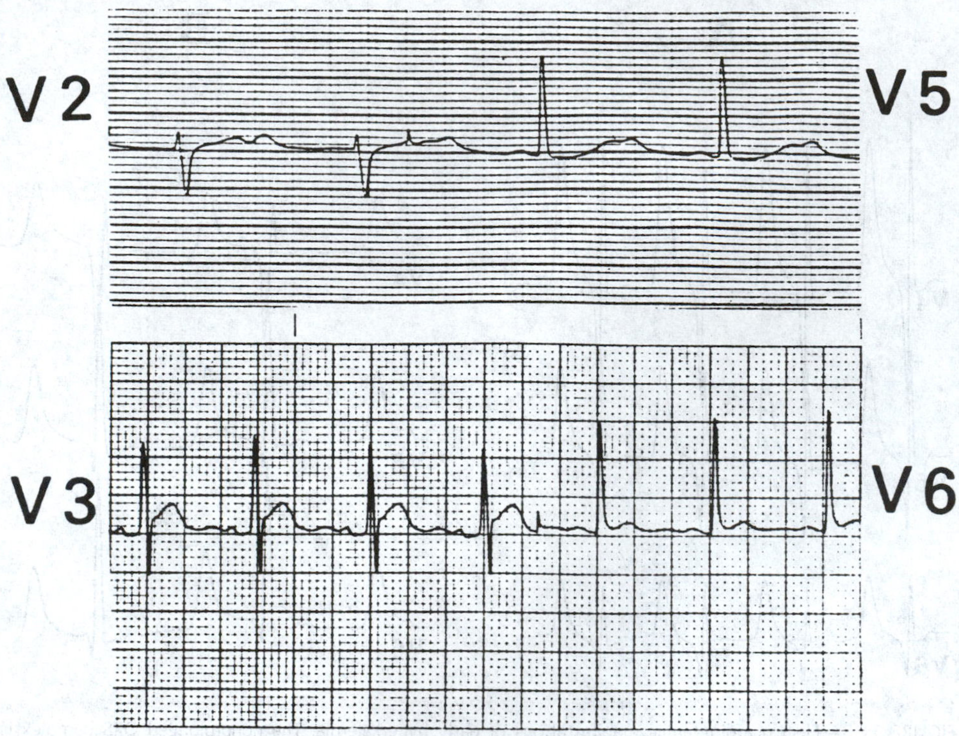

FIGURE 11-36 Electrocardiographic manifestations of hypokalemia (*upper strip*) and hypercalcemia (*lower strip*).

The role played by the intramyocardial M cells in its genesis has been discussed previously.[14]

ARTIFACTS

During the last few years, the number and types of instruments used for noninvasive and invasive (electrical and nonelectrical) study of cardiac functions have multiplied. Naturally, physicians and hospital administrators have concentrated their attention on them. Technicians have been more interested in working in these more lucrative services. Such factors, and others, have downgraded the importance of recording 12-lead ECGs, relegating them to less qualified personnel. Not surprisingly, the quality of technicians and of the ECG that they record has deteriorated in many centers. Optimal quality can only be achieved if the parties involved understand what is happening. The following are some of the artifacts commonly seen in current routine 12-lead ECGs. They are important because they can confound the interpreter and, worse, the computer program.

TABLE 11-8 Acquired QT Prolongation Usually Bradycardia-and(or) Pause-Dependent

1. Electrolyte disturbances
   a. Hypokalemia
   b. Hypocalcemia
   c. Hypomagnesemia
2. Drugs
   a. Class IA antiarrhythmic agents (quinidine, disopyramide, procainamide)
   b. Class III antiarrhythmic agents (amiodarone, sotalol)
   c. Psychotropic drugs
3. Central nervous system diseases
   a. Subarachnoid hemorrhage
   b. Ruptured berry aneurysm
   c. Cryptococcal meningitis
4. Congenital syndromes
5. Electrocardiographic ischemia
6. Arrhythmias
   a. Posttachycardia syndrome
   b. Cardiac arrest of any etiology
   c. Chronic idioventricular rhythms
7. Hypothermia

Muscle Tremor and Alternating-Current Interference

These are the most frequently encountered artifacts because some patients will continue to have disease processes producing tremor and because the amount of electronic equipment causing interference in a hospital environment has increased.

Improper Limb-Lead Positioning

This has become more frequent after relaxation of quality control, especially in hospitals with inadequate standards for hiring technicians and with poor on-site training. Mixing up the cables from the ECG machine has gone beyond switching the right arm and left arm cables.[11] Various types of misplacements of only one cable are illustrated in Fig. 11-38. The method depicted in this illustration, based on the use of unipolar extremity leads only, is simpler than those incorporating the analysis of bipolar standard leads.[11] Not frequently recognized in ECG textbooks is the incontrovertible fact that in some centers even the "sanctity" of the attachment of the right leg (ground) cable to the right leg has been violated[136] (Fig. 11-39). In our experience, this error is usually identified as improper lead placement, but determination of the cables involved is usually not made correctly.[136]

Variations in Precordial-Lead Placement

This is a problem more common now than when, in 1961, Simonson noted the considerable variation in chest lead placement in the same patient by different technicians and even by the same technician in several ECGs in the same patient.[137] Simonson also found that in a controlled study, placement of the V_2 electrode varied 10 cm vertically and 8 cm horizontally in 103 healthy subjects.[137] Moreover, Kerwin et al.[138] found a rather

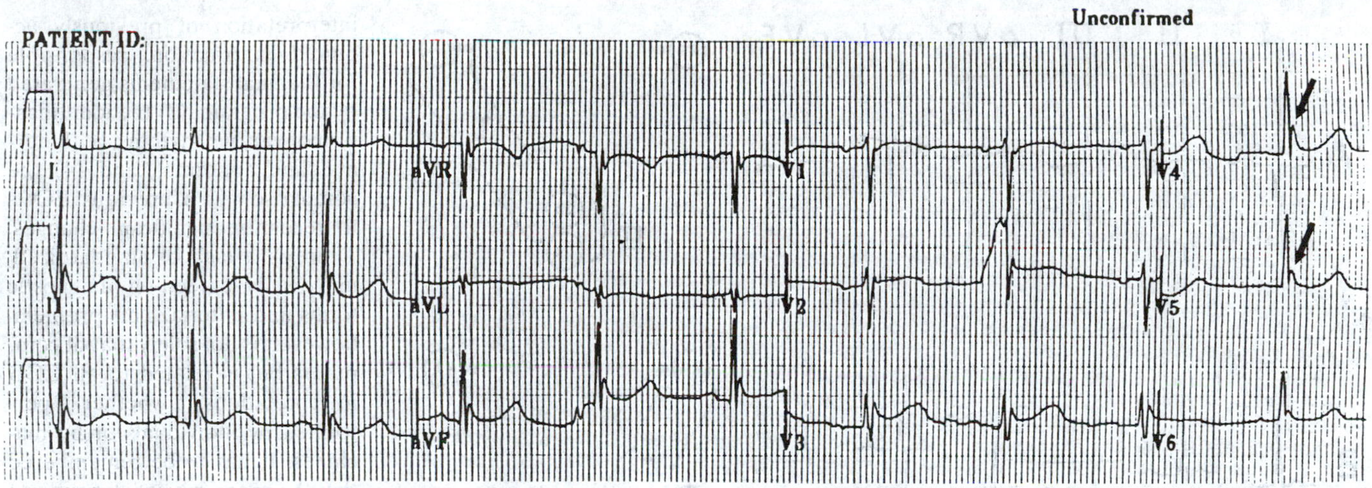

FIGURE 11-37 ECG obtained from a patient with hypothermia. The characteristic Osborn wave (*arrows*) is the terminal deflection inscribed between the slender part of the QRS complexes and the beginning of the ST segment. Note that it is not easy to determine where the ST segment starts. In addition, there is marked prolongation of the QT interval.

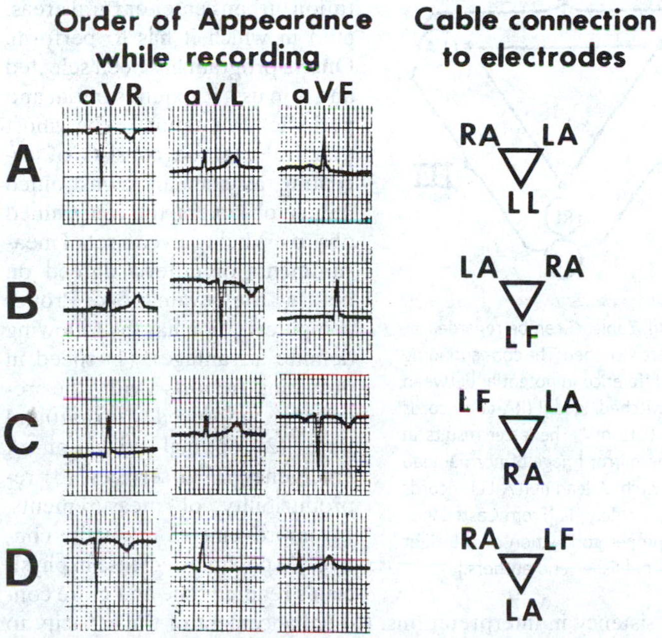

FIGURE 11-38 Identification of improper connections of a single cable from the electrocardiographic machine to the corresponding electrodes placed on the patient's limbs. Note that aV_R, aV_L, and aV_F invariably refer to whatever morphology is recorded when, while the ECG is being obtained, the corresponding knobs are turned in this order (regardless of whether the cables were attached properly or improperly). On the other hand, RA (right arm), LA (left arm), and LL (left leg) or LF (left foot) correspond to the normal morphology recorded by the cables so labeled. This method, based solely on the analysis of the unipolar extremity leads, is simpler than the method based on the study of the bipolar standard leads but is useful only when a single cable is misconnected. *A.* Normal. *B.* Since LA appears in aV_R and RA appears in aV_R (with LF being in its normal position), the right arm and left arm cables must have been switched. *C.* Since LF appears in aV_R and RA appears in aV_F (with LA in its normal position), the right arm and left leg cables must have been switched. *D.* Since LA appears in aV_F and LF appears in aV_L (with RA in its normal position), the left arm and left leg cables must have been switched.

large error in placement of chest electrodes (2 to 3 cm in both the horizontal and vertical directions) in repeated trials in the same patients by the same technicians.[138] Perhaps the frequency of precordial-lead misplacement is greater than that of somatic tremor. In our institution, the most frequent cause of "poor" r-wave progression in the anteroseptal leads (often misinterpreted by the computer as indicative of anteroseptal MI) is misplacements of leads V_2 and V_3.

False Variations in Voltage

Garson[139] noticed how, in several patients, ECGs taken weeks apart showed markedly different QRS voltages. The latter were sometimes of enough magnitude to cause a pseudonormalization of a ventricular hypertrophy pattern. There had been no changes in hemodynamics, but different types of ECGs were used. A study of this problem demonstrated that electrocardiographic data had a different voltage depending on whether they were recorded and displayed on an analog electrocardiograph or on a digital electrocardiograph. Thus, if there is a statistically significant difference among ECGs, the serial comparisons must be done with the same machine. Moreover, criteria for voltage are only applicable to the type of instrument with which the data were gathered.

In addition, overshooting, overdamping, and running down of the standardization battery can cause significant changes in QRS voltage and ST segments.

How Should an ECG Be Performed?

This question is appropriate in view of the many artifacts and technical (machine and human) problems occurring when ECGs are recorded. The Task Force of the American College of Cardiology (ACC)—American Heart Association (AHA) in their *Guidelines for Electrocardiography*[4] have stated that the ECG should be performed and interpreted in accordance with the guidelines for optimal electrocardiography described in the ACC *Tenth Bethesda Conference Report*,[140] the guidelines for training described in the ACC *Seventeenth Bethesda Conference*

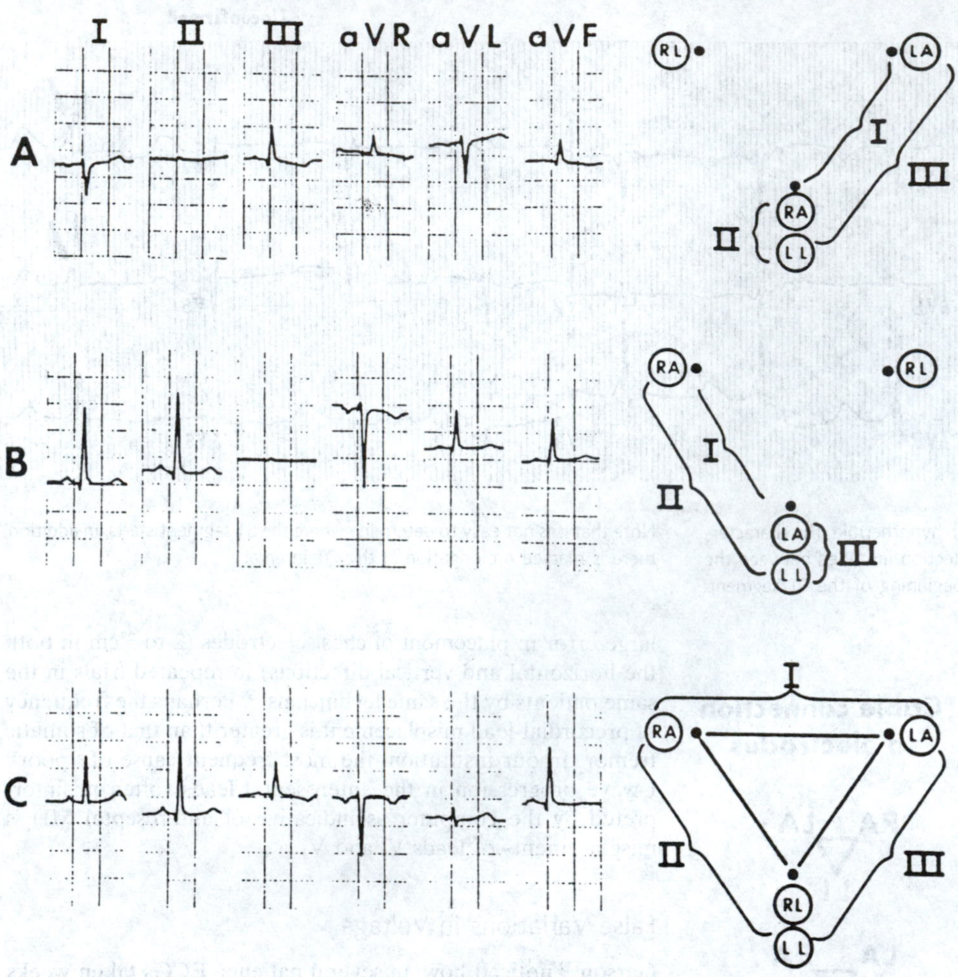

FIGURE 11-39 Identification of improper connections of the right leg (RL) (ground) cable. *C* can be regarded as almost equal to the control tracing because the RL (ground) and left leg (LL) cables were switched. The corresponding morphologies are not identical to the control morphologies because a very small difference in potential between both legs does exist. The latter is seen in *A*. Because the RL and RA cables were switched, lead II (RA-LL) records the difference in potential between both legs, which seems to be approximately 0.15 mV. The latter results in an almost straight line interrupted by a small blip. In addition, lead I represents the mirror image of normal lead III, and lead III is the normal lead III. In *B*, where the LA and RL cables have been switched, lead III (LA-LL) records almost a straight line. In addition, lead I is the normal lead II, and lead II is the normal lead II. [From Castellanos A, Saoudi NC, Schwartz A, et al. Electrocardiographic patterns resulting from improper connection of the right leg (ground) cable. *PACE* 1985; 8:364-368. Reproduced with permission from the publisher and authors.]

Report on Cardiology Training,[141] the recommendations for standardization of leads and specifications for instruments in electrocardiography and vectorcardiography of the AHA,[142] and the recommendations for standardization and specifications for automated electrocardiography of the AHA.[143]

COMPUTER APPLICATIONS

It has been almost 40 years since the first attempts were made to apply computer technology to the interpretation of ECGs.[144] Today its use is universal.[1,144-147] In general, computer systems for true analysis of ECGs have, as their main component, a program usually having the following four basic functions: (1) the measuring of ECG parameters, which includes an automatic wave-front-recognition section and a measurement section that extracts the wave fronts, a set of values, and control, (2) the interpretation of previously acquired information, responsible for the final statements generated by the program, (3) the identification of various rhythms, both normal and abnormal, and (4) the comparison with previous ECGs to recognize significant changes. There is a lack of standardized, universally agreed-on diagnostic terms and criteria. This problem, however, is not solely that of computers but is related to all ECG interpretations, whether performed by individuals or by machines. It has to be remembered that the program used depends on criteria imposed on it by human programmers. Physicians should insist that the program selected has to be "tuned in" with the operational environment (e.g., community hospital or teaching institution, urban center or rural areas, etc.) in which it has to perform. Once a program has been selected and is in use, it requires initial and periodic evaluation. The most practical method consists of accepting as standard constrained human observers, the constrained observers being given a set of measurements or criteria agreed on before the evaluation. Proper computerization has the following definite advantages: (1) speed in providing reports with the resulting improved turnaround time, (2) optimal utilization of emergency ECG services, (3) reproducibility of measurements, (4) improvements in quality control, (5) possible decrease in physician's reading time and more consistency in interpretations, (6) enhancement of the capacity to handle large volumes of ECGs, and (7) substantial improvement in record storage and retrieval with better comparison with previous tracings.

Administrators are usually the ones selecting equipment, and frequently they know nothing about its medical performance. They usually use standard cost-effective, not medically-effective methods. That is, the economics involved—initial investment, operational costs, payroll, overhead, and professional fees—become priorities. This is important because it was estimated that even 10 years ago more than 40 percent of all ECGs recorded in the United States were obtained by some type of automatic system.[144] Presently, however, this figure is reaching 100 percent. Finally, emphasis should be placed on the obvious: All computer ECG interpretations, particularly those of rhythm disturbances, must be checked by a physician qualified to interpret ECGs and with an in-depth knowledge of the program

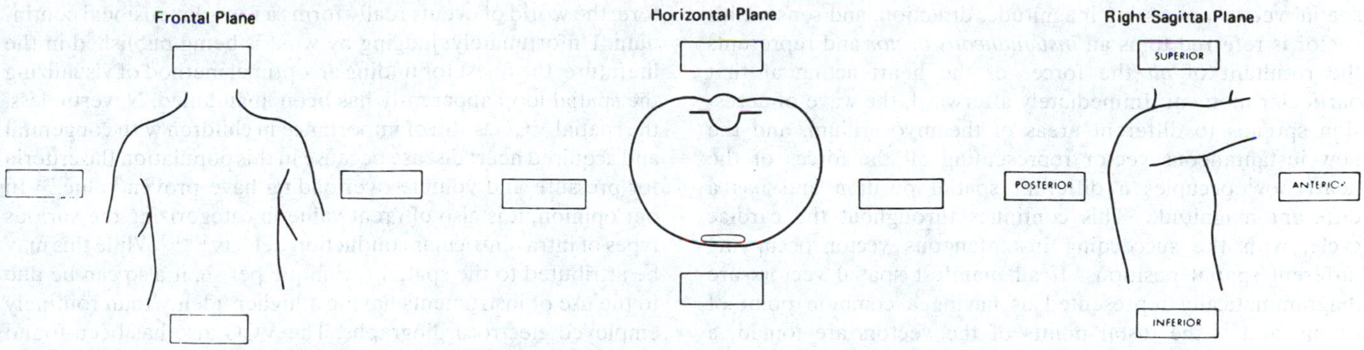

FIGURE 11-40 The spatial vectorcardiographic loops cannot be analyzed routinely in space with presently available techniques. Therefore, it is customary to study their projections in three planes seen as depicted in this figure. Note that (1) the frontal plane conforms to Einthoven's view of his equilateral triangle, (2) the horizontal plane is seen in such a way that the anterior surfaces of the heart and sternum are displayed in the inferior portions of the paper (in contrast to other noninvasive, nonelectrical methods), and (3) the sagittal plane is viewed from the right side of the patient. (From Lemberg and Castellanos.[151] Reproduced with permission from the publisher and authors.)

used. Decisions based on a computerized interpretation may, on occasion, lead to improper patient care. This also can have medicological implications. Of clinical importance was the report finding that computer interpretations of ECGs obtained 1 min apart were grossly different in 36 of 92 (39 percent) unselected pairs of tracings.[148] The latter refers to only one program but nevertheless should be an impetus to designers and manufacturers to improve their product and a warning to those who rely, exclusively, on computer interpretations.[148] The ACC/AHA Task Force on Guidelines for Electrocardiography states: "There is no computer program that can replace the skilled physician."[4] Finally, cardiology fellows in training should interpret ECGs without a printed computer interpretation rather than by having to evaluate the latter.

SPATIAL VECTORCARDIOGRAPHY

Generalities

The following statements, which need reemphasis, should not be considered redundant: (1) Since the ECG deals with electrical forces, it follows that very strictly speaking, electrocardiography can be considered vectorial.[149–150] (2) Orthodoxically, a scalar quantity only has magnitude, whereas a vector quantity has magnitude, direction, and sense. When analyzing the vectorcardiogram (VCG), one should consider the activation of each muscle cell as producing an electrical force that can be represented by a vector depicting the spatial orientation and magnitude of this force.[149]

During the spread of the activation process, innumerable electrical forces are generated. These multiple forces vary in magnitude and differ in direction. At any given moment, the resultant of these electrical forces can be represented by a

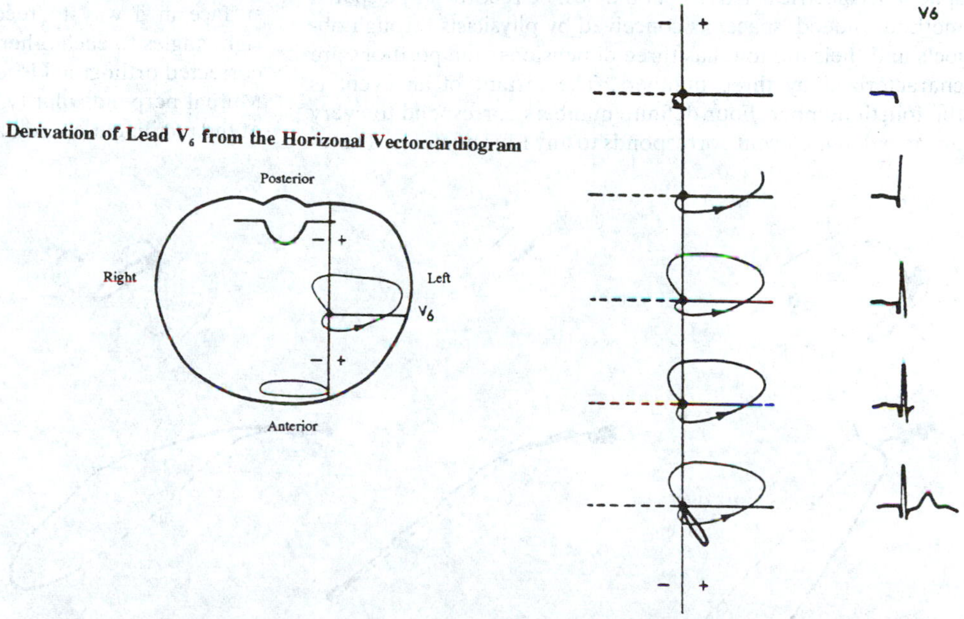

FIGURE 11-41 Method used to derive the morphology of a unipolar precordial lead (in this example lead V_6) from the planar projection of the spatial QRS and ST-T loops on the horizontal plane. First (*left panel*), a line is drawn from the estimated location of the corresponding electrode to the point of origin of the loops. Thereafter, a perpendicular to this line passing from the point of origin is drawn. This divides the thorax into a negative area (for V_6) that is located beyond the perpendicular line and a positive area that is located between the perpendicular line and the electrode. Thus, in the top right schematic, the small part of the loop located beyond the perpendicular line produces the small q wave in V_6. The other schematics show how progression of depolarization and repolarization produces parts of the QRS loop (and the entire ST-T loop), which are positive in lead V_6. The S wave occurs because the terminal part of the QRS loop is located beyond the perpendicular line. When using this type of lead derivation, any precordial lead will only record forces moving in an anteroposterior (or posteroanterior) and in a left-to-right or right-to-left direction. Forces moving up or down will not be recorded. This contrasts with scalar concept of precordial leads which can, especially when misplaced, record forces moving in any direction. (From Lemberg and Castellanos.[151] Reproduced with permission from the publisher and authors.)

spatial vector possessing magnitude, direction, and sense. This vector is referred to as an *instantaneous vector* and represents the resultant of *all* the forces of the heart acting at that particular moment. Immediately afterward, the wave of accession spreads to different areas of the myocardium, and the new instantaneous vector representing all the forces of the heart now occupies a different spatial position and has a different magnitude. This continues throughout the cardiac cycle, with the succeeding instantaneous vector occupying different spatial positions. If all manifest spatial vectors are diagrammatically represented as having a common point of origin, and if the distal points of the vectors are joined, a single spatial loop is formed for ventricular depolarization (QRS), ventricular repolarization (ST-T), and the atrial complex (P). The VCG consists of four different loops. The electrical activity of the atria is recorded as a small loop designated the *P loop,* the depolarization of the ventricles is recorded as a large loop designated the *QRS loop,* while the repolarization of the ventricles is recorded as a smaller loop designated the *ST-T loop*. Finally, at high magnifications, even a small *U loop* also can be recorded.[149–153]

Space: The Final Frontier

The theory of the truly spatial VCG is theoretically attractive. Because the heart is a tridimensional structure (located in space), its electrical activity should best be recorded by a spatial method. Indeed, space, as conceived by physicists through objects and their motion, has three dimensions, and positions are characterized by three numbers. The instant of an event is the fourth number. Four definite numbers correspond to every event; a definite event corresponds to any four numbers. Therefore, the world of events really forms a four-dimensional continuum. Unfortunately, judging by what is being published in the literature, the quest for finding an optimal method of visualizing the spatial loop apparently has been abandoned. Nevertheless, the spatial VCG is still of importance in children with congenital and acquired heart disease because in this population the criteria for pressure and volume overloading have proven value.[151] In our opinion, it is also of great value in categorizing the various types of intraventricular conduction defects.[151–153] While this may be attributed to the spatial technique per se, it also can be due to the use of instruments having a higher fidelity than routinely employed electrocardiographs. The VCG also has been found useful in detecting MI and certain types of RV enlargement.[151–153] In practice, it has not been proven that the VCG gives more information than the routine 12-lead ECG,[151] although some computer programs may still use the Frank orthogonal leads *X, Y,* and *Z*. These programs thus constitute a 15-lead system. In addition, the time required to obtain a VCG is longer than the time required to record a 12-lead ECG. These are the main reasons for the decrease in the use of spatial vectorcardiography during recent decades. Other reasons are nonreimbursement and the continuously increasing interest in other noninvasive methods of recording electrical activity (such as signal averaging, body surface mapping, and heart rate variability) or nonelectrical activity (such as echocardiography or magnetic resonance imaging, which looks at planes from *different* views). To obtain the spatial VCG, electrodes are placed on the body surface in a way to record three leads whose planes are at right angles to each other. The true spatial VCG requires three corrected orthogonal leads with the following features[151–154]: (1) Mutual perpendicularity, with each lead being parallel to one of the rectilinear coordinate axes of the human body. Such axes are the horizontal, *X* (left-to-right and right-to-left) axis; the vertical, *Y* (inferosuperior or superoinferior) axis; and sagittal, *Z* (anteroposterior or posteroanterior) axis. (2) Equal amplitude from the vectorial viewpoint. (3) Retention of the same magnitude and direction for all points where cardiac electromotive forces are generated. For example, even if the leads forming Einthoven's frontal plane were to be spatially correct, Einthoven's theory itself would make any electrodes placed for the purpose of obtaining the horizontal and sagittal planes (such as the tetrahedral system) spatially incorrect. The most widely used, corrected spatial VCG method probably is the one introduced by Frank.[154] Since the spatial loop cannot be analyzed tridimensionally, it is customary to study its planar projections (Fig. 11-40). By proper attachment to the oscilloscope, the *X* and *Y* leads are used for the frontal plane, the *X* and *Z* leads for the horizontal plane, and

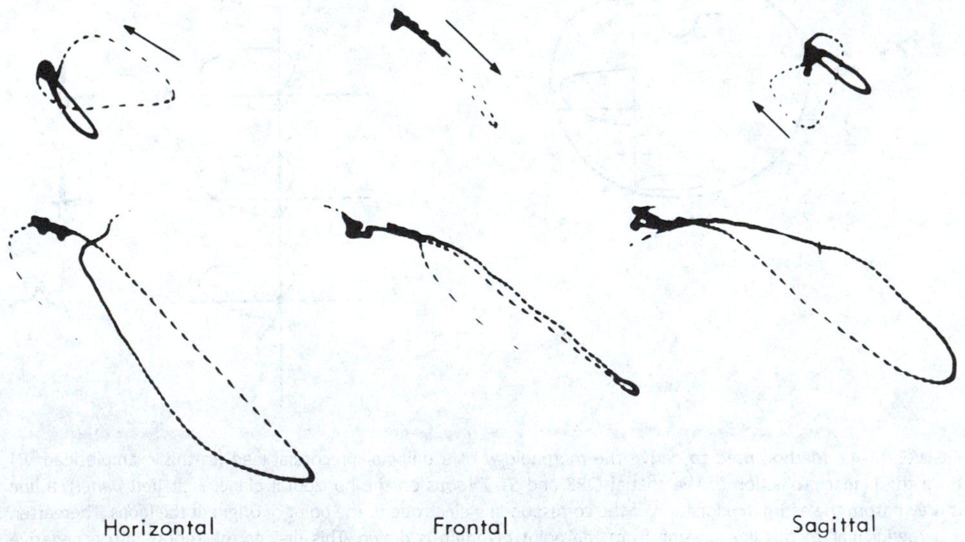

FIGURE 11-42 Planar projections of normal spatial VCG obtained with the Frank method. The ST-T loops are enlarged in the bottom view. In the horizontal plane, the QRS loop shows the expected, normal, counterclockwise (CCW) rotation (indicated by arrows). Although the narrow frontal plane QRS loop has clockwise (CW) rotation, in this plane either CCW, CW, or figure-eight rotations can be normal. In the right sagittal plane, the QRS loop displays its normal (CW) rotation. Enlargement of the ST-T loop clearly shows that its first half is inscribed more slowly. Therefore, the dashes (each representing 0.0025 s, or 25 ms) are closer together. Note that the rotation of the ST-T loop is similar to the rotation of the QRS loop in all planes. (From Lemberg and Castellanos.[151] Reproduced with permission from the publisher and authors.)

the Z and Y leads for the sagittal plane (of which the right side has been the most popular).

Differences between Electrovectorcardiography and Spatial Vectorcardiography

Spatial vectorcardiography is distinctly different from the various vectorial methods of ECG interpretation, such as those of Sodi-Pallares et al.[7] and Grant.[56,57] In clinical practice and in teaching, both seem to be considered equal, but this is so only for pragmatic and didactic reasons. Although the spatial VCG and the ECG should each be studied as distinct methods, most electrocardiographers either memorize loop patterns or attempt to derive the leads with which they are familiar from the corresponding QRS loops. Thus bipolar standard and unipolar extremity leads are derived from the frontal plane more or less as when, in clinical ECG, they are derived from the electrical axis. To do this in spatial vector loops, the electrical axis is equated with the maximal QRS vector that extends from the point of origin of the loop to its farthest point. The unipolar precordial leads are derived from the horizontal plane loops. Leads thus derived are different from the usual precordial ECG leads. The latter, as mentioned previously, record electrical forces moving toward or away from them, including local potentials that can be of different duration in different precordial leads.[13,35,133] In the 12-lead ECG (especially when the precordial electrodes are misplaced), however, these forces can move spatially not only in a left-to-right and anteroposterior direction but also in an inferosuperior direction as in leads V_5 and V_6 in patients with a very superior and leftward deviation of the EA. On the other hand, the theory of spatial vectorcardiography states that the horizontal plane and unipolar leads derived from them just record left-to-right and anteroposterior forces and that they do not record local potentials so that any difference in the duration of intervals is merely an illusion[133,151] (Fig. 11-41). In spatial vectorcardiography, electrical forces oriented superiorly or inferiorly cannot be reflected in the horizontal plane but only in the frontal and sagittal planes. Most of the information contained in the sagittal plane is present in the frontal and horizontal planes. In practice, the sagittal plane is useful to act as a "judge" in cases of apparent discrepancy between the other two planes. For example, it serves to determine if a localized delay present in one of the two planes is "real" or is due to perpendicularity of vectors. It also serves for a better evaluation of the upward or downward direction of the initial 0.01- and 0.02-s vectors than the frontal plane. Projections of normal spatial QRS and ST-T loops in the corresponding planes are depicted in Fig. 11-42.

References

1. Macfarlane PW, Lawrie TDV, eds. *Comprehensive Electrocardiology: Theory and Practice in Health and Disease*. New York: Pergamon Press; 1989.
2. Myerburg RJ, Castellanos A. Resolution of nonspecific repolarization patterns from body surface signals: A new horizon of clinical electrocardiography. *J Am Coll Cardiol* 1989; 14:703–704.
3. Einthoven W, Fahr G, de Waart A. uber die Richtung und die manifeste Grosse der Pontetialschwankungen in menchlichen Herzen und uber den Einfluss der Herzlage auf die Form des Elecktrokardiogramms. *Arch Physiol* 1913; 150:275–315.
4. Task Force Report of the American College of Cardiology and the American Heart Association. ACC/AHA Guidelines for Electrocardiography. *Circulation* 1992; 19:473–481.
5. Castellanos A, Myerburg RJ. Electrocardiography. In: Schlant RC, Alexander RW, Lipton MJ, eds. *Diagnostic Atlas of the Heart*. New York: McGraw-Hill; 1996.
6. Sodi-Pallares D, Calder RM. *New Bases of Electrocardiography*. St. Louis: Mosby; 1956:169, 373.
7. Sodi-Pallares D, Medrano GA, Bisteni A, et al. *Deductive and Polyparametric Electrocardiography*. Mexico City: Inst Nac Cardiol Mexico; 1970:36, 136.
8. Rosenbaum MB, Elizari MV, Lazzari JO. *The Hemiblocks*. Oldsmar, FL: Tampa Tracings; 1970.
9. Lipman BS, Massie E, Kleiger RE. *Clinical Scalar Electrocardiography*, 6th ed. Chicago: Year Book Medical Publishers; 1972:210–215.
10. Schamroth L. *The Electrocardiology of Coronary Artery Disease*, 2d ed. Oxford, England: Blackwell Scientific; 1984.
11. Marriott HJL. *Practical Electrocardiography*, 8th ed. Baltimore: Williams & Wilkins; 1988.
12. Cabrera E, Gaxiola A. *Teoria y Practica de la Electrocardiografia*, 2d ed. Mexico City: La Prensa Medica Mexicana; 1966.
13. Barker JM. *The Unipolar Electrocardiogram: A Clinical Interpretation*. New York: Appleton-Century-Crofts; 1952.
14. Antzelevitch C, Shimizu W, Yan GX, et al. The M cell: Its contribution to the ECG and to normal and abnormal electrical function of the heart. *J Cardiovasc Electrophysiol* 1999; 10:1124–1152.
15. Castellanos A, Myerburg RJ. *The Hemiblocks in Myocardial Infarction*. New York: Appleton-Century-Crofts; 1976.
16. Castellanos A Jr, Lemberg L. *A Programmed Introduction to the Electrical Axis and Action Potential*. Oldsmar, FL: Tampa Tracings; 1974:34, 114.
17. Wilson FN, MacLeod AG, Barker PS, et al. The determination and significance of the areas of the ventricular deflections of the electrocardiogram. *Am Heart J* 1934; 10:46–61.
18. Rosenbaum MB, Blanco HH, Elizari MV, et al. Electrotonic modulation of ventricular repolarization and cardiac memory. In: Rosenbaum MB, Elizari MV, eds. *Frontiers of Cardiac Electrophysiology*. Boston: Martinus Nijhoff; 1983:67–99.
19. Goyal R, Syed ZA, Mukhopadhyay PS, et al. Changes in cardiac repolarization following short periods of ventricular pacing. *J Cardiovasc Electrophysiol* 1998; 9:269–280.
20. Surawicz B. Transient T wave abnormalities after cessation of ventricular preexcitation: Memory of what? *J Cardiovasc Electrophysiol* 1996; 7:51–59.
21. Bayley RH. An interpretation of injury and the ischemic effects of myocardial infarction in accordance with the laws which determine the flow of electric current in homogenous volume conductors and in accordance with relevant pathologic changes. *Am Heart J* 1942; 24:514–528.
22. Bruyneel KJJ. Use of moving epicardial electrodes in defining ST-segment changes after acute coronary occlusion in the baboon: Relation to primary ventricular fibrillation. *Am Heart J* 1975; 89:731–741.
23. Holland RP, Brooks H. TQ-ST segment mapping: Critical review and analysis of current concepts. *Am J Cardiol* 1977; 40:110–129.
24. Janse MJ. Electrophysiology and electrocardiology of acute myocardial ischemia. *Can J Cardiol* 1986; 2(suppl A):46A–52A.
25. Tzivoni D, Chenzbraun A. The significance of ST abnormalities in myocardial infarction. *Cardiol Clin* 1987; 5:419–426.
26. Mills RM, Young E, Gorlin R, et al. Natural history of ST-segment elevation after acute myocardial infarction. *Am J Cardiol* 1975; 35:609–614.
27. Arvan S, Varat MA. Persistent ST-segment elevation and left ventricular wall abnormalities: A 2-dimensional echocardiographic study. *Am J Cardiol* 1984; 53:1542–1546.

28. Wasserburger RH, Alt WJ. The normal RS-T segment elevation variant. *Am J Cardiol* 1961; 8:184–192.
29. Goldberger AL. ST-segment elevation: normal variants: Benign (functional ST-segment elevation, "early repolarization variant." In: Goldberger AL, ed. *Myocardial Infarction: ECG Differential Diagnosis*, 3d ed. St. Louis: Mosby; 1984:1970–1978.
30. Morace G, Padeletti L, Porciani MC, et al. Effect of isoproterenol on the carly repolarization syndrome. *Am Heart J* 1979; 97:343–347.
31. Miyazaki T, Mitamura H, Miyoshi S, et al. Autonomic and antiarrhythmic drug modulation of ST segment elevation in patients with Brugada syndrome. *J Am Coll Cardiol* 1996; 27:1061–1070.
32. Brugada P, Brugada J. Right bundle branck block, persistent ST segment elevation and sudden cardiac death: A distinct clinical and electrocardiographic syndrome. *J Am Coll Cardiol* 1992; 20:1391–1396.
33. Corrado D, Nava A, Buja G, et al. Familial cardiomyopathy underlies syndrome of right bundle branck block, ST segment elevation and sudden death. *J Am Coll Cardiol* 1996; 27:443–448.
34. Fujiki A, Usui M, Nagasawa H, et al. ST segment elevation in the right precordial leads induced with class IC antiarrhythmic drugs: Insight into the mechanism of Brugada syndrome. *J Cardiovasc Electrophysiol* 1999; 10:214–218.
35. Fontaine G, Fontaliran F, Lascault P, et al. In: Zipes DP, Jalife J, eds. *Cardiac Electrophysiology: From Cell to Bedside*, 2nd ed. Philadelphia: Saunders; 1995:754–768.
36. Phibbs B, Marcua F, Marriott HJC, et al. Q-wave versus non-Q wave myocardial infarction: A meaningless distinction. *J Am Coll Cardiol* 1999; 33:576–582.
37. Barold SS, Falkoff MD, Ong LS, et al. Significance of transient electrocardiographic Q waves in coronary artery disease. *Cardiol Clin* 1987; 5:367–380.
38. Timmis GC. Electrocardiographic effects of reperfusion. *Cardiol Clin* 1987; 5:427–446.
39. Braunwald E, Kloner RA. The stunned myocardium: Prolonged postischemic ventricular dysfunction. *Circulation* 1982; 66:1146–1149.
40. Bashour TT, Kabbani SS, Brewster HP, et al. Transient Q waves and reversible cardiac failure during myocardial ischemia: Electrical and mechanical stunning of the heart. *Am Heart J* 1983; 106:780–783.
41. Rahimtoola SH. A perspective on the three large multicenter randomized clinical trials of coronary bypass surgery for chronic stable angina. *Circulation* 1985; 72(suppl 5):123–135.
42. Braunwald E, Rutherford JD. Reversible ischemic left ventricular dysfunction: Evidence for the "hibernating myocardium." *J Am Coll Cardiol* 1986; 8:1467–1470.
43. Dunn MI, Starr SK. False-positive electrocardiographic findings mimicking myocardial infarction. *ACC Curr J Rev* 1993; Nov/Dec:74–76.
44. Nelson SD, Kou WH, Annesley T, et al. Significance of ST segment depression during paroxysmal supraventricular tachycardia. *J Am Coll Cardiol* 1988; 12:383–387.
45. Fisch C. Electrocardiography and vectorcardiography. In: Braunwald E, ed. *Heart Disease*, 4th ed. Philadelphia: Saunders; 1992:116–160.
46. Friedberg CK, Zager A. Nonspecific ST and T-wave changes. *Circulation* 1961; 23:655–661.
47. Spodick DH. Q wave infarction versus SS-T infarction: Nonspecificity of electrocardiographic criteria for differentiating transmural and nontransmural lesion. *Am J Cardiol* 1983; 913–915.
48. Gersh B, Rahimtoola SH. *Acute Myocardial Infarction*. New York: Elsevier; 1991:144.
49. Bayes de Luna A. *Clinical Electrocardiography: A Textbook*. Mt. Kisco, NY: Futura; 1993:450.
50. Califf RM, Mark DB, Wagner GS. *Acute Coronary Care in the Thrombolytic Era*. Chicago: Year Book Medical Publishers; 1988.
51. Shah PK, Zahger D, Ganz W. Streptokinase in acute myocardial infarction. In: Francis GS, Alpert JS, eds. *Coronary Care*, 2d ed. Boston: Little, Brown; 1995:409–450.
52. Fernandez AR, Sequeira RF, Chakko S, et al. ST segment tracking for rapid determination of patency of the infarct-related artery in acute myocardial infarction. *J Am Coll Cardiol* 1995; 26:675–683.
53. Veldkamp RF, Simoons ML, Pope JE, et al. Continuous multilead ST-segment monitoring in acute myocardial infarction. In: Clements IP, ed. *The Electrocardiogram in Acute Myocardial Infarction*. Mt. Kisco, NY: Futura; 1998.
54. Goodman S. Q wave and non-Q wave myocardial infarction after thrombolysis (Letter). *J Am Coll Cardiol* 1996; 27(7):1817–1819.
55. Sclarovsky S. Acute ischaemic syndrome: The pre-infarction ischaemic syndrome. In: Sclarovsky S, ed. *Electrocardiography of Acute Myocardial Ischaemic Syndromes*. London: Martin Dunitz; 1999:31–63.
56. Grant RP. Spatial vector electrocardiography: A method for calculating the spatial electrical vectors of the heart from conventional leads. *Circulation* 1950; 2:676–695.
57. Grant RP, Estes EH Jr. *Spatial Vector Electrocardiography*. New York: Blakiston; 1951.
58. Kracoff OH, Adelman AG, Marquis JF, et al. Twelve-lead electrocardiogram recording during percutaneous transluminal coronary angioplasty: Analysis of reciprocal changes. *J Electrocardiol* 1990; 23:191–198.
59. Wagner GS. *Marriott's Practical Electrocardiography*, 9th ed. Baltimore: Williams & Wilkins; 1994:141.
60. Braat SH, Brugada P, den Dulk K, et al. Value of lead V_{4R} for recognition of the infarct coronary artery in acute inferior myocardial infarction. *Am J Cardiol* 1984; 53:1538–1541.
61. Castellanos A, Pina IL, Zaman L, et al. Recent advances in the diagnosis of fascicular blocks. *Cardiol Clin* 1987; 5:469–488.
62. Rosenbaum MB, Corrado G, Oliveri R, et al. Right bundle branch block with left anterior hemiblock surgically induced in tetralogy of Fallot. *Am J Cardiol* 1970; 26:12–19.
63. Cohen SI, Lau SH, Stein E, et al. Variations of aberrant ventricular conduction in man: Evidence of isolated and combined block within the specialized conduction system. *Circulation* 1968; 38:899–916.
64. Milliken JA. Isolated and complicated left anterior fascicular block: A review of suggested electrocardiographic criteria. *J Electrocardiol* 1983; 16:199–211.
65. Warner RA, Hill NE, Mookerjee S. Improved electrocardiographic criteria for the diagnosis of left anterior hemiblock. *Am J Cardiol* 1983; 51:723–726.
66. Rosenbaum MB, Elizari MV, Lazzari JO. The differential electrocardiographic manifestations of hemiblocks, bilateral bundle branch blocks and trifascicular blocks. In: Schlant RC, Hurst JW, eds. *Advances in Electrocardiography*. New York: Grune & Stratton; 1972:145–161.
67. Rosenbaum MB, Elizari MV, Lazzari JO, et al. The clinical causes and mechanisms of intraventricular conduction disturbances. In: Schlant RC, Hurst JW, eds. *Advances in Electrocardiography*. New York: Grune & Stratton; 1972:183–220.
68. Grant RP. Peri-infarction block. *Prog Cardiovasc Dis* 1959; 27:237–247.
69. Oppenheimer BS, Rothschild MA. Electrocardiographic changes associated with myocardial involvement: With special reference to prognosis. *JAMA* 1917; 69:429–431.
70. Castle CH, Keane WM. Electrocardiographic "peri-infarction block": A clinical and pathologic correlation. *Circulation* 1965; 31:403–408.
71. Cotne RA, Parkin TW, Brandenburg RO, et al. Peri-infarction block: Postmyocardial-infarction intraventricular conduction disturbance. *Am Heart J* 1965; 69:150–153.

72. First SR, Bayley RH, Bedford DR. Peri-infarction block. *Circulation* 1950; 2:31–36.
73. Wilson FN, Herrmann GR. Bundle branch block and arborization block. *Arch Intern Med* 1920; 26:153–191.
74. Wilson FN, Hill IGW, Johnston FD. The form of electrocardiogram in experimental myocardial infarction: III. The later effects produced by ligation of the anterior descending branch of the left coronary artery. *Am Heart J* 1935; 10:903–915.
75. Castellanos A Jr. Diagnosis of left anterior hemiblock and left posterior hemiblock in the presence of inferior wall myocardial infarction. *Bull NY Acad Med* 1971; 47:923–930.
76. Jacobson LB, Scheinman M. Catheter-induced intra-Hisian and intrafascicular block during recording of His bundle electrograms: A report of two cases. *Circulation* 1974; 49:579–584.
77. Luck JC, Engel TR. Transient right bundle branch block with "Swan-Ganz" catheterization. *Am Heart J* 1976; 92:263–264.
78. Narula OS. Longitudinal dissociation in the His bundle: Bundle branch block due to asynchronous conduction within the His bundle in man. *Circulation* 1977; 56:996–1006.
79. El-Sherif N, Amat-y-Leon F, Schonfield C, et al. Normalization of bundle branch block patterns by distal His bundle pacing: Clinical experimental evidence of longitudinal dissociation in the pathologic His bundle. *Circulation* 1978; 57:473–483.
80. Scherlag BJ, El-Sherif N, Hope RR, et al. The significance of dissociation of conduction in the canine His bundle: Electrophysiological studies in vivo and in vitro. *J Electrocardiol* 1978; 4:343–354.
81. Nakaya Y, Hiasa Y, Murayama Y, et al. Prominent anterior QRS forces as a manifestation of left septal fascicular block. *J Electrocardiol* 1978; 11:39–46.
82. Gambetta M, Childers RW. Rate-dependent right precordial Q waves: "Septal focal block." *Am J Cardiol* 1973; 32:196–201.
83. Dhala A, Gonzalez-Zuelgaray J, Deshpande S, et al. Unmasking the trifascicular left intraventricular conduction system by ablation of the right bundle branch. *Am J Cardiol* 1996; 77:706–712.
84. Wilson FN, Herrmann GR. An experimental study of incomplete bundle branch block and of the refractory period of the heart of the dog. In: Johnston FD, Lepeschkin E, eds. *Selected Papers of Dr. Frank N. Wilson*. Ann Arbor, MI: Edwards Brothers; 1954:749–810.
85. Barker JM, Valencia F. The precordial electrocardiogram in incomplete right bundle branch block. In: Johnson FD, Lepeschkin E, eds. *Selected Papers of Dr. Frank N. Wilson*. Ann Arbor, MI: Edwards Brothers; 1954:884–914.
86. Blount SG, Munyan EA Jr, Hoffman MS. Hypertrophy of the right ventricular outflow tract: A concept of the electrocardiographic findings in atrial septal defect. *Am J Med* 1957; 22:784–790.
87. Moore EN, Hoffman BF, Patterson DF, et al. Electrocardiographic changes due to delayed activation of the wall of the right ventricle. *Am Heart J* 1964; 68:347–361.
88. Sung RJ, Tamer DM, Agha AS, et al. Etiology of the electrocardiographic pattern of "incomplete right bundle branch block" in atrial septal defect: An electrophysiologic study. *J Pediatr* 1975; 87:1182–1186.
89. Castellanos A, Ramirez AV, Mayorga-Cortes A, et al. Left fascicular blocks during right-heart catheterization using the Swan-Ganz catheter. *Circulation* 1981; 64:1271–1276.
90. Pickoff AS, Wolff GS, Tamer D, et al. Arrhythmias and conduction system disturbances in infants and children: Recent advances and contributions of intracardiac electrophysiology. In: Castellanos A, Brest AN, eds. *Cardiac Arrhythmia—Mechanisms and Management. Cardiovasc Clin* 1980; 11:203–219.
91. Garcia OL, Castellanos A, Sung RJ, et al. Exposure of concealed right bundle branch block in Wolff-Parkinson-White type B by pacing from the vicinity of the A-V node. *Am Heart J* 1978; 96:662–668.
92. Sgarbossa EB. Recent advances in the electrocardiographic diagnosis of myocardiol infarction: Left bundle branch block and pacing. *PACE* 1998; 21:120–131.
93. Kindwall KE, Brown JP, Josephson ME. Predictive accuracy of criteria for chronic myocardial infarction in pacing-induced left bundle branch block. *Am J Cardiol* 1986; 57:1255–1260.
94. Wackers FJT. The diagnosis of myocardial infarction in the presence of left bundle branch block. *Cardiol Clin* 1987; 5:393–401.
95. Wolff L, Parkinson J, White PD. Bundle-branch block with short P-R interval in healthy young people prone to paroxysmal tachycardia. *Am Heart J* 1930; 5:685–704.
96. Castillo CA, Castellanos A Jr. His bundle recordings in patients with reciprocating tachycardias and Wolff-Parkinson-White syndrome. *Circulation* 1970; 42:271–285.
97. Rosenbaum FF, Hecht HH, Wilson FN, et al. The potential variations of the thorax and esophagus in anomalous atrioventricular excitation (Wolff-Parkinson-White syndrome). *Am Heart J* 1945; 29:281–326.
98. Wallace AG, Sealy WC, Gallagher JJ, et al. Ventricular excitation in Wolff-Parkinson-White syndrome. In: Wellens HJJ, Lie KI, Janse MJ, eds. *The Conduction System of the Heart: Structure, Function and Clinical Implications*. Leiden: HE Stenfert Kroese; 1976:613–630.
99. Befeler B, Castellanos A, Castillo CA, et al. Arrival of excitation at the right ventricular apical endocardium in Wolff-Parkinson-White syndrome type B. *Circulation* 1973; 48:655–660.
100. Castellanos A, Agha AS, Portillo B, et al. Usefulness of vectorcardiography combined with His bundle recordings and cardiac pacing in evaluation of the pre-excitation (Wolff-Parkinson-White) syndrome. *Am J Cardiol* 1972; 30:623–628.
101. Wellens HJJ. Contribution of cardiac pacing to our understanding of the Wolff-Parkinson-White syndrome. *Br Heart J* 1975; 37:231–241.
102. Milstein S, Sharma AD, Guiraudon GM, et al. An algorithm for the electrocardiographic localization of accessory pathways in the Wolff-Parkinson-White syndrome. *PACE* 1987; 10:555–563.
103. Gallagher JJ, Smith WM, Kasell JH, et al. Role of Mahaim fibers in cardiac arrhythmias in man. *Circulation* 1971; 64:176–189.
104. Basiouny T, De Chillou D, Fareh S, et al. Accuracy and limitations of published algorithms using the twelve-lead electrocardiogram to localize overt atrioventricular accessory pathways. *J Cardiovasc Electrophysiol* 1999; 10:1340–1349.
105. Chiang CE, Chen SA, Teo WS, et al. An accurate stepwise electrocardiographic algorithm for localization of accessory pathways in patients with Wolff-Parkinson-White syndrome from a comprehensive analysis of delta waves and r/s ratio during sinus rhythm. *Am J Cardiol* 1995; 76:40–46.
106. Castellanos A Jr, Ortiz JM, Pastis N, et al. The electrocardiogram in patients with pacemakers. *Prog Cardiovasc Dis* 1970; 13:190–209.
107. Castellanos A Jr, Lemberg L, Salhanick L, et al. Pacemaker vectorcardiography. *Am Heart J* 1968; 75:6–18.
108. Cosio FG, Anderson RH, Kuck KH, et al. ESCWGA/NASPE/P experts consensus statement: Living anatomy of the atrioventricular junctions. A guide to electrophysiologic mapping. *J Cardiovasc Electrophysiol* 1999; 10:1162–1170.
109. Munuswamy K, Alpert MA, Martin RH, et al. Sensitivity and specificity of commonly used electrocardiographic criteria for left atrial enlargement determined by M-mode echocardiography. *Am J Cardiol* 1984; 53:829–832.
110. Josephson ME, ed. *Clinical Cardiac Electrophysiology: Techniques and Interpretations*, 2d ed. Philadelphia: Lea & Febiger; 1993.
111. Surawicz B. Electrocardiographic diagnosis of chamber enlargement. *J Am Coll Cardiol* 1986; 8:711–724.
112. Reichet N, Devereaux RB. Left ventricular hypertropy: Relation-

ship of anatomic echocardiographic and electrocardiographic findings. *Circulation* 1981; 63:1391–1399.

113. Bommer K, Weinert L, Neumann A, et al. Determinations of right atrial and right ventricular size by two-dimensional echocardiography. *Circulation* 1980; 60:91–98.
114. Doxandabaratz J, Fort de Ribot R, Trilla E, et al. Miocardiopatia hipertrofica apical. *Rev Latina Cardiol* 1982; 3:35–41.
115. Romhilt D, Estes E. A point score system for the ECG diagnosis of left ventricular hypertrophy. *Am Heart J* 1968; 75:752.
116. Casale PN, Devereaux R, Alonso D, et al. Autopsy validation of improved ECG criteria of left ventricular hypertrophy. *J Am Coll Cardiol* 1985; 5:511–517.
117. Talbot S, Kilpatrick D. Diagnostic criteria for left ventricular hypertrophy. In: McFarlane PW, ed. *Progress in Electrocardiology*. London: Pittman Medical; 1979:534–541.
118. Koito H, Spodick D. Electrocardiographic RV_6/RV_1 voltage ratio for diagnosis of left ventricular hypertrophy. *Am J Cardiol* 1989; 63:352–359.
119. Hernandez Padial L. Usefulness of total 12-lead QRS voltage for determining the presence of left ventricular hypertrophy in systemic hypertension. *Am J Cardiol* 1991; 68:261–262.
120. Kafka H, Burggraf GW, Milliken JA. Electrocardiographic diagnosis of left ventricular hypertrophy in the presence of left bundle branch block: An echocardiographic study. *Am J Cardiol* 1985; 55:103–106.
121. Gertsch M, Theler A, Foglia E. Electrocardiographic detection of left ventricular hypertrophy in the presence of left anterior fascicular block. *Am J Cardiol* 1988; 61:1089–1101.
122. Vander Ark CR, Ballantyne F III, Reynolds EW Jr. Electrolytes and the electrocardiogram. *Cardiovasc Clin* 1973; 5:269–294.
123. Levine HD, Wanzer SH, Merrill JP. Dialyzable currents of injury in potassium intoxication resembling acute myocardial infarction or pericarditis. *Circulation* 1956; 13:29–36.
124. Mosseri M, Porath A, Ovsyshcher I, et al. Electrocardiographic manifestations of combined hypercalcemia and hypermagnesemia. *J Electrocardiol* 1990; 23:235–241.
125. Kulick DL, Hong R, Ryzen E, et al. Electrophysiologic effects of intravenous magnesium in patients with normal conduction systems and no clinical evidence of significant cardiac disease. *Am Heart J* 1988; 148:367–373.
126. Tzivoni D, Keren A, Cohen AM, et al. Magnesium therapy for torsades de pointes. *Am J Cardiol* 1984; 53:528–530.
127. Lepeschkin E. *Modern Electrocardiography*, Vol 1: *The P-Q-R-S-T-U Complex*. Baltimore: Williams & Wilkins; 1951.
128. Kligfield P, Lax KG, Okin PM. QT_c behavior during treadmill exercise as a function of the underlying QT-heart rate relationship. *J Electrocardiol* 1996; 30:206–210.
129. Day CP, McComb JM, Campbell RWF. QT dispersion: An indication of arrhythmia risk in patients with long QT intervals. *Br Heart J* 1990; 63:342–344.
130. Zabel M, Klingenheben T, Franz MR, et al. Assessment of QT dispersion for prediction of mortality or arrhythmic events after myocardial infarction: Results of a prospective long-term follow-up study. *Circulation* 1998; 97:2543–2550.
131. Kautzner J, Gang Y, Kishore AGR, et al. Interobserver reproducibility of QT interval and QT dispersion in patients after acute myocardial infarction. *Ann Noninvas Electrocardiol* 1996; 1:363–374.
132. Mirvis DM. Spatial variation of QT intervals in normal persons and patients with acute myocardial infarction. *J Am Coll Cardiol* 1985; 5:625–631.
133. Coumel P, Maison-Blanche P, Badilini F. Dispersion of ventricular repolarization: Reality? Illusion? Significance? *Circulation* 1998; 97:2491–2493.
134. Hashiba K, Moss AJ, Schwartz PJ. QT prolongation and ventricular arrhythmias. *Ann NY Acad Sci* 1992; 644:1–247.
135. Osborn JJ. Experimental hypothermia: Respiratory and blood pH changes in relation to cardiac function. *Am J Physiol* 1953; 175:389–398.
136. Castellanos A, Saoudi NC, Schwartz A, et al. Electrocardiographic patterns resulting from improper connections of the right leg (ground) cable. *PACE* 1985; 8:364–368.
137. Simonson E. *Differentiation between Normal and Abnormal in Electrocardiography*. St. Louis: Mosby; 1961:262.
138. Kerwin AJ, McLean R, Tegelaar H. A method for the accurate placement of chest electrodes in the taking of serial electrocardiographic tracings. *Can Med Assoc J* 1960; 82:258–261.
139. Garson A Jr. Clinically significant differences between the "old" analog and the "new" digital electrocardiograms. *Am Heart J* 1987; 114:194–197.
140. Tenth Bethesda Conference of the American College of Cardiology. Optimal electrocardiography. *Am J Cardiol* 1978; 41:111–191.
141. Seventeenth Bethesda Conference of the American College of Cardiology. Adult cardiology training. *J Am Coll Cardiol* 1986; 7:1192–1218.
142. AHA Committee Report. Recommendations for standardization of leads and of specifications for instruments in electrocardiography and vectorcardiography. Report of the Committee on Electrocardiography, American Heart Association. *Circulation* 1975; 52:11–31.
143. Bailey JJ, Berson AS, Garson A Jr, et al. Recommendations for standardization and specifications in automated electrocardiography: Bandwith and digital signal processing. A report for health professionals by an ad hoc writing group of the Committee on Electrocardiography and Cardiac Electrophysiology of the Council on Clinical Cardiology, American Heart Association. *Circulation* 1990; 81:730–739.
144. Taback L, Marden E, Mason HL, et al. Digital recording of electrocardiographic data for analysis by a digital computer. *IRE Trans Med Elect* 1959; 6:167–171.
145. Pipberger HV, Cornfeld J. What ECG computer program to choose for clinical application: The need for consumer protection. *Circulation* 1973; 47:918–920.
146. Laks MM, Ginzton L. Computerized electrocardiographic interpretation: A practical adjunct to the electrocardiographer. *Pract Cardiol* 1979; 5:127–144.
147. Proceedings of the Engineering Foundation Conference "Computerized Interpretation of the Electrocardiogram XII." *J Electrocardiol* 1987; 20(suppl):Preface.
148. Spodick DH, Bishop RL. Computer treason: Intraobserver variability of an electrocardiographic computer system. *Am J Cardiol* 1997; 80:102–103.
149. Wilson FN, Johnston FD. The vectorcardiogram. *Am Heart J* 1938; 16:14–28.
150. Mann H. A method of analyzing the electrocardiogram. *Arch Intern Med* 1920; 25:238–294.
151. Lemberg L, Castellanos A Jr. *Vectorcardiography*, 2d ed. New York: Appleton-Century-Crofts; 1975.
152. Massie E, Walsh TJ. *Clinical Vectorcardiography and Electrocardiography*. Chicago: Year Book Medical Publishers; 1960.
153. Chou TC, Helm RA, Kaplan S. *Clinical Vectorcardiography*, 2d ed. New York: Grune & Stratton; 1974.
154. Frank E. An accurate, clinically practical system for spatial vectorcardiography. *Circulation* 1956; 13:737–749.

C H A P T E R 12

THE CHEST ROENTGENOGRAM AND CARDIAC FLUOROSCOPY

James T. T. Chen

On November 8, 1895, Wilhelm Conrad Roentgen discovered x-rays[1] and ushered in a new era of diagnostic roentgenology. With wavelengths only 1/10,000 those of visible light, x-rays can penetrate the human body to produce roentgenograms, which revolutionized the field of medical diagnosis. Chest roentgenography in particular has since become a routine part of medical workup because of the invaluable information it can provide.

Familiarity with the altered anatomy and understanding of the underlying pathophysiology of a diseased heart are the cornerstones to appropriate interpretation of its roentgen manifestations. The conventional four-view cardiac series is tabulated in Table 12-1 and the views are illustrated in Fig. 12-1*C* to *F*.

The approach to the chest roentgenogram should be thorough and objective so that no clue is overlooked and no bias is incorporated in the process of radiographic analysis.[2–5] Rib notching (see Fig. 12-1*A*, *B*), for example, offers important clues to the diagnosis of coarctation of the aorta.[4,6] To prevent occasional erroneous clinical information from misleading the radiographic interpretation, films should at first be read without any knowledge about the patient. A patient may be referred, for instance, because of "bronchial asthma" refractory to therapy, only to be found later to suffer from cardiac asthma due to critical mitral stenosis. In this case, the classic radiographic manifestations of severe mitral stenosis should help clarify the confusion and prompt a change in patient management.

On other occasions, a secundum atrial septal defect may be misinterpreted as mitral stenosis because of similar physical signs. The split second sound may be misinterpreted as the opening snap. The diastolic rumble due to increased flow through a normal tricuspid valve may mimic the diastolic murmur of mitral stenosis. The x-ray signs of the two entities, however, are quite different (Fig. 12-2*B* versus Fig. 12-3*A*).

The final radiologic conclusion, however, should be drawn only after correlating the x-ray findings with clinical information and other laboratory parameters.

The radiologic examination for heart disease consists of six major steps. They are (1) roentgenographic examination for anatomy; (2) fluoroscopic examination for dynamics, (3) comparison, (4) statistical guidance, (5) clinical correlation, and (6) conclusion (Table 12-2).

ROENTGENOGRAPHIC EXAMINATION FOR ANATOMY

An Overview

The first step is to survey the roentgenogram and assess the entire situation, searching particularly for noncardiac conditions that may reflect heart disease. For instance, a right-sided stomach with an absent image of the inferior vena cava may suggest the possibility of congenital interruption of the inferior vena cava with azygos continuation[7,8] (Fig. 12-4). A narrowed anteroposterior diameter of the thorax may be the cause of an innocent murmur[9] (Fig. 12-5).

Pulmonary Vasculature

The lung may often reflect the underlying pathophysiology of the heart. By careful evaluation of the pulmonary vasculature,

TABLE 12-1 Conventional Four-View Cardiac Series

Posteroanterior (PA) view	With barium
Left lateral (lateral) view	With barium
45° Right anterior oblique (RAO) view	With barium
60° Left anterior oblique (LAO) view	Without barium

one may narrow down the diagnostic possibilities to a manageable level. For example, if uniform dilatation of all pulmonary vessels is present, the diagnosis of a left-to-right shunt (see Fig. 12-2*B*) is more likely than a left-sided obstructive lesion. The latter typically shows a cephalic pulmonary blood flow pattern (see Fig. 12-3*A*). More detailed analysis of the pulmonary vascularity will be discussed separately below.

Lung Parenchyma

With right-sided heart failure, the lungs become unusually radiolucent because of decreased pulmonary blood flow (PBF). On the other hand, significant failure on the left side of the heart is characterized by the presence of pulmonary edema and/or a cephalic blood flow pattern (Fig. 12-6). Long-standing, severe pulmonary venous hypertension may lead to hemosiderosis and/or ossification of the lung.[10,11] When right-sided heart failure results from severe left-sided heart failure, the preexisting pulmonary congestion may improve because of the decreased pulmonary blood flow (see Fig. 12-6*B*).

Cardiac Size

A significantly enlarged heart is always abnormal; however, mild cardiomegaly may reflect a higher than average cardiac output from a normal heart, as seen in athletes in active training. The cardiothoracic ratio remains the simplest and most practical yardstick for assessment of cardiac size.[2] The mean value for adults in an upright position in the posteroanterior (PA) view is 44 percent. More accurate roentgen measurements of cardiac size have been well documented[12,13] but are beyond the scope of the present discussion.

The nature of cardiomegaly usually can be determined by the specific roentgen appearance. As a rule, when the PBF pattern remains normal, cardiac lesions with volume overload tend to present a greater degree of cardiomegaly than lesions with pressure overload alone. For example, patients with aortic stenosis typically show features of left ventricular hypertrophy without dilatation. On the other hand, the left ventricle both dilates and hypertrophies in the case of aortic regurgitation, producing a much larger heart even before the development of congestive heart failure.

Both right- and left-sided heart failure can cause gross cardiac enlargement. The associated vascular abnormality in each case, however, is drastically different (see "Pulmonary Vascularity," below).

A smaller than average heart is encountered in patients with chronic obstructive pulmonary disease (Fig. 12-7*A*), Addison's disease, anorexia nervosa, and starvation. An abnormally small heart, however, is difficult to define except in a retrospective fashion, when the heart has returned to its normal capacity following successful therapy. For example, in patients with Addison's disease, the heart may become significantly larger following appropriate steroid therapy.

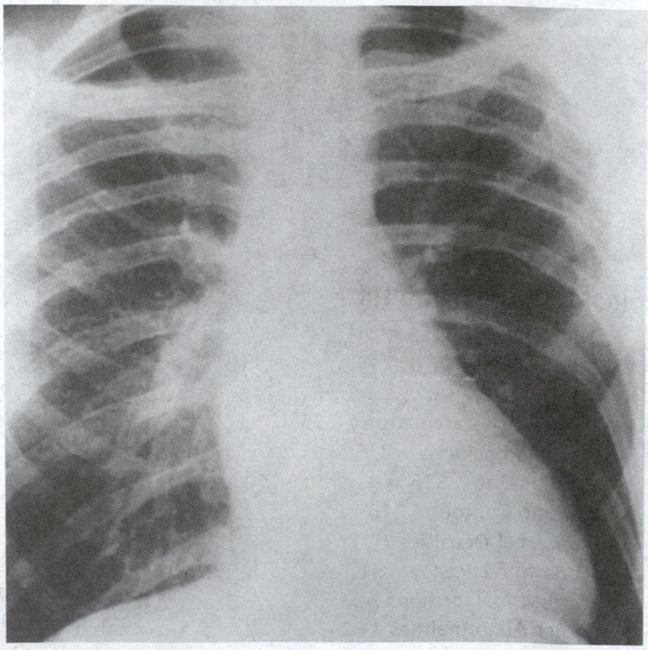

A

FIGURE 12-1 Practical application of four-view cardiac series. *A.* Posteroanterior view in a patient with coarctation of the aorta showing areas of rib notching bilaterally and left ventricular enlargement in the inferior and leftward direction. *B.* Magnified view of the left upper thorax of the same patient showing multiple areas of rib notching (*arrows*). The sclerotic margin of each represents a reparative process by which new bone is laid down in the defect. *C.* Posteroanterior view of another patient with aortic coarctation showing "3 sign" of the deformed descending aorta and "E sign" on the barium-filled esophagus. The upper arrow (on the patient's left) points to the level of coarctation. The lower arrow (on the patient's left) marks the apex of the enlarged left ventricle. The arrow on the patient's right indicates the dilated ascending aorta. *D.* Lateral view of a third patient with the same disease showing a barium-filled esophagus to be pushed forward (*upper arrow*) by the poststenotic dilatation of the descending aorta and pushed backward (*middle arrow*) by the enlarged left atrium. The very large left ventricle (*lower arrow*) simply casts a shadow behind the esophagus without displacing it. The oblique arrow points to the calcified stenotic bicuspid aortic valve. *E.* Right anterior oblique view of same patient whose posteroanterior view is shown in Fig. 12-7*D*. Note the huge right atrium casting a triangular density (*lower horizontal arrow*) behind the esophagus without displacing it. The esophagus is deviated posteriorly by the enlarged left atrium (*upper horizontal arrow*). The upper oblique arrows indicate the direction of the enlarging pulmonary trunk and right ventricle. The lower oblique arrow points to the normal left ventricle with the undisturbed left costophrenic sulcus. *F.* Left anterior oblique view of a patient with valvular aortic stenosis. The dilated ascending aorta (*upper white arrow*) is immediately above the flat anterior border of normal right ventricle. The black arrow points to the calcified aortic valve. The lower white arrow marks the enlarged left ventricle.

Cardiac Contour

Any significant deviation from the normal cardiovascular contour may serve as a clue to the correct diagnosis. For instance, *coeur en sabot*, a "boot-shaped heart" (see Fig. 12-2*C*), is characteristic of tetralogy of Fallot. A bulge along the left cardiac border with a retrosternal double density is virtually diagnostic of left ventricular aneurysm (Fig. 12-8). A markedly widened right cardiac contour in association with a straightened left cardiac border is seen frequently in patients with severe mitral stenosis leading to tricuspid regurgitation (see Fig. 12-7*D*).

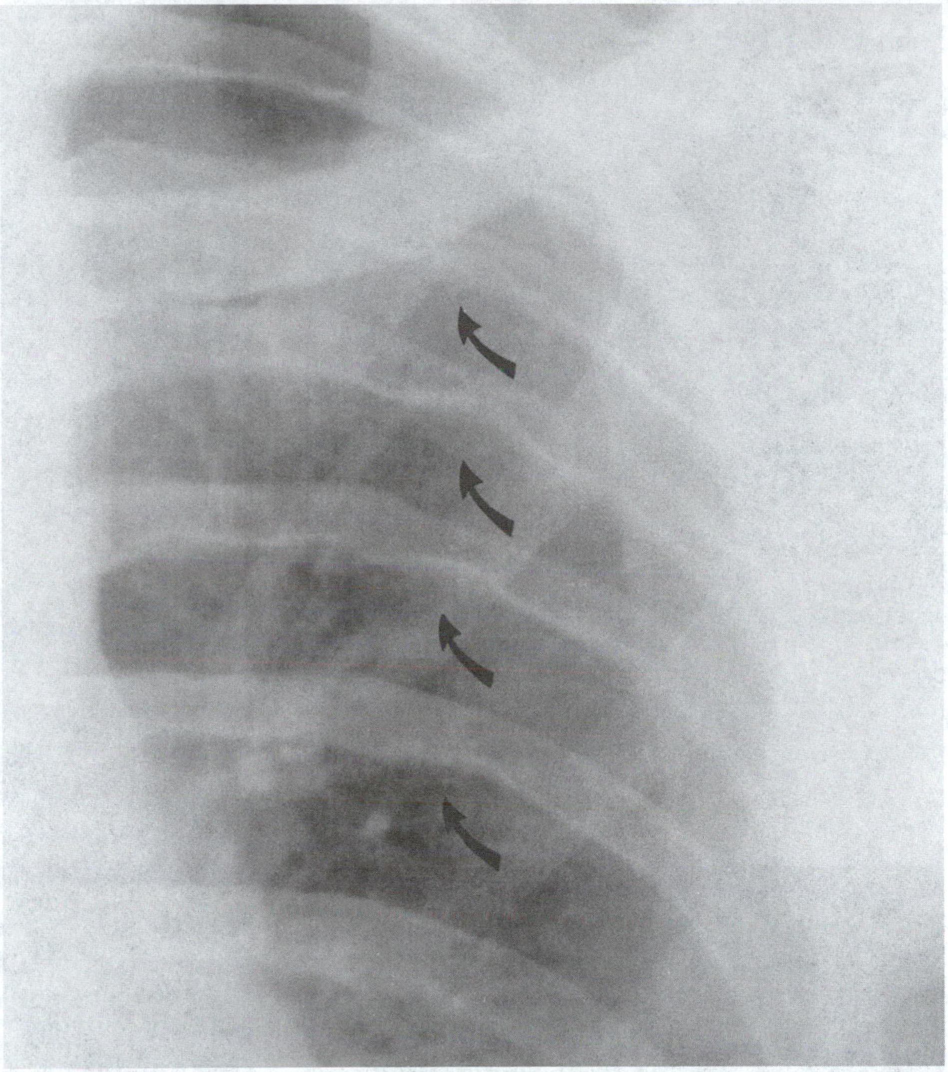

B

FIGURE 12-1 (*Continued*)

Abnormal Densities

Besides the familiar double density cast by an enlarged left atrium, other increased densities may be found within the confines of the heart, indicating a variety of dilated vascular structures, e.g., tortuous descending aorta, aortic aneurysm, coronary artery aneurysm, pulmonary varix, etc.[3] Furthermore, large cardiac calcifications are seen easily, particularly in lateral and oblique views. If smaller calcific deposits are suspected, they should be verified promptly or ruled out by cardiac fluoroscopy or computed tomographic (CT) scanning (see Chap. 17). Any radiologically detectable calcification in the heart is of clinical importance. The heavier the calcification, the more significant it becomes (see Fig. 12-1*F*). The extent of valvular calcification tends to be proportionate to the severity of the valve stenosis regardless of the other roentgen signs of the disease.[2,3,14,15] Calcification of the coronary artery is almost always atherosclerotic in nature. Mönckeberg's medial calcification of the coronary system is extremely rare. A fluoroscopically detectable coronary calcification is correlated with major vessel occlusion in 94 percent of patients with chest pain;[16] however, the sensitivity of the test is only 40 percent (see "Cardiac Fluoroscopy," below).

Recently, electron-beam CT scanning has proved to be a sensitive tool for the detection and quantification of coronary calcifications (see Chap. 17). A negative result may indicate no need for further testing in asymptomatic individuals. A positive result, however, does not necessarily denote obstructive coronary artery disease. The sensitivity for detecting any coronary calcifications is greater than 95 percent with a *specificity of less than 65 percent* for significant coronary artery disease. Another use of this method is to identify high-risk patients with calcific nonobstructive atherosclerotic lesions. By vigorous therapeutic intervention, one may be able to halt progression or even cause regression of their disease. In fact, the results of such interventions can be correlated with the increase or decrease in coronary calcific plaques[15] (see Chap. 17).

A calcified ascending aortic aneurysm with aortic regurgitation is highly suggestive of syphilitic aortitis[14] (Fig. 12-9).

Abnormal Lucency

The abnormal lucent areas in and about the heart include (1) displaced subepicardial fat stripes caused by effusion or thickening of the pericardium (Fig. 12-10), (2) pneumopericardium (Fig. 12-11), and (3) pneumomediastinum. Pneumomediastinum is differentiated from pneumopericardium by the fact that the former shows a superior extension of the air strip beyond the confines of the pericardium.

Cardiac Malposition

According to Elliott and Schiebler, "cardiac malpositions" are diagnosed only when either the heart or the stomach is out of the normal left-sided position. This definition is crucial in distinguishing an isolated right-sided aortic arch from a cardiac malposition.[7,8]

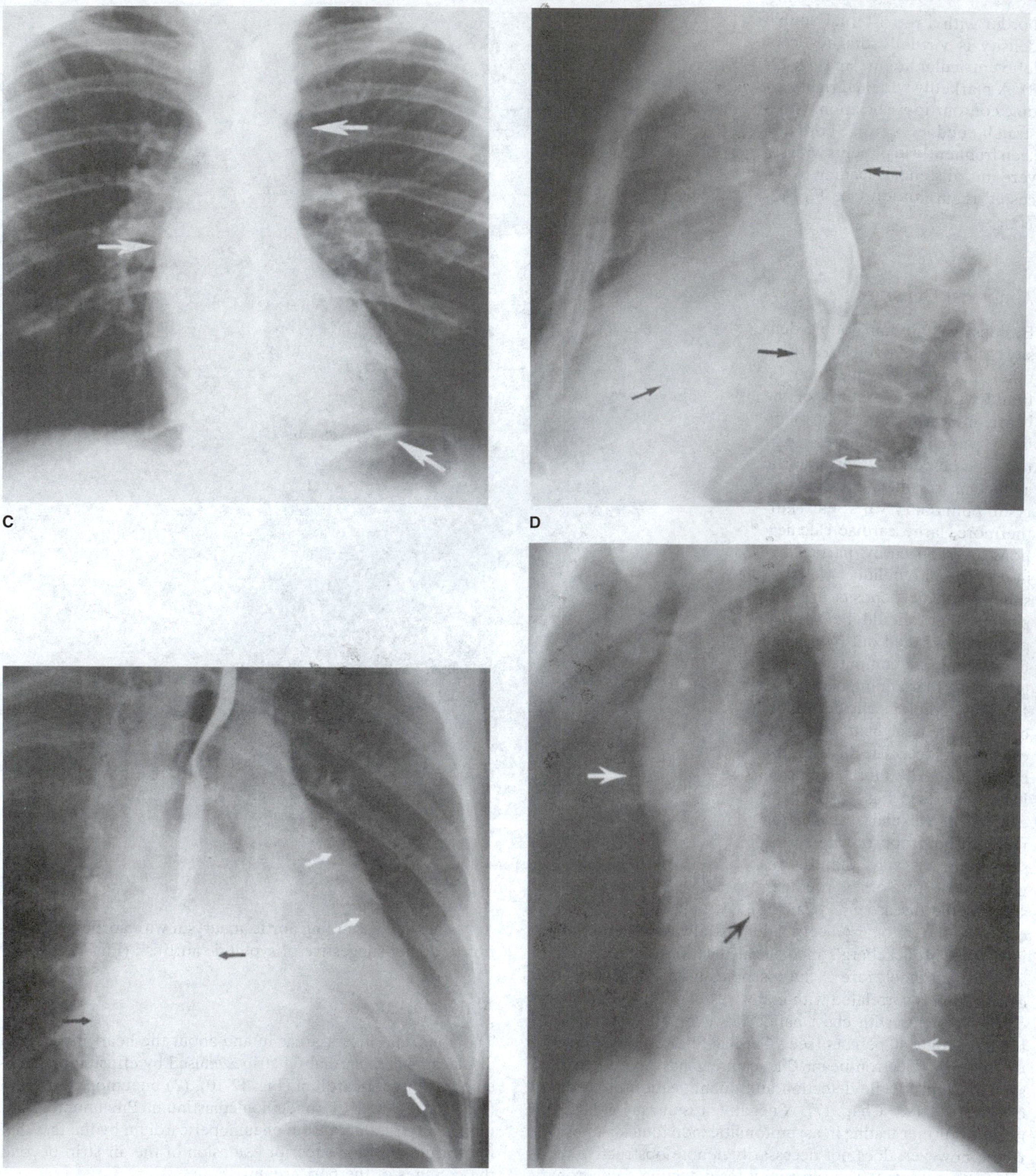

C D E F

FIGURE 12-1 (*Continued*)

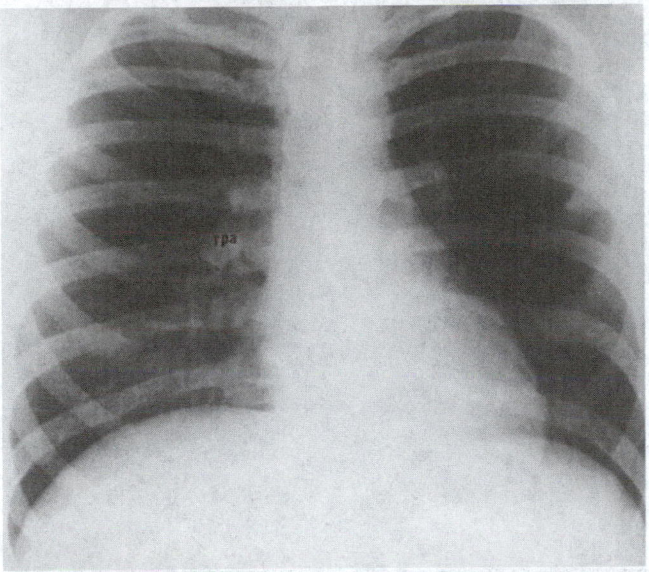

A

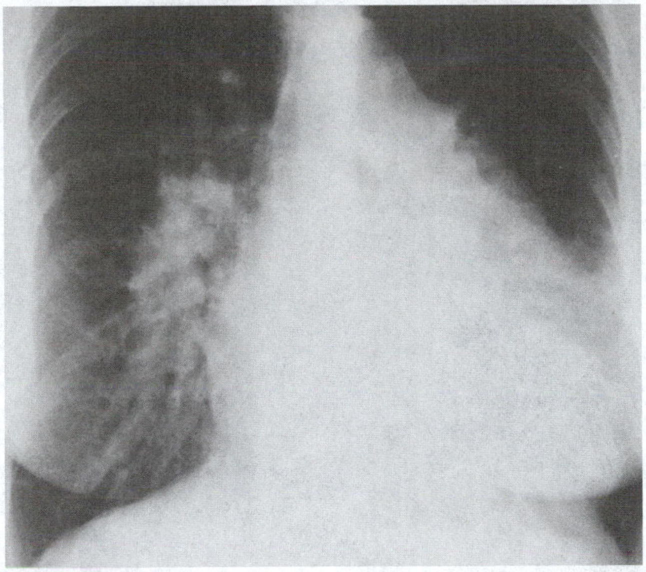

B

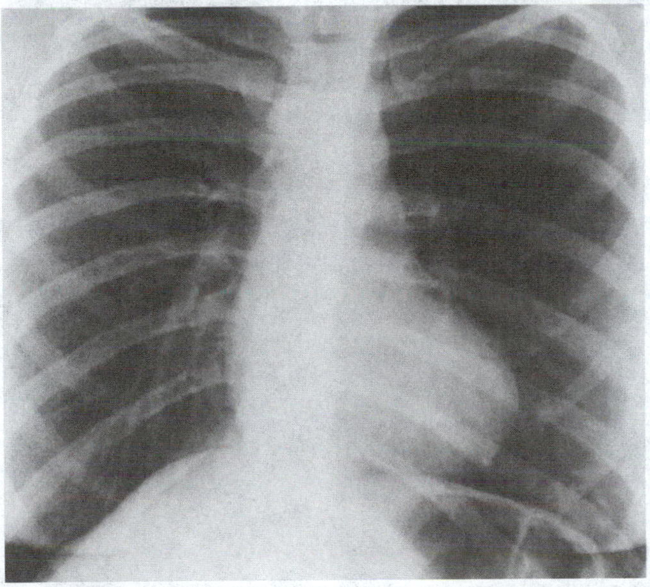

C

FIGURE 12-2 Roentgenographic assessment of the volume of pulmonary blood flow. *A.* Normal. There is caudalization of the pulmonary vascularity due to gravity. The right descending pulmonary artery (rpa) measures 13 mm in diameter in this young man. *B.* Increased. Patient with a secundum atrial septal defect showing uniform increase in pulmonary vascularity bilaterally. The right descending pulmonary artery is markedly enlarged, measuring 27 mm. *C.* Decreased. Patient with tetralogy of Fallot showing a boot-shaped heart and uniform decrease in pulmonary vascularity. The right descending pulmonary artery is much smaller than normal, measuring 6 mm in diameter.

DEXTROCARDIA WITH SITUS INVERSUS

Recently, the term *dextrocardia* has been used to indicate any congenital right-sided heart regardless of the position of abdominal viscera. To specify the kind of dextrocardia under test, one must affix the status of the abdominal viscera. *Dextrocardia with situs inversus* means the mirror image of normal. In this situation, the incidence of congenital heart disease is only 5 percent, which is a ninefold increase over the general population. The combination of dextrocardia, sinusitis, and bronchiectasis is known as *Kartagener's triad*.

DEXTROCARDIA WITH SITUS SOLITUS

This represents an anomaly with normal situs but a right-sided heart. Radiographically, normal situs (situs solitus) is a certainty when both the aortic knob and the gastric air bubble are on the left side. *Situs solitus* also means that both the abdominal viscera and the atria are in the normal position. Under these circumstances, if the ventricles fail to swing from the primitive right-sided position to the normal left-sided position, abnormal relationships between the ventricles and the rest of the cardiovascular structures are bound to develop. This entity was formerly termed *dextroversion*.

In patients with dextroversion, the incidence of congenital heart disease has been estimated at 98 percent. More than 80 percent have congenitally corrected (or L-loop) transposition of great arteries. The next most commonly associated lesions are a combination of ventricular septal defect and pulmonary stenosis, a tetralogy-like pathophysiology (Fig. 12-12). Therefore, from a statistical point of view, it is important to be able to differentiate this entity from dextrocardia with situs inversus, which is associated with a much lower incidence of congenital heart disease (see above and also Chap. 63).

LEVOCARDIA WITH SITUS INVERSUS

This is a mirror image of dextroversion, and it is associated with an extremely high incidence (nearly 100 percent) of cyanotic congenital cardiac lesions similar to those seen in dextroversion. This entity was formerly termed *levoversion*.

LEVOCARDIA WITH SITUS SOLITUS

This is entirely normal.

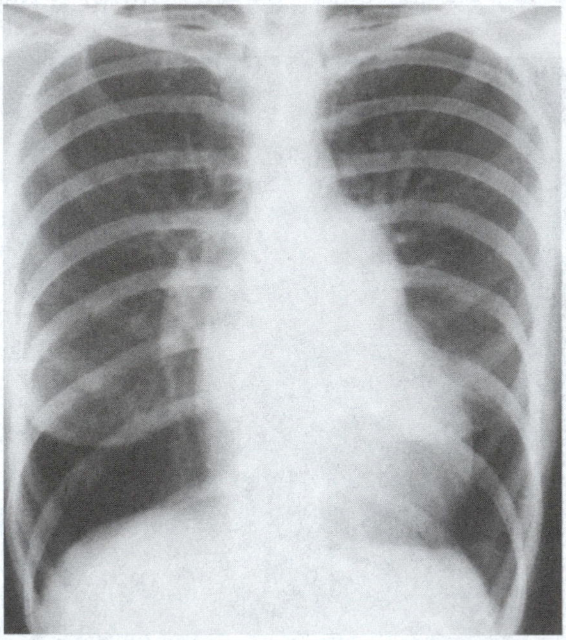

A

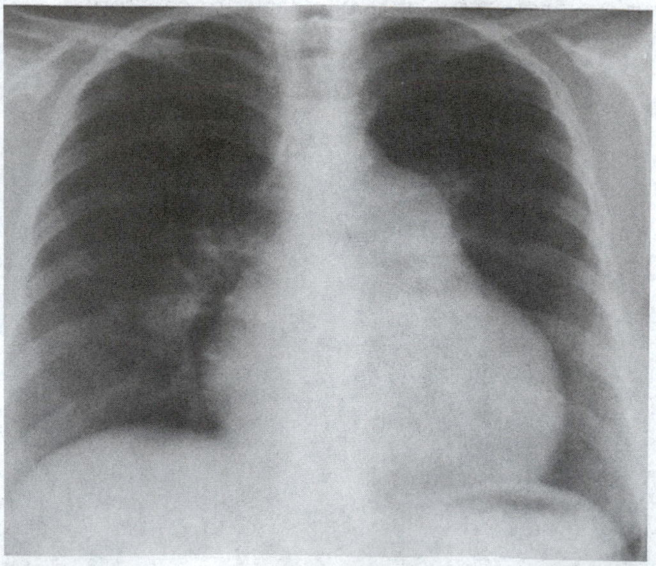

B

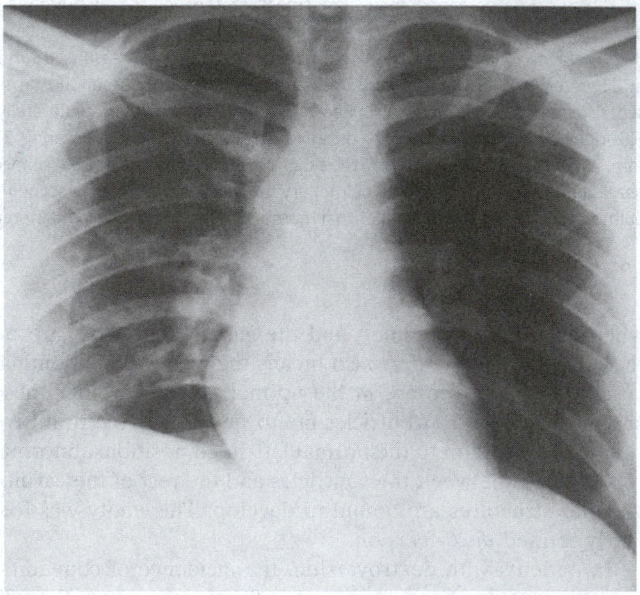

C

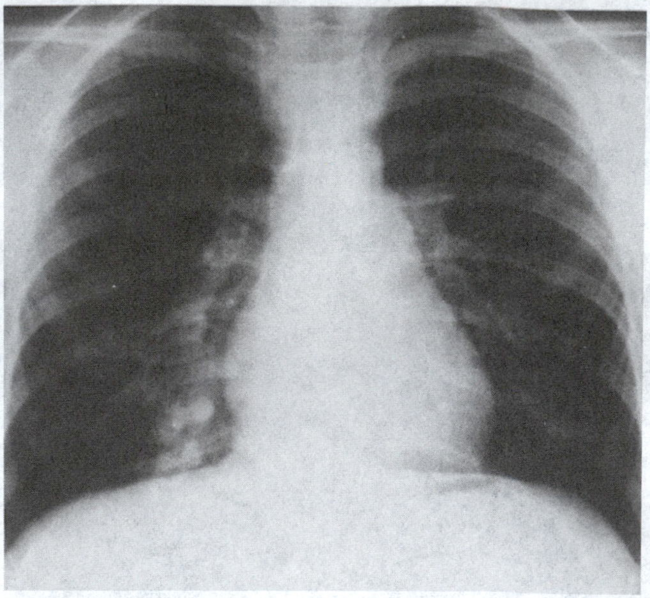

D

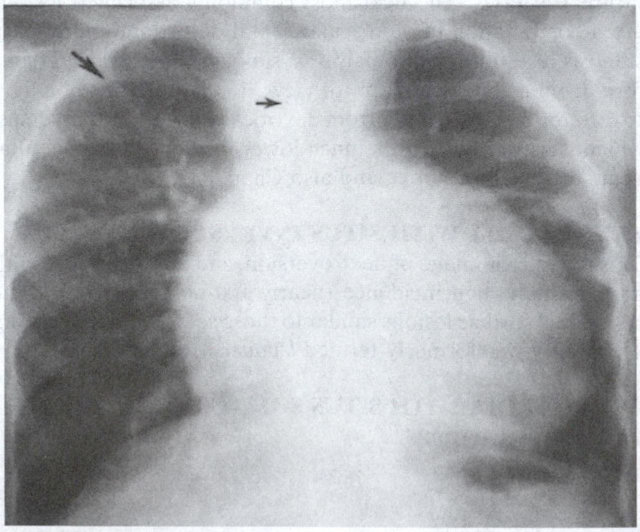

E

FIGURE 12-3 Abnormal pulmonary blood flow patterns. *A.* Cephalization. Patient with severe mitral stenosis showing dilatation of the upper vessels with constriction of the lower vessels. *B.* Centralization. Patient with primary pulmonary hypertension showing marked dilatation of the pulmonary trunk and the central segments of both pulmonary arteries with pruning of the peripheral branches. *C.* Lateralization. Patient with massive pulmonary embolism obstructing the left main pulmonary artery. Note the uneven distribution of pulmonary blood flow between the two lungs in favor of the right. *D.* Localization. A cyanotic child showing localized vascular changes representing a large pulmonary arteriovenous fistula in the right lower lobe. *E.* Collateralization. A child with pseudotruncus arteriosus with cardiomegaly and a right aortic arch (*small arrow*). Note severe pulmonary oligemia with numerous small tortuous vessels (*large arrow*) in upper medial lung zones, representing bronchial arterial collaterals.

TABLE 12-2 Major Steps of Roentgenologic Examination

Roentgenographic examination for anatomy
Overview, e.g., rib notching
Pulmonary vascularity, e.g., shunt vascularity in ASD
Lung parenchyma, e.g., ossification in critical MS
Cardiac size, e.g., huge right heart in Ebstein's anomaly
Cardiac contour, e.g., boot-shaped heart in TOF
Abnormal densities, e.g., calcification of LV aneurysm
Abnormal lucency, e.g., conspicuous fat stripes in PE
Cardiac malpositions, e.g., dextrocardia with SS
Other abnormalities, e.g., Holt-Oram syndrome
Fluroscopic observation for dynamics
Comparison
Statistical guidance
Clincal correlation
Conclusion

ABBREVIATIONS: ASD = atrial septal defect; MS = mitral stenosis; TOF = tetralogy of Fallot; LV = left ventricle; PE = pericardial effusion; SS = situs solitus.

CARDIAC MALPOSITIONS WITH SITUS AMBIGUUS

In this group, the patient's heart may be either left- or right-sided. The situs is ambiguous because the aortic arch and the stomach are not on the same side. Under these circumstances, we are dealing with either asplenia or polysplenia syndrome. Patients with polysplenia syndrome tend to be acyanotic, running a milder clinical course, and frequently survive into adulthood. The associated lesions are bilateral left-sidedness, interruption of the inferior vena cava with azygos continuation (see Fig.12-4), polysplenia, and a left-to-right shunt, most frequently an atrioventricular septal defect.[17] Patients with asplenia syndrome, on the other hand, tend to be cyanotic and critically ill and die in infancy. The associated lesions are bilateral right-sidedness, asplenia, midline liver, and pulmonary stenosis or atresia with oligemic lungs. It is noteworthy that interruption of inferior vena cava has never been reported in patients with asplenia.

Other Abnormalities

GREAT VESSELS

The roentgen appearance of the great vessels often provides valuable information for the diagnosis of heart disease.[2,3,18,19] For example, selective dilatation of the ascending aorta is the hallmark of valvular aortic stenosis (Fig. 12-13); generalized dilatation of the entire thoracic aorta (Fig. 12-14), on the other hand, favors the diagnosis of aortic regurgitation, systemic hypertension, or both, depending on the size of the left ventricle. A larger left ventricle is associated with aortic regurgitation because of volume overload. In atrial septal defect and mitral stenosis, the pulmonary trunk is quite large, and the aortic knob

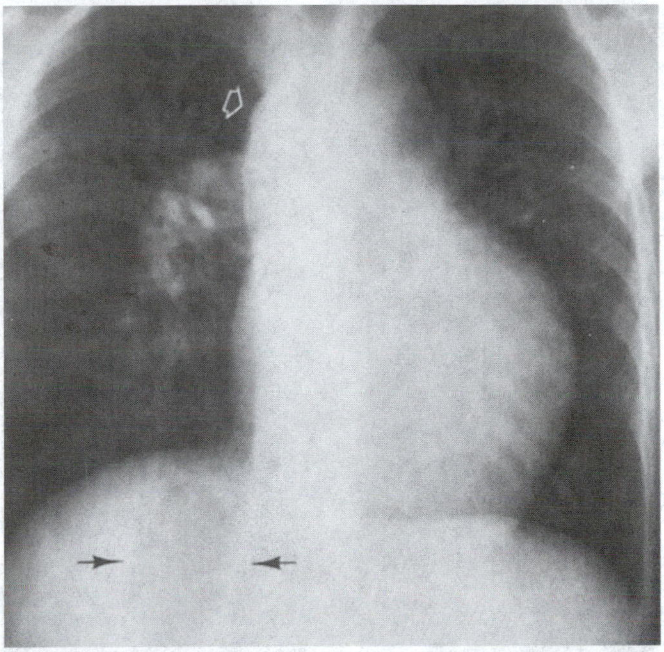

A

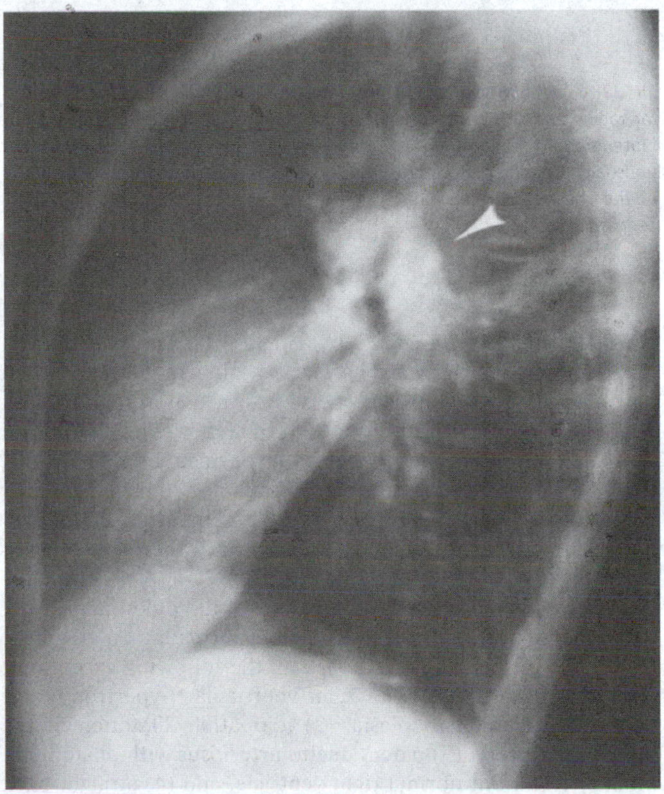

B

FIGURE 12-4 Patient with situs ambiguous, interruption of the inferior vena cava, ventricular septal defect, and polysplenia. *A*. Posteroanterior view shows that the aortic arch and the heart are left-sided and the stomach (*lower arrows*) is right-sided. The azygos vein (*upper arrow*) is markedly enlarged. The heart is mildly enlarged, and there is a moderate increase in pulmonary vascularity. *B*. Lateral view shows an absent image of the inferior vena cava. The azygos arch (*arrow*) is markedly dilated.

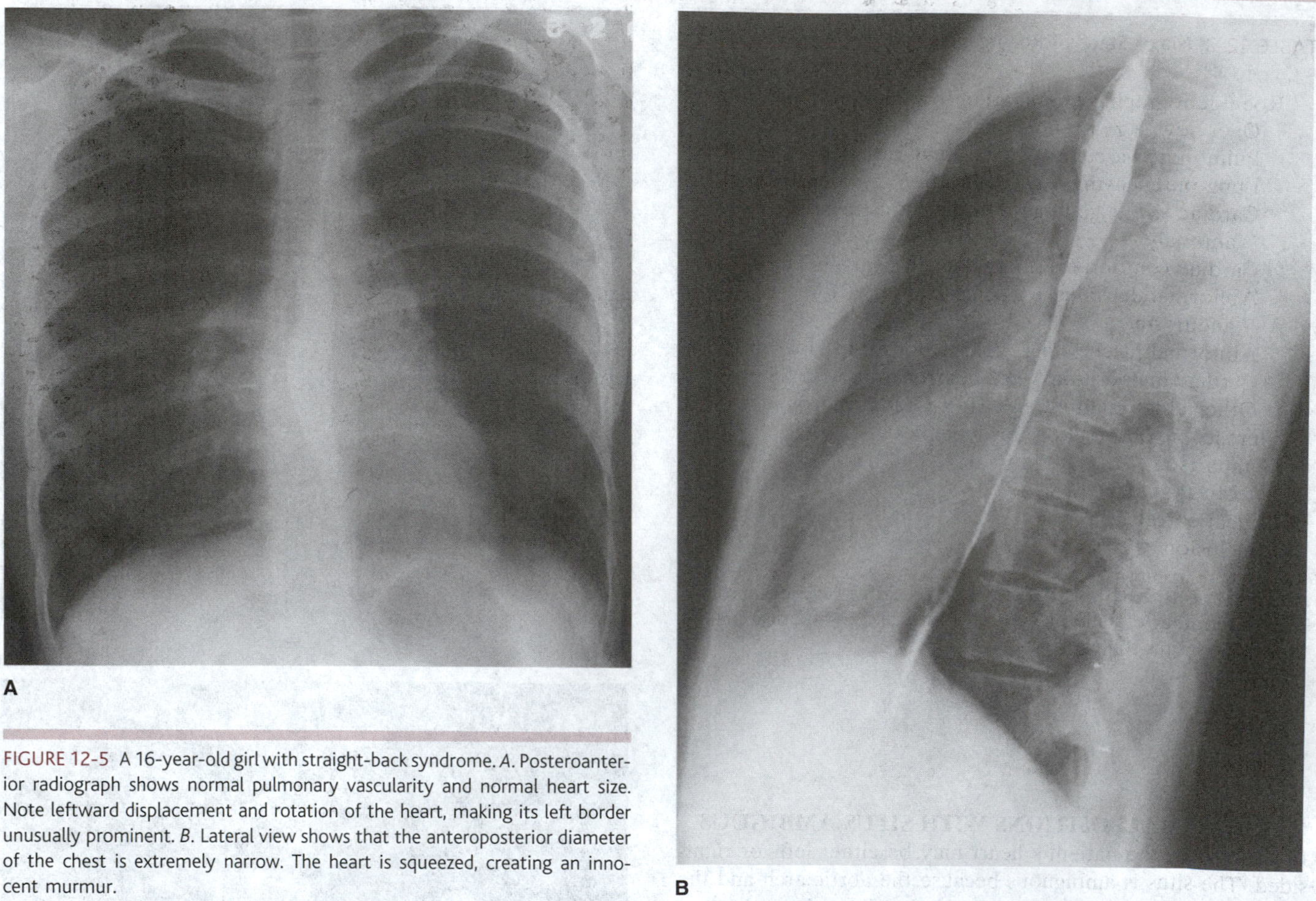

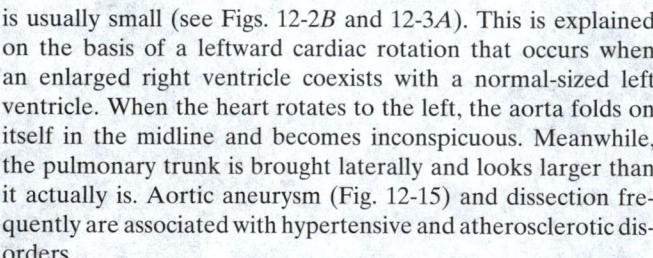

FIGURE 12-5 A 16-year-old girl with straight-back syndrome. *A*. Posteroanterior radiograph shows normal pulmonary vascularity and normal heart size. Note leftward displacement and rotation of the heart, making its left border unusually prominent. *B*. Lateral view shows that the anteroposterior diameter of the chest is extremely narrow. The heart is squeezed, creating an innocent murmur.

is usually small (see Figs. 12-2*B* and 12-3*A*). This is explained on the basis of a leftward cardiac rotation that occurs when an enlarged right ventricle coexists with a normal-sized left ventricle. When the heart rotates to the left, the aorta folds on itself in the midline and becomes inconspicuous. Meanwhile, the pulmonary trunk is brought laterally and looks larger than it actually is. Aortic aneurysm (Fig. 12-15) and dissection frequently are associated with hypertensive and atherosclerotic disorders.

As already mentioned, prominence of the pulmonary trunk is a reliable secondary sign of right ventricular enlargement (Fig. 12-16; also see Fig. 12-2*B*), with the following exceptions: (1) tetralogy of Fallot with right ventricular hypertrophy but pulmonary trunk hypoplasia, (2) idiopathic dilatation of the pulmonary artery, (3) patent ductus arteriosus with dilated pulmonary trunk but normal right ventricle, and (4) straight-back syndrome, pectus excavatum, and scoliosis with narrowed anteroposterior diameter of the chest. Under the latter conditions, the heart is compressed, displaced, and rotated to the left, giving rise to a falsely enlarged pulmonary artery.

In coarctation of the aorta, the engorged aortic knob and the poststenotic dilatation of the descending aorta may cause a "3 sign" on the aorta and an "E sign" on the barium-filled esophagus, both depicting the site of coarctation[6] (see Fig. 12-1*C*).

The abnormal size and distribution of both the pulmonary and systemic veins are important clues to the presence of certain conditions, e.g., anomalous pulmonary venous connections, pulmonary arteriovenous fistulas, pulmonary varix, persistent left superior vena cava, and interruption of inferior vena cava with azygos continuation (see Fig. 12-4).

The significance of aortic arch anomalies is discussed under "Statistical Guidance," below.

MEDIASTINAL STRUCTURES

The mediastinal organs frequently are affected by the cardiovascular structures because of their close spatial interrelationships. An enlarged left atrium not only displaces the esophagus (see Fig. 12-1*C–E*) and the descending aorta but also elevates and compresses the left mainstem bronchus. A double aortic arch may compress both the trachea and the esophagus. On the other hand, malignant processes may invade the heart and great vessels, causing cardiac tamponade or the superior vena cava syndrome, for example. Usually, these mediastinal changes are evident on the chest roentgenogram and should be recognized promptly.[18–22]

PLEURA

A right-sided pleural effusion often is present with left-sided heart failure. A bilateral hydrothorax, on the other hand, suggests bilateral heart failure or a noncardiac etiology of the effusion. Congestive heart failure is also known to be associated

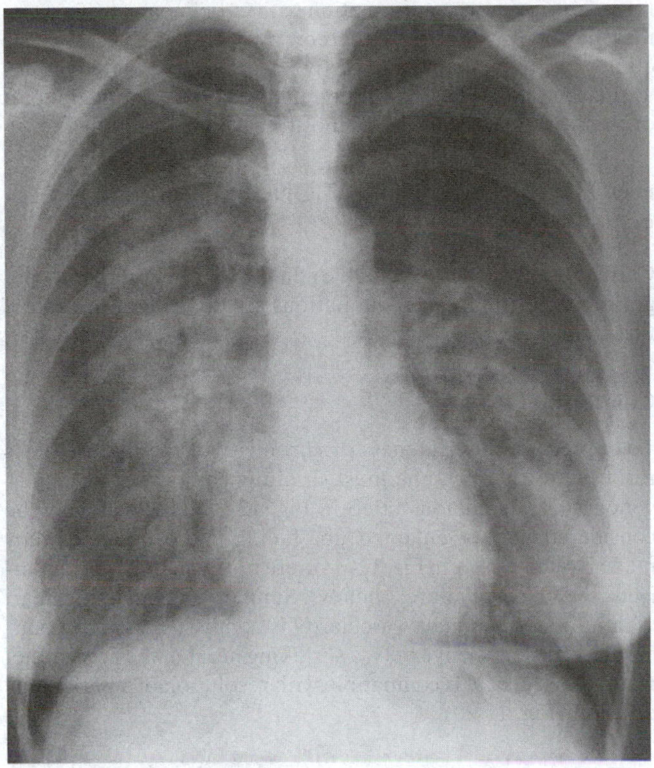

A

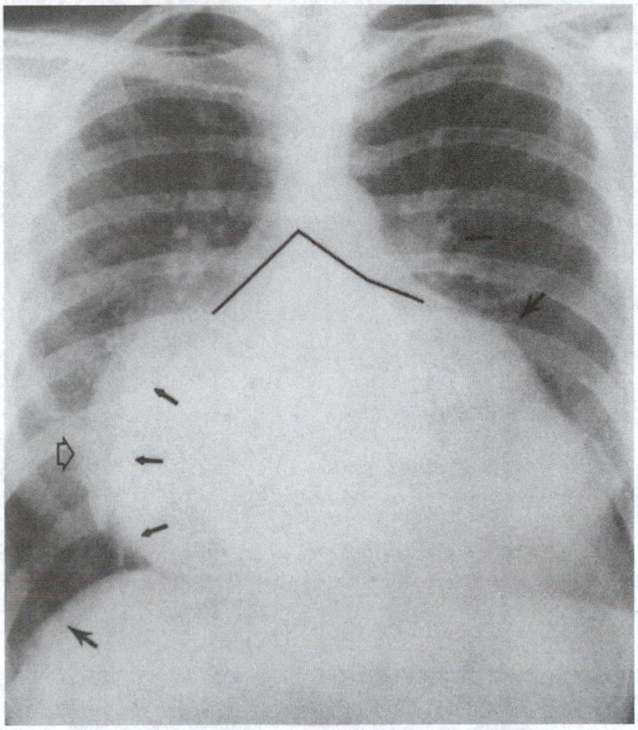

B

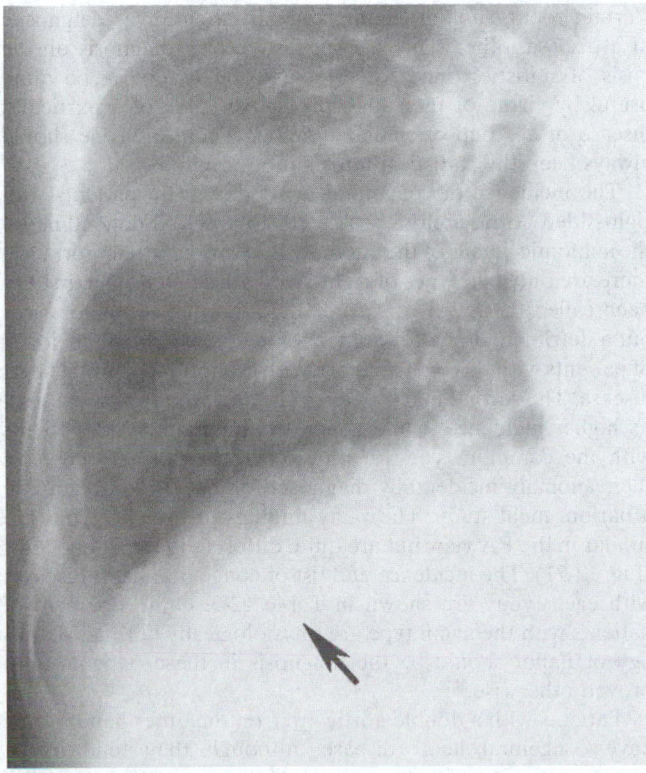

C

FIGURE 12-6 Roentgen appearance of left-sided heart failure. *A*. Acute. Patient with acute mitral regurgitation due to rupture of chordae tendineae showing "bat wings" appearance of severe alveolar type of pulmonary edema and a normal-sized heart. *B*. Chronic. Patient with severe mitral and tricuspid regurgitation and mild aortic regurgitation. This is a predominantly left-sided failure pattern. Note gross cardiomegaly with striking cephalization and interstitial pulmonary edema. The giant left atrium forms the right cardiac border (*open arrow*), makes its appendage bulge outward on the left side (*upper large arrow*), and splays the mainstem bronchi wide apart (*solid lines*). The huge right atrium forms a double density within the right cardiac border (*three small arrows*). The upper small arrow marks the peribronchial cuffing of edema fluid. The lower large arrow points to multiple Kerley B lines. *C*. Magnified view of right costophrenic sulcus showing multiple Kerley B lines (*arrow*). *D*. A 44-year-old woman with severe mitral stenosis. Her radiograph shows a diffuse stippling with fine nodules representing hemosiderosis. Hemosiderin-laden macrophages were found in her sputa. *E*. Posteroanterior radiograph of a 63-year-old man with severe mitral stenosis, status post mitral valve replacement, shows multiple scattered bony nodules (*arrows*) 2 to 10 mm in diameter throughout the lower two-thirds of both lungs, compatible with pulmonary ossification.

with a pseudotumor or "vanishing" tumor, representing an interlobar collection of pleural fluid (Fig. 12-17). As congestive heart failure improves, the "tumor" disappears.

BONES AND JOINTS

Notching of the ribs has many origins. Basically, any of the three major intercostal structures can enlarge, compress, and erode the lower borders of the ribs, producing areas of notching. They are intercostal arteries, veins, and nerves. Coarctation of the aorta[6] (see Fig. 12-1*A*) represents the most common cause of rib notching due to dynamic dilatation and tortuosity of the arteries. Superior vena cava syndrome may cause a similar

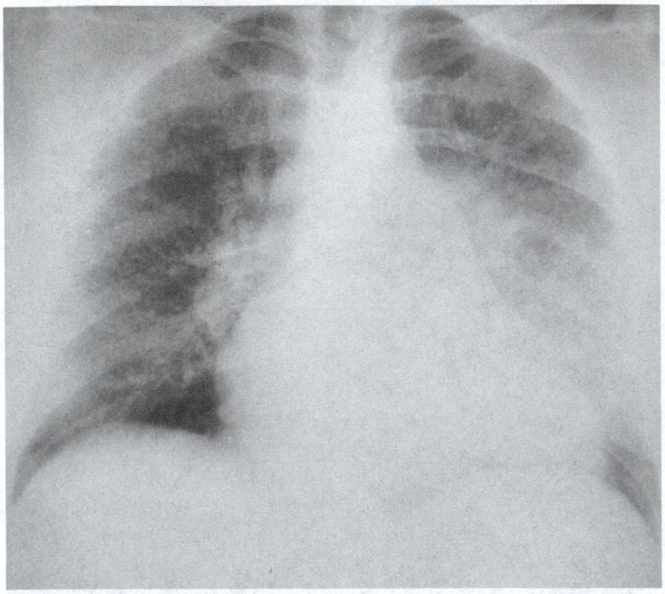

D

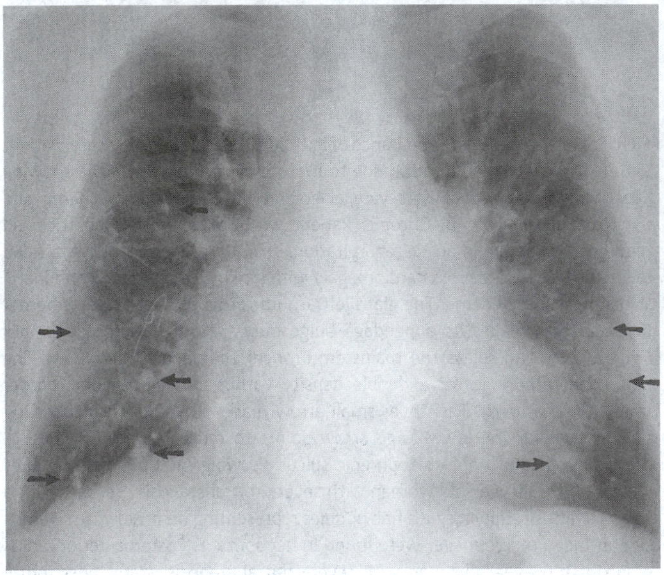

E

FIGURE 12-6 (*Continued*)

phenomenon of venous origin. Neurofibromatosis also can produce rib notching by numerous intercostal neurofibromas.

SOFT TISSUES OVER THE CHEST

Patients with renal failure may show severe edema in the soft tissues over the chest as part of the picture of general anasarca (Fig. 12-18).

EXTRATHORACIC STRUCTURES

In Holt-Oram syndrome (Fig. 12-19), the upper extremity abnormalities may be evident in a chest roentgenogram or on other films in the patient's x-ray folder (see also Chap. 63). A large arteriovenous malformation with curvilinear calcifications may be seen in the neck, thereby providing a clue as to the etiology of the patient's congestive heart failure. Radiographic evaluation of the patient's abdominal viscera is an integral part of the workup for cardiac malpositions.[7,8]

FLUOROSCOPIC OBSERVATION FOR DYNAMICS

Cardiac fluoroscopy is a valuable adjunct to the chest roentgenogram.[2] Its advantages and limitations are detailed at the end of this chapter.

COMPARISON

To appreciate the acuteness or chronicity of the disease or its response to therapy, one must carefully compare serial roentgenograms. As demonstrated in Fig. 12-7*B*, the heart may be considered neither enlarged nor failing if the baseline study made 3 years earlier in Fig. 12-7*A* were not available for comparison (see "Heart Failure," below). Similarly, an enlarging heart with normal pulmonary vascularity is highly suggestive of pericardial effusion. Conversely, a shrinking heart in the presence of normal vascularity is compatible with resolution of a pericardial effusion (Fig. 12-20).

STATISTICAL GUIDANCE

Certain roentgenologic findings are by themselves diagnostic of a disease; other signs are suggestive of a diagnosis on the basis of statistics only. Nevertheless, the latter can be quite useful by virtue of their high predictive value of a particular disease or a group of similar diseases. Therefore, one should always keep the statistical information in mind.

The incidence of congenital heart disease in patients with right-sided aortic arch increases 10- to 100-fold depending on the anatomic details of the anomaly.[21,22] Of practical importance, there are only two types of right-sided aortic arch. The first has been called the *avian type*, implying a normal status for birds but a detrimental one for humans. The overwhelming majority of patients with this type are born with cyanotic congenital heart disease. The second may be called the *common type* because of its higher incidence in the general population. Most patients with the common type are physiologically normal and have their anomaly incidentally diagnosed on chest radiographs or a barium meal study. The x-ray findings of the two types are similar in the PA view but are quite different in the lateral view (Fig. 12-21). The incidence and list of congenital heart diseases with each type[20] are shown in Table 12-3. Only 2 percent of patients with the avian type are physiologically normal. Tetralogy of Fallot should be the diagnosis in these patients until proved otherwise.[21,22]

Patients with a double aortic arch, on the other hand, rarely have congenital heart disease, although they tend to be symptomatic in infancy because of a compressing vascular ring.[21]

CLINICAL CORRELATION

The next step in the examination is to correlate the roentgenologic findings with the clinical information and other laboratory

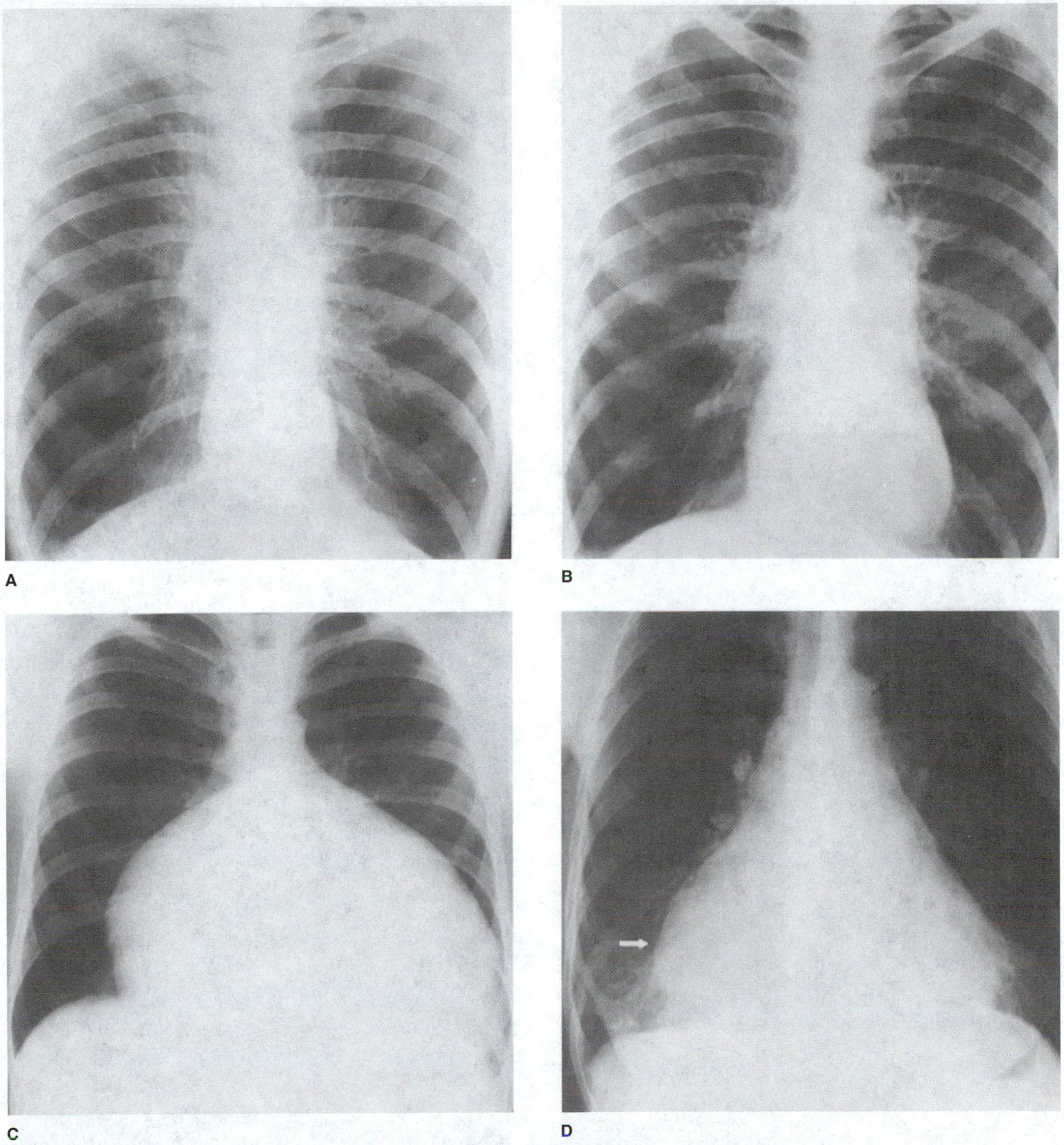

FIGURE 12-7 Roentgen appearance of right-sided heart failure. *A.* Patient with severe obstructive emphysema showing overaeration of the lungs, centralized flow pattern, and a small heart size. *B.* Three years later, the patient was in frank right-sided heart failure. Note that the heart got bigger as his emphysema got worse. The centralized flow pattern became more severe. *C.* Patient with Ebstein's anomaly showing gross cardiomegaly with severe decrease in pulmonary vascularity. The right cardiac border represents the huge right atrium, and the left cardiac border represents the giant right ventricle. *D.* Patient with mitral stenosis showing a giant right atrium (*arrow*) representing severe functional tricuspid regurgitation due to unrelenting left-sided failure. The pulmonary venous congestion had improved following the onset of right-sided heart failure.

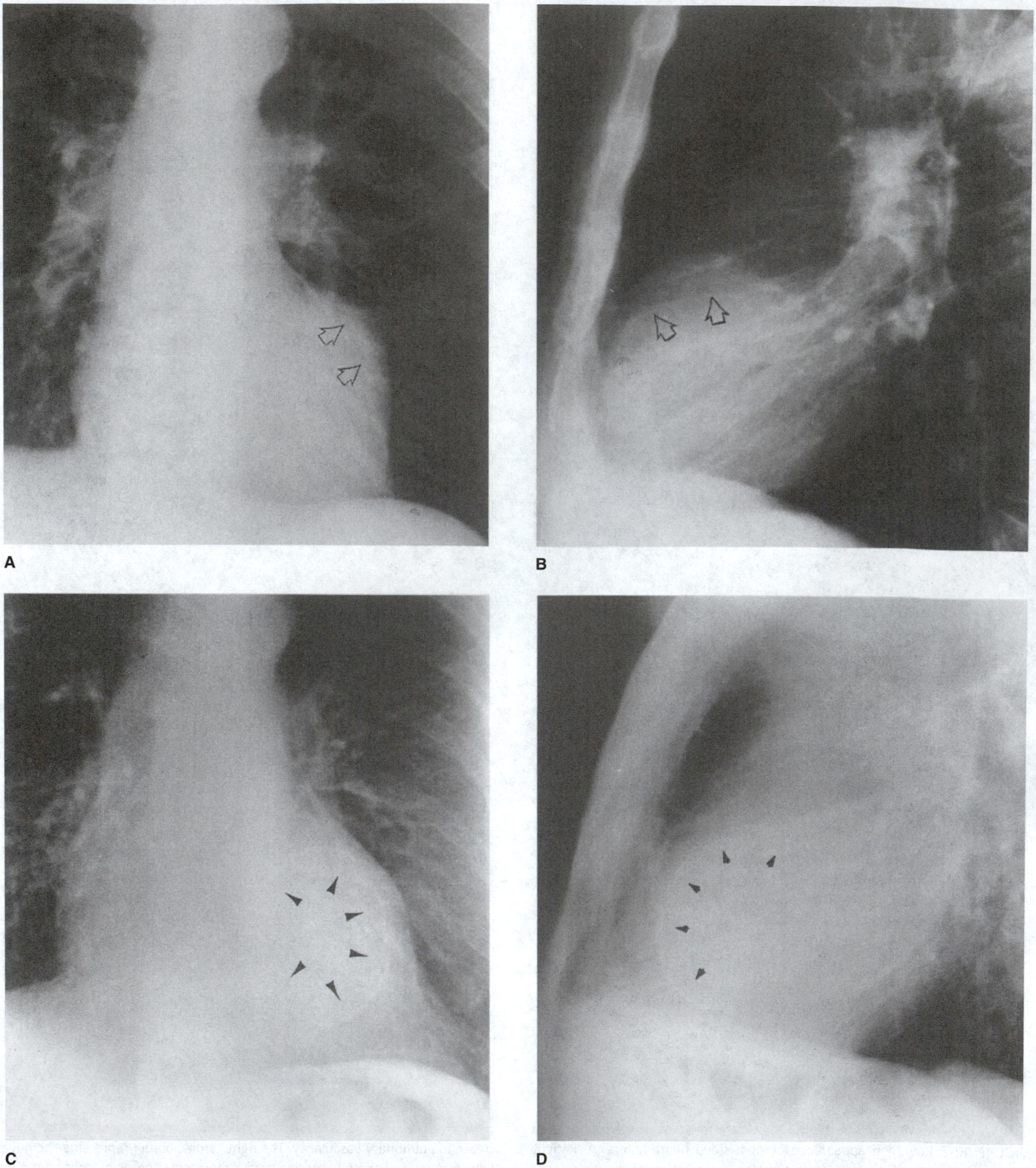

FIGURE 12-8 Left ventricular aneurysms. *A*. Posteroanterior view of patient 1 shows a localized bulge (*arrows*) along the left cardiac border representing a left ventricular aneurysm from the anterolateral wall. *B*. Lateral view shows a double density with sharp borders anteriorly and superiorly (*arrows*). This is the left ventricular aneurysm that casts a shadow on the normal right ventricle. Fluoroscopically, it is easy to confirm its origin and to separate it from the right ventricle by rotating the patient under direct vision. *C*. Posteroanterior view of patient 2, a 69-year-old man, shows total calcification of an anterolateral apical left ventricular aneurysm (*arrows*). *D*. Lateral view shows the same (*arrows*).

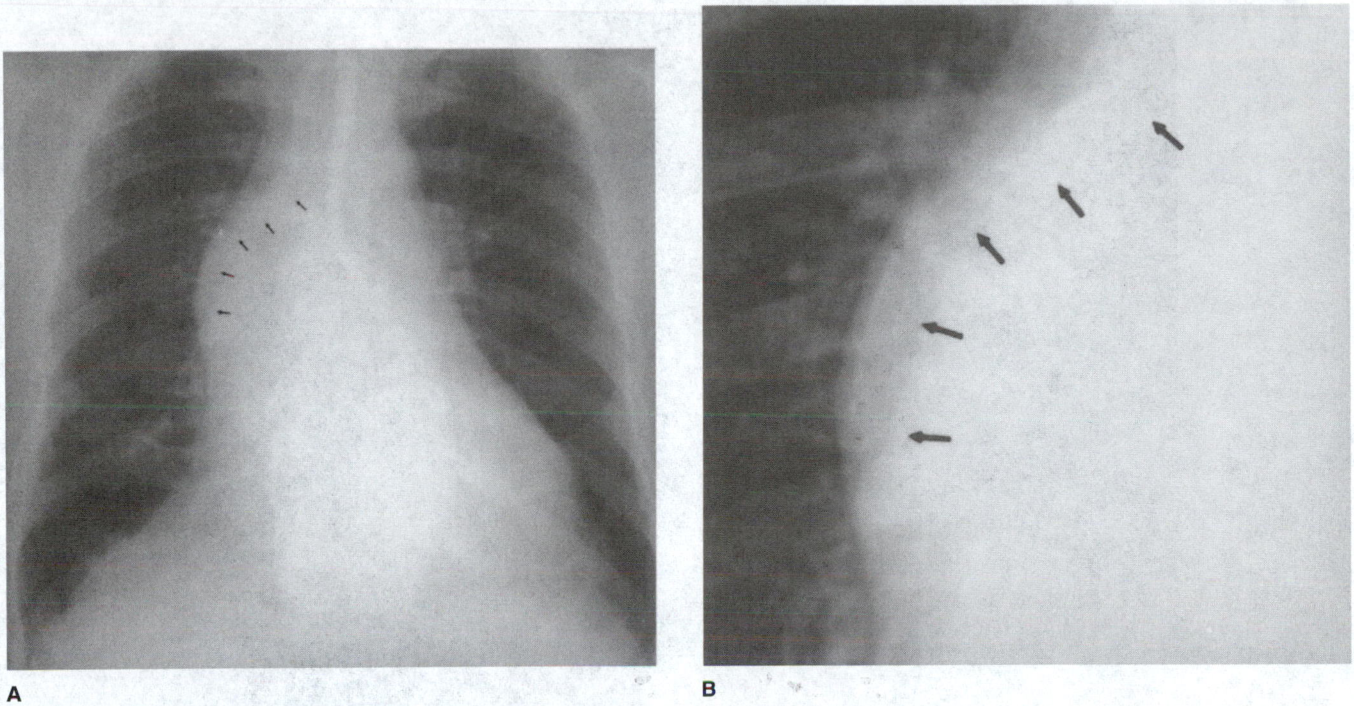

FIGURE 12-9 A 71-year-old woman with syphilitic aortitis. Her posteroanterior radiograph (*A*) shows a huge, calcified ascending aortic aneurysm (*arrows*). In addition, the entire aorta and the left ventricle are markedly dilated, compatible with severe aortic regurgitation (From Chen,[14] with permission.) A magnified view of the ascending aorta (*B*) shows the calcified aneurysm to better advantage.

parameters for a final conclusion. It may become necessary at this point to reexamine the radiograph or review the fluoroscopic observation or both. After detailed analysis of some finer points, a wrong impression may be corrected or a correct diagnosis reinforced[2] (see Table 12-2).

PULMONARY VASCULARITY

Normal

The normal roentgen appearance of the pulmonary vasculature of an upright human being is typified by a caudal flow pattern because of gravity. The pressure differential between the apex and the base of the lung is approximately 22 mmHg in adults in the upright position.[2,23] Therefore, more flow under higher distending pressure is expected in the lower-lobe vessels than in the upper. Normally, one sees very little vascularity above the hilum, whereas more and larger vessels are found below the hilum. Since the pulmonary resistance is normal, all vessels taper gradually in a treelike manner from the hilum toward the periphery of the lung. The right descending pulmonary artery measures 10 to 15 mm in diameter in males and 9 to 14 mm in females[2,24] (see Fig. 12-2).

Abnormal

Abnormal pulmonary vascularity can be classified into two categories, either in terms of volume or in terms of distribution[2,10,25] (Table 12-4).

Abnormalities in Volume

In the evaluation of pulmonary vasculature, the caliber of the vessels is more important than the length or the number. As long as the PBF pattern remains normal, with a greater amount of flow to the bases than to the apices, the volume of the flow is proportional to the caliber of the pulmonary arteries (see Fig. 12-2). In addition to measuring the right descending pulmonary artery, one also may assess the pulmonary blood volume by comparing the size of the pulmonary artery with that of the accompanying bronchus where they are viewed on end. Normally, the two structures have approximately equal diameters.[2,26] When the artery-bronchus ratio is greater than unity, increased blood flow is suggested. Conversely, when the ratio is smaller than unity (see Fig. 12-2), decreased flow is likely.

INCREASED PBF

In the case of mild to moderate left-to-right shunts, for example, the vessels dilate in proportion to the increased flow with no significant change in pressure, resistance, or flow pattern. This phenomenon is also called *shunt vascularity* or *equalization*. Equalization of PBF between the upper and lower lung zones is only apparent rather than real, however; the lower lobes still receive a great deal more blood than the upper lobes, although the ratio of PBF between the two zones has changed—e.g., from 5:1 to 4:1 or 3:1. A mild increase in pulmonary vascularity with slight cardiomegaly is commonly found in pregnant women and trained athletes with increased cardiac output and supernormal performance of the heart (see Chaps. 82 and 85).

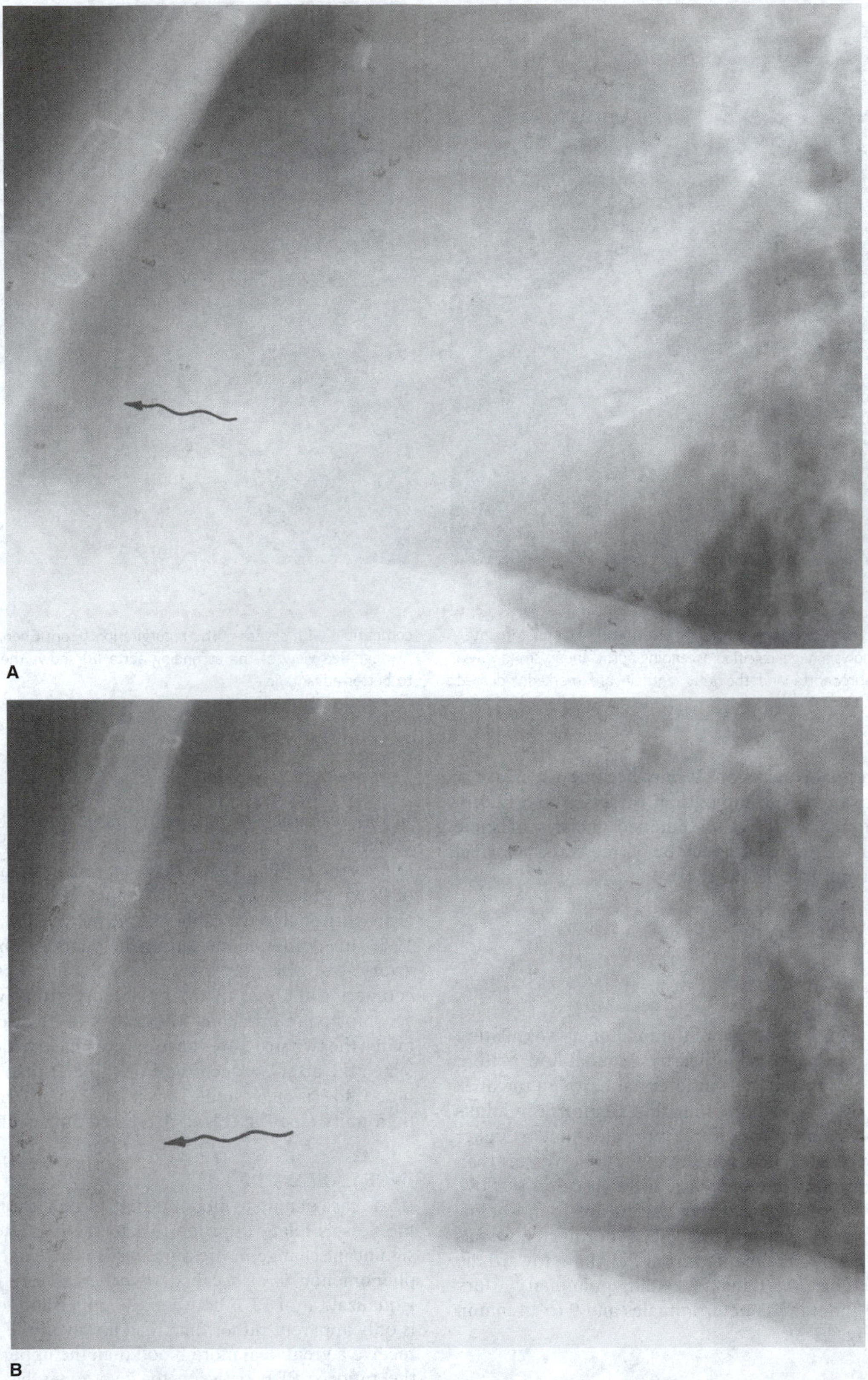

FIGURE 12-10 Developing pericardial effusion in 2 weeks. *A.* A magnified view of the retrosternal area showing the hairlike normal pericardium (*arrow*) sandwiched between the subepicardial fat stripe interiorly and the mediastinal fat stripe exteriorly. The maximal width of normal pericardium is 2 mm. *B.* The same patient 2 weeks later, with moderate pericardial effusion. The pericardial cavity now measured more than 1 cm in width (*arrow*).

TABLE 12-3 Cardiac Defects Associated with Each Type of Right-Sided Aortic Arch

	Type of Anomaly	
	Avian	Common
Anatomic details	With mirror-image branching; the arch is anterior to the trachea	With aberrant left subclavian artery arising from a large aortic diverticulum that is posterior to the esophagus
Patients with cardiac defects, %	98	12
Type of defects, %		
Tetralogy of Fallot	90	71
Truncus arteriosus	2.5	
Transposition of great arteries	1.5	
Atrial septal defect and/or ventricular septal defect	0.5	21
Coarctation of aorta		7
Others	5.5	1

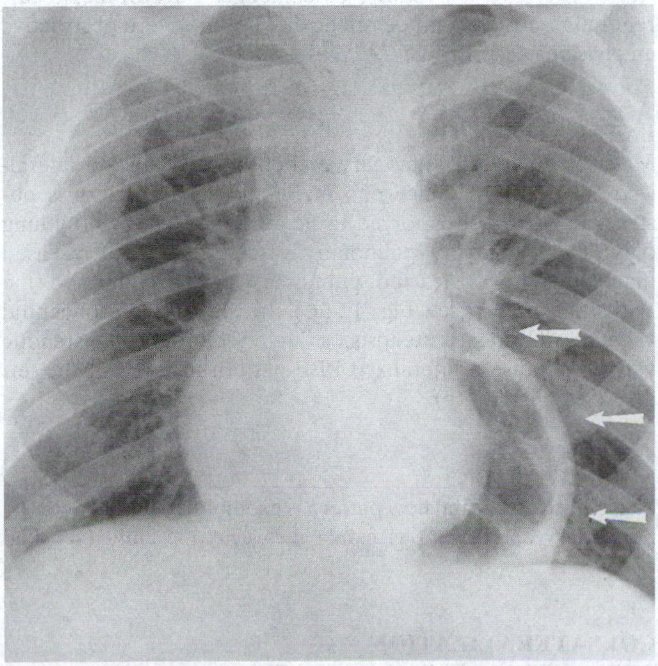

FIGURE 12-11 Traumatic constrictive-effusive pericarditis in a young man. Following emergent pericardiocentesis and injection of air, a radiograph was taken in the supine position. Air is confined to the left side of the pericardium. Note markedly thickened parietal layer (*arrows*).

TABLE 12-4 Pulmonary Vascularity

- Normal
  - Caudal PBF pattern in upright position (PBF controlled by gravity)
  - Gradual branching, treelike
  - RDPA = 10–15 mm in males
  - RDPA = 9–14 mm in females
  - A/B ratio = 1
- Abnormal
  - Volume with normal PBF pattern (distribution)
    - Increased, larger vessels, e.g., ASD
    - Decreased, smaller vessels, e.g., TOF
  - Distribution with abnormal PBF pattern
    - Cephalic, e.g., MS
    - Centralized, e.g., Eisenmenger syndrome
    - Lateralized, e.g., Westermark sign
    - Localized, e.g., pulmonary AV fistulas
    - Collateralized, e.g., severe TOF
- Combined
  - Decreased volume and cephalization, e.g., cricitcal MS
  - Lateralization and localization, e.g., scimitar syndrome

Abbreviations: RDPA = right descending pulmonary artery; A/B = artery/bronchus; PBF = pulmonary blood flow; ASD = atrial septal defect; TOF = tetralogy of Fallot; AV = arteriovenous; MS = mitral stenosis.

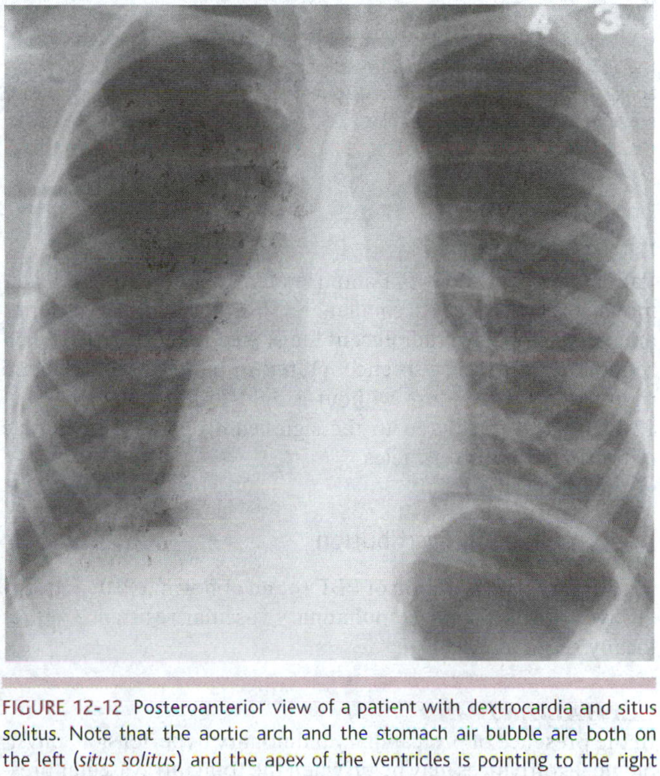

FIGURE 12-12 Posteroanterior view of a patient with dextrocardia and situs solitus. Note that the aortic arch and the stomach air bubble are both on the left (*situs solitus*) and the apex of the ventricles is pointing to the right inferiorly. According to statistics and proved by cardiac catheterization, this patient had the typical combination of congenitally corrected transposition of the great arteries, ventricular septal defect, and pulmonary stenosis. He was cyanotic. The pulmonary vascularity appears decreased.

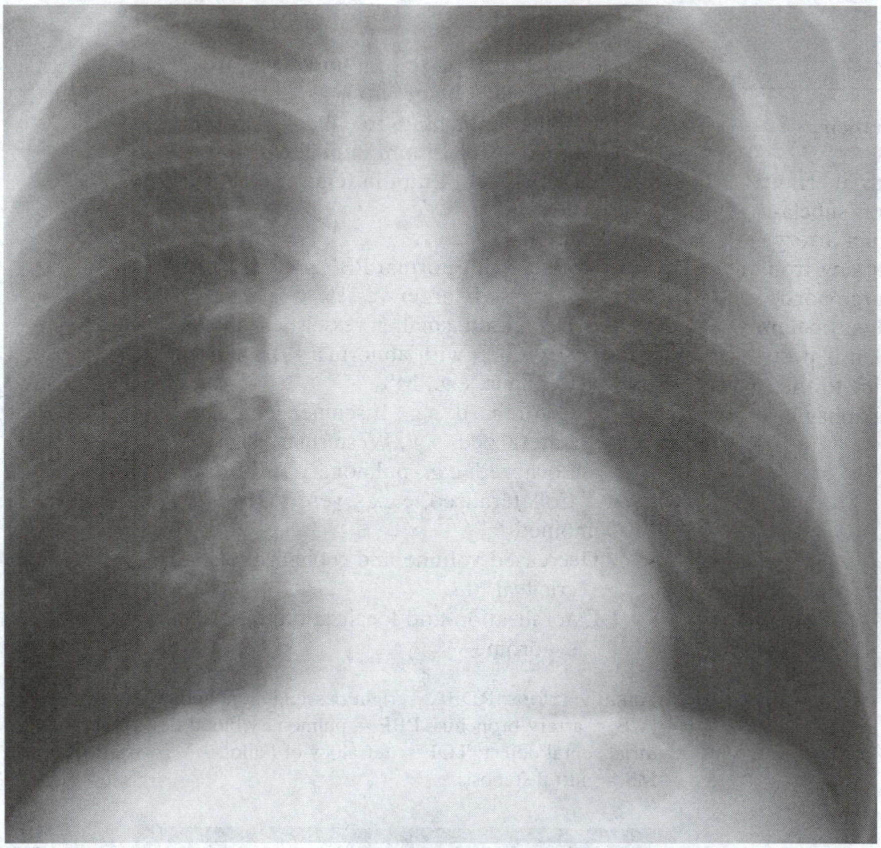

FIGURE 12-13 A 17-year-old boy with congenital aortic valve stenosis. Note dilatation of the ascending aorta, increased convexity of the left ventricle, and normal pulmonary vascularity. The systolic aortic pressure gradient was 100 mmHg.

DECREASED PBF

Patients with tetralogy of Fallot frequently show decreased pulmonary vascularity with smaller and shorter pulmonary arteries and veins and more radiolucent lungs (see Fig. 12-2*C*). Marked reduction in PBF is also encountered in patients with isolated right-sided heart failure without a right-to-left shunt (see Fig. 12-7). This is attributed to the significant decrease in cardiac output from both ventricles.

Abnormalities in Distribution

An abnormal distribution of PBF (or an abnormal PBF pattern) always reflects a changed pulmonary vascular resistance, either locally or diffusely.

CEPHALIZATION

In the presence of postcapillary pulmonary hypertension, physiologic disturbances may begin when the total intravascular pressure exceeds the oncotic pressure of the blood. As a result, fluid leaks out of the vessels and collects in the interstitium before pouring into the alveoli.

Pulmonary edema interferes with gas exchange, resulting in a state of hypoxemia. Alveolar hypoxia has a profound influence on the pulmonary vessels, causing them to constrict. Since there is greater alveolar hypoxia in the lung bases than in the apices, the basilar vessels constrict significantly, forcing the blood to flow upward. This phenomenon actually represents a reversal of the normal PBF pattern: redistribution or cephalization of the pulmonary vascularity.

Cephalization occurs in any of three conditions: (1) left-sided obstructive lesions, e.g., mitral stenosis[24] (see Fig. 12-3*A*) or aortic stenosis, (2) left ventricular failure, e.g., coronary heart disease or cardiomyopathies, and (3) severe mitral regurgitation even before pump failure of the left ventricle occurs. It should be emphasized that unless there is obvious constriction of the lower-lobe vessels, the diagnosis of cephalization should not be made. Dilatation of the upper-lobe vessels is of secondary importance and can be found without narrowing of the basilar vessels in a number of entities, most noticeably left-to-right shunts.

CENTRALIZATION

In the presence of precapillary pulmonary hypertension, the pulmonary trunk and central pulmonary arteries dilate, whereas the distal pulmonary arteries constrict in a concentric fashion from the periphery of the lung toward the hilum. This phenomenon is called *centralization of the pulmonary vascularity*. It occurs in patients with primary pulmonary hypertension (see Fig. 12-3*B*), Eisenmenger's syndrome, recurrent pulmonary thromboembolic disease, or severe obstructive emphysema (see Fig. 12-7*A*, *B*).

LATERALIZATION

Massive unilateral pulmonary embolism may cause a lateralized PBF pattern. Since one major pulmonary artery is obstructed, the blood is forced to flow through the healthy lung only. The paucity of pulmonary vascularity in the diseased lung with the obstructed pulmonary artery is termed the *Westermark sign* (see Fig. 12-3*C*). In the case of congenital valvular pulmonary stenosis, a jet effect from the stenotic valve can cause a lateralized PBF pattern in favor of the left side (see Fig. 12-16).

LOCALIZATION

A localized abnormal flow pattern is exemplified by a congenital pulmonary arteriovenous fistula in a cyanotic child (see Fig. 12-3*D*).

COLLATERALIZATION

Patients with markedly decreased PBF (e.g., severe tetralogy of Fallot) tend to show numerous small and tortuous bronchial arterial collaterals in the upper medial lung zones near their

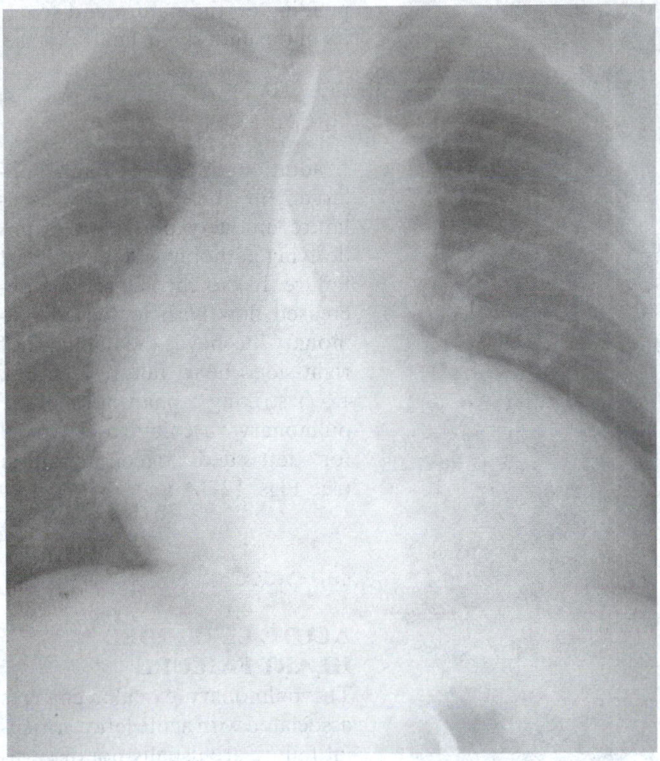

A

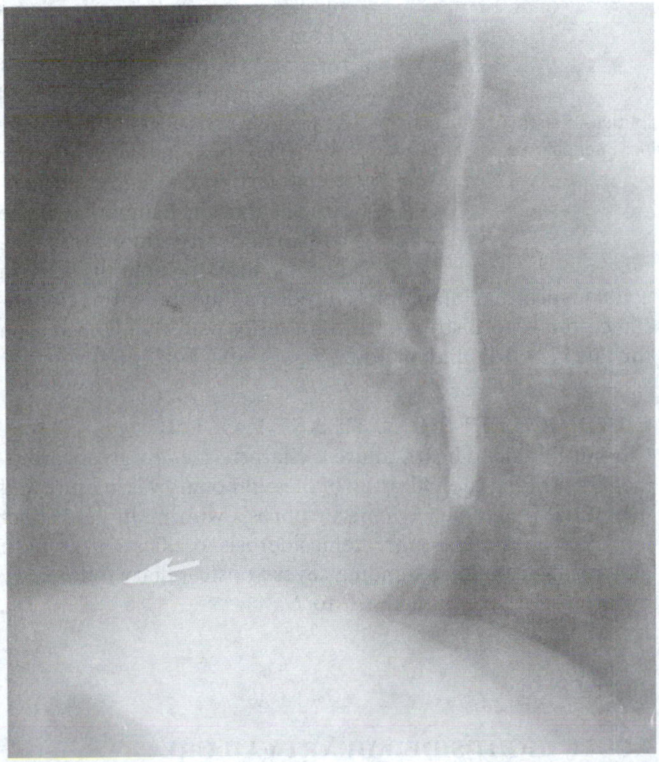

B

FIGURE 12-14 A 45-year-old man with Marfan's syndrome, severe aortic regurgitation, and proximal aortic dissection into the pericardial cavity. *A*. Posteroanterior view shows a huge left ventricular and aneurysmal dilatation of the ascending aorta. There is no sign of heart failure. *B*. Lateral view shows a small pericardial effusion (*arrow*).

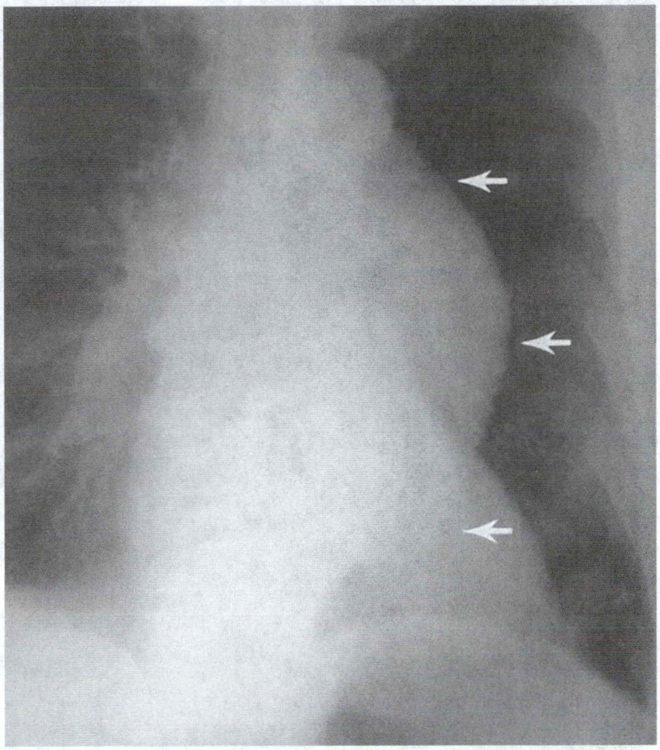

FIGURE 12-15 Posteroanterior view of a 77-year-old man shows a huge descending aortic aneurysm (*arrows*).

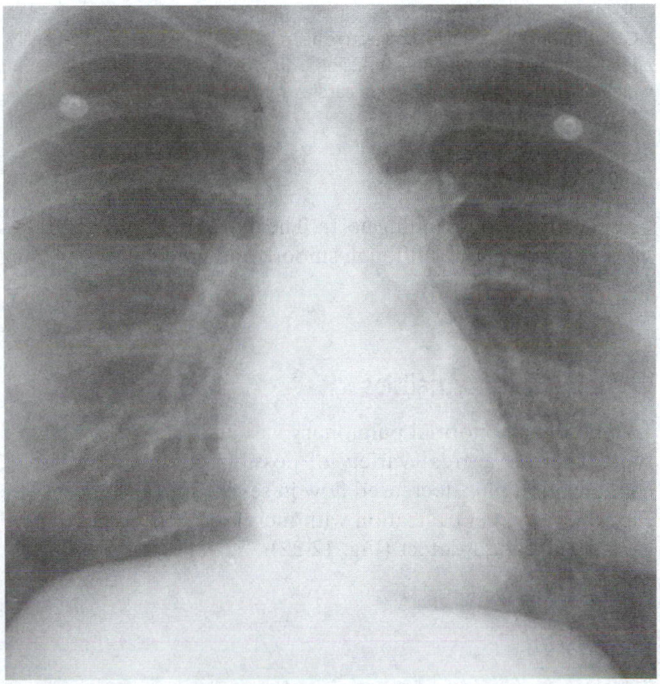

FIGURE 12-16 A 37-year-old woman with congenital valvular pulmonary stenosis. Note enlarged pulmonary trunk and left pulmonary artery versus diminished right pulmonary artery. Also note increased pulmonary blood flow on the left side and decreased pulmonary blood flow on the right side.

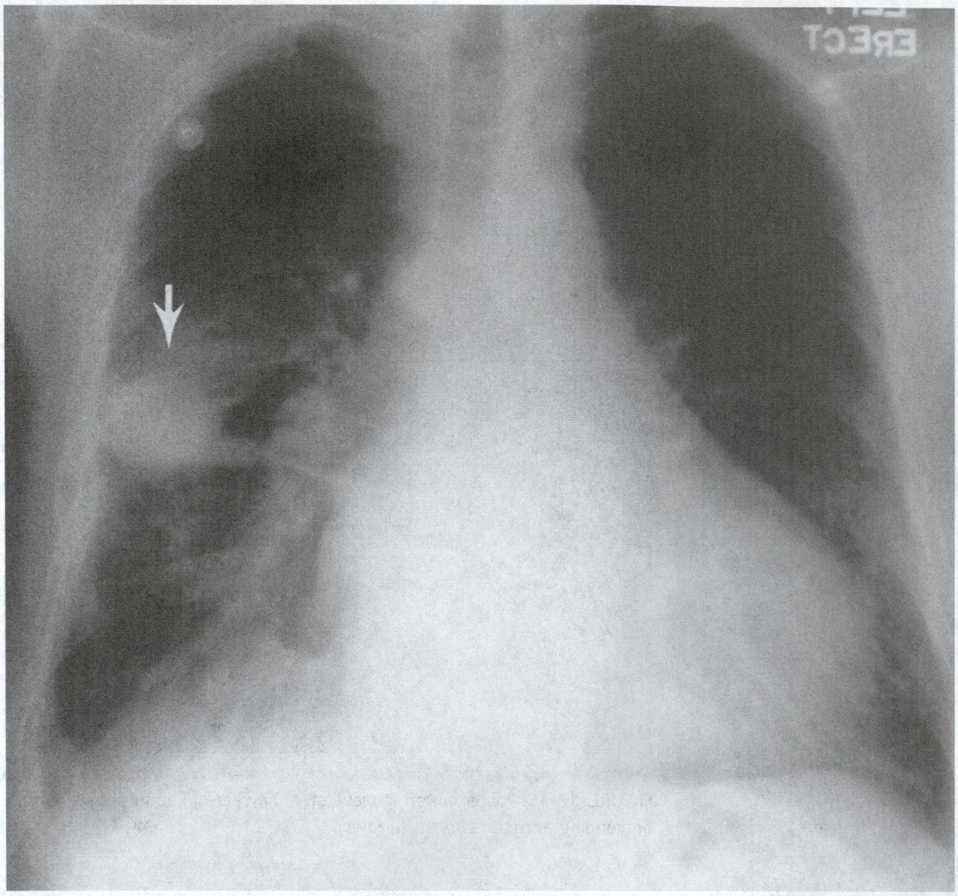

FIGURE 12-17 Patient with congestive heart failure. Note gross cardiomegaly, cephalization, interstitial pulmonary edema, and right-sided pleural effusion. Some of the fluid was loculated in the minor interlobar fissure (*arrow*), which disappeared with improved cardiac function.

origin from the descending aorta. The native pulmonary arteries are extremely small, although smooth and gracefully branching (see Fig. 12-3*E*).

Combined Abnormalities

In reality, an abnormal pulmonary vascularity is often a mixed type. There is a great variety of possible combinations—e.g., cephalization plus decreased flow in severe mitral stenosis (see Fig. 12-3*A*) or centralization with increased PBF in Eisenmenger's atrial septal defect (Fig. 12-22).

Summary

Roentgen analysis of the pulmonary vasculature is accomplished in two steps. First, the volume of the pulmonary flow can be estimated by the degree of pulmonary arterial enlargement as long as the PBF pattern remains normal. Second, the distribution of the pulmonary flow is assessed by the presence of an abnormal flow pattern. The volume and the distribution of pulmonary blood flow may change singly or in combination depending on the nature and severity of the underlying heart disease.

HEART FAILURE

In addition to specific chamber enlargement, the pulmonary vasculature uniquely portrays the underlying pathophysiology of heart failure. In the chronic setting, decreased flow with increased pulmonary lucency is the hallmark of right-sided heart failure (see Fig. 12-7); striking cephalization of the pulmonary vasculature is typical for left-sided decompensation (see Figs. 12-3*A* and 12-6*B*).

Left-Sided

ACUTE LEFT-SIDED HEART FAILURE

The pulmonary vascular changes associated with acute left ventricular failure are usually not discernible for two reasons: (1) the resulting severe pulmonary edema obscures the pulmonary vasculature, and (2) the redistribution of PBF secondary to acute left-sided heart failure is usually relatively mild. The combination of alveolar pulmonary edema and a normal-sized heart is the hallmark of acute left-sided heart failure[10] (see Fig. 12-6*A*), most commonly seen in acute myocardial infarction. The edema fluid under this circumstance tends to distribute in a butterfly pattern.[27] The reason for this is poorly understood.

CHRONIC LEFT-SIDED HEART FAILURE

Chronic left-sided heart failure is characterized by gross cardiomegaly, striking cephalization of the pulmonary vasculature and interstitial pulmonary edema or fibrosis with multiple distinct Kerley B lines. Pulmonary hemosiderosis, ossification, or both may result from long-standing severe postcapillary pulmonary hypertension (see Figs. 12-6*B* to *E*).

Right-Sided

ACUTE RIGHT-SIDED HEART FAILURE

Acute right-sided heart failure most commonly results from massive pulmonary embolism. The typical radiographic signs are rapidly developing centralization of the pulmonary vasculature and dilatation of the right-sided cardiac chambers and venae cavae. In addition, the lungs may show localized or lateralized oligemia (see Fig. 12-3*C*). Eventually, opacities in either or both lungs may develop as a result of pulmonary infarction.

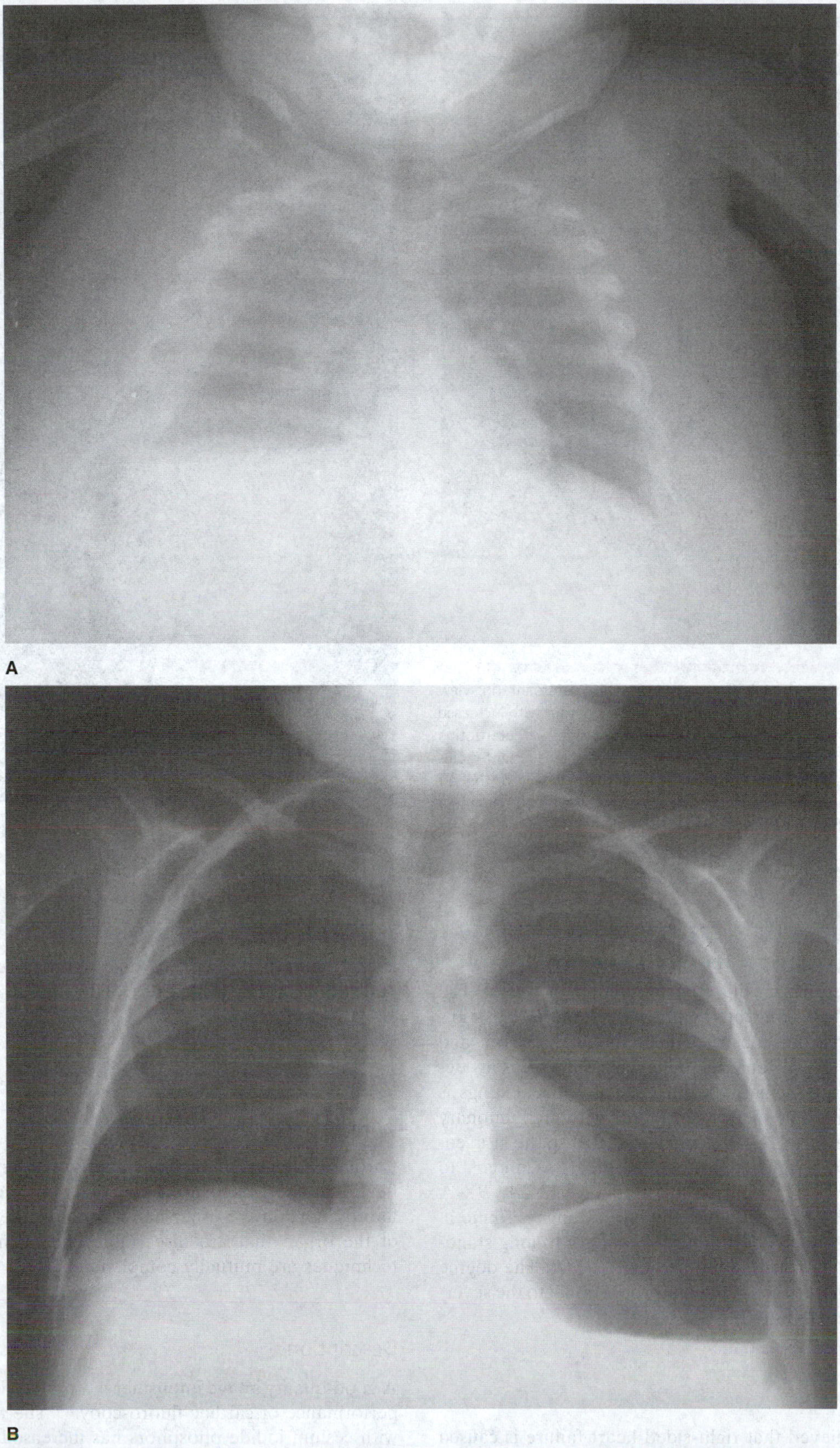

FIGURE 12-18 A child suffering from nephrotic syndrome, which was treated successfully. *A*. Posteroanterior view during the worst period of his disease shows general anasarca, pulmonary edema, and pleural effusion. Note considerable soft tissue edema in the chest wall. *B*. With proper treatment, everything returned to normal in 2 weeks.

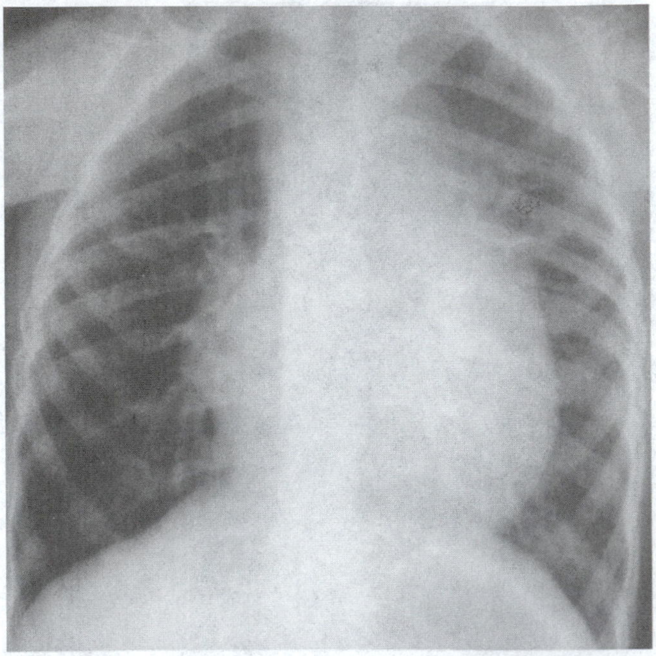

A

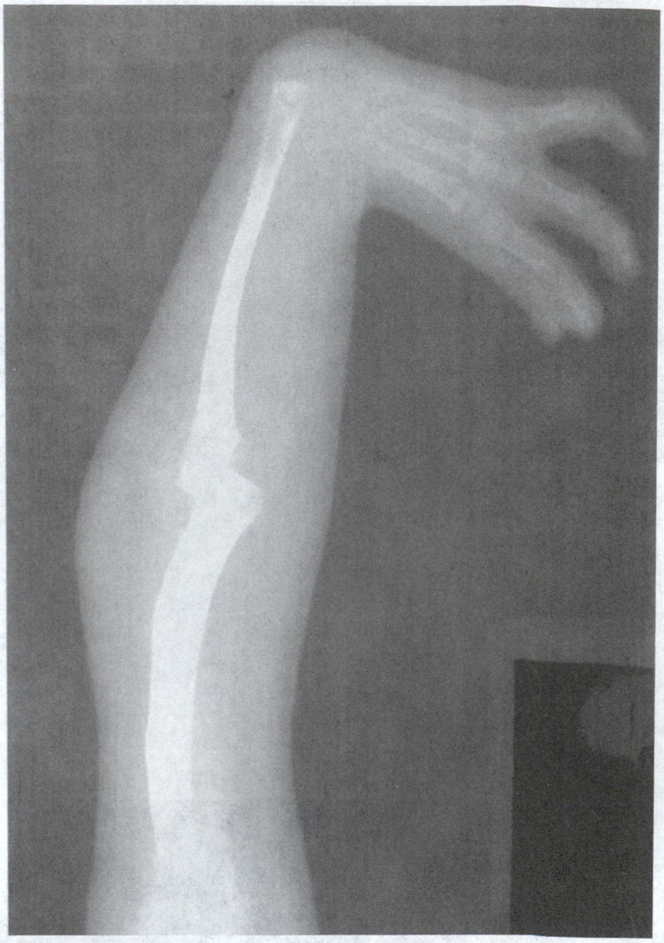

B

FIGURE 12-19 Patients with Holt-Oram syndrome. *A*. Posteroanterior view of patient 1, a 7-year-old girl, shows a globular cardiac contour with increased pulmonary blood flow. The aortic arch is on the right side. Catheterization diagnosis: secundum atrial septal defect. *B*. Her left arm shows absent radius and thumb with radial clubhand. Her right arm is a mirror image of the left (not shown). *C*. Forearms of patient 2, a 33-year-old woman with secundum atrial septal defect, show bilateral absence of thumb.

CHRONIC RIGHT-SIDED HEART FAILURE

Chronic right-sided heart failure has a number of causes. The common ones include congenital pulmonary stenosis, Ebstein's anomaly, severe chronic obstructive pulmonary disease, and recurrent pulmonary thromboembolic disease. Diffusely decreased pulmonary vascularity with unusually lucent lungs is seen in patients with right-sided heart failure without pulmonary hypertension (see Fig. 12-7*C*). Centralized PBF pattern is encountered when the right-sided heart failure is secondary to precapillary pulmonary hypertension (see Fig. 12-7*A*, *B*). A cephalized flow pattern with unusually lucent lungs is found in patients with right-sided heart failure secondary to long-standing severe left-sided heart failure (see Fig. 12-7*D*). The degree of right-sided chamber enlargement is proportional to the severity of tricuspid regurgitation.

Combined

It is generally believed that right-sided heart failure is caused most often by severe left-sided heart failure. This is exemplified by patients with severe mitral stenosis leading to severe tricuspid regurgitation (see Fig. 12-7*D*). Other examples of bilateral heart failure are cardiac tamponade and constrictive pericarditis, when both sides of the heart are affected (Fig. 12-23).

CARDIAC FLUOROSCOPY

Cardiac radiography deals primarily with anatomic details by filming at short exposure times that stop the motion. Cardiac fluoroscopy, on the other hand, explores the dynamic features of the organ that are discernible only in motion.[28] The two techniques are mutually complementary.

Description

A good-quality image intensifier is a prerequisite for the proper performance of cardiac fluoroscopy.[2,19] The modern intensifier with cesium iodide phosphors has increased the brightness of the fluoroscopic image at least 10,000 times. Television viewing permits cone vision under dim light with better perception of detail. The attached videotape or videodisk recorder provides a means for instant playback as well as future analysis of the fluoroscopic observations.

The milliamperage and kilovoltage of the fluoroscope should be adjusted according to the patient's size in different projections. The milliamperage ranges from 1.5 to 3.5 mA, and the kilovoltage varies between 90 and 120 kV. Too high a kilovoltage tends to reduce the contrast, and excessive milliamperage blurs the margin of the image. The shortest fluoroscopic time and the smallest shutter opening are employed to keep the dose of radiation to the patient to the minimum. The average examining time for this author is 3 min.

The patient is routinely examined in the erect position with four views. The patient should be asked to stop breathing during the brief moment of fluoroscopy. A barium meal is given only after a thorough search for cardiac calcifications is completed. Occasionally, a recumbent position is used for better visualization of small calcifications, as well as for a critical evaluation of cardiac asynergy. The cardiac output increases and the heart rate decreases on assuming recumbency, thereby giving a truer and more representative picture of the left ventricular contractility. In obese patients, the thick layer of soft tissue over the thorax is compressed and pushed aside, thereby improving the fluoroscopic image significantly.

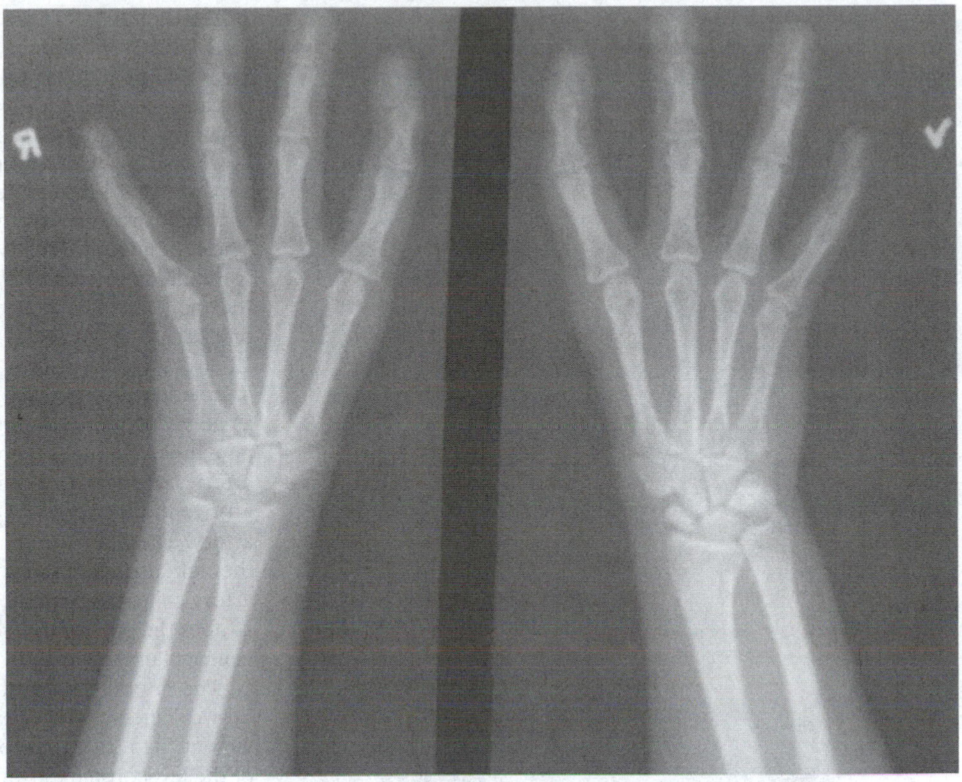

C

FIGURE 12-19 (*Continued*)

Results

When performed properly, cardiac fluoroscopy is useful in the following areas of investigation: (1) assessment of cardiovascular dynamics, (2) detection of small cardiovascular calcifications, (3) visualization of important anatomic landmarks, e.g., subepicardial fat stripes, (4) differentiation of cardiac from noncardiac disease, and (5) evaluation of cardiac valve prostheses, pacemakers, and radiopaque foreign bodies.

Precautions

Although no complication from modern fluoroscopy has been reported, both the patient and the examiner should be protected from excessive radiation. Even with an image intensifier, a routine cardiac fluoroscopy still involves more radiation than does two-view chest roentgenography. Therefore, the fluoroscopist should accomplish the task within the shortest possible period of time. Although all aspects of the heart are surveyed briefly, one should emphasize special areas of interest for each patient, as suggested by the baseline radiographs. If coarctation of the aorta is suspected in a patient older than 40 years of age, for instance, particular attention should be paid to finding calcium in a stenotic bicuspid aortic valve.

Applications

ASSESSMENT OF CARDIOVASCULAR DYNAMICS

The chest roentgenogram that is taken at random largely records the diastolic image of the heart. Fluoroscopy, on the other hand, provides a continuous vision of the pulsating organ through the entire cardiac cycle. On becoming familiar with the normal cardiovascular movements, the fluoroscopist will find that any deviation from the norm will be obvious.[2,29–32]

The telltale x-ray signs of many cardiac lesions manifest themselves only in ventricular systole. Therefore, what may be missed on the film is often readily seen and diagnosed under the fluoroscope. For instance, left ventricular enlargement may be the only radiographic abnormality of severe aortic regurgitation in children or young adults. On fluoroscopy, however, the aorta is vigorously expanding in systole and rapidly collapsing in diastole. This dynamic alternation is characteristic of aortic regurgitation (Fig. 12-24). Other examples include mild mitral regurgitation, mitral valve prolapse, left ventricular dyskinesia, and broad-based left ventricular aneurysm.

In valvular pulmonary stenosis, vigorous pulsation of the pulmonary trunk and its left branch is in bold contrast to the diminished pulsation of the right pulmonary artery.[31] Increased pulsation of diffusely enlarged pulmonary arteries is characteris-

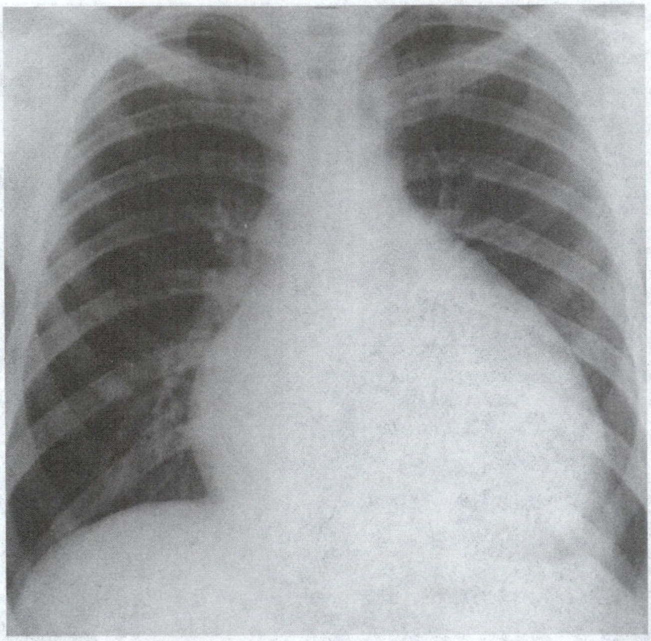

A

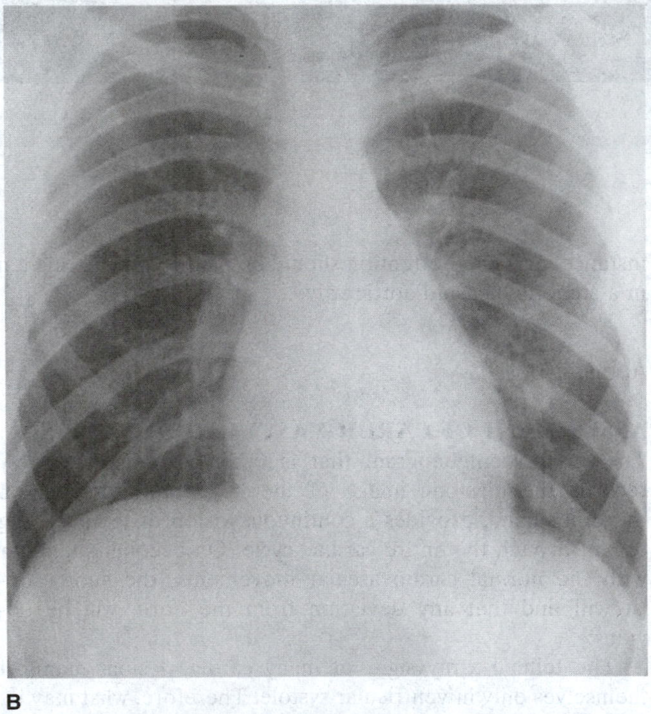

B

FIGURE 12-20 Young man with acute pericarditis with effusion. *A*. Posteroanterior view shows a water bottle–shaped cardiomegaly, clear lungs, and normal pulmonary vascularity. *B*. Repeat film taken 5 days later shows excellent response to therapy.

tic of left-to-right shunts. When marked discrepancy in size and pulsation is noted between the central and peripheral vessels, Eisenmenger's syndrome should be considered. Exaggerated left atrial expansion in ventricular systole is a reliable sign of mitral regurgitation.[32]

DETECTION OF CARDIOVASCULAR CALCIFICATIONS

Heavy calcifications of the heart and vessels are easily detected by chest roentgenography, particularly in the lateral and oblique views (Fig. 12-25). Small calcifications, on the other hand, can be registered only by fluoroscopy by virtue of their rhythmic movements from the pulsating heart.[3,8] Detection of even tiny coronary artery calcifications is of vital practical importance. The combination of chest pain and coronary calcification results from major vascular obstruction 94 percent of the time.[16] Since the major coronary arteries are embedded in the subepicardial fat stripes in the grooves between cardiac chambers (Fig. 12-26), such fat stripes can be used effectively to locate the calcified arteries. Under the fluoroscope, the fat stripes present as pulsating radiolucent (bright) lines, in contrast to the accompanying pulsating radiopaque (dark) lines of calcified coronary arteries. If the artery coincides with the fat line within the left atrioventricular groove (aL), it portrays the circumflex coronary artery. The right coronary artery is moving synchronously with the right atrioventricular groove (aR). The anterior descending artery coincides with the anterior interventricular groove (vA), as does the posterior descending artery with the posterior interventricular groove (vP).

The lateral view is the best or the only view for detection of a calcified right coronary artery. The left anterior oblique view at 20 to 30° is the most suitable for localizing the bifurcation of the left coronary artery. In this view, the left coronary artery is brought into relief between the hilar shadow anteriorly and the spinal column posteriorly. A ringlike density is seen frequently in this view, representing the end-on image of the calcified anterior descending artery. The right anterior oblique angle is used to view a calcified left main coronary artery. If both the anterior descending and the circumflex branches are also calcified, a Y-shaped density may be seen. The calcified cardiac valves, the myocardium, and the pericardium are easily confirmed by fluoroscopy.[2,29]

VISUALIZATION OF SUBEPICARDIAL FAT STRIPES

The subepicardial fat lines are important landmarks in the diagnosis of heart disease. The fat stripe is a cushion-like structure separating the myocardium from the pericardium. Normally, it is difficult to see the fat line because of the adjacent similar radiolucency of the air-filled lung. The in-between hairline density of the normal pericardium is delicate and also difficult to see except in the left lateral view (Fig. 12-10*A*). In the presence of pericardial effusion or thickening, the subepicardial fat line is displaced interiorly and becomes more visible because of the added background of water density (see Fig. 12-10*B*). The subepicardial fat pulsates with the contracting myocardium within the immobile band of pericardial fluid. This is diagnostic of pericardial effusion.[33] In contrast, when pericardial thickening alone is present, the exterior border of the heart pulsates with the fat line. This, in turn, suggests the diagnosis of pericardial constriction.

Although the displaced subepicardial fat stripe is visualized only in the lateral radiograph (see Fig. 12-10*B*), fluoroscopically, the pulsating fat line is clearly visible in all four views throughout the entire cardiac cycle (Fig. 12-27).

DIFFERENTIATION OF CARDIAC FROM NONCARDIAC DISEASE

When respiration is suspended, any structures that are moving are likely to be cardiovascular in nature. Conversely, noncardiac

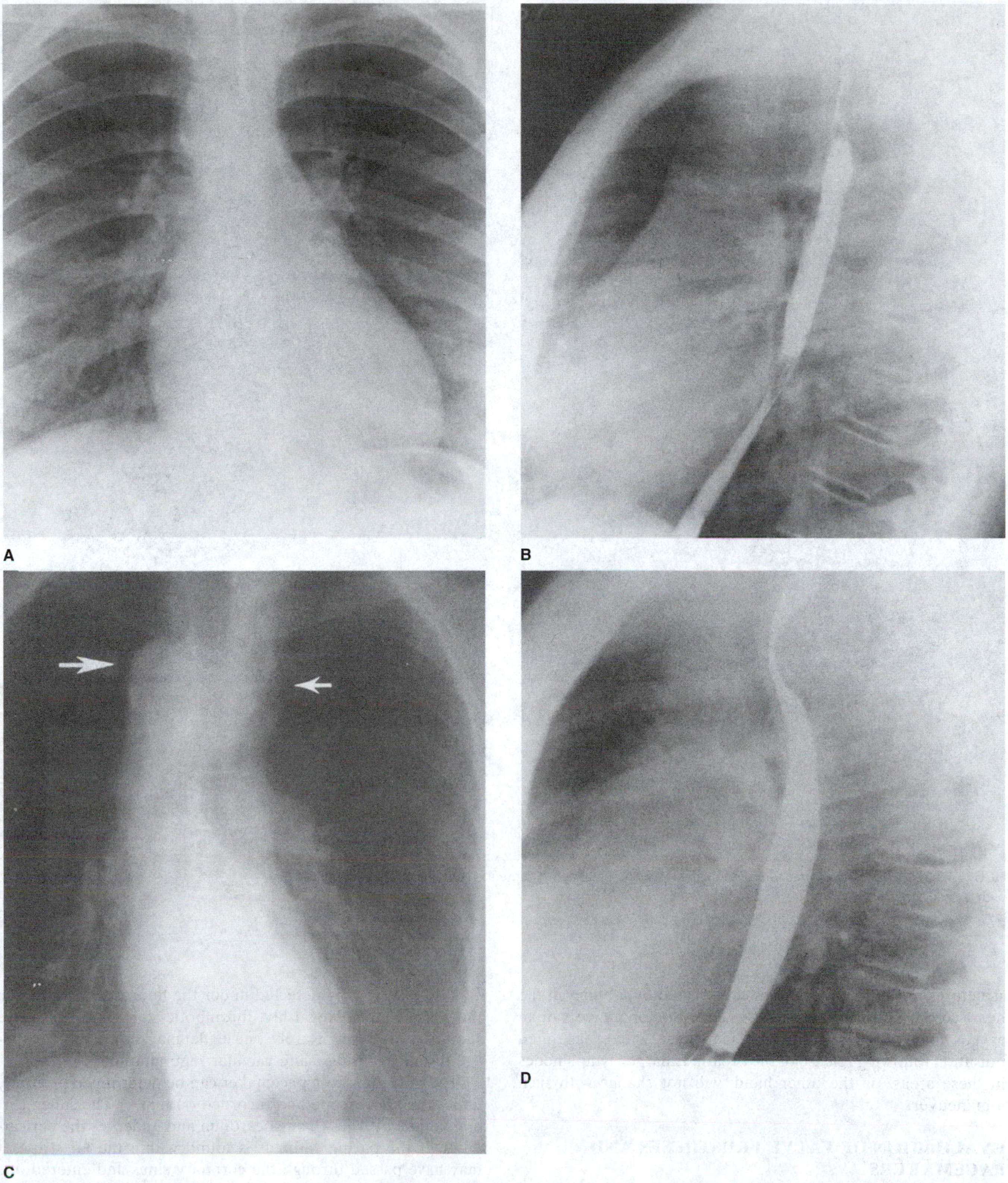

FIGURE 12-21 Statistical guidance focusing on the best diagnostic possibilities. *A*. Posteroanterior view of a patient with tetralogy of Fallot showing a right aortic arch, avian type. Note that the esophagus and trachea are deviated to the left. The cardiovascular structures are otherwise within normal limits. *B*. Lateral view of the same patient showing the aortic arch normally situated, in front of the trachea and esophagus. *C*. Posteroanterior radiograph of a healthy woman shows a right aortic arch (*large arrow*) with a large aortic diverticulum (*small arrow*) that protrudes to the left of the midline. The distal segment of the trachea is deviated to the left side by the right arch. Unlike double aortic arch, the left lateral margin of the trachea is not indented because the diverticulum is posterior and not lateral in position. *D*. Lateral view of similar patient, a healthy man. Note that both the esophagus and the trachea are markedly displaced anteriorly by a huge diverticulum, which invariably gives rise to the aberrant left subclavian artery.

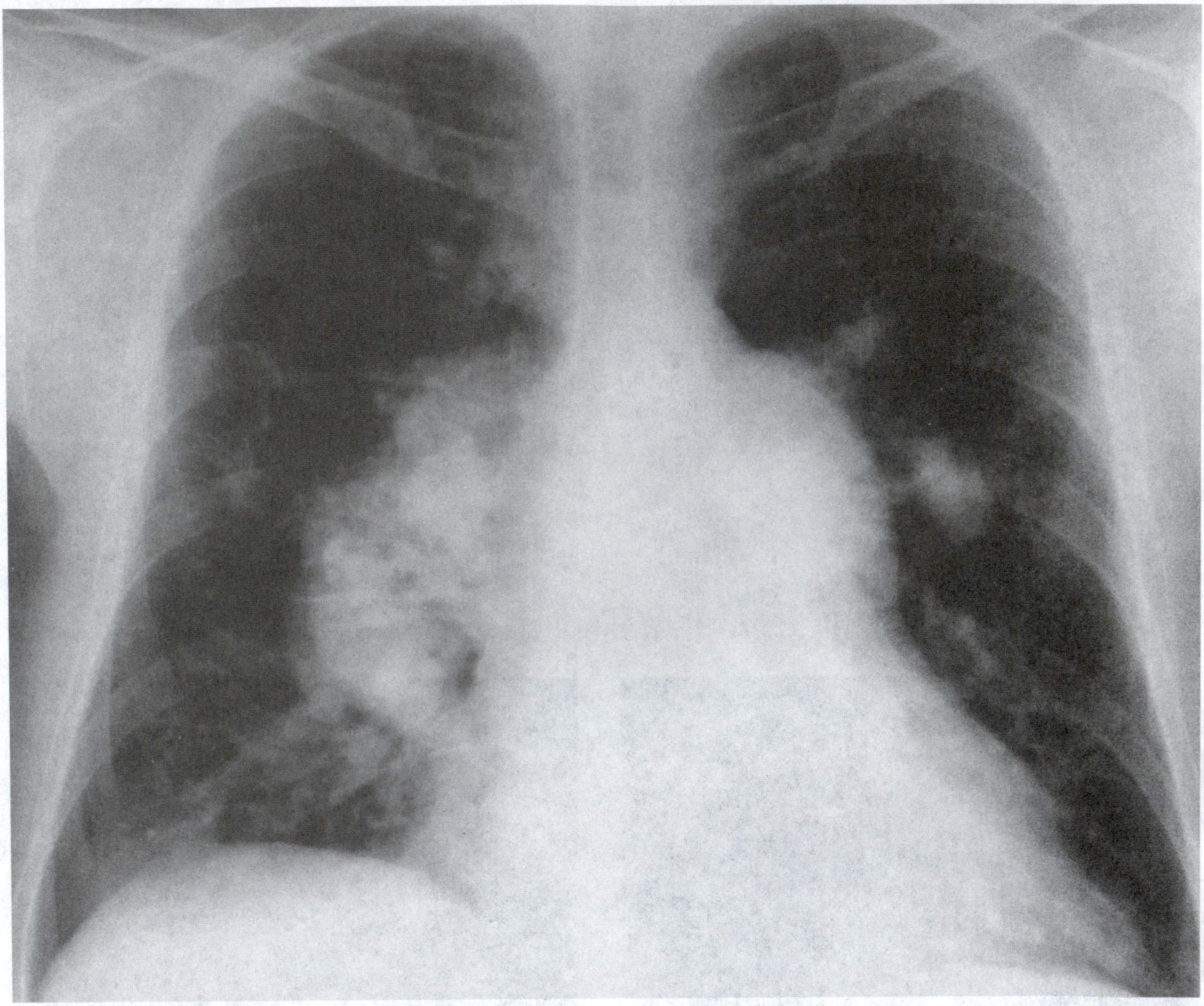

FIGURE 12-22 A 42-year-old man with Eisenmenger's atrial septal defect. Note increased pulmonary blood flow with a centralized pattern.

structures are immobile. This is exemplified by a bullet in the heart versus another in the chest wall. A pulmonary varix or an azygos vein collapses on Valsalva maneuver, with exaggerated pulsation following release of the breath. Enlarged lymph nodes in these areas, on the other hand, will not change with such a maneuver.

EVALUATION OF VALVE PROSTHESES AND PACEMAKERS

The normal movements of cardiac valve prostheses are parallel between the two phases of the cardiac cycle. If a significant angle of tilt (more than 12°) is formed between the two phases, instability of the valve with associated regurgitation is nearly always present.[2,29,32,34]

The bileaflet St. Jude valve[35] is used in both mitral and aortic positions. The valve is difficult to see radiographically (Fig. 12-28) but is readily detected under the fluoroscope.[1,2,35] When the leaflets move sluggishly, thrombotic stenosis of the valve should be suspected. Rarely, one leaflet may dislodge and embolize distally, causing acute valvular regurgitation.[35]

The position of the pacemaker can be determined promptly under the fluoroscope and recorded on film.[2,36] The subepicardial fat line overlies the myocardium and underlies the pericardium. If the pacing catheter is found within the fat stripe, it may have passed through the coronary sinus and entered one of the major cardiac veins. If the tip of the catheter is seen outside the fat stripe, however, it may have perforated the myocardium and thus be lying in the pericardium or beyond.[2] Although the wires and electrodes of a transmediastinal pacemaker may look normal on the films, minor breakage can be appreciated only in ventricular systole with the aid of fluoroscopy.[36]

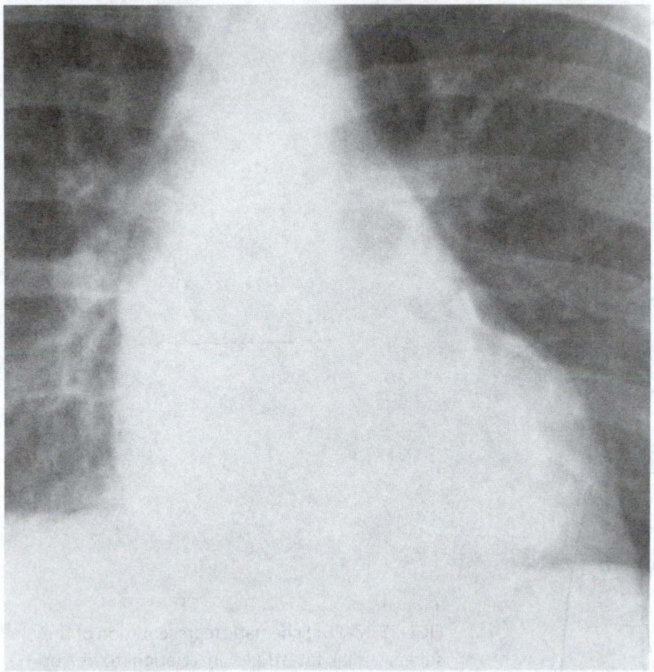

A

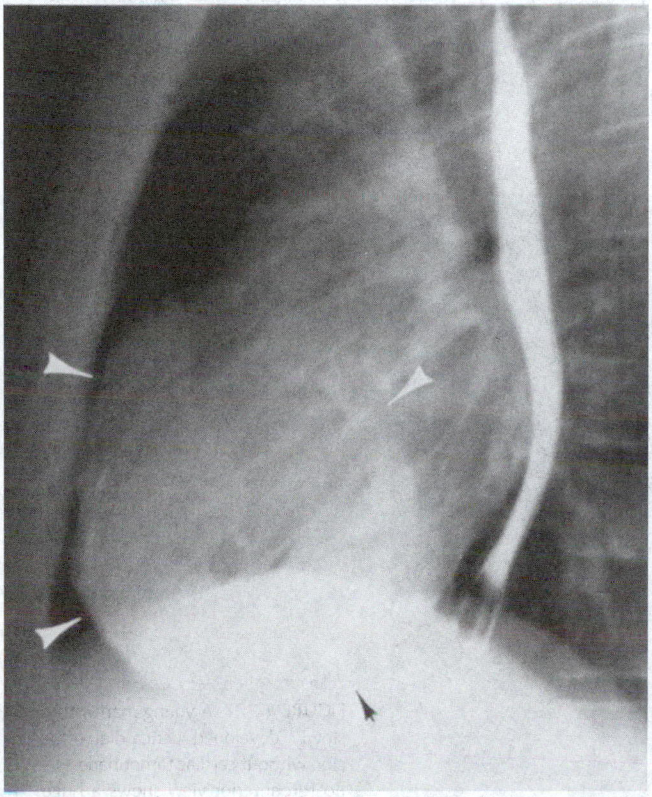

B

FIGURE 12-23 Patient with calcific constrictive pericarditis. Typically there is only mild postcapillary pulmonary hypertension due to left-sided constriction. Severe pulmonary venous congestion is prevented by the concurrent right-sided constriction. *A*. Posteroanterior view shows moderate cardiomegaly and mildly cephalic pulmonary blood flow pattern. *B*. Lateral view shows heavy calcification of the pericardium (*arrows*) and left atrial enlargement deviating the barium-filled esophagus posteriorly.

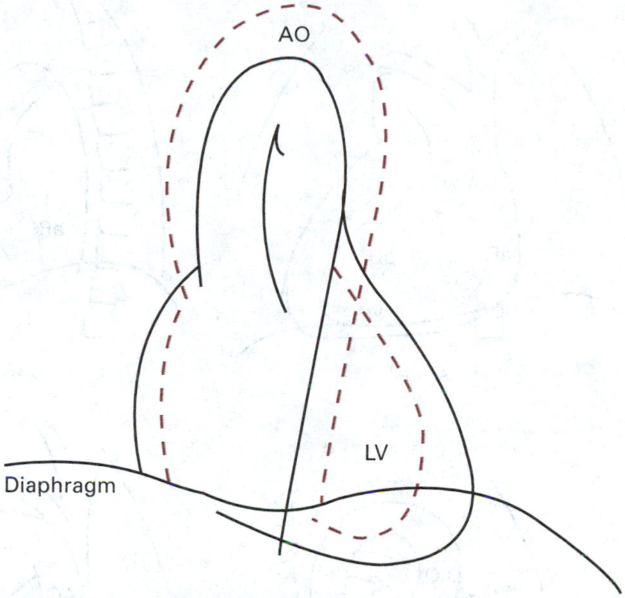

FIGURE 12-24 Schematic representation of dynamic changes of aortic regurgitation. Blue interrupted lines represent images in systole; solid lines, those in diastole.

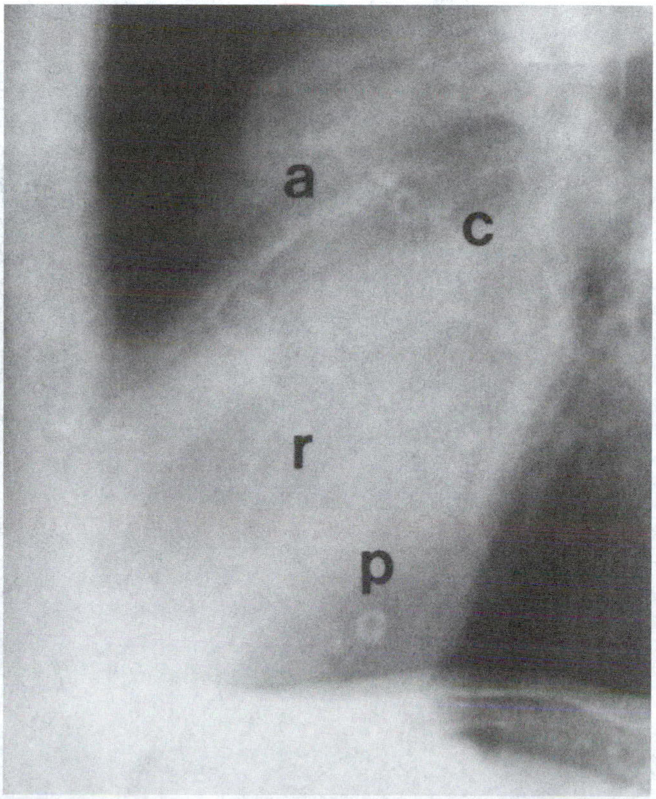

FIGURE 12-25 Lateral view shows heavy railroad track-like calcification of all three major coronary arteries. r, right coronary artery; a, anterior descending; c, circumflex; p, posterior descending. Note the ringlike densities representing vessels viewed on end.

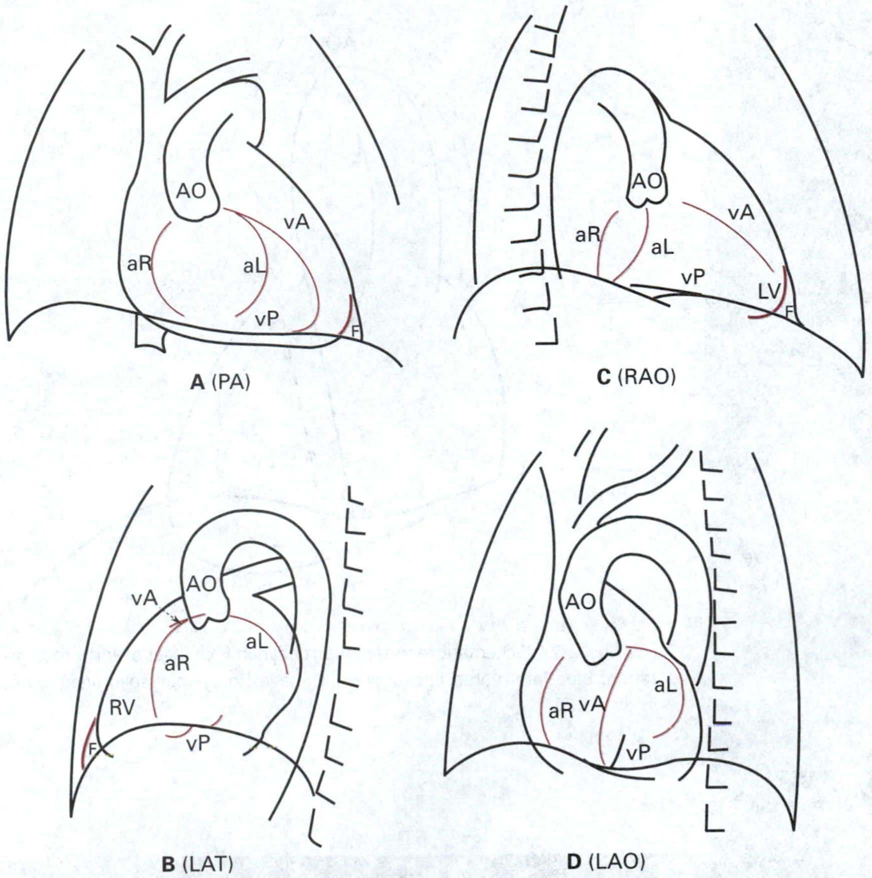

FIGURE 12-26 Schematic representation of the subepicardial fat stripes in relation to major coronary arteries. *A*. Posteroanterior view. *B*. Lateral view. *C*. Right anterior oblique view. *D*. Left anterior oblique view. aL, left atrioventricular groove (circumflex); aR, right atrioventricular groove (right); vA, anterior interventricular groove (anterior descending); vP, posterior interventricular groove (posterior descending); F, apical fat pad; AO, aorta; LV, left ventricle.

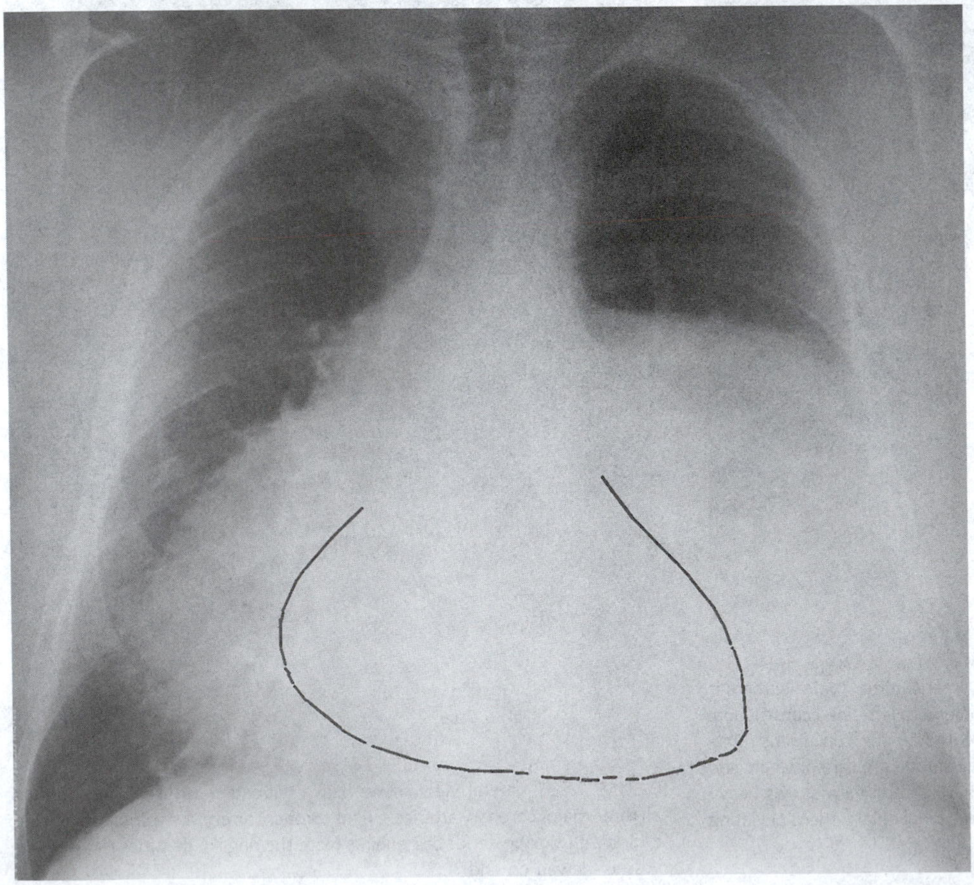

FIGURE 12-27 A young man with a slowly developed pericardial effusion without cardiac tamponade. His posteroanterior view shows a huge water bottle-like cardiac silhouette. Note the lungs are clear and the PBF pattern is normal. The subepicardial fat stripe (black curvilinear line) within the immobile pericardial effusion was clearly visible and bouncing vigorously under the fluoroscope. The amplitude of excursion of the fat stripe reflected the normally functioning myocardium.

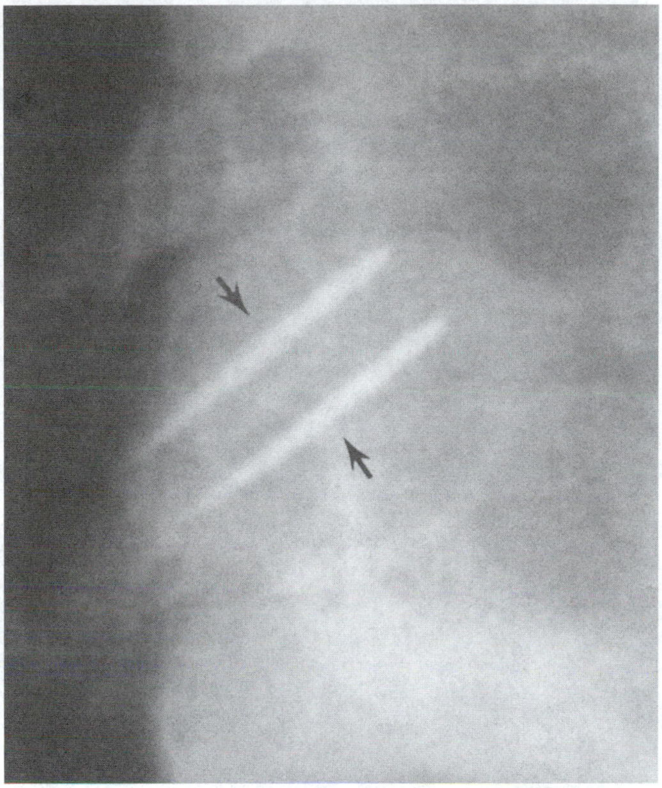

FIGURE 12-28 Patient with congenitally corrected transposition of the great arteries. The left-sided atrioventricular valve was replaced with a St. Jude prosthesis. The valve was caught in the opened position (in diastole), when both leaflets were seen as a pair of parallel lines (*arrows*). The same valve was invisible in the closed position (*not shown*).

References

1. Roentgen WB. *New Forms of Radiation*. Würzburg, Germany: Würzburger Physical Medical Society; December 28, 1895.
2. Chen JTT. *Essentials of Cardiac Imaging*, 2d ed. Philadelphia: Lippincott-Raven; 1997.
3. Chen JTT. The plain radiograph in the diagnosis of cardiovascular disease. In: Putman C, ed. Symposium on cardiopulmonary imaging. *Radiol Clin North Am* 1983; 21:609–621.
4. Juhl JH, Grummy AB. *Essentials of Radiologic Imaging*, 6th ed. Philadelphia: Lippincott; 1993:1065–1138.
5. Meschan I, Formanek A. Roentgenology of the heart inclusive of major vessels. In: Meschan I, ed. *Roentgen Signs in Diagnostic Imaging*, 2d ed. Philadelphia: Saunders; 1987:784–925.
6. Figley M. Accessory roentgen signs of coarctation of the aorta. *Radiology* 1954; 62:671–686.
7. Elliott LP, Jue KL, Amplatz K. A roentgen classification of cardiac malpositions. *Invest Radiol* 1966; 1:17–28.
8. Elliott LP, Schiebler GL. *X-ray Diagnosis of Congenital Cardiac Disease*, 2d ed. Springfield, IL: Charles C Thomas; 1979.
9. deLeon AC, Perloff JK, Twigg HL. The straight back syndrome: Clinical and cardiovascular manifestations. *Circulation* 1965; 32:193–203.
10. Chen JTT, Capp MP, Johnsrude IS, Goodrich JK, Lester RG. Roentgen appearance of pulmonary vascularity in the diagnosis of heart disease. *AJR* 1971; 112:559–570.
11. Woodley K, Stark P. Pulmonary parenchymal manifestations of mitral valve disease. *Radiographics* 1999; 19:965–972.
12. Keats TE. *Atlas of Roentgenographic Measurement*, 6th ed. St Louis: Mosby–Year Book; 1990:393–450.
13. Chickos PM, Figley MM, Fisher L. Correlation between chest film and angiographic assessment of left ventricular size. *AJR* 1977; 128:367–373.
14. Chen JTT. The significance of cardiac calcifications. *Appl Radiol* 1992; 21:11–19.
15. Stanford W, Rumberger JA. *Ultrafast Computed Tomography in Cardiac Imaging: Principles and Practice*. Mt. Kisco, NY: Futura; 1992.
16. Margolis JR, Chen JTT, Kong Y, et al. The diagnostic and prognostic significance of coronary artery calcification: A report of 800 cases. *Radiology* 1980; 137:609–616.
17. Applegate KE, Goske MJ, Pierce G, Murphy D. Situs revisited: Imaging of the heterotaxy syndrome. *Radiographics* 1999; 19:837–852.
18. Meszaros WT. *Cardiac Roentgenology*. Springfield, IL: Charles C Thomas; 1969.
19. Cooley RN. *Radiology of the Heart and Great Vessels*, 3d ed. Baltimore: Williams & Wilkins; 1978.
20. Swischuck LE. *Plain Film Interpretation in Congenital Heart Disease*, 2d ed. Baltimore: Williams & Wilkins; 1979.
21. Shuford WH, Sybers RG. *The Aortic Arch and Its Malformations*. Springfield, IL: Charles C Thomas; 1974:18.
22. Stewart JR, Kincaid OW, Titus JL. Right aortic arch: Plain film diagnosis and significance. *AJR* 1966; 97:377–389.
23. Fraser RG, Pare JAP, Pare PD, et al. Factors influencing pulmonary circulation. In: Fraser RG, Pare JAP, Pare PD, et al, eds. *Diagnosis of Diseases of the Chest*, 3d ed: Vol I. Philadelphia: Saunders; 1988:128–129.
24. Chen JTT, Behar VS, Morris JJ, et al., Correlation of roentgen findings with hemodynamic data in pure mitral stenosis. *AJR* 1968; 102:280–292.
25. Milne ENC, Pistolesi M. *Reading the Chest Radiograph: A Physiologic Approach*. St Louis: Mosby; 1993:164–241, 343–369.
26. Wojtowicz J. Some tomographic criteria for an evaluation of the pulmonary circulation. *Acta Radiol [Diagn] (Stockh)* 1964; 2:215–224.
27. Fleischner FG. The butterfly pattern of acute pulmonary edema. *Am J Cardiol* 1967; 20:39–46.
28. Jeffers K, Rees S, eds. *Clinical Cardiac Radiology*, 2d ed. London: Butterworths; 1980.
29. Chen JTT. Cardiac fluoroscopy. In: Kelley MJ, ed. Symposium on chest radiography for the cardiologist. *Cardiol Clin* 1983; 1:565–573.
30. Chen JTT, McIntosh HD, Capp MP, et al. Intercalative angiocardiography: A method for recording cardiovascular dynamics on a single film. *Radiology* 1969; 93:499–506.
31. Chen JTT, Robinson AE, Goodrich JK, Lester RG. Uneven distribution of pulmonary blood flow between left and right lungs in isolated valvular pulmonary stenosis. *AJR* 1969; 107:343–350.
32. Chen JTT, Lester RG, Peter RH. Posterior wedging sign of mitral insufficiency. *Radiology* 1974; 113:451–453.
33. Jorgens J, Kundel R, Lieber A. The cinefluorographic approach to the diagnosis of pericardial effusion. *AJR* 1962; 87:911–916.
34. Gimenez JL, Soulen RL, Davila JC. Prosthetic valve detachment: Its roentgenographic recognition: Report of cases. *AJR* 1968; 103:595–600.
35. Kotler MN, Panidis J, Mintz GS, et al. The role of noninvasive technique in the evaluation of the St. Jude cardiac prosthesis. In: DeBakey ME, ed. *Advances in Cardiac Valves: Clinical Perspectives*. New York: Yorke; 1983:213–226.
36. Sorkin RP, Schuurmann BJ, Simon AB. Radiographic aspects of permanent cardiac pacemakers. *Radiology* 1976; 119:281–286.

CHAPTER 13

THE ECHOCARDIOGRAM

Anthony N. DeMaria / Daniel G. Blanchard

INTRODUCTION

The term *echocardiography* refers to the evaluation of cardiac structure and function with images and recordings produced by ultrasound. In the past three decades it has rapidly become a fundamental component of the cardiac evaluation. Currently, echocardiography provides essential (and sometimes unexpected) clinical information and has become the second most frequently performed diagnostic procedure after electrocardiography.[1] What began as a one-dimensional method performed from the precordial area to assess cardiac anatomy has evolved into a two-dimensional (2D) modality performed from either the thorax or from within the esophagus, capable of also delineating flow and deriving hemodynamic data.[2] Newly evolving technical developments likely will extend the capacity of ultrasound to routine 3D visualization[3] as well as to the assessment, in conjunction with contrast agents,[4] of myocardial perfusion.

The development of echocardiography is usually credited to Elder and Hertz in 1954.[5] Primitive cross-sectional images of the excised human heart were produced in 1957[6]; however, for nearly two additional decades, clinical echocardiography consisted primarily of 1D time-motion (M-mode) recordings, as popularized by Feigenbaum.[7] In the mid-1970s, Bom and associates developed a multielement linear-array scanner that could produce spatially correct images of the beating heart.[8] 2D images of superior quality were soon achieved by mechanical sector scanners[9,10] and ultimately by phased-array instruments as developed by Thurston and Von Ramm, which are the present-day standard.[11] In the past several years, 3D instruments capable of real-time volumetric imaging have been developed.

Although efforts to use the Doppler principle to measure flow velocity by ultrasound were begun in the early 1970s by Baker et al.,[12] clinical application of this technique did not thrive until the work of Hatle in the early 1980s.[13,14] Pulsed and continuous-wave Doppler recordings soon were expanded to full 2D color-flow imaging.[15] Most recently, miniaturization of ultrasound transducers has led to their incorporation into gastroscopes and cardiac catheters to achieve transesophageal and intravascular images.[16,17]

PRINCIPLES OF ECHOCARDIOGRAPHY

Physics and Instrumentation

Sound is an energy form that travels through a medium as a series of alternating compressions and rarefactions of the molecules (Fig. 13-1). Sound is typically characterized by its wavelength, which is the distance between any two consecutive phases of the cycle (e.g., peak compression to peak compression), and by its frequency, which is the number of wavelengths per unit time [customarily expressed as cycles per second, or hertz (Hz)]. The velocity of sound is the product of wavelength and frequency; thus there is an inverse relationship between these two characteristics: the greater the frequency, the shorter the wavelength. Ultrasound is sonic energy with a frequency above the audible range of the human ear (greater than 20,000 Hz) and is useful for diagnostic imaging, since, like light, it can be directed as a beam that will obey the laws of reflection and refraction.[14–18] Thus, an ultrasound beam will travel in a straight line through a homogeneous medium. If the beam meets an interface of different acoustic impedance, however, part of the energy will be reflected, and the remaining attenuated signal will be transmitted. The reflected energy, or echo, is used to construct an image—in the case of echocardiography, an image of the heart (Fig. 13-2).

The most fundamental component of any echocardiographic instrument is the transducer, which is responsible for both transmitting and receiving the ultrasound signal. The transducer consists of electrodes and a piezoelectric crystal whose ionic structure results in deformation of shape when exposed to an electric current.[18] Thus, piezoelectric crystals are composed of synthetic materials, such as barium titanate, that, when exposed to electric current from the electrodes, alternately expand and contract to create sound waves. When subjected to the mechanical energy of sound returning from a reflecting surface, the same piezoelectric element changes shape, thereby generating an electrical signal detected by the electrodes (Fig. 13-3). Thus the transducer both produces and receives ultrasonic signals.

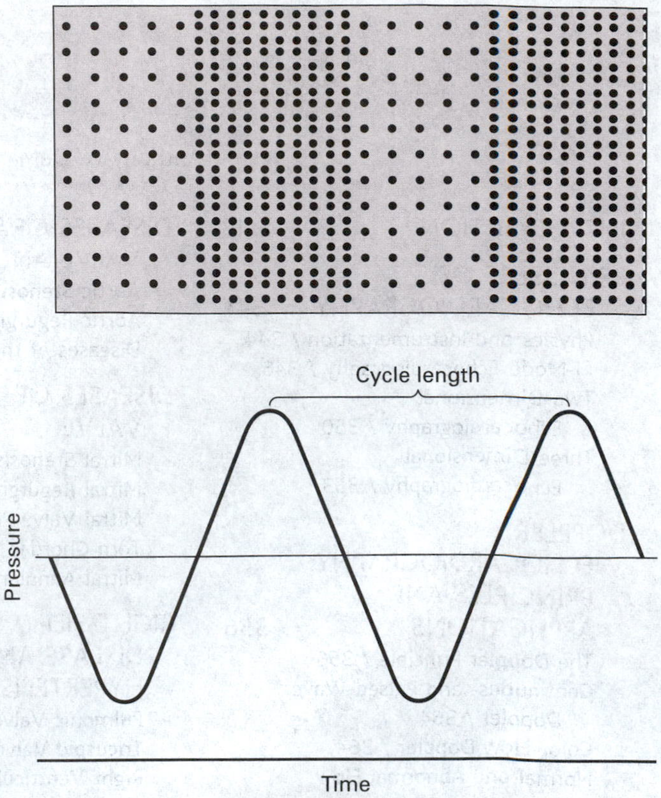

FIGURE 13-1 Sound energy results in alternating compression and rarefaction of particles in a conducting medium. This alternation, which can be plotted against time (or distance), conforms to a sine-wave pattern (*bottom panel*). (Modified from Hagan AD, DeMaria AN. *Clinical Applications of Two-Dimensional Echocardiography and Cardiac Doppler.* Boston: Little, Brown; 1989, with permission.)

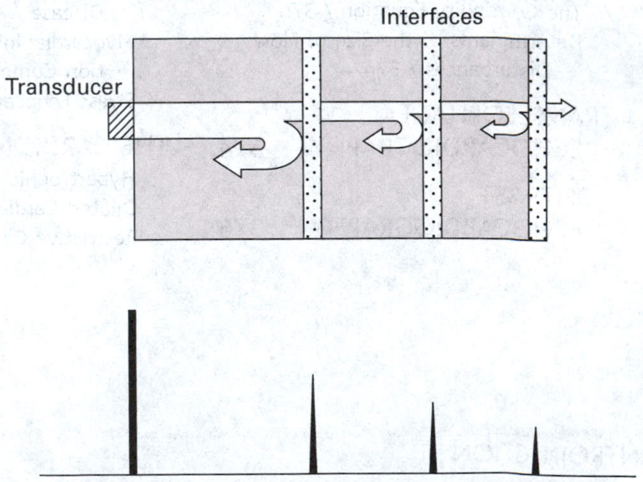

FIGURE 13-2 *Upper panel:* Attenuation of an ultrasound beam emitted from a transducer. There is reflection and progressive loss of energy at each interface encountered. *Lower panel:* the reflected wavefronts are recorded as signals of varying amplitudes (A mode) via the piezoelectric crystal. (Upper panel modified from Hagan AD, DeMaria AN. *Clinical Applications of Two-Dimensional Echocardiography and Cardiac Doppler.* Boston: Little, Brown; 1989, with permission.)

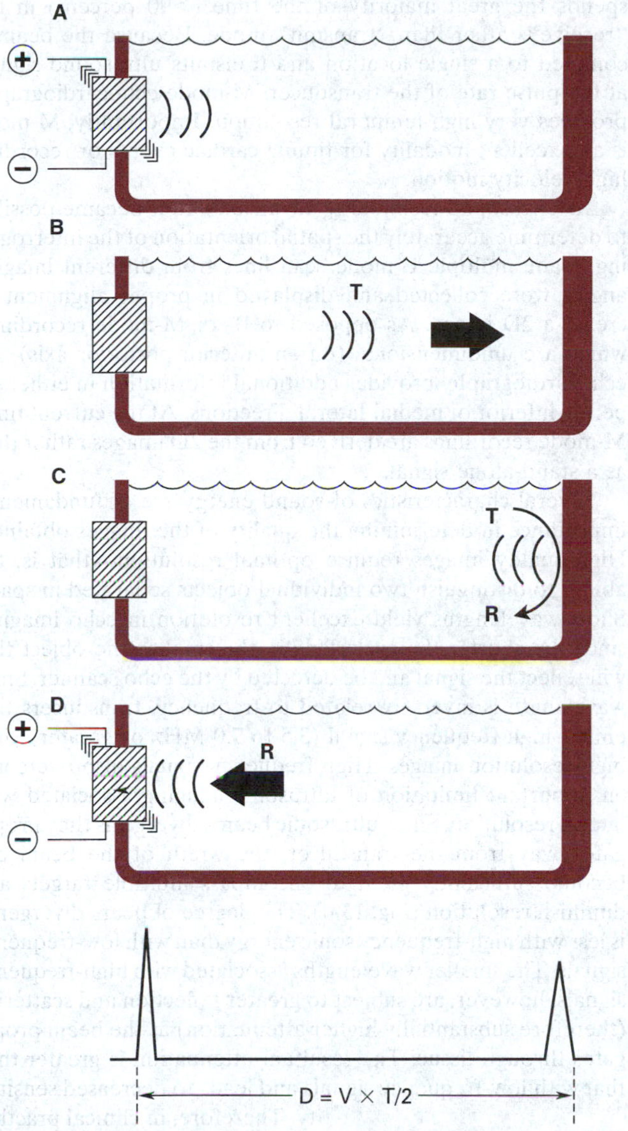

FIGURE 13-3 *A* through *D:* the basic principle of ultrasonic imaging. The piezoelectric crystal is activated, producing a transmitted pulse (T), which reflects off the interface. The reflected pulse (R) excites the crystal, producing an electric current. As the velocity of the pulse is constant, distance can be calculated based on the transit time. (Because the pulse must travel back and forth from the interface, the time is divided by 2.) (Modified from Weyman AE. *Principles and Practice of Echocardiography,* 2d ed. Philadelphia: Lea & Febiger; 1994, with permission.)

In the past, echographs have both transmitted and received signals of the same frequency. Recently, *harmonic imaging* has been implemented, in which ultrasound energy is transmitted at one frequency (fundamental) and received at a higher harmonic of that frequency (usually the first). Tissue harmonic signals are created by alteration of the frequency of the wave as it propagates through the structure.[18a] Contrast microbubbles produce harmonics by virtue of resonating (expanding/constricting) in the ultrasound field.[18b] The net effect of harmonic imaging is to reduce the signal intensity of background noise and enhance that from true tissue (or microbubble) structure, although some blooming of the signals from valves may be observed.[18a]

As an imaging modality, ultrasound carries with it several unique technical difficulties. Sound energy is poorly transmitted through air and bone, and the ability to record adequate images is dependent upon a thoracic window that gives the interrogating beam adequate access to cardiac structures. The degree to which ultrasonic energy will be reflected when striking an interface of differential impedance is dependent upon how perpendicular the interrogating beam is to the interface. When the ultrasound beam is directed parallel or near parallel to the interface, little or no sound energy will be reflected to the transducer. Therefore poor signal transmission, a nonorthogonal orientation of the ultrasound beam to the surface, and energy attenuation can result in failure to record signals from cardiac structures—a phenomenon referred to as *echo dropout.*[19] Conversely, some structures may be such strong ultrasonic reflectors—being perpendicular to the beam or extremely dense—that sufficient energy returns to the transducer to be reflected and again transmitted into the field. This phenomenon can lead to reverberations, or the reproduction of the echoes of anatomic structures at multiple locations within the image.[20] In addition, background noise artifacts, or signals generated from the system rather than tissue, can also be encountered. Finally, since the ultrasound beam diverges with distance from the transducer and always has a finite width, targets lying on the periphery of the beam may be recorded and displayed as if they were located along the central scan line (Fig. 13-4). This problem may be accentuated in the setting of very strong reflectors that result in the formation of *side lobes.*[21] In either case, beam-width problems associated with ultrasound may result in the depiction of targets in erroneous locations and create problems in interpreting the images.[22]

The construction of a cardiac image from ultrasound signals is based upon computation of the distance between an anatomic structure and the transducer (Fig. 13-3). Thus, an ultrasound beam is produced by a hand-held transducer positioned on the thorax and directed into the heart. This beam will travel in a straight line until it reaches an interface between structures of

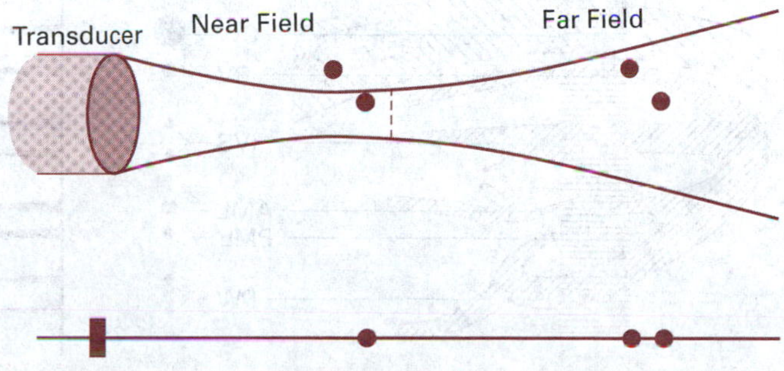

FIGURE 13-4 *Upper panel:* The transducer emits an ultrasonic beam that has a near field (where the beam is relatively focused) and a far field (where the beam width increases). *Lower panel:* B-mode diagram showing the effect of beam width. In the near field, the beam reflects off only one of two objects in close proximity to each other. In the far field, however, two similarly positioned objects are both within the beam width. Therefore, lateral resolution is compromised and the objects' positions are misrepresented.

different acoustic impedance, such as blood and myocardium. At this point, some ultrasonic energy will be reflected (depending on the density of interface), some will be scattered, and some will continue forward. The amplitude of the propagating signal will be attenuated because of the reduction in energy at the interface (Fig. 13-2). The reflected sound waves return to the transducer and form the basis of the echogram. Electronic circuitry within the echograph measures the time interval required for the transit of the ultrasound beam from the transducer to the interface and back again. Since the velocity of sound in soft tissue is constant (approximately 1540 m/s), the instrument can calculate the total distance traveled to and from the reflecting surface as the product of transit time and velocity of sound. Interface location is derived as one-half of the total transit distance, and a signal is depicted on an oscilloscope or video monitor at that point (Fig. 13-3). The amplitude of ultrasonic energy reflected from each target interface is represented by the brightness of the signal that is displayed.

The one-dimensional ultrasonic B- (or brightness) mode scan line resulting from a single transmitted beam is the cornerstone of echocardiographic imaging. In the most basic form of echocardiography, a single scan line produced by a piezoelectric crystal is passed through the heart (Fig. 13-5). At each structural interface, ultrasonic energy is reflected back and displayed at the appropriate distance as a signal, whose amplitude represents the acoustic impedance or density of the material encountered. These signals are subsequently displayed as dots, whose brightness is proportional to the amplitude of reflected ultrasonic energy. The distance from the transducer of these B-mode dots changes as the cardiac structures move during the cardiac cycle. Accordingly, if repetitive B-mode scan lines are produced and swept across the screen over time, the movement of the heart can be obtained as a time-motion (or M-mode) recording,[23] providing dynamic rather than merely static cardiac images (Fig. 13-5). In clinical use, the piezoelectric crystal within the transducer is activated by alternating electric current to transient at a rate of approximately 1000 pulses per second. This same crystal also receives the returning echo reflections and actually spends the great majority of the time (>90 percent) in the "receive" rather than "transmit" mode. Because the beam is confined to a single location and transmits ultrasound signals at the pulse rate of the transducer, M-mode echocardiography provides very high temporal resolution. Importantly, M mode is an excellent modality for timing cardiac events or recording high-velocity motion.

As ultrasound technology advanced and it became possible to determine accurately the spatial orientation of the interrogating beam, multiple B-mode scan lines from different imaging angles were collected and displayed in proper alignment to create a 2D image. As opposed to B- or M-mode recordings, which are unidimensional (on an anterior-posterior axis), 2D echocardiography provides additional information in either superior-inferior or medial-lateral directions. At the current time, M-mode recordings are derived from the 2D images rather than as a stand-alone signal.

Several characteristics of sound energy are of fundamental importance in determining the quality of the images obtained. High-quality images require optimal resolution—that is, the ability to distinguish two individual objects separated in space. Short wavelengths yield excellent resolution in echo imaging, since the shorter the cycle length, the smaller the object that will reflect the signal and be detected by the echo scanner. Since wavelength is inversely related to frequency, transducers that emit a high-frequency signal (3.5 to 7.0 MHz or greater) yield high-resolution images. High-frequency signals also overcome an important limitation of ultrasonic imaging associated with lateral resolution. Since ultrasonic beams diverge as they propagate away from the transducer, the width of the beam can become sufficiently great to encompass multiple targets and diminish resolution (Fig. 13-4). The degree of beam divergence is less with high-frequency sonic energy than with low-frequency signals. The smaller wavelengths associated with high-frequency signals, however, are subject to greater reflection and scattering (therefore substantially higher attenuation) as the beam propagates through tissue. The resultant attenuation is greater than that with low-frequency signals and leads to decreased sensitivity. Therefore, in clinical practice, echocardiographic examinations are performed utilizing the highest-frequency transducer capable of obtaining signals from all potential targets within the ultrasound field.[23]

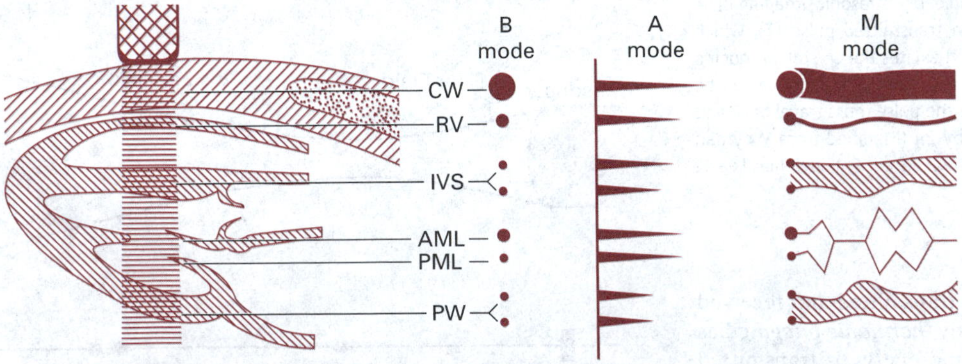

FIGURE 13-5 Formation of A-mode, B-mode, and M-mode echocardiograms. The transducer emits an ultrasound beam, which reflects at each anatomic interface. The reflected wavefronts can be represented as dots (B mode) or spikes (A mode). The dot brightness and spike magnitude vary with the amplitude of the reflected wave. If the B-mode scan is swept from left to right with time, an M-mode image is produced. CW = chest wall; RV = right ventricle; IVS = interventricular septum; AML = anterior mitral leaflet; PML = posterior mitral leaflet; and PW = posterior wall. (Modified from Hagan AD, DeMaria AN. *Clinical Applications of Two-Dimensional Echocardiography and Cardiac Doppler.* Boston: Little, Brown; 1989, with permission.)

M-Mode Echocardiography

THE STANDARD M-MODE EXAMINATION

Although largely supplanted by 2D imaging, M-mode echocardiography remains a useful part of a complete ultrasound examination. Figure 13-6*A* through *D* shows the typical views obtained when the transducer is placed at the left parasternal area and rocked through the heart from apex to

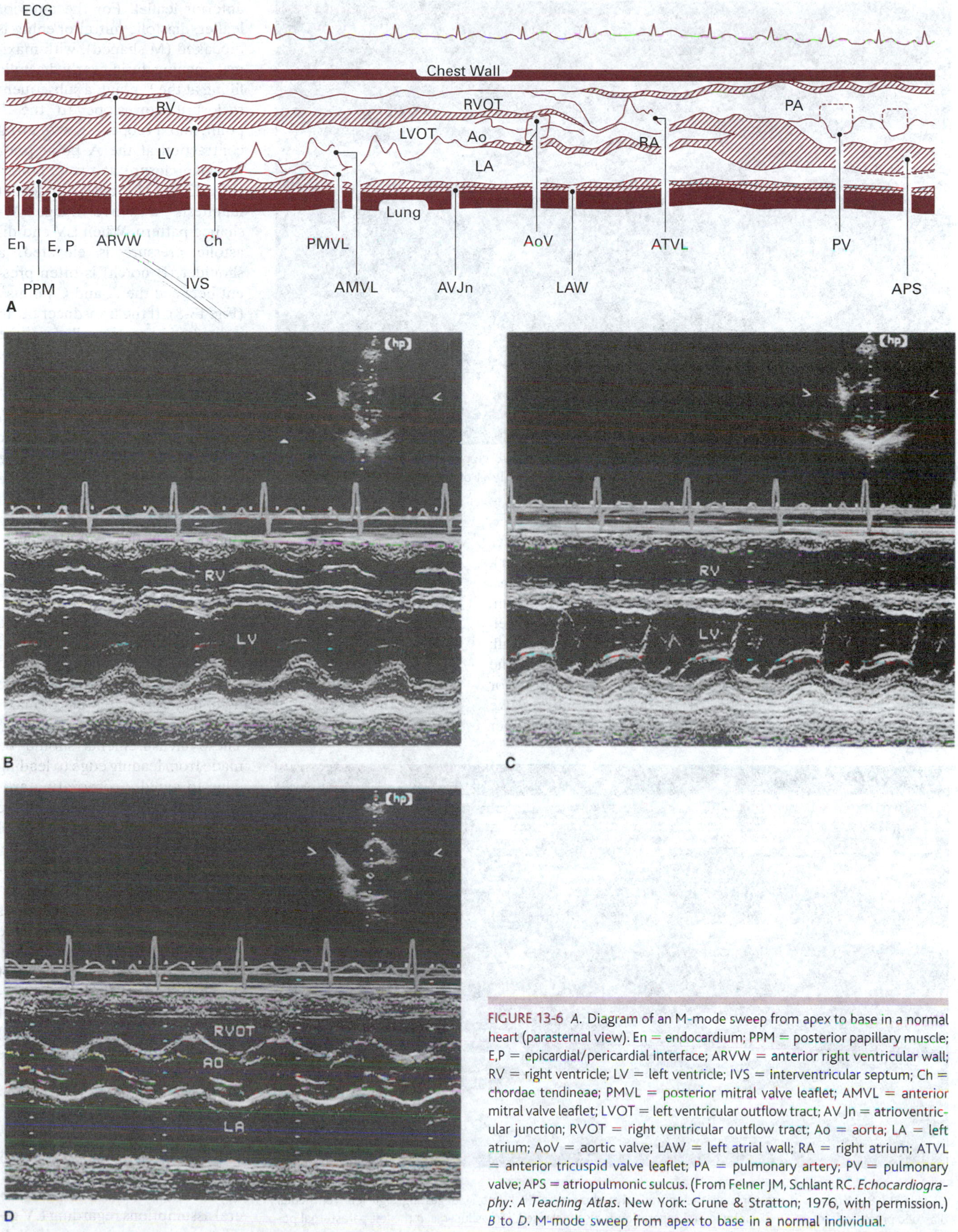

FIGURE 13-6 *A*. Diagram of an M-mode sweep from apex to base in a normal heart (parasternal view). En = endocardium; PPM = posterior papillary muscle; E,P = epicardial/pericardial interface; ARVW = anterior right ventricular wall; RV = right ventricle; LV = left ventricle; IVS = interventricular septum; Ch = chordae tendineae; PMVL = posterior mitral valve leaflet; AMVL = anterior mitral valve leaflet; LVOT = left ventricular outflow tract; AV Jn = atrioventricular junction; RVOT = right ventricular outflow tract; Ao = aorta; LA = left atrium; AoV = aortic valve; LAW = left atrial wall; RA = right atrium; ATVL = anterior tricuspid valve leaflet; PA = pulmonary artery; PV = pulmonary valve; APS = atriopulmonic sulcus. (From Felner JM, Schlant RC. *Echocardiography: A Teaching Atlas*. New York: Grune & Stratton; 1976, with permission.) *B* to *D*. M-mode sweep from apex to base in a normal individual.

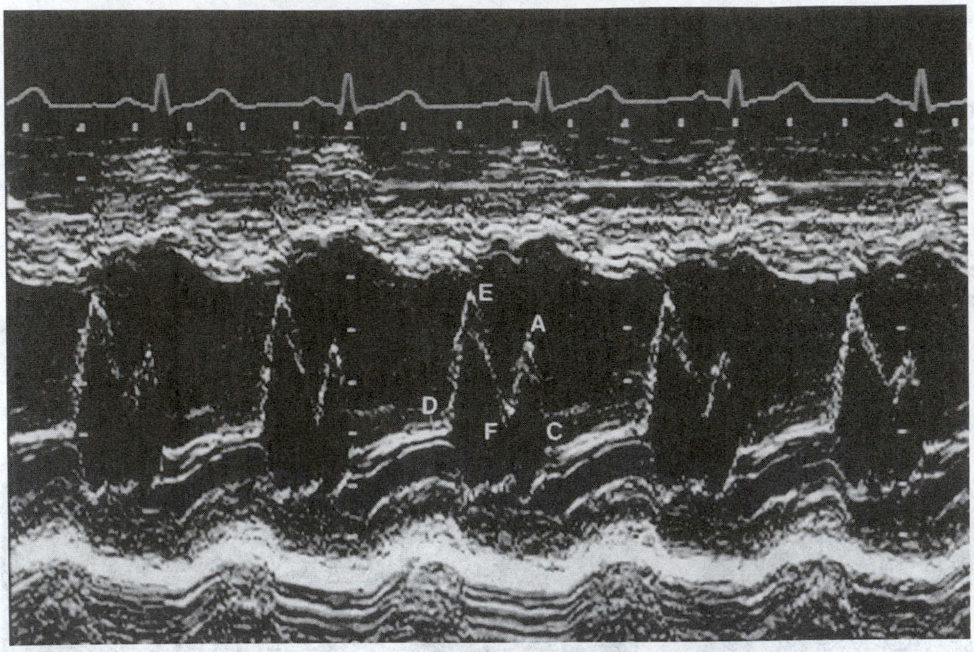

FIGURE 13-7 Standard M-mode image through the left ventricle at the level of the mitral valve. See text for discussion of nomenclature.

base. Tissue typically reflects ultrasound at its surface (specular reflectors) and from internal inhomogenicity (backscatter), while blood is homogenous and does not produce reflections. Thus, blood is free of ultrasonic signals on the echocardiogram. At the mitral valve level (Fig. 13-6*C*), the cardiac structure seen closest to the transducer is the right ventricular (RV) free wall; it is followed by the RV cavity, the interventricular septum, the mitral valve apparatus, and the left ventricular (LV) posterior wall as the beam travels backward. At this level, mitral valve excursion is well seen and is more easily recorded for the longer anterior leaflet. For the anterior leaflet, diastolic mitral opening is bipeaked (M-shaped), with maximal opening during early diastolic filling at the E point, a subsequent reclosure downslope to the F point, and a reopening with atrial contraction at the A point prior to valve closure at the C point[24] (Fig. 13-7). The posterior leaflet manifests a mirror-image W-shaped pattern. When LV end-diastolic pressure is elevated, a shoulder (B notch) is often present between the A and C points[25] (Fig. 13-8). If the transducer beam is directed inferolaterally from the mitral valve level, the papillary muscles and LV apex will be imaged (Fig. 13-6*A*). With superior and medial angulation, the left atrium, aortic valve, and aortic root are seen. The tricuspid valve can be imaged by angulating the transducer inferomedially and the pulmonic valve by angulating slightly superiorly and laterally.

ASSESSMENT OF SYSTOLIC FUNCTION BY M-MODE ECHOCARDIOGRAPHY

Measurements of the LV cavity dimension and wall thickness can be readily derived from M-mode recordings (Fig. 13-9) and are usually made according to the recommendations of the American Society of Echocardiography at end diastole (the onset of the QRS complex) and end systole (the point of maximum upward motion of the LV posterior wall endocardium).[26] These measurements should be made from leading edge to leading edge to avoid incorporating artifacts and reverberations; they are accurate if the beam is orthogonal to the long axis of the ventricle. By convention, left atrial (LA) dimension is measured at end systole and aortic root diameter is recorded at end diastole at the level of the base of the heart (Fig. 13-9). During systole, opening of the aortic leaflets appears as a parallelogram produced by motion of the right coronary and (usually) the noncoronary aortic valve cusps.[27]

The M-mode LV cavity dimensions can be used to estimate ventricular volumes and ejection fraction (EF) if desired, most simply by merely cubing the value (D^3); but these calculations involve several assumptions regarding LV geometry that are not uniformly

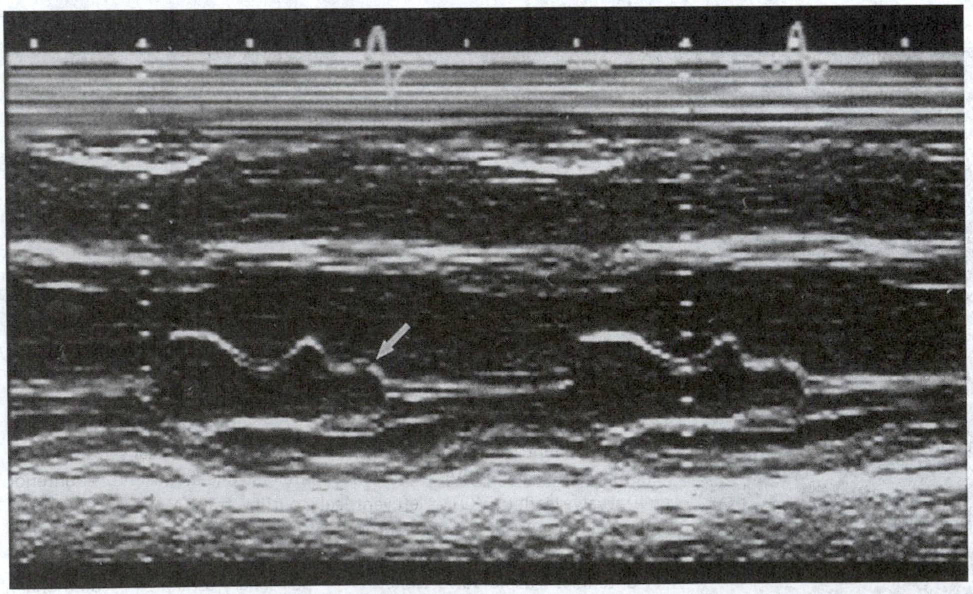

FIGURE 13-8 M-mode image through the mitral valve showing a "B bump," suggesting high left ventricular diastolic pressure (*arrow*). The E-point septal separation is also increased. (Transducer is in the left parasternal position.)

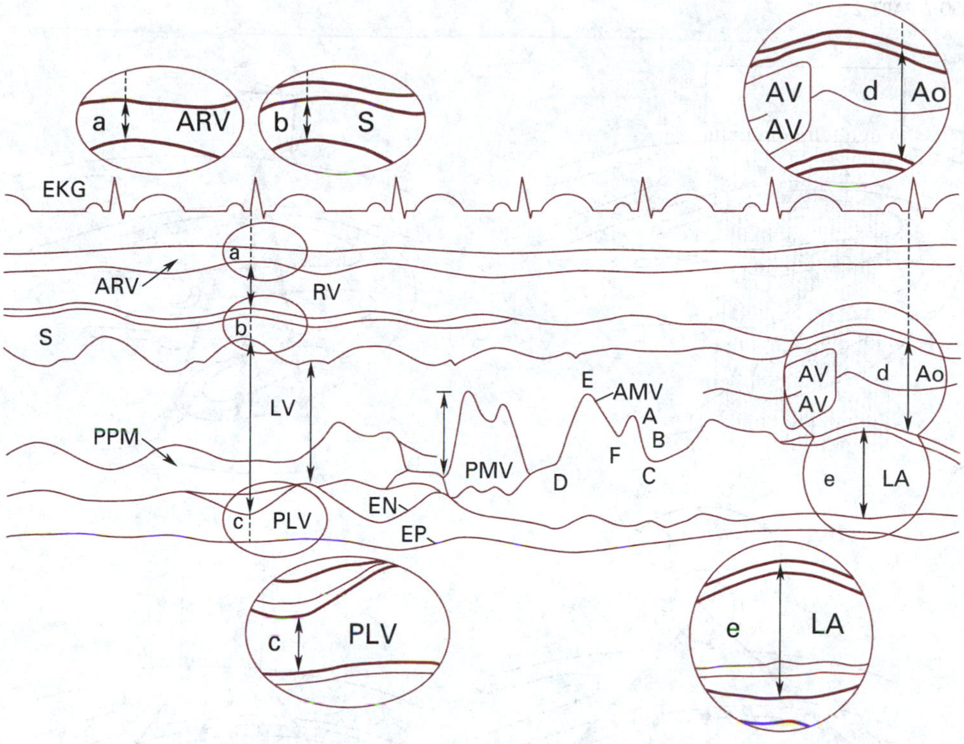

FIGURE 13-9 Recommended criteria for M-mode measurement of cardiac dimensions (see text for details). The figure and the elliptical inserts (*a, b, c, d,* and *e*) illustrate the leading-edge method. ARV = anterior right ventricular wall; RV = right ventricle; LV = left ventricle; PLV = posterior left ventricular wall; S = septum; PPM = papillary muscle; AMV and PMV = anterior and posterior mitral valve leaflets, EN: endocardium, EP: epicardium; AV = aortic valve; Ao = aorta; LA = left atrium. (Reproduced with permission from Sahn DJ, DeMaria AN, Kisslo J, Weyman AE. Recommendations regarding quantitation in M-mode echocardiography: Results of a survey of echocardiographic measurements. *Circulation* 1978; 58;1072, with permission.)

TABLE 13-1 Normal Values

	Mean ± Standard Deviation	Range	Mean ± Standard Deviation	Range
No. of patients	25	—	50	—
Age, years	10 ± 3	4–18	24 ± 6	1.10–2.53
BSA, m²	1.33 ± 0.38	0.72–2.04	1.81 ± .34	1.10–2.53
$LVID_d$, mm	44 ± 6	32–50	50 ± 3	42–60
$LVID_s$, mm	28 ± 7	32–50	50 ± 3	22–43
FSLV	34 ± 4	25–42	33 ± 3	28–37
IVS thickness, mm	8 ± 2	5–10	9 ± 1	7–12
IVS excursion, mm	7 ± 1	5–9	9 ± 1	7–12
PW_d thickness, mm	7 ± 2	4–9	9 ± 1	7–12
PW_s thickness, mm	12 ± 3	8–17	16 ± 2	13–20
Δ thickening PW	0.70 ± 0.25	0.41–0.95	0.50 ± 0.19	0.32–0.69
PW excursion, mm	9 ± 2	7–14	11 ± 2	9–17
RVD_d supine, mm	—	—	15 ± 6	7–22
RVD_d left lateral, mm	—	—	20 ± 8	10–37
$Aorta_d$ mm	23 ± 4	15–27	28 ± 5	26–36
LAD_s mm	25 ± 5	20–31	27 ± 6	12–35

ABBREVIATIONS: BSA = Body surface area; $LVID_d$ = left ventricular internal diameter, end diastole; $LVID_s$ = left ventricular internal diameter, end systole; FSLV = fractional shortening of left ventricle; PWV = posterior wall velocity; IVS = interventricular septum; PW = posterior wall; RVD = right ventricular dimension; LAD = left atrial dimension.

SOURCE: Felner JM, Schlant RC. *Echocardiography: A Teaching Atlas.* New York: Grune & Stratton; 1976. Reproduced with permission from the publisher and authors.

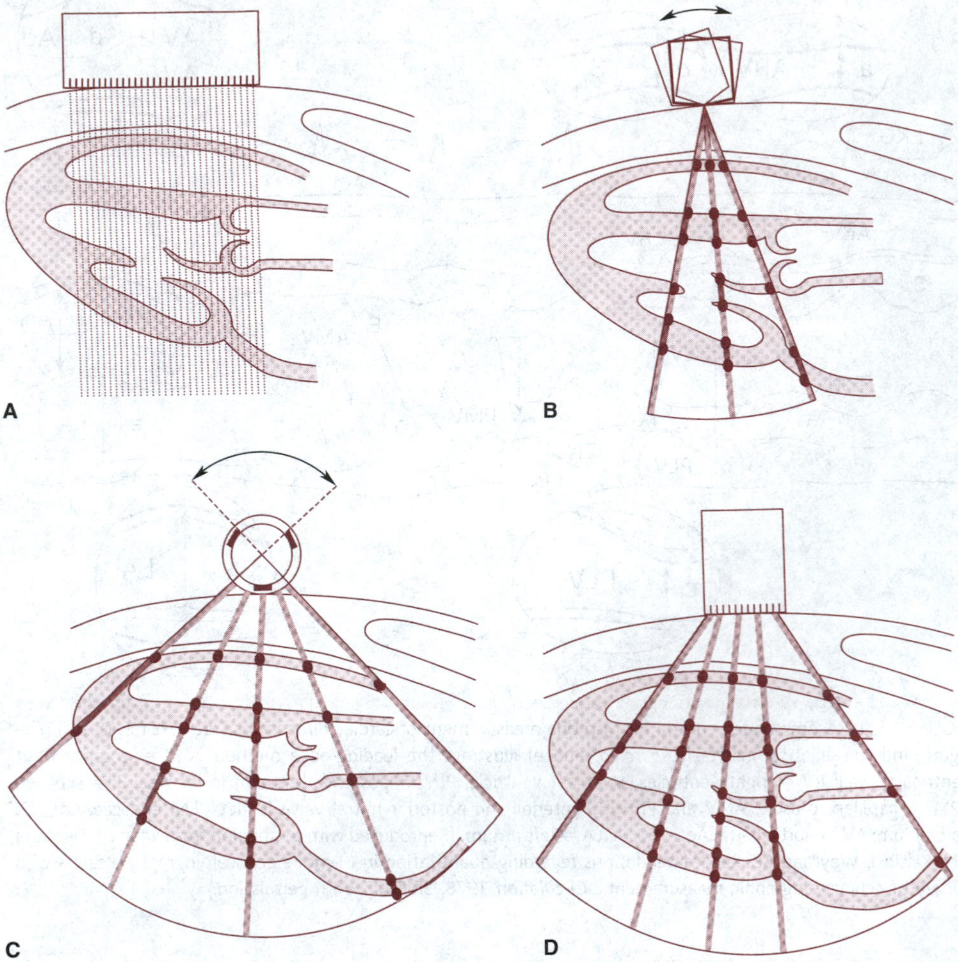

FIGURE 13-10 The four major types of ultrasonic scanners used to acquire 2D echocardiographic images. *A.* Linear-array scanner. *B.* Oscillating scanner. *C.* Rotating mechanical scanner. *D.* Phased-array scanner. (From Hagan AD, DeMaria AN. *Clinical Applications of Two-Dimensional Echocardiography and Cardiac Doppler*. Boston: Little, Brown; 1989, with permission.)

valid.[28,29] In addition, the M-mode dimension may not be representative of the entire ventricle. The fractional shortening can also be determined.[30] This value is often helpful in assessing systolic function, but it reflects the function of the LV in one chord and in one plane and can be misleading with asynchronous contraction [for example, left bundle branch block (LBBB)] or segmental dyssynergy.[31] An additional M-mode marker of systolic function is *E point–septal separation* (EPSS), or the distance between the anterior mitral valve leaflet at its most anterior opening excursion (the E point) and the interventricular septum. A value of 8 mm or greater is abnormal.[32] The normal M-mode measurements are seen in Table 13-1.

Two-Dimensional Echocardiography

A number of technical approaches exist by which multiple individual B-mode scan lines can be rapidly transmitted, received, and displayed in appropriate spatial orientation to construct a 2D image of the heart. The initial approach simply utilized a linear array of 20 piezoelectric crystals placed side by side, each of which transmitted and received signals independently[8] (Fig. 13-10*A*). The resulting scan lines were displayed simultaneously to yield rectangular images. Unfortunately, transducer size and interaction between the elements resulted in images of unsatisfactory quality.

Current 2D scanners utilize B-mode scan lines that are independently transmitted and received and are directed through a wedge-shaped sector of cardiac anatomy by means of mechanical or electrical beam steering (Fig. 13-10*B* to *D*). A variety of motorized devices are available that, by rapidly oscillating or rotating one or more ultrasonic crystals through space, can mechanically direct multiple scan lines through a sector arc of the cardiovascular system.[9,10] The position of the beam in space is derived by determining the orientation of the piezoelectric crystal. A majority of current 2D scanners utilize a phased-array approach, where multiple ultrasonic crystals are employed in concert to create individual B-mode scan lines.[11] The piezoelectric crystals are activated in a closely coordinated temporal sequence such that the individual wavelets produced by each element merge to form a single beam whose direction is determined by the sequence of crystal firing (Fig. 13-11). Since the direction of the resultant beam is determined by the sequence of activation of the individual elements, the beam can be electrically swept throughout a 90-degree sector arc. In addition to electronic beam steering, a firing sequence can be employed that results in dynamic focusing of the beam along its length to achieve minimal beam width and increased resolution. Phased-array 2D scanners employ small transducers without moving parts that could require repair. The increased complexity of these scanners, however, makes the systems more costly.

Originally, echocardiographic data were displayed in analog form on a standard oscilloscope, transferred to a video monitor by a television camera, and hard-copied onto videotape or paper. Currently, computerized analog-to-digital scan conversion is standard, so that the polar signals of individual scan lines are converted to a series of numerical gray-level values for individual box-like picture elements (pixels) aligned along *X*-*Y* coordinates.[33] The ability of a digital step-gradation technique to reproduce the continuous gradation of analog methods is a function of the density of pixels in the matrix and the shades of gray levels available. No loss of data can be detected in current digitally converted images, and the digital format provides the opportunity for image processing, enhancement, and quantitation. More importantly, storage in digital format can avoid the image degradation inherent in videotape, provide

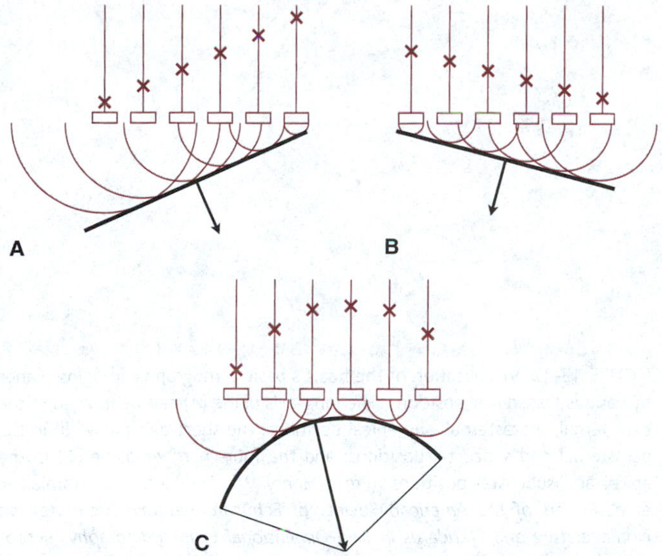

FIGURE 13-11 Electronic "steering" of a phased-array ultrasound beam. *A.* Elements are fired in sequence from left to right, resulting in a beam directed to the left. *B.* Elements are fired in sequence opposite to those in (*A*), producing a beam directed to the right. *C.* Elements are fired from the periphery toward the center, producing a beam that converges on a given focal point. (From Hagan AD, DeMaria AN. *Clinical Applications of Two-Dimensional Echocardiography and Cardiac Doppler.* Boston: Little Brown; 1989, with permission.)

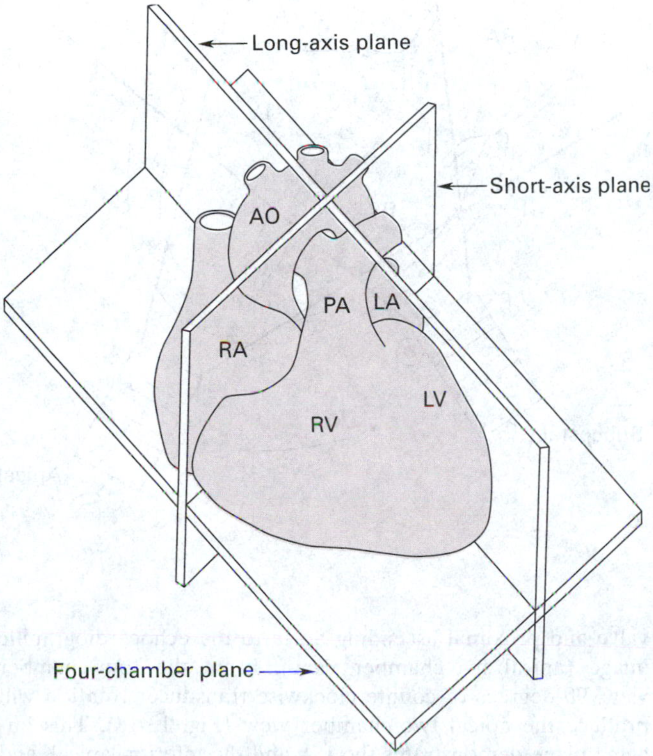

FIGURE 13-12 The three basic tomographic imaging planes used in echocardiography: long-axis, short-axis, and four-chamber. LV = left ventricle; LA = left atrium; RV = right ventricle; RA = right atrium; PA = pulmonary artery; AO = aorta. (From Hagan AD, DeMaria AN. *Clinical Applications of Two-Dimensional Echocardiography and Cardiac Doppler.* Boston: Little, Brown; 1989, with permission.)

random access and easy comparison of studies, enable rapid image transmission, and prevent deterioration with image copying and prolonged storage. Technology for fully digital echocardiography is now becoming available, and fully digital acquisition and storage of echocardiograms will be commonplace in the near future, replacing analog videotape recordings.

THE STANDARD TWO-DIMENSIONAL EXAMINATION

The heart can be imaged through a multitude of planes with 2D echocardiography. To help standardize the 2D examination, the American Society of Echocardiography has recommended that cardiac imaging be performed in three orthogonal planes: long-axis (from aortic root to the apex), short-axis (perpendicular to long axis), and four-chamber (traversing both ventricles and atria through the mitral and tricuspid valves)[34] (Fig. 13-12). It is important to recognize that the long and short axes are those of the heart, not the body. These three planes can be visualized using four basic transducer positions: parasternal, apical, subcostal, and suprasternal[35,36] (Figs. 13-13*A*, *B*, and *C*). In general, the long-axis plane is best imaged from parasternal, apical, and occasionally the suprasternal positions, while the short-axis plane is best imaged in the parasternal and subcostal positions. The four-chamber views are obtained from the apical and subcostal positions. The American Society of Echocardiography recognizes that these basic positions and planes may be modified somewhat and recommends that an image obtained within 45 degrees of a basic orthogonal plane be identified with that orthogonal plane. Table 13-2 lists the standard transducer positions and transthoracic echocardiographic views. Anatomic drawings of the various imaging planes are seen in Figs. 13-13 through 13-20.

As opposed to other types of cardiac imaging, such as chest radiography, which are well standardized, the echocardiographic examination is iterative and largely determined by the anatomic characteristics of the patient and manual manipulation of the transducer by the operator. Of paramount importance is the identification of a thoracic site (window) that enables transmission of the ultrasound signal to the heart. In actual practice, the echocardiographic examination is performed with the operator either to the patient's left or right. The patient is in the left lateral decubitus position for most of the examination, with the head of the bed elevated 20 to 30 degrees. Alternate positioning may be employed for individual patients and views. Use of a thick foam rubber mattress (made expressly for echocardiography) that has a removable section under the area of the cardiac apex may facilitate the examination.

The examination customarily begins with the transducer in the left parasternal position in the long-axis view (Fig. 13-14). This provides excellent images of the left ventricle, aorta, left atrium, and the mitral and aortic valves. By angling the beam slightly rightward and inferiorly (right ventricular inflow view), the right atrium, right ventricle, and tricuspid valve are visualized (Fig. 13-15). If the beam is turned slightly leftward and rotated clockwise from the standard parasternal long-axis view, the right ventricular outflow tract, pulmonic valve, and main pulmonary artery appear (right ventricular outflow view).

A 90-degree clockwise turn of the transducer produces the parasternal short-axis view. Slight axial angulation of the trans-

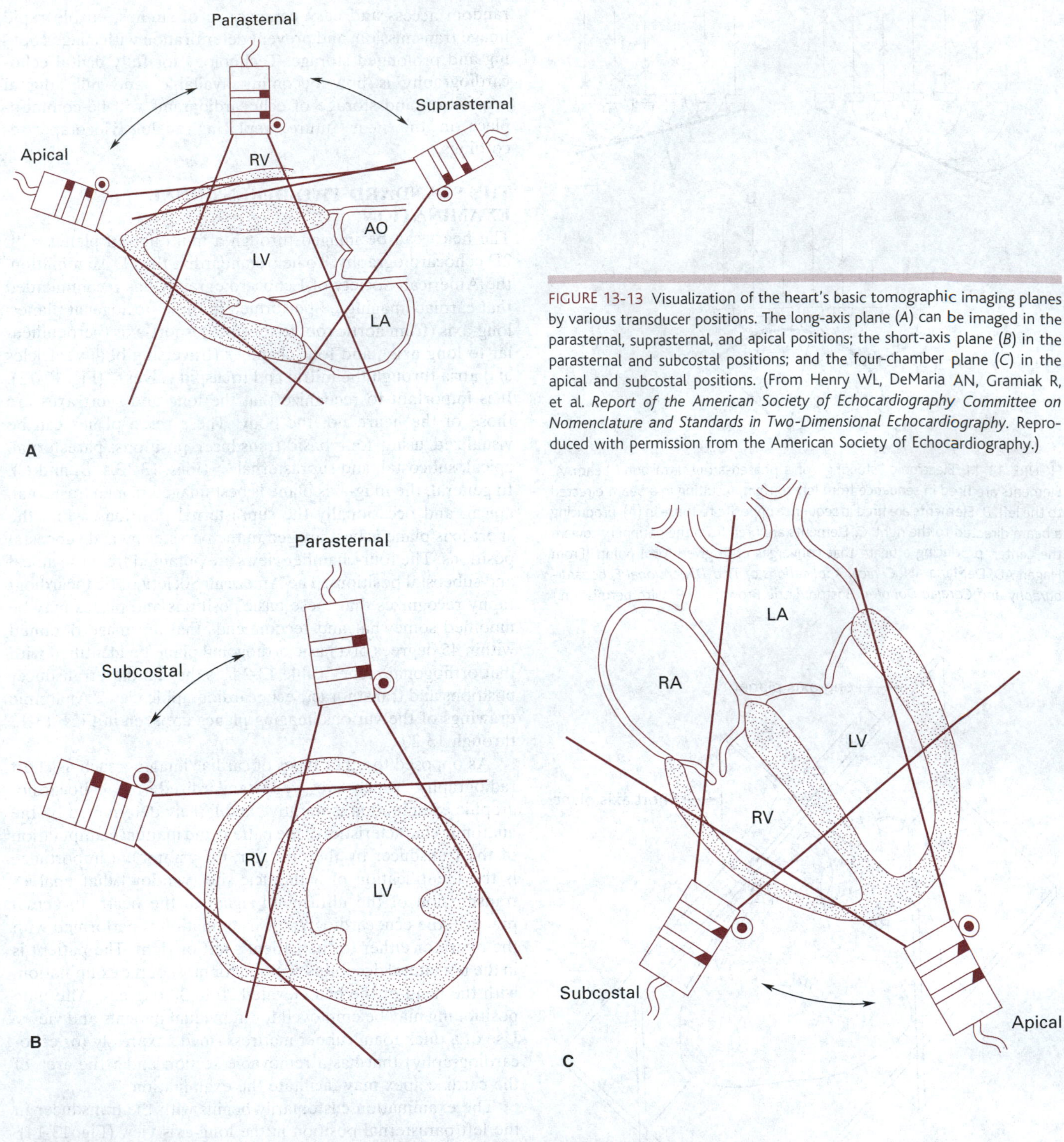

FIGURE 13-13 Visualization of the heart's basic tomographic imaging planes by various transducer positions. The long-axis plane (*A*) can be imaged in the parasternal, suprasternal, and apical positions; the short-axis plane (*B*) in the parasternal and subcostal positions; and the four-chamber plane (*C*) in the apical and subcostal positions. (From Henry WL, DeMaria AN, Gramiak R, et al. *Report of the American Society of Echocardiography Committee on Nomenclature and Standards in Two-Dimensional Echocardiography*. Reproduced with permission from the American Society of Echocardiography.)

ducer enables visualization of the LV at various levels of the short axis, including the papillary muscle, mitral leaflets, and aortic valve (Fig. 13-16). With angulation toward the base, the LA right heart structures, main pulmonary artery, and occasionally the left atrial appendage are also recorded.

The apical views are best acquired with the patient in a steep left lateral decubitus position and the transducer at the point of the apical impulse. The four-chamber view is obtained by turning the transducer so that both ventricles, atrioventricular valves, and atria are visualized (Fig. 13-17). In this view, the septal, apical, and lateral walls of the LV are visualized. Slight superior angulation of the transducer will add the aortic valve and proximal ascending aorta to the echocardiographic image (apical five-chamber view). From the four-chamber view, 90 degrees of counterclockwise transducer rotation will produce the apical two-chamber view (Fig. 13-18). This imaging plane demonstrates the LA and the inferior, apical, and anterior wall segments of the LV (the right heart structures are absent). If the transducer is rotated slightly back toward the four-chamber plane, a three-chamber view similar to the parasternal long-axis view is produced (Fig. 13-18) and provides images of the posterior, apical, and anteroseptal LV wall segments as well as the LA, aorta, and mitral and aortic valves.

TABLE 13-2 Standard Two-Dimensional Echocardiographic Transducer Positions

Parasternal Position
Long axis
Left ventricular long axis
Right ventricular long
Right ventricular outflow
Short axis
Short axis through the plane of
The cardiac base
The mitral valve
The chordae tendineae
The papillary muscles
The apex
Apical Position
Four-chamber plane
Five-chamber plane
(Four-chamber plane angled superiorly to include the aorta)
Two-chamber plane
Three-chamber plane
Subcostal Position
Four-chamber plane
Short-axis through the plane of
The mitral valve
The papillary muscles
The cardiac base
Posteriorly directed planes through the venae cavae and atria
Suprasternal Position
Long axis (through the ascending and descending aorta)
Short axis

To facilitate subcostal imaging, the patient is moved into a supine position. The subcostal four-chamber view is much like the apical four-chamber view (Fig. 13-19), but because the ultrasound beam is now more perpendicular to the interventricular and interatrial septa, subcostal imaging is often helpful in the examination of these structures. A 90-degree rotation of the transducer will record a subcostal short-axis view. The transducer can also be angled to image the RV outflow and pulmonary artery as well as the inferior vena cava (Fig. 13-19).

The long-axis suprasternal imaging plane is shown in Fig. 13-20. In adult echocardiography, the LV is usually not visualized satisfactorily from the suprasternal position, but these imaging planes are well suited for examination of the thoracic aorta, pulmonary artery, and great vessels. Normal values for 2D echocardiographic measurements are shown in Table 13-3.

Three-Dimensional Echocardiography

Several approaches exist to obtaining 3D echocardiographic images. The simplest approach is to merely move the transducer through a defined space and align the tomographic slices appropriately. A variety of spatial locator devices can be attached to the transducer to provide spatial orientation. This enables the acquisition of data from many transducer positions. Recently, two orthogonally positioned crystal arrays have been applied in conjunction with rapid parallel signal processing to achieve real-time 3D volumetric imaging. A pyramid-shaped ultrasound beam is produced that can often encompass the entire heart from one transducer location and acquire an entire data set in a single cardiac cycle (Fig. 13-20*C*). The resultant 3D data sets from any approach can be displayed as 2D tomographic cuts with 3D spatial orientation, as wire runs, or with surface rendering. 3D images have been particularly of value in providing accurate quantitation, in assessing congenital heart disease, and in evaluating structures of complex geometry such as the right ventricle.[36a,36b]

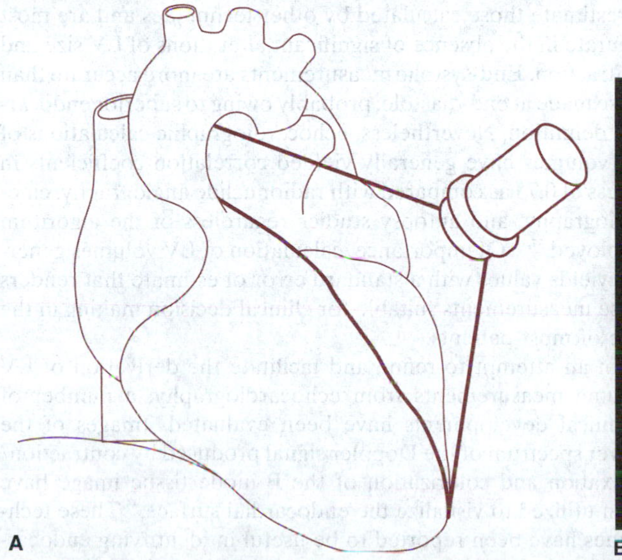

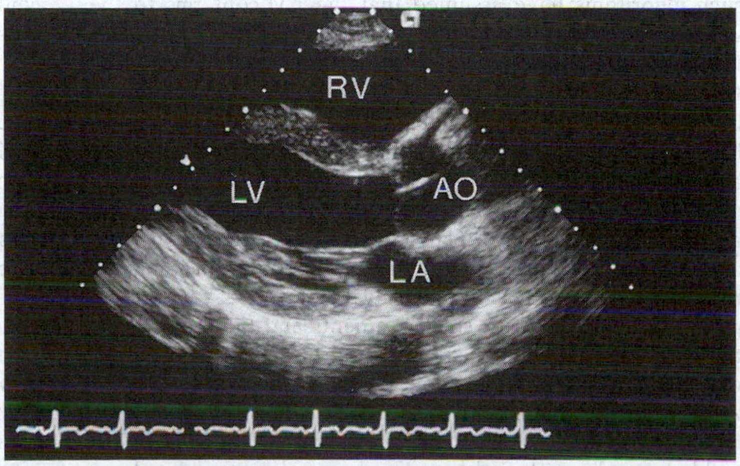

FIGURE 13-14 *A.* Orientation of the sector beam and transducer position for the parasternal long-axis view of the left ventricle. *B.* 2D image of the heart, parasternal long-axis view. LV = left ventricle; LA = left atrium; AO = aorta; RV = right ventricle.

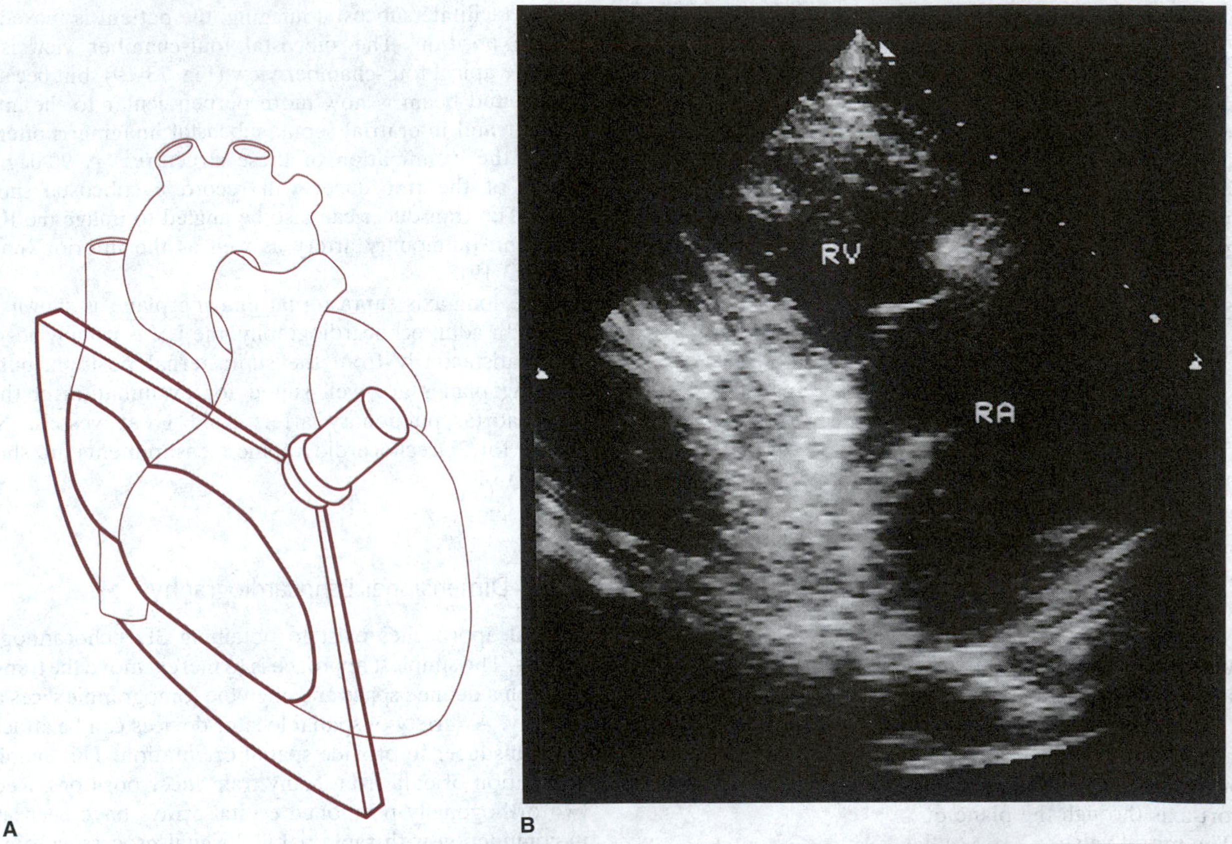

FIGURE 13-15 *A.* Orientation of the sector beam and transducer position for the parasternal RV inflow plane. (From Hagan AD, DeMaria AN. *Clinical Applications of Two-Dimensional Echocardiography and Cardiac Doppler.* Boston: Little, Brown; 1989, with permission.) *B.* Two-dimensional image of right ventricular inflow plane. RA = right atrium, RV = right ventricle.

ASSESSMENT OF SYSTOLIC FUNCTION BY TWO-DIMENSIONAL ECHOCARDIOGRAPHY

Because 2D echocardiography enables visualization of the entire LV perimeter in multiple planes, it is significantly superior to M-mode approaches for the measurement of cardiac chamber volumes and EF.[37–40] Numerous algorithms have been applied to calculate LV volumes by echocardiography (Fig. 13-21). Most such algorithms have assumed that the LV conforms to the shape of a prolate ellipsoid and calculated volume by diameter-length or area-length formulas.[38,41] Multiple studies comparing LV volume calculated by area-length methods to those obtained by other techniques have yielded good correlations, with the best results obtained utilizing biplane apical views.[41,42] Other algorithms have assumed an LV cavity configuration that is a combination of geometric shapes, such as a cylinder-cone or a cylinder-hemiellipse.[41,43] Currently, the most commonly used algorithm to calculate LV volumes is based upon the Simpson rule, which derives measurements by dividing the LV by parallel planes into a number of small segments and then summating the area of the individual disks. This approach has the advantage of making no assumptions about the geometry of the ventricle. A number of modifications of the basic Simpson rule method have been applied to calculate LV volumes. Although all have yielded good results, the optimal correlations have been achieved with a modification that separately quantifies the volume of the apex as an ellipsoid.[40–45]

Regardless of the methodologic approach used, accurate calculations of LV volumes by echocardiography require attention to detail and are critically dependent upon high-quality images to delineate the endocardium and image the entire LV perimeter. As a rule, echocardiographic estimates of LV volumes underestimate those calculated by other techniques and are most accurate in the absence of significant alterations of LV size and contraction. End-systolic measurements are more accurate than those made at end-diastole, probably owing to superior endocardial definition. Nevertheless, echocardiographic calculations of LV volumes have generally yielded correlation coefficients in excess of 0.75 as compared with radionuclide angiography, cineangiography, and autopsy studies regardless of the algorithm employed.[37–45] Of importance, calculation of LV volumes generally yields values with a standard error of estimate that renders these measurements suitable for clinical decision making in the care of most patients.

In an attempt to refine and facilitate the derivation of LV volume measurements from echocardiography, a number of technical developments have been evaluated. Images of the power spectrum of the Doppler signal produced by contraction/relaxation and colorization of the B-mode tissue image have been utilized to visualize the endocardial surface.[46] These techniques have been reported to be useful in identifying endocardial signals, particularly in patients with suboptimal tissue images. Greater enhancement of endocardial border delineation

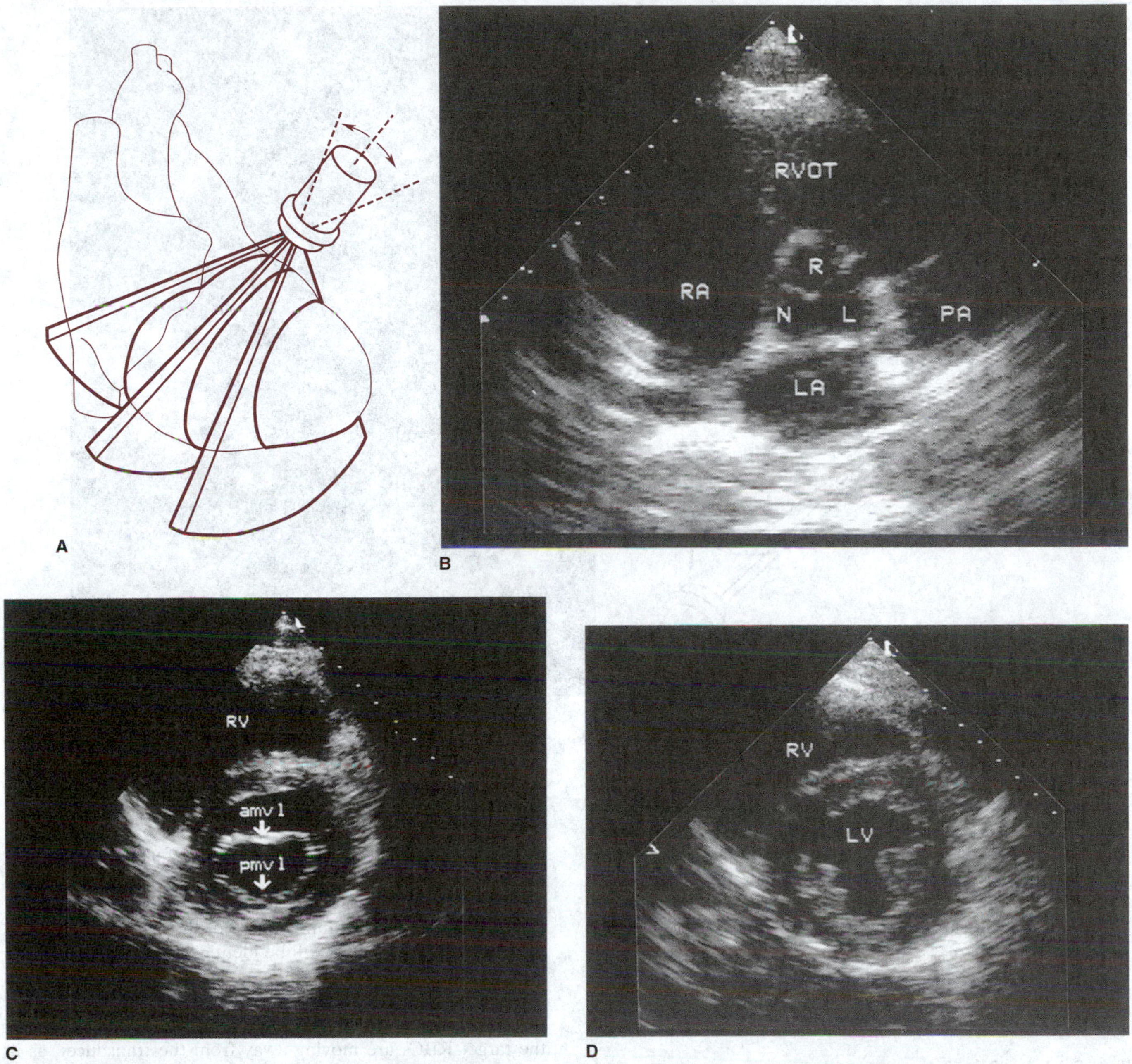

FIGURE 13-16 *A.* Orientation of various short-axis sector beams through the left ventricle obtained by angling the transducer in the parasternal position. (From Hagan AD, DeMaria AN. *Clinical Applications of Two-Dimensional Echocardiography and Cardiac Doppler.* Boston: Little, Brown; 1989, with permission.) *B.* Short-axis plane through the base of the heart. *C.* At the level of the mitral valve leaflets. *D.* At the papillary muscle level. LV = left ventricle; RV = right ventricle; LA = left atrium; RA = right atrium; RVOT = right ventricular outflow tract; PA = pulmonary artery; R, L, N = right, left, and noncoronary cusps of the aortic valve. RV = right ventricle; LV = left ventricle; amvl = anterior mitral valve leaflet; pmvl = posterior mitral valve leaflet.

and improvement of the reliability of measures of LV size and contraction has been achieved through utilization of tissue harmonic imaging and by the injection of ultrasonic contrast agents to produce LV cavity opacification.[18a,46a] A software package that provides instantaneous and automated endocardial border delineation throughout the cardiac cycle has been developed based upon the display of tissue signals as backscatter rather than specular reflection.[47] This technique of automated quantitation can yield continuous measurements of LV volume throughout the cardiac cycle and can derive values for ejection fraction, ejection rate, and rate of filling during diastole (Fig. 13-22). This same technology has been utilized to display endocardial excursion throughout systolic contraction or diastolic expansion in a color format superimposed upon the tissue image (Fig. 13-23, Plate 53). This technique has proved to be of value in the recognition of abnormalities of LV contraction and regional disturbances of LV diastolic function.[48,49,49a] Finally, studies employing 3D echocardiography have reported improved repro-

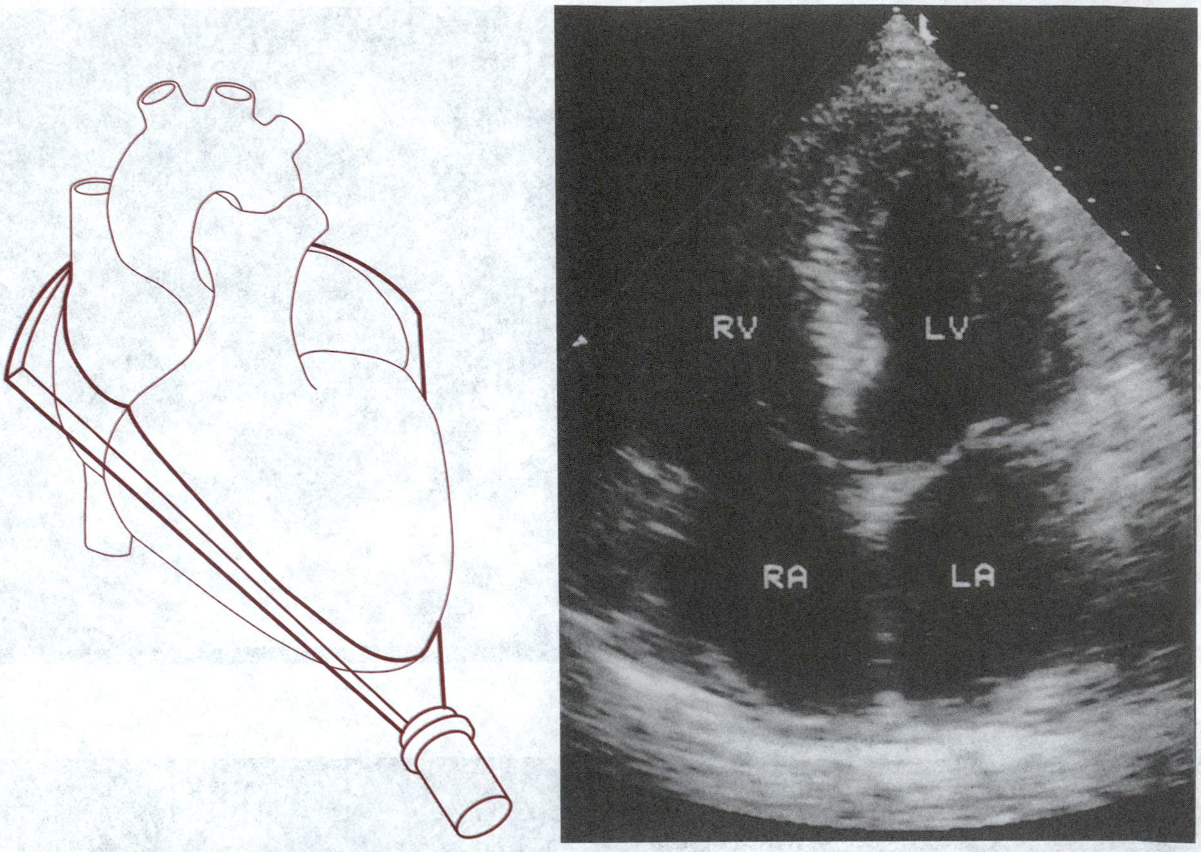

A B

FIGURE 13-17 *A.* Orientation of the sector beam and transducer position for the apical four-chamber plane. (From Hagan AD, DeMaria AN. *Clinical Applications of Two-Dimensional Echocardiography and Cardiac Doppler.* Boston: Little, Brown; 1989, with permission.) *B.* 2D image of the apical four-chamber plane. RA = right atrium; RV = right ventricle; LV = left ventricle; LA = left atrium.

ducibility of measures over 2D methods. Although these technical developments are relatively untested, they promise to facilitate the quantitative assessment of LV size and function from routine echocardiograms.

DOPPLER ECHOCARDIOGRAPHY: PRINCIPLES AND APPLICATIONS

The Doppler Principle

Although 2D and M-mode echocardiography provide abundant information about cardiac structure and movement, they supply no direct data concerning blood flow. This is a significant limitation, as the presence and severity of conditions such as valvular regurgitation and intracardiac shunting can be suspected or inferred only indirectly by 2D imaging. Using the principle first delineated by the physicist Johann Christian Doppler,[50] one can use ultrasound to determine the velocity and direction of blood flow by measuring the change in frequency produced when sound waves are reflected from red blood cells.[51–53] In this way, information regarding the presence, direction, velocity, and turbulence of blood flow can be acquired by cardiac ultrasound.[54]

The Doppler principle states that when a sound (or light) signal strikes a moving object, the frequency of that signal will be altered, and the increase or decrease in frequency will be proportional to the velocity and direction at which the object is moving. This is illustrated in Fig. 13-24. If a stationary transducer at the apex emits a sound wave with a transmitted frequency of *fo* and the wave is reflected by nonmoving red blood cells (RBCs) in an isovolumic phase of the cardiac cycle, then the received frequency *fr* will be identical to *fo*. If the signal is reflected by RBCs that are moving toward the transducer, as through the mitral valve in diastole, the returning waves will be compressed so that *fr* will be greater than *fo*. Conversely, if the target RBCs are moving away from the transducer, as in the outflow tract in systole, the returning sound waves will be elongated and the received frequency will be decreased. Of importance, the magnitude of change in the received frequency is directly related to the velocity at which blood is flowing toward or away from the transducer.[53] If the velocity of sound and the angle θ between the direction of RBC flow and the beam path are known, then the velocity of the RBCs is described by the Doppler equation:

$$V = fd(c)/2fo(\cos\theta)$$

where *fd* is the frequency shift recorded, *fo* the transmitted frequency, and *c* the velocity of sound. Note that the denominator is doubled because the sound wave does not originate with the RBC but must travel back and forth from the transducer. By measuring Doppler shift frequencies, the velocity and direction of blood flow can be calculated, displayed, and recorded.

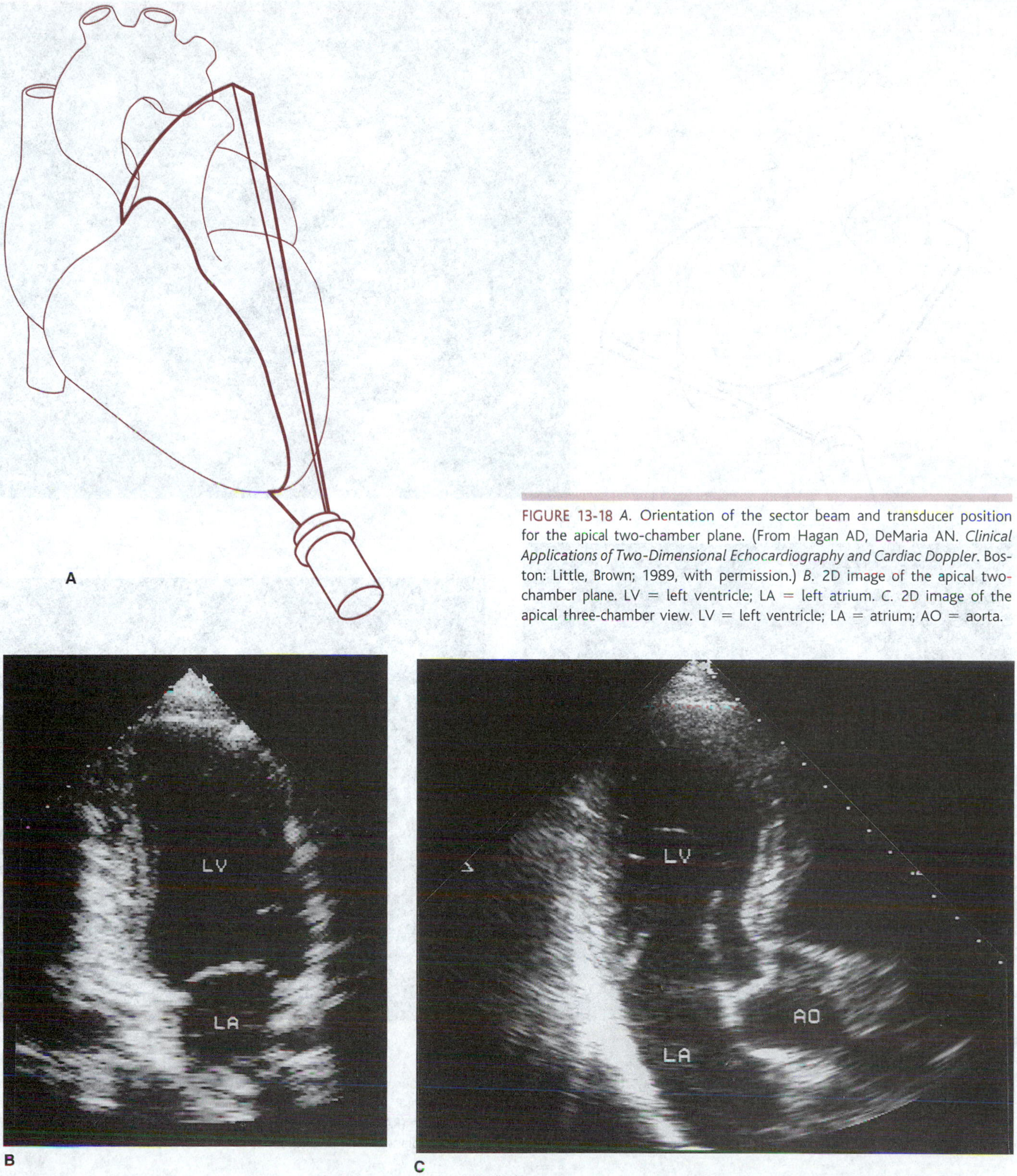

FIGURE 13-18 *A.* Orientation of the sector beam and transducer position for the apical two-chamber plane. (From Hagan AD, DeMaria AN. *Clinical Applications of Two-Dimensional Echocardiography and Cardiac Doppler*. Boston: Little, Brown; 1989, with permission.) *B.* 2D image of the apical two-chamber plane. LV = left ventricle; LA = left atrium. *C.* 2D image of the apical three-chamber view. LV = left ventricle; LA = atrium; AO = aorta.

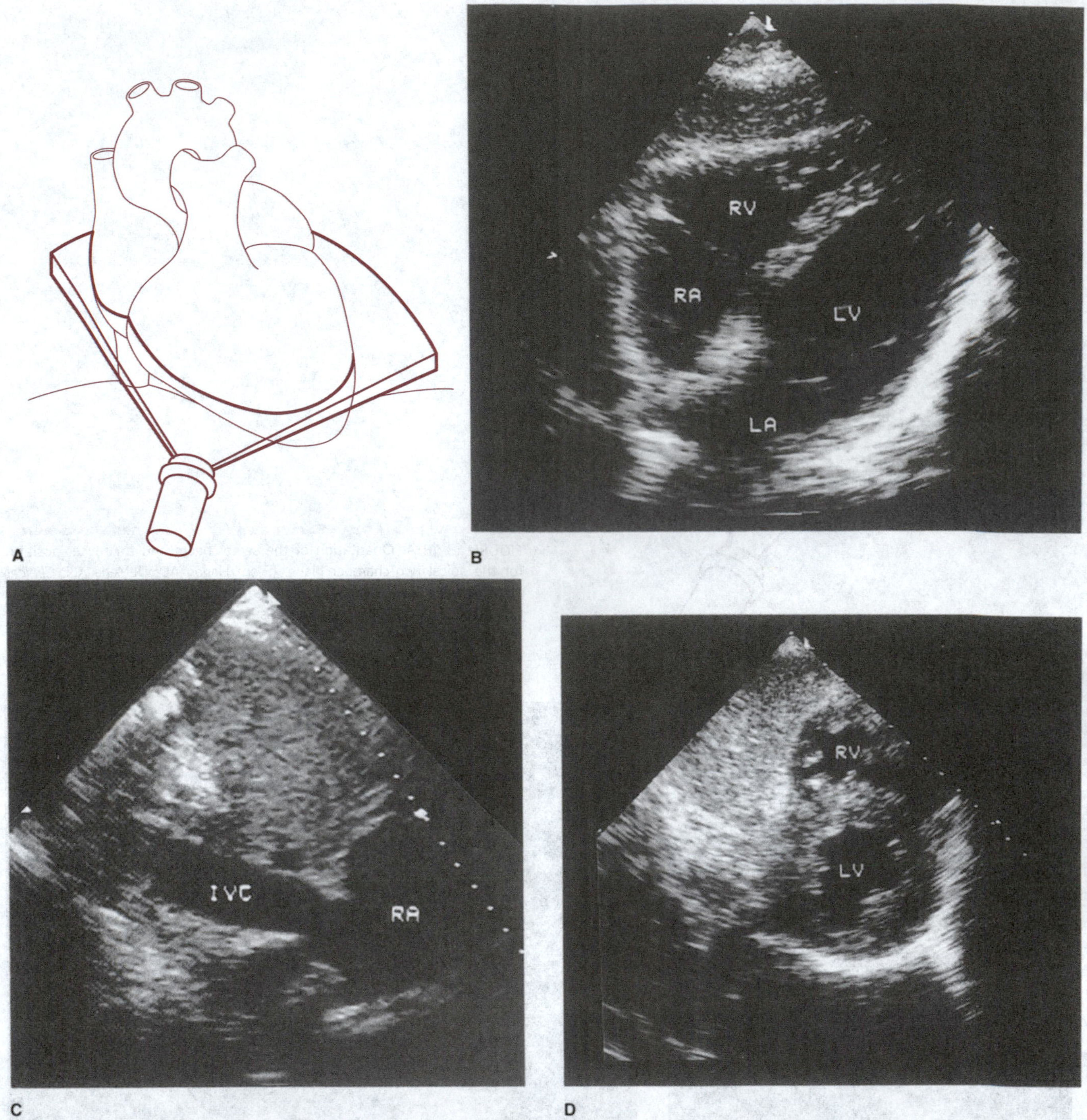

FIGURE 13-19 *A.* Orientation of the sector beam and transducer position for the subcostal four-chamber plane. (From Hagen AD, DeMaria AN. *Clinical Applications of Two Dimensional Echocardiography and Cardiac Doppler.* Boston: Little, Brown; 1989, with permission.) *B.* Two-dimensional image of the subcostal four-chamber plane. LV = left ventricle; LA = left atrium; RA = right atrium; RV = right ventricle. *C.* Subcostal 2D image demonstrating the right atrium (RA) and inferior vena cava (IVC). *D.* 2D image of the subcostal short-axis plane. LV = left ventricle; RV = right ventricle.

The angle between the direction of blood flow and the course of the sound beam is a most important factor in Doppler ultrasound (Fig. 13-25). Velocity is a vectorial entity, having magnitude and direction, and Doppler will detect only those velocities parallel or near parallel to the interrogating signal. Since the relationship between velocity and the angle is a cosine function and the cosine of angles up to 20 degrees is 0.9, little error is introduced within this range.[53] Because the processor that calculates blood velocity assumes that the angle is 0 degrees, however, considerable errors occur when it is greater than 20 degrees. Moreover, the angle of incidence in 3D space usually cannot be determined with certainty from 2D echocardiographic

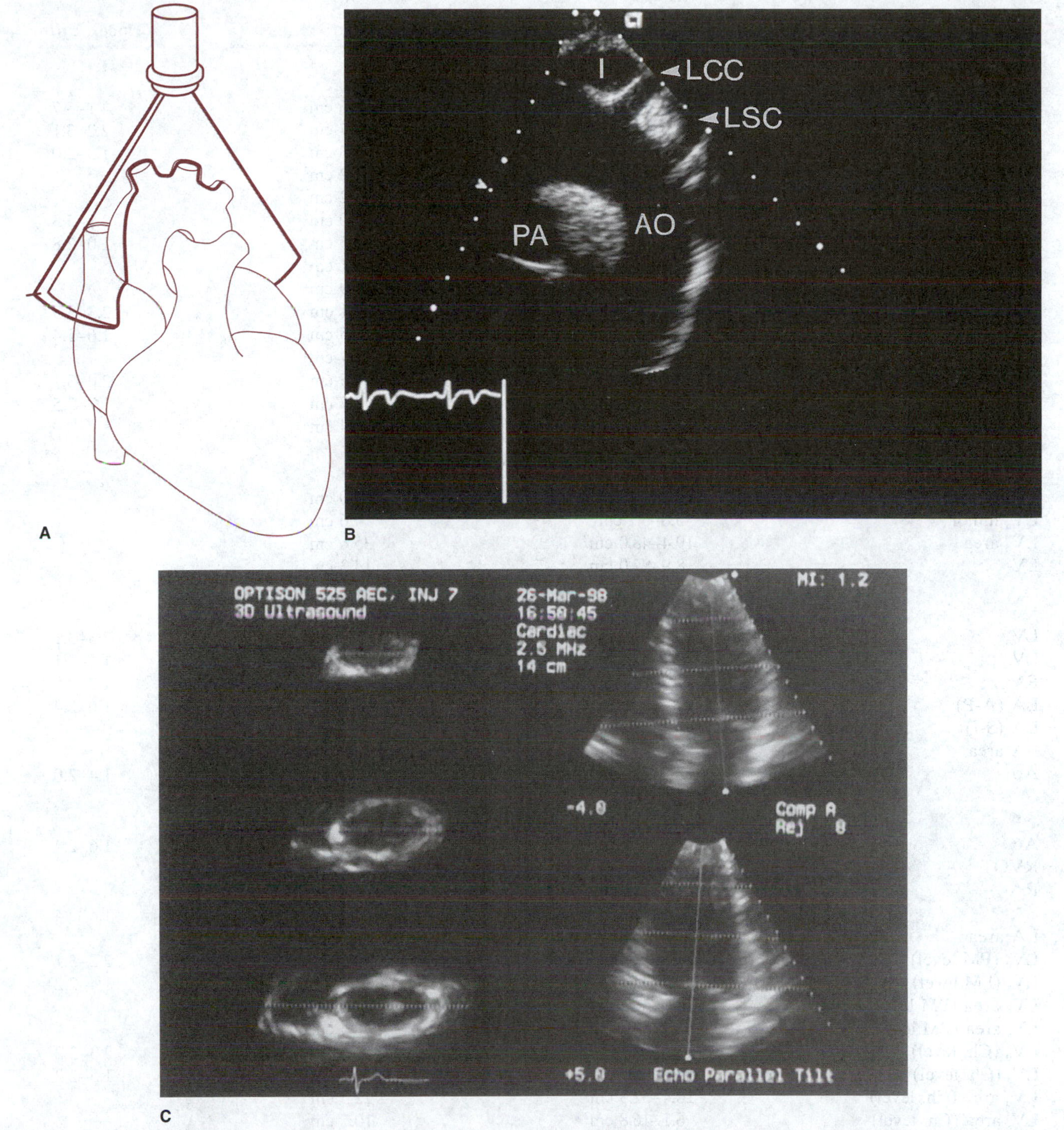

FIGURE 13-20 *A.* Orientation of the sector beam and transducer position for long axis plane through the aorta from the suprasternal position. *B.* 2D image of the suprasternal long axis view of the thoracic aorta. AO = aorta; PA = right pulmonary artery; I = innominate artery; LCC = left common carotid artery; LSC = left subclavian artery. *C.* Short-axis, apical four-chamber, and apical two-chamber images acquired simultaneously with a pyramidal 3D transducer system.

TABLE 13-3 Cardiac Dimensions by Two-Dimensional Echocardiography

Cardiac Feature	Range	Mean	Index, cm/m^2
Apical Four-Chamber View			
LV_d major	6.9–10.3 cm	8.6 cm	4.1–5.7
LV_d minor	3.3–6.1 cm	4.7 cm	2.2–3.1
LV_s minor	1.9–3.7 cm	2.8 cm	1.3–2.0
LV_d area	21.2–40.2 cm^2	31.2 cm^2	
LV_s area	8.0–21.1 cm^2	14.2 cm^2	
RV major	6.5–9.5 cm^2	8.0 cm	3.8–5.3
RV minor	2.2–4.4 cm^2	3.3–3.5 cm	1.0–2.8
RV_d area	12.0–22.2 cm^2	18.6–2.1 cm^2	
RV_s area	5.4–14.6 cm^2	9.9 cm^2	
LA major	4.1–6.1 cm	5.1 cm	2.3–3.5
LA minor	2.8–4.3 cm	3.5 cm	1.6–2.4
LA area	10.2–17.8 cm^2	14.7 cm^2	
RA major (inf-sup)	3.5–5.5 cm	4.3–4.5 cm	2.0–3.1
RA minor	2.5–4.9 cm	3.7 cm	1.7–2.5
RA area	11.3–16.7 cm^2	13.8–14 cm^2	
Apical Two-Chamber View			
LV_d major	6.8–9.4 cm	8.0 cm	
LV_d minor	3.8–5.7 cm	4.6 cm	
LV_d area	19.4–48.0 cm^2	35.6 cm^2	
LV_s	8.9–27.0 cm	14.3 cm	
Parasternal Long-Axis View			
LV_d	3.5–6.0 cm	4.8 cm	2.3–3.1
LV_s	2.1–4.0 cm	3.1 cm	1.4–2.1
RV	1.9–3.8 cm	2.8 cm	1.2–2.0
LA (A-P)	2.7–4.5 cm	3.6 cm	1.6–2.4
LA (S-I)	3.1–5.5 cm	4.4 cm	
LA area	9.0–19.3 cm^2	13.8 cm^2	
Ao	2.2–3.6 cm	2.9 cm	1.4–2.0
Parasternal Short-Axis View			
Ao	2.3–3.7 cm	3.0–2.3 cm	1.6–2.4
RVOT	1.9–2.2 cm	2.7 cm	
RA	1.5–2.5 cm	1.9–2.2 cm	
LA	2.6–4.5 cm	3.6 cm	1.6–2.4
LA area	7.2–13.0 cm^2	10.8 cm^2	
LV_d (PM level)	3.5–5.8 cm	4.7 cm	2.2–3.1
LV_s (PM level)	2.2–4.0 cm	3.1 cm	1.4–2.2
LV_d area (PM level)	16.0–31.2 cm^2	22.2 cm^2	
LV_s area (PM level)	5.2–13.4 cm^2	8.5 cm^2	
LV_d (Ch. level)	3.5–6.2	4.8 cm	2.3–3.2
LV_s (Ch. level)	2.3–4.0	3.2 cm	1.5–2.2
LV_d area (Ch. level)	16.4–32.3 cm^2	22.5 cm^2	
LV_s area (Ch. level)	6.1–16.8 cm^2	10.7 cm^2	
Subcostal View			
IVC diameter		1.8 cm	

Abbreviations: LV = left ventricle; LV_d = left ventricle, end diastole; LV_s = left ventricle, end systole; RV = right ventricle; RV_d = right ventricle, end diastole; RV_s = right ventricle, end systole; LA = left atrium; RA = right atrium; Ao = aorta; RVOT = right ventricular outflow tract; PA = pulmonary artery; IVC = inferior vena cava; PM = papillary muscle; Ch = chordal.

Source: The values shown in this table represent a compilation of data from three sources: Schnittinger I, Gordon EP, Fitzgerald PJ, et al. Standardized intracardiac measurements of two-dimensional echocardiography. *J Am Coll Cardiol* 1983; 5:934. Triulzi M, Weyman A. Normal cross-sectional measurements in adults. In: Weyman A, ed. *Echocardiography.* Philadelphia: Lea & Febiger; 1982;497. Hagan AD, DiSessa TG, Bloor CM, et al. *Two-Dimensional Echocardiography: Clinical-Pathological Correlations in adult and Congenital Heart Disease.* Boston: Little, Brown; 1983;553.

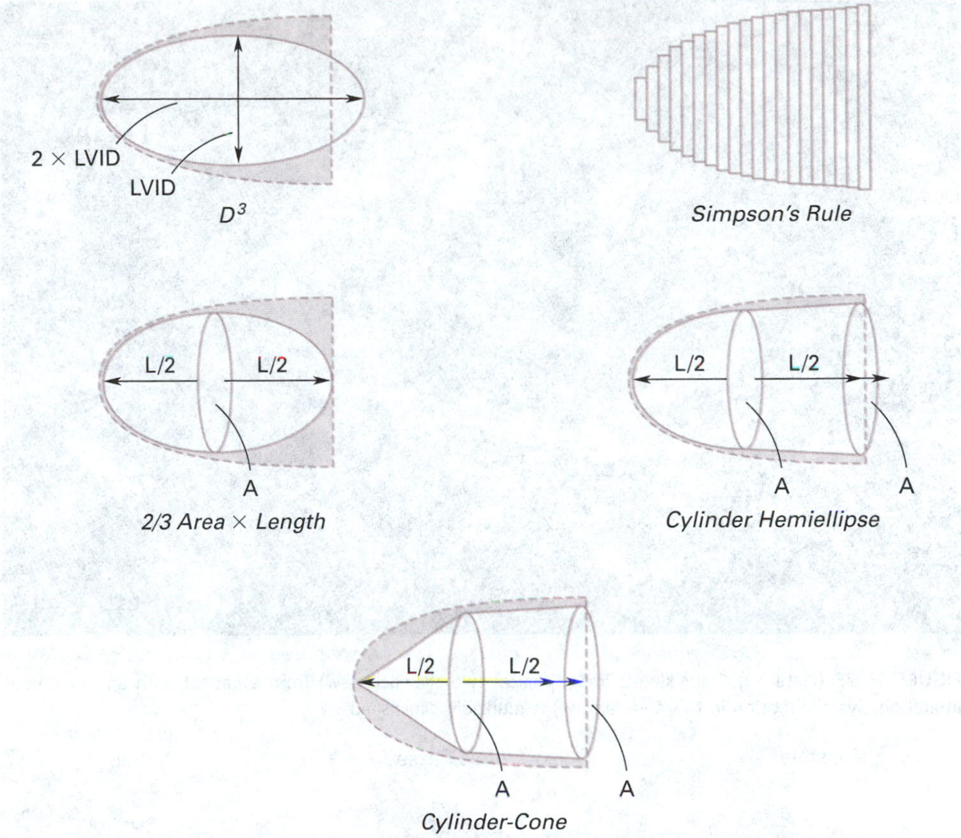

FIGURE 13-21 Various models used to estimate left ventricular volume. *A.* "D-cubed." *B.* Two-thirds area × length. *C.* Simpson's rule. *D.* Cylinder-hemiellipse. *E.* Cylinder-cone. A = cross-sectional area; LVID = left ventricular internal dimension (minor axis); L = length of LV major axis.

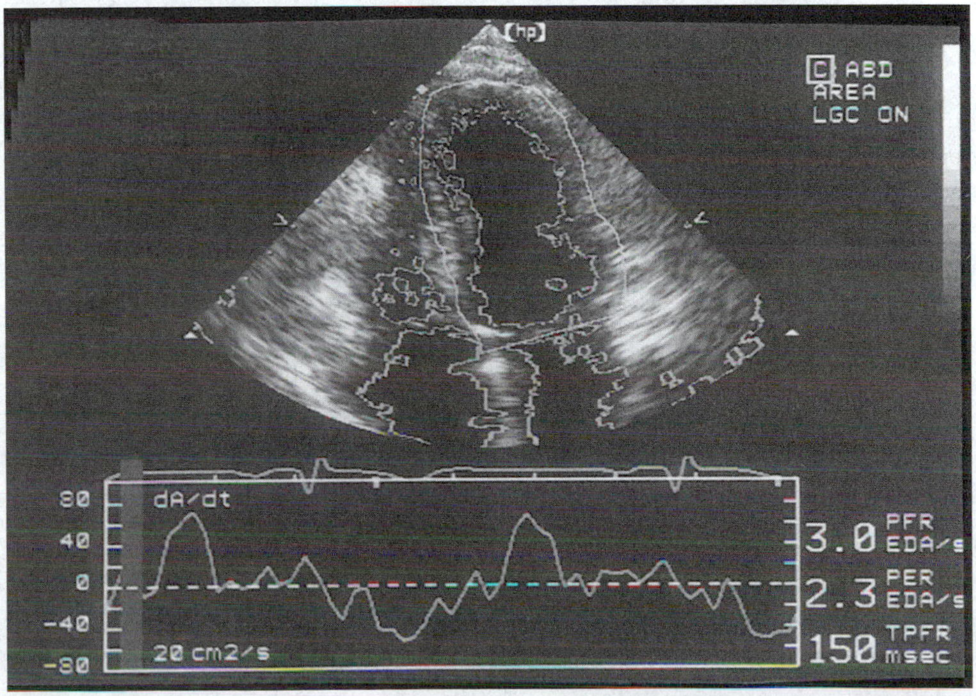

FIGURE 13-22 Example of endocardial border detection and on-line calculation of change in area over time (*dA/dt*).

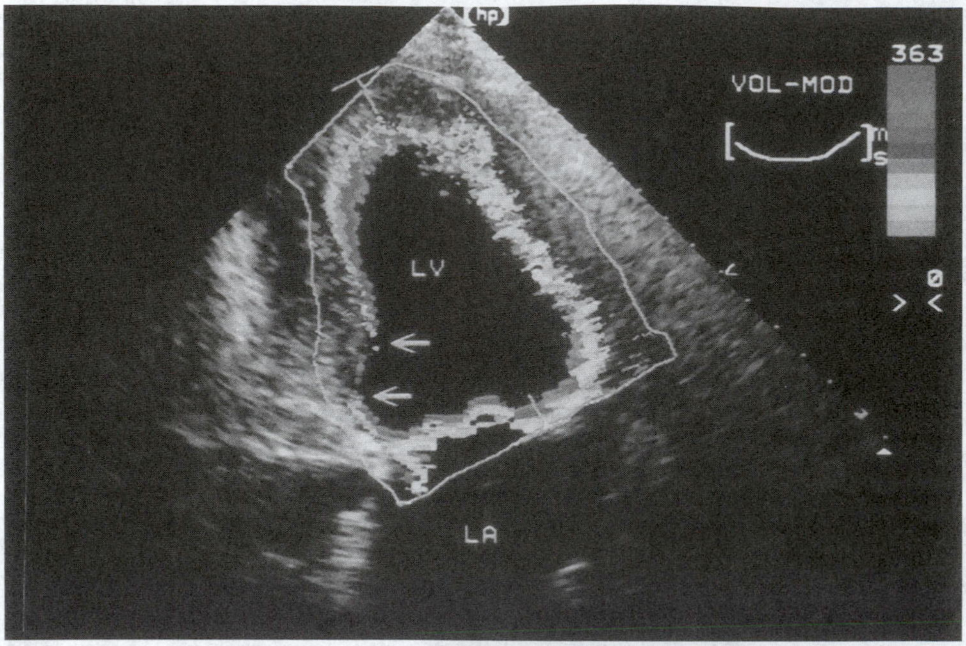

FIGURE 13-23 (Plate 53) Color kinesis image (apical two-chamber view) from a patient with an inferobasal infarction. Systolic motion in this area (*arrows*) is markedly diminished.

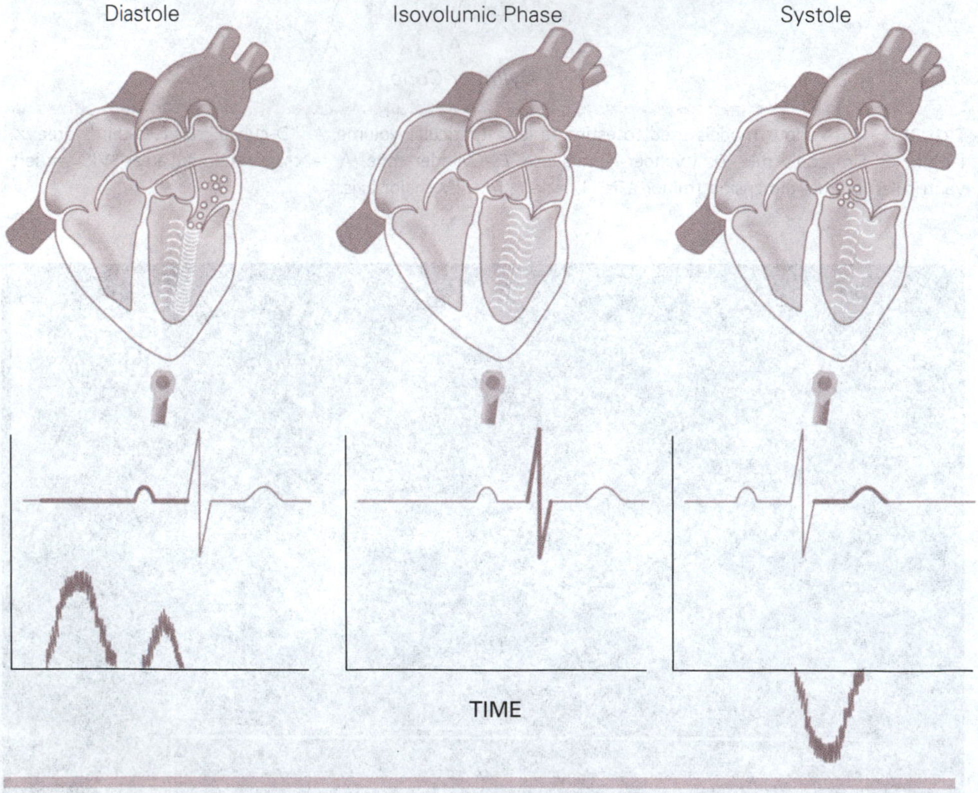

FIGURE 13-24 Basic principle of the Doppler shift. During diastole (*left panel*), an ultrasound beam directed toward the junction of the mitral and aortic annuli is reflected by red blood cells moving toward the transducer. The frequency of the received ultrasound is greater than that of the transmitted beam, and the spectral tracing is recorded above the baseline (i.e., flow is toward the transducer). During the isovolumic phase (*middle panel*), both the mitral and aortic valves are closed and little flow occurs within the left ventricle. Therefore, there are no significant changes in the transmitted and received frequencies of the Doppler beam and no spectral tracing is recorded. During systole (*right panel*), the transmitted beam is reflected by red blood cells moving away from the transducer. Therefore, the frequency of the received ultrasound is lower than that of the transmitted beam, and the spectral tracing is recorded below the baseline.

images. Therefore, in order to obtain accurate velocity determination by Doppler, it is crucial to position and direct the transducer so that the beam is as parallel to flow as possible.

In clinical use, the frequency of transmitted ultrasound is in the range of 2 to 7 MHz, the velocity of sound in tissue is approximately 1540 m/s, and the Doppler shift frequency is relatively small (approximately 1 to 4 kHz) as compared with the transmitted frequency. As the Doppler shift frequencies are in the audible range, a speaker integrated into the Doppler echocardiography system can present them as an audible signal. Normal signals are tonal or musical. The Doppler shift also can be presented graphically to provide a hard copy printout and enable measurement.

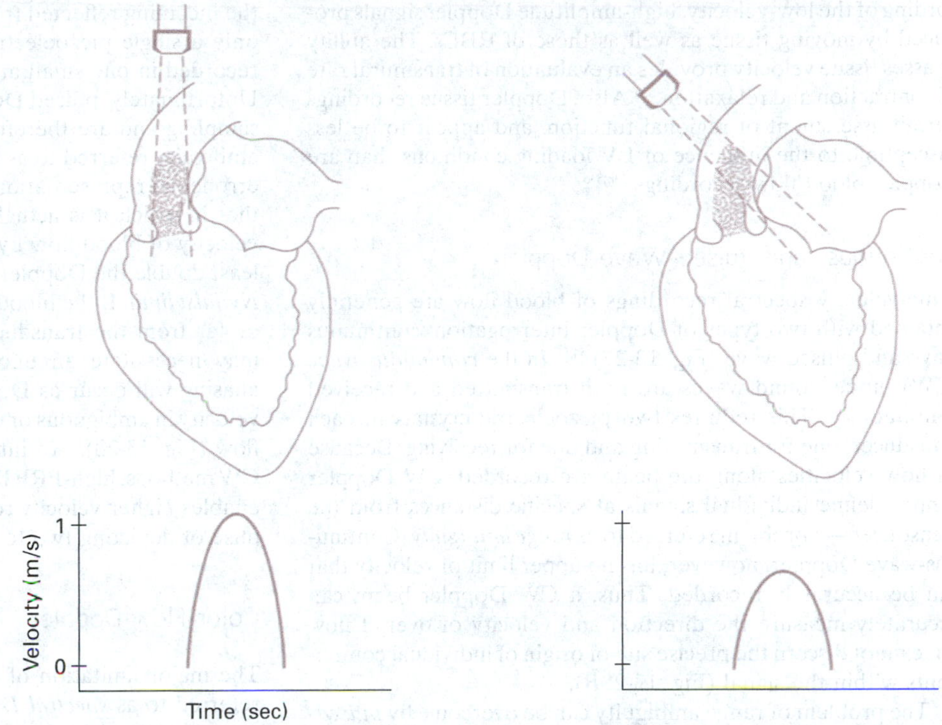

FIGURE 13-25 Effect of the angle of incidence on the velocity recorded with Doppler analysis. The true velocity is underestimated when the ultrasound beam is not parallel to the direction of blood flow. (From Hagan AD, DeMaria AN. *Clinical Applications of Two-Dimensional Echocardiography and Cardiac Doppler*. Boston: Little, Brown; 1989, with permission.)

Figure 13-26 shows the typical graphic pulsed Doppler pattern of normal systolic blood flow through the RV outflow tract into the pulmonary artery, with flow velocity on the *y* axis and time on the *x* axis. The location and size of the area from which Doppler recordings are derived is determined by the operator by positioning a sample volume on the echo image. The absence of flow is represented by the zero or no-flow line, termed the *baseline*. By convention, flow toward the transducer is displayed above the baseline and flow away from the transducer is displayed below the baseline. The velocities above and below baseline represent flow toward or away from the transducer and not forward or backward in the circulation. Because of the effects of viscous friction, the sample volume almost invariably includes RBCs flowing at slightly different velocities. Even normal laminar blood flow in the great vessels varies in velocity across the lumen, as RBCs in the center of the vessel move at higher velocity than those exposed to viscous friction at the wall, and this creates a parabolic rather than a flat flow profile. Therefore, any returning Doppler shifted signal contains a spectrum of velocities, each of which can be displayed by means of fast Fourier transform analysis. The graphic output of the Doppler signal displays the range of velocities within the sample volume site at any time in gray scale and the number of RBCs moving at any velocity as relative intensity. Normal laminar flow is characterized by a uniformity of velocity and direction of individual RBCs, and therefore a narrowly dispersed signal, while disturbed or turbulent flow is manifest by marked variability in velocity and direction and therefore a broad signal, which is multitoned, dissonant, and harsh.

Recently, echographs have been modified to enable re-

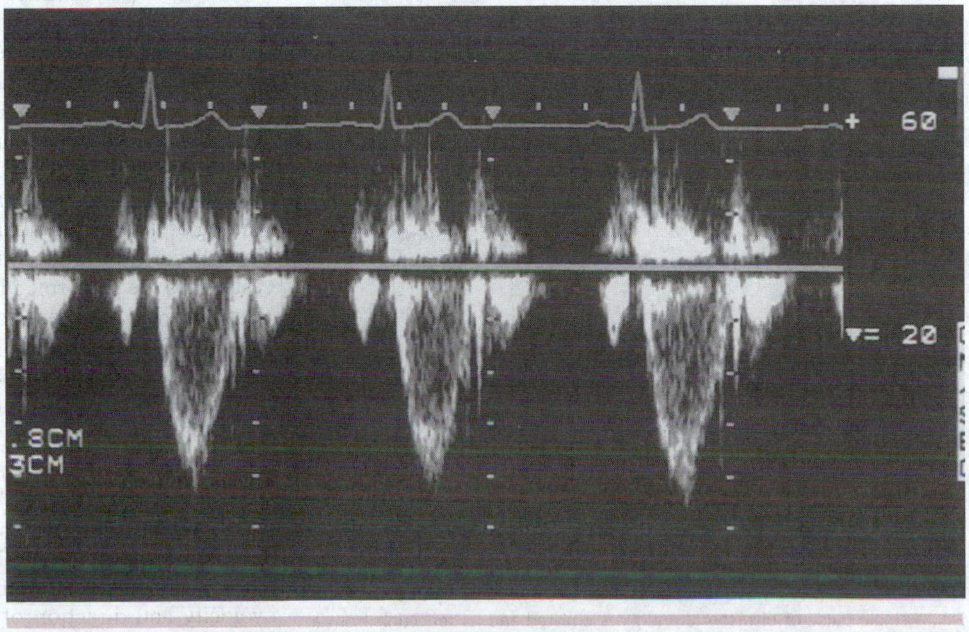

FIGURE 13-26 Doppler spectral envelope of normal blood flow through the RV outflow tract during systole. The transducer is in the parasternal position and the sample volume is placed just proximal to the pulmonic valve.

cording of the low-velocity, high-amplitude Doppler signals produced by moving tissue as well as those of RBCs. The ability to asses tissue velocity provides an evaluation of transmural rate of contraction and relaxation.[53a] Also, Doppler tissue recordings permit assessment of regional function, and appear to be less susceptible to the influence of LV loading conditions than are Doppler blood flow recordings.[53b,53c]

Continuous- and Pulsed-Wave Doppler

Time-velocity spectral recordings of blood flow are generally obtained with two types of Doppler interrogation: continuous wave and pulsed wave (Fig. 13-27).[54,55] In the *continuous-wave* (CW) mode, sound waves are both transmitted and received continuously. This requires two piezoelectric crystals in each transducer, one for transmitting and one for receiving. Because all flow velocities along the beam are recorded, CW Doppler cannot define individual signals at specific distances from the transducer—a problem referred to as *range ambiguity*. Continuous-wave Doppler, however, has no upper limit of velocity that can be accurately recorded. Thus, a CW Doppler beam can accurately measure the direction and velocity of overall flow but cannot discern the precise site of origin of individual components within the signal (Fig. 13-28*B*).

The problem of range ambiguity can be overcome by *pulsed-wave* Doppler. In this mode, short bursts of signal are transmitted from the transducer at a given *pulse-repetition frequency* (PRF). The instrument then receives the signal for only a brief period—an interval that corresponds to the time required for sound energy to travel and return from a specific site along the beam path. In practice, the operator selects the location at which flow is to be examined by positioning a sample volume, and the instrument determines the period during which to receive

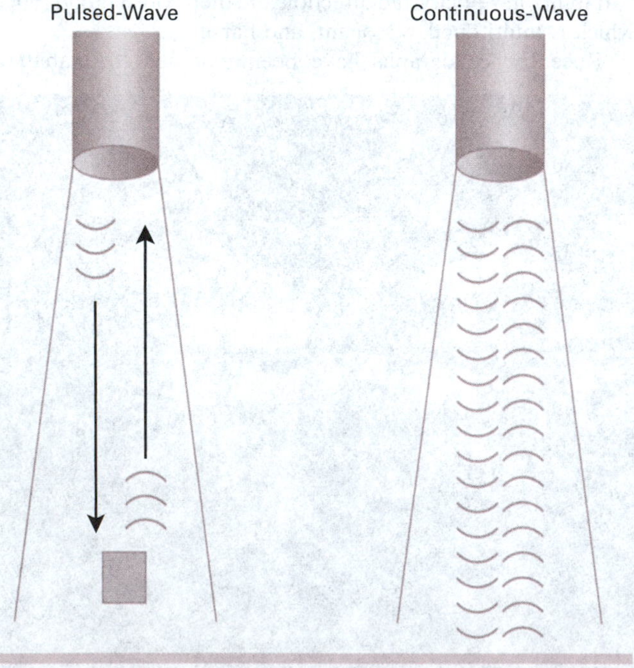

FIGURE 13-27 Pulsed-wave (PW) and continuous-wave (CW) Doppler. With PW, a single pulse of ultrasound energy is emitted and its reflection from a sample volume is received before the following pulse is transmitted. With CW, there is continuous transmission and reception of ultrasound energy.

the incoming reflected frequencies. With pulsed-wave Doppler, only a single piezoelectric crystal is needed and flow can be recorded in one small area within the heart or vasculature.[54,55] Unfortunately, pulsed Doppler techniques employ intermittent sampling and are therefore susceptible to a problem of range ambiguity referred to as *aliasing*.[56] By definition, aliasing is the erroneous representation of flow in the direction opposite to that in which it is actually occurring. To correctly record the velocity of blood flow by pulsed Doppler, the PRF must be at least double the Doppler shift frequency, a value known as the *Nyquist limit.* If the blood flow examined is of very high velocity or far from the transducer (requiring a long transit time), it may necessitate an unobtainably high PRF. In such cases, aliasing will occur as Doppler signals that depict flow at high velocity in ambiguous or opposite directions compared to actual flow (Fig. 13-28). An intermediate mode between pulsed and CW methods, high-PRF Doppler, is also available.[57,58] This mode enables higher-velocity recordings to be obtained at a compromise of depicting two to four sample sites simultaneously.

Color-Flow Doppler

The major limitation of pulsed and CW Doppler (sometimes referred to as *spectral Doppler*) is that no spatial information regarding the size, shape, and 2D direction of flow is provided. An extension of pulsed-wave Doppler techniques, *color-flow Doppler* (CFD), provides real-time M-mode or 2D imaging of blood flow by presenting the velocity and direction of RBC movement as shades of color superimposed upon gray-level 2D tissue structure. Standard pulsed Doppler yields flow signals from a single site along a single scan line. In CFD, rapid pulsed-wave interrogations are performed at multiple sites for multiple scan lines to create a spatially correct and dynamic display of moving blood within the heart and vasculature[59–61] (Fig. 13-29). Doppler signals are presented as colors assigned to individual sites (Fig. 13-30, Plate 54). Blood flow moving toward the transducer is displayed in red, flow away from the transducer is displayed in blue, and increasing velocity is depicted in brighter shades of each color. The variance within each signal is calculated as a statistical marker of turbulence and is presented by adding green to the image (Fig. 13-31, Plate 55). Therefore, turbulent flow jets appear as a mosaic mix of colors. CFD also can be superimposed onto M-mode tracings (Fig. 13-32, Plate 56), often termed *M/Q imaging,* and is helpful in clarifying the timing of flow phenomena. Given the time constraints imposed by collecting the large volume of data required by CFD, velocity estimates are performed by autocorrelation techniques that are less accurate than fast Fourier transform analysis.[62] Nevertheless, CFD technology is a major advance that has improved the rapid detection of cardiac pathology, especially valvular regurgitation and intracardiac shunts.

Normal and Abnormal Flow Dynamics

The clinical application of Doppler recordings is based on the fundamental differences between normal and disturbed blood flow. Normal flow is laminar, with all RBCs exhibiting the same velocity and direction of flow. Although some abnormalities, such as atrial septal defects, involve laminar flow, most pathologic conditions involve disturbed or turbulent flow and share a common hydrodynamic basis for the resultant flow dynamics. Specifically, nearly all circulatory disturbances (stenosis, regurgitation, shunt) involve blood flow from a high-pressure chamber to a lower-pressure chamber through a restricted orifice.[53] Aortic valve disease is a perfect example. Aortic stenosis is a forward flow disturbance in which turbulent blood travels from a high-pressure LV to a lower-pressure aorta through a restricted aortic orifice in systole. Aortic regurgitation is a retrograde flow disturbance in which turbulent blood regurgitates from a high-pressure aorta to a lower-pressure left ventricle through a small regurgitant orifice in diastole. In each case, the pressure gradient results in a high-velocity jet coursing through a restricted orifice, reaching its maximal velocity at a site just distal to the orifice, designated the *vena contracta,* at which time shear forces produce vortices resulting in flow of varying direction and velocity (Fig. 13-33). In each case, the velocity of the jet is related to the pressure gradient across the orifice. Thus, the hallmark of disturbed flow is a very high velocity jet with adjacent vortices of varying direction and velocity of flow. On pulsed Doppler recordings, these hemodynamic abnormalities cause broadening of the spectral signal and aliasing. On CW recordings, high velocity represents the primary abnormality. By color-flow imaging, the disturbance is manifest by the increased variance and higher velocities in the signal. With any of these techniques, of course, inappropriate timing of flow serves to highlight the abnormality (e.g., high-velocity LA flow during systole in mitral regurgitation).

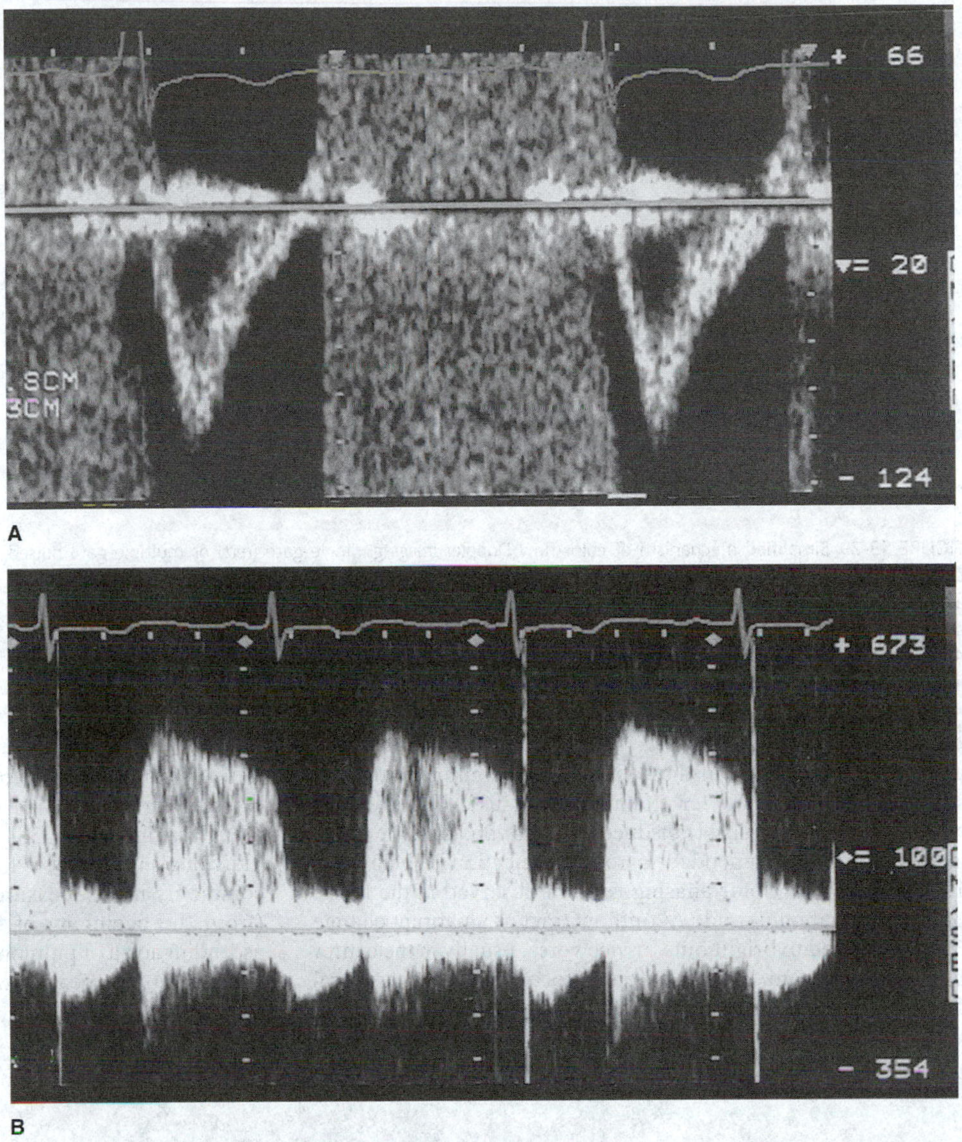

FIGURE 13-28 *A.* Pulsed-wave Doppler tracing from a patient with aortic regurgitation. The transducer is in the apical position and the sample volume is in the left ventricular outflow tract. A laminar envelope is seen during systole, while aliased flow is present during diastole because of high-velocity flow. *B.* Continuous-wave Doppler tracing through the left ventricular outflow tract (with transducer in the apical position). The maximal velocity of the aortic regurgitation is now measurable, but all other velocities along the Doppler beam are recorded as well.

The Standard Doppler Examination

A clinical Doppler examination must be performed with full consideration of the three different Doppler modalities available, the types of information each can provide, the multiple sites for flow interrogation, and the spectrum of pathologic lesions that produces flow disturbances. In light of these considerations, it is understandable that the Doppler examination may not be as standardized as the format for 2D cardiac imaging; however, a number of usual practices have emerged. A vast majority of echocardiographic examinations include screening for flow disturbances by CFD. Since Doppler signals are best recorded with the ultrasound beam parallel to flow, screening is typically performed in long-axis or apical views. Any flow disturbances visualized are subsequently examined by CW spectral recordings and, in most laboratories, by pulsed-wave Doppler. Although CW examination is typically reserved for flow disturbances, pulsed-wave Doppler also may be of value in quantifying flow dynamics in the setting of laminar flow. In this regard, pulsed Doppler recordings obtained at the mitral, tricuspid, and aortic valve orifices, pulmonary artery, and pulmonary veins constitute part of a standard echocardiogram in many laboratories (Figs. 13-26 and 13-34 to 13-37).

The normal Doppler examination is characterized by uniformity of flow velocity and the absence of high-velocity turbulent flow. CFD recordings demonstrate laminar flow through the

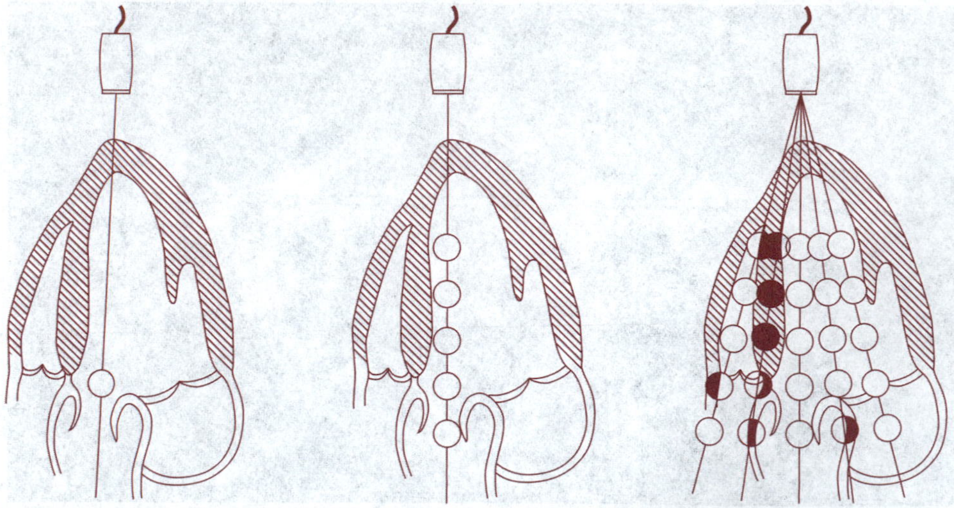

FIGURE 13-29 Simplified mechanism of color-flow Doppler imaging. Single-gate (*left*) or multiple-gate pulsed Doppler (*center*) can evaluate flow at points along a single ultrasound beam path. Color-flow imaging (*right*) assesses the velocity and direction of flow for multiple sample volumes along multiple beam paths and assigns a color indicative of velocity and direction at each sample volume site. (From Hagan AD, DeMaria AN. *Clinical Applications of Two-Dimensional Echocardiography and Cardiac Doppler.* Boston: Little, Brown; 1989, with permission.)

atrioventricular valves in diastole and the semilunar valves in systole. Since the Doppler examination is usually performed with a long-axis or apical transducer orientation, diastolic filling is characteristically encoded in red and ejection in blue (Fig. 13-30, Plate 54). Color aliasing is often observed at the levels of the mitral annulus and LV outflow tract as an abrupt change from bright red to bright blue or vice versa, usually in the center of the flow stream. Pulsed Doppler recordings of transmitral flow velocities are often recorded at the level of both the leaflet tips and annulus. Velocities are higher at the tips, while recordings at the annulus offer the ability to calculate flow through a cross-sectional area that is relatively uniform throughout the cardiac cycle. A sample volume positioned in the right upper pulmonary vein reveals systolic and diastolic emptying flow of nearly equal magnitude followed by a short, low-velocity reversal of flow into the pulmonary veins following atrial contraction (Fig. 13-36). Flow in the LV outflow tract and aortic annulus area is characterized by a progressive increase of velocity peaking in early systole, followed by a more gradual deceleration of flow (Fig. 13-35). Minimal if any flow velocities are detected in the mitral valve orifice and LV outflow tract in systole and diastole, respectively, in normal examinations. Examinations of the tricuspid and pulmonic valves give qualitatively similar results to those of the mitral and aortic valves (Figs. 13-26 and 13-37). Normal values for forward flow velocity are given in Table 13-4. As can be seen, velocity in normal individuals is highest in the aorta and is less than 2 m/s.[63] Other commonly made measurements include the acceleration time (from the beginning of flow to peak velocity of flow in the ascendingaorta or pulmonary artery); and the deceleration time, from LV inflow peak E-wave velocity extrapolated to baseline zero velocity.

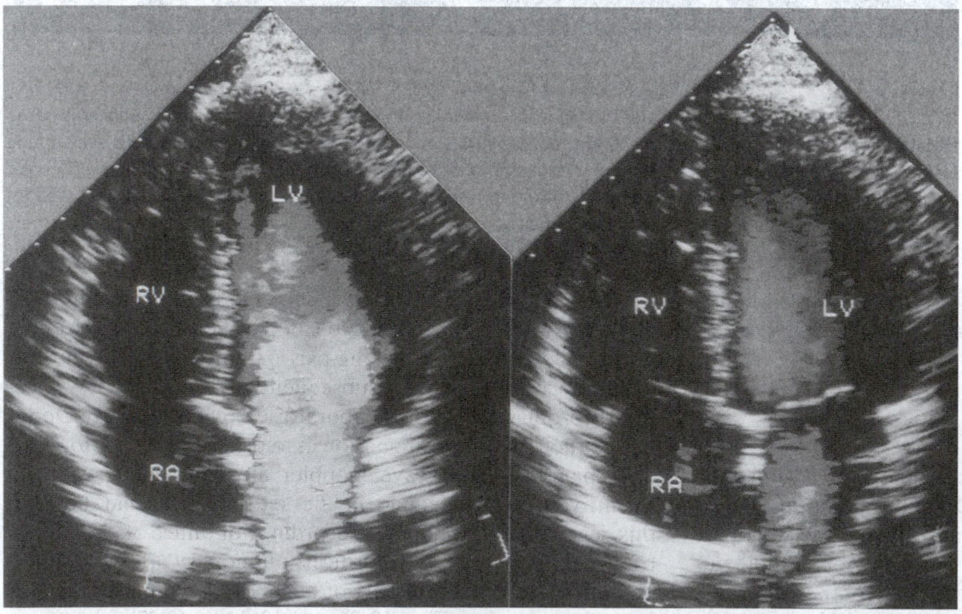

FIGURE 13-30 (Plate 54) Apical four-chamber images with color-flow Doppler during diastole and systole. Red flow indicates movement toward the transducer (diastolic filling); blue flow indicates movement away from the transducer (systolic ejection).

Doppler Assessment of Diastolic Function

In recent years, there has been a great deal of interest in using mitral inflow velocity patterns to evaluate LV diastolic properties.[64–74,74a] Transmitral filling velocities reflect the pressure gradient between the LA and LV during diastole[65] (Fig. 13-34). In early diastole, pressure in the LV normally falls below that in the LA, producing an increase in velocity due to rapid transmitral inflow (E wave). Flow decelerates as the pressures equilibrate in middiastole. In late diastole, LA contraction restores a small gradient, causing transmitral flow to accelerate to a second peak (A wave) that is of less magnitude than the E wave. In individuals in whom early LV relaxation is im-

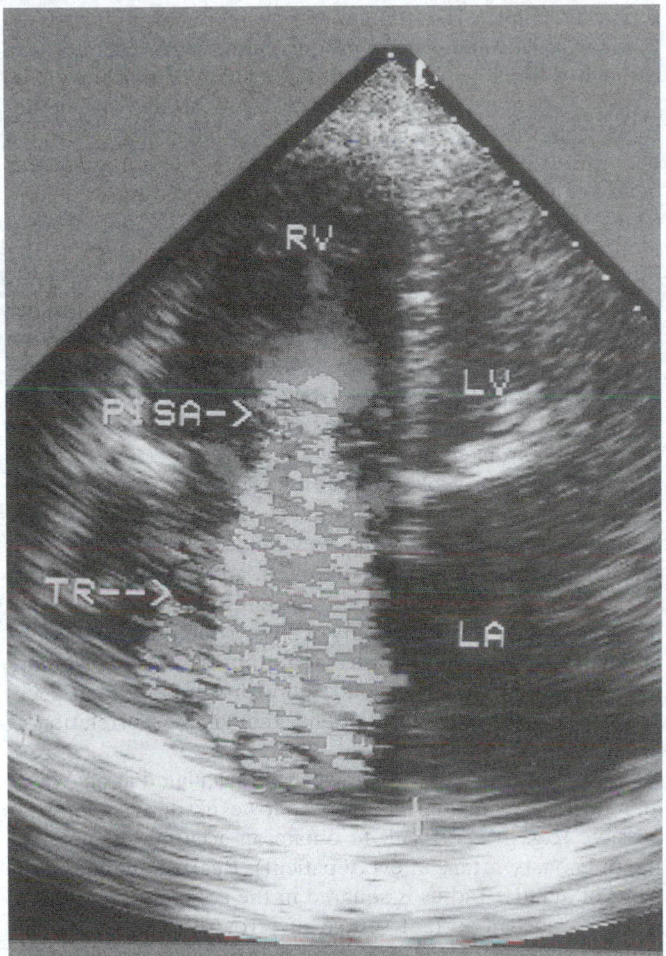

FIGURE 13-31 (Plate 55) Apical four-chamber view of severe tricuspid regurgitation. The Doppler color jet fills the RA. PISA = proximal isovelocity surface area; LV = left ventricle; LA = left atrium; RV = right ventricle.

paired, the transmitral pressure gradient is blunted, resulting in a decrease in both the velocity of early filling and rate of E-wave deceleration[66,68,70] (Fig. 13-38). Conversely, in patients with marked increases of LA pressure and LV stiffness, early diastolic filling velocities are high, deceleration is rapid, and late filling following atrial contraction is markedly reduced. This is the so-called restrictive pattern of LV filling (Fig. 13-39). Accordingly, an E-wave velocity that is substantially less than the A-wave velocity and is accompanied by a prolonged deceleration time represents evidence of impaired early diastolic relaxation by Doppler, while an increased E-wave velocity and decreased A-wave velocity (E/A ratio greater than 2.5 or 3 to 1) accompanied by a diminished deceleration time (less than 100 ms) is indicative of a noncompliant LV with markedly elevated lef atrial pressures.[69,70,73,73a] Although a restrictive pattern can be seen with restrictive cardiomyopathy or advanced LV dysfunction of any cause, it also occurs in pericardial disease.[75] Of significance, a restrictive pattern of LV filling has been associated with an increased mortality rate in patients with advanced congestive heart failure,[76] and persistence of this pattern despite changes in loading condition is an additional poor prognostic sign.[76a,76b]

These abnormal mitral inflow patterns can be clinically useful and, when they are markedly distorted, are generally reliable in identifying and characterizing diastolic dysfunction. A number of variables other than diastolic function, however, are capable of influencing transmitral filling velocities. It has been shown that transmitral Doppler filling dynamics are affected by the age of the patient,[77,78] changes in heart rate,[79,80] respiration,[81] and even the position of the Doppler sample volume within the mitral valve orifice.[82–84] Of greatest significance, transmitral inflow is very sensitive to loading conditions, and reductions in LV preload induced by nitroglycerin and/or lower-body negative pressure can induce a striking decrease in early transmitral filling velocities independent of changes in diastolic properties.[85,86] The influence of LV loading upon transmitral filling is most striking when an increase in LA pressure due to cardiac dysfunction restores early diastolic filling velocities and obscures impaired relaxation, thus inducing "pseudonormalization."[68] Therefore, as Doppler transmitral filling dynamics have many limitations in assessing diastolic function, particular filling patterns should not be interpreted as "pathognomonic" findings of diastolic dysfunction but rather as a component of a complete clinical and echocardiographic evaluation.

Recently, attention has focused upon ancillary Doppler techniques to evaluate LV diastolic dysfunction and LA pressure. An impaired systolic filling wave and increased A-wave flow reversal in the velocity recordings from pulmonary veins in the setting of a relatively normal transmitral pattern of diastolic

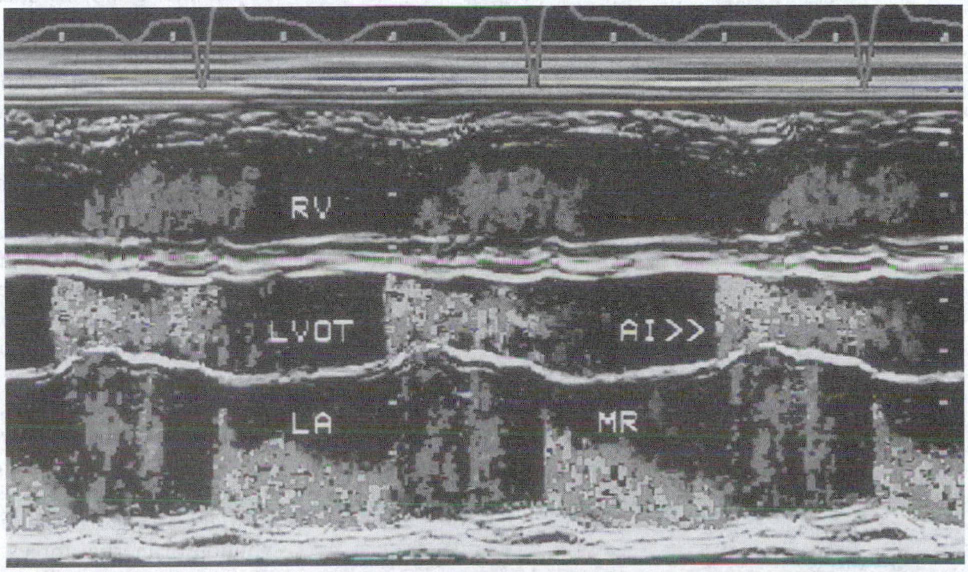

FIGURE 13-32 (Plate 56) Color-flow Doppler superimposed on an M-mode image. The transducer is in parasternal position, and the cursor is directed through the left ventricular outflow tract (LVOT) and left atrium (LA). The patient under study has both aortic insufficiency (AI) and mitral regurgitation (MR). RV = right ventricle.

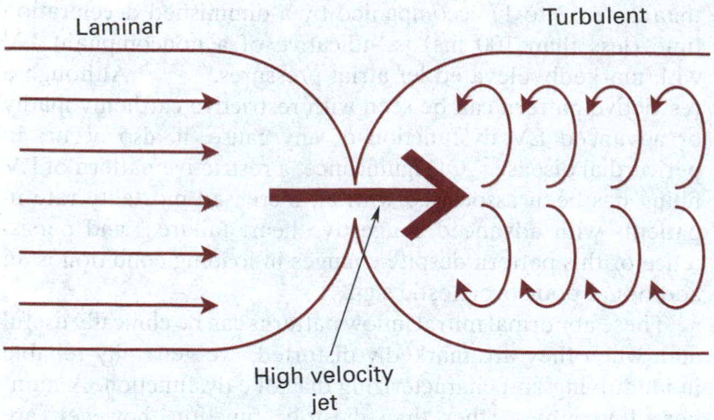

FIGURE 13-33 Flow characteristics through a stenotic orifice. Proximal to the stenosis, the flow is laminar. Near the point of maximal stenosis, the flow velocity is markedly increased. Turbulent flow is present distal to the stenosis.

filling suggests elevated LV filling pressures and may be useful in distinguishing normal from pseudonormal mitral inflow pattern (Fig. 13-36). In addition, an increased amplitude of the pulmonary vein A-wave reversal in comparison with the forward transmitral A-wave velocity, especially in regard to duration, has been found to be of value in detecting elevated LV filling pressures by Doppler.[87,88] Tissue Doppler recordings also yield early diastolic and late atrial velocity signals which are altered in a similar fashion to transmitral filling in the setting of diastolic dysfunction.[53a] Tissue Doppler recordings are less influenced by LV loading, and may be of value in distinguishing pseudonormalization.[53c] The rate of propagation of the transmitral LV filling stream into the LV may also be utilized to detect impaired diastolic function as well as constrictive pericarditis.[53a]

Doppler Assessment of Systolic Function and Cardiac Output

Although measurements of LV volumes and ejection fraction can be obtained by 2D echocardiography, Doppler interrogation provides a unique and complementary noninvasive assessment of systolic function. Thus, LV systolic dysfunction often results in decreased aortic velocity and acceleration time.[89–91] As discussed below, in the presence of *mitral regurgitation* (MR), the acceleration of the MR jet can provide information regarding contractile function.[92]

One of the most important applications of Doppler is in the calculation of the stroke volume.[93] The theory involved is relatively simple. The volume of flow through any orifice or tube can be calculated as the product of the cross-sectional area through which flow occurs and the velocity of that flow (Fig. 13-40). Measures of anatomic cross-sectional area can be derived from echocardiographic images, while velocity can be determined by Doppler. As the annulus of the aortic valve is nearly circular, its cross-sectional area can be estimated from a measurement of diameter, as $\pi(\text{diameter}/2)^2$. The pulsed-wave Doppler envelope also can be recorded at the same level. The *mean* flow velocity through the orifice is calculated by integrating velocity over time. (that is, by measuring the area under the Doppler curve). This velocity-time integral, often called the *stroke distance,* is then multiplied by the cross-sectional area at the level of the Doppler interrogation to obtain the stroke volume.[93–96] The product of the stroke volume and heart rate then yields cardiac output.

TABLE 13-4 Normal Intracardiac Doppler Velocities

	Velocity, m/s
Right ventricle	
Tricuspid flow	0.3–0.7
Pulmonary artery	0.6–0.9
Left ventricle	
Mitral flow	0.6–1.3
Aorta	1.0–1.7

SOURCE: Hatle L, Angelsen B. *Doppler Ultrasound in Cardiology,* 2d ed. Philadelphia: Lea & Febiger; 1985.

Calculation of stroke volume by the Doppler method involves a number of assumptions. The orifice must be circular and constant in size, and the flow velocity must be uniform throughout the cross-sectional area. In addition, the angle between flow and the interrogating beam must be less than 20 degrees. Despite the uncertainty of these assumptions, Doppler-derived measurements of cardiac output and stroke volume have been shown to correspond well with thermodilution, Fick, and the angiographic calculations, though the correlation is not perfect.[93–99]

Theoretically, stroke volume can be calculated at any valve annulus.[96,97,100–102] In clinical practice, however, this is not always possible (e.g., it is difficult to obtain an accurate diameter of the pulmonary artery in every patient). Because the measurement of annular radius is squared in the computation of area, it is the most important source of error of Doppler stroke-volume analyses. Stroke-volume analysis through the mitral annulus is cumbersome; it is uncertain whether the mitral annulus is best described as a circle or an ellipse, and the cross-sectional area of the annulus probably changes slightly during diastole. Calculations using the tricuspid annulus are hampered by similar problems. Despite these limitations, measurements of stroke volume through the various cardiac valves are clinically useful and can be used to calculate pulmonary-to-systemic shunt ratios, regurgitant volumes,[103–110] and orifice areas of stenotic valves by the continuity equation[111–115] (see below).

The Bernoulli Equation

An important application of Doppler echocardiography is the calculation of pressure gradients within the cardiovascular system using a modification of the Bernoulli equation.[116–118] This theorem states that the pressure drop across a discrete stenosis in the heart or vasculature occurs because of energy loss due to three processes: (1) acceleration of blood through the orifice (*convective acceleration*), (2) inertial forces (*flow acceleration*), and (3) resistance to flow at the interfaces between blood and the orifice (*viscous friction*).[119] Therefore, the pressure drop across any orifice can be calculated as the sum of these three variables (Fig. 13-41). In most clinical situations, the contribution of inertial forces and viscous friction are minimal and can be discounted. Since convective acceleration is determined by velocity, the pressure gradient can be calculated from the velocities of blood proximal to and at the level of an orifice as gradient = $4[(\text{orifice velocity})^2 - (\text{proximal velocity})^2]$. If the

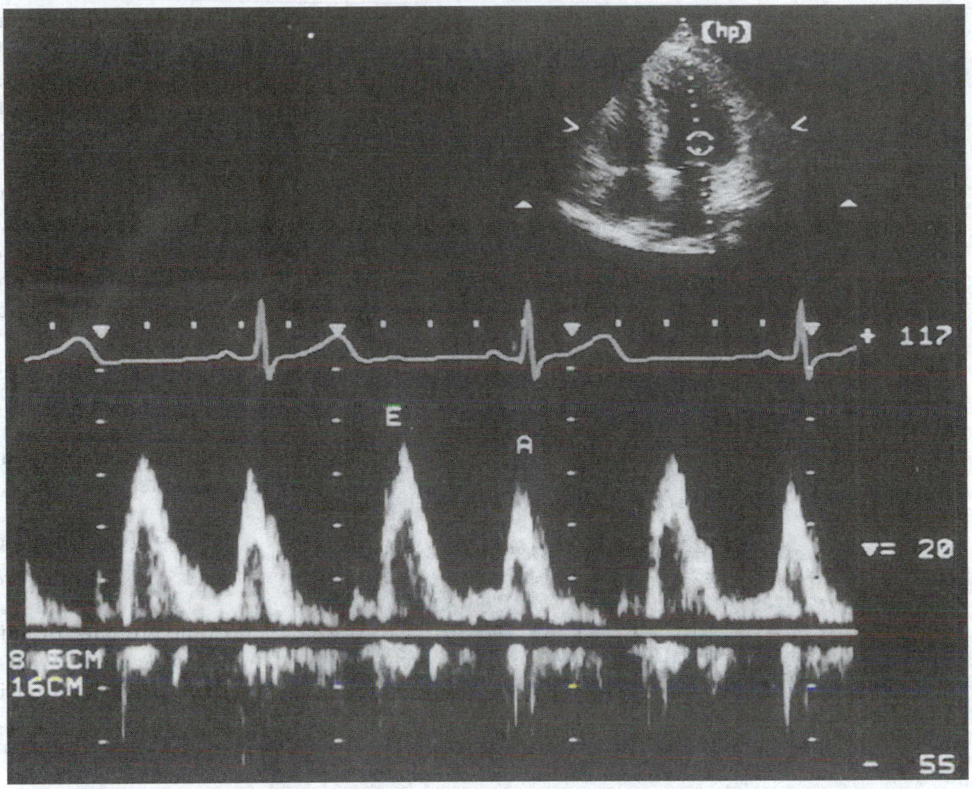

FIGURE 13-34 Normal pulsed-wave Doppler tracing from the left ventricular inflow tract, displaying the early rapid filling (E) and atrial contraction (A) phases of diastolic flow. The transducer is in the apical position and the sample volume is at the mitral leaflet tips.

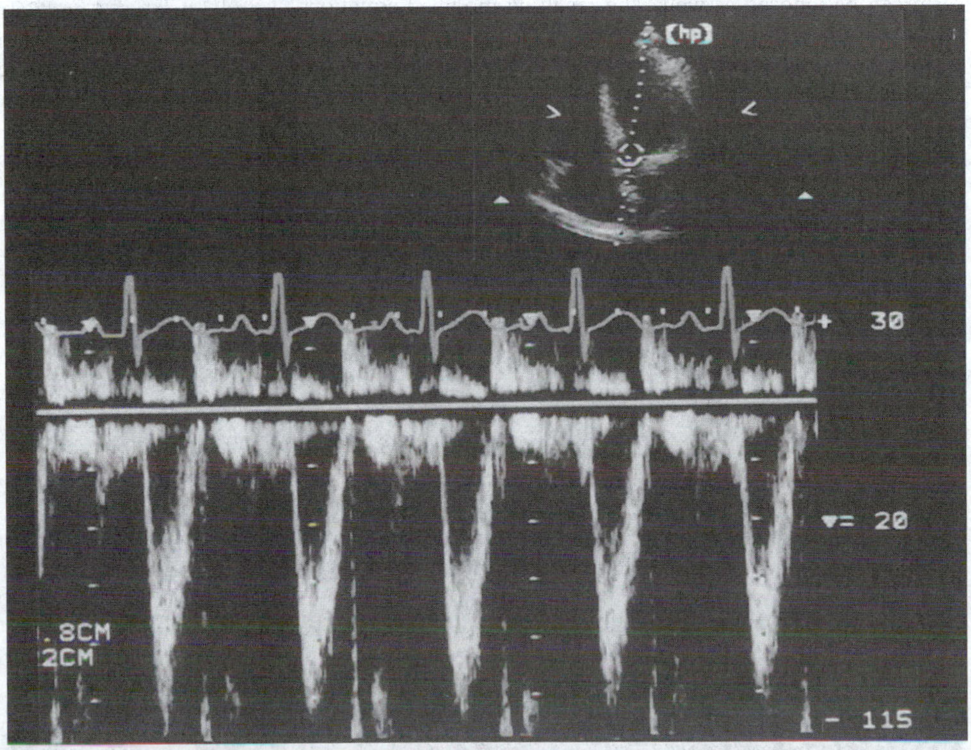

FIGURE 13-35 Normal pulsed-wave Doppler tracing with the sample volume in the left ventricular outflow tract (apical transducer position).

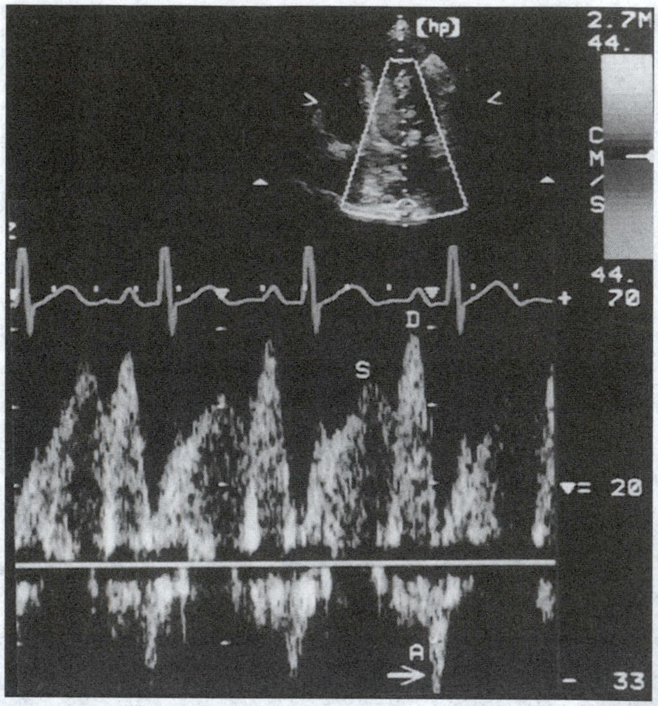

FIGURE 13-36 Pulsed-wave Doppler tracing from the right upper pulmonary vein (recorded from the apical transducer position). Flow toward the heart is biphasic, with peaks in systole (S) and diastole (D). A small amount of reversed flow is seen during atrial contraction (A).

blood velocity proximal to the stenosis is low (<1.0 m/s), this term can be ignored as well. The resulting modified equation states that the pressure gradient across a discrete orifice is equal to four times the square of the peak velocity (*V*) through the stenosis (PG = $4V^2$).[116–119]

The modified Bernoulli equation can be used to calculate pressure gradients across any flow-limiting orifice and has been validated against invasive measurements.[116–122] The method was originally applied to aortic, mitral, and pulmonic stenosis, but further uses have been identified. If at least trivial valvular regurgitation is present, systolic gradients across the tricuspid and end-diastolic gradients across the pulmonic valve can be calculated.[123,124] If the RV diastolic pressure is known (or estimated as the right atrial or central venous pressure), peak RV and pulmonary artery pressure (assuming pulmonic stenosis is absent) can be computed as follows[125,126]:

$$\text{Peak pulmonary artery pressure} = 4(\text{TR velocity})^2 + \text{RA pressure}$$

End-diastolic pulmonary artery pressure (PAD) also can be calculated:

$$\text{PAD} = 4(\text{end-diastolic pulmonary regurgitation velocity})^2 + \text{RA pressure}$$

In the presence of mitral regurgitation, a variety of calculations can be made. With measurement of peak systolic arterial pressure, systolic left atrial pressure can be estimated[127]:

$$\text{Left atrial systolic pressure} = \text{systolic blood pressure} - 4(\text{MR velocity})^2$$

Further, the acceleration of the MR jet can be used to estimate LV systolic *dP/dt*.[128] Thus, from the Bernoulli equation, the LA-to-LV pressure gradients at regurgitant velocities of 1 and 3 m/s are 4 and 36 mmHg, respectively. Therefore, *dP/dt* can be calculated as 32 mmHg divided by the time (in seconds) required for the mitral regurgitant jet to accelerate from 1 to 3 m/s. In the case of ventricular septal defects or aortopulmonary shunts, measurements of the peak systolic arterial pressure and the peak Doppler velocity across the defect allows calculation of the right ventricular (or pulmonary arterial) systolic pressure.

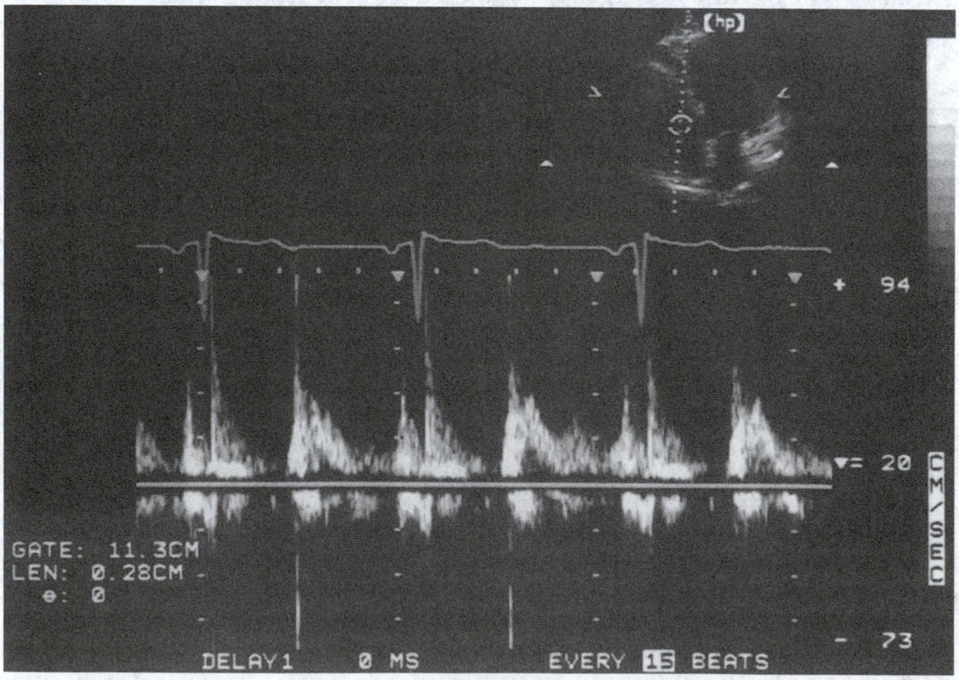

FIGURE 13-37 Pulsed-wave Doppler tracing from the right ventricular inflow tract (apical transducer position).

The Continuity Equation

Although transvalvular pressure gradients can be calculated from CW Doppler recordings using the modified Bernoulli equation, gradients sometimes can be misleading in the evaluation of valvular stenosis. The transvalvular gradient is determined by both the size of the stenotic orifice and the stroke volume traversing it. Severe aortic stenosis and accompanying LV systolic dysfunction may produce a low transvalvular gradient despite a small valve area, while coexistent aortic regurgitation may result in a large gradient with only mild aortic stenosis. The

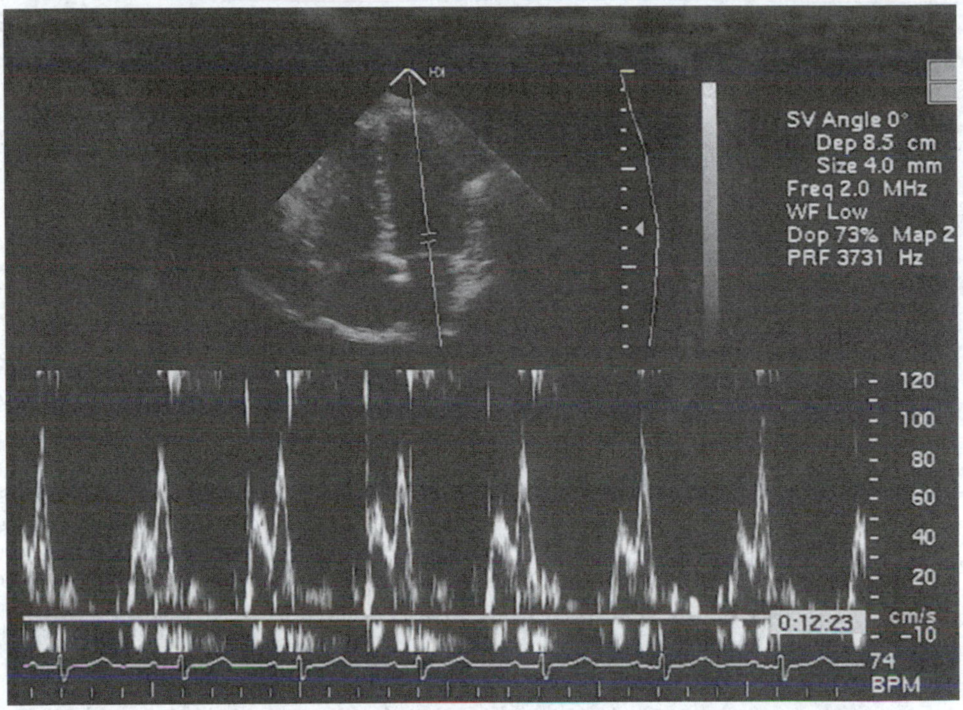

FIGURE 13-38 Pulsed-wave Doppler tracing of diastolic relaxation abnormality (see text for details).

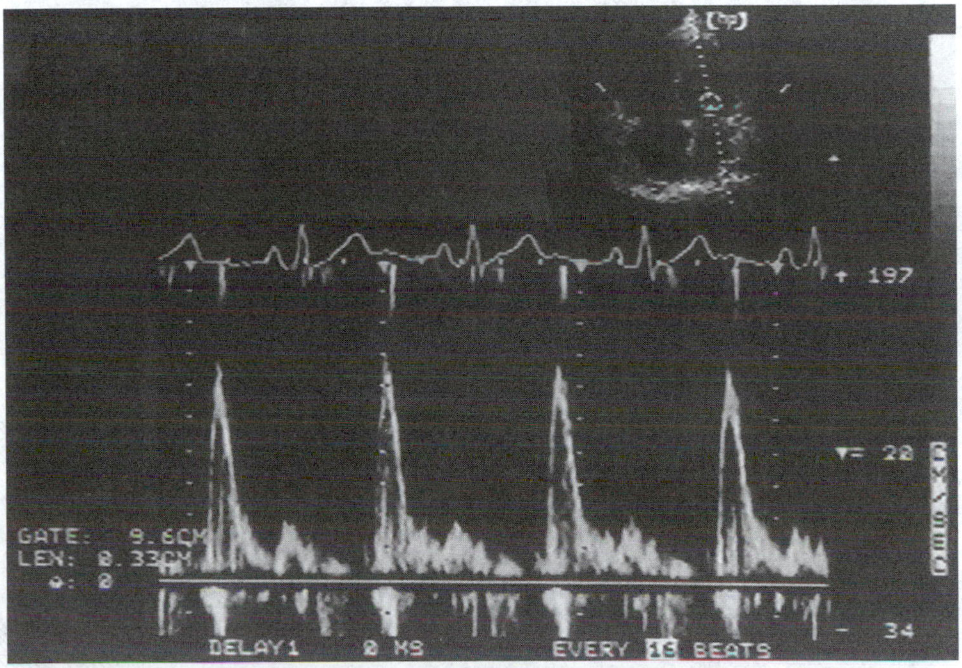

FIGURE 13-39 Pulsed-wave Doppler tracing of diastolic restrictive abnormality (see text for details).

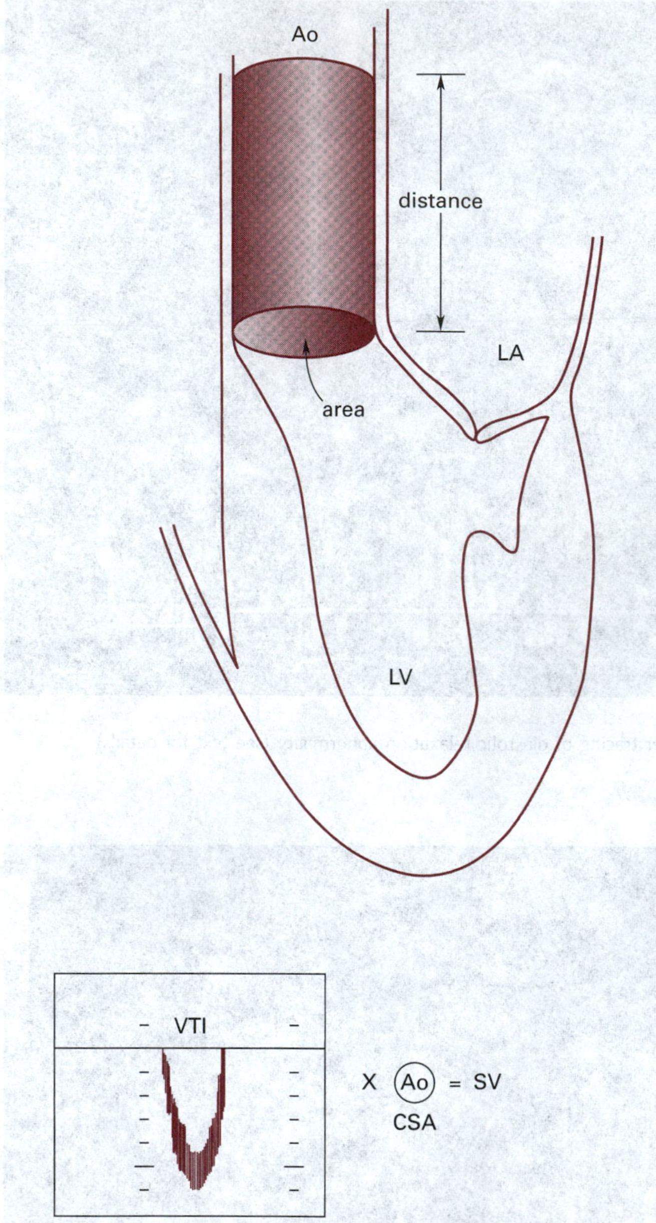

FIGURE 13-40 Calculation of stroke volume. Multiplying the cross-sectional area (CSA) of the blood column in the ascending aorta by the distance the column moves during a single cardiac contraction yields the stroke volume (SV). The velocity-time integral (VTI), expressed in units of length, represents the "stroke distance." (Modified from Pearlman AS. Technique of Doppler and color flow Doppler in the evaluation of cardiac disorders and function. In: Schlant RC, Alexander RW, eds. *The Heart, Arteries, and Veins*, 8th ed. New York: McGraw-Hill; 1994:2229, with permission.)

calculation of orifice area by Doppler echocardiography employs the *continuity equation*, which is derived from the law of the conservation of mass and states that the product of cross-sectional area and velocity is constant in a closed system of flow[129] (Fig. 13-42). Thus, in the case of aortic stenosis, the product of the area and velocity of the left LV outflow tract equals the product of the area and velocity of the aortic valve orifice. Annulus diameter and integrated velocity measurements are derived by the standard volumetric approach, while the velocity across the stenotic orifice is derived by CW Doppler. The equation is then solved for the valve area.[111–116]

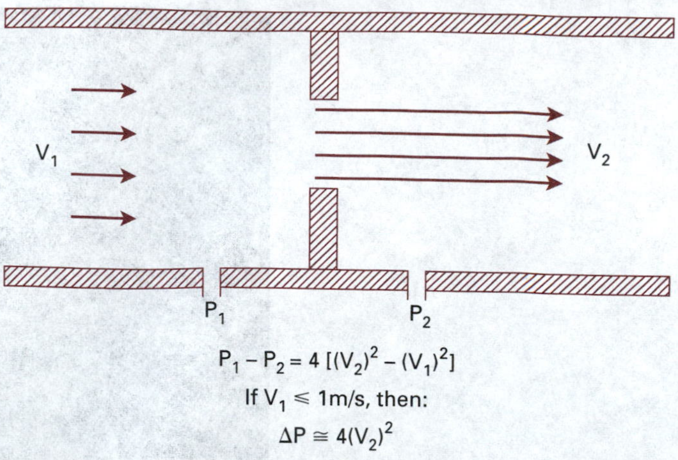

FIGURE 13-41 The modified Bernoulli equation. Pressure drop across a small orifice can be estimated as four times the square of the peak velocity (if the proximal velocity is less than 1 m/s). V_1 and P_1 = proximal velocity and pressure; V_2 and P_2 = distal velocity and pressure. (Modified from Pearlman AS. Technique of Doppler and color flow Doppler in the evaluation of cardiac disorders and function. In: Schlant RC, Alexander RW, eds. *The Heart, Arteries, and Veins,* 8th ed. New York: McGraw-Hill; 1994:2229, with permission.)

The continuity equation is simple and the constituent factors are readily measured, but a number of potential errors can occur. The most common pitfall is an inaccurate estimation of

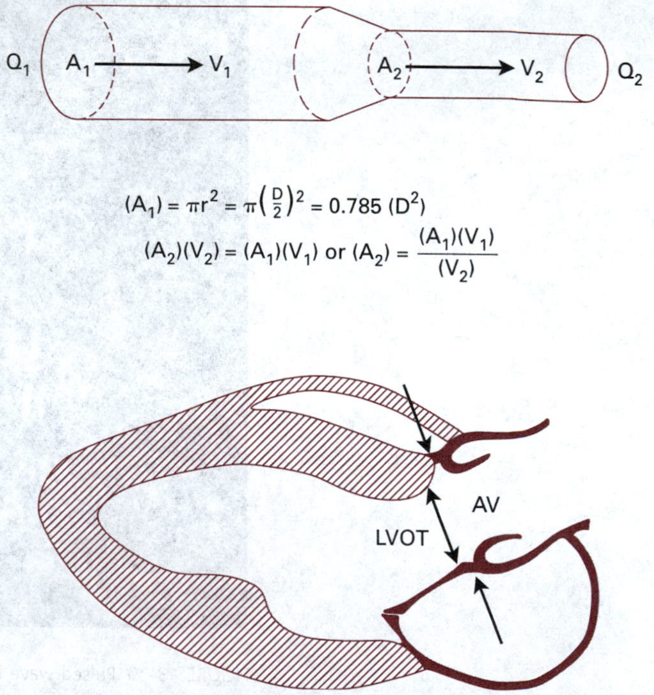

FIGURE 13-42 The continuity equation. In a closed system (*top*) with constant flow, $Q_1 = Q_2$. Therefore, $A_1 \times V_1$ must equal $A_2 \times V_2$. Determination of any three of the variables allows calculation of the fourth. Clinically (*bottom*), the area of the left ventricular outflow tract (LVOT) can be estimated and used to determine aortic valve area. (From Hagan AD, DeMaria AN. *Clinical Applications of Two-Dimensional Echocardiography and Cardiac Doppler.* Boston: Little, Brown; 1989, with permission.)

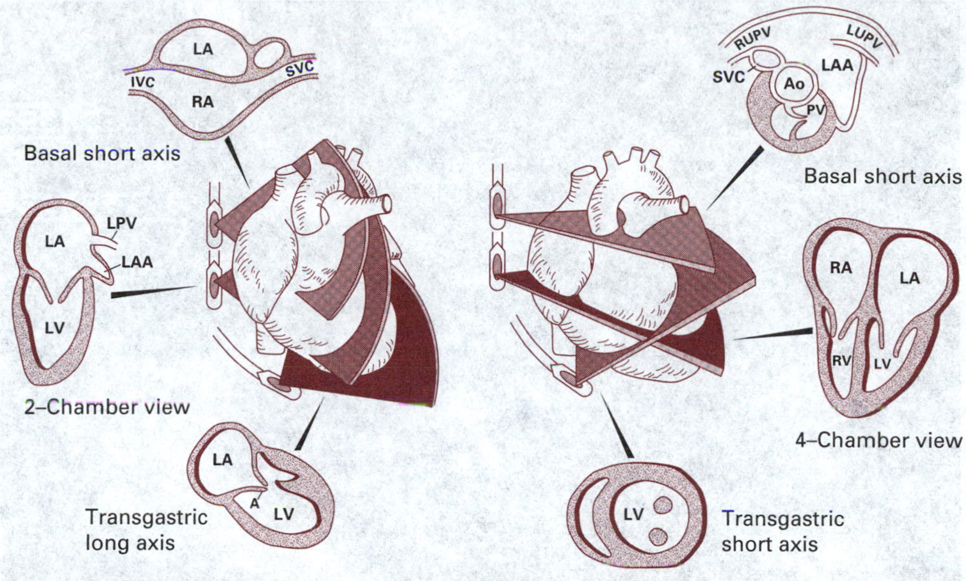

FIGURE 13-43 Standard TEE imaging planes in transverse and longitudinal axes. (From Fisher EA, Stahl JA, Budd JH, Goldman ME. Transesophageal echocardiography: Procedures and clinical applications. *J Am Coll Cardiol* 1991; 18:1333–1348, with permission.)

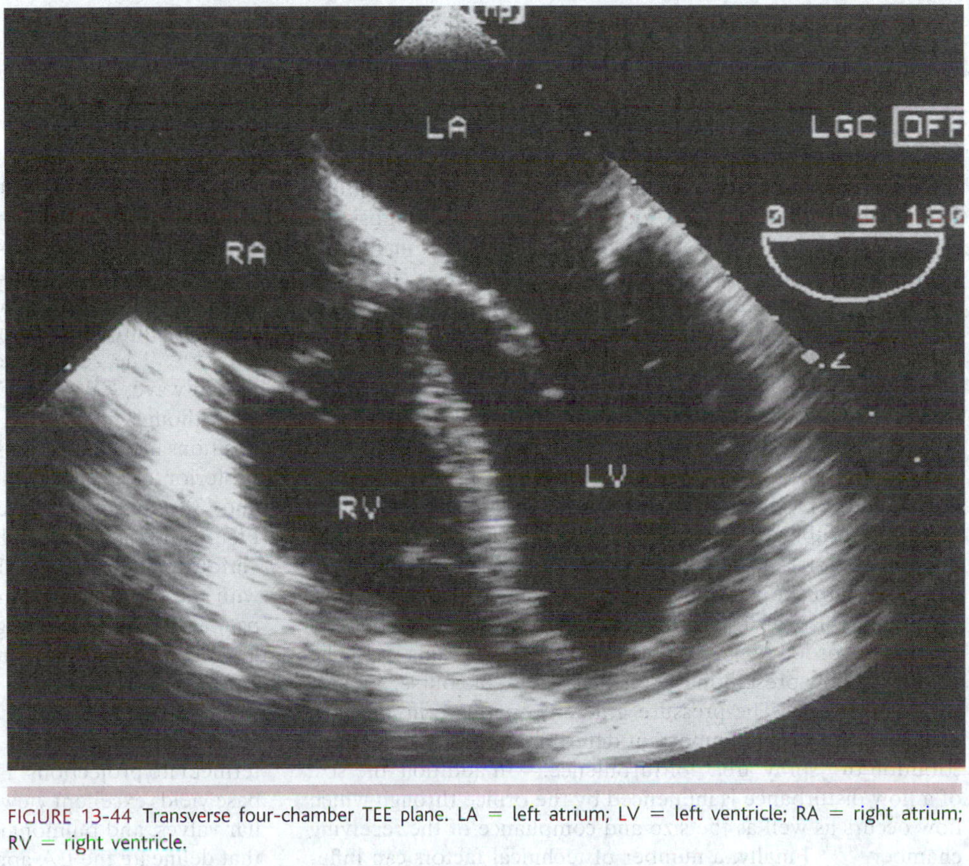

FIGURE 13-44 Transverse four-chamber TEE plane. LA = left atrium; LV = left ventricle; RA = right atrium; RV = right ventricle.

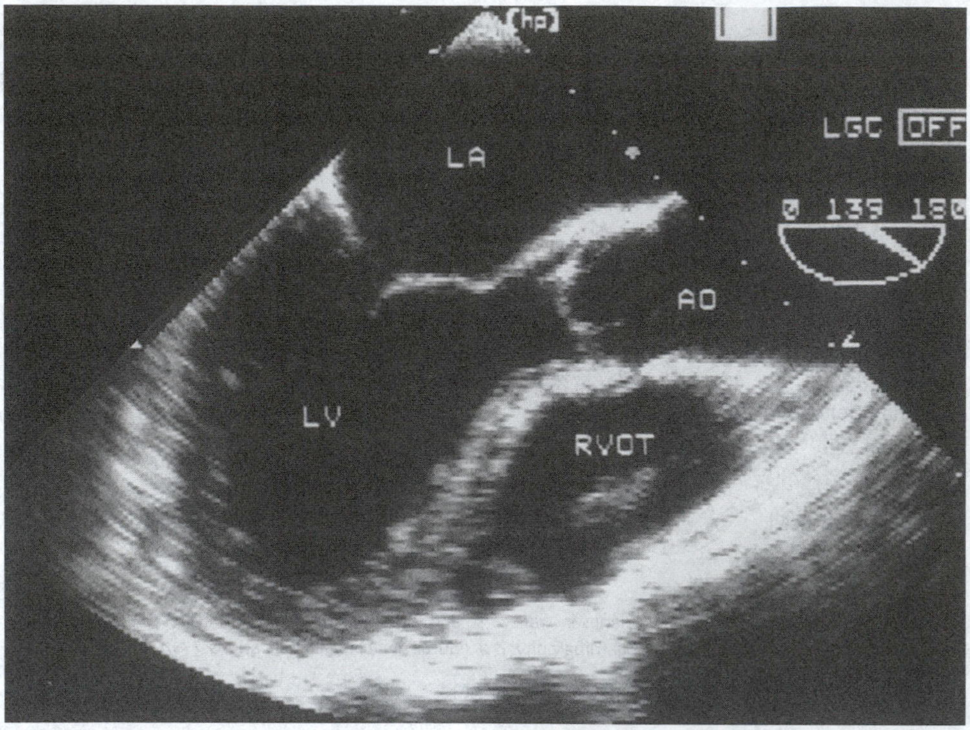

FIGURE 13-45 Modified longitudinal TEE plane (with transducer rotated to approximately 140 degrees), demonstrating a TEE apical "three-chamber" view. AO = ascending aorta; RVOT = right ventricular outflow tract; LA = left atrium; LV = left ventricle.

the cross-sectional area proximal to the stenosis. In addition, it is essential that blood velocity proximal to a stenosis be measured outside the area of flow acceleration. Finally, the continuity equation actually solves for the area of the vena contracta, which is usually just distal to the stenotic orifice. Although this area is very similar to the area of the stenotic orifice, occasional discrepancies occur.

Determinants of the Size of Flow Disturbances

Although CFD yields primarily qualitative information, it is unique in its ability to provide measurements of the size of flow disturbances. It is logical that the size of a turbulent jet should correlate with the volume of blood contained within the flow disturbance. Regardless of the lesion, however, the area of turbulence recorded by CFD has multiple determinants.[130–134] The volume of flow present in the disturbance is, of course, a major factor in its size. The pressure gradient operative in any flow disturbance is also an important determinant of the spatial distribution or "spray area" of turbulence.[134] In addition, the size of a flow disturbance is influenced by the orifice through which flow occurs as well as the size and compliance of the receiving chamber.[130–136] Finally, a number of technical factors can influence jet size as imaged by CFD, including instrument gain, the angle of incidence of the interrogating beam, the frequency and pulse repetition rate of the transducer, and the temporal sampling rate.[137] Therefore, measurements derived from the size of the turbulent jet recorded by color Doppler, are at best semiquantitative and should not be expected to correlate with the volume of blood contained in the flow disturbance.

TRANSESOPHAGEAL ECHOCARDIOGRAPHY

Transthoracic echocardiography (TTE) usually defines cardiac anatomy and function satisfactorily, often obviating the need for further cardiac imaging. Occasionally, however, TTE does not provide complete or adequately detailed information. This is especially true in the evaluation of posterior cardiac structures (e.g., the LA, the left atrial appendage, the interatrial septum, the aorta distal to the root), in the assessment of prosthetic cardiac valves, and in the delineation of cardiac structures less than 3 mm in size (e.g., small vegetations or thrombi). Ultrasonic imaging from the esophagus is uniquely suited to these situations, as the esophagus is adjacent to the LA and the thoracic aorta for much of its course[138,139] and affords excellent access of the interrogating beam to these structures.

Over the past decade, a number of technologic advances have occurred in the field of *transesophageal echocardiography* (TEE), and flexible transesophageal ultrasound probes capable of multiplanar imaging of the heart are now widely available.[140–142] The current generation of probes also provide full pulsed-wave, CW, and CFD capabilities.

Although images can be recorded from a variety of probe positions most authorities recommend three basic positions: (1) posterior to the base of the heart, (2) posterior to the left atrium, and (3) inferior to the heart (transgastric position; Fig. 13-43). Figures 13-44 through 13-47 show TEE images obtained in various planes through the heart. It must be emphasized that, with the transducer in the esophagus, posterior structures appear at the top of the image. With the transducer in the stomach, a short-axis view is standardly obtained, with long-axis and apical views available to a variable degree. Upon withdrawing the transducer to the esophagus, one usually obtains apical-equivalent four-chamber and long-axis views, with multiple intermediate projections. Further withdrawal of the probe to the base yields excellent views of the atria, great vessels and semilunar valves, and pulmonary veins. Of particular value are views that delineate the LA appendage, all three leaflets of the aortic valve in short axis, and the transverse and descending aorta.[143]

TEE has become an important imaging modality for the diagnosis and management of infective endocarditis and its complications, including valvular vegetations, chordal rupture, fistulas, perivalvular abscesses, and mycotic aneurysms.[143–148] TEE

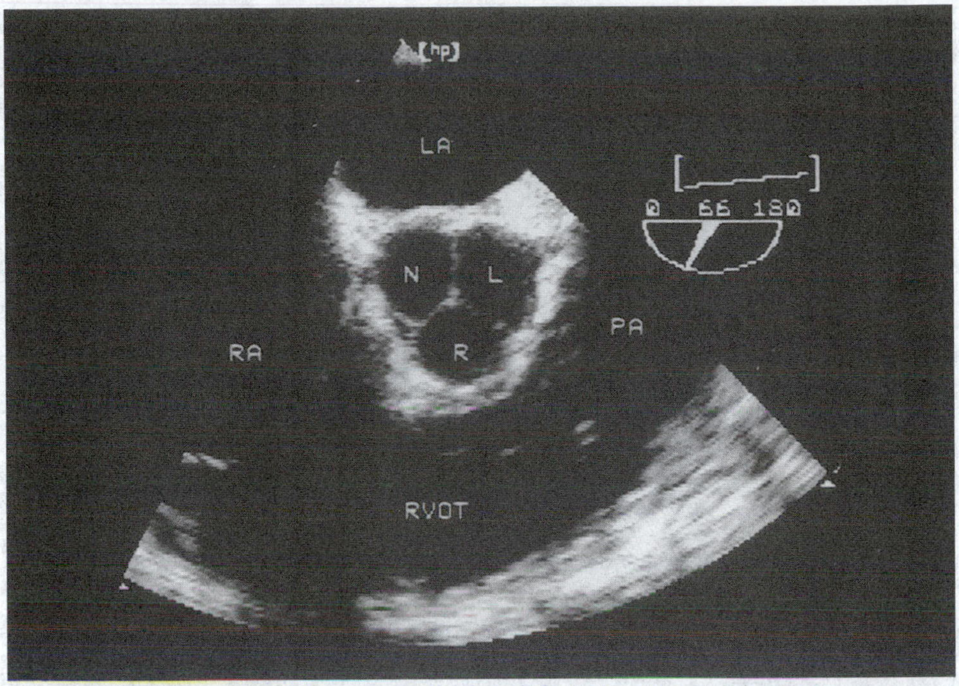

A

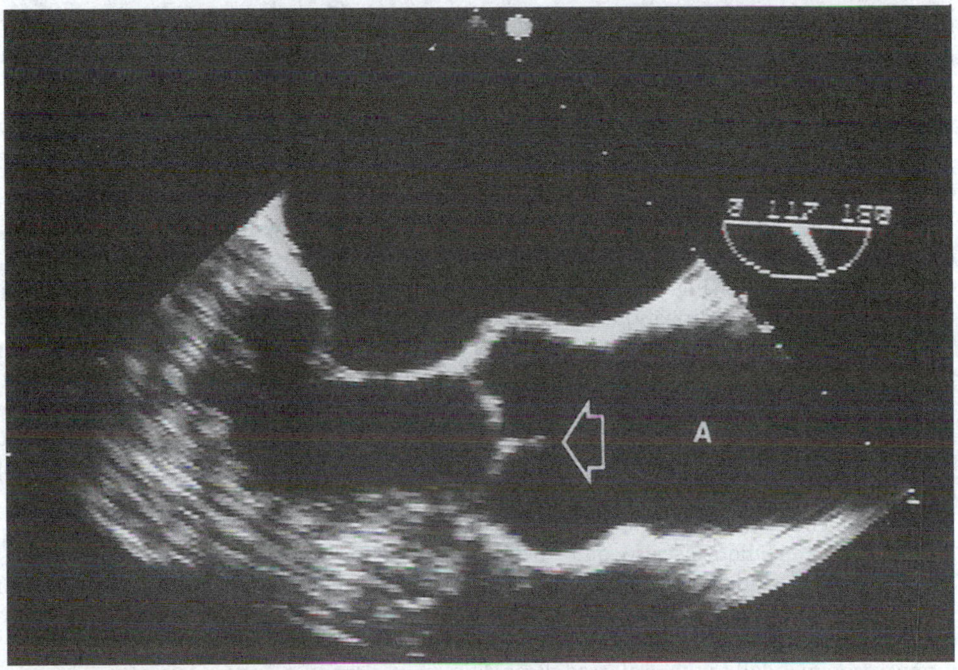

B

FIGURE 13-46 *A.* Modified short-axis view through the level of the aortic valve, demonstrating the left (L), right (R), and noncoronary (N) valvular cusps. LA = left atrium; RA = right atrium; RVOT = right ventricular outflow tract; PA = pulmonary artery. *B.* Magnified longitudinal view of the aortic valve (*arrow*) showing the coaptation of the cusps and the sinuses of Valsalva. A = aorta. (From Blanchard DG, Kimura BJ, Dittrich HC, DeMaria AN. Transesophageal echocardiography of the aorta. *JAMA* 1994; 272:546–551, with permission.)

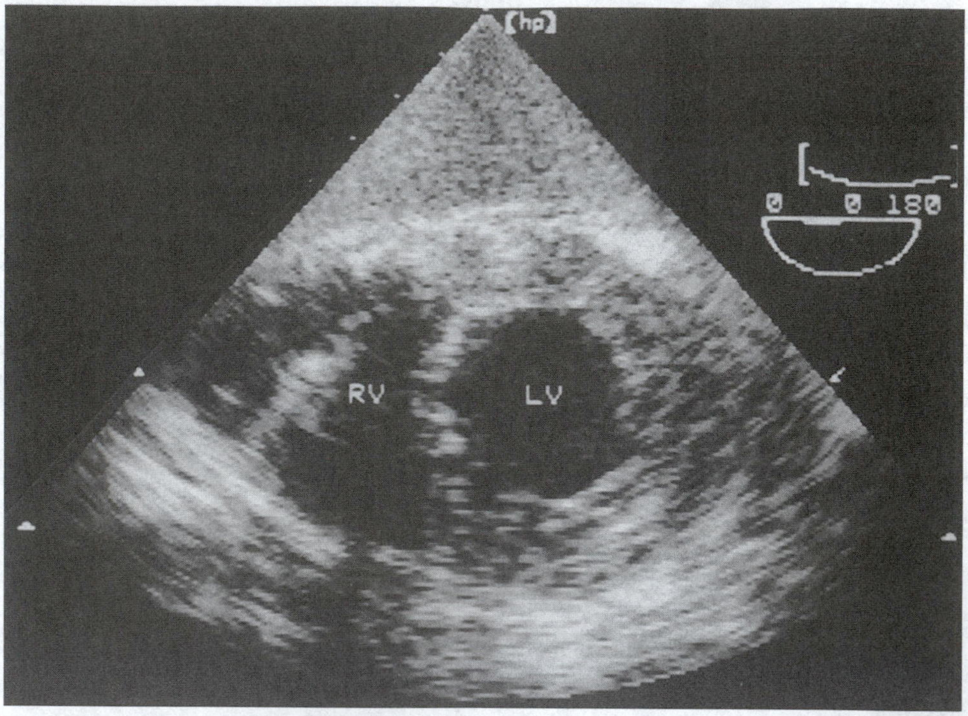

FIGURE 13-47 Short-axis TEE plane through the left ventricle from transgastric position. The inferior wall is closest to the transducer, the anterior wall farthest. The interventricular septum is to the reader's left, the lateral wall to the right. LV = left ventricle; RV = right ventricle.

is more accurate in detecting vegetations and abscesses than TTE[143,149,150] and provides prognostic information as well[150] (Fig. 13-48). In addition, TEE imaging may aid in accurate quantification of valvular disease (particularly mitral regurgitation) if TTE is inconclusive[151] (Fig. 13-49, Plate 57). TEE is especially useful for Doppler interrogation of the pulmonary veins (Fig. 13-50, Plate 58). Flow patterns in these vessels reflect LA pressure, and systolic reversal of pulmonary venous flow has been identified as an accurate marker of mitral regurgitation.[152,153] Although mitral regurgitant color jets are easier to see with TEE than TTE, they are usually larger, and care must be exercised not to overestimate severity of the regurgitation.[154] Multiplane TEE can be used to planimeter the orifice area in AS.[155,155a] The technique is also quite helpful in detection of aortic disease, including dissection, aneurysm, congenital malformations, and atherosclerosis.[139,156,157] Because of its portability, accuracy, and short preparation and procedural times, TEE is now recommended as the preferred diagnostic study in many cases of suspected aortic dissection (Fig. 13-51, Plate 59).[139,158]

Thromboemboli may originate from posterior cardiac structures such as the left atrium (LA) and appendage, interatrial septum, and aorta[159–168]; therefore, TEE has received wide application in the evaluation of possible cardiogenic embolization. Since the most common site of LA thrombi is the appendage, the ability of TEE to visualize this structure is of particular value (Fig. 13-52). TEE can also detect spontaneous contrast signals (that appear to represent transient rouleaux formation and predispose to thromboemboli).[169] In addition, TEE has provided unique real-time images of mobile, pedunculated, atherosclerotic "debris" in the thoracic aorta (Fig. 13-53). Although the optimal therapy for this disorder is currently unknown, warfarin may be helpful and mobile or protruding aortic atheromas appear to be significant risk factors for embolic events.[167,168,170,171,171a,171b] The optimal role for TEE in the detection of intracardiac sources of emboli is controversial, and clinical trials are ongoing to evaluate the effect of treatment after discovery of potential embolic sources.

One of the proven applications of TEE is the evaluation of prosthetic valve dysfunction, particularly mechanical valves in the mitral position.[172–174] Since the materials used in artificial valves are strong reflectors and often cause ultrasonic shadowing, the areas behind prosthetic valves are usually hidden from view when transthoracic imaging is used. Because of its unique window on the heart, TEE is clearly superior to TTE imaging for detection of prosthetic regurgitation, infection, tissue ingrowth, and thrombosis[172,174] (Fig. 13-54).

TEE has also become an important intraoperative tool for the detection of cardiac ischemia, the evaluation of valve function after repair or replacement, and the delineation of congenital heart disease.[175–183] Cardiac surgeons often request intraoperative TEE for evaluation of cardiac anatomy and confirmation of a success of surgical repair before closing the chest. In this regard, TEE has almost completely replaced epicardial echocardiography. When TEE images are inadequate, TEE is helpful in managing critically ill patients[184–187] and also can be used to monitor or guide interventional procedures, such as transseptal catheterization,[185–190] mitral valvuloplasty, pericardiocentesis, and endomyocardial biopsy.[191]

CONTRAST ECHOCARDIOGRAPHY

Opacification of the right heart cavities with dense ultrasonic reflectances during intravenous contrast injection was first applied clinically in 1968.[192] Subsequently, it became clear that the origin of the dense intracavitary echoes were microbubbles within the injectate, and that any agitated liquid injected intravenously caused the effect.[193] Since room-air microbubbles with the diameter of pulmonary capillaries persist in blood for less than 1 s before dissolving, agitated agents injected intravenously cannot cross the lungs and enter the left-sided cardiac chambers. Thus, the presence of echocardiographic contrast entering left heart chambers after intravenous injection of an agitated liquid indicates the presence of a right-to-left shunt.[194,195]

Identification of intracardiac shunts, particularly patent foramen ovale in patients with unexplained cerebral ischemia (Fig. 13-55), remains the most frequent indication for contrast echocardiography.[196] Simple agitated normal saline solution remains the most commonly used contrast agent for such studies.

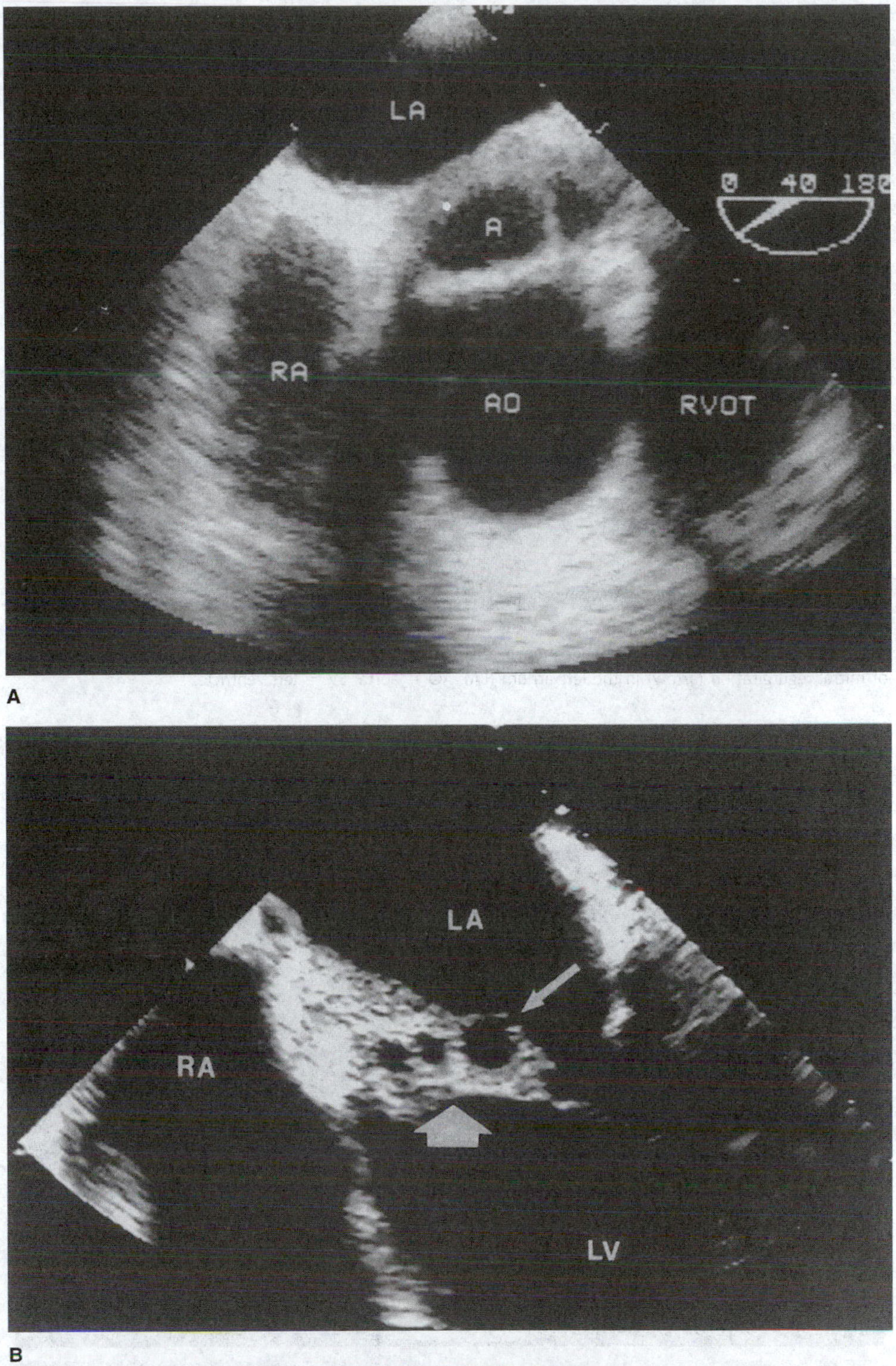

FIGURE 13-48 *A*. Short-axis TEE plane through the cardiac base. A large septated abscess cavity (A) is present between the aortic root (AO) and the left atrium (LA). RA = right atrium; RVOT = right ventricular outflow tract. *B*. Modified transverse four-chamber TEE plane showing a large abscess with several cavitations (*arrows*) involving the anterior mitral valve leaflet and the intervalvular fibrosa. RA = right atrium; LA = left atrium; LV = left ventricle. (From Sobel J, Maisel AS, Tarazi R, Blanchard DG. Gonococcal endocarditis: Assessment by transesophageal echocardiography. *J Am Soc Echocardiogr* 1997; 10:367–370.)

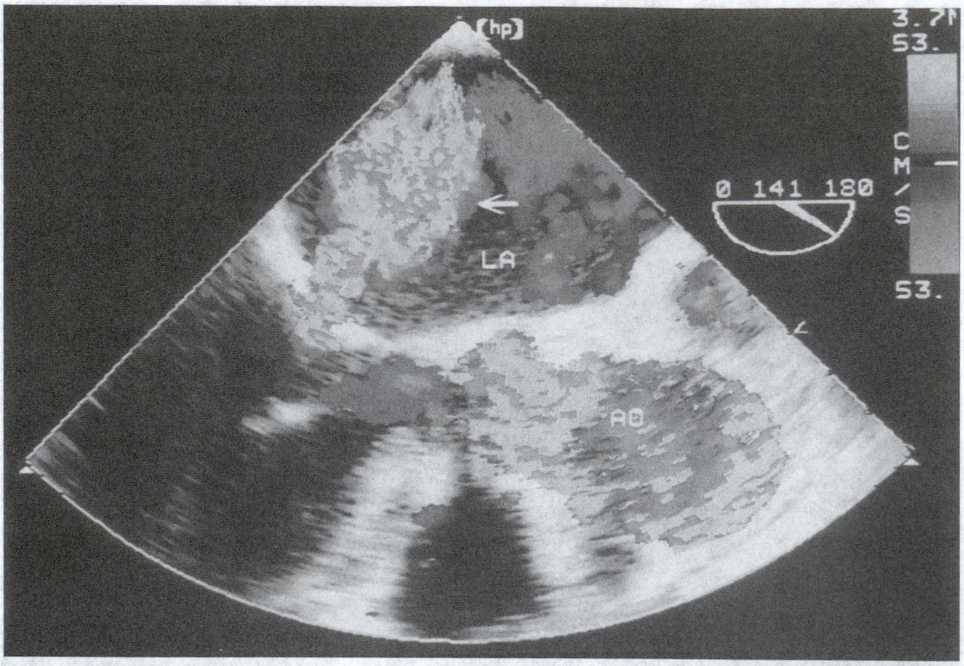

FIGURE 13-49 (Plate 57) Transesophageal echocardiography image (three-chamber plane) demonstrating a jet of mitral regurgitation (*arrow*) in the left atrium (LA). AO = aorta; LV = left ventricle.

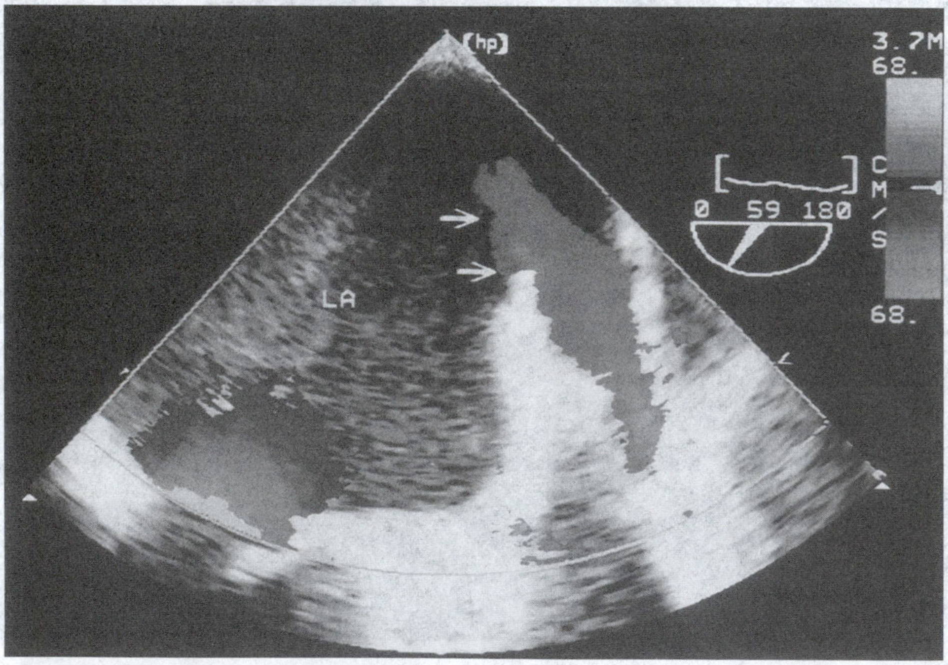

FIGURE 13-50 (Plate 58) Transesophageal echocardiography image of pulmonary venous flow (*arrows*) entering the left atrium (LA) during diastole.

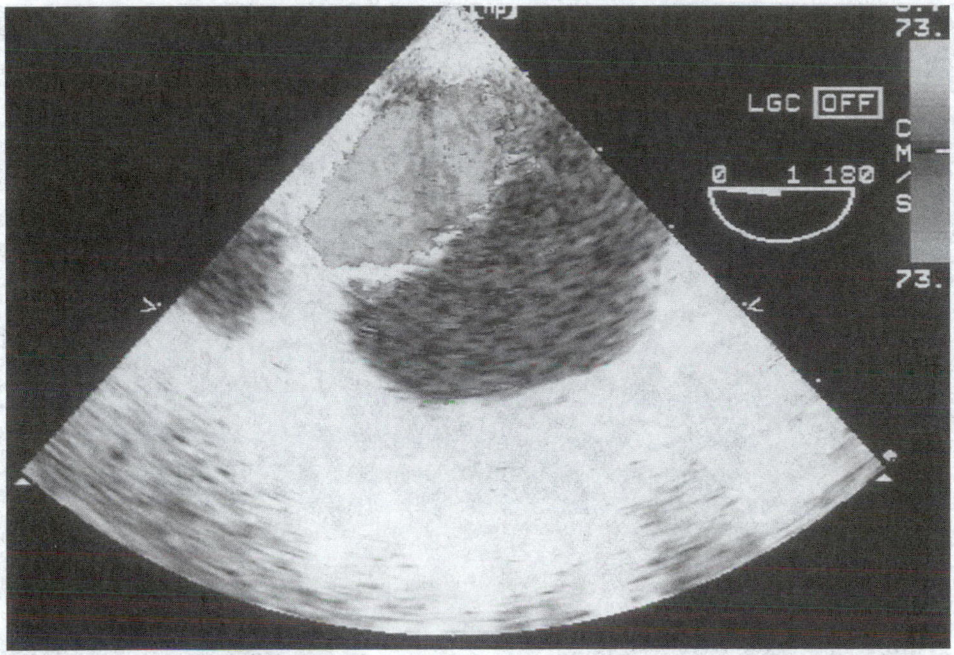

FIGURE 13-51 (Plate 59) Transverse TEE image of a descending aortic dissection. The true lumen is color-coded orange. The false lumen is mostly devoid of flow, but a small blue jet of communication between the two channels is present.

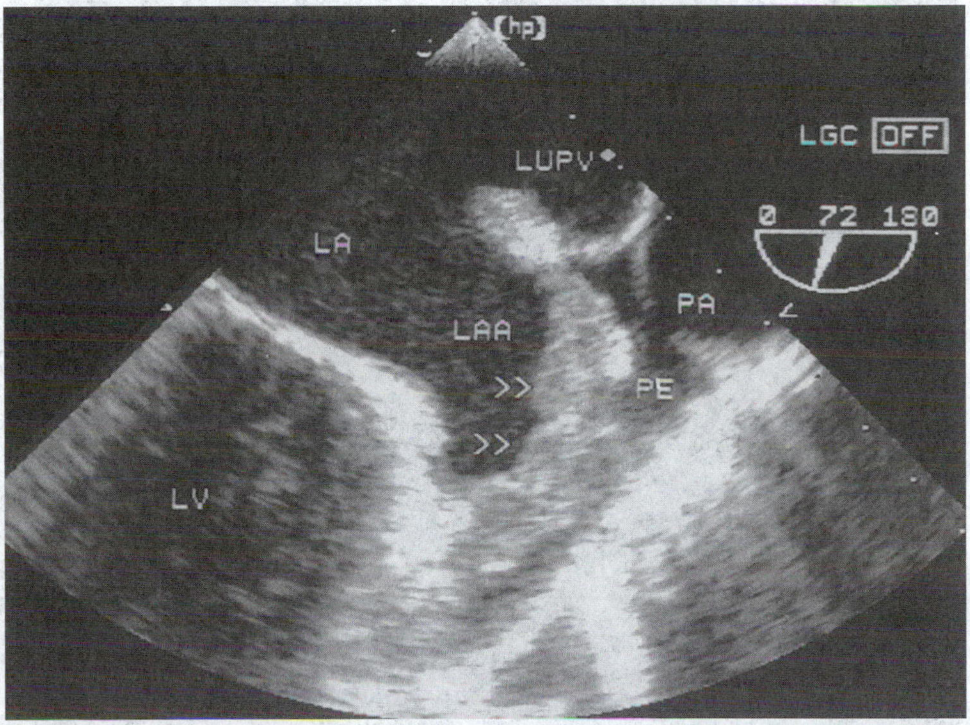

FIGURE 13-52 Transesophageal echocardiography image of a laminar thrombus (*arrows*) within the left atrial appendage (LAA). This thrombus was not visible with transthoracic echocardiography. LA = left atrium; LV = left ventricle; LUPV = left upper pulmonary vein; PA = pulmonary artery; PE = small pericardial effusion.

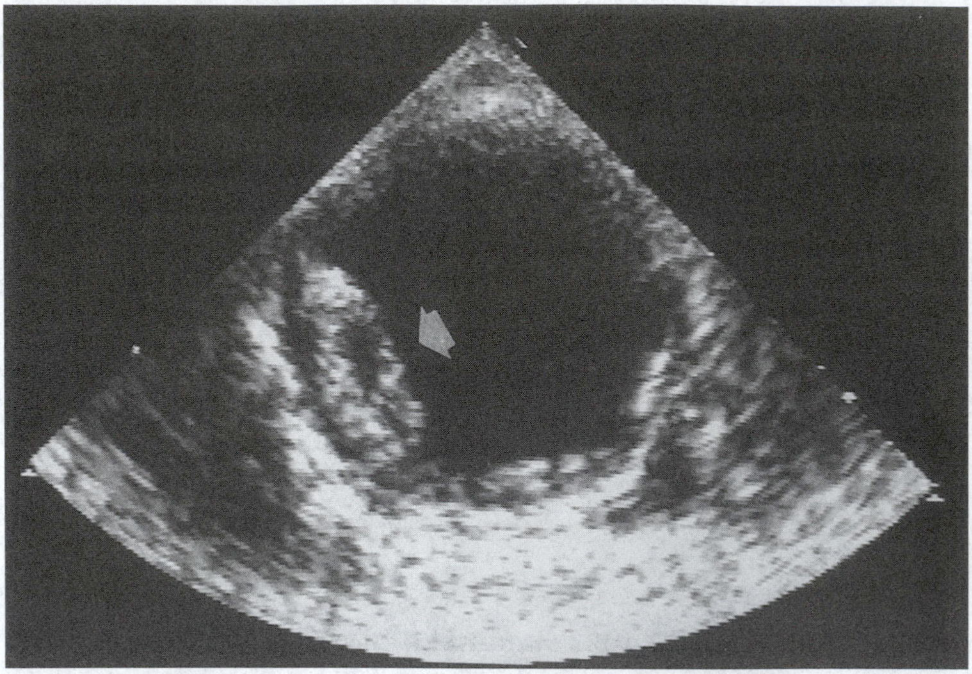

FIGURE 13-53 Transverse TEE image of the descending aorta, demonstrating extensive atherosclerosis and a large atheroma (*arrow*).

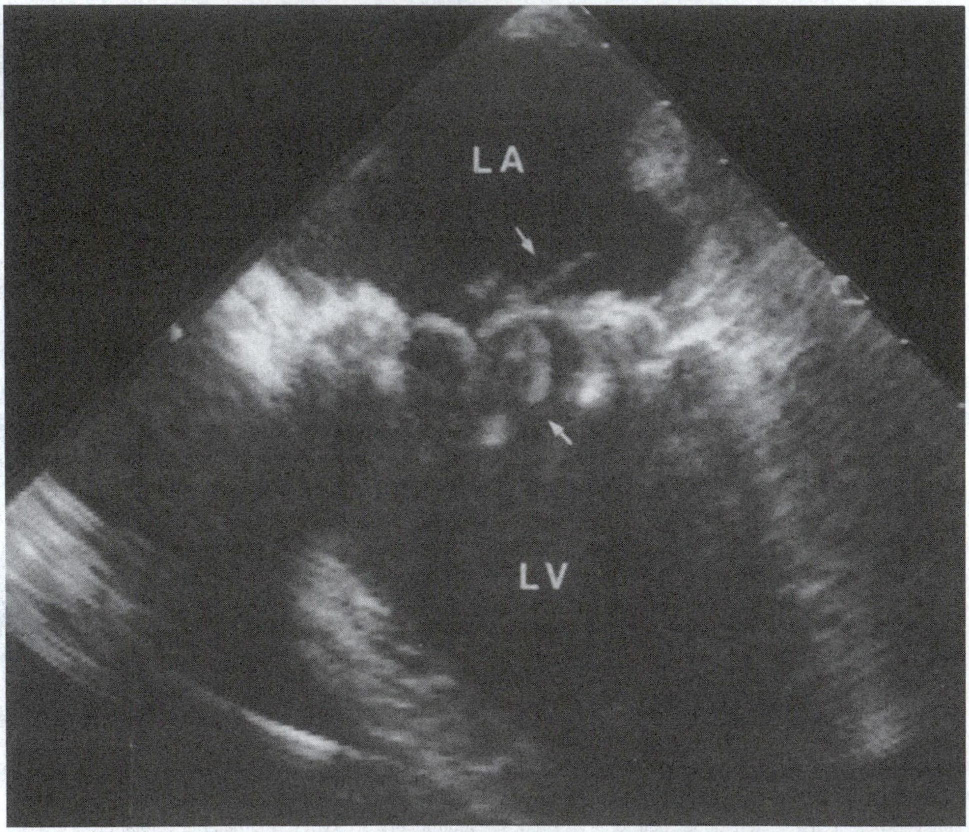

FIGURE 13-54 Transverse four-chamber TEE image of infective vegetations (*arrows*) on a porcine prosthesis in the mitral position. LA = left atrium; LV = left ventricle.

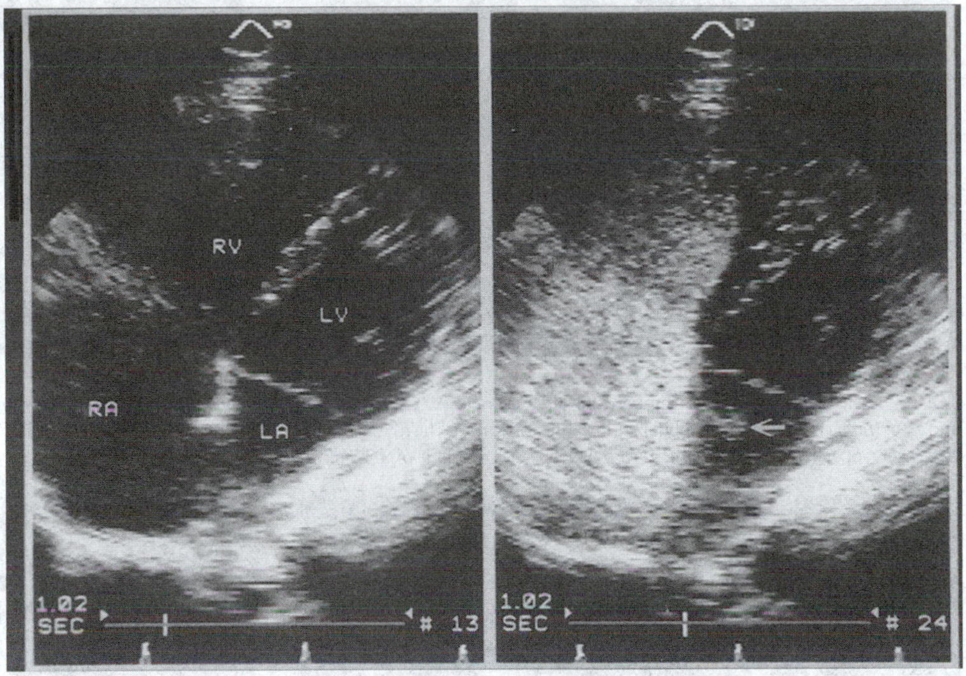

FIGURE 13-55 Contrast microbubble injection demonstrating a shunt (*arrow*) from the right atrium (RA) to left atrium (LA). RV = right ventricle; LV = left ventricle.

In recent years, many attempts have been made to achieve echocardiographic opacification of the LV cavity and myocardium.[197–200] Initial attempts utilized direct left-sided administration. Injection of agitated saline or other fluids into the LV or aorta causes echocardiographic opacification of those chambers and has been used as an alternative to angiography to evaluate mitral and aortic regurgitation.[194] In addition, injection of sonicated radiographic contrast agents into the aortic root or coronary arteries can produce myocardial opacification[201] (Fig. 13-56). The presence of echocardiographic contrast within the myocardium after such injections reflects the spatial distribution of coronary blood flow (CBF)[198] and is valuable in identifying collateral CBF and the absence of reflow following reperfusion therapy of acute myocardial infarction (MI).[202–210] Of significance, the presence of microcirculatory flow and integrity in these studies was a reliable predictor of viable myocardium.[207–209]

Direct injection of coronary contrast into the left heart is limited by its invasive nature. Therefore, stabilized solutions of microbubbles have been developed which can traverse the pulmonary capillary bed in high concentration after intravenous injection. These new ultrasonic contrast agents have been designed to achieve prolonged bubble persistence or survival after injection into blood. The persistence time of a bubble prior to disolving in blood can be increased by utilizing a shell or surface modifying of gas across the bubble surface. Alternatively, prolonged bubble survival can be achieved by utilizing a dense, high-molecular-weight gas with a reduced capacity to diffuse across the bubble shell and a low saturation constant in blood, which favors return of gas back into the bubble. Therefore, the new ultrasonic contrast agents utilize shells made of human serum albumin, liposomes, or even biodegradable poliment materials, and the fluorocarbon gases, which are dense and poorly soluble. These new microbubble agents are all capable of producing dense, high-intensity signals not only within the LV but also within the myocardium following intravenous injection.[210a,210b]

Efforts to produce stabilized solutions of microbubbles have now resulted in a commercially available agent, Optison, which is composed of a perfluorocarbon gas in an albumin shell. Intravenous injection of Optison opacifies the left ventricle in nearly all patients, thereby facilitating identification of the endomyocardial border. This capacity has found its greatest application in stress echocardiography, where detection of the endocardium is of fundamental importance in recognizing abnormal contraction produced by ischemia. By intensifying backscatter within the intracardiac cavities, new ultrasonic agents also enhance Doppler recording of flow abnormalities.[211] Marginal Doppler spectral tracings in cases of mitral regurgitation, tricuspid regurgitation, and aortic stenosis often improved dramatically after contrast injection, facilitating the quantitation of valvular lesions and pulmonary hypertension.[212–216] In addition to new contrast agents, novel imaging technology directed to the amplification of contrast signals are also available. Second harmonic imaging enhances the ultrasonic backscatter from contrast microbubbles (which resonate in an ultrasonic field) while decreasing the returning signal from myocardium (which does not resonate).[217–219] (Fig. 13-57). Power Doppler imaging is a method that correlates signals between successfully transmitted pulses to derive images of moving blood or cardiac structures. Power Doppler techniques are especially well delineated to detect the changing signals produced by movement and/or dissolution of contrast microbubbles.[46] Finally, since exposure to ultrasound energy can produce microbubble destruction, intermittent electrocardiography (ECG) gated rather than continuous ultrasound transmission can also prolong microbubble persistence and amplify contrast signals.[220–221] When combined with the new ultrasonic contrast agents, these refined imaging modalities can achieve visualization of myocardial opacification following intravenous drug administration, thereby delineating myocardial perfusion. Initial studies indicate that myocardial contrast echocardiography can yield information regarding myocardial perfusion comparable to that obtainable by radionuclide techniques and can be of value in delineating coronary artery stenoses.[221a,221b] Intravenous injection of new contrast agents may actually permit visualization of intramyocardial vessels (Fig. 13-58).[214–217,221c] The ability to delineate regional myocardial perfusion is a major step forward in noninvasive imaging and can be expected to provide important information regarding coronary artery disease (CAD) in the near future.

In addition to new contrast agents, novel imaging technologies directed to the amplification of contrast signals are also available. For example, second-harmonic imaging enhances the

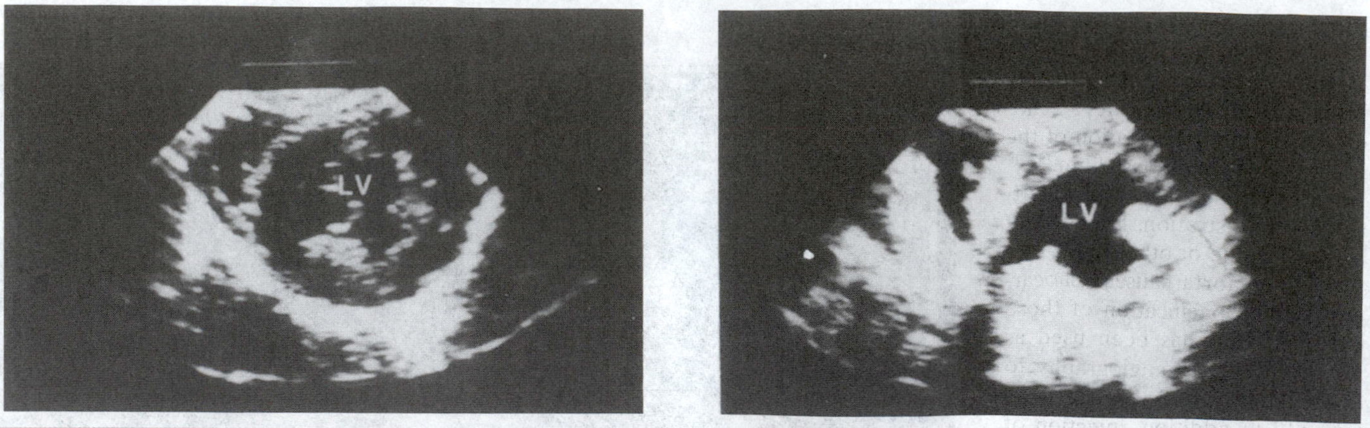

FIGURE 13-56 Short-axis plane through the left ventricle (LV) before (*left*) and after (*right*) injection of microbubbles into the aortic root. The myocardium is densely opacified on the right. (From Hagan AD, DeMaria AN. *Clinical Applications of Two-Dimensional Echocardiography and Cardiac Doppler*. Boston: Little, Brown; 1989, with permission.)

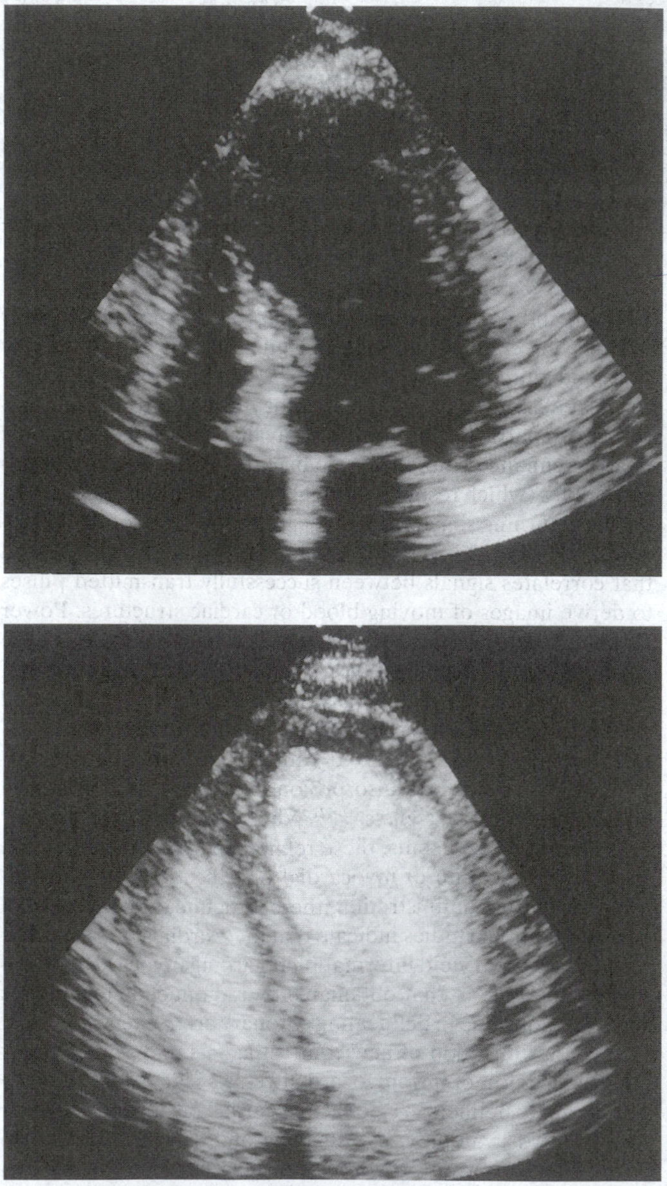

FIGURE 13-57 Harmonic imaging with second-generation echocardiographic contrast. Endocardial border definition before injection is fair (*upper panel*) but is markedly improved with harmonic imaging following contrast injection (*lower panel*).

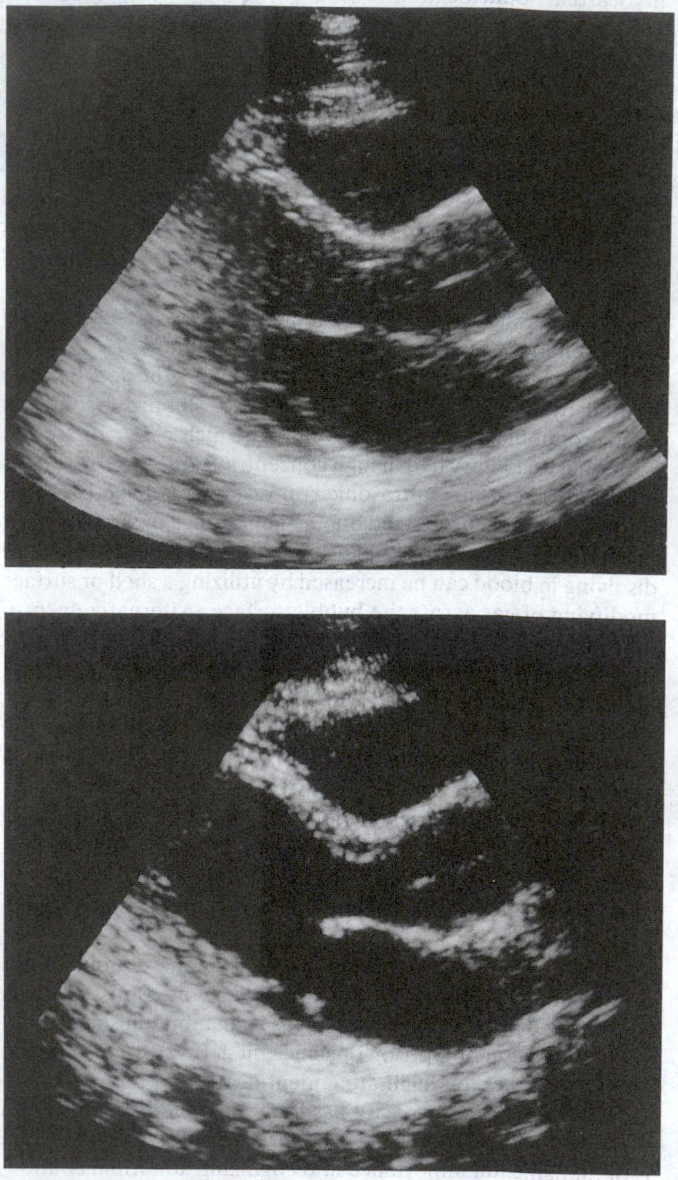

A

FIGURE 13-58A Tissue harmonic imaging. The upper panel shows a parasternal long-exis new figure view obtained with standard (fundamental) imaging. Endocardial definition is poor, but is markedly enhanced with tissue harmonic imaging (*lower panel*).

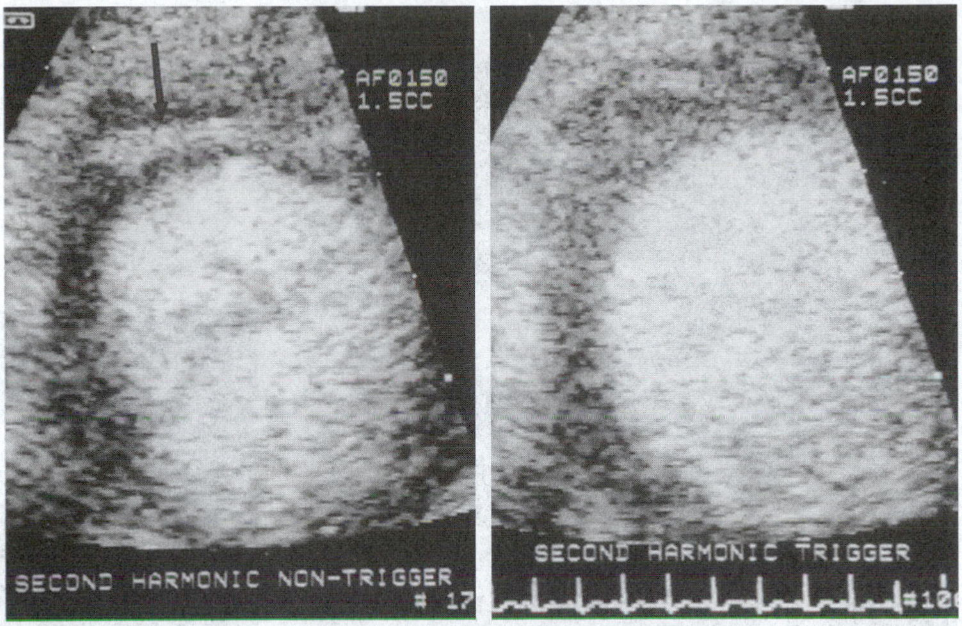

B

FIGURE 13-58B Transthoracic short-axis views (with second-harmonic imaging) after intravenous injection of a second-generation echocardiography contrast agent. Imaging was continuous on the left and gated ("triggered") on the right. With continuous imaging, an intramyocardial vessel (*arrow*) is visualized.

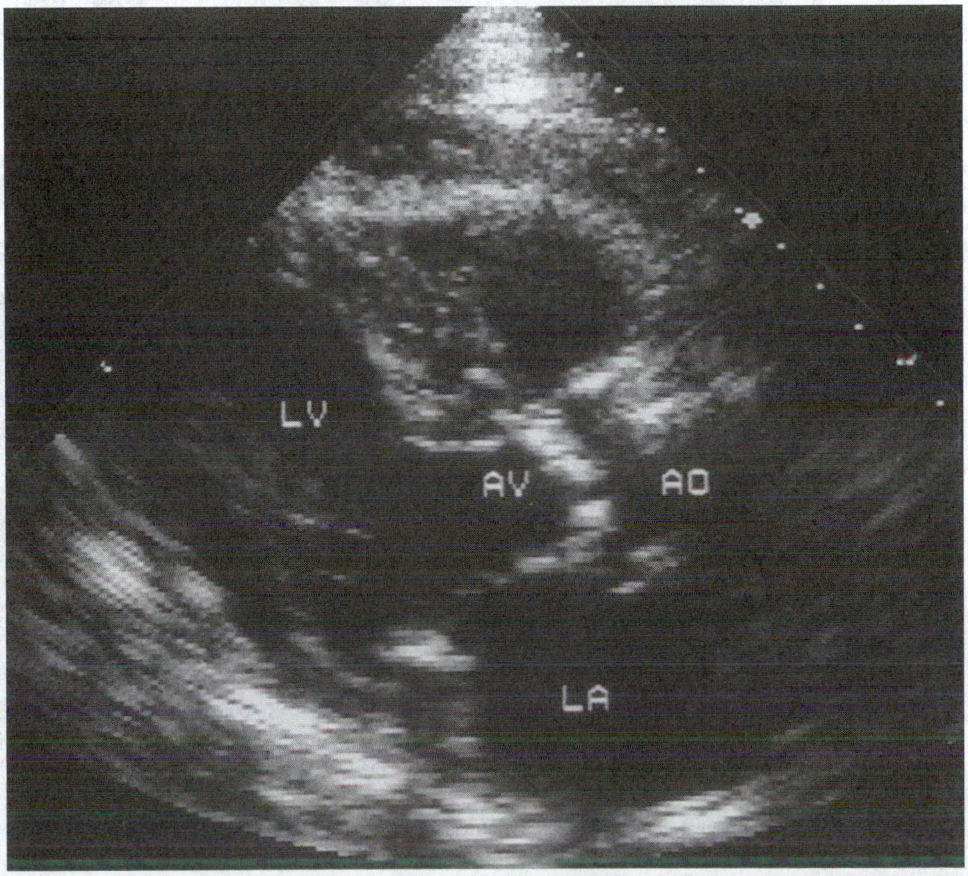

FIGURE 13-59 Parasternal long-axis plane demonstrating a thickened, stenotic aortic valve (AV). AO = aorta; LV = left ventricle; LA = left atrium.

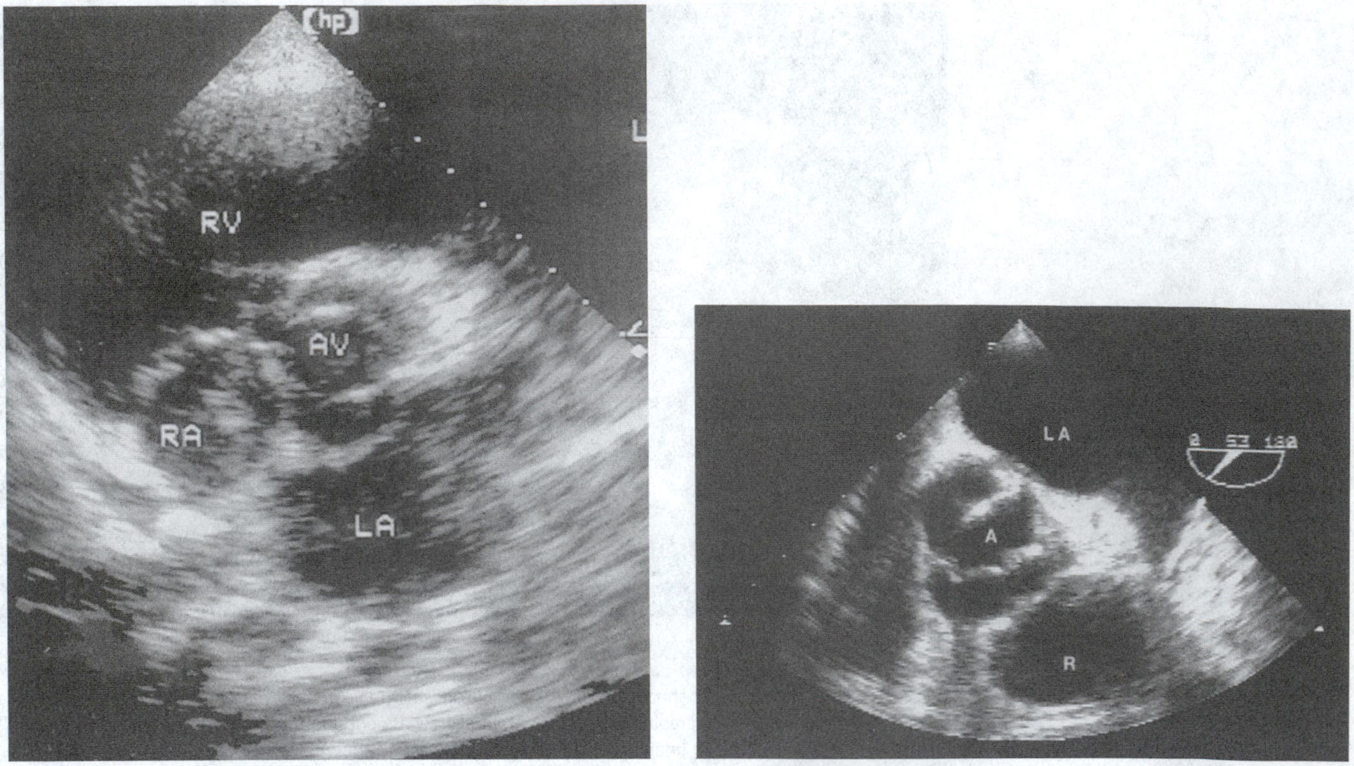

A

B

FIGURE 13-60 *A*. Parasternal short-axis image of a bicuspid aortic valve (AV) during systole. RV = right ventricle; RA = right atrium; LA = left atrium. *B*. Transesophageal image of a bicuspid aortic valve (A). LA = left atrium, R = right ventricular outflow tract. (From Blanchard DG, Kimura BJ, Dittrich HC, DeMaria AN. Transesophageal echocardiography of the aorta. *JAMA* 1994; 272:546–551, with permission.)

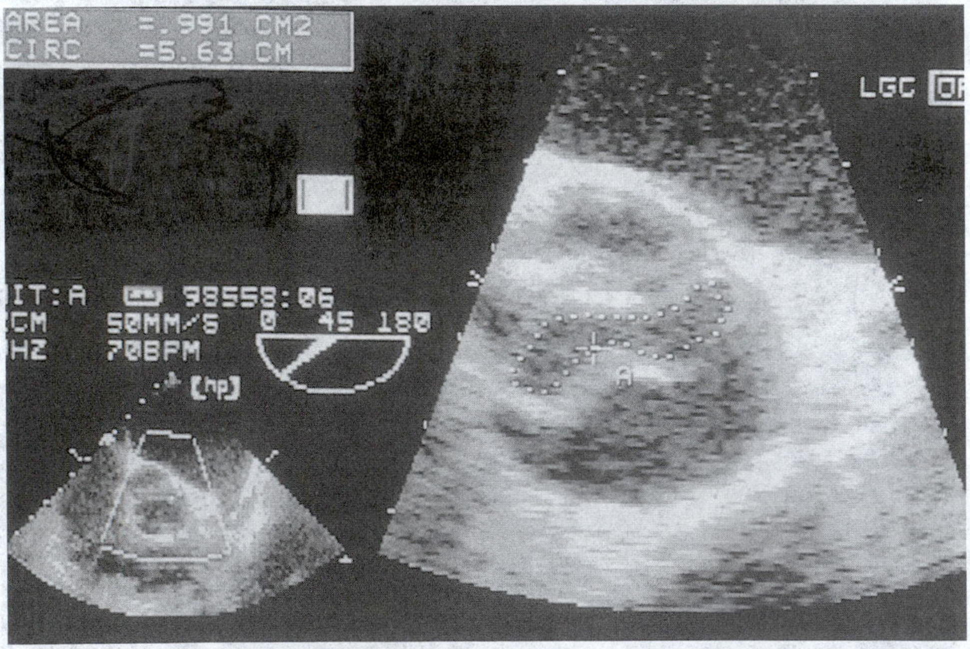

FIGURE 13-61 Transesophageal image of a stenotic bicuspid aortic valve (*A*) with superimposed planimetry of the valve area (approximately 1 cm^2).

ultrasonic backscatter from contrast microbubbles (which resonate in an ultrasonic field) while decreasing the returning signal from myocardium (which does not resonate)[217–219] (Fig. 13-57). Early after contrast injection, second-harmonic imaging increases the cavity-to-myocardium contrast intensity ratio, improving visualization of the left ventricular cavity. Second-harmonic imaging may also enhance the myocardial contrast phase, which follows LV cavity opacification with second-generation contrast agents.[217–219] As exposure to ultrasound energy can produce microbubble destruction, intermittent rather than continuous ultrasound transmission can also prolong microbubble persistence and amplify contrast signals.[220,221,210b] In recent years, harmonic imaging has been used to visualize cardiac structures in the absence of contrast injection. This tissue harmonic imaging decreases clutter and other artifacts, often improving endocardial definition (Fig. 13-58*A*).

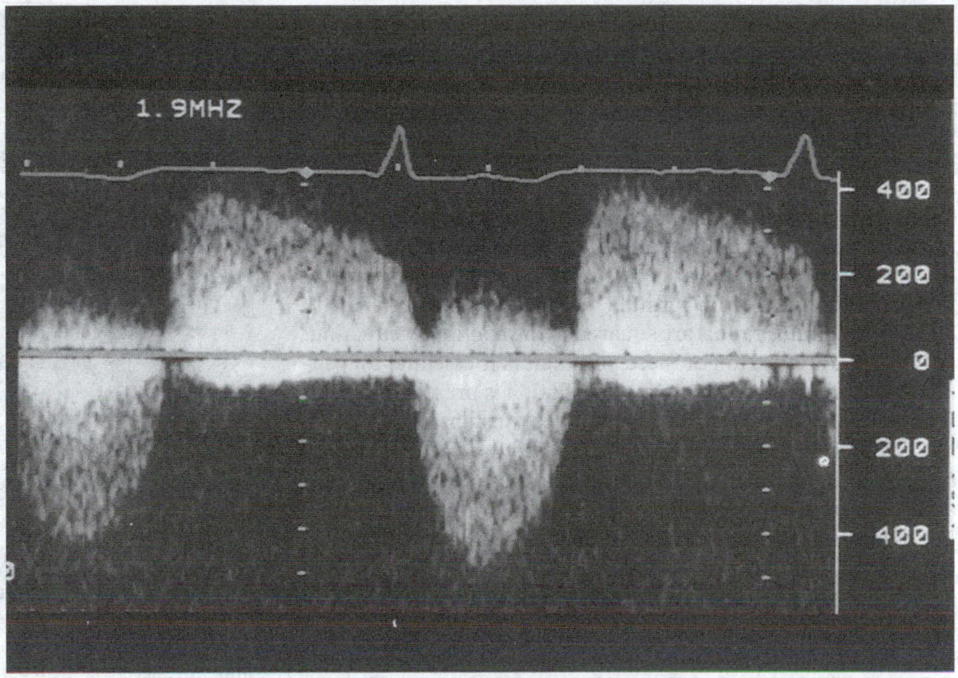

FIGURE 13-62 Continuous-wave Doppler tracing (from the apical transducer position) through the aortic valve in a case of combined aortic stenosis and insufficiency. The peak systolic velocity approaches 5 m/s.

DISEASES OF THE AORTIC VALVE AND AORTA

Aortic Stenosis

The aortic valve is best imaged in the parasternal views.[222] The leaflets are thin, linear structures. All three can be visualized in the short-axis view and produce a triangular orifice during systolic opening. The long-axis view exhibits the right and usually the noncoronary leaflets, which normally open to the walls of the aorta. Mild thickening and reduction of mobility is often observed in the elderly (aortic sclerosis) and is associated with an increased risk of CAD. In older adults, acquired aortic stenosis (AS) is manifested by markedly thickened, often calcified, immobile aortic valve leaflets,[223] while doming of the leaflets suggests congenital aortic stenosis and is usually encountered in younger patients (Fig. 13-59).[224] Echocardiography can distinguish valvular from sub- and supravalvular AS, can accurately identify bicuspid valves, and can delineate the presence of LV hypertrophy.[225,226] Subaortic stenosis may be caused by asymmetrical septal hypertrophy with systolic anterior mitral motion, a subaortic membrane, or (less commonly) a subaortic tunnel. Bicuspid valves exhibit an oval rather than triangular orifice (Fig. 13-60). Although the severity of stenosis can be assessed semiquantitatively by 2D and M-mode image echocardiography, valvular calcification may shadow the leaflets or produce reverberations and obscure their motion.[223] Therefore, attempts to measure valve area by transthoracic planimetry have been unsuccessful, although multiplane TEE has been of greater value[155] (Fig. 13-61). Thus, 2D-echocardiographic imaging accurately detects the presence and etiology of AS but not the severity. Likewise, CFD demonstrates turbulent flow through the aortic valve and may guide continuous wave interrogation but provides little quantitative data.[227] The use of Doppler echocardiography and the modified Bernoulli and continuity equations have now made noninvasive calculation of aortic gradients and valve area routine and have affected utilization of cardiac catheterization in AS patients.[228] (See also Chap. 56).

The cornerstone of the ultrasound evaluation of AS is CW Doppler interrogation through the aortic valve. The calculated gradient using the peak Doppler velocity [4(AS velocity)^2] correlates closely with the peak instantaneous gradient measured at catheterization[117–119] (Fig. 13-62). In interpreting echocardiographic studies, it is important to distinguish between the peak instantaneous pressure gradient, the mean gradient, and the peak-to-peak gradient. The first two physiologic parameters represent simultaneous pressure differences between LV and aorta and can be measured accurately by Doppler echocardiography. The *peak-to-peak gradient,* commonly used in the catheterization laboratory, compares the highest pressures reached in the LV and aorta (even though not simultaneous) and is uniformly lower than the peak instantaneous gradient recorded by Doppler. Therefore, the maximal Doppler gradient does not correlate with the peak-to-peak catheterization gradient, and comparisons between the two should be avoided (Chap. 56).

A number of potential sources of error exist in the estimation of the transvalvular aortic gradient by CW Doppler recordings. It is imperative that Doppler signals from the stenotic jet be obtained with an angle of incidence of less than 20 degrees. Since the direction of the jet rarely can be known with precision from 2D techniques, each examination must employ all possible windows and angulations, including apical, parasternal, and suprasternal transducer positions. Also, one must be careful to account for the proximal flow velocity in the Bernoulli equation if it is 1.5 m/s or greater. Finally, since some degree of pressure recovery occurs distal to the aortic valve leaflets, it is important to record continuous wave signals as close to these structures as possible.

Values for aortic valve area can be calculated using the continuity equation by measuring the velocity of the jet across the aortic valve with CW Doppler, the velocity in the LV outflow tract just proximal to the valve with PW Doppler, and by deriving the area of the outflow tract from the diameter of the aortic annulus. Results from the continuity equation have been found to correlate well with the area calculations based on catheterization data and the Gorlin formula.[111–115] As both AS jet velocity and aortic annulus radius are squared in the continuity equation, accurate determination of these parameters is essential for reliable measurements. When atrial fibrillation is present, the peak Doppler velocity still correlates with peak instantaneous gradient through the aortic valve, but *calculations of valve area may be problematic*, as the outflow tract and peak aortic velocities are not measured simultaneously.

In summary, a comprehensive echocardiographic examination in a patient with AS should establish both the presence and severity of disease. Echocardiographic imaging should identify the structural abnormality involving either the subvalvular, valvular, or supravalvular area; distinguish congenital from acquired etiologies; and evaluate the state of LV hypertrophy and function. CW Doppler recordings should provide accurate measurements of instantaneous and mean transaortic valvular gradients, and the continuity equation should provide reliable estimates of aortic valve area. In cases where the relative roles of orifice stenosis and LV dysfunction are uncertain, TEE imaging or Doppler recordings during inotropic stimulation with dobutamine may be of value.[155,229] Cardiac catheterization is still necessary for the delineation of coronary anatomy.

Aortic Regurgitation

In contrast to AS, the aortic valve leaflets are often anatomically normal by echocardiography in patients with aortic regurgitation (AR).[230,231] 2D and M-mode echocardiography often provide indirect evidence of the presence of AR, including signs of LV volume overload, diastolic fluttering of the anterior mitral valve leaflet, aortic root enlargement, and incomplete coaptation of the aortic valve leaflets.[232,233] The important M-mode finding of premature diastolic closure of the mitral valve prior to the onset of systole due to LV filling by the regurgitant jet signifies acute, severe AR[234] (Fig. 13-63) and the need for surgery (Chap. 56).

Perhaps the most important contribution of echocardiographic tissue imaging to the assessment of AR is in identifying the etiology.[235] Thus, thickened leaflets that are restricted in movement are observed in patients with acquired AS, while oval doming of two functional leaflets will be observed in the presence of a bicuspid aortic valve (Fig. 13-60). AR due to infectious endocarditis can be identified by the presence of valvular vegetations, while regurgitation due to diseases of the aorta are manifest by anatomic changes of the vessel. Less common etiologies of AR, such as those associated with subvalvular pathology or ventricular septal defect, may also be recognized by echocardiographic imaging.

Although the findings yielded by echocardiographic imaging are useful, Doppler interrogation is necessary to obtain direct evidence of the presence and severity of AR. Screening with

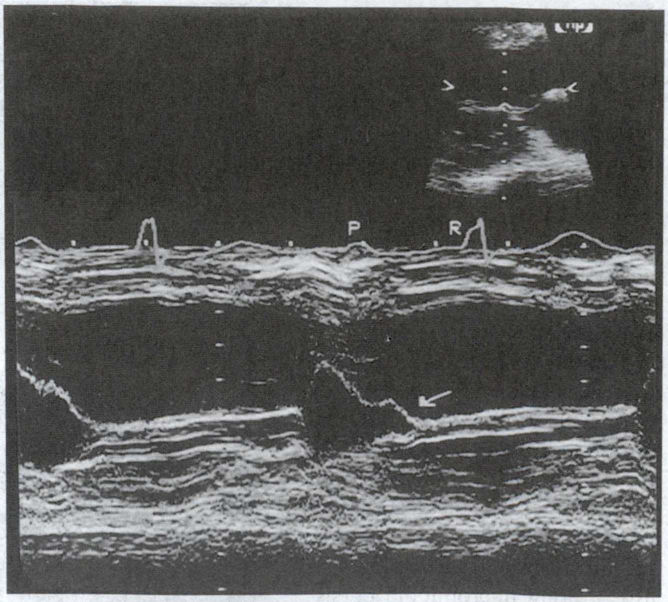

FIGURE 13-63 M-mode tracing (from the parasternal position) in a patient with acute severe aortic regurgitation. The mitral valve leaflets close (*arrow*) before ventricular contraction begins. P = p wave, R = QRS complex.

CFD demonstrates turbulent flow in the LV outflow tract during diastole in virtually all views[236] (Fig. 13-64*A*, *B*, and *C*, Plate 60). The jet is typically elliptical and may be located anywhere in the LV outflow tract. CW Doppler spectral recordings from this jet yield a high-velocity diastolic signal directed toward the apex[237] (Fig. 13-62). Since AR jet velocity accurately reflects the diastolic pressure gradient between aorta and LV, it is maximum at the point of valve closure and decreases throughout diastole.[238] The flow pattern of AR may be readily distinguished from mitral inflow in that it is higher in velocity, begins immediately after aortic valve closure, generally has a much slower deceleration, and does not have an increased velocity following atrial contraction.

Several approaches exist for the quantitation of AR by echocardiography. Conventional echocardiographic imaging can provide evidence of the presence and extent of LV volume overload. More direct evidence of the severity of AR can be derived from the deceleration rate of the jet recorded by CW Doppler (Fig. 13-65).[237–240] In the presence of mild degrees of AR, the transvalvular pressure gradient will be maintained throughout diastole, creating a high-velocity jet with a minimal deceleration rate. Conversely, severe AR reduces aortic pressures and increases LV pressures in diastole, eliminating the pressure gradient and creating a rapid jet deceleration to a low velocity (Fig. 13-65). Severe, acute AR can also cause diastolic MR (Fig. 13-64*C*, Plate 60). The most common approach to assessing the deceleration rate of the AR jet is by calculating the time required for the velocity to fall to one-half of the maximal pressure equivalent, a technique similar to the pressure half-time measurements performed in the quantitation of mitral stenosis (MS). Previous studies have demonstrated that a pressure half-time of less than 250 ms reliably identifies patients with severe degrees of aortic regurgitation as assessed by invasive methods.[240] Application of the pressure half-time approach to

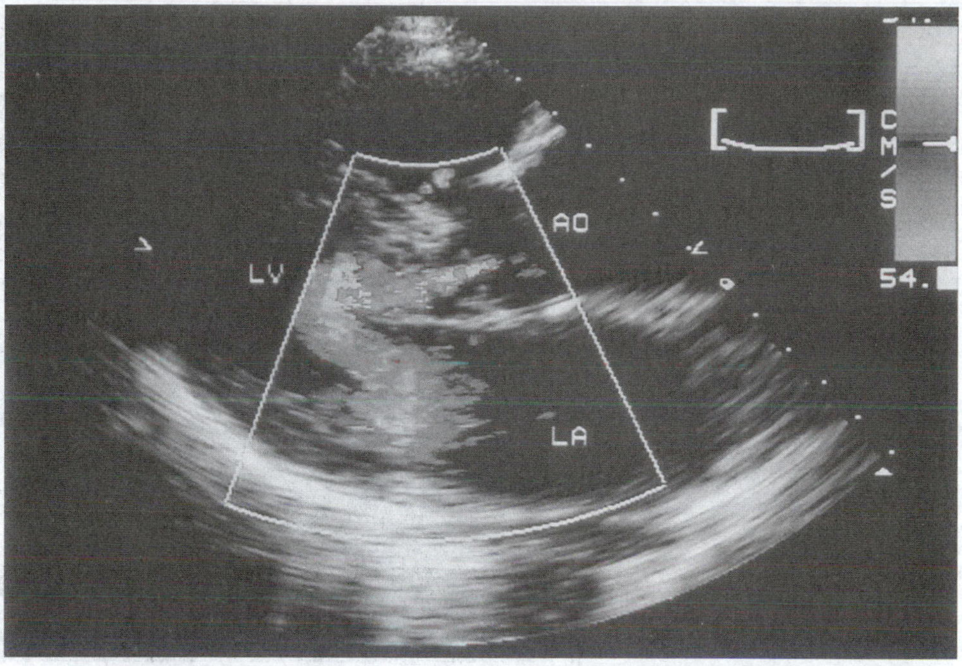

A

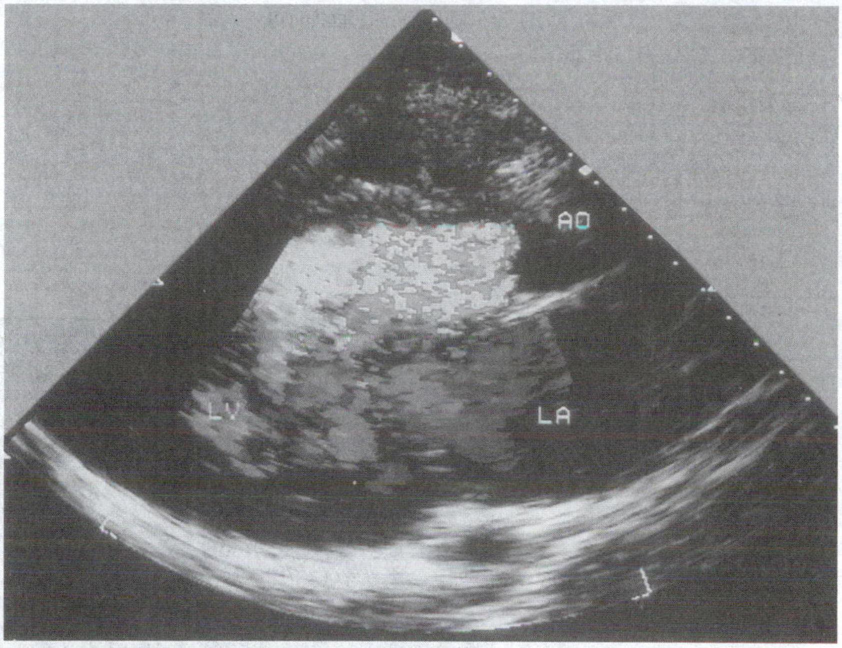

B

FIGURE 13-64 (Plate 60) *A*. Parasternal long-axis plane showing a multicolor jet (indicating turbulent flow) of aortic regurgitation in the left ventricular outflow tract. The jet is narrow in width, suggesting mild regurgitation. AO = aorta; LA = left atrium; LV = left ventricle. *B*. Parasternal long-axis plane with color-flow Doppler imaging. The aortic regurgitant (AR) color jet is as wide as the left ventricular outflow tract, suggesting severe AR. AO = aorta; LA = left atrium; LV = left ventricle. *C*. Parasternal long-axis image of acute severe aortic insufficiency (AI). The accompanying marked elevation of left ventricular (LV) diastolic pressure causes diastolic mitral regurgitation (MR). AO = aorta; LA = left atrium.

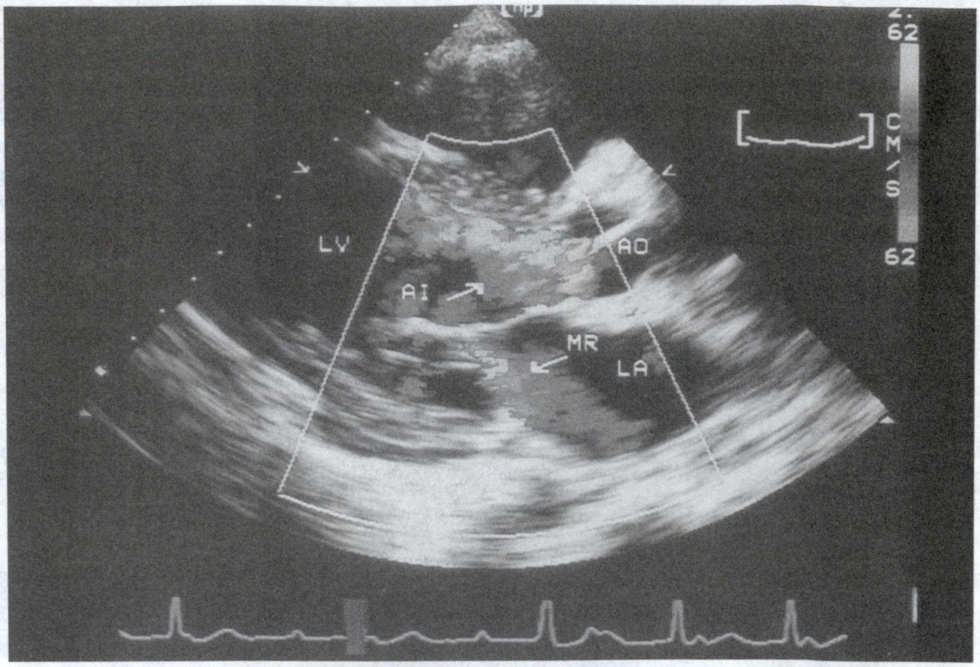

C

FIGURE 13-64 (*Continued*)

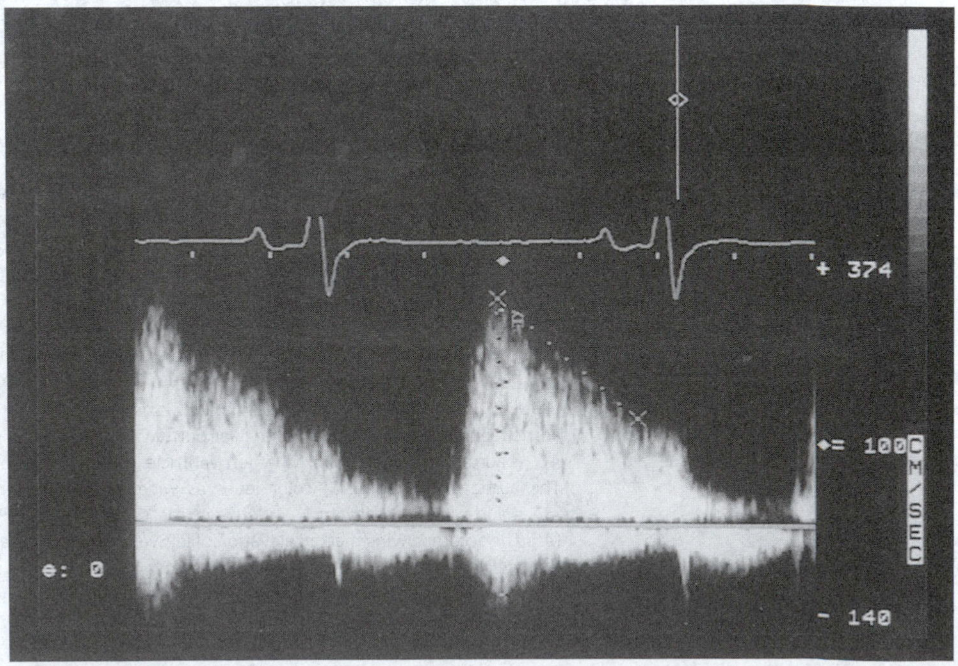

FIGURE 13-65 Continuous-wave Doppler tracing (from the apical transducer position) of severe AR. The pressure half-time of the AR envelope is approximately 200 ms.

quantifying AR must take into account that, since the deceleration rate is a reflection of pressure gradient, it is determined by both the volume of AR and the compliance of the left ventricle. Accordingly, ventricles that vary greatly in stiffness or distensibility will yield different AR deceleration rates for the same regurgitant volume.

The estimate of severity most commonly derived from echocardiography is the size of the AR jet by CFD.[236] Conceptually, jets that are distributed over a small area of the LV outflow tract represent lesser degrees of AR than jets that penetrate widely and to the level of the papillary muscles. Some studies have demonstrated a general correlation between jet length and severity of AR.[241] The optimal results have been obtained when the width of the AR jet just proximal to the valve was expressed as a percentage of the width of the LV outflow tract; a jet occupying 50 percent or more of the outflow tract correlates with severe regurgitation by angiography.[236] Quantitation of AR based upon the size of the flow disturbance is subject to errors induced by the other factors that influence jet area: transvalvular pressure gradient, volume and compliance of the receiving chamber, regurgitant orifice, the Coanda effect (wall effect), and technical factors relating to the operator and instrument settings. In addition, entrainment and displacement of RBCs in the LV outflow tract also influence the size of the regurgitant jet. Finally, convergence of AR with normal transmitral filling may obscure the flow disturbance. Therefore, assessment of the severity of AR by analysis of the size and shape of the flow disturbance *is at best semiquantitative.*

The AR volume can be estimated by comparing volumetric measurements of LV inflow and LV outflow calculated from annular velocity and cross-sectional area (derived from pulsed Doppler and 2D images respectively).[110] This method is contingent upon the absence of valvular stenosis and of other regurgitant lesions. In the setting of AR, the volume ejected through the aortic annulus represents both systemic flow and regurgitant volume, while the volume coursing through the mitral annulus represents only systemic flow. Thereby, LV outflow will exceed LV inflow by the amount of the regurgitant volume.[110,242–244] This technique can provide useful estimates of regurgitant volume, but with any flow volume calculation by echocardiography, errors in technique and the assumptions involved in volume calculation can result in significant errors. An alternate *quantitative approach* derives estimates of regurgitant fraction from reverse diastolic flow in the aorta.[245] Assuming a constant cross-sectional aortic area, comparison of integrated flow velocities during forward systolic flow and retrograde diastolic flow should yield an estimate of regurgitant fraction. Although this is somewhat imprecise, the presence of a significant flow reversal in the aorta visualized by color or spectral Doppler is a reliable marker of severe AR (Fig. 13-66).

Determination of the optimal timing of surgical intervention in patients with AR remains a difficult problem in clinical medicine (see also Chap. 56). Several criteria derived from echocardiographic recordings have been proposed to guide this decision.[246–249] Most prominently, an LV end-systolic dimension of 55 mm or greater with a shortening fraction of 25 percent or less have been advocated as sufficient criteria for surgical intervention in the absence of symptoms.[250] Considerable debate continues regarding this issue, however, and no universally accepted echocardiographic criteria exist by which to determine the optimal role for surgical treatment.

Diseases of the Aorta

The thoracic aorta is best visualized from the left and right parasternal positions and from the suprasternal notch.[251] The descending aorta may also be imaged from subcostal and modified apical views. Normally, short-axis images of the aortic root yield a circular structure, while long-axis images exhibit two parallel linear walls with a maximal diameter of 35 mm.[252] Although 2D imaging is used most commonly, M-mode recordings of the aortic root facilitate precise measurement of its dimensions.

AORTIC DISSECTION

In recent years, 2D echocardiography has dramatically changed the diagnostic approach to aortic dissection. TTE is a convenient screening test (Fig. 13-67) and often enables accurate detection of ascending aortic dissection.[253] The diagnostic findings include a dilated aorta with a mobile intimal flap that presents as a thin, linear signal within the lumen. Transthoracic imaging is unreliable for detection of descending aortic dissection,[254] although it occasionally visualizes the complete length of the thoracic aorta (see also Chap. 88).

Although several noninvasive methods exist to diagnose aortic dissection, TEE has become the procedure of choice in many hospitals because of its accuracy, portability, rapid procedural time, and ability to provide data regarding valvular regurgitation and LV function.[139,158,255–257] Except for *a short portion of the proximal aortic arch,* which is obscured by the bronchus, multiplane TEE provides excellent visualization of the entire thoracic aorta and high accuracy in detecting aortic enlargement, intimal tears, and false lumen thrombus (Fig. 13-68). CFD may reveal communications between true and false channels (Fig. 13-51, Plate 59; Fig. 13-69, Plate 61). TEE also appears useful for the diagnosis of aortic intramural hematoma, an increasingly recognized disorder which has a clinical prognosis similar to that of classic dissection.[258,259]

AORTIC ANEURYSM

Aneurysms of the aorta may be saccular or fusiform and are recognized as localized or circumferential areas of aortic enlargement, often with thin walls. TTE is especially useful in detecting ascending aortic dilatation but can also visualize descending thoracic and abdominal aortic aneurysms.[252,260] Echocardiography has been used extensively to assess aortic pathology in patients with Marfan syndrome.[261] The nature of the lesion is relatively specific in that there is symmetrical dilatation of the annulus, sinuses of Valsalva, and aortic root (Fig. 13-70, Plate 62). Aortic leaflet coaptation may be compromised leading to AR. Echocardiography is helpful in determining prognosis and optimal timing of aortic root replacement.[262–264]

Sinus of Valsalva aneurysms are also well visualized by both TTE and TEE.[265,266] These lesions cause asymmetrical dilatation of the aortic root and seem to affect the right coronary sinus most frequently. They are prone to rupture, often into the right heart[267] (Fig. 13-70*A*). Doppler echocardiography in such settings demonstrates fluttering of the tricuspid valve, a color jet crossing from the aortic root into the right heart, and occasionally diastolic opening of the pulmonic valve.

Congenital aortic disease, such as supravalvular aortic stenosis (SAS), aortic coarctation, patent ductus arteriosus, and truncus arteriosus also can be detected with echocardiography (see

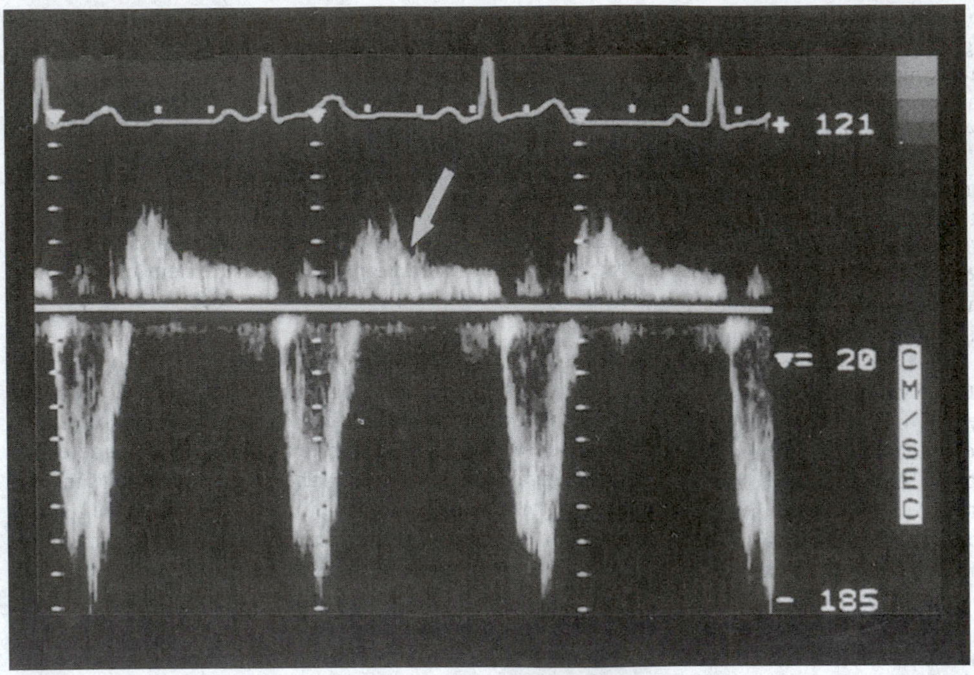

FIGURE 13-66 Pulsed-wave Doppler tracing (from the suprasternal transducer position) in a case of severe aortic regurgitation. The sample volume is in the descending thoracic aorta, and holodiastolic flow reversal (*arrow*) is present.

Chaps. 63 and 64).[225,268] In these conditions, suprasternal and transesophageal imaging are often helpful. SAS is recognized as an "hourglass" narrowing just distal to the leaflets, while coarctation presents a more localized, abrupt luminal reduction in the descending aorta. Patent ductus arteriosus and truncus arteriosis are often best identified by virtue of the accompanying flow disturbance on CFD.[269,270]

AORTIC ATHEROSCLEROSIS

As mentioned in the section on TEE, recent studies suggest that aortic atherosclerosis is an important cause of stroke and embolic events.[167,168] Mobile and protruding intimal plaques have been detected by TEE (Fig. 13-53) in patients with stroke with a prevalence greater than in controls, a finding not previously appreciated by other imaging techniques.[271] Optimal treatment for extensive aortic atherosclerosis is currently unknown; although warfarin appears useful.[171b] It appears that detection of large aortic arch plaques prior to cardiopulmonary bypass should prompt adjustment of cannula placement to avoid dislodging the aortic debris.[272]

Penetrating aortic ulceration, which affects the descending aorta and mimics the clinical syndrome of acute aortic dissection, may also be diagnosed by TEE (Fig. 13-71, Plate 63).[273,273a] The diagnosis is based upon visualization of a localized defect with protrusion of the ulcer into the vessel wall (in the absence of dissection). This disease entity, which occurs in the setting of atherosclerosis, warrants urgent surgery to avoid aortic rupture. Aortic tears induced by trauma are also accurately detected by TEE[273b,273c] (Fig. 13-72).

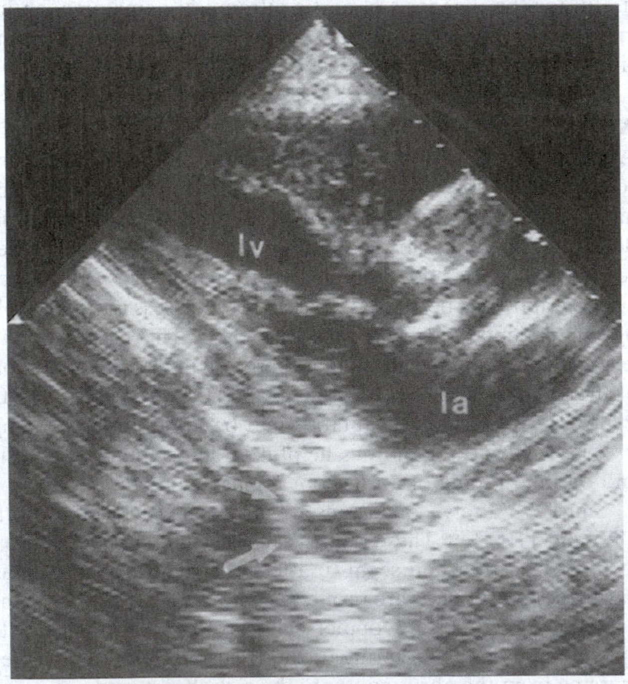

FIGURE 13-67 Transthoracic parasternal long-axis plane demonstrating a dissection of the descending thoracic aorta. The aortic root is dilated, the aortic valve is thickened, and an intimal flap is present in the descending aorta (*arrows*). LV = left ventricle; LA = left atrium.

DISEASES OF THE MITRAL VALVE

Mitral Stenosis

Detection of *mitral stenosis* (MS) was one of the earliest clinical applications of echocardiography[274] (see Chap. 57). In most individuals, the mitral valve leaflets are easily visualized and yield thin linear echoes that exhibit wide bipeaked excursions as they open in early and late diastole.[24] The characteristic 2D ultrasound findings of MS are seen clearly in nearly all patients with this disorder.[275] The mitral valve leaflets are thickened and often present bright high-intensity reflections indicating calcification. The process may involve thickening and shortening of the chordal apparatus as well. There are varying degrees of commissural fusion restricting mitral leaflet separation, especially at the distal tips.[276,277] This leads to diastolic "doming" or a right-angle bend of the anterior mitral valve leaflet, as high LA pressure creates a bulge in the leaflet's midportion (which

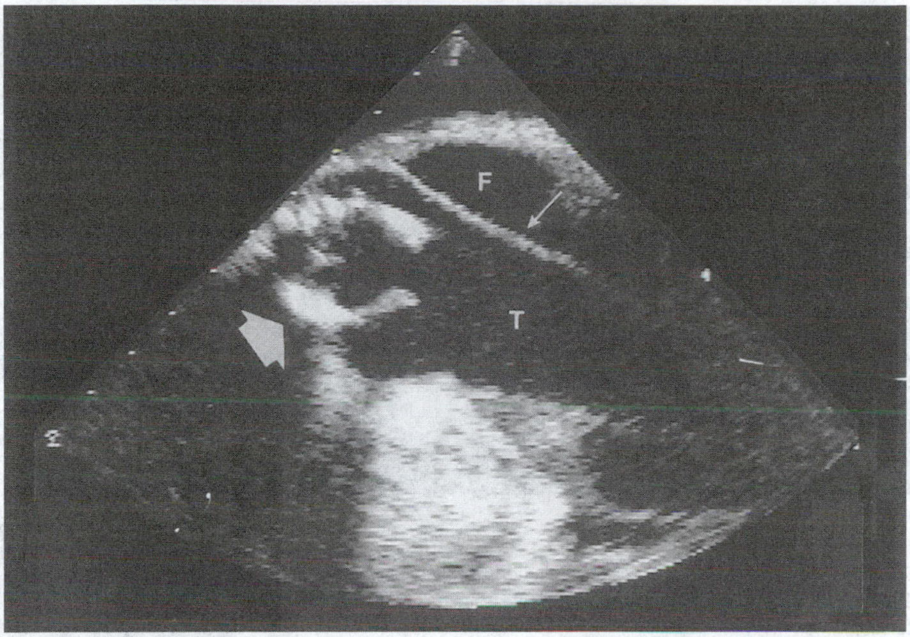

FIGURE 13-68 Longitudinal TEE view of an ascending aortic dissection in a patient with a porcine prosthetic valve in the aortic position (*large arrow*). The false (F) and true (T) lumens are separated by an intimal flap (*small arrow*). (From Blanchard DG, Kimura BJ, Dittrich HC, DeMaria AN. Transesophageal echocardiography of the aorta. *JAMA* 1994; 272:546–551, with permission.)

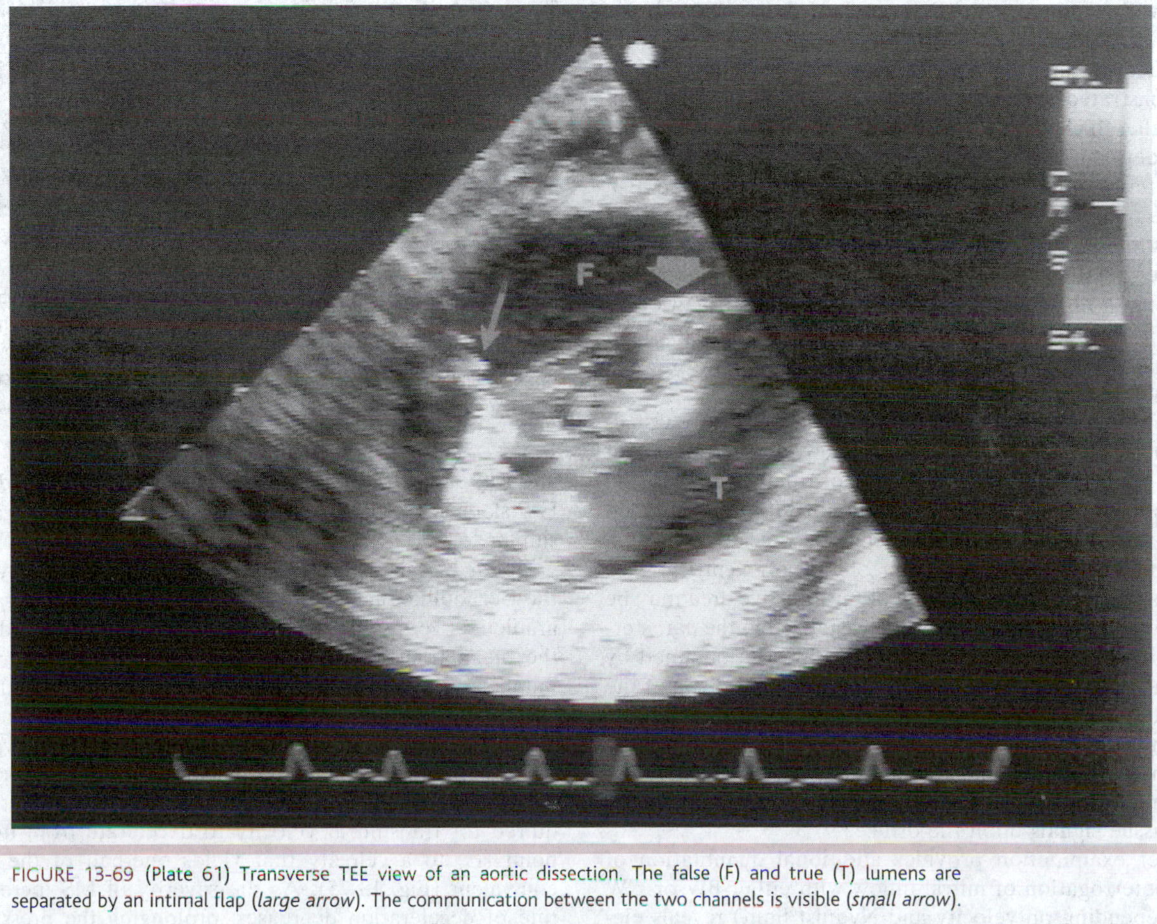

FIGURE 13-69 (Plate 61) Transverse TEE view of an aortic dissection. The false (F) and true (T) lumens are separated by an intimal flap (*large arrow*). The communication between the two channels is visible (*small arrow*).

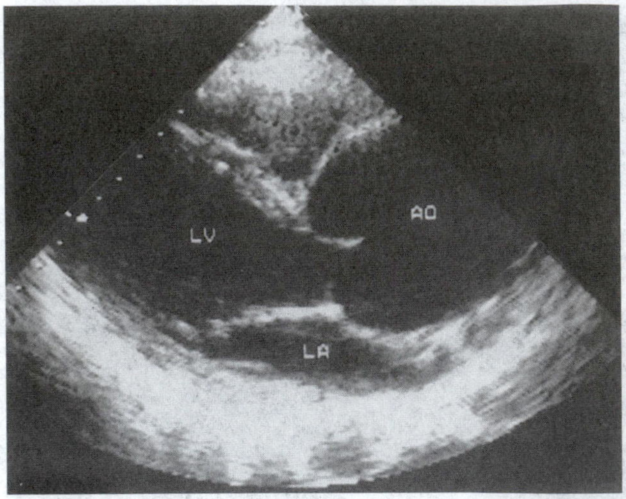

A

FIGURE 13-70A Parasternal long-axis plane demonstrating severe aortic root (AO) enlargement. LV = left ventricle; LA = left atrium. (Courtesy of Kirk L. Peterson, MD.)

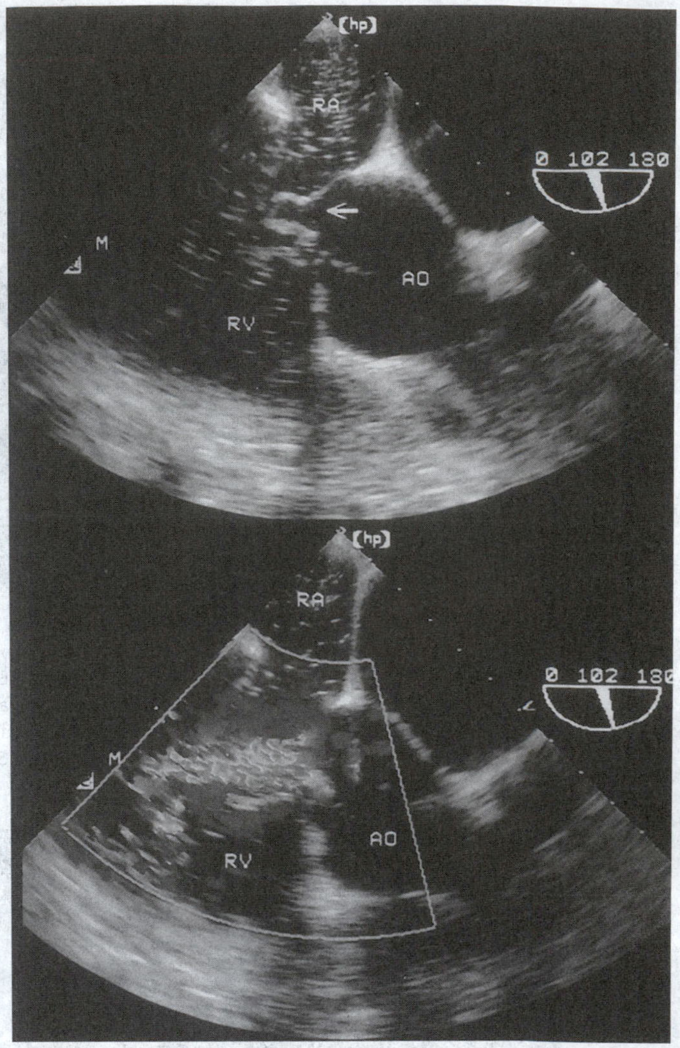

B

FIGURE 13-70B (Plate 62) TEE image of a ruptured sinus of Valsalva aneurysm. The upper image shows focal aneurysmal dilatation of the right coronary sinus with the appearance of a "windsock." Color Doppler (*lower image*) reveals a high-velocity flow jet from the aorta into the right ventricle. Agitated saline was injected intravenously to highlight right heart structures.

is generally more pliable than the distal portion) (Fig. 13-73). The posterior leaflet actually may be pulled anteriorly during diastole because of commissural fusion with the longer anterior leaflet.[278] Mitral doming may also occur in congenital valvular disease, but it is not seen when mitral leaflet opening is reduced due to low-flow states[32] or AR jets. The LA is nearly always enlarged with MS.

The effects of stenosis upon mitral valve motion are often best demonstrated by M-mode recordings (Fig. 13-74). In addition to leaflet thickening and reduced excursion, M-mode tracings also depict a characteristic decrease in the reclosure rate of the anterior mitral leaflet in early diastole (reduced E-F slope) due to a persistent LA-LV pressure gradient and a slow rate of LV filling.[276-279] The decrease of the E-F slope has been found to correlate grossly with the severity of mitral stenosis. This finding is not specific for MS, however, and may occur whenever early diastolic filling is reduced.[24,280] Attempts to calculate mitral valve orifice area using the E-F slope have proved unsatisfactory.[281]

The entire perimeter of the mitral valve orifice can be visualized in the 2D parasternal short-axis view, and mitral leaflet excursion normally approaches the endocardial borders of the LV at the mitral tip level. In the setting of MS, the thickened leaflets form a fish-mouth orifice, which occupies only a small portion of the cross-sectional area of the left ventricle (see also Chap. 57).[275,282] Measurements of mitral valve area may be obtained by planimetry of the orifice visualized in the parasternal short-axis view and correlate well with those obtained by cardiac catheterization (Fig. 13-73).[282-284] Since the shape of the mitral valve resembles a funnel, it is crucial to identify the smallest cross-sectional area and obtain recordings with orthogonal beam orientation at that point in order to avoid overestimation. Optimal gain settings must be employed to avoid encroachment of tissue signals upon the orifice.[285]

Doppler examination provides additional quantitation of MS.[286,287] Interrogation of mitral inflow with either PW or CW modes (depending on velocity and Nyquist limit) reveals elevated diastolic velocities, with a reduction in the rate of deceleration in early diastole yielding a pattern similar to decreased E-F slope seen with M-mode in MS (Fig. 13-75). In a fashion similar to that of AS, the maximal gradient across the mitral valve can be calculated from the peak diastolic velocity utilizing the Bernoulli equation.[286,288] But since the maximal transmitral gradient is very sensitive to changes in heart rate and loading, the mean transmitral gradient obtained as the average of a number of individual gradients derived throughout diastole is customarily utilized to assess the severity of MS.[288] In addition, Doppler technique may provide estimates of mitral valve area (MVA) by means of the calculation of the pressure half-time.[284,287] The pressure half-time represents the interval required for transmitral velocity to decelerate from its highest point (E) to a velocity that yields one-half of the pressure equivalent (Fig. 13-75). As the severity of MS increases, the rate of deceleration decreases, prolonging the pressure half-time. Further, dividing an empiric constant of 220[289] by the

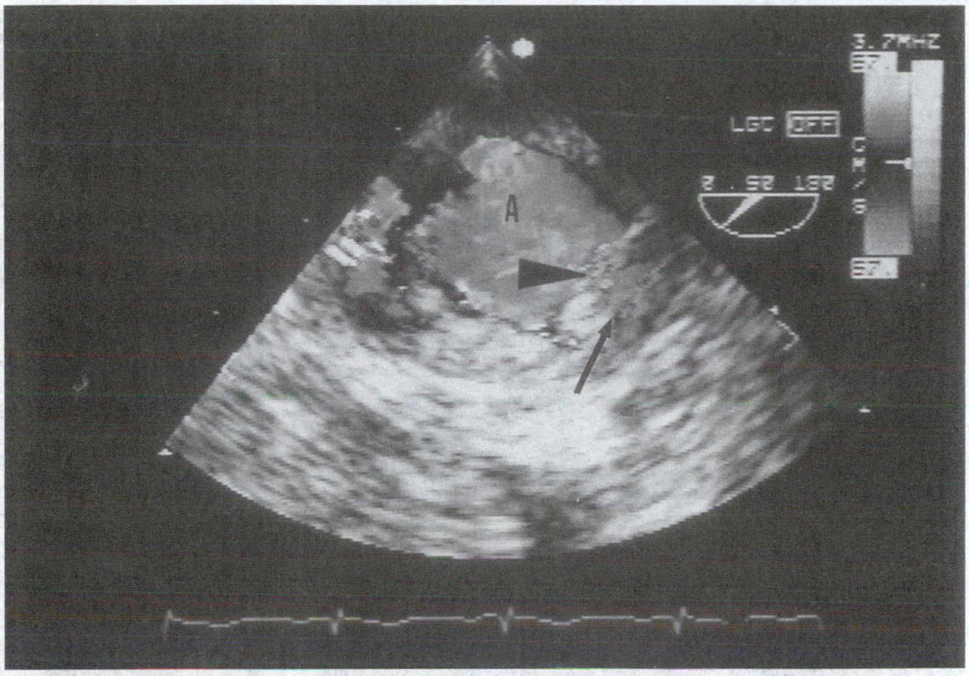

FIGURE 13-71 (Plate 63) Transverse TEE view of penetrating ulceration in the proximal portion of the descending aorta (A). The mouth of the ulcer crater is visible (*large arrowhead*), as is blood flow within the atheroma (*arrow*).

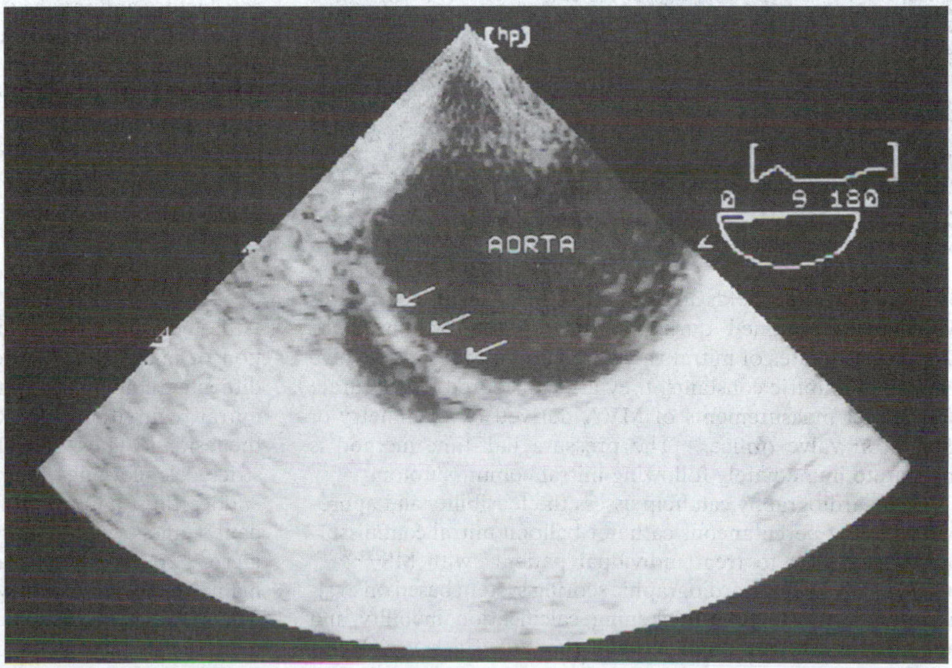

FIGURE 13-72 Transverse TEE image of traumatic aortic disruption and partial transection (*arrows*) involving the distal portion of the aortic arch.

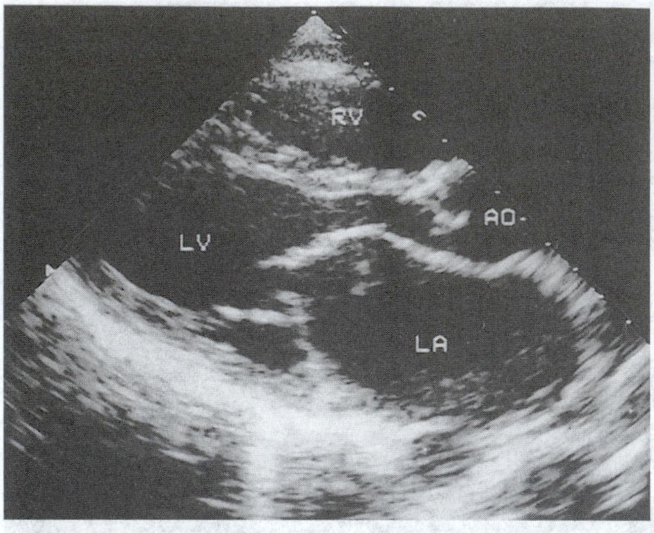

A

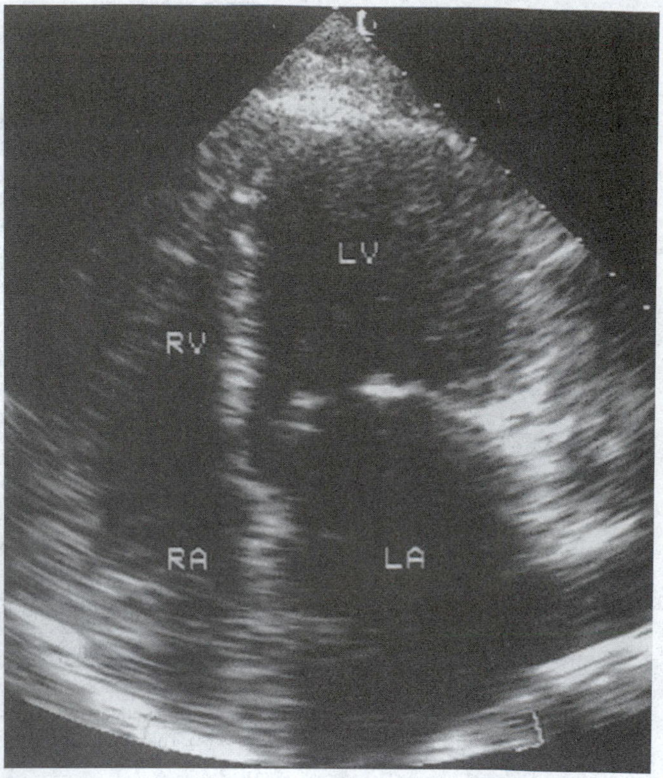

B

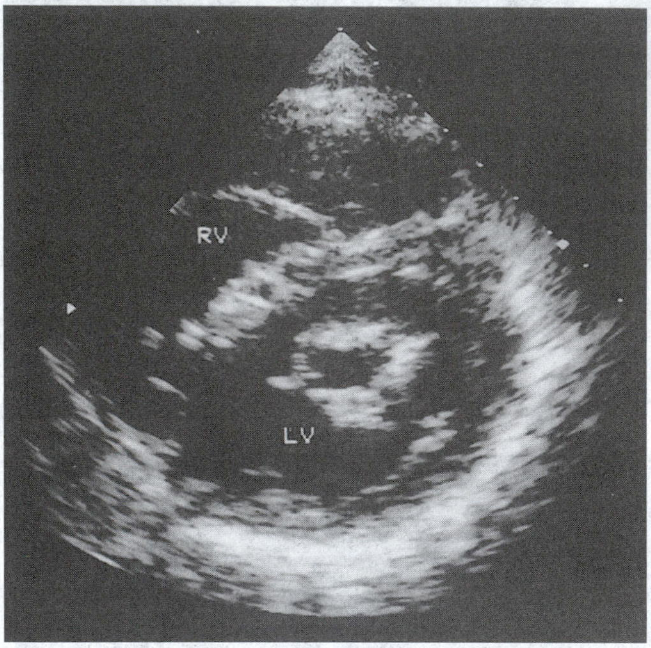

C

FIGURE 13-73 *A.* Parasternal long-axis view of mitral stenosis. The left atrium (LA) is enlarged, mitral opening is limited, and "doming" of the anterior mitral leaflet is present. LV = left ventricle; RV = right ventricle; AO = aorta. *B.* Apical four-chamber view in mitral stenosis. The left artium is markedly dilated. RA = right atrium. *C.* Parasternal short-axis plane in mitral stenosis.

pressure half-time yields an estimate of MVA, which correlates with values obtained during cardiac catheterization. Since Doppler estimates of mitral valve area are indirect and involve the use of empiric constants, they are considered less accurate than direct measurements of MVA derived by planimetry of the mitral valve orifice.[290] The pressure half-time method is inaccurate immediately following mitral commissurotomy.[291,292]

Echocardiography can help assess the feasibility and appropriateness of percutaneous catheter balloon mitral commissurotomy (CBMC) to treat individual patients with MS[293,294,294a] (Chap. 37). An echocardiographic scoring system based on evaluation of mitral valvular thickening, calcification, mobility, and subvalvular involvement has been devised. Each variable is assigned a grade of 1 (minimal involvement) to 4 (severe), with a maximal score of 16. Although the prognostic capability of this method is limited, the outcome of balloon valvuloplasty in patients with higher scores, particularly greater than 12, is less satisfactory and involves a higher risk of complications than in patients with lower scores.[293,294,294b] Therefore, echocardiographic analysis is an important part of the decision-making process prior to CBMC. Preprocedural TEE is also often performed to detect left atrial thrombi, which can embolize during transseptal catheterization.[295,296] Following CBMC, echocardiography can identify complications including mitral regurgitation[297] and atrial septal defect.[298]

Mitral Regurgitation

Although echocardiography is extremely accurate in the detection of mitral (and aortic) regurgitation, *quantitation* is more difficult. 2D imaging alone does not provide direct evidence of mitral regurgitation (MR) but usually reveals the etiology of the lesion.[299] Thus, 2D echocardiography reveals thickened, restricted leaflets in rheumatic disease, vegetations in infective endocarditis, flail mitral leaflets with torn chordae, and redundant leaflets with abnormal coaptation in mitral valve prolapse.[300] 2D echocardiography can also detect LA and LV abnormalities associated with MR, such as myxoma, papillary muscle dysfunction, and dilated cardiomyopathy. In addition, enlargement of these chambers offers indirect evidence of MR severity. In cases of chronic, severe MR, 2D echocardiography can also discern the presence of depressed LV function and decreased ejection fraction (see also Chap. 57).

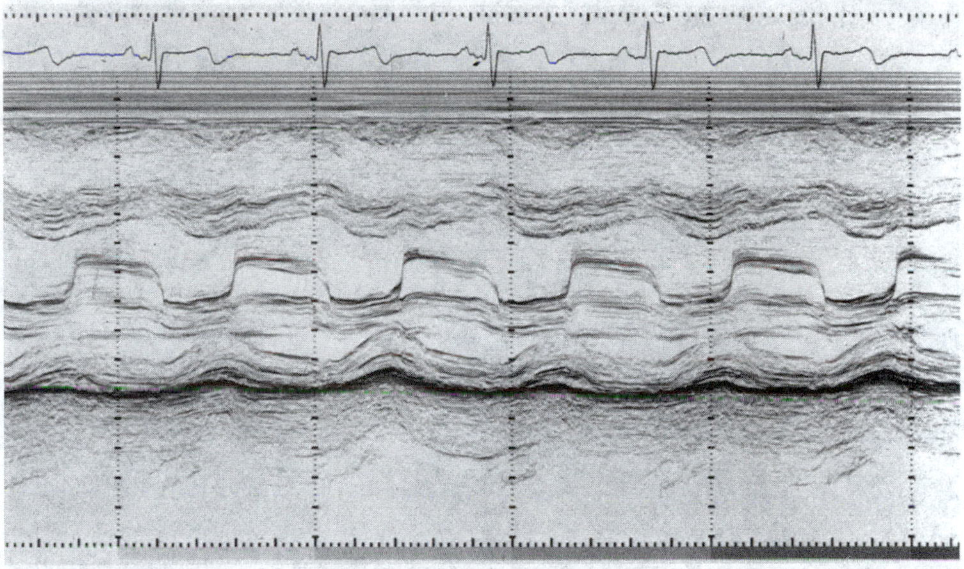

FIGURE 13-74 Parasternal M-mode image through the mitral valve in a patient with mitral stenosis. The normal rapid downslope of the anterior mitral leaflet after early rapid diastolic filling is absent.

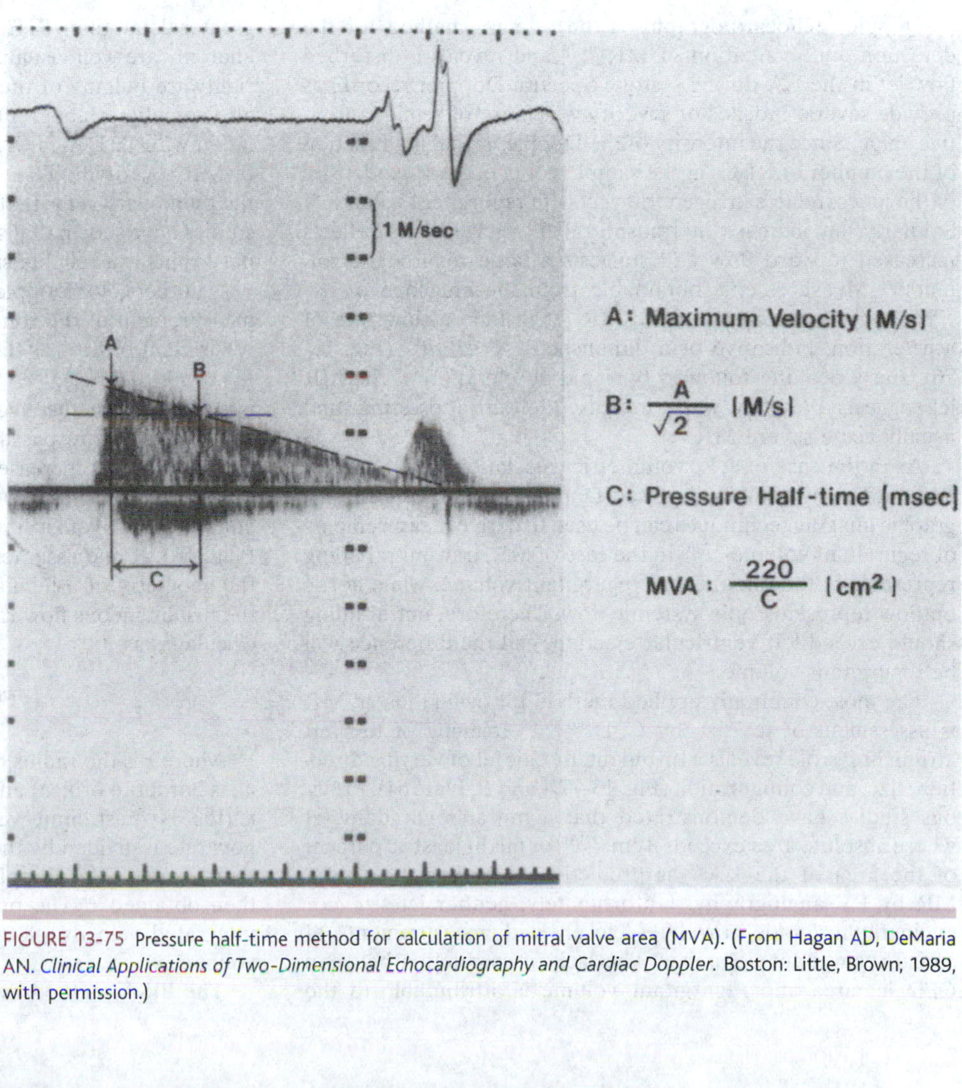

FIGURE 13-75 Pressure half-time method for calculation of mitral valve area (MVA). (From Hagan AD, DeMaria AN. *Clinical Applications of Two-Dimensional Echocardiography and Cardiac Doppler*. Boston: Little, Brown; 1989, with permission.)

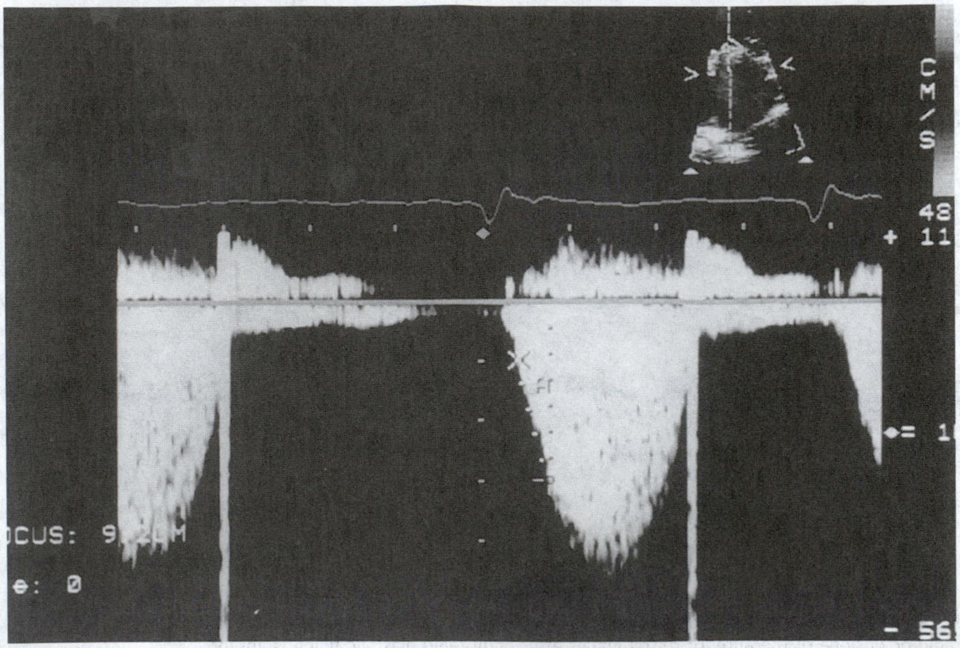

FIGURE 13-76 Continuous-wave tracing of mitral regurgitation with calculation of *dP/dt* (apical transducer position). The time period between velocities of 1 and 3 m/s is 0.07 s; the calculated *dP/dt* is approximately 460 mmHg/s. See text for details.

Doppler echocardiography is the primary method for the detection and evaluation of MR[301–303] and reveals a disturbed flow jet in the LA during systole. Spectral Doppler recordings provide several indexes of severity which are of semiquantitative value. Since the intensity of the Doppler signal is a function of the number of RBCs in the sample volume, the videodensity of the jet correlates in a general way with regurgitant volume.[304] Similarly, an increase in transmitral filling velocities reflects increased forward flow and suggests a large regurgitant volume.[304a] Measurements obtainable from the envelope of the CW Doppler recording of the MR jet include a slow rate of acceleration, indicative of a diminished LV *dP/dt*[305] (Fig. 13-76). Early peaking followed by rapid deceleration of the MR jet suggests a large V wave, increased left atrial pressure, and usually acute severe MR.[306]

As in the case of AR, volumetric calculations of LV inflow and outflow by combined pulsed Doppler and 2D-echocardiographic imaging techniques can be used to derive measurements of regurgitant volume.[307,308] In the case of MR, transmitral filling represents both systemic and regurgitant volume, while aortic outflow represents only systemic flow. Therefore, mitral filling should exceed left ventricular ejection, and the difference will be regurgitant volume.

The most commonly applied method for evaluation of MR is assessment of jet size by CFD.[303,309,310] Imaging of the left atrium in systole reveals a turbulent, mosaic jet of varying direction, size, and configuration (Fig. 13-77*A* and *B*, Plate 64). Previous studies have demonstrated that a mitral regurgitant jet whose absolute area exceeds 8 cm^2 [303,310] or fills at least 40 percent of the area of the LA[309] is predictive of finding 3+ to 4+ MR by LV angiography. Unfortunately, neither jet size nor angiographic grade correlates closely with measurements of actual regurgitant volume.[310] The lack of correlation between CFD jet area and regurgitant volume is attributable to the additional variables that influence the distribution of the flow disturbance, such as pressure gradient and the volume and compliance of the LA, as well as technical limitations. The Coanda effect is of particular significance in regard to MR, since jets into the left atrium are often eccentric (for example, in cases of mitral valve prolapse and torn chordae tendineae). Due to differential frictional forces and resistance to flow, eccentric MR jets are drawn along the walls of the LA, resulting in cross-sectional jet areas that are smaller than centrally directed flow disturbances of comparable regurgitant volume (Figs. 13-77 and 13-78). This effect can lead to underestimation of severity of regurgitation.[311,312]

TEE is also useful for assessment of MR, as the close proximity of the probe and its higher-frequency interrogating beam permit imaging of regurgitant jets in greater detail than TTE.[313–315] Eccentric jets and mitral valvular anatomy are well visualized (Fig. 13-78*A* and *B*, Plate 65), and rightward bulging of the interatrial septum with severe MR is also sometimes apparent. As the regurgitant jets often appear larger with TEE than with TTE, one must avoid overestimation of MR severity.[154] TEE often yields Doppler interrogation of the pulmonary veins that is superior to TTE, and several recent studies have shown that systolic reversal of flow into the pulmonary veins is a reliable sign of severe MR[152,315a,315b] (Fig. 13-79).

Another color Doppler method of flow quantitation involves measurement of the zone of flow convergence proximal to the regurgitant orifice (or the *proximal isovelocity surface area, referred to as PISA*).[316–319] The mechanism for this phenomenon is derived from the hydrodynamic principle that blood flow accelerates before passing through a small orifice under high pressure. If this increase in flow velocity exceeds the Nyquist limit, color aliasing occurs and the velocity aliasing border is equal to the Nyquist limit (Fig. 13-31 and Fig. 13-80*A* and *B*; Plate 66). If one assumes that the aliasing border conforms to the geometry of a hemisphere around the mitral orifice, then the instantaneous flow rate of blood through the orifice can be calculated as:

$$\text{Flow} = 2\pi r^2 \cdot V_r$$

where r is the radius of the hemisphere shell (distance from alias border to orifice) and V_r is the velocity of blood at distance r (the Nyquist limit velocity).[316] If the maximal calculated flow rate is divided by the peak regurgitant flow velocity (measured with CW Doppler), the regurgitant orifice area is then obtained.[320] The product of regurgitant orifice area and integrated velocity of the MR jet by CW yields regurgitant volume.

The PISA method avoids the variables associated with jet

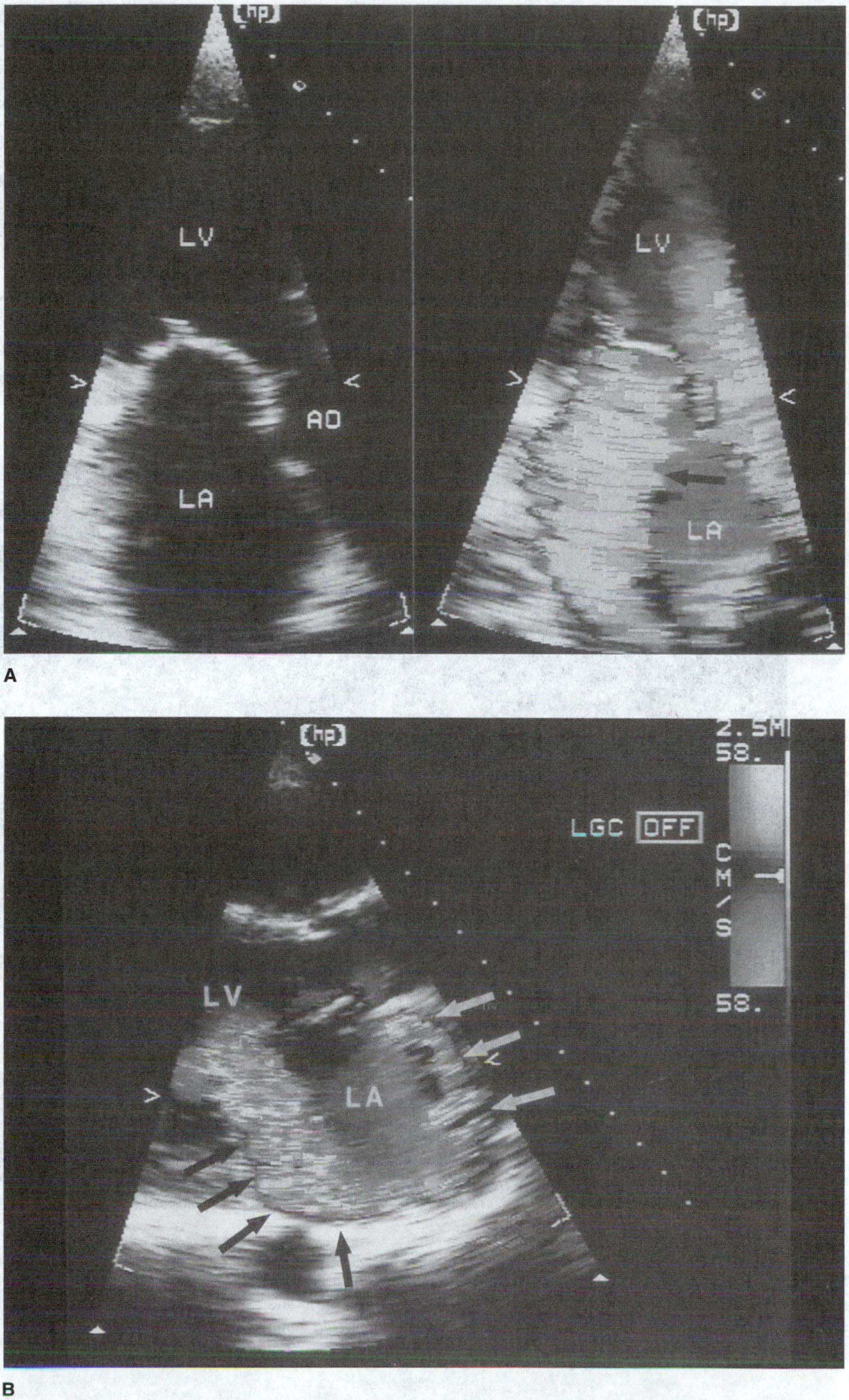

FIGURE 13-77 (Plate 64) *A*. Mitral regurgitation. *Left:* apical three-chamber plane. Right: same plane with color Doppler imaging. A large jet of mitral regurgitation (*arrow*) is present. AO = aorta; LA = left atrium; LV = left ventricle. *B*. Parasternal long-axis view from a patient with angiographically proved severe mitral regurgitation. The color Doppler jet in this case is directed posteriorly and eccentric (*black arrows*). The jet hugs the wall of the left atrium (LA) and wraps around all the way to the aortic root (*white arrows*). LV = left ventricle.

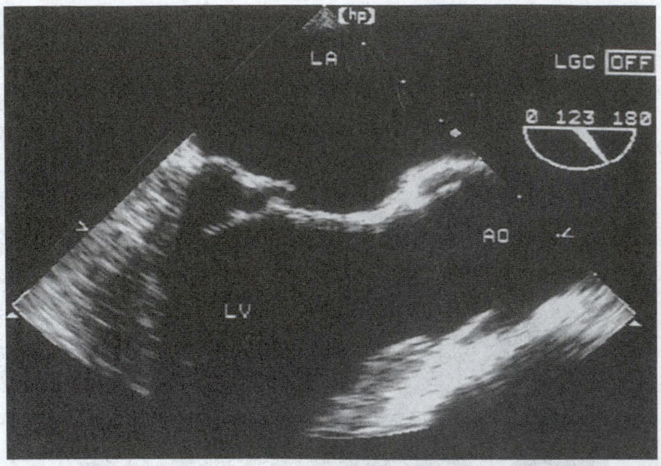

A

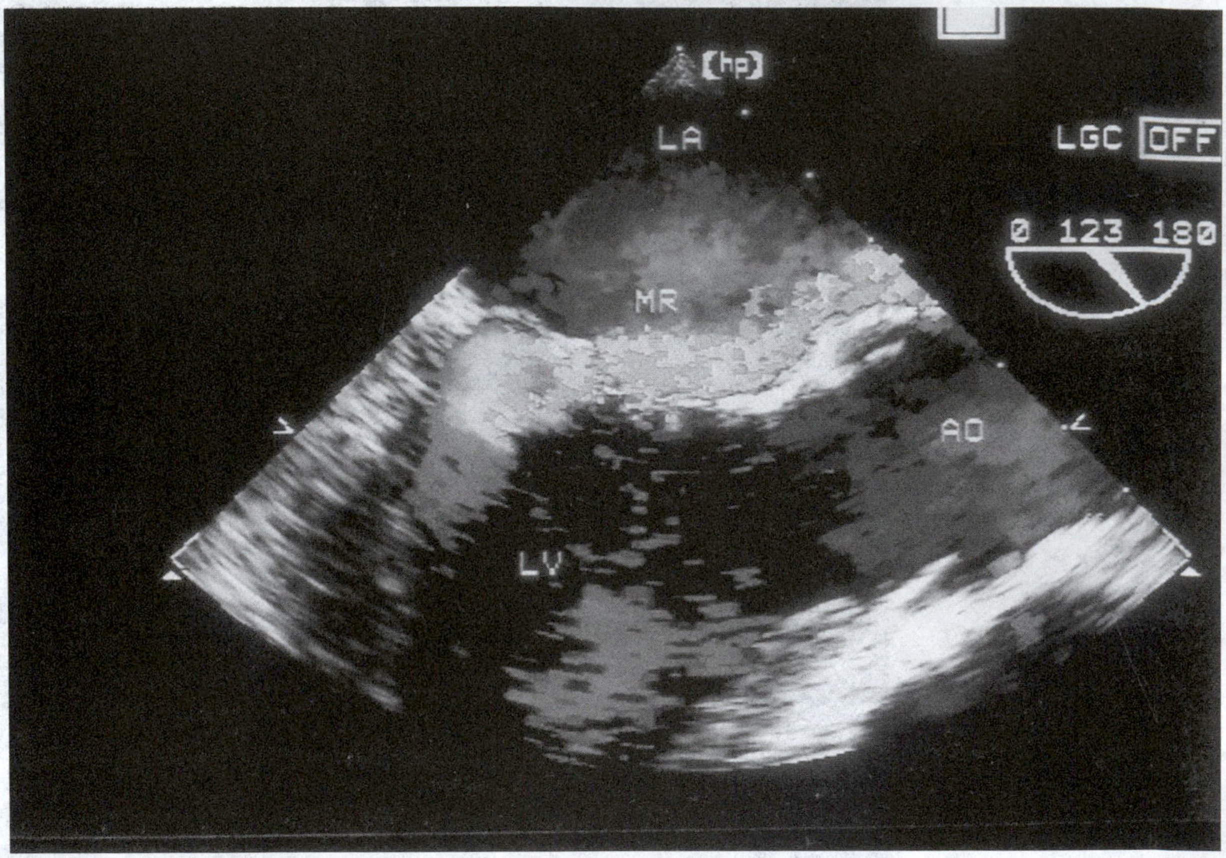

B

FIGURE 13-78 (Plate 65) TEE images from a case of severe mitral regurgitation secondary to a flail posterior mitral valve leaflet. *A.* abnormal coaptation and prolapse of the posterior leaflet is apparent. *B.* Color Doppler imaging demonstrates an eccentric jet of MR directed anteriorly toward the aortic root (AO). LA = left atrium; LV = left ventricle.

size and the assumptions and technical limitations of volumetric calculations. Numerous studies have shown a correlation between both flow rate and regurgitant orifice area calculated by PISA and the severity of MR assessed by standard methods.[316,320] In addition, flow convergence calculations have been applied to other valvular lesions, including AR and MS[321,322] (Fig. 13-81, Plate 67), ventricular septal defect,[323] and prosthetic heart valves.[324] The proximal flow convergence assumes a hemispheric geometry for the PISA signal and that the plane of the mitral leaflets is flat, two sources of potential error.[325] Despite these limitations, the method holds considerable promise for the clinical evaluation of valvular regurgitation.

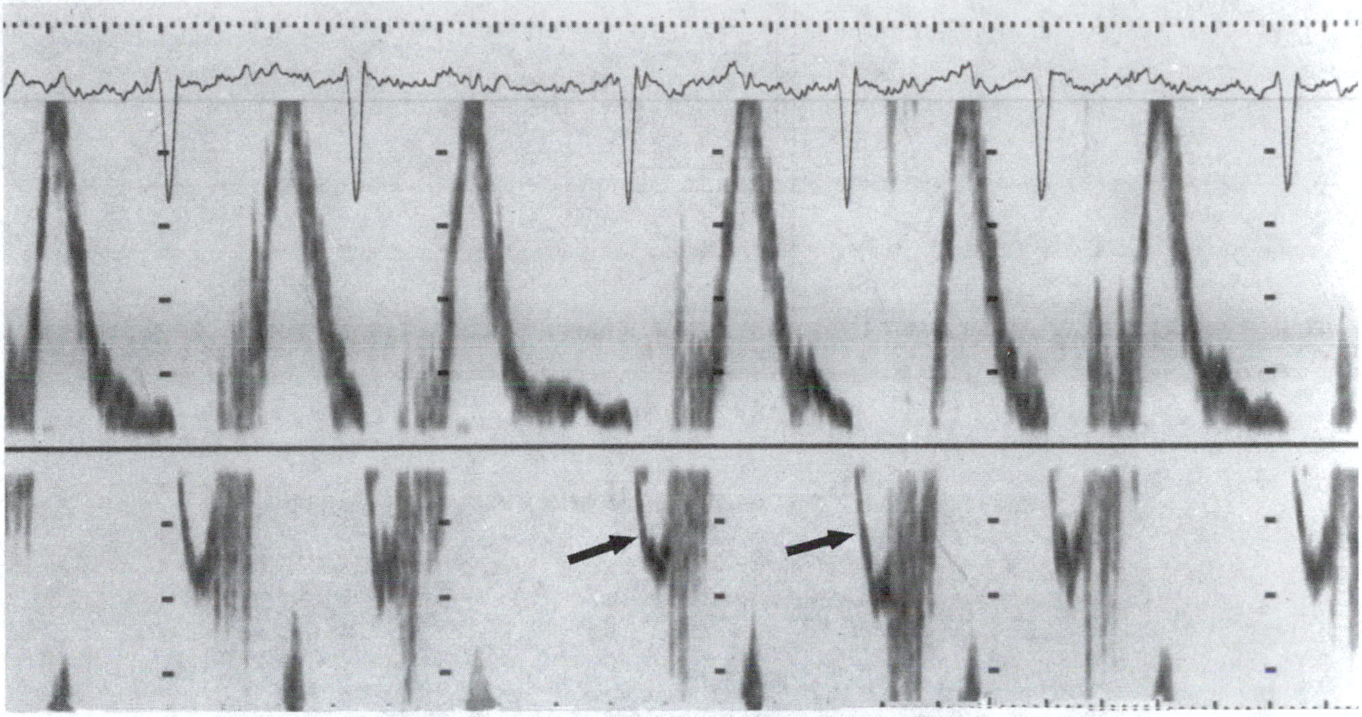

FIGURE 13-79 Pulmonary venous pulsed-wave Doppler in severe mitral regurgitation. Systolic flow reversal (i.e., systolic flow into the pulmonary vein) is present (*arrows*).

Mitral Valve Prolapse

As is true of so many aspects of mitral valve prolapse (MVP),[326] the echocardiographic findings in this disorder have been controversial for many years.[327] Recent insights into the anatomy of the mitral annulus and the significance of abnormal leaflet structure have established a central role for echocardiography in the diagnosis and prognosis of MVP.[328] The classic echocardiographic findings in overt MVP syndrome consists of mid- to late-systolic bulging of one or both mitral leaflets across the plane of the mitral valve annulus into the LA (Fig. 13-82*A* to *C*).[329] The leaflets are often observed to be structurally abnormal, with thickening, elongation, and hooding.[330] Mid- to late-systolic MR is sometimes present, often eccentric, and generally directed away from the prolapsing leaflet.[326] The chordae tendineae may be thickened and elongated, the aortic root may be dilated, and the tricuspid valve leaflets may prolapse as well. LV function is usually normal, although the LA and LV may be enlarged if MR is significant. The greater temporal resolution of M-mode over 2D echocardiography often yields striking evidence of abrupt midsystolic posterior/superior motion of the mitral valve leaflets in prolapse patients[331] (Fig. 13-82*C*). Although such M-mode findings, which resemble a question mark on its side, are specific for mitral valve prolapse, patients with classic MVP occasionally may demonstrate diagnostic findings only with 2D imaging (Chap. 58).

Although the diagnosis of classic, fully expressed MVP is straightforward by echocardiography, identification of mild prolapse is more difficult, and no absolute diagnostic criteria currently exist.[329] This is largely related to the absence of any "gold standard" with which to validate findings, including auscultation, angiography, and even pathology.[326] For prolapse to be present, the mitral valve leaflets must cross the plane of the mitral valve annulus after initial systolic coaptation. Recent studies have established that the mitral valve annulus is not flat but rather saddle-shaped.[332] The annulus reaches its nadir in the apical four-chamber view, and even normally coapting mitral valve leaflets may appear to prolapse in this projection. Therefore, current criteria require that MVP be diagnosed only when one or both of the mitral leaflets clearly bulge past the plane of the mitral valve annulus in the parasternal long-axis view.[328] Unfortunately, the degree to which the mitral leaflets must break the plane of the annulus is unclear. The greater the portion of the mitral valve leaflets entering the LA, the more likely the existence of signs and symptoms related to this disorder; a peak distance behind the annulus of 2 mm almost invariably establishes the presence of MVP.[329] The diagnosis of mild MVP may be assisted by examination of the structure of the leaflets and chordae tendineae, since it has been demonstrated that patients with redundant or thickening valve leaflets (greater than 5 mm in midleaflet) are at increased risk of complications, including severe MR and infective endocarditis[333] (Chap. 73).

Torn Chordae Tendineae

Rupture of chordae tendineae may occur spontaneously or in conjunction with MVP or endocarditis. This can result in a flail mitral leaflet and severe MR. Although TTE often detects these

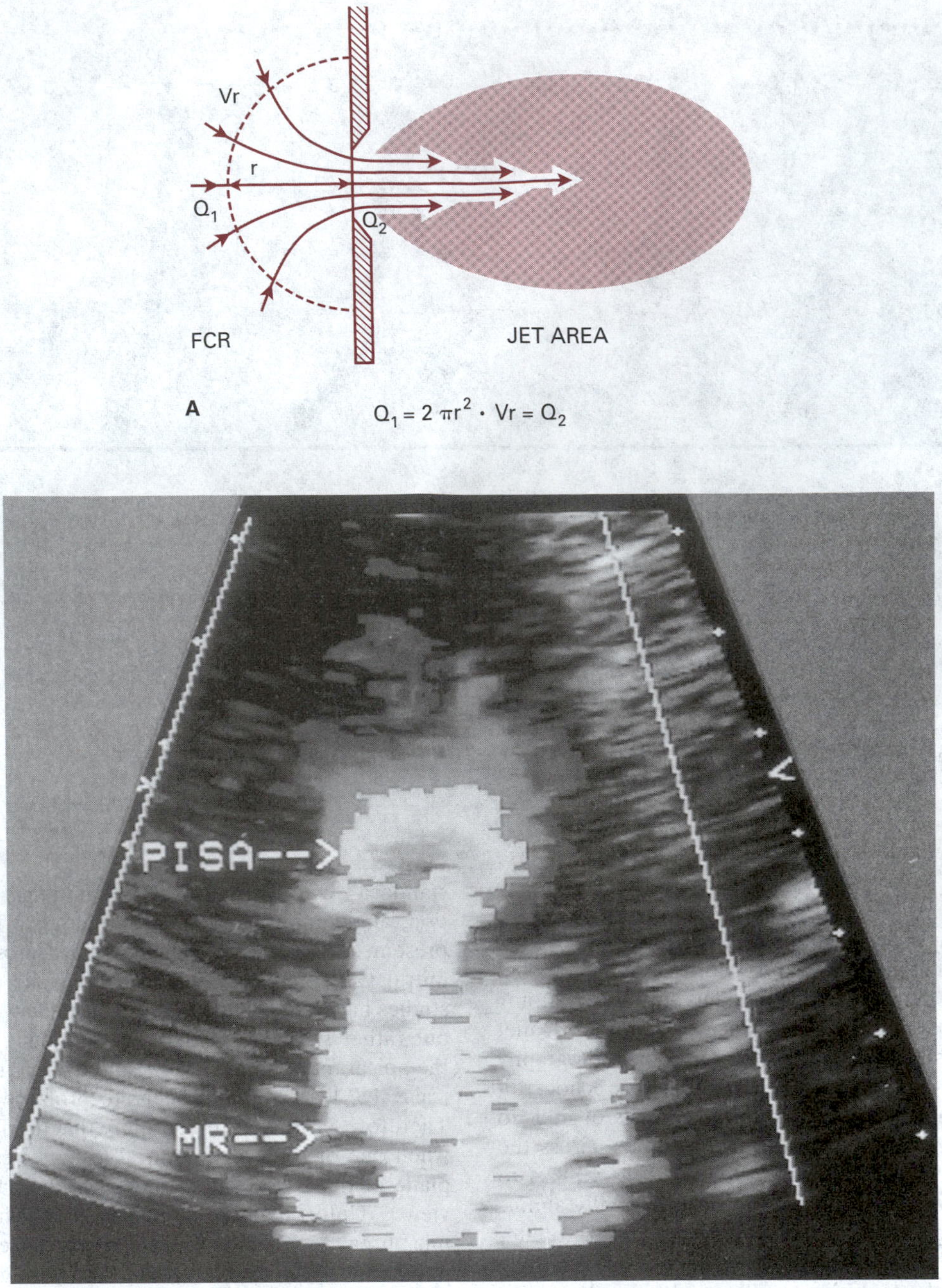

FIGURE 13-80 (Plate 66) *A*. Proximal isovelocity surface area (PISA). See text for details. Q = flow; FCR = flow convergence region; r = radius of isovelocity hemisphere; Vr = velocity of flow at distance r from the orifice. (From Bargiggia GS, Tronconi L, Sahn DJ, et al. A new method for quantitation of mitral regurgitation based on color flow Doppler imaging of flow convergence proximal to regurgitant orifice. *Circulation* 1991; 84:1481–1489, with permission.) *B*. Magnified view (from the apical four-chamber plane) of mitral regurgitation (MR) demonstrating color Doppler flow convergence proximal to the mitral valve (PISA).

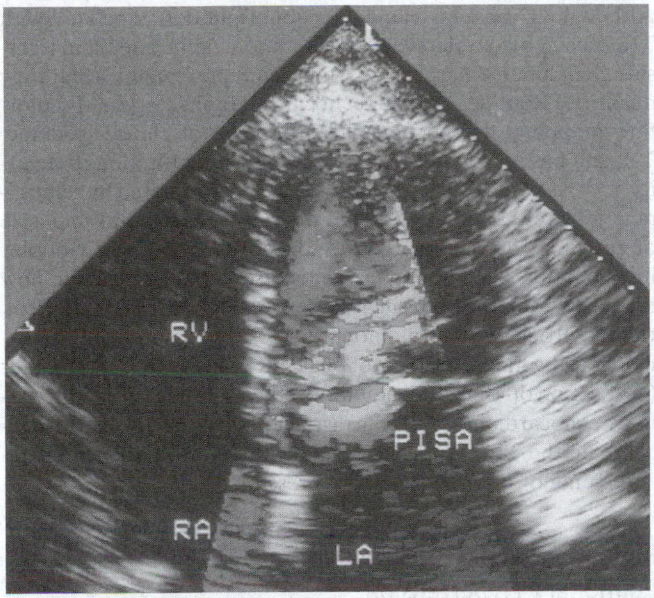

FIGURE 13-81 (Plate 67) Apical four-chamber plane in mitral stenosis. Color flow imaging in the mitral valve region shows flow convergence (PISA) proximal to the valve during diastole. LA = left atrium; RA = right atrium; RV = right ventricle.

lesions, TEE is especially sensitive and accurate and often demonstrates free motion of the leaflet and ruptured chord into the LA even when the TTE is equivocal (Fig. 13-83*A* and *B*).[334] As with MVP, the MR jet in this condition is usually eccentric and directed away from the affected leaflet, often "hugging" the adjacent left atrial wall (Coanda effect). Therefore, the jet's cross-sectional area may be misleadingly small. The findings of mitral valvular anatomy on TEE may also be helpful in predicting the feasibility and success of valve repair surgery.[335]

In the setting of ischemic heart disease, both LV enlargement and papillary muscle dysfunction (from infarction or transient ischemia) may cause MR.[336] Both the MR and the contractile abnormality responsible for it are usually well visualized by 2D echocardiography. In rare cases, papillary muscle rupture (partial or complete) occurs in the postinfarction period.[337] Rapid echocardiographic diagnosis often requires TEE and may be lifesaving in these cases.[334]

Mitral Annular Calcification

The finding of mitral annular calcification (MAC) is fairly common in adults and occurs more frequently with advancing age. Although ultrasound cannot discern histology, calcification typically appears as thickened, extremely high-intensity ("bright") signals (Fig. 13-84). The posterior portion of the mitral annulus is affected much more commonly than the anterior segment, and calcification often extends into the posterior mitral leaflet, sometimes restricting its motion.[338–340] The abnormality, best visualized in the parasternal long- and short-axis views, is seen as a bright calcific density at the junction of the posterior mitral leaflet and the annulus. In the short-axis view, the posterior band of calcification often appears crescentic. Rarely, the calcification is extensive enough to cause marked valvular thickening and clinically significant mitral stenosis.[339] MAC has also been implicated as a source of cardiogenic embolization.[341]

RIGHT-SIDED VALVULAR DISEASE AND PULMONARY HYPERTENSION

Pulmonic Valve

Major structural abnormalities of the pulmonic valve are relatively rare. *Pulmonic stenosis* (PS) is usually congenital in origin and resembles congenital AS in many respects. The stenotic valve does not open fully and exhibits characteristic thickening and systolic doming on 2D imaging[342] (Fig. 13-85). M-mode recordings of the pulmonic valve often show a large a wave, since right ventricular diastolic pressure is often so high and pulmonary artery (PA) pressure so low that the atrial "kick" is sufficient to open the pulmonic valve.[343] Doppler interrogation reveals turbulent flow distal to the valve, and CW measurements can be used to calculate gradients and valve areas with the Bernoulli and continuity equations much as in aortic stenosis.[344]

Although severe *pulmonic regurgitation* (PR) is rare, mild PR is common and appears as a flame shaped flow disturbance in the *right ventricular outflow tract* (RVOT) in diastole.[345] Many individuals have trivial PR on color Doppler examination; this is a physiologic, normal variant (Fig. 13-86). Hemodynamically significant PR is uncommon; when present, it is usually due to congenital heart disease, valvular tumors, endocarditis, or carcinoid heart disease (Chap. 59). The echocardiographic grading of PR is semiquantitative, based on the density of the CW envelope, area of the color Doppler jet, and width of the jet at the valve.[346,347] The PR pressure half-time by CW Doppler may be shorter with more severe PR, but this is not as well investigated as in the case of aortic regurgitation. Measurements derived from the CW Doppler recording also provide estimates of end-diastolic pulmonary artery pressure using the Bernoulli equation as follows[348]: $[4(\text{PR end-diastolic velocity})^2 + \text{central venous pressure (CVP)}$.

Tricuspid Valve

Tricuspid stenosis (TS) is usually rheumatic in origin, and coexistent mitral and aortic valvular disease is the rule. Congenital or acquired (nonrheumatic) causes of TS are quite uncommon. On rare occasions, tricuspid stenosis may be caused by carcinoid heart disease or by leaflet adhesions to permanent pacemaker leads. Because of the large size of the tricuspid annulus, obstruction by masses, even multiple vegetations, is unlikely to cause stenosis (Chap. 59).

Regardless of the etiology, diastolic doming of the valve leaflets suggests stenosis.[349,350] CW Doppler interrogation is also helpful and mimics the findings of MS (high diastolic velocity with prolonged pressure half-time).[349] The pressure half-time equation of mitral valve area calculation cannot be applied directly to the tricuspid valve, and large studies comparing Doppler echocardiography with right heart catheterization in TS are not available.

Tricuspid regurgitation (TR) is much more common than TS, and like PR is present to a mild degree in many normal individuals (Chap. 59). Hemodynamically significant TR may be caused by endocarditis, rheumatic valvular disease, pulmonary

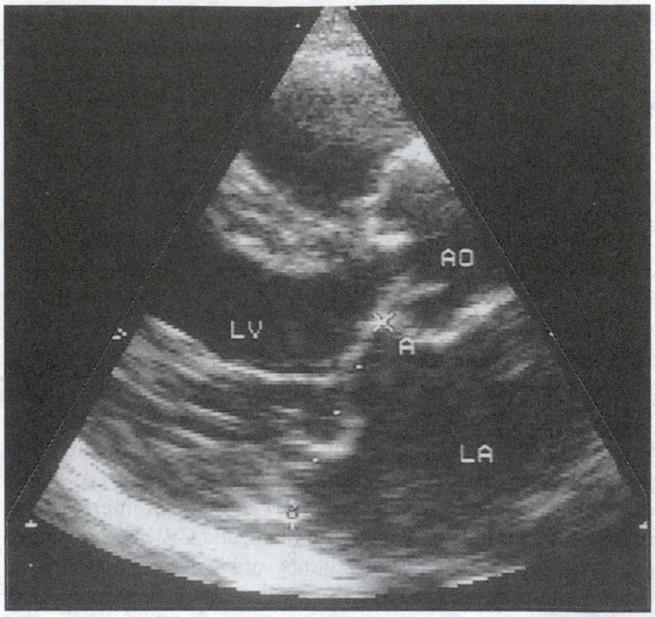

A

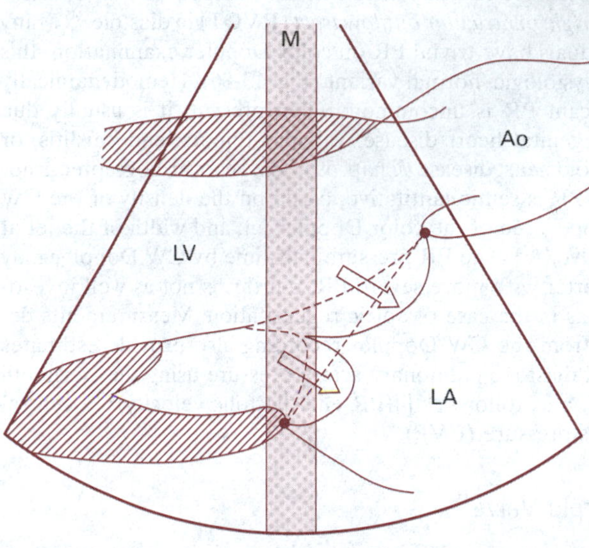

B

FIGURE 13-82 *A*. Parasternal long-axis plane through the mitral valve in late systole. The plane of the mitral annulus (A) is drawn in a dotted line. The posterior mitral leaflet prolapses past the level of the annulus into the left atrium (LA). AO = aorta; LV = left ventricle. *B*. Diagram of true mitral valve prolapse. The mitral leaflets clearly prolapse (*arrows*) posterior to the plane of the mitral annulus (*straight dotted line*). Ao = aorta; LV = left ventricle; LA = left atrium; M = m-mode imaging beam. (From Devereux RB, Kramer-Fox R, Kligfield P. Mitral valve prolapse: Causes, clinical manifestations, and management. *Ann Intern Med* 1989; 111:305–317, with permission.) C. M-mode image through the plane of the mitral valve demonstrating posterior prolapse of the leaflets during systole (*arrow*). E = early diastolic filling; A = atrial component.

hypertension, congenital heart disease (for example, Ebstein's anomaly), carcinoid heart disease, flail TR leaflet (which can occur as a complication of cardiac trauma or endomyocardial biopsy), and tricuspid valve prolapse. Echocardiographic findings in patients with TR generally mirror those found in MR.[351]

Although 2D imaging can detect abnormalities associated with TR, such as incomplete leaflet coaptation, flail leaflet, and right-sided chamber enlargement, the technique cannot accurately quantify TR grade. Doppler echocardiography, especially color-flow mapping, has become the procedure of choice to detect TR, and has reasonable accuracy for semiquantitation of severity.[352,353] As with MR, severity of TR can be estimated by regurgitant jet area, ratio of jet area to right atrial area, and size of proximal flow convergence zones[354] (Fig. 13-31). Doppler interrogation of the hepatic vein is also useful, as systolic flow reversal within the vein suggests severe TR[355] (Fig. 13-87). Peak right ventricular (and pulmonary artery) pressure can be estimated using measurements of peak TR velocity by CW Doppler (see section on Bernoulli equation, above). If necessary, intravenous echocardiographic contrast agents can be injected to accentuate the TR Doppler jet and facilitate more accurate measurements of pulmonary artery pressure.[352–354]

Right Ventricular Function and Pulmonary Hypertension

Right ventricular (RV) enlargement and pulmonary hypertension can be diagnosed and assessed by echocardiography[355,356] (Fig. 13-88*A* and *B*). Because of the asymmetrical and crescentic shape of the RV, accurate volume calculations are difficult.[357,358] Nonetheless, 2D imaging provides useful general information regarding RV size and function. In the apical four-chamber view, the RV should appear somewhat smaller than the LV; therefore RV enlargement can be diagnosed qualitatively when the RV cross-sectional area exceeds that of the LV. RV chamber area measurements in the apical four-chamber imaging plane can also be compared to standardized normal values.[359] Although not well standardized, measurements of RV wall thickness can be performed from the parasternal view; a value of 5 mm is generally accepted as the upper limit of normal.[360,361] Systolic motion of the RV free wall and LV lateral wall toward the interventricular septum should be similar and roughly symmetrical in normal situations. Asymmetrical hypokinesis of the RV free wall indicates RV dysfunction.[362]

RV volume overload can lead to RV hypertrophy, chamber enlargement, and, in advanced stages, depressed RV systolic function. TR can result from or cause RV overload, and the TR Doppler velocity allows estimation of the peak RV systolic pressure. The interventricular septum also becomes abnormal in RV overload and tends to flatten or even bulge toward the LV (Fig. 13-89).[363] The pattern of septal movement can help distinguish between volume and pressure overload: in pure volume overload, the RV diastolic pressure may equal or exceed that of the LV, while the systolic pressure of the LV greatly exceeds that of the RV. Therefore, the interventricular septum flattens during diastole and returns to its normal curvature during systole.[363,364] With RV pressure overload, however, the abnormally high RV pressures persist through the entire cardiac cycle and the interventricular septum remains deformed during both systole and diastole.[364]

The hallmark of pulmonary hypertension by Doppler echocardiography is a high-velocity TR jet in the absence of PS. Peak TR jet velocity can be converted to peak systolic PA pressure as follows[365]:

$$4(\text{TR velocity})^2 + \text{CVP}$$

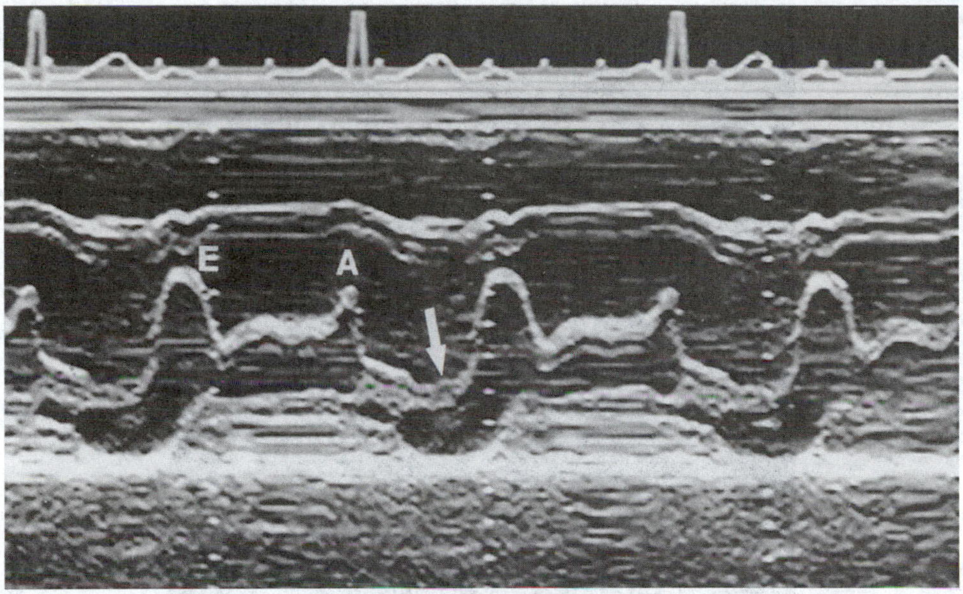

C

FIGURE 13-82 (*Continued*)

In the setting of severe pulmonary hypertension, the main PA and the inferior vena cava are often dilated. If RA pressure is elevated, the inferior vena cava (IVC) does not decrease in diameter with inspiration as normally expected.[366] M-mode examination of the pulmonic valve in pulmonary hypertension may show a characteristic W-shaped motion of the valve leaflet during systole[367–369] (Fig. 13-90) and loss of the normal a dip caused by partial opening of the valve during atrial contraction. The loss of the a wave is probably due to the large pressure difference between the RV and pulmonary artery during late diastole and the resulting inability of the atrial contraction to partially open the pulmonic valve. The midsystolic closure of the valve and partial reopening in late systole (sometimes called the *flying W*) may be caused by elevated pulmonary vascular resistance and oscillation of a pressure wavefront within the pulmonary artery.[370]

Characteristic pulsed-wave Doppler abnormalities in pulmonary hypertension include a decrease in the velocity-time integral of flow through the pulmonic valve (secondary to depressed RV stroke volume) and a shortening of the acceleration time (measured from beginning of flow through the pulmonic valve to peak velocity). The acceleration time (in milliseconds) can be used to estimate the mean pulmonary artery (PA) pressure[371] as:

$$\text{Mean PA pressure} = 80 = (\text{acceleration time}/2)$$

Pulmonic regurgitation is also common in the setting of pulmonary hypertension and is usually well recorded by pulsed Doppler. As discussed above, the end-diastolic PR velocity can be used to estimate PA end-diastolic pressure by the Bernoulli equation.

PROSTHETIC CARDIAC VALVES

Echocardiography is a critically important tool in the evaluation and serial follow-up of mechanical and bioprosthetic valves.[372] Unfortunately, the increased echo reflectivity of prosthetic valves (especially the mechanical models) causes extensive distal shadowing and reverberations that markedly limit the utility of transthoracic 2D echocardiography (Figs. 13-91 and 13-92). TTE imaging may detect partial ring dehiscence manifest as abnormal "rocking" motion of a prosthetic valve. TTE may also identify reduced movement of the valve disks or leaflets and may occasionally visualize adherent thrombi, tissue ingrowth, and vegetations.[373–375] Leaflet thickening, detachment, and flail motion also may be visualized for bioprosthetic valves.

Doppler interrogation is the cornerstone of the echocardiographic assessment of prosthetic valvular stenosis and regurgitation.[376–379] Color-flow imaging can document the presence, direction, and size of the forward flow stream. Color-flow Doppler can also detect regurgitant flow jets, but like 2D imaging, is limited by acoustic shadowing distal to the prosthesis. Doppler color jets due to prosthetic AR can be readily visualized from the transthoracic apical view, but jets produced by prosthetic mitral and tricuspid regurgitation are often obscured.[380,381] Therefore, although detection of prosthetic regurgitation by transthoracic Doppler is usually feasible, quantitation is often difficult. A small flow signal shortly after valve closure may be observed frequently with prosthetic valves and is likely related to the blood caught behind the occluder as it closes.[382]

Doppler flow velocities and gradients (calculated by the Bernoulli equation) through normal prosthetic valves vary depending upon the type, position, and diameter of the prosthesis.[376–379] The velocities and gradients across prosthetic valves are flow-dependent as well[383] and therefore related to LV function. Given these variables, it is not surprising that a wide range of transvalvular gradients exists for normally functioning prosthetic valves. Nevertheless, "normal" ranges have been reported for various valve types and can be used as a guide to recognize malfunction. High prosthetic valvular gradients due to increased flow volume rather than stenosis can be recognized by high flow velocity across the remaining native valves, a short pressure half-time for mitral prostheses, and a short ejection time for aortic prostheses. With aortic valve prostheses, peak systolic Doppler velocities may indicate higher systolic pressure gradients than those actually found during cardiac catheterization.[384,385] This problem may be more prevalent with Starr-Edwards (ball-in-cage) and St. Jude (bileaflet tilting disks) valves than with Medtronic-Hall (single tilting disk) and bioprosthetic valves. The inaccuracies with Starr-Edwards and St. Jude valves are probably due to the presence of multiple flow channels (with various orifice areas) and the phenomenon of flow recovery.[385,386] Because of these variabilities, an echocardiographic examination is warranted following prosthetic valve

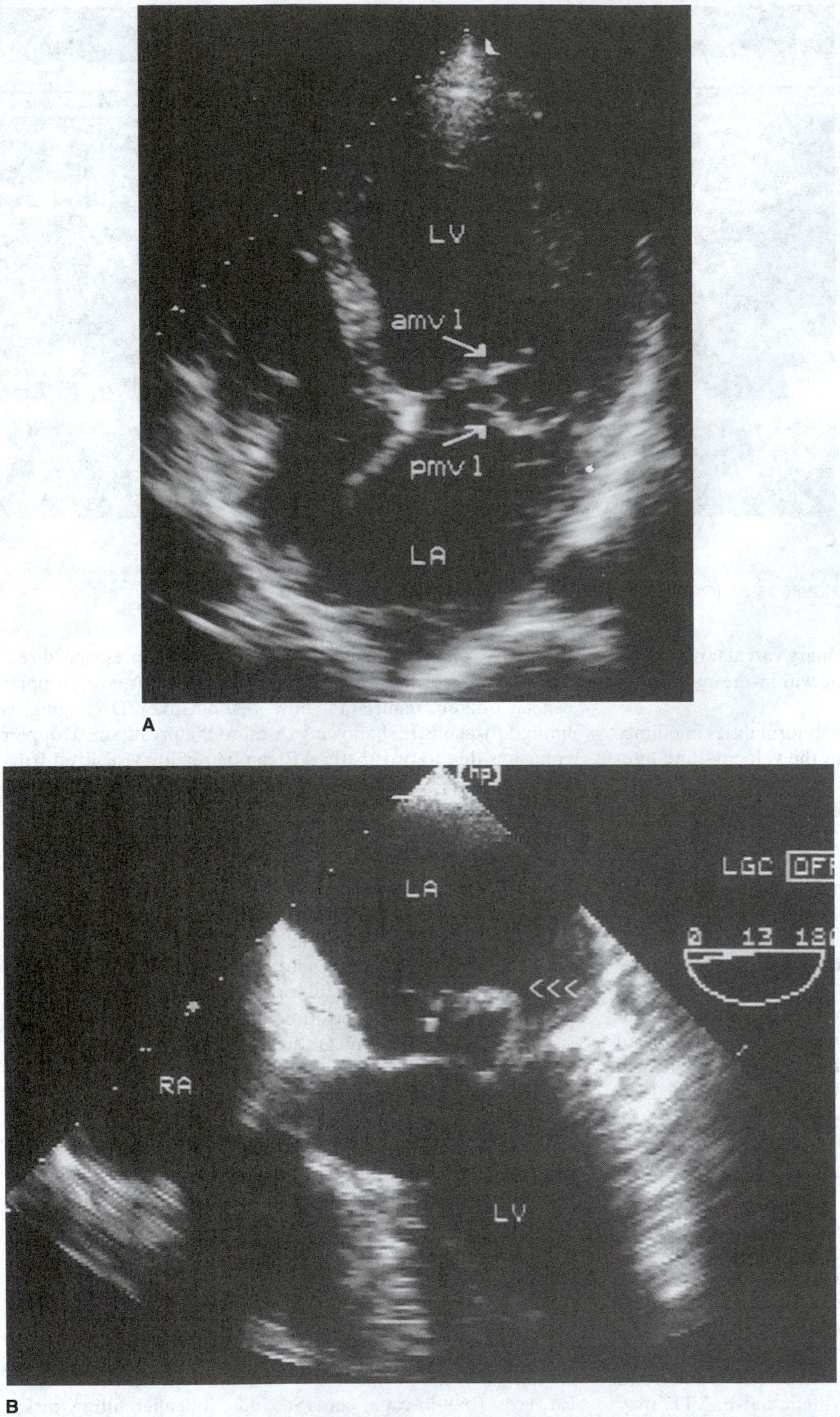

FIGURE 13-83 *A.* Apical four-chamber image of a flail posterior mitral valve leaflet (pmvl). The mitral valve is thickened and myxomatous. amvl = anterior mitral valve leaflet. *B.* Transesophageal echocardiography image (transverse four-chamber plane) of a flail posterior mitral valve leaflet (*arrows*) secondary to ruptured chordae. LA = left atrium; RA = right atrium; LV = left ventricle.

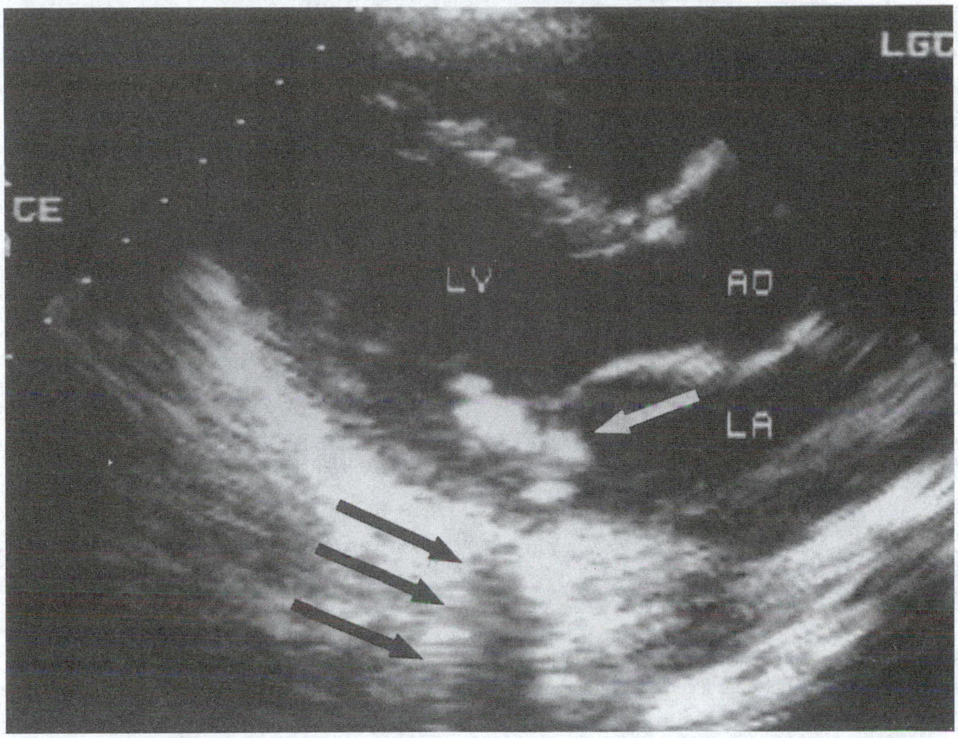

FIGURE 13-84 Parasternal long-axis plane demonstrating mitral annular calcification (*white arrow*) with ultrasonic shadowing posteriorly (*black arrows*). AO = aorta; LV = left ventricle; LA = left atrium. (From Blanchard DG, DeMaria AN. Cardiac and extracardiac masses: Echocardiographic evaluation. In: Skorton DJ, Schelber HR, Wolf GL, Brundage BH, eds. *Marcus' Cardiac Imaging*, 2d ed. Philadelphia: Saunders; 1996:452–480, with permission.)

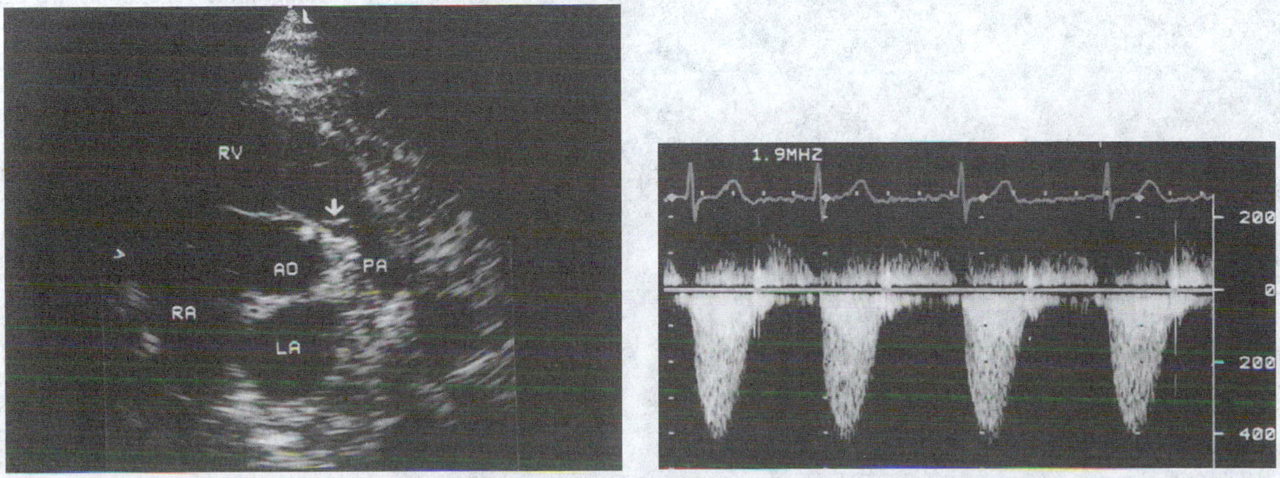

A B

FIGURE 13-85 *A.* Pulmonic stenosis. The pulmonic valve leaflet is thickened and echo-reflective (*arrow*). RA = right atrium; LA = left atrium; AO = aorta; PA = pulmonary artery; RV = right ventricle. *B.* Doppler interrogation reveals increased flow velocity (4 m/s) through the valve orifice.

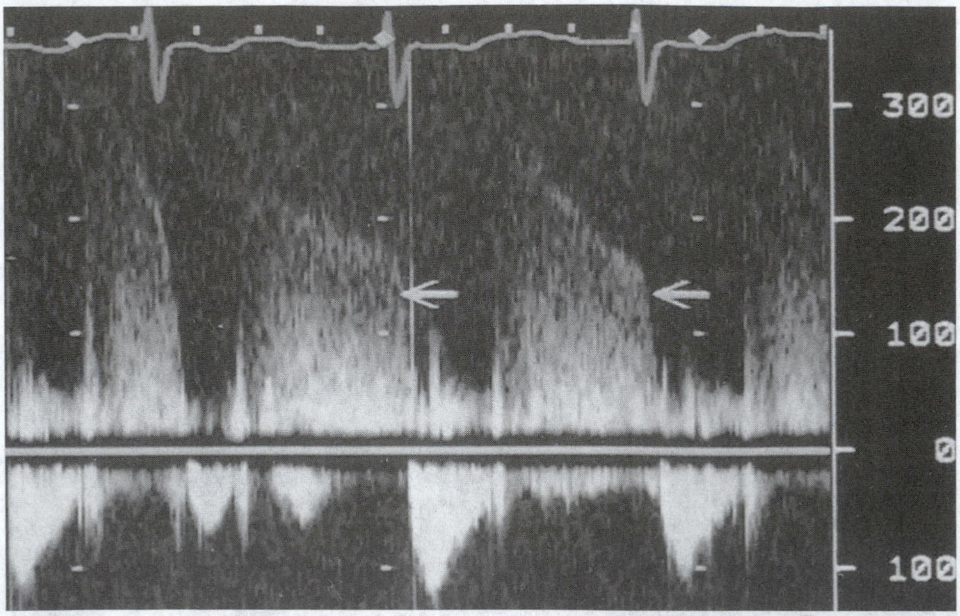

FIGURE 13-86 Continuous-wave Doppler tracing through the right ventricular outflow tract and pulmonary artery (left parasternal transducer position). Mild pulmonic regurgitation is present (*arrows*).

implantation to establish its baseline Doppler characteristics.[387] As opposed to peak gradients, mean transvalvular gradients calculated by Doppler correlate reasonably well with direct catheter measurements.

TEE has dramatically changed the diagnostic approach to prosthetic valve dysfunction,[380,381] and is especially useful for assessing mitral prostheses, as it overcomes the problem of left atrial shadowing and reverberation (Fig. 13-93). TEE is extremely accurate in the detection of prosthetic regurgitation and impaired movement of the valve occluder, and it is the diagnostic procedure of choice in most cases of suspected prosthetic valve endocarditis.[388–390] Small thrombi, tissue ingrowth, infected or sterile vegetations, and even sutures in the sewing ring usually can be readily visualized. The enhanced sensitivity of TEE requires operator experience and judgment, as nearly all mechanical prostheses exhibit a normal small amount of regurgitation, which should not be misinterpreted as pathologic.[382] TEE may also visualize thin fibrinous strands sometimes attached to prosthetic valves; these structures appear to be a potential source of cardiogenic embolization.[391,392] The technique is quite accurate in the diagnosis of prosthetic valve thrombosis, a potentially fatal medical emergency, and can assist clinical decision making in this disorder.[393–395]

INFECTIVE ENDOCARDITIS

Infective endocarditis remains an all too common illness, with a significant risk of morbidity and mortality (see also Chap. 78). Traditionally, the diagnosis has been based on either the cumulative results of blood cultures, physical examination, and laboratory findings or on pathologic proof of infected valvular vegetations at surgery or autopsy. Echocardiography may play an important role in infective endocarditis in regard to diagnosis, detection of associated cardiac abnormalities and hemodynamic dysfunction, prognosis, and the need for surgery. Vegetations can now be visualized noninvasively in many (but not all) cases of endocarditis and have become the echocardiographic hallmark of this disorder.[396–398] Thus, even though TTE cannot exclude endocarditis, abnormal findings may strongly suggest the disorder, even in the presence of negative blood cultures. Since no single abnormality has 100 percent diagnostic accuracy for infective endocarditis, strategies for diagnosis have been devised based upon a number of criteria,[399,399a,399b] and definite echocardiographic vegetations are designated as a major criterion. Both TTE and TEE are valuable in the detection of perivalvular abscesses and prosthetic-valve endocarditis.[147,400] Although there is considerable debate concerning the most accurate diagnostic criteria for endocarditis, echocardiography has become one of the most commonly used techniques for the evaluation of potentially affected patients.[401] Echocardiography (both TTE and TEE) is also useful for evaluation of patients with systemic lupus erythematosus complicated by Libman-Sacks endocarditis.[402,403]

Even though M-mode recordings produced the first echocardiographic description of vege-

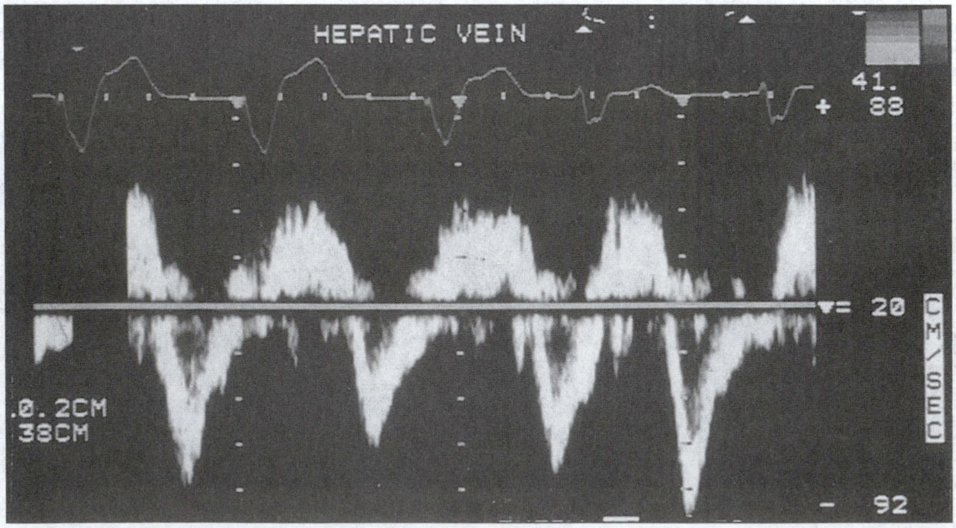

FIGURE 13-87 Pulsed-wave Doppler tracing of the hepatic vein in severe tricuspid regurgitation (TR) (subcostal transducer position). Systolic flow reversal into the hepatic vein is present.

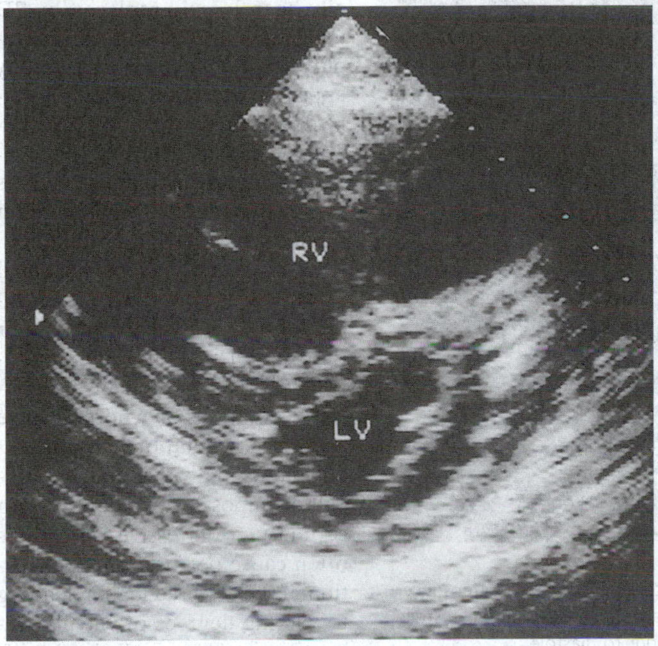

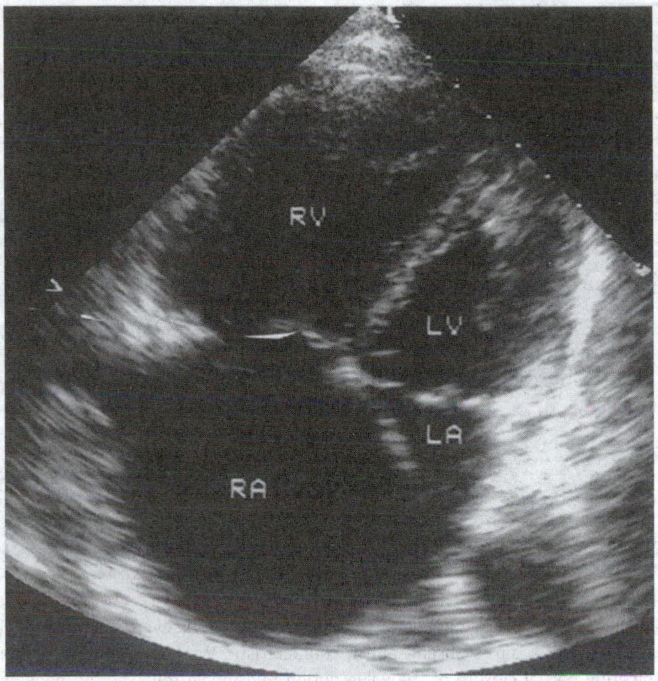

FIGURE 13-88 *A.* Parasternal short-axis view in severe pulmonary hypertension with marked enlargement of the right ventricle (RV). The left ventricle (LV) is small, and the interventricular septum is flattened. *B.* Apical four-chamber view in pulmonary hypertension. The right atrium (RA) and right ventricle (RV) are much larger than the left-sided chambers. LA = left atrium; LV = left ventricle.

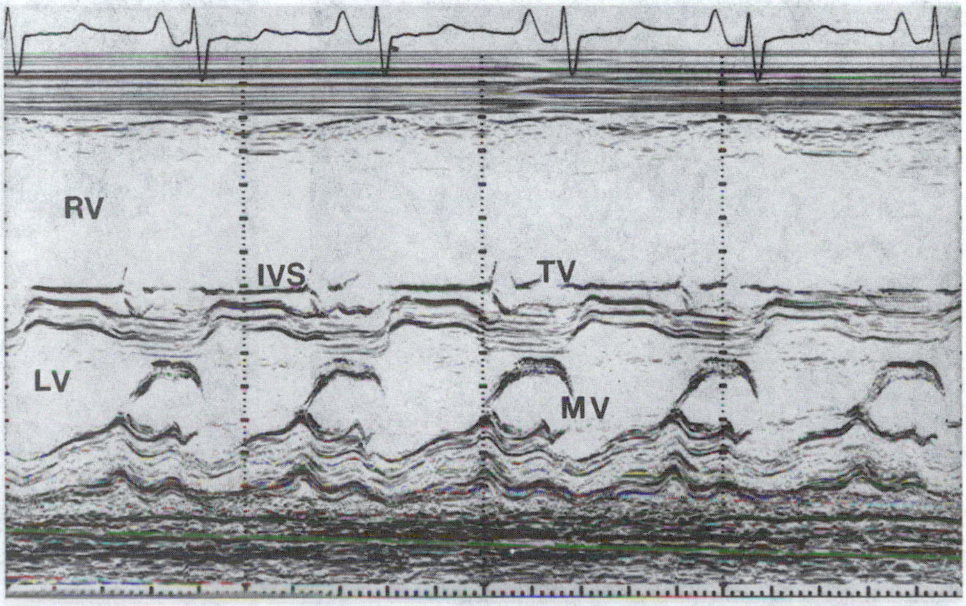

FIGURE 13-89 M-mode in severe pulmonary hypertension. The dimension of the right ventricle (RV) is larger than that of the left ventricle (LV). The interventricular septum (IVS) moves paradoxically—i.e., *toward* the mitral valve (MV) during diastole rather than away. TV = tricuspid valve.

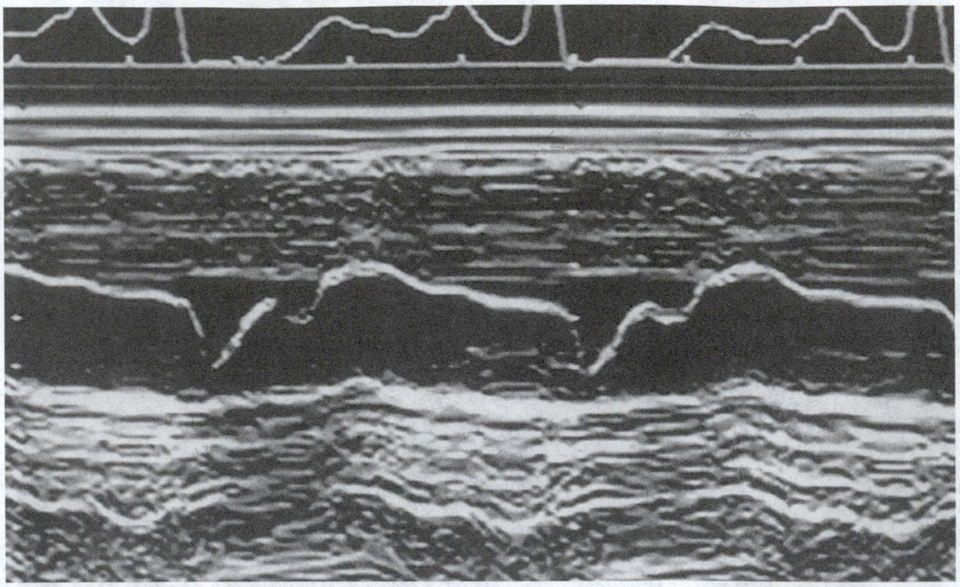

FIGURE 13-90 M-mode image of the pulmonic valve in severe pulmonary hypertension (parasternal transducer position). The a dip is absent, and a characteristic W-shaped motion of the leaflet is present during systole, indicating partial closure of the valve during midsystole followed by reopening prior to diastole.

tations,[396] this modality has gradually been largely replaced by 2D imaging. With 2D echocardiography, valvular vegetations typically appear as irregular, usually localized masses of varying echocardiographic density attached to valvular or perivalvular structures (Figs. 13-94 and 13-95) without significantly altering their mobility. The vegetations may be small or quite large and may attach directly to the valve leaflets or the supporting chordal apparatus.[397,398,404,405] Both small, nonmobile vegetations on a normal valve and large vegetations on a markedly abnormal valve may be difficult or impossible to identify with certainty. Aggressive infections often cause perforation or distortion of the affected leaflet, leading to varying degrees of valvular regurgitation. This is distinctly different from most cases of nonbacterial thrombotic (marantic) endocarditis, where the valvular vegetations are usually nondestructive.[406] In cases of infective endocarditis, the presence of vegetations by TTE increases the risk of heart failure, embolic events, and the ultimate necessity of valve replacement.[407–411] Unfortunately, TTE is not 100 per-

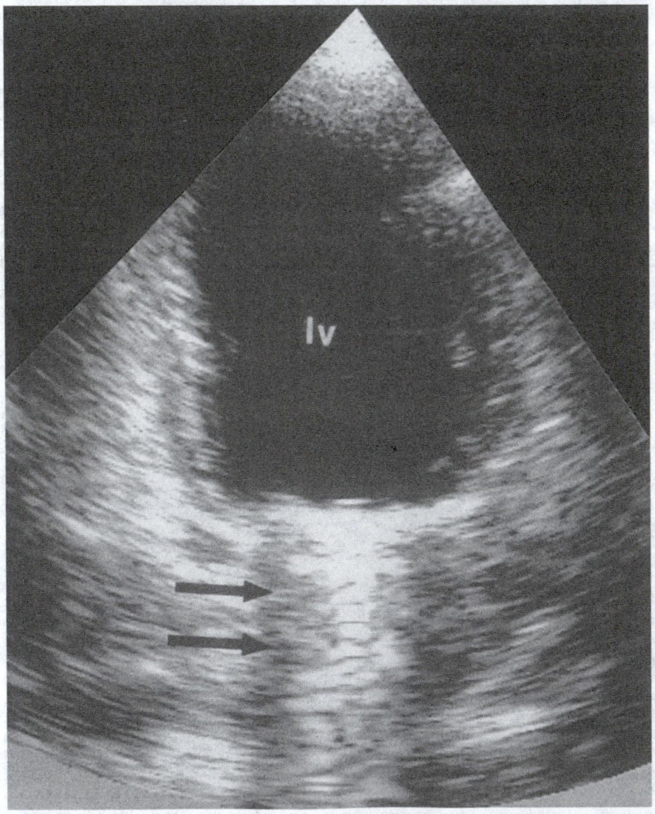

FIGURE 13-91 Apical two-chamber view of a mechanical prosthetic valve (mitral position) during systole. The left atrium is completely obscured by ultrasonic shadowing (*arrows*). LV = left ventricle.

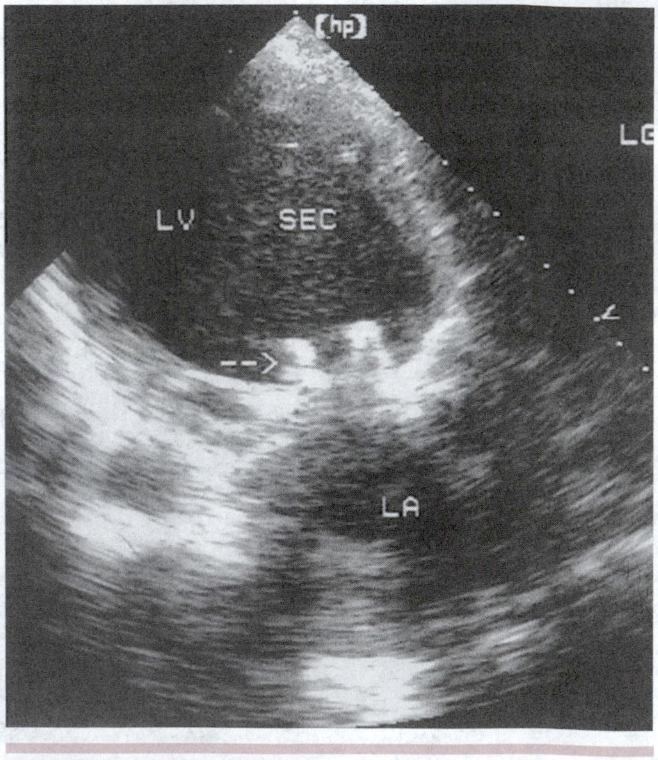

FIGURE 13-92 Apical view of a bioprosthetic valve (*arrow*) in the mitral position (two of the three prosthetic valve struts are apparent). Spontaneous echo contrast (SEC) is also present, secondary to systolic dysfunction and enlargement of the left ventricle (LV); LA = left atrium.

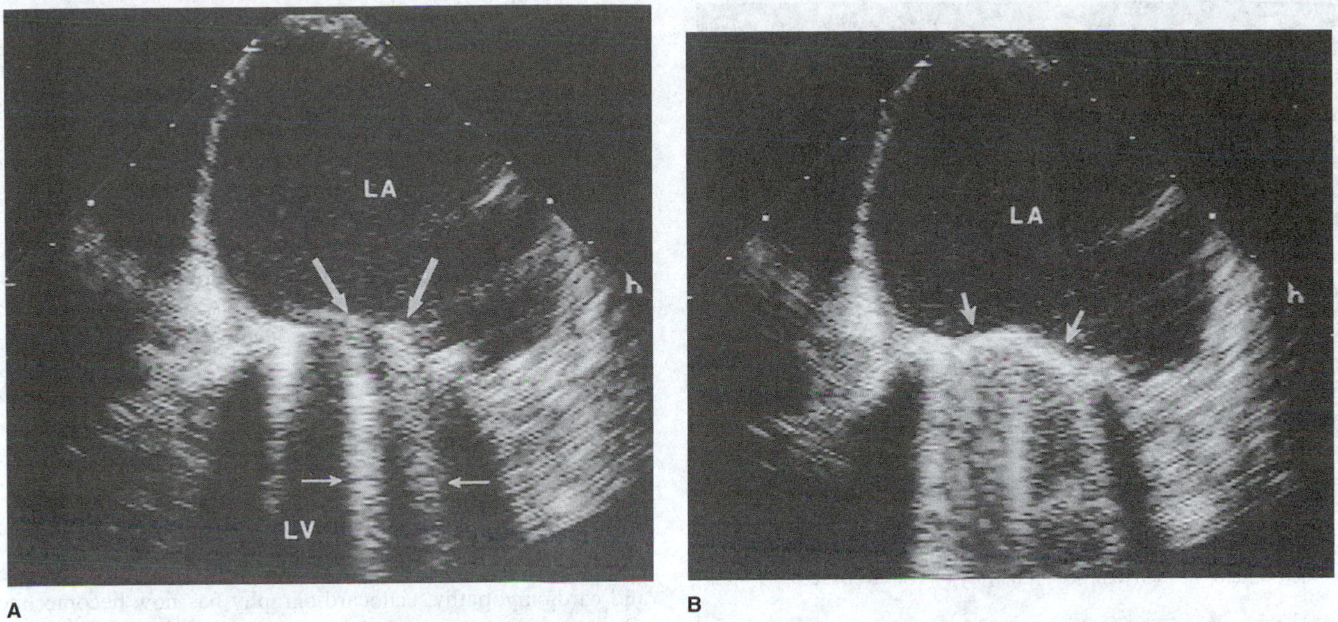

FIGURE 13-93 TEE images from a patient with a St. Jude prosthetic valve in the mitral position. *A*. Diastolic image. The two struts of the open valve are seen (*large arrows*) as well as their ultrasonic shadows (*small arrows*). LA = left atrium; LV = left ventricle. *B*. Systolic image. The two prosthetic leaflets are closed (*arrows*) and cast a dense ultrasonic shadow, obscuring the left ventricle.

cent sensitive in detecting vegetations, and up to 20 percent of patients with proved native-valve endocarditis may have unremarkable examinations.[412] The sensitivity of TTE in prosthetic valve endocarditis has been found to be even lower (approximately 60 percent) due to technical limitations in imaging.[400]

TEE has proved significantly more sensitive than TTE for detection of infective vegetations and is extremely helpful for the diagnosis of perivalvular abscesses, mycotic diverticula, and prosthetic valve involvement.[147,413] The technique is also useful for assessing valvular regurgitation, fistulas (Fig. 13-96), and other hemodynamic complications of endocarditis.[414] Although a negative TEE examination cannot completely exclude infective endocarditis, it confers a relatively good prognosis in those cases where the diagnosis is eventually confirmed.

The optimal use of TEE in suspected endocarditis remains controversial: some authorities recommend routine TEE in all

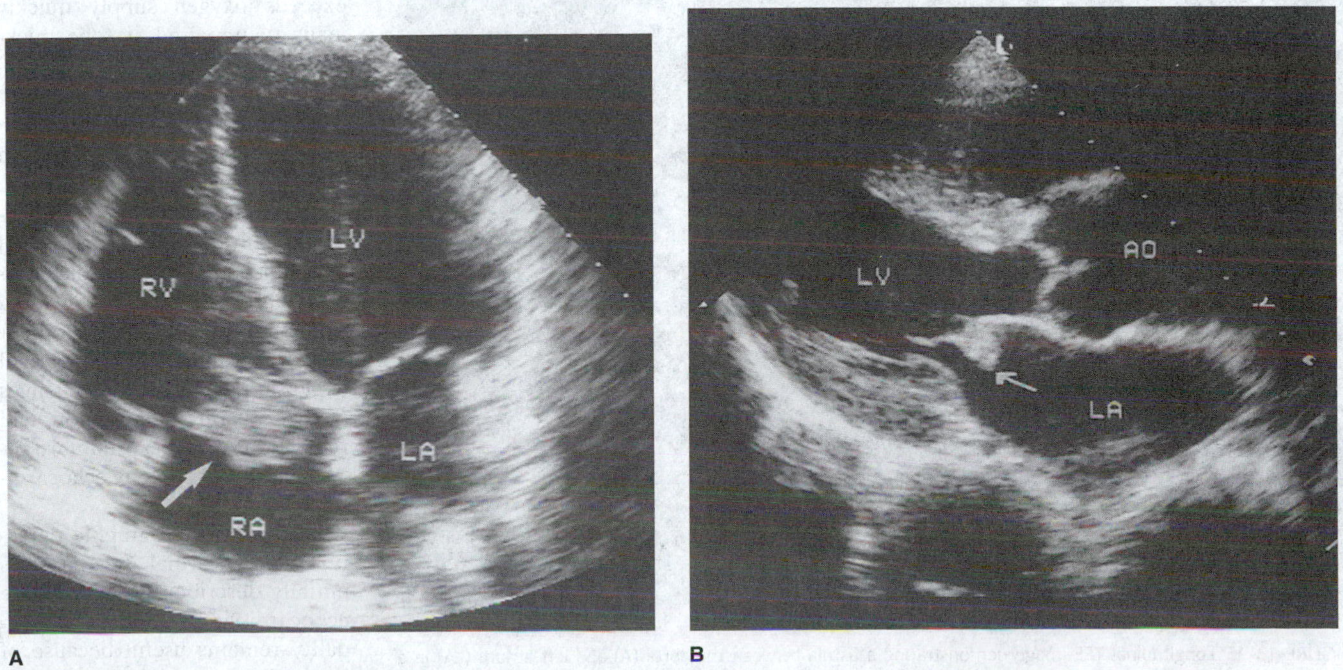

FIGURE 13-94 *A*. Apical four-chamber view demonstrating a large tricuspid valve vegetation (*arrow*). RA = right atrium; LA = left atrium; LV = left ventricle; RV = right ventricle. *B*. Parasternal long axis view demonstrating a vegetation (*arrow*) on the anterior valve leaflet; AO = aorta.

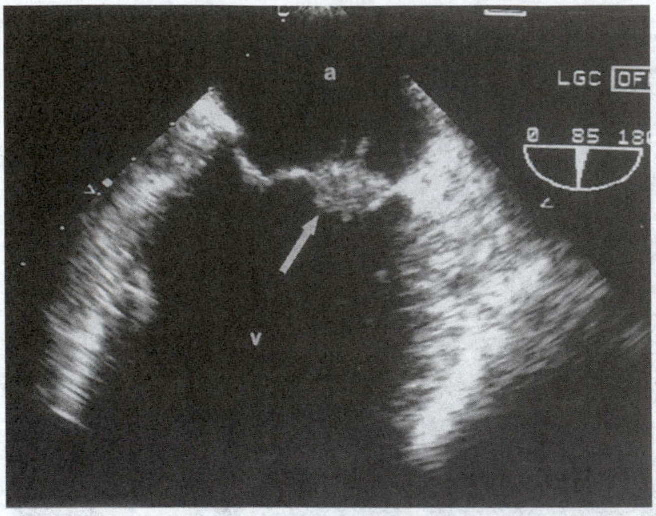

FIGURE 13-95 Longitudinal TEE view of a large mitral valve vegetation (*arrow*). a = left atrium; v = left ventricle. (Courtesy of William D. Keen, Jr., MD.)

cases, but many do not.[415] A reasonable approach may be to perform TTE as the first screening test in patients with suspected endocarditis. If the study is technically difficult, equivocal, or detects vegetations in patients at high risk for perivalvular complications or hemodynamic compromise, TEE should be performed. If TTE is unremarkable or detects vegetations in patients at low risk for complications, TEE may not be necessary.[149] Exceptions to this last recommendation might include patients with prior antibiotic treatment or those with persistent bacteremia or fever of unknown etiology. In high-risk patients (i.e., with possible prosthetic valve involvement, congenital heart disease, or infection with especially virulent organisms), TEE is recommended even if TTE is normal.[149]

Echocardiographic evaluation of suspected endocarditis is not without pitfalls. It may be quite difficult to detect active vegetations in patients with preexisting valvular abnormalities such as calcification, myxomatous change, rheumatic involvement, and healed vegetations. Despite recent technologic advances, the diagnosis of infective endocarditis remains a clinical one, and over-reliance on echocardiography may cause mistakes. Therefore, *echocardiographic results should be integrated with other clinical information* to diagnose this disorder accurately.[416]

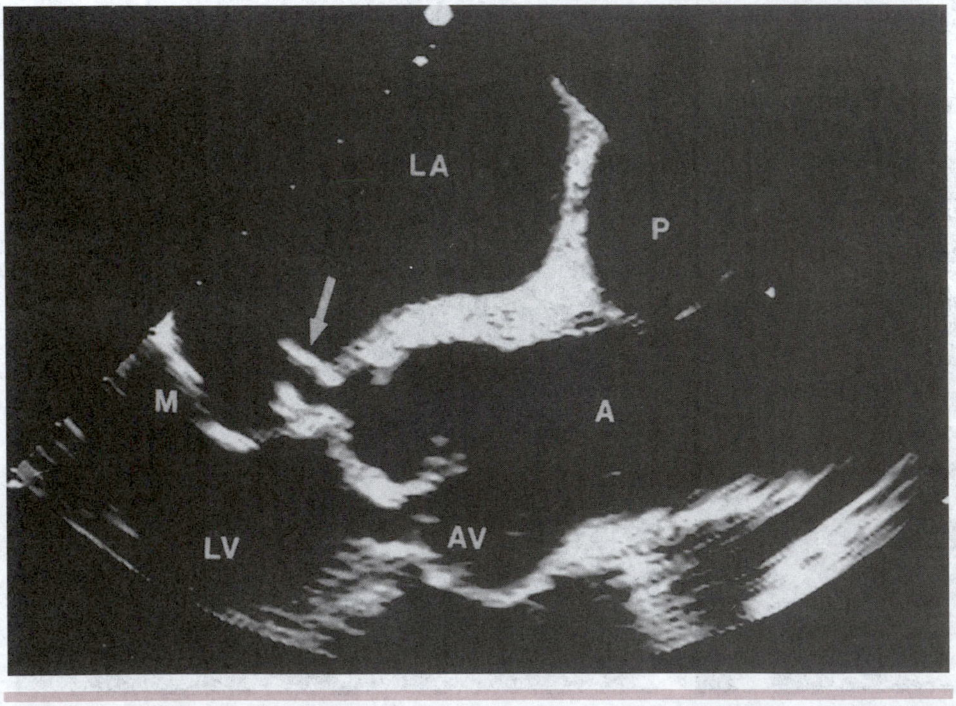

FIGURE 13-96 Longitudinal TEE image demonstrating a fistula between the aorta (A) and left atrium (LA) in a patient with endocarditis. AV = aortic valve; P = pulmonary artery; LV = left ventricle; M = mitral valve. (From Sobel J, Maisel AS, Tarazi R, Blanchard DG. Gonococcal endocarditis: Assessment by transesophageal echocardiography. *J Am Soc Echocardiogr* 1997; 10:367–370.)

ISCHEMIC HEART DISEASE

Echocardiography in Coronary Heart Disease

Although originally of greatest value in valvular heart disease and cardiomyopathy, echocardiography has now become one of the most important techniques for the detection and quantitative assessment of myocardial ischemia and infarction. Cardiac ultrasound—because it is rapid, portable, noninvasive, and inexpensive—is especially well suited to the evaluation of ischemic heart disease. Although visualization of coronary artery structure and flow has been achieved by echocardiography,[417–420] the application of this technique in ischemic heart disease continues to revolve primarily about the assessment of LV function.

Currently, the primary application of echocardiography in patients with coronary heart disease is based upon the detection of the effects of myocardial ischemia and/or infarction upon LV structure and function. Interruption of coronary flow or imposition of an oxygen demand that exceeds oxygen supply quickly leads to impaired systolic thickening and excursion of the affected myocardium. If flow is not restored and transmural infarction occurs, the affected myocardium may become akinetic or dyskinetic and eventually thinned and fibrotic. In addition, myocardial ischemia produces diastolic dysfunction, which may be detected by analysis of transmitral Doppler flow recordings or endocardial expansion profiles. These changes in the structure, contraction, and relaxation of myocardium are often readily detected by echocardiography.

The echocardiographic detection of myocardial ischemia was initially described using M-mode echocardiography, and this modality remains useful because of its excellent sensitivity and temporal resolution.[421] 2D imaging, however, has now become the primary technique for the examination of LV size, wall thickness, myocardial thickening, and regional wall motion, since it enables visualization of all LV wall segments. Thereby, in patients with CAD, standard echocardiographic approaches can be utilized to calculate LV diastolic and systolic volumes as well as ejection fraction.

The echocardiographic manifestations of CAD consist of one or more of the following: reduction in systolic thickening, abnormal segmental wall motion during systole or diastole, and alterations in the acoustic properties of the myocardium (usually termed *tissue characterization*).[422] These abnormalities may be expressed as a disturbance in global LV size and function, an increase in LV volume, and a decrease in LVEF calculated by standard approaches. In addition, using the standard tomographic planes, the LV can be divided into 16 wall segments according to the format recommended by the American Society of Echocardiography (Fig. 13-97).[423] By grading the contraction of each of the 16 segments as hyperkinetic, normal, hypokinetic, akinetic, or dyskinetic (and assigning a numerical value to each grade), a semiquantitative wall motion score can be calculated as the mean numerical value for all segments. Wall motion scores of this kind have been used to assess prognosis in both acute myocardial infarction[424] and chronic coronary artery disease.[425] When LV dysfunction is detected echocardiographically, the specific coronary artery responsible can often be inferred based upon the dyssynergy region(s).[426,427] The echocardiographic findings of akinesis with segmental myocardial thinning can also be used to distinguish CAD from dilated cardiomyopathy, which typically manifests global hypokinesis and decreased wall thickness. There is overlap in the echocardiographic findings between these two groups, however, as severe ischemic disease may cause global hypokinesis and nonischemic cardiomyopathy may sometimes cause heterogeneous dysfunction.[428]

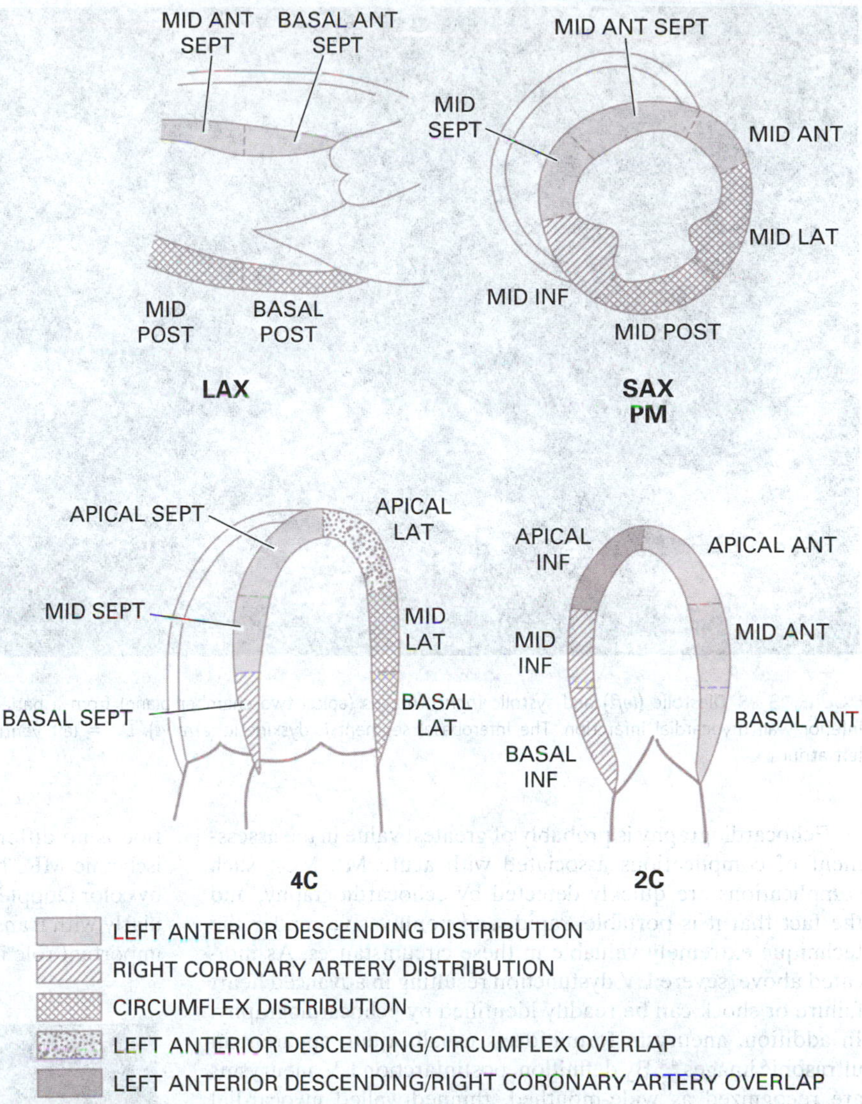

FIGURE 13-97 Sixteen-segment format for identification of left ventricular wall segments. Coronary arterial territories are also included. LAX = parasternal long axis; SAX PM = short axis at papillary muscle level; 4C = apical four-chamber; 2C = apical two-chamber; ANT = anterior; SEPT = septal; POST = posterior; LAT = lateral; INF = inferior. (From Segar D, Brown S, Sawada S, et al. Dobutamine stress echocardiography: Correlation with coronary lesion severity as determined by quantitative angiography. *J Am Coll Cardiol* 1992; 19:1197, with permission.)

Myocardial Infarction and Postinfarction Complications

Cardiac ultrasound has achieved an important role in the evaluation of patients with acute myocardial infarction (MI) and is frequently used for diagnosis, quantitative functional assessment, risk stratification, and detection of complications[424,429–432] (see also Chap. 47). Echocardiography is especially valuable in *excluding* transmural infarctions, as these are almost always associated with regional akinesis or dyskinesis (Figs. 13-98 to 13-100).[433,434] Non-Q-wave infarctions are more difficult to diagnose with certainty, however, as the echocardiogram may show subtle regional hypokinesis or even normal wall motion in some cases. Thus, echocardiography has been used to evaluate chest pain in the emergency department and appears to have a reasonable sensitivity and specificity in the diagnosis of MI.[433,434] It may also help select patients for thrombolytic therapy.[435] In addition, patients without contractile abnormalities who ultimately exhibit signs of MI have a low incidence of complications.[434]

Echocardiography is now the most commonly utilized approach to assess the effects of MI upon LV function. Ultrasound imaging studies of LV remodeling have demonstrated that infarct expansion occurs commonly with anterior infarctions, often beginning within the first 10 days, and conveys an adverse prognosis.[436,437] Similarly, calculation of the wall motion score has identified a cohort of post-MI patients at markedly increased risk for in-hospital complications.[434] This prognostic marker appears superior to conventional clinical criteria in predicting events.[434]

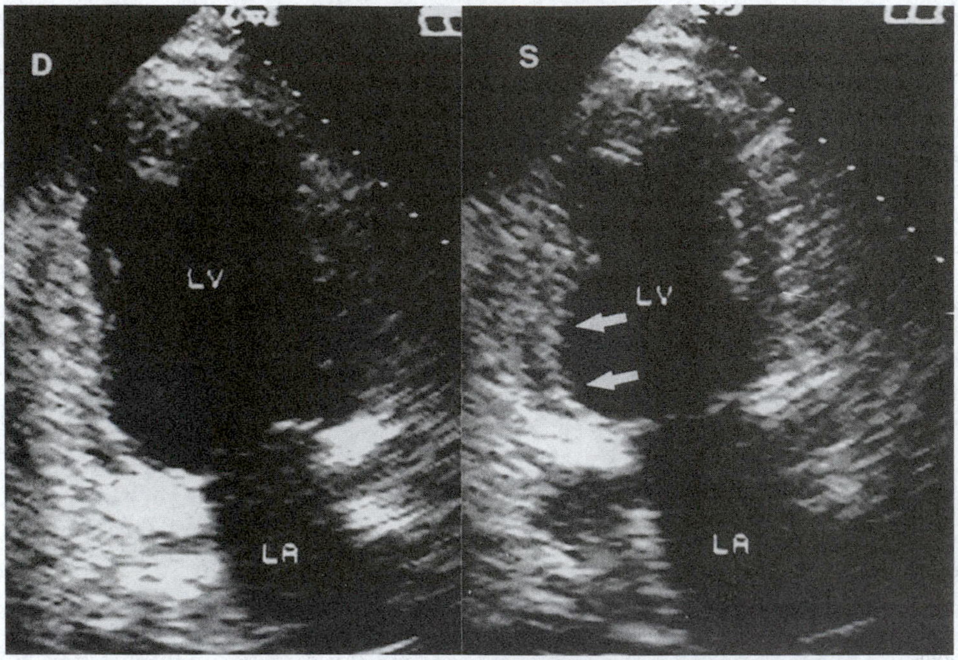

FIGURE 13-98 Diastolic (*left*) and systolic (*right*) images (apical two-chamber plane) from a patient with an inferior wall myocardial infarction. The inferobasal segment is dyskinetic (*arrows*). LV = left ventricle; LA = left atrium.

of myocardium and distinct flow jets communicating between the LV and RVs (Fig. 13-102, Plate 68).[444] These color jets are typically high-velocity and aliased, coursing from the septum into the RV. The echocardiographic location of the defect and jet correlate well with the location by cineangiography, surgery, or autopsy, and an apical location is most amenable to surgical correction.[444]

MR is a common sequela of acute MI; if severe, it may result in profound congestive heart failure and shock. Several mechanisms may be responsible for the occurrence of postinfarction MR including dilation of the LV cavity and mitral annulus, papillary muscle dysfunction, and partial or complete rupture of a papillary muscle (Fig. 13-103).[445–447] MR from papillary dysfunction may lead to eccentric color jets within the LA. In general, the recognition and quantitation of MR occurring in the postinfarction period is no different from that of any other type of MR. Acute ischemic MR, however may cause a smaller flow disturbance by color Doppler than comparable grades of chronic MR, particularly with transthoracic imaging. Therefore, TEE may play an important role in the identification and quantitative assessment

Echocardiography is probably of greatest value in the assessment of complications associated with acute MI. Most such complications are quickly detected by echocardiography, and the fact that it is portable, rapid, and noninvasive render the technique extremely valuable in these circumstances. As indicated above, severe LV dysfunction resulting in advanced heart failure or shock can be readily identified by echocardiography. In addition, aneurysm formation is usually quite apparent in ultrasonic images.[438] By definition, postinfarction LV aneurysms are recognized as wide-mouthed, thinned-walled myocardial segments that display dyskinetic expansion during systole. Aneurysms are a favored site for development of LV thrombi, which are discussed in detail in the discussion of cardiac masses, below. A less frequent complication is rupture of the LV free wall, which is usually rapidly fatal and therefore rarely imaged by echocardiography.[439] However, the presence of significant pericardial effusion on echocardiography in patients with hemodynamic compromise in the postinfarction period should suggest this condition. If a free wall rupture is sealed off by clot and pericardial inflammation, a pseudoaneurysm is formed[440,441] (Fig. 13-101). This lesion is distinguished from a true aneurysm by its highly localized nature and the presence of a narrow neck connecting it with the ventricle. Pseudoaneurysms frequently have multilayered thrombi within them and exhibit characteristic Doppler flow signals at the junction with the ventricle.[441] Since the risk of rupture is high, accurate diagnosis and prompt surgical repair of pseudoaneurysms is important.

Although postinfarction free wall rupture does not lend itself well to echocardiographic detection, acquired defects of the interventricular septum are more commonly delineated by cardiac ultrasound.[442,443] Acquired ventricular septal defects often consist of a latticework of tissue rather than a discrete orifice, but nevertheless echocardiographic images can depict absence

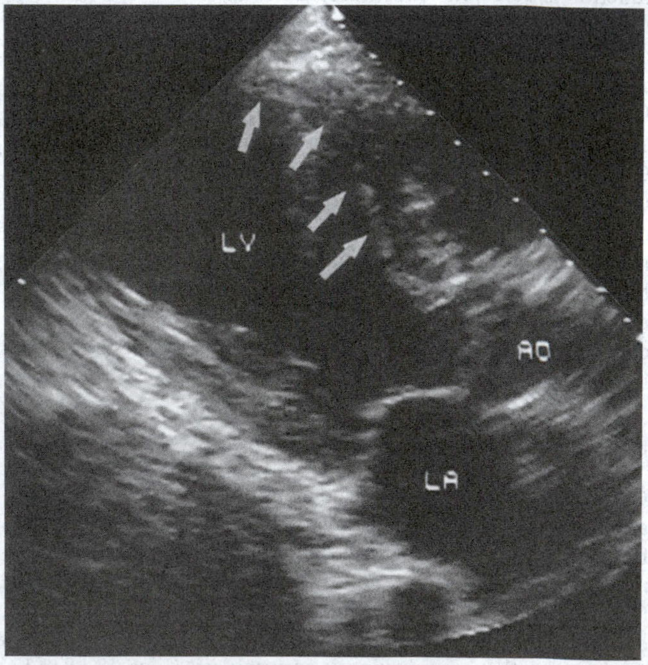

FIGURE 13-99 Parasternal long-axis view of a large anteroseptal myocardial infarction, with thinning and dyskinesis of the anteroseptal wall (*arrows*). LV = left ventricle; LA = left atrium; AO = aorta.

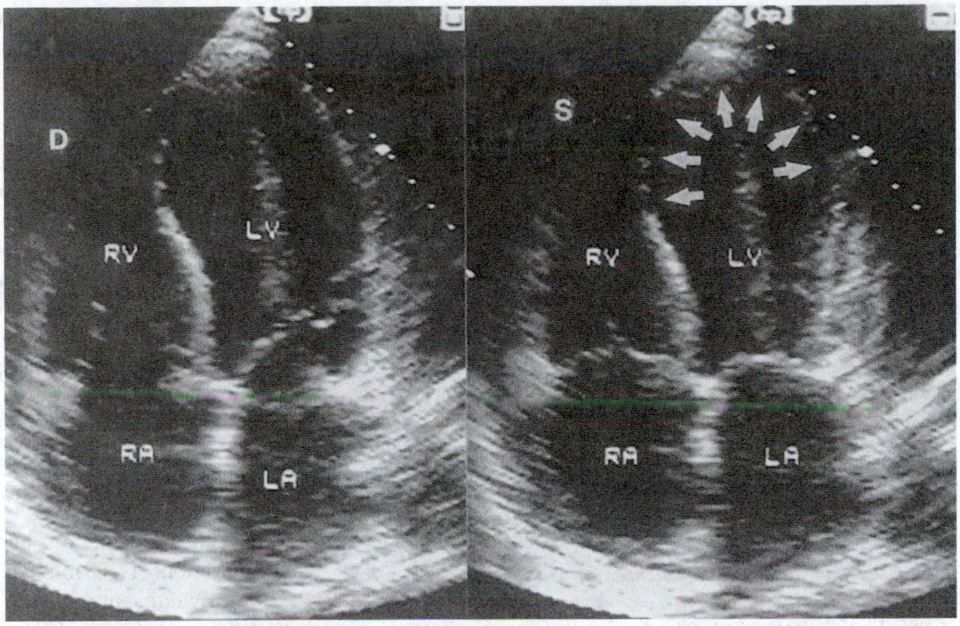

FIGURE 13-100 Apical four-chamber images of a large apical infarction. Diastole (D) is displayed on the left, systole (S) on the right. During systole, the base of the ventricle contracts, but the apex is dyskinetic (*arrows*).

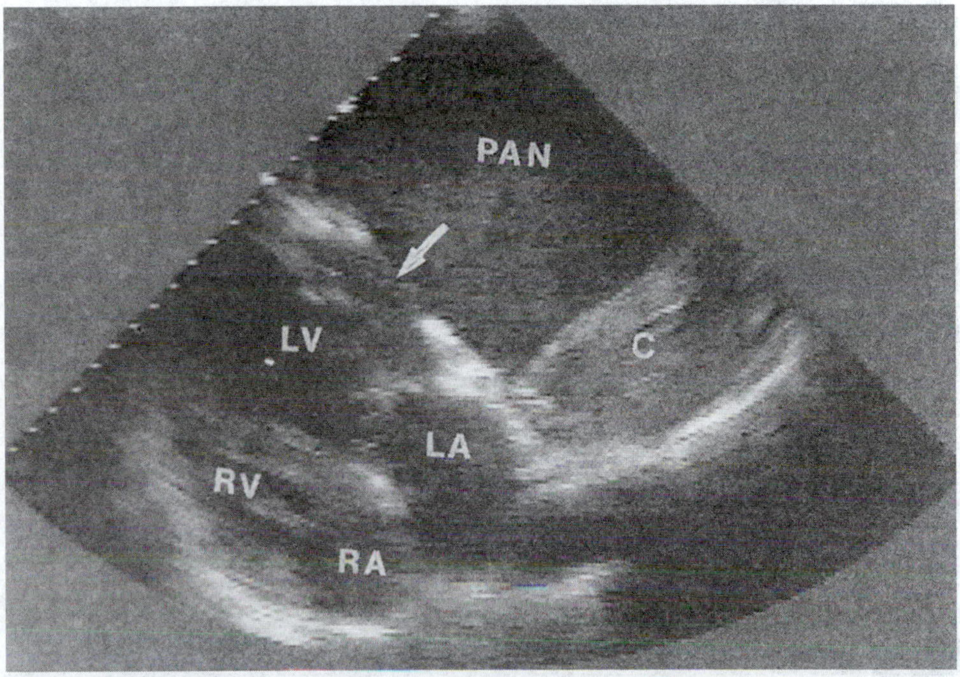

FIGURE 13-101 Modified apical four-chamber view of a large pseudoaneurysm (PAN) communicating with the left ventricle (LV). The rupture site is apparent (*arrow*); clot (C) is present within the aneurysm. (From Yucel G, Steinberg E, O'Reilly M, Kronzon I. Giant left ventricular pseudoaneurysm. *Circulation* 1996; 94:848, with permission.)

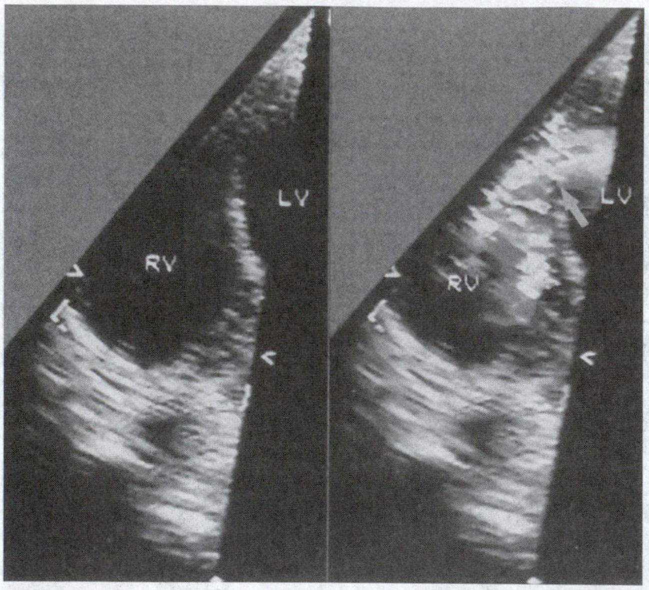

FIGURE 13-102 (Plate 68) Modified apical four-chamber image of a distal septal ventricular septal rupture. With 2D imaging (*left*), the distal septum is incompletely visualized. With color Doppler imaging, however, a high-velocity aliased color jet is seen in the right ventricle (RV). In addition, an area of flow convergence is seen on the left ventricular (LV) side of the rupture (*arrow*).

of this complication, as well as in ensuring adequate operative repair.[447]

In the setting of inferior wall infarction due to occlusion of the proximal right coronary artery, right ventricular MI may occur. The most specific echocardiographic sign of right ventricular infarction is a regional wall motion abnormality, which is usually best visualized in the RV free wall (Fig. 13-104).[448] RV infarction is typically accompanied by RV enlargement and tricuspid regurgitation; associated inferior or posterior left ventricular wall motion abnormalities are virtually always present.

Pericarditis is a common complication of acute MI, typically occurring during the acute phase of the illness and much less often in the late phases as part of Dressler syndrome. Postinfarction pericarditis, however, is not typically associated with marked echocardiographic abnormalities. If a pericardial effusion is present at all, the amount of fluid is usually quite small. Therefore, the absence of pericardial fluid on ECG cannot rule out pericarditis, and the presence of a large effusion with tamponade should raise the suspicion of a LV free wall rupture.

TEE has recently assumed a central role in the evaluation of patients with significant hemodynamic abnormalities in the postinfarction period. When TTE is technically suboptimal, transesophageal images can rapidly identify LV dyssynergy, valvular dysfunction, and other abnormalities associated with infarction. TEE may enable direct visualization of acquired ventricular septal defects when the lesion is not obvious or seen only as a disturbed flow stream in the RV with transthoracic imaging. Perhaps of greatest significance, TEE can provide definitive identification of a ruptured papillary muscle and a quantitative assessment of postinfarction mitral regurgitation.

Echocardiography has been used to evaluate the extent of reperfusion after thrombolytic or interventional therapy for acute MI. Several reports have demonstrated that LV systolic function assessed by 2D imaging improved within 24 h to 10 days of successful thrombolysis.[449,450] More recently, contrast echocardiograms obtained by direct intracoronary injection have shown that reperfusion of the infarct-related epicardial coronary artery by angiography is not necessarily accompanied by evidence of normal flow in the downstream microcirculation. In addition, this "no-reflow" phenomenon on echocardiography heralds a poor prognosis, including failure of improvement of LV performance as well as increased late complications.[208–210,450a]

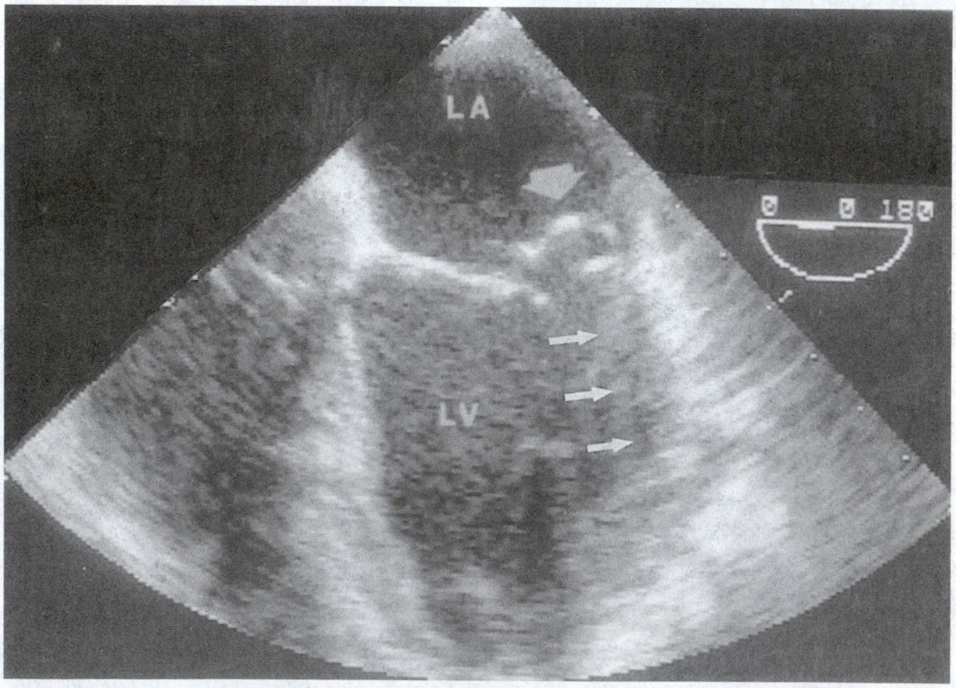

FIGURE 13-103 Transverse four-chamber TEE image of a posterolateral infarction causing posterior papillary muscle ischemia and partial rupture. The posterior mitral leaflet (*large arrow*) is poorly supported (but not actually flail) and prolapses into the left atrium (LA). The basal lateral wall segment (*small arrows*) of the left ventricle (LV) is dyskinetic.

Stress Echocardiography

Recently, the combination of stress testing and echocardiography (stress echocardiography) has found an important role in the diagnosis of CAD[451–453] (see also Chap. 42). The utility of this technique improved dramatically when technologic advances permitted side-by-side viewing of rest and stress images together in a cine-loop format.[454] The application of stress echocardiography is based upon the concept that a stress-induced imbalance in the

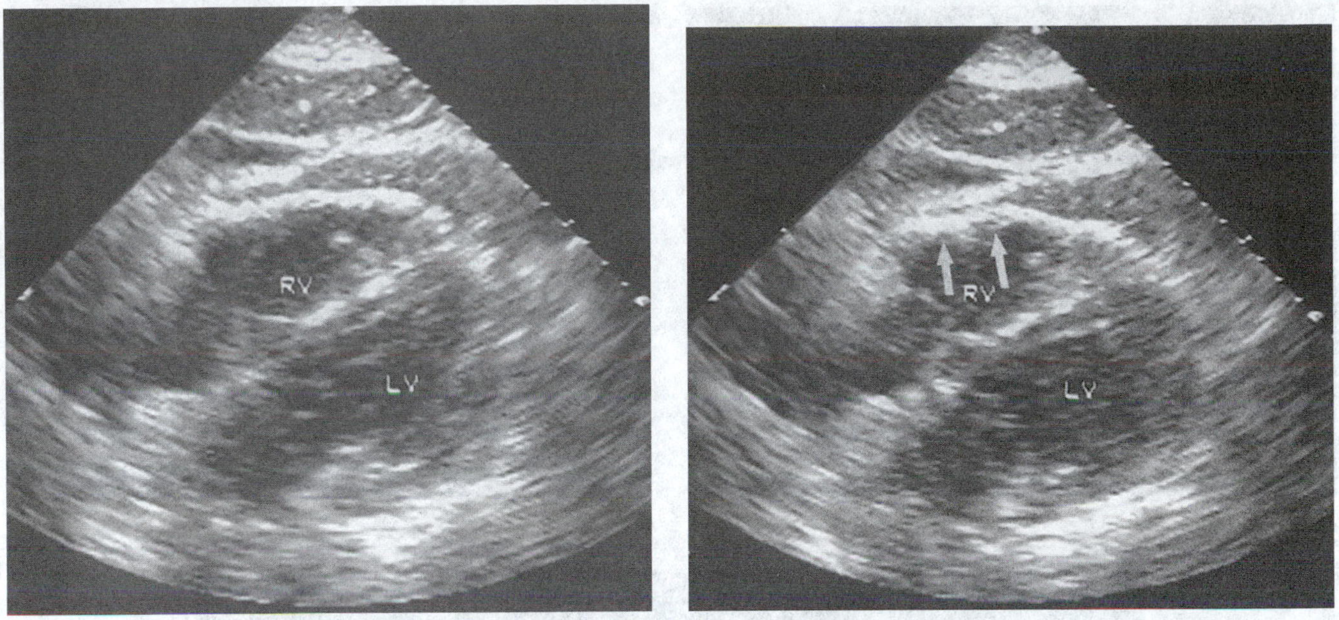

A B

FIGURE 13-104 Diastolic (*A*) and systolic (*B*) subcostal four-chamber images of right ventricular (RV) myocardial infarction. The RV free wall is dyskinetic (*arrows*) during systole (*B*).

myocardial supply/demand ratio will produce regional ischemia and resultant abnormalities of regional contraction, which can be readily identified by echocardiography (Fig. 13-105). The location of wall motion abnormalities may be used to predict the stenosed coronary vessel(s), while the ratio of dyssynergic to normal myocardium can provide a quantitative assessment of LV ischemia.[426,427] Although the digital techniques currently employed limit the number of views available and restrict the examination to eight frames during systole, this process does not seem to impair the ability to identify contractile dysfunction.[455,456]

The types of stress employed fall into two basic groups, exercise and pharmacologic.[426,427] Other forms, such as mental stress and atrial pacing, are not widely used. Exercise testing can be performed either on a treadmill or a stationary bicycle (either upright or supine).[457] Treadmill testing involves a familiar activity, uses equipment that is widely available, and achieves a greater oxygen consumption than bicycle ergometry. Echo imaging usually can be accomplished only before and after treadmill exercise, however, whereas bicycle exertion facilitates the acquisition of images during the exercise protocol. Thus far, treadmill has been the preferred exercise modality. Of importance, all postexertional images should be obtained within a 2-min window following exercise to avoid recording normal contractile function after recovery from ischemia.

Pharmacologic stress has the advantages of reducing the motion artifact of exercise, enabling continuous imaging throughout the protocol, and assessing myocardial viability.[458–469] Pharmacologic stress echocardiography can employ vasodilator agents such as dipyridamole or adenosine, which induce a heterogeneity of myocardial perfusion in ischemic heart disease, or inotropic agents such as dobutamine and arbutamine, which increase myocardial oxygen demand and directly produce ischemia.[458–469] As with exercise stress, diagnostic criteria include induction of regional wall motion abnormalities and LV dilatation. It is important to recognize that the normal response to exercise is hyperkinesis, and wall motion abnormalities may take the form of a lesser degree of hyperkinesis of a given segment in comparison with the rest of the LV myocardium. Dobutamine stress echocardiography appears to be of particular value in detecting myocardial viability.[455–463,466–469,469a,469b]

The safety and accuracy of stress echocardiography for the diagnosis of myocardial ischemia has been examined in a number of studies.[453,469–472] Both exercise and pharmacologic stress carry an extremely low risk of arrhythmia or infarction, although dobutamine can result in hypotension or *systolic anterior motion of the mitral valve* (SAM) with resultant LV outflow obstruction.[453,473,474] In general, stress echocardiography and nuclear scintigraphy yield similar results, although stress echocardiography may be slightly less sensitive and slightly more specific than scintigraphy.[455,464,475] In a study performed in an institution with high volumes and expertise in both ultrasound and radionuclide stress imaging, the two techniques were found to be comparable in their accuracy of detecting coronary artery disease.[455]

The most common clinical application of stress echocardiography is in the diagnosis of CAD, and it appears especially useful in cases where exercise *electrocardiography* (ECG) may be inaccurate or falsely positive (e.g., abnormal baseline ECG, LV hypertrophy, or chronic digitalis administration).[453,472,476,477] In this regard, stress echocardiography appears especially useful for detection of ischemia in women,[478,478a,478b] in whom stress ECG yields a high incidence of false-positive results. Stress echocardiography also adds independent prognostic information to exercise ECG, even in multivessel CAD.[479] Dobutamine echocardiography may aid in the detection of ischemia in patients with cardiac transplantation and allograft vasculopathy (chronic rejection).[480] In patients with known CAD, exercise echocardiography may facilitate localization and quantitation of ischemia, guide revascularization procedures, and assess the functional severity of coronary artery stenoses.[481] Stress echo-

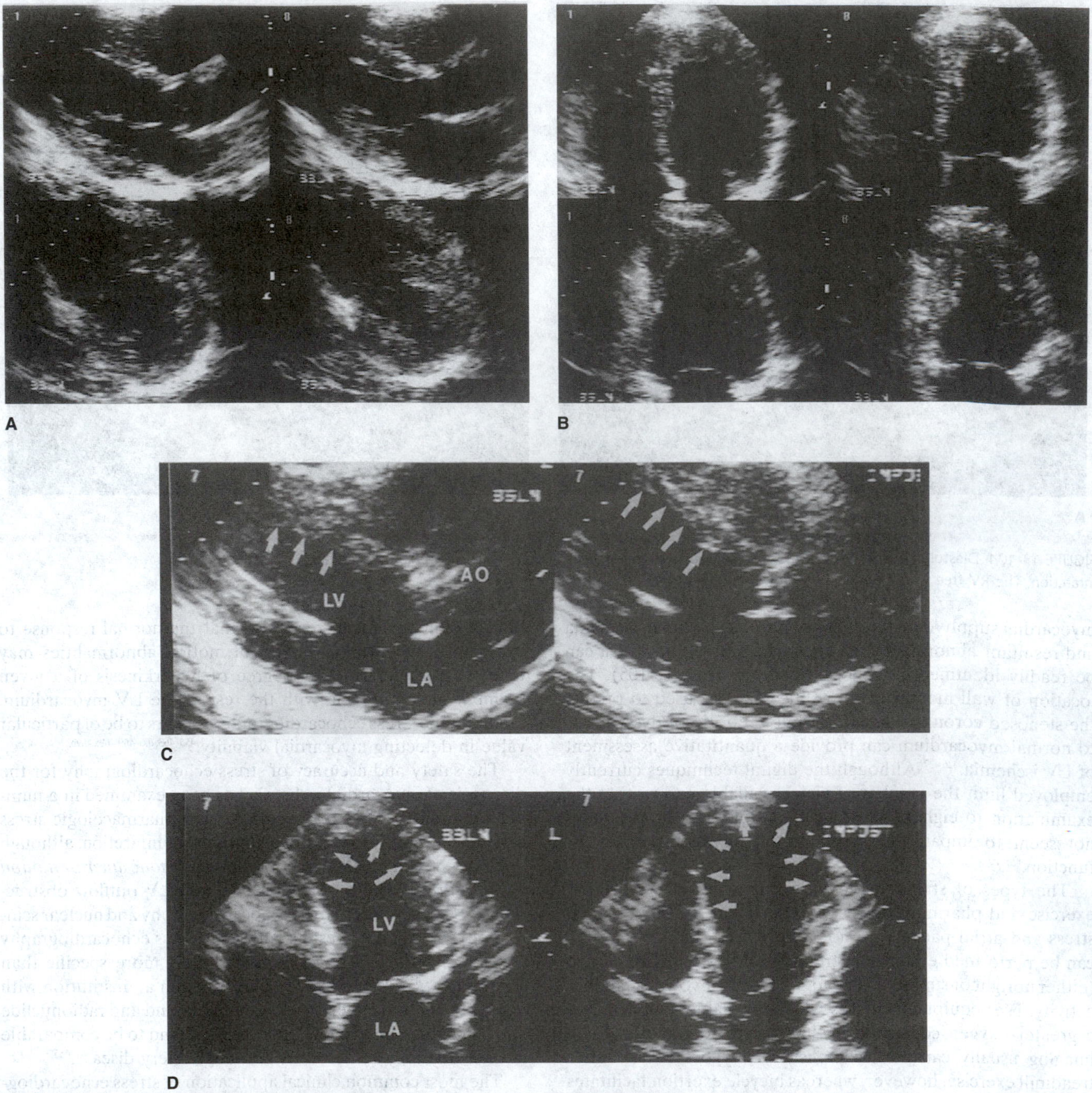

FIGURE 13-105 *A.* Digitized parasternal views during diastole (*left*) and systole (*right*) from a normal individual. *Upper panels:* long-axis plane; *lower panels:* short-axis plane. *B.* Digitized apical views during diastole (*left*) and systole (*right*) from a normal individual. *Upper panels:* four-chamber plane; *lower panels:* two-chamber plane. *C.* Digitized parasternal long-axis views at peak systole before (*left*) and immediately after exercise (*right*). The anteroseptal wall moves normally at rest (*arrows*) but becomes dyskinetic with exercise. LV = left ventricle; LA = left atrium; AO = aorta. *D.* Digitized apical four-chamber views at peak systole before (*left*) and immediately after exercise (*right*). The apical septal, apical, and apical lateral walls become dyskinetic with exercise, suggesting inducible ischemia in the left anterior descending artery territory. LA = left atrium; LV = left ventricle. *E.* Digitized parasternal short-axis views (all recorded at peak systole) during dobutamine echocardiography in a patient with three-vessel coronary artery disease. At baseline (*upper left panel*), the left ventricular systolic function is normal. With low-dose dobutamine (5 μg/kg/min, *upper right panel*), function improves. With 10 μg/kg/min, however (*lower left panel*), function is similar to that at baseline. At 20 μg/kg/min (*lower right panel*), systolic function deteriorates and the left ventricle dilates. This response suggests global ischemia induced by dobutamine infusion.

cardiography can also demonstrate resolution of regional ischemia after successful coronary artery bypass surgery or angioplasty.[482–485]

Stress echocardiography can play an important role in determining the prognosis of patients with CAD.[486–494,494a,494b,494c] Both exercise and pharmacologic stress echocardiography appear superior to exercise ECG for identification of patients at high risk of recurrent ischemic events after MI.[486–491] In addition, dobutamine stress echocardiography is useful in predicting perioperative ischemic complications in patients undergoing noncardiac surgery and appears to have a very strong negative predictive value.[492–494]

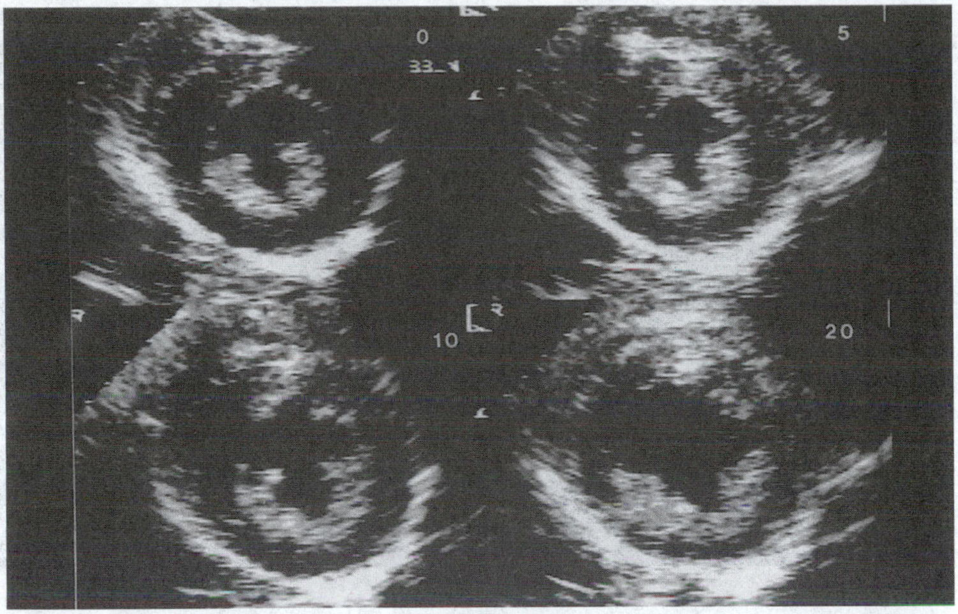

E

FIGURE 13-105 (*Continued*)

In patients with chronic CHD, dobutamine stress echocardiography can identify hypokinetic yet viable myocardium and predicts improvement in function after successful revascularization.[457–463,467,469a,469b,470] Functional improvement in a hypokinetic segment with low-dose dobutamine infusion which then progresses to hypokinesis or akinesis with higher dobutamine dose (the so-called biphasic response) correlates well with the presence of ischemic yet viable ("hibernating") myocardium. Studies have suggested that dobutamine stress echocardiography compares well with positron emission tomography and thallium single-photon emission computed tomography (SPECT) imaging in this regard.[466–468,495–505,501a,501b] It is likely that this application of echocardiography will continue to evolve over time, particularly for pharmacologic stress testing (Chap. 48).

There is evidence that exercise echocardiography can provide useful information regarding the hemodynamic status and functional severity of valvular heart disease.[502–505] Specifically, stress echocardiography has been used to assess the degree of obstruction in patients with MS[503] and to quantitate the severity of AS in patients with advanced LV dysfunction.[505] These data may help guide the timing of surgical valve repair or replacement.

As is true of all diagnostic modalities, stress echocardiography has certain limitations. High-quality ultrasound images may be difficult to acquire in some patients—a situation that may be exacerbated by exertion and the time constraints inherent to exercise stress testing. In addition, considerable expertise is required to interpret stress echocardiographic images accurately, and this learning curve precludes the use of stress echocardiography by all but experienced echocardiographers. Nevertheless, stress echocardiography has many advantages over alternate diagnostic approaches such as radionuclide scintigraphy and coronary angiography, including its noninvasive and relatively inexpensive nature, rapid acquisition and interpretation times, and freedom from ionizing radiation. Harmonic imaging (both with and without intravenous echocardiographic contrast) has also enhanced endocardial border definition, facilitating stress echo studies in many patients with suboptimal fundamental (nonharmonic) echo images. Therefore it is anticipated that the use of stress echocardiography will continue to increase in the foreseeable future.

THE CARDIOMYOPATHIES

The evaluation of cardiomyopathy is complicated by the fact that few specific diagnostic criteria exist, and identification is often a process of exclusion. Further, many potential etiologies may be responsible for the myopathic process, and it may be possible to identify a specific etiology in only the minority of patients. Accordingly, a diagnostic strategy has evolved that initially seeks to place patients into one of three pathophysiologic categories: dilated, hypertrophic, or restrictive; then, the specific etiologies recognized as producing the individual pathophysiologic state are pursued.[506] Thus, dilated cardiomyopathies are associated with myocyte loss and necrosis, a marked increase in LV volume, thinning of the myocardium, and profound systolic dysfunction.[507] *Hypertrophic cardiomyopathy* (HCM) is recognized by increased myocardial thickness, particularly involving the interventricular septum, with preserved systolic function.[508] Restrictive cardiomyopathies may be due to infiltration of the myocardium by abnormal substances or fibrotic tissue; these cause symmetrical degrees of wall thickening with modest or no diminution of systolic function and little change in cavity size.[509] Echocardiography customarily serves as the cornerstone of such evaluations and provides data on cavity size, wall thickness, and systolic function. Thus, on echocardiogram, patients with dilated cardiomyopathy exhibit a marked increase in left LV and volume, little change in wall thickness, and severe contractile dysfunction.[507] Patients with HCM exhibit a dramatic increase in LV wall thickness, with the septum characteristically disproportionate to the posterior wall, and often subaortic stenosis induced by systolic anterior motion of the anterior mitral

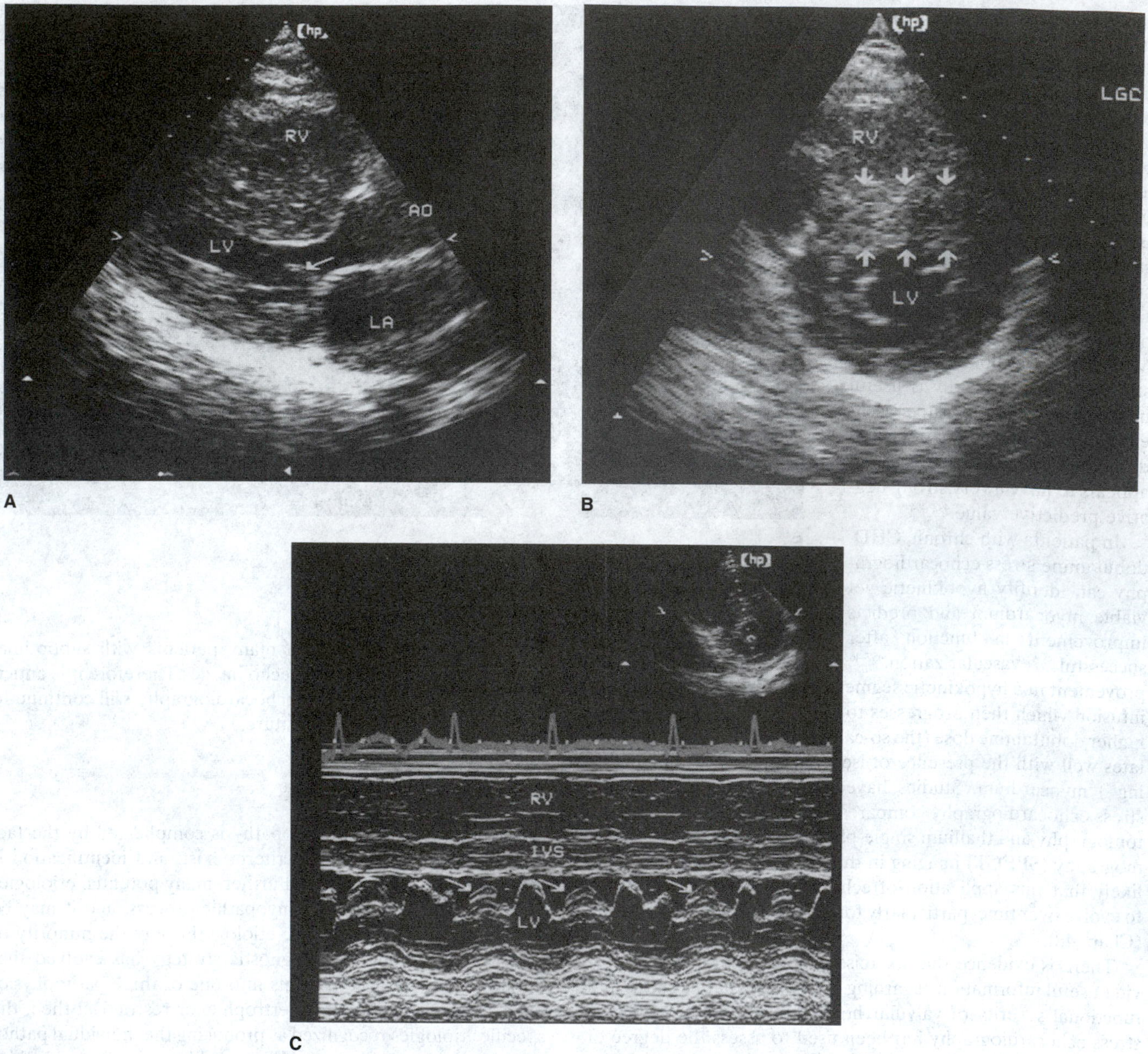

FIGURE 13-106 *A.* Parasternal long-axis view (during systole) of hypertrophic cardiomyopathy (HCM). Asymmetrical septal hypertrophy is present, as is systolic anterior motion of the anterior mitral valve leaflet (*arrow*). LV = left ventricle; LA = left atrium; RV = right ventricle; AO = aorta. *B.* Parasternal short-axis view of HCM. Asymmetrical septal hypertrophy is present (*arrows*). RV = right ventricle; LV = left ventricle. *C.* Parasternal M-mode image from a patient with HCM, demonstrating systolic anterior motion of the anterior mitral valve leaflet (*arrows*). RV = right ventricle; IVS = interventricular septum; LV = left ventricle.

valve leaflet. Patients with restrictive cardiomyopathy are identified by a symmetrical increase in wall thickness accompanied by modest changes in contractile function and LV cavity size.[509]

Hypertrophic Cardiomyopathy

HCM is a primary abnormality of the myocardium that exhibits myocyte disarray and unprovoked hypertrophy, often affecting the septum disproportionately[508] (see also Chap. 74). The disorder, which is often transmitted in an autosomal dominant pattern, has been linked to a number of abnormalities in genes that code for myocardial proteins.[510,511] A number of classic echocardiographic findings occur in HCM (Fig. 13-106). The fundamental abnormality on echocardiogram in HCM is LV hypertrophy, which is often severe. Although the hypertrophy may be confined to the septum, it may be concentric or involve any other portion of the LV.[512] The customary classic finding is *asymmetrical septal hypertrophy* (ASH), defined as a disproportionate thickness of the interventricular septum compared to the posterobasal wall with a ratio of greater than 1.3 to 1.[513,514] In some cases the entire septum is hypertrophied, while in others the thickening may be localized to the proximal, mid-, or distal (apical) septum.[515] Asymmetric hypertrophy of the proximal interventricular septum may lead to dynamic LV outflow tract obstruction—*hypertrophic obstructive cardiomyopathy* (HOCM) or *idiopathic hypertrophic subaortic stenosis* (IHSS). Although ASH is almost always present in cases of dynamic LV outflow tract obstruction, it is not a specific marker for HCM and may occur in some patients with RV hypertrophy, inferior MI, and a minority with hypertensive LV hypertrophy.[516] In general, the more extensive the hypertrophic process, the more severe the symptoms. Extent of hypertrophy, however, does not appear to correlate well with risk of sudden death, as patients with minimal hypertrophy may still be at significant risk.[517]

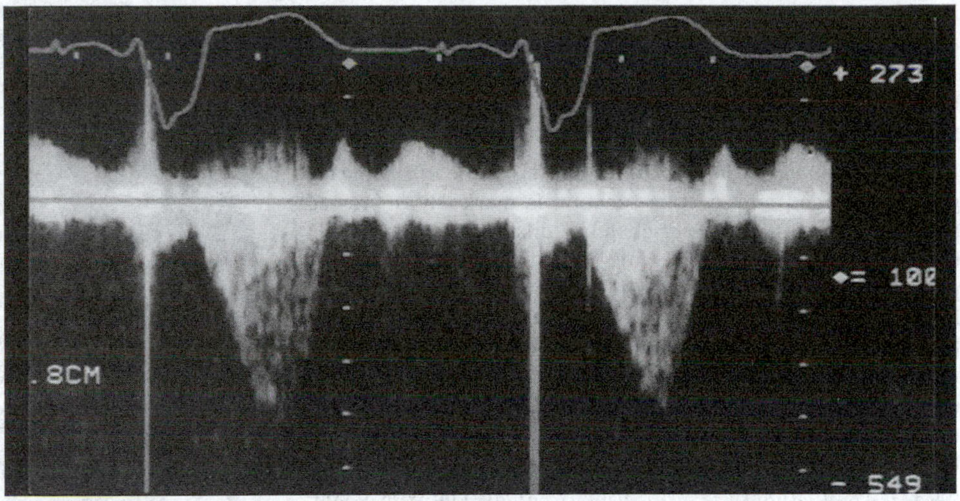

FIGURE 13-107 Continuous-wave Doppler tracing through the left ventricular outflow tract (from the apical transducer position) in hypertrophic obstructive cardiomyopathy (HOCM). In comparison to valvular aortic stenosis, the rise in velocity is delayed (reflecting dynamic rather than fixed outflow obstruction).

The second characteristic finding of HCM is systolic anterior motion of the mitral valve, or SAM, which usually involves the anterior mitral valve leaflet. Posterior-leaflet SAM also has been reported in HCM, as have a variety of mitral valve deformities.[518,519] Encroachment of the pathologically thickened septum upon the LV outflow tract creates a pressure drop by a Venturi effect, which draws the mitral leaflets toward the septum, creating dynamic (subaortic) LV outflow obstruction (Fig. 13-106). Recent work has also demonstrated the important effects of papillary muscle position and chordal tension on systolic mitral morphology and SAM.[520] Because of distorted mitral coaptation during systole, SAM generally causes MR of variable severity. The severity and duration of SAM directly influence the degree of both outflow tract obstruction and mitral regurgitation.[521] Like asymmetrical septal hypertrophy, SAM (especially systolic motion of the chordae) is not pathognomonic for HCM, having been reported in other conditions such as hypovolemia, anemia, and states where LV outflow tract narrowing and hyperdynamic contraction are present.[522,523]

The third manifestation of classic HCM is midsystolic closure of the aortic valve.[524] This finding is best seen on M-mode recordings, occurs only in the presence of outflow tract obstruction, and is probably a manifestation of the sudden pressure drop during mid- and late systole caused by SAM. As with ASH and SAM, midsystolic aortic closure is not specific for HCM and can occur in MR, aortic root dilatation, ventricular septal defect, and discrete subaortic stenosis.[525,526] When HCM is present, however, midsystolic aortic valve closure suggests significant outflow tract obstruction.

The fourth important abnormality of HCM is observed on Doppler examination of the LV outflow tract (LVOT). Normally, Doppler interrogation of this area produces a spectral tracing that peaks early in systole and has a maximum velocity of less than 1.7 m/s. In many patients, HCM creates a high-pressure gradient coincident with SAM, which is detected by Doppler as a high-velocity systolic jet in the LVOT. As opposed to valvular aortic stenosis, however, the maximal velocity in obstructive HCM peaks late in systole, creating a characteristic "saber-tooth" pattern (Fig. 13-107).[527–530] Although the subaortic gradient can be estimated using the modified Bernoulli equation,[529,530] the assumptions used in this equation may not apply to HCM, as intraventricular gradient calculations can be spuriously high because of the phenomenon of pressure recovery.[531] Similar Doppler patterns also may be seen occasionally within the LV in patients with HCM if systolic obliteration of the hypertrophied LV causes localized areas of high flow velocity in the more distal portions of the ventricular cavity.[527]

Diastolic dysfunction has been long recognized in HCM. Doppler interrogation of LV inflow often reveals a relaxation abnormality, with a reduced early diastolic (E) velocity, a prolonged deceleration slope of the E wave, and an increased velocity of the atrial systolic (A) component.[532,533] Color Doppler

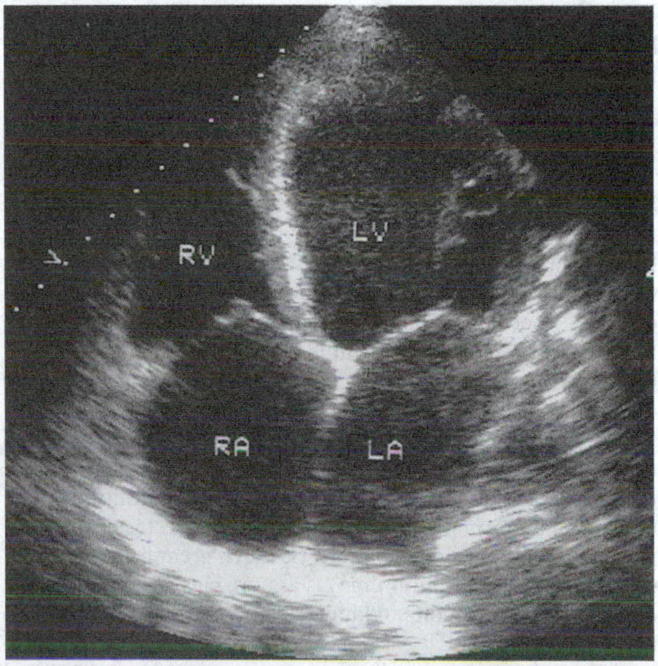

FIGURE 13-108 Apical four-chamber image of dilated cardiomyopathy. There is four-chamber enlargement as well as left ventricular (LV) spontaneous echo contrast. RV = right ventricle; RA = right atrium; LA = left atrium.

imaging can be used to demonstrate intraventricular flow characteristics.[534]

Dilated Cardiomyopathy

In cases of *dilated cardiomyopathy* (DCM), the heart is typically greatly enlarged and systolic function is markedly depressed (see also Chap. 66).[535] Four-chamber dilatation is a common but not uniform finding, as some patients may have relatively preserved RV size (this may confer an improved prognosis).[536] Marked LV enlargement and generalized dysfunction can also be caused by severe ischemic heart disease, chronic alcohol abuse, various infectious myocarditides, anthracyclines and other cardiotoxic agents, nutritional deficiencies, and hereditary myopathies.[537,538] Severe ischemic disease is often segmental and has been reported to spare the posterior wall frequently,[539] while the LV dysfunction of DCM is usually global. The typical constellation of echocardiographic findings in DCM include an increased LV end-diastolic diameter and volume with decreased fractional shortening, thinning of the LV walls (Fig. 13-108), increased E point-septal separation, LA enlargement, and limited mitral and aortic valve opening (due to low stroke volume).[535,540] Intracardiac thrombi are frequently observed and are most often found in the LV apex.[540] M-mode imaging of the mitral leaflets may demonstrate a "B bump," or notch just before systolic valve closure, indicating elevated LV diastolic pressure (Fig. 13-8). The cardiac valves are usually normal, but mitral annular dilatation and secondary MR are common.

Doppler echocardiography often reveals an abnormally low-velocity time integral in the LV outflow or inflow tracts.[541] Diastolic MR due to elevated LV diastolic pressure also may be present. Diastolic dysfunction is common, and pulsed-wave Doppler interrogation of mitral inflow may show an abnormal relaxation, restrictive, or pseudonormal pattern depending on LV diastolic pressures and loading conditions.[541,541a] A restrictive pattern of mitral inflow Doppler confers a poor prognosis in patients with DCM.[542,543]

Restrictive Cardiomyopathy

Restrictive cardiomyopathy may be idiopathic or secondary to infiltrative diseases such as amyloidosis, hemochromatosis, hypereosinophilic syndrome and Loeffler endocarditis, sarcoidosis, radiation toxicity, glycogen storage diseases, and Gaucher disease[544] (see also Chap. 75). Typical 2D echocardiographic features of these diseases include (1) a diffuse increase of ventricular thickness in the absence of marked ventricular chamber dilation and (2) marked biatrial enlargement[509,545–549] (Fig. 13-109). Systolic function is often modestly decreased. As with the other cardiomyopathies, these echocardiographic findings are nonspecific. Doppler examination may show a mitral inflow relaxation abnormality early in the course of restrictive cardiomyopathy, but restrictive pattern (E much greater than A, with shortened E deceleration time) is a more classic finding, which often evolves with time and indicates both a high LA pressure and poor prognosis.[550]

Amyloidosis is generally the most commonly encountered restrictive cardiac disease. In addition to biventricular hypertrophy, amyloidosis is also associated with diffuse thickening of the interatrial septum and cardiac valves.[549] In advanced disease, depressed systolic function is also common. An abnormal "speckled" pattern or "ground-glass" appearance of the myocardium has been described on 2D echocardiography, but this sign is absent in many cases and therefore has minimal clinical usefulness.[547,549] The finding of a restrictive mitral inflow pattern (and an abnormally high diastolic component of pulmonary vein inflow) on Doppler echocardiography has been identified as a marker of advanced disease and poor prognosis.[551,552] In addition to increased myocardial thickness, endocardial thickening and fibrosis and restricted atrioventricular leaflet motion are common features of Loeffler endocarditis and endomyocardial fibroelastosis.[548] Intraventricular thrombi are also common in these processes.[553]

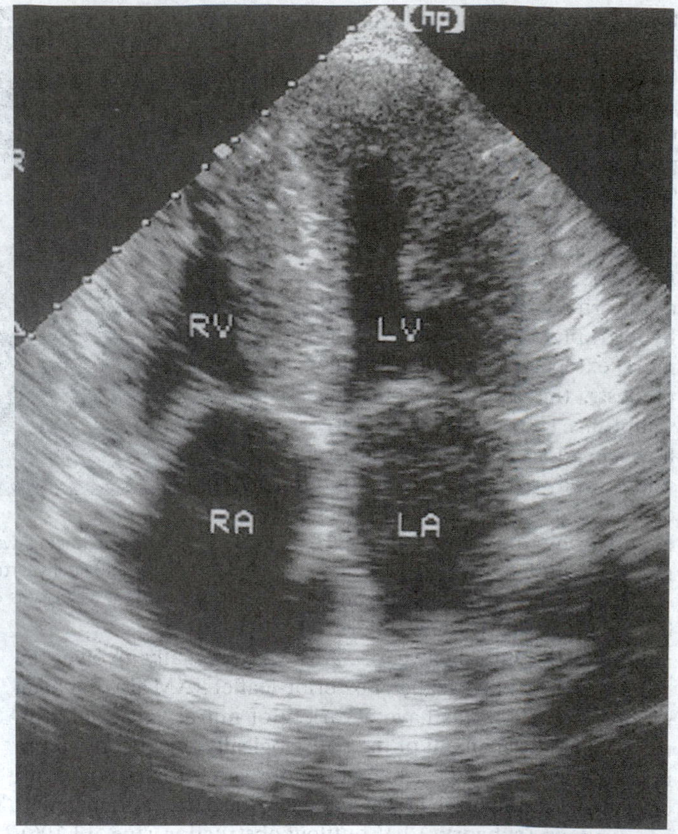

FIGURE 13-109 Apical four-chamber image of cardiac amyloid. RV = right ventricle; RA = right atrium; LA = left atrium; LV = left ventricle.

CONGENITAL HEART DISEASE

Echocardiographic Identification of Congenital Cardiac Anomalies

2D and Doppler echocardiography has had a major impact on the diagnosis and management of patients with congenital heart disease (see also Chaps. 63 and 64). From isolated congenital lesions to complex, extensive cardiac malformations, echocardiographic imaging (often with intravenous contrast injection) is usually sufficient to delineate cardiac anatomy. TEE is an important adjunctive technique as well[554]; in many cases, a thorough echocardiographic evaluation may obviate the need for cardiac catheterization and angiography.[555–557]

The ultrasound diagnosis of a simple intracardiac shunt is usually straightforward, but the task of defining complex congenital cardiac abnormalities can be daunting. In these cases, it is useful to remember a few basic anatomic rules. The venae cavae and pulmonary veins generally empty into the morphologic right atrium and LA, respectively. The atrioventricular valves uniformly follow their ventricles through embryologic development: a tricuspid valve accompanies the morphologic right ventricle and a mitral valve accompanies the left. Similarly, the semilunar valves follow the great vessels. The aorta and pulmonary artery can be distinguished, regardless of their position, by the bifurcation of the pulmonary artery.

Several features aid identification of the morphologic right and left ventricles. The right ventricle has a tricuspid atrioventricular valve; in comparison with the mitral annulus, the tricuspid annulus is positioned slightly closer to the cardiac apex.[558] The right ventricle also has a moderator band, coarser trabeculations than those in the left ventricle, and an infundibulum that separates the inlet area from the right ventricular outflow tract.

Cardiovascular Shunts

ATRIAL SEPTAL DEFECT

Most secundum and primum *atrial septal defects* (ASD) are easily visualized by echocardiography, although sinus venous defects are often difficult to detect without TEE.[559,560] Apical echocardiographic views often show artifactual "dropout" in the region of the fossa ovalis, since the interatrial septum is thin in this area and runs parallel to the ultrasound beam. Therefore, the subcostal view provides the optimal imaging plane to detect lesions of the atrial septum.[561] Ostium secundum defects are the most common form of ASD, and 2D imaging shows a localized absence of septal tissue in the midportion of the interatrial septum (Fig. 13-110*A*, Plate 69). Lack of any interatrial septal tissue between the defect and the base of the interventricular septum characterizes an ostium primum defect (Figure 13-110*B*). Although ostium secundum defects are usually isolated, ostium primum (or partial AV canal) defects are often accompanied by other lesions, such as cleft anterior mitral valve leaflet, MR, and atrioventricular canal ventricular septal defect.[562] Sinus venosus defects are strongly associated with partial anomalous pulmonary venous return (for example, drainage of the right upper pulmonary vein into the right atrium or superior vena cava) (Fig. 13-111). Rarely, the atrial septum may be completely absent (Fig. 13-112). With all but small ASDs, the right atrium is enlarged and RV volume overload is present, with a dilated RV and paradoxical septal motion.[563]

Intravenous contrast injection generally demonstrates shunting across the ASD, frequently with bidirectional flow.[564] Therefore, "negative jets" of unopacified flow from the left atrium into the contrast-filled right atrium may alternate with the appearance of contrast bubbles flowing through the defect into the LA. When an ASD is present, contrast should appear quickly (within three to five heartbeats) in the LA after entering the right atrium. Delayed appearance of contrast in the LA may indicate an intrapulmonary shunt rather than an ASD.

Color Doppler imaging is also useful for detecting flow through ASDs (Fig. 13-110*A*, Plate 69), although the pressure drop between atria often does not produce turbulence. Inflow from the inferior vena cava and right-sided pulmonary veins may be prominent in normals and can be misinterpreted as a shunt.[565,566] Pulsed-wave Doppler recordings usually reveal continuous flow, which peaks in late systole. Pulmonary-to-systemic flow ratios can be estimated in ASD (and ventricular septal defects) by comparing volumetric flow measurements through the LV and RV outflow tracts. Such calculations are only moderately accurate in adults.[567,568]

VENTRICULAR SEPTAL DEFECT

Ventricular septal defects (VSDs) may be classified as perimembranous, inlet, outlet, or trabecular. Echocardiography is quite useful for the detection and classification of VSDs.[569–571] The defect itself is sometimes visible with 2D imaging alone (Fig. 13-113*A*), but smaller VSDs are easily missed. Complete absence of the interventricular septum (single ventricle) is quite rare (Fig. 13-113*B*). Pulsed- or continuous-wave Doppler interrogation often reveals discrete areas of high-velocity flow across the interventricular septum. Measurement of the peak CW velocity through the shunt allows calculation of the interventricular pressure gradient (via the modified Bernoulli equation); subtraction of this gradient from the systolic blood pressure (in the absence of aortic valve disease) approximates the RV systolic pressure.

Overall, color-flow imaging is the most useful Doppler technique for the diagnosis of VSDs.[571] Typically, a high-velocity systolic color jet is seen traversing the interventricular septum, although the velocity is lower with large defects and in the presence of pulmonary hypertension (Fig. 13-114, Plate 70). The appearance of the color jet in the standard imaging planes can be used to determine the type of VSD. Intravenous contrast injection may reveal a negative contrast jet in the right ventricle, and contrast may cross the defect and partially opacify the left ventricle. In the absence of MR, contrast will not enter the left atrium, distinguishing an isolated VSD from an ASD. Doppler echocardiography can also be used to detect abnormalities associated with VSDs, such as ventricular septal aneurysm, MR and TR, ASD (especially with inlet VSDs), aortic insufficiency—with outlet (supracristal) VSDs—and "straddling" of the defect by the mitral or tricuspid valve.[572,573] Accurate detection of such lesions is especially critical before surgical intervention.

PATENT DUCTUS ARTERIOSUS

The ductus arteriosus originates just to the left of the PA bifurcation and inserts into the aorta slightly distal to and opposite from the ostium of the left subclavian artery. Given this posterior location, it is difficult to image a *patent ductus arteriosus* (PDA) itself with 2D TTE alone, and TEE is usually superior for direct visualization of the lesion[574] (Fig. 13-115*A* and *B*, Plate 71). In most cases, 2D imaging of the communication is not essential, as color-flow Doppler reliably detects high-velocity diastolic flow within the PA in nearly all non-Eisenmenger patients.[575–577] The flow jet characteristically enters the distal left region of the main PA and streams anterior along the medial wall of the vessel (Fig. 13-115*B*, Plate 42*B*). With large shunts, volume overload and subsequent dilation of the left ventricle occurs. Aortopulmonary window is a much rarer shunt involving the great vessels which presents as a communication anteriorly between the ascending aorta and proximal PA.[578,579] It is embryo-

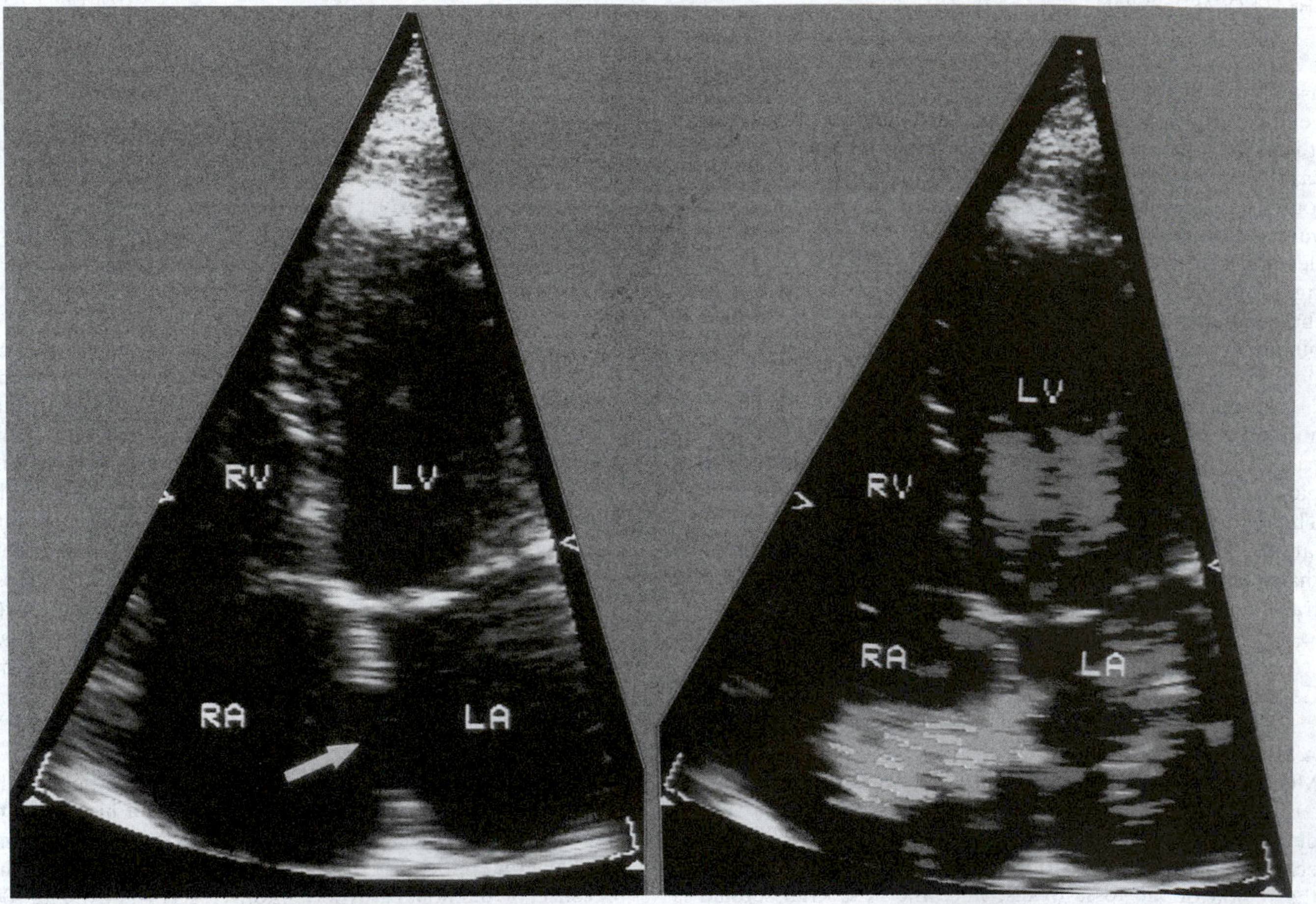

A

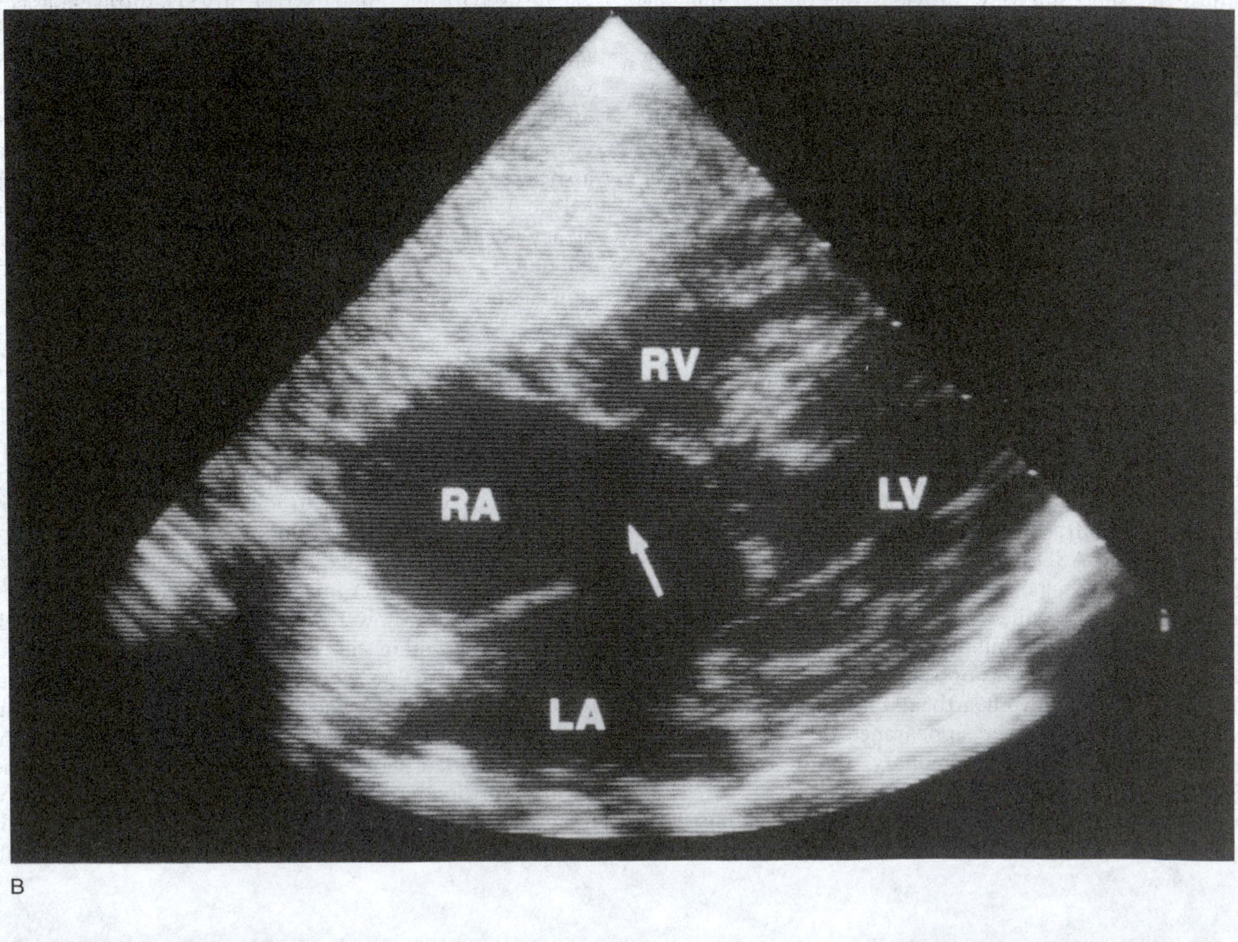

B

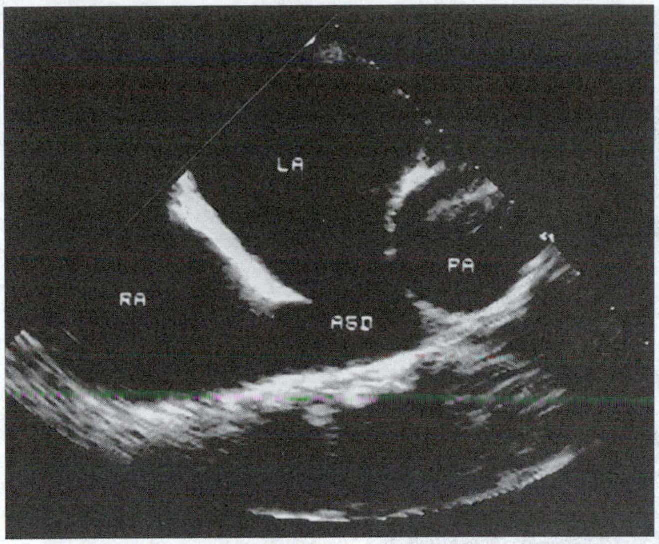

FIGURE 13-111 Transesophageal image of a sinus venosus atrial septal defect (ASD) (longitudinal plane). The defect is present in the superior portion of the interatrial septum. RA = right atrium; LA = left atrium; ASD = atrial septal defect; PA = pulmonary artery.

logically distinct from a PDA and more closely related to a truncus arteriosus defect.

Venous Inflow Abnormalities

Anomalous pulmonary venous return (APVR) may be partial or total. Partial APVR is present in 80 percent of sinus venosus ASD cases and is a feature of the Scimitar syndrome.[580,581] The usual finding on TTE is RV volume overload. TEE is quite useful in detecting these abnormal venous connections. In total APVR, the pulmonary veins may empty directly into the right atrium or into a common posterior chamber or vein. This structure and its connection with the right atrium may be visualized echocardiographically, along with the obligatory ASD.[582–585] In some cases, the collecting chamber posterior to the left atrium may mimic the appearance of *cor triatriatum*, an entity characterized by a membrane in the posterior left atrium which may obstruct pulmonary venous inflow, causing symptoms similar to those of mitral stenosis[586] (Fig. 13-116).

Persistent left superior vena cava occurs in 0.5 percent of the normal population.[587,588] In most cases, the anomalous vein empties into the coronary sinus, which then drains into the right atrium (Fig. 13-117). Unless the coronary sinus is unroofed and drains into the left atrium, no shunting occurs. The typical echocardiographic finding is a large coronary sinus, which is especially well seen on transesophageal or parasternal transthoracic views. The diagnosis may be confirmed by intravenous contrast injection from the left arm, as this will opacify the coronary sinus shortly before filling the right atrium.[587,588]

Conotruncal and Aortic Abnormalities

Tetralogy of Fallot is one of the more common conotruncal abnormalities, and affected individuals may sometimes survive to adulthood without surgical intervention. The classic echocardiographic features include a large perimembranous VSD, an anteriorly displaced aorta which overrides the VSD, RV enlargement and dysfunction, and pulmonic stenosis (either infundibular, valvular, or suprevalvular) (Fig. 13-118).[589,590] The VSD and aorta are well visualized in the parasternal long-axis view, while the RV outflow tract and proximal PA are best seen in the parasternal short-axis view at the base of the heart. Doppler interrogation can provide evaluation of the severity of pulmonic stenosis, both before and after surgery. Echocardiography may aid detection of infants with tetralogy who will require early surgical intervention as well as patients who are at high risk for sudden death after surgical repair.[591,592]

Although *double-outlet right ventricle* (DORV) shares several clinical characteristics with tetralogy of Fallot (VSD and anterior aortic displacement are invariably present, and pulmonic valvular stenosis and ASD are common in both), it is morphologically distinct (Fig. 13-119). Normal continuity of the posterior aortic wall with the anterior mitral valve leaflet (always present in tetralogy of Fallot) is absent in DORV, and an interposed mass of fibrous tissue between the left atrium and the nearest great vessel is seen on 2D imaging.[593,594] In addition, the great vessels may be transposed in DORV, resulting in a characteristic side-by-side appearance of the aorta and PA on parasternal short-axis images.[595]

Echocardiography has become a valuable tool for detection, management, and postoperative follow-up of patients with *transposition of the great arteries.* Attention to the anatomic rules mentioned earlier is essential for accurate diagnosis of both D (classic) and L ("congenitally corrected") transposition. In D-transposition, the aorta arises from the RV, the PA arises from the LV, and one or more obligatory shunts are present. With L-transposition, the morphologic right and left ventricles are switched, and associated anomalies such as VSD and pulmonic stenosis are common. In both types of transposition, the normal echocardiographic orientation of the great vessels on parasternal short-axis images (a sausage-shaped RVOT and PA draped over a circular aorta) is no longer present, and the two great vessels are typically side by side and parallel (Fig. 13-120).[596,597] In general, the aorta is anterior and to the right of the PA in D-transposition and anterior and to the left in L-transposition. Both TTE and TEE are an important part of continuing care after surgical repair or palliation of transposition; they can detect valvular regurgitation, outflow tract narrowing, and stenosis of the atrial baffle systems used to palliate D-transposition surgically.[598–600]

FIGURE 13-110 (Plate 69) *A.* Apical four-chamber view of an ostium secundum atrial septal defect (ASD). On the left, a defect in the mid atrial septum is apparent (*arrow*). On the right, there is color flow through the shunt. RV = right ventricle; RA = right atrium; LA = left atrium; LV = left ventricle. *B.* Subcostal four-chamber view of a large ostium primum atrial septal defect (*arrow*). RA = right atrium; LA = left atrium; LV = left ventricle; RV = right ventricle. (Reproduced with permission of Joseph A. Kisslo, MD.)

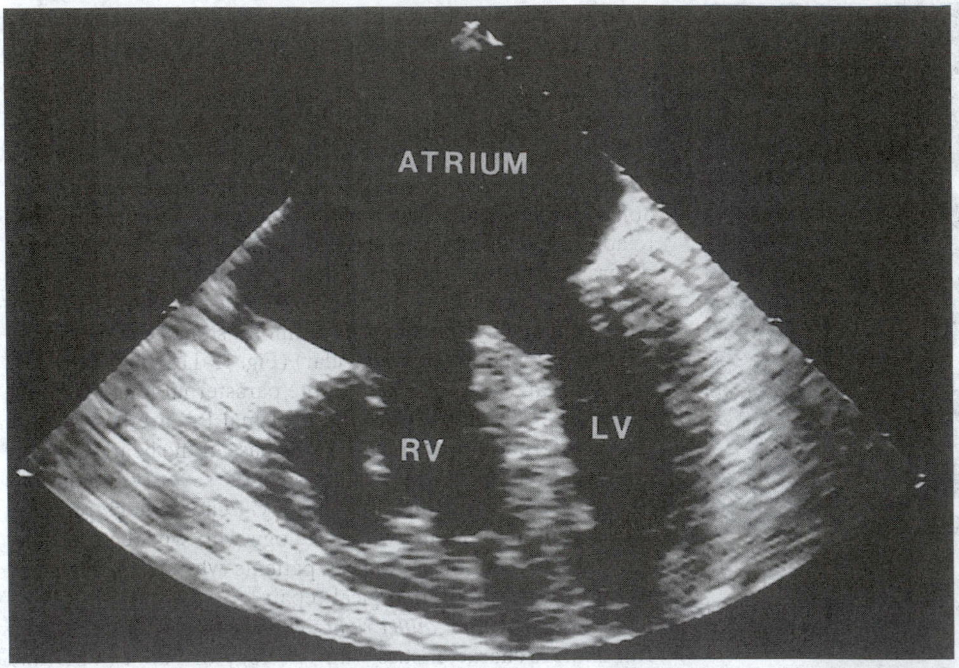

FIGURE 13-112 Transverse transesophageal image of single atrium. RV = right ventricle; LV = left ventricle. (From Blanchard DG, Scott ED. Single atrium. *Circulation* 1997; 95:273, with permission.)

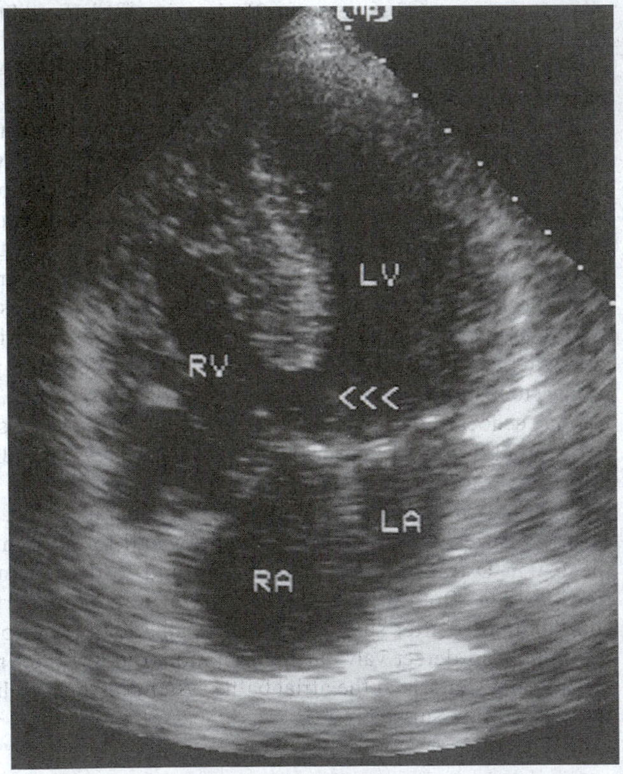

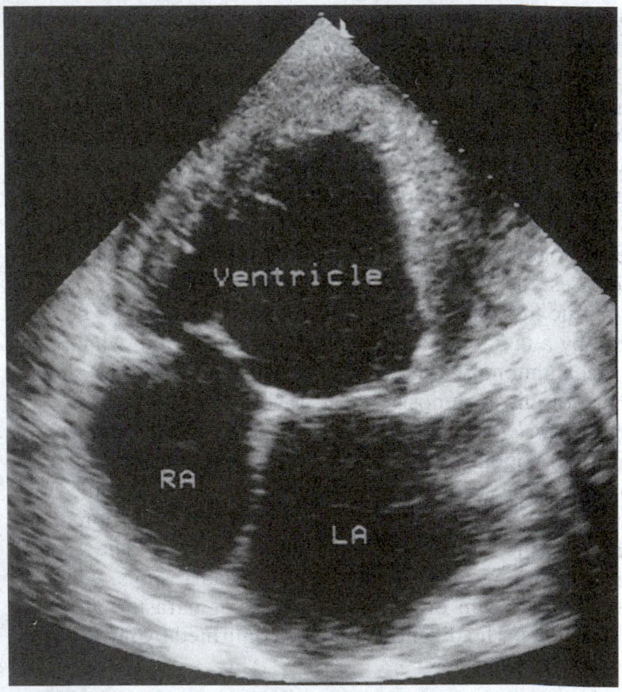

FIGURE 13-113 *A.* Apical four-chamber image of an inlet ventricular septal defect (VSD). The defect (*arrows*) is situated more inferiorly than the typical position of a perimembranous VSD. RV = right ventricle; RA = right atrium; LA = left atrium; LV = left ventricle. *B.* Apical image of single ventricle. RA = right atrium; LA = left atrium.

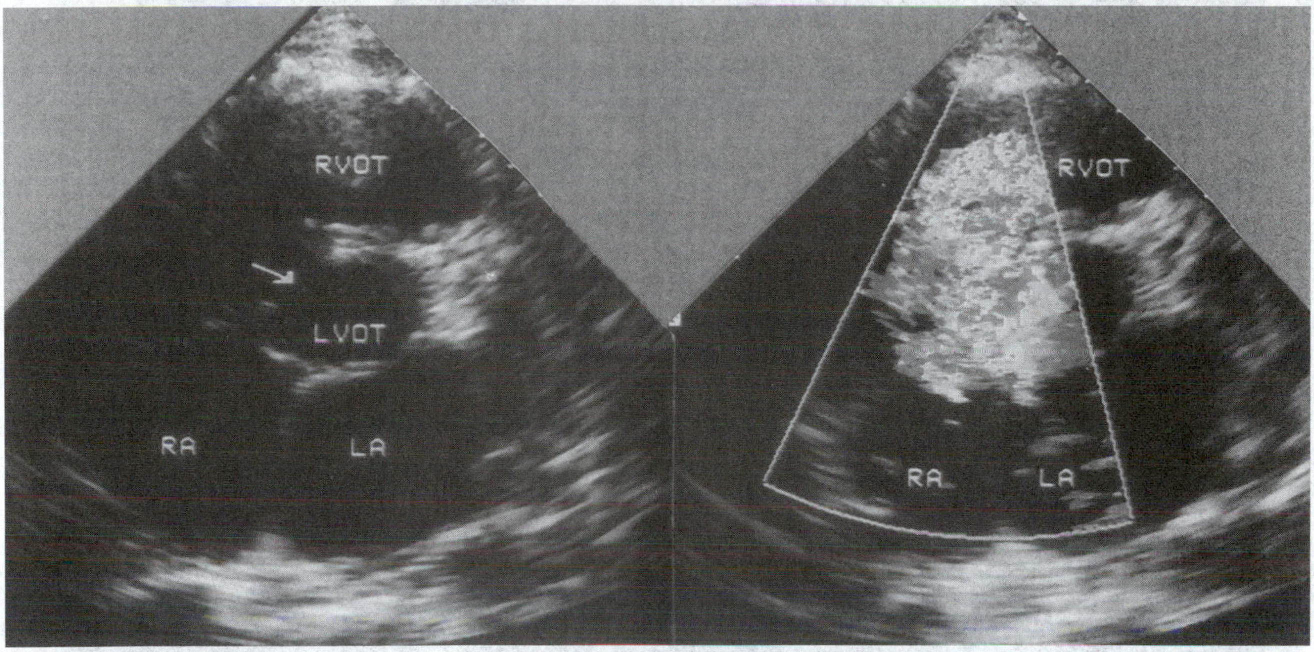

FIGURE 13-114 (Plate 70) Parasternal short-axis images of a large perimembranous ventricular septal defect (VSD) (*arrow*) without (*left*) and with (*right*) superimposed color flow Doppler. A large, turbulent color jet crosses the VSD during systole (*right*). RVOT = right ventricular outflow tract; RA = right atrium; LA = left atrium; LVOT = left ventricular outflow tract.

Truncus arteriosus is a rare anomaly characterized by a large VSD, a single semilunar valve, and a single great vessel that divides into the ascending aorta and PA.[601,602] Ultrasound imaging can determine the anatomy of the great vessels and assist in defining the various subsets of truncus arteriosus.

Coarctation of the aorta is associated with a bicuspid aortic valve and is best visualized from the suprasternal position. 2D imaging may identify the site of coarctation, but the natural mild curving of the descending aorta can occasionally lead to a false-positive diagnosis. Clear visualization of narrowing in the proximal descending aorta with poststenotic dilatation, however, is pathognomonic of coarctation.[603,604] Doppler interrogation from the suprasternal notch demonstrates increased systolic velocity in the descending aorta and may also reveal a persistent flow gradient throughout diastole in cases of severe coarctation (Fig. 13-121).[605] Color imaging often displays flow acceleration and aliasing proximal to the site of coarctation. The maximum velocity through the coarctation can be used to estimate the pressure gradient, and this measurement can be particularly valuable for the detection of restenosis after surgical repair or percutaneous balloon aortic dilatation.[606,607]

Supravalvular aortic stenosis, either isolated or associated with Williams syndrome (Chap. 10), is generally imaged best from the suprasternal and superior parasternal positions. Echocardiography reveals either an hourglass-shaped stenosis of the aorta above the sinuses of Valsalva, diffuse hypoplasia of the ascending aorta, or a focal fibrous ridge at the sinotubular junction.[608] Doppler imaging can help estimate the gradient across the stenosis, and marked aliasing of color-flow imaging in the ascending aorta should raise suspicion of the diagnosis. Thickening of the aortic valve leaflets and stenoses of the coronary ostia are important associated findings that may be detectable by echocardiography.

Ventricular Outflow Tract and Semilunar Valve Abnormalities

RIGHT VENTRICLE

Infundibular stenosis is rare outside the setting of tetralogy of Fallot and is much less common than valvular PS. On 2D imaging, muscular hypertrophy is often visualized proximal to the pulmonary artery, while Doppler interrogation reveals increased flow velocities through the infundibulum.[609] PS is reasonably common and may be either isolated or associated with other congenital lesions (such as VSD, transposition, and tetralogy of Fallot). Typical echocardiographic features include thickening of the leaflets, restricted leaflet motion, systolic doming of the valve, and elevated systolic flow velocity on Doppler[610] (Fig. 13-85). As with other stenotic lesions, the gradient can be estimated using the modified Bernoulli equation. The pulmonic valve is best visualized in the parasternal short-axis view through the base (or a modified parasternal view of the RVOT). In children, the subcostal position frequently provides excellent visualization of the RVOT and pulmonic valve. When TTE is suboptimal, TEE can provide detailed images of the pulmonic valve. In pulmonic stenosis, the valve leaflets may calcify over

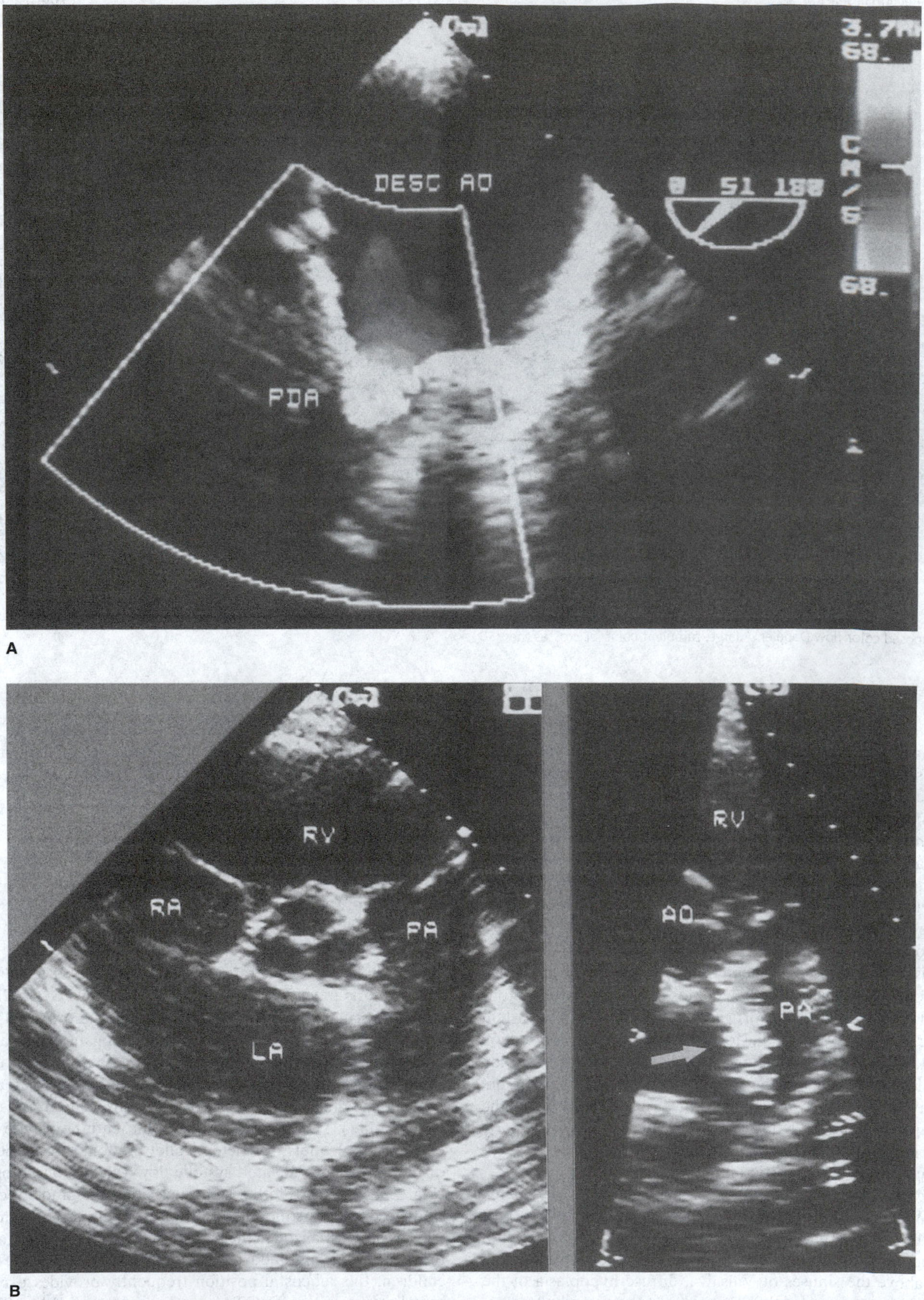

FIGURE 13-115 (Plate 71) *A.* Transesophageal image of a patent ductus arteriosus (PDA). Color Doppler imaging shows flow from the descending aorta (DESC AO) into the PDA. (Courtesy of Bruce J. Kimura, M.D.) *B.* Parasternal short-axis images at the aortic valve level. On the left, the pulmonary artery (PA) is somewhat enlarged. On the right, color imaging reveals diastolic flow within the PA, consistent with a patent ductus arteriosus. RV = right ventricle; RA = right atrium; LA = left atrium; AO = aorta.

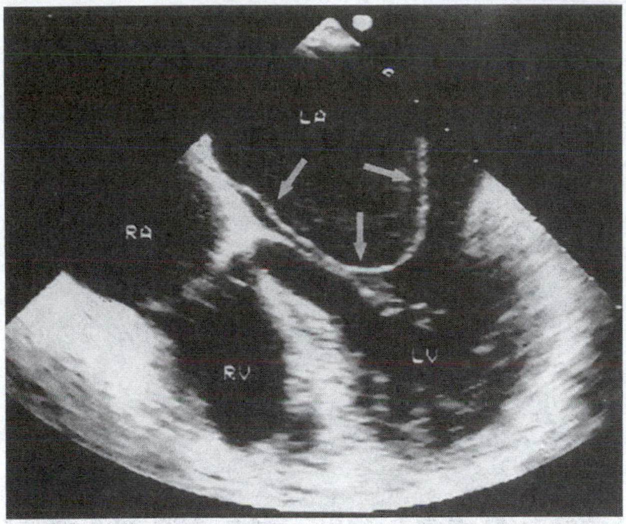

FIGURE 13-116 Transverse transesophageal image of cor triatriatum. A membrane (*arrows*) is present in the left atrium. RV = right ventricle; RA = right atrium; LA = left atrium; LV = left ventricle. (From Blanchard DG, DeMaria AN. Cardiac and extracardiac masses: Echocardiographic evaluation. In: Skorton DJ, Schelbert HR, Wolf GL, Brundage BH, eds. *Marcus' Cardiac Imaging,* 2d ed. Philadelphia: Saunders; 1996:452–480, with permission.)

time, and poststenotic dilatation of the pulmonary artery is often present.

LEFT VENTRICLE

Subvalvular obstruction may be dynamic or fixed. *Hypertrophic cardiomyopathy,* which may present at any age, is discussed earlier in this chapter. Discrete *subaortic stenosis* may be caused by a thin membrane in the LV outflow tract, a fibromuscular ridge, or diffuse muscular narrowing of the outflow tract (Figs. 13-122*A* and *B*, Plate 72).[611] 2D echocardiographic imaging can distinguish these various forms of discrete subvalvular stenosis, and Doppler analysis permits estimation of the systolic gradient.[612] Color-flow imaging demonstrates increased turbulence in the LVOT as well as aortic valvular regurgitation in about 50 percent of cases. Apical views are sometimes more useful for detecting thin subaortic membranes, as these structures are parallel to the ultrasound beam on parasternal images (Fig. 13-122). Subaortic fibromuscular ridges are sometimes associated with anomalous mitral valve chordae connecting the papillary muscles or the anterior mitral valve leaflet to the septum.[613,614] M-mode imaging may reveal midsystolic partial closure of the aortic valve, differentiating subvalvular from valvular AS.

Bicuspid aortic valve is the most common congenital cardiac lesion in adults and is present in 1 to 2 percent of all individuals (men are affected more often than women).[615,616] Initially, eccentric diastolic coaptation of the aortic cusps was reported on M-mode in patients with bicuspid valves. However, M-mode findings are less accurate than 2D imaging, and the parasternal short-axis view is generally best for defining the fish-mouthed systolic aortic valvular anatomy (Figs. 13-60 and 13-61). Bicuspid valves are sometimes easy to detect in diastole as well, but raphes and remnants of commissures may obscure the diagnosis and mimic a trileaflet valve. In general, asymmetry of the aortic leaflets suggests congenital deformation. In equivocal cases, multiplane TEE is usually diagnostic (Fig. 13-61).

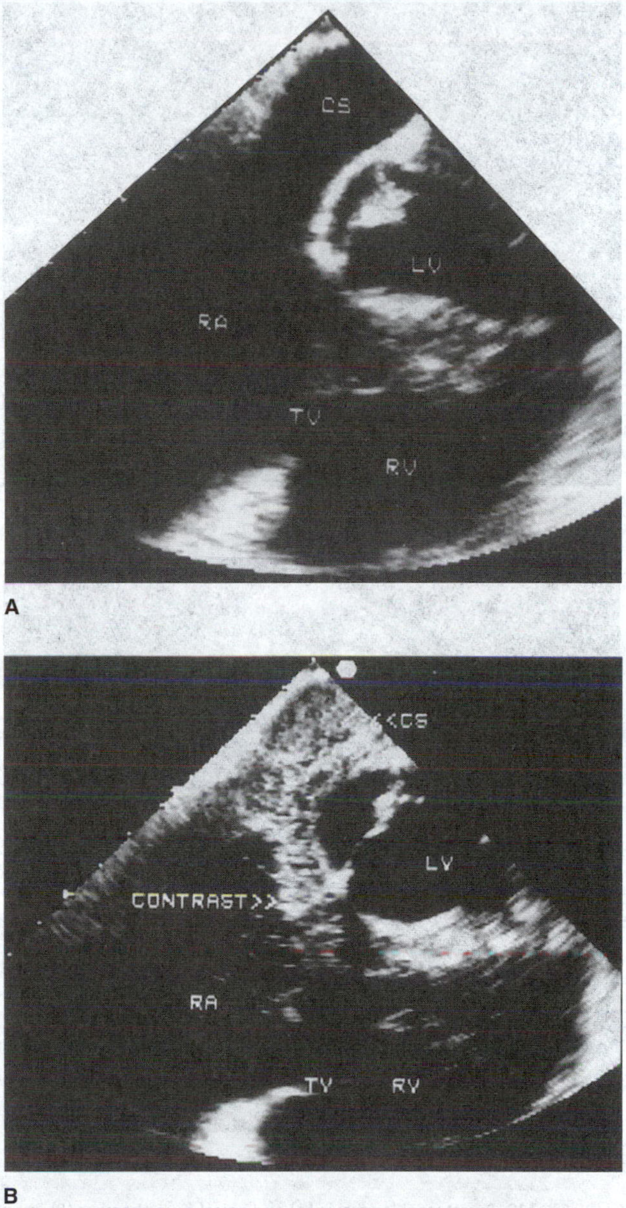

FIGURE 13-117 *A.* Transesophageal image (transverse plane) from a patient with persistent left superior vena cava. The coronary sinus (CS) is dilated. *B.* After injection of agitated saline into the left antecubital vein, contrast is seen entering the right atrium (RA) via the CS. TV = tricuspid valve; RV = right ventricle; LV = left ventricle. (From Blanchard DG, DeMaria AN. Cardiac and extracardiac masses: Echocardiographic evaluation. In: Skorton DJ, Schelbert HR, Wolf GL, Brundage BH, eds. *Marcus' Cardiac Imaging,* 2d ed. Philadelphia: Saunders; 1996:452–480, with permission.)

Ventricular Inflow Tract Abnormalities

Ebstein's anomaly is a congenital deformity of the tricuspid valve in which the leaflets are displaced into the right ventricle. Associated findings include TR, right atrial enlargement, and ASD.[617,618] 2D imaging typically shows abnormal apical displacement of the septal leaflet insertion, with variable deformity of

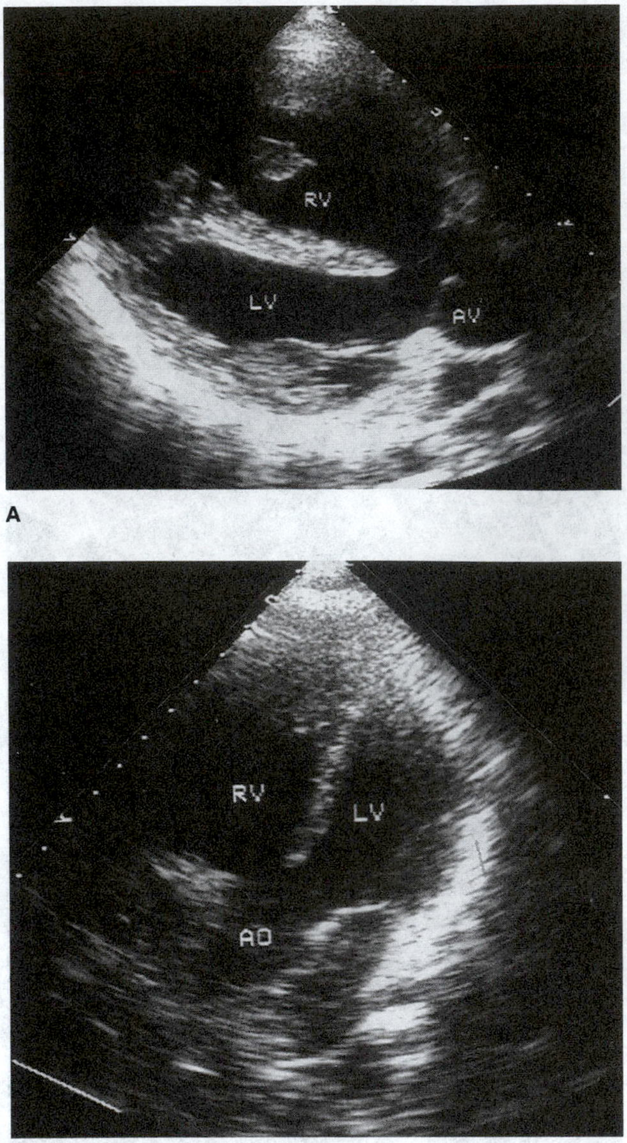

FIGURE 13-118 Parasternal long-axis (*A*) and apical four-chamber (*B*) images of tetralogy of Fallot. The right ventricle (RV) is enlarged, and a large VSD is present. The aorta (AO) overrides the interventricular septum. LV = left ventricle. (Courtesy of Reinaldo W. Beyer, MD.)

the leaflet (Fig. 13-123). The anterior leaflet originates from the tricuspid annulus but is elongated and often tethered to the RV free wall by abnormal chordal attachments. The tricuspid deformity and regurgitation are best visualized in the apical four-chamber view, although the subcostal and modified parasternal views also may be helpful.

Atrioventricular valvular atresia is usually accompanied by hypoplasia of the corresponding ventricle. Echocardiographic images of tricuspid atresia characteristically show a small, nonfunctional right ventricle, an interatrial communication of variable size, and a normally developed left ventricle. Associated lesions include VSD, transposition, and RV outflow obstruction. Echocardiography is an important tool in the management of patients with tricuspid atresia after palliation with the Fontan procedure. Mitral atresia is associated with a hypoplastic LV.

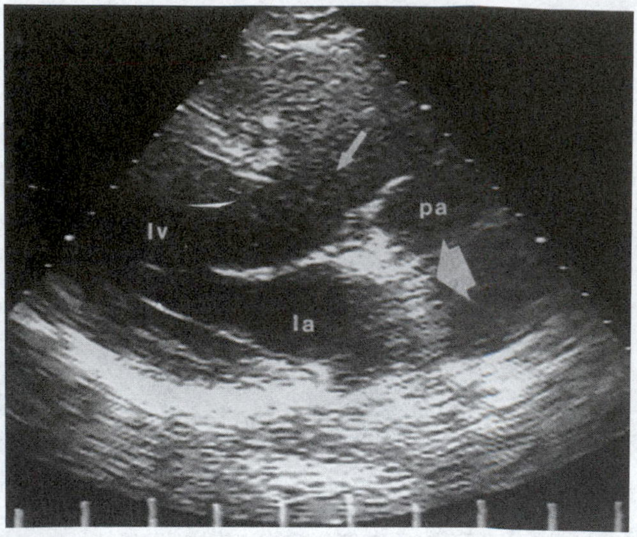

FIGURE 13-119 Parasternal long-axis image of double-outlet right ventricle. A large VSD is present (*small arrow*) and the normal continuity between the posterior aortic wall and the anterior mitral leaflet is absent. Fibrous tissue is seen (*large arrow*) between the left atrium (LA) and the nearest great vessel (in this case, the pulmonary artery (PA). LV = left ventricle.

Additional rare congenital mitral anomalies imaged by echocardiography include parachute mitral valve and congenital MS.

Fetal Echocardiography

The average risk for significant heart disease in the fetus is approximately 0.4 to 0.8 percent. Fetal echocardiography has evolved over the past 14 years into a sophisticated method for intrauterine detection of cardiac abnormalities[619] (Fig. 13-124). The technique has been advocated for the preterm diagnosis of congenital heart disease, especially in higher-risk cases [for example, maternal congenital heart disease or diabetes mellitus, maternal teratogen exposure or *t*oxoplasmosis, *o*ther intrauterine infections, *r*ubella, *c*ytomegalovirus, and *h*erpes virus (TORCH) infection, and familial syndromes that may affect

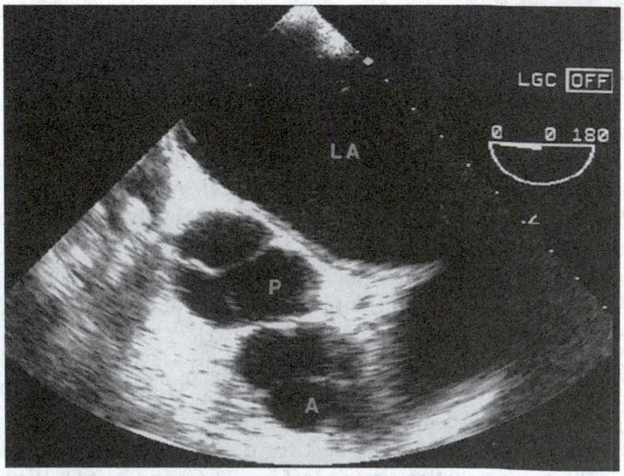

FIGURE 13-120 Transverse transesophageal image through the semilunar valves in L-transposition. The aortic valve (A) is anterior and to the left of the pulmonic valve (P). LA = left atrium.

the heart].[620] Fetal echocardiography has successfully identified a variety of congenital lesions including atrial and ventricular septal defect, pulmonic stenosis, transposition, tetralogy of Fallot, hypoplastic left heart, Ebstein's anomaly, and tricuspid atresia.[621] Prenatal detection of these lesions may improve prognosis and guide therapy. Although some have recommended routine limited fetal echocardiography during the second or third trimester,[620] recent reports have suggested a low yield and limited diagnostic accuracy.[622–624] Like many imaging techniques, fetal echocardiography is evolving, and further study is required to define its optimal clinical use.

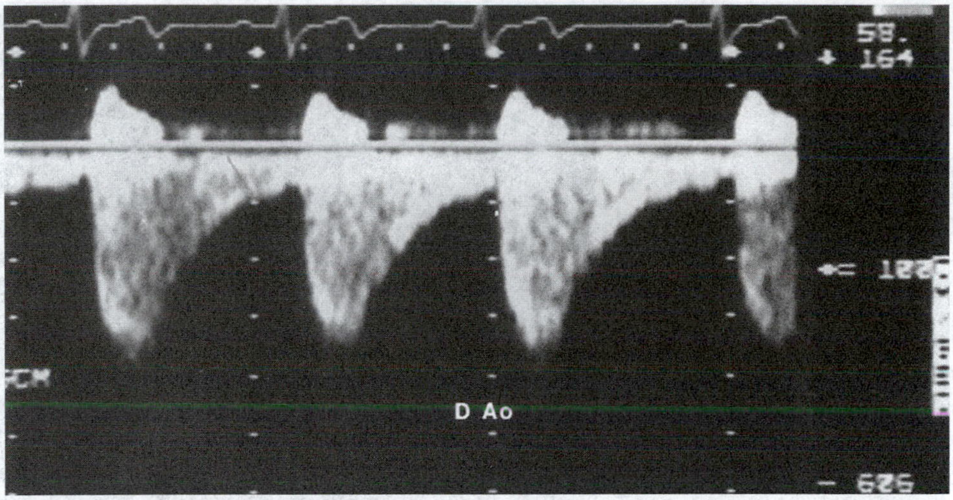

FIGURE 13-121 Continuous-wave Doppler tracing of the descending aorta (from the suprasternal position) in aortic coarctation. Peak systolic velocity is approximately 3.6 m/s, and there is persistent flow during diastole, suggesting severe coarctation. D Ao = descending aorta.

CARDIAC MASSES, THROMBI, AND TUMORS

Normal Variants and Masses of Uncertain Significance

When an abnormally localized accumulation of dense reflectances appears on the echocardiogram, it is said to represent a mass. Echocardiographic masses may be caused by technical artifacts or anomalous structures, but they are of greatest significance in representing true lesions of the heart such as tumors, thrombi, and vegetations. Echocardiography is the procedure of choice for the detection and evaluation of cardiac mass lesions; often, it is the only modality capable of delineating small lesions such as papillary fibroelastomas.[625] Accordingly, echocardiographic examinations are commonly performed to search for embolic sources, particularly in patients with cerebral ischemic events.

A number of technical artifacts are capable of appearing as masses on echocardiogram. For example, side lobe signals, reverberations, and noise artifact may lead to accumulations of ultrasonic reflectance within the cavities or adjacent to the myocardium of the heart.[20,21] Such structures usually lack distinct borders, do not move appropriately through the cardiac cycle, lack identifiable attachments to endocardial surfaces, and cannot be visualized in all views and at all depth settings. In seeking a way to distinguish artifacts from LV thrombi (a common clinical dilemma) the absence of wall motion abnormalities is of particular value.[626]

Several benign normal variant findings can be observed during echocardiographic examination and must be distinguished from pathologic lesions. Thus, many adults manifest persistence of the eustachian valve (Fig. 13-125), a thin ridge of tissue at the junction of the inferior vena cava and right atrium.[627,628] The eustachian valve appears as a long, linear, freely mobile structure in the right atrium at the mouth of the inferior vena cava and is nearly always benign (although infective involvement has been reported).[629,630] An additional embryonic remnant that may be seen in the posterior right atrium is the Chiari network, which typically appears as a weblike mobile structure.[631,632] In some individuals, RV hypertrophy may produce significant enlargement of the RV moderator band coursing along the interventricular septum to the apex of the RV.[633] Similarly, false chordae tendineae ("heartstrings") can occasionally be visualized as linear structures spanning the LV cavity attached to endomyocardium at both ends (Fig. 13-126).[634,635] Neither of the foregoing lesions has been conclusively associated with morbidity or mortality. On occasion, LV hypertrophy or hypertrophied papillary muscles may simulate cardiac mass lesions.[633] Although TEE provides enhanced sensitivity and resolution in the delineation of cardiac mass lesions, this technique may be associated with variants and artifacts of its own.[636,637]

A variety of foreign bodies and iatrogenically induced anatomic alterations may be visualized on echocardiogram and must be distinguished from pathologic lesions. Intracardiac catheters, pacemaker leads (Fig. 13-127), prosthetic valves or patches, and atrial suture lines after cardiac transplantation can be visualized during echocardiographic examination.[638,639] These structures are usually easily recognized due to the highly reflective properties of the foreign material, which result in bright echoes, reverberations, and shadowing behind the structures. In this regard, endomyocardial biotomes and pericardiocentesis catheters can be readily visualized by cardiac ultrasound, and echocardiography can be employed to guide procedures utilizing these instruments in lieu of fluoroscopy.[640,641] Last, a variety of manufactured objects that have penetrated the heart have been described on echocardiography, including bullets, pellets, and nails.[642]

Several morphologic changes involving the interatrial septum are often considered under the classification of cardiac mass lesions of uncertain significance. Aneurysms of the interatrial septum have been reported in about 1 percent of the population and are recognized on echocardiogram as a protrusion of the interatrial septum of at least 1.5 cm from its longitudinal plane dividing the left and right atrium (Fig. 13-128).[643,644] Although usually benign, interatrial septal aneurysms are often associated with a patent foramen ovale and have been implicated as a source of cardiogenic emboli.[645] Interatrial septal aneurysms may be detected by TTE, but they are more readily imaged by

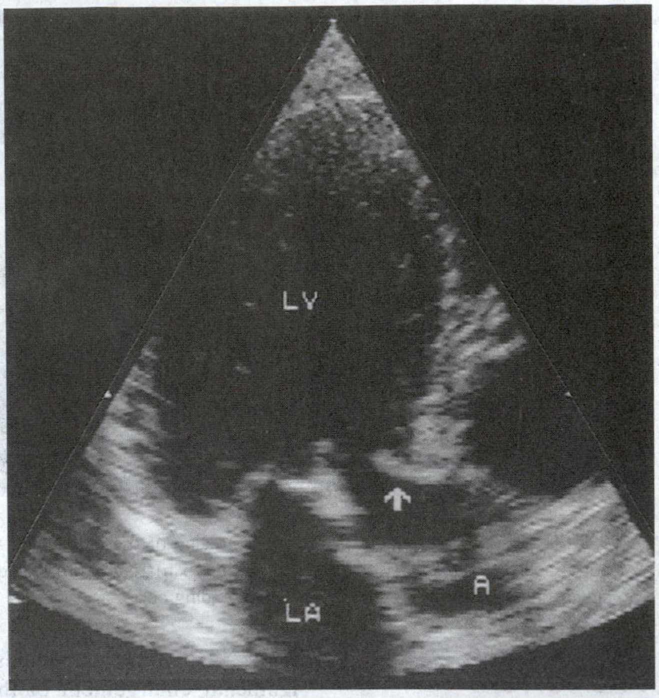

A

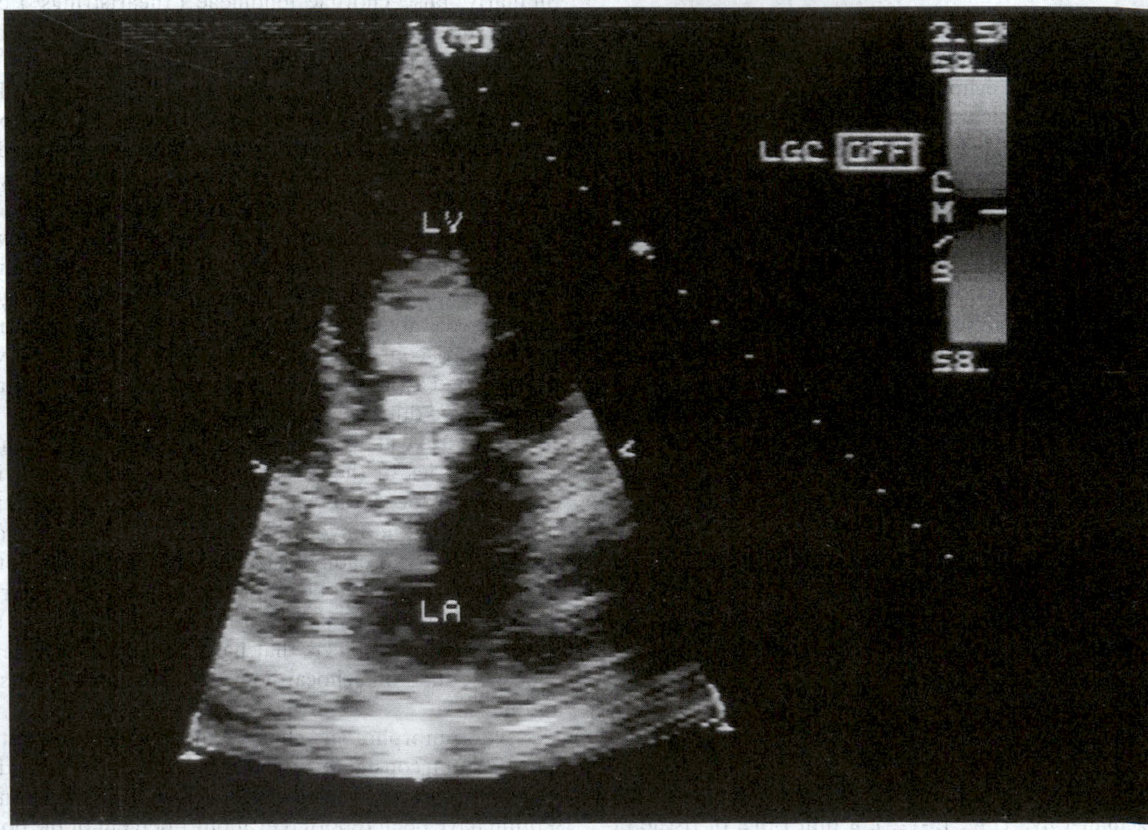

B

FIGURE 13-122 (Plate 72) Apical three-chamber view of discrete subaortic stenosis. *A.* Fibromuscular ridge (*arrow*) is present in the left ventricular outflow tract. LV = left ventricle; LA = left atrium; A = aortic root. *B.* Apical five-chamber view of discrete subaortic stenosis with color-flow Doppler, demonstrating aliasing and proximal flow convergence in the left ventricular outflow tract. LV = left ventricle; LA = left atrium.

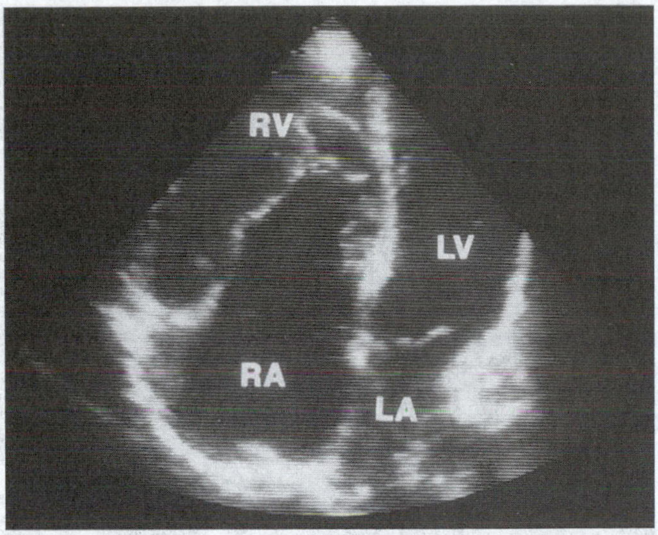

FIGURE 13-123 Apical four-chamber image of Ebstein's anomaly. The right heart is enlarged, and the insertion of the septal leaflet of the tricuspid valve is displaced apically. The anterior tricuspid leaflet (to the patient's right) is abnormally elongated. RV = right ventricle; RA = right atrium; LA = left atrium; LV = left ventricle. (Reproduced with permission of Joseph A. Kisslo, MD.)

the transesophageal approach.[644] Lipomatous hypertrophy of the interatrial septum, or accumulation of adipose tissue within this structure, is not an uncommon finding in elderly individuals. Lipomatous hypertrophy appears as a highly reflective thickening of the interatrial septum that typically spares the foramen ovale, thereby creating a characteristic dumbbell echocardiographic appearance.[646,647] No significant consequences or sequelae have been attributed to lipomatous infiltration of the interatrial septum.

Intracardiac Thrombi

Intracardiac thrombi occur commonly in a variety of cardiovascular disorders, may be visualized in any chamber of the heart, and frequently result in embolic events.[648] The major factors that predispose to the formation of intracardiac thrombi include localized stasis of flow, low cardiac output, and cardiac injury. In addition, migration of venous thrombi may also result in intracardiac clots.[649,650] The appearance of intracardiac thrombi may vary considerably, and although they are typically attached to the endocardium, unrestricted and freely mobile thrombi occasionally may be encountered (particularly in the setting of valvular stenosis which prevents exit of the thrombus from the heart).[651] Thrombi typically have identifiable borders and may be layered and homogeneous or heterogeneous, with areas of central liquefaction (Figs. 13-129 and 13-130).[651,652]

RIGHT HEART

Thrombi within the right heart chambers may form locally or migrate from the venous circulation; they are found most commonly in the RA.[653] As opposed to the laminar, relatively immobile nature of RA thrombi that form in situ, venous thromboemboli trapped in the RA tend to be serpentine and mobile.[649] The potential for pulmonary embolism is high.[654] Thrombi also can be seen within the main pulmonary arteries, although they are less well visualized by TTE than TEE.[655] RV thrombi are rare but may occur with RV infarction and endomyocardial fibrosis.[656,657] Their appearance is similar to that of LV thrombi.

LEFT ATRIUM

Left atrial thrombi occur in the setting of low cardiac output, mitral valvular disease (particularly mitral stenosis), atrial fibrillation, and LA enlargement. Both TTE and TEE can detect thrombi within the main cavity of the left atrium (Fig. 13-131), but TEE is clearly superior for visualizing thrombi within the left atrial appendage.[658–660] Since approximately 50 percent of LA thrombi are limited to the appendage, TEE is the diagnostic procedure of choice to detect this lesion.[652,661] LA thrombi appear as discrete masses, either fixed or mobile, and are usually of homogeneous echo density[659] (Fig. 13-52). On TEE, normal pectinate muscular ridges in the appendage must be distinguished from small thrombi. In addition, the left atrial appendage may occasionally be multilobed. Although this anatomic variant may be a risk factor for appendage thrombi, the atrial tissue separating the lobes should not be mistaken for clot.[662]

Left atrial thrombi are often accompanied by spontaneous echo contrast (or "smoke") within the LA. This finding, proba-

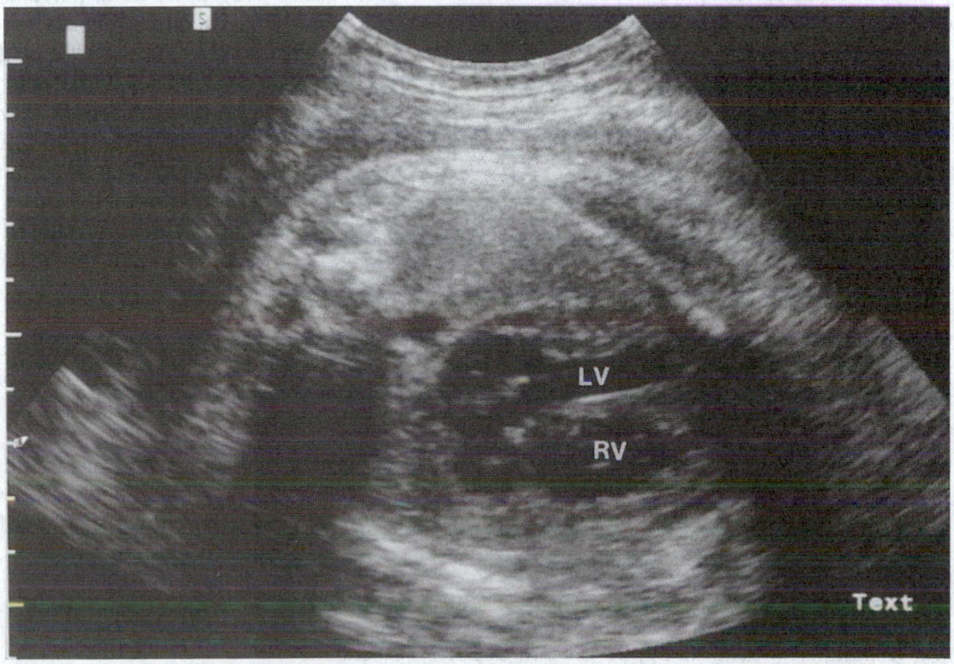

FIGURE 13-124 Fetal echocardiogram (four-chamber view). LV = left ventricle; RV = right ventricle.

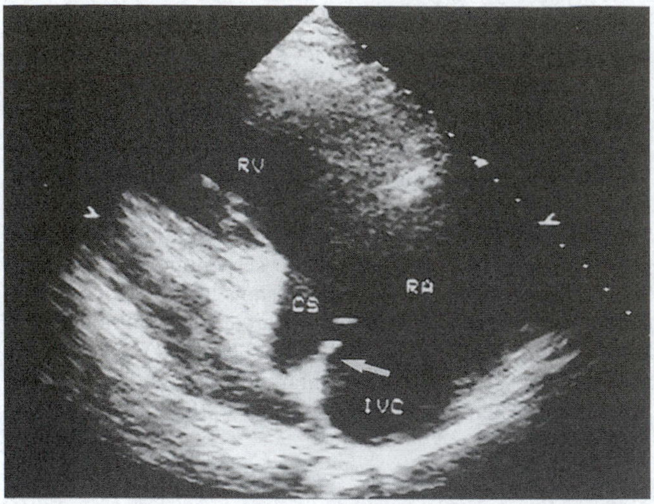

FIGURE 13-125 Right ventricular inflow view showing a prominent eustachian valve (*arrow*) at the junction of the inferior vena cava (IVC) and the right atrium (RA). RV = right ventricle; CS = coronary sinus. (From Blanchard DG, DeMaria AN. Cardiac and extracardiac masses: Echocardiographic evaluation. In: Skorton DJ, Schelbert HR, Wolf GL, Brundage BH, eds. *Marcus' Cardiac Imaging,* 2d ed. Philadelphia; Saunders; 1996:452–480, with permission.)

bly produced by transient aggregation of erythrocytes and plasma proteins,[663] indicates stagnant blood flow and can occur in any cardiac chamber or the aorta. Left atrial spontaneous echo contrast, like LA thrombus, has been associated with embolic events[664,665] and may be a marker of regional prothrombotic activity.[666] On 2D imaging, the contrast signals are in constant motion and can be missed if gain settings are inappropriately low.

LEFT VENTRICLE

Most LV thrombi occur in settings of abnormal systolic contraction (dilated cardiomyopathy, acute myocardial infarction, and chronic LV ventricular aneurysm).[667–669] LV thrombi have been

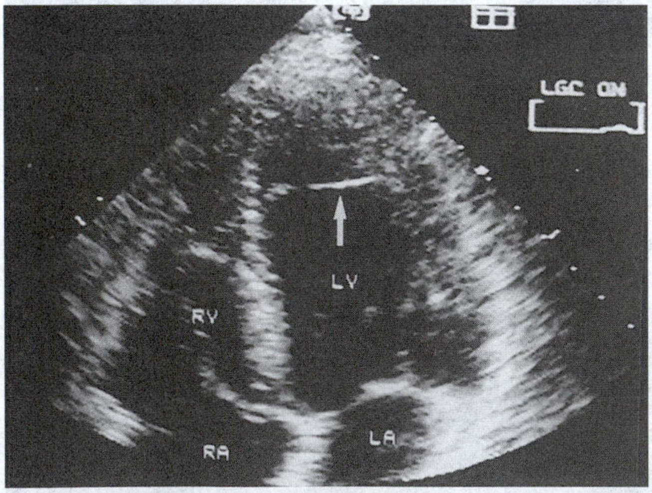

FIGURE 13-126 Apical four-chamber view demonstrating a false chord (*arrow*) within the left ventricle (LV). LA = left atrium; RA = right atrium; RV = right ventricle. (From Blanchard DG, DeMaria AN. Cardiac and extracardiac masses: Echocardiographic evaluation. In: Skorton DJ, Schelbert HR, Wolf GL, Brundage BH, eds. *Marcus' Cardiac Imaging,* 2d ed. Philadelphia: Saunders; 1996:452–480, with permission.)

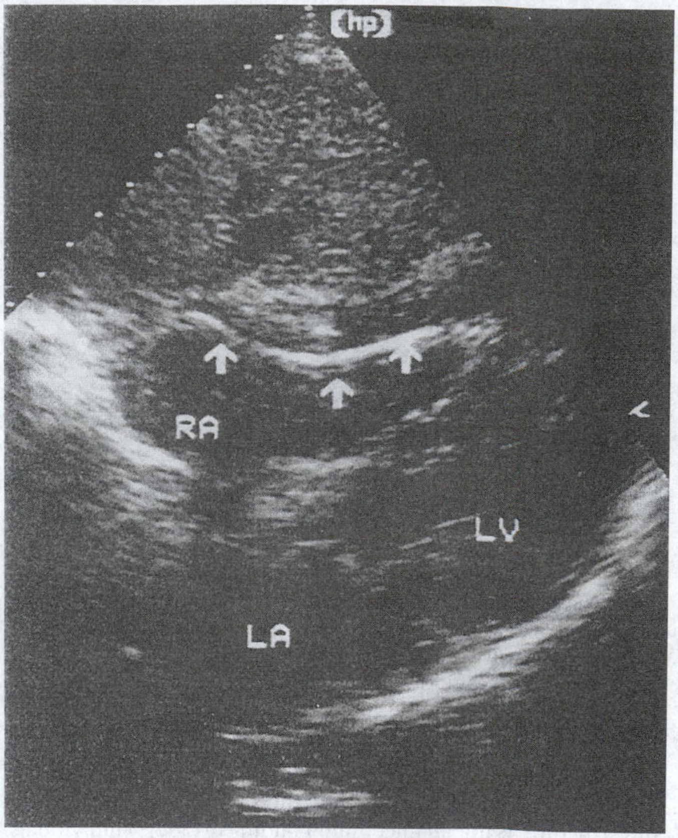

FIGURE 13-127 Subcostal four-chamber image demonstrating a pacemaker wire (*arrows*) in the right heart. RA = right atrium; LA = left atrium; LV = left ventricle.

reported in up to one-half of patients with large myocardial infarctions and occur more frequently in anterior infarctions (up to 30 to 40 percent of such patients).[668] Most thrombi are located in the apex[626] and thus are best visualized in the apical views (Fig. 13-129). Although echocardiography is the procedure of choice for detecting LV thrombi,[669] the technique's true sensitivity and specificity remains uncertain, since most patients included in validating studies had LV aneurysms and the echocardiographic criteria applied were subjective.[668–670]

LV thrombi may be laminar and fixed or protruding and mobile, and they may have a heterogeneous echo density (Figs. 13-129 and 13-130). Studies suggest that "immature" thrombi are often filamentous, with irregular borders, while older thrombi tend to be echodense and fixed.[626,648,671] The echocardiographic characteristics of thrombi may influence the risk of cardiogenic embolization, as irregularly shaped, mobile, and protruding thrombi are more likely to embolize than laminar, immobile clots.[648] True LV thrombi have a density distinct from the underlying myocardium, appear in multiple imaging planes, and move concordantly with the underlying myocardium.[669] Suspected masses in areas of normally functioning myocardium are rarely thrombi.

CARDIAC TUMORS

Although diagnosed infrequently, cardiac tumors often are included in the differential diagnosis of cardiac problems because of their protean clinical manifestations. Cardiac tumors may be intracavitary or intramural, and the location determines their echocardiographic appearance. Intracavitary tumors appear as sessile or mobile echo densities attached to the mural endocardium while intramural tumors appear as localized thickening of the LV wall.[672] The pericardium also may be involved with cardiac tumors, with or without the presence of concomitant effusion (Chap. 77).

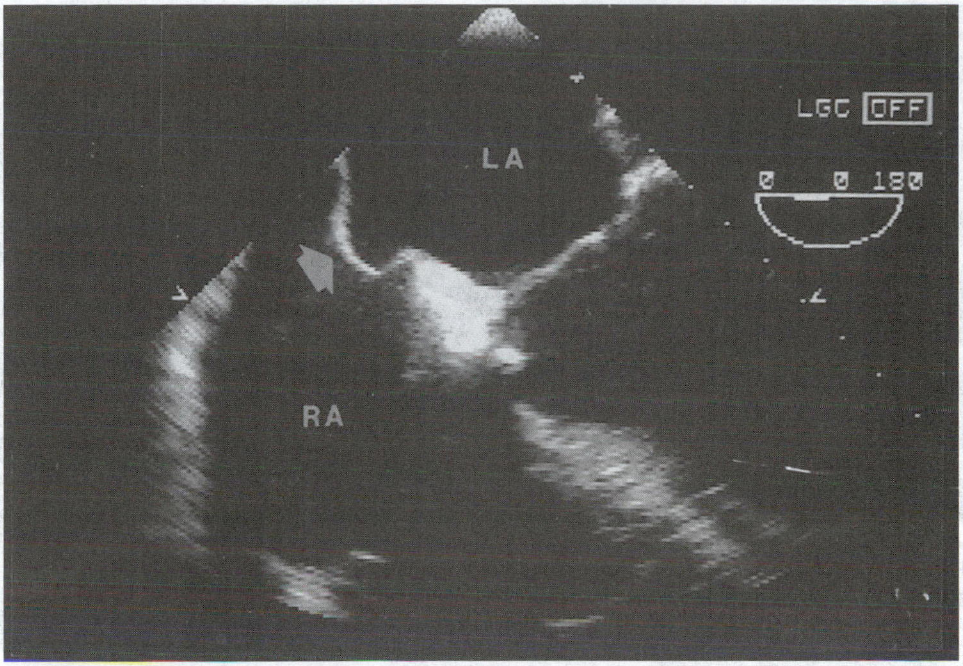

FIGURE 13-128 Transverse transesophageal image of an interatrial septal aneurysm (*arrow*). RA = right atrium; LA = left atrium. (From Blanchard DG, DeMaria AN. Cardiac and extracardiac masses: Echocardiographic evaluation. In: Skorton DJ, Schelbert HR, Wolf GL, Brundage BH, eds. *Marcus' Cardiac Imaging*, 2d ed. Philadelphia: Saunders; 1996:452–480, with permission.)

Myxomas

Myxomas are the most common primary cardiac tumors, accounting for about 25 percent of all such lesions.[673-675] Myxomas can occur in any cardiac chamber, but 75 percent are found in the LA.[675] On 2D imaging, myxomas usually appear as gelatinous, speckled, sometimes globular masses with frond-like projections (Figs. 13-132 and 13-133). Tissue heterogeneity is common, but calcification is rare.[673] Although they may be sessile, myxomas are usually attached to the endocardial surface by a pedicle. Typically, they are attached to the interatrial septum, but they can originate from the posterior or anterior atrial wall, the appendage, or even the cardiac valves.[676,677] Large tumors are almost always mobile to some degree, and a sizable left atrial mass that appears fixed in position is therefore less likely to be a myxoma. Large left atrial myxomas may move back and forth into the mitral valve annulus during the cardiac cycle, entering the orifice in diastole and the left atrium in systole. Accordingly, Doppler interrogation may demonstrate either obstruction of flow, valvular regurgitation, or both.[678,679] Most myxomas are visible on TTE, but TEE is superior for the delineation of tumor attachments and detection of small myxomas.[680] Since approximately 5 percent of myxomas are biatrial, careful evaluation of the RA is mandatory.[675]

Additional Primary Tumors

Benign Rhabdomyomas are rare cardiac tumors associated with tuberous sclerosis.[681,682] There is a strong tendency for multiple tumors to occur within an affected heart (90 percent of cases).[681,683] Fibromas are found most often in children and affect the left ventricle most frequently. The tumor may grow within the myocardium rather than expanding into a cardiac chamber.[684,685] Papillary fibroelastomas are usually quite small in size (less than 1 cm in diameter) and often grow on cardiac valves or chordae. These rare tumors typically have multiple small fronds that tend to embolize.[625,686,687] Echocardiographic differentiation from vegetations can be difficult (Chap. 77).

Malignant Primary malignant cardiac tumors are quite rare and confer a very poor prognosis. Angiosarcoma is the most common and occurs most often in the right atrium. Rhabdomyosarcoma is an additional primary cardiac malignancy.[688] Echocardiography can be useful in monitoring response to therapy, but its diagnostic utility is limited, as most findings are nonspecific.

Metastatic and Secondary Tumors of the Heart and Pericardium

Metastatic tumors to the pericardium and heart occur 20 to 40 times more often than primary cardiac tumors (Fig. 13-134).[689]

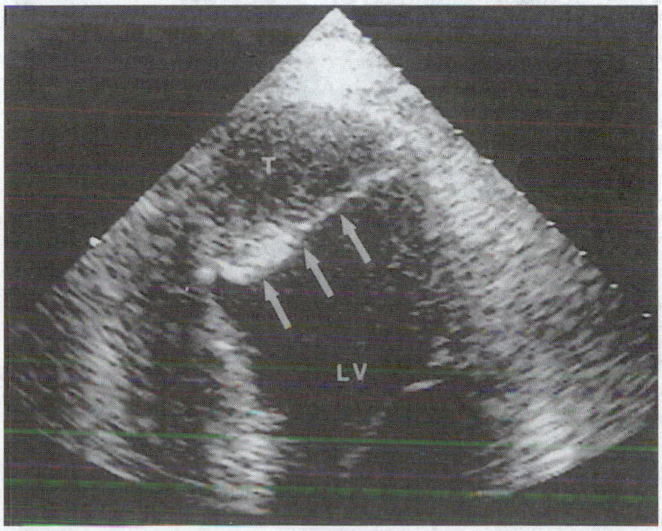

FIGURE 13-129 Magnified apical view of a large thrombus (T) in the apex of the left ventricle (LV). Although the thrombus is fairly homogeneous, its border is more echo-dense (*arrows*).

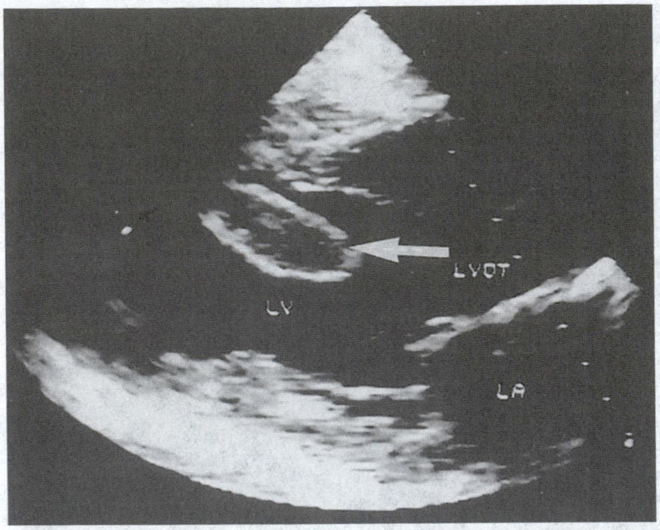

FIGURE 13-130 Parasternal long-axis view of a large mobile thrombus (*arrow*) attached to the anteroseptal segment of the left ventricle (LV). LVOT = left ventricular outflow tract; LA = left atrium. (From Blanchard DG, DeMaria AN. Cardiac and extracardiac masses: Echocardiographic evaluation. In: Skorton DJ, Schelbert HR, Wolf GL, Brundage BH, eds. *Marcus' Cardiac Imaging,* 2d ed. Philadelphia: Saunders; 1996:452–480, with permission.)

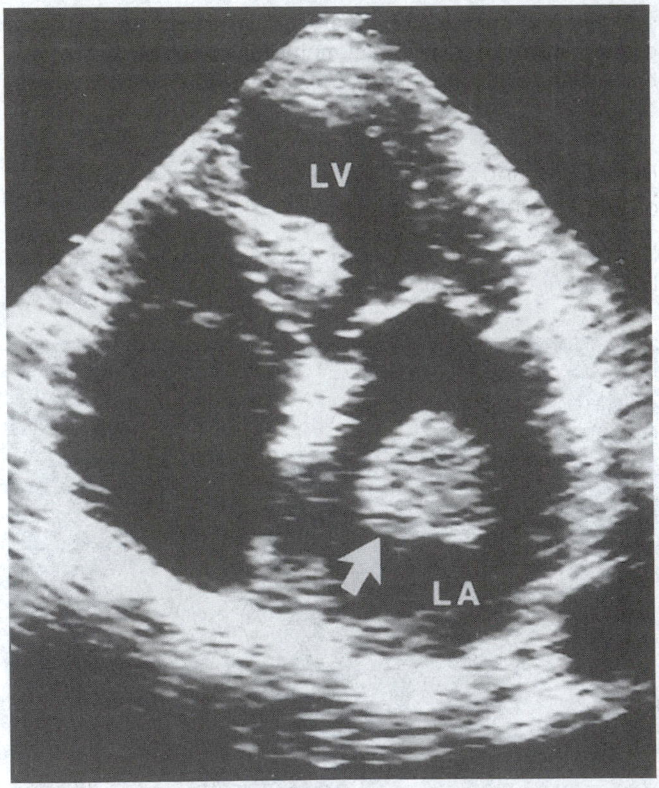

FIGURE 13-131 Apical four-chamber image of a large mobile "ball" thrombus (*arrow*) in the left atrium (LA). LV = left ventricle. (From Blanchard DG, DeMaria AN. Cardiac and extracardiac masses: Echocardiographic evaluation. In: Skorton DJ, Schelbert HR, Wolf GL, Brundage BH, eds. *Marcus' Cardiac Imaging,* 2d ed. Philadelphia: Saunders; 1996:452–480, with permission.)

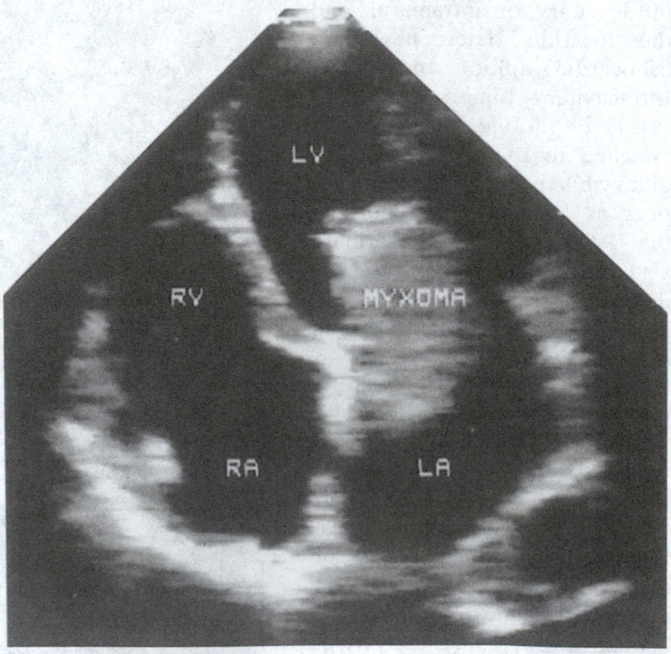

FIGURE 13-132 Apical four-chamber image of a left atrial myxoma which is attached to the interatrial septum and prolapses through the mitral valve. LA = left atrium; RA = right atrium; RV = right ventricle; LV = left ventricle. (From Blanchard DG, DeMaria AN. Cardiac and extracardiac masses: Echocardiographic evaluation. In: Skorton DJ, Schelbert HR, Wolf GL, Brundage BH, eds. *Marcus' Cardiac Imaging,* 2d ed. Philadelphia: Saunders, 1996:452–480, with permission.)

Tumors that commonly involve the heart and pericardium include breast and lung carcinoma, melanoma, and lymphoma. Involvement may be secondary to hematogenous, lymphatic, or contiguous spread. Tumors such as hepatoma and renal carcinoma can also extend to the heart via the venae cavae.[690] In these cases, tumor is often visible in the inferior vena cava and RA. Metastatic disease affects the pericardium more frequently than the heart itself, and pericardial effusion is the most common echocardiographic manifestation in patients with cardiac metastases.[689,691,692] Intracavitary and pericardial masses are easily visualized with 2D imaging, although intramural tumors are sometimes difficult to image. Echocardiographic findings are nonspecific, and metastatic tumors may be mistaken for primary cardiac neoplasms, vegetations, thrombi, or even prominent muscular trabeculations (Chap. 77).

Additional Cardiac Masses

The heart is rarely involved in echinococcal disease (<2 percent of cases), but intracardiac or intrapericardial rupture of a cyst can lead to anaphylaxis and cardiac tamponade, respectively.[693] Echocardiographic detection of a multiseptated cyst in the left ventricle or interventricular septum suggests cardiac echinococcal disease.[694]

Simple pericardial cysts usually occur in the right costophrenic angle (posterior to the right atrium) and have a benign prognosis. The structures are nonseptated and fluid-filled; they do not compress the cardiac chambers.[695]

PERICARDIAL DISEASE

In normal subjects, the pericardium is difficult to visualize since the pericardial cavity is only a potential space and visceral and parietal pericardial layers appear as a single echo.[696] In the setting of pericardial effusion, the fluid appears as a sonolucent area (or clear space) separating epicardium from pericardium.[697] Pericarditis may be unaccompanied by pericardial effusion and in such cases may be undetectable by echocardiography.[698] In addition, although thickening and/or calcification of the pericardium may be detectable by echocardiography in patients with constrictive pericarditis, cardiac ultrasound is limited in this capability.[699–700a] Therefore, the evaluation of constrictive pericarditis by echocardiography, primarily involves Doppler flow recordings.[701]

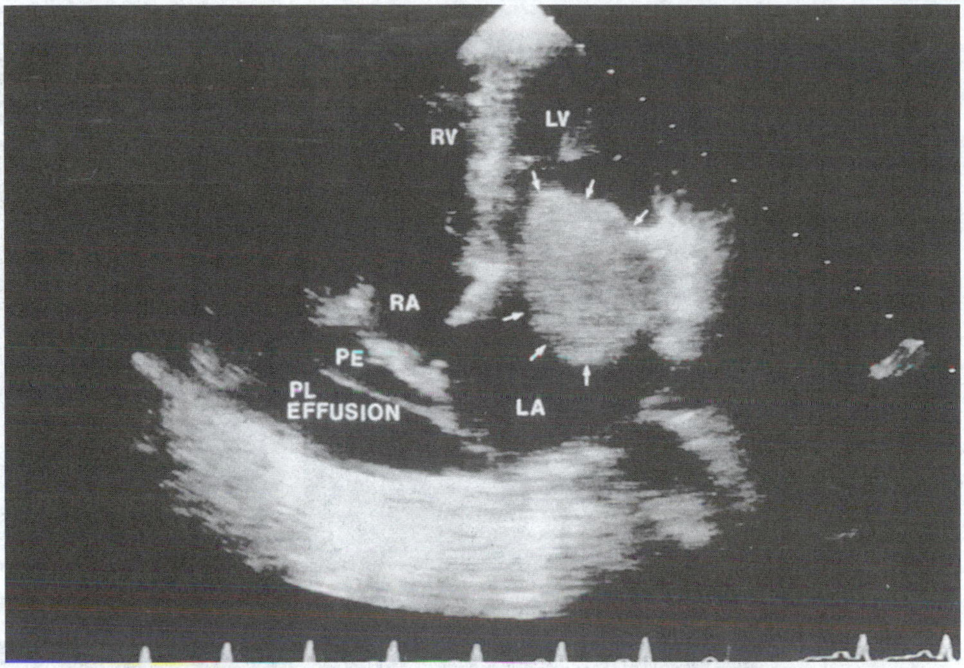

FIGURE 13-133 Apical four-chamber image of a large left atrial myxoma (*arrows*), which is attached to the lateral wall of the atrium. LA = left atrium; RA = right atrium; RV = right ventricle; LV = left ventricle; PE = pericardial effusion; PL = pleural.

Pericardial Effusion

Echocardiography is the diagnostic procedure of choice for detection of pericardial fluid[696,697] (Fig. 13-135), and early M-mode studies demonstrated that volumes as small as 20 to 30 mL could be detected reliably.[702] As both myocardium and pericardium are echo-reflective and pericardial fluid is not, a sonolucent area between the epicardium and pericardium is diagnostic of a pericardial effusion. Although epicardial-pericardial separation may be seen during systole in normal cases, separation throughout the cardiac cycle is abnormal.[702] Descending aorta, coronary sinus, pleural effusion, pericardial cyst, and LV pseudoaneurysm occasionally may be mistaken for pericardial effusion.[703]

Echocardiography can be used to identify pericardial loculations, fibrous strands, and pericardial tumors as well as to assess the size of effusions[692,696,697,699,700] (Fig. 13-136). Pericardial effusions may be concentric or loculated (the latter type is especially common with postoperative, infective, and malignant effusions). As pericardial tissue reflects upon itself behind the left atrium between the pulmonary veins (the oblique sinus), fluid is rarely seen in this area. Small, nonloculated effusions may move depending on patient position and thus are often drawn posteriorly and inferiorly by gravity during routine imaging. A rim of pericardial fluid surrounding the heart is evidence of a moderate or large effusion, and the heart can sometimes be seen "swinging" back and forth within the pericardial space, creating the mechanism of *electrical alternans.*[704] In general, small effusions are seen posteriorly rather than anteriorly on supine imaging.[696] Moderate-sized (100 to 500 mL) nonloculated effusions are present both anterior and posterior to the heart.[696] Large nonloculated effusions (>500 mL) are circumferential and frequently allow free motion of the heart within the fluid-filled space.[696,697]

Distinguishing between pericardial and pleural effusions is occasionally difficult with echocardiography.[705] If these conditions coexist, the pericardium usually can be identified as a linear density separating fluid in the two spaces. The parasternal long-axis view is often helpful in differentiating the disorders. The descending aorta is a mediastinal structure; therefore peri-

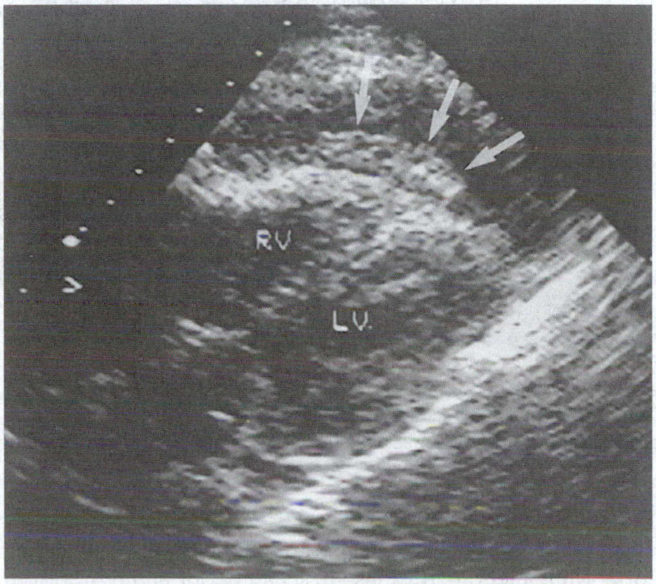

FIGURE 13-134 Modified subcostal image showing a metastatic tumor on the epicardium (*arrows*) and a malignant pericardial effusion. RV = right ventricle; LV = left ventricle. (From Blanchard DG, DeMaria AN. Cardiac and extracardiac masses: Echocardiographic evaluation. In: Skorton DJ, Schelbert HR, Wolf GL, Brundage BH, eds. *Marcus' Cardiac Imaging*, 2d ed. Philadelphia: Saunders; 1996:452–480, with permission.)

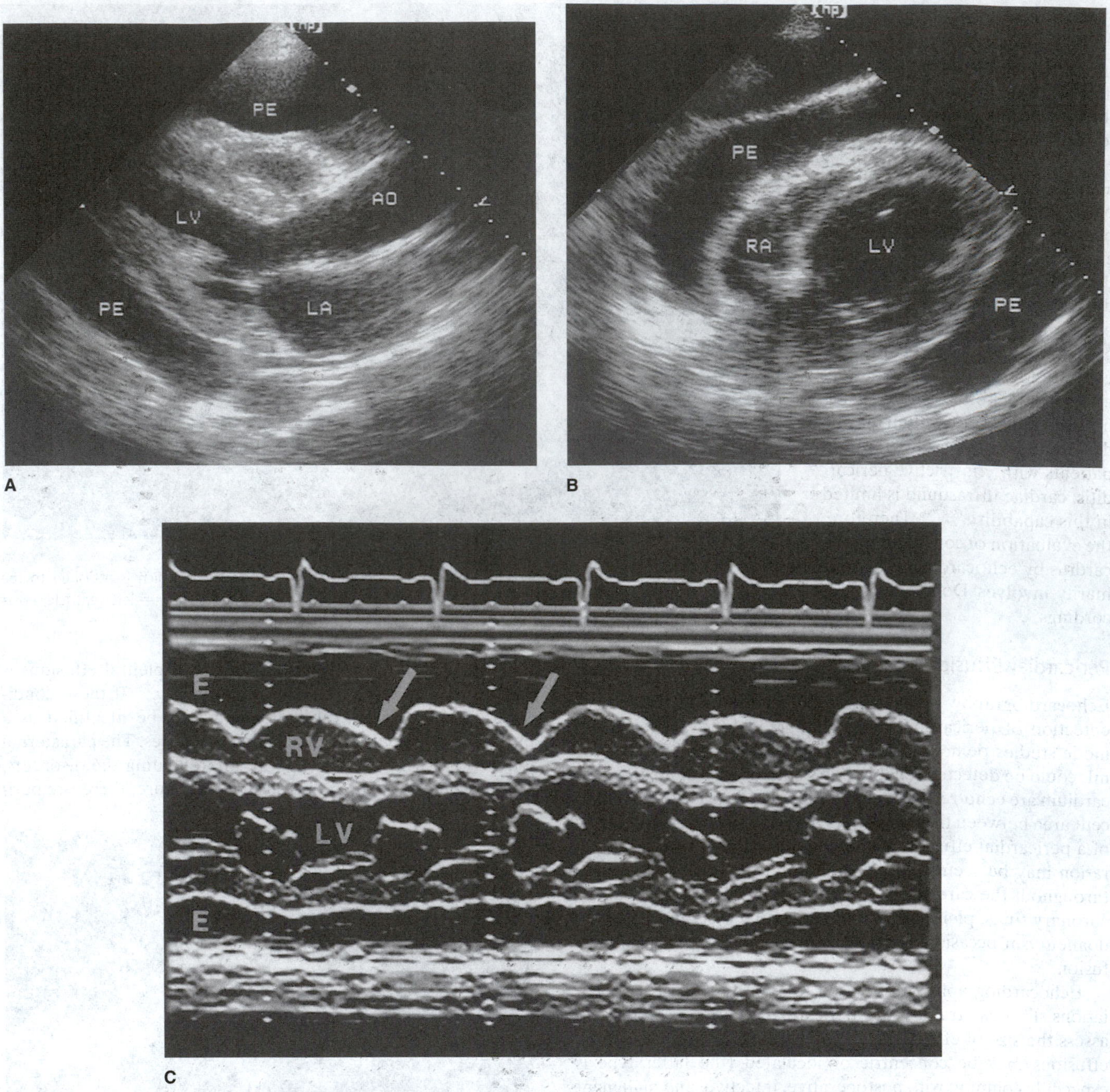

FIGURE 13-135 *A.* Moderate pericardial effusion (PE) on parasternal long-axis imaging. AO = aorta; LV = left ventricle; LA = left atrium. *B.* Right ventricular compression in cardiac tamponade (subcostal plane). RA = right atrium; LV = left ventricle; PE = pericardial effusion. *C.* M-mode image of cardiac tamponade and right ventricular diastolic collapse. The right ventricular (RV) free wall (*arrows*) moves posteriorly toward the interventricular septum during diastole. E = effusion; LV = left ventricle.

cardial effusions will often separate the heart and descending aorta, while pleural effusions are seen inferior and posterior to the aorta[705] (Fig. 13-137). In cases of large pleural effusions, atelectatic lung tissue also may be present (Fig. 13-137). Subcostal views are often valuable and may yield the only satisfactory transthoracic images in postoperative or posttraumatic cases. The inferior vena cava also can be imaged in this view; if the vessel does not display inspiratory collapse greater than 50 percent of its maximum diameter, elevated RA pressure is present.[366]

On parasternal images, an echolucent space is sometimes visualized anterior to the RV.[706] Although this finding may represent pericardial fluid, it usually is caused by epicardial fat (without effusion) and has no pathologic significance. Therefore the diagnosis of pericardial effusion based solely on the presence of this anterior clear space should be avoided.

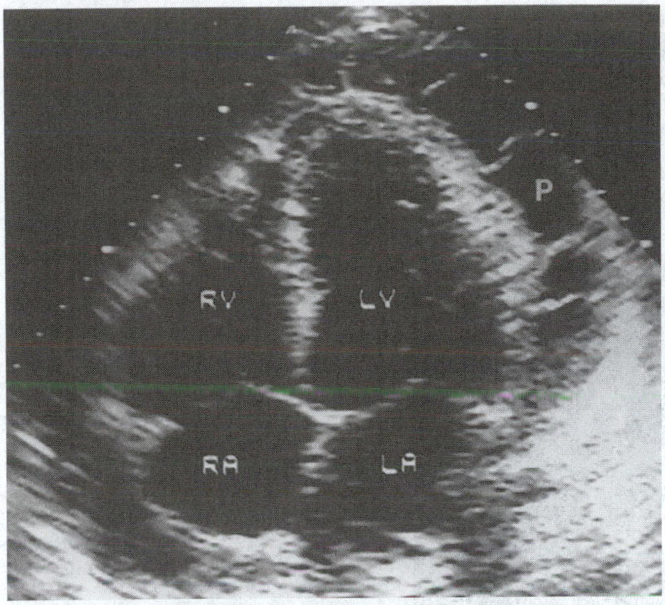

FIGURE 13-136 Apical four-chamber image in a case of malignant pericardial effusion (P). Numerous fibrinous strands are seen within the effusion. LA = left atrium; RA = right atrium; RV = right ventricle; LV = left ventricle. (From Blanchard DG, DeMaria AN. Cardiac and extracardiac masses: Echocardiographic evaluation. In: Skorton DJ, Schelbert HR, Wolf GL, Brundage BH, eds. *Marcus' Cardiac Imaging*, 2d ed. Philadelphia: Saunders, 1996:452–480, with permission.)

Cardiac Tamponade

As the pericardium is a relatively noncompliant membrane that adapts slowly to volume changes, pericardial effusions (especially those that accumulate rapidly) may limit cardiac filling and cause cardiac tamponade. Echocardiography can help diagnose this condition by detecting (1) morphologic signs of increased intrapericardial pressure and (2) abnormal intracardiac flow patterns caused by tamponade and enhanced ventricular interdependence.[707,708]

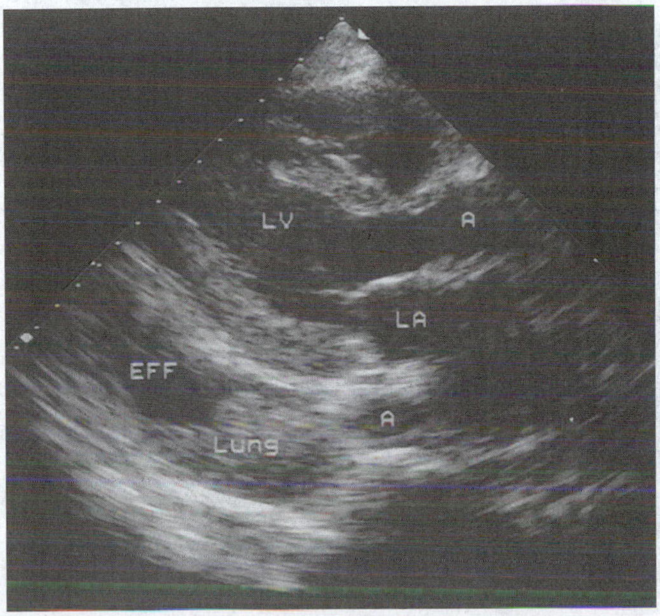

FIGURE 13-137 Parasternal long-axis view in a patient with a pleural effusion (EFF) posterior to the heart. Atelectatic lung tissue is present within the effusion. LA = left atrium; LV = left ventricle; A = aorta.

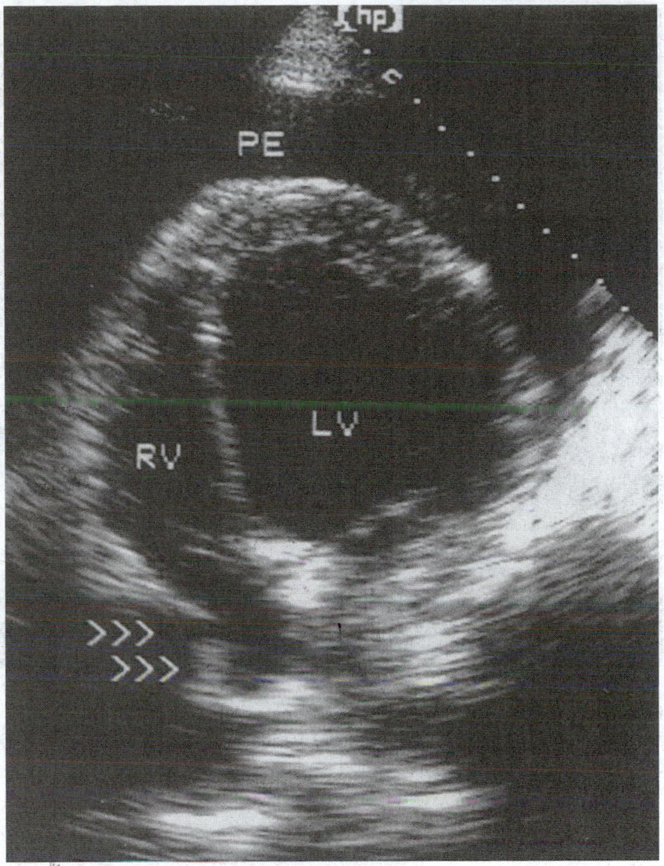

FIGURE 13-138 Right atrial collapse (*arrows*) in cardiac tamponade. PE = pericardial effusion; LV = left ventricle; RV = right ventricle.

As diastolic pressures are slightly lower in the right heart than the left, the RA and RV are usually the first chambers to exhibit evidence of increased intrapericardial pressure. High intrapericardial pressure can cause compression or collapse of right heart chambers.[707,709,710] Invagination of the right atrial wall during atrial systole is a sensitive (but not specific) sign of tamponade (Fig. 13-138).[709] Diastolic collapse or "buckling" of the RV free wall is a more specific sign of tamponade, and can be visualized both on 2D and M-mode imaging[707,710] (Fig. 13-135*B* and *C*). In cases of localized tamponade or severe RV hypertrophy, left atrial or ventricular diastolic collapse may be the first sign of tamponade.[711,712]

Doppler echocardiographic recordings in patients with tamponade have demonstrated an enhancement or exaggeration of the normal respiratory variation in ventricular inflow and outflow.[708,713] Thus, transmitral and LVOT velocities decrease significantly with inspiration, probably because of enhanced ventricular interdependence and a marked decrease in the transmitral diastolic gradient during inspiration (Fig. 13-139). The latter is caused both by high intrapericardial pressure as well as leftward motion of the interventricular septum from increased RV filling.[708] Although cardiac tamponade remains a clinical diagnosis, echocardiography has significantly improved the detection of hemodynamic effects from pericardial fluid,

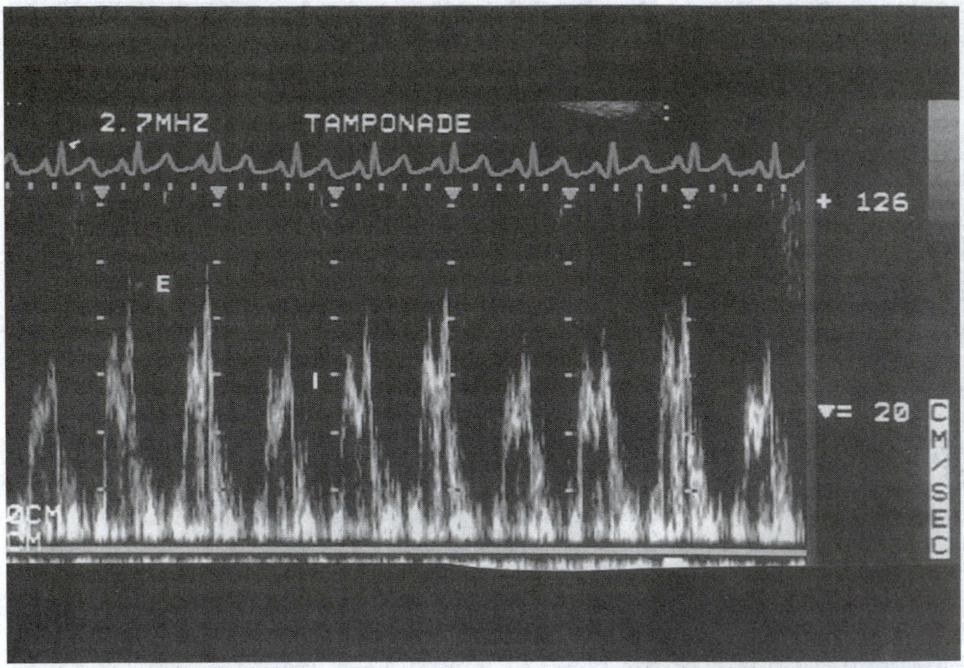

FIGURE 13-139 Pulsed-wave Doppler tracing of left ventricular inflow in cardiac tamponade (apical transducer position). There is abnormal respiratory variation in the peak E wave velocity (which varies from 60 to 80 cm/s). E = expiration; I = inspiration.

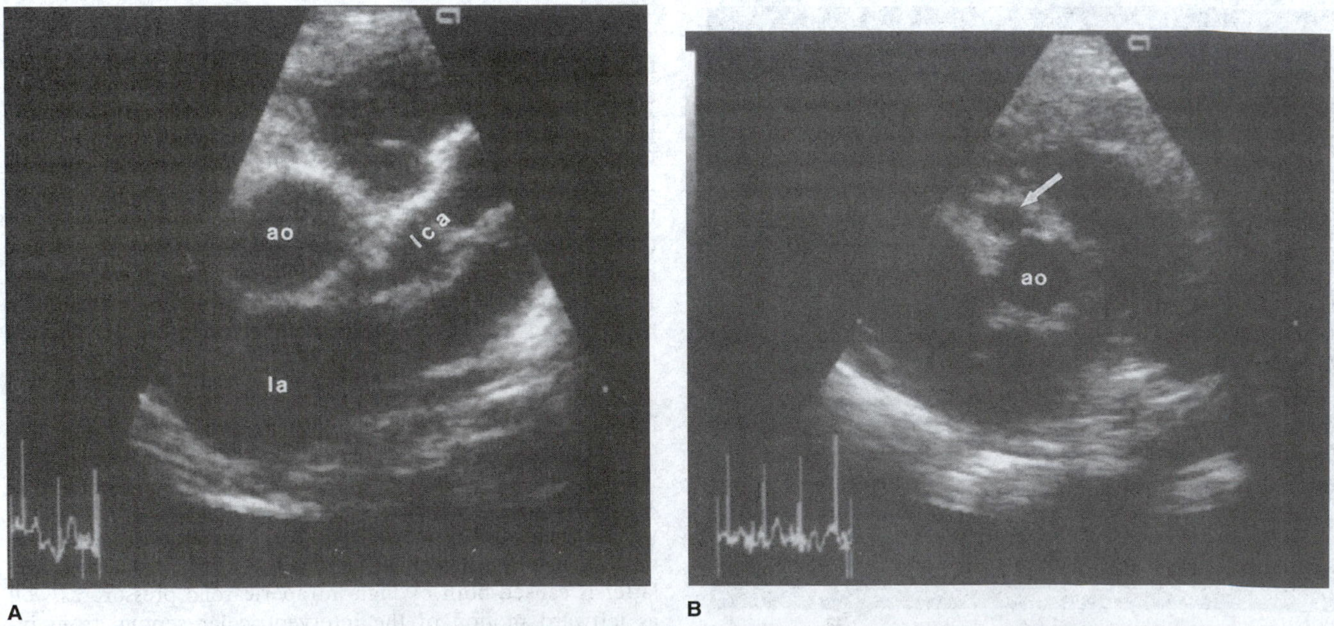

FIGURE 13-140 Parasternal short-axis images of coronary artery aneurysms associated with Kawasaki's disease. *A.* The proximal left coronary artery (LCA) is seen to be diffusely dilated and aneurysmal. *B.* A proximal right coronary artery aneurysm (*arrow*) is shown. AO = aorta, LA = left atrium. (Courtesy of Victor Lucas, MD and Paul Grossfeld, MD.)

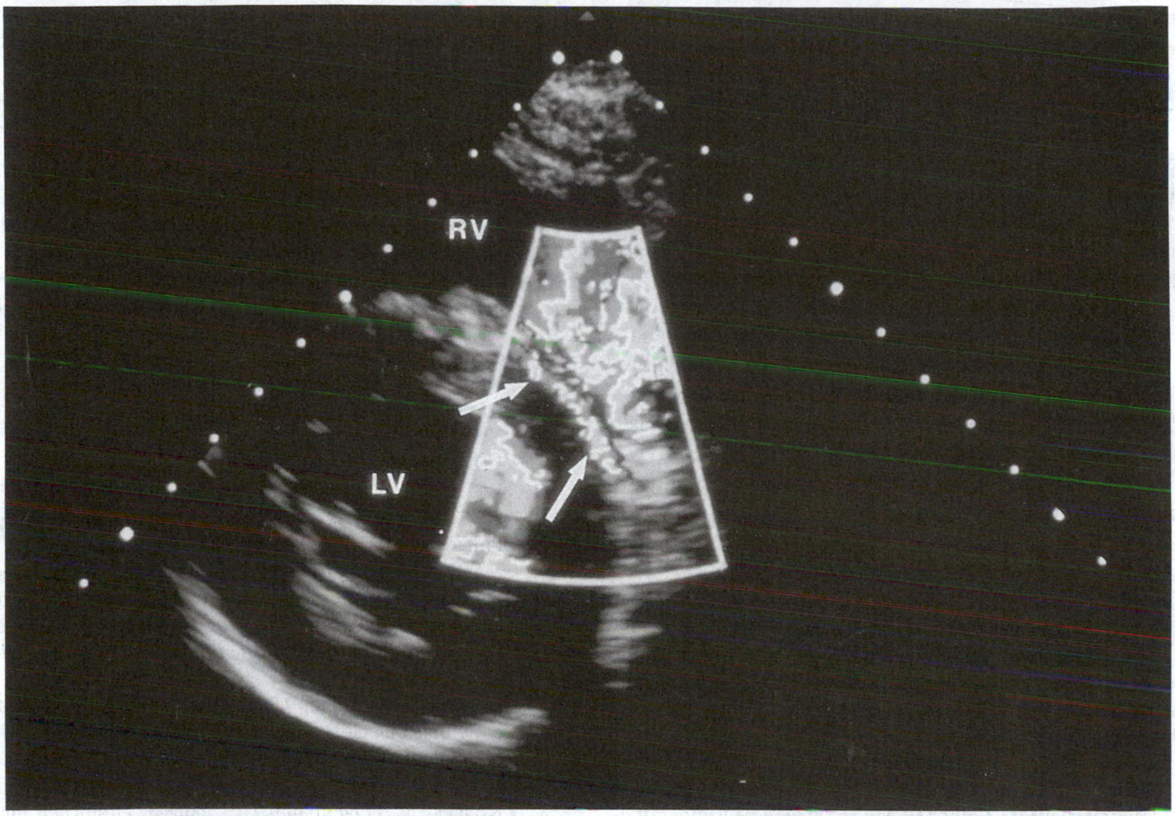

FIGURE 13-141 (Plate 73) Transthoracic short-axis image of a coronary artery within the interventricular septum (*arrows*). LV= left ventricle; RV = right ventricle.

especially in early and equivocal cases. Studies have also indicated that when echocardiography is used to direct pericardiocentesis to the site of greatest fluid accumulation, the risks associated with blind pericardial puncture are decreased.[714]

Constrictive Pericarditis

The diagnosis of constrictive pericarditis is sometimes difficult to establish, even by cardiac catheterization. 2D and M-mode echocardiography may provide evidence of thickened pericardial tissue by demonstrating increased reflectivity and multiple parallel moving echoes in the area of the pericardium.[699,700] The criteria for pericardial thickening on echocardiogram are imperfect, however, as the normal pericardium is an echodense, highly reflective structure with a gain-dependent signal.[715] Paradoxical septal motion may be seen on M-mode with constriction, as can an abnormal inspiratory interventricular septal "bounce"[716] and limited diastolic motion of the posterior LV wall.[717] A dilated inferior vena cava that does not collapse on deep inspiration is indicative of high RA pressure and may be observed on 2D imaging in constrictive pericarditis.[716]

The utility of Doppler recordings in evaluating constrictive pericarditis has been shown in several recent studies.[550,701,718–723,723a,723b] As with cardiac tamponade, pericardial constriction produces exaggerated respiratory variation in the isovolumic relaxation time and in flow velocities within right and left ventricles, pulmonary veins, and hepatic vein.[701,718,722] A respiratory variation of >20 percent in peak mitral E velocity favors the diagnosis of constriction over restrictive cardiomyopathy, while little respiratory variation and a shortened E deceleration time favor restrictive physiology.[701] Doppler echocardiographic criteria for constriction have been validated prospectively and may help predict clinical response to pericardiectomy.[721] Unfortunately, exaggerated respiratory flow variation is not specific for pericardial constriction and also can be seen in chronic obstructive pulmonary disease and asthma.[724] In these cases, Doppler examination of superior vena cava flow is useful: patients with asthma will have increased flow toward the heart during inspiration, while limited forward flow will be seen in constriction (the echocardiographic equivalent of Kussmaul's sign).[724,724a] Recently, respiratory variation in the peak velocity and duration of continuous-wave Doppler TR spectral envelopes has been shown to reflect accurately the enhanced ventricular interaction seen in constrictive pericarditis.[725]

IMAGING OF THE CORONARY ARTERIES

The ability to visualize the proximal segments of the left and right coronary arteries was initially demonstrated by Weyman et al.[417] Subsequent studies established the ability of color and spectral Doppler examination to image and record the velocity of flow from TTE and TEE approaches, particularly with regard to the left anterior descending coronary artery.[418–420] However, visualization of the coronary arteries by echocardiography has not achieved a significant role in clinical practice because the resolution of the technique is at the limit of vessel size and the vessels are circuitous and move vigorously, often coursing in and out of the beam path. Despite these limitations, transthoracic

..g has proven useful for the diagnosis and follow-up of ..ents with Kawasaki disease and coronary involvement[726–728] (Fig. 13-140) and may also help distinguish normal from atherosclerotic coronary arteries.[729]

The coronary arteries are routinely imaged with TEE, which can detect proximal stenoses, atherosclerosis, and congenital abnormalities of the coronaries more accurately than surface imaging.[730–732] Doppler TEE analysis also has been used to determine coronary low reserve.[733,734]

Visualization of mid- and distal coronary arteries is problematic with both TTE and TEE. Recent advances in technology and contrast agents, however, may significantly improve capabilities in this area. Figure 13-141 (Plate 73) shows color flow within a septal coronary artery. This image was produced by an instrument utilizing a carrier frequency range of 5 to 7 MHz, rather than the more commonly used range of 2.5 to 3.5 MHz. This area of echocardiography is expanding rapidly and clinical applications will grow in the future.[735,736]

References

1. ACC/AHA Guidelines for the Clinical Application of Echocardiography: Executive Summary. A Report of the American College of Cardiology/American Heart Association Task Force on Practice Guidelines (Committee on Clinical Application of Echocardiography). *J Am Coll Cardiol* 29:862–879, 1997.
2. Daniel WG, Mügge A. Transesophageal echocardiography. *N Engl J Med* 1995; 332:1268–1279.
3. Handschumacher MD, Lethor JP, Siu SC, et al. A new integrated system for three-dimensional echocardiographic reconstruction: Development and validation for ventricular volume with application in human subjects. *J Am Coll Cardiol* 1993; 21:743–753.
4. Rovai D, DeMaria AN, L'Abbate A. Myocardial contrast echo effect: The dilemma of coronary blood flow and volume. *J Am Coll Cardiol* 1995; 26:12–17.
5. Elder I, Hertz CH. The use of ultrasonic reflectoscope for the continuous recording of movement of heart walls. *Kungl Fysiorgr Sallski Fund Forhandl* 1954; 24:40–45.
6. Wild JJ, Crawford HD, Reid JM. Visualization of the excised human heart by means of reflected ultrasound or echocardiography. *Am Heart J* 1958; 54:903–906.
7. Feigenbaum H, Zaky A. Use of diagnostic ultrasound in clinical cardiology. *J Indiana State Med Assoc* 1966; 49:140–152.
8. Bom N, Lancee CT Jr, Van Zwieten G, et al. Multiscan echocardiography: I. Technical description. *Circulation* 1973; 48;1066–1073.
9. Griffith JM, Henry WL. A sector scanner for real time two-dimensional echocardiography. *Circulation* 1974; 49:1147–1152.
10. Eggelton RC, Johnston KW. Real time mechanical scanning system compared with array techniques. *IEEE Proc Sonics Ultrasounds* 1974; Cat. No. 74-CH0896-1:16.
11. VonRamm OT, Thurstone FL. Cardiac imaging using a phased array ultrasound system: I. System design. *Circulation* 1976; 53:258–262.
12. Baker DW. Pulsed ultrasonic Doppler blood-flow sensing. *IEEE Trans Sonics Ultrasonics* 1970; SU-17(3).
13. Hatle L, Angelsen B, Tromsdal A. Noninvasive assessment of atrioventricular pressure half-time by Doppler ultrasound. *Circulation* 1979; 60:1096–1104.
14. Hatle L, Angelsen BA, Tromsdal A. Noninvasive assessment of aortic stenosis by Doppler ultrasound. *Br Heart J* 1980; 3:284–292.
15. Omoto R. *Color Atlas of Real-Time Two-Dimensional Doppler Echocardiography*, 2d ed. Tokyo: Sindan-to-Chiryo; 1987.
16. Hanrath P, Kremer P, Langenstein BA, et al. Transoesophageale Eckokardiographie: Ein neues Verfahren zur dynamischen Ventrikelfunktionsanalyse. *Dtsch Med Wochenschr* 1981; 106: 523–525.
17. Seward JB, Khanderia BK, Oh JK, et al. Transesophageal echocardiography: Technique, anatomic correlations, implementation and clinical applications. *Mayo Clin Proc* 1988; 63:649–680.
18. Wells PNT. *Ultrasonics in Clinical Diagnosis*, 2d ed. New York: Churchill Livingstone; 1977.

18a. Thomas JD, Rubin DN. Tissue harmonic imaging: Why does it work? *J Am Soc Echocardiogr* 1998; 11:803–808.

18b. Main ML, Asher CR, Rubin DN, et al. Comparison of tissue harmonic imaging with contrast (sonicated albumin) echocardiography and Doppler myocardial imaging for enhancing endocardial border resolution. *Am J Cardiol* 1999; 83:218–222.

19. Kremkau FW, Taylor KJW. Artifacts in ultrasound imaging. *J Ultrasound Med* 1986; 15:227–237.
20. Yeh E. Reverberations in echocardiograms. *J Clin Ultrasound* 1977; 5:84–86.
21. Weyman AE. Physical principles of ultrasound. In: Weyman AE, ed. *Principles and Practice of Echocardiography*, 2d ed. Philadelphia: Lea & Febiger; 1994:3–28.
22. Mann DL, Gillam LD, Weyman AE. Cross-sectional echocardiographic assessment of regional left ventricular performance and myocardial perfusion. *Prog Cardiovac Dis* 1986; 29:1–52.
23. Rose JL, Goldberg BB. *Basic Physics in Diagnostic Ultrasound*. New York: Wiley; 1979.
24. DeMaria AN, Miller RR, Amsterdam EA, et al. Mitral valve early diastolic closing velocity in the echocardiogram: Relation to sequential diastolic flow and ventricular compliance. *Am J Cardiol* 1976; 37:693–700.
25. Konecke L, Feigenbaum H, Chang S. Abnormal mitral valve motion in patients with elevated left ventricular end diastolic pressure. *Circulation* 1973; 47:989–996.
26. Sahn DJ, DeMaria A, Kisslo J, Weyman AE. Recommendations regarding quantitation in M-mode echocardiography: Results of a survey of echocardiographic measurements. *Circulation* 1978; 58:1072–1083.
27. Nanda NC, Gramiak R, Manning EB. Echocardiographic recognition of the congenital bicuspid aortic valve. *Circulation* 1974; 49:870–875.
28. Rasmussen S, Corya BC, Phillips JF, Black MJ. Unreliability of M-mode left ventricular dimensions for calculating stroke volume and cardiac output in patients without heart disease. *Chest* 1982; 81:614–619.
29. Teichholz LE, Kreulen T, Herman MV, Gorlin R. Problems in echocardiographic volume determinations: Echocardiographic-angiographic correlations in the presence or absence of synergy. *Am J Cardiol* 1976; 37:7–11.
30. McDonald IG, Feigenbaum H, Chang S. Analysis of left ventricular wall motion by reflected ultrasound: Application to assessment of myocardial function. *Circulation* 1972; 46:14–25.
31. Feigenbaum H: Echocardiographic examination of the left ventricle. *Circulation* 1975; 51:1–7.
32. Massie BM, Schiller NB, Ratshin RA, Parmley WW. Mitral-septal separation: New echocardiographic index of left ventricular function. *Am J Cardiol* 1977; 39:1008–1016.
33. Ophir J, Maklad NF. Digital scan converters in diagnostic ultrasound imaging. *Proc IEEE* 1979; 67–75.
34. Henry WL, DeMaria A, Gramiak R, et al. Report of the American Society of Echocardiography: Nomenclature and standards in two-dimensional echocardiography. *Circulation* 1980; 62:212–217.
35. Feigenbaum H. The echocardiographic examination. In: Feigenbaum H. *Echocardiography*, 5th ed. Philadelphia: Lea & Febiger; 1994:68–133.
36. Weyman AE. *Principles and Practice of Echocardiography*, 2d ed. Philadelphia: Lea & Febiger; 1994.

36a. Sapin PM, Clarke GB, Gopal AS, et al. Validation of three-dimensional echocardiography for quantifying the extent of dyssynergy in canine acute myocardial infarction: Comparison with two-dimensional echocardiography. *J Am Coll Cardiol* 1996; 27:1761–1770.

36b. Shiota T, Jones M, Chikada M, et al. Real-time three-dimensional echocardiography for determining right ventricular stroke volume in an animal model of chronic right ventricular volume overload. *Circulation* 1998, 97:1896–1900.

37. Teichholtz LE, Kreulen T, Herman MV, Gorlin R. Problems in echocardiographic volume determinations: Echocardiographic-angiographic correlations in the presence or absence of asynergy. *Am J Cardiol* 1976; 37:7–11.

38. Wyatt HL, Heng MK, Meerbaum S, et al. Cross-sectional echocardiography: II. Analysis of mathematic models for quantifying volume of formalin fixed left ventricle. *Circulation* 1980; 61:1119–1125.

39. Wyatt HL, Meerbaum S, Heng MK, et al. Cross-sectional echocardiography: III. Analysis of mathematic models for quantifying volume of symmetric and asymmetric left ventricles. *Am Heart J* 1980; 100:821–828.

40. Schiller NB, Acquatella H, Ports TA, et al. Left ventricular volume from paired biplane two-dimensional echocardiography. *Circulation* 1979; 60:547–555.

41. Folland ED, Parisi AF, Moynihan PF, et al. Assessment of left ventricular ejection fraction and volumes by real-time, two-dimensional echocardiography and radionuclide techniques. *Circulation* 1979; 60:760–766.

42. Stamm RB, Carabello BA, Mayers DL, Martin RP. Two-dimensional echocardiographic measurement of left ventricular ejection fraction: Prospective analysis of what constitutes an adequate determination. *Am Heart J* 1982; 104:136–144.

43. Gueret P, Corday E. Etude quantitative de la fonction ventriculaire gauche par l'echocardiographie bidimensionnelle. *Arch Mal Coeur* 1981; 74:329–336.

44. Starling MR, Crawford MH, Sorensen SG, et al. Comparative accuracy of apical biplane cross-sectional echocardiography and gated equilibrium radionuclide angiography for estimating left ventricular size and performance. *Circulation* 1981; 63:1075–1084.

45. Erbel R, Schweizer P, Lambertz H, et al. Echoventriculography—A simultaneous analysis of two-dimensional echocardiography and cineventriculography. *Circulation* 1983; 67:205–215.

46. Becher H, Tiemann K, Schlief R, et al. Harmonic power Doppler contrast echocardiography: Preliminary clinical results. *Echocardiography* 1997; 14:637–642.

46a. Spencer KT, Bednarz J, Rafter PG, et al. Use of harmonic imaging without echocardiographic contrast to improve two-dimensional image quality. *Am J Cardiol* 1998; 82:794–799.

47. Perez JE, Waggoner AD, Barzilai B, et al. On-line assessment of ventricular function by automatic boundary detection and ultrasonic backscatter imaging. *J Am Coll Cardiol* 1992; 19:313.

48. Lang RM, Vignon P, Weinert L, et al. Echocardiographic quantification of regional left ventricular wall motion with color kinesis. *Circulation* 1996; 93:1877–1885.

49. Duong AM, Blanchard DG, Cotter B, et al. Endomyocardial movement in patients with disturbed diastolic filling dynamics: Assessment by acoustic quantitation color kinesis (abstr). *J Am Soc Echocardiogr* 1996; 9:365.

49a. Godoy IE, Mor-Avi V, Weinert L, et al. Use of color kinesis for evaluation of left ventricular filling in patients with dilated cardiomyopathy and mitral regurgitation. *J Am Coll Cardiol* 1998;31:1598–606.

50. Doppler JC. Ueber das farbige Licht der Dopplesterne und einiger anderer Gestirne des Himmels. *Abhandlungen der Konigl, Bohmischen Gesellschaft der Wissenschaften*, 5th ser. 1842; 2:465.

51. Franklin DL, Schlegal W, Rushmer RF. Blood flow measured by Doppler frequency shift of backscattered ultrasound. *Science* 1961; 134:564.

52. Baker DW. Pulsed ultrasonic Doppler flow sensing. *IEEE Trans Sonics Ultrasonics* 1970; 17:170.

53. Hatle L, Angelsen B. *Doppler Ultrasound in Cardiology: Physical Principles and Clinical Applications*, 2d ed. Philadelphia: Lea & Febiger; 1984.

53a. Garcia MJ, Thomas JD, Klein AL. New Doppler echocardiographic applications for the study of diastolic function. *J Am Coll Cardiol* 1998; 32:865–875.

53b. Nagueh SF, Middleton KJ, Kopelen HA, et al. Doppler tissue imaging: A noninvasive technique for evaluation of left vertricular relaxation and estimation of filling pressures. *J Am Coll Cardiol* 1997; 30:1527–1533.

53c. Garcia MJ, Smedira NG, Greenberg NL, et al. Color M-mode Doppler flow propagation velocity is a preload insensitive index of left ventricular relaxation: Animal and human validation. *J Am Coll Cardiol* 2000; 35:201–208.

54. Baker DW, Rubenstein SA, Lorch GS. Pulsed Doppler echocardiography: Principles and applications. *Am J Med* 1977; 63:69–80.

55. Burns PM. The physical principles of Doppler and spectral analysis. *J Clin Ultrasound* 1987; 15:567–590.

56. Bom K, deBoo J, Rijsterborgh H. On the aliasing problem in pulsed Doppler cardiac studies. *J Clin Ultrasound* 1984; 12:559–567.

57. Steward WJ, Galvin KA, Gillam LD, et al. Comparison of high pulse repetition frequency and continuous wave Doppler echocardiography in the assessment of high flow velocity in patients with valvular stenosis and regurgitation. *J Am Coll Cardiol* 1985; 6:565–571.

58. Otto CM, Pearlman AS. Measurement of high flow velocities using pulsed Doppler echocardiography. *Echocardiography* 1985; 2:141–152.

59. Omoto R. *Color Atlas of Real-Time Two-Dimensional Doppler Echocardiography*, 2d ed. Tokyo: Shindan-to-Chiryo; 1987.

60. Bommer W, Miller L. Real time two-dimensional color flow Doppler-enhanced imaging in the diagnosis of cardiovascular disease. (abstr). *Am J Cardiol* 1982; 49:944.

61. Stevenson JG. Appearance and recognition of basic concepts in color flow imaging. *Echocardiography* 1989; 6:451.

62. Omoto R, Kasai C. Physics and instrumentation of Doppler color flow mapping. *Echocardiography* 1987; 4:467.

63. Feigenbaum H. Appendix: Echocardiographic measurements and normal values. In: Feigenbaum H, ed. *Echocardiography*, 5th ed. Philadelphia: Lea & Febiger, 1994:658–683.

64. Rakowski H, Appleton C, Chan K-L, et al. Canadian consensus recommendations for the measurement and reporting of diastolic dysfunction by echocardiography. *J Am Soc Echocardiogr* 1996; 9:736–760.

65. Nishimura RA, Housmans PR, Hatle LK, Tajik AJ. Assessment of diastolic function of the heart: Background and current applications of Doppler echocardiography: Part I. Physiologic and pathophysiologic features. *Mayo Clin Proc* 1989; 64:71–81.

66. Nishimura RA, Hatle LK, Abel MD, Tajik AJ. Assessment of diastolic function of the heart: Background and current applications of Doppler echocardiography: Part II. Clinical studies. *Mayo Clin Proc* 1989; 4:181–204.

67. Stoddard MF, Pearson AC, Kern MJ, et al. Left ventricular diastolic function: Comparison of pulsed Doppler echocardiographic and hemodynamic indexes in subjects with and without coronary artery disease. *J Am Coll Cardiol* 1989; 13:327–336.

68. Klein AL, Hatle L, Burstow DJ, et al. Doppler characterization of left ventricular diastolic function in cardiac amyloidosis. *J Am Coll Cardiol* 1989; 13:1017–1026.

69. Cohen GI, Pietrolungo JF, Thomas JD, Klein AL. A practical

guide to assessment of ventricular diastolic function using Doppler echocardiography. *J Am Coll Cardiol* 1996; 27;1753–1760.

70. Thomas JD, Weyman AE. Echocardiographic Doppler evaluation of left ventricular diastolic function: Physics and physiology. *Circulation* 1991; 84:977–990.

71. Chen C, Rodriguez L, Levine RA, et al. Noninvasive measurement of the time constant of left ventricular relaxation using the continuous-wave Doppler velocity of mitral regurgitation. *Circulation* 1992; 86:272–278.

72. Nishimura RA, Schwartz RS, Tajik AJ, Holmes DR Jr. Noninvasive measurement of rate of left ventricular relaxation by Doppler echocardiography: Validation with simultaneous cardiac catheterization. *Circulation* 1993; 88:146–155.

73. Pai RG, Suzuki M, Heywood JT, et al. Mitral A velocity wave transit time to the outflow tract as a measure of left ventricular diastolic stiffness: Hemodynamic correlations in patients with coronary artery disease. *Circulation* 1994; 84:553–557.

73a. Nishimura RA, Tajik AJ. Evaluation of diastolic filling of left ventricle in health and disease: Doppler echocardiography is the clinician's rosetta stone. *J Am Coll Cardiol* 1997; 30:8–18.

74. Yamamoto K, Masuyama T, Doi Y, et al. Noninvasive assessment of left ventricular relaxation using continuous-wave Doppler aortic regurgitant velocity curve: Its comparative value to the mitral regurgitation method. *Circulation* 1995; 91:192–200.

74a. DeMaria AN, Blanchard D. The hemodynamic basis of diastology. *J Am Coll Cardiol* 1999; 34:1659–1662.

75. Appleton CP, Hatle LK, Popp RL. Cardiac tamponade and pericardial effusion: Respiratory variation in transvalvular flow velocities studied by Doppler echocardiography. *J Am Coll Cardiol* 1988; 11:1020–1030.

76. Xie G-Y, Berk MR, Smith MD, et al. Prognostic value of Doppler transmitral flow patterns in patients with congestive heart disease. *J Am Coll Cardiol* 1994; 24:132–139.

76a. Pozzoli M, Traversi E, Cioffi G, et al. Loading manipulations improve the prognostic value of Doppler evaluation of mitral flow in patients with chronic heart failure. *Circulation* 1997; 95:1222–1230.

76b. Temporelli PL, Corra U, Imparato A, et al. Reversible restrictive left ventricular diastolic filling with optimized oral therapy predicts a more favorable prognosis in patients with chronic heart failure. *J Am Coll Cardiol* 1998; 31:1591–1597.

77. Miyatake K, O'Kamoto M, Knoshita N, et al. Augmentation of atrial contribution to left ventricular inflow with aging as assessed by intracardiac Doppler flowmetry. *Am J Cardiol* 1984; 53:586–589.

78. Bryg RJ, Williams GA, Labovitz AJ. Effect of aging on left ventricular diastolic filling in normal subjects. *Am J Cardiol* 1987; 59:971–974.

79. Harrison M, Clifton G, Pennell A, DeMaria A. Effect of heart rate on left ventricular diastolic transmitral flow velocity patterns assessed by Doppler echocardiography in normal subjects. *Am J Cardiol* 1991; 67:622–627.

80. Appleton C, Carucci M, Henry C, Olajos M. Influence of incremental changes in heart rate on mitral flow velocity: Assessment of lightly sedated, conscious dogs. *J Am Coll Cardiol* 1991; 17:227–236.

81. Dabestani A, Takenaka K, Allen B, et al. Effects of spontaneous respiration on left ventricular filling assessed by pulsed Doppler echocardiography. *Am J Cardiol* 1988; 61:1356–1358.

82. Drinkovic N, Smith MD, Wisenbaugh T, et al. Influence of sampling site upon the ratio of atrial to early diastolic transmitral flow velocities by Doppler (abstr). *J Am Coll Cardiol* 1987; 9:16A.

83. Pearson AC, et al. Effect of sample volume location on pulsed Doppler-echocardiographic evaluation of left ventricular filling. *Am J Cardiac Imaging* 1988; 24:40.

84. Dittrich HC, Blanchard DG, Wheeler K, et al. Influence of Doppler sample location on the assessment of changes in mitral inflow velocity profiles. *J Am Soc Echocardiogr* 1990; 3:303–309.

85. Choong CY, Abascal VM, Thomas JD, et al. Combined influence of ventricular loading and relaxation on the transmitral flow velocity profile in dogs measured by Doppler echocardiography. *Circulation* 1988; 78:672–683.

86. Berk MR, Xie G, Kwan OL, et al. Reduction of left ventricular preload by lower body negative pressure alters Doppler transmitral filling patterns. *J Am Coll Cardiol* 1990; 16:1387–1392.

87. Appleton CP, Galloway JM, Gonzalez MS, et al. Estimation of left ventricular filling pressures using two dimensional and Doppler echocardiography in adult patients with cardiac disease: Additional value of analyzing left atrial size, left atrial ejection fraction and the difference in duration of pulmonary venous and mitral flow velocity at atrial contraction. *J Am Coll Cardiol* 1993; 22:1972–1982.

88. Rossvoll O, Hatle LK. Pulmonary venous flow velocities recorded by transthoracic Doppler ultrasound: Relation to left ventricular diastolic pressures. *J Am Coll Cardiol* 1993; 21:1687–1696.

89. Gardin JM. Doppler measurements of aortic blood flow velocity and acceleration: Load-independent indexes of left ventricular performance? *Am J Cardiol* 1989; 64:935–936.

90. Harrison MR, Smith ND, Nissen SE, et al. Use of exercise Doppler echocardiography to evaluate cardiac drugs: Effects of propranolol and verapamil on aortic blood flow velocity and acceleration. *J Am Coll Cardiol* 1988; 11:1002–1009.

91. Gardin JM, Tobis J, Henry WL. Evaluation of dilated cardiomyopathy by pulsed Doppler echocardiography. *Am Heart J* 1983; 106:1057–1065.

92. Chen C, Rodriguez L, Guerrero JL, et al. Noninvasive estimation of the instantaneous first derivative of left ventricular pressure using continuous-wave Doppler echocardiography. *Circulation* 1991; 83:2101–2110.

93. William GA, Labovitz AJ. Doppler estimation of cardiac output: Principles and pitfalls. *Echocardiography* 1987; 4:355–374.

94. Huntsman LL, Stewart DK, Barnes SR, et al. Noninvasive Doppler determination of cardiac output in man—Clinical validation. *Circulation* 1983; 67:593–602.

95. Ihlen H, Amlie JP, Dale J, et al. Determination of cardiac output by Doppler echocardiography. *Br Heart J* 1984; 51:54–60.

96. Sahn DJ. Determination of cardiac output by echocardiographic Doppler methods: Relative accuracy of various sites for measurement. *J Am Coll Cardiol* 1985; 6:663–664.

97. Lewis JF, Kuo KC, Nelson JG, et al. Pulsed Doppler echocardiographic determination of stroke volume and cardiac output: Clinical validation of two new methods using the apical window. *Circulation* 1984; 70:425–431.

98. Huntsman LL, Stewart DK, Barnes SR, et al. Noninvasive Doppler determination of cardiac output in man—Clinical validation. *Circulation* 1983; 67:593–602.

99. Looyenga DS, Liebson PR, Bone RC, et al. Determination of cardiac output in critically ill patients by dual beam Doppler echocardiography. *J Am Coll Cardiol* 1989; 13:340–347.

100. Meijboom EJ, Horowitz S, Valdes-Cruz LM, et al. A Doppler echocardiographic method for calculating volume flow across the tricuspid valve: Correlative laboratory and clinical studies. *Circulation* 1985; 71:551–556.

101. Zhand Y, Nitter-Hauge N, Ihlen H, Myhre E. Doppler echocardiographic measurement of cardiac output using the mitral orifice method. *Br Heart J* 1985; 53:130–136.

102. Valdes-Cruz LM, Horowitz S, Goldberg SJ, Allen HD. The mitral valve orifice method for noninvasive two-dimensional echo Doppler determinations of cardiac output. *Circulation* 1983; 67:872–877.

103. Kitabatake A, Inoue M, Asao M, et al. Noninvasive evaluation

of the ratio of pulmonic to systemic flow in atrial septal defect by duplex Doppler echocardiography. *Circulation* 1984; 69:73–79.
104. Kurokawa S, Takahashi M, Katoh Y, et al. Noninvasive evaluation of the ratio of pulmonary to systemic flow in ventricular septal defect by means of Doppler two-dimensional echocardiography. *Am Heart J* 1988; 116:1033–1044.
105. Barron JV, Sahn DJ, Valdes-Cruz LM, et al. Clinical utility of two-dimensional Doppler echocardiographic techniques for estimating pulmonary to systemic flow ratios in children with left to right shunting, atrial septal defect, ventricular septal defect and patent ductus arteriosus. *J Am Coll Cardiol* 1984; 3:169–178.
106. Cloez JL, Schmidt KG, Birk E, Silverman NH. Determination of pulmonary to systemic blood flow ratio in children by a simplified Doppler echocardiographic method. *J Am Coll Cardiol* 1988; 11:825–830.
107. Nichol PM, Boughner DR, Persaud J. Noninvasive assessment of mitral insufficiency by Doppler ultrasound. *Circulation* 1976; 54:656–661.
108. Zhang Y, et al. Quantification of mitral regurgitation by Doppler echocardiography. *Eur Heart J* 1987; 8:59–62.
109. Blumlein S, Bouchard A, Schiller NB, et al. Quantitation of mitral regurgitation by Doppler echocardiography. *Circulation* 1986; 74:306–314.
110. Xie G-Y, Berk MR, Smith ND, DeMaria AN. A simplified method for determining regurgitant fraction by Doppler echocardiography in patients with aortic regurgitation. *J Am Coll Cardiol* 1994; 24:1041–1045.
111. Skjaerpe T, Hegrenaes L, Hatle L. Noninvasive estimation of valve area in patients with aortic stenosis by Doppler ultrasound and two-dimensional echocardiography. *Circulation* 1985; 72:810–818.
112. Warth DC, Stewart WJ, Block PC, Weyman AE. A new method to calculate aortic valve area without left heart catheterization. *Circulation* 1984; 70:978–983.
113. Oh JK, Taliercio CP, Holmes DR, et al. Prediction of the severity of aortic stenosis by Doppler aortic valve area determination: Prospective Doppler-catheterization correlation in 100 patients. *J Am Coll Cardiol* 1988; 11:1227–1234.
114. Richards KL, Cannon SR, Miller JF, Crawford MH. Calculation of aortic valve area by Doppler echocardiography: A direct application of the continuity equation. *Circulation* 1986; 73:964–969.
115. Zoghbi WA, Farmer KL, Soto JG, et al. Accurate noninvasive quantitation of stenotic aortic valve area by Doppler echocardiography. *Circulation* 1986; 73:452–459.
116. Hegrenaes L, Hatle L. Aortic stenosis in adults: Non-invasive estimation of pressure differences by continuous wave Doppler echocardiography. *Br Heart J* 1985; 54:396–404.
117. Currie PJ, Seward JB, Reeder GS, et al. Continuous wave Doppler echocardiographic assessment of severity of calcific aortic stenosis: A simultaneous Doppler-catheter correlative study in 100 adult patients. *Circulation* 1985; 71:1162–1169.
118. Smith MD, Dawson PL, Elion JL, et al. Correlation of continuous wave Doppler velocities with cardiac catheterization gradients: An experimental model of aortic stenosis. *J Am Coll Cardiol* 1985; 6:1306–1314.
119. Holen J, Waag RC, Gramiak R, et al. Doppler ultrasound in orifice flow: In vitro studies of the relationship between pressure difference and fluid velocity. *Ultrasound Med Biol* 1985; 11:261–266.
120. Currie PJ, Hagler DJ, Seward JB, et al. Instantaneous pressure gradient: A simultaneous Doppler and dual catheter correlative study. *J Am Coll Cardiol* 1986; 7:800–806.
121. Hatle L, Brubakk A, Tromsdal A, Angelsen B. Noninvasive assessment of pressure drop in mitral stenosis by Doppler ultrasound. *Br Heart J* 1978; 40:131–140.
122. Stamm RB, Martin RP. Quantification of pressure gradients across stenotic valves by Doppler ultrasound. *J Am Coll Cardiol* 1983; 2:707–718.
123. Perez JE, Ludbrook PA, Ahumada GG. Usefulness of Doppler echocardiography in detecting tricuspid valve stenosis. *Am J Cardiol* 1985; 55:601–602.
124. Lee RT, Lord CP, Plappert T, Sutton MS. Prospective Doppler echocardiographic evaluation of pulmonary artery diastolic pressure in the medical intensive care unit. *Am J Cardiol* 1989; 64:1366–1370.
125. Berger M, Haimowitz A, van Tosh A, et al. Quantitative assessment of pulmonary hypertension in patients with tricuspid regurgitation using continuous wave Doppler ultrasound. *J Am Coll Cardiol* 1985; 6:359–365.
126. Yock PG, Popp RL. Noninvasive estimation of right ventricular systolic pressure by Doppler ultrasound in patients with tricuspid regurgitation. *Circulation* 1984; 70:657–662.
127. Nishimura RA, Tajik AJ. Determination of left-sided pressure gradients by utilizing Doppler aortic and mitral regurgitant signals: Validation by simultaneous dual catheter and Doppler studies. *J Am Coll Cardiol* 1988; 11:317–321.
128. Pai RG, Bansal RC, Shah PM. Doppler-derived rate of left ventricular pressure rise: Its correlation with the postoperative left ventricular function in mitral regurgitation. *Circulation* 1990; 84:514–520.
129. Requarth JA, Goldberg SJ, Vasko SD, et al. In vitro verification of Doppler prediction of transvalve pressure gradient and orifice area in stenosis. *Am J Cardiol* 1984; 53:1369–1373.
130. Krabill KA, Tamura T, Phil C, et al. The shape of regurgitant jets: In vitro flow visualization and color flow Doppler studies (abstr). *J Am Coll Cardiol* 1987; 9:110A.
131. Thomas JD, Davidoff R, Wilkins GT, et al. The volume of a color flow jet varies directly with flow rate and inversely with orifice size: A hydrodynamic in vitro assessment (abstr). *J Am Coll Cardiol* 1988; 11:19A.
132. Thomas JD, O'Shea JP, Rodriguez L. The impact of orifice geometry on the shape of jets: An in vitro color Doppler flow study. *J Am Coll Cardiol* 1991; 17:901–908.
133. Wong M, Matsumura M, Suzuki K, Omoto R. Technical and biologic sources of variability in the mapping of aortic, mitral and tricuspid color flow jets. *Am J Cardiol* 1987; 60:847–851.
134. Simpson IA, Valdes-Cruz LM, Sahn DJ. Color Doppler flow mapping of simulated in vitro regurgitant jets: Evaluation of the effects of orifice size and hemodynamic variables. *J Am Coll Cardiol* 1989; 13:1195.
135. Chao K, Moises VA, Shandas R, et al. Influence of the Coanda effect on color Doppler jet area and color encoding; In vitro studies using color Doppler flow mapping. *Circulation* 1992; 85:333–341.
136. Chen C, Thomas JD, Anconina J, et al. Impact of impinging wall jet on color Doppler quantification on mitral regurgitation. *Circulation* 1991; 84:712–720.
137. Matsumura M, Wong M, Omoto R. Assessment of Doppler color flow mapping in quantification of aortic regurgitation—Correlations and influencing factors. *Jpn Circ J* 1989; 53:735–746.
138. Dittrich HC, ed. *Clinical Transesophageal Echocardiography*. St. Louis: Mosby–Year Book; 1992.
139. Blanchard DG, Kimura BJ, Dittrich HC, DeMaria AN. Transesophageal echocardiography of the aorta. *JAMA* 1994; 272:546–551.
140. Freeman WK, Seward JB, Khanderia BK, Tajik AJ, eds. *Transesophageal Echocardiography*. Boston: Little, Brown; 1994.
141. Seward JB, Khanderia BK, Edwards WD, et al. Biplanar transesophageal echocardiography: Anatomic correlations, image orientation, and clinical applications. *Mayo Clin Proc* 1990; 65:1193–1213.

142. Roelandt JRTC, Thomsom IR, Vletter WB, et al. Multiplane transesophageal echocardiography: Latest evolution in an imaging revolution. *J Am Soc Echocardiogr* 1992; 5:361–367.
143. Daniel WG, Mügge A. Transesophageal echocardiography. *N Engl J Med* 1995; 332:1268–1279.
144. Taams MS, Gussenhoven EJ, Bos E, et al. Enhanced morphological diagnosis in infective endocarditis by transesophageal echocardiography. *Br Heart J* 1990; 63:109–113.
145. Shively BK, Gurule FT, Roldan CA, et al. Diagnostic value of transesophageal compared with transthoracic echocardiography in infective endocarditis. *J Am Coll Cardiol* 1991; 18:391–397.
146. Bansal RC, Graham BM, Jutzy KR, et al. Left ventricular outflow tract to left atrial communication secondary to rupture of mitral-aortic intervalvular fibrosa in infective endocarditis: Diagnosis by transesophageal echocardiography and color flow imaging. *J Am Coll Cardiol* 1990; 15:499–504.
147. Daniel WG, Mügge A, Martin RP, et al. Improvement in the diagnosis of abscesses associated with endocarditis by transesophageal echocardiography. *N Engl J Med* 1991; 324:795–800.
148. Erbel R, Rohmann S, Drexler M, et al. Improved diagnostic value of echocardiography in patients with infective endocarditis by transesophageal approach: A prospective study. *Eur Heart J* 1988; 9:43–53.
149. Yvorchuk KJ, Chan K-L. Application of transthoracic and transesophageal echocardiography in the diagnosis and management of infective endocarditis. *J Am Soc Echocardiogr* 1994; 14:294–308.
150. Mügge A, Daniel WG, Frank G, Lichtlen PR. Echocardiography in infective endocarditis: Reassessment of prognostic implications of vegetation size determined by the transthoracic and the transesophageal approach. *J Am Coll Cardiol* 1989; 14:631–638.
151. Yoshida K, Yoshikawa J, Yamaura Y, et al. Assessment of mitral regurgitation by biplane transesophageal color Doppler flow mapping. *Circulation* 1990; 82:1121–1126.
152. Klein AL, Obarski TP, Stewart WJ, et al. Transesophageal Doppler echocardiography of pulmonary venous flow: A new marker of mitral regurgitation severity. *J Am Coll Cardiol* 1991; 18:518–526.
153. Castello R, Pearson AC, Lenzen P, Labovitz AJ. Effect of mitral regurgitation on pulmonary venous velocities derived from transesophageal echocardiography and color-guided pulsed Doppler imaging. *J Am Coll Cardiol* 1991; 17:1499–1605.
154. Smith MD, Harrison MR, Pinton R, et al. Regurgitant jet size by transesophageal compared with transthoracic Doppler color flow imaging. *Circulation* 1991; 83:79–86.
155. Hoffmann R, Flachskampf FA, Hanrath P. Planimetry of orifice area in aortic stenosis using multiplane transesophageal echocardiography. *J Am Coll Cardiol* 1993; 22:529–534.
155a. Tardif JC, Rodrigues AG, Hady JF, et al. Simultaneous determination of aortic valve area by the Gorlin formula and by transesophageal echocardiography under different transvalvular flow conditions. *J Am Coll Cardiol* 1997;29:1296–1302.
156. Freeman WK. Diseases of the thoracic aorta: utility of transesophageal echocardiography. In: Freeman WK, Seward JB, Khanderia BK, Tajik AJ, eds. *Transesophageal Echocardiography*. Boston: Little, Brown; 1994:425–467.
157. Keren A, Kim CB, Hu BS, et al. Accuracy of biplane and multiplane transesophageal echocardiography in diagnosis of typical acute aortic dissection and intramural hematoma. *J Am Coll Cardiol* 1996; 28:627–636.
158. Cigarroa JE, Isselbacher EM, DeSanctis RW, Eagle KA. Diagnostic imaging in the evaluation of suspected aortic dissection. *N Engl J Med* 1993; 328:35–43.
159. Pearson AC. Transthoracic echocardiography vs. transesophageal echocardiography in detecting cardiac source of embolism. *Echocardiography* 1993; 10:397–403.
160. Hoffman T, Kasper W, Meinertz T, et al. Echocardiographic evaluation of patients with clinically suspected arterial emboli. *Lancet* 1990; 336:1421–1424.
161. DeRook FA, Comess KA, Albers GW, Popp RL. Transesophageal echocardiography in the evaluation of stroke. *Ann Intern Med* 1992; 117:922–932.
162. Manning WJ, Weintraub RM, Waksmonski CA, et al. Accuracy of transesophageal echocardiography for identifying left atrial thrombi: A prospective, intraoperative study. *Ann Intern Med* 1995; 123:817–822.
163. Kronzon I, Tunick PA. Transesophageal echocardiography as a tool in the evaluation of patients with embolic disorders. *Prog Cardiovasc Dis* 1993; 36:39–60.
164. Daniel WG, Kronzon I, Mügge A, eds. *Cardiogenic Embolism*. Baltimore: Williams & Wilkins; 1996.
165. Click RL, Espinosa RE, Khanderia BK. Source of embolism: Utility of transesophageal echocardiography. In: Freeman WK, Seward JB, Khanderia BK, Tajik AJ, eds. *Transesophageal Echocardiography*. Boston: Little, Brown; 1994:469–499.
166. Zenker G, Erbel R, Krämer G, et al. Transesophageal two-dimensional echocardiography in young patients with cerebral ischemic events. *Stroke* 1988; 19:345–348.
167. Amarenco P, Cohen A, Tzourio C, et al. Atherosclerotic disease of the aortic arch and the risk of ischemic stroke. *N Engl J Med* 1994; 331:1474–1479.
168. Amarenco P, Duyckaerts C, Tzourio C, et al. The prevalence of ulcerated plaques in the aortic arch in patients with stroke. *N Engl J Med* 1992; 326:221–225.
169. Merino A, Haupman P, Badimon L, et al. Echocardiographic "smoke" is produced by an interaction of erythrocytes and plasma proteins modulated by shear forces. *J Am Coll Cardiol* 1992; 20:1661–1668.
170. The French Study of Aortic Plaques in Stroke Group. Atherosclerotic disease of the aortic arch as a risk factor for recurrent ischemic stroke. *N Engl J Med* 1996; 334:1216–1221.
171. Khatibzadeh M, Mitusch R, Stierle U, et al. Aortic atherosclerotic plaques as a source of systemic embolism. *J Am Coll Cardiol* 1996; 27:664–669.
171a. Vaduganathan P, Ewton A, Nagueh SF, et al. Pathologic correlates of aortic plaques, thrombi and mobile "aortic debris" imaged in vivo with transesophageal echocardiography. *J Am Coll Cardiol* 1997;30:357–363.
171b. Dressler FA, Craig WR, Castello R, Labovitz AJ. Mobile aortic atheroma and systemic emboli: Efficacy of anticoagulation and influence of plague morphology on recurrent stroke. *J Am Coll Cardiol* 1998; 31:134–138.
172. Dittrich HC, McCann HA, Walsh TP, et al. Transesophageal echocardiography in the evaluation of prosthetic and native aortic valves. *Am J Cardiol* 1990; 66:758–760.
173. Van den Brink RBA, Visser CA, Basart DCG, et al. Comparison of transthoracic and transesophageal color Doppler flow imaging in patients with mechanical prostheses in the mitral valve position. *Am J Cardiol* 1989; 63:1471–1474.
174. Nellessen U, Schnittger I, Appleton CP, et al. Transesophageal two-dimensional echocardiography and color Doppler flow velocity mapping in the evaluation of cardiac valve prostheses. *Circulation* 1988; 78:848–855.
175. Kronzon I, Tunick PA, Freedberg RS, et al. Transesophageal echocardiography is superior to transthoracic echocardiography in the diagnosis of sinus venous atrial septal defect. *J Am Coll Cardiol* 1991; 17:537–542.
176. Fyfe DA. Transesophageal echocardiography for congenital heart disease. *J Invasive Cardiol* 1992; 4;459–467.
177. Joffe II, Jacobs LE, Lampert C, et al. Role of echocardiography in perioperative management of patients undergoing open heart surgery. *Am Heart J* 1996; 131:162–176.
178. Dan M, Bonato R, Mazzucco A, et al. Value of transesophageal

echocardiography during repair of congenital heart defects. *Ann Thorac Surg* 1990; 50:637–643.

179. Fyfe DA, Kline CH. Transesophageal echocardiography for congenital heart disease. *Echocardiography* 1991; 8:573–586.
180. Mehta RH, Helmcke F, Nanda NC, et al. Transesophageal Doppler color flow mapping assessment of atrial septal defect. *J Am Coll Cardiol* 1990; 16:1010–1016.
181. Kremer P, Calahan M, Beaupre P, et al. Intraoperative monitoring by two-dimensional echocardiography. *Anesthetist* 1985; 34:111–117.
182. Smith JS, Cahalan MK, Benefiel DJ, et al. Intraoperative detection of myocardial ischemia in high risk patients: Electrocardiography versus two-dimensional transesophageal echocardiography. *Circulation* 1985; 72:1015–1021.
183. Dahm M, Iverson S, Schmidt FS, et al. Intraoperative evaluation of reconstruction of the atrioventricular valves by transesophageal echocardiography. *Thorac Cardiovasc Surg* 1987; 35(special issue 2):140–142.
184. Chan KL, Seward JB, Khandheria BK, et al. Transesophageal echocardiography in critically ill patients. *Am J Cardiol* 1990; 61:1492–1495.
185. Alam M. Transesophageal echocardiography in critical care units: Henry Ford hospital experience and review of the literature. *Prog Cardiovasc Dis* 1996; 38:315–328.
186. Foster E, Schiller NB. The role of transesophageal echocardiography in critical care: The UCSF experience. *J Am Soc Echocardiogr* 1992; 5:368–374.
187. Oh JK, Seward JB, Khanderia BK, et al. Transesophageal echocardiography in critically ill patients. *Am J Cardiol* 1990; 66;1492–1495.
188. Hellenbrand WE, Fahey JT, McGowan FX, Transesophageal echocardiographic guidance of transcatheter closure of atrial septal defect. *Am J Cardiol* 1990; 66:207–213.
189. Tong AD, Rothman A, Shiota T, et al. Interventional cardiac catheterization under transesophageal echocardiographic guidance. *Am Heart J* 1995; 129:827–831.
190. Ballal RS, Mahan EF III, Nancy NC, Dean LS. Utility of transesophageal echocardiography in interatrial septal puncture during percutaneous mitral balloon commissurotomy. *Am J Cardiol* 1990; 66:230–232.
191. Jaarsma W, Visser CA, Suttorp MJ, et al. Transesophageal echocardiography during percutaneous balloon mitral valvuloplasty. *J Am Soc Echocardiogr* 1990; 3:384–391.
192. Gramiak R, Shah PM: Echocardiography of the aortic root. *Invest Radiol* 1968; 3:356–366.
193. Meltzer RS, Tichner EG, Shaines TP, Popp RL. The source of ultrasonic contrast effect. *J Clin Ultrasound* 1980; 8:121–127.
194. Kerber RE, Kioschos JM, Lauer RM: Use of an ultrasonic contrast method in the diagnosis of valvular regurgitation and intracardiac shunts. *Am J Cardiol* 1974; 34:722–727.
195. Valdes-Cruz LM, Sahn DJ: Seminar on contrast two-dimensional echocardiography: Applications and new developments: Part II. *J Am Coll Cardiol* 1984; 3:978–985.
196. Lechat P, Mas JL, Lascault G, et al. Prevalence of patent foramen ovale in patients with stroke. *N Engl J Med* 1988; 318:1148–1152.
197. DeMaria AN. Echocardiographic visualization of myocardial perfusion by left heart and intracoronary injection of echo contrast agents (abstr). *Circulation* 1980; 60(suppl 3):II–143.
198. Armstrong WF, Mueller TM, Kinney EL, et al. Assessment of myocardial perfusion abnormalities with contrast enhanced two-dimensional echocardiography. *Circulation* 1982; 66:166–173.
199. Kaul S, Jayaween AR, Glasheen WP, et al. Myocardial contrast echocardiography and the transmural distribution of flow: A critical appraisal during myocardial ischemia not associated with infarction. *J Am Coll Cardiol* 1992; 20:1005–1016.
200. Crouse LJ, Cheirif J, Hanly DE, et al. Opacification and border delineation improvement in patients with suboptimal endocardial border definition in routine echocardiography: Results of the phase III Albunex multicenter trial. *J Am Coll Cardiol* 1993; 22:1494–1500.
201. Moore CA, Smucker ML, Kaul S. Myocardial contrast echocardiography in humans: I. Safety—a comparison with routine coronary arteriography. *J Am Coll Cardiol* 1986; 8:1066–1072.
202. Sabia PJ, Powers ER, Jayaweera AR, et al. Functional significance of collateral blood flow in patients with recent acute myocardial infarction. *Circulation* 1992; 85:2080–2089.
203. Lim Y-J, Nanto S, Masuyama T, et al. Visualization of subendocardial myocardial ischemia with myocardial contrast echocardiography in humans. *Circulation* 1989; 79:233–244.
204. Agati L, Voci P, Bilotta F, et al. Influence of residual perfusion within the infarct zone on the natural history of left ventricular dysfunction after acute myocardial infarction: A myocardial contrast echocardiographic study. *J Am Coll Cardiol* 1994; 24:336–342.
205. Perchet H, Dupouy P, Duval-Moulin A-M, et al. Improvement of subendocardial myocardial perfusion after percutaneous transluminal coronary angioplasty: A myocardial contrast echocardiography study with correlation between myocardial contrast reserve and Doppler coronary reserve. *Circulation* 1995; 91:1419–1426.
206. Ismail S, Jayaweera AR, Goodman NC, et al. Detection of coronary stenoses and quantification of the degree and spatial extent of blood flow mismatch during coronary hyperemia with myocardial contrast echocardiography. *Circulation* 1995; 91:821–830.
207. Sabia PJ, Powers ER, Ragosta M, et al. An association between collateral blood flow and myocardial viability in patients with recent myocardial infarction. *N Engl J Med* 1992; 327:1825–1831.
208. Ito H, Tomooka T, Sakai N, et al. Lack of myocardial perfusion immediately after successful thrombolysis: A predictor of poor recovery of left ventricular function in anterior myocardial infarction. *Circulation* 1992; 85:1699–1705.
209. Ito H, Maruyama A, Iwakura K, et al. Clinical implications of "no reflow" phenomenon: A predictor of complications and left ventricular remodeling in reperfused anterior wall myocardial infarction. *Circulation* 1996; 93:223–228.
210. Villanueva FS, Camarano G, Ismail S, et al. Coronary reserve abnormalities in the infarcted myocardium: Assessment of myocardial viability immediately versus late after reflow by contrast echocardiography. *Circulation* 1996; 94:748–754.
210a. Price RJ, Skyba DM, Kaul S, Skalak TC. Delivery of colloidal particles and red blood cells to tissue through microvessel ruptures created by targeted microbubble destruction with ultrasound. *Circulation* 1998; 98:1264–1267.
210b. Porter TR, Li S, Kricsfeld D, Armbruster RW. Detection of myocardial perfusion in multiple echocardiographic windows with one intravenous injection of microbubbles using transient response second harmonic imaging. *J Am Coll Cardiol* 1997; 29:791–799.
211. vonBibra H, Becher H, Firschke C, et al. Enhancement of mitral regurgitation and normal left atrial color Doppler flow signals with peripheral venous injections of a saccharide-based contrast agent. *J Am Coll Cardiol* 1993; 22:521–528.
212. Himelman RB, Stulbarg MS, Lee E, et al. Noninvasive evaluation of pulmonary artery systolic pressure during dynamic exercise by saline-enhanced Doppler echocardiography. *Am Heart J* 1990; 119:685–688.
213. Nakatani S, Imanishi T, Terasawa A, et al. Clinical application of transpulmonary contrast enhanced Doppler technique in the assessment of severity of aortic stenosis. *J Am Coll Cardiol* 1992; 20:973–975.
214. Cotter B, Kwan OL, Cha YM, et al. Dose-response characteristics, time-course, and hemodynamic responses to QW3600, an

ultrasonic contrast agent capable of myocardial opacification by intravenous injection (abstr). *J Am Coll Cardiol* 1994; 23:393A.
215. Dittrich HC, Bales GL, McFerran BA, et al. Reproducibility of myocardial opacification using FS069, a new intravenously administered ultrasound contrast agent (abstr). *J Am Coll Cardiol* 1995; 25:204A.
216. Porter TR, Xie F, Kresfeld A, Kilzer K. Noninvasive identification of acute myocardial ischemia and reperfusion with contrast ultrasound using intravenous perfluoropropane-exposed sonicated dextrose albumin. *J Am Coll Cardiol* 1995; 26:33–40.
217. Mulvagh SL, Foley DA, Aeschbacher BC, et al. Second harmonic imaging of in intravenously administered echocardiographic contrast agent: Visualization of coronary arteries and measurement of coronary blood flow. *J Am Coll Cardiol* 1996; 27;1519–1525.
218. Cotter B, Kwan OL, Cha YM, et al. Augmentation of contrast enhancement by second harmonic imaging: Experimental studies with new agents (abstr). *J Am Soc Echocardiogr* 1995; 8:345.
219. Porter TR, Xie F, Kricsfeld D, Armbruster RW. Improved myocardial contrast with second harmonic transient ultrasound response imaging in humans using intravenous perfluorocarbon-exposed sonicated dextrose albumin. *J Am Coll Cardiol* 1996; 27:1497–1501.
220. Ohmori K, Cotter B, Kwan OL, DeMaria AN. Relation of flow velocity and signal intensity to the amplification of contrast opacification produced by intermittent ultrasound emission (abstr). *J Am Soc Echocardiogr* 1996; 9:384.
221. Mottley JG, Giakoumopoulos M, Porter T, et al. Acoustic bubble destruction is a possible mechanism for transient response imaging (abstr). *J Am Soc Echocardiogr* 1996; 9:385.
221a. Kaul S, Senior R, Dittrich H, et al. Detection of coronary artery disease with myocardial contrast echocardiography: Comparison with ^{99m}Tc-sestamibi single-photon emission computed tomography. *Circulation* 1997; 96:785–792.
221b. Galiuto L, DeMaria AN, May-Newman K, et al. Evaluation of dynamic changes in microvascular flow during ischemia-reperfusion by myocardial contrast echocardiography. *J Am Coll Cardiol* 1998; 32:1096–1101.
221c. Mulvagh SL, Foley DA, Aeschbacher BC, et al. Second harmonic imaging of an intravenously administered echocardiographic contrast agent. *J Am Coll Cardiol* 1996;27:1519–1525.
222. Tajik AJ, Seward JB, Hagler DJ, et al. Two-dimensional real-time ultrasonic imaging of the heart and great vessels: Technique, image orientation, structures, identification, and validation. *Mayo Clin Proc* 1978; 53:271–303.
223. DeMaria AN, Bommer W, Joye JA, et al. Value and limitations of cross-sectional echocardiography of the aortic valve in the diagnosis and quantification of valvular aortic stenosis. *Circulation* 1980; 62:304–312.
224. Nanda NC, Gramiak R. Evaluation of bicuspid valves by two-dimensional echocardiography. (abstr). *Am J Cardiol* 1978; 41:372.
225. Weyman AE, Feigenbaum H, Hurwitz RA. Localization of left ventricular outflow obstruction by cross-sectional echocardiography. *Am J Med* 1976; 60:33–38.
226. Williams DE, Sahn DJ, Friedman WF. Cross-sectional echocardiographic localization of sites of left ventricular outflow obstruction. *Am J Cardiol* 1976; 37:250–255.
227. Fan PH, Kapur KK, Nanda NC. Color-guided Doppler echocardiographic assessment of aortic valve stenosis. *J Am Coll Cardiol* 1988; 12:441–449.
228. Roger VL, Tajik AJ, Reeder GS, et al. Effect of Doppler echocardiography on utilization of hemodynamic cardiac catheterization in the preoperative evaluation of aortic stenosis. *Mayo Clin Proc* 1996; 71:141–149.
229. DeFilippi CR, Willett DL, Brickner ME, et al. Usefulness of dobutamine echocardiography in distinguishing severe from nonsevere valvular aortic stenosis in patients with depressed left ventricular function and low transvalvular gradients. *Am J Cardiol* 1995; 75:191–194.
230. Ciobanu M, Abbasi AS, Allen M, et al. Pulsed Doppler echocardiography in the diagnosis and estimation of severity of aortic insufficiency. *Am J Cardiol* 1982; 49:339–343.
231. Klein AL, Davison MB, Vonk G, Tajik AJ. Doppler echocardiographic assessment of aortic regurgitation: Uses and limitations. *Cleve Clin J Med* 1992; 59:359–368.
232. Robertson WS, Stewart J, Armstrong WF, et al. Reverse doming of the anterior mitral leaflet with severe aortic regurgitation. *J Am Coll Cardiol* 1984; 3:431–436.
233. Grayburn PA, Smith MD, Handshoe R, et al. Detection of aortic insufficiency by standard echocardiography, pulsed Doppler echocardiography and auscultation. *Ann Intern Med* 1986; 104:599–605.
234. Pridie RB, Beham R, Oakley CM. Echocardiography of the mitral valve in aortic valve disease. *Br Heart J* 1971; 33:296–304.
235. Guiney TE, Davies MJ, Parker DJ, et al. The etiology and course of isolated severe aortic regurgitation: A clinical, pathological and echocardiographic study. *Br Heart J* 197; 53:358–368.
236. Perry GJ, Nelmcke F, Nanda NC, et al. Evaluation of aortic insufficiency by Doppler color flow mapping. *J Am Coll Cardiol* 1987; 9:952–959.
237. Masuyama T, Kodama K, Kitabatake A, et al. Noninvasive evaluation of aortic regurgitation by continuous-wave Doppler echocardiography. *Circulation* 1986; 73:460–466.
238. Grayburn PA, Handshoe R, Smith MD, et al. Quantitative assessment of the hemodynamic consequences of aortic regurgitation. *J Am Coll Cardiol* 1987; 10:135–141.
239. Beyer RW, Ramirez M, Josephson MA, Shah PM. Correlation of continuous wave Doppler assessment of chronic aortic regurgitation with hemodynamics and angiography. *Am J Cardiol* 1987; 60:852–856.
240. Samstad SO, Hegrenaes L, Skjaerpe T, Hatle L. Half time of the diastolic aortoventricular pressure difference by continuous wave Doppler ultrasound: A measure of the severity of aortic regurgitation? *Br Heart J* 1989; 61:336–343.
241. Omoto R, Yokote Y, Takamoto S, et al. The development of real-time two-dimensional Doppler echocardiography and its clinical significance in acquired valvular disease. *Jpn Heart J* 1984; 25:325–340.
242. Quinones MA, Young JB, Waggoner AD, et al. Assessment of pulsed Doppler echocardiography in detection and quantification of aortic and mitral regurgitation. *Br Heart J* 1980; 44:612–620.
243. Touch T, Prasquier R, Nitenberg A, et al. Assessment and follow-up of patients with aortic regurgitation by an updated Doppler echocardiographic measurement of the regurgitant fraction in the aortic arch. *Circulation* 1985; 72:819–824.
244. Takenaka K, Dabelstani A, Gardin JM, et al. A simple Doppler echocardiographic method for estimating severity of aortic regurgitation. *Am J Cardiol* 1986; 57:1340–1343.
245. Perlman AS, Otto CM. Quantification of valvular regurgitation. *Echocardiography* 1987; 4:271–287.
246. Fioretti P, Roelandt J, Sclavo M, et al. Postoperative regression of left ventricular dimensions in aortic insufficiency: A long-term echocardiographic study. *J Am Coll Cardiol* 1985; 5:856–861.
247. Siemienzuk D, Greenberg B, Morris C, et al. Chronic aortic insufficiency: Factors associated with progression to aortic valve replacement. *Ann Intern Med* 1989; 110:587–592.
248. Bonow RO, Dodd JT, Maron BJO, et al. Long-term serial change in left ventricular function and reversal of ventricular dilatation after valve replacement for chronic aortic regurgitation. *Circulation* 1988; 78:1108–1120.
249. Kodas E, Enriquez-Sarano M, Tajik AJ, et al. Surgery for aortic

regurgitation in women: Contrasting indications and outcomes compared with men. *Circulation* 1996; 94:2472–2478.

250. Henry WL, Bonow RO, Borer JS, et al. Observations on the optimum time for operative intervention for aortic regurgitation: I. Evaluation of the results of aortic valve replacement in symptomatic patients. *Circulation* 1980; 61:471–483.

251. Seward JB, Tajik AJ. Non-invasive visualization of the entire thoracic aorta: A new application of wide-angle two dimensional sector echocardiographic technique (abstr). *Am J Cardiol* 1979; 43:387.

252. DeMaria AN, Bommer W, Newmann A, et al. Identification and localization of aneurysms of the ascending aorta by cross-sectional echocardiography. *Circulation* 1979; 59:755–761.

253. Granato JE, Dee P, Gibson RS. Utility of two-dimensional echocardiography in suspected aortic dissection. *Am J Cardiol* 1985; 56:123–129.

254. Eagle KA, DeSanctis RW. Aortic dissection. *Curr Prob Cardiol* 1989; 14:231–278.

255. Ballal RS, Nanda NC, Gatewood R, et al. Usefulness of transesophageal echocardiography in assessment of aortic dissection. *Circulation* 1991; 84:1903–1914.

256. Nienaber CA, Spielman RP, von Kodolitsch Y, et al. Diagnosis of thoracic aortic dissection: Magnetic resonance imaging versus transesophageal echocardiography. *Circulation* 1992; 85: 434–447.

257. Nienaber CA, von Kodolitsch Y, Nicolas V, et al. The diagnosis of thoracic aortic dissection by noninvasive imaging procedures. *N Engl J Med* 1993; 328:1–9.

258. Robbins RC, McManus RP, Mitchell RS, et al. Management of patients with intramural hematoma of the thoracic aorta. *Circulation* 1993; 88(part 2):1–10.

259. Nienaber CA, von Kodolitsch Y, Petersen B, et al. Intramural hemorrhage of the thoracic aorta: Diagnostic and therapeutic implications. *Circulation* 1995; 92:1465–1472.

260. Eisenberg MJ, Geraci SJ, Schiller NB. Screening for abdominal aortic aneurysms during transthoracic echocardiography. *Am Heart J* 1995; 130:109–115.

261. Come PC, Fortuin NJ, White RI Jr, McKusick VA. Echocardiographic assessment of cardiovascular abnormalities in the Marfan syndrome. *Am J Med* 1983; 74:465–474.

262. Roman MJ, Rosen SE, Kramer-Fox R, Devereux RB. Prognostic significance of the pattern of aortic root dilation in the Marfan syndrome. *J Am Coll Cardiol* 1993; 22:1470–1476.

263. Shores J, Berger KR, Murphy EA, Pyeritz RE. Progression of aortic dilatation and the benefit of long-term beta-adrenergic blockade in Marfan's syndrome. *N Engl J Med* 1994; 30:1335–1341.

264. Recchia D, Sharkey AM, Bosner MS, et al. Sensitive detection of abnormal aortic architecture in Marfan syndrome with high-frequency ultrasonic tissue characterization. *Circulation* 1994; 91:1036–1043.

265. Kiefaber RW, Tabakin BS, Coffin LH, Gibson TC. Unruptured sinus of Valsalva aneurysm with right ventricular outflow obstruction diagnosed by two-dimensional and Doppler echocardiography. *J Am Coll Cardiol* 1986; 7:438–442.

266. Lewis RS, Agathangelou NE. Echocardiographic diagnosis of unruptured sinus of Valsalva aneurysm. *Am Heart J* 1984; 107:1025–1027.

267. Chia BL, Ee BK, Choo MH, Yan PC. Ruptured aneurysm of sinus of Valsalva: Recognition by Doppler color flow mapping. *Am Heart J* 1988; 115:686–688.

268. Alboliras E, Seward J, Hagler D, et al. Impact of two-dimensional and Doppler echocardiography on care of children aged two years and younger. *Am J Cardiol* 1988; 61:166–169.

269. Rice MJ, Seward JB, Hagler DJ, et al. Definitive diagnosis of truncus arteriosus by two-dimensional echocardiography. *Mayo Clin Proc* 1982; 57:476–481.

270. Swensson RE, Valdes-Cruz LM, Sahn DJ, et al. Real-time Doppler color flow mapping for detection of patent ductus arteriosus. *J Am Coll Cardiol* 1986; 8:1105–1112.

271. Tunick PA, Perez JL, Kronzon I. Protruding atheromas in the thoracic aortic and systemic embolization. *Ann Intern Med* 1991; 115:423–427.

272. Katz ES, Tunick PA, Rusinek H, et al. Protruding atheromas predict stroke in elderly patients undergoing cardiopulmonary bypass: Experience with intraoperative transesophageal echocardiography. *J Am Coll Cardiol* 1992; 20:70–77.

273. Cooke JP, Kazmeier FJ, Orszulak TA. The penetrating aortic ulcer: Pathologic manifestations, diagnosis, and management. *Mayo Clin Proc* 1988; 63:718–725.

273a. Atar S, Ngai T, Birnbaum Y, et al. Transesophageal echocardiographic Doppler findings in patients with penetrating aortic ulcers. *Am J Cardiol* 1999; 83:133–135.

273b. Smith MD, Cassidy M, Souther S, et al. Transesophageal echocardiography in the diagnosis of traumatic rupture of the aorta. *N Engl J Med* 1995; 332:356–362.

273c. Vignon P, Gueret P, Vedrinne J-M, et al. Role of transesophageal echocardiography in the diagnosis and management of traumatic aortic disruption. *Circulation* 1995; 92:2959–2968.

274. Edler I. The diagnostic use of ultrasound in heart disease. *Acta Med Scand* 1955; 308:32.

275. Nichol PM, Gilbert BW, Kisslo JA. Two-dimensional echocardiographic assessment of mitral stenosis. *Circulation* 1977; 55:120–128.

276. Zaky A, Nasser WK, Feigenbaum H. Study of mitral valve action recorded by reflected ultrasound and its application in the diagnosis of mitral stenosis. *Circulation* 1988; 37:789–799.

277. Glover MU, Warren SE, Vieweg WVR, et al. M-mode and two-dimensional echocardiographic correlation with findings at catheterization and surgery in patients with mitral stenosis. *Am Heart J* 1983; 105:98–102.

278. Duchak JM Jr, Chang S, Feigenbaum H. The posterior mitral valve echo and the echocardiographic diagnosis of mitral stenosis. *Am J Cardiol* 1972; 29:628–632.

279. Segal BL, Likoff W, Kingsley B. Echocardiography: Clinical application in combined mitral stenosis and mitral regurgitation. *Am J Cardiol* 1967; 19:42–49.

280. Quinones MA, Gaasch WH, Waisser E, Alexander J. Reduction in the rate of diastolic descent of the mitral valve echogram in patients with altered left ventricular diastolic pressure-volume relations. *Circulation* 1974; 49:246–254.

281. Gustafson A. The correlation between ultrasound cardiology, hemodynamics and surgical findings in mitral stenosis. *Am J Cardiol* 1967; 19:32–41.

282. Henry WL, Griffith JM, Michaelis LL, McIntosh CL. Measurement of mitral orifice area in patients with mitral valve disease by real-time two-dimensional echocardiography. *Circulation* 1975; 51:827–831.

283. Wann LS, Weyman AE, Feigenbaum H, et al. Determination of mitral valve area by cross-sectional echocardiography. *Ann Intern Med* 1978; 88:337–341.

284. Smith MD, Handshoe R, Handshoe S, et al. Comparative accuracy of two-dimensional echocardiography and Doppler pressure half-time methods in assessing severity of mitral stenosis in patients with and without prior commissurotomy. *Circulation* 1986; 73:100–107.

285. Martin RP, Rakowski H, Kleinman JH, et al. Reliability and reproducibility of two-dimensional echocardiography measurement of the stenotic mitral valve orifice area. *Am J Cardiol* 1979; 43:560–568.

286. Holen J, Simonsen S. Determination of pressure gradient in mitral stenosis with Doppler echocardiography. *Br Heart J* 1979; 41:529–535.

287. Hatle L, Angelsen B, Tromsdal A. Noninvasive assessment of

atrioventricular pressure half-time by Doppler ultrasound. *Circulation* 1979; 60:1096–1104.

288. Hatle A, Brubakk A, Tromsdal A, Angelsen B. Noninvasive assessment of pressure drop in mitral stenosis by Doppler ultrasound. *Br Heart J* 1978; 40:131–140.
289. Libanoff AJ, Rodbard S. Atrioventricular pressure half-time: Measure of mitral valve area. *Circulation* 1968; 38:144.
290. Loyd D, Ask P, Wranne B. Pressure half-time does not always predict mitral valve area correctly. *J Am Soc Echocardiogr* 1988; 1:313–321.
291. Thomas JD, Wilkins GT, Choong CYP, et al. Inaccuracy of mitral pressure half-time immediately after percutaneous mitral valvulotomy. *Circulation* 1988; 78:980–993.
292. Chen C, Wang Y, Guo B, Lin Y. Reliability of the Doppler pressure half-time method for assessing effects of percutaneous mitral balloon valvuloplasty. *J Am Coll Cardiol* 1989; 13:1309–1313.
293. Wilkins GT, Weyman AE, Abascal VM, et al. Percutaneous balloon dilatation of the mitral valve: An analysis of echocardiographic variables related to outcome and the mechanism of dilatation. *Br Heart J* 1988; 60:299–308.
294. Palacios IF, Block PC, Wildins GT, Weyman AE. Follow-up of patients undergoing percutaneous mitral balloon valvotomy. *Circulation* 1989; 79:573–579.
294a. Cannon CR, Nishimura RA, Reeder GS, et al. Echocardiographic assessment of commissural calcium: A simple predictor of outcome after percutaneous mitral balloon valvotomy. *J Am Coll Cardiol* 1997; 29:175–180.
294b. Hernandez R, Banuelos C, Alfonso F, et al. Long-term clinical and echocardiographic follow-up after percutaneous mitral valvuloplasty with the Inoue balloon. *Circulation* 1999; 99:1580–1586.
295. Manning WJ, Reis GJ, Douglas PS. Use of transesophageal echocardiography to detect left atrial thrombi before percutaneous balloon dilation of the mitral valve: A prospective study. *Br Heart J* 1992; 67:170–173.
296. Chen W-J, Chen MF, Liau C-S, et al. Safety of percutaneous transvenous balloon mitral commissurotomy in patients with mitral stenosis and thrombus in the left appendage. *Am J Cardiol* 1992; 70:117–119.
297. Abascal VM, Wilkins GT, Choong CY, et al. Mitral regurgitation after percutaneous balloon valvuloplasty in adults: Evaluation by pulsed Doppler echocardiography. *J Am Coll Cardiol* 1988; 11:257–263.
298. Yoshida K, Yoshikawa J, Akasaka T, et al. Assessment of left-to-right atrial shunting after percutaneous mitral valvuloplasty by transesophageal color Doppler flow-mapping. *Circulation* 1989; 80:1521–1526.
299. Roberts WC, Perloff JK. Mitral valvular disease: A clinicopathologic survey of the conditions causing the mitral valve to function abnormally. *Ann Intern Med* 1972; 77:939–975.
300. Mintz GS, Kotler MN, Segal BL, Parry WR. Two-dimensional echocardiographic evaluation of patients with mitral insufficiency. *Am J Cardiol* 1979; 44:670–678.
301. Abbasi AS, Allen MW, DeCristofara D, Ungar T. Detection and estimation of the degree of mitral regurgitation by range-gated pulsed Doppler echocardiography. *Circulation* 1980; 61:143–147.
301a. Thomas L, Foster E, Schiller NB. Peak mitral inflow velocity predicts mitral regurgitation severity. *J Am Coll Cardiol* 1998; 31:174–179.
302. Matsuo H, Morita H, Senda S, et al. Detection and visualization of regurgitant flow in valvular diseases by pulsed Doppler technique. *Jpn Circ J* 1982; 46:377–388.
303. Miyatake K, Izumi S, Okamoto M, et al. Semiquantitative grading of severity of mitral regurgitation by real-time two-dimensional Doppler flow imaging. *J Am Coll Cardiol* 1986; 7:82–88.
304. Utsunomiya T, Patel D, Doshi R, et al. Can signal intensity of the continuous wave Doppler regurgitant jet estimate severity of mitral regurgitation? *Am Heart J* 1992; 123:166–171.
305. Pai RG, Bansal RC, Shah PM. Doppler-derived rate of left ventricular pressure rise: Its correlation with the postoperative left ventricular function in mitral regurgitation. *Circulation* 1990; 84:514.
306. Kisanuki A, Tei C, Minagoe S, Natsugoe K, et al. Continuous wave Doppler echocardiographic evaluations of the severity of mitral regurgitation. *J Cardiol* 1989; 19:831.
307. Rokey R, Sterling LL, Zoghbi WA, et al. Determination of regurgitant fraction in isolated mitral or aortic regurgitation by pulsed Doppler two-dimensional echocardiography. *J Am Coll Cardiol* 1986; 7:1273.
308. Enriques-Sarano M, Bailey KR, Seward JB, et al. Quantitative Doppler assessment of valvular regurgitation. *Circulation* 1993; 87:841–848.
309. Helmeke R, Nanda N, Hsiung MC, et al. Color Doppler assessment of mitral regurgitation with orthogonal planes. *Circulation* 1987; 75:175.
310. Spain MG, Smith MD, Grayburn PA, et al. Quantitative assessment of mitral regurgitation by Doppler color flow imaging: Angiographic and hemodynamic correlations. *J Am Coll Cardiol* 1989; 13:585.
311. Chao K, Moises VA, Shandas R, et al. Influence of the Coanda effect on color Doppler jet area and color encoding: In vitro studies using color Doppler flow mapping. *Circulation* 1992; 85:333–341.
312. Chen C, Thomas JD, Anconina J, et al. Impact of impinging wall jet on color Doppler quantification on mitral regurgitation. *Circulation* 1991; 84:712–720.
312a. Enriquez-Sarano M, Dujardin KS, Tribouilloy CM, et al. Determinants of pulmonary venous flow reversal in mitral regurgitation and its usefulness in determining the severity of regurgitation. *Am J Cardiol* 1999; 83:535–541.
312b. Seiler C, Aeschbacher BC, Meier B. Quantitation of mitral regurgitation using the systolic/diastolic pulmonary venous flow velocity ratio. *J Am Coll Cardiol* 1998; 31:1383–1390.
313. Klein AL, Stewart WJ, Bartlett J, et al. Effects of mitral regurgitation on pulmonary venous flow and left atrial pressure: An intraoperative transesophageal echocardiographic study. *J Am Coll Cardiol* 1992; 20:1345–1352.
314. Castello R, Lenzen P, Aguirre F, Labovitz AJ. Quantitation of mitral regurgitation by transesophageal echocardiography with color flow mapping: Correlation with cardiac catheterization. *J Am Coll Cardiol* 1992; 19;1516–1521.
315. Pieper EPG, Hamer HPM, Sluijs RAP, et al. Usefulness of multiplane transesophageal echocardiography to improve the assessment of severity of mitral regurgitation. *Am J Cardiol* 1996; 78:1132–1139.
316. Bargiggia GS, Tronconi L, Sahn DJ, et al. A new method for quantitation of mitral regurgitation based on color flow Doppler imaging of flow convergence proximal to regurgitant orifice. *Circulation* 1991; 84:1481–1489.
317. Xie G-Y, Berk MB, Hixson CS, et al. Quantification of mitral regurgitation volume by the color Doppler proximal isovelocity surface area method: A clinical study. *J Am Soc Echocardiogr* 1995; 8:48–54.
318. Enriquez-Sarano M, Miller FA, Hayes SN, et al. Effective mitral regurgitant orifice area: Clinical use and pitfalls of the proximal isovelocity surface area method. *J Am Coll Cardiol* 1995; 25:703–709.
319. Utsunomiya T, Doshi R, Patel D, et al. Regurgitant volume estimation in patients with mitral regurgitation: Initial studies using the color Doppler "proximal isovelocity surface area" method. *Echocardiography* 1992; 9:63–70.
320. Vandervoort PM, Rivera JM, Mele D, et al. Application of color

Doppler flow mapping to calculate effective regurgitant orifice area: An in vitro study and initial clinical observations. *Circulation* 1993; 88:1150–1156.

321. Rodriguez L, Thomas JD, Monterroso V, Weyman AE, Harrison P, Mueller LN, Levine RA. Validation of the proximal flow convergence method: Calculation of orifice area in patients with mitral stenosis. *Circulation* 1993; 88:1157–1165.
322. Rivera JM, Vandervoort PM, Mele D. Quantification of tricuspid regurgitation using proximal flow convergence methods: Clinical validation (abstr). *J Am Soc Echocardiogr* 1992; 5:318.
323. Moises VA, Maciel BC, Hornberger LK, et al. A new method for noninvasive estimation of ventricular septal defect shunt flow by Doppler color flow mapping: Imaging of the laminar convergence region on the left septal surface. *J Am Coll Cardiol* 1991; 18:824–832.
324. Yoshida K, Yoshikawa J, Akasaka T, et al. Value of acceleration flow signals proximal to the leaking orifice in assessing the severity of prosthetic mitral valve regurgitation. *J Am Coll Cardiol* 1992; 19:333–338.
325. Simpson IA, Shiota T, Gharib M, Sahn DJ. Current status of flow convergence for clinical applications: Is it a leaning tower of "PISA"? *J Am Coll Cardiol* 1996; 27:504–509.
326. Devereux RB, Kramer-Fox R, Kligfield P. Mitral valve prolapse: Causes, clinical manifestations, and management. *Ann Intern Med* 1989; 111:305–317.
327. DeMaria AN, King JF, Bogren HG, et al. The variable spectrum of echocardiographic manifestations of the mitral valve prolapse syndrome. *Circulation* 1974; 50:33–41.
328. Levine RA, Triulzi MO, Harrigan P, Weyman AE. The relationship of mitral annular shape to the diagnosis of mitral valve prolapse. *Circulation* 1987; 75:756–767.
329. Levine RA, Stathogiannis E, Newell JB, et al. Reconsideration of echocardiographic standards for mitral valve prolapse: Lack of association between leaflet displacement isolated to the apical four-chamber view and independent echocardiographic evidence of abnormality. *J Am Coll Cardiol* 1988; 11:1013–1019.
330. Chun PKC, Sheehan MW. Myxomatous degeneration of mitral valve M-mode and two-dimensional echocardiographic findings. *Br Heart J* 1982; 47:404–408.
331. Dillon JC, Haine CL, Chang S, Feigenbaum H. Use of echocardiography in patients with prolapsed mitral valve. *Circulation* 1971; 43:503–507.
332. Levine RA, Handschumacher MD, Sanfilippo AJ, et al. Three-dimensional echocardiographic reconstruction of the mitral valve with implications for the diagnosis of mitral valve prolapse. *Circulation* 1989; 80:589–598.
333. Nishimura RA, McGowon MD, Shub C, et al. Echocardiographically documented mitral valve prolapse: Long term follow-up of 232 patients. *N Engl J Med* 1985; 313:1305–1309.
334. Himelman RB, Kusumoto R, Oken K, et al. The flail mitral valve: Echocardiographic findings by precordial and transesophageal imaging and Doppler color flow imaging. *J Am Coll Cardiol* 1991; 17:272–279.
335. Marwick TH, Stewart WJ, Currie PJ, et al. Mechanisms of failure of mitral valve repair: An echocardiographic study. *Am Heart J* 1991; 122:149–156.
336. Boltwood CM, Tei C, Wong M, Shah PM. Quantitative echocardiography of the mitral complex in dilated cardiomyopathy: The mechanism of functional mitral regurgitation. *Circulation* 1983; 68:498–508.
337. Nishimura RA, Shub C, Tajik AJ. Two dimensional echocardiographic diagnosis of partial papillary muscle rupture. *Br Heart J* 1982; 48:598–600.
338. D'Cruz I, Panetta F, Cohen H, Glock G. Submitral calcification or sclerosis in elderly patients: M-mode and two-dimensional echocardiography in "mitral annulus calcification." *Am J Cardiol* 1979; 44:31–38.
339. Nair CK, Aronow WS, Sketch MH, et al. Clinical and echocardiographic characteristics of patients with mitral annular calcification. *Am J Cardiol* 1983; 51:992–995.
340. Nair CK, Thompson W, Ryschon K, et al. Long-term follow-up of patients with echocardiographically detected mitral annular calcium and comparison with age- and sex-matched control subjects. *Am J Cardiol* 1989; 63:465–470.
341. Benjamin EJ, Plehn JF, D'Agostino RB, et al. Mitral annular calcification and the risk of stroke in an elderly cohort. *N Engl J Med* 1992; 327:374–379.
342. Weyman AE, Hurwitz RA, Gilrod DA, et al. Cross-sectional echocardiographic visualization of the stenotic pulmonary valve. *Circulation* 1977; 56:769–774.
343. Weyman AE, Dillon JC, Feigenbaum H, Chang S. Echocardiographic patterns of pulmonic valve motion in pulmonic stenosis. *Am J Cardiol* 1974; 34:644–651.
344. Johnson GL, Kwan OL, Handshoe S, et al. Accuracy of combined two-dimensional echocardiography and continuous wave Doppler recordings in the estimation of pressure gradient in right ventricular outlet obstruction. *J Am Coll Cardiol* 1984; 3:1013–1018.
345. Chandraratna PA, Wilson D, Imaizumi T, et al. Invasive and noninvasive assessment of pulmonic regurgitation: Clinical, angiographic, phonocardiographic, echocardiographic, and Doppler ultrasound correlations. *Clin Cardiol* 1982; 5:360–365.
346. Waggoner AD, Quinones MA, Young JB, et al. Pulsed Doppler echocardiographic detection of right-side valve regurgitation. *Am J Cardiol* 1981; 47:279–286.
347. Miyatake K, Okamoto M, Kinoshita N, et al. Pulmonary regurgitation studied with the ultrasonic pulsed Doppler technique. *Circulation* 1982; 65:969–976.
348. Lee RT, Lord CP, Plappert T, Sutton MS. Prospective Doppler echocardiographic evaluation of pulmonary artery diastolic pressure in the medical intensive care unit. *Am J Cardiol* 1989; 64:1366–1370.
349. Parris TM, Panidis IP, Ross J, Mintz GS. Doppler echocardiographic findings in rheumatic tricuspid stenosis. *Am J Cardiol* 1987; 60:1414–1416.
350. Guyer DE, Gillam LD, Foale RA, et al. Comparison of the echocardiographic and hemodynamic diagnosis of rheumatic tricuspid stenosis. *J Am Coll Cardiol* 1984; 3:1135–1144.
351. Miyatake K, Okamoto M, Kinoshita N, et al. Evaluation of tricuspid regurgitation by pulsed Doppler and two-dimensional echocardiography. *Circulation* 1982; 66:777–784.
352. Curtius MM, Thyssen M, Breuer HWM, Loogen F. Doppler versus contrast echocardiography for diagnosis of tricuspid regurgitation. *Am J Cardiol* 1985; 56:333–336.
353. Suzuki Y, Kambara H, Kadota K, et al. Detection and evaluation of tricuspid regurgitation using a real-time, two-dimensional, color-coded, Doppler flow imaging system: Comparison with contrast two-dimensional echocardiography and right ventriculography. *Am J Cardiol* 1986; 57:811–815.
354. Skjaerpe T, Hatle L. Diagnosis of tricuspid regurgitation: Sensitivity of Doppler ultrasound compared with contrast echocardiography. *Eur Heart J* 1985; 6:429–436.
355. Pennestri F, Loperfido F, Salvatori MP, et al. Assessment of tricuspid regurgitation by pulsed Doppler ultrasonography of the hepatic veins. *Am J Cardiol* 1984; 54:363–368.
356. Dittrich HC, McCann HA, Blanchard DG. Cardiac structure and function in chronic thromboembolic pulmonary hypertension. *Am J Cardiac Imaging* 1994; 8:18–27.
357. Levine R, Gibson T, Aretz T, et al. Echocardiographic measurement of right ventricular volume. *Circulation* 1984; 69:497–505.
358. Gibson TC, Miller SW, Aretz T, et al. Method for estimating right ventricular volume by planes applicable to cross-sectional echocardiography: Correlation with angiographic formulas. *Am J Cardiol* 1985; 15:1584–1588.

359. Weyman AE. Appendix A: Normal cross-sectional echocardiographic measurements. In: Weyman AE, ed. *Principles and Practice of Echocardiography*, 2d ed. Philadelphia: Lea & Febiger; 1994:1289–1298.
360. Cacho A, Prakash R, Sarma R, Kaushik VS. Usefulness of two-dimensional echocardiography in diagnosing right ventricular hypertrophy. *Chest* 1983; 84:154–157.
361. Baker BJ, Scovil JA, Kane JJ, Murphy MG. Echocardiographic detection of right ventricular hypertrophy. *Am Heart J* 1983; 105:611–614.
362. D'Arcy B, Nanda NC. Two-dimensional echocardiography features of right ventricular infarction. *Circulation* 1982; 65: 167–173.
363. Weyman AE, Wann LS, Feigenbaum H, Dillon JC. Mechanism of abnormal septal motion in patients with right ventricular volume overload. *Circulation* 1976; 54:179.
364. Ryan T, Petrovic O, Dillon J, et al. An echocardiographic index for separation of right ventricular volume and pressure overload. *J Am Coll Cardiol* 1985; 5:918–924.
365. Yock PG, Popp RL. Noninvasive estimation of right ventricular systolic pressure by Doppler ultrasound in patients with tricuspid regurgitation. *Circulation* 1984; 70:657–662.
366. Himelman RB, Kircher B, Rockey DC, Schiller NB. Inferior vena cava plethora with blunted respiratory response: A sensitive echocardiographic sign of cardiac tamponade. *J Am Coll Cardiol* 1988; 12:470–477.
367. Weyman AE, Dillon JC, Feigenbaum H, Chang S. Echocardiographic patterns of pulmonary valve motion with pulmonary hypertension. *Circulation* 1974; 50:905–910.
368. Tukelvich D, Groves BM, Micco A, et al. Early partial systolic closure of the pulmonic valve relates to severity of pulmonary hypertension. *Am Heart J* 1988; 115:409–418.
369. Hirshfeld S, Meyer R, Schwartz DC, et al. The echocardiographic assessment of pulmonary artery pressure and pulmonary vascular resistance. *Circulation* 1975; 52:642–650.
370. Tahara M, Tanaka H, Nakao S, et al. Hemodynamic determinants of pulmonary valve motion during systole in experimental pulmonary hypertension. *Circulation* 1981; 64:1249–1256.
371. Beard JT, Newman JH, Loyd JE, Byrd BF III. Doppler estimation of changes in pulmonary artery pressure during hypoxic breathing. *J Am Soc Echocardiogr* 1991; 4:121–130.
372. Zabalgoitia M. Echocardiographic assessment of prosthetic heart valves. *Curr Prob Cardiol* 1992; 17:271–325.
373. Mehta A, Kessler KM, Tamer D, et al. Two-dimensional echocardiographic observations in major detachment of a prosthetic aortic valve. *Am Heart J* 1981; 101:231–233.
374. Ledain LD, Onayon JP, Colle JP, et al. Acute thrombotic obstruction with disc valve prostheses: Diagnostic considerations and fibrinolytic treatment. *J Am Coll Cardiol* 1986; 7:743–751.
375. Come PC, Riley MF. Echocardiographic recognition of perivalvular infection complicating aortic bacterial endocarditis. *Am Heart J* 1984; 108:166–168.
376. Williams GA, Labovitz AJ. Doppler hemodynamic evaluation of prosthetic (Starr-Edwards and Bjork-Shiley) and bioprosthetic (Hancock and Carpentier-Edwards) cardiac valves. *Am J Cardiol* 1985; 56:325–332.
377. Cooper DM, Stewart WJ, Schiavone WA, et al. Evaluation of normal prosthetic valve function by Doppler echocardiography. *Am Heart J* 1987; 114:576–582.
378. Reisner SA, Meltzer RS. Normal values of prosthetic valve Doppler echocardiographic parameters: A review. *J Am Soc Echocardiogr* 198; 1:201–210.
379. Panadis IP, Ross J, Mintz GS. Normal and abnormal prosthetic valve function as assessed by Doppler echocardiography. *J Am Coll Cardiol* 1986; 8:317–326.
380. Nellessen U, Schnittger I, Appleton CP, et al. Transesophageal two-dimensional echocardiography and color Doppler flow velocity mapping in the evaluation of cardiac valve prostheses. *Circulation* 1988; 78:848–855.
381. Khandheria BK, Seward JB, Oh JK, et al. Value and limitations of transesophageal echocardiography in assessment of mitral valve prostheses. *Circulation* 1991; 83:1956–1968.
382. Flachskampf FA, O'Shea JP, Griffin BP, et al. Patterns of normal transvalvular regurgitation in mechanical valve prostheses. *J Am Coll Cardiol* 1991; 18:1493–1498.
383. Baumgartner H, Khan S, DeRobertis M, et al. Effect of prosthetic aortic valve design on the Doppler-catheter gradient correlation: An in vitro study of normal St. Jude, Medtronic-Hall, Starr-Edwards and Hancock valves. *J Am Coll Cardiol* 1992; 19:324–332.
384. Burstow DJ, Nishimura RA, Bailey KR, et al. Continuous wave Doppler echocardiographic measurement of prosthetic valve gradients: A simultaneous Doppler-catheter correlative study. *Circulation* 1980; 8:504–514.
385. Vandervoort PM, Greenberg NL, Pu M, et al. Pressure recovery in bileaflet heart valve prostheses: Localized high velocities and gradients in central and side orifices with implications for Doppler-catheter gradient relation in aortic and mitral position. *Circulation* 1995; 92:3464–3472.
386. Voelker W, Reul J, Stelzer T, et al. Pressure recovery in aortic stenosis: An in vitro study in a pulsatile flow model. *J Am Coll Cardiol* 1992; 20:1585–1593.
387. Wiseth R, Hegrenaes L, Rossvoll O, et al. Validity of an early postoperative baseline Doppler recording after aortic valve replacement. *Am J Cardiol* 1991; 7:869–872.
388. Dittrich HC, McCann HA, Walsh T, et al. Transesophageal echocardiography in the evaluation of prosthetic and native aortic valves. *Am J Cardiol* 1990; 66:758–761.
389. Alam M, Serwin JB, Rosman HS, et al. Transesophageal echocardiographic features of normal and dysfunctioning bioprosthetic valves. *Am Heart J* 1991; 121:1149–1155.
390. Alam M, Serwin JB, Rosman HS, et al. Transesophageal color flow Doppler and echocardiographic features of normal and regurgitant St. Jude medical prostheses in the mitral valve position. *Am J Cardiol* 1990; 66:871–873.
391. Orsinelli DA, Pearson AG. Detection of prosthetic valve strands by transesophageal echocardiography: Clinical significance in patients with suspected cardiac source of embolism. *J Am Coll Cardiol* 1995; 26:1713–1718.
392. Freedberg RS, Goodkin GM, Perez JL, et al. Valve strands are strongly associated with systemic embolization: A transesophageal echocardiographic study. *J Am Coll Cardiol* 1995; 26:1709–1712.
393. Dzavik V, Cohen G, Chan KL. Role of transesophageal echocardiography in the diagnosis and management of prosthetic valve thrombosis. *J Am Coll Cardiol* 1991; 18:1829–1833.
394. Currie P, Sutherland GR, Starkey IR. Thrombolysis as an emergency treatment for a thrombosed prosthetic mitral valve diagnosed by transesophageal echocardiography. *Br Heart J* 1993; 70:198–200.
395. Hurrell DG, Schaff HV, Tajik AJ. Thrombolytic therapy for obstruction of mechanical prosthetic valves. *Mayo Clin Proc* 1996; 71:605–613.
396. Dillon LC, Feigenbaum H, Konecke LL, et al. Echocardiographic manifestations of valvular vegetations. *Am Heart J* 1973; 86:698–704.
397. Wann LS, Dillon JC, Weyman AE, Feigenbaum H. Echocardiography in bacterial endocarditis. *N Engl J Med* 1976; 295:135–139.
398. Gilbert BW, Haney RS, Crawford F, et al. Two-dimensional echocardiographic assessment of vegetative endocarditis. *Circulation* 1977; 55:346–353.
399. Durack DT, Lukes AS, Bright DK. New criteria for diagnosis of

infective endocarditis: Utilization of specific echocardiographic findings. *Am J Med* 1994; 96:200–209.

399a. Bayer AS, Bolger AF, Taubert KA, et al. Diagnosis and management of infective endocarditis and its complications. *Circulation* 1998; 98:2936–2948.

399b. Habib G, Derumeaux G, Avierinos JF, et al. Value and limitations of the Duke criteria for the diagnosis of infective endocarditis. *J Am Coll Cardiol* 1999; 33:2023–2029.

400. Pedersen WR, Walker M, Olson JD, et al. Value of transesophageal echocardiography as an adjunct to transthoracic echocardiography in evaluation of native and prosthetic valve endocarditis. *Chest* 1991; 100:351–356.

401. von Reyn CF, Arbeit RD. *Case definitions for infective endocarditis. Am J Med* 1994; 96:220–222.

402. Galve E, Candell-Riera J, Pigrau C, et al. Prevalence, morphologic types, and evolution of cardiac valvular disease in systemic lupus erythematosus. *N Engl J Med* 1988; 319:817–823.

403. Roldan CA, Shively BK, Crawford MH. An echocardiographic study of valvular heart disease associated with systemic lupus erythematosus. *N Engl J Med* 1996; 335:1424–1430.

404. Martin RP, Meltzer RS, Chia BL, et al. Clinical utility of two-dimensional echocardiography in infective endocarditis. *Am J Cardiol* 1980; 46:379–385.

405. Stewart JS, Silimpert D, Harris P, et al. Echocardiographic documentation of vegetative lesions in infective endocarditis: Clinical implications. *Circulation* 1980; 61:374–380.

406. Blanchard DG, Ross RS, Dittrich HC. Nonbacterial thrombotic endocarditis: Assessment by transesophageal echocardiography. *Chest* 1992; 102:954–956.

407. Mügge A, Daniel WG. Echocardiographic assessment of vegetations in patients with infective endocarditis: Prognostic implications. *Echocardiography* 1995; 12:651–661.

408. Buda AJ, Zotz RJ, LeMire MS, Bach DS. Prognostic significance of vegetations detected by two-dimensional echocardiography in infective endocarditis. *Am Heart J* 1986; 112:1291–1296.

409. Sanfillipo AJ, Picard MH, Newell JB, et al. Echocardiographic assessment of patients with infectious endocarditis: Prediction of risk for complications. *J Am Coll Cardiol* 1991; 18:1191–1199.

410. Jaffe WM, Morgan DE, Perlman AS, Otto CM. Infective endocarditis, 1983–1988: Echocardiographic findings and factors influencing morbidity and mortality. *J Am Coll Cardiol* 1990; 15:1127–1233.

411. Steckelberg JM, Murphy JG, Ballard D, et al. Emboli in infective endocarditis: The prognostic value of echocardiography. *Ann Intern Med* 1991; 114:635–640.

412. Klodas E, Edwards WD, Khanderia BK. Use of transesophageal echocardiography for improving detection of valvular vegetations in subacute bacterial endocarditis. *J Am Soc Echocardiogr* 1989; 2:386–389.

413. Birmingham GD, Rahko PS, Ballantyne F. Improved detection of infective endocarditis with transesophageal echocardiography. *Am Heart J* 1992; 123:774–781.

414. Karalis DG, Bansal RC, Hauck AJ, et al. Transesophageal echocardiographic recognition of subaortic complications in aortic valve endocarditis: Clinical and surgical implications. *Circulation* 1992; 86:353–362.

415. Khanderia BK. Suspected bacterial endocarditis: To TEE or not to TEE. *J Am Coll Cardiol* 1993; 21:222–224.

416. Lindner JR, Case RA, Dent JM, et al. Diagnostic value of echocardiography in suspected endocarditis: An evaluation based on pretest probability of disease. *Circulation* 1996; 93:730–736.

417. Weyman AE, Feigenbaum H, Dillon JL, et al. Noninvasive visualization of the left main coronary artery by cross-sectional echocardiography. *Circulation* 1976; 54:169.

418. Raisinghani A, Ohmori K, Cotter B, et al. Does flow reversal within intramyocardial coronary vessels occur systole? Detection of biphasic flow in intramyocardial vessels by transthoracic echo (abstr). *J Am Coll Cardiol* 1997; 29:365A.

419. Ryan T, Armstrong WF, Feigenbaum H. Prospective evaluation of the left main coronary artery using digital two-dimensional echocardiography. *J Am Coll Cardiol* 1986; 7:807–812.

420. Yamagishi M, Miyatake K, Beppu S, et al. Assessment of coronary blood flow by transesophageal two-dimensional pulsed Doppler echocardiography. *Am J Cardiol* 1988; 62:641–644.

421. Kerber R, Abboud F. Echocardiographic detection of regional myocardial infarction. *Circulation* 1973; 47:997.

422. Franklin TD Jr, Cuddeback JK, Sanghn NT, et al. Differentiation of A-mode ultrasound signals from normal and ischemic myocardium by multivariate discriminant analysis of waveform parameters. (abstr). *Am J Cardiol* 1980; 45:403.

423. Bourdillon PDV, Broderick TM, Sawada SG, et al. Regional wall motion index for infarct and noninfarct regions after reperfusion in acute myocardial infarction: Comparison with global wall motion index. *J Am Soc Echocardiogr* 1989; 2:398–407.

424. Nishimura RA, Tajik AJ, Shub C, et al. Role of two-dimensional echocardiography in the prediction of in-hospital complications after acute myocardial infarction. *J Am Coll Cardiol* 1984; 4:1080–1087.

425. Feigenbaum H. Coronary artery disease. In: *Echocardiography*, 5th ed. Philadelphia: Lea & Febiger; 1994:452.

426. Crouse LJ, Harbrecht JJ, Vacek JL, Exercise echocardiography as a screening test for coronary artery disease and correlation with coronary arteriography. *Am J Cardiol* 1991; 67:1213–1218.

427. Segar DS, Brown SC, Sawada SG, et al. Dobutamine stress echocardiography: Correlation with coronary lesions severity as determined by quantitative angiography. *J Am Coll Cardiol* 1992; 19:1197–1202.

428. Corya BC, Feigenbaum H, Rasmussen S, Black MJ. Echocardiographic features of congestive cardiomyopathy compared with normal subjects and patients with coronary artery disease. *Circulation* 1974; 49:1153–1159.

429. Heger J, Weyman AE, Wann S, et al. Cross-sectional echocardiographic analysis of the extent of left ventricular asynergy in acute myocardial infarction. *Circulation* 1980; 61:1113–1118.

430. Weiss JL, Buckley BH, Hutchins GM, Mason SJ. Two-dimensional echocardiographic recognition of myocardial injury in man: Comparison with postmortem studies. *Circulation* 1981; 63:401–408.

431. Horowitz RS, Morganroth J, Parrotto C, et al. Immediate diagnosis of acute myocardial infarction by two-dimensional echocardiography. *Circulation* 1982; 65:323–329.

432. Gibson RS, Bishop HL, Stamm RB, et al. Value of early two-dimensional echocardiography in patients with acute myocardial infarction. *Am J Cardiol* 1982; 49:1110–1119.

433. Peels CH, Visser CA, Kupper AJF, et al. Usefulness of two-dimensional echocardiography for immediate detection of myocardial ischemia in the emergency room. *Am J Cardiol* 1990; 65:687–691.

434. Sabia P, Abbott RD, Afrookteh A, et al. Importance of two-dimensional echocardiographic assessment of left ventricular systolic function in patients presenting to the emergency room with cardiac-related symptoms. *Circulation* 1991; 84:1615–1624.

435. Oh JK, Miller FA, Shub C, et al. Evaluation of acute chest pain syndromes by two-dimensional echocardiography: Its potential application in the selection of patients for acute reperfusion therapy. *Mayo Clin Proc* 1987; 62:59–66.

436. Eaton L, Weiss JL, Bulkley BH, et al. Regional cardiac dilatation after acute myocardial infarction. *N Engl J Med* 1979; 300:57–62.

437. Picard MH, Wilkins GT, Ray PA, Weyman AT. Progressive changes in ventricular structure and function during the year after acute myocardial infarction. *Am Heart J* 1992; 124:24–31.

438. Matsumoto M, Watanabe F, Gotto A, et al. Left ventricular aneurysm and the prediction of left ventricular enlargement

studied by two-dimensional echocardiography: Quantitative assessment of aneurysm size in relation to clinical course. *Circulation* 1985; 72:280–286.

439. VanTassel RA, Edwards JE. Rupture of the heart complicating myocardial infarction: Analysis of 40 cases including nine examples of left ventricular false aneurysms. *Chest* 1972; 61:104–116.

440. Catherwood E, Mintz GS, Kotler MN, Two-dimensional echocardiographic recognition of left ventricular pseudoaneurysm. *Circulation* 1980; 62:294–303.

441. Roelandt J, Sutherland GR, Yoshida K, Yoshikawa J. Improved diagnosis and characterization of left ventricular pseudoaneurysm by Doppler color imaging. *J Am Coll Cardiol* 1988; 12:807–811.

442. Miyatake K, Okamoto M, Kinoshita N, et al. Doppler echocardiographic features of ventricular septal rupture in myocardial infarction. *J Am Coll Cardiol* 1985; 5:182–187.

443. Helmcke F, Mahan EF, Nanda NC, et al. Two-dimensional echocardiography and Doppler color flow mapping in the diagnosis and prognosis of ventricular septal rupture. *Circulation* 1990; 81:1775–1783.

444. Harrison MR, MacPhail B, Gurley JC, et al. Usefulness of color Doppler flow imaging to distinguish ventricular septal defect from acute mitral regurgitation complicating acute myocardial infarction. *Am J Cardiol* 1989; 64:697–701.

445. Kono T, Sabbah HN, Rosman H, et al. Mechanism of functional mitral regurgitation during acute myocardial infarction. *J Am Coll Cardiol* 1992; 9:1101–1105.

446. Nishimura RA, Schaff HV, Shub C, et al. Papillary muscle rupture complicating acute myocardial infarction: Analysis of 17 patients. *Am J Cardiol* 1983; 51:373–377.

447. Stoddard MF, Keedy DL, Kupersmith J. Transesophageal echocardiographic diagnosis of papillary muscle rupture complicating acute myocardial infarction. *Am Heart J* 1990; 120:690–692.

448. D'Arcy B, Nanda NC. Two-dimensional echocardiographic features of right ventricular infarction. *Circulation* 1982; 65: 167–173.

449. Otto CM, Stratton JR, Maynard C, et al. Echocardiographic evaluation of segmental wall motion early and late after thrombolytic therapy in acute myocardial infarction: The Western Washington issue plasminogen activator emergency room trial. *Am J Cardiol* 1990; 65:132–138.

450. Bourdillon PDV, Broderick TM, Williams ES, et al. Early recovery of regional left ventricular function after reperfusion in acute myocardial infarction assessed by serial two-dimensional echocardiography. *Am J Cardiol* 1989; 63:641–642.

450a. Porter TR, Li S, Oster R, Deligonul U. The clinical implications of no reflow demonstrated with intravenous perfluorocarbon containing microbubbles following restoration of Thrombolysis in Myocardial Infarction (TIMI) 3 flow in patients with acute myocardial infarction. *Am J Cardiol* 1998; 82:1173–1177.

451. Wann LS, Faris JV, Childress RH, et al. Exercise cross-sectional echocardiography in ischemic heart disease. *Circulation* 1979; 60:1300–1308.

452. Armstrong WF, O'Donnell J, Ryan T, Feigenbaum H. Effect of prior myocardial infarction and extent and location of coronary disease on accuracy of exercise echocardiography. *J Am Coll Cardiol* 1987; 10:531–538.

453. Marwick T, Nemec J, Pashkow F, et al. Accuracy and limitations of exercise echocardiography in a routine clinical setting. *J Am Coll Cardiol* 1992; 19:74–81.

454. Feigenbaum H. Exercise echocardiography. *J Am Soc Echocardiogr* 1988; 1:161–166.

455. Quinones MA, Verani MS, Haichin RM, et al. Exercise echocardiography versus T1–201 single photon emission computerized tomography in evaluation of coronary artery disease: Analysis of 292 patients. *Circulation* 1992; 85:1026–1031.

456. Roger VL, Pellikka PA, Oh JK, et al. Identification of multivessel coronary artery disease by exercise echocardiography. *J Am Coll Cardiol* 1994; 24:109–114.

457. Ryan T, Segar DS, Sawada SG, et al. Detection of coronary artery disease with upright bicycle exercise echocardiography. *J Am Soc Echocardiogr* 1993; 6:186–197.

458. Cigarroa CG, deFilippi CR, Brickner ME, et al. Dobutamine stress echocardiography identifies hibernating myocardium and predicts recovery of left ventricular function after coronary revascularization. *Circulation* 1993; 88:430–436.

458a. Geleijnse ML, Floretti PM, Roelandt J. Methodology, feasibility, safety and diagnostic accuracy of dobutamine stress echocardiography. *J Am Coll Cardiol* 1997; 30:595–606.

458b. Secknus MA, Marwick TH. Evolution of dobutamine echocardiography protocols and indications: Safety and side effects in 3,011 studies over 5 Years. *J Am Coll Cardiol* 1997; 29:1234–1240.

459. Marcowitz P, Armstrong WF. Accuracy of dobutamine stress echocardiography in detecting coronary artery disease. *Am J Cardiol* 1992; 69:1269–1273.

460. Sawada SG, Segar DS, Ryan T, et al. Echocardiographic detection of coronary artery disease during dobutamine infusion. *Circulation* 1991; 83:1605–1614.

461. Picano E. Stress echocardiography: From pathophysiologic toy to diagnostic tool. *Circulation* 1992; 85:1604–1612.

462. Sun KT, Czernin J, Krivokapich J, et al. Effects of dobutamine stimulation on myocardial blood flow, glucose metabolism, and wall motion in normal and dysfunctional myocardium. *Circulation* 1996; 94:3146–3154.

463. Pierard LA, De Landsheere CM, Berthe C, et al. Identification of viable myocardium by echocardiography during dobutamine infusion in patients with myocardial infarction after thrombolytic therapy: Comparison with positron emission tomography. *J Am Coll Cardiol* 1990; 15:1021–1031.

464. Smart SC, Sawada S, Ryan T, et al. Low-dose dobutamine echocardiography detects reversible dysfunction after thrombolytic therapy of acute myocardial infarction. *Circulation* 1993; 88:405–415.

465. Forster T, McNeill AJ, Salustri A, et al. Simultaneous dobutamine stress echocardiography and echocardiography and technetium-99m isonitrile single-photon emission computed tomography in patients with suspected coronary artery disease. *J Am Coll Cardiol* 1993; 21:1591–1596.

466. Attenhoffer CH, Pellikka PA, Oh JK, et al. Comparison of ischemic response during exercise and dobutamine echocardiography in patients with left main coronary artery disease. *J Am Coll Cardiol* 1996; 27:1171–1177.

467. Bax JJ, Cornel JH, Visser FC, et al. Prediction of recovery of myocardial dysfunction after revascularization: Comparison of fluorine-18 fluorodeoxyglucose/thallium-201 SPECT, thallium-201 stress-reinjection SPECT and dobutamine echocardiography. *J Am Coll Cardiol* 1996; 28:558–564.

468. Afridi I, Main ML, Grayburn PA. Accuracy of dobutamine echocardiography for detection of myocardial viability in patients with occluded left anterior descending coronary artery. *J Am Coll Cardiol* 1996; 28:455–459.

469. Vanoverschelde J-LJ, D'Hount A-M, Marwick T, et al. Head-to-head comparison of exercise-redistribution-reinjection thallium single-photon emission computed tomography and low dose dobutamine echocardiography for prediction of reversibility of chronic left ventricular ischemic dysfunction. *J Am Coll Cardiol* 1996; 28:432–442.

469a. Cornel JH, Bax JJ, Elhendy A, et al. Diphasic response to dobutamine predicts improvement of global left ventricular function after surgical revascularization in patients with stable coronary artery disease. *J Am Coll Cardiol* 1998; 31:1002–1010.

469b. Afridi I, Grayburn PA, Panza JA, et al. Myocardial viability during dobutamine echocardiography predicts survival in pa-

tients with coronary artery disease and severe left ventricular systolic dysfunction. *J Am Coll Cardiol* 1998; 32:921–926.
470. Baer FM, Voth E, Deutsch HJ, et al. Assessment of viable myocardium by dobutamine transesophageal echocardiography and comparison with fluorine-18 fluorodeoxyglucose positron emission tomography. *J Am Coll Cardiol* 1994; 24:343–353.
471. Mertes H, Sawada SG, Ryan T, et al. Symptoms, adverse effects, and complications associated with dobutamine stress echocardiography: Experience in 1118 patients. *Circulation* 1993; 88:15–19.
472. Bach DS, Muller D, Gros BJ, Armstrong WF. False positive dobutamine stress echocardiograms: Characterization of clinical, echocardiographic, and angiographic findings. *J Am Coll Cardiol* 1994; 24:928–933.
473. Anthopoulos LP, Bonou MS, Kardaras FG, et al. Stress echocardiography in elderly patients with coronary artery disease. *J Am Coll Cardiol* 1996; 28:52–59.
474. Pellikka PA, Oh JK, Bailey KR, et al. Dynamic intraventricular obstruction during dobutamine stress echocardiography: A new observation. *Circulation* 1992; 86:1429–1432.
475. Tanimoto M, Pai RG, Jintapakorn W, Shah PM. Mechanisms of hypotension during dobutamine stress echocardiography in patients with coronary artery disease. *Am J Cardiol* 1995; 76:26–30.
476. Marwick T, Wilemart B, D'Hondt AM, et al. Selection of the optimal non-exercise stress for the evaluation of ischemic regional myocardial dysfunction and malperfusion: Comparison of dobutamine and adenosine using echocardiography and Tc-99m MIBI single photon emission computerized tomography. *Circulation* 1993; 87:345–354.
477. Mairesse GH, Marwick TH, Arnese M, et al. Improved identification of coronary artery disease in patients with left bundle branch block by use of dobutamine stress echocardiography and comparison with myocardial perfusion tomography. *Am J Cardiol* 1995; 76:321–325.
477a. Spes CH, Klauss V, Mudra H, Schnaack, SD, et al. Diagnostic and prognostic value of serial dobutamine stress echocardiography for noninvasive assessment of cadiac allograft vasculopathy: A comparison with coronary angiography and intravascular ultrasound. *Circulation* 1999; 100:509–515.
478. Sawada SG, Ryan T, Feinberg NS, et al. Exercise echocardiographic identification of coronary artery disease in women. *J Am Coll Cardiol* 1989; 14:1440–1447.
478a. Marwick TH, Anderson T, Williams J, et al. Exercise echocardiography is an accurate and cost-effective technique for detection of coronary artery disease in women. *J Am Coll Cardiol* 1995; 26:335–341.
478b. Heupler S, Mehta R, Lobo A, et al. Prognostic implications of exercise echocardiography in women with known or suspected coronary artery disease. *J Am Coll Cardiol* 1997; 30:414–420.
479. Roger VL, Pellikka PA, Oh JK, et al. Identification of multivessel coronary artery disease by exercise echocardiography. *J Am Coll Cardiol* 1994; 24:109–114.
480. Spes CH, Mudra H, Schnaak SD, et al. Dobutamine stress echocardiography for noninvasive diagnosis of cardiac allograft vasculopathy: A comparison with angiography and intravascular ultrasound. *Am J Cardiol* 1996; 78:168–174.
481. Davila-Roman VG, Wong AK, Li D, et al. Usefulness of dobutamine stress echocardiography for the prospective identification of the physiological significance of coronary narrowings of moderate severity in patients undergoing evaluation for percutaneous transluminal coronary angioplasty. *Am J Cardiol* 1995; 76:245–249.
482. Kafka H, Leach AJ, Fitzgibbon GM. Exercise echocardiography after coronary artery bypass surgery: Correlation with coronary angiography. *J Am Coll Cardiol* 1995; 25:1019–1023.
483. Elhendy A, Geleijnse ML, Roelandt J, et al. Assessment of patients after coronary artery bypass grafting by dobutamine stress echocardiography. *Am J Cardiol* 1996; 77:1234–1237.
484. Labovitz AJ, Lewen M, Kern WJ, et al. The effects of successful PTCA on left ventricular function: Assessment by exercise echocardiography. *Am Heart J* 1989; 117:1003–1008.
485. Crouse LJ, Vacek JL, Beauchamp GD, et al. Exercise echocardiography after coronary artery bypass grafting. *Am J Cardiol* 1992; 70:572–576.
486. Ryan T, Armstrong WF, O'Donnell JA, Feigenbaum H. Risk stratification after acute myocardial infarction by means of exercise two-dimensional echocardiography. *Am Heart J* 1987; 114:1305–1316.
487. Picano E, Pingitore A, Sicari R, et al. Stress echocardiographic results predict risk of reinfarction early after uncomplicated acute myocardial infarction: Large-scale multicenter study. *J Am Coll Cardiol* 1995; 26:908–913.
488. Quintana M, Lindvall K, Ryden L, Brolund F. Prognostic value of predischarge exercise stress echocardiography after acute myocardial infarction. *Am J Cardiol* 1995; 76:1115–1121.
489. Williams MJ, Odabashian J, Lauer MS, et al. Prognostic value of dobutamine echocardiography in patients with left ventricular dysfunction. *J Am Coll Cardiol* 1996; 27:132–139.
490. Smart SC, Sawada S, Ryan T, et al. Low-dose dobutamine echocardiography detects reversible dysfunction after thrombolytic therapy of acute myocardial infarction. *Circulation* 1993; 88:405–415.
491. Kamaran M, Teague SM, Finkelhor RS, et al. Prognostic value of dobutamine stress echocardiography in patients referred because of suspected coronary artery disease. *Am J Cardiol* 1995; 76:887–891.
492. Davila-Roman VG, Waggoner AD, Sicard GA, et al. Dobutamine stress echocardiography predicts surgical outcome in patients with an aortic aneurysm and peripheral vascular disease. *J Am Coll Cardiol* 1993; 21:957–963.
493. Poldermans D, Fioretti PM, Forster T, et al. Dobutamine stress echocardiography for assessment of perioperative cardiac risk in patients undergoing major vascular surgery. *Circulation* 1993; 87:1506–1512.
494. Lane RT, Sawada SG, Segar DS, et al. Dobutamine stress echocardiography for assessment of cardiac risk before noncardiac surgery. *Am J Cardiol* 1991; 68:976–977.
494a. Poldermans D, Arnese M, Floretti PM, et al. Sustained prognostic value of dobutamine stress echocardiography for late cardiac events after major noncardiac vascular surgery. *Circulation* 1997; 95:53–58.
494b. Carlos ME, Smart SC, Wynsen JC, Sagar KB. Dobutamine stress echocardiography for risk stratification after myocardial infarction. *Circulation* 1997; 95:1402–1410.
494c. Pingitore A, Picano E, Varga A, et al. Prognostic value of pharmacological stress echocardiography in patients with known or suspected coronary artery disease. *J Am Coll Cardiol* 1999; 34:1769–1777.
495. Chen C, Li L, Chen LL, et al. Incremental doses of dobutamine induce a biphasic response in dysfunctional left ventricular regions subtending coronary stenoses. *Circulation* 1995; 92: 756–766.
496. Afridi I, Kleiman NS, Raizner AE, Zoghbi WA. Dobutamine echocardiography in myocardial hibernation: Optimal dose and accuracy in predicting recovery of ventricular function after coronary angioplasty. *Circulation* 1995; 91:663–670.
497. Perrone-Filardi P, Pace L, Prastaro M, et al. Dobutamine echocardiography predicts improvement of hypoperfused dysfunctional myocardium after revascularization in patients with coronary artery disease. *Circulation* 1995; 91:2556–2565.
498. Arnese M, Cornel JH, Salustri A, et al. Prediction of improvement of regional left ventricular function after surgical revascularization: A comparison of low-dose dobutamine echocardiog-

raphy with thallium-201 single-photon emission computed tomography. *Circulation* 1995; 91:2748–2752.
499. Watada H, Ito H, Oh H, et al. Dobutamine stress echocardiography predicts reversible dysfunction and quantitates the extent of irreversibly damaged myocardium after reperfusion of anterior myocardial infarction. *J Am Coll Cardiol* 1994; 24:624–630.
500. La Canna G, Alfieri O, Giubbini R, et al. Echocardiography during infusion of dobutamine for identification of reversible dysfunction in patients with chronic coronary artery disease. *J Am Coll Cardiol* 1994; 23:617–626.
501. Baer FM, Voth E, Deutsch HJ, et al. Predictive value of low dose dobutamine transesophageal echocardiography and fluorine-18 fluorodeoxyglucose positron emission tomography for recovery of regional left ventricular function after successful revascularization. *J Am Coll Cardiol* 1996; 28:60–69.
501a. Bax JJ, Poldermans D, Elhendy A, et al. Improvement of left ventricular ejection fraction, heart failure symptoms and prognosis after revascularization in patients with chronic coronary artery disease and viable myocardium detected by dobutamine stress echocardiography. *J Am Coll Cardiol* 1999; 34163–34169.
501b. Senior R, Kaul S, Lahiri A. Myocardial viability on echocardiography predicts long-term survival after revascularization in patients with ischemic congestive heart failure. *J Am Coll Cardiol* 1999; 33:1848–1854.
502. Tischler MD, Plehn JF. Applications of stress echocardiography: Beyond coronary artery disease. *J Am Soc Echocardiogr* 1995; 8:185–197.
503. Leavitt JI, Coats MH, Falk RH. Effects of exercise on transmitral gradient and pulmonary artery pressure in patients with mitral stenosis or a prosthetic mitral valve: A Doppler echocardiographic study. *J Am Coll Cardiol* 1991; 17:1520–1526.
504. Tunick PA, Freedberg RS, Gargiulo A, Kronzon I. Exercise Doppler echocardiography as an aid to clinical decision making in mitral valve disease. *J Am Soc Echocardiogr* 1992; 5:225–230.
505. deFilippi CR, Willett DL, Brickner ME, et al. Usefulness of dobutamine echocardiography in distinguishing severe from nonsevere valvular aortic stenosis in patients with depressed left ventricular function and low transvalvular gradients. *Am J Cardiol* 1995; 75:191–194.
506. Abelmann WH. Classification and natural history of primary myocardial disease. *Prog Cardiovasc Dis* 1984; 27:73–94.
507. Rihal CS, Nishimura RA, Hatle LK, et al. Systolic and diastolic dysfunction in patients with clinical diagnosis of dilated cardiomyopathy: Relation to symptoms and prognosis. *Circulation* 1994; 90:2772–2779.
508. Wigle ED, Rakowski H, Kimball BP, Williams WG. Hypertrophic cardiomyopathy: Clinical spectrum and treatment. *Circulation* 1995; 92:1680–1692.
509. Siegel RJ, Shah PK, Fishbein MC. Idiopathic restrictive cardiomyopathy. *Circulation* 1984; 70:165–169.
510. Watkins H, McKenna WJ, Thierfelder L, et al. Mutations in the genes for cardiac troponin T and atropomyosin in hypertrophic cardiomyopathy. *N Engl J Med* 1995; 332:1058–1064.
511. Solomon S, Wolff S, Watkins H et al. Left ventricular hypertrophy and morphology in familial hypertrophic cardiomyopathy associated with mutations of the beta-myosin heavy chain gene. *J Am Coll Cardiol* 1993; 22:498–505.
512. Louie EK, Maron BJ. Apical hypertrophic cardiomyopathy: Clinical and two-dimensional echocardiographic assessment. *Ann Intern Med* 1987; 106:663–670.
513. Maron BJ. Asymmetry in hypertrophic cardiomyopathy: The septal to free wall ratio revisited. *Am J Cardiol* 1985; 55:835–838.
514. Henry WL, Clark CE, Epstein SE. Asymmetric septal hypertrophy (ASH): Echocardiographic identification of the pathognomonic anatomic abnormality of IHSS. *Circulation* 1973; 47:225–233.
515. Maron BJ, Gottdiener JS, Epstein SE. Patterns and significance of distribution of left ventricular hypertrophy in hypertrophic cardiomyopathy: A wide angle, two dimensional echocardiographic study of 125 patients. *Am J Cardiol* 1981, 48:418–428.
516. Maron BJ, Epstein SE. Hypertrophic cardiomyopathy: Recent observations regarding the specificity of three hallmarks of the disease: Asymmetric septal hypertrophy, septal disorganization and systolic anterior motion of the anterior mitral leaflet. *Am J Cardiol* 1980; 45:141.
517. Blanchard DG, Ross J Jr. Hypertrophic cardiomyopathy: Prognosis with medical or surgical therapy. *Clin Cardiol* 1991; 14:11–19.
518. Maron BJ, Harding AM, Spirito P, et al. Systolic anterior motion of the posterior mitral leaflet: A previously unrecognized cause of dynamic subaortic obstruction in patients with hypertrophic cardiomyopathy. *Circulation* 1983; 68:282–293.
519. Klues HG, Roberts WC, Maron BJ. Morphologic determinants of echocardiographic patterns of mitral valve systolic anterior motion in obstructive hypertrophic cardiomyopathy. *Circulation* 1993; 87:1570–1579.
520. Jiang L, Levine RA, King ME, Weyman AE. An integrated mechanism for systolic anterior motion of the mitral valve in hypertrophic cardiomyopathy based on echocardiographic observations. *Am Heart J* 1987; 113:633–644.
521. Henry WL, Clark CE, Griffith JM, Epstein SE. Mechanism of left ventricular outflow obstruction in patients with obstructive asymmetric septal hypertrophy (idiopathic hypertrophic subaortic stenosis). *Am J Cardiol* 1975; 35:337–345.
522. Gardin JM, Talano JV, Stephanides L, et al. Systolic anterior motion in the absence of asymmetric septal hypertrophy: A buckling phenomenon of the chordae tendineae. *Circulation* 1981; 63:181–188.
523. Maron BJ, Gottdiener JS, Perry LW. Specificity of systolic anterior motion of anterior mitral leaflet for hypertrophic cardiomyopathy. *Br Heart J* 1981; 45:206–212.
524. Gilbert BW, Pollick C, Adelman AG, Wigle ED. Hypertrophic cardiomyopathy: Subclassification by M mode echocardiography. *Am J Cardiol* 1980; 45:861–872.
525. Gardin J, Tommaso CL, Talano JV. Echocardiographic early systolic partial closure (notching) of the aortic valve in congestive cardiomyopathy. *Am Heart J* 1984; 107:135–142.
526. Eldar M, Motro M, Rath S, et al. Systolic closure of aortic valve in patients with prosthetic mitral valves. *Br Heart J* 1982; 48:48–53.
527. Zoghbi WA, Haichin RN, Quinones MA. Mid-cavity obstruction in apical hypertrophy: Doppler evidence of diastolic intraventricular gradient with higher apical pressure. *Am Heart J* 1988; 116:1469–1474.
528. Maron BJ, Gottdiener JS, Arce J, et al. Dynamic subaortic obstruction in hypertrophic cardiomyopathy: Pulsed Doppler echocardiography. *J Am Coll Cardiol* 1985; 6:1–15.
529. Sasson Z, Yock PG, Hatle LK, et al. Doppler echocardiographic determination of the pressure gradient in hypertrophic cardiomyopathy. *J Am Coll Cardiol* 1988; 11:752–756.
530. Panza JA, Petrone RK, Fananapazir L, Maron BJ. Utility of continuous wave Doppler echocardiography in the noninvasive assessment of left ventricular outflow tract pressure gradient in patients with hypertrophic cardiomyopathy. *J Am Coll Cardiol* 1992; 19:91–99.
531. Baumgartner H, Schima H, Tulzer G, Kühn P. Effect of stenosis geometry on the Doppler-catheter gradient relation in vitro: A manifestation of pressure recovery. *J Am Coll Cardiol* 1993; 21:1018–1025.
532. Spirito P, Maron BJ. Relation between extent of left ventricular hypertrophy and diastolic filling abnormalities in hypertrophic cardiomyopathy. *J Am Coll Cardiol* 1990; 15:808–813.
533. Keren A, Popp RL. Assignment of patients into the classification of cardiomyopathies. *Circulation* 1992; 86:1622–1633.

534. Hoit BD, Penonen E, Dalton N, Sahn DJ. Doppler color flow mapping studies of jet formation and spatial orientation in obstructive hypertrophic cardiomyopathy. *Am Heart J* 1989; 117:1119.
535. Douglas PS, Morrow R, Ioli A, Reichek N. Left ventricular shape afterload in survival in idiopathic dilated cardiomyopathy. *J Am Coll Cardiol* 1989; 13:311–315.
536. Lewis JF, Webber JD, Sutton LL, et al. Discordance in degree of right and left ventricular dilation in patients with dilated cardiomyopathy: Recognition and clinical implications. *J Am Coll Cardiol* 1993; 21:640–654.
537. Blanchard DG, Hagenhoff C, Chow LC, et al. Reversibility of cardiac abnormalities in human immunodeficiency virus (HIV) infected individuals: A serial echocardiographic study. *J Am Coll Cardiol* 1991; 17:1270–1276.
538. Frishman WH, Sung HM, Yee HCM, et al. Cardiovascular toxicity with cancer chemotherapy. *Curr Probl Cardiol* 1996; 21:225–288.
539. Corya BC, Feigenbaum H, Rasmussen S, Black MJ. Echocardiographic features of congestive cardiomyopathy compared with normal subjects and patients with coronary artery disease. *Circulation* 1974; 49:1153–1159.
540. Shah PM. Echocardiography in congestive or dilated cardiomyopathy. *J Am Soc Echocardiogr* 1988; 1:20–27.
541. Rihal CS, Nishimura RA, Hatle LK, et al. Systolic and diastolic dysfunction in patients with clinical diagnosis of dilated cardiomyopathy: Relation to symptoms and prognosis. *Circulation* 1994; 90:2772–2779.
541a. Nishimura RA, Appleton CP, Redfield MM, et al. Noninvasive Doppler echocardiographic evaluation of left ventricular filling pressures in patients with cardiomyopathies: A simultaneous Doppler echocardiographic and cardiac catheterization study. *J Am Coll Cardiol* 1996; 28:1226–1233.
542. Pinamonti B, Di Lenarda A, Sinagra G, Camerini F. Restrictive left ventricular filling pattern in dilated cardiomyopathy assessed by Doppler echocardiography: Clinical, echocardiographic, and hemodynamic correlations and prognostic implications. *J Am Coll Cardiol* 1993; 22:808–815.
543. Nishimura RA, Tajik AJ. Quantitative hemodynamics by Doppler echocardiography: A noninvasive alternative to cardiac catheterization. *Prog Cardiovasc Dis* 1994; 36:309–342.
544. Shabetai R. The role of the pericardium in the pathophysiology of heart failure. In: Hosenpud JD, Greenberg BH, eds. *Congestive Heart Failure: Pathophysiology, Diagnosis, and Comprehensive Approach to Management*. New York: Springer-Verlag; 1994:95–125.
545. Borer JS, Henry WL, Epstein SE. Echocardiographic observations in patients with systemic infiltrative disease involving the heart. *Am J Cardiol* 1977; 39:184–188.
546. Gross DM, Williams JC, Caprioli CC, et al. Echocardiographic abnormalities in the mucopolysaccharide storage diseases. *Am J Cardiol* 1988; 61:170–176.
547. Picano E, Pinamonti B, Ferdeghini EM, et al. Two-dimensional echocardiography in myocardial amyloidosis. *Echocardiography* 1991; 8:253–262.
548. Acquatella H, Schiller NB, Puigbo JJ, et al. Value of two dimensional echocardiography in endomyocardial disease with and without eosinophilia. *Circulation* 1983; 67:1219–1226.
549. Siqueira-Filho AG, Cunha CLP, Tajik AJ, et al. M-mode and two-dimensional echocardiographic features in cardiac amyloidosis. *Circulation* 1981; 63:188–196.
550. Klein AL, Cohen GI. Doppler echocardiographic assessment of constrictive pericarditis, cardiac amyloidosis, and cardiac tamponade. *Cleve Clin J Med* 1992; 59:278–290.
551. Klein AL, Hatle LK, Taliercio CP, et al. Serial Doppler echocardiographic follow-up of left ventricular diastolic function in cardiac amyloidosis. *J Am Coll Cardiol* 1990; 16:1135–1141.
552. Klein AL, Hatle LK, Taliercio CP, et al. Prognostic significance of Doppler measures of diastolic function in cardiac amyloidosis. *Circulation* 1991; 83:808–816.
553. Acquatella H, Schiller NB. Echocardiographic recognition of Chagas' disease and endomyocardial fibrosis. *J Am Soc Echocardiogr* 1988; 1:60–68.
554. Fyfe DA, Kline CH. Transesophageal echocardiography for congenital heart disease. *Echocardiography* 1991; 8:573–586.
555. Huhta JC, Glasow P, Murphy DJ, et al. Surgery without catheterization for congenital heart defects: Management of 100 patients. *J Am Coll Cardiol* 1987; 9:823–829.
556. Lipschulz SE, Sanders SP, Mayer JE, et al. Are routine preoperative cardiac catheterization and angiography necessary before repair of ostium primum atrial septal defect? *J Am Coll Cardiol* 1988; 11:373–378.
557. Shub C, Tajik J, Seward JB, et al. Surgical repair of uncomplicated atrial septal defect without "routine" operative cardiac catheterization. *J Am Coll Cardiol* 1985; 6:49–54.
558. Hagler DJ, Tajik AJ, Seward JB, et al. Aterioventricular and ventriculoarterial discordance (corrected transposition of the great arteries): Wide-angle two-dimensional echocardiographic assessment of ventricular morphology. *Mayo Clin Proc* 1981; 56:591–600.
559. Nasser FN, Tajik AJ, Stewart JB, Hagler DJ. Diagnosis of sinus venous atrial septal defect by two-dimensional echocardiography. *Mayo Clin Proc* 1981; 6:568–572.
560. Mehta RH, Helmcke F, Nanda NC, et al. Transesophageal Doppler color flow mapping assessment of atrial septal defect. *J Am Coll Cardiol* 1990; 16:1010–1016.
561. Shub C, Dimopoulos IN, Seward JB, et al. Sensitivity of two-dimensional echocardiography in the direct visualization of atrial septal defect utilizing the subcostal approach: Experience with 154 patients. *J Am Coll Cardiol* 1983; 2:127–135.
562. Hagler DJ, Tajik AJ, Seward JB, et al. Real-time wide-angle sector echocardiography: Atrioventricular canal defects. *Circulation* 1979; 59:140–150.
563. Mehta RH, Helmcke F, Nanda NC, et al. Uses and limitations of transthoracic echocardiography in the assessment of atrial septal defect in the adult. *Am J Cardiol* 1991; 67:288–294.
564. Franker TD, Harris PJ, Behar VS, Kisslo JA. Detection and exclusion of interatrial shunts by two-dimensional echocardiography and peripheral venous injections. *Circulation* 1979; 59:379–384.
565. Pollick C, Sullivan H, Cujec B, Wilansky S. Doppler color-flow imaging assessment of shunt size in atrial septal defect. *Circulation* 1988; 78:522–528.
566. Minagoe S, Tei C, Kisanuki A, et al. Noninvasive pulsed Doppler echocardiographic detection of the direction of shunt flow in patients with atrial septal defect. *Circulation* 1985; 71:745–753.
567. Dittman H, Jacksch R, Voelker W, et al. Accuracy of Doppler echocardiography in quantification of left to right shunts in adult patients with atrial septal defect. *J Am Coll Cardiol* 1988; 11:338–342.
568. Jenni R, Ritter M, Vieli A, et al. Determination of the ratio of pulmonary blood flow to systemic blood flow by deviation of amplitude weighed mean velocity from continuous wave Doppler spectra. *Br Heart J* 1989; 61:167–171.
569. Sutherland GR, Godman MJ, Smallhorn JF, et al. Ventricular septal defects: Two-dimensional echocardiographic and morphological correlations. *Br Heart J* 1982; 47:316–328.
570. Capelli H, Andrade JL, Somerville J. Classification of the site of ventricular septal defect by two-dimensional echocardiography. *Am J Cardiol* 1983; 51:1474–1488.
571. Linker DT, Rossvoll O, Chapman JV, Angelsen B. Sensitivity and speed of color Doppler flow mapping compared with continuous wave Doppler for the detection of ventricular septal defects. *Br Heart J* 1991; 65:201–203.

572. Baron JV, Sahn DJ, Valdes-Cruz LM, et al. Two-dimensional echocardiographic features of ventricular septal aneurysm paradoxically bulging into the left ventricular outflow tract. *Am Heart J* 1982; 104:156–158.
573. Schmidt KG, Cassidy SC, Silverman NH, Stanger P. Doubly committed subarterial ventricular septal defects: Echocardiographic features and surgical implications. *J Am Coll Cardiol* 1988; 12:1538–1546.
574. Takenaka K, Sakmoto T, Shiota T, et al. Diagnosis of patent ductus arteriosus in adults by biplane transesophageal color Doppler flow mapping. *Am J Cardiol* 1991; 68:691–693.
575. Snider AR, Silverman NH. Suprasternal notch echocardiography: A two-dimensional technique for evaluating congenital heart disease. *Circulation* 1982; 63:165–173.
576. Liao P-K, Su W-J, Hung J-S. Doppler echocardiographic flow characteristics of isolated patent ductus arteriosus: Better delineation by Doppler color flow mapping. *J Am Coll Cardiol* 1988; 12:1285–1291.
577. Swensson RE, Valdes-Cruz LM, Sahn DJ, et al. Real-time Doppler color flow mapping for detection of patent ductus arteriosus. *J Am Coll Cardiol* 1896; 8:1105–1112.
578. Alboliras ET, Chin AJ, Barbar G, et al. Detection of aortopulmonary window by pulsed and color Doppler echocardiography. *Am Heart J* 1988; 115:900–902.
579. Balaji S, Burch M, Sullivan ED. Accuracy of cross-sectional echocardiography in diagnosis of aortopulmonary window. *Am J Cardiol* 1991; 67:650–653.
580. Gao Y-A, Burrows PE, Benson LN, et al. Scimitar syndrome in infancy. *J Am Coll Cardiol* 1993; 22:873–882.
581. Oakley D, Naik D, Verel D, Rajan S. Scimitar vein syndrome: Report of nine new cases. *Am Heart J* 1984; 107:596–598.
582. Huhtas JC, Gutgesell HP, Nihill MR. Cross-sectional echocardiographic diagnosis of total anomalous pulmonary venous connection. *Br Heart J* 1985; 53:525–534.
583. Sahn DJ, Allen HD, Lange LW, Goldberg SJ. Cross-sectional echocardiographic diagnosis of the sites of total anomalous pulmonary venous drainage. *Circulation* 1979; 60:1317–1325.
584. Smallhorn JF, Burrows P, Wilson G, et al. Two-dimensional and pulsed Doppler echocardiography in the postoperative evaluation of total anomalous pulmonary venous connection. *Circulation* 1987; 76:289–305.
585. Sreeram N, Walsh K: Diagnosis of total anomalous pulmonary venous drainage by Doppler color flow imaging. *J Am Coll Cardiol* 1992; 19:1577–1582.
586. Lengyel M, Arvay A, Biro V. Two-dimensional echocardiographic diagnosis of cor triatriatum. *Am J Cardiol* 1987; 59: 484–485.
587. Snider AR, Port TA, Silverman NH. Venous anomalies of the coronary sinus: detection by M-mode, two-dimensional, and contrast echocardiography. *Circulation* 1979; 60:721–727.
588. Chaudhry F, Zabalgoitia M: Persistent left superior vena cava diagnosed by contrast transesophageal echocardiography. *Am Heart J* 1991; 122:1175–1177.
589. Flanagan MF, Foran RB, VanPraagh R, et al. Tetralogy of Fallot with obstruction of the ventricular septal defect: Spectrum of echocardiographic findings. *J Am Coll Cardiol* 1988; 11:386–395.
590. Musewe NN, Smallhorn JF, Moes CAF, et al. Echocardiographic evaluation of obstructive mechanism of tetralogy of Fallot with restrictive ventricular septal defect. *Am J Cardiol* 1988; 61:664–668.
591. Geva T, Ayres NA, Pac FA, Pignatelli R. Quantitative morphometric analysis of progressive infundibular obstruction in tetralogy of Fallot: A prospective longitudinal echocardiographic study. *Circulation* 1995; 9:886–892.
592. Bricker JT. Sudden death and tetralogy of Fallot: Risks, markers, and causes. *Circulation* 1995; 92:158–159.
593. Macartney FJ, Rigby ML, Anderson RH, et al. Double outlet right ventricle: Cross-sectional echocardiographic findings—their anatomical explanation and surgical relevance. *Br Heart J* 1984; 52:164–177.
594. DiSessa TG, Hagman AD, Pope C, et al. Two-dimensional echocardiographic characteristics of double outlet right ventricle. *Am J Cardiol* 1979; 44:1146–1154.
595. Roberson DA, Silverman NH. Malaligned outlet septum with subpulmonary ventricular septal defect and abnormal ventriculoarterial connection: A morphologic spectrum defined echocardiographically. *J Am Coll Cardiol* 1990; 16:459–468.
596. Chin AJ, Yeager SB, Sanders SP, et al. Accuracy of prospective two-dimensional echocardiographic evaluation of left ventricular outflow tract in complete transposition of the great arteries. *Am J Cardiol* 1985; 55:759–764.
597. Daskalopoulos DA, Edwards WD, Driscoll DJ, et al. Correlation of two-dimensional echocardiographic and autopsy findings in complete transposition of the great arteries. *J Am Coll Cardiol* 1983; 3:1151–1157.
598. Smallhorn J, Grow R, Freedom R, et al. Pulsed Doppler echocardiographic assessment of the pulmonary venous pathway after the Mustard or Senning procedure for transposition of the great arteries. *Circulation* 1986; 73:765–774.
599. Kaulitz R, Stümper OFW, Geuskens R, et al. Comparative values of the precordial and transesophageal approaches in the echocardiographic evaluation of atrial baffle function after an atrial correction procedure. *J Am Coll Cardiol* 1990; 16:686–694.
600. Mahoney LT, Knoedel DI, Skorton DJ. Echocardiographic postoperative assessment of patients with transposition of the great arteries. *Echocardiography* 1995; 12:545–557.
601. Rice MJ, Seward JB, Hagler DJ, et al. Definitive diagnosis of truncus arteriosus by two-dimensional echocardiography. *Mayo Clin Proc* 1982; 57:476–481.
602. Marin-Garcia J, Tonkin ILD. Two-dimensional echocardiographic evaluation of persistent truncus arteriosus. *Am J Cardiol* 1982; 50:1376–1379.
603. Simpson IA, Sahn DJ, Valdes-Cruz LM, et al. Color Doppler flow mapping in patients with coarctation of the aorta: New observations and improved evaluation with color flow diameter and proximal acceleration as predictors of severity. *Circulation* 1988; 77:736–744.
604. Rao PS, Carey P. Doppler ultrasound in the prediction of pressure gradients across aortic coarctation. *Am Heart J* 1989; 118:299–307.
605. Shaddy RE, Snider AR, Silverman NH, Lutin W. Pulsed Doppler findings in patients with coarctation of the aorta. *Circulation* 1986; 73:82–88.
606. Nihoyannopoulos P, Karas S, Sapsford RN, et al. Accuracy of two-dimensional echocardiography in the diagnosis of aortic arch obstruction. *J Am Coll Cardiol* 1987; 10:1072–1077.
607. Marx GR, Allen HD. Accuracy and pitfalls of Doppler evaluation of the pressure gradient in aortic coarctation. *J Am Coll Cardiol* 1986; 7:1379–1385.
608. Vogt J, Rupprath G, Grimm T, Beuren AJ. Qualitative and quantitative evaluation of supravalvular aortic stenosis by cross-sectional echocardiography: A report of 80 patients. *Pediatr Cardiol* 1982; 3:13–17.
609. Johnson GL, Kwan OL, Handshoe S, et al. Accuracy of combined two-dimensional echocardiography and continuous wave Doppler recordings in the estimation of pressure gradient in right ventricular outlet obstruction. *J Am Coll Cardiol* 1984; 3:1013–1018.
610. Weyman AE, Hurwitz RA, Girod DA, et al. Cross-sectional echocardiographic visualization of the stenotic pulmonary valve. *Circulation* 1977; 56:769–774.
611. Choi JY, Sullivan ID. Fixed subaortic stenosis: Anatomical spectrum and nature of progression. *Br Heart J* 1991; 65:280–286.
612. Valdes-Cruz LM, Jones M, Scagnelli S, et al. Prediction of gradi-

ents in fibrous subaortic stenosis by continuous wave two-dimensional Doppler echocardiography: Animal studies. *J Am Coll Cardiol* 1985; 5:1363–1367.
613. Wu JR, Huang TY, Chen YF, et al. Aortico-left ventricular tunnel: Two-dimensional echocardiographic and angiocardiographic features. *Am Heart J* 1989; 117:697–699.
614. Zielinsky P, Rossi M, Haertel JC, et al. Subaortic fibrous ridge and ventricular septal defect: Role of septal malalignment. *Circulation* 1987; 75:1124–1129.
615. Zema JJ, Caccavano M. Two-dimensional echocardiograpic assessment of aortic morphology: Feasibility of bicuspid valve detection. *Br Heart J* 1982; 48:428–433.
616. Brandenberg J, Tajik AJ, Edwards WD, et al. Accuracy of two-dimensional echocardiographic diagnosis of congenitally bicuspid aortic valve: Echocardiographic-anatomic correlation in 115 patients. *Am J Cardiol* 1983; 51:1469–1473.
617. Shiina A, Seward JB, Edwards WD, et al. Two-dimensional echocardiographic spectrum of Ebstein's anomaly: Detailed anatomic assessment. *J Am Coll Cardiol* 1984; 3:356–370.
618. Quaegebeur JM, Sreeram N, Fraser AG, et al. Surgery for Ebstein's anomaly: The clinical and echocardiographic evaluation of a new technique. *J Am Coll Cardiol* 1991; 17:722–728.
619. Copel JA, Pilu G, Green J, et al. Fetal echocardiographic screening for congenital heart disease: The importance of the four-chamber view. *Am J Obstet Gynecol* 1987; 157:648–655.
620. Tan A, Kleinman C, Copel J. Does prenatal diagnosis of congenital heart disease make a difference? *Ultrasound Obstet Gynecol* 1995; 6:76S.
621. Sharland GK, Chita SK, Allan LD. The use of color Doppler in fetal echocardiography. *Int J Cardiol* 1990; 28:229–236.
622. Ewingman BG, Crane JP, Frigoletto F, et al. Effect of prenatal ultrasound screening on perinatal outcome. *N Engl J Med* 1993; 329:821–827.
623. Buskens E, Grobbee DE, Frohn-Mulder IME, et al. Efficacy of routine fetal ultrasound screening for congenital heart disease in normal pregnancy. *Circulation* 1996; 94:67–72.
624. Chang AC, Huhta JC, Yoon GY, et al. Diagnosis, transport, and outcome in fetuses with left ventricular outflow tract obstruction. *J Thorac Cardiovasc Surg* 1991; 102:841–848.
625. Hicks KA, Kovack JA, Frishberg DP, et al. Echocardiographic evaluation of papillary fibroelastoma: A case report and review of the literature. *J Am Soc Echocardiogr* 1996; 9:353–360.
626. DeMaria AN, Bommer W, Neumann A, et al. Left ventricular thrombi identified by cross-sectional echocardiography. *Ann Intern Med* 1979; 90:14–18.
627. Limacher M, Gutgesell HP, Vick GW, et al. Echocardiographic anatomy of the eustachian valve. *Am J Cardiol* 1986; 57:363–365.
628. Orita Y, Meno H, Kanarck M, et al. Echocardiographic features of persistent right sinus venosus valve in adults. *J Clin Ultrasound* 1982; 10:461.
629. Georgeson R, Liu M, Bansal RC. Transesophageal echocardiographic diagnosis of eustachian valve endocarditis. *J Am Soc Echocardiogr* 1996; 9:206–208.
630. Palakodeti V, Keen WD, Rickman L, Blanchard DG. Eustachian valve endocarditis: Detection by transesophageal echocardiography. *Clin Cardiol* 1997; 20:579–580.
631. Panidis IP, Kotler MN, Mintz GS, Ross J. Clinical and echocardiographic features of right atrial masses. *Am Heart J* 1984; 107:745–758.
632. Werner JA, Cheitlin MD, Gross BW, et al. Echocardiographic appearance of the Chiari network: Differentiation from right-heart pathology. *Circulation* 1981; 63:1104–1109.
633. Keren A, Billingham ME, Popp RL. Echocardiographic recognition and implications of ventricular hypertrophic trabeculations and aberrant bands. *Circulation* 1984; 70:836–842.
634. Perry LW, Ruckman RN, Shapiro SR, et al. Left ventricular false tendons in children: Prevalence as detected by two dimensional echocardiography and clinical significance. *Am J Cardiol* 1983; 52:1264–1266.
635. Vered Z, Melzer RS, Benjamin P, et al. Prevalence and significance of false tendons in the left ventricle as determined by echocardiography. *Am J Cardiol* 1984; 53:330–332.
636. Seward JB, Khanderia BK, Oh JK, et al. Critical appraisal of transesophageal echocardiography: Limitations, pitfalls, and complications. *J Am Soc Echocardiogr* 1992; 5:288–305.
637. Blanchard DG, Dittrich HC, Mitchell M, McCann HA. Diagnostic pitfalls in transesophageal echocardiography. *J Am Soc Echocardiogr* 1992; 5:525–540.
638. Starling RC, Baker PB, Hirsch SC, et al. An echocardiographic and anatomic description of the donor-recipient atrial anastomosis after orthotopic cardiac transplantation. *Am J Cardiol* 1989; 64:109–111.
639. Drinkovic N. Subcostal echocardiography to determine right ventricular pacing catheter position and control advancement of electrode catheters in intracardiac electrophysiologic studies: M-mode and two-dimensional studies. *Am J Cardiol* 1981; 47:1260–1265.
640. Bierard L, Allaf DE, D'Orio V, et al. Two-dimensional echocardiographic guiding of endomyocardial biopsy. *Chest* 1984; 85:759–762.
641. French JW, Popp RL, Pitlick PT. Cardiac localization of transvascular biotome using two-dimensional echocardiography. *Am J Cardiol* 1983; 51:219–223.
642. Reeves WC, Movahed A, Chitwood R, et al. Utility of precordial, epicardial and transesophageal two-dimensional echocardiography in the detection of intracardiac foreign bodies. *Am J Cardiol* 1989; 64:406–409.
643. Hanley PC, Tajik AJ, Hynes JK, et al. Diagnosis and classification of atrial septal aneurysm by two-dimensional echocardiography: Report of 80 consecutive cases. *J Am Coll Cardiol* 1985; 6:1370–1382.
644. Pearson AC, Nagelhout D, Castello R, et al. Atrial septal aneurysm and stroke: A transesophageal echocardiographic study. *J Am Coll Cardiol* 1991; 18:1223–1229.
645. Zabalgoitia-Reyes M, Herrera C, Gandhi DK, et al. A possible mechanism for neurologic ischemic events in patients with atrial septal aneurysm. *Am J Cardiol* 1990; 66:761–764.
646. Fyke III FE, Tajik AJ, Edwards WD, Seward JB. Diagnosis of lipomatous hypertrophy of the interatrial septum by two-dimensional echocardiography. *J Am Coll Cardiol* 1983; 1:1352–1357.
647. Pochis WT, Saeian K, Sager KB. Usefulness of transesophageal echocardiography in diagnosing lipomatous hypertrophy of the atrial septum with comparison to transthoracic echocardiography. *Am J Cardiol* 1992; 70:396–398.
648. Haugland JM, Asinger RW, Mikell FL, et al. Embolic potential of left ventricular thrombi detection by two-dimensional echocardiography. *Circulation* 1984; 70:588–598.
649. Hunter JJ, Johnson KR, Karagianes TG, Dittrich HC. Detection of massive pulmonary embolus-in-transit by transesophageal echocardiography. *Chest* 1991; 100:1210–1214.
650. Pasierski TJ, Alton ME, Van Fossen DB, Pearson AC. Right atrial mobile thrombus: Improved visualization by transesophageal echocardiography. *Am Heart J* 1991; 123:802–803.
651. Armbruster RW, Labovitz AJ. Mitral stenosis. In: Daniel WG, Kronzon I, Mügge A, eds. *Cardiogenic Embolism.* Baltimore: Williams & Wilkins; 1996:81–92.
652. Aschenberg W, Schluter M, Kremer P, et al. Transesophageal two-dimensional echocardiography for the detection of left atrial appendage thrombus. *J Am Coll Cardiol* 1986; 7:163–166.
653. Torbicki A, Pasierski T, Uchman B, Miskiewicz A. Right atrial mobile thrombi: Two-dimensional echocardiographic diagnosis and clinical outcome. *Cor Vasa* 1987; 29:293–303.
654. Goldberg SM, Pizzarello RA, Goldman MA, Padmanabhan VT.

Echocardiographic diagnosis of right atrial thromboembolism resulting in massive pulmonary embolization. *Am Heart J* 1984; 108:1371–1372.

655. Klein AL, Stewart WC, Cosgrove DM III, et al. Visualization of acute pulmonary emboli by transesophageal echocardiography. *J Am Soc Echocardiogr* 1990; 3:412–415.
656. Wiseman MN, Giles MS, Camm AJ. Unusual echocardiographic appearance of intracardiac thrombi in a patient with endomyocardial fibrosis. *Br Heart J* 1986; 56:179–181.
657. Stowers SA, Leiboff RH, Wasserman AG, et al. Right ventricular thrombus formation in association with acute myocardial infarction: Diagnosis by 2-dimensional echocardiography. *Am J Cardiol* 1983; 52:912–913.
658. Herzog CA, Bass L, Kane M, Asinger R. Two-dimensional echocardiographic imaging of left atrial appendage thrombi. *J Am Coll Cardiol* 1984; 3:1340–1344.
659. Manning WJ, Reis GJ, Douglas PS. Use of transesophageal echocardiography to detect left atrial thrombi before percutaneous balloon dilatation of the mitral valve: A prospective study. *Br Heart J* 1992; 67:170–173.
660. Olson JD, Goldenberg IF, Pedersen W, et al. Exclusion of atrial thrombus by transesophageal echocardiography. *J Am Soc Echocardiogr* 1992; 5:52–56.
661. Feltes TF, Friedman RA. Transesophageal echocardiographic detection of atrial thombi in patients with nonfibrillation atrial tachyarrhythmias and congenital heart disease. *J Am Coll Cardiol* 1994; 24:1365–1370.
662. Galzerano D, Tucillo B, Lama D, et al. Does multilobularity of left atrial appendage represent an additional risk for thrombus formation in atrial fibrillation? (abstr). *J Am Coll Cardiol* 1997; 29:212A.
663. Merino A, Haupman P, Badimon L, et al. Echocardiographic "smoke" is produced by an interaction of erythrocytes and plasma proteins modulated by shear forces. *J Am Coll Cardiol* 1992; 20:1661–1668.
664. Castello R, Pearson AC, Labovitz AJ. Prevalence and clinical implications of atrial spontaneous contrast in patients undergoing transesophageal echocardiography. *Am J Cardiol* 1990; 65:1149–1153.
665. Daniel WG, Nellessen U, Schroder E, et al. Left atrial spontaneous echo contrast in mitral valve disease: An indicator for an increased thromboembolic risk. *J Am Coll Cardiol* 1988; 11:1204–1211.
666. Peverill RE, Harper RW, Gelman J, et al. Determinants of increased regional left atrial coagulation activity in patients with mitral stenosis. *Circulation* 1996; 94:331–339.
667. Keating EC, Gross SA, Schalmatitz RA, et al. Mural thrombi in myocardial infarctions: Prospective evaluations by two-dimensional echocardiography. *Am J Med* 1983; 74:989–995.
668. Asinger RW, Mikell FL, Elsperger J, Hodges M. Incidence of left ventricular thrombosis after acute transmural myocardial infarction: Serial evaluation by two-dimensional echocardiography. *N Engl J Med* 1981; 305:297–302.
669. Visser CA, Kan G, David G, et al. Two-dimensional echocardiography in the diagnosis of left ventricular thrombus: A prospective study of 67 patients with anatomic validation. *Chest* 1983; 83:228–232.
670. Takamoto T, Kim D, Murie P, et al. Comparative recognition of left ventricular thombi by echocardiography and cineangiography. *Br Heart J* 1985; 53:36–42.
671. Meltzer RS, Visser CA, Kan G, Roelandt J. Two-dimensional echocardiographic appearance of left ventricular thombi with systemic emboli after myocardial infarction. *Am J Cardiol* 1984; 53:1511–1513.
672. Edwards LC III, Louie EK. Transthoracic and transesophageal echocardiography for the evaluation of cardiac tumors, thrombi, and valvular vegetations. *Am J Cardiac Imaging* 1994; 8:45–58.
673. Meller J, Teichholz LE, Pichard AD, et al. Left ventricular myxoma: Echocardiographic diagnosis and review of the literature. *Am J Med* 1977; 63:816.
674. Peters MN, Hall RJ, Cooley DA, et al. The clinical syndrome of atrial myxomas. *JAMA* 1974; 230:695.
675. Reynen K. Cardiac myxomas. *N Engl J Med* 1995; 1610–1617.
676. Gosse P, Herpin D, Roudault R, et al. Myxoma of the mitral valve diagnosed by echocardiography. *Am Heart J* 1986; 111:803–805.
677. Suri RK, Pattnkar VL, Singh H, et al. Myxoma of the tricuspid valve. *Aust NZ J Surg* 1978; 48:429–432.
678. Goli VD, Thadani U, Thomas SR, et al. Doppler echocardiographic profiles in obstructive right and left atrial myxomas. *J Am Coll Cardiol* 1987; 9:701–703.
679. Gorcsan J III, Blanc MS, Reedy PS, Marrone GC. Hemodynamic diagnosis of mitral valve obstruction by left atrial myxoma with transesophageal continuous wave Doppler. *Am Heart J* 1992; 124:1109–1112.
680. Obeid AI, Marvasti M, Parker F, Rosenberg J. Comparison of transthoracic and transesophageal echocardiography in diagnosis of left atrial myxoma. *Am J Cardiol* 1989; 63:1006–1008.
681. Nir A, Tajik AJ, Freeman WK, et al. Tuberous sclerosis and cardiac rhabdomyoma. *Am J Cardiol* 1995; 76:419–421.
682. Fenoglio JJ, McAllister HA, Fernas VJ. Cardiac rhabdomyoma: A clinicopathologic and electron microscopic study. *Am J Cardiol* 1976; 38:241–251.
683. Smythe JF, Dick JD, Smallhorn JF, Freedon RM. Natural history of cardiac rhabdomyoma in infancy and childhood. *Am J Cardiol* 1990; 66:1247–1249.
684. deRuiz M, Potter JL, Stavinoha J. Real-time ultrasound diagnosis of cardiac fibroma in a neonate. *J Ultrasound Med* 1985; 4:367–369.
685. Parmley LF, Salley RK, William JP, Head GB. The clinical spectrum of cardiac fibroma with diagnostic and surgical considerations: Noninvasive imaging enhances management. *Ann Thorac Surg* 1988; 45:455–465.
686. Topol EJ, Biern RO, Reitz BA. Cardiac papillary fibroelastoma and stroke. *Am J Med* 1986; 80:129–132.
687. Brown RD, Khanderia BK, Edwards WD. Cardiac papillary fibroelastoma: A treatable cause of transient ischemic attack and ischemic stroke detected by transesophageal echocardiography. *Mayo Clin Proc* 1995; 70:863–868.
688. Hui KS, Green LK, Schmidt WA. Primary cardiac rhabdomyosarcoma: Definition of a rare entity. *Am J Cardiovasc Pathol* 1988; 2:19–29.
689. Hanfling SM. Metastatic cancer to the heart. *Circulation* 1960; 22:474.
690. Riggs T, Paul MH, DeLeon S, Ilbawi M. Two-dimensional echocardiography in evaluation of right atrial masses: Five cases in pediatric patients. *Am J Cardiol* 1981; 48:961–966.
691. Roberts WC, Glancy DL, DeVita VT. Heart in malignant lymphoma (Hodgkins' disease, lymphosarcoma, reticulum cell sarcoma and mycosis fungoides): A study of 196 autopsy cases. *Am J Cardiol* 1968; 22:85–107.
692. Chandraratna PAN, Arnow WS. Detection of pericardial metastases by cross-sectional echocardiography. *Circulation* 1981; 63:197–199.
693. Limacher MC, McEntee CW, Attart M, et al. Cardiac echinococcal cyst: Diagnosis by two dimensional echocardiography. *J Am Coll Cardiol* 1983; 2:574–577.
694. Rey M, Alfonso F, Torricella EG. Diagnostic valve of two-dimensional echocardiography in cardiac hydatid disease. *Eur Heart J* 1991; 12:1300.
695. McAllister HA Jr. Primary tumors and cysts of the heart and pericardium. *Curr Probl Cardiol* 1979; 4:1–51.
696. Martin RP, Rakowski H, French J, Popp RL. Localization of

pericardial effusion with wide angle phased-array echocardiography. *Am J Cardiol* 1978; 42:904–912.

696a. Ling LH, OH JK, Tei C, et al. Pericardial thickness measured with transesophageal echocardiography: Feasibility and potential clinical usefulness. *J Am Coll Cardiol* 1997; 29:1317–1323.

697. Martin RP, Bowden R, Filly K. Intrapericardial abnormalities in patients with pericardial effusion: Findings by two-dimensional echocardiography. *Circulation* 1980; 61:568–572.

698. Luft FC, Gilman JK, Weyman AE. Pericarditis in the patient with uremia: Clinical and echocardiographic evaluation. *Nephron* 1980; 25:160–166.

699. Schnittger I, Bowden RE, Abrams J, Popp RL. Echocardiography: Pericardial thickening and constrictive pericarditis. *Am J Cardiol* 1978; 42:388–395.

700. Lewis BS. Real time two dimensional echocardiography in constrictive pericarditis. *Am J Cardiol* 1982; 49:1789–1793.

701. Hatle LK, Appleton CP, Popp RL. Differentiation of constrictive pericarditis and restrictive cardiomyopathy by Doppler echocardiography. *Circulation* 1989; 79:357–370.

702. Horowitz MS, Schultz CS, Stinson EB. Sensitivity and specificity of echocardiographic diagnosis of pericardial effusion. *Circulation* 1974; 50:239–247.

703. Come PC, Riley MF, Fortuin NJ. Echocardiographic mimicry of pericardial effusion. *Am J Cardiol* 1981; 47:365–370.

704. Gabor GE, Winsberg F, Bloom HS. Electrical and mechanical alternation in pericardial effusion. *Chest* 1971; 59:341–344.

705. Haaz WS, Mintz GS, Kotler MN, et al. Two dimensional echocardiographic recognition of the descending thoracic aorta: Value in differentiating pericardial from pleural effusion. *Am J Cardiol* 1980; 46:739–743.

706. Isner JM, Carter BL, Roberts WC, Bankoff MS. Subepicardial adipose tissue producing echocardiographic appearance of pericardial effusion. *Am J Cardiol* 1983; 51:565–569.

707. Schiller NB, Botvinick EH. Right ventricular compression as a sign of cardiac tamponade: An analysis of echocardiographic ventricular dimensions and their clinical implications. *Circulation* 1977; 56:774–779.

708. Appleton CP, Hatle LK, Popp RL. Cardiac tamponade and pericardial effusion: Respiratory variation in transvalvular flow velocities studied by Doppler echocardiography. *J Am Coll Cardiol* 1988; 11:1020–1030.

709. Gillam LD, Guyer DE, Gibson TC, et al. Hydrodynamic compression of the right atrium: A new echocardiographic sign of cardiac tamponade. *Circulation* 1983; 68:294–301.

710. Armstrong WF, Schilt BF, Helper DJ, et al. Diastolic collapse of the right ventricle with cardiac tamponade: An echocardiographic study. *Circulation* 1982; 65:1491–1503.

711. Conrad SA, Byrnes TJ. Diastolic collapse of the left and right ventricles in cardiac tamponade. *Am Heart J* 1988; 115:475–478.

712. Brodyn NE, Rose MR, Prior FP, Haft JI. Left atrial diastolic compression in a patient with a large pericardial effusion and pulmonary hypertension. *Am J Med* 1990; 88:1–8.

713. Leeman DE, Levine MJ, Come PC. Doppler echocardiography in cardiac tamponade: Exaggerated respiratory variation in transvalvular blood flow velocity integrals. *J Am Coll Cardiol* 1988; 11:572–578.

714. Callahan JA, Seward JB, Tajik AJ. Cardiac tamponade: Pericardiocentesis directed by two-dimensional echocardiography. *Mayo Clin Proc* 1985; 60:344–347.

715. Pandian NG, Skorton DJ, Kieso RA, Kerber RE. Diagnosis of constrictive pericarditis by two-dimensional echocardiography: Studies in a new experimental model and in patients. *J Am Coll Cardiol* 1984; 4:1164–1173.

716. Himelman RB, Lee S, Schiller NB. Septal bounce, vena cava plethora, and pericardial adhesion: Informative two-dimensional echocardiographic signs in the diagnosis of pericardial constriction. *J Am Soc Echocardiogr* 1988; 1:333–340.

717. Morgan JM, Raposo L, Clague JC, et al. Restrictive cardiomyopathy and constrictive pericarditis: Non-invasive distinction by digitized M mode echocardiography (abstr). *Br Heart J* 1988; 59:629.

718. Schiavone WA, Calafiore PA, Currie PJ, Lytle BW. Doppler echocardiographic demonstration of pulmonary venous flow velocity in three patients with constrictive pericarditis before and after pericardioectomy. *Am J Cardiol* 1989; 63:145–147.

719. vonBibra H, Schober K, Jenni R, et al. Diagnosis of constrictive pericarditis by pulsed Doppler echocardiography of the hepatic vein. *Am J Cardiol* 1989; 63:483–488.

720. Schiavone WA, Calafiore PA, Salcedo EE. Transesophageal Doppler echocardiographic demonstration of pulmonary venous flow velocity in restrictive cardiomyopathy and constrictive pericarditis. *Am J Cardiol* 1989; 63:1286–1288.

721. Oh JK, Hatle LK, Seward JB, et al. Diagnostic role of Doppler echocardiography in constrictive pericarditis. *J Am Coll Cardiol* 1994; 23:154–162.

722. Klein AL, Cohen GI, Pietrolungo JF, et al. Differentiation of constrictive pericarditis from restrictive cardiomyopathy by Doppler transesophageal echocardiographic measurements of respiratory variations in pulmonary vein flow. *J Am Coll Cardiol* 1993; 22:1935–1943.

723. Garcia MJ, Rodriquez L, Ares M, et al. Differentiation of constrictive pericarditis from restrictive cardiomyopathy: Assessment of left ventricular diastolic velocities in longitudinal axis by Doppler tissue imaging. *J Am Coll Cardiol* 1996; 27:108–114.

723a. Oh JK, Tajik AJ, Appleton CP, et al. Preload reduction to unmask the characteristic Doppler features of constrictive pericarditis: A new observation. *Circulation* 1997; 95:796–799.

723b. Akasaka T, Yoshida K, Yamamuro A, et al. Phasic coronary flow characteristics in patients with constrictive pericarditis: Comparison with restrictive cardiomyopathy. *Circulation* 1997; 96:1874–1881.

724. Izumi S, Mariyama K, Kobayashi S, et al. Phasic venous return abnormality in chronic pulmonary diseases: Pulsed Doppler echocardiographic study. *Intern Med* 1994; 33:326–333.

724a. Boonyaratavej S, Oh JK, Tajik AJ, et al. Comparison of mitral inflow and superior vena cava Doppler velocities in chronic obstructive pulmonary disease and constrictive pericarditis. *J Am Coll Cardiol* 1998; 32:2043–2048.

725. Kodas E, Nishimura RA, Appleton CP, et al. Doppler evaluation of patients with constrictive pericarditis: Use of tricuspid regurgitation velocity curves to determine enhanced ventricular interaction. *J Am Coll Cardiol* 1996; 28;652–657.

726. Capannari TE, Daniels SR, Meyer RA, et al. Sensitivity, specificity, and predictive value of two-dimensional echocardiography in detecting coronary artery aneurysms in patients with Kawasaki disease. *J Am Coll Cardiol* 1986; 7:355–360.

727. Noto N, Ayusawa M, Karasawa K, et al. Dobutamine stress echocardiography for detection of coronary artery stenosis in children with Kawasaki disease. *J Am Coll Cardiol* 1996; 27:1251–1256.

728. Burns JC, Shike H, Gordon JB, et al. Sequelae of Kawasaki disease in adolescents and young adults. *J Am Coll Cardiol* 1996; 28:253–257.

729. Petrovic O, Elsner GB, Wilensky RL, et al. Transthoracic echocardiographic detection of coronary atherosclerosis. *Am J Cardiol* 1996; 77:569–574.

730. Fernandes F, Alam M, Smith S, Khaja F. The role of transesophageal echocardiography in identifying anomalous coronary arteries. *Circulation* 1993; 88:2532–2540.

731. Samdarshi TE, Nanda NC, Gatewood RP Jr, et al. Usefulness and limitations of transesophageal echocardiography in the assessment of proximal coronary artery stenosis. *J Am Coll Cardiol* 1992; 19:572–580.

732. Yamagishi M, Yasu T, Ohara K, et al. Detection of coronary blood flow associated with left main coronary artery stenosis by transesophageal Doppler color flow echocardiography. *J Am Coll Cardiol* 1991; 17:87–93.

733. Redberg RF, Sobol Y, Chou TM, et al. Adenosine-induced coronary vasodilatation during transesophageal Doppler echocardiography: Rapid and safe measurement of coronary flow reserve ratio can predict significant left anterior descending coronary stenosis. *Circulation* 1995; 92:190–196.

734. Zehetgruber M, Mundigler F, Christ G, et al. Estimation of coronary flow reserve by transesophageal coronary sinus Doppler measurements in patients with syndrome X and patients with significant left coronary artery disease. *J Am Coll Cardiol* 1995; 25:1039–1045.

735. Raisinghani A, Ohmori K, Blanchard D, et al. Non-invasive visualization and measurement of coronary blood flow by transthoracic Doppler echocardiography: Initial results (abstr). *Circulation* 1996; 94(I):I-561.

736. Raisinghani A, Cotter B, Ohmori K, et al. Assessment of the effects of sublingual NTG upon intramyocardial blood flow velocity in normals by transthoracic echocardiography (abstr). *Circulation* 1996; 94(I):I-503.

CHAPTER 14

ECG EXERCISE TESTING

Victor F. Froelicher

The exercise test continues to have an integral place in cardiovascular medicine because of its high yield of diagnostic, prognostic, and functional information.[1] When conducting an exercise test, the method and analysis of the data should be determined by the objective of the test. In the clinical setting, the major indications for exercise testing are the diagnosis and prognostication of heart disease. The determination of exercise capacity is helpful in quantifying disability, estimating prognosis, and monitoring the disease state of patients with chronic obstructive pulmonary disease, chronic heart disease, and known coronary heart disease. However, the major emphasis is on the analysis of the electrocardiogram (ECG) in the majority of clinical tests. Also, the reproduction of symptoms such as angina or presyncope is vital for clinical purposes.

METHODS

Excellent guidelines have been updated by organizations such as the American Heart Association, the American Association of Cardiovascular and Pulmonary Rehabilitation, and the American College of Sports Medicine that are based on a multitude of research studies over the last 20 years and have led to greater uniformity in methods.[2-4] These should be followed as closely as possible. General concerns prior to performing an exercise test include safety precautions and equipment needs, patient preparation, choosing a test type, choosing a test protocol, patient monitoring, reasons to terminate a test, and posttest monitoring.

Safety Precautions and Equipment

The safety precautions outlined by the American Heart Association are very explicit in regard to the requirements for exercise testing. Everything necessary for cardiopulmonary resuscitation must be available, and regular drills should be performed to ascertain that both personnel and equipment are ready for a cardiac emergency. The first survey of clinical exercise facilities by Rochmis and Blackburn[5] showed exercise testing to be a safe procedure, with approximately 1 death and 5 nonfatal complications per 10,000 tests. Perhaps due to an expanded knowledge concerning indications, contraindications, and end points, maximal exercise testing appears safer today than 20 years ago.[6] Gibbons et al.[7] reported the safety of exercise testing in 71,914 tests conducted over a 16-year period. The complication rate was 0.8 per 10,000 tests. The authors suggested that the low complication rate may be due to a cool-down walk, but we have observed a low complication rate despite laying patients supine immediately after the test and exercising higher-risk patients.[7]

Besides emergency equipment, the safety and accuracy of the testing equipment should be considered. The treadmill should have front and side rails for subjects to steady themselves. It should be calibrated monthly. Some models can be greatly affected by the weight of the subject and will not deliver the appropriate workload to heavy individuals. An emergency stop button should be readily available to the staff only. A small platform or stepping area at the level of the belt is advisable so that the subject can start the test by "pedaling" the belt with one foot prior to stepping on.

Although numerous clever devices have been developed to automate blood pressure measurement during exercise, none can be recommended. The time-proven method of holding the subject's arm with a stethoscope placed over the brachial artery remains most reliable. The subject's arm should be free of the handrails so that noise is not transmitted up the arm. It is sometimes helpful to mark the brachial artery. An anesthesiologist's auscultatory piece or an electronic microphone can be fastened to the arm. A device that inflates and deflates the cuff on the push of a button can be helpful also.

Exercise Testing

PRETEST PREPARATIONS

During the pretest evaluation, the physician should establish an understanding of any patterns of cardiopulmonary compromise associated with exercise and the patient's usual level of exercise tolerance. The patient should be asked whether he or she has ever become light-headed or fainted while exercising and whether anyone in the family has died suddenly during exercise. The physician also should ask about family history and general medical history, making note of any conditions that may increase the risk of sudden death.

A brief physical examination always should be performed prior to testing to rule out significant outflow obstruction. In some instances, such as when asymptomatic, apparently healthy subjects are being tested for exercise capacity or a repeat treadmill test is being done on a patient whose condition is stable and established, a physician need not be present but should be in close proximity and prepared to respond promptly. The response to signs or symptoms should be moderated by the information the patient gives regarding his or her usual activity. If abnormal findings occur at levels of exercise that the patient usually performs, then it may not be necessary to stop the test because of them. Also, the patient's activity history should help determine appropriate target workload for testing.

Table 14-1 lists the absolute and relative contraindications to performing an exercise test, as well as the factors to consider in assessing the degree of exercise.

Preparations for exercise testing include the following:

1. The subject should be instructed not to eat or smoke at least 2 hours prior to the test and to come dressed for exercise.
2. A brief history and physical examination (particularly noting systolic murmurs) should be accomplished to rule out any contraindications to testing (see Table 14-1).
3. Specific questioning should determine which drugs are being taken, and potential electrolyte abnormalities should be considered. The labeled medication bottles should be brought along so that medications can be identified and recorded. Because of a greater potential for cardiac events with the sudden cessation of β blockers, they should not be automatically stopped prior to testing but done so gradually under physician guidance, only after consideration of the purpose of the test.
4. Pretest standard 12-lead ECGs are necessary in both the supine and standing positions. Good skin preparation must cause some discomfort but is necessary for good conductance and to avoid artifacts. The changes caused by exercise electrode placement can be kept to a minimum by keeping the arm electrodes off the chest, placing them on the shoulders, and by recording the baseline ECG supine[8] (Fig. 14-1). In this situation, the modified exercise limb lead placement can serve well as the reference resting ECG prior to an exercise test.
5. Hyperventilation is not necessary prior to testing. Subjects both with and without disease may or may not exhibit ST-segment changes with hyperventilation; the value of this procedure in lessening the number of false-positive responders is no longer considered useful.

TABLE 14-1 Contraindications to Exercise Testing

ABSOLUTE
Acute myocardial infarction (within 2 d)
Unstable angina not previously stabilized by medical therapy*
Uncontrolled cardiac arrhythmias causing symptoms or hemodynamic compromise
Symptomatic severe aortic stenosis
Uncontrolled symptomatic heart failure
Acute pulmonary embolus or pulmonary infarction
Acute myocarditis or pericarditis
Acute aortic dissection
RELATIVE†
Left main coronary artery stenosis
Moderate stenotic valvular heart disease
Electrolyte abnormalities
Severe arterial hypertension‡
Tachyarrhythmias or bradyarrhythmias
Hypertrophic cardiomyopathy and other forms of outflow tract obstruction
Mental or physical impairment leading to inability to exercise adequately
High-degree atrioventricular block

*Appropriate timing of testing depends on level of risk of unstable angina, as defined by the Agency for Health Care Policy and Research Unstable Angina Guidelines.

†Relative contraindications can be superseded if the benefits of exercise outweigh the risks.

‡In the absence of definitive evidence, the committee suggests a systolic blood pressure of >200mmHg and/or diastolic blood pressure of >110 mmHg.

SOURCE: Modified from Fletcher GF, Balady G, Froelicher VF, et al. Exercise standards: A statement for healthcare professionals from the American Heart Association. Special report. *Circulation* 1995; 91:580–615.

DURING THE TEST

Most problems can be avoided by having an experienced physician, nurse, or exercise physiologist standing next to the subject, measuring blood pressure, and assessing appearance during the test. The exercise technician should operate the recorder and treadmill, take the appropriate tracings, enter data on a form, and alert the physician to any abnormalities that may appear on the monitor scope.

Subjects should be reminded not to grasp the front or side rails because this decreases the work performed and creates noise in the ECG. Hanging on increases exercise time, resulting in an overestimation of exercise capacity.

Target heart rates based on age should not be used because the relationship between maximal heart rate and age is poor, and a wide scatter exists around the many different recommended regression lines. Such heart rate targets result in a submaximal test for some individuals, a maximal test for some, and an unrealistic goal for others. The Borg scales are an excellent means of quantifying an individual's effort. At 1- to 2-min intervals, subjects should be monitored for perceived effort level by using the 6 to 20 Borg scale or the nonlinear 1 to 10 scale of perceived exertion.[9,10]

INDICATIONS FOR TEST TERMINATION

The absolute and relative indications for termination of an exercise test listed in Table 14-2 have been derived from clinical experience. Absolute indications are clear-cut, whereas relative indications sometimes can be disregarded if good clinical judgment is used. Absolute indications include a drop in systolic blood pressure despite an increase in workload, anginal chest pain becoming worse than usual, central nervous system symptoms, signs of poor perfusion (such as pallor, cyanosis, and cold skin), serious dysrhythmias, technical problems with monitoring the patient, patient's request to stop, and marked electrocardiographic changes, e.g., more than 0.3 mV of horizontal or downsloping ST-segment depression or 0.2 mV of ST-segment elevation. Relative indications for termination include other worrisome ST-segment or QRS changes such as excessive junctional depression; increasing chest pain; fatigue, shortness of breath, wheezing, leg cramps, or intermittent claudication; and worrisome appearance, hypertensive response (systolic pressure >260 mmHg, diastolic pressure >115 mmHg), and less serious dysrhythmias including supraventricular tachycardias. If more information is required, the test can be repeated later after symptoms have been stabilized.

AFTER EXERCISE

If maximal sensitivity for ischemic markers is to be achieved with an exercise test, patients should be supine during the postexercise period. It is advisable to record about 10 s of electrocardiographic data while the patient is standing motionless but still experiencing near-maximal heart rate and then have the patient lie down. Having the patient perform a cool-down walk after the test can delay or eliminate the appearance of ST-segment depression.[11] According to the law of LaPlace, the increase in venous return and thus ventricular volume in the supine position increases myocardial oxygen demand. Data from our laboratory[12] demonstrate that having patients lie down enhances ST-segment abnormalities in recovery.

Monitoring should continue for at least 5 min after exercise or until changes stabilize. An abnormal response occurring only in the recovery period is not unusual. All such responses are not false-positive results, as has been suggested. Experiments confirm mechanical dysfunction and electrophysiologic abnormalities in the ischemic ventricle following exercise. A cool-down walk can be helpful when performing tests on patients with an established diagnosis undergoing testing for other than diagnostic reasons, when testing athletes, or when testing patients with dangerous dysrhythmias. When this is the case, it may be preferable to walk slowly (1.0–1.5 mi/h) or continue cycling against zero or minimal resistance (0–25 W when testing with a cycle ergometer) for several minutes following the test.

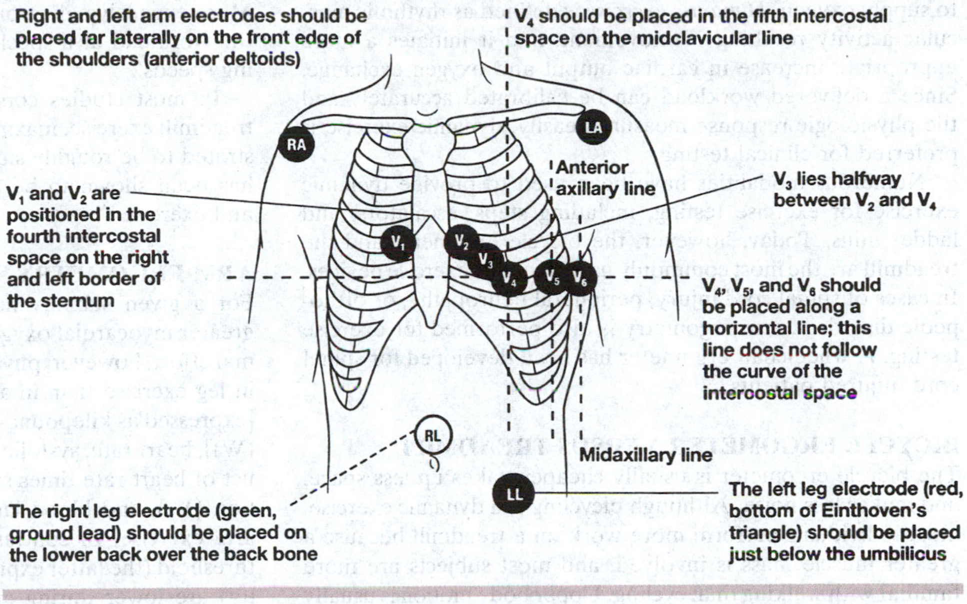
Right and left arm electrodes should be placed far laterally on the front edge of the shoulders (anterior deltoids)
V_4 should be placed in the fifth intercostal space on the midclavicular line
RA
LA
Anterior axillary line
V_3 lies halfway between V_2 and V_4
V_1 and V_2 are positioned in the fourth intercostal space on the right and left border of the sternum
V_1
V_2
V_3
V_4
V_5
V_6
V_4, V_5, and V_6 should be placed along a horizontal line; this line does not follow the curve of the intercostal space
RL
Midaxillary line
LL
The right leg electrode (green, ground lead) should be placed on the lower back over the back bone
The left leg electrode (red, bottom of Einthoven's triangle) should be placed just below the umbilicus

FIGURE 14-1 The correct placement for the 12-lead ECG electrodes during exercise.

Exercise Test Modalities

Three types of exercise can be used to stress the cardiovascular system: isometric, dynamic, and a combination of the two. *Isometric exercise*, defined as constant muscular contraction without movement (such as handgrip), imposes a disproportionate pressure load on the left ventricle relative to the body's ability

TABLE 14-2 Indications for Terminating Exercise Testing

ABSOLUTE INDICATIONS
Drop in systolic blood pressure (persistently below (baseline) despite an increase in workload
Onset of new or increasing anginal chest discomfort
Central nervous system symptoms (ataxia, dizziness, or near syncope)
Evidence of poor peripheral perfusion (cyanosis or pallor)
Serious arrhythmias (i.e., high-grade ventricular, such as multiform complexes, triplets, and runs)
Technical difficulties in monitoring the ECG or systolic blood pressure
Patient's request to stop
RELATIVE INDICATIONS
ST or QRS changes such as excessive (≥3–4 mm) St-segment displacement, junctional depression, or marked QRS axis shift
Increasing chest discomfort
Fatigue, shortness of breath, wheezing, leg cramps, or intermittent claudication
General appearance (see discussion)
Less serious arrhythmias, including supraventricular tachycardias
Development of bundle branch block thar cannot be distinguished from ventricular tachycardia

to supply oxygen. *Dynamic exercise* is defined as rhythmic muscular activity resulting in movement, and it initiates a more appropriate increase in cardiac output and oxygen exchange. Since a delivered workload can be calibrated accurately and the physiologic response measured easily, dynamic exercise is preferred for clinical testing.

Numerous modalities have been used to provide dynamic exercise for exercise testing, including steps, escalators, and ladder mills. Today, however, the bicycle ergometer and the treadmill are the most commonly used dynamic exercise devices. In cases of spinal cord injury, peripheral neuropathy, or orthopedic disorders, arm ergometry is also performed for exercise testing. A wheelchair ergometer has been developed for spinal cord–injured patients.[13]

BICYCLE ERGOMETER VERSUS TREADMILL

The bicycle ergometer is usually cheaper, takes up less space, and makes less noise. Although bicycling is a dynamic exercise, most individuals perform more work on a treadmill because a greater muscle mass is involved, and most subjects are more familiar with walking than cycling. Upper body motion is usually reduced, but care must be taken so that the arms do not perform isometric exercise. The workload administered by the simple bicycle ergometer is not well-calibrated and depends on pedaling speed. It is too easy for a subject to slow pedaling speed during exercise testing and decrease the administered workload. More expensive electronically braked bicycle ergometers keep the workload at a specified level over a wide range of pedaling speeds.

In most studies comparing upright cycle ergometer with treadmill exercise, maximal heart rate values have been demonstrated to be roughly similar, whereas maximal oxygen uptake has been shown to be 6 to 25 percent greater during treadmill exercise.[14–16]

ARM ERGOMETRY

For a given submaximal workload, arm exercise requires a greater myocardial oxygen demand than leg exercise. At maximal effort, however, physiologic responses generally are greater in leg exercise than in arm exercise. At a given power output [expressed as kilopound-meters per minute (kpm/min) or watts (W)], heart rate, systolic and diastolic blood pressure, the product of heart rate times systolic blood pressure, minute ventilation (V_E), and blood lactate concentration are higher during arm exercise. In contrast, stroke volume and the ventilatory threshold (the latter expressed as a percentage of aerobic capacity) are lower during arm exercise compared with leg exercise.[17–20] Since cardiac output is nearly the same in arm and leg exercise at a given oxygen uptake,[21] the elevated blood pressure during arm exercise is due to increased peripheral vascular resistance. Maximal oxygen uptake ($\dot{V}_{O_2max}$) during arm ergometry in men generally varies between 64 and 80 percent of leg

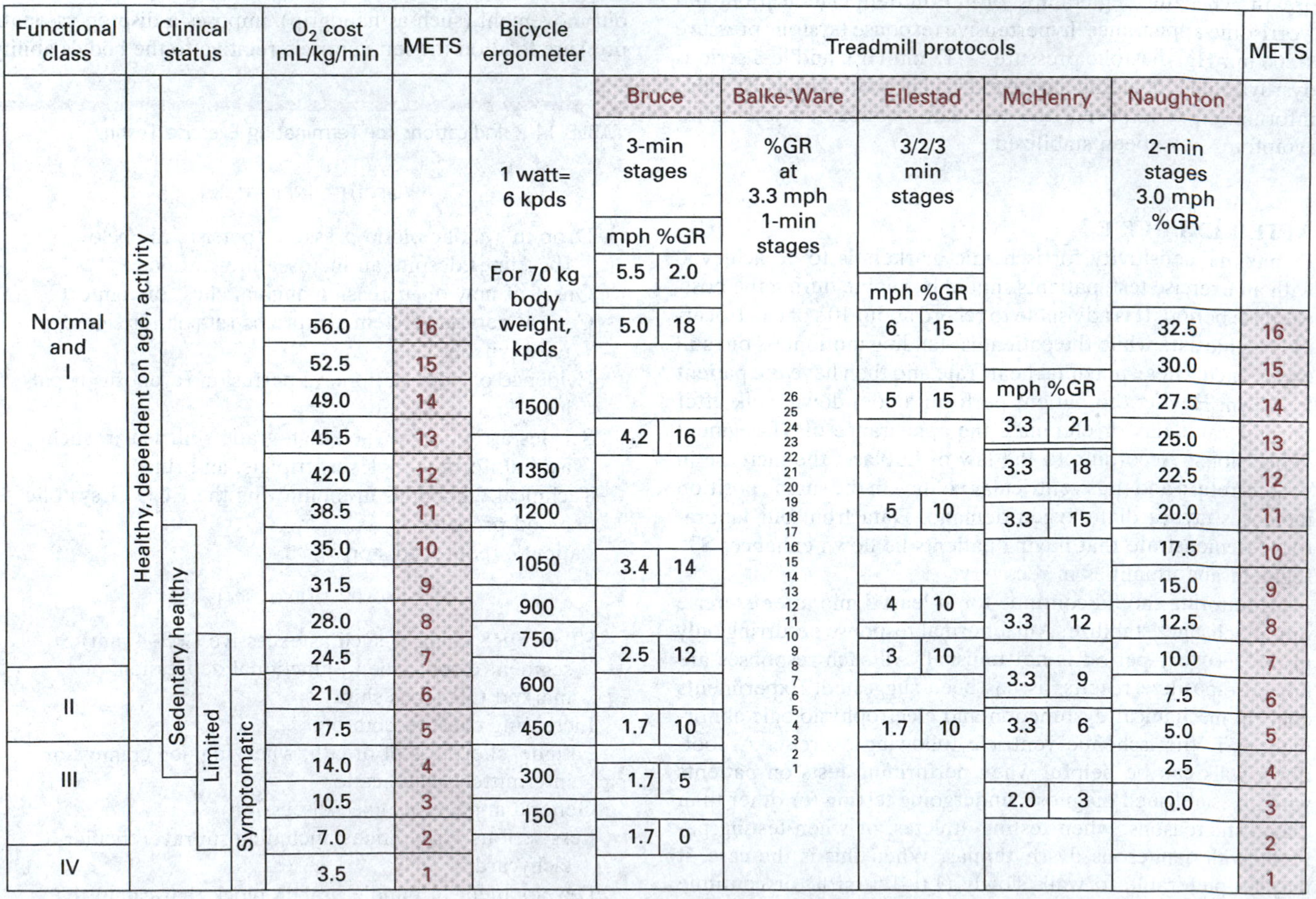

Functional class
Clinical status
O2 cost mL/kg/min
METS
Bicycle ergometer
Treadmill protocols
METS
Normal and I
II
III
IV
Healthy, dependent on age, activity
Sedentary healthy
Limited
Symptomatic
56.0
52.5
49.0
45.5
42.0
38.5
35.0
31.5
28.0
24.5
21.0
17.5
14.0
10.5
7.0
3.5
16 15 14 13 12 11 10 9 8 7 6 5 4 3 2 1
1 watt= 6 kpds
For 70 kg body weight, kpds
1500
1350
1200
1050
900
750
600
450
300
150
Bruce
3-min stages
mph %GR
5.5 2.0
5.0 18
4.2 16
3.4 14
2.5 12
1.7 10
1.7 5
1.7 0
Balke-Ware
%GR at 3.3 mph 1-min stages
26 25 24 23 22 21 20 19 18 17 16 15 14 13 12 11 10 9 8 7 6 5 4 3 2 1
Ellestad
3/2/3 min stages
mph %GR
6 15
5 15
5 10
4 10
3 10
1.7 10
McHenry
mph %GR
3.3 21
3.3 18
3.3 15
3.3 12
3.3 9
3.3 6
2.0 3
Naughton
2-min stages 3.0 mph %GR
32.5
30.0
27.5
25.0
22.5
20.0
17.5
15.0
12.5
10.0
7.5
5.0
2.5
0.0

FIGURE 14-2 The most common protocols, their stages, and the predicted oxygen cost of each stage.

ergometry $\dot{V}_{O_2max}$. Similarly, maximal cardiac output is lower during arm exercise compared with leg exercise, whereas maximal heart rate, systolic blood pressure, and rate-pressure product are comparable[22] or slightly lower[23] during arm exercise.

Exercise Protocols

The many different exercise protocols in use have led to some confusion regarding how physicians compare tests between patients and serial tests in the same patient. The most common protocols, their stages, and the predicted oxygen cost of each stage are illustrated in Fig. 14-2. When treadmill and cycle ergometer testing were first introduced into clinical practice, practitioners adopted protocols used by major researchers.[24–28] The large and uneven work increments in some of these protocols have been shown to result in a tendency to overestimate exercise capacity.[29] Investigators have since recommended protocols with smaller and more equal increments.[30,31] Recent guidelines suggest that protocols should be individualized for each subject such that test duration is approximately 8 to 12 min.

RAMP TESTING

An approach to exercise testing that has gained interest is the ramp protocol, in which work increases constantly and continuously (Fig. 14-3). The recent call for "optimizing" exercise testing would appear to be facilitated by the ramp approach, since work increments are small, and since it allows for increases in work to be individualized, a given test duration can be targeted.

To investigate this, our laboratory compared ramp treadmill and bicycle tests with protocols used more commonly clinically.[32] Ten patients with chronic heart failure, 10 with coronary artery disease who were limited by angina during exercise, 10 with coronary artery disease who were asymptomatic during exercise, and 10 age-matched normal subjects performed three bicycle tests (25 W/2-min stage, 50 W/2-min stage, and ramp) and three treadmill tests (Bruce, Balke, and ramp) in randomized order on different days. Maximal oxygen uptake was significantly higher (18 percent) on the treadmill protocols versus the bicycle protocols collectively, confirming previous observations. Only minor differences in maximal oxygen uptake, however, were observed among the treadmill protocols themselves or among the cycle ergometer protocols themselves. Our observations suggest that (1) oxygen uptake is overestimated from tests that contain large increments in work, and (2) the variability in estimating oxygen uptake from work rate is markedly greater on these tests than for an individualized ramp treadmill test.

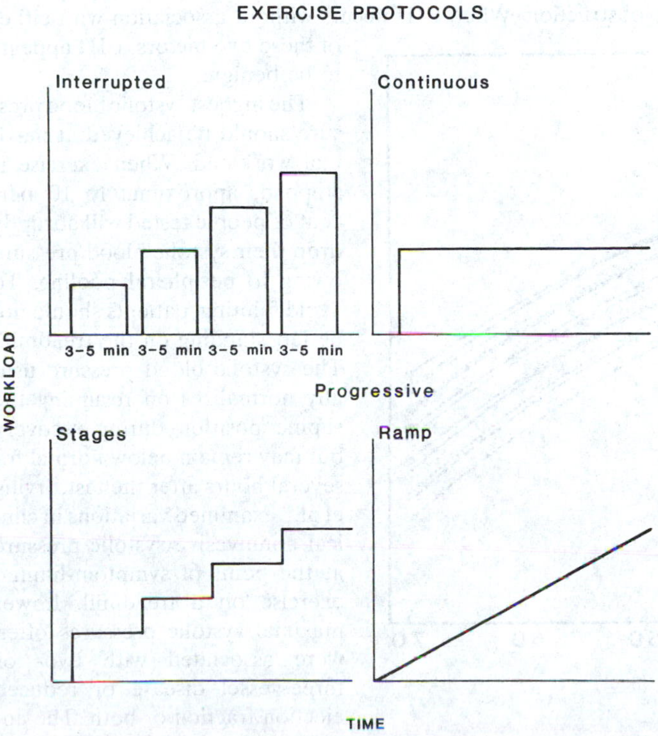

FIGURE 14-3 An approach to exercise testing that has gained interest is the ramp protocol, in which work increases constantly and continuously, as shown in this illustration.

HEMODYNAMIC RESPONSES

Monitoring hemodynamic responses while conducting a treadmill test is vital to assessing the patient's response to exercise. Measurements are used for diagnosis and prognosis and can necessitate test termination.

Maximal Heart Rate

METHODS OF RECORDING

Although measuring a patient's maximal heart rate (HR_{max}) should be a simple matter, the different ways of recording rate and differences in the type of exercise used may affect its measurement. Heart rate drops quickly in recovery and can climb steeply even in the last seconds of exercise. Premature beats can affect averaging and must be eliminated in order to obtain the actual heart rate. Cardiotachometers are incorporated into most exercise test devices but may fail to trigger or may trigger inappropriately on T waves, artifacts, or aberrant beats, thus yielding inaccurate results.

FACTORS LIMITING MAXIMAL HEART RATE

Several factors may affect the HR_{max} during dynamic exercise. HR_{max} declines with advancing years and is affected by gender. Height, weight, and even lean body weight apparently do not affect HR_{max} very much. The physiologic limits on HR_{max} in normal men are determined by rapidity of sinus node recovery, cardiac dimensions, left ventricular filling, and contractile state. Systole has a relatively fixed time interval; in contrast, relatively less time of the cardiac cycle is spent in diastole when heart rate increases. Many studies have reported HR_{max} during treadmill testing in a variety of patients. Regressions with age have varied depending on the population studied and other factors. Figure 14-4 summarizes these studies of HR_{max}.[33,34] In an effort to clarify the relationship between HR_{max} and age, Londeree and Moeschberger[35] performed a comprehensive review of the literature compiling over 23,000 subjects aged 5 to 81 years. A stepwise multiple regression revealed that age alone accounted for 75 percent of the variability; other factors added only about 5 percent and included mode of exercise, level of fitness, and continent of origin but not sex. The 95 percent confidence interval, even when accounting for these factors, was 45 beats per minute (Fig. 14-5). Heart rates at maximal exercise were lower on bicycle ergometry than on the treadmill and lower still with

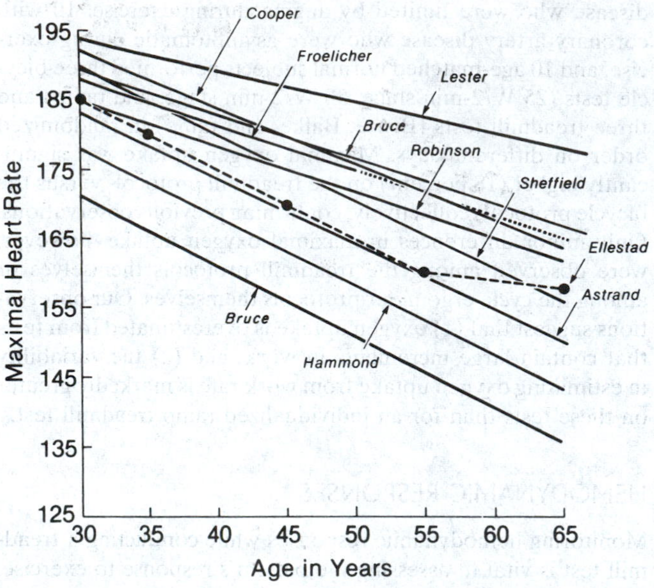

FIGURE 14-4 Many studies, as shown in this illustration, have reported HR_{max} during treadmill testing in a variety of patients. Regressions with age have varied depending on the population studied and other factors.

swimming. Their analysis revealed that trained individuals had significantly lowered maximal heart rates. Graettinger et al.[36] from our laboratory presented clinical, echocardiographic and functional determinants of HR_{max}. Despite controlling for age, activity status, sex, and hypertension, measures of cardiac size and function added little to the prediction of HR_{max}. Most of the variance in HR_{max} was accounted for simply by age. Given the large degree of individual variability in cardiac variables, as well as the HR_{max}/age relationship, HR_{max} always may be a difficult variable to explain.

Another factor that affects HR_{max} and which is important to clinical medicine is bed rest.[37] Altitude may affect the heart rate response to exercise.[38] Some investigators report substantially lower maximal heart rates in well-trained athletes. A final factor determining maximal exercise heart rate is motivation to exert oneself maximally. Older patients may be restrained by poor muscle tone, pulmonary disease, claudication, orthopedic problems, and other noncardiac causes of limitation. The usual decline in HR_{max} with age is not as steep in people who are free from myocardial disease and stay active, but it still occurs. Recent work from the Cleveland Clinic emphasizes the prognostic importance of chronotropic incompetence or heart rate impairment and demonstrates that such a response does not make a test "inadequate."[39]

Blood Pressure Response

Systolic blood pressure should rise with increasing treadmill workload, whereas diastolic blood pressure usually remains about the same (Fig. 14-6). A rising diastolic blood pressure can be associated with coronary heart disease; however, it is more likely a marker for labile hypertension, which leads to coronary disease. A drop in systolic blood pressure below preexercise values is the most ominous criterion, whereas a drop of 20 mmHg or more without a fall below preexercise values appears to have less predictive value.[40] Exercise-induced hypotension (EIH) can be due to either left ventricular dysfunction (as reflected by myocardial infarction status), ischemia, or outflow obstruction. When EIH occurs without association with either of these two factors, EIH appears to be benign.

The highest systolic blood pressure should be achieved at maximal workload. When exercise is stopped, approximately 10 percent of people tested will abruptly drop their systolic blood pressure owing to peripheral pooling. To avoid fainting, patients should not be left standing on the treadmill. The systolic blood pressure usually normalizes on resuming the supine position during recovery but may remain below normal for several hours after the test. Irving et al.[41] examined variations in clinical noninvasive systolic pressure at the point of symptom-limited exercise on a treadmill. Lower maximal systolic pressures often were associated with two- or three-vessel disease or reduced ejection fraction or both. The annual rate of sudden cardiac death decreased from 98 per 1000 men to 25 and 7 per 1000 men as the range of maximal systolic pressure

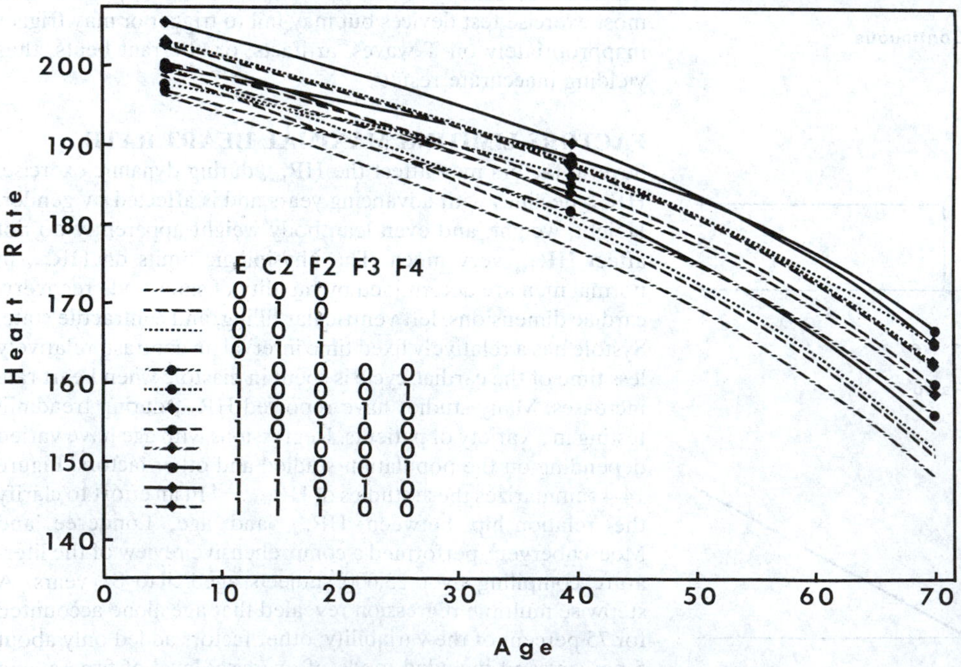

FIGURE 14-5 Plots from literature review of studies involving multiple different types of dynamic exercise by Londeree and Moeschberger. Under E (ergometer), 0 = bicycle and 1 = treadmill; under C2 (European), F2 (sedentary), F3 (active), and F4 (endurance trained), 1 = class inclusion (i.e., a member of that category) and 0 = class exclusion.

increased from less than 140 to 140 to 199 to 200 mmHg or more, respectively.

The 3-min systolic blood pressure ratio is a useful and readily obtainable measure that can be applied in all patients who are undergoing exercise testing for the evaluation of known or suspected ischemic heart disease.[42] The ratio is calculated by dividing the systolic blood pressure 3 min into the recovery phase of a treadmill exercise test by the systolic blood pressure at peak exercise. A 3-min systolic blood pressure ratio greater than 0.90 is considered abnormal. Higher values for the ratio are associated with more extensive coronary artery disease, as well as an adverse prognosis after myocardial infarction.

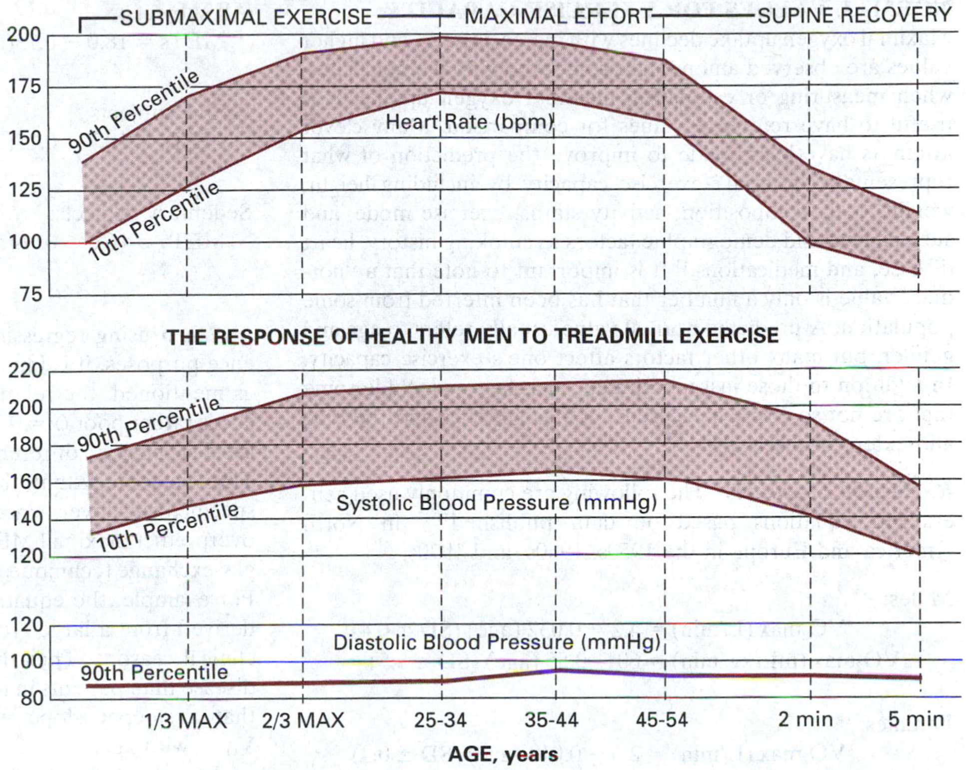

FIGURE 14-6 The results of a large number of normal individuals who underwent a progressive treadmill test shows the response of heart rate and blood pressure according to age.

EXERCISE CAPACITY

Maximal ventilatory oxygen uptake ($\dot{V}_{O_2max}$) is the greatest amount of oxygen that a person can extract from inspired air while performing dynamic exercise involving a large part of the total-body muscle mass. Since maximal ventilatory oxygen uptake is equal to the product of cardiac output and arteriovenous oxygen difference (aV_{O_2}), it is a measure of the functional limits of the cardiovascular system. Maximal a V_{O_2} difference is physiologically limited to roughly 15 to 17 mL/dL. Thus maximal a V_{O_2} difference behaves more or less as a constant, making maximal oxygen uptake an indirect estimate of maximal cardiac output.

Maximal oxygen uptake depends on many factors, including natural physical endowment, activity status, age, and sex, but it is the best index of exercise capacity and maximal cardiovascular function. As a rough reference, the maximal oxygen uptake of the normal sedentary adult is often considered approximately 30 mL O_2/kg per minute, and the minimal level for physical fitness is often considered roughly 40 mL O_2/kg per minute. In general, aerobic training can increase maximal oxygen uptake by up to 25 percent. This increase depends on the initial level of fitness and age as well as the intensity, frequency, and length of training sessions. Individuals performing aerobic training such as distance running can have maximal oxygen uptakes as high as 60 to 90 mL O_2/kg per minute. For convenience, oxygen consumption is often expressed in multiples of basal resting requirements. The metabolic equivalent (MET) is a unit of basal oxygen consumption equal to approximately 3.5 mL O_2 per kilogram of body weight per minute. This is the amount of oxygen required to sustain life in the resting state. Table 14-3 lists clinically meaningful METs for exercise, prognosis, and maximal performance.

It is preferable to estimate an individual's maximal oxygen uptake from the workload reached while performing an exercise test. Maximal oxygen uptake is, of course, most precisely determined by direct measurement using ventilatory gas-exchange techniques. Thus, if quantifying work with precision is an important objective, such as in athletics, research studies, and patients considered for cardiac transplantation, a direct measurement is essential. *Clinical exercise test results always should be reported in METs and not minutes of exercise.* In this way, the results from different protocols and exercise modalities can be compared directly.

TABLE 14-3 Clinically Significant Metabolic Equivalents for Maximum Exercise

1 MET*	Resting
2 METs	Level walking at 2 mi/h
4 METs	Level walking at 4 mi/h
<5 METs	Poor prognosis; usual limit immediately after myocardial infarction, peak cost of basic activities of daily living
10 METs	Prognosis with medical therapy as good as coronary artery bypass surgery
13 METs	Excellent prognosis regardless of other exercise responses
18 METs	Elite endurance athletes
20 METs	World-class athletes

*MET = metabolic equivalent, or a unit of sitting resting oxygen uptake. 1 MET = 3.5 mL/kg/min oxygen uptake.

SOURCE: From Fletcher GF, Balady G, Froelicher VF, et al. Exercise standards: A statement for health professionals from the American Heart Association Writing Group. *Circulation* 1995; 91:580–615. Reproduced with permission from the publisher and authors.

NORMAL VALUES FOR EXERCISE CAPACITY

Maximal oxygen uptake declines with increasing age, and higher values are observed among men compared with women. Thus, when measuring or estimating maximal oxygen uptake, it is useful to have reference values for comparison. Many clever attempts have been made to improve the prediction of what represents a "normal" exercise capacity by including height, weight, body composition, activity status, exercise mode, and such clinical and demographic factors as smoking history, heart disease, and medications.[43] It is important to note that a "normal" value is only a number that has been inferred from some population. A predicted normal value usually refers to age and gender, but many other factors affect one's exercise capacity. In addition to those just mentioned, such factors include some that are not so easily measured, such as genetics and the type and extent of disease.

Regression Equations The following are commonly used generalized equations based on data published[44–47] in North America and Europe in the 1950s, 1960s, and 1970s:

Males:

$$\dot{V}O_2\text{max (L/min)} = 4.2 - 0.032\text{ (age) (SD} \pm 0.4)$$
$$\dot{V}O_2\text{max (mL/kg/min)} = 60 - 0.55\text{ (age) (SD} \pm 7.5)$$

Females:

$$\dot{V}O_2\text{max (L/min)} = 2.6 - 0.014\text{ (age) (SD} \pm 0.4)$$
$$\dot{V}O_2\text{max (mL/kg/min)} = 48 - 0.37\text{ (age) (SD} \pm 7.0)$$

Application of Nomograms Morris et al.[48] developed a nomogram from 1388 male veteran patients (Fig. 14-7). The regression equations derived from the group were:

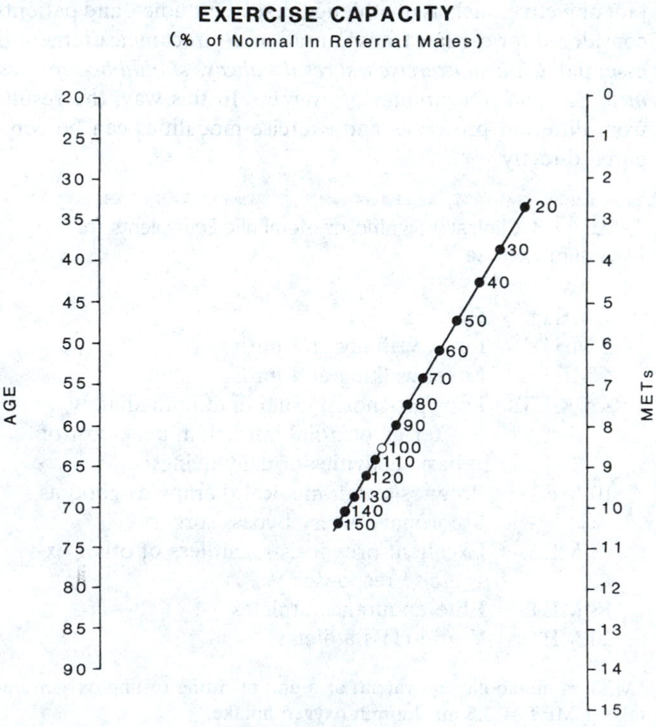

FIGURE 14-7 The exercise capacity nomogram providing a relative estimate of normal for age, with 100 percent being as expected for age in a clinical population.

All subjects:

$$\text{METs} = 18.0 - 0.15(\text{age}),\ \text{SEE} = 3.3,\ r = -0.46,\ p < 0.001$$

Active subjects:

$$\text{METs} = 18.7 - 0.15(\text{age}),\ \text{SEE} = 3.0,\ r = -0.49,\ p < 0.001$$

Sedentary subjects:

$$\text{METs} = 16.6 - 0.16(\text{age}),\ \text{SEE} = 3.2,\ r = -0.43,\ p < 0.001$$

When using regression equations or nomograms for reference purposes, it is important to consider several points. First, as mentioned, the relationship between exercise capacity and age is rather poor ($r = 0.30$ to 0.60). Second, nearly all equations are derived from different populations using different protocols. Thus, to some extent, they are both population- and protocol-specific. Moreover, since treadmill time or workload tends to overpredict maximal METs, it is important to consider whether gas-exchange techniques were used in developing the equations. For example, the equations developed by Morris et al.[48] were derived from a large group of veterans referred for testing for clinical reasons. Thus they had a greater prevalence of heart disease than patients in the other studies, and it is not surprising that a steeper slope was present with a faster decline in $\dot{V}_{O_2max}$ with age.

To account for the differences in measured versus predicted oxygen uptake, a nomogram also was developed using measured oxygen uptake among 244 active or sedentary apparently healthy males (Fig. 14-8). The MET values are shifted downward roughly 1.0 to 1.5 METs for any given age, reflecting the lower but more precise measures of exercise capacity:

All subjects:

$$\text{METs} = 14.7 - 0.11(\text{age})$$

Active subjects:

$$\text{METs} = 16.4 - 0.13(\text{age})$$

Sedentary subjects:

$$\text{METs} = 11.9 - (-0.07)(\text{age})$$

Thus such scales are specific to both the population tested and to whether oxygen uptake was measured directly or predicted. Within these limitations, these equations and the nomograms derived from them can provide reasonable references for normal values and can facilitate communication with patients and between physicians regarding their level of exercise capacity in relation to their peers.

ECG INTERPRETATION

ST Analysis

ST-segment depression is a representation of global subendocardial ischemia, with a direction determined largely by the placement of the heart in the chest. ST-segment depression does not localize coronary artery lesions. V_5 is the lead predomi-

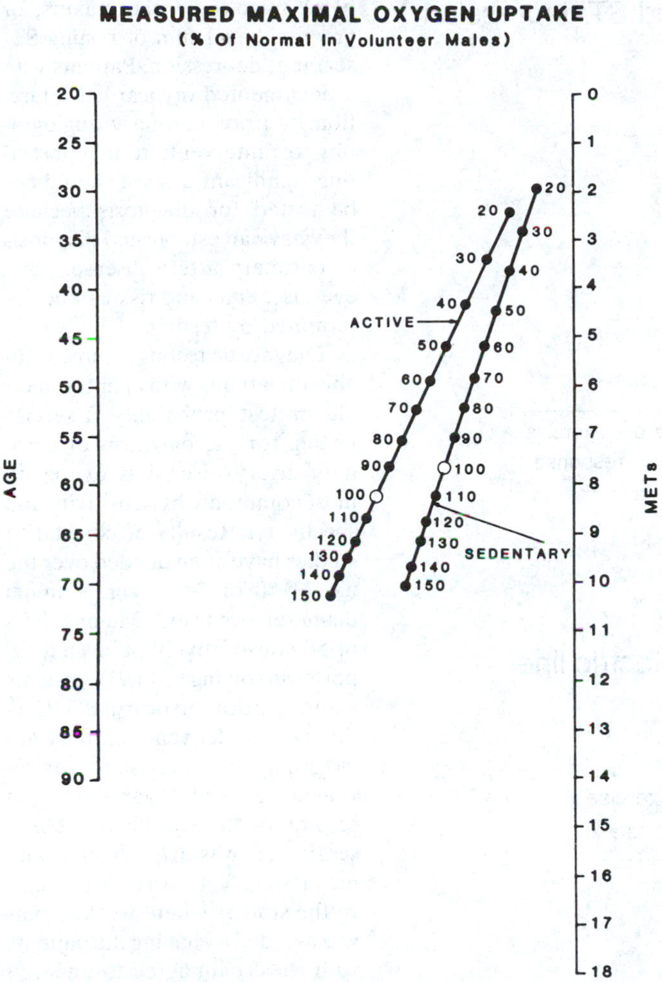

FIGURE 14-8 The exercise capacity nomogram for estimating aerobic impairment in normal male volunteers.

nating in significant ST-segment depression. Depression isolated to other leads is usually due to Q-wave distortion of the resting ECG. ST-segment depression in the inferior leads (II, aV_F) is most often due to the atrial repolarization wave that begins in the PR segment and can extend to the beginning of the ST segment. When ST-segment depression is isolated to these leads and there are no diagnostic Q waves, it is usually a false-positive response.[48] ST-segment depression limited to the recovery period does not generally represent a false-positive response. Inclusion of analysis during this time period increases the diagnostic yield of the exercise test.

When the resting ECG shows Q waves of an old myocardial infarction, ST-segment elevation is due to wall-motion abnormalities, whereas accompanying ST-segment depression can be due to a second area of ischemia or reciprocal changes. When the resting ECG is normal, exercise-induced ST-segment elevation is due to severe ischemia (spasm or a critical lesion), although accompanying ST-segment depression is reciprocal. Such ST-segment elevation is uncommon and very arrhythmogenic, and it localizes the involved coronary artery. Exercise induced ST-segment elevation (not over diagnostic Q waves) and ST-segment depression both represent ischemia, but they are quite distinctive: Elevation is due to transmural ischemia, is arrhythmogenic, has a 0.1 percent prevalence, and localizes the artery where there is spasm or a tight lesion, whereas depression is due to subendocardial ischemia, is not arrhythmogenic, has a 5 to 50 percent prevalence, is rarely due to spasm, and does not localize. Figure 14-9 illustrates the various patterns. The standard criterion for abnormal is 1 mm of horizontal or downsloping ST-segment depression below the PR isoelectric line or 1 mm further depression if there is baseline depression. While computer analysis can help interpretation, the raw data always should be considered first because processing can cause artifacts.[49] Also, though numerous computerized ST-segment scores have been recommended, they only appear to be equivalent to visual interpretation using standard criteria. Most information is available in lead V_5, with maximal exercise and 3 min of recovery being the most important times to look for ST-segment depression.[50] ECG recordings should continue for 5 min in recovery or until any new changes from baseline stabilize.

Nonsustained ventricular tachycardia is uncommon during routine clinical treadmill testing (prevalence <2 percent) and is well tolerated, and its prognosis is determined by the accompanying ischemia and left ventricular damage.[51]

THE ACC/AHA GUIDELINES FOR THE USE OF THE STANDARD EXERCISE TEST

The task force to establish guidelines for the use of exercise testing produced guidelines in 1986 and 1997.[52] The most recent publication had some dramatic changes from the first, including the recommendation that the standard exercise test be the first diagnostic procedure in women and in most patients with resting ECG abnormalities rather than performing imaging studies. The following classifications were used to summarize the indications for exercise testing:

Class I: Conditions for which there is evidence and/or general agreement that the exercise test is useful and effective (appropriate).

Class II: Conditions for which there is conflicting evidence and/or a divergence of opinion about the usefulness/efficacy of the exercise test.

Class IIa: Weight of evidence/opinion is in favor of usefulness/efficacy (probably appropriate).

Class IIb: Usefulness/efficacy is less well established by evidence/opinion (maybe appropriate).

Class III: Conditions for which there is evidence and/or general agreement that the exercise test is not useful/effective and in some cases may be harmful (not appropriate).

Patients who are candidates for exercise testing may have stable symptoms of chest pain, may be stabilized by medical therapy following symptoms of unstable chest pain, or may be postmyocardial infarction or postrevascularization patients. The indications provided in the guidelines are summarized below.

For Diagnosis of Coronary Artery Disease

Exercise testing for the diagnosis of obstructive coronary artery disease is one of the most common uses of exercise testing. Most relative evidence for this use has been gathered in patients presenting with chest pain, although it has been logically extended to those with other symptomology or ECG changes

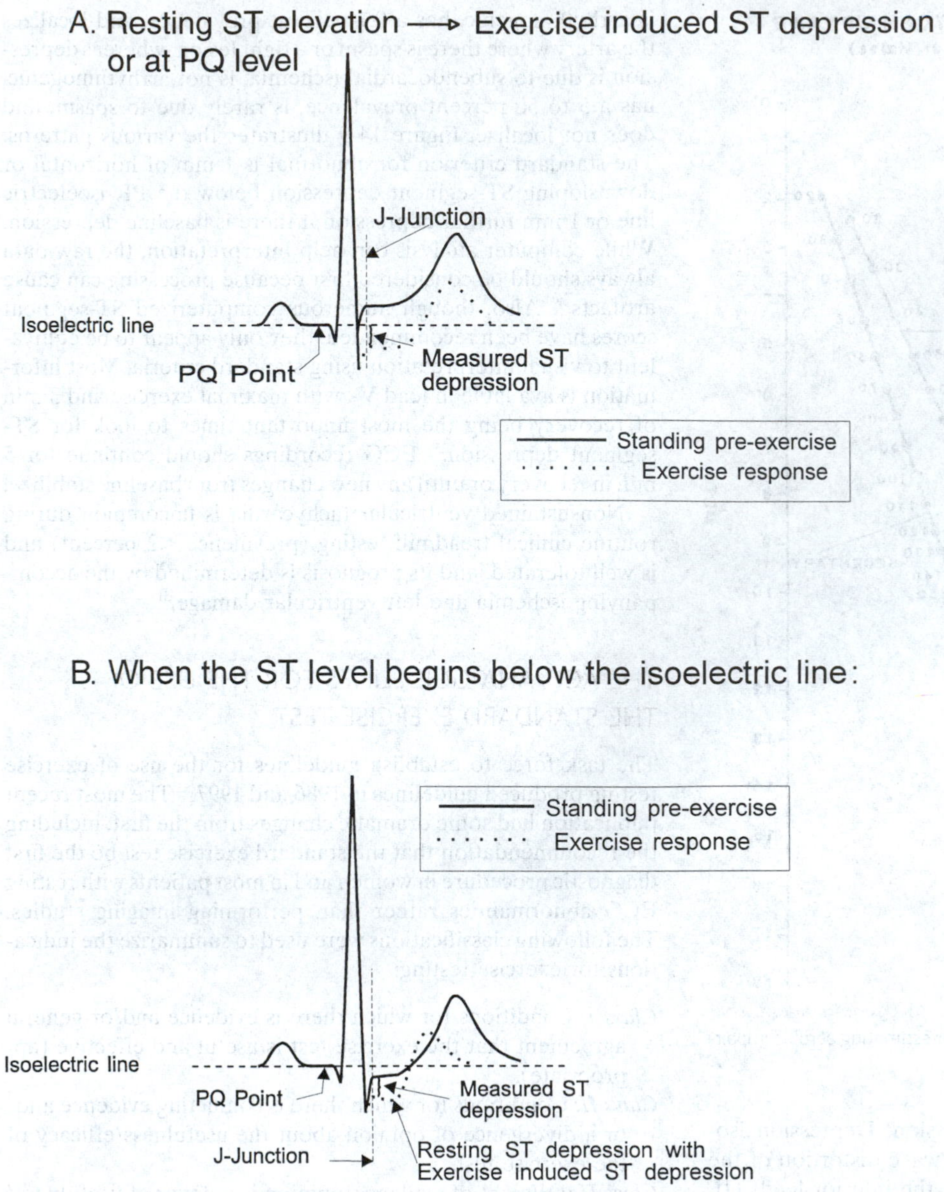

FIGURE 14-9 The various patterns of ST-segment shift. The standard criterion for abnormal is 1 mm of horizontal or downsloping ST-segment depression below the PR isoelectric line or 1 mm further depression if there is baseline depression.

possibly due to coronary artery disease. Appropriate evidence-based use of the test for this application (class I) is in adult patients (including those with complete right bundle branch block or less than 1 mm of resting ST-segment depression) with an intermediate pretest probability of coronary artery disease based on gender, age, and symptoms (Table 14-4) (see also Chap. 40). A probable diagnostic use of the test (less evidence) is in patients with vasospastic angina (class IIa). The efficacy is less well established by evidence/opinion (class IIb) in patients with a low or high pretest probability of coronary artery disease by age, symptoms, and gender and in patients with less than 1 mm of baseline ST-segment depression and taking digoxin or with left ventricular hypertrophy. The exercise ST-segment analysis should not be used for diagnosis (class III) in patients with Wolff-Parkinson-White syndrome, left bundle-branch block, electronic pacemakers, or greater than 1 mm of resting ST-segment depression. Patients with a documented myocardial infarction or prior coronary angiography or intervention demonstrating significant disease should not be tested for diagnosis because they have an established diagnosis of coronary artery disease; however, ischemia and risk can be determined by testing.

Diagnostic testing is most valuable in patients with an intermediate pretest probability. Exercise testing for the diagnosis of coronary artery disease is expressed most commonly by sensitivity and specificity. Results of correlative studies have been divided over the use of 50 or 70 percent luminal diameter occlusion. Metaanalysis of 58 consecutively published reports involving 11,691 patients without prior myocardial infarction who underwent coronary angiography and exercise testing revealed a wide variability in sensitivity and specificity.[53] Mean sensitivity was 67 percent, and mean specificity was 72 percent. In the studies where workup bias was avoided by having the patients with chest pain agree to undergo both procedures, the approximate sensitivity and specificity of 1 mm of horizontal or downsloping ST-segment depression for diagnosis of coronary artery disease were 50 and 90 percent, respectively.[54] The true diagnostic value of the exercise ECG lay in its relatively high specificity, but the sensitivity can be enhanced by consideration of clinical and hemodynamic variables in scores.

Screening for Silent Coronary Artery Disease in Asymptomatic Individuals

A diagnostic test such as the exercise ECG can be used to screen asymptomatic individuals for coronary artery disease. As mentioned previously, there are 12 studies using the exercise test to do such.[55] Patients were screened for silent heart disease using the exercise test and followed for 5 to 10 years for cardiac events. Considerably different results were obtained in these studies according to the end points considered. When angina is included as an end point, nonspecific symptoms in a subject with an abnormal test are more likely to be called coronary artery disease during the follow-up period. Hard end points, such as death or myocardial infarction, eliminate this misclassification and are more appropriate. The first eight screening studies included angina as an end point; the last four have used only hard end points. In Table 14-5, the first eight studies tested 5000 subjects and ranged in size from 113 to 1390 individuals. Sensitivity was 50 percent, specificity was 90 percent, the risk ratio was 9, and the predictive value of a positive response was 25 percent. This means that 1 of 4 patients with abnormal tests went on to have a cardiac event. Remember that some of these events will be angina, which probably was not actually due to coronary artery disease or truly angina. The last four studies have been larger in size and have included only hard end points. The sensitivity of the test has been about 25 percent, specificity about 90 percent, the risk ratio was 4, and the predictive value of a positive response was only 5 percent. This means that only 1 of 20 people with an abnormal test went on to a cardiac event. Because of this very limited predictive value, in any asymptomatic population, screening has not been recommended. It will lead to many other unnecessary tests. Attempts to raise the pretest probability by considering risk factors have not been able to limit the false-positive results and improve the predictive value. Theoretically, this should be possible by using a risk factor score.

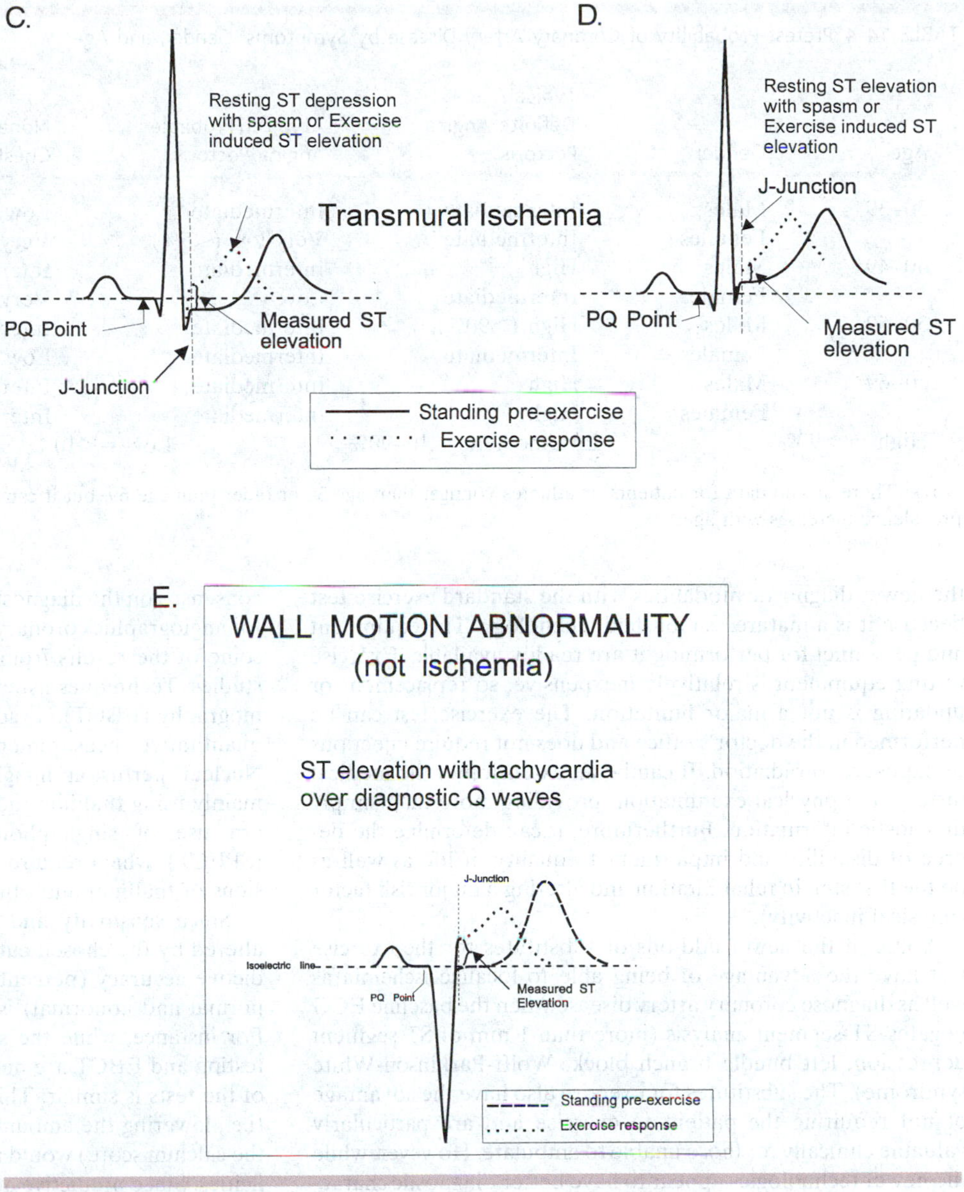

FIGURE 14-9 (*Continued*)

Using soft end points exaggerates the sensitivity and predictive value of the test. This could be avoided by blinding all parties to the test result, but this has been considered unethical. Since some of the asymptomatic individuals developing chest pain really have angina due to coronary artery disease, the sensitivity probably lies between the 25 and 50 percent obtained in the studies that used respectively hard and hard plus soft end points. While soft end points are very appropriate for intervention studies, they can result in important prediction errors in studies of diagnostic procedures.

Screening studies have other important population selection considerations. First, the population should truly be asymptomatic and should represent a random sample of the target population. Volunteers are not appropriate because they usually represent the extremes of the population: the healthiest and those who are concerned for personal reasons regarding their health (i.e., family history, symptoms they chose to deny, etc.). Volunteers represent a subtle form of limited challenge.

There is no class I indication for the use of the exercise test in asymptomatic persons without known coronary artery disease because the available evidence demonstrates a large number of false-positive results in low-prevalence populations.

The efficacy of using the exercise test in evaluation of persons with multiple risk factors or of asymptomatic men older than 40 years and women older than 50 years who plan to start vigorous exercise (especially if sedentary) or who are involved in occupations in which impairment may have an impact on public safety or who are at high risk for coronary artery disease due to other diseases (e.g., chronic renal failure) is possibly but not definitely supported by evidence (class IIb).

The test should not be used for routine screening (class III) of asymptomatic men or women.

COMPARISON WITH OTHER DIAGNOSTIC TESTS

While the studies of the standard exercise test have been helpful in illustrating the problems in demonstrating test characteristics, newer technologies often have been evaluated by studies with the same limitations. Nonetheless, it is appropriate to compare

TABLE 14-4 Pretest Probability of Coronary Artery Disease by Symptoms, Gender, and Age

Age	Gender	Typical/ Definite Angina Pectoris	Atypical/Probable Angina Pectoris	Nonanginal Chest Pain	Asymptomatic
30–39	Males	Intermediate	Intermediate	Low (<10%)	Very low (<5%)
	Females	Intermediate	Very low (<5%)	Very low	Very low
40–49	Males	High	Intermediate	Intermediate	Low
	Females	Intermediate	Low	Very low	Very low
50–59	Males	High (>90%)	Intermediate	Intermediate	Low
	Females	Intermediate	Intermediate	Low	Very low
60–69	Males	High	Intermediate	Intermediate	Low
	Females	High	Intermediate	Intermediate	Low

High = >90% Intermediate = 10–90% Low =<10% Very Low = <5%

NOTE: There are no data for patients or athletes younger than age 30 or older than age 69, but it can be assumed that coronary artery disease prevalence increases with age.

the newer diagnostic modalities with the standard exercise test because it is a mature, established technology. The equipment and personnel for performing it are readily available. Exercise testing equipment is relatively inexpensive, so replacement or updating is not a major limitation. The exercise test can be performed in the doctor's office and does not require injections or exposure to radiation. It can be an extension of the medical history and physical examination, providing more than simply diagnostic information. Furthermore, it can determine the degree of disability and impairment to quality of life as well as be the first step in rehabilitation and altering a major risk factor (physical inactivity).

Some of the newer add-ons or substitutes for the exercise test have the advantage of being able to localize ischemia as well as diagnose coronary artery disease when the baseline ECG negates ST-segment analysis (more than 1 mm of ST-segment depression, left bundle branch block, Wolff-Parkinson-White syndrome). The substitutes for exercise also have the advantage of not requiring the patient to exercise and are particularly valuable clinically for those unable to ambulate. However, while the newer technologies appear to have better diagnostic characteristics, this is not always the case, particularly when more than the ST segments from the exercise test are used in scores.

Test evaluation has been advanced by the critical analysis of Feinstein[56,57] and Guyatt.[58] A number of researchers have applied these guidelines along with meta-analyses to reach a consensus on the diagnostic characteristics of the available tests for angiographic coronary artery disease.[59,60] Table 14-6 presents some of the results from meta-analyses and from multicenter studies. Techniques listed include electron-beam computed tomography (EBCT), a radiographic technique that can make a quantitative measurement of coronary artery calcification.[61,62] Nuclear perfusion imaging includes both the early studies mainly using thallium radiographic images and the more modern use of single-photon-emission computed tomography (SPECT), which requires computer enhancement of the emissions of thallium and other agents.

Since sensitivity and specificity are inversely related and altered by the chosen cut point for normal/abnormal, the predictive accuracy (percentage of patients correctly classified as normal and abnormal) is a convenient way to compare tests. For instance, while the sensitivity and specificity for exercise testing and EBCT are nearly opposite, the predictive accuracy of the tests is similar. This means that altering their cut points (i.e., lowering the amount of ST-segment depression or raising the calcium score) would result in similar sensitivities and specificities. Since predictive accuracy can be thought of as the number of individuals correctly classified out of 100 tested, simply subtracting predictive accuracy provides an estimate of how many more patients are classified by substituting one test for another test. However, this does assume a disease prevalence of 50 percent that is the intermediate probability for appropriate use of diagnostic tests (i.e., predictive accuracy is affected by disease prevalence).

While the nonexercise stress tests are very useful, the results shown in Table 14-6 are probably better than their actual performance because of patient selection. For studies of diagnostic characteristics, patients with a prior myocardial infarction should be excluded because diagnosis of coronary artery disease is already known to be present.

TABLE 14-5 The Twelve Screening Studies

Study	No. of Patients	Sensitivity	Specificity	Relative Risk	Predictive Value (+)
First 8 (soft end points)	5526	50%	90%	9×	25%
Last 4 (hard end points)	12,212	25%	90%	4×	5%

TABLE 14-6 Comparison of Exercise Testing and Add-Ons or Other Test Modalities

Grouping	No. of Studies	Total No. of Patients	Sensitivity	Specificity	Predictive Accuracy
Meta-analysis of standard exercise ECG	147	24,047	68%	77%	73%
Excluding myocardial infarction patients	58	11,691	67%	72%	69%
Limiting workup bias	2	>1,000	50%	90%	69%
Meta-analysis of exercise test scores	24	11,788			80%
Thallium scintigraphy	59	6,038	85%	85%	85%
SPECT without myocardial infarction	27	2,136	86%	62%	74%
Exercise ECHO	58	5,000	84%	75%	80%
Exercise ECHO excluding myocardial infarction patients	24	2,109	87%	84%	85%
Nonexercise stress tests					
Persantine thallium	11	<1,000	85%	91%	87%
Dobutamine ECHO	5	<1,000	88%	84%	86%
Electron-beam computed tomography (EBCT)	5	2,373	90%	45%	61%

EXERCISE TEST SCORES

The exercise testing studies that have considered additional information besides the ST-segment response have been reviewed and demonstrate the improved test characteristics obtained using this approach.[63] Recent publications have extended the Duke prognostic score to diagnosis,[64] and a consensus approach that uses a number of equations appears to make the scores more applicable to other populations.[65]

EXERCISE NUCLEAR PERFUSION AND ECHOCARDIOGRAPHY

A review of the contemporary literature compared the diagnostic performance of exercise echocardiography and exercise nuclear perfusion scanning in the diagnosis of coronary artery disease (see Chaps. 13 and 16).[66] Studies published between January 1990 and October 1997 were identified from MEDLINE search, bibliographies of reviews and original articles, and suggestions from experts in each area. Articles were included if they discussed exercise echocardiography and/or exercise perfusion imaging for detection and/or evaluation of coronary artery disease, if data on coronary angiography were presented as the reference test, and if the absolute numbers of true-positive, false-negative, true-negative, and false-positive observations were available or derivable from the data presented. Studies performed exclusively in patients after myocardial infarction, with coronary interventions, or with recent unstable coronary syndromes were excluded. Two reviewers used a standardized spreadsheet to independently extract data with discrepancies and resolve them by consensus. Forty-four articles met inclusion criteria: 24 reported exercise echocardiography results in 2637 patients with a weighted mean age of 59 years, 69 percent men, 66 percent with angiographic coronary artery disease, and 20 percent with prior myocardial infarction, and 27 reported exercise SPECT in 3237 patients, 70 percent men, 78 percent with angiographic coronary artery disease, and 33 percent with prior myocardial infarction. In pooled data weighted by the sample size of each study, exercise echocardiography had a sensitivity of 85 percent (95% CI, 83–87 percent) with a specificity of 77 percent (95% CI, 74–80 percent). Exercise perfusion yielded a similar sensitivity of 87 percent (95% CI, 86–88 percent) but a lower specificity of 64 percent (95% CI, 60–68 percent).

ELECTRON-BEAM COMPUTED TOMOGRAPHY

Of the angiographic correlative studies of EBCT, we selected the five with more than 200 subjects without overlapping populations. One hundred and sixty men and women with coronary artery disease (45–62 years of age), of whom 138 had obstructive coronary artery disease and 22 had normal coronary arteries, and 56 age-matched healthy control subjects underwent double-helix CT.[67] Sensitivity in detecting obstructive coronary artery disease was high (91 percent); however, specificity was low (52 percent) because of calcification in nonobstructive lesions. A multicenter study evaluated patients referred for angiography.[68] Four hundred and ninety-one symptomatic patients underwent coronary angiography and EBCT at five different centers between 1989 and 1993. Sensitivity of any detectable calcification by EBCT as an indicator of significant stenosis (>50 percent narrowing) was 92 percent, and specificity 43 percent. When these CT images were reinterpreted in a blinded and standardized manner, however, specificity was only 31 percent. In another multicenter study[69] of 710 enrolled patients, 427 had significant angiographic coronary artery disease, and coronary artery calcification was detected in 404, yielding a sensitivity of 95 percent. Of the 283 patients without angiographically significant disease, 124 had negative EBCT studies, for a specificity of 44 percent. Ultrafast CT was used to detect and quantify coronary artery calcium levels in 584 subjects, 19 percent of whom had clinical coronary artery disease.[70] Sensitivity, specificity, and predictive values for clinical coronary artery disease were calculated for several total calcium scores in each decade. For age groups 40 to 49 and 50 to 59 years, a total score of 50 resulted in sensitivities of 71 and 74 percent, respectively, and specificities of 91 and 70 percent, respectively. For the age group 60 to 69 years, a total score of 300 gave a sensitivity of 74 percent and a specificity of 81 percent. Three hundred and sixty-eight symptomatic patients underwent coronary angiography and EBCT at four different centers between April 1989 and December 1993.[71] One hundred and fifty-eight patients (43 percent) had angiographically obstructive coronary artery disease (>50 percent), and 297 (81 percent) had coronary calcification. It appears that even the best studies of EBCT suffer from limited challenge and workup bias so that the true characteristics of this procedure are not known. However, the five studies averaged in the table demonstrated a high sensitivity and a low specificity, with a predictive accuracy of about 61 percent. While adjusting the cut point for calcium density can alter the sensitivity and specificity, EBCT is not more diagnostic for angiographic coronary artery disease than the standard exercise test (see Chaps. 17 and 40).

For Risk Assessment and Prognosis

Risk assessment (prognostication) and postmyocardial infarction are the next two applications of the standard exercise ECG. The test should not be performed in these situations in patients with severe comorbidity likely to limit life expectancy and/or candidacy for revascularization (class III).

The second major application of the exercise ECG test is for assessment of risk and prognosis in patients with symptoms or a prior history of coronary artery disease. Appropriate evidence-based use of the test for this application (class I) is in patients undergoing initial evaluation or in patients with significant change in clinical status with suspected or known coronary artery disease.

Exercise testing may be useful for prognostic assessment of patients on digoxin or with abnormal resting ECGs, but its usefulness is less well established in this setting (class IIb). Also, the exercise test may still provide prognostic information (particularly exercise capacity) in patients with preexcitation, ventricular paced rhythm, more than 1 mm of ST-segment depression, and left bundle-branch block but cannot be used to identify ischemia. The test also may be used in patients with a stable clinical course who undergo periodic monitoring to guide treatment. The Duke treadmill score (see nomogram in Fig. 14-10) incorporates two of the major prognostic markers (i.e., exercise capacity[72] and exercise-induced ischemia) and was strongly recommended.[73]

After Myocardial Infarction

The third major application of the exercise ECG is for patients within 2 months of a myocardial infarction.[74] Appropriate evidence-based uses of the test for prognostic assessment, activity prescription, evaluation of medical therapy, and cardiac rehabilitation of these patients (class I) are (1) before discharge for prognostic assessment, activity prescription, or evaluation of medical therapy (submaximal at about 4–7 days), (2) early after discharge if the predischarge exercise test was not done (symptom-limited, about 14–21 days), and (3) late after discharge if the early exercise test was submaximal (symptom-limited, about 3–6 weeks). A probable postmyocardial infarction use of the test (less evidence) is for activity counseling and/or exercise training as part of cardiac rehabilitation in patients who have undergone coronary revascularization (class IIa). The efficacy is less well established by evidence/opinion (class IIb) before discharge in patients who have undergone cardiac catheterization to identify ischemia in the distribution of a coronary lesion of borderline severity or in those with the above-mentioned ECG abnormalities that interfere with the recognition of ischemia or for periodic monitoring in patients who continue to participate in exercise training or cardiac rehabilitation.

A meta-analysis of 28 studies involving 15,613 patients found that markers of ventricular dysfunction were more accurate predictors of adverse cardiac events after myocardial infarction than measures of exercise-induced ischemia.[75] A similar study in the postthrombotic age considered other test modalities and validated these conclusions.[76–78]

Exercise Testing Using Ventilatory Gas Analysis

Evidence supports the addition of ventilatory gas analysis to the exercise test (class I) for the evaluation of exercise capacity and response to therapy in patients with heart failure who are being considered for heart transplantation and when assistance is needed in differentiating cardiac versus pulmonary limitations as a cause of exercise-induced dyspnea or impaired exercise capacity.

A probable reason to add gas analysis to the exercise test (less evidence, class IIa) is for the evaluation of exercise capacity when indicated for medical reasons in patients in whom subjective assessment of maximal exercise is unreliable.

The efficacy of adding gas analysis is less well established by evidence/opinion (class IIb) for evaluation of the patient's response to specific therapeutic interventions in which improvement of exercise tolerance is an important goal or end point or for deter-

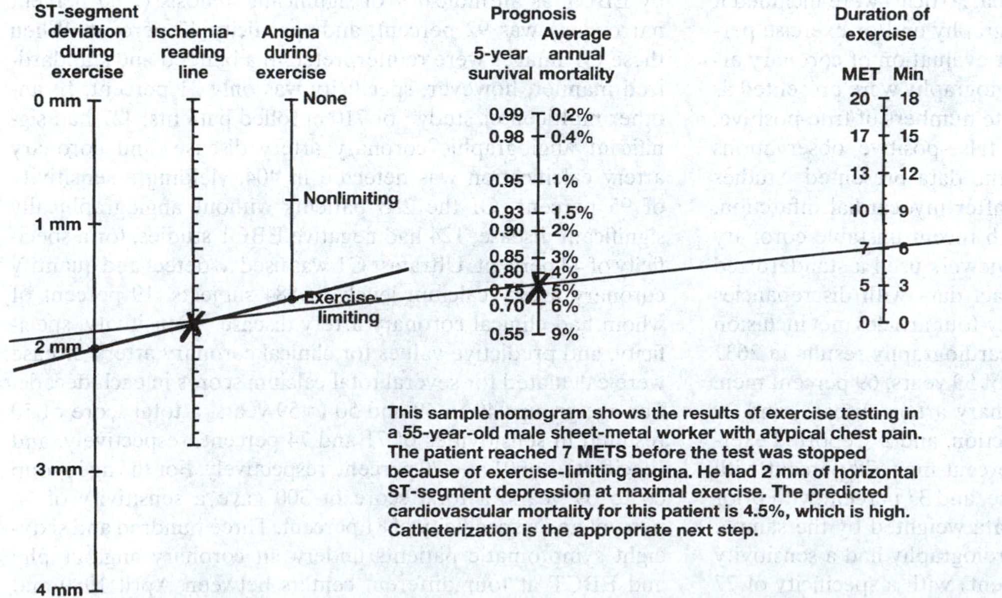

FIGURE 14-10 The Duke treadmill score nomogram for predicting cardiovascular mortality from treadmill testing.

mination of the intensity for exercise training as part of comprehensive cardiac rehabilitation.

Expired gas analysis is not indicated (class III) routinely to evaluate exercise capacity.

Valvular Heart Disease

There is no evidence-based class I indication for testing patients with valvular heart disease. The test possibly can be used, although there are no convincing data to evaluate exercise capacity in patients with valvular heart disease (class IIb). The exercise ECG should not be used to diagnose coronary artery disease in patients with valvular heart disease (class III).

Before and After Revascularization

The evidence supports the use of the exercise ECG test to demonstrate ischemia before revascularization and to evaluate patients with recurrent symptoms suggesting ischemia after revascularization (class I).

A probable use of the test (less evidence) is after discharge for activity counseling and/or exercise training as part of cardiac rehabilitation in patients who have undergone coronary revascularization (class IIa). The efficacy is less well established by evidence/opinion (class IIb) for detection of restenosis in selected high-risk asymptomatic patients within the first months after angioplasty or for periodic monitoring of selected high-risk asymptomatic patients for restenosis, graft occlusion, or disease progression.

The test should not be used to localize ischemia for determining the site of intervention or for routine periodic monitoring of asymptomatic patients after percutaneous transluminal coronary angioplasty (PTCA) or coronary artery bypass grafting without specific indications (class III).

Since the guidelines were published, investigators have found nuclear perfusion exercise testing to be important in prognostication in patients after coronary artery bypass grafting.[78]

Investigation of Heart Rhythm Disorders

The exercise test should be used to identify the appropriate settings in patients with rate-adaptive pacemakers (class I).

A probable use of the test (less evidence) is for evaluation of patients with known or suspected exercise-induced arrhythmias or for evaluation of medical, surgical, or ablative therapy in patients with exercise-induced arrhythmias (including atrial fibrillation) (class IIa). The efficacy is less well established by evidence/opinion for investigation of isolated ventricular ectopic beats in middle-aged patients without other evidence of coronary artery disease (class IIb).

The test should not be used to investigate isolated ectopic beats in young patients (class III).

SUMMARY

While cardiologists are frequently relinquishing the performance of the standard exercise test to internists and family practitioners, it is important that the latter be properly trained to do it correctly and have expertise in its interpretation. However, the addition of echocardiography or myocardial perfusion imaging does not negate the importance of the ECG or clinical and hemodynamic responses to exercise. The exercise test complements the medical history and the physical examination, and it remains the second most commonly performed cardiologic procedure next to the routine ECG. The renewed efforts to control costs undoubtedly will support the role of the exercise test. Convincing evidence that treadmill scores enhance the diagnostic and prognostic power of the exercise test certainly has cost-efficacy implications. In addition, there is also evidence that measurement of expired gases improves the prognostic power of the test in certain groups of patients and helps to determine if exercise intolerance is due to the heart or the lungs.

Use of proper methodology is critical for safety and obtaining accurate and comparable results. The use of specific criteria for exclusion and termination, interaction with the subject, and appropriate emergency equipment are essential. The exercise protocol should be progressive, with even increments in speed and grade whenever possible.

The following rules are important to follow for getting the most information from the standard exercise test:

- The treadmill protocol should be adjusted to the patient, and one protocol is not appropriate for all patients; consider using a manual or automated ramp protocol.
- Report exercise capacity in METs, not minutes of exercise.
- Hyperventilation prior to testing is not indicated.
- ST-segment measurements should be made at ST0 (J-junction) and ST-segment depression should only be considered abnormal if horizontal or downsloping.
- Raw ECG waveforms should be considered first and then supplemented by computer-enhanced (filtered and averaged) waveforms when the raw data are acceptable.
- Patients should be placed supine as soon as possible after exercise, with a cool-down walk avoided in order for the test to have its greatest diagnostic value.
- The 3-min recovery period is critical to include in analysis of the ST-segment response.
- Measurement of systolic blood pressure during exercise is extremely important, and exertional hypotension is ominous; at this point, only manual blood pressure measurement techniques are valid.
- Age-predicted heart rate targets are largely useless because of the wide scatter for any age; a relatively low heart rate can be maximal for a patient of a given age and submaximal for another. Thus a test should not be considered nondiagnostic if a percentage of age-predicted maximal heart rate (i.e., 85 percent) is not reached. In fact, chronotropic incompetence or heart rate impairment has important prognostic implications.
- Calculation of the Duke treadmill score for every patient should be considered.
- Other predictive equations should also be considered as part of the treadmill report.

To ensure the safety of exercise testing, the following list of the most dangerous circumstances in the exercise testing laboratory should be recognized:

- Testing patients with aortic valvular disease should be done with great care because they may develop severe cardiovascular complications. Thus, a physical examination including assessment of systolic murmurs should be done before all exercise tests. If a significant murmur is heard, an echocardiogram should be considered.

- When patients exhibit ST-segment elevation without diagnostic Q waves due to transmural ischemia, this can be associated with dangerous arrhythmias and infarction. The incidence is about 1 in 1000 clinical tests and usually occurs in V_2 or aV_F rather than V_5.
- When a patient with an ischemic cardiomyopathy exhibits severe chest pain due to ischemia (angina pectoris), a cool-down walk is advisable because the ischemia can worsen in the recovery period.
- When a patient develops exertional hypotension accompanied by ischemia (angina or ST-segment depression) or when it occurs in a patient with a history of congestive heart failure, cardiomyopathy, or recent myocardial infarction, safety is a serious issue.
- When a patient with a history of sudden death or collapse during exercise develops premature ventricular contractions that become frequent, a cool-down walk is advisable because the premature ventricular contractions can increase in recovery, particularly after an abrupt cessation of exercise.

The ACC/AHA guidelines for exercise testing clearly indicate the correct uses of exercise testing. Since the last guidelines, it has been extended as the first diagnostic test in women and in individuals with right bundle branch block and resting ST-segment depression. The Duke prognostic nomogram and scores increase the value of the exercise test. In fact, the use of scores results in test characteristics that approach the nuclear and echocardiographic add-ons to the exercise test.

References

1. Froelicher VF, Myers J. *Exercise and the Heart*, 4th ed. Philadelphia: Saunders; 1999.
2. American Association of Cardiovascular and Pulmonary Rehabilitation. *Guidelines for Cardiac Rehabilitation Programs.* Champaign, IL: Human Kinetics; 1998.
3. American College of Sports Medicine. *Guidelines for Exercise Testing and Exercise Prescription*, 6th ed. Philadelphia: Lea & Febiger; 1999.
4. Fletcher GF, Froelicher VF, Hartley LH, et al. Exercise standards: A statement for health professionals from the American Heart Association. *Circulation* 1990; 82:2286–2321. *Revised Circulation* 1995; 91:580–632.
5. Rochmis P, Blackburn H. Exercise tests: A survey of procedures, safety, and litigation experience in approximately 170,000 tests. *JAMA* 1971; 217:1061–1066.
6. Franklin BA, Gordon S, Timmis GC, O'Neill WW. Is direct physician supervision of exercise stress testing routinely necessary? *Chest* 1997; 111(2):262–265.
7. Gibbons L, Blair SN, Kohl HW, Cooper K. The safety of maximal exercise testing. *Circulation* 1989; 80:846–852.
8. Yang JC, Wesley RC, Froelicher VF. Ventricular tachycardia during routine treadmill testing. *Arch Intern Med* 1991; 151:349–353.
9. Gamble P, McManus H, Jensen D, Froelicher VF. A comparison of the standard 12-lead electrocardiogram to exercise electrode placement. *Chest* 1984; 85:616–622.
10. Borg G. *Borg's Perceived Exertion Scales.* Champaign, IL: Human Kinetics; 1998.
11. Myers JN. Perception of chest pain during exercise testing in patients with coronary artery disease. *Med Sci Sports Exerc* 1994; 26(9):1082–1086.
12. Gutman RA, Alexander ER, Li YB, et al. Delay of ST depression after maximal exercise by walking for two minutes. *Circulation* 1970; 42:229–233.
13. Lachterman B, Lehmann KG, Abrahamson D, Froelicher VF. "Recovery only" ST segment depression and the predictive accuracy of the exercise test. *Ann Intern Med* 1990; 112:11–16.
14. Phillips W, Kiratli J, Sarkarati M, et al. The effect of spinal cord injury on the heart and cardiovascular fitness. *Curr Probl Cardiol* 1998; 23:641–720.
15. Myers J, Froelicher VF. Optimizing the exercise test for pharmacological investigations. *Circulation* 1990; 82:1839–1846.
16. Hambrecht RP, Schuler GC, Muth T, et al. Greater diagnostic sensitivity of treadmill versus cycle exercise testing of asymptomatic men with coronary artery disease. *Am J Cardiol* 1992; 70(2):141–146.
17. Buchfuhrer MJ, Hansen JE, Robinson TE, et al. Optimizing the exercise protocol for cardiopulmonary assessment. *J Appl Physiol* 1983; 55:1558–1564.
18. Astrand P, Ekblom B, Messin R, et al. Intra-arterial blood pressure during exercise with different muscle groups. *J Appl Physiol* 1965; 20:253–256.
19. Bevegard S, Freyschuss U, Strandell T. Circulatory adaptation to arm and leg exercise in supine and sitting positions. *J Appl Physiol* 1966; 21:37–46.
20. Bobbert AC. Physiological comparison of three types of ergometry. *J Appl Physiol* 1960; 15:1007–1014.
21. Davis JA, Vodak P, Wilmore JH, et al. Anaerobic threshold and maximal aerobic power for three modes of exercise. *J Appl Physiol* 1976; 41:544–550.
22. Asmussen E, Nielsen M. Regulation of body temperature during work performed with arms and legs. *Acta Physiol Scand* 1947; 14:373–382.
23. Balady GJ, Weiner DA, McCabe CH, Ryan TJ. Value of arm exercise testing in detecting coronary artery disease. *Am J Cardiol* 1985; 55(1):37–39.
24. DeBusk RF, Valdez R, Houston N, Haskell W. Cardiovascular responses to dynamic and static effort soon after myocardial infarction: Application to occupational work assessment. *Circulation* 1978; 58:368–375.
25. Balke B, Ware R. An experimental study of physical fitness of air force personnel. *US Armed Forces Med J* 1959; 10:675–688.
26. Astrand PO, Rodahl K. *Textbook of Work Physiology.* New York: McGraw-Hill; 1986:331–365.
27. Bruce RA. Exercise testing of patients with coronary heart disease. *Ann Clin Res* 1971; 3:323–330.
28. Ellestad MH, Allen W, Wan MCK, Kemp G. Maximal treadmill stress testing for cardiovascular evaluation. *Circulation* 1969; 39:517–522.
29. Froelicher VF, Brammel H, Davis G, et al. A comparison of three maximal treadmill exercise protocols. *J Appl Physiol* 1974; 36:720–725.
30. Sullivan M, McKirnan MD. Errors in predicting functional capacity for postmyocardial infarction patients using a modified Bruce protocol. *Am Heart J* 1984; 107:486–491.
31. Webster MWI, Sharpe DN. Exercise testing in angina pectoris: The importance of protocol design in clinical trials. *Am Heart J* 1989; 117:505–508.
32. Panza JA, Quyyumi AA, Diodati JG, et al. Prediction of the frequency and duration of ambulatory myocardial ischemia in patients with stable coronary artery disease by determination of the ischemic threshold from exercise testing: Importance of the exercise protocol. *J Am Coll Cardiol* 1991; 17:657–663.
33. Myers J, Buchanan N, Walsh D, et al. Comparison of the ramp versus standard exercise protocols. *J Am Coll Cardiol* 1991; 17:1334–1342.

34. Bruce RA, Gey GO Jr, Cooper MN, et al. Seattle Heart Watch: Initial clinical, circulatory and electrocardiographic response to maximal exercise. *Am J Cardiol* 1974; 33:459.
35. Cooper KH, Purdy JG, White SR, et al. Age-fitness adjusted maximal heart rates. *Med Sport* 1977; 10:78–88.
36. Londeree BR, Moeschberger ML. Influence of age and other factors on maximal heart rate. *J Cardiac Rehabil* 1984; 4:44–49.
37. Graettinger W, Smith D, Neutel J, et al. Influence of LV chamber size on maximal heart rate. *Circulation* 1991; 84:II–187.
38. Convertino V, Hung J, Goldwater D, et al. Cardiovascular responses to exercise in middle-aged man after 10 days of bed rest. *Circulation* 1982; 65:134–140.
39. Hartley LH, Vogel JA, Cruz JC. Reduction of maximal exercise heart rate at altitude and its reversal with atropine. *J Appl Physiol* 1974; 36:362–365.
40. Lauer M, Mehta R, Pashkow F, et al. Association of chronotropic incompetence with echocardiographic ischemia and prognosis. *J Am Coll Cardiol* 1998; 32(5):1280–1286.
41. Dubach P, Froelicher VF, Klein J, et al. Exercise-induced hypotension in a male population: Criteria, causes, and prognosis. *Circulation* 1988; 78:1380–1387.
42. Irving JB, Bruce RA, DeRouen TA. Variations in and significance of systolic pressure during maximal exercise (treadmill) testing. *Am J Cardiol* 1977; 39(6):841–848.
43. Taylor AJ, Beller GA. Postexercise systolic blood pressure response: Clinical application to the assessment of ischemic heart disease. *Am Fam Phys* 1998; 58(5):1126–1130.
44. Wasserman K, Hansen JE, Sue DY, Whipp BJ. *Principles of Exercise Testing and Interpretation.* Philadelphia: Lea & Febiger; 1999:72–86.
45. Shephard RJ. *Endurance Fitness*. Toronto: University of Toronto Press; 1969.
46. Astrand P. Human physical fitness, with special reference to sex and age. *Physiol Rev* 1956; 36(suppl 2):307–335.
47. Astrand I. Aerobic work capacity in men and women with special reference to age. *Acta Physiol Scand* 1960; 49(suppl 196):1–92.
48. Morris CK, Myers J, Kawaguchi T, et al. A nomogram based on metabolic equivalents and age for aerobic exercise capacity in men. *J Am Coll Cardiol* 1993; 22:175–182.
49. Miranda CP, Liu J, Kadar A, et al. Usefulness of exercise-induced ST-segment depression in the inferior lead. *Am J Cardiol* 1992; 69(4):303–307.
50. Milliken JA, Abdollah H, Burggraf GW. False-positive treadmill exercise tests due to computer signal averaging. *Am J Cardiol* 1990; 65:946–948.
51. Lachterman B, Lehmann KG, Abrahamson D, Froelicher VF. "Recovery only" ST-segment depression and the predictive accuracy of the exercise test. *Ann Intern Med* 1990; 112(1):11–16.
52. Yang JC, Wesley RC, Froelicher VF. Ventricular tachycardia during routine treadmill testing: Risk and prognosis. *Arch Internal Med* 1991; 151:349–353.
53. Gibbons RJ, Balady GJ, Beasley JW, et al. ACC/AHA guidelines for exercise testing: A report of the American College of Cardiology/American Heart Association Task Force on Practice Guidelines (Committee on Exercise Testing). *J Am Coll Cardiol* 1997; 30(1):260–311.
54. Gianrossi R, Detrano R, Lehmann K, et al. Exercise-induced ST depression in the diagnosis of coronary artery disease: A meta-analysis. *Circulation* 1989; 80:87–98.
55. Froelicher VF, Lehmann KG, Thomas R, et al. The electrocardiographic exercise test in a population with reduced workup bias: Diagnostic performance, computerized interpretation, and multivariable prediction. Veterans Affairs Cooperative Study in Health Services No. 016 (QUEXTA) Study Group (Quantitative Exercise Testing and Angiography). *Ann Intern Med* 1998; 128(12 pt 1):965–974.
56. Froelicher VF, Quaglietti, S. *Handbook of Exercise Testing.* Boston: Little, Brown; 1995.
57. Philbrick JT, Horowitz, Feinstein AR. Methodological problems of exercise testing for coronary artery disease: Groups, analysis and bias. *Am J Cardiol* 1989; 64:1117–1122.
58. Reid M, Lachs M, Feinstein A. Use of methodological standards in diagnostic test research. *JAMA* 1995; 274:645–651.
59. Guyatt GH. Readers' guide for articles evaluating diagnostic tests: What ACP Journal Club does for you and what you must do yourself. *ACP Journal Club* 1991; 115:A-16.
60. Gianrossi R, Detrano R, Columbo A, Froelicher VF. Cardiac fluoroscopy for the diagnosis of coronary artery disease: A meta-analytic review. *Am Heart J* 1990; 120(5):1179–1188.
61. Detrano R, Janosi A, Marcondes G, et al. Factors affecting sensitivity and specificity of a diagnostic test: The exercise thallium scintigram. *Am J Med* 1988; 84:699–710.
62. Wexler L, Brundage B, Crouse J, et al. Coronary artery calcification: Pathophysiology, epidemiology, imaging methods, and clinical implications. A statement for health professionals from the American Heart Association Writing Group. *Circulation* 1996; 94(5):1175–1192.
63. Fiorino AS. Electron-beam computed tomography, coronary artery calcium, and evaluation of patients with coronary artery disease. *Ann Intern Med* 1998; 128(10):839–847.
64. Yamada H, Do D, Morise A, Froelicher V. Review of studies utilizing multi-variable analysis of clinical and exercise test data to predict angiographic coronary artery disease. *Prog Cardiovasc Dis* 1997; 39:457–481.
65. Shaw LJ, Peterson ED, Shaw LK, et al. Use of a prognostic treadmill score in identifying diagnostic coronary disease subgroups. *Circulation* 1998; 98(16):1622–1630.
66. Do D, West JA, Morise A, Froelicher V. A consensus approach to diagnosing coronary artery disease based on clinical and exercise test data. *Chest* 1997; 111(6):1742–1749.
67. Fleischmann KE, Hunink MG, Kuntz KM, Douglas PS. Exercise echocardiography or exercise SPECT imaging? A meta-analysis of diagnostic test performance. *JAMA* 1998; 280(10):913–920.
68. Shemesh J, Apter S, Rozenman J, et al. Calcification of coronary arteries: Detection and quantification with double-helix CT. *Radiology* 1995; 197(3):779–783.
69. Detrano R, Hsiai T, Wang S, et al. Prognostic value of coronary calcification and angiographic stenoses in patients undergoing coronary angiography. *J Am Coll Cardiol* 1996; 27(2):285–290.
70. Budhoff MJ, Georgiou D, Brody A, et al. Ultrafast computed tomography as a diagnostic modality in the detection of coronary artery disease: A multicenter study. *Circulation* 1996; 93:898–904.
71. Agatston AS, Janowitz WR, Hildner FJ, et al. Quantification of coronary artery calcium using ultrafast computed tomography. *J Am Coll Cardiol* 1990; 15(4):827–832.
72. Kennedy J, Shavelle R, Wang S, et al. Coronary calcium and standard risk factors in symptomatic patients referred for coronary angiography. *Am Heart J* 1998; 135(4):696–702.
73. Morris CK, Ueshima K, Kawaguchi T, et al. The prognostic value of exercise capacity: A review. *Am Heart J* 1991; 122:1423–1431.
74. Mark DB, Hlatky MA, Harrell FE, et al. Exercise treadmill score for predicting prognosis in coronary artery disease. *Ann Intern Med* 1987; 106:793–800.
75. Ryan TJ, Anderson JL, Antman EM, et al. ACC/AHA guidelines for the management of patients with acute myocardial infarction: Executive summary. A report of the American College of Cardiology/American Heart Association Task Force on Practice Guidelines. *Circulation* 1996; 94(9):2341–2350.

76. Froelicher VF, Perdue S, Pewen W, Risch M. Application of meta-analysis using an electronic spread sheet to exercise testing in patients after myocardial infarction. *Am J Med* 1987; 83:1045–1054.
77. Shaw LJ, Peterson ED, Kesler K, et al. A metaanalysis of predischarge risk stratification after acute myocardial infarction with stress electrocardiographic, myocardial perfusion, and ventricular function imaging. *Am J Cardiol* 1996; 78(12):1327–1337.
78. Lauer MS, Lytle B, Pashkow F, et al. Prediction of death and myocardial infarction by screening with exercise-thallium testing after coronary-artery-bypass grafting. *Lancet* 1998; 351(9103): 615–622.

CHAPTER 15

CARDIAC CATHETERIZATION, CORONARY ARTERIOGRAPHY, AND CORONARY BLOOD FLOW AND PRESSURE MEASUREMENTS

Robert H. Franch / John S. Douglas, Jr. / Spencer B. King III / Morton J. Kern

In 1929, Werner Forssman, a resident surgeon at Eberswalde, catheterized his right atrium from a left antecubital vein cutdown using self-fluoroscopy with a mirror. The position of the catheter tip was verified by a roentgenogram.[1] The extensive use of the right heart catheter by Cournand in the early 1940s in the study of human cardiovascular physiology led his group and others to explore the use of this technique for the study of heart disease.[2] In 1945, Brannon, Weens, and Warren described the hemodynamics of atrial septal defect in four patients. From these beginnings, steady advances in methods occurred.[3,4] Catheterization then spread from the laboratory to the bedside, to yield physiologic data and to guide treatment.[5] Now, palliative and corrective interventions involving valves, arteries, veins, and septal defects may accompany the catheterization study.[6]

PREPARATIONS FOR CARDIAC CATHETERIZATION

A relaxed meeting with the patient and the patient's family serves to lessen apprehension, correct any misunderstanding, and establish rapport. Since catheterization is frequently the first major step on the road to cardiac surgery, a tolerable experience fosters an optimistic attitude in the patient and family toward future events. The patient should be examined, and the history, a current chest x-ray, an electrocardiogram, and past catheterizations should be reviewed, along with surgical records, angiocardiograms, and echocardiograms. The site of optimal vascular access is chosen. Nearly all balloon catheters and many gloves contain latex, and it should be added to the list of allergens sought in the history.[7] Old operative notes are examined, especially for complex palliation or repair. A clinical diagnosis is made, and a catheterization protocol is designed to answer pertinent specific questions. The catheterization protocol also may be modified as data become available during the procedure. The patient's education booklet about the procedure is usually read by the patient and the family prior to securing informed consent. Absolute contraindications include the refusal of a competent adult or the absence of a qualified operator and/or a suitable facility[8] (Table 15-1). Anticoagulants are stopped, and the prothrombin time is brought to less than

TABLE 15-1 Contraindications to Cardiac Catheterization

THE ONLY ABSOLUTE CONTRAINDICATIONS

1. Refusal of a mentally competent adult (>16 years of age) patient, or of the parent(s) (guardians) of children, infants, or neonates to consent to the procedure
2. Absence of an experienced cardiac angiography and/or suitable laboratory facilities

RELATIVE CONTRAINDICATIONS TO BE CAUTIOUSLY APPLIED TO INDIVIDUAL PATIENT

1. Significant electrolyte abnormalities or digitalis toxicity
2. Uncontrolled hypertension
3. Febrile illness (not related to endocarditis)
4. Decompensated congestive heart failure
5. Bleeding diathesis: includes patients receiving anticoagulation therapy whose prothrombin time is >18 s (INR >2)
6. Presence of a noncardiac disease that precludes long-term survival
7. Refusal to undergo surgical or interventional curvative or palliative procedures regardless of the outcome of the catheterization (angiogram)
8. Previous history of severe contrast reaction
9. Active gastrointestinal bleeding
10. Pregnancy, especially during first trimester

SOURCE: From Ruiz et al.,[8] with permission from the authors and publisher.

18 s (INR <2) before a percutaneous arterial catheterization. Dimethyl biguanide, an oral hypoglycemic drug, is not given for 2 days prior to angiography. Serum levels of creatinine, urea nitrogen, and potassium are noted. A patient with chronic renal disease is hydrated; prophylaxis for past allergy to contrast material is given.[9] Breakfast is withheld for a morning procedure; for an afternoon procedure, coffee or juice is permitted, and lunch is withheld. In our experience, prophylactic antibiotics are not necessary. Conscious sedation for diagnostic catheterization involves the incremental use of intravenous drugs that are titrated to each patient's response. Pulse oximeter monitors require accuracy to within 3 percent in the 70 to 100 percent saturation range. Diazepam (Valium) or midazolam (Versed) is given intravenously; intravenous fentanyl may be added for more sedation. Intravenous hydromorphone (Dilaudid) is used if analgesia is required. Subcutaneous 1% lidocaine (Xylocaine) is used locally. If there is a history of allergy, intradermal or subcutaneous testing is done with serial dilutions of a preservative-free local anesthetic agent.[10] Occasionally, particularly in adults, vagal slowing of the pulse, nausea, and perspiration are noted, for which intravenous atropine is the antidote. Systemic anticoagulation is achieved via a bolus of heparin at the start of a diagnostic study that uses the brachial artery but not routinely if the femoral artery is used.

It is desirable that the laboratory be fully involved daily in diagnostic work. General efficiency is increased, costly equipment and space are used, and most important, all personnel become confident and knowledgeable with experience. Certainly the most important ingredient in the laboratory is the thoroughly experienced technical-professional team. The primary objective is to make an accurate diagnosis at one sitting, with the least possible risk and discomfort to the patient. After the procedure, a preliminary, labeled single-page diagram in the patient's chart can accurately present the essence of the catheterization findings.

Outpatient left-sided heart and coronary artery studies require careful selection of patients and an experienced support team.[11,12] The clinical profiles of patients who are not suitable candidates for outpatient catheterization have been published.[13] Others have stated that if a patient is stable enough to be at home before cardiac catheterization, an outpatient catheterization can be considered and a decision following the procedure can be made based on the patient's tolerance of the procedure and the catheterization findings. This approach is most relevant when a catheterization laboratory is in or adjacent to a hospital. The cost savings per patient with outpatient procedures remain significant. Although some physicians have performed cardiac catheterization of stable, low-risk patients in freestanding facilities, the lack of support in this environment is a potential liability, and thus the procedure is not recommended.

TECHNIQUES

Catheterization of the Right Side of the Heart: Percutaneous Venous

Percutaneous femoral or median cubital vein catheterization usually permits reuse of the vein. The femoral vein is entered medial to the common femoral artery pulse. Puncture may be facilitated by a Valsalva maneuver to increase femoral vein size. To extend the range of the percutaneous technique, a thin tubular sheath is advanced over a short introducer catheter into the lumen of the vein. This temporary conduit then may be used to introduce a variety of catheters. Two catheters can be inserted through a single femoral vein puncture site by initially placing two guidewires through the femoral vein sheath; the maneuver is repeated to insert an additional catheter. If the hepatic portion of the inferior vena cava (IVC) is absent, the azygos vein channels the catheter tip into the right superior vena cava (SVC) and then into the right atrium (Fig. 15-1), or the azygos vein may enter a persistent left SVC and then through the coronary sinus to the right atrium (Fig. 15-2). In order to cross the tricuspid valve from the IVC, bending the catheter tip against the right atrial wall may be required. If atrial ectopy occurs, the catheter tip can be looped in a hepatic vein and then advanced into the right atrium. The tip is then rotated from the lateral right atrial wall clockwise across the anterior atrial wall and through the tricuspid valve, followed by a slight counterclockwise turn to the anterolateral position in the right ventricle and then clockwise to place the tip via the outflow tract into the main pulmonary artery and then into the left pulmonary artery, its direct continuation. The foramen ovale is entered with the tip pointed leftward and 45° posteriorly. The SVC lies posteriorly and is entered by making a 60° counterclockwise turn from the lateral right atrial border with a straight catheter tip. The foramen ovale is probe-patent in approximately 20 to 35 percent of adults.

The internal jugular vein or the subclavian vein also may be

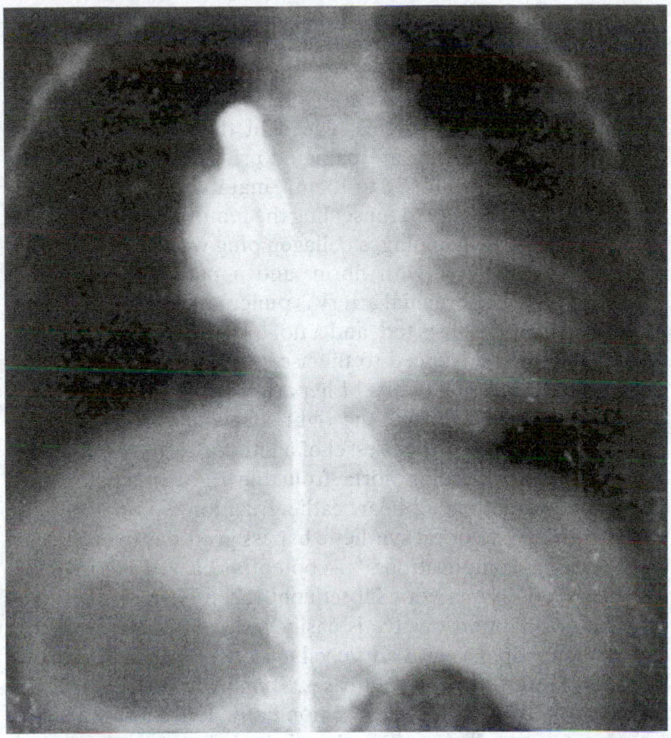

FIGURE 15-1 Selective injection of a right azygos vein. The hepatic portion of the IVC is absent. The catheter tip enters the right atrium superiorly through the right SVC via the azygos vein.

used to insert a balloon catheter percutaneously. The latter catheter produces little ectopy because the advancing force is distributed over the surface of the balloon. The tricuspid valve is crossed easily with this approach. If a right-to-left shunt is present, the balloon should be filled with CO_2 and the sidearm of the sheath flushed regularly. In children who lack conventional venous access, transhepatic venous catheterization via a right midaxillary approach is safe and effective.[14]

Rarely, if a venous cutdown is necessary, the right basilic or right median cubital (but not the cephalic) vein is preferred. Care should be taken not to mistake the superficial radial, ulnar, or accessory brachial arteries for veins. From the left arm, the catheter tip may enter a persistent left SVC, exiting via the coronary sinus into the right atrium in an awkward position for entering the right ventricle. A deep inspiration often enables the catheter tip to pass the subclavian vein–brachiocephalic vein junction. The seating of a conventional catheter tip in the pulmonary artery wedge position may be difficult if severe pulmonary artery hypertension or extreme enlargement of the right side of the heart is present. A flow-directed balloon catheter may then be used. Clues to inadvertent coronary sinus catheterizations are (1) the acute angle that the catheter shaft makes as it enters the coronary sinus, especially in the right anterior oblique position, (2) the marked desaturation of coronary sinus blood, and (3) the posterior position of the catheter in the lateral view.

In order to enter the pulmonary artery in patients with transposition of the great arteries and an intact ventricular septum, a balloon catheter is passed across the inevitably present interarterial communication to the left atrium and then superiorly looped in the left ventricular (LV) outflow tract, from which it enters the pulmonary artery readily. In postoperative patients with pulmonary valve atresia, the pulmonary artery also may be entered via a subclavian (Blalock) or aorticopulmonary (Waterston or Potts) shunt.

Catheterization of the Left Side of the Heart

PERCUTANEOUS TECHNIQUE

In 1953, Seldinger described the use of a flexible metal leader to introduce a polyethylene tube into the artery. The Seldinger technique is used in the common femoral and less often in the axillary radial or brachial arteries in carrying out catheterization of the left side of the heart.[15] The common femoral artery, 4 cm in length, begins at the inguinal ligament and ends at its bifurcation into the deep and superficial femoral arteries at the inferior cortical margin of the head of the femur. The inguinal

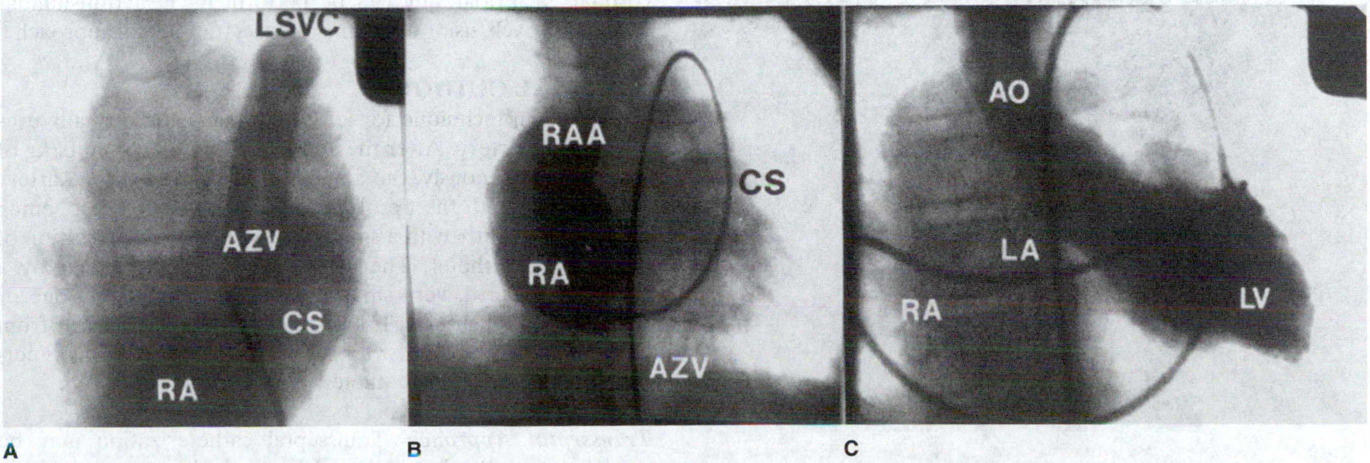

FIGURE 15-2 *A–C.* Progression of a catheter from the femoral vein. The hepatic portion of the IVC is absent. The systemic venous return is via a left azygos vein (AZV) to the left superior vena cava (LSVC) and then via the coronary sinus (CS) to the right atrium (RA). The catheter tip passes from the RA to the left atrium (LA) via an atrial septal defect and then across the mitral valve into the left ventricle (LV). RAA, right atrial appendage.

crease, especially in an obese patient, tends to be inferior to the ligament. In this case, a puncture at or below the crease may involve the superficial femoral artery, and lack of posterior bony support results in poor compression with the chance of bleeding and pseudoaneurysm formation[16] (Fig. 15-3). A skin puncture site chosen 3 cm below the inguinal ligament (not the crease) allows the common femoral artery to be entered at a point where it is compressible against the head of the femur. External rotation of the leg and slight adduction help fixate the artery. The artery is punctured with a nonstylet needle at a 45° angle, transfixing the anterior wall. The guidewire is inserted only when the needle spurt is maximal. Resistance to insertion usually indicates an intramural or extravascular position of the needle or entry into a side branch artery by the guide. The catheter is inserted into the artery over the guidewire, or a sheath assembly may be used, facilitating catheter introduction in a very obese patient or if scar tissue is superficial to the artery. The catheter sheath reduces bleeding during manipulation and reduces discomfort during catheter changes. Arterial pressure may be monitored through a side port in the sheath. Guidewires with torsional control of a flexible distal tip aid passage through a tortuous iliac artery, as does a right Judkins catheter, alone or with a guide. The guide tip is kept at the level of the diaphragm, and the catheter is advanced to this level. The catheter is aspirated and then flushed with heparinized saline solution. To avoid added manipulation of the catheter tip in the transverse arch, the guidewire is placed in the aortic root.[17] The femoral and foot pulses are palpated prior to withdrawal. The artery is compressed for 10 to 15 min, maintaining normal ankle pulses. Devices deployed for sealing the femoral artery puncture site include a collagen plug, a collagen plug with anchor, thrombin with collagen or with fibrin, and a percutaneous suture technique.[18,19] The brachial artery is punctured with an 18-gauge needle, a sheath is inserted, and a no. 6 French 80-cm multipurpose catheter is advanced to the ascending aorta over a 0.032-in. J-guide. Then 5000 units of heparin is given. An arm board is applied for 6 h. Rarely, the right subclavian artery will rise aberrantly as the last root vessel of a left aortic arch, precluding access to the ascending aorta from the right brachial artery. Percutaneous left-sided heart catheterization via an aortofemoral or axillary-femoral synthetic bypass graft has been surprisingly free of complications.[20] A potential hazard is disruption of the pseudointima with subsequent thrombosis.

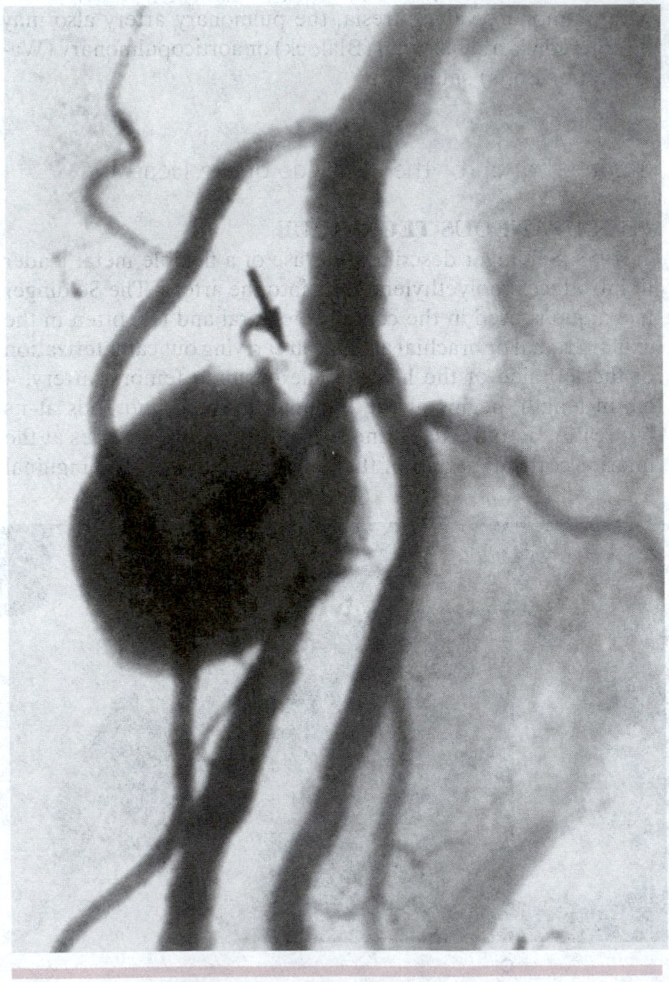

FIGURE 15-3 The femoral arteriogram shows the neck (*arrow*) of an oval pseudoaneurysm (pulsating hematoma) arising from the right superficial femoral artery (*arrow*) at the site of the previous catheter entry. (Reproduced with permission from Rapoport et al.[16] and the Radiological Society of North America, Inc.)

The normal aortic valve is easily crossed retrogradely with the catheter tip. Even in aortic valve stenosis, the left ventricle can be entered in nearly all cases. By slowly withdrawing the catheter tip from its looped position in the left aortic sinus, one may perform wall-to-wall exploration of the severely stenotic valve. A straight-tip guidewire may enhance this maneuver. Left and right Judkins, left Amplatz, and pigtail catheters have all been used to center the guidewire in the aortic root to achieve more effective probing of the stenotic orifice.[21,22]

In selected patients who have aortic and mitral valve disk or ball-valve prostheses, a brief direct percutaneous puncture through the palpable apex of the left ventricle is surprisingly free of complications.[23] LV angiography can be performed through the sheath or a catheter. Retrograde catheterization of the left ventricle via a prosthetic aortic disk valve should be avoided. Valvular incompetence is induced, and the catheter may become entrapped in the disk valve mechanism. In contrast, tissue valves can be crossed without significant hazard. In patients with both femoral and axillary artery disease, selective coronary arteriography can be performed via a translumbar aortic approach, using a sheath,[24] or via a transseptal approach.[25]

ARTERIAL CUTDOWN

The cutdown technique for left-sided heart study usually uses the brachial artery. After the administration of 100 units/kg of heparin intravenously, the anterior wall of the exposed artery is punctured with the tip of an 18-gauge needle. The opening is enlarged slightly with a small forceps, permitting insertion of the tapered catheter. The arteriotomy is closed either by a previously placed, very small purse-string loop or by one or two interrupted sutures. If brisk bleeding does not occur from both proximal and distal artery segments, thrombectomy is performed with a balloon catheter.

Transseptal Approach Transseptal catheterization may be used to enter the left atrium.[26] From the right femoral vein percutaneously, a 71-cm-long needle is advanced inside a dilator catheter-sheath system to a position beneath the ledge of the limbus fossae ovalis in the right atrium. The needle is then bared to puncture the atrial septum.[27–29] Entry into the left atrium is confirmed by a clear continuous pressure tracing. The dilator is then pushed across the septum. The needle tip is pulled back into the dilator, and when both are well in the left atrium (Fig. 15-4), the sheath is slid over them to also enter the left atrium; needle and dilator are then withdrawn. The sheath permits various preformed open- or closed-tip catheters or large guidewires to be passed into the left atrium and left ventricle. A CO_2-filled balloon catheter may be passed from the left atrium to the left ventricle to the ascending aorta. Biplane fluoroscopy, continuous pressure recording, a catheter in the aortic root, and knowledge of the size and position of the left atrium following pulmonary artery angiography are helpful in positioning the transseptal needle. The left atrium is difficult to enter if there is deformity of the thoracic or lumbar spine or if there is a very large right atrium. Other relative contraindications to transseptal catheterization include marked dilatation of the aortic root and other anatomic distortions of the IVC or atria. The procedure is not done if there is intraatrial thrombus or tumor.

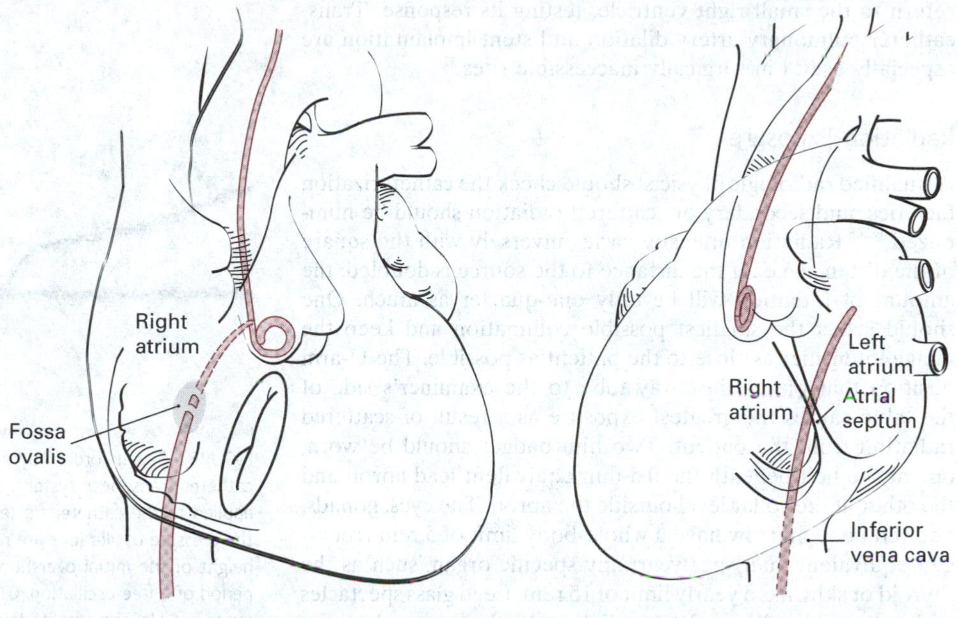

FIGURE 15-4 Anteroposterior (*left*) and lateral (*right*) views of a sheath and dilator positioned in the left atrium following needle puncture of the interatrial septum. The aortic root is defined by a pigtail catheter. Note that the septum is safely crossed posterior and inferior to the aortic valve. (Reproduced with permission from the publisher and authors from Roelke M, Conrad-Smith AJ, Palacios IF. The technique and safety of transseptal left heart catheterization. *Cathet Cardiovasc Diagn* 1994; 32:332–339.)

Retrograde catheterization of the left atrium from the left ventricle in the right anterior oblique (RAO) projection uses a tapered flexible catheter that forms a clockwise loop in the left ventricle as it passes to the left atrium. A pigtail catheter has been used similarly.[29]

EQUIPMENT

Catheters

Disposable single-use catheters in a wide range of sizes, shapes, and lengths with end and/or side holes are available for diagnostic use. The ideal nonpreformed catheter is soft enough to permit bending as required, has "memory" to hold its shape, and has enough strength or body to permit the curve of the tip to be advanced intact. Torque control is improved by incorporating a thin wire braid in the walls. Transmission of torque to the catheter tip in the ascending aorta is damped by a tortuous iliac artery. The torque is received instead by the proximal part of the catheter, resulting in coiling or potential knotting in the iliac artery. Preformed catheters are made to serve a specific function with a minimum of manipulation. Catheters should have smooth, regular surfaces to reduce thrombogenicity. Atrial septostomy with a fluid-filled balloon catheter or with a controlled folding surgical blade at the catheter tip improves shunting and increases systemic arterial saturation in patients with transposition of the great arteries.[30] A precompressed Ivalon plug or thrombogenic coils inserted by catheter have been used to close the patent ductus arteriosus. Loop-snare or jawed biopsy catheters are used for nonthoracotomy retrieval of intraluminal cardiovascular foreign bodies. A small Doppler crystal mounted on a thin guidewire serves as an intraluminal probe to measure coronary artery blood flow velocity.[31] A catheter-tip electromagnetic probe can be used to measure aortic blood flow velocity. A Doppler pulmonary artery catheter can provide continuous instantaneous stroke output values,[32] assuming a flat velocity profile. An intracoronary artery ultrasound imaging catheter system can provide a cross-sectional, two-dimensional image of good anatomic detail (see Chap. 47). The coronary artery lumen also may be visualized by fiberoptic angioscopic catheters.[33] Inhaled hydrogen gas is detected within 4 s of inhalation with extreme sensitivity by a pacing catheter electrode positioned at the site of a left-to-right shunt or downstream from it.

Used in treating valvular pulmonic stenosis and coarctation of the aorta,[34,35] pulmonary valvuloplasty and aortic angioplasty balloons up to 4 cm long with an inflation diameter up to 20 mm are made of high-tensile-strength polyethylene. Inflation to 3 to 4 atm with a 20-mL plastic syringe is usual. The lumen between the no. 8 or 9 French catheter and the balloon is large, permitting deflation in less than 7 s, decreasing the occlusion time. A short bilobed balloon catheter (two layers with a polyester micromesh between) permits stable positioning across the stenotic valve, stepwise dilation, and a short deflation time.[36] A catheter can be used to deliver a device to close a secundum atrial septal defect as large as 2 cm. Test balloon occlusion of aortopulmonary collaterals mimics the effects of planned surgical closure. In patients with pulmonary atresia and an intact ventricular septum who have had surgical relief of the pulmonary atresia, the atrial septal defect can be closed temporarily with a balloon catheter in order to direct all the systemic venous return to the small right ventricle, testing its response. Transcatheter pulmonary artery dilation and stent implantation are especially useful in surgically inaccessible sites.[37]

Radiation Exposure

A qualified radiologic physicist should check the catheterization facilities, and secondary or scattered radiation should be minimized.[38–40] Radiation intensity varies inversely with the square of the distance; i.e., if the distance to the source is doubled, the amount of radiation will be only one-quarter as much. One should select the smallest possible collimation and keep the image intensifier as close to the patient as possible. The U-arm position that places the x-ray tube to the examiner's side of the table causes the greatest exposure as a result of scattered radiation from the patient. Two film badges should be worn, one at the belt beneath the 0.5-mm equivalent lead apron and the other at the collar level outside the apron. The eyes, gonads, and red bone marrow have a whole-body limit of 5 rem (roentgen equivalent man) per year; any specific organ, such as the thyroid or skin, has a yearly limit of 15 rem. Lead glass spectacles and a thyroid collar reduce radiation to the eye and to the thyroid. Both a floating and a table-to-floor screen are needed for added shielding. The maximal permissible dose, or "safe" exposure, for catheterization laboratory personnel is 100 mrem per week monitored by an unshielded left collar badge. If possible, women of childbearing age should have studies done within 10 days after the onset of menstruation.

Pressure-Recording System

If the heart rate is 60 to 120 beats per minute, the fundamental frequency of the basic wave is 1 to 2 per s. The tenth harmonic or sine-wave component of the pressure wave then occurs at a frequency of 10 to 20 Hz; it is important to detect these components without phase lag or amplitude distortion because their sum represents the rising and falling contours of the native pressure curve. A properly responding pressure-recording system should have a high natural frequency and optimal damping. A high natural frequency is obtained by using a bubble-free, saline solution–filled system of minimum length whose catheter and connector tubings have stiff walls and wide bores. Many catheter-tubing transducer systems are underdamped. To achieve optimal damping, a damping needle or tube is placed between the catheter and the transducer. This extends the output-input ratio of the pressure wave in a nearly uniform manner (unity + 5 percent) to as close as possible to the natural frequency of the system. The values for both frequency response and damping coefficient are obtained by introducing a square-wave pressure input to the catheter system and by measuring the amplitude ratio of any two successive peak pressure amplitudes and the time interval between peaks (Fig. 15-5). For clinical cardiac catheterization, a manometer system with a uniform dynamic response of greater than 20 Hz is desirable.

Clinically, the zero position for an external pressure transducer is set at the lateral midchest level. Specifically, hydrostatic zero is considered to be at the level of most anterior surfaces of the LV blood pool.[41] An additional limiting factor in pressure recording is the superimposition of artifacts on the pressure pulse by the accelerating and decelerating movements imparted to the fluid-filled cardiac catheter by the beating heart. Distortion of the catheter-obtained phasic pressure waveform by motion or damping artifact can be avoided with the use of a catheter-tip, side-mounted, ultraminiature semiconductor gauge. This manometer system is required for first- or second-derivative measurements of the pressure curve.

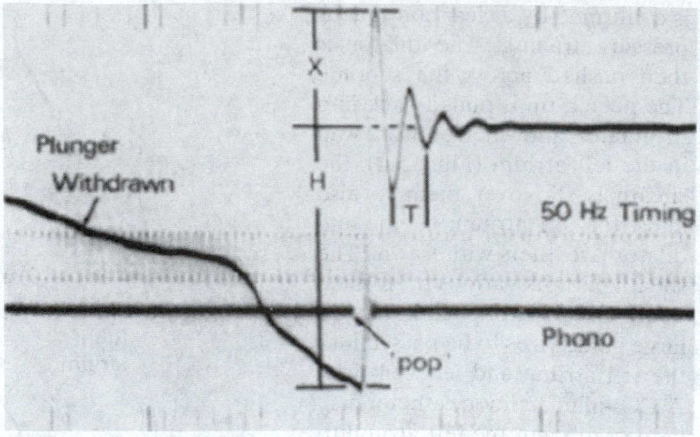

FIGURE 15-5 In order to measure the dynamic frequency response of a catheter transducer system, an abrupt transient input dynamic pressure is applied to the catheter tip (a plunger is pulled free of an air-filled syringe); the pressure oscillations are recorded at a fast paper speed and measured. X, height of the initial overshoot; H, end height of the recorded deflection; T, period of a free oscillation, 0.08 s. The natural frequency is 13 Hz; the useful range is 4 Hz. The amplitude ratio of two successive peak amplitudes is 0.59, and the damping coefficient is 0.17. This underdamped system is optimally damped to a coefficient around 0.64 by the addition of a narrow-bore tube between catheter and transducer. (Reproduced with permission of Irex Corporation.)

Oxygen Analysis

The total oxygen content of the blood, once determined by the classic Van Slyke manometric technique, is now obtained by gas chromatography or mass spectrometry. The percent oxyhemoglobin saturation is measured from a small sample of whole blood in a disposable plastic curvette by direct photooximetry or, after hemolysis, by a precision spectrophotometer.[42] Analysis of expired air, from collecting bag or breath by breath, for oxygen and carbon dioxide may be made by gas analyzers or infrared or mass spectroscopy. Oxygen consumption also can be measured throughout the procedure using a flow-through hood technique.[43] Oxygen consumption also can be estimated with a 10 to 25 percent variation from measured values.

DATA OBTAINED AT CATHETERIZATION

Pressure Measurements

High-fidelity phasic pressure curves are not obtained from the ventricles or great arteries by fluid-filled catheter recording systems. The underdamped curve gives falsely high systolic and falsely low diastolic readings, and the overdamped curve has a smooth shape with disappearance of the incisura. The shape of the ventricular or great artery pressure trace is occasionally of diagnostic aid. An abrupt fall in pressure in early diastole (early diastolic dip) followed by a sudden rise to a high end-diastolic pressure plateau occurs in both ventricles in abnormal compliance states such as constrictive pericarditis and restrictive cardiomyopathy. In patients with constriction, the LV and right ventricular (RV) pressures have a respiratory reciprocal (discordant) relationship, whereas with heart failure, the relationship is concordant.[44,45] In isolated pulmonary stenosis, the configuration of the RV pressure curve is frequently peaked or triangular.

In valvular pulmonary stenosis, the pulse pressure is frequently greater in the left pulmonary artery than in the right pulmonary artery because flow is preferentially directed into the left pulmonary artery and kinetic energy is translated into lateral pressure. A systolic dip is noted in the main pulmonary artery due to pressure loss from the Bernoulli effect (Fig. 15-6). In bilateral branch pulmonary artery stenosis, the proximal main pulmonary artery shows a wide pulse pressure with a low dicrotic notch. In supravalvular aortic stenosis, the coanda effect makes the right brachial and right carotid artery peak pressures greater than those on the left. A large *a* wave in the right atrium is characteristic of valvular pulmonary stenosis but not of tetralogy of Fallot. A large *v* wave on the pulmonary artery wedge ("pulmonary capillary") pressure tracing may or may not mean that severe mitral regurgitation is present.[46]

Left ventricular end-diastolic pressure (LVEDP) is recorded on a high-sensitivity scale and is measured where the downslope of the *a* wave in the left ventricle coincides with the initial upstroke of the LV pressure. The LVEDP also may be measured at the peak of the R wave of the electrocardiogram. An elevated LVEDP reflects an alteration in the ventricular pressure-volume relation or a decrease in diastolic compliance of the ventricle. An increased LVEDP occurs commonly with a dilated failing left ventricle but also may be noted in a small ventricular cavity with thick walls or in a normal-size LV cavity during an acute ischemic attack.

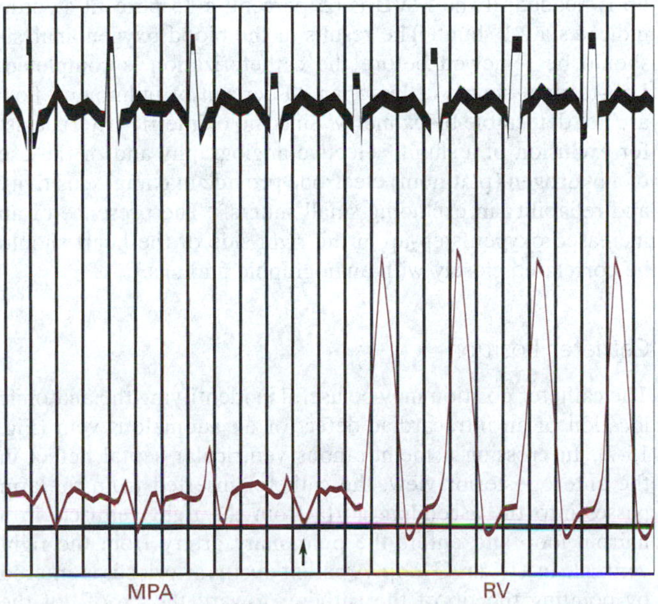

FIGURE 15-6 Pullback continuous pressure tracing from the main pulmonary artery (MPA) to the right ventricle (RV) recorded in a 27-year-old male with moderate valvular pulmonic stenosis. RV systolic pressure is 84 mmHg. MPA pressure is 16/7 mmHg. Note the systolic dip (*arrow*) in the MPA pressure tracing, due to the pressure loss from the Bernoulli effect. (From Franch RH. Recognition and management of valvular pulmonic stenosis. *Heart Dis Stroke* 1994; 3:365–370. Reproduced with permission from the author and publisher.)

In order to measure the maximal rate of rise of LV pressure, or peak dP/dt, a high-fidelity pressure record is needed, obtained ideally via a catheter-tip transducer. This value is influenced by preload and afterload in addition to the contractile state. The preejection phase index $(dP/dt)/P$, where P is the LV pressure during isovolumic systole, reflects the velocity of shortening of contractile elements but also responds to changes in preload. In daily practice, ejection-phase indexes derived from the conventional LV angiogram are used to assess LV function.[47] The ejection fraction is commonly employed as an index of ventricular contractility but is sensitive to changes in preload and afterload as well (see Chap. 22).

A satisfactory pulmonary artery wedge mean pressure provides a good estimate of left atrial mean pressure. Some damping in waveform and phase shift (0.06-s time delay) occurs in the transmitted wedge pressure when compared with the direct left atrial pressure record. During diastole, pulmonary artery wedge diastolic mean pressure tends to be higher than the left atrial diastolic mean pressure, especially in the presence of a prosthetic or abnormal mitral valve. End-expiratory pulmonary artery diastolic pressure agrees within 2 to 4 mmHg with mean pulmonary artery wedge pressure in the absence of increased pulmonary arteriolar resistance. In contrast, pulmonary vein wedge pressure does not give an accurate estimate of the pulmonary artery pressure in the presence of pulmonary artery hypertension.

Pressure recording permits measurement of either the peak or the mean pressure differential across a stenotic semilunar or atrioventricular (AV) valve or a segmentally narrowed blood vessel. If possible, simultaneous pressure recordings across a valve should be obtained, especially if there is atrial fibrillation. If the pulmonary artery wedge is used as an estimate of left atrial mean pressure, the waveform and amplitude should be confirmed at a second site. The error in assessing the mitral valve area in mitral stenosis can be large when the measured pressure differential is small. Because of the slow fall of the *y* descent in the wedge position, the mitral valve gradient may be overestimated by 3 to 4 mmHg when compared with the gradient obtained with a direct left atrial pressure.[48,49] A pullback record across the semilunar valve performed with a catheter having multiple paired side holes may show a false zone of composite ventricular and great artery pulses resulting from the simultaneously recorded pressures through proximal and distal side holes. Occasionally, a gradient may be overlooked if the catheter tip cannot be advanced well into the ventricle so that it washes into the aorta in systole and falls into the left ventricle in diastole. The ascending aortic pressure should be recorded at the level of the coronary ostia to avoid the effects of pressure recovery,[50,51] i.e., the increase in lateral pressure downstream from a stenosis as the narrow, high-velocity flow field broadens and slows, losing kinetic energy.[52–54] The LV pressure in aortic valve stenosis is recorded well in the LV cavity to avoid systolic pressure loss due to tapering high-velocity flow in the subaortic area. In a case of proximal infundibular pulmonary stenosis, if the pullback is at the cranial aspect of the tricuspid valve, the catheter may fall back into the right atrium from the RV outflow tract very quickly, missing the gradient.

LV cavity obliteration with catheter entrapment may result in spurious pressure gradient. To detect an intraventricular gradient, the LV pressure should be checked in the inflow and outflow (i.e., submitral and subaortic) positions simultaneously and in the apical versus the inflow or outflow positions simultaneously. These recordings enable one to detect any delay in the fall of LV systolic pressure that may occur when the catheter is entrapped.

Interventions during Catheterization

We use a bicycle ergometer that provides loads of 0 to 450 W in steps of 5 W; the level of effort remains constant by maintaining a monitor pointer at a neutral position. The regression equation for oxygen consumption in milliliters per minute for a given load in watts on this ergometer is $V_{O_2} = 13.16\ W + 254$ mL. An increase in cardiac output of 0.6 L/min or greater for each 100 mL of oxygen consumed presumes a normal response. If the oxygen consumption is increased 200 to 250 mL/min by supine use of a bicycle ergometer, an increase in arteriovenous oxygen content difference greater than 30 mL/L is considered abnormal. When the pulmonary artery oxygen saturation falls to substantially less than 30 percent during exercise, the upper limit of circulatory stress is being approached. Normally, during moderate exercise, LVEDP actually falls, and stroke work increases; if LV performance is only moderately impaired, LVEDP rises, and stroke work rises; but in severe dysfunction, stroke work fails to increase despite an increase in LVEDP. Isometric hand-grip exercise increases heart rate, systemic mean pressure, and cardiac output. A fall in LV stroke work and a sharp rise in LVEDP during the grip test is evidence of poor LV reserve. All patients with mitral stenosis who have normal or mildly increased pulmonary artery and wedge pressures at rest should have the mitral gradient and cardiac output rechecked during exercise. In normal patients during exercise, pulmonary artery pressure rises minimally, usually no higher than 25 mmHg mean. In a patient with a repaired ventricular septal defect and residual pulmonary vascular disease, the pulmonary artery pressure may be at the upper limits of normal or slightly increased at rest but may double with low-level exercise.

Rapid atrial pacing also may be used as a stress intervention. In normal individuals, LVEDP falls as the heart rate is increased. If a paced patient with coronary artery disease is unable to meet the increased myocardial oxygen demand, the LVEDP rises in the early postpacing period, and excess lactate is noted in coronary sinus blood. In patients with tetralogy of Fallot, spontaneous or drug-induced increases in heart rate or atrial pacing produce a drop in arterial oxygen saturation and an increase in right-to-left shunting by increasing dynamic RV outflow tract obstruction.

In hypertrophic obstructive cardiomyopathy, isoproterenol, amyl nitrite, exercise, tilting, and the Valsalva maneuver, which tends to decrease diastolic ventricular volume, can intensify or provoke a systolic outflow tract pressure gradient, whereas a purely vasopressor amine, phenylephrine, which enlarges ventricular volume, tends to decrease the outflow tract pressure gradient[53] (see Chap. 67).

The response of cardiac output to vasodilator drugs in a patient with heart failure can be assessed. In patients with primary pulmonary artery hypertension (see Chap. 59), a 30 percent decrease in pulmonary vascular resistance and a 10 percent decrease in mean pulmonary artery pressure are the usual criteria for a positive response to pulmonary vasodilator drugs.[55]

Blood Oxygen Measurements

An increase in the oxygen content of blood from the chambers of the right side of the heart in excess of the normal variation in oxygen content on serial sampling is used as evidence of a left-to-right shunt.[56] Thus an oxygen step-up from the SVC to the right atrium of more than 1.9 vol% indicates shunting into the right atrium; a step-up from the right atrium to the right ventricle of 0.9 vol% or more and a step-up from the right ventricle to the pulmonary artery of 0.5 vol% or more indicates a left-to-right shunt at the RV and pulmonary artery levels, respectively. By these criteria, false-positive results are rare, but false-negative results can occur in patients with small shunts. In an anemic or polycythemic patient, the detection of shunting is best reflected by the step-up in percentage oxygen saturation rather than the step-up in volume percent, since the latter depends on the hemoglobin concentration.[57]

Studies show that sensitivity in detecting left-to-right shunts is improved if numerous serial blood samples are withdrawn in rapid succession for oximetry. If two sets of interrupted samples are taken from the SVC, right atrium, right ventricle, and pulmonary artery, a 9 percent saturation increase between the SVC and the right atrium indicates a large atrial shunt, a 5 percent saturation increase between the right atrium and the right ventricle indicates a ventricular shunt, and a 3 percent saturation increase between the right ventricle and the pulmonary artery indicates a pulmonary artery shunt. Sensitivity can be improved if blood samples are obtained in multiple pairs in a rapid serial sweep without flushing with saline solution between samples. The rise in oxygen saturation step-up for a given left-to-right shunt is related to the saturation of mixed venous blood (MVB). For example, if the MVB is 85 percent, a 5 percent step-up represents a 2:1 shunt; if MVB is 75 percent, a 10 percent step-up is needed; if the MVB is 65 percent, a 15 percent step-up indicates a 2:1 shunt. The results of the blood oxygen analysis should be reviewed before the catheterization is completed. Left-to-right shunts of less than 20 percent of pulmonary flow are not detectable by oximetry. Since no oximetric criteria exist for exclusion of a shunt, selective angiography and/or the use of a hydrogen (platinum) electrode provide maximal sensitivity and reliability in excluding small shunts.[58] The presence of an increased oxygen step-up in the right side of the heart should be correlated closely with angiographic findings.

Catheter Position

The catheter position may be useful in identifying the anatomic location of an intracardiac defect or an anomalous vein (Fig. 15-7). In crossing a membranous ventricular septal defect in the anteroposterior view, the catheter inserted from the arm passes into the ascending aorta from the right ventricle in a hairpin loop and enters the pulmonary artery from the right ventricle in a wider U loop. A patent ductus arteriosus is entered by pointing the tip of the catheter toward the "roof" of the junction of the main and left pulmonary arteries. Failing direct catheter passage, a flexible-spring guidewire, introduced while the venous catheter tip rests in the main pulmonary artery, readily passes through the ductus into the descending aorta; in aorticopulmonary septal defect, the tip passes directly up the ascending aorta from the main pulmonary artery. When the catheter tip enters a pulmonary vein within the heart shadow,

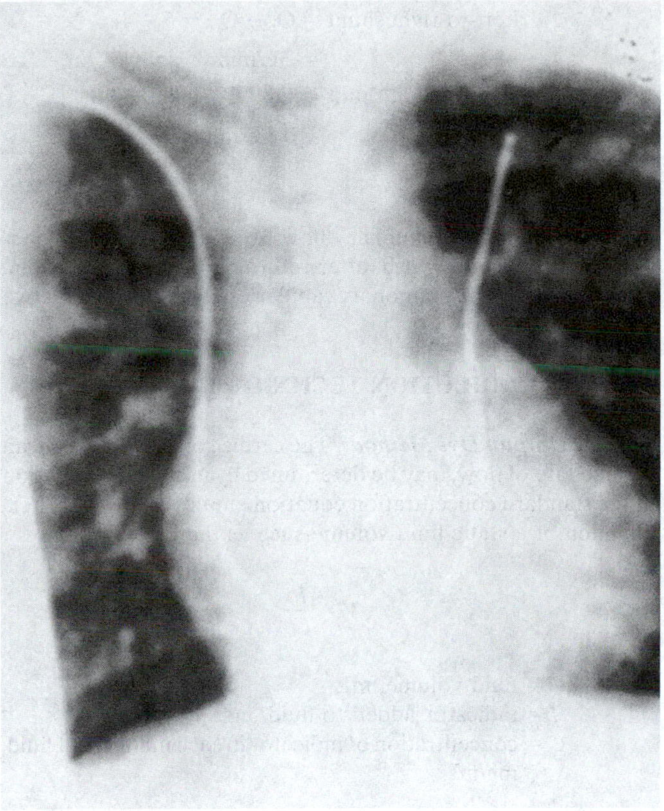

FIGURE 15-7 The catheter tip passes from the right SVC to the right atrium and then to the coronary sinus, the left SVC, and an anomalous left upper lobe pulmonary vein.

angiography is necessary to ascertain whether the pulmonary vein drains into the left or the right atrium. A secundum atrial septal defect is more easily crossed from the leg approach, a sinus venosus defect from an arm approach, and an ostium primum defect from either approach. If the tricuspid valve is congenitally displaced into the right ventricle, the pressure transition from the right ventricle to the right atrium may occur while the catheter tip is far to the left of the spine. Simultaneous intracardiac electrocardiography is confirmatory (see also Chap. 70).

Flow and Shunt Calculations

FICK METHOD: CARDIAC OUTPUT

In 1870, Adolph Fick expounded a theory for the measurement of blood flow that he never used in the laboratory: "The total uptake or release of a substance by an organ is the product of the blood flow to the organ and of the arteriovenous concentration of the substance." In the following example, the cardiac output may be calculated given the following three values: total oxygen consumption of 300 mL/min, arterial blood oxygen content of 19 mL per 100 mL of blood, and mixed venous blood oxygen content of 14 mL per 100 mL of blood. The cardiac output, in liters per minute, is equal to the oxygen consumption divided by the arteriovenous oxygen difference multiplied by 10 (to convert the latter to liters). In this case, the cardiac output equals 6.0 L/min. Cardiac output may be related to the body surface area (BSA) as the *cardiac index*. If one assumes a BSA of 2.0 m^2, the cardiac index would be 3 L/min per square meter. Because of laminar flow from the coronary sinus and the cavae and in the right atrium, MVB is best obtained from the pulmonary artery. Under conditions of exercise, a minimum of 3 min is usually required to obtain a steady-state preliminary to expired air and blood collection. In a given person, repeated measurements of the cardiac output at rest by the Fick technique may vary to a maximum of ±17 percent, presuming a continued steady state.

SHUNT CALCULATIONS

Shunt calculations using the Fick principle tend to be approximations, since complete mixing of venous and shunted blood may not occur. Also, as the arteriovenous oxygen narrows, small errors in the analysis or in the collection of blood samples make large variations in the calculated pulmonary blood flow possible. The calculation of shunt flow, however, is useful; it provides a quantitative index that is combined with clinical findings to determine whether or not surgery is advisable.

Numerous formulas have been developed, but those listed below are the ones used most often. The *oxygen capacity* is the maximal amount of oxygen that will combine with hemoglobin and that will be dissolved in plasma at a high P_{O_2}. One gram of hemoglobin can combine with 1.36 mL of oxygen. The amount of oxygen dissolved in plasma depends on the solubility coefficient of oxygen, the temperature, and the partial pressure of oxygen. At 37°C, the solubility coefficient is such that the amount of oxygen dissolved in plasma is 0.03 mL/mmHg per liter. With an oxygen tension of about 100 mmHg, about 3 mL of oxygen is dissolved per liter of blood. This small amount is usually ignored, although when the patient is breathing 100% oxygen, a considerable amount of oxygen can be dissolved in plasma. Oxygen content is related to both the hemoglobin concentration and the oxygen saturation. The oxygen content equals 1.36 × Hb (g/dL) × Sa_{O_2} (%)/100.

1. A sample calculation of left-to-right shunt:

Total oxygen consumption (V_{O_2})	240 mL/min
Pulmonary artery blood oxygen content (PA_{O_2})	17 mL/100 mL
Mixed venous blood oxygen content (MV_{O_2})	15 mL/100 mL
Arterial blood oxygen content (Sa_{O_2}) (assumed to equal pulmonary venous oxygen content)	19 mL/100 mL

$$\text{Pulmonary flow } (Q_p) = \frac{V_{O_2}}{Sa_{O_2} - PA_{O_2}} = \frac{240}{19 - 17(10)} = 12 \text{ L/min}$$

$$\text{Systemic flow } (Q_s) = \frac{V_{O_2}}{Sa_{O_2} - MV_{O_2}} = \frac{240}{19 - 15(10)} = 6 \text{ L/min}$$

a. Pulmonary flow/systemic flow ratio = $Q_p/Q_s = 12/6 = 2$.

b. If one substitutes for Q_s and Q_p in the preceding formula and reduces to a common denominator, the *pulmonary flow–systemic flow* ratio is obtained from a formula requiring only the oxygen saturation. Assuming an oxygen capacity of 20 vol%, the following blood oxygen saturations for the preceding samples are Sa = 95 percent, PA = 85 percent, and MV = 75 percent.

c. Left-to-right shunt also may be expressed as the percentage of total pulmonary flow that is shunted blood. The 2:1 Q_p/Q_s ratio above then represents a 50 percent left-to-right shunt.

2. Calculation of right-to-left shunt:

$$\frac{Q_p}{Q_s} = \frac{Sa_{O_2}\% - MV_{O_2}\%}{Sa_{O_2}\% - Pa_{O_2}\%} = \frac{95 - 75}{95 - 85} = 2$$

$$V_{O_2} = 240 \text{ mL/min}$$
$$MV_{O_2} = 13 \text{ mL/100 mL blood}$$
$$Sa_{O_2} = 17 \text{ mL/100 mL blood}$$

Pulmonary vein blood oxygen content is as follows:

$$PV_{O_2} = 19 \text{ mL/100 mL blood}$$

(assumed to be 98 percent of oxygen capacity + 0.3 mL of dissolved oxygen).

$$Q_p = \frac{V_{O_2}}{PV_{O_2} - MV_{O_2}} = \frac{240}{19 - 13(10)}$$
$$= 4 \text{ L/min}$$

$$Q_s = \frac{V_{O_2}}{Sa_{O_2} - MV_{O_2}} = \frac{240}{17 - 13(10)}$$
$$= 6 \text{ L/min}$$

Pulmonary/systemic flow ratio = $Q_p/Q_s = 0.7$. Right-to-left shunt also may be expressed as the percentage of total systemic flow that is shunted blood. The 0.66 Q_p/Q_s ratio above represents a 33 percent right-to-left shunt.

3. Calculation of bidirectional shunt:

$$V_{O_2} = 240 \text{ mL/min}$$
$$PA_{O_2} = 15 \text{ mL/100 mL blood}$$
$$MV_{O_2} = 13 \text{ mL/100 mL blood}$$
$$Sa_{O_2} = 18 \text{ mL/100 mL blood}$$
$$PV_{O_2} = 19 \text{ mL/100 mL blood}$$

$$Q_p = \frac{V_{O_2}}{PV_{O_2} - PA_{O_2}} = \frac{240}{19 - 15(10)}$$

$$Q_s = \frac{V_{O_2}}{Sa_{O_2} - MV_{O_2}} = \frac{240}{18 - 13(10)}$$
$$= 4.8 \text{ L/min}$$

$$Q_{ep} = \frac{V_{O_2}}{PV_{O_2} - MV_{O_2}} = \frac{240}{19 - 13(10)}$$
$$= 4.0 \text{ L/min}$$

$$\text{Left-to-right shunt} = Q_p - Q_{ep} = 6 - 4$$
$$= 2 \text{ L/min}$$
$$\text{Right-to-left shunt} = Q_s - Q_{es} = 4.8 - 4.0$$
$$= 0.8 \text{ L/min}$$

Note that effective pulmonary flow Q_{ep} is that volume of systemic venous blood which, after returning to the right atrium, actually reaches the pulmonary capillaries. It is equal to effective systemic blood flow Q_{es}.

INDICATOR-DILUTION TECHNIQUE

Cardiac Output: Dye Method The cardiac output, or the mean volume rate of flow, may be determined by using a modification of the standard concentration equation employed for the determination of a static fluid volume such as the blood volume:

$$V = \frac{I}{C}$$

where V = fluid volume, mL
I = indicator added to fluid, mg
C = concentration of indicator in each milliliter of fluid, mg/mL

For determination of a moving fluid volume,

$$\text{Cardiac output} = \frac{I}{Ct}$$

where t = time required for all indicator-fluid mixture to pass sampling site once

If the indicator particles are injected into the circulation as a bolus and measured in the initial passage at a downstream site, they distribute themselves in a time-concentration plot of grossly predictable form called an *indicator-dilution curve* (Fig. 15-8). The descending limb of the indicator-dilution curve is distorted by indicator-blood mixture that has begun a second circulation. To exclude recirculating indicator, the concentration is plotted logarithmically against time. The early portion of the disappearance slope is extrapolated linearly on semilogarithmic paper to obtain a primary curve, on the premise that if indicator-blood mixing is complete, the washout of indicator is an exponential function of time. A cuvette densitometer is used to obtain a continuous arterial time-concentration curve. Thus

$$\text{Cardiac output (in L/min)} = \frac{I \times 60 \text{ s}}{Ct}$$

where C = mean concentration of indicator in one circulator passage, mg/L
t = time, s

The cardiac output is falsely high if an indicator is lost. If an indicator is counted twice, i.e., if undetected recirculation occurs, the cardiac output is falsely low. An analogue computer provides rapid calculation of cardiac output from dye-dilution curves and detects whether or not logarithmic decay of indicator concentration has occurred. The Stewart-Hamilton formula assumes constant heart rate and stroke volume and a linear runoff in the pulmonary artery. Values for cardiac output obtained with the indicator-dilution technique compare closely with those obtained by the Fick method.[59]

In the absence of shunt, the indicator-dilution curve shows an uninterrupted buildup slope, a sharp concentration peak, a steep disappearance slope, and a prominent recirculation peak. Two major types of distortion are produced by central shunting. In a left-to-right shunt, there is decreased peak concentration of dye, a gentle disappearance slope (prolonged disappearance time), and absence of the recirculation peak. These alterations are produced by the recirculation of indicator particles through the lungs, resulting in a slow release of indicator to the peripheral circulation. The typical curve produced by a venoarterial, or right-to-left, shunt shows deformity of the buildup slope by an abnormal or early-appearing hump, or reflection, representing indicator that has been shunted from right to left. The distortion in contour of the indicator-dilution curve in valvular regurgitation is similar to that occurring with left-to-right shunts. Efforts have been made to predict all or part of the curve from certain other curve components. The cardiac output obtained by the forward-triangle method compares favorably with the classic Hamilton method. In this technique, the initial portion of the indicator-dilution curve is considered to be a triangle. The area of this triangle multiplied by a constant gives the area of the primary dilution curve. Intracardiac shunts can be detected and quantified by indicator-dilution curves.[61]

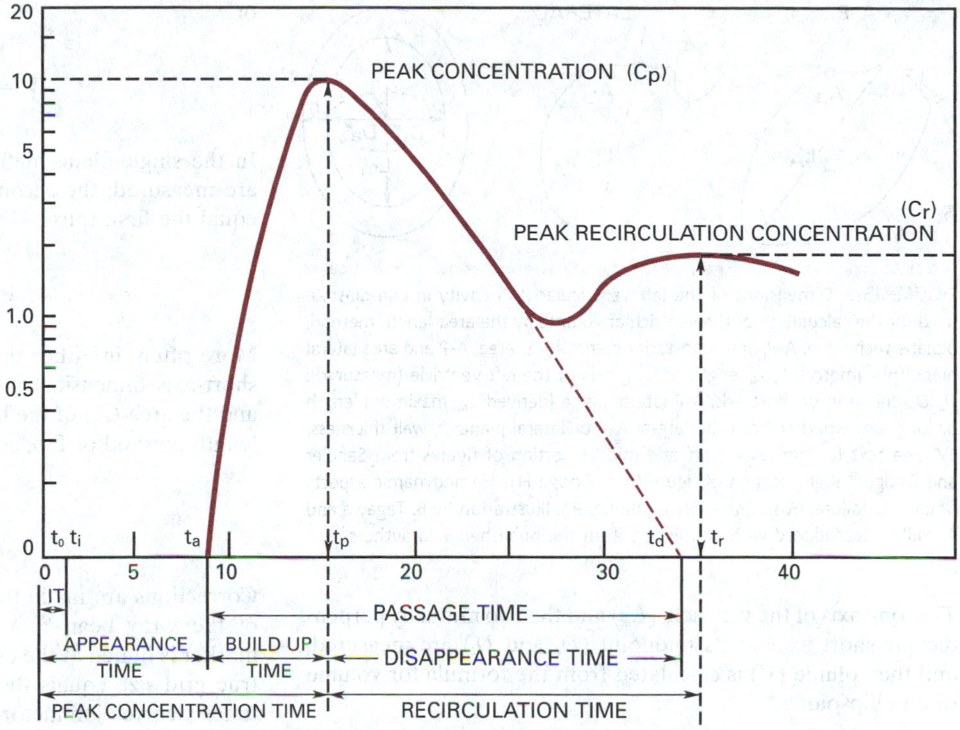

FIGURE 15-8 Time and concentration components of a normal indicator-dilution curve that has been replotted semilogarithmically, with extrapolation of the declining slope of concentration to eliminate the effect of recirculated indicator. The logarithm of the concentration on the ordinate is plotted against time on the abscissa. t_o, time of onset of injection of the indicator slug; t_i, time from t_o to the end of the injection; t_a, time from t_o to the first detectable appearance of indicator at the sampling site; t_p, time from t_o to the peak (maximal) concentration of the indicator; t_d, time when the declining concentration of indicator reaches a minimally detectable value; t_r, time from t_o to the time of the secondary concentration peak due to systemic recirculation of indicator; IT, the injection time. (From Wood EH, Swan HJC. Definition of terms and symbols for description of circulatory dilution curves. *J Appl Physiol* 1954; 6:797. Modified and reproduced with permission from the publisher and authors.)

Cardiac Output: Thermodilution Technique The thermodilution technique was introduced by Fegler in 1953 to measure volume flow rate.[61,62] A multiple-lumen, balloon-tipped flow-directed thermistor catheter is placed in the pulmonary artery. Ten milliliters of room-temperature (22°C) 5% dextrose or normal saline solution is injected rapidly (<4 s) through a second lumen into the right atrium. As the injectate blood mixture initially passes from the right ventricle, the pulmonary artery blood temperature drops maximally and then progressively rises in a beat-to-beat disappearance slope as the residual injectate-blood mixture is washed out of the right ventricle. The recirculation phase is negligible. Recording the curve allows assessment of the technical adequacy of the study. The area under the time-temperature curve is electronically integrated, and the cardiac output is computed by the Stewart-Hamilton formula. The difference between successive determinations should be less than 10 percent. Since there is no "gold standard" for cardiac output, the results have been compared with the dye-dilution and Fick techniques and have been noted to correlate well, except in low cardiac output states, where the Fick method is preferable. If severe tricuspid or pulmonary regurgitation or significant left-to-right shunting is present, the peak is attenuated and the downslope of the curve is prolonged, so the thermal dilution cardiac output likely will be unreliable.[63] In general, when one uses thermal dilution, a true directional change in cardiac output is reflected by an observed change of ±10 percent.

Ventricular Volume Measurements

LV volume is estimated by selective injection of contrast medium into the left ventricle or left atrium. The image of the opacified LV cavity is obtained by cineventriculography. Biplane view image pairs used include frontal and lateral, right and left anterior oblique, or half-axial left anterior oblique and conventional RAO.[64,65] A single-plane mode using the frontal or RAO projection often is adequate.[66,67] In the classic biplane technique, each shadow of the LV cavity is treated as an ellipse.

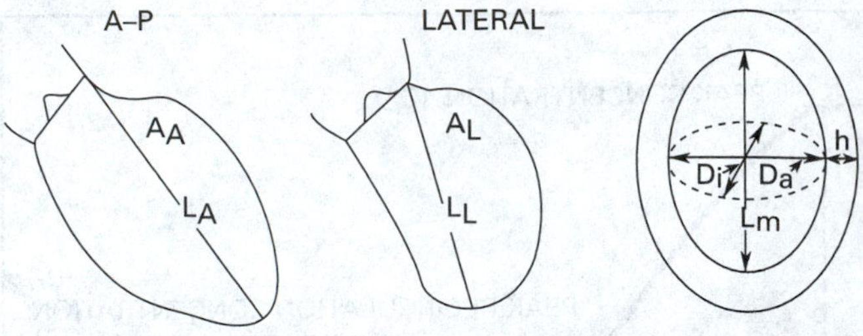

FIGURE 15-9 Dimensions of the left ventricular (LV) cavity in end-diastole used for the calculation of the ventricular volume by the area-length method, biplane technique. A-P, anteroposterior plane; A_a, A_l, area, A-P and area lateral plane (planimetry); L_a, L_l, length or long axis of the left ventricle (measured); D_a, D_l, diameter of short axis, A-P lateral plane (derived; L_m, maximum length or long axis whether from the lateral A-P or lateral plane; h, wall thickness, LV. See text for formulas. (Left and middle portion of figures from Sandler and Dodge.[66] Right portion of figure from Dodge HT. Hemodynamic aspects of cardiac failure. *Hosp Pract* 1971; January:91. Illustration by B. Tagawa and A. Miller. Reproduced with permission from the publishers and authors.)

The long axis of the ventricle (L_m) and the two mutually perpendicular short axes at its midpoint (D_a and D_l) are measured, and the volume (V) is calculated from the formula for volume of an ellipsoid:

$$V = \frac{4}{3}\pi \times \frac{D_a}{2} \times \frac{D_l}{2} \times \frac{L_m}{2}$$

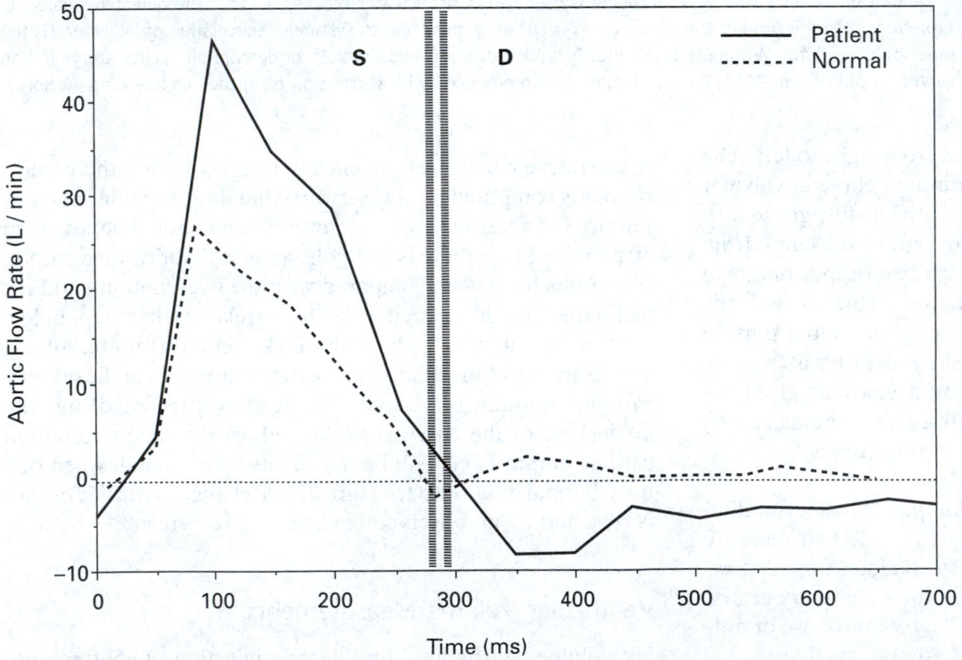

FIGURE 15-10 Using magnetic resonance phase-velocity mapping, aortic flow waveforms are obtained from an imaging slice placed in the aortic root. In a patient with moderate aortic valve regurgitation, increased forward flow occurred in systole and significant negative (regurgitant) flow rate occurred in diastole. The regurgitant volume was 32 mL per beat. No significant reverse flow is seen in the normal subject. (Used with permission of Chatzimavroudis GP, Walker PG, Oshinski JN, Franch RH, Pettigrew RI, and Yoganathan AP, Institute for Bioengineering and Biosciences, Georgia Institute of Technology, and F. Phillips Magnetic Resonance Research Center, Emory University Hospital, Atlanta, GA.)

or

$$V = \frac{\pi}{6} \times D_a \times D_l \times L_m$$

In the single-plane method, the long axis and one short axis are measured; the second nonvisible short axis is assumed to equal the first; thus

$$V = \frac{\pi}{6} \times L_m \times D_l^2$$

More often, in either the biplane or single-plane method, the short-axis dimension is derived from the measured long axis and the area (A) of the LV shadow, treated as an ellipse (area-length method of Dodge) (Fig. 15-9):

$$A = \pi L_m \frac{D}{4}$$

Corrections are made for magnification due to the divergence of the x-ray beam.[68] A calibrated grid or circular reference marker is filmed at the estimated level of the left ventricle. The true grid size equals the size measured on the projected film times a correction factor. More magnification may occur in the periphery than in the center of the field (pincushion effect) due to spherical aberration in the lens system. Digital ventriculography provides rapid, computer-derived ventricular volumes. Geometric and nongeometric count-based radionuclide techniques for calculation of ventricular volumes are well validated.

By the use of magnetic resonance imaging (MRI) in each case, LV volume obtained by the biplane long-axis method and LV volume obtained from multiple short-axis plane images (using Simpson's rule) agree closely.[69] If the left ventricle of a postmortem heart specimen is filled with contrast material and filmed, the calculated estimate of the volume of the left ventricle is higher than the known volume of the left ventricle. An appropriate regression equation for both single-plane[66,67] and biplane[64,65] techniques has been derived to adjust for this initial overestimate. The LVEDV is normally 70 ± 20 mL/m^2, and the end-systolic volume is 24 ± 10 mL/m^2. The forward stroke volume obtained by left ventriculography agrees well with indicator-dilution and Fick determinations. The ejection fraction of the left ventricle is 0.67 ± 0.08; values below 0.55 are usually considered abnormal. Diastolic LV wall thickness measured by angiography is 9 mm for women and 12 mm for men, and LV wall mass is 76 g/m^2 for women and 99 g/m^2 for men.[70]

The total stroke volume obtained by left ventriculography is used to assess the severity of mitral and aortic valve regurgitation. Total stroke volume minus forward stroke volume equals regurgitant stroke volume. The regurgitant fraction equals regurgitant stroke volume divided by total stroke volume. Severe valvular regurgitation has a regurgitant fraction of 0.50 or greater. Direct measurement of aortic regurgitation in milliliters per stroke in a pulsatile circulation model agrees closely with MRI-derived phase velocity encoding data in the model. The technique is clinically applicable (Fig. 15-10).

RV volume is estimated by applying Simpson's rule or the area-length method to the cavity silhouettes after biplane angiography.[71] The end-diastolic volume of the right ventricle in normal persons is 81 ± 12 mL/m^2. The opacified left atrial shadow is represented as an ellipsoid, so the left atrial volume also can be calculated in the biplane mode; the normal left atrial maximal volume is 63 ± 16 mL with a mean volume of 35 ± 8.7 mL.

Resistance

By Poiseuille's law, the flow varies directly with the fourth power of the radius of a tube; resistance varies inversely with the fourth power of the radius. Vascular resistance to blood flow in systemic, pulmonary, or regional vascular beds is estimated by analogy to Ohm's law:

$$\text{Resistance} = \frac{\text{pressure (or volts)}}{\text{mean blood flow (or amperes)}}$$

or resistance = mean pressure differential across the vascular bed divided by the blood flow (see also Chap. 3).

To obtain the pressure difference across the pulmonary bed, subtract the pulmonary artery wedge (or left atrial) pressure from the pulmonary artery mean pressure; for the systemic pressure difference, subtract the mean central venous or right atrial pressure from the mean aortic pressure. Conversion into centimeter-gram-second (cgs) units (dyn·s/cm^5) is usual, but it does not add to the intrinsic significance of the measurements. Resistance also can be expressed simply as R in units = mean pressure difference (mean flow in millimeters of mercury) divided by the cardiac output (in liters per minute). In infants and children, the pressure drop is related to the flow index; thus R in units × m^2 = pressure difference divided by cardiac index. Pulmonary resistance calculations in adults are usually not indexed, although there is an increasing tendency to do so. The normal pulmonary vascular resistance index is 1 to 2 units. Generally, 1 resistance unit is approximately equal to 80 dyn·s/cm^5. In a physiologic sense, the term *resistance* avoids specific definition. A change in resistance usually implies a change in a cross-sectional area of the vascular bed but does not indicate the mechanism behind the change. Passive widening of the vessels by increases in intravascular flow as well as the opening of previously closed channels may produce changes in resistance similar to those of active vasomotion. Subnormal calculated pulmonary vascular resistance is found in the patient who has a large atrial septal defect with normal pulmonary artery pressure. Clinically, the resistance figure is useful in quantitating the extent of pulmonary vascular disease; thus a patient with a pulmonary vascular resistance of 10 units/m^2 probably would not benefit from closure of a septal defect (see Chap. 70). The total resistance to blood flow in a pulsatile system is defined as *impedance*. Its clinical use is limited, however, since the accurate calculation of impedance requires high-fidelity pressure and velocity or flow recordings.

Calculation of Valve Areas

The equation for calculation of valve area (Torricelli's orifice equation) uses a standard hydrokinetic formula for a rounded-edge orifice or a short tube. When flow occurs across a narrow orifice, the pressure differential is related to the conversion of pressure energy into kinetic energy. The Gorlin formula for calculation of valve area is derived by combining two standard orifice formulas, one describing the volume rate of flow and the second, the velocity of flow.[72,73]

FORMULA I

$$F = AVC_c$$

where F = volume rate of flow during the time the valvular orifice is open, mL/s of diastole or systole
A = area of fixed orifice, cm^2
V = velocity flow, cm/s
C_c = coefficient of orifice contraction compensating for the physical phenomenon of reduction of the orifice stream to an area less than the area of the actual orifice

FORMULA II

$$V^2 = C_v^2\, 2gh \quad \text{or} \quad V = C_v\sqrt{2gh}$$

where V = as above
C_v = coefficient of velocity (allowing for some loss in conversion of pressure energy to velocity)
g = gravity acceleration (980 cm/s per second)
h = pressure head or differential across the orifice, cmH$_2$O

COMBINING I AND II

$$A = \frac{F}{C_c \times C_v\sqrt{2gh}} \qquad A = \frac{F}{C \times 44.3\sqrt{P_1 - P_2}}$$

where C = discharge coefficient (an orifice constant obtained by comparing calculated with measured valve areas at postmortem, which combines C_c, C_v, conversion factor, mmHg to cmH$_2$O, other unknown factors)

$44.3 = \sqrt{2g} = \sqrt{1960}$
$h = P_1 - P_2$
= pressure differential across the orifice, mmHg

The duration of ventricular filling or emptying is calculated in seconds per minute from pullback or simultaneous pressure records obtained immediately upstream and downstream from the valve. The systolic or diastolic time per beat multiplied by the heart rate gives the number of seconds in each minute during which either filling or emptying occurs across the AV or semilunar valve, respectively. Thus the volume rate of flow in milliliters per second of systole or diastole is the mean volume rate of flow (cardiac output in milliliters per minute) divided by the filling or emptying time in seconds per minute. A sample calculation of mitral valve area is as follows:

Cardiac output (CO) = 5000 mL/min
Diastolic filling period (DFP) beat = 0.38 s/beat
Pulse rate = 90 beats/min
DFP/min = 34 s/min
Left atrial mean diastolic pressure (LAP) = 30 mmHg

Left ventricular mean diastolic pressure (LVDP) = 5 mmHg
C = 0.85 (orifice constant for the mitral valve)[77]

$$\text{Mitral valve flow (MVF)} = \frac{\text{CO}}{\text{DFP/min}} = \frac{5000 \text{ mL/min}}{34 \text{ s/min}} = 147 \text{ mL/s of diastole}$$

$$\text{Mitral valve orifice area (MAV)} = \frac{\text{MVF}}{0.85 \times 44.5\sqrt{\text{LAP} - \text{LVDP}}} = \frac{147}{38\sqrt{25}} = 0.8 \text{ cm}^2$$

The calculation for the aortic valve area is as follows:

$$\text{AVA (in cm}^2) = \frac{F}{C \times 44.5\sqrt{P_1 - P_2}} = \frac{\text{aortic valve flow (mL/s of systole)}}{1 \times 44.5\sqrt{\text{LVS} - \text{ASP}}}$$

where LVS = left ventricular systolic mean pressure, mmHg
ASP = aortic systolic mean pressure, mmHg
C = orifice constant coefficient (value of 1 for the aortic valve)

If the femoral artery is used, the aortic gradient from the simultaneous left ventricular–femoral artery pressure tracing should be averaged with the gradient obtained from the tracing that is realigned to correct for the central to peripheral time lag of the femoral pulse.[74] Other modifications also have been proposed.[75,76]

Similarly, orifice areas may be calculated for the tricuspid and pulmonary valves, using an orifice constant of 1.0. In a pulsatile flow model, the Gorlin valve area predicted the severity of aortic stenosis better than valvular resistance or stroke-work loss measurements.[77] The approximations and systemic errors in the formula do not detract from its usefulness in providing objectivity in the classification of patients with valvular disease.[78] The valve orifice, and thus the calculated valve area, may not be fixed and may be flow- and pressure-dependent. The orifice constant, too, may vary with the square root of the mean pressure gradient. Modifications of the widely used Gorlin formula have been made. To estimate aortic valve area, the Bache formula uses either the peak-to-peak or the maximum systolic gradient, thus avoiding planimetry.[79] Hakki omits the ejection or filling period and the empirical constant. He uses the square root of either the mitral mean, aortic mean, or aortic peak pressure gradients divided into the cardiac output. The Hakki mitral or aortic valve area generally agrees with the Gorlin areas[80]; a correction factor for heart rate has been proposed.[81] If flow is normal, reducing a valve orifice diameter to less than half or the cross-sectional area to one-fourth is generally required to offer significant obstruction. A significantly reduced mitral valve area is 1 cm^2; aortic valve area is 0.7 cm^2 (see Chap. 57). The transmitral pressure gradient is somewhat overestimated if the pulmonary artery wedge pressure is used rather than the left atrial pressure.[82] Calculation of the orifice area of a stenotic valve in the presence of associated valvular regurgitation must take into consideration the added regurgitant flow or the severity of the stenosis will be overestimated. To obtain an estimate of mitral or aortic regurgitant volume, the forward stroke volume should be subtracted from total angiographic LV stroke volume.

SELECTIVE ANGIOGRAPHY

Contrast medium was first injected through a rubber catheter placed in the right ventricle by Chavez in 1947. The technique of selective angiography has been continually refined. In the patient with valvular or congenital heart disease, the diagnosis is often made initially by noninvasive imaging. Catheterization and angiography are then performed as directed studies to provide histologic data and additional anatomic detail. A catheter with a large lumen facilitates rapid low-pressure delivery of a single bolus of the contrast agent. A catheter with a coiled open tip and multiple laterally directed openings reduces recoil. A balloon-tipped angiographic catheter with proximal side holes is easy to manipulate and induces less ectopy than do conventional catheters. A power injector delivers the desired volume of contrast medium at a preselected maximal flow rate. In adults with complex cyanotic congenital heart disease, a large closed-end catheter with multiple side holes inserted via the femoral vein can deliver 70 mL of contrast medium in 2 s without recoil. Positioning the catheter in the apex of the right ventricle is done by using a guidewire or a tip deflector wire when a large-diameter catheter is used.

Contrast Media

In 1923, Osborn noted that the urinary bladder of luetic patients treated with oral and intravenous sodium iodide became opaque to x-rays because of the absorption of photons by iodine. All contrast media contain three iodine molecules attached to a fully substituted benzene ring. The fourth position in the standard ionic agent is taken up by sodium or methylglucamine as cation; the remaining two positions of the benzene ring have side chains of diatrizoate, metatrizoate, or iothalamate. All media are excreted predominantly by glomerular filtration. The normal half-time of excretion is 20 min; biliary excretion is 1 percent. A dose of 0.5 to 1.0 mL/kg of medium may be scaled up or down in relation to total body weight, size of the heart chambers, systemic blood flow, degree of left-to-right shunting, severity of pulmonary vascular disease, and clinical status of the patient. If significant hemodynamic changes rapidly follow the administration of contrast medium, subsequent large-volume injections ideally should be spaced in time as the clinical status of the patient dictates. The vasodilator effect and the transient decrease in systemic vascular resistance are directly related to the degree of osmolality of the contrast medium used. Transient hypervolemia and depressed contractility are in part responsible for the elevation of left atrial and LV end-diastolic pressure.

To reduce the osmotic effects of contrast medium, the number of dissolved particles must be decreased or the molal concentration of iodine per particle must be increased (Fig. 15-11). New-generation, nonionic, monomer, and ionic dimer contrast agents have approximately the same viscosity and iodine concentration but have only one-half or less of the osmolality of the ionic agents, e.g., iopamidol and ioxaglic acid (ioxaglate), 796 and 560 mosmol/kg H_2O, respectively, versus 1689 mosmol/kg H_2O for diatriozate sodium.[83] The advantages of the new agents include less hemodynamic loading,[84] patient discomfort, binding of ionic calcium, depression of myocardial function and blood pressure,[85] and possibly fewer anaphylactoid reactions. A disadvantage is the high cost that leads to a policy of selected use.[86] Also, while standard contrast media have a moderate anticoagulant effect, some nonionic media have only a slight anticoagulant effect, and the catheter and syringe containing them should thus be kept free of blood.[87] The principal use of the new agents may be in very ill patients, especially in adults

CONTRAST MEDIA

	Standard Agents	New Generation Agents	
	High Osmolality	Low Osmolality	
Structure	Ionic Monoacid Monomer	Non-Ionic Monomer	Ionic Monoacid Dimer
Benzene Rings	One	One	Two
Cation	One	None	One
Moles of Iodine	Three	Three	Six
Particles in Solution	Two	One	Two
Molal Concentration Of Iodine Per Particle	1.5	3.0	3.0
Side Chains	Ditrizoate[1] Metrizoate[2] Iothalamate[3]	Metrizamide[4] Iopamidol[5] Iohexol[6]	Ioxaglate[7]
Proprietary Names	[1]Renografin 76 Angiovist Hypaque [2]Isopaque [3]Conray	[4]Amipaque [5]Isovue [6]Omnipaque	[7]Hexabrix

FIGURE 15-11 Comparison of structure, iodine per particle, and side chain between standard and new contrast media. The number next to the proprietary name identifies the side chain it contains.

with extremely poor LV function, in patients with renal disease, especially those with diabetes, and in patients with a history of serious reaction to contrast media or with multiple allergies. If standard high-osmolality agents are used, those which are non-calcium binding may produce less negative inotropic effect and less ventricular fibrillation.[88]

Filming Methods

Cineangiography uses intensification and amplification fluoroscopy and filming by a 35-mm movie camera as well as television monitoring and disk recording.[89] Perfection in image quality is achieved when each point in the object is recorded as a point on the film. In practice, this reproduction is hindered by the diffusion of light by intensifying screens interfering with sharpness and resolving power. Although the detail of the individual cine frame lacks the spatial resolution of the cut-film screen angiogram, the motion itself increases visual perception by noise averaging and use of the integrating (5 frames per second) or persistence ability of the eye (0.2 s). The circular image of the phosphor is usually overframed on relatively slow 35-mm film with an 18 × 24 mm useful film area. Meticulous attention to film processing and the film type is essential to obtain the desired contrast and image detail. Radiographic contrast, or the difference in density or grayness between areas, depends in part on the proper x-ray photon penetration of the subject, film contrast, and scatter radiation. The latter is minimized by a collimation of the x-ray beam. For coronary angiography, short-scale, high-contrast, sharp white images on a dark gray background are desired; in the congenital heart patient, a long scale of shades of gray helps to define the entire cardiac anatomy. Biplane cineangiography is highly desirable in the study of complex congenital heart defects, especially in infancy. The total amount of contrast medium is significantly reduced, and chamber and great vessel relations are better defined.

To perform computer-enhanced digital angiography, the catheterization laboratory image intensifier and video camera are linked to an analogue-to-digital converter, computer system, and digital storage device. The analogue video signal is digitized into a series of discrete numerical values that represent continuous voltage fluctuation and can be stored on disks. The images are acquired in the standard cineradiographic mode and simultaneously are stored on film via the cine camera and digitized from the video image. The digital information is enhanced for display by a real-time image processor and is stored on a digital disk for further processing. In single-plane acquisition, exposure rates of 15, 30, and 60 frames per second in a 512 × 512 or 1024 × 1024 matrix are available. In simultaneous biplane acquisition, 7.5, 15, and 30 frames per second are possible. Enhanced images can be recalled and reviewed to allow selection of a freeze frame. The selected image can be stored and displayed on a separate monitor. A real-time image processor enhances and smooths the fluoroscopic image. For difficult projections, pulsed fluoroscopy is available on demand at approximately half the cine dose level, the last 5 s of which can be stored on digital disk for instant review. Varying degrees of enhancement, frame rates, and exposure times can be selected from a preprogrammed push-button module. Analytical programs include subtraction capabilities, ventricular ejection fraction, edge enhancement, and regional and global wall motion. An image mask is made electronically by reversing the polarity of the

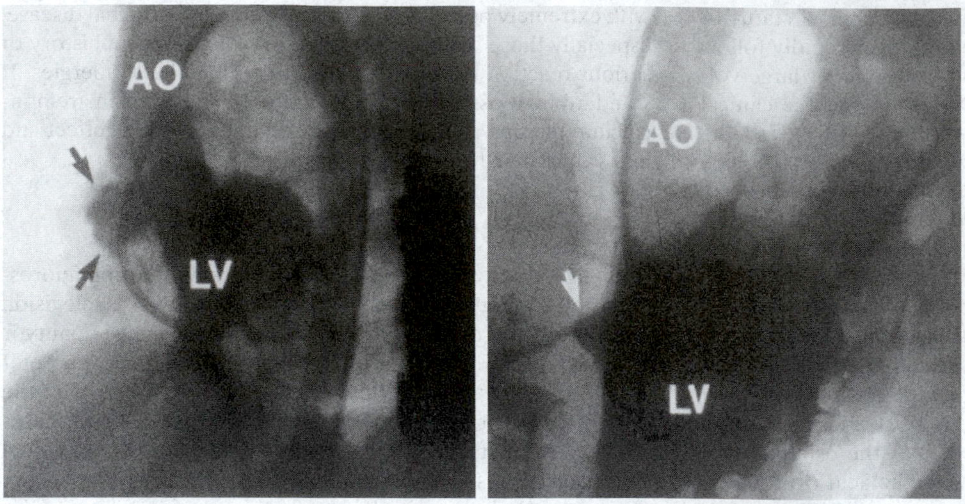

A B

FIGURE 15-12 Selective left ventricular angiography. *A.* 60° LAO and 30° cranial position demonstrates closed membranous ventricular septal defect (VSD) at the site of a large septal aneurysm (*arrows*). *B.* 40° LAO and 30° cranial position outlines a closing muscular VSD. A jet of contrast media exits the funnel-shaped defect (*arrow*).

background image of bone and tissue. The mask is then superimposed on the angiographic image. The positive and negative images of the competing tissue background cancel, leaving the digital subtraction angiogram. Arterial stenosis quantification and 2× zoom magnification can be performed in postprocessing. A hand-held infrared control device permits image review and freeze-frame storage during the study. It can be placed in a sterile bag and operated by the cardiologist at tableside. Post-case review and additional image processing are accomplished via the view panel. Hard-copy images of selected frames, which are particularly useful for interventional procedures, can be recorded via video paper, x-ray film, or laser copier. In practice, the resolution of the digital arteriogram from the hard disk approaches that of cine film. Unacceptable image degradation occurs when the digital angiogram is transferred to videocassette tape. Thus, once a practical way of permanent digital image archiving is established and if a standard compatible system for exporting image data is developed, digital angiography is likely to replace film in the catheterization laboratory.[90] The compact disc-recordable (CD-R) format and a universal interchange standard set by users and makers, i.e., Digital Imaging and Communications in Medicine (DICOM), appears promising.

Positioning

Universal positioning capability of the x-ray and intensifier tubes by using stands of L-, U-, or C-arm configuration permits angled views of a supine patient. Two profile views of the curved ventricular septum are needed. They are made in degrees of axial obliquity and cranial angulation as follows: (1) The 40° left anterior oblique (LAO) and 30° cranial position (four-chamber view) outlines the posterior third of the ventricular septum, the valve plane in AV canal defects, and the four heart chambers without superimposition. (2) The 60° LAO and 30° cranial position (long-axial view) outlines the anterior two-thirds of the ventricular septum, the membranous ventricular septal defect, and the LV outflow tract (Fig. 15-12*A*,*B*). An elongated RAO view, which is useful for seeing the RV infundibulum and supracristal ventricular septal defect, is obtained by 30° axial RAO and 40° cranial angulation. The main pulmonary artery and its bifurcation are seen in the frontal position with 30° of cranial angulation; a steep LAO position with marked cranial angulation is also used.[91]

A successful procedure results when a rapid injection of the proper volume of contrast medium is made through an adequate-sized catheter, properly positioned, with detailed attention to radiologic technique and to the position of the x-ray tube or tubes. Complete opacification of the LV cavity without inducing ventricular ectopy defines a satisfactory LV angiogram.[92]

Uses of Angiography

Right atrial angiography is useful in defining the following: (1) the tricuspid valve in Ebstein's anomaly and tricuspid atresia or stenosis, (2) myxoma or thrombus, (3) juxtaposition of right atrial appendage in cyanotic congenital heart disease, (4) the right atrial border in pericardial effusion or tumor, and (5) atrial septal defect with right-to-left shunting or occasionally the site entrance of an anomalous pulmonary vein by reflux. In the lateral position, an RV injection is used to study the caliber and the level of obstruction to RV outflow and the relation of the great vessels to the right ventricle (Fig. 15-13). A pulmonary artery injection may be used to fill the left side of the heart to detect a left-to-right shunt and to detect the site of partial (Fig. 15-14) or total anomalous venous drainage of the pulmonary veins and to visualize the pulmonary artery and its branches (Fig. 15-15). An atrial septal defect is best defined by selectively injecting the right upper-lobe pulmonary vein rather than the left atrium itself. In patients with an endocardial cushion defect and an ostium primum atrial defect, selective LV angiography shows relative elongation (Swan's neck) of the LV outflow tract and shortening of the LV inflow tract due to deficiency of the upper part of the inlet ventricular septum (Fig. 15-16). To identify the pulmonary arteries in cases of pulmonary atresia with ventricular septal defect or to identify one pulmonary artery in cases where a shunt procedure has inadvertently produced discontinuity between right and left branches, a hand injection of contrast medium into an end-hole balloon catheter occluding a pulmonary vein or into a conventional catheter in the pulmonary vein wedge position frequently will opacify the ipsilateral pulmonary artery retrogradely back to its main confluence.[93] The size and origin of systemic artery-to-pulmonary artery collaterals arising from the descending aorta, the patent ductus, and the subclavian arteries should be defined in the patient with pulmonary atresia (Fig. 15-17).

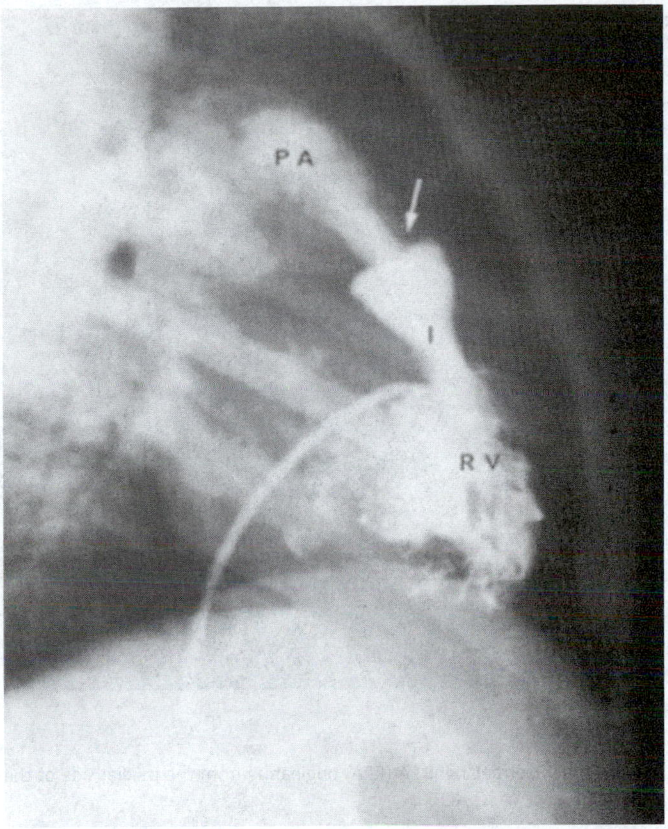

FIGURE 15-13 Valvular pulmonary stenosis (lateral view). Right ventricular injection of opaque medium. Contrast material exits through central orifice of pulmonary valve in form of a jet (*arrow*). RV, right ventricle; I, infundibulum of right ventricle; PA, pulmonary artery.

Valve Regurgitation

Injections made above the aortic valve serve to detect and qualitatively assess aortic regurgitation. In milder degrees of aortic regurgitation, a fine regurgitant jet or puff is noted; opacification is limited to the LV outflow tract, clearing with each systole (grade 1), or faint, persistent, incomplete opacification of the LV cavity (grade 2) occurs. In grades 3 and 4, no distinct jet is seen, and dense complete opacification of the left ventricle occurs either progressively or in one or two diastolic cycles, and LV density exceeds aortic density in the severe case. After an aortic injection, the size and mobility of a stenotic aortic valve may be visualized by negative-contrast washout of the opacified aorta with nonopaque ventricular blood. In the LAO view, the mouthlike opening of a bicuspid aortic valve is seen when fusion of the commissure between the right and the left aortic sinus leaflets occurs. An LV injection may display the level of subaortic obstruction to LV outflow. In patients with endocardial cushion defect, the frontal view may show a radiolucent notch in the anterior mitral valve leaflet or between the superior and inferior bridging leaflets of the AV valve.

LV injection in the RAO view is used to detect and grossly quantitate mitral regurgitation. Forty-five milliliters of contrast medium is delivered at 15 mL/s via a pigtail catheter positioned to avoid ventricular ectopy. The angiographic criteria for grading mitral regurgitation are somewhat subjective, so disagreement may arise between observers in assessing the degree of reflux. In grades 1 and 2 mitral regurgitation, a narrow- to moderate-width regurgitant jet of slight to moderate density is noted; minimum to moderate opacification of the left atrium clears quickly. In grades 3 and 4, a well-defined jet is absent, and left atrial opacification is intense, immediate, and lingering; thus the left atrium appears denser than the left ventricle or

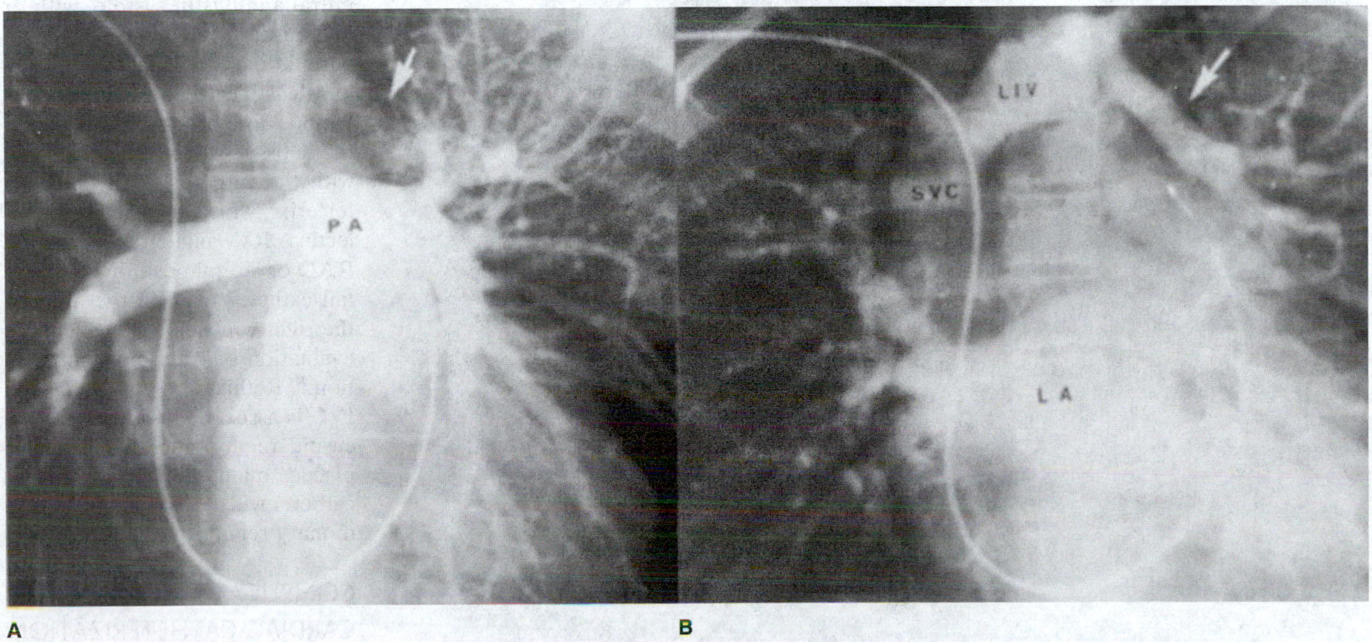

FIGURE 15-14 Partial anomalous drainage of pulmonary veins (frontal view). *A.* The catheter has been introduced into the right atrium and ventricle and positioned in the main pulmonary artery (PA), where selective injection is performed. *B.* Pulmonary venous phase. A large pulmonary vein (*arrow*) drains the upper lobe of the left lung, with anomalous venous return to the left innominate vein (LIV). SVC, superior vena cava; LA, left atrium.

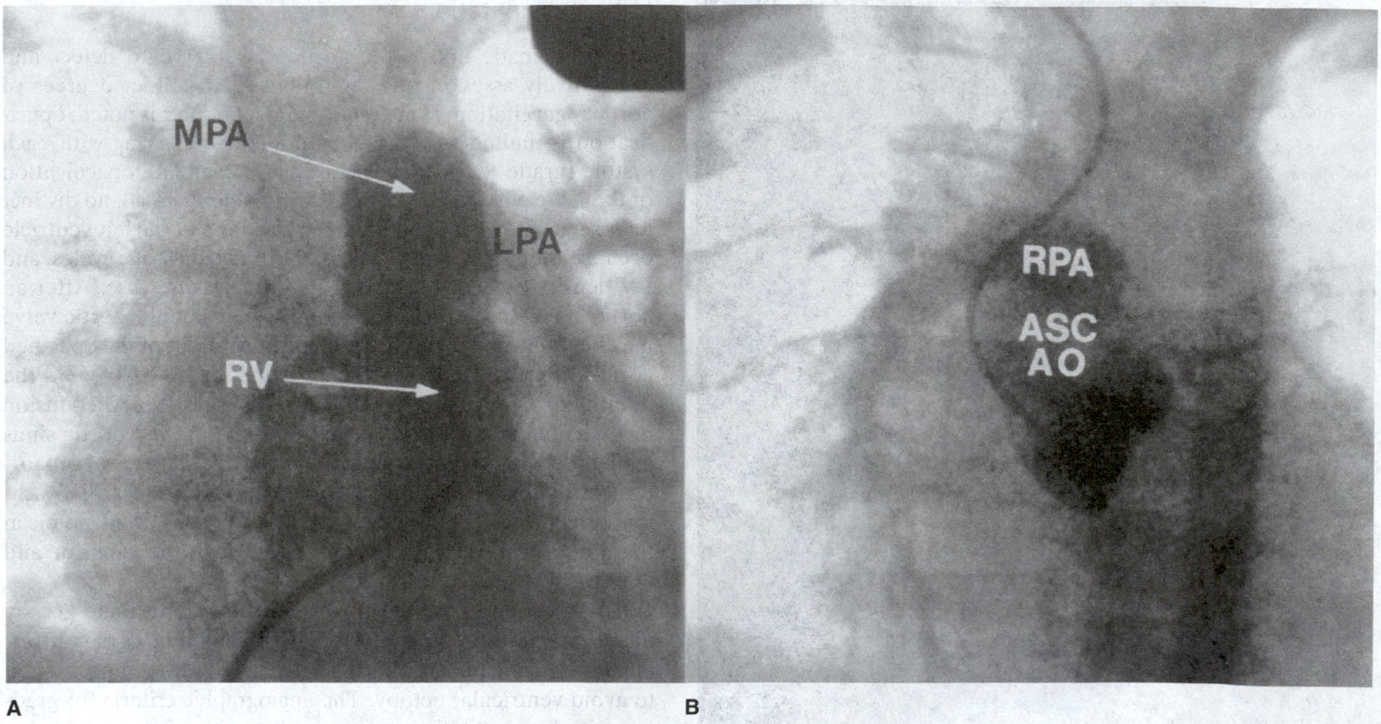

FIGURE 15-15 *A*. Selective right ventricular (RV) injection, frontal view opacifying the main pulmonary artery (MPA) and the left PA (LPA). The right PA does not opacify. *B*. Selective injection of the aortic root in the frontal view opacifies the aberrant right PA (RPA) originating from the medial side of the ascending aorta (ASC AO).

aorta in grade 4 mitral regurgitation. In mitral valve prolapse, which is shown best in a lateral projection with slight cranial angulation, all or a portion of one or both leaflets balloons above the mitral annulus in systole, with or without associated mitral valve regurgitation. A normal mitral valve may leak if ectopic beating occurs. Unlike disk or ball valves, prosthetic tissue valves can be crossed with the catheter tip without interfering with valve function. Selective RV angiography in the RAO or lateral position via a pigtail catheter lying in the apex of the right ventricle gives adequate evaluation of tricuspid regurgitation.[94] Reflux into the SVC and IVC is associated with severe tricuspid regurgitation. A properly placed main pulmonary artery catheter will detect significant pulmonary regurgitation.

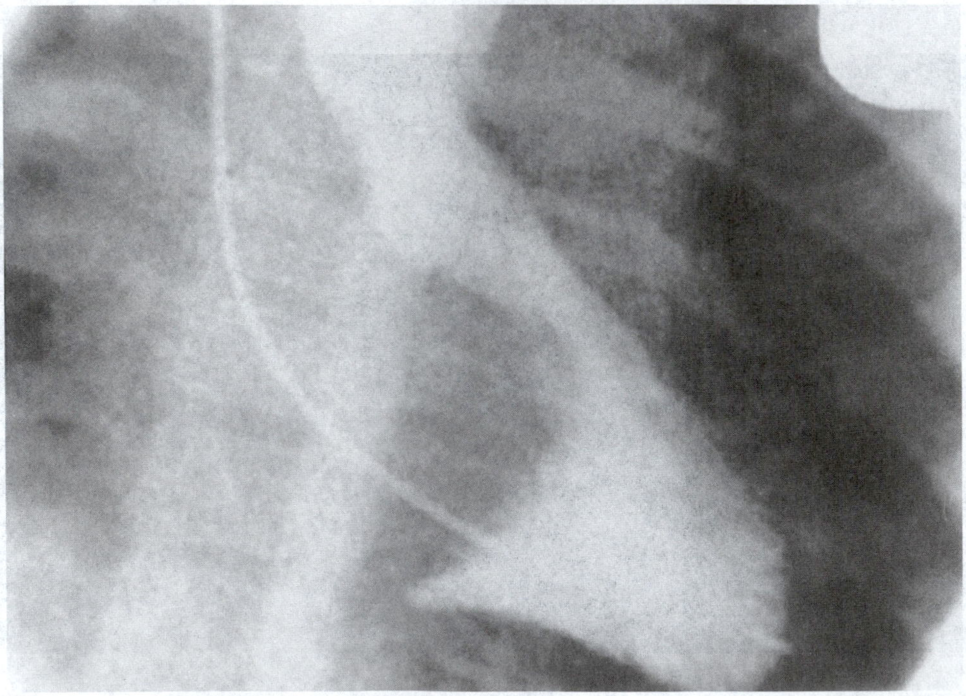

FIGURE 15-16 The frontal view of the left ventricular (LV) cineangiogram of a young girl with partial AV canal shows the typical swan's neck contour of the LV outflow tract. Note the shorter than normal mitral valve annulus to LV apex distance (the LV inflow tract) in comparison with the LV apex to aortic valve distance (LV outflow tract).

COMPLICATIONS OF CARDIAC CATHETERIZATION AND ANGIOGRAPHY

An experienced operator can carry out catheterization of the

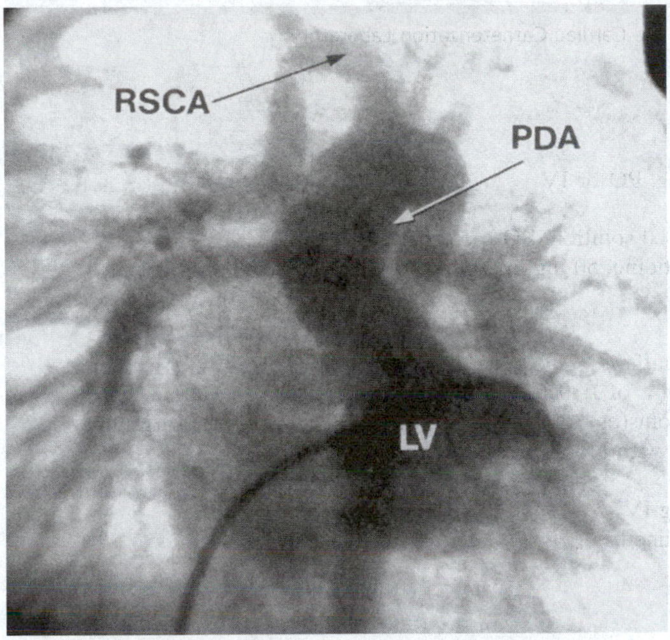

FIGURE 15-17 Selective LV angiogram in a patient with ventricular septal defect and pulmonary atresia, frontal view. The right and left pulmonary arteries are supplied by a patent ductus arteriosus (PDA). A branch from the right subclavian artery (RSCA) fills a separate right pulmonary artery supplying the right middle and upper lobe.

right side of the heart without difficulty in practically all cases. Complications may include knotting of the catheter; breakage of the guidewire; perforation of the atrium, ventricle, or coronary vein; and pulmonary infarction or pulmonary artery rupture associated with balloon catheter inflation.[95] Complete heart block may be induced if left bundle-branch block is already present or if prolonged catheter manipulation is required in a cyanotic patient. Prolonged ventricular or atrial arrhythmia may occur.

In the catheterization of the left side of the heart, thrombosis or hematoma may occur at the percutaneous arterial puncture site, and blood may migrate into fascial and retroperitoneal planes.[96] Perforation may occur at a tortuous subclavian or pelvic arterial site. The most common vascular complication is femoral arterial pseudoaneurysm or pulsating hematoma, in part due to the increased use of heparin after catheterization (see Fig. 15-3). Pseudoaneurysm following catheterization may be detected by color Doppler flow imaging. In systole, a high-velocity flow signal moves into the sac of the pseudoaneurysm from the small puncture site in the superficial or common femoral artery; in diastole, there is a low flow velocity from the sac into the femoral artery retrogradely. In the presence of the femoral artery-to-femoral vein fistula, there is a constant-flow signal from the artery to the vein.[97,98] Ultrasound-guided compression obliteration of these communications has been helpful. Among approximately 23,000 patients (72 percent males) at Emory University Hospital who had coronary artery angiography via the percutaneous femoral approach using a no. 8 French multipurpose catheter, 14 patients (12 females and 2 males) required femoral artery thrombectomy. The smaller femoral artery of the female is more prone to thrombotic occlusion than is that of the male. Cerebral embolism results primarily from plaque material dislodgment in the ascending aorta and less often from a fibrin clot on catheters.[99] Isolated persistent diplopia or hemianopia may occur. In 30,000 coronary artery and LV catheterizations, 35 patients had central nervous system complications (carotid distribution in 15, vertebrobasilar in 20, and diffuse encephalopathy in 2). The deficit resolved in one-half of all patients and persisted in one-half. There were two deaths. Cholesterol crystal embolization shower syndrome may follow catheter manipulation in the aorta and can result in progressive renal failure. Transseptal puncture may result in inadvertent perforation of the aorta or the free wall of the atrium, with resulting cardiac tamponade.

Nausea with or without vomiting may develop immediately after the initial injection of contrast medium, probably related to direct stimulation of serotonin receptors in the brain. Adverse reactions also include sneezing, chills, low-grade fever, hives, itching, angioedema, bronchospasm, and shock. Since no anti-contrast medium immunoglobulin E (IgE) is found, these reactions are anaphylactoid rather than being true anaphylaxis. The mechanism may be related to activation of the kallikrein, classic or alternate complement, or intrinsic coagulation systems or to direct hyperosmolar or chemical cytotoxicity.[100] Rare reactions include parotitis (iodide mumps), glossitis, and pancreatic edema. A two-dose oral glucocorticoid regimen (methylprednisolone, 32 mg) given 12 and 2 h before standard contrast medium injection significantly reduces acute allergic reactions. Diphenhydramine hydrochloride, cimetidine hydrochloride, epinephrine, and hydrocortisone, singly or combined, have been added to a treatment protocol outlined in Table 15-2. Patients at high risk for contrast medium nephropathy usually have preexisting renal insufficiency and diabetes. An increase in serum creatinine levels of 0.5 to 1.0 mg/dL or a rise of 25 to 50 percent over baseline at 24 to 48 h after angiography is noted in 2 to 7 percent of an unselected population and is considered to reflect contrast medium-induced renal injury. Good hydration is essential in preventing or diminishing renal injury: 0.45% normal saline at a rate of 1 mL/kg per hour is begun 12 h before and is continued for 12 h after the procedure.[101] The mechanism of contrast nephrotoxicity is related in part to renal cortical vasoconstriction and to tubular cell toxicity[102,103] (Fig. 15-18). Renal insult in a high-risk-group subset in a randomized trial was diminished with the use of low-osmolality media. There is little difference in the rate in serum creatinine levels after angiography in low-risk groups whether ionic or nonionic contrast media are used.[104,105] Pulmonary edema following angiography may be caused by volume overload and a negative inotropic effect.

In desperately ill patients and in those with marked ventricular dysfunction or severe valvular obstruction, the desire for films that display the cardiac anatomy spectacularly should be tempered by the potential consequences of large doses of contrast medium in this setting.[106]

CORONARY ARTERIOGRAPHY AND LEFT VENTRICULOGRAPHY

Coronary arteriography remains the standard by which all methods of diagnosing coronary artery disease are measured. It is the primary method of defining coronary anatomy in living patients. To accomplish this in a safe, reliable, and reproducible manner, adherence to certain principles of performance and interpretation is required.[107–109]

TABLE 15-2 Guidelines for Management of Anaphylacioid Reactions in the Cardiac Catheterization Laboratory

Condition	Therapy
Urticaria and skin itching	1. No treatment 2. Diphenhydramine. 25–50 mg, PO or IV 3. Unresponsive to therapy: Epinephrine, 0.3 mL of 1:1000 solution, SQ q 15 min up to 1 mL Cimetidine, 300 mg, or ranitidine, 50 mg in 20 mL normal saline, IV over 15 min
Bronchospasm	1. O_2 by mask Oximetry 2. *Mild:* albuterol inhaler—2 puffs *Moderate:* epinephrine, 0.3 mL of 1:1000 solution, SQ q 15 min up to 1 mL *Severe:* epinephrine IV as bolus(es)[a] of 10 μg/min, then infusion[b] of 1 to 4 μg/min; observe for desired effect with blood pressure and ECG monitoring 3. Diphenhydramine, 50 mg IV 4. Hydrocortisone, 200–400 mg IV 5. Optional; H_2 blocker as outlined
Facial and laryngeal edema	1. Call anesthesia 2. Assess airway O_2 Intubation Tracheostomy tray 3. *Mild:* epinephrine SQ as outlined *Moderate/severe:* epinephrine IV as outlined above 4. Diphenhydramine, 50 mg IV 5. Oximetry/arterial blood gases 6. H_2 blocker as outlined
Hypotension/shock	1. Simultaneous administration a. Epinephrine IV as bolus(es) of 10 μg/min until desired blood pressure response obtained, then infusion of 1–4 μg/min to maintain desired blood pressure b. Large volumes of 0.9% normal saline IV (1–3 L in the first hour) 2. O_2 by mask Intubation 3. Diphenhydramine, 50–100 mg IV 4. Hydrocortisone, 400 mg IV 5. Central venous pressure/Swan-Ganz 6. Oximetry/arterial blood gases 7. Unresponsive to therapy: H_2 blocker as outlined Dopamine, 2–15 μg/kg per min IV Advanced cardiac life support

[a]Bolus dose: 0.1 mL of 1:1000 solution or 1 mL of 1:10,000, diluted to 10 mL (10 μg/mL).
[b]Infusion dose: 1 mL of 1:1000 or 10 mL in 250 mL normal saline (4 μg/mL).
NOTE: ECG, electrocardiographic, IV, intravenous; PO, by mouth; SQ, subcutaneous.
Source: From Gross JE, Chambers CE, Heupler FA, members of the Laboratory Performance Standards Committee of the Society for Cardiac Angiography and Interventions. *Cathet Cardiovasc Diagn* 1995; 34: 99–104. With permission of the authors and publisher.

Coronary arteriography provides not only an anatomic map of the coronary arteries, including the site, severity, and shape of stenotic lesions, but also the characteristics of distal vessels in terms of size, presence of atherosclerotic disease, mass of myocardium served, a rough index of differential coronary flow, identification of collateral vessels, and an estimate of their functional importance.[110–113] Intracoronary thrombi can be recognized, although it is clear from angioscopic studies that coronary arteriography is relatively insensitive in the detection of thrombi. In addition, the presence of coronary spasm can be ascertained by using provocative maneuvers.[114–116] The functional significance of a coronary stenosis can be assessed by measuring coronary flow directly, both at rest and during an intense coronary dilator stimulus. The difference between resting and maximal coronary flow is the coronary flow reserve capacity of the coronary bed. Coronary flow reserve can be measured in the coronary arteriography laboratory by using digital subtraction or intracoronary Doppler techniques.[117]

LV catheterization makes possible measurements of LV pressure at rest, with exercise, or after pharmacologic agents. Left ventriculography enables one to make a visual analysis of wall motion. Ventricular systolic and diastolic volume and

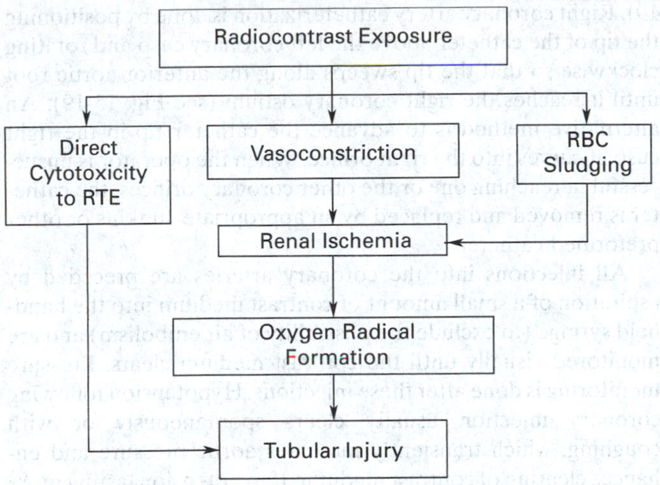

FIGURE 15-18 Proposed mechanisms of contrast media-induced acute renal injury. RBC, red blood cells; RTE, renal tubular epithelial cells. (From Rocher.[102] Reproduced with permission of the author and publisher.)

ejection fraction can be calculated. Careful correlation of the coronary arteriogram and left ventriculogram permits identification of stenotic and potentially bypassable arteries serving viable myocardium. LV wall motion can be further evaluated by the addition of stress such as atrial pacing, pharmacologic agents, or exercise. Augmenting LV contraction by the use of nitrates, catecholamines, or postextrasystolic beats may permit the identification of LV wall segments that have a potential for improved function after revascularization surgery.[118–120] The presence of associated valvular heart disease may be determined. In patients who have previously undergone surgery, patency of grafts and status of the native coronary arteries can be ascertained. In certain children with congenital heart disease, the location of the coronary arteries can be determined as an aid to planning surgical correction.[121]

Techniques of Coronary Arteriography

Sones ushered in the modern era of coronary arteriography in 1958 when he developed a safe and reliable method of selective coronary arteriography.[110] The Sones technique uses an antecubital incision over the brachial artery. The artery is exposed, and a woven Dacron catheter (Sones USCI) is passed into the brachial artery and maneuvered through the axillary and subclavian arteries into the ascending aorta. Manipulation techniques depend on deflecting the soft, tapered catheter tip off the aortic valve cusps up to the coronary orifices. The Sones technique has stood the test of time. The advantages are that it requires only one catheter, aortoiliac disease is avoided, and the operator is close to the aortic root and therefore has a good feel of the catheter tip. The disadvantages of antecubital dissection, arteriotomy, and arterial closure have been nearly entirely overcome by percutaneous entry of the brachial artery and, in recent years, the radial artery. Manipulation skills and precise knowledge of the aortic root anatomy are required. A detailed description of the Sones technique has been published.[122]

Percutaneous arterial catheterization, described in 1953 by Seldinger,[123] was first used to study the coronary arteries, as reported by Ricketts and Abrams in 1962.[124] Modification of catheters was made by Amplatz et al.[125] and by Judkins[126] in 1967. The Judkins technique requires three preformed catheters: one for each coronary artery and a pigtail catheter for the LV injection. The Judkins technique is much easier to learn; paradoxically, this may be its major drawback. The femoral artery is punctured below the inguinal ligament, and a left coronary artery catheter is passed over the guidewire into the aorta. After the catheter is flushed and good pressure tracings are obtained from the tip, the catheter is advanced until it engages the left coronary orifice. The preformed shape of the catheter holds it against the inside of the aortic curve, enabling the tip to spring into the left coronary orifice. The tip is made in four lengths for use with different-sized aortic roots. After the left catheter is removed, the appropriate-sized right coronary catheter is inserted over a guidewire and positioned above the right coronary orifice, where it is rotated clockwise. The tip will descend and will be held against the outside curve of the aorta, causing it to spring into the right coronary orifice. LV studies are performed by replacing the coronary catheters with the pigtail catheter. A detailed description of the Judkins technique also has been published.[127]

This technique has the advantages of a percutaneous approach; the disadvantages are the requirement for multiple catheter exchanges and a potential increased risk of emboli to the coronary or cerebral circulation. Complications may arise from the ease of entry of the catheter tip into the coronary arteries. Some poorly trained angiographers have applied this technique without proper appreciation of the devastating consequences of catheter obstruction of the left main coronary artery. Methods of avoiding serious complications of catheter emboli, including systemic heparinization and catheter-debriding techniques, have reduced complications in active centers. In an attempt to combine the advantages of the Sones and Judkins techniques, the single-catheter percutaneous femoral approach was first applied by Schoonmaker in 1968, and use of this technique was reported by Schoonmaker and King.[128] This technique has been employed at Emory University Hospital in over 80,000 studies since 1972.

Performance of Coronary Arteriography

The description of our technique of coronary arteriography is brief; a more detailed description has been published.[129] It is our belief that one cannot become expert in performing coronary arteriography by reading. Only through training in an active laboratory and performing hundreds of coronary arteriograms under close supervision can the physician gain a proper appreciation of the potential hazards of coronary arteriography so that they can be avoided.[130] A close physician-patient relationship is essential to reduce fear of the examination. The patient is seen before the procedure, and a thorough history, physical examination, and description of the procedure are completed. Patients with mild or stable symptoms may undergo coronary arteriography as outpatients, unless noninvasive studies indicate the likely presence of severe anatomic problems such as left main coronary artery stenosis. In most laboratories, outpatient catheterization studies are performed with smaller-diameter catheters of a no. 5 or no. 6 French size. Cardiac medications are usually continued up to and through the procedure. An intravenous line is routinely started for administration of midazolam for conscious sedation. The intravenous line is also essential as a port for the administration of additional drugs during the procedure, as needed, if pain or hypotension occurs or if congestive failure is aggravated. Electrocardiographic and pulse oximetry monitoring is performed throughout the procedure. Atropine, lidocaine, propranolol, furosemide, glucocorticoids, an antihistamine, nitroglycerin, epinephrine and other vasopressors, and a narcotic should be readily available for intravenous administration. Heparin and antibiotics are not administered routinely in our laboratory. Patients with a history of anaphylactoid reactions to contrast media are pretreated with antihistamines and glucocorticoids.

A three-way stopcock manifold is connected to lines for pressure monitoring, contrast medium, and heparinized saline solution. A clear catheter is maintained by intermittent flushing with saline solution and contrast medium. The femoral artery is catheterized by the Seldinger technique, and a multipurpose polyurethane catheter is inserted into the descending aorta, where it is flushed before being advanced around the aortic arch without a guidewire. The catheter is advanced to the left ventricle, where, following pressure measurements and test injections to exclude catheter-tip entrapment, 10 to 20 mL of contrast medium is injected over 3 s. This slow injection allows adequate visualization without recoil of the end-hole and side-hole catheter. Filming is done routinely in the RAO view or in a biplane mode using RAO and LAO views.

Essential to any coronary arteriographic technique is a thorough knowledge of aortic root anatomy (Fig. 15-19). Usually the left coronary orifice arises from the left sinus of Valsalva, which is posterior and to the left. The right coronary artery usually arises from the right sinus of Valsalva, which is anterior. Because of extensive variation in the position, size, and number of orifices, considerable experience is required to avoid failure to identify and study one of the arteries. Left coronary cannulation is performed in the following manner: The tip of the catheter is placed in the noncoronary cusp, which lies posterior and to the left (toward the spine in the RAO view). As the catheter is advanced with a slight clockwise rotation, the tip flips up into the left coronary ostium or into the left cusp. From the left coronary cusp, the catheter tip can be rotated posteriorly and advanced superiorly into the left coronary ostium (see Fig. 15-19). Right coronary artery catheterization is done by positioning the tip of the catheter above the left coronary cusp and rotating clockwise so that the tip sweeps along the anterior aortic root until it reaches the right coronary ostium (see Fig. 15-19). An alternative method is to advance the catheter tip in the right cusp; it curves into the right orifice. When the operator is unsuccessful in reaching one or the other coronary orifices, the catheter is removed and replaced by an appropriate Judkins or other preformed catheter.

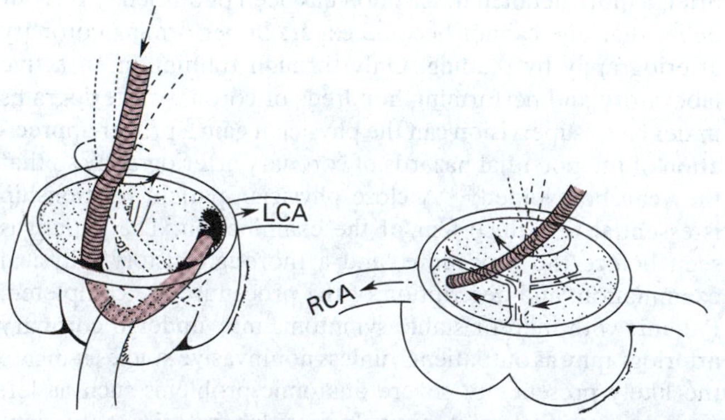

FIGURE 15-19 (*Left*) A 30° RAO view of the aortic root demonstrating the left coronary orifice. (*Right*) A 60° LAO view of the aortic root demonstrating location of the right coronary orifice. (From Schoonmaker and King.[128] Reproduced with permission from the American Heart Association, Inc., and the authors.)

All injections into the coronary arteries are preceded by aspiration of a small amount of contrast medium into the hand-held syringe (to exclude the possibility of air embolism) and are monitored visually until the contrast medium clears. Pressure monitoring is done after these injections. Hypotension following coronary injection usually clears spontaneously or with coughing, which transiently increases aortic pressure and enhances clearing of contrast medium. If hypotension lasting more than a few seconds occurs, especially in a patient with severe proximal coronary artery disease, a pressor agent in an adequate dose to obtain a quick response is started promptly. Adequate coronary perfusion pressure is essential. If congestive heart failure is aggravated by the effect of contrast medium, the first drug used is sublingual nitroglycerin; furosemide may be needed, however. When chest pain occurs, nitrates are given sublingually or intravenously, and the catheter is repositioned in the left ventricle to monitor LVEDP. If pain continues or ST-segment elevation occurs, coronary injection may reveal coronary spasm. Intracoronary nitroglycerin usually provides prompt relief. If severe elevation of end-diastolic pressure occurs, the patient may be propped up and given additional nitrates and oxygen. When tachycardia accompanied by adequate or elevated blood pressure develops during angina, 1-mg increments of propranolol or metroprolol may be given intravenously, producing dramatic relief. Narcotics are used for pain that is not relieved promptly by nitroglycerin and propranolol. Ventricular fibrillation, a rare occurrence, is corrected promptly with the defibrillator. All laboratory personnel must be thoroughly trained in cardiopulmonary resuscitation, since unstable patients may develop life-threatening arrhythmias before, during, and after angiography.[130] Minor anaphylactoid reactions are treated with antihistamines; more serious reactions are treated with the addition of epinephrine and glucocorticoids.[131] Maximal safety is obtained when an expert angiographer performs a brief but complete study, obtaining all clinically pertinent information with a minimal number of injections. Because of the osmotic diuresis induced by the contrast media, intravenous and oral fluid supplements are required after catheterization, and postural hypotension must be checked for when the patient is allowed up.

Interpretation of the Coronary Arteriogram

Once of interest to angiographers and surgeons only, the viewing and interpretation of coronary arteriograms should now be of vital interest to cardiologists if they are to make informed decisions about their patients. The coronary arteriogram should be viewed in a systematic fashion. Because coronary anatomy can be quite variable, one needs to view the films with an eye toward making sure the entire LV epicardial surface and septum are adequately supplied and that no gaps exist. If significant gaps are found, an occluded or anomalous artery is likely. The

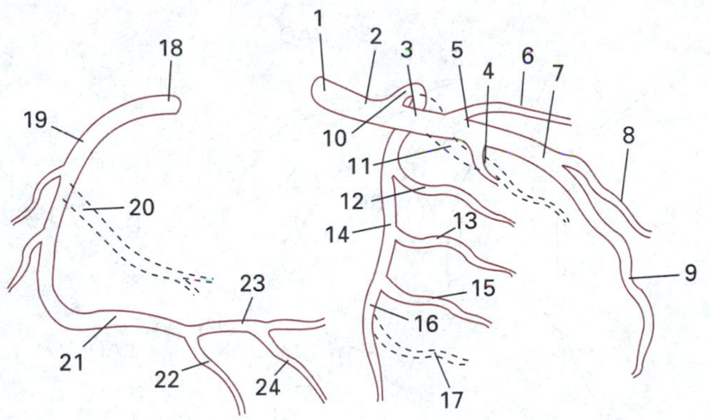

FIGURE 15-20 Diagram of the coronary circulation. Each arterial segment is evaluated carefully in all views and the degree of stenosis is determined. Left main coronary artery, 1, 2; left anterior descending coronary artery, 3, 5, 7, 9; diagonal branches, 6, 8; major septal perforating branch, 4; circumflex coronary artery in the atrioventricular groove, 10, 14, 16; ramus intermedius, 11; obtuse marginal branches, 12, 13, 15; posterior descending branch of the circumflex coronary artery, if present, 17; right coronary artery in the atrioventricular groove, 18, 19, 21, 23; large right ventricular branch of the right coronary artery, 20; posterior descending branch of the right coronary artery, 22; left ventricular branch of the right coronary artery, 24. (From King SB III, Douglas JS Jr. *Coronary Arteriography and Angioplasty*. New York: McGraw-Hill; 1985:363. Reproduced with permission from the publisher and authors.)

coronary arteries should be viewed one at a time, and some division of arterial segments such as the one suggested by the American Heart Association[132] should be made (Fig. 15-20). Areas of foreshortening and overlap should be examined in other views to convince the observer that there is not a hidden lesion. It is helpful for several observers to study the arteriogram. As each segment is viewed, a systematic scoring and recording system is mandatory if consistency is to be maintained and no segments are to be overlooked.

Angiographic Views

Filming is done in a number of projections so that all coronary arteries can be visualized throughout their lengths and significant disease can be detected and quantified. Multiple views in the transverse plane (Figs. 15-21 to 15-23) were used until 1973, when Bunnell reported the advantages of obtaining views incorporating sagittal angulation of the x-ray beam along the long axis of the body (Fig. 15-24). Use of these views (Figs. 15-25 and 15-26) greatly enhances the ability to visualize the proximal left coronary artery, unmasking lesions that otherwise would be missed in up to 20 percent of patients and significantly improving diagnosis in an additional 30 to 40 percent.[133–135] The evolution of a new generation of x-ray equipment to obtain these views has revolutionized coronary arteriography. In most laboratories, standard views of the left coronary artery are the frontal view, 30° RAO, 45° LAO, 45° LAO with 30° of cranial angulation, 30° RAO with 30° of cranial angulation, and 30° RAO with 15° of caudal angulation. Other views may be needed to separate overlapping vessels or to focus on a particular problem area. The right coronary artery usually is visualized in the right and left oblique projections, and sagittally angulated views frequently are helpful in evaluating the proximal posterior descending artery (Figs. 15-27 and 15-28). The use of sagittally angulated views also provides for improved visualization of LV wall motion and mitral valve motion and for evaluation of the LV outflow tract.[136]

THE LEFT CORONARY ARTERY

The ostium of the left coronary artery originates from the left sinus of Valsalva near the sinotubular ridge. The main left coronary artery usually courses to the left and slightly anterior. After a quite variable length, it gives rise at near right angles to the circumflex artery and continues in a straight line as the anterior descending artery (Figs. 15-29 and 15-30). The left orifice and the left main coronary artery are best seen in a direct frontal view or in a shallow LAO or RAO projection or a shallow LAO with 30° of cranial angulation. The diagonal artery may arise between the circumflex and anterior descending arteries as a trifurcation of the left main coronary artery, or the diagonal branch may originate from the anterior descending artery and course over the anterolateral free wall of the left ventricle. The diagonal branches are seen on the side in the RAO view; however, the origin is obscured by overlap with the anterior descending artery (see Figs. 15-29 and 15-30). The LAO view separates the anterior descending artery and diagonals somewhat; however, because of the frequent horizontal orientation of these arteries, there may be considerable foreshortening. Cranial angulation of the overhead intensifier with shallow LAO or RAO rotation is most helpful in separating the proximal anterior descending artery and its diagonal branches (see Figs. 15-25 and 15-26). The anterior descending artery continues in the interventricular groove toward the apex, giving rise at nearly right angles to the septal perforating arteries that go deep into the muscular septum. The first septal perforator may arise before or after the first diagonal and is usually the largest septal artery. The septal vessels differ from the epicardial arteries in that they are straighter and move little with cardiac action, in contrast to the buckling of epicardial arteries that frequently occurs with systole. The left anterior descending artery usually continues around the apex but may end short of the apex in association with an unusually long posterior descending artery. The anterior descending artery is usually best visualized in the RAO view and in a cranially angulated shallow oblique view unless the orientation of the anterior descending artery is unusually superior, in which case a caudally angulated LAO view or a straight lateral view may be helpful.

The circumflex coronary artery, after its right-angle origin from the left anterior descending artery, travels in the AV groove. Its course is quite variable. The artery may terminate in one or more large, obtuse marginal branches that course over the lateral to posterolateral LV free wall, or it may continue as a large artery in the interventricular groove and, in 10 to 15 percent of cases, give rise to a posterior descending artery, which more often arises from the right coronary artery (Fig. 15-31). When the circumflex artery supplies the major posterior descending artery, it is commonly referred to as a *dominant* circumflex artery. The circumflex artery in the AV groove is best seen in the LAO view, but surgically more important marginal branches are visualized best in the RAO view. Occasionally, proximal stenoses in the circumflex artery are best viewed in an RAO view with 15° of caudal angulation, which produces a view as though looking from the superior aspect of the liver toward the left shoulder.

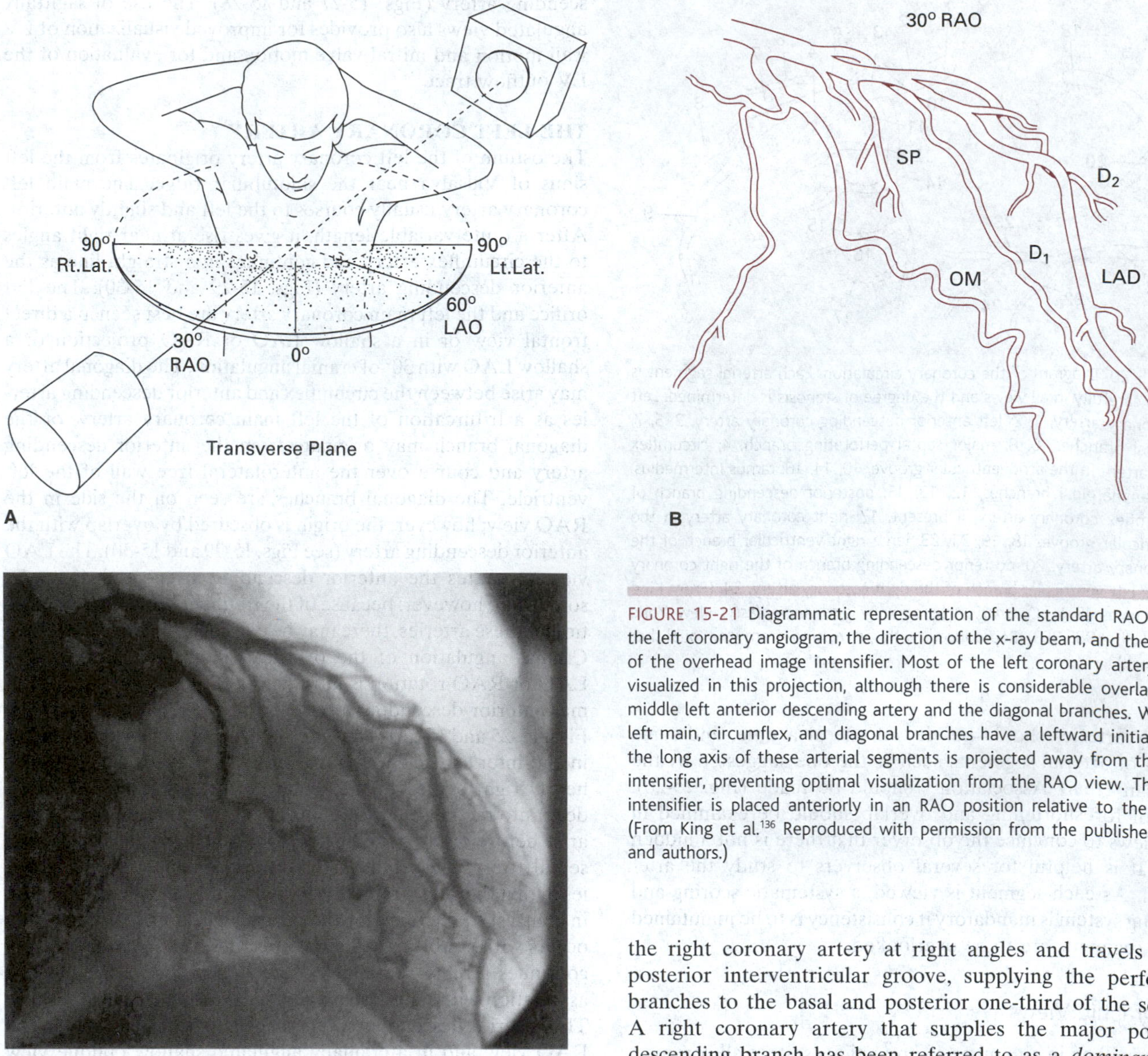

FIGURE 15-21 Diagrammatic representation of the standard RAO view of the left coronary angiogram, the direction of the x-ray beam, and the position of the overhead image intensifier. Most of the left coronary artery is well visualized in this projection, although there is considerable overlap of the middle left anterior descending artery and the diagonal branches. When the left main, circumflex, and diagonal branches have a leftward initial course, the long axis of these arterial segments is projected away from the image intensifier, preventing optimal visualization from the RAO view. The image intensifier is placed anteriorly in an RAO position relative to the patient. (From King et al.[136] Reproduced with permission from the publisher, editor, and authors.)

THE RIGHT CORONARY ARTERY

The right coronary artery orifice normally is located in the right sinus of Valsalva. It may be high near the sinotubular ridge or above it, in the midsinus, or occasionally low near the aortic valve. The artery commonly courses upward from the plane of the aortic valve and then travels in the right AV groove as a conduit to reach the posterior LV wall (Figs. 15-32 and 15-33). Along the way, several vessels arise. The conus branch and sinus node branches arise first, followed by small RV branches. At the acute margin of the heart, there is usually a large branch that courses over the right ventricle. In some cases this may supply the apical portion of the interventricular septum and therefore be of greater importance. The posterior descending artery usually arises before the right coronary artery reaches the crux of the heart (junction of the interventricular and interatrial septa). The posterior descending artery arises from the right coronary artery at right angles and travels in the posterior interventricular groove, supplying the perforating branches to the basal and posterior one-third of the septum. A right coronary artery that supplies the major posterior descending branch has been referred to as a *dominant* right coronary artery. The posterior descending artery usually stops before reaching the apex, but it may curl around the apex in association with a short anterior descending artery to form the loop previously described. After giving rise to the posterior descending artery, the right coronary artery becomes intramyocardial at the crux, gives rise to the AV node artery, and subsequently returns to the surface, making an inverted U curve (see Fig. 15-33). The LV branches of the right coronary artery are variable and cover the same area as the posterolateral branches of a large circumflex system. The proximal conduit portion of the right coronary artery is well seen in standard RAO and LAO views. Because of its horizontal orientation, however, the origin of the posterior descending artery is well seen in the RAO view but foreshortened in the LAO view; to overcome this, cranial angulation of the intensifier is necessary. Pathologic studies indicate that lesions at the takeoff of the posterior descending artery frequently are overlooked if standard oblique views in the transverse plane are used.

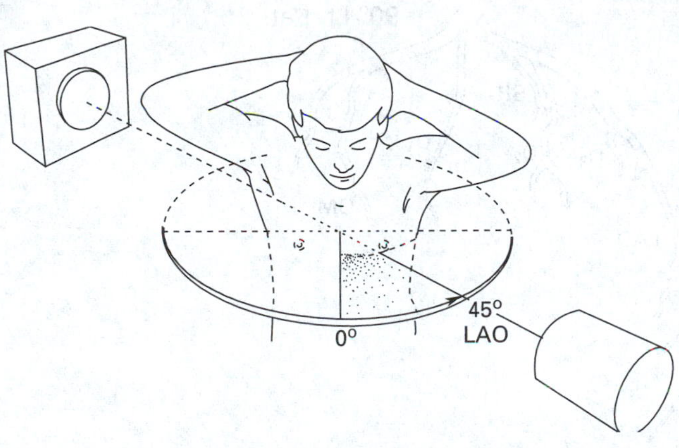

A

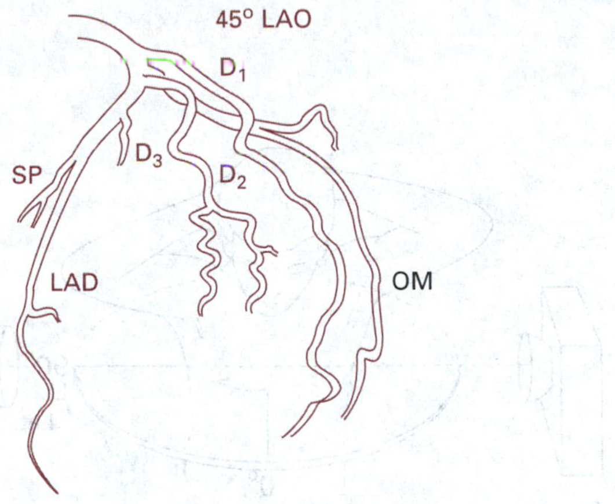

B

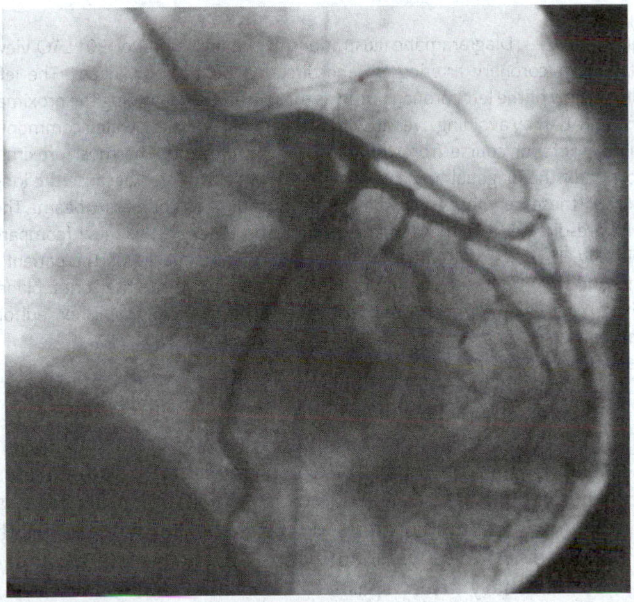

C

FIGURE 15-22 Diagrammatic representation of the LAO left coronary angiogram and the direction of the x-ray beam in this view. The value of this view depends in large part on the orientation of the long axis of the heart. When the heart is relatively horizontal, the left anterior descending (LAD) coronary artery and diagonal branches are seen end-on throughout much of the course. In this illustration, the longitudinal axis is an intermediate position and there is moderate foreshortening of the anterior descending and diagonal branches in their proximal portions (compare with Fig. 15-25). The LAO projection is frequently inadequate to visualize the proximal LAD and its branches; the left main segment, which is directed toward the image tube and therefore foreshortened, and the proximal circumflex coronary artery, which may be obscured by overlapping vessels, as in this illustration. The LAO projection is frequently used to visualize the distal LAD and its branches, the mid-circumflex coronary artery in the AV groove, and the distal right coronary artery that is filling via collaterals from the left coronary artery. The image intensifier is above the patient in an LAO position. (From King et al.[136] Reproduced with permission from the publisher, editor, and authors.)

Grading Stenoses

Visual inspection of the coronary arteriogram traditionally has been used to assess the severity of coronary artery stenosis. In our laboratory, a system of analyzing each arterial segment has been used, and the degree of stenosis is recorded as a reduction in lumen diameter expressed as a percentage, with total occlusion being 100 percent. Measurement of cineangiograms has been done with a programmable digital caliper system. In each available projection, the frame showing the most severe stenosis in end-diastole is chosen for measurement. The percentage of diameter stenosis recorded is a mean value of the measurements from two or three available projections. This method has been shown to reduce observer variability. Although cross-sectional area reduction is the measurement of greatest physiologic importance, use of diameter stenosis is in keeping with the American Heart Association recommendation that the diameter method be adopted for grading coronary artery stenoses.[132] A 50 percent reduction in diameter is equivalent to a 75 percent reduction in cross-sectional area, and a 75 percent reduction in diameter is equal to a 90 percent reduction in cross-sectional area. It is of great importance to identify which method of expressing stenosis is being used. From the standpoint of surgically significant lesions, it has been our practice to consider stenoses with greater than 50 percent diameter reduction, or greater than 75 percent cross-sectional area reduction, as lesions that may produce myocardial ischemia. Lesions in series and long stenoses are of added importance. Quantitative computerized methods for calculating coronary artery stenosis are used for clinical investigations and are also increasingly used for routine clinical coronary arteriography.[137] Techniques employing edge-detection algorithms are often applied clinically.

Pitfalls in Coronary Arteriography

There are a number of pitfalls in coronary arteriography that should be looked for and avoided.

1. *Short left main or double left coronary orifices*. When the left main orifice is very short or absent, selective injection of the anterior descending or circumflex arteries may be done (Fig. 15-34). If, on viewing an arteriogram, no circumflex or anterior descending artery is seen filling either primarily or through collaterals from the right coronary artery,

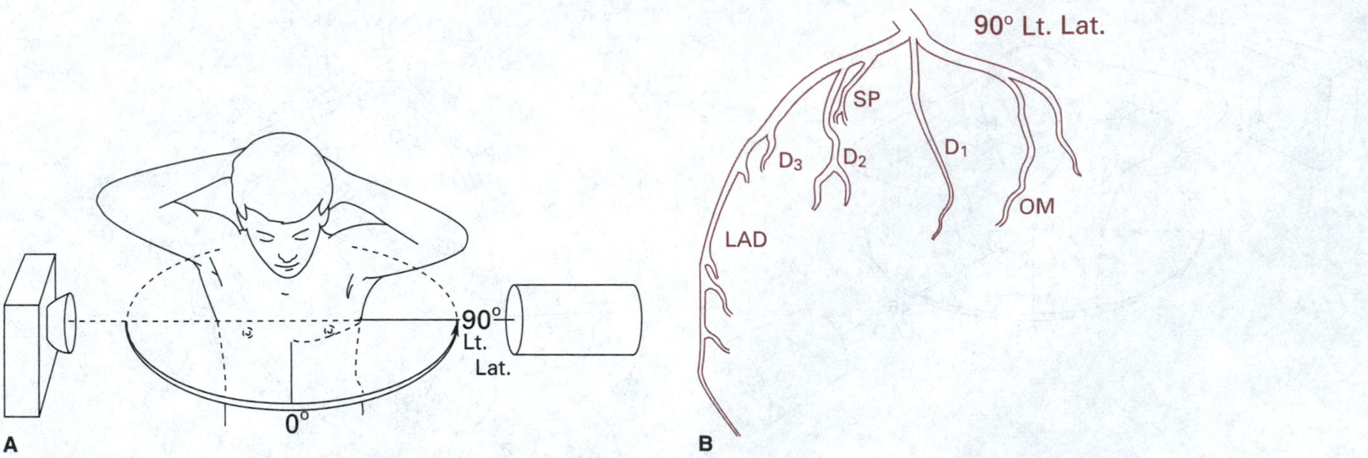

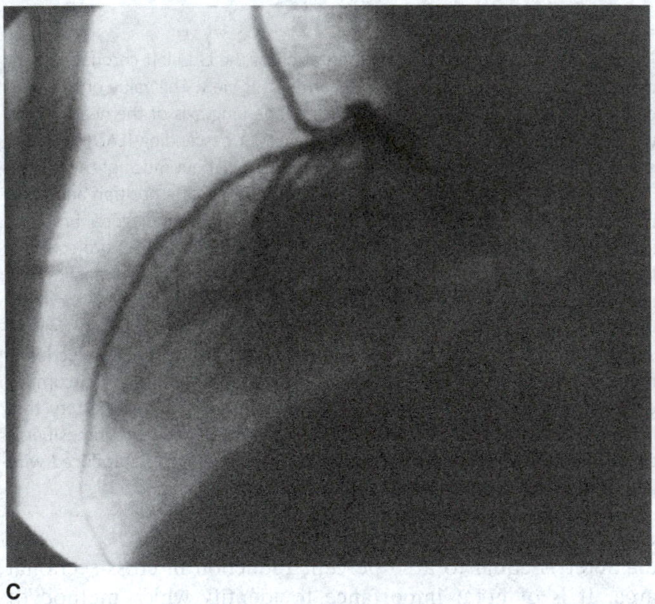

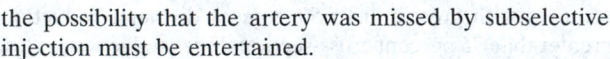

FIGURE 15-23 Diagrammatic illustrations of the left lateral or 90° LAO view of the left coronary arteriogram and direction of the x-ray beam. The left lateral view of the left coronary artery is most useful for analyzing the proximal and mid-LAD by avoiding overlap with the diagonal branches, which commonly take an inferior course from the LAD in this projection. The most proximal portion of the diagonal branches may not be well visualized because the long axis of these segments may be in the direction of the x-ray beam. The leftward-directed left main segment is foreshortened in this view (compare with Fig. 15-22). In this view, the image intensifier is placed on the patient's left, and the x-ray beam has a right-to-left direction in the horizontal plane. (From King et al.[136] Reproduced with permission from the publisher, editor, and authors.)

the possibility that the artery was missed by subselective injection must be entertained.

2. *Orifice lesions*. The left and right coronary artery orifices need to be seen on a tangent with the aortic sinuses. Some backflow from the orifices is needed if the catheter is lying within the left main or proximal right coronary artery to avoid missing an orifice lesion.
3. *Myocardial bridges*. The anterior descending, diagonal, and marginal branches not uncommonly dip intramyocardially, and the overlying myocardium may act to compress the artery during systole (Fig. 15-35). If the coronary artery is not viewed carefully in diastole, this bridging may give the appearance of an area of stenosis.[138]
4. *Foreshortening*. When possible, avoid reading lesions in segments that are seen only coming toward or away from the image intensifier. Dense opacification of segments seen end-on may produce the appearance of a lesion in an intervening segment.
5. *Coronary spasm*. Catheter-induced spasm may give the appearance of a lesion (Fig. 15-36). When spasm is suspected (usually at the catheter tip in the right coronary artery), nitrates should be given, and the injection should be repeated in 5 to 10 min. Spontaneous coronary artery spasm is a separate problem, and when this is suspected, nitrates and atropine are avoided because the atropine may play a role in blocking coronary artery spasm. Provocation with ergot derivatives will identify most patients with spontaneous coronary artery spasm.[114–116]

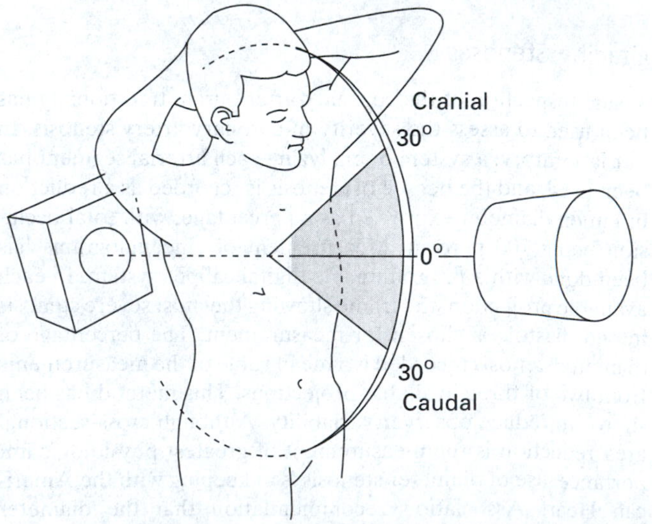

FIGURE 15-24 Illustration of sagittal angulation of x-ray beam in coronary arteriography. (From King et al.[136] Reproduced with permission from the publisher, editor, and authors.)

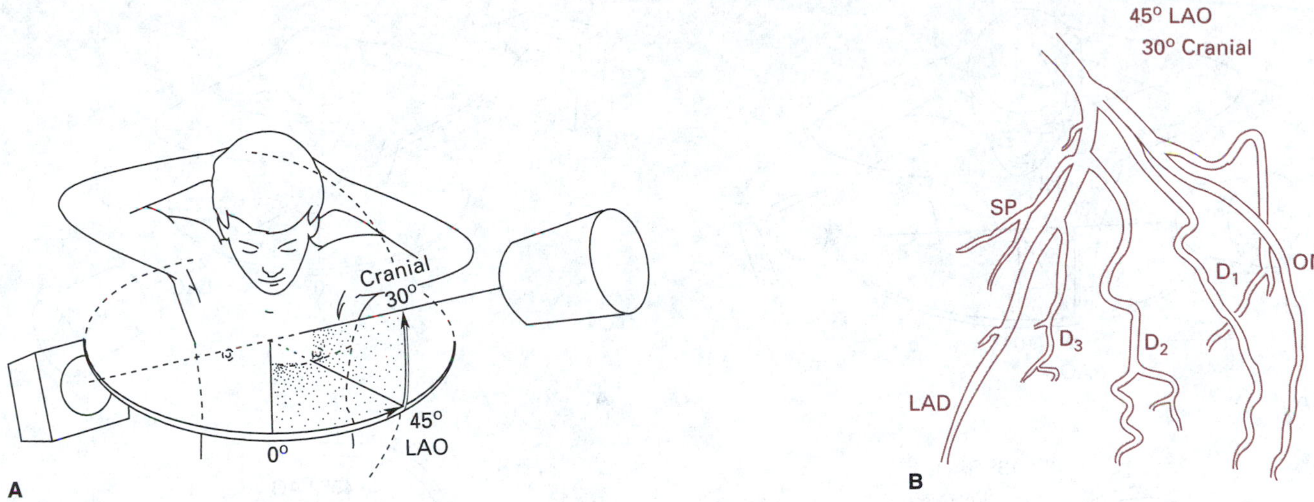

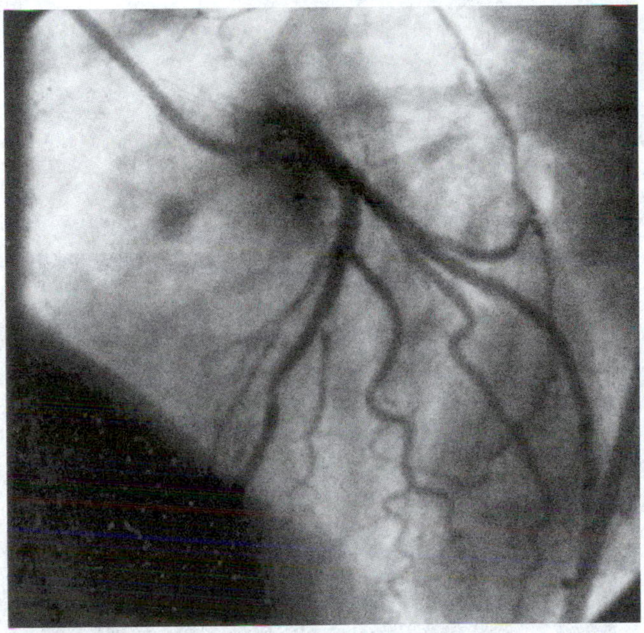

C

FIGURE 15-25 Diagrammatic illustration of the left coronary angiogram in the 45° LAO with 30° cranial angulation and the direction of the x-ray beam used to produce this view. This is the most valuable view of the left coronary artery in most patients. Foreshortening of the left main and proximal left anterior descending and diagonal branches present in the LAO view is usually overcome by cranial angulation of the image intensifier. The proximal left coronary arterial segments are frequently visualized at an angle almost perpendicular from their long axis. The ostium of the left main coronary artery, the most proximal portion of the LAD, and the origin of the diagonal branches are usually well visualized without overlap (compare with Fig. 15-22). Some overlap may occur with branches of the proximal circumflex coronary artery, and this is frequently overcome by using a 60° LAO with 30° of cranial angulation. The value of the LAO with cranial angulation is considerably less when the proximal left coronary artery is superiorly directed, in which case caudal angulation of the image intensifier is frequently helpful. The direction of the x-ray beam in the 45° LAO with 30° of angulation is demonstrated. (From King et al.[136] Reproduced with permission from the publisher, editor, and authors.)

6. *Anomalous coronary arteries.* Coronary arteries may arise from ectopic locations, or a single coronary artery may be present.[139] Only by ensuring that the entire epicardial surface has an adequate arterial supply can one be confident that all branches have been visualized.
7. *Totally occluded arteries or vein grafts.* Absence of vascularity in a portion of the heart may indicate total occlusion of its arterial supply. Usually, however, collateral channels permit visualization of the distal occluded artery unless it is an acute occlusion. Vessels filled solely by collaterals have very little pressure supporting their walls and may appear smaller than their actual lumen size, giving a false sense of pessimism about the possibilities for surgical anastomosis.

Limitations of Coronary Arteriography

Despite significant improvements in the quality of coronary arteriographic studies as a result of improved x-ray imaging systems, there remain a number of limitations of the method. Film interpretation is subjective. Different angiographers may interpret the same film differently, and the same angiographer may render a different interpretation at a time remote from the first reading.[140–141] It has been reported that the average standard deviation of estimation of any segmental stenosis by experienced angiographers may be as high as 20 percent and that disagreement about the number of major vessels with 70 percent stenosis may occur 30 percent of the time.[142] These reported studies, however, used only views in the transverse plane, imposing greater interpretive burdens than are encountered when sagittally angulated views are obtained. Further studies using sagittally angulated views would be expected to show less variability in interpreting coronary arteriograms. Inter- and intraobserver variability in interpreting coronary arteriograms is not unlike interpretive differences in chest x-rays

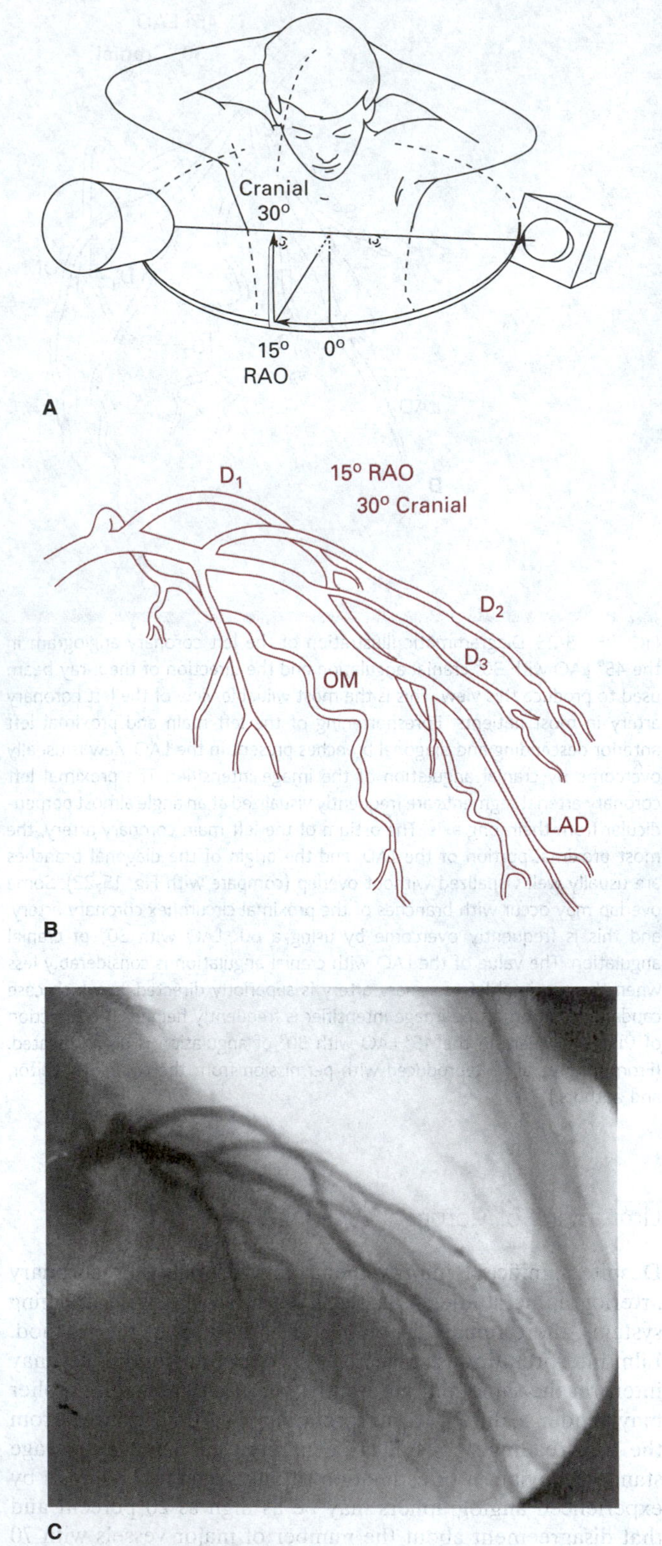

FIGURE 15-26 Diagrammatic illustration of the direction of the x-ray beam and the left coronary angiogram in the 15° RAO with 30° of cranial angulation. This view is particularly helpful in analyzing the mid-left anterior descending artery and the diagonal branch points. Overlap with diagonal branches is usually avoided. The origin of the circumflex artery may be well seen, as in this illustration. (From King et al.[136] Reproduced with permission from the publisher, editor, and authors.)

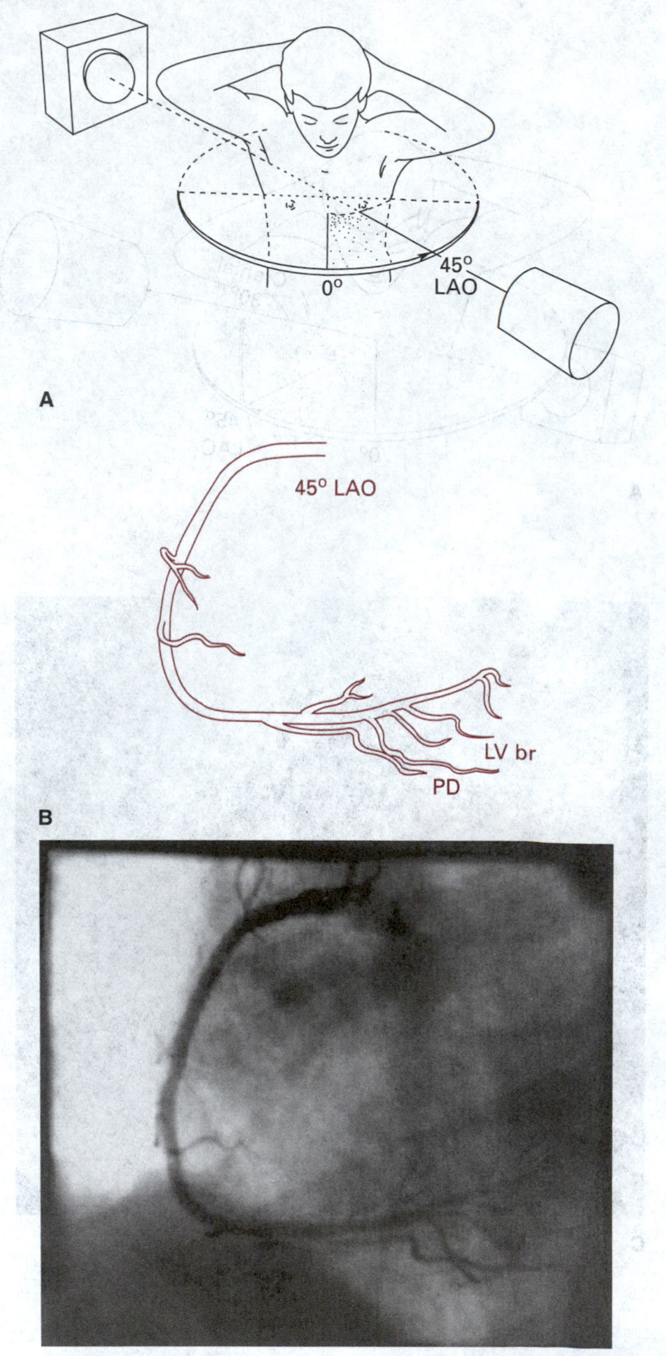

FIGURE 15-27 Diagrammatic illustration of the direction of the x-ray beam and the right coronary artery in the 45° LAO projection. This view is excellent for visualizing the proximal mid and distal right coronary artery in the AV groove since the direction of the x-ray beam is perpendicular to these arterial segments. Ostial lesions of the right coronary artery are now well visualized if the proximal right coronary artery takes an anterior direction from the aorta and therefore originates in a direction parallel to the x-ray beam. This usually can be overcome by turning to a more severe left oblique projection. The posterior descending and LV branches of the right coronary artery, which pass down the posterior aspect of the heart toward the apex, are severely foreshortened because the long axis of these vessels is in the same direction as the x-ray beam. The proximal posterior descending branches can be visualized by cranial angulation of the overhead intensifier (see Fig. 15-28) or from a right oblique view. The image intensifier is in the standard LAO position. (From King et al.[136] Reproduced with permission from the publisher, editor, and authors.)

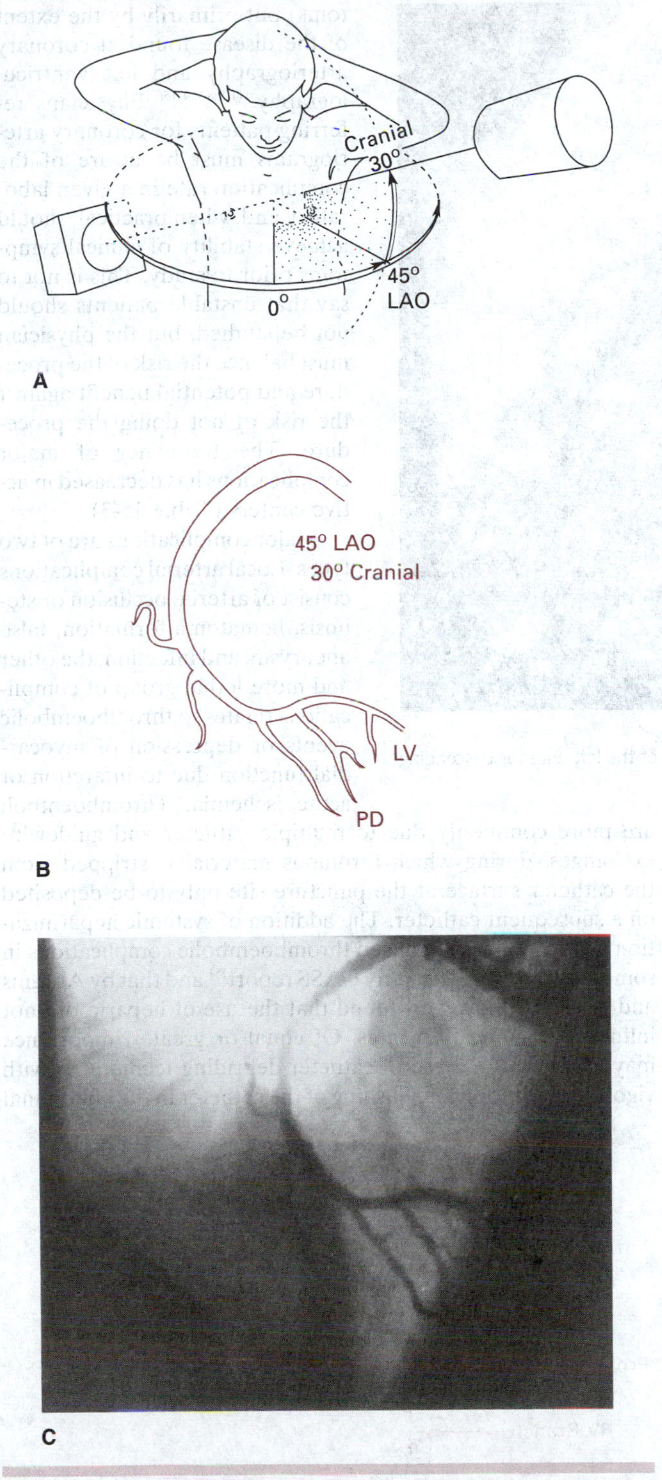

FIGURE 15-28 Diagrammatic illustration of the direction of the x-ray beam and the right coronary artery in 30° LAO with 30° of cranial angulation. Cranial angulation of the image intensifier overcomes the problem of foreshortening of the posterior descending and left ventricular branches observed in Fig. 15-27. Lesions in the posterior descending or LV branches can be well visualized. When the right coronary artery originates anteriorly from the aorta, the proximal portion of the vessel is frequently well seen in this projection. With anomalous origin of the left anterior descending artery from the right coronary artery, this view is helpful because the standard LAO view produces considerable foreshortening of the anomalous artery. The direction of the x-ray beam is the same as in Fig. 15-25. (From King et al.[136] Reproduced with permission from the publisher, editor, and authors.)

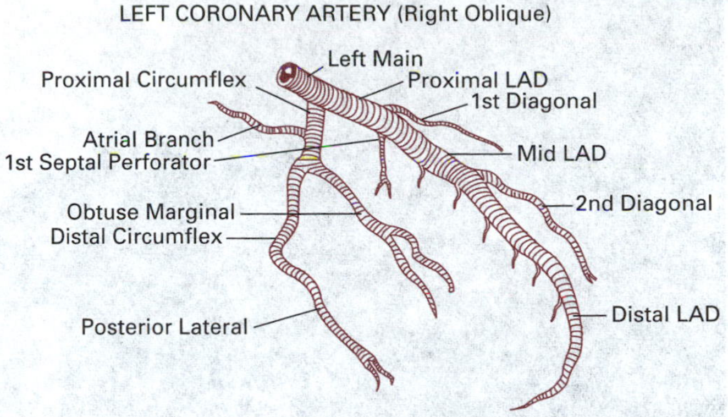

FIGURE 15-29 Anatomy of the left coronary tree in the right oblique view.

or other diagnostic studies involving human error and judgment. Routine use of several readers has been shown to reduce interpretive error.[141] Although correlation of angiography with postmortem findings has been acceptable in most studies,[142–148] certain coronary pathologic-anatomic factors may favor angiographic underestimation of the degree of stenosis present in any arterial segment. In large part, this is due to the tendency for diffuse atheromatous narrowing of the coronary arteries to occur. In attempting to grade stenosis of an obviously narrow segment, one may not have a normal segment for comparison or may choose for comparison an apparently normal segment that in fact has diffuse tubular narrowing.[145–147] This leads to underestimation of the degree of stenosis present. Pathologic studies currently available probably overestimate the frequency of this problem, since the pathologic material available for study represents the severest end of the spectrum of the disease. Eccentric atherosclerotic plaques also may be underestimated unless the minor axis of the stenotic lumen is visualized. Sagittally angulated views are particularly valuable in this regard. Very discrete membrane-like lesions, which fortunately are rare, may be missed unless they are visualized directly in the plane of the lesion. Pathologic studies have shown poor correlation between left main coronary stenosis at autopsy and that at angiography, especially in the presence of a short left main coronary artery, and point out the importance of sufficient angiographic views and excellent interpretive skills in evaluating this critical portion of the coronary circulation.[148] Quantitative computer techniques have shown excellent correlation between the cross-sectional luminal area of stenotic lesions at arteriography and direct planimetered measurements of distended postmortem specimens.[149] Dynamic phenomena that are not active at the time of the study may be important. "Hit and run" events such as coronary embolization or thrombosis with subsequent resolution, coronary artery spasm, and even primary coronary artery dissection may leave LV scars but not result in coronary angiographic findings.

Risk of Coronary Arteriography

As with any invasive procedure, there is a finite risk to patients undergoing coronary arteriography. The magnitude of the risk is influenced by certain factors definable prior to the procedure (e.g., skill of the angiographer and instability of clinical symp-

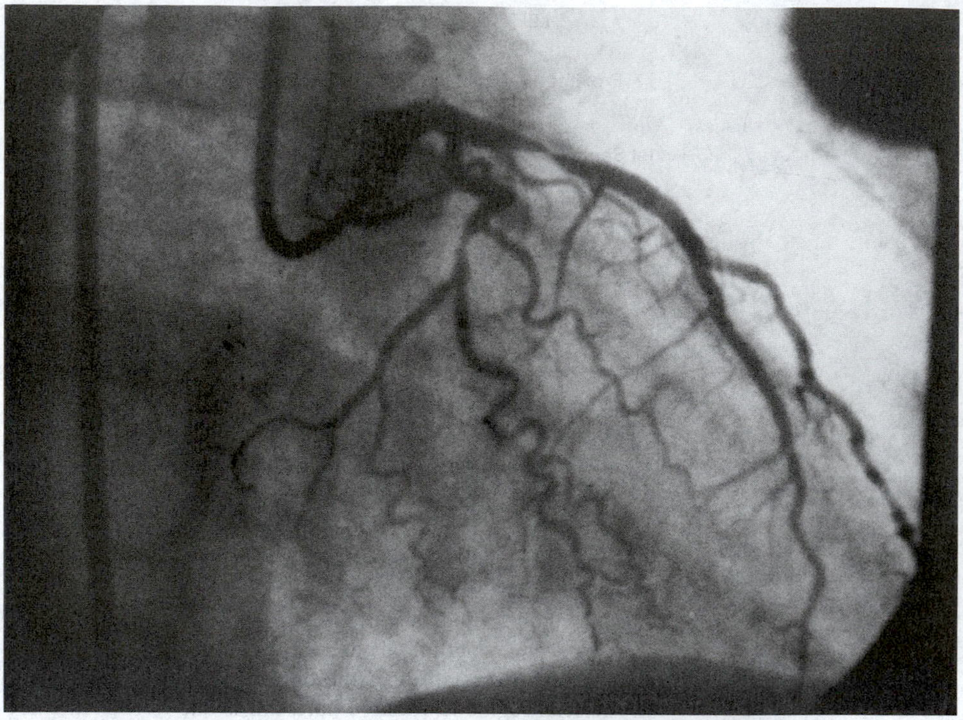

FIGURE 15-30 RAO view of the left coronary artery showing high-grade stenosis of the left anterior descending proximal to the first septal perforating branch.

toms) but primarily by the extent of the disease found at coronary arteriography and left ventriculography.[111,128,150–156] Physicians referring patients for coronary arteriograms must be aware of the complication rate in a given laboratory and, when practical, should achieve stability of clinical symptoms prior to study. This is not to say that unstable patients should not be studied, but the physician must balance the risk of the procedure and potential benefit against the risk of not doing the procedure. The frequency of major complications has decreased in active centers (Table 15-3).

Major complications are of two types: Local arterial complications consist of arterial occlusion or stenosis, hematoma formation, false aneurysm, and infection; the other and more lethal group of complications relates to thromboembolic events or depression of myocardial function due to infarction or acute ischemia. Thromboemboli are more commonly due to multiple catheter and guidewire exchanges, during which thrombus material is stripped from the catheter surface at the puncture site only to be deposited on a subsequent catheter. The addition of systemic heparinization was felt to have reduced thromboembolic complications in some laboratories. The early CASS report[151] and that by Abrams and Adams,[150] however, found that the use of heparin did not influence complication rates. Of equal or greater importance may be the routine use of catheter debriding techniques, with vigorous aspiration and flushing of the catheter in the abdominal

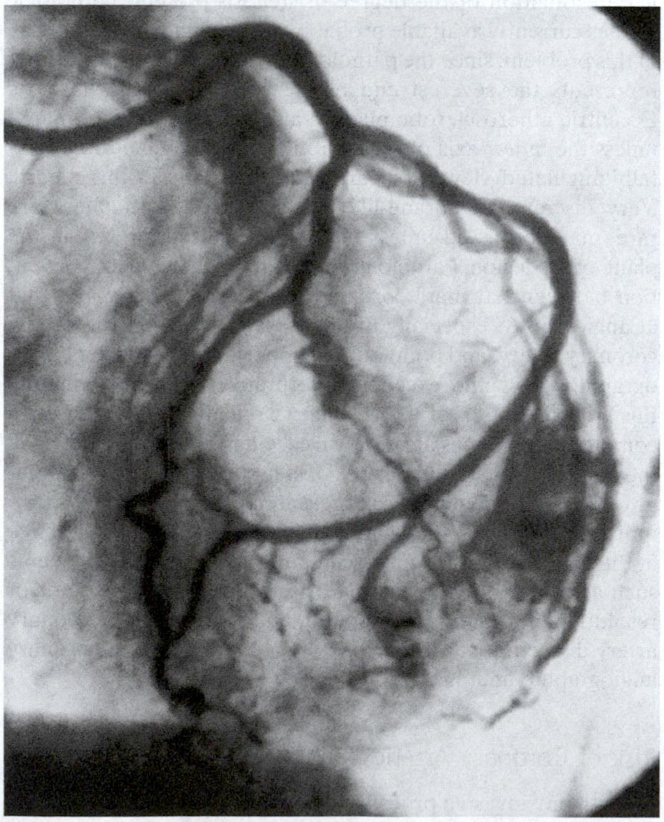

FIGURE 15-31 LAO view of the left coronary artery demonstrating dominant circumflex coronary artery giving rise to the posterior descending artery.

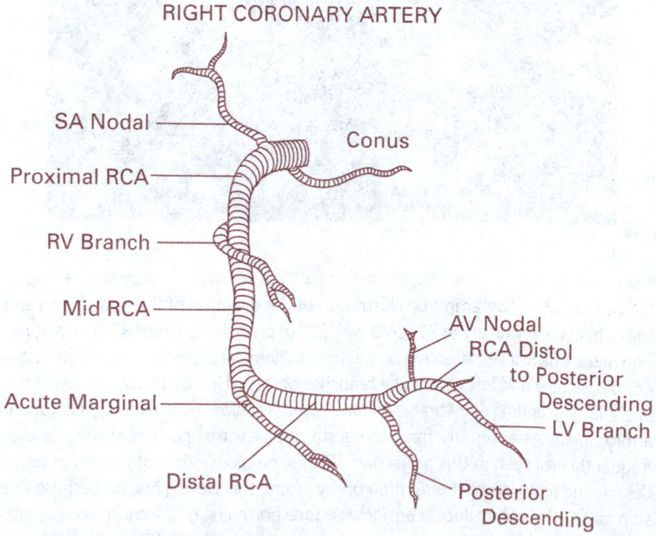

FIGURE 15-32 Anatomy of the right coronary tree.

TABLE 15-3 Complications of Coronary Arteriography

	CASS[a]		
	1979[151]	1983[154]	SCAI,[b] 1990–1995[155]
Death	0.0020	0.0007	0.001 each year
Myocardial infarction	0.0025	0.0027	<0.001 each year
Cerebral emboli	0.0003	0.0007	<0.001 each year
Arterial complications	0.0080	0.0082	—
Ventricular fibrillation	0.0063	0.0038	0.003 (0.002 in 1995)

[a]Coronary Artery Surgery Study.
[b]Society for Coronary Angiography and Interventions.

aorta to dislodge any retained thrombus material. Minor allergic reactions to contrast media in the form of urticaria occur commonly, but anaphylactic and pyrogenic reactions are exceedingly rare. Radiation exposure to the patient, estimated as 20 to 45 rem, has little risk unless multiple restudies are needed.

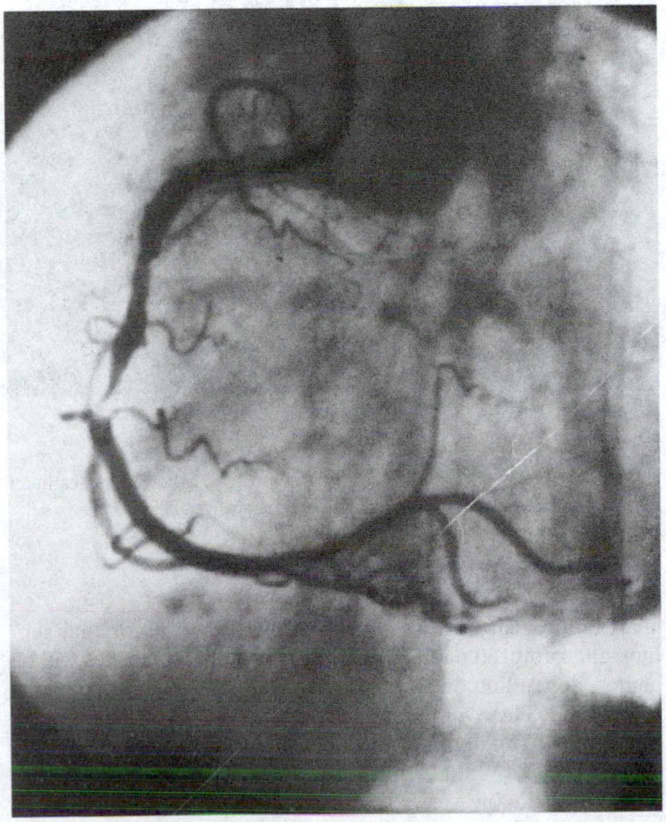

FIGURE 15-33 LAO view of the right coronary artery (RCA) with high-grade lesion in its midportion.

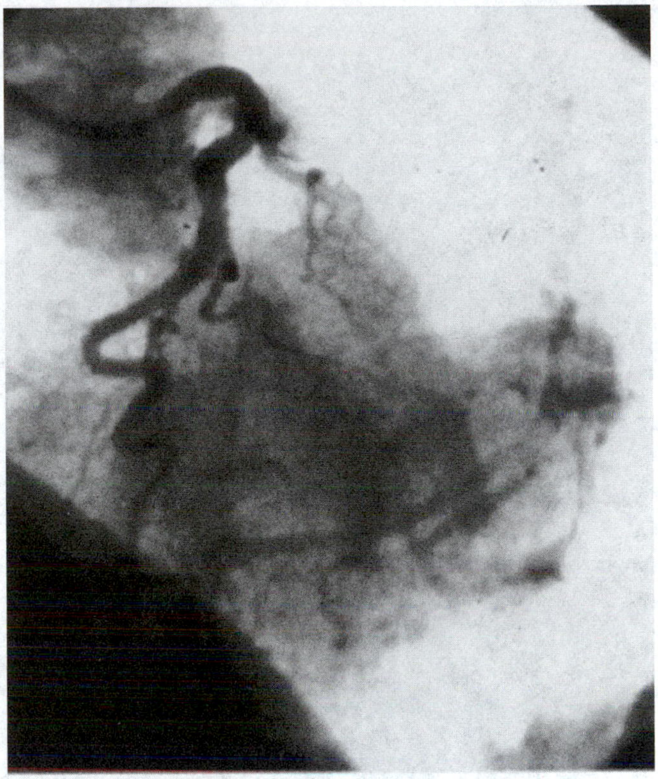

A

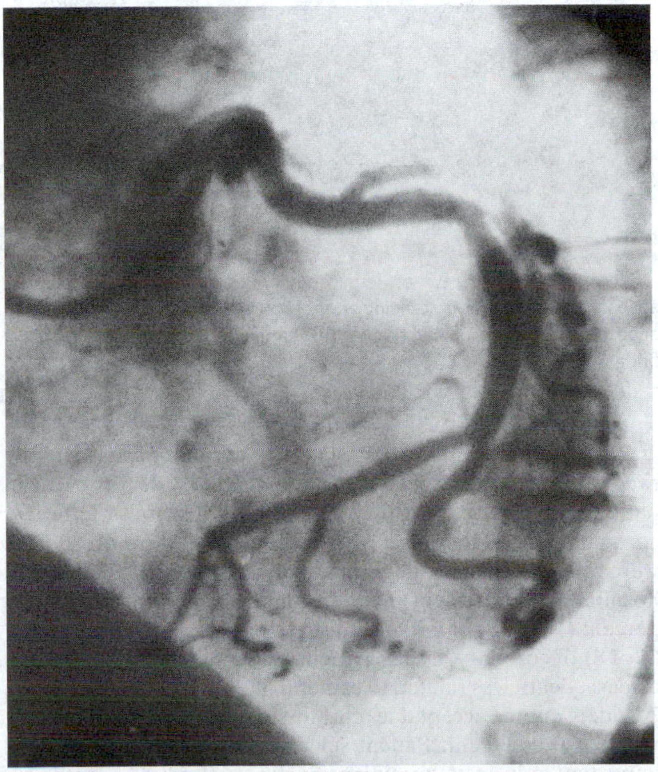

B

FIGURE 15-34 *A.* LAO view of selective injection into left anterior descending (LAD) artery. *B.* LAO view of selective injection into circumflex artery.

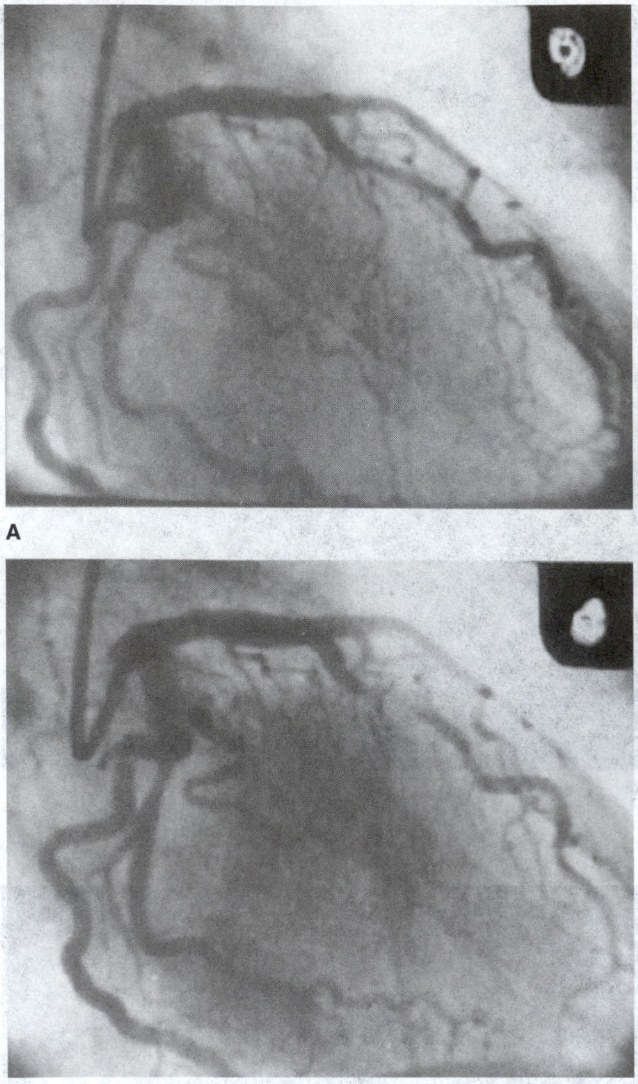

A

B

FIGURE 15-35 RAO view of left coronary artery system. *A*. Diastolic appearance of anterior descending artery showing smooth lumen. *B*. Systolic appearance showing obliteration of the lumen by an overriding muscular bridge.

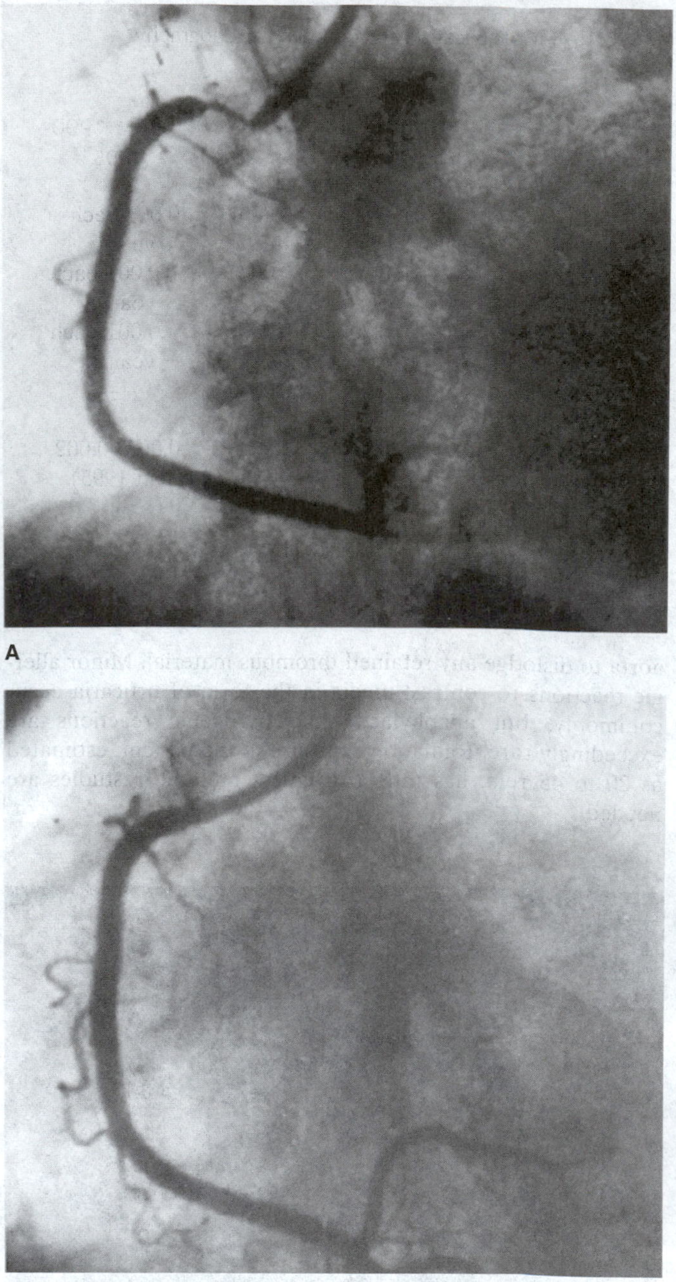

A

B

FIGURE 15-36 *A*. LAO view of right coronary injection showing pericatheter spasm. *B*. Same view following nitroglycerin, showing relief of spasm.

Reported mortality rates related to coronary arteriography range from 0.05 to 4 percent, and virtually all deaths occur in patients with severe, multivessel coronary disease or left main coronary artery stenosis.[126,150–153] Of 30 patients whose deaths were related to diagnostic cardiac catheterization at the Toronto hospital, 18 (60 percent) had left main coronary disease. In 89 percent (16 of 18) of left main disease patients and in 50 percent (4 of 8) of coronary disease patients without apparent left main disease, death was related to catheter-induced left main trauma. A widely quoted acceptable mortality rate for coronary arteriography is 0.1 percent. Patient selection, however, may play an important role in determining mortality. Studies in predominantly stable patients will result in a very low mortality rate. On the other hand, if a broad spectrum of patients is studied—including those with preinfarction angina, acute myocardial infarction, and complications of myocardial infarction such as heart failure, cardiogenic shock, ruptured interventricular septum, and ruptured papillary muscle—complication rates will be higher, depending on the frequency with which sicker patients are studied. The overall mortality rate in the CASS and Society for Cardiac Angiography and Interventions reports was 0.07 to 0.1 percent. It was 0.05 percent for single-vessel disease, 0.07 percent for double-vessel disease, 0.12 percent for triple-vessel disease, and 0.8 percent in patients with left main coronary artery stenosis.[151,154] The point to be made is that laboratory and surgical teams must be prepared to act in the best interest of

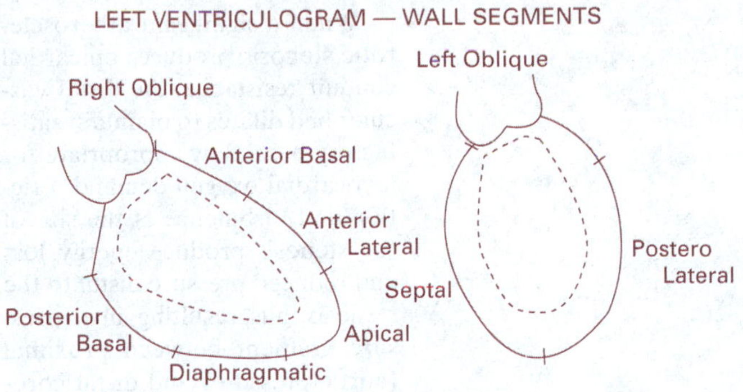

FIGURE 15-37 LV wall silhouette in RAO and LAO views.

severely ill patients and not be overly concerned with an arbitrary mortality figure.

Left Ventriculography

Left ventriculography is the standard method for evaluating LV performance in the coronary angiography laboratory. The normal pattern of LV contraction is a uniform and almost concentric inward movement of all points along the endocardial surface during systole. Harrison introduced the term *asynergy*, which has been used to indicate a disturbance of the normal contraction pattern. The Ad Hoc Committee for Grading of Coronary Artery Disease of the American Heart Association[132] has recommended that five RAO segments and two LAO left ventricular segments be defined and characterized as to wall motion (Fig. 15-37). Herman and coworkers classified LV asynergy according to the severity of the contractile abnormality, and a similar classification of LV wall motion was recommended by the Ad Hoc Committee:

Normal: Normal wall motion of the indicated ventricular segment
Reduced: Reduced velocity and/or amplitude of indicated wall segment
None: Absence of appropriate wall motion of indicated ventricular segment
Dyskinetic: Paradoxical wall motion of the indicated segment
Aneurysmal: Bulging during systole and diastole with sharply defined margins of indicated ventricular segment
Undefined

Many angiographers use the term *akinesis* when no wall motion is present and the term *hypokinesis* when wall motion is reduced.

The ability of the left ventricle to function as a pump is best analyzed by LV volume determinations. Single-plane and biplane volume determinations may differ significantly in patients with coronary artery disease and nonhomogeneous contraction patterns. In particular, the single-plane RAO or lateral left ventriculogram frequently underestimates overall LV contraction because it selectively visualizes the anterior and inferior free walls of the left ventricle, which are most commonly involved in myocardial infarction. Vogel et al.[157] found that the single-plane RAO left ventriculogram underestimated ejection fraction in 70 percent of patients with coronary artery disease. For this reason, biplane left ventriculography frequently is desirable in evaluating patients with coronary artery disease.

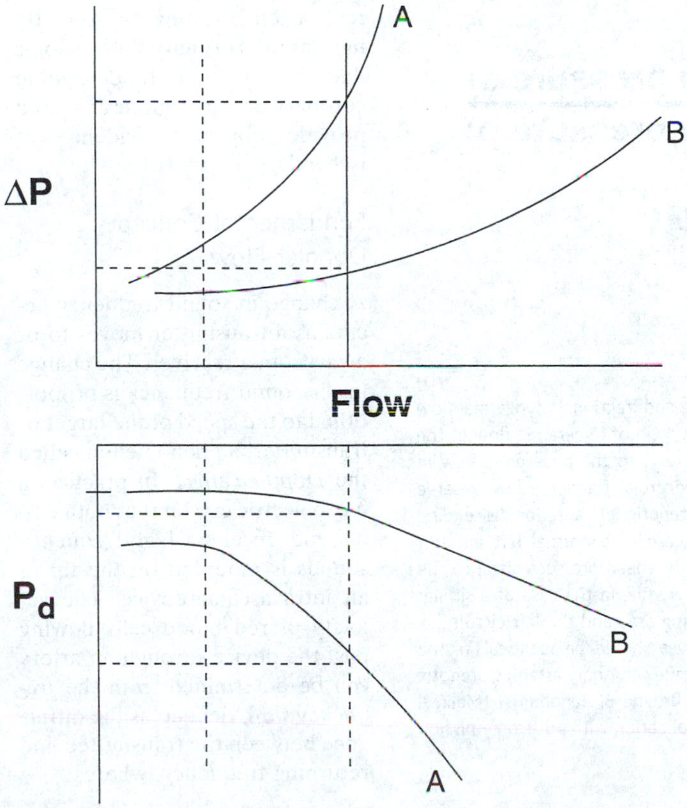

FIGURE 15-38 Coronary pressure-flow relationships for two stenoses of the same angiographic severity. (*Top*) P_a = aortic P = pressure gradient (aortic-distal coronary pressure, P_d) versus coronary flow. (*Bottom*) Absolute P_d versus flow. Increasing flow produces marked loss of P_d as well as an increase in P_d = distal coronary P. The loss of P_d in absolute terms determines myocardial perfusion pressure (P_d − venous pressure) and the potential for inducible ischemia.

MEASUREMENTS OF CORONARY BLOOD FLOW AND PRESSURE

Coronary artery disease affects the vessel wall with a highly variable influence on the configuration of the lumen and subsequent resistance to blood flow. The functional characterization of a coronary stenosis identified on angiography remains a well-recognized limitation,[158–160] repeatedly documented by intravascular ultrasound (IVUS) imaging and ischemic testing. Measurements of coronary flow and pressure can be obtained directly using Doppler and pressure sensor angioplasty guidewires.[161]

Coronary Physiology

Coronary blood flow increases from a resting level to a maximum depending on myocardial oxygen demand and other hyperemic stimuli. Normally, epicardial resistance to flow is trivial, with flow normally controlled by the precapillary arteriolar resistance vessels. Coronary blood flow in a normal artery supply-

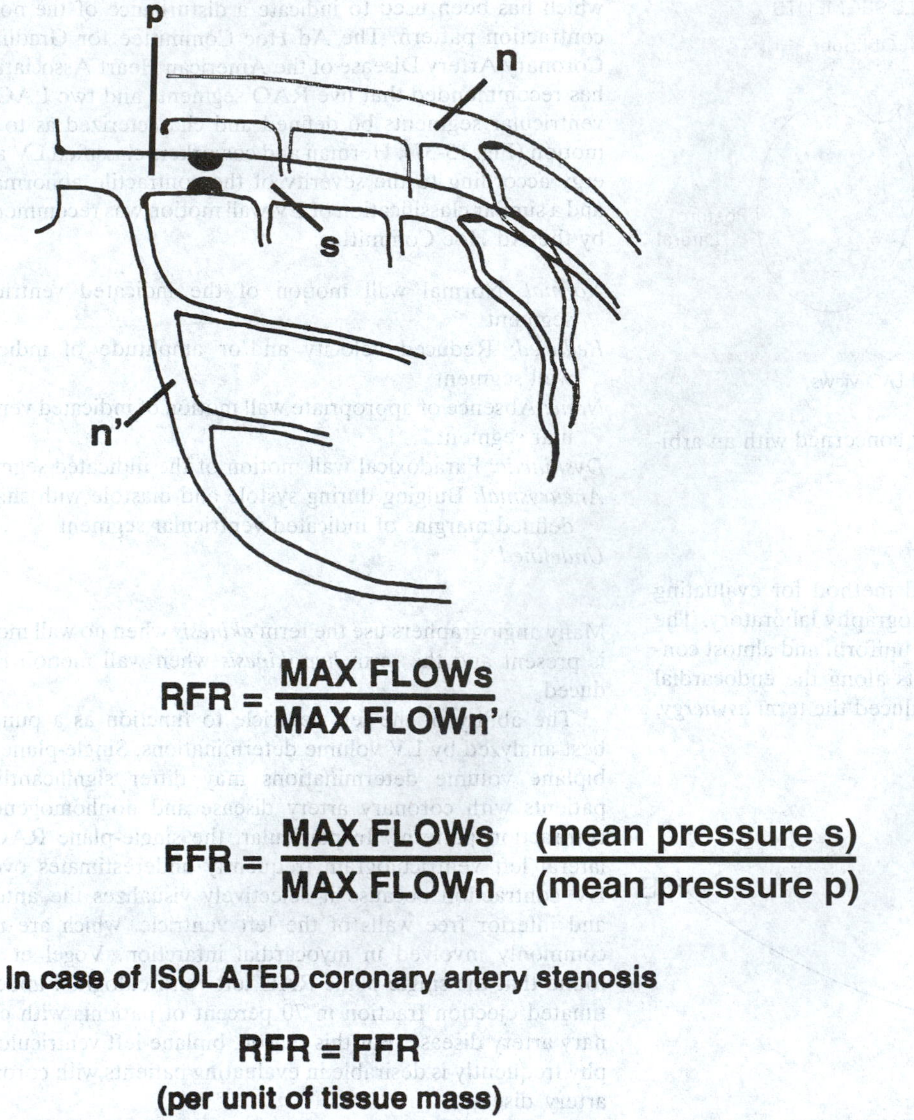

p
n
s
n'
RFR = MAX FLOWs / MAX FLOWn'
FFR = MAX FLOWs / MAX FLOWn (mean pressure s) / (mean pressure p)
In case of ISOLATED coronary artery stenosis
RFR = FFR
(per unit of tissue mass)

FIGURE 15-39 Schematic drawing illustrating the rationale of comparing relative and fractional myocardial flow reserve in this particular group of patients. The relative flow reserve (RFR) is the ratio of hyperemic flow in the anterior region (depending on the stenotic left anterior descending coronary artery) to the hyperemic flow in the normal region (depending on the left circumflex coronary artery). The myocardial fractional flow reserve (FFR) is the ratio of hyperemic flow in the anterior region (depending on the stenotic left anterior descending coronary artery) to hyperemic flow in that same region in the hypothetical case of a normal left anterior descending coronary artery (*faint lines*). These measurements are derived from the mean pressure distal to the stenosis divided by the mean pressure proximal to the stenosis at maximal hyperemia. In the case of a similar decrease of myocardial resistance during hyperemia in the left anterior descending area and the left circumflex area, the value of both the relative and the fractional myocardial flow reserves should be identical. n, the hypothetical normal left anterior descending coronary artery; n', normal left circumflex coronary artery; s, stenotic left anterior descending coronary artery. (Reproduced with permission from de Bruyne B, Banohuin T, Melin J, et al. Coronary flow reserve calculated from pressure measurements in humans. Validation with positron emission tomography. *Circulation* 1994; 89:1013–1022.)

ing normal myocardium can increase more than threefold in adults. However, some patients may have conditions affecting the microcirculation (LV hypertrophy, myocardial ischemia, diabetes, or other conditions impairing the microcirculatory responses) that can blunt the normal increase in coronary flow.

When a significant atherosclerotic stenosis produces epicardial conduit resistance, the distal vascular bed dilates to maintain satisfactory basal flow appropriate for myocardial oxygen demand. Friction and turbulence at the site of the stenosis produce energy loss and reduced pressure distal to the stenosis,thus resulting in a pressure gradient between proximal (aortic pressure) and distal coronary artery segments. As coronary flow increases across the stenosis, the distal pressure decreases along a curvilinear pressure-flow relationship of coronary stenosis resistance as described by Gould et al.[162–163] From this relationship, both coronary flow reserve (CFR) and pressure-derived fractional flow reserve (see below) can be elucidated and applied for coronary lesion assessment (Fig. 15-38). Because of the strong association of coronary flow with indirect ischemia testing,[164–167] directly measured coronary physiologic data can be used to determine coronary lesion significance and provide objective evidence of ischemia.

Fundamental Concepts: Doppler Flow

A change in sound frequency occurs as a transmitter moves to or away from a receiver. The change in the sound frequency is proportional to the speed of the target or transmitter, a phenomenon called the *Doppler effect*. In practice, a piezoelectric crystal that both emits and receives high-frequency sounds is mounted on the tip of an intravascular device. The velocity of red blood cells flowing past the device through an artery can be determined from the *frequency shift*, defined as the difference between the transmitted and returning frequency, where

$$\text{Velocity} = (F_1 - F_0)(C)/(2F_0)(\cos\theta)$$

where V = velocity of blood flow
F_0 = transmitting (transducer) frequency
F_1 = returning frequency
C = constant (speed of sound in blood)
θ = angle of incidence

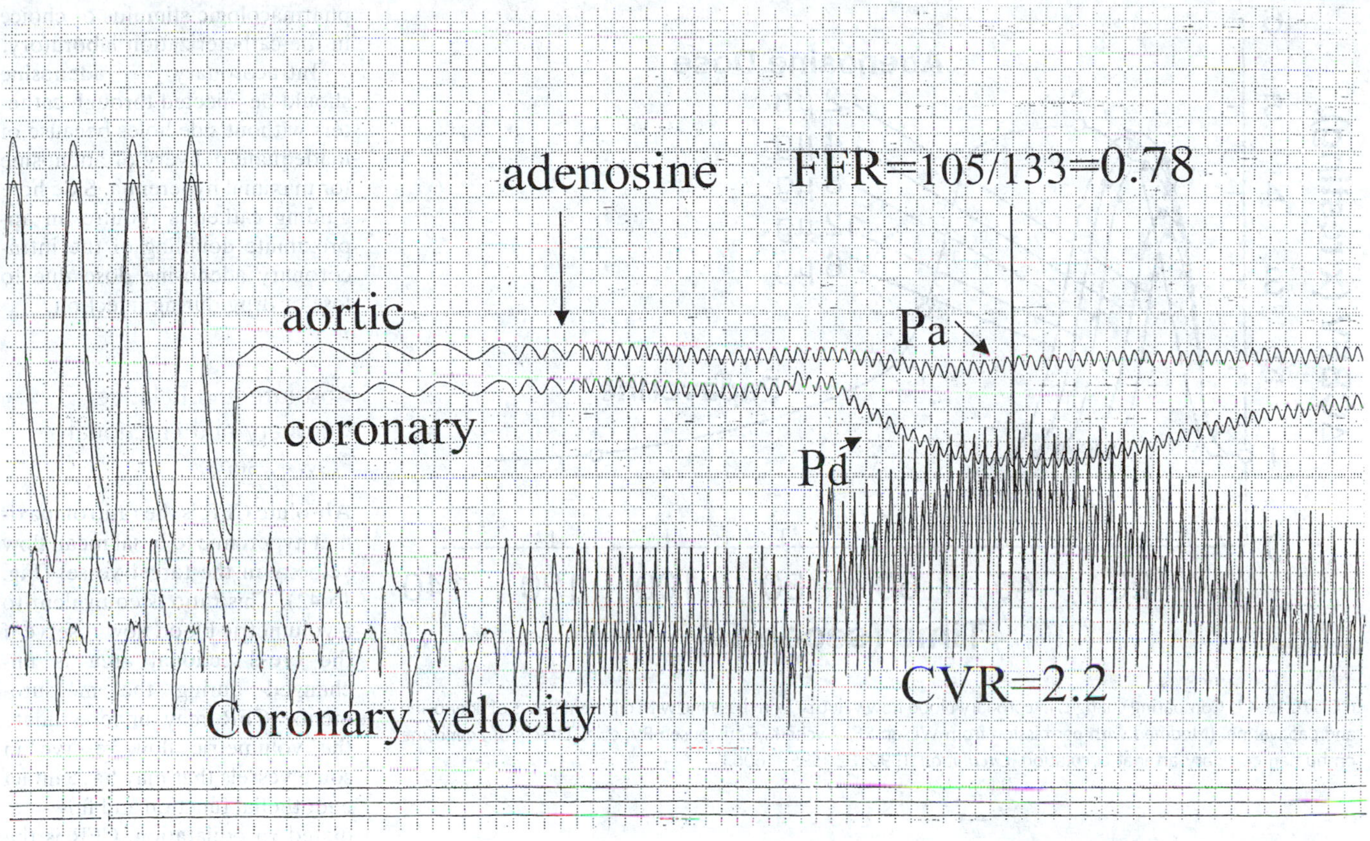

FIGURE 15-40 Hemodynamic and coronary flow velocity tracings demonstrating coronary flow reserve (CFR) and fractional flow reserve (FFR) data collection. Aortic (P_a) and distal coronary pressure (P_d) at baseline and during adenosine hyperemia (*at vertical line*). Coronary velocity shows a 2.2-fold increase with adenosine. FFR = 0.78.

Volumetric flow can be determined as the product of vessel area (cm^2) and flow velocity (cm/s), yielding a value in cubic centimeters per second. Absolute Doppler flow velocities represent changes in volumetric coronary flow when the vessel cross-sectional area remains constant over the measurement period. The Doppler guidewire velocity and volumetric relationship has been validated during intravascular measurement by Doucette et al.[168] and Labovitz et al.[169]

Fundamental Concepts: Fractional Flow Reserve

Pressure gradients (aortic-coronary mean pressure) at rest do not accurately characterize the ischemic potential of a stenosis.[170,171] Resting translesional pressure gradients measured during the early years of angioplasty were not accepted because of inadequate devices (nos. 3–4 French catheters) used under inappropriate circumstances (i.e., not during maximal hyperemia). The translesional gradient was incompletely interpreted (i.e., resting gradients rather than hyperemia-induced fractional flow reserve). A new concept based on the pressure-derived measurement of coronary perfusion, called *fractional flow reserve* (FFR),[170,171] is a measure of the fraction of maximal coronary blood flow that traverses the stenotic vessel as a percentage of blood flow through the same artery in the theoretical absence of the stenosis. This measurement is derived from the mean pressure distal to the stenosis divided by the mean pressure proximal to the stenosis at maximal hyperemia. The FFR reflects the true reduction in myocardial perfusion resulting from a stenosis rather than merely a stenosis pressure gradient. During maximal hyperemia, resistance is minimal across both the epicardial and microvascular beds. Because the ratio of the absolute distal coronary to aortic pressures is measured when myocardial resistance is minimal, the status of the microcirculation does not, in theory, affect the FFR. Unlike CFR, FFR is independent of hemodynamic and microcirculatory factors.[172,173] The normal value for FFR is 1.0 for each patient, coronary artery, myocardial distribution, and microcirculatory status (Figs. 15-39 and 15-40).

Pharmacologic Hyperemic Stimuli

Stenosis severity always should be assessed using flow measurements during maximal hyperemia. The most widely used maximal vasodilator agents are adenosine, papaverine, and dipyridamole.[174–176] The hyperosmolar ionic and low-osmolar nonionic contrast media do not produce maximal vasodilatation.

Intracoronary and intravenous adenosine produces hyperemia equivalent to papaverine[18] but has a much shorter half-life (Fig. 15-41). Intravenous adenosine produces similar hyperemia equal to that of intracoronary adenosine but in a sustained fashion. Both intracoronary and intravenous adenosine has an extremely high safety profile in low doses and has become the

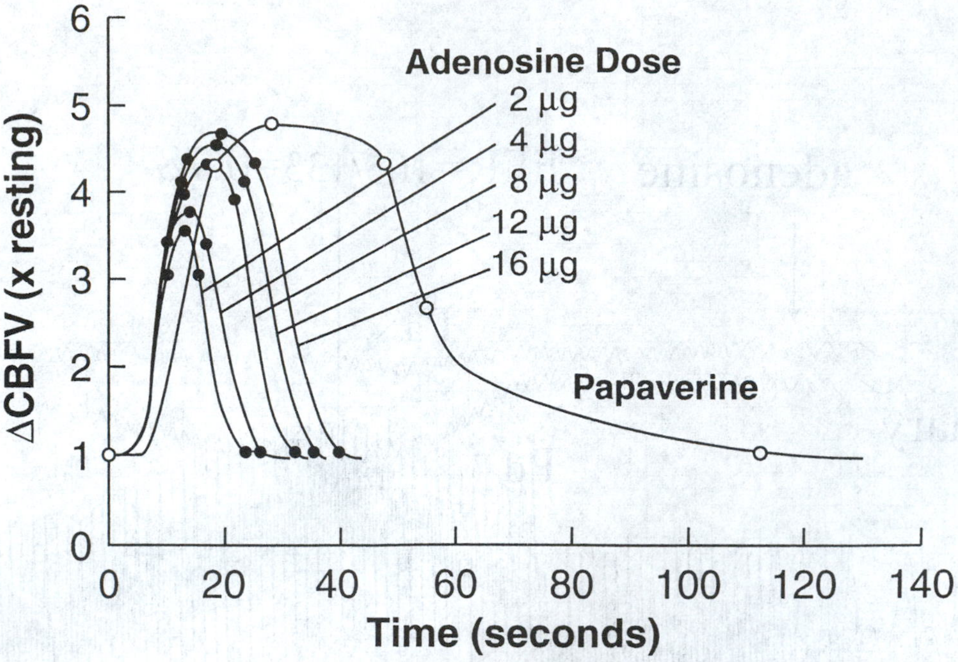

FIGURE 15-41 Comparing changes in coronary blood flow velocity from baseline with different doses of adenosine and papaverine. (Modified with permission from Wilson RF, Wyche K, Christensen BV, et al. Effects of adenosine on human coronary arterial circulation. *Circulation* 1990; 82:1595–1606.)

pharmacologic stimulus of choice in the catheterization laboratory.

Intracoronary adenosine should be injected through catheters without side holes because of inadequate delivery of adenosine for maximal hyperemia. Side hole guiding catheters require an approximate doubling of the intracoronary adenosine dose due to loss of drug during injection.[177]

Absolute and Relative Coronary and Fractional Flow Reserve

Absolute CFR is the ratio of maximal hyperemic to basal mean flow velocity in the target vessel (Fig. 15-42). This ratio is equivalent to a volumetric blood flow reserve if the cross-sectional area is unchanged during the measurements. CFR may underestimate the volumetric flow reserve in some vessels that may have intact endothelial function and flow-mediated vasodilatation. CFR is the summed response of flow through

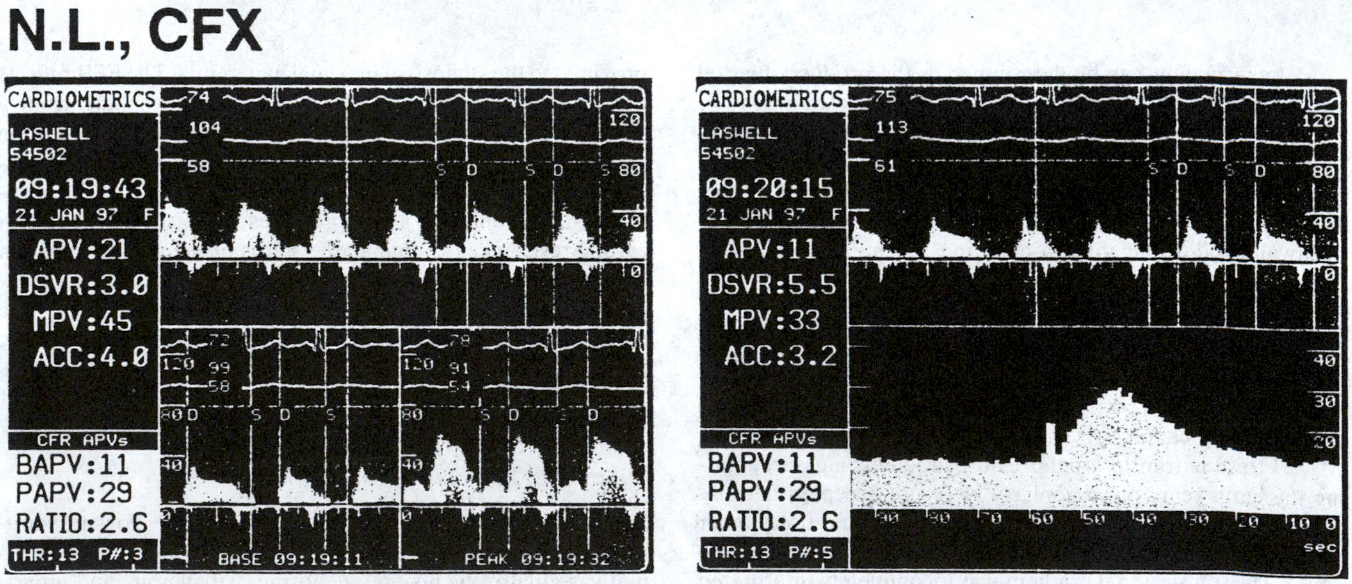

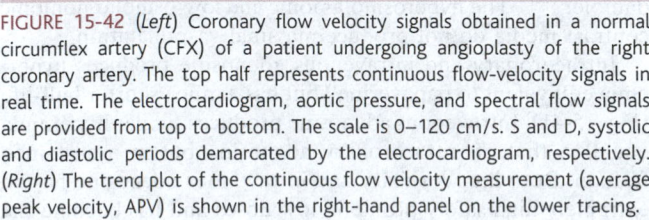

FIGURE 15-42 (*Left*) Coronary flow velocity signals obtained in a normal circumflex artery (CFX) of a patient undergoing angioplasty of the right coronary artery. The top half represents continuous flow-velocity signals in real time. The electrocardiogram, aortic pressure, and spectral flow signals are provided from top to bottom. The scale is 0–120 cm/s. S and D, systolic and diastolic periods demarcated by the electrocardiogram, respectively. (*Right*) The trend plot of the continuous flow velocity measurement (average peak velocity, APV) is shown in the right-hand panel on the lower tracing. After intracoronary adenosine administration, APV increased from 11 to 29 cm/s, producing a coronary flow ratio (CFR) of 2.6. The duration of hyperemia is 45 s. The trend velocity scale is 0 to 40 cm/s. The time base is 90 s. (Reproduced with permission from Kern MJ, de Bruyne B, Pijls NHJ, et al. From Research to clinical practice: Current role of physiologically based decision making in the catheterization laboratory. *J Am Coll Cardiol* 1997; 30:613–620.)

the conduit and the myocardial bed; thus an abnormal CFR does not separate a significant stenosis from an abnormal microcirculation (Fig. 15-43). Measurement of CFR in an angiographically normal vessel can serve as a reference value against which to compare the results in a target vessel. The relative CFR (rCFR), the ratio of CFR_{target} to $CFR_{reference}$, in theory, should identify whether an impaired target CFR is the result of a flow-limiting stenosis or microvascular abnormalities (Fig. 15-44). The normal absolute CFR is 2.7 ± 0.6[178] in adults in the cardiac catheterization laboratory with chest pain syndromes. Absolute CFR appears reproducible among angiographically normal vessels within a 10 percent variance. The average CFR measured using the flow-velocity technique in patients with normal coronary arteries undergoing cardiac catheterization differs little between patients who have had cardiac transplantation and those who have chest pain syndromes and angiographically normal arteries, with approximately 12 percent of patients having a CFR of less than 2.0. rCFR relies on the assumption that the microvascular circulatory response is uniformly distributed among the myocardial beds. The normal range for rCFR is 0.8 to 1.0.[179–180] The major limitations of rCFR include patients with three-vessel coronary disease who have no suitable reference vessel, patients in whom the target vessel supplies an area of myocardial infarction with LV regional dysfunction, or patients in whom the microcirculatory responses are heterogeneous.

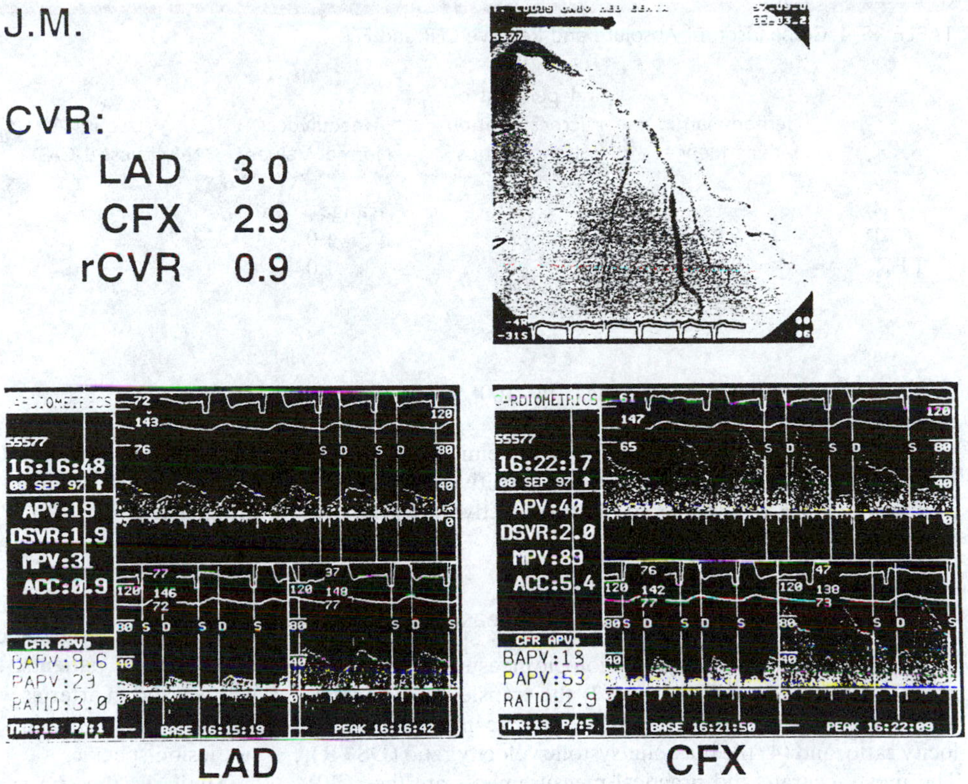

FIGURE 15-44 Measurements of absolute and relative coronary flow (velocity) reserve (CFR) used to assess long 60 percent mid-left anterior descending (LAD) coronary stenosis in patient J.M. (*top right*). Left anterior descending CFR_{target} is 2.9, CFR_{ref} in the circumflex (CFX) artery is 3.0. Relative CFR (rCFR) is 0.9. Angioplasty was deferred.

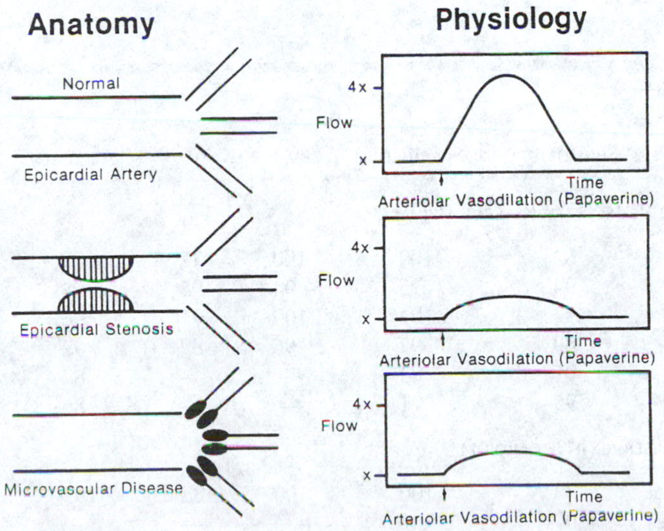

FIGURE 15-43 Comparison of coronary flow reserve (CFR) in arteries with normal (*top*) epicardial stenosis (*middle*) and abnormal microcirculation (*bottom*).

rCFR and FFR are more specific for flow limitations due to a stenosis than CFR. FFR, rCFR, and CFR were determined in 21 patients in 24 target vessels for stenosis severity ranging from 40 to 95 percent, with an average of 74 ± 15 percent.[179] Absolute CFR did not correlate with percentage area stenosis or FFR. FFR, as well as rCFR, showed a curvilinear relationship with percentage area stenosis (r = 0.89 and r = 0.79; $p < 0.0001$), with a close linear relationship between FFR and rCFR (0.91; $p < 0.0001$). rCFR closely correlated with FFR and percentage area stenosis. Absolute CFR, as expected, varied due to the influence of microvascular flow status (Table 15-4).

Intracoronary Blood Flow Measurements and Ischemia Testing

Several single-center studies[164–166,181–183] and one multicenter trial[167] have reported strong correlations with myocardial stress perfusion imaging and post-stenotic coronary flow velocity reserve. An abnormal distal hyperemic flow velocity reserve (<2.0) corresponded with reversible myocardial perfusion imaging defects with high sensitivity (86–92 percent), specificity (89–100 percent), predictive accuracy (89–96 percent), and posi-

TABLE 15-4 Comparison of Absolute and Relative CFR and FFR

	Hemodynamic Independence	Independent of Microcirculation Abnormalities	Unequivocal Normal Values	Use in Multivessel CAD
CFR	−	−	Range > 2.0	+
rCFR	+	+	1.0	−
FFR	+	+	1.0	+

of proximal-to-distal flow) can be used as a marker of lesion-specific disease within the artery. In normal arteries, the proximal-to-distal flow velocity ratio should be 1.0.[184] A strong correlation exists between translesional pressure gradients and the ratios of the proximal-to-distal total flow velocity integrals ($r = 0.8, p < 0.001$), with a weaker relationship between pressure gradients and QCA ($r = 0.6$, $p < 0.001$).[184] In angiographically intermediate stenoses (50–70 percent), angiography was a poor predictor of translesional gradients ($r = 0.2$, $p =$ ns), whereas the flow velocity ratios continued to have a strong correlation with such gradients ($r = 0.8$, $p < 0.0001$). The proximal-to-distal flow velocity ratio demonstrated highly significant differences between patients with and without significant stenoses. A proximal-to-distal flow velocity integral ratio of less than 1.7 was associated with a gradient of less than 30 mmHg in more than 85 percent of patients. However, the proximal-to-distal ratio will be valid in arteries without branches or in those with ostial stenoses. The proximal-to-distal flow ratio index is sensitive but not lesion-specific.

Similarly, the phasic pattern of coronary flow (DSVR) reflects stenosis resistance. As a stenosis becomes more severe, diastolic flow is impaired first; then, as the stenosis increases, systolic flow is diminished. The normal DSVR is less than 1.8, 1.5, and 1.2 for the left anterior descending, circumflex, and proximal right coronary arteries, respectively.[185] A reduction in the normal DSVR generally indicates an important stenosis but is only a weak index for lesion-specific flow impairment. The relationship between DSVR and lesion severity requires a normally contracting myocardium in the region of the target stenosis to be accurate.

tive and negative predictive values (94–100 and 77–95 percent), respectively.

The sensitivity of FFR for reversible ischemia (FFR < 0.75) was 88 percent, specificity 100 percent, positive and negative predictive values 100 and 88 percent, respectively, with a predictive accuracy of 93 percent (Table 15-5).

Other Lesion-Specific Flow-Velocity Measurements

There are four lesion-specific physiologic measurements: (1) the rCFR ratio ($CFR_{target}/CFR_{normal}$), (2) the translesional pressure gradient at hyperemia (FFR_{myo}), (3) the proximal-to-distal velocity ratio, and (4) the diastolic/systolic velocity ratio (DSVR). The most accurate and practical measurements are the rCFR and FFR, as discussed earlier.

The proximal-to-distal flow velocity ratio depends on coronary arterial branching, which results in decremental volumetric flow and cross-sectional vessel area from the proximal to the distal myocardial regions. Because both volume and cross-sectional area diminish along the course of the vessel, velocity remains relatively constant (usually within 10 to 15 percent of the proximal velocity in vessel segments of more than 2 mm diameter). Maintenance of the flow velocity (but not volume) from the proximal to the distal part of the artery (i.e., the ratio

TABLE 15-5 Stress Testing and Directly Measured Coronary Hemodynamics

Author	Ref	*n*	Ischemic Test	CFR	Sensitivity	Specificity	PV+	PV−	Accuracy
			POSTSTENOTIC CORONARY FLOW VELOCITY RESERVE (CFR)						
Miller	7	33	Adeno/dipy MIBI	<2.0	82	100	100	77	89
Joye	10	30	Exercise thallium	<2.0	94	95	94	95	94
Deychak	9	17	Exercise thallium	<1.8	94	94	100	91	96
Heller	8	100	Exercise thallium	<1.8	89	92	96	89	92
Danzi	25	30	Dipy echo	<2.0	91	84	—	—	87
Schulman	26	35	Exercise ECG	<2.0	95	71	—	—	86
			FRACTIONAL FLOW RESERVE, MYOCARDIUM						
Pijls	14	45	Four-test standard	<0.75	88	100	100	88	93
de Bruyne	15	60	Exercise ECG	<0.72	100	87	—	—	—
Bartunek	24	37	Dobu/exercise echo	<0.68	95	90	—	—	—

NOTE: Adeno/dipy MIBI, adenosine or dipyridamole sestamibi scan; CFR, coronary vasodilatory reserve; Dobu, dobutamine; PV +/PV−, predictive value positive/negative.

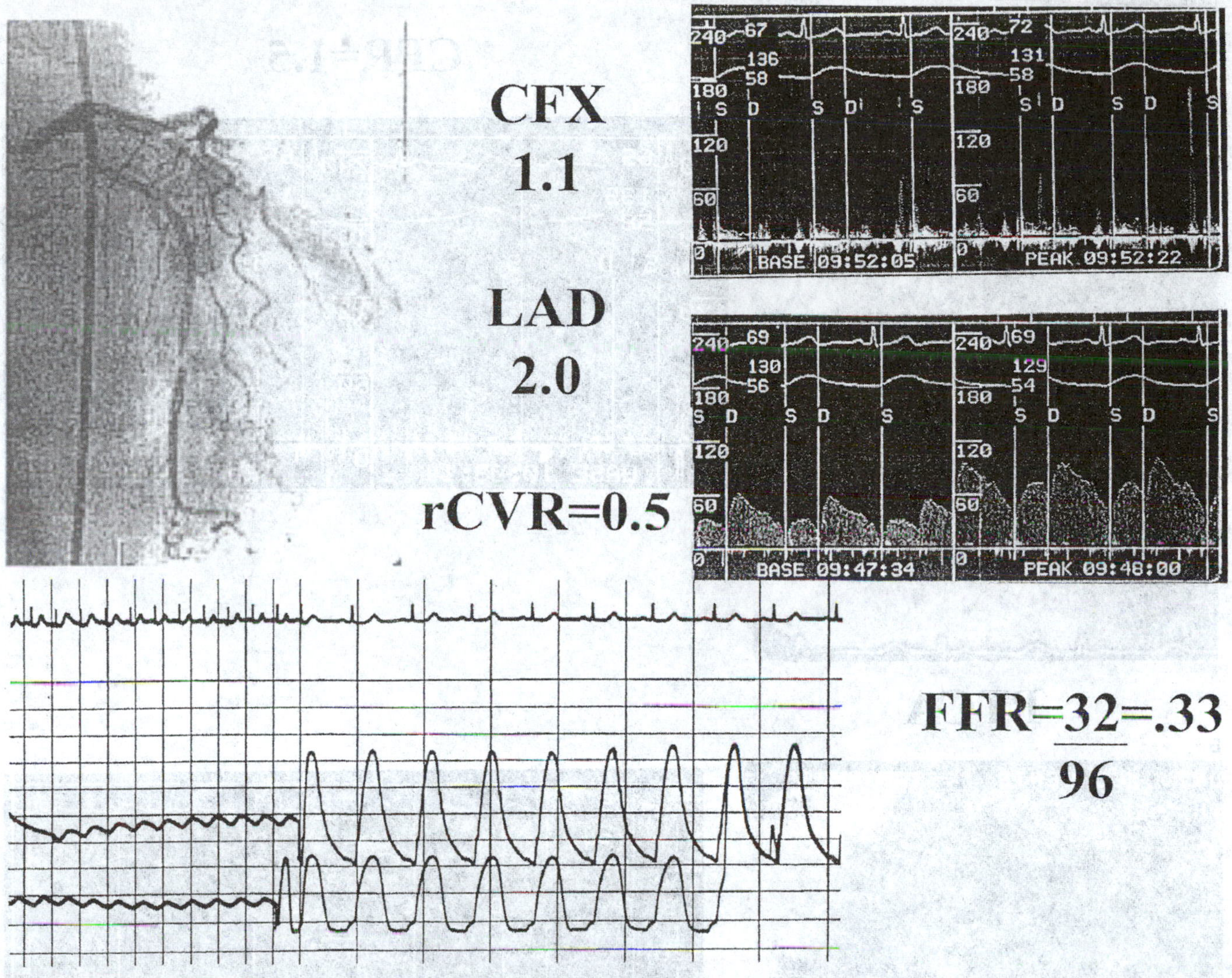

A

FIGURE 15-45 *A.* Coronary angiography, relative coronary flow velocity reserve (rCFR), and fractional flow reserve (FFR) before angioplasty of a circumflex (CFX) coronary lesion in a 78-year-old woman. LAD, left anterior descending artery. *B, C.* Results of coronary angioplasty (PTCA) and eight-stent placement with measurements of coronary flow reserve (CFR) and fractional flow reserve (FFR), as well as relative coronary flow reserve (rCFR) after the procedure.

Case Example: Physiologic Assessment of Critical Circumflex Lesion

A 78-year-old woman presented with unstable angina. Coronary arteriography revealed a nondominant right coronary artery, a 90 percent midcircumflex lesion, and a mildly and diffusely diseased left anterior descending coronary artery (Fig. 15-45*A*, top left). CFR and translesional pressure were measured to demonstrate the effect of angioplasty on the coronary physiologic parameters and use these variables as an end point. Coronary angioplasty was performed using a Doppler flow wire. Before angioplasty, circumflex CFR was 1.1, left anterior descending CFR was 2.0, and rCFR was 0.5 (see Fig. 15-45*A*, top right and bottom). The FFR was measured before angioplasty using a pressure guidewire (see Fig. 15-45*A*, bottom). The FFR was 0.33. A pressure transducer pullback to verify gradient location is shown at the far right of the tracing (see Fig. 15-8*A*, far right). After angioplasty (see Fig. 15-45*B*, left), the angiographic result appears satisfactory; however, the CFR in the circumflex (CFR_{CFX}) is still impaired at 1.5 (see Fig. 15-45*B*, right). After stent placement for the impaired CFR_{CFX}, the angiogram is somewhat improved with a 0 percent residual stenosis, but the CFR_{CFX} is now 2.0, rCFR is 1.0, and FFR is 1.0 (see Fig. 15-45*C*, top right and bottom right), indicating a highly successful and correlative physiologic result for this angioplasty.

Summary

Coronary pressure and flow describe coronary lesion resistance. The strong correlation of directly measured coronary flow and pressure to indirect ischemia testing can facilitate clinical in-lab decisions. Use of in-lab physiology strongly complements coronary lumenology and continues to have important clinical

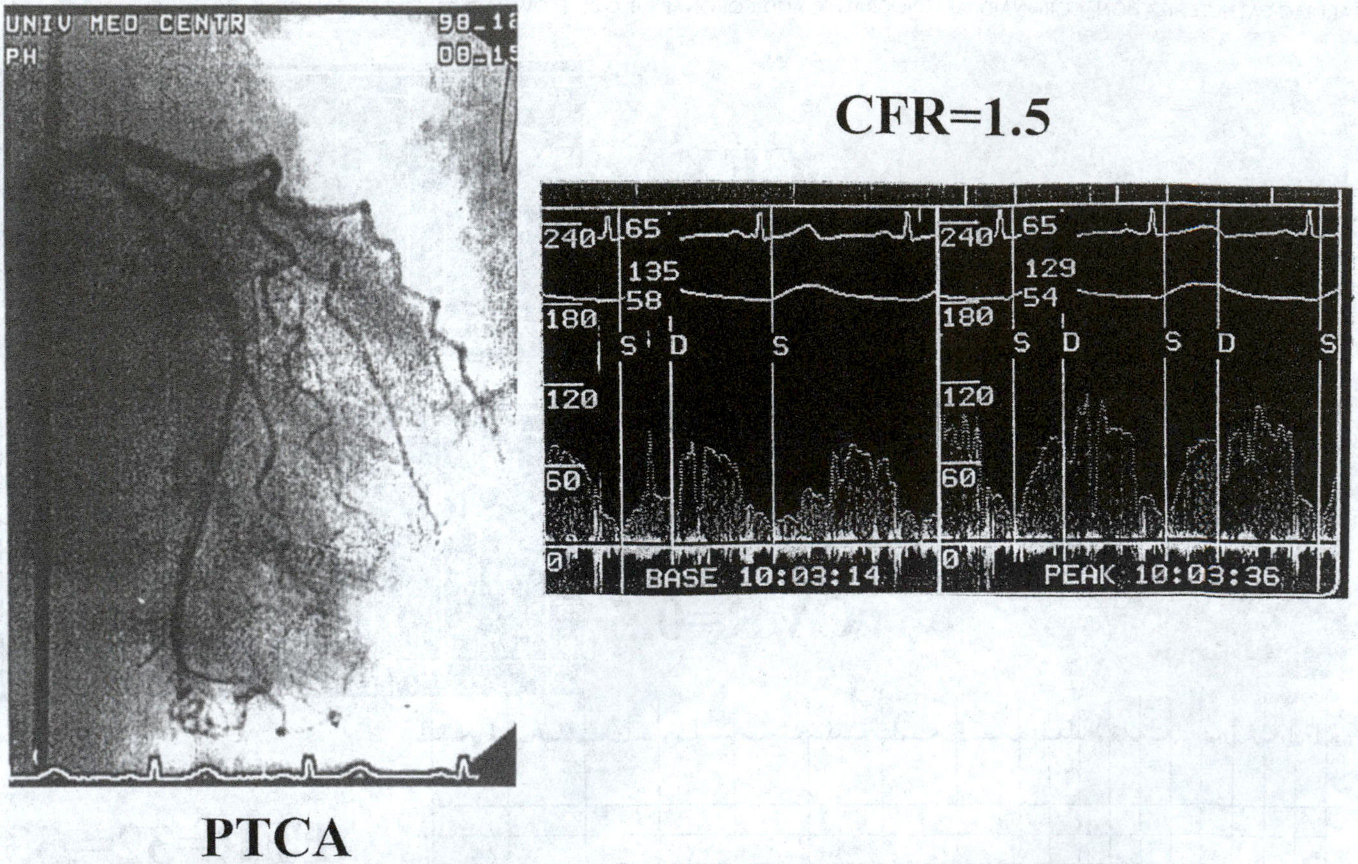

B

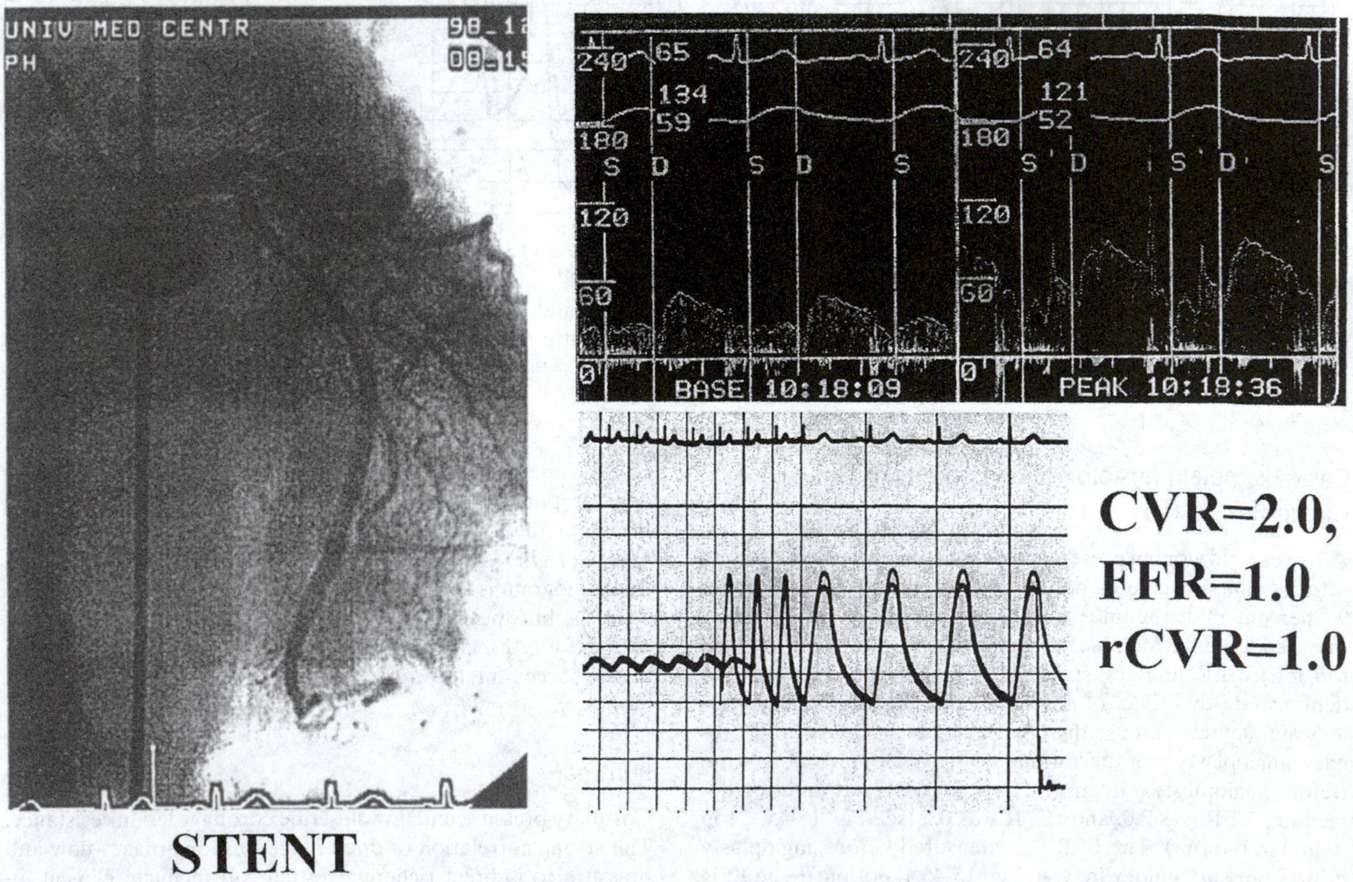

C

FIGURE 15-45 (*Continued*)

and economic implications for and research into the coronary circulation of patients.

References

1. Forssman W. Die Sondierung des rechten Herzens. *Berl Klin Wochenschr* 1929; 8:2085–2087.
2. Cournand A. Cardiac catheterization: Development of the technique, its contribution to experimental medicine and its initial application to man. *Acta Med Scand* 1975; 579(suppl):7–32.
3. Grossman W, Baim DS, eds. *Cardiac Catheterization, Angiography and Intervention*, 5th ed. Baltimore: Williams & Wilkins; 1996.
4. Pepine CJ, Hill JA, Lambert CR. *Diagnostic and Therapeutic Cardiac Catheterization*, 3d ed. Baltimore: Williams & Wilkins; 1998.
5. Mueller HS, Chatteryee K, Davis KB, et al. Present use of bedside right heart catheterization in patients with cardiac disease. *J Am Coll Cardiol* 1998; 32:840–864.
6. Allen HD, Beekman RH III, Garson A Jr, et al. AHA statement: Pediatric therapeutic cardiac catheterization. *Circulation* 1998; 97:609–625.
7. Myers GE, Crick WF, King WS, et al. Latex versus iodinated contrast media anaphylaxis in the cardiac cath lab. *Cathet Cardiovasc Diagn* 1995; 35:228–231.
8. Ruiz CE, Mullins CE, Rochini AP, et al. Core curriculum for the training of pediatric invasive interventional cardiologists. *Cathet Cardiovasc Diagn* 1996; 37:409.
9. Lasser EC, Berry CC, Talner LB, et al. Pretreatment with corticosteroids to alleviate reactions to intravenous contrast material. *New Engl J Med* 1987; 317:845–849.
10. Feldman T, Moss J, Teplinsky K, Carroll JD. Cardiac catheterization in the patient with a history of allergy to local anesthesia. *Cathet Cardiovasc Diagn* 1990; 20:165–167.
11. Clements SD, Gatlin S. Outpatient cardiac catheterization: A report of 3000 cases. *Clin Cardiol* 1991; 14:477–480.
12. Ad Hoc Task Force, Pepine CJ (chairman). ACC/AHA guidelines for cardiac catheterization and cardiac catheterization laboratories. *J Am Coll Cardiol* 1991; 18:1149–1182.
13. Scanlon PJ, Faxon DP, Audet A, et al. ACC/AHA guidelines for coronary angiography. *J Am Coll Cardiol* 1999; 33:1756–1824.
14. Shim D, Lloyd TR, Beekman RH III. Transhepatic therapeutic cardiac catheterization. *Cathet Cardiovasc Intervent* 1999; 47:41–45.
15. Louvard Y, Krol M, Pezzano M, et al. Feasibility of routine transradial coronary angiography: A single operative experience. *J Invas Cardiol* 1999; 11:543–544.
16. Rapoport S, Sniderman KW, Morse SS, et al. Pseudoaneurysm: A complication of faulty technique in femoral artery puncture. *Radiology* 1985; 154:529–530.
17. Montgomery DH, Veveris JJ, McGorisk G, et al. Natural history of severe atheromatous disease of the thoracic aorta: A transesophageal echocardiographic study. *J Am Coll Cardiol* 1996; 27:95–101.
18. Silber S. Rapid hemostasis of arterial puncture sites with collagen in patients undergoing diagnostic and interventional cardiac catheterization. *Clin Cardiol* 1997; 20:981–982.
19. Chamberlin JA, Lardi AB, McKeever LS, et al. Use of vascular sealing devices (Vasoseal and Perclose) versus assisted manual compression (Femostop) in transcatheter coronary interventions requiring abciximab (ReoPro). *Cathet Cardiovasc Intervent* 1999; 47:143–147.
20. Lesnefsky EJ, Carrea FP, Groves BM. Safety of cardiac catheterization via peripheral vascular grafts. *Cathet Cardiovasc Diagn* 1993; 29:113–116.
21. Laskey WK. Percutaneous retrograde left ventricular catheterization in aortic valve stenosis. *Cathet Cardiovasc Diagn* 1986; 12: 75–79.
22. MacDonald RG, Feldman RL, Pepine CJ. A modified catheter system for retrograde left ventricular catheterization in aortic valve stenoses. *Cathet Cardiovasc Diagn* 1985; 11:433–439.
23. Ommen SR, Higano ST, Nishimura RA, et al. Summary of the Mayo Clinic experience with direct left ventricular puncture. *Cathet Cardiovasc Diagn* 1998; 44:175–178.
24. Henry GA, Williams B, Pollak J, et al. Placement of an intracoronary stent via translumbar puncture. *Cathet Cardiovasc Intervent* 1999; 46:340–342.
25. Pearce AC, Schwengal RH, Simione LM, et al. Antegrade selective coronary angiography via the transseptal approach in a patient with severe vascular disease. *Cathet Cardiovasc Diagn* 1992; 26:300–303.
26. O'Keefe JH, Vlietstra RE, Hanley PC, Seward JB. Revival of the transseptal approach for catheterization of the left atrium and ventricle. *Mayo Clin Proc* 1985; 60:790–795.
27. Mullins CE. Transseptal left heart catheterization: Experience with a new technique in 520 pediatric and adult patients. *Pediatr Cardiol* 1983; 4:239–246.
28. Laskey WK, Kusiak V, Untereker WJ, Hirshfeld JW. Transseptal left heart catheterization: Utility of a sheath technique. *Cathet Cardiovasc Diagn* 1982; 8:535–542.
29. Croft CH, Lipscomb K. Modified technique of transseptal left heart catheterization. *J Am Coll Cardiol* 1985; 5:904–910.
30. Ali Kahn MA, Bucher JT, Mullins CE, et al. Blade atrial septostomy: Experience with the first 50 procedures. *Cathet Cardiovasc Diagn* 1991; 23:257–262.
31. Doucette JW, Corl PD, Payne HM. Validation of a Doppler guidewire for intravascular measurement of coronary artery. *Circulation* 1992; 85:1899–1911.
32. Segal J, Nasse M, Ford AJ Jr, Schuenemeyer TD. Instantaneous and continuous cardiac output in humans obtained with a Doppler pulmonary artery catheter. *J Am Coll Cardiol* 1990; 16:1398–1407.
33. Mizuno K, Satomura K, Miyamoto A. Angioscopic evaluation of coronary artery thrombi in acute coronary artery syndromes. *New Engl J Med* 1992; 326:287–291.
34. Rocchini AP, Kveselis DA, Crowley D, et al. Percutaneous balloon valvuloplasty for treatment of congenital pulmonary valvular stenosis in children. *J Am Coll Cardiol* 1984; 3:1005–1012.
35. Chen CR, Chen TO, Huang T, et al. Percutaneous balloon valvuloplasty for pulmonic stenosis in adolescents and adults. *New Engl J Med* 1996; 335:21–25.
36. Mitchell SE, White RI Jr, Kan J, Tolkoff J. Improved balloon catheters for large vessel and valvular angioplasty. *AJR* 1984; 142:571–572.
37. Grifka RG. Transcatheter intervention for the treatment of congenital cardiac defects. *Texas Heart Inst J* 1997; 24:293–300.
38. Limacher ML, Douglas PS, Germano G, et al. Radiation safety in the practice of cardiology. *J Am Coll Cardiol* 1998; 31:892–893.
39. Cusma JT, Bell MR, Wondrow MA, et al. Real time measurement of radiation exposure during diagnostic coronary angiography and percutaneous interventional procedures. *J Am Coll Cardiol* 1999; 33:427–435.
40. Balter S. Radiation safety in the cardiac catheterization laboratory. *Cathet Cardiovasc Intervent* 1999; 47:347–353.
41. Courtois M, Faltal PG, Kovacs SJ, et al. Anatomically and physiologically based reference levels for measurement of intracardiac pressures. *Circulation* 1995; 92:1994–2000.
42. Shepherd AP, McMahan CA. Role of oximeter error in the diagnosis of shunts. *Cathet Cardiovasc Diagn* 1996; 37:435–446.
43. Lange RA, Dehmer GJ, Wells PJ. Limitations of the metabolic rate meter for measuring oxygen consumption and cardiac output. *Am J Cardiol* 1989; 64:783–786.
44. Hurrell DG, Nishamura RA, Higano ST, et al. Value of dynamic respiratory changes in left and right ventricular pressures for the

diagnosis of constrictive pericarditis. *Circulation* 1996; 93:2007–2013.
45. Higano ST, Azrak F, Tahirkheli NK, et al. Hemodynamics of construction physiology: Influence of respiratory dynamics on ventricular pressures. *Cathet Cardiovasc Intervent* 1999; 46: 473–486.
46. Snyder RW II, Glamann DB, Lange RA, et al. Predictive value of prominent pulmonary arterial wedge V waves on assessing the presence and severity of mitral regurgitation. *Am J Cardiol* 1994; 73:568–570.
47. Dodge HT, Sheehan FH. Quantitative contrast angiography for assessment of ventricular performance in heart disease. *J Am Coll Cardiol* 1983; 1:73–81.
48. Lange RA, Moore DM Jr, Cigarroa RG, Hillis LD. Use of pulmonary capillary pressure to assess severity of mitral stenosis. Is true left atrial pressure needed in this condition? *J Am Coll Cardiol* 1989; 13:825–829.
49. Nishimura R, Rihal CS, Tajik AJ, Holmes DR. Accurate measurement of the transmitral gradient in patients with mitral stenosis: A simultaneous catheterization and Doppler echocardiographic study. *J Am Coll Cardiol* 1994; 24:152–158.
50. Assey ME, Zile MR, Usher BW, et al. Effect of catheter positioning on the variability of measured gradient in aortic stenosis. *Cathet Cardiovasc Diagn* 1993; 30:287–292.
51. Laskey WK, Kussmoul WG. Pressure recovery in aortic stenosis. *Circulation* 1994; 89:116–121.
52. Vandervoort DM, Greenberg NL, Pu M, et al. Pressure recovery in bileaflet heart valve prosthesis. *Circulation* 1995; 92:3464–3472.
53. Niederberger J, Schima H, Mauver G, et al. Importance of pressure recovery for the assessment of aortic stenosis by doppler ultrasound. *Circulation* 1996; 94:1934–1940.
54. Lemler MS, Valdey-Cruz LM, Shandas RS, et al. Insights into catheter/Doppler discrepancies in congenital aortic stenosis. 1999; 83:1447–1450.
55. Palevsky HI, Long W, Crow J, Fishman AP. Prostacyclin and acetylcholine as screening agents for acute pulmonary vasodilator responsiveness in primary pulmonary hypertension. *Circulation* 1990; 82:2018–2026.
56. Hillis DL, Firth BG, Winniford MD. Variability of right-sided cardiac oxygen saturations in adults with and without intracardiac left-to-right shunting. *Am J Cardiol* 1986; 58:129–132.
57. Freed MD, Miettinen OS, Nadas AS. Oximetric detection of intracardiac left-to-right shunts. *Br Heart J* 1979; 42:690–694.
58. Glamman DB, Lange RA, Willard JE, et al. Hydrogen inhalation for detecting intracardiac left-to-right shunting in adults. *Am J Cardiol* 1993; 72:711–714.
59. Bloomfield DA. *Dye Curves: The Theory and Practice of Indicator Dilution.* Baltimore: University Park Press; 1974.
60. Hillis DL, Winniford MD, Jackson JA, Firth BG. Measurement of left-to-right intracardiac shunting in adults: Oximetric versus indicator dilution techniques. *Cathet Cardiovasc Diagn* 1985; 11: 467–472.
61. Levett JM, Replogle RL. Thermodilution cardiac output: A critical analysis and review of the literature. *J Surg Res* 1979; 27: 392–404.
62. Lehmann KG, Platt MS. Improved accuracy and precision of thermodilation cardiac output measurement using a dual thermistor catheter system. *J Am Coll Cardiol* 1999; 33:883–891.
63. Hamilton MA, Stevenson LW, Woo RN, et al. Effect of tricuspid regurgitation on the reliability of the thermodilution cardiac output technique in congestive heart failure. *Am J Cardiol* 1989; 64:945–948.
64. Dodge HT, Sandler H, Ballew DW, Lord JD Jr. The use of biplane angiocardiography for the measurement of left ventricular volume in man. *Am Heart J* 1960; 60:762–776.
65. Wynne J, Green LH, Mann T, et al. Estimation of left ventricular volumes in man from biplane cineangiograms filmed in oblique projections. *Am J Cardiol* 1978; 41:726–732.
66. Sandler H, Dodge HT. The use of single plane angiocardiograms for the calculation of left ventricular volume in man. *Am Heart J* 1968; 75:325–334.
67. Kennedy JW, Trenholme SE, Kasser IS. Left ventricular volume and mass from single plane cineangiocardiograms. *Am Heart J* 1970; 80:343–352.
68. Sheehan FH, Mitten-Lewis S. Factors influencing accuracy in left ventricular volume determination. *Am J Cardiol* 1989; 64: 661–664.
69. Lawson MA, Blackwell GG, Doves ND, et al. Accuracy of biplane long-axis left ventricular volume determined by cine magnetic resonance imaging in patients with regional and global dysfunction. *Am J Cardiol* 1996; 77:1098–1104.
70. Kennedy JW, Baxley WA, Figley MM, et al. Quantitative angiocardiography: I. The normal left ventricle in man. *Circulation* 1966; 34:272–278.
71. Shimazaki Y, Kawashima Y, Mori T, et al. Angiographic volume estimation of right ventricle. *Chest* 1980; 77:390–395.
72. Gorlin R, Gorlin G. Hydraulic formula for calculation of area of stenotic mitral valve, other cardiac valves and central circulatory shunts. *Am Heart J* 1951; 41:1–29.
73. Cohen MV, Gorlin R. Modified orifice equation for the calculation of mitral valve area. *Am Heart J* 1972; 84:839–840.
74. Folland ED, Parisi AF, Carbone C. Is peripheral arterial pressure a satisfactory substitute for ascending aortic pressure when measuring aortic valve gradients? *J Am Coll Cardiol* 1984; 4:1207–1212.
75. Vaitkus PT, Higgins C, Watkins MW, et al. Accuracy of quantitation of aortic stenosis using femoral artery recording corrected for both temporal delay and systolic amplification. *Am J Cardiol* 1995; 76:725–728.
76. Krueger SK, Orme EC, King CS, Barry WH. Accurate determination of the transaortic valve gradient using simultaneous left ventricular and femoral artery pressure. *Cathet Cardiovasc Diagn* 1989; 16:202–206.
77. Voelker W, Reul H, Niehaus G, et al. Comparison of valvular resistance, stroke work loss and Gorlin valve area for quantification of aortic stenosis. *Circulation* 1995; 91:1196–1204.
78. Roger VL, Tajik AJ, Reeder GS, et al. Effect of Doppler echocardiography on utilization of hemodynamic cardiac catheterization in the preoperative evaluation of aortic stenosis. *Mayo Clin Proc* 1996; 71:141–149.
79. Bache RJ, Jorgensen CR, Wany Y. Simplified estimation of aortic valve area. *Br Heart J* 1972; 34:408–411.
80. Hakki AH. A simplified valve formula for the calculation of stenotic cardiac valve areas. *Circulation* 1981; 63:1050–1055.
81. Angel J, Soler-Soler J, Anivarro I, Domingo E. I. Hemodynamic evaluation of stenotic cardiac valves. II. Modification of the simplified formula for mitral and aortic valve area calculation. *Cathet Cardiovasc Diagn* 1985; 11:127–138.
82. Hosenpud JD, McAnulty JH, Morton MJ. Overestimation of mitral valve gradients obtained by phasic pulmonary artery wedge pressure. *Cathet Cardiovasc Diagn* 1983; 9:283–290.
83. Bettmann MA. Angiographic contrast agents: Conventional and new media compared. *AJR* 1982; 139:787–794.
84. Kern MJ. Selection of radiocontrast media in cardiac catheterization: Comparative physiology and clinical effects of nonionic and ionic dimeric formulations. *Am Heart J* 1991; 122:195–201.
85. Werner GS, Schmidt T, Scholz KH, et al. Comparison of hemodynamic and Doppler echocardiographic effects of new low osmolar non-ionic and a standard ionic contrast agent after left ventriculography. *Cathet Cardiovasc Diagn* 1994; 33:11–19.
86. McClennan BL. Ionic and nonionic iodinated contrast media: Evolution and strategies for use. *AJR* 1990; 155:225–233.
87. Brogan WC III, Hillis LD, Lange RA. Contrast agents for cardiac

catheterization: Conceptions and misconceptions. *Am Heart J* 1991; 122:1129–1135.
88. Hirshfield JW Jr. Cardiovascular effects of contrast agents. *Am J Cardiol* 1990; 66(suppl):9F-17P.
89. Curry III TS, Dowdey JE, Murray RC Jr, eds. *Christensen's Physics of Diagnostic Radiology*, 4th ed. Philadelphia: Lea & Febiger; 1990:77.
90. Holmes DR, Wondrow MA, Bell MR, et al. Cine film replacement digital archival requirements and remaining obstacles. *Cathet Cardiovasc Diagn* 1998; 44:346–356.
91. Soto B, Pacifico AD. *Angiocardiography in Congenital Heart Malformations*. Mount Kisco, NY: Futura; 1990.
92. Delegonul U, Jones S, Shurmur S, Oskarsson H. Contrast cine left ventriculography. *Cathet Cardiovasc Diagn* 1996; 37:428–433.
93. Nihill MR, Mullins CE, McNamara DG. Visualization of the pulmonary arteries in pseudotruncus by pulmonary vein wedge angiography. *Circulation* 1978; 58:140–147.
94. McGrath LB, Chen C, Bailey BN, et al. Determination of the need for tricuspid valve replacement value of preoperative right ventricular angiography. *J Invas Cardiol* 1991; 3:35–40.
95. Fraser RS. Catheter-induced pulmonary artery perforation: Pathologic and pathogenic features. *Hum Pathol* 1987; 18:1246–1251.
96. Trerotola SO, Kuhlman JE, Fishman EK. Bleeding complications of femoral catheterization: CT evaluation. *Radiology* 1990; 174: 37–40.
97. Cohen GI, Chan KL. Physical examination and echo Doppler study in the assessment of femoral artery complications following cardiac catheterization. *Cathet Cardiovasc Diagn* 1990; 21: 137–143.
98. Chatterjee T, Do D, Kaufmann U, et al. Ultrasound-guided repair for treatment of femoral artery pseudoaneurysm. *Cathet Cardiovasc Diagn* 1996; 38:335–340.
99. Lazar JM, Uretsky BF, Denys BG, et al. Predisposing risk factors and natural history of acute neurologic complications of left-sided cardiac catheterization. *Am J Cardiol* 1995; 75:1056–1060.
100. Bettmann MA. Safety and efficacy of iodinated contrast agents. *Invest Radial* 1994; 29:533–536.
101. Solomon R, Wenner C, Mann D, et al. Effects of saline, mannitol, and furosemide on acute decreases in renal function induced by radiocontrast agents. *New Engl J Med* 1994; 331:1416–1420.
102. Rocher L. Radiocontrast-induced acute renal failure. *Am Coll Cardiol Curr J Rev* 1996; 5:75–78.
103. Barrett BJ. Contrast nephrotoxicity. *J Am Soc Nephrol* 1994; 125–137.
104. Parfrey PS, Griffiths SM, Barrett MB, et al. Contrast material-induced renal failure in patients with diabetes mellitus, renal insufficiency or both. *New Engl J Med* 1989; 320:143–149.
105. Schwab SJ, Hlatky MA, Pieper KS. Contrast nephrotoxicity: A randomized controlled trial of a nonionic and an ionic contrast agent. *New Engl J Med* 1989; 320:149–153.
106. Tworetzky W, McElhinney DB, Brook MM, et al. Echocardiographic diagnosis alone for the complete repair of major congenital heart defects. *J Am Coll Cardiol* 1999; 33:228–233.
107. Stanlon PJ, Faxon DP (cochairs). Guidelines for coronary angiography: A report of the American College of Cardiology/American Heart Association Task Force on assessment of diagnostic and therapeutic cardiovascular procedures (Committee on Coronary Angiography). *J Am Coll Cardiol* 1999; 33:1756–1824.
108. Pepine CJ, Allen HD, Bashore TM, et al. ACC/AHA guidelines for cardiac catheterization laboratories. *Circulation* 1991; 84: 2213–2247.
109. Bashore TM. State of the art of coronary angiography. *J Invas Cardiol* 1991; 3(suppl B):47B-59B.
110. Sones FM Jr, Shirey EK. Cine coronary arteriography. *Mod Concepts Cardiovasc Dis* 1962; 31:735–738.
111. Conti ER. Coronary arteriography. *Circulation* 1977; 55:227–237.
112. Nohara R, Kambara H, Murakami T, et al. Collateral function in early acute myocardial infarction. *Am J Cardiol* 1983; 52:955–959.
113. Helfant RH, Vokonas PS, Gorlin R. Functional importance of the human coronary collateral circulation. *New Engl J Med* 1971; 284:1277–1281.
114. Heupler FA Jr. Syndrome of symptomatic coronary arterial spasm with nearly normal coronary arteriograms. *Am J Cardiol* 1980; 45:873–881.
115. Conti CR, Curry RC, Christie LG, Pepine CJ. Clinical use of provocative pharmacoangiography in patients with chest pain. *Adv Cardiol* 1979; 26:44–54.
116. Waters DD, Szlachcic J, Bonan R. Comparative sensitivity of exercise, coldpressor and ergonovine testing in provoking attacks of variant angina in patients with active disease. *Circulation* 1983; 67:310–315.
117. Donohue TJ, Kern MJ, Aguirre FV, et al. Assessing the hemodynamic significance of coronary artery stenoses: Analysis of translesional pressure-flow velocity relations in patients. *J Am Coll Cardiol* 1993; 22:449–458.
118. Helfant RH, Pine R, Meister SG, et al. Nitroglycerin to unmask reversible asynergy: Correlation with post coronary bypass ventriculography. *Circulation* 1974; 50:108–113.
119. Horn HR, Teichholz LE, Cohn PF, et al. Augmentation of left ventricular contraction pattern in coronary artery disease by inotropic catecholamine: The epinephrine ventriculogram. *Circulation* 1974; 49:1063–1071.
120. Dyke SH, Cohn PF, Gorlin R, Sonnenblick EH. Detection of residual myocardial function in coronary artery disease using post extrasystolic potentiation. *Circulation* 1974; 50:694–699.
121. Formanek A, Nath PH, Zollikofer C, Moller JH. Selective coronary arteriography in children. *Circulation* 1980; 61:84–95.
122. Heupler FA Jr. Coronary arteriography and left ventriculography: Sones technique. In: King SB III, Douglas JS Jr, eds. *Coronary Arteriography*. New York: McGraw-Hill; 1984:137–181.
123. Seldinger SI. Catheter replacement of the needle in percutaneous arteriography: A new technique. *Acta Radiol* 1953; 39:368–376.
124. Ricketts HJ, Abrams HL. Percutaneous selective coronary cine arteriography. *JAMA* 1962; 181:620–626.
125. Amplatz K, Formanek G, Stranger P, Wilson W. Mechanics of selective coronary artery catheterization via femoral approach. *Radiology* 1967; 89:1040–1047.
126. Judkins MP. Selective coronary arteriography: I. A percutaneous transfemoral technique. *Radiology* 1967; 89:815–824.
127. Judkins MP, Judkins EJ. The Judkins technique. In: King SB III, Douglas JS Jr, eds. *Coronary Arteriography*. New York: McGraw-Hill; 1984:182–217.
128. Schoonmaker FW, King SB III. Coronary arteriography by the single catheter percutaneous femoral techniques: Experience with 6800 cases. *Circulation* 1974; 50:735–740.
129. King SB III, Douglas JS Jr. Catheterization techniques in coronary arteriography and left ventriculography: Multipurpose techniques: In: King SB III, Douglas JS Jr, eds. *Coronary Arteriography*. New York: McGraw-Hill; 1984:239–274.
130. Heupler FA, Chambers CE, Dear WE, et al. Guidelines for internal peer review in the cardiac catheterization laboratory. *Cathet Cardiovasc Diagn* 1997; 40:21–32.
131. Douglas JS Jr, King SB III. Complications of coronary arteriography: Management during and following the procedure. In: King SB III, Douglas JS Jr, eds. *Coronary Arteriography*. New York: McGraw-Hill; 1984:302–313.
132. Austin WG, Edwards JE, Frye RL, et al. A reporting system on patients evaluated for coronary artery disease: Report of the ad hoc committee for grading coronary artery disease, Council on Cardiovascular Surgery, American Heart Association. *Circulation* 1975; 51(suppl 4):5–40.
133. Bunnell IL, Greene DG, Tandom RN, Arani DT. The half-axial

projection: A new look at the proximal left coronary artery. *Circulation* 1973; 48:1151–1156.

134. Aldridge HE, McLoughlin MJ, Taylor KW. Improved diagnosis in coronary cine arteriography with routine use of oblique views and cranial and caudal angulations. *Am J Cardiol* 1975; 36: 468–473.

135. Frederick PR, Fry WH, Russell JG, Marshall HW. Longitudinal angulation in coronary arteriography: Apparatus and evaluation. *Cathet Cardiovasc Diagn* 1977; 3:305–311.

136. King SB III, Douglas JS Jr, Morris DC. New angiographic views for coronary arteriography. In: Hurst JW, ed. *The Heart, Update IV*. New York: McGraw-Hill; 1980:275–287.

137. Hermiller JB, Cusma JT, Spero LA, et al. Quantitative and qualitative coronary angiographic analysis: Review of methods, utility and limitations. *Cathet Cardiovasc Diagn* 1992; 25:110–131.

138. Kramer JR, Kitazume H, Proudfitt WL, Sones FM Jr. Clinical significance of isolated coronary bridges: Benign and frequent condition involving the left anterior descending artery. *Am Heart J* 1982; 103:283–288.

139. Douglas JS Jr, Franch RH, King SB III. Coronary artery anomalies. In: King SB III, Douglas JS Jr, eds. *Coronary Arteriography and Angioplasty*. New York: McGraw-Hill; 1985:33–85.

140. Zir LM, Miller SW, Dinsmore RE, et al. Interobserver variability in coronary arteriography. *Circulation* 1976; 53:627–630.

141. DeRouen TA, Murray JA, Owen W. Variability in the analysis of coronary arteriograms. *Circulation* 1977; 55:324–328.

142. Schwartz JN, King Y, Hackel DB, Bartel AG. Comparison of angiographic and postmortem findings in patients with coronary artery disease. *Am J Cardiol* 1975; 36:174–178.

143. Kemp HG, Evans H, Elliott WC, Gorlin R. Diagnostic accuracy of selective coronary cinearteriography. *Circulation* 1967; 36: 526–533.

144. Grandin CM, Dyrda I, Pastemac A, et al. Discrepancies between cineangiographic and postmortem findings in patients with coronary artery disease and recent myocardial revascularization. *Circulation* 1974; 49:703–708.

145. Roberts WC. The coronary arteries and left ventricle in clinically isolated angina pectoris: A necropsy analysis. *Circulation* 1976; 54:388–390.

146. Arnett EN, Isner JM, Redwood DR, et al. Coronary artery narrowing in coronary heart disease: Comparison of cine angiographic and necropsy findings. *Ann Intern Med* 1979; 91:350–356.

147. Roberts CS, Roberts WC. Cross-sectional area of the proximal portions of the three major epicardial coronary arteries in 98 patients with different coronary events: Relationship to heart, weight, age, and sex. *Circulation* 1980; 62:953–959.

148. Isner JM, Kishel J, Kent KM, et al. Inaccuracy of angiographic determination of left main coronary arterial narrowing: Angiographic-histologic correlative analysis of 29 patients. *Circulation* 1979; 59,60(suppl 2):ii–161.

149. Brown BG, Bolson E, Frimer M, Dodge HT. Quantitative coronary arteriography: Estimation of dimensions, hemodynamic resistance, and atheroma mass of coronary artery lesions using the arteriogram and digital computation. *Circulation* 1977; 55: 329–337.

150. Abrams HL, Adams DF. The complications of coronary arteriography (abstr). *Circulation* 1975; 52(suppl 2):27.

151. Davis K, Kennedy JW, Kemp HG, et al. Complications of coronary arteriography from the Collaborative Study of Coronary Artery Surgery (CASS). *Circulation* 1979; 59:1105–1112.

152. Johnson LW, Lozner EC, Johnson S, et al. Coronary arteriography 1984–1987: A report of the Registry of the Society for Cardiac Angiography and Interventions. 1. Results and complications. *Cathet Cardiovasc Diagn* 1989; 17:5–10.

153. Devlin G, Lazzam LM, Schwartz L. Current mortality rate of diagnostic cardiac catheterization: The importance of left main coronary artery disease and catheter-induced trauma (abstract). *Circulation* 1995; 92(suppl I):i–602.

154. Gersh BJ, Kronmal RA, Frye RL, et al. Coronary arteriography and coronary bypass surgery: Morbidity and mortality in patients ages 65 years or older: A report from the coronary artery surgery study. *Circulation* 1983; 67:483–491.

155. Krone RJ, Johnson L, Noto T. Five year trends in cardiac catheterization: A report from the Registry of the Society for Cardiac Angiography and Interventions. *Cathet Cardiovasc Diagn* 1996; 39:31–35.

156. Takaro T, Hultgren HN, Littmann D, Wright EC. An analysis of deaths occurring in association with coronary arteriography. *Am Heart J* 1973; 86:587–597.

157. Vogel JHK, Cornish D, McFadden RB. Underestimations of ejection fraction with single plane angiography in coronary artery disease: Role of biplane angiography. *Chest* 1973; 64:217–221.

158. De Feyter PJ, Serruys PW, Davies MJ, et al. Quantitative coronary angiography to measure progression and regression of coronary atherosclerosis: Value, limitations, and implications for clinical trials. *Circulation* 1991; 84:412–423.

159. White CW, Wright CB, Doty DB, et al. Does visual interpretation of the coronary arteriogram predict the physiologic importance of a coronary stenosis? *New Engl J Med* 1984; 310:819–824.

160. Harrison DG, White CW, Hiratzka LF, et al. The value of lesion cross-sectional area determined by quantitative coronary angiography in assessing the physiologic significance of proximal left anterior descending coronary arterial stenoses. *Circulation* 1984; 69:1111–1119.

161. Kern MJ, de Bruyne B, Pijls NHJ. From research to clinical practice: Current role of physiologically based decision making in the catheterization laboratory. *J Am Coll Cardiol* 1997; 30: 613–620.

162. Gould KL, Kirkeeide RL, Buchi M. Coronary flow reserve as a physiologic measure of stenosis severity. *J Am Coll Cardiol* 1990; 15:459–474.

163. Gould KL, Lipscomb K, Hamilton GW. Physiologic basis for assessing critical coronary stenosis: Instantaneous flow response and regional distribution during coronary hyperemia as measures of coronary flow reserve. *Am J Cardiol* 1974; 33:87–94.

164. Miller DD, Donohue TJ, Younis LT, et al. Correlation of pharmacologic ^{99m}Tc-sestamibi myocardial perfusion imaging with poststenotic coronary flow reserve in patients with angiographically intermediate coronary artery stenoses. *Circulation* 1994; 89:2150–2160.

165. Heller LI, Cates C, Popma J, et al., for the FACTS study group. Intracoronary Doppler assessment of moderate coronary artery disease: comparison with ^{201}Tl imaging and coronary angiography. *Circulation* 1997; 96:484–490.

166. Deychak YA, Segal J, Reiner JS, et al. Doppler guide wire flow-velocity indexes measured distal to coronary stenoses associated with reversible thallium perfusion defects. *Am Heart J* 1995; 129:219–227.

167. Joye JD, Schulman DS, Lasorda D, et al. Intracoronary Doppler guide wire versus stress single-photon emission computed tomographic thallium-201 imaging in assessment of intermediate coronary stenoses. *J Am Coll Cardiol* 1994; 24:940–947.

168. Doucette JW, Corl PD, Payne HM, et al. Validation of a Doppler guide wire for intravascular measurement of coronary artery flow velocity. *Circulation* 1992; 85:1899–1911.

169. Labovitz AJ, Anthonis DM, Cravens TL, Kern MJ. Validation of volumetric flow measurements by means of a Doppler-tipped coronary angioplasty guide wire. *Am Heart J* 1993; 126:1456–1461.

170. Pijls NH, van Son JA, Kirkeeide RL, et al. Experimental basis of determining maximum coronary, myocardial, and collateral

blood flow by pressure measurements for assessing functional stenosis severity before and after percutaneous transluminal coronary angioplasty. *Circulation* 1993; 87:1354–1367.
171. Pijls NHJ, de Bruyne B, Peels K, et al. Measurement of myocardial fractional flow reserve to assess the functional severity of coronary artery stenosis. *New Engl J Med* 1996; 334:1703–1708.
172. de Bruyne B, Bartunek J, Sys SU, et al. Simultaneous coronary pressure and flow velocity measurements in humans: Feasibility, reproducibility, and hemodynamic dependence of coronary flow velocity reserve, hyperemic flow versus pressure slope index, and fractional flow reserve. *Circulation* 1996; 94:1842–1849.
173. de Bruyne B, Paulus WJ, Pijls NHJ. Rationale and application of coronary transstenotic pressure gradient measurements. *Cathet Cardiovasc Diagn* 1994; 33:250–261.
174. Wilson RF, White CW. Intracoronary papaverine: An ideal coronary vasodilator for studies of the coronary circulation in conscious humans. *Circulation* 1986; 73:444–451.
175. Wilson RF, Wyche K, Christensen BV, et al. Effects of adenosine on human coronary arterial circulation. *Circulation* 1990; 82: 1595–1606.
176. Caracciolo EA, Wolford TL, Underwood RD, et al. Influence of intimal thickening on coronary blood flow responses in orthotopic heart transplant recipients: A combined intravascular Doppler and ultrasound imaging study. *Circulation* 1995; 92(suppl II):II-182–II-190.
177. Abizaid A, Kornowski R, Mintz GS, et al. Influence of guiding catheter selection on the measurement of coronary flow reserve. *Am J Cardiol* 1997; 79:703–704.
178. Kern MJ, Bach RG, Mechem CJ, et al. Variations in normal coronary vasodilatory reserve stratified by artery, gender, heart transplantation and coronary artery disease. *J Am Coll Cardiol* 1996; 28:1154–1160.
179. Baumgart D, Haude M, Goerge G, et al. Improved assessment of coronary stenosis severity using the relative flow velocity reserve. *Circulation* 1998; 98:40–46.
180. Kern MJ, Donohue TJ, Bach. RG, et al. Assessment of intermediate coronary stenosis by relative coronary flow velocity reserve (abstract). *J Am Coll Cardiol* 1997; 29(suppl A):21A.
181. Bartunek J, Van Schuerbeeck E, de Bruyne B. Comparison of exercise electrocardiography and dobutamine echocardiography with invasively assessed myocardial fractional flow reserve in evaluation of severity of coronary arterial narrowing. *Am J Cardiol* 1997; 79:478–481.
182. Danzi GB, Pirelli S, Mauri L, et al. Which variable of stenosis severity best describes the significance of an isolated left anterior descending coronary artery lesion? Correlation between quantitative coronary angiography, intracoronary Doppler measurements and high dose dipyridamole echocardiography. *J Am Coll Cardiol* 1998; 31:526–533.
183. Schulman DS, Lasorda D, Farah T, et al. Correlations between coronary flow reserve measured with a Doppler guide wire and treadmill exercise testing. *Am Heart J* 1997; 134:99–104.
184. Donohue TJ, Kern MJ, Aguirre FV, et al. Assessing the hemodynamic significance of coronary artery stenoses: Analysis of translesional pressure-flow velocity relationships in patients. *J Am Coll Cardiol* 1993; 22:449–458.
185. Ofili EO, Kern MJ, Labovitz AJ, et al. Analysis of coronary blood flow velocity dynamics in angiographically normal and stenosed arteries before and after endolumen enlargement by angioplasty. *J Am Coll Cardiol* 1993; 21:308–316.

C H A P T E R 16

NUCLEAR CARDIOLOGY

Daniel S. Berman / Leslee J. Shaw / Guido Germano

OVERVIEW

During the last three decades, a number of noninvasive testing modalities have become widely available in clinical cardiology. Since the early 1970s, there has been a sustained growth of nearly 15 percent per year in the field of nuclear cardiology. Today, state-of-the-art nuclear cardiology allows for the measurement of both myocardial function and relative regional perfusion at rest and stress, providing accurate risk assessment in a wide variety of patient subsets. This chapter provides a synopsis of published evidence on the role of nuclear cardiology procedures in diagnosis and risk assessment with a view to effective clinical management of patients with suspected or known coronary artery disease (CAD). Positron emission tomography (PET) is discussed in Chap. 19.

Major Advances in Clinical Cardiology

Important experimental and clinical research has led to a substantial reduction in the risk of coronary artery disease events in westernized countries.[1] Current evidence from randomized trials notes a 35 to 50 percent reduction in mortality associated with ischemic heart disease and stroke.[2] A comparison of mortality statistics from 1973 to 1993 reveals a decrease in the total number of deaths, mostly affecting the young and middle-aged population (see Chap. 38). Improved outcomes were the result of improved diagnosis and effective risk-reducing therapies.[3,4] New therapies aimed at reducing blood pressure and cholesterol levels are effective strategies for the prevention of cardiovascular disease.[5] In the case of cholesterol lowering, a linear relationship between serum levels and CAD risk has been established, a 10 percent reduction in cholesterol levels being associated with a 30 percent reduction in disease incidence; and the widespread availability of effective, low-risk drugs has made major cholesterol reduction feasible.[6] An overview of randomized trials for coronary artery bypass surgery (CABS) indicates that the appropriate surgical treatment has resulted in an overall mortality reduction as compared with medical treatment.[7] These effective therapies have increased the importance of accurate risk assessment, ideally more accurately and quantitatively based than is feasible from historical information alone or nonimaging treadmill stress testing.

Despite the abundance of high-quality evidence on the effectiveness of medical and surgical management of patients, the body of evidence on the effectiveness of noninvasive testing in guiding management decisions is less well established. Nonetheless, evidence-based medicine is now the standard serving for the evaluation of new technologies and their assimilation into daily clinical practice. Nuclear cardiology is a well-established modality with large observational series available to provide the basis for effective medical management of patients with suspected or known CAD.

Era of Cost Containment in Medical Practice

Declining reimbursement levels coupled with an ever-increasing emphasis on cost containment has led many to advocate development of a body of evidence to justify use of any medical procedure. For a nonivasive test, justification may be defined as assessing its economic and clinical incremental value as compared with other modalities. A synthesis of evidence reviewed in the recent ACC/AHA/ACP-ASIM guidelines for the management of patients with chronic stable angina revealed an abundance of data on the clinical incremental value of nuclear cardiology procedures.[8] Selected reports are also available on economic data for nuclear cardiology procedures as compared with other noninvasive tests used in cardiology.[9]

Historical Perspectives in Nuclear Cardiology

Continuous growth in the field of nuclear cardiology over the last three decades has been facilitated by the development of improved perfusion tracers, enhancements in scintillation cameras, and dramatic improvements in computer technology and specialized computer hardware and software, allowing for rapid assessment of patient data. In 1999, nearly 5 million myocardial perfusion studies were performed in the United States, a rate nearly threefold higher than other stress imaging tests. Major growth in procedure use has occurred in the outpatient setting, with an ever-increasing proportion of tests being performed in nonhospital facilities. The Anger scintillation camera, the imaging device used today for virtually all of nuclear cardiology except PET, became clinically available in the late 1960s. In the 1990s, the principal advances were the wide use of dual and triple detector cameras that improved image quality and shortened acquisition time as well as dramatic increases in the speed of computer systems that decreased processing time and made gated single-photon emission tomography (SPECT) clinically feasible. In 1973, Liebowitz et al. introduced thallium 201 (^{201}Tl) for medical use.[10] Following its commercial availability, ^{201}Tl quickly became the myocardial perfusion imaging agent of choice, a position it maintained until the technetium 99m (^{99m}Tc) perfusion agents became widely accepted. In 1990, ^{99m}Tc sestamibi was approved for use in the United States. Owing to its more favorable physical properties and better image quality, this agent has become the most frequently used radiopharmaceutical in the United States. Another ^{99m}Tc-based agent, tetrofosmin, was approved in the United States in 1997 and has also demonstrated widespread growth. By 1998, some 72 percent of nuclear cardiology tests used a ^{99m}Tc myocardial perfusion imaging agent.

State-of-the-Art Nuclear Cardiology

With the recent widespread availability of powerful computer systems as well as multidetector SPECT systems, gated myocardial perfusion scintigraphy has become routine; it was performed in 66 percent of myocardial perfusion SPECT studies in the United States in 1999, providing objective assessments of global and regional myocardial function in addition to traditional perfusion assessment. The increasing acceptance of the gated myocardial perfusion SPECT technique is a consequence of its becoming a powerful clinical tool to address a variety of clinical questions arising in the assessment of patients with known or suspected CAD. Although radionuclide angiography played a prominent role in noninvasive testing in decades past, in the 1990s the use of this modality became largely replaced by echocardiography and gated perfusion SPECT. Some important clinical applications of this modality remain, however, and are discussed in the latter portion of this chapter.

MYOCARDIAL PERFUSION SINGLE PHOTON EMISSION COMPUTED TOMOGRAPHY

A large number of acquisition protocols and techniques are used in nuclear cardiology today. Most of them are based on the Anger scintillation camera or a variation of it. The Anger scintillation camera (or gamma camera) consists of one or more scintillation detectors, typically made of high-density materials such as NaI, sodium iodide. Myocardial perfusion scintigraphy can be performed with either planar or SPECT approaches. With the planar technique, generally three two-dimensional (2D) images are obtained, usually 10 to 15 min each. Myocardial perfusion SPECT consists of imaging the 3D distribution of a radioactive perfusion agent in the myocardium. For SPECT acquisition, the camera detectors rotate around the patient in a circular or elliptical fashion, collecting a "projection image" at every few degrees. The 3D distribution of radioactivity is then mathematically "reconstructed" from the 2D projection images, usually using a process called "filtered-backprojection" and incorporating a variety of filters that enhance the images.

Multidetector cameras have come to be more commonly purchased than single-detector systems, and their increasing diffusion is an important factor supporting the increasing utilization of gated SPECT. Dual-detector cameras with the two detectors positioned at 90 degrees allow completion of 180-degree SPECT acquisitions in half the time taken by a single detector system for the same count level, or collection of twice the counts in the same time, and are therefore highly efficient for gated cardiac SPECT for imaging perfusion and function. A gated SPECT acquisition is similar to a standard SPECT acquisition, since in both cases the camera detector(s) rotates around the long axis of the patient, acquiring a number of planar ("projection") images at regular angular intervals (Fig. 16-1). What distinguishes the gated from the nongated technique is that, in the former, a number (8 or 16) of projection images is acquired at each projection angle, with each image (also called an interval or frame) corresponding to a specific portion of the cardiac cycle. A gated SPECT acquisition results in a standard SPECT data set ("summed" gated SPECT), from which perfusion is assessed, and a larger gated SPECT data set, from which function is evaluated. Gated SPECT has become the most commonly performed perfusion SPECT protocol as a direct consequence of the ease and modest expense with which perfusion assessment is "upgraded" to perfusion/function assessment and of the documentation of incremental information by the combined measurements.

As long as adequate count statistics are achieved, there is no limitation as to the specific perfusion agent that can be imaged with the gated SPECT technique. The quality of the gated SPECT study is directly related to the number of counts in its individual frames. Count statistics are influenced by numerous factors, including injected dose, acquisition time, patient size, number of detectors, collimation, number of frames, and count acceptance criteria.

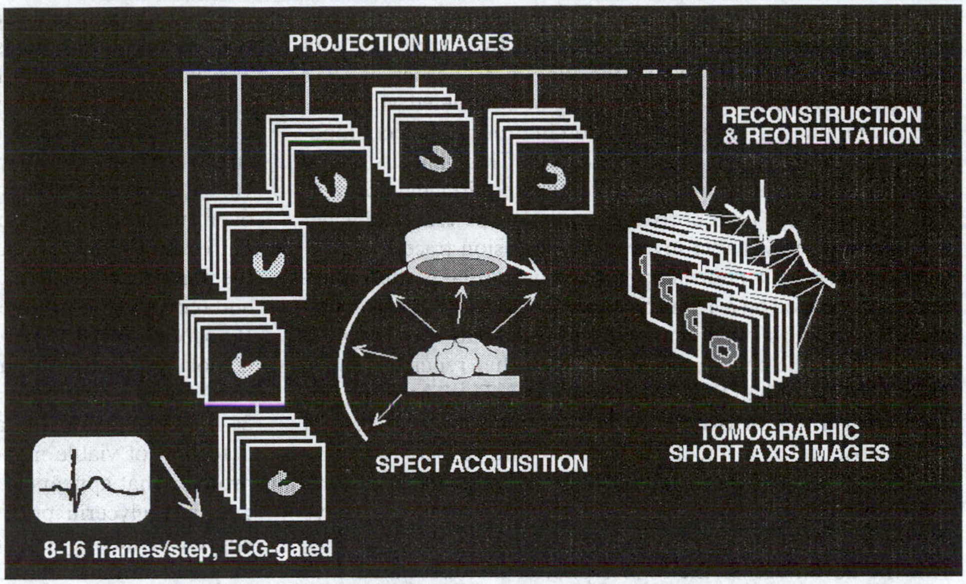

FIGURE 16-1 Schematic representation of ECG-gated perfusion SPECT acquisition and processing.

Radiopharmaceuticals

THALLIUM 201

A cyclotron-generated radionuclide with a half-life of 73 h, ^{201}Tl emits gamma rays from 68 to 80 kev (94 percent abundant) and at 167 kev (10 percent abundant). Owing to its relatively long half-life, the absorbed radiation dose is such that recommended injected doses are limited to 2 to 4 mCi. ^{201}Tl has excellent physiologic properties for myocardial perfusion imaging. Importantly for stress myocardial perfusion scintigraphy, a linear relationship between blood flow to viable myocardium and ^{201}Tl uptake is maintained during exercise[11] up to very high levels of flow (e.g., vasodilator stress, >3 mL/min/g), where a "roll-off" in uptake occurs.[12] After intravenous injection, thallium is rapidly extracted throughout the body roughly in proportion to the distribution of cardiac output.[13] As an unbound potassium analog, ^{201}Tl redistributes over time. At equilibrium its distribution of ^{201}Tl is proportional to the regional potassium pool, reflecting the amount of viable myocardium. Thus, following intravenous injection and initial myocardial uptake, approximately half of the ^{201}Tl washes out of the normal myocardium over 5 to 8 h.[14] Differential washout rates between hypoperfused but viable myocardium and normal zones and washin to initially hypoperfused zones are the fundamental mechanisms of ^{201}Tl redistribution.

A factor governing the washout rate of ^{201}Tl is the concentration gradient between the myocardial cell and the blood. There is slower blood clearance of ^{201}Tl following resting or low-level exercise injection. Diffuse slow washout rates, mimicking diffuse ischemia, may be observed in normal patients who do not achieve adequate levels of stress. Hyperinsulinemic states slow redistribution, leading to an underestimation of viable myocardium; thus, fasting is recommended prior to and for 4 h following ^{201}Tl injection.[15]

An inverse relationship between the degree of coronary stenosis and subsequent redistribution of ^{201}Tl (i.e., late redistribution) has been reported.[16] Redistribution may occur early in areas with minor stenoses (where hyperemia postexercise would be expected), and late in regions with critical stenoses (in which poststress hyperemia is unlikely and resting hypoperfusion slows the delivery of thallium to the region).[17]

^{99m}Tc SESTAMIBI AND TETROFOSMIN

^{99m}Tc is produced from a molybdenum-99m generator, has a half-life of 6 h, and emits monoenergetic gamma rays at 140 kev. The whole-body radiation dose is estimated to be 16 mrad/mCi, in contrast to 240 mrad/mCi associated with ^{201}Tl. Owing to this more favorable dosimetry, larger doses of ^{99m}Tc myocardial perfusion imaging agents are used than with ^{201}Tl, usually in the range of 30 mCi. ^{99m}Tc sestamibi belongs to a class of compounds called *isonitriles* and is a complex organic compound that behaves physiologically as a monovalent cation. Following its extraction from the blood, ^{99m}Tc sestamibi is bound by mitochondria, and only a limited amount of myocardial washout (or washin) occurs over time.[18,19] As with ^{201}Tl, the initial uptake of ^{99m}Tc sestamibi is a function of myocardial perfusion to viable tissue. In general, ^{201}Tl has a higher myocardial uptake (as measured by the percent injected dose per gram of myocardium) throughout the range of flow, secondary to a higher extraction fraction than ^{99m}Tc sestamibi (approximately 85 percent compared with 65 percent).[20,21] At very low levels of flow, extraction of these tracers appears to increase, affecting ^{99m}Tc sestamibi more than ^{201}Tl.[22]

^{99m}Tc tetrofosmin is extracted by the myocardium and bound in mitochondria, like sestamibi. The extraction fraction of this agent is slightly lower than that of sestamibi.[23] There is less hepatic uptake with this tracer than with ^{99m}Tc sestamibi, resulting in more favorable heart/liver ratios early following resting injection.[24,25]

OTHER ^{99m}Tc MYOCARDIAL PERFUSION AGENTS

^{99m}Tc teboroxime belongs to another class of ^{99m}Tc myocardial perfusion agents, which are neutral lipophilic complexes of boronic acid called BATO compounds. ^{99m}Tc teboroxine appears to have a higher extraction fraction than ^{201}Tl. The high extraction fraction with this agent plateaus at a higher flow rate than any other agent.[26,27] These highly desirable extraction characteristics of teboroxime are counterbalanced by a rapid washout from the myocardium.[28] Thus, the kinetic properties of ^{99m}Tc teboroxime require that initial imaging be completed within the first few minutes after tracer injection in order to reflect blood-flow distribution at the time of injection. This limits its use to multiple-detector systems.[29] Due to the requirement for very rapid imaging, ^{99m}Tc teboroxime is the most technically demanding of the available myocardial perfusion tracers.

^{99m}Tc NOET is a neutral lipophilic myocardial perfusion imaging agent based on a Tc-nitrido core.[30] Although an extraction fraction as high as 76 percent with this tracer has been reported under hyperemic conditions,[31] there are other reports of much lower extraction than that associated with ^{201}Tl.[32] There appears to be redistribution over time of this tracer, related in part to the absence of intracellular binding and in part to higher circulating blood levels of radioactivity with this tracer as compared with ^{99m}Tc sestamibi.[31] ^{99m}Tc NOET overall may have kinetic and imaging properties very similar to those of ^{201}Tl, with the advantage of the higher photon flux associated with the higher injected dose that is possible with a ^{99m}Tc agent.[33] The redistribution of ^{99m}Tc NOET appears to be almost complete after 90 min of reflow, potentially shortening the clinical protocols applicable for assessment of myocardial viability with this tracer. A disadvantage of this tracer, like that of ^{201}Tl, is the lack of flexibility in the timing of postexercise imaging and the ability to repeat imaging.

^{99m}Tc furifosmin appears to be very similar to ^{99m}Tc tetrofosmin,[34,35] with an extraction fraction lower than that of ^{99m}Tc sestamibi. Neither ^{99m}Tc NOET nor ^{99m}Tc furifosmin have been approved for clinical use in the United States at this time.

Imaging Protocols and Image Interpretation

^{201}Tl PROTOCOLS

With ^{201}Tl, a variety of SPECT acquisition protocols are available (Fig. 16-2). When ^{201}Tl alone is employed as the radiopharmaceutical, the usual acquisition protocol uses some combination of stress with redistribution and/or reinjection imaging. The latter, as initially described, involved obtaining an additional image in patients with nonreversible ("fixed") perfusion defects following reinjection of one-half of the dose used at stress, with imaging performed immediately thereafter[36] (Fig. 16-2*A*). This protocol improves detection of viable myocardium over standard-stress 4-h redistribution imaging.[37] Since it requires three image acquisitions and a decision as to whether the reinjection is needed, a two-acquisition sequence with stress and redistribution/reinjection imaging is commonly performed. If no fixed defects are noted, with this approach further imaging is not required. If, on the other hand, following the 4-h reinjection/redistribution image, fixed defects are present, 24-h imaging results in a small but significant improvement in detection of viable myocardium[16,37] (Fig. 16-2*B*). An alternate protocol that appears to be gaining popularity is to give sublingual nitroglycerin prior to the reinjection of ^{201}Tl. With this approach, the frequency of further improvement at 24-h imaging may be substantially reduced; i.e., we consider it likely that a stress- and nitrate-augmented early reinjection protocol will reduce the benefit of, and thus the need for, 24-h imaging.[38] The other form of thallium imaging in frequent use is the rest/redistribution protocol, considered to be the most effective ^{201}Tl protocol for the assessment of viable myocardium[39,40] (Fig. 16-2*C*).

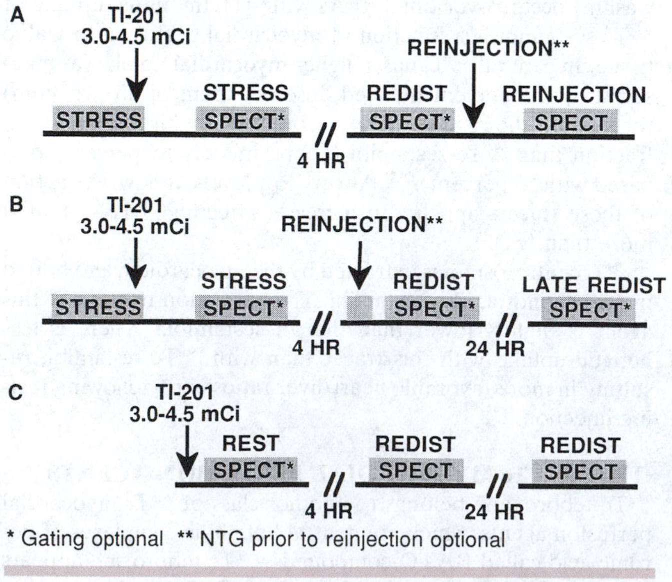

FIGURE 16-2 ^{201}Tl protocols. *A.* Stress/redistribution (redist), reinjection. *B.* Stress/reinjection/late redistribution. *C.* Rest/redistribution.

With a ^{201}Tl SPECT protocol, most investigators utilize all-purpose rather than high-resolution collimators,[41] although some prefer high-resolution collimators.[42,43] If high-resolution collimators are used, lengthening of the time of acquisition for ^{201}Tl SPECT should be considered—compared with ^{99m}Tc-based SPECT protocol—to provide adequate SPECT count statistics. This is particularly relevant for late redistribution imaging, because of the lower count rate due to radioactive decay. The timing of the initial poststress acquisition is particularly important with thallium, since excessive delay could result in decreased sensitivity for detection of coronary artery disease, owing to early redistribution of the radiopharmaceutical. However, SPECT acquisition of either the ^{201}Tl or the ^{99m}Tc myocardial perfusion agent should begin $\geq$10 min following exercise injection because of the frequent observation of an artifactual perfusion defect due to "upward creep of the heart."[44] This phenomenon is related to the increased depth of respiration very early postexercise, which is associated with an average lower position of the diaphragm in the chest compared with the normal ventilatory state. This causes the heart to gradually move cephalad during the early portion of SPECT acquisition, resulting in a form of motion artifact after reconstruction. By delaying acquisition until 10 to 15 min after exercise stress, this "upward creep" artifact is avoided. Although initially described with ^{99m}Tc sestamibi, gated SPECT can also be performed with ^{201}Tl, particularly with multidetector system. LVEF measurement with gated ^{201}Tl SPECT correlates highly with that of ^{99m}Tc sestamibi SPECT.[45]

^{99m}Tc SESTAMIBI OR TETROFOSMIN PROTOCOLS

Owing to the absence of clinically significant redistribution, separate rest and stress injections are standard with ^{99m}Tc sestamibi or tetrofosmin SPECT (Fig. 16-3).[46,47] A benefit of the absence of redistribution is that image acquisition can be repeated if imaging artifact is suspected. In this regard, imaging

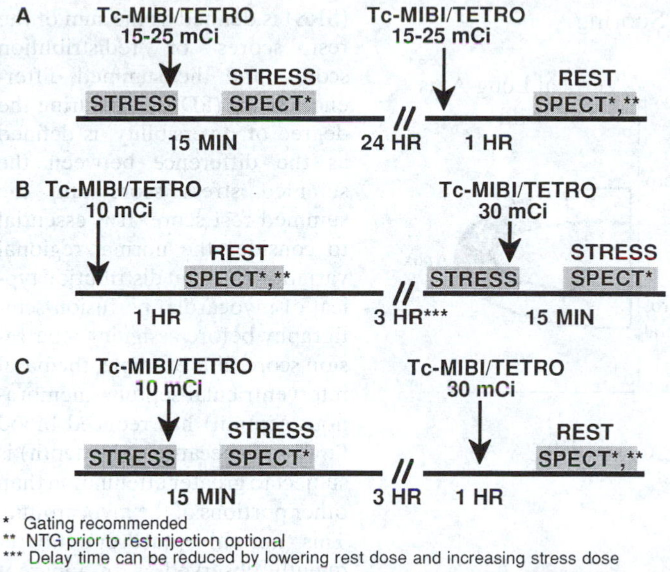

FIGURE 16-3 Two day (*A*), same-day rest-stress (*B*), and same-day stress-rest (*C*), ^{99m}Tc sestamibi or tetrofosmin protocols. Tc = ^{99m}Tc; MIBI = sestamibi; Tetro = tetrofosmin.

in the prone position, as well as in the supine position, increases the specificity of myocardial perfusion SPECT with ^{99m}Tc sestamibi or tetrofosmin.[47] A variety of protocols can be used with these agents, including 2-day stress/rest, same-day rest/stress, same-day stress/rest, and dual isotope. From the standpoint of defect contrast and optimal image quality, the 2-day stress/rest protocol is ideal (Fig. 16-3*A*). With the 2-day stress/rest protocol, both the stress and the rest study are obtained following the injection of high doses of ^{99m}Tc sestamibi or tetrofosmin, allowing the acquisition of high-quality, high-count images for the accurate assessment of perfusion and function. The principal drawback of this protocol is its requirement for two imaging days, resulting in a delay in the delivery of final information to be used in patient management. The same-day low-dose rest/high-dose stress protocol[48] (Fig. 16-3*B*) has the disadvantage of causing a reduction in stress defect contrast, as approximately 15 percent of the radioactivity observed at the time of stress imaging comes from the preexisting resting myocardial distribution. The same-day low-dose stress/high-dose rest sequence[49,50] (Fig. 16-3*C*), on the other hand, has the advantage of requiring image acquisition times essentially identical to those used for ^{201}Tl imaging, making it easy for a laboratory to alternate between the two protocols. The principal drawback of this approach is that less than ideal count rates are associated with the most important stress image set, and it is difficult to assess defect reversibility accurately.[51] With respect to the assessment of myocardial viability, all stress/rest or rest/stress ^{99m}Tc sestamibi or tetrofosmin imaging protocols have theoretical limitations in distinguishing severely hibernating myocardium from infarction. These constraints do not apply to ^{201}Tl because of its redistribution properties.[52,53] Viability assessment with ^{99m}Tc sestamibi or tetrofosmin may be improved by the administration of nitroglycerin prior to the rest-injection study.[54,55]

A common alternative to the standard ^{99m}Tc sestamibi or tetrofosmin protocols is a rest ^{201}Tl/stress ^{99m}Tc sestamibi dual-isotope SPECT (Fig. 16-4).[56] Dual isotope imaging takes advantage of the Anger camera's ability to collect data in different energy windows and can be performed with simultaneous or separate rest/stress acquisitions. The separate acquisition approach using rest ^{201}Tl/stress ^{99m}Tc sestamibi or tetrofosmin does not require correction for cross-contamination between the two radioisotopes,[56] whereas this correction is likely to be required with the simultaneous dual-isotope approach.[57] Of note, with this protocol, if defects are present on the rest ^{201}Tl study, redistribution ^{201}Tl SPECT can be performed before or 24 h after the ^{99m}Tc sestamibi or tetrofosmin injection.[58]

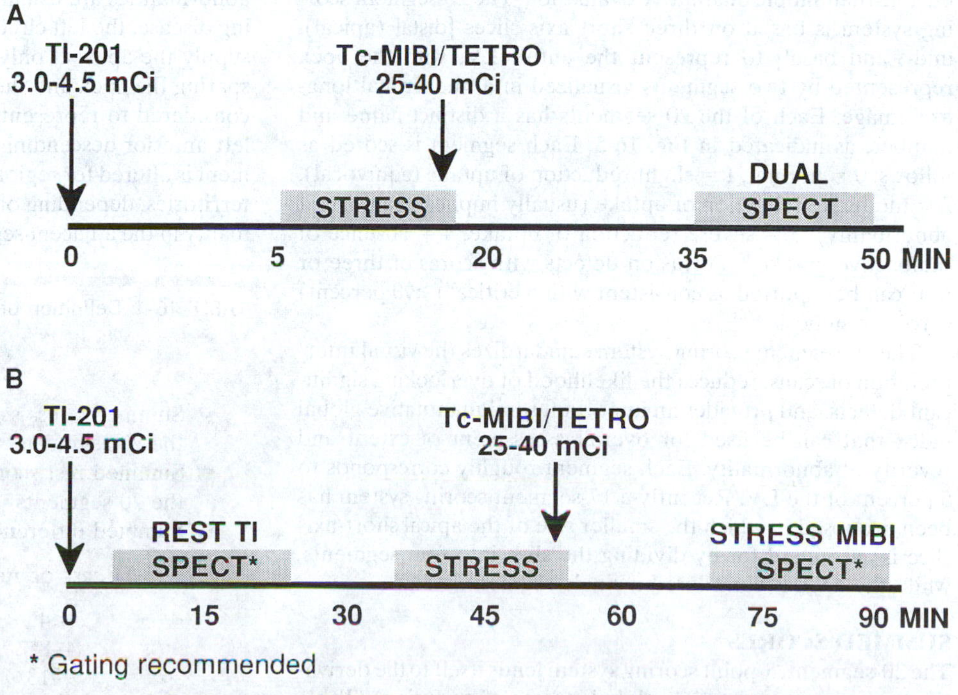

FIGURE 16-4 Simultaneous (*A*) and separate acquisition (*B*) dual-isotope rest ^{201}Tl/stress ^{99m}Tc sestamibi or tetrofosmin SPECT protocols.

ATTENUATION CORRECTION

Several camera manufacturers have recently provided hardware and software implementation of attenuation correction protocols, and these have undergone preliminary validation.[59,60] In general, these attenuation corrections are imperfect, reducing but not eliminating apparent perfusion defects due to soft tissue attenuation in normal patients. At times, true perfusion defects might be obscured or eliminated by the application of these

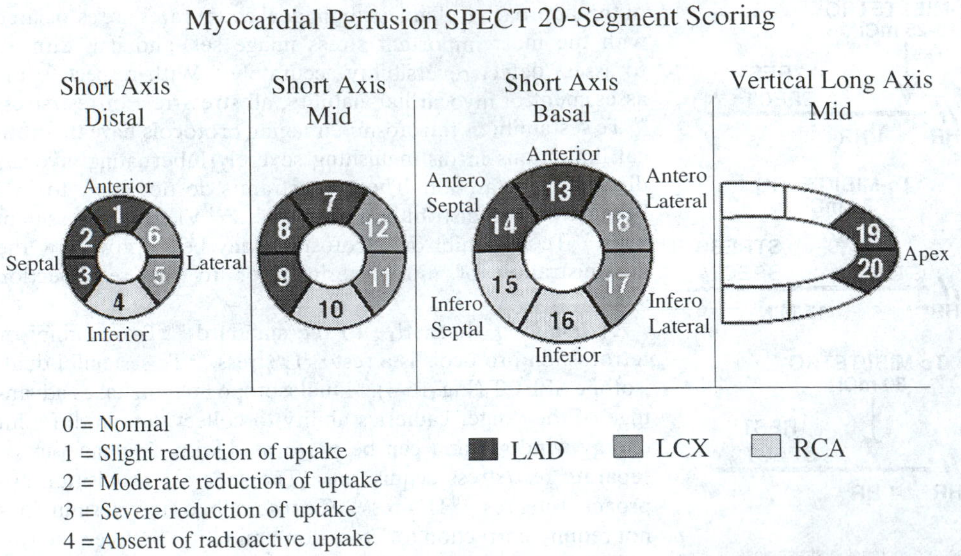

FIGURE 16-5 Diagrammatic representation of the segmental division of the SPECT slices and assignment of individual segments to individual coronary arteries using the 20-segment model. LAD = left anterior descending coronary artery; LCX = left circumflex coronary artery; RCA = right coronary artery.

approaches. The artifactual elimination of perfusion defects is usually due to filtering or to scatter from adjacent organs, which becomes more apparent after attenuation correction. It is prudent to visualize attenuation-corrected tomographic data sets simultaneously with noncorrected datasets.

20-SEGMENT VISUAL ANALYSIS

The use of a semiquantitative scoring system in which each of 20 segments is scored according to a 5-point scheme provides an approach to interpretation that is more systematic and reproducible than simple qualitative evaluation. The 20-segment scoring system is based on three short axis slices [distal (apical), mid-, and basal] to represent the entire LV, with the apex represented by two segments visualized in a midvertical long-axis image. Each of the 20 segments has a distinct name and number, as indicated in Fig. 16-5. Each segment is scored as follows: 0 = normal, 1 = slight reduction of uptake (equivocal), 2 = moderate reduction of uptake (usually implies a significant abnormality), 3 = severe reduction of uptake, 4 = absence of radioactive uptake.[61] Perfusion defects with scores of three or four can be reported as consistent with a critical (≥90 percent) coronary stenosis.[62,63]

The 20-segment scoring system standardizes the visual interpretation of scans, reduces the likelihood of overlooking significant defects, and provides an important semiquantitative global index that can be used for overall assessment of extent and severity of abnormality. Each segment roughly corresponds to 5 percent of the LV. Recently a 17-segment scoring system has been proposed in which the smaller size of the apical short-axis slice is accounted for by dividing the slice into four segments, while the apex is considered a single segment.[64]

SUMMED SCORES

The 20-segment, 5-point scoring system lends itself to the derivation of summed scores (i.e., global indices of perfusion) (Table 16-1).[65] The summed stress score (SSS) is defined as the sum of the stress scores for the 20 segments. The summed rest score (SRS) is defined as the sum of the rest scores or redistribution scores, and the summed differences score (SDS), measuring the degree of reversibility, is defined as the difference between the summed stress score and the summed rest score. It is essential to consider the normal regional variation of count distribution typical of myocardial perfusion scintigraphy before assigning a perfusion score. For example, the basal interventricular septum (membranous septum) has reduced blood flow, and (because of its depth) is subject to greater attenuation than other portions of the myocardium. This "normal septal dropout," frequently observed as an apparent defect on the basal septal slices, should be assigned a score of 0 rather than a score suggesting the presence of abnormality. Risk groups may be defined using the SSS,[66,67] where a score <4 is considered normal or nearly normal, scores of 4 to 8 are mildly abnormal, scores of 9 to 13 moderately abnormal, and summed stress scores >13 severely abnormal.

The 20 myocardial segments can be ascribed to individual coronary territories.[56,68] The inferior and basal septal segments are ascribed to the PDA (posterior descending artery), the lateral segments to the left circumflex coronary artery, and the mid- and distal septal as well as all anterior slices to the left anterior descending coronary artery. Although isolated apical abnormalities are usually associated with left anterior descending disease, the left circumflex or right coronary artery can also supply the apex. If only anterior wall segments are abnormal, sparing the apex and the septum, the abnormalities are usually considered to represent disease of the diagonal branch of the left anterior descending coronary artery. The coronary assignment is altered for regions at the border between specific vessels territories, depending on the pattern of perfusion defect abnormality in the adjacent segments. At times, a dominant perfusion

TABLE 16-1 Definition of Scintigraphic Indices

SUMMED SCORES

- Summed stress score (SSS):* Sum of stress scores of the 20 segments
- Summed rest score (SRS):* Sum of rest scores of the 20 segments
- Summed difference score (SDS):* SSS − SRS

DEGREE OF ABNORMALITY BY SSS CATEGORY

<4	Normal
4–8	Mildly abnormal
9–13	Moderately abnormal
>13	Severely abnormal

*Incorporates extent and severity of defects.

defect in a specific vascular territory will "tail" into a contiguous territory of another vessel. In these circumstances, the defect would generally be attributed to the vessel associated with the dominant defect. This pertains most commonly to the inferoseptal and inferolateral walls, but also to the anterolateral wall. Regarding the septum, if an inferoseptal defect is present (excluding the basal inferoseptal segment, which is generally a right coronary artery territory), the septal abnormalities would be assigned to the left anterior descending or right coronary artery, depending on which of these vessels had a perfusion defect. Similarly, if an inferolateral or anterolateral defect but not both were present in patients with adjacent defects in either the anterior or inferior wall, the lateral wall defect would be assigned to the vessel attributed to the neighboring defect. In general, isolated septal defects (without anterior wall or inferior wall involvement) are rare; isolated lateral wall defects (in the absence of anterior wall or inferior wall defects) would be attributed to the left circumflex coronary artery.[56]

GATED SPECT

Gated perfusion SPECT can be used to quantify a variety of global function parameters, including LVEF, end-diastolic volumes, and end-systolic volumes. Diastolic function assessment is generally not performed with gated SPECT, since it requires too large a number of gating intervals.[69] Regional parameters of function that can be quantitated from gated perfusion SPECT images include LV myocardial wall motion and thickening. Quantitation of gated perfusion SPECT images can be performed by employing algorithms adapted from other imaging modalities, including methods resembling equilibrium radionuclide angiography data processing[70,71] and biplane Simpson's rule analogs or by fully 3D algorithms. The most common algorithms are fully 3D and are based on the automatic detection of endocardial and epicardial surface points.[72–76]

In validation studies of gated perfusion SPECT LVEF published to date,[77] it is apparent that the agreement between gated SPECT and gold standard measurements of LVEF is generally very good to excellent. Indeed, it has been pointed out that 2D "gold standards" may be intrinsically less accurate than gated SPECT algorithms operating in the 3D space because of geometric assumptions required by the former.[72] The normal threshold for the global LVEF measured from gated SPECT images is slightly lower than that measured using other imaging modalities, or approximately 45 percent, due to an approximate 3–4 point underestimation of true LVEF associated with the use of only eight gating intervals.[77] Normal limits for eight-frame LVEF and LV volumes have been recently reported.[78–80] LVEFs can be slightly overestimated in analyzing gated SPECT images of small hearts.[81] Figure 16-6 illustrates an example of perfusion SPECT quantitative perfusion analysis (including the 20-segment scores) and quantitative gated SPECT from a patient with severe disease of the left anterior descending coronary artery.

ASSESSMENT OF MYOCARDIAL VIABILITY

The presence of myocardial viability is implied with the myocardial perfusion tracers if the degree of uptake at rest, redistribution, or following nitrate-augmented rest injection[82–86] is normal. If a region has severely reduced or absent uptake of radioactivity in these settings, it is considered to be nonviable. Areas with moderate reduction of counts in these conditions (score 2 at redistribution or nitrate-augmented rest) are usually partially viable, and patients in this group have a variable response in terms of postoperative improvement. Some have utilized a cutoff percentage of maximal counts in the myocardium for predicting viability in a region in question[87,88]; others use the number of standard deviations below normal. An example of rest-redistribution imaging of myocardial viability is illustrated in Fig. 16-7 for a patient with poor LVEF (<35 percent) evaluated for CABS.

OTHER ABNORMALITIES

In addition to perfusion defects, several nonperfusion abnormalities can be observed with myocardial perfusion SPECT including size of the LV, transient ischemic dilation (TID) of the LV,[89,90] RV myocardial uptake pattern, RV size, and abnormalities of lung uptake or other abnormal extracardiac activity.

Transient Ischemic Dilation of the Left Ventricle TID is considered present when the LV cavity appears to be significantly larger in the poststress images than at rest (Fig. 16-6)[89,90] and may actually be an apparent cavity dilation secondary to diffuse subendocardial ischemia (obscuring the endocardial border). This explains why TID may be seen for several hours following stress, when true cavity dilation is probably no longer present.[91] The correlation between TID of LV and lung uptake is weak, suggesting that there may be different pathophysiologic mechanisms for each; their measurements may be complementary in assessing the extent and severity of CAD for risk stratification.[92] TID was initially reported to be moderately sensitive and highly specific for critical stenosis (greater than 90 percent narrowing) in vessels supplying a large portion of the myocardium (i.e., proximal left anterior descending or multivessel 90 percent lesions).[89,90] Dipyridamole-induced TID has similar implications as those associated with exercise.[91] TID can easily be measured by slight modifications of the quantitative gated SPECT algorithms. The upper limits of normal for the TID ratio in dual-isotope imaging has been reported to be 1.22. Patients who have TID of the LV (TID > 1.22) are likely to have severe and extensive CAD (>90 percent stenosis of the proximal left anterior descending coronary artery, or of multiple vessels).[90]

Increased Lung Uptake of Radioactivity Increased lung uptake of ^{201}Tl was first described by Boucher et al., as noted on the anterior view of planar thallium images.[93] It is generally accepted that increased pulmonary uptake of thallium reflects increased pulmonary capillary wedge pressure. When noted at rest, it reflects increased pulmonary capillary wedge pressure at rest,[94] and when noted with stress (either exercise or pharmacologic), it indicates the presence of increased pulmonary capillary wedge pressure during stress.[95] Nonischemic causes of increased pulmonary capillary wedge pressure, such as mitral regurgitation, mitral stenosis, etc., are also associated with increased pulmonary thallium uptake. Increased thallium lung uptake after exercise has been shown to have incremental prognostic information over myocardial perfusion defect assessment.[96] Only a few studies have examined the implications of increased pulmonary uptake of ^{99m}Tc sestamibi, with differing results.[95,97–99] It is possible that the differences among these reports are largely explained by the frequent greater delay in imaging of ^{99m}Tc sestamibi following stress than is associated with imaging of ^{201}Tl. The impact of the starting time of poststress acquisition of ^{99m}Tc sestamibi studies on lung uptake

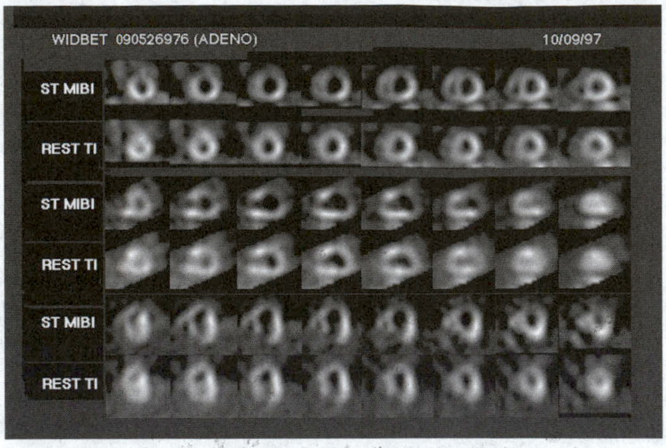

A

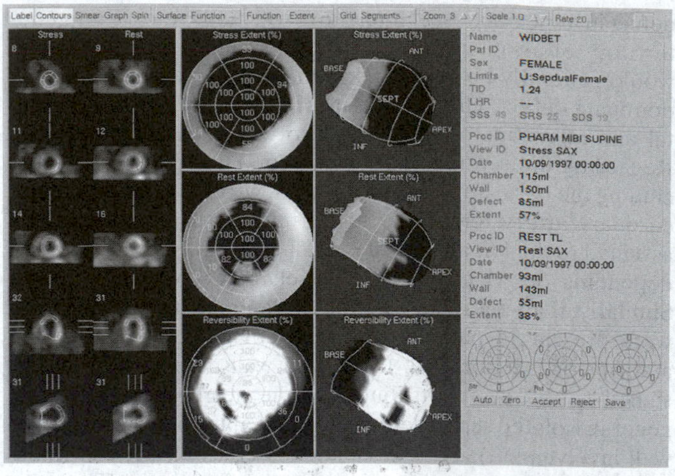

B

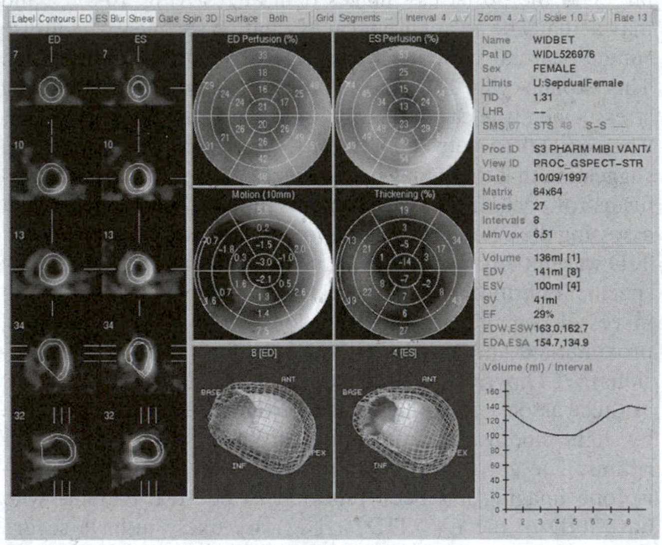

C

FIGURE 16-6 *A.* Adenosine stress ^{99m}Tc sestamibi/rest ^{201}Tl-myocardial perfusion SPECT images in an 83-year-old female with typical angina. There is evidence of a severe and extensive reversible defect throughout the LAD coronary artery and transient ischemia dilation of the left ventricle. Angiography revealed proximal 95 percent stenosis of LAD. *B.* Quantitative perfusion SPECT (QPS) analysis of the patient shown in Fig. 16-6*A*. The right panel illustrates the three-dimensional images viewed from the septal surface. The summed stress score is very high at 34 as is the perfusion defect extent (57 percent). There is quantitative transient ischemia dilation of the left ventricle (1.31). Due to the severe perfusion defect (as well as TID), the study is interpreted as indicating the presence of a critical (> than 90 percent) stenosis of the proximal LAD. *C.* Quantitative gated SPECT (QGS) analysis of the patient illustrated in Fig. 16-6*A* and *B*. The left ventricular fraction is severely reduced at 29 percent and left ventricular and diastolic volume is elevated at 141 mL.

has been confirmed by Hurwitz et al.,[98] who found a good correlation between lung-heart ratio and angiographic findings on immediate images (4 min after stress), whereas no such correlation was found on the late images. By delaying 1 to 2 h following stress, increased pulmonary uptake that would have been present initially might no longer be present at the time of imaging. The prognostic implications of increased exercise sestamibi lung uptake as well as the findings of increased uptake in pharmacologic stress with this tracer have not yet been explored.

EXERCISE PROTOCOLS

Exercise stress is the most commonly performed form of stress for myocardial perfusion SPECT. Exercise stress allows assessment of exercise capacity and symptoms as well as ST-segment response, providing additional clinical information that can be useful in daily clinical decision making (see Chap. 14). For exercise nuclear imaging, (1) an indwelling intravenous line for injection of the tracer at peak exercise is inserted, (2) injection of the tracer is performed at maximal stress, and (3) exercise is continued for an additional minute to allow optimal myocardial tracer concentration.

PHARMACOLOGIC STRESS PROTOCOLS

For patients who cannot achieve an adequate level of stress, pharmacologic stress testing is generally performed.[100–104] Generally, if the patient cannot perform ≥5 METs or more of exertional stress or fails to achieve ≥85 percent of maximal predicted heart rate a pharmacologic stress protocol should be encouraged. The preferred form of pharmacologic stress for myocardial perfusion SPECT is the use of coronary vasodilators—dipyridamole or adenosine, providing a three- to fivefold increase in coronary flow. Dipyridamole blocks the cellular reuptake of adenosine, increasing the extracellular adenosine concentration. Increased extracellular adenosine, either with adenosine infusion or dipyridamole, causes coronary vasodilation. The comparative effects of the vasodilators, exercise, and dobutamine are illustrated in Fig. 16-8. In general, the diagnostic accuracy of myocardial perfusion scintigraphy using pharmacologic stress is equivalent to that of exercise, despite the differences in flow rates.[100]

Importantly, methylxanthines, such as theophylline or caffeine, block adenosine binding and can eliminate the effects of dipyridamole or adenosine on coronary vasodilation. Since the half-life of caffeine is variable[105] with either dipyridamole or adenosine, it has been recommended that patients be off caffeine-containing compounds for 24 h prior to imaging. There is no currently available means of identifying patients in whom the pharmacologic effects of adenosine or dipyridamole have

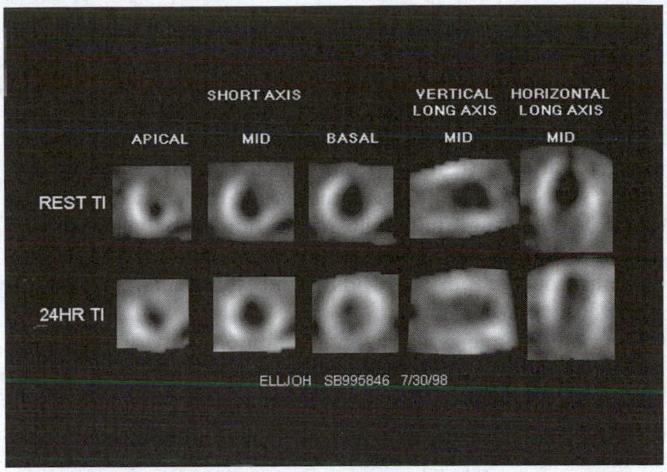

FIGURE 16-7 Rest and 24-h redistribution ^{201}Tl SPECT images showing large partially reversible defect in the anterior and anterolateral walls associated with LVEF at 24 percent. These findings are consistent with myocardial viability and predict functional improvement with revascularization.

been blocked by caffeine; in contrast to exercise, the heart rate or blood pressure does not provide accurate information regarding response.[106]

Dipyridamole is usually infused at 0.142 mg/kg/min for 4 min, although some investigators have recommended increasing the dose by 50 percent.[100,101] The maximal effect occurs approximately 3 to 4 min after termination of the infusion. Side effects are common and transient, including nonspecific chest pain, shortness of breath, dizziness, and flushing. Severe side effects are rare, being noted that in only 1 of 10,000 in the largest study to date.[102] The side effects can usually be reversed by intravenous administration of aminophylline, usually 75 to 125 mg, although additional administration of nitroglycerin may occasionally be needed. Due to the potential side effect of severe bronchospasm, dipyridamole is contraindicated for patients with asthma. Adenosine is infused intravenously, usually at a dose of 140 mg/kg/min over 6 min, with administration of the radiopharmaceutical at the midpoint of the infusion.[107] Minor and transient side effects occur more frequently with adenosine, than with

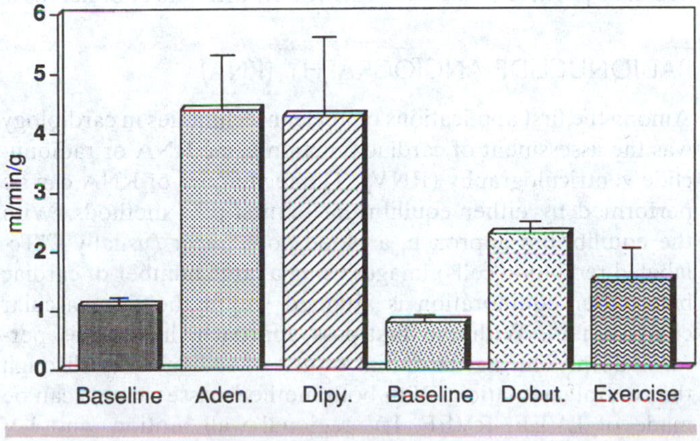

FIGURE 16-8 Coronary blood flow at baseline, exercise, dobutamine (Dobut.), adenosine (Aden.), and dipyridamole (Dipy.) stress measured with 13*N*-labeled ammonia. Baseline results are listed twice because of slight differences in absolute results. (Reproduced with permission from Iskandrian et al.[111])

dipyridamole.[107] With adenosine, there is an increased incidence of advanced atrioventricular (AV) block. As the half-life of adenosine is very short (several seconds), side effects usually remit quickly within termination of the infusion. Adenosine is considered contraindicated for patients with equal to or greater than first-degree AV block, sick sinus syndrome, or bronchospasm.

COMBINED PHARMACOLOGIC AND EXERCISE TESTING

It has become increasingly common to combine vasodilator stress with low-level exercise. This is generally accomplished by beginning exercise at the end of the dipyridamole infusion. With adenosine stress, exercise is initiated during the adenosine infusion.[108]

DOBUTAMINE STRESS

An alternative to vasodilator stress is inotropic stress, usually performed with dobutamine.[109,110] At the present time, dobutamine stress is usually reserved for patients with asthma or those who have recently ingested caffeine. Dobutamine stress is associated with a lower rate pressure product and a lower degree of hyperemia in the myocardial bed than with exercise[111,112] or vasodilator stress (Fig. 16-8). Side effects are more common than with the vasodilator stress, including, more commonly, premature ventricular contractions serious side effects are rare.[113] Thus, dobutamine is not considered the agent of first choice for myocardial perfusion scintigraphy. Arbutamine, another inotropic agent, is not currently available in the United States.[114,115]

LEFT BUNDLE-BRANCH BLOCK

Patients with LBBB may frequently demonstrate reversible defects in the interventricular septum in the absence of CAD.[116] The mechanism has been postulated to be a true septal ischemia that occurs in LBBB in the presence of marked tachycardia. This perfusion defect may indicate a decrease in flow resulting from an increase in early diastolic compressive resistance, in turn caused by delayed ventricular relaxation.[117] In view of this pathophysiology, stress techniques that do not increase heart rate as markedly as exercise are preferred in LBBB; i.e., adenosine or dipyridamole testing without walking is generally considered preferable in LBBB patients.[118,119]

Nonperfusion Myocardial SPECT

Radionuclide imaging has an inherent advantage over other cardiac imaging techniques for assessment of myocardial metabolic and biochemical processes. Two nonperfusion myocardial scintigraphic applications in common use in other countries are fatty-acid imaging and imaging of myocardial innervation. The most commonly used radionuclide for these purposes is iodine 123 (^{123}I). From a biochemical standpoint, ^{123}I is an excellent metabolic imaging tracer, since it is easily incorporated into a wide variety of compounds by a halogen exchange reaction in which the iodine replaces a methyl group. Unfortunately, none of the ^{123}I-labeled compounds is currently commercially available for routine use in the United States.

FATTY ACID IMAGING

A comprehensive review of this subject has recently been provided by Tamaki.[120] Two principal types of fatty acid compounds have been described for myocardial imaging. Straight-chain fatty acid imaging has been most commnly performed with ^{123}I iodophenyl pentadecanoic acid (IPPA). With this tracer, initial uptake allows assessment of myocardial perfusion at rest or exercise.[121] The washout of ^{123}I IPPA appears to be related to fatty-acid metabolism (primarily beta oxidation) and can provide information about myocardial ischemia and myocardial viability. In ischemic but viable myocardium, IPPA washout is slower than normal but faster than in infarcted tissue.[122] This intermediate range of IPPA washout has been shown to be predictive of improvement in LV function after revascularization. Iskandrian et al.[123] have suggested that defect reversibility was more commonly seen with IPPA SPECT than with rest/redistribution ^{201}Tl SPECT. Despite these promising features for assessment of myocardial perfusion and viability through sequential SPECT acquisitions, this radiopharmaceutical has not yet become commercially available in the United States.

The other major class of fatty-acid compounds for SPECT are modified branched-chain fatty acids. These agents provide superior imaging quality with the Anger scintillation camera, since the washout of the modified branched-chain fatty acid is slower than that of the straight-chain agents due to partial metabolic trapping in the myocardium. Betamethyl iodophenylpentadecanoic acid (BMIPP), first introduced by Knapp et al.,[124] has become widely used in Japan and Europe. This tracer appears to uncover an "ischemic memory" and may have unique capability for the assessment of previously severely ischemic myocardium. Discordant radiopharmaceutical uptake, with less BMIPP uptake than with ^{201}Tl, has been described in patients with unstable angina and those with acute myocardial infarction who were acutely revascularized.[125] This finding likely represents a persistent metabolic abnormality out of proportion to the perfusion abnormality at the time of injection. Furutani et al.[126] have suggested that this finding allows assessment of the amount of myocardium at risk in the subacute phase of the myocardial infarction (MI). For patients revascularized during acute MI, the size of the BMIPP defect 1 week after revascularization reflects the area of risk measured by ^{99m}Tc perfusion imaging before revascularization.[126a] In 50 consecutive patients with MI receiving BMIPP and thallium scans (average follow-up 23 months), discordant BMIPP uptake compared with ^{201}Tl was the best predictor of future cardiac events, followed by the number of coronary stenoses. In unstable angina, a decrease in BMIPP has been reported under resting conditions, even after chest pain has resolved.[127]

IMAGING OF MYOCARDIAL INNERVATION

Imaging of myocardial innervation is another application of the tracer technique to cardiac imaging recently reveiwed by Dae.[128] The sympathetic nerves of the myocardium take up exogenously administered catecholamines with high affinity.[129] An analog of a false nerve transmitter is meta-^{125}I-iodobenzylguanidine (MIBG). MIBG is taken up in myocardial sympathetic nerve endings in a manner similar to norepinephrine,[130] but it is not metabolized. In regionally denervated myocardium, MIBG uptake is decreased while perfusion is unchanged.[131] In the setting of ischemic heart disease, it is generally held that ischemia must be severe enough to cause myocardial necrosis before regional denervation (and subsequent decreased MIBG uptake) occurs.[132] In "syndrome X," abnormal cardiac MIBG uptake has been reported in 75 percent of patients, with the abnormality out of proportion to perfusion defects supporting the cardiac origin of chest pain in this syndrome.[133] Furthermore, in diabetic patients, assessment of myocardial MIBG uptake may be useful in defining autonomic dysfunction early in the course of type I disease.[134] Asymmetric uptake of MIBG has been shown for patients with ventricular tachycardia and no CAD.[135,136] Regional decreases of MIBG uptake in the basal left ventricle have also been demonstrated in a high proportion of patients with arrhythmogenic RV cardiomyopathy,[137] and abnormal MIBG uptake has been reported in idiopathic ventricular tachycardia and ventricular fibrillation.[138]

In nonischemic cardiomyopathy, abnormality of MIBG distribution and washout has been reported.[139] Generally, in congestive heart failure, excessive stimulation of the cardiac nervous system is believed to lead to further depression of cardiac function and may play a role in sudden death.[140] Recent studies have suggested that impaired cardiac sympathetic innervation in heart failure patients can be assessed by MIBG.[141] The late myocardial-to-mediastinal MIBG uptake 4 h after injection was shown to be the most powerful predictor of cardiac death, providing incremental information over clinical variables in a large clinical study. Furthermore, MIBG imaging may be useful in predicting the effectiveness of beta-blocker therapy for patients with dilated myocardial myopathies.[142,143] The pattern of a low heart-to-mediastinal ratio on 4-h delayed MIBG images appears to be predictive of a poor response to beta-blocker therapy.[128]

INFARCT-AVID IMAGING

Hot-spot (infarct-avid) imaging methods for detecting acute MI are among the oldest techniques in nuclear cardiology. These techniques have included ^{99m}Tc pyrophosphate myocardial scintigraphy,[144–148] indium 111 (^{111}In) antimyosin antibody scintigraphy,[149] and ^{99m}Tc glucarate imaging.[150] Although these methods have been documented to be sensitive and specific for the detection of myocardial necrosis, they are not widely utilized owing to the needed delay between injection and imaging. Antimyosin antibody, not available in the United States, is highly specific for myocardial necrosis and has been shown to be useful in the assessment of myocarditis[151] and the necrosis associated with cardiac transplant rejection.[151a] A new agent, ^{99m}Tc glucarate, a small molecule similar to glucose with rapid blood pool clearance, is taken up acutely in the necrotic myocardium[150,152] and becomes positive in the very early hours after onset of necrosis.

RADIONUCLIDE ANGIOGRAPHY (RNA)

Among the first applications of nuclear techniques in cardiology was the assessment of cardiac function using RNA or radionuclide ventriculography (RNV). The techniques of RNA can be performed by either equilibrium or first-pass methods. With the equilibrium approach, a blood-pool tracer (usually ^{99m}Tc-labeled red blood cells) images using a large number of cardiac beats after equilibration is attained within the intravascular compartment. With the first-pass approach, imaging is performed only during the initial transit of radioactivity through the central circulation. With both methods, assessments can be made of LVEF, RVEF, LV regional wall motion, and LV volumes.

The first-pass technique is a type of dynamic acquisition that uses rapid temporal sampling (20 to 100 frames per second) to look at the initial transit of a radionuclide bolus through the central circulation. This form of imaging is limited to the planar approach. The perfusion agents ^{99m}Tc sestamibi and ^{99m}Tc tetrofosmin can be used with success in first-pass studies.[153] Acquisition is completed in less than 1 min and can be performed in any desired view; in practice, however, these studies are usually limited to a single acquisition and are most commonly performed in either the anterior or right anterior oblique view.

Equilibrium RNA uses ECG-gated acquisitions, in which each frame corresponds to a specific portion (interval or gate) of the cardiac cycle, identified relative to the R wave on the patient's ECG. Because of the use of a multiple-gated acquisition, the term *MUGA scan* has also been applied to this technique. The cardiac cycle is divided in as many as 8 to 64 intervals and data from multiple cardiac cycles are averaged to ensure adequate count statistics. For equilibrium-gated RNA, the imaged radiopharmaceutical must stay within the vascular compartment during the imaging period. Although labeled proteins such as ^{99m}Tc albumin could be employed for blood pool imaging, labeled red blood cells are most commonly employed, labeled either through in vivo or in vitro methods. The latter provides the highest target-to-background ratio. Acquisition typically takes 5 to 10 min per view and multiple planar views are obtained. For exercise RNA, image acquisition can be as brief as 2 min.

Because of the ability to image the blood pool radiopharmaceuticals for a substantial time period, SPECT acquisition is also practical with equilibrium radionuclide angiography.[154,155] It has recently been shown that equilibrium blood pool SPECT acquisition and processing are essentially the same as for myocardial perfusion SPECT, and thus can be easily adopted in the laboratory where myocardial perfusion SPECT is being performed. Methods for automatically assessing LVEF from gated blood pool SPECT have been developed and validated.[156] Since the SPECT approach avoids the overlap of cardiac chambers inherent in planar imaging, it enhances assessment of regional function and may well become the method of choice for radionuclide angiography.

For exercise RNA, again either equilibrium or first-pass techniques can be employed. With the first-pass technique for exercise radionuclide angiography, a multicrystal camera has been most commonly used.[157] The advantage of first-pass over equilibrium RNA is that ventricular function assessments at the true peak of exercise can be obtained, since the procedure is accomplished in less than 30 s. For this purpose, patients can use either bicycle[157] or treadmill[158,159] exercise. At the peak of exercise, the patient's chest is placed against the surface of the scintillation camera and a bolus injection is made, usually with 15 to 30 mCi of ^{99m}Tc radiopharmaceutical; most commonly, a 40-frames-per-second acquisition is used for the 30 s. Subsequently LVEF is computed, most commonly in a semiautomatic fashion using a count-based technique applied to motion-corrected, background-corrected scintigraphic data. LVEF is computed from the portion of the first pass of radionuclide through the central circulation that corresponds to the left ventricular filling and emptying phase. In a similar fashion, the first-pass scintigraphic data can be used to evaluate RVEF by processing the data acquired during the RV phase of the first pass.

For the equilibrium RNA, EFs of the LV[160–162] or RV[163] can be measured. The preferred method for measurement of EF from equilibrium RNA is referred to as the "area-counts" technique. This method takes advantage of the proportionality between the volume of a cardiac chamber and the number of counts emitted from that chamber following injection of a blood-pool radiopharmaceutical. Thus, a background-corrected curve of ventricular activity versus time is a curve of relative volume versus time of the corresponding ventricle. From this curve, EF can be measured as a function of the peak (relative end-diastolic) and the nadir (relative end-systolic) volume by the formula EDC − ESC/EDC, where EDC and ESC represent background-corrected counts in the end-diastolic and end-systolic frames, respectively. It is generally accepted that for most accurate measurement of LVEF, 16 frames or more per cardiac cycle are required. For measurement of RVEF, it has been demonstrated that carefully placed regions of interest over the RV at end-diastole and end-systole, using a left periventricular background region of interest, provide an effective method for assessment of RVEF. Very high degrees of correlation have been reported between LVEF and contrast ventriculography. Good correlation has been demonstrated between RVEF measurements using equilibrium RNA and RV first pass measurements.[163] RNA is considered one of the "gold standards" for assessing LVEF on the basis of its accuracy and reproducibility.[164,165]

CLINICAL APPLICATIONS OF NUCLEAR CARDIOLOGY

The principles of diagnostic and prognostic accuracy outlined below are followed by a review of the evidence for the most common indications for nuclear cardiology procedures in the outpatient and inpatient cardiology settings.

Selecting the Appropriate Test Candidates

BAYESIAN THEORY: INTEGRATION OF PRETEST PROBABILITY ASSESSMENT INTO TEST INTERPRETATION

The central premise underlying patient selection for nuclear imaging is the ability to determine clinically an individual patient's likelihood of CAD or risk of important cardiac outcomes. The accurate evaluation of pretest clinical risk allows for the appropriate selection of patients who would most likely benefit from referral to nuclear imaging. The clinical pretest risk assessment may be estimated using published nomograms or from available computerized programs (see Chaps. 14, 38, and 40). Integrated predictive models based on clinical history and physical examination parameters have been developed from large patient registries and are published in the form of a nomogram for estimating the likelihood of CAD as well as cardiac survival. A review of models indicating the likelihood of clinical disease, aimed for use in varying populations, is presented in Chap. 38. For patient populations, several models have been developed with a large proportion of symptomatic patients designed to predict significant and extensive CAD as well as cardiac survival.[166–171] One of these approaches uses a validated computer algorithm to determine CAD likelihood based on age, sex, symptom classification, and conventional cardiac risk factors (resting systolic blood pressure, smoking history, glucose intolerance, resting ECG ST-segment abnormalities, and family history of early CAD).[171]

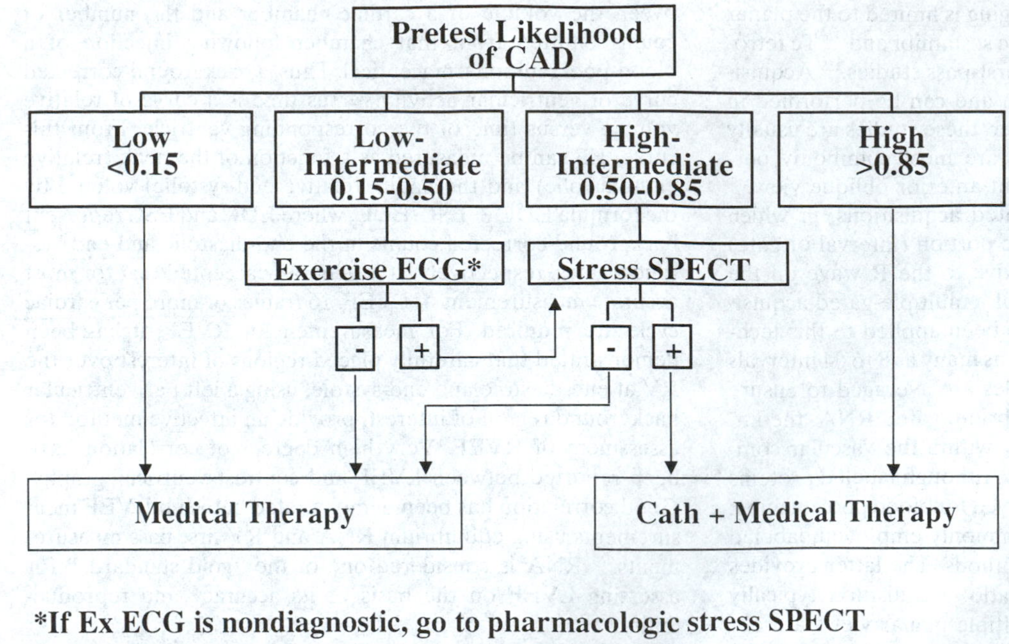

FIGURE 16-9 Role of nuclear testing in coronary artery disease diagnosis.

The rationale for selection of patients for noninvasive diagnostic and prognostic testing is based upon Bayesian theory (Chaps. 14 and 40), by which the posttest probability is a function of the patient's pretest clinical risk and the sensitivity and specificity of the test. The ability to shift posttest probabilities is directly related to pretest probability of disease or event risk. The greatest shift in posttest probabilities of disease occurs in those patients with an intermediate pretest probability of CAD.

Diagnostic Accuracy

Detection of CAD is one of the most common indications for performing myocardial perfusion SPECT. This referral is most appropriate in patients who are at intermediate risk of CAD, often including those with an abnormal rest electrocardiogram (ECG) where interpretation of exertional ST-segment changes is problematic.

A clinical algorithm for the purpose of simple detection of CAD based on these concepts, including the known sensitivity and specificity of treadmill ECG testing, is illustrated in Fig. 16-9.[172] Patients with a low probability (<0.15) of having angiographically significant (>50 percent stenosis) CAD can be identified even before standard exercise tolerance test (ETT) is performed. Patients with a low pre-ETT likelihood of CAD do not require further diagnostic testing, although continued medical follow-up or a "watchful waiting" approach is recommended. Patients with a low-intermediate pre-ETT likelihood of CAD (0.15 to 0.50) would undergo standard ETT as the next diagnostic step. Those who continue to have an intermediate likelihood of CAD after ETT (or those with an indeterminate ETT, as with LBBB, LVH, perfusion, ejection, etc.) and those whose pre-ETT likelihood of CAD is in the 0.50 to 0.85 range (in these patients even a negative ETT would not result in a low likelihood of CAD) will benefit from stress nuclear testing. Patients with a high pre-ETT likelihood of CAD (>0.85) are generally considered to have an established diagnosis of CAD and would not need nuclear stress testing for diagnostic purposes. A variation of this approach was recently published in the "ACC/AHA/ACP-ASIM Guidelines for Management of Patients with Chronic Stable Angina."[8] The application of nuclear testing for diagnosis and the intermediate likelihood of CAD has been given a class I indication (condition for which there is general agreement that a given procedure is useful and effective).[8]

Table 16-2 presents uncorrected sensitivities and specificities of myocardial perfusion SPECT for the detection of angiographically significant (≥50 to 70 percent stenosis) CAD. From the ACC/AHA/ACP-ASIM stable angina guidelines (Chaps. 14 and 40), in populations referred to nuclear SPECT (i.e., a large proportion with uninterpretable ST segments), there is an improved predictive accuracy—defined as [(true positives + true negatives)/total]—by nuclear testing over pretest information and ECG stress testing.[8,173] Despite the differences in the extraction characteristics of the various nuclear tracers, there have been few reports that reveal marked differences in test sensitivity. Owing principally to a reduction in soft tissue artifact, there is an increase in test specificity with ^{99m}Tc-based agents as compared with ^{201}Tl imaging in women.[174] SPECT acquisition can be repeated with ^{99m}Tc-based agents when either attenuation or motion artifact is suspected further increasing specificity. A major limitation to the use of test statistics such as sensitivity and specificity for CAD is that they require referral to cardiac catheterization for calculation. In estimating the true sensitivity and specificity of noninvasive testing, referral or workup bias must be taken into account.[47,175] Sensitivity is the proportion of patients with disease who are correctly detected as abnormal by the test, and specificity is the proportion of patients

TABLE 16-2 Sensitivity and Specificity of Stress Myocardial Perfusion SPECT for Detecting CAD (≥50% stenosis), Without Correction for Referral Bias Results from the ACC/AHA/ACP/ASIM Guidelines for Chronic Stable Angina*

	Publication Years	No. of Studies	Sensitivity†	Specificity†
Exercise SPECT	1984–1997	16	0.88	0.72
Adenosine SPECT	1991–1997	9	0.89	0.81

*From Ref. 8.
†Average of reported sensitivities and specificities.

without disease who are correctly detected as normal by the test. As routine patient workup results in preferential catheterization of patients with abnormal test results, the resulting observed test sensitivity is enhanced and the specificity is decreased. In general, referral bias leads to an overestimation in test sensitivity and a lowering in test specificity.[176] Once the test becomes used as a "gatekeeper" to catheterization, sensitivity and specificity can no longer be accurately measured. Thus, due to referral bias, test specificity becomes a poor measure of the ability of a test to exclude disease.

The normalcy rate has been advocated as an improved measure for this purpose.[47] This has been defined as the percentage of patients with normal test results in a population with a low likelihood of disease. A synthesis of data on nuclear SPECT normalcy rates has been reported to be in the range of 80 to 90 percent with ^{201}Tl testing and generally greater than 90 percent with ^{99m}Tc sestamibi SPECT; it would be expected to be similar to the latter for ^{99m}Tc tetrofosmin SPECT (Table 16-3).

Principles of the Use of Nuclear Cardiology for Risk Stratification/Patient Management

The most rapidly growing area of application of myocardial perfusion SPECT is risk stratification based on increased acceptance of a new paradigm in patient management. A risk-based approach to patients with suspected CAD appears better suited to the modern environment of cost containment and dramatic improvements in medical therapy than the approach focusing on simple diagnosis, in which the patient with suspected disease undergoes coronary angiography and then is frequently revascularized. With the risk-based approach, the focus is not on predicting who has CAD but on identifying and separating patients at risk for cardiac death, patients at risk for nonfatal myocardial infarction, and patients at low risk for either event.

The basic concept in the use of nuclear tests for risk stratification is that they are best applied to patients with an intermediate risk of a subsequent cardiac event, analogous to the optimal diagnostic application of nuclear testing of patients with an intermediate likelihood of having CAD. For prognostic testing, patients known to be at high or low risk for event would not be appropriate patients for cost-effective risk stratification with nuclear imaging since they are already stratified in the era of cost containment, the intensity of management and the effectiveness of therapy is tailored to patient risk. For low-risk patients, minimal further diagnostic testing results in the avoidance of excessive downstream costs. In contrast, high-risk patients are appropriately aggressively managed and usually undergo coronary angiography with consideration of revascularization. In chronic CAD, it has been suggested that a greater than 3 percent per year mortality rate can be used to identify patients with minimal symptoms whose mortality rate can be improved by coronary artery bypass grafting.[7] For purposes of risk assessment, it has been proposed that low risk be defined as a less than 1 percent cardiac mortality rate per year. Thus, intermediate-risk could be defined by patients in whom the cardiac mortality is in the range of 1 to 3 percent per year.[8] Since the mortality risk for patients undergoing either coronary artery bypass grafting or angioplasty is greater than 1 percent per year,[177] mildly symptomatic patients with a less than 1 percent mortality rate would not be candidates for revascularization to improve survival and would be appropriately classified by this rate as at a low risk of death. Note that while, for diagnostic testing, nuclear imaging would be most appropriate in patients with an intermediate likelihood of CAD, for risk stratification this appropriateness extends to the groups of patients with a high likelihood of CAD.

PHYSIOLOGIC BASIS FOR RISK ASSESSMENT IN MYOCARDIAL PERFUSION SPECT

The basis for the power of nuclear testing for risk stratification is found in the fact that the major determinants of prognosis in CAD can be assessed by measurements of stress-induced perfusion or function. These measurements include the amount of infarcted myocardium, the amount of jeopardized myocardium (supplied by vessels with hemodynamically significant stenosis), and the degree of jeopardy (severity of the individual

TABLE 16-3 Normalcy Rate of Stress SPECT in Patients with a Low Likelihood of CAD (<5 to 10%)

Year	Author	Reference	Stress	Isotope	Normalcy Rate	%
1989	Maddahi	(176A)	exercise	Tl	24/28	86
1989	Iskandrian	(176B)	exercise	Tl	123/131	94
1990	Kiat	(176C)	exercise	MIBI	7/8	88
1990	Van Train	(176D)	exercise	Tl	62/76	82
1992	Kiat	(176E)	exercise	Tl	49/55	89
1993	Berman	(56)	exercise	Tl/MIBI	102/107	95
1994	Heo	(176F)	exercise or adenosine	Tl/MIBI	33/34	97
1994	Van Train	(176G)	exercise	MIBI	30/37	81
1995	Zaret	(176H)	exercise	Tetrofosmin	56/58	97
1995	Kiat	(176I)	arbutamine	Tl	52/58	90
1996	Hendel	(35)	exercise	Furifosmin	39/39	100
1996	Amanullah	(176J)	adenosine	MIBI	66/71	93
1997	Heo	(176K)	exercise	MIBI	58/61	95
Total					701/763	92

ABBREVIATIONS: CAD = coronary artery disease; MIBI = ^{99m}Tc-sestamibi; Tl = Tl-201; tetrofosmin = ^{99m}Tc-tetrofosmin; furifosmin = ^{99m}Tc-furifosmin.

coronary artery stenosis). An additional important factor in prognostic assessment is the stability (or instability) of the CAD process. This last consideration may help to interpret what appears to be a paradox: nuclear tests, which in general are expected to be positive only in the presence of hemodynamically significant stenosis, are associated with a very low risk of either cardiac death of nonfatal MI when normal; in contrast, it has been observed that most MIs occur in regions with pre-MI lesions causing less than 50 percent stenosis.[178,179] It has been postulated that this paradox may be explained by the different response to stress of mild stenoses associated with stable and unstable plaque. Thus, beyond the ability to define anatomic stenosis, nuclear tests (by virtue of their physiologic assessments) may be able to discern abnormalities of endothelial function associated with high risk, even in the absence of significant stenosis.

To maximally extract the information regarding these prognostic determinants in CAD, it is necessary to consider the full extent and severity of abnormality, either quantitatively[180,181] or semiquantitatively,[56] rather than simply determining that the nuclear study is normal or abnormal. Furthermore, there appears to be incremental value in measuring both perfusion and function for the purposes of risk stratification, thus leading to increased prognostic utility of gated cardiac SPECT over standard myocardial perfusion SPECT.

ASSESSMENT OF STABLE OUTPATIENT POPULATIONS

Suspected Chronic Coronary Artery Disease

The most frequent reason for referral to the nuclear laboratory is the evaluation of known or suspected CAD. In outpatient populations, this often includes the evaluation of the presence and extent of cardiac ischemia. Stress nuclear imaging is an integral part of the evaluation of symptomatic patients for CAD. An imaging modality is commonly used in intermediate-risk patients or those with resting ECG abnormalities that preclude evaluation with the routine treadmill test. In this patient population, nuclear imaging most commonly includes myocardial perfusion SPECT performed to evaluate stress-induced defects and, more recently, gated SPECT to also allow assessment of ventricular function. If the ECG could not be interpreted for purposes of stress testing (e.g., LBBB, LV hypertrophy, digoxin therapy, Wolff-Parkinson-White syndrome), direct nuclear testing is highly effective in prognostic stratification (Chap. 14).

A synthesis of available data reveals that a normal scan is uniformly associated with a <1% annual risk of cardiac death or MI.[8,67,182,183,183a] Abnormal scans are associated with an increased risk of cardiac events.[8,67,182] Characteristics of low-, intermediate-, and high-risk scans are listed in Table 40-4.

Normal Perfusion Scan

The event rate associated with a normal or low-risk perfusion scan has been shown by numerous investigators to be <1 percent per year of follow-up and to be isotope-independent—similar to the data from exercise and pharmacologic stress SPECT.[65–67,182] A recent meta-analysis of the prognostic value of a normal stress perfusion scan reveals that the annual risk of MI or cardiac death after a normal perfusion scan is 0.7 percent (95 percent CI 0.5 to 0.9 percent).[183] This uniformly low event rate is critical when applying nuclear test information to risk stratification. In the absence of limiting symptoms in patients who are at low risk of major cardiac events with normal perfusion scans, a conservative approach to posttest patient management would be appropriate. This conservative approach includes medical follow-up for signs of clinical worsening and treatment of cardiac risk factors and related cardiac symptoms (see Chap. 40).

Mild-Risk Perfusion Scans

Multiple randomized trials have demonstrated that revascularization can reduce the risk of cardiac death in selected high-risk subsets. However, since the annual mortality rate of patients undergoing revascularization is at least 1 percent,[177] patients predicted to have a rate of cardiac death of less than 1 percent per year do not warrant revascularization for purposes of improving survival. Recently, Hachamovitch et al. analyzed 5183 patients undergoing stress perfusion SPECT testing.[67] A total of 158 nonfatal MIs and 119 cardiac deaths were observed during follow-up of 646 ± 226 days. The nonfatal MI and cardiac death rates as a function of the summed stress perfusion scores are illustrated in Fig. 16-10. Patients with moderately and severely abnormal scans were at intermediate risk for both cardiac death and MI. Importantly, however, patients with mildly abnormal summed stress scores were at intermediate risk for MI (2.7 percent risk of MI per year of follow-up), but at low risk for subsequent mortality (0.8 percent annual cardiac death rate). Based on the results of this study, patients with a mildly abnormal scan (summed stress score between 4 and 8) could be considered as having "flow-limiting" CAD and intermediate risk of MI but to be at low risk of cardiac death. These patients would be candidates for aggressive risk-factor modification using secondary prevention guidelines. Medical therapy known to reduce a patient's risk of acute ischemic syndromes or cardiac

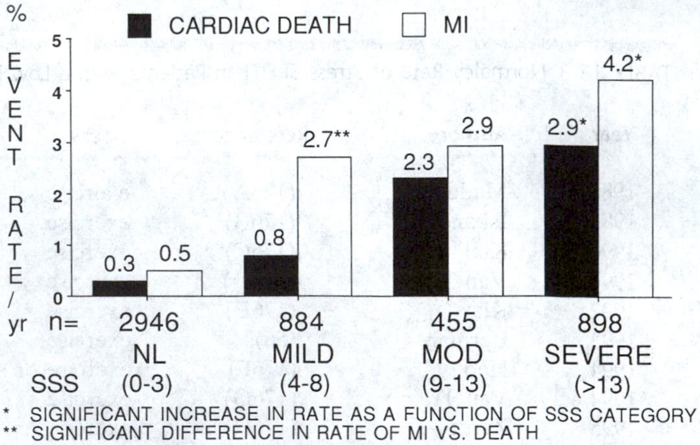

FIGURE 16-10 Rates of cardiac death (*solid bars*) and myocardial infarction (*open bars*) per year as a function of scan result. The numbers of patients within each scan category are shown underneath each pair of columns. *Statistically significant increase as a function of scan result. **Statistically significant increase in rate of MI versus cardiac death with scan category. NL = normal, MILD = mildly abnormal, MOD = moderately abnormal, SEVERE = severely abnormal. (Reproduced with permission from Hachamovitch et al.[67])

hospitalizations [e.g., statins, acetylsalicylic acid, angiotensin converting enzyme (ACE) inhibitors, etc.] would then be indicated.[184–193]

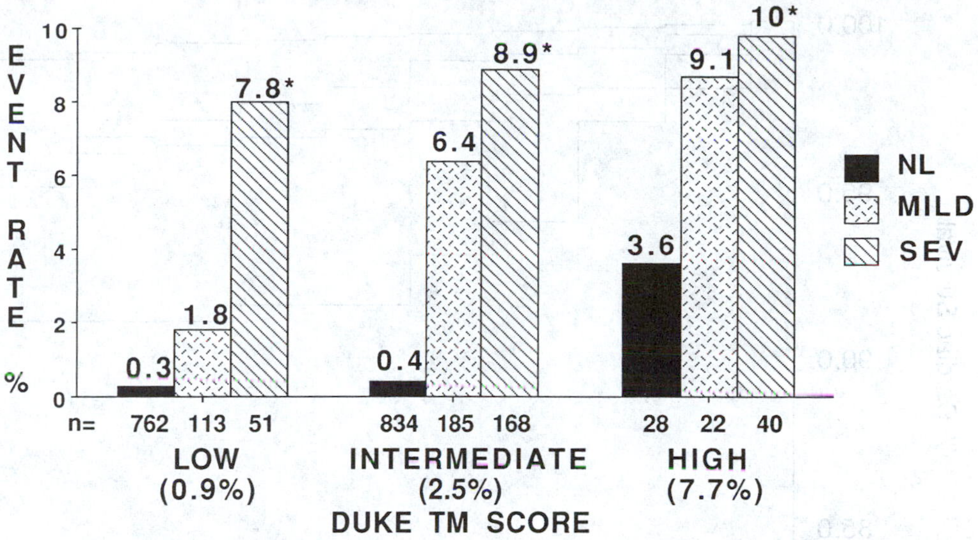

FIGURE 16-11 Duke treadmill (TM) score category and nuclear scan result versus hard event rate. Rates of hard (myocardial infarction or cardiac death) events over the follow-up period in patients in low, intermediate, and high Duke treadmill score categories with normal (NL), mildly abnormal (MILD), and severely abnormal (SEV) nuclear scans. Parentheses under Duke treadmill subgroups show hard event rates in these groups. *$p < 0.05$ across scan results. (Adapted and reproduced with permission from Hachamovitch et al.[66])

Moderately to Severely Abnormal Perfusion Scans

The relationship of varying extent and severity of perfusion abnormalities with cardiac outcomes has been reported in a variety of patient subsets.[66,67] Although both reversible and fixed stress perfusion defects are predictors of prognosis, those at highest risk of cardiac events include patients with extensive multizone abnormalities. Prognosis is also dependent on both the severity of perfusion defects (a correlate of the magnitude of stenosis) and their extent (a correlate of the amount of myocardium supplied by vessels with significant disease).[67] The combination of both of these factors is predictive of cardiac event rates. That is, as the severity and extent of defects worsens, there is an increase in the rate of major cardiac outcomes (Fig. 16-9). Annual cardiac event rates have been reported to range from 0.3 to 4.2 percent for patients with a normal, mild, moderate, and severely abnormal perfusion scans.[67]

Evidence Supporting Nuclear Imaging for Patients with an Intermediate/Indeterminate Treadmill Test

Several recent reports support nuclear testing in patients with uninterpretable or intermediate exercise ECG response.[66,195] An initial report from Cedars-Sinai (Fig. 16-11) demonstrated that myocardial perfusion SPECT was most effective in risk stratification and governing management of patients with intermediate treadmill test result (i.e., Duke treadmill score, a composite score integrating ST-segment changes, chest pain, and exercise time).[66] Patients with a low Duke treadmill score had a hard event rate of less than 1 percent, perhaps not needing nuclear testing.[194] Those with a high Duke treadmill score (representing less than 5 percent of the population) overall had a high event rate of 7.7 percent over the 18-month follow-up, and could have been directly catheterized. The majority of the patients in the study, however, fell into the category of an intermediate Duke treadmill score with an intermediate event rate of 2.5 percent. Within this category, those patients with a normal scan had a very low event rate and were infrequently catheterized; those with moderately abnormal scans had intermediate event rates and an intermediate rate of catheterization; and those with moderately to severely abnormal scans had higher event rates with higher rates of catheterization. Thus, the nuclear tests were able to stratify patients who could not be differentiated according to risk by Duke treadmill score alone. Similar results were shown by Shaw et al. in a large multicenter publication reporting event rates in 2498 patients with intermediate Duke treadmill scores undergoing stress myocardial perfusion SPECT (Fig. 16-12).[195]

Guidelines for Management of Patients with Stable Chest Pain by SPECT Results

Thus, patients with mildly abnormal scans (summed stress score between 4 and 8) could be considered as having CAD and intermediate risk of MI, but low risk of cardiac death[67] (Fig. 16-13). In the absence of refractory symptoms, these patients would be candidates for aggressive risk-factor modification without catheterization, using secondary prevention guidelines. Unlike the case with revascularization, a variety of medical therapies have been shown by randomized trials to reduce the risk of MI.[184–193] For patients with very abnormal summed stress scores, early revascularization resulted in a favorable survival benefit when compared with medical therapy from a recent observational assessment.[67] O'Keefe et al. reported similar results with medical versus invasive strategy.[196] As noted below, these recommendations for guiding patient management may now be further influenced by combining perfusion and poststress ventricular function variables from gated SPECT (LVEF and systolic volume). It is noteworthy that the above-described application of nuclear testing for risk stratification and prognosis in patients with an intermediate or high probability of CAD has been given class I recommendations in the ACC/AHA/ACP-ASIM guidelines.[8]

It appears that for patients who are appropriately referred to testing in the first place (patients with intermediate to high likelihood of CAD), a normal scan result is associated with a very low risk for approximately 2 years. After that time the risk rises, suggesting that repeat testing after 2 years should be considered in most patients for prognostic purposes.[197]

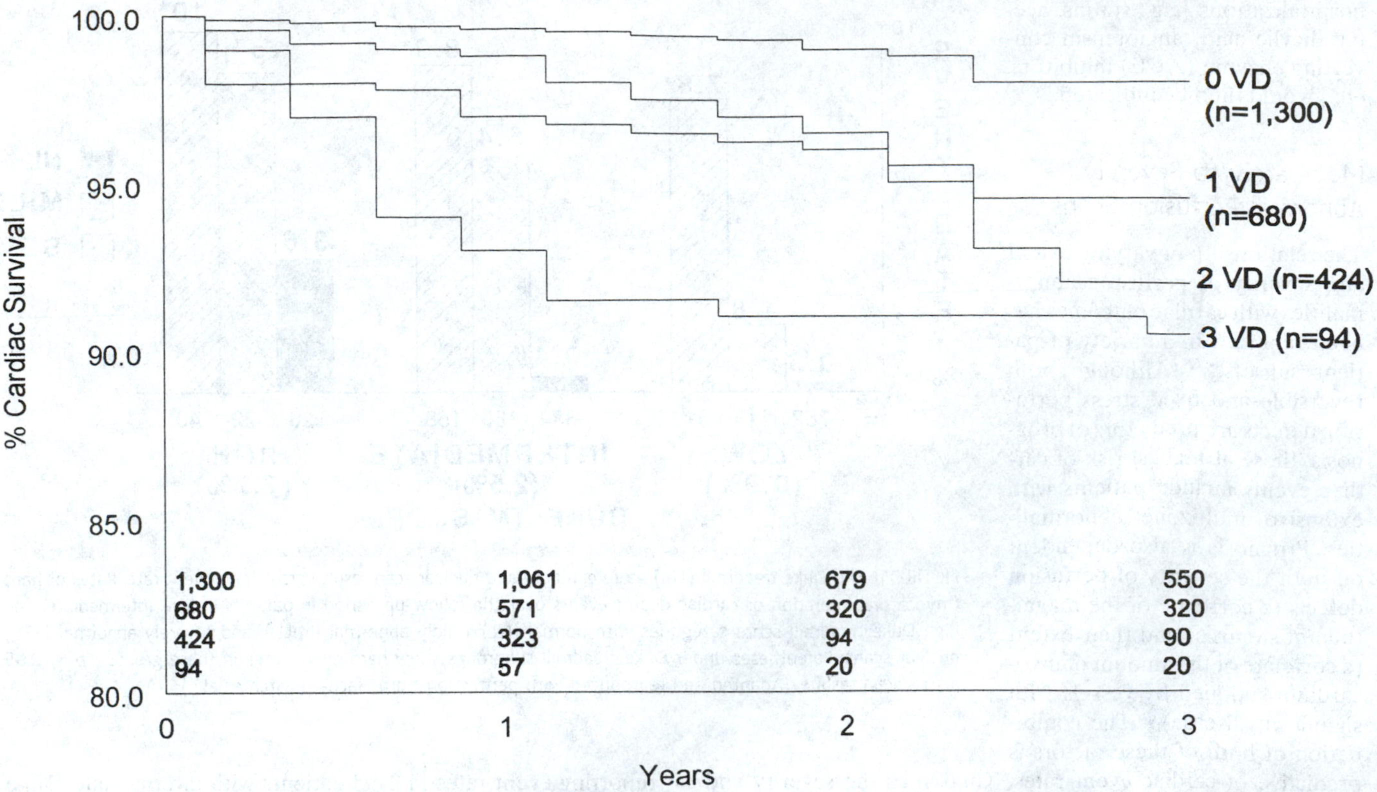

FIGURE 16-12 Kaplan-Meier survival curves by number of ischemic vascular territories on myocardial perfusion SPECT in 2498 patients with intermediate Duke treadmill likelihood score. Overall 3-year survival was 98, 95, 92, and 90 percent for patients with no, one, two, and three vascular territories with ischemia, respectively ($p < 0.001$). (Adapted with permission from Shaw et al.[194])

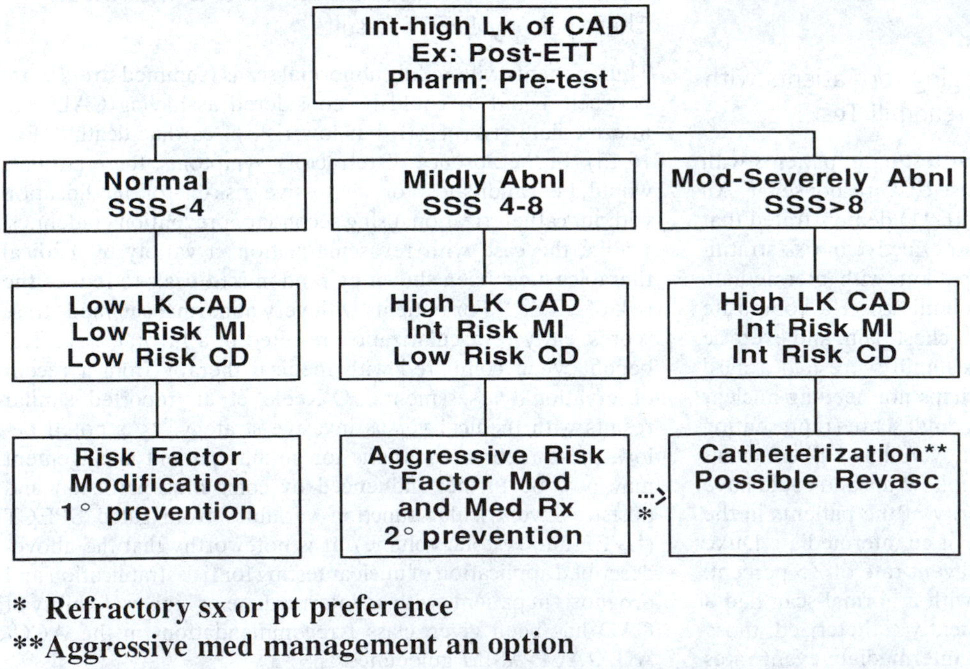

FIGURE 16-13 Strategy for management of coronary artery disease based on the results of myocardial perfusion SPECT (developed from Hachamovitch et al.[67]). INT–high LK of CAD = intermediate to high likelihood of coronary artery disease (≥0.15). For exercise, this represented the postexercise tolerance test (ETT) likelihood; for pharmacologic stress, the pretest likelihood; SSS = summed stress score; MI = myocardial infarction; CD = cardiac death; MOD = moderately; ABNL = abnormal; SX = symptoms; PT = patient. (Adapted with permission from Berman et al.[68])

Current Data May Underestimate the True Prognostic Value of SPECT

The foregoing information provides compelling evidence that ^{99m}Tc sestamibi or ^{201}Tl myocardial perfusion SPECT is effective in the prognostic stratification of patients. Preliminary data have also been reported suggesting that ^{99m}Tc tetrofosmin is effective in risk stratification in chronic CAD.[198] It would appear, however, that current data on risk stratification by myocardial perfusion SPECT may actually underestimate the strength of this modality. In all the data quoted above, patients referred for early revascularization following nuclear testing were excluded (censored) from consideration in the prognostic studies. Although there is a reason for this censorship—namely, that the event rate may have been altered by the revascularization procedure—the exclusion results in the published data's inability to reflect the prognostic information derived from scans performed in the highest risk patient subset. A similar effect occurs to the extent that physicians and patients alter therapy and modify risk factors on the basis of the scan information, thereby probably reducing the event rate that might be observed for a given abnormal scan pattern in a natural history study. In other words, if patients with high-risk abnormalities are treated medically, they are likely to be treated aggressively in a manner that would lower their observed event rates.

Additionally, recent technical advances in the field of myocardial perfusion SPECT have typically not been included in the prognostic assessments. For example, the impact of quantitative analysis on prognosis has not been studied in any detail, although it has been reported to be equal to that of semiquantitative analysis, potentially improving the ability to generalize the findings to less experienced laboratories.[199]

ADDED VALUE OF GATED SPECT

The potent information contained in the ejection fraction assessed from gated SPECT is likely to enhance the prognostic content of myocardial perfusion SPECT. Since gated SPECT has become routine only recently, there are few reports of its incremental value over perfusion in assessing prognosis. Evidence that gated SPECT is likely to add to prognostic assessment is provided by prior ejection fraction data. LV ejection fraction has been shown to risk-stratify suspected disease patients according to their risk of subsequent cardiac death. In a series of reports from the Duke databank using rest and exercise first-pass radionuclide angiography, patients with suspected disease could be risk-stratified using a diagnostic threshold of 50 percent EF.[200–205]

In a preliminary communication, Hachamovitch et al. demonstrated that after risk adjustment for pretest likelihood of CAD and results of perfusion SPECT, EF provided significant incremental value in prediction of cardiac death or nonfatal myocardial infarction in patients with known or suspected chronic CAD.[206] Sharir et al.,[207] studying 1680 patients, demonstrated that poststress LVEF, as measured by gated SPECT, provided significant information over the extent and severity of perfusion defect as measured by the summed stress score (Fig. 16-14). Furthermore, these authors demonstrated that LV end-systolic volume provided added information over poststress LVEF in prediction of cardiac death (Fig. 16-15). The relatively low cardiac death rate in patients with abnormal perfusion and normal LV function in this study is probably explained by a referral bias in which patients with greatest ischemia by SSS were preferentially sent for early revascularization and thus censored from assessment of the prognostic value of the test. In a subsequent preliminary report of 2600 patients, Sharir et al. have shown that while poststress EF provides incremental information over prescan and perfusion variables in prediction of cardiac death, the perfusion variables are stronger predictors of nonfatal MI. Once prescan and perfusion variables were known, poststress EF did not provide incremental information with respect to the risk of nonfatal MI.[208]

In the future, complex algorithms will need to be developed that incorporate all of the information from gated SPECT for purposes of guiding patient management. In this regard, it is likely that poststress EF (related predominately to the size of MI) and summed difference score (an expression of the amount of stress-induced ischemia) will provide the greatest complementary information. As an initial approach, Sharir et al. have reported the combination of the ejection fraction and reversible ischemia in the prediction of cardiac events. If poststress EF is less than 30 percent, cardiac death or nonfatal MI rates appear to be high regardless of the amount of ischemia as assessed by the summed difference score. In patients with poststress EF from 30 to 50 percent, mild amounts of ischemia were associated with relatively high cardiac event rates. In patients with ejection fractions of greater than 50 percent, only patients with moderately extensive ischemia were at high risk of cardiac events.

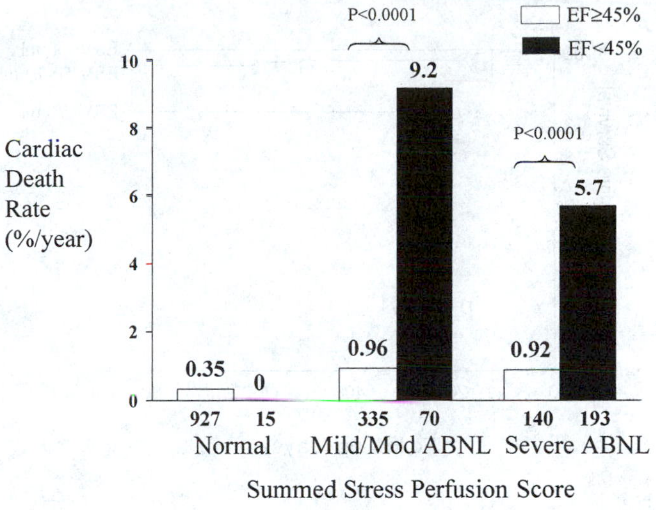

FIGURE 16-14 Cardiac death (percent per year) as a function of perfusion abnormality and poststress EF by gated SPECT. The number of patients within each category is indicated below ech column. MOD = moderate; ABNL = abnormality. The categories for summed stress score are normal (0–3), mild/moderate (4–13), severe (greater than 13). (Adapted with permission from Sharir et al.[207])

Other important information that can be derived from myocardial perfusion scintigraphy and may be related to risk has not been widely included in the prognostic assessment. Such information includes the assessment of poststress wall motion abnormalities on gated SPECT, a sign of exercise-induced stunning and a marker of severe CAD.[209,210] Additionally, transient ischemic dilation of the LV[89,90] and pulmonary uptake of radioactivity as determined by the measurement of lung/heart ratios of radioactivity[95,211,212] have been shown to be of prognostic importance[96,212,213] but are not yet part of most analyses of myocardial perfusion SPECT for purposes of risk stratification. Extensive resting defect reversibility rest ^{201}Tl/stress ^{99m}Tc sestamibi, evaluated by 24-h ^{201}Tl imaging, has been shown to be predictive of a higher mortality rate than would be predicted by rest or stress perfusion defect abnormalities alone.[213]

NUCLEAR TESTING AS THE GATEKEEPER TO CARDIAC CATHETERIZATION

The major clinical decisions after nuclear testing include the decision to initiate new medical therapy, to refer a patient to cardiac catheterization, or to provide a conservative, watchful waiting approach to care. Among patients with normal scans, only a small proportion will require cardiac catheterization as a result of clinical symptomatology.[65] In a population of 2203 patients[66] (follow-up, 18 months), by multivariate analysis, the

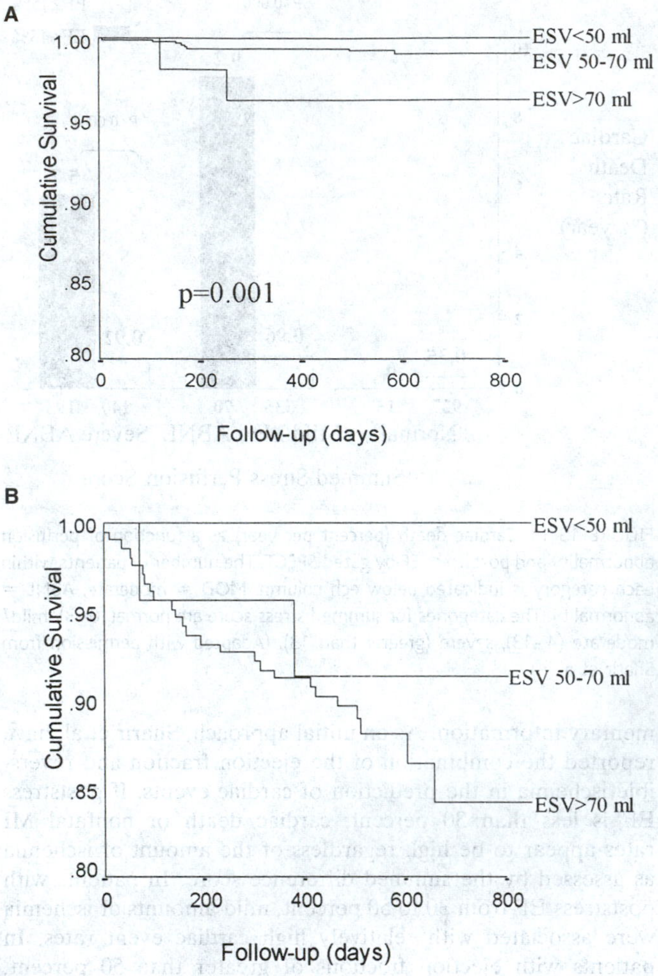

FIGURE 16-15 Cumulative survival of patients with poststress EF by quantitative gated SPECT greater than or equal to 45 percent (*left*) and less than 45 percent (*right*) stratified by end-systolic volume (ESV), also measured by gated SPECT. (Adapted with permission from Sharir et al.[207])

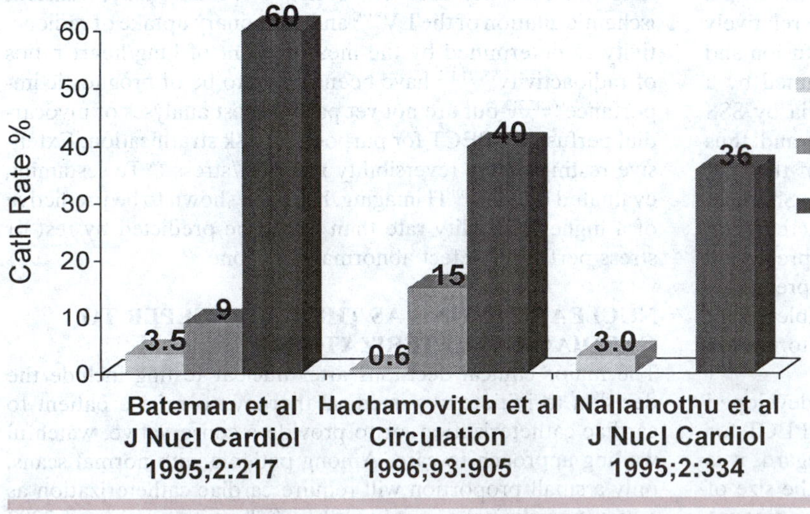

FIGURE 16-16 Comparative relationship between myocardial perfusion SPECT results and rates of subsequent catheterization in three separate trials.

nuclear result was the dominant factor determining the referral to catheterization. This relationship between the results of myocardial perfusion SPECT and catheterization rates have also been reported by Bateman et al.[214] and Nallamothu et al.[215] (Fig. 16-16). Hachamovitch et al.[67] reported that when catheterization was limited to patients with moderate to severe perfusion abnormalities (i.e., summed stress score >8), significant cost savings (17 percent reduction in cardiac catheterization rate) could be achieved for 5183 patients undergoing dual isotope stress SPECT imaging.

In the era of cost containment, it becomes increasingly important to determine whether noninvasive testing can result in substantial cost savings in the diagnosis of CAD. Shaw et al.[216] evaluated a total of 11,249 consecutive stable angina patients, including our own, in a large multicenter study. In a matched cohort study of patients with chronic stable angina comparing direct catherization to myocardial perfusion SPECT with selective catheterization, there was a substantial reduction (31 to 50 percent) in costs for all levels of pretest clinical risk using the myocardial perfusion SPECT plus selective catheterization approach. This cost reduction was seen in both the diagnostic (early) and follow-up (late) costs, which included costs of revascularization (Fig. 16-17). The rates of subsequent nonfatal MI and cardiac death were virtually identical in comparisons of direct catheterization and myocardial perfusion imaging with selective catheterization approaches in all patient risk subsets of stable chestpain patients (Fig. 16-18). What was significantly different was the rate of revascularization, which was reduced by nearly 50 percent in the cohort receiving myocardial perfusion imaging with selective catheterization. In fact, patients with normal perfusion results had a reduced rate of cardiac catheterization as well as a reduced frequency of normal coronary angiographic findings at the time of catheterization.

The Role of RNA in Chronic CAD

In chronic CAD, the principal applications of RNA at the present time are at rest. Resting RNA using either equilibrium or first-pass techniques can be effective in defining the presence of a reduced LVEF, and thereby a patient population for whom ACE inhibitors can be effective. Following initial observations in patients with MI,[217] subsequent randomized trials in patients with chronic CAD demonstrated that patients who have reduced LVEF obtain a distinct beneficial effect from the long-term administration of ACE inhibitors. Thus, the available evidence would suggest that patients with suspected acute or chronic CAD are candidates for ACE inhibitor therapy if LVEF is low.[5,8,218,219] The other manner in which patients with CAD can benefit from RNA is with serial assessment of ventricular function. This is important in assessing the efficacy of treatments such as ACE

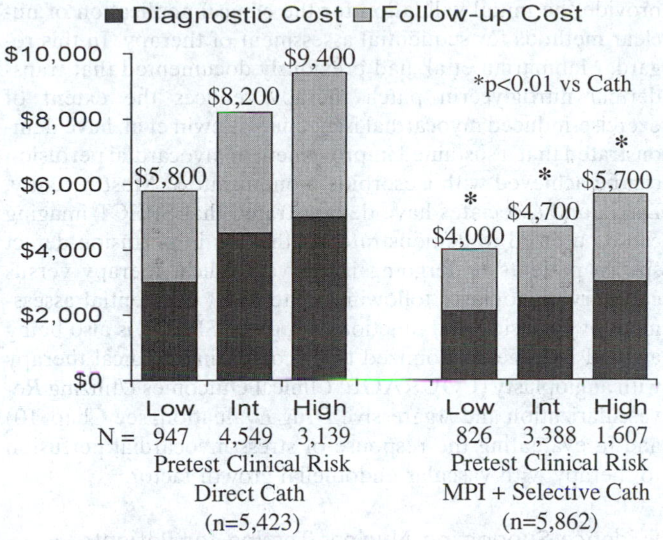

FIGURE 16-17 Comparative cost between screening strategies employing direct catheterization (Cath) and myocardial perfusion imaging (MPI) with selective Cath. Low, Int, and High represent low-, intermediate-, and high-risk subsets of the patients with stable angina. Shown are the initial diagnostic costs (*solid bars*) and follow-up costs including costs of revascularization (*gray bars*). A 30 to 41 percent reduction in costs was noted in each category. (Adapted with permission from Shaw et al.[216])

inhibitor therapy and has been used in many trials of a variety of approaches to patients with severe reductions of LVEF. Commonly, a measurement of LVEF by equilibrium RNA is required as a method of documenting severe reduction of LVEF prior to admission into heart failure trials.

For the detection of CAD and management of patients with this condition, exercise RNA continues to play a role in some centers. The most commonly utilized measurement derived from RNA for these decisions is the peak exercise LVEF, whether from first-pass or equilibrium techniques. Many studies have reported the prognostic power of exercise EF as measured by the first-pass technique for subsequent cardiovascular death or nonfatal MI.[200–205,220] Similar reports have emerged from equilibrium RNA.[221–226] In a recent report by Shaw et al., the prognostic value of LV function during exercise was examined in 863 consecutive patients undergoing exercise gated equilibrium RNA within 90 days of catheterization who were followed up for subsequent events, with 99 percent of survivors completing five years of follow-up.[222] In a multivariable analysis, the resting or exercise EF contained significant predictive information ($p <$ 0.0001). The rest or exercise EF contained similarly predictive information (exercise EF provided 63 percent of the information of the exercise model and resting EF provided 60 percent). When considering the addtion of the presence and extent of CAD observed at catheterization rest and exercise RNA data still provided significant improvement in the prediction of cardiac death.[222] There was aninverse relationship between peak exercise LVEF and survival.[219,222]

Bonow et al., using equilibrium RNA, documented the complementary role of exercise RNA and coronary angiography.[224] In this study, patients with triple-vessel disease and preserved LVEF at rest could be divided into a group in which mortality was negligible when exercise ejection fraction was normal and a high-risk group with an annual mortality of 7 percent when exercise ejection fraction was <50 percent.[224] Similarly, among patients with one- or two-vessel disease and reduced resting LVEF, those with normal EF responses did not exhibit any mortality over a 5-year follow-up, whereas 26 percent of patients with an abnormal EF response at exercise died in this time frame. Recently, Supino et al.[228] reported a 9-year follow-up of 167 stable patients with triple-vessel disease who had undergone rest and exercise RNA. Change in the LVEF from rest to exercise was the strongest predictor of major cardiac events and also predicted which patients would benefit from CABS. Patients whose LV ejection fraction decreased 8 percent or more with exercise had survival-prolonging benefit from bypass surgery performed less than 1 month after testing. Thus, data from several studies indicate that patients with chronic CAD can be accurately assessed with respect to prognosis by exercise RNA and that such assessment contains information that is complementary to that provided by standard clinical assessment as well as by coronary angiography.

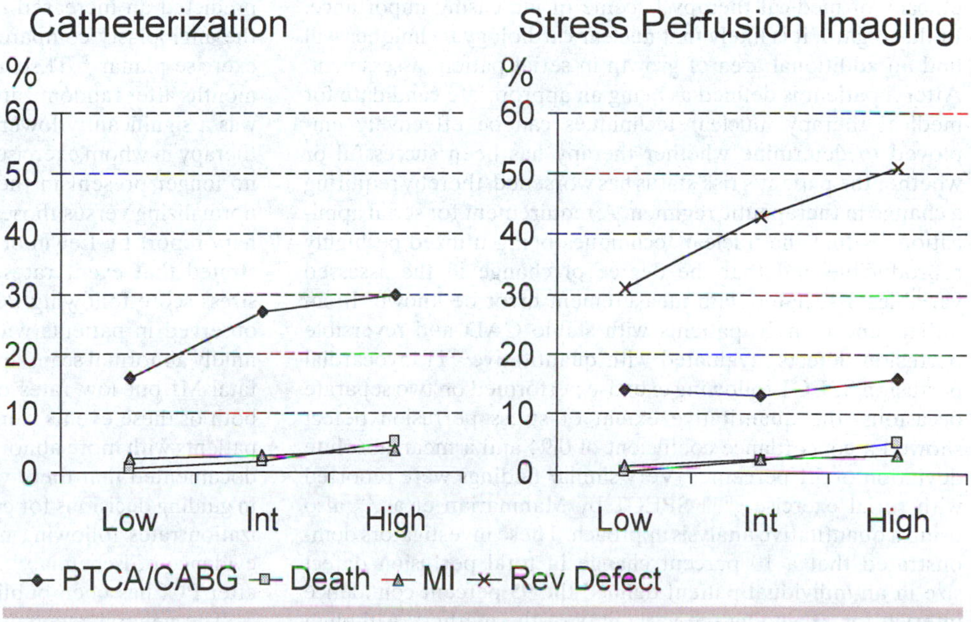

FIGURE 16-18 Subsequent event rates in the patient populations illustrated in Fig. 16-17. The rates of myocardial infarction and cardiac death were identical between the populations. The difference between the populations was an approximate 50 percent reduction in revascularization in the group approached with myocardial perfusion imaging and selective catheterization. Abbreviations as in Fig. 16-17. PTCA = percutaneous transluminal coronary angioplasty; CABG = coronary artery bypass graft; Death = cardiac death; MI = myocardial infarction; Rev defect = reversible defect. (Adapted with permission from Shaw et al.[216])

Postcatheterization Patients

Although coronary angiography provides detail of coronary anatomy, the functional implications of coronary stenoses are not always evident from the angiographic data. High-grade stenoses in the absence of collaterals are appropriately considered lesions of clinical significance; frequently, however, lesions of lesser grade are observed, or the implications of higher-grade lesions may be unclear due to presence of excellent collateral vessels. In these cases, the application of stress nuclear testing can supplement risk assessment for patients on the basis of the extent of stress-induced ischemia. Legrand et al. used exercise planar nuclear procedures to demonstrate that coronary flow reserve was normal in patients with 0 to 25 percent lesions and abnormal in patients with stenoses greater than 75 percent.[229] For patients in those extreme ranges, the data from nuclear testing were concordant with the angiographic results, supporting the concept that when angiographic results are clear, nuclear testing is not needed for functional assessment. In the range of 25 to 75 percent stenosis, however, there was an intermediate coronary flow reserve, unpredictable on the basis of coronary stenosis alone. In those patients, nuclear tests effectively separated the patients with low coronary flow reserve from those with normal coronary flow reserve. Therefore, the data on these patients with intermediate stenoses support the concept that nuclear testing can be useful with respect to functional significance in further assessment of such lesions. Similar data have been observed using sestamibi by Miller et al.[230]

Assessment of Therapy

With the broadening of the application of aggressive medical therapy (as an alternative to revascularization) to various subgroups of patients with CAD, methods for evaluation of the efficacy of medical therapy become of increasing importance. In this regard, it is likely that nuclear cardiology techniques will find an additional area of growth in serial patient assessment. After a patient is defined as being an appropriate candidate for medical therapy, nuclear techniques can be effectively employed to determine whether therapy has been successful or whether the patient's risk status has worsened, thereby requiring a change in therapeutic regimen. A requirement for serial applications is that the nuclear techniques being utilized be highly reproducible and that the degree of change in the assessed variables associated with measurement error be known. In an initial report on 16 patients with stable CAD and reversible perfusion defects, evaluated with quantitative ^{201}Tl myocardial perfusion SPECT following exercise performed on two separate occasions, the quantitative extent of stress perfusion defect showed a concordance coefficient of 0.94 and a mean absolute deviation of 5.1 percent.[231] Very similar findings were reported with serial exercise ^{201}Tl SPECT by Mahmarian et al.,[232] also using a quantitative analysis approach. These investigators demonstrated that a 10 percent change in total perfusion defect size in an individual patient defined the 95 percent confidence interval for exceeding the variability of the method. Although the statistical analyses were different between these studies, the results are very similar. More recently, high repeatability of exercise ^{99m}Tc sestamibi SPECT has been demonstrated using quantitative analysis approaches.[233] The summed stress score has also been shown to be highly reproducible.[233] These data provide the initial validation for the clinical application of nuclear methods for sequential assessment of therapy. In this regard, Mahmarian et al. had previously documented that transdermal nitroglycerin patch therapy reduces the extent of exercise-induced myocardial ischemia.[234] Lewin et al. have demonstrated that a sustained improvement in myocardial perfusion can be achieved with isosorbide mononitrate.[235] Most recently, Dakik and associates have demonstrated that SPECT imaging can be utilized to demonstrate a reduction in perfusion defect size in patients undergoing intensive medical therapy versus coronary angioplasty following acute MI.[236] Sequential assessment of perfusion and function with gated SPECT is also being applied in large randomized trials comparing medical therapy with angioplasty (COURAGE: *C*linical *O*utcomes *U*tilizing *R*e-vascularization and *A*ggressive *D*rug *E*valuation, see Chap. 10) and in evaluating the response of stress myocardial perfusion to therapy with vascular endothelial growth factor.[237]

Evidence Supporting Nuclear Testing for Patients after Percutaneous Coronary Intervention (PCI)

Nuclear testing is useful following PCI owing to the frequent occurrence of significant restenosis. Although recurrent symptoms often herald the presence of restenosis, clinically significant restenosis is frequently silent.[238] Exercise ^{201}Tl SPECT data obtained by Hecht et al.[239] have demonstrated that nuclear testing is accurate in defining the presence of restenosis. Subsequent work by Hecht et al. demonstrated this accurate detection of restenosis in asymptomatic as well as symptomatic patients.[240] Recent data suggest that nuclear testing remains effective in detecting restenosis for patients undergoing angioplasty with coronary stenting.[241,242] Pfisterer et al., using planar ^{201}Tl scintigraphy, demonstrated that silent and symptomatic ischemia in patients undergoing exercise scintigraphy 6 months following PCI, predicted an increased risk of recurrent ischemic events.[238] In the angioplasty compared to medical therapy study (ACME), exercise planar ^{201}Tl scintigraphy was performed before and 6 months after randomization to medical therapy or PCI.[243] There was a significantly lower mortality rate in patients with either therapy in whom exercise-induced ischemia by scintigraphy was no longer present in the 6-month study (6 versus 18 percent, normalizing versus those nonnormalizing, $p = 0.02$). A preliminary report by Lewin et al. from our institution[244] has demonstrated that event rates are strongly related to the summed stress score following PCI, with a pattern very similar to that observed in patients with no known CAD; i.e., patients with mildly abnormal scans appeared to have increased rates of nonfatal MI but low rates of cardiac death, whereas the rates of both of these events were in the intermediate to high range in patients with more abnormal scans. This preliminary report also documented that there was an appropriate use of nuclear scan in guiding decisions for catheterization, with low early catheterization rates following nuclear scanning in patients with little evidence of ischemia.[244] A review of the use of nuclear testing after PCI has been published.[245,246]

The general recommended approach of nuclear testing in the post-PCI patient would therefore be as follows: in patients with single vessel CAD and angina or interpretable ST segment depression pre-PCI, post-PCI assessment could be performed on a clinical or standard exercise testing basis. In other patients, when symptoms develop, nuclear testing can be helpful in defining the culprit vessel and assessing the extent of ischemic abnormality. For patients with no symptoms, nuclear testing between 3 and 6 months after angioplasty has been recommended. Whenever moderate to severe ischemia is found by nuclear testing, consideration should be given to repeat catheterization.

Evidence Supporting Nuclear Testing after Coronary Bypass Surgery

Nuclear testing has become central in the assessment of the post-CABS patient. It is known that 75 percent of vein grafts can be expected to be occluded or severely stenosed by 10 years after surgery, particularly in patients undergoing saphenous vein CABS.[247,248] Due to an increased incidence of graft closure, a 5-year cutoff point to evaluate the postbypass patient may be considered appropriate.[246,249–251] Kaplan-Meier survival and MI-free survival for post-CABS patients undergoing exercise ^{201}Tl imaging from a recent study is depicted in Fig. 16-19.[250] This study also demonstrated that exercise ^{201}Tl SPECT is predictive of hard cardiac events even in the asymptomatic postbypass patient.[250] Moreover, we have reported findings using ^{99m}Tc sestamibi, illustrating that nuclear stress testing is effective in predicting subsequent events and determining need for catheterization in the post-CABS population.[251] In general, the recommendations for the post-CABS patient are that when symptoms develop, SPECT imaging is useful in determining the presence and extent of CAD. In the asymptomatic patient, SPECT perfusion imaging should be considered in the 5 to 7 years postoperative time frame. Whenever moderate to severe ischemia is present, consideration of repeat catheterization arises.[246,251]

Nuclear Testing for Risk Stratification in Special Populations

One of the principal strengths of nuclear cardiology is that a very large database has been accumulated, far larger than for any other noninvasive modality, documenting clear effectiveness of myocardial perfusion SPECT in risk stratification of

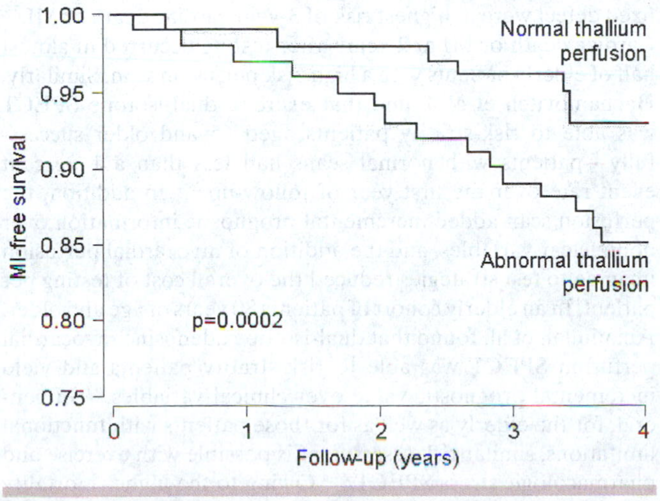

FIGURE 16-19 Kaplan-Meier plot for post-CABS patients associates reversible thallium defects with MI-free survival. Patients with reversible thallium perfusion defects had higher event rates. (From Lauer et al.,[250] with permission.)

appropriately selected patients with suspected chronic CAD. These large databases have now made it possible to evaluate risk in subsets of chronic CAD. Several of these applications are separately described below.

DIABETES

Myocardial perfusion SPECT has now been reported to be highly effective in risk stratification of patients with diabetes.[252,253] For example, in a study of 1271 patients with diabetes and 5862 without, Kang et al. demonstrated that a normal scan was similarly predictive of low cardiac event rates in both groups. Risk-adjusted event-free survival in patients with mildly and moderately abnormal scans, as defined by the SSS, was worse in patients with diabetes than in those without[252] (Fig. 16-20). A recent multicenter series reported that the extent of perfusion deficits and cardiac symptoms is more predictive of cardiac mortality in diabetics.[254] In a preliminary report, Lewin et al. have shown that in patients without diabetes, those with a moderately abnormal SSS had a cardiac mortality rate similar to that of patients with a mildly abnormal or normal SSS, whereas diabetics with moderately abnormal SSS had increased mortality rates. These findings suggest that in nondiabetic patients with known or suspected chronic CAD, the group with relatively low risk for cardiac death may be extended beyond that observed in general populations, potentially increasing the group of patients appropriately defined for noninvasive strategies (see also Chap. 78).[253]

LEFT BUNDLE-BRANCH BLOCK

Myocardial perfusion SPECT is highly useful for risk stratification in patients with LBBB. In a long-term follow-up of 245 patients with LBBB, Wagdy et al.[255] demonstrated that myocardial perfusion SPECT with vasodilator stress was an excellent predictor of cardiac events, with high risk being defined by a large, severe, fixed defect, a large reversible defect, cardiac enlargement and increased pulmonary uptake, or low resting EF. The 3-year survival was 57 percent in the high-risk group, versus 87 percent in the low-risk group ($p < 0.0001$). Similar findings have been reported by Nallamothu et al. in 293 medically treated patients with LBBB followed for 33 months.[256]

GENDER-BASED DIFFERENCES IN THE PROGNOSTIC VALUE OF PERFUSION IMAGING

For women, CAD incidence lags 10 years behind that of men. With the onset of menopause, the prevalence of CAD increases, achieving equivalence in disease prevalence at age 70 years.[257] In nondiabetic women before the age of 45 years, the likelihood of CAD is exceedingly low. In addition to differences in disease prevalence, a number of studies of small series of female patients have reported technical limitations and diminished accuracy in exercise treadmill testing, ^{201}Tl imaging, and in echocardiography.[174,258,259] With a perception on the part of clinicians of diminished accuracy of test results, reports have described sex-related bias in referral to cardiac catheterization after noninvasive testing.[260,261] When ^{201}Tl is used as the radiopharmaceutical in women, false-positive test results may be due to soft-tissue (breast) attenuation in the anterior and anterolateral segments.[174,262] In a small randomized trial comparing the diagnostic accuracy of ^{201}Tl with that of ^{99m}Tc sestamibi, test specificity was 67 versus 92 percent, respectively,[174] suggesting that gated

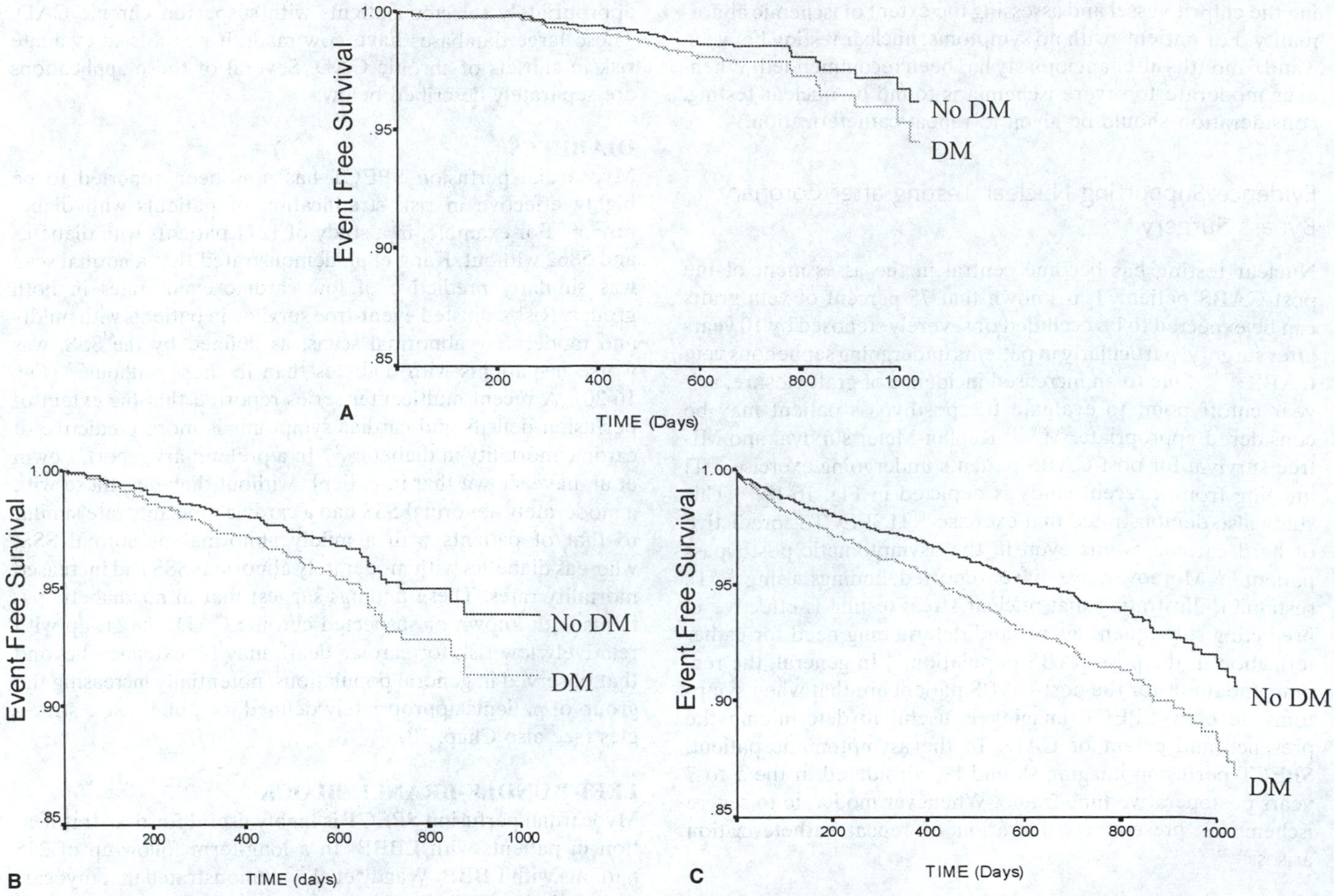

FIGURE 16-20 Risk-adjusted event-free survival curves for prediction of hard events among patients with diabetes (DM) and without diabetes (No DM) with normal scan results (SSS < 4) *A*, mildly abnormal scan results (SSS 4-8) *B*, and moderately to severely abnormal scan results as defined by SSS 78 *C*. All $p > 0.001$. (Adapted with permission from Kang et al.[252])

SPECT with a ^{99m}Tc perfusion agent may be the preferred form of SPECT in women. Reports from large female populations indicate that for both ^{99m}Tc sestamibi (rest and exercise) and dual-isotope myocardial perfusion SPECT, there is an added incremental prognostic value of myocardial perfusion data as compared to clinical and exercise variables in women.[66,263,264] From a recent multicenter registry of 3402 women with stable chest pain symptoms, risk stratification was similar by gender (84 percent underwent ^{99m}Tc sestamibi SPECT).[264] By the number of vascular territories with ischemia, 3-year survival ranged from 98.5 to 85 percent for none to three vascular territories abnormal by SPECT.[264] Amanullah and colleagues reported on 130 women undergoing adenosine ^{99m}Tc sestamibi SPECT, revealing that a moderately to severely abnormal perfusion scan (i.e., SSS >8) was associated with a sensitivity and specificity of 91 and 70 percent for the detection of multivessel CAD.[265]

PROGNOSTIC VALUE OF PERFUSION IMAGING IN THE ELDERLY

Patients over age 65 years have a higher disease prevalence and risk of major cardiac events as well as more frequent comorbid diseases. Exercise duration, heart rate, and total workload decrease with increasing age of our screened population. The prognostic value of perfusion scintigraphy has been reported in several recent series.[266,267] In an ambulatory population over age 70 years, abnormal exercise thallium imaging was accurate in identifying a high-risk population.[266] In a consecutive series of elderly patients, those with evidence of reversibility and a fixed defect were at highest risk of 3-year cardiac death or MI.[266] Cardiac death or MI at 2 years after testing occurred in almost half of elderly patients with a high-risk perfusion scan. Similarly, Hachamovitch et al. found that exercise dual-isotope SPECT was able to risk-stratify patients aged 65 and older successfully—patients with normal scans had less than a 1 percent event rate over the first year of follow-up.[266a] In addition, the perfusion scan added incremental prognostic information over nonnuclear variables, and the addition of myocardial perfusion imaging to test strategies reduced the overall cost of testing per patient. In an elderly cohort of patients 80 years of age and older, Amanullah et al. found that dual-isotope adenosine myocardial perfusion SPECT was able to risk-stratify patients and yield incremental prognostic value over clinical variables.[267] In general, for the elderly as well as for those patients with functional limitations, similar risk assessment is possible with exercise and pharmacologic stress SPECT.[267a] Owing to the higher mortality rate of the general population in this age group, upward adjustment of the "intermediate-risk" group to levels higher than the 1 to 3 percent used for general populations may be appropriate.

In this regard, Hayes et al. evaluated 1848 consecutive patients ≥80 years of age undergoing rest ^{201}Tl/stress ^{99m}Tc sestamibi dual isotope myocardial perfusion SPECT. Annualized cardiac death rates ranged from 1.9 percent in 722 patients with normal summed stress score to 9.3 percent in 401 patients with severely abnormal summed stress score (SSS ≥13).[267b]

PREOPERATIVE RISK ASSESSMENT IN NONCARDIAC SURGERY PATIENTS

Preoperative risk assessment is a common reason for cardiology consultation. Although clinical history, physical examination, and the resting ECG are highly useful, in many clinical settings these tools are inadequate. In contrast, assessment of LV function and/or jeopardized myocardium provides an accurate method to complement clinical assessment. Patients with peripheral vascular disease are at increased risk of having CAD. A large coronary angiographic study of asymptomatic patients revealed that 44 percent of patients undergoing peripheral vascular surgery have angiographically significant CAD.[268] It has furthermore been shown that peripheral vascular surgery, with its associated marked hemodynamic stresses, carries at least a moderate risk of perioperative events for patients with known CAD. Since these patients frequently cannot exercise, they are ideal candidates for the utilization of vasodilator stress in conjunction with myocardial perfusion imaging, and a large body of literature exists documenting the effectiveness of nuclear stress testing in this context. Although some have advocated the routine application of stress nuclear testing in this patient group, recent guidelines have been developed suggesting that nuclear testing is best reserved for patients with an intermediate risk of a cardiac event at the time of the procedure. Data supporting this approach were first presented by Eagle et al.[269] and then expanded in 1996 to include 3368 operations.[270] A metanalysis of the comparative value of the vasodilator myocardial perfusion scintigraphy and dobutamine echocardiography in risk stratification before vascular surgery has been published.[271] Together with other data sets, these data led to the guidelines for perioperative cardiovascular evaluation, published by the ACC/AHA task force (see Chap. 74). From these guidelines, candidates for vasodilator myocardial perfusion SPECT (or dobutamine echo) include patients with two of three high-risk factors (Table 16-4). In general, this includes patients who are at intermediate risk for cardiac events.

TABLE 16-4 Shortcut to Noninvasive Testing Based on Guidelines*,†

- Intermediate clinical predictors are present (Canadian class 1 or 2 angina, prior myocardial infarction based on history or pathologic Q waves, compensated or prior CHF, or diabetes)
- Poor functional capacity (<4 METS)
- High surgical risk procedure (emergency major operations; aortic repair or peripheral vascular; prolonged surgical procedures with large fluid shifts and or blood loss)

*Based on Leppo JA, American Society of Nuclear Cardiology, Tutorial in Nuclear Cardiology, Sept. 30–Oct. 3, Washington, D.C., 1999.
†Noninvasive testing is useful in preoperative patients if any two factors are present.

Assessment of Myocardial Viability

Mortality associated with LV dysfunction in the setting of severe CAD is quite high.[272–275] Patients with LV dysfunction who undergo CABS receive a greater proportional risk reduction compared to patients with preserved function.[8] The clinical setting in which viability assessment is most commonly used is the evaluation of patients with poor LV function, when the likelihood of improvement after revascularization is being considered. This information can be useful in determining the appropriateness of medical management, revascularization, or cardiac transplantation. Excellent reviews of radionuclide techniques for assessment of myocardial viability have recently been provided by Bonow[272,273] and Dilsizian.[274]

As early as 1989, positron emission tomographic (PET) imaging was studied to examine the differential benefit of identifying viable from nonviable myocardium (see Chap. 19). Improved regional function postsurgery would occur more often in the setting of some modicum of myocardial viability. In addition to PET imaging, various protocols utilizing combinations of rest, redistribution, and reinjection thallium imaging have been devised, validated, and compared to assess the presence of hibernating myocardium optimally. When reversibility of defects is noted on stress/rest or stress/redistribution studies, the likelihood of postrevascularization improvement of regions with abnormal ventricular function is high. The likelihood of improvement is also high for patients in whom reversibility is noted on rest/redistribution myocardial perfusion scintigraphy. Improvement would also be expected in patients with very severe angiographic CAD (virtually certain to cause severe flow restriction with stress) if normal, mildly reduced, or even moderately reduced tracer uptake is noted on rest or redistribution scintigraphy, since it could be predicted that such patients would show clear reversibility if stress-rest or stress-redistribution imaging were feasible. This inference is commonly made for patients with known coronary anatomy, unstable angina, and physician reluctance to perform stress imaging. When severe reduction in uptake of radioactivity is noted on redistribution ^{201}Tl imaging, the likelihood of improvement in regional ventricular function is low. When a moderate defect is noted at rest (or redistribution), the likelihood of improvement is intermediate.

Many studies have demonstrated thallium protocols using either rest-redistribution or stress-redistribution-reinjection to be nearly as accurate as PET in assessing myocardial viability.[274] Recent studies have also examined the predictive value of ^{99m}Tc sestamibi for functional recovery post-CABS. Summary data of the positive and negative predictive value of ^{201}Tl and ^{99m}Tc sestamibi in estimating functional recovery following CABS (using 2- to 3-month post-RNA or echocardiographic imaging) have shown that the positive predictive value (either weighted average or pooled) ranged from 69 to 79 percent and was similar by radioisotope. The negative predictive value (either by pooled or weighted average) ranged from 72 to 85 percent and was also similar by radioisotope. These accuracy statistics are dependent upon underlying risk (with higher predictive values noted for higher-risk populations); average patient samples were 25 to 30 for ^{201}Tl and ^{99m}Tc sestamibi.[272–275]

Currently there is controversy as to whether resting myocardial perfusion scintigraphy with ^{99m}Tc sestamibi (particularly if augmented by preinjection administration of nitroglycerin)[85,86] is as effective as redistribution ^{201}Tl scintigraphy in assessing myocardial viability. Without nitroglycerin, however, in principle it would be expected that rest/redistribution ^{201}Tl myocardial perfusion scintigraphy would be a more accurate approach than ^{99m}Tc sestamibi imaging for detection of viability in patients with severe hibernation (severe reduction in resting blood flood, downregulation of ventricular function, but preservation of the ability to improve ventricular function with restoration of blood flow).[277,278] Of note, it has been suggested for both ^{99m}Tc sestamibi[88] and ^{99m}Tc tetrofosmin[24] that an increase in extraction fraction at low flow may make the resting study with the ^{99m}Tc agent more like a redistribution thallium than a resting thallium study, potentially explaining the observed excellent ability of these tracers, even without nitroglycerin administration, to predict postrevascularization improvement in ventricular function.

Several technical improvements could improve the use of myocardial perfusion SPECT in the assessment of myocardial viability. As mentioned above for ^{99m}Tc sestamibi and tetrofosmin, the possibility of further enhancing the viability information of reinjection ^{201}Tl through the administration of nitroglycerin has been described.[38,276] Furthermore, in many of the studies assessing viability, a single cutoff point for myocardial counts in the region in question compared to the maximal observed value is employed: e.g., 50 or 60 percent of the maximal counts.[87,88] Of note, however, is the fact that the inferior wall in non-attenuation-corrected SPECT studies has far fewer counts than the other myocardial regions. This observation would suggest that the ability to predict viability for myocardial perfusion SPECT would be enhanced by approaches that take into account the number of standard deviations below normal in a given region rather than a single percentage of maximal count uptake. Finally, the use of combined rest-redistributioned ^{201}Tl/stress ^{99m}Tc sestamibi or tetrofosmin dual isotope SPECT may be particularly effective in assessing myocardial viability, since the protocol can combine what may be the optimal rest SPECT protocol (rest and redistribution ^{201}Tl) with a stress imaging assessment.[56,213]

Table 16-5 illustrates conceptually the relationship between several different myocardial states associated with chronic CAD and the patterns that might be observed on myocardial perfusion SPECT. In the presence of myocardial hibernation, resting blood flow would be expected to be mildly to even severely reduced, with corresponding reductions in resting ^{201}Tl or ^{99m}Tc perfusion agent uptake.[277,278] With ^{201}Tl, the equilibrium uptake of radioactivity would also be expected to be normal or potentially slightly reduced if true equilibrium was not achieved or if prolonged hibernation had resulted in cellular degeneration.[278] Thus these patients often demonstrate resting reversibility of perfusion defects.[213] For the ^{99m}Tc agents, resting perfusion (and thus viability assessment) can be enhanced by nitroglycerin administration prior to the resting injection of the tracer.[85,86] If patients with hibernation are subjected to stress, an even greater degree of reduction in flow would be expected, causing a greater degree of defect reversibility in most cases. The likelihood of improvement with revascularization is great in these patients.

Stunning occurs in the setting of a prolonged episode of severe ischemia[279] with subsequent restoration of flow. It is usually associated with acute CAD and is most often seen in the setting of aborted MI (either by thrombolytic therapy, direct revascularization, or spontaneous thrombolysis). Stunning can also occur in the setting of chronic CAD, such as following prolonged exercise in patients with high-grade coronary lesions.[209,280] In these circumstances, resting myocardial perfusion scintigraphy is generally normal or minimally reduced, reflecting the return of normal or nearly normal perfusion. Equilibrium ^{201}Tl concentration would be normal, and there would be no evidence of resting reversibility. However, patients with exercise-induced stunning would be expected to demonstrate marked perfusion defects on the stress study.[209] In these patients, the likelihood of improvement in exercise flow and function, as well as postexercise function following revascularization, would be high. It should be noted that stunning observed in conjunction with stress is not generally associated with an abnormality of true resting ventricular function but is discovered as a consequence of measuring ventricular function early after using stress testing.[209,280] For this type of stunning abnormality to improve, revascularization is usually necessary; in contrast, improvement in ventricular function occurs spontaneously over time with the stunning associated with an aborted acute coronary syndrome.

A great deal of attention has recently been placed on the remodeled LV, usually occurring as a consequence of extensive

TABLE 16-5 Scintigraphic and Clinical Characteristics of Hypocontractile Regions According to Their Viability Status

Viability Status	Rest	Redistribution (Tl-201)	Rest Reversibility	Stress/Rest/RI Reversibility	Likelihood of Improvement with Revasc
Q MI	↓↓↓	↓↓↓	—	—	—
Non Q MI	↓–↓↓	↓–↓↓	—	±*	±*
Hibernation	↓ to ↓↓↓	→ to ↓	+	+++	+++
Stunning (with exercise)	→	→	→	+++	+++
Remodeled	→	→	→	→	→
Nonischemic CM with incidental CAD	→	→	→	→	→

*Depends on stenosis of IRA.

ABBREVIATIONS: Q = Q wave; MI = myocardial infarction; CM = cardiomyopathy; RI = reinjection; Revasc = revascularization.

prior MI.[281,282] In this circumstance, LV function can become diffusely abnormal, even in areas remote from the infarct zone. The area of abnormal contraction associated with remodeling in these patients would be expected to have normal resting ^{99m}Tc perfusion tracer or ^{201}Tl uptake, normal equilibrium ^{201}Tl uptake, no evidence of reversibility on either stress or rest imaging, and little likelihood of improvement following revascularization. Patients with remodeled LVs may have very profoundly reduced ventricular function. Given the differential response to revascularization of the remodeled LV and the hibernating LV, this ability of nuclear scanning to differentiate between them becomes important.

TABLE 16-6 Guidelines for Monitoring Patients Receiving Doxorubicin*

Perform baseline radionuclide angiocardiography at rest for calculation of left ventricular ejection fraction (LVEF) prior to administration of 100 mg/m² doxorubicin. Subsequent studies are performed at least three weeks after the indicated total cumulative doses have been given, before consideration of the next dose.

PATIENTS WITH NORMAL BASELINE LVEF (≥50%)

Perform the second study after 250 to 300 mg/m²

Repeat study after 400 mg/m² in patients with known heart disease, radiation exposure, abnormal electrocardiographic results, or cyclophosphamide therapy; or after 450 mg/m² in the absence of any of these risk factors.

Perform sequential studies thereafter prior to each dose.

Discontinue doxorubicin therapy once functional criteria for cardiotoxicity develop, i.e., absolute decrease in LVEF ≥10% (EF units)

PATIENTS WITH ABNORMAL BASELINE LVEF (≤50%)

Doxorubicin therapy should not be initiated with baseline LVEF ≤30%.

In patients with LVEF >30% and <50%, sequential studies should be obtained prior to each dose.

Discontinue doxorubicin with cardiotoxicity: absolute decrease in LVEF ≥10% (EF units) and/or final LVEF ≥30%.

*From Ref. 284.

Nuclear Cardiology Applications Unique to RNA

ASSESSMENT OF ANTHRACYCLINE CARDIOTOXICITY

RNA, using either the equilibrium or first-pass approach has become the method of choice for evaluating the effects of doxorubicin and other anthracyclines on LV function in patients with suspected cardiotoxicity. In an early report, Alexander and colleagues demonstrated that patients with normal LVEF that had not fallen by more than 15 points did not develop cardiotoxicity with continued doxorubicin therapy; however, once EF fell below 45 percent or by more than 15 percent, continued doxorubicin therapy was commonly associated with irreversible cardiac failure.[283] In a subsequent report of a large high-risk population from the same group, guidelines were established for the use of continued doxorubicin therapy.[284] These recommendations are summarized in Table 16-6. In a group of 70 high-risk patients in whom these guidelines were strictly followed, 2.9 percent developed subsequent congestive heart failure (CHF) that responded to therapy. Of 212 high-risk patients in whom the recommendations were not closely followed, 21 percent developed CHF ($p < .001$ versus the strict-guideline group). The CHF in the majority of these patients was considered moderate to severe. Similar findings have been reported by other groups.[285,286]

DETERMINING THE TIME FOR VALVE REPLACEMENT IN AORTIC REGURGITATION

It has been demonstrated that resting LVEF, as measured by equilibrium RVA, provides an excellent method for the sequential follow-up of asymptomatic patients with aortic regurgitation. For patients with chronic aortic regurgitation, a fall in LVEF has been shown to be strongly predictive of the development of subsequent progressive severe deterioration in LV function.[287,288] These investigators have suggested that asymptomatic patients with severe aortic regurgitation whose EFs at rest fall below normal should be considered for elective valve replacement. Using a combination of rest/exercise RNA and rest/echo, a recent study by Borer et al.[289] demonstrated in asymptomatic patients with severe aortic insufficiency that if a change in LVEF from rest to exercise, normalized for the change in end-systolic stress from rest to exercise, is abnormal, even patients with normal resting LVEF and no symptoms were likely to develop future complications. Cheitlin[290] suggested, however, that the more commonly available, less complex periodic assessment of rest LVEF or end-systolic volume may be as good an approach for determining the time for operative intervention in this condition.

ACUTE CORONARY ISCHEMIC SYNDROMES

Acute coronary ischemic syndromes have been categorized as acute transmural (Q) MI, nontransmural (non-Q) MI, and unstable angina pectoris. More recently, unstable angina and non-ST-segment elevation MI have been linked since flow preservation strategies and treatment are similar in these conditions (see Chap. 41). In general, all of these syndromes have the underlying pathophysiology of the presence of severe obstruction or closure of a coronary artery secondary to acute thrombus formation or spasm in a segment of an artery. Because of this relationship to closure of a vessel, myocardial perfusion/function scintigraphy is an effective means of detecting patients with acute ischemic syndromes. Acute coronary syndromes represent a wide array of clinical presentations from worsening chest pain in patients seen in the outpatient clinic to acute MI. Annually, there are a total of 1.5 million admissions to coronary care units in the United States, with half of these patients ruling in for ischemia or MI (Chaps. 41 and 42). A number of guidelines have described the advantages of postinfarction stratification afforded by nuclear testing.[218,219,291] While less dramatic than with chronic CAD, there has been continued growth in the application of nuclear cardiology to the assessment of patients with acute ischemic syndromes.

Evaluation of Acute Chest Pain

Although the diagnosis of acute MI is frequently straightforward, in many patients it is not. For example, the ECG is diagnostic in only two-thirds of patients with MI at the time of their initial presentation to the emergency department (ED). In non-Q-wave MI, and particularly in left circumflex MI, the ECG is frequently normal.[292,293] Furthermore, the ECG is frequently nondiagnostic even when abnormal (e.g., with LBBB, nonspecific ST- or T-wave changes, pacemakers).[294] From the emergency physician's standpoint, the problem of missed MIs in the ED is of particular importance. It is has been estimated that up to 50,000 patients per year in the United States have MIs that are missed, representing approximately 4 percent of all patients with MIs who present to the ED.[218,219,291,295] Approximately 25 to 40 percent of malpractice claims against emergency physicians arise from patients with missed MI.[295] It has also been demonstrated that patients discharged from the ED with missed MIs have a substantially higher mortality rate than patients in whom MI is appropriately detected and results in admission.[294,296] Therefore, with respect to patients with normal or nondiagnostic initial ECGs on presentation to the ED, an important clinical problem is how to distinguish those with acute coronary syndromes, who may benefit from early intervention, from those who may require less intensive care, can be discharged, or undergo immediate stress testing (see Chaps. 41 and 42).

For patients without ST-segment elevation, clinical management is not defined. The reasons are multifold, including the fact that only a small portion of patients presenting with an acute onset of chest pain symptoms are eligible for thrombolysis (i.e., 9 to 39 percent).[218,291] Of the remaining cohort of chest pain patients presenting to the ED, the outcome of patients with only minor ST-T-wave changes is variable. Evidence from the recent GUSTO IIa trial revealed that the outcome of patients with presenting ST-segment depression was 6.8 percent for 30-day mortality and 12.4 percent for death or MI at 1 year. Of the non-ST-segment elevation candidates, 28 percent have three-vessel CAD and half have an MI during the index hospitalization. As such, in nonthrombolytic candidates the risk of CAD and major cardiac complications varies and may be high in a large proportion of patients.[297]

Because many of these patients are subsequently ruled out for MI, chest pain units have been instituted for the acute evaluation of chest pain patients presenting to the ED.[298,299] The chest pain units provide an integrated approach to the diagnosis and treatment of patients at risk for CAD. This includes laboratory tests, cardiac imaging, and early and aggressive treatment vis-à-vis a dedicated staff of nurses and physicians. A number of reports have documented the economic savings that have been realized by the introduction of these dedicated facilities.[298,299] The ROMIO study randomized 100 low-risk patients to an ED-based rapid-rule-out protocol or to routine hospital care.[299] The results revealed that the hospital stay was shorter and charges were lower with the rapid protocol than with routine care ($p = 0.001$). Among patients in whom ischemia was ruled out, those assigned to the rapid protocol had a shorter hospital stay (median 11.9 versus 22.8 h, $p = 0.0001$) and lower initial ($893 versus $1349, $p = 0.0001$) and 30-day ($898 versus $1522, $p = 0.0001$) hospital charges than did patients given routine care.

^{99m}Tc sestamibi or tetrofosmin SPECT, with injection during chest pain, provides an excellent opportunity to reduce clinical indecision in the acute evaluation of chest pain[300–302] (Fig. 16-21). Investigations have demonstrated a role for myocardial perfusion imaging in the initial evaluation of these patients. Hilton and colleagues performed acute sestamibi imaging for patients presenting to their ED with typical angina and normal or nondiagnostic ECGS.[300] Only one patient of 70 in this cohort with a normal scan experienced a subsequent cardiac event on follow-up (cardiac death, MI, PCI, CABS, thrombolysis). Patients with equivocal or abnormal scans had event rates of 13 and 71 percent, respectively. The nuclear scan provided incremental risk stratification over clinical and ECG data. Based on these data, nuclear imaging can be used to assist in the risk stratification of patients with ongoing symptoms whose diagnosis cannot be clearly determined in an ED setting. In patients with ongoing symptoms, a normal perfusion scan can identify patients who can either be discharged early or admitted to non-intensive-care beds.

A number of larger series have been reported.[303–307] Tatum et al.[303] developed a triage evaluation strategy in which patients with a very high, high, or very low probability of an acute ischemic syndrome did not undergo nuclear testing, but those with a moderate to low probability of an acute ischemic syndrome did. It was found that 338 of 438 patients had normal studies and 100 patients had abnormal studies. Subsequent deaths and MIs over the following year were found to occur only in the patients with abnormal ^{99m}Tc sestamibi studies, while none of the 338 patients with normal ^{99m}Tc sestamibi studies developed subsequent MI (these studies included assessment of perfusion as well as myocardial function using gated SPECT). This group subsequently demonstrated, in a study of 620 patients with acute chest pain, that early myocardial perfusion SPECT and serial cardiac troponin I measurements have comparable sensitivities for identifying MI. This study also demonstrated that the two tests provide complementary information for identifying patients at risk for acute coronary syndromes.[304] In another report of 218 patients, this group demonstrated that

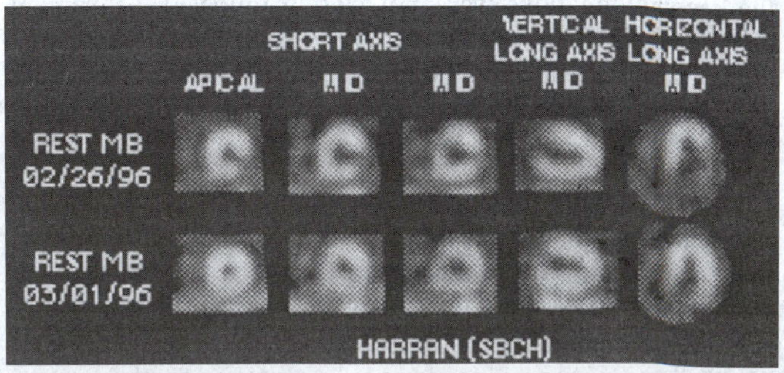

FIGURE 16-21 Resting sestamibi (MB) injected during chest pain in emergency department (*top*) and 3 days post-PCI of the left circumflex coronary artery (LCX) (*bottom*) in patient with no EGG or enzyme abnormalities. Clear evidence of extensive myocardial salvage in LCX territory is shown.

myocardial perfusion scintigraphy is useful in assessing chest pain associated with cocaine use, with abnormal studies being very infrequent in this population.[305] A multicenter series employing ^{99m}Tc tetrofosmin of 357 patients presenting to six centers with symptoms suggestive of myocardial ischemia was recently published.[306] This study examined the predictive value of rest ^{99m}Tc tetrofosmin SPECT at the time of ED admission for patients with a nondiagnostic ECG upon presentation. Of this study cohort, 20 patients had an acute MI, with a test sensitivity of 90 percent and a specificity of 60 percent. Most of the missed MIs were small inferior wall MIs mistaken as attenuation artifacts. The slightly lower sensitivity for acute MI in this series might be attributed to not using gated SPECT, which helps distinguish true resting perfusion defect from attentuation artifacts in these patients. In the analysis of these authors, using a normal SPECT image to decide not to admit a patient to the hospital would result in a 57 percent reduction in hospital admissions with a mean cost savings per patient of $4258.

A synthesis of published reports on acute use of myocardial perfusion imaging reveals an average sensitivity and specificity of 98 and 69 percent, respectively, for patients who are admitted with an abnormal perfusion scan.[302,303,306–308] A predictive model of index MI or revascularization based on multivariable risk-adjusted logistic regression has been reported in a cohort of 532 patients with acute chest pain revealed the following predictors: abnormal ^{99m}Tc sestamibi scan [odds ratio (OR) = 14-fold], diabetes (OR = 2.8-fold), typical angina (OR = 2.1-fold), and male gender (OR = twofold).[307] A very recent randomized clinical trial in 2300 patients tested the incremental value of historical, ECG, and sestamibi parameters in the decision to admit a patient presenting with acute chest pain (multicenter trial sponsored by the Agency for Healthcare Policy Research).[309] This trial randomized patients without a prior CAD history but with symptoms suggestive of acute ischemia, and a nondiagnostic ECG, to a nuclear scan versus no scan strategy. This study compared the ability of the scan to correctly classify patients who should be admitted as well as the costs associated with each comparative management strategy and demonstrated a 20 percent reduction in hospital admissions of patients subsequently shown not to have acute ischemic syndromes, no change in admission rates of patients with acute ischemic syndromes, and modest cost savings associated with nuclear scanning. Among 2127 patients whose final confirmed diagnosis was not acute cardiac ischemia, 52 percent of the patients randomized to the usual-care strategy were admitted to hospital or observation in what could be classified in retrospect as unnecessary admissions. Among the patients randomized to have a sestamibi scan as part of their evaluation strategy, however, the unnecessary admission rate was reduced to 42 percent. These data suggest that incorporating perfusion imaging into an ED strategy for patients with chest pain and a nondiagnostic ECG can improve the effectiveness of ED triage. Furthermore, projecting data on total direct costs from one site to the entire trial, we estimate that the added cost of the perfusion scan was more than overridden by the savings accrued from the reduction in unnecessary admissions in patients without acute ischemia.

Guidelines for SPECT Imaging in the ED

Several considerations are important for the most effective application of acute nuclear imaging. If the patient has had prior MI, the studies are generally not useful. The principal exception to this rule occurs in patients who had previously undergone myocardial perfusion scintigraphy, the results of which are immediately available to compare with the results of the new study performed during acute chest pain. Also, combined assessment of perfusion and function should be routinely performed in order to minimize the false negative rate. Of note, ^{99m}Tc-based myocardial perfusion imaging agents (^{99m}Tc sestamibi or tetrofosmin) are preferable in this acute ischemic syndrome application, since they may be injected during chest pain in the emergency department and imaged 30 min to 4 h later. Thus, the absence of redistribution with these myocardial perfusion imaging agents provides an advantage for acute imaging applications.

The accuracy of this approach for detecting an acute ischemic syndrome is probably related to the timing of injection with respect to the patient's chest pain. Ideally, the agent would be administered during chest pain or the first hour after chest pain; however, the importance of this timing has not been widely studied. In this regard, patients with unstable angina could conceivably have intermittent coronary occlusion, with normalization of myocardial perfusion at the time the vessel is open.

Because of this consideration, a protocol suggested by Ziffer et al.[310] is recommended for the assessment of those patients in whom chest pain has been relieved prior to injection (Fig. 16-22). In this protocol, patients with ongoing chest pain and resolved chest pain are managed differently. The former are injected with ^{99m}Tc sestamibi, as noted above; a normal study in this cohort may result in either discharge or referral for immediate stress testing, depending on the clinical likelihood of an acute ischemic syndrome. On the other hand, patients with abnormal initial studies are admitted with a presumptive acute ischemic syndrome.

Unique to the protocol described by Ziffer is the handling of a patient with resolved chest pain in the ED. In this case, a resting ^{201}Tl injection would be performed instead of resting ^{99m}Tc sestamibi or ^{99m}Tc tetrofosmin. If the resting ^{201}Tl SPECT is abnormal, the patient would be admitted and therapy for an acute ischemic syndrome begun, including consideration of early coronary angiography. Redistribution imaging may be useful for the assessment of myocardial viability. If the resting ^{201}Tl study is normal, the patient would not be discharged, since the possibility of resolved chest pain secondary to unstable angina would not yet have been evaluated. The patient would instead be submitted to a stress ^{99m}Tc sestamibi study (after a series of negative enzyme studies) employing the resting ^{201}Tl/stress ^{99m}Tc sestamibi protocol described at the beginning of Chap. 56. Based on these combined assessments, patient management would range from discharge (with a normal scan or mildly abnormal scan) to admission (with a clearly abnormal scan). In this latter case, the presumptive diagnosis would be that unstable angina caused the resting chest pain that had led to the emergency room presentation.

Ziffer et al. have recently published preliminary data on 2737 patients undergoing this protocol.[310] In 32 percent of the patients only resting imaging was performed, while in the remaining 68 percent rest and subsequent stress imaging were performed. Overall, 77 percent of all patients imaged were discharged without admission, and 23 percent were admitted. When the success of this protocol was evaluated, two aspects

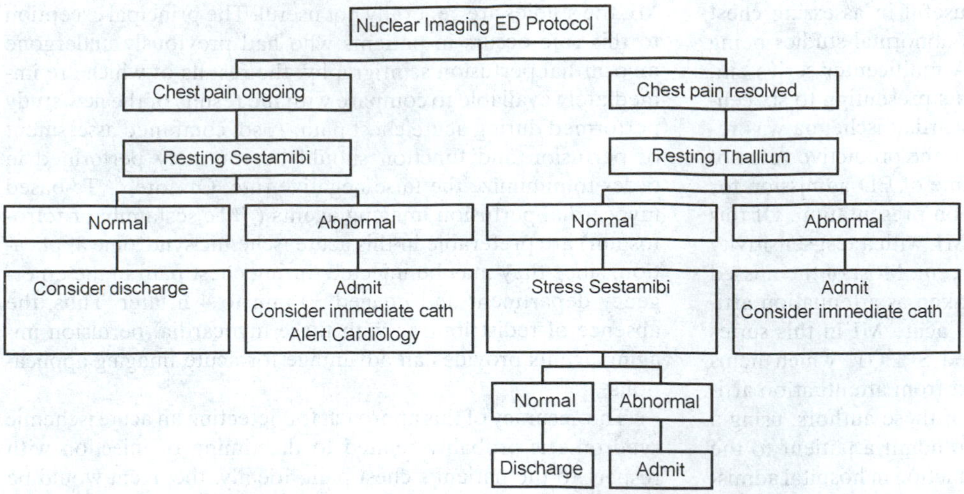

FIGURE 16-22 Nuclear imaging protocol for emergency department (ED) patients with low to intermediate risk of acute coronary syndrome.

were of particular importance. The investigators compared the event rates for patients who were discharged from the hospital following imaging to the event rates that had previously been observed for patients discharged from the emergency room before the myocardial perfusion imaging protocol had been instituted. With the chest pain center and the myocardial perfusion imaging protocol, the annualized event rate for patients discharged from the emergency room was 0.17 percent. In the patients discharged in the period immediately prior to the opening of the chest pain center, the annualized cardiac event rate was 2.7 percent. Thus, use of myocardial perfusion scintigraphy in the chest pain center was associated with a 16-fold reduction in the event rate (death or nonfatal MI) for patients discharged. In a subsequent preliminary communication, Ziffer et al. demonstrated clear cost savings by applying myocardial perfusion scintigraphy to appropriately selected patients.[311] Application of this modified protocol to patients in whom acute chest pain has resolved is illustrated in Fig. 16-23, in which a patient with unstable angina was correctly classified by the combination of rest and stress scintigraphy but would have been misclassified by the use of resting scintigraphy alone.

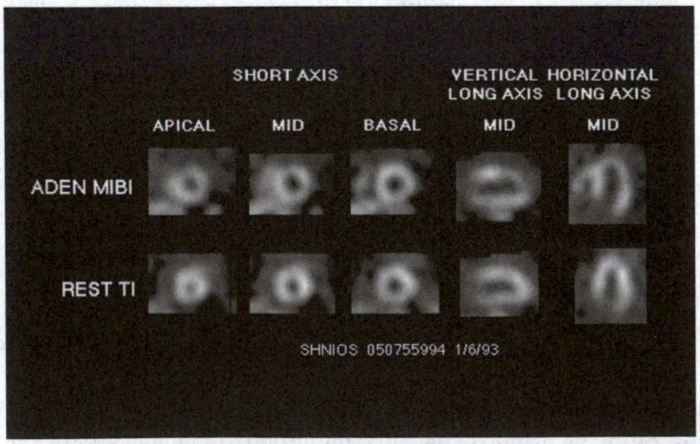

FIGURE 16-23 Normal rest ^{201}Tl SPECT (*bottom*) followed by adenosine ^{99m}Tc sestamibi (ADEN MIBI) (*top*) in a patient with intermittent chest pain which had resolved prior to injection with ^{201}Tl at rest. Reversible defects are seen in the left arterior descending and left circumflex territories. Angiography revealed 50 percent left main, 100 percent left anterior descending, 90 percent left circumflex, and 50 percent right coronary artery stenoses.

Assessment during Early Hospitalization for Acute Coronary Syndromes

Early (i.e., within 24 h) risk assessment has included perfusion or ventricular function imaging. Miller et al.[312] have documented that there is a strong relationship between the size of a very early myocardial perfusion defect (an indicator of infarct size) and subsequent mortality in the setting of acute MI. Overall a 3 percent mortality rate was observed in patients following acute MI. However, 7 percent of patients with myocardial perfusion defects (infarct size) greater than 12 percent of the myocardium had died at the end of a 2-year follow-up, compared to zero percent of the patients with infarct size less than 12 percent.[312] Christian et al.[313] have shown that rest myocardial perfusion SPECT, when combined with resting LV function, can provide information on myocardial stunning. In patients with acute MI, when there was a mismatch (with LVEF lower than would be expected from admission myocardial perfusion SPECT defect size), late improvement in LV function could be predicted.[313]

Radionuclide angiography has also been applied in the coronary care unit setting for assessing prognosis in patients with acute MI,[314,315] establishing the diagnosis of RV infarction,[314,315] and differentiating causes of cardiogenic shock.[314,315] A strong inverse relationship between resting EF and 1-year cardiac mortality has been demonstrated in large multicenter trials[316] (Fig. 16-24). At the other end of the clinical spectrum, resting RNA can aid in the assessment of the cause of low cardiac output in the acute setting. The approach can accurately distinguish patients with LV dysfunction, RV dysfunction, mitral regurgitation, cardiac tamponade, and ventricular septal defect. Those with LV dysfunction would have substantially reduced LVEF and concomitant severe wall motion abnormalities. The syndrome with predominant RV dysfunction is easily recognized by RV enlargement and a greater reduction in RVEF than LVEF.[314,315] Mitral regurgitation severe enough to allow low cardiac output in the setting of acute MI would be detectable through the LV/RV stroke-count ratio which can be derived from the regions of interest utilized to calculate RVEF and LVEF. Similarly, if a pericardial effusion, with or without bleeding, is large enough to cause hemodynamic compromise, it would easily be detected by equilibrium RNA as a halo surrounding the left cardiac chambers. Furthermore, in the postoperative setting, RNA allows identification of pericardial bleeding.[317,318] By combining a first-pass and equilibrium acquisition (with acquisition of one to two frames per cardiac cycle), one can also assess the presence of a ventricular septal defect through analyzing the pulmonary time–activity curve.

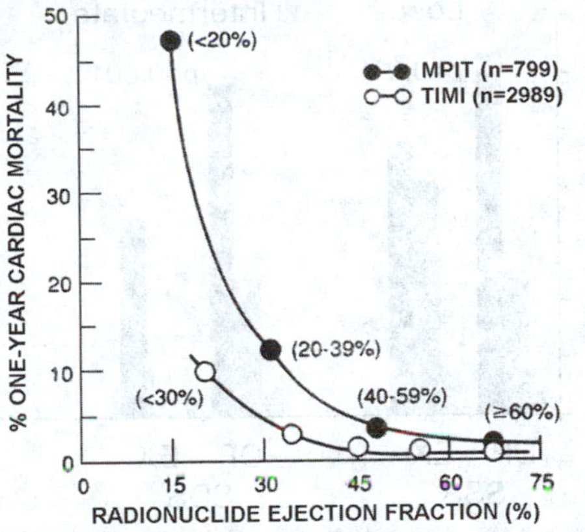

FIGURE 16-24 One-year mortality rates after acute myocardial infarction as function of left ventricular ejection fraction at rest. Data are shown from Multicenter Postinfarction Trial (MPIT) a decade ago and compared with more recent Thrombolysis in Myocardial Infarction (TIMI) II Trial. (From the Multicenter Postinfarction Research Group,[316] with permission.)

SELECTION OF INITIAL THERAPY

An important application of myocardial perfusion scintigraphy in acute ischemic syndromes is the selection of the appropriate therapy for patients with a known ischemic syndrome. For example, in patients presenting late (greater than 12 h) after onset of symptoms and acute MI, Christian et al. have suggested that not all patients will benefit from reperfusion therapy but that the benefit might be predictable based on the myocardial perfusion imaging pattern at the time of admission.[318] In this regard, thrombolytic therapy or angioplasty may not be beneficial in patients with severely reduced or absent myocardial perfusion late following symptoms, but these therapies may be successful for patients with preserved myocardial perfusion (and therefore preserved myocardial viability).

It has been suggested that considerations as to whether thrombolytic therapy or PCI should be performed can be elucidated by resting myocardial perfusion scintigraphy in the following conditions: (1) patients presenting late after chest pain, as noted above, (2) patients with ST-segment depression in whom injection can be made during chest pain (those with severe reduction in flow would be candidates for thrombolytic therapy or PCI, whereas those without decrease in flow would not be good candidates). Additionally, (3) patients with LBBB, in whom thrombolytic therapy or PCI are generally recommended, could most likely be better classified for therapy on the basis of resting myocardial perfusion scintigraphy rather than through the use of clinical criteria alone. None of these applications have been well studied by randomized trials, but they remain interesting potential clinical applications.

EVALUATION OF THERAPY

It has by now been well demonstrated that myocardial perfusion scintigraphy is useful in the assessment of therapeutic efficacy for patients undergoing thrombolytic therapy or percutaneous transluminal coronary angioplasty (PTCA). Maddahi et al. first demonstrated this application using ^{201}Tl planar scintigraphy in the early 1980s.[319,320] Subsequently, Gibbons et al.[321] reported similar findings using ^{99m}Tc sestamibi. On the basis of extensive work by that group of investigators, myocardial perfusion scintigraphy can be used in patients with acute MI before and after therapy (or even simply after therapy) and represents an efficient, less expensive endpoint for examining the efficacy of a variety of therapies compared to conventional mortality endpoints.

ASSESSMENT OF MYOCARDIAL VIABILITY

In the setting of acute MI, at times it becomes clinically important to assess the viability of abnormally contracting segments. In this regard, it has become important to recognize the high frequency of myocardial stunning that occurs in the setting of an aborted acute MI. Since the earliest thrombolytic trials, it has been clear that severe and extensive wall motion abnormalities and severe reduction of LV function can be associated with the stunned myocardium when thrombolytic therapy or PTCA is applied early enough to abort the development of myocardial necrosis. Although the return of ventricular function may be delayed by up to several months, the degree of improvement in ventricular function can be dramatic. In this regard, the finding of normal or nearly normal perfusion after initial therapy (thrombolytic therapy or PTCA) can be used to accurately predict the return of ventricular function in a patient with an acute ischemic syndrome, whereas ongoing resting ischemia might indicate the need for urgent revascularization.[321a]

Discharge Planning Post–Unstable Angina

Guidelines developed under the sponsorship of the Agency for Health Care Policy Research (AHCPR) have indicated a clear role for the use of nuclear testing in patients admitted with unstable angina.[291] Although at the present time most patients admitted with unstable angina are referred to catheterization, the guidelines suggest that a significant number of these patients should be medically treated after appropriate risk stratification. This strategy is applicable to patients who respond quickly to medical therapy, particularly in the presence of concomitant conditions that increase the risk of or decrease the likelihood of using an invasive strategy (e.g., very advanced age or debilitation). In these medically stabilized patients, either exercise or pharmacologic stress testing with perfusion imaging can effectively stratify patients into low- and high-risk subsets, as demonstrated by a number of studies.[291] Failure of medical treatment to control ischemia or the presence of hemodynamic instability would result in referral to catheterization. Hemodynamically stable patients with medically controlled ischemia would be candidates for a noninvasive management approach. Within this approach, those patients at low risk by clinical factors (patients who probably did not have unstable angina initially) can be managed as outpatients and referred to stress testing within 72 h of initial admission. Patients at intermediate to high risk who have been pain-free for 48 h and have no recurrent angina, LV dysfunction, or significant ventricular dysrhythmias are also candidates for in-hospital noninvasive risk stratification. The initial test on these patients could be treadmill ECG testing in those individuals with normal resting ECGs who are not on digoxin and are able to perform exercise. Patients with abnormal rest ECGs or on digoxin would undergo exercise or pharmacologic stress imaging; those patients unable to exercise would undergo pharmacological stress imaging. Either of these latter two groups are also potential candidates for stress echocardiographic studies. The decision between stress echocardiography and stress perfusion imaging would be guided by test availability and local expertise. For hospitalized patients with acute unstable angina, the 1994 AHCPR guidelines reported annual rates of cardiac death or MI of 3 percent for patients with normal test results as compared with 18 percent event rates for patients with high-risk nuclear scan results.[291]

Discharge Planning after Uncomplicated Acute MI

Practice guidelines in the United States have indicated that stress testing (with or without imaging) can be effective in risk stratification and guiding subsequent management of hospitalized patients without acute MI in whom the clinical indications of high risk are not present.[291] This suggestion is based on the results of several clinical trials. For example, in the TIMI-IIB study of 1681 patients assigned to early catheterization and 1658 patients assigned to "watchful waiting" strategies following acute MI with thrombolysis, there was no significant difference with respect to cardiac death, MI, or anginal status. Of importance, these excellent outcomes with "watchful waiting" were obtained without any standardized approach to the use of noninvasive testing.[218] Recently, the results of the VANQWISH trial (Veterans Affairs non Q-Wave Infarction Strategies in Hospital) provided similar data for patients with non Q-wave MI.[322] Common clinical thought had been that patients with non-Q-wave MIs were more likely to have a subsequent acute event and should require more aggressive management when compared to patients with Q-wave MIs. Nonetheless, this supposition was not borne out by the VANQWISH study. A total of 920 patients were randomly assigned to "invasive" (462 patients) versus "conservative" (458 patients) management. The invasive management included early catheterization performed a median of 2 days following MI (see Chap. 41). The conservative management included the use of RNA and predischarge symptom-limited exercise ^{201}Tl study or dipyridamole ^{201}Tl study. Catheterization was recommended if recurrent angina developed with ECG changes (>2-mm ST-segment depression on exercise testing), if there were two or more reversible defects on the ^{201}Tl study, or if increased ^{201}Tl uptake was observed.[355] The probability of event-free survival was higher in patients undergoing conservative therapy than in patients undergoing the invasive therapy approach.

Despite these findings, there is discordance between the practice guidelines and the actual practice in the United States. Mark et al. reported that 72 percent of patients following acute MI underwent early catheterization in the United States, compared to only 25 percent of patients in Canada. Interestingly, there was no significant difference in 1-year mortality rates between the two countries.[323] Topol et al. have noted that only 9 percent of patients undergoing PTCA after a recent MI had stress testing prior to their angioplasty.[324a]

Both exercise[324a] and pharmacologic stress testing postmyocardial infarction has also shown to effectively identify patients at low and high risk of subsequent events.[325,326] With respect to perfusion scintigraphy, it should be noted here that the post-MI application is one in which the use of pharmacologic stress over low-level nuclear stress testing may be particularly advantageous. Although either type of stress would be recommended by the guidelines, our preference is to use pharmacologic stress. The reasons are as follows: (1) pharmacologic stress does not require that the patient be able to exercise; (2) it can be easily and safely employed as early as 2 days following MI[327,328]; (3) it lowers rather than raises blood pressure, avoiding the potential problem of myocardial rupture; and (4) it produces a maximal hyperemic stimulus, thereby obviating the need for maximal stress testing after recovery.

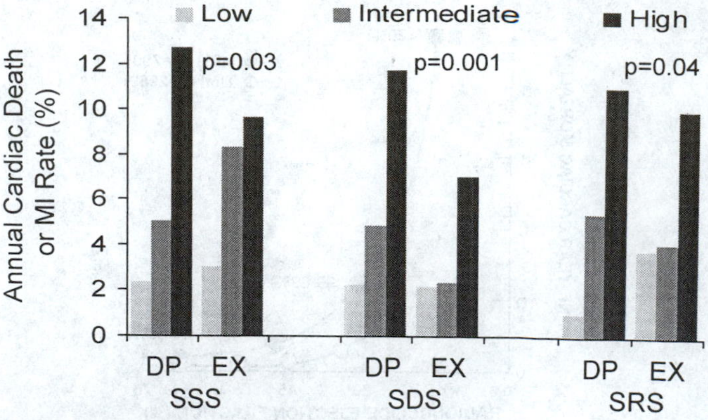

FIGURE 16-25 Annual cardiac death rate or recurrent MI rate as a function of SSS, SDS, and SRS for dipyridamole (DP) and submaximal exercise (EX) ^{99m}Tc sestamibi SPECT imaging. Event rate increased as scores increased. The ability to predict cardiac events was better for dipyridamole studies than for exercise studies for each summed score (p value depicted). All event rates are derived from risk-adjusted Cox survival curves. Intermed indicates intermediate. (From Brown et al.,[321] with permission.)

In studies performed in the postthrombolytic era by Mahmarian and colleagues suggested that adenosine thallium SPECT is effective in stratifying patients in the post-MI period.[325,329] In the most recent study, they also showed that there is incremental value in knowing the LVEF as well as the extent of jeopardized myocardium, as determined by equilibrium radionuclide angiography and adenosine ^{201}Tl myocardial perfusion SPECT.[329] These same investigators have demonstrated the value of adding LVEF to exercise myocardial perfusion SPECT.[325] As described above, these assessments can now be made with a single study using gated myocardial perfusion SPECT. Assessment of increased lung uptake of radioactivity during myocardial perfusion scintigraphy has also been shown to be of prognostic significance in patients with acute syndromes of unstable angina and non-Q-wave MI.[330] Overall, myocardial perfusion test results which have been demonstrated to indicate

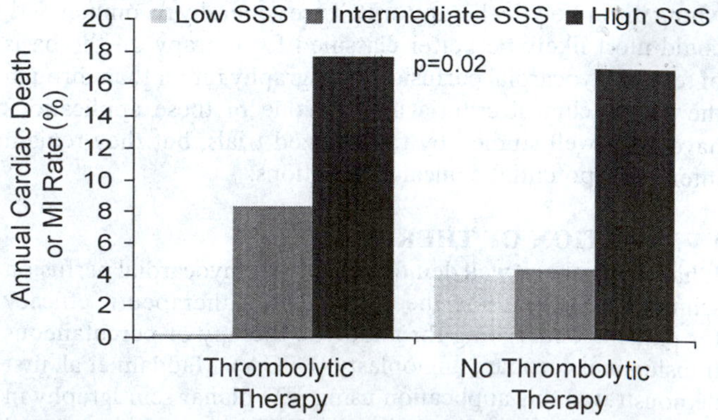

FIGURE 16-26 Annual cardiac death or MI rate as a function of SSS and thrombolytic therapy. The predictive value of SSS was greater for patients receiving thrombolysis (p = 0.02). (From Brown et al.,[331] with permission.)

high risk (and thus the need for angiography) in the predischarge patient include reversible defects in the MI zone, a multivessel defect pattern, large nonreversible defects, transient left ventricular dilation, increased lung uptake, and reduced left ventricular ejection fraction.[330a]

A recent landmark multicenter randomized trial has been reported comparing submaximal ^{99m}Tc sestamibi SPECT at discharge to early dipyridamole ^{99m}Tc sestamibi SPECT performed 2 to 4 days after acute MI.[331] A total of 451 patients presenting with first acute MI were randomized in a 3:1 ratio to either (1) an early (days 2 to 4) dipyridamole ^{99m}Tc sestamibi SPECT and a predischarge (days 6 to 12) submaximal exercise ^{99m}Tc sestamibi SPECT or (2) only the predischarge study. The very early use of dipyridamole testing was associated with no adverse events, indicating the safety of this approach in appropriately selected post-MI patients. Multivariate predictors of in-hospital events included the summed stress score and summed reversibility scores, derived using a 17-segment model with the same 0-to-4 scale described above,[56,66] as well as peak creatine kinase levels. For postdischarge cardiac events, the multivariate predictors in patients undergoing dipyridamole sestamibi SPECT were the SSS, the summed reversibility score, the summed rest score, and anterior MI. Dipyridamole sestamibi imaging showed better risk stratification than submaximal exercise myocardial perfusion imaging (Fig. 16-25). Importantly, the submaximal exercise ECG had no significant predictive value for cardiac events. Interestingly, the ability to separate low- and high-risk subsets by use the of the SSS in early dipyridamole sestamibi SPECT was significantly better for patients who received thrombolysis than for those who did not (Fig. 16-26).

The investigators found a significant interaction between the degree of reversibility on dipyridamole sestamibi imaging (SDS) and the overall stress perfusion defect size (SSS) (Fig. 16-27). In the low and intermediate summed stress score groups, the annual cardiac death or nonfatal infarction rate was low when the SDS was low (0 to 2). The event rate in patients with intermediate SSS (5 to 8) increased to 6 percent in patients with intermediate SDS (3 to 7) and to 17 percent in patients with high SDS (greater than 7). In patients with high SSS (greater than 8), the cardiac event rate was high regardless of the extent of defect reversibility by SDS. The authors concluded

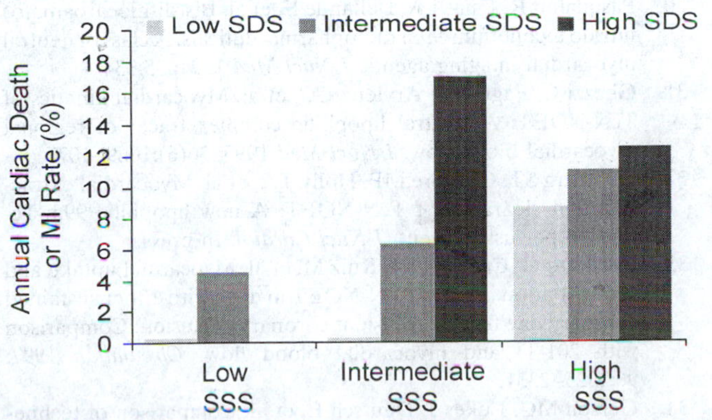

FIGURE 16-27 Annual cardiac death or MI rate as a function of SDS for a given SSS. For each SSS subgroup, cardiac event risk increased as SDS increased. The effect of SDS was greatest in the intermediate (intermed) SSS group. (From Brown et al.,[331] with permission.)

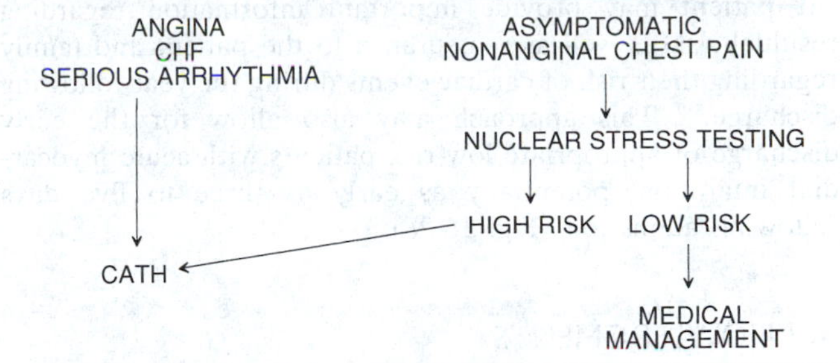

FIGURE 16-28 Management strategy for the use of nuclear stress testing in patients recovering from acute MI. Cath = catheterization; CHF = congestive heart failure.

that the dipyridamole sestamibi scanning very early after MI predicts early and late cardiac events, with superior prognostic value compared with submaximal exercise testing. They suggested that the technique can allow management decisions to be made earlier in patients with acute MI, with potentially significant cost implications associated with earlier discharge of low-risk patients.[331]

The potential of this early hospital discharge summary was discussed in an accompanying editorial.[332] The editorial points out that intervenous adenosine may be preferable to dipyramole in the very early post-MI patient owing to its very brief half-life; it also suggests that if a management strategy based on the results of this study were widely adopted, substantial cost savings could be realized in appropriate patients populations. Recent work of Dakik et al.[236] suggests that the approach to medical therapy might safely be extended to patients considered to be at moderate to even high risk following acute MI, with serial nuclear studies providing the basis for initial selection of therapy as well as for subsequent assessment of its effectiveness and consideration for therapeutic change.

It is anticipated that these results will be integrated into the future guidelines for the management of patients with acute MI.

One of the major dilemmas in post-MI patient management is the timing and use of cardiac catheterization. Conceptually, a conservative patient management approach of "watchful waiting" for provocative ischemia or recurrent symptoms could result in worse outcomes, while at the same time an aggressive approach to care (i.e., early and direct catheterization) might result in more expensive care without an improvement in outcomes.[218] In fact, the challenge for clinicians caring for acute MI patients is to identify the balance between extra clinical benefits and extra costs. Currently, routine catheterization is performed in the vast majority of patients with acute MI.[218] An alternate strategy that has been advocated in several recent national guidelines is to refer to catheterization (with consideration of early revascularization) only when clinically necessary and to use noninvasive testing to selectively identify patients for catheterization.[219] From the recent American College of Physicians (ACP) guidelines for risk stratification after MI, a 3 to 5 day assessment of ventricular function for patients with an uncomplicated hospital course is recommended.[219] For patients with preserved systolic function, a vasodilator stress myocardial perfusion SPECT early (i.e., days 2 to 4)[331] in the course of care of the uncomplicated

MI patient may provide important information regarding residual risk as well as reassurance to the patient and family regarding their risk of cardiac events during the year following discharge.[219] This approach may also allow for the early discharge of appropriate low-risk patients with acute myocardial infarction, potentially as early as three to five days following admission (Fig. 16-28).

ACKNOWLEDGMENTS

The authors gratefully acknowledge the excellent efforts of Sean Hayes, M.D., in contributing to the medical content; Suzanne Ridgway and Terry Tripodi for editorial assistance and manuscript preparation; and Xingping Kang, M.D., and James Gerlach for research and technical assistance.

References

1. Pearson T, Fuster V. Executive Summary, 27th Bethesda Conference, Matching the intensity of risk factor management with the hazard for coronary disease events. *J Am Coll Cardiol* 1996; 27(5):957–963.
2. Fuster V. Epidemic of cardiovascular disease and stroke: The three main challenges, in *American Heart Association 71st Scientific Session*. Dallas: American Heart Association, 1999.
3. Wright J, Weinstein M. Gains in life expectancy from medical interventions: Standardizing data and outcomes. *N Engl J Med* 1998; 339:380–385.
4. AHA. *1999 Heart and Stroke Statistical Update*. Dallas: American Heart Association; 1999.
5. Lonn E, Yusuf S. Evidence based cardiology: Emerging approaches in preventing cardiovascular disease. *BMJ* 1999; 318:1337–1341.
6. Law M, Wald N, Thompson S. By how much and how quickly does reduction in serum cholesterol concentration lower risk of ischemic heart disease. *BMJ* 1994; 308:367–373.
7. Yusuf S, Zucker D, Peduzzi P, et al. Effect of coronary artery bypass graft surgery on survival: Overview of 10-year results from randomized trials by the Coronary Artery Bypass Graft Surgery Trialists Collaboration. *Lancet* 1994; 344:563–570.
8. Gibbons R, Chatterjee K, Daley J, et al. ACC/AHA/ACP-ASIM guidelines for the management of patients with chronic stable angina. *J Am Coll Cardiol* 1999; 33(7):2092–2197.
9. Shaw L, Hachamovitch R. Papatheofanis. *Outcomes and Technology Assessment in Nuclear Medicine*. Society of Nuclear Medicine; Reston, VA. In press.
10. Lebowitz E, Greene M, Bradley-Moore P, et al. Tl-201 for medical use (abstr). *J Nucl Med* 1973; 14:421.
11. Nielsen AP, Morris KG, Murdock BS, et al. Linear relationship between the distribution of thallium-201 and blood flow in ischemic and nonischemic myocardium during exercise. *Circulation* 1980; 61:797–801.
12. L'Abbate A, Biagin A, Michelassic, et al. Myocardial kinetics of thallium and potassium in man. *Circulation* 1979; 60:776.
13. Strauss HW, Harrison BS, Pitt B. Thallium-201: Noninvasive determination of the regional distribution of cardiac output. *J Nucl Med* 1977; 18:1167.
14. Bradley-Moore PR, Lebowitz E, Greene M, et al. Tl-201 for medical use: II. Biologic behavior. *J Nucl Med* 1975; 16:156.
15. Angello DA, Wilson RA, Palac RT. Effect of eating on thallium-201 myocardial redistribution after myocardial ischemia. *Am J Cardiol* 1987; 60(7):528–533.
16. Berman D, Maddahi J, Charuzi Y, et al. Rate of redistribution in Tl-201 exercise myocardial scintigraphy: Inverse relationship to degree of coronary stenosis (abstr). *Circulation* 1978; 58(suppl 2):II-63.
17. Gutman J, Berman DS, Freeman M, et al. Time to completed redistribution of thallium-201 in exercise myocardial scintigraphy: Relationship to the degree of coronary artery stenosis. *Am Heart J* 1983; 106(5 pt 1):989–995.
18. Li Q-S, Frank TL, Franceschi D, et al. Technetium-99m methoxyisobutyl isonitrile (RP30) for quantification of myocardial ischemia and reperfusion in dogs. *J Nucl Med* 1988; 29: 1539.
19. Sinusas AJ, Bergin JD, Edwards NC, et al. Redistribution of ^{99m}Tc-sestamibi and ^{201}Tl in the presence of a severe coronary artery stenosis. *Circulation* 1994; 89:2332.
20. Leppo JA, Meerdink DJ. Comparison of the myocardial uptake of a technetium-labeled isonitrile analogue and thallium. *Circ Res* 1989; 65(3):632–639.
21. Hurwitz GA, Blais M, Powe JE, et al. Stress/injection protocols for myocardial scintigraphy with 99Tcm-sestamibi compared with 201Tl: Implications of early post-stress kinetics. *Nucl Med Commun* 1996; 17(5):400–409.
22. Udelson JE. Choosing a thallium-201 or technetium 99m sestamibi imaging protocol. *J Nucl Cardiol* 1994; 1(5 pt 2):S995–S108.
23. Dahlberg ST, Leppo JA. Myocardial kinetics of radiolabeled perfusion agents: Basis for perfusion imaging. *J Nucl Cardiol* 1994; 1(2 pt 1):189–97.
24. Jain D, Wackers FJ, Mattera J, et al. Biokinetics of technetium-99m-tetrofosmin: Myocardial perfusion imaging agent: Implications for a one-day imaging protocol. *J Nucl Med* 1993; 34(8):1254–1259.
25. Wackers FJ, Berman DS, Maddahi J, et al., Technetium-99m hexakis 2-methoxyisobutyl isonitrile: Human biodistribution, dosimetry, safety, and preliminary comparison to thallium-201 for myocardial perfusion imaging. *J Nucl Med* 1989; 30(3): 301–311.
26. Meerdink DJ, Leppo JA. Experimental properties of technetium-99m agents: Myocardial transport of perfusion imaging agents. *Am J Cardiol* 1990; 66:9E–15E.
27. Leppo JA, Meerdink DJ. Comparative myocardial extraction of two technetium-labeled BATO derivatives (SQ30217, SQ30214) and thallium. *J Nucl Med* 1990; 31:67–74.
28. Chua T, Kiat H, Germano G, et al. Technetium-99m teboroxime regional myocardial washout in subjects with and without coronary artery disease. *Am J Cardiol* 1993; 72(9):728–734.
29. Chua T, Kiat H, Germano G, et al., Rapid back to back adenosine stress/rest technetium-99m teboroxime myocardial perfusion SPECT using a triple-detector camera. *J Nucl Med* 1993; 34(9):1485–1493.
30. Pasqualini R, Duatti A, Bellande E, et al. Bis(dithiocarbamato) nitrido technetium-99m radiopharmaceuticals: A class of neutral myocardial imaging agents. *J Nucl Med* 1994; 35:334.
31. Ghezzi C, Fagret D, Arvieux CC, et al. Myocardial kinetics of TcN-NOET: A neutral lipophilic complex tracer of regional myocardial blood flow. *J Nucl Med* 1995; 36(6):1069–1077.
32. Dahlberg ST, Gilmore MP, Holly TA, et al. Myocardial extraction and clearance of TcN-NOET: A new lipophilic 99m-Tc-labeled perfusion agent. *J Nucl Cardiol*. In press.
33. Vanzetto G, Calnon DA, Ruiz M, et al. Myocardial uptake and redistribution of 99m-Tc-N-NOET in dogs with either sustained coronary low flow or transient coronary occlusion: Comparison with 201-Tl and myocardial blood flow. *Circulation* 1997; 96:2325–2331.
34. Gerson MC, Lukes J, Deutsch E, et al. Comparison of technetium 99m Q12 and thallium 201 for detection of angiographically documented coronary artery disease in humans. *J Nucl Cardiol* 1994; 1(6):499–508.
35. Hendel RC, Verani MS, Miller DD, et al. Diagnostic utility of tomographic myocardial perfusion imaging with technetium

99m furifosmin (Q12) compared with thallium 201: Results of a phase III multicenter trial. *J Nucl Cardiol* 1996; 3(4):291–300.
36. Dilsizian V, Rocco TP, Freedman NM, et al. Enhanced detection of ischemic but viable myocardium by the reinjection of thallium after stress-redistribution imaging. *N Engl J Med* 1990; 323(3):141–146.
37. Dilsizian V, Smeltzer WR, Freedman NM, et al. Thallium reinjection after stress-redistribution imaging: Does 24-hour delayed imaging after reinjection enhance detection of viable myocardium? *Circulation* 1991; 83(4):1247–1255.
38. Basu S, Senior R, Raval U, et al. Superiority of nitrate-enhanced 201Tl over conventional redistribution 201Tl imaging for prognostic evaluation after myocardial infarction and thrombolysis. *Circulation* 1997; 96(9):2932–2937.
39. Pohost GM, Zir LM, Moore RH, et al. Differentiation of transiently ischemic from infarcted myocardium by serial imaging after a single dose of thallium-201. *Circulation* 1977; 55(2): 294–302.
40. Pagley PR, Beller GA, Watson DD, et al. Improved outcome after coronary artery bypass surgery in patients with ischemic cardiomyopathy and residual myocardial viability. *Circulation* 1997; 96(3):793–800.
41. Bateman TM. Nuclear cardiology in private practice. *J Nucl Cardiol* 1997; 4(2 Pt 2):S184–S188.
42. Mahmarian JJ, Boyce TM, Goldberg RK, et al. Quantitative exercise thallium-201 single photon emission computed tomography for the enhanced diagnosis of ischemic heart disease. *J Am Coll Cardiol* 1990; 15(2):318–329.
43. Mahmarian J. State of the art for coronary artery disease detection: thallium-201. In: Zaret BL, Beller G, eds. *Nuclear Cardiology: State of the Art and Future Directions,* 2nd ed. St. Louis: Mosby; 1998:237–272.
44. Friedman J, Van Train K, Maddahi J, et al. "Upward creep" of the heart: A frequent source of false-positive reversible defects during thallium-201 stress-redistribution SPECT. *J Nucl Med* 1989; 30(10):1718–1722.
45. Germano G, Erel J, Kiat H, et al. Quantitative LVEF and qualitative regional function from gated thallium-201 perfusion SPECT. *J Nucl Med* 1997; 38(5):749–754.
46. Berman DS, Kiat H, Maddahi J. The new 99mTc myocardial perfusion imaging agents: 99mTc-sestamibi and 99mTc-teboroxime. *Circulation* 1991; 84(3 suppl):17–21.
47. Berman D, Kiat H, Germano G, et al. 99m Tc-sestamibi SPECT. In DePuey EG, Berman DS, Garcia EV, *Cardiac SPECT Imaging.* New York: Raven Press; 1995: 121–146.
48. Van Train KF, Areeda J, Garcia EV, et al. Quantitative same-day rest-stress technetium-99m-sestamibi SPECT: Definition and validation of stress normal limits and criteria for abnormality. *J Nucl Med* 1993; 34(9):1494–1502.
49. Buell U, Dupont F, Uebis R, et al. 99Tcm-methoxy-isobutylisonitrile SPECT to evaluate a perfusion index from regional myocardial uptake after exercise and at rest: Results of a four hour protocol in patients with coronary heart disease and in controls. *Nucl Med Commun* 1990; 11(2):77–94.
50. Heo J, Kegel J, Iskandrian AS, et al. Comparison of same-day protocols using technetium-99m-sestamibi myocardial imaging. *J Nucl Med* 1992; 33(2):186–191.
51. Taillefer R, Gagnon A, Laflamme L, et al. Same day injections of Tc-99m methoxy isobutyl isonitrile (hexamibi) for myocardial tomographic imaging: Comparison between rest-stress and stress-rest injection sequences. *Eur J Nucl Med* 1989; 15(3):113–117.
52. Marzullo P, Parodi O, Reisenhofer B, et al. Value of rest thallium-201/technetium-99m sestamibi scans and dobutamine echocardiography for detecting myocardial viability. *Am J Cardiol* 1993; 71(2):166–172.
53. Berman DS, Kiat HS, Van Train KF, et al. Myocardial perfusion imaging with technetium-99m-sestamibi: Comparative analysis of available imaging protocols. *J Nucl Med* 1994; 35(4):681–688.
54. Sciagrà R, Bisi G, Santoro GM, et al. Comparison of baseline-nitrate technetium-99m sestamibi with rest-redistribution thallium-201 tomography in detecting viable hibernating myocardium and predicting postrevascularization recovery. *J Am Coll Cardiol* 1997; 30(2):384–391.
55. He Z, Verani M. Evaluation of myocardial viability by myocardial perfusion imaging: Should nitrates be used? *J Nucl Cardiol* 1998; 5:527–532.
56. Berman DS, Kiat H, Friedman JD, et al. Separate acquisition rest thallium-201/stress technetium-99m sestamibi dual-isotope myocardial perfusion single-photon emission computed tomography: A clinical validation study. *J Am Coll Cardiol* 1993; 22(5):1455–1464.
57. Nakamura M, Takeda K, Ichihara T, et al. Feasibility of simultaneous stress 99m-Tc-sestamibi/rest 201-Tl dual isotope myocardial perfusion SPECT in the detection of coronary artery disease. *J Nucl Med* 1999; 40:895–903.
58. Berman D. Imaging in cardiovascular disease. In: Pohost G, Berman DS, Germano G, eds. *Myocardial Perfusion Single Photon Approaches.* Philadelphia: Lippincott Williams, & Wilkins; 2000. In press.
59. Ficaro EP, Fessler JA, Shreve PD, et al. Simultaneous transmission/emission myocardial perfusion tomography: Diagnostic accuracy of attenuation-corrected 99mTc-sestamibi single-photon emission computed tomography. *Circulation* 1996; 93(3):463–473.
60. Cullom S, Hendel R, Liu L, et al. Diagnostic accuracy and image quality of a scatter, attenuation and resolution compensation method for Tc-99m cardiac SPECT: Preliminary results (abstr). *J Nucl Med* 1996; 37(5):81P.
61. Berman DS, Kiat H, Van Train K, et al. Technetium 99m sestamibi in the assessment of chronic coronary artery disease. *Semin Nucl Med* 1991; 21(3):190–212.
62. Reisman S, Berman D, Maddahi J, et al. The severe stress thallium defect: An indicator of critical coronary stenosis. *Am Heart J* 1985; 110(1 pt 1):128–134.
63. Matzer L, Kiat H, Van Train K, et al. Quantitative severity of stress thallium-201 myocardial perfusion single-photon emission computed tomography defects in one-vessel coronary artery disease. *Am J Cardiol* 1993; 72(3):273–279.
64. Port SC. Imaging guidelines for nuclear cardiology procedures: Part 2. *J Nucl Cardiol* 1999; 6(2):G49–G84.
65. Berman DS, Hachamovitch R, Kiat H, et al. Incremental value of prognostic testing in patients with known or suspected ischemic heart disease: A basis for optimal utilization of exercise technetium-99m sestamibi myocardial perfusion single-photon emission computed tomography. *J Am Coll Cardiol* 1995; 26(3):639–647.
66. Hachamovitch R, Berman DS, Kiat H, et al. Exercise myocardial perfusion SPECT in patients without known coronary artery disease: Incremental prognostic value and use in risk stratification. *Circulation* 1996; 93(5):905–914.
67. Hachamovitch R, Berman DS, Shaw LJ, et al. Incremental prognostic value of myocardial perfusion single photon emission computed tomography for the prediction of cardiac death: Differential stratification for risk of cardiac death and myocardial infarction. *Circulation* 1998; 97(6):535–543.
68. Berman DS, Germano G. Clinical applications of nuclear cardiology. In: Germano G, Berman DS, eds. *Clinical Gated Cardiac SPECT.* Armonk, NY: Futura: 1991:1–71.
69. Germano G, Van Train K, Kiat H, et al. Digital techniques for the acquisition, processing, and analysis of nuclear cardiology images. In: Sandler MP, *Diagnostic Nuclear Medicine.* Baltimore: Williams & Wilkins; 1995; 347–386.
70. Smith WH, Kastner RJ, Calnon DA, et al. Quantitative gated

single photon emission computed tomography imaging: A counts-based method for display and measurement of regional and global ventricular systolic function. *J Nucl Cardiol* 1997; 4(6):451–463.
71. Calnon DA, Kastner RJ, Smith WH, et al. Validation of a new counts-based gated single photon emission computed tomography method for quantifying left ventricular systolic function: Comparison with equilibrium radionuclide angiography. *J Nucl Cardiol* 1997; 4(6):464–471.
72. Germano G, Kiat H, Kavanagh PB, et al. Automatic quantification of ejection fraction from gated myocardial perfusion SPECT. *J Nucl Med* 1995; 36(11):2138–2147.
73. Faber TL, Cooke CD, Folks RD, et al. Left ventricular function and perfusion from gated SPECT perfusion images: An integrated method. *J Nucl Med* 1999; 40(4):650–659.
74. Faber TL, Akers MS, Peshock RM, et al. Three-dimensional motion and perfusion quantification in gated single-photon emission computed tomograms. *J Nucl Med* 1991; 32(12):2311–2317.
75. Faber TL, Stokely EM, Peshock RM, et al. A model-based four-dimensional left ventricular surface detector. *IEEE Trans Med Imaging* 1991; 10(3):321–329.
76. Goris ML, Thompson C, Malone LJ, et al., Modelling the integration of myocardial regional perfusion and function. *Nucl Med Commun* 1994; 15(1):9–20.
77. Germano G, Berman DS. Quantitative gated perfusion SPECT. In: Germano G, Berman DS, eds. *Clinical Gated Cardiac SPECT.* Armonk, NY: Futura; 1999:115–146.
78. Kang X, Berman D, Germano G, et al. Normal parameters of left ventricle volume and ejection fraction measured by gated myocardial perfusion SPECT (abstr). *J Am Coll Cardiol* 1999; 33(2 suppl.A):409A.
79. Case J, Bateman T, Moutray K, et al. Establishing normal limits for LVEF from ECG-gated resting Tl-201 myocardial perfusion SPECT imaging (abstr). *J Nucl Cardiol* 1999; 6(1, part 2):S116.
80. Fujino S, Masuyama K, Kanayama S, et al. Early and delayed technetium-99m labeled sestamibi myocardial ECG-gated SPECT by QGS program in normal volunteers (abstr). *J Nucl Med* 1999; 40(5):180P.
81. Case J, Cullom S, Bateman T et al. Overestimation of LVEF by gated MIBI myocardial perfusion SPECT in patients with small hearts (abstr). *J Am Coll Cardiol* 1998; 31(2, suppl.A):43A.
82. Bisi G, Sciagra R, Santoro GM, et al. Sublingual isosorbide dinitrate to improve technetium-99m-teboroxime perfusion defect reversibility. *J Nucl Medi* 1994; 35:1274–1278.
83. He ZX, Darcourt J, Guignier A, et al. Nitrates improve detection of ischemic but viable myocardium by thallium-201 reinjection SPECT [published erratum appears in *J Nucl Med* 1993; 34(11):1909]. *J Nucl Med* 1993; 34(9):1472–1477.
84. Sciagra R, Bisi G, Santoro GM, et al. Comparison of baseline-nitrate technetium-99m sestamibi with rest-redistribution thallium-201 tomography in detecting viable hibernating myocardium and predicting post-revasularization recovery. *J Am Coll Cardiol* 1997; 30:384–391.
85. Galli M, Marcassa C, Imparato A, et al. Effects of nitroglycerin by technetium-99m sestamibi tomoscintigraphy on resting regional myocardial hypoperfusion in stable patients with healed myocardial infarction. *Am J Cardiol* 1994; 74(9):843–848.
86. Maurea S, Cuocolo A, Soricelli A, et al. Enhanced detection of viable myocardium by technetium-99m-MIBI imaging after nitrate administration in chronic coronary artery disease. *J Nucl Med* 1995; 36(11):1945–1952.
87. Bonow R. Assessment of myocardial viability with thallium-201. In: Zaret BL, Beller G, eds. *Nuclear Cardiology: State of the Art and Future Directions,* 2d ed. St. Louis: Mosby; 1998:503–512.
88. Udelson JE, Coleman PS, Metherall J, et al. Predicting recovery of severe regional ventricular dysfunction: Comparison of resting scintigraphy with 201Tl and 99mTc-sestamibi. *Circulation* 1994; 89(6):2552–2561.
89. Weiss AT, Berman DS, Lew AS, et al. Transient ischemic dilation of the left ventricle on stress thallium-201 scintigraphy: A marker of severe and extensive coronary artery disease. *J Am Coll Cardiol* 1987; 9(4):752–759.
90. Mazzanti M, Germano G, Kiat H, et al. Identification of severe and extensive coronary artery disease by automatic measurement of transient ischemic dilation of the left ventricle in dual-isotope myocardial perfusion SPECT. *J Am Coll Cardiol* 1996; 27(7):1612–1620.
91. Chouraqui P, Rodrigues EA, Berman DS, et al. Significance of dipyridamole-induced transient dilation of the left ventricle during thallium-201 scintigraphy in suspected coronary artery disease. *Am J Cardiol* 1990; 66(7):689–694.
92. Hansen CL, Sangrigoli R, Nkadi E, et al. Comparison of pulmonary uptake with transient cavity dilation after exercise thallium-201 perfusion imaging. *J Am Coll Cardiol* 1999; 33(5):1323–1327.
93. Boucher CA, Zir LM, Beller GA, et al. Increased lung uptake of thallium-201 during exercise myocardial imaging: Clinical, hemodynamic and angiographic implications in patients with coronary artery disease. *Am J Cardiol* 1980; 46(2):189–96.
94. Tamaki N, Itoh H, Ishii T, et al. Hemodynamic significance of increased lung uptake. *Am J Roentgenol* 1982; 138(2):223–228.
95. Bacher-Stier C, Sharir T, Kavanagh P, et al. Post-exercise lung uptake of Tc-99m sestamibi determined by a new automatic technique: Validation and application in detection of severe and extensive coronary ariery disease and reduced left ventricular function. *J Nucl Med.* In press.
96. Gill JB, Ruddy TD, Newell JB, et al. Prognostic importance of thallium uptake by the lungs during exercise in coronary artery disease. *N Engl J Med* 1987; 317(24):1486–1489.
97. Hurwitz G, Fox S, Driedger A, et al. Pulmonary uptake of sestamibi on early post-stress images: Angiographic relationships, incidence and kinetics. *Nucl Med Commun* 1993; 14:15–22.
98. Hurwitz G, Ghali S, Husni M. Pulmonary uptake of technetium-99m sestamibi induced by dipyridamole-based stress or exercise. *J Nucl Med* 1998; 39:339–345.
99. Giubbini R, Campini R, Milan E. Evaluation of technetium-99m sestamibi lung uptake: Correlation with left ventricular function. *J Nucl Med* 1995; 36:58–63.
100. Iskandrian A. State of the art for pharmacologic stress imaging. In: Zaret BL, Beller G, eds. *Nuclear Cardiology: State of the Art and Future Directions,* 2d ed. St. Louis: Mosby; 1998: 312–330.
101. Picano E, Marini C, Pirelli S, et al. Safety of intravenous high-dose dipyridamole echocardiography. *Am J Cardiol* 1992; 70:252–258.
102. Lette J, Tatum JL, Fraser S, et al. Safety of dipyridamole testing in 73,806 patients: The Multicenter Dipyridamole Safety Study. *J Nucl Cardiol* 1995; 2(1):3–17.
103. Verani MS, Mahmarian JJ. Myocardial perfusion scintigraphy during maximol coronary artery vasodilation with adenosine. *Am J Cardiol* 1991; 67:12D–17D.
104. Verani MS, Mahmarian JJ, Hixson JB, et al. Diagnosis of coronary artery disease by controlled coronary vasodilation with adenosine and thallium-201 scintigraphy in patients unable to exercise. *Circulation* 1990; 82:80–87.
105. Smits P, Thien T, van't Laar A. Circulation effects of coffee in relation to the pharmacokinetics of caffeine. *Am J Cardiol* 1985; 56:958–963.
106. Amanullah AM, Berman DS, Kiat H, et al. Usefulness of hemodynamic changes during adenosine infusion in predicting the diagnostic accuracy of adenosine technetium-99m sestamibi single-photon emission computed tomography (SPECT). *Am J Cardiol* 1997; 79(10):1319–1322.
107. Cerqueira MD, Verani MS, Schwaiger M, et al. Safety profile of

adenosine stress perfusion imaging: Results from the Adenoscan Multicenter Trial Registry. *J Am Coll Cardiol* 1994; 23:384–389.
108. Pennell DJ, Mavrogeni SI, Forbat SM, et al. Adenosine combined with dynamic exercise for myocardial perfusion imaging. *J Am Coll Cardiol* 1995; 25(6):1300–1309.
109. Mason JR, Palac RT, Freeman ML, et al. Thallium scintigraphy during dobutamine infusion: Nonexercise-dependent screening test for coronary disease. *Am Heart J* 1984; 107(3):481–485.
110. Pennell DJ, Underwood SR, Swanton RH, et al. Dobutamine thallium myocardial perfusion tomography. *J Am Coll Cardiol* 1991; 18(6):1471–1479.
111. Iskandrian AS, Verani MS, Heo J. Pharmacologic stress testing: Mechanism of action, hemodynamic responses, and results in detection of coronary artery disease. *J Nucl Cardiol* 1994; 1(1):94–111.
112. Cerqueira MD. Pharmacologic stress versus maximal-exercise stress for perfusion imaging: Which, when, and why? *J Nucl Cardiol* 1996; 3(6 pt 2):S10–S14.
113. Elhendy A, Valkema R, van Domburg RT, et al. Safety of dobutamine-atropine stress myocardial perfusion scintigraphy. *J Nucl Med* 1998; 39:162–166.
114. Dennis CA, Pool PE, Perrins EJ, et al. Stress testing with closed-loop arbutamine as an alternative to exercise. *J Am Coll Cardiol* 1995; 26:1151–1158.
115. Kiat H, Iskandrian AS, Villegas BJ, et al. Arbutamine stress thallium-201 single-photon emission computed tomography using a computerized closed-loop delivery system: Multicenter trial for evaluation of safety and diagnostic accuracy. *J Am Coll Cardiol* 1995; 26:1159–1167.
116. Hirzel HO, Senn M, Nuesch K, et al. Thallium-201 scintigraphy in complete left bundle branch block. *Am J Cardiol* 1984; 53(6):764–769.
117. Skalidis EI, Kochiadakis GE, Koukouraki SI, et al. Phasic coronary flow pattern and flow reserve in patients with left bundle branch block and normal coronary arteries. *J Am Coll Cardiol* 1999; 33:1338–1346.
118. Rockett J, Wood W, Moinuddim M. Intravenous dipyridamole thallium-201 SPECT imaging in patients with left bundle branch block. *Clin Nucl Med* 1990; 15:401.
119. O'Keefe J, Bateman T, Barnhart C. Adenosine thallium-201 is superior to exercise thallium-201 for detecting coronary artery disease in patients with left bundle branch block. *J Am Coll Cardiol* 1993;21:1332–1338.
120. Tamaki N. Fatty acid imaging. In: Pohost G, et al., eds. *Imaging in Cardiovascular Disease.* Philadelphia: Lippincott Williams & Wilkins: In press.
121. Caldwell JH, Martin GV, Link JM. Iodophenylpentadecanoic acid-myocardial blood flow relationship during maximal exercise with coronary occlusion. *J Nucl Med* 1990; 31:99–105.
122. Hansen CL, Heo J, Oliner CM, et al. Prediction of improvement in left ventricular function with iodine-123-IPPA after coronary revascularization. *J Nucl Med* 1995; 36:1987–1993.
123. Iskandrian AS, Power J, Cave V, et al. Assessment of myocardial viability by dynamic tomographic 123-I-iodophenylpentadecanoic acid imaging: Comparison to rest-redistribution thallium imaging. *J Nucl Cardiol* 1995; 2:101–109.
124. Knapp FF Jr, Goodman MM, Callahan AP, et al. Radioiodinated 15-(p-iodophenyl)-3, 3-dimethylpentadecanoic acid: A useful new agent to evaluate myocardial fatty acid uptake. *J Nucl Med* 1986; 27:521–531.
125. Saito T, Yasuda T, Gold HK, et al. Differentiation of regional perfusion and fatty acid uptake in zones of myocardial injury. *Nucl Med Commun* 1991; 12:663–675.
126. Furutani Y, Shiigi T, Nakamura Y, et al. Quantification of area at risk in acute myocardial infarction by tomographic imaging. *J Nucl Med* 1997; 38:1875–1882.
126a. Kawai Y, Tsukamoto E, Nozaki Y, et al. Use of 123I-BMIPP single-photon emission tomography to estimate areas at risk following successful revascularization in patients with acute myocardial infarction. *Eur J Nucl Med* 1998; 25:1390–1395.
127. Tateno M, Tamaki N, Kudoh T, et al. Assessment of fatty acid uptake in patients with ischemic heart disease without myocardial infarction. *J Nucl Med* 1996; 37:1981–1985.
128. Dae MW. Imaging of myocardial innervation. In: Pohost G, et al., eds. *Imaging in Cardiovascular Disease.* Philadelphia: Lippincott Williams & Wilkins. In press.
129. Whitby LG, Axelrod J, Weil-Malherbe H. The fate of 3H-norepinephrine in animals. *J Pharm Exp Ther* 1961; 132:193–201.
130. Wieland DM, Brown LE, Roger WL, et al. Myocardial imaging with a radioiodinated norepinephrine storage analog. *J Nucl Med* 1981; 22:22–31.
131. Dae MW, O'Connell JW, Botvinick EH, et al. Scintigraphic assessment of regional cardiac adrenergic innervation. *Circulation* 1989; 79(3):634–644.
132. Dae M, O'Connell J, Botvinick E, et al. Acute and chronic effects of transient myocardial ischemia on sympathetic nerve activity, density, and norepinephrine content. *Cardiovasc Res* 1995; 30:270–280.
133. Lanza GA, Giordano A, Pristipino C, et al. Abnormal cardiac adrenergic nerve function in patients with syndrome X detected by 123I metaiodobenzylguanidine myocardial scintigraphy. *Circulation* 1997; 96:821–826.
134. Schnell O, Muhr D, Dresel S, et al. Partial restoration of scintigraphically assessed cardiac sympathetic denervation in newly diagnosed patients with insulin-dependent (type 1) diabetes mellitus at one-year follow-up. *Diabetic Med* 1997; 14:57–62.
135. Mitrani R, Klein L, Miles W, et al. Regional cardiac sympathetic denervation in patients with ventricular tachycardia in the absence of coronary artery disease. *J Am Coll Cardiol* 1993; 22:1344–1353.
136. Gill J, Hunter G, Gane J, et al. Asymmetry of cardiac 123I metaiodobenzylguanidine scans in patients with ventricular tachycardia and a "clinically normal" heart. *Br Heart J* 1993; 69:6–13.
137. Wichter T, Hindricks G, Lerch H, et al. Regional myocardial sympathetic dysinervation in arrhythmogenic right ventricular cardiomyopathy—An analysis using 123 I-meta-iodobenzylguanidine scintigraphy. *Circulation* 1994; 89:667–683.
138. Schafers M, Wichter T, Lerch H, et al. 123 I-MIBG uptake in idiopathic ventricular tachycardia and fibrillation. *J Nucl Med* 1999; 40:1–5.
139. Henderson EB, Kahn JK, Corbett JK, et al. Abnormal I-123 metaidobenzylguanidine myocardial washout and distribution may reflect myocardial adrenergic derangement in patients with congestive cardiomyopathy. *Circulation* 1988; 78:1192–1199.
140. Eichhorn E, Hjalmarson A. Beta-blocker treatment for chronic heart failure. *Circulation* 1994; 90:2153–2156.
141. Nakata T, Miyamoto K, Doe A, et al. Cardiac death prediction and impaired cardiac sympathetic innervation assessed by MIBG in patients with failing and nonfailing hearts. *J Nucl Cardiol* 1998. 5:579–590.
142. Fukukoa S, Hayashida K, Hirose Y, et al. Use of iodine-123 metaiodobenzylguanidine myocardial imaging to predict the effectiveness of beta-blocker therapy in patients with dilated cardiomyopathy. *Eur J Nucl Med* 1997; 24:523–529.
143. Suwa M, Otake Y, Moriguchi A, et al. Iodine-123 metaiodobenzylguanidine myocardial scintigraphy for prediction of response to beta-blocker therapy in patients with dilated cardiomyopathy. *Am Heart J* 1997; 133:353–358.
144. Krause T, Joseph A, Kutzner C, et al. Acute myocardial infarction delineated by noninvasive thallium-201/technetium-99m pyrophosphate tomography. *Nucl Med Commum* 1990; 11(9): 617–629.
145. Krause T, Kasper W, Zeiher A, et al. Relation of technetium-

99m pyrophosphate accumulation to time interval after onset of acute myocardial infarction as assessed by a tomographic acquisition technique. *Am J Cardiol* 1991; 68(17):1575–1579.

146. Bonte FJ, Parkey RW, Graham KD, et al. A new method for radionuclide imaging of myocardial infarcts. *Radiology* 1974; 110(2):473–474.

147. Willerson JT, Parkey RW, Bonte FJ, et al. Acute subendocardial myocardial infarction in patients. Its detection by Technetium 99-m stannous pyrophosphate myocardial scintigrams. *Circulation* 1975; 51(3):436–441.

148. Berman DS, Amsterdam EA, Hines HH, et al. New approach to interpretation of technetium-99m pyrophosphate scintigraphy in detection of acute myocardial infarction: Clinical assessment of diagnostic accuracy. *Am J Cardiol* 1977; 39(3):341–346.

149. Tamaki N, Yamada T, Matsumori A, et al. Indium-III-antimyosin antibody imaging for detecting different stages of myocardial infarction: Comparison with technetium-99m-pyrophosphate imaging. *J Nucl Med* 1990; 31(2):136–142.

150. Gerson MC, McGoron AJ. Technetium 99m glucarate: What will be its clinical role? (editorial). *J Nucl Cardiol* 1997; 4(4): 336–340.

151. Narula J, Khaw BA, Dec GW, et al. Diagnostic accuracy of antimyosin scintigraphy in suspected myocarditis (abstr). *J Nucl Cardiol* 1996; 3(5):371–381.

151a. Ballester M, Bordes R, Tazelaar HD, et al. Evaluation of biopsy classification for rejection: Relation to detection of myocardial damage by monoclonal antimyosin antibody imaging. *J Am Coll Cardiol* 1998; 31:1357–1361.

152. Narula J, Petrov A, Pak K, et al. Very early noninvasive detection of acute experimental nonreperfused myocardial infarction with 99m-Tc-labeled glucarate. *Circulation* 1997; 95:1577–1584.

153. Bisi G, Sciagra R, Bull U, et al. Assessment of ventricular function with first-pass radionuclide angiography using technetium 99m hexakis-2-methoxyisobutylisonitrile: A European multicentre study. *Eur J Nucl Med* 1991; 18(3):178–183.

154. Moore ML, Murphy PH, Burdine JA. ECG-gated emission computed tomography of the cardiac blood pool. *Radiology* 1980; 134(1):233–235.

155. Tamaki N, Mukai T, Ishii Y, et al. Multiaxial tomography of heart chambers by gated blood-pool emission computed tomography using a rotating gamma camera. *Radiology* 1983; 147(2):547–554.

156. Van Krienkinge SD, Berman DS, Germano G. Automatic quantification of left ventricular ejection fraction from gated blood pool SPECT. *J Nucl Cardiol* 1999; 6:498–506.

157. Jones RH. Use of radionucline measurements of left ventricular function for prognosis in patients with coronary artery disease. *Semin Nucl Med* 1987; 12:95–103.

158. Borges-Neto S, Coleman RE, Jones RH. Perfusion and function at rest and treadmill exercise using technetium-99m-sestamibi: Comparison of one- and two-day protocols in normal volunteers. *J Nucl Med* 1990; 31(7):1128–1132.

159. Friedman JD, Berman DS, Kiat H, et al. Rest and treadmill exercise first-pass radionuclide ventriculography: Validation of left ventricular ejection fraction measurements. *J Nucl Cardiol* 1994; 1(4):382–388.

160. Borer JS, Bacharach SL, Green MV, et al. Real-time radionuclide cineangiography in the noninvasive evaluation of global and regional left ventricular function at rest and during exercise in patients with coronary artery disease. *N Engl J Med* 1977; 296(15):839–844.

161. Bourguignon MH, Douglass KH, Links JM, et al. Fully automated data acquisition, processing, and display in equilibrium radioventriculography. *Eur J Nucl Med* 1981; 6:343–347.

162. Hains ADB, Al-Khawaja I, Hinge DA, et al. Radionuclide left ventricular ejection fraction: A comparison of three methods. *Br Heart J* 1987; 57:242–246.

163. Maddahi J, Berman DS, Matsuoka DT, et al. A new technique for assessment of right ventricular ejection fraction by multiple gated equilibrium scintigraphy: Description, validation and findings in chronic coronary artery disease. *Circulation* 1979; 60:581–589.

164. Hains ADB, Al-Khawaja IM, Hinge DA. Radionuclide left ventricular function ejection fraction. A comparison of three methods. *Br Heart J* 1986; 57(3):242.

165. Maddahi J, Berman DS, Silverberg R, et al. Validation of a two-minute technique for multiple gated scintigraphic assessment of left ventricular ejection fraction and regional wall motion. *J Nucl Med* 1978; 19:669.

166. Diamond GA, Forrester JS. Analysis of probability as an aid in the clinical diagnosis of coronary artery disease. *N Engl J Med* 1979; 300(24):1350–1358.

167. Grundy SM, Pasternak R, Greenland P, et al. Assessment of cardiovascular risk by use of multiple-risk-factor assessment equations: A statement for healthcare professionals from the American Heart Association and the American College of Cardiology. *Circulation* 1999; 100(13):1481–1492.

168. Pryor DB, Harrell FE, Lee KL, et al. Estimating the likelihood of significant coronary artery disease. *Am J Med* 1983; 73: 771–780.

169. Pryor DB, Shaw L, Harrell FE Jr, et al. Estimating the likelihood of severe coronary artery disease. *Am J Med* 1991; 90(5): 553–562.

170. Pryor DB, Shaw L, McCants CB, et al. Value of the history and physical in identifying patients at increased risk for coronary artery disease. *Ann Intern Med* 1993; 118:81–90.

171. Diamond GA, Staniloff HM, Forrester JS, et al. Computer-assisted diagnosis in the noninvasive evaluation of patients with suspected coronary artery disease. *J Am Coll Cardiol* 1983; 1(2 pt 1):444–455.

172. Berman D, Hachamovitch R, Lewin H, et al. Risk stratification in coronary artery disease: Implications for stabilization and prevention. *Am J Cardiol* 1997; 79(12B):10–16.

173. Fleischmann KE, Hunink MG, Kuntz KM, et al. Exercise echocardiography or exercise SPECT imaging? A meta-analysis of diagnostic test performance. *JAMA* 1998; 280(10):913–920.

174. Taillefer R, DePuey EG, Udelson JE, et al. Comparative diagnostic accuracy of Tl-201 and Tc-99m sestamibi SPECT imaging (perfusion and ECG-gated SPECT) in detecting coronary artery disease in women. *J Am Coll Cardiol* 1997; 29(1):69–77.

175. Rozanski A, Diamond GA, Berman D, et al. The declining specificity of exercise radionuclide ventriculography. *N Engl J Med* 1983; 309(9):518–522.

176a. Roger VL, Pellikka PA, Bell MR, et al. Sex and test verification bias: Impact on the diagnostic value of exercise echocardiography. *Circulation* 1997; 95(2):405–410.

176b. Maddahi J, Van Train K, Prigent F, et al. Quantitative single photon emission computed thallium-201 tomography for detection and localization of coronary artery disease: Optimization and prospective validation of a new technique. *J Am Coll Cardiol* 1989; 14(7):1689–1699.

176c. Iskandrian AS, Heo J, Kong B, et al. Effect of exercise level on the ability of thallium-201 tomographic imaging in detecting coronary artery disease: Analysis of 461 patients. *J Am Coll Cardiol* 1989; 14:1477–1486.

176d. Kiat H, Van Train KF, Maddahi J, et al. Development and prospective application of quantitative 2-day stress-rest Tc-99m methoxy isobutyl isonitrile SPECT for the diagnosis of coronary artery disease. *Am Heart J* 1990; 120:1255–1266.

176e. VanTrain KF, Maddahi J, Berman DS, et al. Quantitative analysis of tomographic stress thallium-201 myocardial scintigrams: A multicenter trial. *J Nucl Med* 1990; 31:1168–1179.

176f. Kiat H, Van Train KF, Friedman JD, et al. Quantitative stress-redistribution thallium-201 SPECT using prone imaging: Methodologic development and validation. *J Nucl Med* 1992; 33(8):1509–1515.

176g. Heo J, Wolmer I, Kegel J, et al. Sequential dual-isotope SPECT imaging with thallium-201 and technetium-99m-sestamibi. *J Nucl Med* 1994; 35:549–553.

176h. Van Train KF, Garcia EV, Maddahi J, et al. Multicenter trial validation for quantitative analysis of same-day rest-stress technetium-99m-sestamibi myocardial tomographs. *J Nucl Med* 1994; 35:609–618.

176i. Zaret BL, Rigo P, Wackers FJT, et al. Myocardial perfusion imaging with 99mTc tetrofosmin. *Circulation* 1995; 91:313–319.

176j. Kiat H, Iskandrian AS, Villegas BJ, et al. Arbutamine stress thallium-201 single-photon emission computed tomography using a computerized closed-loop delivery system. *J Am Coll Cardiol* 1995; 26:1159–1167.

176k. Amanullah AM, Kiat H, Friedman JD, et al. Adenosine technetium-99m sestamibi myocardial perfusion SPECT in women: Diagnostic efficacy in detection of coronary artery disease. *J Am Coll Cardiol* 1996; 27(4):803–809.

176l. Heo J, Powers J, Iskandrian AE. Exercis-rest same-day SPECT sestamibi imaging to detect coronary artery disease. *J Nucl Med* 1997; 38(2):200–203.

177. Comparison of coronary bypass surgery with angioplasty in patients with multivessel disease: The Bypass Angioplasty Revascularization Investigation (BARI) Investigators. [published erratum appears in *N Engl J Med* 1997; 9;336(2):147] *N Engl J Med* 1996; 335(4):217–225.

178. Little WC, Constantinescu M, Applegate RJ, et al. Can coronary angiography predict the site of a subsequent myocardial infarction in patients with mild-to-moderate coronary artery disease? *Circulation* 1988; 78(5 pt 1):1157-1166.

179. Ambrose JA, Tannenbaum MA, Alexopoulos D, et al. Angiographic progression of coronary artery disease and the development of myocardial infarction. *J Am Coll Cardiol* 1988; 12(1):56–62.

180. Garcia EV. Quantitative myocardial perfusion single-photon emission computed tomographic imaging: Quo vadis? (Where do we go from here?). *J Nucl Cardiol* 1994; 1(1):83–93.

181. Sharir T, Germano G, Waechter PB, et al. A new algorithm for the quantitation of myocardial perfusion SPECT II: Validation and diagnostic yield. *J Nucl Med* 2000; 41:720–727.

182. Iskander S, Iskandrian AE. Risk assessment using single-photon emission computed tomographic technetium-99m sestamibi imaging. *J Am Coll Cardiol* 1998; 32:57–62.

183. Hachamovitch R, Schnipper J, Young-Xu Y. Are patients with known or suspected coronary artery disease and normal stress imaging studies at low risk for adverse outcomes? Meta-analysis of stress echocardiography and SPECT. *J Am Coll Cardiol* 2000.

183a. Soman P, Parson A, Lahiri N, et al. The prognostic value of a normal Tc-99m sestamibi SPECT study in suspected coronary artery disease. *J Nucl Cardiol* 1999; 6:252–256.

184. Randomized trial of cholesterol lowering in 4444 patients with coronary heart disease: The Scandinavian Simvastatin Survival Study (4S). *Lancet* 1994; 344(8934):1383–1389.

185. Kjekshus J, Pedersen TR. Reducing the risk of coronary events: Evidence from the Scandinavian Simvastatin Survival Study (4S). *Am J Cardiol* 1995; 76(9):64C–68C.

186. Shepherd J, Cobbe SM, Ford I, et al. Prevention of coronary heart disease with pravastatin in men with hypercholesterolemia: West of Scotland Coronary Prevention Study Group. *N Engl J Med* 1995; 333(20):1301–1307.

187. Pfeffer MA, Sacks FM, Moyé LA, et al. Cholesterol and recurrent events: A secondary prevention trial for normolipidemic patients. CARE Investigators. *Am J Cardiol* 1995; 76(9):98C–106C.

188. Pasternak RC, Brown LE, Stone PH, et al. Effect of combination therapy with lipid-reducing drugs in patients with coronary heart disease and "normal" cholesterol levels: A randomized, placebo-controlled trial. Harvard Atherosclerosis Reversibility Project (HARP) Study Group. *Ann Intern Med* 1996; 125(7): 529–540.

189. Borzak S, Cannon CP, Kraft PL, et al. Effects of prior aspirin and anti-ischemic therapy on outcome of patients with unstable angina. TIMI 7 Investigators: Thrombin Inhibition in Myocardial Ischemia. *Am J Cardiol* 1998; 81(6):678–681.

190. Køber L, Torp-Pedersen C, Carlsen JE, et al. A clinical trial of the angiotensin-converting-enzyme inhibitor trandolapril in patients with left ventricular dysfunction after myocardial infarction: Trandolapril Cardiac Evaluation (TRACE) Study Group. *N Engl J Med* 1995; 333(25):1670–1676.

191. Haim M, Shotan A, Boyko V, et al. Effect of beta-blocker therapy in patients with coronary artery disease in New York Heart Association classes II and III: The Bezafibrate Infarction Prevention (BIP) Study Group. *Am J Cardiol* 1998; 81(12):1455–1460.

192. de Lorgeril M, Salen P, Caillat-Vallet E, et al. Control of bias in dietary trial to prevent coronary recurrences: The Lyon Diet Heart Study. *Eur J Clin Nutr* 1997; 51(2):116–122.

193. Ornish D, Brown SE, Scherwitz LW, et al., Can lifestyle changes reverse coronary heart disease? The Lifestyle Heart Trial. *Lancet* 1990; 336(8708):129–133.

194. Shaw LJ, Hachamovitch R, Peterson ED, et al. Using an outcomes-based approach to identify candidates for risk stratification after exercise treadmill testing. *J Gen Intern Med* 1999; 14:1–9.

195. Mark DB, Hlatky MA, Harrell FE Jr, et al. Exercise treadmill score for predicting prognosis in coronary artery disease. *Ann Intern Med* 1987; 106(6):793–800.

196. O'Keefe JH Jr, Bateman TM, Ligon RW, et al. Outcome of medical versus invasive treatment strategies for non-high-risk ischemic heart disease. *J Nucl Cardiol* 1998; 5:28–33.

197. Hachamovitch R, Berman D, Kiat H, et al. What is the warranty period for a normal scan? Temporal changes in risk in patients with normal exercise sestamibi SPECT (abstr). *Circulation* 1995; 92(8):I-130.

198. Galassi AR, Azzarelli S, Rodi G, et al. Exercise 99m-technetium tetrofosmin tomography for cardiac risk stratificcation of patients with suspected or known coronary artery disease (abstr). *J Nucl Cardiol* 1999; 6(1):S93.

199. Berman DS, Kang X, Van Train KF, et al. Comparative prognostic value of automatic quantitative analysis versus semiquantitative visual analysis of exercise myocardial perfusion single-photon emission computed tomography. *J Am Coll Cardiol* 1998; 32(7):1987–1995.

200. Johnson SH, Bigelow C, Lee KL, et al. Prediction of death and myocardial infarction by radionuclide angiocardiography in patients with suspected coronary artery disease. *Am J Cardiol* 1991; 67(11):919–926.

201. Lee KL, Pryor DB, Pieper KS, et al. Prognostic value of radionuclide angiography in medically treated patients with coronary artery disease: A comparison with clinical and catheterization variables. *Circulation* 1990; 82(5):1705–1717.

202. Upton MT, Palmeri ST, Jones RH. Assessment of left ventricular function by resting and exercise radionucline angiocardiography following acute myocardial infarction. *Am Heart J* 1982; 104:1232–1243.

203. Pryor DB, Harrell FE Jr, Lee KL, et al. Prognostic indicators from radionuclide angiography in medically treated patients with coronary artery disease. *Am J Cardiol* 1984; 53(1):18–22.

204. Jones RH, Johnson SH, Bigelow C, et al. Exercise radionuclide angiocardiography predicts cardiac death in patients with coronary artery disease. *Circulation* 1991; 84(3 suppl):I52–I58.

205. Morris KG, Palmeri ST, Califf RM, et al. Value of radionuclide

angiography for predicting specific cardiac events after acute myocardial infarction. *Am J Cardiol* 1985; 55:318–324.

206. Hachamovitch R, Berman D, Lewin H, et al. Incremental prognostic value of gated SPECT ejection fraction in patients undergoing dual-isotope exercise or adenosine stress SPECT (abstr). *J Am Coll Cardiol* 1998; 31(2, suppl. A):441A.

207. Sharir T, Germano G, Kavanaugh PB, et al. Incremental prognostic value of post-stress left ventricular ejection fraction and volume by gated myocardial perfusion single photon emission computed tomography. *Circulation* 1999; 100:1035–1042.

208. Sharir T, Germano G, Lewin HC, et al. Prognostic value of myocardial perfusion and function by gated SPECT in the prediction of non-fatal myocardial infarction and cardiac death (abstr). In: American Heart Association 72d Scientific Sessions. 1999. Atlanta.

209. Sharir T, Bacher-Stier C, Lewin HC, et al. Identification of severe and extensive coronary artery disease by post-exercise regional wall motion abnormalities in Tc-technetium-99m sestamibi gated single photon emission computed tomography. *Am J Cardiol.* In press.

210. Ambrosio G, Betocchi S, Pace L, et al. Prolonged impairment of regional contractile function after resolution of exercise-induced angina: Evidence of myocardial stunning in patients with coronary artery disease. *Circulation* 1996; 94:2455–2464.

211. Morise AP. An incremental evaluation of the diagnostic value of thallium single-photon emission computed tomographic imaging and lung/heart ratio concerning both the presence and extent of coronary artery disease. *J Nucl Cardiol* 1995; 2(3):238–245.

212. Bacher-Stier C, Kavanagh P, Sharir T, et al. Post-exercise Tc-99m sestamibi lung uptake determined by a new automatic technique (abstr). *J Nucl Med* 1998; 39(5):104P.

213. Sharir T, Berman DS, Lewin HC, et al. Incremental prognostic value of rest-redistribution 201-Tl single photon emission computed tomography. *Circulation* 1999; 100:1964–1970.

214. Bateman TM, O'Keefe JH Jr, Dong VM, et al. Coronary angiographic rates after stress single-photon emission computed tomographic scintigraphy. *J Nucl Cardiol* 1995; 2(3):217–223.

215. Nallamothu N, Pancholy SB, Lee KR, et al. Impact on exercise single-photon emission computed tomographic thallium imaging on patient management and outcome. *J Nucl Cardiol* 1995; 2(4):334–338.

216. Shaw LJ, Hachamovitch R, Berman DS, et al. The economic consequences of available diagnostic and prognostic strategies for the evaluation of stable angina patients—An observational assessment of the value of precatheterization ischemia: Economics of Noninvasive Diagnosis (END) Multicenter Study Group. *J Am Coll Cardiol* 1999; 33(3):661–669.

217. Sharp N, Murphy J, Smith H, et al. Treatment of patients with symptomless left ventricular dysfunction after myocardial infarction. *Lancet* 1988; 6:255.

218. Ryan TJ, Anderson JL, Antman EM, et al. ACC/AHA guidelines for the management of patients with acute myocardial infarction: A report of the American College of Cardiology/American Heart Association Task Force on Practice Guidelines (Committee on Management of Acute Myocardial Infarction). *J Am Coll Cardiol* 1996; 28(5):1328–1428.

219. Peterson ED, Shaw LJ, Califf RM. Risk stratification after myocardial infarction. *Ann Intern Med* 1997; 126(7):561–582.

220. Jones RH, McEwan P, Newman GE, et al. Accuracy of diagnosis of coronary artery disease by radionuclide management of left ventricular function during rest and exercise. *Circulation* 1981; 64(3):586–601.

221. Moriel M, Rozanski A, Klein J, et al. The differing prognostic utility of exercise radionuclide ventriculography in coronary artery disease patients with and without prior myocardial infarction. *Int J Cardiac Imaging* 1997; 13:403–413.

222. Shaw LJ, Heinle SK, Borges-Neto S, et al. Prognosis by measurements of left ventricular function during exercise. Duke Noninvasive Research Working Group. *J Nucl Med* 1998; 39(1):140–146.

223. Mazzotta G, Bonow RO, Pace L, et al. Relation between exertional ischemic and prognosis in nmildly symptomatic patients with single- or double-vessel coronary artery disease and left ventricular dysfunction at rest. *J Am Coll Cardiol* 1989; 13:567–573.

224. Bonow RO, Bacharach SL, Green MV, et al. Prognostic implications of symptomatic versus asymptomatic (silent) myocardial ischemia induced by exercise in mildly symptomatic and asymptomatic patients angiographically documented coronary artery disease. *Am J Cardiol* 1987; 60:778–783.

225. Iqbal A, Gibbon RJ, Zinsmeister AR, et al. Prognostic value of exercise radionuclide angiography in a population-based cohort of patients with known or suspected coronary artery disease. *Am J Cardiol* 1994; 74:119–124.

226. Iskandrian AS, Hakki AH, Goel IP, et al. The use of rest and exercise radionucline ventriculography in risk stratification in patients with suspected coronary artery disease. *Am Heart J* 1985; 110:864–872.

227. Coronary Artery Surgery Study (CASS): A randomized trial of coronary artery bypass surgery—Survival data. *Circulation* 1983; 68(5):939–950.

228. Supino PG, Borer JS, Herrold EM, et al. Prognostication in 3-vessel coronary artery disease based on left ventricular ejection fraction during exercise: Influence of coronary artery bypass grafting. *Circulation* 1999; 100:924–932.

229. Legrand V, Mancini GB, Bates ER, et al. Comparative study of coronary flow reserve, coronary anatomy and results of radionuclide exercise tests in patients with coronary artery disease. *J Am Coll Cardiol* 1986; 8(5):1022–1032.

230. Miller DD, Donohue TJ, Younis LT, et al. Correlation of pharmacological 99mTc-sestamibi myocardial perfusion imaging with poststenotic coronary flow reserve in patients with angiographically intermediate coronary artery stenoses. *Circulation* 1994; 89(5):2150–2160.

231. Prigent FM, Berman DS, Elashoff J, et al. Reproducibility of stress redistribution thallium-201 SPECT quantitative indexes of hypoperfused myocardium secondary to coronary artery disease. *Am J Cardiol* 1992; 70(15):1255–1263.

232. Mahmarian JJ, Moyé LA, Verani MS, et al. High reproducibility of myocardial perfusion defects in patients undergoing serial exercise thallium-201 tomography. *Am J Cardiol* 1995; 75(16):1116–1119.

233. Lewin H, Sharir T, Germano G, et al. Reproducibility of dual isotope myocardial perfusion SPECT using a new quantitative perfusion SPECT (QPS) approach (abstr). *J Am Coll Cardiol* 1999; 33(2, suppl. A):483A.

234. Mahmarian JJ, Fenimore NL, Marks GF, et al. Transdermal nitroglycerin patch therapy reduces the extent of exercise-induced myocardial ischemia: Results of a double-blind, placebo-controlled trial using quantitative thallium-201 tomography. *J Am Coll Cardiol* 1994; 24(1):25–32.

235. Lewin HC, Hachamovitch R, Harris AG, et al. Sustained reduction of exercise perfusion defect extent and severity with isosorbide mononitrate (Imdur) as demonstrated by Tc-99m sestamibi (SPECT). *J Nucl Cardiol* In press.

236. Dakik H, Kleiman N, Farmer J, et al. Intensive medical therapy versus coronary angioplasty for suppression of myocardial ischemia in survivors of acute myocardial infarction. *Circulation* 1998; 98(19):2017–2023.

237. Henry T, Annex B, Azrin M, et al. Double blind, placebo controlled trial of recombinant human vascular endothelial growth factor—*the* VIVA trial (abstract). *J Am Coll Cardiol* 1999; 33(2, suppl. A):384A.

238. Pfisterer M, Rickenbacher P, Kiowski W, et al. Silent ischemia

after percutaneous transluminal coronary angioplasty: Incidence and prognostic significance. *J Am Coll Cardiol* 1993; 22:1446–1454.

239. Hecht HS, Shaw RE, Bruce TR, et al. Usefulness of tomographic thallium-201 imaging for detection of restenosis after percutaneous transluminal coronary angioplasty. *Am J Cardiol* 1990; 66(19):1314–1318.

240. Hecht HS, Shaw RE, Chin HL, et al. Silent ischemia after coronary angioplasty: Evaluation of restenosis and extent of ischemia in asymptomatic patients by tomographic thallium-201 exercise imaging and comparison with symptomatic patients. *J Am Coll Cardiol* 1991; 17(3):670–677.

241. Milavetz JJ, Miller TD, Hodge DO, et al. Accuracy of single-photon emission computed tomography myocardial perfusion imaging in patients with stents in native coronary arteries. *Am J Cardiol* 1998; 82:857–861.

242. Kosa I, Blasini R, Schneider-Eicke J, et al. Myocardial perfusion scintigraphy to evaluate patients after coronary stent implantation. *J Nucl Med* 1998; 39:1307–1311.

243. Parisi AF, Hartigan PM, Folland ED. Evaluation of exercise thallium scintigraphy versus exercise electrocardiography in predicting survival outcomes and morbid cardiac events in patients with single- and double-vessel disease: Findings from the Angioplasty Compared to Medicine (ACME) Study. *J Am Coll Cardiol* 1997; 30(5):1256–1263.

244. Lewin H, Hachamovitch R, Cohen I, et al. Stress SPECT in patients following recent PTCA: Incremental prognostic value and risk stratification (abstr). *J Nucl Med* 1997; 38(5):130P.

245. Miller DD, Verani MS. Current status of myocardial perfusion imaging after percutaneous transluminal coronary angioplasty. *J Am Coll Cardiol* 1994; 24(1):260–266.

246. Zellweger M, Berman DS, Shaw LJ, et al. Evaluation of patients after intervention. In: Pohost G, et al., eds. *Imaging in Cardiovascular Disease.* Philadelphia: Lippincott Williams & Wilkins; 2000.

247. Grondin CM, Campeau L, Lespérance J, et al. Comparison of late changes in internal mammary artery and saphenous vein grafts in two consecutive series of patients 10 years after operation. *Circulation* 1984; 70(3 pt 2):I208–I212.

248. FitzGibbon GM, Leach AJ, Kafka HP, et al. Coronary bypass graft fate: Long-term angiographic study. *J Am Coll Cardiol* 1991; 17(5):1075–1080.

249. Palmas W, Bingham S, Diamond GA, et al. Incremental prognostic value of exercise thallium-201 myocardial single-photon emission computed tomography late after coronary artery bypass surgery. *J Am Coll Cardiol* 1995; 25(2):403–409.

250. Lauer MS, Lytle B, Pashkow F, et al. Prediction of death and myocardial infarction by screening with exercise-thallium testing after coronary-artery-bypass grafting. *Lancet* 1998; 351 (9103):615–622.

251. Zellweger MJ, Lewin HC, Lai S, et al. Risk stratification in patients early and late post-CABG using stress myocardial perfusion SPECT: Implications of appropriate clinical strategies. *J Am Coll Cardiol.* In press.

252. Kang X, Berman D, Lewin HC, et al. Incremental prognostic value of myocardial perfusion single photon emission computed tomography in patients with diabetes mellitus. *Am Heart J* 1999; 138:1025–1032.

253. Lewin HC, Berman DS, Shaw LJ, et al. Noninvasive risk assessment of diabetic and non-diabetic patients with suspected ischemic heart disease (abstr). *J Am Coll Cardiol* 1999; 33:447A.

254. Giri S, Shaw LJ, Miller DD, et al. Stress SPECT myocardial perfusion imaging for predicting cardiac events in diabetic women (abstr). *J Am Coll Cardiol* 2000; 35(2):338A.

255. Wagdy HM, Hodge D, Christian TF, et al. Prognostic value of vasodilator myocardial perfusion imaging in patients with left bundle-branch block. *Circulation* 1998; 97:1563–1570.

256. Nallamothu N, Bagheri B, Acio ER, et al. Prognostic value of stress myocardial perfusion single photon emission computed tomography imaging in patients with left ventricular bundle branch block. *J Nucl Cardiol* 1997; 4(6):487–493.

257. Kannel WB. Prevalence, incidence, and hazards of hypertension in the elderly. *Am Heart J* 1986; 112(6):1362–1363.

258. Hlatky MA, Pryor DB, Harrell FE, et al. Factors affecting sensitivity and specificity of exercise electrocardiography: Multivariable analysis. *Am J Med* 1984; 77:64–71.

259. Sketch MH, Mohiuddin SM, Lynch JD, et al. Significant sex differences in the correlation of electrocardiographic exercise testing and moronary arteriograms. *Am J Cardiol* 1975; 36:169–173.

260. Mark DB, Shaw LK, DeLong ER, et al. Absence of sex bias in the referral of patients for cardiac catheterization. *N Engl J Med* 1994; 330(16):1101–1106.

261. Shaw LJ, Miller DD, Romeis JC, et al. Gender differences in the noninvasive evaluation and management of patients with suspected coronary artery disease. *Ann Intern Med* 1994; 120(7):559–566.

262. Detrano R, Janosi A, Lyons KP, et al. Factors affecting sensitivity and specificity of a diagnostic test: The exercise thallium scintigram. *Am J Med* 1988; 84(4):699–710.

263. Hachamovitch R, Berman DS, Kiat H, et al. Effective risk stratification using exercise myocardial perfusion SPECT in women: Gender-related differences in prognostic nuclear testing. *J Am Coll Cardiol* 1996; 28(1):34–44.

264. Marwick TH, Shaw LJ, Lauer MS, et al. The noninvasive prediction of cardiac mortality in men and women with unknown or suspected coronary artery disease. *Am J Med* 1999; 106:172–178.

265. Amanullah AM, Berman DS, Hachamovitch R, et al. Indentification of severe or extensive coronary artery disease in women by adenosine Tc-99m sestamibi SPECT. *Am J Cardiol* 1997; 80:132–137.

266. Hilton TC, Shaw LJ, Chaitman BR, et al. Prognostic significance of exercise thallium-201 testing in patients aged greater than or equal to 70 years with known or suspected coronary artery disease. *Am J Cardiol* 1992; 69(1):45–50.

266a. Hachamovitch R, Diamond GA, Kiat H, et al. Noninvasive risk stratification of the elderly patient: Use of nuclear testing to identify high-risk patient populations. *Circulation* 1994; 90:I-102.

267. Amanullah AM, Hachamovitch R, Erel J, et al. Prognostic value of exercise and adenosine myocardial perfusion SPECT in the very elderly (abstr). *J Am Coll Cardiol* 1997; 29:362A.

267a. Hachamovitch R, Berman DS, Kiat H, et al. Incremental prognostic value of adenosine stress myocardial perfusion single photon emission computed tomography and impact on subsequent management in patients with or suspected of having myocardial ischemia. *Am J Cardiol* 1997; 80:426–433.

267b. Hayes SW, Lewin HC, Friedman JD, et al. Prognostic significance of rest Tl-201/stress Tc-technetium-99m sestamibi dual-isotope myocardial perfusion SPECT in very elderly patients (abstr). *J Am Coll Cardiol* 2000; 35:455A.

268. Cutler BS. Prevention of cardiac complications in peripheral vascular surgery. *Surg Clin North Am* 1986; 66(2):281–292.

269. Eagle KA, Coley CM, Newell JB, et al. Combining clinical and thallium data optimizes preoperative assessment of cardiac risk before major vascular surgery. *Ann Intern Med* 1989; 110 (11):859–866.

270. Eagle KA, Charanjit SR, Mickel MC, et al. Cardiac risk of noncardiac surgery: Influence of coronary disease and type of surgery in 3368 operations. *Circulation* 1997; 96(6):1882–1887.

271. Shaw L, Eagle KA, Gersh BJ, et al. Meta-analysis of intravenous dipyridamole-thallium-201 imaging (1985 to 1994) and dobutamine echocardiography (1991 to 1994) for risk stratification before vascular surgery. *J Am Coll Cardiol* 1996; 27(4):787–798.

272. Bonow RO. Identification of viable myocardium. *Circulation* 1996; 94(11):2674–2680.
273. Bonow RO. Clinical value of combined assessment of perfusion and function for the evaluation of myocardial viability. In: Germano G, Berman DS, eds. Clinical Gated Cardiac SPECT. Armonk, NY: Futura; 1999:307–324.
274. Arrighi A, Dilsizian V. In: Pohost G, et al., eds. *Imaging in Cardiovascular Disease.* Philadelphia: Lippincott Williams & Wilkins. In press.
275. Bax JJ, Wijns W, Cornel JH, et al. Accuracy of currently available techniques for prediction of functional recovery after revascularization in patients with left ventricular dysfunction due to chronic coronary artery disease: Comparison of pooled data. *J Am Coll Cardiol* 1997; 30:1451–1460.
276. He ZX, Medrano R, Hays JT, et al. Nitroglycerin-augmented 201Tl reinjection enhances detection of reversible myocardial hypoperfusion. A randomized, double-blind, parallel, placebo-controlled trial. *Circulation* 1997; 95(7):1799–1805.
277. Tubau JF, Rahimtoola SH. Hibernating myocardium: A historical perspective. *Cardiovasc Drugs Ther* 1992; 6(3):267–271.
278. Elsässer A, Schlepper M, Klövekorn WP, et al. Hibernating myocardium: an incomplete adaptation to ischemia. *Circulation* 1997; 96(9):2920–2931.
279. Braunwald E, Kloner RA. The stunned myocardium: Prolonged, postischemic ventricular dysfunction. *Circulation* 1982; 66(6): 1146–1149.
280. Johnson LL, Verdesca SA, Aude WY, et al. Postischemic stunning can affect left ventricular ejection fraction and regional wall motion on post-stress gated sestamibi tomograms. *J Am Coll Cardiol* 1997; 30(7):1641–1648.
281. Rumberger JA. Ventricular dilatation and remodeling after myocardial infarction. *Mayo Clin Proc* 1994; 69(7):664–674.
282. Gaudron P, Eilles C, Kugler I, et al. Progressive left ventricular dysfunction and remodeling after myocardial infarction. Potential mechanisms and early predictors. *Circulation* 1993; 87 (3):755–763.
283. Alexander J, Dainiak N, Berger HJ, et al. Serial assessment of doxorubicin cardiotoxicity with quantitative radionuclide angiocardiography. *N Engl J Med* 1979; 300(6):278–283.
284. Schwartz RG, McKenzie WB, Alexander J, et al. Congestive heart failure and left ventricular dysfunction complicating doxorubicin therapy: Seven-year experience using serial radionuclide angiocardiography. *Am J Med* 1987; 82:1109.
285. Ritchie JL, Singer JW, Thorning D, et al. Anthracycline cardiotoxicity: Clinical and pathologic outcomes assessed by radionuclide ejection fraction. *Cancer* 1980; 46:1109.
286. Morgan GW, McIlveen BM, Freedman A, et al. Radionuclide ejection fraction in doxorubicin cardiotoxicity. *Cancer Treat Rep* 1981; 65:629.
287. Bonow RO, Rosing DR, Kent KM, et al. Timing of operation for chronic aortic regurgitation. *Am J Cardiol* 1982; 50:3251.
288. Bonow RO, Rosing DR, Mason BJ, et al. Reversal of left ventricular dysfunction after aortic valve replacement for chronic aortic regurgitation: Influence of duration of preoperative left ventricular dysfunction. *Circulation* 1984; 70:570.
289. Borer JS, Hochreiter C, Herrold EM, et al. Prediction of indications for valve replacement among asymptomatic or minimally symptomatic patients with chronic aortic regurgitation and normal left ventricular performance. *Circulation* 1998; 97:525–534.
290. Cheitlin MD. Finding "just the right moment" for operative intervention in the asymptomatic patient with moderate to severe aortic regurgitation (editorial). *Circulation* 1998; 97: 518–520.
291. Braunwald E, Jones RH, Mark DB, et al. Diagnosing and managing unstable angina. *Circulation* 1994; 90(1):613–622.
292. Bell MR, Montarello JK, Steele PM. Does the emergency room electrocardiogram identify patients with suspected myocardial infarction who are at low risk of acute complications? *Aust NZ J Med* 1990; 20(4):564–569.
293. Karlson BW, Herlitz J, Wiklund O, et al. Early prediction of acute myocardial infarction from clinical history, examination and electrocardiogram in the emergency room. *Am J Cardiol* 1991; 68(2):171–175.
294. Lee TH, Rouan GW, Weisberg MC, et al. Clinical characteristics and natural history of patients with acute myocardial infarction sent home from the emergency room. *Am J Cardiol* 1987; 60(4):219–224.
295. Karcz A, Holbrook J, Auerbach BS, et al. Preventability of malpractice claims in emergency medicine: a closed claims study. *Ann Emerg Med* 1990; 19(8):865–873.
296. Pelberg AL. Missed myocardial infarction in the emergency room. *Quality Assur Utili Rev* 1989; 4(2):39–42.
297. Ohman EM, Armstrong PW, Christenson RH, et al. Cardiac troponin T levels for risk stratification in acute myocardial ischemia: GUSTO IIA Investigators. *N Engl J Med* 1996; 335(18):1333–1341.
298. Graff LG, Dallara J, Ross MA, et al. Impact on the care of the emergency department chest pain patient from the chest pain evaluation registry (CHEPER) study. *Am J Cardiol* 1997; 80(5):563–568.
299. Gomez MA, Anderson JL, Karagounis LA, et al. An emergency department-base protocol for rapidly ruling out myocardial ischemia reduces hospital time and expense: results of a randomized study (ROMIO). *J Am Coll Cardiol* 1996; 28(1):25–33.
300. Hilton TC, Thompson RC, Williams HJ, et al. Technetium-99m sestamibi myocardial perfusion imaging in the emergency room evaluation of chest pain. *J Am Coll Cardiol* 1994; 23(5):1016–1022.
301. Hilton TC, Fulmer H, Abuan T, et al. Ninety-day follow-up of patients in the emergency department with chest pain who undergo initial single-photon emission computed tomographic perfusion scintigraphy with technetium 99m-labeled sestamibi. *J Nucl Cardiol* 1996; 3(4):308–311.
302. Varetto T, Cantalupi D, Altieri A, et al. Emergency room technetium-99m sestamibi imaging to rule out acute myocardial ischemic events in patients with nondiagnostic electrocardiograms. *J Am Coll Cardiol* 1993; 22(7):1804–1808.
303. Tatum JL, Jesse RL, Kontos MC, et al. Comprehensive strategy for the evaluation and triage of the chest pain patient. *Ann Emerg Med* 1997; 29(1):116–125.
304. Kontos MC, Jesse RL, Anderson FP, et al. Comparison of myocardial perfusion imaging and cardiac troponin I in patients admitted to the emergency department with chest pain. *Circulation* 1999; 99:2073–2078.
305. Kontos MC, Schmidt KL, Nicholson CS, et al. Myocardial perfusion imaging with technetium-99m sestamibi in patients with cocaine-associated chest pain. *Ann Emerg Med* 1999; 33: 639–645.
306. Heller GV, Stowers SA, Hendel RC, et al. Clinical value of acute rest technetium-99m tetrofosmin tomographic myocardial perfusion imaging in patients with acute chest pain and nondiagnostic electrocardiograms. *J Am Coll Cardiol* 1998; 31:1011–1017.
307. Kontos MC, Jesse RL, Schmidt KL, et al. Value of acute rest sestamibi perfusion imaging for evaluation of patients admitted to the emergency department with chest pain. *J Am Coll Cardiol* 1997; 30(4):976–982.
308. Radensky PW, Hilton TC, Fulmer H, et al. Potential cost effectiveness of initial myocardial perfusion imaging for assessment of emergency department patients with chest pain. *Am J Cardiol* 1997; 79(5):595–599.
309. Udelson. Late-breaking trials. Presented at the 72d Annual Scientific Sessions of the American Heart Association, Atlanta, GA, 1999.

310. Ziffer J, Nateman D, Janowitz W, et al. Myocardial perfusion imaging is a routinely effective triage tool to evaluate ongoing and recently resolved chest pain in a dedicated center (abstr). *J Nucl Med* 1997; 38(5):131P.
311. Ziffer J, Nateman D, Janowitz W, et al. Improved patient outcomes and cost effectiveness of utilizing nuclear cardiology protocols in an emergency department chest pain center: Two-year results in 6,548 patients (abstr). *J Nucl Med* 1998; 39(5):139P.
312. Miller TD, Christian TF, Hopfenspirger MR, et al. Infarct size after acute myocardial infarction measured by quantitative tomographic 99mTc sestamibi imaging predicts subsequent mortality. *Circulation* 1995; 92(3):334–341.
313. Christian TF, Gitter MJ, Miller TD, et al. Prospective identification of myocardial stunning using technetium-99m sestamibi-based measurements of infarct size. *J Am Coll Cardiol* 1997; 30:1633–1640.
314. Rodrigues EA, Dewhust NG, Smart LM, et al. Diagnosis and prognosis of right ventricular infarction. *Br Heart J* 1986; 56:19.
315. Shah PK, Maddahi J, Staniloff HM, et al. Scintigraphically detected predominant right ventricular dysfunction in acute myocardial infarction: Clinical and hemodynamic correlates and implications for therapy and prognosis. *J Am Coll Cardiol* 1985; 6:1264.
316. Group MPR. Risk stratification and survival after myocardial infarction. *N Eng J Med* 1983; 309:331.
317. Bateman T, Czer LSC, Gray R, et al. Detection of occult pericardial hemorrhage early after open-heart surgery using technetium-99m red blood cell radionuclide ventriculography. *Am Heart J* 1984; 108:1198.
318. Bateman T, Czer LSC, Kass RM, et al. Cardiac causes of shock early after open heart surgery: Eriologic classification by radionuclide ventriculography. *Circulation* 1985; 71:1153.
319. Christian TF, Schwartz RS, Gibbons RJ. Determinants of infarct size in reperfusion therapy for acute myocardial infarction. *Circulation* 1992; 86(1):81–90.
320. O'Keefe JH Jr, Grines CL, DeWood MA, et al. Factors influencing myocardial salvage with primary angioplasty. *J Nucl Cardiol* 1995; 2(1):35–41.
321. Gibbons RJ, Verani MS, Behrenbeck T, et al. Feasibility of tomographic 99mTc-hexakis-2-methoxy-2-methylpropyl-isonitrile imaging for the assessment of myocardial area at risk and the effect of treatment in acute myocardial infarction. *Circulation* 1989; 80(5):1277–1286.
321a. Lew A, Maddahi J, Shah PK, et al. Critically ischemic myocardium in clinically stable patients following thrombolytic therapy for acute myocardial infarction: Potential implications for early coronary angioplasty in selected patients. *Am Heart J* 1990; 120:1015–1025.
322. Boden WE, O'Rourke RA, Crawford MH, et al. Outcomes in patients with acute non-Q-wave myocardial infarction randomly assigned to an invasive as compared with a conservative management strategy. Veterans Affairs Non-Q-Wave Infarction Strategies in Hospital (VANQWISH) Trial Investigators. *N Engl J Med* 1998; 338(25):1785–1792.
323. Mark DB, Naylor CD, Hlatky MA, et al. Use of medical resources and quality of life after acute myocardial infarction in Canada and the United States. *N Engl J Med* 1994; 331(17): 1130–1135.
324. Topol EJ, Ellis SG, Cosgrove DM, et al. Analysis of coronary angioplasty practice in the United States with an insurance-claims data base. *Circulation* 1993; 87(5):1489–1497.
324a. Gibson RS, Watson DD, Craddock GB, et al. Prediction of cardiac events after uncomplicated myocardial infarction: A prospective study comparing predischarge exercise thallium 201 scintigraphy and coronary angiography. *Circulation* 1983; 68:321–336.
325. Dakik HA, Mahmarian JJ, Kimball KT, et al. Prognostic value of exercise ^{201}Tl tomography in patients treated with thrombolytic therapy during acute myocardial infarction. *Circulation* 1996; 94(11):2735–2742.
326. Shaw LJ, Peterson ED, Kesler K, et al. A meta-analysis of predischarge risk stratification after acute myocardial infarction with stress electrocardiographic, myocardial perfusion, and ventricular function imaging. *Am J Cardiol* 1996; 78:1327–1337.
327. Santos-Ocampo CD, Herman SD, Travin MI, et al. Comparison of exercise, dipyridamole, and adenosine by use of technetium 99m sestamibi tomographic imaging. *J Nucl Cardiol* 1994; 1(1):57–64.
328. Heller GV, Brown KA, Landin RJ, et al. Safety of early intravenous dipyridamole technetium 99m sestamibi SPECT myocardial perfusion imaging after uncomplicated first myocardial infarction: Early Post MI IV Dipyridamole Study (EPIDS). *Am Heart J* 1997; 134(1):105–111.
329. Mahmarian JJ, Mahmarian AC, Marks GF, et al. Role of adenosine thallium-201 tomography for defining long-term risk in patients after acute myocardial infarction. *J Am Coll Cardiol* 1995; 25(6):1333–1340.
330. Jain D, Thompson B, Wackers FJ, et al. Relevance of increased lung thallium uptake on stress imaging in patients with unstable angina and non-Q-wave myocardial infarction: Results of the Thrombolysis in Myocardial Infarction (TIMI)-IIIB Study. *J Am Coll Cardiol* 1997; 30(2):421–429.
330a. Beller GA, Zaret BL. Contributions of nuclear cardiology to diagnosis and prognosis of patients with coronary artery disease. *Circulation* 2000; 101:1465–1478.
331. Brown KA, Heller GV, Landin RS, et al. Early dipyridamole Tc-99m SPECT imaging after acute myocardial infarction predicts in-hospital and post-discharge cardiac events: Comparison with submaximal exercise imaging. *Circulation* 1999; 100:2060–2066.
332. Wackers JT, Zaret BL. Risk stratification soon after acute infarction (editorial). *Circulation* 1999; 100:2040–2042.

CHAPTER 17

COMPUTED TOMOGRAPHY OF THE HEART

John J. Mahmarian

Computed tomography has emerged as a technique that can fully evaluate both cardiac structure and function. Recent advances in imaging speed have allowed for more complete evaluation of relatively stationary structures, such as the thoracic aorta, and rapidly moving structures, such as the myocardium. When combined with electrocardiographic (ECG) gating, literally "freeze frame" images of the heart can be obtained, obviating most of the blur caused by motion artifact during systole and diastole. This is particularly important when obtaining contrast-enhanced images of the coronary arteries or quantifying coronary artery calcium.

Two types of computed tomographic (CT) scanners are currently available for performing cardiac evaluations. Continuously rotating spiral CT scanners can acquire images within 500 ms, whereas exposure times have been markedly reduced to 50 ms with the advent of electron-beam computed tomography (EBCT).

TECHNICAL CONSIDERATIONS

Spiral Computed Tomography

Traditional CT scanners produce images by rotating an x-ray tube around a circular gantry through which the patient passes on a table. With spiral CT scanners, the x-ray tube rotates continuously as the table moves through the gantry without the need for incremental stops. The x-ray tube can make one revolution around the patient in less than 1 s, and the table can advance through the gantry to acquire up to two slices per second. Further improvements in spiral CT technology have increased the number of images that can be obtained through each revolution of the x-ray beam, thus shortening total acquisition times at any given slice thickness.

The actual rotation of the x-ray tube is limited, however, by its mechanical movement around the patient. Therefore, imaging time is still currently limited to at best 500 ms. When imaging the constantly moving myocardium and coronary arteries, faster acquisition times are required to avoid image blur, even when ECG gating is employed.

EBCT

EBCT uses an electron beam of 130 kV that is deflected via a magnetic coil and focused to strike a series of four tungsten targets located beneath the patient (Fig. 17-1). The electron beam is magnetically swept along the tungsten targets at a 210° arc. Each target ring is separated by a distance of 4 mm. The resulting x-rays generated beneath the patient are then attenuated as they pass through the thorax and recorded by a series of two twin fixed detector arrays arranged in a semicircle above the patient. Imaging is complete within 50 ms, which is the time required for the electron beam to sweep along the tungsten targets. With a 100-ms acquisition time, a "freeze frame" image of the myocardium and coronary arteries in end-diastole can be achieved with little, if any, motion blur.

EBCT is commonly operated using three different acquisition modes. The *cine mode* creates real-time cross-sectional views of the beating heart and is commonly used to assess both global and regional right ventricular (RV) and left ventricular (LV) function (Fig. 17-2). The *volume mode* allows acquisition of a single image with each preselected movement of the patient

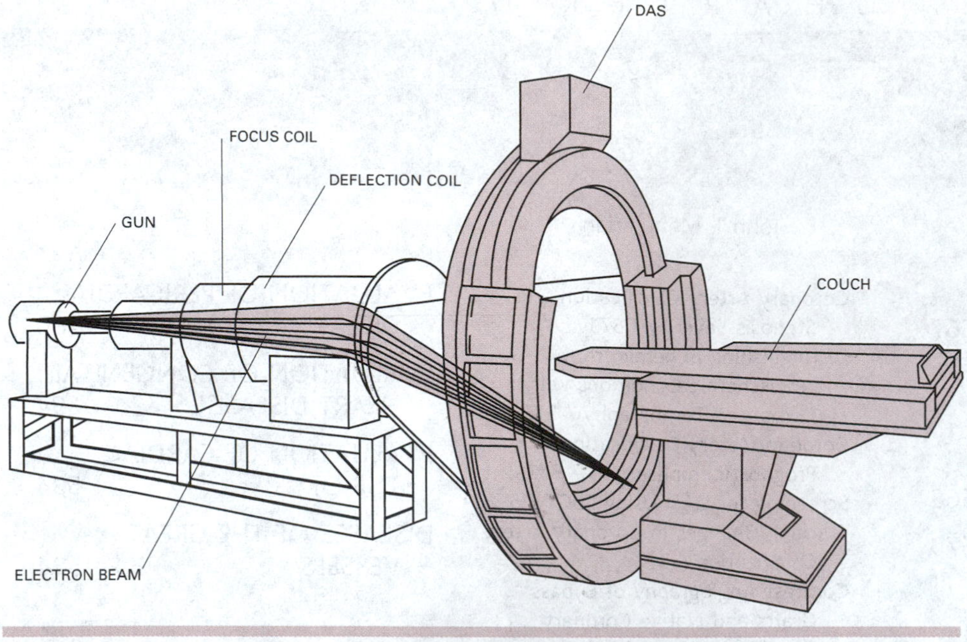

FIGURE 17-1 Diagram of the EBCT scanner. The electron beam is emitted from the electron gun and focused onto the tungsten targets by the magnetic deflection coil. DAS, immediate memory.

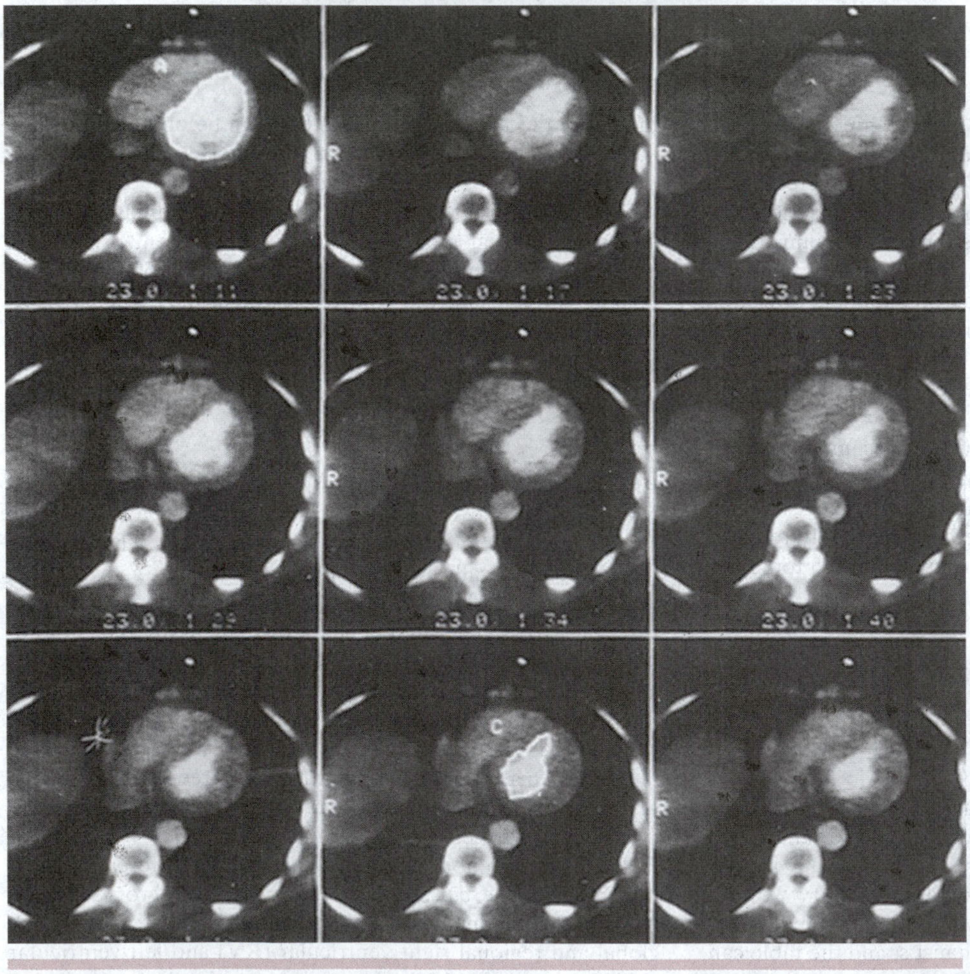

FIGURE 17-2 An 8-mm-thick CT slice of the mid-left ventricle imaged for one complete cardiac cycle at 58-ms intervals. *A*, end-diastole; *C*, end-systole.

couch. Up to 40 continuous slices can be obtained scanning 12 to 32 cm of anatomy (Fig. 17-3). This imaging mode is commonly gated to the electrocardiogram to obtain high-resolution static images for detailed evaluation of cardiovascular anatomy, such as coronary artery calcification (see also Chap. 40). The *triggered* (*flow*) *mode* is used to assess blood flow through specific cardiac chambers and the myocardium itself. This mode allows acquisition of some 20 to 40 consecutive scans, where imaging occurs at a designated time during each cardiac cycle. From these consecutive scans, time-density curves can be constructed that can estimate blood flow through specific cardiac chambers and within the myocardium.

EVALUATION OF MYOCARDIAL STRUCTURE AND FUNCTION

Both the left and right ventricles are well visualized by spiral computed tomography and EBCT, allowing excellent spatial separation between the two structures. Delineation of the epicardial and endocardial surfaces allows accurate and reproducible measurement of LV and RV wall thickness and myocardial mass.[1-3] LV hypertrophy can be quantified and serially assessed. RV dysplasia is accurately diagnosed based on the characteristic EBCT findings of an enlarged right ventricle with a scalloped appearance, trabeculations with low attenuation characteristics, and abundant epicardial adipose tissue.[4]

EBCT can assess LV and RV hemodynamics[5] as well as regional myocardial wall motion and thickening.[6-8] The cine mode is used to acquire multiple gated images of the right and left ventricles during maximal contrast enhancement of the cavities.[7,8] This affords accurate and reproducible quantification of LV and RV end-diastolic and end-systolic volumes and ejection fraction.[5,7] EBCT is comparable with first-pass radionuclide angiography for calculation of left ventricular ejection fraction (LVEF) in patients with myocardial infarction[9] (Fig. 17-4). Serial changes in RV and LV volumes and diastolic parameters are well defined in patients following acute myocardial infarction.[10–12] Ventricular remodeling can be assessed by using EBCT in a similar fashion to gated blood pool radionuclide angiography[13,14] and echocardiography.[15] Cine EBCT can identify wall thinning and impaired LV thickening in an area of previous myocardial infarction[16] and delineate the presence of anterior and posterior LV aneurysms and associated mural thrombus[17,18] (Fig. 17-5).

Stress-rest EBCT imaging has been used to detect underlying ischemic heart disease based on changes in global LVEF and regional wall motion. One *small* study compared semisupine bicycle exercise contrast-enhanced EBCT with ^{99m}Tc myocardial perfusion single-photon-emission computed tomography (SPECT) in patients with suspected coronary artery disease (CAD), all of whom underwent angiography.[7] An abnormal EBCT study was defined as a less than 5 percent increase in LVEF during exercise. The sensitivity and specificity of exercise EBCT for detecting CAD were 81 and 76 percent, respectively, when using the global LVEF criteria for abnormalcy but improved to 88 and 100 percent when regional wall motion abnormalities were considered. EBCT was as accurate as ^{99m}Tc SPECT in the diagnosis of CAD.

Although echocardiography generally is used to assess valvular heart disease, EBCT is an alternative modality in patients with poor acoustic windows. In patients with mitral or aortic regurgitation, EBCT can accurately determine LV and RV stroke volumes and thereby calculate valvular regurgitant fractions.[5,19] When contemplating possible need for valvular surgery, EBCT can delineate the important parameters of LV chamber size, wall thickness, and LVEF. As with gated blood pool radionuclide angiography, EBCT

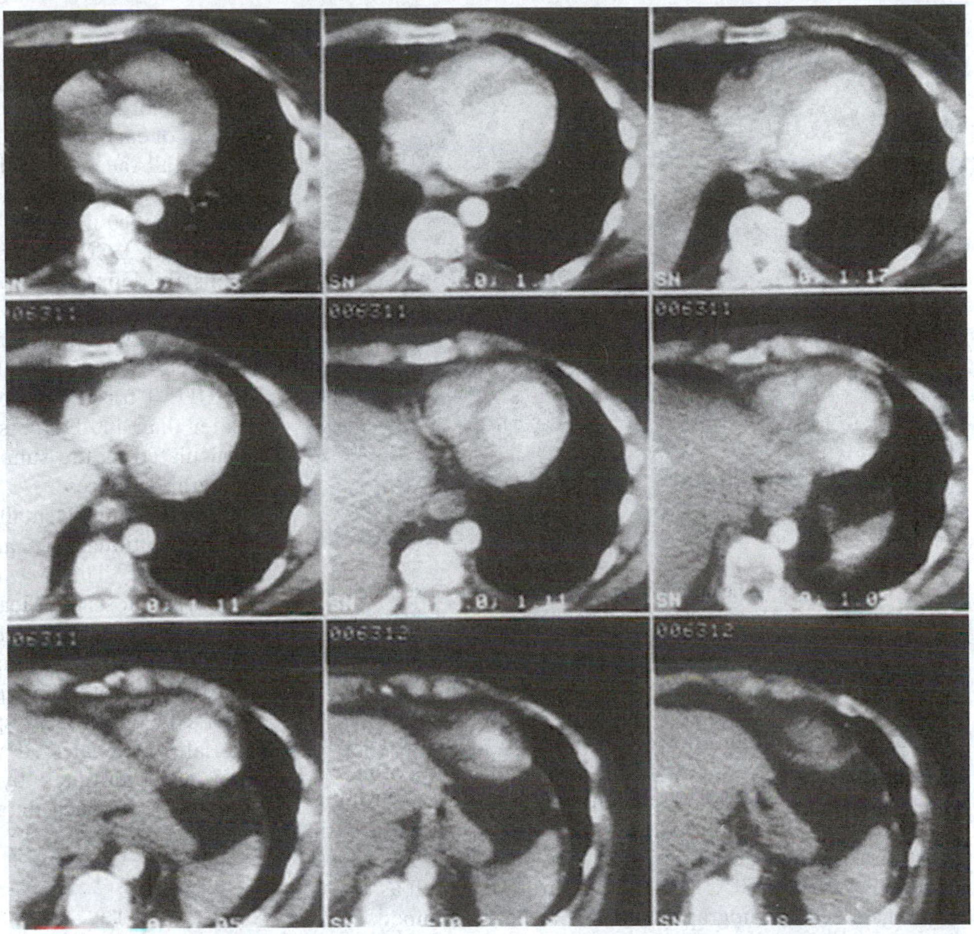

FIGURE 17-3 Fifty-millisecond contrast-enhanced EBCT images gated to end-diastole include the left ventricle from base (*top left*) to apex (*bottom right*). (From Brundage BH, Chomka E. Evaluation of acute myocardial infarction by computed tomography. In: Brundage BH, ed. *Comparative Cardiac Imaging*. Rockville, MD, Aspen, 1990:223–229. Reproduced with permission from the publisher and the authors.)

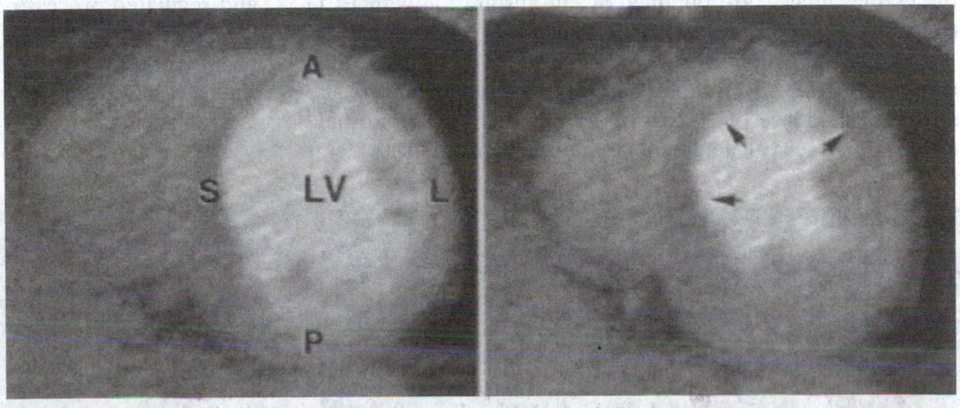

FIGURE 17-4 EBCT image of a mid-left ventricular (LV) slice in diastole (*left*) and systole (*right*), with an area of anteroseptal dyskinesis (*arrows*). The LVEF by EBCT was 37 percent versus 39 percent by first-pass radionuclide angiography. A, anterior; L, lateral; P, posterior; S, septal LV wall. (From Gerber TC, Behrenbeck T, Allison T, et al. Comparison of measurement of left ventricular ejection fraction by Tc-99m sestamibi first-pass angiography with electron beam computed tomography in patients with anterior wall acute myocardial infarction. *Am J Cardiol* 1999; 83:1022–1026. Reproduced with permission from the publisher and authors.)

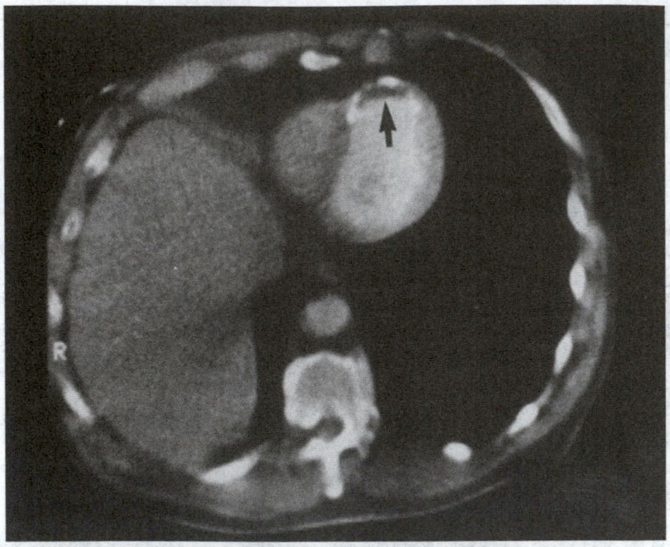

FIGURE 17-5 A single frame from a contrast-enhanced cine CT scan demonstrates thrombus in a LV aneurysm. Also note that the wall of the aneurysm is calcified.

cannot distinguish mitral from aortic regurgitation and cannot calculate the regurgitant fraction if significant right-sided valvular regurgitation is present. One of the complications of mitral valve disease is the development of left atrial thrombi. *One study* showed greater accuracy of EBCT as compared with transthoracic echocardiography in demonstrating left atrial thrombi.[20] Whether EBCT can detect thrombi as well as transesophageal echocardiography remains to be determined.

EVALUATION OF CAD

Detection of Coronary Artery Calcification

For the detection of coronary artery calcium with EBCT, typically 40 consecutive 3-mm-thick images are acquired at a rate of 100 ms per image from the base of the heart to just below the carina. Images are obtained at end-inspiration with ECG triggering at 80 percent of the RR interval (end-diastole). A calcified lesion generally is defined as either two or three adjacent pixels (0.68–1.02 mm^2 for a 512^2 reconstruction matrix and a camera field size of 30 cm) of greater than 130 Hounsfield units (HU). Each calcified lesion is multiplied by a density factor as follows: 1 for lesions with a maximal density between 130 and 199 HU, 2 for lesions between 200 and 299 HU, 3 for lesions between 300 and 399 HU, and 4 for lesions greater than 400 HU. The total coronary artery calcium score (CACS) is calculated as the sum of each calcified lesion in the four main coronary arteries over all the consecutive tomographic slices (Fig. 17-6).

With spiral computed tomography, consecutive 3-mm-thick images are acquired at a rate of two contiguous 2.5-mm slices per second. ECG gating generally is not employed. Calcified lesions are defined as those with a tomographic density greater than 90 HU (2 standard deviations above blood density) with an area greater than 0.5 mm^2. A modified density factor is used: 1 for lesions of 90 to 199 HU, 2 for lesions of 200 to 299 HU, 3 for lesions of 300 to 399 HU, and 4 for lesions greater than 400 HU. As with EBCT scoring, the total CACS is calculated as the sum of each calcified plaque over all the tomographic slices.

To date, only 1 small study has directly compared EBCT with conventional CT scanning in patients referred for coronary angiography.[21] Thirty-seven of 42 patients had significant (>50 percent) stenosis in at least one coronary artery. A close linear correlation was observed between the CACS derived from EBCT versus conventional CT scanning ($r = 0.98$; $p < 0.0001$). There are no other published studies comparing EBCT with either conventional or spiral CT. The EBCT-derived CACS correlates with calcified areas found in individual coronary arteries as determined by histomorphometric measurements[22] (Fig. 17-7). No such data are available using conventional or spiral CT.

Coronary Artery Calcification and Atherosclerotic Plaque Burden

The presence of coronary artery calcification is clearly indicative of coronary atherosclerosis.[23,24] Furthermore, the CACS severity, as assessed by EBCT, is directly related to the total atherosclerotic plaque burden present in the epicardial coronary arteries.[23,24] Coronary calcification begins early in life but progresses more rapidly in older individuals who have further advanced atherosclerotic lesions.[25] Calcification is an active, organized, and regulated process occurring during atherosclerotic plaque development, where calcium phosphate in the form of hydroxyapatite precipitates in atherosclerotic coronary arteries in a similar fashion as observed in bone mineralization.[26–28] Although lack of calcification does not categorically exclude the presence of atherosclerotic plaque, calcification occurs exclusively in ath-

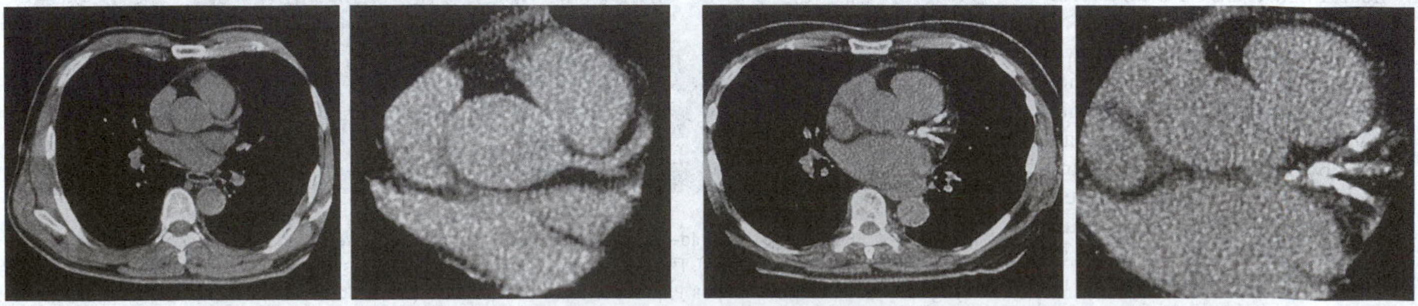

FIGURE 17-6 Single-level noncontrast EBCT scan of a normal subject (*left*) and an individual with severe coronary artery calcification (*right*). Calcium is shown as intensely white areas within the coronary arteries.

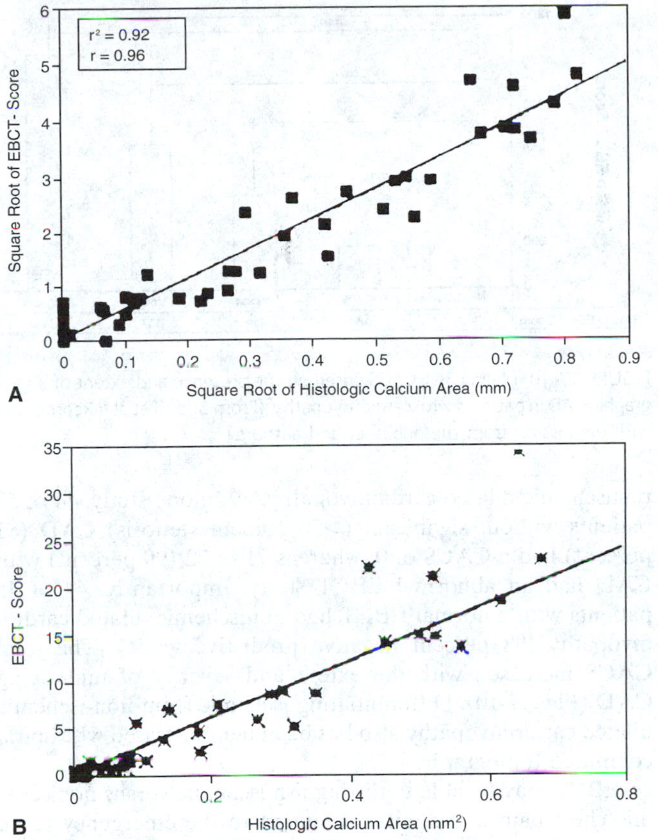

FIGURE 17-7 Linear regression comparing the EBCT CACS [square root transformation (*A*) and actual data (*B*)] versus the calcium area measured at histomorphometric examination. There is an apparent high positive correlation between the EBCT calcium score and histomorphometric calcium area ($r^2 = 0.92, r = 0.96; p < 0.0001$). (From Mautner et al.[22] Reproduced with permission from the publisher and authors.)

erosclerotic arteries and is not found in normal coronary arteries. However, it does not necessarily correlate with the presence or extent of coronary artery luminal stenosis (Chap. 40).

The presence and extent of histologically determined plaque area have been compared with the total calcium area as assessed by EBCT in individual coronary arteries derived from autopsied hearts.[23] A strong linear correlation exists between total coronary artery plaque area and the extent of coronary artery calcification as found in individual hearts ($r = 0.93; p < 0.001$) and in individual coronary arteries ($r = 0.90; p < 0.001$) (Fig. 17-8). However, the total calcium area underestimates total plaque area, with approximately five times as many noncalcified as calcified plaques.[23]

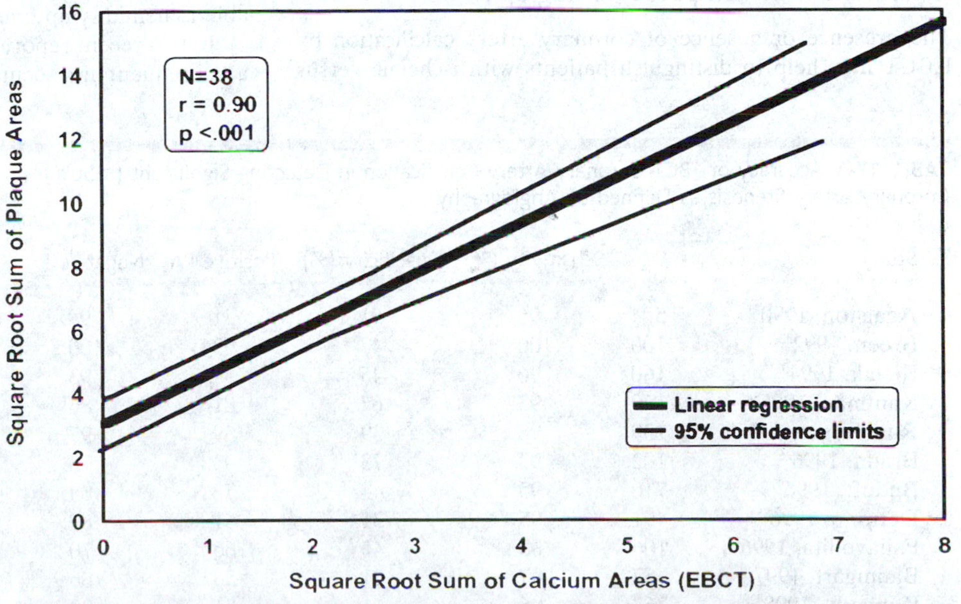

FIGURE 17-8 Comparison of the square root sum of total coronary calcium area (mm²) by EBCT with the actual atherosclerotic plaque area (mm²) for 38 individual coronary arteries. The linear regression line and 95 percent confidence intervals are shown. (From Rumberger et al.[23] Reproduced with permission from the publisher and authors.)

Coronary Artery Calcification and Stenosis Severity

Significant (>50 percent) coronary artery stenosis by angiography is associated with the presence of coronary artery calcium as assessed by EBCT. *Stenosis severity is not directly related to the total CACS, however.* A recent study compared calcium extent with coronary artery luminal diameter stenosis determined by morphologic examination of 723 coronary artery segments.[24] Although coronary stenosis severity increased with increasing coronary artery calcification, this relationship was poor and could not be used to estimate angiographic stenosis severity on a segment-by-segment basis (Fig. 17-9). One explanation is that coronary artery diameter increases with increasing plaque burden so as to maintain luminal patency.[29,30] Noncalcified plaques are usually associated with less than 50 percent diameter stenosis and typically less than 20 percent stenosis.[24] These data indicate that lack of coronary calcification predicts a very low likelihood of obstructive CAD.

Clinical angiographic trials confirm the relationship between CACS severity and the presence of significant (≥50 percent) CAD.[31–42] Although the diagnostic accuracy of EBCT improves with age, most younger patients (<50 years) with obstructive CAD also have coronary calcification (85 percent).[37,39] To date, there are 12 studies evaluating EBCT with coronary angiography where obstructive CAD was defined as greater than 50 percent luminal diameter stenosis[31–42] (Table 17-1). In these studies, the overall sensitivity and specificity for detecting obstructive CAD are 95 and 43 percent, respectively. *The poor specificity* of EBCT can be reconciled by the fact that the presence of coronary artery calcification confirms the presence of atherosclerotic plaque that may not necessarily be obstructive in nature. The CACS severity may be a better barometer of obstructive CAD than the mere presence of calcium. Budoff et al.[37] observed that specificity increased with the number of calcified

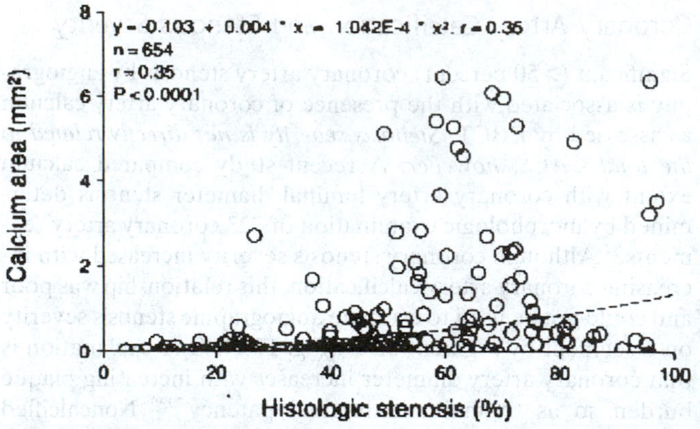

FIGURE 17-9 Graph showing the polynomial regression analysis of coronary calcium area (mm^2) versus percent histologic stenosis for 654 coronary artery segments with calcium greater than 0 mm^2. (From Sangiorgi et al.[24] Reproduced with permission from the publisher and authors.)

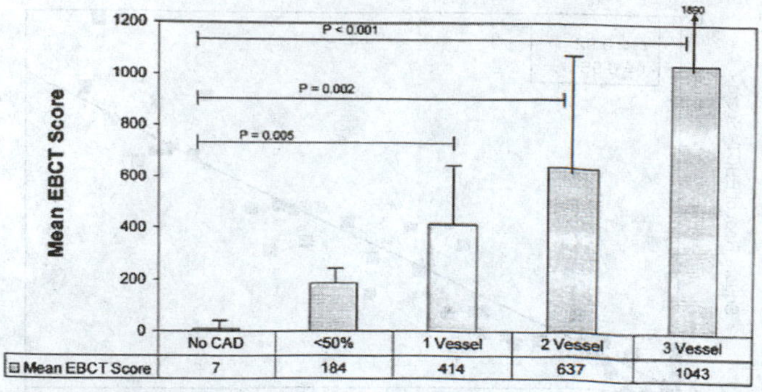

FIGURE 17-10 Mean EBCT CACS based on the presence and extent of angiographic CAD in patients with cardiomyopathy. (From Budoff et al.[45] Reproduced with permission from the publisher and authors.)

coronary arteries (i.e., high calcium scores). Two separate reports in patients referred for coronary angiography found that a CACS of more than 100 best predicted obstructive CAD with an equally high sensitivity and specificity of 80 percent.[43,44] There appears to be a threshold CACS above which most patients will have significant coronary artery stenosis. However, despite the relationship between obstructive CAD and CACS severity, *the latter is still too imprecise in itself to be used as a definitive criterion for proceeding directly to coronary angiography*. The current ACC/AHA guidelines on coronary angiography do not recommend coronary angiography on the basis of a positive EBCT.

Distinguishing Ischemic from Nonischemic Conditions with Computed Tomography

The presence or absence of coronary artery calcification by EBCT may help to distinguish patients with ischemic versus nonischemic dilated cardiomyopathy.[45,46] In one study, 44 of 53 patients without significant (>50 percent stenosis) CAD (83 percent) had a CACS of 0, whereas 71 of 72 (99 percent) with CAD had an abnormal EBCT study. Importantly, 44 of 45 patients with a normal EBCT had nonischemic dilated cardiomyopathy (98 percent negative predictive value). The total CACS increased with the extent and severity of underlying CAD (Fig. 17-10). Differentiating ischemic from non-ischemic dilated cardiomyopathy also has been demonstrated with spiral computed tomography.[46]

EBCT may be able to distinguish ischemic versus nonischemic chest pain in patients presenting to the emergency room with nondiagnostic electrocardiograms.[47] In one series, none of 47 patients with a normal EBCT had a subsequent cardiac event over a 1-month period. Conversely, 7 of 86 patients (8 percent) who had coronary calcification had a subsequent myocardial infarction ($n = 4$) or revascularization procedure ($n = 3$). The high negative predictive value of EBCT, despite its low positive predictive value, may improve triage of patients with questionable ischemic symptoms.

In two recent reports, most asymptomatic patients who had a subsequent first acute myocardial infarction had coronary calcification by EBCT (96 percent).[41,48] Since many acute myocardial infarctions occur following rupture of nonobstructive plaques, it is not surprising that the CACS will be mild (<100) in a large percentage (34 percent) of patients and severe (>400) in relatively few (27 percent).[48] In one study evaluating survivors of a first myocardial infarction with spiral CT, 19 percent lacked coronary artery calcification.[49] This higher percentage of normal studies may reflect the lower sensitivity of spiral CT as compared to EBCT for detecting calcium. Patients without calcium generally are younger in age and tend to be active smokers.[48,50] With the exception of young smokers, a normal EBCT defines a population at low likeli-

TABLE 17-1 Accuracy of EBCT Coronary Artery Calcification in Detecting Significant (>50%) Coronary Artery Stenosis as Defined by Angiography

Study	N	Sensitivity (%)	Specificity (%)	Positive PA	Negative PA
Agatston, 1990[31]	584	96	51	31	98
Breen, 1992[32]	100	100	47	63	100
Bielak, 1994[33]	160	96	45	57	93
Kaufman, 1995[34]	160	93	67	81	86
Rumberger, 1995[35]	139	98	39	59	97
Braun, 1996[36]	102	93	73	93	73
Budoff, 1996[37]	710	95	44	72	84
Detrano, 1996[38]	491	95	31	51	89
Fallavollita, 1996[39]	106	85	45	66	70
Baumgart, 1997[40]	57	97	21	56	86
Kennedy, 1998[42]	368	96	31	51	90
Schmermund, 1997[41]	118	95	88	99	58
TOTAL	3095	95	43	60	90

ABBREVIATIONS: PA = predictive accuracy.

hood for significant CAD and subsequent acute cardiac events. *Larger prospective trials in patients with acute coronary syndromes are needed to further delineate the role of EBCT in this population.*

Coronary Artery Calcification: Prognostic Implications

The likelihood of plaque rupture and the development of acute cardiovascular events is related to the total atherosclerotic plaque burden.[51,52] Since there is a direct relationship between the CACS severity and the extent of atherosclerotic plaque, the calcium score should predict risk for subsequent cardiovascular events among otherwise heterogeneous patient populations with cardiac risk factors even though most plaques vulnerable to erosion or fissure resulting in plaque rupture contain minimal calcium.[52a] In a study by He et al.,[53] the CACS severity identified a high-risk group of asymptomatic subjects who had silent myocardial ischemia. In fact, the total CACS was the best single predictor of an abnormal stress SPECT study. Many studies have now demonstrated an increased risk for cardiac events in asymptomatic patients who have extensive silent myocardial ischemia.[54–58] Since the total CACS severity predicts the presence of significant anatomic CAD and myocardial ischemia, it could be useful for risk assessment of asymptomatic individuals and potentially guide therapeutics.

Several recent trials have studied whether the extent of coronary artery calcification as assessed by EBCT can predict subsequent patient outcome. In an early series by Secci et al.,[59] 324 initially asymptomatic subjects were followed for 32 ± 4 months. Eleven patients died or had a nonfatal myocardial infarction (3.3 percent), and an additional 12 patients (3.7 percent) underwent coronary revascularization. A threefold higher event rate was observed in patients in the highest quartile of CACS (>506). In another report from the same group, 1196 asymptomatic patients were followed for 41 ± 5 months after undergoing EBCT.[60] Subjects with a CACS of greater than 44 (median value in this trial) were 2.3 times more likely to suffer myocardial infarction or cardiovascular death as compared with subjects with lower scores. Patients were enrolled only if they had greater than 10 percent risk for developing cardiovascular events over an 8-year period, as determined by the Framingham risk model. In this group at relatively high pretest clinical risk for cardiovascular events, the CACS results did not add to the Framingham risk model for predicting patient outcome.

Arad et al.[61] followed 1173 asymptomatic patients for 19 months after an initial screening EBCT. During follow-up, 18 patients (1.53 percent) had 26 cardiac events, including *1 death, 7 nonfatal myocardial infarctions,* and 17 coronary revascularization procedures. No events occurred in patients with a normal study, and the negative predictive value was 99.8 percent in patients with a CACS of less than 100. The positive predictive accuracy for cardiac events increased as the CACS increased from greater than 100 (5.5 percent) to 160 (7.1 percent) to greater than 680 (14 percent). Callister et al.[48] also reported similar data on 632 asymptomatic patients who were *referred* for a screening EBCT and then followed for 32 ± 7 months. In this study, both the absolute CACS and the age- and gender-adjusted relative CACS percentiles predicted subsequent hard cardiac events of death and nonfatal myocardial infarction. Hard cardiac events occurred in only 0.3 percent of subjects

TABLE 17-2 Cardiac Event Rates in Asymptomatic Subjects Based on Absolute and Relative Coronary Artery Calcium Scores

Absolute Calcium Score	Event Rate, Death/NFMI
0	0.3% (1/292)
1–99	5.5% (12/219)
100–400	10.8% (8/74)
>400	12.8% (6/47)
Calcium Score Percentile	
<50th	1.1% (4/351)
>50th	8.2% (23/281)
>75th	10.5% (19/181)
>90th	11.8% (11/93)

ABBREVIATIONS: NFMI = nonfatal myocardial infarction.
SOURCE: From Callister et al.[48] Adapted with permission of the publisher and authors.

with a normal EBCT, but this increased to 13 percent in those with a CACS of greater than 400. Likewise, in patients in the lower 50th percentile for CACS severity based on age and gender, the total cardiac event rate was only 1.1 percent compared with 8.2 percent for patients with a CACS greater than the 50th percentile (Table 17-2). In the studies of both Arad et al. and Callister et al., there were no adjusted estimates of outcome.[52,61a]

The exceedingly low cardiac event rate in subjects with a CACS of less than 100 is consistent with angiographic studies indicating a comparably low likelihood of significant CAD and an extremely low incidence of stress-induced myocardial ischemia (1.5 percent) in such individuals.[53] The increasing number of cardiac events with an ever-increasing CACS is also consistent with the dramatic increase in the incidence of stress-induced myocardial ischemia when scores are greater than 100 and particularly greater than 400.[53] All these data in asymptomatic patients indicate a potential role of EBCT in screening subjects for subclinical CAD. However, enrollment in prognostic studies primarily has been limited to Caucasian men. Whether the CACS severity has similar prognostic value in other patient populations remains unclear.[62] Since cardiac event rates are known to be very low in asymptomatic individuals with cardiac risk factors[57,61,63–66] (Table 17-3), large prospective trials in patients of greater ethnic diversity, followed for a longer period of time, will be needed to further clarify the value of EBCT in risk stratification.[67]

Screening for CAD Using EBCT

One of the most novel applications of EBCT may be as a screening test for identifying subjects with subclinical CAD based on the presence and severity of coronary artery calcification (for contrary view see Chap. 40). This is particularly true in view of recent primary prevention trials demonstrating that aggressive risk factor modification, including treatment of hyperlipidemia, reduces the incidence of subsequent cardiac events.[64,68]

TABLE 17-3 Cardiac Event Rates in Asymptomatic Patients

Study	N	% Men	Age (yrs)	F/U	Total Deaths/yr	CV Deaths/yr	Nonfatal MIs/yr	Angina Pectoris/yr
Arad et al.[61]	1173	71%	53 ± 11	1.6 yrs	—	0.05%	0.37%	2.3%
Shepherd et al.[66]	6595	100%	55 ± 5 (45–64)	5 yrs	0.73%	0.27%	1.0%	—
Detrano et al.[63]	1462	88%	63 ± 8 (≥45)	1 yr	—	0.40%	0.7%	2.5%
Ekelund et al.[57]	3806	100%	48 (35–59)	7.4 yrs	0.49%	0.24%	1.0%	—
MRFIT[65]	12,866	100%	46 (35–57)	7.0 yrs	0.58%	0.31%	0.7%	1.6%
Gordon et al.[66]	3640	100%	(30–70)	8.5 yrs	0.58%	0.27%	—	—
TOTAL	29,541	98%	—		0.60%	0.28%	0.8%	1.74%

ABBREVIATIONS: CV = cardiovascular; MI = myocardial infarction

RISK FACTOR ANALYSIS

Traditional risk factor analysis is commonly used to identify individuals who are at increased risk for developing cardiovascular disease based on standard clinical criteria.[69,70] Implicit to this risk model is the assumption that a certain combination of risk factors will promote atherosclerosis, which, in turn, will result in cardiovascular events. However, among individuals with a similar risk factor profile, the presence and severity of atherosclerosis will vary enormously; thereby overestimating risk in certain subjects and underestimating risk in others. This discrepancy will be most apparent among individuals with several risk factors who are members of a more heterogeneous population at risk compared with those without risk factors (a more uniformly low-risk group) or those with multiple risk factors (a more uniformly high-risk group). The imprecision of risk factor analysis for identifying patients with significant atherosclerosis is probably related to the fact that traditional risk factor analysis fails to incorporate presently unknown biochemical, environmental, and genetic factors that promote the development of CAD.

Since the development of symptomatic cardiovascular disease occurs almost exclusively in patients with atherosclerosis, it would seem advantageous in risk assessment to use a technique that directly measures the presence and severity of atherosclerotic burden rather than estimate its presence through indirect measures. For example, although there is a clear relationship between the number of cardiac risk factors and the presence of coronary artery calcification by EBCT, in one recent series, 40 percent of men and 30 percent of women without risk factors had coronary artery calcification, whereas 26 percent of men and 36 percent of women with greater than three traditional risk factors did not.[71] Similarly, in the Healthy Women Study, risk factor analysis was imprecise at predicting coronary calcification in postmenopausal women.[72] Although the combination of a high low-density lipoprotein (LDL) cholesterol level, a low high-density lipoprotein (HDL) cholesterol level, and a history of cigarette smoking was a strong predictor of coronary artery calcification, this risk factor profile was observed in only 6 percent of all women studied. Furthermore, only 6 of 21 women with the highest calcium scores (>101) had this risk factor profile. Conversely, 20 percent of women in the lowest risk profile (i.e., nonsmokers, LDL cholesterol < 130 mg/dL, and HDL cholesterol > 60 mg/dL) had calcium by EBCT. The incorporation of EBCT calcium results into traditional risk factor analysis may improve accuracy for identifying significant obstructive CAD in symptomatic patients[44,73] and also may be helpful in excluding extensive three-vessel or left main CAD in others.[74]

SUBCLINICAL CAD DETECTION AND STRESS TESTING

Noninvasive techniques, such as exercise treadmill testing and myocardial perfusion imaging, can identify patients with coronary atherosclerosis. However, unlike EBCT, which can detect coronary atherosclerosis at its earliest stages, these techniques can only identify patients with advanced CAD who manifest myocardial ischemia. Although the presence and extent of ischemia can accurately identify asymptomatic individuals at high risk for cardiac events[55–57] (Fig. 17-11), the very low prevalence of a positive test result (<5 percent) precludes their use as primary screening tests for the early detection and treatment of CAD. In fact, both exercise treadmill testing and myocardial perfusion imaging have received a class III indication (no justification for their use) for screening asymptomatic individuals (see Chap. 40).[75,76]

EBCT AND MYOCARDIAL PERFUSION IMAGING

A recent trial explored the complementary role of EBCT and myocardial perfusion SPECT for identifying both subclinical CAD and silent myocardial ischemia in a generally asymptomatic population who had risk factors for CAD development.[53] The purpose of this study was to identify (1) patients with subclinical CAD who might benefit from aggressive risk factor modification and (2) those who are at relatively higher short-term risk for cardiac events based on the presence of silent myocardial ischemia. Among the 3895 subjects who had EBCT, 411 also underwent stress SPECT within a close temporal period (median 17 days). The mean CACS was significantly higher in the 81 subjects (20 percent) who had an abnormal (1065 ± 983) as compared with a normal (286 ± 394; $p < 0.00001$) SPECT. The likelihood of an abnormal SPECT increased dramatically with the total CACS. Whereas only 1 percent of subjects with a total CACS of less than 100 had an abnormal SPECT, this was observed in 46 percent of those with scores of 400 or higher. Only 10 percent of all 3895 subjects scanned with EBCT had a CACS of 400 or higher. Large ischemic perfusion defects were virtually confined to subjects who had a CACS of 400 or higher. Patients with large ischemic perfusion defects by SPECT are known to be at high risk for subsequent cardiac events, whereas patients with small perfusion defects or those with normal scans

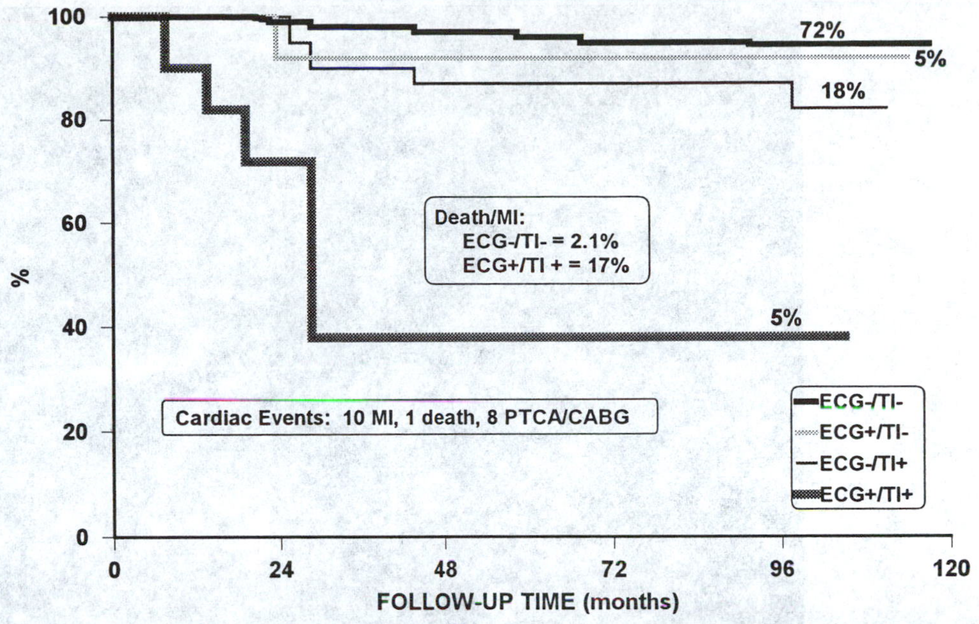

FIGURE 17-11 Kaplan-Meier survival curves based on exercise electrocardiogram and thallium-201 (Tl) scan results. The highest event rate is observed in patients with ischemia (+) by both tests. The percentage of patients with each test combination is shown above the curves. CABG, coronary artery bypass surgery; MI, myocardial infarction; PTCA, percutaneous transluminal coronary angioplasty. (From Blumenthal et al.[55] Reproduced with permission from the publisher and authors.)

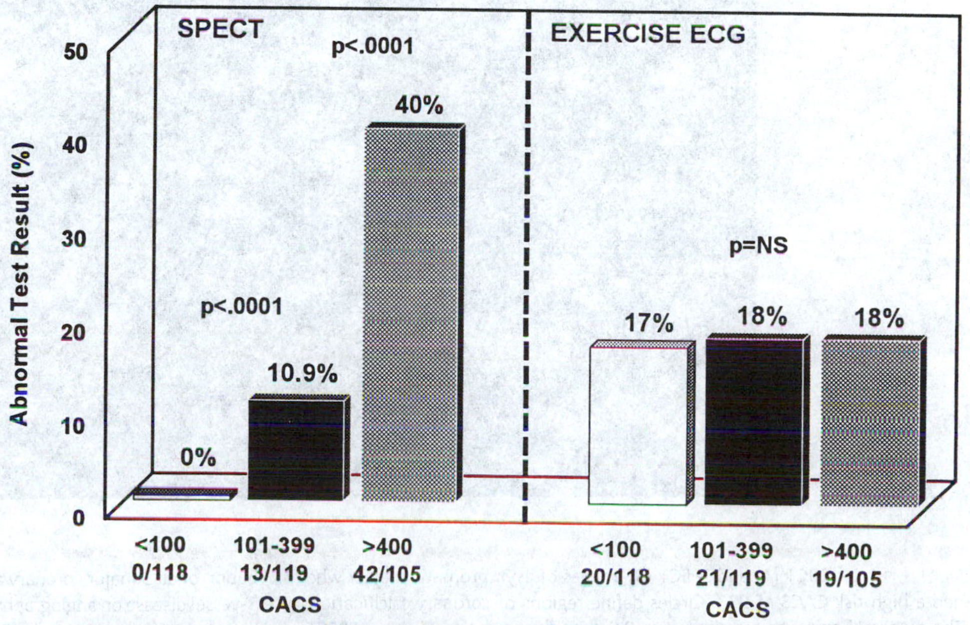

FIGURE 17-12 Exercise SPECT and ECG results based on total CACS. (From He et al.[53] Reproduced with permission from the publisher and authors.)

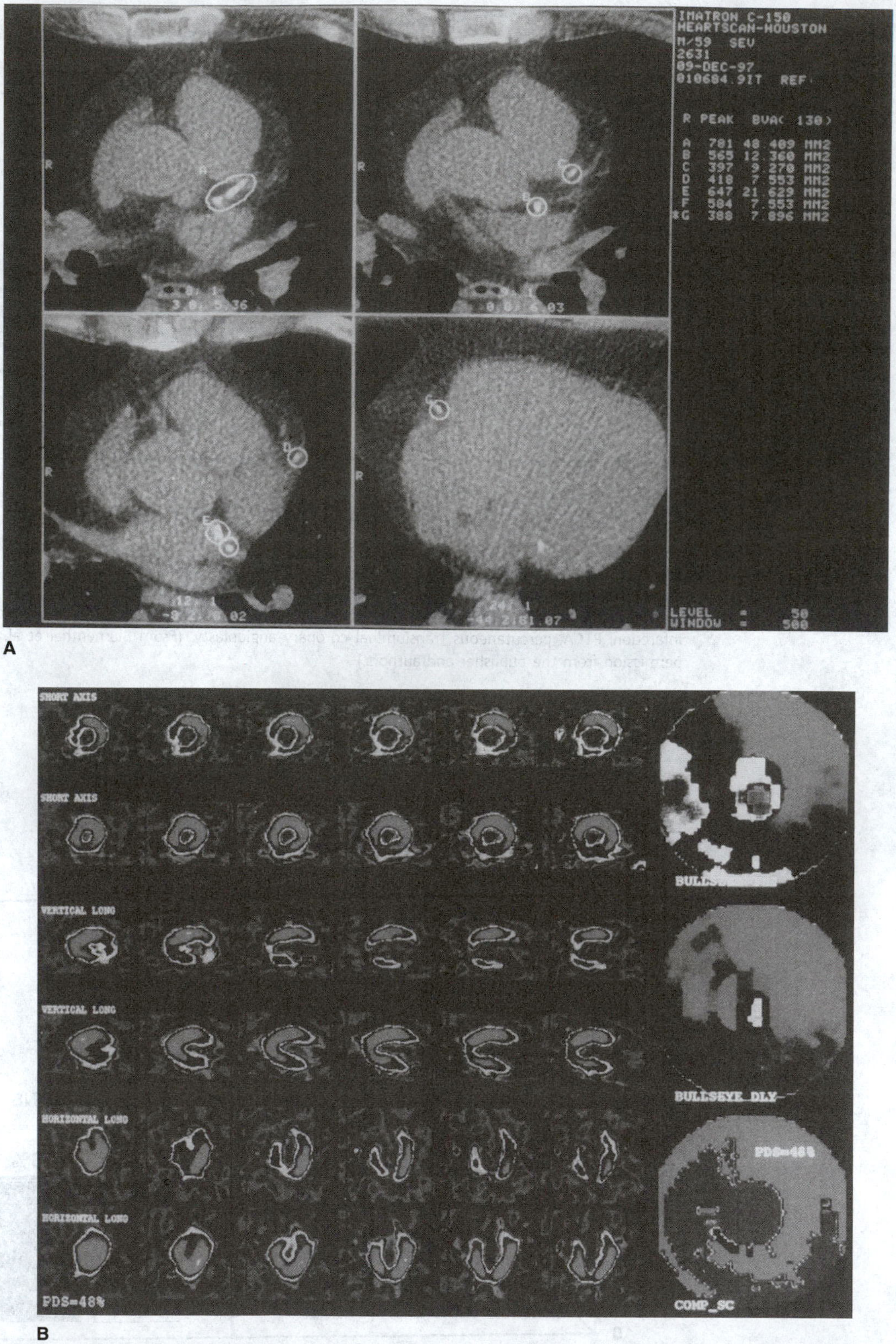

FIGURE 17-13 EBCT (*A*) and SPECT (*B*) images of asymptomatic subject who had a high-risk CACS of 937. Circles define regions of coronary calcification. The treadmill test was terminated at 9.0 min due to patient fatigue. SPECT demonstrated a large, reversible 48 percent perfusion defect within the distribution of all 3 major coronary arteries (COMP-SC) (*B*). This patient had severe 3-vessel disease on angiography and underwent CABG. PDS indicates perfusion defect size. (From He et al.[53] Reproduced with permission from the publisher and authors.)

have an exceedingly low cardiac event rate.[55–56,77–79] Although a similar percentage of subjects had an abnormal SPECT (16.1 percent) or stress electrocardiogram (17.5 percent; p = NS), only the former was related to the total CACS (Fig. 17-12), further illustrating the poor predictive accuracy of treadmill testing for detecting CAD in asymptomatic subjects (see also Chap. 14).

In the author's opinion, the results of this study support the role of EBCT as an initial screening test for identifying subjects with varying degrees of coronary atherosclerosis and emphasize the effectiveness of selectively combining SPECT with EBCT in the anticipated small percentage of subjects who will have a high (>400) CACS so as to specifically identify those with silent myocardial ischemia (Fig. 17-13). *These results need further confirmation.* Although the cost-effectiveness of using EBCT as a screening test requires further clinical investigation, it has been proposed that the CACS may be used to guide therapeutics and recommend the need for additional diagnostic testing.[80] This approach has not been sanctioned by the ACC/AHA expert consensus document on EBCT for the diagnosis and prognosis of CAD[81] or by the AHA Prevention V Conference[82] (see Chap. 40).

Tracking Changes in Coronary Artery Calcification

Sequential testing with EBCT may be useful in determining the rate of progression of coronary atherosclerosis[83] or in identifying treatment effects based on regression of coronary artery calcification.[84] In order for sequential testing to have any clinical relevance, the biologic changes being studied need to be greater than the intrinsic variability of the test result. Thus, if a CACS increased from 300 to 400, only by knowing the variability inherent to the test result could one determine whether this was a true patient change.

EBCT REPRODUCIBILITY

The reproducibility of EBCT has been evaluated using both the traditional Agatston scoring system[33,85–87] and a more recent volumetric calcium scoring system.[88] With the Agatston method, good inter- and intraobserver reproducibility is reported for recalculating the CACS on a single scan.[31,86] However, significant variability exists when comparing the results of two separate studies on the same patient. Devries et al.[85] studied 91 subjects who had two EBCT scans performed 24 h apart using an identical acquisition protocol. The variability in CACS observed in the 42 subjects who were abnormal on both scans was 49 ± 45 percent. Variability was inversely related to the absolute value of the CACS, being particularly great when the initial score was less than 10 (72 ± 54 percent). In a report by Bielak et al.,[33] 256 patients had two EBCT studies performed minutes apart. The mean CACS was 73 ± 233 (scan 1) versus 75 ± 242 (scan 2). Linear regression analysis showed that the two scores were highly correlated ($r = 0.962$; $p = 0.0001$). However, CACS variability was greatest particularly in patients with low scores. These studies indicate that large changes in initial CACS may be needed to be confident that a real change has occurred beyond chance alone. If one considers that the rate of progression of CACS in patients with known CAD may be less than the observed variability of the test,[83] EBCT assessments using the Agatston scoring system may not be able to track changes in atherosclerotic plaque burden.

The volumetric calcium scoring method proposed by Callister et al.[88] calculates the volume of calcified plaque area rather than generating a CACS based on an arbitrary plaque attenuation coefficient (i.e., Agatston method). This method has been shown in one study to be more reproducible than the Agatston method, with an approximately 40 percent reduction in overall variability.[88]

TRACKING CALCIUM PROGRESSION/REGRESSION

If the reproducibility of EBCT using the volumetric method is adequate, an important question is whether EBCT can be used to track the effects of pharmacologic therapy on plaque progression.[84] In a recent *retrospective* analysis with all of its limitations, Callister et al.[84] studied 149 asymptomatic hyperlipidemic patients who had no history of prior CAD or treatment of hyperlipidemia and who underwent a baseline screening EBCT. Following EBCT, treatment with a statin drug was begun at the discretion of the referring physician. Serial measurements of LDL cholesterol were obtained and correlated with the change in calcified plaque volume. Sixty-five treated patients achieved an LDL cholesterol level of less than 120 mg/dL (mean 100 ± 17 mg/dL), whereas 40 did not (mean 139 ± 18 mg/dL). In the 44 untreated patients, the mean LDL cholesterol level was 147 ± 22 mg/dL. Importantly, in the 44 untreated patients and in the 40 treated patients with an LDL cholesterol level of greater than 120 mg/dL, the calcium score increased by 52 ± 36 and 25 ± 22 percent, respectively. However, in the treated patients who achieved an LDL cholesterol level of less than 120 mg/dL, the calcium score decreased by 7 ± 23 percent. Sixty-three percent of the patients in this group had a net decrease in their calcium volume score, whereas none of the other patients had a reduction in calcium score.

These data suggest that aggressive treatment with cholesterol-lowering medication can reduce *calcified plaque burden* as assessed by EBCT. The reduction in calcified plaque burden presumably indicates a reduction in total atherosclerotic plaque, which is consistent with prior angiographic studies showing a small, albeit significant, reduction in coronary artery stenosis severity with long-term statin therapy.[89,90]

Contrast Angiography of Bypass Grafts and Native Coronary Arteries

BYPASS GRAFTS

Contrast-enhanced EBCT can visualize both coronary artery bypass grafts[91–93] and native coronary arteries.[94–97] Initial studies using conventional CT angiography reported a sensitivity and specificity of 93 and 95 percent, respectively, for detecting graft patency when compared with coronary angiography.[98] More recently, spiral CT also has been studied for identifying bypass graft patency.[99] The sensitivity, specificity, and diagnostic accuracy for detecting graft patency were 92, 97, and 93 percent, respectively.[99] Positive predictive accuracy for graft closure was 78 percent, and the negative predictive accuracy for graft patency was 99 percent. The accurate detection of internal mammary artery grafts was somewhat lower than that for vein grafts, as was the detection of distal anastomotic sites. Studies using EBCT have likewise reported high sensitivity (89 percent), spec-

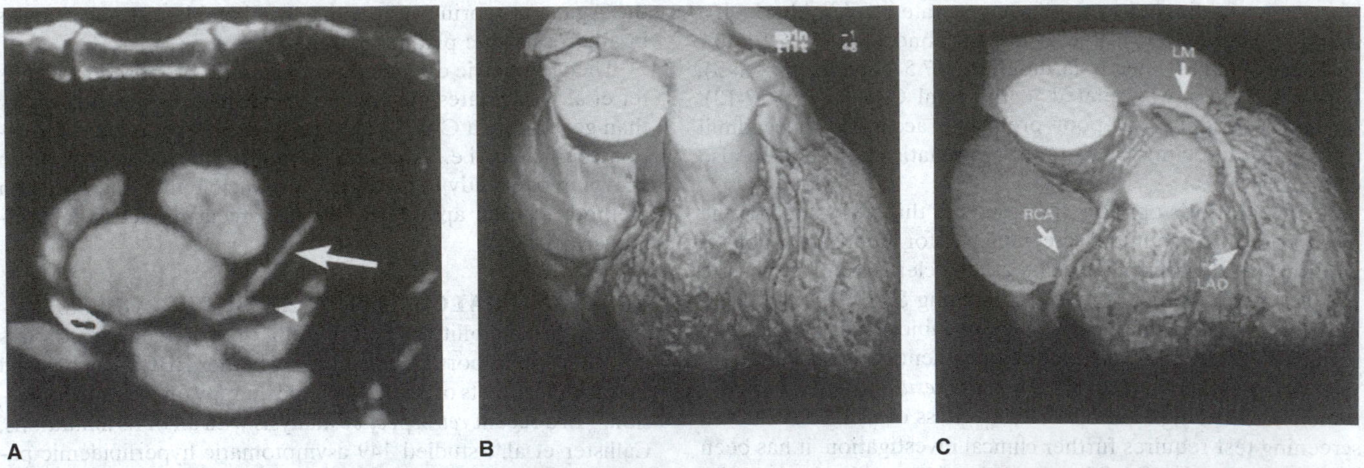

FIGURE 17-14 EBCT images of the heart. *A.* A cross section of the heart at the level of the aortic root depicts the origin of the left main (LM), proximal left anterior descending (LAD) (*arrow*), and left circumflex (*arrowhead*) coronary arteries. *B.* A contrast-enhanced three-dimensional reconstruction of the entire heart. *C.* The main stem of the pulmonary artery and the atrial appendages have been removed to show the LM, LAD, and right (RCA) coronary arteries. (From Achenbach et al.[94] Reproduced with permission from the publisher and authors.)

ificity (93 percent), and overall diagnostic accuracy (92 percent) for detecting bypass graft patency.[91] However, as with spiral computed tomography, EBCT cannot distinguish partially obstructive versus nonobstructed grafts, and the accuracy for assessing graft patency is worse for the right and circumflex arteries as compared with the left anterior descending coronary artery.

NATIVE CORONARY ARTERIES

EBCT also has been established as a noninvasive method for visualizing the epicardial coronary arteries.[94–97] The imaging technique is similar to that used for scanning for coronary artery calcification but requires intravenous contrast material injection. A scout scan is first performed to localize the position of the heart in the chest. The time from contrast material injection to peak contrast enhancement of the aortic root is then determined. The amount of dye administered is based on the heart rate and the number of slices desired. Forty contrast-enhanced cross-sectional images of the heart of 3-mm thickness are then obtained during full inspiration at an acquisition rate of 100 ms per image (one image per cardiac cycle). Image acquisition is gated to the electrocardiogram in a standard fashion. Using the preceding parameters and depending on the heart rate, the total imaging time is between 30 and 50 s (Fig. 17-14).

Several small series have compared EBCT with standard coronary angiography for detecting CAD[94–97] (Table 17-4). The overall sensitivity of EBCT for detecting significant (>50 percent) stenosis is 83 percent and increases to 92 percent for detecting high-grade (>75 percent) stenosis (Fig. 17-15). Specificity is also comparably high at 92 percent.

EBCT can detect high-grade restenosis after previous coronary artery angioplasty with high sensitivity (94 percent) and specificity (82 percent).[100] Most patients (96 percent) without restenosis by EBCT have comparable normal angiographic findings (Fig. 17-16).

These reports are encouraging, but several points must be emphasized. EBCT *cannot* assess approximately 20 to 25 percent of all coronary arteries due to technical factors, such as respiration artifact, the presence of severe coronary calcification, and motion artifacts. Respiration artifacts can be avoided

TABLE 17-4 Diagnostic Accuracy of Contrast Enhanced EBCT as Defined by Coronary Angiography

Study	No. of Pts	CAD Definition	ARI	Sensitivity	Specificity	Positive PA	Negative PA	Overall Accuracy
Achenbach et al.[94]	125	>75%	376/500 (75%)	69/75 (92%)	282/301 (94%)	69/88 (78%)	282/288 (98%)	351/376 (93%)
Schmermund et al.[95]	28	>50%	237/330* (72%)	31/38 (82%)	176/199 (88%)	31/54 (57%)	176/183 (96%)	207/237 (87%)
Rensing et al.[96]	37	>50%	211/259* (81%)	25/33 (76%)	168/178 (94%)	25/35 (71%)	168/176 (95%)	193/211 (91%)
Budoff et al.[97]	52	>50%	185/208 (89%)	43/55 (78%)	118/130 (91%)	43/55 (78%)	118/130 (91%)	161/185 (87%)
TOTAL	242		1009/1297 (78%)	168/201 (83%)	744/808 (92%)	168/232 (72%)	741/777 (96%)	912/1009 (90%)

ABBREVIATIONS: ARI = arteries (segments*) interpretable by EBCT; PA = predictive accuracy.

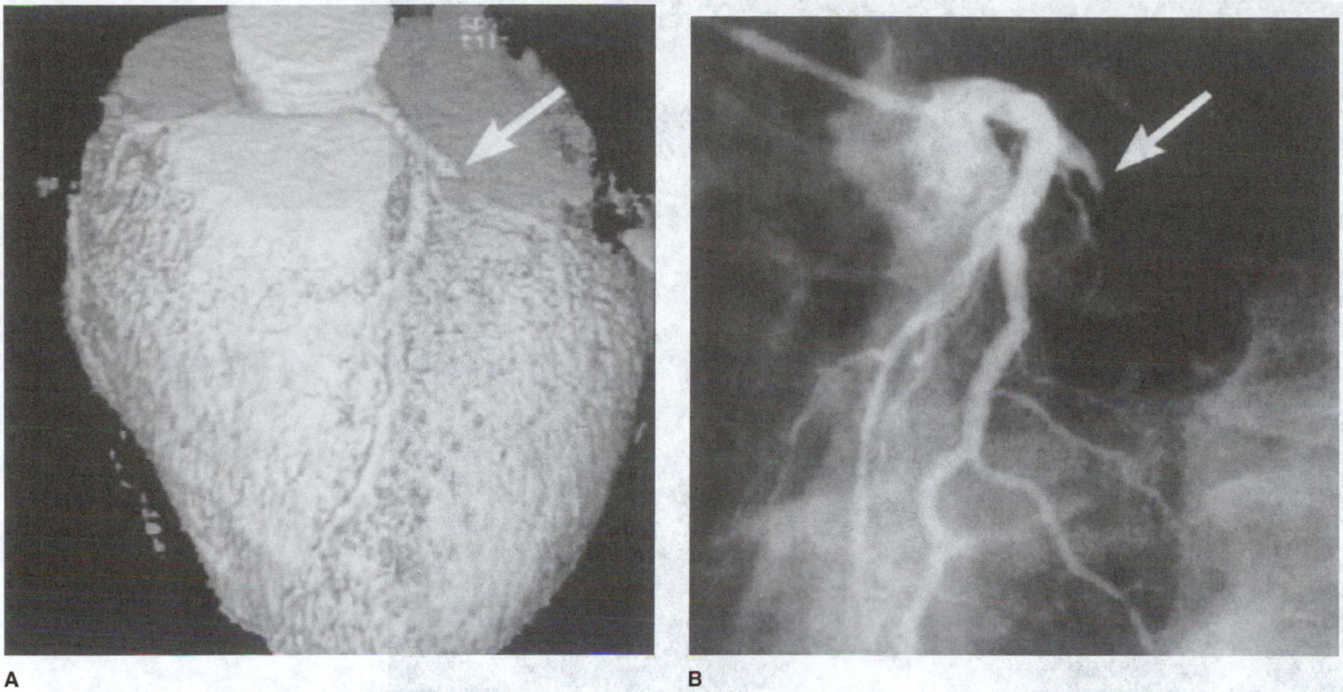

FIGURE 17-15 EBCT (*A*) and coronary angiography (*B*) of a patient with complete occlusion of the left circumflex coronary artery (*arrow*). (From Achenbach et al.[94] Reproduced with permission from the publisher and authors.)

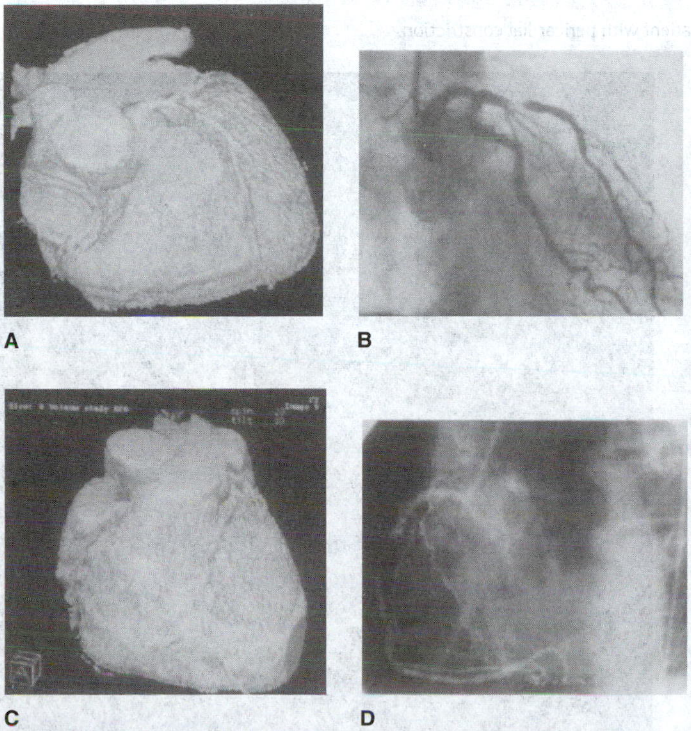

FIGURE 17-16 Three-dimensional EBCT reconstruction and coronary angiography depicting high-grade restenosis after coronary angioplasty of the proximal left anterior descending coronary artery (*A, B*) and right coronary artery (*C, D*). (From Achenbach et al.[100] Reproduced with permission from the publisher and authors.)

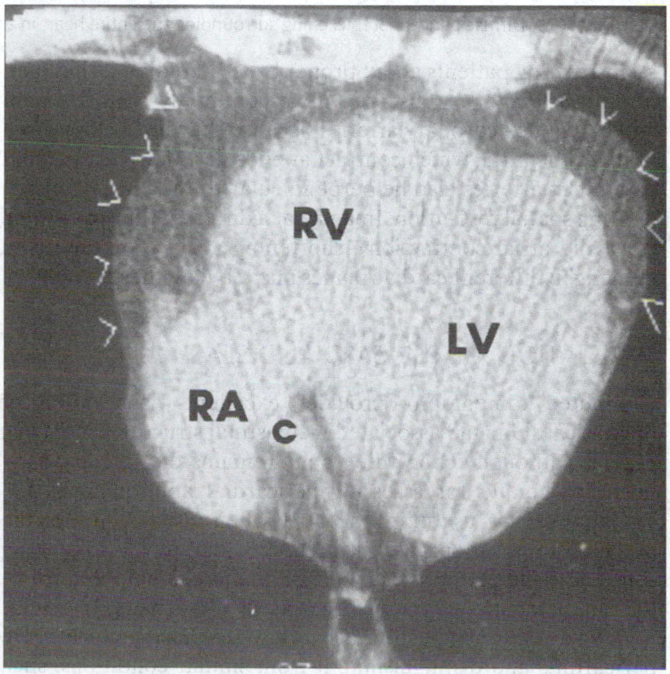

FIGURE 17-17 The fat that resides both inside and outside (*arrowheads*) the pericardium provides sufficient contrast to outline the normal pericardium, which is only 1- to 2-mm thick. Contrast enhancement with iodine agents is unnecessary. C, coronary sinus; LV, left ventricle; RA, right atrium; RV, right ventricle. (From Brundage BH, Mao SS. In: Schlant RC et al., eds. *Diagnostic Atlas of the Heart*. New York: McGraw-Hill; 1996:243. Reproduced with permission from the publisher and authors.)

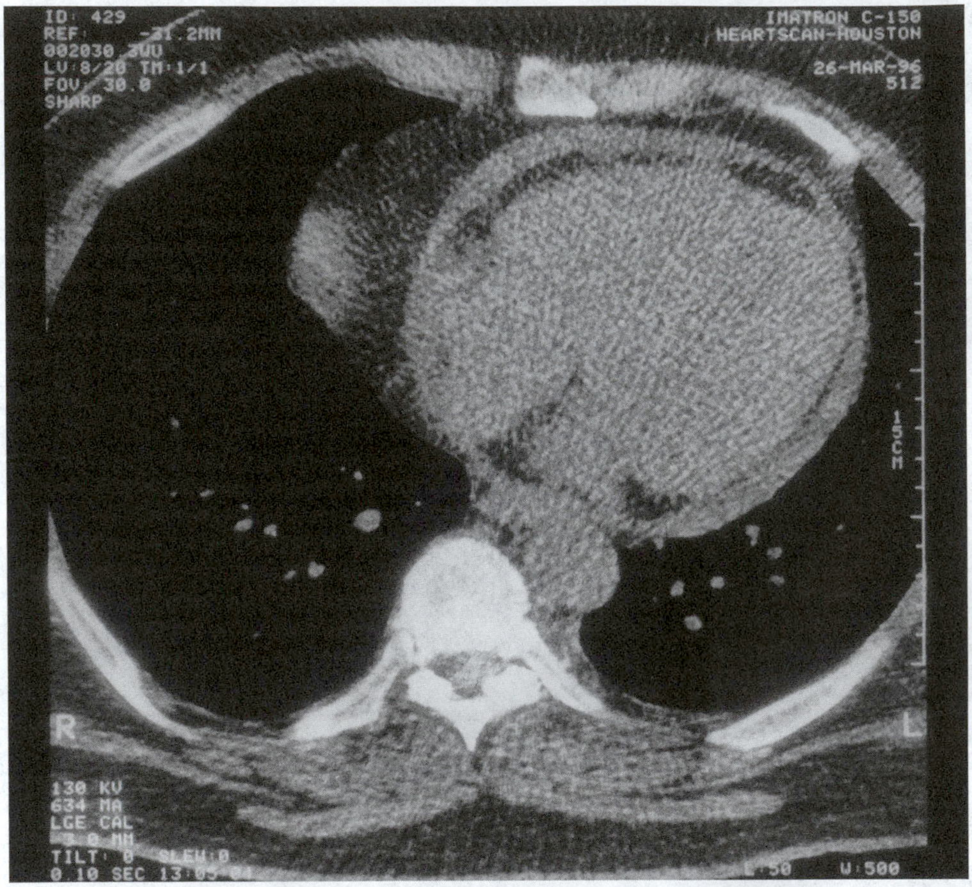

FIGURE 17-18 Diffuse pericardial thickening surrounding the entire heart in a patient with pericardial constriction.

by instructing patients about proper breath-holding techniques. *Motion artifacts* are observed most commonly with the right and circumflex coronary arteries because they lie in close proximity to the atria, which contract at end-diastole. The right and circumflex arteries also lie perpendicular to the imaging plane, limiting spatial resolution. Imaging at a different time in diastole (to avoid atrial contraction), shortening acquisition time, and imaging in different cardiac planes may obviate these problems.

EVALUATION OF PERICARDIAL DISEASE

Computed tomography provides excellent visualization of the pericardium and associated mediastinal structures[101–104] (Fig. 17-17). Although echocardiography remains the primary diagnostic technique for assessing pericardial abnormalities, CT scanning can be useful, particularly when visualization of the pericardium is suboptimal with echocardiography. CT scanning can readily detect pericardial effusion and can help determine the characteristics of the fluid based on CT density.[105]

CT scanning is useful in accurately diagnosing constrictive pericarditis and distinguishing it from similar conditions, such as restrictive myopathy.[102] Based on the presence of pericardial thickening (Fig. 17-18) or calcification (Fig. 17-19), cine EBCT can assess both the anatomic and functional abnormalities associated with pericardial constriction.[103] A pericardial thickness of more than 4 mm in a patient with typical abnormal rapid early LV diastolic filling is diagnostic of pericardial constriction.

CT scanning can assess congenital abnormalities such as absence of the pericardium[106] or pericardial cyst.[107] CT scanning

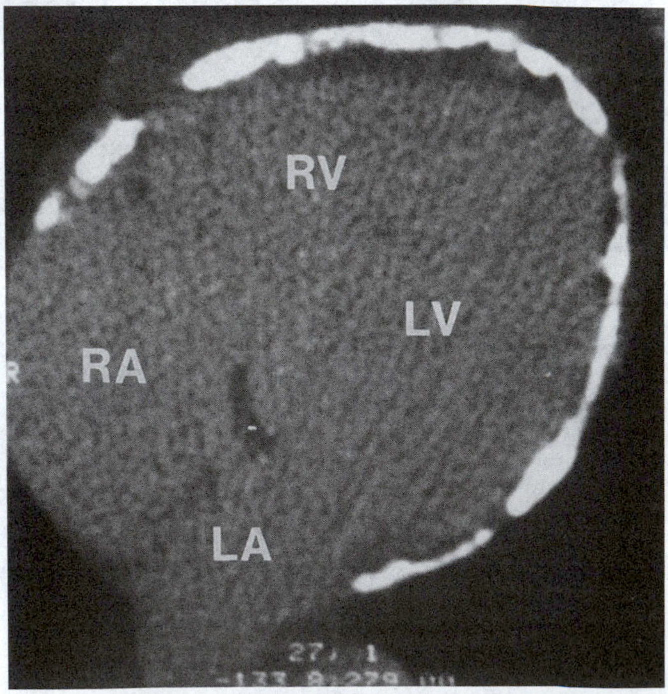

FIGURE 17-19 Densely calcified pericardium is easily identified in this scan of the midheart. LA, left atrium; LV, left ventricle; RA, right atrium; RV, right ventricle. (From Brundage BH, Mao SS. In: Schlant RC et al., eds. *Diagnostic Atlas of the Heart*. New York: McGraw-Hill; 1996:243. Reproduced with permission from the publisher and authors.)

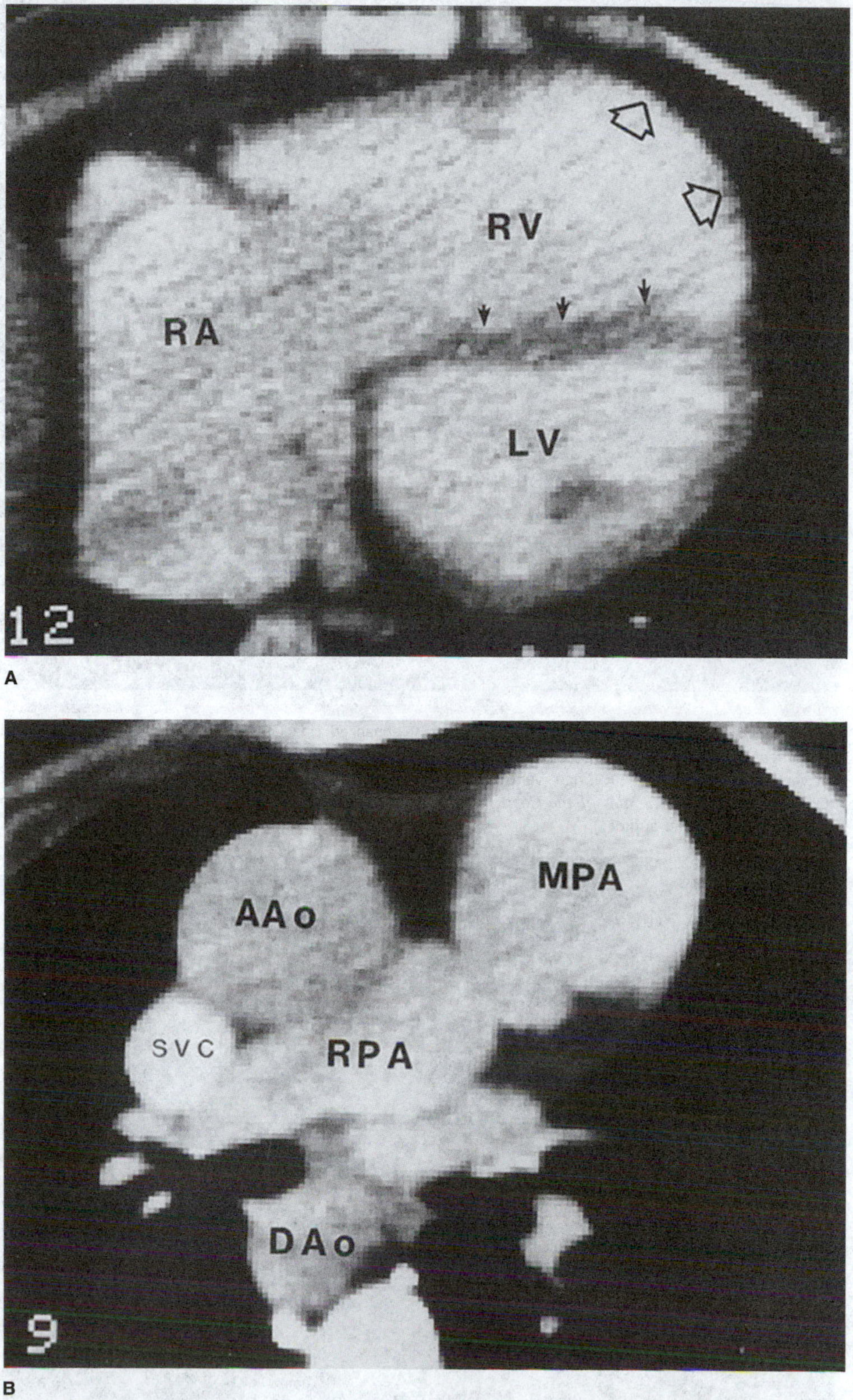

FIGURE 17-20 Postoperative EBCT study of a patient operated for tetralogy of Fallot demonstrates (*A*) RV dilatation and aneurysm (*open arrows*) with paradoxical diastolic flattening of the interventricular septum due to severe tricuspid regurgitation. The same study (*B*) revealed residual stenosis of the right pulmonary artery (RPA). Aao, ascending aorta; Dao, descending aorta; LV, left ventricle; MPA, main pulmonary artery; RA, right atrium; SVC, superior vena cava.

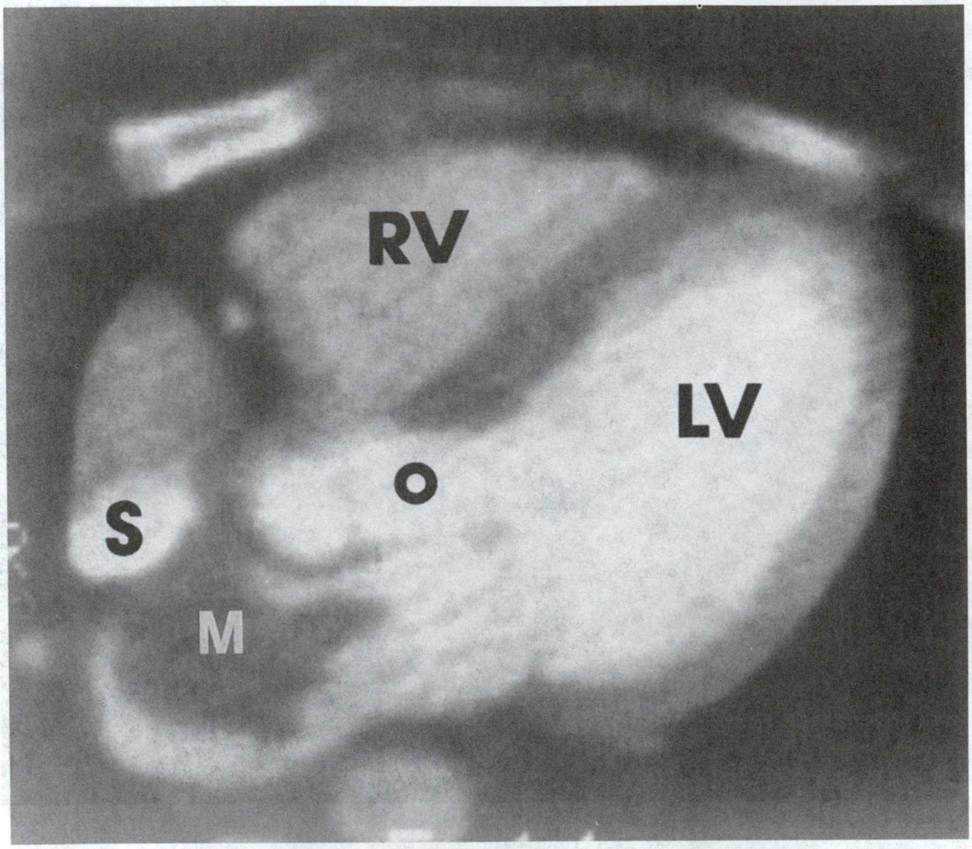

FIGURE 17-21 A single diastolic frame from a contrast-enhanced cine CT scan defines the left atrial septal attachment of a myxoma (M). The frondlike excrescences are characteristic of this tumor. LV, left ventricle; O, left ventricular outflow tract; RV, right ventricle; S, superior vena cava. (From Brundage BH, Mao SS. In: Schlant RC et al., eds. *Diagnostic Atlas of the Heart*. New York: McGraw-Hill; 1996:244. Reproduced with permission from the publisher and authors.)

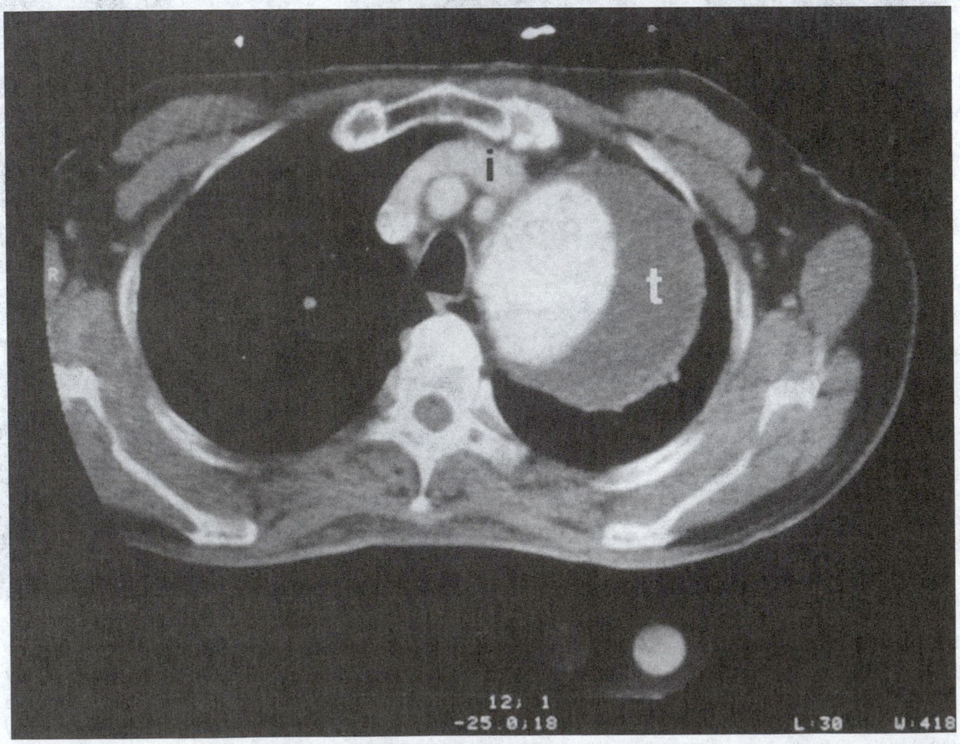

FIGURE 17-22 A large thrombus (t)-filled aneurysm of the aortic arch occupies most of the upper left thoracic cavity. The innominate vein (i) courses anterior to the innominate and left common carotid artery.

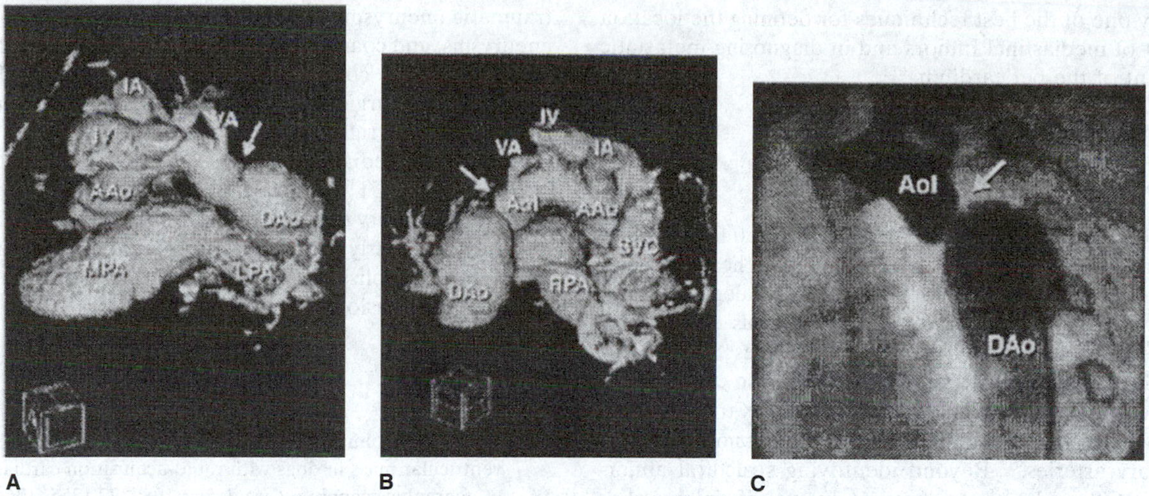

FIGURE 17-23 Three-dimensional EBCT reconstructions of aortic arch, innominate vein (IV), main (MPA), left (LPA), and right (RPA) pulmonary arteries in a patient with recurrent coarctation of the aorta. The upper panel (*A*) shows a possible web along the upper surface of the aortic isthmus (AoI) (*arrow*) with aneurysmal dilatation of the descending aorta (DAo) below the coarctation site. The lower panel (*B*) shows a well-defined web (*arrow*). The corresponding aortogram (*C*) (*right*) shows a discrete web below AoI with a DAo aneurysm. Aao, ascending aorta; IA, innominate artery; SVC, superior vena cava; VA, vertebral artery. (From Pitlick PT, Anthony CL, Moore P, et al. Three-dimensional visualization of recurrent coarctation of the aorta by electron-beam tomography and MRI. *Circulation* 1999; 99:3086–3087. Reproduced with permission from the publisher and authors.)

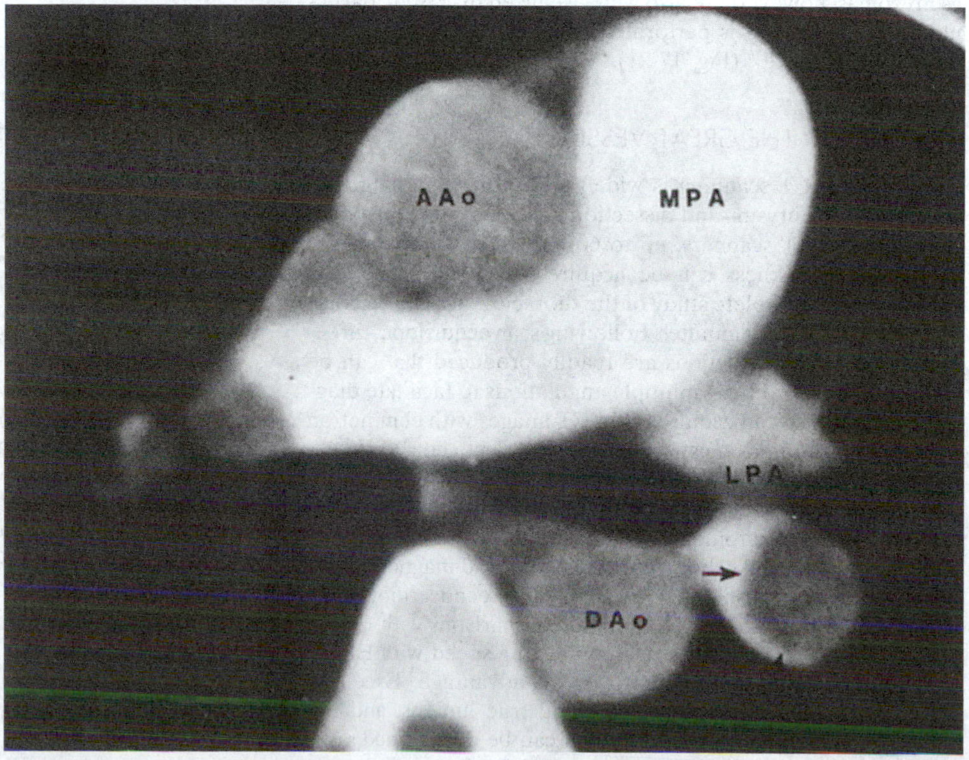

FIGURE 17-24 Large left pulmonary artery (LPA) chronic thrombus (*arrows*) is outlined by contrast medium on this high-resolution ultrafast CT scan. Aao, ascending aorta; Dao, descending aorta; MPA, main pulmonary artery.

is currently one of the best techniques for defining the location and extent of mediastinal tumors and in diagnosing metastatic involvement of the pericardium.[107,108]

EVALUATION OF CONGENITAL HEART DISEASE

Standard CT scanning and EBCT are both useful techniques in the evaluation of patients with congenital heart disease. Anomalies of the aortic arch, septal defects, tetralogy of Fallot, Ebstein's anomaly, and abnormal arteriovenous connections can all be carefully evaluated with CT techniques[109,110] (Fig. 17-20). EBCT, due to its high spatial resolution, also can evaluate the atrioventricular valves in conditions such as tricuspid and mitral valve atresia,[111,112] and detect congenital abnormalities of the coronary arteries.[113] Beyond identifying structural abnormalities, EBCT can be used to accurately quantify intracardiac shunts,[114,115] assess RV and LV function,[5,7] measure myocardial mass,[1-3] and evaluate valvular function. Despite the applications of CT scanning in evaluating congenital heart disease, magnetic resonance imaging is the modality of choice because it does not require x-ray exposure or the need for intravenous contrast material for both structural and functional delineation.

EVALUATION OF CARDIAC TUMORS

The presence and extent of intracardiac tumors (Chap. 77) can be well defined with either conventional CT scanning or EBCT. CT scanning also can delineate metastatic tumor within the myocardial wall. Intracardiac tumors are readily detected by noninvasive two-dimensional echocardiography. Tumors such as myxomas, however, are also well visualized by EBCT, particularly when imaging is performed following intravenous contrast enhancement[116] (Fig. 17-21).

DISEASES OF THE GREAT VESSELS

Conventional CT scanning is widely used for diagnosing thoracic aortic aneurysms and dissections.[117-119] With the introduction of spiral CT scanners, up to 60 images of approximately 2- to 3-mm thickness can be acquired within a single 30-s breathhold. A complete study of the thoracic aorta can be completed in only several minutes. Following scan acquisition, three-dimensional reconstructions are readily produced that can be rotated and viewed from multiple angulations to facilitate diagnosis. EBCT also can acquire rapid CT images with elimination of aortic pulsation as a cause for potential artifact.[120]

Aortic dissection is readily diagnosed with CT angiography with greater than 90 percent accuracy. In a recent study comparing spiral computed tomography, magnetic resonance imaging, and two-dimensional echocardiography, CT and magnetic resonance imaging were shown to be superior to echocardiography in their diagnostic accuracy.[119] Similar comparisons with EBCT are not available, but the increased imaging speed with EBCT over spiral CT would appear to be an advantage. Excellent definition of the intimal flap, false and true lumens, and the amount of intraaneurysmal thrombus can be determined.

CT scanning is also an effective method for diagnosing aortic aneurysm, defining its maximal diameter, and monitoring its expansion over time[120] (Fig. 17-22). CT scanning can diagnose traumatic aneurysms of the thoracic aorta,[118] sinus of Valsalva aneurysms, and coarctation of the aorta (Fig. 17-23). In patients undergoing redo coronary artery bypass surgery, CT scanning may guide the surgical approach by defining the position of the sternum to the right ventricle and aorta and thereby avoid unnecessary bleeding.[121]

Both spiral CT[122,123] and EBCT[124] can diagnose acute and chronic pulmonary thromboembolism (Fig. 17-24). CT scanning may be particularly useful in confirming the diagnosis of acute pulmonary embolism in patients with an intermediate nuclear ventilation-perfusion scan.[123]

References

1. Feiring AJ, Rumberger JA, Reiter SJ, et al. Determination of left ventricular mass in dogs with rapid-acquisition cardiac computed tomographic scanning. *Circulation* 1985; 72:1355–1364.
2. Hajduczok ZD, Weiss RM, Stanford W, et al. Determination of right ventricular mass in humans and dogs with ultrafast cardiac computed tomography. *Circulation* 1990; 82:202–212.
3. Roig E, Deorgiou D, Chomka EV, et al. Reproducibility of left ventricular myocardial volume and mass measurements by ultrafast computed tomography. *J Am Coll Cardiol* 1991; 18:990–996.
4. Tada H, Shimizu W, Ohe T, et al. Usefulness of electron-beam computed tomography in arrhythmogenic right ventricular dysplasia: Relationship to electrophysiological abnormalities and left ventricular involvement. *Circulation* 1996; 94:437–444.
5. Reiter SJ, Rumberger JA, Feiring AJ, et al. Precision of measurements of right and left ventricular volume by cine computed tomography. *Circulation* 1986; 74:890–900.
6. Roig E, Chomka EV, Castaner A, et al. Exercise ultrafast computed tomography for the detection of coronary artery disease. *J Am Coll Cardiol* 1989; 13:1073–1081.
7. Budoff MJ, Gillespie R, Georgiou D, et al. Comparison of exercise electron beam computed tomography and sestamibi in the evaluation of coronary artery disease. *Am J Cardiol* 1998; 81:682–687.
8. Feiring AJ, Rumberger JA, Reiter SJ, et al. Sectional and segmental variability of left ventricular function: Experimental and clinical studies using ultrafast computed tomography. *J Am Coll Cardiol* 1988; 12:415–425.
9. Gerber TC, Behrenbeck T, Allison T, et al. Comparison of measurement of left ventricular ejection fraction by Tc-99m sestamibi first-pass angiography with electron beam computed tomography in patients with anterior wall acute myocardial infarction. *Am J Cardiol* 1999; 83:1022–1026.
10. Hirose K, Reed JE, Rumberger JA. Serial changes in left and right ventricular systolic and diastolic dynamics during the first year after an index left ventricular Q wave myocardial infarction. *J Am Coll Cardiol* 1995; 25:1097–1104.
11. Hirose K, Reed JE, Rumberger JA. Serial changes in regional right ventricular free wall and left ventricular septal wall lengths during the first 4 to 5 years after index anterior wall myocardial infarction. *J Am Coll Cardiol* 1995; 26:394–400.
12. Chareonthaitawee P, Christian TF, Hirose K, et al. Relation of initial infarct size to extent of left ventricular remodeling in the year after acute myocardial infarction. *J Am Coll Cardiol* 1995; 25:567–573.
13. Konstam MA, Rousseau MF, Kronenberg MW, et al. Effects of the angiotensin converting enzyme inhibitor enalapril on the long-term progression of left ventricular dysfunction in patients with heart failure. *Circulation* 1992; 86:431–438.
14. Mahmarian JJ, Moye LA, Chinoy DA, et al. Transdermal nitroglycerin patch therapy improves left ventricular function and prevents remodeling after acute myocardial infarction: Results of a

multicenter prospective randomized double-blind placebo controlled trial. *Circulation* 1998; 97:2017–2024.
15. St. John Sutton M, Pfeffer MA, Plappert T, et al. Quantitative two-dimensional echocardiographic measurements are major predictors of adverse cardiovascular events after acute myocardial infarction: The protective effects of captopril. *Circulation* 1994; 89:68–75.
16. Lipton MJ, Farmer DW, Killebrew EJ, et al. Regional myocardial dysfunction: Evaluation of patients with prior myocardial infarction with fast CT. *Radiology* 1985; 157:735–740.
17. Tomoda H, Hoshiai M, Furuya H, et al. Evaluation of intracardiac thrombus with computed tomography. *Am J Cardiol* 1983; 51:843–852.
18. Lessick J, Sideman S, Azhari H, et al. Regional three-dimensional geometric ventricle with fibrous aneurysms: A cine computed tomography study. *Circulation* 1991; 84:1172–1186.
19. Reiter SJ, Rumberger JA, Stanford W, et al. Quantitative determination of aortic regurgitant volume in dogs by ultrafast computed tomography. *Circulation* 1987; 76:728–735.
20. Helgason CM, Chomka E, Louie E, et al. The potential role for ultrafast cardiac computed tomography in patients with stroke. *Stroke* 1989; 20:465–472.
21. Becker CR, Knez A, Jakobs TF, et al. Detection and quantification of coronary artery calcification with electron-beam and conventional CT. *Eur Radiol* 1999; 9:620–624.
22. Mautner GC, Mautner SL, Froehlich J, et al. Coronary artery calcification: Assessment with electron beam CT and histomorphometric correlation. *Radiology* 1994; 192:619–623.
23. Rumberger JA, Simons DB, Fitzpatrick LA, et al. Coronary artery calcium area by electron-beam computed tomography and coronary atherosclerotic plaque area: A histopathologic correlative study. *Circulation* 1995; 92:2157–2162.
24. Sangiorgi G, Rumberger JA, Severson A, et al. Arterial calcification and not lumen stenosis is highly correlated with atherosclerotic plaque burden in humans: A histologic study of 723 coronary artery segments using nondecalcifying methodology. *J Am Coll Cardiol* 1998; 31:126–133.
25. Janowitz WR, Agatston AS, Kaplan G, et al. Differences in prevalence and extent of coronary artery calcium detected by ultrafast computed tomography in asymptomatic men and women: Relation to age and risk factors. *Am J Cardiol* 1993; 72:247–254.
26. Ikeda T Shirasawa T, Esaki Y, et al. Osteopontin mRNA is expressed by smooth muscle-derived foam cells in human atherosclerotic lesions of the aorta. *J Clin Invest* 1993; 92:2814–2820.
27. Fitzpatrick LA, Severson A, Edwards WD, et al. Diffuse calcification in human coronary arteries: Association of osteopontin with atherosclerosis. *J Clin Invest* 1994; 94:1597–1604.
28. Hirota S, Imakita M, Kohri K, et al. Expression of osteopontin messenger RNA by macrophages in atherosclerotic plaques: A possible association with calcification. *Am J Pathol* 1993; 143:1003–1008.
29. Glagov S, Weisenberg BA, Zarins CK, et al. Compensatory enlargement of human atherosclerotic coronary arteries. *New Engl J Med* 1987; 316:1371–1375.
30. Clarkson TB, Prichard RW, Morgan TM, et al. Remodeling of coronary arteries in human and nonhuman primates. *JAMA* 1994; 271:289–294.
31. Agatston AS, Janowitz WR, Hildner FJ, et al. Quantification of coronary artery calcium using ultrafast computed tomography. *J Am Coll Cardiol* 1990; 15:827–832.
32. Breen JF, Sheedy PF, Schwartz RS, et al. Coronary artery calcification detected with ultrafast CT as an indication of coronary artery disease. *Radiology* 1992; 185:435–439.
33. Bielak LW, Kaufmann RB, Moll PP, et al. Small lesions in the heart identified at electron beam CT: Calcification or noise? *Radiology* 1994; 192:631–636.
34. Kaufmann RB, Sheedy PF, Maher JE, et al. Quantity of coronary artery calcium detected by electron beam computed tomography in asymptomatic subjects and angiographically studied patients. *Mayo Clin Proc* 1995; 70:223–232.
35. Rumberger JA, Sheedy PF, Breen JF, et al. Coronary calcium, as determined by electron beam computed tomography, and coronary disease on arteriogram: Effect of patient's sex on diagnosis. *Circulation* 1995; 91:1363–1367.
36. Braun J, Oldendorf M, Moshage W, et al. Electron beam computed tomography in the evaluation of cardiac calcification in chronic dialysis patients. *Am J Kidney Dis* 1996; 27:394–401.
37. Budoff MJ, Georgiou D, Brody A, et al. Ultrafast computed tomography as a diagnostic modality in the detection of coronary artery disease: A multicenter study. *Circulation* 1996; 93:898–904.
38. Detrano R, Hsiai T, Wang S, et al. Prognostic value of coronary calcification and angiographic stenoses in patients undergoing coronary angiography. *J Am Coll Cardiol* 1996; 27:285–290.
39. Fallavollita JA, Brody AS, Bunnell IL, et al. Fast computed tomography detection of coronary calcification in the diagnosis of coronary artery disease: Comparison with angiography in patients <50 years old. *Circulation* 1994; 89:285–290.
40. Baumgart D, Schmermund A, George G, et al. Comparison of electron beam computed tomography with intracoronary ultrasound and coronary angiography for detection of coronary atherosclerosis. *J Am Coll Cardiol* 1997; 30:57–64.
41. Schmermund A, Baumgart D, Gorge D, et al. Coronary artery calcium in acute coronary syndromes: A comparative study of electron-beam computed tomography, coronary angiography, and intracoronary ultrasound in survivors of acute myocardial infarction and unstable angina. *Circulation* 1997; 96:1461–1469.
42. Kennedy J, Shavelle R, Wang S, et al. Coronary calcium and standard risk factors in symptomatic patients referred for coronary angiography. *Am Heart J* 1998; 135:696–702.
43. Rumberger JA, Sheedy PF, Breen JF, et al. Electron beam computed tomographic coronary calcium score cutpoints and severity of associated angiographic lumen stenosis. *J Am Coll Cardiol* 1997; 29:1542–1548.
44. Guerci AD, Spadaro LA, Goodman KJ, et al. Comparison of electron beam computed tomography scanning and conventional risk factor assessment for the prediction of angiographic coronary artery disease. *J Am Coll Cardiol* 1998; 32:673–679.
45. Budoff MJ, Shavelle DM, Lamont DH, et al. Usefulness of electron beam computed tomography scanning for distinguishing ischemic from nonischemic cardiomyopathy. *J Am Coll Cardiol* 1998; 32:1173–1178.
46. Shemesh J, Tenenbaum A, Fisman EZ, et al. Coronary calcium as a reliable tool for differentiating ischemic from nonischemic cardiomyopathy. *Am J Cardiol* 1996; 77:191–194.
47. McLaughlin VV, Balogh T, Rich S. Utility of electron beam computed tomography to stratify patients presenting to the emergency room with chest pain. *Am J Cardiol* 1999; 84:327–8, A8.
48. Callister TQ, Raggi P, Cooil B, et al. Identification of patients at increased risk of first unheralded acute myocardial infarction by electron beam computed tomography. *Circulation* 2000; 101: 850–855.
49. Shemesh J, Stroh CI, Tenenbaum A, et al. Comparison of coronary calcium in stable angina pectoris and in first acute myocardial infarction utilizing double helical computerized tomography. *Am J Cardiol* 1998; 81:271–275.
50. Schmermund A, Baumgart D, Adamzik M, et al. Comparison of electron-beam computed tomography and intracoronary ultrasound in detecting calcified and noncalcified plaques in patients with acute coronary syndromes and no or minimal to moderate angiographic coronary artery disease. *Am J Cardiol* 1998; 81: 141–146.
51. Ringqvist I, Fisher LD, Mock M, et al. Prognostic value of angiographic indices of coronary artery disease from the Coronary Artery Surgery Study (CASS). *J Clin Invest* 1983; 71:1854–1866.

52. Emond M, Mock MB, David KR, et al. Long-term survival of medically treated patients in the Coronary Artery Surgery Study (CASS) Registry. *Circulation* 1994; 90:2645–2657.

52a. Detrano R, Staly H, Doherty T, et al. Predicting coronary events with coronary calcium: Patho-physiologic clinical and political problems. June 2000. *Current Problems in Cardiology* 2000; 37–402.

53. He Z-X, Hedrick TD, Pratt CM, et al. Severity of coronary artery calcification by electron beam computed tomography predicts silent myocardial ischemia. *Circulation* 2000; 101:244–251.

54. Weiner DA, Ryan TJ, McCabe CH, et al. Significance of silent myocardial ischemia during exercise testing in patients with coronary artery disease. *Am J Cardiol* 1987; 59:725–729.

55. Blumenthal RS, Becker DM, Moy TF, et al. Exercise thallium tomography predicts future clinically manifest coronary heart disease in a high-risk asymptomatic population. *Circulation* 1996; 93:915–923.

56. Fleg JL, Gerstenblith G, Zonderman AB, et al. Prevalence and prognostic significance of exercise-induced silent myocardial ischemia detected by thallium scintigraphy and electrocardiography in asymptomatic volunteers. *Circulation* 1990; 81:428–436.

57. Ekelund L-G, Suchindran CM, McMahon RP, et al. Coronary heart disease morbidity and mortality in hypercholesterolemic men predicted from an exercise test: The Lipid Research Clinics Coronary Primary Prevention Trial. *J Am Coll Cardiol* 1989; 14: 556–563.

58. Heller LI, Tresgallo M, Sciacca RR, et al. Prognostic significance of silent myocardial ischemia on a thallium stress test. *Am J Cardiol* 1990; 65:718–721.

59. Secci A, Wong N, Tang W, et al. Electron beam computed tomographic coronary calcium as a predictor of coronary events: Comparison of two protocols. *Circulation* 1997; 96:1122–1129.

60. Detrano RC, Wong ND, Doherty TM. Coronary calcium does not accurately predict near-term future coronary events in high-risk adults. *Circulation* 1999; 99:2633–2638.

61. Arad Y, Spadaro LA, Goodman K, et al. Predictive value of electron beam computed tomography of the coronary arteries: 19-month follow-up of 1173 asymptomatic subjects. *Circulation* 1996; 93:1951–1953.

61a. Shaw LJ, O'Rourke RA. The challenge of improving risk assessment in asymptomatic individuals: The additive prognostic value of electron beam tomography? *JACC.* August 2000 (in press).

62. Doherty TM, Tang W, Detrano RC. Racial differences in the significance of coronary calcium in asymptomatic black and white subjects with coronary risk factors. *J Am Coll Cardiol* 1999; 34:787–794.

63. Detrano RC, Wong ND, Tang W, et al. Prognostic significance of cardiac cinefluoroscopy for coronary calcific deposits in asymptomatic high risk subjects. *J Am Coll Cardiol* 1994; 24:354–358.

64. Shepherd J, Cobbe SM, Ford I, et al. Prevention of coronary heart disease with pravastatin in men with hypercholesterolemia. *New Engl J Med* 1995; 333:1301–1307.

65. Multiple Risk Factor Intervention Trial Research Group. Coronary heart disease death, nonfatal acute myocardial infarction and other clinical outcomes in the Multiple Risk Factor Intervention Trial. *Am J Cardiol* 1986; 58:1–13.

66. Gordon DJ, Ekelund L-G, Karon JM, et al. Predictive value of the exercise tolerance test for mortality in North American men: The Lipid Research Clinics Mortality Follow-Up Study. *Circulation* 1986; 74:252–261.

67. O'Malley PG, Taylor AJ, Gibbons RV, et al. Rationale and design of the Prospective Army Coronary Calcium (PACC) Study: Utility of electron beam computed tomography as a screening test for coronary artery disease and as an intervention for risk factor modification among young, asymptomatic, active-duty United States Army personnel. *Am Heart J* 1999; 137:932–941.

68. Downs JR, Clearfield M, Weis S, et al. Primary prevention of acute coronary events with lovastatin in men and women with average cholesterol levels: Results of AFCAPS/TexCAPS. Air Force/Texas Coronary Atherosclerosis Prevention Study. *JAMA* 1998; 279;1615–1622.

69. Califf RM, Armstrong PW, Carver JR, et al. Task Force 5: Stratification of patients into high, medium and low risk subgroups for purposes of risk factor management. *J Am Coll Cardiol* 1996; 27:1007–1019.

70. Wilson PWF, D'Agostino RB, Levy D, et al. Prediction of coronary heart disease using risk factor categories. *Circulation* 1998; 97:1837–1847.

71. Wong ND, Kouwabunpat D, Vo AN, et al. Coronary calcium and atherosclerosis by ultrafast computed tomography in asymptomatic men and women: Relation to age and risk factors. *Am Heart J* 1994; 127:422–430.

72. Kuller LH, Matthews KA, Sutton-Tyrrell K, et al. Coronary and aortic calcification among women 8 years after menopause and their premenopausal risk factors. The Healthy Women Study. *Arterioscler Thromb Vasc Biol* 1999; 19:2189–2198.

73. Schmermund A, Denktas AE, Rumberger JA, et al. Independent and incremental value of coronary artery calcium for predicting the extent of angiographic coronary artery disease: Comparison with cardiac risk factors and radionuclide perfusion imaging. *J Am Coll Cardiol* 1999; 34:777–786.

74. Schmermund A, Bailey KR, Rumberger JA, et al. An algorithm for noninvasive identification of angiographic three-vessel and/or left main coronary artery disease in symptomatic patients on the basis of cardiac risk and electron-beam computed tomographic calcium scores. *J Am Coll Cardiol* 1999; 33:444–452.

75. Gibbons RJ, Balady GJ, Beasley JW, et al. ACC/AHA guidelines for exercise testing: a report of the American College of Cardiology/American Heart Association Task Force on Practice Guidelines (Committee on Exercise Testing). *J Am Coll Cardiol* 1997; 30:260–315.

76. Ritchie JL, Cheitlin MD, Garson A Jr, et al. Guidelines for clinical use of cardiac radionuclide imaging: Report of the American College of Cardiology/American Heart Association Task Force on Assessment of Diagnostic and Therapeutic Cardiovascular Procedures (Committee on Radionuclide Imaging), developed in collaboration with the American Society of Nuclear Cardiology. *J Am Coll Cardiol* 1995; 25:521–547.

77. Olmos LI, Dakik H, Gordon R, et al. Long-term prognostic value of exercise echocardiography compared with exercise Tl-201, ECG, and clinical variables in patients evaluated for coronary artery disease. *Circulation* 1998; 98:2679–2686.

78. Iskandrian AS, Chae SC, Heo J, et al. Independent and incremental prognostic value of exercise single-photon emission computed tomographic (SPECT) thallium imaging in coronary artery disease. *J Am Coll Cardiol* 1993; 22:665–670.

79. Hachamovitch R, Berman DS, Kiat H, et al. Exercise myocardial perfusion SPECT in patients without known coronary artery disease: Incremental prognostic value and use in risk stratification. *Circulation* 1996; 93:905–914.

80. Rumberger JA, Brundage BH, Rader DJ, et al. Electron beam computed tomographic coronary calcium scanning: A review and guidelines for use in asymptomatic persons. *Mayo Clin Proc* 1999; 74:243–252.

81. O'Rourke RA, Brundage BH, Froelicher VF, et al. American College of Cardiology/American Heart Association Expert Consensus Document on Electron Beam Computed Tomography for the Diagnosis of Coronary Artery Disease (Committee on Electron Beam Computed Tomography). *Circulation* 2000; 126–140.

82. Smith SC, Greenland P, Scott SM. Prevention V Conference. *Circulation* 2000; 101:111–116.

83. Janowitz WR, Agatston AS, Viamonte M Jr. Comparison of serial quantitative evaluation of calcified coronary artery plaque by ul-

trafast computed tomography in persons with and without obstructive coronary artery disease. *Am J Cardiol* 1991; 68:1–6.
84. Callister TQ, Raggi P, Cooil B, et al. Effect of HMG-CoA reductase inhibitors on coronary artery disease as assessed by electron-beam computed tomography. *New Engl J Med* 1998; 339:1972–1978.
85. Devries S, Wolfkiel C, Shah V, et al. Reproducibility of the measurement of coronary calcium with ultrafast computed tomography. *Am J Cardiol* 1995; 75:973–975.
86. Kajinami K, Seki H, Takekoshi N, et al. Quantification of coronary artery calcification using ultrafast computed tomography: Reproducibility of measurements. *Coronary Artery Dis* 1993;4:1103–1108.
87. Wang, S, Detrano RC, Secci A, et al. Detection of coronary calcification with electron-beam computed tomography: Evaluation of interexamination reproducibility and comparison of three image-acquisition protocols. *Am Heart J* 1996; 132:550–558.
88. Callister TW, Cooil B, Raya SP, et al. Coronary artery disease: Improved reproducibility of calcium scoring with an electron-beam CT volumetric method. *Radiology* 1998; 208:807–814.
89. Blankenhorn DH, Azen SP, Kramasch DM, et al. Coronary angiographic changes with lovastatin therapy: The Monitored Atherosclerosis Regression Study (MARS). *Ann Intern Med* 1993; 119:969–976.
90. Jukema JW, Bruschke AVG, van Boven AJ, et al. Effects of lipid lowering by pravastatin on progression and regression of coronary artery disease in symptomatic men with normal to moderately elevated serum cholesterol levels: The Regression Growth Evaluation Statin Study (REGRESS). *Circulation* 1995; 91:2528–2540.
91. Stanford W, Brundage BH, MacMillan R, et al. Sensitivity and specificity of assessing coronary bypass graft patency with ultrafast computed tomography: Results of a multicenter study. *J Am Coll Cardiol* 1988; 12:1–7.
92. Bateman TM, Gray RJ, Whiting JS, et al. Ultrafast computed tomographic evaluation of aortocoronary bypass graft patency. *J Am Coll Cardiol* 1986; 8:693–698.
93. Bateman TM, Gray RJ, Whiting JS, et al. Prospective evaluation of ultrafast CT for determination of coronary bypass graft patency. *Circulation* 1987; 75:1018–1024.
94. Achenbach S, Moshage W, Ropers D, et al. Value of electron-beam computed tomography for the noninvasive detection of high-grade coronary-artery stenoses and occlusions. *New Engl J Med* 1998; 339:1964–1971.
95. Schmermund A, Rensing BJ, Sheedy PF, et al. Intravenous electron-beam computed tomographic coronary angiography for segmental analysis of coronary artery stenoses. *J Am Coll Cardiol* 1998; 31:1547–1554.
96. Rensing BJ, Bongaerts A, van Geuns RJ, et al. Intravenous coronary angiography by electron beam computed tomography: A clinical evaluation. *Circulation* 1998; 98:2509–2512.
97. Budoff MJ, Oudiz RJ, Zalace CP, et al. Intravenous three-dimensional coronary angiography using contrast enhanced electron beam computed tomography. *Am J Cardiol* 1999; 83:840–845.
98. Brundage B, Lipton MJ, Herfkens RJ, et al. Detection of patent coronary artery bypass grafts by computed tomography: A preliminary report. *Circulation* 1980; 61:826–831.
99. Tello R, Costello P, Ecker C, et al. Spiral CT evaluation of coronary artery bypass graft patency. *J Comput Assist Tomogr* 1993; 17:253–259.
100. Achenbach S, Moshage W, Bachmann K, et al. Detection of high-grade restenosis after PTCA using contrast-enhanced electron beam CT. *Circulation* 1997; 96:2785–2788.
101. Ling LH, Oh JK, Tei C, et al. Pericardial thickness measured with transesophageal echocardiography: Feasibility and potential clinical usefulness. *J Am Coll Cardiol* 1997; 29:1317–1323.
102. Isner JM, Carter BL, Bankoff MS, et al. Differentiation of constrictive pericarditis from restrictive cardiomyopathy by computed tomographic imaging. *Am Heart J* 1983; 105:1019–1025.
103. Oren RM, Grover-McKay M, Stanford W, et al. Accurate preoperative diagnosis of pericardial constriction using cine computed tomography. *J Am Coll Cardiol* 1993; 22:832–838.
104. Doppman JL, Rienmuller R, Lissner J, et al. Computed tomography in constrictive pericardial disease. *J Comput Assist Tomgr* 1981; 5:1–11.
105. Tomoda H, Hoshiai M, Furuya H, et al. Evaluation of pericardial effusion with computed tomography. *Am Heart J* 1980; 99:701–706.
106. Baim RS, MacDonald IL, Wise DJ, et al. Computed tomography of absent left pericardium. *Radiology* 1980; 135:127–128.
107. Moncada R, Baker M, Salinas M, et al. Diagnostic role of computed tomography in pericardial heart disease: Congenital defects, thickening, neoplasms and effusions. *Am Heart J* 1982; 103:263–282.
108. Glazer GM, Gross BH, Oringer MB, et al. Computed tomography of pericardial masses. *J Comput Assist Tomogr* 1984; 8:895–899.
109. Farmer DW, Lipton MJ, Webb WR, et al. Computed tomography in congenital heart disease. *J Comput Assist Tomogr* 1984; 8:677–687.
110. Webb WR, Gamsu G, Speckman JM, et al. CT demonstration of mediastinal aortic arch anomalies. *J Comput Assist Tomogr* 1982; 6:445–451.
111. Eldridge WJ. Comprehensive evaluation of congenital heart disease using ultrafast computed tomography. In: Marcus ML, Schelbert HR, Skorton DJ, et al., eds. *Cardiac Imaging*. Philadelphia: Saunders; 1991:714.
112. Eldridge WJ, Flicker S, Steiner RM. Cine CT in the anatomical evaluation of congenital heart disease. In: Pohost G, Higgins CB, Morgenroth J, et al., eds. *New Concepts in Cardiac Imaging*, Vol 3. Chicago: Year Book Medical; 1987:265.
113. MacMillan RM, Shakriari A, Sumithisena F, et al. Contrast enhanced cine computed tomography for the diagnosis of right coronary to coronary sinus arteriovenous fistulae. *Am J Cardiol* 1985; 56:997–998.
114. MacMillan RM, Rees MR, Eldredge WJ, et al. Quantitation of shunting at the atrial level using rapid acquisition computed tomography with comparison to cardiac catheterization. *J Am Coll Cardiol* 1986; 7:946–948.
115. Skotvicki R, Maranhao V, Clark D, et al. Detection of atrial septal defect by cine CT scanning. *Cathet Cardiovasc Diagn* 1986; 12:103–106.
116. Bateman TM, Sethna DH, Whiting JS, et al. Comprehensive non-invasive evaluation of left atrial myxoma using cardiac cine-computed tomography. *J Am Coll Cardiol* 1987; 9:1180–1183.
117. Nienaber CA, von Kodolitsch Y, Nicolas V. The diagnosis of thoracic aortic dissection by noninvasive imaging procedures. *New Engl J Med* 1993; 328:1–9.
118. Reardon MJ, Hedrick TD, Letsou GV, et al. CT reconstruction of an unusual chronic posttraumatic aneurysm of the thoracic aorta. *Ann Thorac Surg* 1997; 64:1480–1482.
119. Sommer T, Fehske W, Holzknecht N, et al. Aortic dissection: A comparative study of diagnosis with spiral CT, multiplanar transesophageal echocardiography, and MR imaging. *Radiology* 1996; 199:347–352.
120. Stanford W. Ultrafast computed tomography in the diagnosis of aortic aneurysms and dissections. *J Thorac Imaging* 1990; 5:32–39.
121. Cremer J, Teebken OE, Simon A, et al. Thoracic computed tomography prior to redo coronary surgery. *Eur J Cardiothorac Surg* 1998; 13:650–654.
122. Remy-Jardin M, Remy J, Deschildre F, et al. Diagnosis of pulmonary embolism with spiral CT: Comparison with pulmonary angiography and scintigraphy. *Radiology* 1996; 200:699–706.
123. Mayo JR, Remy-Jardin M, Muller NL, et al. Pulmonary embolism: Prospective comparison of spiral CT with ventilation perfusion scintigraphy. *Radiology* 1997; 205:447–452.
124. Teigen CL, Maus TP, Sheedy PF, et al. Pulmonary embolism diagnosis with contrast-enhanced electron-beam CT and comparison with pulmonary angiography. *Radiology* 1995; 194:313–319.

CHAPTER 18A

MAGNETIC RESONANCE IMAGING OF THE HEART

Mark Doyle / Gerald M. Pohost

INTRODUCTION

The phenomenon of nuclear magnetic resonance (NMR) was discovered more than 60 years ago, and NMR spectroscopic methods were initially applied by physicists and chemists to explore molecular structure and composition.[1,2] Although NMR spectroscopy has proved invaluable in providing metabolic information in a variety of different myocardial physiologic and pathologic states, it is still used primarily as a research tool. The concept of using NMR to obtain images was propounded by Lauterbur[3] and was introduced independently by Mansfield in the early 1970s, when it was discovered that an inhomogeneous magnetic field can localize nuclei in space and thus produce an image. Advances in computer technology and superconducting magnets now allow routine clinical NMR imaging. Images are obtained with exquisite morphologic detail, in any tomographic orientation, in a nondestructive and noninvasive manner. As NMR entered mainstream clinical practice, the potential for public concern about "nuclear" technology was avoided by using the less descriptive term *magnetic resonance imaging* (MRI). It is important to note that there are types of magnetic resonance in addition to NMR, including electron spin resonance and Mossbauer spectroscopy.

Physicians and patients have become aware of the great versatility of MRI, and that knowledge has allowed the modality to become the "gold standard" of noninvasive imaging for many diagnostic and management areas in noncardiac diseases. Similarly, MRI has the potential to become an invaluable tool for evaluating cardiovascular morphology, function, perfusion, and viability. Even diagnostic imaging of the coronary arteries promises to become a reality in the near future. In addition, investigations of the clinical characteristics of plaque promise an exciting future in this area of MRI.

This chapter focuses on the basic principles and practices of applying MRI for the evaluation of normal cardiovascular structures and the diagnosis of diseases that affect the heart.

PRINCIPLES OF NMR

Magnetism and Vectors

To fully understand NMR, one must have extensive knowledge of quantum and nuclear physics; fortunately, the basic theory of NMR can be explained by using concepts drawn mostly from classical physics. An intrinsic property of atomic nuclei is that of *spin*. The combination of nuclear spin and electric charge is analogous to an electric current circulating in a small wire loop, producing a small magnetic field (Fig. 18A-1). The strength of the magnetic field produced by the nucleus is expressed in terms of a magnetic moment.

Within the body, nuclei orient randomly in space and do not produce any net magnetization; however, positioning the body within a strong magnetic field produces a net magnetic moment within the body. Intuitively, one might expect all nuclei to align parallel to the magnetic field (B_0); however, two energy states are created: parallel and antiparallel to B_0. Since the parallel alignment is at a lower energy level, slightly more nuclei become aligned parallel to B_0, causing the body to become weakly magnetized (Fig. 18A-2). The strength of the magnetization vector is proportional to the strength of B_0, the energy difference between spin states, and temperature. The fractional excess in the lower-energy state is extremely small [i.e., about 3 per million for hydrogen nuclei at a field of strength 1.5 tesla (T) at body temperature].

In equilibrium, the magnetic moment does not yield a detectable signal. Signal can be generated by perturbing the system, causing its net magnetization to deviate from alignment with B_0. When tilted from alignment, the magnetization vector experiences a torque that causes it to precess. The phenomenon of nuclear precession is analogous to the precession exhibited by a spinning gyroscope tilted from alignment with the earth's gravitational field. Importantly, the precession frequency (ω_0) is much lower than the spinning frequency and is proportional

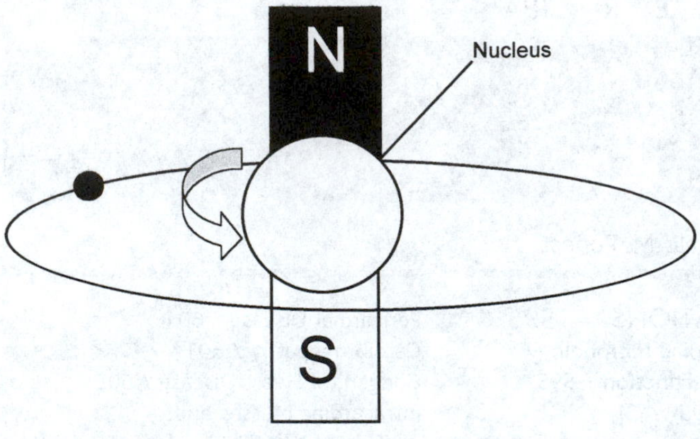

FIGURE 18A-1 The positively charged nucleus of a hydrogen atom spins and creates a magnetic field.

to the field strength B_0. The frequency ω_0 is related to B_0 by a constant (γ) termed the *gyromagnetic ratio,* and these valves are related by the Larmor equation:

$$\omega_0 = \gamma B_0$$

The gyromagnetic ratio (γ) is unique for each nuclear isotope.

The Resonance Phenomenon

To displace spins from alignment with B_0, a magnetic field of much lower strength (B_1) is applied so that B_1 rotates in a plane perpendicular to B_0. If the B_1 field rotates at the Larmor frequency, it will maximally affect the net magnetization of the body by virtue of being on resonance (Fig. 18A-3). The resonance frequency of the B_1 field is in the radiofrequency (RF) range and contributes the term *resonance* to NMR and MRI. The angle (θ) of rotation from B_0 is proportional to the time (t) of application of the rotating field and the strength, $|B_1|$:

$$\theta = \gamma |B_1| t$$

When B_1 is turned off, the spins are free to precess under the influence of the extrinsic static magnetic field. It is during this time of free precession that the spins give off a detectable electromagnetic signal, again in the RF frequency range. The

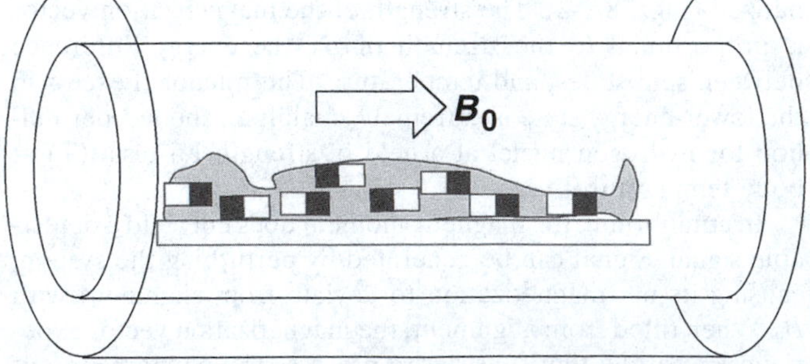

FIGURE 18A-2 The nuclei of the hydrogen atoms within the body (represented by the black and white bar magnets) align with the magnetic field (B_0), both parallel and antiparallel. Slightly more nuclei align parallel to the B_0, creating a net magnetization vector (*open arrow*).

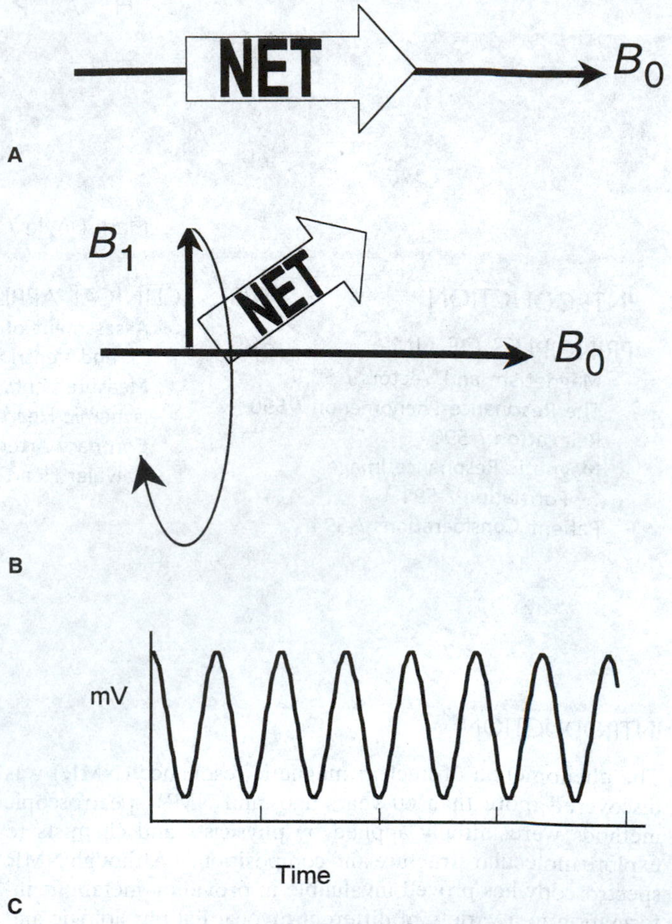

FIGURE 18A-3 The net magnetization vector (NET) aligns with B_0 (*A*). A rotating magnetic field (B_1) applied as a radiofrequency (RF) pulse causes the vector to precess out of B_0 alignment (*B*). The RF pulse is then discontinued, and the vector precesses, producing a signal (*C*) with a characteristic frequency, which depends on the field strength (B_0) of the magnet and the atomic species producing the signal (usually hydrogen).

spin signal decays over a matter of tens of milliseconds and is known as *a free induction decay* (FID) (Fig. 18A-4).

Relaxation

The spin signal gradually decays as a result of "relaxation" phenomena, that is, the gradual return of nuclei to their equilib-

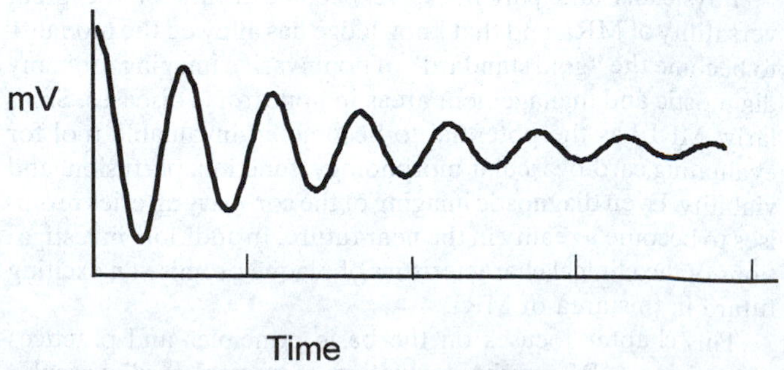

FIGURE 18A-4 The signal detected from the freely precessing nuclei decay, typically in a matter of milliseconds.

rium energy states. Two distinct relaxation parameters are used frequently: T1 and T2; these parameters can be exploited to enhance image contrast.

T1 RELAXATION

Nuclei in the body are surrounded by a network of structures collectively known as the *lattice*. The lattice and the spin system constantly exchange energy; hence, nuclei lose the energy initially imparted by the RF pulse, resulting in a decrease in the net magnetic moment as spins realign along the B_0 axis. The realignment occurs in an exponential manner, and T1 relates to the time constant of this exponential decay. The time constant, T1, for a particular sample is the time needed for 63 percent of the nuclei to return to their equilibrium value. T1 frequently is referred to as the spin-lattice relaxation time. After a perturbation of the spin system, a time period of 5 T1 is regarded as necessary for the spins to return to equilibrium. Since spin-lattice relaxation requires an exchange of energy, the process is field-strength-dependent. The T1 of myocardium is approximately 900 ms at a field strength of 1.5 T and is less at lower fields.

T2 RELAXATION

Aside from the lattice, the interaction of neighboring spins contributes to the relaxation process. These interactions are referred to as *spin-spin relaxation* or *T2 relaxation*. Spin-spin relaxation occurs in the so-called transverse plane, i.e., the plane orthogonal to the B_0 direction in which the spins precess. The spin-spin interaction does not require any net energy exchange but instead can be envisioned as a loss of coherence of the precessing spins. As the spins gradually lose phase coherence, their net signal diminishes exponentially. The T2 for a sample is the time interval for the transverse magnetization to decay to 37 percent of its initial value. Additionally, in practice, B_0 fields are not perfectly homogeneous. Thus, nuclei within a sample are exposed to slightly different magnetic fields and, as a result, precess at slightly different frequencies. The free induction decay in such a field occurs more rapidly than is indicated by purely T2 considerations. This more rapid rate of decay is termed T2* ("T2 star"). The T2 process does not involve an exchange of energy with the lattice and is essentially independent of field strength. The T2 of myocardium is approximately 80 ms.

Each type of tissue has characteristic T1 and T2 relaxation properties that are influenced by a variety of conditions, including the proximity and mobility of molecules in the surrounding environment, the hydrogen concentration of the tissue, and exposure to the local magnetic fields at the molecular level. MR image contrast can be made sensitive to these conditions through the use of specialized pulse sequences that can be implemented by using the computer in the MR system. Image contrast generally is described in terms of the level of T1 or T2 "weighting" (described later in this chapter). Additionally, image contrast can be sensitive to motion of either the blood or the myocardium. These different contrast mechanisms can be understood in terms of the image-forming process of MRI techniques used clinically to image cardiovascular structures.

Magnetic Resonance Image Formation

MRI is the most complex of all the medical imaging modalities, and it is important in regard to optimal image interpretation to have an understanding of the technical aspects of image formation. While scanner technology is constantly improving, certain basic system features remain constant. The following paragraphs describe the basic elements of an MR system.

A general misconception exists that clinical MR systems, which are used commonly for brain and musculoskeletal imaging, cannot perform cardiovascular imaging and thus a dedicated cardiovascular system is needed. In fact, specialized software can produce a means for cardiovascular imaging in most clinical systems. Typically, the only additional hardware requirements are cardiac and respiratory gating devices, which are available for most systems. However, optimal cardiovascular magnetic resonance (CMR) requires a specialized system dedicated to cardiovascular applications. Clinical MR systems use superconducting magnets with field strengths typically ranging from 0.5 to 1.5 T. A tesla is the equivalent of 10,000 gauss (G). To put this into perspective, the earth's magnetic field is between 0.3 and 0.7 G, and a household magnet is about 100 G (0.01 T). Higher-field-strength magnets result in an increased signal-to-noise ratio and, as a consequence, clearer images; however, these higher field strengths often exaggerate artifacts because of cardiac, respiratory, and blood flow motion. Most clinical systems operate at 1.5 T, but clinical magnets with field strengths as high as 8 T are being used for research.

Systems tailored for cardiac applications generally acquire data rapidly to "freeze" cardiac motion and produce images with minimal blur. In an attempt to decrease scan times, the signal-to-noise ratio generally is reduced. Thus, of particular importance to cardiac systems is the requirement to obtain data with a high signal-to-noise ratio. Thus, cardiac systems typically are supplied with specialized receiver coils. Signal reception is optimal when the coil is closest to the heart. Typically, a cardiac coil comes in two parts: one positioned posteriorly and one positioned anteriorly over the heart. These coils are usually of the efficient phased-array design.[4]

As a result of its lesser regularity, respiratory motion is more difficult to compensate for than is normal cardiac motion. Cardiac motion is accommodated by synchronizing the acquisitions with the electrocardiogram. However, for general cardiac imaging, simultaneous triggering with the respiratory cycle is generally time-prohibitive. To accommodate the requirements for respiratory compensation, a number of rapid cardiac scan approaches have been developed that can be applied in combination with respiratory compensation. One method of respiratory compensation is to have the patient voluntarily suspend breathing temporarily (typically for 15 to 30 s). During this interval, the scan is performed. Other methods involve tracking the respiratory excursion of the heart by means of a belt and bellows apparatus secured around the patient's waist. Alternatively, an MRI-derived "navigator" signal (analogous to an M-mode echocardiogram) can be used to track the position of the diaphragm and allow synchronization with the respiratory cycle.[5,6]

GRADIENTS

To produce an image, spatial discrimination must be encoded in the NMR signal. Within a homogeneous B_0 field, all nuclei resonate at the same frequency; thus, after the application of an RF pulse, a single frequency signal is produced with no spatial information. To generate an image, the magnetic field must vary over the field of interest. This is best accomplished by applying a linear magnetic field gradient over the sample. Three orthogonal gradients are incorporated into the scanner system: in the craniocaudal direction (z), in the right-to-left direction (x), and in the anterior-posterior direction (y). These gradients are controlled by the scanner's computer system. The first step in spatial resolution is to select a slice at a specified location. Slice selection is accomplished by the application of a linear gradient orthogonal to the desired slice direction. This gradient generates a range of resonant frequencies along the direction of the gradient. When the B_1 RF pulse is applied at a specific frequency (corresponding to the resonance frequency of the desired slice position), only spins in a narrow frequency range experience the effect of the RF pulse (Fig. 18A-5*A*). In this way, a slice can be selected with programmable orientation and thickness. To generate an image of the slice, it is necessary to apply gradients in two dimensions. Unfortunately, the application of two such gradients simultaneously results in a single gradient vector. Hence, image generation in two dimensions requires that the two gradients be applied at separate times. This feature is responsible for the relatively long acquisition times associated with cardiovascular MRI. It is important to realize that the MRI signal does not directly relate to an image. Instead, an image is formed by the mathematical process known as a Fourier transform (Fig. 18A-5*B*). The MRI signal is acquired and assembled into a matrix that is termed k-space, and an image is produced when the Fourier transform is applied. In Fig. 18A-5*C*, the process of acquiring lines in k-space is illustrated. The data are read in the presence of one imaging gradient termed the *frequency encoding* or *measurement* gradient. To step between lines of k-space, a "phase-encoding" gradient is applied as indicated in Fig. 18A-5*C*.

PULSE SEQUENCES

A pulse sequence is a set of RF and gradient waveforms that are required for image generation. Different pulse sequences highlight different features in an MR image.

Gated Spin Echo On slice selection using the gradient and RF pulse combination, the signal is maximal immediately at the end of the RF pulse. However, relatively few sequences can use the signal at this time, since the signal generally requires some form of preparation before it can be useful. However, as time from the RF pulse elapses, the signal loses coherence because of the combined effects of T2 and magnet inhomogeneities.

The application of a second pulse of 180° causes the spins to reverse direction and realign (or refocus), resulting in a so-called spin echo. This refocused echo signal is corrected for the effects of field inhomogeneity (but not for the effects of T2 relaxation). The time from the RF pulse to the maximal signal is called the *echo time* (TE). The time interval between each "phase-encoding" step in the image-generating process is called the *repetition time* (TR). The imaging computer can vary TE and TR to affect the degree of T1 and T2 "weighting" in the images; i.e., for a short TE and TR the image becomes T1-weighted, and for a long TE and TR the image becomes T2-weighted. However, much of the contrast in such spin-echo images occurs as a result of rapidly flowing blood. Since blood moves between applications of the two RF pulses, the signal emanating from the region with flowing blood is related to the

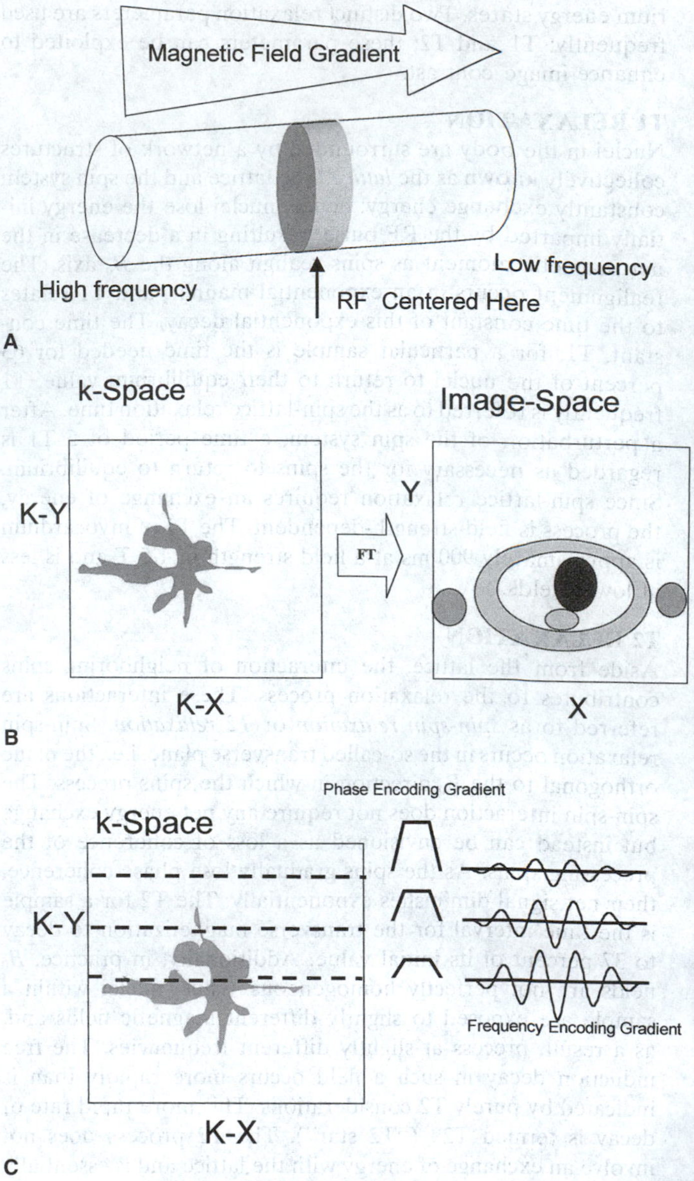

FIGURE 18A-5 A combination of gradient and RF energy is used to select a slice in the sample (*A*). The gradient imposes a range of frequencies over the sample, and the B_1 field is applied at the frequency needed to select the slice. The data sampled by MRI are in the so-called k-space of the frequency domain (*B*). Images in this domain are converted into images in the spatial domain by performing a Fourier transform (FT). Each line of k-space is sampled by application of a "frequency-encoding" gradient (typically for 2–3 ms) (*C*). To step between each line of k-space, a "phase-encoding" gradient is applied (typically in 1 ms).

blood flow. In the presence of rapid blood flow that is directed out of the imaging plane, there is no signal, since the blood does not experience the refocusing pulse. As blood flow decreases, its signal increases. Thus, within vascular lumens and cardiac chambers, signal voids generally are seen in spin-echo images (also termed dark blood images). This sequence highlights cardiovascular wall morphology (Fig. 18A-6).

Gated Gradient Echo Another widely used method for generating clinical images involves applying a magnetic gradient to

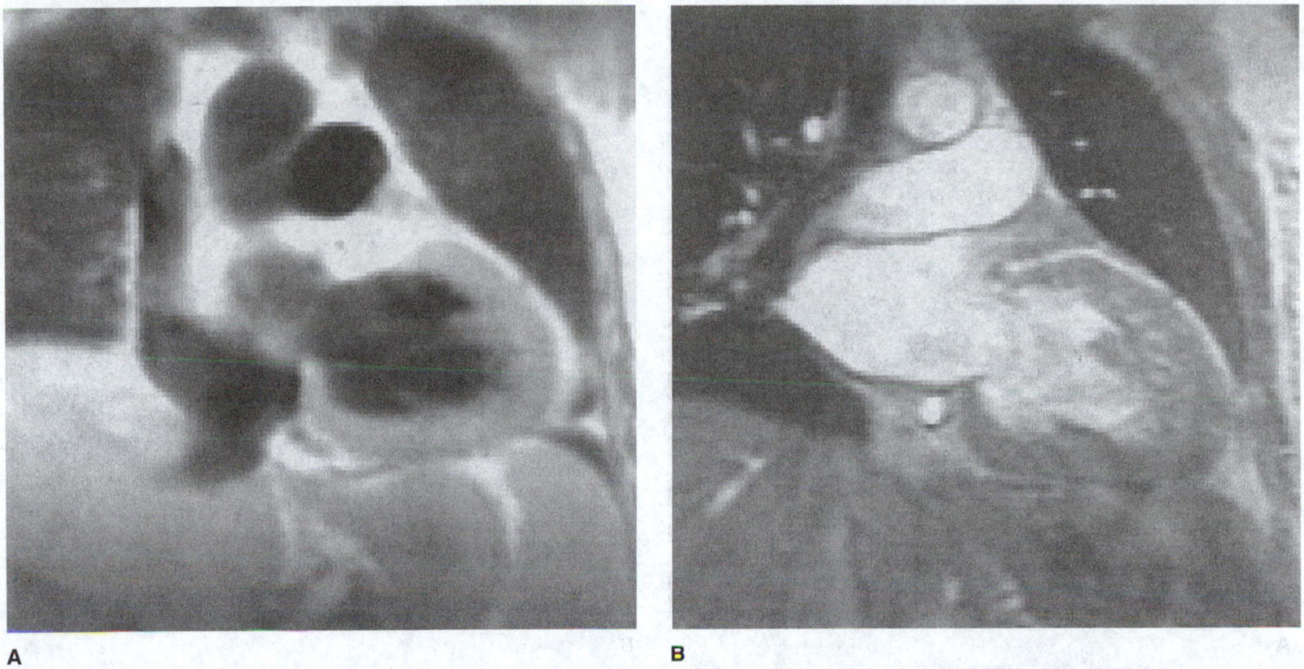

FIGURE 18A-6 A coronal image of the heart using spin-echo (SE) (*A*) and gradient-recalled-echo (GRE) techniques (*B*). Note the lack of blood signal in the SE image ("dark blood" approach) and the presence of blood signal in the GRE image ("bright blood" approach).

recall a signal echo. After the RF pulse used in slice selection, an additional gradient is applied and then reversed after several milliseconds. This refocuses the spins into an echo. The major difference between this "gradient-echo" approach and the "spin-echo" approach is that with gradient-echo approach, only one RF pulse is applied. Thus, gradient-echo images can be made sensitive to flowing blood (since even moving blood experiences the signal-refocusing properties of the gradient echo sequence). This method typically uses rapidly repeated RF pulses and causes partial "saturation" (i.e., heavy T1 weighting) of spins. Thus, decreased signal from static tissues results from the rapid repetition rates of the RF pulse. However, blood flowing into the imaging plane will not have been exposed to the slice-selective train of RF pulses and thus will not be "saturated," resulting in an intense blood signal relative to the static tissue signal with low intensity (Fig. 18A-6). Consequently, flowing blood appears bright. Thus, the gradient-echo-type sequence also is known as the *bright blood sequence*. This imaging approach is quite useful, since the resultant images may be displayed in a cine/movie to allow visualization of cardiac and blood pool motion. One should note that turbulent flow causes dephasing of spins as a result of chaotic motion, resulting in signal loss. Therefore, this technique is useful for visualizing regurgitant, stenotic, and shunt lesions.

Rapid Imaging Of particular importance to cardiovascular imaging are rapid imaging sequences, since the gated approaches result in a prolongation of the basic scan time. A two-dimensional (2D) image of a stationary object can be generated in a matter of seconds (e.g., with a TR of 7 ms, an image with 128 lines can be generated in less than 1 s). With the requirement of cardiac triggering, the scan time will be extended to the time of 128 cardiac cycles. Thus, methods for producing cardiac images in shorter times have been an active area of research.[7–9]

One such rapid sequence is echo-planar imaging (EPI).[10–13] EPI is based on the gradient-echo approach, but instead of just one echo being recalled, a number of echoes are recalled, speeding up the sequence. The main disadvantage of the EPI approach is that the echo train can be quite long (i.e., greater than 50 ms) and thus the images are heavily T2-weighted. An approach that avoids the T2 weighting of EPI is the segmented or turbo imaging approach. This involves the acquisition of a series of single gradient echoes that are acquired rapidly in a group and assigned to one cardiac phase.[14–17] Further modification and variants continue to be developed to allow the production of cardiac images in shorter scan times.

One rapid technique that merits special mention is spiral imaging. This approach does not encode data in an orthogonal matrix (as is done in the techniques described above) but acquires data in a curved matrix. This approach exploits the fact that it is physically easier to drive the imaging gradients by using a waveform with gradually increasing amplitude as opposed to abruptly switching the polarity of the gradients (as is required for the gradient-echo and spin-echo approaches). Spiral approaches have been used to produce high-resolution images of the coronary arteries. The disadvantage of this technique is that high system performance is required.[18]

SPECIALIZED PULSE SEQUENCES

An imaging sequence that can be used in conjunction with many of the approaches described above is that of tagging[19–22] (Fig. 18A-7). Typically, tagging involves applying a set of parallel lines or a grid of orthogonal lines at the time of the electrocardiogram (ECG) R wave. Once they are applied, these lines or grids then move with the heart to highlight motion. Naturally, since the lines or grids are composed of tagged signal regions, they cannot interfere with cardiac function. Such RF tagging allows quantification of cardiac function on a regional basis.

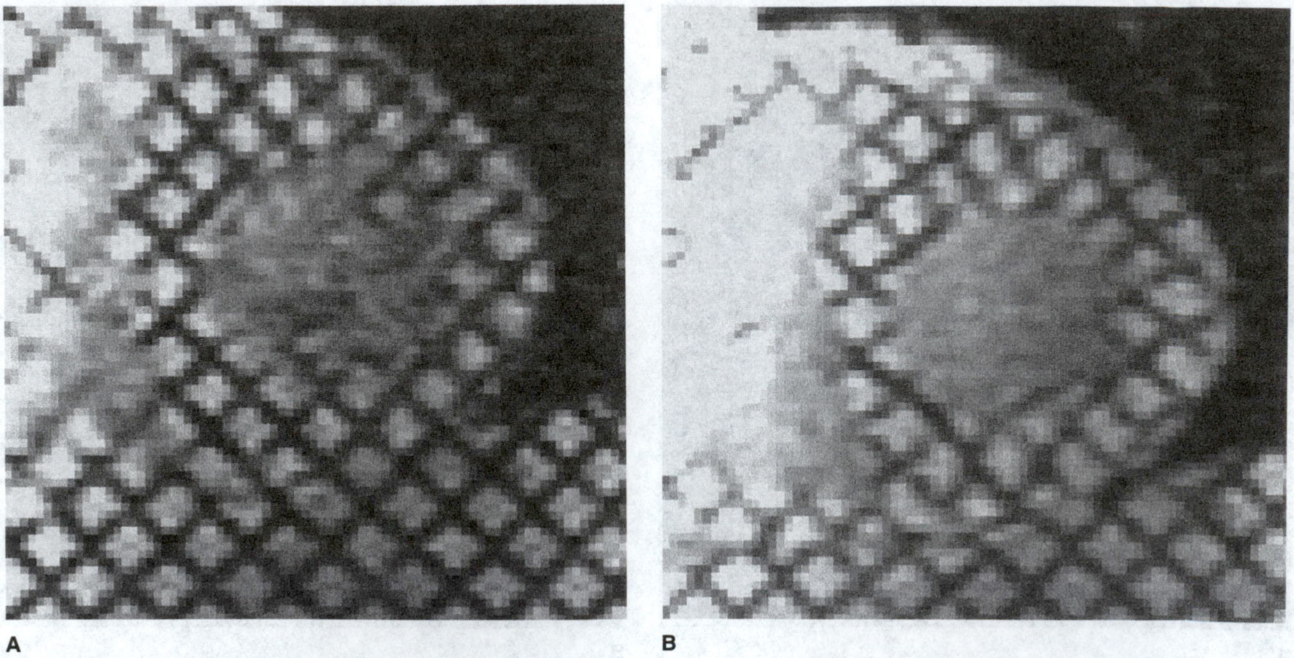

FIGURE 18A-7 Tagged short-axis images showing mainly a tomographic cut through the left ventricle at end diastole (*A*) and end systole (*B*). The tag lines are applied at end diastole and thus have a linear grid pattern in panel *A*. At end systole, the grid lines are deformed because of myocardial contractile motion, yielding information about regional wall function.

A specialized sequence known as phase-velocity mapping (PVM) is used to measure blood flow and myocardial motion. PVM uses NMR signal phase (as opposed to signal amplitude) that is made sensitive to motion.[23–27] With PVM, two image sets are required to generate a velocity map, and this doubles the scan time compared with conventional MRI. However, the advantage of generating such "phase-velocity maps" is that the velocity in any selectable direction can be encoded.

It can be appreciated that many creative pulse sequences can be used to highlight morphology, function, blood flow, perfusion, and even diffusion. These include techniques applied to MR angiography (MRA), quantification of cardiac function, quantification and visualization of blood flow velocity, and cardiac perfusion imaging. Clinical application of these techniques will be discussed in detail later in this chapter.

Patient Considerations

PATIENT COMFORT

Most patients tolerate the MRI procedure without the need for sedation. However, claustrophobia limits scan completion in approximately 5 percent of patients. Although rarely necessary, gentle sedation may be required so that the patient can relax and then remain motionless during the scan acquisition. Methods more commonly used to decrease anxiety include removing the patient from the magnet bore between scans and allowing a friend or family member to be positioned at the head of the bore to talk to the patient during scanning. Earphones are placed on the patient to minimize the acoustic noise, allowing many patients to sleep during the scan. However, for protocols that require the patient to perform breath holds, it is necessary for the patient to remain conscious throughout the examination. For these scans, some systems allow the patient to view movies through special MRI-compatible virtual reality systems. Newer magnets are shorter and may reduce the incidence of claustrophobia. Scan preparation and imaging time vary with the complexity of the clinical question to be answered. For example, if only ventricular function is assessed, the study can be performed in approximately 20 min; however, if the patient is being assessed for complex congenital heart disease, imaging times of 1 h or more may be required. As scanner technology and software have improved, imaging times have decreased. However, as the capabilities of MRI have increased, the amount of clinical data that can be acquired during an MRI session has increased. Thus, typically an MRI scan session can last 30 to 45 min. However, during this time a great deal of clinical information can be acquired.

PATIENT SAFETY

As with any diagnostic medical technique, safety is a critical issue, and safety procedures and rules should be familiar to the physicians ordering the scan and the technicians performing the scan. MR techniques can be contraindicated in a patient because of (1) the potential of the magnetic field to move or dislodge an object or device, (2) the possibility that the RF field will heat a conductor such as a pacemaker electrode, (3) the potential for inducing electric currents in a conductor such as a pacing electrode, and (4) the generation of artifacts by metallic objects that can confound diagnoses. The most common implanted devices that exclude a patient from having an MRI study are pacemakers (permanent or temporary) and automated implantable cardiovascular defibrillators. At least six deaths have occurred in patients with pacemakers, and those deaths were thought to be related to an MRI procedure.[28] Prosthetic heart valves are generally MR-compatible, with the possible exception of the pre-6000 series Starr-Edwards valve, a caged ball device used clinically several decades ago. To the authors' knowledge, there has never been a report of an untoward incident with a heart valve prosthesis. The presence of sternal wires and bypass graft clips is not hazardous to the patient but results in MR signal artifact. Properly installed intravascular coils, stents, and filters are unlikely to dislodge but result in MR signal loss in the region of the metallic device.[29] Commonly encountered implanted devices that are potentially MR-hazardous include intracranial aneurysm clips and certain metallic ocular, cochlear, and penile prostheses. Technicians also must be aware of the potential danger associated with metallic devices that may accompany the patient, such as wheelchairs, intravenous (IV) poles, oxygen tanks, and iron-shot-filled hemostatic "sandbags." These devices may become dangerous projectiles in the vicinity of an MR system. A useful resource is the Web site that lists current devices and their degree of MR compatibility: http://MRIsafety.com/index.html.

A static magnetic field is not the only potential source of hazard. The rapidly changing magnetic gradients required for imaging can induce strong currents in conducting objects such as wires and cables. Further, the RF fields also can induce electric currents to flow. External devices that may cause harm to a patient by causing skin burns include pulse oximetry and ECG cables. MR-compatible cables, i.e., those designed to reduce the incidence of heating or induced currents, are available and must be used in an MR facility. In addition, all non-MRI-compatible metal cables and detection devices must be removed from the patient before the scan is performed.

CLINICAL APPLICATIONS

There are many applications of MR to the cardiovascular system, both clinical and research.[30] The current clinical indications are for assessment of function and morphology of the heart and great vessels. However, MR methods also have the potential ability to image perfusion (using the first transit of a paramagnetic contrast agent), assess viability after a myocardial infarction (MI), image the coronary arteries, and image and characterize atherosclerotic plaque.

Since MRI can generate images in any tomographic orientation, it can provide information for comprehensive assessment of the heart with excellent spatial resolution. The three-dimensional imaging ability of MRI allows accurate assessment of global and regional function. Such assessment in theory should be more accurate than methods that are predominantly two-dimensional, such as echocardiography and x-ray angiography, and methods with lower resolution, such as radionuclide approaches.

Assessment of Cardiac Morphology and Ventricular Function

The standard cardiac MRI exam begins with spin-echo images in the orthogonal planes of the body: transverse, coronal, and sagittal. To evaluate ventricular function, image planes should be oriented in relation to the intrinsic axes of the heart. Accordingly, cine cardiac MR images are obtained in the two-chamber (right anterior oblique), four-chamber, and short-axis views (Fig. 18A-8). Consequently, the resultant image orientation is comparable to that of other imaging modalities. Both static spin-echo (dark blood) and dynamic cine MR (bright blood) imaging allow comprehensive assessment of a wide variety of cardiac dimensions and volumes.

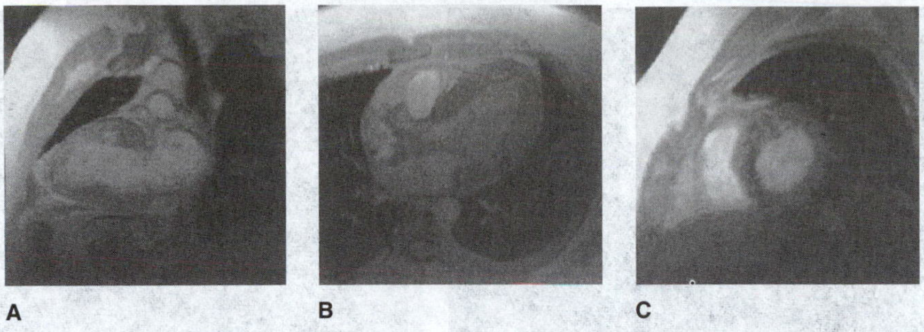

FIGURE 18A-8 Gradient-echo images acquired in a two-chamber (*A*), a four-chamber (*B*), and a midventricular short-axis tomographic plane (*C*).

Measurements

"Computer calipers" are a standard feature of the software available on clinical MR systems. Linear point-to-point measurements of distances similar to that used on echocardiographic equipment provide a means to report standard dimensions. Since spin-echo images highlight morphologic detail, these images are used to evaluate the diameter of the great vessels and the cardiac chambers,[31–33] ventricular wall thickness,[34] left ventricular (LV) mass, pericardial thickness, cardiac and paracardiac masses, and congenital anomalies.

MRI generally provides images with excellent definition of endocardial surfaces, allowing ready measurement of left and right ventricular end-diastolic and end-systolic size within each myocardial slice. When area-length calculations are used for orthogonal long- and short-axis slices or for summing serial short-axis slices (Simpson's rule), end-systolic, end-diastolic, and stroke volumes of the left and right ventricles can be determined accurately. From these volumes, one can calculate cardiac output and ejection fraction. These volumetric parameters correlate well with other imaging techniques.[35–43] MRI allows routine quantitative assessment of regional ventricular function with visualization of all myocardial segments. In a similar fashion, the epicardial contour also may be outlined, and thus the volume of the myocardium, i.e., the volume between the epicardial and endocardial surfaces, can be calculated. Myocardial mass can be determined without geometric assumptions by multiplying the myocardial volume by the assumed value for the density of myocardial tissue.[44–48]

When the technique of phase-contrast imaging (PVM, velocity-flow mapping, or velocity-encoded cine MR is used), blood flow velocity can be determined (Fig. 18A-9). This method has been validated in a variety of in vivo models.[49–53] With this technique, blood flow in both the ascending aorta and the pulmonary artery can be determined simultaneously, allowing calculation of the ratio of pulmonary to systemic flow (Q_p/Q_s) for

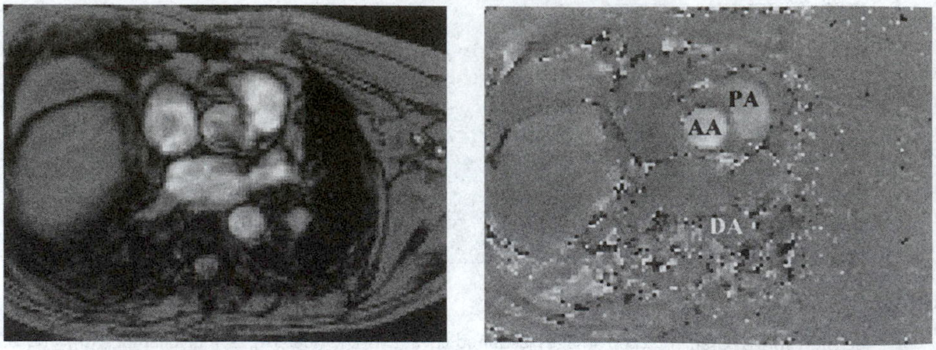

A B

FIGURE 18A-9 *A.* Conventional gradient-echo MR tomograph in the transverse plane at the level of the right pulmonary artery (PA). *B.* Corresponding velocity-encoded image, with bright signals representing velocity toward the viewer, e.g., ascending aorta (AA), and low signal representing velocity away from the viewer, e.g., descending aorta (DA). In this case, as is the convention, the viewer is looking into the plane from a cranial perspective.

assessment of shunt size[54] or regurgitant volumes. Myocardial contractile velocity also has been determined by using PVM.

Ischemic Heart Disease

Several MR approaches are useful for detecting various aspects of ischemic heart disease. These include myocardial tissue characterization, postinfarct imaging of the intensity of contrast agents (e.g., hyperenchancement), stress-induced segmental dysfunction, perfusion imaging, and ischemia-induced changes in high-energy phosphate metabolism using spectroscopic methods (Table 18A-1). This section is divided into two main components: evaluation of stable and acute ischemic syndromes.

STABLE ISCHEMIC HEART DISEASE

A number of MR methods are useful for detecting and evaluating the severity of stable ischemic heart disease. Some of these methods have been applied widely and should be considered as the standard of care, some are promising but still under development, and some are still considered research (Table 18A-1).

Stress-Induced Segmental Dysfunction Stress-induced impairment of regional LV function is an early and reliable sign of ischemia associated with significant coronary artery stenosis, preceding ST-segment depression, and angina pectoris.[55,56] Dobutamine can be used as a pharmacologic means of inducing stress and provides a way to induce ischemia-related wall motion abnormalities. Dobutamine infusion generally begins at 10 μg/min and is increased 5 μg every 2 min until angina occurs. ECGs are distorted in MR systems by the magnetic and RF fields. Thus, reliable ECG monitoring is not possible during MRI. Nevertheless, with symptoms, blood pressure, and pulse closely monitored, the test has been performed without life-threatening complications. Regional abnormalities of wall motion can be observed by using radionuclide cineangiography[57] and echocardiography.[58-61] MRI offers a noninvasive imaging approach with high spatial resolution and three-dimensional imaging for optimally accurate evaluation of regional LV function.[62,63] Van Rugge and colleagues used graded dobutamine infusion in conjunction with MRI in 45 patients with chest pain. Thirty-seven patients had angiographically significant coronary artery disease;[64] with peak dobutamine infusion, segmental dysfunction was observed in 30 patients, yielding an overall sensitivity for detection or coronary artery disease of 81 percent. None of the eight patients without significant coronary artery stenoses had abnormal wall motion; i.e., the specificity in this very small series was 100 percent. Furthermore, the sensitivity for detecting single-, double-, and triple-vessel disease was 75 percent, 80 percent, and 100 percent, respectively. The total duration of the examination is approximately 1 h.

Myocardial Perfusion Imaging Using MR Contrast Agents Myocardial perfusion imaging (MPI) is used widely with radionuclides. However, it is now clear that MPI with MR methods

TABLE 18A-1 Ischemic Heart Disease Assessment by MR

Method	Established for Clinical Application	Ready for Clinical Application	Under Development (Emerging)	Research
Regional wall motion at rest	Cine, tagging			
Global ventricular function	Cine, tagging			
Regional and global stress		Cine, tagging		
Myocardial perfusion			Contrast agent	
Myocardial viability			Contrast agent Delayed hyperenhancement	
Myocardial metabolism				Spectroscopy (e.g., ^{31}P, ^{1}H)
Coronary artery disease			Angiography Plaque characterization	

can provide higher-resolution imaging without ionizing radiation. Although a substantial body of data has been acquired using MR MPI, this procedure should be considered developmental until a larger-scale multicenter study is done.

Paramagnetic substances such as gadolinium and dysprosium cause a reduction in both T1 and T2. The magnitude of the decrease is related to the magnetic field strength and the concentration of the paramagnetic agent.[65] When a paramagnetic agent (e.g., gadolinium DTPA or gadoteridol) is given intravenously as a bolus, generally using a power injector, regional myocardial perfusion can be assessed. Currently, there are three classes of paramagnetic agents: extracellular, blood pool, and intracellular. The most commonly used is extracellular gadolinium diethylenetriamine pentaacetic acid (Gd-DTPA), which actually distributes in the blood pool and extracellular space.

MRI records the first pass of the paramagnetic agent through the myocardium. A pulse sequence that markedly diminishes (or "nulls") the signal intensity of the myocardium is used. Thus, myocardium with the greatest concentration of contrast agent is assumed to be normally perfused. The portion of the myocardium with reduced signal is presumed to be underperfused or ischemic (Fig. 18A-10). The authors' initial experience in over 200 patients compared MR and radionuclide perfusion imaging using acquisitions at rest with thallium-201 or low dose ^{99m}Tc sestamibi and then with the first bolus injection of the gadolinium-based agent. A dipyridamole infusion was then initiated using this standard dose of 0.56 mg/kg over a 4-min interval. Two minutes after the infusion, practically simultaneous infusion of ^{99m}Tc sestamibi and gadoteridol was given. In the first 50 patients, sensitivity and specificity were significantly better with radionuclides. In the second 50 patients, radionuclides and MR showed equivalent sensitivity and specificity (probably related to a "learning curve").

Reading MR perfusion images requires some experience, since the approach is dynamic rather than static as it is with radionuclides.[66] One must evaluate the homogeneity with which the myocardium enhances as the paramagnetic agent enters the myocardium. One pitfall that it is essential to know about is that the lower portion of the interventricular septum frequently demonstrates reduced signal in patients without significant coronary artery disease. Accordingly, if this territory is the only one with a "defect," one should not assume abnormal perfusion but instead an artifact of the MR method. Manning and associates[67] used Gd-DTPA to assess myocardial perfusion at rest in patients with severe coronary artery disease. As was anticipated, the time to peak signal intensity was delayed, and peak signal intensity was reduced in regions of the myocardium perfused by a severely stenotic coronary artery. An alternative approach to detecting regions of compromised myocardium has been developed by Hundley and colleagues,[68] utilizing the ability of MRI to measure flow.

Using dipyridamole, Matheijssen and coworkers[69] compared perfusion MRI with sestamibi single photon emission computed tomography (SPECT). Agreement in localization of the artery with significant occlusive disease was 80 percent between angiography and SPECT, 70 percent between angiography and MRI, and 90 percent between SPECT and MRI. MR perfusion studies have been limited by the need to use first-pass acquisition, resulting in the depiction of only one or two slices at the level of the mid-left ventricle. Walsh and associates have developed a method called the block regional interpolation scheme for k-space (BRISK) to acquire up to four tomographic slices

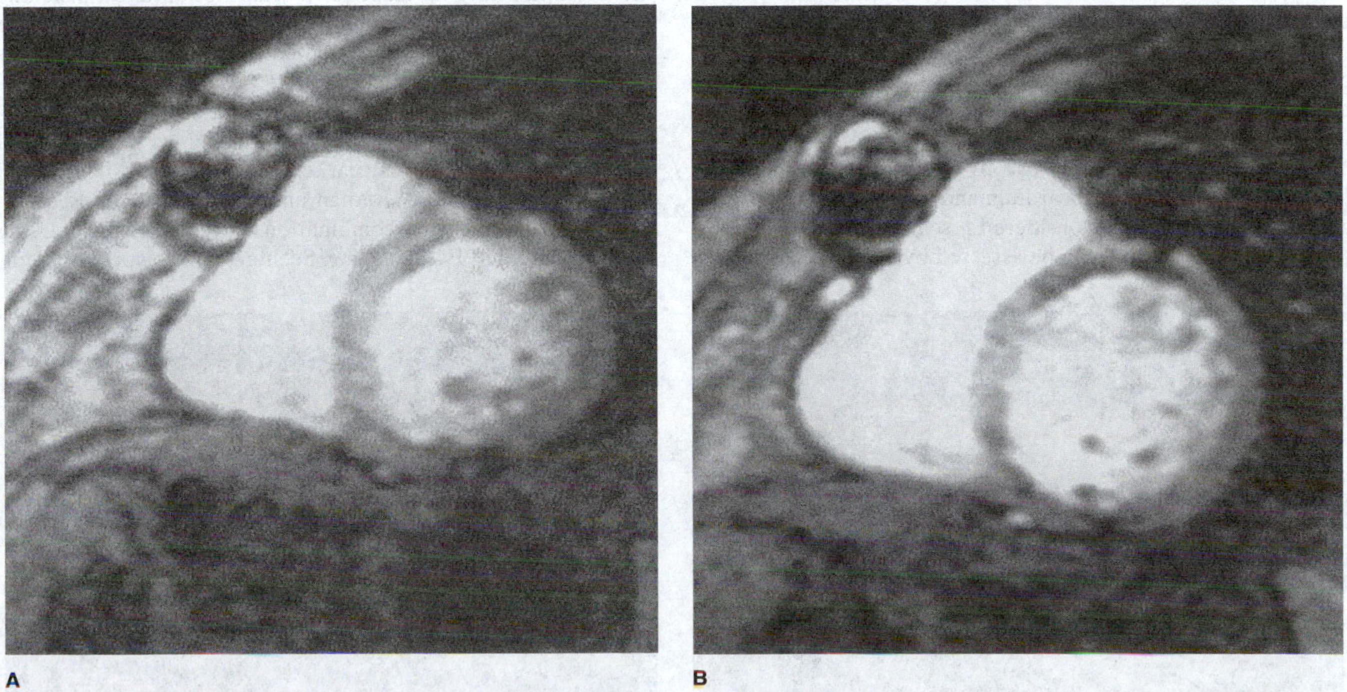

FIGURE 18A-10 First-pass contrast perfusion images at (*A*) rest and (*B*) peak stress. The patient has coronary artery disease with restenosis of an LAD stent (visualized as a small signal void artifact localized to the anterior wall). At rest, there is little evidence of a perfusion defect, but at stress, a moderate, primarily subendocardial defect is seen directly around the stent. Also seen is a small fixed inferior defect. (Images provided courtesy of Andrew Arai, MD, Laboratory of Cardiac Energetics, National Heart, Lung and Blood Institute.)

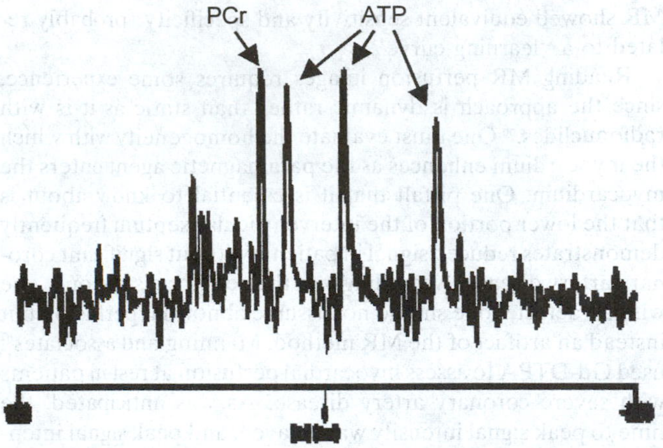

FIGURE 18A-11 Myocardial spectrum acquired from a healthy person, indicating the phosphocreatine (PCr) and adenosine triphosphate (ATP) peaks.

through the ventricle by using a conventional MR scanner. This approach represents a great step forward, allowing a more extensive evaluation of perfusion within the short duration of the first pass of the paramagnetic bolus.[70-72] New contrast agents are under development. One strategy includes blood pool agents such as iron particles and a gadolinium agent that binds to albumin. Contrast agents that remain within the blood pool are less complex to analyze since they involve only one compartment. Iron particles have been under investigation, since they remain within the blood pool.[73] Another, more long-range approach for perfusion imaging was reported by Simor and coworkers.[74] This group described an agent that appears to enter and remain within the myocardium, as thallium-201 or sestamibi.[74] Such agents, when clinically available, should allow myocardial perfusion imaging over many cardiac cycles rather than only one, as is the case with the "first-pass" approach. The use of such myocardial localizing agents should provide the highest-resolution perfusion images available by any technology.

MR Spectroscopy MR spectroscopy provides another perspective for evaluating the myocardium and defining ischemia. This approach should still be considered research. Cardiac metabolism and energy reserve can be assessed by using spectroscopic methods to assess baseline and changes in the high-energy phosphates within the myocardium (Fig. 18A-11).[75-78] Studies in laboratory animals have demonstrated a rapid decrease in phosphocreatine (PCr) after coronary occlusion. The PCr-to-adenosine triphosphate (ATP) ratio is used frequently to express changes in bioenergetics, particularly with myocardial ischemia.[79-81] Typically, a surface coil is placed on the anterior chest wall and ^{31}P spectroscopic imaging is performed before, during, and after hand-grip exercise stress. The patient is asked to grip as hard as possible. This is said to be the maximal level. Then, during the study, the grip is maintained at 30 percent of maximum.[82,83] Localized spectroscopic methods then examine PCr/ATP in the anterior myocardium. Using isometric handgrip stress, Weiss and coinvestigators[84] and Yabe and associates[85] reported significant decreases in PCr/ATP ratios in patients with angiographically documented left anterior descending (LAD) coronary artery disease. In the NHLBI-supported WISE (Women with Ischemia Syndrome Evaluation) study, 20 to 30 percent of women with no significant coronary artery disease (CAD) but chest pain had a significant reduction in PCr/ATP compared with age-matched controls. Such data suggest the importance of the PCr/ATP stress test in detecting ischemia.

ACUTE ISCHEMIC SYNDROMES

MR imaging can be used to differentiate between angina and acute MI. Morphology, function, perfusion, and coronary angiography may all be useful to differentiate reversible ischemia syndromes from MI. Infarct size, regional and global function, and viability can be evaluated. Further, the sequelae of myocardial infarction can be assessed.

Global and Regional Function Wall motion and thickening can be readily assessed using a cine technique or a real-time approach[86-89] (Fig. 18A-12). Regional wall motion abnormalities and wall thickening by MRI correlate well with sites of dysfunction by x-ray cineventriculography.[90] End-diastolic wall thickness and the degree of systolic wall thickening demonstrated by MRI may be used as markers for predicting myocardial viability (Fig. 18A-13). Hofman and coworkers proposed employing cardiac pacing in combination with MR imaging.[91] Using ^{99m}Tc sestamibi SPECT imaging, Sechtem and coworkers[92] dem-

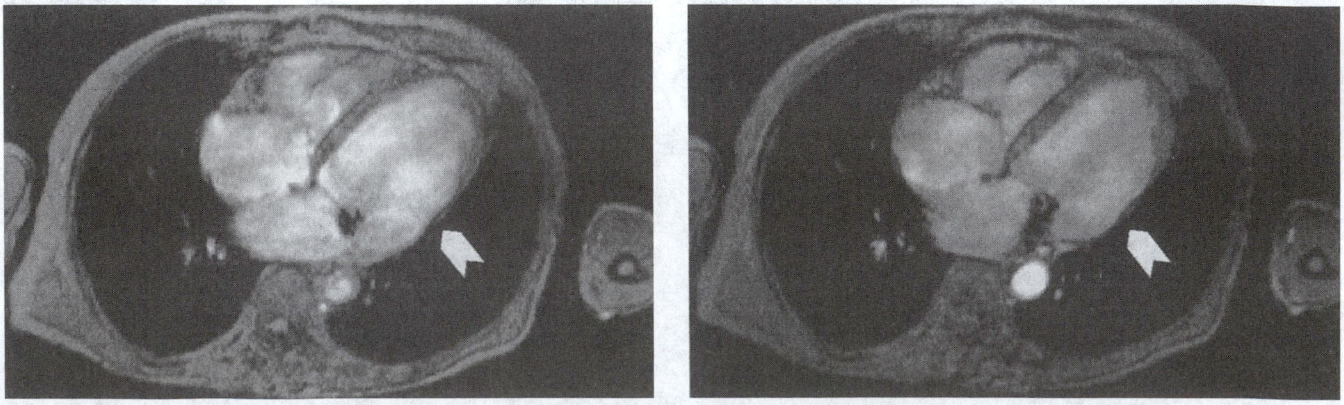

A B

FIGURE 18A-12 Regional left ventricular dysfunction. Midventricular long-axis tomographic gradient-echo sections in end diastole (*A*) and end systole (*B*). Note some thickening of the interventricular septum but akinesis and marked thinning of the posterior and posterolateral segments (*arrows*).

onstrated that an end-diastolic wall thickness greater than 6 mm or a systolic wall thickening greater than 1 mm correlated with viable myocardium. This was supported by positron emission tomography (PET) imaging with ^{18}F-fluorodeoxyglucose and cine MR imaging of wall thickness and wall thickening to define viability.[93,94] Normal MR values of left ventricular dimensions have been reported by Lorenz and colleagues.[95] Wall function can be assessed quantitatively by using MR cine tagging approaches.[96,97]

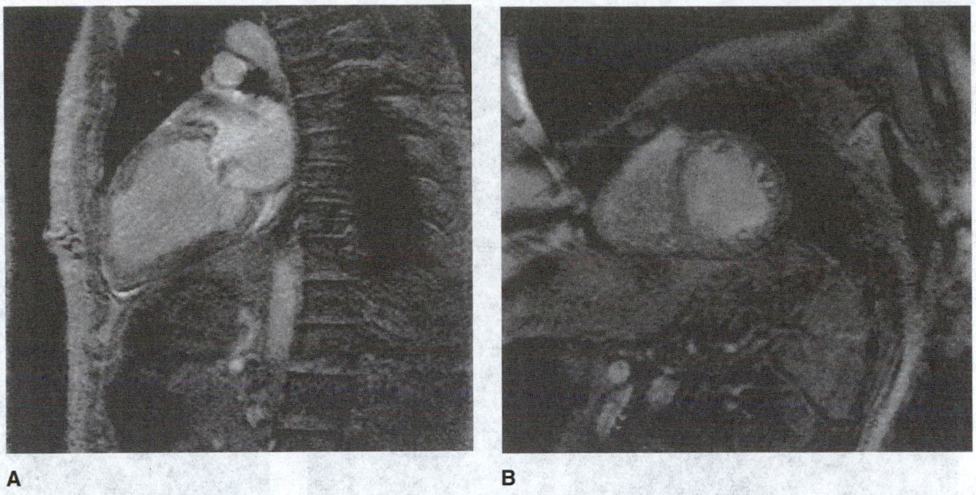

FIGURE 18A-13 Long-axis (*A*) and short-axis (*B*) views of the heart. Note the generalized myocardial thinning of the dilated left ventricle and dilation of the right ventricle (*B*). The mid-left ventricular anterilateral wall and the interventricular septum are particularly thin.

Infarct Size Within an hour of the onset of an MI, T1 and T2 relaxation times generally increase within infarcted myocardium; such prolongation of relaxation times provide a means to determine the location and extent of the infarction.[98–100] Whereas some investigators have claimed that infarct imaging with T1 and T2 is not specific,[101] others have demonstrated a good correlation between thallium-201 scintigraphy and T1 and T2 MR imaging in examining infarct size and location.[102,103] Using spin-echo imaging to emphasize T2 has demonstrated increased signal intensity in regions of infarcted tissue and provides a means to determine infarct size.[104,105] Furthermore, wall thinning and asynergy may be of value in assessing the extent of myocardial tissue infarction.[106]

Paramagnetic contrast agents such as a chelate of gadolinium have been reported to be of value in differentiating between infarcted and noninfarcted myocardium. A phenomenon termed *delayed hyperenhancement* has been observed 3 to 15 min after contrast administration and has been found to correlate with zones of irreversible myocardial damage, whereas the absence of delayed hyperenhancement indicated reversible damage.[107] However, this observation may be controversial in view of the recent study of Rogers and coinvestigators.[108] In that study, delayed enhancement occurred in regions in which myocardial injury was reversible, while hypoenhancement occurred in regions with irreversible myocardial injury. The hyperenhancement phenomenon most likely is related to a delay in the uptake of the paramagnetic agent within the injured territory as a result of reduced blood flow and edema (Fig. 18A-14).[109] The ultimate significance of this finding awaits further study.

Myocardial Tissue Characterization Changes in the biophysical properties of ischemic myocardium during an ischemic insult can be detected readily by using MR imaging. The relaxation times, T1 and T2, increase with several ischemic insults and are related largely to an increase in water content.[110–113] In animal models, the largest increase in relaxation times occurs in ischemic zones with moderate to severely reduced blood flow, whereas in zones in which the ischemia is total, there is little, if any, increase in myocardial T1 and T2. Other factors of less importance than edema that contribute to such changes in relaxation times include the presence of free radicals, the change in magnetic susceptibility related to the paramagnetic effects of deoxyhemoglobin as a result of hemorrhage, and lipid accumulation.[114,115] Spin-echo images with long echo times will emphasize T1 increases, depicting them as zones of increased intensity.

Complications of Myocardial Infarction MR imaging provides exquisite morphologic and functional detail. Thus, it can be used to sensitively detect short- and long-term complications of myocardial infarction, including ventricular aneurysm, mitral regurgitation caused by papillary muscle necrosis, perforation of the interventricular septum, LV thrombus, and pericardial effusion. In addition to the regional wall thinning of infarcted myocardium, compensatory hypertrophy and LV chamber enlargement (remodeling) also may be demonstrated. Furthermore, pericardial effusions after infarction are readily demonstrated and quantified.

Coronary Artery Disease

It is possible, using MR angiography methods, to perform coronary artery imaging. In addition, several investigators have demonstrated the feasibility of characterizing the stability of atherosclerotic plaque by using MR methods. These topics are described in detail in Chap. 18B.

Valvular Heart Disease

The ideal approach for evaluating patients with valvular heart disease must include an accurate assessment of the valve morphology and function and a means to assess myocardial structure and function and potentially energetics (e.g., using ^{31}P spectroscopy). Structural and functional changes related to valve dysfunction include atrial and/or ventricular chamber enlargement, ventricular wall thickening, poststenotic dilatation of the aorta and/or pulmonary artery, and atrial and/or ventricular thrombus.

MORPHOLOGY

Normal valve leaflets are 1 to 2 mm in thickness and are highly mobile throughout the cardiac cycle. Echocardiography pro-

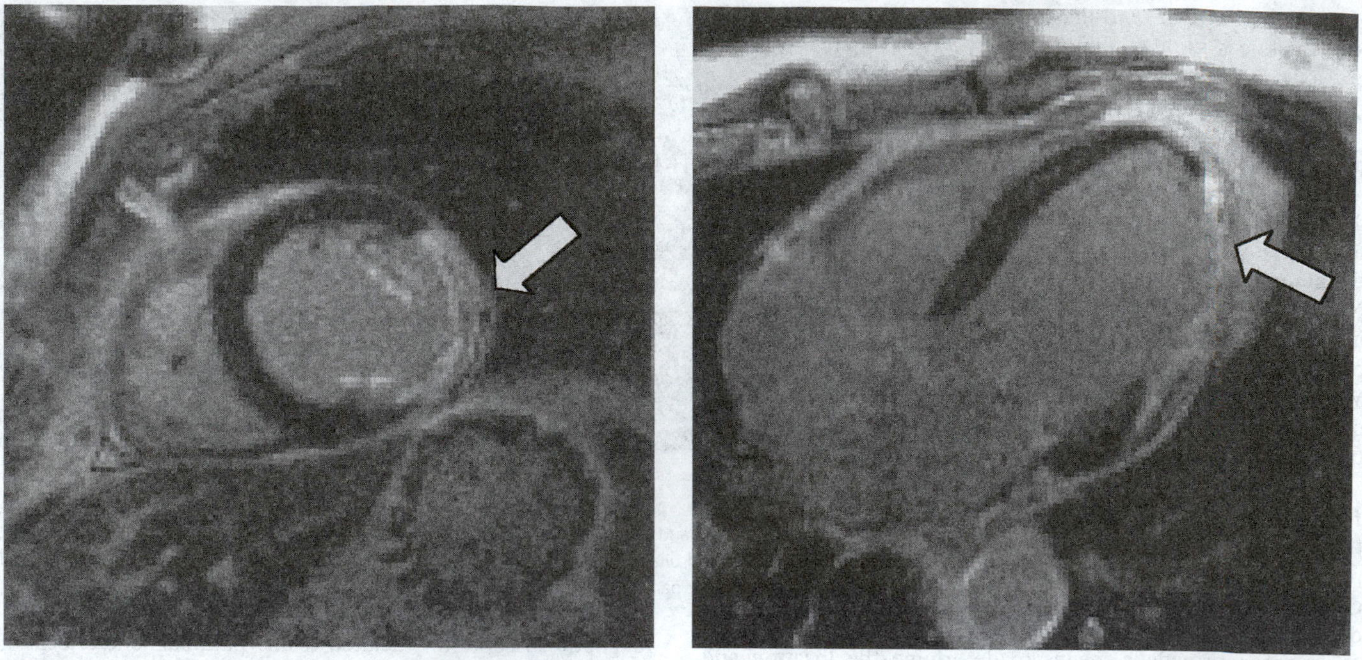

A B

FIGURE 18A-14 A patient with an occluded left circumflex coronary artery that was opened by percutaneous transluminal coronary angioplasty (PTCA) and stented. The MRI was performed 2 weeks after an acute MI. Images are seen in the short-axis (*A*) and long-axis views (*B*), and the regions of delayed hyperenhancement are arrowed. (Images provided courtesy of Robert M. Judd.)

vides high spatial and temporal resolution of the valve leaflets. Since the slice thickness of clinical MR images ranges from 5 to 10 mm, the spatial resolution is not adequate to assess the valve leaflets accurately and reproducibly. Nevertheless, spin-echo and gradient-echo images provide a reasonable approach for determining the number of leaflets, the degree of excursion, and approximate leaflet thickness.

With MRI, because of dimensional accuracy, high resolution, and three-dimensional aspects, the ventricular and atrial morphology and function can be assessed accurately without employing geometric assumptions. When the resultant information is used, MR imaging can be helpful in determining the approximate time for surgical intervention by defining chamber volumes and function. It has been demonstrated that preoperative LV size and ejection fraction are good predictors of LV function after surgical intervention for aortic and mitral regurgitation.

VALVE FUNCTION

The severity of valvular dysfunction can be assessed by two MR methods: cine gradient-echo imaging and phase-velocity imaging. In the former method, the chaotic motion of turbulent flow results in dephasing and consequently in a reduction of MR signal. Thus, a signal void is present within a normally signal-intense blood pool. The territory of MR signal void corresponds to the area of color Doppler signal by echocardiography[116–119] (Fig. 18A-15). The reduction in signal can be altered by changing acquisition parameters such as TE, TR, sampling size of the imaged volume element (voxel), and/or orientation of the imaging plane relative to the flow jet.[120,121] Thus, consistency of these factors must be maintained to assure appropriate interpretation. Similar to echocardiography, the volume of proximal flow convergence, which appears as a small cone-shaped MR signal void on the side of the valve opposite to the direction of regurgitant flow, is predictive of the severity of regurgitation.[122,123] MR has been used to measure regurgitant volumes and regurgitant fraction by measuring right ventricular (RV) and LV stroke volumes and thus determining the severity of regurgitation, assuming that regurgitant lesions involve only one side (RV or LV).[124–126]

In addition, gradient-echo imaging can be used to approximate the degree of aortic stenosis by observing the extent of turbulent flow (signal loss) in the ascending aorta.[127] However, it is possible to

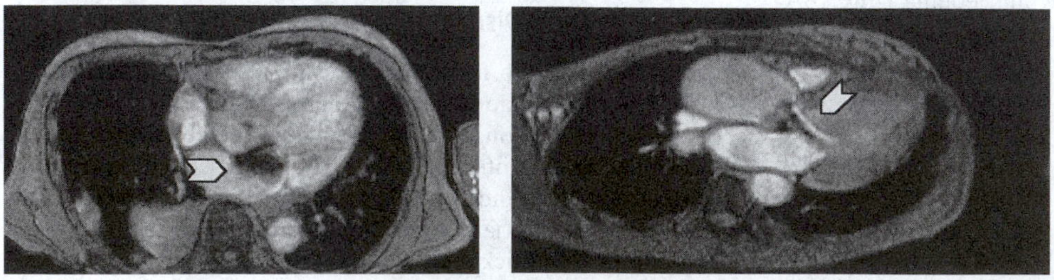

A B

FIGURE 18A-15 Transverse gradient-echo images are shown depicting mitral (*A*) and aortic regurgitation (*B*). In each case, turbulent flow caused by the regurgitant lesion results in loss of MR signal (*arrow*). Note reduced signal on the side of the valve opposite the direction of regurgitation. This in part is consistent with proximal flow convergence.

use phase-velocity imaging to assess flow velocities to 5 m/s.[128] In this way, the severity of aortic stenosis can be assessed more reliably.

In summary, MRI represents a reliable noninvasive means for assessing valvular and ventricular function to assist in determining the appropriate timing for valve replacement. PVM may be useful for the quantification of valve dysfunction.

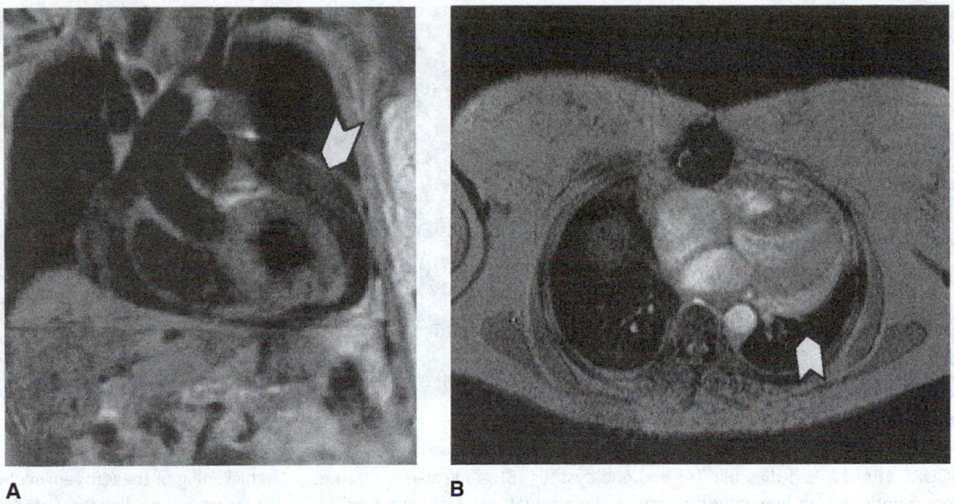

FIGURE 18A-16 *A.* A coronal spin-echo image depicting a large pericardial effusion (*arrow*) *B.* A gradient-echo image depicting bright signal from a pericardial effusion (*arrow*). Also note the circular region of reduced signal intensity related to postoperative sternal wire.

Pericardial Disease

Normal pericardium on multislice spin-echo MR images appears as a thin, low-intensity signal (<3 mm) between the high-intensity signal of mediastinal and epicardial fat and the medium-intensity signal of myocardium.[129,130] The lower signal intensity of the normal pericardium results from the amount of fibrous tissue (with long T1 and short T2 relaxation times). Sechtem and associates reported that the pericardium adjacent to the right ventricle could be visualized by MR in 100 percent of the subjects studied, whereas the pericardium along the lateral wall of the left ventricle could be visualized in only 61 percent of the subjects.[131]

PERICARDIAL EFFUSION

Normal pericardial fluid has a low signal intensity on spin-echo images. Such fluid leads to a zone of reduced signal intensity separating the pericardium from the myocardium and the epicardial fat. It has been postulated that the appearance is dark because of the nonlaminar flow of fluid within the pericardial sac as a consequence of cardiac motion. Such nonlaminar flow changes the spin phase and causes MR signal loss.[132] In gradient-echo images, the pericardial fluid appears bright as a result of this flow, clearly separating the parietal pericardium from the myocardium (Fig. 18A-16).

The ability of MRI to detect moderate or large pericardial effusions is comparable to that of echocardiography. However, MRI is able to detect small fluid collections better than echocardiography can. This is especially noteworthy in areas at the medial border of the right atrium or posterior to the LV apex.[133] Because of its lower cost and portability, echocardiography should be used as the first-line approach in assessing patients for pericardial effusion; however, MRI should be performed when a clinically suspected pericardial effusion is not detected on echocardiography. MRI is also useful for demonstrating loculated pericardial effusions.

PERICARDIAL THICKENING

In both MRI and computed x-ray tomography, a pericardial thickness of more than 4 mm is considered abnormal.[134] Pericardium visualized by MRI varies in thickness in different regions of the heart; thus, a standard imaging plane must be established. For this reason, transverse imaging at the levels of the right atrium and the right and left ventricles is recommended.

By demonstrating the presence or absence of a thickened pericardium, MRI can help distinguish between constrictive pericarditis and restrictive cardiomyopathy. Patients examined by MRI who had proven constrictive pericarditis had a pericardial thickening greater than 5 mm.[135] In addition, calcification of the pericardium, which demonstrates reduced signal intensity, also aids in the diagnosis of a pericardial rather than cardiomyopathic restrictive disease.

Cardiomyopathy

Evaluation of global and regional wall thickness and thickening, wall excursion, and chamber size is helpful in diagnosis and prognostication in cardiomyopathy. For example, a dilated cardiomyopathic ventricle with substantial regional wall motion abnormalities suggests an "ischemic" process. Further, valve dysfunction, ventricular outflow tract obstruction, and vena caval dilatation are readily detectable signs of cardiomyopathy. As was stated above, MRI is an optimal means for detecting these conditions with excellent reproducibility.

HYPERTROPHIC CARDIOMYOPATHY

The diagnosis of hypertrophic cardiomyopathy is most sensitively made by visualizing the entire myocardium in view of its wide phenotypic variability. The most common pattern is associated with asymmetric hypertrophy. Nevertheless, a wide variety of patterns of wall thickening can be seen, from extensive and diffuse to limited and segmental, with no single morphologic expression considered typical.[136] Serial short-axis MR images systematically slice the ventricles from base to apex, allowing comprehensive evaluation of wall thickness (Fig. 18A-17). Cardiac MRI using this approach correlates well with echocardiography and x-ray cineventriculography in delineating the precise site and extent of hypertrophy.[137–139] Hypertrophy confined to the apex is a variant of hypertrophic cardiomyopathy that may be difficult to visualize by conventional echocardiography but is readily distinguished by MRI.[140–142] When the extent of turbulent flow (signal loss) in the LV outflow tract is defined, a semiquantitative assessment of the degree of dynamic LV outflow tract obstruction can be made with gradient-echo MRI.

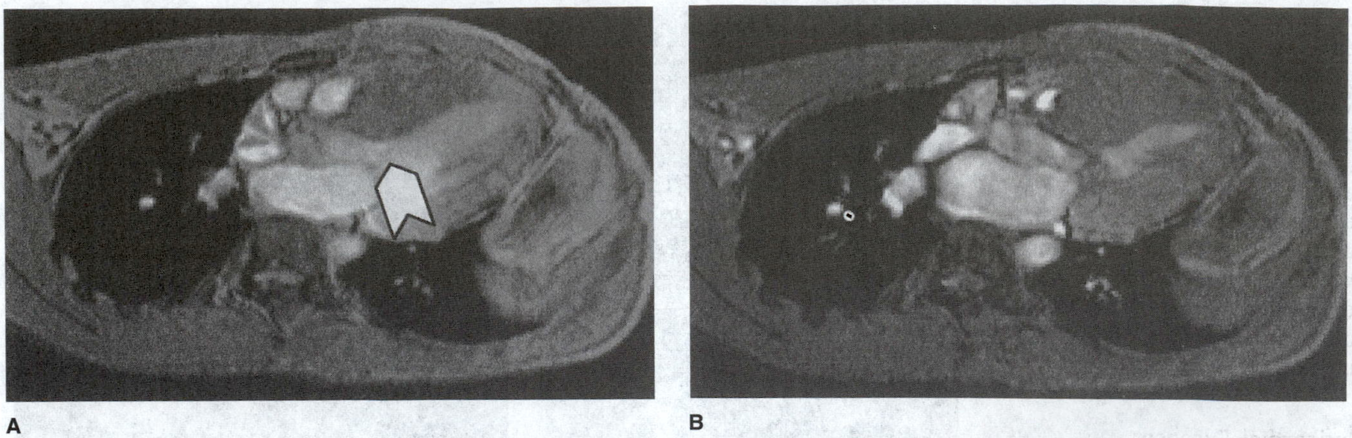

FIGURE 18A-17 End-diastolic (*A*) and end-systolic (*B*) gradient-echo frames from a patient with hypertrophic cardiomyopathy (HCM). Note the marked thickening of the left ventricular myocardium, particularly the interventricular septum (*arrow*). In late systole, the left ventricular cavity becomes very small.

DILATED CARDIOMYOPATHY

Typically, dilated cardiomyopathy is characterized by biventricular enlargement with depressed systolic function. MRI provides a noninvasive method for accurately determining RV and/or LV end-systolic and end-diastolic volumes, stroke volume, ejection fraction, thrombus, and/or valve dysfunction. Segmental wall thinning and regional dysfunction suggest a coronary artery disease etiology. However, one must be cautious in evaluating regional LV function, since the apex is frequently akinetic in dilated cardiomyopathy.

RESTRICTIVE CARDIOMYOPATHY

Restrictive cardiomyopathy is characterized by myocardial thickening with normal to reduced chamber volumes and frequently depressed LV systolic function. In addition, because of restricted diastolic ventricular filling, the atria and vena cavae commonly are dilated.[143] In patients with restrictive/constrictive hemodynamics, MRI frequently can distinguish between restrictive cardiomyopathy, which is managed medically, and constrictive pericarditis, which is managed surgically. The pericardium is thickened in constrictive pericarditis but usually is not thickened in restrictive cardiomyopathy. Occasionally, restrictive cardiomyopathy is caused by hemochromatosis. This condition frequently is characterized by a reduced or absent signal from the liver and spleen, since the reticuloendothelial system is laden with iron.

ARRHYTHMOGENIC RIGHT VENTRICULAR DYSPLASIA

Because of the geometric shape of the right ventricle, segmental analysis is exceedingly difficult using current imaging technologies. The segmental morphology and function of the right ventricle can be evaluated extensively by using serial contiguous tomographic slices through the heart from base to apex, for example, by spin-echo and gradient-echo imaging. The hallmark of arrhythmogenic RV dysplasia is fatty infiltration with extreme thinning and akinesis of the RV free wall. Fat is identified readily by its increased intensity on T1-weighted MR images. The RV free wall is normally 3 mm in thickness, and thinning is more difficult to detect because of limitations of spatial resolution on traditionally gated cine MR studies. Also, it can be difficult to distinguish between the intramyocardial fat and the epicardial fat adjacent to the RV wall.[144] Analysis of RV function using gradient-echo or echo-planar MRI provides a means of observing focal RV free wall aneurysms and segmental dyskinesis[145] (Fig. 18A-18). Nevertheless, the resolution afforded by MRI allows other characteristics of arrhythmogenic RV dysplasia, such as conspicuous trabeculations and scalloping of the RV free wall, to be visualized.

Congenital Heart Disease

Transthoracic echocardiography is an ideal approach for noninvasive assessment of congenital cardiovascular anomalies in infants and young children, since this technique often requires no sedation and the ultrasound beam is not obstructed by calcified bone and has a nearer target than it does in older children, adolescents, and adults. As a child approaches adolescence or has a surgical repair, the echo assessment may become more difficult and sometimes incomplete. More often, invasive techniques must be performed to assess cardiac, vascular, conduit, or baffle structures adequately. Because of the morpho-

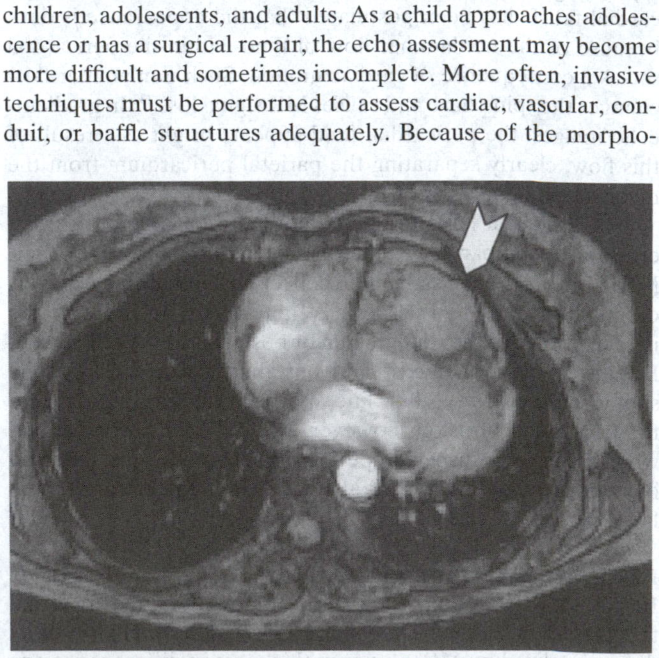

FIGURE 18A-18 Gradient-echo image of a patient with arrythmogenic RV dysplasia (ARVD). Note the focal region of thinning of the right ventricular free wall (*arrow*). Another sign of ARVD is the appearance of lipid infiltrating the involved segment. However, this is not the case here.

logic detail afforded by MRI and MRA, virtually all common congenital anomalies have been reported in the literature.[146–149] Hence, many patients do not require cardiac catheterization to identify complex congenital anatomy accurately.

MR approaches can image the five necessary anatomic parameters for the initial evaluation of a patient with complex congenital heart disease: situs, ventricular loop, atrioventricular connection, location of the apex, and ventriculoarterial connections. Since MR methods are not influenced by body habitus or scar tissue, deep vascular structures such as the central pulmonary arteries and the ductus arteriosus are well visualized even in a postoperative patient. Baffles and conduit size and function can be evaluated fully by MR provided that no metallic (conductor or ferromagnetic) materials were used at the sites, which would interfere with image integrity because of substantial signal loss.[150] As was described previously, RV size and function are determined more accurately by MRI, which is most relevant in the management of patients with disorders such as transposition of the great vessels and interventricular and interatrial shunts or after repair of tetralogy of Fallot. In patients with coarctation of the aorta with or without aortic hypoplasia, angiography is no longer required unless knowledge of coronary anatomy also is desired.[151–154] Measurements of flow and velocity across shunts and within baffles and conduits also can be made by using PVM. By using such phase-velocity measurements, one can determine the magnitude of the shunt severity or the severity of stenosis noninvasively.[155,156] Furthermore, when phase-contrast cine MR is used, the size of an atrial septal defect can be defined accurately, thus assisting in determining the timing for optimal operative intervention.[157]

Intracardiac Masses and Thrombi

Masses within a heart chamber can be identified with either spin-echo (dark blood) or gradient-echo (bright blood) imaging. The MR intensity of the mass in the spin-echo image also may help characterize its pathology on the basis of T1 relaxation time. For example, cysts and lipomas have very high signal intensity, whereas lymphomas and myxomas have less intensity[158–162] (Fig. 18A-19). Thrombus is more difficult to identify since it is usually present in a dysfunctional ventricular segment or in the atrial appendages.[163] Within a cardiac chamber, slow-moving blood within the area of the akinesis or dyskinesis will contain signal and sometimes artificially appear as a mass. Gradient-echo and/or phase-velocity imaging can be used to differentiate clot from blood stasis. The contents of the atrial appendages, especially in patients with atrial fibrillation, also may resemble thrombus since the blood movement is typically sluggish. The most definitive assessment of atrial thrombi continues to be transesophageal echocardiography (TEE).

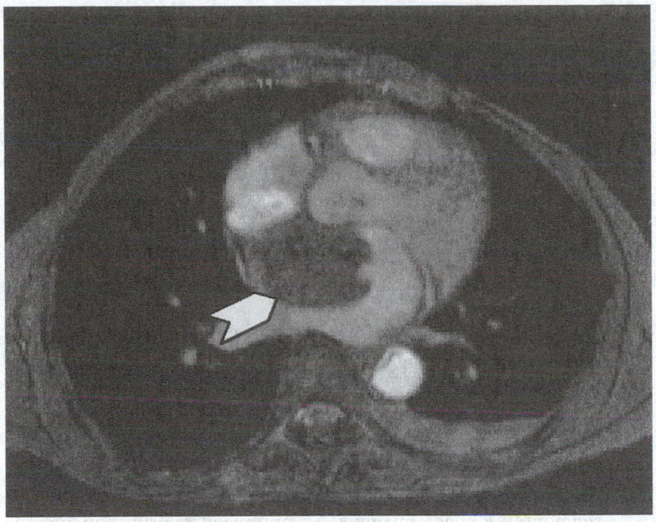

FIGURE 18A-19 A two-chamber gradient-echo image of a patient with a large left atrial mass (arrow points to region with reduced signal). Note that the mass occupies about half the left atrial cavity.

SUMMARY

Cardiovascular MR methods have gone beyond the status of a research tool to become the diagnostic method of choice for many conditions involving the cardiovascular system. This is a noninvasive modality that can generate unlimited tomographic planes, and operator interaction is not necessary. Further, there is no exposure to ionizing radiation. Resolution is high and real-time imaging is normally possible with new-generation MR systems. Also, it can generate spectra showing important metabolites such as ATP within the myocardium. Weaknesses include the lack of portability, the maintenance expense of the instrument, and the risk of the magnetic and RF fields that can displace or heat implanted devices. Despite its technical superiority, reimbursement for cardiac MRI is only somewhat higher than that for a two-dimensional echo/Doppler TEE study. Currently, MRI and MRA are most cost-effective when they replace an invasive procedure (e.g., aortography or TEE) or are performed when multiple diagnostic techniques would otherwise be required. For complex congenital heart disease in adults, aortic pathology, and cardiac or paracardiac masses, MRI is the imaging modality of choice. As physicians become more conversant with MRI in clinical practice, they will discover a diagnostic technology capable of answering questions that previously were unanswerable and improving the information provided by other technologies. If one generates images depicting ventricular and valve function, myocardial perfusion, viability, and coronary anatomy within a single time period, there is no better way to evaluate a patient with suspected cardiovascular pathology. This goal is imminently achievable.

References

1. Bloch R, Hensen WW, Packard ME. Nuclear induction. *Phys Rev* 1946; 69:127.
2. Purcell EM, Torrey HC, Pound RV. Resonance absorption by nuclear magnetic moments in a solid. *Phys Rev* 1946; 69:37–38.
3. Lauterbur PC. Image formation by induced local interactions: Examples employing nuclear magnetic resonance. *Nature* 1973; 242:190–191.
4. Foo TK, MacFall JR, Hayes CE, et al. Pulmonary vasculature: Single breath-hold MR imaging with phased-array coils. *Radiology* 1992; 183(2):473–477.
5. Botnar RM, Stuber M, Danias PG, et al. Improved coronary artery definition with T2-weighted, free-breathing, three-dimensional coronary MRA. *Circulation* 1999; 99(24):3139–3148.
6. Molinari G, Sardanelli F, Zandrino F, et al. Magnetic resonance assessment of coronary artery bypass grafts. *Rays* 1999; 24(1):131–139.
7. Rasche V, Holz D, Proksa R. MR fluoroscopy using projection

reconstruction multigradient-echo (prMGE) MRI. *Magn Reson Med* 1999; 42(2):324–334.
8. Yang PC, Kerr AB, Liu AC, et al. New real-time interactive cardiac magnetic resonance imaging system complements echocardiography. *Coll Cardiol* 1998; 32(7):2049–2056.
9. Bloomgarden DC, Fayad AZ, Ferrari VA, et al. Global cardiac function using fast breath-hold MRI: Validation of new acquisition and analysis techniques. *Magn Reson Med* 1997; 37(5):683–692.
10. Rzedzian R, Doyle M, Mansfield P, et al. Echo planar imaging in paediatrics: Real-time-nuclear magnetic resonance. *Ann Radiol (Paris)* 1984; 27(2–3):182–186.
11. Doyle M, Rzedzian R, Mansfield P, Coupland RE. Dynamic NMR cardiac imaging in a piglet. *Br J Radiol* 1983; 56(672):925–930.
12. Chrispin A, Small P, Rutter N, et al. Echo planar imaging of normal and abnormal connections of the heart and great arteries. *Pediatr Radiol* 1986; 16(4):289–292.
13. Reeder SB, Atalar E, Faranesh AZ, McVeigh ER. Multi-echo segmented k-space imaging: An optimized hybrid sequence for ultrafast cardiac imaging. *Magn Reson Med* 1999; 41(2):375–385.
14. Atkinson DJ, Edelman RR. Cineangiography of the heart in a single breath hold with a segmented turboFLASH sequence. *Radiology* 1991; 178(2):357–360.
15. Pennell DJ, Keegan J, Firmin DN, et al. Magnetic resonance imaging of coronary arteries: Technique and preliminary results. *Br Heart J* 1993; 70(4):315–326.
16. Hernandez RJ, Aisen AM, Foo TK, Beekman RH. Thoracic cardiovascular anomalies in children: Evaluation with a fast gradient-recalled-echo sequence with cardiac-triggered segmented acquisition. *Radiology* 1993; 188(3):775–780.
17. Reeder SB, Atalar E, Faranesh AZ, McVeigh ER, Multi-echo segmented k-space imaging: An optimized hybrid sequence for ultrafast cardiac imaging. *Magn Reson Med* 1999; 41(2):375–385.
18. Thedens DR, Irarrazaval P, Sachs TS. et al. Fast magnetic resonance coronary angiography with a three-dimensional stack of spirals trajectory. *Magn Reson Med* 1999; 41(6):1170–1179.
19. Axel L, Dougherty L. Heart wall motion: Improved method of spatial modulation of magnetization for MR imaging. *Radiology* 1989; 172(2):349–350.
20. Doyle M, Walsh EG, Foster RE, Pohost GM. Common k-space acquisition: A method to improve myocardial grid-tag contrast. *Magn Reson Med* 1997; 37(5):754–763.
21. Stuber M, Fischer SE, Scheidegger MB, Boesiger P. Toward high-resolution myocardial tagging. *Magn Reson Med* 1999; 41(3):639–643.
22. Denney TS Jr, McVeigh ER. Model-free reconstruction of three-dimensional myocardial strain from planar tagged MR images. *J Magn Reson Imaging* 1997; 7(5):799–810.
23. Gatehouse PD, Firmin DN, Collins S, Longmore DB. Real time blood flow imaging by spiral scan phase velocity mapping. *Magn Reson Med* 1994; 31(5):504–512.
24. Keegan J, Firmin D, Gatehouse P, Longmore D. The application of breath hold phase velocity mapping techniques to the measurement of coronary artery blood flow velocity: Phantom data and initial in vivo results. *Magn Reson Med* 1994; 31(5):526–536.
25. Oshinski JN, Parks WJ, Markou CP, et al. Improved measurement of pressure gradients in aortic coarctation by magnetic resonance imaging. *J Am Coll Cardiol* 1996; 28(7):1818–1826.
26. Bogren HG, Buonocore MH. Complex flow patterns in the great vessels: A review. *Int J Card Imaging* 1999; 15(2):105–113.
27. Davis CP, Liu PF, Hauser M, et al. Coronary flow and coronary flow reserve measurements in humans with breath-held magnetic resonance phase contrast velocity mapping. *Magn Reson Med* 1997; 37(4):537–544.
28. Shellock FG. *Pocket Guide to MR Procedures and Metallic Objects: Update 1999*. Philadelphia: Lippincott Williams & Wilkins; 1999.
29. Strohm O, Kivelitz D, Gross W, et al. Safety of implantable coronary stents during 1h-magnetic resonance imaging at 1.0 and 1.5 T. *J Cardiovasc Magn Reson* 1999; 1(3)239–245.
30. Budinger T, Berson A, McVeigh E, et al. NHLBI working group in cardiovascular magnetic resonance: Magnetic resonance imaging of the cardiovascular system. *J Cardiovasc Magn Reson* 1999; 1(1):53–58.
31. Byrd BF III, Schiller NB, Botvinick EH, Higgins CB. Normal cardiac dimensions by magnetic resonance imaging. *Am J Cardiol* 1985; 55:1440–1442.
32. Byrd BF III, Schiller NB, Botvinick EH, Higgins CB. Normal cardiac dimensions by magnetic resonance imaging. *Am J Cardiol* 1985; 55:1440–1442.
33. Kaul S, Wismer G, Brady TJ, et al. Measurements of normal left heart dimensions using optimally oriented MR images. *AJR* 1986; 146:75–79.
34. Fisher MR, von Schulthess GK, Higgins CB. Multi-phase cardiac magnetic resonance imaging: Normal regional left ventricular wall thickening. *AJR* 1985; 145:27–30.
35. Van Rossum AC, Visser FC, Sprenger M, et al. Evaluation of magnetic resonance imaging for determinations of left ventricular ejection fraction and comparison with angiography. *Am J Cardiol* 1988; 62:628–633.
36. Buser PT, Auffermann W, Holt WW, et al. Noninvasive evaluation of global left ventricular function with use of cine nuclear magnetic resonance. *J Am Coll Cardiol* 1989; 13:1294–1300.
37. Dilworth LR, Aisen AM, Mancini J, et al. Determination of left ventricular volumes and ejection fraction by nuclear magnetic resonance imaging. *Am Heart J* 1987; 113:24–32.
38. Cranney GB, Lotan CS, Dean L, et al. Left ventricular volume measurement using cardiac axis nuclear magnetic resonance imaging: Validation by calibrated ventricular angiography. *Circulation* 1990; 82:154–163.
39. Matsouka H, Hamada M, Honda T, et al. Measurement of cardiac chamber volumes by cine magnetic resonance imaging. *Angiology* 1993; 44(4):321–327.
40. Buser PT, Auffermann W, Holt WW, et al. Noninvasive evaluation of left global left ventricular function with use of cine nuclear magnetic resonance. *J Am Coll Cardiol* 1989; 13:1294–1300.
41. Rehr RB, Malloy CR, Filichuck NG, Peshock RM. Left ventricular volumes measured by MR imaging. *Radiology* 1985; 156:717–719.
42. Semeika RC, Tomei E, Wagner S, et al. Normal left ventricular dimensions and functions: Interstudy reproducibility of measurements of cine MR imaging. *Radiology* 1990; 174:763–768.
43. Van Rossum AC, Visser FC, Sprenger M, et al. Evaluation of magnetic resonance imaging for determinations of left ventricular ejection fraction and comparison with angiography. *Am J Cardiol* 1988; 62:628–633.
44. Ostrzega E, Maddahi J, Honma H, et al. Quantification of left ventricular myocardial mass in humans by nuclear magnetic resonance imaging. *Am Heart J* 1989; 117:444–452.
45. Yamaoka O, Yabe T, Okada M, et al. Evaluation of left ventricular mass: Comparison of ultrafast computed tomography, magnetic resonance imaging, and contrast left ventriculography. *Am Heart J* 1993; 126:1372–1379.
46. Aurigemma G, Davidoff A, Silver K, Boehmer J. Left ventricular mass quantitation using single-phase cardiac magnetic resonance imaging. *Am J Cardiol* 1992; 70:259–262.
47. Keller A, Peshock R, Mally C, et al. In vivo measurements of myocardial mass using MR imaging. *J Am Coll Cardiol* 1986; 8:113–117.
48. Allison JD, Flickinger FW, Wright JC, et al. Measurement of left ventricular mass in hypertrophic cardiomyopathy using MRI:

Comparison with echocardiography. *Magn Reson Imaging* 1993; 11(3):329–334.
49. Bryant DJ, Payne JA, Firmin DN, Longmore DB. Measurement of flow with NMR imaging using gradient pulses and phase difference technique. *J Comput Assist Tomogr* 1984; 8:588–593.
50. Firmin DN, Nayler GL, Klipstein RH, et al. In vivo validation of MR velocity imaging. *J Comput Assist Tomogr* 1987; 11:751–756.
51. Van Rossum A, Sprenger KH, Peels FC. In vivo validation of quantitative flow imaging in arteries and veins using magnetic resonance phase-shift techniques. *Proceedings of the Society of Magnetic Resonance in Medicine*, Amsterdam, 1989:205.
52. Kondo C, Caputo GR, Semelka R, et al. Right and left ventricular slope volume measurements with velocity encoded cine and MR imaging: In vitro and in vivo evaluation. *AJR* 1991; 157:9–16.
53. Hundley WG, Li HF, Hillis LD, et al. Quantitation of cardiac output with velocity-encoded, phase-difference magnetic resonance imaging. *Am J Cardiol* 1995; 75(17):1250–1255.
54. Brenner LD, Caputo GR, Mostbeck G, et al. Quantification of left to right atrial shunts with velocity-encoded cine nuclear magnetic resonance imaging. *J Am Coll Cardiol* 1992; 20:1246–1250.
55. Sugishita J, Koscki S, Matsido M, et al. Dissociation between regional myocardial dysfunction and EKG changes during myocardial ischemia induced by exercise in patients with angina pectoris. *Am Heart J* 1993; 106:1–8.
56. Upton MT, Rerych SK, Newman GE, et al. Detecting abnormalities in left ventricular function during exercise before angina, and ST segment depression. *Circulation* 1980; 62:341–349.
57. Freeman ML, Palac RT, Mason J, et al. A comparison of dobutamine infusion and supine bicycle exercise for radionuclide cardiac stress testing. *Clin Nucl Med* 1984; 9:251–255.
58. Cohen JL, Green TO, Ottenweller J, et al. Dobutamine digital echocardiography for detecting coronary artery disease. *Am J Cardiol* 1991; 67:1311–1318.
59. Marcovitz PA, Armstrong WF. Accuracy of dobutamine stress echocardiogrphy in detecting coronary artery disease. *Am J Cardiol* 1992; 69:1269–1273.
60. Sawada SG, Segar DS, Ryan T, et al. Echocardiography detection of coronary disease during dobutamine infusion. *Circulation* 1991; 83:1605–1614.
61. Mazeika PK, Nadazdin A, Oakley CM. Dobutamine stress echocardiography for detection and assessment of coronary disease. *J Am Coll Cardiol* 1992; 19:1203–1211.
62. Lotan CS, Cranney CB, Bouchard A, et al. The value of cine magnetic resonance imaging for assessing regional ventricular function. *J Am Coll Cardiol* 1989; 14:1721–1729.
63. Marcus JT, Gotte MJ, Van Rossum AC, et al. Myocardial function in infarcted and remote regions early after infarction in man: Assessment by magnetic resonance tagging and strain analysis. *Magn Reson Med* 1997; 38(5):803–810.
64. Van Rugge FP, van der Wall EE, de Roos A, Bruschke AVG. Dobutamine stress magnetic resonance imaging for detection of coronary artery disease. *J Am Coll Cardiol* 1993; 22:431–439.
65. Brown JJ, Higgins CB. Myocardial paramagnetic contrast agents for MR imaging. *AJR* 1988; 151:865–872.
66. Vallee JP, Sostman HD, MacFall JR, et al. MRI quantitative myocardial perfusion with compartmental analysis: A rest and stress study. *Magn Reson Med* 1997; 38(6):981–989.
67. Manning WJ, Atkinson DJ, Grossman W, et al. First-pass nuclear magnetic resonance imaging studies using gadolinium-DTPA in patients with coronary artery disease. *J Am Coll Cardiol* 1991; 18:59–65.
68. Hundley WG, Lange RA, Clarke GD, et al. Assessment of coronary arterial flow and flow reserve in humans with magnetic resonance imaging. *Circulation* 1996; 93(8):1502–1508.
69. Matheijssen NA, Louwerenburg HW, van Rugge FP, et al. Comparison of ultrafast dipyridamole magnetic resonance imaging with dipyridamole sestamibi SPECT for detection of profusion abnormalities in patients with one-vessel coronary artery disease: Assessment by quantitative model fitting. *Magn Reson Med* 1996; 35:221–228.
70. Walsh EG, Doyle M, Lawson MA, et al. Multislice first-pass myocardial perfusion imaging on a conventional clinical scanner. *Magn Reson Med* 1995; 34:39–47.
71. Walsh EG, Doyle M, Lawson MA, Pohost GM. Multislice myocardial perfusion imaging using BRISK (abstr). *Proceedings of the Society of Magnetic Resonance*, Fourth Scientific Meeting, Vancouver, 1996.
72. Kraitchman DL, Young AA, Bloomgarden DC, et al. Integrated MRI assessment of regional function and perfusion in canine myocardial infarction. *Magn Reson Med* 1998; 40(2):311–326.
73. Taylor AM, Panting JR, Keegan J, et al. Use of the intravascular contrast agent nc100150 injection in spin-echo and gradient-echo imaging of the heart. *J Cardiovasc Magn Reson* 1999; 1(1):23–32.
74. Simor T, Chu W-J, Johnson L, et al. In vivo MRI visualization of acute myocardial ischemia and reperfusion in ferrets by the persistent action of contrast agent Gd (BME-DTTA). *Circulation* 1995; 92:3549–3559.
75. Pohost GM. The next horizon in CNR spectroscopy. *J Cardiovasc Magn Reson* 1999; ix-x.
76. Okada M, Mitsunami K, Inubushi T, Kinoshita M. Influence of aging or left ventricular hypertrophy on the human heart: Contents of phosphorus metabolites measured by 31P MRS. *Magn Reson Med* 1998; 39(5):772–782.
77. Pluim BM, Lamb HJ, Kayser HW, et al. Functional and metabolic evaluation of the athlete's heart by magnetic resonance imaging and dobutamine stress magnetic resonance spectroscopy. *Circulation* 1998; 97(7):666–672.
78. Farrall AJ, Thompson RT, Wisenberg G, et al. Myocardial infarction in a canine model monitored by two-dimensional 31P chemical shift spectroscopic imaging. *Magn Reson Med* 1997; 38(4):577–584.
79. Flaherty JT, Weisfeldt ML, Bulkley BH, et al. Mechanisms of ischemic myocardial damage assessed by phosphorous-31 nuclear magnetic resonance. *Circulation* 1982; 65:561–570.
80. Nunnally RL, Bottomley PA. Assessment of pharmacological treatment of myocardial infarction by phosphorous-31 NMR with surface coils. *Science* 1981; 211:177–180.
81. Jacobus WE, Taylor GJ, Hollis DP, Nunnally RL. Phosphorous nuclear magnetic resonance of perfused working rat hearts. *Nature* 1977; 265:756–758.
82. Bottomley PA, Herfkins RJ, Smith LS, et al. Noninvasive detection of monitoring of regional myocardial ischemia in situ using depth-resolved ^{31}P NMR spectroscopy. *Proc Natl Acad Sci USA* 1985; 82:8747–8751.
83. Bottomley PA. Noninvasive study of high-energy phosphate metabolism in human heart by depth-resolved ^{31}P NMR spectroscopy. *Science* 1985; 229:769–772.
84. Weiss RG, Bottomley PA, Hardy CJ, Gerstenblith G. Regional metabolism of high-energy phosphates during isometric exercise in patients with coronary artery disease. *N Engl J Med* 1990; 323:1593–1600.
85. Yabe T, Mitsunami K, Okada M, et al. A detection of myocardial ischemia by ^{31}P magnetic resonance spectroscopy during handgrip exercise. *Circulation* 1994; 89:1709–1716.
86. Higgins CB, Sakuma H. Heart disease: Functional evaluation with MR imaging. *Radiology* 1996; 199:307–315.
87. Sechtem U, Sommerhoff BA, Markiewicz W, et al. Regional left ventricular wall thickening by magnetic resonance imaging: Evaluation in normal persons and persons with global and regional dysfunction. *Am J Cardiol* 1987; 59:145–151.
88. Pflugfelder PW, Sechtem UP, White RD, Higgins CB. Quantification of regional myocardial function by rapid cine MR imaging. *AJR* 1988; 150:523–529.
89. Dubach P, Myers J, Dziekan G, et al. Effect of exercise training on

myocardial remodeling in patients with reduced left ventricular function after myocardial infarction: Application of magnetic resonance imaging. *Circulation* 1997; 95(8):2060–2067.
90. Underwood SR, Rees RSO, Savage PE, et al. Assessment of regional left ventricular function by magnetic resonance. *Br Heart J* 1986; 56:334–340.
91. Hofman MB, de Cock CC, van der Linden JC, et al. Transesophageal cardiac pacing during magnetic resonance imaging: Feasibility and safety considerations. *Magn Reson Med* 1996; 35(3):413–422.
92. Sechtem U, Baer F, Voth E, et al. Assessment of residual viability in patients with myocardial infarction using magnetic resonance imaging. *Int J Cardiac Imaging* 1993; 9:931–940.
93. Baer FM, Smolarz K, Jungehulsing M, et al. Chronic myocardial infarction: Assessment of morphology, function and perfusion by gradient echo magnetic resonance imaging and ^{99m}Tc-methoxyisobutyl-isonitrile SPECT. *Am Heart J* 1992; 123:636–645.
94. Baer FM, Voth E, Schneider CA, et al. Comparison of low-dose dobutamine-gradient-echo magnetic resonance imaging and positron emission tomography with [^{18}F] fluorodeoxyglucose in patients with chronic coronary artery disease. *Circulation* 1995; 91:1006–1015.
95. Lorenz CH, Walker ES, Morgan VL, et al. Normal human right and left ventricular mass, systolic function, and gender differences by cine magnetic resonance imaging. *J Cardiovasc Magn Reson* 1999; 1(1):7–21.
96. Moore CC, McVeogh ER. Noninvasive measurement of three-dimensional myocardial deformation with tagged magnetic resonance imaging during graded local ischemia. *Cardiovasc Magn Reson* 1999; 1(3):207–222.
97. Walsh EG, Doyle M, Kortright E, et al. Recent progress in radio-frequency-tagged left ventricular function studies. *Cardiovasc Magn Reson* 1999; 1(2):185–193.
98. Fisher MR, McNamara MT, Higgins CB. Acute myocardial infarction: MR evaluation in 29 patients. *AJR* 1987; 148:247–251.
99. Johnston DL, Thompson RC, Liu P, et al. Magnetic resonance imaging during acute myocardial infarction. *Am J Cardiol* 1986; 57:1059–1065.
100. Tian G, Shen JF, Dai G, et al. An interleaved T1-T2* imaging sequence for assessing myocardial injury. *J Cardiovasc Magn Reson* 1999; 1(2):145–151.
101. Ahmad M, Johnson RF, Fawcett HD, Schreiber MH. Magnetic resonance imaging in patients with unstable angina: Comparison with acute myocardial infarction and normals. *Magn Reson Imaging* 1988; 6:527–534.
102. Krauss XH, van der Wall EE, Doornbos J, et al. The value of nuclear magnetic resonance imaging in patients with a recent myocardial infarction: Comparison with planar thallium-201 scintigraphy. *Cardiovasc Intervent Radiol* 1989; 12:119–124.
103. Krauss XH, van der Wall EE, van der Laarse A, et al. Magnetic resonance imaging of myocardial infarction: Correlation with enzymatic angiographic and radionuclide findings. *Am Heart J* 1991; 122:1274–1283.
104. Johns JA, Leavitt MB, Newell JB, et al. Quantitation of acute myocardial infarction size by nuclear magnetic resonance imaging. *J Am Coll Cardiol* 1990; 15:143–149.
105. Turnbull LW, Ridgeway JP, Nicoll JJ, et al. Estimating the size of myocardial infarction by magnetic resonance imaging. *Br Heart J* 1991; 66:359–363.
106. White RD, Holt WW, Cheitlin MD, et al. Estimation of the functional and anatomic extent of myocardial infarction using magnetic resonance imaging. *Am Heart J* 1988; 115:740–748.
107. Ramani K. Judd RM, Holly TA, et al. Contrast magnetic resonance imaging in the assessment of myocardial viability in patients with stable coronary artery disease and left ventricular dysfunction. *Circulation* 1998; 98(24):2687–2694.
108. Rogers WJ Jr, Kramer CM, Geskin G, et al. Early contrast-enhanced MRI predicts late functional recovery after reperfused myocardial infarction. *Circulation* 1999; 99(6):744–750.
109. Kim RJ, Chen EL, Lima JA, Judd RM. Myocardial Gd-DTPA kinetics determine MRI contrast enhancement and reflect the extent and severity of myocardial injury after acute reperfused infarction. *Circulation* 1996; 94(12):3318–3326.
110. Canby RC, Reeves RC, Evanochko WT, et al. Proton nuclear magnetic resonance relaxation times in severe myocardial ischemia. *J Am Coll Cardiol* 1987; 10:412–420.
111. Scholz TD, Martins JB, Skortin DJ. NMR relaxation times and acute myocardial ischemia: Relative influence of tissue water and fat content. *Magn Reson Med* 1992; 23:89–95.
112. Higgins CB, Herfkins R, Lipton MJ, et al. Nuclear magnetic resonance imaging of acute myocardial infarction in dogs: Alterations in magnetic relaxation times. *Am J Cardiol* 1983; 52:184–188.
113. Williams ES, Kaplan JI, Thatcher F, et al. Prolongation of proton spin lattice times in regionally ischemic tissue from dog hearts. *J Nucl Med* 1980; 21:449–453.
114. Pflugfelder PW, Wisenberg G, Prato FS, Carrol SE. Serial imaging of canine myocardial infarction by in vivo nuclear magnetic resonance. *J Am Coll Cardiol* 1986; 7:843–849.
115. Lotan CS, Miller SK, Bouchard A, et al. Detection of intramyocardial hemorrhage using high-field proton nuclear magnetic resonance imaging. *Cathet Cardiovasc Diagn* 1990; 20:205–211.
116. Schiebler N, Axel L, Reichek N, et al. Correlation of cine MR imaging with two-dimensional pulse Doppler echocardiography in valvular insufficiency. *J Comput Assist Tomogr* 1987; 11: 627–632.
117. Utz JA, Herfkens RJ, Heinsimer JA, et al. Valvular regurgitation: Dynamic MR imaging. *Radiology* 1988; 168:91–94.
118. Pflugfelder PW, Landzberg JS, Cassidy MN, et al. Comparison of cine MR imaging with Doppler echocardiography for the evaluation of aortic regurgitation. *AJR* 1989; 152:729–735.
119. Underwood SR, Klepstein RH, Firmin DN, et al. Magnetic resonance assessment of aortic and mitral regurgitation. *Br Heart J* 1986; 56:455–462.
120. Bryant DJ, Payne JA, Firman DN, Longmore DB. Measurement of flow with NMR imaging using a gradient pulse and phase difference technique. *J Comput Assist Tomogr* 1984; 8:588.
121. Podolak MJ, Hedlund LW, Evans AJ, Herfkens RJ. Evaluation of flow through simulated vascular stenosis with gradient echo magnetic resonance imaging. *Invest Radiol* 1989; 24:184.
122. Recusani F, Bargiggia G, Yaganathan AP, et al. Color flow quantitation of regurgitant flow using flow convergence proximal to the orifice of the regurgitant jet. *Circulation* 1991; 83:594–604.
123. Shandas R, Golebiovski P, Elkadi T, et al. Influence of complex "valve" surface geometry on flow convergence methods for calculating flow rate by color Doppler (abstr). *Circulation* 1990; 82(suppl III):III-63.
124. Hundley WG, Li HF, Willard JE, et al. Magnetic resonance imaging assessment of the severity of mitral regurgitation: Comparison with invasive techniques. *Circulation* 1995; 92:1151–1158.
125. Fugita N, Chazauilleres AF, Hartiala JJ, et al. Quantification of mitral regurgitation by phase-encoded cine nuclear magnetic resonance imaging. *J Am Coll Cardiol* 1994; 23:951–958.
126. Sechtem U, Pflugfelder PW, Cassidy MM, et al. Mitral and aortic regurgitation: Quantification of regurgitant volumes with cine MR imaging. *Radiology* 1988; 167:425–430.
127. De Roos A, Reichek N, Axel L, Kressel HY. Cine MR imaging in aortic stenosis. *J Comput Assist Tomogr* 1989; 13:421–425.
128. Kilner JP, Manzara KG, Mohaiddin RH, et al. Magnetic resonance jet velocity mapping in mitral and aortic stenosis. *Circulation* 1993; 87:1279–1298.
129. Stark DD, Higgins CB, Lanzer P, et al. Magnetic resonance imaging of the pericardium: Normal and pathologic findings. *Radiology* 1984; 151:469–474.

130. White CS. MR evaluation of the pericardium. *Top Magn Reson Imaging* 1995; 7(4):258–266.
131. Sechtem U, Tscholakoff D, Higgins CB. MRI of the normal pericardium. *AJR* 1986; 147:239.
132. VonSchulthess GK, Higgins CB. Blood flow imaging with MR: Spin phase phenomena. *Radiology* 1985; 157:687.
133. Mulvagh SL, Rokey R, Vick GW, Johnston DL. Usefulness of nuclear magnetic resonance imaging for evaluation of pericardial effusions, in comparison with two-dimensional echocardiography. *J Am Coll Cardiol* 1989; 64:1002–1009.
134. Sechtem U, Tscholakoff D, Higgins CB. MRI of the abnormal pericardium. *AJR* 1986; 147:245.
135. Soulen RL, Stark DD, Higgins CB. Magnetic resonance imaging of constrictive pericardial disease. *Am J Cardiol* 1995; 55:480–484.
136. Klues HG, Schiffers A, Maron BJ. Phenotypic spectrum and patterns of left ventricular hypertrophy and hypertrophic cardiomyopathy: Morphologic observations and significance as assessed by 2-dimensional echocardiography in 600 patients. *J Am Coll Cardiol* 1995; 26:1699–1708.
137. Thompson RC, Lavine RA, Mille S, Dinsmore RE. Magnetic resonance imaging along the left ventricular axis in hypertrophic heart disease: Accurate characterization of cardiac hypertrophy. *Circulation* 1985; 72(suppl III):122.
138. Higgins CB, Byrd BF III, Stark D, et al. Magnetic resonance imaging in hypertrophic cardiomyopathy. *Am J Cardiol* 1985; 55:1121–1126.
139. Higgins CB, Byrd BF III, Stark D, et al. Magnetic resonance imaging in hypertrophic cardiomyopathy. *Am J Cardiol* 1985; 55:1121–1126.
140. Webb JG, Sasson Z, Rakowski H, et al. Apical hypertrophic cardiomyopathy: Clinical follow-up and diagnostic correlates. *J Am Coll Cardiol* 1990; 15:83–90.
141. Suzuki J, Watanabe F, Takenaka K, et al. New subtype of apical hypertrophic cardiomyopathy identified with nuclear magnetic resonance imaging as an underlying cause of markedly inverted T waves. *J Am Coll Cardiol* 1993; 22:1175–1181.
142. Guado C, Pelliccia FTA, Nzilli G, et al. Magnetic resonance imaging for assessment of apical hypertrophy in hypertrophic cardiomyopathy. *Clin Cardiol* 1992; 15:164–168.
143. Sechtem U, Higgins CB, Summerhoff BA, et al. Magnetic resonance imaging of restrictive cardiomyopathy. *Am J Cardiol* 1987; 59:480–482.
144. Blake LM, Scheinman MM, Higgins CB. MR features of arrhythmogenic right ventricular dysplasia. *AJR* 1994; 162:809–812.
145. Ricci C, Longo R, Pagnan L, et al. Magnetic resonance imaging in right ventricular dysplasia. *Am J Cardiol* 1992; 70:1589–1595.
146. Higgins CB, Byrd BF, Farmer D, et al. Magnetic resonance imaging in patients with congenital heart disease. *Circulation* 1984; 70(5):851–860.
147. Didier D, Higgins CB, Fisher MR, et al. Congenital heart disease: Gated MR imaging in 72 patients. *Radiology* 1986; 158:227.
148. Kersting-Summerhoff BA, Sechtem UP, Fisher MR, Higgins CB. MR of congenital anomalies of the aortic arch. *AJR* 1987; 149:9.
149. Fletcher BD, Jacobstein MD, Nelson AD, et al. Gated magnetic resonance imaging of congenital cardiac malformations. *Radiology* 1984; 150:137–140.
150. Be'eri E, Maier SE, Landzberg MJ, et al. In vivo evaluation of Fontan pathway flow dynamics by multidimensional phase-velocity magnetic resonance imaging. *Circulation* 1998; 98(25):2873–2882.
151. vonSchulthess G, Higashino SM, Higgins SS, et al. Coarctation of the aorta: MR imaging. *Radiology* 1986; 158:469–474.
152. Amparo EG, Higgins CB, Shafton EP. Demonstration of coarctation of the aorta by magnetic resonance imaging. *AJR* 1984; 143:1192–1194.
153. Gomes AS, Lois JF, George B, et al. Congenital abnormalities of the aortic arch: MR imaging. *Radiology* 1987; 165:691–695.
154. Nyman R, Hallberg M, Sunnegardh J, et al. Magnetic resonance imaging and angiography in the assessment of coarctation of the aorta. *Acta Radiol* 1989; 30:481–485.
155. Rees S, Firmin D, Mohiaddin R, et al. Application of flow measurements and magnetic resonance velocity mapping to congenital heart disease. *Am J Cardiol* 1989; 64:953–956.
156. Brenner LD, Caputo GR, Mostbeck G, et al. Quantitation of left to right atrial shunts with velocity-encoded cine nuclear magnetic imaging. *J Am Coll Cardiol* 1992; 20:1246–1250.
157. Holmvang G, Palacios I, Vlahakes G, et al. Imaging and sizing of atrial septal defects by magnetic resonance. *Circulation* 1995; 92:3473–3480.
158. Go R, O'Donnell JK, Underwood DA, et al. Comparison of gated cardiac MRI and 2D echocardiography of intracardiac neoplasm. *AJR* 1985; 145:21–25.
159. Freedberg RS, Krozon I, Runnancik WN, Liebeskind D. The contribution of magnetic resonance imaging to the evaluation of intracardiac tumors, diagnosed by echocardiography. *Circulation* 1988; 77:96–103.
160. Lund JT, Ehman RL, Julsrud PR, et al. Cardiac masses: Assessment by MR imaging. *AJR* 1989; 152:469–473.
161. Casolo F, Biasi S, Balzarii L, et al. MRI as an adjunct to echocardiography for the diagnostic imaging of cardiac masses. *Eur J Radiol* 1988; 88:226–230.
162. Winkler M, Higgins CB. Suspected intracardiac masses: Evaluation with MR imaging. *Radiology* 1987; 165:117–122.
163. Dooms GC, Higgins CB. MR imaging of cardiac thrombi. *J Comput Assist Tomogr* 1986; 10:415–420.

C H A P T E R 18B

MAGNETIC RESONANCE IMAGING OF THE VASCULAR SYSTEM

Zahi A. Fayad / Stephen G. Worthley / Gerard Helft / Thomas K. F. Foo / Valentin Fuster

INTRODUCTION

Over the last decade, there has been substantial growth in the role of cardiovascular magnetic resonance (CMR) imaging in evaluating cardiovascular structure and function in both clinical practice and research. CMR is an excellent diagnostic tool because of its noninvasive nature, lack of ionizing radiation, high spatial resolution, tomographic acquisition in any plane, and unique tissue contrast. This chapter reviews technical considerations in CMR, describes the established clinical CMR applications, and describes novel and promising approaches for the diagnosis of cardiovascular disease.

CMR relies on the same principles as do other MR techniques.[1-4] Since hydrogen (^1H) is the simplest and most abundant element in the human body, most MR studies are of hydrogen nuclei (protons) in water. During the examination, the patient is subjected to a strong local magnetic field, usually 1.5 tesla, that aligns the protons in the patient's body. These protons or spins are excited by a radiofrequency (RF) pulse and subsequently are detected with receiver coils. The detected signals are influenced by relaxation times (T1 and T2), proton density, motion and flow, molecular diffusion, magnetization transfer, changes in susceptibility, and so forth. Three additional magnetic fields (gradient fields) are applied during MR imaging: one to select the slice and two to encode spatial information. The timing of the excitation pulses and the successive magnetic field gradients determine the image contrast.

TECHNICAL CONSIDERATIONS

Introduction

In MR imaging, an image is encoded into its constituent spatial frequency components. To generate an image of a specific spatial resolution and image field of view (FOV), data for a minimal set of spatial frequencies, or k-space lines, must be sampled so that the object's spatial frequency distribution can be determined. With a single k-space line sampled after a single RF excitation pulse, the number of k-space lines in an image directly determines the total image acquisition time.

In CMR, cardiac motion and respiratory motion present unique challenges in obtaining images of the heart at specific time points in the cardiac cycle. To freeze the motion of the heart, image acquisition time must be shorter than 50 to 100 ms. Longer data acquisition periods lead to increased cardiac motion artifacts. If all the data (k-space data) needed to reconstruct an image cannot be acquired with a single R-R interval, data acquisition must be partitioned across several cardiac cycles, with each data segment being acquired at the same cardiac phase. This synchronization of data acquisition to the cardiac cycle [electrocardiogram (ECG)-gating] ensures that the heart is in the same spatial position or cardiac state for each data acquisition (k-space phase encoding) segment.

Similar to cardiac gating, acquisitions can be triggered by the respiratory cycle, hence the use of a device (e.g., respiratory bellows or belt) or method (e.g., navigator echoes[5]) that indicates expiration and inspiration. Therefore, data acquisition is performed only during a certain phase of the respiratory cycle. Cardiac and respiratory gating may be combined, but image acquisition is therefore increased.

Cardiac MR images can depict the anatomy of the vasculature at a single phase of the cardiac cycle and at multiple spatial locations (multislice imaging) or can be acquired at the same spatial location but at different temporal cardiac phases (multiphase imaging or cine). The multislice techniques can generate projectional angiograms similar to those of conventional x-ray angiography and provide structural anatomic information. Images acquired at multiple phases of the cardiac cycle then can be played back in a movie loop to provide a dynamic representation of the flowing blood[6] (see also Chap. 18A).

Black Blood Imaging Techniques

CONVENTIONAL ECG-GATED SPIN ECHO

The conventional single-phase, multiple-slice ECG-gated spin echo (SE) is the most common imaging sequence traditionally used for CMR. The SE technique generates images in which

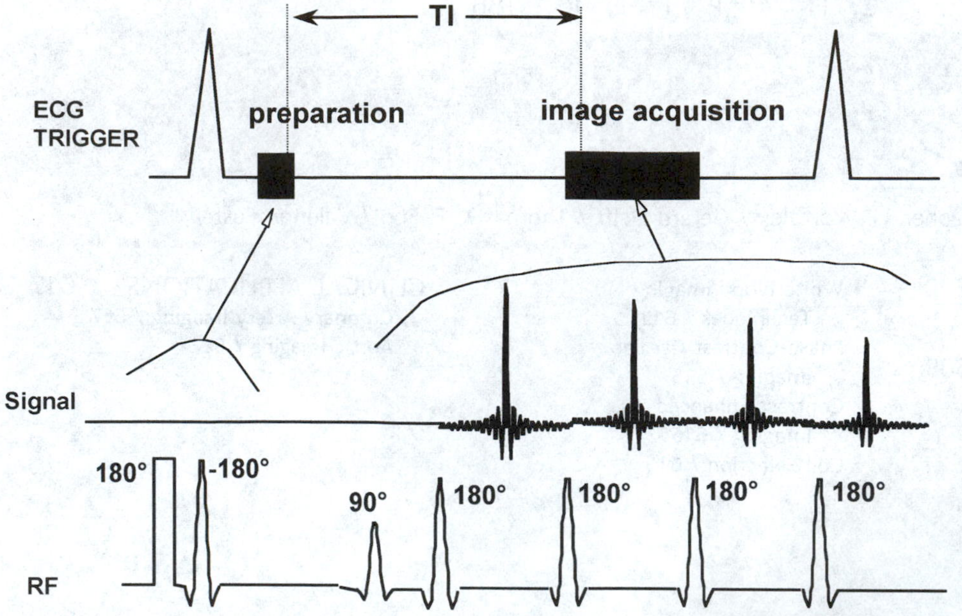

FIGURE 18B-1 Pulse sequence timing diagram of the double-inversion recovery fast spin-echo sequence. The double-inversion recovery preparatory pulses are used to null signal from blood. Also, the inversion time (TI) is calculated to null signal from blood.

the blood signal appears dark ("black blood" images) because of the requirement that any spins excited by the initial 90° RF pulse dephase and are rephased by the subsequent 180° RF pulse. Flowing spins (such as blood) transiting through the imaged slice are affected by one but not both of the RF pulses. Hence, the spins flowing through the slice will not refocus and return a signal; i.e., the signal appears dark in the image. However, slow-flowing blood will not appear dark in SE images as it may remain within the imaged slice and thus see both the 90° and 180° RF pulses. Saturation RF pulses usually are placed above and below the image planes to ensure that the blood signal is dark.

Long scan times make gated SE images extremely sensitive to respiratory motion and dependent on consistent ECG gating. To minimize the image artifacts from respiratory motion, respiratory view ordering (respiratory compensation) often is used.[7] However, this further extends the total scan time (10 to 20 min) and is sometimes ineffective.

ECG-GATED FAST SPIN ECHO

Conventional SE, with its acquisition of a single line of k-space data per slice excitation, is susceptible to respiratory artifacts, but this can be overcome by using techniques that provide shorter imaging times. When multiple k-space lines are encoded after a single 90° RF excitation pulse with a train of refocusing 180° RF pulses, the fast spin-echo (FSE), or turbo spin echo, sequence provides shorter imaging with reduced respiratory motion artifacts. The number of echoes acquired after the 90° excitation is called *echo train length* (ETL), or turbo factor. With an ETL of 8, the scan time for a T2-weighted sequence [repetition time (TR) = 2 R-R] is reduced to 32 heartbeats for a 128-phase-encoding image.

To ensure that signal from blood is suppressed adequately, a double-inversion recovery magnetization preparation pulse ("velocity-selective" inversion) is used.[8] As shown in Fig. 18B-1, a nonselective inversion pulse inverts all spins in the body. This is followed quickly by a slice-selective inversion pulse that restores the magnetization within the imaged slice. An inversion time (TI = ~600 ms) is selected to null signal from blood when the 90° RF excitation pulse is applied. To minimize image-blurring artifacts from T2 decay in a long echo train, the acquisition is segmented over to several heartbeats and the spacing between echoes [echo spacing (ESP)] is minimized. With an ETL of 32, a gated T2-weighted FSE image can be acquired in 16 heartbeats for 256 k-space lines. This allows fast data acquisition during suspended respiration and provides artifact-free images of the cardiovascular anatomy (Fig. 18B-2). One of the disadvantages of the current double-inversion recovery FSE sequence is that images are acquired a single slice at a time to avoid affecting the effectiveness of the inversion pulses used to null signal from blood.

A recent extension of the FSE sequence is the single- or segmented-shot (half Fourier turbo spin-echo (HASTE) tech-

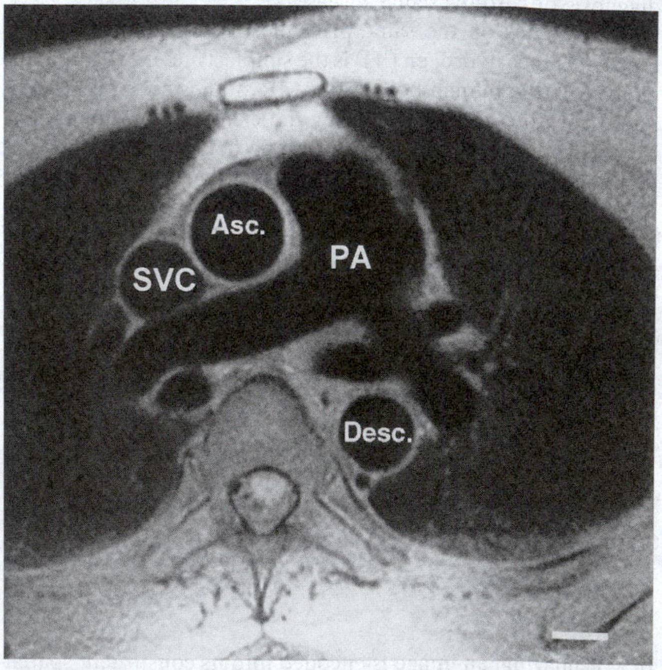

FIGURE 18B-2 Double-inversion recovery, fast spin-echo, proton-density-weighted magnetic resonance image from a normal subject. The signal from blood is suppressed, and therefore, the lumen is dark. The aortic wall of the ascending (Asc.) and descending (Desc.) aorta is clearly seen. PA = pulmonary artery; SVC = superior vena cava.

nique.[9,10] Image acquisition can be acquired in as a short a time as a single heartbeat.

White Blood Imaging Techniques

INTRODUCTION

So-called white blood imaging techniques refer primarily to gradient-recalled echo pulse sequences, which provide images that are T1-weighted. These techniques are characterized by short sequence TRs, flip angles less than 90°, and substantially greater signal intensity of the ventricular blood pool compared with that of the myocardium. The latter effect is due to the in-flow refreshment phenomenon, in which fresh unsaturated blood continues to course through the imaged slice and experience fewer RF pulses than does stationary tissue that remains in the imaged slice throughout the data acquisition period. Bright blood techniques can be subcategorized into time-of-flight (TOF) and phase-contrast techniques.

TIME OF FLIGHT

Conventional Gradient Echo (Cine) Short TR-gated gradient echo-pulse sequence are used to generate cine images at multiple time frames in the cardiac cycle. Conventional cine pulse sequences run asynchronously to the cardiac cycle, with the spatial frequency (phase)-encoding value updated on detection of the R-wave trigger. Each RF excitation pulse is applied at the same spatial location and is repeated at intervals of TR in the cardiac cycle. Since the sequence runs asynchronously, the RF excitation pulses may occur at varying time delays from the R wave from one cardiac cycle to the next. On detection of the next cardiac R wave, the k-space encoding value is updated and the acquired temporal data from the previous R-R interval are resorted and interpolated into evenly distributed time frames within each cardiac cycle. This method of gating also is known as retrospective gating because data from the current R-R interval are resorted only after the next R-wave trigger is detected.

As was noted earlier, conventional gradient-echo cine pulse sequences acquire only one k-space encoding view per heartbeat. The total image acquisition time is then of the order of 128 heartbeats. As this time is beyond the ability of patients to maintain an effective breath hold, conventional cine scans are subject to respiratory motion artifacts and require some form of respiratory gating or an intelligent k-space acquisition view reordering to maintain an artifact-free image. These measures, however, are only marginally effective and cannot substitute for a breath-held acquisition.

Segmented K-Space Techniques Faster CMR techniques have been able to dramatically reduce the image acquisition time to as little as 10 to 15 heartbeats, making breath holding a feasible option to reduce respiratory motion artifacts. Faster scan times have been achieved by segmenting k-space and acquiring multiple k-space lines per R-R interval.[11] The scan time is speeded up by a factor equal to that of the number of k-space lines acquired per image per R-R interval. In this manner, a typical cine acquisition with a matrix size of 128 pixels in the phase-encoding direction can be completed in as little as 16 heartbeats, with eight k-space lines per segment (or views per segment). K-space is divided into several segments, with each k-space line in a segment acquired in a single R-R interval.

Because of the need to acquire data rapidly for several k-space lines to minimize motion-blurring artifacts, segmented k-space techniques are used almost exclusively with fast gradient-echo pulse sequences that have very short TR. Fast gradient-recalled echo acquisition also can be RF-phase spoiled to achieve better tissue–blood pool contrast. However, shorter TRs require smaller flip angles, and as a consequence, image signal-to-noise ratio is lower than that in conventional gradient-echo cine acquisitions.

Multiple phases of the cardiac cycle can be visualized by means of repeated acquisition of the same k-space segment within an R-R interval but assigning the data acquired at different time points in the cardiac cycle to different temporal phases.

In segmented k-space scans, the total scan time is inversely proportional to the number of views per segment (vps). The larger the number of views acquired per segment, the shorter the scan time. However, the reduction in scan time is obtained at the expense of reducing the image's temporal resolution. Significant motion of the heart during data segment acquisition time will result in a loss of spatial resolution from cardiac motion–related blurring. Minimizing artifacts from cardiac motion by decreasing the number of views per segment, conversely, would lead to an increase in the total scan time, reducing the ability to breath hold and reintroducing respiratory-related motion artifacts.

Fortunately, the minimum temporal resolution needed to sample cardiac motion, especially during systole, is about 40 ms. With fast gradient-echo pulse sequences, TR can be reduced to about 5 to 8 ms, permitting the collection of at least 5 to 8 k-space lines per segment. Similar to conventional cine acquisition, a higher effective temporal resolution can be obtained by means a simple interpolation or nearest neighbor view-sharing process.[12]

Each temporal phase image represents the cardiac motion at specific delays from the cardiac R-wave trigger, averaged over the acquisition time per segment. In Fig. 18B-3, it is clear that intermediate cardiac phases can be synthesized or interpolated by sharing k-space views between adjacent time segments to generate images averaged over different time points. The true image temporal resolution is unchanged, but the effective temporal resolution is doubled. View sharing thus can increase the number of phases reconstructed without affecting the manner in which the k-space data are acquired (Fig. 18B-3).

In addition to the acquisition of images at the same spatial location at different time points in the cardiac cycle (cine), a single-phase multislice acquisition can be performed. A segmented k-space gradient-echo multiplanar acquisition would then acquire images at different spatial locations, each at a different phase of the cardiac cycle. Although the image quality is somewhat limited, a wide range of pathologies can be detected on these images. Major structures such as the aorta, main pulmonary arteries, liver, spleen, and spine are viewed. Another application of this technique is the imaging of uncooperative and sedated patients for whom breath holding is not possible.

Fast Hybrid Imaging Very fast imaging techniques such as echo-planar imaging (EPI) and spiral imaging (see below) can achieve short scan times by acquiring a larger portion of k-space in each TR compared with conventional imaging. As will

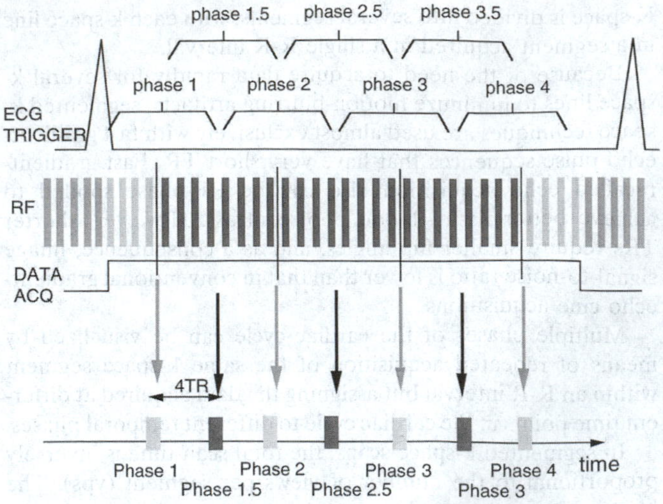

FIGURE 18B-3 Segmented k-space acquisition and view sharing. View sharing increases the effective temporal resolution by reconstructing images at different time points in the cardiac cycle, similar to the linear interpolation scheme applied to conventional cine scans. The true temporal resolution remains unchanged even though the effective (reconstructed) temporal resolution is doubled.

be discussed in this section, these techniques are prone to image artifacts. When multishot hybrid EPI and interleaved spiral techniques with relatively short echo train length and short echo spacing and sampling times are used, image artifacts are reduced while significant fast scan times are achieved compared with conventional imaging techniques. New gradient and receiver MR subsystems have substantially improved the performance of EPI and spiral imaging. Several CMR applications, such as real-time interactive scanning, coronary imaging, first-pass myocardial perfusion, and fast functional cardiac imaging, are now possible with these techniques.

Conventional, Interleaved, and Hybrid EPI In fast segmented k-space cardiac acquisitions, only one k-space line or view is acquired per RF excitation pulse. EPI is an acquisition technique that collects all lines (single-shot imaging) or several k-space lines (multishot imaging) per RF excitation.[13] As is shown in Fig. 18B-4, this is accomplished by effecting rapid gradient reversals of the readout gradient, generating a series of gradient echoes with each readout echo acquiring data for a single k-space line or view.[14] The number of gradient echoes after a single RF pulse is known as an ETL. As segmented k-space acquisitions reduced the scan time corresponding to a factor equal to the number of k-space lines acquired per R-R interval, interleaved EPI scans further reduce the scan time by a factor equal to ETL. The most significant benefit from using interleaved EPI sequences is that breath-holding times can be further reduced from 16s to 4s with comparable image spatial resolution.

Unlike conventional EPI scans, not all the k-space lines necessary to reconstruct an image are acquired after a single RF excitation pulse. The data acquisition is interleaved between several RF excitation pulses, with between four and eight echoes acquired per RF excitation pulse.[15] The result is a hybrid EPI sequence that is inherently more efficient than conventional segmented k-space fast-gradient echo because multiple phase-

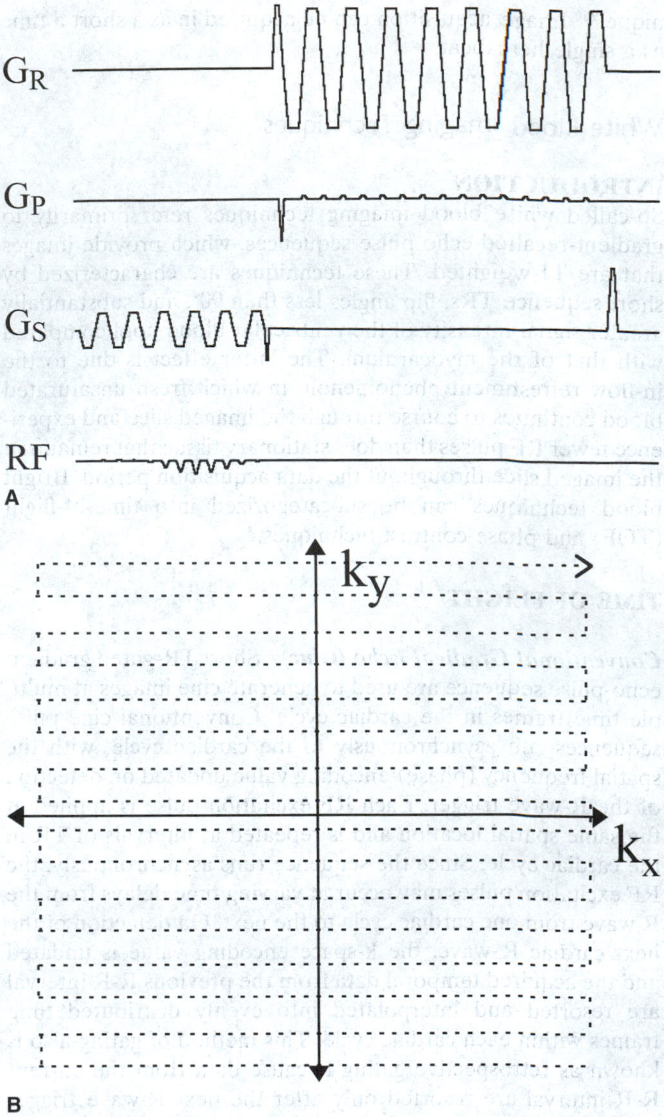

FIGURE 18B-4 *A.* Pulse sequence timing diagram for multishot echo-planar imaging. Note the spectral-spatial RF pulse used for fat suppression. *B.* K-space trajectory traversed by one repetition of the pulse sequence shown in (*A*).

encode lines are acquired in each TR. The smaller number of ETLs in a cardiac interleaved EPI acquisition significantly improves image quality, as there is less image blurring from changes in signal intensity across the multiple gradient echoes from T2* relaxation.

Different versions of EPI have been proposed for CMR applications. Single-shot EPI and dual-shot EPI have been used to multislice first-pass myocardial perfusion imaging.[14,16] Similarly, single-shot and multishot EPI and hybrid EPI have been used for faster functional cardiac imaging (multislice and phase imaging)[15,17] and for fast flow quantification.[18] Finally, three-dimensional (3D) multishot EPI also has been used for coronary imaging.[19]

Spiral Imaging A different approach to cardiac imaging involves the use of spiral rather than rectilinear sampling of k-space.[20] In spiral imaging, the k-space trajectory usually starts at the center of k-space for each RF excitation pulse and pro-

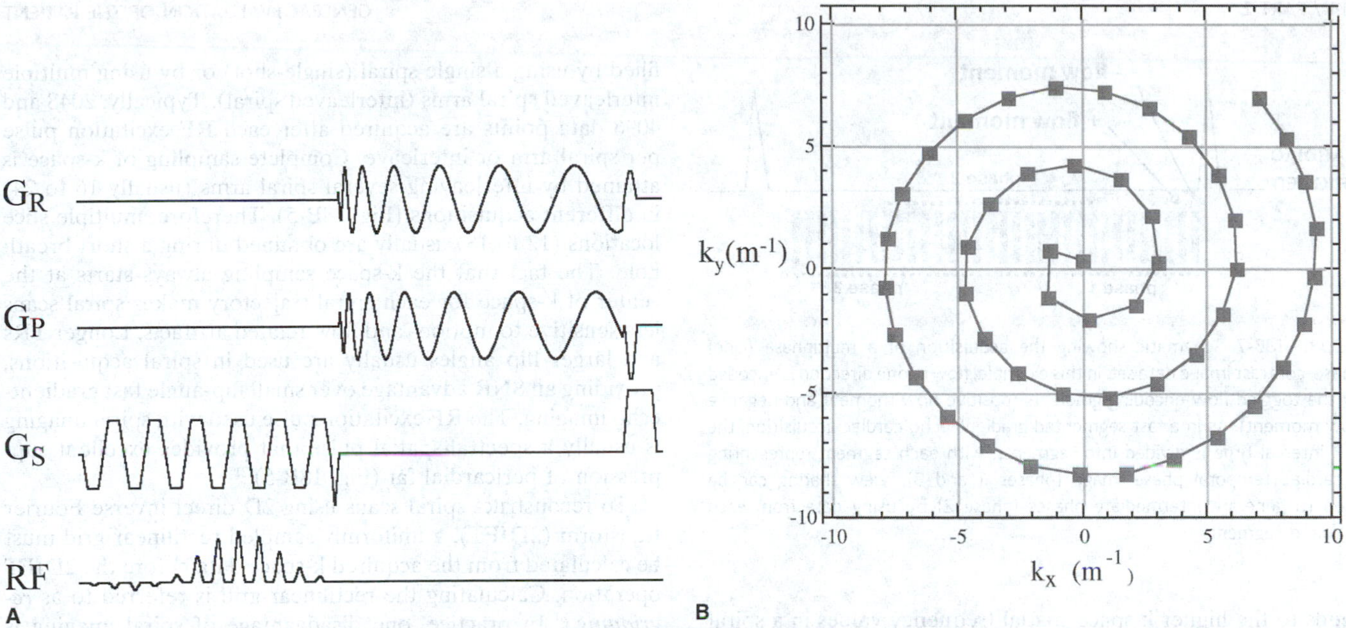

FIGURE 18B-5 *A*. Pulse sequence timing diagram for an interleaved spiral scan. Note the spectral-spatial RF pulse used for fat saturation. *B*. K-space trajectory traversed by one repetition of the pulse sequence shown in (*A*).

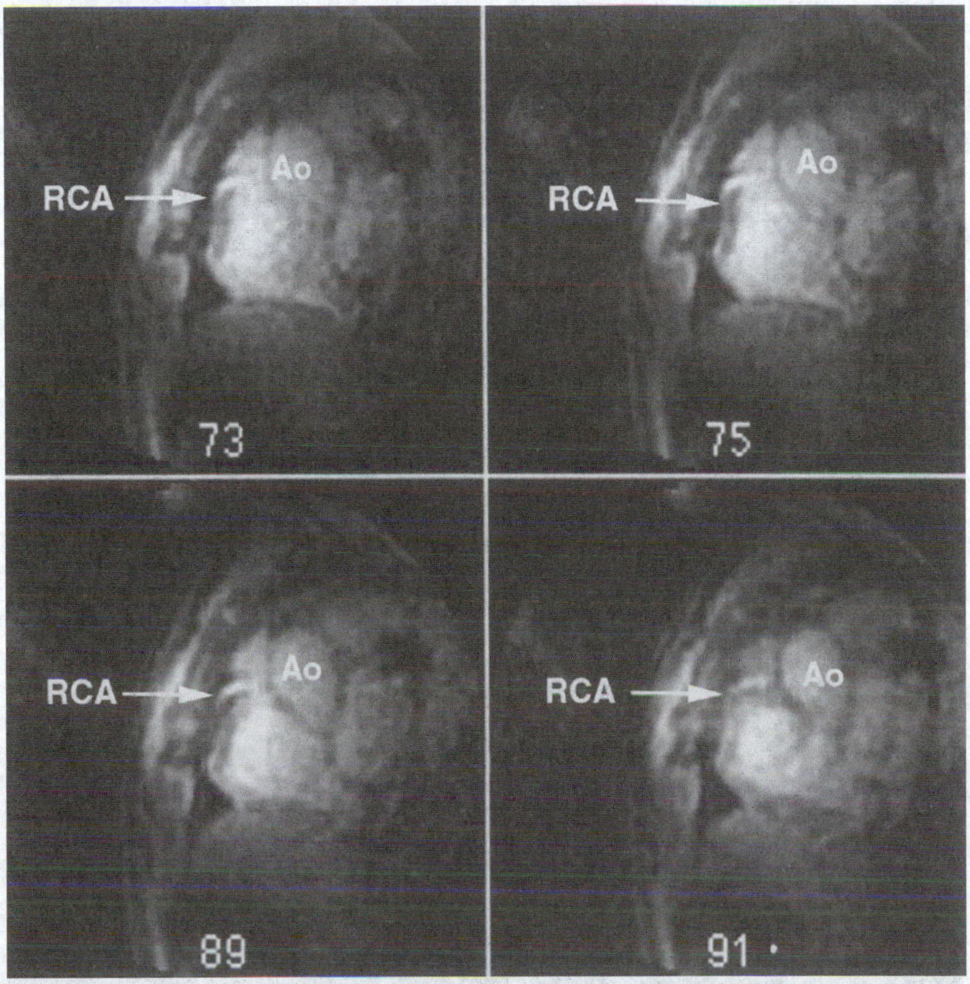

FIGURE 18B-6 A long segment of the right coronary artery (RCA) (indicated by the arrowhead) on several frames during the cardiac cycle. The free breathing images were obtained using the real-time imaging spiral sequence and acquired at a rate of 12 images per second. No cardiac gating was used. The spatial resolution is ~2mm. Ao = aorta.

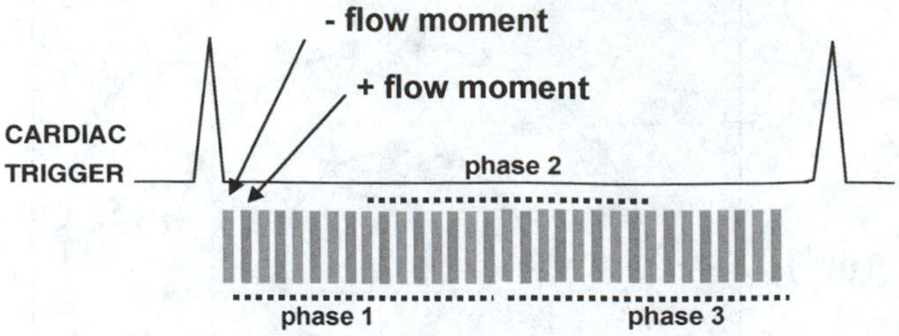

FIGURE 18B-7 Schematic showing the acquisition of a multiphase (cine) phase-contrast image data set. In this example, flow in one direction is encoded by the toggled flow-encoding gradients (positive flow moment and negative flow moment). As in a fast segmented gradient-echo cardiac acquisition, the R-R interval time is divided into segments, with each segment representing a cardiac temporal phase image (phases 1 and 3). View sharing can be used to generate intermediate phases (phase 2) by using data from each acquired segment.

ceeds to the higher k-space spatial frequency values in a spiral fashion. This imaging technique has the advantage of acquiring a greater number of data points than are acquired in a conventional rectilinear two-dimensional (2D) Fourier transform acquisition per RF excitation. A complete k-space matrix can be filled by using a single spiral (single-shot) or by using multiple interleaved spiral arms (interleaved spiral). Typically, 2048 and 4096 data points are acquired after each RF excitation pulse per spiral arm or interleave. Complete sampling of k-space is attained by interleaving several spiral arms (usually 16 to 24) in different acquisitions (Fig. 18B-5). Therefore, multiple slice locations (12 to 18) usually are obtained during a short breath hold. The fact that the k-space sampling always starts at the center of k-space for each spiral trajectory makes spiral scans less sensitive to motion- and flow-related artifacts. Longer TRs and larger flip angles usually are used in spiral acquisitions, providing an SNR advantage over small flip-angle fast gradient-echo imaging. The RF excitation pulse used with spiral imaging is usually a spectral-spatial pulse that provides excellent suppression of pericardial fat (Fig. 18B-5).[21]

To reconstruct spiral scans using 2D direct inverse Fourier transform (2DIFT), a uniformly sampled rectilinear grid must be calculated from the acquired k-space data before the 2DIFT operation. Calculating the rectilinear grid is referred to as *regridding*.[20] In practice, one disadvantage of spiral imaging is that the regridding process increases the time required for image reconstruction.

The primary and distinctive image artifact for spiral imaging is spatially localized blurring caused by off-resonance effects (e.g., the chemical shift of fat and magnetic field inhomogeneities). These artifacts are minimized by using the spectral-spatial RF excitation pulse, short sampling times, and deblurring postprocessing methods.[22] The sampling time can be kept short by increasing the number of interleaves and using a high sampling bandwidth (64 to 125 kHz).

Studies have shown that spiral imaging can provide excellent high-resolution depiction of the coronary arteries[20] (see the section on coronary artery imaging, below) and cardiac cine imaging.[23]

Real-Time Imaging The short scan times afforded by spiral trajectories and EPI imaging have enabled fast real-time imaging of cardiac motion. The images are acquired with no ECG gating and during free breathing at a frame rate of about 12 to 24 images per second at an in-plane resolution of ~2 mm.[24,25] The combination of higher-performance gradient subsystems and fast compute engines permits fast data acquisition and image reconstruction with minimal lag time.

This real-time imaging capability allows the user to change and localize scan planes of the heart and coronary arteries rapidly (Fig. 18B-6).

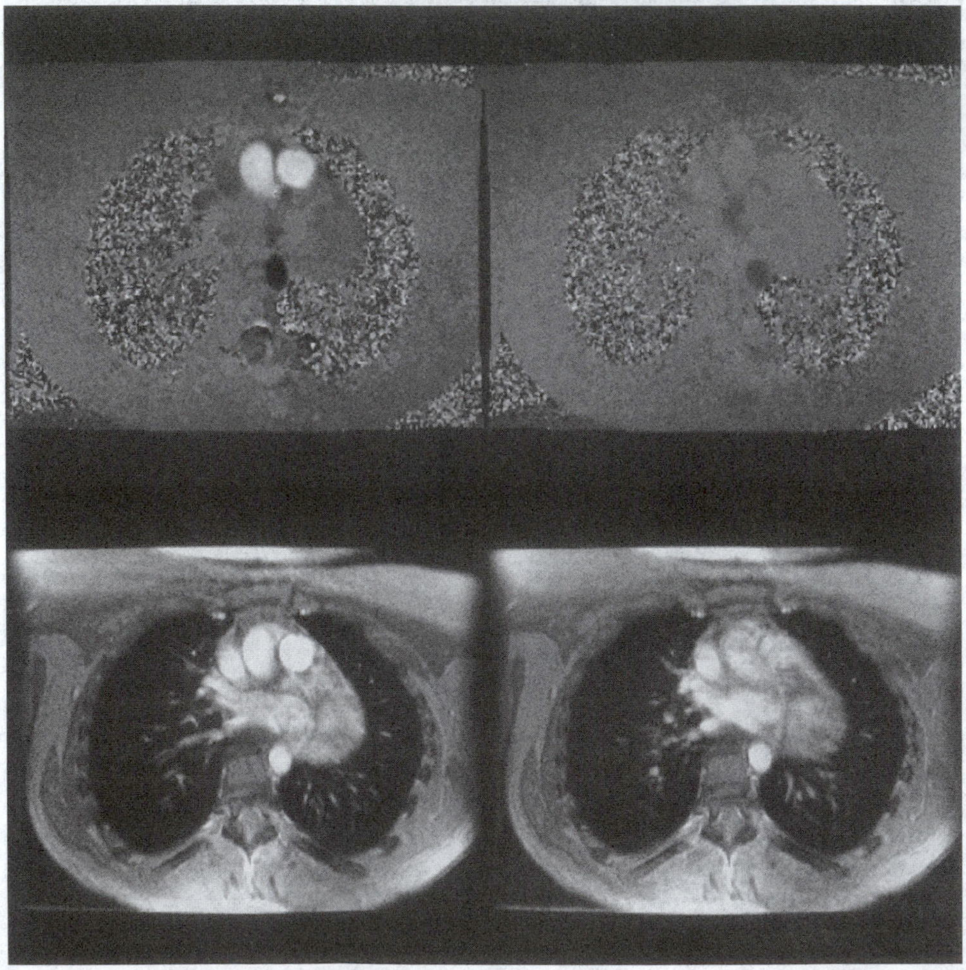

FIGURE 18B-8 Phase-contrast (*top row*) and the corresponding magnitude images (*bottom row*) from a phase-contrast acquisition. Images at systole (*first column*) and diastole (*second column*) are shown. Note the changes in flow velocities between systole and diastole.

Phase-Contrast Cardiac Imaging

PRINCIPLES

Phase-contrast (PC) MR angiography[26] offers a different contrast mechanism to discriminate between flowing spins and stationary tissue. Rather than depending on the relative saturation of flowing blood and tissue, PC angiography derives image contrast from the differences in the phase accumulated by stationary and moving spins in a magnetic field gradient. The amount of phase accumulated is directly proportional to the flow velocity, allowing quantitative measurement of flow velocities, with stationary tissue having zero value for the phase. In addition, PC angiography allows discrimination of flow direction. Spins moving in the direction of a magnetic field gradient accumulate positive phase, while spins moving in the opposite direction accumulate negative phase. Hence, the magnitude of the phase determines the velocity, while the sign of the accumulated phase determines flow direction.

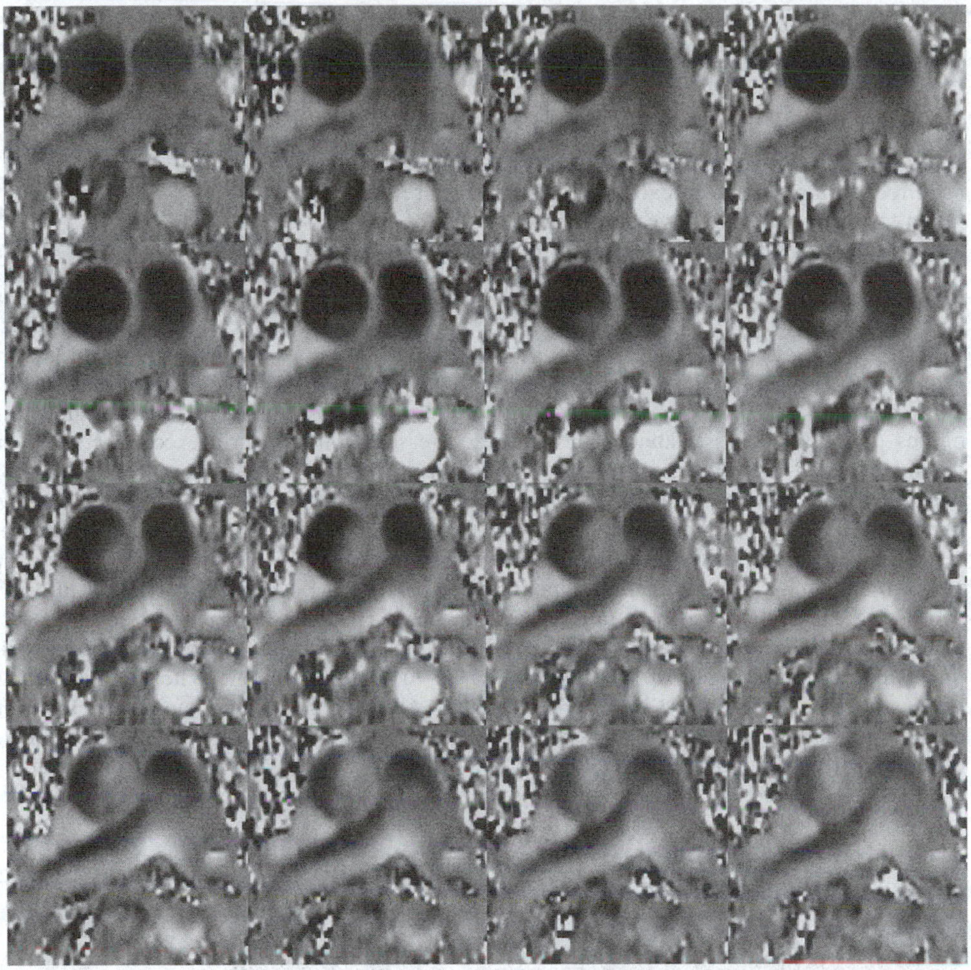

FIGURE 18B-9 Phase-contrast cine images at the level of the pulmonary artery outflow tract in a healthy volunteer. At this level, both the ascending and descending sections of the aorta can be seen clearly, together with the right and left pulmonary arteries. In this figure, 16 different time frames are shown with an effective temporal resolution of 35 ms (interpolated). Actual temporal resolution is defined as the acquisition time per segment [number of views per segment × TR toward the feet are represented by negative signal intensities (*black*)]. Imaging parameters were 40-cm field of view, 256 × 160 matrix, 4 views per segment, TE/TR/flip = 3.1/8.7 m/15°, 8-mm-thick sections.

TIME-RESOLVED QUANTITATIVE FLOW MEASUREMENT

Time-resolved flow information can be obtained by using an ECG-gated fast gradient-echo acquisition and linear interpolation, similar to conventional cine pulse sequences. The difference here is that a pair of flow-encoding acquisitions must be acquired for each k-space view to quantify flow in a single direction (Fig. 18B-7). In a PC acquisition, two images are generated. The phase image contains information about the direction and magnitude of the velocity, and the magnitude image provides T1-weighted image contrast (Fig. 18B-8). When played in a cine loop, the multiple temporal PC images can provide visualization of changes in the flow (direction and velocity) as a function of the cardiac cycle (Fig. 18B-9).

Plots of the phase velocity as a function of time also can be made across a cross-sectional area of the vessel. If the cross-sectional area of the vessel is known and the flow-velocity time profile is integrated, an average measure of flow in milliliters per minute can be calculated. However, in these measurements, care must be taken to ensure that there are sufficient pixels across the target vessel to minimize errors in the flow measurement from partial volume inclusion of stationary spins.[27]

As in conventional cine acquisitions, the acquisition time for a gated cine phase-contrast scan (cine-PC) is a function of the patient's heart rate and the spatial resolution. A typical cine-PC scan can be completed in about 2 min. The respiratory deficiencies encountered in conventional cine scans are also present in cine-PC acquisitions.

Aortic flow and pulmonary arterial flow also can be measured and assessed against left and right ventricular function, respectively. The assessment of flow across valve leaflets in patients with valvular abnormalities also has been proposed. PC imaging has been shown to provide discriminate flow between the true lumen and the false lumen in aortic dissections and to separate thrombus and flow.

FAST CARDIAC PHASE CONTRAST

Segmented fast gradient-echo techniques also can be applied to PC (Fastcard-PC) scans to reduce the total scan time substantially.[12] Rather than acquiring one flow-encoded k-space view per cardiac cycle, several k-space views can be acquired with flow-encoding gradients, generating a series of flow-sensitized images at different temporal phases with substantially reduced total scan time.

Fastcard-PC scans have been used to evaluate flow in the great vessels and also in the measurement of coronary flow reserve.[28–30] With shorter scan times, PC-cine images can be acquired during a single breath hold. However, care must be taken to avoid using too large of a number of vps, as this may lead to low pass filtering or blunting of the temporal response of the PC measurements.[31]

Contrast-Enhanced 3D Imaging

Conventional and breath-hold SE and gradient-echo techniques define most vessel abnormalities; these are situations in which vessel anatomy is not seen with sufficient clarity because of artifacts. Contrast (e.g., gadolinium-chelates)-enhanced (CE) imaging is advantageous in displaying detailed vessel anatomy and reducing artifacts.[32] The high signal provided by vascular contrast enhancement makes 3D image processing easier than it is with unenhanced images. CE MR angiography requires very short TR and echo time (TE) times and timing imaging to coincide with the arterial or venous phase of the contrast bolus. The resulting MR images can be rendered in multiple projections. If the patient is incapable of performing breath holding, a slower acquisition can be done over several minutes with a longer and/or slower infusion of contrast agent. However, the vessels may be degraded by respiratory motion.

Coil Selection

Early on, CMR was performed using a body coil, which has the primary advantage of a large FOV and uniform signal intensity. Conventional surface or phased-array coils that were not specifically optimized for cardiac imaging also have been used because of the lack of a cardiac-specific coil. These conventional receiver coils are optimized for general body-imaging purposes (spine, pelvis, etc.); therefore, they have poor sensitivity at larger depths and do not address the specific geometry of the heart within the chest. For example, a standard quatradure surface coil for spine imaging provides adequate images at depths of penetration of only up to 7 cm from the surface of the coil. When such a coil is placed on the anterior chest wall, the deep structures, such as the posterior wall of the left ventricle (located approximately 10 to 15 cm from the anterior chest wall) or the distal coronary arteries, can be well visualized.

Dedicated cardiac coils[33] are becoming commercially available. The FOV is somewhat smaller, and the signal intensity is not uniform. However, the cardiac coils are necessary for improved SNR and for good coverage of the heart and coronaries. Coil placement is very important for adequate SNR, and care must be taken to center the coil around the heart.

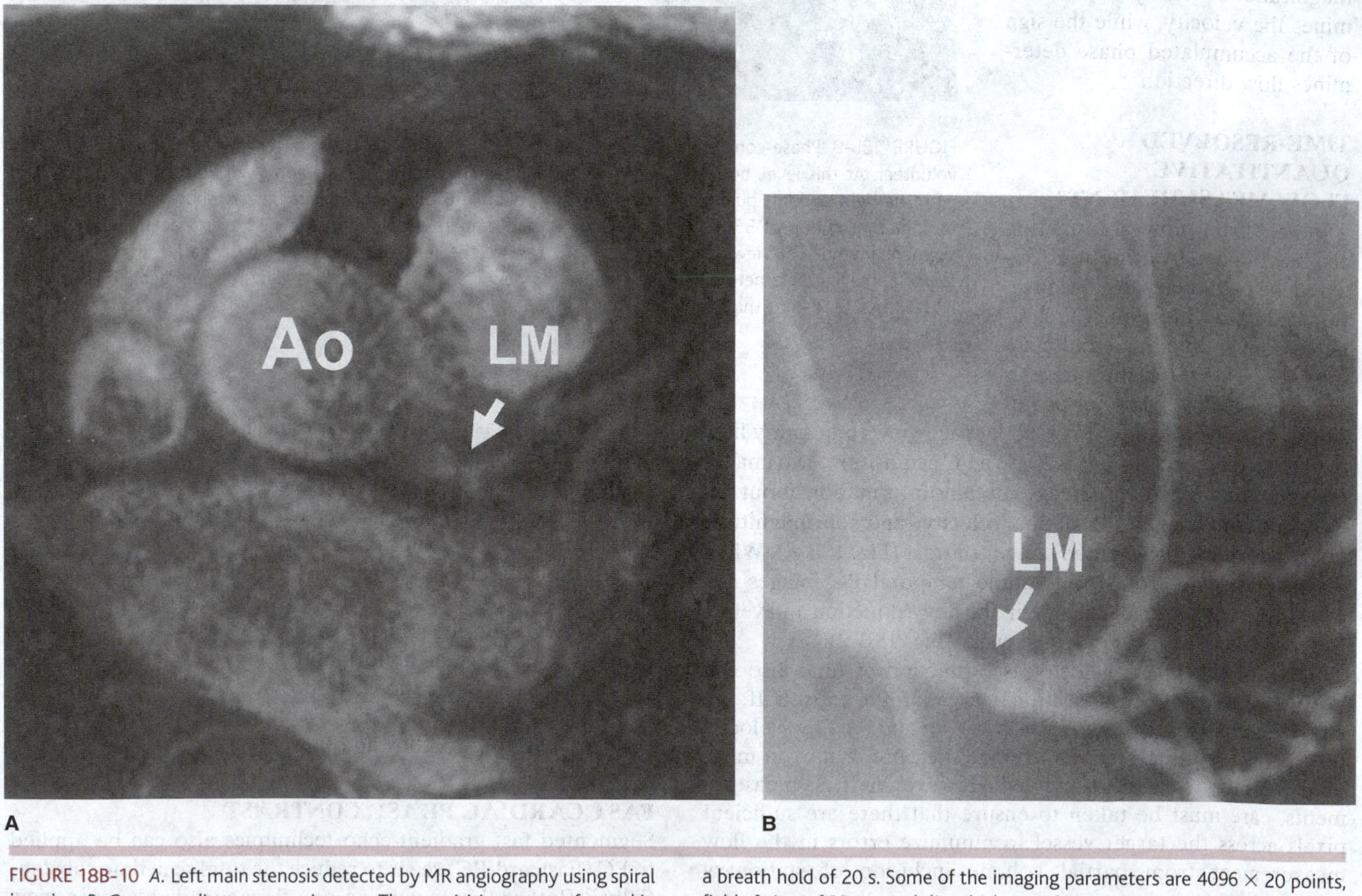

A B

FIGURE 18B-10 *A.* Left main stenosis detected by MR angiography using spiral imaging. *B.* Corresponding x-ray angiogram. The acquisition was performed in a breath hold of 20 s. Some of the imaging parameters are 4096 × 20 points, field of view of 22 cm, and slice thickness of 3 mm. Ao = aorta; LM = left main.

CLINICAL APPLICATIONS

Coronary Artery Imaging

INTRODUCTION

Coronary artery magnetic resonance imaging (MRI) is considered a very challenging area and often is referred to as one of the "holy grails" of CMR. Coronary arteries are small structures (3 to 4 mm in diameter), follow a tortuous course, and are intimate with many surrounding structures, making them difficult to visualize. Motion artifacts from cardiac and respiratory motion provide a further challenge to image quality. Existing coronary MR angiography (MRA) techniques[34–36] can visualize the proximal and middle portions of most coronary artery segments and some branches. Clinical applications include determining patency and direction of flow in native coronary arteries, evaluating the patency of coronary artery bypass grafts and native vessels after intervention, evaluating anomalous coronary arteries, and following up after surgical or medical therapy. The blind prospective detection of coronary artery lesions with coronary MRA is being evaluated with several MRI techniques. No single technique has emerged that can provide the sensitivity and specificity of catheter-based x-ray contrast angiography, although preliminary clinical studies appear promising. At this stage of development, coronary MRA can be used to exclude or confirm suspected clinically important coronary stenoses in patients referred for diagnostic contrast x-ray angiography. As techniques continue to improve, coronary MRA may become an integral part of the clinical evaluation and screening of patients with ischemic heart disease.

CORONARY MR IMAGING TECHNIQUES

Early Imaging Early attempts at coronary MRA using conventional SE were inadequate. Reports by Lieberman and associates[37] and Paulin and coworkers[38] demonstrated the difficulty of visualizing long portions of artery as well as any stenosis that existed. Since that time, advances in MR technology have allowed more reliable visualization of the proximal epicardial vessels. In an attempt to improve image quality, current techniques combine ECG gating, suppression of respiratory motion (e.g., respiratory gating and compensation), fast image acquisition, and the suppression of signal from surrounding tissues.

2D Segmented K-Space Breath-Hold Methods The most widely studied modality uses 2D segmented k-space gradient-echo imaging.[39] This method allows image acquisition (100 to 150 ms) during middiastole, a period of bulk cardiac diastasis and high coronary blood flow. Each cardiac cycle typically contains eight interleaved phase-encoding steps (vp = 8) and generates a single 2D image on a 128 × 256 matrix in a breath hold of 16 heartbeats (~15 to 20 s, depending on the heart rate) to minimize interference from respiratory motion. Typical parameters are a slice thickness of 3 to 5 mm, an FOV of 240 mm, and in-plane spatial resolution of 1.9 × 0.9 mm. To complete a study, 40 or more breath holds may be required. In this white blood technique, laminar blood flow appears "bright" (inflow of unsaturated spins) in normal regions and turbulent blood flow appears "dark" (dephasing of signal) in areas of possible stenosis.[39–41] Coronary arteries usually are embedded in fat, which has high signal intensity on T1-weighted images. Suppression of the high signal from fat offers improved coronary visualization. This technique is called *fat suppression* and suppresses the signal from the pericardial and epicardial fat.

Other Methods Segmented k-space methods require repetitive excitation of the same slice of slab within each cardiac

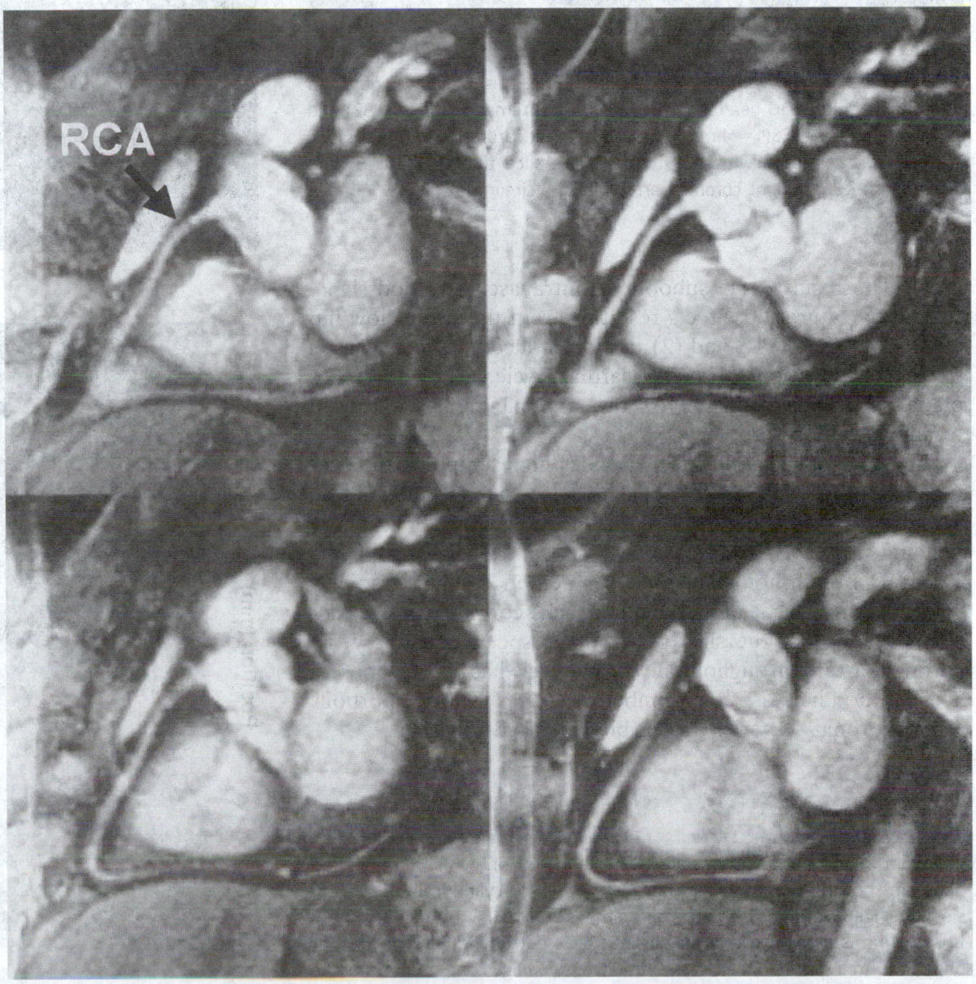

FIGURE 18B-11 A 2D multislice segmented k-space gradient-echo image of the right coronary artery (RCA). The imaging was performed using automated vessel tracking and increased the number of images in which portions of the right coronary artery were visible. Imaging was performed after the injection of gadolinium (0.10 mmol/kg).

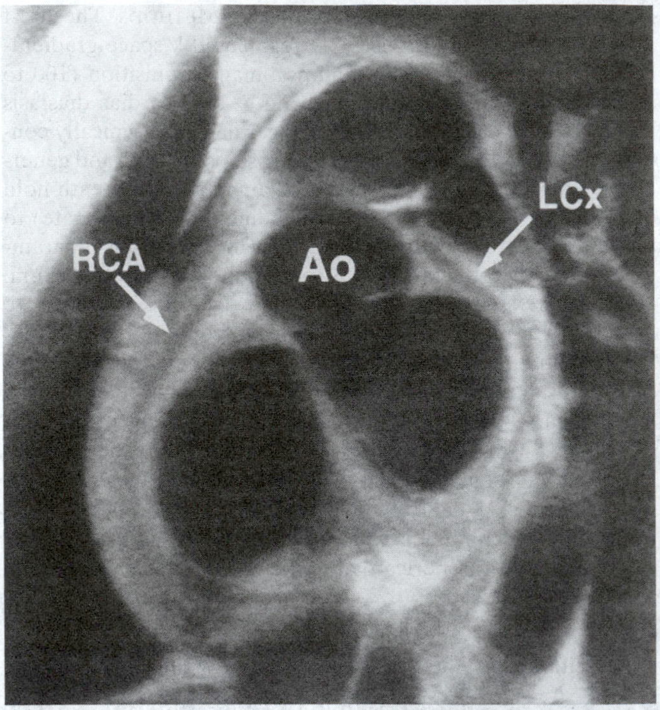

FIGURE 18B-12 Black blood imaging of the coronary arteries using a 2D double-inversion recovery fast spin-echo sequence. This image was obtained in a breath hold of 16 heartbeats. Long-echo train imaging (ETL = 32) and short echo spacing (ESP = 4 ms) were used. No fat saturation was necessary. The in-plane resolution was 0.5 mm, and the slice thickness was 3 mm. Ao = aorta; RCA = right coronary artery; LCx = circumflex.

cycle. The result is (1) suboptimal intravascular blood signal caused by saturation effects resulting from the use of low flip angles and short TRs and (2) motion-induced artifacts caused by long acquisition times per cardiac cycle. Multishot echo-planar breath-hold imaging for coronary imaging has been used to alleviate these problems.[42]

Interleaved spiral imaging provides high temporal and spatial resolution with relative insensitivity to flow and motion artifacts.[20] This technique has shown great promise for coronary imaging (Fig. 18B-10).

A 2D breath-hold multislice segmented k-space gradient-echo technique that automatically tracks coronary artery motion by adjusting the slice offset to prospectively follow the coronary artery throughout the cardiac cycle has been proposed. This method increases the number of images in which portions of the coronary arteries are visible (Fig. 18B-11).[43]

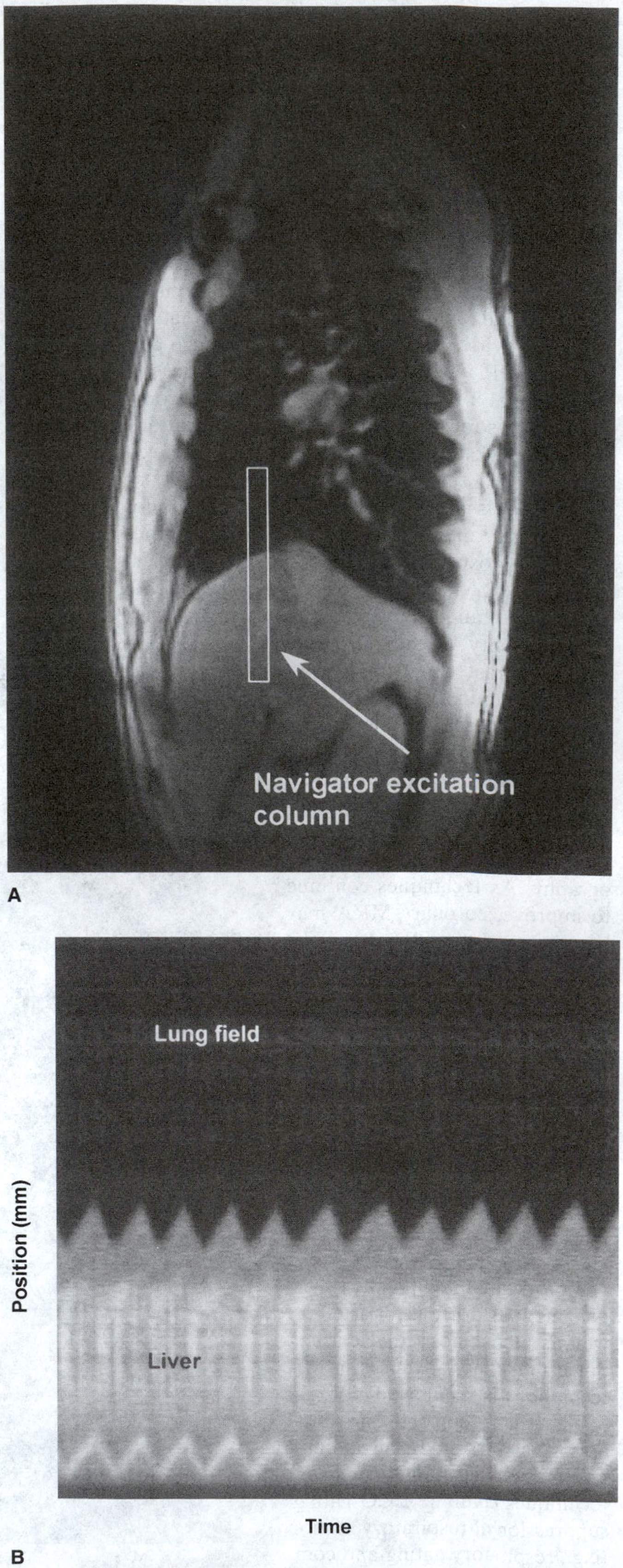

FIGURE 18B-13 *A.* A sagittal scout image in the region of the right hemidiaphragm showing the placement of a rectangular or cylindrical two-dimensional navigator echo column. The one-dimensional profile of the signal from this column is used to determine the displacement of the edge of the diaphragm from a specified reference position. *B.* An image composed of stacked one-dimensional navigator profiles as a function of time. The vertical axis has units of distance, and the horizontal axis is a function of time. The region of bright signal is the dome of the liver, and the lung field is indicated by the noise.

Using the black blood fast spin-echo sequence with "velocity-selective" inversion preparatory pulses[8] to null the signal from flowing blood high-resolution imaging of the coronary arteries also can be performed in a breath hold (Fig. 18B-12). The advantage of this sequence versus bright blood imaging techniques is being investigated.

Contrast preparation mechanisms such as magnetization transfer,[44] inversion recovery,[45] and T2 preparation[46] also can be employed to improve the delineation between the coronary artery and the surrounding myocardial tissue, especially for the left coronary artery distribution. These contrast preparation techniques are important because they improve vessel visualization by reducing partial volume effects.

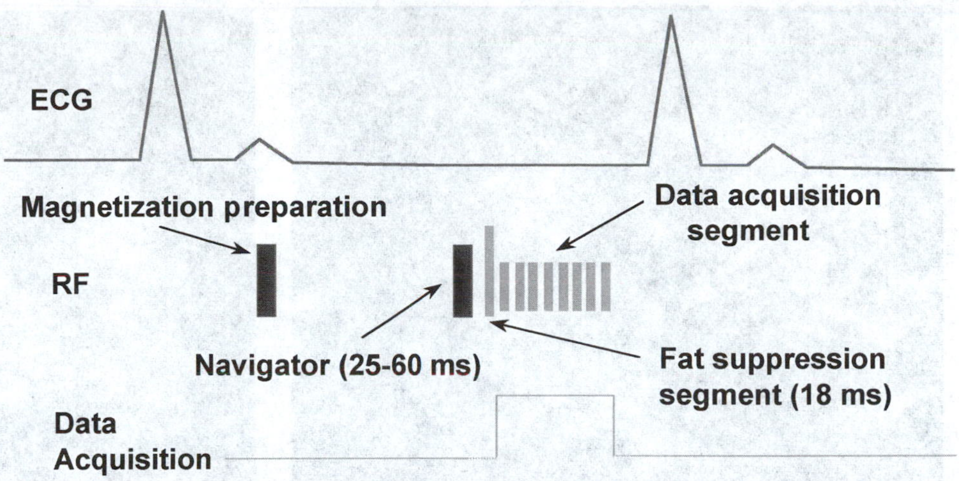

FIGURE 18B-14 Diagram showing the timing of the 3D navigator echo pulse sequence for imaging the coronary arteries. As shown in this figure, the navigator echo segment precedes the fat suppression segment and the image data acquisition segments. Each data acquisition segment consists of an RF excitation pulse to encode for one value of the k-space view in the slice or phase-encoding direction. A magnetization preparation segment also can be implemented into the sequence without affecting the navigator echo acquisition. In this scheme, prospective determination to enable or disable data acquisition for the current R-R interval depends on the ability of the MR imaging system to calculate the diaphragm displacement and arrive at an accept-reject decision within the time period of the navigator echo segment.

3D Imaging Three-dimensional imaging offers enhanced signal reception[47] with reconstruction capabilities used for visualizing tortuous vessels.[48] 3D imaging is prone to blurring and requires scan times that far exceed that of a breath hold.[49]

Attempts have been made to improve the free breathing 3D acquisition methods. Signal averaging,[50] respiratory feedback,[51] a respiratory monitoring belt,[52] and coached breathing[53] have all been used. New thin 3D slab acquisition is allowing imaging of the coronary arteries in a breath hold.[19]

Navigator Echo Imaging Techniques used to suppress motion artifact may eliminate the difficult task of breath holding. Real-time navigator echo[5] has been successful in limiting respiratory motion artifacts. When the lung-heart or lung-diaphragm interface is interrogated (Fig. 18B-13*A*), positional changes can be monitored through the respiratory cycle (Fig. 18B-13*B*) and image acquisition can be gated to respiratory motion according to the superoinferior position of the diaphragm (Fig. 18B-14).[54] The navigator data then are used to perform image correction prospectively[55,56] or retrospectively.[44,57] The navigator data also can be used to prospectively correct the slice position, allowing the use of wider gating windows with improved time efficiency.[45,46,58] Irregular breathing patterns may be problematic, and the accuracy with which the diaphragm is tracked determines to a great extent whether the coronary arteries are imaged at a constant position.[54]

Typically, the acquisition parameters for a coronary MR study have an image FOV of 20 to 24 cm, with 1- to 1.5-mm sections. Since the volume acquisition is targeted over a specific vessel, the use of 16 to 20 partitions allows a 15- to 30-mm-thick region to be imaged, with the coronary artery approximately in the plane of acquisition. Scan times may range from 5 to 10 min for visualizing a single coronary artery distribution. The scan planes can be targeted for the different coronary artery structures (Fig. 18B-15).

Contrast-Enhanced Coronary Angiography Contrast-enhanced MRA has dramatically affected aortic, renal, and peripheral MRA through the use of both conventional extravascular (e.g., gadolinium-chelates) and new intravascular contrast agents. The latter include iron particle-based (e.g., iron particle–based AMI-227, Advanced Magnetics; iron particle and NC100150, Nycomed-Amersham; gadolinium-chelate, which binds to plasma albumin IS325, EPIX, and gadomer-17, Shering) contrast agents. Intravascular agents have several advantages over extravascular contrast agents: (1) higher T1 relaxivity, (2) higher concentration within the blood, (3) reduction of extravasation into the myocardium, and (4) blood signal remaining enhanced for a relatively long time. Early studies suggest that CE coronary MRA may play a role in improving coronary imaging (Fig. 18B-11).[59–61] The potential clinical applications of these agents awaits the results of large-scale multicenter clinical trials.

ANOMALOUS CORONARY ARTERIES

Not only is coronary MRA a noninvasive method, conventional x-ray angiography often may not be able to determine the exact pathway of an anomalous vessel. Both 2D and 3D coronary MR methods are proving to be well suited for the characterization of anomalous coronary arteries. Although rare, coronary anomalies must be defined accurately, as certain varieties carry the risk of sudden cardiac death (Fig. 18B-16). MRA is an excellent way to identify anomalies and in some cases is superior to coronary angiography.[62,63] Coronary MRA should be considered a diagnostic tool in any suspected case.

CORONARY BYPASS GRAFTS

Conventional ECG-gated spin echo and gradient echo have been used to evaluate coronary bypass grafts. The more stationary position and the straight path of internal mammary and

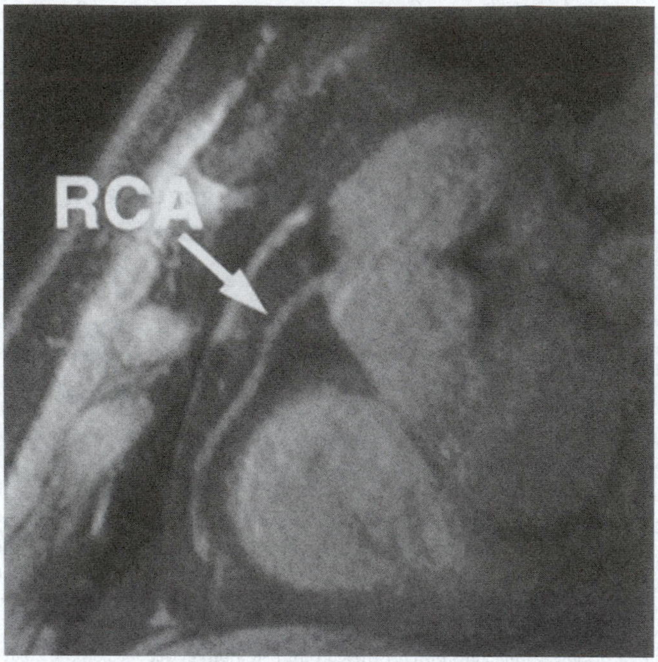

A

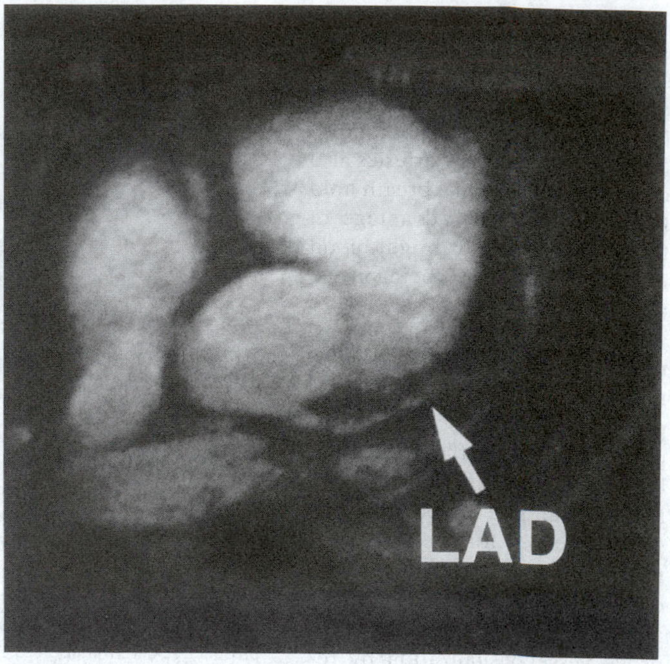

B

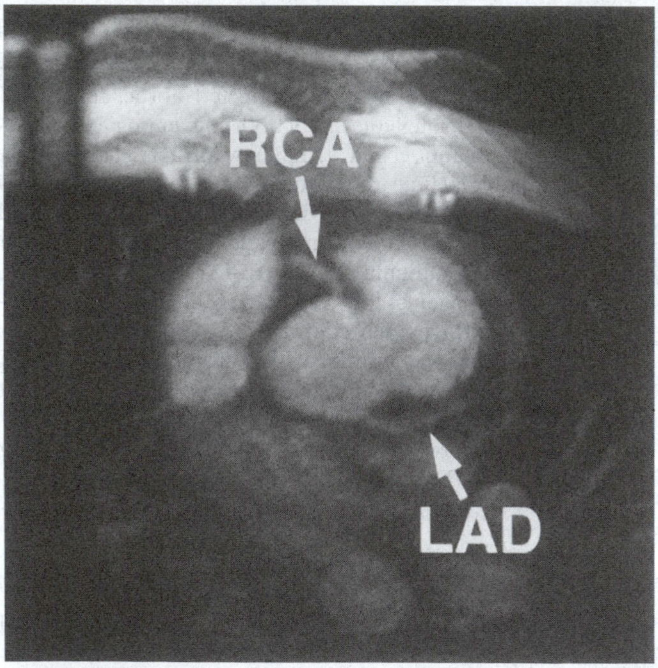

C

FIGURE 18B-15 Prospective navigator echo three-dimensional coronary artery images in double oblique planes after planar reformation in a healthy volunteer. In two separate acquisitions, the right coronary artery (RCA) (*A*) and the left main coronary artery/left anterior descending (LAD) artery (*B* and *C*) can be visualized clearly. Acquisition parameters were 24-cm field of view, 20 1.5-mm sections, and 256 × 224 matrix with partial Fourier reconstruction in the phase-encoding direction. Average scan times for both scans were approximately 5 to 6 min.

saphenous vein grafts contribute to the relative ease at which these vessels may be visualized by MRA. Routinely, contiguous transverse images are obtained through the area expected to contain each graft. The graft is deemed patent if laminar flow is detected by signal void (spin echo) or bright signal (gradient echo) in at least two contiguous anatomic levels. Laminar flow on only one level is considered indeterminate. The absence of laminar signal means the vessel is occluded. SE and gradient-echo methods have demonstrated equal accuracy.[64–66] Contrast-enhanced MRA has demonstrated improved accuracy in bypass graft evaluation.[67,68]

As with intravascular stents (see below), a major obstacle for bypass graft imaging is the local signal loss and artifact associated with implanted metallic objects such as ostial graft rings and homeostatic clips. These artifacts may make signal voids related to blood flow through a stenosis in the bypass graft indistinguishable. In addition, grafts with tight stenoses may result in insufficient contrast penetration to characterize graft patency. Therefore, identification of focal stenoses within a graft may be extremely difficult and limited. The possible use of more MR-"friendly" materials may help alleviate this problem in the future.

STENTS

Since the introduction of coronary stents,[69] coronary stenting has been used commonly to treat obstructive coronary artery disease. Coronary stents typically are made of stainless steel or tantalum.[70] After implantation, they are endothelialized and incorporated into the vessel wall. Because of the strong magnetic field required by current MRI systems, there has been concern about the possible heating or even dislocation of previously implanted coronary stents in patients undergoing MRI. The current recommendation is to wait several weeks (~6 weeks) after stent placement before doing an MRI.[71] Addition-

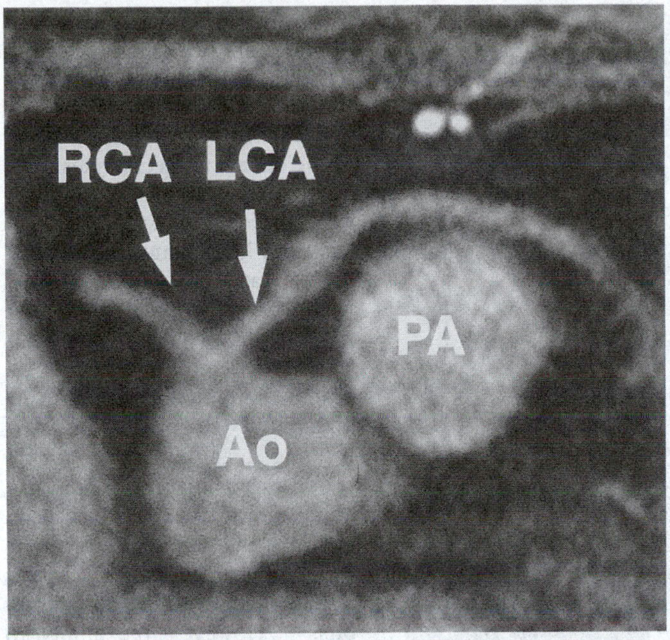

FIGURE 18B-16 A 53-year-old woman with multiple cardiac risk factors and recent onset of chest discomfort suggestive of angina. Thallium stress test was suggestive of reversible ischemia. 3-D navigator triggered MR angiogram (curved reformat) shows anomalous left coronary artery (LCA) originating from right cusp and passing anterior to pulmonary artery (PA). Ao = aorta; RCA = right coronary artery. (Courtesy Dr. Christine H. Lorenz, Barnes-Jewish Hospital at Washington University Medical Center, St. Louis, MO.)

ally, the implanted stent may cause imaging artifacts and signal loss[72] because of its metallic nature[73] at the implantation site, prohibiting the visualization of the underlying structures (Fig. 18B-17).

Despite these challenges and limitations, coronary MRA after stent placement has been found to be safe[74] and possible for the assessment of coronary artery patency.[75] The use of more MR-"friendly" and artifact-free stents may provide a way to minimize this problem in the future.[76]

CORONARY BLOOD FLOW ASSESSMENT

Assessment of coronary blood flow with MR at rest and under pharmacologic stress offers the potential to identify noninvasively areas of the myocardium that merit revascularization in coronary artery disease (CAD) patients. MR flow measurement is based on modification of the MR signal of the flowing blood as it traverses the imaging plane. The use of phase-contrast MR imaging (velocity-encoded cine) is based on the principle that protons in the bloodstream experience a net change in the phase of precession proportionally to their velocity as they travel in a magnetic field gradient. The region of interest around the vessel perimeter is defined, and flow-velocity values are analyzed.

The main technical challenge for coronary flow determinations is the small diameter of the coronary arteries. Partial volume averaging results in overestimation of the flow velocity. Furthermore, cardiac motion and the currently limited spatial resolution of MR imaging introduce potential error in the measurement of coronary artery cross-sectional area and quantification of absolute coronary blood flow. Measurement of flow in the coronary sinus[29] and proximal aorta[77] can overcome the

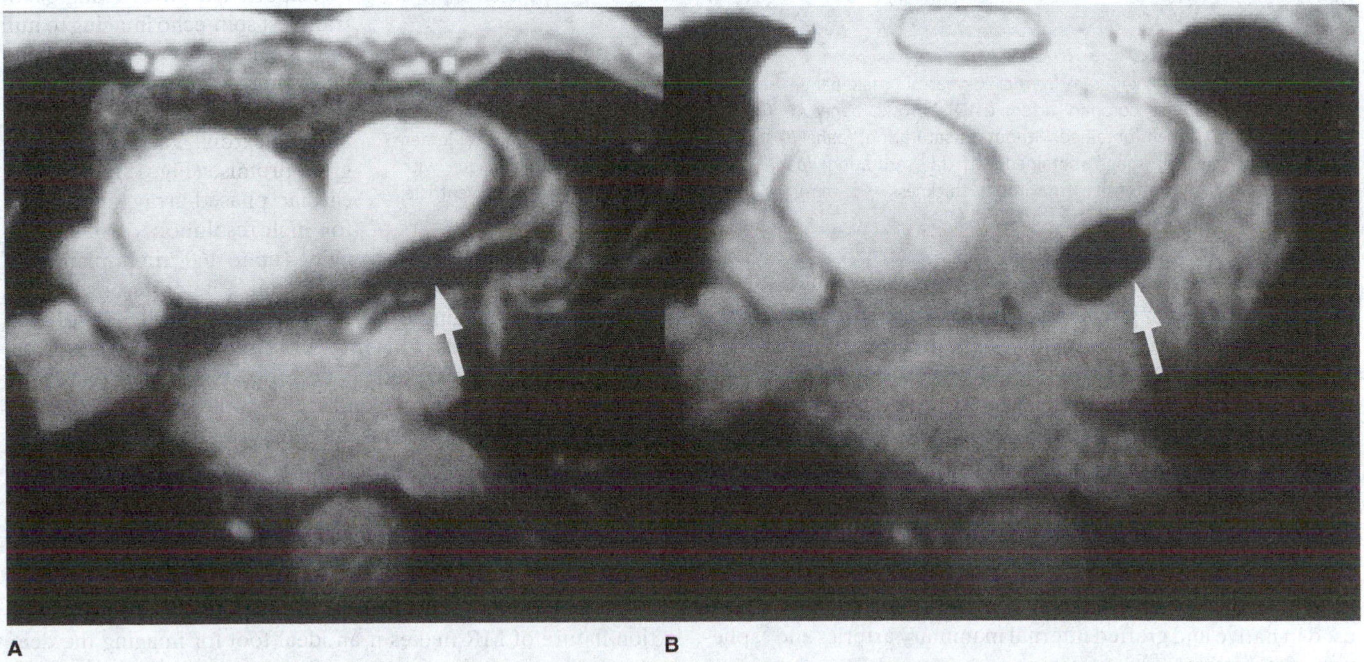

FIGURE 18B-17 A 55-year-old man with a single stent in the proximal left anterior descending artery (LAD). *A.* Oblique transaxial images with fat suppression. An area of signal void caused by the susceptibility artifact of the stent is visualized (*arrow*). *B.* Oblique transaxial images without fat suppression. The area of signal void caused by the susceptibility artifact of the stent is better visualized. The mid-LAD is seen only faintly (*arrow*). (From Duerinckx AJ, with permission. Duerinckx AJ, et al.[75])

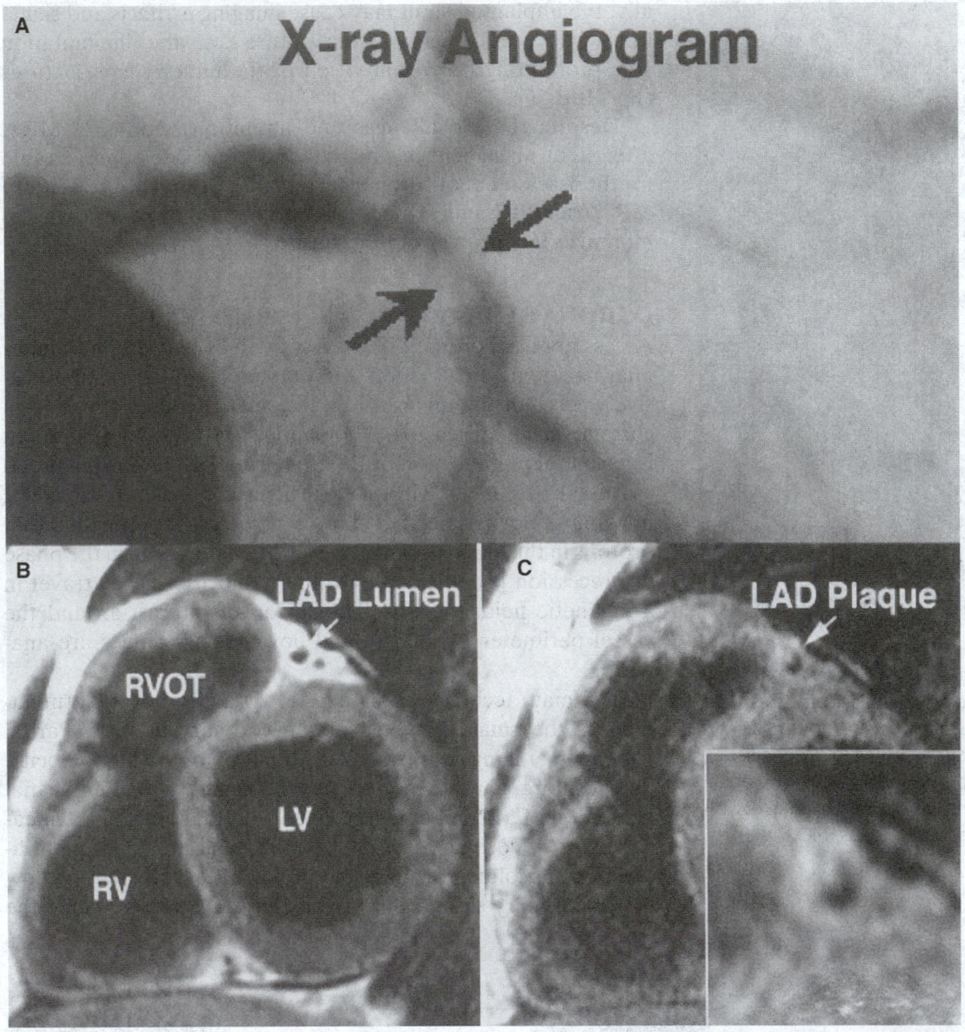

FIGURE 18B-18 X-ray angiogram from a 76-year-old male patient showing high-grade stenosis in the proximal left anterior descending coronary artery (LAD) (*arrows, panel A*). The in vivo cross-sectional black blood MR image of the LAD lumen (obtained without fat saturation) (*panel B*) shows an obstructed lumen (elliptical lumen shape), while the wall image (obtained with fat saturation) (*panel C*) shows a large eccentric plaque with heterogeneous signal intensity (maximum thickness ~6 mm). LV = left ventricle; RV = right ventricle; RVOT = right ventricular outflow tract.

problems of partial volume averaging, motion, and low resolution. However, such global assessment of the coronary circulation is of little help in the study of focal coronary stenoses.

Various modifications of the phase-contrast approach[30,78,79] have been used to measure coronary flow at rest and after intravenous injection of adenosine or dipyridamole and after isometric exercise in patients with CAD.[80,81] A threefold to fivefold increase over resting blood flow and velocity can be measured after pharmacologic vasodilatation.[78,79] In patients with significant stenoses, the impaired coronary flow reserve has less than a twofold increase.

Similarly, MR coronary blood flow measurement has been used in native and grafted internal mammary arteries and saphenous vein grafts.[65,66,82]

CORONARY WALL IMAGING AND PLAQUE CHARACTERIZATION

The ability to define the components of a complex coronary atherosclerotic lesion (i.e., fibrous cap, lipid core, calcium, and hemorrhage) accurately could potentially allow risk stratification of patients for future acute coronary syndromes.[83] Given the excellent soft tissue contrast provided by CMR imaging techniques, the ability of MR to differentiate between these plaque components has been investigated.[84–87] Experimental data have shown that MR is effective in identifying both the normal vessel wall components and atherosclerotic plaque in research conditions, often using high-field MR systems and performing imaging ex vivo to improve the spatial resolution.[88,89] In animal models, MR has been shown to be able to characterize the components of atherosclerotic lesions in transgenic mice and rabbits.[90–92] However, the ability to translate these techniques to the human coronary arteries in vivo has the same limitations that initially faced MR coronary angiography: motion (cardiac and respiratory), small vessel size, and tortuousity of the vessels. However, to visualize the components of a coronary atherosclerotic lesion, submillimeter resolution will be required.[93]

Experience with long-echo-train fast spin-echo imaging to null the signal from flowing blood and an optimized chemical shift pulse to null signal from perivascular and epicardial fat have shown great promise (Fig. 18B-18).[94,95] A cardiac phased-array surface coil for high-resolution coronary imaging (up to 460-μm in-plane spatial resolution) is used.[33] Normal and atherosclerotic human coronary wall imaging can be performed with high-resolution black blood methods. This may allow the identification of atherosclerotic disease before it becomes symptomatic. Further studies are necessary to identify the different plaque components and assess lesions in asymptomatic patients and their outcomes.

Aortic Imaging

CMR has been shown to be useful in both acquired and congenital abnormalities of the aorta. The noninvasive and high-resolution nature of MR makes it an ideal tool for imaging the deep structures of the thorax.

AORTIC DISSECTION

Among all the imaging modalities currently clinically available for the detection of aortic dissection, CMR appears to have the highest accuracy.[96,97] Furthermore, because of its noninvasive

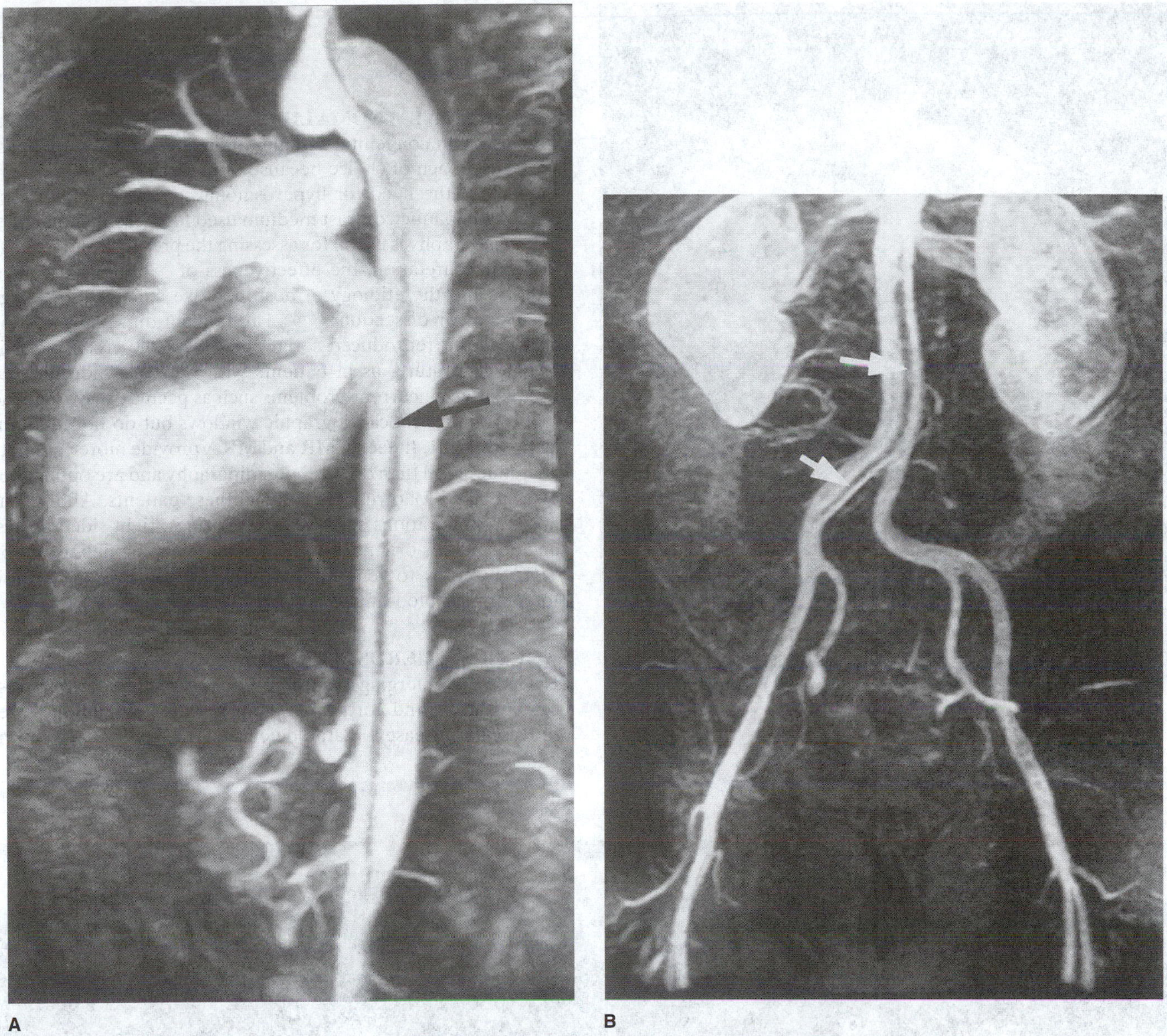

FIGURE 18B-19 Maximum intensity projection images. Dynamic 3D imaging after the administration of gadolinium. Patient had a history of ascending aortic dissection repair. Images show a residual aortic dissection (*arrow*) extending from near the origin of the right subclavian artery through the thoracic (*A*) and abdominal aorta into the right common iliac arrows (*B*). (Courtesy of Dr. Steven D. Wolff, Integrated Cardiovascular Therapeutics, Woodbury, NY.)

nature, it permits sequential imaging over time and thus allows patients at risk of and those who already have had an aortic dissection to be monitored. Using CMR, one can assess not only the intimal flap and site of tear with contrast-enhanced 3D MRA (Fig. 18B-19) but other important associated abnormalities, such as aortic wall thrombus/hematoma, aortic regurgitation, pericardial effusion, and branch vessel involvement.[98,99] It is the investigation of choice in hemodynamically stable patients. However, because of potential delays in patient access, transesophageal echocardiography (TEE) is indicated for unstable patients. Despite a high sensitivity for aortic dissection detection with TEE, it has a reduced specificity compared with MRI.[96]

The ability to detect aortic wall thrombus/hematoma has clinical implications, as it is considered a precursor for dissection.[100] MRI can accurately identify aortic wall thrombus/hematoma, as determined by aortic wall thickening (>7 mm), with a smooth surface and often areas of high signal intensity on T1-weighted images because of the presence of methemoglobin.[101]

AORTIC ANEURYSM

When contrast-enhanced three-dimensional MRA is used, high-quality imaging of the thoracic aorta can be performed (Fig. 18B-20), allowing not only detection of aortic dissection, as described above, but also visualization of aneurysms irrespective of the site or etiology; thus, it can assist in determining the appropriate timing for surgery.[102] CMR appears to be better able to accurately define complex aneurysm anatomy and branch vessel involvement than ultrasound for abdominal aortic aneurysms.[103] Furthermore, CMR is able to detect mural thrombus (gradient- and spin-echo sequences) complicating an aortic aneurysm.[104,105] However, the advantage of CMR over simpler

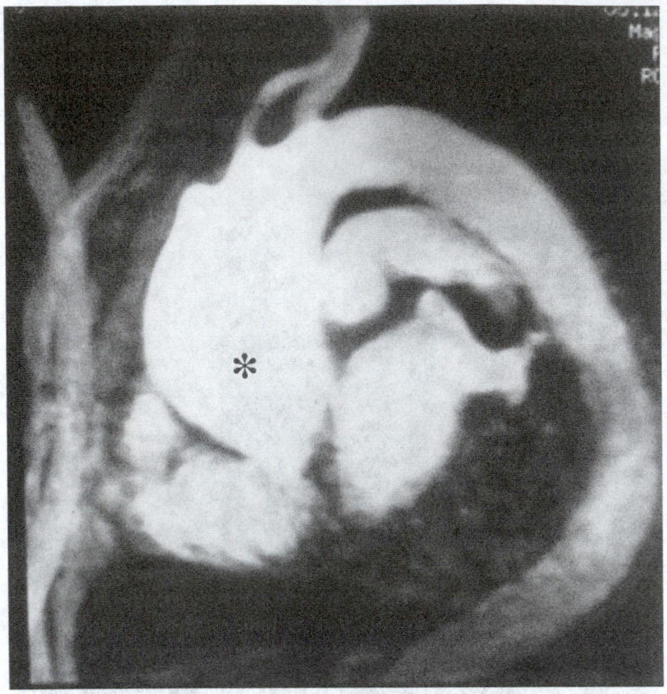

FIGURE 18B-20 Dynamic 3D imaging after the administration of Gd-DTPA. This MR image shows a severe aortic aneurysm in the ascending aorta (*asterisk*).

techniques (ultrasound and computed topography) in determining the timing of surgery in patients with aortic aneurysms is unclear.

CONGENITAL ANOMALIES

In adults with congenital vascular anomalies, CMR is the diagnostic approach of choice because of its large field of view and the lack of the need for hyperosmolar contrast medium such as the radiopaque contrast medium used for x-ray angiography. MR angiography is useful for assessing the presence and severity of aortic coarctation, the effectiveness of balloon aortic angioplasty, and the etiology of postoperative complications, e.g., aneurysms or dissections.[106–108] The luminal dimensions of the aorta can be reproduced serially to assess the risk for aortic aneurysm rupture, as in patients with Marfan syndrome.[109,110] Frequently, concurrent problems such as pectus excavatum and scoliosis limit echocardiographic windows but do not limit imaging with MR. In fact, CMR and MRA provide more complete anatomic detail than does echocardiography and are optimal for assessing and following virtually all these patients. Anomalous aortic configurations such as vascular rings, right-sided aortas, and anomalous origins of branch vessels may be delineated by MRA not only to generate morphologic information but also to determine blood flow.

AORTIC ATHEROSCLEROSIS

Evidence is emerging confirming an association between ascending aortic and aortic arch plaque and atheroembolic cerebrovascular disease.[111] Pathologic and TEE studies have shown

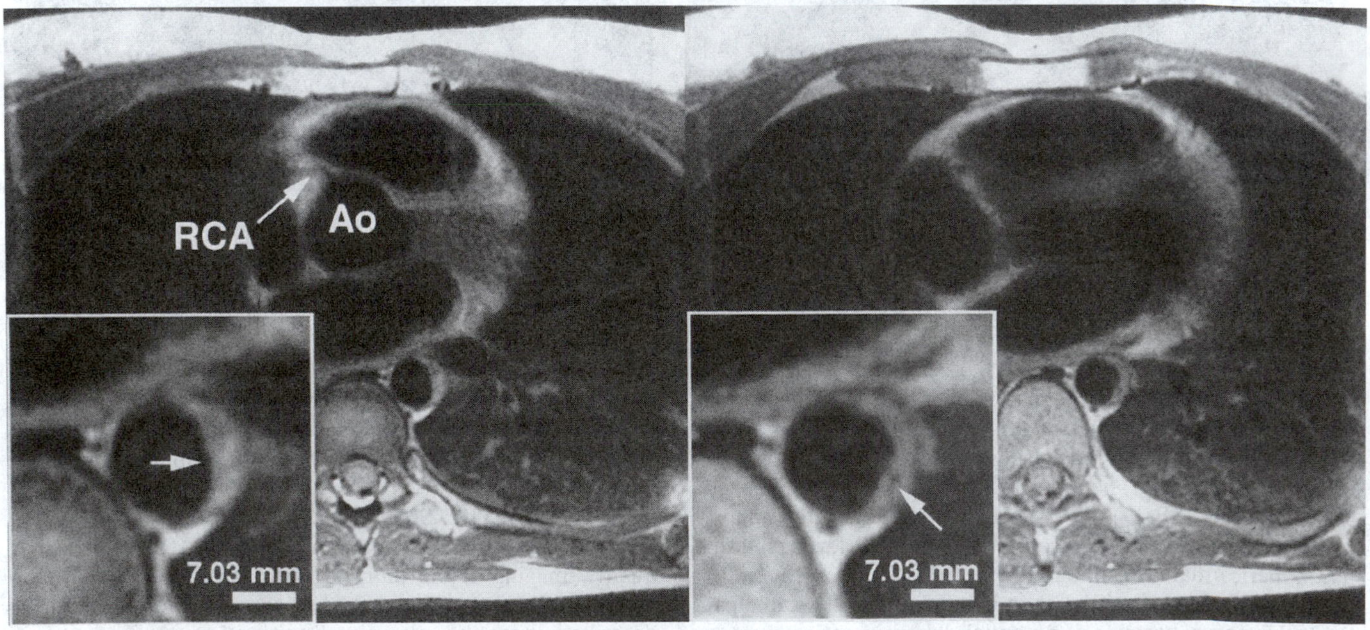

A B

FIGURE 18B-21 T2-weighted CMR images from a patient with severe diffuse disease in the descending thoracic aorta. The plaques are different in appearance and characteristics from one location to another. Plaque characterization was based on the information obtained from T1-, proton-density-, and T2-weighted MR images. The inserts in each panel represent a magnified view of the descending thoracic aorta. Panel A shows a type Vc (fibrocellular) plaque. Panel B shows a lipid-rich plaque (type Va). MR images are 5 mm thick, were acquired with no interslice gap, and are displayed cephalad (*panel A*) to caudal (*panel B*). The origin of the right coronary artery (RCA) is clearly seen taking off from the aortic root (Ao).

that aortic atheroma in these regions is an important cause of embolic cerebral infarction.[111] The risk of atherosclerotic plaque rupture and subsequent thrombogenicity appears to be modulated by the composition of aortic atheroma.[83] The ability to document noninvasively the size and composition (i.e., lipidic versus fibrotic components) of aortic atheroma could permit stratification of risk and allow monitoring of therapeutic approaches such as lipid lowering on the aortic atheroma. However, TEE is semi-invasive, and ultrasound techniques may be limited in their ability to differentiate the various components of complex atherosclerotic lesions.[112]

MR has been shown to accurately differentiate atherosclerotic plaque components in experimental and human models.[84,85,88–90,92] Furthermore, with black blood double-inversion recovery fast spin-echo sequences, there is the potential to visualize the aortic wall with submillimeter resolution, providing noninvasive data about atheroma size and composition (Fig. 18B-21).[86,87] This use for CMR remains under investigation and is an area of ongoing research.

References

1. Bogaert J, Duerinckx AJ, Rademakers FE. *Magnetic Resonance of the Heart and Great Vessels: Clinical Applications*. Berlin: Springer-Verlag; 1999.
2. Hashemi RH, Bradley WGJ. *MRI: The Basics*. Baltimore: Williams & Wilkins; 1997.
3. Mitchell DG. *MRI Principles*. Philadelphia: Saunders; 1999.
4. Wood ML, Wehrli FW. Principles of magnetic resonance imaging. In: *Magnetic Resonance Imaging*, 3d ed. St. Louis: Mosby; 1999.
5. Ehman RL, Felmlee JP. Adaptive technique for high-definition MR imaging of moving structures. *Radiology* 1989; 173:255–263.
6. Yucel EK, Anderson CM, Edelman RR, et al. AHA scientific statement: Magnetic resonance angiography: Update on applications for extracranial arteries. *Circulation* 1999; 100:2284–2301.
7. Bailes DR, Gilderdale DJ, Bydder GM, et al. Respiratory ordered phase encoding (ROPE): A method for reducing respiratory motion artefacts in MR imaging. *J Comput Assist Tomogr* 1985; 9:835–838.
8. Simonetti OP, Finn JP, White RD, et al. "Black blood" T2-weighted inversion-recovery MR imaging of the heart. *Radiology*. 1996; 199:49–57.
9. Le Roux P, Gilles RJ, McKinnon GC, et al. Optimized outer volume suppression for single-shot fast spin-echo cardiac imaging. *J Magn Reson Imaging* 1998; 8:1022–1032.
10. Pislaru SV, Ni Y, Pislaru C, et al. Noninvasive measurements of infarct size after thrombolysis with a necrosis-avid MRI contrast agent. *Circulation* 1999; 99:690–696.
11. Atkinson DJ, Edelman RR. Cineangiography of the heart in a single breath hold with a segmented turboFLASH sequence. *Radiology* 1991; 178:357–360.
12. Foo TK, Bernstein MA, Aisen AM, et al. Improved ejection fraction and flow velocity estimates with use of view sharing and uniform repetition time excitation with fast cardiac techniques. *Radiology* 1995; 195:471–478.
13. Schmitt F, Stehling MK, Turner R. *Echo-Planar Imaging: Theory, Technique and Application*. Berlin: Springer-Verlag; 1998.
14. Ding S, Wolff SD, Epstein FH. Improved coverage in dynamic contrast-enhanced cardiac MRI using interleaved gradient-echo EPI. *Magn Reson Med* 1998; 39:514–519.
15. Epstein FH, Wolff SD, Arai AE. Segmented k-space fast cardiac imaging using an echo-train readout. *Magn Reson Med* 1999; 41:609–613.
16. Schwitter J, Debatin JF, von Schulthess GK, et al. Normal myocardial perfusion assessed with multishot echo-planar imaging. *Magn Reson Med* 1997; 37:140–147.
17. Lamb HJ, Doornbos J, van der Velde EA, et al. Echo planar MRI of the heart on a standard system: Validation of measurements of left ventricular function and mass. *J Comput Assist Tomogr* 1996; 20:942–949.
18. Mckinnon GC, Debatin JF, Wetter DR, et al. Interleaved echo planar flow quantitation. *Magn Reson Med* 1994; 32:263–267.
19. Wielopolski PA, van Geuns RJ, de Feyter PJ, et al. Breath-hold coronary MR angiography with volume-targeted imaging. *Radiology* 1998; 209:209–219.
20. Meyer CH, Hu BS, Nishimura DG, et al. Fast spiral coronary artery imaging. *Magn Reson Med* 1992; 28:202–213.
21. Meyer CH, Pauly JM, Macovski A, et al. Simultaneous spatial and spectral selective excitation. *Magn Reson Med* 1990; 15:287–304.
22. Irarrazabal P, Meyer CH, Nishimura DG, et al. Inhomogeneity correction using an estimated linear field map. *Magn Reson Med* 1996; 35:278–282.
23. Liao JR, Sommer FG, Herfkens RJ, et al. Cine spiral imaging. *Magn Reson Med* 1995; 34:490–493.
24. Hardy CJ, Darrow RD, Pauly JM, et al. Interactive coronary MRI. *Magn Reson Med* 1998; 40:105–111.
25. Yang PC, Kerr AB, Liu AC, et al. New real-time interactive cardiac magnetic resonance imaging system complements echocardiography. *J Am Coll Cardiol* 1998; 32:2049–2056.
26. Pelc NJ, Herfkens RJ, Shimakawa A, et al. Phase contrast cine magnetic resonance imaging [review]. *Magn Reson Q* 1991; 7:229–254.
27. Bernstein MA, Ikezaki Y. Comparison of phase-difference and complex-difference processing in phase-contrast MR angiography. *J Magn Reson Imaging* 1991; 1:725–729.
28. Lund GK, Sakuma H, Higgins CB. Coronary flow reserve: Assessment by magnetic resonance imaging. *Rays* 1999; 24:119–130.
29. Kawada N, Sakuma H, Yamakado T, et al. Hypertrophic cardiomyopathy: MR measurement of coronary blood flow and vasodilator flow reserve in patients and healthy subjects. *Radiology* 1999; 211:129–135.
30. Wedding KL, Grist TM, Folts JD, et al. Coronary flow and flow reserve in canines using MR phase difference and complex difference processing. *Magn Reson Med* 1998; 40:656–665.
31. Polzin JA, Frayne R, Grist TM, et al. Frequency response of multi-phase segmented k-space phase-contrast. *Magn Reson Med* 1996; 35:755–762.
32. Prince MR. Gadolinium-enhanced MR aortography. *Radiology* 1994; 191:155–164.
33. Fayad ZA, Connick TJ, Axel L. An improved quadrature or phased-array coil for MR cardiac imaging. *Magn Reson Med* 1995; 34:186–193.
34. Duerinckx AJ. Coronary MR angiography. *Radiol Clin North Am* 1999; 37:273–318.
35. Danias PG, Edelman RR, Manning WJ. Coronary MR angiography. *Cardiol Clin* 1998; 16:207–225.
36. Woodard PK, Li D, Zheng J, et al. Coronary MR angiography. *Magn Reson Imaging Clin North Am* 1999; 7:365–378.
37. Lieberman LM, Botti RE, Nelson AD. Magnetic resonance of the heart. *Radiol Clin North Am* 1994; 22:847–858.
38. Paulin S, von Schulthess GK, Fossel E, et al. MR imaging of the aortic root and proximal coronary arteries. *AJR* 1987; 148:665–670.
39. Manning WJ, Li W, Edelman RR. A preliminary report comparing magnetic resonance coronary angiography with conventional angiography. *N Engl J Med* 1993; 328:828–832.
40. Pennell DJ, Bogren HG, Keegan J, et al. Assessment of coronary artery stenosis by magnetic resonance imaging. *Heart* 1996; 75:127–133.
41. Duerinckx AJ, Urman MK. Two-dimensional coronary MR angi-

ography: Analysis of initial clinical results. *Radiology* 1994; 193:731–738.
42. Slavin GS, Riederer SJ, Ehman RL. Two-dimensional multishot echo-planar coronary MR angiography. *Magn Reson Med* 1998; 40:883–889.
43. Foo TKF, Ho VB, Hood MN. A novel method for improved visualization of coronary arteries: Prospective slice selective adjustment for coronary artery positional variation over the cardiac cycle. In: *Proceedings of the International Society for Magnetic Resonance in Medicine*, 6th Scientific Meeting. Sydney, Australia, 1998:862.
44. Li D, Kaushikkar S, Haacke EM, et al. Coronary arteries: Three-dimensional MR imaging with retrospective respiratory gating. *Radiology* 1996; 201:857–863.
45. Stuber M, Botnar RM, Danias PG, et al. Double-oblique free-breathing high resolution three-dimensional coronary magnetic resonance angiography. *J Am Coll Cardiol* 1999; 34:524–531.
46. Botnar RM, Stuber M, Danias PG, et al. Improved coronary artery definition with T2-weighted, free-breathing, three-dimensional coronary MRA. *Circulation* 1999; 99:3139–3148.
47. Li D, Paschal CB, Haacke EM, et al. Coronary arteries: Three-dimensional MR imaging with fat saturation and magnetization transfer contrast. *Radiology* 1993; 187:401–406.
48. Cline HE, Thedens DR, Irarrazaval P, et al. 3D MR coronary artery segmentation. *Magn Reson Med* 1998; 40:697–702.
49. Hofman MB, Paschal CB, Li D, et al. MRI of coronary arteries: 2D breath-hold vs 3D respiratory-gated acquisition. *J Comput Assist Tomogr* 1995; 19:56–62.
50. Paschal CB, Haacke EM, Adler LP. Three-dimensional MR imaging of the coronary arteries: Preliminary clinical experience. *J Magn Reson Imaging* 1993; 3:491–500.
51. Wang Y, Grimm RC, Rossman PJ, et al. 3D coronary MR angiography in multiple breath-holds using a respiratory feedback monitor. *Magn Reson Med* 1995; 34:11–16.
52. Oshinski JN, Hofland L, Mukundan S Jr, et al. Two-dimensional coronary MR angiography without breath holding. *Radiology* 1996; 201:737–743.
53. Bornert P, Jensen D. Coronary artery imaging at 0.5 T using segmented 3D echo planar imaging. *Magn Reson Med* 1995; 34:779–785.
54. Taylor AM, Keegan J, Jhooti P, et al. Differences between normal subjects and patients with coronary artery disease for three different MR coronary angiography respiratory suppression techniques. *J Magn Reson Imaging* 1999; 9:786–793.
55. Lethimonnier F, Furber A, Morel O, et al. Three-dimensional coronary artery MR imaging using prospective real-time respiratory navigator and linear phase shift processing: Comparison with conventional coronary angiography. *Magn Reson Imaging* 1999; 17:1111–1120.
56. McConnell MV, Khasgiwala VC, Savord BJ, et al. Comparison of respiratory suppression methods and navigator locations for MR coronary angiography. *AJR* 1997; 168:1369–1375.
57. Muller MF, Fleisch M, Kroeker R, et al. Proximal coronary artery stenosis: Three-dimensional MRI with fat saturation and navigator echo. *J Magn Reson Imaging* 1997; 7:644–651.
58. Stuber M, Botnar RM, Danias PG, et al. Submillimeter three-dimensional coronary MR angiography with real-time navigator correction: Comparison of navigator locations. *Radiology* 1999; 212:579–587.
59. Goldfarb JW, Edelman RR. Coronary arteries: Breath-hold, gadolinium-enhanced, three-dimensional MR angiography. *Radiology* 1998; 206:830–834.
60. Kessler W, Laub G, Achenbach S, et al. Coronary arteries: MR angiography with fast contrast-enhanced three-dimensional breath-hold imaging—Initial experience. *Radiology* 1999; 210:566–572.
61. Li D, Zheng J, Bae KT, et al. Contrast-enhanced magnetic resonance imaging of the coronary arteries: A review. *Invest Radiol* 1998; 33:578–586.
62. White CS, Laskey WK, Stafford JL, et al. Coronary MRA: Use in assessing anomalies of coronary artery origin. *J Comput Assist Tomogr* 1999; 23:203–207.
63. Oshinski JN, Franch R, Shirazi SH, et al. Use of navigator-echo-gated MRI to diagnose a coronary shunt involving an anomalous origin of the right coronary artery from the pulmonary artery. *J Magn Reson Imaging* 1999; 9:738–740.
64. Duerinckx AJ, Lewis BS, Louie HW, et al. MRI of pseudoaneurysm of a brachial venous coronary bypass graft. *Cathet Cardiovasc Diagn* 1996; 37:281–286.
65. Galjee MA, van Rossum AC, Doesburg T, et al. Quantification of coronary artery bypass graft flow by magnetic resonance phase velocity mapping. *Magn Reson Imaging* 1996; 14:485–493.
66. Hoogendoorn LI, Pattynama PM, Buis B, et al. Noninvasive evaluation of aortocoronary bypass grafts with magnetic resonance flow mapping. *Am J Cardiol* 1995; 75:845–848.
67. Wintersperger BJ, Engelmann MG, von Smekal A, et al. Patency of coronary bypass grafts: Assessment with breath-hold contrast-enhanced MR angiography—Value of a non-electrocardiographically triggered technique. *Radiology* 1998; 208:345–351.
68. Brenner P, Wintersperger B, von Smekal A, et al. Detection of coronary artery bypass graft patency by contrast enhanced magnetic resonance angiography. *Eur J Cardiothorac Surg* 1999; 15:389–393.
69. Sigwart U, Puel J, Mirkovitch V, et al. Intravascular stents to prevent occlusion and restenosis after transluminal angioplasty. *N Engl J Med* 1987; 316:701–706.
70. Ruygrok PN, Serruys PW. Intracoronary stenting: From concept to custom. *Circulation* 1996; 94:882–890.
71. Shellock FG. *Pocket Guide to MR Procedures and Metallic Objects: Update 1998.* Philadelphia: Lippincott-Raven; 1998.
72. Bernardino ME, Steinberg HV, Pearson TC, et al. Shunts for portal hypertension: MR and angiography for determination of patency. *Radiology* 1986; 158:57–61.
73. New PF, Rosen BR, Brady TJ, et al. Potential hazards and artifacts of ferromagnetic and nonferromagnetic surgical and dental materials and devices in nuclear magnetic resonance imaging. *Radiology* 1983; 147:139–148.
74. Strohm O, Kivelitz D, Gross W, et al. Safety of implantable coronary stents during 1H-magnetic resonance imaging at 1.0 and 1.5 T. *J Cardiol Magn Res* 1999; 1:239–245.
75. Duerinckx AJ, Atkinson D, Hurwitz R. Assessment of coronary artery patency after stent placement using magnetic resonance angiography. *J Magn Reson Imaging* 1998; 8:896–902.
76. Hilfiker PR, Quick HH, Debatin JF. Plain and covered stent-grafts: In vitro evaluation of characteristics at three-dimensional MR angiography. *Radiology* 1999; 211:693–697.
77. Bogren HG, Buonocore MH. Measurement of coronary artery flow reserve by magnetic resonance velocity mapping in the aorta. *Lancet* 1993; 342:899–900.
78. Grist TM, Polzin JA, Bianco JA, et al. Measurement of coronary blood flow and flow reserve using magnetic resonance imaging. *Cardiology* 1997; 88:80–89.
79. Sakuma H, Saeed M, Takeda K, et al. Quantification of coronary artery volume flow rate using fast velocity-encoded cine MR imaging. *AJR* 1997; 168:1363–1367.
80. Hundley WG, Hamilton CA, Clarke GD, et al. Visualization and functional assessment of proximal and middle left anterior descending coronary stenoses in humans with magnetic resonance imaging. *Circulation* 1999; 99:3248–3254.
81. Hundley WG, Clarke GD, Landau C, et al. Noninvasive determination of infarct artery patency by cine magnetic resonance angiography. *Circulation* 1995; 91:1347–1353.
82. Sakuma H, Globits S, O'Sullivan M, et al. Breath-hold MR measurements of blood flow velocity in internal mammary arteries

and coronary artery bypass grafts. *J Magn Reson Imaging* 1996; 6:219–222.
83. Fuster V, Fayad ZA, Badimon JJ. Acute coronary syndromes: Biology. *Lancet* 1999; 353(suppl 2):SII5–SII9.
84. Fayad ZA, Fuster V. Characterization of atherosclerotic plaques by magnetic resonance imaging. *Ann NY Acad Sci* 2000; 902:173–188.
85. Toussaint JF, LaMuraglia GM, Southern JF, et al. Magnetic resonance images lipid, fibrous, calcified, hemorrhagic, and thrombotic components of human atherosclerosis in vivo. *Circulation* 1996; 94:932–938.
86. Fayad ZA, Nahar T, Badimon JJ, et al. In-vivo MR characterization of plaques in the thoracic aorta. *Circulation* 1998; 98:S-515.
87. Fayad ZA, Nahar T, Fallon JT, et al. In vivo MR evaluation of atherosclerotic plaques in the human thoracic aorta: A comparison with TEE. *Circulation* 2000; 101:2503–2509.
88. Shinnar M, Fallon JT, Wehrli S, et al. The diagnostic accuracy of ex vivo magnetic resonance imaging for human atherosclerotic plaque characterization. *Arterioscler Thromb Vasc Biol* 1999; 19:2756–2761.
89. Worthley SG, Helft G, Fuster V, et al. High resolution ex vivo magnetic resonance imaging of in situ coronary and aortic atherosclerotic plaque in a porcine model. *Atherosclerosis* 2000; 150:321–329.
90. Skinner MP, Yuan C, Mitsumori L, et al. Serial magnetic resonance imaging of experimental atherosclerosis detects lesion fine structure, progression and complications in vivo. *Nat Med* 1995; 1:69–73.
91. Worthley SG, Heft G, Fuster V, et al. Serial in vivo magnetic resonance imaging documents arterial remodeling in experimental atherosclerosis. *Circulation* 2000; 101:586–589.
92. Fayad ZA, Fallon JT, Shinnar M, et al. Noninvasive in vivo high-resolution magnetic resonance imaging of atherosclerotic lesions in genetically engineered mice. *Circulation* 1998; 98:1541–1547.
93. Worthley SG, Helft G, Fuster V, et al. In vivo high-resolution MRI non-invasively defines coronary lesion size and composition in a porcine model. *Circulation* 1999; 100:I-521.
94. Fayad ZA, Fuster V, Fallon JT, et al. Human coronary atherosclerotic wall imaging using in vivo high resolution MR. *Circulation* 1999; 100:I-520–I-521.
95. Fayad ZA, Fuster V, Fallon JT, et al. Noninvasive in vivo human coronary artery lumen and wall imaging using black blood magnetic resonance. *Circulation* 2000; (August 8):102.
96. Nienaber CA, von Kodolitsch Y, Nicolas V, et al. The diagnosis of thoracic aortic dissection by noninvasive imaging procedures. *N Engl J Med* 1993; 328:1–9.
97. Laissy JP, Blanc F, Soyer P, et al. Thoracic aortic dissection: Diagnosis with transesophageal echocardiography versus MR imaging. *Radiology* 1995; 194:331–336.
98. Nienaber CA, von Kodolitsch Y, Brockhoff CJ, et al. Comparison of conventional and transesophageal echocardiography with magnetic resonance imaging for anatomical mapping of thoracic aortic dissection: A dual noninvasive imaging study with anatomical and/or angiographic validation. *Int J Card Imaging* 1994; 10:1–14.
99. Link KM, Lesko NM. Magnetic resonance angiography: Great vessels and abdomen. In: *Magnetic Resonance Imaging.* St. Louis: Mosby; 1999:373.
100. Nienaber CA, von Kodolitsch Y, Petersen B, et al. Intramural hemorrhage of the thoracic aorta: Diagnostic and therapeutic implications. *Circulation* 1995; 92:1465–1472.
101. Wolff KA, Herold CJ, Tempany CM, et al. Aortic dissection; Atypical patterns seen at MR imaging. *Radiology* 1991; 181:489–495.
102. Webb WR, Sostman HD. MR imaging of thoracic disease: Clinical uses. *Radiology* 1992; 182:621–630.
103. Lee JK, Ling D, Heiken JP, et al. Magnetic resonance imaging of abdominal aortic aneurysms. *AJR* 1984; 143:1197–1202.
104. White EM, Edelman RR, Wedeen VJ, et al. Intravascular signal in MR imaging: Use of phase display for differentiation of blood-flow signal from intraluminal disease. *Radiology* 1986; 161: 245–249.
105. Von Schulthess GK, Augustiny N. Calculation of T2 values versus phase imaging for the distinction between flow and thrombus in MR imaging. *Radiology* 1987; 164:549–554.
106. Fellows KE, Weinberg PM, Baffa JM, et al. Evaluation of congenital heart disease with MR imaging: Current and coming attractions. *AJR* 1992; 159:925–931.
107. Hartnell GC. Great vessels of the chest. In: Bogaert J, Duerinckx AJ, Rademakers FE, eds. *Magnetic Resonance of the Heart and Great Vessels: Clinical Applications*. Berlin: Springer-Verlag; 1999:245.
108. Fawzy ME, Sivanandam V, Galal O, et al. One- to ten-year follow-up results of balloon angioplasty of native coarctation of the aorta in adolescents and adults. *J Am Coll Cardiol* 1997; 30:1542–1546.
109. Hartnell GG, Meier RA. MR angiography of congenital heart disease in adults. *Radiographics* 1995; 15:781–794.
110. Kawamoto S, Bluemke DA, Traill TA, et al. Thoracoabdominal aorta in Marfan syndrome: MR imaging findings of progression of vasculopathy after surgical repair. *Radiology* 1997; 203:727–732.
111. Atherosclerotic disease of the aortic arch as a risk factor for recurrent ischemic stroke: The French Study of Aortic Plaques in Stroke Group. *N Engl J Med* 1996; 334:1216–1221.
112. Montauban van Swijndregt AD, Elbers HR, Moll FL, et al. Ultrasonographic characterization of carotid plaques. *Ultrasound Med Biol* 1998; 24:489–493.

CHAPTER 19

POSITRON EMISSION TOMOGRAPHY FOR THE NONINVASIVE STUDY AND QUANTIFICATION OF BLOOD FLOW AND METABOLISM IN HUMAN CARDIAC DISEASE

Heinrich R. Schelbert

The study of the human heart with conventional radionuclide techniques remains confined to primarily ventricular function and relative distributions of regional myocardial blood flow (MBF). Positron emission tomography (PET) exceeds these capabilities. It offers the probing and defining regional functional processes in absolute units in the human heart spanning from MBF to biochemical reaction rates, substrate fluxes, and neuronal activity. The many positron-emitting, biologically active tracers, the quantitative imaging capability, and the in vivo application of tracer kinetic principles are unique to PET and account for this capability. The human heart's physiology and pathophysiology thus can be characterized more comprehensively. Also, novel insights into the function of the human heart can be gained, while, at the same time, PET can have a decisive impact on patient diagnosis and management. This chapter describes the key ingredients of PET and the tools for the evaluation and/or quantification of local functional processes in the human heart. It then examines how these tools can be applied to the diagnosis and characterization of coronary artery disease (CAD) and its consequences on regional myocardial function and discusses the impact of PET findings on patient management.

TOOLS FOR PROBING MYOCARDIAL TISSUE FUNCTION

Fundamental to the uniqueness of PET are (1) the quantitative imaging and high temporal resolution capability, (2) the in vivo application of tracer kinetic principles, and (3) the large number of physiologically active radiotracers.

Imaging with Positron-Emitting Radiopharmaceuticals

DEDICATED PET SYSTEMS

The quantitative imaging capability results from the physical properties unique to positrons. After losing their kinetic energy, they combine with an electron and "annihilate." The annihilation represents a conversion of mass into energy; i.e., the combined mass of the positron and the electron converts into two 511-keV photons that leave the site of the annihilation in diametrically opposed directions. If both strike two scintillation detectors connected by a coincidence circuitry at the same time, an annihilation event is registered. Its location in space can be defined by circular arrays of scintillation detectors. The near-simultaneous arrival of two 511-keV photons at the two scintillation detectors positioned in opposite directions allows the use of tomographic reconstruction algorithms analogous to those used with x-ray computed tomography. Accordingly, the spatial resolution throughout the image plane is rather homogeneous, unlike that obtainable with single-photon-emission computed tomography (SPECT), where the spatial resolution declines as a function of the distance between the imaged object and the scintillation detectors. Further, by acquiring "transmission" images with external rotating or circular sources of positron-emitting isotopes, the images of the tracer tissue concentrations ("emission" images) can be corrected for photon attenuation so that the resulting tomographic images represent accurately the true regional radioactivity concentrations (mCi or MBq/cm^3). Current PET systems offer spatial resolutions of as high as 4 to 5 mm full-width half-maximum (FWHM). Further, because modern tomographs are stationary circular devices, images can be acquired at sampling rates in the range of seconds. It is therefore possible with PET to rapidly measure changing radiotracer concentrations in tissues.

COMBINED SPECT AND PET

Several institutions use SPECT and PET for the evaluation of cardiovascular disease. For example, the distribution of MBF is determined with ^{201}Tl- or ^{99m}Tc-labeled tracers of MBF and SPECT and then compared with the distribution of myocardial glucose use by imaging [^{18}F]deoxyglucose with dedicated PET systems.[1-3] While this approach yields a diagnostic accuracy comparable with that achieved with dedicated PET systems, diagnostic difficulties can arise due to differences in the geometry of the heart and spatial resolution on SPECT and PET images, as well as artifacts on the SPECT images due to photon attenuation, especially of the inferior wall and the interventricular septum.[4,5]

MULTIPURPOSE IMAGING SYSTEMS

Most clinical applications of PET do not require assessment of functional processes in absolute units. This is particularly true for the identification of myocardial viability and, to some extent, for the detection of CAD. In view of the high cost of dedicated PET systems, lower-cost "hybrid" or "multipurpose" imaging systems are now available. Generally, two types of systems have emerged (Fig. 19-1). One is a SPECT-like system equipped with ultra-high-energy general-purpose collimators to accommodate the 511-keV photons of positrons instead of the 70- to 160-keV photon energies of conventional radiotracers. When used together with ^{201}Tl- or ^{99m}Tc-labeled flow tracers, the [^{18}F]deoxyglucose images provide diagnostic information comparable with that available with dedicated PET systems.[6-11] The second type of system entails a SPECT-like dual-head device with coincidence detection. While highly promising because of its superior spatial resolution, its use is still evolving, and clinical studies are scarce.[12] Initial studies demonstrate a spatial and contrast resolution that is superior to the high-energy-collimator SPECT system and approaches that of dedicated PET systems. Critical, however, is appropriate correction for photon attenuation that now seems feasible with 511-keV photon sources.[13] Both camera types also can be used for conventional single-photon-emitting tracers, hence the name *hybrid* or *multipurpose* systems.

Tracer Kinetic Principles

Positron-emitting isotopes of elements that constitute major parts of living matter such as carbon-11 (^{11}C), nitrogen-13 (^{13}N), and oxygen-15 (^{15}O) are inserted into biomolecules without disturbing their very physiologic properties. Their high specific activity (radioactivity per mass) permits administration of true tracer quantities without exerting a mass effect and perturbing

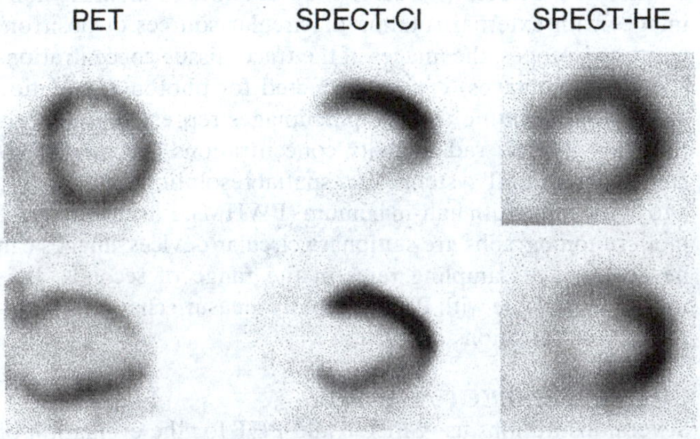

FIGURE 19-1 Examples of myocardial [^{18}F]deoxyglucose images obtained with PET (*left*), a SPECT-like system with coincidence detection (CI, *middle panel*) (courtesy Dr. R. Henkins, Chicago, IL), and a SPECT system equipped with an ultra-high-energy-photon general-purpose collimator (HE). For the SPECT-CI images, the non-attenuation-corrected image is shown on top and the corrected image at the bottom.

the very process to be studied. Since their physical half-life is short, functional processes can be measured repeatedly or different aspects of the myocardial tissue function can be explored within the same study session. The radioactivity concentrations of these tracers in tissues such as arterial blood and myocardium and their changes over time can be determined noninvasively. The time-activity curves derived from serially acquired tomographic images at sampling rates of 1 to 10 s are fitted with operational equations that are derived from tracer kinetic models and yield quantitative estimates of regional functional processes. Tracer compartment models describe the distribution of the tracer radiolabel in tissue and its time-dependent changes. Because only the activity concentration of the tracer radiolabel can be measured externally, these models relate the externally derived signal to the metabolic fate of the tracer label and its relationship to the functional process under study. Such tracer kinetic models typically consist of functional rather than anatomic pools or compartments that contain the radiotracer or its metabolites. Exchange of radiotracers between compartments is described typically by first-order rate constants. Flux of a radiotracer through a given compartment depends on the flux rate of tracer or of its metabolite and on the size of the compartment. Tracer compartment models provide the basis for developing operational equations; applied to the externally derived radioactivity signal as, for example, tissue time-activity curves, estimates of regional functional processes are derived in absolute units.

Positron-Emitting Tracers of Myocardial Tissue Function

BLOOD VOLUME AND TISSUE CHARACTERIZATION

Blood can readily be radiolabeled with minute quantities of ^{15}O or ^{11}C carbon monoxide (CO). Once inhaled, the radiolabeled CO binds to hemoglobin, thereby tagging red blood cells. The latter serve to define the components of the myocardium in terms of vascular space, viable and normal myocytes, and scar tissue. One such characterization assumes that only living myocytes exchange water rapidly.[14] Transmission images represent the densities of the various tissues in the chest. They resemble low-spatial-resolution x-ray computed tomographic (CT) images and delineate the volume of the myocardium together with the blood in its cavities. The true extravascular volume is obtained by subtracting blood pool images from the transmission images. The fraction of the extravascular volume that exchanges water rapidly is then estimated with ^{15}O-labeled water and is referred to as the *water perfusable tissue index* (PTI). If all the extravascular volume does indeed rapidly exchange water, then the PTI approaches unity.[14] If a portion of the myocardium is injured irreversibly and scar tissue has formed, this fraction becomes less than unity.[15,16] Further, the PTI also will be reduced in diffuse interstitial fibrosis. Initial clinical investigations demonstrated that the fraction of irreversibly injured myocardium or of regional scar tissue formation does indeed indicate whether an impairment in contractile function is irreversible or whether a postrevascularization improvement is likely.[15] If functionally compromised but viable myocardium exchanges water as rapidly as normal myocardium, this may limit the predictive value of the PTI. In recent observations, a reduced PTI had a high negative predictive value, but a near-normal PTI predicted less accurately than [^{18}F]deoxyglucose an improvement in contractile dysfunction.[17] Moreover, the sum of viable and normal myocytes in a given myocardial segment also serves as a reference to which transmural estimates of MBF or substrate metabolism can be related.[18]

MYOCARDIAL BLOOD FLOW

Several approaches exist for measurements of regional MBF in absolute units. Tracers such as ^{82}Rb or [^{13}N]ammonia are retained in myocardium in proportion to MBF.[19,20] Images of their regional activity concentrations in the myocardium depict the relative distribution of MBF at the time of tracer injection. Each tracer offers advantages and disadvantages. For example, ^{82}Rb is available through a generator based pushbutton-operated infusion system and hence is easy to use clinically.[21] Its physical half-life of only 75 s affords repeat studies at only 10-min time intervals, enabling evaluation of changes in regional MBF in response to physiologic or pharmacologic interventions. The short physical half-life, however, can result in low-count and, thus, statistically noisy images. The longer physical half-life of [^{13}N]ammonia (10 min), by contrast, produces images of higher count rates and higher diagnostic quality but requires 40- to 50-min time intervals between studies.[20]

The various approaches yield comparable estimates of MBF in the human myocardium during rest and during pharmacologically induced hyperemia.[22-27] Some variability between studies probably derives from methodologic differences but also from intergroup differences in the hemodynamic state. Importantly, MBF in the normal myocardium depends largely on oxygen demand and thus on cardiac work as estimated from the rate pressure product.[28] Thus individual flow measurements should be interpreted within the context of the rate-pressure product.[29] Finally, gender-related differences in MBF have been reported. Compared with an age-matched group of males, women demonstrated higher MBFs both at rest and during hyperemia, which the authors attributed to higher high-density lipoprotein (HDL) cholesterol and lower triglyceride plasma levels in females.[30]

Repeat studies in the same normal volunteers report a 10 ± 11 percent *reproducibility* (average percentage difference of flows normalized to the rate pressure product) for rest MBF and a 12 ± 9 percent reproducibility for hyperemic MBFs.[31] Other studies report similar values for both, [^{13}N]ammonia and for [^{15}O]water.[32,33] Furthermore, the validity of the noninvasive measurements of MBF has been extensively established in animal experiments,[22,27,34-36] as well as in humans, using intracoronary flow velocity probes.[37]

MYOCARDIAL SUBSTRATE METABOLISM

Figure 19-2 depicts the major aspects of the myocardial substrate metabolism. According to this simplified depiction, the myocardium chooses between various substrates; foremost are free fatty acid (FFA), glucose, lactate, and ketone bodies. Selection of a given fuel substrate depends largely on its concentration in plasma and the overall hormonal milieu.[38,39] These in turn are governed by the dietary state, the level of physical activity, and the plasma concentrations of catecholamines, insulin, and glucagon. In the fasting state, circulating FFA levels are high and insulin levels are low so that as much as 70 to 80 percent of the myocardium's oxygen consumption can be accounted for by oxidation of FFA.[40] Conversely, oral glucose

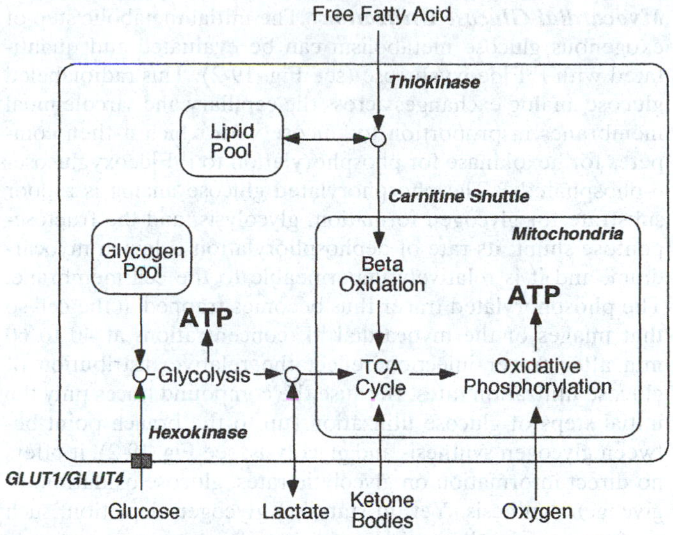

FIGURE 19-2 Highly simplified depiction of the myocardium's substrate metabolism (TCA, tricarboxylic acid; ATP, adenosine triphosphate; GLUT1 and GLUT4, glucose transporters 1 and 4).

intake elevates the plasma glucose level and thus insulin levels while lowering FFA levels so that myocardium shifts its fuel selection to glucose.[39] Strenuous physical exercise increases plasma levels of lactate, which then becomes the major fuel substrate.[41,42] In fact, as much as 60 percent of the O_2 consumption can be accounted for by oxidation of lactate. On the other hand, catecholamines accelerate lipolysis so that circulating FFA levels increase, shifting the heart's substrate selection to FFA.

Glucose enters the cell via facilitated transport systems, the largely insulin-independent glucose transporter GLUT1 and the largely insulin-dependent glucose transporter GLUT4. The hexokinase reaction phosphorylates glucose to glucose-6-phosphate. This compound then may be synthesized to glycogen or, alternatively, enter glycolysis with pyruvate as its end product. Converted to lactate, it may leave the myocardium or, if activated to acetyl-CoA, enters the tricarboxylic acid (TCA) cycle as the final oxidative pathway shared by most fuel substrates. Exogenous lactate can be converted via NAD^+ to pyruvate, which then again after esterification to acyl-CoA enters the TCA cycle. FFA also may enter two different metabolic pathways. On entering the cells, it is esterified by the thiokinase reaction to acetyl-CoA. This compound then enters an endogenous lipid pool, consisting mostly of glycerides and phospholipids, and/or proceeds via the carnitine shuttle to the inner mitochondrial membrane. It is there where β-oxidation cleaves of the long-chain acyl-CoA units' two-carbon fragments, which then engage in the TCA cycle. The TCA cycle metabolizes the two-carbon units into CO_2 and H_2O. The rate of flux through the TCA cycle is coupled closely with oxidative phosphorylation, where the energy resulting from the synthesis of oxygen and hydrogen ions is stored in the high-energy phosphate bonds of adenosine triphosphate (ATP). The latter is shuttled into the cytosol with transfer of energy to the high-energy phosphate bond of creatine phosphate. Other sites of high-energy production include glycolysis. The energy yields relative to oxygen differ between the various substrates; e.g., for 1 mol of oxygen, glucose yields 6.3, lactate 6, and FFA 5.7 mol ATP.[43]

Myocardial Glucose Utilization The initial metabolic step of exogenous glucose metabolism can be evaluated and quantitated with [^{18}F]deoxyglucose (see Fig. 19-2). This radiolabeled glucose analog exchanges across the capillary and sarcolemmal membranes in proportion to glucose with which it then competes for hexokinase for phosphorylation to [^{18}F]deoxyglucose-6-phosphate.[44,45] The phosphorylated glucose analog is a poor substrate for glycogen formation, glycolysis, and the fructose-pentose shunt; its rate of dephosphorylation is low in myocardium, and it is relatively impermeable to the cell membrane. The phosphorylated tracer thus becomes trapped in the cell so that images of the myocardial ^{18}F concentrations at 40 to 60 min after tracer injection reflect the relative distribution of glucose utilization rates. Because the compound traces only the initial steps of glucose utilization (up to the branch point between glycogen synthesis and glycolysis; see Fig. 19-2), it offers no direct information on glycolytic rates, glucose oxidation, or glycogen synthesis. Yet, in states of glycogen depletion, such as, for example, during ischemia, exogenous glucose serves as the major source of glycolytic flux so that [^{18}F]deoxyglucose may offer an estimate of the rate of glycolysis.

Myocardial Fatty Acid Metabolism This aspect of the substrate metabolism can be evaluated with 1-[^{11}C]palmitate. The labeled long-chain FFA participates fully in the metabolic fate of its natural counterpart (see Fig. 19-2). Once esterified to acyl-CoA, a fraction of tracer label proceeds via the carnitine shuttle into mitochondria, where β-oxidation catabolizes the long-chain fatty acid into two-carbon fragments that are oxidized via the TCA cycle. The label is released from the myocardium in the form of $^{11}CO_2$. The remaining fraction of the initially extracted and activated tracer enters intracellular lipid pools, mostly those of di- and triglycerides and phospholipids. The biexponential morphology of the myocardial time-activity curve reflects the metabolic fate of the tracer. The slow turnover rate of the intracellular lipid pools accounts for the slow clearance phase, whereas the rapid clearance curve component corresponds to the fraction of tracer that enters β-oxidation and its rate of oxidation. Ischemia reduces the rate of FFA oxidation and of TCA cycle activity. The relative size and rate of the rapid clearance curve component on the ^{11}C myocardial time-activity curve typically decline during acute myocardial ischemia.[46,47] A disproportionately greater fraction of tracer label then enters the slower-turnover endogenous lipid pool. Used mostly as a tracer for the qualitative evaluation of regional myocardial fatty acid metabolism, recent studies suggest the possibility of quantitating myocardial fatty acid oxidation in milliequivalents of FFA per gram of myocardium per minute.[48]

Preferential use of a given fuel substrate (e.g., glucose, lactate, or FFA) depends on its concentration in arterial blood, which, in turn, depends on dietary state, serum levels or insulin resistance, and physical stress.[49] A change in the myocardium's preferential substrate use can be demonstrated with either [^{11}C]palmitate and [^{18}F]deoxyglucose or both.[49–51] In the presence of high FFA and low glucose and insulin levels, use of FFA as the preferred substrate is reflected on the [^{11}C]palmitate curve by the large relative size of the rapid clearance phase and its steep slope (both corresponding to increased fatty acid oxidation) and the low or even undetectable [^{18}F]deoxyglucose uptake. Ingestion of carbohydrates raises plasma glucose levels, stimulates insulin secretion, and depresses FFA levels. The shift to glucose use is reflected by a decline in the size and slope of the rapid-clearance phase of [^{11}C]palmitate and by an increase in myocardial [^{18}F]deoxyglucose uptake.

Myocardial Oxygen Consumption (MVO_2) While molecular ^{15}O oxygen is available for measurements of the (MVO_2,[52,53] the more widely applied approach entails rapid serial imaging with [^{11}C]acetate. The radiotracer clears rapidly from blood into the myocardium and produces high signal-to-background images.[54–57] It directly traces the rate of substrate flux through the TCA cycle as the final oxidative pathway common to most fuel substrates. The rate of clearance of ^{11}C activity from the myocardium on serially acquired images corresponds to the TCA cycle activity and, because of its close coupling to oxidative phosphorylation, to oxidative metabolism and MVO_2. Of note, the tracer yields rate constants only, which can be converted into units of O_2 per minute per gram. Unlike [^{11}C]palmitate or [^{18}F]deoxyglucose, the clearance rate of [^{11}C]acetate from myocardium is relatively insensitive to changes in myocardial substrate utilization.[54] A tracer compartment model, based on biochemical assays of the tracer tissue kinetics of [^{14}C]acetate in isolated rat hearts[58] forms the base for estimating MVO_2 in absolute units in the human heart and, at the same time, of regional MBFs.[59,60]

CLINICAL APPLICATIONS

Clinical imaging of positron-emitting radionuclides with PET or PET-like devices is gaining momentum because of research showing the considerable potential for contributing to diagnosis, characterization, treatment, and monitoring of disease. New, lower-cost positron imaging devices and the availability of positron-emitting tracers through regional distribution centers have accelerated the pace of dissemination. Foremost in cardiology have been (1) the identification and characterization of CAD and (2) the detection of myocardial viability.

Identification and Characterization of CAD

GENERAL CONSIDERATIONS

Most studies with PET, such as, for example, those performed with [^{13}N]ammonia or ^{82}Rb, evaluate the relative distribution of MBF from the retention of tracer in the myocardium. More recent investigations use PET's quantitative capability for estimating regional MBF in milliliters of blood per minute per gram of myocardium in order to demonstrate abnormalities in vasomotion of the human coronary circulation during the early stages of coronary atherosclerosis.

Unlike other radionuclide approaches, PET employs almost exclusively pharmacologic stress for the detection of CAD and determination of its extent and functional significance. The transmission images, essential for correction of photon attenuation, must be acquired with the patient in exactly the same position as during the emission images. Both dipyridamole and adenosine afford the determination of the myocardial flow reserve as the ratio of hyperemic to rest MBFs. The now classic studies by Gould et al.[61] demonstrated a curvilinear, inverse correlation between stenosis severity and hyperemic flows or flow reserve. Thus the attenuation of the MBF response to dipyridamole induced hyperemia depends on the functional stenosis severity. As demonstrated by flow measurements with either [^{15}O]water or [^{13}N]ammonia, dipyridamole and adenosine as direct vascular smooth muscle dilators evoke interindividually variable hyperemic responses but induce on average four- to fivefold increases in MBF.[22,23,25,62] The magnitude of the hyperemic flow response is similar for dipyridamole (at a dose of 0.56 mg/kg over 4 min) and for adenosine (140 μg/kg/min).[26] Increases in the dipyridamole dose by 50 percent do not produce higher flows, nor do they reduce the interpatient variability in flow responses.[63] Additionally, the values of the normal flow reserve were derived from studies in young normal volunteers with an average age of 34 ± 16 years. This is important as evidence accumulates that flow reserve declines progressively with age[64–66] (Fig. 19-3). Contributing factors include an age-dependent *decline* in the vasodilator capacity and an age-dependent *increase* in baseline MBF due to higher rate-pressure products as a major determinant of MBF. A progressive decline in vascular compliance is another possible explanation. Surprisingly, increases in the mean arterial blood pressure due to either isometric handgrip exercise or supine bicycle exercise attenuated the maximum flow response, most likely because of increased vascular resistance due to greater extravascular resistive forces.[63,67] These factors also may contribute to lesser flow increases during physical exercise when flow increases in proportion to MVO_2. Thus pharmacologically induced hyperemia may not necessarily prove to be more accurate in identifying functionally significant coronary stenoses. Even though flows in remote myocardium may rise less with exercise depending on the level of cardiac work, higher intracavitary left ventricular (LV) pressures and regional wall stresses in ischemic or dysfunctional myocardium may enhance extravascular resistive forces so that flow responses in stenosis-dependent myocardium in fact may be even more attenuated. Because of differences between pharmacologically and physically stressed-induced ischemia, the vasodilator reserve as determined pharmacologically may not necessarily reflect truly the myocardium's ability to raise flow during physical exercise. An example is hypertrophic cardiomyopathy, where MBF during exercise failed to increase despite some residual flow reserve demonstrated with dipyridamole.[68]

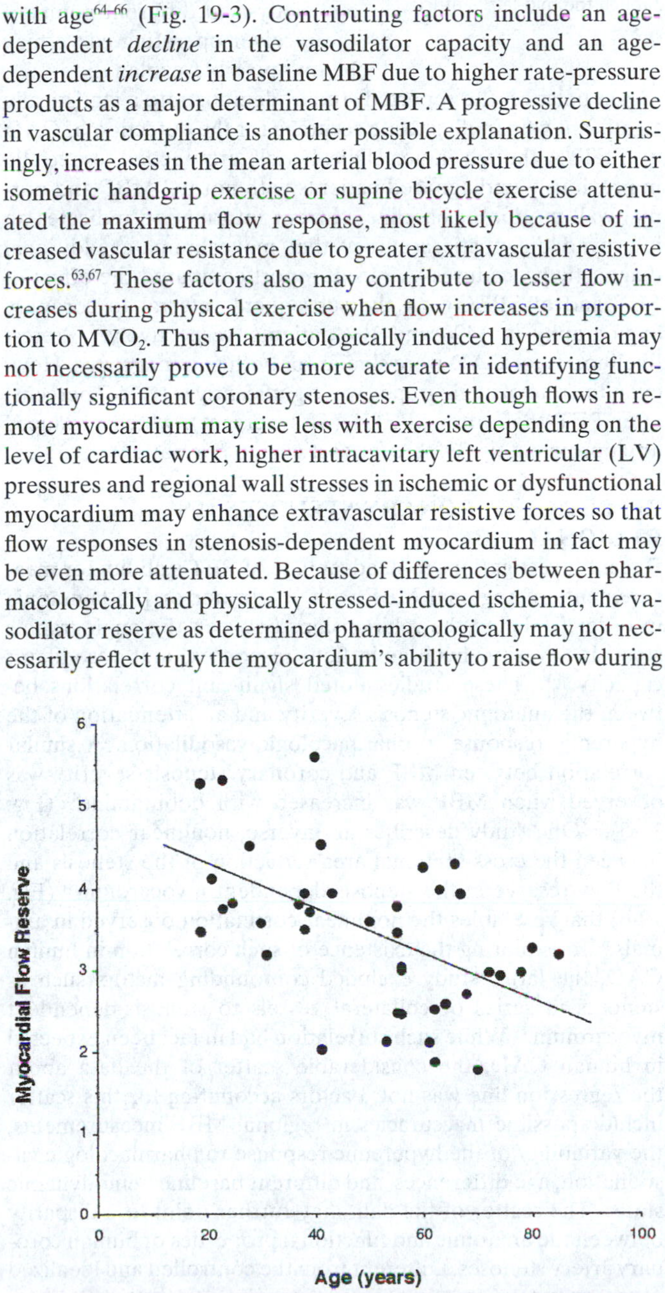

FIGURE 19-3 Progressive decline in myocardial perfusion reserve as a function of age in 40 normal volunteers. (Reproduced with permission of the American Heart Association from Czernin et al.[29])

Another important consideration with regard to pharmacologic stress is the variability of the hyperemic response. In normal individuals, responses range from about two- to sixfold increases in MBF. Several factors may account for this variability. Among these are (1) the coronary driving pressure, best reflected by the mean arterial blood pressure, (2) extravascular resistive forces as a function of wall tension and tension development, which in turn depend on the diastolic volume and the myocardium's contractile state, (3) β- and especially α-adrenergic control of the basic vasomotor tone,[69] (4) endothelial-dependent vasomotion, and (5) pharmacologic effects on vascular smooth muscle relaxation. The latter may be altered by antagonists of dipyridamole and adenosine, such as, for example, caffeine or theophylline-containing agents.[70] It thus is imperative that patients refrain from these substances for at least 24 h prior to a pharmacologic stress study.

Positive inotropic agents also are used for stress interventions. Dobutamine raises MBF in proportion to increases in cardiac work, as evidenced by increases in the rate pressure product.[71] In one study, intravenous infusion of dobutamine in normal volunteers at a rate of 40 μg/kg of body weight per minute increased the rate-pressure product by about 200 percent, which was paralleled by a 225 percent increase in MBF.[71] Lower infusion rates produced lesser increases in the rate-pressure product and thus in MBF.[72]

ASSESSMENT OF HEMODYNAMICALLY SIGNIFICANT CAD

For the detection of CAD, the relative distribution of MBF is examined at rest and during pharmacologic vasodilation. Either ^{82}Rb or [^{13}N]ammonia is used. Both are retained in myocardium in proportion to MBF so that the resulting images depict the distribution of MBF at rest and during hyperemia. The approach identifies flow defects at rest as well as attenuated responses of regional MBF to hyperemia as a consequence of a coronary stenosis (Fig. 19-4). The baseline and hyperemia flow images are analyzed by visual inspection combined with circumferential activity profile techniques or polar map approaches. While most studies rely on visual analysis, several laboratories employ quantitative image analysis. The regional tracer activity concentrations in a patient are compared with databases of normal displayed graphically in various cartographic forms, such as polar (or azimuthal) or cylindrical (Mercator-like) projections or surface rendered three-dimensional displays of the LV myocardium.[73–76]

Clinical investigations confirmed PET's high diagnostic performance for the detection of CAD.[77–83] Sensitivities range from 87 to 97 percent; and specificities from 78 to 100 percent. Most studies compared rest or stress-induced flow defects to arteriographic findings by visual analysis, and most defined a 50 to 70 percent diameter luminal narrowing as significant stenosis. Given the well-known limitation of visual analysis, Gould et al.[84] and, subsequently, Demer et al.[79] graded stenosis severity by estimates of coronary flow reserve by quantitative arteriography. Coronary arteries were classified as moderately to severely stenosed if the predicted coronary flow reserve was less than 3, as intermediate if the coronary flow reserve ranged from 3 to 4, and as minimal for coronary flow reserve values of greater

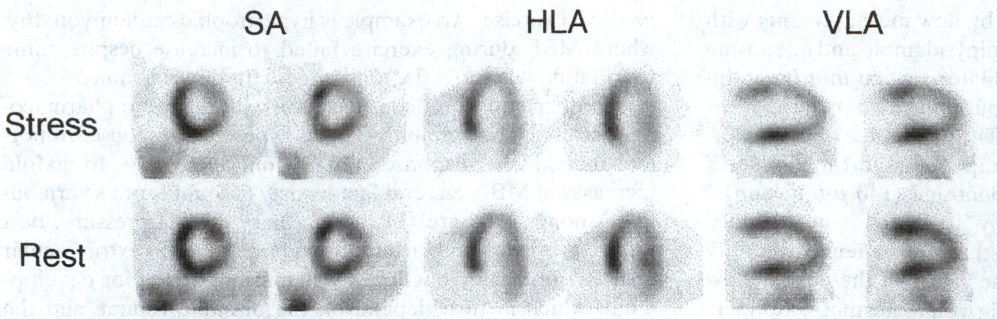

FIGURE 19-4 Stress induced perfusion defect in the lateral wall of the left ventricle, depicted each on two contiguous short- (SA), horizontal long- (HLA), and vertical long-axis slices (VLA) through the mid-left ventricle. Note the normalization of myocardial perfusion on the rest images.

than 4. According to this classification, 94 percent of vessels with moderate to severe, 49 percent of vessels with intermediate, and 5 percent of vessels with minimal stenosis were accurately identified with PET and pharmacologic vasodilator stress.

COMPARISON OF PET WITH CONVENTIONAL TECHNIQUES

The diagnostic accuracy of PET must be directly compared with that of more conventional approaches in order to define the diagnostic gain. (See also Chap. 16.) Demer et al.[79] indirectly compared their findings with those by another laboratory using ^{201}Tl SPECT but an identical angiographic approach for defining stenosis severity.[85] In this comparison, PET outperformed SPECT. Both studies defined stenosis severity by the angiographically predicted coronary flow reserve. Moderate to severe coronary stenoses were detected with a 95 percent sensitivity by PET and a 72 percent sensitivity by ^{201}Tl SPECT; intermediate stenoses were detected with a 49 percent sensitivity by PET, whereas none were detected by SPECT.

Other studies compared the PET with the SPECT approach in the same patients. An early study used supine bicycle stress and [^{13}N]ammonia in 48 patients with CAD and reported comparable diagnostic performances for PET and SPECT.[78] In another investigation of 202 patients, MBF was evaluated with ^{82}Rb at rest and again 4 min after the dipyridamole infusion.[80] About 8 to 9 min later, or a total of 12 to 13 min after the end of the dipyridamole infusion, ^{201}Tl was injected and SPECT imaging performed within 10 min. PET and SPECT exhibited comparable specificities, while PET demonstrated a significantly higher sensitivity than SPECT. The results were similar when only 132 of the 202 patients without prior cardiac events were analyzed. A third study reported somewhat different findings in 81 patients.[81] Again, all patients underwent rest and dipyridamole stress imaging with ^{82}Rb and PET; for the ^{201}Tl SPECT study, 38 (or 47 percent) of the patients underwent treadmill testing, and the remaining 43 (or 53 percent) underwent pharmacologic stress with dipyridamole. In that study, PET and SPECT exhibited comparable sensitivities; however, the specificity was higher for PET than for SPECT. The diagnostic accuracies were similar for patients submitted to treadmill stress testing and patients with pharmacologically induced hyperemia for SPECT imaging with ^{201}Tl.

Thus both studies demonstrate the high diagnostic accuracy for PET but differ in terms of higher sensitivities and specificities. The average decay half-time of 33 min for the hyperemic response amounts to an only 10 percent decline in the hyperemic response over a 4-min period[86] that is unlikely to fully explain the lower sensitivity of ^{201}Tl SPECT. The gain in specificity in the study by Stewart et al.[81] most likely resulted from the adequate correction of photon attenuation and thus a reduction of falsely positive findings. Although the reasons for the observed differences between both studies remain unclear, image analysis at different points of the receiver operating curve may be one possible explanation.

On balance, the reported studies demonstrate a statistically significant gain in diagnostic accuracy for the detection of CAD by PET. Although larger clinical trials are needed, especially in previously undiagnosed patients with normal MBF and normal wall motion at baseline, current information indicates an improved diagnostic accuracy that may eliminate additional diagnostic procedures. A recent report compared the effect of PET and of SPECT on the subsequent referral to coronary angiography in 1490 and 102 patients, respectively.[87] Pretest likelihoods for CAD were similar for both patient groups. However, the rate of angiography was significantly less (16.7 percent) after PET than after SPECT (31.4 percent), which produced an approximately 23 percent cost saving per patient.

EFFECT OF CORONARY STENOSES ON REGIONAL MBF

Recent investigations took advantage of PET's ability for measurements of regional MBF with [^{15}O]water or [^{13}N]ammonia in order to define the relationships between the angiographic stenosis severity, hyperemic flow responses, and vasodilator capacity.[88–90] These studies noted significant correlations between the anatomic stenosis severity and an attenuation of the hyperemic response to pharmacologic vasodilation. A similar correlation between MBF and coronary stenosis severity was observed when MBF was increased with dobutamine[41] (Fig. 19-5).[91] One study describes an inverse, nonlinear correlation between the cross-sectional area reduction of the stenosis and the flow reserve in the stenosis-dependent myocardium[84] (Fig. 19-6) that resembles the nonlinear correlation observed in animals.[61] In exploring the existence of such correlation in human CAD, the latter study excluded confounding factors such as stenoses in series or collateral vessels to stenosis-dependent myocardium.[89] While such correlation had in fact been expected in human CAD, the considerable scatter of the data about the regression line was not. Factors accounting for this scatter include possible inaccuracies in regional MBF measurements, the variability of the hyperemic response to pharmacologic vasodilation, age differences, and different baseline hemodynamic states. The scatter of the data may further point to a disparity between the anatomic and functional properties of human coronary artery stenoses. Different from the controlled and idealized coronary artery stenoses in the experimental setting, human coronary artery stenoses are of remarkably greater morphologic complexity, including eccentricity, variable stenosis inflow and outflow angles, and different lengths and irregular surfaces, that

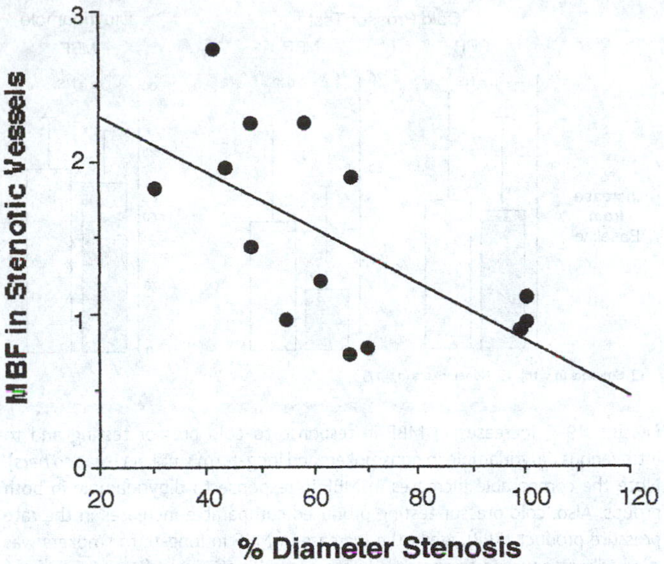

FIGURE 19-5 Correlation between coronary artery stenosis severity as determined by quantitative angiography and MBF in the stenosis-dependent myocardium during intravenous dobutamine infusion. (Reproduced with permission from Krivokapich et al.[228])

may not be fully appreciated by angiography nor be adequately accounted for by assumptions underlying model-based estimates of stenosis severity. It thus seems probable that the evaluation of flow, either semiquantitatively or quantitatively, renders more accurate functional information on the stenosis severity and, more broadly, on CAD. Moreover, estimates of an attenuated flow reserve obtained from static images of the relative distribution of MBF during hyperemic stress clearly offer invaluable information on the functional significance of coronary artery stenosis. Yet, in view of the nonlinear response in flow tracer uptake to increases in blood flow, such "semiquantitative" estimates would tend to be less accurate than those available through true measurements of MBF.

ASSESSMENT OF CORONARY VASOMOTION AND PRECLINICAL CAD

Noninvasive measurements of regional MBF offer the intriguing possibility to uncover vasomotor abnormalities of the human coronary circulation. If such abnormalities exist already during the early stages of CAD, it then may become possible to detect the disease during its evolutionary and preclinical stages. Such measurements further offer the prospect of monitoring disease progression as well as the responses to interventions aiming at regression of disease or slowing or halting its progression. Several lines of evidence support such possibility.

The now well-established beneficial effects of cholesterol lowering and especially of HMG-CoA reductase inhibitors have shifted the emphasis to the assessment of function rather than to the morphology of the human coronary circulation. Dietary and/or pharmacologic cholesterol lowering affect the anatomic stenosis severity only little, if at all, at least over the time periods studied, but strikingly reduced cardiac morbidity and mortality.[92] Hence the beneficial effects are attributed to plaque stabilization and improvements in endothelial function.[93]

Invasive studies of the human coronary circulation, performed during cardiac catheterization with intracoronary administration of direct vascular smooth muscle dilator agents such as adenosine or papavarine and of acetylcholine as a pharmacologic probe of predominantly endothelial-mediated coronary vasomotion, emphasize the importance of endothelial dysfunction early during the development of atherosclerosis (see Chaps. 36 and 37). For example, human coronary arteries with minimal atherosclerotic changes but no flow-limiting stenoses or even without any structural changes but in the presence of coronary risk factors alone revealed normal, predominantly vascular smooth muscle–mediated vasodilator capacities but attenuated or even highly abnormal endothelial-mediated flow responses.[94–96] These invasive studies test endothelial function at two sites of the coronary circulation, the large epicardial conduit and the coronary resistance vessel.[94–96] Measurements of regional MBF by PET offer the opportunity to probe the function of the human coronary circulation entirely noninvasively and mostly at the level of the resistance vessels.

PET-based measurements of MBF in asymptomatic patients with hypercholesteremia revealed an approximately 32 percent reduction in myocardial flow reserve or an approximately 18 percent reduction in hyperemic flow during adenosine administration.[97–102] In fact, the myocardial flow reserve was correlated with the ratio of plasma total cholesterol over HDL cholesterol.[97] Subsequent investigations confirmed these observations but also noted that elevated plasma triglycerides or, in young individuals, a family history of CAD alone or of hypertension was associated with diminished vasodilator capacities and myocardial flow reserves.[103–105] Other studies again observed diminished hyperemic responses in patients with diabetes,[104,106–108] and one study found a correlation between the hyperemic MBF response and the therapeutic control of the diabetic state.[109]

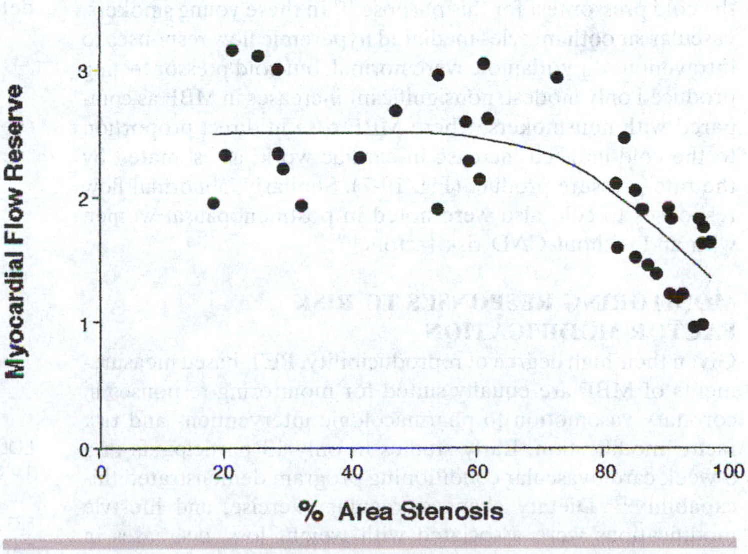

FIGURE 19-6 Myocardial flow reserve and coronary artery stenosis severity by quantitative angiography. Note the curvilinear relationship between the myocardial flow reserve as determined quantitatively from hyperemic and rest MBF measurements with [^{13}N]ammonia. (Reproduced with permission of the American Heart Association from Di Carli et al.[89])

To some extent, these observations differ from those made by invasive techniques, where frequently the predominantly vascular smooth muscle–mediated vasodilator response to, for example, intracoronary papavarine or adenosine was preserved despite the presence of coronary risk factors, while primarily endothelial-mediated responses were markedly abnormal.[110] As Bache suggests,[111] however, the major resistance to flow through the coronary circulation resides at vessels in the diameter range of 100 to 400 μm. If increases in flow exert shear stresses on the endothelium of the 400-μm vessels, then primarily endothelial-dependent mechanisms augment the flow response to predominantly vascular smooth muscle vasodilators. Conversely, as forearm blood flow measurements have shown, pharmacologic impairments of endothelial function reduce the maximal flow response to intravascular adenosine by about 25 to 35 percent.[112] Consequently, coronary risk factors such as low-density lipoprotein (LDL) cholesterol, triglycerides, and diabetes interfere with endothelial function and account for the diminished hyperemic response to adenosine or dipyridamole.

Another potentially important new concept for identifying diffuse coronary artery narrowing without discrete stenoses has been introduced recently.[113,114] Diffuse luminal narrowing causes a greater decline in pressure along the coronary artery. This then is associated with a progressive decrease in myocardial perfusion from the proximal to the distal portion of the coronary arterial system and hence in a longitudinal base-to-apex perfusion gradient. A similar longitudinal perfusion gradient likely exists during hyperemia in patients without CAD but with coronary risk factors.[115]

The predominantly endothelial-mediated coronary vasomotion can be assessed by the cold pressor test. In invasive studies, cold pressor testing evoked paradoxical changes in the diameter of the conduit vessels comparable with those evoked by intracoronary acetylcholine and, further, alterations at the level of the resistance vessels that correlated with those produced by intracoronary acetylcholine.[116–118] Observations with PET-based measurements of MBF in long-term smokers support the use of the cold pressor test for this purpose.[119] In these young smokers, vascular smooth muscle–mediated hyperemic flow responses to intravenous dipyridamole were normal, but cold pressor testing produced only modest, nonsignificant increases in MBF as compared with nonsmokers, where MBF rose in direct proportion to the cold-induced increase in cardiac work, as estimated by the rate-pressure product (Fig. 19-7). Similarly, abnormal flow responses to cold also were noted in postmenopausal women with and without CAD risk factors.[120]

MONITORING RESPONSES TO RISK FACTOR MODIFICATION

Given their high degree of reproducibility, PET-based measurements of MBF are equally suited for monitoring responses in coronary vasomotion to pharmacologic interventions and risk factor modification. Early studies in only 13 participants in a 6-week cardiovascular conditioning program demonstrated this capability.[121] Dietary changes, regular exercise, and lifestyle modifications were associated with weight loss, decreases in heart rate and blood pressure at rest, and significant decreases in plasma total and LDL cholesterol. A 12 percent decline in MBF at rest was proportionate to the decrease in resting cardiac work. Cardiovascular conditioning also produced a 9 percent increase in hyperemic flow, and MBF reserve increased by a total of 20 percent. Rigorous lifestyle and risk factor modification had been shown previously with PET to result in smaller and less severe stress-induced perfusion defects.[122,123] More recent studies with PET-based measurements of MBF have demonstrated beneficial effects of cholesterol lowering by HMG-CoA reductase inhibitors.[124,125] In one study, a 6-month course of fluvastatin treatment produced a 26 percent increase in hyperemic MBFs (at 6 months but not at 2 months) and thus in vasodilator capacity.[124] Of interest was the delayed improvement in vasodilator capacity (Fig. 19-8). In these patients with CAD, the cumulative coronary function improved in myocardial territories subtended by both diseased and nondiseased coronary arteries. These observations differ with those of another study that demonstrated a significant improvement in vasodilator capacity only in territories with stress-induced perfusion defects but not in apparently normal myocardium,[126] whereas

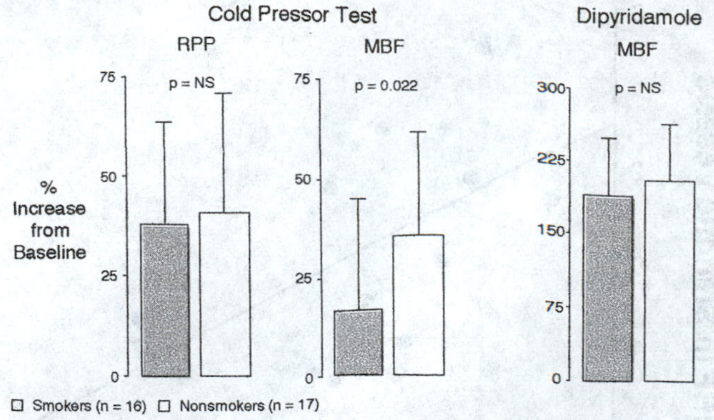

FIGURE 19-7 Increases in MBF in response to cold pressor testing and to intravenous dipyridamole in nonsmokers and long-term smokers (*shaded bars*). Note the comparable increases in MBF in response to dipyridamole in both groups. Also, cold pressor testing produced comparable increases in the rate pressure product (RPP), while the increase in MBF in long-term smokers was markedly attenuated as compared with normal individuals. (Data taken from Campisi et al.[119])

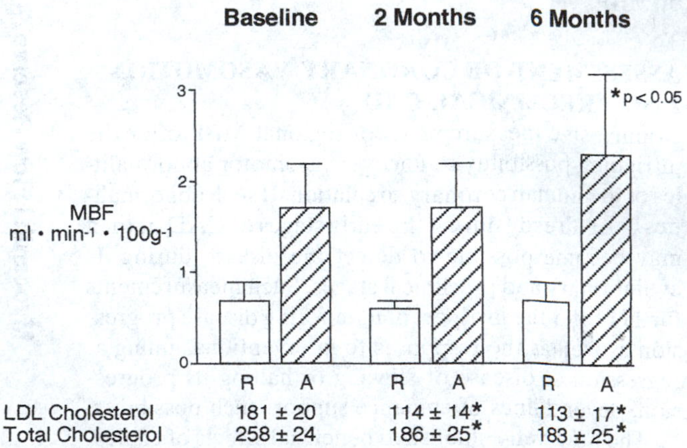

FIGURE 19-8 Changes in coronary artery vasodilator function in patients with CAD on a 6-month course of fluvastatin. The upper panel shows the MBF at rest and during adenosine hyperemia (A, *shaded bars*); the lower panel, the plasma levels for cholesterol in milligrams per deciliter. Note the delayed improvement of hyperemic MBF despite the significant decline in plasma total and LDL cholesterol at 2 months (*$p < 0.05$ versus baseline). (Data after Guethlin et al.[124])

a third study demonstrated again a 20 percent improvement of hyperemic flows in remote myocardium.[125] Another study reported immediate (within 24 h) improvements in hyperemic MBFs following LDL cholesterol plasma apheresis.[127] In the latter study, however, plasma LDL cholesterol apheresis reduced total cholesterol by 42 percent and LDL cholesterol by 58 percent, which was greater than in the fluvastatin study with total and LDL cholesterol reductions of 29 and of 37 percent, respectively.[124]

Other investigations explored pharmacologic effects on predominantly endothelial-dependent coronary vasomotion. For example, intravenous L-arginine (30 g) as the substrate of nitric oxide synthase (NOS) in long-term smokers normalized the MBF response to cold pressor testing, suggesting that endothelial function or, at least, the bioactivity of nitric oxide had normalized.[128] Whether increases in the substrate for NOS accelerate production of nitric oxide remains uncertain, especially in view of the low K_m, which renders the reaction relatively substrate-independent.[129] One possibility could be a nonspecific effect, perhaps on the oxidative stress, as recently demonstrated with cold pressor testing in response to acute administration of vitamin C.[130] Other possible mechanisms include competitive displacement of asymmetric dimethylarginine, an inhibitor of NOS with elevated plasma levels in hypercholesteremic patients.[131] An insulin-dependent mechanism is also possible, especially because L-arginine infusions prompted three- to fourfold increases in plasma insulin concentrations.[128] Similarly, hormone-replacement therapy in postmenopausal women without coronary risk factors can normalize the MBF response to cold, while the responses remain abnormal in postmenopausal women with coronary risk factors despite hormone-replacement therapy.[120]

Assessment of Myocardial Viability

Myocardial viability pertains to an impairment of myocardial contractile function that is potentially reversible. Distinction of such potentially reversible from irreversible impairment of contractile function often is of considerable clinical importance but remains diagnostically challenging. Both types of tissue injury share several features, including similar degrees of abnormal systolic wall motion, of reduced MBF, and of electrocardiographic abnormalities. Persistence of metabolic activity for sustaining vital, energy-requiring processes, however, including cellular homeostasis, depends on some residual MBF for removal of inhibitory metabolites as well as for supply of fuel substrates. Hence key features of viable myocardium include

- Impairment of systolic wall motion at rest
- Normal or reduced, but not absent, blood flow
- Preservation of cellular homeostasis
- Persistent metabolic activity for high-energy phosphate production
- Recruitable contractile reserve

GENERAL CONSIDERATIONS

Research studies in animals provided the base for the detection of myocardial viability. Known alterations in substrate metabolism during acute myocardial ischemia were demonstrated noninvasively with positron-emitting tracers of myocardial substrate metabolism.[132] Consistent with an impaired FFA oxidation was the diminished initial uptake of [^{11}C]palmitate and its delayed clearance from the myocardium.[46,47] Additionally, the known increase in glucose extraction and use was reflected by a regional increase in [^{18}F]deoxyglucose uptake.[133] Initial studies in patients with acute myocardial ischemia revealed blood flow and glucose metabolism patterns that were virtually identical to those in animals, e.g., enhanced [^{18}F]deoxyglucose uptake in hypoperfused dysfunctional myocardial regions. Unexpectedly, the same pattern existed in patients with chronic CAD but no signs of acute ischemia (Fig. 19-9). This raised the question of whether the observed blood flow–metabolism pattern was unique to acute ischemia or represented a more general metabolic pattern in chronically dysfunctional and hypoperfused myocardium. Also intriguing were observations in other CAD patients with regionally reduced [^{18}F]deoxyglucose uptake that paralleled the reduction in regional MBF[134] (see Fig. 19-9). A more systematic study in patients scheduled for surgical revascularization confirmed the hypothesis that the regionally enhanced [^{18}F]deoxyglucose uptake, in contrast to a reduction, reflected metabolic activity as evidence of viability in myocardium with complete or partial loss of contractile function.[135] Restoration of tissue perfusion was followed by improved contractile function in myocardium with but not in myocardium without persistent glucose metabolic activity.

Possible Mechanisms of the Blood Flow Metabolism Pattern

The preceding observations established the clinical utility of these PET findings, but the underlying mechanisms remained uncertain. Patients with CAD revealed after supine bicycle exercise in stress-induced flow defects an augmented [^{18}F]deoxyglucose uptake when the radiotracer was administered 20 to 30 min after exercise and after the stress-induced flow defect had already resolved.[136] This implicated *myocardial stunning* as one possibility, subsequently supported by observations in animal experiments and in patients with either collaterized myocardium or unstable angina.[137–139] These studies demonstrated the evolution of a blood flow–metabolism pattern in chronically reperfused myocardium: An immediate postreperfusion decrease in glucose uptake was followed by an increase that subsequently declined to normal as contractile function returned.[137] The enhanced [^{18}F]deoxyglucose uptake was attributed to increased lactate release and thus anaerobic glycolysis that persisted even after blood flow had been restored.[140] The evolution of such metabolic pattern also may pertain to early postinfarction patients[141] but does not fully explain all observations in patients with chronic CAD. Another possibility includes *repetitive stunning*[142] as the reason for the persistent increase in [^{18}F]deoxyglucose uptake in dysfunctional myocardium. An impairment in contractile function associated with enhanced glucose use was noted in collateral-dependent myocardium only if the flow reserve was markedly restricted.[138] It limits the coronary circulation's ability to respond appropriately to transient and frequent increases in oxygen demand during daily life, leading to transient ischemic episodes, each followed by stunning and preventing recovery of contractile function.

Myocardial hibernation serves as another explanation.[143] The postulated downregulation of contractile function in response to diminished rest MBF is thought to be associated with an alteration of the myocardium's substrate metabolism with a dominant role for the more oxygen-efficient glucose. Hibernation in its truest sense then implies that the downregulated

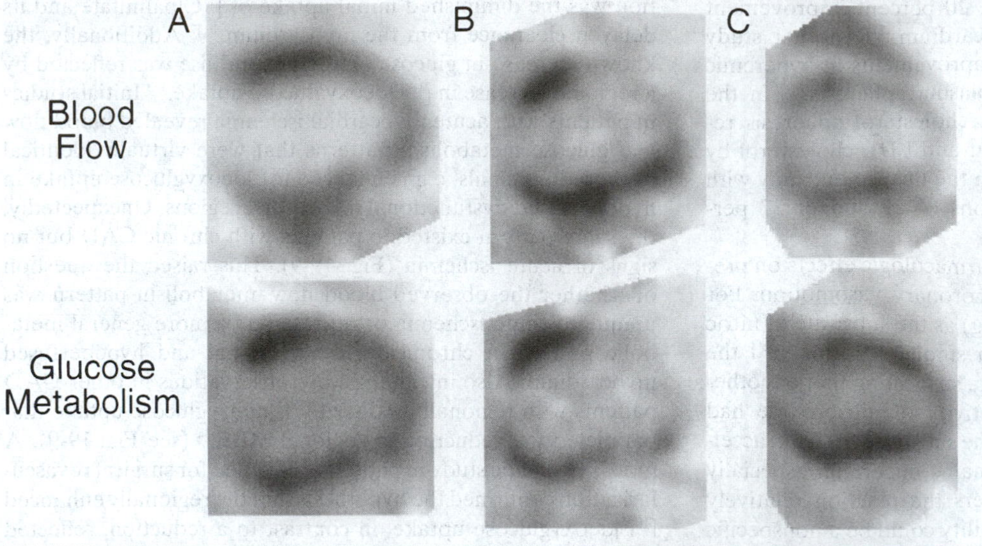

FIGURE 19-9 Patterns of MBF and glucose metabolism (with [^{13}N]ammonia, [^{18}F]deoxyglucose, and PET) in three patients with ischemic cardiomyopathy and poor LV function. Only vertical long-axis cuts through the mid-left ventricle are shown. Patient A demonstrates an enlarged LV cavity with a mild decrease in perfusion in the anterior wall, apex, and distal inferior wall. Glucose metabolism parallels the distribution of MBF ("mild match"). In patient B, a severe perfusion defect in the akinetic anterior wall is matched on the glucose metabolic images by a decreased uptake of [^{18}F]deoxyglucose (severe "match" pattern). In contrast, in patient C, the extensive perfusion defect in the anterior wall and apex is associated with near normally preserved [^{18}F]deoxyglucose uptake ("blood flow metabolism mismatch").

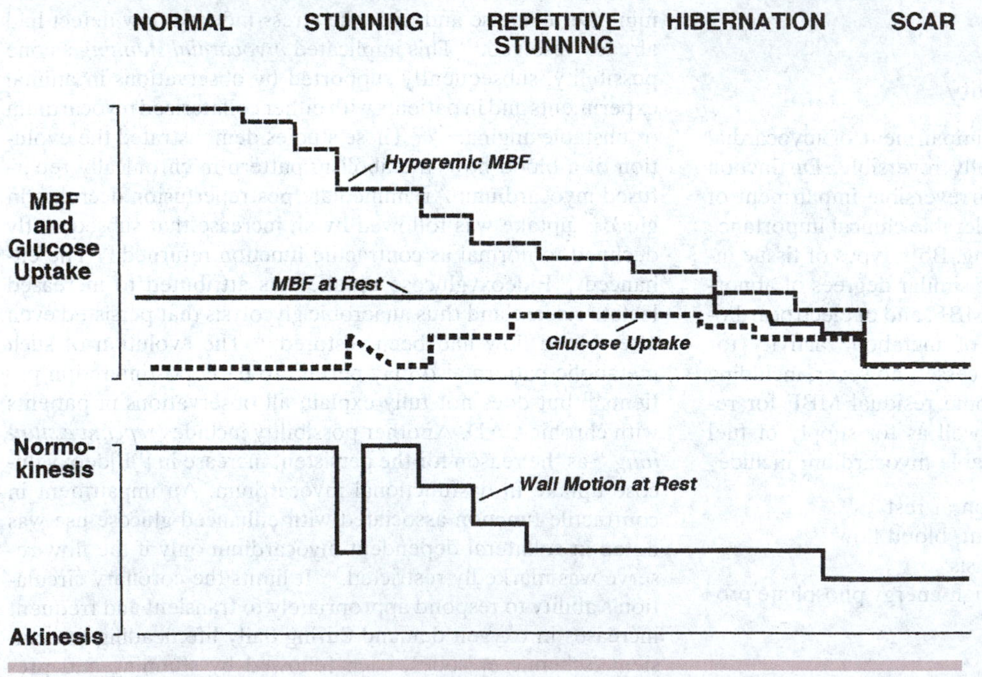

FIGURE 19-10 Possible time-dependent spectrum of various types of reversible contractile dysfunction as a function of myocardial flow reserve and resting MBF. The spectrum proceeds from normal to scar tissue or loss of viability. As the coronary flow reserve declines, occasional episodes of ischemia and stunning lead to intermittent dysfunction of stunning associated with enhanced glucose uptake. More severe reductions in flow reserve are then associated with repetitive ischemia and repetitive stunning leading to chronically reduced contractile function but increased glucose uptake. With progression of the coronary artery stenosis, resting MBF may decline, while the increased glucose uptake is maintained until the amount of fibrosis increases and more myocytes undergo necrosis and metabolic activity ceases.

energy requirements match the available energy supply. A new supply-demand imbalance is established, but at a lower level. Such a new balance, however, will be a precarious one because even moderate increases in demand or decreases in supply disturb the steady state and cause ischemia. It is thus possible and likely that both *hibernation* and *stunning* coexist to varying extents in many patients. Observations in experimental animals suggest that sustained reductions in both blood flow and contractile function can be maintained for some time without significant necrosis, but development of structural alterations resembling those in patients with chronic CAD[144–148] supports the concept of hibernation.

Both concepts, repetitive stunning and hibernation, may, in their purest form, represent the two ends of a spectrum. As Fig. 19-10 illustrates, the spectrum begins with a reduction in myocardial flow reserve, where increased demand can no longer be matched by an appropriate increase in supply and which ends with a loss of the flow reserve and a decline in regional MBF at rest, associated with a downregulation of contractile function and adaptation of substrate metabolism. Such a spectrum could represent a temporal progression in coronary artery stenosis severity. Recent findings in chronically instrumented animals with a progressive decline in and ultimately loss of regional flow reserve associated with a decrease in rest blood flow support such a scenario.[148–151] Reductions in flow or flow reserve also may occur suddenly in view of the high incidence of blood flow metabolism mismatches in early postinfarction patients.[134,141,152] In acute animal studies, sudden moderate reductions in regional MBF are associated initially with evidence of acute ischemia (e.g., release of lactate and enhanced glucose uptake). An apparent resetting or adjustment of demand follows, and lactate release converts to uptake, high-energy phosphate stores are replenished, and a new supply-demand balance seems to have returned.[144,153,154] Some debate focused on the issue of whether MBF at rest can indeed be chronically reduced.[155] Nevertheless, findings in chronic animal experiments, as well as substantial improvements in resting MBF following surgical revascularization, argue in favor of the possibility of a true chronic regional hypoperfusion.[148,150,151,156,157]

Ultrastructural and Histochemical Observations Other attempts to gain mechanistic insights into the enhanced [^{18}F]deoxyglucose uptake include morphometric and histochemical analyses of biopsy specimens harvested from dysfunctional human myocardium during surgical revascularization. Prior autopsy studies indicated a general correlation between the degree of regional myocardial fibrosis and the severity of the impairment of regional contractile function. Yet there were exceptions.[158] In some instances, dyskinetic myocardium was free of fibrosis at autopsy, or conversely, some normally contracting myocardium contained as much as 40 percent fibrosis.[159] It also was known that "abnormal" myocytes (Fig. 19-11) existed in chronically dysfunctional myocardium.[160] More recent investigations noted correlations between the externally determined relative blood flows and relative [^{18}F]deoxyglucose concentrations with the morphometrically determined fractions of fibrosis, abnormal myocytes, and normal myocardium.[138,161,162] The various studies agree on a general correlation between relative blood flow and the percentage of tissue fibrosis (Fig. 19-12) but differ on the fraction of abnormal myocytes. In one study, this fraction is the same in reversibly and irreversibly dysfunctional myocardium,[161] whereas a second study notes a significantly greater fraction in reversibly than in irreversibly dysfunctional myocardium.[162] Because the centrally located glycogen granules are key features of such abnormal myocytes and a significant correlation exists between the fraction of such abnormal myocytes and the relative [^{18}F]deoxyglucose uptake, these abnormal myocytes have been considered the ultrastructural correlate of enhanced [^{18}F]deoxyglucose uptake in chronically dysfunctional myocardium. Other observations argue against this notion. Again, electron microscopy and histochemistry of biopsy samples from the center of the dysfunctional myocardial wall demonstrate highly different degrees of severity of morphologic alterations in myocardial regions with blood flow–metabolism mismatches.[163] Despite identical flow and glucose metabolism findings on PET, nearly half the patients in this study revealed only minimal, if any, morphologic changes, whereas the other half demonstrated severe structural abnormalities. Such variability in morphologic alterations argues against the structurally abnormal myocyte and especially the glycogen granules as an explanation of the enhanced [^{18}F]deoxyglucose uptake. More likely explanations include translocation and possibly upregulation of GLUT1[164] as a flux-generating step, uncoupling of glycolysis from glucose oxidation, regulated probably by malonyl-CoA and carnitine palmitate transferase I,[165,166] and possibly an ischemia-related loss of adrenergic innervation or function[167] associated with increased exogenous glucose use. In cardiac allografts, glucose use was about 70 percent higher in denervated than in reinnervated myocardium.[168]

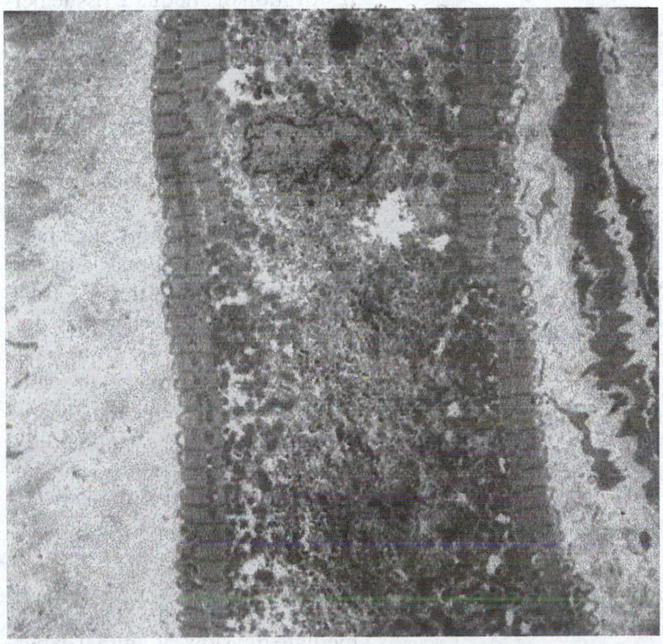

FIGURE 19-11 Abnormal myocyte in human chronically dysfunctional myocardium. Note the irregularly shaped nucleus, the loss of sarcomeres in the center of the myocyte, and the extensive deposition of glycogen. (Courtesy of M. Borgers, Maastricht, The Netherlands.)

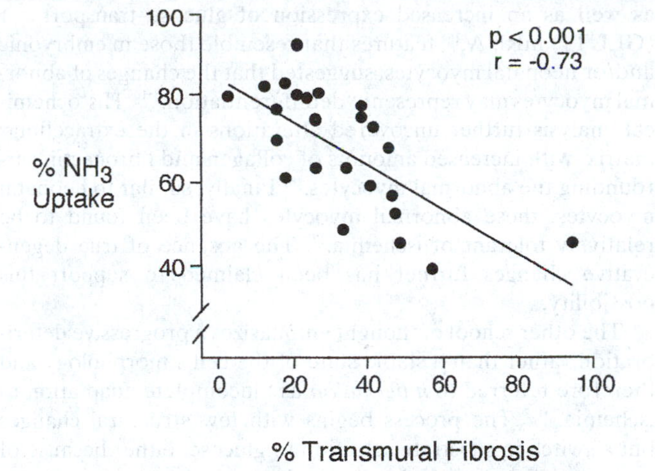

FIGURE 19-12 Inverse correlation between the fractional amount of tissue fibrosis by morphometry and MBF by relative [^{13}N]ammonia tissue concentration (%NH_3 uptake). (Reproduced with permission of the American Heart Association from Depré at al.[162])

Myocytes in Chronically Dysfunctional Myocardium Whether abnormal myocytes as described initially by Flameng et al.[160] and subsequently observed in biopsy material from mismatched myocardium point specifically in the direction of or are ingredients unique to any particular pathophysiologic mechanism underlying the chronic, though potentially reversible, impairment of contractile function remains uncertain. Two schools of thought exist. One holds that the morphologic alterations result from (1) contractile unloading, (2) increased wall stress (stretch), and (3) a metabolic substrate switch to preferential glucose use.[169] In fact, contractile unloading recently has been demonstrated to result in virtually identical structural changes.[170,171] The expression and distribution patterns of other features such as of α-smooth muscle actin, cardiotin, and titin,[169] as well as an increased expression of glucose transporter 1 (GLUT1) mRNA,[164] features that resemble those in embryonic and/or neonatal myocytes, suggested that the changes of abnormal myocytes may represent "dedifferentiation."[169] Histochemical analysis further uncovered alterations in the extracellular matrix, with increased amounts of collagen and fibronectin surrounding the abnormal myocytes.[169] Finally, similar to neonatal myocytes, these abnormal myocytes have been found to be relatively tolerant of ischemia.[172] The absence of true degenerative changes further has been claimed to support this possibility.

The other school of thought emphasizes a progressive deterioration rather than a stable state of the cell's morphology and therefore referred to *hibernation* as "incomplete adaptation to ischemia."[173] The process begins with few structural changes but a switch in substrate selection to glucose, either because of its greater oxygen efficiency or, alternatively, because of loss of enzymes essential for fatty acid oxidation, followed by loss of contractile protein and accumulation of glycogen and mitochondrial and nuclear alterations, ultimately leading to cell death and scar tissue formation (Fig. 19-13).[163] Other studies again report reduced expression of contractile and cytoskeletal proteins associated with increased expression of extracellular matrix proteins,[173] implying a progressive loss of contractile protein and of the cell structure that is paralleled by accelerated formation of tissue fibrosis and hence a progressive loss of viability that was further found to be associated with apoptosis and replacement fibrosis. Biopsies from patients with preoperatively viable myocardium but without a postrevascularization improvement in contractile dysfunction demonstrated an about threefold increase in mRNA of caspase-3, a promoter of apoptosis, together with an about 50 percent reduction in the expression of the antideath genes *Bcl-2* and *p53,* again consistent with continued cell death and replacement fibrosis.[174] Chronic animal experimental studies similarly have demonstrated significant increases in apoptotic myocytes in hibernating myocardium with reduced rest MBF and critically reduced or absent flow reserve.[151] The fact that myocyte apoptosis in these studies occurred scattered and not in clusters raises the question of whether apoptosis is indeed the end point of the progressively deteriorating abnormal myocyte or such apoptosis represents a process that occurs in parallel. To some extent this may depend on the duration and severity of the ischemic compromise. For instance, other animal studies with more sudden reductions in flow and shorter time periods report higher rates of myocyte apoptosis occurring in clusters.[175]

A progressive deterioration of reversibly dysfunctional myocardium is also consistent with clinical observations that point to the high prevalence of mismatch patterns in patients with prior myocardial infarctions[134,176] but note a declining incidence of blood flow–metabolism mismatches as a function of time after an acute myocardial infarction.[152] Moreover, the loss of the capability to improve global LV function if revascularization was delayed by more than 6 months[177] or an increase in fibrosis and loss of functional recovery after revascularization as a function of the duration of clinical symptoms[178] seem to support such progression. The blood flow–metabolism mismatch may represent a transient rather than a permanent state of reversibly dysfunctional myocardium. It is possible that reversibility can be maintained up to a certain point. Once this critical point has been reached, myocytes become committed to irreversibility and cell death.

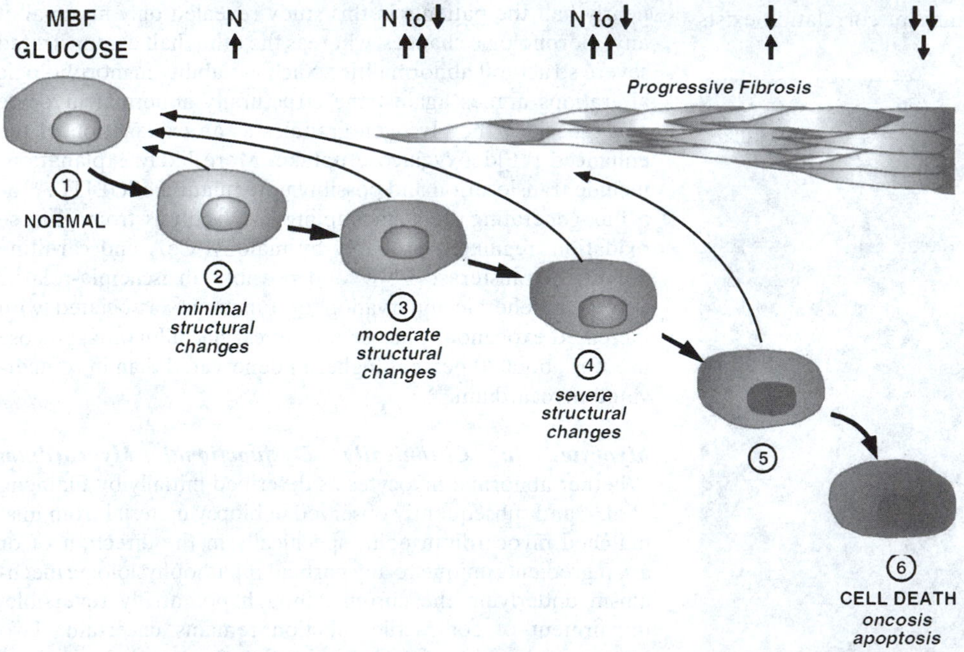

FIGURE 19-13 Progressive deterioration of myocytes in chronically dysfunctional myocardium beginning with few, if any, changes in morphology, followed by loss of contractile proteins and glycogen accumulation with continued deterioration of the cytoskeleton and progressive interstitial fibrosis with coagulation necrosis or, more likely, aptotic cell death as the ultimate end point. Possible myocyte recovery and rate of recovery are likely to depend on the severity of morphologic and functional changes, which may, however, reach a point beyond which recovery is no longer possible.

In the clinical setting, prompt restoration of adequate tissue perfusion through interventional revascularization therefore will be essential, regardless of whether abnormal myocytes represent dedifferentiation or degeneration. It would seem that ultimately the return of contractile function will depend on the amount of connective tissue. Once fibrosis and scar tissue occupy more than 35 to 40 percent of the myocardium, dysfunction has been shown to be irreversible.[15,16] Also, the presence of structural changes in viable myocardium, as demonstrated with blood flow–metabolism imaging, implies that if the contractile machinery in abnormal or dedifferentiated myocytes can be reconstructed, the recovery of contractile function will not be immediate but slow, as animal experimental[179] and clinical investigations have indeed demonstrated.[180] The delay in cell repair also may explain the persistence of increased [^{18}F]deoxyglucose uptake after successful revascularization.[181]

Viability Assessment in the Clinical Setting The classic and now most widely applied approach entails evaluation of the relative distribution of blood flow and exogenous glucose use with [^{18}F]deoxyglucose. Initial studies uncovered three distinct patterns:

- Normal blood flow and normal or enhanced glucose uptake
- Reduced blood flow but normal glucose uptake in excess of blood flow (mismatch)
- Reduced blood flow and proportionately reduced glucose uptake (match)[135]

While these terms are purely operational, they infer, at least to some extent, the underlying pathophysiology accounting for the contractile dysfunction. Normal flow and/or metabolism may represent *stunned* myocardium, whereas the classic mismatch may be consistent with *hibernating* myocardium. Both patterns predict a postrevascularization improvement in contractile function, whereas the concordant reduction in blood flow and metabolism predicts that function will not improve.[135,182,183] It should be emphasized that the reduction in regional flow for both matches and mismatches may vary considerably between patients.

Because of the observed correlation between tissue fibrosis and relative flow tracer uptake, the evaluation of regional MBF alone can provide information on the presence of reversible contractile dysfunction (Fig. 19-12). [162] Severe reductions to less than 25 percent of normal or complete absence of blood flow reflects complete or nearly complete transmural scar tissue formation and hence nonreversiblity.[184] In another study, flow reductions of more than 60 percent were highly accurate in predicting nonreversiblity of contractile dysfunction.[185] Conversely, completely normal or only mild reductions (<20 percent) of MBF in dysfunctional myocardium argue against the presence of significant amounts of tissue fibrosis; it possibly reflects myocardial stunning and thus indicates functional reversibility. Mild to moderate flow reductions are less reliable discriminators. If combined with a metabolic study, the [^{18}F]deoxyglucose uptake in the case of a small nontransmural/infarction with otherwise normal myocardium would be reduced in proportion to blood flow.[186] Conversely, an increase in glucose uptake would indicate the coexistence of reversibly dysfunctional myocardium with scar tissue and predict an improvement in contractile function.

Another, again limited approach for identifying reversible contractile dysfunction is the use of [^{18}F]deoxyglucose alone. This approach assumes that regional reductions in [^{18}F]deoxyglucose greater than 50 percent relative to remote myocardium represent irreversible contractile function, whereas mildly reduced or normal uptake indicates the presence of reversible dysfunction.[187,188] While used for some time as a benchmark for defining the accuracy of ^{201}Tl-based techniques for assessing myocardial viability,[187] only recently has the validity of this particular approach been tested against the postrevascularization outcome in regional contractile function.[189] Electrocardiographic gated image acquisition affords simultaneous evaluation of regional function and metabolism and thus can further augment the predictive accuracy of the [^{18}F]deoxyglucose standalone approach.[190,191] A more recent report emphasizes the utility of measurements of exogenous glucose use in absolute units. Using a threshold value of 0.25 μmol/g per minute offered a 93 percent positive and a 95 percent negative predictive accuracy for the improvement of contractile dysfunction.[192] Nevertheless, this approach is severely limited when glucose use and hence [^{18}F]deoxyglucose uptake cannot be controlled sufficiently. In such instances, it may be difficult to distinguish between scar tissue, normal myocardium, and reversibly contractile dysfunction, which then could be readily clarified by evaluating the distribution of regional MBF.[193]

The pattern of normal blood flow and glucose metabolism in mildly to severely hypokinetic myocardium of severely depressed left ventricles is a difficult clinical problem. One study reports that of 32 such myocardial regions, only 8 regions (or 25 percent) improved following surgical revascularization.[194] Such regions therefore may represent remodeled LV myocardium. Conversely, an improvement in wall motion may be consistent with myocardial stunning. If suspected, careful evaluation of the coronary anatomy or, if unavailable, the addition of a pharmacologic stress study can aid in distinguishing between stunned and remodeled LV myocardium (Fig. 19-14).

Alternate Approaches to Blood Flow and Glucose Metabolism Imaging Several institutions use SPECT myocardial perfusion imaging with either ^{201}Tl or ^{99m}Tc-sestamibi and metabolic imaging with [^{18}F]deoxyglucose with dedicated PET systems. The reported predictive accuracies for segmental and global LV function approach those obtained with dedicated PET systems.[1] Nevertheless, such combined PET/SPECT approaches present at times with diagnostic limitations, especially because of considerable differences in contrast and spatial resolutions as well as

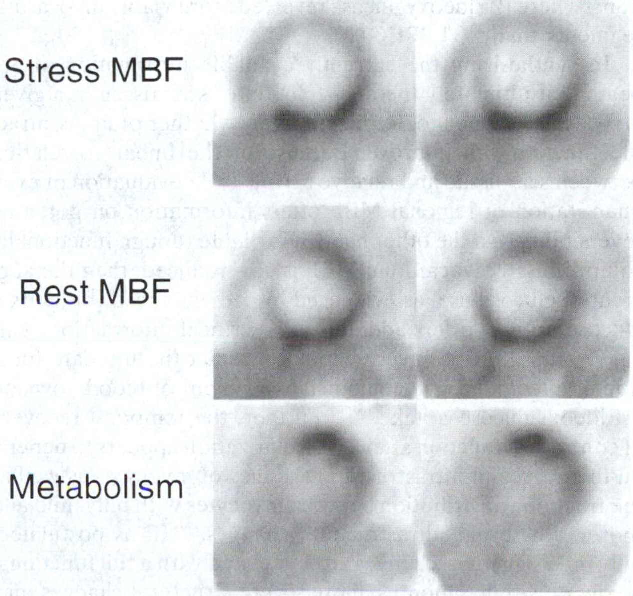

FIGURE 19-14 Two contiguous short-axis images through the mid-left ventricle in a patient with ischemic cardiomyopathy. The MBF images at rest (*middle panel*) reveal in the interventricular septum reduced but relatively well preserved flow in the anterior and anterolateral wall associated with regionally increased [^{18}F]deoxyglucose uptake in the same portion of the left ventricle as seen in the lower panel (metabolism). The stress induced flow defect in the anterior and anterolateral wall (as seen in the upper panel) implicates stunning as the cause of the enhanced [^{18}F]deoxyglucose uptake.

artifactual reductions in tracer concentrations due to photon attenuation.[4,5] This can limit the ability to accurately estimate the extent of a blood flow–metabolism mismatch.

More recent approaches rely solely on the use of multipurpose SPECT-like systems, either equipped with ultra-high-photon-energy general-purpose collimators or with coincidence-detection systems (see also Fig. 19-1). Little information thus far has become available on the clinical performance of coincidence-detection systems, whereas systematic studies with ultra-high-photon-energy general-purpose collimator SPECT systems using ^{201}Tl- or ^{99m}Tc-labeled flow tracers and [^{18}F]deoxyglucose report predictive accuracies that are comparable with those reported with dedicated PET systems.[195,196]

Further, ^{201}Tl rest-redistribution imaging has been useful for identifying myocardial viability and for predicting the postoperative outcome of ischemic cardiomyopathy, although with a somewhat lower predictive accuracy (see Chap. 17). This approach suffers from instrumentation-related shortcomings, especially in patients with poor LV function, and consequently, poor signal-to-noise ratios. Thallium-201 offers a negative signal (reduced tracer uptake) as compared with [^{18}F]deoxyglucose, with a positive signal (enhanced tracer uptake) that is more readily accessible to visual analysis.[193] One study reporting that [^{18}F]deoxyglucose and PET identified myocardial viability in 18 of 20 patients with an average LV ejection fraction of 23 percent and only fixed ^{201}Tl defects on SPECT[197] is consistent with a more recent report of viability by [^{18}F]deoxyglucose in 17 of 33 patients (LV ejection fraction <35 percent) with fixed or minimally redistributing ^{201}Tl defects.[198] Further, a comparison study of ^{201}Tl and [^{18}F]deoxyglucose SPECT reports a generally excellent agreement between both approaches but observed disparities in patients with severely depressed LV ejection fractions, where [^{18}F]deoxyglucose revealed more viable myocardial segments than ^{201}Tl SPECT.[11]

In synthesizing the currently available information, it appears that ultimately the total fraction of scar tissue in a given myocardial segment determines largely whether or not contractile function will improve. Because of the linear correlation between scar tissue and relative MBF,[138,161,162] evaluation or even quantitation of regional MBF offers information on potential reversibility. On the other hand, if in viable though functionally compromised myocardium MBF is also reduced, then the augmented glucose use, as evidenced by the enhanced [^{18}F]deoxyglucose uptake, offers additional and critical information. This has prompted most investigators to predict the ultimate functional outcome from a combined assessment of blood flow and [^{18}F]deoxyglucose uptake.[199,200] Further, the temporal recovery of contractile function after revascularization appears to depend on the degree of ultrastructural changes of myocytes as well as the fractional distribution between myocytes with only mild and those with severe ultrastructural changes.[199] If, as postulated, only mild structural changes are associated with a full functional recovery within 3 months, more severe structural changes may require substantially longer time periods and, further, may account for the persistence of increased [^{18}F]deoxyglucose uptake even for many months following revascularization.[181]

CLINICAL ROLE OF PET VIABILITY ASSESSMENT

Among the various PET approaches, the blood flow and glucose metabolism approach has gained the greatest clinical acceptance. Viability assessments with PET can decisively affect therapeutic strategies in patients with advanced CAD and ischemic cardiomyopathy. The therapeutic options in these patients range from aggressive medical management to surgical revascularization and cardiac transplantation. While conservative pharmacologic approaches to the management of such patients has improved markedly over the past decade, the long-term survival of medically treated patients remains relatively poor.[201] Cardiac transplantation as another approach offers a better long-term survival and an improvement in the quality of life, but the supply of donor hearts has not kept pace with the increasing demand, so this therapeutic option remains limited (see Chap. 22). At present, the prevalence of ischemic cardiomyopathy in the United States alone amounts to about 2.5 million cases, thus affecting roughly 1 percent of the U.S. population. The decision to revascularize frequently depends on the answers to several questions. First, what is the leading cause of poor LV function? Second, if CAD has been identified as the culprit, is there enough viable myocardium so that surgical revascularization produces an improvement in LV performance and/or congestive heart failure symptoms? Third, will revascularization avert future catastrophic cardiac events and prolong survival? And finally, can the surgical risk be predicted, since this will influence the preoperative risk-benefit ratio?

Ischemic versus Idiopathic Dilated Cardiomyopathy In addition to heart failure symptoms, ischemic cardiomyopathy shares several other features with idiopathic dilated cardiomyopathy, such as, for example, the LV enlargement, the often diffuse hypokinesis, the markedly depressed LV ejection fraction, and frequently, mitral regurgitation. Biventricular enlargement has been thought of as a feature characteristic of idiopathic dilated cardiomyopathy but also can be present in ischemic cardiomyopathy. Conduction abnormalities often limit the accuracy of electrocardiographic criteria to distinguish between both entities. Additionally, an intrinsic myopathic process including LV remodeling also may exist in a number of patients with CAD so that the major cause of the poor LV function may remain unknown or difficult to elucidate. Importantly, however, the therapeutic approach to both disease entities will differ strikingly (see Chap. 66).

Both disease entities, however, reveal remarkably different patterns of blood flow and substrate metabolism on PET. A comparative study in patients with ischemic cardiomyopathy and idiopathic dilated cardiomyopathy found the distribution of MBF to be characteristically homogeneous in idiopathic cardiomyopathy as compared with distinct flow reductions clearly corresponding in ischemic cardiomyopathy to the coronary vascular territories.[202] Similarly, uptake of [^{18}F]deoxyglucose was noted to be homogeneous in dilated cardiomyopathy, whereas matches and/or mismatches between blood flow and [^{18}F]deoxuglucose uptake were present in ischemic cardiomyopathy (Fig. 19-15). Combined imaging of blood flow and glucose metabolism distinguished with an overall accuracy of 85 percent between both disease entities.

Prediction of the Outcome in Global LV Function Numerous clinical investigations have reported the high accuracy of [^{18}F]deoxyglucose imaging with PET in predicting the postrevascularization outcome in regional LV wall motion.[1,135,182,183,188,189,203–205] Even though some of these investigations employed permutations of the initially described blood flow–

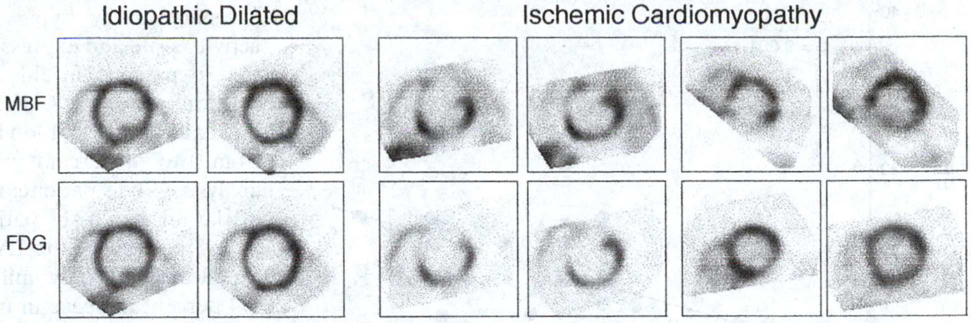

FIGURE 19-15 Patterns of MBF and [^{18}F]deoxyglucose uptake in idiopathic dilated (*left*) and ischemic cardiomyopathy (*right*) (see text). Short-axis images are shown. Note the homogeneous blood flow and glucose uptake in idiopathic dilated cardiomyopathy (*left*) and the highly heterogeneous blood flow and glucose uptake in ischemic cardiomyopathy (*center* and *right*). Of the two patient examples of ischemic cardiomyopathy, one shows a "mismatch" (*right*) and the other one a "match."

metabolism approach or relied only on the evaluation of regional [^{18}F]deoxyglucose uptake in dysfunctional myocardium,[188,189] the predictive accuracy, both positive and negative, continued to be high. Such studies have been important because they prove the concept of blood flow–metabolism patterns as accurate predictors of the outcome of regional wall motion after restoration of MBF. More relevant in the clinical setting is whether blood flow–metabolism patterns can predict the postrevascularization outcome in global LV function.

Initial semiquantitative studies demonstrated some correlation between the extent of the blood flow–metabolism mismatch and the postrevascularization gain in LV ejection fraction.[135] Patients with blood flow–metabolism mismatches that occupied at least two or more of seven total myocardial segments revealed a statistically significant increase in the LV ejection fraction following coronary bypass grafting.[135] No such improvement was observed in patients with only one mismatch segment or with only matches. Subsequent studies reported significant gains in LV function in patients with blood flow–metabolism mismatches as compared with no improvement in those patients without metabolic evidence of viability. Fig. 19-16 summarizes the findings in 19 investigations including a total of 570 patients.[1,3,156,161–163,177,183,194,195,198,205–211] The gain in global LV function is most striking in patients with an LV ejection fraction of less than 35 percent, who had a 34 percent postoperative increase in the LV ejection fraction as compared with a 19 percent ($p < 0.02$) improvement in patients with an LV ejection fraction of more than 35 percent. Additionally, recent studies reported significant correlations between the percentage of the left ventricle with a blood flow–metabolism mismatch and the postrevascularization increase in the LV ejection fraction.[212,213] Thus the extent of a blood flow–metabolism mismatch has some predictive value on the postoperative gain in global LV performance[194,211] (Fig. 19-17). The absence of such improvement in one specific laboratory may be attributable to differences in the imaging and analysis approach used.[181,205] MBF is evaluated with ^{82}Rb at rest and during pharmacologic stress, and the distribution of MBF during stress is compared with the myocardial glucose uptake at rest. This approach identifies both stress induced ischemia and "viable myocardium" at rest. Hence blood flow and possibly wall motion at rest may be normal in some patients so that revascularization predominately improves the capacity of the left ventricle to respond to exercise.[205,214]

The improvement in regional and especially global LV function may not occur immediately but slowly though progressively following revascularization. In a highly selected patient group, blood flow had been shown to recover promptly following revascularization by angioplasty, whereas contractile function remained initially unchanged.[180] On reexamination 67 ± 19 days later, no further improvements in regional MBF had occurred, but systolic wall motion had now significantly improved. The disparity between recovery of MBF and contractile function may be attributed to stunning and/or to rebuilding of the contractile machinery that had been lost in abnormal myocytes. Preliminary observations suggest a correlation between severity of the mismatch and the rate of recovery of contractile function. The rate of recovery appears to be faster when flow is relatively well preserved as compared with segments with more severe flow reductions and possibly more severe ultrastructural changes. Segments with largely preserved flows recovered faster than segments with more severe flow reductions.[215] The contractile function appears to recover or improve more promptly in myocardial regions without marked ultrastructural abnormalities or a lesser fraction of abnormal myocytes.[199] Finally, in addition to a slow recovery of contractile function in reversibly dysfunctional myocardium, other studies describe an associated decline in end-diastolic and end-systolic volumes, suggesting the possibility of a reversal of LV remodeling.[216]

Effect on Congestive Heart Failure–Related Symptoms A related clinical question is whether such improvement is also

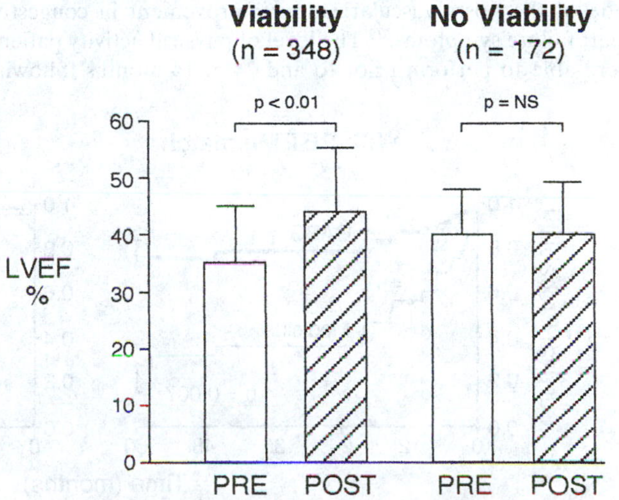

FIGURE 19-16 Summary of changes in LV ejection fraction from baseline (PRE) to following revascularization (POST) as reported for a total of 570 patients in 19 clinical investigations.[1,3,135,156,161–163,177,183,194,195,198,205–211] Patients with metabolic evidence of reversible contractile dysfunction are shown on the left and those without on the right. The average LV ejection fractions are shown at baseline (PRE) and following surgical revascularization (POST).

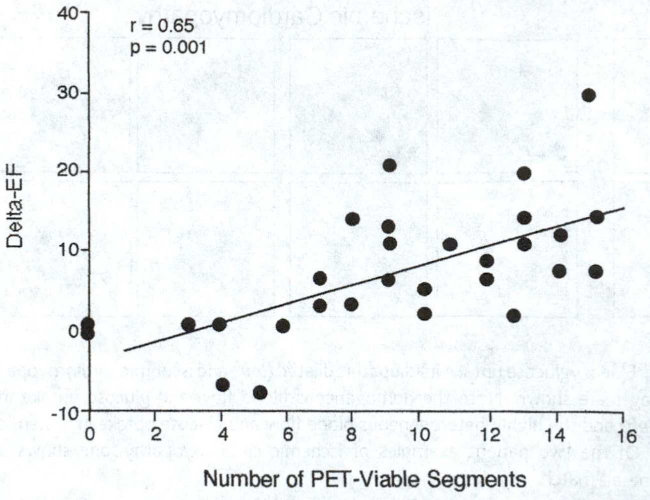

FIGURE 19-17 Postrevascularization improvement in LV ejection fraction as a function of the number of viable myocardial segments as determined by PET. (Reproduced with permission Pagano et al.[211])

associated with relief or amelioration of congestive heart failure symptoms. Several retrospective studies indicate such possible symptomatic improvement. Two investigations concluded that patients with blood flow–metabolism mismatches undergoing surgical revascularization demonstrated a significantly higher incidence of improvement in NYHA functional class than patients without mismatches or patients with matches but not submitted to regional revascularization.[217,218] Among the 52 patients with mismatches and congestive heart failure class III or IV, 81 percent of the 26 patients undergoing revascularization revealed a significant improvement in congestive heart failure class as compared with only 23 percent of 26 patients treated conservatively.[218]

The amount of viable myocardium on blood flow and [^{18}F]deoxyglucose imaging contains information on the magnitude of the postrevascularization improvement in congestive heart failure symptoms.[219] The level of physical activity patients were able to perform prior to and 24 ± 14 months following coronary artery bypass grafting was graded on a specific activity scale and expressed in metabolic equivalents.[220] Among the 36 patients in this study with an average LV ejection fraction of only 28 ± 6 percent prior to revascularization, the extent of the blood flow–metabolism mismatch ranged from 0 to 74 percent (mean 23 ± 22 percent) on polar map analysis. When patients were grouped according to the extent of the mismatch, 11 patients with a mismatch occupying less than 5 percent of the LV myocardium revealed a statistically significant but only mild improvement in functional status (34 percent increase in metabolic equivalents) (see Chap. 17). Intermediate-sized mismatches (5 to 17 percent) in 8 patients were associated with a 42 percent increase in metabolic equivalents, whereas large mismatches, i.e., greater than 18 percent, in 17 patients were followed after revascularization by an average increase of 107 percent in metabolic equivalents. Furthermore, the improvement in functional status was linearly correlated with the anatomic extent of the blood flow–metabolism mismatch. Lastly, blood flow–metabolism mismatches of 18 percent or more were 70 percent sensitive and 78 percent specific in predicting an improvement in physical activity or functional status following successful surgical revascularization.

Impact on Long-Term Survival Several studies examined the long-term fate of patients after being evaluated for MBF and metabolism with PET.[217,218,221,222] These studies presented compelling evidence for an increased prevalence of cardiac events in patients with blood flow–metabolism mismatches not submitted to interventional revascularization. They also implied that revascularization of blood flow–metabolism mismatches may avert future cardiac events.

Despite this general agreement, important differences emerged from these studies. One study in 129 chronic CAD patients followed for a time period of 17 ± 19 months found the presence of mismatches in the absence of revascularization to be independent predictors of the 17 nonfatal ischemic events.[221] Nevertheless, the LV ejection fraction and the patient's age contained the highest predictive values for the 13 cardiac deaths in this patient group. In patient series with more homogeneously depressed LV function, the predictive value of a low LV ejection fraction applied equally to all groups. As shown in Fig. 19-18, the cumulative long-term survival was lowest in the patient subgroup with blood flow–metabolism mismatches who were on medical treatment. Of note, all four subgroups were similar with regard to age and clinical and hemodynamic findings. There were no significant intergroup differences in the LV ejection fraction, which for the whole patient group averaged only 25 ± 7 percent. Of note, patients with mismatches who underwent revascularization revealed a significantly better cumulative survival that no longer differed significantly from that of

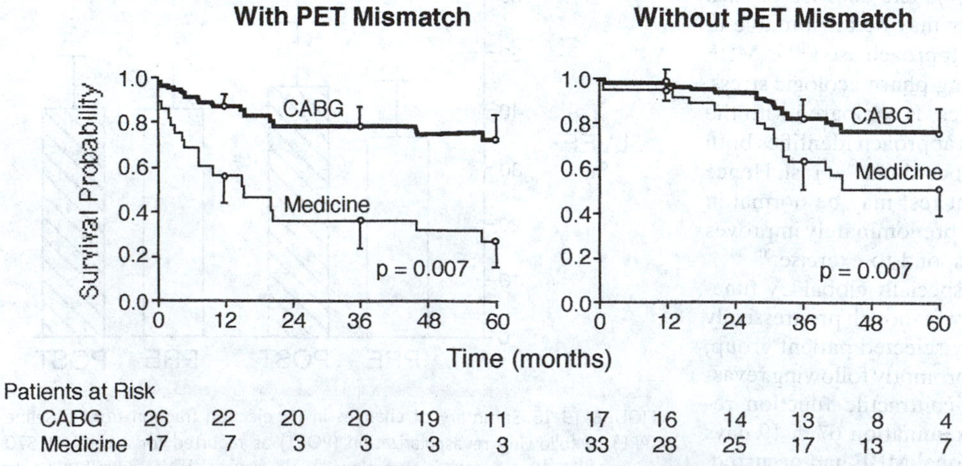

FIGURE 19-18 Estimated survival probabilities by Kaplan-Meyer analysis for patients with LV function treated medically (medicine) and with surgical revascularization (CABG) based on the absence or presence of viability as determined by PET blood flow–metabolism imaging. (Reproduced with permission from Di Carli et al.[229])

the groups without mismatches (Fig. 19-18). In this study, the LV ejection fraction was without significant predictive value, whereas by Cox model analysis the extent of a mismatch had a significant negative effect on survival ($p < 0.02$), and revascularization of mismatch patients had a significant positive effect on survival ($p < 0.04$).[218] A second study in patients with similar uniform depression of LV ejection fraction reached similar conclusions.[217]

Assessment of Perioperative Risk Surgical revascularization of patients with ischemic cardiomyopathy is associated with high perioperative mortality and morbidity. Two investigations have explored the contribution of PET to the surgical risk assessment.[208,223] Both studies together include a total of 317 patients with ischemic cardiomyopathy and LV ejection fractions of less than 35 percent. The patients were categorized into two groups. Group one (35 and 88 patients, respectively, in each study) underwent coronary artery bypass grafting based on standard clinical criteria including LV size or ejection fraction, the suitability of the coronary anatomy for surgical revascularization, and the presence of comorbidities. The same criteria also were applied to the second group (41 and 153 patients per study), which, however, underwent blood flow metabolism imaging with PET in addition. Thirty-four of 41 patients (83 percent) in one and 110 of 153 patients (72 percent) in the other group demonstrated evidence of reversibly dysfunctional myocardium involving at least 20 to 30 percent of the left ventricle and subsequently underwent bypass grafting. Both studies consistently demonstrated lower perioperative mortalities in those patients who had undergone PET imaging (30-day mortalities of 0 and 0.9 percent) as compared with mortalities of 11.4 and 19.8 percent in the patients not evaluated by PET. Additionally, 1-year cardiac mortalities were lower for the PET-selected patients (3 and 10 percent, respectively) than for those not evaluated with PET (21 and 30 percent, respectively). PET-selected patients required less inotropic support or intraaortic balloon pumping and had better cardiac output and shorter stays in the intensive care unit. If further confirmation of such short-term benefits is established, PET evaluations of patients with ischemic cardiomyopathies would then offer important and possibly critical prognostic information on the immediate and long-term risks of cardiovascular surgery in patients with severe ischemic cardiomyopathy.

Lastly, the prevalence of reversibly dysfunctional myocardium is high. A survey of 283 patients with ischemic cardiomyopathy revealed a 55 percent prevalence of blood flow and glucose metabolism mismatches.[224] Half these mismatches involved 25 percent or more of the LV myocardium and thus would lead to significant gains in LV function and clinical symptoms after revascularization. The remainder of mismatches were smaller but, if not revascularized, may be associated with an increased long-term cardiac morbidity and mortality. Indeed, in the setting of ischemic cardiomyopathy, inclusion of PET in the diagnostic algorithm can be cost-effective and, at the same time, cost saving.[225,226] Clinical criteria for deciding on coronary artery bypass grafting in patients with ischemic cardiomyopathy have already been developed.[227] In addition to the diastolic dimension, the LV ejection fraction, and suitable target vessels, the criteria include the presence of viable myocardium affecting at least 15 to 20 percent of the LV myocardium.

ACKNOWLEDGMENTS

This work was supported in part by the Director of the Office of Energy Research, Office of Health and Environmental Research, Washington, DC, by Research Grant Nos. HL 29845 and HL 33177, National Institutes of Health, Bethesda, MD, and by an Investigative Group Award by the Greater Los Angeles Affiliate of the American Heart Association, Los Angeles, CA.

References

1. Lucignani G, Paolini G, Landoni C, et al. Presurgical identification of hibernating myocardium by combined use of technetium-99m hexakis 2-methoxyisobutylisonitrile single photon emission tomography and fluorine-18 fluoro-2-deoxy-D-glucose positron emission tomography in patients with coronary artery disease. *Eur J Nucl Med* 1992; 19:874–881.
2. Altehoefer C, Kaiser H-J, Dörr R, et al. Fluorine-18 deoxyglucose PET for assessment of viable myocardium in perfusion defects in ^{99m}Tc-MIBI SPECT: A comparative study in patients with coronary artery disease. *Eur J Nucl Med* 1992; 19:334–342.
3. vom Dahl J, Eitzman D, Al-Aouar A, et al. Relation of regional function, perfusion, and metabolism in patients with advanced coronary artery disease undergoing surgical revascularization. *Circulation* 1994; 90:2356–2366.
4. Sawada S, Allman K, Muzik O, et al. Positron emission tomography detects evidence of viability in rest technetium-99m sestamibi defects. *J Am Coll Cardiol* 1994; 23:92–98.
5. Sand NP, Bottcher M, Madsen MM, et al. Evaluation of regional myocardial perfusion in patients with severe left ventricular dysfunction: Comparison of ^{13}N-ammonia PET and ^{99m}Tc sestamibi SPECT. *J Nucl Cardiol* 1998; 5:4–13.
6. Bax J, Visser F, van Lingen A, et al. Feasibility of assessing regional myocardial uptake of ^{18}F-fluorodeoxyglucose using single photon emission computed tomography. *Eur Heart J* 1993; 14:1675–1682.
7. Martin WH, Delbeke D, Patton JA, et al. FDG-SPECT: Correlation with FDG-PET. *J Nucl Med* 1995; 36:988–995.
8. Burt R, Perkins O, Oppenheim B, et al. Direct comparison of fluorine-18-FDG SPECT, fluorine-18-FDG PET and rest thallium-201 SPECT for detection of myocardial viability. *J Nucl Med* 1995; 36:176–179.
9. Bax J, Visser F, Blanksma P, et al. Comparison of myocardial uptake of fluorine-18-fluorodeoxyglucose imaged with PET and SPECT in dyssynergic myocardium. *J Nucl Med* 1996; 37:1631–1636.
10. Chen EQ, MacIntyre WJ, Go RT, et al. Myocardial viability studies using fluorine-18-FDG SPECT: A comparison with fluorine-18-FDG PET. *J Nucl Med* 1997; 38:582–586.
11. Srinivasan G, Kitsiou AN, Bacharach SL, et al. [^{18}F]fluorodeoxyglucose single photon emission computed tomography: Can it replace PET and thallium SPECT for the assessment of myocardial viability? (see comments). *Circulation* 1998; 97:843–850.
12. Hasegawa S, Uehara T, Yamaguchi H, et al. Vilidity of ^{18}F-fluorodeoxyglucose imaging with a dual-head coincidence camera for detection of myocardial viability. *J Nucl Med* 1999; 40:1884–1892.
13. Pirich C, Wetzel D, Odaka K, et al. Feasibility of myocardial metabolic imaging with F-18 deoxyglucose using a gamma camera in coincidence mode. *Circulation* 1999; 100(suppl I):I-865.
14. Iida H, Rhodes C, de Silva R, et al. Myocardial tissue fraction: Correction for partial volume effects and measure of tissue viability. *J Nucl Med* 1991; 32:2169–2175.
15. Yamamoto Y, De Silva R, Rhodes C, et al. A new strategy for the assessment of viable myocardium and regional myocardial

blood flow using ^{15}O-water and dynamic positron emission tomography. *Circulation* 1992; 86:167–178.
16. de Silva R, Yamamoto Y, Rhodes CG, et al. Preoperative prediction of the outcome of coronary revascularization using positron emission tomography. *Circulation* 1992; 86:1738–1742.
17. Bax JJ, Fath-Ordoubadi F, Wijns W, Camici PG. Water-perfusable tissue fraction for the assessment of myocardial viability: Comparison with F18-fluorodeoxyglucose. *Circulation* 1999; 100(suppl I):I-865.
18. Marinho N, Keogh B, Costa D, et al. Pathophysiology of chronic left ventricular dysfunction. *Circulation* 1996; 93:737–744.
19. Budinger TF, Yano Y, Derenzo SE, et al. Rb-82 myocardial positron emission tomography. *J Nucl Med* 1979; 20:P603.
20. Schelbert HR, Phelps ME, Hoffman EJ, et al. Regional myocardial perfusion assessed with N-13 labeled ammonia and positron emission computerized axial tomography. *Am J Cardiol* 1979; 43:209–218.
21. Gould KL. Identifying and measuring severity of coronary artery stenosis: Quantitative coronary arteriography and positron emission tomography. *Circulation* 1988; 78:237–245.
22. Bergmann SR, Herrero P, Markham J, et al. Noninvasive quantitation of myocardial blood flow in human subjects with oxygen-15-labeled water and positron emission tomography. *J Am Coll Cardiol* 1989; 14:639–652.
23. Araujo L, Lammertsma A, Rhodes C, et al. Noninvasive quantification of regional myocardial blood flow in coronary artery disease with oxygen-15-labeled carbon dioxide inhalation and positron emission tomography. *Circulation* 1991; 83:875–885.
24. Krivokapich J, Smith GT, Huang SC, et al. N-13 ammonia myocardial imaging at rest and with exercise in normal volunteers: Quantification of absolute myocardial perfusion with dynamic positron emission tomography. *Circulation* 1989; 80:1328–1337.
25. Hutchins G, Schwaiger M, Rosenspire K, et al. Noninvasive quantification of regional blood flow in the human heart using N-13 ammonia and dynamic positron emission tomographic imaging. *J Am Coll Cardiol* 1990; 15:1032–1042.
26. Chan S, Brunken R, Czernin J, et al. Comparison of maximal myocardial blood flow during adenosine infusion with that of intravenous dipyridamole in normal men. *J Am Coll Cardiol* 1992; 20:979–985.
27. Bellina C, Parodi O, Camici P, et al. Simultaneous in vitro and in vivo validation of nitrogen-13-ammonia for the assessment of regional myocardial blood flow. *J Nucl Med* 1990; 31: 1335–1343.
28. Holmberg S, Serzysko W, Varnauskas E. Coronary circulation during heavy exercise in control subjects and patients with coronary heart disease. *Acta Med Scand* 1971; 190:465–480.
29. Czernin J, Müller P, Chan S, et al. Influence of age and hemodynamics on myocardial blood flow and flow reserve. *Circulation* 1993; 88:62–69.
30. Duvernoy CS, Meyer C, Seifert-Klauss V, et al. Gender differences in myocardial blood flow dynamics: Lipid profile and hemodynamic effects. *J Am Coll Cardiol* 1999; 33:463–470.
31. Nagamachi S, Czernin J, Kim AS, et al. Reproducibility of measurements of regional resting and hyperemic myocardial blood flow assessed with PET. *J Nucl Med* 1996; 37:1626–1631.
32. Sawada S, Muzik O, Beanlands RS, et al. Interobserver and interstudy variability of myocardial blood flow and flow-reserve measurements with nitrogen 13 ammonia-labeled positron emission tomography. *J Nucl Cardiol* 1995; 2:413–422.
33. Kaufmann PA, Gnecchi-Ruscone T, Yap JT, et al. Assessment of the reproducibility of baseline and hyperemic myocardial blood flow measurements with ^{15}O-labeled water and PET. *J Nucl Med* 1999; 40:1848–1856.
34. Kuhle WG, Porenta G, Huang SC, et al. Quantification of regional myocardial blood flow using ^{13}N-ammonia and reoriented dynamic positron emission tomographic imaging. *Circulation* 1992; 86:1004–1017.
35. Bol A, Melin JA, Vanoverschelde J-L, et al. Direct comparison of [^{13}N]ammonia and [^{15}O]water estimates of perfusion with quantification of regional myocardial blood flow by microspheres. *Circulation* 1993; 87:512–525.
36. Muzik O, Beanlands RSB, Hutchins GD, et al. Validation of nitrogen-13-ammonia tracer kinetic model for quantification of myocardial blood flow using PET. *J Nucl Med* 1993; 34:83–91.
37. Merlet P, Mazoyer B, Hittinger L, et al. Assessment of coronary reserve in man: Comparison between positron emission tomography with oxygen-15-labeled water and intracoronary Doppler technique. *J Nucl Med* 1993; 34:1899–1904.
38. Opie LH. Metabolism of the heart in health and disease. *Am Heart J* 1968; 76:685–698.
39. Liedtke AJ. Alterations of carbohydrate and lipid metabolism in the acutely ischemic heart. *Prog Cardiovasc Dis* 1981; 23:321–336.
40. Bing RJ. *The Metabolism of the Heart* (Harvey Lecture Series). New York: Academic Press; 1954:27–70.
41. Keul J, Doll E, Steim H, et al. Über den Stoffwechsel des menschlichen Herzens: I. Substratversorgung des gesunden Herzens in Ruhe, während und nach körperlicher Arbeit. *Pfluegers Arch* 1965; 282:1–27.
42. Keul J, Doll E, Steim H, et al. Über den Stoffwechsel des menschlichen Herzens: III. Der oxidative Stoffwechsel des menschlichen Herzens unter verschiedenen Arbeitsbedingungen II. *Pfluegers Arch* 1965; 282:43–53.
43. Taegtmeyer H. Myocardial metabolism. In: Phelps M, Mazziotta J, Schelbert H, eds. *Positron Emission Tomography and Autoradiography: Principles and Applications for the Brain and Heart.* New York: Raven Press; 1986:149–195.
44. Sokoloff L, Reivich M, Kennedy C, et al. The [^{14}C]deoxyglucose method for the measurement of local cerebral glucose utilization: Theory, procedure and normal values in the conscious and anesthetized albino rat. *J Neurochem* 1977; 28:897–916.
45. Ratib O, Phelps ME, Huang SC, et al. Positron tomography with deoxyglucose for estimating local myocardial glucose metabolism. *J Nucl Med* 1982; 23:577–586.
46. Schelbert HR, Henze E, Schön HR, et al. C-11 palmitic acid for the noninvasive evaluation of regional myocardial fatty acid metabolism with positron computed tomography: IV. In vivo demonstration of impaired fatty acid oxidation in acute myocardial ischemia. *Am Heart J* 1983; 106:736–750.
47. Schön HR, Schelbert HR, Najafi A, et al. C-11 labeled palmitic acid for the noninvasive evaluation of regional myocardial fatty acid metabolism with positron computed tomography: II. Kinetics of C-11 palmitic acid in acutely ischemic myocardium. *Am Heart J* 1982; 103:548–561.
48. Bergmann S, Weinheimer C, Markham J, Herrero P. Quantitation of myocardial fatty acid metabolism using PET. *J Nucl Med* 1996; 37:1723–1730.
49. Schelbert HR, Henze E, Schön HR, et al. C-11 palmitate for the noninvasive evaluation of regional myocardial fatty acid metabolism with positron computed tomography. III. In vivo demonstration of the effects of substrate availability on myocardial metabolism. *Am Heart J* 1983; 105:492–504.
50. Cohen MB. Synthesis and utilization of ^{13}N compounds for positron scanning. *Int J Nucl Med Biol* 1978; 5:201.
51. Choi Y, Brunken R, Hawkins R, et al. Factors affecting myocardial 2-[F-18]fluoro-2-deoxy-D-glucose uptake in positron emission tomography studies of normal humans. *Eur J Nucl Med* 1993; 20:308–318.
52. Iida H, Rhodes C, Araujo L, et al. Noninvasive quantification of regional myocardial metabolic rate for oxygen by use of $^{15}O_2$ inhalation and positron emission tomography: Theory, error analysis, and application in humans. *Circulation* 1996; 94:792–807.
53. Yamamoto Y, de Silva R, Rhodes C, et al. Noninvasive quantifi-

cation of regional myocardial metabolic rate of oxygen by $^{15}O_2$ inhalation and positron emission tomography: Experimental validation. *Circulation* 1996; 94:808–816.
54. Buxton DB, Nienaber CA, Luxen A, et al. Noninvasive quantitation of regional myocardial oxygen consumption in vivo with [1-^{11}C]acetate and dynamic positron emission tomography. *Circulation* 1989; 79:134–142.
55. Armbrecht JJ, Buxton DB, Brunken RC, et al. Regional myocardial oxygen consumption determined noninvasively in humans with [1-^{11}C]acetate and dynamic positron tomography. *Circulation* 1989; 80:863–872.
56. Henes C, Bergmann S, Walsh M, et al. Noninvasive quantification of myocardial metabolic reserve by positron emission tomography (PET) with C-11 acetate and dobutamine. *Circulation* 1989; 80:II-312.
57. Armbrecht JJ, Buxton DB, Schelbert HR. Validation of [1-^{11}C] acetate as a tracer for noninvasive assessment of oxidative metabolism with positron emission tomography in normal, ischemic, postischemic and hyperemic canine myocardium. *Circulation* 1991; 81:1594–1605.
58. Ng NCK, Huang SC, Schelbert HR, Buxton DB. Validation of a model for [1-^{11}C]acetate as a tracer of cardiac oxidative metabolism. *Am J Physiol* 1994; 266:H1304–H1315.
59. Sun K, Chen K, Huang S-C, et al. Compartment model for measuring myocardial oxygen consumption using [1-^{11}C]acetate. *J Nucl Med* 1997; 38:459–466.
60. Sun KT, Yeatman LA, Buxton DB, et al. Simultaneous measurement of myocardial oxygen consumption and blood flow using [1-carbon-11]acetate. *J Nucl Med* 1998; 39:272–280.
61. Gould KL, Lipscomb K, Hamilton GW. Physiologic basis for assessing critical coronary stenosis: Instantaneous flow response and regional distribution during coronary hyperemia as measures of coronary flow reserve. *Am J Cardiol* 1974; 33:87–94.
62. Chan S, Kobashigawa J, Stevenson L, et al. Myocardial blood flow at rest and during pharmacologic vasodilation in cardiac transplants during and after successful treatment of rejection. *Circulation* 1994; 90:204–212.
63. Czernin J, Auerbach M, Sun K, et al. Effects of modified pharmacologic stress approaches on hyperemic myocardial blood flow. *J Nucl Med* 1995; 36:575–580.
64. Czernin J, Muller P, Chan S, et al. Influence of age and hemodynamics on myocardial blood flow and flow reserve. *Circulation* 1993; 88:62–69.
65. Senneff M, Geltman E, Bergmann S, Hartman J. Noninvasive delineation of the effects of moderate aging on myocardial perfusion. *J Nucl Med* 1991; 32:2037–2042.
66. Uren N, Camici P, Melin J, et al. Effect of aging on myocardial perfusion reserve. *J Nucl Med* 1995; 36:2032–2036.
67. Müller P, Czernin J, Choi Y, et al. Effect of exercise supplementation during adenosine infusion on hyperemic blood flow and flow reserve. *Am Heart J* 1994; 128:52–60.
68. Nienaber CA, Gambhir SS, Mody FV, et al. Regional myocardial blood flow and glucose utilization in symptomatic patients with hypertrophic cardiomyopathy. *Circulation* 1993; 87:1580–1590.
69. Czernin J, Sun K, Brunken R, et al. Effect of acute and long-term smoking on myocardial blood flow and flow reserve. *Circulation* 1995; 91:2891–2897.
70. Böttcher M, Czernin J, Sun K, et al. Effect of caffeine on myocardial blood flow at rest and during pharmacological vasodilation. *J Nucl Med* 1995; 36:2016–2021.
71. Krivokapich J, Huang S-C, Schelbert H. Assessment of the effects of dobutamine on myocardial blood flow and oxidative metabolism in normal human subjects using nitrogen-13 ammonia and carbon-11 acetate. *Am J Cardiol* 1993; 71:1351–1356.
72. Sun K, Czernin J, Krivokapich J, et al. Effects of dobutamine stimulation on myocardial blood flow, glucose metabolism and wall motion in normal and dysfunctional myocardium. *Circulation* 1996; 94:3146–3154.
73. Gould K. *Coronary Artery Stenosis*. New York: Elsevier; 1990.
74. Porenta G, Kuhle W, Czernin J, et al. Semiquantitative assessment of myocardial viability and perfusion utilizing polar map displays of cardiac PET images. *J Nucl Med* 1992; 33:1623–1631.
75. Laubenbacher C, Rothley J, Sitomer J, et al. An automated analysis program for the evaluation of cardiac PET studies: Initial results in the detection and localization of coronary artery disease using nitrogen-13-ammonia. *J Nucl Med* 1993; 34:968–978.
76. Nekolla SG, Miethaner C, Nguyen N, et al. Reproducibility of polar map generation and assessment of defect severity and extent assessment in myocardial perfusion imaging using positron emission tomography. *Eur J Nucl Med* 1998; 25:1313–1321.
77. Schelbert HR, Wisenberg G, Phelps ME, et al. Noninvasive assessment of coronary stenoses by myocardial imaging during pharmacologic coronary vasodilation. VI. Detection of coronary artery disease in man with intravenous N-13 ammonia and positron computed tomography. *Am J Cardiol* 1982; 49:1197–1207.
78. Tamaki N, Yonekura Y, Senda M, et al. Value and limitation of stress thallium-201 single photon emission computed tomography: Comparison with nitrogen-13 ammonia positron tomography. *J Nucl Med* 1988; 29:1181–1188.
79. Demer LL, Gould KL, Goldstein RA, et al. Assessment of coronary artery disease severity by positron emission tomography. Comparison with quantitative arteriography in 193 patients. *Circulation* 1989; 79:825–835.
80. Go R, Marwick T, MacIntyre W, et al. A prospective comparison of rubidium-82 PET and thallium-201 SPECT myocardial perfusion imaging utilizing a single dipyridamole stress in the diagnosis of coronary artery disease. *J Nucl Med* 1990; 31:1899–1905.
81. Stewart R, Schwaiger M, Molina E, et al. Comparison of rubidium-82 positron emission tomography and thallium-201 SPECT imaging for detection of coronary artery disease. *Am J Cardiol* 1991; 67:1303–1310.
82. Simone G, Mullani N, Page D, Anderson B Sr. Utilization statistics and diagnostic accuracy of a nonhospital-based positron emission tomography center for the detection of coronary artery disease using rubidium-82. *Am J Physiol Imaging* 1992; 7:203–209.
83. Williams B, Millani N, Jansen D, Anderson B. A retrospective study of the diagnostic accuracy of a community hospital-based PET center for the detection of coronary artery disease using rubidium-82. *J Nucl Med* 1994; 35:1586–1592.
84. Gould KL, Goldstein RA, Mullani NA, et al. Noninvasive assessment of coronary stenoses by myocardial perfusion imaging during pharmacologic coronary vasodilation: VIII. Clinical feasibility of positron cardiac imaging without a cyclotron using generator-produced rubidium-82. *J Am Coll Cardiol* 1986; 7:775–789.
85. Zijlstra F, Fioretti P, Reiber J, Serruys P. Which cineangiographically assessed anatomical variable correlates best with functional measurements of stenosis severity? A comparison of quantitative analysis of the coronary cineangiogram with measured coronary flow reserve and exercise/redistribution thallium-201 scintigraphy. *J Am Coll Cardiol* 1988; 12:686–691.
86. Brown BG, Josephson MA, Peterson RB, et al. Intravenous dipyridamole combined with isometric handgrip for near maximal acute increase in coronary flow in patients with coronary artery disease. *Am J Cardiol* 1981; 48:1077–1085.
87. Merhige ME, Houston T, Shalton V, et al. PET myocardial perfusion imaging reduces the cost of coronary disease management by eliminating unnecessary invasive diagnostic and therapeutic procedures. *Circulation* 1999; 100(suppl I):I-26.
88. Uren N, Melin J, De Bruyne B, et al. Relation between myocardial blood flow and the severity of coronary-artery stenosis. *New Engl J Med* 1994; 330:1782–1788.
89. Di Carli M, Czernin J, Hoh C, et al. Relation among stenosis

severity, myocardial blood flow, and flow reserve in patients with coronary artery disease. *Circulation* 1995; 91:1944–1951.
90. Beanlands R, Schwaiger M. Changes in myocardial oxygen consumption and efficiency with heart failure therapy measured by ^{11}C acetate PET. *Can J Cardiol* 1995; 11:293–300.
91. Krivokapich J, Czernin J, Schelbert HR. Dobutamine positron emission tomography: Absolute quantitation of rest and dobutamine myocardial blood flow and correlation with cardiac work and percent diameter stenosis in patients with and without coronary artery disease. *J Am Coll Cardiol* 1996; 28:565–572.
92. Smith SC Jr. Risk-reduction therapy: The challenge to change. Presented at the 68th scientific sessions of the American Heart Association, November 13, 1995, Anaheim, California. *Circulation* 1996; 93:2205–2211.
93. Libby P. Molecular bases of the acute coronary syndromes. *Circulation* 1995; 91:2844–2850.
94. Zeiher S, Drexler H, Wollschläger H, Just H. Modulation of coronary vasomotor tone: Progressive endothelial dysfunction with different early stages of coronary atherosclerosis. *Circulation* 1991; 83:391–401.
95. Zeiher A, Drexler H, Saurbier B, Just H. Endothelium-mediated coronary blood flow modulation in humans. Effects of age, atherosclerosis, hypercholesterolemia, and hypertension. *J Clin Invest* 1993; 92:652–662.
96. Egashira K, Inou T, Hirooka Y, et al. Impaired coronary blood flow response to acetylcholine in patients with coronary risk factors and proximal atherosclerotic lesions. *J Clin Invest* 1993; 91:29–37.
97. Dayanikli F, Grambow D, Muzik O, et al. Early detection of abnormal coronary flow reserve in asymptomatic men at high risk for coronary artery disease using positron emission tomography. *Circulation* 1994; 90:808–817.
98. Yokoyama I, Murakami T, Ohtake T, et al. Reduced coronary flow reserve in familial hypercholesterolemia. *J Nucl Med* 1996; 37:1937–1942.
99. Yokoyama I, Ohtake T, Momomura S, et al. Reduced coronary flow reserve in hypercholesterolemic patients without overt coronary stenosis. *Circulation* 1996; 94:3232–3238.
100. Rönnemaa T, Viikari J, Taskinen MR, et al. Coronary flow reserve in young men with familial combined hyperlipidemia. *Circulation* 1999; 99:1678–1684.
101. Raitakari OT, Pitkänen OP, Lehtimeaki T, et al. In vivo low density lipoprotein oxidation relates to coronary reactivity in young men. *J Am Coll Cardiol* 1997; 30:97–102.
102. Pitkänen OP, Raitakari O, Niinikoski H, et al. Coronary flow reserve is impaired in young men with familial hypercholesterolemia. *J Am Coll Cardiol* 1996; 28:1705–1711.
103. Pitkänen OP, Raitakari OT, Ronnemaa T, et al. Influence of cardiovascular risk status on coronary flow reserve in healthy young men. *Am J Cardiol* 1997; 79:1690–1692.
104. Yokoyama I, Ohtake T, Momomura S, et al. Impaired myocardial vasodilation during hyperemic stress with dipyridamole in hypertriglyceridemia. *J Am Coll Cardiol* 1998; 31:1568–1574.
105. Yokoyama I, Ohtake T, Momomura S, et al. Altered myocardial vasodilatation in patients with hypertriglyceridemia in anatomically normal coronary arteries. *Arterioscler Thromb Vasc Biol* 1998; 18:294–299.
106. Yokoyama I, Momomura S, Ohtake T, et al. Reduced myocardial flow reserve in non-insulin-dependent diabetes mellitus (see comments). *J Am Coll Cardiol* 1997; 30:1472–1477.
107. Pitkänen OP, Nuutila P, Raitakari OT, et al. Coronary flow reserve is reduced in young men with IDDM. *Diabetes* 1998; 47:248–254.
108. Di Carli MF, Bianco-Batlles D, Landa ME, et al. Effects of autonomic neuropathy on coronary blood flow in patients with diabetes mellitus. *Circulation* 1999; 100:813–819.
109. Yokoyama I, Ohtake T, Momomura S, et al. Hyperglycemia rather than insulin resistance is related to reduced coronary flow reserve in NIDDM. *Diabetes* 1998; 47:119–124.
110. Reddy K, Nair R, Sheehan H, Hodgson JM. Evidence that selective endothelial dysfunction may occur in the absence of angiographic or ultrasound atherosclerosis in patients with risk factors for atherosclerosis. *J Am Coll Cardiol* 1994; 23:833–843.
111. Bache RJ. Vasodilator reserve: A functional assessment of coronary health (editorial, comment). *Circulation* 1998; 98:1257–1260.
112. Smits P, Williams S, Lipson D, et al. Endothelial release of nitric oxide contributes to the vasodilator effect of adenosine in humans. *Circulation* 1995; 92:2135–2141.
113. Gould KL. *Coronary Artery Stenosis and Reversing Atherosclerosis*. New York: Oxford University Press; 1998.
114. Gould KL, Nakagawa Y, Nakagawa K, et al. Frequency and clinical implications of fluid dynamically significant diffuse coronary artery disease manifest as graded, longitudinal, base to apex, myocardial perfusion abnormalities by noninvasive positron emission tomography. *Circulation* 2000; 101:1931–1939.
115. Schelbert HR, Keng F, Pampaloni MH, Kudo T. Abnormal longitudinal base to apex myocardial perfusion gradient by quantitative blood flow measurements in patients with coronary risks. *Circulation* 1999; 100(suppl I):I-88.
116. Nabel E, Ganz P, Gordon J, et al. Dilation of normal and constriction of atherosclerotic coronary arteries caused by the cold pressor test. *Circulation* 1988; 77:43–52.
117. Zeiher AM, Drexler H, Wollschläger H, et al. Coronary vasomotion in response to sympathetic stimulation in humans: Importance of the functional integrity of the endothelium (see comments). *J Am Coll Cardiol* 1989; 14:1181–1190.
118. Zeiher A, Drexler H, Wollschläger H, Just H. Endothelial dysfunction of the coronary microvasculature is associated with impaired coronary blood flow regulation in patients with early atherosclerosis. *Circulation* 1991; 84:1984–1992.
119. Campisi R, Czernin J, Schöder H, et al. Effects of long-term smoking on myocardial blood flow, coronary vasomotion, and vasodilator capacity. *Circulation* 1998; 98:119–125.
120. Campisi R, Nathan L, Pampaloni MH, et al. Effect of chronic hormone replacement therapy on coronary vasomotion in postmenopausal women. *Circulation* 1999; 100(suppl I):I-221.
121. Czernin J, Barnard J, Sun K, et al. Effect of short-term cardiovascular conditioning and low fat diet on myocardial blood flow and flow reserve. *Circulation* 1995; 92:197–204.
122. Gould K, Martucci J, Goldberg D, et al. Short-term cholesterol lowering decreases size and severity of perfusion abnormalities by positron emission tomography after dipyridamole in patients with coronary artery disease: A potential noninvasive marker of healing coronary endothelium. *Circulation* 1994; 89:1530–1538.
123. Gould K, Ornish D, Scherwitz L, et al. Changes in myocardial perfusion abnormalities by positron emission tomography after long-term, intense risk factor modification. *JAMA* 1995; 274:894–901.
124. Guethlin M, Kasel AM, Coppenrath K, et al. Delayed response of myocardial flow reserve to lipid-lowering therapy with fluvastatin. *Circulation* 1999; 99:475–481.
125. Yokoyama I, Momomura S, Ohtake T, et al. Improvement of impaired myocardial vasodilatation due to diffuse coronary atherosclerosis in hypercholesterolemics after lipid-lowering therapy. *Circulation* 1999; 100:117–122.
126. Huggins GS, Pasternak RC, Alpert NM, et al. Effects of short-term treatment of hyperlipidemia on coronary vasodilator function and myocardial perfusion in regions having substantial impairment of baseline dilator reverse (see comments). *Circulation* 1998; 98:1291–1296.
127. Mellwig KP, Baller D, Gleichmann U, et al. Improvement of coronary vasodilatation capacity through single LDL apheresis. *Atherosclerosis* 1998; 139:173–178.
128. Campisi R, Czernin J, Schöder H, et al. L-Arginine normalizes

coronary vasomotion in long-term smokers. *Circulation* 1999; 99:491–497.
129. Harrison DG. Endothelial control of vasomotion and nitric oxide production: A potential target for risk factor management. *Cardiol Clin* 1996; 14:1–15.
130. Jeserich M, Schindler T, Olscheski M, et al. Vitamin C improves endothelial function of epicardial coronary arteries in patients with hypercholestaemia or essental hypertension-assessed by cold pressor testing. *Eur Heart J* 1999; 20:1676–1680.
131. Böger RH, Bode-Böger SM, Szuba A, et al. Asymmetric dimethylarginine (ADMA): A novel risk factor for endothelial dysfunction: Its role in hypercholesterolemia. *Circulation* 1998; 98:1842–1847.
132. Opie LH. Myocardial ischemia: Metabolic pathways and implications of increased glycolysis. *Cardiol Drugs Ther* 1990; 4:777–790.
133. Schelbert HR, Phelps ME, Selin C, et al. Regional myocardial ischemia assessed by ^{18}fluoro-2-deoxyglucose and positron emission computed tomography. In: Kreuzer H, Parmley W, Rentrop P, Heiss H, eds. *Quantification of Myocardial Ischemia*, Vol I. New York: Gehard Witzstrock Publishing House; 1980:437–447.
134. Marshall RC, Tillisch JH, Phelps ME, et al. Identification and differentiation of resting myocardial ischemia and infarction in man with positron computed tomography ^{18}F-labeled fluorodeoxyglucose and N-13 ammonia. *Circulation* 1983; 67:766–778.
135. Tillisch J, Brunken R, Marshall R, et al. Reversibility of cardiac wall motion abnormalities predicted by positron tomography. *New Engl J Med* 1986; 314:884–888.
136. Camici P, Araujo LI, Spinks T, et al. Increased uptake of ^{18}F-fluorodeoxyglucose in postischemic myocardium of patients with exercise-induced angina. *Circulation* 1986; 74:81–88.
137. Schwaiger M, Schelbert HR, Ellison D, et al. Sustained regional abnormalities in cardiac metabolism after transient ischemia in the chronic dog model. *J Am Coll Cardiol* 1985; 6:336–347.
138. Vanoverschelde J-L, Wijns W, Depré C, et al. Mechanisms of chronic regional postischemic dysfunction in humans: New insights from the study of noninfarcted collateral-dependent myocardium. *Circulation* 1993; 87:1513–1523.
139. Gerber BL, Wijns W, Vanoverschelde JJ, et al. Myocardial perfusion and oxygen consumption in reperfused noninfarcted dysfunctional myocardium after unstable angina: Direct evidence for myocardial stunning in humans. *J Am Coll Cardiol* 1999; 34:1939–1946.
140. Schwaiger M, Neese RA, Araujo L, et al. Sustained nonoxidative glucose utilization and depletion of glycogen in reperfused canine myocardium. *J Am Coll Cardiol* 1989; 13:745–754.
141. Schwaiger M, Brunken R, Grover-McKay M, et al. Regional myocardial metabolism in patients with acute myocardial infarction assessed by positron emission tomography. *J Am Coll Cardiol* 1986; 8:800–808.
142. Bolli R, Triana F, Jeroudi MO. Postischemic mechanical and vascular dysfunction (myocardial "stunning" and microvascular "stunning") and the effects of calcium-channel blockers on ischemia/reperfusion injury. *Clin Cardiol* 1989; 12:III-16–III-25.
143. Rahimtoola SH. The hibernating myocardium. *Am Heart J* 1989; 117:211–221.
144. Schulz R, Rose J, Martin C, et al. Development of short-term myocardial hibernation: Its limitation by the severity of ischemia and inotropic stimulation. *Circulation* 1993; 88:684–695.
145. Chen C, Gillam L, Chen L, et al. Temporal hierarchy in functional and ultrastructural recoveries between short-term and chronic hibernating myocardium after reperfusion. *Circulation* 1995; 92:I-552.
146. Chen C, Chen L, Fallon J, et al. Functional and structural alterations with 24-hour myocardial hibernation and recovery after reperfusion. *Circulation* 1996; 94:507–516.
147. Fallavollita J, Bryan P, Canty J. ^{18}F-2-deoxyglucose deposition and regional flow in pigs with chronically dysfunctional myocardium: Evidence for transmural variations in chronic hibernating myocardium. *Circulation* 1997; 95:1900–1909.
148. Fallavollita JA, Canty JM Jr. Differential ^{18}F-2-deoxyglucose uptake in viable dysfunctional myocardium with normal resting perfusion: Evidence for chronic stunning in pigs. *Circulation* 1999; 99:2798–2805.
149. Fallavollita JA, Perry BJ, Canty JM Jr. ^{18}F-2-deoxyglucose deposition and regional flow in pigs with chronically dysfunctional myocardium: Evidence for transmural variations in chronic hibernating myocardium. *Circulation* 1997; 95:1900–1909.
150. Shivalkar B, Flameng W, Szilard M, et al. Repeated stunning precedes myocardial hibernation in progressive multiple coronary artery obstruction. *J Am Coll Cardiol* 1999; 34:2126–2136.
151. Lim H, Fallavollita JA, Hard R, et al. Profound apoptosis-mediated regional myocyte loss and compensatory hypertrophy in pigs with hibernating myocardium. *Circulation* 1999; 100:2380–2386.
152. Fragasso G, Chierchia S, Lucignani G, et al. Time dependence of residual tissue viability after myocardial infarction assessed by [^{18}F]fluorodeoxyglucose and positron emission tomography. *Am J Cardiol* 1993; 72:131G–139G.
153. Fedele FA, Gewortz J, Capone RJ, et al. Metabolic response to prolonged reduction of myocardial blood flow distal to a severe coronary artery stenosis. *Circulation* 1988; 78:729–735.
154. Schaefer S, Schwartz G, Wisneski J, et al. Response of high-energy phosphates and lactate release during prolonged regional ischemia in vivo. *Circulation* 1992; 85:342–349.
155. Camici P, Wijns W, Borgers M, et al. Pathophysiological mechanisms of chronic reversible left ventricular dysfunction due to coronary artery disease (hibernating myocardium). *Circulation* 1997; 96:3205–3214.
156. Maes A, Vlameng W, Borgers M, et al. Regional myocardial blood flow, glucose utilization and contractile function before and after revascularization and ultrastructural findings in patients with chronic coronary artery disease. *Eur J Nucl Med* 1995; 22:1299–1305.
157. Wolpers H, Burchert W, van den Hoff J, et al. Assessment of myocardial viability by use of ^{11}C-acetate and positron emission tomography. *Circulation* 1997; 95:1417–1424
158. Stinson EB, Griepp RB, Bieber CP, Shumway NE. Changes in coronary blood flow during rejection of orthotopically transplanted canine hearts. *J Cardiovasc Surg* 1987; 63:854–864
159. Cabin HS, Clubbs KS, Vita N, Zaret BL. Regional dysfunction by equilibrium radionuclide angiography: A clinicopathologic study evaluating the relation of degree of dysfunction to the presence and extent of myocardial infarction. *J Am Coll Cardiol* 1987; 10:743–747.
160. Flameng W, Suy R, Schwarz F, et al. Ultrastructural correlates of left ventricular contraction abnormalities in patients with chronic ischemic heart disease: Determinants of reversible segmental asynergy post-revascularization surgery. *Am Heart J* 1981; 102:846–857.
161. Maes A, Flameng W, Nuyts J, et al. Histological alterations in chronically hypoperfused myocardium: Correlation with PET findings. *Circulation* 1994; 90:735–745.
162. Depré C, Vanoverschelde J-LJ, Melin J, et al. Structural and metabolic correlates of the reversibility of chronic left ventricular ischemic dysfunction in humans. *Am J Physiol* 1995; 268:H1265–H1275.
163. Schwarz E, Schaper J, vom Dahl J, et al. Myocyte degeneration and cell death in hibernating human myocardium. *J Am Coll Cardiol* 1996; 27:1577–1585.
164. Schwaiger M, Sun D, Deeb G, et al. Expression of myocardial glucose transporter (GLUT) mRNAs in patients with advanced coronary artery disease (CAD). *Circulation* 1994; 90:I-113.
165. Lopaschuk G, Stanley W. Glucose metabolism in the ischemic heart. *Circulation* 1997; 95:313–315.
166. Lopaschuk GD. Treating ischemic heart disease by pharmacologi-

cally improving cardiac energy metabolism. *Am J Cardiol* 1998; 82:14K–17K.
167. Allman K, Wieland D, Muzik O, et al. Carbon-11 hydroxyephedrine with positron emission tomography for serial assessment of cardiac adrenergic neuronal function after acute myocardial infarction in humans. *J Am Coll Cardiol* 1993; 22:368–375.
168. Bengel F, Ueberfuhr P, Ziegler SI, et al. Effect of cardiac sympathetic innervation on metabolism of the human heart by positron emission tomography. *Circulation* 1999; 100(suppl I):I-201.
169. Borgers M, Ausma J. Structural aspects of the chronic hibernating myocardium in man. *Basic Res Cardiol* 1995; 90:44–46.
170. Ausma J, Wijffels M, van Eys G, et al. Dedifferentiation of atrial cardiomyocytes as a result of chronic atrial fibrillation. *Am J Pathol* 1997; 151:985–997.
171. Depré C, Shipley GL, Chen W, et al. Unloaded heart in vivo replicates fetal gene expression of cardiac hypertrophy. *Nature Med* 1998; 4:1269–1275.
172. Ausma J, Thonae F, Dispersyn GD, et al. Dedifferentiated cardiomyocytes from chronic hibernating myocardium are ischemia-tolerant. *Mol Cell Biochem* 1998; 186:159–168.
173. Elsässer A, Schlepper M, Klövekorn W-P, et al. Hibernating myocardium: An incomplete adaptation to ischemia. *Circulation* 1997; 96:2920–2931.
174. Elsaesser A, Greiber S, Hein S, et al. Hibernating myocardium: Upregulation of caspase-3 gene and reduction of *bcl-2*. *Circulation* 1999; 100(suppl I):I-758.
175. Chen C, Lijie M, Linfert D, et al. Myocardial cell death and apoptosis in hibernating myocardium. *J Am Coll Cardiol* 1997; 30:1407–1412.
176. Brunken R, Mody F, Hawkins R, et al. Metabolic imaging with positron emission tomography detects viable tissue in myocardial segments with persistent defects on twenty-four hour tomographic thallium-201 scintigraphy. *Circulation* 1992; 86:1357–1369.
177. Beanlands RS, Hendry PJ, Masters RG, et al. Delay in revascularization is associated with increased mortality rate in patients with severe left ventricular dysfunction and viable myocardium on fluorine 18-fluorodeoxyglucose positron emission tomography imaging. *Circulation* 1998; 98:II51–II56.
178. Schwarz E, Schoendube F, Kostin S, et al. Prolonged myocardial hibernation exacerbates cardiomyocyte degeneration and impairs recovery of function after revascularization. *J Am Coll Cardiol* 1998; 31:1018–1026.
179. Ausma J, Duimel H, Wouters L, et al. Structural atrial remodeling in the goat by 16 weeks of atrial fibrillation is not reversed 8 weeks after cardioversion. *Circulation* 1999; 100(suppl I):I-10.
180. Nienaber C, Brunken R, Sherman C, et al. Metabolic and functional recovery of ischemic human myocardium after coronary angioplasty. *J Am Coll Cardiol* 1991; 18:966–978.
181. Marwick T, MacIntyre W, Lafont A, et al. Metabolic responses of hibernating and infarcted myocardium to revascularization: A follow-up study of regional perfusion, function, and metabolism. *Circulation* 1992; 85:1347–1353.
182. Tamaki N, Yonekura Y, Yamashita K, et al. Positron emission tomography using fluorine-18 deoxyglucose in evaluation of coronary artery bypass grafting. *Am J Cardiol* 1989; 64:860–865.
183. Carrel T, Jenni R, Haubold-Reuter S, et al. Improvement of severely reduced left ventricular function after surgical revascularization in patients with preoperative myocardial infarction. *Eur J Cardiothorac Surg* 1992; 6:479–484.
184. Gewirtz H, Fischman A, Abraham S, et al. Positron emission tomographic measurements of absolute regional myocardial blood flow permits identification of nonviable myocardium in patients with chronic myocardial infarction. *J Am Coll Cardiol* 1994; 23:851–859.
185. Duvernoy CS, vom Dahl J, Laubenbacher C, Schwaiger M. The role of nitrogen-13 ammonia positron emission tomography in predicting functional outcome after coronary revascularization. *J Nucl Cardiol* 1995; 2:499–506.
186. Bax JJ, Poldermans D, Elhendy A, et al. Improvement of left ventricular ejection fraction, heart failure symptoms and prognosis after revascularization in patients with chronic coronary artery disease and viable myocardium detected by dobutamine stress echocardiography. *J Am Coll Cardiol* 1999; 34:163–169.
187. Bonow R, Dilsizian V, Cuocolo A, Bacharach S. Identification of viable myocardium in patients with chronic coronary artery disease and left ventricular dysfunction: Comparison of thallium scintigraphy with reinjection and PET imaging with F-18-fluorodeoxyglucose. *Circulation* 1991; 83:26–37.
188. Knuuti M, Saraste M, Nuutila P, et al. Myocardial viability: Fluorine-18-deoxyglucose positron emission tomography in prediction of wall motion recovery after revascularization. *Circulation* 1994; 90:2356–2366.
189. Baer F, Voth E, Deutsch H, et al. Predictive value of low-dose dobutamine transesophageal echocardiography and fluorine-18 fluorodeoxyglucose positron emission tomography for recovery of regional left ventricular function after successful revascularization. *J Am Coll Cardiol* 1996; 28:60–69.
190. Buvat I, Bartlett M, Srinivasan G, et al. Can gated FDG PET assess LV function as well as gated bloodpool SPECT? *J Nucl Med* 1996; 37:39P.
191. Buvat I, Kitsiou A, Srinivasan G, et al. Relationship between metabolism and function in CAD patients using gated FDG PET. *J Nucl Med* 1996; 37:161P.
192. Fath-Ordoubadi F, Beatt KJ, Spyrou N, Camici PG. Efficacy of coronary angioplasty for the treatment of hibernating myocardium. *Heart* 1999; 82:210–216.
193. DePuey EG, Ghesani M, Schwartz M, et al. Comparative performance of gated perfusion SPECT wall thickening, delayed thallium uptake, and F-18 fluorodeoxyglucose SPECT in detecting myocardial viability. *J Nucl Cardiol* 1999; 6:418–428.
194. Schöder H, Campisi R, Ohtake T, et al. Blood flow-metabolism imaging with positron emission tomography in patients with diabetes mellitus for the assessment of reversible left ventricular contractile dysfunction. *J Am Coll Cardiol* 1999; 33: 1328–1337.
195. Bax J, Cornel J, Visser F, et al. Prediction of improvement of global function after revascularization in patients with ischemic left ventricular dysfunction: Detection by F18-fluorodeoxyglucose SPECT. *J Am Coll Cardiol* 1997; 29:377A.
196. Bax J, Cornel J, Visser F, et al. Prediction of improvement of contractile function in patients with ischemic ventricular dysfunction after revascularization by fluorine-18 fluorodeoxyglucose single-photon-emission computed tomography. *J Am Coll Cardiol* 1997; 30:377–383.
197. Dreyfus G, Duboc D, Blasco A, et al. Myocardial viability assessment in ischemic cardiomyopathy: Benefits of coronary revascularization. *Ann Thorac Surg* 1994; 57:1402–1408.
198. Akinboboye OO, Idris O, Cannon PJ, Bergmann SR. Usefulness of positron emission tomography in defining myocardial viability in patients referred for cardiac transplantation. *Am J Cardiol* 1999; 83:1271–1274.
199. Shivalkar B, Maes A, Borgers M, et al. Only hibernating myocardium invariably shows early recovery after coronary revascularization. *Circulation* 1996; 94:308–315.
200. Grandin C, Wijns W, Melin J, et al. Delineation of myocardial viability with PET. *J Nucl Med* 1995; 36:1543–1552.
201. Stevenson W, Stevenson L, Middlekauff H, et al. Improving survival for patients with advanced heart failure: A study of 737 consecutive patients. *J Am Coll Cardiol* 1995; 26:1417–1423.
202. Vaghaiwalla Mody F, Brunken R, Warner-Stevenson L, et al. Differentiating cardiomyopathy of coronary artery disease from nonischemic dilated cardiomyopathy utilizing positron tomography. *J Am Coll Cardiol* 1991; 17:373–383.

203. Tamaki N, Ohtani H, Yamashita K, et al. Metabolic activity in the areas of new fill-in after thallium-201 reinjection: Comparison with positron emission tomography using fluorine-18-deoxyglucose. *J Nucl Med* 1991; 32:673–678.
204. Gropler RJ, Geltman EM, Sampathkumaran K, et al. Comparison of carbon-11-acetate with fluorine-18-fluorodeoxyglucose for delineating viable myocardium by positron emission tomography. *J Am Coll Cardiol* 1993; 22:1587–1597.
205. Marwick T, Nemec J, Lafont A, et al. Prediction by postexercise fluoro-18-deoxyglucose positron emission tomography of improvement in exercise capacity after revascularization. *Am J Cardiol* 1992; 69:854–859.
206. Paolini G, Lucignani G, Zuccari M, et al. Identification and revascularization of hibernating myocardium in angina-free patients with left ventricular dysfunction. *Eur J Cardiothorac Surg* 1994; 8:139–144.
207. vom Dahl J, Altehoefer C, Sheehan F, et al. Recovery of regional left ventricular dysfunction after coronary revascularization: Impact of myocardial viability assessed by nuclear imaging and vessel patency at follow-up angiography. *J Am Coll Cardiol* 1996; 28:948–958.
208. Haas F, Haehnel C, Picker W, et al. Preoperative positron emission tomographic viability assessment and perioperative and postoperative risk in patients with advanced ischemic heart disease. *J Am Coll Cardiol* 1997; 30:1693–1700.
209. Flameng WJ, Shivalkar B, Spiessens B, et al. PET scan predicts recovery of left ventricular function after coronary artery bypass operation. *Ann Thorac Surg* 1997; 64:1694–1701.
210. Fath-Ordoubadi F, Pagano D, Marinho NV, et al. Coronary revascularization in the treatment of moderate and severe postischemic left ventricular dysfunction. *Am J Cardiol* 1998; 82:26–31.
211. Pagano D, Townend JN, Littler WA, et al. Coronary artery bypass surgery as treatment for ischemic heart failure: The predictive value of viability assessment with quantitative positron emission tomography for symptomatic and functional outcome. *J Thorac Cardiovasc Surg* 1998; 115:791–799.
212. Czernin J, Porenta G, Brunken R, et al. Perfusion defect extent on PET polar maps is linearly related to left ventricular function. *J Nucl Med* 1991; 32:999.
213. Yoshida K, Gould K. Quantitative relation of myocardial infarct size and myocardial viability by positron emission tomography to left ventricular ejection fraction and 3-year mortality with and without revascularization. *J Am Coll Cardiol* 1993; 22: 984–997.
214. Marwick TH, Zuchowski C, Lauer MS, et al. Functional status and quality of life in patients with heart failure undergoing coronary bypass surgery after assessment of myocardial viability. *J Am Coll Cardiol* 1999; 33:750–758.
215. Haas F, Haebnel N, Augustin N, et al. Prevalence and time-course of functional improvements in stunned and hibernating myocardium in patients with coronary artery disease (CAD) and congestive heart failure (CHF). *J Am Coll Cardiol* 1997; 29:376A.
216. Vanoverschelde J, Melin J, Depré C, et al. Time-course of functional recovery of hibernating myocardium after coronary revascularization. *Circulation* 1994; 90:I-378.
217. Eitzman D, Al-Aouar Z, Vom Dahl J, et al. Clinical outcome of patients with advanced coronary artery disease after viability studies with positron emission tomography. *J Am Coll Cardiol* 1992; 20:559–565.
218. Di Carli M, Davidson M, Little R, et al. Value of metabolic imaging with positron emission tomography for evaluating prognosis in patients with coronary artery disease and left ventricular dysfunction. *Am J Cardiol* 1994; 73:527–533.
219. Di Carli M, Asgarzadie F, Phelps M, Schelbert H. Can myocardial viability be assessed by quantitative measurements of myocardial perfusion at rest and during pharmacologic stress? *J Nucl Med* 1995; 36:66P.
220. Goldman L, Hashimoto B, Cook E, Loscalzo A. Comparative reproducibility and validity of systems for assessing cardiovascular functional class: Advantages of a new specific activity scale. *Circulation* 1981; 64:1227–1234.
221. Lee K, Marwick T, Cook S, et al. Prognosis of patients with left ventricular dysfunction, with and without viable myocardium after myocardial infarction. *Circulation* 1994; 90:2687–2694.
222. Tamaki N, Kawamoto M, Takahashi N, et al. Prognostic value of an increase in fluorine-18-deoxyglucose uptake in patients with myocardial infarction: Comparison with stress thallium imaging. *J Am Coll Cardiol* 1993; 22:1621–1627.
223. Landoni C, Lucignani G, Paolini G, et al. Assessment of CABG-related risk in patients with CAD and LVD: Contribution of PET with [^{18}F]FDG to the assessment of myocardial viability. *J Cardiovasc Surg* 1999; 40:363–372.
224. Auerbach MA, Schöder H, Hoh C, et al. Prevalence of myocardial viability as detected by positron emission tomography in patients with ischemic cardiomyopathy. *Circulation* 1999; 99:2921–2926.
225. Duong T, Hendi P, Fonarow G, et al. Role of positron emission tomographic assessment of myocardial viability in the management of patients who are referred for cardiac transplantation. *Circulation* 1995; 92:I-123.
226. Duong T, Fonarow G, Laks H, et al. Cost effectiveness of positron emission tomography (PET) in the management of ischemic cardiomyopathy patients who are referred for cardiac transplantation. *J Am Coll Cardiol* 1996; 27:144A.
227. Louie H, Laks H, Milgalter E, et al. Ischemic cardiomyopathy: Criteria for coronary revascularization and cardiac transplantation. *Circulation* 1991; 84:III-290–III-295.
228. Krivokapich J, Schelbert H, Czernin J. Dobutamine positron emission tomography: Absolute quantitation of rest and dobutamine myocardial blood flow and correlation with cardiac work and percent diameter stenosis in patients with and without coronary artery disease. *J Am Coll Cardiol* 1996; 28:565–572.
229. Di Carli MF, Maddahi J, Rokhsar S, et al. Long-term survival of patients with coronary artery disease and left ventricular dysfunction: Implications for the role of myocardial viability assessment in management decisions. *J Thorac Cardiovasc Surg* 1998; 116:997–1004.

PART THREE

HEART FAILURE

CHAPTER 20

PATHOPHYSIOLOGY AND DIAGNOSIS OF HEART FAILURE

Gary S. Francis / John P. Gassler / Edmund H. Sonnenblick

DEFINITION OF TERMS AND CLASSIFICATION

Heart failure is a broad term that encompasses multiple etiologies, pathophysiologic mechanisms, and clinical presentations. There has been and continues to be much confusion regarding the definition and classification of heart failure. The definition of heart failure has changed remarkably throughout the years,[1] undoubtedly related to the difficulties integrating many simple bedside observations (water retention, scant and concentrated urine, distended neck veins, and enlarged heart) with intellectual elaborations of the laboratory. For the practitioner, heart failure is a clinical syndrome in which structural or functional alterations of the heart lead to secondary phenomena such as exertional dyspnea and circulatory congestion. The diseased heart is the centerpiece of the syndrome. It is perhaps useful to think of heart failure as a continuum that begins with structural or functional abnormalities of the heart that have few or no clinical manifestations. This is followed by an often slow progression, with changes such as chamber enlargement, hypertrophy, or in some cases impairment of ejection phase indices, leading eventually to the clinical manifestations that are apparent by history and physical examination. There is often an important time element between the very beginnings of impaired cardiac structure or function and the clinical manifestations of heart failure that are observed weeks, months, or years later. In some cases, such as in severe hypertrophic cardiomyopathy or mitral stenosis, left ventricular (LV) systolic function may be intact, and there may be no LV chamber enlargement. In acute myocardial infarction, structural and functional changes occur swiftly, and symptoms of heart failure may appear suddenly. Such patients may then recover and have a long latency period of few symptoms, only to manifest substantial chamber enlargement, impaired LV function, and clinical heart failure many months or even years after the index event. There is an important time domain that spans the onset of cardiac structural and functional changes (often asymptomatic) to the clinical syndrome that the physician recognizes at the bedside or in the office as "heart failure." Although it is the clinical manifestations such as cardiomegaly, exertional dyspnea, and circulatory congestion that define the syndrome to the clinician, the student of heart failure knows that the disorder often has its roots in more fundamental structural and functional impairment that begins long before the patient experiences signs and symptoms of dyspnea and circulatory congestion.

The clinical syndrome of heart failure must be distinguished from other causes of circulatory congestion where the heart is not the culprit. It is worth considering the definition of heart failure put forth by Professor Ludwig W. Eichna in his George E. Brown Memorial Lecture at the American Heart Association meeting in Philadelphia in 1959.[2] This definition makes the important distinction between *circulatory congestion* (which can be due to noncardiac causes such as renal failure) and *congestive heart failure* (CHF), where the myocardium is at fault. Eichna opined that "circulatory (venous) congestion is the hemodynamic disturbance responsible for the symptoms usually associated with congestive heart failure; removal of the congestion, regardless of how accomplished, relieves the symptoms. Circulatory congestion is a nonspecific hemodynamic disturbance and may arise when the heart does not fail as a pump. This is noncardiac circulatory congestion. The term *congestive heart failure* should be reserved for those states of circulatory congestion in which there is myocardial failure." Basically, Eichna is making the important distinction between circulatory congestion of noncardiac cause (e.g., acute renal failure) and circulatory congestion due to "myocardial failure." The implication is that in *heart failure* there must be something structurally or functionally abnormal with the heart.

Heart failure remains largely a clinical or bedside diagnosis. There is no "gold standard" laboratory test. The combination of a careful history (breathlessness, fatigue, fluid retention) and physical examination (congested lungs, distended neck veins, tachypnea, gallop rhythm, and fluid retention) is how one makes the diagnosis. There should be some direct evidence of structural heart disease, and the echocardiogram is most useful in this regard. However, it remains a clinical, bedside diagnosis. One makes the diagnosis by a careful bedside or office examination and confirms the diagnosis by chest x-ray and/or echocardiography.

The bedside diagnosis of heart failure has been made somewhat more subtle in the past 20 years by the widespread contemporary use of potent loop diuretics. Some of the cardinal clinical features of heart failure may be unimpressive or even lacking.[3,4] Patients may present with a history of breathlessness and fatigue who have clear lungs, no venous distention, and no edema. The "congestion" may be lacking in some patients with "congestive heart failure," thus rendering the term *heart failure* more appropriate than *congestive heart failure*. Moreover, with the gradual erosion of bedside skills and more reliance placed recently on echocardiography, we have allowed the less sophisticated physician to equate the clinical syndrome of heart failure with the finding of a low ejection fraction. A low ejection fraction is *not* heart failure. No single laboratory test fulfills all diagnostic purposes. The heart may be small on chest x-ray. Echocardiography and cardiac catheterization may indicate normal systolic function. Impaired relaxation of the left ventricle may be the primary mechanism, emphasizing the need to perform echocardiography. Heart failure is a clinical syndrome with multiple etiologies, heterogeneity, and great plasticity. This is why it has been difficult to clearly define. The following definitions, though imperfect, have been used in the past by various authors.

Circulatory Failure

Circulatory failure is a nonspecific older term that is sometimes used to describe heart failure and includes the condition of *circulatory shock*. The basic concept of circulatory failure implies that there is inadequacy of the cardiovascular system in providing nutrition and blood flow to the cells of the body and inadequacy in removing metabolic products from cells. Circulatory failure can be due to cardiac and noncardiac causes. *Myocardial failure*, from acute or chronic injury, would be a cardiac cause of circulatory failure. Examples of cardiac circulatory failure would include acute myocardial infarction, acute inflammatory conditions such as lymphocytic myocarditis, chronic cardiomyopathy, and severe valvular heart disease. Noncardiac circulatory failure would include inadequate blood volume and insufficient oxyhemoglobin.

Circulatory overload or *congestion* is also an older general term referring to excess blood volume from either cardiac or noncardiac causes,[2] but it still carries some important conceptual considerations. *Noncardiac circulatory overload* may be divided into two categories: (1) conditions where the primary defect appears to be an increase in blood volume, as may occur with the accumulation of excess salt and water due to salt-retaining steroids, excess blood or fluid administration, acute glomerulonephritis, oliguria, or anuria, and (2) conditions where the primary defect appears to be an increased venous return and/or decreased peripheral resistance, as may occur with arteriovenous fistulas, beriberi, cirrhosis, or severe anemia, in which the increase in blood volume is secondary. Many patients with noncardiac circulatory overload eventually develop secondary "high output" heart failure.

Heart Failure

Heart failure also has been defined as a complex clinical syndrome that arises from a process of ventricular dysfunction (acute or chronic) where the heart is unable to pump sufficient blood to meet the metabolic needs of the body at normal filling pressures, provided the venous return to the heart is normal. Ventricular systolic dysfunction is characterized by a loss of contractile strength of the myocardium accompanied by the compensations of ventricular hypertrophy and/or dilatation (ventricular remodeling). This syndrome, however, involves more than a circulatory disorder caused by impaired pump function. As ventricular dysfunction proceeds, there is activation of numerous neuroendocrine systems that, although "designed" to protect blood pressure, are directly toxic to the heart and contribute to progressive cardiomegaly and sodium retention. Heart failure is also generally associated with a very poor prognosis, even when symptoms are mild.[5,6] *Systolic LV dysfunction* or *failure* reflects a decrease in normal emptying capacity [usually with an ejection fraction (EF) of 45 percent or less] that is usually associated with a compensatory increase in diastolic volume. *Isolated diastolic ventricular dysfunction* or *failure* is present when the filling of one or both ventricles is impaired, while the emptying capacity is normal. It may be due to a thickened (hypertrophied) ventricular wall, infiltrative cardiomyopathies, and/or tachycardia, which limits the time for diastolic filling, resulting in increased ventricular filling pressures and eventually pulmonary edema.

Congestive heart failure denotes a clinical syndrome with complex and variable signs and symptoms, including dyspnea and increased fatigability, tachypnea, tachycardia, pulmonary rales, cardiomegaly, ventricular gallop sounds, and peripheral edema. In most patients, CHF and abnormal circulatory congestion occur as a result of both heart failure and subsequent changes in the peripheral circulation, accompanied by activation of the sympathetic nervous system and the renin-angiotensin system. In most patients with clinical CHF due to mechanical or myocardial abnormalities, the heart (pump) failure is preceded by a substantial period of *myocardial* dysfunction during which cardiac *pump* function and cardiac output (at least while at rest) may be maintained by compensatory mechanisms that include myocardial hypertrophy and ventricular dilatation. For this reason, in the early stages the patient may have little or no limitations or symptoms. Initially, the cardiac output may be within the range of normal at rest but fails to increase or may even decline during exercise or stress. Ultimately, the cardiac output is decreased even at rest. Associated changes include an increase in systemic vascular resistance (SVR) at rest and a failure of the SVR to decrease with increased metabolic needs.

When the intravascular circulatory congestion is present for any length of time with elevation of LV diastolic and pulmonary venous pressures, fluid transudation from the capillaries into the interstitial spaces increases. In the pulmonary circulation, pulmonary edema develops if the rate of transudation exceeds the rate of lymphatic drainage. Pulmonary edema is often detected initially by x-ray examination, and only later are audible rales detected on physical examination. In the systemic venous system, elevated jugular venous pressure is often visible and may be accompanied by dependent peripheral edema and hepatomegaly. In the majority of patients, CHF develops chronically and is associated with the retention of sodium and water by the kidneys.

Acute heart failure can develop during acute ischemia of the ventricle (i.e., a myocardial infarction), secondary tachycardia, or due to the rupture of a cardiac valve or structure. An acute shift of blood from the systemic to the pulmonary circulation can occur before the retention of significant sodium or water. The term *congestive heart failure* should not be used unless there is congestion of cardiac origin. When the cause of the pulmonary or peripheral congestion is not clear, however, it is usually preferable to describe the symptoms or signs, which are nonspecific, and to avoid improperly diagnosing heart failure.

CLASSIFICATION AND STAGES OF HEART FAILURE

Numerous classification schemes and definitions have evolved over the years (Table 20-1), including the antiquated "forward heart failure" and "backward heart failure" concepts that are no longer very useful. Even the New York Heart Association classification system, though widely used, lacks precision.

New York Heart Association Functional Classification

I. *Patients with cardiac disease but without resulting limitations of physical activity.* Ordinary physical activity does not cause undue fatigue, palpitation, dyspnea, or anginal pain.

II. *Patients with cardiac disease resulting in slight limitation of physical activity.* These patients are comfortable at rest. Ordinary physical activity results in fatigue, palpitation, dyspnea, or anginal pain.

III. *Patients with cardiac disease resulting in marked limitation of physical activity.* These patients are comfortable at rest. Less than ordinary physical activity causes fatigue, palpitation, dyspnea, or anginal pain.

IV. *Patients with cardiac disease resulting in inability to carry on any physical activity without discomfort.* Symptoms of cardiac insufficiency or of the anginal syndrome may be present even at rest. If any physical activity is undertaken, discomfort is increased.

A more recent and useful "staging" scheme of heart failure is now being used more commonly by guideline committees and regulatory agencies and is more closely intertwined with prevention and therapy:

TABLE 20-1 Classifications and Definitions of Some Common Types of Heart Failure

Heart failure A clinical syndrome with classic symptoms of breathlessness, fatigue, and exercise intolerance that are attributable to impaired myocardial function.

Congestive heart failure Similar to the preceding but with features of circulatory congestion such as jugular venous distention, rales, peripheral edema, and ascites.

Noncardiac circulatory congestion A syndrome that is clinically indistinguishable from congestive heart failure where there is no reason to ascribe the condition to structural heart disease. There must be a noncardiac cause such as acute renal failure.

Systolic heart failure A clinical syndrome with classic symptoms of breathlessness, fatigue, and exercise intolerance whereby the dominant cardiac feature is a large, dilated heart and impaired systolic performance. There may or may not be concomitant valvular disease.

Heart failure with normal systolic function Sometimes referred to as *diastolic heart failure,* this is a clinical syndrome characterized by breathlessness, fatigue, and exercise intolerance whereby the dominant cardiac feature is impaired diastolic function (usually diagnosed by echo) and normal or near-normal ejection phase indices. There is often LV hypertrophy and impaired filling of the heart due to altered LV stiffness or other evidence of diastolic dysfunction. Often, severe systemic hypertension is present. There may or may not be concomitant valvular disease, such as mitral insufficiency. This form of heart failure may coexist with systolic heart failure.

Right-sided heart failure A clinical syndrome characterized by tissue congestion including jugular venous distention, peripheral edema, ascites, and abdominal organ engorgement. There is marked impairment of right ventricular systolic performance, usually with right ventricular dilatation and severe tricuspid regurgitation. There are multiple causes of this syndrome, including severe left-sided heart failure, severe lung disease with chronic hypoxemia and pulmonary hypertension (so-called cor pulmonale), right ventricular myocardial infarction, and primary pulmonary hypertension.

Stages of Heart Failure

Stage A. Patients at risk of developing heart failure because of comorbid conditions that are strongly associated with the development of HF. Such patients have no signs or symptoms of HF and have never manifested signs or symptoms of HF. There are no structural or functional abnormalities of the valves or ventricles. Examples: systemic hypertension, coronary artery disese, diabetes mellitus.

Stage B. Patients who have developed structural heart disease that is strongly associated with the development of HF, but

TABLE 20-2 The Differential Diagnosis of Systolic Heart Failure and Heart Failure with Normal Systolic Function (Diastolic Heart Failure)

Systolic Heart Failure	Diastolic Heart Failure
Large, dilated heart	Small LV cavity, concentric LV hypertrophy
Normal or low blood pressure	Systemic hypertension
Broad age group; more common in men	Elderly women more common
Low ejection fraction	Normal or increased ejection fraction
S_3 gallop	S_4 gallop
Systolic and diastolic impairment by echo	Diastolic impairment by various echo measurements
Treatment well established	Treatment not well established
Poor prognosis	Prognosis not as poor
Role of myocardial ischemia important in selected cases	Myocardial ischemia common

have no symptoms of HF and have never manifested signs or symptoms of HF. Examples: left ventricular hypertrophy (LVH); enlarged, dilated ventricles asymptomatic valvular heart disease; previous myocardial infarction.

Stage C. Patients who have current or prior symptoms of HF associated with underlying structural heart disease.

Stage D. Patients with marked symptoms of heart failure at rest despite maximal medical therapy and who require specialized interventions. Examples include patients who cannot be safely discharged from the hospital; recurrently hospitalized; are in the hospital awaiting heart transplantation; are in a hospice setting; at home receiving continuous intravenous support for symptom relief; are being supported with a mechanical circulator assist device.

This newer staging scheme is very clinically oriented and allows physicians to target therapy in a more focused manner toward specific subsets of patients. In general, patients only progress forward in this schema, although occasionally patients may go from D to C.

Systolic and Diastolic Dysfunction

A useful distinction in ventricular failure is that between systolic and diastolic dysfunction (Table 20-2 and Fig. 20-1). These terms, however, are most appropriately defined in terms of altered ventricular architecture rather than systemic hemodynamics. *Systolic dysfunction* describes a large, dilated ventricle

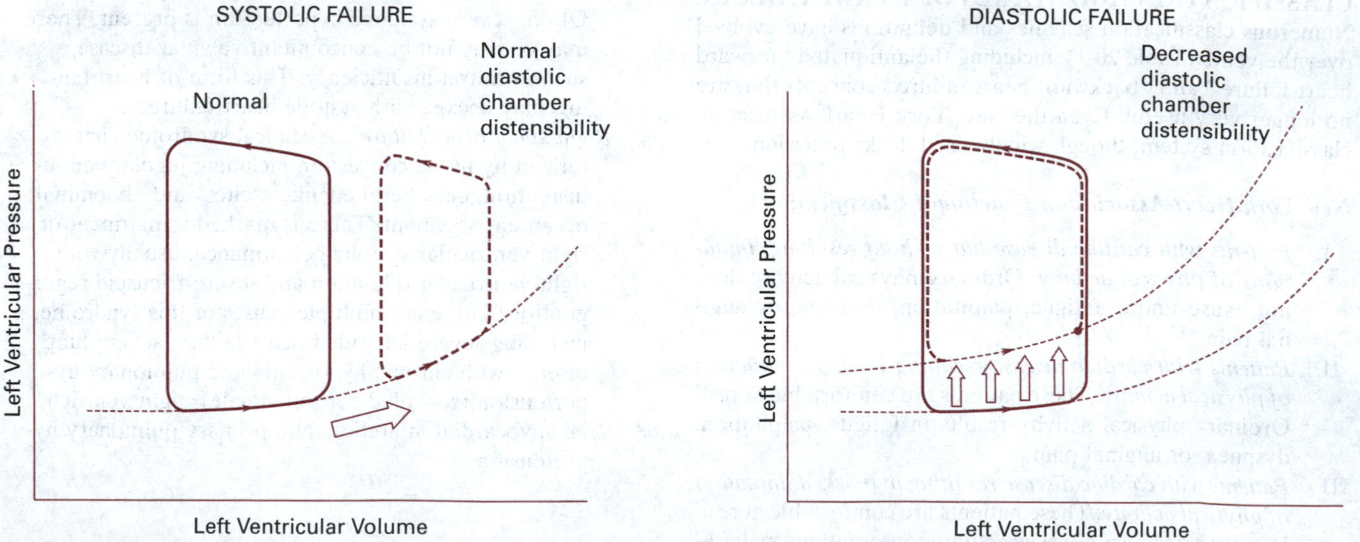

FIGURE 20-1 The left panel shows a schematized left ventricular pressure-volume loop from a patient with primary systolic failure. A normal left ventricular pressure-volume loop (*solid loop*) is shown on the left portion of the curve, and the transition to inotropic failure (*dashed loop*) is shown on the right. Systolic failure is manifested as an increase in LV end-systolic volume and as a reduction in the extent of shortening (stroke volume). LVEDP is increased because left ventricular volume is increased. As indicated by the arrow, the diastolic portion of the pressure-volume loop has simply shifted to the right along the same diastolic pressure-volume relationship, thus no change in the distensibility of the left ventricle has occurred. The right panel shows a left ventricular pressure-volume loop from a patient with primary diastolic failure (*dashed loop*). Note that the LVEDP is the same as that in the patient with primary inotropic failure, as denoted by the heavy dot on both pressure-volume loops. In the right panel, however, this is caused by an upward shift of the left ventricular diastolic pressure-volume relationship (*arrows*), which indicates a decrease in left ventricular diastolic distensibility such that a higher diastolic pressure is required to achieve the same diastolic volume. In this patient, no change in end-diastolic volume or systolic shortening has occurred. (From Lorell BH: Left ventricular diastolic pressure-volume relations: Understanding and managing congestive heart failure. *Heart Failure* 1988; 4:206–223. Reproduced with permission from the publisher and author.)

whose output is limited by impaired ejection, whereas *diastolic dysfunction* refers to a thickened, small cavity ventricle in which filling is limited. It is appropriate to reserve the term *systolic dysfunction* for a dilated, often eccentrically hypertrophied ventricle and *diastolic dysfunction* for a thick-walled, concentrically hypertrophied ventricle with a normal or small cavity, highlighting the important architectural differences between these two entities.

Diastolic heart failure (or heart failure with preserved LV systolic function) is increasingly recognized as a major and growing epidemiologic clinical problem.[7,8] As many as 40 percent of patients presenting with heart failure have preserved LV systolic function, and it may be an even higher proportion in hospitals caring for more elderly and inner-city patients. Diastolic heart failure often coexists with poorly controlled systemic hypertension. Factors contributing to altered LV diastolic function include myocardial fibrosis, hypertrophy, ischemia, and increased afterload.[9] Myocardial ischemia is an especially important mechanism to identify[10] because, like hypertension, it is usually treatable.

It is important to recognize that systolic and diastolic dysfunction frequently coexist in patients with heart failure and that systolic events can influence diastolic function.[11,12] The diagnosis of diastolic dysfunction can be challenging, but advancing echocardiographic techniques for this purpose have improved substantially. Limitations imparted by loading conditions, heart rate, and age to some extent have been overcome by new applications of continuous-wave Doppler, color Doppler M-mode, and Doppler tissue imaging.[13–15]

Women seem to be overrepresented in the group of patients with diastolic heart failure,[16] especially elderly women with hypertension, diabetes mellitus, and LV hypertrophy. For any given afterload stress, women seem to develop more hypertrophy than men. Patients with heart failure and normal systolic function have a lower mortality risk than patients with a reduced EF,[17] but they still have a fourfold mortality risk compared with control subjects who are free of heart failure.[18] Assessing LV architecture and function by echocardiography is important before initiating therapy in a patient with heart failure, since treatment for systolic dysfunction may be ineffective or even counterproductive if symptoms are due to abnormal diastolic properties with preserved systolic function. Knowledge of renal function and renal vasculature also may be important, especially in patients with severe hypertension. For example, many elderly patients with heart failure and severe hypertension have associated renal vascular stenosis.[19] Institution of an angiotensin-converting enzyme inhibitor in such a patient could lead to severe renal insufficiency. Likewise, prolonged aggressive use of diuretics in patients with severe LV hypertrophy and a small LV cavity may lead to a reduced stroke volume and hypotension. It is important, therefore, to have knowledge of myocardial architecture, anatomy, and function when planning therapy and in determining prognosis.

Generally, systolic ventricular dysfunction is characterized by an increase in end-diastolic volume (EDV) and a normal or somewhat reduced stroke volume (SV), resulting in a decrease in EF. This relationship of SV to EDV is normally described by the Frank-Starling relationship (Fig. 20-2). The increase in EDV is associated with an increase in ventricular end-diastolic pressure (EDP) in consonance with the resting pressure-volume curve. The filling pressures may be further elevated for a given

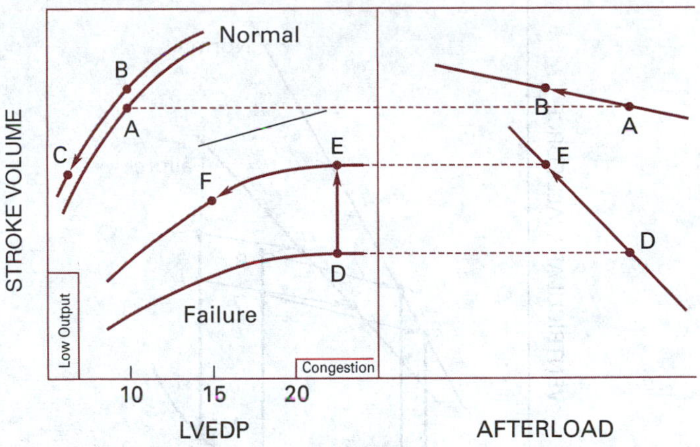

FIGURE 20-2 Relationship between stroke volume and left ventricular end-diastolic pressure (LVEDP) (*left*) and afterload (*right*). Normally, the ventricle operates on a sharply rising Frank-Starling curve with an LVEDP less than 12 mmHg (point *A*), where small changes in filling pressure yield large changes in stroke volume. Further, stroke volume is largely independent of the afterload. When failure occurs, ventricular function is characterized by a shift of the curve relating stroke volume to LVEDP to the right and downward. Low output may ensue if the curve is sufficiently depressed, while pulmonary congestion occurs as the LVEDP is increased. At the same time, this failing ventricle is now highly afterload-dependent, in that small changes in afterload produce large changes in stroke volume. When afterload is reduced in the normal heart (point *A* to point *B, right*), stroke volume rises very slightly. If, at the same time, venodilation reduces filling pressure, stroke volume falls to point *C* (*left*). The net result is a decrease in cardiac output. On the contrary, when afterload is reduced in the presence of severe ventricular failure, stroke volume is increased (point *D* to point *E, right*). Since the Frank-Starling curve is relatively flattened, a simultaneous decrease in filling pressure leads to a decrease in LVEDP with only a small decrease in stroke volume (point *E* to point *F, left*). The net reult of these opposing consequences can increase stroke volume. These results are observed clinically when a vasodilator is administered along with a diuretic in treating the failing ventricle.

EDV by concentric hypertrophy or a fibrotic wall. Conversely, they actually may be decreased by chronic overdistention (eccentric hypertrophy). The relation between LV wall force and fiber length is depicted in Fig. 20-3.

In patients with mild heart failure, the ventricular EDP and the cardiac output may be normal at rest, but the former may become elevated to abnormal levels during stress such as exercise or an increase in afterload. The ability to increase the cardiac output in response to the increase in oxygen consumption is also reduced (see below and Chap 3). In patients with more severe systolic dysfunction, both the early pressure and the EDP may be elevated even at rest. The elevated LV diastolic pressure increases pulmonary venous and capillary pressures and contributes to increased dyspnea as a result of changes in pulmonary compliance due to pulmonary congestion and edema. It is also apparent that before one reaches this stage of clinical heart failure, the body has used many compensatory mechanisms after the onset of the initial abnormality or stress and that these compensatory mechanisms eventually have failed to maintain the needs for cardiac output (see below).

Low-Output Heart Failure

The causes of overall heart pump failure may be classified in four main categories: (1) failure primarily related to work over-

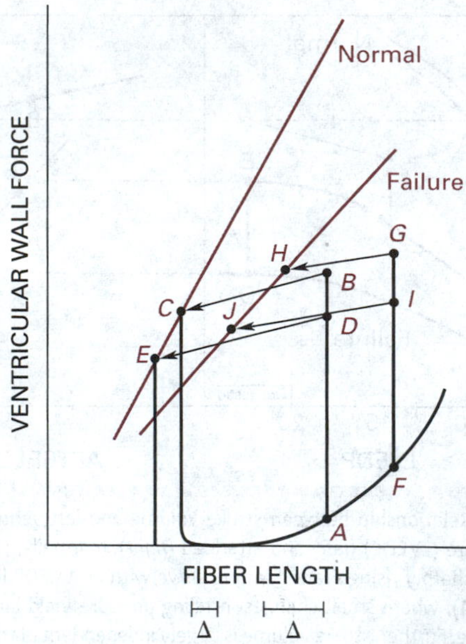

FIGURE 20-3 Relationship between LV wall force and fiber length. Hypothetical contractile cycles have been portrayed for the normal and failing ventricle. In the normal heart, contraction starts at point *A*, LV pressure rises until the aortic valve is opened (point *B*), the ventricle empties (point *B* to *C*), and relaxation ensues. When arterial pressure (afterload) is reduced (e.g., to point *D*), ejection starts at point *D* and proceeds to point *E*, which increases stroke volume. When the ventricle fails, the fiber length in diastole is increased, and ventricular contraction starts at point *F*. With systolic contraction, ventricular pressure rises to point *G*, and with ventricular emptying, fiber length decreases to point *H*. With a similar decrease in the afterload, wall force only needs to reach point *I* when ventricular emptying occurs to point *J*. As a result, for the same relative change in afterload, the increase in shortening is greater in the failing ventricle (Δ*H–J*) than in the normal heart (Δ*C–E*).

loads or mechanical abnormalities, (2) failure mostly related to primary myocardial abnormalities, (3) failure related to abnormal cardiac rhythm or conduction disturbances, and (4) myocardial ischemia/infarction. Myocardial infarction resulting in a quantitative loss of myocardium creates a special type of work overload. During the acute infarction, the EF falls as the EDV is increased to sustain a reduced SV, and the fall in EF is approximately proportional to the amount of myocardium lost. With time, the EF tends to remain at this reduced level. With healing of the infarction, the akinetic infarcted region becomes a scar that not only cannot contribute to ventricular emptying but may even contribute to the load. Thus the entire load falls on the remaining nonischemic myocardium. This load is further increased by the increased diastolic volume, which causes wall tension to be increased for any given pressure, even though the nonischemic myocardium hypertrophies in proportion to the amount of myocardium that is lost. Heart failure may ensue months or years later as a so-called ischemic cardiomyopathy resulting from progressive ventricular dilatation and reactive hypertrophy, termed *ventricular remodeling,* in the remaining nonischemic myocardium.

Cardiomyopathy

Virtually any form of heart disease eventually can lead to heart failure, and there are many causes of both "primary" and "secondary" heart failure. However, these distinctions are quite arbitrary and of little clinical value. *Primary heart failure* usually refers to "cardiomyopathy," a vague term that can include idiopathic dilated cardiomyopathy, familial dilated cardiomyopathy (an increasingly recognized cause of dilated cardiomyopathy), and hypertrophic cardiomyopathy. It simply depends on how one defines the term *cardiomyopathy*. Familial dilated cardiomyopathy is more common than previously believed.[20] It cannot be predicted by clinical or phenotypic techniques and requires family screening for identification. It is important to always consider familial dilated cardiomyopathy when evaluating patients with "idiopathic dilated cardiomyopathy" because it has a more unpredictable natural history and can present with a very rapid downhill course necessitating early referral to a heart transplant center.[21] Cardiac abnormalities are common in asymptomatic relatives of patients with dilated cardiomyopathy.[22] As many as 30 percent or more of patients with dilated cardiomyopathy may have an inherited disorder.[23] Single-gene defects may be important in the disease pathogenesis.[24]

Hypertrophic obstructive cardiomyopathy (HOCM) and nonobstructive hypertrophic cardiomyopathy are also often familial, affecting about 1 in 500 people in the general population. Most cases are inherited in an autosomal dominant manner with variable clinical penetrance and expression. Many different mutations have been described for at least seven abnormal sarcomeric proteins. Late-onset expression of HOCM may be a distinct clinical entity. Unfortunately, the genetic heterogeneity of this disease has made routine genetic testing impractical. Clinical screening may be warranted for members of families characterized by hypertrophic cardiomyopathy.

Unlike familial dilated or hypertrophic cardiomyopathy, alcoholic cardiomyopathy and "viral" cardiomyopathy (e.g., secondary to inflammatory myocarditis) may be overdiagnosed by clinicians. There are no specific clinical markers for so-called alcoholic cardiomyopathy, and there is no good evidence indicating an alcohol dose-response relationship. Apparently, a broad segment of the alcoholic population remains somehow immune to this complication. Nevertheless, patients believed to be "heavy" users of alcohol who present with dilated cardiomyopathy in whom heart failure resolves on cessation of alcohol use probably have "alcoholic cardiomyopathy." This observation should be a strong reason to encourage abstinence in patients with dilated cardiomyopathy of uncertain or possibly alcoholic origin.

Viral myocarditis can only be diagnosed by examining myocardial tissue (e.g., myocardial biopsy), since we now know that the "clinical" diagnosis of viral myocarditis is notoriously inaccurate. Only 5 to 10 percent of biopsies taken from the hearts of patients suspected clinically of having inflammatory myocarditis are actually "positive." Physicians should refrain from telling patients that their heart failure was due to a virus unless there is tissue verification. There are, of course, patients with mild or subclinical acute myocarditis who progress to heart failure and present with "dilated cardiomyopathy." The prognosis of patients with proven inflammatory myocarditis may be somewhat better than that of patients with idiopathic dilated cardiomyopathy, since spontaneous improvement in LV ejection fraction is not uncommon.[25] However, others have found no difference in the 5-year survival between patients with myocarditis and idiopathic dilated cardiomyopathy (56 versus 54 percent, respectively).[26] Patients with active inflammatory myocarditis may suffer severe rejection earlier and more commonly after heart transplantation. Idiopathic giant-cell myocarditis is important to distinguish from inflammatory lymphocytic myocarditis because it has a worse survival rate and may respond better to heart transplantation.[27]

Anthracycline-induced heart failure is now increasingly recognized as a form of "toxic" heart failure.[28] It is clearly a dose-related phenomenon and may present as a "cardiomyopathy." A rapidly growing number of persons, including a fraction of the 150,000 adults in the United States who have survived childhood cancers, will develop anthracycline-induced cardiomyopathy.[29,30] There may be a long latency period (years) between treatment and onset of symptoms. Recently, Herceptin (recombinant humanized anti-HER2 antibody) has been approved for the treatment of breast cancer. About 27 percent of patients receiving both Herceptin and doxorubicin or Paclitaxel experience cardiac dysfunction,[31] which is a far greater percentage than those receiving anthracycline or Paclitaxel alone. Cardiac toxicity should be a major concern for patients receiving Herceptin, which is often used in conjunction with an anthracycline. Heart failure induced by these drugs is not a simple complication that can be "managed" by drug therapy but is a potentially lethal complication that requires skillful care. Other causes of toxic cardiomyopathy include cocaine, other cytostatic agents, interferons, interleukin-2, anabolic steroids, and a host of miscellaneous agents.[31]

The cause of LV systolic dysfunction in patients with chronic obstructive lung disease is unknown, although the combination of hypoxia and hypercapnia may be important. LV diastolic dysfunction in such patients is, in part, secondary to the pronounced right ventricular hypertrophy and dilatation with secondary elevation of LV diastolic pressure due to ventricular interdependence. The latter phenomenon is also important in the pathophysiology of acute pulmonary edema occasionally encountered in patients with acute pulmonary embolus.

Myocardial "Overload"

Myocardial failure may develop from many causes of "overload." It may evolve from pressure overloads in which myocytes hypertrophy to meet the load. Hypertrophied cells contract and relax more slowly[32] and may be subject to metabolic limitations. In addition, hypertrophied myocardial cells may have a shortened life span.[33,34] This is of considerable prognostic importance because cardiac myocytes appear to have little or no capacity to proliferate. When age-related myocyte loss is added to the picture, particularly in association with a late decrease in myocyte contractile activity, failure may ensue with ventricular dilatation. Loss of myocytes—whether segmental, as in acute myocardial infarction, or diffuse, as in myocarditis—sets up a vicious cycle that leads to reactive hypertrophy in remaining myocytes. As compensatory hypertrophy becomes more marked in some disease states, the unit contractility of the myocardium often declines because of molecular changes in the heart's contractile proteins and activation system. This is especially likely to occur in response to pressure overload, as in systemic arterial hypertension or aortic stenosis, but also ensues when myocytes are lost.

Ultimately, the myocardial failure (plus mechanical abnormalities that may be present) often leads to a decrease in systolic pump function that is sufficient to produce overall pump or heart failure. In most patients, significant dysfunction and failure of the myocardium occur before the clinical syndrome of CHF becomes apparent.

High-Output Failure

Some patients with high-output states or primary noncardiac circulatory overload may develop pulmonary congestion and edema secondary to an abnormal elevation of ventricular diastolic pressure at a time when the total cardiac output (systolic, or pump, function) and EF of the left ventricle are normal or even increased. The latter syndrome also can occur in conditions associated with an increase in blood volume from the accumulation of excess salt and water due to salt-retaining steroids, excess blood or fluid administration, acute glomerulonephritis, oliguria, or anuria. In other patients, it may occur with an abnormally increased venous return and/or decreased peripheral resistance, as might occur in patients with arteriovenous fistulas, beriberi, hyperthyroidism, cirrhosis, severe anemia, and large vascular tumors. Under such conditions, the chronic volume and/or pressure overload on the ventricle eventually may produce myocardial and ventricular systolic (pump) dysfunction or failure. Ultimately, this can both increase diastolic pressures and reduce cardiac output to abnormally low levels. When symptoms of pulmonary congestion or pulmonary edema secondary to elevated diastolic pressure occur while the cardiac output is still normal or elevated, the syndrome is sometimes referred to as *high-output failure*.

High-output heart failure is rare in the United States. For example, to have high-output heart failure from chronic anemia, a hematocrit of about 13 percent (9–16 percent) typically would be necessary.[35] This is an uncommon presentation in North America. However, this condition may be found in areas of the world where chronic parasite infestation can lead to severe, chronic anemia. As with low-output heart failure, patients with high-output heart failure have salt and water retention, reduced renal blood flow, and neuroendocrine activation.[35] Low concentration of hemoglobin in patients with anemia may lead to a relative inability to degrade nitric oxide (NO), leading to the vasodilation that is so typical of high-output heart failure. Low blood pressure may in turn activate neuroendocrine activity. Various conditions that increase cardiac output are depicted in Table 20-3.

TABLE 20-3 Conditions That Increase Cardiac Output

Bacteremia/sepsis	Fibrous dysplasia (Albright's syndrome)
Anemia (acquired or congenital)	Renal disease (acute or chronic)
Hyperthyroidism	Hepatic disease
Beriberi	Environmental temperature extremes
Arteriovenous fistulas (acquired or congenital)	Polycythemia vera
Pregnancy	Carcinoid syndrome
Paget's disease	Dermatologic abnormalities
Hyperdynamic heart syndrome	Erythroderma syndrome
Arterial hypertension	Kaposi's sarcoma

Left and Right Heart Failure

Left heart (*left-sided*) *failure* and *right heart* (*right-sided*) *failure* are clinical terms for conditions in which the primary impairment is of the left side of the heart or of the right side of the heart, respectively. Since both sides of the heart are in a circuit, it is apparent that one side cannot pump significantly more blood than the other side for any length of time in the absence of abnormal shunts, communications, or regurgitation. Furthermore, experimentally produced failure of one ventricle may produce significant hemodynamic and biochemical abnormalities of the other ventricle, even without the usual hemodynamic manifestations of ventricular failure. Abnormal function of the left ventricle not only overloads the right ventricle from augmented pulmonary pressures but also may affect the right ventricle via the shared septum and the phenomenon of ventricular interdependence or interaction (see below). Altered elastic recoil of the left ventricle in diastole also may affect the right ventricle. Accordingly, when the pumping ability of one ventricle is primarily impaired, the output of the contralateral ventricle can be secondarily decreased; the biochemistry and hemodynamics of the contralateral ventricle also can be abnormal even in "pure" one-sided failure.

Right-sided heart failure commonly follows left-sided heart failure. In most situations, the expression *left-sided heart failure* is used clinically in reference to symptoms and signs of elevated pressure and congestion in the pulmonary veins and capillaries, whereas the term *right-sided heart failure* is used clinically in reference to symptoms and signs of elevated pressure and congestion in the systemic veins and capillaries. Actually, significant amounts of sodium and water retention, with subsequent peripheral edema formation, may occur with pure left-sided heart failure without hemodynamic evidence of right-sided heart failure. As noted previously, an increase in the diastolic pressure in either ventricle can increase the diastolic pressure or decrease the distensibility of the contralateral ventricle, especially if the pericardium is intact.

Compensated Heart Failure

Compensated heart failure is that condition in which the symptoms of heart failure are relieved, usually by therapy or compensatory mechanisms, although the EDV and EDP often remain elevated, and the EF remains reduced. As noted below and in Table 20-4, the usual "compensatory" mechanisms include increased sympathetic adrenergic stimulation of the heart, activation of the renal renin-angiotensin system, increased vasoconstriction, fluid retention by the kidney, increased venous return, increased ventricular preload, and cardiac dilatation and hypertrophy. Clinically, myocardial compensation and a decrease in congestion may be produced by improved ventricular performance. The term *compensated heart failure* frequently is used in reference to patients with CHF whose symptoms and signs of pulmonary or peripheral congestion have been relieved by therapy. In many such patients, reduced myocardial function and low cardiac output persist, although symptoms are relieved by an improvement in peripheral circulation and the reduction in edema and congestion.

MECHANISMS OF HEART FAILURE

Since virtually any form of heart disease can lead to heart failure, there can be no single causative mechanism. At the organ and the cellular level, there is likewise no single mechanism that is consistently operative. Identification of fundamental mechanisms remains an area of very active investigation (Table 20-5). Multiple alterations in organ and cellular physiology contribute to heart failure under various circumstances and at different points in time. Adaptive processes occur that affect the myocardium, kidneys, smooth and skeletal muscles, endothelium, peripheral vasculature, and multiple reflex control mechanisms, adding to the complexity of the syndrome (Tables 20-6 and 20-7). The schema of the sequence of events in heart failure is daunting (Fig. 20-4). Distinguishing primary etiologic forces from secondary epiphenomena has been very difficult. Identification of the precise mechanisms whereby heart failure evolves and quantifying the contributions of individual components (e.g., apoptosis) have remained elusive. Major gaps in our knowledge, such as what triggers the early activation of the sympathetic nervous system and withdrawal of vagal tone or how spontaneous resolution of heart failure occurs, have persisted despite in-

TABLE 20-4 Compensatory Mechanisms Initiated by Low Cardiac Output[a]

Mechanism	Short-Term Adaptive Response	Long-Term Maladaptive Response
Salt and water retention	⇑ Preload ⇑ Cardiac output[b]	Edema, anasarca, pulmonary congestion
Vasoconstriction	⇑ Afterload Maintained blood pressure	⇓ Cardiac output, ⇑ ardiac energy expenditure Cell death[b]
⇑ Cardiac, adrenergic drive	⇑ Contractility, ⇑ relaxation, ⇑ heart rate ⇑ Cardiac output[b]	Arrhythmias, ⇑ cardiac energy expenditure Cell death[b]
Transcription factor activation, cell growth	Adaptive hypertrophy ⇑ Sarcomere number ⇑ Cardiac output[b]	Maladaptive hypertrophy Apoptosis, mitochondrial DNA abnormalities Cell death[b]

[a]The compensatory mechanisms initiated by a short-term fall in cardiac output, as occurs following hemorrhage, generate an adaptive response. However, when sustained, as in the chronically overloaded heart, these same mechanisms cause maladaptive responses that further reduce cardiac output, exacerbate symptoms, and appear to accelerate cell death.
[b]Secondary responses.
SOURCE: Adapted with permission from Katz AM.[34]

TABLE 20-5 Possible Mechanisms of Myocardial Failure

- Loss of myocytes
- Hypertrophy of remaining myocytes
- Energy production and utilization
  - Oxygen and energy supply
  - Substrate utilization and energy storage
  - Inadequate mitochondria mass and function
- Ventricular remodeling
- Contractile proteins
  - Abnormal myofibrillar or myosin ATPase
  - Abnormal myocardial proteins
  - Defective protein synthesis
  - Nonuniformity of contraction and function
- Activation of contractile elements
  - Membrane Na^+,K^+-ATPase defects
  - Abnormal sarcoplasmic reticulum function
    - Abnormal Ca^{2+} release
    - Abnormal Ca^{2+} uptake
- Abnormal myocardial receptor function
  - Downregulation of beta adrenoreceptors
  - Decreased β_1 receptors
  - Decreased G_s protein
  - Increased G_1 protein
- Autonomic nervous system
  - Abnormal myocardial norepinephrine function or kinetics
  - Abnormal baroreceptor function
- Increased myocardial fibroblast growth and collagen synthesis
- Aging changes, presbycardia
- Sustained tachycardia
- Miscellaneous

TABLE 20-6 Compensatory Mechanisms in Heart Failure

- Autonomic nervous system
  - Heart
    - Increased heart rate
    - Increased myocardial contractile stimulation
    - Increased rate of relaxation
  - Peripheral circulation
    - Arterial vasoconstriction (increased afterload)
    - Venous vasoconstriction (increased preload)
- Kidney (renin-angiotensin-aldosterone)
  - Arterial vasoconstriction (increased afterload)
  - Venous vasconstriction (increased preload)
  - Sodium and water retention (increased preload and afterload)
  - Increased myocardial contractile stimulation
- Endothelin-1 (increased preload and afterload)
- Arginine vasopressin (increased preload and afterload)
- Atrial and brain natriuretic peptides (decreased afterload)
- Prostaglandins
- Peptides
- Frank-Starling law of the heart
  - Increased end-diastolic fiber length, volume, and pressure (increased preload)
- Hypertrophy
- Peripheral oxygen delivery
  - Redistribution of cardiac output
  - Altered oxygen-hemoglobin dissociation
  - Increased oxygen extraction by tissues
- Anaerobic metabolism

TABLE 20-7 Neurohumoral Changes in Heart Failure

- Increased sympathetic nervous system activity (increased norepinephrine, epinephrine)
- Increased endothelin
- Increased arginine vasopressin
- Increased renin and angiotensin II
- Increased aldosterone
- Increased neuropeptide Y
- Increased atrial and brain natriuretic peptides
- Increased
  - Insulin
  - Cortisol
  - Growth hormone
  - Tumor necrosis factor-α
  - Interleukin 6
  - Vasoactive intestinal peptide
  - Adrenomedullin
  - Urodilatin
- Increased dopamine
- Increased prostaglandins (PGI_2, PGE_2)
- Increased vasodilator peptides, (e.g., bradykinin)

NOTE: Measurements in individual patients vary significantly, and changes may not always be present.

tense investigation. Nevertheless, enough information has accrued to construct a reasonably coherent working hypothesis.

To understand heart failure, it is useful to think in terms of evolutionary theory.[36] The cell, the organ, and the organism each has evolved adaptive responses to offset hostile environments, thus allowing a survival advantage. In many cases, heart failure may begin as an acute injury to the heart, such as an acute myocardial infarction or severe inflammatory myocarditis. In other cases, there may be a phenotypically silent mutation that is finally expressed (for unknown reasons), leading to structural and functional perturbations of such magnitude that the heart eventually fails. Valvular heart disease may lead to unusual loading conditions, forcing the myocytes to adapt by increasing their size (hypertrophy). In essence, there is an *index event* that in many cases is not clinically visible or may occur secondary to unknown toxins or an unusual mechanical load on the heart. The heart and its circulary physiology must somehow "adapt" to this "hostile" new environment.

In response to increased load, whether created by increased pressure or loss of myocytes, hypertrophy occurs that tends to normalize the load per cell. With an increased volume load, myocytes elongate and in rare cases may undergo division.[37,38] It is believed that hyperplasia and apoptosis involves less than 1 percent of the cardiac myocytes. Reprogramming of the cardiac myocytes occurs, resulting in a more fetal-like response leading

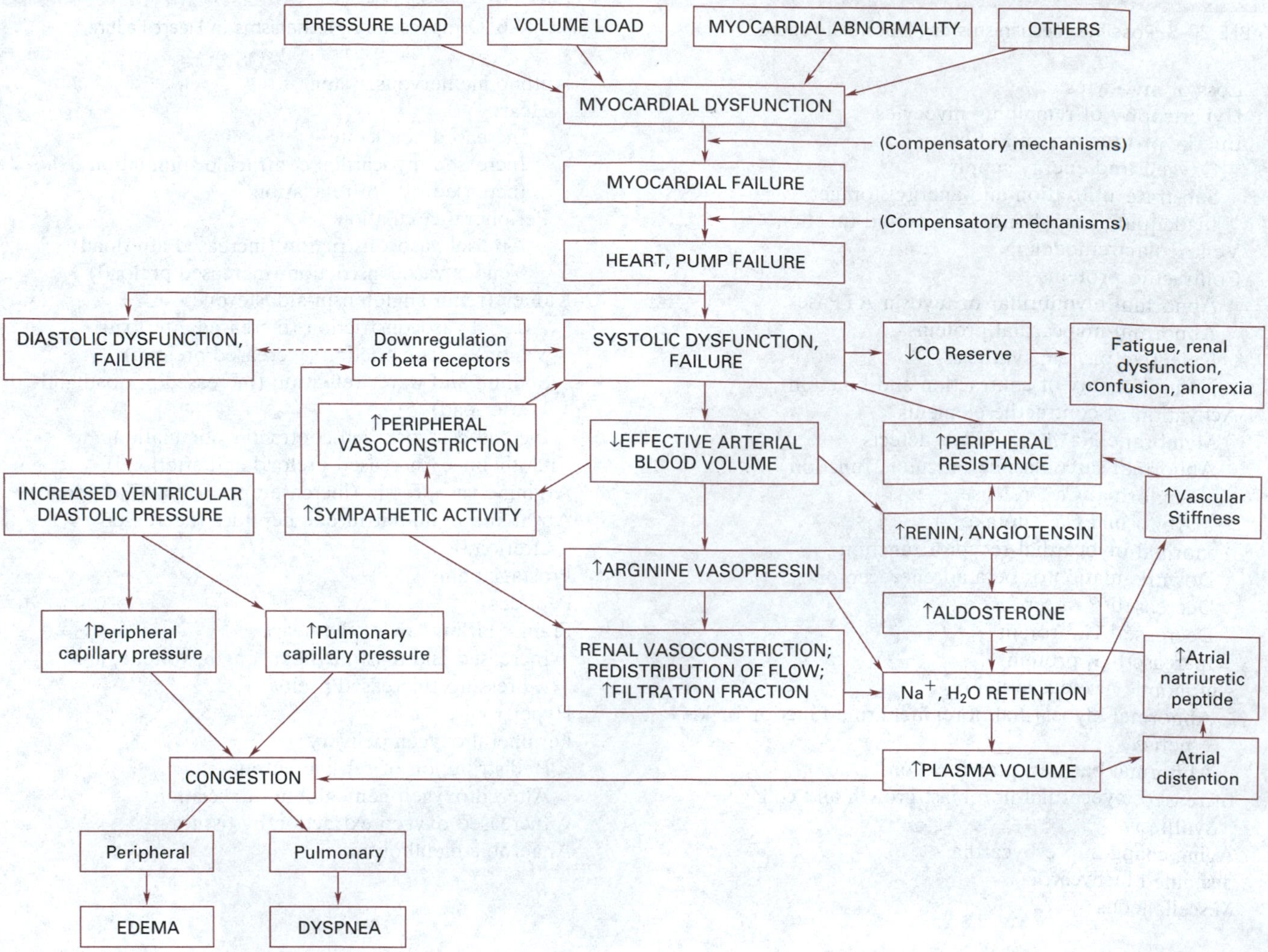

FIGURE 20-4 Schema of the sequence of events in heart failure. An increased load or myocardial abnormality leads to myocardial failure and eventually to heart failure. This results in increased sympathetic activity, increased levels of renin-angiotensin-aldosterone, pulmonary and peripheral congestion and edema, and decreased cardiac output reserve. Endothelial dysfunction also occurs, with decreased endothelial-dependent vasodilatation and with increased plasma levels of endothelin-1, a very strong vasoconstrictor. See text for details.

to an increase in the size of the cardiac myocyte,[39,40] presumably rendering the surviving myocytes a short-term structural and functional advantage. The reprogramming requires altered signals, both mechanical and "chemical," to reach the nucleus of the cardiac myocyte in order to set into motion "new" gene transcription.[41] Ultimately, there is a transition from hypertrophy to heart failure,[42] which has been recognized for more than 100 years but is still not well understood.[34] In a sense, this "unnatural growth response" of myocyte hypertrophy leads to the obvious structural changes of LV remodeling, thus creating a large, dilated, and poorly functioning heart. The processes of cellular remodeling and subsequent architectural changes in cell and chamber size and shape are highly complex[41] and include many components other than myocardial cell hypertrophy. There is myocardial fibrosis, cell dropout, and myocyte slippage. As cardiac output falls, multiple neurohormones including renin and norepinephrine are "released" in an attempt to protect blood pressure and organ perfusion,[43] while atavistic counter-regulatory natriuretic peptides are "released" in an attempt to offset vasoconstriction, hypertrophy, and volume conservation.[44] The story is undoubtedly much more complex than this[45] and includes a cornucopia of molecular mechanisms,[41,46] some of which primarily affect the cardiac interstitium and others the cardiac myocytes. The pathophysiologic changes observed in heart failure are partially depicted in Table 20-6 and Fig. 20-5.

Maladaptive remodeling of cardiac myocyte size and shape begins long before clinical heart failure begins.[47-50] Alterations in myocyte proteins and mitochondria size and number and changes in myocardial interstitium and collagen content/architecture are seen in response to a variety of "injuries" including pressure overload,[51-53] volume overload,[54] and myocardial ischemia.[55,56] Additional phenotypic changes in heart failure include apoptosis[57,58] and side-to-side slippage of myocytes.[59] It is important to recognize that much of the neuroendocrine activation that occurs in a primordial attempt to conserve organ perfusion appears to facilitate this myriad of phenotypic change in the heart at the cellular level,[45] thereby possibly accounting for the success of neuroendocrine blockers as therapy for heart failure. Lastly, there is no single phenotypic change, protein expression, or signal-transduction pathway that is dominant. Rather, there is extraordinary redundancy in these mechanisms. This observation has important implications for therapy. For example, blocking one neuroendocrine system may lead to enhanced overactivity of other neuroendocrine systems. Blocking one signal-transduction pathway may lead the cell to hypertrophy through alternative pathways. Thus it is likely that polypharmacy will always be necessary in the treatment of heart failure.

In summary, heart failure often begins with an index event that results in loss of myocardium (e.g., acute myocardial infarction) or excessive overload (e.g., valvular heart disease, acute myocardial infarction, mutation leading to dilated or hypertrophic cardiomyopathy, etc.). Where hypertrophy cannot sustain the increased load, ventricular dilatation occurs, and the ventricle assumes a more globular shape (i.e., eccentric hypertrophy), thus allowing for maintenance of stroke volume despite a reduced EF. This provides short-term benefit. Absence of some dilatation probably would lead to shock and early death. Neuroendocrine activation presumably occurs in response to a perceived need to protect perfusion pressure, but neurohormones also facilitate the LV remodeling process, thus contributing importantly to the pathogenesis and progression of heart failure. Despite the presumed coherency of this oversimplified working hypothesis, many gaps in our knowledge remain to be filled in, particularly with regard to the quantitative contribution that each phenotypic change makes toward the progression of heart failure. We still have much to learn.

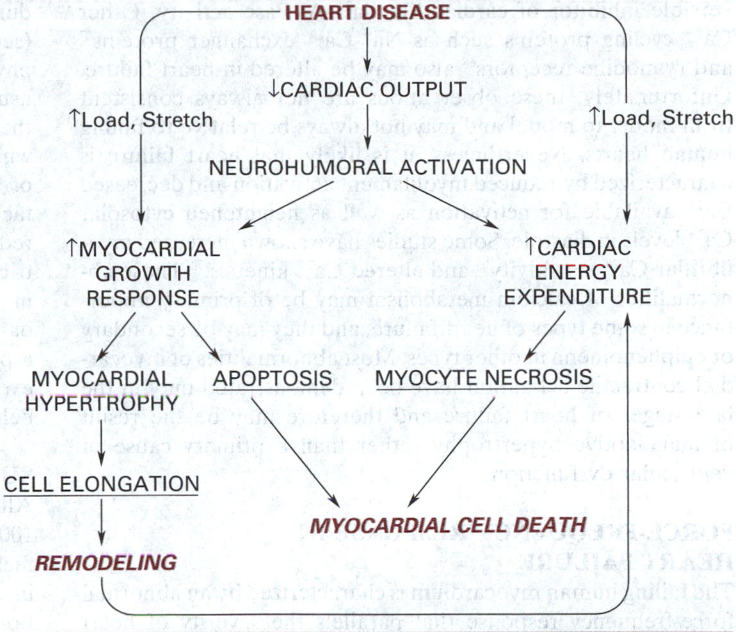

FIGURE 20-5 Possible mechanisms by which overloading can cause progressive deterioration of the heart ("cardiomyopathy of overload"). Several mechanisms, including myocyte stretch, activate a growth response that initiates myocardial hypertrophy in the overloaded heart (*left*). The same growth response may also activate signal transduction systems that cause programmed cell death (apoptosis). The hypertrophic response to overload, by causing sarcomeres to be added in series, can also lead to cell elongation and so accelerate remodeling; the resulting increase in wall tension, along with the overload itself (*right*), increases cardiac energy expenditure that, in the overloaded heart, can accelerate myocyte necrosis. Reduced cardiac output activates neurohumoral responses (*center*), which, by increasing afterload and β-adrenergic stimulation of the heart, also increase cardiac energy expenditure. Because many mediators of the neurohumoral response to a fall in cardiac output promote myocardial cell growth, neurohumoral activation can also accelerate both apoptosis and remodeling.

Molecular, Physiologic, and Biochemical Alterations Occurring with Hypertrophy and the Progression to Heart Failure

Alterations are found in the failing heart in numerous contractile proteins, especially in heredity-based idiopathic dilated cardiomyopathies. In the latter situation, these alterations can be the sole cause of heart failure. Such alterations have been found in myosin, troponin T, and actin. These alterations in protein structure likely contribute to diminished myocardial performance. Alterations in gross cardiac structure and cellular components in heart failure resulting from systolic overloads are much more complex. Findings in animal models of overload-produced heart failure may vary from model to model, and observations made in human failing hearts may be different from those made in animal models. In the human failing heart, many changes in gene expression at the mRNA or protein level have been found in hearts harvested at the time of cardiac transplantation. These are hearts with end-stage myocardial disease in which many factors (such as receiving multiple inotropic drugs) may obscure actual pathogenesis. Despite these caveats, we have learned much from these studies, only some of which will be discussed here.

β-MYOSIN HEAVY CHAIN

Two myosin heavy chain (MHC) isoforms are present in mammalian heart, α- and β-MHC. The α-MHC is cardiac-specific and is more enzymatically active. The less active β-MHC is present in heart and also in slow-twitch skeletal muscle. The distribution of α- and β-MHC is developmentally and hormonally regulated. Mechanical stress, such as pressure overload, induces an α- to β-MHC transition in the ventricles of experimental animals, thus imparting a slower but more economical type of work for the overloaded heart. Either way, myosin remains the principal structural and contractile unit of muscle fiber. Lowes et al.[60] recently have demonstrated downregulation of α-MHC and upregulation of β-MHC using mRNA measurements from right ventricular endomyocardial biopsies from nonfailing hearts and failing human hearts. This alteration, if translated into protein expression, would decrease myosin ATPase enzyme velocity and slow the speed of contraction. Although such adaptive changes could be viewed to have an "economical" survival advantage in the face of increased load, slower contraction and relaxation may contribute to diastolic dysfunction.

SARCOPLASMIC RETICULUM FUNCTION

There is substantial evidence that defects in sarcolemma Ca^{2+} uptake (sarcolemmal transport via Na^+,K^+-ATPase) and release by the sarcoplasmic reticulum (SR) are present in heart failure, especially at later stages.[61-63] Alternatively, uptake of Ca^{2+} by the SR may remain intact.[64] These alterations in Ca^{2+} transport may be secondary to quantitative alterations of gene expression of SR Ca^{2+} transport proteins, especially the sarco(endo)plasmic reticulum Ca^{2+}-ATPase (SERCA)[65] and phospholamban,[66] a reversible inhibitor of cardiac SR Ca^{2+}-ATPase activity. Other Ca^{2+} cycling proteins such as Na^{+}-Ca^{2+} exchanger proteins[67] and ryanodine receptors[68] also may be altered in heart failure. Unfortunately, these observations are not always consistent from model to model and may not always be relative to failing human hearts. Nevertheless, it is likely that heart failure is characterized by reduced myofilament activation and decreased Ca^{2+} available for activation as well as heightened cytosolar Ca^{2+} levels in diastole. Some studies have shown increased myofibrillar Ca^{2+} sensitivity[69] and altered Ca^{2+} kinetics.[70] These abnormalities of calcium metabolism may be of primary importance in some types of heart failure, and they may be secondary or epiphenomena in other types. Most abnormalities of myocardial contractile activation have been demonstrated only in the late stages of heart failure and therefore may be the result of maladaptive hypertrophy rather than a primary cause of ventricular dysfunction.

FORCE-FREQUENCY RESPONSE IN HEART FAILURE

The failing human myocardium is characterized by an abnormal force-frequency response that parallels the severity of heart failure. Normally, increase in frequency of stimulation is accompanied by an enhanced force of contraction (Bowditch effect). In heart failure, an increase in heart rate by pacing an additional 50 beats per minute is accompanied by about a 30 percent decrease in myocardial performance as measured by dP/dt_{max}. It is likely that some impairment of systolic function in response to increased heart rate may be related to impaired LV filling, although a negative inotropic effect, as shown in isolated muscle to be due to alterations in intracellular Ca^{2+} handling, cannot be excluded. This feature of heart failure may help explain some impairment of cardiac function during exercise.[71,72]

ENERGY PRODUCTION AND USE

Oxygen deprivation, which is most often due to coronary artery disease, results in impaired relaxation and weakened contraction, as may be seen in angina pectoris. When transient, these are readily reversible. With prolonged ischemia, decreased contraction (dyskinesis) may persist for hours beyond return of blood flow and is termed stunning. If coronary blood flow is chronically reduced, myocardium may fail to contract normally (*hibernation*), even if necrosis does not ensue. With more serious loss of flow, infarction can occur. All these stages may produce substantial dyskinesia for which the remaining myocardium must sustain this load. The result is hypertrophy of the nonischemic portion of the ventricle; if this is inadequate, an increase in ventricular volume occurs using the Frank-Starling mechanism to sustain stroke volume.

In patients with heart failure, the total amount of oxygen consumed by the heart may be increased significantly because of the increased total mass, the increase in myocardial systolic wall tension due to the Laplace relationship, and perhaps some wasted contractile energy. This increase may result in the extraction of a greater amount of oxygen from each unit of coronary blood flow and a widening of the coronary arteriovenous oxygen difference. Many patients with heart failure are able to increase coronary blood flow during exercise; however, some patients with a dilated ventricle that increases in diameter during exercise may have a further widening of the coronary arteriovenous oxygen difference during exercise and a decrease in coronary blood flow reserve (see Chaps. 3 and 37). In the presence of severe LV hypertrophy, coronary blood flow per unit mass of myocardium is usually normal at rest. On the other hand, the capacity of the coronary vascular bed to dilate during reactive hyperemia, which is normally four- to fivefold, is reduced. In the presence of severe hypertrophy where filling pressures are elevated, tachycardia such as may occur with atrial fibrillation may reduce diastolic coronary perfusion, producing ischemic ventricular failure. While reduced perfusion is probably common in end-stage heart failure, a deficit in coronary blood flow or oxygen delivery has not been clearly demonstrated to be a primary cause of heart failure associated with hypertrophy, except in the presence of obstructive coronary disease (see below).

SUBSTRATE USE AND ENERGY STORAGE

Although the myocardial uptake of fatty acids and glucose per 100 g of myocardium is normal in heart failure,[73] there is conflicting evidence on whether or not there is a primary decrease in energy liberation by mitochondrial oxidative phosphorylation.[33,34,73–77] The reductions in stores of myocardial high-energy phosphate, creatine phosphate, and/or adenosine triphosphate (ATP) generally found in heart failure usually are thought to be secondary and to be the consequence of the failure rather than the primary cause of the failure.[73–82] There also may be reduced levels of creatine kinase and changes in the isoenzymes of creatine kinase in heart failure.[82]

The major consequences of the state of energy starvation that is probably seen in many, if not most, failing hearts are due to attenuation of important allosteric (regulatory) effects of ATP rather than reduction in the supply of substrate for the many energy-consuming reactions involved in contraction, relaxation, and excitation-contraction coupling. Because the normal systolic ATP concentration is around 5 to 10 mM, whereas the substrate-binding sites of most ATP-hydrolzing systems are saturated at ATP concentrations less than 1 mM, it is unlikely that ATP concentrations fall to levels below those needed to saturate known energy-consuming reactions except in the dying heart. These allosteric effects of high ATP concentrations, which do not require that the nucleotide be hydrolyzed, resemble those of a "lubricant" in that ATP accelerates ion pumps, ion exchangers, and passive ion fluxes through membrane channels. By facilitating the many calcium fluxes involved in excitation-contraction coupling and relaxation, these allosteric effects of ATP exert both inotropic and lusitropic effects.[76]

MITOCHONDRIAL MASS AND FUNCTION

There are conflicting data on whether or not there is a significant decrease in the mass of mitochondria relative to the mass of myofibrils that occurs in experimental cardiac hypertrophy.[80–82] It is possible that this is one of the limitations of severe hypertrophy. Defects in mitochondrial oxidative phosphorylation and in mitochondrial calcium metabolism also may be associated with myocardial failure.[83] Except in circumstances where coronary flow is limited, such as with large vessel obstructive disease (see Chap. 40) or purported microvascular obstructive or vasospastic disease, a primary role of energy limitation in the evolution of heart failure has yet to be demonstrated.[74] It is possible that it may play a role during periods of higher metabolic demand, such as tachycardia,[77] as noted previously.[84,85]

VENTRICULAR REMODELING (HYPERTROPHY AND DILATATION)

When one portion of the ventricle is disabled, an increase in intraventricular volume slowly occurs, presumably in response to a sustained venous return. This involves increased myocyte length, with the limit being at the level of the sarcomere at 2.2 μm. With systolic overloads, compensatory hypertrophy occurs with the addition of sarcomeres in parallel, leading to a lateral thickening of the myocyte while sarcomere length does not change.

Acute dilatation is also limited by the sarcomere, which at 2.2 μm attains maximum force. Beyond this point, stiffness of the sarcomere and the myocardium becomes very large, and resting tension rises to high levels. Such acute dilatation may lead to relative "side to side" slippage of myocytes. When distending forces become chronic, addition of new sarcomeres occurs in series. Dilatation of the ventricle also adds to the load by the Laplace relation, whereby tension in the wall rises with increased volume at the same pressure. This results in some lateral growth of myocytes, although elongation is the major alteration. In addition, functional mitral regurgitation may occur from excessive ventricular volume that adds to the volume overload. When increased systolic tension occurs, myocyte hypertrophy that occurs by laying down of sarcomeres in parallel is accomplished by biochemical alterations in both the contractile proteins and activating membrane systems (see Chap. 5).

In addition to the synthesis of sarcomeres in series with preexisting sarcomeres, "slippage" of myofibrils and myocardial fibers and rearrangement of myocardial fibers along cleavage planes of the left ventricle occur.[59] Thus, although overstretch of sarcomeres rarely may be present very transiently, it does not appear to be an important primary mechanism of chronic heart failure. There is evidence, however, that excessive stretch of myocytes can lead to myocyte death, apparently by the process of apoptosis (programmed cell death), which may lead to further heart failure. The effects of the law of Laplace with ventricular dilatation were noted earlier. Nonuniformity of myocardial contraction and functional mitral regurgitation also contribute to heart failure.

MYOCARDIAL RECEPTOR FUNCTION

One of the hallmarks of heart failure is decreased myocardial inotropic function. Although it is clear that no single mechanism accounts for the depressed inotropic state, reduction in myocardial β-adrenergic receptors and its subsequent second messenger cAMP may play an important role in this regard.[86] β-Adrenergic stimulation contributes importantly to the cardiac response to exercise,[87] and β-adrenergic desensitization and uncoupling may be at least partially responsible for the reduced chronotropic and inotropic response to peak exercise commonly found in patients with heart failure.[87] The β-adrenergic receptor abnormalities in heart failure appear to be due to desensitization and uncoupling of the β_1 receptor produced by local and not systemic alterations in catecholamines.[88] In severe heart failure, the norepinephrine (NE) stores in sympathetic nerve endings are well known to be depleted. In a sense, the failing myocardium becomes functionally denervated. cAMP responses are reduced by about 30 to 35 percent, leading to further contractile dysfunction.[79] It is possible that with rather selective downregulation of the β_1 receptor, there remains a relatively high proportion of β_2 receptors to mediate chronotropic and inotropic responses.[89] However, there is mild uncoupling of the β_2 receptor from its G protein and a mild upregulation of the $G_{\alpha i}$ subunit, further contributing to a depressed response to chronotropic and inotropic stimuli.[90–92] There is also a profound decrease in cardiac β-adrenergic responsiveness with aging,[93] which has clinical implications because heart failure is heavily concentrated in the aging population.

The desensitization and uncoupling of β-adrenergic receptors occurs early with mild to moderate ventricular dysfunction. It is related to the degree of heart failure and is associated with a very reduced response to β-adrenergic stimulation with drugs such as dobutamine.[94] Long-term stimulation of β-adrenergic receptors may enhance myocardial β-adrenergic receptor kinase (β-ARK) activity,[95] leading to further desensitization and uncoupling of the β-adrenergic receptor. These observations generally support the previously counterintuitive concept of using β-adrenergic blocking drugs to treat patients with heart failure. Of some interest, β-adrenergic blockade with metoprolol, a relatively cardioselective β_1 blocker, upregulates the β_1 receptor, whereas carvedilol, a nonselective β_1 and β_2 blocker with additional α_1 blocking activity, does not increase β_1 receptor density.[96] Both drugs can improve LV function. This suggests that the improvement in cardiac function seen with chronic β blocker use is not simply due to upregulation of β-adrenergic receptors. Moreover, high plasma norepinephrine levels do not predict benefit from carvedilol,[97] suggesting that there is not a simple relation between activation of the sympathetic nervous system and β-adrenergic receptor function in heart failure.

AUTONOMIC NERVOUS SYSTEM DYSFUNCTION

Heart failure is characterized by many abnormal reflex control mechanisms. Peripheral vascular resistance is increased, there is defective cardiac parasympathetic control,[98] an abnormal response to upright tilt,[99] altered baroreceptor function,[100–103] and reduced cardiac sympathetic activity in response to a variety of stimuli.[104–106] Indeed, an early sign of heart failure is increased sympathetic tone accompanied by reduced vagal tone resulting in an increased heart rate even at rest.

The increase in systemic vascular resistance observed in well-established heart failure, a therapeutic target for short-term hemodynamic treatment with nitroprusside, is likely due to a combination of locally active heightened vasoconstrictors (norepinephrine, angiotensin II, endothelin, vasopressin, neuropeptide Y) and to structural changes in blood vessels related to fluid retention and reduced endothelial-dependent vasodilation. Early in heart failure there may be a fall in cardiac output, arterial pressure, and baroreceptor activity, leading to an "adaptive" increase in excessive neuroendocrine drive. The sympathetic nervous system and the renin-angiotensin-aldosterone axis are activated. Arginine vasopressin is released. Sodium and water retention occur, hypervolemia restores cardiac output and arterial pressure, and neuroendocrine activity may reach a steady state. However, as heart failure progresses, there is impaired cardiosensory activity that fails to reduce neuroendocrine drive. Cardiac afferent activity to the central nervous system, for unclear reasons, is reduced, leading to unhindered, efferent excitatory responses from the brain to the periphery. Reflex vasoconstrictor responses to unloading the heart are paradoxically blunted.[99,106] There are abnormal vascular responses to postural change.[107] Some of these changes lead to alterations in regional blood flow that accompany heart failure.[108] Heart rate variability is markedly reduced and is a hallmark in defining congestive failure. Further, decreased heart rate variability may provide independent prognostic value in the identification of patients at risk for premature death.[109]

Although the genesis of these abnormal reflex control mechanisms is still not clearly understood, the changes may be more functional than structural in origin. Heart transplantation reverses cardiopulmonary baroreflex control mechanisms to some extent,[110,111] but the improvement may be absent[112] or delayed[113] in some cases. The role that abnormal reflex control mechanisms plays in the progression of heart failure, like other neuroendocrine alterations, has been difficult to quantitate. Nevertheless, it is now increasingly clear that the sympathetic nervous system and the renin-angiotensin-aldosterone system greatly influence the progression and natural history of heart failure. The therapeutic implications derived from these observations have proven to be very important.[114,115]

MECHANICAL AND HEMODYNAMIC FEATURES OF HEART FAILURE

The term *heart failure* implies structural heart disease. The central problem of heart failure remains impaired cardiac performance, although many of the secondary "adaptive" responses become maladaptive and contribute substantially to progression of heart failure. An understanding of how these changes occur can provide insight into the pathophysiology of the syndrome.

As ventricular function becomes impaired, the Frank-Starling law of the heart becomes operative (see Fig. 20-2). Inadequate emptying of the ventricle leads to increased EDVs. This is referred to as *increased preload,* and it produces an increase in SV during the next contraction. The Frank-Starling law simply states that the increase in contractile force (i.e., contractility) is related to sarcomere lengthening (up to 2.2 μm). For any given amount of Ca^{2+} released into the myocyte, there is increased crossbridge formation and enhanced sensitivity of the myofilament to Ca^{2+} as the sarcomeres lengthen.

In the failing ventricle, the extent of shortening for a given diastolic fiber length and load (afterload) is reduced. The ventricle can maintain a normal or near-normal SV with an increased EDV and thus maintain end-diastolic fiber length for a period of time. Eventually, the filling pressure rises inordinately, limiting this compensation (see Fig. 20-1). Further, the clinically dilated ventricle tends to "give" like an overstretched elastic band, and end-diastolic volume may increase somewhat with no increase in LV end-diastolic pressure, reflecting a shift in the passive pressure-volume curve to the right. An obligatory reduction in ejection fraction occurs when SV is maintained in the face of a large EDV (EF = SV/EDV; normal EF = 0.62 ± 0.12). Eventually, further increases in EDP produce little change in EDV, thus flattening the SV-EDP curve (see Fig. 20-1). There is no true descending limb to Starling curve because increasing preload indefinitely ultimately will lead to mitral regurgitation.[116,117] As the heart dilates, the increase in wall stress according to the Laplace relationship also will increase afterload, which may account for any observed reduction in SV as the heart dilates further (i.e., the perception of a descending limb). It is important to keep in mind that LV performance depends not only on systolic pump function but also on active relaxation, passive diastolic properties, and vascular loading conditions. It is likely that at high LV end-diastolic pressure, valvular incompetence (mitral regurgitation) is a major cause of a decrease in cardiac output. Thus, in end-stage heart failure in the intact circulation, the Starling curve flattens out. It is possible under certain experimental conditions that the severely failing heart is able to utilize the Frank-Starling mechanism,[118] but a hallmark of heart failure is the inability of the chamber to respond robustly to an increase in preload.

Afterload and the Concept of the Laplace Relation

A characteristic feature of the dilated, failing heart is that it gradually becomes less sensitive to preload (EDV and fiber length) and more sensitive to afterload stress. At very high LV filling pressures (>30 mmHg) when the sarcomeres are fully extended and the preload reserve is exhausted, the SV becomes exquisitely sensitive to alterations in the afterload.[119] The impedance to ejection includes blood viscosity, vascular resistance, vascular distensibility, and myocardial wall tension. The afterload is the total load that the heart must work against during contraction. Much of the afterload is made up of ventricular myocardial wall tension. In the ventricle, the tension on the walls increases as ventricular chamber volume increases, even if intraventricular pressure remains constant. Calculations of myocardial wall tension are defined by the Laplace equation and are expressed in terms of tension T per unit of cross-sectional area (dynes per centimeter).

Within a cylinder, the law of Laplace states that wall tension is equal to the pressure within the cylinder times the radius of curvature of the wall:

$$T = P \times R$$

where T is wall tension (dyn/cm), P is pressure (dyn/cm^2), and R is the radius (cm). Basically, wall tension is proportional to radius. Because the heart has thick ventricular walls, wall tension is distributed over a large number of muscle fibers, thereby reducing tension on each. The equation for a thick-walled cylinder such as the heart is:

$$T = \frac{P \times R}{h}$$

where h is wall thickness. The equation is sometimes stated as:

$$T = \frac{P \times R}{2h}$$

Since the geometry of the ventricles is more complex than a cylinder, ventricular wall tension cannot be measured with precision. Wall stress, the force distributed across an area, is actually more correct but is seldom measured.

There are two fundamental principles that stem from the relationship between the geometry of the ventricular cavity and the tension on its muscular walls:

1. *Dilation of the ventricles leads directly to an increase in tension on each muscle fiber.*
2. *An increase in wall thickness reduces the tension on any individual muscle fiber. Therefore, ventricular hypertrophy*

reduces afterload by distributing tension among more muscle fibers.

The wall tension is highest in the inner surface of the heart. The endocardial surfaces must do more work and therefore are also more vulnerable to reductions in coronary blood flow. Dilatation of the heart decreases cardiac efficiency, unless hypertrophy is sufficient to normalize wall stress. In heart failure, wall tension (or stress) is high, and thus afterload is increased. The energetic consequences of the law of Laplace may have some role in progressive deterioration of energy-starved cardiac myocytes in the failing heart.

Another major disadvantage of the dilated ventricle is the inability to decrease the average radius during contraction. In the normal heart, wall tension falls during ventricular ejection as the volume decreases, even though pressure is rising. In heart failure, given the dilated heart with reduced ejection, the average tension in the myocardial fibers actually may continue to increase from the beginning of the ejection until peak systolic pressure is reached,[120–122] adding additional afterload during ejection. The rate of myocardial fiber shortening is reduced, further contributing to diminished myocardial performance. It is difficult to overstate the importance of the law of Laplace when considering the syndrome of heart failure. This contrast is apparent in mitral insufficiency. With preserved contractility and a relatively small EDV, mitral insufficiency leads to rapid unloading of volume and reduced tension. When ventricular dilatation occurs with decreased ventricular contractility, ejection is reduced, and tension remains high during systole, leading to an unsteady state that cannot be maintained for long.

Ventricular dilatation, though initially adaptive as an attempt to sustain SV, eventually becomes a substantial disadvantage and contributes importantly to impaired myocardial performance. As the left and right ventricles dilate, functional mitral and tricuspid regurgitation can occur, adding to circulatory congestion. Stretched myocardial cells can induce programmed cell death (apoptosis), thereby contributing to further disease progression.[123] Any treatment that slows progressive dilatation of the heart, such as angiotensin-converting enzyme inhibitors or β-adrenergic blockers, will likely have a powerful role in the treatment of heart failure. The plasticity of the process of progressive dilatation is now more apparent, with remarkable reversal of dilatation observed under specific circumstances such as cessation of alcohol use in patients with alcoholic cardiomyopathy and spontaneous improvement in patients with inflammatory myocarditis.

Myocardial Hypertrophy

Hypertrophy of myocardial myocytes occurs to meet the demand of increased rate of use of mechanical energy. It is basically a response to sustained hemodynamic overloading of the heart, be it a volume or pressure overload or a combination of the two. Ischemic heart disease leads to a reduction of contractile tissue, ventricular dilatation, and a volume overload on the remaining viable myocytes. In this sense, it is a form of volume overload hypertrophy. Up to a point, the increased mass of cardiac muscle is beneficial in that it tends to normalize wall stress and provides for a larger number of contractile elements (sarcomeres).

Experimentally, evidence of hypertrophy (e.g., synthesis of new mRNA) occurs within hours of imparting a new load on the heart.[124,125] Pressure- and volume-induced hypertrophy are associated with distinct myocyte phenotypes and differential induction of peptide growth factors.[126] The heart demonstrates remarkable plasticity in response to a variety of growth factors and hemodynamic loads.[41] Isolated cell deformation is a sufficient stimulus for induction of hypertrophic growth, but the modulating role of angiotensin II, norepinephrine, altered membrane ion channels, and numerous growth factors is of obvious importance. The changing mechanical loading conditions appear to be the primary driving force behind myocardial hypertrophy in heart failure, and other factors likely act more as important modulators or facilitators of the process. Hyperplasia, or an increase in new myocardial cells, may occur to some extent under conditions of excessive loading or myocyte loss.[127,128] However, the capacity for new cardiac myocytes to form is limited, and whether they are functionally useful is unknown. Rather, the primary response to altered load is the assembly of new working units or sarcomeres per myocardial cell. In general, pressure overload results in replication of sarcomeres in parallel, whereas volume overload leads to new sarcomeres both in parallel and in series.[129] There is, however, significant hyperplasia of fibroblasts,[130–136] which outnumber cardiac myocytes by 3:1 to 4:1. It is the fibroblasts that are the major source of the reparative and replacement collagen when myocytes are lost in the evolution of heart failure.

Classically, pressure overload induces a form of *concentric hypertrophy,* whereas volume overload causes a form of *eccentric hypertrophy*. Concentric hypertrophy typically occurs with aortic stenosis or severe hypertension and causes a thickened ventricular wall, usually with no increase in chamber diameter. Myocytes primarily are increased in diameter. Capillary growth to these thickened myocytes may be diminished.[137,138] In eccentric hypertrophy, usually a consequence of volume overload, there is a proportional increase in wall thickness and chamber diameter. Myocytes primarily elongate from new sarcomeres assembled in series.

There also may be *reactive hypertrophy* of remaining myocytes in response to myocardial infarction.[139] In actuality, such myocardial hypertrophy is often hybrid, with both myocyte elongation and increased thickness of individual cardiac myocytes being observed. Local activation of autocrine/paracrine angiotensin II may play a role in the regulation of the hypertrophic process[140] but may not be an essential component of this complex system.[141]

There is now evidence from animal experiments that cell elongation may contribute importantly to chamber dilatation.[142,143] However, other factors such as myocyte slippage and increased interstitial tissue also may help to explain the increase in heart size frequently encountered in patients with heart failure. It should be pointed out that the original increase in heart size is geared to maintain stroke volume and normal wall tension. When decompensated heart failure occurs, it is apparent that the increase in wall thickness is insufficient to normalize wall tension. Afterload rises and performance worsens, contributing to decompensation.

Of course, other changes in the myocardium are occurring simultaneously, and hypertrophy is only one factor, albeit an important one. Biochemical changes, phenotypic changes in protein synthesis, altered excitation-contraction, slower velocity

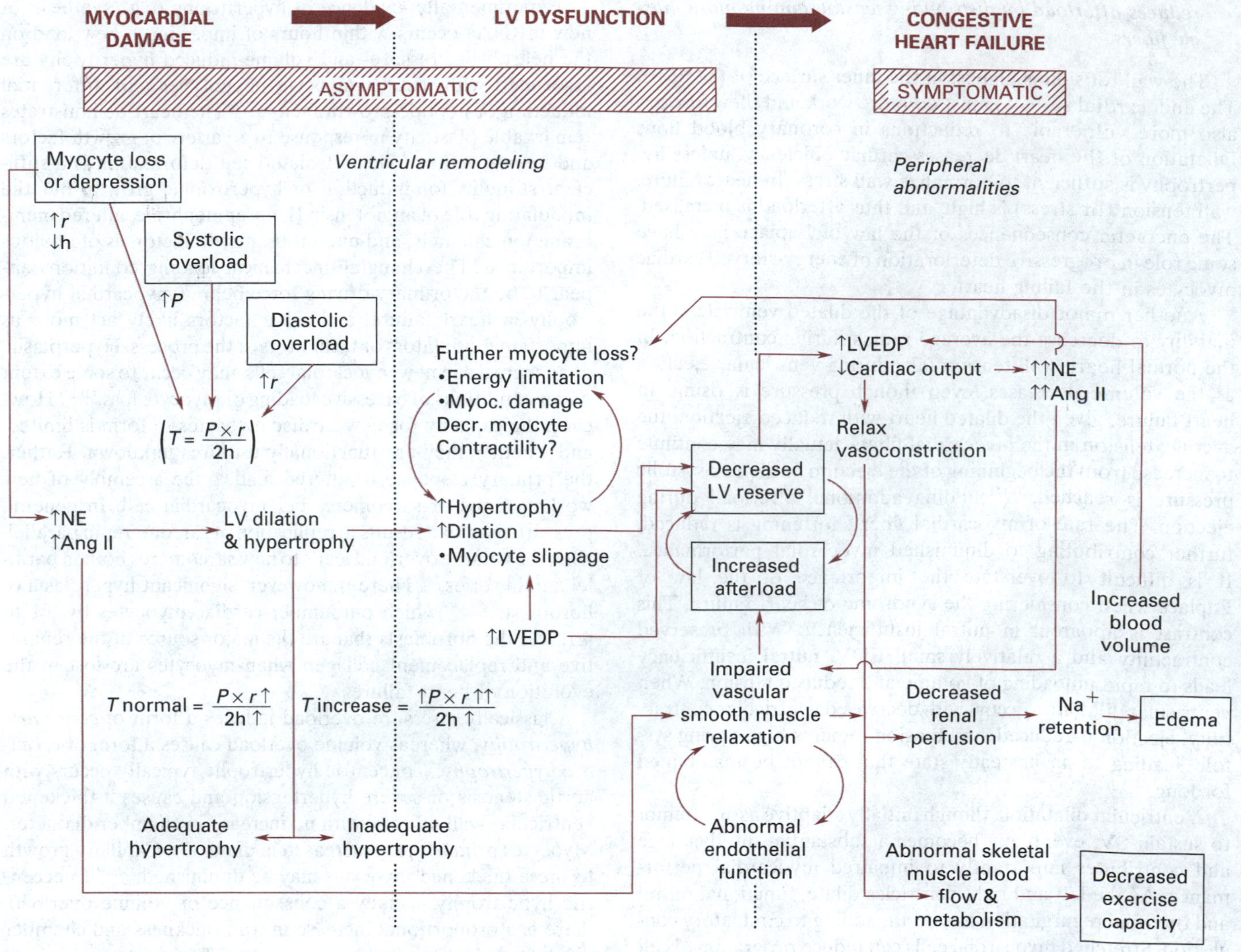

FIGURE 20-6 Evolution of myocardial damage to left ventricular function and ultimate congestive heart failure. The syndrome of congestive heart failure is the end result of processes that evolve in response to initial myocardial damage and/or cardiac overloads. The initiating event may be myocyte loss, either segmental, as with acute myocardial infarction, or diffuse, as with idiopathic cardiomyopathies and myocarditis; systolic overload, such as hypertension or aortic stenosis; or diastolic overload, such as mitral regurgitation or aortic regurgitation. Major loss of myocytes may also stimulate the renin-angiotensin and adrenergic systems, which may contribute to ventricular and vascular remodeling. All of these overloads create an increased workload for the heart, as characterized by Laplace relationship, where tension (T) is equal to the product of pressure (P) and ventricular radius (r) divided by twice the wall of thickness (h). The initial adaptations to these overloads, termed *ventricular remodeling*, are an increase in both myocyte length and diameter as well as an increase in ventricular volume to maintain adequate stroke volume and hence cardiac output. If hypertrophy is adequate to normalize the tension load, a relatively steady state may be maintained. Myocytes continue to be lost as a function of aging per se, however, and this tends to lead to further myocyte hypertrophy and cardiac dilatation. Moreover, the aging process may be amplified by hypertrophy. Should there be a sudden increase in end-diastolic pressure within the ventricle, an added factor of relative myocyte slippage within the wall tends to occur, which may lead to a further decrease in myocytes across the ventricular wall, further increasing ventricular wall tension. This may create a downward spiral in which progressive cell loss leads to further ventricular remodeling and continued ventricular dilation. As noted above, the entire process of ventricular remodeling may occur asymptomatically, and myocardial damage progresses to left ventricular dysfunction, which is characterized by an increasing diastolic volume and thus a reduced ventricular ejection fraction. Symptoms associated with congestive heart failure occur when decreased left ventricular reserve limits cardiac output response to exercise. As the process of heart failure evolves, abnormalities of endothelial function in the peripheral arterioles lead to reduced ability of the peripheral vasculature to dilate in response to metabolic need. As these abnormalities occur, abnormal skeletal muscle blood flow occurs in response to exercise and decreased exercise tolerance. In addition decreased renal perfusion leads to further activation of the renin-angiotensin-aldosterone system (RAAS), with increased aldosterone secretion and sodium retention. The combination of these two events leads to decreased exercise capacity and peripheral edema, important components of the symptom complex of congestive heart failure. Decreased cardiac performance promotes neurohumoral responses characterized by activation of the sympathetic nervous system and the renin-angiotensin-aldosterone system, leading to peripheral vasoconstriction and sodium accumulation. These factors feed back to increase the ventricular remodeling process and to amplify cardiac damage. Thus, initial myocardial damage progresses to ventricular dysfunction and ultimately to congestive heart failure. It is important to note that the myocardial damage and left ventricular dysfunction are often asymptomatic, and by the time symptomatic heart failure ensues, the disease process is far advanced. [Revised from LeJemtel TH, Sonnenblick EH. Heart failure and maladaptive processes: Introduction. *Circulation* 1993; 87(suppl VII):VII1–VII4. Reproduced with permission from the American Heart Association and the authors.]

of shortening due to a slower acting myosin heavy chain, and reduced β-adrenergic receptor density are all occurring simultaneously. Mechanically, reduced velocity of contraction, delayed time to peak tension, and slower relaxation are observed in the myocardium of failing hearts. All these factors likely converge to produce clinical decompensation. Delayed ventricular relaxation may limit filling, leading to heightened filling pressure, pulmonary congestion, and shortness of breath. Force development and shortening capacity remain intact in the face of hypertrophy, and only in very late failure does contractility or contractile force decline. What ultimately happens to the patient may depend on the acuteness or chronicity of the load, the extent of hypertrophy and fibrosis, the amount of myocyte loss, the heart rate and synchrony of atrioventricular contraction, and a host of invisible perturbations occurring at the level of the cell (Fig. 20-6).

Diastolic Heart Failure

Diastolic heart failure is often present when there is limitation of exercise tolerance and dyspnea that cannot be explained by lung disease or the extent of underlying LV systolic dysfunction. Diastole is usually divided into several mechanical phases (Fig. 20-7). Investigation of patients with heart failure and normal systolic function, usually by echo, often indicates LV hypertrophy and abnormal diastolic function. Unfortunately, there is no agreement as to what constitutes abnormal diastolic function. Disturbances include alterations in relaxation (reduced rate of decline in wall tension), an upward shift of the LV diastolic pressure-volume relationship (a decrease in LV diastolic distensibility) (see Fig. 20-1), incoordinate wall motion during isovolumic relaxation, and altered ventricular inflow velocity. These measurements are influenced by loading conditions, ischemia, heart rate, and age, making it difficult to determine the actual contribution of diastolic dysfunction to heart failure. This is why some prefer the phrase "heart failure with intact or normal systolic function." Nevertheless, disturbances in diastolic function are common in patients with heart failure and are multifactorial. Diastolic impairment is frequently symptomatic in patients with LV hypertrophy, coronary artery disease, and diabetes mellitus. There also may be impairment of diastolic function due to an infiltrative process such as amyloid. For any given EDV, there is often a higher LV end-diastolic pressure, indicating increased chamber stiffness and a smaller cavity size.

As the population ages, one can expect to see more diastolic heart failure.[144] The development of atrial fibrillation with resulting reduced diastolic ventricular filling time commonly produces pulmonary edema in such patients. Although not as lethal as heart failure with a reduced ejection fraction, the prognosis of diastolic heart failure is poor. Diastolic abnormalities usually coexist with alterations in systolic function in patients with dilated cardiomyopathy.[145] The recognition, evaluation, and treatment of diastolic heart failure remain an obvious challenge,[146,147] but diastolic heart failure is an important component of the syndrome of heart failure and must be considered by all who care for patients with heart failure.

Hibernating and Stunned Myocardium

There is now a considerable body of evidence indicating that the myocardium can adapt its activity successfully to prevailing energetic circumstances.[148,149] *Hibernating* myocardium is a condition of reduced myocardial blood flow and impaired myocardial function that improves with revascularization. Myocardial *stunning* is the mechanical dysfunction that persists after reperfusion despite the absence of irreversible damage. Hibernation is particularly important to recognize, diagnose, and treat because revascularization may be associated with a lower cardiovascular event rate.[150] The most commonly used tests for diagnosing hibernating myocardium are dobutamine echocardiography, thallium and sestamibi single-photon-emission computed tomographic (SPECT) myocardial perfusion imaging, positron-emission tomography, and magnetic resonance imaging (MRI) with gadolinium (see Chaps. 16, 18, and 19). Essentially, these imaging techniques are used to define myocardial viability.[151] Many large referral centers have developed their preferred method of assessment. LV function often improves or normalizes with revascularization when there is a "significant" amount of hibernating, but viable, myocardium as the major cause of LV dysfunction. When hibernating myocardium is documented, revascularization rather than heart transplantation is the appropriate therapy, provided the coronary arteries are suitable for revascularization.

Although the precise mechanism of hibernating myocardium has not been determined, the concept is very attractive to clinicians. It is as though the heart downgrades its myocardial function to the extent that blood flow and function are once again in equilibrium. There is no myocardial necrosis or symptoms of ischemia. These observations suggest that the heart can adapt to chronically low myocardial blood flow and that a new steady state between perfusion and contraction can be achieved and maintained. The pathophysiology is undoubtedly highly complex and is accompanied by phenotypic changes and morphologic alterations.[152] It is likely that hibernating myocardium represents a precarious though reversible state, and failure to revascularize it may lead to an increased rate of adverse events and a poor prognosis. Hibernating myocardium may be the end result of repetitive myocardial stunning, perpetuated by renewed episodes of ischemia.

The Cardiac Interstitium

Collagen and the interstitium are normally in a steady state but increase during hypertrophy and following loss of myocytes due to myocardial injury. In heart failure the interstitial space includes reparative and interstitial fibrosis. Contrary to previous concepts, the interstitium is a very dynamic structure, with both matrix removal and synthesis occurring simultaneously at all times. Connective tissue remodeling, either physiologic or pathologic, is in most cases a homeostasis between collagen synthesis and collagen degradation by matrix metalloproteases (MMPs). The matrix of the heart is a very complex scaffolding composed of fibrillar and ground substance proteins (collagen) that pattern around and between myocytes in a very precise and organized pattern. The matrix likely plays a very important role in maintaining an ideal ventricular shape.[153] Changes in the cardiac "skeleton" can contribute to impairment of both diastolic and systolic function.[154] In the failing human heart with advanced coronary disease (so-called ischemic cardiomyopathy), fibrosis is the major force of LV remodeling. Infarct scars may account for 30 percent of fibrosis, whereas microscopic fibrosis remote from the infarct may account for 70 percent of

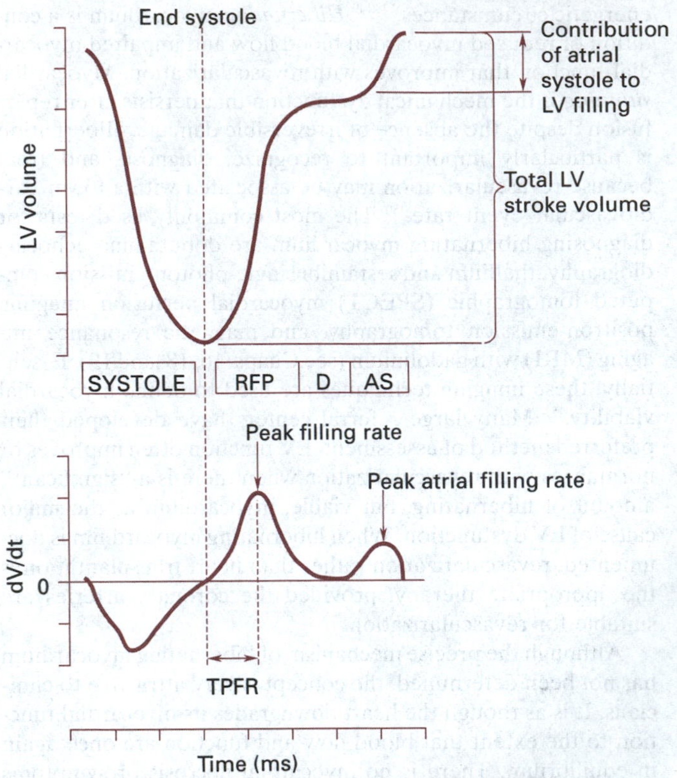

FIGURE 20-7 Idealized plot of left ventricular volume versus time (*top*) and the rate of change of volume (*dV/dt*) versus time (*bottom*), such as might be obtained from contrast or radionuclide ventriculographic studies. The representative cardiac cycle begins at end diastole. Subsequent events as depicted by the bars in the center of the figure are (1) systole, during which left ventricular volume decreases to a minimum and −*dV/dt* reaches its maximum; and (2) diastole, the beginning of which is signaled by the opening of the mitral valve and the onset of left ventricular filling. Diastole has three distinct phases in normal individuals: (1) the rapid filling phase (RFP), during which the left ventricle fills rapidly but passively and the peak filling rate occurs; (2) diastasis (D), during which relatively little left ventricular volume change occurs; and (3) atrial systole (AS), in which active atrial contraction fills the left ventricle to its end-diastolic volume. The diastolic parameters that have been derived from such analysis are the peak filling rate, the time to peak filling rate (TPFR), the percent contribution of atrial systole, and the first third filling fraction. (From Labovitz AJ, Pearson AC. Evaluation of left ventricular diastolic function: Clinical relevance and recent Doppler echocardiographic insights. *Am Heart J* 1987; 114:836–849. Reproduced with permission from the publisher and authors.)

the total fibrous tissue found in the ventricles.[155] In general, interstitial loci of fibrosis are the "tombstones" of lost myocytes. It is likely that increased MMPs contribute to ventricular dilatation in heart failure.[156] Tissue inhibitors of MMPs (TIMPS) exist in the myocardium and are regulated independently of MMPs,[156] an observation with potentially important therapeutic implications. Enhanced protease activity in heart failure contributes to fibrillar collagen degradation, setting the stage for weakened connective tissue and disrupted organ integrity, myocyte slippage, and ventricular remodeling.

The growth of the interstitium in response to pressure and volume overload is highly complex and involves fibroblasts and their ability to sense altered mechanical forces. Hormones, including the renin-angiotensin-aldosterone system[157] and endothelin,[158] also facilitate the production of collagen via their interaction with fibroblasts. Once abnormal loading conditions are removed, connective tissue hypertrophy regresses more slowly than myocyte hypertrophy. It is rather striking how the importance of this once considered inert ground substance has emerged over the past 15 years, previously hidden to investigators largely because it was essentially invisible by the usual techniques of light microscopy. It is now clear that the cardiac interstitium is very important in the syndrome of heart failure and contributes in many ways to the structural and functional alterations.

NONCARDIAC "ADAPTATIONS" IN HEART FAILURE

The Neurohumoral Hypothesis

A large number of neurohormones have been found to circulate in abnormal quantities in heart failure (Table 20-7). The natriuretic peptides [atrial natriuretic peptide (ANP), brain natriuretic peptide (BNP), and clearance natriuretic peptide(CNP)] are considered counterregulatory because they tend to reduce right atrial pressure, systemic vascular resistance, aldosterone secretion, sympathetic nerve stimulation, and hypertrophy of cells and can enhance sodium excretion.[159] The predominant consequence of most neurohormone "release" in heart failure, however, is vasoconstriction coupled with salt and water retention. The regulation of body fluid volume is very complex but has a primitive relation to many of the neurohormones and their propensity to facilitate retention of sodium and water while at the same time protecting perfusion pressure. The integrity of the arterial circulation as a function of cardiac output and SVR is also determined by flexibility in renal sodium and water excretion.[160] Underfilling of the arterial bed by low cardiac output or vasodilation activates neuroendocrine reflexes that stimulate sodium and water retention. Sodium and water retention cease to be major problems after heart transplantation, indicating that there is no intrinsic renal dysfunction in heart failure. The kidney responds to a perceived reduction in arterial filling in an appropriate manner by retaining volume.

Decreases in blood pressure, stroke volume (pulse pressure), and perfusion (flow) in heart failure are sensed by mechanoreceptors in the left ventricle, carotid sinus, aortic arch, and renal afferent arterioles. When there is diminished activation of these receptors, as in heart failure, there is augmentation of sympathetic outflow, activation of the renin-angiotensin-aldosterone system, and nonosmotic release of arginine vasopressin (AVP).[160] Heightened peripheral vasoconstriction occurs along with increased blood volume, thereby "restoring" circulatory integrity and perfusion pressure. Of course, neuroendocrine activation has many important consequences at the cellular level, including facilitation of myocyte hypertrophy[41] and collagen synthesis.[136] Activation of the sympathetic nervous system contributes to tachycardia and arrhythmias and can be directly toxic to the myocardium.[161,162] Cardiac myocyte necrosis also occurs in response to low levels of angiotensin II.[163] Although neuroendocrine responses are not the primary cause of heart failure under most circumstances, they clearly contribute to the pathogenesis of the syndrome[164] (Fig. 20-8). The overly simplistic view that neuro-

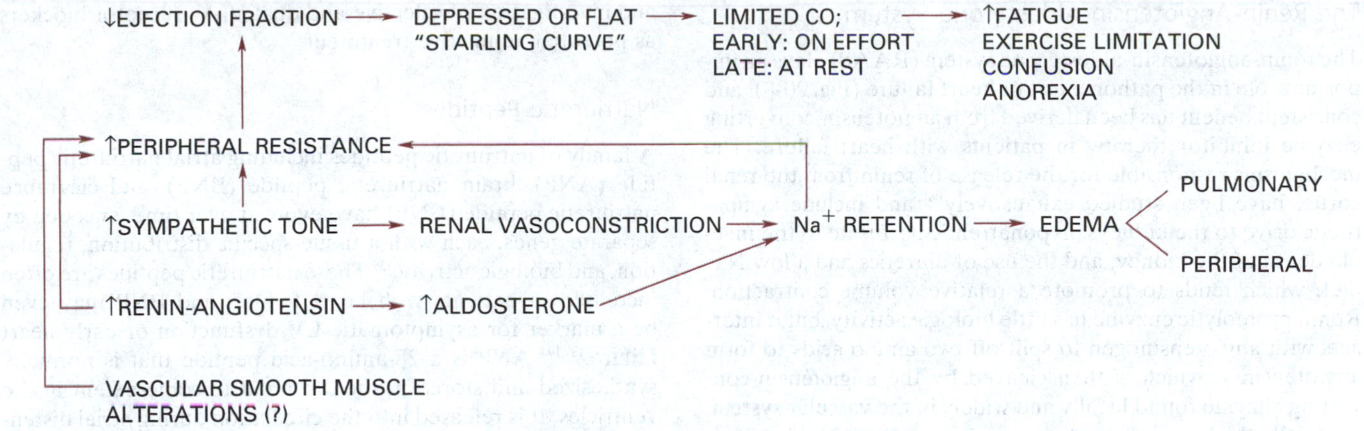

FIGURE 20-8 Schema of events in congestive heart failure leading to symptoms. Note that fatigue and other symptoms of limited cardiac output are primarily related to decreased ejection, whereas peripheral and pulmonary edema are related to Na^+ and water retention from increased sympathetic tone and increased renin-angiotensin-aldosterone. See text for details.

hormones in heart failure are a response to perceived "hypovolemia" is clearly incorrect.[165] Neuroendocrine mechanisms are now the targets of several important and successful therapeutic interventions in heart failure and hypertension[166] and have a key role in determining prognosis.[167] Angiotensin-converting enzyme inhibitors, β-adrenergic blockers, and aldosterone antagonists now have a prominent role in the treatment of heart failure, and new, more innovative neuroendocrine-blocking agents are being developed rapidly, adding strong support to the neurohumoral hypothesis.[164]

Norepinephrine

It has been recognized since the time of Starling that patients with heart failure manifest signs of a hyperadrenergic state. Vascular constriction, tachycardia, diaphoresis, and oliguria are clear signs of increased sympathetic drive. Starling's observations in 1897[168] were amplified in the early 1960s by the group from the National Institutes of Health (NIH), who verified increased plasma norepinephrine (NE) levels in patients with heart failure.[169] Myocardial stores of NE were found to be depleted.[170] Later studies by various investigators using the more sensitive radioenzymatic technique measured plasma NE levels in patients with heart failure and described a correlation with functional class[171] and extent of hemodynamic dysfunction.[172]

NE synthesis begins in the body of the neuron with the synthesis of enzymes necessary to go from tyrosine to NE. The enzymes are transported down the neuron to the dendrites of the cell, where the actual synthetic steps take place. Dopamine is synthesized and transported into storage vesicles, where the final synthetic steps occur. These storage vesicles are both large and small, the large vesicles containing additional peptides such as neuropeptide Y. Following discharge of an axonal action potential, exocytosis occurs, allowing the vesicle contents to be released into the synaptic cleft. The vast majority of the NE is then taken back up into the cell for storage and rerelease (uptake 1). Some NE is taken up by effector organs and metabolized (uptake 2), and only a small quantity is released into the plasma (≈5 percent), where it circulates as plasma NE. There are now microneurographic techniques than can be used to directly measure sympathetic traffic direction[173] and "spillover" techniques that can measure specific organ sympathetic activity.[174] It now seems clear that increased cardiac sympathetic traffic precedes more generalized sympathetic activation in the course of heart failure.[175] However, the plasma NE level has served as a useful research and prognostic guide for the study of patients with heart failure.[176]

It is overly simplistic to consider NE to be "good" or "bad" for patients with heart failure. Those with severe New York Heart Association (NYHA) class IV heart failure may be quite dependent on catecholamine support[177] and often require a continuous dobutamine infusion to maintain suitable organ perfusion prior to heart transplantation. However, there is no question that NE is toxic to the myocardium and is responsible in part for progressive LV remodeling.[178,179] The favorable and detrimental effects of sympathetic drive are depicted in Table 20-8. These observations imply that blocking the sympathetic nervous system effects are most likely to benefit NYHA class I-III patients, whereas such action potentially could worsen the condition of class IV patients who manifest congestion.

TABLE 20-8 Favorable and Detrimental Effects of Sympathetic Drive in Patients with Heart Failure

FAVORABLE	
↑ HR, improved cardiac output ↑ contractility, improved cardiac output maintenance of perfusion pressure	NYHA class IV
DETRIMENTAL	
Progressive LV remodeling LV hypertrophy → failure ↑ myocardial MV_{O_2} arrhythmias ↑ SVR → ↑ afterload Na^+ and H_2O retention, facilitation of renin release, oliguria	NYHA class I-III

The Renin-Angiotensin-Aldosterone System

The renin-angiotensin-aldosterone system (RAAS) plays an important role in the pathogenesis of heart failure (Fig. 20-8), and consistent benefit has been derived from angiotensin-converting enzyme inhibitor therapy in patients with heart failure. The mechanisms responsible for the release of renin from the renal cortex have been studied exhaustively[180] and include sympathetic drive to the kidneys, hyponatremic perfusate to the macula densa of the kidney, and the use of diuretics and a low Na^+ diet, which tends to promote a relative volume contraction. Renin proteolytic enzyme has little biologic activity, but it interacts with angiotensinogen to split off two amino acids to form angiotensin I, which is then cleaved by the angiotensin-converting enzyme found locally and widely in the vascular system, especially the lungs, to produce angiotensin II, a peptide with a vast range of biologic activities. Angiotensin II in turn stimulates release of aldosterone from the adrenal cortex, which also has an array of biologic effects, including Na^+ and H_2O retention and kaliuresis.

There now are at least four recognized angiotensin II (AT) receptors, but much of the activity is subserved by the AT_1 receptor. The AT_1 actions include arterial vasoconstriction, cell growth (hypertrophy), apoptosis in myocytes, polydypsia, NE release, sensitization of blood vessels to NE, AVP release, and aldosterone release. The AT_2 receptor appears to subserve somewhat counterregulatory effects, including antigrowth/antiremodeling, apoptosis in vasculature, vasodilation, and activation of the kinin–nitric oxide–cGMP system.[181] Since AT_1 receptor-blocking drugs (so-called ARBs) increase angiotensin II levels, they may enhance unoccupied AT_2 receptor activity. Angiotensin II levels tend to "escape" the pharmacologic effects of chronic angiotensin-converting enzyme inhibition and may stimulate AT_2 and AT_2 receptor activity. It is also now clear that the RAAS is not solely a classic endocrine system but has autocrine and paracrine activity that may be particularly important in cardiovascular, brain, and renal tissue. With our current knowledge that angiotensin-converting enzyme inhibitors remarkably reduce all cardiovascular events and the onset of new diabetes mellitus in patients with cardiovascular disease, it is difficult to overstate the role of the RAAS in the pathogenesis of heart and vascular disease, including progressive heart failure.[182–184]

Arginine Vasopressin

Patients with heart failure sometimes may have water retention in excess of Na^+ retention, which leads to hyponatremia. The hyponatremia is due in part to nonosmotic release of AVP, which acts on the kidney to reduce clearance of free water.[185] Release of AVP in heart failure probably occurs via activation of carotid baroreceptors.[160] Plasma AVP levels are often but not always increased in patients with LV dysfunction[186] and heart failure.[187] AVP acts on the V_2 receptors in the collecting duct of the kidney via adenylate cyclase to translocate aquaporin-2 water channels from cytoplasmic vesicles to the apical surface of the collecting duct. AVP also increases aquaporin channel-2 synthesis. Activation of V_1 receptors in vascular tissue contributes to heightened vascular resistance and myocardial dysfunction in heart failure.[188] Recognition of the role of AVP in the pathogenesis of heart failure has led to the development and investigation of selective and dual V_1-V_2 receptor blockers as potential adjunctive treatment.

Natriuretic Peptides

A family of natriuretic peptides including atrial natriuretic peptide (ANP), brain natriuretic peptide (BNP), and clearance natriuretic peptide (CNP) have evolved over time, encoded by separate genes, each with a tissue-specific distribution, regulation, and biologic activity.[159] These natriuretic peptides are often increased in patients with heart failure, and BNP may even be a marker for asymptomatic LV dysfunction or early heart failure.[189,190] ANP is a 28-amino-acid peptide that is normally synthesized and stored in the atria and to some extent in the ventricles. It is released into the circulation during atrial distention. BNP is synthesized mainly by the ventricles and is released in LV dysfunction or early heart failure. For the most part, these peptides act via guanylate cyclase receptors to promote vasodilation (ANP, BNP, CNP) and natriuresis (ANP, BNP). They also may attenuate NE release, RAAS activity, and the growth/hypertrophy of target cells—hence the term *counterregulatory hormones*.

Patients with heart failure are relatively resistant to the natriuretic effects of these peptides when they are administered exogenously, perhaps due to decreased Na^+ delivery to the collecting duct as a result of diminished glomerular filtration or increased Na^+ reabsorption in the proximal tubule.[160] Nevertheless, BNP infusion has a remarkable positive hemodynamic effect in patients with heart failure,[191] and drugs designed to inhibit degradation of natriuretic peptides (so-called neutral endopeptidase inhibitors) have been combined with angiotensin-converting enzyme inhibitor activity as potential therapy for hypertension and heart failure. The role of natriuretic peptides as potential therapy continues to evolve.

Endothelin

Endothelins are a family of vasoconstrictor peptides produced by vascular endothelial cells[192,193] whose normal function is as yet unclear. Although blood levels are increased in patients with heart failure,[194,195] endothelin-1 (ET-1) is more of a paracrine than an endocrine hormone. In heart failure, myocardial tissue ET-1 levels are increased, possibly more due to decreased clearance by the lungs than to increased synthesis.[196] Endothelial cells synthesize ET-1 rapidly and convert so-called big endothelin-1 into endothelin by an endothelin-converting enzyme. The synthesis of ET-1 is enhanced by angiotensin II, NE, growth factors, insulin, hypoxia, oxidized low-density lipoproteins (LDLs), shear stress, and thrombin.[193] Its synthesis is antagonized by ANP and prostaglandins.

Endothelin acts on at least two types of G protein-coupled receptors, A and B. The ET-A receptor subserves smooth muscle vasoconstriction and cell proliferation/hypertrophy and mainly resides on vascular smooth muscle cells. The ET-B receptor, which is mainly endothelial, subserves vasodilation that is probably mediated by a variety of mechanisms including increased production of nitric oxide and prostaglandins and activation of potassium channels. ET-1 also can act on the heart to cause hypertrophy, on the adrenal gland to release aldosterone, and on the kidney to promote Na^+ and H_2O retention.[193] The importance of ET-1 in the pathogenesis of heart failure is highlighted by the development and clinical testing of several new endothelin antagonists.[197] Endothelin-blocking agents are believed to hold promising vasodilator, natriuretic, and antiremodeling effects.

Additional Neurohormones

Many other neurohormones are believed to be important in the pathogenesis of heart failure, including neuropeptide Y, vasointestinal peptide, bradykinin, prostaglandins, adrenomedullin, and urodilatin. As we grow to better understand heart failure, some of them may emerge as "systems" to block or enhance, depending on their primary function.

Cytokines

In 1990 it was reported by Levine et al.[198] that circulating tumor necrosis factor alpha (TNF-α), a proinflammatory cytokine, was increased in cachectic patients with chronic heart failure. Since then, a large body of work has emerged indicating that proinflammatory cytokines such as TNF-α may play a fundamentally important role in modulating abnormal myocardial structure and function in late stages of heart failure.[199–201] This group of proinflammatory cytokines also includes interleukin 1 (IL-1) and interleukin 6 (IL-6). These proteins, largely products of macrophages and lymphocytes, are also expressed under some circumstances by myocardial tissue. Each of these cytokines can influence the expression of the other two, and each can modulate cardiovascular performance when expressed at sufficiently high levels. Experimentally, a continuous infusion of TNF-α leads to time-dependent depression in LV function[202] and provokes a hypertrophic growth response in adult cardiac myocytes.[203] When there are large quantities being produced, TNF-α spills over into the circulation and acts as an endocrine "hormone" leading to metabolic wasting and cachexia.[204,205] Overexpression of TNF-α in a transgenic mouse model leads to a phenotype consistent with cardiomyopathy.[206] TNF-α acts via two different membrane receptors. The transduction signal pathways are not fully understood, but in the heart they may mediate cell growth, negative inotropy, and apoptosis. The emergence of these important observations has lead to the launching of a clinical trial with etanercept (a fusion molecule that binds circulating TNF-α) for the treatment of patients with late-stage heart failure.

Renal Retention of Salt and Water

Since its earliest clinical descriptions, a hallmark of heart failure has been renal retention of Na^+ and H_2O, resulting in signs and symptoms of fluid retention. The precise mechanism whereby the heart signals the kidney in the early stages of heart failure to retain Na^+ and H_2O is still unknown, although in the late stages reduced cardiac output and impaired renal blood flow likely play a major role. In early heart failure, when normal cardiac output is maintained via compensatory mechanisms and renal blood flow is not reduced, there is still some Na^+ retention. Curiously, some patients with advanced heart failure rarely demonstrate peripheral edema or ascites. This suggests that in some cases counterregulatory natriuretic peptides may be acting to maintain natriuresis. Perhaps release of ANP and BNP in the early stages of heart failure offsets the tendency to retain Na^+, thereby maintaining Na^+ balance. Salt and water retention usually becomes evident in the syndrome of heart failure as adequate perfusion and protection of blood pressure become more imperative.[207] The RAAS is dominant in this regard.[208] Angiotensin II preserves glomerular filtration rate in patients with heart failure even when renal perfusion is severely compromised, and this effect is achieved independently of this hormonal system's propensity to support systemic blood pressure.[209] Intraglomerular hydraulic pressure and therefore glomerular filtration are preserved by the constriction of glomerular efferent arterioles via angiotensin II.[210] Increased intrarenal formation of angiotensin II during a reduction in renal artery pressure maintains efferent arteriolar tone and, consequently, the effective filtration pressure.[211] The resulting high level of filtration fraction favors changes in the postglomerular circulation that promote avid proximal fluid reabsorption via elevated peritubular capillary oncotic pressure.[212] Increased aldosterone acts principally on the cortical collecting tubules to conserve Na^+. Because the plasma volume and blood pressure vary considerably from day to day, there is no consistent relation between the RAAS and fluid retention.

The mechanisms of Na^+ and H_2O retention in heart failure are complex and determined by multiple other factors. Sympathetic nervous system traffic to the kidney favors sodium retention. Increased AVP activity diminishes free water clearance. The prostaglandins normally dilate afferent glomerular arterioles to enhance intraglomerular flow and pressure, and their inhibition by nonsteroidal anti-inflammatory agents may lead to a marked reduction in filtration and sodium retention. Enhanced Na^+ reabsorption of heart failure also occurs in the ascending loop of Henle, as well as in the cortical and medullary collecting ducts. Eventually, the "goal" of plasma volume expansion is met, but at the expense of circulatory and tissue congestion.

Endothelial Dysfunction, Nitric Oxide, Exercise Intolerance, and Sleep Disorders

Data from many animal and human studies indicate that endothelium-dependent vasodilation is abnormal in a number of disease states, including atherosclerosis, hypertension, heart failure, hyperhomocysteinemia, insulin resistance, and hypercholesterolemia. Treasure et al.[213] observed abnormal endothelial-dependent dilatation of the coronary arteries in patients with dilated cardiomyopathy. Peripheral resistance vessels in both experimental animals[214] and patients with heart failure[215] demonstrate endothelial dysfunction. Data collected to date would suggest that the endothelial dysfunction in heart failure (i.e., failure to vasodilate in response to a specific endothelial-dependent vasodilator) may be due to a reduced release of nitric oxide during stimulation.[216] The basal release of nitric oxide may be preserved or even enhanced in heart failure[217] and may be compensatory by antagonizing neuroendocrine vasoconstrictor forces. However, impairment of endothelium-dependent peripheral vasodilation may be a factor contributing to exercise intolerance in patients with chronic heart failure, perhaps by limiting nutritive skeletal muscle flow during exercise.[218] This dysfunction of the endothelium may be related to deconditioning in later stages of heart failure, and with training, it is largely reversible. Further, abnormal endothelium-dependent responses in heart failure are reversible following heart transplantation.[219]

The roles of nitric oxide and nitric oxide synthase in the failing heart are much more complex.[220,221] Nitric oxide inhibits the positive inotropic response to β-adrenergic stimulation in the failing heart. While smaller physiologic amounts of constitutive nitric oxide (cNOS) are necessary for normal function and have an antioxidant effect to protect cells, high levels of nitric oxide in the heart may exert proapoptotic and cytotoxic effects. The inducible isoform of nitric oxide synthase (iNOS) is overexpressed in human heart failure[222] and therefore may contribute to worsening heart failure. On the other hand, there is decreased myocardial nitric oxide synthesis during decompensation of experimental heart failure.[223] The relative roles of nitric oxide also may differ at different stages in the evolution of heart failure.

In addition to a reduced myocardial force-frequency response, inability to fully use the Starling effect, chronotropic incompetence and diminished myocardial β-receptor density, endothelial dysfunction, reduced nutritive blood flow, and disuse atrophy of skeletal muscles limits exercise tolerance in patients with heart failure. The latter effects appear to be excessively dependent on a glycolytic metabolism,[224] in part due to reduced metabolic efficiency in performing external work. Possible mechanisms include changes in muscle fiber recruitment, selective atrophy of oxidative fibers, and physical deconditioning. The mitochondrial content of skeletal muscle is reduced[225] in heart failure. Increased expression of the inducible isoform of nitric oxide synthase in skeletal muscle is correlated with reduced mitochondrial creatine kinase expression and exercise intolerance.[226] Apoptosis is frequently found in skeletal muscle of patients with heart failure and is associated with exercise impairment.[227] Exercise capacity and EF are very poorly correlated in heart failure, suggesting that impairment in nutritive blood flow is not the dominant reason for exercise intolerance.

Pulmonary dysfunction is common in patients with heart failure and also may contribute to exercise intolerance. The amount of intrathoracic space available for ventilation may be decreased by alveolar and interstitial edema, by pleural effusions, or by an increase in blood volume. Increased pulmonary vascular congestion decreases lung compliance and increases the work of breathing. Excessive ventilation during exercise is a hallmark of heart failure. Acute reduction in pulmonary capillary wedge pressure has no effect on the augmented ventilatory response, and the extent of excessive ventilation does not relate to either resting or exercise pulmonary capillary wedge pressure.

The potential mechanisms resonsible for exercise intolerance, a uniform feature of heart failure, are numerous (Table 20-9). Exercise intolerance is clearly multifactorial and is a potent prognostic indicator used the to help determine the optimal timing of heart transplantation (e.g., $\dot{V}_{O_{2,max}}$ of less than 50 percent predicted for size and age). Exertional symptoms generally correlate with maximal exercise capacity,[228] although exertional symptoms frequently underestimate the severity of functional disability. Although EF does not correlate with exercise performance ($\dot{V}_{O_2}$ if the latter is markedly reduced (e.g., ($\dot{V}_{O_2}$ <12 mL/kg/min) along with a low EF, the prognosis is especially grave. Cardiopulmonary exercise testing should be done in patients with heart failure to assess functional capacity. Importantly, exercise tolerance can improve with training, which should be encouraged in patients with classes I to III heart failure symptoms.

TABLE 20-9 Mechanisms of Exercise Intolerance in Heart Failure

Inability of endothelium to respond to vasodilator stimulus
Reduced nutritive blood flow to skeletal muscle
Inability to increase stroke volume in response to exercise
Chronotropic incompetence
Reduced myocardial force-frequency response
Diminished myocardial β-adrenergic receptor density
Skeletal muscle atrophy
Shift from slow- to fast-twitch fiber types
Atrophy of fast-twitch type II fibers
Reduced level of skeletal muscle mitochondrial enzymes
Reduced skeletal muscle mitochondrial size
Increased skeletal muscle apoptosis
Reduced lung compliance
Excessive ventilatory response to exercise
Generalized deconditioning

Periodic breathing (Cheyne-Stokes) is common in patients with heart failure. It can be caused by lung edema, which can excite carbon dioxide responses through vagal reflexes. Enhanced sensitivity to carbon dioxide may predispose some patients with heart failure to the development of central sleep apnea.[229] Cheyne-Stokes respiration in heart failure is associated with a poor prognosis.[230] Successful treatment of Cheyne-Stokes respiration with nocturnal nasal oxygen improves sleep, exercise tolerance, and cognitive function in patients with heart failure.[231] Severe untreated sleep-disordered breathing can further impair LV function, leading to arterial oxyhemoglobin desaturation and arrhythmias.[232] Central sleep apnea may occur in as many as 40 percent of patients with heart failure, and 10 percent suffer from obstructive sleep apnea.[233] Obstructive sleep apnea increases afterload and heart rate during sleep but is responsive to continuous positive airway pressure.[234]

DIAGNOSIS AND EVALUATION OF PATIENTS WITH HEART FAILURE

History

The dominant and most recognizable symptom of congestive heart failure is "shortness of breath." The clinical term for this shortness of breath is *dyspnea,* and it is described by patients as the sensation of being unable to get enough air with each inspiration. Frequently, dyspnea is first noted by the patient on exertion and often dismissed by the patient as part of aging. As the heart failure progresses, the sensation of dyspnea occurs with less and less exertion, until the patient experiences symptoms at rest.

Despite all the advances in the field of cardiology, the mechanism of dyspnea remains poorly understood. When patients develop acute heart failure, they are often hypoxemic secondary to pulmonary edema and a resulting decrease in oxygen diffusing capacity. Patients with chronic stable heart failure, even if clinically compensated, still experience dyspnea, despite a lack of overt pulmonary edema. The explanation for the dyspnea in this latter group of patients is likely multifactorial, including increased physiologic dead space, increased airway resistance, reduced lung compliance, and fatigue of the respiratory muscles. Additionally, there may be some as yet undefined signals from the pulmonary J-receptors and respiratory muscles that contribute centrally to the sensation of dyspnea.[235,236]

The classic respiratory symptom triad of heart failure includes dyspnea, orthopnea and paroxysmal nocturnal dyspnea (PND). Orthopnea is the sensation of shortness of breath in the supine position. Patients may describe the need for more pillows under their head to sleep or even needing to prop the head of the bed up. PND relates to sudden, nocturnal dyspnea, often awakening the patient from sleep and requiring the patient to sit or stand up and ambulate to improve breathing. Onset of these symptoms indicates progression of the underlying heart failure and may culminate in a Cheyne-Stokes respiratory pattern.

The other typical complaint of patients with heart failure is fatigue. Since everyone feels fatigued at some time, this a vague, subjective complaint that does not easily lend itself to measurement. Often, the interviewer must inquire about specific tasks or ask the patient to provide examples of how the fatigue occurs. The patient often will describe being physically exhausted by activities that presented no difficulty weeks or months prior to the interview. Some may be able to separate fatigue from dyspnea, but the two complaints frequently coexist. Like dyspnea, the underlying mechanism of fatigue remains unclear. It is likely multifactorial and may be in part due to a reduced cardiac output with resulting poor tissue perfusion, excessive activity of the neuroendocrine system, elevated cytokine levels, or deconditioning of skeletal muscles.

Wheezing and cough are additional common complaints of patients with heart failure. Symptoms of circulatory and organ congestion also can occur and include nausea, vomiting, and discomfort from hepatic and bowel edema. Right upper quadrant abdominal pain can be severe in acute heart failure and is due to distention of the hepatic capsule. Peripheral edema is also a frequent complaint of patients with heart failure, though, curiously, some patients never manifest it. Along with dyspnea, ankle swelling is a common early symptom that often brings the patient for treatment. This is generally more prominent at day's end; with sleeping, fluid reabsorption with redistribution into the chest may lead to orthopnea.

The initial evaluation of the patient suspected of having heart failure should include a thorough past medical history and review of systems. This can be beneficial in defining the etiology of the patient's cardiac dysfunction. Since ischemic heart disease is the most frequent cause of heart failure in the United States, coronary risk factors such as diabetes mellitus, hypertension, cigarette smoking, hyperlipidemia, and family history need to be assessed and vigorously treated. Poorly controlled hypertension can cause heart failure that is unrelated to coronary artery disease. Relatively mild hypertension in the diabetic may result in a specific cardiomyopathy. Excessive alcohol or illicit drug use also can lead to cardiomyopathy. A comprehensive list of cardiomyopathies, though far from exhaustive, is found in Table 20-10. Dietary needs and therapeutic compliance need to be assessed in all patients. They must know that excessive salt intake can lead to diuretic resistance and acute decompensation. Patient education regarding signs, symptoms, treatment, and prognosis is critical for the well-being of the patient. End-of-life wishes regarding resuscitation and intubation also should be discussed at a time when the patient is stable and can participate in meaningful dialogue.

TABLE 20-10 Classification of Cardiomyopathies

Dilated cardiomyopathy (idiopathic)
Hypertrophic, cardiomyopathy
Restrictive cardiomyopathy
Arrhythmogenic right ventricular cardiomyopathy
Unclassified cardiomyopathy
Ischemic cardiomyopathy
Valvular cardiomyopathy
Hypertensive cardiomyopathy
Inflammatory cardiomyopathy
Metabolic cardiomyopathy
Infiltrative cardiomyopathy
Muscular dystrophy–associated cardiomyopathy
Neuromuscular disorder–associated cardiomyopathy
Toxic cardiomyopathy
Peripartum cardiomyopathy

SOURCE: Adapted from Richardson P, McKenna W, Bristow M, et al. Report of the 1995 World Health Organization/International Society and Federation of Cardiology Task Force on the Definition and Classification of Cardiomyopathies *Circulation* 1996; 93:841–842.

Physical Examination

The physical examination in heart failure is not relegated solely to the cardiovascular examination. A complete examination is necessary because peripheral findings can provide additional insight into the extent and chronicity of the disease process. The patient's overall appearance can be very enlightening. A generalized wasting with skeletal muscle loss, referred to as *cardiac cachexia,* is usually indicative of severe and late-stage heart failure.

A complete cardiovascular examination encompasses both peripheral and cardiac findings (see Chap. 10). On palpation of the heart, the point of maximal impulse is often laterally displaced and diffuse. An LV heave often can be appreciated, as can a right ventricular heave if the pulmonary artery pressures are elevated or if right-sided heart failure has begun. In the case of severe valvular aortic stenosis, a palpable thrill, LV heave, and radiation of the murmur into the carotids is often present. On cardiac auscultation of the apex, an S_3 gallop rhythm is indicative of decompensated heart failure. An S_4 gallop in a patient with coronary artery disease, hypertension, or aortic valve stenosis makes the examiner consider a stiff ventricle due to cardiac hypertrophy. A pericardial knock can be found in constrictive pericarditis, an unusual cause of circulatory congestion. The systolic murmur of mitral regurgitation can be found in either primary (organic valve disease) or secondary (due to LV dilatation) mitral valve incompetence. Severe mitral regurgitation can occur with no or little audible murmur. Additionally, the murmurs of aortic stenosis, aortic insufficiency, tricuspid regurgitation, and less commonly, a ventricular septal defect can provide further evidence of the etiology and extent of CHF.

A loud P_2 (i.e., audible at the apex of the heart) can indicate elevated pulmonary artery pressures in either the acute or chronic setting.

The vascular examination provides important information. An increased resting heart rate is common. An new irregular pulse in a previously compensated patient can implicate new-onset atrial fibrillation as the source of an unexplained decompensation. Bilateral carotid "bruits" radiating from the heart with a decreased and delayed (*parvus et tardus*) pulse can indicate severe aortic stenosis. However, in the absence of the bruit and any aortic stenosis murmur, a decreased pulse waveform may indicate a poor stroke volume and therefore low cardiac output. This is also usually reflected by a narrow pulse pressure. Poor capillary refill and cool extremities can indicate a severely restricted cardiac output. An elevated jugular venous pressure is an indicator of high right-sided pressure and volume overload. Careful examination of the jugular venous pressure is most useful when determining diuretic dosage. A prominent *v* wave can be seen in severe tricuspid regurgitation, which is often accompanied by a pulsatile liver. Pedal edema is often observed in heart failure, and scaly, discolored, and ulcerated lower legs denote a chronic edematous state (*stasis dermatitis and ulceration*).

The pulmonary examination can be relatively normal in chronic compensated heart failure. However, rales due to alveolar fluid accumulation accompanied by hypoxemia often are found in acute or decompensated heart failure. Decreased breath sounds at the bases and dullness to percussion are found with pleural effusions. On occasion, wheezing rather than rales will be heard, which is termed *cardiac asthma*.

Diagnostic Studies

Routine blood work sometimes can provide some insight into the etiology of heart failure and the extent of decompensation. Noncardiac factors may increase failure or make it initially evident. Fever or anemia may help to explain decompensation in a previously stable patient with severe coronary disease. A low serum sodium level (hyponatremia) often is observed in patients with advanced heart failure and can be a poor prognostic sign. Prerenal azotemia is found in patients with poor cardiac output and resulting renal hypoperfusion, whereas a rise in the creatinine level may indicate renal dysfunction that can be primary or secondary to heart failure. Other laboratory values of import are noted in Table 20-11.

The standard 12-lead electrocardiogram should be part of the routine evaluation. Pathologic Q waves can indicate previous myocardial infarction. Evidence of LV hypertrophy can be found in patients with aortic stenosis or chronic systemic hypertension. New atrial fibrillation in a patient with previously compensated heart failure may explain recent decompensation. The chest x-ray also provides information beyond radiographic pulmonary edema and pleural effusions. An enlarged cardiac silhouette is usually found in dilated cardiomyopathy or can be due to a large pericardial effusion. Taking note of the various chambers can provide insight into valvular involvement and can indicate the presence of right-sided heart failure.

The echocardiogram is the most important imaging tool for evaluating patients with symptoms of heart failure. The overall systolic function and chamber size can be evaluated quickly. Global LV dysfunction can be differentiated from the regional abnormalities more commonly found in ischemic cardiomyopathy. Valvular stenosis and incompetence can be defined and graded. Furthermore, mitral regurgitation can be evaluated to determine if it is a primary valvular problem or secondary to the LV dilatation and related to LV chamber enlargement. This information may provide insight into the potential benefit of mitral valve repair or replacement, as well as the type of surgical technique required. Importantly, diastolic function of the heart can be evaluated by echocardiography. Abnormalities of diastolic function are a component of all cardiomyopathies but are particularly important in patients with normal *systolic* function. Finally, dobutamine stress echocardiography can help to define ischemic and hibernating myocardium, which may be necessary when considering coronary revascularization. The use of coronary angiography in patients with heart failure, however, is still somewhat controversial. It should be strongly considered when there is angina.

Radionuclide imaging is sometimes preferred when evaluating patients with heart failure. It is perhaps more quantitative than echocardiography. Additionally, positron-emission tomographic (PET) scanning is useful in distinguishing nonviable myocardial scar from dysfunctional but viable myocardium (Table 20-12) when considering coronary revascularization.

METABOLIC EXERCISE TESTING

The addition of gas-exchange measurements to exercise stress testing creates a noninvasive test that provides a wealth of information and can be performed safely in a symptom-limited fashion in patients with heart failure.[235] In addition to the evaluation of potential ischemia and objective assessment of functional capacity, the patient's maximal oxygen consumption at peak exercise ($\dot{V}_{O_{2,max}}$) and anaerobic threshold can be evaluated.[236-239] As an initial evaluation, metabolic exercise testing can provide insight into the patient's functional disability and allow the physician to council the individual patient on physical limitations and rehabilitation. When a patient's maximal oxygen consumption is less than 50 percent of expected for age and body size and/or if the $\dot{V}_{O_{2,max}}$ is below 14 mL/kg per minute, the patient may be a candidate for heart transplant evaluation.[240,241]

CARDIAC CATHETERIZATION

Swan-Ganz (right-sided heart) catheterization is performed frequently in patients with heart failure. Even so, its use in this patient population remains a point of contention among experts in the field. In general, the diagnosis of heart failure can be made on physical examination. Prognosis also can be estimated reasonably by noninvasive means.[242] The major benefit of right-sided heart catheterization (RHC) resides in the ability of the physician to demonstrate hemodynamic changes in response to pharmacologic treatment. The primary use of RHC should be in patients with worsening heart failure requiring intravenous agents in an intensive care unit setting. Sometimes it is necessary to use RHC when LV filling pressure is uncertain and the patient is clearly deteriorating.

The need for coronary angiography in patients with heart failure is controversial. It should be strongly considered if angina is present. In a country where ischemic heart disease is rampant and post-myocardial infarction patients are surviving more frequently to develop ischemic cardiomyopathy, diagnostic coronary angiography is performed frequently. It may not be possible to distinguish clinically ischemic cardiomyopathy from

TABLE 20-11 Recommended Tests for Patients with Signs or Symptoms of Heart Failure

Test Recommendation	Findings	Suspected Diagnosis
Electrocardiogram	Acute ST-T-wave changes	Myocardial ischemia
	Atrial fibrillation, other tachyarrhythmia	Thyroid disease or heart failure due to rapid ventricular rate
	Bradyarrhythmias rate	Heart failure due to low heart
	Previous myocardial infarction (e.g., Q waves), left ventricular performance	Heart failure due to reduced contractile tissue
	Low voltage	Pericardial effusion
	Left ventricular hypertrophy	Diastolic dysfunction
Complete blood count	Anemia	Heart failure due to or aggravated by decreased oxygen-carrying capacity
Urinalysis	Proteinuria	Nephrotic syndrome
	Red blood cells or cellular casts	Glomerulonephritis
Serum creatinine	Elevated in renal failure	Volume overload due to renal dysfunction
Serum albumin	Decreased	Increased extravascular volume due to hypoalbuminemia
T_4 and TSH (obtain only if atrial fibrillation, evidence of thyroid disease, or patient age >65)	Abnormal T_4 or TSH	Heart failure due to or aggravated by hypo/hyperthyroidism

SOURCE: From Konstam M, Dracup K, Baker D, et al. *Heart Failure: Management of Patients with Left-Ventricular Systolic Dysfunction. Quick Reference Guide for Clinicians No. 11.* AHCPR Publication No. 94-0613. Rockville, MD: Agency for Health Care Policy and Research, Public Health Service, U.S. Department of Human Services; June 1994.

nonischemic dilated cardiomyopathy. The prognosis of patients with heart failure is worse when there is underlying coronary artery disease and is related to the extent of coronary artery disease.[243]

CONCLUSIONS

Heart failure is a complex clinical syndrome that is growing in magnitude as the population ages. It is difficult to define but relatively straightforward to diagnose. Heart failure implies underlying structural and functional changes in the heart that contribute importantly to the clinical syndrome. Although the molecular underpinnings of heart failure are still incompletely understood, the importance of pathophysiologic principles such as reduced preload reserve and enhanced sensitivity to afterload is now well recognized. Neuroendocrine and inflammatory responses are common in patients with heart failure and serve as important therapeutic targets. There is no single cause or unifying mechanism of heart failure. There can be a diversity of signs and symptoms, most of which can be evaluated at the bedside.

TABLE 20-12 Echocardiography and Radionuclide Ventriculography Compared in Evaluation of Left Ventricular Performance

Test	Advantages	Disadvantages
Echocardiogram	Permits concomitant assessment of valvular disease, left ventricular hypertrophy, and left atrial size	Difficult to perform in patients with lung disease
	Less expensive than radionuclide ventriculography in most areas	Usually only semiquantitative estimate of ejection fraction provided
	Able to detect pericardial effusion and ventricular thrombus	Technically inadequate in up to 18% of patients under optimal circumstances
	More generally available	
Radionuclide ventriculogram	More precise and reliable measurement of EF	Requires venipuncture and radiation exposure
	Better assessment of right ventricular function	Limited assessment of valvular heart disease and left ventricular hypertrophy

SOURCE: From Konstam M, Dracup K, Baker D, et al. *Heart Failure: Management of Patients with Left-Ventricular Systolic Dysfunction. Quick Reference Guide for Clinicians No. 11.* AHCPR Publication No. 94-0613. Rockville, MD: Agency for Health Care Policy and Research, Public Health Service, U.S. Department of Health and Human Services; June 1994.

The echocardiogram in conjunction with a careful history and physical examination remains the primary diagnostic test. Ancillary evaluation includes use of the chest x-ray, electrocardiogram, exercise test, and in some cases, cardiac catheterization with coronary angiography.

References

1. Harris P. The problem of defining heart failure. *Cardiovasc Drugs Ther* 1994; 8:447–452.
2. Eichna LW. The George E. Brown memorial lecture: Circulatory congestion and heart failure. *Circulation* 1960; 22:864–886.
3. Stevenson LW, Perloff JK. The limited reliability of physical signs for estimating hemodynamics in chronic heart failure. *JAMA* 1989; 261:884–888.
4. Badgett RG, Lucey CR, Mulrow CD. Can the clinical examination diagnose left-sided heart failure in adults? *JAMA* 1997; 277:1712–1719.
5. Cowie MR, Mosterd A, Wood DA, et al. The epidemiology of heart failure. *Eur Heart J* 1997; 18:208–225.
6. Ho KKL, Anderson KM, Kannel WB, et al. Survival after the onset of congestive heart failure in Framingham heart study objects. *Circulation* 1993; 88:107–115.
7. Vasan RS, Benjamin EJ, Levy D. Prevalence, clinical features and prognosis of diastolic heart failure: An epidemiologic perspective. *J Am Coll Cardiol* 1995; 26(7):1565–1574.
8. Vasan RS, Benjamin EJ, Levy D. Congestive heart failure with normal left ventricular systolic function. *Arch Intern Med* 1996; 156:146–157.
9. Bonow RO, Udelson JE. Left ventricular diastolic dysfunction as a cause of congestive heart failure. *Ann Intern Med* 1992; 117:502–510.
10. Kunis R, Greenberg H, Yeoh CB, et al. Coronary revascularization for recurrent pulmonary edema in elderly patients with ischemic heart disease and preserved ventricular function. *N Engl J Med* 1985; 313:1207–1210.
11. Eichorn EJ, Willard JE, Alvarez L, et al. Are contraction and relaxation coupled in patients with and without congestive heart failure? *Circulation* 1992; 85:2132–2139.
12. Rihal CS, Nishimura RA, Hatle LK, et al. Systolic and diastolic dysfunction in patients with clinical diagnosis of dilated cardiomyopathy. *Circulation* 1994; 90:2772–2779.
13. Cohen GI, Bietrolungo JF, Thomas JD, Klein AL. A practical guide to assessment of ventricular diastolic function using Doppler echocardiograph *J. Am Coll Cardiol* 1996; 27:1753–1760.
14. Nishimura RA, Tajik AJ. Evaluation of diastolic filling of left ventricle in health and disease: Doppler echocardiography is the clinician's Rosetta stone. *J Am Coll Cardiol* 1997; 30:8–18.
15. Douglas PS. Diastolic dysfunction: Old dog, new tricks. *Am Heart J* 1999; 137:777–778.
16. Lindenfeld J, Krause-Steinrauf H, Salerno J. Where are all the women with heart failure? *J Am Coll Cardiol* 1997; 30:1417–1419.
17. Cohn JN, Johnson G. Heart failure with normal ejection fraction. *Circulation* 1990; 81(suppl III):III-48–III-53.
18. Vasan RS, Larson MG, Benjamin EJ, et al. Congestive heart failure in subjects with normal versus reduced left ventricular ejection fraction. *J Am Coll Cardiol* 1999; 33:1948–1955.
19. MacDowell P, Kalra PA, O'Donoghue DJ, et al. Risk of morbidity from renovascular disease in elderly patients with congestive cardiac failure. *Lancet* 1998; 352:13–16.
20. Mestroni L, Rocco C, Gregori D, et al. Familial dilated cardiomyopathy: Evidence for genetic and phenotypic heterogeneity. *J Am Coll Cardiol* 1999; 34:181–190.
21. Valentine HA, Hunt SA, Fowler MB, et al. Frequency of familial nature of dilated cardiomyopathy and usefulness of cardiac transplantation in this subset. *Am J Cardiol* 1989; 63:959–963.
22. Baig MK, Goldman JH, Caforio AL, et al. Familial dilated cardiomyopathy: Cardiac abnormalities are common in asymptomatic relatives and may represent early disease. *J Am Coll Cardiol* 1998; 31:195–201.
23. Grjnig E, Tasman JA, Kjcherer H, et al. Frequency and phenotypes of familial dilated cardiomyopathy. *J Am Coll Cardiol* 1998; 31:186–194.
24. Olson TM, Keating MT. Defining the molecular genetic basis of idiopathic dilated cardiomyopathy. *Trends Cardiovasc Med* 1997; 7:60–63.
25. Mason JW, O'Connell JB, Herkowitz A, et al. A clinical trial of immunosuppressive therapy for myocarditis. *N Engl J Med* 1995; 333:269–275.
26. Grogan M, Redfield MM, Bailey KR, et al. Long-term outcome of patients with biopsy-proved myocarditis: Comparison with idiopathic dilated cardiomyopathy. *J Am Coll Cardiol* 1995; 26:80–84.
27. Cooper LT, Berry GJ, Shabetal R. Idiopathic giant-cell myocarditis: Natural history and treatment. *N Engl J Med* 1997; 336:1860–1866.
28. Singal PK, Iliskovic N. Doxorubicin-induced cardiomyopathy. *N Engl J Med* 1998; 339:900–906.
29. Shan K, Lincoff AM, Young JB. Anthracycline-induced cardiotoxicity. *Ann Intern Med* 1996; 125:47–58.
30. Singal PK, Iliskovic N, Li T, Kuman D. Adriamycin cardiomyopathy: Pathophysiology and prevention. *FASEB J* 1997; 11:931–936.
31. Feenstra J, Grobbee DE, Remme WJ, Stricker BH. Drug-induced heart failure. *J Am Coll Cardiol* 1999; 33:1152–1162.
32. Skelton CL, Sonnenblick EH. Heterogeneity of contractile function in cardiac hypertrophy. *Circ Res* 1974; 35(suppl 2):83–96.
33. Katz AM. Cardiomyopathy of overload: A major determinant of prognosis in congestive heart failure. *N Engl J Med* 1990; 322:100–110.
34. Katz AM. Cardiomyopathy of overload: An unnatural growth response in the hypertrophied heart. *Ann Intern Med* 1994; 121:363–371.
35. Anand IS, Chandrashekhar Y, Ferrari R, et al. Pathogenesis of oedema in chronic severe anaemia: Studies of body water and sodium, renal function, hemodynamic variables, and plasma hormones. *Br Heart J* 1993; 70:357–362.
36. Harris P. Evolution of the cardiac patient. *Cardiovasc Res* 1983; 17(6–8):313–319, 373–378, 437–445.
37. Kajstura J, Leri A, Finato N, et al. Myocyte proliferation in end-stage cardiac failure in humans. *Proc Natl Acad Sci USA* 1998; 95:8801–8805.
38. Anversa P, Kajstura, J. Ventricular myocytes are not terminally differentiated in the adult mammalian heart. *Circ Res* 1998; 83:1–14.
39. Linzbach AJ. Heart failure from the point of view of quantitative anatomy. *Am J Cardiol* 1960; 5:370–382.
40. Gerdes AM, Kellerman SE, Moore JA, et al. Structural remodeling of cardiac myocytes in patients with ischemic cardiomyopathy. *Circulation* 1992; 86:426–430.
41. Hunter JJ, Chien KR. Signaling pathways for cardiac hypertrophy and failure. *N Engl J Med* 1999; 341(17):1276–1283.
42. Lorell BH. Transition from hypertrophy to failure. *Circulation* 1997; 96:3824–3827.
43. Harris P. Congestive cardiac failure: Central role of the arterial blood pressure. *Br Heart J* 1987; 58:190–203.
44. DeBold AJ. Atrial natriuretic factor: A hormone produced by the heart. *Science* 1985; 20:767–770.
45. Francis GS. Changing the remodeling process in heart failure: Basic mechanisms and laboratory results. *Curr Opin Cardiol* 1998; 13(3):156–161.
46. Swynghedauw B. Molecular mechanisms of myocardial remodeling. *Physiol Reviews* 1999; 79(1):215–262.
47. Onodera T, Tamura T, Said S, et al. Maladaptive remodeling of

cardiac myocyte shape begins long before failure in hypertension. *Hypertension* 1998; 32:753–575.
48. Francis GS, McDonald KM. Left ventricular hypertrophy: An initial response to myocardial injury. *Am J Cardiol* 1992; 69:3G–9G.
49. Francis GS, McDonald KM, Cohn JN. Neurohumoral activation in preclinical heart failure. *Circulation* 1993; 87(5):IV90–IV96.
50. Francis GS, Carlyle WC. Hypothetical pathways of cardiac myocyte hypertrophy response to myocardial injury. *Eur Heart J* 1993; 14(suppl):49–56.
51. Gerdes AM, Onedera T, Wang X, McCune SA. Myocyte remodeling during the progression to failure in rats with hypertension. *Hypertension* 1996; 28(4):609–614.
52. Tamura T, Onodera T, Said S, Gerdes MA. Correlation of myocyte lengthening to chamber dilation in the spontaneously hypertensive heart failure (SHHF) rat. *J Mol Cell Cardiol* 1998; 30:2175–2181.
53. Wang X, Li F, Geres AM. Chronic pressure overload cardiac hypertrophy and failure in guinea pigs: I. Regional hemodynamics and myocyte remodeling. *J Mol Cell Cardiol* 1999; 31:307–317.
54. Liu Z, Hilbelink DR, Crockett WB, Gerdes AM. Regional changes in hemodynamics and cardiac myocyte size in rats with aortocaval fistulas. *Circulation* 1991; 69:52–58.
55. Anversa P, Loud AV, Levicky V, Guideri G. Left ventricular failure induced by myocardial infarction. *Am J Physiol* 1985; 248(17):H883–H889.
56. Anversa P, Li P, Zhang X, et al. Ischaemic myocardial injury and ventricular remodelling. *Cardiovasc Res* 1993; 27:145–157.
57. Olivetti G, Abbi R, Quaini F, et al. Apoptosis in the failing human heart. *N Engl J Med* 1997; 336:1131–1141.
58. Williams RS. Apoptosis and heart failure. *N Engl J Med* 1999; 341(10):759–760.
59. Olivetti G, Capasso JM, Sonnenblick EH, Anversa P. Side-to-side slippage of myocytes participates in ventricular wall remodeling acutely after myocardial infarction in rats. *Circ Res* 1990; 67:23–34.
60. Lowes BD, Minobe W, Abraham WT, et al. Change in gene expression in the intact human heart. *J Clin Invest* 1997; 100:2315–2324.
61. Mercadier J, Lompré A, Duc P, et al. Altered sarcoplasmic reticulum Ca^{2+}-ATPase gene expression in the human ventricle during end-stage heart failure. *J Clin Invest* 1990; 85:305–309.
62. Gwathmey JK, Copelas L, MacKinnon R, et al. Abnormal intracellular calcium handling in myocardium from patients with end-stage heart failure. *Circ Res* 1987; 61:70–76.
63. Meyer M, Schillinger W, Pieske B, et al. Alterations of sarcoplasmic reticulum proteins in failing human dilated cardiomyopathy. *Circulation* 1995; 92:778–784.
64. Movsesian MA, Bristow MR, Krall J. Ca^{2+} uptake by cardiac sarcoplasmic reticulum from patients with idiopathic dilated cardiomyopathy. *Circ Res* 1989; 65:1141–1144.
65. Arai M, Matsui H, Periasamy M. Sarcoplasmic reticulum gene expression in cardiac hypertrophy and heart failure. *Circ Res* 1994; 74(4):555–564.
66. Kiss E, Ball NA, Kranias EG, Walsh RA. Differential changes in cardiac phospholamban and sarcoplasmic reticular Ca^{2+}-ATPase protein levels effects on Ca^{2+} transport and mechanics in compensated pressure-overload hypertrophy and congestive heart failure. *Circ Res* 1995; 77:759–764.
67. Hasenfuss G, Schillinger W, Lehnart SE, et al. Relationship between Na^+-Ca^{2+}-exchanger protein levels and diastolic function of failing human myocardium. *Circulation* 1999; 99:641–648.
68. Brillantes A, Allen P, Takahashi T, et al. Differences in cardiac calcium release channel (ryanodine receptor) expression in myocardium from patients with end-stage heart failure caused by ischemic versus dilated cardiomyopathy. *Circ Res* 1992; 71:18–26.
69. Wolff MR, Buck SH, Stoker SW, et al. Myofibrillar calcium sensitivity of isometric tension is increased in human dilated cardiomyopathies. *J Clin Invest* 1996; 98(1):167–176.
70. Pèrez NG, Hashimoto K, McCune S, et al. Origin of contractile dysfunction in heart failure: Calcium cycling versus myofilaments. *Circulation* 1999; 99:1077–1083.
71. Hajar RJ, DiSalvo TG, Schmidt U, et al. Clinical correlates of the myocardial force-frequency relationship in patients with end-stage heart failure. *J Heart Lung Transplant* 1997; 16:1157–1167.
72. Bhargava V, Shabetai R, Mathiäsen RA, et al. Loss of adrenergic control of the force-frequency relation in heart failure secondary to idiopathic or ischemic cardiomyopathy. *Am J Cardiol* 1998; 81:1130–1137.
73. Scheuer J. Metabolism of heart failure. *Prog Cardiovasc Dis* 1970; 13:24–54.
74. Schwartz A, Sordahl LA, Entman ML, et al. Abnormal biochemistry in myocardial failure. In: Mason DT, ed. *Congestive Heart Failure: Mechanisms, Evaluation and Treatment.* New York: Yorke Medical; 1976:25–44.
75. Badeer HS. *Cardiovascular Physiology*. Basel: Karger; 1984: 1–276.
76. Katz AM. *Physiology of the Heart*, 2d ed. New York: Raven Press; 1995:1–687.
77. Katz AM. Is the failing heart an energy-starved organ? (editorial). *J Cardiac Failure* 1996; 2:267–272.
78. Alpert NR, Hamrell BB. Cardiac hypertrophy: A compensatory and anticompensatory response to stress. In: Vassalle M, ed. *Cardiac Physiology for the Clinician.* New York: Academic Press; 1976:174–201.
79. Feldman MD, Copelas L, Gwathmey JK, et al. Deficient production of cyclic AMP: Pharmacologic evidence of an important case of contractile dysfunction in patients with end-stage heart failure. *Circulation* 1987; 75:331–339.
80. Rabinowitz M, Zak R. Mitochondria and cardiac hypertrophy. *Circ Res* 1975; 36:367–376.
81. Sievers R, Parmley WW, James T, Wilkman-Coffelt J. Energy levels at systole and diastole in normal hamster hearts vs. myopathic hamster hearts. *Circ Res* 1983; 53:759–766.
82. Ingwall JS, Kramer MF, Fifer MA, et al. The creatine kinase system in normal and diseased human myocardium. *N Engl J Med* 1985; 313:1050–1054.
83. Lentz RW, Harrison CE Jr, Dewey JD, et al. Functional evaluation of cardiac sarcoplasmic reticulum and mitochondria in human pathologic states. *J Mol Cell Cardiol* 1978; 10:3–30.
84. Scheuer J. Metabolic factors in myocardial failure. *Circulation* 1993; 87(suppl VII):VII54–VII57.
85. Markiewicz W, Wu S, Sievers R, et al. Influence of heart rate on metabolic and hemodynamic parameters in the Syrian hamster cardiomyopathy. *Am Heart J* 1987; 114:362–368.
86. Bristow MR, Ginsburg R, Minobe W, et al. Decreased catecholamine sensitivity and β-adrenergic-receptor density in failing human hearts. *N Engl J Med* 1982; 307:205–211.
87. White M, Yanowitz F, Gilbert EM, et al. Role of β-adrenergic receptor down-regulation in the peak exercise response in patients with heart failure due to idiopathic dilated cardiomyopathy. *Am J Cardiol* 1995; 76:1271–1276.
88. Bristow MR, Minobe W, Rasmussen R, et al. β-Adrenergic neuroeffector abnormalities in the failing human heart are produced by local rather than systemic mechanisms. *J Clin Invest* 1992; 89:803–815.
89. Bristow MR, Ginsburg R, Umans V, et al. β_1- and β_2-adrenergic-receptor subpopulations in non-failing and failing human ventricular myocardium: Coupling of both receptor subtypes to muscle contraction and selective β_1-receptor down-regulation in heart failure. *Circ Res* 1986; 59:297–309.
90. Feldman AM, Cates AE, Veazey WB, et al. Increase of the 40,000-mol wt pertussis toxin substrate (G protein) in the failing human heart. *J Clin Invest* 1988; 82:189–197.

91. Feldman AM, Cates AE, Bristow MR, Van Dop C. Altered expression of α-subunits of G proteins in failing human hearts. *J Mol Cell Cardiol* 1989; 21:359–365.
92. Vatner DE, Sato N, Galper JB, Vatner SF. Physiological and biochemical evidence for coordinate increases in muscarinic receptors and G_i during pacing-induced heart failure. *Circulation* 1996; 94:102–107.
93. White M, Roden R, Minobe W, et al. Age-related changes in β-adrenergic neuroeffector systems in human heart. *Circulation* 1994; 90:1225–1238.
94. Fowler MB, Laser JA, Hopkins GL, et al. Assessment of the β-adrenergic receptor pathway in the intact failing human heart: Progressive receptor down-regulation and subsensitivity to agonist response. *Circulation* 1986; 74(6):1290–1302.
95. Iaccarino G, Tomhave ED, Leftkowitz RJ, Koch WJ. Reciprocal in vivo regulation of myocardial G protein-coupled receptor kinase expression by β-adrenergic receptor stimulation and blockade. *Circulation* 1998; 98:1783–1789.
96. Gilbert EM, Abraham WT, Olsen S, et al. Comparative hemodynamic, left ventricular functional, and antiadrenergic effects of chronic treatment with metoprolol versus carvedilol in the failing heart. *Circulation* 1996; 94:2817–2825.
97. Richards AM, Doughty R, Nicholls MG, et al. Neurohumoral prediction of benefit from carvedilol in ischemic left ventricular dysfunction. *Circulation* 1999; 99:786–792.
98. Eckberg DL, Drabinski M, Braunwald E. Defective cardiac parasympathetic control in patients with heart disease. *N Engl J Med* 1971; 265:877–883.
99. Levine TB, Francis GS, Goldsmith SR, et al. The neurohumoral and hemodynamic response to orthostatic tilt in patients with congestive heart failure. *Circulation* 1983; 67(5):1070–1075.
100. Hirsch AT, Dzau VJ, Creager MA. Baroreceptor function in congestive heart failure: Effect on neurohumoral activation and regional vascular resistance. *Circulation* 1987; 75(suppl IV): IV36–IV48.
101. Zucker IH, Wang W, Brändle M. Baroreflex abnormalities in congestive heart failure. *NIPS* 1993; 8:87–90.
102. Thames MD, Kinugawa T, Smith ML, Dibner-Dunlap ME. Abnormalities of baroflex control in heart failure. *J Am Coll Cardiol* 1993; 22(suppl A):56A–60A.
103. Mortara A, La Rovere MT, Pinna GD, et al. Arterial baroflex modulation of heart rate in chronic heart failure. *Circulation* 1997; 96:3450–3458.
104. Dibner-Dunlap ME, Thames MD. Control of sympathetic nerve activity by vagal mechanoreflexes is blunted in heart failure. *Circulation* 1992; 86:1929–1934.
105. Grassi G, Seravalle G, Cattaneo BM, et al. Sympathetic activation and loss of reflex sympathetic control in mild congestive heart failure. *Circulation* 1995; 92:3206–3211.
106. Newton GE, Parker JD. Cardiac sympathetic responses to acute vasodilation. *Circulation* 1996; 94:3161–3167.
107. Goldsmith SR, Francis GS, Levine TB, Cohn JN. Regional blood flow response to orthostatis in patients with congestive heart failure. *J Am Coll Cardiol* 1983; 6:1391–1395.
108. Zelis R, Nellis SH, Longhurst J, et al. Abnormalities in the regional circulations accompanying congestive heart failure. *Prog Cardiovasc Dis* 1975; 18(3):181–199.
109. Brouwer J, Van Veldhuisen DJ, Man Veld AJ, et al. Prognostic value of heart rate variability during long-term follow-up in patients with mild to moderate heart failure. *J Am Coll Cardiol* 1996; 28:1183–1189.
110. Levine TB, Olivari MT, Cohn JN. Effects of orthotopic heart transplantation on sympathetic control mechanisms in congestive heart failure. *Am J Cardiol* 1986; 58:1035–1040.
111. Ellenbogen KA, Mohanty PK, Szentpetery S, Thames MD. Arterial baroreflex abnormalities in heart failure. *Circulation* 1989; 79:51–58.
112. Mohanty PK, Thames MD, Arrowood JA, et al. Impairment of cardiopulmonary baroreflex after cardiac transplantation in humans. *Circulation* 1987; 75(4):914–921.
113. Sinoway LI, Minotti JR, Davis D, et al. Delayed reversal of impaired vasodilation in congestive heart failure after heart transplantation. *Am J Cardiol* 1988; 61:1076–1079.
114. Ferguson DW, Abboud FM, Mark AL. Selective impairment of baroreflex-mediated vasoconstrictor responses in patients with ventricular dysfunction. *Circulation* 1984; 69(3):451–460.
115. Francis GS, Cohn JN. The autonomic nervous system in congestive heart failure. *Annu Rev Med* 1986; 37:235–247.
116. Katz AM. The descending limb of the Starling curve and the failing heart. *Circulation* 1965; 32:871–875.
117. MacGregor DC, Covell JW, Mahler F, et al. Relations between afterload, stroke volume, and the descending limb of Starling's curves. *Am J Physiol* 1974; 227:884–890.
118. Holubarsch C, Ruf T, Goldstein DJ, et al. Existence of the Frank-Starling mechanism in the failing human heart. *Circulation* 1996; 94:683–689.
119. Ross J Jr. Afterload mismatch and preload reserve: A conceptual framework for the analysis of ventricular function. *Prog Cardiovasc Dis* 1976; 18(4):255–264.
120. Badeer HS. Contractile tension in the myocardium. *Am Heart J* 1963; 66:432–434.
121. LaKatta EG. Starling's law of the heart is explained by an intimate interaction of muscle length and myofilament calcium activation. *J Am Coll Cardiol* 1987; 10:1157–1164.
122. Hoh JF, Rossmanith GH, Kwan LJ, Hamilton AM. Adrenaline increases the rate of cycling of crossbridges in rat cardiac muscle as measured by pseudo-random binary noise–modulated pertubation analysis. *Circ Res* 1988; 62:452–461.
123. Cheng W, Li B, Kajstura J, et al. Stretch-induced programmed myocyte cell death. *J Clin Invest* 1995; 96:2247–2259.
124. Komuro I, Kurabyashi M, Takaku F, Yazaki Y. Expression of cellular oncogenes in the myocardium during the developmental stage and pressure-overloaded hypertrophy of the rat heart. *Circ Res* 1988; 62:1075–1079.
125. Komuro I, Kaida T, Shibazaki Y, et al. Stretching cardiac myocytes stimulates protooncogene expression. *J Biol Chem* 1990; 265(7):3595–3598.
126. Calderone A, Takahashi N, Izzo NJ Jr, et al. Pressure- and volume-induced left ventricular hypertrophies are associated with distinct myocyte phenotypes and differential induction of peptide growth factor mRNAs. *Circulation* 1995; 92:2385–2390.
127. Anversa P, Ricci R, Olivetti G. Quantitative structural analysis of the myocardium during physiological growth induced cardiac hypertrophy: A review. *J Am Coll Cardiol* 1986; 7:1140–1149.
128. Anversa P, Capasso JM, Olivetti G, Sonneblick EH. Cellular basis of ventricular remodeling in hypertensive cardiomyopathy. *Am J Hypertens* 1992; 5:758–770.
129. Grossman W, Jones D, McLaurin LP. Wall stress and patterns of hypertrophy in the human left ventricle. *J Clin Invest* 1975; 56:56–64.
130. Weber KT, Clark WA, Janicki JS, Shroff SG. Physiologic versus pathologic hypertrophy and the pressure-overloaded myocardium. *J Cardiovasc Pharmacol* 1987; 10(suppl 6):537–550.
131. Weber KT, Janicki JS, Shroff SG, et al. Collagen compartment remodeling in the pressure overloaded left ventricle. *J Appl Cardiol* 1988; 3:37–46.
132. Weber KT, Janicki JS, Shroff SG, et al. Collagen remodeling of the pressure-overload hypertrophied nonhuman primate myocardium. *Circ Res* 1988; 62:757–765.
133. Weber KT. Cardiac interstitium in health and disease: The fibrillar collagen network. *J Am Coll Cardiol* 1989; 13:1637–1652.
134. Zhao M, Zhang H, Robinson TF, et al. Profound structural alterations of the extracellular collagen matrix in post-ischemic dys-

functional but viable myocardium. *J Am Coll Cardiol* 1987; 10:1322–1334.
135. Weber KT, Pick R, Silver MA, et al. Fibrillar collagen and remodeling of dilated canine left ventricle. *Circulation* 1990; 82:1387–1401.
136. Weber KT, Brilla CG. Pathological hypertrophy and cardiac interstitium: Fibrosis and renin-angiotensin-aldosterone system. *Circulation* 1991; 83:1849–1865.
137. Breish EA, Houser SR, Carey RA, et al. Myocardial blood flow and capillary density in chronic pressure overload of the feline left ventricle. *Cardiovasc Res* 1980; 14:469–475.
138. Tomanek RJ, Palmer PJ, Peiffer GL, et al. Morphometry of canine coronary arteries, arterioles, and capillaries during hypertension and left ventricular hypertrophy. *Circ Res* 1986; 58:26–37.
139. Anversa P, Sonnenblick EH. Ischemic cardiomyopathy: Pathophysiologic mechanisms. *Prog Cardiovasc Dis* 1990; 33:49–70.
140. Sadoshima J, Malhotra R, Izumo S. The role of the cardiac renin-angiotensin system in load-induced cardiac hypertrophy. *J Cardiac Failure* 1996; 2(suppl 4):S1–S6.
141. Harada K, Komuro I, Shiojima I, Hayashi D, Kudoh S, Mizuno T, et al. Pressure overload induces cardiac hypertrophy in angiotensin II type 1a receptor knockout mice. *Circulation* 1998; 97:1952–1959.
142. Tamura T, Onodera T, Said S, Gerdes AM. Correlation of myocyte lengthening to chamber dilation in the spontaneously hypertensive heart failure (SHHF) rat. *J Mol Cell Cardiol* 1998; 30:2175–2181.
143. Wang X, Li F, Gerdes AM. Chronic pressure overload cardiac hypertrophy and failure in guinea pigs: Regional hemodynamics and myocyte remodeling. *J Mol Cell Cardiol* 1999; 31:307–317.
144. Kelly DT. Our future society: A global challenge. *Circulation* 1997; 95:2459–2464.
145. Grossman W, McLaurin LP, Rollet EL. Alterations in left ventricular relaxation and diastolic compliance in congestive cardiomyopathy. *Cardiovasc Res* 1979; 13:514–522.
146. Staufer GC, Gaasch WH. Recognition and treatment of left ventricular diastolic dysfunction. *Prog Cardiovasc Dis* 1990; 32(5): 319–332.
147. Little WC, Downes TR. Clinical evaluation of left ventricular diastolic performance. *Prog Cardiovasc Dis* 1990; 32(4):273–290.
148. Bolli R. Mechanism of myocardial "stunning." *Circulation* 1990; 82:723–738.
149. Marban E. Myocardial stunning and hibernation: The physiology behind the colloquialisms. *Circulation* 1991; 83(2):681–688.
150. Rahimtoola SH. Importance of diagnosing hibernating myocardium: How and in whom? *J Am Coll Cardiol* 1997; 30(7):1701–1706.
151. Marwick TH. The viable myocardium: Epidemiology, detection, and clinical implications. *Lancet* 1998; 351:815–819.
152. Vanoverschelde JJ, Wijns W, Borgers M, et al. Chronic myocardial hibernation in humans: From bedside to bench. *Circulation* 1997; 95:1961–1971.
153. Weber KT, Brilla CG, Janicki JS. Myocardial fibrosis: Functional significance and regulatory factors. *Cardiol Res* 1993; 27:341–348.
154. Weber KT. Cardiac interstitium in health disease: The fibrillar collagen network. *J Am Coll Cardiol* 1989; 13:1637–1652.
155. Weber KT. Monitoring tissue repair and fibrosis from a distance. *Circulation* 1997; 96:2488–2492.
156. Thomas CV, Coker ML, Zellner JL, et al. Increased matrix metalloproteinase activity and selective upregulation in LV myocardium from patients with end-stage dilated cardiomyopathy. *Circulation* 1998; 97:1708–1715.
157. Weber LT, Brilla CG. Pathological hypertrophy and cardiac interstitium: Fibrosis and renin-angiotensin-aldosterone system. *Circulation* 1991; 83:1849–1865.
158. Harada M, Itoh H, Nakagawa S, et al. Significance of ventricular myocytes and nonmyocytes interaction during cardiocyte hypertrophy: Evidence for endothelin-1 as a paracrine hypertrophic factor from cardiac nonmyocytes. *Circulation* 1997; 96:3737–3744.
159. Levin ER, Gardner DG, Samson WK. Natriuretic peptides. *N Engl J Med* 1998; 339(5):321–328.
160. Schrier RW, Abraham WT. Hormones and hemodynamics in heart failure. *N Engl J Med* 1999; 341(8):577–585.
161. Rona G. Catecholamine cardiotoxicity. *J Mol Cell Cardiol* 1985; 17:291–306.
162. Mann DL, Kent RL, Parsons B, Cooper G IV. Adrenergic effects on the biology of the adult mammalian cardiocyte. *Circulation* 1992; 85:790–804.
163. Tan L, Jalil JE, Pick R, et al. Cardiac myocyte necrosis induced by angiotensin II. *Circulation* 1991; 69:1185–1195.
164. Francis GS, Goldsmith SR, Levine B, et al. The neurohumoral axis in congestive heart failure. *Ann Intern Med* 1984; 101: 370–377.
165. Packer M. Neurohormonal interactions and adaptations in congestive heart failure. *Circulation* 1988; 77(4):721–730.
166. Packer M. The neurohormonal hypothesis: A theory to explain the mechanism of disease progression in heart failure. *J Am Coll Cardiol* 1992; 20:248–254.
167. Packer M, Lee WH, Kessler PD, et al. Role of neurohormonal mechanisms in determining survival in patients with severe chronic heart failure. *Circulation* 1987; 75(suppl 4):IV80–IV92.
168. Starling EH. Points on pathology of heart disease. *Lancet* 1897; 1:569–572.
169. Chidsey CA, Harrison DC, Braunwald E. Augmentation of the plasma norepinephrine response to exercise in patients with congestive heart failure. *N Engl J Med* 1962; 267:650–654.
170. Braunwald E, Chidsey CA, Pool PE, et al. Congestive heart failure: Biochemical and physiological considerations. *Ann Intern Med* 1966; 64:904–941.
171. Thomas JA, Marks BH. Plasma norepinephrine in congestive heart failure. *Am J Cardiol* 1978; 41:233–243.
172. Levine TB, Francis GS, Goldsmith SR, et al. Activity of the sympathetic nervous system and renin-angiotensin system assessed by plasma hormone levels and their relation to hemodynamic abnormalities in congestive heart failure. *Am J Cardiol* 1982; 49:1659–1666.
173. Leimbach WN, Wallin G, Victor RG, et al. Direct evidence from intraneural recordings for increased central sympathetic outflow in patients with heart failure. *Circulation* 1986; 73(5):913–919.
174. Hasking GJ, Esler MD, Jennings GL, et al. Norepinephrine spillover to plasma in patients with congestive heart failure: Evidence of increased overall and cardiorenal sympathetic nervous activity. *Circulation* 1986; 73(4):615–621.
175. Rundqvist B, Elam M, Bergmann-Sverrisodottir Y, et al. Increased cardiac adrenergic drive precedes generalized sympathetic activation in human heart failure. *Circulation* 1997; 95:169–175.
176. Cohn JN, Levine TB, Olivari MT, et al. Plasma norepinephrine as a guide to prognosis in patients with chronic congestive heart failure. *N Engl J Med* 1984; 311:819–823.
177. Gafney TE, Braunwald E. Importance of the adrenergic nervous system in the support of circulatory function in patients with congestive heart failure. *Am J Med* 1963; 34:320–324.
178. Hall SA, Cigarroa CG, Marcoux L, et al. Time course of improvement in left ventricular function, mass and geometry in patients with congestive heart failure treated with beta-adrenergic blockade. *J Am Coll Cardiol* 1995; 25:1554–1161.
179. Eichhorn EJ, Bristow MR. Medical therapy can improve the biological properties of the chronically failing heart: A new era in the treatment of heart failure. *Circulation* 1996; 94(9):2285–2296.
180. Keeton TK, Campbell WB. The pharmacologic alteration of renin release. *Pharmacol Rev* 1981; 31:81–227.
181. Matsubara H. Pathophysiological role of angiotensin II type 2

receptor in cardiovascular and renal diseases. *Circ Res* 1998; 83:1182–1191.
182. Francis GS. The renin-angiotensin system. In: Parmley W and Chatterjee K, eds. *Cardiology.* New York: Lippincott-Raven; 1997:1–16.
183. Gibbons GH, Pfeffer MA. The role of angiotensin in cardiovascular disease: Pathophysiologic insights and therapeutic implications. In: Topol EJ, ed. *Textbook of Cardiovascular Medicine.* New York: Lippincott-Raven; 1998:1–12.
184. Pitt B, Zannad F, Remme WJ, et al. The effect of spironolactone on morbidity and mortality in patients with severe heart failure. *N Engl J Med* 1999; 341(10):709–755.
185. Szatalowicz VL, Arnold PE, Chaimovitz C, et al. Radioimmunoassay of plasma arginine vasopressin in hyponatremic patients with congestive heart failure. *N Engl J Med* 1981; 305(5): 263–266.
186. Francis GS, Benedict C, Johnstone DE, et al. Comparison of neuroendocrine activation in patients with left ventricular dysfunction with and without congestive heart failure. *Circulation* 1990; 82:1724–1729.
187. Goldsmith SR, Francis GS, Cowley AW, et al. Increased plasma arginine vasopressin levels in patients with congestive heart failure. *J Am Coll Cardiol* 1983; 1(6):1385–1390.
188. Goldsmith SR, Francis GS, Cowley AW Jr, et al. Hemodynamic effects of infused arginine vasopressin in congestive heart failure. *J Am Coll Cardiol* 1986; 8:779–783.
189. Cowie MR, Struthers AD, Wood DA, et al. Value of natriuretic peptides in assessment of patients with possible new heart failure in primary care. *Lancet* 1997; 350:1347–1351.
190. Niinuma H, Nakamura Mo, Hiramori K. Plasma B-type natriuretic peptide measurement in a multiphasic health screening program. *Cardiology* 1998; 90:89–94.
191. Mills RM, LeJemtel TH, Horton DP, et al. Sustained hemodynamic effects of an infusion of nesiritide (human b-type natriuretic peptide) in heart failure. *J Am Coll Cardiol* 1999; 34: 155–162.
192. Yanagisawa M, Kurihara H, Kimura S, et al. A novel potent vasoconstrictor peptide produced by vascular endothelial cells. *Nature* 1988; 332:411–415.
193. Levin ER. Mechanisms of disease. *N Engl J Med* 1995; 333(6):356–363.
194. Rodehefer RJ, Lerman A, Heublein DM, Burnett JC. Increased plasma concentrations of endothelin in congestive heart failure in humans. *Mayo Clin Proc* 1992; 67:719–724.
195. McMurray JJ, Ray SG, Abdullah I, et al. Plasma endothelin in chronic heart failure. *Circulation* 1992; 85:1374–1379.
196. Zolk O, Quattek J, Sitzler G, et al. Expression of endothelin-1, endothelin-converting enzyme, and endothelin receptors in chronic heart failure. *Circulation* 1999; 99:2118–2123.
197. Benigni A, Remuzzi G. Endothelin antagonists. *Lancet* 1999; 353:133–138.
198. Levine B, Kalman J, Mayer L, et al. Elevated circulating levels of tumor necrosis factor in severe chronic heart failure. *N Engl J Med* 1990; 323(4):236–241.
199. Torre-Amione G, Kapadia S, Lee J, et al. Tumor necrosis factor-a and tumor necrosis factor receptors in the failing human heart. *Circulation* 1996; 93:704–711.
200. Torre-Amione G, Kapadia S, Benedict C, et al. Proinflammatory cytokine levels in patients with depressed left ventricular ejection fraction: A report from the studies of left ventricular dysfunction. *J Am Coll Cardiol* 1996; 27:1201–1206.
201. Bristow MR. Tumor necrosis factor-α and cardiomyopathy. *Circulation* 1998; 97:1340–1341.
202. Bozkurt B, Kribbs SB, Clubb FJ Jr, et al. Pathophysiologically relevant concentrations of tumor necrosis factor-α promote progressive left ventricular dysfunction and remodeling in rats. *Circulation* 1998; 97:1382–1391.
203. Yokoyama T, Nakano M, Bednarczyk JL, et al. Tumor necrosis factor-α provokes a hypertrophic growth response in adult cardiac myocytes. *Circulation* 1997; 95:1247–1252.
204. Anker SD, Chua TP, Ponikowski P, et al. Hormonal changes and catabolic/anabolic imbalance of chronic heart failure and their importance for cardiac cachexia. *Circulation* 1997; 96: 526–534.
205. Anker SD, Clark AL, Kemp M, et al. Tumor necrosis factor and steroid metabolism in chronic heart failure: Possible relation to muscle wasting. *J Am Coll Cardiol* 1997; 30:97–1001.
206. Bryant D, Becker L, Richardson J, et al. Cardiac failure in transgenic mice with myocardial expression of tumor necrosis factor-α. *Circulation* 1998; 97:1375–1381.
207. Cannon PJ. The kidney in heart failure. *N Engl J Med* 1977; 296:26–32.
208. Dzau VJ. Renin-angiotensin system and renal circulation in clinical congestive heart failure. *Kidney Int* 1987; 31(suppl 20):S203–S209.
209. Packer M, Lee WH, Kessler PD. Preservation of glomerular filtration rate in human heart failure by activation of the renin-angiotensin system. *Circulation* 1986; 74(4):766–774.
210. Ichikawa I, Yoshioka T, Fogo A, Kon V. Role of angiotensin II in altered glomerular hemodynamics in congestive heart failure. *Kidney Int* 1990; 38(suppl 30):S123–S126.
211. Hall JE, Guyton AC, Jackson TE, et al. Control of glomerular filtration rate by renin-angiotensin system. *Am J Physiol* 1977; 235(5):F366–F372.
212. Ichikawa I, Pfeffer JM, Pfeffer MA, et al. Role of angiotensin II in the altered renal function of congestive heart failure. *Circ Res* 1984; 55:669–675.
213. Treasure CB, Vita JA, Cox DA, et al. Endothelium-dependent dilation of the coronary microvasculature is impaired in dilated cardiomyopathy. *Circulation* 1990; 81:772–779.
214. Drexler H, Lu W. Endothelial dysfunction of hindquarter resistance vessels in experimental heart failure. *Am J Physiol* 1992; 262(*Heart Circ Physiol* 31):H1640–H1645.
215. Kubo SH, Rector TS, Bank AJ, et al. Endothelium-dependent vasodilation is attenuated in patients with heart failure. *Circulation* 1991; 84:1589–1596.
216. Drexler H, Hayoz D, Münzel T, et al. Endothelial function in chronic congestive heart failure. *Am J Cardiol* 1992; 69:1596–1601.
217. Winlaw DS, Smythe GA, Keogh AM, et al. Increased nitric oxide production in heart failure. *Lancet* 1994; 344:373–374.
218. Nakamura M, Ishikawa M, Funakoshi T, et al. Attenuated endothelium-dependent peripheral vasodilation and clinical characteristics in patients with chronic heart failure. *Am Heart J* 1994; 128:1164–1169.
219. Kubo SH, Rector TS, Bank AJ, et al. Effects of cardiac transplantation on endothelium-dependent dilation of the peripheral vasculature in congestive heart failure. *Am J Cardiol* 1993; 71:88–93.
220. Kelly RA, Balligand JL, Smith TW. Nitric oxide and cardiac function. *Circ Res* 1996; 79:363–380.
221. Drexler H. Nitric oxide synthases in the failing human heart: A double edged sword. *Circulation* 1999; 99:2972–2975.
222. Haywood GA, Tsao PS, von der Leyen HE, et al. Expression of inducible nitric oxide synthase in human heart failure. *Circulation* 1996; 93:1087–1094.
223. Recchia RA, McConnell PI, Bernstein RD, et al. Reduced nitric oxide production and altered myocardial metabolism during the decompensation of pacing-induced heart failure in the conscious dog. *Circ Res* 1998; 83:969–979.
224. Massie BM. Exercise tolerance in congestive heart failure: Role of cardiac function, peripheral blood flow, and muscle metabolism and effect of treatment. *Am J Med* 1988; 84(suppl 3A):75–82.
225. Massie BM, Simonini A, Sahgal P, et al. Relation of systemic and

local muscle exercise capacity to skeletal muscle characteristics in men with congestive heart failure. *J Am Coll Cardiol* 1996; 27:140–145.

226. Hambrecht R, Adams V, Gielen S, et al. Exercise intolerance in patients with chronic heart failure and increased expression of inducible nitric oxide synthase in the skeletal muscle. *J Am Coll Cardiol* 1999; 33:174–179.
227. Adams V, Jiang H, Yu J, et al. Apoptosis in skeletal myocytes of patients with chronic heart failure is associated with exercise intolerance. *J Am Coll Cardiol* 1999; 33:959–965.
228. Wilson JR, Hanamanthu S, Chomsky DB, Davis SF. Relationship between exertional symptoms and functional capacity in patients with heart failure. *J Am Coll Cardiol* 1999; 33:1943–1947.
229. Javaheri S. A mechanism of central sleep apnea in patients with heart failure. *N Engl J Med* 1999; 341:949–954.
230. Lanfranchi PA, Braghiroli AL, Bosimini E, et al. Prognostic value of nocturnal Cheyne-Stokes respiration in chronic heart failure. *Circulation* 1999; 99:1435–1440.
231. Andreas S, Clemens C, Sandholzer H, et al. Improvement of exercise capacity with treatment of Cheyne-Stokes respiration in patients with congestive heart failure. *J Am Coll Cardiol* 1996; 27:1486–1490.
232. Javaheri S, Parker TJ, Wexler L, et al. Occult sleep-disordered breathing in stable congestive heart failure. *Ann Intern Med* 1995; 122:487–492.
233. Javaheri S, Parker TJ, Liming JD, et al. Sleep apnea in 81 ambulatory male patients with stable heart failure: Types and their prevalences, consequences, and presentations. *Circulation* 1998; 97:2154–2159.
234. Tkacova R, Rankin F, Fitzgerald FS, et al. Effects of continuous positive airway pressure on obstructive sleep apnea and left ventricular afterload in patients with heart failure. *Circulation* 1998; 98:269–2275.
235. Tristani FE, Hughes CV, Archibald DG, et al. Safety of graded symptom-limited exercise testing in patients with congestive heart failure. *Circulation* 1987; 76:51–54.
236. Myers J, Foelicher VF. Hemodynamic determinants of exercise capacity in chronic heart failure. *Ann Intern Med* 1991; 115: 377–386.
237. Myers J, Salleh A, Buchanan N, et al. Ventilatory mechanisms of exercise intolerance in chronic heart failure. *Am Heart J* 1992; 124:7–10.
238. Weber KT, Kinasewitz GT, Janicki JS, Fishman AP. Oxygen utilization and ventilation during exercise in patients with chronic cardiac failure. *Circulation* 1982; 65:1213–1223.
239. Aaronson KD, Mancini DM. Is the percentage of predicted maximal exercise oxygen consumption a better predictor of survival than peak exercise oxygen consumption for patients with severe heart failure? *J Heart Lung Transplant* 1995; 14:981–989.
240. Mancini DM, Eisen H, Kussmaul W, et al. Value of peak exercise oxygen consumption for optimal timing of cardiac transplantation in ambulatory patients with heart failure. *Circulation* 1991; 83(3):778–786.
241. Stelken AM, Younis LT, Jennison SH, et al. Prognostic value of cardiopulmonary exercise testing using percent achieved of predicted peak oxygen uptake for patients with ischemic and dilated cardiomyopathy. *J Am Coll Cardiol* 1996; 27:345–352.
242. Aaronson KD, Schwartz S, Chen TM, et al. Development and prospective validation of a clinical index to predict survival in ambulatory patients referred for cardiac transplant evaluation. *Circulation* 1997; 95:2660–2667.
243. Bart BA, Shaw LK, McCants CB Jr, et al. Clinical determinants of mortality in patients with angiographically diagnosed ischemic or nonischemic cardiomyopathy. *J Am Coll Cardiol* 1997; 30:1002–1008.

CHAPTER 21

DIAGNOSIS AND MANAGEMENT OF HEART FAILURE

Thierry H. LeJemtel / Edmund H. Sonnenblick / William H. Frishman

The management of patients with chronic heart failure is increasingly complex, since congestive heart failure (CHF) represents the end result of many cardiovascular, pulmonary, and systemic diseases that require specific and aggressive therapy.[1–3] Moreover, ventricular dysfunction generally precedes clinical symptoms by months or years.[4] Thus, the initial aim of therapy is to treat the primary etiology and prevent or slow the progression of or even reverse left ventricular (LV) systolic dysfunction independent of symptoms. This goal most often is achieved on an outpatient basis. Once symptoms of CHF occur, their control becomes a primary focus. Ultimately, the severity of symptoms may require hospitalization with parenteral therapy. Overall, successful management of patients with CHF rests on in-depth knowledge and treatment of the processes responsible for ventricular dysfunction and ultimately the symptoms that evolve. Despite the diversity of the initial processes, three guiding principles remain central.

The first guiding principle in CHF management is the concomitant, continuous, and aggressive pursuit and treatment of the underlying disease or diseases that led to the development of CHF. For example, hypertension requires vigorous and adequate therapy. When CHF is due to obstruction of the coronary arteries, a demonstration of reversible myocardial ischemia, even in the absence of angina, can lead to a coronary revascularization procedure that in turn can lead to an improvement in myocardial function. Similarly, slowing the progression of coronary artery disease through the use of both antithrombotic and lipid-lowering therapies along with cessation of cigarette smoking is as important as is the treatment of the clinical symptoms of ischemic CHF.

The second guiding principle in managing patients with CHF is to define precisely the stage of the disease when therapy begins. The syndrome of CHF is a dynamic process, and the therapeutic goals and end points vary as the process evolves. Symptoms, even as judged by exercise testing,[5] do not correlate with the severity of ventricular dysfunction as judged by measurement of the ejection fraction.[6] Thus, symptoms should not be used to guide therapy in the early stages of the disease. Minimal serial measurement of the ejection fraction remains the guide to advancement of the primary diseases, and symptoms and their relief may not predict survival. Prevention of sudden death is an important therapeutic outcome in patients with asymptomatic or mildly asymptomatic LV systolic dysfunction. It may be a limited therapeutic goal in extremely symptomatic patients who are not candidates for cardiac transplantation or LV assist devices, in whom symptom relief becomes a primary concern.

The third guiding principle in managing patients with severe CHF is the recognition that a key determinant of successful therapy is the intensity of care; this requires frequent visits, in-home monitoring, and meticulous attention to management details such as diet, daily activity level, daily weight, and the doses of the medications being used, with an appreciation of their adverse effects.[7,8] The importance of this principle is illustrated by the careful approach that is required to both successfully initiate and increase the dosage of beta-adrenergic blockade therapy in patients with symptomatic LV systolic dysfunction.

To plan an appropriate therapy, an accurate clinical diagnosis is necessary, with an understanding of the pathophysiology involved. Details of diagnostic approaches are presented elsewhere (see Chap. 20).

PREVENTION OR REVERSAL OF LV DILATATION AND HYPERTROPHY

Besides primary prevention of the processes that are associated with LV systolic dysfunction and the development of CHF (coronary artery atherosclerosis, hyperlipidemias, hypertension, diabetes), secondary prevention of LV dilatation has been achieved most successfully over the past decade by modulating heightened activity of the neurohumoral activity of the sympathetic and renin-angiotensin-aldosterone systems. As will be discussed, below deactivation of both systems has led to attenuation or reversal of the remodeling process that accompanies the syndrome of CHF. However, the extent to which these systems should be deactivated is still poorly understood, especially late in the syndrome of CHF. Of interest, the dissociation between LV systolic performance and functional capacity that is present at baseline in patients with CHF seems also to be observed during therapeutic interventions. Further, the substantial improvement in LV ejection fraction that frequently occurs during long-term beta-adrenergic blockade does not necessarily translate into improved functional capacity. Current therapeutic investigations regarding the progression of LV dilatation and hypertrophy are focusing on cytokine receptor antagonists and endothelin receptor antagonists.[9,10]

PATHOPHYSIOLOGY AND DIAGNOSIS OF CONGESTIVE HEART FAILURE

The dynamic process by which ventricular dysfunction evolves into CHF can be conveniently described in three phases[11] (Fig. 21-1). The clinical characteristics of each phase and its duration depend heavily on the specific primary etiology involved. Myocardial damage with massive myocyte loss and fibrotic repair may be rapid, as occurs with an acute transmural myocardial infarction or a viral myocarditis, or may evolve over years, as occurs with overloads resulting from systemic hypertension or valvular disease.[12,13] In the absence of overt clinical symptoms, such as chest pain with a myocardial infarction or sudden (flash) pulmonary edema, the initial damage may go undiagnosed. In this situation, a two-dimensional echocardiogram can be helpful in documenting the presence and extent of LV dysfunction and segmental wall motion abnormalities. Ventricular dilatation is not uncommon in largely asymptomatic patients.

The second stage in the evolution of heart failure involves an adaptation to myocardial damage termed *ventricular remodeling*. This involves myocardial hypertrophy in response to myocardium that is lost or overloaded and ventricular dilatation, which helps sustain cardiac output (Fig. 21-1). In general, heart failure begins with increased loading of the ventricle with pressure or volume or with loss of myocardium leading to ventricular dysfunction. In a sense, loss of myocardium, whether segmental as occurs with myocardial infarction or diffuse as occurs with cardiomyopathies, creates an overload for the myocardium in that less myocardium must maintain the work of the heart. Once an overload is created, the myocardium responds with changes in growth and architecture that constitute ventricular remodeling. This includes increases in myocyte length as well as lateral dimension. With an increased pressure load, myocytes respond by laying down more contractile units in parallel, thus increasing the lateral dimensions of the myocyte and its force potential. This form of hypertrophy tends to normalize the tension in the ventricular wall. When volume is increased, whether because of increased flow from an insufficient valve or increased diastolic filling pressure that results as a compensation for lost myocardium, myocytes elongate in order to maintain force and shortening. Acutely, this occurs within the limits created by the physiological lengthening of the sarcomere, i.e., the Frank-Starling length-tension curve. With a sustained diastolic load, sarcomeres are added in series, resulting in increased myocyte length. Since augmented diastolic volume itself results in increased ventricular wall tension [wall tension (T) = pressure (P) × dimension (r)/wall thickness (h)], lateral growth (hypertrophy) of myocytes commonly accompanies myocyte lengthening. In addition to hypertrophy of myocytes, other dynamic events occur in the myocardium.

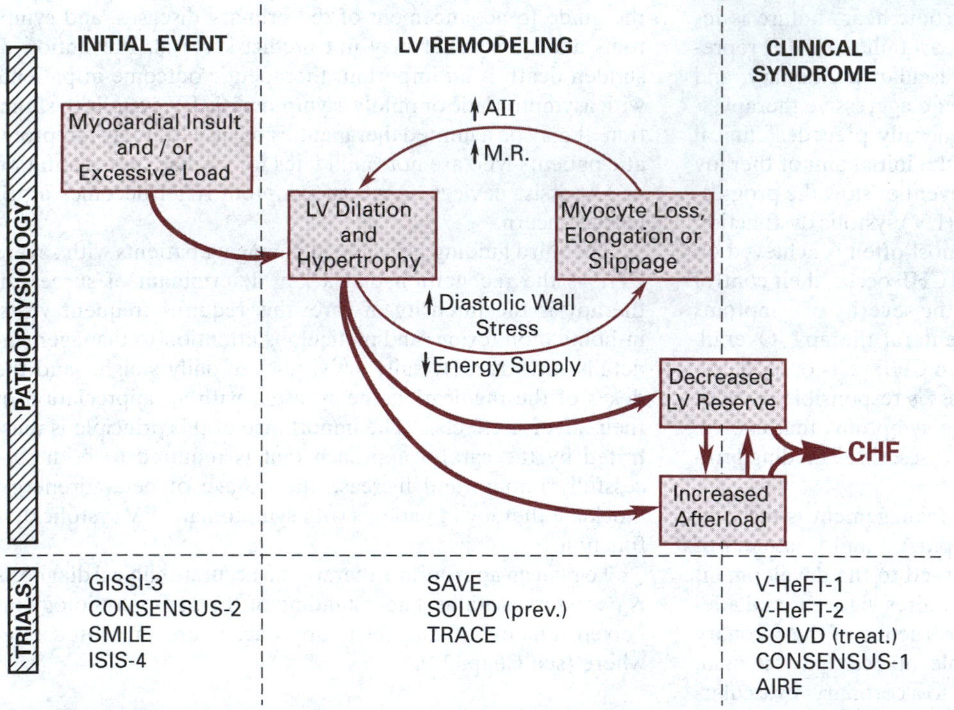

FIGURE 21-1 The pathophysiology of heart failure progressing with time from the initial event, related to a loss of myocardium and/or a persistent overload, to the adaptive responses, including myocardial hypertrophy, and ultimately ventricular dilatation. Left ventricular (LV) dilatation augments diastolic wall stress that produces deformations of the ventricular wall and functional mitral regurgitation (MR) as well as further myocyte loss (apoptosis). Neurohumoral responses become activated with increased sympathetic tone, reduced parasympathetic tone, and activation of the renin-angiotensin system. These structural alterations constitute what is termed *ventricular remodeling*. With progression of these latter processes and with decreased ventricular capacity to augment cardiac output as required along with renal retention of sodium, central and peripheral edema ensue, with limitation of exercise performance. Thus, the syndrome of congestive heart failure (CHF) finally becomes manifest. Shown at the bottom of the figure are various studies addressing these phases of heart failure in terms of morbidity and mortality. GISSI, Gruppo Italiano per lo Studio dell a Sopravivenza nell'Infarcto Miocardio; CONSENSUS, Cooperative North Scandinavian Enalapril Study; SMILE, Survival of Myocardial Infarction; ISIS, International Study of Infarct Survival; SAVE, Survival and Ventricular Enlargement Trial; SOLVD, Studies of Left Ventricular Dysfunction; TRACE, Trandolapril Cardiac Evaluation: V-HeFT, Veterans Administration Cooperative Vasodilator Heart Failure Trial; AIRE, Acute Infarction Ramipril Efficacy Study.

Myocytes may be lost diffusely when excessive overloads occur through the process of apoptosis and focal necrosis with replacement fibrosis. With sustained diastolic loads, ventricular dilatation proceeds with not only marked myocyte lengthening but also with apparent displacement of myocytes or groups of myocytes one to the other, a process labeled *myocyte slippage.* While hypertrophy of myocytes is readily demonstrable, hyperplasia of myocytes also may be observed.[14,15] Taken together, hypertrophy, myocyte hypertrophy, further myocyte loss, and hyperplasia, along with ventricular wall restructuring, constitute ventricular remodeling. With systolic overloads, this generally is characterized by increased ventricular wall thickness with normal intraventricular volumes (e.g., normal ejection fraction). When the hypertrophy cannot sustain required systolic tension, whether because of a primary decrease in force production by a given myocyte[16] or because of loss of myocytes, ventricular dilatation occurs and a fall in the ejection fraction is observed. Generally, it proceeds silently unless it is heralded by an acute myocardial infarction. Thus, except for clinical symptoms, such as dyspnea and exertion, that may reflect an increased diastolic filling pressure resulting from a thickened ventricular wall, ventricular remodeling generally progresses unobserved.

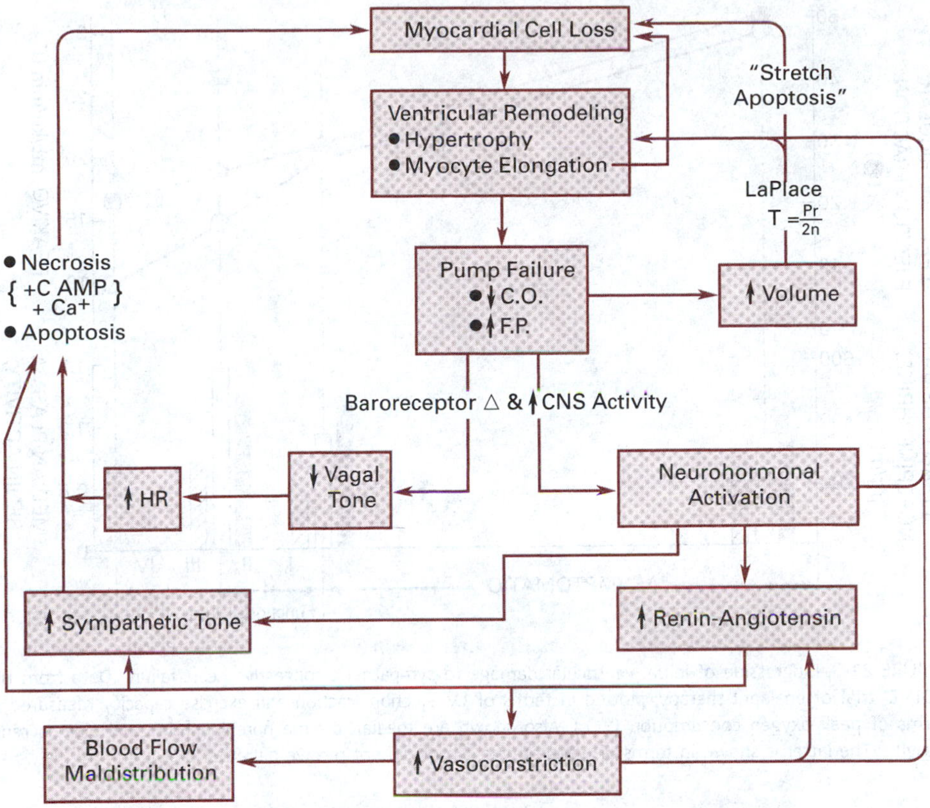

FIGURE 21-2 Ventricular remodeling and progression of ventricular dysfunction. Myocardial cell loss leads to ventricular remodeling, characterized by myocyte hypertrophy and elongation. An increase in ventricular volume (the Starling effect) helps maintain cardiac output (CO), but at the cost of increasing ventricular filling pressures. The increase in diastolic stretch and pressure produces further damage, including stretch-induced myocyte death (apoptosis), which amplifies the process of remodeling. With inadequate pump function, neurohumoral activation occurs with decreased vagal tone and enhanced sympathetic tone. With activation of the renin-angiotensin system and increased sympathetic tone, arterial vasoconstriction occurs with resultant maldistribution of blood flow. Decreased vagal and increased sympathetic stimulation induce tachycardia, and the latter system, along with the activated renin-angiotensin system, via angiotensin II can produce further myocyte death. In this manner, the process is self-perpetuating in that ventricular damage leads to remodeling, which in turn leads to further damage. These interrelated cycles thus provide therapeutic opportunities.

The factors that mediate progressive ventricular remodeling (hypertrophy) are both physical forces and hormonal factors (e.g., angiotensin). During this evolution of ventricular remodeling, neurohumoral activation occurs.[17] Activation of the sympathetic nervous system with parasympathetic withdrawal leads to tachycardia and peripheral vasoconstriction. Activation of the renin-angiotensin system causes further vasoconstriction and salt accumulation through stimulated aldosterone secretion. Both of these latter factors, along with excessive stretch of the myocardium, can lead to further myocyte loss, with fibrosis along with further myocyte hypertrophy, while ventricular dilatation may induce functional mitral and/or tricuspid insufficiency, creating an additional hemodynamic load (Fig. 21-2).[18]

The third phase in the evolution of heart failure evolves from these adaptive changes, with development of symptoms of CHF, characterized by decreased exercise tolerance, pulmonary and systemic congestion, and central and peripheral edema. The interval between the initiation of ventricular dysfunction and the onset of symptoms, during which ventricular remodeling occurs, may extend over a long period, but if the damage is related to an acute myocardial infarction, this period can be very short. With more chronic processes, such as those which occur with hypertension or idiopathic cardiomyopathies, this period may extend over months or years. Indeed, when patients were first identified with asymptomatic LV dysfunction in the Studies of Left Ventricular Dysfunction (SOLVD) trial (discussed below), their average ejection fraction was already reduced to 28 percent, indicating that extensive ventricular damage had already occurred (Fig. 21-3). At this point, exercise performance, as represented by peak oxygen consumption, was moderately reduced, but not to an extent that limited exercise performance or produced symptoms. Circulating norepinephrine was increased slightly, while plasma renin levels (slashed lines) were not, except when diureties had been administered (open bars). Once symptoms occurred, there was a progressive increase in circulating norepinephrine and plasma renin. A progressive decline in exercise capacity was documented as patients

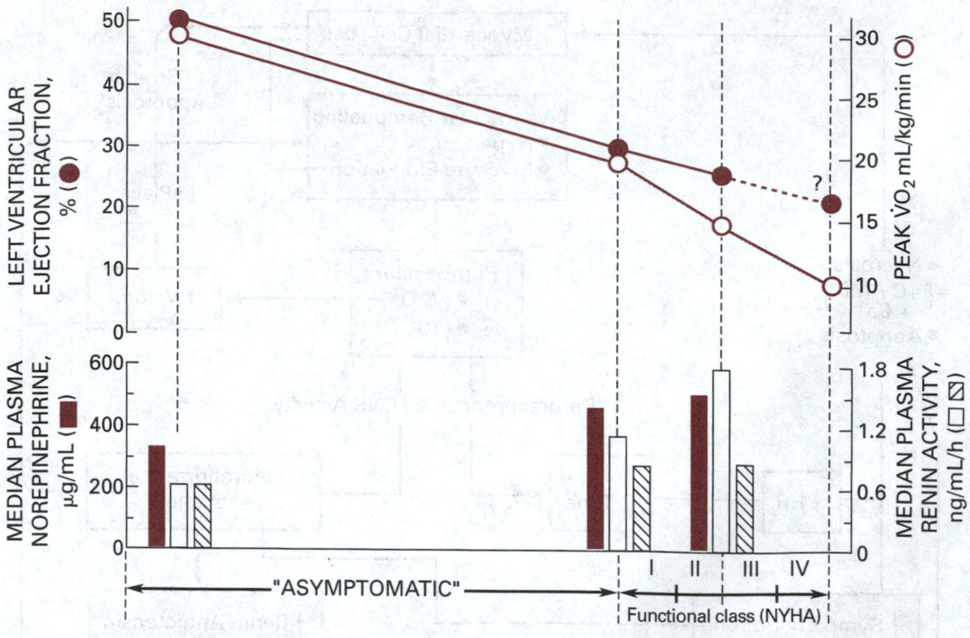

FIGURE 21-3 Progression of initial ventricular damage to sympathetic congestive heart failure. Data from the SOLVD trial of enalapril therapy, plotted in terms of LV ejection fraction and exercise capacity measured in terms of peak oxygen consumption (VO_2). Also shown are median plasma norepinephrine and plasma renin activity. The latter is shown in terms of patients who did or did not receive diuretics.

progressed from New York Heart Association (NYHA) class I to class IV. The reduction in exercise performance was relatively greater than the decrease in the ejection fraction. This relates to the finding that with inactivity, the capacity for peripheral vasodilatation is reduced, limiting skeletal muscle performance. Ventricular dysfunction may involve the left ventricle, the right ventricle, or both. In addition, such abnormalities may be amplified by overloads created by valvular insufficiency (e.g., mitral or tricuspid) or systolic overloads (e.g., aortic stenosis, arterial or pulmonary hypertension). Separating the effects of myocardial dysfunction from such imposed overloads is difficult. Moreover, functional mitral and/or tricuspid insufficiency resulting from ventricular dilatation imposes a further volume load on an already damaged myocardium.

Abnormalities of ventricular function can be usefully divided into problems of ventricular filling (diastole) and problems of ventricular emptying (systole). Even in the presence of normal systolic ventricular performance, abnormalities of ventricular filling, termed *diastolic ventricular dysfunction,* may be observed, and these abnormalities require specific diagnostic consideration (Fig. 21-4). This is characterized by an increased ventricular filling pressure for any end-diastolic volume (EDV) resulting from reduced compliance of the ventricle. Thus, with normal EDV and stroke volume (SV), filling pressures may be markedly increased, leading to signs of pulmonary congestion despite a normal ejection fraction. Such a situation may occur with LV hypertrophy, especially when associated with a rapid heart rate, which further limits the time for ventricular filling. It also can occur with an aging heart, where diffuse myocyte loss can occur with replacement fibrosis and reactive myocyte hypertrophy.[19]

Systolic ventricular dysfunction is characterized by a reduced ability to generate pressure isovolumically and a decreased capacity to eject blood in systole. As is known from classic physiology, the SV depends on the diastolic volume as well as the afterload, which is directly related to the arterial pressure. If the afterload is reasonably normal, there is a linear relation between SV and EDV, and the resultant slope (SV/EDV) is termed the *ejection fraction.* If the slope of the relation linking end-systolic pressure and LV volume is reduced, as occurs when the ventricle is depressed, the SV at any EDV is reduced, resulting in a decreased ejection fraction. If the afterload is approximately normal, this reduced ejection fraction can serve as a measure of *reduced systolic ventricular performance.* Since the extent of shortening of myocardium is reduced as afterload is increased, an increased systolic ventricular pres-

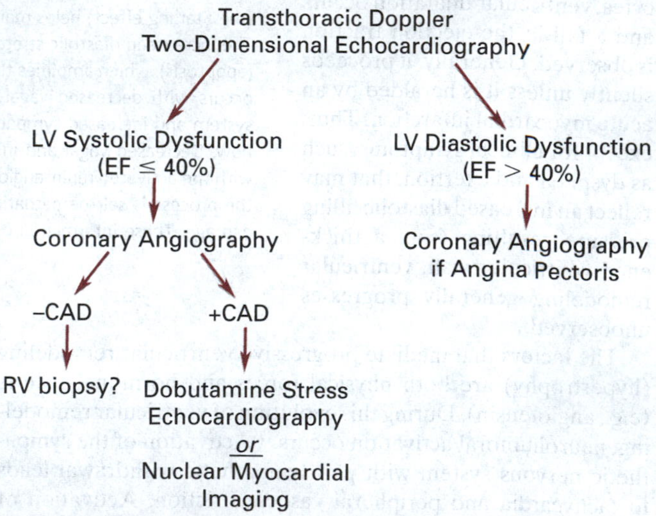

FIGURE 21-4 Evaluation of patients with congestive heart failure. Transthoracic Doppler and two-dimensional echocardiography provide a central modality to evaluate ventricular function and valvular abnormalities. Ventricular wall thickness and both end-diastolic and end-systolic volumes can be determined. With an ejection fraction (EF) more than 40 percent, coronary angiography is indicated in the presence of angina pectoris or evidence of significant ischemia. With an EF less than 40 percent, coronary arteriography is indicated since the underlying ischemic depression may be amenable to reperfusion by angioplasty or coronary bypass surgery. Nuclear imaging techniques are used to define viable ischemic myocardium, while stimulation of such myocardium with dobutamine or extrasystolic potentiation may indicate recoverable hibernating myocardium. Right ventricular biopsy may be indicated in the absence of coronary artery disease to rule out processes such as amyloid or sarcoid.

sure can by itself reduce SV and hence tend to decrease EF, as can occur in severe aortic stenosis. Similarly, with severe mitral insufficiency, which decreases afterload through a low-impedance pathway into the left atrium, an increased SV tends to occur, yielding an artificially increased ejection fraction. Thus, with these considerations in mind, the ejection fraction can provide a useful indicator of systolic ventricular performance.

Although complex indices of systolic ventricular function have been described on the basis of myocardial muscle function,[20] the measurement of the ejection fraction has served as the clinical standard, whether determined noninvasively by echocardiography and nuclear imaging techniques or invasively with angiography. In addition to an overall depression of myocardial function, focal abnormalities of ventricular wall motion, described in terms of hypokinesis and akinesis, may produce major alterations in overall LV function, as seen in coronary artery disease. While a segment of the LV wall may be replaced by fibrotic scar, focal abnormalities of contraction may occur in viable myocardium when coronary perfusion is transiently reduced, leading to a prolonged decrease in contraction; this is termed *stunning*. Alternatively, with a sustained reduction in coronary blood flow that is still adequate to sustain viability, contraction can be persistently reduced or absent; this is termed *hibernation*.[21,22] These important alterations can occur simultaneously in a given patient and are hard to separate.[22] Defining these abnormalities in coronary heart disease with heart failure is extremely important, since reversal of transient or persistent ischemia with vascular reperfusion may be vital for restoring segmental contraction and improving overall ventricular function.[21,23] Various techniques have been employed to identify such tissue, including echocardiographic studies using a catecholamine stress[24–28] and angiographic studies using nitroglycerin[29] or extrasystolic potentiation after a premature ventricular contraction.[21,30,31]

Once ventricular dysfunction is manifest, abnormalities of reflex control of the circulation ensue. As CHF progresses, decreased baroreceptor sensitivity occurs with augmented sympathetic tone and reduced parasympathetic tone (Fig. 21-2).[32] This results in an increase in heart rate along with reduced beat-to-beat heart rate variability and loss of the Valsalva overshoot. These changes also help establish the diagnosis of heart failure.

With reduced ventricular function, exercise performance tends to be reduced as measured by a reduced maximum O_2 uptake on a treadmill (VO_2). However, this reduction in exercise performance does not always correlate with a reduced ejection fraction,[5] since it also reflects the *training* state of the peripheral circulation.

Clinical Assessment in Directing Therapy

Clinically, the initial diagnosis of heart failure is made by the patient's history, physical findings on clinical examination, and data obtained from routine chest x-rays and electrocardiography (ECG). The history obtained from patients tends to reflect pulmonary or systemic congestion or both, with complaints of shortness of breath, initially with effort and on lying down, generally associated with easy fatigability and, commonly, peripheral edema. Common factors in the history often include diabetes mellitus, ischemic events, and hypertension. On physical examination, peripheral vasoconstriction and tachycardia are common, along with the presence of pulmonary rales and physical signs of pleural effusion. Cardiac findings may include a fourth heart sound (S_4), reflecting a stiffened or hypertrophied ventricle, and a third heart sound (S_3), reflecting more profound LV failure. Murmurs can be auscultated that may relate to valvular organic abnormalities, although functional mitral and tricuspid insufficiency can occur as a function of LV and/or right ventricular (RV) dilatation per se. Peripheral venous engorgement and an enlarged liver, along with peripheral edema, are detected as RV failure ensues. If RV failure is severe, clinical symptoms associated with LV failure, such as severe shortness of breath, actually may be lessened.

Precipitating factors for developing CHF should be looked for, such as anemia, infection, dietary indiscretion, acute arrhythmias (especially atrial fibrillation), poor compliance with treatment, pulmonary embolism, and occult myocardial infarction.

Nuclear imaging techniques, computed tomography, and magnetic resonance imaging have been useful in assessing ventricular volume, shapes, and motion and have provided an excellent assessment of ventricular function. However, two-dimensional echocardiography provides much of the necessary information in a practical and cost-effective manner and remains the clinical standard. Its accuracy and usefulness depend on the care expended in performing the procedure and the professional oversight utilized in both detecting and interpreting the findings that are obtained. Echo-Doppler examination not only provides information about systolic and diastolic volumes, and thus ejection fraction, but also allows for the evaluation of valve structure and function, including regurgitation and stenosis. Reasonably accurate measurements of gradients, and thus valvular orifices, can be made, and this can help direct therapy.

In defining the etiology of heart failure, segmental wall motion abnormalities with hypokinetic and contralateral hyperkinetic segments suggest an ischemic etiology. Indeed, after an acute myocardial infarction, a two-dimensional echocardiogram obtained within a few days is essential. The finding of ventricular dilatation within a few days of an acute anterior wall infarction tends to predict progressive LV dilatation with a falling ejection fraction. Among patients sustaining an anterior wall infarction without initial ventricular dilatation, approximately one-third will show ventricular dilatation at 3 months. In contrast, ventricular dilatation rarely occurs after inferior wall infarctions, except when the region involved is large, extending from the base of the heart to the apex. After an acute myocardial infarction,[33] LV enlargement, as measured by two-dimensional echocardiography, is associated with an increased incidence of adverse cardiovascular events. When LV diastolic volumes of patients with an infarction are divided into quartiles, patients in the fourth quartile have a mortality rate of 45.5 percent, while patients in the third quartile have a mortality rate of 21.1 percent and those in the first and second quartiles both have a mortality rate of 16.7 percent.[34] If LV dilatation occurs much later, however, two-dimensional echocardiography will not differentiate between the causes of heart failure, i.e., coronary artery disease or other etiologies. Moreover, patients with a primary cardiomyopathy also may exhibit segmental wall motion abnormalities. As was noted above, stimuli that elicit latent contraction, such as low-dose dobutamine, stress, and premature ventricular contractions, may help identify patients with dilated left ventricles and severe coronary artery disease who also have *hibernating* or *stunned* myocardium.[22,35,36]

THE TREATMENT OF CONGESTIVE HEART FAILURE

As was noted initially, the treatment of heart failure requires close attention to both the primary etiology and the relief of symptoms while attempting to reduce the risk of death from the process. This includes vigorous control of hypertension, if present, and an evaluation for treatment of myocardial ischemia. As was noted above and discussed further relative to surgical approaches to heart failure, noncontractile but viable myocardium, whether resulting from stunning or from hibernation, requires definition with consideration of coronary reperfusion.[22,37] Valvular disease that imposes an excessive volume or pressure overload must be considered relative to the need for surgical correction. For example, critical aortic stenosis with heart failure is an urgent indication for aortic valve replacement, when possible, not medical therapy. To those ends, there is a multifactorial approach to therapy[38] that varies with the etiology and stage of the heart failure process (Fig. 21-5).

General Principles in the Pharmacologic Treatment of CHF

Therapy is tailored to the phase of heart failure. In the initial phase, where ventricular damage is a primary concern, identification of etiology is essential with appropriate therapy. This might be termed treatment of ventricular dysfunction and its causes. Hypertension must be controlled aggressively. Even mild hypertension should be treated in the presence of the diabetic state to attempt to prevent large- and small-vessel coronary disease. Overt or silent ischemia should be identified and treated. Early inhibition of the neurohumoral responses to initial cardiac damage with both beta-adrenergic blockade and inhibition of the activated renin-angiotensin-aldosterone system (RAAS) requires consideration. This is particularly the case as one moves into the phase of ventricular remodeling in which inhibition of progressive ventricular damage is essential. It is important to remember that what bothers the patient, such as edema and shortness of breath, is generally not life-threatening, while therapy that may reduce mortality, such as beta blockers, may do nothing to alleviate symptoms. Thus, both agendas must be addressed. In general, mortality has been used to measure efficacy. Improvement in symptoms has been difficult to assess, and a combined end point of mortality and the need for hospitalization has been useful. As the syndrome of CHF ensues, pharmacologic treatment is directed to three demonstrable hemodynamic end points: (1) reducing volume overloads and maintaining a stable volume state, (2) reducing preload and afterload to enhance ventricular performance, and (3) improving ventricular contractility when necessary. An additional pharmacologic aim is to reduce heightened neurohumoral activity, which is seen in patients with heart failure, with the hope of limiting abnormal loading created by these systems and preventing the progression of the heart failure process. The ultimate aim is to reduce morbidity and perhaps extend life.

INACTIVATION OF THE RENIN-ANGIOTENSIN SYSTEM AND ALTERNATIVE THERAPIES

Neurohumoral activation plays an important role in the progression of the syndrome of chronic LV systolic dysfunction/heart failure. After initial increases in sympathetic tone and decreases in parasympathetic tone, the renin-angiotensin system is activated.[39] This generally occurs when diuretics are initiated or, in their absence, with the onset of the clinical symptoms of CHF. With release of renin from the kidneys, angiotensinogen, which is circulating in the blood, is converted to inactive angiotensin

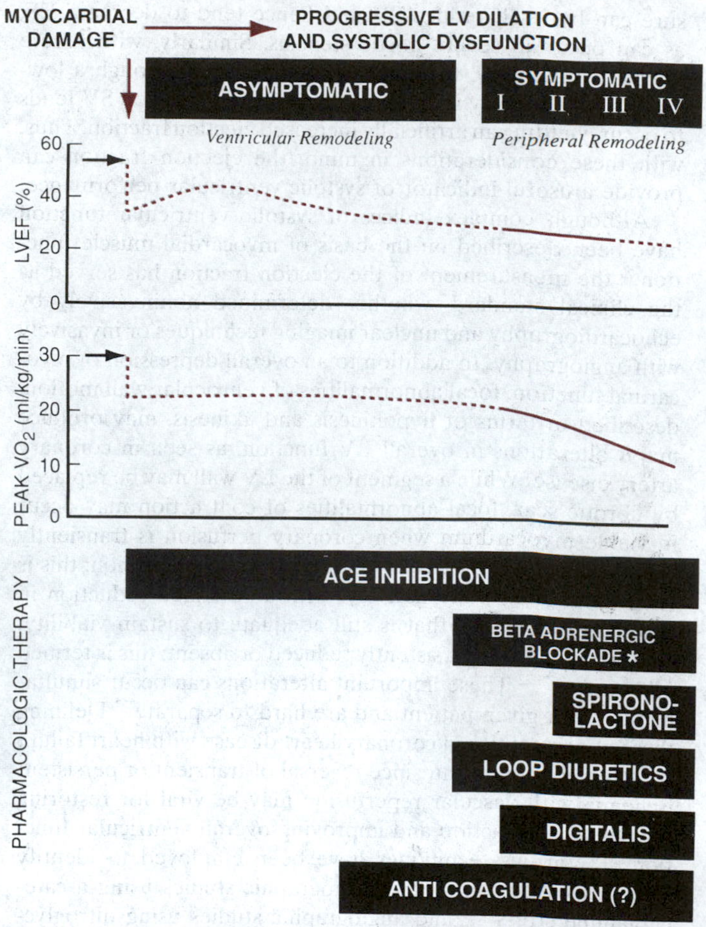

FIGURE 21-5 Staged use of therapeutic agents in heart failure. Initial approaches include control of factors that may cause progression of heart failure and/or augment its manifestations. Hypertension requires control. Unanticipated tachycardia may augment oxygen needs while reducing the time in diastole for coronary flow to take place. The reduction in the diastolic time can lead to marked elevations of left ventricular (LV) diastolic pressure as well as increased ischemia. Moreover, atrial fibrillation will deprive ventricular filling of the "atrial kick" and lead to further elimination of diastolic pressures. These considerations are of special importance with ventricular hypertrophy and resultant diastolic dysfunction. During the "remodeling" phase of ventricular failure, the patient may be asymptomatic. Nevertheless, inhibition of the renin-angiotensin system is indicated to reduce the rate of ventricular remodeling and slow ventricular dilation. Beta-adrenergic blockade reverses ventricular remodeling and improves survival in patients with class II to III symptoms. * Reflects the inconsistent effects of beta-adrenergic blockade in patients with class IV symptoms. In the Copernicus trial, carvedilol was beneficial, while in the BEST trial, bucindolol appears to be detrimental. Once symptoms ensue, loop diuretics generally are needed for fluid control. Digitalis glycosides also are indicated for neurohumoral benefits in reducing sympathetic tone and enhancing parasympathetic tone while providing modest inotropic support. These actions appear to improve morbidity without necessarily altering mortality.

I, which in turn is converted to the highly active angiotensin II by a converting enzyme that is ubiquitously located along vascular walls. Angiotensin II in turn stimulates aldosterone secretion by the adrenals, which results in sodium accumulation and also produces marked arteriolar constriction, which augments peripheral vascular resistance. Both phenomena, which increase ventricular preload (filling pressure) and afterload (systolic pressure), contribute to the clinical picture of CHF. In addition to these actions, angiotensin II serves as a growth factor, adding to myocardial hypertrophy and apparently fostering fibrosis. It also may contribute to subtle myocyte loss by enhancing apoptosis.[40]

TABLE 21-1 FDA-Approved Indications for ACE Inhibitors

ACE Inhibitor	Hypertension	CHF	Acute MI	LV Dysfunction	Diabetic Nephropathy
Benazepril	+				
Captopril	+	+		+[a]	+
Enalapril	+	+		+[b]	
Fosinopril	+	+			
Lisinopril	+	+	+		
Moexipril	+				
Perindopril	+				
Quinapril	+	+			
Ramipril	+	+[c]			
Trandolapril	+	+[d]		+[d]	

[a]Captopril is indicated in clinically stable patients with left ventricular (LV) dysfunction (ejection fraction ≤40 percent) after myocardial infarction (MI) to improve survival and reduce the incidence of overt heart failure.

[b]Enalapril is indicated in clinically stable asymptomatic patients with LV dysfunction (ejection fraction ≤35 percent) to decrease the rate of development of overt heart failure and decrease the incidence of hospitalization from congestive heart failure (CHF).

[c]Ramipril is indicated in stable patients who have demonstrated clinical signs of CHF within the first few days after sustaining acute MI to decrease mortality and progression to severe heart failure.

[d]Trandolapril is indicated for treatment of heart failure after MI and LV dysfunction after MI.

SOURCE: Reproduced with permission from Cheng A, Frishman WH. Use of angiotensin converting enzyme inhibitors as monotherapy and in combination with diuretics and calcium channel blockers. *J Clin Pharmacol* 1998; 38:477–491.

ANGIOTENSIN-CONVERTING ENZYME INHIBITORS

The initial impetus toward the use of angiotensin-converting enzyme (ACE) inhibitors for the treatment of patients with CHF was the desire to duplicate with one agent the hemodynamic effects produced by the combination of nitrate and hydralazine.[41] In the late 1970s, combined administration of nitrate and hydralazine was shown to enhance LV systolic performance and alleviate symptoms in patients with CHF.[42] In severe heart failure, this resulted from the combined action of nitrates to reduce diastolic filling pressures (preload) and hydralazine to reduce peripheral arterial resistance (afterload). The result was reduced filling pressures accompanied by an increased cardiac output. Initial hemodynamic studies with captopril (Table 21-1) demonstrated substantial lowering of ventricular filling pressures, a modest increase in cardiac output, and a reduction in systemic arterial pressure without tachycardia.[41] In a landmark randomized, placebo-controlled study, the administration of captopril for 3 months produced sustained improvement in LV performance, improvement in the functional class, and increased duration of maximal exercise,[43] resulting in U.S. Food and Drug Administration (FDA) approval of captopril for the treatment of CHF. In the first weeks of the study, exercise duration also improved in patients on placebo. This initial improvement in exercise duration on placebo probably is due to familiarization with exercise equipment and increased patient motivation.

Several aspects of long-term therapy with ACE inhibitors in patients with CHF are worthy of mention:

1. The magnitude of the initial hemodynamic change does not predict the long-term clinical response. Some of the beneficial effects of lower ventricular filling and systemic arterial pressures may relate to increased levels of kinins, resulting from decreased enzymatic destruction that also is mediated by ACE inhibitors.[44] Whether sustained elevation in kinin levels exerts long-term clinical benefits is uncertain. The dissociation between acute hemodynamic effects and long-term clinical benefit suggests that the mechanisms underlying the benefits of ACE inhibitors may be related to structural and functional changes in the peripheral vasculature. Improvement in peak aerobic capacity (VO_2) has been directly related to enhanced perfusion of skeletal muscle at maximal exercise.[45] The exact mechanisms that mediate the benefits of ACE inhibitors on the vasculature are poorly understood. The time differential between the acute, immediate hemodynamic and the more delayed functional benefits suggests that the cellular alterations produced by ACE inhibitors, rather than just the relief from heightened vasoconstriction, may mediate the clinical benefits. Improvement of vascular endothelial function, which is reversibly depressed in CHF, as through the response to local administration of acetylcholine, is so far the best documented vascular effect of ACE inhibitors in patients with CHF.[46,47] Improved vascular endothelial function during long-term ACE inhibition may be mediated in part via the kinins pathway. Whether lowering tissue levels of angiotensin II (AII) affects vascular smooth muscle structure and function is unknown. However, AII is a smooth muscle growth factor, and its reduction may reduce smooth muscle mass and thus affect vascular tone and compliance.[48]
2. The impact of long-term ACE inhibition on LV systolic function appears to be modest. Thus, the absolute increase in LV ejection fraction observed in large multicenter randomized trials ranged from 1 to 3 absolute units.[49] With long-term use of ACE inhibitors, LV end-diastolic and systolic volumes are only modestly altered and somewhat disparate in patients with CHF. Initial reduction in LV end-diastolic

volume during long-term ACE inhibition appears to be related largely to decreased loading of the failing ventricle rather than structural cardiac alterations, since LV volume increases within a few days after the withdrawal of ACE inhibition.[50] More recently, LV end-diastolic volume was noted to increase steadily during long-term ACE inhibition in patients with CHF while remaining unchanged in patients treated with AII type 1 receptor blockade (ARB) in addition to ACE inhibition.[51] However, persistent diastolic unloading with these agents may reduce the progression of dilatation.

3. Long-term use of ACE inhibitors has significant natriuretic effects. From a hormonal point of view, a decrease in AII tends to reduce aldosterone secretion, with a resultant lessening of sodium accumulation and a reduced potassium loss. However, aldosterone synthesis is modulated by factors other than AII, such as potassium levels, corticotropin, and endothelin, among others.[52] During long-term treatment with ACE inhibitors, levels of aldosterone remain elevated in up to 38 percent of patients of with CHF.[53] Thus, one cannot assume that long-term ACE inhibition alone can reliably lower plasma aldosterone levels. Increased diuresis with the consequent reduction in the dose of loop diuretics has been reported during long-term therapy with captopril.[54] This natriuretic effect of captopril may be related to the increase in renal blood flow demonstrated after the administration of captopril, despite the concomitant reduction in systemic arterial pressure.[55]

A major impetus for an increasing use of ACE inhibitors in patients with LV systolic dysfunction and CHF derives from the experimental work of Pfeffer and associates.[56] Ligation of the left anterior descending coronary artery in rats resulted in a large infarction and progressive ventricular dilatation. Long-term therapy with captopril reduced LV dilatation and shifted the pressure-volume curve favorably to the left. The process of LV enlargement in those experiments was largely dependent on the size and location of the myocardial infarct as well as the patency of the infarct-related artery. It was theorized that by lowering LV diastolic wall stress, long-term therapy with ACE inhibitors could favorably alter the loading conditions of the left ventricle and reduce LV enlargement, thus enhancing the survival of patients after a myocardial infarction.[57] A short-term trial in humans with acute myocardial infarction suggested that ventricular dilation could be attenuated with ACE inhibition (captopril).[58] A subsequent study with postinfarction patients with an ejection fraction less than 40 percent demonstrated a 21 percent reduction in mortality after 4 years.[58a] Of note, a similar reduction in reinfarction was observed.

In addition to the work of Pfeffer and associates,[56] several large survival trials were launched and completed exploring the effects of ACE inhibitors in patients with heart failure.[59] Beneficial effects of an ACE inhibitor on mortality in patients with CHF was first demonstrated with enalapril. The results of the Cooperative North Scandinavian Enalapril Study (CONSENSUS) involving 253 patients with symptoms compatible with NYHA functional class IV showed that after an average follow-up of 188 days, 68 of the 126 patients randomized to placebo died, while only 50 of 127 patients randomized to enalapril died, a reduction in mortality of 27 percent ($p = .003$).[60] The entire reduction in total mortality was found to occur among patients with progressive heart failure, whereas no difference was observed in the incidence of sudden death. After the initial dose of enalapril was reduced from 10 to 2.5 mg, only 3.2 percent of the patients could not tolerate enalapril because of symptomatic hypotension.

The second Veterans Administration Cooperative Vasodilator Heart Failure Trial (V-HeFT II) randomized 804 men with peak aerobic capacity <25 mL/kg per minute to enalapril or to hydralazine plus isosorbide dinitrate. At 2 years, the mortality was lower in the enalapril group than it was in the hydralazine plus isosorbide dinitrate group (18 percent versus 25 percent, $p = .016$; reduction in mortality, 28 percent).[61] The reduction in mortality, particularly in patients with less severe symptoms (NYHA classes I and II), was attributable to a reduction in sudden death. V-HeFT II also confirmed previous findings that treatment with long-term ACE inhibitor was associated with a minimal absolute increase in the LV ejection fraction, i.e., 2 percent with enalapril and 45 percent with hydralazine plus nitrate.

The SOLVD Study assessed the effect of ACE inhibition with enalapril in patients with symptomatic and asymptomatic LV systolic dysfunction as evidenced by an ejection fraction <35 percent.[62,63] Two thousand five hundred sixty-nine patients who had CHF as defined by the need for therapy and a mean ejection fraction of 24.8 percent were enrolled in the treatment arm of SOLVD and randomized to placebo or enalapril. Over a period of 48 months, 510 of the 1284 patients randomized to placebo died, while only 452 of the 1285 patients randomized to enalapril died [risk reduction, 10 percent; 95 percent confidence interval (CI), 5 to 26 percent; $p = .0036$]. The chief difference in mortality was due mostly to progressive heart failure, as the number of deaths classified as arrhythmogenic without worsening CHF was similar in the placedo and enalapril arms. Four thousand two hundred twenty-eight patients who were not treated for CHF and thus were considered asymptomatic had a mean ejection fraction of 28 percent and were enrolled in the prevention arm of SOLVD. Over a period of 37.4 months, 334 of the 2117 patients randomized to placebo and 313 of the 2111 patients randomized to enalapril died (risk reduction, 8 percent; 95 percent CI, 8 to 21 percent; $p = .030$). In the placebo group, 818 patients developed heart failure or died compared with only 630 patients in the enalapril group, i.e., 38.1 versus 29.8 percent (risk reduction, 29 percent; 95 percent CI, 21 to 30 percent; $p < .001$).

Of great note was a common effect of enalapril in both the treatment and prevention arms of the SOLVD trials to reduce the incidence of recurrent myocardial infarction, i.e., 288 in the enalapril group versus 362 in the placebo group (risk reduction, 23 percent; 95 percent CI, 11 to 34 percent; $p < .001$).[64] Similarly, 499 patients in the enalapril group and 595 in the placebo group developed unstable angina (risk reduction, 20 percent; 95 percent CI, 9 to 29 percent; $p < .001$). Whether this reduction in the incidence of acute coronary events in patients with coronary artery disease is associated with long-term ACE inhibition with enalapril or is related to the improvement in endothelium vasomotor dysfunction, which was subsequently demonstrated with quinapril, another ACE inhibitor, is not known.[46,65] It is also possible that ACE inhibition plays a role in stabilizing atherosclerotic plaques, perhaps by reducing smooth muscle growth. Importantly, as is noted below, the same considerations have been raised by the Survival and Ventricular Enlargement

(SAVE) trial of ACE inhibition in the depressed heart after myocardial infarction.

The impetus for an earlier use of an ACE inhibitor in patients with LV dysfunction and heart failure also has been provided by the results of the Heart Outcomes Prevention Evaluation (HOPE) study.[66] Therapy with ACE inhibitors traditionally has been recommended in patients with CHF related to LV systolic dysfunction, as defined by an LV ejection fraction <40 percent (to 35 percent) in most clinical trials. By demonstrating that long-term administration of ramipril, a tissue-specific ACE inhibitor, improved life expectancy in patients with vascular disease or diabetes and one cardiovascular factor who did not have any evidence of LV systolic dysfunction, the findings of the HOPE trial indirectly but strongly argued for the use of ACE inhibitors at a pre-LV dysfunction stage in patients with clinical conditions known to be associated with the development of chronic heart failure.[67] These results also emphasize the vascular benefits of ACE inhibitors, since other morbid vascular events, such as stroke, were reduced significantly. Since the conditions that lead to LV systolic and diastolic dysfunction are similar, the early use of ACE inhibitors is warranted in patients with both LV systolic and diastolic dysfunction. Besides the already mentioned effects of ACE inhibitors on skeletal muscle vasculature and the prevention of subsequent acute coronary events by ACE inhibitors in patients enrolled in the SOLVD and SAVE trials, the results of the HOPE trial point out the importance of the vascular effects of ACE inhibitors in mediating their clinical benefits. To a large extent, in the majority of patients with CHF, deterioration of LV function is related to progressive systemic and coronary vascular processes that now can be altered favorably by ACE inhibitors. The vascular benefits of ACE inhibitors appear to be additional to those provided by aspirin, beta-adrenergic blockers, and lipid-lowering agents.[66]

The fact that ramipril exerted vascular benefits in patients who were receiving aspirin is of particular importance, as the attenuations of the hemodynamic effects of ACE inhibitors have been reported in patients receiving aspirin.[68] The negative interaction between ACE inhibitors and aspirin presumably is due to interference with kinin-mediated synthesis of prostaglandin. The loss of benefit from ACE inhibitors noted in patients treated with aspirin in some large trials contrasts with the findings of the HOPE trials and others.[69] In view of the importance of the kinin pathway in vascular biology, one would expect that if a negative interaction exists between ACE inhibitors and aspirin, it would have been observed in patients enrolled in the HOPE trial. Whether the use of ticlopidine or clopidogrel is preferable in a subset of patients with LV dysfunction, CHF, and renal insufficiency who are treated with ACE inhibitors is unknown.

By preventing events related to myocardial ischemia and the progression of atherosclerosis, ACE inhibitors are becoming the cornerstone of both treatment and prevention in patients with LV dysfunction, independent of the presence or absence of symptoms. Whether patients should be treated for vascular protection with ACE inhibitors other than those specifically approved for the treatment of LV systolic dysfunction and CHF is unclear. So far no study has included clinical end points to show an advantage of one ACE inhibitor over another. Tissue-specific ACE inhibitors appear more apt to exert vascular benefits than do ACE inhibitors with low tissue specificity.[47] Tissue specificity is probably most relevant at low doses of ACE inhibitors; at maximally recommended doses of ACE inhibition, tissue specificity is less likely to be relevant. Overall, in several clinical trials and in daily practice the dose of ACE inhibitors is strikingly low.[62,63] The patients randomized to ACE inhibition in the SOLVD trial received only 11 mg of enalapril daily.[62] Several small studies and one large study [Assessment of Treatment with Lisinopril and Survival (ATLAS)] randomized patients to 2.5 to 3.5 mg or to 32.5 to 35 mg of lisinopril and showed that high doses of ACE inhibitors produce greater hemodynamic and clinical benefits.[70] Moreover, recent data suggest that even what is currently considered a maximal dose of ACE inhibitors may in fact be insufficient to completely block formation of AII via the ACE pathway, independent of the possible contribution of enzymatic pathways other than ACE to the generation of AII.[71] Thus, every effort should be made to increase the dose of ACE inhibitors to the maximally recommended or tolerated dose in every patient with LV systolic dysfunction and CHF. Unfortunately, this practice is not followed routinely.

In view of the clear benefits observed, all patients with documented LV dilatation should be treated with ACE inhibitors. The only patients with LV dysfunction who should not be treated with ACE inhibitors are pregnant women, patients with documented angioedema or anuria during earlier exposure to ACE inhibitors, and patients with severe bilateral artery stenosis. The benefits of ACE inhibitors have not been looked for in patients with serum creatinine levels >2.5 mg/dL, since those patients have been excluded from clinical trials. The important effects of ACE inhibitors on cardiovascular protection that are independent of any renal effects argue in favor of a trial of ACE inhibitors in patients with CHF with severe chronic renal insufficiency as defined by a serum creatinine level >3.0 mg/dL. However, patients with serum levels of creatinine >3.0 mg/dL require careful follow-up, including daily monitoring of renal function after the initiation of ACE inhibitors at the lowest possible dose. Since inhibition of AII production leads to dilatation of the efferent artery of the glomerulus, a decrease in glomerular perfusion pressure occurs and a modest rise in serum creatinine (0.5 to 1.9 mg/L) is anticipated. This poses no problem unless the creatinine continues to rise, in which case ACE inhibition needs to be reduced. Indeed, in the presence of diabetes, renal protection is afforded by ACE inhibition, and the rise in creatinine, which is reversible, does not reflect ACE inhibitor–induced renal damage.[72] Moreover, ACE inhibitors that are in part excreted by the liver are preferable in this clinical situation. Overall, it is always recommended to avoid prescribing nonsteroidal anti-inflammatory drugs (NSAIDs) in patients with CHF, but this is particularly important in patients with decreased renal function. Renal function is likely to deteriorate further after the initiation of ACE inhibitor therapy in patients treated with NSAIDs. Patients with plasma levels of potassium >5.0 mmol/L at baseline, particularly if they are diabetic with renal tubular acidosis, require daily measurement of electrolytes and renal function at the initiation of ACE inhibitor therapy.

A potential drug-drug interaction with aspirin and ACE inhibitors has been described, with a potential loss of the protective effects of ACE inhibition on patient survival in heart failure. However, this finding has not been substantiated in recent analyses of large clinical data bases.[69]

ALTERNATIVES TO ACE INHIBITORS

Angiotensin II Receptor Antagonists Several ARBs are approved by the FDA for the treatment of hypertension (losartan, valsartan, irbesartan, candesartan, telmisartan and eprosartan) (Fig. 21-6). Although trials are in progress involving the use of ARBs alone or in combination with ACE inhibitors in heart failure, none have been approved for this purpose. The first comparison of ACE inhibition with captopril (150 mg daily) and ARB (losartan 50 mg daily) was undertaken in 722 patients with CHF who were over 65 years old. The results suggested that losartan may be preferable to captopril.[73] The rate of death and hospitalization for heart failure was 9.4 percent in patients randomized to losartan and 13.2 percent in patients randomized to captopril (risk reduction 32 percent; 95 percent CI, 4 to 55 percent, $p = .075$). The results of ELITE I were not confirmed by a subsequent study of identical design that included over 3000 patients, ELITE II.[74] In fact, while the number of deaths or hospitalizations was similar during the first 12 months of the study, thereafter fewer patients randomized to captopril died or were hospitalized for heart failure compared with patients randomized to losartan. Thus, the results of ELITE II failed to confirm the hypothesis derived from ELITE I, suggesting that ARBs may be superior to ACE inhibition for the treatment of patients with CHF. Of note, the design of ELITE II and the number of patients studied do not allow one to conclude that the two interventions are equal, based on a lack of statistical difference between the number of events noted in patients randomized to captopril and that in patients randomized to losartan. The ELITE II trial also must be viewed as inconclusive since there remains a question of adequate dosage and, as noted below, the potential for the concomitant use of ACE inhibition and ARBs.

The present use of ARBs for the treatment of CHF is limited to patients who experience intolerable cough or angioedema while receiving ACE inhibitors. Patients who cannot tolerate ACE inhibitors because of worsening renal function or hyperkalemia are likely to experience similar side effects with ARBs.

Another potential use of ARBs for the management of CHF is to counteract the attenuation of the benefits of ACE inhibition that may occur with time, a phenomenon often referred to as *ACE escape*. After long-term (1 year) ACE inhibition, plasma AII levels rise above initial values and LV antiremodeling and the decrease in norepinephrine levels effects attenuate.[75–77] Whether this is due to ACE inhibition becoming partial with time or whether AII is generated via pathways other than the converting enzyme is controversial.[78] Independent of the underlying mechanisms that mediate ACE escape, the addition of ARB to ACE inhibition negates the detrimental effects of elevated levels of tissue and circulating angiotensin.[79]

Several experimental and small studies have clearly demonstrated the added benefits of combined ARB and ACE inhibition on LV performance, functional capacity, and safety.[80–84] The safety of combining ARB and ACE inhibition has been well documented in the Valsartan Heart Failure Trial (Val-HeFT), which has safely randomized 4000 patients treated with adequate doses of ACE inhibitors to 320 mg daily of valsartan or to placebo. The results of Val-HeFT are not yet known, but enrollment and maintenance into the trial were uneventful. The addition of ARBs to ACE inhibitors is extremely well tolerated even in patients who do not tolerate high doses of ACE inhibitors because of symptomatic hypotension.[82] This may be explained by the fact that ARBs are specific vasodilators that lower vascular resistance primarily to essential organs such as the heart, brain, and kidneys. In contrast, as a result of the concomitant increases in kinin levels, ACE inhibitors are also nonspecific vasodilators that lower vascular resistance to cutaneous tissues and splanchnic beds.[85] In addition, ARBs are associated with a greater improvement in plasma fibrinolytic parameters than that achieved by ACE inhibitors.[86] Whether the beneficial effects of combined ARB and ACE inhibition on functional capacity and LV performance and dimensions will

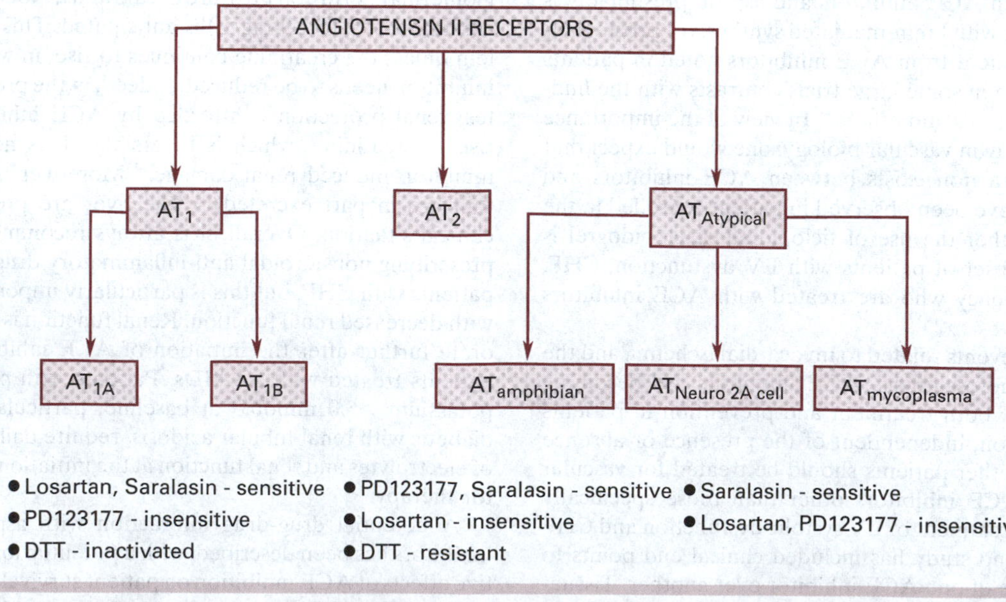

FIGURE 21-6 The classification and characteristics of angiotensin II receptors. DTT, dithiothreitol. (From Kang PM, Landau AJ, Eberhardt RT, Frishman WH. Angiotensin II receptor antagonists: A new approach to blockade of the renin-angiotensin system. *Am Heart J* 1994; 127:1388–1401.)

translate into added benefits in life expectancy over those provided by ACE inhibition alone is being evaluated in the Val-HeFT trial with valsartan and the CHARM trial with candesartan.

Other Vasodilators Vasodilator agents may be used as adjunctive therapy in the management of heart failure. The combination of hydralazine and isosorbide dinitrate is an alternative therapy when ACE inhibitors are contraindicated or cannot be tolerated. Daily doses of hydralazine up to 300 mg in combination with isosorbide dinitrate 160 mg in the presence of cardiac glycosides and diuretics probably have some effect in reducing mortality in patients with chronic heart failure but not in reducing hospitalization for heart failure.[87] At these doses, the combination increased exercise performance more than enalapril did.[61] The effects of hydralazine and nitrates, alone or in combination, when added to ACE inhibitors are unknown. There is no evidence of proven benefit when either nitrates or hydralazine is used alone, but nitrates often are prescribed without hydralazine. Nitrates also may be used effectively for the treatment of concomitant angina. Early development of hemodynamic tolerance (tachyphylaxis) to nitrates may occur with frequent dosing (every 4 to 6 h) but is less with intervals of 8 to 12 h[88] or in conjunction with ACE inhibition. Also, hemodynamic tolerance may be less during coadministration with hydralazine.[89]

Prostacyclin, which is a potent systemic vasodilator used in the treatment of primary pulmonary hypertension, has not been shown to improve mortality outcomes in patients with heart failure despite improvements in hemodynamics. Similarly, alpha blockers, despite their potent vasodilatory activity, have not shown benefit in patients with chronic heart failure; this probably is related to hemodynamic tolerance with prolonged drug treatment.

Calcium Antagonists Calcium antagonists are not recommended for the treatment of CHF because of their negative inotropic effects. However, second-generation dihydropyridine-type calcium antagonists such as amlodipine and felodipine may be considered for the treatment of concomitant arterial hypertension or angina. Some second-generation calcium antagonists are still under investigation with respect to their long-term effect on mortality in chronic heart failure, in addition to baseline therapy including ACE inhibition. Preliminary data indicate either no effect[90] or a positive outcome in restricted patient populations, i.e., in patients with idiopathic dilated cardiomyopathy.[91] Although in these studies the second-generation dihydropyridine agents evaluated appeared to be safe and seemed not to increase mortality, there are no reasons to recommend these agents for the treatment of heart failure caused by systolic dysfunction; rather, they can be recommended as adjunctive medication for ischemia. As a result of the potential benefits noted below, however, beta blockers should be preferable to calcium blockers for patients with CHF and ischemia.

A study is in progress evaluating the dihydropyridine agent amlodipine as an adjunctive therapy for patients with congestive cardiomyopathy. Similarly, the selective T-channel calcium antagonist mibefradil, a drug that has no apparent effect on myocardial function,[92] has been studied. No beneficial effects of mibefradil on survival were demonstrated in patients with heart failure, and unfavorable drug-drug interactions, especially with amiodarone, led to the withdrawal of mibefradil from the market.[93] The use of calcium blockers in patients with diastolic dysfunction (e.g., verapamil) has been reported, but there are no long-term outcome studies with this form of treatment. The use of verapamil in the treatment of patients with hypertrophic cardiomyopathy has been well defined.[92]

BETA-ADRENERGIC BLOCKADE

In view of the marked benefits afforded by beta-adrenergic blockade in patients with heart failure after a myocardial infarction, beta-adrenergic blockade was advocated 25 years ago by Waagstein and colleagues for the treatment of patients with dilated cardiomyopathies.[94] In the BHAT trial, in which propranolol was begun 7 to 21 days after an acute MI and continued for 24 months, 5 lives per 100 were saved when heart failure was present, and only 2 lives when heart failure was absent.[95] Just as the use of ACE inhibitors in patients with CHF did not become widely accepted until the positive results of large survival trials such as CONSENSUS I, SOLVD, and V-HeFT II were known, the use of beta-blocking agents did not gain broad acceptance until large survival trials demonstrated the benefits of beta-adrenergic blockade on survival in patients with CHF.[96,97] The Cardiac Insufficiency Bisoprolol Study II (CIBIS II) evaluated the effects of bisoprolol, a beta$_1$-selective adrenergic blocker, on mortality from all causes in patients with CHF treated with standard medical regimens, including ACE inhibitors.[98] This multicenter placebo-controlled trial was conducted in Europe and enrolled 2647 patients with CHF characterized by functional class III–IV according to the NYHA and an LV ejection fraction <40 percent. Treated patients received up to 10 mg of bisoprolol. The trial was discontinued prematurely because mortality from all causes was significantly lower in the bisoprolol group than it was in the placebo group. Of the 1320 patients receiving bisoprolol, 156 died; of the 1327 patients randomized to placebo, 228 died. The estimated annual mortality rate was 8.8 percent in the bisoprolol group and 13.2 percent in the placebo group (hazard ratio, 0.66; 95 percent CI, 0.54–0.81 percent). The most common dose of bisoprolol was 10 mg in 564 patients, followed by 5 mg in 176 patients and 7.5 mg in 152 patients. Sudden death and hospitalization for worsening CHF were 42 percent and 32 percent lower in patients randomized to bisoprolol, respectively. In summary, in a trial that did not include a run-in period and thus did not select patients who tolerated beta-adrenergic blockade, bisoprolol lowered the risk of mortality from all causes by 32 percent. Bisoprolol was equally efficacious in patients with ischemic cardiomyopathy and patients in functional classes II and IV. However, in view of the overall low mortality rate of patients randomized to placebo, one may question how many patients were really in functional class IV before prerandomization.

In the Metoprolol CR/XL Randomised Intervention Trial (MERIT-HF), the effects of a controlled-release/extended-release formulation of metoprolol (CR/XL) on mortality was studied in patients with CHF treated with a standard medical regimen, including ACE inhibitors.[99] The 3991 patients with LV ejection fractions <40 and functional class II–IV were randomized to metoprolol (target dose 200 mg) for 2 months or to placebo after a 2-week single-blind placebo period. The study was terminated prematurely on the recommendation of the safety committee after a mean follow-up of 12 months. One hundred forty-five of the 1990 patients randomized to metoprolol died, and 217 of the 2001 patients randomized to placebo died ($p = .0062$). The mortality rates were 7.2 percent and 22 percent per patient-year of follow-up, respectively, with a relative risk of 0.66 (95 percent CI, 0.53–0.81 percent). Sudden death and death from aggravated heart failure were less frequent among treated patients: 79 versus 132, 0.59 (0.45–0.78), $p < .0002$, and 30 versus 58, 0.51 (0.33–0.79), $p = .0023$. The mean daily dose of metoprolol was 159 mg, with 87 percent of patients receiving more than 100 mg and 64 percent receiving the target dose of 200 mg. In summary, as demonstrated with bisoprolol, metoprolol CR/XL lowered mortality from all causes by 34 percent in patients with CHF already treated with ACE inhibitors and diuretics. As was noted in the CIBIS II trial, most of the patients enrolled in the MERIT-HF trial had moderate CHF, as evidenced by the low mortality of patients in the placebo group. Few patients in functional class IV participated in MERIT-HF. Thus, too few patients in functional class IV were randomized to active therapy in both the CIBIS II and MERIT-HF trials to assess the safety and efficacy of bisoprolol and metoprolol in this population. Both the CIBIS II and MERIT-HF trials demonstrated that mortality from all causes can be reduced by a selective $beta_1$-adrenergic agent in patients with mild to moderate CHF. Metoprolol is about 80-fold more selective for the human $beta_1$ than for the $beta_2$ receptor, and bisoprolol is approximately 120-fold more selective.[100]

While both $beta_1$ and $beta_2$ receptors are present in the normal human myocardium, $beta_2$ receptors predominate in the human failing myocardium, since $beta_1$ receptors are downregulated.[101] Thus, selection of a nonselective beta-blocking agent may seem preferable when the therapeutic aim is to protect the heart from beta-adrenergic stimulation. In the United States, most of the experience in treating patients with beta-adrenergic blockers has been gained with nonselective agents such as carvedilol and bucindolol. In addition to being a nonselective beta-adrenergic blocker, carvedilol has alpha-blocking and antioxidant properties, while bucindolol has direct vasodilating properties.[102]

Carvedilol is the only beta blocker currently approved by the FDA for the treatment of patients with CHF.[102] Since a long-term survival trial has not been conducted with carvedilol, its approved use is for delaying the progression of myocardial disease and heart failure. The U.S. Carvedilol Program was composed of four trials and was stopped prematurely by the safety committee because of a highly significant reduction in mortality in treated patients (65 percent, $p < .0001$) compared with placebo.[102–107] The four trials were the Multicenter Oral Carvedilol in Heart Failure Assessment (MOCHA), the Prospective Randomized Evaluation of Carvedilol in Symptoms and Exercise (PRECISE), and the "mild" and "severe" heart failure trials.[103–106] The intended duration of these trials was 6 months. The primary end points were submaximal exercise for the MOCHA and PRECISE trials; a composite end point of death, reduction in cardiovascular hospitalizations, and a need to increase heart failure medications for the "mild" heart failure trial; and quality-of-life evaluation for the "severe" heart failure trial. The MOCHA and PRECISE trials had completed enrollment by the time the program was interrupted. Whereas primary end points were not reached expect in the "mild" heart failure trial, the average LV ejection fraction increased substantially in patients randomized to carvedilol in all the trials, while LV ejection fraction remained unaltered in patients randomized to placebo.[103–106] The improvement in LV ejection fraction was noted in patients who were already receiving optimal standard therapy, including ACE inhibitors. A dose-related reduction in mortality and enhancement of LV ejection fraction was noted in the MOCHA trial.[103] Cardiovascular hospitalizations were fewer and symptoms were alleviated in patients randomized to carvedilol in the PRECISE trials.[104] Lastly, global heart failure assessments were improved in patients randomized to carvedilol in the "severe" heart failure trial.[106] Thus, although the primary end points were different, the carvedilol trials demonstrated substantial reduction in mortality and dose-dependent improvement in the ejection fraction. This improvement was present in both ischemic and nonischemic cardiomyopathies, although it was greater in the latter group.

The Australia–New Zealand (ANZ) trial included an initial phase of 6 months and a longer phase with an average follow-up of 19 months.[108] Submaximal exercise, the end point of the initial phase, remained unchanged in patients randomized to carvedilol. During the second phase of the ANZ trial, fewer patients randomized to carvedilol died or were hospitalized.

The effects of beta-adrenergic blockade on LV function and dimensions are unique. No other pharmacologic intervention has been shown to reverse LV remodeling and improve LV ejection fraction so consistently in patients with CHF caused by LV systolic dysfunction. In all clinical trials in which patients received beta-blocking agents for at least 3 months, LV ejection fraction increased.[102] Long-term administration of selective and nonselective beta-blocking agents increases LV ejection fraction consistently to a much greater extent than is achieved by vasodilator therapy. The long-term benefits of beta-adrenergic blockade on LV performance are in contrast with the deterioration that may be observed initially. The time course of the effects of beta-adrenergic blockade includes an initial reduction in LV ejection fraction during the first weeks of treatment, a return to the initial ejection fraction at 4 weeks, and a substantial increase ranging from 5 to 10 absolute units at 3 months.[109] Thereafter, from 4 to 12 months, LV end-systolic and end-diastolic volumes and mass steadily decrease, a phenomenon often referred to as *reversed remodeling*.[110] Reversal of LV remodeling has been documented with carvedilol at 12 months in a substudy of the ANZ trial.[111] At 1 year, LV ejection fraction was greater and LV end-diastolic volume index was 14 mL/m^2 smaller in patients randomized to carvedilol than was the case in patients randomized to placebo.[111]

Not every patient benefits from long-term adrenergic blockade. In those who benefit, the rise in ejection fraction averages 10 percent. Increases in LV ejection fraction up to 15 to 20 percent with a normalization of LV volumes have been observed in individual patients. Systolic blood pressure and myocardial contractility, as evaluated by LV maximal rate of rise of pressure (dp/dt), are predictors of the response to long-term beta-adrenergic blockade in terms of LV ejection fraction.[112] The higher systolic blood pressure and LV dp/dt are, the more likely the ejection fraction is to increase during long-term beta-adrenergic blockade. Thus, patients with mild to moderate CHF and LV systolic dysfunction are the optimal candidates for beta-adrenergic blockade. Conversely, beta-adrenergic blockade is unlikely to benefit, and at present is not recommended for, patients in functional class IV with extremely reduced ejection fractions. Despite the fact that patients in functional class IV are the least likely to benefit from long-term beta-adrenergic blockade, they are the most likely to decompensate at the initiation of therapy as a result of their lack of cardiac reserve. Exacerbation of LV dysfunction at the initiation of therapy often leads to worsening CHF and hospitalization. The Beta Blocker Estimation of Survival Trial (BEST), a large randomized, placebo-controlled study of the effect of bucindolol, a third-generation beta-adrenergic blocking agent with direct vasodilating properties, on the survival of 2708 patients with NYHA functional class III and IV, was stopped because of the lack of benefit seen. A preliminary report indicates that whereas bucindolol reduced mortality in patients in functional class III, it did not do so in patients in functional class IV.

The long-term and acute effects of beta-adrenergic blockade on LV performance have important therapeutic and pathophysiologic implications. First, the deterioration in LV performance that is observed routinely during the first weeks of therapy mandates that beta-adrenergic blockade be initiated at the lowest dose possible of a given agent in stable patients with CHF. Since beta-adrenergic blockade is aimed at altering the progression of the syndrome of CHF and not at providing acute relief of symptoms, effective beta blockade can be reached progressively by increasing doses of beta blocker agents every 2 to 3 weeks. When CHF is associated with angina or excessive tachycardia and effective beta blockade is needed for control of symptoms, the doses of beta blockers can be increased every few days under close in-hospital monitoring. An important unresolved issue concerning beta-adrenergic blockade in CHF is the treatment of patients whose symptoms worsen to functional class IV while they are being treated with beta-blocking agents. No data are available to provide guidelines to manage these patients. A pragmatic approach is to hospitalize patients who decompensate while receiving beta blockade and treat them with temporary inotropic support with a specific phosphodiesterase inhibitor, such as milrinone, which does not require beta receptors for its activity. Patients who improve are kept on a beta-adrenergic blocker, and inotropic support is discontinued after a few days. Beta-adrenergic blockade should be tapered off and withdrawn in patients who fail to improve. The pathophysiologic implication of successful beta-adrenergic blockade is that the process of LV dysfunction can be reversed by pharmacologic means even in patients with markedly reduced LV function. Thus, a certain amount of plasticity that was previously unrecognized remains in dilated fibrotic left ventricles. The cellular and molecular mechanisms that reverse myocyte dysfunction, thereby enhancing global LV performance, are poorly understood (Table 21-2). Since patients with both ischemic and nonischemic cardiomyopathy benefit from long-term beta-adrenergic blockade, dysfunction of surviving myocytes is a common characteristic of CHF independent of its etiology.[113] Patients with nonischemic cardiomyopathy were initially thought to experience greater benefit from long-term beta blockade compared with patients with ischemic cardiomyopathy. Since it is practically impossible to compare patients with different etiologies of CHF at a similar stage of their disease process, definite conclusions concerning the effects of long-term beta-adrenergic blockade as a function of the etiology probably should not be drawn.

The selection of a beta-adrenergic blocker for the treatment of CHF is at the present time somewhat academic, since carvedilol is the only beta blocker approved by the FDA for this indication in the United States. The rationale for selecting a nonselective agent over a selective $beta_1$ antagonist has been mentioned previously. Studies comparing a selective versus a nonselective agent are few and have enrolled small numbers of patients. Their results are controversial. In a 6-month study of 67 patients randomized to carvedilol or metoprolol, Kukin and associates demonstrated no significant difference between these agents.[114] In contrast, carvedilol was reported to enhance LV function and reverse LVE remodeling in patients with dilated cardiomyopathy who were failing metoprolol therapy.[115] Similarly, compared with metoprolol, carvedilol was found by Gilbert and colleagues to produce greater improvement in functional class and LV performance in patients with idiopathic dilated cardiomyopathy.[116] Lastly, the antioxidant properties of carvedilol were recently documented in vivo by demonstrating an inhibition of reactive oxygen species generation by leukocytes.[117] The clinical relevance of the antioxidant action of carvedilol remains to be determined in patients with CHF. A large trial comparing the respective benefits of carvedilol and metoprolol in patients with CHF is under way [Carvedilol or Metoprolol Evaluation Trial (COMET)]. Whether enough events will occur in the patients enrolled in the COMET trial to detect a meaningful difference between these agents is uncertain. In addition, a trial is in place [Carvedilol Prospective Randomized Cumulative Survival Trial (COPERNICUS)] that is examining the effects of carvedilol in class IV patients.

TABLE 21-2 Possible Mechanisms by Which Beta-Adrenergic Blockers Improve Ventricular Function in Chronic Congestive Heart Failure

1. Upregulation of beta receptors
2. Direct myocardial protective action against catecholamine toxicity
3. Improved ability of noradrenergic sympathetic nerves to synthesize norepinephrine
4. Decreased release of norepinephrine from sympathetic nerve endings
5. Decreased stimulation of other vasoconstrictive systems, including renin-angiotensin-aldosterone, vasopression, and endothelin
6. Potentiation of kalikrein-kinin system and natural vasodilatation (increase in bradykinin)
7. Antiarrhythmic effects raising ventricular fibrillation threshold
8. Protection against catecholamine-induced hypokalemia
9. Increase in coronary blood flow by reducing heart rate and improving diastolic perfusion time; possible coronary dilation with vasodilator–beta blocker
10. Restoration of abnormal baroreflex function
11. Prevention of ventricular muscle hypertrophy and vascular remodeling
12. Antioxidant effects (carvedilol?)
13. Shift from free fatty acid to carbohydrate metabolism (improved metabolic efficiency)
14. Vasodilation (e.g., bucindolol, carvedilol)
15. Antiapoptosis effect
16. Improved left atrial contribution to left ventricular filling

In summary, in the absence of an indication such as reversible airways obstructive disease, advanced heart block, or episodic decompensation, all symptomatic patients with CHF, except those in functional class IV, should be treated with long-term beta-adrenergic blockade.[3,101,102] Treatment should be initiated at the lowest possible dose and advanced to full beta blockade over 1 to 2 months as tolerated. Patients who do not tolerate the full dose should be kept on intermediate doses that still result in substantial improvement in LV function and a reduction in mortality.[102] Beta-adrenergic blockade is the only pharmacologic intervention that reverses LV remodeling, whereas ACE inhibition is the only intervention that improves the vascular processes. Thus, beta-adrenergic blockade is not an exclusive intervention but a complementary intervention. Both ACE inhibition and beta-adrenergic blockade are essential interventions for the treatment of CHF.

DIURETICS

Sodium accumulation tends to occur in the early stages of CHF, with peripheral edema accompanied by weight gain. Diuretics, along with salt restriction, remain the best therapeutic tool for treating the edematous state in heart failure. Despite the advent of new agents for treating symptomatic CHF, diuretics continue to be among the most commonly prescribed drugs in the world.

The mechanism for edema is generally multifactorial and includes renal vasoconstriction, increased aldosterone and vasopressin activity, and/or increased venous pressures. Increased sympathetic nervous system activity (tone) tends to occur early in the course of heart failure. Activation of the renin-angiotensin axis tends to occur somewhat later, commonly when diuretics are begun.[39] This leads to increased aldosterone, leading to sodium accumulation and potassium loss. Even with asymptomatic LV dysfunction, avidity of the kidneys for sodium and water is enhanced greatly, and peripheral edema constitutes an early physical sign that brings the problem of CHF to the physician's attention. Salt and water retention leads to an expanded intravascular volume, with an increase in LV filling pressures to maintain cardiac output.[118] With continued worsening of LV function, progressive volume expansion continues and LV end-diastolic pressure rises along with venous hydrostatic pressure in both the systemic and pulmonary beds. This alteration in Starling forces favors transudation of intravascular fluid into the interstitial compartment, culminating in edema formation.[119] Eventually a point is reached at which additional increases in LV filling pressure fail to augment cardiac output, and with progressive increases in peripheral arterial vasoconstriction, renal perfusion is reduced. By this time, overt heart failure is established, and the kidney's ability to excrete a salt load is severely impaired.[118] Important mediators in this process are (1) activation of the renin-angiotensin-aldosterone axis, (2) stimulation of the sympathetic nervous system, (3) increased levels of antidiuretic hormone leading to water retention and hyponatremia, and (4) resistance to atrial natriuretic peptide (ANP), which is an endogenous hormonal vasodilator and diuretic.

The appropriate use of diuretics depends on the stage of disease and severity. With mild fluid accumulation characterized by peripheral edema, pulmonary rales, and weight gain, oral diuretics are indicated. Long-acting but less potent diuretics, such as hydrochlorothiazide and chlorthalidone, may be adequate. Intermittent use of more potent loop diuretics, such as furosemide, bumetanide, and torsemide, may allow one to regain dry weight more rapidly. Efficacy can be assessed by daily weights, and diuretic regimens can be adjusted appropriately.

Loop Diuretics The most potent diuretics are those whose action occurs in the medullary thick ascending limb of Henle because of the percentage of filtrate reabsorption that occurs at this segment of the nephron. In the euvolemic state, about 20 percent of filtered sodium load is reabsorbed in the thick ascending limb, compared with only 7 percent in the distal tubule and 5 percent in the collecting duct.[120] Drugs in this diuretic class include furosemide, bumetanide, torsemide, and ethacrynic acid. The loop diuretics are more than 98 percent protein-bound and therefore are not freely filtered by the glomerulus. Rather, they access the tubular lumen, where they act by secretion via an organic anion transporter.[121] This secretion of loop diuretic may be impaired and their action may be limited by the presence of elevated levels of endogenous organic acids, as occurs in renal failure, and by probenecid, salicylates, and NSAIDs. Once in the lumen of the tubule, the loop diuretics compete with chloride for binding to the $Na^+/K^+/2Cl$ contransporter situated on the apical membrane of cells of the medullary thick ascending limb, thus inhibiting the reabsorption of both sodium and chloride.[122] The urinary diuretic concentration best represents the fraction of drug delivered to the thick ascending limb and significantly correlates with the natriuretic response after diuretic administration.[123]

Furosemide is the most widely used loop diuretic. In normal patients, the oral bioavailability of furosemide is 50 percent. After an oral dose, the onset of action occurs within 30 to 60 min, peaks at 1 to 2 h, and has a duration of action of 6 h, with a half-life of 50 min.[121,124] Furosemide may be given intravenously over 1 to 2 min; after intravenous administration, diuresis begins within 15 min and peaks at 30 to 60 min. The duration of action is up to 2 h when the drug is given intravenously. Sixty percent of furosemide is excreted unchanged in the urine; the rest is conjugated with glucuronic acid in the kidney.[121,124] In renal insufficiency [glomerular filtration rate (GFR) >30 mL/min)], the elimination half-life is prolonged, although the diuretic response is impaired, largely owing to reduced drug delivery to its site of action within the tubule.[125]

In CHF, the pharmacokinetics of oral furosemide are also altered; furosemide absorption is delayed, which leads to a delay in the time at which peak concentration occurs.[123] Altered pharmacodynamic properties of furosemide occur independent of the route of administration, resulting from adaptations within the glomerular microcirculation and renal tubule that are present during chronic diuretic administration.[123] Bumetanide is 40 times more potent than furosemide and is available in both oral and intravenous formulations. In normal patients, the bioavailability is 80 percent after an oral dose, and the onset of diuretic effect occurs within 30 min and peaks within 1 h. The duration of action of oral bumetanide is between 3 and 6 h, with a half-life between 1 and 3.5 h.[124,126] Similar to furosemide, the delayed absorption of oral bumetanide in heart failure results in lower peak concentrations as well as a delayed time to peak concentration.

Torsemide is a newer loop diuretic that differs from others in its class in that 80 percent of a dose undergoes hepatic metabolism. Because only 20 percent of the drug is excreted unchanged in the urine, its half-life is altered minimally in renal failure.[127]

Torsemide is absorbed rapidly and is 80 to 90 percent bioavailable. In patients with chronic renal insufficiency or with cirrhosis, the natriuretic response after torsemide is unaffected by the route of administration.[128] Maximal sodium excretion occurs within the first 2 h after either routine. In healthy individuals, the half-life of torsemide is 3.3 h, but it is prolonged to 8 h in cirrhosis.[127,129] When selecting an oral agent in patients with heart failure, the physician may find oral torsemide to be advantageous since its absorption is unimpaired and is less variable than that of oral furosemide.[130] In fact, the pharmacokinetics of torsemide in CHF patients are comparable to those in normal persons. As is the case with all loop diuretics, however, dose-response curves for torsemide in patients with CHF are shifted downward and to the right, suggesting altered drug pharmacodynamics and a diminished diuretic response. The efficacy of loop diuretics often is reduced significantly in patients with decompensated heart failure. Impaired drug absorption has been implicated as one cause of variable efficacy. Reduced gastric and intestinal motility, an edematous bowel wall, and decreased splanchnic blood flow may delay absorption. The total amount of furosemide absorbed over 24 h, however, is similar to that found in normal individuals.[131–133]

In patients with stable, compensated heart failure who are given oral furosemide, the time to peak urinary excretion is prolonged to about 190 min (normal, 90 min) and peak urinary excretion rate is reduced by 50 percent.[123] Furosemide and bumetanide, when given in doses of equivalent potency, induce a similar natriuretic response in patients with heart failure.[123] The pharmacokinetic properties of intravenous furosemide are unaltered in heart failure patients compared with normal individuals.[134]

The effectiveness of loop diuretics is limited by two phenomena in patients with chronic heart failure and normal renal function. The *rebound phenomenon* consists of a decrease in sodium excretion below baseline after the effect of the loop diuretic has worn off. The *braking phenomenon* refers to an increase in tubular sodium reabsorption by the distal tubule that occurs during long-term administration of loop diuretics.

In decompensated heart failure, the intravenous route of administration is preferable when possible, since the onset of diuresis is shorter and more predictable (Fig. 21-7). In patients with CHF that is refractory to standard doses of intravenous furosemide, higher doses may be efficacious. In 20 patients with severe CHF that was previously resistant to lower intravenous doses of furosemide,[135] intravenous furosemide was administered at doses of 500 to 2000 mg daily for a mean of 10 days, with increased diuresis, weight reduction, and symptomatic improvement. Other investigators observed a similar clinical improvement, as assessed by NYHA classification criteria, in 17 of 21 patients using high-dose oral furosemide (>500 mg daily) for 1 month.[136]

Continuous intravenous rather than intermittent administration of loop diuretics is an effective method of overcoming diuretic resistance in heart failure. In a randomized crossover study comparing continuous versus bolus bumetanide in patients with chronic renal failure (mean GFR, 17 mL/min), a greater net sodium excretion was observed during continuous infusion despite comparable drug excretion.[137] In CHF, continuous infusion of furosemide produces a similar natriuresis at serum concentrations 20 times lower than those after a comparable effective bolus dose.[138] Only one prospective, randomized crossover study is available that compares the continuous infusion of furosemide (loading dose 30 to 40 mg followed by infusion at a rate of 2.5 to 3.3 mg/h for 48 h) with intermittent intravenous bolus administration (30 to 40 mg every 8 h for 48 h) in NYHA class III and IV heart failure.[139] When it was infused continuously, furosemide's pattern of delivery produced more effective drug utilization, that is, sodium excretion relative to total furosemide excretion, whereas with intermittent bolus furosemide, wide fluctuations in urine output and sodium excretion were observed. Theoretically, an infusion of furosemide at a constant rate may be safe than using intermittent intravenous dosing, although a larger study is needed to confirm this.[140]

In summary, loop diuretics with salt restriction monitored by weight measurement by scale remain the basis for the treatment of edema. As CHF progresses, increasing oral doses of loop diuretics tend to be needed. In severe CHF with hospitalization, intravenous loop diuretics, commonly at higher doses, become essential. As will be discussed below, other agents, such as metolazone, may be required as well to increase and sustain sodium loss. Limitations to diuretic use remain hyponatremia

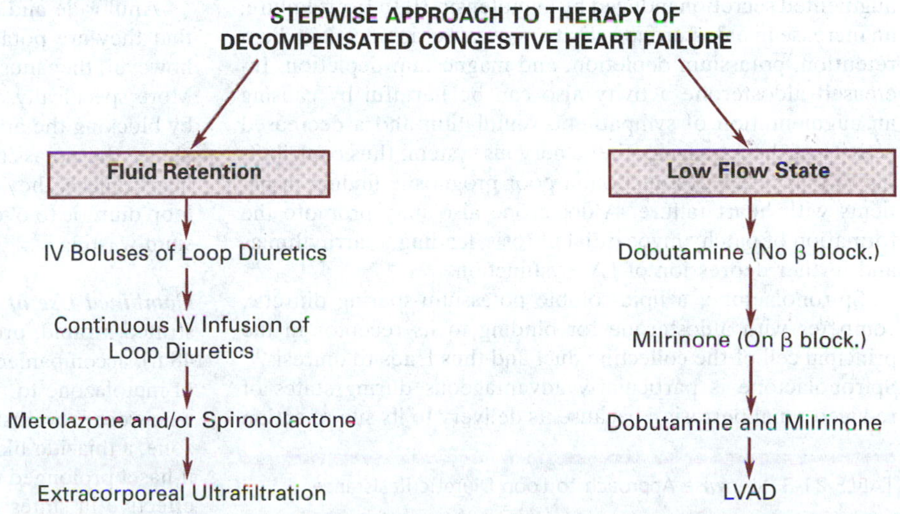

FIGURE 21-7 Treatment of congestive heart failure is directed toward controlling salt and water retention (central or peripheral edema) and/or relieving a low-flow state by increasing cardiac output while reducing very increased filling pressures. Dobutamine is useful to augment cardiac output except when $beta_1$-adrenergic blockade is present. Milrinone, which stimulates the adenyl cyclase system beyond the beta receptor, acts well in this circumstance to augment the effects of dobutamine while serving as an arterial and venous dilator. When inadequate cardiac output can no longer be maintained, surgical implantation of a left ventricular assist device (LVAD) may be used to pump blood from the left ventricle to the aorta as a temporary support or bridge to transplantation.

and a progressive increase in serum creatinine, which may require careful dose reductions (Table 21-3).

Thiazides The thiazide diuretics may be reasonable first-line natriuretic agents in early LV dysfunction when renal perfusion is not yet significantly compromised. In overt ventricular failure, however, thiazides are usually ineffective or inadequate. Thiazides are 50 percent protein-bound, and more than 95 percent of the dose is excreted unchanged in the urine.[124] They gain access into the tubular lumen through both glomerular filtration and tubular secretion. In the kidney, they inhibit sodium chloride reabsorption in the early distal tubule, where they compete for the chloride site on the apically located Na^+/Cl cotransporter.[141,142]

Hydrochlorothiazide is the most widely prescribed drug in this class of diuretics. Seventy-one percent of an oral dose is absorbed. The onset of diuresis occurs within 2 h, peaks between 3 and 6 h, and continues for up to 12 h.[124] Hydrochlorothiazide's pharmacokinetics follow a two-compartment model of elimination (α phase, 5 h; β phase, 6 to 15 h), and the half-life is prolonged in patients with decompensated heart failure and those with renal insufficiency.

Metolazone is a quinazoline diuretic and is similar to the thiazides in structure and mechanism of action.[124,143] Although its major effect occurs in the cortical diluting segment, metolazone has a minor inhibitory effect on proximal tubular sodium reabsorption. Metolazone is lipid-soluble and easily accesses the tubular lumen during states of renal insufficiency, unlike the thiazides.[144] Another advantage of metolazone is its longer duration of action (12 to 24 h).[124,143]

Potassium-Sparing Diuretics Aldosterone, an endogenous adrenal hormone, normally increases sodium reabsorption with the simultaneous excretion of potassium. Aldosterone levels are increased in heart failure, to some degree because of its augmented secretion induced by angiotensin II. In heart failure, an increase in aldosterone activity may cause significant sodium retention, potassium depletion, and magnesium depletion. Increased aldosterone activity also can be harmful by causing an augmentation of sympathetic stimulation and a decreased activity of the parasympathetic nervous system, thus contributing to baroreflex dysfunction, a poor prognostic finding in patients with heart failure. Aldosterone also may promote the formation of patchy myocardial fibrosis, leading to arrhythmias and further depression of LV dysfunction.

Spironolactone, a lipid-soluble potassium-sparing diuretic, competes with aldosterone for binding to its receptor in the principal cell of the collecting duct and thus leads to diuresis.[124] Spironolactone is particularly advantageous during states of reduced renal perfusion because its delivery to its site of action is not dependent on GFR. Spironolactone may be a useful adjunct to hydrochlorothiazide in offsetting its effect of producing hypokalemia resulting from sodium-potassium exchange. Since the exchange of sodium for potassium is reduced, potassium loss is reduced and hypokalemia may be corrected. Indeed, potassium supplements given for hypokalemia generally should be stopped to avoid hyperkalemia. If the use of spironolactone is warranted in a severe heart failure patient receiving an ACE inhibitor, therapy may be initiated at a dose of 25 mg a day. Because of the risk of hyperkalemia, serum potassium concentration should be monitored closely not only during concomitant therapy with ACE inhibitors or AII receptor blockers but also during periods of declining renal function. If the serum potassium concentration exceeds 5.5 meq/L, the spironolactone dose should be reduced to 25 mg every other day. Alternatively, after 8 weeks, the spironolactone dose may be increased to 50 mg a day in patients with stable serum potassium concentrations who are experiencing worsening heart failure symptoms. Maintenance doses of 50 mg a day or greater should be limited to patients with refractory or severe heart failure who have evidence of pulmonary or peripheral edema caused by an increased incidence of hyperkalemia. In this particular patient population, however, doses as high as 200 mg a day may be necessary. However, once a patient's condition has stabilized, the dose of spironolactone should be decreased to the maintenance level (25 to 50 mg a day) used before the heart failure exacerbation.[145]

The use of spironolactone also has been associated with reduced mortality in CHF, perhaps by helping to maintain potassium levels, thus reducing the risk of arrhythmic death in patients with heart failure,[146] or by inhibiting other pathologic processes influenced by aldosterone.[147] Spironolactone also has been shown to improve endothelial dysfunction, increase nitric oxide bioactivity, and inhibit the conversion of angiotensin I to angiotensin II, providing additional mechanisms for its beneficial effects on cardiovascular mortality.[148]

Amiloride and triamterene are similar to spironolactone in that they are potassium-sparing and act on the principal cell; however, they must be delivered intralumenally to be effective. More specifically, they reduce sodium flux into principal cells by blocking the apically located sodium channel.[124] When used alone, the potassium-sparing diuretics are relatively weak. In heart failure, they are useful when used in combination with a loop diuretic to overcome diuretic resistance and reduce potassium wasting.[149]

Combined Use of Diuretics Numerous reports have demonstrated a rapid, profound diuresis (1 to 2 L daily within 24 to 48 h), accompanied by clinical improvement, after the addition of metolazone to furosemide in patients with CHF (Fig. 21-7) who were previously resistant to furosemide alone.[150–157] Metolazone, a thiazide-like diuretic, is particularly advantageous since it has a prolonged duration of action, is lipophilic, and remains effective in states of renal impairment. In a study comparing metolazone with a thiazide, however, when either was used in combination with a loop diuretic, no significant difference in sodium excretion or urine output was observed between the two drugs.[157] Spironolactone, when used in combination with a loop diuretic (Fig. 21-7), also has been associated with an improvement in diuretic response in patients with CHF previously resistant to loop diuretics.[149]

In summary, thiazides, potassium-sparing diuretics, and aldo-

TABLE 21-3 Stepwise Approach to Loop Diuretic Resistance

1. Enforcement of strict low-sodium diet
2. Use of effective doses of loop diuretics
3. Combination administration of long-acting thiazide with loop diuretic to offset the antinatriuretic rebound effect observed after administration of short-acting loop diuretics
4. Constant intravenous infusion of loop diuretic

sterone inhibitors (e.g., spironolactone), along with loop diuretics, provide potent tools to reduce salt accumulation in CHF. Early in CHF, their use is mainly to reduce or eliminate peripheral edema and help relieve pulmonary congestion. Once dry weight is approximated, intermittent and reduced diuretic use is advisable to avoid electrolyte problems. Daily weights are the best guide to the adequacy of this therapy. Early in CHF, thiazides with potassium-sparing diuretics may be all that is necessary, although loop diuretics provide increased diuresis. Indeed, loop diuretics can be used intermittently on top of thiazides when needed. It is possible that the early use of diuretics can hasten the evolution of CHF by increasing reflex neurohumoral responses that may have adverse consequences, such as activation of the renin-angiotensin system.[39] As CHF progresses, the loop diuretics in increasing amounts are generally required. Here again, a scale for weight provides guidance for the dose. With excessive diuresis in very severe CHF, increasing renal insufficiency may be induced by hypovolemia, and this in itself may increase loop diuretic dose, its used intravenously, and the need for the concomitant use of thiazides (metolazone) or spironolactone.

INOTROPIC AGENTS

The use of inotropic agents in the treatment of CHF is predicated on the finding that a major contributing factor in reducing ventricular performance results from depression of myocardial contractility and that this can be reversed, or at least improved, by inotropic drugs. The fact that there is reduced myocardial contractility in failing heart muscle, whether from a sustained work overload of pressure or in response to losing myocardium, has been well demonstrated and appears to be due largely to inadequate Ca^{2+} availability for activation. All currently available inotropic agents act to increase Ca^{2+} for activation in both normal and failing myocardium. This is the case whether the mechanism of action is via cyclic AMP system excitation (e.g., catecholamines) or occurs by sarcolemmal Na^+-K^+-ATPase inhibition (e.g., digitalis glycosides). The problem remains whether this increase in intracellular Ca^{2+} can benefit pump function while doing no harm, such as enhancing the propensity for arrhythmia or theoretically producing further myocyte loss. Moreover, agents that reduce afterload may enhance ventricular emptying without these potential hazards. In end-stage, severely decompensated CHF, inotropic agents (e.g., dobutamine) may be temporarily lifesaving (Fig. 21-7), and at somewhat earlier stages, they may reduce morbidity (e.g., digitalis glycosides). In earlier stages of CHF, the benefits of inotropic agents may not outweigh the risk, and their use is relegated to later stages in the disease process (Figs. 21-5 and 21-7).

Digitalis Glycosides Digitalis glycosides have had a long and venerable history in the treatment of CHF and are the only oral inotropic agents available currently for this purpose (Fig. 21-8). In 1785, William Withering[158] reported on his use of the digitalis leaf as a purported diuretic agent to treat anasarca, presumably caused by CHF. Indeed, the major effects of digitalis initially were thought to be on the kidneys, although important effects on heart rate were noted. Only during the latter part of the nineteenth century did it become apparent that there was a direct action of digitalis glycosides to increase cardiac contractility,[159] while in the earlier part of the twentieth century the effects of digitalis on the peripheral circulation and the autonomic nervous system were noted.[160] Despite this long history, the risks and benefits of digitalis administration in patients with sinus rhythm have remained controversial. The controversy was partially addressed in a large randomized, placebo-controlled clinical trial of digoxin use in CHF.[161] Overall, digoxin was shown to be safe with a significant reduction in morbidity, expressed in terms of less need for hospitalization, but not in mortality. The benefit in terms of hospitalization for heart failure appears greatest in those with lower ejection fractions. As will be discussed later, with serum digoxin levels below 1 μg/mL, the neurohumoral and autocrine effects of digoxin predominate over the inotropic effects.

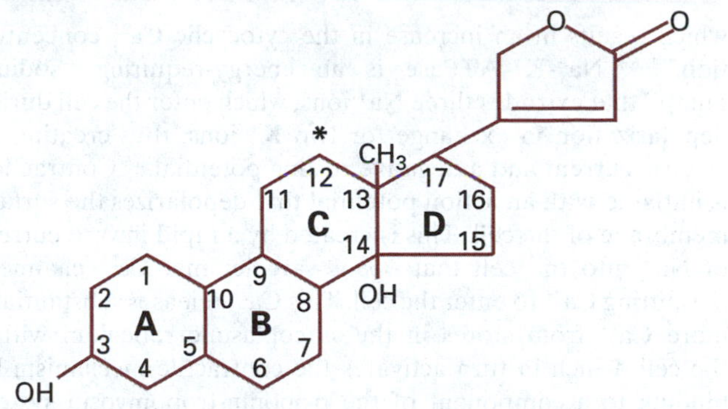

FIGURE 21-8 Structure of digitalis molecule. * Digitoxin becomes digoxin with OH placement at C_{12}. (From Sonnenblick EH, LeJemtel TH, Frishman WH. Digitalis preparations and other inotropic agents. In: Frishman WH, Sonnenblick EH, eds. *Cardiovascular Pharmacotherapeutics*. New York, McGraw-Hill; 1997:241. Reproduced with permission from the publisher and authors.)

Digitalis glycosides have important effects on multiple systems in addition to augmenting the contractility of the myocardium.[162,163] Electrophysiologically, digitalis glycosides speed conduction in the atrium while inhibiting conduction at the atrioventricular node. This has made them useful for rate control in atrial fibrillation. In the normal circulation, digitalis glycosides also produce generalized arteriolar vasoconstriction while affecting the central nervous system to enhance parasympathetic tone and reduce sympathetic nervous system activation. Digitalis glycosides sensitize baroreflexes to decrease efferent sympathetic activity, which acts to reduce sinus node activity and thus reduce heart rate. The precise mechanism for these effects is unclear. The increase in baroreflex sensitization also increases parasympathetic tone, even in mild heart failure, while central vagal nuclei also are stimulated. The broad enhancement of parasympathetic activity with digitalis glycosides helps explain the sinus heart rate slowing observed after digitalis glycosides even with sinus rhythm as well as their therapeutic efficacy in controlling supraventricular arrhythmias. As is discussed below, in the failing state, the effects of sympathetic withdrawal may be dominant, leading to reduced arterial vascular resistance, while in the normal circulation, arterial vasoconstriction may be dominant. Integration of these various actions adds to the inotropic activity and the therapeutic usefulness of digitalis glycosides.

The positive inotropic action of digitalis glycosides to increase the contractility and alter the electrophysiology of heart muscle occurs through binding to and inhibition of the enzyme Na^+-K^+-ATPase on the surface membrane of myocardial cells, which results in an increase in the cytocyclic Ca^{2+} concentration.[164,165] Na^+-K^+-ATPase is an energy-requiring "sodium pump" that extrudes three Na^+ ions, which enter the cell during depolarization in exchange for two K^+ ions, thus creating an electric current and a negative resting potential.[166] Contraction is initiated with an action potential that depolarizes the surface membrane of the cell. This is created by a rapid inward current of Na^+ into the cell that opens sarcolemmal Ca^{2+} channels, permitting Ca^{2+} to enter the cell. This Ca^{2+} releases substantially more Ca^{2+} from stores in the sarcoplasmic reticulum within the cell, which in turn activates the contractile mechanism by binding to a component of the troponin-tropomyosin system that had been maintaining the resting state. With Ca^{2+} bound to troponin, actin and myosin can interact to produce force and shortening. The greater the amount of activating Ca^{2+}, the greater the force and the shortening.[165,166] When Ca^{2+} is released from troponin and taken up by the sarcoplasmic reticulum, relaxation occurs.[165] The relatively small amount of Ca^{2+} that enters the cell with activation ultimately is removed by an electrogenic Na^+/Ca^{2+} exchange that extrudes one Ca^{2+} for three Na^+ ions. When intracellular Na^+ is increased, less exchange occurs and the net amount of intracellular Ca^{2+} is increased. Thus, by inhibiting the Na^+-K^+-ATPase, digitalis glycosides produce a decrease in intracellular K^+ and an increase in intracellular Na^+ that increases intracellular Ca^{2+} (Fig. 21-9).[165,166] In general, the main way in which all inotropic agents, including digitalis glycosides, increase contractility is by increasing the amount of Ca^{2+} available for activation.[167] This is the case in both normal and failing myocardium. In the failing heart, there is also a decrease in the Ca^{2+} released into the cytosol with activation.[168,169] Digitalis glycosides increase this intracellular Ca^{2+} that augments Ca^{2+} stores in the sarcoplasmic reticulum, resulting in a subsequent increase in previously reduced myocyte contraction.

Digoxin Although there are numerous digitalis glycosides with varying durations of action and metabolic fates, digoxin has a relatively rapid onset and an intermediate duration of action. Digoxin has its most beneficial hemodynamic actions when substantial ventricular depression is evident along with CHF. In this circumstance, it augments myocardial performance while reflexly reducing peripheral resistance.[170] Acutely, digoxin also reduces cardiac norepinephrine spillover and reduces efferent sympathetic nerve activity in skeletal muscles in patients with CHF.[170] Slowing of the heart rate, whether via enhanced parasympathetic tone and reduced sympathetic activity to reduce sinus rate or via control of heart rate in atrial fibrillation (as discussed below), greatly benefits ventricular filling and reduces pulmonary congestion.[171] In the treatment of CHF, digoxin generally is employed along with diuretics and vasodilator agents. Thus, by reducing peripheral resistance, digoxin and peripheral vasodilators act in a complementary manner.

In acute heart failure, either caused by massive sudden loss of myocardium, as may occur with a myocardial infarction, or with increasing decompensation in severe chronic CHF, characterized by acute pulmonary edema, severe limitations of cardiac output, and perhaps hypotension, more rapidly acting inotropic agents such as intravenous dobutamine and milrinone (dis-

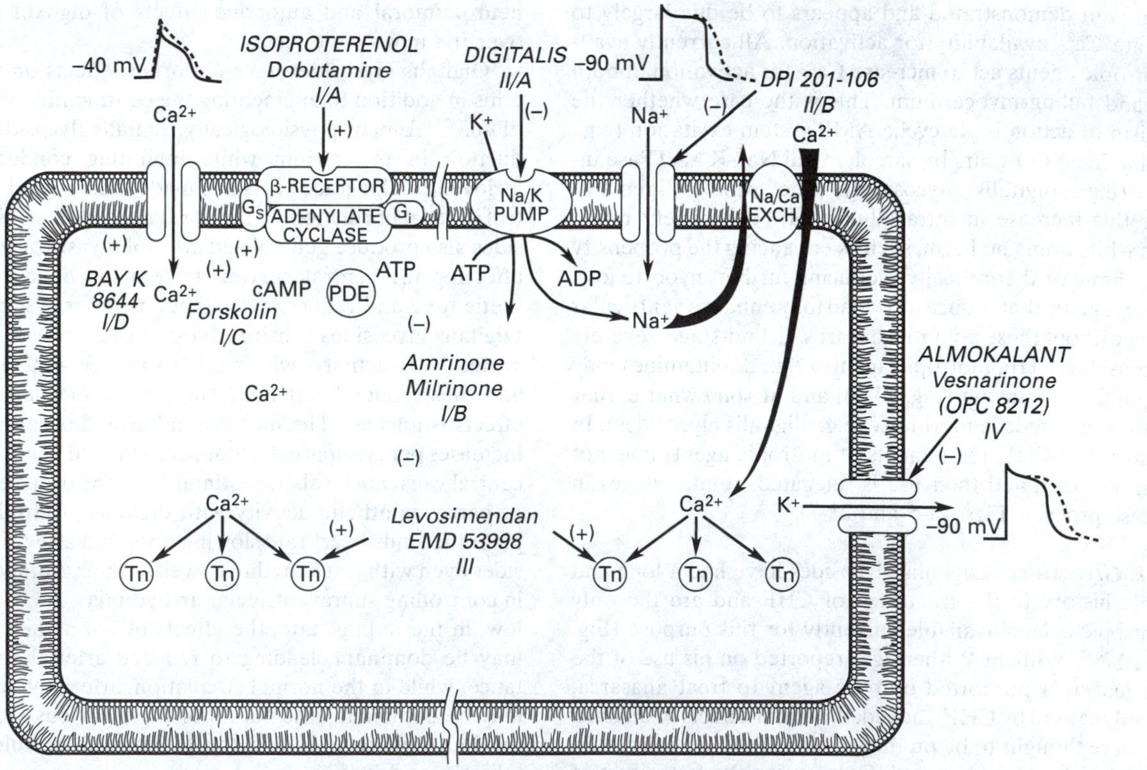

FIGURE 21-9 Diagram of various inotropic sites of action on and within the cardiac cell. While catecholamines act at cell surface receptors, agents such as amrinone and milrinone (PDE III inhibitors) act within the cell to augment adenylate cyclase. Calcium sensitizers increase Ca^{2+} sensitivity of troponin (Tn) in the contractile system itself. (From Varro A, Papp JG. Classification of positive inotropic actions based on electrophysiologic characteristics: Where should calcium sensitizers be placed? *J Cardiovasc Pharmacol* 1995; 26(suppl 1):S32. Reproduced with permission from the publisher and authors.)

cussed below) may be required (Fig. 21-7), together with loop diuretics and vasodilators. This situation may occur in the setting of rapid deterioration of a patient with more chronic heart failure or after a large myocardial infarction.[172] In this circumstance, the main aim is to increase cardiac output and reduce filling pressures as a setting for longer-term stabilization. While rapidly acting inotropic agents are being used, digitalis may be administered cautiously for its longer-term effects. In the setting of myocardial infarction, the situation is more complex. Because of a fear that arrhythmias may be induced or oxygen consumption may be increased, which might be detrimental, digoxin generally is avoided in the first few days after infarction,[172] although in a longer-term treatment of CHF, digitalis, especially if dosing is carefully controlled, may be of value along with other agents, especially ACE inhibitors.

For chronic CHF, digoxin is of use over the long term when administered in association with loop diuretics and ACE inhibitors. Benefits are most evident in patients with NYHA class III or IV CHF. In this circumstance, the response of the circulation is characterized by a decrease in venous pressures and ventricular filling pressures and an increase in cardiac output. Heart rate is slowed, and the ejection fraction tends to rise, while peripheral resistance falls with little or no change in arterial pressure. These salutary effects are attributed to a combination of augmented myocardial contractility and restoration of baroreceptor sensitivity, which results in enhanced parasympathetic and decreased sympathetic tone. Whereas myocardial oxygen consumption may increase in the normal heart from the increased contractility, in heart failure it tends to be reduced as a result of a decrease in heart size, and thus ventricular wall tension, and a slowing of heart rate. Earlier concepts supported the view that digoxin is of greatest benefit when atrial fibrillation is present and controlled. It is now clear that efficacy is also present when a patient with heart failure is in sinus rhythm.[173] Withdrawal of digoxin from such patients led to rapid deterioration even when both diuretics and ACE inhibitors were used.[174,175] While digoxin has been associated with an increase in the ejection fraction, vasodilators have been shown to cause more significant increments in exercise performance.[176] These considerations would justify the combined use of these agents. Whereas the use of ACE inhibitors may be indicated when the ejection fraction is reduced and symptoms are limited (class I, II), digoxin probably should be reserved for use with more overt symptoms (class III, IV).

While digoxin can be given once a day without tolerance or tachyphylaxis, the dose is a matter at issue.[177] In general, a serum level of 0.5 to 1.5 mg/L is felt to be therapeutic.[178] This level may vary from patient to patient, and a clear dose-response relation has not been established. Indeed, some of the greatest benefits may be gained from lower doses (e.g., 0.125 mg/day), which may induce the neurohumoral benefits of lower sympathetic and higher parasympathetic tone while reducing the incidence of possible toxic side effects,[177] as is discussed below. There appear to be no adverse effects from digoxin usage in terms of mortality in patients with CHF,[161] and the substantially increased morbidity noted when the drug is withdrawn[174,179,180] suggests such a result. Effects on mortality with digoxin are complicated by the fact that the nature and progression of the underlying process, which led to failure in the first place, may be the ultimate determinant of mortality. If morbidity is reduced substantially with digoxin, as has been demonstrated,[161] a neutral effect on ultimate mortality would be acceptable. This was demonstrated in the Digitalis Investigation Group (DIG) Study (sponsored by the National Institutes of Health), a controlled trial in patients with CHF that showed no effect on survival compared to placebo, a reduction in hospitalizations, and a low incidence of digoxin toxicity.[161]

Digoxin has been shown to be of limited value in the treatment of right-sided heart failure, which can occur in cor pulmonale or with left-to-right shunts. Digoxin also has limited value in acute LV failure caused by acute myocardial infarction, although it is useful in the subsequent treatment of ischemia-related CHF. Nevertheless, since mortality may be increased after infarction by digoxin, especially when clear evidence of heart failure is absent, its use is best reserved for patients with overt CHF.

Toxicities from digitalis glycosides can be numerous and are somewhat dependent on the serum level. Central nervous symptoms include loss of appetite and nausea, and visual changes may be seen. Cardiac limitations include atrioventricular block, premature ventricular extra systoles, and ultimately ventricular tachycardia and fibrillation. Monitoring serum levels may be useful in a patient with sinus rhythm, while the ventricular rate provides an adequate guide to dosing in the presence of atrial fibrillation. Except in dire circumstances, such as a suicide attempt, cessation of therapy is adequate. In the former circumstances, antibodies to digoxin may be indicated.

Catecholamines As was noted above, positive inotropism is based on enhancing the delivery of Ca^{2+} to the contractile system to increase force and shortening. Increasing Ca^{2+} in the serum effects this transiently, while digitalis glycosides increase Ca^{2+} for activation by inhibiting sarcolemmal Na^+-K^+-ATPase. Catecholamines increase activating Ca^{2+} via beta-adrenergic receptors and the adenyl cyclase system (Fig. 21-9).

Beta receptors are located in the sarcolemma and constitute a complex structure that spans the membrane.[181] The beta receptor is connected with G proteins (Fig. 21-9) that either activate (G_s) or inhibit (G_i) a secondary enzyme system, adenylate cyclase, which, when activated by G_s, induces the formation of 3′–5′ cyclic adenosine-monophosphate (cyclic AMP). Cyclic AMP in turn activates certain protein kinases, which lead to intracellular phosphorylation of proteins that enhance both the entry and the removal of intracellular Ca^{2+}.[182] When more Ca^{2+} is provided to the troponin-tropomyosin system, a greater interaction between actin and myosin occurs, increasing force and shortening. Increasing the rate of Ca^{2+} removal from the cytoplasm speeds the rate of relaxation.

In a normal heart, norepinephrine is synthesized and stored in the sympathetic nerve endings that invest the entire heart, including the atria, conduction system, and ventricle.[183] When these nerve endings are depolarized, norepinephrine is released from granules in nerve endings into myocardial clefts containing beta-adrenergic receptors, which, when activated, turn on the sequence of events noted above. Not only does this enhance Ca^{2+} entry into the myocyte to augment contraction, it also phosphorylates phospholamban, which enhances relaxation.[182] Subsequently, most of the released norepinephrine is taken back up and restored in the sympathetic nerve endings. Released norepinephrine also is inactivated by two enzymes, catechol *O*-methyltransferase (COMT) and monoamine oxidase (MAO), and the products are excreted largely by the kidneys.[182]

In very severe heart failure, stores of norepinephrine in the ventricle are largely depleted and the sympathetic nerve endings fail to take up norepinephrine normally.[184] Rapid turnover of whatever norepinephrine stores remain is suggested by increased cardiac norepinephrine spillover in CHF. At the same time, circulating norepinephrine released from peripheral sympathetic nerve endings may be increased, especially in severe failure.[185] In less severe heart failure, the serum norepinephrine levels tend to be normal despite increased sympathetic nerve activity.[186]

In both normal and failing myocardium, activation of the adenyl cyclase system can augment contractility. Agents that do this may be divided into two categories. The first category consists of the catecholamines (e.g., norepinephrine, epinephrine) and their synthetic derivatives (e.g., dobutamine, isoproterenol), which act via cell-surface adrenergic receptors (Fig. 21-9).[182] The second includes agents that inhibit the breakdown of cyclic AMP by inhibiting phosphodiesterase type III (e.g., amrinone, milrinone, and pimobendan), resulting in an increase in cyclic AMP.[186] Some of these agents, such as pimobendan, also may increase myofibril sensitivity to calcium and then further augment contraction.[187]

Catecholamines constitute an endogenous hormonal system that exerts reflex control of the heart and circulation. Their effects depend on localized, controlled neural release and receptor specificity in terms of action. Dopamine is the naturally occurring precursor of both norepinephrine and epinephrine (Fig. 21-10).[188] While epinephrine is released from the adrenal medulla, norepinephrine is the primary mediator in the heart and the peripheral circulation.[182]

The actions of both endogenous and exogenous catecholamines depend on their activation of specific alpha- and beta-adrenergic receptors (Tables 21-4 and 21-5).[182] Alpha receptors include $alpha_1$ receptors, which are postsynaptic and are located

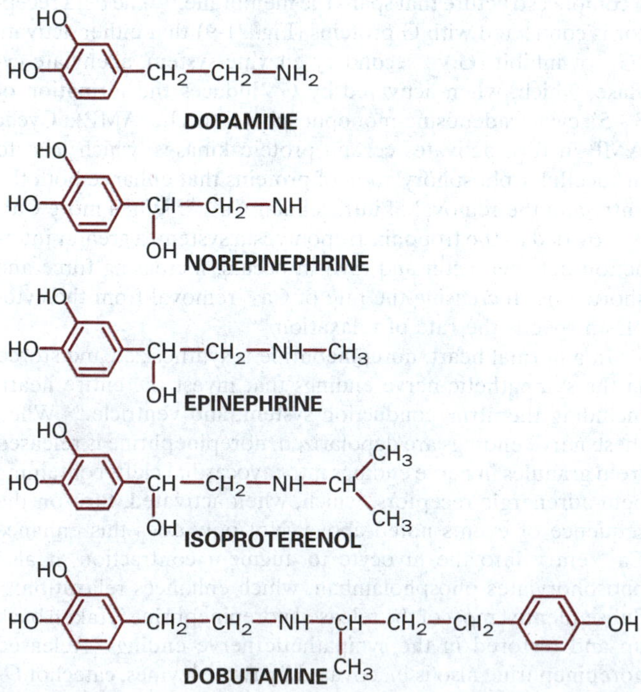

FIGURE 21-10 Structure of catecholamines.

in vascular smooth muscle and in the myocardium. In smooth muscle, they mediate vasoconstriction; in the heart, weak positive inotropic and negative chronotropic effects. $Alpha_2$ receptors are presynaptic and, when stimulated, decrease norepinephrine release from peripheral nerve endings as well as sympathetic outflow from the central nervous system. $Alpha_2$ receptors also may mediate vasoconstriction in specific peripheral vascular beds.

Beta-adrenergic receptors can be divided into $beta_1$ and $beta_2$ subtypes. $Beta_1$ receptors are located in the myocardium, where they mediate positive inotropic, chronotropic, and dromotropic effects.[186] Their activation occurs primarily through norepinephrine released from neurons in the heart. $Beta_2$ receptors are located in vascular smooth muscle, where they mediate vasodilatation, and in the sinoatrial node, where they are chronotropic. In general, $beta_2$ receptors are activated by circulating catecholamines released from peripheral sites such as the adrenal medulla.

Another type of receptor, which has been termed the *dopaminergic receptor,* is localized to the mesenteric and renal circulation and mediates arterial vasodilatation. The physiologic and pharmacologic actions of various catecholamines depend on which receptor they activate, both in the heart and in the periphery (Tables 21-4 and 21-5).

Norepinephrine has potent $alpha_1$ and $beta_1$ activity. When norepinephrine is released from cardiac nerve endings, as occurs in normal exercise, myocardial contractility and heart rate are augmented. When norepinephrine is administered exogenously, its major action is to stimulate $alpha_1$ receptors, leading to marked peripheral arterial vasoconstriction. Thus, norepinephrine has been used to increase arterial blood pressure in the presence of severe hypotension to maintain blood flow to vital organs. Long-term renal vasoconstriction from continued norepinephrine administration may produce ischemic renal damage, including acute tubular necrosis, so that prolonged use, i.e., for more than 24 to 48 h, is usually untenable. For a failing heart, this peripheral vasoconstriction also provides an undesirable added pressure load (afterload), which tends to vitiate the potential benefits of $beta_1$ stimulation.

Dopamine[188] has both $alpha_1$ and $beta_1$ activity but also stimulates dopaminergic receptors in the renal vasculature to produce arterial dilation and increased renal blood flow. Its $beta_1$ effects in the heart occur largely through the release of endogenous norepinephrine, which may be largely depleted in a failing heart. As doses of dopamine are increased, conversion to norepinephrine also occurs, which tends to produce relatively more pressor effects than myocardial inotropic stimulation (Table 21-4). As such, the benefits of dopamine administration, if any, occur at low doses (e.g., 0.02 mg/kg per minute), where it may induce renal arterial vasodilatation. In general, it is employed in association with more potent inotropic agents (e.g., dobutamine).

Dobutamine[189,190] is a synthetic variant of the catecholamines whose structure has been altered to optimize the hemodynamic response in the dog, characterized by an increase in cardiac output and a decrease in ventricular filling pressure with little change in heart rate. Since arterial pressure also rises modestly, peripheral vascular resistance must of necessity fall. The positive inotropic activity of dobutamine is mediated by direct stimulation of $beta_1$-adrenergic receptors in the myocardium (Table 21-4). It is unclear why a concomitant increase in heart rate

TABLE 21-4 Adrenergic Receptor Activity of Sympathomimetic Amines

	$Alpha_1$	$Beta_1$	$Beta_2$	Dopaminergic	Dose
Dopamine	+++	++	+	++++	<2 (μg/kg)/min: vasodilation effects on peripheral dopaminergic receptors 2–10 (μg/kg)/min: inotropic effects, $beta_1$ receptor activation; 5–20 (μg/kg)/min: peripheral vasoconstriction, alpha effects
Norepinephrine	++++	++++	0	0	Initiate with 8–12 μg/min; maintain 2–4 μg/min
Epinephrine	+++	++++	++	0	
Isoproterenol	0	++++	++++	0	0.5–5 μg/min
Dobutamine	+++	++++	++	0	Start at 2–3 (μg/kg)/min and titrate upward

SOURCE: From Sonnenblick EH, LeJemtel TH, Frishman WH. Digitalis preparations and other inotropic agents. In: Frishman WH, Sonnenblick EH, eds. *Cardiovascular Pharmacotherapeutics.* New York: McGraw-Hill; 1997:246. Reproduced with permission from the publisher and authors.

does not always occur. One possibility is that an increase in cardiac output that increases arterial pressure serves to buffer any increase in heart rate reflexly. Given its capacity to increase cardiac output and reduce filling pressures without substantial changes in heart rate, dobutamine has been used widely to treat severe acute LV failure in the absence of profound hypotension, which is poorly responsive to diuretics and vasodilators (Fig. 21-7). This may be seen after a very large myocardial infarction or in acute decompensation in the course of chronic CHF. In the presence of severe hypotension, the $beta_2$ stimulation of dobutamine may be harmful, and the administration of an $alpha_1$-stimulating vasoconstrictor such as norepinephrine or higher-dose dopamine also may be necessary to increase arterial peripheral resistance.

Dobutamine infusion generally is begun at 2 μg/kg per minute and titrated to optimize cardiac output while reducing LV filling pressure. Tachycardia is avoided carefully to avoid increasing myocardial oxygen demands and inducing ischemia. The effects on myocardial oxygen consumption (MVO_2) are complex.[190] While the increase in contractility will increase MVO_2, a decrease in heart size will tend to reduce it. The end result is generally a modest increase in MVO_2 induced by dobutamine. With a better maintained arterial pressure and reduced LV diastolic pressure in the absence of tachycardia, coronary perfusion pressure also may be increased. The major side effects of dobutamine are an excessive increase in heart rate with high doses and ventricular arrhythmias, both of which may mandate dose reduction and even drug discontinuation. Tachyphylaxis also may occur to a variable degree. In general, once hemodynamic benefits are attained, dobutamine is withdrawn slowly. In some cases this has not been possible, and sustained administration becomes necessary, which may require portable pumps for administration at home. The outcome in this circumstance is generally dire.

In chronic CHF, the patient commonly is maintained on vasodilators such as ACE inhibitors, loop diuretics, and digoxin. Nevertheless, episodes of acute decompensation may intervene, characterized by increased pulmonary congestion and edema and reduced renal function with increasing fluid accumulation (Fig. 21-7). The in-hospital addition of dobutamine, with or without milrinone (see below), using a Swan-Ganz catheter to monitor hemodynamics, provides for an increase in cardiac output with a decrease in filling pressures, which, with added diuretics, may help restore a steady state for a variable period. Dopamine, at a low dose, commonly is used concomitantly to augment renal blood. This generally requires a short hospitalization and temporary hemodynamic monitoring. In CHF, norepinephrine is used only for a limited time to treat severe hypoten-

TABLE 21-5 Physiologic and Pharmacologic Actions of Catecholamine Receptors

Receptor	Receptor Activity	Primary Location
$Beta_1$	Positive inotropic and chronotropic action; increased AV conduction	Heart (atria, ventricle, AV node)
$Beta_2$	Peripheral vasodilation	Arterioles, arteries, veins, bronchioles
$Alpha_1$	Arteriolar vasoconstriction	Arterioles
$Alpha_2$	Presynaptic inhibition of norepinephrine release	Sympathetic nerve endings, CNS
Dopaminergic-1	Renal and mesenteric vasodilation, natriuresis, diuresis	Kidneys

NOTE: AV = atrioventricular; CNS = central nervous system.
SOURCE: From Sonnenblick EH, LeJemtel TH, Frishman WH. Digitalis preparations and other inotropic agents. In: Frishman WH, Sonnenblick EH, eds. *Cardiovascular Pharmacotherapeutics.* New York: McGraw-Hill; 1997:246. Reproduced with permission from the publisher and authors.

sion and shock unresponsive to dopamine and dobutamine, and then the outcome is generally very poor.

Phosphodiesterase Inhibitors and Other Agents The adenyl cyclase—cyclic AMP system also can be activated beyond the beta receptor. Hormones such as glucagon activate the system and can increase myocardial contractility acutely despite $beta_1$ blockade.[191] While intravenous glucagon administration is useful in overcoming beta-adrenergic blockade when necessary, glucagon may induce gastric atony and nausea, and this has limited its more generalized use.

Amrinone and milrinone are prototypes of cardiotonic agents that activate the adenyl cyclase system through inhibition of the enzyme that breaks down cyclic AMP, phosphodiesterase (PDE) III.[192,193] Type III PDE inhibitors decrease the breakdown of cyclic AMP in the myocardium and increase cyclic guanidine monophosphate (cyclic GMP) in vascular smooth muscle, resulting in an increase in myocardial contractility as well as arterial and venous vasodilatation. Other members of this class of drugs include enoximone and pimobendan, although only intravenous amrinone and milrinone have been approved by the FDA for the treatment of acute heart failure. The mechanisms by which vasodilatation occurs are not completely understood. Increased cyclic GMP induces phosphorylation of myosin light-chain kinase, which decreases sensitivity to calcium and calmodulin. In the heart, inotropism may relate not only to increased cyclic AMP–mediated calcium availability for contraction and increased rates of its removal for relaxation but also to increased sensitivity of the contractile system for calcium.[194] Both amrinone and milrinone,[193] which are available as intravenous agents, have substantial ability to augment cardiac output while reducing both RV and LV filling pressures. The lowering of filling pressures is greater than that seen with dobutamine. Dilatation of the pulmonary arterial vasculature is also a very useful therapeutic effect. Arterial pressure tends to be reduced, while an increase in heart rate may occur. Since dobutamine increases cyclic AMP and milrinone reduces its breakdown, the combination of these agents is substantially more potent than is either agent alone.[193] When either dobutamine or milrinone is utilized, ectopic activity may be increased; this requires careful supervision in their use. PDE III inhibitors are also orally active and produce the same hemodynamic improvement seen with intravenous use. In longer-term oral use, however, increased mortality was seen with the use of milrinone, especially in the presence of class IV heart failure.[195] This increased mortality might have been due to the relatively short action of this agent (90-min half-life), which leads to large peaks and valleys in dosing and concomitant arrhythmias. For the time being, this has vitiated clinical study of these agents in oral formulations, but more stringent control of the use of this class of agents as adjuncts to other agents ultimately may increase their value, especially in improving quality of life in the terminal and short-term outcome of very severe CHF.

NEWER INOTROPIC AGENTS

Agents under investigation include the inodilatory benzimidazoline PDE inhibitors, such as levosimendan, which acutely increase cardiac output and reduce filling pressure while improving exercise tolerance in patients with CHF.[196] Levosimendan and other drugs in this class (MCI-154, EMD 53998, EMD 57033) may have additional effects to enhance calcium binding to troponin-C, a calcium-sensitizing action (Fig. 21-9).[196–198] Theoretically, this could enhance the contractile response for a given amount of cytolytic Ca^{2+}, which could lead to less arrhythmogenicity. This may be an important consideration since the activation of the cyclic AMP system may be detrimental in inducing tachycardia and arrhythmias. Clinical trials evaluating the efficacy and safety of levosimendan are in progress. Preliminary results from one study that compared levosimendan to dobutamine [Levosimendan versus Dobutamine (LIDO)] demonstrated comparable hemodynamic activities with less chest pain and arrhythmia with levosimendan. The critical issues to be addressed, now that acute efficacy is apparent, are whether these agents will improve symptoms, i.e., reduce morbidity, and/or improve mortality.

ADJUNCTIVE THERAPIES

As was mentioned earlier, patients with heart failure require treatment of underlying disease processes that may be aggravating the myopathic process. Systemic hypertension should be treated vigorously. In diabetes, hyperglycemia should be controlled. Aspirin prophylaxis and cholesterol-lowering drugs should be used in patients with coronary artery disease. It is not known whether estrogen replacement therapy in postmenopausal women can modify the course of heart failure.[199]

Heart failure patients with mental depression have an increased mortality risk. The tricyclic antidepressant drugs have been associated with myocardial depression and probably are contraindicated in heart failure patients. However, the selective serotonin reuptake inhibitors have a favorable risk profile in cardiac patients and could be considered an adjunctive treatment for relieving mental depression. However, many of these drugs interfere with the hepatic cytochrome P450 system, and that might affect the metabolism of drugs being used to treat heart failure (see Chap. 81).

Beta blockers should be considered in all patients who survive a myocardial infarction with or without ventricular dysfunction. As was described earlier, carvedilol, metoprolol, and bisoprolol should probably be the beta blockers of choice in patients with symptomatic mild to moderate CHF of ischemic or nonischemic origin. Propranolol, metoprolol, atenolol, or timolol should be used in myocardial infarction survivors who are asymptomatic with and without LV dysfunction.

Patients with CHF are liable to develop venoembolic disease and systemic emboli from intracardiac mural thrombi. These embolic events are major causes of morbidity and mortality in CHF. In patients with atrial fibrillation and CHF, with and without mitral stenosis, anticoagulation is indicated. In patients with normal sinus rhythm and cardiomyopathy, the role of prophylactic anticoagulation with warfarin is not well defined.[3] A cohort analysis of the SOLVD population focused on the relation between warfarin use and the risk of all-cause mortality and found a beneficial effect with an anticoagulant.[200] Most of this benefit appeared to relate to reduced ischemic events. It is more difficult to anticoagulate patients with CHF because of drug–drug interactions, malabsorption of medications, varying perfusion of the liver, and malnutrition.[201] Patients with CHF who have developed a phlebothrombotic process or who have definite evidence of ventricular mural thrombi and systemic embolism should receive warfarin despite the potential problems with the regulation of anticoagulation in these patients.

Patients with heart failure have a markedly increased prevalence of ventricular ectopy and incidence of sudden death. These patients should be assessed for hypokalemia, hypomagnesemia, hypoxia, infection, and the use of antidepressant drugs. Many antiarrhythmic drug regimens have negative inotropic actions and may aggravate the heart failure process. Amiodarone and beta blockers have been used in patients with LV dysfunction with less risk involved and are probably the drugs of choice when treatment of ventricular ectopy is considered.[202,203] There is little evidence to show that antiarrhythmic drug therapy changes the natural history of advanced CHF.[203] Amiodarone also can be used to treat atrial arrhythmias with and without digoxin and calcium channel blockers.

DIASTOLIC DYSFUNCTION

Diastolic dysfunction of the left and right ventricles often leads to all the signs and symptoms of systolic dysfunction, but the therapeutic approach varies for these two conditions. Often, there is significant LV hypertrophy present, and aggressive management of systemic hypertension is required.[202,204] These patients develop significant congestion, and so diuretics are often necessary. With hypovolemia from other diseases, however, patients are prone to develop hypotension. The effects of diuretics in these patients should be monitored carefully. Digoxin is probably of no use unless the patient is in atrial fibrillation, and vasodilating drugs with peripheral venodilator actions may cause hypotension. The role of ACE inhibitors, angiotensin II receptor blockers, and other vasodilator drugs are not well defined in this condition, and they may cause hypotension. Large clinical trials have begun to include patients who have diastolic dysfunction as the primary cause for clinical heart failure. Studies with the ACE inhibitor perindopril and the angiotensin receptor blocker candesartan are in progress.

Tachycardia must be avoided. Rate-lowering calcium blockers (verapamil, diltiazem) are useful drugs of choice for reducing elevated blood pressure, keeping the heart rate under control, and improving ventricular compliance.[205] Beta-adrenergic blockers are first-line therapy for maintaining relative bradycardia to maintain time for diastolic ventricular filling. However, their effects on ventricular compliance are not as well defined. Both verapamil and beta blockers can be used with caution in patients with heart failure caused by hypertrophic cardiomyopathy.

DRUG THERAPIES UNDER INVESTIGATION

Natriuretic Peptides and Their Enhancers Conventional diuretics are associated with undesirable stimulation of the renin-angiotensin axis, sympathetic nervous system, and vasopressin. ANP and brain natriuretic peptide (BNP), by contrast, induce diuresis and natriuresis while concomitantly suppressing the renin-angiotensin axis with dilation of peripheral vascular beds.[206–210] In heart failure, despite high endogenous ANP and BNP levels, a state of intense sodium avidity prevails.[206,207,210,211] Attempts at restoring the efficacy of ANP in heart failure include infusing ANP intravenously and administering a neutral endopeptidase inhibitor. Prolonged infusion of ANP in patients with moderate CHF (NYHA class II to III) has been associated with doubling of the urine flow rate and a three- to fourfold increase in sodium excretion.[212] When ANP is infused in patients with moderate to severe CHF (NYHA class II to IV), however, the natriuretic and diuretic response is attenuated.[207,208]

Favorable hemodynamic responses have been observed after ANP infusion, including a fall in pulmonary capillary wedge pressure (PCWP), plasma renin activity, and systemic vascular resistance and an increase in cardiac output.[207,208,213] When ANP and furosemide are administered concomitantly, urine volume and sodium excretion are not augmented, although in this setting ANP does maintain its inhibitory effect on the renin-angiotensin axis and on sympathetic discharge.[214]

Neutral endopeptidase (NEP) inhibitor administration is associated with a rise in endogenous ANP levels resulting from the inhibition of ANP metabolism.[210,215–219] In a canine model of CHF, Cavero and coworkers reported that at similar ANP levels, NEP inhibitor treatment was associated with a better diuretic and natriuretic effect than was an ANP infusion.[215] In human studies, however, the two modalities appear to have similar natriuretic and diuretic effects. In 1989, Northridge and colleagues were the first to report diuresis after NEP inhibitor infusion in six patients with mild CHF (mean ejection fraction, 37 percent).[218] A 60 percent increase in the 4-h urine sodium excretion was observed, associated with a three- to fivefold rise in ANP levels.[218] The same investigators compared the renal and hemodynamic effects of NEP inhibitor administration to low-dose furosemide in mild CHF.[220] Eighteen patients were randomized to receive an NEP inhibitor, candoxatrilat 200 mg twice daily, candoxatrilat 400 mg twice daily, or furosemide 20 mg twice daily. The administration of a NEP inhibitor was associated with diuresis; however, the change in urine flow rate and sodium excretion from baseline was greater in the low-dose furosemide group. Although its diuretic effect was modest, the NEP inhibitor was associated with desirable hemodynamic effects, including marked preload reduction (PCWP decreased 40 percent), and with no stimulation of plasma renin activity. In comparison, the group given furosemide experienced only a 15 percent reduction in PCWP and a threefold rise in plasma renin activity.

The natriuretic properties of NEP inhibitors are mediated by inhibition of sodium reabsorption within the renal tubule, since they do not alter renal hemodynamics (GFR or renal plasma flow) significantly. This is supported by their association with an increased fractional excretion of lithium, a marker of proximal tubular reabsorption.[215,217] In addition to inhibiting ANP degradation, the NEP inhibitors inhibit the breakdown of bradykinin and BNP. They also have been shown to enhance prostacyclin synthesis, another mechanism by which they may exert a natriuretic effect.[221,222] In the most severe stages of CHF (NYHA class III to IV; ejection fraction, 22 percent), an impaired renal response to NEP inhibitor treatment can be expected. Munzel and colleagues[209] reported an unpredictable natriuretic response to candoxatrilat in nine patients with severe CHF. Three patients had no diuresis, five had a minimal response, and one (cardiac index > 2.5 L/min) had a good diuresis. The natriuretic response correlated closely with the cardiac output, which theoretically was most likely related to renal perfusion status.

In contrast to ANP, the natriuretic effect of BNP infusion is surprisingly and significantly more pronounced in patients with CHF than in normal patients, even when similar BNP levels are infused.[210] Yoshimura and colleagues infused BNP in normal patients and in those with NYHA class II to IV CHF and observed a fivefold rise in urine flow rate and a tenfold increase in sodium excretion in the CHF group.[210] In normal patients, diuresis and natriuresis were only three- to fourfold that of baseline, respectively. BNP infusion also was associated with a reduction in PCWP, systemic vascular resistance, and aldosterone levels as well as a rise in ANP levels.

It is unclear why high-dose BNP infusion is not associated with an attenuated natriuretic response in CHF, as is seen with ANP infusion. Like the process in ANP, inhibition of NEP 24.11 with candoxatril prevents the metabolism of BNP, increasing BNP levels by about 50 percent.[222] Because of its enhanced natriuretic effect at high infusion rates and prolonged duration of action compared with ANP, BNP appears to be the most promising natriuretic peptide candidate for future investigation and potential clinical therapeutic use.

When the BNP nesiritide is infused in patients with CHF, it reduces pulmonary capillary wedge pressure and systemic vascular resistance while increasing stroke volume and cardiac index. It suppresses plasma aldosterone but does not change plasma renin, norepinephrine, or epinephrine. It increases renal plasma flow and GFR as well as insulin excretion without affecting blood pressure and heart rate.[223] Nesiritide was recently considered by the FDA for intravenous clinical use in the treatment of acute heart failure, but excessive hypotension caused by treatment in studies has delayed its approval.[224] A recent study demonstrated that twice-daily subcutaneous injections of nesiritide can improve hemodynamics in patients with CHF, and this may provide a new therapeutic approach to chronic therapy.[225]

It is believed that the attenuation of responsiveness to endogenous ANPs with endopeptidase inhibition is due to activation of the RAAS. This has prompted the development of agents that both augment the action of ANP and block the RAAS, the dual NEP-ACE inhibitor drugs (e.g., omapatrilat, sampatrilat), which are now being examined in patients with systemic hypertension and CHF.[226]

In patients with heart failure, omapatrilat has been shown to be more effective in improving symptoms and reducing the combined risk of death and hospitalization than is the ACE inhibitor lisinopril (IMPRESS trial). In addition, fewer omapatrilat-treated patients exhibited signs of renal dysfunction. Results from a substudy showed that omapatrilat caused a greater improvement in arterial compliance.[227] Omapatrilat is being compared to enalapril in a long-term survival study (OVERTURE Study).

Another naturally occurring natriuretic peptide being evaluated for the treatment of patients with heart failure is adrenomedullin,[223,228] a hypotensive peptide originally isolated from human pheochromocytoma.

Endothelin Inhibitors Endothelin-1 exhibits potent inotropic activity in isolated hearts, cardiac muscle strips, isolated cells, and instrumented intact animals.[229] High-affinity receptors for endothelin have been demonstrated in both the atria and the ventricles.[230-232] Intravenous endothelin-1 produces a delayed prolonged augmentation of LV performance in addition to its biphasic vasoactive effects of transient vasodilation followed by sustained vasoconstriction.[229]

Endothelin is also a potent secretagogue of atrial natriuretic factor, which is a naturally occurring antagonist of endothelin that acts by inhibiting its release.[233] The endothelin-A receptor appears to mediate endothelin's actions of vasoconstriction and the stimulation of the ANP secretion, and the endothelin-B receptor mediates endothelin-induced vasodilatation and activation of the RAAS. Urinary water excretion is mediated through both receptors, but sodium excretion is mediated through the endothelin-A receptor.

Increased endothelin levels have been described in patients with CHF[234-239] that are predictive of increased mortality risk.[235] It also has been suggested that increased endothelin levels may play an important role in the increased systemic vascular resistance observed in CHF.[234,240,241] Endothelin-1 levels decrease with therapy and have been found to correlate significantly with symptomatic improvement. It therefore appears that endothelin-1 is an independent, noninvasive predictor of functional and hemodynamic response to therapy in patients with CHF.[242] Increased endothelin levels also have been observed in the plasma and hearts of cardiomyopathic Syrian hamsters[243] and in the cells of endothelial cells infected with *Trypanosoma cruzi* in experimental Chagas' cardiomyopathy.[244]

There is early clinical evidence that treatment with endothelin-A receptor antagonists and endothelin-converting enzyme inhibitors can influence the course of human heart failure favorably.[245] Some of these agents are being investigated in clinical heart failure trials (bosentan, BMS193884, LU135252).[246,247] ACE inhibitors also may benefit patients with heart failure because of their antiendothelin actions.[248,249]

Vasopressin Antagonists Vasopressin, which usually is elevated in patients with heart failure, correlates with the severity of disease and the incidence of hyponatremia. In human beings, this aquaretic hormone is released in response to the level of plasma osmotic pressure or osmolality. Its release also is influenced by hemodynamics in the setting of heart failure, a decrease in mean arterial pressure, a decrease in cardiac output, a decrease in atrial pressure, hormones such as angiotensin II, increased sympathetic nervous system activation, and a variety of less common stimuli.[250]

Two physiologically important subtypes of vasopressin receptors are the V1 and V2 receptors. V1 is found primarily in vascular smooth muscle and promotes vasoconstriction. The V2 receptor is found in renal collecting duct cells and promotes reabsorption of free water in the kidney. Vasopressin elevations in heart failure could induce vasoconstriction and increase renal water retention and thirst.

The first peptide vasopressin antagonists (V2 receptor specific) were developed in the 1980s.[251] More recently, combined V1A/V2 receptor antagonists have become available. In human studies vasopressin antagonists have been shown to reverse the impaired urinary diluting capacity seen in chronic heart failure, increase sodium free water excretion, correct dilutional hyponatremia, decrease urinary aquaporin-2 (AQP-2) excretion, promote peripheral vasodilation, and improve cardiac output.

Two orally active V2 receptor antagonists (WAY-VPA985 and SR49-059) and a combined V1A/V2 receptor antagonist YM087 are being evaluated in clinical trials in patients with class III and IV heart failure who are currently on standard treatment that includes continuous inotropic drug infusion.

Adenosine Receptor Antagonism Blockade of adenosine (A1) receptors in animals can induce a brisk natriuresis without a kaliuretic effect,[252] an observation that has been confirmed in humans in short-term studies using FK 4531, a selective A1 receptor antagonist.[253-255] The mechanism for this lack of kaliuretic action has not been elucidated; neither has the safety and efficacy of this drug class in long-term clinical trials.

Oral Dopamine Receptor Agonists The unique, selective vasodilatory and inotropic actions of intravenous dopamine are limited by the lack of an oral formulation. This has led investigators to develop newer dopamine agonists that are orally effective. Unlike L-dopa, which has been used in heart failure, these new drugs do not cross the blood-brain barrier but maintain most of the pharmacologic activity of dopamine.[256]

Ibopamine, which is an orally active derivative of dopamine, has dopaminergic D_1 and D_2 activity with alpha- and beta-adrenergic actions. In therapeutic doses, it is a peripheral vasodilator and appears to have favorable cardiovascular and renovascular actions in patients with heart failure. The results of the Prospective Randomized Study of Ibopamine on Mortality and Efficacy in Heart Failure (PRIME-2), however, raised serious questions about the safety of ibopamine and agents of this class[257] in patients with heart failure. Fenoldopam is a selective D_1 agonist that has been used to treat patients with CHF and hypertension. Because of bioavailability problems with the oral formulation, only the intravenous form is used in patients with severe hypertension.[258] Dopexamine is an intravenous D_1 and beta$_2$-receptor agonist that is being studied in patients with CHF and low cardiac output states.

Inhibition of Immune Activation Cytokines are a group of small pleiotropic endogenous peptides produced by a variety of cell types in response to a variety of different stimuli. Tumor necrosis factor-alpha (TNFα), interleukin-1α and -1β, and interleukin-6 are classified as "proinflammatory" cytokines. These substances are responsible for initiating the primary host response to bacterial infections as well as initiating the repair of injured tissues.[259]

Cytokines are involved in augmenting the expression of adhesion molecules and the enhanced cell-to-cell interactions involved in inflammation. In addition, the proinflammatory cytokines are able to affect cardiovascular functioning by promoting LV remodeling, causing ventricular dysfunction, and uncoupling myocardial beta receptors.[259] They are elevated in the serum in various cardiovascular disorders and are often a marker of the severity of disease.[260]

TNFα was originally discovered in 1975 as a protein with necrotizing effects in certain transplantable mouse tumors.[261] More recently, this cytokine has been shown to exert a spectrum of pleiotropic effects in many different cell types.[262] The major biological role of TNFα is thought to be a host response to systemic infections, most notably gram-negative sepsis.[263] In fact, TNFα levels are elevated considerably in patients with septic shock, and TNFα has been implicated as an important mediator in the lethal effect of endotoxin, possibly causing the symptoms characteristic of the "shock state."

Many experimental and clinical studies have shown an association between depressed myocardial function and elevated levels of TNFα.[264] The basis of this association is not clear; however, there are studies suggesting that elevated levels of TNFα play a major role in causing myocardial depression, whereas other studies have concluded that TNFα is likely to play a role in the alleviation of this condition.[265] A third school of thought suggests that the elevated levels of TNFα are merely a marker that may indicate the stage of progression of the disease. Thus, although it is clear that there are elevated levels of TNFα in various cardiac diseases, the reasons for these increased levels and the mechanisms of their effects are not agreed on. Since there is a strong association and possibly a causative relationship between TNFα and CHF, various drug trials are looking at TNFα and its possible metabolic pathways as a therapeutic target in the treatment of heart disease.[266]

The drugs thalidomide and pentoxifylline have been shown in small studies to suppress the production of TNFα in patients with heart failure, with favorable effects on hemodynamics being reported.

A study is in progress evaluating the effects of a soluble recombinant human TNF-R fusion protein (etanercept) on the clinical course of patients with advanced heart failure.[267–269] Preliminary results suggest that etanercept will suppress the cardioinflammatory cytokines IL-1β and IL-6 while increasing the anti-inflammatory cytokine IL-10. These effects appeared to be associated with impaired clinical functioning and regression of ventricular remodeling. Other inflammatory cytokines may be therapeutic targets in the future.

A recent clinical trial evaluated the use of the intravenous immunoglobulin IgG in patients with a new onset of dilated cardiomyopathy, with no apparent benefit compared to placebo. In experimental studies, the cytokine interleukin-10 has been used successfully to treat viral myocarditis.[270]

Studies with prednisone and cyclosporine have shown no clinical benefit in the treatment of patients with dilated cardiomyopathy and myocarditis.[271–273]

Other approaches under consideration for attenuating the heightened inflammatory responses observed in patients with heart failure include monoclonal antibodies that interfere with complement activation and those which interfere with neutrophil adhesion and migration.

Nitric Oxide Preliminary work is being done investigating inhaled nitric oxide, a vasodilator substance produced by the endothelium, as a possible treatment for CHF.[274–277] Arginine, a nitric oxide precursor, and agents that potentiate nitric oxide synthesis, are now potential directions for new heart failure therapies. To date, results with L-arginine use in patients with heart failure have been inconclusive. Nitric oxide donor substances are also being evaluated.[277]

Imidazoline Receptor Agonists The drugs rilmenidine and moxonidine are centrally acting antihypertensive agents that decrease sympathetic outflow by stimulating nonadrenergic imidazole-l receptors in the brain. These drugs are similar to clonidine in their pharmacologic activities but cause less sedation. Modulation of the sympathetic nervous system by decreasing central catecholamine release has been proposed as a therapeutic approach to prolonging life in patients with CHF. However, the results of a recent study using moxonidine in heart failure patients did not show any benefit on survival.[278]

Matrix Metalloproteinase Inhibitors Matrix metalloproteinases and their inhibitors are biological proteins that are involved with the formation and breakdown of collagen and interstitial tissue. Matrix metalloproteinase activity is elevated in patients with heart failure, suggesting that these proteins may be contributors to myocardial remodeling and the worsening of symptoms.

Matrix metalloproteinase inhibitors are being considered as treatments for heart failure.[279]

Supplementary Hormones and Antioxidants Increasing experimental evidence and preliminary clinical data suggest that growth hormones may have beneficial effects in the treatment of heart failure. However, the mechanisms behind these favorable actions are not well understood.[280,281] Growth hormone exerts its effects either directly or indirectly through insulin growth factors.

In experimental studies, growth hormone has been shown to increase the force of contraction by increasing the number of myocardial cross-bridges and the amount of available calcium. Growth hormone also can enhance peripheral blood flow and increase skeletal muscle mass. Growth hormone has been shown to attenuate pathologic remodeling without inducing LV hypertrophy.

In patients with heart failure, growth hormone has been shown to improve LV systolic function and exercise tolerance while normalizing plasma levels of BNP. Long-term morbidity and mortality studies in patients with heart failure remain to be done.

Anabolic steroids have been evaluated in patients with heart failure. They have been shown to improve left myocardial performance, increase skeletal muscle, and improve the patient's sense of well being. However, there is little long-term morbidity and mortality experience with this treatment.

Metabolic Enhancers and Antimetabolites Abnormalities of energy metabolism often are cited as key elements in the progression of the worsening LV dysfunction that characterizes heart failure. Ranolazine is one of a class of partial inhibitors of fatty oxidation (pFOX inhibitors). By shifting adenosine triphosphate production away from fatty acid oxidation and toward carbohydrate oxidation, ranolazine reduces oxygen demand without decreasing cardiac work and maintaining coupling of glycolysis to pyruvate oxidation, which minimizes lactate accumulation. Ranolazine may be useful as an antianginal drug, and in experimental heart failure studies it has been shown to improve LV performance.

Carnitine is a biological substance that plays an important role in the oxidation of long-chain fatty acids. It also allows for the removal of short- and medium-chain fatty acids from the cell. Carnitine also has been shown to facilitate the aerobic metabolism of carbohydrates.[282]

It has been demonstrated by investigators that myocardial carnitine levels are decreased in many pediatric and adult cardiomyopathies in which myocardial fatty acid metabolism is impaired. It has been proposed that the restoration of normal carnitine levels through the administration of exogenous L-carnitine would be of therapeutic value in heart failure through its ability to stimulate fatty acid metabolism.

The usefulness of oral L-carnitine for the treatment of pediatric cardiomyopathy is well established.[283] A few small studies in patients with heart failure have examined the effects of L-carnitine and have demonstrated improvements in hemodynamics, functional capacity, and survival.[282] A large randomized, placebo-controlled trial is still required to adequately assess the usefulness of L-carnitine in heart failure.

Coenzyme Q10(CoQ10), or ubiquinone, is an endogenous cellular membrane constituent that has been shown to have antioxidant properties. Its central physiologic role is in mediating electron transport between nicotinamide adenine dinucleotide and succinate dehydrogenases and the cytochrome system.

CoQ10 has been suggested as a treatment for CHF in which low levels of the substance in the myocardium have been observed. Despite a theoretical benefit in patients with heart failure, trials with CoQ10 supplementation have not demonstrated any effectiveness.

Heart failure also has been associated with the accumulation of oxygen free radicals, which can cause cellular damage in the heart. At this juncture, treatments with various nutritive antioxidants (vitamins and minerals) and naturally occurring enzymatic free radical scavengers have not been associated with efficacy in patients with heart failure.

Antiapoptosis Therapy An innovative approach to preserving myocardial function involves interventions that can interfere with programmed myocardial cell death (apoptosis), a natural process that is accelerated by aging, myocardial ischemia, hypertension, diabetes mellitus, and myocardial cell stretch (LV dilation). Utilization of AII receptor blockers and the infusion of insulin growth factor in rats can inhibit the amount of myocardial apoptosis by 50 percent and suggests future therapeutic approaches in human beings. Caspase, an enzyme essential to the apoptotic process, can be inhibited pharmacologically, with evidence of enhanced myocardial preservation in experimental animals.

Gene Therapy

In experimental studies, gene therapy has been shown to improve failing human cardiac myocyte function.[284,285] It was demonstrated that the abnormal contraction, relaxation, and contraction amplitude-frequency relationship of isolated myocytes obtained from patients with dilated cardiomyopathy could be normalized by transfection of the myocytes in vitro with an adenovirus expressing the sarcoplasmic reticulum Ca^{2+}-ATPase, SERCA2a; transfection increased Ca^{2+}-ATPase activity 80 percent. The enhanced function of the myocytes was associated with corresponding improvements in the kinetics of the Ca^{2+} transient. The isolated myocyte results confirm previous in vitro findings by Meyer and associates in normal rabbit myocytes that indicated that adenoviral transfection of SERCA2a can improve contraction and relaxation.[286]

Nonpharmacologic Aspects of Treatment

Nonpharmacologic factors contribute to the overall efficacy of care. Weight reduction by dieting is generally advisable when obesity is present. Often, however, nutritional status is compromised and cachexia is present.[287] Limitation of salt intake is important and may delay the time when diuretics may be necessary as well as reduce the amount required. In advanced heart failure, strict salt limitation is essential, although it is difficult to maintain. A diet containing less than 20 g/day of salt is desirable. Intake of fluids should be reduced to 1 to 1.5 L every 24 h in patients with advanced heart failure, with or without hyponatremia, except in warm climates. As will be stressed in relation to the use of diuretics, a readable weight scale is essential, and daily weights are of great value in judging therapy.

Smoking should be discouraged strongly in all patients, especially in the presence of obstructive vascular disease. Alcohol is a cardiac depressant in general and should be forbidden if an alcoholic cardiomyopathy is suspected. In all other cases, daily intake of alcohol probably should not exceed 40 g/day in men and 30 g/day in women, although there are insufficient data on the effects of alcohol in patients with mild heart failure to support these recommendations.[288]

Patients should routinely receive vaccinations against influenza and pneumococcal pneumonia.

Deconditioning related to muscular inactivity in association with muscular atrophy and decreased metabolic vascular dilatation is a major factor in reducing exercise performance as heart failure progresses.[289] The 6-min walk test is a semiquantitative assessment tool for assessing functional capacity before and after treatment.[290] Low-level exercise, such as walking, should be encouraged, whereas strenuous isometric activities should be discouraged. Specific exercise training needs to be tailored to the appropriate level of the patient's disease and always should be performed under medical guidance. Isometric exercise should be avoided. In patients with stable heart failure, there is evidence that appropriate physical exercise and exercise training can lead to improvements in both exercise capacity and the quality of life of the patient, although the effect of this intervention on the prognosis is unknown.[291–293] Specific recommendations include dynamic aerobic exercise (walking) three to five times a week for 20 to 30 min and cycling for 20 min at 70 to 80 percent of the peak heart rate five times a week.[291,292]

In patients with acute heart failure and in those with exacerbations of chronic heart failure, rest is advisable. Prolonged rest, however, should not be encouraged in patients with stable chronic heart failure.

Surgical Treatment

BIVENTRICULAR CARDIAC PACING

The use of dual-chamber pacemaker technology to treat patients with chronic heart failure remains controversial.[294–300] It has been proposed that by altering the timing, sequence, and site of cardiac electrical activation in patients with heart failure, hemodynamic abnormalities may be favorably altered.

The subgroups of patients with heart failure who might benefit include (1) those with an atrial contraction too early in relation to the onset of ventricular contraction during native conduction, (2) patients with long atrioventricular (AV) conduction and significant shortening of the diastolic filling period because of presystolic mitral or tricuspid regurgitation or both, and (3) certain patients with ECG PR intervals >200 ms in whom dual-chamber pacing at an optimal AV delay eliminates diastolic mitral regurgitation and improves cardiac output.[294]

In patients with heart failure, it was shown that single-site pacing at the site of greatest intraventricular conduction delay was as beneficial in improving hemodynamics as was biventricular pacing[300]

A blinded randomized clinical trial is in progress [The Multicenter InSync Randomized Clinical Evaluation (MIRACLE)] evaluating a new biventricular myocardial conduction resynchronization device (InSync) in 300 patients with class III and IV heart failure. End points include measures of functional status, quality of life, and effects on peak oxygen consumption and echocardiographic indices of both systolic and diastolic function.

IMPLANTABLE CARDIOVERTER DEFIBRILLATORS

In patients with documented sustained ventricular tachycardia or ventricular fibrillation, an implantable cardioverter defibrillator is highly effective in treating recurrences of these arrhythmias by antitachycardia pacing or cardioversion-defibrillation, reducing morbidity and the need for rehospitalization. There is some evidence that the efficacy of this device in terminating ventricular tachycardia or ventricular fibrillation may translate into improved survival[3,301] in patients with heart failure, but no definite proof exists. Studies are in progress that are designed to address this issue.[302,303]

The benefit of implantable cardioverter defibrillation therapy may decrease with increasing degrees of heart failure.[304] Preliminary data suggest improved survival compared with conventional antiarrhythmic therapy, including amiodarone, in patients with asymptomatic LV dysfunction or mild to moderate heart failure.[305,306] For patients with severe heart failure and documented sustained ventricular tachyarrhythmias, implantable cardioverter defibrillators at present should be considered a bridge to transplantation, but their effectiveness in this setting has not been proved.

LEFT VENTRICULAR ASSIST DEVICES

In a patient who cannot be sustained with medical therapy and for whom ultimate cardiac transplantation is anticipated, an LV mechanical support device (LVAD) has been successful in serving to maintain ventricular function as a bridge to transplantation. With two portable devices now approved by the FDA, the question remains whether they eventually can be used as long-term destination therapy for patients with end-stage heart disease. Preliminary results from randomized studies have demonstrated a 100 percent increase in survival at 2 years in patients with class IV heart failure who are ineligible for heart transplantation and are maintained on standard medical therapy. However, recent data have shown that LVAD implantation in heart failure patients is associated with activation-induced T-cell death and immune dysfunction, putting recipients at risk of serious infection.[307]

HEART TRANSPLANTATION

Heart transplantation is now an accepted mode of treatment for end-stage CHF. Transplantation significantly increases survival, exercise capacity, return to work, and quality of life compared with conventional treatment provided that proper selection criteria are applied. Recent results in patients on triple immunosuppressive therapy have shown a 5-year survival of approximately 70 to 80 percent[308] and a return to full- or part-time work or seeking employment after 1 year in about two-thirds of the patients in the best series.[309]

Patients who should be considered for transplantation are those with severe CHF with no alternative form of treatment. Predictors of poor survival are taken into account. The patient must be willing and able to undergo intensive medical treatment and be emotionally stable to withstand the many uncertainties that are likely to occur both before and after transplantation.

Besides a shortage of donor hearts, the main problem in heart transplantation is rejection of the allograft, which is responsible for a considerable percentage of deaths in the first postoperative year. The long-term outcome is limited predominantly by the consequences of immunosuppression (infection, hypertension, renal failure, malignancy, accelerated progression

TABLE 21-6 Chronic Heart Failure—Choice of Pharmacologic Therapy

	ACE Inhibitor	Diuretic	Potassium-Sparing Diuretic	Cardiac-glycosides	Vasodilator (Hydralazine/ISDN)	Beta Blocker
Systolic dysfunction						
Asymptomatic LV dysfunction	Indicated in some	Not indicated (unless ↑ BP)	Not indicated	Only with atrial fibrillation	Not indicated	After MI
Symptomatic HF (NYHA-II)	Indicated			(a) When atrial fibrillation is present or (b) when improved from more severe HF in sinus rhythm[a]	If ACE inhibitors are not tolerated	Indicated (under specialist care)
− Fluid retention		Indicated in some	Not indicated			
+ Fluid retention		Indicated	Persisting hypokalemia			
Worsening/severe HF (NYHA III–IV)	Indicated	Indicated, combinations of diuretics	Persisting hypokalemia; spironolactone for efficacy	Indicated	If ACE inhibitors are not tolerated or insufficient	Indicated (under specialist care)
End-stage HF (persisting NHYA IV)	Indicated	Indicated, combinations of diuretics	Persisting hypokalemia; spironolactone for efficacy	Indicated	If ACE inhibitors are not tolerated or insufficient	Indicated (under specialist care)

[a]Preliminary data from the DIG (Digitalis Investigation Group) trial suggest that digoxin also may be indicated in NYHA II heart failure and sinus rhythm.

NOTE: ACE, angiotensin-converting enzyme; BP, blood pressure; HF, heart failure; ISDN, isosorbide dinitrate; LV, left ventricular; MI, myocardial infarction; NYHA, New York Heart Association.

SOURCE: From Task Force of the Working Group on Heart Failure of the European Society of Cardiology. The treatment of heart failure. *Eur Heart J* 1997; 18:748. Reproduced with permission from the publisher and authors.

of atherosclerotic vascular disease) and by transplant coronary artery disease.

Experimental work is under way looking at xenotransplantation of myocardial cells and entire organs (pig hearts) as potential heart failure treatment. The humoral immune response of the recipient against the graft remains a preeminent hurdle. There is also limited information regarding the physiology of the pig heart as a replacement for the human heart.

CORONARY REVASCULARIZATION SURGERY

A major and important surgical approach to ischemic cardiomyopathies is reperfusion of ischemic tissue by coronary bypass surgery.[310] This is based on the concept that transiently ischemic myocardium (stunning) and myocardium with reduced flow (hibernating) have reduced contractility, which may return to normal with restoration of adequate coronary blood flow. Moreover, revascularization of ischemic regions of the ventricle may prevent recurrent infarction in this area and thus help prevent further deterioration of ventricular function. In such patients, it is necessary to establish that significant amounts of viable tissue remain in an akinetic or hypokinetic zone; this can be accomplished with nuclear techniques such as a 24-h thallium perfusion study and positron emission tomographic scanning.[311] If contractile activity also can be elicited, as shown in echo studies with low-dose dobutamine stimulation[22] or postextrasystolic potentiation, coronary bypass surgery provides a good chance to stabilize or improve ventricular function[310,312,313] and enhance survival.[314] In this era, every patient with ischemic cardiomyopathy should be evaluated for possible revascularization and assumed to be a candidate until proved otherwise.

OTHER PROCEDURES

Other surgical approaches to the dilated heart have included the recent concept of removing a segment of the left ventricular wall, the "Battista operation," to reduce LV volume and thus wall stress. The surgical risk is immense, and specific benefits have not been established.[315]

Enhanced external counterpulsation is a noninvasive therapy consisting of gated diastolic sequential leg compression, producing hemodynamic effects similar to those from an intraaortic

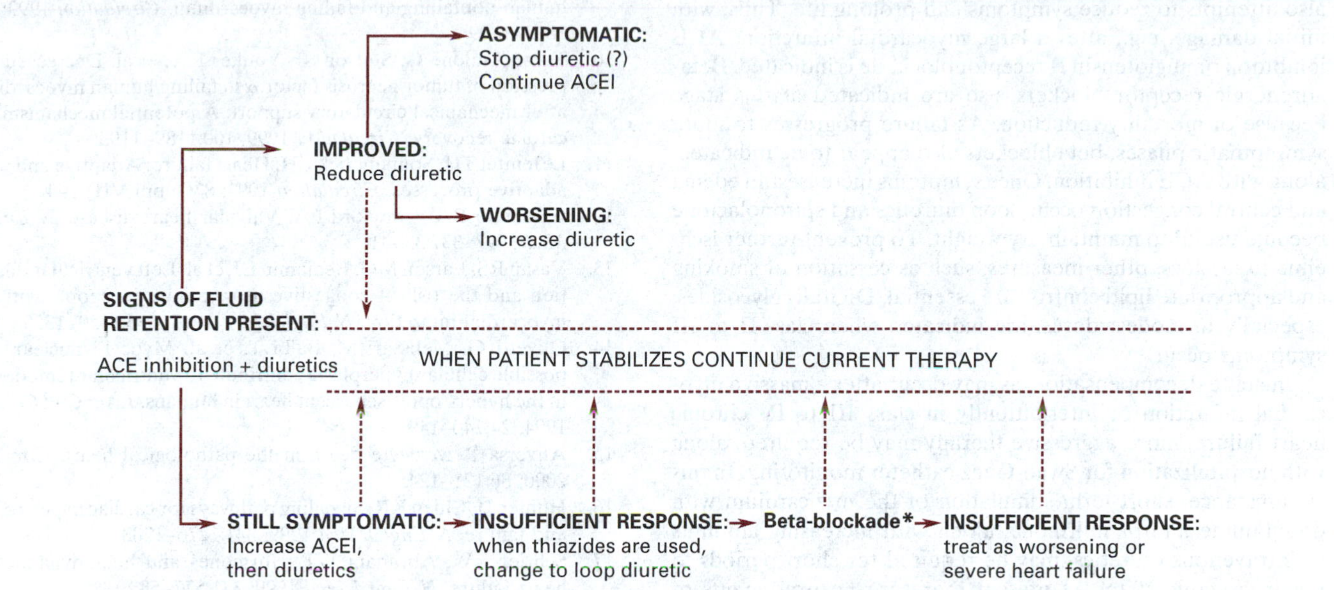

FIGURE 21-11 Flowchart of pharmacologic treatment of mild symptomatic systolic left ventricular (LV) dysfunction, NYHA II, and signs of fluid retention. * Data available only for carvedilol. (From Task Force of the Working Group on Heart Failure of the European Society of Cardiology. The treatment of heart failure. *Eur Heart J* 1997; 18:746. Reproduced with permission from the publisher and authors.)

balloon pump. The procedure has been shown to improve exercise capacity and LV failure in patients with heart failure who already are receiving medical therapy.[316]

Immunoabsorption procedures have been directed against beta$_1$-adrenergic receptor antibodies, with clinical improvement found in patients with heart failure.[317]

The General Approach to Therapy in Congestive Heart Failure

Appropriate therapy in CHF depends on the stage of the disease process (Table 21-6 and Figs. 21-11 and 21-12). While one seeks to define and treat the factors that initiated the process, one

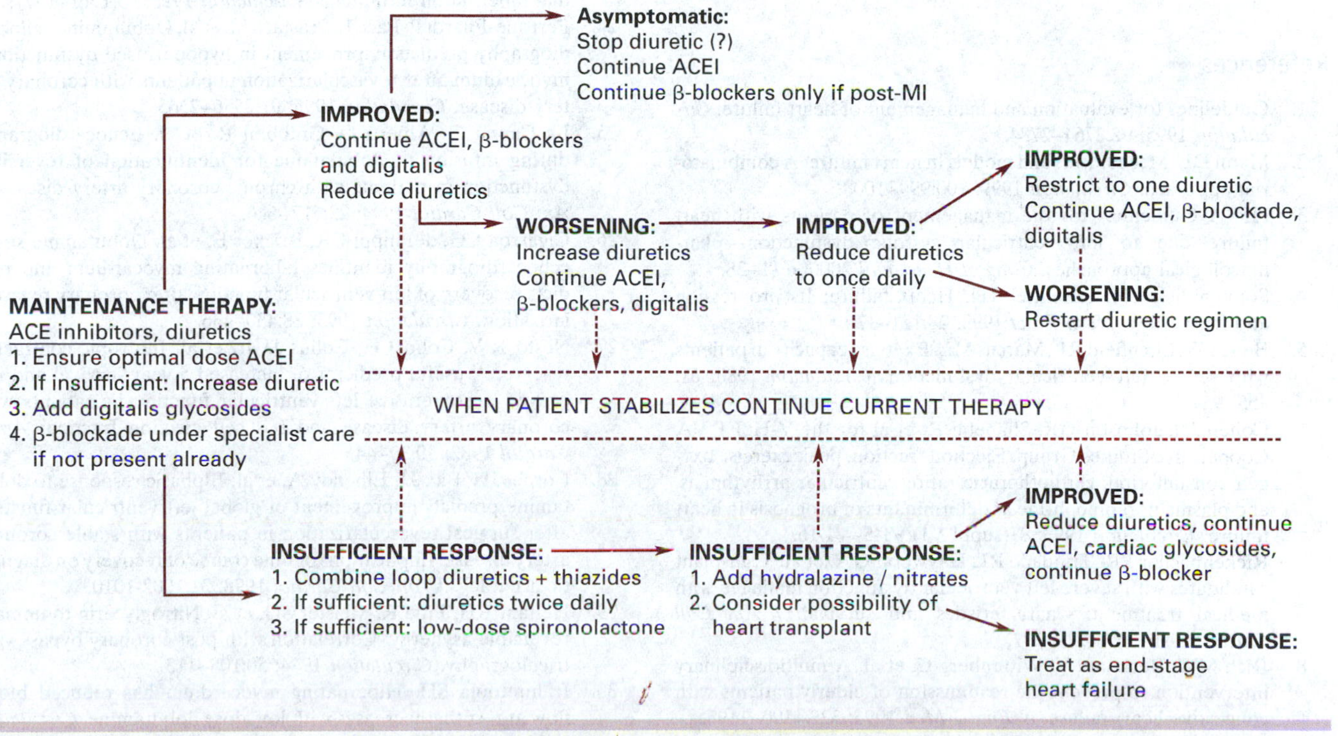

FIGURE 21-12 Flowchart of pharmacologic treatment of symptomatic left ventricular dysfunction and worsening heart failure (NYHA III to IV). (From Task Force of the Working Group on Heart Failure of the European Society of Cardiology. The treatment of heart failure. *Eur Heart J* 1997; 18:747. Reproduced with permission from the publisher and authors.)

also attempts to reduce symptoms and prolong life. Thus, with initial damage, e.g., after a large myocardial infarction, ACE inhibition or angiotensin II receptor blockade is indicated. Beta-adrenergic receptor blockers also are indicated at this stage because of mortality reduction. As failure progresses to more symptomatic phases, beta blockers also appear to be indicated, along with ACE inhibition. Once symptoms increase and edema and central congestion occur, loop diuretics and spironolactone become useful to maintain dry weight. To prevent further ischemic tissue loss, other measures, such as cessation of smoking and appropriate lipid control, are essential. Digitalis glycosides, especially in modest doses, are indicated when class II to III symptoms occur.

In acute decompensation, as may occur after a massive myocardial infarction or intermittently in class III to IV chronic heart failure, more aggressive therapy may be required, along with hospitalization for Swan-Ganz catheter monitoring. In this circumstance, short-term stimulation of the myocardium with dobutamine and/or milrinone, along with increasing amounts of intravenous diuretics, may be required for short periods to regain a stable state. At present there are no oral agents of this nature available to extend this care to outpatients, and if dobutamine cannot be withdrawn, occasional administration by an external pump is required. Such therapy presents a short outcome of days or months.

In summary, therapy for heart failure seeks the reversal or attenuation of the processes that initiated the syndrome while treating the patient to relieve symptoms and prolong life. The latter end is best achieved early in the disease process through prevention of further loss of myocardium (e.g., reperfusion) or reduction of loading (e.g., appropriate valve surgery or treatment of hypertension). In very late stages of the disease, relief of symptoms can now be accomplished with modest gains in life expectancy.

References

1. Guidelines for evaluation and management of heart failure. *Circulation* 1995; 92:2764–2784.
2. Mann DL. Mechanisms and models in heart failure: A combinatorial approach. *Circulation* 1999; 100:999–1008.
3. HFSA Guidelines for the management of patients with heart failure due to left ventricular systolic dysfunction—pharmacological approaches. *Congest Heart Fail* 2000; 6:11–38.
4. Sonnenblick EH, LeJemtel TH. Heart failure: Its progression and its therapy. *Hosp Pract* 1993; 28:121–130.
5. Benge W, Litchfield RL, Marcus ML. Exercise capacity in patients with severe left ventricular dysfunction. *Circulation* 1980; 61: 955–959.
6. Cohen JN, Johnson GR, Shabetai R, et al for the V-HeFT VA Cooperative Studies Group. Ejection fraction, peak exercise oxygen consumption, cardiothoracic ratio, ventricular arrhythmias, and plasma norepinephrine as determinants of prognosis in heart failure. *Circulation* 1993; 87(suppl VI):VI-5–VI-16.
7. Rickenbacher PR, Trindade PT, Haywood GA, et al. Transplant candidates with severe left ventricular dysfunction managed with medical treatment: Characteristics and survival. *J Am Coll Cardiol* 1996; 27:1192–1197.
8. Rich MW, Beckham V, Wittenberg C, et al. A multidisciplinary intervention to prevent the readmission of elderly patients with congestive heart failure. *N Engl J Med* 1995; 333:1190–1195.
9. Pieske B, Beyermann B, Breu V, et al. Functional effects of endothelin and regulation of endothelin receptors in isolated human nonfailing and failing myocardium. *Circulation* 1999; 99: 1802–1809.
10. Torre-Amione G, Stetson SJ, Youker KA, et al. Decreased expression of tumor necrosis factor-α in failing human myocardium after mechanical circulatory support: A potential mechanism for cardiac recovery. *Circulation* 1999; 100:1189–1193.
11. LeJemtel TH, Sonnenblick EH. Heart failure: Adaptive and maladaptive processes. *Circulation* 1993; 87(suppl VII):1–4.
12. Carabello BA, Crawford FA. Valvular heart disease. *N Engl J Med* 1997; 337:32–41.
13. Vasan RS, Larson MG, Benjamin EJ, et al. Left ventricular dilatation and the risk of congestive heart failure in people without myocardial infarction. *N Engl J Med* 1997; 336:1350–1355.
14. Olivetti G, Melissari M, Balbi T, et al. Myocyte nuclear and possible cellular hyperplasia contribute to ventricular remodeling in the hypertrophic senescent heart in humans. *J Am Coll Cardiol* 1994; 24:140–149.
15. Anversa P. Myocyte death in the pathological heart. *Circ Res* 2000; 86:121–124.
16. Hunter JJ, Chien KR. Signaling pathways for cardiac hypertrophy and failure. *N Engl J Med* 1999; 341:1276–1283.
17. Schrier RW, Abraham WT. Hormones and hemodynamics in heart failure. *N Engl J Med* 1999; 341:577–585.
18. Olivetti G, Abbi R, Quaini F, et al. Apoptosis in the failing human heart. *N Engl J Med* 1997; 336:1131–1141.
19. LeJemtel TH, Sonnenblick EH. Heart failure in elderly patients. In: Aronow W, Tresch DD, eds. *Cardiovascular Disease in the Elderly Patient.* New York: Marcel Dekker; 1993:473.
20. Brutsaert DL, Sonnenblick EH. Cardiac muscle mechanics in the evaluation of myocardial contractility and pump function: Problems, concepts and directions. *Prog Cardiovasc Dis* 1973; 16:337–361.
21. Hendel RC, Chandhry FA, Bonow RO. Myocardial viability. *Curr Probl Cardiol* 1996; 21:145–224.
22. Bonow RO. Identification of viable myocardium. *Circulation* 1996; 94:2674–2680.
23. Vanoverschelde J-LJ, Wijns W, Borgers M, et al. Chronic myocardial hibernation in humans. *Circulation* 1996; 95:1961–1971.
24. Perrone-Filardi P, Pace L, Prastaro M, et al. Dobutamine echocardiography predicts improvement in hypoperfused dysfunctional myocardium after revascularization in patients with coronary artery disease. *Circulation* 1995; 91:2556–2565.
25. La Canna G, Alfiero O, Giubbini R, et al. Echocardiography during infusion of dobutamine for identification of reversible dysfunction in patients with chronic coronary artery disease. *J Am Coll Cardiol* 1994; 23:617–626.
26. Cigarroa CG, deFilippi CR, Bricker E, et al. Dobutamine stress echocardiography identifies hibernating myocardium and predicts recovery of left ventricular function after coronary revascularization. *Circulation* 1993; 88:430–436.
27. Nesto RW, Cohn LH, Colins JJ Jr, et al. Inotropic contractile reserve: A useful predictor of increased 5 year survival and improved postoperative left ventricular function in patients with coronary artery disease and reduced ejection fraction. *Am J Cardiol* 1982; 50:39–44.
28. Cornel JH, Bax JJ, Elhendy A, et al. Biphasic response to dobutamine predicts improvement of global left ventricular function after surgical revascularization in patients with stable coronary artery disease: Implications of time course of recovery on diagnostic accuracy. *J Am Coll Cardiol* 1998; 31:1002-1010.
29. Helfant RH, Pine R, Meister SG, et al. Nitroglycerin to unmask reversible asynergy: Correlation with post coronary bypass ventriculography. *Circulation* 1974; 50:108–113.
30. Rahimtoola SH. Hibernating myocardium has reduced blood flow at rest that increases with low-dose dobutamine. *Circulation* 1996; 94:3055–3061.
31. Popio KA, Gorlin R, Bechtel D, Levine JA. Postextrasystolic

potentiation as a predictor of potential myocardial viability: Preoperative analyses compared with studies after coronary bypass surgery. *Am J Cardiol* 1977; 39:944–953.

32. Floras JS. Clinical aspects of sympathetic activation and parasympathetic withdrawal in heart failure. *J Am Coll Cardiol* 1993; 22(suppl A):72A–84A.
33. Picard MH, Wilkins GT, Ray PA, Weyman AE. Natural history of left ventricular size and function after actue myocardial infarction: Assessment and prediction by echocardiographic endocardial surface mapping. *Circulation* 1990; 82:484–494.
34. St. John Sutton M, Pfeffer MA, Plappert T, et al for the SAVE Investigators. Quantitative two-dimensional echocardiographic measurements are major predictors of adverse cardiovascular events after acute myocardial infarction: The protective effects of captopril. *Circulation* 1994; 89:68–75.
35. Marmor A, Raphael T, Marmor M, Blondheim D. Evaluation of contractile reserve by dobutamine echocardiography: Noninvasive estimation of the severity of heart failure. *Am Heart J* 1996; 132:1195–1201.
36. Horn HR, Teichholz LE, Cohn PF, et al. Augmentation of left ventricular contraction pattern in coronary artery disease by an inotropic catecholamine: The epinephrine ventriculogram. *Circulation* 1974; 49:1063–1071.
37. Gheorghiade M, Bonow RO. Chronic heart failure in the United States: A manifestation of coronary artery disease. *Circulation* 1998; 97:282–289.
38. Packer M, Cohn JN (eds) on behalf of the Steering Committee and Membership of the Advisory Council to Improve Outcomes Nationwide in Heart Failure. Consensus recommendations for the management of chronic heart failure. *Am J Cardiol* 1999; 3(suppl 2A):1–38.
39. Francis GS, Benedict C, Johnstone DE, et al. Comparison of neuroendocrine activation in patients with left ventricular dysfunction with and without congestive heart failure: A substudy of the Studies of Left Ventricular Dysfunction (SOLVD). *Circulation* 1990; 82:1724–1729.
40. Kajstura J, Cigola E, Malhotra A, et al. Angiotensin II induces apoptosis of adult ventricular myocytes in vitro. *J Mol Cell Cardiol* 1997; 29:859–870.
41. Davis R, Ribner HS, Keung E, et al. Treatment of chronic congestive heart failure with captopril, an oral inhibitor of angiotensin-converting enzyme. *N Engl J Med* 1979; 301:117–121.
42. Remme WJ. Vasodilator therapy without converting-enzyme inhibition in congestive heart failure—usefulness and limitations. *Cardiovasc Drugs Ther* 1989; 3:375–396.
43. Captopril Multicenter Research Group. A placebo-controlled trial of captopril in refractory chronic congestive heart failure. *J Am Coll Cardiol* 1983; 2:755–763.
44. Massie BM, Kramer BL, Topic N. Lack of relationship between the short-term hemodynamic effects of captopril and subsequent clinical responses. *Circulation* 1984; 69:1135–1141.
45. Drexler H, Banhardt U, Meinertz T, et al. Contrasting peripheral short-term and long-term effects of converting enzyme inhibition in patients with congestive heart failure: A double-blind, placebo-controlled trial. *Circulation* 1989; 79:491–502.
46. Mancini GBJ, Henry GC, Macaya C, et al. Angiotensin converting enzyme inhibition with quinapril improves endothelial vasomotor dysfunction in patients with coronary artery disease: The TREND (Trial on Reversing ENdothelial Dysfunction) Study. *Circulation* 1996; 94:258–265.
47. Hornig B, Arakawa N, Haussmann D, Drexler H. Differential effects of quinaprilat and enalaprilat on endothelial function of conduit arteries in patients with chronic heart failure. *Circulation* 1998; 98:2842–2848.
48. Griendling KK, Berk BC, Ganz P, et al. Angiotensin II stimulation of vascular smooth muscle phosphoinositide metabolism: State of the art lecture. *Hypertension* 1987; 9(suppl III):III-181–III-185.
49. Giles TD, Katz R, Sullivan JM, et al. Short- and long-acting angiotensin converting enzyme inhibitors: A randomized trial of lisinopril versus captopril in the treatment of congestive heart failure. *J Am Coll Cardiol* 1989; 13:1240–1247.
50. Konstam MA, Rousseau MF, Kronenberg MW, et al. Effects of the angiotensin converting enzyme inhibitor enalapril on the long-term progression of left ventricular dysfunction in patients with heart failure. *Circulation* 1992; 86:431–438.
51. McKelvie RS, Yusuf S, Pericak D, et al. Comparison of candesartan, enalapril, and their combination in congestive heart failure: Randomized Evaluation of Strategies for Left Ventricular Dysfunction (RESOLVD) pilot study: The RESOLVD pilot study investigators. *Circulation* 1999; 100:1056–1064.
52. Zannad F. Aldosterone and heart failure. *Eur Heart J* 1995; 16(suppl N):98–102.
53. MacFadyen RJ, Lee AFC, Morton JJ, et al. How often are angiotensin II and aldosterone concentrations raised during chronic ACE inhibitor treatment in cardiac failure? *Heart* 1999; 82:57–61.
54. Volpe M, Tritto C, DeLuca N, et al. Angiotensin converting enzyme inhibition restores cardiac and hormonal responses to volume overload in patients with dilated cardiomyopathy and mild heart failure. *Circulation* 1992; 86:1800–1809.
55. LeJemtel TH, Maskin CS, Chadwick B. Effect of acute angiotensin converting enzyme inhibition on renal blood flow in patients with stable congestive heart failure. *Am J Med Sci* 1986; 292: 123–127.
56. Pfeffer MA, Braunwald E. Ventricular remodeling after myocardial infarction: Experimental observations and clinical implications. *Circulation* 1990; 81:1161–1172.
57. Lonn EM, Yusuf S, Jha P, et al. Emerging role of angiotensin-converting enzyme inhibitors in cardiac and vascular protection. *Circulation* 1994; 90:2056–2069.
58. Pfeffer MA, Lamas GA, Vaughan DE, et al. Effect of captopril on progressive ventricular dilatation after anterior myocardial infarction. *N Engl J Med* 1988; 319:80–86.
58a. Pfeffer MA, Braunwald E, Moyé LA, et al. Effect of captopril on mortality and morbidity in patients with left ventricular dysfunction after myocardial infarction. *N Engl J Med* 1992; 327:669–677.
59. ACE Inhibitor Myocardial Infarction Collaborative Group. Indications for ACE inhibitors in the early treatment of acute myocardial infarction: Systematic overview of individual data from 100,000 patients in randomized trials. *Circulation* 1998; 97:2202–2212.
60. The CONSENSUS Trial Study Group. Effect of enalapril on mortality in severe congestive heart failure: Results of the Cooperative North Scandinavian Enalapril Survival Study (CONSENSUS). *N Engl J Med* 1987; 316:1429–1435.
61. Cohn JN, Johnson G, Ziesche S, et al. A comparison of enalapril with hydralazine-isosorbide dinitrate in the treatment of chronic congestive heart failure. *N Engl J Med* 1991; 325:303–310.
62. The SOLVD Investigators. Effect of enalapril on survival in patients with reduced left ventricular ejection fraction and congestive heart failure. *N Engl J Med* 1991; 325:293–302.
63. The SOLVD Investigators. Effect of enalapril on mortality and the development of heart failure in asymptomatic patients with reduced left ventricular ejection fractions. *N Engl J Med* 1992; 327:685–691.
64. Yusuf S, Pepine CJ, Garces C, et al. Effect of enalapril on myocardial infarction and unstable angina in patients with low ejection fractions. *Lancet* 1992; 340:1173–1178.
65. Rajagopalan S, Harrison DG. Reversing endothelial dysfunction with ACE inhibitors: A new TREND? *Circulation* 1996; 94:240–243.
66. The Heart Outcomes Prevention Evaluation Study Investigators.

Effects of an angiotensin-converting-enzyme inhibitor, ramipril, on cardiovascular events in high-risk patients. *N Engl J Med* 2000; 342:145–153.

67. Heart Outcomes Prevention Evaluation (HOPE) study investigators. Effects of ramipril on cardiovascular and microvascular outcomes in people with diabetes mellitus: Results of the HOPE study and MICRO-HOPE substudy. *Lancet* 2000; 355:253–259.
68. Hall D, Zeitler H, Rudolph W. Counteraction of the vasodilator effects of enalapril by aspirin in severe heart failure. *J Am Coll Cardiol* 1992; 20:1549–1555.
69. Latini R, Santoro E, Masson S, et al on behalf of the GISSI-3 Investigators. Aspirin does not interact with ACE inhibitors when both are given early after acute myocardial infarction: Results of the GISSI-3 trial. *Heart Disease* 2000, in press.
70. Packer M, Poole-Wilson PA, Armstrong PW, et al on behalf of the ATLAS Study Group. Comparative effects of low and high doses of the angiotensin-converting inhibitor, lisinopril, on morbidity and mortality in chronic heart failure. *Circulation* 1999; 100:2312–2318.
71. Jorde UP, Ennezat PV, Lisker J, et al. Maximally recommended doses of angiotensin-converting enzyme (ACE) inhibitors do not completely prevent ACE-mediated formation of angiotensin II in chronic heart failure. *Circulation* 2000; 101:844–846.
72. Ruggenenti P, Perna A, Gherardi G, et al. Renal function and requirement for dialysis in chronic nephropathy patients on long-term ramipril: REIN follow-up trial. *Lancet* 1998; 352:1252–1256.
73. Pitt B, Segal R, Martinez FA, et al on behalf of ELITE Study Investigators. Randomised trial of losartan versus captopril in patients over 65 with heart failure (Evaluation of Losartan in the Elderly Study, ELITE). *Lancet* 1997; 349:747–752.
74. Pitt B, Poole-Wilson P, Segal R, et al. Effects of losartan versus captopril on mortality in patients with symptomatic heart failure: Rationale, design, and baseline characteristics of patients in the Losartan Heart Failure Survival Study—ELITE II. *J Cardiac Fail* 1999; 5:146–154.
75. St. John Sutton M, Pfeffer MA, Moye L, et al for the SAVE Investigators. Cardiovascular death and left ventricular remodeling two years after myocardial infarction: Baseline predictors and impact of long-term use of captopril: Information from the Survival and Ventricular Enlargement (SAVE) trial. *Circulation* 1997; 96:3294–3299.
76. Francis GS, Cohn JN, Johnson G, et al for the V-HeFT VA Cooperative Studies Group. Plasma norepinephrine, plasma renin activity, and congestive heart failure: Relations to survival and the effects of therapy in V-HeFT II. *Circulation* 1993; 87(suppl VI):VI-40–VI-48.
77. Rousseau MF, Konstam MA, Benedict CR, et al. Progression of left ventricular dysfunction secondary to coronary artery disease, sustained neurohormonal activation and effects of ibopamine therapy during long-term therapy with angiotensin-converting enzyme inhibitor. *Am J Cardiol* 1994; 73:488–493.
78. Kokkonen JO, Saarinen J, Kovanen PT. Regulation of local angiotensin II formation in the human heart in the presence of interstitial fluid: Inhibition of chymase by protease inhibitors of interstitial fluid and of angiotensin-converting enzyme by Ang-(1-9) formed by heart carboxypeptidase A-like activity. *Circulation* 1997; 95:1455–1463.
79. Ménard J, Campbell DJ, Azizi M, Gonzales M-F. Synergistic effects of ACE inhibition and Ang II antagonism on blood pressure, cardiac weight, and renin in spontaneously hypertensive rats. *Circulation* 1997; 96:3072–3078.
80. Spinale FG, Iannini JP, Mukherjee R, et al. Angiotensin AT1 receptor inhibition, angiotensin-converting enzyme inhibition, and combination therapy with developing heart failure: Cellular mechanisms of action. *J Cardiac Fail* 1998; 4:325–332.
81. Krombach RS, Clair MJ, Hendrick JW, et al. Angiotensin converting enzyme inhibition, AT1 receptor inhibition, and combination therapy with pacing induced heart failure: Effects on left ventricular performance and regional blood flow patterns. *Cardiovasc Res* 1998; 38:631–645.
82. Hamroff G, Blaufarb I, Mancini D, et al. Angiotensin II receptor blockade further reduces afterload safely in patients maximally treated with angiotensin converting enzyme inhibitors for heart failure. *J Cardiovasc Pharmacol* 1997; 30:533–536.
83. Baruch L, Anand I, Cohen IS, et al for the Vasodilator Heart Failure Trial (V-HeFT) Study Group. Augmented short- and long-term hemodynamic and hormonal effects of an angiotensin receptor blocker added to angiotensin converting enzyme inhibitor therapy in patients with heart failure. *Circulation* 1999; 99: 2658–2664.
84. Hamroff G, Katz SD, Mancini D, et al. Addition of angiotensin II receptor blockade to maximal angiotensin-converting enzyme inhibition improves exercise capacity in patients with severe congestive heart failure. *Circulation* 1999; 99:990–992.
85. Gainer JV, Morrow JD, Loveland A, et al. Effect of bradykinin-receptor blockade on the response to angiotensin-converting-enzyme inhibitor in normotensive and hypertensive subjects. *N Engl J Med* 1998; 339:1285–1292.
86. Goodfield NER, Newby DE, Ludlam CA, Flapan AD. Effects of acute angiotensin II type 1 receptor antagonism and angiotensin converting enzyme inhibition on plasma fibrinolytic parameters in patients with heart failure. *Circulation* 1999; 99:2983–2985.
87. Cohn JN, Archibald DG, Ziesche S, et al. Effect of vasodilator therapy on mortality in chronic congestive heart failure: Results of a Veterans Administration Cooperation study. *N Engl J Med* 1986; 314:1547–1552.
88. Packer M, Lee WH, Kessler PD, et al. Prevention and reversal on nitrate tolerance in patients with congestive heart failure. *N Engl J Med* 1987; 317:799–804.
89. Gogia H, Mehra A, Parikh S, et al. Prevention of tolerance to hemodynamic effects of nitrates with concomitant use of hydralazine in patients with chronic heart failure. *J Am Coll Cardiol* 1995; 26:1575–1580.
90. Cohn JN, Ziesche SM, Loss LE, Anderson GT. Effects of felodipine on short-term exercise and neurohormones and long-term mortality in heart failure: Results of V-HeFT III (abstr). *Circulation* 1995; 92(suppl I):I-143.
91. O'Connor CM, Belkin RN, Carson PE, et al for PRAISE Investigators. Effect of amlodipine on mode of death in severe chronic heart failure: The PRAISE trial (abstr). *Circulation* 1995; 92(suppl I):I-143.
92. Frishman W. Calcium channel blockers. In: Frishman WH, Sonnenblick EH, eds. *Cardiovascular Pharmacotherapeutics.* New York: McGraw-Hill; 1997:101.
93. Levine TB, Bernink PJLM, Caspi A, et al. Effect of mibefradil, a T-type channel blocker, on morbidity and mortality in moderate to severe congestive heart failure: The MACH-1 Study. *Circulation* 2000; 101:758–764.
94. Waagstein F, Hjalmarson A, Varnauskas E, Wallentin I. Effect of chronic beta-adrenergic receptor blockade in congestive cardiomyopathy. *Br Heart J* 1975; 37:1022–1036.
95. Frishman WH, Furberg CD, Friedewald WT. β-Adrenergic blockade in survivors of acute myocardial infarction. *N Engl J Med* 1984; 310:830–837.
96. The CIBIS Investigators and Committees. A randomized trial of beta blockade in heart failure: The Cardiac Insufficiency Bisoprolol Study. *Circulation* 1994; 90:1765–1773.
97. Lechat P, Escolano S, Golmard JL, et al on behalf of the CIBIS Investigators. Prognostic value of bisoprolol-induced hemodynamic effects in heart failure during the Cardiac Insufficiency Bisoprolol Study (CIBIS). *Circulation* 1997; 96:2197–2205.
98. CIBIS-II Investigators and Committees. The Cardiac Insufficiency Bisoprolol Study II (CIBIS-II): A randomised trial. *Lancet* 1999; 353:9–13.

99. MERIT-HF Study Group. Effect of metoprolol CR/XL in chronic heart failure: Metoprolol CR/XL randomised intervention trial in congestive heart failure (MERIT-HF). *Lancet* 1999; 353:2001–2007.
100. Frishman WH. Alpha- and beta-adrenergic blocking drugs. In: Frishman WH, Sonnenblick EH, eds. *Cardiovascular Pharmacotherapeutics*. New York: McGraw-Hill; 1997:59.
101. Bristow MR. β-Adrenergic receptor blockade in chronic heart failure. *Circulation* 2000; 101:558–569.
102. Frishman WH. Carvedilol. *N Engl J Med* 1998; 339:1759–1765.
103. Bristow MR, Gilbert EM, Abraham WT, et al for the MOCHA Investigators. Carvedilol produces dose-related improvements in left ventricular function and survival in subjects with chronic heart failure. *Circulation* 1996; 94:2807–2816.
104. Packer M, Colucci WS, Sackner-Bernstein JD, et al for the PRECISE Study Group. Double-blind, placebo-controlled study of the effects of carvedilol in patients with moderate to severe heart failure: The PRECISE trial. *Circulation* 1996; 94:2793–2799.
105. Colucci WS, Packer M, Bristow MR, et al for the U.S. Carvedilol Heart Failure Study Group. Carvedilol inhibits clinical progression in patients with mild symptoms of heart failure. *Circulation* 1996; 94:2800–2806.
106. Cohn JN, Fowler MB, Bristow MR; et al. Safety and efficacy of carvedilol in severe heart failure: *J Cardiac Fail* 1997; 3:173–179.
107. Packer M, Bristow MR, Cohn JN, et al for the U.S. Carvedilol Heart Failure Study Group. The effect of carvedilol on morbidity and mortality in patients with chronic heart failure. *N Engl J Med* 1996; 334:1349–1355.
108. Australia/New Zealand Heart Failure Research Collaborative Group. Randomised, placebo-controlled trial of carvedilol in patients with congestive heart failure due to ischaemic heart disease. *Lancet* 1997; 349:375–380.
109. Hall SA, Cigarroa CG, Marcoux L, et al. Time course of improvement in left ventricular function, mass and geometry in patients with congestive heart failure treated with beta-adrenergic blockade. *J Am Coll Cardiol* 1995; 25:1154–1161.
110. LeJemtel TH, Galvao M, Sonnenblick EH. Beta-adrenergic blockade reverses, while ACE inhibition attenuates, left ventricular remodeling in patients with chronic heart failure. *Heart Fail* 1998; 14:57–63.
111. Doughty RN, Whalley GA, Gamble G, et al on behalf of the Australia-New Zealand Heart Failure Research Collaborative Group. Left ventricular remodeling with carvedilol in patients with congestive heart failure due to ischemic heart disease. *J Am Coll Cardiol* 1997; 29:1060–1066.
112. Packer M. Effects of beta-adrenergic blockade on survival of patients with chronic heart failure. *Am J Cardiol* 1997; 80(11A):46L–54L.
113. Schmidt U, del Monte F, Miyamoto MI, et al. Restoration of diastolic function in senescent rat hearts through adenoviral gene transfer of sarcoplasmic reticulum Ca^{2+}-ATPase. *Circulation* 2000; 101:790–796.
114. Kukin ML, Kalman J, Charney RH, et al. Prospective, randomized comparison of effect of long-term treatment with metoprolol or carvedilol on symptoms, exercise, ejection fraction, and oxidative stress in heart failure. *Circulation* 1999; 99:2645–2651.
115. DiLenarda A, Sabbadini G, Sulvatore L, et al and the Heart-Muscle Disease Study Group. Long-term effects of carvedilol in idiopathic dilated cardiomyopathy with persistent left ventricular dysfunction despite chronic metoprolol. *J Am Coll Cardiol* 1999; 33:1926–1934.
116. Gilbert EM, Abraham WT, Olsen S, et al. Comparative hemodynamic, left ventricular functional, and antiadrenergic effects of chronic treatment with metoprolol versus carvedilol in the failing heart. *Circulation* 1996; 94:2817–2825.
117. Dandona P, Karne R, Ghanim H, et al. Carvedilol inhibits reactive oxygen species generation by leukocytes and oxidative damage to amino acids. *Circulation* 2000; 101:122–124.
118. Schlant RC, Sonnenblick EH. Pathophysiology of heart failure. In: Hurst JW, Schlant RC, Rackly CE, eds. *The Heart*, 7th ed. New York: McGraw-Hill; 1990:387.
119. Bichet DG, Schrier RW. Cardiac failure, liver disease and nephrotic syndrome. In: Schrier RW, Gottschalk CW, eds. *Diseases of the Kidney*, 5th ed. Boston: Little, Brown; 1993:2453.
120. Koeppen BM, Stanton BA. Regulation of extracellular fluid volume. In: Koeppen BM, Stanton BA, eds. *Renal Physiology*. St. Louis: Mosby Year Book; 1992:91.
121. Boles Ponto LL, Schoenwald RD. Furosemide: A pharmacokinetic/pharmacodynamic review. *Clin Pharmacokinet* 1990; 18:381–408.
122. O'Grady SM, Palfrey HC, Field M. Characteristics and function of Na-K-2Cl cotransport in epithelial tissues. *Am J Physiol* 1987; 253(2, part 1):C177–C192.
123. Brater DC, Day B, Burdette A, Anderson S. Bumetidine and furosemide in heart failure. *Kidney Int* 1984; 26:183.
124. Knoben JE, Anderson PO, eds. Diuretics. In: *Clinical Drug Data*, 6th ed. IL: Drug Intelligence Publications; 1988.
125. Voelker JR, Brown-Cartwright D, Anderson S, et al. Comparison of loop diuretics in patients with chronic renal insufficiency: Mechanism of difference in response. *Kidney Int* 1987; 32:572–578.
126. Ward A, Heel RC. Bumetadine: A review of its pharmacokinetic and pharmacodynamic properties and therapeutic use. *Drugs* 1984; 28:426–464.
127. Brater DC. Clinical pharmacology of loop diuretics in health and disease. *Eur Heart J* 1992; 13(suppl G):10–14.
128. Rudy DW, Gehr TWB, Matzke GR, et al. The pharmacodynamics of IV and oral torsemide in patients with chronic renal insufficiency. *Clin Pharmacol Ther* 1994; 56:39–47.
129. Schwartz S, Brater C, Pound D, et al. Bioavailability, pharmacokinetics, and pharmacodynamics of torsemide in patients with cirrhosis. *Clin Pharmacol Ther* 1993; 54:90–97.
130. Vargo DL, Kramer WG, Black PK, et al. Bioavailability, pharmacokinetics, and pharmacodynamics of torsemide and furosemide in patients with congestive heart failure. *Clin Pharmacol Ther* 1995; 57:601–609.
131. Benet LZ, Greither A, Meister W. Gastrointestinal absorption of drugs in patients with cardiac failure. In: Benet LZ, ed. *The Effect of Disease States on Drug Pharmacokinetics*. Washington, DC: American Pharmaceutical Association Academy of Pharmaceutical Sciences; 1976:33.
132. Vasko MR, Brown-Cartwright D, Knochel JP, et al. Furosemide absorption altered in decompensated congestive heart failure. *Ann Intern Med* 1985; 102:314–318.
133. Van Meyel JJM, Gerlag PGG, Smits P, et al. Absorption of high dose furosemide in congestive heart failure. *Clin Pharmacokinet* 1992; 22:308–318.
134. Brater DC. Resistance to loop diuretics: Why it happens and what to do about it. *Drugs* 1985; 30:427–443.
135. Marangoni E, Oddone A, Surian M, et al. Effect of high-dose furosemide in refractory congestive heart failure. *Angiology* 1990; 41:862–868.
136. Kuchar DL, O'Rourke MF. High dose furosemide in refractory cardiac failure. *Eur Heart J* 1985; 6:954–958.
137. Rudy DW, Voelker JR, Greene PK, et al. Loop diuretics for chronic renal insufficiency: A continuous infusion is more efficacious than bolus therapy. *Ann Intern Med* 1991; 115:360–366.
138. Lawson DH, Gray J, Henry DA, Tilstone WJ. Continuous infusion of frusemide in refractory oedema. *Br Med J* 1978; 2:476.
139. Lahav M, Regev A, Ra'Anani P, Theodor E. Intermittent administration of furosemide vs continuous infusion preceded by a loading dose for congestive heart failure. *Chest* 1992; 102:725–731.

140. Rybak LP. Pathophysiology of furosemide ototoxicity. *J Otolaryngol* 1982; 11:127–133.
141. Tran JM, Farrell MA, Fanestil DD. Effect of ions on binding of the thiazide-type diuretic metolazone to kidney membrane. *Am J Physiol* 1990; 258:F908–F915.
142. Ellison DH, Morrisey J, Desir GV. Solubilization and partial purification of the thiazide diuretic receptor from rabbit renal cortex. *Biochem Biophys Acta* 1991; 1069:241.
143. Stern A. Metolazone, a diuretic agent. *Am Heart J* 1976; 91: 262–263.
144. Craswell PW, Ezzat E, Kopstein J, et al. Use of metolazone, a new diuretic, in patients with renal disease. *Nephron* 1973; 12:63–73.
145. Aull MJ, Sanoski CA. Optimizing inhibition of aldosterone: Use of spironolactone in chronic heart failure. *Formulary* 1999; 34: 752–763.
146. Cooper HA, Dries DL, Davis CE, et al. Diuretics and risk of arrhythmic death in patients with left ventricular dysfunction. *Circulation* 1999; 100:1311–1315.
147. Pitt B, Zannad F, Remme WJ, et al. The effect of spironolactone on morbidity and mortality in patients with severe heart failure. *N Engl J Med* 1999; 341:709–717.
148. Farquharson CAJ, Struthers AD. Spironolactone increases nitric oxide bioactivity, improves endothelial vasodilator dysfunction, and suppresses vascular angiotensin I/angiotensin II conversion in patients with chronic heart failure. *Circulation* 2000; 101: 594–597.
149. Van Vliet AA, Donker AJM, Nauta JJP, Verheught FWA. Spironolactone in congestive heart failure refractory to high-dose loop diuretic and low-dose angiotensin converting enzyme inhibitor. *Am J Cardiol* 1993; 71:21A–28A.
150. Epstein M, Lepp BA, Hoffman DS, Levinson R. Potentiation of furosemide by metolazone in refractory edema. *Curr Ther Res* 1977; 21:656–667.
151. Olesen KH, Sigurd B. The supra-additive natriuretic effect addition of quinethazone or bendroflumethiazide during long-term treatment with furosemide and spironolactone. *Acta Med Scand* 1971; 190:233–240.
152. Asscher AW. Treatment of frusemide resistant oedema with metolazone. *Clin Trials* 1974; 11:134–137.
153. Ram CVS, Reichgott MJ. Treatment of loop diuretic resistant edema by the addition of metolazone. *Curr Ther Res* 1977; 22: 686–691.
154. Furrer J, Hess OM, Kuhlmann U, et al. Furosemid und Metolazon: Eine hochwirksame Diuretikakombination. *Schweiz Med Wochenschr* 1980; 110:1825–1829.
155. Channer KS, Richardson M, Crook R, Jones JV. Thiazides with loop diuretics for severe congestive heart failure. *Lancet* 1990; 335:922–923.
156. Kiyingi A, Field MJ, Pawsey CC, et al. Metolazone in treatment of severe refractory congestive cardiac failure. *Lancet* 1990; 335: 29–31.
157. Channer KS, McLean KA, Lawson-Matthew P, Richardson M. Combination diuretic treatment in severe heart failure: Randomized controlled trial. *Br Heart J* 1994; 71:146–150.
158. Withering W. *An Account of the Foxglove, and Some of Its Medical Uses: With Practical Remarks on Dropsy and Other Diseases.* London: G.G.J. and J. Robinson; 1785.
159. Fothergill JM. *Digitalis: Its Mode of Action.* London, 1871.
160. Dock W, Tainter ML. The circulatory changes after full therapeutic doses of digitalis, with critical discussion of views on cardiac output. *J Clin Invest* 1929; 8:467–484.
161. The Digitalis Investigation Group. The effect of digoxin on mortality and morbidity in patients with heart failure. *N Engl J Med* 1997; 336:525–533.
162. Fisch C, Withering W: An account of the foxglove and some of its medical uses, 1785–1985. *J Am Coll Cardiol* 1985; 5:1A–2A.
163. Gillis RA, Quest JA. The role of the nervous system in the cardiovascular effects of digitalis. *Pharmacol Rev* 1980; 31:19–97.
164. Skou JC. Enzymatic basis for active transport of Na^+ and K^+ across cell membrane. *Physiol Rev* 1965; 45:596–617.
165. Fozzard HA, Sheets MF. Cellular mechanism of action of cardiac glycosides. *J Am Coll Cardiol* 1985; 5:10A–15A.
166. Charlemagne D. Molecular and cellular level of action of digitalis. *Herz* 1993; 18:79.
167. Scholz H. Inotropic drugs and their mechanisms of action. *J Am Coll Cardiol* 1984; 4:389–397.
168. Siri FM, Krueger JW, Nordin C, et al. Depressed intracellular calcium transients and contraction in myocytes from hypertrophied and failing guinea pig hearts. *Am J Physiol* 1991; 261: H514–H530.
169. Li P, Park C, Micheletti R, et al. Myocyte performance during evolution of myocardial infarction in rats: Effects of propionyl-L-carnitine. *Am J Physiol* 1995; 268:H1702–H1713.
170. Mason DT, Braunwald E, Karsh RB, Bullock FA. Studies on digitalis. X: Effects on ouabain on forearm vascular resistance and venous tone in normal subjects and in patients with heart failure. *J Clin Invest* 1964; 43:532–543.
171. Van Veldhuisen DJ, de Graeff PA, Remme WJ, Lie KI. Value of digoxin in heart failure and sinus rhythm: New features of an old drug? *J Am Coll Cardiol* 1996; 28:813–819.
172. Muller JE, Turi ZG, Stone PH, et al for the MILIS Group. Digoxin therapy and mortality following confirmed or suspected myocardial infarction: Experience in the MILIS Study. In: Erdmann E, Greeff JC, Skou JC, eds. *Update in Cardiac Glycosides 1785–1985*. New York: Springer-Verlag; 1986:493.
173. Kraus F, Rudolph C, Rudolph W. Efficacy of digitalis in patients with chronic congestive heart failure and sinus rhythm: An overview of randomized, double-blind, placebo-controlled studies. *Herz* 1993; 18:95.
174. Packer M, Gheorghiade M, Young JB, et al. Withdrawal of digoxin from patients with chronic heart failure treated with angiotensin-converting-enzyme inhibitors: RADIANCE Study. *N Engl J Med* 1993; 329:1–7.
175. Adams KF Jr, Gheorghiade M, Uretsky BF, et al. Patients with mild heart failure worsen during withdrawal from digoxin therapy. *J Am Coll Cardiol* 1997; 30:42–48.
176. Captopril-Digoxin Multicenter Research Group. Comparative effects of therapy with captopril and digoxin in patients with mild to moderate heart failure. *JAMA* 1988; 259:539–544.
177. Slatton ML, Irani WN, Hall SA, et al. Does digoxin provide additional hemodynamic and autonomic benefit at higher doses in patients with mild to moderate heart failure and normal sinus rhythm? *J Am Coll Cardiol* 1997; 29:1206–1213.
178. Wirth KE. Relevant metabolism of cardiac glycosides. In: Erdmann E, Greeff K, Skou JC, eds. *Update in Cardiac Glycosides, 1785–1985*. New York: Springer-Verlag; 1986:257.
179. Uretsky BF, Young JB, Shahidi FE, et al. Randomized study assessing the effect of digoxin withdrawal in patients with mild to moderate chronic congestive heart failure: Results of the PROVED Trial. *J Am Coll Cardiol* 1993; 22:955–962.
180. Tauke J, Goldstein S, Gheorghiade M. Digoxin for chronic heart failure: A review of the randomized controlled trials with special attention to the PROVED and RADIANCE Trials. *Prog Cardiovasc Dis* 1994; 37:49–58.
181. Benovic JL, Bouvier M, Caron MG, Lefkowitz RJ. Regulation of adenylyl cyclase–coupled β-adrenergic receptors. *Am Rev Cell Biol* 1988; 4:405–428.
182. Lefkowitz RJ, Hoffman BB, Taylor P. Neurotransmission. In: Hardman JG, Limbird LE, eds. *Goodman & Gilman's The Pharmacological Basis of Therapeutics*, 9th ed. New York: McGraw-Hill; 1996:105.
183. Kelley RB. Storage and release of neurotransmitters. *Cell/Neuron* 1993; 72/10(suppl):43–53.

184. Spann JF, Sonnenblick EH, Cooper T, et al. Cardiac norepinephrine stores and the contractile state of the heart. *Circ Res* 1966; 19:317–325.
185. Francis GS, Goldsmith SR, Levine TB, et al. The neurohumoral axis in congestive heart failure. *Ann Intern Med* 1984; 101:370–377.
186. Insel PA. Adrenergic receptors—evolving concepts and clinical implications. *N Engl J Med* 1996; 334:580–585.
187. Haikala H, Linden I. Mechanisms of action of calcium-sensitizing drugs. *J Cardiovasc Pharmacol* 1995; 26(suppl 1):S10–S19.
188. Goldberg LI, Raifer SI. Dopamine receptors: Applications in clinical cardiology. *Circulation* 1985; 72:245–248.
189. Ruffolo RR Jr. Review: The pharmacology of dobutamine. *Am J Med Sci* 1987; 294:244–248.
190. Sonnenblick EH, Frishman WH, LeJemtel TH. Dobutamine: A new synthetic cardioactive sympathetic amine. *N Engl J Med* 1979; 300:17–22.
191. Parmley WW, Sonnenblick EH. A role for glucagon in cardiac therapy (editorial). *Am J Med Sci* 1969; 258:224–229.
192. Braunwald E, Sonnenblick EH, Chakrin LW, Schwarz RP Jr, eds. *Milrinone Investigation: A New Inotropic Therapy for Congestive Heart Failure*. New York: Raven; 1984.
193. Grose R, Strain J, Greenberg M, LeJemtel TH. Systemic and coronary effects of intravenous milrinone and dobutamine in congestive heart failure. *J Am Coll Cardiol* 1986; 7:1107–1113.
194. Nielsen-Kudsk JE, Aldershville J. Will calcium sensitizers play a role in the treatment of heart failure? *J Cardiovasc Pharmacol* 1995; 26(suppl 1):S77–S84.
195. Packer M, Carver JR, Rodeheffer RJ, et al for the PROMISE Study Research Group. Effect of oral milrinone on mortality in severe chronic heart failure. *N Engl J Med* 1991; 325:1468–1475.
196. Rector TW, Cohn JN with the Pimobendan Multicenter Research Group. Assessment of patient outcome with the Minnesota Living with Heart Failure questionnaire: Reliability and validity during a randomized, double-blind, placebo-controlled trial of pimobendan. *Am Heart J*. 1992; 124:1017–1025.
197. Lilleberg J, Sundberg S, Nieminen MS. Dose-range study of a new calcium sensitizer, levosimendan, in patients with left ventricular dysfunction. *J Cardiovasc Pharmacol* 1995; 26(suppl 1):S63–S69.
198. Pagel PS, Haikala H, Pentikainen PJ, et al. Pharmacology of levosimendan: A new myofilament calcium sensitizer. *Cardiovasc Drug Rev* 1996; 14:286–316.
199. Gomberg-Maitland M, Frishman WH, Karch S, et al. Hormones as cardiovascular drugs: Estrogens, progestins, thyroxine, growth hormone, corticosteroids, and testosterone. In: Frishman WH, Sonnenblick EH, eds. *Cardiovascular Pharmacotherapeutics*. New York: McGraw-Hill; 1997:787.
200. Al-Khadra AS, Salem DN, Rand WM, et al. Warfarin anticoagulation and survival: A cohort analysis from the Studies of Left Ventricular Dysfunction. *J Am Coll Cardiol* 1998; 31:749–753.
201. Sokol SI, Cheng-Lai A, Frishman WH, Kaza CS. Cardiovascular drug therapy in patients with hepatic diseases and patients with congestive heart failure. *J Clin Pharmacol* 2000; 40:11–30.
202. McAlister FA, Teo KT. The management of congestive heart failure. *Postgrad Med J* 1997; 73:194–200.
203. Singh SN, Fletcher RD, Fisher SG, et al. Amiodarone in patients with congestive heart failure and asymptomatic ventricular arrhythmia. *N Engl J Med* 1995; 333:77–82.
204. Gottdiener JS, Reda DJ, Massie BM, et al for the VA Cooperative Study Group of Antihypertensive Agents. Effect of single-drug therapy on reduction of left ventricular mass in mild to moderate hypertension: Comparison of six antihypertensive agents: The Department of Veterans Affairs Cooperative Study Group on Antihypertensive Agents. *Circulation* 1997; 95:2007–2014.
205. Nul DR, Doval HC, Grancelli HO, et al. Heart rate is a marker of amiodarone mortality reduction in severe heart failure. *J Am Coll Cardiol* 1997; 29:1199–1205.
206. Cogan MG. Atrial natriuretic peptide. *Kidney Int* 1990; 37:1148–1160.
207. Cody RJ, Atlas SA, Laragh JH, et al. Atrial natriuretic factor in normal subjects and heart failure patients: Plasma levels and renal, hormonal, and hemodynamic responses to peptide infusion. *J Clin Invest* 1986; 78:1362–1374.
208. Molina CR, Fowler MB, McCrory S, et al. Hemodynamic, renal and endocrine effects of atrial natriuretic peptide infusion in severe heart failure. *J Am Coll Cardiol* 1988; 12:175–186.
209. Munzel T, Kurz S, Holtz J, et al. Neurohumoral inhibition and hemodynamic unloading during prolonged inhibition of ANP degradation in patients with severe chronic heart failure. *Circulation* 1992; 86:1089–1098.
210. Yoshimura M, Yasue H, Morita E, et al. Hemodynamic, renal and hormonal responses to brain natriuretic peptide infusion in patients with congestive heart failure. *Circulation* 1991; 84:1581–1588.
211. Frishman WH. Recent advances in cardiovascular pharmacology. *Curr Probl Cardiol* 2000; 25(4):221–296.
212. Elsner D, Muders F, Muntze A, et al. Efficacy of prolonged infusion of urodilatin [ANP (95-126)] in patients with congestive heart failure. *Am Heart J* 1995; 129:766–773.
213. Giles TD, Quiroz AC, Roffidal LE, et al. Prolonged hemodynamic benefits from a high-dose bolus injection of human atrial natriuretic factor in congestive heart failure. *Clin Pharmacol Ther* 1991; 50:557–563.
214. Connelly TP, Francis GS, Williams RN, et al. Interaction of intravenous atrial natriuretic factor with furosemide in patients with heart failure. *Am Heart J* 1994; 127:392–399.
215. Cavero PG, Margulies KB, Winaver J, et al. Cardiorenal actions of neutral endopeptidase inhibition in experimental congestive heart failure. *Circulation* 1990; 82:196–201.
216. Northridge DB, Jardine AG, Findlay IN, et al. Inhibition of the metabolism of atrial natriuretic factor causes diuresis and natriuresis in chronic heart failure. *Am J Hypertens* 1990; 3:682–687.
217. Good JM, Peters M, Wilkins M, et al. Renal response to candoxatrilat in patients with heart failure. *J Am Coll Cardiol* 1995; 25: 1273–1281.
218. Northridge DB, Jardine AG, Alabaster CT, et al. Effects of UK 69 578: A novel atriopeptidase inhibitor. *Lancet* 1989; 2:591–593.
219. Frishman WH, Goldman A. Inhibitors of neutral endopeptidase. In: Frishman WH, Sonnenblick EH, eds. *Cardiovascular Pharmacotherapeutics*. New York: McGraw-Hill; 1997:611.
220. Northridge DB, Jackson NC, Metcalfe MJ, et al. Effects of candoxatril, a novel endopeptidase inhibitor, compared with frusemide in mild chronic heart failure: Proceedings of the British Pharmacological Society, University of Glasgow, July 10–12, 1991. *Br J Clin Pharmacol* 1991; 32:645.
221. Ura N, Carretero OA, Erdos EG. Role of renal endopeptidase 24.11 in kinin metabolism in vitro and in vivo. *Kidney Int* 1987; 32:507–513.
222. Lang CC, Motwani J, Coutie W, Struthers AD. Influence of candoxatril on plasma brain natriuretic peptide in heart failure. *Lancet* 1991; 338:255.
223. Frishman WH, Weisner M, Somer BG, et al. Natriuretic peptides and other vasoactive peptides: Implications for future drug therapy. In: Frishman WH, Sonnenblick EH, eds. *Cardiovascular Pharmacotherapeutics*. New York: McGraw-Hill; 1997:573.
224. Cho Y, Somer GB, Amatya A. Natriuretic peptides and their therapeutic potential. *Heart Dis* 1999; 1:305–328.
225. Burger AJ, Horton DP, Elkayam U, et al. Nesiritide is not associated with the pro-arrhythmic effects of dobutamine in the treatment of decompensated CHF: The PRECEDENT Study. *Circulation* 1999; 100(suppl):I-647.
226. Rajan V, Frishman WH, Goldman A. Vasopeptidase inhibitors: Inhibitors of neutral endopeptidase and dual inhibitors of angio-

tensin converting enzyme and neutral endopeptidase. *Heart Dis*, in press.
227. Mitchell GF, Block AJ, Hartley HL, et al. The vasopeptidase inhibitor, omapatrilat, has a favorable, pressure-independent effect on conduit vessel stiffness in patients with congestive heart failure (abstr). *Circulation* 1999; 100(suppl I):I-646.
228. Nagaya N, Satoh T, Nishikimi T, et al. Hemodynamic, renal and hormonal effects of adrenomedullin infusion in patients with congestive heart failure. *Circulation* 2000; 101:498–503.
229. Ohno M, Li W, Cheng C-P. Effects of endothelin-1 on left ventricular performance in conscious dogs: Assessment by pressure-volume analysis (abstr). *Circulation* 1994; 90(4, part 2):I-16.
230. Gu X-H, Casley D, Nayler W. Specific high affinity binding sites for 125I-labelled porcine endothelin in rat cardiac membranes. *Eur J Pharmacol* 1989; 167:281–290.
231. Galron R, Kloog Y, Bdolah A, Sokolovsky M. Functional endothelin/sarafotoxin receptors in rat heart myocytes: Structure activity relationships and receptor subtypes. *Biochem Biophys Res Commun* 1989; 163:936–943.
232. Hirata Y. Endothelin-1 receptors in cultured vascular smooth muscle cells and cardiocytes of rats. *J Cardiovasc Pharmacol* 1989; 13:s157–s158.
233. Moe GW, Ferrazzi S, Naik G, Howard RJ. Endothelin in heart failure: Temporal evolution, source of production and interaction with atrial natriuretic peptide (abstr). *Circulation* 1994; 90(4, part 2):I-592.
234. Teerlink JR, Hess P, Clozel M, et al. Role of endothelin in conscious rats with chronic heart failure (abstr). *Circulation* 1994; 90(4, part 2):I-261.
235. Galatius-Jensen S, Wroblewski H, Emmeluth C, et al. Plasma endothelin-1 in chronic heart failure—a predictor of cardiac death? *Circulation* 1994; 90(4, part 2):I-379.
236. Pacher R, Stanek B, Hulsmann M, et al. Prognostic impact of big endothelin-1 plasma concentrations compared with invasive hemodynamic evaluation in severe heart failure. *J Am Coll Cardiol* 1996; 27:633–641.
237. Colucci WS. Myocardial endothelin. Does it play a role in myocardial failure? (editorial). *Circulation* 1996; 93:1069–1072.
238. Sakai S, Miyauchi T, Sakurai T, et al. Endogenous endothelin-1 participates in the maintenance of cardiac function in rats with congestive heart failure: Marked increase in endothelin-1 production in the failing heart. *Circulation* 1996; 93:1214–1222.
239. Nootens M, Kaufman E, Rector T, et al. Neurohormonal activation in patients with right ventricular failure from pulmonary hypertension: Relation to hemodynamic variables and endothelin levels. *J Am Coll Cardiol* 1995; 26:1581–1585.
240. Webb DJ. Evidence for endothelin-1-mediated vasoconstriction in severe chronic heart failure: Endothelin antagonism in heart failure. *Circulation* 1995; 92:3372.
241. Cannan CR, Burnett JC Jr, Lerman A. Enhanced coronary vasoconstriction to endothelin-B-receptor activation in experimental congestive heart failure. *Circulation* 1996; 93:646–651.
242. Krum H, Gu A, Wilshire Clement M, et al. Changes in plasma endothelin-1 levels reflect clinical response to beta blockade in chronic heart failure. *Am Heart J* 1996; 131:337–341.
243. Inada T, Tanaka M, Hasegawa K, et al. Increased levels of endothelin-1 in plasma and heart tissue of cardiomyopathic Syrian hamsters (abstr). *Circulation* 1994; 90(4, part 2):I-260.
244. Wittner M, Morris SA, Christ GJ, et al. Infection of cultured human endothelial cells increases endothelin levels (abstr). *Circulation* 1994; 90(4, part 2):I-293.
245. Love MP, Haynes WG, Webb DJ, McMurray JJV. Anti-endothelin therapy is of potential benefit in heart failure (abstr). *Circulation* 1994; 90(4, part 2):I-547.
246. Teerlink JR, Loffler BM, Hess P, et al. Role of endothelin in the management of blood pressure in conscious rats with chronic heart failure: Acute effects of the endothelin receptor antagonist RO 47-0203 (bosentan). *Circulation* 1994; 90:2510–2518.
247. Frishman WH, Tamirisa P, Kumar A. Endothelin and endothelin antagonism. In: Frishman WH, Sonnenblick EH, eds. *Cardiovascular Pharmacotherapeutics*. New York: McGraw-Hill; 1997:689.
248. Galatius-Jensen S, Wroblewski H, Emmeluth C, et al. Plasma endothelin in congestive heart failure: Effect of the ACE inhibitor, fosinopril. *Cardiovasc Res* 1996; 32:1148–1154.
249. Clavell AL, Mattingly MM, Nir A, et al. Angiotensin converting enzyme inhibition modulates circulating and tissue endothelin activity in experimental heart failure (abstr). *Circulation* 1994; 90(4, part 2):I-452.
250. Frishman WH, Mayerson AB: Vasopressin and vasopressin receptor antagonists in cardiovascular disease. In: Frishman WH, Sonnenblick EH, eds. *Cardiovascular Pharmacotherapeutics*. New York: McGraw-Hill; 1997:769.
251. Manning M, Sawyer WH. Discovery, development and some uses of vasopressin and oxytocin antagonists. *J Lab Clin Med* 1989; 114:617–632.
252. Kuan CJ, Herzer WA, Jackson EK. Cardiovascular and renal effects of blocking A1 adenosine receptors. *J Cardiovasc Pharmacol* 1993; 21:822–828.
253. Balakrishnan VS, Coles, GA, Williams JD. A potential role for endogenous adenosine in control of human glomerular and tubular function. *Am J Physiol* 1993; 265:F504–F510.
254. VanBuren M, Bijlsma JA, Boer P, et al. Natriuretic and hypotensive effect of adenosine-1 blockade in essential hypertension. *Hypertension* 1993; 22:728–734.
255. Somer BG, Frishman WH. Adenosine and its pharmacologic manipulation in cardiovascular disease. In: Frishman WH, Sonnenblick EH, eds. *Cardiovascular Pharmacotherapeutics*. New York: McGraw-Hill; 1997:703.
256. Frishman WH, Hotchkiss H. Selective and non-selective dopamine receptor agonists: An innovative approach to cardiovascular disease treatment. *Am Heart J* 1996; 132:861–870.
257. Frishman WH, Hotchkiss H. Selective and nonselective dopamine receptor agonists. In: Frishman WH, Sonnenblick EH, eds. *Cardiovascular Pharmacotherapeutics*. New York: McGraw-Hill; 1997:727.
258. Post JB IV, Frishman WH. Fenoldopam: A new dopamine agonist for the treatment of hypertensive urgencies and emergencies. *J Clin Pharmacol* 1998; 38:2–13.
259. Mann DL, Young JB. Basic mechanisms in congestive heart failure: Recognizing the role of proinflammatory cytokines. *Chest* 1994; 105:897–904.
260. Biasucci LM, Vitelli A, Liuzzo G, et al. Elevated levels of interleukin-6 in unstable angina. *Circulation* 1996; 94:874–877.
261. Carswell EA, Old LJ, Kassel RL, et al. An endotoxin-induced serum factor that causes necrosis of tumors. *Proc Natl Acad Sci USA* 1975; 72:3666–3670.
262. Yokoyama T, Vaca L, Rossen RD, et al. Cellular basis for the negative inotropic effects of tumor necrosis factor-alpha in the adult mammalian heart. *J Clin Invest* 1993; 92:2303–2312.
263. Bazzoni F, Beutler B. The tumor necrosis factor ligand and receptor families. *N Engl J Med* 1996; 334:1717–1725.
264. Frishman WH, Weisen S, Lerro KA, et al. Innovative drug targets for treating cardiovascular disease: Adhesion molecules, cytokines, neuropeptide Y and bradykinin. In: Frishman WH, Sonnenblick EH, eds. *Cardiovascular Pharmacotherapeutics*. New York: McGraw-Hill; 1997:881.
265. Katz SD, Rao R, Berman JW, et al. Pathophysiological correlates of increased serum tumor necrosis factor in patients with congestive heart failure: Relation to nitric oxide dependant vasodilation in the forearm circulation. *Circulation* 1994; 90:12–16.
266. Mohler ER III, Sorensen LC, Ghali JK, et al. Role of cytokines in the mechanism of action of amlodipine: The PRAISE Heart Failure Trial. *J Am Coll Cardiol* 1997; 30:35–41.

267. Herrera-Garza EH, Stetson SJ, Cubillos-Garzon A, et al: Tumor necrosis factor-α: A mediator of disease progression in the failing human heart. *Chest* 1999; 115:1170–1174.
268. Bozkurt B, Torre-Amione G, Deswal A, et al. Regression of left ventricular remodeling in chronic heart failure after treatment with ENBREL® (etanercept p75 TNF receptor Fc fusion protein) (abstr). *Circulation* 1999; 100(suppl I): I-645.
269. Bozkurt B, Torre-Amione G, Soran OZ, et al. Safety and efficacy of ENBREL® (etanercept) in the treatment of chronic heart failure (abstr). *J Am Coll Cardiol* 2000; 35(suppl A):240A.
270. Nishio R, Matsumori A, Shioi T, et al. Treatment of experimental viral myocarditis with interleukin-10. *Circulation* 1999; 100:1102–1108.
271. Parrillo JE, Cunnion RE, Epstein SE, et al. A prospective, randomized, controlled trial of prednisone for dilated cardiomyopathy. *N Engl J Med* 1989; 321:1061–1068.
272. Latham RD, Mulrow JP, Virmani R, et al. Recently diagnosed idiopathic dilated cardiomyopathy: Incidence of myocarditis and efficacy of prednisone therapy. *Am Heart J* 1989; 117:876–881.
273. Mason JW, O'Connell JB, Herskowitz A, et al. A clinical trial of immunosuppressive therapy for myocarditis. *N Engl J Med* 1995; 333:269–275.
274. Hayward CS, Kalnins WV, Rogers P, et al. Effect of inhaled nitric oxide on normal human left ventricular function. *J Am Coll Cardiol* 1997; 30:49–56.
275. Hare JM, Sherman SK, Body SC, et al. Influence of inhaled nitric oxide on systemic flow and ventricular filling pressure in patients receiving mechanical circulatory assistance. *Circulation* 1997; 95: 2250–2253.
276. Matsumoto A, Momomura S, Hirata Y, et al. Inhaled nitric oxide and exercise capacity in congestive heart failure. *Lancet* 1997; 349: 999–1000.
277. Helisch A, Frishman WH, Hays RM, Loskove JA. Nitric oxide donors in the treatment of cardiovascular disease. In: Frishman WH, Sonnenblick EH, eds. *Cardiovascular Pharmacotherapeutics*. New York: McGraw-Hill; 1997:739.
278. Palkhiwala SA, Yu A, Frishman WH. Imidazoline receptor agonist drugs for treatment of systemic hypertension and congestive heart failure. *Heart Dis* 2000; 2:83–92.
279. Sinha S, Frishman WH. Matrix metalloproteinases and abdominal aortic aneurysms: A potential therapeutic target. *J Clin Pharmacol* 1998; 38:1077–1088.
280. Gomberg-Maitland M, Frishman WH, Karch S, et al. Hormones as cardiovascular drugs: Estrogens, progestins thyroxine, growth hormone, corticosteroids and testosterone. In: Frishman WH, Sonnenblick EH, eds. *Cardiovascular Pharmacotherapeutics*. New York: McGraw-Hill; 1997:787.
281. Gomberg-Maitland M, Frishman WH. Recombinant growth hormone: A new cardiovascular drug therapy. *Am Heart J* 1996; 132:1244–1262.
282. Retter A. Carnitine and its role in cardiovascular disease. *Heart Dis* 1999; 1:108–113.
283. Frishman WH, Greenberg S, Goldschmidt M, et al. Innovative pharmacologic approaches for the treatment of myocardial ischemia. In: Frishman WH, Sonnenblick EH, eds. *Cardiovascular Pharmacotherapeutics*. New York: McGraw-Hill; 1997:837.
284. Barry WH. Molecular inotropy: A future approach to the treatment of heart failure? *Circulation* 1999; 100:2303–2304.
285. Del Monte F, Harding SE, Schmidt U, et al. Restoration of contractile function in isolated cardiomyocytes from failing human hearts by gene transfer of SERCA2a. *Circulation* 1999; 100:2308–2311.
286. Meyer M, Bluhm WF, He H, et al. Phospholamban-to-SERCA2 ratio controls the force-frequency relationship. *Am J Physiol* 1999; 276:H779–H785.
287. Ankers S, Ponikowski P, Varney S, et al. Wasting as an independent risk factor for mortality in chronic heart failure. *Lancet* 1997; 349:1050–1053.
288. DelVecchio A, Frishman WH, Fadel A, Ismail A. Cardiovascular manifestations of substance abuse. In: Frishman WH, Sonnenblick EH, eds. *Cardiovascular Pharmacotherapeutics*. New York: McGraw-Hill; 1997:1115.
289. Mancini DM, Davis L, Wexler JP, et al. Dependence of enhanced maximal exercise performance on increased peak skeletal muscle perfusion during long-term captopril therapy in heart failure. *J Am Coll Cardiol* 1987; 10:845–850.
290. Guyatt GH, Sullivan MJ, Thompson PJ, et al. The six-minute walk: A new measure of exercise capacity in patients with chronic heart failure. *Can Med Assoc J* 1985; 132:919–923.
291. Coats AJS, Adamopoulos S, Meyer TE, et al. Effects of physical training in chronic heart failure. *Lancet* 1990; 335:63–66.
292. Coats AJS, Adamopoulos S, Radeaelli A, et al. Controlled trial of physical training in chronic heart failure: Exercise performance, hemodynamics, ventilation and autonomic function. *Circulation* 1992; 85:2119–2131.
293. Hambrecht R, Niebauer J, Fiehn E, et al. Physical training in patients with stable chronic heart failure: Effects on cardiorespiratory fitness and ultra-structural abnormalities of leg muscles. *J Am Coll Cardiol* 1995; 25:1239–1249.
294. Jeanrenaud X, Goy JJ, Kappenberger L. Effects of dual-chamber pacing in hypertrophic obstructive cardiomyopathy. *Lancet* 1992; 339:1318–1323.
295. Fananapazir L, Cannon RO III, Tripodi D, Panza JA. Impact of dual-chamber permanent pacing in patients with obstructive hypertrophic cardiomyopathy with symptoms refractory to verapamil and beta adrenergic blocker therapy. *Circulation* 1992; 85:2149–2161.
296. Slade AK, Sadoul N, Shapiro L, et al. DDD pacing in hypertrophic cardiomyopathy: A multicenter clinical experience. *Heart* 1996; 75:44–49.
297. Fananapazir L, Epstein ND, Curiel RV, et al. Long-term results of dual-chamber (DDD) pacing in obstructive hypertrophic cardiomyopathy: Evidence for progressive symptomatic and hemodynamic improvement and reduction of left ventricular hypertrophy. *Circulation* 1994; 90:2731–2742.
298. Nishimura RA, Hayes DL, Ilstrup DM, et al. Effect of dual-chamber pacing on systolic and diastolic function in patients with hypertrophic cardiomyopathy: Acute Doppler echocardiographic and catheterization hemodynamic study. *J Am Coll Cardiol* 1996; 27:421–430.
299. Hochleitner M, Hörtnagl H, Hörtnagl H, et al. Long-term efficacy of physiologic dual-chamber pacing in the treatment of end-stage idiopathic dilated cardiomyopathy. *Am J Cardiol* 1992; 70:1320–1325.
300. Auricchio A, Sommariva L, Salo RW, et al. Improvement of cardiac function in patients with severe congestive heart failure and coronary artery disease by dual chamber pacing with shortened AV delay. *PACE* 1993; 16:2034–2043.
301. Bocker D, Block M, Isbruch F, et al. Do patients with an implantable defibrillator live longer? *J Am Coll Cardiol* 1993; 21:1638–1644.
302. Moss AJ, Cannon DS, Daubert JP, et al for the MADIT II Investigators. Multicenter Automatic Defibrillator Implantation Trial II (MADITT II): Design and clinical protocol. *Ann Noninvas Electrocardiol* 1999; 4:83–91.
303. Klein H, Auricchio A, Reek S, et al. New primary prevention trials of sudden cardiac death in patients with left ventricular dysfunction: SCD-HEFT and MADIT-II. *Am J Cardiol* 1999; 87(suppl):91D–97D.
304. Breithardt G, Camm AJ, Campbell RWF. Guidelines for the use of implantable cardioverter defibrillators. *Eur Heart J* 1992; 13:1304–1310.
305. Moss AJ, Hall WJ, Cannom DS, et al on behalf of the MADIT

Investigators. Multicenter Automatic Defibrillator Implantation Trial (abstr). *Circulation* 1996; 94:I-567.

306. Goldberger JJ. Prevention of sudden cardiac death. *Heart Disease*, in press July/Aug 2000.
307. Ankersmit HJ, Tugulea S, Spanier T, et al. Activation-induced T-cell death and immune dysfunction after implantation of left ventricular assist device. *Lancet* 1999; 354:550–555.
308. The Registry of the International Society of Heart and Lung Transplantation. Ninth Official Report 1992. *J Heart Lung Transplant* 1992; 11:599–606.
309. Paris W, Woodbury A, Thompson S, et al. Returning to work after heart transplantation. *J Heart Lung Transplant* 1993; 12:46–54.
310. Milano CA, White WD, Smith LR, et al. Coronary artery bypass in patients with severely depressed ventricular function. *Ann Thorac Surg* 1993; 56:487–493.
311. Maddahi J, Schelbert H, Brunken R, DiCarli M. Role of thallium-201 and PET imaging in evaluation of myocardial viability and management of patients with coronary artery disease and left ventricular dysfunction. *J Nucl Med* 1994; 35:707–715.
312. Kern JA, Kron I. Ischemic cardiomyopathy: High risk revascularization vs transplantation. *ACC Curr J Rev* 1999; 8(1): 40–43.
313. Samady H, Elefteriades JA, Abbott BG, et al. Failure to improve left ventricular function after coronary revascularization for ischemic cardiomyopathy is not associated with worse outcome. *Circulation* 1999; 100:1298–1304.
314. Elefteriades JA, Tolis G Jr, Levi E, et al. Coronary artery bypass grafting in severe left ventricular dysfunction: Excellent survival with improved ejection fraction and functional state. *J Am Coll Cardiol* 1993; 22:1411–1417.
315. Thomas B, Batista RJV. Left ventricular reduction surgery. *Heart Disease*, in press May/June 2000.
316. Gorcsan J III, Crawford L, Soran O, et al. Improvement in left ventricular performance by enhanced external counterpulsation in patients with heart failure. *J Am Coll Cardiol* 2000; 35(suppl A):230A.
317. Dörffel WV, Felix SB, Wallukat G, et al. Short-term hemodynamic effects of immunoabsorption in dilated cardiomyopathy. *Circulation* 1997; 95:1994–1997.

C H A P T E R 22

CARDIAC TRANSPLANTATION, MECHANICAL VENTRICULAR SUPPORT, AND ENDOMYOCARDIAL BIOPSY

Sharon A. Hunt / John S. Schroeder / Gerald J. Berry

HISTORY AND OVERVIEW

Although a number of advances in therapy for failing myocardium have saved or at least prolonged the lives of many patients with previously terminal myocardial dysfunction, a sizable number of young patients are fated to die or be severely disabled because of irreversible myocardial disease. In patients with such end-stage disease, biological replacement of the heart has come to be a standard therapy and is currently widely accepted as a modality for prolonging life and improving its quality in carefully selected patients. As technological and engineering advances occur, mechanical replacement of the heart and xenotransplantation (transplantation of animal organs) may become very competitive or complementary modalities for the treatment of such patients, but biological replacement with human donor hearts is the current standard of therapy.

Interest in developing surgical techniques to interpose a functioning heart into a recipient's circulation dates back at least to the early part of the 20th century. In 1905, Carrel and Guthrie[1] described the heterotopic transplantation of a functioning donor heart into the neck of a dog. The heart in that model functioned in sequence with the recipient's heart in the circulation and was not actually capable of supporting the circulation. Although the exact anatomic connections were not described in detail, this apparently nonworking model of heterotopic transplantation beat regularly for approximately 2 h before the blood clotted in all the chambers. Carrel's initial interest was in the concept of performing vascular anastomoses, an interest reportedly stimulated by his distress at the inability of the best French surgeons of that time to avert the death by exsanguination from a severed portal vein of the president of the French republic.[2] Carrel and his colleague Guthrie developed innovative surgical techniques for vascular anastomoses at the University of Chicago, and those advances set the stage for anastomoses leading to organ transplantation. This work was a major part of the body of work for which Carrel was awarded the Nobel Prize for Medicine and Physiology in 1912.

Work in the field lay dormant until Mann and coworkers from the Mayo Clinic published their seminal report in 1933 of a technique for heterotopic heart transplantation with circulatory loading of the right ventricle.[3] Presumably because this was a working model, the chambers did not clot immediately, and the hearts in their dogs beat for a mean of 4 days. Mann perceived several important surgical points, including the importance of avoiding ventricular distention and air embolism and the prevention of thrombosis by heparin, but his most incisive and critical observation was that failure of a transplanted heart was in fact due not always to faulty surgical technique "but to some biologic factor which is probably identical to that which prevents survival of other homotransplanted tissues and organs." In what was undoubtedly the first description of acute allograft rejection, Mann recounts: "When the heart was removed just before it became quiescent . . . the surface of the heart was covered with mottled areas of ecchymoses . . . histologically the heart was completely infiltrated by large mononuclears and polymorphonuclears." Although various other animal models for surgical techniques for heterotopic heart transplantation were described in subsequent years,[4-7] it took another 30 years to better understand and manipulate the "biologic factor" Mann described as limiting the survival of allografted organs. In 1960,

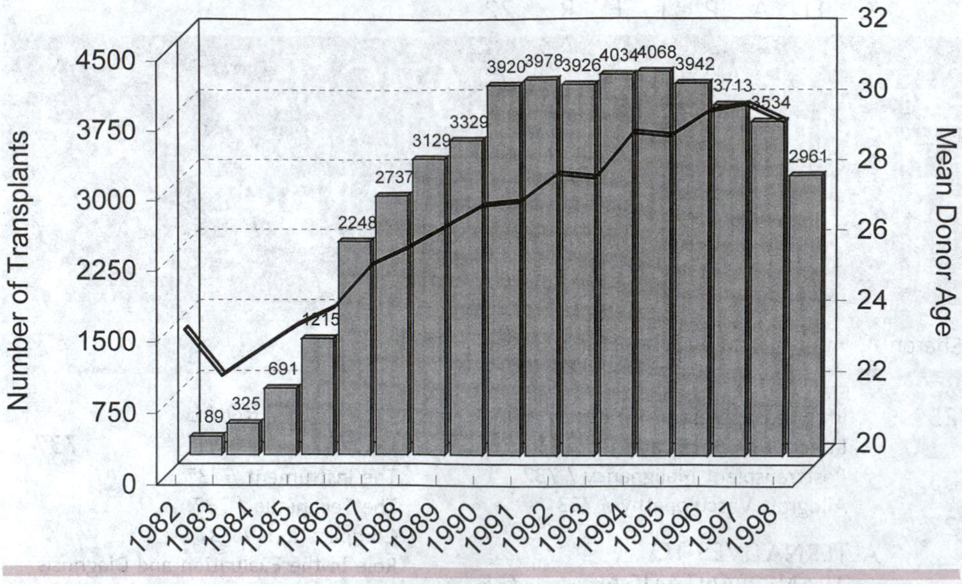

FIGURE 22-1 Data from the International Society for Heart and Lung Transplantation: numbers of heart transplant procedures per calendar year. (From Hosenpud et al.,[13] with permission.)

Shumway and Lower performed orthotopic heart transplants in dogs using cardiopulmonary bypass and topical hypothermia for donor heart preservation.[8] The dogs survived between 6 and 21 days and died of rejection. Shumway and Lower also recognized the limiting "biologic factor" and stated that "if the immunologic mechanisms of the host were prevented from destroying the graft, in all likelihood it would continue to function adequately for the normal lifespan of the animal." Their technique, involving anastomoses at the midatrial level and the supravalvular level in the great vessels, remained the basis of cardiac transplant technique in the 1990s.

In the early 1960s, the concept of pharmacologic immunosuppression was introduced; it ushered in the marriage of surgical and medical technology that is known today as the field of organ transplantation. Immunosuppression was, of course, seen as a means to mitigate the "biologic factor" that otherwise limited organ graft survival. The first clinical transplants were of the kidney, a logical choice since hemodialysis was then available as a backup system if the graft failed, and the field has flourished since the early 1960s.[9]

The first human heart allograft procedure was performed in South Africa in 1967,[10] followed shortly by the first U.S. transplant by Shumway at Stanford in 1968 and then by a flurry of transplant activity in many centers. This initial enthusiasm subsided as it became evident that postoperative survival was limited by a variety of complex medical problems, including opportunistic infections and graft rejection. Most major centers discontinued performing heart transplantation in the early 1970s, and it was not until the introduction of cyclosporine-based immunosuppression at Stanford in 1980 and the demonstration of the attendant improvement in survival rates[11] that the procedure reemerged as a widely accepted therapy for end-stage heart disease. In the 1990s, many tertiary care centers provided programs for heart transplantation, and most medical care payers in the United States, including the federal government, provided coverage for such care.

Cardiopulmonary transplantation was introduced at Stanford in 1981,[12] and subsequent experience with heart and lung and with both single- and double-lung transplantation in many centers has proved that these procedures are valid therapies for a wide variety of primary lung diseases and end-stage cardiopulmonary disorders.[13]

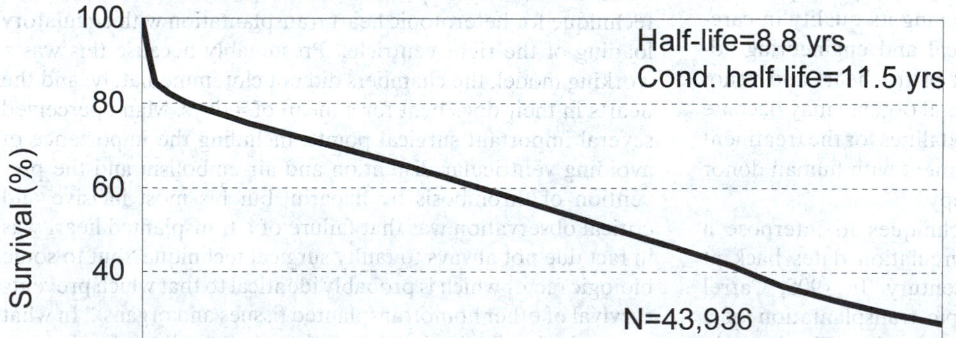

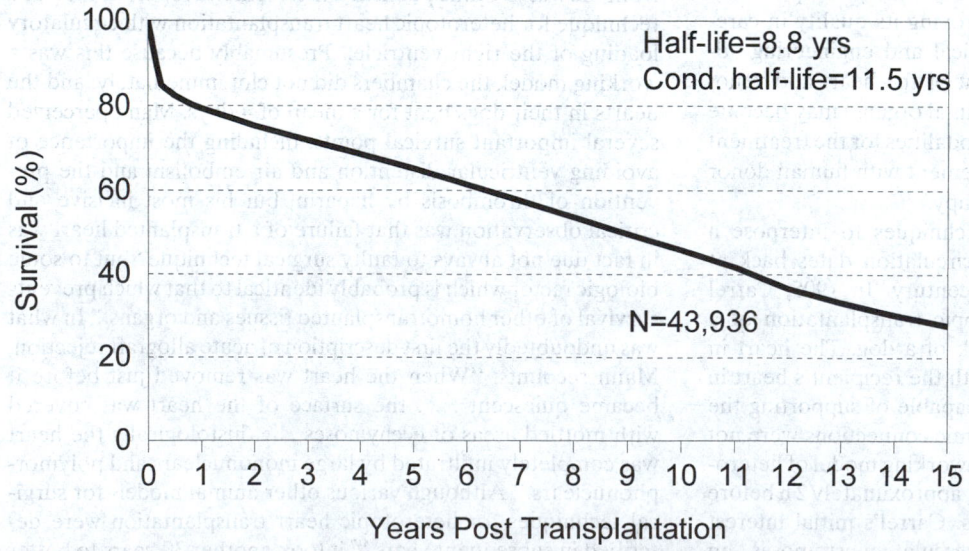

FIGURE 22-2 Data from the International Society for Heart and Lung Transplantation: overall cardiac transplant recipient postoperative survival rates. (From Hosenpud et al.,[13] with permission.)

Current Status

The most accurate data on volume and outcomes of thoracic organ transplantation are provided by the Registry of the International Society for Heart and Lung Transplantation and are updated yearly and published in the journal of that society. Since 1994, the Registry has been administered by the U.S. donor allocation organization, the United Network for Organ Sharing (UNOS), but it includes data on the vast majority of non-U.S. programs as well as all U.S. programs. As of the most recent Registry report,[13] there has been a plateau of heart transplant operations at approximately 3500 procedures worldwide on an annual basis since the late 1980s, a level generally accepted to be due to limitations of donor availability (Fig. 22-1). This most recent report includes data on 48,541 transplant procedures reported since the Registry's inception in 1982 and documents overall patient survival rates of 79, 71, and 63 percent, at 1, 3, and 5 years, respectively (Fig. 22-2). After the first year, there is a linear attrition rate of 4 percent per year to a survival of about 40 percent at 10 years.

According to this Registry, there are currently 304 programs in clinical heart transplantation, of which 165 are in the United States. According to data published in 1994, a large number of these U.S. programs have very low volume, and low volume is associated with inferior survival rates.[14,15] Thus, the survival rates to be expected at major, high-volume programs should be somewhat in excess of the overall reported rates.

RECIPIENT SELECTION AND MANAGEMENT

As is the case with any surgical procedure, careful selection of patients for heart transplantation results in optimum postoperative survival rates. In contrast, however, to the quality-of-life or prolongation-of-life issues involved in decisions regarding more conventional heart surgery, decisions regarding candidacy for heart transplantation must take into consideration a limited donor supply and the necessity of following a highly complex medical regimen for the rest of the patient's posttransplant life. These considerations can make selecting recipients most difficult. Major guidelines for recipient selection have been developed and are intended to provide the maximum benefit from the limited resource of donor organs.[16] Selection criteria are in a state of change worldwide, and criteria for acceptance at one center may not match exactly those at another center. The criteria generally reflect experience with the selection of patients who are most likely to survive and benefit, with a return to a normal life after the transplant.

Some basic or general criteria can be described that are universally accepted; these criteria are summarized in Table 22-1. They include the most basic criterion: the existence of end-stage cardiac disease irremediable by other, more conventional forms of medical or surgical therapy. The term *end stage* is, of course, difficult to define exactly, but in general it refers to cardiac disease associated with New York Heart Association (NYHA) functional class IV symptomatic status despite optimum medical management. In the past, one criterion was an estimated life expectancy of 6 months or less; however, the increasingly long waiting times for a suitable donor caused by increased patient numbers on the transplant waiting list now require the much more difficult task of estimating 1- to 2-year mortality in potential candidates. *With the recent major advances in heart failure therapy has come the realization that many transplant operations in patients referred for transplantation can be avoided by utilizing aggressive medical therapies.* Many transplant centers have found that as many as 30 to 50 percent of patients referred for heart transplants can be stabilized or even have their heart failure reversed by an aggressive, well-organized medical approach using angiotensin-converting enzyme (ACE) inhibitors or angiotensin II receptor blockade, combination diuretics, beta blockers, and meticulous monitoring of the patient's weight, general status, electrolytes, and renal function.[17,18] Thus, most heart transplant centers have evolved into centers for heart failure management as well as transplantation. Table 22-2 lists a typical drug regimen for a patient with advanced heart failure who is waiting for a donor. The frequency of clinic visits for monitoring ranges from every week to every 4 weeks, depending on the status of the patient. Furthermore, the introduction of transvenously placed antitachycardia/defibrillation devices and the increasing use of new beta blockers have contributed to this ability to stabilize patients in order to avoid or delay heart transplantation. It also has been realized that a small percentage of patients may have their left ventricular dysfunction reversed by high-risk percutaneous interventional procedures or coronary bypass surgery in order to restore blood flow to areas of "hibernating myocardium." Positron emission tomography (see Chap. 19) or 24-h thallium scanning (see Chap. 16) is utilized to identify potential candidates for such procedures. It is also important to identify potentially reversible causes of cardiomyopathy as summarized in Table 22-3 (see Chaps. 66 and 69). Cessation of excessive alcohol

TABLE 22-1 Criteria for Acceptance of Cardiac Transplant Recipients

- Unacceptable heart failure that has not responded to an aggressive medical or surgical regimen
- Unacceptable prognosis for survival of 1–2 years
- Biological age less than 55–60 years
- Absence of irreversible pulmonary hypertension
- Absence of other systemic diseases that would limit long-term survival
- Medically compliant, with the ability to follow a complex medical regimen
- Adequate psychosocial support to assure compliance with medical directions and office visits
- Absence of self-abusive behavior that would interfere with postoperative course

TABLE 22-2 Typical Pharmacologic Regimen for Advanced Heart Failure Patients

ACE inhibitor/angiotensin II blocker
Loop diuretic
Triamterene/hydrochlorothiazide
Digoxin (low dose)
Coumadin
Enteric-coated aspirin if CAD
HMG-CoA reductase inhibitor if CAD
Beta-blocker trial

ABBREVIATIONS: ACE = angiotensin-converting enzyme; CAD = coronary artery disease.

TABLE 22-3 Identification of Potentially Reversible Causes of Congestive Heart Failure

Ischemic left ventricular dysfunction reversible with interventional or surgical reperfusion
Cardiomyopathy secondary to
- Lymphocytic myocarditis
- Sarcoidosis
- Tachycardia
- Ethanol

intake or slowing of the ventricular rate with drugs or atrioventricular (AV) nodal ablation in patients with rapid heart rates occasionally results in a dramatic reversal of the heart failure.[19] Although it is more controversial, some centers continue to treat biopsy-proven acute lymphocytic myocarditis with high-dose steroids. This approach also is used for sarcoid cardiomyopathy. Finally, the introduction of beta blockers has resulted in dramatic improvement in survival statistics. Their use is associated with improved left ventricular ejection fraction over time as well[20–25] (see Chap. 21).

Age limits for cardiac transplant recipients are a second criterion for acceptance, and those limits have been expanded considerably in both directions over the past several years. In the early years of experience with cardiac transplantation, older patients experienced very inferior survival rates and the upper limit of eligibility was set at age 50. Since the advent of cyclosporine-based immunosuppression in 1980, it has become apparent that survival rates are no longer inferior in older age groups.[24] In the most recent year in which such data were analyzed in the Registry of the International Society for Heart Transplantation, the 30-day mortality rates according to age were identical (at 10 percent) for all ages between 10 and 69,[25] and in the current Registry data, 1- and 5-year mortality risk increases only slightly over age 65. Reports from several individual centers also have attested to the excellence of both early and late postoperative survival rates in older patients.[26–29] On the basis of those data, most centers have now advanced the official age of acceptability to 60 and may accept patients up to age 65 as well as highly selected patients over age 65. The lower age limits for transplantation eligibility also have been expanded recently, with a number of major centers embarking on programs involving neonates and young children.

Potential cardiac transplant recipients also are screened for the existence of any other systemic disease that independently is likely to limit their survival. The coexistence of an active malignancy and the potentially increased tendency for its advancement in the presence of immunosuppression are an obvious problem, and such patients are routinely excluded. How to deal with a patient with end-stage heart disease and a remote history of malignancy is a more difficult problem. Edwards and associates[30] reported a small group of patients with a prior history of malignancy who were considered to have been cured of their malignant disease and were otherwise candidates for cardiac transplantation. Seven such patients underwent transplantation; six had a remote history of lymphoproliferative disease, and one had had adenocarcinoma of the colon. Only the patient with colon cancer has had recurrence of malignancy during follow-up averaging over 2 years. Thus, cautious acceptance of such patients may be justified.

The coexistence of one other major systemic disease—insulin-requiring diabetes—had been considered a contraindication to cardiac transplantation in otherwise acceptable patients. The rationale for this was the well-known increase in the incidence of early peripheral and cerebrovascular disease and nephropathy in these patients as well as their generally poor ability for wound healing and the difficulty of diabetic control during the period of constantly varying steroid doses in the early postoperative period. As steroid requirements have become lower, this requirement generally has been relaxed to allow the inclusion of stable (as opposed to "brittle") insulin-requiring diabetic patients, and in recent years several reports have attested to the safety and efficacy of heart transplantation in very carefully selected diabetic patients.[31–33]

Human immunodeficiency virus (HIV) positivity generally is considered an absolute contraindication to heart transplantation. Other comorbid conditions must be considered on an individual basis, but irreversible organ dysfunction such as emphysema, severe peripheral vascular disease, and hepatic or renal dysfunction out of proportion to that predictable as a consequence of severe congestive heart failure are strong relative contraindications. The presence of an active infection is an often temporary absolute contraindication to transplantation because of the mandatory posttransplant institution of immunosuppression. Early in the years of clinical experience with heart transplantation, it was found that a normal donor right ventricle is unable to increase its external workload acutely to overcome elevated pulmonary vascular resistance (PVR). Because of this, patients who have end-stage heart disease with an elevated PVR often experience acute right-sided heart failure and cardiogenic shock after the transplantation of a normal heart with a right ventricle that has not been conditioned to pump against high resistance. This problem was a major cause of intraoperative deaths in the early years of transplantation and led to the setting of an upper limit of 4 Wood units of PVR (approximately 320 dynes·s/cm^5) as the cutoff point or fourth criterion for suitability for cardiac transplantation. In recent years, the concept of reactivity of the pulmonary vasculature and the potential reversibility of elevated PVR has gained acceptance. Because of this, potential candidates with PVR greater than 4 Wood units (320 dynes·s/cm^5) at baseline usually are subjected to pharmacologic maneuvers during hemodynamic monitoring, using nitroprusside and/or prostaglandin E_1 or inhaled nitric oxide to determine whether the elevated PVR is reversible; such patients are accepted as candidates for transplantation if the PVR can be reduced to acceptable levels while systemic arterial pressure remains adequate.

The last criterion that is accepted by most centers is the absence of unresolved pulmonary infarction. In spite of systemic anticoagulation, pulmonary infarcts that are due to emboli from the dilated right ventricle or the leg or pelvic veins are common complications in patients with biventricular congestive heart failure who are awaiting transplantation. *Experience has shown that pulmonary infarcts have a high probability of becoming pulmonary abscesses after the institution of immunosuppression.* For this reason, waiting recipients who sustain a pulmonary infarction usually are removed temporarily from the waiting list until the infarct resolves radiographically. Unfortunately, such resolution can be quite slow in this severely ill group of patients, and many never survive to return to the waiting list.

On the basis of these criteria, a group of patients is selected who are believed to have the best chance of benefiting from the operation and the attendant substantial commitment of medical resources. The type of underlying heart disease in the adult population selected for the procedure is nearly evenly split between idiopathic cardiomyopathy and ischemic disease; in the pediatric population, predictably, there is a higher percentage with congenital heart disease.

DONOR SELECTION AND MANAGEMENT

Acceptance of the concept of brain death, both legally and medically, has been central to the emergence of organ transplantation (particularly transplantation of unpaired organs such as the heart) in the modern era. The mandatory warm ischemic time that would be involved if cardiopulmonary death were the only accepted criterion of death would make heart transplantation impossible. Acceptance of the concept of irreversible brain death has been a perhaps surprisingly recent phenomenon. In 1970, Kansas became the first state in the United States to pass legislation recognizing the legal concept of brain death. Several states followed suit, and the medical and legal criteria for brain death have been refined over the years. The most recent and widely accepted set of guidelines was set out in the President's Commission Report in 1980.[34] It has been estimated that only 15 to 20 percent of persons who qualify as brain-dead and have usable or transplantable organs become organ donors in the United States.[35] The reasons for this are complex and include a lack of public awareness of the potential to donate organs as well as reticence among medical staff to make a request for donation. Efforts are being made in many areas to improve the percentage of organs recovered for transplantation from potential donors, but even with much higher recovery rates, heart transplantation probably will be a donor-limited field for the foreseeable future.

To be considered suitable donors for cardiac transplantation, brain-dead individuals must meet certain minimum criteria. Age criteria vary in different programs, but most cardiac donors have been under age 40. The donor obviously should not have had any significant cardiac disease, malignant disease, or acute or chronic infection. Risk factors for cardiovascular disease such as diabetes and severe hypertension or hypercholesterolemia are relative exclusion factors. Donors routinely are screened serologically for HIV and hepatitis B and C. Baseline serology for a number of other infectious diseases, such as cytomegalovirus (CMV), is obtained in many programs but usually is not used prospectively in donor-recipient matching. If there is any suspicion of cardiac disease in the donor, appropriate diagnostic studies (including echocardiography, cardiac catheterization, and coronary angiography) to assure the normality of the potential cardiac graft are pursued.

Once a potential donor is identified, the procurement process is initiated by contacting and referring to the local organ procurement organization (OPO), which maintains a registry of waiting recipients and coordinates equitable distribution of donor organs within a geographic area. Donor-recipient matching is fairly straightforward and requires ABO blood group compatibility as well as overall body size comparability, with ±20 percent body weight considered an acceptable discrepancy. Human leukocyte antigen (HLA) matching is not attempted prospectively because of the difficulty of obtaining HLA typing promptly as well as the relatively small numbers of donors and recipients, which severely limits choices.

Most donor hearts currently are "harvested," or removed, from the donor by a transplant donor team from a transplantation center and transported back to the center for implantation. A cold ischemic time of 4 h in adults generally is considered safe; this requirement limits the distance from which hearts can be transported and leads to the rationale for geographic subdivision into OPOs for cardiac allografts despite the drive for a "national" list for other organs.

SURGICAL TECHNIQUE

As was noted above, the surgical technique used in most centers today differs little from that described by Lower and Shumway in 1960.[8] With this procedure, both the donor and recipient hearts are removed by transecting the atria at the midatrial level, leaving the multiple pulmonary venous connections to the left atrium intact in the posterior wall of the left atrium, and then transecting the aorta and pulmonary artery just above their respective semilunar valves (Fig. 22-3).

As was noted above, the donor heart usually is explanted, or harvested, by a surgical team at a hospital remote from the transplant center, and this surgery most often needs to be coordinated with the requirements of other surgical teams procuring nonthoracic organs for transplantation at other centers. The donor heart is arrested with cold crystalloid or blood cardioplegic solution, and the explanted heart then is cooled topically by being placed in an iced preservation solution; it then is placed in a secure container and transported expeditiously to the transplant center. Ischemic times average 3 to 4 h. Implantation of the heart in the orthotopic position begins with reanastomosis at the midatrial level, beginning with the atrial septum (Fig. 22-4). Efforts are made to include a generous cuff of donor right atrium so that the sinoatrial node will be included. The great vessels are reanastomosed just above the semilunar valves.

In recent years, there has been a move to alter the surgical technique by leaving the donor atria intact and making anastomoses at the level of the superior and inferior venae cavae and pulmonary veins[36]; this is known as the *technique of bicaval anastomosis.*[37,38] There is evidence that this modified technique is associated with a decreased requirement for pacemaker placement for donor sinus node malfunction and with less AV valve

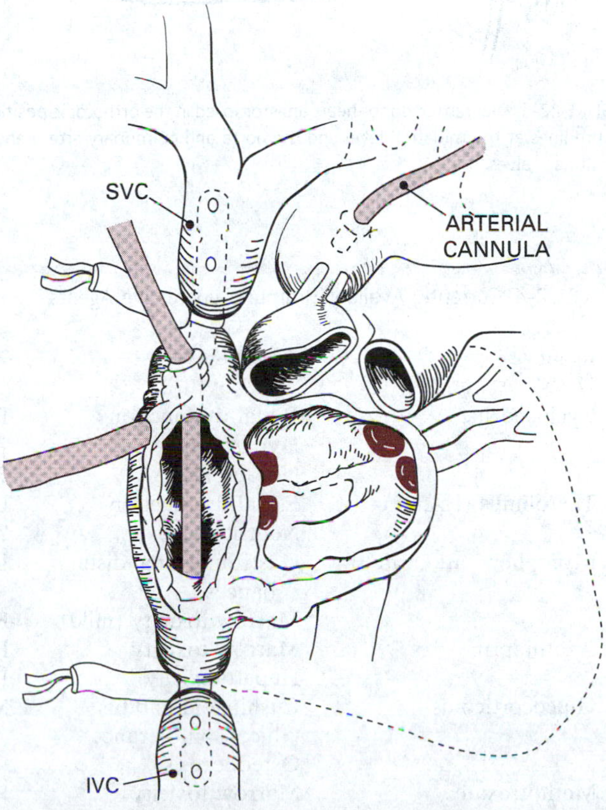

FIGURE 22-3 Diagram of recipient's mediastinum with heart resected and arterial and venous cannulas in place.

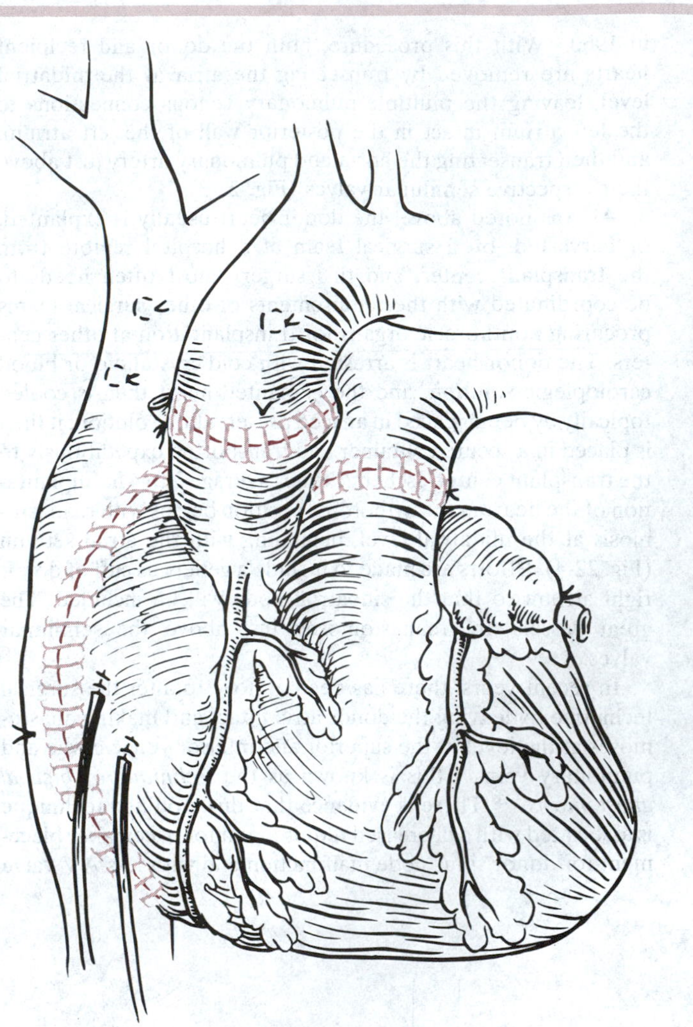

FIGURE 22-4 Diagram of donor heart anastomosed in the orthotopic position. Suture lines at the midatrial level and the aorta and pulmonary artery above semilunar valves.

regurgitation,[39,40] most likely as a result of preservation of the geometric configuration and anatomic size of the atria and the preserved integrity of the sinoatrial node.

Immediate postoperative care differs little from that after more routine heart surgery except for the institution of immunosuppression (described below) and the need for chronotropic support of the donor sinoatrial node for the first 2 to 3 postoperative days, usually with temporary pacemaker support but occasionally with infusion of isoproterenol. Uncomplicated patients may be discharged from the hospital 7 to 10 days postoperatively.

POSTOPERATIVE MANAGEMENT

Immunosuppression

GENERAL

The need to suppress the normal immune response in the presence of a solid organ allograft begins immediately at the time of surgery and continues for the life of the graft, which is generally concurrent with the life of the patient in the field of cardiac transplantation. Historically, most clinically used immunosuppressive regimens have consisted of a combination of several agents used concurrently and sequentially. This multiple-drug approach continues to be considered the state of the art. The number of drugs and the timing of their administration vary from institution to institution, but several general principles are commonly adhered to.

The first general principle is that immune reactivity and the tendency toward graft rejection are highest early after graft implantation and decrease with time, although they probably never disappear entirely. Thus, most regimens employ the highest levels of immunosuppression immediately after surgery and decrease those levels later, eventually settling on the lowest maintenance levels of suppression that are compatible with preventing recurrent graft rejection. The second general principle is reminiscent of that originated in oncology chemotherapy regimens, using low doses of several drugs without overlapping toxicities in preference to higher (and more toxic) doses of fewer drugs whenever feasible. The third general principle is that too much or too intense immunosuppression is undesirable because it leads to myriad undesirable effects, such as susceptibility to infection and malignancy, but too little is equally undesirable because it permits graft rejection. Finding the right balance between over- and underimmunosuppression in an individual patient is truly an art that utilizes science. As newer immunosuppressive agents and modalities are developed, the possible array of drug regimens can be expected to multiply accordingly, but these principles probably will remain, and the

TABLE 22-4 Currently Available Immunosuppressive Agents

Agent	Toxicities	Avoid Toxicity
Cyclosporine	Renal dysfunction	Follow blood levels
	Hypertension	Antihypertensive medication
	Neurotoxicity	?
Tacrolimus (FK506)	Renal dysfunction	Follow blood levels
	Neurotoxicity	?
Mycophenolate mofetil	Gastrointestinal disturbances	Reduce dose
	Marrow toxicity (mild)	Follow CBC
Azathioprine	Marrow toxicity	Follow CBC
	Hepatotoxicity	Discontinue drug
Glucocorticoids	Cushingoid habitus	Minimize dose
	Glucose intolerance	
	Osteoporosis	
Methotrexate	Marrow toxicity	Follow CBC

ABBREVIATIONS: CBC = complete blood count.

process of tailoring an individual patient's immunosuppressive regimen probably will continue to be an art as well as a science.

There is currently a relatively limited repertoire of approved agents for immunosuppression after organ transplantation, but their numbers can be expected to increase. Most programs employ a long-term two- or three-drug regimen, and roughly half additionally use a brief early postoperative course of "induction" cytolytic therapy. Most programs employ glucocorticoids as one of the agents, usually in relatively high doses early postoperatively and then tapering to low doses or discontinuing the drug during the first postoperative year. The commonly used drugs and their toxicities are outlined in Table 22-4.

In managing patients on these drugs, it is most important to be aware of the potential for drug interactions when other agents are added to or deleted from the patient's regimen. A list of the most common and clinically important drug interactions is shown in Table 22-5. It is also important to keep in mind the potential for changing drug concentrations in the face of intercurrent hepatic or renal dysfunction.

SURVEILLANCE AND THERAPY FOR REJECTION

There are rarely any striking physical signs or symptoms of rejection until it is far advanced. Cardiac allograft rejection is diagnosed almost exclusively by examining histologic findings in surveillance right ventricular endomyocardial biopsies. The technique used and the pathologic criteria for diagnosis are

TABLE 22-5 Drug Interactions with Azathoprine and/or Cyclosporine

Medication	Effects	Mechanism	Management	Onset	Severity
Allopurinol	Neutropenia 2° bone marrow suppression	Competitive inhibition of azathioprine metabolism	1. *Don't use* allopurinol unless absolutely necessary 2. If used, monitor WBC count and adjust azathioprine dose accordingly	Delayed 2–3 weeks	Major
Amphotericin	Increased nephrotoxicity	Possible synergism with cyclosporine	Follow renal function; titrate dose accordingly	Delayed 1–2 weeks	Moderate
Barbiturates	Decreased cyclo levels	Increased hepatic metabolism	Follow cyclo levels carefully; increase cyclo doses PRN	Delayed 1 week	Moderate
Diltiazem (?? other Ca^{2+} antagonists)	Increased cyclo levels	Unknown	Follow cyclo levels carefully; decrease cyclo doses PRN	Delayed 1–2 weeks	Moderate
Erythromycin	Increased cyclo levels	Decreased hepatic metabolism	Decrease cyclo dose by approximately *half;* follow levels carefully during and after therapy	Rapid	Major
Hydantoins	Decreased cyclo levels	Increased hepatic metabolism	Increase cyclo dose 25%, follow levels carefully	Rapid	Major
Imipenem	Increased CNS effects	Unknown	Avoid the antibiotic	Rapid	Moderate
Ketoconazole or itraconazole	Increased cyclo levels	Unknown	Follow levels carefully; decrease cyclo doses PRN	Delayed 1–2 weeks	Moderate
Metoclopramide	Increased cyclo levels	Increased cyclo bioavailability	Follow cyclo levels carefully; decrease cyclo doses PRN	Delayed 1–2 weeks	Moderate
Rifampin	Decreased cyclo levels	Increased hepatic metabolism	Increase cyclo dose by 100% follow levels carefully	Delayed 1 week	Major
Sulfamethoxazole/trimethoprim	Increased nephrotoxicity Increased marrow suppression Neutropenia	Unknown	Follow WBC count and renal function; adjust cyclo and azathioprine doses PRN	Delayed 2–3 weeks	Moderate

ABBREVIATIONS: WBC = white blood cells; cyclo = cyclosporine; 2° = secondary.

described below. A wide variety of noninvasive methods to diagnose rejection have been investigated, but none has been determined to have sufficient sensitivity and specificity to replace the biopsy. Protocols for the timing of surveillance endomyocardial biopsies generally are chosen to match the observed frequency of rejection episodes, which is clearly highest in the early postoperative period. Most programs perform surveillance biopsies on a weekly basis for the first 4 to 6 postoperative weeks and then with diminishing frequency in a stable patient but at a minimum every 3 months for the first postoperative year. The need for continued surveillance biopsies after the first year in clinically stable patients has been questioned,[41,42] but most centers continue to do them every 4 to 6 months.

Rejection episodes are treated with augmented immunosuppression, the intensity of which is matched to the histologic, or occasionally clinical, severity of the episode. Early or first rejection episodes usually are treated with methylprednisolone given intravenously in a dose of 1 g daily for 3 days followed by a repeat biopsy in 7 to 10 days. Episodes after 3 months that are not clinically severe can be treated safely with an increase in the oral steroid dose.[43] More severe rejection is treated with glucocorticoids and the addition of cytolytic therapy with either polyclonal antithymocyte globulin (commonly of rabbit or equine origin) or the murine monoclonal anti-CD3 preparation OKT3. Such treatment is highly effective,[44] but sensitization can limit its use.[45]

Several strategies are employed as adjunctive therapy for repetitive or recalcitrant rejection episodes. They include the use of two modalities with proven efficacy in therapy for autoimmune disease: total lymphoid irradiation[46] and low-dose methotrexate.[47] Both have been shown to be of benefit in patients with frequent or difficult-to-treat cardiac allograft rejection.[48–51] An analysis from 1997 suggests that the two modalities are both reasonably effective in this setting.[52] Tacrolimus (FK506), when substituted for cyclosporine, has been reported to benefit several heart transplant recipients with resistant rejection[53] as well as to be safe and effective as a primary agent in a cohort of patients[54]; there is a larger body of experience with its use in resistant renal graft rejection.[55] Similar success has been reported with the use of mycophenolate mofetil in therapy for recalcitrant rejection.[56] Studies are under way to evaluate several other drugs, modalities, and immunologic manipulations in the setting of resistant graft rejection.

If all these strategies fail and severe graft dysfunction supervenes, retransplantation is the only remaining option and is offered in many centers. The results of retransplantation in this setting are, however, disappointing, with only 33 percent 1-year survival in one registry[57] and consistently inferior survival in the international registry.[13]

Infectious Complications

Although their incidence has decreased in the cyclosporine "era," infections, often with unusual and opportunistic organisms, are the major cause of death during the first postoperative year and remain a threat throughout the life of a chronically immunosuppressed patient. Effective therapy demands an extremely aggressive approach to obtaining a specific diagnosis and a background of experience in recognizing the more common clinical presentations of CMV, *Aspergillus,* and other opportunistic infectious agents. Transplant cardiologists generally have expertise in infectious disease management but usually require the availability of both infectious disease consultation for the more unusual problems and a high-quality infectious disease laboratory. Several well-proven regimens for infection prophylaxis are commonly used and are outlined in Table 22-6. Infection surveillance is mainly clinical, but routine chest radiography often detects infections, especially fungal and mycobacterial ones, at an early and asymptomatic stage.

TABLE 22-6 Infection Prophylaxis Regimens

Pathogen/Disease	Strategy
Aspergillus	? Air filtration ? Prophylactic antifungals
Bacterial endocarditis	Standard subacute bacterial endocarditis prophylaxis
Cytomegalovirus	Blood product selection Prophylactic ganciclovir Prophylactic immunoglobulin
Influenza	None recommended
Pneumococcus	Preoperative vaccine
Pneumocystis	Sulfamethoxazole/trimethoprim Inhaled pentaminide
Toxoplasma	Pyrimethamine if donor seropositive

Posttransplant Malignancy

Any program of chronic immunosuppression is associated with a subsequent increased risk of lymphoproliferative malignancy; the earliest cases were noted after a period of immunosuppressive therapy for chronic hepatitis.[58] Organ transplantation has proved to be no exception, and the incidence of posttransplant lymphoproliferative disease (PTLD) has been documented in a registry based at the University of Cincinnati. The incidence of PTLD in heart transplant recipients is somewhat higher than that in kidney transplant recipients but not as high as that in liver recipients (Table 22-7); this probably is related to the intensity of immunosuppression required after the various allograft procedures.[59] According to the most recent registry report, malignancy accounts for 18.6 percent of deaths 4 years after heart transplantation.[13]

There is convincing evidence that most PTLDs are related to infection (either primary or reactivation) with the Epstein-

TABLE 22-7 Posttransplant Lymphoproliferative Disorder Incidence in Organ Transplantation

Organ	Incidence, %
Kidney	1.0
Heart	1.8
Liver	3.0
Heart/lung	4.6

SOURCE: Reproduced from Penn I. Roundtable report: Immunosuppression and lymphoproliferative disorders, 1992. (With permission of the author and Pro/Com International, Parsippany, NJ.)

Barr virus (EBV).[60–62] They frequently occur in unusual, extranodal locations and may respond to reduction in immunosuppression,[63] although such reduction is clearly a "double-edged sword" with a cardiac allograft for which there is no alternative system, such as dialysis in renal transplantation, if the graft is rejected. PTLDs are usually quite radiosensitive, and both radiotherapy and surgical resection can play a major role in therapy when there is a single lesion.

There is anecdotal evidence that the use of the antiviral agent acyclovir may be useful in therapy for PTLD,[64] and most centers employ it as an adjunctive therapy. In recent years, there has been interest in the use of interferon for these malignancies,[65] and a multicenter oncology group protocol is under way to evaluate its efficacy. Recently, there has been interest in the use of infusions of donor leukocytes[66] and donor-derived EBV-specific cytotoxic lymphocytes for this disease in bone marrow transplant recipients.[67] The technology may well be transferred to organ transplant recipients but would require the maintenance of donor tissue lines prospectively.

Allograft Vasculopathy

INCIDENCE

When clinical heart transplantation was introduced, the complications discussed above were all anticipated problems in light of the nonspecific nature of available immunosuppression, but the frequent development of diffuse and often rapidly progressive obliterative coronary artery disease in young donor hearts was not expected. It occurs angiographically in approximately 10 percent of cardiac transplant recipients by the first postoperative year and in 50 percent by 5 years postoperatively,[68,69] and its incidence did not decrease after the introduction of cyclosporine-based immunosuppression in the early 1980s.[70] *The ischemic sequelae of this vasculopathy account for the vast majority of late posttransplant deaths, and it is currently the main factor limiting truly long-term survival.*[13]

MORPHOLOGY

The angiographic morphology of cardiac allograft vasculopathy has been well described,[71,72] and its main features are summarized in Table 22-8. The very diffuseness of the disease makes it easy to underestimate angiographically even when, as is usually recommended, similar angiographic views from serial angiograms are reviewed simultaneously with side-by-side projectors.

In recent years, the use of intravascular ultrasound has gained acceptance as a sensitive and early detector of the intimal thickening that characterizes graft vasculopathy.[73–75] Intravascular ultrasound measurements of the extent of coronary intimal thickening currently serve as surrogate end points for the prevention of vasculopathy in several trials of new immunosuppressive agents that have shown promise of lessening the incidence of vasculopathy in animal models.

TABLE 22-8 Angiographic Features of Cardiac Allograft Coronary Artery Disease

Distribution: diffuse, distal, concentric, longitudinal obliterative lesions
May coexist with focal proximal lesions
Collateral vessel formation uncommon

PATHOLOGY

The morphologic features of accelerated transplant vasculopathy and the principal differences from conventional atherosclerosis have been described.[76–78] In transplant arteriopathy, the major epicardial vessels, their branches, and often the intramyocardial divisions display uniform, diffuse involvement extending along their entire length. The arteries are cordlike in texture, and cross sections show uniform, concentric luminal narrowing (Fig. 22-5). The asymmetric and calcified plaques or lesions composed of cholesterol that are characteristic of conventional atherosclerosis are not found in uncomplicated lesions of vessels affected by transplant vasculopathy. Histopathologic sections show a thickened intimal layer composed of modified smooth muscle cells, foamy macrophages, and variable numbers of histiocytes and lymphocytes within a connective tissue matrix that ranges from loose, edematous, and myxoid in early lesions to densely hyalinized and fibrotic in older lesions (Fig. 22-6). The internal elastic membrane is usually preserved, with only focal interruptions and reduplications. The medial layer is generally intact but may show atrophy in advanced lesions. Intraluminal thrombosis is uncommon. While these changes rarely are seen

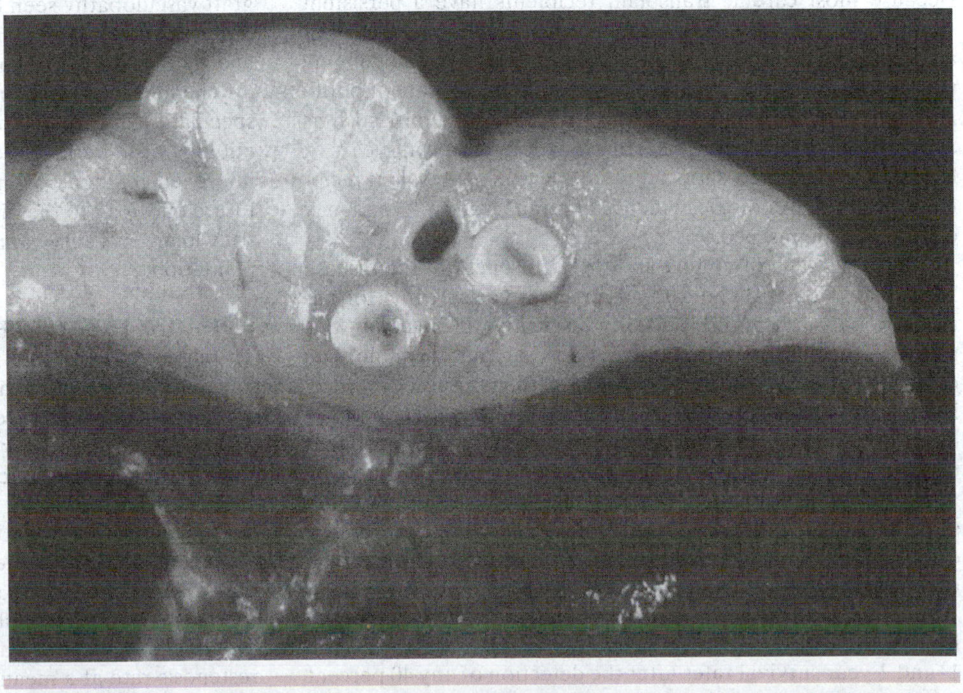

FIGURE 22-5 The mid-left anterior descending artery at autopsy in a 63-year-old man with advanced graft coronary disease.

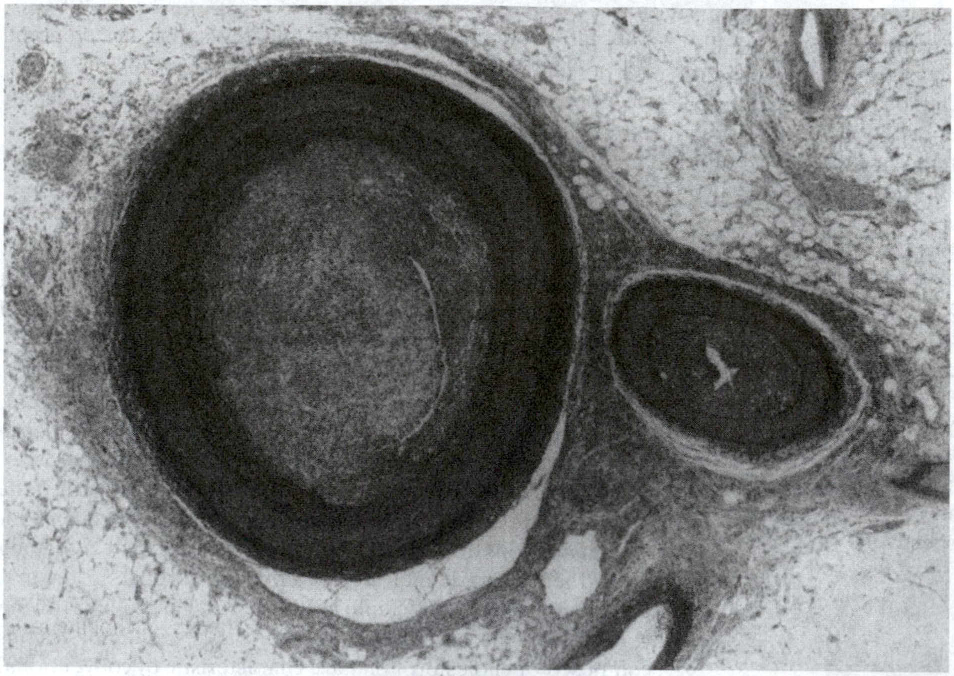

FIGURE 22-6 A main epicardial artery and division vessel showing occlusive graft coronary disease. Note the concentric intimal proliferation with a slitlike lumen. The internal elastica of both vessels is intact. (EUG ×10)

on endomyocardial biopsy samples, signs of ischemia or infarction seen in the endomyocardial biopsy should alert the pathologist and the clinician to the possibility of the insidious presence of graft coronary disease.[79]

CLINICAL PRESENTATION, SCREENING, AND PROGNOSIS

Because most cardiac transplant recipients have a persistent state of both afferent and efferent cardiac denervation, most are incapable of experiencing the subjective sensation of angina pectoris. Clinical presentations of ischemia in this patient population usually are related to sequelae of the ischemia, such as arrhythmias or left ventricular dysfunction. In recent years, it has been convincingly shown that some cardiac transplant recipients do have physiologic evidence of reinnervation[80–83] and may experience angina pectoris.[84]

The usual lack of angina and the diffuseness of the disease have made standard clinical and noninvasive screening for native coronary artery disease fairly insensitive in detecting this form of coronary vasculopathy.[85] Most of this technology is designed to detect uneven myocardial perfusion caused by focal lesions and is less effective in detecting the global ischemia of diffuse obliterative disease. Several reports have suggested that dobutamine stress echocardiography may in fact be the one noninvasive technique that offers reasonable sensitivity and specificity as well as prognostic value in screening for this disease,[86–88] and it offers an attractive alternative to the usual annual coronary angiography performed in these patients.

The prognosis for survival once significant graft vasculopathy is detected angiographically is generally poor. In one study, the 1- and 2-year survival rates after the detection of any 40 percent coronary artery stenosis were 67 and 44 percent, respectively.[89] After an ischemic event such as congestive heart failure or myocardial infarction, 1-year survival was only 18 to 20 percent in this study.

APPROACHES TO PREVENTION

A number of approaches to the prevention of allograft vasculopathy have been proposed, and several show promise. As was noted above, a decreased incidence of vasculopathy is one of the desired end points in all preclinical and clinical trials of new immunosuppressive agents, and several such trials are in progress. In addition, two studies have shown some decrease in the incidence and sequelae of vasculopathy with the use of other agents: one with a calcium channel blocker added to the patient regimen early after surgery and another with the lipid-lowering agent pravastatin added. In the former study, diltiazem was used in a randomized study involving a total of 106 patients, and those taking diltiazem had little change in overall coronary diameter on quantitative angiography over a 3-year follow-up period and displayed a trend toward a decreased incidence of angiographic coronary stenosis and clinical events resulting from ischemia.[90] In the other study,[91] also randomized and involving a total of 97 patients, the use of pravastatin (regardless of lipid levels) was associated with improved survival and a markedly decreased incidence of allograft vasculopathy seen both at angiography and at autopsy. A more recent study[92] documented similar results with simvastatin, and this benefit is probably a class effect.

The mechanism of action for either of these agents remains speculative. It is to be hoped that since, as described below, the etiology of allograft vasculopathy is most likely immunologic, improved methods of inducing specific graft tolerance in the future may lead to the disappearance of this disease and permit truly long-term survival rates after heart and other organ transplantation.

APPROACHES TO THERAPY

The choice of treatment for established cardiac allograft vasculopathy is often difficult and controversial. No agent or modality has been shown to reverse the process. Its very diffuseness makes the disease only infrequently amenable to otherwise standard revascularization procedures such as angioplasty and surgical bypass grafting. A registry of revascularization procedures performed on heart transplant recipients in 13 large transplant centers in the United States documented 97 balloon angioplasty procedures in 66 patients before November 1991.[93] There was an angiographic 94 percent success rate and an acceptable complication rate. There was, however, a 55 percent restenosis rate at a mean of 8 months after angioplasty, and 19 patients underwent 31 repeat angioplasty procedures for 24 restenoses and 30 new lesions. Only 61 percent of these patients were alive without retransplantation at a mean of 19 months after coronary angioplasty. In the same registry, 12 surgical coronary bypass procedures were reported; 4 of these patients died in the hospital, a fifth died suddenly 2 months postoperatively, and a sixth has required further palliative angioplasty. Revascularization is clearly, at best, short-term palliation for this highly lethal disease.

The most definitive form of therapy for graft failure resulting from severe vasculopathy is obviously retransplantation, and this procedure has been offered in many centers to highly selected patients with advanced allograft vasculopathy. Survival rates after retransplantation, however, are clearly inferior to those after primary transplants, averaging only 52 percent at 1 year in the most recent registry data.[13] In data analyzed from a group of the highest-volume U.S. centers, even the most ideal retransplant candidates had only 68 percent 1-year postoperative survival.[57] While this clearly represents an improvement in the individual patient's prognosis, these lower survival rates, along with the increased costs involved,[94] have led some to question the ethics of performing retransplantation.[95] Nevertheless, most large programs continue to offer the option to highly selected patients.

ALTERNATIVES TO TRANSPLANTATION

Mechanical Support

TEMPORARY: PERCUTANEOUS INTRAAORTIC BALLOON PUMP

When aggressive medical therapy for severe heart failure no longer provides adequate organ perfusion in either the acute or the chronic setting, several mechanical devices are available to support the failing circulation on a temporary basis until myocardial recovery ensues or an appropriate cardiac donor for transplantation is procured. The intraaortic balloon pump (IABP), which first was described by Mouloupoulos in 1962,[96] is the most widely used device for such mechanical circulatory assistance. The device consists of a nonocclusive balloon catheter positioned in the descending aorta, with the balloon cyclically inflated during diastole (to provide diastolic pressure augmentation and increase coronary blood flow) and deflated during systole (to provide reduced arterial impedance or afterload reduction during ejection), a rhythmic sequence termed *counterpulsation*. These devices are widely used for circulatory support in acute situations, such as cardiogenic shock and refractory ischemia after myocardial infarction or cardiac surgery, as well as to support patients awaiting cardiac transplantation who become refractory to pharmacologic therapy.

Technique A number of IABP systems are commercially available for surgical or percutaneous insertion. Most have a second lumen that permits balloon insertion over a guidewire and later provides monitoring of central aortic pressure. Percutaneous insertion systems generally require 9F femoral introducer sheaths. Retrograde insertion of the IABP system through a sheath in the femoral artery is the most commonly used method of insertion and can be accomplished under local anesthesia in the intensive care unit. When femoral pulses are absent or when percutaneous femoral cannulation is considered hazardous, surgical exposure of the common femoral artery enables the operator to cannulate the artery under direct vision. The existence of severe aortoiliac occlusive disease occasionally mandates insertion of the IABP from the upper extremities or from a graft attached to the ascending aorta.

Timing Proper timing of inflation and deflation is necessary for IABP counterpulsation to provide effective ventricular assistance. Ideally, the balloon should inflate immediately after aortic valve closure and deflate at the onset of the subsequent systole. When initiating support, it is often helpful to begin with the balloon augmenting every other beat (the 2:1 mode) to be able to compare an unaugmented beat with an augmented beat as one adjusts the timing of the balloon. The aim here is to maximize the height of the augmented diastolic peak and minimize the height of the systolic peak after the augmented diastole.

Weaning The balloon generally is used for augmentation of all beats (1:1 mode) until the patient's ventricular function improves and allows stepwise reduction of the assist mode to the 2:1 and later the 3:1 mode over a period of 6 to 12 h.[97] When hemodynamic independence from the IABP is established, the balloon may be removed.

Complications Complications have been reported to occur in 5 to 35 percent of IABP insertions.[98,99] Ischemia of the extremity distal to the femoral insertion site is the most common complication and may be more common when the percutaneous technique is used.[100] Severe ischemia requiring amputation of the toes, foot, or lower leg has been reported in 1 to 2 percent of cases.[97–99] Wound infection at the groin insertion site is the second most common complication, occurring in 3 to 4 percent of patients and usually presenting several days after catheter removal. Most of these complications resolve with topical care and systemic antibiotics. Other reported complications of IABP use include dissection or perforation of the distal aorta or its branches and peripheral or visceral embolization caused by thrombus formation. The incidence of the latter is decreased by the routine use of therapeutic doses of heparin.

TEMPORARY: VENTRICULAR ASSIST DEVICES

Mechanical support for a failing heart that becomes refractory even to IABP support is available in the form of ventricular assist devices (VADs) or replacement artificial ventricles. Since the first report of successful use of a VAD in 1965,[101] the technology has progressed a great deal. Most of these assist devices function by diverting blood out of the left ventricle through a large inflow conduit inserted into the left ventricular apex, into a pump-drive system, and back through a large outflow conduit into the ascending aorta. Figure 22-7 shows a typical VAD system in situ.

In the United States, VADs are currently approved for two indications. The first is temporary support of potentially reversible cardiac dysfunction, and substantial myocardial salvage has been achieved in postcardiotomy[102,103] and, less frequently, postinfarction[104] cardiogenic shock. The second approved indication for VAD support is as a "bridge" to transplantation in waiting transplant recipients (who, by definition, have irreversible myocardial dysfunction) who deteriorate severely before a donor becomes available. Successful bridging with a VAD was first reported in 1984, using the Novacor implantable electrical VAD (Novacor Division, Baxter Healthcare Corporation, Oakland,

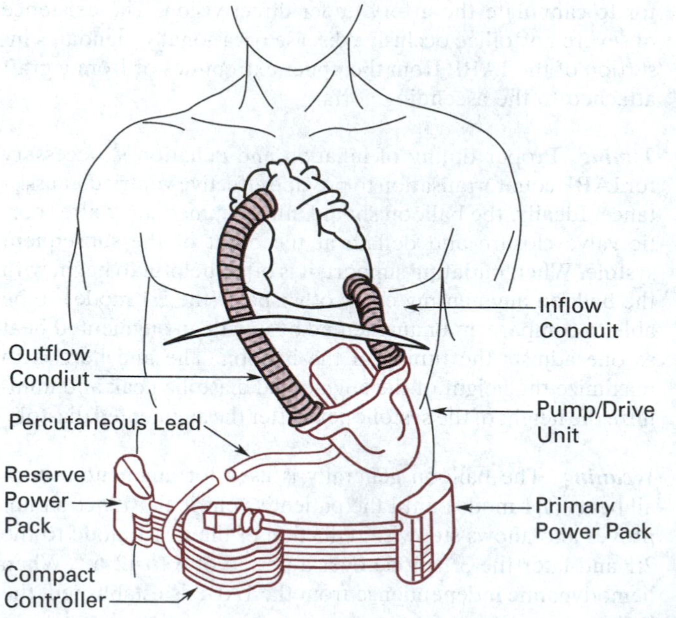

FIGURE 22-7 Diagram of a wearable Novacor left ventricular assist device in situ, showing inflow conduit inserted in apex of left ventricle leading to body of electrically driven pump, with outflow conduit returning blood to the ascending aorta. (Courtesy of Novacor Division, Baxter Healthcare Corporation, Oakland, CA.)

CA) in a patient with end-stage ischemic heart disease.[105] Success with replacement artificial ventricles (an orthotopic artificial heart) was reported a year later in a patient with cardiomyopathy.[106] The artificial heart technology, however, was fraught with high complication rates and has not been used for a number of years. There has been some resurgence of interest in the use of total artificial hearts as bridges to transplantation[107] and their future is uncertain.

Because of the progressive "mismatch" between the increasing demand for donor hearts and the stable donor supply rate, increasing numbers of patients on transplant waiting lists are deteriorating and requiring the use of such bridge devices to survive until a donor becomes available. The use of mechanical technology in this situation is associated with excellent posttransplant survival rates for supported patients,[108,109] but it does add a substantial level of pretransplant expense and of course does not increase the overall size of the donor pool.

The Future: Permanent Ventricular Assist Devices

With the growing shortage of donor organs, there is an increasing need for a mechanical device as an alternative to the biological transplantation of a failing heart. The ultimate goal of the evolving technology first used for temporary ventricular assistance has been to develop a completely implantable electrical system with rechargeable batteries (allowing the patient freedom from tethering to a power supply) to serve as a permanent assist to left ventricular function. The first clinical trials of such devices have commenced and involve patients with end-stage heart disease who, for reasons of age or other comorbid conditions, are not considered transplant candidates.[110] If their safety and efficacy are established in this patient population, clinical trials comparing VAD support directly with transplantation can proceed and address many end points, such as quality of life, in addition to survival.

The Future: Xenotransplantation

Work on the development of a mechanical alternative to biological cardiac transplantation has proceeded simultaneously with immunologic research aimed at making it possible to use animal organs in humans, a field known as *xenotransplantation*. Formidable anatomic, physiologic, and immunologic barriers must be overcome before xenotransplantation can become a solution to the shortage of donor organs.[111] Anatomically, transplanted organs must be of the appropriate size and structure to replace the native organ. Physiologically, the transplanted organ must perform a complex set of tasks that require it to receive and often send appropriate hormonal and metabolic signals. Such needs require reasonable homology of both the involved hormones and the cell surface receptors between the human and donor species. Technically and biologically, primates are the obvious choice for a donor species. However, the supply of primates is much too small to fill the potential demand; ethical considerations also are a drawback to the use of primates as organ donors. The pig has emerged as the most likely species to provide the appropriate size, anatomic structure, and available numbers for human organ transplantation. Unfortunately, swine are quite phylogenetically distant from humans, and this distance is associated with a formidable immunologic barrier. Humans universally possess so-called natural antibodies directed against swine antigens, primarily against carbohydrate moieties that are present on endothelial and other cells. These antibodies lead to hyperacute rejection of a swine organ through activation of the complement system initiated by the antibodies binding to donor endothelial cells, a process that occurs within an hour after implantation and leads to rapid destruction of the graft.[112,113]

Several means have been investigated to prevent hyperacute rejection. Depletion of xenogeneic natural antibodies against the donor organ as a way of modifying the host's humoral immunity is one approach.[114,115] Transient inhibition of complement activity with cobra venom factor or a soluble complement receptor delays hyperacute rejection and attests to the central role of the complement system in this process.[116] The activation and activity of complement are ordinarily regulated and limited by several endothelial cell–associated proteins. These proteins may function less effectively against heterologous than against native complement, making xenografts potentially more susceptible to complement-mediated injury. The production of transgenic swine bred to express human complement regulatory proteins to decrease the xenograft's susceptibility to complement-mediated injury has been an area of active research.[117,118] Such genetic alterations of the donor species hold some promise, at least for overcoming this first immunologic barrier to xenotransplantation. The later occurrences of acute and chronic rejection, however, are problems that remain to be solved. With current technology, the prevention of acute rejection of xenografts would require unacceptably intense regimens of immunosuppression, and prevention of chronic rejection, as was noted earlier, is inadequate with current technology, even in allografts.

The prospect of using animal tissues in transplantation has raised concern about the potential for the transmission of zoonotic pathogens from animal to human.[119] Since the likelihood of an organism causing disease in humans may be independent of its disease-causing potential in the donor species, the issue becomes a major one for the individual recipient and potentially has wide public health implications. When clinical trials begin, it will be extremely important to monitor recipients of xenogeneic tissue for the occurrence of unexplained illness; it has been suggested that the creation of a national or international registry of exposure to xenogeneic tissue would facilitate identification of clusters of events or illness.[119,120]

ENDOMYOCARDIAL BIOPSY

The Instrument

A percutaneous transvascular approach to biopsy of the beating heart was first described by Sakakibara and Konno in Japan in 1962,[121] and modifications of their instrument are still widely used. They generally are introduced from a femoral or brachial vein. This technology to permit nonsurgical biopsy of the myocardium was further developed in response to the need to obtain tissue from a transplanted heart to assess the presence and severity of graft rejection and monitor the response to antirejection therapy. Cardiac allograft rejection initially had been recognized by means of clinical observation of phenomena such as the emergence of heart failure, a gallop rhythm, or declining electrocardiographic voltage. Such phenomena often did not occur, however, until rejection was quite severe, and biopsy offered a means of early and objective assessment of rejection. In 1973, Caves and associates at Stanford introduced a new, shorter (and therefore more controllable) bioptome, which was introduced from the jugular rather than the femoral vein and allowed easy and repeated serial biopsy procedures under fluoroscopic guidance.[122] The Caves-Schultz-Scholten instrument was improved by Mason[123] and for years was the most commonly used bioptome in the United States. This bioptome is reusable, but its cleaning procedure is costly and labor-intensive, and several disposable instruments have been developed and have gained widespread use in recent years. An example of one of the most widely used is shown in Fig. 22-8 with the standard percutaneous approach from the right internal jugular vein. Longer bioptomes are also available for use from the femoral approach (usually through a long guiding sheath) in patients without internal jugular access.

The Technique

The right ventricle is usually the ventricle of choice for obtaining biopsy material because of the relative convenience and safety of approach to the right, as opposed to the left, ventricle as well as the usually homogeneous distribution of myocardial inflammatory and rejection processes. The procedure is performed with the patient supine, usually in a cardiac catheterization laboratory or in a procedure room or in the operating room if facilities are available. For the internal jugular approach, positioning with the feet elevated increases central venous pressure and facilitates cannulation of the vein. After the introduction of an intravascular sheath with the standard percutaneous technique, the bioptome can be advanced through it down to the right atrium, across the tricuspid valve, and into the right ventricle, pointed toward the septal wall. The stimulation of premature ventricular contractions by the instrument serves as confirmation of its presence in the ventricular chambers. Once it is safely within the ventricle and directed toward the septum, the jaws of the bioptome are opened, the instrument is advanced gently against the wall, and the jaws are closed, "biting off" a piece of septal myocardium 1 to 3 mm in diameter. The bioptome is then withdrawn, and the specimen is retrieved and placed in an appropriate medium for pathologic examination. The process is repeated until three to five adequate specimens are obtained.

Endomyocardial biopsy procedures generally are performed on an outpatient basis without the requirement for sedation or concomitant measurement of right-sided heart pressures unless they are clinically indicated. The procedure usually is done under fluoroscopic guidance,[124] but many centers perform it safely[125] and potentially with less cost[126] under echocardiographic guidance.

Complications

Large series have documented the low morbidity and mortality of endomyocardial biopsy, with major complications such as cardiac perforation and tamponade occurring in <0.5 percent of procedures.[127,128] More minor and generally transient complications include bundle branch block and arrhythmias. Fistulas between the coronary artery and the right ventricle have been described in a number of transplant patients who have had multiple biopsy procedures but generally seem to have no hemodynamic consequence.[129,130] With increasing lengths of survival of cardiac transplant recipients and the continued use of surveillance myocardial biopsies, complications related to the sheer

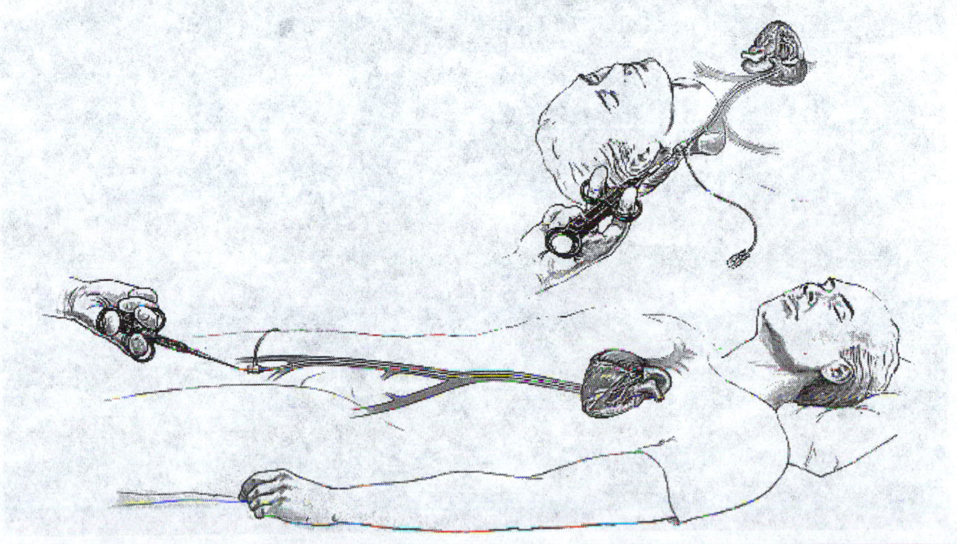

FIGURE 22-8 Diagrams of bioptomes inserted from right internal jugular or femoral approach. (Courtesy of Cordis Corporation, Miami, FL.)

TABLE 22-9 Possible Indications for Endomyocardial Biopsy

Diagnosis and grading of acute rejection
Diagnosis of myocarditis
Evaluation of idiopathic cardiomyopathy
Diagnosis of specific heart muscle diseases
Distinguish restrictive versus constrictive heart disease
Evaluation and grading of anthracycline cardiotoxicity
Diagnosis of primary and secondary cardiac neoplasms
Evaluation of idiopathic arrhythmias
Evaluation of atypical chest pain

numbers of biopsies performed are becoming more apparent. Chief among these complications is damage to the tricuspid valve and its subvalvular structures. This complication was first reported in 1990,[131] when a series of five patients with tricuspid valve chordal rupture as a complication of endomyocardial biopsy was reported. None of those patients had hemodynamically significant tricuspid regurgitation. Subsequently, there have been reports suggesting that signs of right-sided heart failure eventually appear in some patients, and several patients are known to have required tricuspid valve replacement because of intractable right heart failure. The incidence of tricuspid valve injury may be decreased with the use of a sheath across the valve during biopsy.[132]

Role in the Evaluation and Diagnosis of Cardiac Disease

TISSUE HANDLING AND PROCESSING

Correct handling of retrieved biopsy specimens is essential for obtaining accurate histopathologic results and interpretability. To limit crush distortion of the tissue, the biopsy specimen should be teased gently from the bioptome with a needle and immediately placed in an appropriate fixative. Neutral buffered 10% formalin is the standard fixative for light microscopy, and gluteraldehyde-based solutions are used for transmission electron microscopy (TEM). The specific clinical circumstances usually determine how the specimen will be fixed and processed and which histochemical stains will be selected. For the evaluation of myocarditis, cardiomyopathy, and specific heart muscle diseases, at least four biopsy pieces are recommended for light microscopy; one piece may be retained for TEM, and an unfixed piece may be frozen for immunofluorescence or immunohistochemical studies (optional). At least four pieces are required for light microscopy for adequate sampling in the grading of acute rejection; one piece may be frozen for immunofluorescence studies if acute vascular rejection is suspected. All the tissue samples (four to five pieces) should be placed in gluteraldehyde when grading of anthracycline cardiotoxicity is the clinical issue.

INDICATIONS FOR ENDOMYOCARDIAL BIOPSY

Since the successful application of an endomyocardial biopsy for the diagnosis and monitoring of acute rejection in the early 1970s, the indications for the procedure have expanded. The right ventricle usually is selected for technical reasons, including safety, although left ventricular biopsy occasionally is performed for the diagnosis of endomyocardial fibrosis, infantile fibroelastosis, left-sided irradiation effects, and cardiac involvement by scleroderma. The current indications for endomyocardial biopsy are listed in Table 22-9.

Myocarditis As an inflammatory or immunologic process, myocarditis is defined by the presence of an inflammatory infiltrate in association with nonischemic damage or necrosis of the adjacent myocytes;[133] these features are termed *the Dallas criteria* (see Chap. 69). The different types of inflammatory cells help define possible etiologies in myocarditis. Lymphocytes are the predominant cell type seen in idiopathic (postviral) myocarditis (Fig. 22-9), sarcoidosis, Lyme disease, Kawasaki's disease, polymyositis, and AIDS myocarditis (see Chap. 70). Eosinophils are commonly found in drug hypersensitivity but also may indicate parasitic infection or a hyper-eosinophilic syndrome. Myocyte necrosis associated with multinucleated giant cells is characteristic of giant-cell myocarditis[134] (Fig. 22-10). Epithelioid histiocytes forming granulomas are seen in cardiac sarcoidosis.[135]

Idiopathic Cardiomyopathy The morphologic diagnosis of idiopathic dilated cardiomyopathy, including familial and postpartum types, is primarily one of exclusion, as a variety of storage and

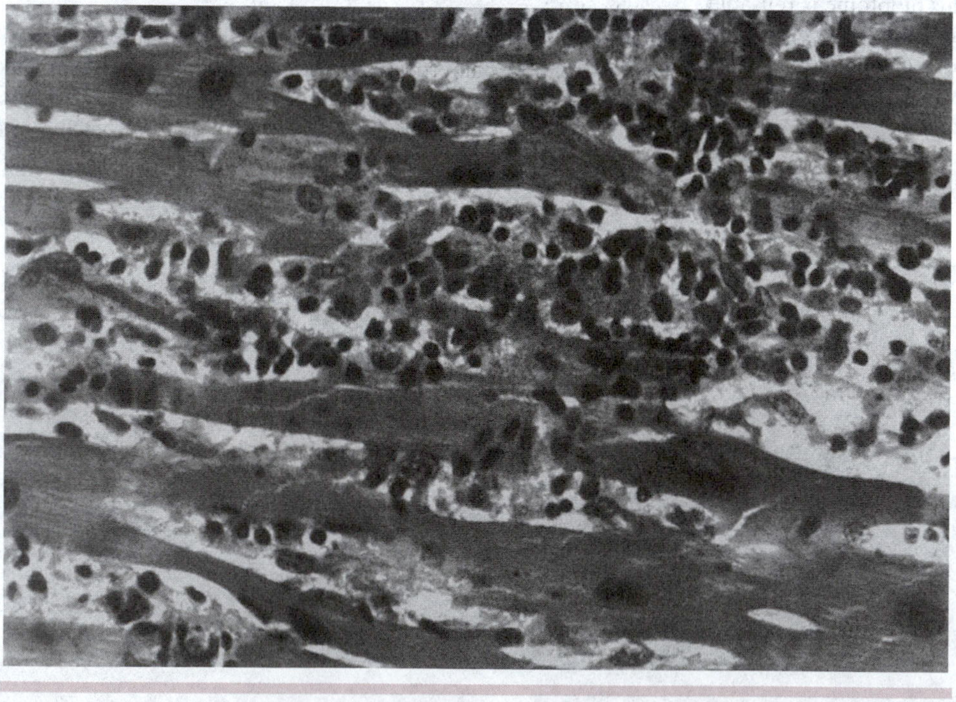

FIGURE 22-9 Lymphocytic myocarditis in a young man presenting with sudden-onset congestive heart failure. Dense interstitial infiltrates of lymphocytes are seen in association with myocyte damage. (H&E ×400)

infiltrative heart muscle diseases and myocarditis may mimic dilated cardiomyopathy (see Chaps. 62, 66–69, and 82). Hypertensive, ischemic, and valvular heart disease also must be excluded. Endomyocardial biopsy is used routinely in some institutions in evaluating dilated cardiomyopathy of unknown causes. The morphologic features of idiopathic cardiomyopathy are nonspecific and include myocyte hypertrophy and interstitial fibrosis (Fig. 22-11). Hypertrophic cardiomyopathy is the second most common type of cardiomyopathy. It cannot be diagnosed reliably by endomyocardial biopsy since the characteristic histologic features are found mainly in the midportion of the ventricular septum.[136] Mimics of hypertrophic cardiomyopathy such as amyloidosis can be delineated by biopsy.

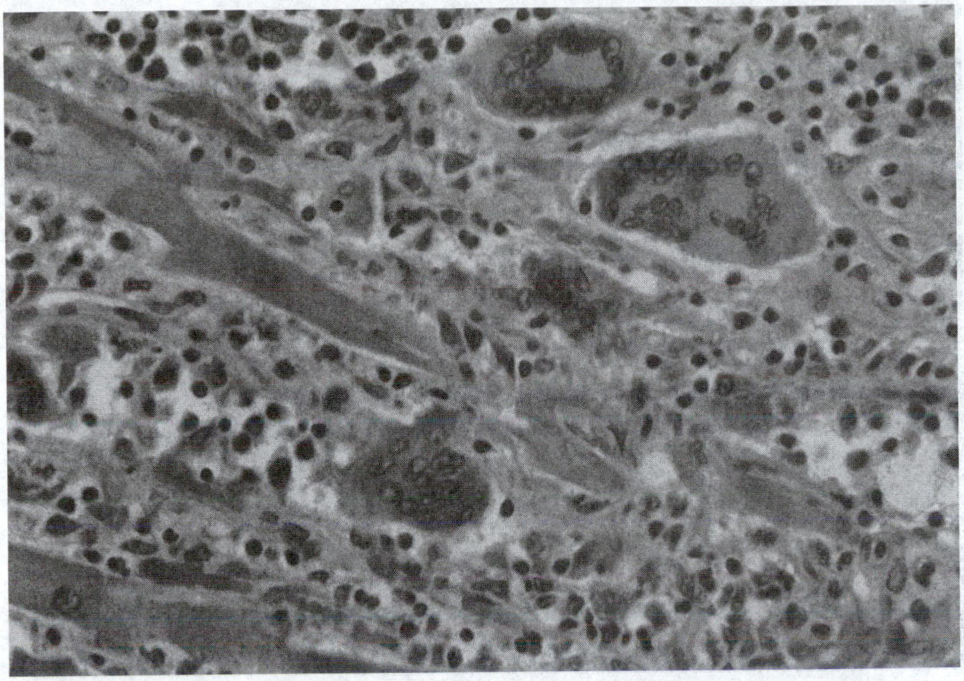

FIGURE 22-10 Giant-cell myocarditis showing an inflammatory infiltrate composed of lymphocytes, histiocytes, and eosinophils admixed with multinucleated giant cells. Myocyte damage is conspicuous in this case. (H&E ×400)

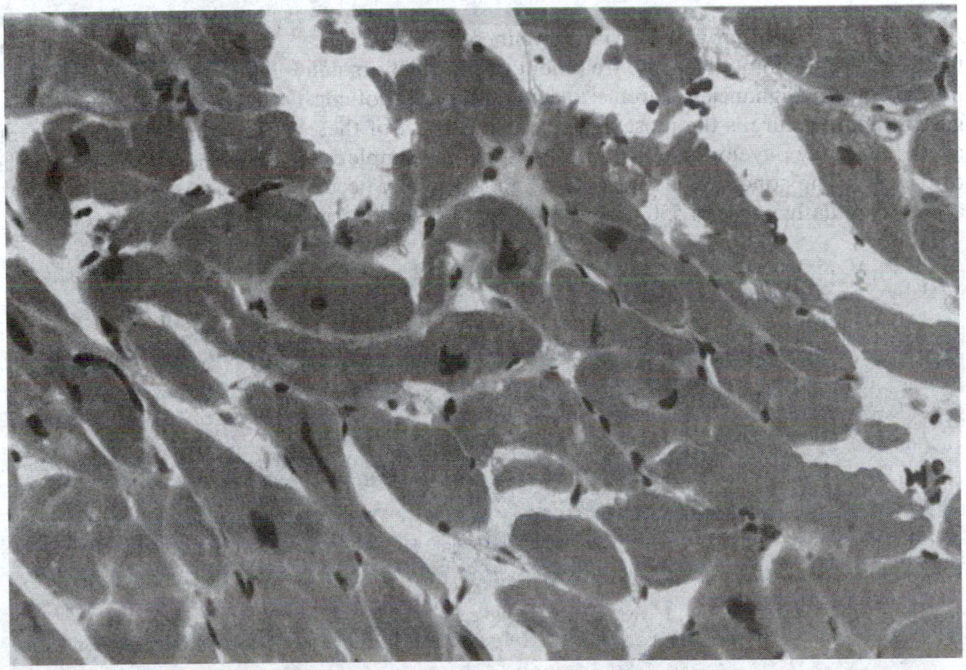

FIGURE 22-11 A young woman presenting with congestive heart failure. Myocyte hypertrophy characterized by large, irregular nuclei is seen. The findings are compatible with dilated cardiomyopathy. (H&E ×400)

Specific Heart Muscle Diseases A variety of infiltrative diseases and storage disorders of the myocardium can be readily diagnosed by endomyocardial biopsy (see Chap. 68). Cardiac amyloidosis may be seen with primary amyloidosis, plasma cell dyscrasias, and chronic inflammatory conditions and in elderly patients (senile amyloid). The histologic appearance includes interstitial, subendocardial, or vascular deposits of finely fibrillar, eosinophilic material (Fig. 22-12). Senile amyloid often is characterized by nodular deposits of transthyretin. Histochemical stains such as Congo red and trichrome are useful in distinguishing amyloid from collagen.[137]

Disorders of iron metabolism (hemochromatosis) and iron overload states (hemosiderosis) result in perinuclear accumulations of iron pigment within the myocytes. Special stains such as Prussian blue highlight the pigment (Fig. 22-13). In advanced disease, marked myocyte hypertrophy and interstitial fibrosis are found. The diagnosis of metabolic enzyme deficiencies, including glycogen storage diseases, Gaucher's disease, and Fabry's disease (see Chap. 62), also may be established by endomyocardial biopsy.

Restrictive versus Constrictive Heart Disease The clinical distinction of restrictive heart disease from constrictive pericardial disease can be difficult, and the therapeutic implications are significant. In some cases, imaging and hemodynamic studies may not provide a definitive diagnosis. Specific heart muscle diseases resulting in restrictive physiologic profiles, including amyloidosis, carcinoid heart disease, endocardial fibrosis, and radiation-induced interstitial fibrosis, can be diagnosed by biopsy[138] (see Chaps. 68 and 72).

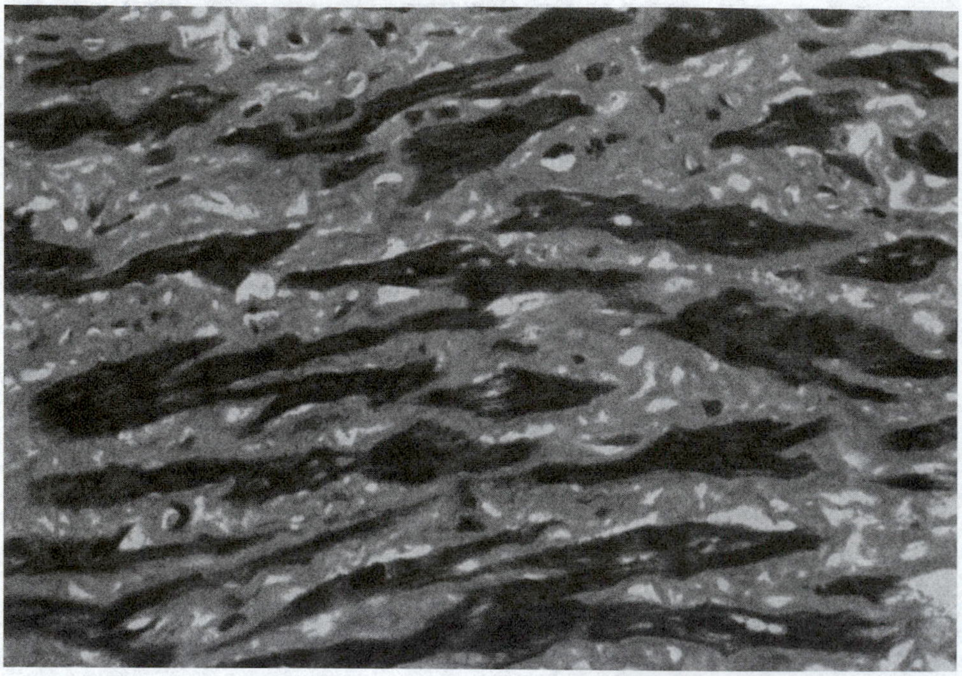

FIGURE 22-12 Severe interstitial amyloidosis showing fibrillar deposits along the sarcolemma with constriction of the myocytes. (H&E ×400)

Anthracycline Cardiotoxicity Anthracyclines such as doxorubicin are used commonly in the treatment of solid tumors and hematologic malignancies. Cardiac toxicity in the form of congestive heart failure is the most significant side effect of these agents and may develop months to years after the completion of therapy. The condition is dose-related and generally occurs after a cumulative dose of 550 mg/m^2. Individual patient variation and factors such as prior mediastinal irradiation, hypertension, and increased age may potentiate cardiotoxicity at lower cumulative doses.[139] TEM of heart biopsies remains the "gold standard" for the diagnosis and grading of doxorubicin toxicity.[140]

The Billingham grading scheme for doxorubicin toxicity is based on the percentage of myocytes that demonstrate doxorubicin effect. Grades 0 through 3 are used and are associated with specific therapeutic recommendations.[141] The characteristic changes include myofibrillar loss with Z-band remnants and sarcotubular dilatation within the myocytes (Fig. 22-14). This approach to drug toxicity has provided a valuable method of monitoring patients and preventing irreversible cardiac failure.[142]

Primary and Metastatic Neoplasms Endomyocardial biopsy has been used to provide morphologic confirmation and classification of benign and malignant primary cardiac tumors and to document the presence of metastatic malignancies[143] (see Chap. 77). Cardiac myxomas, fibromas, and rhabdomyomas as well as sarcoma, lymphoma, leukemia, and malignant mesothelioma have been diagnosed. Secondary neoplasms such as metastatic carcinoma and melanoma also may be found in right ventricular specimens (Fig. 22-15).

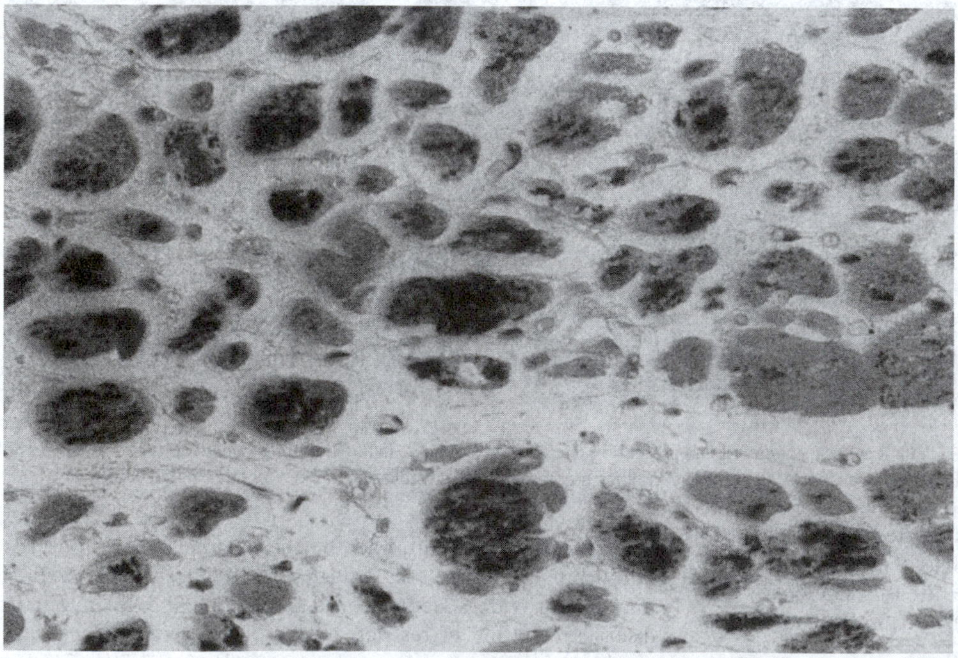

FIGURE 22-13 Cardiac hemochromatosis in a young man. Dense accumulations of iron pigment are seen in a perinuclear location. (Prussian blue ×400)

Idiopathic Arrhythmias In the absence of a documented anatomic abnormality such as ischemic heart disease, cardiomyopathy, or mitral valve prolapse as an explanation for ventricular or supraventricular rhythm disturbances, an endomyocardial biopsy may be helpful. Lesions of the conduction system can result in nonspecific myocyte hypertrophy and interstitial fibrosis. Lymphocytic myocarditis, sarcoidosis, and giant-cell myocarditis all may present with arrhythmias. In a recent study of 80 patients with unexplained arrhythmias 88 percent of the biopsies revealed pathologic changes. Among these patients, 56 percent of the biopsies showed features of cardiomyopathy, 19 percent had clinically unsuspected myocarditis, 10 percent had small vessel disease, 3 percent had amyloidosis, and 1 percent showed an intravascular organizing thrombus.[144] An uncommon cause of arrhythmia is arrhythmogenic right ventricular dysplasia (see Chap. 33). It should be suspected in biopsy specimens showing hypertrophy and fibrosis in association with abundant myocardial deposits of adipose tissue. Clinicopathologic correlation is required for the diagnosis, as myocardial accumulations of fat normally are found in the right ventricle.

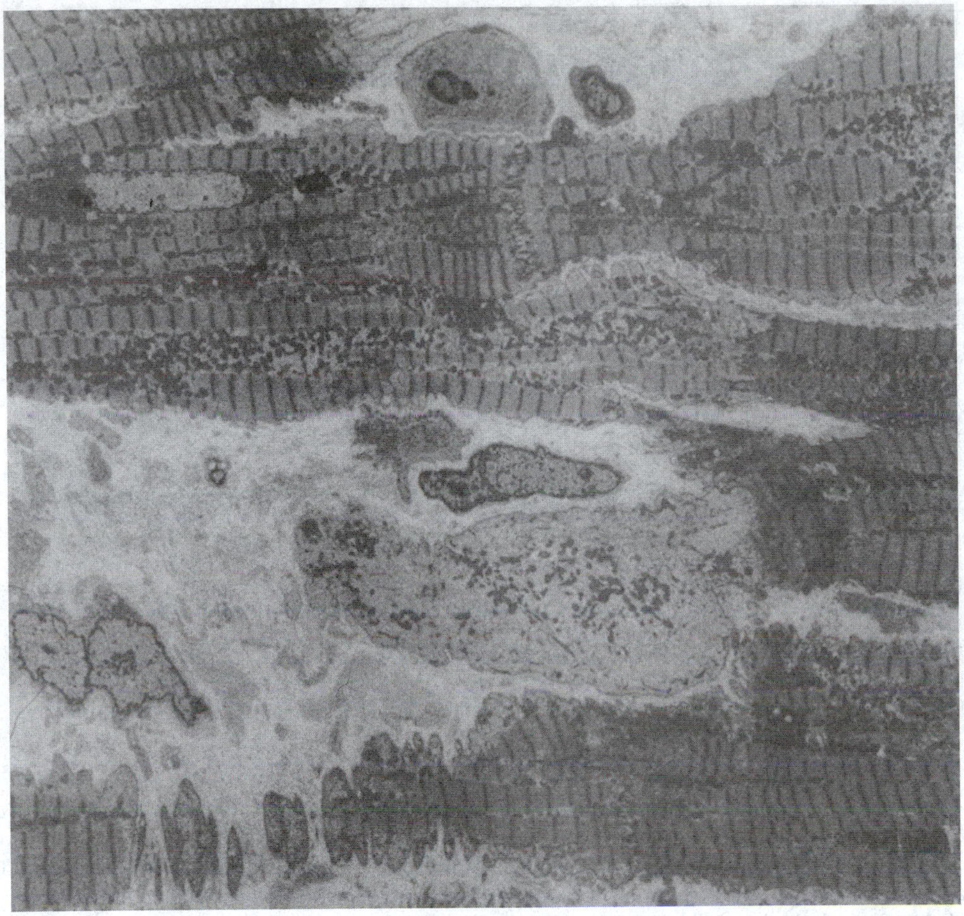

FIGURE 22-14 Transmission electron micrograph of adriamycin cardiotoxicity. Note the atrophic myocyte with myofibrillar loss surrounded by normal myocytes. (TEM ×3200)

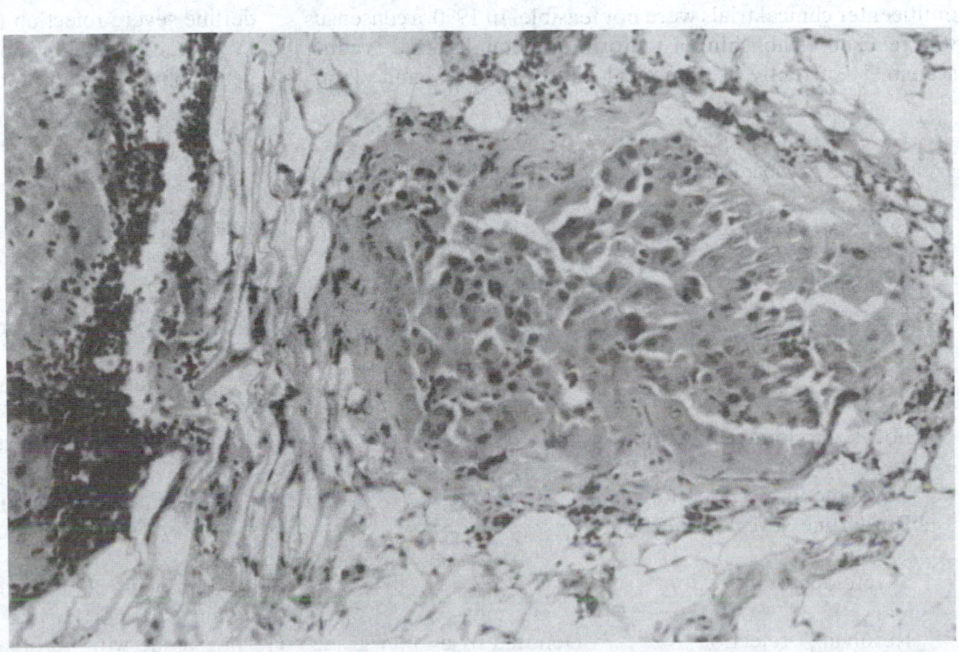

FIGURE 22-15 Metastatic adenocarcinoma in a 51-year-old woman with sudden-onset congestive heart failure and tamponade. (H&E ×400)

Pathology of Acute Rejection

MACROSCOPIC PATHOLOGY

In advanced cardiac rejection, the heart is larger than normal, stiff, and noncompliant. In the early posttransplant period, a fibrinous pericarditis may be seen. The heart appears edematous and hemorrhagic with a dark plum color. Along the atrial sutures a sharp tinctorial delineation between the hemorrhagic myocardium of the donor heart and the pale tan myocardium of the recipient heart is a characteristic of severe rejection. Less commonly, the valves may be swollen and turgid. The trabecular muscles are prominent and often demonstrate subendocardial hemorrhages.

MICROSCOPIC PATHOLOGY

Hyperacute Rejection This rare pattern of allograft rejection occurs in the setting of preformed circulating antibodies such as ABO blood group incompatibility or, rarely, antibodies against specific endothelial antigens or HLA.[145] The myocardium is globally edematous and hemorrhagic as a result of diffuse interstitial hemorrhages. Neutrophils and fibrin thrombi may be seen within the microvasculature (Fig. 22-16). Hyperacute rejection manifests as severe graft failure immediately or within the first few hours after transplantation. Without mechanical cardiopulmonary support, plasmapheresis, and emergent retransplantation, the recipient usually does not survive.

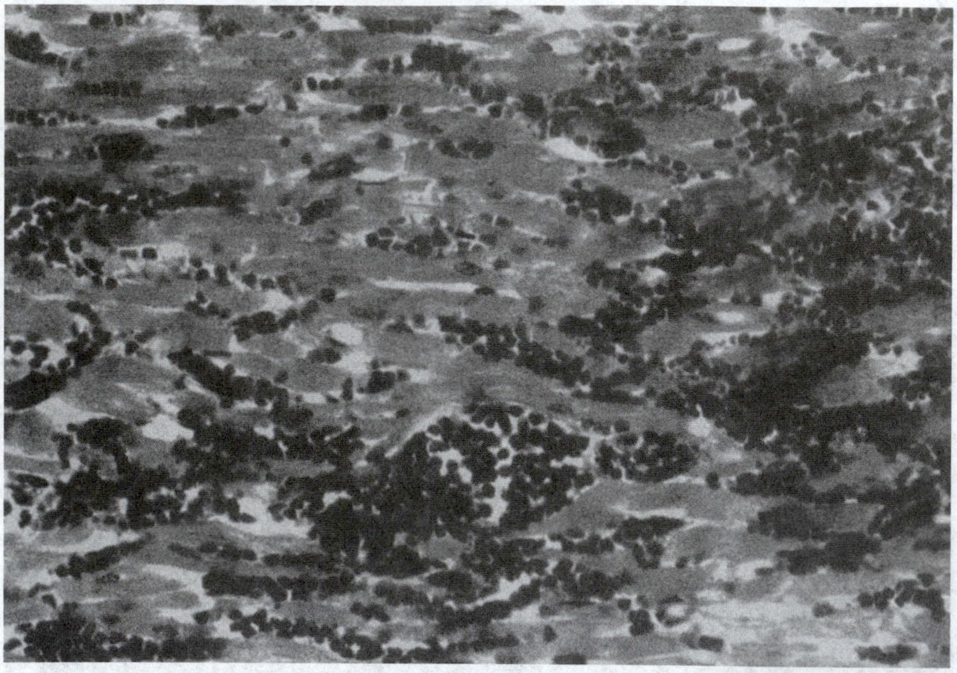

FIGURE 22-16 Hyperacute rejection is characterized by diffuse interstitial hemorrhage. (H&E ×400)

Acute Cellular Rejection The principal histopathologic features of acute cellular rejection are the distribution and extent of inflammation and the presence or absence of myocyte damage. The severity of the rejection process reflects these features along a morphologic continuum. In 1973, the Stanford grading scheme of mild-moderate-severe rejection was introduced,[146] and modifications were developed by other programs.[147–149] As a result, comparisons of results between institutions and in multicenter clinical trials were not feasible. In 1990, a consensus was reached establishing a uniform and standardized grading system.[150] Currently, a numerical and descriptive grade is assigned to each biopsy sample. This scheme requires at least four pieces of myocardium using a standard bioptome, 50 percent of which must be evaluable myocardium, i.e., not a biopsy site or scar. If a smaller bioptome (7F or smaller) is used, at least six pieces of myocardium are required.

Six patterns of acute cellular rejection have been described (Table 22-10). Mild acute rejection is divided into two patterns on the basis of the cytoarchitectural features. Focal mild rejection (grade IA) represents a circumscribed, usually perivascular arrangement of lymphocytes in one or more sites that is not associated with myocyte damage. In diffuse mild rejection (grade IB), the infiltrates are arranged in a more diffusely interstitial architectural pattern; myocyte damage is not found. Focal moderate rejection (grade II) is characterized by a solitary, sharply circumscribed inflammatory focus that is associated with myocyte damage. The other biopsy pieces may be free of rejection or have a lower grade. In multifocal moderate rejection (grade IIIA), at least two foci of inflammatory infiltrate display myocyte damage. These foci are often in different pieces of myocardium. Diffuse moderate rejection (grade IIIB) is represented by diffuse interstitial infiltrates in most or all of the biopsy pieces. Myocyte damage is significant, and the findings may be classified as borderline severe rejection (Fig. 22-17). In severe rejection (grade IV), a dense polymorphous infiltrate that includes lymphocytes, neutrophils, and eosinophils is present diffusely in the inter-

TABLE 22-10 Standardized Cardiac Biopsy Grading (Modified)

"Old" Nomenclature	Grade	"New" Nomenclature
No rejection	0	No rejection
Mild rejection	I	A = Focal (perivascular or focal interstitial infiltrate without myocyte damage)
		B = Sparse focal interstitial infiltrate without myocyte damage
"Focal" moderate rejection	II	One focus only with activated lymphocytes and myocyte damage
"Low" moderate rejection	III	A = Multifocal lymphocytic infiltrates with myocyte damage
"Borderline/severe" rejection		B = Diffuse (sometimes polymorphous) inflammatory process
"Severe/acute" rejection	IV	Diffuse, polymorphous infiltrate with myocyte necrosis ± edema ± hemorrhage ± vasculitis
"Resolving" rejection	Denoted by a lower grade	Healing tissue with fibroblasts and pigmented macrophages
"Resolved" rejection	0	Mature scar tissue

SOURCE: From Billingham ME, Carey NRB, Hammond EH, et al. A working formulation for the standardization of nomenclature in the diagnosis of heart and lung rejection: Heart rejection study group. *J Heart Transplant* 1990; 9:587–592, with permission.

stitium. Myocyte damage, edema, and hemorrhage are conspicuous as a result of injury of the microvasculature. Resolving or resolved acute rejection is denoted by a lower grade on the biopsy than was denoted on the previous biopsy.

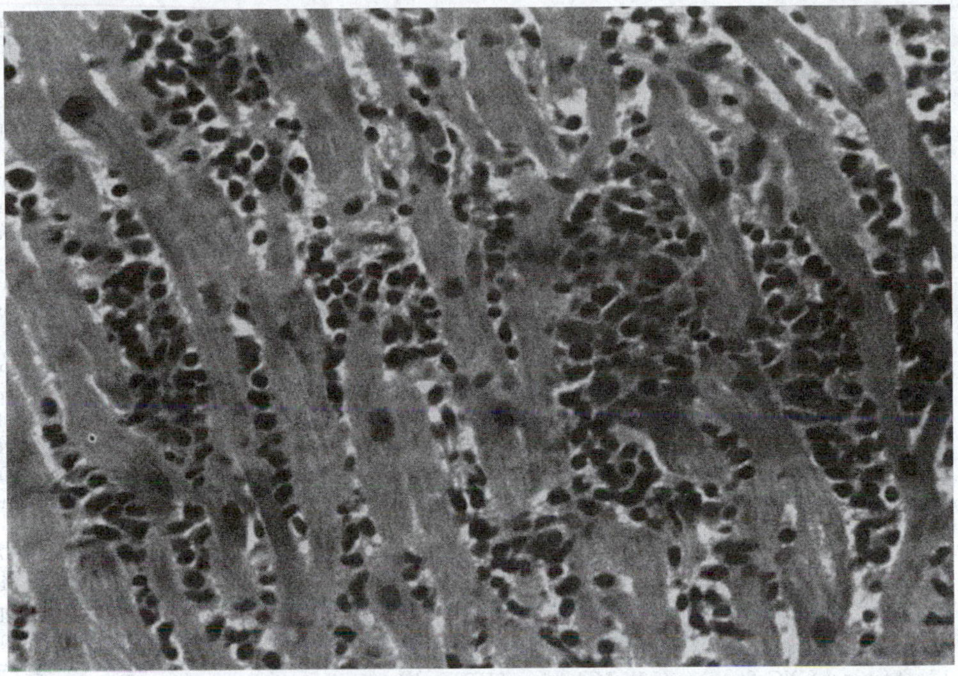

FIGURE 22-17 Diffuse moderate acute rejection (grade IIIB) showing activated lymphocytes within the interstitium and myocyte damage. (H&E ×400)

Morphologic Mimics of Acute Rejection Inflammatory infiltrates and myocyte damage of the allograft may be found in conditions other than cardiac rejection. The diagnosis of acute rejection should be made after the careful exclusion of these histologic mimics (Table 22-11). Within the first 3 weeks after transplantation, biopsies often show evidence of ischemia or preservation injury. Reperfusion of the allograft contributes to myocyte damage. Likewise, the use of pressor agents for hemodynamic support either before or after transplantation may result in small circumscribed foci of myocyte damage. The infiltrates are composed of neutrophils in the initial stages and are replaced by granulation tissue. Sharply delineated endocardial infiltrates composed of lymphocytes and a delicate vascular stroma have been designated the "Quilty effect" and may be confused with rejection when the infiltrate extends into the subadjacent myocardium. Infectious myocarditis, particularly toxoplasmic and CMV myocarditis, can resemble acute rejection. The infiltrates are usually polymorphous (lymphocytes, neutrophils, and eosinophils), and the organisms may be found. Immunohistochemical or molecular techniques are useful in difficult cases.[151] The granulation tissue and inflammation associated with previous biopsy sites may be confused with acute rejection. PTLDs uncommonly involve a cardiac allograft. Both polyclonal and monoclonal lesions have been reported, and histopathologic analysis and clonality studies are essential for classification and prognosis.[152] The presence of atypical lymphocytes, plasmacytoid or immunoblastic cell infiltrates, abundant tissue necrosis, and frequent mitotic figures should suggest the possibility of PTLD.[153]

Acute Vascular (Humoral) Rejection Most episodes of rejection in the posttransplant period are mediated by lymphocytes and histiocytes and are examples of "cellular" rejection. Hammond and colleagues found cases of allograft dysfunction occurring in the first 6 weeks after transplantation in which the classic features of cellular rejection were absent.[154] Immunofluorescence studies on fresh-frozen myocardial samples demonstrate the presence of immunoglobulin, complement, and fibrinogen, suggesting a humoral immune response mediated by endothelial and B cells. The myocardium displays large prominent endothelial cells in venules and capillaries, perivascular and interstitial edema. Currently, the diagnosis requires both the histologic and immunofluorescence findings. Infection and ischemic changes also must be excluded. A number of studies have suggested that these patients are at higher risk for developing accelerated graft coronary disease.[155] The etiology, incidence, optimum treatment strategies, and natural history of this form of rejection warrant further clinical studies.

TABLE 22-11 Histopathologic Mimics of Acute Rejection

Reperfusion/ischemic injury
Quilty effect
Infectious myocarditis (cytomegalovirus/toxoplasmic)
Previous biopsy site
Posttransplant lymphoproliferative disorder

References

1. Carrel A, Guthrie CC. The transplantation of veins and organs. *Am J Med* 1905; 10:1101.
2. Edwards WS, Edwards PD. *Alexis Carrel: Visionary Surgeon.* Springfield, IL: Charles C Thomas; 1974.
3. Mann FC, Priestly JT, Markowitz J, Yater WM. Transplantation of the intact mammalian heart. *Arch Surg* 1933; 26:219–224.
4. Marcus E, Wong SNT, Luisida AA. Homologous heart grafts: Transplantation of the heart in dogs. *Surg Forum* 1951; 2:212–214.
5. Neptune WB, Cookson BA, Bailey CP. Complete homologous heart transplantation. *Arch Surg* 1953; 66:174–177.
6. Downie HG. Homotransplantation of the dog heart. *Arch Surg* 1953; 66:624–626.
7. Demikhov VP. *Experimental Transplantation of Vital Organs*, Haigh B (trans). New York: Consultants Bureau; 1962.
8. Lower RR, Shumway NE. Studies of orthotopic homotransplantation of the canine heart. *Surg Forum* 1960; 11:18–19.
9. Starzl TE, Marchioro RI, Waddell WR. The reversal of rejection

in human renal homografts with subsequent development of homograft tolerance. *Surg Gynecol Obstet* 1963; 117:385–395.
10. Barnard CN. The operation. *S Afr Med J* 1967; 41:1271–1274.
11. Oyer PE, Stinson EB, Jamieson SW, et al. Cyclosporine A in cardiac allografting: A preliminary experience. *Transplant Proc* 1983; 15:1247–1252.
12. Reitz BA, Wallwork JL, Hunt SA, et al. Heart-lung transplantation: Successful therapy for patients with pulmonary vascular disease. *N Engl J Med* 1982; 306:557–564.
13. Hosenpud JD, Bennett LE, Keck BM, et al. The Registry of the International Society for Heart and Lung Transplantation: Thirteenth official report—1999. *J Heart Lung Transplant* 1999; 18:611–626.
14. Laffel GL, Barrett AI, Finkelstein S, Kaye ML. The relation between experience and outcome in heart transplantation. *N Engl J Med* 1992; 327:1220–1225.
15. Hosenpud JD, Breen TJ, Edwards EB, et al. The effect of transplant center volume on cardiac transplant outcome. A report of the United Network for Organ Sharing Scientific Registry. *JAMA* 1994; 271:1844–1849.
16. Costanzo MR, Augustine S, Bourge R, et al. Selection and treatment of candidates for heart transplantation: A statement for health professionals from the Committee on Heart Failure and Cardiac Transplantation of the Council on Clinical Cardiology, American Heart Association. *Circulation* 1995; 92:3593–3612.
17. Stevenson WG, Stevenson LW, Middlekauff HR, et al. Improving survival for patients with advanced heart failure: A study of 737 consecutive patients. *J Am Coll Cardiol* 1995; 26:1417–1423.
18. Stevenson LW. Heart transplant centers: No longer the end of the road for heart failure. *J Am Coll Cardiol* 1996; 27:1198–2000.
19. Packer DL, Bardy GH, Worley SJ, et al. Tachycardia-induced cardiomyopathy: A reversible form of left ventricular dysfunction. *Am J Cardiol* 1986; 57:563–570.
20. Olsen SL, Gilbert EM, Renlund DG, et al. Carvedilol improves left ventricular function and symptoms in chronic heart failure: A double-blind randomized study. *J Am Coll Cardiol* 1995; 25:1225–1231.
21. Australia-New Zealand Heart Failure Research Collaborative Group. Effects of carvedilol, a vasodilator-β-blocker, in patients with congestive heart failure due to ischemic heart disease. *Circulation* 1995; 92:212–218.
22. Packer M, Bristow MR, Cohn JN, et al. The effect of carvedilol on morbidity and mortality in patients with chronic heart failure. *N Engl J Med* 1996; 334:1349–1355.
23. Macdonald PS, Keogh AM, Aboyoun CL, et al. Tolerability and efficacy of carvedilol in patients with New York Heart Association class IV heart failure. *J Am Coll Cardiol* 1999; 33:924–931.
24. Bull DA, Karwande SV, Hawkins JA, et al. Older transplant recipients still do less well. *J Thorac Cardiovasc Surg* 1996; 111:423–428.
25. Heck CF, Shumway SJ, Kaye MP. The Registry of the International Society for Heart Transplantation: Sixth official report, 1989. *J Heart Transplant* 1989; 8:271–276.
26. Aravot DJ, Banner NR, Khanghani A, et al. Cardiac transplantation in the seventh decade of life. *Am J Cardiol* 1989; 63:90–93.
27. Olivari MT, Antolick A, Kaye MP, et al. Heart transplantation in elderly patients. *J Heart Transplant* 1988; 7:258–264.
28. Miller LW, Vitale-Naedel N, Pennington G, et al. Heart transplantation in patients over age fifty-five years. *J Heart Transplant* 1988; 7:254–257.
29. Carrier M, Emery RW, Riley JE, et al. Cardiac transplantation in patients over 50 years of age. *J Am Coll Cardiol* 1986; 8:285–288.
30. Edwards BS, Hunt SA, Fowler MB, et al. Cardiac transplantation in patients with preexisting malignant disease. *Am J Cardiol* 1990; 65:501–504.
31. Rhenman MJ, Rhenman B, Icenogle T, et al. Diabetes and heart transplantation. *J Heart Transplant* 1988; 7:356–358.
32. Badellino MM, Cavarocchi B, Narins M, et al. Cardiac transplantation in diabetic patients. *Transplant Proc* 1990; 22:2384–2388.
33. Ladowski JS, Kormos RL, Uretsky BP, et al. Heart transplantation in diabetic patients. *Transplantation* 1990; 49:303–305.
34. Report of the medical consultants on the diagnosis of death to the President's Commission for the Study of Ethical Problems in Medicine and Biomedical and Behavioral Research: Guidelines for the determination of death. *JAMA* 1981; 246:2184–2186.
35. Evans RW, Manninen DL, Garrison LP, Maier MA. Donor availability as the primary determinant of the future of heart transplantation. *JAMA* 1986; 255:1892–1898.
36. Dreyfus G, Jebara V, Mihaileanu MD, Carpentier A. Total orthotopic heart transplantation: An alternative to the standard technique. *Ann Thorac Surg* 1991; 52:1181–1184.
37. Yacoub M, Mankad P, Ledingham S. Donor procurement and surgical techniques for cardiac transplantation. *Semin Thorac Cardiovasc Surg* 1990; 2:153–161.
38. El Gamel A, Yonan NA, Grant S, et al. Orthotopic cardiac transplantation: A comparison of standard and bicaval Wythenshawe techniques. *J Thorac Cardiovasc Surg* 1995; 109:721–730.
39. Traversi E, Pozzoli M, Grande A, et al. The bicaval anastomosis technique for orthotopic heart transplantation yields better atrial function than the standard technique: An echocardiographic automatic boundary detection study. *J Heart Lung Transplant* 1998; 17:1065–1074.
40. Beniaminovitz A, Savoia MT, Oz M, et al. Improved atrial function in bicaval versus standard orthotopic techniques in cardiac transplantation. *Am J Cardiol* 1997; 80:1631–1637.
41. Sethi GK, Kosaraju S, Arabia FA, et al. Is it necessary to perform surveillance endomyocardial biopsies in heart transplant recipients? *J Heart Lung Transplant* 1995; 14:1047–1051.
42. White JA, Guiraudon C, Pflugfelder PW, Kostuk WJ. Routine surveillance myocardial biopsies are unnecessary beyond one year after heart transplantation. *J Heart Lung Transplant* 1995; 14:1052–1056.
43. Michler RE, Smith CR, Drusin RE. Reversal of cardiac transplant rejection without massive immunosuppression. *Circulation* 1986; 74(suppl III):III68–III74.
44. Costanzo-Nordin MR, Silver MA, O'Connell JB. Successful reversal of cardiac allograft rejection with OKT3 monoclonal antibody. *Circulation* 1987; 76(suppl V):V71–V79.
45. Macris MP, Frazier OH, Lammermeier D, et al. Clinical experience with Muromonab-CD3 monoclonal antibody (OKT3) in heart transplantation. *J Heart Transplant* 1989; 8:281–287.
46. Strober S. Total lymphoid irradiation in alloimmunity and autoimmunity. *J Pediatr* 1987; 111(6, part 2):1051–1055.
47. Weinblatt ME. Methotrexate for chronic diseases in adults. *N Engl J Med* 1995; 332:330–331.
48. Hunt SA, Strober S, Hoppe RT, Stinson EB. Total lymphoid irradiation for treatment of intractable cardiac allograft rejection. *J Heart Lung Transplant* 1991; 10:211–216.
49. Levin B, Bohannon L, Warvariv V, et al. Total lymphoid irradiation (TLI) in the cyclosporine era-use of TLI in resistant cardiac allograft rejection. *Transplant Proc* 1989; 21:1793–1795.
50. Costanzo-Nordin MR, Grusk BB, Silver MA. Reversal of recalcitrant cardiac allograft rejection with methotrexate. *Circulation* 1988; 78(suppl III):III47–III57.
51. Bouchart F, Gundry SR, Van Schaack-Gonzales J, et al. Methotrexate as rescue/adjunctive immunotherapy in infant and adult heart transplantation. *J Heart Lung Transplant* 1993; 12:427–433.
52. Ross HJ, Gullestad L, Pak J, et al. Methotrexate or total lymphoid irradiation for treatment of persistent or recurrent allograft cellular rejection: A comparative study. *J Heart Lung Transplant* 1997; 16:179–189.
53. Armitage JM, Kormos RL, Griffith BL, et al. A clinical trial

of FK506 as primary and rescue immunosuppression in cardiac transplantation. *Transplant Proc* 1991; 23:1149–1152.

54. Pham SM, Kormos RL, Hattler BG, et al. A prospective trial of tacrolimus (FK506) in clinical heart transplantation: Intermediate term results. *J Thorac Cardiovasc Surg* 1996; 111:1–9.
55. Jordan ML, Shapiro R, Vivas CA, et al. FK506 "rescue" for resistant rejection of renal allografts under primary cyclosporine immunosuppression. *Transplantation* 1994; 57:860–865.
56. Renlund DG, Gopinathan SK, Kfoury AG, Taylor DO. Mycophenolate mofetil (MMF) in heart transplantation: Rejection prevention and treatment. *Clin Transplant* 1996; 10(1, part 2):136–139.
57. Ensley RD, Hunt S, Taylor DO, et al. Predictors of survival after repeat heart transplantation. *J Heart Lung Transplant* 1992; 11:5142–5158.
58. Silvergleid AJ, Schrier S. Acute myelogenous leukemia in two patients treated with azathioprine for non-malignant diseases. *Am J Med* 1974; 57:885–888.
59. Penn I. Cancers after cyclosporine therapy. *Transplant Proc* 1988; 20(suppl I):276–279.
60. Young L, Alfieri C, Hennessy K, et al. Expression of Epstein-Barr virus transformation-associated genes in tissues of patients with EBV lymphoproliferative diseases. *N Engl J Med* 1989; 321:1080–1085.
61. Hanto DW, Frizzera G, Gail-Peczalska KJ, et al. The Epstein-Barr virus (EBV) in the pathogenesis of post transplant lymphoma. *Transplant Proc* 1981; 13:756–760.
62. Hanto DW. Classification of Epstein-Barr virus-associated post transplant lymphoproliferative diseases: Implications for understanding their pathogenesis and developing rational treatment strategies. *Annu Rev Med* 1995; 46:381–394.
63. Starzl TE, Porter FA, Iwatsuki S, et al. Reversibility of lymphoma and lymphoproliferative lesions developing under cyclosporine-steroid therapy. *Lancet* 1984; 1:583–587.
64. Hanto DW, Frizzera G, Gail-Peczalska KJ, et al. Epstein-Barr virus induced B-cell lymphoma after renal transplantation. *N Engl J Med* 1982; 306:913–918.
65. Shapiro RS, Chauvenet A, McGuire W, et al. Treatment of B-cell lymphoproliferative disorders with interferon alpha and intravenous gamma globulin. *N Engl J Med* 1988; 318:1334.
66. Papdopoulos EB, Ladanyi M, Emanuel D, et al. Infusions of donor leukocytes to treat Epstein-Barr virus-associated lymphoproliferative disorders after allogeneic bone marrow transplantation. *N Engl J Med* 1994; 330:1185–1191.
67. Rooney CM, Smith CA, Ng CYC, et al. Use of gene-modified virus-specific T lymphocytes to control Epstein-Barr-virus related lymphoproliferation. *Lancet* 1995; 345:9–13.
68. Gao SZ, Schroeder JS, Alderman EL, et al. Clinical and laboratory correlates of accelerated coronary artery disease in the cardiac transplant patient. *Circulation* 1987; 76(suppl V):56–61.
69. Uretsky BF, Murali S, Reddy PS, et al. Development of coronary artery disease in cardiac transplant patients receiving immunosuppressive therapy with cyclosporine and prednisone. *Circulation* 1987; 76:827–834.
70. Gao SZ, Schroeder JS, Alderman EL, et al. Prevalence of accelerated coronary artery disease in heart transplant survivors: Comparison of cyclosporine and azathioprine regimens. *Circulation* 1989; 80(suppl III):III100–III105.
71. Gao SZ, Alderman EL, Schroeder JS, et al. Accelerated coronary vascular disease in the heart transplant patient: Coronary arteriographic findings. *J Am Coll Cardiol* 1988; 12:334–340.
72. Newton M, Vetrovec G, Hastillo A. Coronary angiographic characteristics of chronic cardiac transplant rejection (abstract). *Circulation* 1984; 70(suppl II):174.
73. St. Goar FG, Pinto FJ, Alderman EL. Intracoronary ultrasound in cardiac transplant recipients: In vivo evidence of "angiographically silent" intimal thickening. *Circulation* 1992; 85:979–987.
74. Heroux AL, Silvermann P, Costanzo MR, et al. Intracoronary ultrasound assessment of morphological and functional abnormalities associated with cardiac allograft vasculopathy. *Circulation* 1994; 89:272–277.
75. Rickenbacher PR, Pinto FJ, Lewis NP, et al. Prognostic importance of intimal thickness as measured by intracoronary ultrasound after cardiac transplantation. *Circulation* 1995; 92:3445–3452.
76. Billingham ME. Cardiac transplant atherosclerosis. *Transplant Proc* 1987; (suppl 5):19–25.
77. Pucci AM, Forbes RDC, Billingham ME. Pathologic features in long-term cardiac allografts. *J Heart Lung Transplant* 1990; 9:385–388.
78. Berry GJ, Rizeq MN, Weiss LM, Billingham ME. Graft coronary disease in pediatric heart and combined heart-lung transplant recipients: A study of 15 cases. *J Heart Lung Transplant* 1993; 12:S309–S319.
79. Palmer DC, Tsai CC, Roodman ST, et al. Heart graft atherosclerosis: An ominous finding on endomyocardial biopsy. *Transplantation* 1985; 39:385–388.
80. Kaye DM, Esler M, Kingwell B, et al. Functional and neurochemical evidence for partial cardiac sympathetic reinnervation after cardiac transplantation in humans. *Circulation* 1993; 88:1110–1118.
81. Bernardi L, Bianchini B, Spadacini G, et al. Demonstrable cardiac reinnervation after human heart transplantation by carotid baroreflex modulation of RR interval. *Circulation* 1995; 92:2895–2903.
82. Givertz MM, Hartley LH, Collucci WS. Long-term sequential changes in exercise capacity and chronotropic responsiveness after cardiac transplantation. *Circulation* 1997; 96:232–237.
83. Bengel FM, Ueberfuhr P, Ziegler SI, et al. Serial assessment of sympathetic reinnervation after orthotopic heart transplantation: A longitudinal study using PET and C-11 hydroxyephedrine. *Circulation* 1999; 99:1866–1871.
84. Stark RP, McGinn AL, Wilson RF. Chest pain in cardiac transplant recipients: Evidence of sensory reinnervation after cardiac transplantation. *N Engl J Med* 1991; 324:1791–1794.
85. Smart FW, Ballantyne CM, Cocanougher B, et al. Insensitivity of noninvasive tests to detect coronary artery vasculopathy after heart transplant. *Am J Cardiol* 1991; 67:243–247.
86. Akosah KO, Mohanty PK, Funai JT. Noninvasive detection of transplant coronary artery disease by dobutamine stress echocardiography. *J Heart Lung Transplant* 1994; 13:1024–1038.
87. Derumeaux G, Redonnet M, Mouton-Schliefer D. Dobutamine stress echocardiography in orthotopic heart transplant recipients. *J Am Coll Cardiol* 1995; 25:1665–1672.
88. Spes CH, Klauss V, Mudra H, et al. Diagnostic and prognostic value of serial dobutamine stress echocardiography for noninvasive assessment of cardiac allograft vasculopathy: A comparison with coronary angiography and intravascular ultrasound. *Circulation* 1999; 100:509–515.
89. Keogh AM, Valantine HA, Hunt SA, et al. Impact of proximal or midvessel discrete coronary artery stenosis on survival after heart transplantation. *J Heart Lung Transplant* 1992; 11:892–901.
90. Schroeder JS, Gao SZ, Alderman EL, et al. A preliminary study of diltiazem in the prevention of coronary artery disease in heart transplant recipients. *N Engl J Med* 1993; 328:164–170.
91. Kobashigawa JA, Katznelson S, Laks H, et al. Effect of pravastatin on outcomes after cardiac transplantation. *N Engl J Med* 1995; 333:621–627.
92. Wenke K, Meiser B, Thiery J, et al. Simvastatin reduces graft vessel disease and mortality after heart transplantation: A four-year randomized trial. *Circulation* 1997; 96:1398–1402.
93. Halle AA, DiSciascio G, Massin EK, et al. Coronary angioplasty, atherectomy and bypass surgery in cardiac transplant recipients. *J Am Coll Cardiol* 1995; 26:120–128.
94. Smith JA, Ribakove GH, Hunt SA, et al. Heart retransplantation:

The 25 year experience at a single institution. *J Heart Lung Transplant* 1995; 14:832–839.
95. Ubel PA, Arnold RM, Caplan AL. Rationing failure: The ethical issues of the retransplantation of scarce vital organs. *JAMA* 1993; 270:2469–2474.
96. Mouloupoulos SD, Topaz S, Kolff WJ. Diastolic balloon pumping (with carbon dioxide) in the aorta: Mechanical assistance to the failing circulation. *Am Heart J* 1962; 63:669–675.
97. Kaplan JA, Grover JM. Assisted circulation. In: Kaplan JA, ed. *Cardiac Anesthesia.* New York: Grune & Stratton; 1979:441.
98. Creswell L, Rosenbloom M, Cox JL, et al. Intraaortic balloon counterpulsation: Patterns of usage and outcome in cardiac surgery patients. *Ann Thorac Surg* 1992; 54:11–20.
99. Miller JF, Dodson TF, Salan AA, Smith RB. Vascular complications following intraaortic balloon pump insertion. *Am Surg* 1992; 58:232–238.
100. McEnany MT, Kay HR, Buckley MJ, et al. Clinical experience with intra-aortic balloon pump support in 728 patients. *Circulation* 1978; 58(suppl I):124–132.
101. Spencer FC, Eiseman UG, Trinkle JK. Assisted circulation for cardiac failure following intracardiac surgery with cardiopulmonary bypass. *J Thorac Cardiovasc Surg* 1965; 45:56–59.
102. Pierce WS, Parr GVS, Myers JL, et al. Ventricular assist pumping in patients with cardiogenic shock after cardiac operations. *N Engl J Med* 1981; 305:1606–1610.
103. Pennington DG, Samuels LD, Williams G, et al. Experience with the Pierce-Donachy ventricular assist device in postcardiotomy patients with cardiogenic shock. *World J Surg* 1985; 9:37–46.
104. Pae WE, Pierce WS. Temporary left ventricular assistance in acute myocardial infarction and cardiogenic shock: Rationale and criteria for utilization. *Chest* 1981; 79:692–695.
105. Portner PM, Oyer PE, McGregor CGA. First human use of an electrically powered implantable ventricular assist system. *Artif Organs* 1985; 9(A):36–38.
106. Copeland JD, Levinson MM, Smith R, et al. The total artificial heart as a bridge to transplantation: A report of two cases. *JAMA* 1986; 256:2991–2995.
107. Copeland JG, Pavie A, Duveau D, et al. Bridge to transplantation with the CardioWest total artificial heart: The international experience 1993 to 1995. *J Heart Lung Transplant* 1996; 15:94–99.
108. Kormos RL, Borovetz HS, Armitage JM, et al. Evolving experience with mechanical circulatory support. *Ann Surg* 1991; 214:471–475.
109. Pifarre R, Sullivan H, Montoya A, et al. Comparison of results after heart transplantation: Mechanically supported versus nonsupported patients. *J Heart Lung Transplant* 1992; 11:235–239.
110. Rose EA, Moskowitz AJ, Packer M, et al. The REMATCH trial: Rationale, design, and end points. *Ann Thoracic Surg* 1999; 67:723–730.
111. Hammer CR. Nature's obstacles to xenotransplantation. *Transplant Rev* 1994; 8:174–184.
112. Dalmasso AP, Vercellotti GM, Fischel RJ, et al. Mechanism of complement activation in the hyperacute rejection of porcine organs transplanted into primate recipients. *Am J Pathol* 1992; 140:1157–1166.
113. Platt JL, Fischel RJ, Matas AJ, et al. Immunopathology of hyperacute xenograft rejection in a swine-to-primate model. *Transplantation* 1990; 52:214–220.
114. Cooper DKC. Depletion of natural antibodies in non-human primates—a step toward successful discordant xenografting in humans. *Clin Transplant* 1992; 6:178–184.
115. Henry ML, Han MK, Davies EA, et al. Antibody depletion prolongs xenograft survival. *Surgery* 1994; 115:355–361.
116. Leventhal JR, Delmasso AP, Cromwell JW, et al. Prolongation of cardiac xenograft survival by depletion of complement. *Transplantation* 1993; 55:857–866.
117. Cary N, Moody J, Yannoutsos N, et al. Tissue expression of human decay accelerating factor, a regulator of complement activation expressed in mice: A potential approach to inhibition of hyperacute xenograft rejection. *Transplant Proc* 1993; 25: 400–401.
118. McCurry KR, Kooyman DL, Alvarado CG, et al. Human complement regulatory proteins protect swine-to-primate cardiac xenografts from humoral injury. *Nature Med* 1995; 1:423–427.
119. Chapman LE, Folks TM, Salomon DR, et al. Xenotransplantation and xenogeneic infections. *N Engl J Med* 1995; 333:1498–1501.
120. Bach FH, Fishman JA, Daniels N, et al. Uncertainty in xenotransplantation: Individual benefit versus collective risk. *Nature Med* 1998; 4:141–144.
121. Sakakibara S, Konno S. Endomyocardial biopsy. *Jpn Heart J* 1962; 3:537–543.
122. Caves PK, Stinson EB, Billingham ME, Shumway NE. Percutaneous transvenous endomyocardial biopsy in human heart recipients (experience with a new technique). *Ann Thorac Surg* 1973; 16:325–336.
123. Mason JW. Techniques for right and left ventricular endomyocardial biopsy. *Am J Cardiol* 1978; 41:887–892.
124. Fowles RE, Anderson JS. Instruments and techniques for cardiac biopsy. In: Fowles RE, ed. *Cardiac Biopsy.* New York: Futura; 1992:71.
125. Miller LW, Labovitz AJ, McBride LA, et al. Echocardiography-guided endomyocardial biopsy: A 5-year experience. *Circulation* 1988; 78(suppl III):III99–III102.
126. Weston MW. Comparison of costs and charges for fluoroscopic- and echocardiographic-guided endomyocardial biopsy. *Am J Cardiol* 1994; 74:839–840.
127. Fowles RE, Mason JW. Endomyocardial biopsy. *Ann Intern Med* 1982; 97:885–894.
128. Deckers JW, Hare JM, Baughman KL. Complications of transvenous right ventricular endomyocardial biopsy in patients with cardiomyopathy: A seven-year survey of 546 consecutive diagnostic procedures in a tertiary referral center. *J Am Coll Cardiol* 1992; 19:43–47.
129. Henslova MJ, Nath H, Bucy RB, et al. Coronary artery to right ventricle fistula in heart transplant recipients: A complication of endomyocardial biopsy. *J Am Coll Cardiol* 1989; 14:258–261.
130. Sandhu JS, Uretsky BF, Zerbe TR, et al. Coronary artery fistula in the heart transplant patient: A potential complication of endomyocardial biopsy. *Circulation* 1989; 79:350–356.
131. Braverman AC, Coplen SE, Mudge GH, Lee RT. Ruptured chordae tendinae of the tricuspid valve as a complication of endomyocardial biopsy in heart transplant patients. *Am J Cardiol* 1990; 66:111–113.
132. Williams MJA, Lee MY, DiSalvo TG, et al. Biopsy-induced flail tricuspid leaflet and tricuspid regurgitation following orthotopic cardiac transplantation. *Am J Cardiol* 1996; 77:1339–1344.
133. Aretz HT, Billingham ME, Edwards WD, et al. Myocarditis: A histopathologic definition and classification. *Am J Cardiovasc Pathol* 1986; 1:3–14.
134. Cooper LT, Berry GJ, Shabetai R. Idiopathic giant cell myocarditis—natural history and treatment: Multicenter giant cell myocarditis study group investigators. *N Engl J Med* 1997; 336:1860–1866.
135. Uemura A, Morinoto S, Hiramitsu S, et al. Histologic diagnostic rate of cardiac sarcoidosis: Evaluation of endomyocardial biopsy. *Am Heart J* 1999; 138:299–302.
136. Tazelaar HD, Billingham ME. The surgical pathology of hypertrophic cardiomyopathy. *Arch Pathol Lab Med* 1987; 111: 257–260.
137. Walley VM, Kisilevesky R, Young ID. Amyloid and the cardiovascular system: A review of pathogenesis and pathology with clinical correlations. *Cardiovasc Pathol* 1995; 4:79–102.
138. Schoenfeld MH, Supple EW, Dec GW, et al. Restrictive cardiomyopathy versus constrictive pericarditis: Role of endomyocar-

dial biopsy in avoiding unnecessary thoracotomy. *Circulation* 1987; 75:1012–1016.

139. Billingham ME, Bristow MR, Glatstein E, et al. Adriamycin cardiotoxicity: Endomyocardial biopsy evidence of enhancement by irradiation. *Am J Surg Pathol* 1977; 1:17–23.
140. Mason JW, Bristow MR, Billingham ME, Daniels JR. Invasive and noninvasive methods of assessing adriamycin cardiotoxic effects in man: Superiority of histopathologic assessment using endomyocardial biopsy. *Cancer Treat Rep* 1978; 2:857–864.
141. Billingham ME, Bristow MR. Evaluation of anthracycline cardiotoxicity: Predictive ability and functional correlation of endomyocardial biopsy. *Cancer Treat Symp* 1984; 3:71–75.
142. Berry GJ, Billingham ME, Alderman E, et al. The use of cardiac biopsy to demonstrate reduced cardiotoxicity in AIDS Kaposi's sarcoma patients treated with pegylated liposomal doxorubicin. *Ann Oncol* 1998; 9:711–716.
143. Tazelaar HD, Locke TJ, McGregor CG. Pathology of surgically excised primary cardiac tumor. *Mayo Clin Proc* 1992; 67:957–965.
144. D'Amati G, Factor SM. Endomyocardial biopsy findings in patients with ventricular arrhythmias of unknown origin. *Cardiovasc Pathol* 1996; 5:139–144.
145. Trento A, Hardesty T, Griffith BP, et al. Role of the antibody to vascular endothelial cells in hyperacute rejection in patients undergoing cardiac transplantation. *J Thorac Cardiovasc Surg* 1988; 95:37–41.
146. Caves PK, Stinson EB, Billingham ME, Shumway NE. Percutaneous transvenous endomyocardial biopsy in human heart recipients (experience with a new technique). *Ann Thorac Surg* 1973; 16:325–336.
147. Kemnitz J, Cohnert T, Schafer H, et al. A classification of acute allograft rejection. *Am J Surg Pathol* 1987; 7:503–515.
148. McAllister HA. Histologic grading of cardiac allograft rejection: A quantitative approach. *J Heart Transplant* 1990; 9:277–282.
149. Zerbe TR, Arena V. Diagnostic reliability of endomyocardial biopsy for assessment of cardiac allograft rejection. *Hum Pathol* 1988; 19:1307–1314.
150. Billingham ME, Carey NRB, Hammond EH, et al. A working formulation for the standardization of nomenclature in the diagnosis of heart and lung rejection: Heart rejection study group. *J Heart Transplant* 1990; 9:587–592.
151. Weiss LM, Movahed LA, Berry GJ, Billingham ME. In situ hybridization studies for CMV viral nucleic acids in heart and lung allograft biopsies. *Am J Clin Pathiol* 1990; 93:675–679.
152. Randhawa PS, Yousem SA, Paradis IL, et al. The clinical spectrum, pathology and clonal analysis of Epstein-Barr virus-associated lymphoproliferative disorders in heart-lung transplant recipients. *Am J Clin Pathol* 1989; 92:177–185.
153. Chadburn A, Chen JM, Hsu DT, et al. The morphologic and molecular genetic categories of posttransplant lymphoproliferative disorders are clinically relevant. *Cancer* 1998; 82:1978–1987.
154. Hammond EH, Hansen JK, Spenser LS, Ensley RD. Vascular rejection in cardiac transplantation: Histologic, immunopathologic and ultrastructural features. *Cardiovasc Pathol* 1993; 2:21–34.
155. Hammond EH, Yowell RI, Price GD, et al. Vascular rejection of human cardiac allografts and the role of humoral immunity in chronic allograft rejection. *Transplant Proc* 1991; 23(suppl 2): 26–30.

PART FOUR

RHYTHM AND CONDUCTION DISORDERS

CHAPTER 23

MECHANISMS OF CARDIAC ARRHYTHMIAS AND CONDUCTION DISTURBANCES

Albert L. Waldo / Andrew L. Wit

OVERVIEW OF MECHANISMS OF CARDIAC ARRHYTHMIAS AND CONDUCTION DISTURBANCES

Introduction

Because of the increasing availability of sophisticated electrophysiologic techniques for the study of cardiac tissues both in vivo and in vitro and the ability to study arrhythmias and conduction disturbances both in experimental models and in patients, knowledge about the mechanisms of arrhythmias and conduction disturbances has increased greatly. Although much is now known, much remains to be understood. Arrhythmias are due to normal or abnormal impulse generation, abnormal impulse conduction, or a combination of simultaneous abnormalities of impulse generation and conduction.[1] This chapter first provides an overview of these mechanisms and identifies the clinical arrhythmias with which they are thought to be associated. This is followed by a much more detailed discussion of these mechanisms as they are currently understood. The detailed discussion requires that the reader have a rudimentary knowledge of the basic cellular electrophysiology of the heart, including the ionic channels and membrane currents causing the resting potential and the cardiac action potential, as well as the mechanisms for automaticity and conduction. However, much of this material is included in a detailed discussion of the mechanisms of arrhythmias, since the chapter considers how alterations in normal electrophysiology lead to abnormal cardiac rhythms.

Causes of Arrhythmias

NORMAL OR ABNORMAL IMPULSE INITIATION

Automatic Rhythms NORMAL MECHANISM Cardiac cells that normally are capable of developing spontaneous diastolic (phase 4) depolarization are called *pacemaker cells*. When pacemaker cells manifest spontaneous diastolic depolarization (Fig. 23-1) and thus are responsible for generating the cardiac rhythm, the rhythm is classified as an *automatic rhythm*. Normally, the dominant pacemaker of the heart is in the sinus node, which in adults fires at a rate of 60 to 100 beats per minute. Cells capable of developing spontaneous diastolic depolarization (i.e., of manifesting automaticity) also are normally found in the specialized fibers in the atria, the atrioventricular (AV) junction, and the His-Purkinje system. The normal rate of impulse formation in adults by these ectopic pacemakers is 40 to 60 beats per minute in the AV junction (the AV node and His bundle). Normal rates of more distally located ectopic pacemakers are probably 20 to 40 beats per minute in the bundle branches. These ectopic (i.e., nonsinus) pacemakers also are called *latent* or *escape* pacemakers for two related reasons: (1) The normal intrinsic rate of these pacemakers is lower than that of the dominant pacemaker, the sinus node, and (2) spontaneous diastolic depolarization of these latent or escape pacemakers normally is suppressed by the more rapid rate of the sinus node pacemaker through the active process of overdrive suppression. Only when the sinus rate slows below the intrinsic rate of these ectopic pacemakers does "the next one in line" warm up and fire (see also "Automaticity," below).

Arrhythmias of the Sinus Node

An arrhythmia occurs when the sinus node pacemaker fires at a rate above 100 beats per minute (sinus tachycardia) (Table 23-1) or at a rate below 60 beats per minute (sinus bradycardia) and is still the dominant pacemaker of the heart. These are called *arrhythmias resulting from normal automaticity*, since the ionic mechanism causing the pacemaker depolarization is unchanged from the normal sinus rhythm. A sinus tachycardia is usually an appropriate response to a precipitating factor (e.g., exercise, fever, hypotension), although on occasion it may be inappropriate, as in the presence of a sympathetic dysautonomia

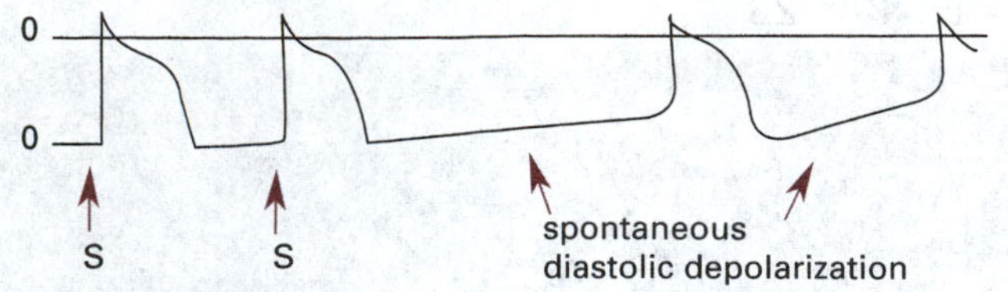

FIGURE 23-1 Arrhythmias may be caused by normal automaticity. Transmembrane potential recorded from a Purkinje fiber stimulated (S) at a regular rate is shown. When the stimulus is turned off, spontaneous diastolic depolarization develops to cause automatic firing by a normal mechanism.

(inappropriate sinus tachycardia). By contrast, sinus bradycardia often reflects an abnormality not only of the sinus node pacemakers (they are too slow) but also of the latent or escape pacemakers (when the sinus rate slows abnormally, they do not escape). Sinus bradycardia may be due to an intrinsic abnormality of pacemaker cells, a parasympathetic dysautonomia (inappropriate sinus bradycardia), or an extrinsic factor such as suppression of automaticity by drug therapy (e.g., a beta blocker, a Ca^{2+} channel blocker, or an antiarrhythmic agent). For some patients, sinus bradycardia, particularly when it is present only at rest, may simply reflect a normal response to increased vagal tone, as in a well-trained athlete. Marked beat-to-beat variations in cycle length of the sinus rhythm, which are due virtually always to the influence of vagal tone on the pacemaker cells of the sinus node, also is considered an arrhythmia (sinus arrhythmia) even if the overall sinus rate is normal.

TABLE 23-1 Types of Tachycardias and Their Selected Characteristics and Documented or Presumed Mechanism

Tachycardia	Mechanism	Origin	Rate Range, bpm	AV or VA Conduction
Sinus tachycardia	Automatic (normal)	Sinus node	≥100	1:1
Sinus nod reentry	Reentry	Sinus node and right atrium	?110–180	1:1 or variable
Atrial fibrillation	Reentry	Atria	260–450	Variable
	Fibrillatory conduction	Pulmonary veins, SVC	?	Variable
Atrial flutter	Reentry	Right atrium, left atrium (infrequent)	240–350, usually 300 ± 20	2:1 or variable
Atrial tachycardia	Reentry	Atria	150–240	1:1, 2:1, or variable
	Automatic (normal or abnormal)	Atria	?	?
	Triggered (DADs) 2° to digitalis toxicity	Atria	150–240	1:1, 2:1, or variable
AV nodal reentry tachycardia	Reentry	AV node with an atrial component	120–250, usually 150–220	1:1
AV reentry (WPW or concealed accessory AV connection)	Reentry	Circuit includes accessory AV connection, atria, AV node, His, Purkinje system, ventricles	140–250, usually 150–220	1:1
Accelerated AV junctional tachycardia	Automatic or ? triggered (? digitalis toxicity)	AV junction (AV node and His bundle)	61–200, usually 80–130	1:1 or variable
Accelerated idioventricular rhythm	Abnormal automaticity	Purkinje fibers	>60–?	Variable, 1:1, or AV dissociation
Ventricular tachycardia	Reentry	Ventricles	120–300, usually 140–240	AV dissociation, variable, or dissociation
	Automatic (rare) (normal or abnormal)	Ventricles	?	Variable, 1:1, or AV dissociation
Bundle branch reentrant tachycardia	Reentry	Bundle branches and ventricular septum	160–250, usually 195–240	AV dissociation, variable, or 1:1
Right ventricular outflow tract	? Triggered (DADs)	Right ventricular outflow tract	120–220	AV dissociation, variable, or 1:1
Torsades de pointes tachycardia	? Triggered (EADs) (with reentry)	Ventricles	>200	AV dissociation

ABBREVIATIONS: DAD = delayed afterdepolarization; WPW = Wolff-Parkinson-White syndrome; EAD = early afterdepolarization; bpm = beats per minute; SVC = superior vena cava.

ECTOPIC AUTOMATIC RHYTHMS

Arrhythmias occur when the site of the dominant pacemaker shifts to a site other than the sinus node (Table 23-1). The site of impulse initiation may shift from the sinus node to an ectopic (latent or escape) pacemaker if any of the following occur: (1) The intrinsic rate of the sinus node decreases, e.g., when pacemaker dysfunction is limited to the sinus node. (2) The intrinsic rate of the ectopic (latent or escape) pacemaker increases, e.g., as a result of enhanced automaticity of latent pacemakers. During such rhythms, the sinus node is normally automatic, but overdrive suppression of the sinus node pacemaker usually occurs because the ectopic pacemaker fires at a more rapid rate. Alternatively, if the rate of the ectopic pacemaker is very fast, there may be entrance block into the sinus node, in which case exit block of the sinus impulses rather than overdrive suppression occurs. (3) The normal sinus impulse is prevented from being the dominant pacemaker of the heart because of sinus node exit block or sinoatrial block (i.e., the impulse cannot exit from the sinus node to excite the atria and subsequently the ventricles) or AV block (the impulse cannot excite the ventricles because of conduction block in the specialized AV conduction system, i.e., the AV node, His bundle, or both bundle branches) (see Chaps. 12 and 27). The automaticity at the ectopic pacemaker site is a result of the normal automatic mechanism; hence, these are arrhythmias caused by normal automaticity.

ABNORMAL MECHANISM

Typically, normal working atrial and ventricular myocardial cells do not develop automaticity. Thus, when they manifest normal transmembrane potentials, no evidence of spontaneous diastolic (phase 4) depolarization is present. Under certain conditions, however, these cardiac muscle fibers, as well as specialized atrial and ventricular fibers, can develop an abnormal type of automatic firing. This occurs when the cell is relatively depolarized so that maximum diastolic potential is reduced to levels much lower than normal, usually by intrinsic cardiac disease. When this occurs, spontaneous diastolic (phase 4) depolarization may occur (Fig. 23-2). Such abnormal automaticity is caused by a pacemaker current that is different from the pacemaker current of normally automatic cells. The transmembrane action potentials associated with abnormal automaticity may be of the slow-response type; i.e., the transmembrane action potential upstroke may depend on the slow inward (L-type) Ca^{2+} current because of inactivation of Na^+ channels at the reduced level of membrane potential. Arrhythmias caused by abnormal automaticity will not be evident unless the rate of the abnormal focus is greater than that of the dominant automatic pacemaker (usually the sinus node) of the heart. They therefore also appear as ectopic automatic rhythms. Accelerated idioventricular rhythms after myocardial infarction sometimes may be caused by abnormal automaticity in Purkinje's cells in the ischemic region (Table 23-1) (see Chap. 47).

Triggered Rhythms These arrhythmias are caused by afterdepolarizations (Table 23-1).

Early afterdepolarizations (*EADs*) are associated with a prolongation of the duration of the action potential and occur during repolarization of a transmembrane action potential that has been initiated from a normal level of membrane potential. They appear as a shift in membrane potential in a positive

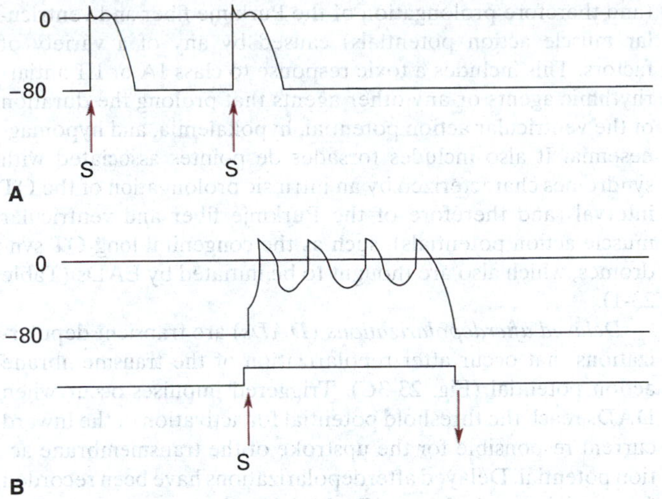

FIGURE 23-2 Arrhythmias may be caused by abnormal automaticity. The figure shows how abnormal automaticity may develop in a ventricular muscle fiber. *A*. Transmembrane potentials recorded from a muscle fiber with a normal resting potential are shown. When the fiber is not stimulated, phase 4 depolarization and automatic firing do not occur (compare with Fig. 23-1). *B*. At the arrow S, the membrane potential is reduced to −50 mV by a current pulse passed through a microelectrode. Automatic firing occurs at this low level of membrane potential. In the heart, certain abnormal states may cause a similar decrease in membrane potential.

direction relative to the membrane potential expected during normal repolarization (Fig. 23-3*A* and *B*). Repetitive depolarizations may originate from the low level of membrane potential that occurs during the afterdepolarization (Fig. 23-3*B*). A clinical example of a rhythm thought to be initiated by EADs is torsades de pointes. This is a polymorphic ventricular tachycardia that is associated with abnormal QT-interval prolongation

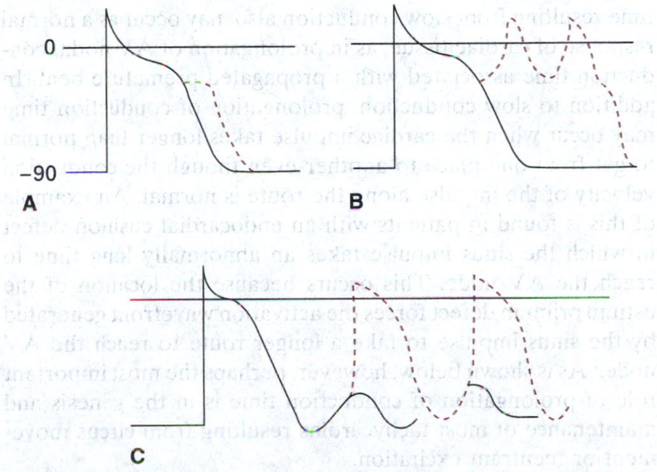

FIGURE 23-3 Triggered activity is caused by afterdepolarizations. *A*. A solid trace shows the normal transmembrane potential from a Purkinje fiber. The dashed trace shows an EAD that is subthreshold. *B*. Early afterdepolarization reached the threshold for the slow inward current, causing repetitive firing during the plateau of the Purkinje fiber action potential (*dashed trace*). *C*. Solid trace shows a transmembrane action potential followed by a subthreshold DAD. The dashed trace shows the triggered action potentials that occur when the afterdepolarization reaches threshold potential.

(and therefore prolongation of the Purkinje fiber and ventricular muscle action potentials) caused by any of a variety of factors. This includes a toxic response to class IA or III antiarrhythmic agents or any other agents that prolong the duration of the ventricular action potential, hypokalemia, and hypomagnesemia. It also includes torsades de pointes associated with syndromes characterized by an intrinsic prolongation of the QT interval (and therefore of the Purkinje fiber and ventricular muscle action potentials), such as the congenital long QT syndromes, which also are thought to be initiated by EADs (Table 23-1).

Delayed afterdepolarizations (*DADs*) are transient depolarizations that occur after repolarization of the transmembrane action potential (Fig. 23-3*C*). Triggered impulses occur when DADs reach the threshold potential for activation of the inward current responsible for the upstroke of the transmembrane action potential. Delayed afterdepolarizations have been recorded from atrial, ventricular, and Purkinje's cells exposed to catecholamines, digitalis, or abnormally high levels of Ca^{2+} and are caused by abnormally high intracellular Ca^{2+}. The ionic mechanism causing DADs is the transient inward current, a current caused by oscillatory changes in intracellular Ca^{2+} concentrations. Some digitalis toxic rhythms are thought to be due to delayed afterdepolarizations as well as some idiopathic ventricular tachycardias originating in the right ventricular outflow tract (Table 23-1).

ABNORMAL IMPULSE CONDUCTION

Prolongation of Conduction Time Prolongation of the conduction time of the cardiac impulse may occur anywhere in the heart. It may result from slow conduction and be generalized, as in response to a class IC antiarrhythmic agent, or the slow conduction may be localized to a portion of the heart, e.g., in a portion of the specialized AV conduction system or in ventricular myocardium injured by a myocardial infarction or by other kinds of cardiac disease. Prolongation of conduction time resulting from slow conduction also may occur as a normal response of cardiac tissue, as in prolongation of AV nodal conduction time associated with a propagated premature beat. In addition to slow conduction, prolongation of conduction time may occur when the cardiac impulse takes longer than normal to get from one place to another even though the conduction velocity of the impulse along the route is normal. An example of this is found in patients with an endocardial cushion defect in which the sinus impulse takes an abnormally long time to reach the AV node. This occurs because the location of the ostium primum defect forces the activation wavefront generated by the sinus impulse to take a longer route to reach the AV node.[2] As is shown below, however, perhaps the most important role of prolongation of conduction time is in the genesis and maintenance of most tachycardias resulting from circus movement or reentrant excitation.

Block of Conduction Block of the propagating impulse may occur for any number of reasons. It may block because the impulse arrives at tissue that is inexcitable either because the tissue is still in its effective refractory period after a recent depolarization or because it has an abnormally low resting potential caused by disease. Block also may occur because the strength of the propagating wavefront is insufficient to excite the tissue ahead of it despite the fact that that tissue is fully excitable (decremental conduction and block). Block also may occur because the propagating impulse encounters tissue that is intrinsically unable to conduct the cardiac impulse, e.g., scar tissue associated with a prior myocardial infarction or surgical incision. If there is conduction block of the cardiac impulse, disturbances of cardiac rhythm may occur in several different ways. If the sinus impulse fails to propagate to the right atrium (sinus node exit block or sinoatrial block), normally an ectopic (latent or escape) pacemaker will emerge and assume the role of cardiac pacemaker. If propagation of the cardiac impulse is impaired in the specialized AV conduction system so that the ventricles are not activated at a sufficiently rapid rate, an ectopic pacemaker (latent or escape) distal to the site of block often will emerge and assume the role of cardiac pacemaker. When either sinoatrial or AV block occurs, however, an ectopic pacemaker may not emerge quickly enough and/or at a clinically adequate rate under some circumstances. Thus, a period of asystole, marked bradycardia, or both may occur. If either or both happen, the clinical problem may be quite serious and even life-threatening. Block also may occur in one of the bundle branches, causing either left or right bundle branch block. Bundle branch block per se is rarely a clinical problem of consequence except when the block occurs simultaneously in both bundle branches.

Unidirectional Block and Reentry During normal sinus rhythm, the conducted impulse from the sinus node pacemaker dies out after orderly and sequential activation of the atria, the specialized AV conduction system, and the ventricles because the impulse is prevented from reactivating the myocardium by the refractoriness of the tissue that has just been activated. The heart then must wait for a new impulse from the sinus node pacemaker for each subsequent activation. The phenomenon of reentry occurs when the propagating impulse does not die out but rather continues to propagate and reactivate the heart, because the activation wavefront continuously encounters excitable cardiac tissue. Most clinically important tachyarrhythmias are due to reentry (Table 23-1). For reentry to occur, several conditions must be met. First, there must be a substrate in the cardiac tissue capable of supporting reentry, i.e., a region in the heart with the appropriate electrical properties in which reentry can occur. Second, the excitation wavefront must encounter unidirectional block. Third, the activation wavefront must be able to circulate around a central area of block.

Figure 23-4*A*, *B*, and *C* illustrates a simple model of reentry in a loop of excitable tissue, as was demonstrated first by Mayer in 1906 in the excitable ring of a jellyfish[3] and later by Mines in rings of cardiac tissue cuts from a tortoise heart.[4] The center of the loop is a hole, and this serves as a central area of block around which the reentrant wavefront can circulate. If the loop of excitable tissue is stimulated at a single point, two wavefronts of excitation circulate in the ring in opposite directions from this point (Fig. 23-4*A*). Since the wavefronts collide, they die out. If block of one of the circulating wavefronts occurs (e.g., in the shaded area), however, an excitation wavefront can circulate in only one direction around the loop; i.e., unidirectional block of the stimulated wavefront has occurred (Fig. 23-4*B*). If either conduction of the nonblocked impulse around the loop is slow enough (e.g., because of a region or regions of slow conduction) or, in the presence of normal conduction, the loop

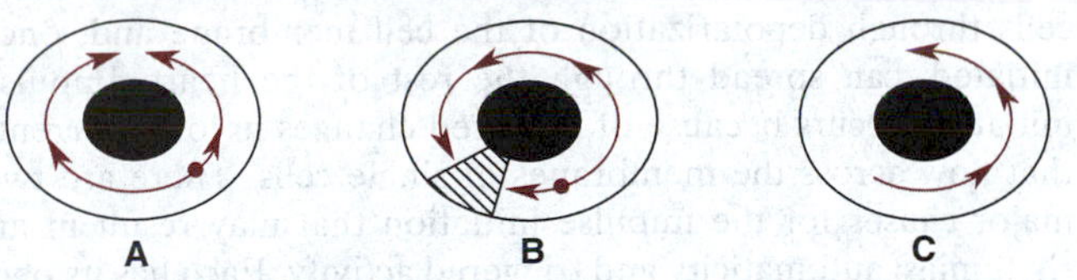

FIGURE 23-4 Schematic representation of reentry in a ring of excitable tissue. *A*. Ring was stimulated in the area indicated by the black dot. Impulses propagated away from the point of stimulation in both directions (*arrows*) and collided; no reentry occurred. *B*. The striped area was compressed while the ring was stimulated, again at the black dot. The impulse propagated around the ring in only one direction, having been blocked in the other direction by the area of compression. Then, immediately after stimulation, the compression was relieved. *C*. Circulating impulse is shown returning to its point of origin and then continuing around the ring. Identical reentry would occur if the striped area in *B* were a region of permanent unidirectional conduction block with block in the right-to-left direction.

is long enough so that by the time the circulating wavefront has returned to its site of origin, this latter region has recovered excitability, the wavefront can then reexcite (i.e., reenter) tissue it has previously excited and continue to circulate (Fig. 23-4*C*). For this to occur, however, the region of block must manifest unidirectional block, i.e., block in the right-to-left direction but conduction in the left-to-right direction (Fig. 23-4*C*). If the region of previous block remains unexcitable, bidirectional block at this site has prevented reentry. Since the block is unidirectional, reentry occurs. In the presence of myocardium manifesting unidirectional block and a central inexcitable area around which an excitation wavefront can circulate, as long as the wavelength (the product of the conduction velocity of the circulating wavefront and the effective refractory period of the tissue of the potentially reentrant circuit) of the circulating wavefront is shorter than the length of the pathway in which it is traveling, the wavefront will continue to circulate. In other words, as long as myocardium in the reentrant circuit ahead of the propagating reentrant excitation wave has sufficient time to recover excitability after its prior excitation, reentry can continue. The result is classical circus movement or reentrant excitation. Thus, an area of slow conduction is not an absolute requisite for reentrant excitation to occur.

Reentry can occur at normal conduction velocities if the path length is sufficiently long. Most reentrant circuits, however, require the presence of an area of slow conduction. This is the case because in most circumstances, despite the presence of unidirectional block, the length of the potential reentrant circuit is too short, so that without the presence of an area or areas of slow conduction, the nonblocked wavefront would otherwise travel around the circuit so quickly that it would arrive at the point of origin of the wavefront (the stimulus site in Fig. 23-4) before that site had recovered sufficiently to become excitable again. In fact, presumably for this very reason, an area or areas of slow conduction is part of the reentrant circuit for virtually all clinical reentrant rhythms. Reentrant circuits may be located almost anywhere in the heart, and they can assume many sizes and shapes.

Reentry in which the circulating wavefront continuously reenters over the same stable pathway to generate the reentrant rhythm is called *ordered reentry*.[1] The circuit may constitute a well-defined anatomic pathway, an anatomic circuit. One example is the reentrant circuit in AV reentrant tachycardia (atrium, AV node, His-Purkinje system, ventricle, accessory AV connection). Functional circuits, which depend on cellular electrophysiologic properties rather than anatomy, also can be associated with ordered reentry if the electrophysiologic properties crucial for reentry are confined to a specific location and reentry occurs only in that location. Ordered reentry also can involve a combination of anatomic and functional pathways. Examples of arrhythmias caused by ordered reentry include atrial flutter, most monomorphic ventricular tachycardias, AV nodal reentrant tachycardia, AV reentrant tachycardia involving an accessory AV connection, and sinus node reentrant tachycardia (Table 23-1) (see Chap. 27). During random reentry,[1] propagation occurs in reentrant pathways that continuously change their size and location with time. For this to occur, circuits must, at least to a significant degree, be functional. Random reentry need not depend on any special electrophysiologic abnormality in the heart, although electrophysiologic abnormalities also may lead to random reentry. Examples of random reentry include some forms of atrial and ventricular fibrillation (Table 23-1).

Reflection The term *reflection* has been used to describe a form of reentry in a linear bundle in which two excitable regions are separated by an area of depressed conduction.[5] During reflection, excitation occurs slowly in one direction along the bundle and is followed by continued propagation and excitation occurring in the opposite direction. One form of reflection may in fact be microreentry based on functional longitudinal dissociation within the depressed segment.[6–8] How this may occur is diagrammed in Fig. 23-5. The diagram at the top of the figure depicts two adjacent fibers in a bundle. The entire shaded area is depressed (reduced membrane potential and slow action po-

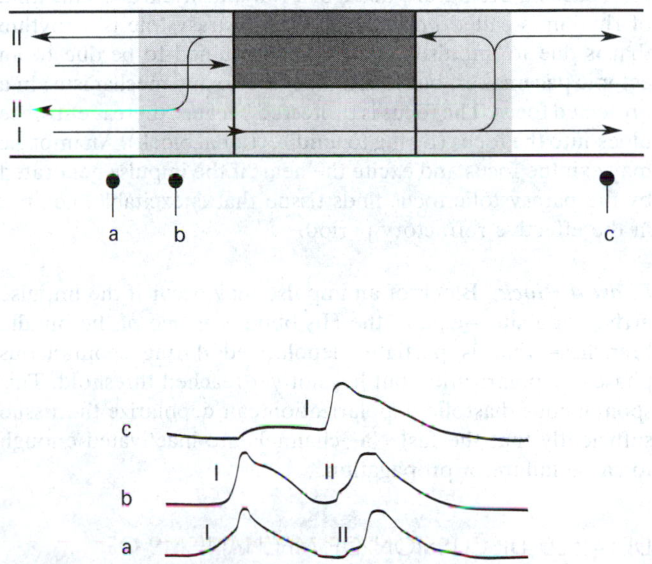

FIGURE 23-5 Diagram of reflection based on microreentry. *Top*: Schematic representation of two adjacent myocardial fibers. The shaded region indicates an area of depressed conduction. Arrows show the pattern of activation: Arrow I is a wavefront conducting in an antegrade direction, and arrow II is a reflected wavefront conducting in a retrograde direction. The action potentials shown below were recorded at sites a, b, and c on the diagram. (Modified from Wit AL, Bigger JT Jr. Possible electrophysiological mechanisms for lethal arrhythmias accompanying myocardial ischemia and infarction. *Circulation* 1975; 52(suppl):III96–III115. Reproduced with permission from the publisher and authors.)

tential upstrokes), with the darker area in the upper fiber indicating more severe depression than the lighter area in the lower fiber. Unidirectional conduction block occurs in the more severely depressed region. Arrows labeled I show the impulse entering the two fibers from the left end. Conduction of the impulse (I) blocks in the fiber at the top, in the severely depressed region, but continues in the fiber at the bottom, which is not as depressed. The impulse conducts transversely from the bottom fiber to the top fiber once it is past the region of severe depression. It then conducts retrogradely through this severely depressed region in the top bundle. Arrows labeled II show the reflected impulse returning to reexcite the left end of the bundle. Action potentials that were recorded from sites a, b, and c in the bottom fiber are shown below: action potentials labeled I were recorded as the impulse conducted from left to right; action potentials labeled II were recorded as the impulse conducted from right to left, returning to its origin. It is thought that such reentry may occur in the His bundle, one of the bundle branches or peripheral branches of Purkinje fiber bundles.

SIMULTANEOUS ABNORMALITIES OF IMPULSE GENERATION AND CONDUCTION

Parasystole At times, an ectopic pacemaker may be connected to the remainder of the heart through tissue or tissues in which there is unidirectional block. The unidirectional block prevents the dominant rhythm, usually a sinus rhythm, from entering the region where the ectopic pacemaker is located. As a result, the ectopic pacemaker is not suppressed by the dominant rhythm of the heart. At the same time, because the block is unidirectional, impulses generated by the ectopic pacemaker can be conducted out to other regions of the heart as long as they are not refractory, causing premature beats or even a tachycardia. This kind of rhythm is called *parasystole*. Thus, parasystole is a rhythm that is due to impulse generation (presumed to be due to an ectopic pacemaker, but it could be due to any mechanism) in a protected focus. The focus is protected because there is entrance block into the focus (owing to unidirectional block). An impulse may exit the focus and excite the heart if the impulse generated by the parasystolic focus finds tissue that is excitable, i.e., not in the effective refractory period.

Phase 4 Block Block of an impulse may occur if the impulse arrives at a site—e.g., in the His bundle or one of the bundle branches—that is partially depolarized during spontaneous phase 4 depolarization but has not yet reached threshold. This spontaneous diastolic depolarization can depolarize the tissue sufficiently that the fast Na^+ channels are inactivated enough to cause failure of propagation.[9]

DETAILED DISCUSSION OF MECHANISMS OF ARRHYTHMIAS AND CONDUCTION DISTURBANCES

Arrhythmias Caused by Impulse Initiation

INTRODUCTION

The term *impulse initiation* is used to indicate that an electrical impulse can arise in a single cell or a group of closely coupled cells through depolarization of the cell membrane and, once initiated, can spread through the rest of the heart. Impulse initiation occurs because of localized changes in ionic currents that flow across the membranes of single cells. There are two major causes for the impulse initiation that may result in arrhythmias: automaticity and triggered activity. Each has its own unique cellular mechanism that results in membrane depolarization.

AUTOMATICITY

It is convenient to subdivide automaticity into two kinds: normal and abnormal. Normal automaticity is found in the primary pacemaker of the heart, the sinus node, as well as in certain subsidiary or latent pacemakers that can become the pacemaker under the conditions described below. Impulse initiation is a normal property of these latent pacemakers. By contrast, abnormal automaticity, whether the result of experimental interventions or of disease, occurs in cardiac cells only when there are major abnormal changes in their transmembrane potentials, in particular in steady-state depolarization of the membrane potential. This property of abnormal automaticity is not confined to any specific latent pacemaker cell type but may occur almost anywhere in the heart.

Normal Automaticity: Pacemaker Mechanisms The normal site of impulse initiation is the sinus node. The cause of normal automaticity in the sinus node is a spontaneous decline in the transmembrane potential during diastole, referred to as the *pacemaker potential, phase 4,* or *diastolic depolarization* (the terms are interchangeable). Diastolic depolarization is the part of the sinus node membrane potential labeled dd in the top panel (*A*) of Fig. 23-6. When the depolarization reaches the threshold potential (dashed line labeled TP), the upstroke of the spontaneous action potential is initiated. In the case of the sinus node this upstroke is caused mainly by an inward-directed calcium current through L-type calcium channels. This fall in membrane potential during phase 4 reflects a gradual shift in the balance between inward and outward membrane currents in the direction of net inward (depolarizing) current.

Studies have been done to elucidate and characterize the membrane currents that cause diastolic (phase 4) depolarization in the sinus node, using voltage clamp techniques in small tissue preparations and in single dissociated sinus node cells. The cause of the pacemaker potential is still controversial. There is some evidence that diastolic depolarization results from the turning on of an inward current, called i_f, which is activated after repolarization of the sinus node action potential. The net inward i_f current is carried largely by Na^+.[10] From the voltage clamp studies, it is known that the i_f channels are inactivated at positive membrane potentials, begin to activate after hyperpolarization to around −40 mV, and are fully activated after hyperpolarization to around −100 mV.[11–13] Since the maximum diastolic potential of the sinus node pacemaker cells is between −60 and −70 mV, the i_f current is turned on during repolarization to this level, although it is not fully activated at the maximum diastolic potential. Activation of the i_f conductance also has a time dependency; therefore, the inward current continues to increase after complete repolarization, causing the progressive fall in the membrane potential during phase 4. Important roles for other membrane currents, including the potassium current i_K and the T and L Ca^{2+} currents that cause spontaneous

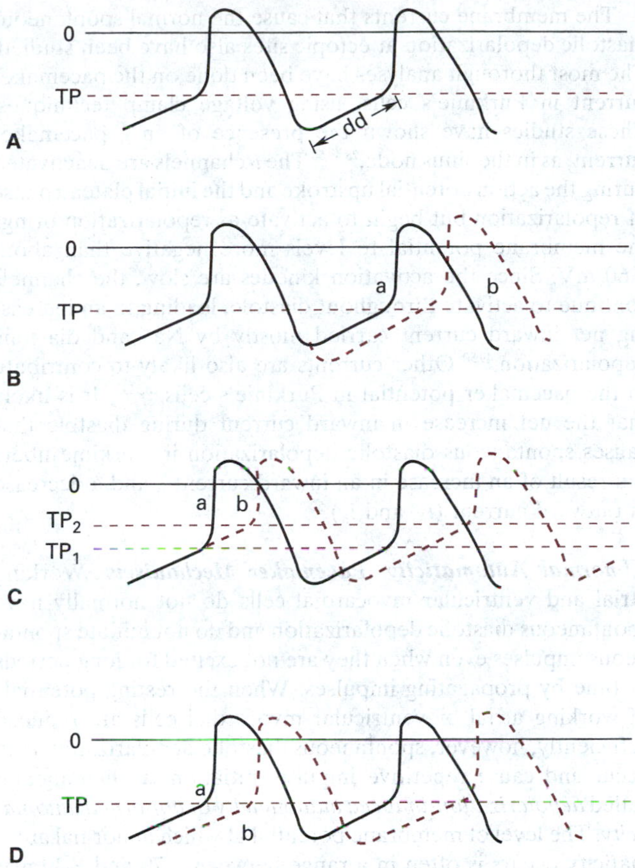

FIGURE 23-6 Diagrams of sinus node action potentials illustrating normal automaticity caused by spontaneous diastolic depolarization and the factors that change the rate of impulse initiation. *A*. Typial sinus node action potential with spontaneous diastolic depolarization (dd). *B*. Change in the rate when the maximum diastolic potential is shifted to a more negative level (from a to b). *C*. Change in rate caused by change in threshold potential to a less negative level (from TP1 to TP2). *D*. Change in rate that occurs when the slope of phase 4 depolarization is decreased (from a to b). (Modified after Wit AL, Janse MJ. *The Ventricular Arrhythmias of Ischemia and Infarction: The Electrophysiological Mechanisms*. Mount Kisco, NY: Futura; 1992:3. Reproduced with permission from the publisher and authors.)

diastolic depolarization, also have been proposed.[14–22] Therefore, there may be no single pacemaker current in the sinus node; rather, a number of currents may contribute to the occurrence of automaticity.[18]

The intrinsic rate at which sinus node pacemaker cells initiate impulses is determined by the interplay of three factors:[23] (1) the maximum diastolic potential, (2) the threshold potential, and (3) the rate or slope of phase 4 depolarization. The third factor is related to the properties of the pacemaker current or currents. A change in any one of these factors will alter the time required for phase 4 depolarization to carry the membrane potential from its maximum diastolic level to threshold and thus alter the rate of impulse initiation. For example, if the maximum diastolic potential increases (becomes more negative) going from the solid trace to the dashed trace in Fig. 23-6*B*, spontaneous depolarization to the threshold potential will take longer and the rate of impulse initiation will fall. Conversely, a decrease in the maximum diastolic potential will tend to increase the rate of impulse initiation (going from dashed trace to solid trace). Similarly, changes in threshold potential or changes in the slope of phase 4 depolarization will alter the rate of impulse initiation. In Fig. 23-6*C*, a change in threshold potential from TP1 to the less negative TP2 causes spontaneous diastolic depolarization to proceed for a longer time (dashed action potential trace) before an impulse is initiated, slowing the rate. In Fig. 23-6*D*, a decrease in the slope of spontaneous diastolic depolarization from a to b also results in a longer interval between action potentials (dashed trace) because of the longer time required for membrane potential to reach the threshold potential. In Fig. 23-6*C* and *D*, changes in the threshold potential or slope of diastolic depolarization in the opposite direction would speed up the rate.

The alterations in the rate of impulse initiation in the sinus node resulting from the factors discussed above may lead to arrhythmias. These arrhythmias are often a result of the actions of the autonomic nervous system on the sinus node. Parasympathetic stimulation and the resultant release of acetylcholine hyperpolarize the membrane potential through stimulation of muscarinic receptors and the activation of a K current (Fig. 23-6*B*).[24,25] Acetylcholine also decreases the inward Ca^{2+} current and the i_f pacemaker current.[26] A combination of these effects slows the rate. Sympathetic stimulation and norepinephrine release increase the slope of diastolic depolarization and therefore sinus rate by increasing L-type Ca^{2+} current[27] and increasing activation of the inward i_f current at the completion of action potential repolarization.[12,13,28] These effects are mediated through beta$_1$-receptor stimulation.

In addition to the sinus node, cells with pacemaking capability in the normal heart are located in some parts of the atria and ventricles, although they are not pacemakers while the sinus node is functioning normally. These are latent or subsidiary pacemakers. Since spontaneous diastolic depolarization is a normal property, the automaticity generated by these cells is classified as normal. In the atria, cells with well-polarized membrane potentials (resting potentials of around −80 mV) and action potentials characterized by fast upstrokes, a plateau phase of repolarization, and spontaneous diastolic depolarization are located along the crista terminalis (Fig. 23-7*A*).[29] Subsidiary atrial pacemakers with somewhat lower maximum diastolic potentials (−75 to −70 mV) and prominent phase 4 depolarization are located at the junction of the inferior right atrium and the inferior vena cava, near or on the eustachian ridge (a remnant of the eustachian valve of the inferior vena cava) (Fig. 23-7*B*).[30–32] Other potential atrial pacemakers are at the orifice of the coronary sinus (Fig. 23-7*C*)[33] and in the atrial muscle that extends into the tricuspid and mitral valves (Fig. 23-7*D*).[34–36] Action potentials of cells in the valves have slow upstrokes that probably are caused to a significant extent by L-type Ca^{2+} current. In the AV junction, AV nodal cells possess the intrinsic property of automaticity (Fig. 23-7*E*),[37] although there is still some uncertainty about the exact location of these pacemakers in the node.[38] The intrinsic rate of the atrial pacemakers is greater than that of AV junctional pacemakers.[39] Both atrial and AV junctional subsidiary pacemakers are under autonomic control, with the sympathetics enhancing pacemaker activity through beta$_1$-adrenergic stimulation and the parasympathetics inhibiting pacemaker activity through muscarinic receptor stimulation.[40–43] In the ventricles, latent or subsidiary pacemakers are found in the His-Purkinje system, where Purkinje fibers have the property of spontaneous diastolic depolarization (Fig.

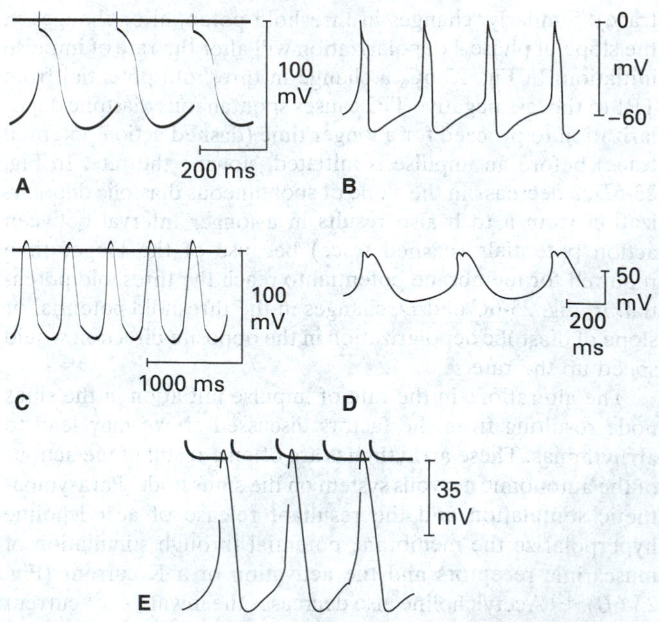

FIGURE 23-7 Transmembrane potentials recorded in isolated superfused preparations from some subsidiary pacemaker cells with the property of normal automaticity. Spontaneous diastolic depolarization that developed in the absence of overdrive suppression is shown in each panel. *A.* Atrial fiber in the crista terminalis in the presence of isoproterenol. *B.* Atrial fiber in the inferior right atrium. *C.* Atrial fiber in the ostium of the coronary sinus in the presence of norepinephrine. *D.* Atrial fiber in stretched mitral valve leaflet. *E.* Atrioventricular nodal fiber of the rabbit heart after the AV node was separated from the atrium. (From Wit AL, Janse MJ. *The Ventricular Arrhythmias of Ischemia and Infarction: The Electrophysiological Mechanisms*. Mount Kisco, NY: Futura; 1992:7. Reproduced with permission from the publisher and authors.)

23-8).[23,44] The intrinsic Purkinje fiber pacemaker rate in general is lower than the rate of atrial and AV junctional pacemakers and decreases from the His bundle to the distal Purkinje branches.[45] The spontaneous diastolic depolarization in this region is also under similar autonomic control. As in the atria, sympathetic activation enhances automaticity,[46] while parasympathetic activation can reduce it, mostly through inhibition of sympathetic influences.[47,48]

The membrane currents that cause the normal spontaneous diastolic depolarization at ectopic sites also have been studied. The most thorough analyses have been done on the pacemaker current in Purkinje's cells, using voltage clamp techniques. These studies have shown the presence of an i_f pacemaker current, as in the sinus node.[28,49,50] The i_f channels are deactivated during the action potential upstroke and the initial plateau phase of repolarization but begin to activate as repolarization brings the membrane potential to levels more negative than about −60 mV. Since the activation kinetics are slow, the channels continue to activate throughout diastole, leading to an increasing net inward current carried mostly by Na^+ and diastolic depolarization.[49,50] Other currents are also likely to contribute to the pacemaker potential in Purkinje's cells.[28,51–53] It is likely that the net increase in inward current during diastole that causes spontaneous diastolic depolarization in Purkinje fibers is a result of an increase in an inward current i_f and a decrease in outward current (i_{K_1} and i_K).[52]

Abnormal Automaticity: Pacemaker Mechanisms Working atrial and ventricular myocardial cells do not normally have spontaneous diastolic depolarization and do not initiate spontaneous impulses even when they are not excited for long periods of time by propagating impulses. When the resting potentials of working atrial or ventricular myocardial cells are reduced sufficiently, however, spontaneous diastolic depolarization may occur and cause repetitive impulse initiation, a phenomenon called *depolarization-induced automaticity* or *abnormal automaticity*. The level of membrane potential at which abnormal automaticity occurs is often in a range between −70 and −30 mV (see Fig. 23-2).[54] Likewise, cells in the Purkinje system, which are normally automatic at high levels of membrane potential, also show abnormal automaticity when the membrane potential is reduced.[55] As was discussed before, the i_f channels that participate in normal pacemaker activity in Purkinje fibers have a gating mechanism controlling channel opening and closing that is dependent on the transmembrane voltage. At membrane potentials that are positive to about −60 mV, as occurs after the upstroke and during the early phases of repolarization, the channels are closed. In response to the negative potentials that occur after complete repolarization, the channels reopen, generating the inward pacemaker current.[49,50] For this reason, when the steady-state membrane potential of Purkinje fibers is reduced to around −60 mV or less, as sometimes may occur in ischemic regions of the heart, these normal pacemaker channels are not functional and automaticity is not caused by the normal pacemaker mechanism. It can, however, be caused by an "abnormal" mechanism (described below).

In Fig. 23-9, the transmembrane potential recorded from a spontaneously firing Purkinje fiber with normal automaticity is shown in panel *A*, and abnormal automatic activity occurring while the membrane potential is depo-

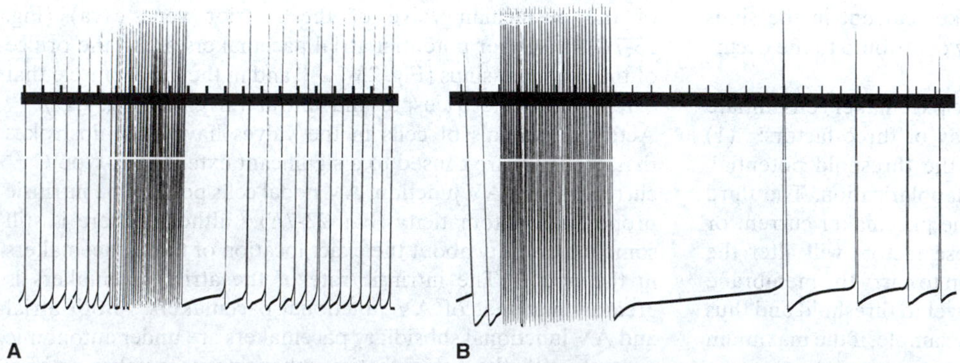

FIGURE 23-8 Overdrive suppression of normal automaticity in a canine Purkinje fiber. The action potentials are displayed at a slow oscilloscopic sweep speed, and so the time course of repolarization cannot be seen. Note the warmup of the spontaneous pacemaker after the termination of pacing. (From Cranefield PF. *The Conduction of the Cardiac Impulse: The Slow Response and Cardiac Arrhythmia*. Mount Kisco, NY: Futura; 1975. Reproduced with permisson from the publisher and author.)

larized to progressively lower membrane potentials is shown in panel *B*, 1, 2, and 3. The abnormal automatic rate increased as membrane potential became more positive. This is a general characteristic of abnormal automaticity in atrial and ventricular cells as well. A low level of membrane potential is not the only criterion for defining abnormal automaticity. If this were so, the automaticity of the sinus node would have to be considered abnormal. Therefore, an important distinction between abnormal and normal automaticity is that the membrane potentials of fibers showing the abnormal type of activity are reduced from their own normal level. For this reason, automaticity in the AV node or valves, where membrane potential is normally low, is not classified as abnormal automaticity. A likely cause of automaticity at depolarized membrane potentials in ventricular muscle is activation and deactivation of the delayed rectifier K current.[56,57] The conductance of this K channel is activated during the normal action potential plateau, and the outward current that flows through it normally contributes to repolarization. The channel then deactivates during diastole. No significant outward current flows through this channel at normal diastolic potentials, since the resting potential lies near the reversal potential and the driving force is negligible.[57] When the membrane potential is depolarized, however, an outward current flows through this channel, which is activated at the depolarized membrane potentials. This current hyperpolarizes the membrane potential. As the channel then deactivates at the hyperpolarized potentials, spontaneous diastolic depolarization occurs. If either Na or Ca channels have been reactivated since the preceding action potential, the spontaneous depolarization caused by K-channel deactivation may lead to an upstroke caused by current flowing through one of these channels (depending on the level of the membrane potential).[57] A similar mechanism may cause abnormal automaticity in partially depolarized Purkinje fibers.

Experiments on depolarized human atrial myocardium from dilated atria indicate that Ca^{2+}-dependent processes also may contribute to abnormal pacemaker activity at low membrane potentials.[58,59] It was proposed that intracellular Ca^{2+} released from the sarcoplasmic reticulum controls membrane permeability to an inward current during diastole, leading to spontaneous diastolic depolarization and abnormal automaticity. The mechanism may be similar to the one that causes the transient inward current responsible for DADs (see "Triggered Rhythms," above). An increase in intracellular Ca^{2+} also is expected to cause an inward Na^+ current through Na^+–Ca^{2+} exchange. In summary, therefore, several different mechanisms probably cause abnormal automaticity, including activation and deactivation of K^+ currents, Ca^{2+}-dependent activation of an inward current, inward Ca^{2+} currents, and even some contribution by the pacemaker current i_f.

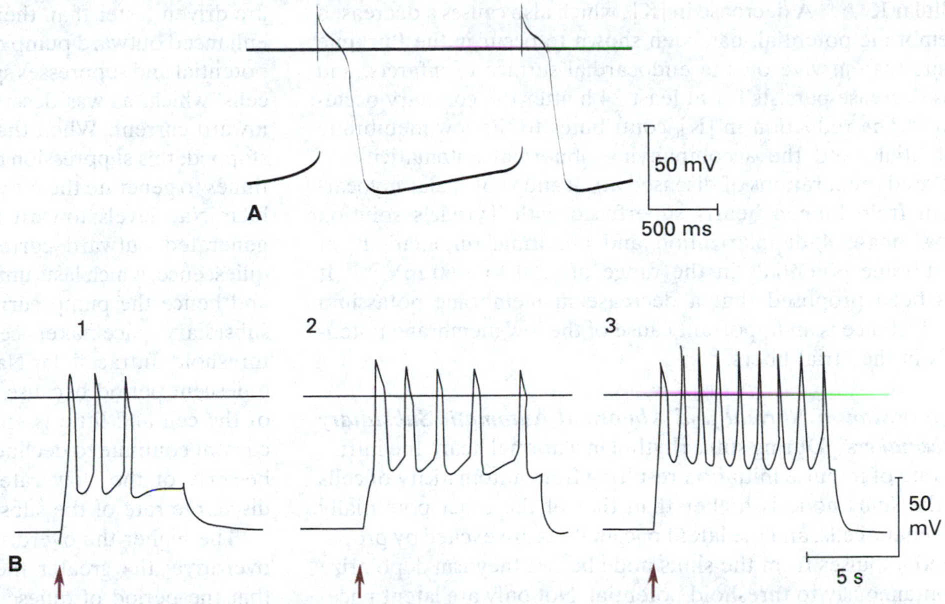

FIGURE 23-9 Normal and abnormal automaticity in a canine Purkinje fiber. *A.* Transmembrane potential recording from a Purkinje fiber with a normal maximum diastolic potential of −85 mV and spontaneous diastolic depolarization. *B.* Abnormal automaticity that occurred when membrane potential was decreased: (1) Fiber was depolarized (*at arrow*) to a membrane potential of −45 mV by the injection of a long-lasting current pulse through a microelectrode, (2) membrane potential was reduced to −40 mV (*at arrow*), (3) membrane potential was reduced to −30 mV (*at arrow*). (Reproduced from Wit AL, Friedman PF. Basis for ventricular arrhythmias accompanying myocardial infarction: Alterations in electrical activity of ventricular muscle and Purkinje fibers after coronary artery occlusion. *Arch Intern Med* 1975; 135:459. Reproduced with permission from the publisher and author.)

It has not been determined which of these mechanisms are operative in the different pathologic conditions in which abnormal automaticity may occur. The upstrokes of the spontaneously occurring action potentials generated by abnormal automaticity may be caused by either Na^+ or Ca^{2+} inward currents or possibly a mixture of the two. In the range of diastolic potentials between approximately −70 and −50 mV, repetitive activity is dependent on extracellular Na^+ concentration and can be decreased or abolished by the Na^+ channel blockers lidocaine and tetrodotoxin, indicating that the Na^+ inward current is involved. In a diastolic potential range of approximately −50 to −30 mV, repetitive activity depends on extracellular Ca^{2+} concentration and is reduced by Ca^{2+} channel blockers, Mn^{2+}, and verapamil, indicating a role for the L-type Ca^{2+} inward current.[5,60] The decrease in the membrane potential of cardiac cells required for abnormal automaticity to occur may be induced by a variety of factors related to cardiac disease. Although an increase in the extracellular potassium concentration can reduce membrane potential, normal or abnormal automaticity in working atrial, ventricular, and Purkinje fibers usually does not occur when $[K]_o$ is elevated because of the increase in K^+ conductance (and hence net outward current) that results from an increase in $[K]_o$.[61,62] This argues against abnormal automaticity being responsible for arrhythmias arising in acutely ischemic myocardium, where cells are partially depolarized by increased extracellular K^+.[63–65] A decrease in $[K]_i$, which also causes a decreased membrane potential, has been shown to occur in the Purkinje fibers that survive on the endocardial surface of infarcts, and this decrease persists for at least 24 h after the coronary occlusion.[66] The reduction in $[K]_i$ contributes to the low membrane potential[67] and the accompanying abnormal automaticity.[68,69] Isolated preparations of diseased atrial and ventricular myocardium from human hearts superfused with Tyrode's solution show phase 4 depolarization and abnormal automaticity at membrane potentials in the range of −50 to −60 mV.[70–72] It has been proposed that a decrease in membrane potassium conductance is an important cause of the low membrane potentials in the atrial fibers.[71]

Suppression of Normal and Abnormal Automatic Subsidiary Pacemakers During sinus rhythm in a normal heart, the intrinsic rate of impulse initiation resulting from automaticity of cells in the sinus node is higher than that of the other potentially automatic cells, and the latent pacemakers are excited by propagated impulses from the sinus node before they can depolarize spontaneously to threshold potential. Not only are latent pacemakers prevented from initiating an impulse because they are depolarized before they have a chance to fire, but the diastolic (phase 4) depolarization of the latent pacemaker cells with the property of normal automaticity is actually inhibited because they are repeatedly depolarized by the impulses from the sinus node.[73,74] This inhibition can be demonstrated by suddenly stopping the sinus node, e.g., by vagal stimulation (vagal stimulation also inhibits subsidiary pacemakers in the atria and AV junction) or in the tissue bath after termination of overdrive pacing (Fig. 23-8). Impulses then usually arise from a subsidiary pacemaker in the ventricular Purkinje system, but that impulse initiation generally is preceded by a long period of quiescence.[75,76] Impulse initiation by the Purkinje fiber pacemaker then begins at a low rate and only gradually speeds up to a final steady rate that is, however, still slower than the original sinus rhythm. The quiescent period after abolition of the sinus rhythm reflects the inhibitory influence exerted on the subsidiary pacemaker by the dominant sinus node pacemaker. This inhibition is called *overdrive suppression*. Similarly, the sinus node also overdrive-suppresses subsidiary atrial pacemakers.[77]

The mechanism of overdrive suppression has been characterized in microelectrode studies of isolated Purkinje fiber bundles exhibiting pacemaker activity.[73] It is mediated mostly by enhanced activity of the Na^+–K^+ exchange pump that results from driving a pacemaker cell faster than its intrinsic spontaneous rate. During normal cardiac rhythm, the sinus node drives the latent pacemakers at a faster rate than their normal (intrinsic) automatic rate. As a result, the intracellular Na^+ of the latent pacemakers is increased to a higher level than would be the case if the pacemakers were firing at their own intrinsic rate. This is the result of Na^+ entering the cells during each action potential upstroke. The rate of activity of the Na^+ pump is determined largely by the level of intracellular Na^+ concentration,[78] so that pump activity is enhanced during high rates of stimulation.[73] The increased pump activity prevents intracellular Na^+ from rising to very high levels, although there is some increase in the steady-state Na^+ concentration at high rates of firing. Since the Na^+ pump moves more Na^+ outward than K^+ inward, it generates a net outward (hyperpolarizing) current across the cell membrane.[79] When subsidiary pacemaker cells are driven faster than their intrinsic rate by the sinus node, the enhanced outward pump current hyperpolarizes the membrane potential and suppresses spontaneous impulse initiation in these cells, which, as was described before, is dependent on the net inward current. When the dominant (overdrive) pacemaker is stopped, this suppression continues because the Na^+ pump continues to generate the outward current as it reduces the intracellular Na^+ levels toward normal. The continued Na^+ pump–generated outward current is responsible for the period of quiescence, which lasts until the intracellular Na^+ concentration, and hence the pump current, becomes small enough to allow subsidiary pacemaker cells to depolarize spontaneously to threshold. Intracellular Na^+ concentration decreases during the quiescent period because Na^+ is constantly being pumped out of the cell and little is entering.[60] Intracellular Na^+ and pump current continue to decline even after spontaneous firing begins because of the slow rate, causing a gradual increase in the discharge rate of the subsidiary pacemaker.

The higher the overdrive rate or the longer the duration of overdrive, the greater the enhancement of pump activity, so that the period of quiescence after the cessation of overdrive is directly related to the rate and duration of overdrive.[73] The sinus node itself also can be overdrive-suppressed if it is driven at a rate more rapid than its intrinsic rate. Thus, there may be a quiescent period after termination of either overdrive pacing or a rapid ectopic arrhythmia before the sinus rhythm resumes.[80–83] When overdrive suppression of the normal sinus node occurs, however, it is of lesser magnitude than that of subsidiary pacemakers overdriven at comparable rates.[30,80] The sinus node action potential upstroke is largely dependent on slow inward current carried by Ca^{2+} through the L-type Ca^{2+} channels, and far less Na^+ enters the fiber during the upstroke than occurs in latent pacemaker cells such as Purkinje fibers. As a result, the activity of the Na^+ pump probably is not increased to the same extent in sinus node cells after a period of overdrive; therefore, there is less overdrive suppression caused by enhanced Na^+ pump current. The relative resistance of the normal sinus node to overdrive suppression may be important in enabling it to remain the dominant pacemaker even when its rhythm is perturbed transiently by external influences such as transient shifts of the pacemaker to an ectopic site. The diseased sinus node, however, may be much more easily overdrive-suppressed.[84]

There is an important distinction between the effects of the dominant sinus pacemaker on the two kinds of automaticity, as abnormal automaticity at reduced levels of membrane potential is not overdrive-suppressed to the same extent as is the normal automaticity that occurs at high levels of membrane potential.[85–87] The amount of suppression of spontaneous diastolic depolarization that causes abnormal automaticity by overdrive is directly related to the level of membrane potential at which the automatic rhythm occurs.[86,87] For example, Purkinje fibers that show automaticity at moderately depolarized membrane potentials of −60 to −70 mV still manifest some overdrive suppression, although less than do fibers with automaticity at −90 mV. Automaticity in Purkinje fibers with membrane potentials less than −60 mV is suppressed only slightly by overdrive, if it is suppressed at all. These differences in the effects of overdrive may be related to the reduction in the amount of Na^+ entering the cell as the membrane potential decreases, as was described for overdrive of the sinus node. At low levels of membrane potential, Na^+ channels are inactivated, decreasing the fast inward Na^+ current; therefore, there is a reduction in the amount of Na^+ entering the cells during overdrive and the degree of stimulation of the sodium-potassium pump.[88]

In addition to overdrive suppression being of paramount importance for maintenance of normal rhythm, the characteristic response of automatic pacemakers to overdrive, as was discussed in the previous paragraphs, is often useful for identifying mechanisms of arrhythmias in the in situ heart, where arrhythmia mechanisms cannot be identified by recording transmembrane potentials because of the technical difficulties. Not all mechanisms of arrhythmogenesis respond in the same way to overdrive that automatic pacemakers do, and the differences in response sometimes can be used to distinguish among mechanisms. These differences are described in detail later in this chapter. In addition to overdrive suppression, a mechanism that may suppress subsidiary pacemakers is the electrotonic interaction between the pacemaker cells and the nonpacemaker cells in the surrounding myocardium.[89] This mechanism may be particularly important in preventing AV nodal automaticity[90,91] or automaticity in the distal Purkinje system, where the pacemaking Purkinje fibers are in contact with nonpacemaking working ventricular muscle.[89,92,93]

Arrhythmias Caused by Automaticity

Arrhythmias caused by normal or abnormal automaticity of cardiac fibers may occur for several different reasons. Such arrhythmias may result simply from an alteration in the rate of impulse initiation by the normal sinus node pacemaker without a shift of impulse origin to a subsidiary pacemaker at an ectopic site. Sinus bradycardia and tachycardia are examples of these arrhythmias. The cellular mechanisms that can change the rate of impulse initiation in the sinus node are described in Fig. 23-6. During alterations in sinus rate, there may be shifts of the pacemaker site within the sinus node.[23,94] A shift in the site of impulse initiation to one of the regions where normal or abnormal subsidiary pacemakers are located also results in arrhythmias. This would be expected to happen when any of the following occurs: (1) The rate at which the sinus node activates subsidiary pacemaker falls considerably below the intrinsic rate of the subsidiary pacemakers, (2) inhibitory electrotonic influences between nonpacemaker cells and pacemaker cells are interrupted, or (3) impulse initiation in subsidiary pacemakers is enhanced.

The rate at which the sinus node activates subsidiary pacemakers may be decreased in a number of situations. Impulse initiation by the sinus node may be slowed or inhibited altogether by heightened activity in the parasympathetic nervous system[95] or as a result of sinus node disease.[96] Alternatively, there may be block of impulse conduction from the sinus node to the atria or block of conduction from the atria to the ventricles. A latent pacemaker also may be protected from being overdriven by the sinus node if it is surrounded by a region in which impulses of sinus origin block (entrance block) before reaching the pacemaker cells. Such block, however, must be unidirectional, so that activity from the pacemaker can propagate into surrounding myocardium whenever the surrounding regions are excitable. Some possible mechanisms for unidirectional block are discussed later in this chapter.

The protected pacemaker is said to be a *parasystolic focus*.[97] In general, under these conditions, a protected focus of automaticity of this type can fire at its own intrinsic frequency. Electronic current flow from surrounding regions also may influence the cycle length of a protected focus, either prolonging or abbreviating it, depending on whether the surrounding activity occurs during the early or late stage of diastolic depolarization.[98–100] Under any of the above conditions (sinus slowing, sinoatrial or AV block, parasystolic focus), there may be "escape" of a subsidiary pacemaker. There is a natural hierarchy of intrinsic rates of subsidiary pacemakers that have normal automaticity, with atrial pacemakers having faster intrinsic rates than do AV junctional pacemakers and AV junctional pacemakers having faster rates than do ventricular pacemakers.[45,74] Once overdrive suppression is removed by sinus node inhibition, the pacemaker with the fastest rate becomes the site of impulse origin.[74] Sometimes mechanisms responsible for the suppression of impulse initiation in the sinus node also suppress pacemaker activity in the atria. In experimental studies in which the sinus node is damaged or removed, the most prevalent atrial pacemaker site is at the junction of the inferior vena cava and the posterior wall of the right atrium.[30,101–103] These atrial pacemakers may cause atrial arrhythmias if the sinus node or its arterial supply is damaged.[104]

Ectopic impulse initiation may occur in the AV junction. In fact, an AV junctional pacemaker may become the dominant rhythm in the absence of normal sinus node function. Atrioventricular junctional pacemakers may be located either in the AV node or in the His bundle. These different sites have somewhat different properties, including their intrinsic rates (faster in the AV node than in the His bundle) and responses to autonomic nerve activity (parasympathetic activity suppresses AV nodal pacemakers to a greater extent than it does His bundle pacemakers). Atrioventricular junctional rhythms may occur during AV block, since the site of block is often proximal to the AV junctional pacemaker location.[38] If AV junctional pacemakers also are suppressed or if the site of disease causing AV block is in the His bundle or bundle branches, the subsidiary pacemaker location is in the His-Purkinje system. The His bundle at the proximal end of the specialized AV conduction system has a faster intrinsic rate than do the more distally located Purkinje fibers.[45] The electrocardiogram (ECG) during idioventricular rhythm in patients with complete heart block often is characterized by a wide, aberrant QRS complex, suggesting impulse initiation in the distal Purkinje system.[105] In acute myocardial ischemia, particularly when it occurs in the inferior wall, parasympathetic activity may be enhanced, depressing the sinus rate, AV conduction, or both.[106] Ectopic impulse initiation then may arise in the ventricular specialized conduction system.[107]

Any event that decreases intercellular coupling between latent subsidiary pacemaker cells and surrounding nonpacemaker cells may remove the inhibitory influence of electrotonic current flow on the latent pacemakers and allow them to fire at their intrinsic rate.[89] Coupling may be reduced by fibrosis, which can separate myocardial fibers. For example, fibrosis in the atrial aspect of the AV junctional region that results in heart block may release nodal pacemakers from electrotonic suppression by surrounding atrial cells and permit them to become the dominant pacemakers driving the ventricles. Uncoupling also may be caused by factors that increase intracellular Ca^{2+},[108] since elevated intracellular Ca^{2+} levels decrease coupling between myocardial cells by decreasing the conductance of gap junction channels (*connexons*). This may result, for example, from treatment with digitalis,[109] which inhibits Na^+ extrusion and thus increases Ca^{2+} levels in the cell.[110] In myocardial infarction, Purkinje fiber pacemakers may be uncoupled from damaged ventricular muscle cells, allowing the Purkinje fibers to fire at their intrinsic rates.

Some inhibition of the sinus node is still necessary for the site of impulse initiation to shift to an ectopic site that is no longer inhibited because of uncoupling from surrounding cells, since, as was explained above, the intrinsic firing rate of subsidiary pacemakers is still slower than that of the sinus node. Subsidiary pacemaker activity also may be enhanced, causing impulse initiation to shift to ectopic sites even when sinus node function is normal. One cause may be enhanced sympathetic nerve activity. Norepinephrine released locally from sympathetic nerves steepens the slope of diastolic depolarization of latent pacemaker cells.[23,33,34,111,112] and diminishes the inhibitory effects of overdrive.[113] The increase in slope of spontaneous diastolic depolarization may result from effects of norepinephrine on the i_f current, as was described above, as well as from an increase in inward Ca^{2+} current in those cells in which this current participates in pacemaker activity. Localized effects on subsidiary pacemakers may occur in the absence of sinus node stimulation.[114] Therefore, sympathetic stimulation may enable the membrane potential of ectopic pacemakers to reach threshold before they are activated by an impulse from the sinus node, resulting in ectopic premature impulses or automatic rhythms. There is evidence that in the subacute phase of myocardial ischemia, increased activity of the sympathetic nervous system may enhance automaticity of Purkinje fibers, enabling them to escape from sinus node domination. Enhanced subsidiary pacemaker activity also may not require sympathetic stimulation. The flow of current between partially depolarized myocardium and normally polarized latent pacemaker cells may enhance automaticity.[115] This mechanism has been proposed to be a cause of some of the ectopic beats that arise at the borders of ischemic areas in the ventricle.[93]

Inhibition of the electrogenic sodium-potassium pump results in a net increase in inward current during diastole because of the decrease in outward current normally generated by the pump and therefore may increase automaticity in subsidiary pacemakers sufficiently to cause arrhythmias. This may occur after adenosine triphosphate (ATP) is depleted during prolonged hypoxia or ischemia or in the presence of toxic amounts of digitalis.[116,117] A decease in the extracellular potassium level also enhances normal automaticity,[75] as does acute stretch.[118] Stretch can induce rapid automatic rates in Purkinje fibers with normal maximum diastolic potentials.[119,120] Stretch of the ventricles also can induce arrhythmias in an intact heart,[121] although the site of origin of the ectopic impulses has not been localized. Stretch of the Purkinje system may occur in akinetic areas after acute ischemia or in ventricular aneurysms in hearts with healed infarcts. At normal sinus rates, there may be little overdrive suppression of pacemakers with abnormal automaticity. As a result of the lack of overdrive suppression, even transient sinus pauses or occasional long sinus cycle lengths may permit an ectopic focus with a slower rate than the sinus node to capture the heart for one or more beats. In contrast, ectopic pacemakers with normal automaticity probably would be quiescent during relatively short, transient sinus pauses because they are overdrive-suppressed.

It is also possible that the depolarized level of membrane potential at which abnormal automaticity occurs may cause entrance block into the focus and prevent it from being overdriven by the sinus node even when impulses initiated in the focus could leave it (unidirectional block).[122] This would lead to parasystole, an example of an arrhythmia caused by a combination of an abnormality of impulse conduction and initiation. All these features of abnormal automaticity are evident in the Purkinje fibers that survive in regions of transmural myocardial infarction and cause ventricular arrhythmias during the subacute phase.[68] The firing rate of an abnormally automatic focus also might be enhanced above that of the sinus node, leading to arrhythmias in the absence of sinus node suppression or conduction block between the focus and the surrounding myocardium. The automatic rate is a direct function of the level of membrane potential: The greater the depolarization, the faster the rate.[5,55,57,123,124] Experimental studies have shown firing rates in muscle and Purkinje fibers of 150 to 200/min at membrane potentials less than −50 mV, and these rates should be sufficiently rapid to enable these pacemakers sometimes to control the rhythm of the heart. Catecholamines also increase the rate of firing caused by abnormal automaticity[125] and therefore may contribute to a shift in the pacemaker site from the sinus node to a region with abnormal automaticity. Among the clinical arrhythmias that are likely to be caused by abnormal automaticity is accelerated idioventricular rhythm after myocardial infarction (see Chap. 47).

TRIGGERED ACTIVITY

Triggered activity is a term used to describe impulse initiation in cardiac fibers that is dependent on afterdepolarizations.[126–128] Afterdepolarizations are oscillations in membrane potential that follow the upstroke of an action potential. Two kinds of afterdepolarizations may cause triggered activity. One occurs early, i.e., during repolarization of the action potential (EADs), and the other is delayed until repolarization is complete or nearly complete (DADs). When either kind of afterdepolarization is large enough to reach the threshold potential for activation of a regenerative inward current, action potentials result that are referred to as "triggered." Therefore, a key characteristic of triggered activity, discriminating it from automaticity, is that for triggered activity to occur, at least one action potential must precede it (the trigger). Automatic rhythms can arise de novo in the absence of any prior electrical activity, such as after long periods of quiescence, whereas triggered activity cannot.[5,128] Triggered activity will cause arrhythmias when the site of impulse initiation shifts from the sinus node to the triggered focus. For this to occur, the rate of triggered impulses should be faster than the sinus rate either transiently or persistently. This may result when firing of the sinus node is slowed or inhibited, when there is block of sinus impulses, or when the rate of triggered activity is faster than normal sinus node impulse initiation. The factors causing the shift in the site of impulse initiation should be very similar to those described in the discussion of automaticity.

Delayed Afterdepolarizations and Triggered Activity Figure 23-10 shows an example of a DAD recorded with a microelectrode in a superfused preparation of atrial muscle exposed to catecholamines. The DAD is an oscillation in membrane potential that occurs after repolarization of the action potential (indicated in the figure by the unfilled arrow). The DAD is caused by events occurring during the action potential that will be

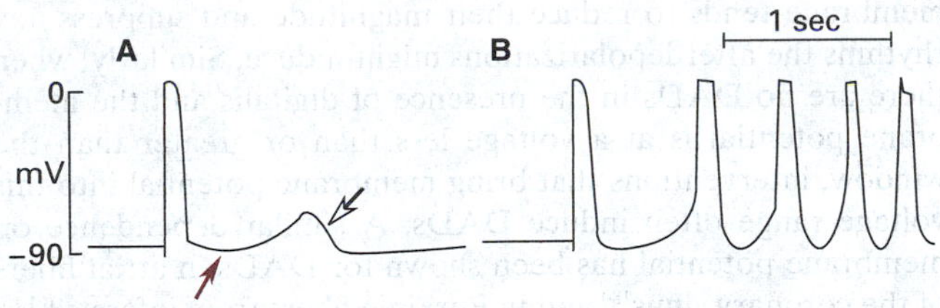

FIGURE 23-10 An example of a DAD (*white arrow*) recorded with a microelectrode from an atrial fiber in the canine coronary sinus. The red arrow indicates an afterhyperpolarization. *B*. The onset of triggered activity is shown. (From Wit AL, Rosen MR. After depolarizations and triggered activity: Distinction from automaticity as an arrhythmogenic mechanism. In: Fozzard HA, Haber E, Jennings RB, et al., eds. *The Heart and Cardiovascular System*. Scientific Foundations, 2d ed. New York, Raven Press; 1991:2113. Reproduced with permission from the publisher and author.)

described below. Figure 23-10*A* also shows that a DAD may be preceded by an afterhyperpolarization (red arrow), in which case the membrane potential transiently becomes more negative after the action potential than it was just before it. Afterhyperpolarizations, however, do not always precede DADs. The transient nature of the DAD clearly distinguishes it from normal spontaneous diastolic (pacemaker) depolarization, during which the membrane potential declines almost monotonically until the next action potential occurs (compare Fig. 23-10*A* with Fig. 23-6). In addition to microelectrode recordings such as the one shown in Fig. 23-10*A*, DADs can be identified by using techniques for recording extracellular potentials.[129,130] A major problem that exists when this technique is used in situ to locate DADs in the heart, however, is discriminating the extracellular voltage deflections caused by afterdepolarizations from deflections that result from the motion of the heart, since movement alone can mimic DADs in extracellular recordings.[131] A second important problem is a possible difficulty in locating focal sites at which afterdepolarizations and triggered activity may be originating. Nevertheless, extracellular electrodes have been used to demonstrate what appear to be DADs occurring in the in situ heart.[132,133]

A triggered impulse is initiated when a DAD depolarizes the membrane potential to the threshold potential for activation of the inward current responsible for the upstroke of the action potential. Triggered impulses are shown in Fig. 23-10*B*. Afterdepolarizations do not always reach threshold, so that triggerable fibers sometimes may be stimulated at a regular rate without becoming rhythmically active, e.g., the stimulated action potential in Fig. 23-10*A*. Probably the most important influence that causes subthreshold DADs to reach threshold is a decrease in the cycle length (an increase in the rate) at which action potentials occur. Therefore, arrhythmias triggered by DADs can be expected to be initiated by either a spontaneous or a pacing-induced increase in the heart rate. A triggered action potential also is followed by an afterdepolarization that may or may not reach threshold. When it does not reach threshold, only one triggered action impulse occurs. Quite often, the first triggered action potential is followed by a short or long "train" of additional triggered action potentials, each arising from the afterdepolarization caused by the previous action potential (Fig. 23-10*B*). The merging of the rising phase of the afterdepolarization with the upstroke of the action potential during triggered activity may be smooth, and as a result, the fiber may show phase 4 depolarization that is indistinguishable from the phase 4 depolarization seen during automatic activity.

CAUSES OF DELAYED AFTERDEPOLARIZATIONS AND TRIGGERED ACTIVITY Delayed afterdepolarizations usually occur under a variety of conditions in which there is an increase in Ca^{2+} in the myoplasm and the sarcoplasmic reticulum above normal levels (sometimes referred to as *Ca overload*). Abnormalities in the sequestration and release of Ca^{2+} by the sarcoplasmic reticulum also may contribute to their occurrence. On depolarization of the membrane during an action potential, the intracellular free Ca^{2+} normally increases, primarily by Ca^{2+} influx through the L-type Ca^{2+} channels. Initially, this rapid rate of change of intracellular Ca^{2+} triggers Ca^{2+} release from the sarcoplasmic reticulum, causing a further rise in intracellular free Ca^{2+} and contraction[134] (see Chap. 3). Repolarization then induces synchronous Ca^{2+} uptake by the sarcoplasmic reticulum in the cell and relaxation. If intracellular Ca^{2+} is very high or if catecholamines or cyclic adenosine monophosphate (AMP) is present, both of which enhance Ca^{2+} uptake by the sarcoplasmic reticulum, the Ca^{2+} in the sarcoplasmic reticulum may rise during repolarization to a critical level, at which time a secondary spontaneous release of Ca^{2+} from the sarcoplasmic reticulum occurs after the action potential and relaxation of contraction.[134] This secondary release of Ca^{2+} generates an aftercontraction as well as the transient inward (TI) current and the afterdepolarization. The TI current is an oscillatory membrane current that is distinct from the pacemaker currents.[135–142] After one or several afterdepolarizations, myoplasmic Ca^{2+} may decrease because Na^+–Ca^{2+} exchange extrudes Ca^{2+} from the cell, and the membrane potential stops oscillating.

The exact mechanism by which the secondary rise in myoplasmic Ca^{2+} after repolarization causes the TI current is unclear. Two possibilities have been considered. The first is that the Ca^{2+} released from the sarcoplasmic reticulum after repolarization acts on the sarcolemma to increase its conductance to ions (mainly Na^+) that flow into the cell down a concentration gradient through membrane channels. The second mechanism proposed for the origin of the TI current is that the rise in Ca^{2+} causes the TI current through an electrogenic (rheogenic) exchange of Ca^{2+} for Na^+. According to this hypothesis, the transient rise in myoplasmic Ca^{2+} released from the sarcoplasmic reticulum after the action potential is expected to result in "transport" of Ca^{2+} out of the cell across the sarcolemma by the Na^+–Ca^{2+} exchanger. Such an efflux is coupled to an Na^+ influx. If more than two Na^+ ions are exchanged for each Ca^{2+} ion, a net inward current occurs.[143–145]

The most widely recognized cause of DAD-dependent triggered activity is digitalis toxicity.[116,117,145–151] Afterdepolarizations caused by digitalis sometimes may reach threshold to cause triggered action potentials, particularly if the rate of stimulation is sufficiently rapid. Ventricular arrhythmias (repetitive responses) caused by digitalis in the heart in situ also can be initiated by pacing at rapid rates.[152] As toxicity progresses, the duration of the trains of repetitive responses induced by pacing increases.[153–155] It is assumed that these arrhythmias are caused by DADs. In addition, spontaneously occurring accelerated ventricular rhythms and ventricular tachycardia that occur during digitalis toxicity are likely to be caused by DADs.

Cardiac glycosides cause DADs by inhibiting the Na^+–K^+ pump. In toxic amounts, this effect results in a measurable increase in intracellular Na^+.[156,157] An increase in intracellular Na^+ in turn causes an increase in intracellular Ca^{2+}.[158] When intracellular Na^+ is increased, the concentration-dependent driving force for Na^+ across the sarcolemma is decreased, and this in turn diminishes Ca^{2+} extrusion from the cell by Na^+–Ca^{2+} exchange. Hence, there is a net inward Ca^{2+} movement.[44,159,160]

Catecholamines are probably the next most widely recognized cause of DADs. Delayed afterdepolarizations and triggered activity caused by catecholamines have been recorded with microelectrodes in atrial fibers of the mitral valve,[161] atrial fibers lining the coronary sinus,[33] atrial fibers in the inferior right atrium,[31] and atrial fibers from hearts with cardiomyopathy.[162] The DADs in Fig. 23-10 were caused by catecholamines in atrial fibers of the canine coronary sinus. Infusion of catecholamines through a catheter into the coronary sinus in the dog causes atrial tachycardia that has all the characteristics of triggered activity;[163] therefore, some naturally occurring atrial tachycardias caused by triggered activity probably are induced by the sympathetic nervous system. Ventricular muscle and Purkinje fibers also can develop DADs in the presence of catecholamines.[164,165] Sympathetic stimulation therefore may also cause triggered ventricular arrhythmias, possibly some of the ventricular arrhythmias that accompany exercise[166] and some ventricular arrhythmias that occur during ischemia and infarction.[167,168]

Catecholamines may cause DADs by increasing the slow inward L-type Ca^{2+} current through stimulation of beta-adrenergic receptors.[169,170] The net effect is an increase in transsarcolemmal Ca^{2+} entry into cardiac cells. In addition to increasing the inward Ca^{2+} current, catecholamines enhance the uptake of Ca^{2+} by the sarcoplasmic reticulum, leading to increased Ca^{2+} stored in the sarcoplasmic reticulum and the subsequent release of an increased amount of Ca^{2+} from the sarcoplasmic reticulum during contraction.[134,171,172] The increased Ca^{2+} in the sarcoplasmic reticulum induced by catecholamines also may lead to the occurrence of DADs. Delayed afterdepolarizations and triggered activity also may occur in the absence of pharmacologic agents, catecholamines, or an increase in extracellular Ca^{2+}. Triggerable fibers have been found in the upper pectinate muscles bordering the crista terminalis in the rabbit heart, branches of the sinoatrial ring bundle or transitional fibers between the ring bundle and ordinary pectinate muscle,[173] apparently normal fibers in human atrial myocardium,[174] human atrial fibers with very low membrane potentials (below −60 mV) and slow response action potentials,[70,71,174] rat ventricular muscle that is hypertrophic secondary to renovascular hypertension,[175] and ventricular myocardium from diabetic rats.[176]

Properties of Delayed Afterdepolarizations The TI current that causes DADs is maximal at around −60 mV and diminishes at more positive and more negative membrane potentials.[138,140,177] As a result of the dependence of the TI current on the level of membrane potential, the amplitude of DADs and therefore the possibility of triggered activity are influenced by the level of membrane potential at which the action potentials occur. In the digitalis-toxic Purkinje system, there is a "window" of membrane voltage for maximum diastolic potential, which is approximately between −75 and −80 mV, at which the amplitude of DADs tend to be greatest.[178,179] When DADs occur at the membrane potentials that favor a maximum amplitude, any intervention that hyperpolarizes or depolarizes the membrane tends to reduce their magnitude and suppress any rhythms the afterdepolarizations might induce. Similarly, when there are no DADs in the presence of digitalis and the membrane potential is at a voltage less than or greater than the window, interventions that bring membrane potential into this voltage range often induce DADs. A similar dependence on membrane potential has been shown for DADs in atrial fibers of the coronary sinus[180] and in Purkinje fibers from infarcts.[181,182]

Delayed afterdepolarizations are influenced by the action potential duration, with longer action potential durations favoring the occurrence of DADs.[180] When the action potential duration is longer, more Ca^{2+} is able to enter the cell. Drugs such as quinidine, which prolong action potential duration, may increase DAD amplitude,[183] while drugs such as lidocaine, which shorten action potential duration, may decrease DAD amplitude.[184] The amplitude of DADs is dependent on the number of action potentials that precede them; i.e., after a period of quiescence, the initiation of a single action potential may be followed by either no afterdepolarization or only a small one. With continued stimulation, the afterdepolarizations increase in amplitude, and triggered activity eventually may occur.[33,117,147,161,185] The amplitude of DADs and their coupling interval to the previous action potentials also are dependent on the cycle length at which action potentials are occurring, and triggered activity can be induced by a critical decrease in the drive cycle length.[117,147,161,168,173,175,176] This is illustrated by the effects of the stimulus cycle length on the amplitude of DADs recorded from an atrial fiber in the canine coronary sinus (Fig. 23-11). The transmembrane potentials at the left were recorded when the stimulus cycle length was 2000 ms; the afterdepolarization amplitude after the last stimulated impulse is 5 mV. In the center, the stimulus cycle length was 1500 ms, and the afterdepolarization amplitude after the last stimulated impulse is 15 mV. At the right, at a stimulus cycle length of 1200 ms, afterdepolarization amplitude reached 20 mV after the third stimulated action potential before triggered activity was initiated. Digitalis-induced DADs occur either singly or as two or more "damped" oscillations after the action potential.[117,147] When two or more afterdepolarizations are present, their relation to the drive cycle

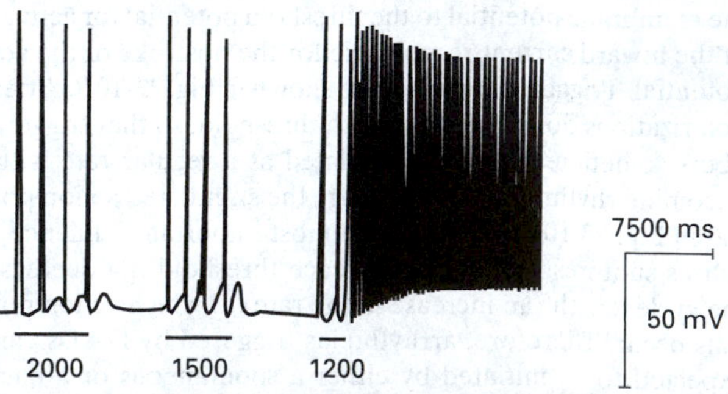

FIGURE 23-11 Effects of stimulation rate on DADs and triggered activity. Transmembrane action potentials were recorded from an atrial fiber in the canine coronary sinus superfused with Tyrode's solution containing norepinephrine. The stimulus cycle lengths and the periods of stimulation are indicated by the black bars. Sustained triggered activity occurred after stimulation at a cycle length of 1200 ms. The rate of triggered activity is so rapid that the individual action potentials cannot be seen at the slow oscilloscopic sweep speed. (From Wit AL, Cranefield PF. Triggered and automatic activity in the canine coronary sinus. *Circ Res* 1977; 41:435. Reproduced with permission from the publisher and author.)

length is complex. As drive cycle length decreases, the amplitude of the first afterdepolarization increases, reaching a peak at a cycle length of about 500 ms, and triggered activity may occur. If it does not, at shorter drive cycle lengths the magnitude of this first afterdepolarization decreases. The second DAD, however, continues to increase in magnitude as drive cycle length shortens further and eventually may reach threshold and induce triggered activity. A decrease in the length of even a single drive cycle (i.e., a premature impulse) also results in an increase in the amplitude of the DAD that follows the premature cycle.

The premature coupling interval at which triggered activity occurs is also dependent on the basic drive cycle length. As the basic drive cycle length decreases, the premature coupling interval needed to induce triggered activity increases.[186] Decreasing the drive cycle length, in addition to increasing amplitude, tends to decrease the coupling interval of DADs to the action potential upstroke or terminal phase of repolarization by increasing the rate of depolarization of the afterdepolarization.[33,117,147,173] As a result, there is a direct relation between the drive cycle length at which triggered impulses are initiated and the coupling interval between the first triggered impulse and the last stimulated impulse that induced them; i.e., as the drive cycle length is reduced, the first triggered impulse occurs earlier with respect to the last driven action potential. This characteristic property forms the basis for one of the indirect ways in which triggered activity induced by a decrease in the drive cycle length in the whole heart sometimes is distinguishable from reentrant activity induced by a decrease in the drive cycle length, since the relationship for reentrant impulses initiated by rapid stimulation is often the opposite; i.e., as drive cycle length is reduced, the first reentrant impulse occurs later with respect to the last driven action potential because of rate-dependent conduction slowing in the reentrant pathway (described in more detail later in this chapter). The increased time during which the membrane is in the depolarized state at shorter stimulation cycle lengths or after premature impulses increases Ca^{2+} in the myoplasm and the sarcoplasmic reticulum, thus increasing the TI current responsible for the increased afterdepolarization amplitude and causing the current to reach its maximum amplitude more rapidly, decreasing the coupling interval of triggered impulses. The repetitive depolarizations can increase intracellular Ca^{2+} because of repeated activation of the inward Ca^{2+} current that flows through L-type Ca^{2+} channels.

This chapter has discussed how triggered activity caused by DADs is initiated by stimulation. These characteristics may be of use in identifying triggered activity in the in situ heart (described below). Also of importance in identifying triggered arrhythmias in situ are the effects of electrical stimulation on established triggered activity. In general, triggered activity is influenced markedly by overdrive pacing (i.e., pacing at a rate faster than the rate of the triggered rhythm). The effects of overdrive pacing on triggered activity have been studied only in several experimental situations: in atrial fibers in which triggered activity is caused by catecholamines and in Purkinje fibers in which triggered activity is caused by digitalis or myocardial infarction. These effects are dependent on both the rate and the duration of overdrive pacing.[187,188] When overdrive pacing is done for a critical duration of time and at a critical rate during a catecholamine-dependent triggered rhythm, the maximum diastolic potential after the overdrive pacing increases to levels more negative than before; during the increase in membrane potential, the rate of triggered activity slows until the triggered rhythm stops. When triggered activity stops after a period of overdrive pacing at a moderate rate, some 10 to 50 impulses may occur after termination of the overdrive pacing before termination of the triggered activity occurs. The increase in maximum diastolic potential and the slowing and termination of triggered activity after a period of overdrive pacing are caused by enhanced activity of the electrogenic Na^+ pump.[187] During a period of overdrive pacing, there is a transient increase in intracellular Na^+ because the increased number of action potentials stimulates the pump to generate increased outward current.[73,189]

In digitalis-toxic Purkinje fibers, overdrive pacing also can terminate triggered activity, and this effect is dependent on the overdrive pacing cycle length but not on the overdrive pacing duration.[186,190] Termination occurs more frequently at more rapid overdrive pacing rates and may not be immediate; i.e., several triggered impulses may continue to occur after stimulation is stopped before triggered activity stops.[186] When overdrive pacing is not rapid enough to terminate the triggered rhythm, it can cause overdrive acceleration. Termination by overdrive pacing is not accompanied by hyperpolarization of the maximum diastolic potential and probably is not caused by increased Na^+–K^+ pump activity, since the pump is partially inhibited by digitalis. The exact mechanism for termination has not been elucidated. Premature stimuli also may terminate triggered rhythms, as shown in digitalis-toxic Purkinje fibers,[186] Purkinje fibers in myocardial infarcts,[191] and atrial fibers exposed to catecholamines,[161,188] although termination is much less common than it is by overdrive pacing.[190] It has not been demonstrated that the premature impulse must occur at a critical point in the cycle length of triggered activity.

Early Afterdepolarizations and Triggered Activity Early afterdepolarizations are manifest as a sudden change in the time course of repolarization of an action potential such that the membrane potential does not follow the trajectory characteristic of normal repolarization but suddenly shifts in a depolarizing direction. This is illustrated in the example of an EAD recorded with an intracellular microelectrode in a superfused Purkinje fiber shown in Fig. 23-12. The normal time course of repolarization of the action potential is shown in panel *A*. The arrow

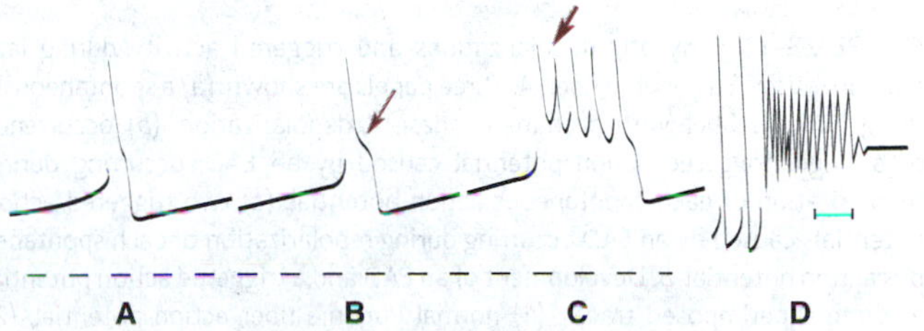

FIGURE 23-12 Early afterdepolarizations and triggered activity during repolarization in a Purkinje fiber. *A*. Transmembrane potential with normal repolarization of a spontaneously active Purkinje fiber. *B*. Early afterdepolarization (*arrow*) occurring during the plateau phase of the action potential. *C*. Triggered action potentials (*arrow*) during the plateau. *D*. Arrest of repolarization at a low level of membrane potential after a period of triggered activity. (From Cranefield PF. Action potentials, afterpotentials and arrhythmias. *Circ Res* 1977; 41:415–425. Reproduced with permission from the publisher and author.)

in panel *B* shows the deviation in membrane potential that constitutes the EAD. Early afterdepolarizations may appear at the plateau level of membrane potential, which is usually more positive than −60 mV, as in Fig. 23-12*B*, or they may appear later, during phase 3 of repolarization. In Fig. 23-13*B*, trace 1 shows the normal time course of repolarization of a Purkinje fiber action potential, while trace 2 shows a deviation from this normal time course late during phase 3, which is the EAD. Early afterdepolarizations occurring late in repolarization occur at membrane potentials more negative than −60 mV in atrial, ventricular, or Purkinje cells that have normal resting potentials. Normally, a net outward membrane current shifts the membrane potential progressively in a negative direction during repolarization of the action potential. An EAD occurs when for some reason the current-voltage relation is altered to cause outward current during repolarization to approach or attain 0, at least transiently. Such a shift can be caused by any factors that either decrease outward current, mostly carried by K^+, or increase inward current, carried by Na^+ or Ca^{2+}. If the change in the current-voltage relation results in a region of net inward current during the plateau range of membrane potentials,[192] it can lead to a secondary depolarization (a triggered action potential) during the plateau or phase 3 by activating a regenerative inward current.

Under certain conditions, EADs can lead to "second upstrokes"[5,127] or action potentials; when an EAD is large enough, the decrease in membrane potential leads to an increase in net inward (depolarizing) current, and a second action potential occurs before complete repolarization of the first, as shown in

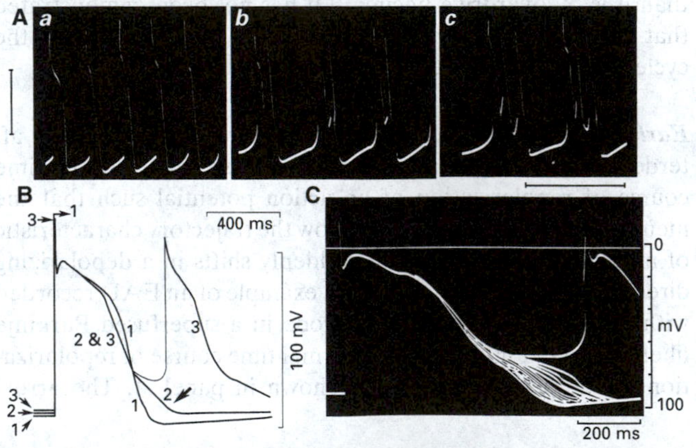

FIGURE 23-13 Early afterdepolarizations and triggered activity during late repolarization in a Purkinje fiber. *A*. Three panels are shown: (*a*) a spontaneously firing Purkinje fiber with prominent phase 4 depolarization, (*b*) occurrence of a single triggered action potential caused by an EAD, occurring during repolarization of each spontaneous action potential, (*c*) two triggered action potentials caused by an EAD occurring during repolarization of each spontaneous action potential. *B*. Development of an EAD and a triggered action potential in three superimposed traces: (1) normal Purkinje fiber action potential, (2) alteration in the time course of late repolarization leading to the occurrence of an EAD (*arrow*), (3) further alteration in late repolarization, leading to a triggered action potential. *C*. Superimposed traces recorded from a Purkinje fiber in the course of developing EADs and a triggered action potential. (From Coulombe A et al. Role of the "Na window" current and other ionic currents in triggering early after-depolarizations and re-exitation in Purkinje fibers. In: Zipes DP, Jalife J, ed. *Cardiac Electrophysiology and Arrhythmias*. New York: Grune & Stratton; 1985:43. Reproduced with permission from the publisher and author.)

panel *C* (arrow) of Fig. 23-12 and trace 3 in panel *B* of Fig. 23-13. The second action potential occurring during repolarization is triggered in the sense that it is evoked by an EAD, which in turn is induced by the preceding action potential. The second action potential also may be followed by other action potentials, all occurring at the low level of membrane potential characteristic of the plateau (Fig. 23-12*C*) or at the higher level of membrane potential of later phase 3 (Fig. 23-13, panels *Ab*, *Ac*, and *B*). Without the initiating action potential, there could be no triggered action potentials. The sustained rhythmic activity may continue for a variable number of impulses and terminates when repolarization of the initiating action potential returns membrane potential to a high level (Fig. 23-12*C*). As repolarization occurs, the rate of the triggered rhythm slows because the rate is dependent on the level of membrane potential in the same way that abnormal automaticity is. Sometimes repolarization to the high level of membrane potential may not occur, and membrane potential may remain at the plateau level or at a level intermediate between the plateau level and the resting potential[62] (Fig. 23-12*D*). The sustained rhythmic activity then may continue at the reduced level of membrane potential and assumes the characteristics of abnormal automaticity.[127]

The level of membrane potential at which the triggered action potentials occur determines both the rate of triggered activity and whether the triggered action potentials can propagate and excite adjacent normal regions.[193] At the more positive membrane potentials of the plateau, the rate of triggered activity is more rapid than it is late during phase 3. Triggered action potentials occurring at the plateau level have slow upstrokes; therefore, conduction of these action potentials sometimes may block,[194,195] while the faster upstrokes of triggered action potentials occurring later during phase 3 enable them to propagate more easily. The ionic current responsible for the upstrokes of the action potentials during triggered activity caused by EADs is determined by the level of membrane potential at which the action potentials occur. Triggered action potentials occurring during the plateau phase and early during phase 3, at a time when most fast Na^+ channels are still inactivated, most likely have upstrokes caused by the inward L-type Ca^{2+} current.[5,196] At higher membrane potentials during late phase 3 of repolarization, where there is partial reactivation of the Na^+ channels, the upstrokes are caused by the fast inward Na^+ current. Current flowing through both L-type Ca^{2+} channels and partially reactivated fast Na^+ channels may be involved over intermediate ranges of membrane potential.

Causes of Early Afterdepolarizations and Triggered Activity Early afterdepolarizations and triggered activity have been produced in experimental studies under a variety of conditions, some of which would never be expected to be associated with naturally occurring arrhythmias in the in situ heart. Most of these conditions somehow delay repolarization of the action potential by increasing inward current or decreasing outward current during the plateau and repolarization phases. Most often, EADs occur more readily in Purkinje fibers than in ventricular or atrial muscle, although EADs can readily occur in the so-called M cells, which are ventricular muscle cells with a prominent plateau phase.[197] Early afterdepolarizations may occur when the rate of stimulation is markedly slowed, reducing the outward current generated by the Na^+–K^+ pump, especially when K^+ in the extracellular environment is lower than normal, also reducing outward current.[128]

At a "physiologic range" of cycle lengths (a range that encompasses the normal sinus rhythm of the adult human heart: 1000 to 700 ms), EADs have rarely occurred in studies of isolated preparations of cardiac fibers. As cycle length is increased and repolarization is prolonged, EADs and triggered activity are more likely to occur.[198] The result is a bradycardia-induced tachycardia during which there may be very slow conduction. Another important characteristic is that the longer the basic drive cycle length, the greater the number of impulses that are triggered by EADs.[198] Once EADs have achieved a steady-state magnitude at a constant drive cycle length, any event that shortens drive cycle length tends to reduce their amplitude.[198] Hence, the initiation of a single premature depolarization, which is associated with an acceleration of repolarization, will reduce the magnitude of the EADs that accompany the premature action potential; as a result, triggered activity is not expected to follow premature stimulation. Polymorphic ventricular tachycardias that sometimes resemble torsades de pointes have been induced in dogs by the infusion of cesium, which blocks i_{K_1} to cause EADs.[199] Occurrence of tachycardia is preceded by QT-interval prolongation, a consequence of delayed repolarization, as is characteristically seen in patients with torsades de pointes.[200] The initial beat of the tachycardia caused by cesium often occurs during repolarization, i.e., during the T wave.

Early depolarizations and triggered activity have been seen in monophasic action potentials recorded from the ventricles in dogs with cesium-induced ventricular tachycardia.[201,202] Because the experimental arrhythmias caused by agents such as cesium, which are known to induce EADs, resemble torsades de pointes, it has been proposed that clinically occurring torsades de pointes sometimes may be caused by EADs. Other agents that can cause EADs and triggered activity are used therapeutically, and therefore, arrhythmias associated with their use may result from triggered activity. Antiarrhythmic drugs that prolong the duration of the action potential of Purkinje fibers or ventricular muscle (e.g., sotalol,[203,204] *N*-acetylprocainamide,[205] and quinidine[206,207]) can cause EADs and triggered activity when administered to isolated preparations, particularly when the rate of stimulation is low and the extracellular K^+ concentration is lower than normal, e.g., <4 m*M*/L.

The mechanisms by which these effects are exerted have been studied in detail for only some of these drugs. Both the d (no beta receptor blockade) and the I (beta-blocking) forms of sotalol prolong the action potential duration by inhibiting the repolarizing K current, i_K.[204] Similarly, the prolongation of the action potential by quinidine, which may lead to EADs, is related to the blocking effect of quinidine on the outward membrane repolarizing K^+ current, not to that drug's well-known blocking effect on the Na^+ channel.[208] It is known that quinidine may cause ventricular tachyarrhythmias in patients undergoing antiarrhythmic therapy with that drug. Interestingly, the arrhythmias may occur at low plasma quinidine concentrations that do not cause widening of the QRS complex in the ECG,[209] consistent with observations in superfused Purkinje fibers that afterdepolarizations caused by quinidine occur without depression of the action potential upstroke. Hypokalemia and bradycardia both predispose to the occurrence of quinidine-induced torsades de pointes,[200,210] and both have been shown to potentiate the induction of EADs in vitro by quinidine.[206,207]

Torsades de pointes also has been associated with the administration to patients of *N*-acetylprocainamide[211] and sotalol.[212] Magnesium has been shown to abolish EAD-dependent triggered activity in experimental studies.[207,213] Magnesium also has been shown to provide effective therapy when used to treat some clinical cases of drug-induced torsades de pointes,[214,215] providing further evidence that this clinical arrhythmia may be a manifestation of triggered activity (see Chap. 27).

Arrhythmias Caused by Reentry

INTRODUCTION

As was discussed previously, the excitation wavefront originating in the sinus node normally activates the cardiac tissues in an orderly sequence and then dies out. Thus, during normal sinus rhythm, each heartbeat is generated by a new pacemaker impulse in the sinus node. There are, however, arrhythmias in which, in the presence of a requisite set of circumstances, an excitation wavefront does not die out but rather can propagate continuously and thus continue to excite the heart because it always encounters excitable tissue. Such an arrhythmia is called reentrant.

REQUISITES FOR REENTRANT EXCITATION

Perhaps the easiest way to illustrate this is to discuss again, but in more detail, the earliest description of reentrant excitation by Mayer[3] in 1906 in the excitable subumbrella ring of tissue of the scyphomedusae (jellyfish), as is shown in Fig. 23-4. This example well illustrates the requisites for reentrant excitation. First, a substrate must be present that will support reentrant excitation, in this case the subumbrella ring of excitable tissue of the jellyfish. Second, the excitation wavefront propagating in this substrate must encounter unidirectional block (Fig. 23-4*B*). Unidirectional block must be present or the excitation wavefronts traveling around the ring will collide and extinguish each other (Fig. 23-4*A*). If the site of unidirectional block instead manifests bidirectional block, reentrant excitation will not occur because the circulating excitation wavefront will be unable to propagate through the area of block to reexcite the tissue that initially was excited. Third, there must be a central area of block around which the reentrant excitation wavefront can circulate. In this example, it is the hole in the center of the ring that clearly is inexcitable. Without a central area of block, the excitation wavefront will not necessarily be conducted around the ring of excitable tissue. Rather, it could take a shortcut, permitting the circulating excitation wavefront to arrive quite early at the site where it originated. If it arrives sufficiently early, the latter tissue will still be refractory, and reentrant excitation will not be possible. But even with the presence of a central area of block and without the presence of a shortcut, the circulating wavefront will manifest reentrant excitation only if the tissue it initially activated has had sufficient time to recover its excitability by the time the reentrant wavefront returns. Thus, conduction of the circulating excitation wavefront in the rest of the circuit must take long enough for this to happen, and there must always be a gap of excitable tissue (either fully or partially excitable) ahead of the circulating wavefront (the so-called excitable gap). In the case of the experiment by Mayer on the subumbrella ring of excitable tissue of the jellyfish, conduction velocity was constant and the length of the ring was long enough that conduction time around the ring was longer than the effective refractory period of the excitable tissue constituting the ring, permitting reentry. If the length of the ring had been critically shorter or if the conduction velocity had been critically faster, the circulating excitation wavefront would have arrived at the site of initial excitation before sufficient recovery of excitability had occurred, preventing reexcitation.

From these sorts of observations grew the concept of the wavelength of the circulating impulse.[4,216,217] The wavelength is the product of the conduction velocity of the circulating excitation wavefront and the effective refractory period of the tissue in which the excitation wavefront is propagating. It quantifies how far the impulse travels relative to the duration of the refractory period. Thus, the wavelength of the reentrant excitation wavefront must be shorter than the length of the pathway of the potential reentrant circuit for reentrant excitation to occur; i.e., the impulse must travel a distance during the refractory period that is less than the complete reentrant path length to give myocardium ahead of it sufficient time to recover excitability.

For virtually all clinically important reentrant arrhythmias resulting from ordered reentry, however, in the presence of uniform, normal conduction velocity along the reentrant pathway, the wavelength would be too long to permit reentrant excitation. Thus, virtually all these arrhythmias must have, and in fact do have, one or more areas of slow conduction as a part of the reentrant circuit. The associated changes in conduction velocity (as well as associated changes in refractory periods) actually cause the wavelength to change in different parts of the circuit. However, the presence of one or more areas of slow conduction permits the average wavelength of reentrant activation to be shorter than the path length.

The fact that the reentrant circuit of virtually all clinically important reentrant arrhythmias has one or more areas of slow conduction serves to emphasize the fact that the electrophysiologic properties of the cardiac tissue making up the reentrant circuit are not uniform. In fact, there may be, and usually are, variations of conduction velocity and refractoriness along the course of the reentrant circuit. An additional requisite for random reentry is the necessity of a critical mass of tissue to sustain the one or usually more simultaneously circulating reentrant excitation wavefronts.[218] Thus, it is essentially not possible to achieve sustained fibrillation of ventricles of very small normal mammalian hearts and equally difficult to achieve sustained fibrillation of the normal atria of humans or smaller mammals.

Finally, another prerequisite for reentrant excitation to occur is often (but not always) the presence of an initiating trigger. The trigger, usually the occurrence of one or more premature beats, frequently is required because it elicits or brings to a critical state one or more of the conditions necessary to achieve reentrant excitation. Thus, a premature impulse initiating reentry may arrive at one site in the potential reentrant circuit sufficiently early that it encounters unidirectional block because that tissue has had insufficient time to recover excitability after excitation by the prior beat (Fig. 23-4). Furthermore, in the other limb of the potential reentrant circuit, the premature arrival of the excitation wavefront either causes slow conduction or results in further slowing of conduction of the excitation wavefront through an area of already slow conduction. The resulting increase in conduction time around this limb of the potential reentrant circuit serves to allow the region of unidirectional block in the tissue in the other limb activated initially by the premature beat to recover excitability. Thus, when the circulating excitation wavefront of the premature beat arrives at these tissue sites, the excitation wavefront can reexcite the tissue, thus manifesting reentrant excitation (Fig. 23-4).

It should be noted that the mechanism causing the premature beat may be different from the reentrant mechanism causing the tachycardia. Thus, the premature beat may be caused by automaticity or triggered activity. An example of the latter may be torsade de pointes, in which the initiating beat (or beats) is the result of triggered activity caused by early afterdepolarization, but the remainder of the beats in this rhythm (it is frequently nonsustained) are now thought to be due to reentry.[219] Another example may occur during cardiac catheterization, in which the premature beat may be due to the catheter forcefully hitting the heart wall, i.e., a mechanical cause. However, the trigger to initiate reentrant excitation need not be a premature beat. The trigger to initiate reentrant excitation may be the normal sinus beat. One example is the rhythm known as permanent nonparoxysmal AV junctional reentrant tachycardia.[220,221] In this example, the potential reentrant circuit contains an area of permanent unidirectional block in an antegrade direction. Moreover, the potential reentrant circuit also has a relatively stable area of very slow conduction, causing the wavelength of the propagating excitation wavefront to be shorter than the path length of the potential reentrant circuit. In this circumstance, the normal sinus beat propagates around the reentrant circuit with sufficient delay that when it arrives in a retrograde direction at the area of permanent antegrade unidirectional block, the tissue at that site has recovered excitability. Furthermore, the conduction time around the reentrant circuit is such that the excitation wavefront continually encounters excitable tissue in the direction in which it is propagating, resulting in continuous reentrant excitation and an incessant tachycardia. Another example where a premature beat is not necessary is reentrant premature ventricular beats, as in ventricular bigeminy (see Chap. 24).

COMPONENTS OF THE REENTRANT CIRCUIT

The Substrate The cardiac tissue that constitutes the substrate for reentrant excitation can be located almost anywhere in the heart. Furthermore, the reentrant circuit may be a variety of sizes and shapes and may include a number of different kinds of myocardial cells, e.g., atrial, ventricular, nodal, and Purkinje. The reentrant circuit may be an anatomic structure such as a loop of fiber bundles in the Purkinje system.[222] The reentrant circuit may be a functionally rather than an anatomically defined pathway, with its existence, size, and shape determined by the electrophysiologic properties of cardiac tissues in which the reentrant wavefront circulates, as has been shown in some patients with atypical atrial flutter.[223,224] Or it may be an anatomic-functional combination, as has been suggested for some intra-atrial reentrant rhythms, such as atrial flutter.[224]

The Area(s) of Slow Conduction As has been discussed, a condition necessary for reentry is that the impulse be delayed sufficiently in the alternative pathway(s) to allow elements proximal to the site of unidirectional block to recover excitability. If reentry is to succeed, the impulse traveling around the reentrant circuit in one direction as a result of the unidirectional block must not return to this site of block before it and regions around it recover excitability. In the presence of normal conduction, sufficient time to allow recovery of excitability may occur if the alternative pathway is sufficiently long. Reentry is facilitated when conduction in all or a part of the alternative pathway is slow, since long pathways that are often not present in the heart are then not necessary. The area(s) of slow conduction may be an anatomic structure normally expected to manifest slow conduction, such as the AV node. Thus, the AV node is the area of slow conduction in AV reentrant tachycardia (a reentrant tachycardia in which the circuit involves the atria, the AV node, the His-Purkinje system, the ventricles, and an accessory AV connection). The area of slow conduction may be in cardiac tissue that normally does not manifest slow conduction. Such an area is not present during sinus rhythm (in contrast to the AV node) but is functionally present during the tachycardia. These areas may develop as a result of premature excitation or may evolve during a rapid transitional rhythm as occurs during atrial flutter.[224,225] An example of a functionally determined area of slow conduction is found in the posterior-inferior right atrium during atrial flutter in patients[226] or in the free wall of the right atrium of the canine sterile pericarditis mode of atrial flutter.[224] Yet another example may be found in tissue that has been damaged, as after a myocardial infarct. Such tissue normally would not manifest slow conduction but after the injury may become an area of slow conduction even during sinus rhythm.[227] Slow conduction can be a consequence of active membrane properties determining the characteristics of inward currents depolarizing the membrane during the action potential, or it can be a consequence of passive properties governing the flow of current between cardiac cells.

Depression of Resting Membrane Potential An important feature of the transmembrane action potential of atrial, ventricular, and Purkinje fibers that governs the speed of propagation is the magnitude of the inward Na^+ current flowing through the fast Na^+ channels in the sarcolemma during the upstroke. The magnitude of this current flow is reflected in the rate at which the cell depolarizes ($\dot{V}_{max}$ of phase 0)[228] and the overshoot of the upstroke (the positive level of depolarization). The depolarization phase or upstroke of the action potential results from the opening of specific membrane channels (fast Na^+ channels) through which Na^+ ions rapidly pass from the extracellular fluid into the cell.

During conduction of the impulse, the inward transmembrane Na^+ current flowing during the depolarization phase (phase 0) of the action potential results in the flow of axial current along the cardiac fiber through the cytoplasm and the gap junctions of the intercalated disks that connect the cardiac cells. The current flows out of the cells through the membrane ahead as resistive and capacitive current. The conduction velocity depends on both how much capacitive current flows out of the cell at unexcited sites ahead of the propagating wavefront and the distance at which the capacitive current can bring membrane potential to threshold. One important factor that influences the amount of current flowing through the sarcoplasm of a muscle fiber (axial current), and therefore capacitive current, is the amount of fast inward current causing the propagating action potential. A reduction in this inward current, leading to a reduction in the rate or amplitude of depolarization during phase 0, may decrease axial current flow, slow conduction, and lead to conduction block. Such a reduction may result from inactivation of Na^+ channels. The intensity of the inward Na^+ current depends on the fraction of Na^+ channels that open when the cell is excited and the size of the Na^+ electrochemical potential gradient (relative concentration of Na^+ in the extracellular space compared with Na^+ concentration inside the cell[229]). The fraction of Na^+ channels available for opening is determined largely by the level of membrane potential at which an action potential is initiated.[229] The Na^+ channels are inactivated either after the upstroke of an action potential or if the steady-state resting membrane potential is reduced. Immediately after the upstroke, cardiac fibers are inexcitable because of Na^+ channel inactivation at the positive level of membrane potential.

During repolarization, progressive removal of inactivation allows increasingly large Na^+ currents to flow through the still partially inactivated Na^+ channels when the cells are excited. The inward Na^+ current, amplitude, and rate of rise of premature action potentials initiated during this relative refractory period are reduced because the Na^+ channels are only partly reactivated.[229] In Fig. 23-14*B*, premature action potentials *a*, *b*, and *c* have low amplitudes and slow rates of depolarization because they were initiated before full repolarization of the action potential. Hence, the conduction velocity of these premature action potentials is low. Premature activation of the heart therefore may induce reentry because premature impulses conduct slowly in regions of the heart where the cardiac fibers are

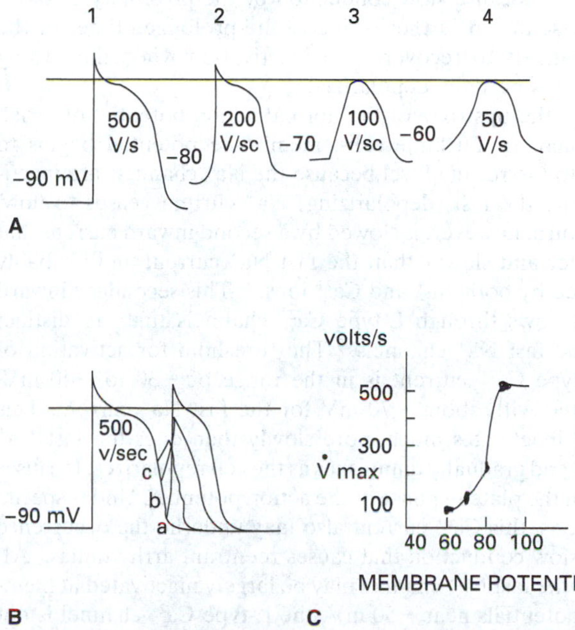

FIGURE 23-14 Diagrammatic representation of the relation between the level of membrane potential at the onset of phase 0 and the maximum rate of depolarization during phase 0 (dv/dt_{max} or $\dot{V}_{max}$). *A*. Fiber has been depolarized by progressively increasing the extracellular potassium concentration. As resting membrane potential decreases, the rate of depolarization of the action potential upstroke decreases. *B*. Fiber is activated by premature stimuli that occur at different times during phase 3 (*a*, *b*, and *c*). The premature action potentials have reduced rates of depolarization because they arise at reduced membrane potentials. *C*. For both types of experiments, the general relationship between $\dot{V}_{max}$ and membrane potential is shown. As the membrane potential becomes smaller (less negative), the rate of phase 0 depolarization ($\dot{V}_{max}$) decreases and therefore conduction velocity decreases.

not completely repolarized (where Na^+ channels are to some extent still inactivated).

Conduction slow enough to facilitate reentry also may occur in cardiac cells with persistently low levels of resting potential (which may be between −60 and −70 mV) caused by disease. At these resting potentials, a significant percentage of the Na^+ channels are inactivated;[229] therefore, they are unavailable for activation by a depolarizing stimulus. Also, at these resting membrane potentials, recovery from inactivation is markedly prolonged and extends beyond complete repolarization.[230] The magnitude of the inward current during phase 0 of the action potential is reduced; consequently, both the speed and the amplitude of the upstroke are diminished (Fig. 23-14*A*, action potentials 2, 3, and 4), decreasing axial current flow and slowing conduction significantly. Such action potentials with upstrokes dependent on inward current flowing via partially inactivated Na^+ channels sometimes are referred to as *depressed fast responses*. Further depolarization of the resting membrane potential and further inactivation of the Na^+ channel may decrease the excitability of cardiac fibers to such an extent that they may become a site of unidirectional conduction block.[231] Thus, in a diseased region with partially depolarized fibers, there may be some areas of slow conduction and some areas of conduction block, depending on the level of resting potential and the amount of Na^+ channels that are inactivated. This combination may cause reentry. The chance for reentry in such fibers is even greater during premature activation or during rhythms at a rapid rate because slow conduction or the possibility of block is increased even further owing to the prolonged time for the Na^+ channels to recover from inactivation when the resting potential is partially depolarized.

After the upstroke of the normal action potential of atrial, ventricular, or Purkinje cells, membrane potential begins to return to the resting level because the Na^+ channels are inactivated and the fast (depolarizing) Na^+ current ceases to flow. This return, however, is slowed by a second inward current that is smaller and slower than the fast Na^+ current and probably is carried by both Na^+ and Ca^{2+} ions.[232] This secondary inward current flows through L-type Ca^{2+} channels that are distinct from the fast Na^+ channels.[20] The threshold for activation of the L-type Ca^{2+} current is in the range of −30 to −40 mV, compared with about −70 mV for the fast Na^+ current. This current inactivates much more slowly than does the fast Na^+ current and gradually diminishes as the cell repolarizes. It causes much of the plateau phase of the action potential. Under special conditions, this Ca^{2+} current also may underlie the occurrence of the slow conduction that causes reentrant arrhythmias.[5] Although the fast Na^+ channel may be largely inactivated at membrane potentials near −50 mV, the L-type Ca^{2+} channel is not inactivated and is still available for activation.[5,232]

Under certain conditions, when the resting potential is reduced to levels lower than −60 mV (as occurs when membrane conductance is very low or when catecholamines are present), this normally weak inward Ca^{2+} current may give rise to regenerative action potentials that propagate very slowly and are prone to block. The propagated action potential, which is dependent on inward Ca^{2+} current, is referred to as the *slow response*.[5] Slow-response action potentials can occur in diseased cardiac fibers with low resting potentials, but they also occur in some normal tissue of the heart, such as cells of the sinus and AV nodes, where the maximum diastolic potential is normally about −60 mV or less.[5,233] In fact, slow conduction is a normal property of both the sinus and the AV nodes. Thus, it should be of no surprise that either of these nodes may be a critical area of slow conduction in some reentrant circuits, e.g., the AV node in AV reentrant tachycardia involving an accessory AV connection.

Anisotropy The slow conduction that facilitates the occurrence of reentry also can be caused by factors other than a decrease in inward current during the upstroke of the transmembrane action potential. An increased resistance to axial current flow, which can be expressed as *effective axial resistance* (defined as resistance to current flow in the direction of propagation[234,235]) decreases the magnitude and spread of axial current of the propagating impulse among the myocardial fibers and may decrease conduction velocity. During conduction of the impulse, axial current flows from one myocardial cell to the adjacent cell through the gap junctions of the intercalated disks, which form a major source of intercellular resistance to current flow between fiber bundles.[228] Therefore, the structure of the myocardium that governs the extent and distribution of these gap junctions has a profound influence on axial resistance and conduction. This influence can be seen in normal atrial or ventricular myocardium, although the structure is different in different regions.

The atria (crista terminalis) and certain regions of the ventricles (except for the subepicardial muscle) are composed of bundles of myocardial cells that have been called *unit bundles* by Sommer and Dolber.[236] Such bundles are made up of 2 to 30 cells surrounded by a connective tissue sheath. Within a unit bundle, cells are tightly connected or coupled to each other through intercalated disks that contain the gap junctions. All the cells of a unit bundle are connected to each other within the space of 30 to 50 μm down the length of a strand.[236] An individual cardiac myocyte may be connected to as many as nine other myocytes through one or more intercalated disks.[237] These connections are mainly at the ends of the myocytes rather than along their sides, but the overlapping nature of the junctions effectively connects myocytes within a bundle in the transverse direction as well as the longitudinal direction. Therefore, as a consequence of the many intercellular connections, the myocytes in a unit bundle are activated uniformly and synchronously as an impulse propagates along the bundle. The unit bundles also are connected to each other. Unit bundles lying parallel to each other in normal atrial and ventricular muscle are connected in a lateral (transverse) direction at intervals in the range of 100 to 150 μm.[236] As a consequence of this structure, the myocardium in regions in which unit bundles occur is better coupled in the direction of the long axis of its cells and bundles (because of the high frequency of the gap junctions within a unit bundle) than in the direction transverse to the long axis (because of the low frequency of interconnections between the unit bundles). This is reflected in a lower axial resistivity in the longitudinal direction than in the transverse direction in cardiac tissues that are composed of many unit bundles.[238,239]

The structure of the interconnections between muscle fibers is somewhat different in the subepicardial regions of the ventricles (and possibly other regions as well) but is still a cause of lower longitudinal axial resistance rather than transverse axial resistance. The subepicardial region is not made up of unit bundles.[240] Each ventricular muscle cell is connected to approximately 11 to 12 other muscle cells in three dimensions. The junctions that connect the cells occur at both the ends and the sides of cells in roughly equivalent numbers; approximately half of all connections are side to side, and half are end to end. Therefore, activation wavefronts can conduct equally well between individual cells in both the longitudinal and transverse directions because there are equal numbers of gap junctions. In the transverse direction, however, a wavefront encounters more gap junctions than it does over an equivalent distance in the longitudinal direction because cell diameter is much smaller than cell length; therefore, the wavefront must traverse more cells transversely. Thus, there is a greater resistance transversely than longitudinally because of the increased number of gap junctions per unit distance traveled.[238]

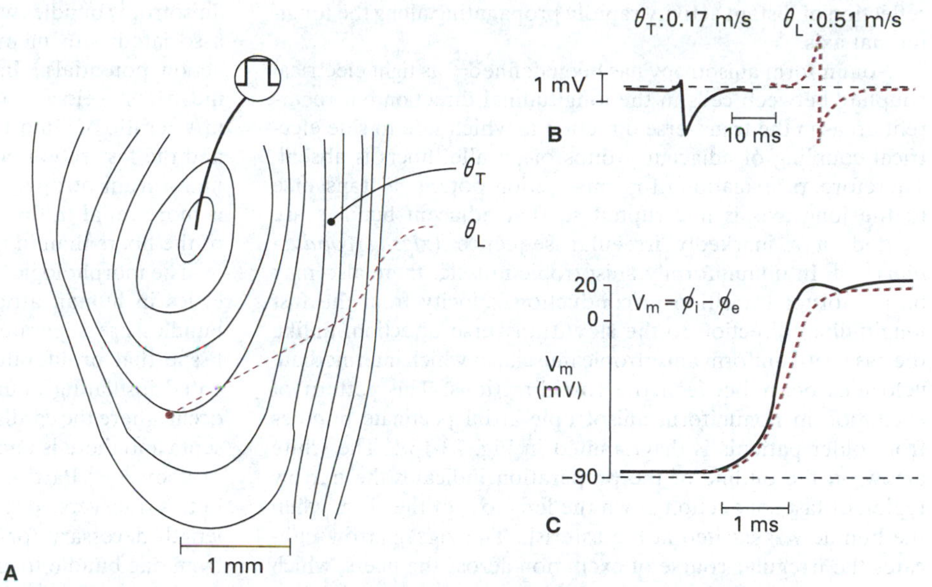

FIGURE 23-15 Relation between the spread of excitation in uniform anisotropic ventricular muscle (*A*) and extracellular (*B*) and transmembrane potential waveforms (*C*). The excitation sequence in *A* was constructed from the extracellular waveforms measured at 100 positions on the endocardial surface of the right ventricular septum. The extracellular waveforms in *B* were measured at the sites indicated by the solid dots superimposed on the isochrones of *A*. The direction of propagation at the single transmembrane recording site was altered by initiating propagation at different locations, one to produce propagation along the longitudinal axis of the impaled fiber and the other to produce propagation along the transverse axis. Panel *C* shows the effects of the different directions of propagation on the upstroke of the action potential. (From Spach MS, Dolber PC. The relation between discontinuous propagation in anisotropic cardiac muscle and the "vulnerable period" of reentry. In: Zipes DP, Jalife J, eds. *Cardiac Electrophysiology and Arrhythmias*. New York: Grune & Stratton, 1985:241. Reproduced with permission from the publisher and author.)

As was stated above, the effective axial resistivity is an important determinant of the conduction velocity; therefore, conduction through atrial and ventricular myocardium is much more rapid in the longitudinal direction, owing to the lower resistivity, than it is in the transverse direction. Thus, cardiac muscle is anisotropic; its conduction properties vary depending on the direction in which they are measured.

Spach and associates.[234,235,241,242] classified anisotropy into two major subdivisions: uniform and nonuniform. Uniform anisotropy is characterized by an advancing wavefront that is smooth in all directions (longitudinal and transverse to fiber orientation), indicating relatively tight coupling between groups of fibers in all directions. Uniform anisotropy is exemplified by the conduction properties of normal septal ventricular muscle, as shown in Fig. 23-15*A*. The muscle in the diagram was stimulated in the center (pulse symbol), and activation spread away from this site in all directions. In the direction of the longitudinal axis of the fibers (from top to bottom), the activation isochrones are widely spaced, indicating rapid conduction—in this case, 0.51 m/s. There is a relatively broad area of fast conduction with an elliptic shape of the isochrones that is characteristic of uniform anisotropy.[241] In the direction transverse to the long axis (to the right and to the left), the isochrones are spaced close together, indicating slower conduction: 0.17 m/s in this example. As the direction of propagation changes between these two axes, the apparent conduction velocity changes monotonically from fast to slow, another characteristic of uniform anisotropy.[234]

The slow conduction in the direction transverse to the longitudinal fiber axis occurs despite action potentials with normal resting potentials and upstroke velocities and is caused by the higher transverse axial resistance. Associated with the differences in conduction velocity that are based on the direction of propagation, however, are unexpected changes in the action potentials. Thus, when going from fast longitudinal conduction to slow transverse conduction, the rate of depolarization during the upstroke of the action potential ($\dot{V}_{max}$) increases and the time constant of the foot of the upstroke decreases without any change in the resting potential, as shown in Fig. 23-15*C*; the upstroke that is dashed was recorded from a cell during longitudinal propagation, while the upstroke indicated by the solid line was recorded from the same cell during transverse propagation.[234] These characteristics are opposite to the changes in the action potentials associated with slowing of conduction when the membrane currents are altered (e.g., by membrane depolarization).[243,244] Despite the increase in $\dot{V}_{max}$, when conduction is slowed in the transverse direction, the slowing of conduction is associated with a decrease in the amplitude of the extracellular electrogram, showing that there is a decrease in the extracellular current flow as a result of the increased axial resistivity.

In uniformly anisotropic tissue, the extracellular unipolar waveform has a large-amplitude, smooth biphasic, positive-negative morphology during propagation in the fast longitudinal direction (Fig. 23-15*B*, dashed line) and a low-amplitude, smooth triphasic (negative-positive-negative) morphology in the transverse direction (Fig. 23-15*B*, solid line). The initial negativity of the electrogram in the transverse direction is a reflection of distant activity rapidly propagating along the longitudinal axis.[245]

Nonuniform anisotropy has been defined[235] as tight electrical coupling between cells in the longitudinal direction but recurrent areas in the transverse direction in which side-to-side electrical coupling of adjacent groups of parallel fibers is absent. Therefore, propagation of normal action potentials transverse to the long axis is interrupted so that adjacent bundles are excited in a markedly irregular sequence (*zigzag conduction*).[235,241] In nonuniformly anisotropic muscle, there also may be an abrupt transition in conduction velocity from the fast longitudinal direction to the slow transverse direction, unlike the case with uniform anisotropic muscle, in which intermediate velocities occur between the two directions. This pattern of excitation in nonuniform anisotropic atrial pectinate bundles from older patients is diagrammed in Fig. 23-16*A*. The white arrow on the outline of the preparation indicates the narrow region of fast conduction down the long axis of the fibers when the bundle was excited at the asterisk. The zigzag arrow indicates the irregular course of excitation across the fibers, which occurred all along the length of the zone of fast conduction. Conduction in the transverse direction in these nonuniformly anisotropic bundles was nearly as slow at the slowest conduction associated with membrane depolarization and slow-response action potentials.[5] In pectinate muscles from older patients, mean fast velocity was 0.69 m/s and slow velocity was 0.07 m/s, a ratio of almost 10,[241] despite the normal resting potential and the fast action potential upstroke of the atrial cells. As in uniform anisotropy, the upstroke velocity of the action potential is more rapid in the slow direction transverse to the long axis of the fibers than in the fast direction parallel to the long axis.

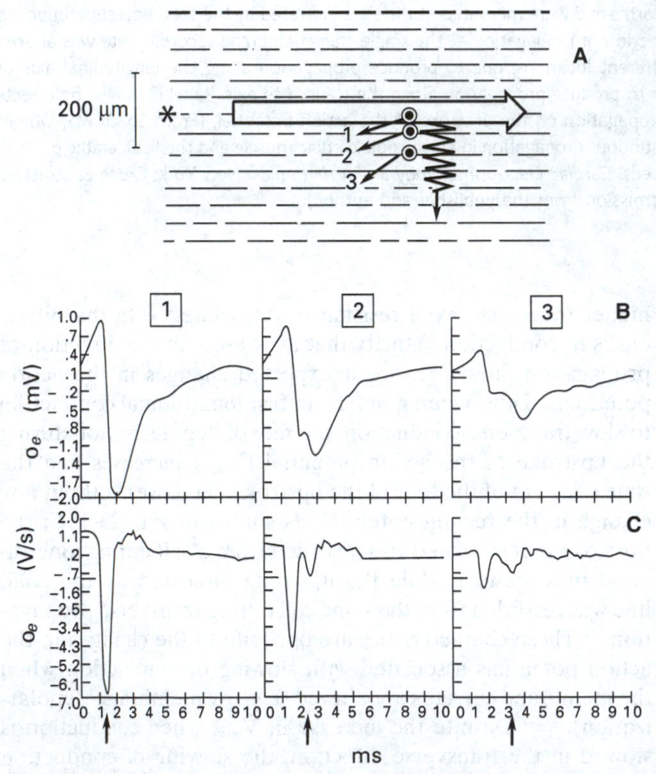

FIGURE 23-16 *A.* Diagram of a nonuniform anisotropic atrial muscle bundle with the long axis of the myocardial fibers indicated by the dashed lines. The bundle was stimulated at the asterisk. Propagation of the longitudinal wavefront is shown by the large white arrow. Transverse propagation occurred as diagrammed by the zigzag arrow. *B.* Electrograms recorded from sites 1, 2, and 3 on the diagram. *C.* The first derivative of these electrograms is shown. (From Spach MS, Dolber PC. Relating extracellular potentials and their derivatives to anisotropic propagation at a microscopic level in human cardiac muscle: Evidence for uncoupling of side-to-side fiber connections with increasing age. *Circ Res* 1986; 58:356. Reproduced with permission from the publisher and author.)

The morphologic basis for the nonuniform anisotropic properties in human atrial muscle is that the fascicles of muscle bundles are separated in the transverse direction by fibrous tissue that proliferates with aging to form longitudinally oriented insulating boundaries. Intercellular connections cannot occur where the cardiac fibers are separated by connective tissue septa and there is uncoupling between parallel-oriented groups of fibers.[235,241] Part of the reduction of the conduction velocity in this transverse direction may be a result of the tortuous path length necessary for the wavefront to propagate transversely from one bundle to another because of these septa, accounting for the zigzag activation pattern. Similar connective tissue septa cause nonuniform anisotropy in other normal cardiac tissues, such as the crista terminalis and the interatrial band in adult atria or ventricular papillary muscle, as well as pathologic situations such as chronic ischemia or a healing myocardial infarction, in which fibrosis in the myocardium occurs.

The irregular activation transversely is evident in the extracellular electrogram, which is characterized by a sequence of multiple deflections, each representing activation of a separate bundle of fibers, with the largest, most rapid intrinsic deflection produced by local excitation and less rapid and lower-amplitude deflections produced by excitation of adjacent fascicles.[235] In Fig. 23-16*B*, the multiple deflections can be seen in electrograms recorded from sites 2 and 3 in the atrial pectinate muscle and are even more prominent in the derivatives of these electrograms (Fig. 23-16*C*). A similarly fractionated electrogram also can be recorded from diseased regions of the ventricles. During longitudinal propagation, large biphasic electrograms are still evident (electrogram at site 1).

Anisotropy on a macroscopic scale also can influence conduction at sites where a bundle of cardiac fibers branches or where separate bundles coalesce. Marked slowing can occur when there is a sudden change in the fiber direction, causing an abrupt increase in the effective axial resistivity.[235] Figure 23-17 illustrates this point. The drawings show a small branch of an atrial pectinate muscle from the crista terminalis. The general direction of the fiber orientation is indicated by the thin broken lines, and the pattern of propagation is illustrated by the thick solid lines with arrows. In *A* (1) at the left, wavefronts initiated by stimulation at the top propagate throughout the crista and its branch along the longitudinal axis of the fibers throughout so that there is no conduction delay entering the branch. At the right in *A* (2), wavefronts initiated by stimulation at the bottom propagate up the crista and into the branch, but they encounter a marked change in the direction of the fibers from longitudinal to transverse while entering the branch, resulting in a slowing of conduction because of the sudden increase in axial resistance. Conduction block, which sometimes may be unidirectional, may occur at such junction sites, particularly when the inward current is decreased, as will be described later.

In addition to the structural features of the cellular interconnections influencing axial current flow and conduction as expressed in the anisotropic properties of cardiac muscle, the intercellular resistance may increase because of an increase in gap junctional resistance that results from a decrease in the conductance of the junctions, i.e., a decrease in the ease with which the ions that carry axial current move through the junctions. In a computer model, conduction velocity can be reduced by a factor of 20 by increasing disk resistance, and decremental conduction and block will result.[246,247]

Perhaps the most important influence on gap junctional resistance in pathologic situations is the level of intracellular Ca^{2+}. A significant rise increases resistance to current flow through the junctions and eventually leads to physiologic uncoupling of the cells.[248,249] Intracellular Ca^{2+} increases during ischemia and may be a factor causing slow conduction and reentry. Thus, there are several causes for slow conduction that may lead to reentry: (1) slow responses that are a normal property of some regions of the heart, such as the sinus and AV node, (2) depressed fast responses or slow responses caused by pathology-induced partial depolarization of the membrane potential, (3) anisotropy, and (4) changes in gap junctional resistance.

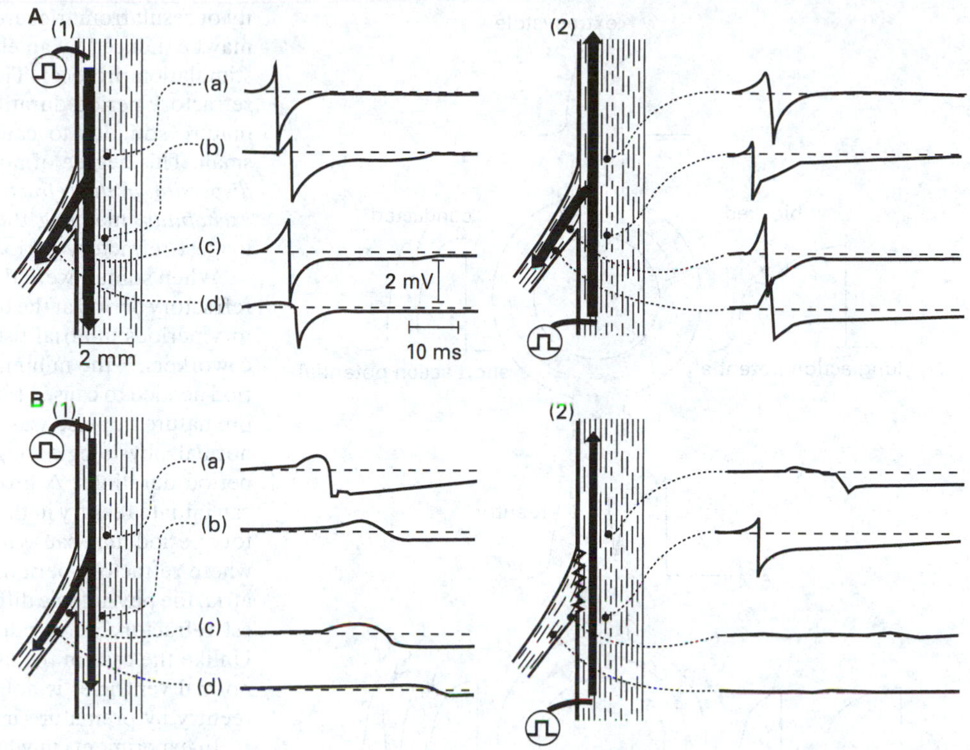

FIGURE 23-17 Conduction characteristics and unidirectional block at branch sites. The drawings represent a small branch formed by the origin of a pectinate muscle from the larger crista terminalis. The general direction of the fiber orientation is indicated by the broken lines. The patterns of propagation are shown by the solid arrows. Extracellular waveforms recorded at sites indicated by the dashed lines also are shown. (From Spach MS et al. The functional role of structural complexities in the propagation of depolarization in the atrium of the dog: Cardiac conduction disturbances due to discontinuities of effective axial resistivity. *Circ Res* 1982; 50:175. Reproduced with permission from the publisher and authors.)

Unidirectional Block Unidirectional block occurs when an impulse cannot conduct in one direction along a bundle of cardiac fibers but can conduct in the opposite direction. This condition is necessary for the occurrence of classical reentrant rhythms. Thus, unidirectional block in part of the circuit leaves a return pathway through which the impulse conducts to reenter previously excited areas. A number of mechanisms, involving both active and passive electrical properties of cardiac cells, may cause unidirectional block.

REGIONAL DIFFERENCES IN RECOVERY OF EXCITABILITY One cause of unidirectional block that allows the initiation of reentry is regional differences in recovery of excitability. When differences in the duration of the effective refractory period occur in adjacent areas, conduction of an appropriately timed premature impulse may be blocked in the region with the longest refractory period, which then becomes a site of unidirectional block, while conduction continues through regions with a shorter refractory period. Figure 23-18 is a schematic representation of the initiation and continuation of circus movement in an anatomically defined circuit, with differences in effective refractory period duration resulting from differences in the time course of action potential repolarization being the cause of unidirectional block in one of the pathways. The action potentials in various parts of the circuit are shown. In the upper panel (*A*), conduction of a premature impulse (extrasystole), which either can be induced by electrical stimulation or may occur "spontaneously," is blocked in the pathway with the long action potential duration and therefore long effective refractory period (to the left), referred to as the *blocked pathway*. The premature impulse, however, conducts in the other pathway with shorter action potential durations and refractory periods (to the right). This pattern of activation is indicated by the arrows. For block to occur, the premature impulse also must arise in a region with a short effective refractory period so that it occurs before repolarization of the action potentials in the left pathway occurs. In the lower panel (*B*), which shows the continuation of these events, the blocked pathway is invaded retrogradely by the impulse conducting from the right, thus causing the second action potential (arrow at the left). The proximal region where the premature impulse originated is then reexcited (reentry) as the impulse once again enters the right pathway and continues around the reentrant circuit, causing another action potential in the right pathway (large arrow). For successful reexcitation to occur in the region where the premature impulse was initiated, elements in the circuit at the region of block and proximal to it (toward the site of origin) must have regained their excitability by the time the cardiac impulse arrives there. Continuation of reentry induced by a premature impulse also is facilitated because the

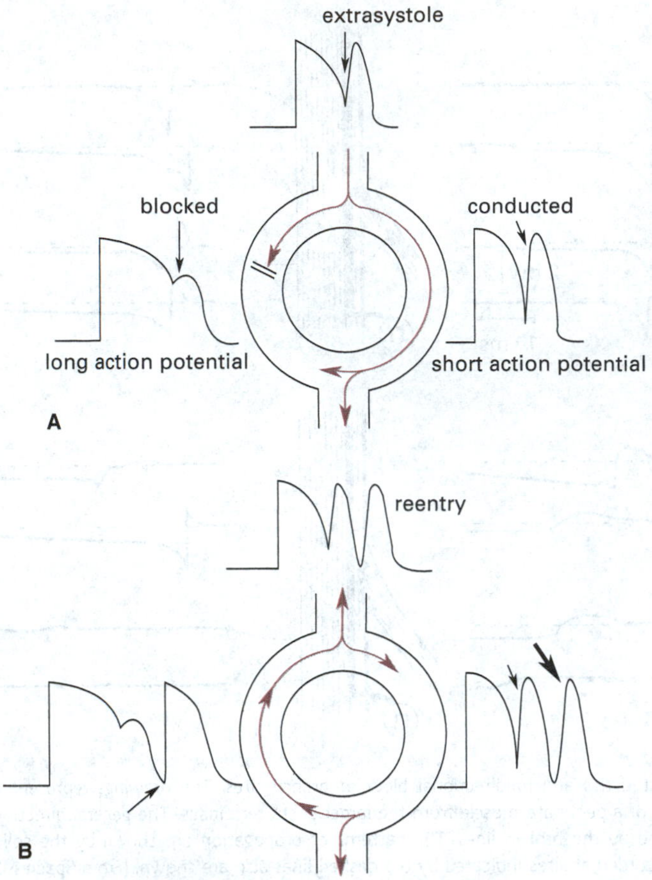

FIGURE 23-18 Diagram of reentry caused by dispersion in refractory periods. A ring of cardiac tissue is shown, and the pattern of conduction is indicated by the arrows. Action potentials with different durations located in different regions of the ring are diagrammed. (From Wit AL, Janse MJ. *The Ventricular Arrhythmia of Ischemia and Infarction: The Electrophysiological Mechanisms.* Mount Kisco, NY: Futura; 1992:86. Reproduced with permission from the publisher and authors.)

duration of the effective refractory period associated with conduction of the premature impulse is shortened. Therefore, on the next excursion of the reentrant impulse around the circuit, conduction occurs in a circuit with a shorter effective refractory period. Finally, the conduction velocity of premature impulses may be decreased, shortening the wavelength[250,251] and facilitating successful excitation of the region proximal to the unidirectional block.

Therefore, unidirectional block caused by regional differences in excitability is actually a result of transient block. Block occurs in the antegrade direction in the left pathway while conduction is successful in the retrograde direction. This kind of unidirectional block can cause the initiation of reentry not only in anatomic circuits, as shown in Fig. 23-18, but also in functional circuits. For reentrant arrhythmias to arise because of regional differences in effective refractory periods, a premature impulse that initiates reentry is as necessary a requirement as are the conditions allowing the perpetuation of reentrant activation. Thus, both a "trigger" (the premature impulse) and a "substrate" (the reentrant circuit) are needed. The mechanism causing the premature impulse may be quite different from the arrhythmia it initiates. It may arise spontaneously by automaticity or result from triggered activity. The premature impulse also may be induced by an electrical stimulus during a programmed stimulation protocol. The degree of nonuniformity in effective refractory period duration necessary for a properly timed premature stimulus to cause unidirectional block may be quite small. This degree of nonuniformity often is referred to as the *dispersion in the refractory periods* or *dispersion in recovery of excitability,* meaning the difference between the shortest and longest refractory periods.

When stimuli were delivered in the region with the shortest refractory period at the border of two areas with different refractory periods in atrial tissue in the experiments of Allessie and coworkers,[252] the minimal difference in effective refractory period needed to cause block of an appropriately timed stimulated premature impulse was between 11 and 16 ms, well within the normal physiologic range of variation of effective refractory period durations. A properly timed single premature stimulus can initiate reentry in the atria because the differences in refractory period may cause unidirectional block.[252] In the ventricles, where refractory periods are much longer than they are in the atria, the physiologic differences between the longest and shortest refractory period durations is on the order of 40 ms.[253,254] Unlike the case in the atria, dispersion of refractory periods in normal ventricles is not sufficiently large to allow initiation of reentry by premature impulses.

In experiments in which the dispersion of refractory periods was increased by local cooling of the ventricles and a critical difference between the shortest and longest effective refractory periods ranging from 95 to 145 ms was reached, premature stimuli delivered at the site with the shortest effective refractory period induced repetitive activity in the canine left ventricle, presumably because block of the premature impulses in the regions with a long effective refractory period created unidirectional block and permitted reentry.[255,256] Similarly, critical increases in the dispersion of refractory periods that are caused by acute or prolonged ischemia result in reentrant arrhythmias. The difference between the longest and shortest refractory periods is not the only factor that determines whether premature stimuli will induce reentry.[252] If the regions of long and short refractory periods are separated by a large distance, an early premature impulse arising in a region of short refractoriness may not be able to arrive in the region of long refractoriness sufficiently early to cause block because conduction between the regions may be slow. Regions of long refractory periods therefore must be relatively close to a region of shorter refractory periods where the premature impulse arises for block to occur. In addition, if block does occur, the size of the area of unidirectional block is of crucial importance, particularly in a functionally determined reentrant circuit. Even in the presence of large differences in effective refractory period duration, reentry may not occur when the area with long effective refractory periods resulting in unidirectional block is small, because the impulse can travel around the area of unidirectional block along an alternative pathway or pathways and will not be delayed sufficiently to allow reexcitation of the point of origin at the end of the latter's effective refractory period. This cannot occur in an anatomic circuit such as the one shown in Fig. 23-18. Thus, *dispersion in recovery of excitability* is by itself not sufficient to describe the propensity for induction of reentrant arrhythmias. The regional differences in recovery of excitability that lead to unidirectional conduction block also may occur in the absence of regional differences in action potential duration. Computer models have shown that the activation sequence of a propagating impulse can lead to asynchronous repolarization and refractoriness even when membrane properties are homogeneous.[89,247] A stimulated premature impulse can block in a region that has been depolarized most recently by a prior wave of excitation and is therefore still refractory, but it may conduct into another region that was excited much earlier by the prior wave of excitation if it has had time to recover excitability. The conducting premature excitation wave then can later return to excite the area of block after it recovers, resulting in reentry.

Asymmetric Depression of Excitability Unidirectional conduction block in a reentrant circuit also can be persistent and independent of premature activation. Persistent unidirectional block often is associated with depression of the transmembrane potentials and excitability of cardiac fibers.[257] There are several possible mechanisms for the persistent unidirectional block in a region where action potentials are depressed. One mechanism is asymmetric depression of excitability. This asymmetric depression may occur because of asymmetric distribution of a pathologic event. As a simple example, the action potential upstrokes in a bundle of fibers may be diminished as a result of a reduction of perfusion after coronary occlusion, but the depression of the upstroke may be more severe toward one end of the bundle than toward the other. This situation is diagrammed in Fig. 23-19. A propagating impulse consisting of an action potential with a normal upstroke velocity (site 1) enters the poorly perfused region (stippled in the diagram) and propagates through this region with decrement (from left to right or from site 1 to 4); i.e., as it conducts from the less depressed end (1) to the more severely depressed end (4), the action potential upstroke velocity and amplitude progressively decrease, as does the axial current flowing toward cells that will be excited by the upstroke (as indicated by the decreasing size of the striped arrows). When the impulse arrives at the opposite end of the depressed segment of the bundle where there is suddenly a normally perfused bundle with normal action potentials (between action potentials 4 and 5), the action potential amplitude is markedly reduced and the weak axial current from site 4 is

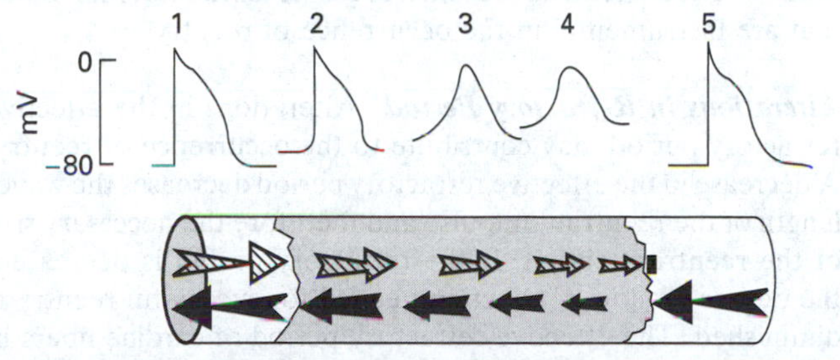

FIGURE 23-19 Asymmetric depression of excitability as a mechanism for unidirectional conduction block in a bundle of cardiac muscle fibers. The action potentials shown above were recorded from sites on the fiber bundle. The shaded part of the bundle is depressed. Conduction from left to right along the bundle is indicated by the striped arrows, conduction from right to left by the black arrows. (Modified from Wit AL, Rosen MR. Cellular electrophysiological mechanisms of cardiac arrhythmias. In: MacFarlane PW, Veitch Lawrie TD, eds. *Comprehensive Electrocardiology: Theory and Practice in Health and Disease*, vol. 2. New York: Pergamon Press; 1989:801. Reproduced with permission from the publisher and authors.)

not sufficient to depolarize the normal membrane to threshold at site 5. Conduction therefore blocks in the left-to-right direction even though the normally perfused region is excitable. Conduction in the opposite direction (from right to left), however, still may succeed. The large axial current generated by the normal action potential at site 5 can flow for a considerable distance through the depressed region and may depolarize to threshold fibers at some distance from the most severely depressed region (perhaps as far as site 3). These cells in turn may be able to excite adjacent fibers in the direction of propagation (from right to left), and as a result, the impulse successfully propagates from site 3 to site 1, as indicated by the black arrows.

Geometric Factors Causing Unidirectional Block Geometric factors related to tissue architecture also may influence impulse conduction and under certain conditions lead to unidirectional block. An impulse can conduct rapidly in either direction along the length of a bundle of atrial, ventricular, or Purkinje fibers with normal electrophysiologic properties. There is usually some asymmetry in the conduction velocity, however, meaning that conduction in one direction may take slightly longer than it does in the other direction.[5,228,231] This is usually of no physiologic significance. The asymmetry of conduction can result from several factors. Bundles of cardiac muscle are composed of interconnecting myocardial fibers with different diameters packed in a connective tissue matrix. These bundles branch frequently (although the individual myocardial fibers do not branch). An impulse conducting in one direction encounters a different sequence of changes in fiber diameter, branching, and frequency and distribution of gap junctions than it does when traveling in the opposite direction. The configuration of pathways in each direction is not the same.[231] These structural features influence conduction by affecting the axial currents that flow ahead of the propagating wavefront.

The results of theoretical analyses indicate that the conduction velocity of an impulse passing abruptly from a fiber of small diameter to one of large diameter transiently slows at the junction because the larger cable results in a larger sink for the longitudinal axial current (there is more membrane for this current to depolarize to threshold if conduction of the impulse is to continue).[228,231,247,258,259] A similar slowing occurs when an impulse conducts into a region where there is an abrupt increase in branching of the myocardial syncytium; conduction transiently slows because of the larger current sink provided by the increased membrane area that must be depolarized.

In the opposite direction, it can be predicted that conduction will speed transiently as the impulse moves from a larger cable to a smaller cable because the small sink for axial current results in more rapid depolarization of the membrane to threshold.[228,258,259] Theoretically, if there is a large enough difference in the diameter of the two cables, an impulse conducting from the small cable to the large cable should block at the junction, while conduction in the opposite direction (from large cable to small cable) is maintained.

A probable example of unidirectional block based on this geometric factor in the normal heart occurs at the junctions between Purkinje's and muscle cells. At certain sites, propagation from muscle to Purkinje fibers is possible, while propagation from Purkinje fibers to muscle is not.[260] This asymmetry of conduction results from the difference in mass between the

Purkinje and muscle layers. The smaller-mass Purkinje fiber bundle is the small-diameter cable, while the larger-mass muscle is the larger-diameter cable. It is unlikely that in normal circumstances these localized sites of unidirectional block predispose to reentry since the myocardium is quickly excited via the many other Purkinje-to-muscle junctions where the geometric differences are not sufficient to cause block. It is possible, however, when conduction in ischemic myocardium is slow and coupling resistance at the junction increases, that such sites of unidirectional block may become important in initiating reentry.[261–263]

It is doubtful that abrupt changes in geometric properties such as fiber diameter of the magnitude required to cause block of the *normal* action potential often exist (except at some Purkinje fiber–muscle junctions, as was described above) because the safety factor for conduction is large; i.e., there is a large excess of activating current over the amount required for propagation.[228] Dodge and Cranefield[231] pointed out that "only if an action potential is a relatively weak stimulus and the unexcited area is not easily excited will plausible changes in membrane resistance, cell diameter, or intercellular coupling produce block." There is a necessity for interaction of abnormal action potentials and decreased excitability with the preexisting anatomic impediments, as occurs in acute ischemia. When the resting potential of fibers in a muscle or Purkinje bundle is decreased, the reduced action potential upstroke results in a decreased axial current, and therefore, the action potential is a weak stimulus. The normal directional differences in conduction are then exaggerated.

At a critical degree of depression of the action potential upstroke, conduction may fail in one direction while being maintained in the other (although it may be slowed markedly). At this critical degree of depression, the reduced axial current may not be sufficient to depolarize the membrane to threshold where the current sink is increased because of the structural changes described above (increased fiber diameter), but the axial current is still more than adequate during conduction in the opposite direction.

The anisotropic properties of cardiac muscle also represent a geometric factor that sometimes may contribute to the occurrence of unidirectional block. Spach and colleagues[234] indicated that in anisotropic muscle, the safety factor for conduction is lower in the longitudinal direction of rapid conduction than it is in the transverse direction of slow conduction (the opposite of that predicted on the basis of continuous cable theory). The low safety factor longitudinally is a result of a large current load on the membrane associated with the low axial resistivity and large membrane capacitance in the longitudinal direction. This low safety factor may result in a preferential conduction block of premature impulses in the longitudinal direction relative to the transverse direction under certain conditions. In uniformly anisotropic muscle, a decrease in inward current during the depolarization phase of an action potential, as may result from premature activation, results in slowing of conduction in the longitudinal direction more than in the transverse direction, but propagation still continues as a spatially smooth process. Conduction block of early premature impulses occurs in both longitudinal and transverse directions nearly simultaneously in uniformly anisotropic muscle.[242]

In nonuniformly anisotropic muscle, however, premature activation can result in conduction block in the longitudinal direction even when the impulse is conducting from a region with a long refractory period into a region with a shorter refractory period while conduction in the transverse direction continues.[242] The site of block in the longitudinal direction can become a site of unidirectional block that leads to reentry, much like the block of premature impulses caused by a sudden increase in action potential duration and effective refractory period. It can be excited by an impulse propagating in the opposite direction, i.e., by the wavefront initially launched successfully in the transverse direction that later propagates to the distal side of the region of the block. In contrast to the propensity of premature impulses to block in the longitudinal direction in nonuniformly anisotropic myocardium because of the decreased depolarizing current and low safety factor, when coupling resistance between cells is increased, conduction of all impulses will block first in the transverse direction. Preferential block in this direction occurs because an increase in coupling resistance will reduce the safety factor below the critical level needed to maintain transverse conduction before the safety factor for longitudinal conduction is reduced to this critical level.[264,265] Unlike longitudinal block of a premature impulse, which is transient block and may lead to reentry, block in the transverse direction caused by increased coupling resistance may be bidirectional and, if so, should not cause reentry.

Anisotropy also can result in unidirectional block at sites of muscle bundle branching or at the junction of muscle bundles.[235] It was shown in Fig. 23-17*A*(2) that when a wavefront propagating in a bundle of parallel fibers enters a branch formed at an acute angle, the direction of propagation is altered quickly from longitudinal to transverse, causing an abrupt increase in the effective axial resistance in the direction of propagation and a slowing of conduction velocity. If the inward current also is reduced by partial depolarization, as occurs after premature stimulation or elevation of extracellular K^+, conduction block may occur.[235] This is shown in Fig. 23-17*B*(2), where the extracellular K^+ concentration was increased from 4.6 to 9.0 meq/L. Failure of the stimulated impulse to enter the branch is shown by the absence of electrical activity at sites c and d. By contrast, as shown in Fig. 23-17*B*(1), propagation from the other direction into the branch does not involve a change in the direction of the wavefront relative to the fiber orientation since it continues in a parallel direction; therefore, there is no block in this direction.[235] These sites can become areas of unidirectional block that are instrumental in the occurrence of reentry.

Alterations in Refractory Period Alterations in the effective refractory period may contribute to the occurrence of reentry. A decrease in the effective refractory period decreases the wavelength of the reentrant impulse and therefore the necessary size of the reentrant circuit. If the refractory period is decreased, the degree of slow conduction needed for successful reentry is diminished. The effective refractory period of cardiac fibers in a reentrant circuit may be decreased during rapid tachycardias because of rate-dependent shortening of the action potential duration.[247,266] The computer model of Quan and Rudy[247] predicts that in circuits with a small or no excitable gap, electrotonic interaction between the head and the tail of the reentrant wavefront also can shorten action potential duration and the refractory period. If the effective refractory period is decreased sufficiently, more than one reentrant circuit can exist at a time in some regions.[267,268] The effective refractory period of atrial muscle, for example, is decreased by the acetylcholine released during vagal stimulation. As a result, reentry in atrial muscle causing atrial fibrillation is more easily induced during vagal stimulation.[269] Several reentrant circuits exist simultaneously during this arrhythmia.[268,270] Action potential duration and effective refractory period are decreased in the ventricle during reperfusion after brief periods of ischemia or in some of the ventricular muscle cells in chronically ischemic areas, probably contributing to the occurrence of reentry.

The Central Area of Block The central area of block around which the reentrant wavefront circulates may be anatomic, functional, or a combination of the two. Anatomic block is the result of a nonconductive medium in the center of the circuit. An example of an anatomically determined central area of block is in the tricuspid ring reentrant circuit found in a canine model of atrial flutter[266] and perhaps present in a clinical counterpart, the atrial flutter found commonly in patients who have previously had a Mustard procedure to repair transposition of the great vessels.[271] The animal model depends critically on large incisions made in the right atrial free wall, which in fact are similar to those made by the surgeon during the Mustard procedure. Functional block at the center of a circuit occurs when there is block of impulses in otherwise excitable cardiac muscle. An example of a functional center of block was first described by Allessie and associates[272] in a model of reentrant excitation in the rabbit left atrium called the leading circle mechanism of reentry. Functional block subsequently has been described in several other models of atrial flutter.[223,224,273,274] The central area of functional block develops during the initiation of the reentrant circuit by the formation of a line of block that most likely is due to refractoriness. When the reentrant circuit forms, the line of block then is sustained by centripetal activation from the circulating reentrant wavefront, which by repeatedly bombarding the central area of block maintains the state of refractoriness of this region. A combination of an anatomic and a functional central area of block in the reentrant circuit has been described in some models of atrial flutter (e.g., the orifice of one or both of the cavae and an area of functional block continuous with or adjacent to either or both of the caval orifices).[224,275]

The Excitable Gap The excitable gap in a reentrant circuit is the region of excitable myocardium that immediately precedes the head of the reentrant wavefront and moves around the circuit in advance of the reentrant wavefront. The occurrence of a gap is dependent on the recovery of excitability of the myocardium from its previous excitation by the reentrant wavefront. There are two different measurements of the excitable gap. One is the spatial gap, which is the distance in the circuit ahead of the wavefront that is excitable. The spatial gap may be composed of either partially excitable or fully excitable myocardium, depending on the time interval between successive excitations of the circuit. The size of the spatial gap changes in different parts of the circuit as the wavelength of the reentrant impulse changes because of changes in conduction velocity, refractory periods, or both, as was described previously.

The second measurement of the excitable gap is the temporal excitable gap. This is the time period during the cardiac cycle in which a stimulus can excite the region ahead of the reentrant wavefront. In regard to the spatial gap, the temporal gap in different parts of the reentrant circuit also can have both partially excitable and fully excitable components and varies in different parts of the circuit because of the changes in the wavelength. The characteristics of the excitable gap may be quite different in reentrant circuits caused by different mechanisms. For example, some anatomically determined circuits have been shown to have large excitable gaps with a fully excitable component, although even in anatomically determined circuits, the gap may be only partially excitable.[276] By comparison, functional reentrant circuits caused by the leading circle mechanism have very small gaps that are only partially excitable,[273] although parts of some functionally determined reentrant circuits may have a small fully excitable gap during part of the reentrant cycle.

TYPES OF REENTRY

It was indicated previously that there are two types of reentry: ordered and random.[1] The reentrant circuits can be anatomically determined, functionally determined, or both. In anatomically determined circuits, the pathway is fixed and the characteristics of the reentrant circuit are determined by the characteristics of the anatomic components of the circuit. Anatomic circuits therefore are associated with ordered reentry. Perhaps the best example is AV reentrant tachycardia, in which the reentrant circuit is composed of atrium, the AV node, the His-Purkinje system, the ventricle, and an accessory AV connection.

In functionally determined circuits, the pathway is formed because of the electrophysiologic properties of the cardiac cells, not by a predetermined anatomic pathway. Functional circuits can be associated with ordered or random reentry. Mechanisms for functionally determined reentrant circuits include the leading circle type of reentry,[272] anisotropic reentry,[277] and spiral wave reentry. Allessie and coworkers[252,272,278] were able to induce stable reentrant tachycardia in small pieces of isolated rabbit left atrium by precisely timed premature impulses in regions that were activated normally at regular rates of stimulation. Initiation of reentry was made possible by the different refractory periods of atrial fibers in close proximity to one another. The premature impulse that initiated reentry blocked in fibers with long refractory periods and conducted in fibers with shorter refractory periods, eventually returning to the initial region of block after excitability recovered there. The impulse then continued to circulate around a central area that was kept refractory because it was bombarded constantly by impulses propagating toward it from all sides of the circuit. This central area provides a functional obstacle that prevents excitation from propagating across the fulcrum of the circuit. No anatomic obstacles or anatomically defined conducting pathways are present in the leading circle, and the reentrant circuit is completely defined by the electrophysiologic properties of the tissue involved. The circumference of the leading circle around a functional obstacle may be as little as 6 to 8 mm and represents a pathway in which the efficacy of stimulation of the circulating wavefront is just sufficient to excite the tissue ahead, which is still in its relative refractory phase. Conduction through the functional reentrant circuit is slowed, therefore, because impulses are propagating in partially refractory tissue (a partially excitable gap). Some of the reentrant excitation that has been mapped in the atria of canine models of atrial flutter may be caused by the leading circle mechanism.[273] The reentrant circuit remains in the same place during the flutter and therefore is ordered reentry. Functional reentrant circuits of the leading circle type also may change their size and location; if they do, they fall under the general category of random reentry. This may occur when leading circle reentry causes fibrillation.

Anisotropy can cause conduction slow enough to result in reentry in small anatomic circuits. Reentrant circuits caused by anisotropy also can occur without well-defined anatomic pathways and may be classified as functional. Unlike the functional characteristic that leads to the leading circle type of reentry (local differences in membrane properties causing a difference in effective refractory periods in adjacent areas), in functional reentry caused by anisotropy, the functional characteristic that is important is the difference in effective axial resistance to impulse propagation dependent on fiber direction. This mechanism has been classified as *anisotropic reentry*.[277] In its pure form, both the unidirectional conduction block and slow conduction in the reentrant circuit result from anisotropic, discontinuous propagation, and there is no need for variations in membrane properties such as regional differences in effective refractory periods or depression of the resting and action potentials.[242]

On the basis of the longitudinal and transverse conduction velocities of premature impulses in nonuniform anisotropic muscle and of measurements of refractory periods in these experiments, Spach and colleagues[242] calculated that circuits in nonuniform anisotropic bundles can be as small as 2 to 4 mm^2 (transverse velocity of 0.5 m/s, dissociated longitudinal velocity of 0.2 m/s) in the absence of nonuniformities in repolarization. Furthermore, anisotropic circuits are elliptical or rectangular because of the directional differences in conduction velocities with the long axis of the ellipse in the fast, longitudinal direction. Circuits with this shape can have a smaller dimension than do circular circuits such as the leading circle.[242] Anisotropic reentrant circuits usually remain in a fixed position to cause ordered reentry.[279] The degree of anisotropy (ratio of longitudinal to transverse conduction velocity) varies in different regions of the heart, and the circuit can reside only in a region where the conduction transverse to the longitudinal axis is sufficiently slow to allow reentry. Stability of anisotropic reentrant circuits also is assisted by the presence of an excitable gap that does not occur in the leading circle functional circuit. The excitable gap is caused by the sudden slowing of conduction velocity and a decrease in the wavelength of excitation as the reentrant impulse turns the corner from the fast longitudinal direction to the slow transverse direction and from the slow transverse direction to the fast longitudinal direction.[280,281]

Another type of functional reentrant excitation, called spiral waves, does not require any inhomogeneities of refractory periods as in leading circle reentry, inhomogeneities in conduction properties as in aniostropic reentry, or a central obstacle, whether functional or anatomic. Spiral waves originally were initiated in computer models of homogeneous elements or in various kinds of homogeneous excitable media (properties do not vary throughout the media), an example of which is molecular diffusion in a chemical system. Under appropriate circumstances, a pulse in two-dimensional, homogeneous, excitable media can be made to circulate as a rotor with a wavelength that is proportional to the square root of the diffusion coefficient of the media.[282–284]

Preexisting functional heterogeneities in conduction (or diffusion) properties or refractoriness (time course of recovery of excitability) are not prerequisites for the initiation of spiral waves in excitable media. The heterogeneity that allows initiation can result from a previous excitation wave and the pattern of recovery from that wave. When heterogeneities in recovery exist, the application of a second stimulus over a large geometric area to initiate a second excitation wave only excites a region where there has been sufficient time for recovery from the previous excitation, not regions that have not yet recovered. An excitation wave is elicited at the excitable site that is in the form of a rotor because the wave cannot move in the direction of the wake of the previous wave but only in the opposite direction, moving into adjacent regions as they in turn recover. The inner tip of the wavefront circulates around a disk of quiescent medium instead of a region of conduction block. The size of this disk expands as the medium is made less excitable.[282–284] The rotor, by definition, has a marked curvature, and this curvature slows down its propagation. A similar pattern of excitation can be induced in cardiac muscle.[285,286]

In the case of a curved depolarization wavefront (rotor) in excitable tissue such as cardiac muscle, slow conduction results from an increased electrical load; e.g., not only must a curved wavefront depolarize cells in front of it in the direction of propagation, but current also flows to cells on its sides. The slow activation by a rotor is not dependent on conduction in relatively refractory myocardium; therefore, there is an excitable gap despite the functional nature of reentry.[282] The location of the rotor can occur anywhere the second stimulated excitation encounters the wake of the first excitation with the appropriate characteristics.[287] Reentrant excitation that occurs during the initiation of ventricular fibrillation by strong electrical shocks[288,289] has characteristics consistent with spiral waves or rotors. These small circulating rotors are not stable and meet the criteria of random reentry. Spiral waves also may cause other kinds of arrhythmias. Even though nonuniform dispersions of refractoriness or anisotropy are not necessary for the initiation of reentrant excitation caused by rotors in excitable media, the myocardium, even when normal, is never homogeneous and the heterogeneities may modify the characteristics of the spiral waves.

Methods to Identify Mechanisms of Arrhythmias

INTRODUCTION

Since the early and classic experiments of Mayer[3,290] on reentry in the Medusa ring and later studies by Mines[4,291] on reentry in ring preparations cut from dogfish auricles or from canine right ventricles, it has been thought that mapping of the sequence of activation of the heart during tachycardia should provide the best evidence for the presence of a reentrant circuit. Even so, the admonition of Mines[291] that "the chief error to be guarded against is that of mistaking a series of automatic beats originating in one point of a ring [substitute "apparent reentrant circuit"] and traveling around it in one direction only owing to a complete block close to the point of origin of the rhythm on one side of this point" for reentrant beats must be kept in mind. The point, of course, is that even sequence of activation mapping may not provide definitive proof of the presence of reentry even though it provides evidence that is consistent with reentry. Mines suggested that severing the ring (again, substitute "the critical portion of the apparent reentrant circuit") and then demonstrating that no further reentrant excitation could occur were required for proof that reentrant excitation had been present. This, of course, has been accomplished in the example of AV reentrant tachycardia, with cure of the arrhythmia following catheter or surgical ablation of the accessory AV connection. Nevertheless, while "severing the ring" is both diagnostic and therapeutic when it can be accomplished to treat a tachyarrhythmia, it is virtually always clinically impractical as a diagnostic tool. Furthermore, until recently, precise sequence of activation cardiac mapping to identify reentry was quite difficult to perform, particularly in patients.

Although it is now possible to obtain remarkably precise maps of the sequence of cardiac activation in vivo by using simultaneous multisite mapping techniques, it is possible only with use of sophisticated recording techniques that require the chest to be open and the heart to be exposed. In fact, for the study of arrhythmias in the in situ heart, it is not routinely possible to obtain the direct electrical recordings (microelectrode studies, simultaneous multisite mapping, etc.) from the arrhythmogenic source that will enable one to determine the electrophysiologic mechanism causing the arrhythmias. A three-dimensional, sequential site-mapping system using a special endocardial catheter system has become available for use in mapping stable reentrant circuits. Indirect approaches have evolved that can provide information that suggests the mechanism of an arrhythmia. These approaches include (1) characterizing the arrhythmia from the ECG, (2) analyzing the response of the arrhythmia to selected forms of cardiac pacing, (3) analyzing the effects of selected pharmacologic agents on the arrhythmia, and (4) analyzing the results of radiofrequency ablation. Since cardiac pacing has long been an important tool in the study of mechanisms of both clinical and experimental arrhythmias and since it is also usually rather easy to apply, the following section presents a discussion of the use of this technique to identify the mechanism of an arrhythmia.

CARDIAC PACING TO DETERMINE ARRHYTHMOGENIC MECHANISMS

The mechanism of an arrhythmia in the in situ heart sometimes can be deduced from the response of the arrhythmia to cardiac pacing. Knowledge about the response of the different arrhythmogenic mechanisms to pacing is based largely on studies in which the effects of electrical stimulation were determined on transmembrane action potentials recorded with microelectrodes in isolated and superfused cardiac tissues. Critical to the ability to use the response to electrical stimulation to determine arrhythmia mechanisms is the requirement that the stimulated impulse(s) reach the site of origin of the arrhythmia. There are many reasons why this may not happen. The stimulated impulse(s) may not reach the site at which the arrhythmia arises because of the electrophysiologic properties of the intervening tissue between the stimulus site and the site of arrhythmia origin. An intervening region of prolonged refractoriness or depressed conduction may cause stimulated impulses to block before they reach the site of origin. If conduction time from the stimulation site to the site of arrhythmia origin is prolonged for any reason, impulses generated in the arrhythmogenic focus also may be able to leave that focus and depolarize large regions of myocardium around it, preventing the stimulated impulse from reaching the site of arrhythmia origin. Even when the stimulation site is close to the site of arrhythmia origin, areas of depressed conduction may prevent the stimulated impulses from reaching the arrhythmogenic cells.

Two basic patterns of stimulation generally are used to study the mechanisms of arrhythmias: (1) overdrive pacing (pacing at a rate or rates faster than the spontaneous rate of the arrhythmia) and (2) introduction of a premature beat or beats by using programmed stimulation. With either technique, the effects of the stimulated impulses on the spontaneous rhythm are observed. Overdrive pacing generally is used during the arrhythmia to determine whether the overdrive can terminate it or, if it does not, to determine the effect of the overdrive on characteristics of the arrhythmia. Overdrive pacing sometimes is used during sinus rhythm to determine whether the period of stimulation can induce an arrhythmia that previously has occurred spontaneously.

The introduction of a premature beat or beats at selected intervals during electrical diastole by programmed stimulation of the heart can be performed either during the spontaneous arrhythmia to test the effects of the premature beats or during sinus rhythm or fixed-rate pacing to see if the arrhythmia can be induced.

EFFECTS OF ELECTRICAL STIMULATION ON ARRHYTHMIAS CAUSED BY AUTOMATICITY

The prior discussion of automaticity as an arrhythmogenic mechanism included a consideration of how the sinus node pacemaker and electrical stimulation (pacing) influence subsidiary pacemakers with different automatic mechanisms. Overdrive either by the sinus node or by electrical stimuli exerts an inhibitory effect on the normal automatic mechanism of subsidiary or latent pacemakers (overdrive suppression) that is primarily the result of enhanced Na^+–K^+ pump activity but has fewer inhibitory effects on the abnormal automatic mechanism of subsidiary pacemakers. These known effects of overdrive on pacemaker mechanisms are sometimes useful in distinguishing automatic arrhythmias from arrhythmias caused by reentry or triggered activity in the in situ heart. The effects of overdrive pacing also can be of use in distinguishing arrhythmias caused by normal automaticity from those caused by abnormal automaticity.[86] From the results of experimental studies, it can be assumed that arrhythmias caused by normal automaticity in the in situ heart cannot be initiated by overdrive pacing. Arrhythmias caused by normal automaticity can be suppressed transiently but cannot be terminated by overdrive pacing. Microelectrode studies on isolated superfused pacemaker tissues indicate that when overdrive pacing is applied during an ongoing arrhythmia caused by normal automaticity, the arrhythmia is expected to be suppressed transiently immediately after the overdrive pacing is stopped. This is manifest by a transient pause after overdrive and should be followed by a gradual speeding up of the rhythm (so-called warmup) until the original rate of the automatic rhythm is resumed. The duration of the transient pause and the time required for resumption of the original rate are expected to be directly related to the rate and duration of the overdrive. This behavior is mainly the result of the increased activity of the Na^+–K^+ pump, which is dependent both on the rate and on the duration of stimulation. This characteristic behavior of normally automatic pacemakers has been demonstrated in some clinical and experimental electrophysiologic studies of both atrial and ventricular tachycardias.[181,292,293]

Like normal automaticity, arrhythmias caused by abnormal automaticity can be neither initiated nor terminated by overdrive pacing. By contrast, arrhythmias caused by abnormal automaticity should not be suppressed by overdrive pacing unless the overdrive period is long and the rate of overdrive is fast.[86] The difficulty in suppressing such arrhythmias stems from the lesser amount of Na^+ entering the cells during the upstroke of the action potential and therefore less intense Na^+ pump stimulation by overdrive. Short periods of overdrive can even result in a transient speeding of the rate of impulse generation (overdrive acceleration).[86] Accelerated idioventricular tachycardia in myocardial infarction is not easily overdrive-suppressed and therefore may be caused by abnormal automaticity.

The response of automatic arrhythmias to premature stimulation also is sometimes useful in distinguishing automaticity from other arrhythmogenic mechanisms. Of major importance, automatic rhythms caused by either normal or abnormal automaticity can be neither initiated nor terminated by premature stimuli, in contrast to reentry and triggered activity (discussed below). Other than that, premature impulses induced at different times during diastole may transiently perturb an automatic rhythm for a few cycles. The characteristics of the perturbation sometimes may distinguish automaticity from other arrhythmogenic mechanisms. The response of normal and abnormal automaticity to premature stimulation may be somewhat similar. The characteristic response of an automatic pacemaker to premature stimulation is best exemplified by the response of the sinus node to atrial premature stimulation.[294] Figure 23-20 plots the normalized return cycle (the cycle after the premature impulse) on the *y* axis versus the normalized premature cycle (test cycle) on the *x* axis for a study in which premature stimuli were applied to the atria of the human heart during sinus rhythm. The solid line (*A*) represents the line of identity; points falling on this line are compensatory (the sum of the premature cycle and the return cycle is equal to the sum of two spontaneous cycles). Premature impulses delivered late in the cycle length are followed by a compensatory pause and fall on this line (as the test cycle shortens, the return cycle lengthens in a reciprocal manner) because the premature impulses collide with the impulse emanating from the sinus node pacemaker without reaching and resetting the pacemaker. Therefore, the pacemaker discharge that follows the premature impulse occurs exactly on time. As the premature coupling interval is decreased, a point is reached in the basic cycle where the premature impulse reaches the pacemaker before it has depolarized spontaneously to threshold and depolarizes it early. The pacemaker is reset. When this occurs, the postextrasystolic cycle (which is a result of the stimulated or reset pacemaker cells spontaneously depolarizing to threshold) is less than compensatory and the points fall below the line of identity. For the most part, the postextrasystolic cycle length is expected to be equal to the unperturbed spontaneous cycle length. The dashed line (*B*) on the graph in Fig. 23-20 indicates the cycle length of the basic rhythm, and so the return cycle length relative to the basic cycle length can be seen to be somewhat longer in this study. The prolonged return cycle has been proposed to result from slowed conduction of both the premature impulse into the pacemaker site and the pacemaker impulse out of this site.[294] It also may result, at least partly, from depression of the rate of spontaneous diastolic depolarization. Further shortening of the premature coupling interval to midcycle results in points parallel to the dashed line and possibly slightly above it; this indicates no change in the postextrasystolic cycle length over a wide range of coupling intervals. Finally, conduction of very early premature impulses may block before reaching the pacemaker, and the next pacemaker discharge will again occur on time and be compensatory. Of course, this relationship might be upset by changes in conduction of impulses into and out of the pacemaker site. This relation between premature and return cycle length found in studies of sinus rhythm also has been shown in studies on some ectopic tachycardias and, when found, indicates that the tachycardias are likely to be caused by automaticity.[292,293,295]

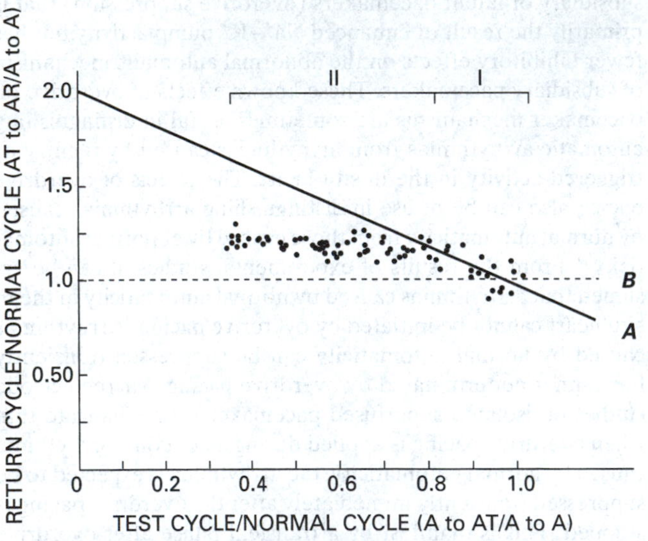

FIGURE 23-20 Return cycles as a function of premature stimulated cycles during premature atrial stimulation in a patient in sinus rhythm. The graph depicts the relation of the normalized return cycle to the degree of prematurity of the test cycle, which also is normalized. Points falling on line *A* represent nonreset of the sinus pacemaker (fully compensatory pause) and are in zone I. Premature stimulated atrial beats introduced earlier in atrial diastole fall in zone II. Line *B*, projected from the *y* axis, is a reference line indicating the spontaneous sinus cycle length. The distance the zone II points (reset points) are above line *B* is interpreted to indicate conduction time into and out of the sinus node, assuming the sinus node pacemaker cycle length immediately after the stimulated premature atrial beat is identical to the preceding sinus node pacemaker cycle length. (From Strauss HC et al. Premature atrial stimulation as a key to the understanding of sinoatrial conduction in man: A presentation of data and critical review of the literature. *Circulation* 1973; 47:86. Reproduced with permission from the publisher and author.)

Ectopic pacemakers also may exist in an extensive region of slow conduction, much as the pacemaker in the sinus node does, and conduction delays into and out of the pacemaker site may influence to some extent the relationship between the return cycle and the premature cycle. Conduction delays may cause some prolongation of the return cycle. When this relationship is seen, however, it is probably indicative of automaticity (either normal or abnormal), since triggered activity and reentry are expected to show a different behavior. In addition to the atrial arrhythmias discussed here, some ventricular arrhythmias are likely to be caused by automaticity. Idioventricular rhythms in patients with complete heart block respond in the manner shown in microelectrode studies of slowly beating Purkinje fibers; the postextrasystolic cycle that follows late premature impulses is longer than the cycle length of the basic rhythm but less than compensatory, while it is shorter than the basic cycle length that follows early premature impulses (and obviously less than compensatory).[296] Some exercise-provoked ventricular tachycardias also may be caused by normal automaticity.[297,298] By contrast, there is some evidence that accelerated idioventricular rhythms in the clinical setting of myocardial infarction may be caused by abnormal automaticity.

EFFECTS OF ELECTRICAL STIMULATION OF REENTRANT EXCITATION

A hallmark feature of a reentrant rhythm is that it usually can be induced and terminated by electrical stimuli (overdrive pacing, introduction of premature stimuli, or both), unlike automaticity. Initially it was thought sufficient to show that an arrhythmia could be initiated or terminated by overdrive pacing or programmed stimulation to demonstrate a reentrant mechanism.[299] That was the case because until the 1970s the only other mechanism that was widely considered a cause of arrhythmias was automaticity, and automatic rhythms can be neither initiated nor terminated by pacing. After the 1970s, when the concept of afterdepolarization-induced arrhythmias was revived and expanded, these criteria alone were no longer sufficient, because triggered activity caused by DADs also can be initiated and terminated by pacing.

The induction of arrhythmias by overdrive pacing or the introduction of a premature beat or beats can be used as an indicator of a reentrant mechanism if other characteristics are also present that eliminate the probability of triggered activity that is dependent on DADs. The ability to demonstrate directly that the induction of an arrhythmia is related to a critical amount of slow conduction in the region where the arrhythmia originates adds credence to the interpretation that the arrhythmia is caused by reentry. The sudden large increase in the A–H interval associated with pacing induction of AV nodal reentrant tachycardia is one example. The induction of triggered activity caused by DADs is not dependent on slowed conduction and should not show this relationship. Also, when a tachycardia is initiated by the introduction of a premature beat over a wide range of coupling intervals, there may be an inverse relation between the coupling interval of the premature impulse and the interval from the premature impulse to the first impulse of tachycardia.[300–302] As the premature impulse occurs earlier in the cycle, its conduction through the reentrant pathway is slower, causing the return cycle to prolong. This too is not found with the induction of triggered activity resulting from DADs. Failure to initiate an arrhythmia by stimulated impulses does not per se eliminate reentry as a mechanism for the arrhythmia.

Another feature of reentrant arrhythmias is that they can be terminated by overdrive pacing or premature stimulation. This is not specific for reentry, since triggered activity caused by DADs also can be terminated. As with initiation, termination by overdrive pacing requires a critical rate and duration of the stimulation train, while termination with stimulated premature impulses requires a critical coupling interval between the premature impulse and the previous impulse of the tachyarrhythmia. Failure to terminate an arrhythmia by stimulated impulses does not by itself eliminate reentry as a mechanism for the arrhythmia. Termination of reentry requires that the stimulated impulse enter the reentrant circuit to cause the block of the reentrant wavefront, and this usually requires that the circuit have a fairly large excitable gap. Some reentrant circuits, particularly if they are caused by the leading circle mechanism of reentry, may not have a gap of excitability large enough to allow a premature impulse to penetrate readily into the circuits. If a tachycardia is very rapid, the excitable gap also may be very small, again preventing ready entry into the circuit by stimulated impulses.

Entrainment In this context, the demonstration of transient entrainment of a tachycardia with or without its subsequent interruption is a relatively easy and reliable way to identify reentry as the mechanism of a tachyarrhythmia. Transient entrainment of a tachycardia was first described in 1977 during rapid pacing to interrupt type I atrial flutter.[303] At that time, although transient entrainment was not well understood, it was recognized as representing an increase in the rate of the tachycardia to the faster pacing rate, with resumption of the intrinsic rate of the tachycardia occuring upon either abrupt cessation of pacing or slowing of the pacing rate below the intrinsic rate of the tachycardia.[303] On the basis of a series of clinical studies during rapid pacing of atrial flutter,[303–306] ventricular tachycardia,[307–309] AV reentrant tachycardia involving an accessory AV connection,[310,311] AV nodal reentrant tachycardia,[312] and intra-atrial reentrant tachycardia,[313] it was proposed that transient entrainment represents capture of a reentrant circuit by wavefronts generated by the pacing impulse without causing interruption of the tachycardia. This was confirmed during studies of transient entrainment in animal models of ventricular tachycardia[314–316] and atrial flutter[317,318] that utilized multiplexing techniques to record simultaneously from large numbers of electrodes in direct contact with cardiac tissue. During transient entrainment of a reentrant tachycardia, the wavefront from each pacing impulse enters into the excitable gap of the reentrant circuit. Once there, it travels in two directions: (1) antidromically, i.e., in the opposite direction of the circulating reentrant wavefront of the spontaneous tachycardia, where it collides with the orthodromic wavefront of the preceding beat, and (2) orthodromically, i.e., in the same direction as the circulating reentrant wavefront of the spontaneous tachycardia, thus both continuing the tachycardia and resetting it to the pacing rate. This explanation is universal for transient entrainment of any tachycardia resulting from reentry with an excitable gap and is diagrammatically illustrated in Fig. 23-21.

The left panel of the figure is a diagrammatic representation of the reentrant circuit during a ventricular tachycardia (VT) at an assumed rate of 145 beats per minute. The *X*s represent the orthodromic wavefronts of the reentrant rhythm. The arrows indicate the direction of spread of the impulse, the box represents an area of slow conduction in the reentrant circuit, the serpentine line indicates slow conduction of the impulse in this latter area, and the dots represent recording sites along the course of the double arc of reentry from which ventricular electrograms (VEGs) are recorded.

The middle panel is a diagrammatic representation of the introduction of the first pacing impulse ($X + 1$) during ventricular pacing at a rate of 150 beats per minute during the VT. The antidromic (anti) wavefronts ($X + 1$) collide with the orthodromic wavefronts from the previous reentrant beat (X), resulting in fusion of ventricular activation. The orthodromic wavefront (ortho) from the pacing impulse ($X + 1$) continues the VT, resetting it to the pacing rate.

The right panel of the figure shows a diagrammatic representation of the introduction of the second pacing impulse ($X + 2$) during ventricular pacing at a rate of 150 beats per minute during the VT. The antidromic wavefronts ($X + 2$) collide with the orthodromic wavefronts from the previous paced beat

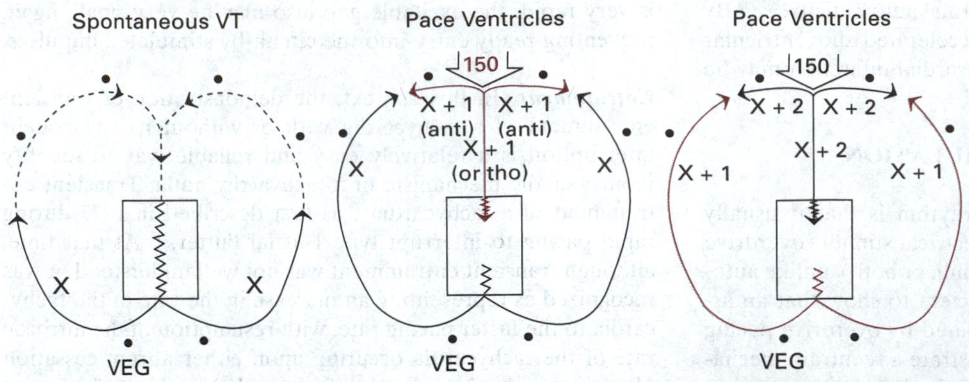

FIGURE 23-21 Diagrammatic representation of the reentrant circuit during spontaneous ventricular tachycardia (VT) and the first two beats of entrainment of the ventricular tachycardia at a rate of 150 beats per minute (*middle and right panels, respectively*). Each *X* represents the orthodromic wavefronts of the reentrant rhythm. In this and subsequent diagrams, the arrows indicate the direction of spread of the impulse, the box represents an area of slow conduction, the serpentine line indicates slow conduction of the impulse in the area of slow conduction, the dots represent recording sites along the course of the double arc of reentry from which ventricular electrograms (VEGs) are recorded, and the large arrow indicates the wavefront from the pacing impulse entering into the ventricular tachycardia reentry circuit, where it is conducted orthodromically (ortho) and antidromically (anti). (From Waldo AL, Henthorn RW. Use of transient entrainment during ventricular tachycardia to localize a critical area in the reentry circuit for ablation. *PACE* 1981; 12:231. Reproduced with permission from the publisher and authors.)

($X + 1$), again resulting in ventricular fusion. Once again, the orthodromic wavefront ($X + 2$) from the pacing impulse continues the VT, resetting it to the pacing rate.

CRITERIA TO ESTABLISH TRANSIENT ENTRAINMENT

Four criteria have been established (Table 23-2), any one of which, if demonstrated, establishes the presence of transient entrainment and thus the presence of a reentrant rhythm with an excitable gap. Figures 23-22 to 23-24 demonstrate the four criteria in diagrammatic fashion for the same ventricular tachycardia illustrated in Fig. 23-21. In Fig. 23-22, which illustrates the first criterion (Table 23-2), the left panel is a diagrammatic representation of the termination of ventricular pacing illustrated in Fig. 23-21. In the left panel, the large arrow indicates the wavefront from the last pacing impulse delivered at a rate of 150 beats per minute entering into the reentrant circuit of the ventricular tachycardia, where it is conducted orthodromically and antidromically. The antidromic wavefronts (X_n[a]) collide with the orthodromic wavefronts (X_n[o]) of the previous beat (X_{n-1}), resulting in the fusion of ventricular activation, but the orthodromic wavefront from the last pacing impulse (X_n[o]) continues and resets the tachycardia. The right panel shows that the orthodromic wavefronts from the last pacing impulse are now unopposed by any antidromic wavefronts because there is no subsequent pacing impulse. Thus, no fusion of ventricular activation occurs despite the presence of transient entrainment. This last entrained beat travels around the reentrant circuit, continuing the tachycardia.

Figure 23-23 is a diagrammatic representation of entrainment in the same ventricular tachycardia during pacing from the same site proximal to the area of slow conduction of the reentrant circuit at rates of 150 (left panel), 155 (middle panel), and 160 beats per minute (right panel), demonstrating both the second and the fourth entrainment criteria. When pacing is at a rate of 155 beats per minute, the pacing cycle length is shorter than it is at 150 beats per minute, so that the antidromic wavefront from each pacing impulse will penetrate the excitable gap

TABLE 23-2 Criteria to Establish the Presence of Transient Entrainment

1. The demonstration of constant fusion beats in the ECG during the period of rapid pacing at a constant rate except for the last captured beat, which is entrained but not fused (i.e., the last entrained beat demonstrates the ECG morphology of the spontaneous tachycardia)
2. The demonstration of constant fusion beats in the ECG during rapid pacing at any constant rate but different degrees of constant fusion at different rapid rates, i.e., progressive fusion
3. Interruption of the tachycardia associated with localized conduction block to a site(s) for one beat, followed by subsequent activation of that site(s) from a different direction, which manifests itself by a change in morphology of the electrogram at the blocked site(s) and with a shorter conduction time
4. A change in conduction time to and electrogram morphology at one recording site when pacing from another site at two different constant pacing rates, each of which is faster than the spontaneous rate of the tachycardia but fails to interrupt it

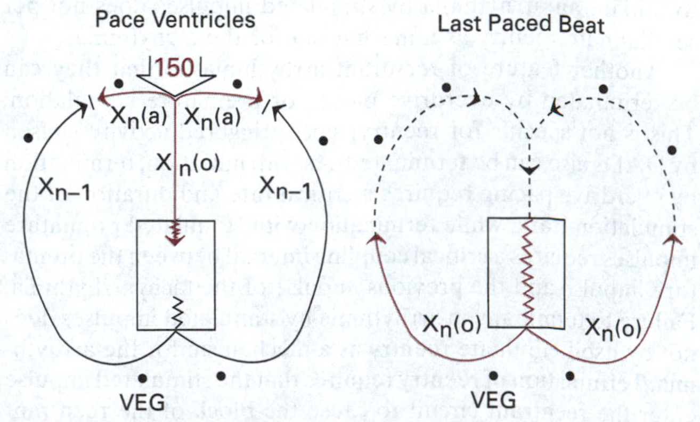

FIGURE 23-22 Diagrammatic representation of the first entrainment criterion during termination of ventricular pacing illustrated in Fig. 23-21. (From Waldo AL, Henthorn RW. Use of transient entrainment during ventricular tachycardia to localize a critical area in the reentry circuit for ablation. *PACE* 1989; 12:231. Reproduced with permission from the publisher and authors.)

of the reentrant circuit to a further degree in an antidromic direction compared to 150 beats per minute, resulting in a degree of fusion of the QRS complex in the ECG different from that which occurs at a rate of 150 beats per minute. As a result, the QRS complex morphology in the ECG during pacing at 155 beats per minute will be different than it is at 150 beats per minute. This, then, is the demonstration of progressive fusion (Table 23-2). When pacing is at 160 beats per minute, once again the antidromic wavefront from each pacing impulse will collide with the orthodromic wavefront, but at yet a different site. This occurs because the pacing cycle length is shorter than pacing at the previous rates, permitting greater penetration of the excitable gap by the antidromic wavefront of the pacing impulse, illustrating yet more progressive fusion.

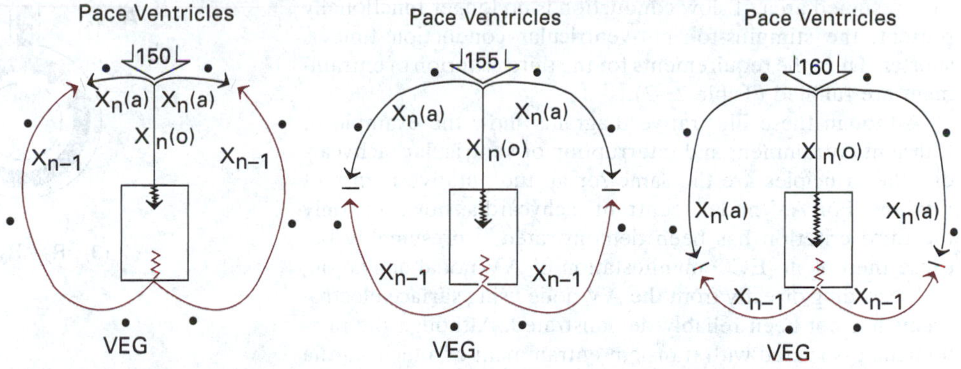

FIGURE 23-23 Diagrammatic representation of the second and fourth entrainment criteria during entrainment of the same spontaneous ventricular tachycardia shown in Fig. 23-21 by ventricular pacing at rates of 150 (*left panel*), 155 (*middle panel*), and 160 (*right panel*) beats per minute. (From Waldo AL, Henthorn RW. Use of transient entrainment during ventricular tachycardia to localize a critical area in the reentry circuit for ablation. *PACE* 1989; 12:231. Reproduced with permission from the publisher and authors.)

These diagrams also illustrate the fourth criterion (Table 23-2): A site or sites activated by the orthodromic wavefront of each pacing impulse during entrainment at one pacing rate will be activated by the antidromic wavefront of each pacing impulse during entrainment at a faster pacing rate. This will be manifest by both a change in the morphology of the electrogram recorded at the site in question (it will have the same morphology during the tachycardia that it has during pacing at the rate that results in activation of the site by the orthodromic wavefront but a different morphology when activated by the antidromic wavefront of the pacing impulse at a faster pacing rate) and a change in conduction time to the recording site from the pacing site (the stimulus-to-recording site interval will be longer when activated by the orthodromic wavefront of each pacing impulse than when activated by the antidromic wavefront of each pacing impulse). Thus, note that the two middle recording sites denoted by black dots on each side of the reentrant circuit become activated in turn from a different direction and with a shorter conduction time when the pacing rate is increased from 150 to 155 beats per minute and then to 160 beats per minute.

Figure 23-24 is a diagrammatic representation of the third criterion and shows the events during interruption of the ventricular tachycardia by ventricular pacing at a rate of 165 beats per minute. In the left panel, the large arrow indicates the wavefront from the pacing impulse delivered at a rate of 165 beats per minute entering into the reentrant circuit of the ventricular tachycardia, where it is conducted orthodromically (X + 1[o]) and antidromically (X + 1[a]). The antidromic wavefronts collide with the orthodromic wavefronts from the previous beat (X), resulting in fusion of ventricular activation. Note that this fusion of ventricular activation is at still a site different from the site during pacing at the previous pacing rates (Fig. 23-23). Thus, initially there is still more progressive fusion of the QRS complex morphology in the ECG. This time, however, the orthodromic wavefront does not reset the tachycardia to the pacing rate. Rather, it too is blocked, presumably in the area of slow conduction, during the same beat. Note that each recording site on each of the two arcs of reentry immediately distal to the area of slow conduction is activated by the orthodromic wave front of the previous beat (X) but is not activated by X + 1 because the orthodromic wavefront (X + 1[o]) never reaches either site (there is localized conduction block for one beat). In the right panel, the large arrows indicate the next pacing impulse (X + 2) delivered at the same pacing rate (165 beats per minute) from the same pacing site described in the left diagram. The dashed lines indicate the reentrant circuit present during the previous periods of ventricular tachycardia and transient entrainment of the ventricular tachycardia. Because the ventricular tachycardia has been interrupted by the previous pacing impulse (X + 1), the sequence of ventricular activation of the next pacing impulse (X + 2) is as one would expect during overdrive pacing of sinus rhythm from that same ventricular pacing site. Therefore, the two electrogram recording sites immediately distal to the previous (but no longer present) area of slow conduction are now activated from a direction different from that during transient entrainment. In addition, because

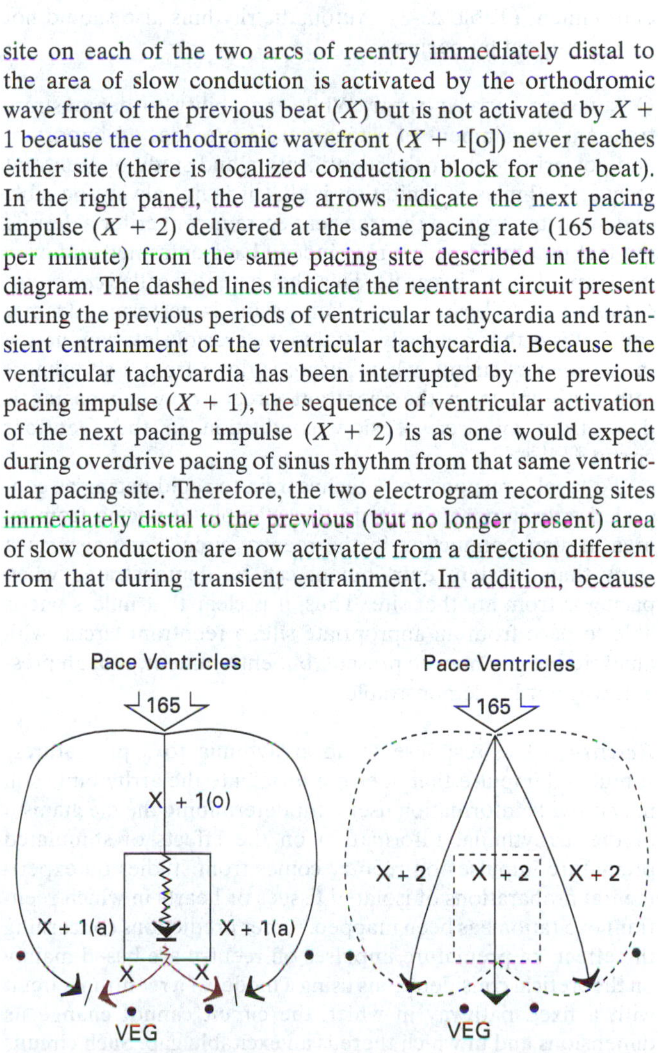

FIGURE 23-24 Diagrammatic representation of the third entrainment criterion during interruption of the ventricular tachycardia by ventricular pacing at a rate of 165 beats per minute. (From Waldo AL, Henthorn RW. Use of transient entrainment during ventricular tachycardia to localize a critical area in the reentry circuit for ablation. *PACE* 1989; 12:231. Reproduced with permission from the publisher and authors.)

the presumed area of slow conduction is no longer functionally present, the stimulus-to-right-ventricular conduction time is shorter. Thus, the requirements for the third criterion of entrainment are fulfilled (Table 23-2).

Although these illustrative diagrams show the example of transient entrainment and interruption of ventricular tachycardia, the principles are the same for all the putative reentrant rhythms. For AV nodal reentrant tachycardia, however, only the third criterion has been demonstrated,[312] presumably because there is no ECG manifestation of AV nodal activation, and recording directly from the AV node using surface electrograms has not been reliably demonstrated. Although the phenomena associated with transient entrainment of a tachycardia with or without its subsequent interruption are best explained by reentry, it still must be asked whether any or all of the criteria for the demonstration of transient entrainment can be explained by another mechanism. Present understanding of the response of automatic and triggered rhythms to rapid pacing is not consistent with the phenomena observed during transient entrainment (Table 23-2). Automatic rhythms also should not be interrupted by pacing.

Concealed Entrainment While the ability to demonstrate transient entrainment of a tachycardia provides an important and powerful tool for the identification and study of reentrant tachyarrhythmias, a limitation is that it is not always possible to demonstrate any of the transient entrainment criteria despite the fact that rapid pacing may indeed have entrained and even interrupted the tachycardia. This phenomenon, called *concealed entrainment*,[309,311] can result when pacing is performed from a site that is orthodromically distal to the area of slow conduction in the reentry circuit, when pacing is done from a site that is rather distant from the reentrant circuit, or when pacing is done from an area of slow conduction in the reentrant circuit.[309,311,319–321]

To label a response of a tachycardia to rapid pacing as concealed entrainment, except in the example of pacing from an area of slow conduction in the reentry circuit, one also must show that transient entrainment can be demonstrated when pacing is from another site. Thus, it is clear that unless one is able to pace from an appropriate site, a reentrant circuit with an excitable gap may be present, but entrainment, though present, will not be demonstrable.

Resetting The response of an arrhythmia to a prematurely stimulated impulse that does not terminate the arrhythmia still may provide information useful for determining the mechanism of the arrhythmia. Information on the effects of stimulated premature impulses on reentry comes from studies on experimental preparations of isolated tissues or hearts in which reentrant excitation has been mapped. Other predictions concerning the effects of premature impulses on reentry are based mainly on theoretical considerations using a model of a reentrant circuit with a fixed pathway in which the circuit cannot change its dimensions and in which there is an excitable gap. Such circuits may have a single entrance and exit pathway leading into and out of the circuit, as illustrated in Fig. 23-25, or the entrance and exit pathways may be separate. These characteristics will influence the characteristics of the resetting response as seen on the ECG.

The theoretically possible responses of a tachycardia caused

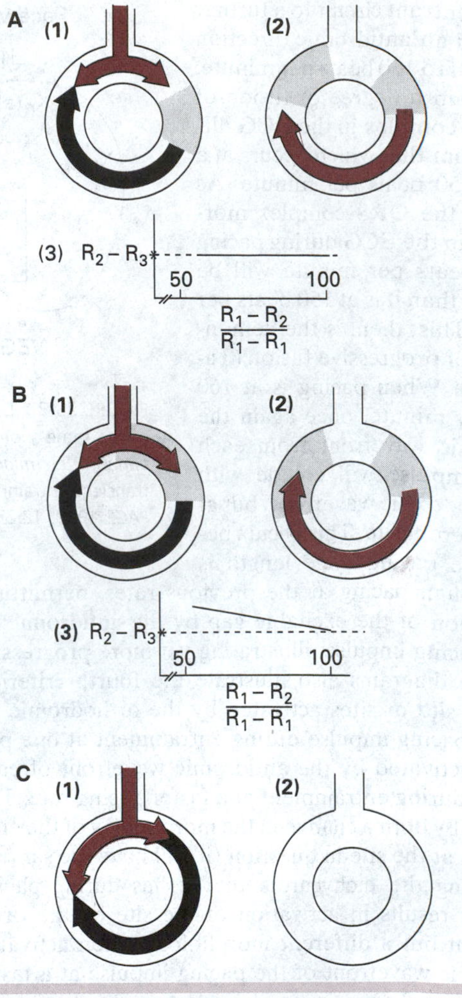

FIGURE 23-25 Effects of premature impulses on reentrant circuit with an excitable gap. In each panel, diagrams are shown of an anatomic circuit with a single entrance route from above. In *A*(1), *B*(1), and *C*(1), red arrows in the circuit represent the reentrant impulse causing tachycardia. The length of the arrow is the wavelength of the impulse and shows the part of the circuit that is completely refractory, The part of the circuit that is stippled is relatively refractory, and the part of the circuit that is clear is completely excitable (the fully excitable gap). Red arrows entering the circuit from above represent a prematurely stimulated impulse initiated outside the circuit. *A*(2) and *B*(2) show conduction of the premature impulse in the circuit. Graphs show the expected relation between the return (premature impulse) cycle length (R_2-R_3) and the premature coupling interval (R_1-R_2/R_1-R_1) for premature impulses conducting in the fully excitable gap *A*(3) and in the relatively refractory tissue of a partially excitable gap *B*(3). (Modified after Wit AL, Janse MJ. *The Ventricular Arrhythmias of Ischemia and Infarction: The Electrophysiological Mechanisms*. Mount Kisco, NY: Futura; 1992:135. Reproduced with permission from the publisher and authors.)

by reentrant excitation to premature stimulation are explained in the diagram in Fig. 23-25. An anatomic circuit with fixed dimensions and a single entrance pathway is diagrammed. In this diagram, the entrance pathway also serves as an exit pathway for the reentrant wavefront to enter surrounding myocardium, but other models may have separate entrance and exit pathways. The black arrow in the reentrant circuit represents the reentrant impulse, with the arrow point being the crest of the depolarizing wave and the end of the arrow being the tail. The length of the arrow is the absolutely refractory part of the circuit, the dotted area that trails it is the relatively refractory part, and the clear region is the fully excitable gap (in some instances there may be no fully excitable gap in the reentrant circuit). The transit time of the reentrant impulse around the circuit determines one cycle length of the tachycardia (the R_1–R_1 interval).

In panel *A*(1), a stimulated premature impulse (R_2) (red arrow from above) is shown to reach the circuit and enter it in the region of the fully excitable gap. The stimulated premature wavefront may then propagate both in the orthodromic (to the right) and antidromic (to the left) directions in the reentrant pathway. In the antidromic direction, it collides with the oncoming reentrant wavefront, extinguishing both stimulated and reentrant impulses at the point of collision. In the orthodromic direction, the stimulated impulse becomes the reentrant impulse and propagates through the circuit in completely excitable tissue of the gap (which also moves around the circuit), as shown in panel *A*(2). This stimulated reentrant wavefront would leave the circuit through the normal exit route and become the next tachycardia impulse.

Since the stimulated impulse traveled through the circuit in completely excitable tissue at a normal conduction velocity, the interval between the stimulated impulse (R_2) and the next impulse of tachycardia (R_3) is equal to the normal transit time around the circuit or the normal tachycardia cycle length (R_1–R_1). The rhythm, however, is reset; i.e., the sum of the curtailed (premature) cycle length and the return cycle length (R_1–R_2 + R_2–R_3) (first poststimulus cycle) is less than two cycle lengths of the tachycardia [2(R_1–R_1)]. This holds throughout the range of premature coupling intervals at which the stimulated premature impulse is able to conduct around the circuit at a normal velocity in completely excitable tissue. Thus, a plot showing the relationship between the premature coupling intervals and the return (poststimulus) cycles over this range appears as a flat line. This plot is shown in Fig. 23-25*A*(3). The poststimulus cycle length is the R_2–R_3 interval on the *y* axis. The normalized premature coupling interval is represented by R_1–R_2/R_1–R_1 on the horizontal axis where R_1–R_1 is the basic cycle length of the tachycardia. In this graph, R_2–R_3 remains constant (and equal to R_1–R_1) over the entire range of premature coupling intervals, indicating conduction of the premature impulse in completely excitable tissue. Premature impulses entering the circuit in the relatively refractory part of the excitable gap (stippled region in the circuit) shown by the red arrow from above in Fig. 23-25*B*(1) also collide with the reentrant impulse in the antidromic direction, extinguishing it while conducting in the orthodromic direction. But conduction around the circuit is slower than normal because the impulse is activating relatively refractory tissue, as indicated by the stippled area in Fig. 23-25*B*(2). Therefore, the return (poststimulus) cycle, which is dependent on the conduction time of the stimulated impulse in the circuit, is longer than the tachycardia cycle.

As the coupling interval of the stimulated premature impulse is decreased and this impulse enters the circuit earlier and earlier in the relatively refractory period of the excitable gap, conduction time around the circuit and the return cycle progressively increase. Thus, a plot showing the relation between the premature coupling interval and the return cycle length appears as shown in Fig. 23-25*B*(3). The line representing the R_2–R_3 interval increases as the normalized premature coupling interval (R_1–R_2/R_1–R_1) decreases. It is also apparent on the graph that the conduction time of the premature impulse around the circuit as measured by the R_2–R_3 interval is greater than the conduction time of the normal tachycardia impulse around the circuit, which is indicated by the dashed line. The sum of the premature and return cycle may be less than or greater than compensatory, depending on how slow conduction of the premature is around the circuit. More often, despite slowing of the conduction of the premature impulse in the circuit, the prolonged return cycle does not compensate for the shortened premature cycle.[322–325]

Panel *C* shows what happens when an earlier premature impulse, indicated by the red arrow from above, reaches the circuit when it is even less excitable. It conducts antidromically into the circuit and collides with the wavefront of the reentrant impulse but cannot excite the orthodromic path because it blocks in refractory tissue (black tail of the reentrant impulse). Thus, reentry is terminated, as shown in *C*(2). The range of coupling intervals over which there is evidence that the premature impulse entered the reentrant circuit to reset the tachycardia before the termination of reentry is a rough measurement of the duration of the excitable gap at the entrance route into the circuit if the premature stimuli are applied close to the circuit.[325] Therefore, fixed reentrant circuits with excitable gaps have patterns of responses to premature stimulation that are characteristic of this mechanism.

In sum, the stable tachycardia cycle length (R_1–R_1) is determined by the time it takes the reentrant wavefront to travel one complete revolution around the circuit and reach an exit pathway to the ventricles. When such a circuit is the cause of a tachycardia, premature depolarizations delivered late in the cycle length often are followed by a postextrasystolic pause that is compensatory for the same reason described for automatic tachycardias; i.e., the stimulated impulse may not be able to reach the reentrant circuit, possibly as a result of collision between the stimulated impulse and the impulse coming from the circuit. The next tachycardia impulse then comes precisely on time. In this case, the tachycardia is not reset since the sum of the premature cycle length and the return cycle length is equal to two successive premature cycle lengths. Over the range of premature coupling intervals that do not reset the tachycardia, the relation between the premature coupling interval and the following (return) cycle falls along the line of identity (see Fig. 23-20).

Premature impulses delivered earlier in the tachycardia cycle may have several different effects that are dependent on some of the characteristics of the reentrant circuit. If there is virtually no excitable gap, as might be expected in some functional circuits, no resetting of the tachycardia will occur, since the stimulated impulse cannot enter the circuit and the return cycle will remain compensatory. If the excitable gap is partially excitable, e.g., composed of relatively refractory tissue, premature impulses that succeed in entering the circuit and traveling around it will do so at reduced conduction velocities, as diagrammed in Fig. 23-25*B*.[326] When they emerge from the circuit, they cause the first postextrasystolic (tachycardia) impulse. As a result of the slowing of conduction of the premature impulse around the circuit, the postextrasystolic cycle is longer than the basic cycle [represented by the dashed line in Fig. 23-25*B*(3)].

The conduction time of the premature impulse around the circuit should continue to increase as the premature impulse is delivered earlier and earlier in the cycle, since the premature impulse conducts in more refractory tissue, causing an inverse relation between the premature coupling interval and the postextrasystolic cycle [Fig 23-25*B*(3)]. In the study of Bigger and Goldreyer[301] on AV nodal reentrant tachycardia, the prolongation of the postextrasystolic cycle over the entire range of premature coupling intervals was sufficient to result in a greater than compensatory pause after the premature impulse. However, the postextrasystolic cycle length can be less than compensatory. An inverse relation between the premature interval and the return cycle interval caused by slowing of the conduction of the premature impulse in the reentrant circuit, as shown in Fig. 23-25*B*(3), is indicative of reentry, since this type of response does not occur with automaticity or triggered activity. Recall that for automatic impulse initiation, the return cycle length is fairly constant over a wide range of premature coupling intervals. If there is a large fully excitable gap, premature impulses reaching the circuit are expected to conduct around the circuit with the same velocity as the reentrant wavefront that is causing the tachycardia, and the postextrasystolic cycle will be equal to the tachycardia cycle and less than compensatory [Fig. 23-25*A*(1) and *A*(2)]. This could occur over a relatively wide range of coupling intervals, resulting in a relationship similar to that expected from a pacemaker over the intermediate range of coupling intervals; the line describing the relationship of the return cycle to the premature cycle would be flat [Fig. 23-25*A*(3)]. Eventually, it is expected that stimulated extrasystoles that are sufficiently premature will invade the circuit when it is relatively refractory, resulting in prolonged return cycles that are inversely related to the premature coupling intervals.

The prolongation of the postextrasystolic cycle after early premature impulses is opposite to that which occurs during automaticity. Thus, a curve might be plotted that consists of a segment that is compensatory at long premature coupling intervals (because the stimulated impulse does not reach the circuit), a segment that is less than compensatory and flat at intermediate premature coupling intervals (when the stimulated impulse is conducting in completely excitable tissue in the circuit), and a segment that is ascending at short premature coupling intervals (when the stimulated impulse is conducting in relatively refractory tissue in the circuit). Still earlier premature impulses might block before reaching a circuit, resulting in interpolation, as described for an automatic focus. A sufficiently early premature impulse also could terminate the tachycardia by blocking in the circuit and causing block of the reentrant wavefront. This is not expected of automatic impulse initiation.

As was mentioned above, the entrance route a stimulated impulse takes into a reentrant circuit and the exit route from the circuit may be separate. When this occurs, the return cycle that follows a premature impulse may be less than the tachycardia cycle because the premature impulse, after entering the circuit, need not conduct around the entire circuit before exiting. The return cycle still may show any of the relationships to the premature cycle described in Fig. 23-25; i.e., it may be flat or show an inverse relationship to the premature coupling interval, depending on whether it is conducting in partially or fully excitable tissue. This expected effect of premature impulses on the cycle length of reentry also may be altered in a functional circuit if the premature impulse somehow can cause a change in the size or shape of the circuit. It is not possible to predict what the effects would be.

In summary, the relation between the postextrasystolic cycle and the curtailed cycle when premature impulses are introduced during a tachycardia caused by reentry may be different from that during automaticity. Therefore, premature stimulation during the study of a tachycardia may provide useful information that helps determine whether reentry is the mechanism. There are, however, a number of confounding influences that, if present, can upset the theoretically predicted relation. They include the absence of a fully excitable gap and properties of intervening tissue between the stimulus site and the site of the circuit that can slow or block conduction of premature impulses into and out of the circuit. Therefore, failure to find the relationships expected for a reentrant mechanism does not necessarily mean that the arrhythmia is caused by a mechanism other than reentry.

EFFECTS OF ELECTRICAL STIMULATION ON ARRHYTHMIAS CAUSED BY TRIGGERED ACTIVITY

Arrhythmias Caused by Delayed Afterdepolarizations The amplitude of DADs increases with a decrease in the cycle length at which the action potentials occur until the afterdepolarizations reach threshold to cause the triggered activity. Therefore, triggered arrhythmias caused by DADs in the in situ heart should be initiated by either overdrive pacing or programmed premature stimulation. Since automatic arrhythmias are not initiated by pacing, they should be distinguished readily from triggered arrhythmias caused by DADs. Reentrant arrhythmias also can be induced by the same stimulation protocols, however, and so whether there are any other characteristics during arrhythmia induction by pacing that might distinguish between triggered activity and reentry is important. An attempt to distinguish between the two mechanisms is further complicated by the fact that triggered activity caused by DADs may be due to different causes, e.g., digitalis and catecholamines, each with somewhat different characteristics.

The following guidelines have been proposed to assist in distinguishing DAD-induced triggered activity from other causes of arrhythmias.[327,328] The guidelines are based on the characteristics of triggered activity determined from in vitro studies with microelectrodes. Triggered activity caused by DADs has been more easily induced by rapid pacing or by several successive premature stimuli than by a single premature stimulus in studies of isolated tissue preparations. This characteristic, which should be expected to occur in the in situ human heart, probably is explained by the fact that rapid pacing or the introduction of a number of premature stimuli is more effective than a single premature stimulus in increasing intracellular Ca^+ levels. The Ca^+ levels control the afterdepolarization amplitude. Also, arrhythmias caused by triggered activity should be more easily induced by premature stimuli superimposed on a rapid drive rate than on a slow one because during rapid pacing, the afterdepolarization amplitude is larger and the membrane potential at the peak of the afterpolarization is closer to threshold. In contrast, ordered reentrant rhythms in humans (with the exception of atrial flutter) seem to be more easily and reproducibly induced by premature impulses than by rapid pacing, although several premature impulses in succession sometimes are necessary. One reason for this may be that premature impulses block more effectively in areas with long refractory periods than do impulses during rapid pacing because rapid pacing can shorten refractory period duration. This, of course, is important because block is a prerequisite for the initiation of reentry.

Both extrasystoles and the first beat of a tachycardia, when caused by DAD-dependent triggered activity initiated by pacing, are predicted to occur late in the cardiac cycle.[327] This proposal is based on experimental data from studies of isolated tissue that show that DADs rarely reach their peak amplitude at less than 50 percent of the cardiac cycle when the drive cycle length is shorter than 1000 ms. In contrast, reentrant beats often occur early in the cycle. One would expect a direct relationship between the pacing cycle length that induces triggered activity resulting from DADs and the coupling interval from the last stimulated impulse to the first beat of the induced tachycardia. As the pacing cycle length decreases, the coupling interval from the last stimulated impulse to the first impulse of tachycardia should decrease because at short cycle lengths, the coupling interval of the afterdepolarizations to the proceeding action potential decreases.

A direct relationship between pacing cycle length and the coupling interval of the first impulse of the tachycardia has been shown to occur in arrhythmias caused by digitalis toxicity.[329] This relationship sometimes may be complicated by the presence of two afterdepolarizations and the possibility of a triggered impulse arising from either one.[330] No comparable data are available from pacing studies on digitalis-toxic human hearts. The direct relation also has been shown in some cases of idiopathic ventricular tachycardia believed to be caused by triggered activity.[166] A direct relation like this is not expected during the initiation of reentrant arrhythmias. Failure to show the direct relation, however, cannot be taken as proof that the arrhythmia is not caused by triggered activity, since slow conduction into or out of the triggerable focus can distort it. In microelectrode studies, during the initiation of triggered activity with premature stimuli, no significant effects of the premature stimulus coupling interval were observed on the relation (coupling interval) of the first triggered impulse to the premature stimulus.[188] On the basis of these data, it is expected that during the initiation of arrhythmias caused by triggered activity in situ with programmed premature stimulation, the coupling interval of the first beat of tachycardia should remain relatively constant over a range of coupling intervals of introduced premature impulses. The response to premature stimulation is also contrary to that expected during the initiation of reentrant arrhythmias, where an inverse relation is expected between the premature stimulus coupling interval and the coupling interval between the premature impulse and the first impulse of tachycardia.

Triggered arrhythmias, unlike automatic arrhythmias but like reentrant arrhythmias, are predicted to be terminated by cardiac pacing. Single premature impulses may terminate triggered arrhythmias, but on the basis of the results of microelectrode studies, termination should be infrequent and not usually reproducible at the same critical premature cycle length. In contrast, single premature impulses often terminate reentrant arrhythmias in a reproducible manner and over a consistent range of premature cycle length in any single individual as long as the reentrant circuit has an excitable gap.[331,332] Therefore, an arrhythmia that is terminated readily by a single prematurely stimulated impulse is more likely to be caused by reentry than by triggered activity.

The effects of premature impulses that do not terminate sustained triggered activity also have been determined.[191] The response is almost identical to that of automaticity. The return cycle length remains fairly constant over a wide range of premature coupling intervals and is nearly the same as the cycle length of the basic triggered rhythm (less than compensatory). By contrast, overdrive pacing should terminate triggered arrhythmias caused by afterdepolarizations. This termination requires a critical rate and duration of overdrive,[186–188] just as it does with reentry.[302,303,307] Overdrive stimulation may cause acceleration of triggered arrhythmias followed by gradual slowing and termination, or rapid overdrive may cause abrupt termination. Although reentrant rhythms may be accelerated by overdrive pacing, a gradual slowing of the rate before termination is not expected. Overdrive pacing that does not terminate triggered activity, as occurs when the cycle length of the overdrive is too long or when the duration of trains of stimuli are too short, does not entrain the arrhythmia either.[333] In fact, none of the characteristics of entrainment are expected during overdrive pacing of triggered activity caused by DADs.

It therefore is apparent that although the response of triggered arrhythmias caused by DADs to stimulation can be predicted from experimental studies, there is no single feature that would positively allow a triggered rhythm to be distinguished from reentry except entrainment. Since the characteristics of initiation and termination of triggered rhythms by stimulation are very different from the characteristics of automatic rhythms, it should be easier to distinguish between these mechanisms by using pacing techniques. This differentiation may be made more difficult when an arrhythmia is persistent and the initiation cannot be studied. Also, entrance block of stimulated impulses into arrhythmogenic foci, whether automatic, triggered, or reentrant, may negate the use of pacing techniques to distinguish between these mechanisms.

The characteristics of some clinical arrhythmias occasionally conform to those expected of DAD-dependent triggered activity.[128,334] In addition to digitalis toxicity, an example is some cases of exercise-induced ventricular tachycardia in patients with no structural heart disease.[166,298] This tachycardia, which occurs spontaneously during exertion, sometimes can be initiated by overdrive pacing or programmed premature stimulation. An isoproterenol infusion during stimulation may be required for successful initiation. Lerman and coworkers[166] proposed that these tachycardias are caused by a catecholamine-induced increase in cyclic AMP, which is known to cause DADs. Evidence supporting this hypothesis is provided by the termination of tachycardias by intravenous injection of adenosine, which antagonizes the electrophysiologic effects of catecholamines mediated through the adenylate cyclase–cyclic AMP system. Jackman and associates[335] proposed that some forms of ventricular tachycardia associated with the congenital long QT syndrome and dependent on adrenergic stimulation result from triggered activity caused by DADs. Cranefield and Aronson[128] provided a detailed review of the clinical arrhythmias that may be caused by triggered activity (see Chap. 27).

Arrhythmias Caused by Early Afterdepolarizations Arrhythmias caused by EADs should not be inducible by overdrive pacing, similar to automatic arrhythmias and unlike arrhythmias caused by DADs or reentry. Similarly, triggered activity dependent on EADs is not expected immediately to follow the short cycle length of one or several prematurely stimulated impulses. As has been shown in experimental studies, the appearance of EAD-induced triggered activity is facilitated by long cycle lengths. Therefore, this kind of triggered activity should be initiated by slowing the basic heart rate. Of course, if an increase in heart rate caused by pacing resulted in entrance block into a focus where EADs occur, the block could cause a prolongation of the cycle length in that focus that might result in triggered activity.[128] Prematurely stimulated impulses also may initiate triggered activity if there is a long compensatory pause after the stimulated impulse. The long cycle might trigger an arrhythmia that would follow it.[128] In the absence of such entrance block, bursts of tachycardia caused by EADs should occur more frequently when the heart rate is slowed, and pacing the heart at rates faster than the basic underlying rhythm is predicted to cause disappearance of the period of tachycardia. Increasing the basic heart rate shortens action potential duration and thereby suppresses EADs. When the pacing is stopped, arrhythmias should reappear, as the action potential returns to its original duration. The reappearance of the arrhythmias may not be immediate, however, since it requires some time for the action potential duration to lengthen owing to the enhanced pump current that follows a period of rapid stimulation.

Many of these characteristics have been shown to apply to the experimental triggered arrhythmias caused by cesium in the in situ canine heart[199] and have been demonstrated in some cases of torsades de pointes in human patients. Acquired forms of the syndrome (e.g., prolonged QT and torsades de pointes by quinidine) exhibit all the features expected of triggered activity caused by EADs, whereas other forms (e.g., congenital) may not be due to this mechanism.[336] Torsades de pointes invariably occurs after a preceding long R–R interval,[200] is unlikely to be initiated by programmed stimulation,[337] and can be prevented from occurring by pacing the heart at a rapid rate.[200,337] Parenthetically, it has been suggested that such rhythms are initiated by EADs but maintained by reentrant excitation.[219] In contrast, triggered arrhythmias caused by DADs may become more frequent as heart rate increases,[327] and the effect of increasing the heart rate on extrasystoles caused by reentry is variable; i.e., reentry may be exacerbated or may stop.[222]

There may be some difficulty in distinguishing EAD-dependent triggered arrhythmias from automatic arrhythmias only on the basis of their response to electrical stimulation, however, since the occurrence of automatic arrhythmias is facilitated by slow heart rates and increasing the basic heart rate by overdrive pacing may cause disappearance of automatic arrhythmias during the periods of pacing. The ECG characteristics of arrhythmias caused by triggered activity resulting from EADs and by automaticity may be of additional help. The triggered rhythms are more likely to occur in bursts or salvos of different lengths, with the first few cycle lengths of a burst decreasing progressively and the last few cycle lengths increasing progressively.

Triggered arrhythmias caused by EADs not only may occur in bursts but also may be sustained. When sustained, their response to single premature stimuli or overdrive pacing can be predicted on the basis of the results of in vitro studies. Some arrhythmias may be terminated by premature stimuli, but this should be a relatively rare occurrence. The effects of premature stimulated impulses that do not terminate the arrhythmia are expected to be the same as their effects on automatic impulse initiation. Some arrhythmias also may be terminated by overdrive pacing, but termination should not be the usual effect. When termination occurs, it is expected to follow the overdrive immediately, whereas termination of triggered activity caused by DADs sometimes may be preceded by up to 10 triggered "afterbeats."[186,187] When termination does not occur, overdrive is not expected to cause any significant effect on the rhythm; the response should be more like that of an arrhythmia caused by abnormal automaticity[191] than one caused by normal automaticity, which is readily overdrive-suppressed.[73] Because of this variability of response, stimulation during a sustained tachycardia caused by EADs is not much help in determining the mechanism.

Therefore, as in the triggered arrhythmias caused by DADs, there is no single feature in the response to cardiac pacing that would positively enable EAD-induced triggered rhythms to be distinguished from other arrhythmogenic mechanisms. Early afterdepolarization-induced nonsustained arrhythmias usually can be differentiated from rhythms induced by DADs or automaticity at high membrane potentials and sometimes from reentry by pacing, but the response of sustained triggered activity to pacing is often indistinguishable from abnormal automaticity at low membrane potentials.

SUMMARY OF EFFECTS OF ELECTRICAL STIMULATION

Despite the fact that there are exceptions and inconsistencies to virtually all the rules that can be proposed to distinguish among the different arrhythmogenic mechanisms using pacing techniques, determining the effects of electrical stimulation is quite useful. The following is a summary of the most important points: (1) Initiation of a tachycardia by stimulation indicates that the arrhythmia is caused by reentry or delayed afterdepolarization-induced triggered activity. Other characteristics of initiation are then useful in distinguishing between the two. Other mechanisms of arrhythmias—such as automaticity and triggered activity caused by early afterdepolarizations—are eliminated when a tachycardia is induced by cardiac pacing. (2) Termination of a tachycardia by overdrive pacing or premature stimulation is expected of reentry or triggered activity caused by delayed afterdepolarizations but not of automaticity and early afterdepolarization-dependent triggered activity. Overdrive suppression is expected of arrhythmias caused by normal automaticity, and overdrive acceleration may occur with arrhythmias caused by abnormal automaticity. (3) Demonstration of entrainment of a tachycardia during overdrive pacing is indicative of a reentrant mechanism and is not expected of other mechanisms. (4) The response to premature stimulation is different during arrhythmias caused by automaticity and those caused by reentry. During automatic arrhythmias, the return cycle length should not increase as the premature coupling interval decreases. The return cycle should be less than compensatory. During reentrant arrhythmias, the return cycle length should increase as the premature impulse occurs earlier in the dominant cycle. The increase sometimes may begin to occur with late coupled premature impulses or may not occur until premature impulses are early coupled. The return cycle length is often less than compensatory.

References

1. Hoffman BF, Rosen MR. Cellular mechanisms for cardiac arrhythmias. *Circ Res* 1981; 49:1–15.
2. Waldo AL, Kaiser GA, Bowman OF Jr, Malm JR. Etiology of

prolongation of the P-R interval in patients with an endocardial cushion defect: Further observations on internodal conduction and the polarity of the retrograde P wave. *Circulation* 1973; 48:19–27.
3. Mayer AG. Rhythmical pulsation in Scyphomedusae. Publication no. 47. Washington, DC: Carnegie Institution of Washington; 1906:1.
4. Mines GR. On dynamic equilibrium in the heart. *J Physiol* (*Lond*) 1913; 46:349–383.
5. Cranefield PF. *The Conduction of the Cardiac Impulse: The Slow Response and Cardiac Arrhythmia*. Mount Kisco, NY: Futura; 1975.
6. Schmitt OF, Erlanger J. Directional differences in the conduction of the impulse through the heart muscle and their possible relation to extrasystolic and fibrillary contractions. *Am J Physiol* 1928–1929; 87:326–347.
7. Wit AL, Hoffman BF, Cranefield PF. Slow conduction and reentry in the ventricular conduction system: I. Return extrasystole in canine Purkinje fibers. *Circ Res* 1972; 30:1–10.
8. Cranefield PF, Wit AL, Hoffman BF. Genesis of cardiac arrhythmias. *Circulation* 1973; 47;190–204.
9. Singer DH, Lazzara R, Hoffman BF. Interrelationships between automaticity and conduction in Purkinje fibers. *Circ Res* 1967; 21:537–558.
10. Di Francesco D. The hyperpolarization-activated current, i_f, and cardiac pacemaking. In: Rosen MR, Janse MJ, Wit AL, eds. *Cardiac Electrophysiology: A Textbook*. Mount Kisco, NY: Futura; 1990:117.
11. Yanagihara K, Irisawa H. Potassium current during the pacemaker depolarization in rabbit sinoatrial node cell. *Pflugers Arch* 1980; 388:255–260.
12. Di Francesco D. Characterization of single pacemaker channels in cardiac sinoatrial node cells. *Nature* 1986; 324:470–473.
13. Di Francesco D, Ferroni A, Massanti M, Tromba C. Properties of the hyperpolarizing-activated current i_f in cells isolated from the rabbit sino-atrial node. *J Physiol* 1986; 37:61–88.
14. Brown HF. Electrophysiology of the sinoatrial node. *Physiol Rev* 1982; 52:505–530.
15. Brown HF, Kimura K, Noble SJ. The relative contributions of various time-dependent membrane currents to pacemaker activity in the sino atrial node. In: Bouman LN, Jongsma HJ, eds. *Cardiac Rate and Rhythm: Physiological, Morphological and Developmental Aspects*. Boston: Martinus-Nijhoff; 1982:53.
16. Nakayama T, Kurachi Y, Noma A. Action potential and membrane currents of single pacemaker cells of the rabbit heart. *Pflugers Arch* 1984; 402:248–257.
17. Shibasaki T. Conductance and kinetics of delayed rectifier potassium channels in nodal cells of the rabbit heart. *J Physiol* 1987; 387:227–250.
18. Irisawa H, Giles WR. Sinus and atrioventricular node cells: Cellular electrophysiology. In: Zipes DP, Jalife J, eds. *Cardiac Electrophysiology: From Cell to Bedside*. Philadelphia: Saunders; 1990:95.
19. Reuter H. Ion channels in cardiac cell membranes. *Annu Rev Physiol* 1984; 46:473–484.
20. Bean BP. Two kinds of calcium channels in canine atrial cells. *J Gen Physiol* 1985; 85:1–30.
21. Hagiwara N, Irisawa H, Kameyama M. Contribution of two types of calcium currents to the pacemaker potentials of rabbit sinoatrial node cells. *J Physiol* 1988; 409:121–141.
22. Doerr T, Denger R, Trautwein W. Calcium currents in single SA nodal cells of the rabbit heart studied with action potential clamp. *Pflugers Arch* 1989; 413:599–603.
23. Hoffman BF, Cranefield PF. *Electrophysiology of the Heart*. New York: McGraw-Hill, 1960.
24. Trautwein W. Effects of acetylcholine on the SA node of the heart. In: Carpenter O, ed. *Cellular Pacemakers: Mechanisms of Pacemaker Generation*. New York: Wiley; 1981:127.
25. Soejma M, Noma A. Mode of regulation of the ACh-sensitive K channel by the muscarinic receptor in rabbit atrial cells. *Pflugers Arch* 1984; 400:424–431.
26. Di Francesco D, Tromba C. Inhibition of the hyperpolarizing-activated current, i_f, induced by acetylcholine in rabbit sino-atrial node myocytes. *J Physiol* 1988; 405:477–491.
27. Noma A, Kotake H, Irisawa H. Slow inward current and its role mediating the chronotropic effect of epinephrine in the rabbit sinoatrial node. *Plfugers Arch* 1980; 388:1–9.
28. Di Francesco D. The cardiac-hyperpolarizing activated current, i_f. Origins and developments. *Prog Biophys Mol Biol* 1985; 46:163–183.
29. Hogan PM, David LD. Evidence for specialized fibers in the canine atrium. *Circ Res* 1968; 23:387–396.
30. Jones SB, Euler DE, Hardie E, et al. Comparison of SA nodal and subsidiary pacemaker function and location in the dog. *Am J Physiol* 1978; 234:H471–H476.
31. Rozanski GJ, Lipsius SL. Electrophysiology of functional subsidiary pacemakers in canine right atrium. *Am J Physiol* 1985; 249:H594–H603.
32. Rozanski GJ, Lipsius SL, Randall WD. Functional characteristics of sinoatrial and subsidiary pacemaker activity in the canine right atrium. *Circulation* 1983; 67:1378–1387.
33. Wit AL, Cranefield PF. Triggered and automatic activity in the canine coronary sinus. *Circ Res* 1977; 41:435–445.
34. Wit AL, Fenoglio JJ Jr, Wagner BM, Bassett AL. Electrophysiological properties of cardiac muscle in the anterior mitral valve leaflet and the adjacent atrium in the dog: Possible implications for the genesis of atrial dysrhythmias. *Circ Res* 1973; 32:731–745.
35. Bassett AL, Fenoglio JJ, Wit AL, et al. Electrophysiologic and ultrastructural characteristics of the canine tricuspid valve. *Am J Physiol* 1976; 230:1366–1377.
36. Rozanski GJ. Electrophysiological properties of automatic fibers in rabbit atrioventricular valves. *Am J Physiol Heart Circ Physiol* 1987; 22:H720–H727.
37. Kokobun S, Nishimura M, Noma A, Irisawa H. The spontaneous action potential of rabbit atrioventricular node cells. *Jpn J Physiol* 1980; 30:529–540.
38. James TN, Isobe JH, Urthaler JH. Correlative electrophysiological and anatomical studies concerning the site of origin of escape rhythm during complete atrioventricular block in the dog. *Circ Res* 1979; 45:108–119.
39. Jones SB, Euler DE, Randall WC, et al. Atrial ectopic foci in the canine heart: Hierarchy of pacemaker automaticity. *Am J Physiol Heart Circ Physiol* 1980; 238:H788–H793.
40. Randall WC, Talano J, Kaye MP, et al. Cardiac pacemakers in the absence of the SA node: Responses to exercise and autonomic blockade. *Am J Physiol* 1978; 234:H465–H470.
41. Wallick DW, Levy MN, Felder DS, Zieske H. Effects of repetitive bursts of vagal activity on atrioventricular junctional rate in dogs. *Am J Physiol* 1979; 237:H275–H281.
42. Spear JF, Moore EN. Influence of brief vagal and stellate nerve stimulation on pacemaker activity and conduction within the atrioventricular conduction system of the dog. *Circ Res* 1973; 32:27–40.
43. Rozanski GJ, Jalife J. Automaticity in atrioventricular valve leaflets of rabbit heart. *Am J Physiol Heart Circ Physiol* 1986; 19:H397–H406.
44. Weidmann S. *Elektrophysiologie Der Herzmuskelfaser*. Bern and Stuttgart: Medizinischer Verlag Hans Huber; 1956.
45. Hope RR, Scherlag BJ, El-Sherif N, Lazzara R. Hierarchy of ventricular pacemakers. *Circ Res* 1976; 39:883–888.
46. Vassalle M, Levine MJ, Stuckey JH. On the sympathetic control of ventricular automaticity: The effects of stellate ganglia stimulation. *Circ Res* 1968; 23:249–258.

47. Levy MN. Sympathetic-parasympathetic interactions in the heart. *Circ Res* 1971; 29:437–445.
48. Levy MN, Blattberg B. Effect of vagal stimulation on the overflow of norepinephrine into the coronary sinus during cardiac sympathetic nerve stimulation in the dog. *Circ Res* 1976; 38:81–85.
49. Di Francesco D. A new interpretation of the pacemaker current in calf Purkinje fibers. *J Physiol* 1981; 314:359–376.
50. Di Francesco D. A study of the ionic nature of the pacemaker current in calf Purkinje fibers. *J Physiol* 1981; 314:377–393.
51. Noble D. The surprising heart: A review of recent progress in cardiac electrophysiology. *J Physiol* 1984; 353:1–50.
52. Vasalle M, Yu H, Cohen IS. The pacemaker current in cardiac Purkinje myocytes. *J Gen Physiol* 1995; 106:559–578.
53. Gintant GA, Cohen IS. Advances in cardiac cellular electrophysiology: Implications for automaticity and therapeutics. *Annu Rev Pharmacol Toxicol* 1988; 28:61–81.
54. Hauswirth O, Noble D, Tsien RW. The mechanism of oscillatory activity at low membrane potentials in cardiac Purkinje fibers. *J Physiol* 1969; 200:255–265.
55. Imanishi S. Calcium-sensitive discharge in canine Purkinje fibers. *Jpn J Physiol* 1971; 21:443–463.
56. Noble D, Tsien RW. The kinetics and rectifier properties of the slow potassium current in cardiac Purkinje fibers. *J Physiol* 1968; 195:185–214.
57. Katzung BG, Morgenstern JA. Effects of extracellular potassium on ventricular automaticity and evidence for a pacemaker current in mammalian ventricular myocardium. *Circ Res* 1977; 40:105–111.
58. Escande D, Coraboeuf E, Planche C. Abnormal pacemaking ismodulated by sarcoplasmic reticulum in partially depolarized myocardium from dilated right atria in humans. *J Mol Cell Cardiol* 1987; 19:231–241.
59. Kimura T, Imanishi S, Atria M, et al. Two differential mechanisms of automaticity in diseased human atrial fibers. *Jpn J Physiol* 1988; 38:851–867.
60. January CT, Fozzard HA. The effects of membrane potential, extracellular potassium and tetrodotoxin on the intracellular sodium ion activity in sheep cardiac muscle. *Circ Res* 1984; 54: 652–665.
61. Carmeliet EE. *Chloride and Potassium in Cardiac Purkinje Fibers*. Thesis, Editions ARSCI, S.A. Brussels: Presses Academiques Europeennes; 1961.
62. Gadsby DC, Cranefield PF. Two levels of resting potential in cardiac Purkinje fibers. *J Gen Physiol* 1977; 70:725–746.
63. Hill JL, Gettes LS. Effects of acute coronary artery occlusion on local myocardial extracellular K^+ activity in swine. *Circulation* 1980; 61:768–778.
64. Hirche HJ, Franz C, Bos L, et al. Myocardial extracellular K^+ and H^+ increase and noradrenaline release as possible cause of early arrhythmias following acute coronary artery occlusion in pigs. *J Mol Cell Cardiol* 1980; 12:579–593.
65. Kleber AG. Resting membrane potential, extracellular potassium activity and intracellular sodium activity during acute global ischemia in isolated perfused guinea-pig hearts. *Circ Res* 1983; 52:442–450.
66. Dresdner KP, Kline R, Wit AL. Intracellular K^+ activity, intracellular Na activity and maximum diastolic potential of canine subendocardial Purkinje cells from one-day-old infarcts. *Circ Res* 1987; 60:122–132.
67. Dresdner KP, Kline RP, Wit AL. Cytoplasmic K^+ and N^+ activity in subendocardial canine Purkinje fibers from one day old infarcts using double-barrel ion sensitive electrodes. *Biophys J* 1985; 47:463.
68. Friedman PL, Stewart JR, Wit AL. Spontaneous and induced cardiac arrhythmias in subendocardial Purkinje fibers surviving extensive myocardial infarction in dogs. *Circ Res* 1973; 33:612–626.
69. Lazzara R, El-Sherif N, Scherlag BJ. Electrophysiological properties of canine Purkinje cells in one day old myocardial infarction. *Circ Res* 1973; 33:722–734.
70. Hordof AJ, Edie R, Malm JR, et al. Electrophysiological properties and response to pharmacological agents of fibers from diseased human atria. *Circulation* 1976; 54:774–779.
71. TenEick RE, Singer DH. Electrophysiological properties from diseased human atria: I. Low diastolic potential and altered cellular response to potassium. *Circ Res* 1979; 44:545–557.
72. Singer DH, Baumgarten CM, TenEick RE. Cellular electrophysiology of ventricular and other dysrhythmias: Studies on diseased and ischemic hearts. *Progr Cardiovasc Dis* 1981; 24:97–156.
73. Vassalle M. Electrogenic suppression of automaticity in sheep and dog Purkinje fibers. *Circ Res* 1970; 27:361–377.
74. Vassalle M. The relationship among cardiac pacemakers: Overdrive suppression. *Circ Res* 1977; 41:269–277.
75. Vassalle M. Cardiac pacemaker potentials at different extra- and intracellular K concentrations. *Am J Physiol* 1965; 208: 770–775.
76. Vassalle M, Caress DL, Slovin AJ, Stuckey JH. On the cause of ventricular asystole during vagal stimulation. *Circ Res* 1967; 20:228–241.
77. Randall WC, Rinkema LE, Jones SB, et al. Overdrive suppression of atrial pacemaker tissues in the alert, awake dog before and chronically after excision of the sinoatrial node. *Am J Cardiol* 1982; 49:1166–1175.
78. Glitsch HG. Characteristics of active Na transport in intact cardiac cells. *Am J Physiol* 1979; 236:H189–H199.
79. Gadsby DC, Cranefield PF. Electrogenic sodium extrusion in cardiac Purkinje fibers. *J Gen Physiol* 1979; 73:819–837.
80. Jordan JL, Yamaguchi I, Mandel WJ, McCullen AE. Comparative effects of overdrive on sinus and subsidiary pacemaker functions. *Am Heart J* 1977; 93:367–374.
81. Kodama I, Goto J, Ando A, et al. Effects of rapid stimulation on the transmembrane action potentials of rabbit sinus node pacemaker cells. *Circ Res* 1980; 46:90–99.
82. Greenberg YJ, Vassalle M. On the mechanism of overdrive suppression in the guinea pig sino-atrial node. *J Electrocardiol* 1990; 37:53–67.
83. Gang ES, Reiffel JA, Livelli FD Jr, Bigger JT Jr. Sinus node recovery times following the spontaneous termination of supraventricular tachycardia and following atrial overdrive pacing: A comparison. *Am Heart J* 1983; 105:210–215.
84. Breithardt G, Seipel L, Loogen F. Sinus node recovery time and calculated sinoatrial conduction time in normal subjects and patients with sinus node dysfunction. *Circulation* 1977; 56:43–50.
85. Carmeliet E. The slow inward current: Non-voltage clamp studies. In: Zipes DP, Bailey JC, Elharrar V, eds. *The Slow Inward Current and Cardiac Arrhythmias*. The Hague: Martinus Nijhoff; 1980:97.
86. Hoffman BF, Dangman KH. Are arrhythmias caused by automatic impulse generation? In: Paes de Carvalho A, Hoffman BF, Lieberman M, eds. *Normal and Abnormal Conduction in the Heart*. Mount Kisco, NY: Futura; 1982:429.
87. Dangman KH, Hoffman BF. Studies on overdrive stimulation of canine cardiac Purkinje fibers: Maximum diastolic potential as a determinant of the response. J Am Coll Cardiol 1983; 2:1183–1191.
88. Falk RT, Cohen IS. Membrane current following activity in canine cardiac Purkinje fibers. *J Gen Physiol* 1984; 83:771–799.
89. Van Capelle FJL, Durer D. Computer simulation of arrhythmias in a network of coupled excitable elements. *Circ Res* 1980; 47:454–466.
90. Wit AL, Cranefield PF. Mechanism of impulse initiation in the atrioventricular junction and the effect of acetylstrophantidin (abstract) *Am J Cardiol* 1982; 49:921.
91. Kirchhof CJ, Bonke FIM, Allessie MA. Evidence for the presence of electrotonic depression of pacemakers in the rabbit atrioven-

tricular node: The effects of uncoupling from the surrounding myocardium. *Basic Res Cardiol* 1988; 83:190–201.
92. Opthof T, van Ginneken ACG, Bouman LN, Jongsma HJ. The intrinsic cycle length in small pieces isolated from the rabbit sinoatrial node. *J Mol Cell Cardiol* 1987; 19:923–934.
93. Janse MJ, Van Capelle FJL. Electrotonic interactions across an inexcitable region as a cause of ectopic activity in acute regional myocardial ischemia: A study in intact porcine and canine hearts and computer models. *Circ Res* 1982; 50:527–537.
94. Boineau JP, Schuessler RB, Mooney CR, et al. Multicentric origin of the atrial depolarization waves: The pacemaker complex: Relation to dynamics of atrial conduction, P wave changes and heart rate control. *Circulation* 1978; 58:1036–1048.
95. Toda N, West TC. Changes in sino-atrial node transmembrane potentials on vagal stimulation of the isolated rabbit atrium. *Nature* 1965; 205:808–809.
96. Ferrer MI: *The Sick Sinus Syndrome*. Mount Kisco, NY: Futura; 1974.
97. Katz LN, Pick A. *Clinical Electrocardiography: The Arrhythmias*. Philadelphia: Lea & Febiger; 1956.
98. Jalife J, Moe GK. Effect of electrotonic potentials on pacemaker activity of canine Purkinje fibers in relation to parasystole. *Circ Res* 1976; 39:801–808.
99. Jalife J, Moe GK. A biologic model of parasystole. *Am J Cardiol* 1979; 43:761–772.
100. Moe GK, Jalife J, Mueller WJ, Moe B. A mathematical model of parasystole and its application to clinical arrhythmias. *Circulation* 1977; 56:968–979.
101. Euler DE, Jones SB, Gunnar WP, et al. Cardiac arrhythmias in the conscious dog after excision of the sinus node and crista terminalis. *Circulation* 1979; 59:468–475.
102. Loeb JM, Euler DE, Randall WC, et al. Cardiac arrhythmias after chronic embolization of the sinus node artery: Alterations in parasympathetic pacemaker control. *Circulation* 1980; 61:192–198.
103. Randall WC, Rinkema LE, Jones SB, et al. Functional characteristics of atrial pacemaker activity. *Am J Physiol* 1982; 242:H98–H106.
104. Gillette PC, Kugler JD, Garson A Jr, et al. Mechanisms of cardiac arrhythmias after the Mustard operation for transposition of the great arteries. *Am J Cardiol* 1980; 45:1225–1230.
105. Klein HO, Lebson R, Cranefield PF, Hoffman BF. Effect of extrasystoles on idioventricular rhythm: Clinical and electrophysiologic correlation. *Circulation* 1973; 47:758–764.
106. Webb SW, Adgey AAJ, Pantridge JF. Autonomic disturbance of onset of acute myocardial infarction. *Br Med J* 1972; 3:89–92.
107. Lie KI, Wellens HJJ, Schuilenburg RM. Mechanism and significance of widened QRS complexes during complete atrioventricular block in acute inferior myocardial infarction. *Am J Cardiol* 1974; 33:833–839.
108. Dahl G, Isenberg G. Decoupling of heart muscle cells: Correlation with increased cytoplasmic calcium activity and with changes of nexus ultrastructure. *J Membr Biol* 1980; 53:63–75.
109. Weingart R. The actions of ouabain on intercellular coupling and conduction velocity in mammalian ventricular muscle. *J Physiol* 1977; 264:341–365.
110. Ellis D. The effects of external cations and ouabain on the intracellular sodium activity of sheep heart Purkinje fibers. *J Physiol* 1977; 273:211–240.
111. Davis LD. Effects of autonomic neurohumors on transmembrane potentials of atrial plateau fibers. *Am J Physiol* 1975; 229:1351–1364.
112. Tsien RW. Effects of epinephrine on the pacemaker potassium current of cardiac Purkinje fibers. *J Gen Physiol* 1974; 64:293–319.
113. Pliam MB, Krellenstein DJ, Vassalle M, Brooks CMcC. The influence of norepinephrine, reserpine and propranolol on overdrive suppression. *J Electrocardiol* 1975; 8:17–24.
114. Armour JA, Hageman GR, Randall WC. Arrhythmias induced by local cardiac nerve stimulation. *Am J Physiol* 1972; 223:1068–1075.
115. Katzung BG, Hondeghem LM, Grant AO. Cardiac ventricular automaticity induced by current of injury. *Pflugers Arch* 1975; 360:193–197.
116. Rosen MR, Gelband H, Hoffman BF. Correlation between the effects of ouabain on the canine electrocardiogram and transmembrane potentials of isolated Purkinje fibers. *Circulation* 1973; 47:65–72.
117. Rosen MR, Gelband H, Merker C, Hoffman BF. Mechanisms of digitalis toxicity: Effects of ouabain on phase four of canine Purkinje fiber transmembrane potentials. *Circulation* 1973; 47:681–689.
118. Deck KA. Aenderungen des Ruhepotentials und der Kabeleigenschaften von Purkinje-Faden bei der Dehnung. *Pflugers Arch* 1964; 280:131–140.
119. Dudel J, Trautwein W. Das Aktionspotential und Mechanogramm des Herzmuskels unter dem Einflusz der Dehnung. *Cardiologia* 1954; 25:344–362.
120. Kaufmann R, Theopile U. Automatie fördernde Dehnungsefekte am Purkinje Faden, Papillarmuskeln und Vorhoftrabekeln von Rhesusaffen. *Pflugers Arch* 1967; 291:174–189.
121. Hansen DE, Craig CS, Hondeghem LM. Stretch-induced arrhythmias in the isolated canine ventricle: Evidence for the importance of mechanoelectrical feedback. *Circulation* 1990; 81:1094–1105.
122. Ferrier GR, Rosenthal JE. Automaticity and entrance block induced by focal depolarization of mammalian ventricular tissues. *Circ Res* 1980; 47:238–248.
123. Imanishi S, Surawicz B. Automatic activity in depolarized guinea-pig ventricular myocardium. *Circ Res* 1976; 39:751–759.
124. Brown HF, Noble SJ. Membrane currents underlying delayed rectification and pacemaker activity in frog atrial muscle. *J Physiol* 1969; 204:717–736.
125. Hume J, Katzung BG. Physiological role of endogenous amines in the modulation of ventricular automaticity in the guinea pig. *J Physiol* 1980; 309:275–286.
126. Cranefield PF, Aronson RS. Initiation of sustained rhythmic activity by single propagated action potentials in canine cardiac Purkinje fibers exposed to sodium-free solution or to ouabain. *Circ Res* 1974; 34:477–481.
127. Cranefield PF. Action potentials, afterpotentials and arrhythmias. *Circ Res* 1977; 41:415–425.
128. Cranefield PF, Aronson RS. *Cardiac Arrhythmias: The Role of Triggered Activity and Other Mechanisms*. Mount Kisco, NY: Futura; 1988.
129. Cramer M, Siegal M, Bigger JT Jr, Hoffman BF. Characteristics of extracellular potentials recorded from the sinoatrial pacemaker of the rabbit. *Circ Res* 1977; 41:292–300.
130. Wit AL, Boyden PA, Gadsby CD, Cranefield PF. Triggered activity as a cause of atrial arrhythmias. In: Narula OS, ed. *Cardiac Arrhythmias: Electrophysiology, Diagnosis and Management*. Baltimore: Williams & Wilkins; 1979:14.
131. Olsson SB, Blomström-Lundqvist C, Wohlfart B. Endocardial monophasic action potentials: Correlations with intracellular electrical activity. *Ann NY Acad Sci* 1990; 601:119–127.
132. Harriman RJ, Holzman R, Gough WB, et al. In vivo demonstration of delayed afterdepolarization as a cause of ventricular rhythms in one day old infarction. *J Am Coll Cardiol* 1984; 3:478.
133. Priori SG, Mantica M, Schwartz PJ. Delayed afterdepolarizations elicited in vivo by left stellate ganglion stimulation. *Circulation* 1988; 78:178–185.
134. Fabiato A, Fabiato F. Contraction induced by a calcium-triggered release of calcium from the sarcoplasmic reticulum of single skinned cardiac cells. *J Physiol* 1975; 249:469–495.
135. Aronson RS, Gelles JM, Hoffman BF. Effect of ouabain on

the current underlying spontaneous diastolic depolarization in cardiac Purkinje fibers. *Nature New Biol* 1973; 245:118–120.
136. Lederer WJ, Tsien RW. Transient inward current underlying arrhythmogenic effect of cardiotonic steroids in Purkinje fibers. *J Physiol* 1976; 263:73–100.
137. Kass RS, Lederer WJ, Tsien RW, Weingart R. Role of calcium ions in transient inward currents and after contractions induced by strophantidin in cardiac Purkinje fibers. *J Physiol* 1978; 281:187–208.
138. Kass RS, Tsien RW, Weingart R. Ionic basis of transient inward current induced by strophantidin in cardiac Purkinje fibers. *J Physiol* 1978; 281:209–226.
139. Karagueuzian HS, Katzung BG. Voltage clamp studies of transient inward current and mechanical oscillations induced by ouabain in ferret papillary muscle. *J Physiol* 1982; 327:255–271.
140. Vassalle M, Mugelli A. An oscillatory current in sheep cardiac Purkinje fibers. *Circ Res* 1981; 48:618–631.
141. Lipsius SL, Gobbins WR. Membrane currents, contractions and aftercontractions in cardiac Purkinje fibers. *Am J Physiol* 1982; 243:H77–H86.
142. Eisner DA, Lederer WJ. Inotropic and arrhythmogenic effects of potassium-depleted solutions on mammalian cardiac muscle. *J Physiol* 1979; 294:255–277.
143. Baker PF, Blaustein MP, Hodgkin AL, Steinhardt RA. The influence of calcium on sodium efflux in squid axons. *J Physiol* 1969; 200:431–458.
144. Mullins LJ. The generation of electrical currents in cardiac fibers by Na/Ca exchange. *Am J Physiol* 1979; 236:C103–C110.
145. Eisner DA, Lederer WJ. Na-Ca exchange: Stoichiometry and electrogenicity. *Am J Physiol* 1985; 248:C189–C202.
146. Davis LD. Effect of changes in cycle length on diastolic depolarization produced by ouabain in canine Purkinje fibers. *Circ Res* 1973; 32:206–214.
147. Ferrier GR, Saunders JH, Mendez C. A cellular mechanism for the generation of ventricular arrhythmias by acetylstrophantidin. *Circ Res* 1973; 32:600–609.
148. Ferrier GR, Moe GK. Effect of calcium on acetylstrophantidin-induced transient depolarizations in canine Purkinje tissue. *Circ Res* 1973; 33:508–515.
149. Hashimoto K, Moe GK. Transient depolarizations induced by acetylstrophantidin in specialized tissue of dog atrium and ventricle. *Circ Res* 1973; 32:618–624.
150. Hogan PM, Wittenberg SM, Kocke FJ. Relationship of stimulation frequency to automaticity in the canine Purkinje fiber during ouabain administration. *Circ Res* 1973; 32:377–384.
151. Aronson RS, Cranefield PF. The effect of resting potential on the electrical activity of canine cardiac Purkinje fibers exposed to Na-free solution or to ouabain. *Pflugers Arch* 1974; 347: 101–116.
152. Zipes DP, Arbel E, Knope RF, Moe GK. Accelerated cardiac escape rhythms caused by ouabain intoxication. *Am J Cardiol* 1974; 33:248–253.
153. Lown B, Cannon RL, Rossi MA. Electrical stimulation and digitalis drugs: Repetitive response in diastole. *Proc Soc Exp Biol Med* 1967; 126:697–701.
154. Lown B. Electrical stimulation to estimate the degree of digitalization: II. Experimental studies. *Am J Cardiol* 1968; 22:251–259.
155. Castellanos A, Lemberg L, Centurion MJ, Berkovits BV. Concealed digitalis-induced arrhythmias unmasked by electrical stimulation of the heart. *Am Heart J* 1967; 73:484–490.
156. Deitmer JW, Ellis D. The intracellular sodium activity of cardiac Purkinje fibers during inhibition and re-activation of the Na-K pump. *J Physiol* 1978; 284:241–259.
157. Lee CO, Dagostino M. Effect of strophantidin on intracellular Na ion activity and twitch tension of constantly driven cardiac Purkinje fibers. *Biophys J* 1982; 40:185–198.
158. Lee CO, Kang DH, Sokol JH, Lee KS. Relation between intracellular Na ion activity and tension of sheep cardiac Purkinje fibers exposed to dihydro-ouabain. *Biophys J* 1980; 29:315–330.
159. Reuter H, Seitz N. The dependence of calcium efflux from cardiac muscle on temperature and external ion composition. *J Physiol* 1968; 195:451–470.
160. Mullins JL. *Ion Transport in Heart.* New York: Raven Press; 1981.
161. Wit A, Cranefield PF. Triggered activity in cardiac muscle fibers of the simian mitral valve. *Circ Res* 1976; 38:85–98.
162. Boyden PA, Tilley LP, Albala A, et al. Mechanisms for atrial arrhythmias associated with cardiomyopathy: A study of feline hearts with primary myocardial disease. *Circ Res* 1984; 69:1036–1047.
163. Malfatto G, Rosen TS, Rosen MR. The response to overdrive pacing of triggered atrial and ventricular arrhythmias in the canine heart. *Circulation* 1988; 77:1139–1148.
164. Belardinelli L, Isenberg G. Actions of adenosine and isoproterenol on isolated mammalian ventricular myocyte. *Circ Res* 1983; 53:287–297.
165. Lazzara R, Marchi S. Electrophysiological mechanisms for the generation of arrhythmias with adrenergic stimulation. In: Brachman J, Schomig A, eds. *Adrenergic System and Ventricular Arrhythmias in Myocardial Infarction.* Heidelberg: Springer Verlag; 1989: 231.
166. Lerman BB, Belardinelli L, West A, et al. Adenosine-sensitive ventricular tachycardia: Evidence suggesting cyclic AMP-mediated triggered activity. *Circulation* 1986; 74:270–280.
167. El-Sherif N, Zeiler R, Gough WB. Effects of catecholamine, verapamil, and tetrodotoxin on triggered automaticity in canine ischemic Purkinje fibers (abstract). *Circulation* 1980; 62:III-281.
168. El-Sherif N, Gough WB, Zeiler RH, Mehra R. Triggered ventricular arrhythmias in one day old myocardial infarction in the dog. *Circ Res* 1983; 52:566–579.
169. Reuter H. Localization of beta adrenergic receptors and effects of noradrenaline and cyclic nucleotides on action potentials, ionic currents and tension in mammalian cardiac muscle. *J Physiol* 1974; 242:429–451.
170. Horn EM, Johnson NJ, Bilezikian JP, Rosen MR. Developmental changes in the electrophysiological properties and the beta-adrenergic receptor-effector complex in atrial fibers of the canine coronary sinus. *Circ Res* 1989; 65:325–333.
171. Morad M, Rolett E. Relaxing effect of catecholamine on mammalian heart. *J Physiol* 1972; 224:537–558.
172. Fabiato A. Calcium-induced release of calcium from the cardiac sarcoplasmic reticulum. *Am J Physiol* 1983; 245:C1–C14.
173. Saito T, Otoguro M, Matsubara T. Electrophysiological studies on the mechanism of electrically induced sustained rhythmic activity in the rabbit right atrium. *Circ Res* 1978; 42:199–206.
174. Mary-Rabine L, Hordof AJ, Danilo P, et al. Mechanisms for impulse initiation in isolated human atrial fibers. *Circ Res* 1980; 47:267–277.
175. Aronson RS. Afterpotentials and triggered activity in hypertrophied myocardium from rats with renal hypertension. *Circ Res* 1981; 48:720–727.
176. Nordin C, Gilat E, Aronson RS. Delayed afterdepolarizations and triggered activity in ventricular muscle from rats with streptozotocin-induced diabetes. *Circ Res* 1985; 57:28–34.
177. Arlock P, Katzung BG. Effects of sodium substitutes on transient inward current and tension in guinea-pig and ferret papillary muscle. *J Physiol* 1985; 360:105–120.
178. Ferrier G. Effects of transmembrane potential on oscillatory afterpotentials induced by acetylstrophantidin in canine ventricular tissues. *J Pharmacol Exp Ther* 1981; 215:332–341.
179. Wasserstrom JA, Ferrier GR. Voltage dependence of digitalis afterpotentials, aftercontractions, and inotropy. *Am J Physiol* 1981; 241:H646–H653.
180. Henning B, Wit AL. Action potential characteristics control after-

depolarization amplitude and triggered activity in canine coronary sinus. *Circulation* 1981; 64:IV–50.

181. LeMarec H, Dangman KH, Danilo P, Rosen MR. An evaluation of automaticity and triggered activity in the canine heart one to four days after myocardial infraction. *Circulation* 1985; 71:1224–1236.
182. Gough WB, El-Sherif N. Dependence of delayed afterdepolarizations on diastolic potentials in ischemic Purkinje fibers. *Am J Physiol* 1989; 257:H770–H777.
183. Wit AL, Tseng G-N, Henning B, Hanna MS. Arrhythmogenic effects of quinidine on catecholamine-induced delayed afterdepolarizations in canine atrial fibers. *J Cardiovasc Electrophysiol* 1990; 1:15–30.
184. Sheu SS, Lederer WJ. Lidocaine's negative inotropic and antiarrhythmic actions: Dependence on shortening of action potential duration and reduction of intracellular sodium activity. *Circ Res* 1985; 57:578–590.
185. Aronson RS. Characteristics of action potentials of hypertrophied myocardium from rats with renal hypertension. *Circ Res* 1980; 47:443–454.
186. Moak JP, Rosen MF. Induction and termination of triggered activity by pacing in isolated canine Purkinje fibers. *Circulation* 1984; 69:149–162.
187. Wit AL, Gadsby DC, Cranefield PF. Electrogenic sodium extrusion can stop triggered activity in the canine coronary sinus. *Circ Res* 1981; 49:1029–1042.
188. Johnson N, Danilo P, Wit A, Rosen MR. Response to pacing of triggered activity occurring in catecholamine-treated canine coronary sinus. *Circulation* 1986; 741:1168–1179.
189. Gadsby DC, Cranefield PF. Direct measurement of changes in sodium pump current in canine cardiac Purkinje fibers. *Proc Natl Acad Sci USA* 1979; 76:1783–1787.
190. Johnson N, Rosen MR. The distinction between triggered activity and other cardiac arrhythmias. In: Brugada P, Wellens HJJ, eds. *Cardiac Arrhythmias: Where to Go from Here*. Mount Kisco, NY: Futura; 1987:129.
191. Dangman KH, Hoffman BF. The effects of single premature stimuli on automatic and triggered rhythms in isolated canine Purkinje fibers. *Circulation* 1985; 71:813–822.
192. Trautwein W. Mechanisms of tachyarrhythmias and extrasystoles. In: Sandoe E, Flenstad-Jenson E, Olesen K, eds. *Symposium on Cardiac Arrhythmias*. Sodertalje, Sweden: AB Astra; 1970:53.
193. January CT, Shorofsky S. Early afterdepolarizations: Newer insights into cellular mechanisms. *J Cardiovasc Electrophysiol* 1990; 1:161–169.
194. Mendez C, Delmar M. Triggered activity: Its possible role in cardiac arrhythmias. In: Zipes DP, Jalife J, eds. *Cardiac Electrophysiology and Arrhythmias*. Orlando, FL: Grune & Stratton, 1985:311.
195. Kupersmith J, Hoff P. Occurrence and transmission of localized repolarization abnormalities in vitro. *J Am Coll Cardiol* 1985; 6:152–160.
196. Wit AL, Wiggins JR, Cranefield PF. Some effects of electrical stimulation on impulse initiation in cardiac fibers: Its relevance for the determination of the mechanisms of clinical cardiac arrhythmias. In: Wellens JH, Lie KI, Janse MJ, eds. *The Conduction System of the Heart*. Philadelphia: Lea & Febiger; 1976:163.
197. Antzelevitch C, Sicouri S. Clinical relevance of cardiac arrhythmias generated by afterdepolarizations: Role of M cells in the generation of U waves, triggered activity and torsade de pointes. *J Am Coll Cardiol* 1994; 23:259–277.
198. Damiano BP, Rosen MR. Effects of pacing on triggered activity induced by early afterdepolarizations. *Circulation* 1984; 69:1013–1025.
199. Brachmann J, Scherlag BJ, Rosenshtraukh LV, Lazzara R. Bradycardia dependent triggered activity: Relevance to drug-induced multiform ventricular tachycardia. *Circulation* 1983; 68:846–856.
200. Kay GN, Plumb VJ, Arciniegas JG, et al. Torsade de pointes: The long-short initiating sequence and other clinical features: Observations in 32 patients. *J Am Coll Cardiol* 1983; 2:806–817.
201. Ben David J, Zipes DP. Differential response to right and left ansae subclaviae stimulation of early afterdepolarizations and ventricular tachycardia induced by cesium in dogs. *Circulation* 1988; 78:1241–1250.
202. Levine JH, Spear JF, Guarnieri T, et al. Cesium chloride-induced long QT syndrome: Demonstration of afterdepolarizations and triggered activity in vivo. *Circulation* 1985; 72:1092–1104.
203. Strauss HC, Bigger JT Jr, Hoffman BF. Electrophysiological and beta-blocking effects of MJ 1999 on dog and rabbit cardiac tissue. *Circ Res* 1970; 26:661–678.
204. Carmeliet E. Electrophysiologic and voltage clamp analyses of the effects of sotalol on isolated cardiac muscle and Purkinje fibers. *J Pharmacol Exp Ther* 1985; 232:817–825.
205. Dangman KH, Hoffman BF. In vivo and in vitro antiarrhythmic and arrhythmogenic effects of N-acetylprocainamide. *J Pharmacol Exp Ther* 1981; 217:851–862.
206. Roden DM, Hoffman BF. Action potential prolongation and induction of abnormal automaticity by low quinidine concentrations in canine Purkinje fibers: Relationship to potassium and cycle length. *Circ Res* 1985; 56:857–867.
207. Davidenko JM, Cohen L, Goodrow R, Antzelevitch C. Quinidine-induced action potential prolongation, early afterdepolarizations, and triggered activity in canine Purkinje fibers: Effects of stimulation rate, potassium, and magnesium. *Circulation* 1989; 79:674–686.
208. Colatsky T. Mechanisms of action of lidocaine and quinidine on action potential duration in rabbit cardiac Purkinje fibers: An effect on steady-state sodium currents. *Circ Res* 1982; 50:17–27.
209. Selzer A, Wray HW. Quinidine syncope: Paroxysmal ventricular fibrillation occurring during treatment of chronic atrial arrhythmias. *Circulation* 1964; 30:17–26.
210. Smith WM, Gallagher JJ. "Les torsades de pointes": An unusual ventricular arrhythmia. *Ann Intern Med* 1980; 93:578–584.
211. Olshansky B, Martins J, Hunt S. *N*-acetyl procainamide causing torsades de pointes. *Am J Cardiol* 1982; 50:1439–1441.
212. Kuck KH, Kunze DP, Roewer N, Bleifield W. Sotalol-induced torsade de pointes. *Am Heart J* 1984; 107:179–180.
213. Bailie DS, Inoue H, Kaseda S, et al. Magnesium suppression of early afterdepolarizations and ventricular tachyarrhythmias induced by cesium in dogs. *Circulation* 1988; 77:1395–1402.
214. Tzivoni D, Keren A, Cohen AM, et al. Magnesium therapy for torsade de pointes. *Am J Cardiol* 1984; 53:528–530.
215. Perticone F, Adinolfi L, Bonaduce D. Efficacy of magnesium sulfate in the treatment of torsade de pointes. *Am Heart J* 1986; 112:847–849.
216. Lewis T. *The Mechanism and Graphic Registration of the Heart Beat*, 3d ed. London: Shaw Sons; 1925.
217. Smeets JLRM, Allessie MA, Lammers WJEP, et al. The wavelength of cardiac impulse and reentrant arrhythmias in isolated rabbit atrium: The role of heart rate, autonomic transmitters, temperature, and potassium. *Circ Res* 1986; 58:96–108.
218. Garrey W. The Nature of fibrillary contraction of the heart: Its relation to tissue mass and form. *Am J Physiol* 1914; 33:397–414.
219. El Sherif N, Carel EB, Yin H, Restivo M. The electrophysiological mechanism of ventricular arrhythmias in the long Q-T syndrome: Tri-dimensional mapping of activation and recovery patterns. *Circ Res* 1996; 79:474–492.
220. Coumel P, Cabrol C, Fabiato A, et al. Tachycardie permanente par rhythme reciproque. *Arch Mal Coeur Vaiss* 1967; 60:1830–1864.
221. Critelli G, Gallagher JJ, Monda V, et al. Anatomic and electrophysiologic substrate of the permanent form of junctional reciprocating tachycardia. *J Am Coll Cardiol* 1984; 4:601–610.
222. Wit AL, Cranefield PF, Hoffman BF. Slow conduction and reen-

try in the ventricular conducting system: II. Single and sustained circus movement in networks of canine and bovine Purkinje fibers. *Circ Res* 1972; 30:11–22.
223. Kall JH, Rubenstein DS, Kopp DE, et al. Atypical atrial flutter originating in the right atrial free wall. *Circulation* 2000; 101: 270–279.
224. Uno K, Kumagai K, Khrestian C, Waldo AL. New insights regarding the atrial flutter reentrant circuit: Studies in the canine sterile pericarditis model. *Circulation* 1999; 100:1354–1360.
225. Shimizu A, Nozaki A, Rudy Y, Waldo AL. Onset of induced atrial flutter in the canine pericarditis model. *J Am Coll Cardiol* 1991; 17:1223–1234.
226. Olshansky B, Okumura K, Hess PG, Waldo AL. Demonstration of an area of slow conduction in human atrial flutter. *J Am Coll Cardiol* 1990; 16:1639–1648.
227. Klein H, Karp RB, Kouchoukus NT, et al. Intraoperative electrophysiological mapping of the ventricles during sinus rhythm in patients with a previous myocardial infarction: Identification of the electrophysiological substrate for the generation of ventricular arrhythmias. *Circulation* 1982; 66:847–853.
228. Fozzard HA. Conduction of the action potential. In: Berne RM, ed. *The Cardiovascular System*. Bethesda, MD: American Physiological Society; 1979:335.
229. Weidmann S. The effect of the cardiac membrane potential on the rapid availability of the sodium carrying system. *J Physiol* 1955; 127:213–224.
230. Gettes LS, Reuter H. Slow recovery from inactivation of inward currents in mammalian myocardial fibers. *J Physiol* 1974; 240: 703–724.
231. Dodge FA, Cranefield PF. Nonuniform conduction in cardiac Purkinje fibers. In: Paes de Carvalho A, Hoffman BF, Lieberman M, eds. *Normal and Abnormal Conduction in the Heart*. Mount Kisco, NY: Futura; 1982:379.
232. Tisen RW. Calcium channels in excitable cell membranes. *Annu Rev Physiol* 1983; 45:341–358.
233. Zipes DP, Mendez C. Action of manganese ions and tetrodotoxin on atrioventricular nodal transmembrane potentials in isolated rabbit hearts. *Circ Res* 1973; 32:447–454.
234. Spach MS, Miller WT, Geselowitz DB, et al. The discontinuous nature of propagation in normal canine cardiac muscle: Evidence for recurrent discontinuities of intracellular resistance that effect membrane currents. *Circ Res* 1981; 48:39–54.
235. Spach MS, Miller WT, Dolber PC, et al. The functional role of structural complexities in the propagation of depolarization in the atrium of the dog: Cardiac conduction disturbances due to discontinuities of effective axial resistivity. *Circ Res* 1982; 50:175–191.
236. Sommer JR, Dolber PC. Cardiac muscle: The ultrastructure of its cells and bundles. In: Hoffman BF, Lieberman M, Paes de Carvallo A, eds. *Normal and Abnormal Conduction of the Heart Beat*. Mount Kisco, NY: Futura; 1982:1.
237. Hoyt RH, Cohen ML, Saffitz JE. Distribution and three-dimensional structure of intercellular junctions in canine myocardium. *Circ Res* 1989; 64:563–574.
238. Roberts DE, Hersh LT, Scher AM. Influence of cardiac fiber orientation on wavefront voltage, conduction velocity and tissue resistivity in the dog. *Circ Res* 1979; 44:701–712.
239. Clerc L. Directional differences of impulse spread in trabecular muscle from mammalian heart. *J Physiol* 1976; 255:335–346.
240. Saffitz JE, Kanter HL, Green KG, et al. Tissue-specific determinants of anisotropic conduction velocity in canine atrial and ventricular myocardium. *Circ Res* 1994; 74:1065–1070.
241. Spach MS, Dolber PC. Relating extracellular potentials and their derivatives to anisotropic propagation at a microscopic level in human cardiac muscle: Evidence for uncoupling of side-to-side fiber connections with increasing age. *Circ Res* 1986; 58:356–371.
242. Spach MS, Dolber PC, Heidlage JF. Influence of the passive anisotropic properties on directional differences in propagation following modification of the sodium conductance in human atrial muscle: A model of reentry based on anisotropic discontinuous propagation. *Circ Res* 1988; 62:811–832.
243. Hunter PJ, McNaughten PA, Noble D. Analytical models of propagation in excitable cells. *Prog Biophys Mol Biol* 1975; 30:99–144.
244. Dominguez C, Fozzard HA. Influence of extracellular K^+ concentration on cable properties and excitability of sheep cardiac Purkinje fibers. *Circ Res* 1970; 26:565–574.
245. Spach MS, Miller WT, Miller-Jones E, et al. Extracellular potentials related to intracellular action potentials during impulse conduction in anisotropic canine cardiac muscle. *Circ Res* 1979; 45:188–204.
246. Rudy Y, Quan W. A model study of the effects of the discrete cellular structure on electrical propagation in cardiac tissue. *Circ Res* 1987; 61:815–823.
247. Quan W, Rudy Y. Unidirectional block and reentry of cardiac excitation: A model study. *Circ Res* 1990; 60:367–382.
248. DeMello WC. Effect of intracellular injection of calcium and strontium in cell communication in heart. *J Physiol* 1975; 250:231–245.
249. Hess SP, Weingart R. Intracellular free calcium modified by pHi in sheep cardiac Purkinje fibres. *J Physiol* 1980; 307:60P–61P.
250. Van Dam RTh. *Experimenteel onderzoek naar het prikkelbaarheidsverloop van de hartspier*. Thesis. Amsterdam: University of Amsterdam, Klein Offsetdrukkerij Poortpers; 1960.
251. Rensma PL, Allessie MA, Lammers WJEP, et al. Length of excitation wave and susceptibility to reentrant atrial arrhythmias in normal conscious dogs. *Circ Res* 1988; 62:395–410.
252. Allessie MA, Bonke FIM, Schopman FJG. Circus movement in rabbit atrial muscle as a mechanism of tachycardia: 2. The role of nonuniform recovery of excitability in the occurrence of unidirectional block as studied with multiple microelectrodes. *Circ Res* 1976; 39:168–177.
253. Han J, Moe GK. Nonuniform recovery of excitability of ventricular muscle. *Circ Res* 1964; 14:44–60.
254. Janse MJ. *The Effects of Changes in Heart Rate on the Refractory Period of the Heart*. Thesis. Amsterdam: University of Amsterdam, Mondeel-Offsetdrukkerij; 1971.
255. Wallace AG, Mignone RS. Physiologic evidence concerning the reentry hypothesis for ectopic beats. *Am Heart J* 1966; 72:60–70.
256. Kuo C-S, Munakata K, Reddy CP, Surawicz B. Characteristics and possible mechanisms of ventricular arrhythmia dependent on the dispersion of action potential durations. *Circulation* 1983; 67:1356–1367.
257. Cranefield PK, Klein HO, Hoffman BF. Conduction of the cardiac impulse: 1. Delay, block and one-way block in the pressed Purkinje fibers. *Circ Res* 1971; 28:199–219.
258. Joyner RW, Overholt ED, Ramza B, Veenstra RD. Propagation through electrically coupled cells: Two inhomogeneously coupled cardiac tissue layers. *Am J Physiol* 1984; 247:H596–H609.
259. Goldstein SS, Rall W. Changes in action potential shape and velocity for changing core conductor geometry. *Biophys J* 1974; 14:731–757.
260. Overholt ED, Joyner RW, Veenstra RD, et al. Unidirectional block between Purkinje and ventricular layers of papillary muscles. *Am J Physiol* 1984; 247:H584–H595.
261. Janse MJ, Wilms-Schopman F, Wilensky RJ, Tranum-Jensen J. Role of the subendocardium in arrhythmogenesis during acute ischemia. In: Zipes DP, Jalife J, eds. *Cardiac Electrophysiology and Arrhythmias*, Orlando, FL: Grune & Stratton, 1985:353.
262. Gilmour RF, Evans JJ, Zipes DP. Purkinje-muscle coupling and endocardial response to hyperkalemia, hypoxia, and acidosis. *Am J Physiol* 1984; 247:H303–H311.
263. Gilmour RF, Evans JJ, Zipes DP. Preferential interruption of impulse transmission across Purkinje-muscle junctions by inter-

ventions that depress conduction. In: Zipes DP, Jalife J, eds. *Cardiac Electrophysiology and Arrhythmias*, Orlando, FL: Grune & Stratton; 1985:287.

264. Delmar M, Michaels DC, Johnson T, Jalife J. Effects of increasing intercellular resistance on transverse and longitudinal propagation in sheep epicardial muscle. *Circ Res* 1987; 60:780–785.
265. Delgado C, Steinhaus B, Delmar M, et al. Directional differences in excitability and margin of safety for propagation in sheep ventricular epicardial muscle. *Circ Res* 1990; 67:97–110.
266. Frame LH, Page RL, Boyden PA, et al. Circus movement in the canine atrium around the tricuspid ring during experimental atrial flutter and during reentry in vitro. *Circulation* 1987; 76: 1155–1175.
267. Moe GK. On the multiple wavelet hypothesis of atrial fibrillation. *Arch Int Pharmacodyn Ther* 1962; 140:180–188.
268. Moe GK, Rheinboldt WC, Abildskov JA. A computer model of atrial fibrillation. *Am Heart J* 1964; 67:200–220.
269. Coumel P. Role of the autonomic nervous system in paroxysmal atrial fibrillation. In: Touboul P, Waldo AL, eds. *Atrial Arrhythmias*. St Louis: Mosby–Year Book; 1990:248.
270. Allessie MA, Lammers WJEP, Bonke FIM, Hollen J. Experimental evaluation of Moe's multiple wavelet hypothesis of atrial fibrillation. In: Zipes DP, Jalife J, eds. *Cardiac Electrophysiology and Arrhythmias*. New York: Grune & Stratton, 1985:265.
271. Waldo AL. Mechanisms of atrial fibrillation, atrial flutter, and ectopic atrial tachycardia—A brief review. *Circulation* 1987; 75-III:37–40.
272. Allessie MA, Bonke FIM, Schopman FJG. Circus movement in rabbit atrial muscle as a mechanism of tachycardia: 3. The "leading circle" concept—A new model of circus movement in cardiac tissue without the involvement of an anatomical obstacle. *Circ Res* 1977; 41:9–18.
273. Allessie MA, Lammers WJEP, Bonke FIM, Hollen J. Intra-atrial reentry as a mechanism for atrial flutter by acetylcholine and rapid pacing in the dog. *Circulation* 1984; 70:123–135.
274. Boyden PA. Activation sequence during atrial flutter in dogs with surgically induced right atrial enlargement: I. Observations during sustained rhythms. *Circ Res* 1988; 62:596–608.
275. Cosio FG. Endocardial mapping of atrial flutter. In: Touboul P, Waldo AL, eds. *Atrial Arrhythmias: Current Concepts and Management*. St Louis: Mosby–Year Book; 1990:229.
276. Spinelli W, Hoffman BF. Mechanisms of termination of reentrant atrial arrhythmias by class I and class III antiarrhythmic agents. *Circ Res* 1989; 65:1565–1579.
277. Wit AL, Dillon SM. Anisotropic reentry. In: Zipes DP, Jalife J, eds. *Cardiac Electrophysiology: From Cell to Bedside*. Philadelphia: Saunders; 1990:353.
278. Allessie MA, Bonke FIM, Schopman FJG. Circus movement in rabbit atrial muscle as a mechanism of tachycardia. *Circ Res* 1973; 32:54–62.
279. Dillon S, Allessie MA, Ursell PC, Wit AL. Influence of anisotropic tissue structure on reentrant circuits and the sub-epicardial border zone of subacute canine infarcts. *Circ Res* 1988; 63:182–206.
280. Schalij MJ. *Anisotropic Conduction and Ventricular Tachycardia*. PhD thesis. Maastricht, the Netherlands: University of Limburg; 1988.
281. Peters NS, Coromilas J, Hanna MS, et al. Characteristics of the temporal and spatial excitable gap in anisotropic reentrant circuits causing sustained ventricular tachycardia. *Circ Res* 1998; 82:279–293.
282. Winfree AT. Electrical instability in cardiac muscle: Phase singularities and rotors. *J Theor Biol* 1989; 138:353–405.
283. Winfree AT. Ventricular reentry in three dimensions. In: Zipes DP, Jalife J, eds. *Cardiac Electrophysiology: From Cell to Bedside*. Philadelphia: Saunders; 1990:224.
284. Courtemanche M, Winfree AT. Re-entrant rotating waves in a Beeler-Reuter based model of two-dimensional cardiac electrical activity. *Int J Bifurc Chaos* 1991; 1:431–444.
285. Davidenko JM, Kent PF, Chialvo DR, et al. Sustained vortex-like waves in normal isolated ventricular muscle. *Proc Natl Acad Sci USA* 1990; 87:8785–8789.
286. Jalife J, Davidenko J, Michaels DC. A new perspective on the mechanisms of arrhythmias and sudden cardiac death: Spiral waves of excitation in heart muscle. *J Cardiovasc Electrophysiol* 1991; 2(suppl 3):S133–S152.
287. Winfree AT. Vortex action potentials in normal ventricular muscle. In: Jalife J, ed. *Mathematical Approaches to Cardiac Arrhythmias. Ann NY Acad Sci* 1990; 591:190–207.
288. Shibata N, Chen P-S, Dixon EG, et al. Influence of shock strength and timing on induction of ventricular arrhythmias in dogs. *Am J Physiol* 1988; 225:H891–H901.
289. Chen P-S, Wolf PD, Dixon EG, et al. Mechanism of ventricular vulnerability to single premature stimuli in open-chest dogs. *Circ Res* 1988; 62:1191–1209.
290. Mayer AG. Rhythmical pulsation in Scyphomedusae: II. *Pap Tortugas Lab Carnegie Inst Wash* 1908; 1:113–131.
291. Mines GR. On circulating excitation in heart muscles and their possible relations to tachycardia and fibrillation. *Trans R Soc Can* 1914; 8(ser III, sec IV):43–52.
292. Goldreyer BN, Gallagher JJ, Damato AN. The electrophysiologic demonstration of atrial ectopic tachycardia in man. *Am Heart J* 1973; 85:205–215.
293. Scheinman MM, Basu D, Holenberg M. Electrophysiologic studies in patients with persistent atrial tachycardia. *Circulation* 1974; 50:266–273.
294. Strauss HC, Saroff AL, Bigger JT Jr, Giardina GV. Premature atrial stimulation as a key to the understanding of sinoatrial conduction in man: Presentation of data and critical review of the literature. *Circulation* 1973; 47:86–93.
295. Gillette PC, Garson A Jr. Electrophysiologic and pharmacologic characteristics of automatic ectopic atrial tachycardia. *Circulation* 1977; 56:571–575.
296. Klein HO, Cranefield PF, Hoffman BF. Effect of extrasystoles on idioventricular rhythm. *Circ Res* 1972; 30:651–665.
297. Palileo EV, Ashley WW, Swiryn S, et al. Exercise provokable right ventricular outflow tract tachycardia. *Am Heart J* 1982; 104:185–193.
298. Sung RJ, Shen EN, Morady F, et al. Electrophysiologic mechanism of exercise-induced sustained ventricular tachycardia. *Am J Cardiol* 1983; 51:525–530.
299. Wellens HJJ. Value and limitations of programmed electrical stimulation of the heart in the study and treatment of tachycardias. *Circulation* 1978; 57:845–853.
300. Goldreyer BN, Bigger JT Jr. Site of reentry in paroxysmal supraventricular tachycardia in man. *Circulation* 1971; 43:15–26.
301. Bigger JT Jr, Goldreyer BN. The mechanism of supraventricular tachycardia. *Circulation* 1970; 42:673–688.
302. Waldo AL. Cardiac pacing: Role in diagnosis and treatment of disorders of cardiac rhythm and conduction. In: Rosen MRR, Hoffman BF, eds. *Cardiac Therapy*. Boston: Martinus Nijhoff; 1983:299.
303. Waldo AL, MacLean WAH, Karp RB, et al. Entrainment and interruption of atrial flutter with atrial pacing: Studies in man following open heart surgery. *Circulation* 1977; 56:737–744.
304. Waldo AL, Plumb VJ, Henthorn RW. Observations on the mechanism of atrial flutter. In: Surawicz B, Reddy CP, Prystowsky EN, eds. *Tachycardias*. The Hague: Martinus Nijhoff; 1984:213.
305. Olshansky B, Okumura K, Henthorn RW, Waldo AL. Characterization of double potentials in human atrial flutter: Studies during transient entrainment. *J Am Coll Cardiol* 1990; 15:833–841.
306. Waldo AL. Some observations concerning atrial flutter in man. *PACE* 1983; 6:1181–1189.
307. MacLean WAH, Plumb VJ, Waldo AL. Transient entrainment

and interruption of ventricular tachycardia. *PACE* 1981; 4:358–366.
308. Waldo AL, Henthorn RW, Plumb VJ, MacLean WAH. Demonstration of the mechanism of transient entrainment and interruption of ventricular tachycardia with rapid atrial pacing. *J Am Coll Cardiol* 1984; 3:422–430.
309. Okumura K, Olshansky B, Henthorn RW, et al. Demonstration of the presence of slow conduction during sustained ventricular tachycardia in man. *Circulation* 1987; 75:369–378.
310. Waldo AL, Plumb VJ, Arciniegas JG, et al. Transient entrainment and interruption of AV bypass pathway type paroxysmal atrial tachycardia: A model for understanding and identifying reentrant arrhythmias in man. *Circulation* 1982; 67:73–83.
311. Okumura K, Henthorn RW, Epstein AE, et al. Further observations on transient entrainment: Importance of pacing site and properties of the components of the reentry circuit. *Circulation* 1985; 72:1293–1307.
312. Brugada P, Waldo AL, Wellens HJJ. Transient entrainment and interruption of atrioventricular tachycardia. *J Am Coll Cardiol* 1987; 9:769–775.
313. Henthron RW, Okumura K, Olshansky B, Waldo AL. A fourth criterion for transient entrainment: The electrogram equivalent of progressive fusion. *Circulation* 1988; 77:1003–1012.
314. Chen P-S, Lowe JE, German LD, et al. Mapping ventricular fusion beats during entrainment. *Circulation* 1986; 74–II:484.
315. El-Sherif N, Gough WB, Restivo M. Reentrant ventricular arrhythmias in the late myocardial infarction period: 14. Mechanisms of resetting, entrainment, acceleration, or termination of reentrant tachycardia by programmed electrical stimulation. *PACE* 1987; 10:341–371.
316. Waldecker B, Coromilas J, Saltman AE, et al. Overdrive stimulation of functional reentrant circuits causing ventricular tachycardia in the infarcted canine heart—Resetting and entrainment. *Circulation* 1993; 87:1286–1305.
317. Boyden PA, Frame LH, Hoffman BF. Activation mapping of reentry around an anatomic barrier in the canine atrium. *Circulation* 1989; 79:406–416.
318. Shimizu A, Nozaki A, Rudy Y, Waldo AL. Multiplexing studies of effects of rapid atrial pacing on the area of slow conduction during atrial flutter in canine pericarditis model. *Circulation* 1991; 83:983–994.
319. Frank R, Tonet JL, Kounde S, et al. Localization of the area of slow conduction during ventricular tachycardia. In: Brugada P, Wellen HJJ, eds. *Cardiac Arrhythmias: Where to Go From Here?* Mount Kisco, NY: Futura; 1987:191.
320. Morady F, Frank R, Kou WH, et al. Identification and catheter ablation of a zone of slow conduction in the reentrant circuit of ventricular tachyardia in humans. *J Am Coll Cardiol* 1988; 11:775–782.
321. Stevenson WG, Weiss JN, Wiener I, et al. Resetting of ventricular tachycardia: Implications for localizing the area of slow conduction. *J Am Coll Cardiol* 1988; 11:522–529.
322. Almendral JM, Rosenthal ME, Stamato NJ, et al. Analysis of the resetting phenomenon in sustained uniform ventricular tachycardia: Incidence and relation to termination. *J Am Coll Cardiol* 1986; 8:294–300.
323. Almendral JM, Stamato NJ, Rosenthal ME, et al. Resetting response patterns during sustained ventricular tachycardia: Relationship to the excitable gap. *Circulation* 1986; 74:722–730.
324. Stamato NJ, Rosenthal ME, Almendral JM, Josephson ME. The resetting response ventricular tachycardia to single and double extrastimuli: Implications for an excitable gap. *Am J Cardiol* 1987; 60:596–601.
325. Bernstein RC, Frame LH. Ventricular reentry around a fixed barrier: Resetting with advancement in an in vitro model. *Circulation* 1990; 81:267–280.
326. Frame LH, Page RL, Hoffman BF. Atrial reentry around an anatomic barrier with a partially refractory excitable gap. *Circ Res* 1986; 58:495–511.
327. Rosen MR, Fisch C, Hoffman BF, et al. Can accelerated atrioventricular junctional escape rhythms be explained by delayed afterdepolarizations? *Am J Cardiol* 1980; 45:1272–1284.
328. Rosen MR, Reder RF. Does triggered activity have a role in the genesis of cardiac arrhythmias? *Ann Intern Med* 1981; 94:794–801.
329. Gorgels APM, Beekman HDM, Brugada P, et al. Extrastimulus-related shortening of the first post pacing interval in digitalis-induced ventricular tachycardia: Observations during programmed electrical stimulation in the conscious dog. *J Am Coll Cardiol* 1983; 1:840–857.
330. Wit AL, Rosen MR. Afterdepolarizations and triggered activity. In: Fozzard HA, Jennings RB, Haber E, et al, eds. *The Heart and Cardiovascular System: Scientific Foundations*. New York: Raven Press; 1986:1449.
331. Akhtar M. Supraventricular tachycardias: Electrophysiologic mechanisms, diagnosis, and pharmacologic therapy. In: Josephson ME, Wellens HJJ, eds. *Tachycardias: Mechanisms, Diagnosis, Treatment*. Philadelphia: Lea & Febiger; 1984:137.
332. Josephson ME, Marchlinski FE, Buxton AE, et al. Electrophysiologic basis for sustained ventricular tachycardia—Role of reentry. In: Josephson ME, Wellens HJJ, eds. *Tachycardias: Mechanisms, Diagnosis, Treatment*. Philadelphia: Lea & Febiger; 1984:305.
333. Vos MA, Gorgels APM, Leunisse JDM, et al. The effect of an entrainment protocol on ouabain-induced ventricular tachycardia. *PACE* 1989; 12:1485–1493.
334. Brugada P, Wellens HJJ. Programmed electrical stimulation of the human heart: General principles. In: Josephson ME, Wellens HJJ, eds. *Tachycardias: Mechanisms, Diagnosis, Treatment*. Philadelphia: Lea & Febiger; 1984:61.
335. Jackman WM, Clark M, Friday KJ, et al. Ventricular tachyarrhythmias in the long QT syndromes. *Med Clin North Am* 1984; 68:107–1109.
336. Schecter E, Freeman CC, Lazzara R. Afterdepolarizations as a mechanism for the long QT syndrome: Electrophysiologic studies of a case. *J Am Coll Cardiol* 1984; 3:1556–1561.
337. Coumel P, LeClercq J, Dessertenne F. Torsades de pointes. In: Josephson ME, Wellens HJJ, eds. *Tachycardia: Mechanisms, Diagnosis, Treatment*. Philadelphia: Lea & Febiger; 1984:325.

CHAPTER 24

RECOGNITION, CLINICAL ASSESSMENT, AND MANAGEMENT OF ARRHYTHMIAS AND CONDUCTION DISTURBANCES

Robert J. Myerburg / E. Martín Kloosterman / Agustin Castellanos

The diagnosis and management of cardiac arrhythmias and conduction disturbances require the coordination of (1) electrocardiographic (ECG) analysis of the rhythm disturbance, (2) assessment of the clinical setting, and (3) identification of an end point and method of therapy.[1]

ECG recognition of arrhythmias requires an organized system of analysis of atrial and ventricular myocardial activation and deduction of atrioventricular (AV) conduction patterns. Forms of arrhythmias are separated into those that cause limited symptoms but may trigger symptomatic sustained arrhythmias under appropriate conditions (e.g., premature atrial or ventricular impulses) and those that are sustained symptomatic and/or potentially fatal arrhythmias [e.g., supraventricular tachycardias (SVTs), ventricular tachycardias (VTs), ventricular fibrillation (VF), or bradycardias] (Table 24-1).

Clinical settings are broadly divided into those that are acute or transient, such as acute ischemia, the acute phase of myocardial infarction, electrolyte disturbances, or proarrhythmic effects of antiarrhythmic drugs, and those that provide a persistent substrate for arrhythmias, such as chronic ischemic heart disease, cardiomyopathies, and anatomic and physiologic substrates for the various paroxysmal supraventricular tachyarrhythmias.[2,3] Analogous to the concept of "triggering" and "sustained" arrhythmias, transient ischemia and hemodynamic disturbances may be viewed as triggering events and chronic ischemic heart disease and the hypertrophied or myopathic heart as sustaining substrates.

The goals, or end points, of therapy of cardiac arrhythmias are dependent on the forms, clinical settings, and mechanisms of arrhythmia. Broadly, goals of treatment may be antiarrhythmic (targeted to the suppression of ambient or triggering arrhythmias or events) or antitachycardiac, antifibrillatory, or heart-rate supporting (in which the goal is prevention or reversion of sustained arrhythmias), whether the arrhythmias are well tolerated, symptomatic, or life-threatening.

PRINCIPLES OF CARDIAC RHYTHM ANALYSIS

The Standard Electrocardiogram

The standard 12-lead ECG and rhythm strips provide a direct and easily accessible method for diagnosing disturbances of

TABLE 24-1 Assessment of Cardiac Arrhythmias

Forms of cardiac arrhythmias
Ambient or triggering arrhythmias (e.g., premature atrial or ventricular impulses)
Sustained or potentially lethal arrhythmias (e.g., supraventricular or ventricular tachycardias, ventricular fibrillation, sustained bradyarrhythmias)
Clinical settings in which arrhythmias occur
Acute, transient (e.g., acute ischemic events, metabolic disturbances)
Chronic, persistent, recurrent (e.g., chronic ischemic heart disease, cardiomyopathy, anatomic or physiologic substrate for paroxysmal supraventricular tachycardia, chronic conducting system disease)
End points of management
Antiarrhythmia (suppress ambient or triggering arrhythmias)
Antitachycardia or antifibrillatory (prevent or revert tachycardias or fibrillation)
Heart rate support (prevent symptomatic bradycardias)

SOURCE: Modified from Myerburg et al.,[1] with permission of the *American Heart Journal.*

cardiac rhythm. The simultaneous-lead rhythm strip accompanying the 12-lead ECG on many current ECG machines, plus the option of recording longer multilead rhythm strips, will yield sufficient information for a prompt and accurate diagnosis of most cardiac rhythm disturbances.

For many arrhythmias, analysis requires only the recognition of P-wave and QRS morphology, their relative timing, and their vectors. Simple inspection of the tracing, with caliper-assisted measurements, may be sufficient; but the analysis of more complex arrhythmias is facilitated by the use of ladder diagrams. First used extensively by Sir Thomas Lewis, they are also referred to as Lewis lines. The ladders are usually constructed with three tiers—A, AV, and V (Fig. 24-1*A*)—but additional tiers may be helpful in depicting events related to sinoatrial (SA) conduction (Fig. 24-1*B*) or ventricular ectopic rhythms (Fig. 24-1*C*). The A and V tiers are used to depict activation of atrial and ventricular muscle, respectively. The middle tier (AV) is used to infer conduction characteristics in the AV junction. Since atrial and ventricular activation are the only direct registrations of cardiac electrical activity on the standard ECG, they are diagrammed first. The A line is drawn from the beginning of the P wave and the V line from the beginning of the QRS. Time is indicated by the slope of the line, and the site within a tier in which impulse propagation begins (upper, middle, or lower) shows the direction the impulse is traveling. The site of origin may be represented by a black dot. A blocked impulse is indicated by a short bar at a right angle to the line indicating direction of conduction, and aberrant intraventricular conduction is shown as a pair of slightly divergent lines. A variety of such examples are shown in Fig. 24-1. In using the diagram, particularly for complex arrhythmias, the first caution is to draw only what can be seen or inferred with certainty. Subsequently, the AV tier can be used to diagram proposed mechanisms of conduction (Fig. 24-2).

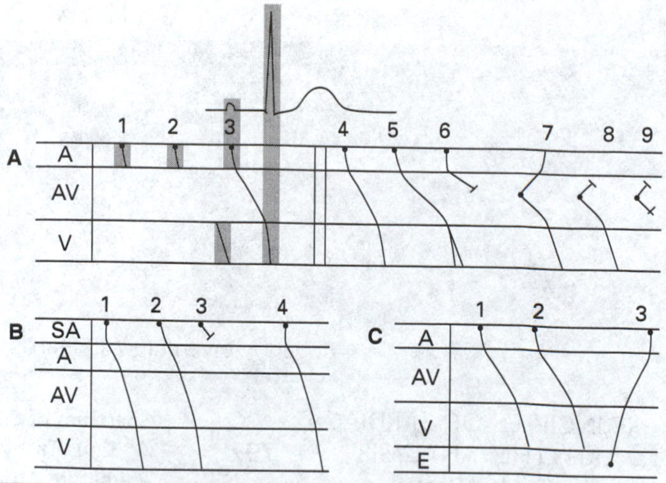

FIGURE 24-1 Ladder diagrams for analysis of cardiac arrhythmias. *A.* Charting of P wave, QRS complexes, and deduction of conduction relationships for a normal sinus impulse are demonstrated in *A1* to *A3*. The diversion of lines shown in the V level in *A5* is used to indicate aberrant intraventricular conduction, and the incomplete cross-hatched line in the AV level in *A6* represents an impulse blocked in the AV junction. The AV junctional impulses with retrograde and antegrade conduction (*A7*), retrograde block and antegrade conduction (*A8*), and block in both directions, resulting in a concealed extrasystole (*A9*), are shown next. *B.* Diagram used to analyze sinoatrial conduction is demonstrated. A sinus impulse that fails to conduct to the atrium is indicated as in *B3*. *C.* Ventricular ectopic activity (E) is depicted as shown in *C3*, which represents a premature ventricular contraction with retrograde conduction to the atrium.

Special Leads

When the standard ECG does not provide sufficient information to establish a diagnosis, usually due to inability to identify P waves, special lead systems may be used. The simplest is the Lewis lead configuration, in which the right and left arm electrodes are deployed as a bipolar lead to the right of the sternum in a superior-inferior orientation.

A bipolar esophageal lead can record left atrial activity, and an intraatrial electrode catheter can record atrial activity from within the right atrium. For both techniques, it is necessary to have at least one standard surface ECG lead recorded simultaneously with the special lead.

Continuous Monitor Recordings

Continuous monitoring of cardiac rhythm may be performed in hospital in special care units or in the ambulatory patient using various types of portable recording devices. Some systems provide the capability for simultaneous multilead recordings that improve diagnostic yield considerably. Long-term storage capabilities for inpatient monitoring permit off-line analysis of complex rhythm disturbances if the physician is not available at the time the arrhythmia occurs. The two most popular leads for use in bedside monitoring are lead II and MCL-I, the latter providing a pattern similar to V_1.

For infrequently occurring arrhythmias, a number of event recorders are now available. They allow the patient to activate the device when an event occurs, providing internal storage that can be transmitted by telephone to a central station for later review. Transtelephonic transmitters also can be used in

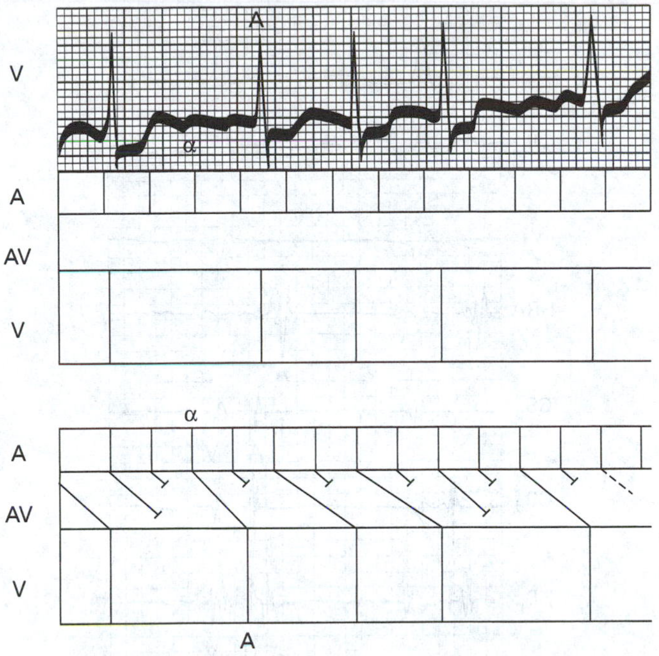

FIGURE 24-2 Construction of ladder diagrams for analyzing specific arrhythmias. *Stage 1:* Draw lines to represent atrial activity (seen and inferred by measurement) and ventricular complexes. *Stage 2:* Since the FR interval in flutter usually ranges between 0.26 and 0.45 s, start by connecting the F wave (α) to the QRS (A) in this example. As successive impulses are diagrammed, it becomes apparent that there is a basic 2:1 AV conduction with a Wenckebach period during the alternate cycles. (From Marriott HJL. *Armchair Arrhythmias.* Tampa, FL: Tampa Tracings; 1966. Reproduced with permission from the publisher and authors.)

real time for more persistent or frequent events. Finally, a small subcutaneous implantable recorder is available for patients with infrequent arrhythmias that warrant an aggressive documentation attempt.[4] The device may be explanted after a diagnosis is established.

Exercise Testing for Cardiac Arrhythmias

Treadmill stress testing may be used to initiate an evanescent arrhythmia, document an exercise relationship to its onset, and evaluate both efficacy and adverse responses to therapy. The standard treadmill is used, and thallium or echocardiographic imaging is not necessary unless an ischemic basis correlating with the onset of arrhythmia is suspected. The procedure is especially useful for eliciting and evaluating therapy of exercise-induced ventricular arrhythmias, for distinguishing autonomic from structural disease mechanisms of sinus or AV node dysfunction, and for evaluating adverse effects of drug therapy, such as rate-dependent proarrhythmic effects, as may occur with strong Na^+-channel blockers, such as flecainide[5] (see below).

Exercise testing may also provide some general insights into the refractory period of an accessory pathway in Wolff-Parkinson-White (WPW) syndrome. Abrupt disappearance of the delta wave during exercise-induced increase in heart rate suggests encroachment on the refractory period, while gradual disappearance may simply be due to enhanced AV nodal conduction.[6]

Signal-Averaged Electrocardiography, Heart Rate Variability, and Baroreceptor Sensitivity

Signal-averaged electrocardiography, heart rate variability, and baroreceptor sensitivity provide information on mortality risk and the probability of life-threatening arrhythmias, whether used separately or combined with other estimates of risk [e.g., premature ventricular contractions (PVCs) and nonsustained VT on 24-h ambulatory monitoring and ejection fraction (EF) measurements]. They have been applied most intensively after myocardial infarction.

Signal-averaged electrocardiography employs amplification of low-amplitude signals occurring after the termination of the standard electrocardiographic QRS complex, as recorded by high-amplification techniques. The low-amplitude signals are repetitive electrical events caused by a delayed activation sequence of part or parts of the ventricular muscle mass. Their repetitive timing allows them to be amplified during signal averaging, while random noise is being canceled out. The resultant signal is a high-gain, high-frequency QRS complex, followed by low-amplitude signals representing the late potentials. The terminal delayed activation pattern represents a pathophysiologic marker for susceptibility to ventricular arrhythmias. It results from fragmented activation in an area of delayed conduction, which is a well-established substrate for reentrant arrhythmias. The characteristics of an abnormal signal-averaged ECG include (1) a prolonged filtered QRS complex (115 ms) with a normal duration of the standard QRS complex, (2) the terminal portion of the filtered QRS complex less than 40 μV for 39 ms, and (3) less than 20 μV of amplitude during the last 40 ms of the filtered QRS complex.[7] At least two of the three criteria must be abnormal to consider the tracing abnormal, and many would require all three to be abnormal (Fig. 24-3). Residual high-frequency

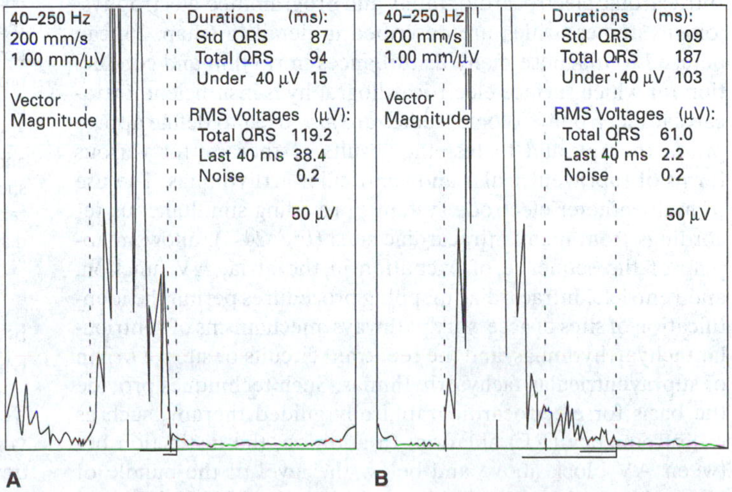

FIGURE 24-3 *A.* Normal signal-averaged vector complex. *B.* Abnormal signal-averaged vector complex. All three signal-averaged measurements are abnormal. The signal-averaged QRS duration is 187 ms, low-amplitude signals are 103 ms in duration, and the root-mean-square voltage is 2.2 μV. (Courtesy of Paul F. Walter, M.D.)

noise content must be less than 1 μV with a 25-Hz high-pass cutoff (less than 0.7 μV with a 40-Hz high-pass cutoff).

Signal-averaged electrocardiography is most useful for demonstrating presence and absence of risk for ventricular arrhythmias and sudden death after myocardial infarction.[8] It is most powerful as a negative predictor of risk, in that a normal signal-averaged ECG after healing of myocardial infarction identifies a greater than 97 percent probability of remaining free of ventricular arrhythmias. The positive predictive accuracy is less powerful and is heavily influenced by other variables, such as EF and ambient ventricular arrhythmias. Signal-averaged electrocardiography alone has a positive predictive value in the range of 20 percent, and combined with a low EF and ambient arrhythmias, the risk may be as high as 50 percent in some subgroups (see "Ventricular Arrhythmias," below).

Heart rate variability studies provide estimates of sympathetic and parasympathetic balance.[9] Blunting of the normal patterns of variability of sinus rate over time in subgroups of myocardial infarction and cardiac arrest survivors appears to increase the risk of life-threatening events.[9,10] As is the case for signal-averaged electrocardiography, the test is used primarily for prognostic information rather than as a therapeutic guide.

Baroreceptor sensitivity estimates the relationship between phenylephrine-induced blood pressure increase and concomitant fall in heart rate as an indication of parasympathetic responsiveness to the pure α-adrenergic stimulus.[11] Following a myocardial infarction, a blunted baroreceptor sensitivity predicts an increased risk of VT and death. A recent large study also demonstrated its power for predicting adverse outcome following a myocardial infarction, which was further enhanced when combined with other risk variables, such as low EF and ambient arrhythmias.[12]

Intracardiac Electrocardiography and Programmed Electrophysiologic Studies

Intracardiac electrocardiography and programmed electrophysiologic studies, which are described in detail in Chap. 26, can be used to diagnose many disturbances in rhythm and conduction for which surface electrocardiography is insufficient. Intracardiac electrophysiologic studies are also used to define appropriate therapy and to test the results of therapy for various forms of supraventricular and ventricular arrhythmias. The use of multicatheter electrode systems, providing simultaneous recordings from many intracardiac sites (Fig. 24-4), allows mapping of the sequence of excitation in the atria, AV junction, and ventricle. Intracardiac mapping procedures permit the identification of sites of accessory pathways, mechanisms of ventricular tachyarrhythmias, and the reentrant circuits or sites of origin of supraventricular tachyarrhythmias. Such techniques provide the basis for electrocardiographically guided therapy, such as radiofrequency (RF) ablation. In addition, the distinction between AV block above and below the level of the bundle of His and between true AV block and pseudo-AV block caused by concealed extrasystoles is also possible. Specific clinical applications are provided in the appropriate sections below and in Chap. 26.

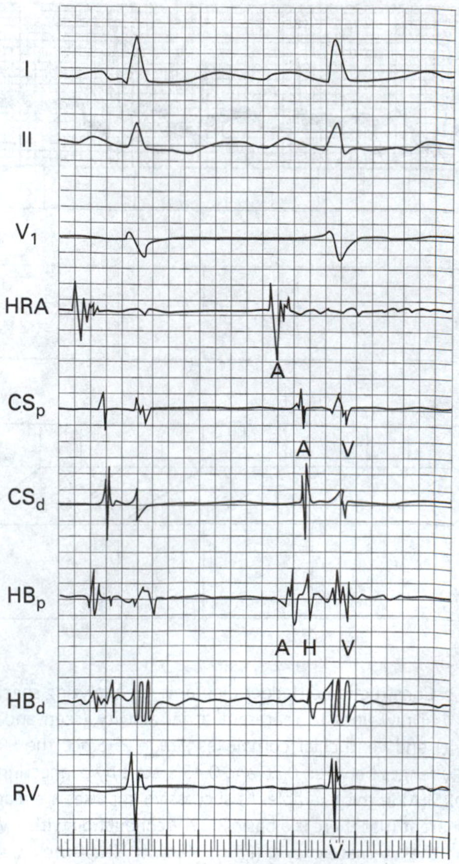

FIGURE 24-4 Intracardiac recordings during electrophysiologic testing. Recordings during sinus rhythm in a multicatheter study are illustrated. The intracardiac study includes the recording of atrial activity (A), the His bundle deflection (H), and ventricular activity (V) used to determine the timing and sequences of activation at various intracardiac sites. A activity is recorded from the high right atrium (HRA); and both A and V activity are recorded from a proximal (HBp) and distal (HBd) site in the His bundle region and from proximal (CSp) and distal (CSd) sites within the coronary sinus. The CS sites record atrial and ventricular activity from the posterior-posteroseptal and posterolateral-lateral areas, respectively. V activity is also recorded from the right ventricle (RV), either the apex or outflow tract, depending upon the positioning of the catheter in the right ventricle. For more detailed mapping procedures, more sites in the coronary sinus or sites around the tricuspid ring can be recorded, or the left ventricle can be mapped by a retrograde recording catheter from the femoral artery. Less extensive studies using fewer catheters and recording sites can be used for different clinical purposes. The configuration shown is standard for studies of supraventricular tachycardias. For ventricular tachycardia studies, three catheters can be used (HRA, HB, and RV) for the diagnostic study.

Endocardial Catheter Mapping and Intraoperative Multiarray Epicardial Mapping

Techniques for mapping pathways and sites of origin for both ventricular and supraventricular tachyarrhythmias, originally developed for intraoperative mapping during antiarrhythmic surgery, have found broad application in catheter-based procedures. Greatly improved catheter-ablation techniques for many arrhythmias, in conjunction with the development of sophisticated computer-based recording, storage, and retrieval systems,[13,14] have limited the role of intraoperative mapping and interventions with the expansion of catheter techniques. The new mapping systems allow simultaneous recordings from many points, generating on-line maps of activation during a procedure. This technology allows the clinical electrophysiologist to identify target areas for delivery of RF energy during an ablation procedure. Figure 24-5 (Plate 74), provides an example of a computer-generated atrial endocardial activation map from such a system, demonstrating a focal atrial tachycardia. The technique of left ventricular (LV) endocardial catheter mapping for identification of sites appropriate for catheter ablation of VT is demonstrated in Fig. 24-6. Computer-generated maps are now also available for ventricular arrhythmias.

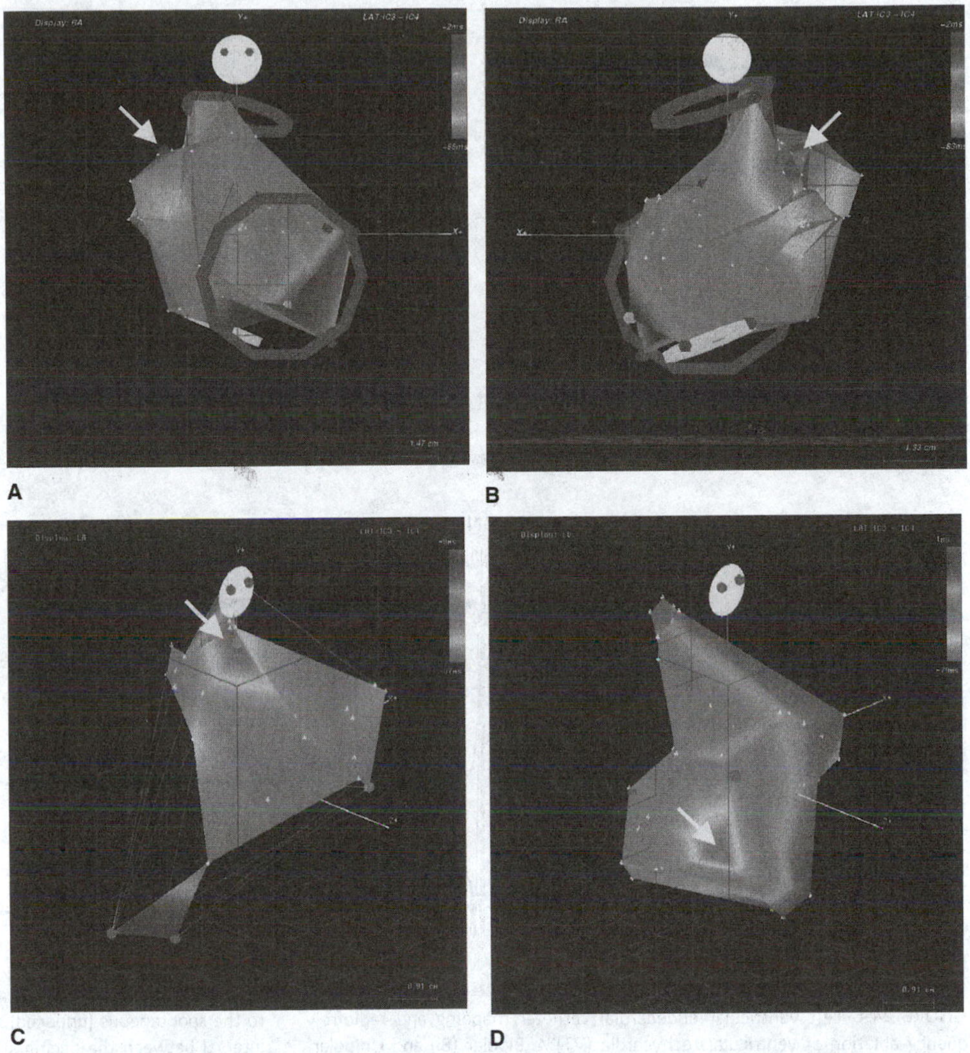

FIGURE 24-5 (Plate 74) Catheter-based mapping of the right atrium using a nonfluoroscopic electroanatomic mapping system that allows computer storage and recall of multisite activation patterns. Panels A and B demonstrate the activation sequence during normal sinus rhythm, with the earliest activation in the region of the sinus node (*arrows*) shown from (*A*) anterior and (*B*) posterior perspectives. The sequence of activation is indicated by the gradation of the color scale, based upon the reference times shown in the spectral bar. *C* and *D* were recorded from another patient who had episodic ectopic atrial tachycardia. In this oblique view, the sequence of activation during sinus rhythm is shown in *C*, with the earliest site of activation in red (*arrow*) representing the region of the sinus node. *D* was recorded during a low right atrial ectopic tachycardia. The earliest site of activation is indicated by the arrow.

OVERVIEW OF MANAGEMENT STRATEGIES

Strategies for the prevention and management of cardiac arrhythmias are based on an understanding of the mechanisms of specific arrhythmias (Table 24-2), in conjunction with systemic and cardiac factors that can be modified to influence predisposition to arrhythmias, and the range of indications for pharmacologic therapy and nonpharmacologic interventions (Table 24-3). Many patients are managed with multiple interventions, one therapeutic mode being complementary to another.

A complete management plan for any arrhythmia must coordinate three spheres of information: (1) the underlying structural etiology (coronary heart disease, cardiomyopathy, WPW syndrome, etc.); (2) transient triggering factors that interact with the underlying structural abnormality (e.g., transient ischemia and hemodynamic, electrolyte, metabolic, and respiratory abnormalities; see Table 24-4),[2,3] and (3) individual patients' preferences and decisions regarding pharmacologic versus interventional approaches. The identification of contributing factors, which interact with underlying etiology as the proximate causes of an arrhythmia, is inherent to any treatment plan. Contributing factors may be systemic or cardiac. The major systemic abnormalities include hemodynamic dysfunction, hypoxia, acidosis, electrolyte disturbances, toxic or proarrhythmic drug effects, and endocrine abnormalities. Central nervous system factors, including fluctuations in autonomic tone, may cause or aggravate specific arrhythmias. Prompt reversal of serious arrhythmias may follow control of these disturbances.

Primary and secondary arrhythmias must be distinguished for both management and prognosis. Medical writings contain conflicting definitions of the term *primary arrhythmia*, which must be clarified for interpretation of investigative data. Historically, a primary arrhythmia was first described as one that resulted from an electrophysiologic disturbance caused by a disease process, in the absence of a significant change in hemodynamic function. An arrhythmia that resulted from an electrical disturbance caused or perpetuated by hemodynamic deterioration or metabolic abnormalities was defined as a sec-

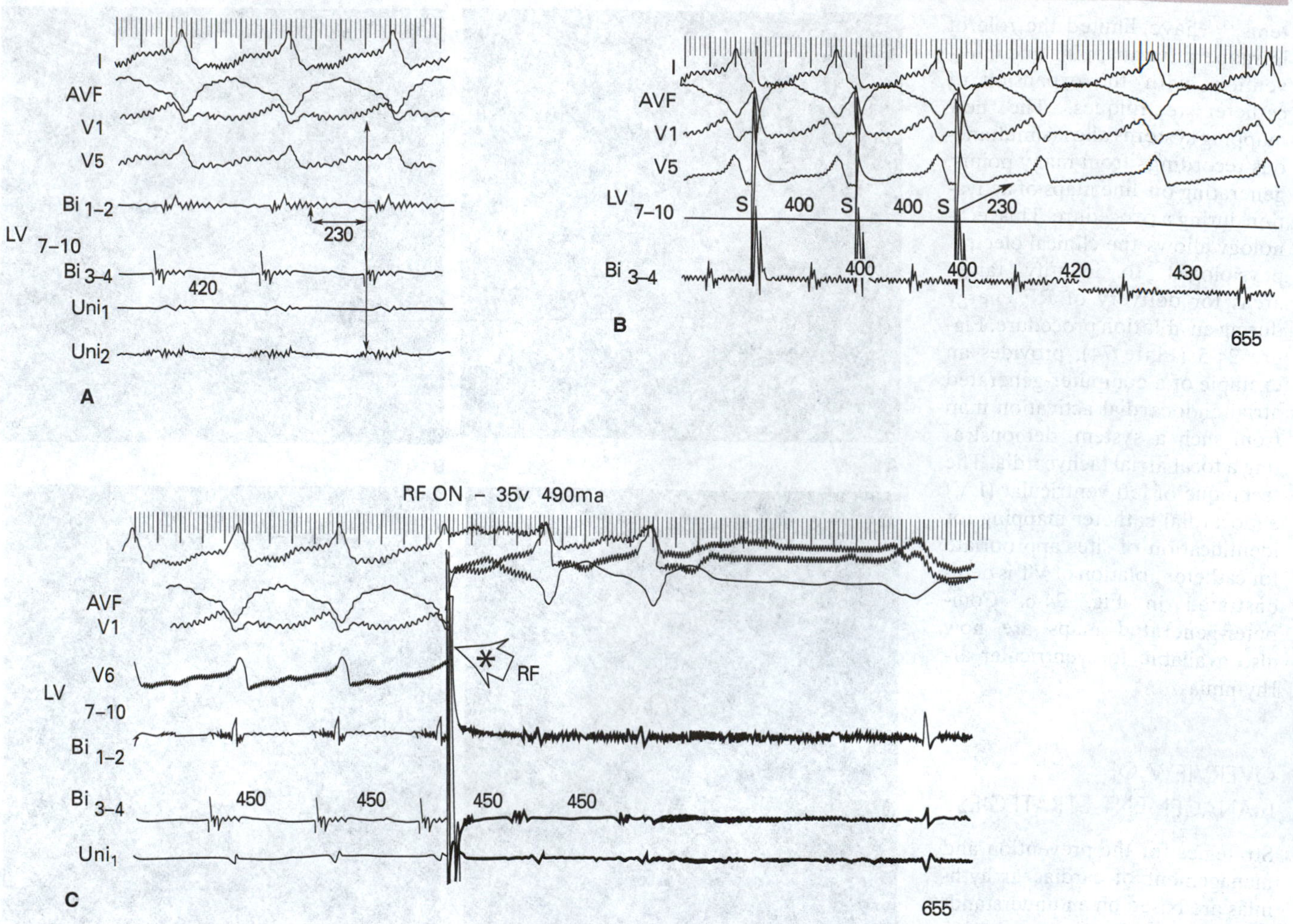

FIGURE 24-6 Left ventricular endocardial catheter mapping and radiofrequency ablation of ventricular tachycardia (VT) *A*. Bipolar (Bi) and Unipolar (Uni) recordings from an LV mapping site. The sustained ventricular tachycardia has a cycle length ranging from 420 to 450 ms. Onset of the VT QRS is indicated by the vertical line. Fractionated electrical activity is recorded from the distal bipolar electrode pair (Bi 1-2). A small potential immediately precedes the QRS onset, and fractionated signals extend 210 ms after the onset. *B*. The tachycardia is entrained during pacing and a cycle length of 400 ms [note the identical morphology of the complexes following pacing stimuli (concealed entrainment, entrainment with concealed fusion)], and a return to the spontaneous (unpaced) VT cycle length after cessation of pacing. The interval between the pacing stimulus and the onset of the responding QRS complex is the same as the interval between the end of the fractionated electrogram in *A* and the onset of the following QRS complex. *C*. RF energy applied through a catheter positioned at the same location results in prompt termination of the tachycardia, loss of fractionated electrograms, and return to sinus rhythm. (From Stevenson WG, et al. Identification of reentry circuits sites during catheter mapping and radiofrequency ablation of ventricular tachycardia late after myocardial infarction. *Circulation* 1993; 88[part 1]:1647–1670. Reproduced with permission from the American Heart Association.)

ondary arrhythmia (Fig. 24-7). In the former, antiarrhythmic drugs alone may be useful, while a secondary arrhythmia requires the concomitant use of hemodynamically active drugs to support the failing circulation. In secondary arrhythmias, antiarrhythmic and hemodynamically active drugs have complementary roles. Subsequent uses of the term *primary arrhythmia* were an arrhythmia that was the first clinical manifestation of disease, such as cardiac arrest due to ventricular fibrillation in coronary heart disease, or an arrhythmia in the absence of structural disease. To avoid confusion, the term primary must be carefully defined with each use.

Direct cardiac interventions for control of arrhythmias include pharmacologic approaches, ablation of specific foci involved in arrhythmogenesis, antiarrhythmic surgical approaches, and implantable devices designed to control tachyarrhythmic events or to prevent symptomatic bradyarrhythmias (Table 24-3). Antiarrhythmic drugs may be classified into groups using the modified Vaughn Williams system, which categorizes them on the basis of electropharmacologic and electrophysiologic properties (see Table 24-5). This classification is useful and practical for the clinician but has shortcomings. These include difficulty categorizing new drugs, exclusion of some drugs with obvious antiarrhythmic properties (e.g., adenosine), and inability to correlate drug class with specific effects as antiarrhythmic agents. Another classification system, the Sicilian gambit,[15] was developed for the purpose of providing deeper insight into drug effects, therapeutic targets, mechanisms of action, and responses (Fig. 24-8). While it is too complex for use as a practical clinical tool, it provides an excellent teaching method for understanding applied pharmacology. The usual dosages and routes of administration for the antiarrhythmic agents approved by the U.S. Food and Drug Administration at the time

TABLE 24-2 Mechanisms of Arrhythmias

Mechanism	Physiology	Tissues	Rhythms
Automaticity Normal	Spontaneous phase-4 depolarization from normal (near-normal) levels of membrane polarization (e.g., −100 to −60 mV) Activating current is I_f; role of $I_{Ca\text{-}T}$, $I_{Ca\text{-}L}$; upstroke generated by Na^+	Sinus node pacemaker cells Atrial muscle (specialized?) AV nodal cells (?) His-Purkinje fibers (His bundle, bundle branches, endocardial Purkinje network, M cells)	Sinus rhythm and variants Focal and multifocal atrial rhythms Atrial parasystole AV nodal (junctional) escape rhythms His, fascicular, and ventricular escape rhythms Ventricular parasystole
Abnormal	Spontaneous depolarization from partially depolarized tissue (e.g., −60 to −30 mV) Upstroke generated by Ca^{2+} ± Na^+	Atrial muscle (partially depolarized) His-Purkinje fibers (His bundle, bundle branches, endocardial Purkinje network, M cells) Ventricular muscle (partially depolarized)	Focal atrial rhythms (pathologic states) Accelerated AV junctional rhythms Accelerated ventricular rhythms
Reentry	Nonuniform conduction and refractory periods Regional slow conduction Local unidirectional block Anatomic basis for circuits Structural barriers to conduction Functional (electrophysiologic) circuit	Reentry may occur *within*: Sinus node Atrial muscle AV junction (?) His-Purkinje system (?) Ventricular muscle Reentry may occur *between*: Sinus node and atrial muscle (?) AV node and its atrial approaches Atrial muscle, accessory pathways, AV node, His-Purkinje system, and ventricular muscle His-Purkinje system and ventricular muscle	Sinoatrial reentrant tachycardia Intraatrial reentrant tachycardia Paroxysmal supraventricular tachycardia, due to: AV nodal reentry WPW Atrionodal, nodofascicular, atriofascicular, nodoventricular tracts: Mahaim variants Permanent junctional reentrant tachycardia Bundle branch reentrant tachycardia Ventricular tachycardia (reentrant)
Triggered activity	Induced by delayed afterdepolarizations: Intracellular Ca^{2+} accumulation → Ca^{2+}-mediated membrane oscillation → triggered responses carried by inward Na^+-current Induced by early afterdepolarizations: Ca^{2+} activation, inactivation, and reactivation (±intracelluar Ca^{2+} accumulation) → Ca^{2+}-mediated membrane oscillation → triggered responses carried by Ca^{2+} ions	Atrial muscle His-Purkinje system Ventricular muscle	Premature atrial contractions Atrial tachyarrhythmias (?) AV junctional tachycardias Premature ventricular contraction (?) Ventricular tachycardia: Polymorphic ventricular tachycardia Torsades de pointes RV outflow tract tachycardia (?)

TABLE 24-3 Summary of Approaches to Arrhythmia Management

General systemic interventions
Respiratory support
Hemodynamic support
Metabolic and electrolyte control
Neurophysiologic control
Electropharmacologic therapy
Control triggering events
Suppress triggering arrhythmias
Prevent or reverse arrhythmogenic factors (e.g., anti-ischemic therapy, or electrolyte replacement)
Control sustained arrhythmias
Acute interventions
Chronic prevention
Control ventricular rate
Catheter ablation procedures
Supraventricular tachycardias
AV nodal reentry
WPW syndrome
AV node ablation in atrial fibrillation
Atrial flutter
Atrial fibrillation, focal mechanisms[a]
Atrial, sinus node, and AV junctional tachycardias
Ventricular tachycardias
Surgical intervention
Antiarrhythmic surgery
Anomalous pathways[a]
Aneurysmectomy, endocardial resection[a]
Cryoablation[a]
Maze procedure for atrial fibrillation[a]
Anti-ischemic surgery
Structural heart disease surgery
Electronic device
Acute applications
Cardioversion
Defibrillation
Temporary pacemakers
Long-term applications
Permanent pacemakers
Implantable cardioverter defibrillators

[a]Limited clinical application at the time of this writing.

of writing are listed in Table 24-6. A number of other drugs are currently at various stages of study for ventricular and supraventricular arrhythmia indications.

SUPRAVENTRICULAR ARRHYTHMIAS

Figure 24-9 compares mechanisms, clinical features, diagnosis, and electrocardiography of the supraventricular arrhythmias described in this section.

Spectrum of Sinus Rhythms and Sinus Tachycardia

The range of rates defining normal sinus rhythm is between 60 and 100 impulses per minute. The rhythm is usually regular, but a rhythmic variation exceeding 0.12 s between the longest and shortest cycles in a sequence on a resting tracing defines sinus arrhythmia (Fig. 24-10*A*). This normal variant is most common in children and decreases with advancing age. It usually has a phasic pattern, in which the cycle lengths shorten with inspiration and lengthen with expiration. If the cycle is unrelated to the respiratory cycle, it is referred to as nonphasic.

A sinus rhythm at a rate below 60 impulses per minute is defined as sinus bradycardia (Fig. 24-10*C*); its significance is largely dependent upon clinical circumstances (see "Sinus Bradycardia," below). It may be normal, even at rates in the mid- to low 30s, in highly trained young athletes at rest, while it is generally considered abnormal, even at rates in the high 40s, in the elderly.

A sinus rate above 100 impulses per minute is defined as sinus tachycardia. Sinus rates in excess of 100 per minute are normal in infants and children under 2 years of age. Occasionally, otherwise normal older children and adults have sinus rates persistently or intermmitently (the latter often positional) in excess of 100 per minute in the absence of normal physiologic or pathologic stimuli for heart rate increases. Such forms of inappropriate sinus tachycardia, apparently mediated by autonomic factors in most cases[16,17] and by electrophysiologic factors in some,[17] may cause disturbing or disabling symptoms.[16,17] If fast enough and persisting for months, it may precipitate a reversible form of tachycardia-induced heart failure.[17,18]

The category of physiologic sinus tachycardias includes the normal sinus rate responses to exercise, excitement, anxiety, and other emotional stresses. Pharmacologic sinus tachycardias result from medications such as epinephrine, ephedrine, amyl nitrate, isoproterenol, and atropine, and may occur upon exposure to alcohol, nicotine, or caffeine. The heart rate responses are a result of the pharmacologic properties of these drugs. Pathologic sinus tachycardia may be secondary to noncardiac systemic factors or due to specific cardiac abnormalities. Among the secondary causes are fever, hypoxemia, hemorrhage, hypotension, thyrotoxicosis, and anemia. Cardiovascular causes include congestive heart failure, myocardial infarction, and pulmonary embolism.

ELECTROCARDIOGRAPHIC FEATURES

The ECG in sinus tachycardia reveals a rate in excess of 100 per minute accompanied by a normal PR relationship and a normal P-wave vector (Fig. 24-10*B*). The upper rate range of sinus tachycardia varies according to the patient's clinical status and factors responsible for the tachycardia. For instance, in the physiologic tachycardia group, the upper limit in the normal adult during exercise testing may range from 160 to 190 per minute, whereas the highly trained athlete may attain a rate of at least 200 per minute under maximal effort. In contrast, the pharmacologic tachycardias do not commonly induce a rate exceeding 140 per minute, whereas rates secondary to pathologic states usually range from just over 100 per minute to 150 per minute (e.g., hypotension, hypovolemia, hemorrhage, or fever) to 160 per minute (hyperthyroidism or severe heart failure). In a persistent sinus tachycardia, the rate characteristically varies during the course of the day, in contrast to the fixed rate that occurs in ectopic tachycardias or AV nodal reentrant tachycardia. Carotid sinus massage usually slows sinus tachycardia transiently.

MANAGEMENT OF SINUS TACHYCARDIA

Sinus tachycardia, except when it is an appropriate response to acute physical or emotional stress, is usually categorized as persistent and is easily recognized. Its management almost always depends on control of exogenous or endogenous systemic factors or of an underlying cardiac disease. Its differentiation from other SVTs at rates of 150 or more a minute may be achieved with carotid sinus massage. Specific therapy is rarely required. When it is required, beta-adrenergic blockade will often achieve at least partial control. In uncomplicated acute myocardial infarction, the sinus rate may be controlled with small doses of propranolol (10 to 20 mg every 6 h). Persistent sinus tachycardia occurs in thyrotoxicosis, and higher doses of propranolol may be required for its control. Sinus tachycardia during heart failure or hypovolemic states will respond promptly to improving hemodynamic status. The chronic or intermittent form of nonparoxysmal inappropriate sinus tachycardia, when symptomatic or associated with tachycardia-induced heart failure, may require RF energy modification or ablation of the sinus node area[19] if it is not controllable by drug therapy.

TABLE 24-4 Causes of Cardiac Arrhythmias: Structure and Function

Structural Abnormalities	Functional Factors
Coronary heart disease	Transient alterations of coronary blood flow
Acute myocardial infarction	Vasomotor dynamics
Chronic ischemic heart disease	Acute ischemia
Ventricular hypertrophy	Reperfusion after ischemia
Secondary left ventricular hypertrophy	Systemic factors
Hypertrophic cardiomyopathy	Hemodynamic fluctuations
Obstructive	Hypoxia, acidosis
Nonobstructive	Electrolyte imbalance
Myopathic ventricles	Neurophysiologic alterations
Dilated cardiomyopathy	Central nervous system influences
Pericarditis, myocarditis	Receptor function
Noninfectious inflammatory diseases	Neurotransmitters
Infiltrative diseases	Toxic substances
Structural electrophysiology abnormalities	Proarrhythmic drugs
Sinus node, AV node, and His-Purkinje disease	Idiosyncratic
Accessory pathways	Dose dependent
Abnormalities of molecular structure (ion channels)	Cardiotoxic substances

SOURCE: Modified from Myerburg et al.,[3] with permission of the *American Journal of Cardiology.*

Premature Atrial Impulses

Atrial extrasystoles or premature atrial contractions (PACs) are extremely common and may occur in normal individuals or in the presence of systemic or cardiac abnormalities. They occur at any age, including infancy. Both endogenous (febrile illnesses, thyrotoxicosis, emotional stress, etc.) and exogenous (alcohol, tobacco, or caffeine consumption) systemic factors may initiate or worsen atrial extrasystolic activity. Among cardiac causes, myopericarditis, ischemia, heart failure, and digitalis intoxication are all precipitating or contributing factors.

ELECTROCARDIOGRAPHIC FEATURES

The PAC is characterized by (1) a P wave that occurs before the next expected sinus impulse and (2) a change in the vector of the premature P wave. For example, a negative P-wave deflection in leads II, III, and aVF suggests an origin from the lower portion of the atrium. The features of the PAC in leads I and V_1 can help distinguish right and left atrial origins. If the premature P wave is positive in lead I and negative in V_1, the impulse is probably of right atrial origin. A negative P wave in leads I and V_6, and a positive P wave in V_1 is consistent with a left atrial origin. If a premature P wave is narrower than in sinus and positive in aVR and aVL, a septal origin is probable. When a premature P wave is negative in aVL and positive in the inferior leads, a right superior pulmonary vein origin should be suspected.

The PR interval of the conducted PAC may be normal or prolonged (see Fig. 24-11). Marked prolongation of the PR

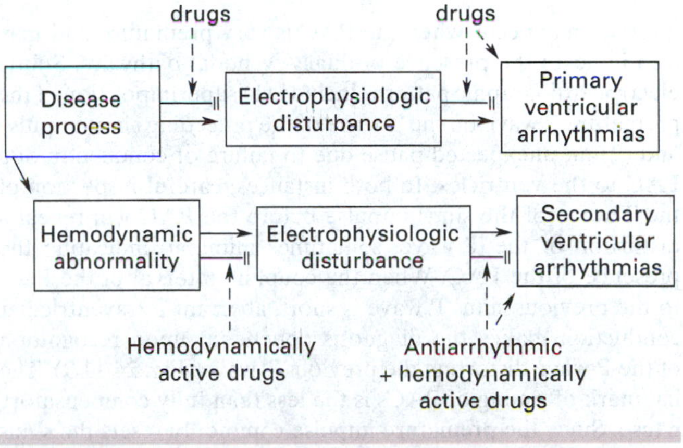

FIGURE 24-7 Primary and secondary arrhythmias. When a disease process directly initiates an electrophysiologic disturbance, the resulting arrhythmia is referred to as primary. In contrast, when the disease process produces a hemodynamic abnormality that in turn initiates the electrophysiologic disturbance, a resulting arrhythmia is referred to as secondary. Antiarrhythmic drugs may be used to prevent the electrophysiologic disturbance, prevent the electrophysiologically unstable heart from developing a manifest arrhythmia, or reverse a primary arrhythmia. In secondary arrhythmias, hemodynamically active drugs are used to prevent or reverse secondary electrophysiologic disturbances, usually in conjunction with antiarrhythmic drugs. Antiarrhythmic drugs alone are less likely to be effective for secondary arrhythmias. (Modified from Myerburg et al.[1] Reproduced with permission from the publisher and authors.)

TABLE 24-5 Modified Vaughn Williams Classification of Drugs Approved for Antiarrhythmic Uses

Examples		Depolarization	Repolarization
Class I: Membrane-active drugs			
IA	Quinidine (Quinaglute, Quinidex, Cardioquin) Procainamide (Pronestyl, Procan-SR) Disopyramide (Norpace) Moricizine (Ethmozine)	Moderate depression of Na^+ current; intermediate kinetics	Prolonged
IB	Lidocaine (Xylocaine) Tocainide (Tonocard) Mexiletine (Mexitil) Phenytoin (Dilantin)	Limited depression of Na^+ current; rapid kinetics	No effect or shortened
IC	Flecainide (Tambocor) Propafenone (Rhythmol)	Marked depression of Na^+ current; slow kinetics	Minimal effect
Class II: Beta-adrenoceptor blocking drugs			
	Propranolol (Inderal) Esmolol (Brevibloc) Acebutolol (Sectral)		
Class III: Drugs that prolong repolarization			
	Amiodarone (Cordarone) Bretylium tosylate (Bretylol) Sotalol (Betapace; Betapace AF) Ibutilide (Corvert) Dofetilide (Tikosyn)		
Class IV: Ca^{2+}-entry blocking drugs			
	Verapamil (Isoptin, Calan) Diltiazem (Cardizem)		
Unclassified in this system			
	Digoxin (Lanoxin) Adenosine (Adenocard)		

NOTE: Drugs identified by name are limited to those approved for antiarrhythmic use by the U.S. Food and Drug Administration at the time of this writing (not necessarily inclusive of all brand names).

interval may occur when the PAC is very premature and may also indicate the presence of dual AV nodal pathways. Subtle electrocardiographic patterns include (1) superimposition of the premature P wave on the T wave of the preceding sinus impulse and (2) an unexpected pause due to failure of conduction of a PAC to the ventricles. In both instances, careful inspection of the T wave of the sinus impulse before the PAC will reveal a distortion of the T wave, sometimes minimal, indicating the presence of the PAC. When the coupling interval of the PAC to the previous sinus P wave is short, aberrant intraventricular conduction makes the diagnosis dependent upon recognition of the P wave distorting the previous T wave (Fig. 24-11*B*). The hallmark of timing of PACs is the less than fully compensatory pause. Since the premature impulse commonly resets the sinus cycle, the PAC is bracketed by a cycle terminated by the early P wave and a return cycle close to the underlying sinus cycle length (Fig. 24-11*A*). The sum of the two cycles will be less than fully compensatory. Occasionally, fully compensatory pauses or longer than compensatory pauses occur because of failure to invade and reset the sinus node cycle or delay of its return because of overdrive suppression.

MANAGEMENT OF PREMATURE ATRIAL CONTRACTIONS

PACs usually do not require treatment, especially when they occur in normal individuals or when due to systemic influences or minor cardiac abnormalities such as mitral valve prolapse and acute viral pericarditis. When PACs may be the triggering events for sustained arrhythmias, their management may become important. Generally, SVT due to AV nodal reentry or the WPW syndrome, paroxysmal atrial fibrillation, or the rare instances of induction of sustained ventricular arrhythmia by supraventricular impulses are best managed by therapy targeted to the prevention of the sustained arrhythmias, but occasionally suppression of triggering PACs is helpful. In recent years, repetitive focal PACs and atrial tachycardia on ambulatory monitor recordings from patients prone to atrial fibrillation have been identified as RF ablation targets during studies in the electrophysiology laboratory. In some patients, these forms of PACs appear to act not only as triggers, but also as drivers, of atrial fibrillation episodes.[20]

Annoying palpitations are a common symptom of PACs in patients who have either no underlying heart disease or mitral valve prolapse. Reassuring the patient of the benign nature of the arrhythmia may suffice, and no therapy is necessary other than removal of inciting factors, such as cigarettes, coffee, alcohol, and excessive fatigue. When the palpitations are sufficiently bothersome to affect on the quality of life, an intervention must be considered. A low dose of a beta-adrenergic blocking agent is preferred to more aggressive (and more dangerous) membrane-active antiarrhythmic agents. Digitalis has been tried, but no systematic studies of its efficacy have been reported.

DRUG	CHANNELS						RECEPTORS				PUMPS	CLINICAL EFFECTS			ECG EFFECTS		
	NA Fast	NA Med	NA Slow	Ca	K	μ	α	β	M_2	P	Na-K ATPase	Left ventricular function	Sinus Rate	Extra-cardiac	PR interval	QRS width	JT interval
Lidocaine	Low											→	→	Moderate			↓
Mexiletine	Low											→	→	Moderate			↓
Tocainide	Low											→	→	High			↓
Moricizine	High (I)											↓	→	Low		↑	
Procainamide		High (A)			Moderate							↓	→	High	↑	↑	↑
Disopyramide		High (A)			Moderate				Low			↓	→	Moderate	↑↓	↑	↑
Quinidine		High (A)			Moderate		Low		Low			→	↑	Moderate	↑↓	↑	↑
Propafenone		High (A)						Moderate				↓	↓	Low	↑	↑	
Flecainide			High (A)		Low							↓	→	Low	↑	↑	
Encainide			High (A)									↓	→	Low	↑	↑	
Bepridil	Low			High	Moderate							?	↓	Low			↑
Verapamil	Low			High			Moderate					↓	↓	Low	↑		
Diltiazem				Moderate								↓	↓	Low	↑		
Bretylium					High		Agonist/Antagonist	Agonist/Antagonist				→	↓	Low			↑
Sotalol					High			High				↓	↓	Low	↑		↑
Amiodarone	Low			Low	High		Moderate	Moderate				→	↓	Low	↑		↑
Alinidine					Moderate	High						?	↓	High			
Nadolol								High				↓	↓	Low	↑		
Propranolol	Low							High				↓	↓	Low	↑		
Atropine									High			→	↑	Moderate	↓		
Adenosine										Agonist		?	↓	Low	↑		
Digoxin									Agonist		High	↑	↓	High	↑		↓

Relative potency of block: ○ Low ◎ Moderate ● High A = Activated state blocker
□ = Agonist ◪ = Agonist/Antagonist I = Inactivated state blocker

FIGURE 24-8 The Sicilian gambit approach to antiarrhythmic drugs. This figure summarizes the important actions of drugs on membrane channels, receptors, and ion pumps in the heart as well as on the ECG, sinus rate, and LV function. Because clinical and ECG effects are diverse, the table unavoidably includes some degree of subjectivity. Accordingly, the shading of the symbols and the direction of the arrows should not be taken as absolute. Moreover, the clinical information presented refers to the patient who does not have significantly compromised LV function prior to the drug administration. For the section on channels, receptors, and pumps, the actions of drugs on the sodium (Na^+), calcium (Ca^{2+}), potassium channels (I_K and I_f) are indicated. Sodium channel blockade is subdivided into three groups of actions characterized by fast (tau less than 300 ms), medium (tau 200 to 1500 ms), and slow (tau greater than 1500 ms) time constants for recovery from block. This parameter is a measure of use dependence and predicts the likelihood that a drug will decrease conduction velocity of normal Na^+-dependent tissues in the heart and perhaps the propensity of a drug for causing bundle-branch block or proarrhythmia. The rate constant for onset of block may be even more clinically relevant. Blockade in the inactivated (I) or activated (A) state is indicated. Drug interaction with receptors [beta-adrenergic, alpha-adrenergic, muscarinic subtype 2 (M_2), and A_1 purinergic (P)] and drug effects on the sodium-potassium pump (Na^+, K^+-ATPase) are indicated. The absence of a symbol indicates lack of effect. The use of a question mark indicates uncertainty concerning effect. The arrows in the clinical effect and ECG section indicate direction; no quantitative differentiation has been made between weak and strong effects. The effects listed for ECG, LV function, sinus rate, and extracardiac are those that may be seen at therapeutic plasma levels. Deleterious effects that may appear with concentrations above the therapeutic range are not listed. [From Schwartz PJ, Zaga A. The Sicilian gambit revisited. *Eur Heart J* 1992; 13(suppl F):23–29. Reproduced with permission from the publisher and authors.]

TABLE 24-6 Antiarrhythmic Drugs: Dosage and Kinetics

Drug	Usual Dosing Range[a]	Half-Life, h	Therapeutic Range, μg/mL	Plasma Protein Binding, %	Major Route of Excretion
Class IA					
Quinidine	Oral sulfate: 200–600 mg q 6 h Oral long acting: 330–660 mg, q 8 h or q 6 h	5–7	2.3–5	80	H
Procainamide	Oral: 250–750 mg, q 4 h or q 6 h Oral long-acting: 500–1500 mg, q 8 h or q 6 h IV: 10–15 mg/kg at 25 mg/min, then 1–6 mg/min	3–5	4–10	15	R[b]
Disopyramide	Oral: 100–200 mg, q 8 h or q 6 h	8–9	2–5	35–95	H/R
Moricizine[c]	Oral: 150–300 mg, q 12 h or q 8 h	6–13	—	95	H
Class IB					
Lidocaine	IV: 1–3 mg/kg at 20–50 mg/min, then 1–4 mg/min	1–2	1–5	60	H
Tocainide	Oral: 400–600 mg q 8–12 h	15	4–10	10	H
Mexiletine	Oral: 200–400 mg q 8 h	10–12	0.5–2.0	55	H
Class IC					
Flecainide	Oral: 100–200 mg q 12 h	20	0.4–1.0	40	H
Propafenone[d]	Oral: 150–300 mg q 8 h	2–10	0.5–1.5[e]	95	H
Class II					
Propanolol	Oral: 10–100 mg q 6 h IV: 0.1 mg/kg in divided 1-mg doses	4–6	0.04–0.10	95	H
Esmolol	IV: 500 mg/kg per min x 1 min followed by 50 mg/kg per min x 4 min, repeat with 50-mg increments to maintenance dose to 200 mg/kg per min	9 min	—	55	H
Acebutolol	Oral: 200-600 mg q 12 h	3–4	—	26	H/R
Class III					
Amiodarone	Oral: 600–1600 mg/day × 1–3 weeks, then 200–400 mg/day	50 days	1–2.5	96	H
	IV: 15 mg/min × 10 min, then 1 mg/min × 6 h, then maintenance at 0.5 mg/min	?	?		
Bretylium	IV: 5–10 mg/kg at 1–2 mg/kg, then 0.5–2.0 mg/min	8–14	0.5–1.5	—	R
Sotalol[d]	Oral: 80–240-mg q 12 h	10–15	—	0	R
Ibutilide	IV: (for >60 kg) 1 mg over 10 min; may repeat × 1 10 min after completion of initial dose[f]	2–12	—	40	H
Dofetilide	Oral: 500 μg q 12 h; creatinine clearance must be calculated and dose adjusted accordingly	10	1.0–3.5 (in ng/mL)	60–70%	R
Class IV					
Verapamil	Oral: 80–32 mg q 6–8 h IV: 5–10 mg in 1–2 min	3–8	0.1–0.15	90	H
Diltiazem	IV: 0.25 mg/kg body wt over 2 min; if response inadequate, wait 15 min, then 0.35 mg/kg over 2 min; maintenance 10–15 mg/h	3.5–5.0	0.1–3.0	70–80	H
Other					
Digoxin	Oral 1.25–1.5 mg in divided doses over 24 h followed by 0.125–0.375 mg/day IV: Approximately 70% of oral dose	36	0.8–1.4 (in ng/mL)	30	R
Adenosine	IV: 6 mg rapidly; if unsuccessful within 1–2 min, 12 mg rapidly	10 s	—	—	—

[a]All dosing should follow FDA-approved guidelines as outlined in package insert or *Physicians' Desk Reference* (see also Chap. 27; does not include pediatric use in infants and young children).
[b]Parent compound metabolized to active metabolite (NAPA) in liver; both active metabolite and unmetabolized parent compound excreted by kidneys.
[c]Shares class IB and IC activities.
[d]Shares class II activity.
[e]Active metabolite limits significance of these measurements.
[f]D/C upon arrhythmia conversion or for ventricular tachycardia or non-pharmacologic prolongation of QT or QTc.
ABBREVIATIONS: H-hepatic; R-renal.

When it is necessary to treat PACs because of intolerable palpitations, conventional antiarrhythmic agents may be effective. Depending upon tolerance and side effects, any of the membrane-active drugs or adrenoceptor-blocking agents may be considered. Few data are available on the efficacy of antiarrhythmic drug therapy for PACs, but clinical experience suggests that it may be effective, particularly in the absence of structural cardiac or pulmonary disease. Antiarrhythmic drugs have not been approved for this indication in the United States, and the threshold for their use for a troublesome but benign arrhythmia is high. Class IC (see Table 24-5) drugs should be avoided for this indication in patients with even the remote possibility of coronary artery disease because of the adverse outcome in the Cardiac Arrhythmia Suppression Trial (CAST).[21,22] Atrial distention in heart failure may induce PACs; they usually disappear as hemodynamics improve and antiarrhythmic drugs are avoided.

Supraventricular Tachyarrhythmias

Supraventricular tachyarrhythmias include all tachyarrhythmias that originate above the bifurcation of the bundle of His or incorporate tissues proximal to the bifurcation of the bundle of His in a reentrant circuit (Fig. 24-9). The diagnosis requires an atrial chamber rate of 100 impulses per minute or more; the ventricular rate may be less when AV conduction is incomplete. SVTs usually have narrow QRS complexes, but they may be wide because of aberrant conduction through the intraventricular conducting tissue, because of participation of a bypass tract in the ventricular depolarization pattern, or when bundle branch block coexists independently.

SVTs may be separated into three groups based on duration: brief paroxysms, persistent, and chronic. Arrhythmias that are paroxysmal in onset and offset [e.g., paroxysmal SVT (PSVT) due to AV nodal reentry or WPW syndrome, paroxysmal atrial fibrillation, and paroxysmal atrial flutter] tend to be recurrent and of short duration, lasting from seconds to hours. Persistent tachycardias [e.g., sinus tachycardia, ectopic atrial tachycardia (nonparoxysmal), multifocal atrial tachycardia, longer episodes of PSVT, or atrial flutter or fibrillation] may last for days or weeks and may be associated with a specific contributing pathophysiologic factor, such as decompensated chronic obstructive pulmonary disease, pulmonary emboli, electrolyte disturbances, or drug toxicity. They tend to be recurrent when an underlying structural cause, such as atrial disease or mitral valve disease, is the dominant pathophysiologic factor. When a transient functional abnormality dominates, such as hypoxemia, heart failure, or an electrolyte abnormality, it may be an isolated clinical event, reappearing only if or when the inciting event occurs. Longstanding or chronic SVTs (e.g., chronic atrial fibrillation or chronic atrial flutter), particularly in the presence of advanced structural heart disease, generally do not revert if untreated, may fail to revert even with attempted treatment, and if reverted will frequently recur despite therapy.

THE REENTRANT PAROXYSMAL SUPRAVENTRICULAR TACHYCARDIAS

PSVT may be due to AV nodal reentry, the WPW syndrome, or intraatrial or sinoatrial reentry. Most of the interventions for SVT listed in Table 24-7 are applicable to these arrhythmias.

PSVT due to AV Nodal Reentry The commonest form of PSVT is due to AV nodal reentry. The underlying disturbance in AV nodal reentry is the presence of dual AV nodal pathway physiology. Previously thought to be restricted to the compact anatomic AV node itself, the dual-pathway physiology is now known to exist in the *region* of the AV node. One pathway is capable of faster conduction and usually has a longer refractory period; the other conducts more slowly and has a shorter refractory period. Both the slow and the fast pathways have components in the low atrial approaches to the AV node as well as in the AV node itself (Fig. 24-12).

In the presence of dual AV nodal physiology, a premature atrial impulse with a coupling interval sho enough to encroach on the refractory period of the fast pathway may block in the fast pathway while allowing conduction to proceed through the slow pathway (Fig. 24-12*B*). This results in slower-than-normal conduction through the AV node, prolonging the PR interval abruptly. The slowly propagating impulse may then reenter the fast pathway in the retrograde direction and arrive at the proximal end after it has recovered excitability. When this occurs, a circuit is completed and the impulse may then reenter the slow pathway if it too has regained excitability (Fig. 24-12*C*). Once established, this reentrant pattern will continue until the relationship between conduction times and refractory periods in the two pathways is disturbed so as to interrupt the cycle. The circulating impulse progresses through the His-Purkinje system to ventricular muscle each time it passes the distal end of the reentrant loop and provides retrograde atrial activation each time it passes the proximal end. Because antegrade conduction is slow and retrograde conduction rapid, atrial activity begins soon after the onset of ventricular activation, usually creating an inability to identify P waves on the standard ECG during AV nodal reentrant tachycardia (Fig. 24-13) because they are within the QRS complex. The characteristic alignment of electrograms recorded during AV nodal reentrant tachycardia is shown in Fig. 24-14*A*. In a much less common form of AV nodal reentry, the circulating wavefront proceeds antegradely down the fast pathway and retrogradely up the slow pathway, creating a sequence of excitation of atria that is delayed relative to ventricular activation because of slow retrograde conduction. This form of AV nodal reentrant tachycardia is characterized by a long RP interval and a short PR interval, with a clearly visible inverted P wave in II, III, and aVF (Fig. 24-9). The electrophysiologic findings in the common and uncommon forms of AV nodal reentry are compared in Figs. 24-14*A* and -14*B* (see also Chap. 23).

Electrocardiographic Features PSVT due to AV nodal reentry is characterized by an abrupt onset and offset, and usually has a narrow QRS complex without clearly discernible P waves. Occasionally, however, P waves can be seen as "pseudo-R" waves, particularly in V_1 and the inferior leads, and more rarely as "pseudo-Q" waves, when the retrograde atrial depolarization precedes ventricular depolarization. Comparison with QRS morphology during sinus rhythm is essential to establish the presence of these waves.

The heart rate during PSVT due to AV nodal reentry is commonly in the range of 160 to 190 per minute but may be as slow as 120 to 130 per minute and occasionally faster than 200 per minute. When preexisting bundle-branch block is present, the tachycardia will reflect the preexisting wide QRS com-

ARRHYTHMIA	MECHANISM	REGULARITY	RATE (bpm)	P Waves PR / RP
SINUS TACHYCARDIA	AUTOMATIC FOCUS	REGULAR	100-180	long RP normal axis P waves
INNAPROPIATE SINUS TACHYCARDIA	AUTOMATIC FOCUS (crista terminalis)	REGULAR	110-190	long RP normal axis P waves
ATRIAL FIBRILLATION	MULTIPLE RE-ENTRANT WAVELETS ——— FOCAL TRIGGER + REENTRY	IRREGULAR IRREGULAR ——— OCCATIONAL REGULARITY	variable ventricular response (40's to 180's)	no define P waves ——— PAC's during SR +/-burst of AT
MULTIFOCAL ATRIAL TACHYCARDIA	MULTIPLE AUTOMATIC FOCI	IRREGULAR IRREGULAR	atrial: 120-180 ventricular: variable response (100's to 180's)	variable, 3 or more P wave morphologies
ATRIAL FLUTTER (TYPICAL)	MACROREENTRY (isthmus dependent) CounterClockWise (CCW) or ClockWise (CW) rotation	REGULAR / IRREGULAR (1:1, 2:1, 3:1...VARIABLE AV BLOCK)	atrial:250-350 ventricular: 150, variable response.	saw tooth pattern, in II, III, AVF,V6 CCW: negative CW:positive
ATRIAL TACHYCARDIA	AUTOMATIC FOCUS MICROREENTRY MACROREENTRY (non isthmus dependent) -including incision-related scar and Atypical Atrial Flutter-	REGULAR (1:1, 2:1)	atrial:180->350 ventricular: variable response (100's to 180's)	short RP/ long RP
ATRIOVENTRICULAR NODAL TACHYCARDIA (TYPICAL 95%)	MICROREENTRY	REGULAR 1:1 (rarely 2:1AV BLOCK)	150-250 (usually 180-200)	short RP
ATRIOVENTRICULAR NODAL TACHYCARDIA (ATYPICAL 5%)	MICROREENTRY	REGULAR 1:1 (rarely 2:1AV BLOCK)	150-250 (usually 180-200)	long RP
ATRIOVENTRICULAR TACHYCARDIA (ORTHODROMIC)	MACROREENTRY	REGULAR (1:1)	170-250	short RP/ long RP
ATRIOVENTRICULAR TACHYCARDIA (ANTIDROMIC)	MACROREENTRY	REGULAR (1:1)	170-250	short RP/ long RP
PJRT Permanent Form Of Junctional Reciprocating Tachycardia	MACROREENTRY	REGULAR (1:1)	170-250	short RP/ long RP
Junctional Tachycardia	Abnormal Automaticity Triggered activity	REGULAR (1:1)	100-120	variable RP relation

FIGURE 24-9 Comparison of mechanisms, electrocardiographic and clinical features, responses to adenosine, activation patterns, and electrocardiographic appearance of the various supraventricular rhythms. See the text for description of the individual arrhythmias.

ADENOSINE RESPONSE	CLINICAL CONCEPTS	
Transient supression. Decreased AV conduction or block without termination.	Secondary to other clinical states (i.e.: fever, excercise, hyperthyroidism, psychological stress, etc.). Non specific therapy; treat the underlying condition.	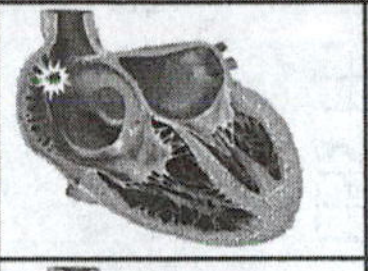
Decreased AV conduction or block without termination.	Diagnosis of exclusion. Exagerated response to sympathetic stimulation. Medical therapy includes beta blockers and calcium channel blockers have uncertain long term success. RFA+G5 is an option.	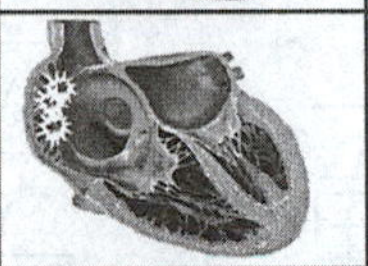
Decreased AV conduction or block without termination.	Variable clinical patterns. Allways consider: 1) Restoration of sinus rhythm 2) Maintenance of sinus rhythm 3) Heart rate control 4) Anticoagulation	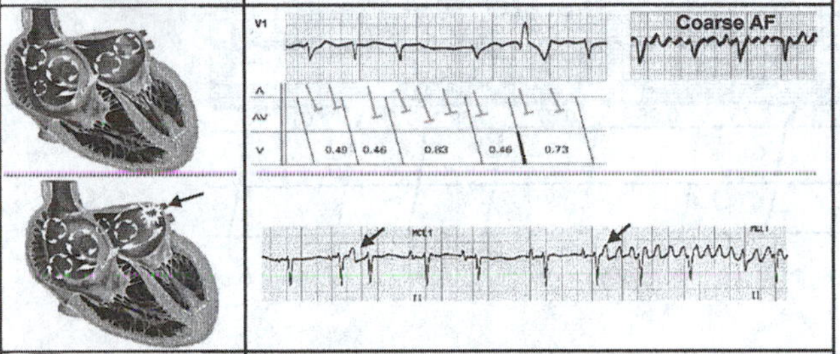
Decreased AV conduction or block without termination. Allows identification of different P waves morphologies.	Common in COPD. Heart rate control with AVN blockers and therapy of triggering condition. No benefit of cardioversion.	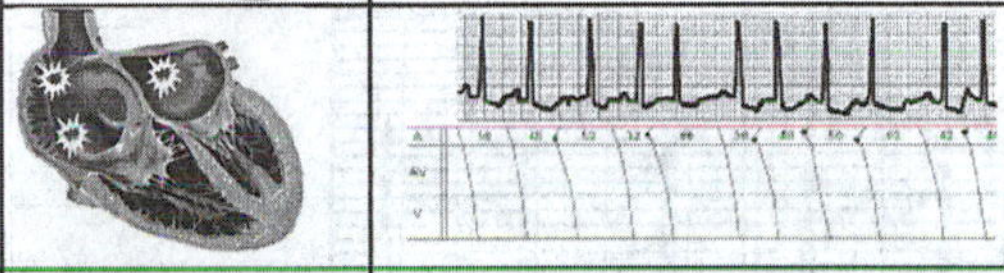
Continuation of atrial flutter with AV block, allows clear visualization of flutter waves.	When recurrent, consider anticoagulation as for atrial fibrillation. RFA primary therapy.	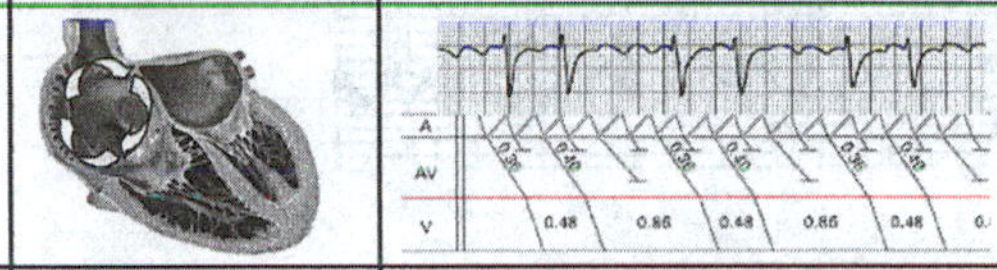
Continuation of atrial tachycardia with AV block, allows visualization of driving P waves. Some atrial tachycardias are adenosine sensitive and may terminate, others may become transintly suppressed.	Variable response to medical therapy. New mapping and ablation techniques have allowed increased cure rates with RFA.	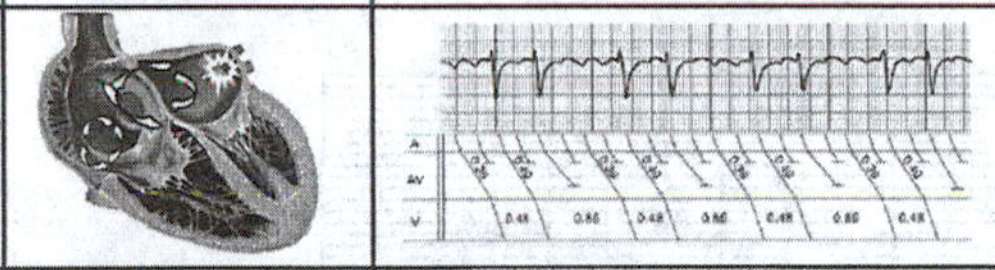
Terminates tachycardia.	RFA curative. Antiarrhythmic therapy palliative.	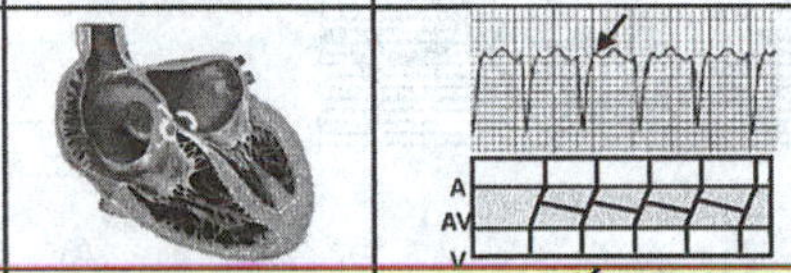
Terminates tachycardia.	RFA curative. Antiarrhythmic therapy palliative.	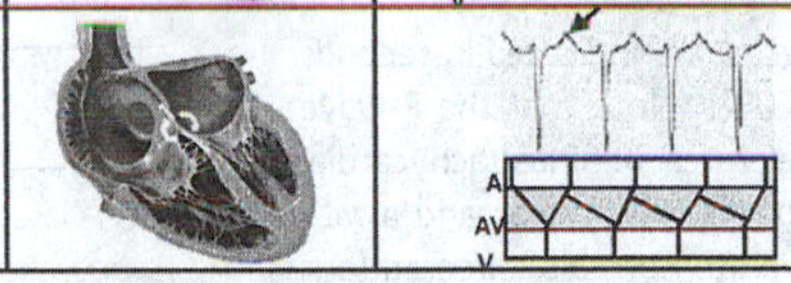
Terminates tachycardia.	RFA curative. Antiarrhythmic therapy palliative.	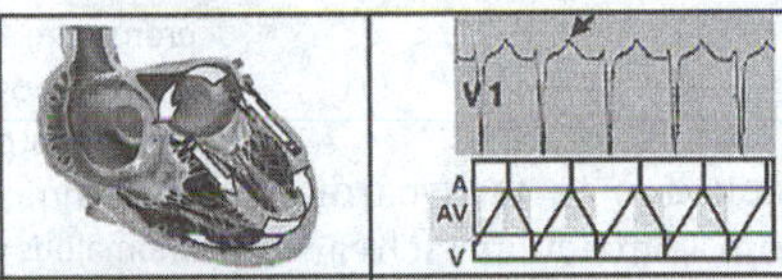
Terminates tachycardia.	Wide complex tachycardia. RFA curative. Antiarrhythmic therapy palliative.	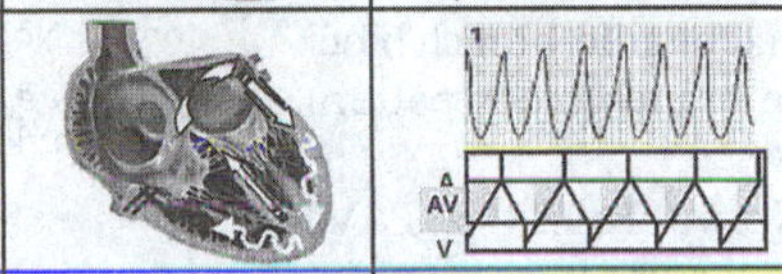
Terminates tachycardia.	Misnomer, involves a posteroseptal concealed accessory pathway with decremental conduction properpties. May produce tachycardia related cardiomyopathy. RFA curative. Antiarrhythmic therapy palliative.	
Variable effect	Adults: associated with valve surgery, acute MI or digitalis toxicity. Children: seen after corrective heart surgery, usually requires RFA for succesful control.	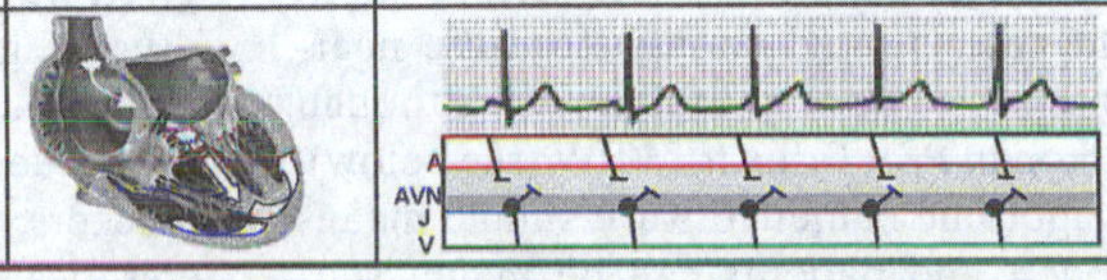

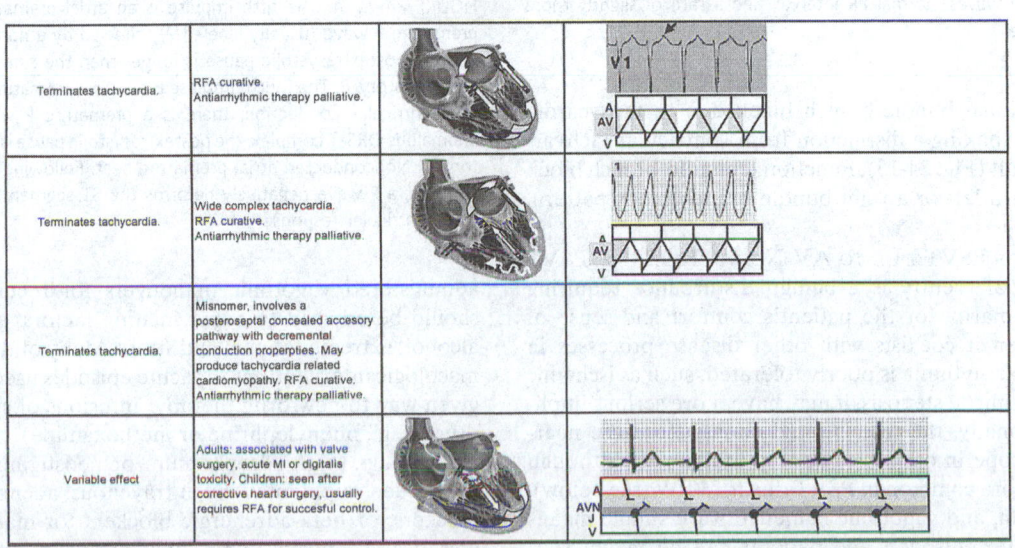

FIGURE 24-9 (*Continued*)

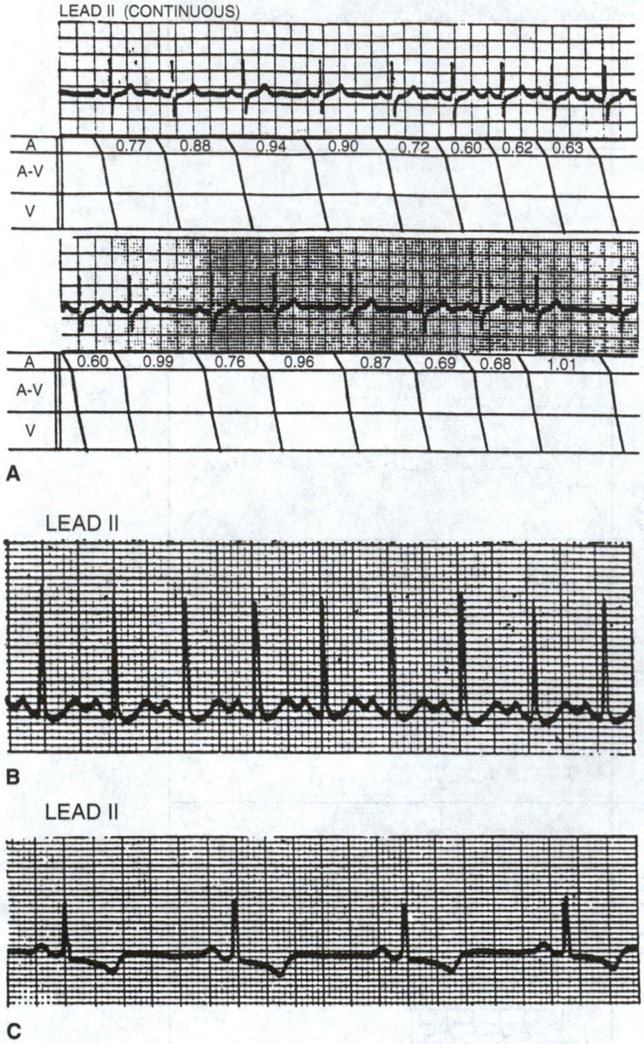

FIGURE 24-10 *A.* Sinus arrhythmia. The sinus cycles are indicated in seconds in the atrial (A) tier; they range from 0.60 to 1.01 s. Note that the P-wave amplitude increases as the sinus pacemaker accelerates. *B.* Sinus tachycardia. Note normally shaped and directed P waves, normal PR interval, and a rate of almost 150 per minute. *C.* Sinus bradycardia. Note normally directed (but abnormally wide) P waves, normal PR interval, and a rate of slightly more than 50 per minute.

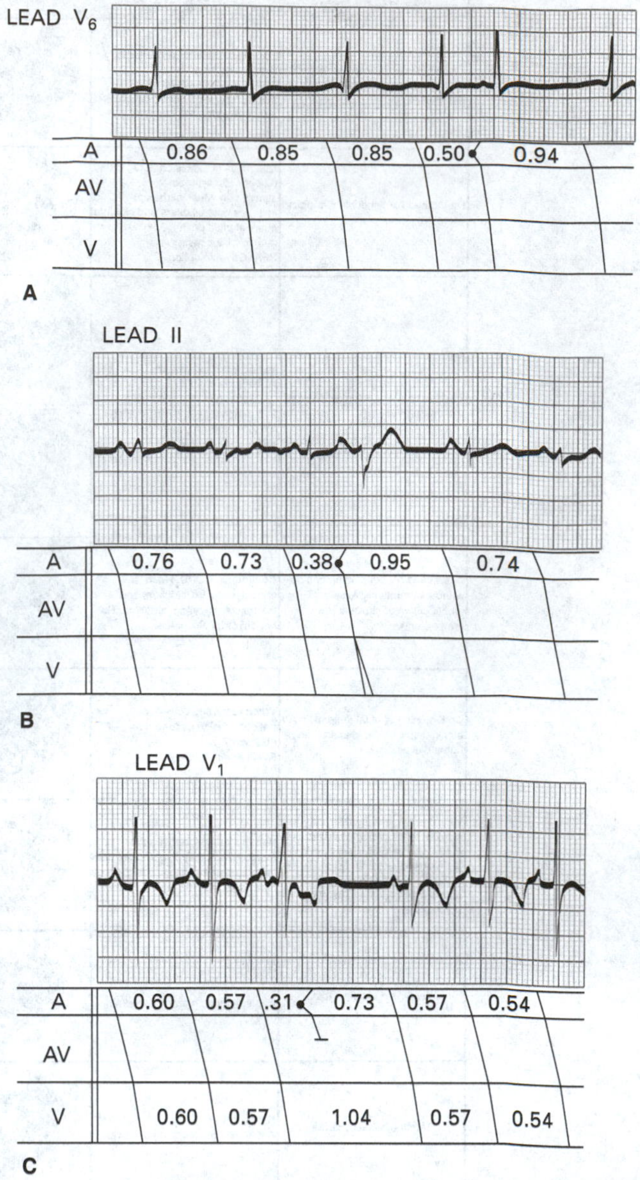

FIGURE 24-11 *A.* The fifth impulse is an atrial premature beat; there is a premature P wave (usually labeled P) followed by a normal QRS-T complex, and the postextrasystolic pause is longer than the sinus cycle but less than compensatory. *B.* The fourth impulse is an atrial premature beat with aberrant intraventricular conduction; there is a premature P wave followed by an anomalous QRS-T complex; the postextrasystolic pause is less than compensatory. *C.* Nonconducted atrial premature beat. Following the third ventricular complex, a P wave negatively deforms the ST segment and is not followed by a ventricular response.

plex, and functional bundle-branch block due to tachycardia may also occur, making a distinction from ventricular tachyarrhythmias difficult (Fig. 24-15). Functional bundle-branch block may have either a left or a right bundle-branch block pattern.

Management of PSVT due to AV Nodal Reentry PSVT due to AV nodal reentry is a benign disturbance requiring intervention primarily for the patient's comfort and sense of well-being. When it coexists with other disease processes in which the tachyarrhythmia is poorly tolerated, such as ischemic heart disease or mitral stenosis, it may have more serious implications. Occasionally, the rate is rapid enough to cause near-syncope or syncope in otherwise normal individuals, although such rates are more common in PSVT due to WPW (see below).

Rest, sedation, and vagotonic maneuvers are simple means of reverting acute episodes, and patients can be taught self-administered vagotonic maneuvers for recurrences. Patients should be advised to avoid inciting factors, such as smoking, alcohol, extreme fatigue, and stress. Many of the effective pharmacologic interventions for acute episodes used in the past have given way to new drug therapy. Infusions of sympathomimetic drugs (e.g., phenylephrine or methoxamine), parasympathomimetic drugs (e.g., edrophonium or neostigmine), and digoxin have been supplanted by intravenous adenosine, Ca^{2+}-entry blockers, or beta-adrenergic blockers for managing the acute episodes. Adenosine, 6 mg given intravenously (see Fig. 24-13),

TABLE 24-7 Management of Paroxysmal Supraventricular Tachycardias

Interventions	Acute	Long-Term
Physiologic interventions	Rest, sedation Valsalva maneuver Carotid sinus massage	Self-administered Valsalva maneuver, carotid sinus massage Avoidance of inciting factors
Pharmacologic therapy	Drugs with direct effect on AV nodal or accessory pathway Drugs that control ventricular rate	Drugs that alter properties of AV node or accessory pathways Drugs that control ventricular rate
Catheter ablation and surgical techniques	—	Ablation of reentrant pathway Modification of AV node
Electronic devices	Temporary pacing Cardioversion	Permanent pacemaker

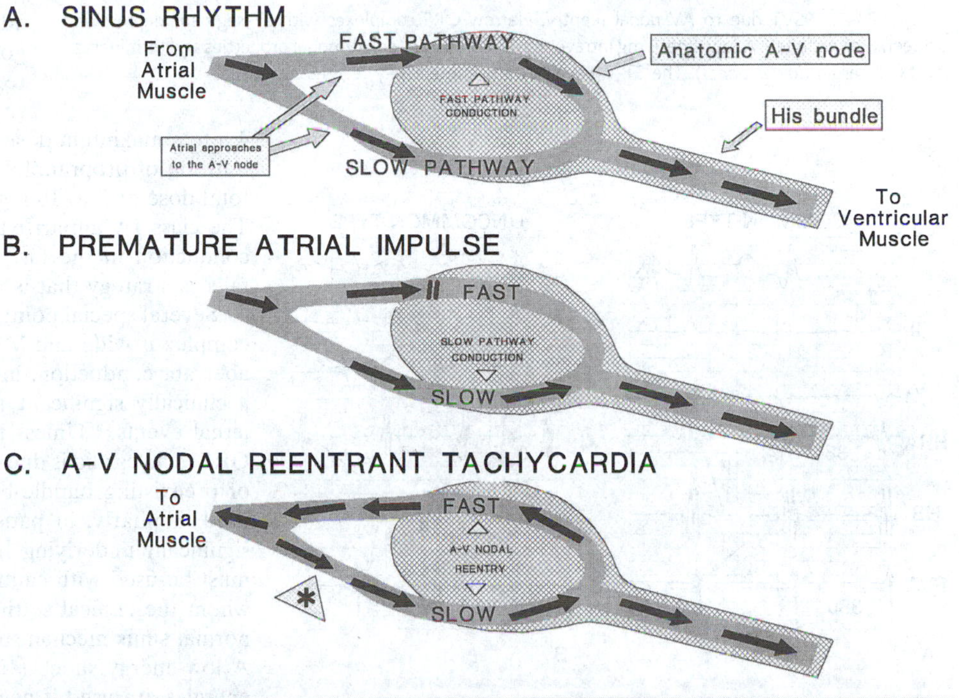

FIGURE 24-12 Mechanism of PSVT due to AV nodal reentry. This arrhythmia is due to the presence of dual AV nodal pathways with different conduction properties and refractory periods. Although the fast and slow pathways were previously thought to be within the anatomic AV node, the pathways are now viewed as having critical components in the atrial approaches to the AV node. Nonetheless, the dual-pathway physiology concept is valid. *A.* During sinus rhythm in the presence of a dual AV nodal pathway, the fast pathway (which generally has a longer refractory period) is primarily responsible for AV transmission because of slower propagation in the other pathway. *B.* A premature atrial impulse blocks in the fast pathway because of its longer refractory period and propagates down the slow pathway, prolonging the PR interval and allowing retrograde invasion of the fast pathway because its tissue remains polarized due to block of the descending impulse. *C.* Echo beats or AV nodal reentrant tachycardia will occur when the time relationships between slow pathway conduction and recovery of excitability at the site of block in the fast pathway allow the impulse to reenter the slow pathway after retrograde fast pathway transmission. The atria are also activated retrogradely. In a much less common form of AV nodal reentry, a shorter refractory period in the fast pathway reverses the loop, with antegrade conduction down the fast pathway and retrograde conduction up the slow pathway (see Fig. 24-13 for examples). RF energy for slow pathway ablation therapy is applied at the site indicated by the asterisk.

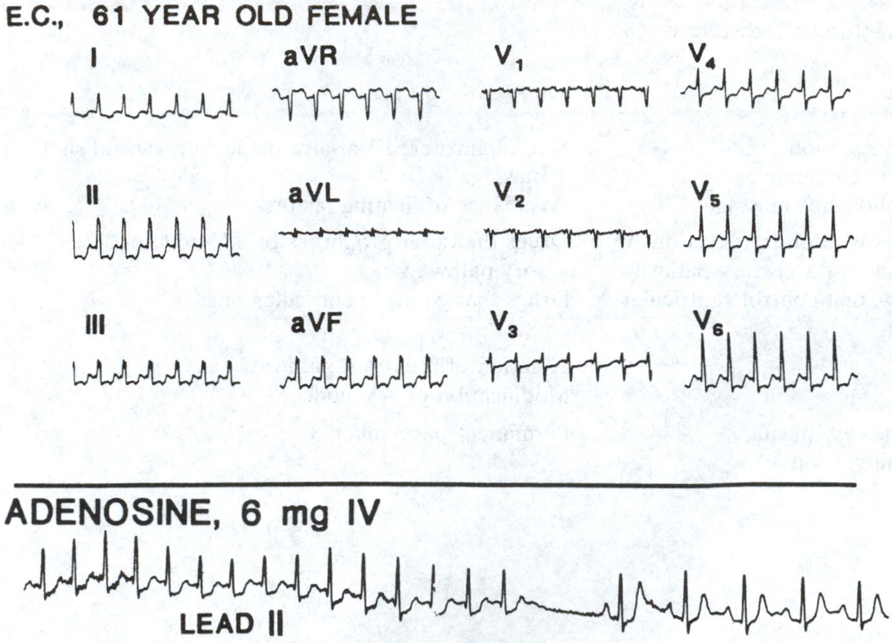

FIGURE 24-13 PSVT due to AV nodal reentry. Narrow QRS complexes with ST-segment depression are seen (*upper panel*). Adenosine, 6 mg intravenously, abruptly alters AV nodal properties and terminates the tachycardia (*lower panel*). The ST-T wave pattern immediately returns to normal.

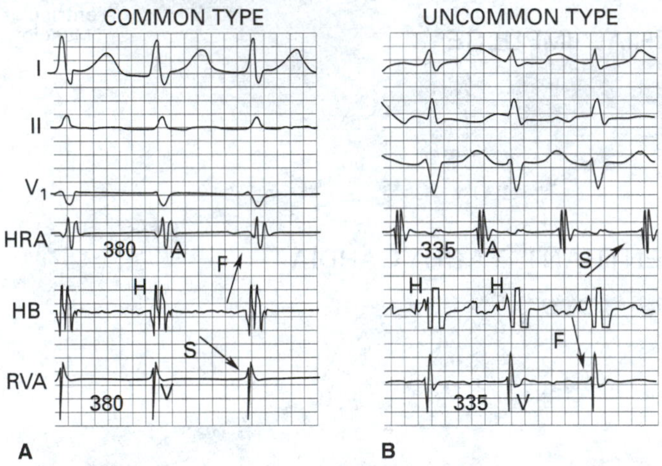

FIGURE 24-14 Common and uncommon forms of AV nodal reentrant tachycardia recorded during electrophysiologic studies. *A*. The common type of AV nodal reentrant tachycardia, antegrade conduction in the slow pathway and retrograde in the fast pathway, results in atrial (A) and ventricular (V) activation that are close to one another in time. Characteristically, intracardiac recordings demonstrate a "lining up" of atrial and ventricular electrograms, indicating that the atria are activated before completion of ventricular activation. *B*. In the uncommon type of AV nodal reentrant tachycardia, antegrade fast pathway and retrograde slow pathway conduction change the relative timing pattern so that atrial activation is delayed relative to ventricular activation, and the electrograms are not in line. In this form of PSVT, the RP interval is longer than the PR interval on the ECG, which results in inscription of the retrograde P wave *after* the ST-T wave of the related ventricular impulse. The uncommon type of AV nodal reentrant tachycardia may be difficult to distinguish from other arrhythmias, such as ectopic atrial tachyarrhythmias or concealed WPW syndrome (see the text).

followed by one or two 12-mg boluses if necessary, is effective and safe[23] for acute treatment. Because of its very short duration of action and lack of the negative inotropic effects of Ca^{2+}-entry blockers, it is now preferred to other acute pharmacologic therapies, especially when managing a patient with concomitant structural heart disease. A 5-mg bolus of verapamil, followed by one or two additional 5-mg boluses 10 min apart if the initial dose does not convert the arrhythmia, has been an effective regimen in up to 90 percent of patients with PSVT due to AV node reentry.[24,25] However, it must not be used for an unknown wide QRS tachycardia because of risk of adverse effects when used in patients who have VT.[26] Intravenous diltiazem is also effective.[27,28] Initial treatment consists of a bolus of 0.25 mg/kg body weight administered over 2 min. If the response is inadequate, a repeat bolus of 0.35 mg/kg over 2 min is administered 15 min later. Intravenous digoxin, 0.5 mg infused over 10 min and repeated if necessary, may convert the arrhythmia. An additional 0.25 mg every 4 h to a maximum dose of 1.5 mg in 24 h may be used. A slow infusion of propranolol may be used;[29] 1 mg/min is given to a total dose of 5 to 10 mg or a significant fall in blood pressure. The class IA antiarrhythmic agents, which appear to depress conduction in the fast pathway, may be tried if other drugs fail,[30] a strategy that is rarely needed.

Several special points must be remembered. When the QRS complex is wide and VT is mistakenly diagnosed as SVT with aberrant conduction, intravenous verapamil frequently causes a clinically significant fall in blood pressure and potentially lethal events.[26] Unless it is known with certainty that a wide QRS tachycardia is due to aberrant intraventricular conduction or preexisting bundle-branch block, verapamil should not be used. Similarly, in patients with coexisting hemodynamically significant underlying heart disease, intravenous propranolol must be used with caution, if at all. For those few patients in whom the clinical setting demands an immediate return to a normal sinus mechanism, DC cardioversion can be employed. A low-energy shock (10 to 50 W · s) may be sufficient; larger energies are used if necessary. If DC cardioversion should be avoided, pacing the right atrium or ventricle via a temporary pacing catheter is usually successful (see Chap. 31).

Long-term prevention of recurrent PSVT due to AV nodal reentry may be achieved with pharmacologic therapy or catheter ablation. Surgical techniques and electronic devices have been used in the past but are now obsolete. Patients who have infrequent, well-tolerated episodes that are short-lived and/or respond to self-administered physiologic maneuvers (Table 24-7) may require no long-term interventions. In many others, pharmacologic therapy is sufficient. Most patients have reduced numbers and severity of attacks with simple medications such as propranolol, verapamil, or digoxin. These drugs act by altering conduction velocities and refractory periods in the AV nodal pathways, disrupting the delicate balance required for initiation

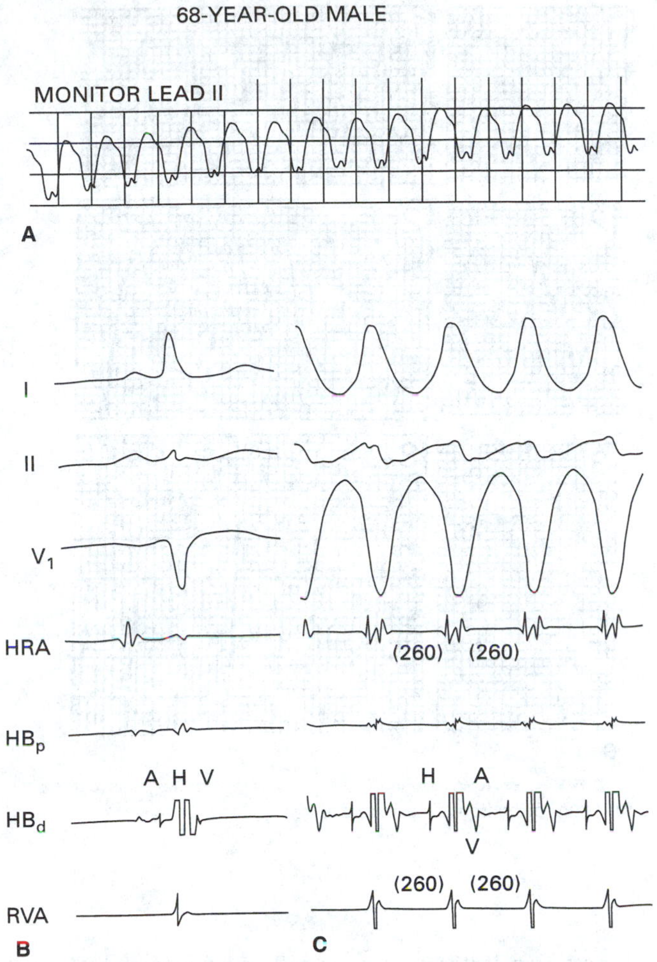

FIGURE 24-15 PSVT due to AV nodal reentry. *A.* The initial presenting rhythm was a wide-QRS tachycardia with a vertical axis and a left bundle-branch block pattern. *B.* A sinus impulse with intracardiac recordings demonstrating normal sequences of AV conduction. *C.* Recording during a wide-QRS tachycardia with a left bundle-branch block pattern. The nearly simultaneous A and V activation patterns in the retrograde and antegrade directions (i.e., atrial activation before the end of ventricular activation) suggest the common form of AV nodal reentry rather than ventricular tachycardia.

or maintenance of sustained arrhythmias. Membrane-active antiarrhythmic drugs may prevent recurrences, both by suppressing triggering premature impulses and by depressing conduction in the anterograde (fast) pathway of the AV nodal reentrant circuit.[30] However, the risk of potentially serious proarrhythmic responses, combined with other troublesome side effects, limits their use for these arrhythmias.

RF catheter ablation is safe and very effective for PSVT due to AV nodal reentrant tachycardia.[31,32] It has therefore emerged as the treatment of choice for patients with frequent arrhythmic episodes and/or poor tolerance of drugs. It is also the preferred option for pharmacologically controllable AV nodal reentrant tachycardia among patients who want to avoid pharmacologic side effects. Among women who have a history of clustering of episodes of AV nodal reentrant tachycardia when perimenstrual, RF ablation procedures should be scheduled when they are premenstrual, in order to maximize the chance of inducing the target arrhythmia during the procedure.[33]

PSVT due to Accessory Pathways: Wolff-Parkinson-White Syndrome As in AV nodal reentry, the pathophysiology of reentrant tachyarrhythmias in WPW syndrome is a consequence of the presence of two pathways between the atria and the ventricles that have different conduction properties and refractory periods. WPW syndrome appears to be the second commonest cause of PSVT. Since it also occurs in a concealed form, in which the standard ECG is normal during sinus rhythm because of inability of the accessory pathway (AP) to conduct in the antegrade direction, the total number of PSVTs that are due to APs may be considerably higher than previous estimates. In the majority of patients, the effective refractory period of the AP exceeds that of the normal AV nodal–His-Purkinje pathway. Therefore, a premature atrial impulse may block at the AP and conduct antegradely in the normal pathway, ultimately entering the AP in the retrograde direction and reentering the atrium to establish a circus movement tachycardia referred to as orthodromic (Fig. 24-16*A*). Since the AP joins ordinary atrial and ventricular muscle and is not composed of specialized conduction tissue, AP conduction is rarely decremental (as it is in the AV node).

Because the normal pathway is responsible for ventricular activation and the AP for return to the atria, the delta wave is absent during orthodromic tachycardia, causing the QRS complex to normalize. In addition, since the AP provides retrograde conduction to the atria, P waves, if seen, are usually inverted in the inferior and lateral leads. The stability of the reentrant circuit depends upon the balance between conduction properties and refractory periods of the two pathways. In a much less common form of PSVT, a shorter refractory period in the anomalous pathway results in block of an initiating premature atrial impulse in the normal pathway, with antegrade conduction down the AP and then retrograde invasion of the normal AV nodal pathway to establish an antidromic tachycardia. The QRS complex is wide, having the characteristics of a ventricular complex originating near the insertion site of the AP (Fig. 24-16*B*). These wide QRS tachycardias may be difficult to distinguish from ventricular tachyarrhythmias if the existence of WPW syndrome is not established prior to presentation with a tachyarrhythmia. In the concealed form of WPW syndrome,[34,35] only orthodromic tachycardias can occur, because of inability of the AP to conduct in the antegrade direction. Distinction between concealed WPW syndrome and AV nodal reentrant tachycardia may be difficult, although a faster rate (greater than 200 per minute) and a visible retrograde P wave after, rather than lost within, the QRS complex favor concealed WPW syndrome. When atrial flutter or fibrillation occurs in patients with WPW syndrome, the risk of potentially lethal arrhythmias due to very rapid conduction across APs must be considered. The risk is particularly treacherous in patients with short-refractory-period APs, since atrial fibrillation may induce ventricular fibrillation in that circumstance.

PSVT in WPW syndrome may begin in childhood or may not appear until middle age. Among women, there appears to be an increased propensity for the first tachyarrhythmic event to occur during pregnancy.[36] In asymptomatic patients, the probability of losing the capacity for antegrade conduction across the AP increases with advancing age.[37] Symptomatic arrhythmias may be due to PSVT, atrial fibrillation or flutter, or both in individual patients. In a series of 212 patients with tachyarrhythmias and WPW, PSVT alone occurred in 64 percent, atrial

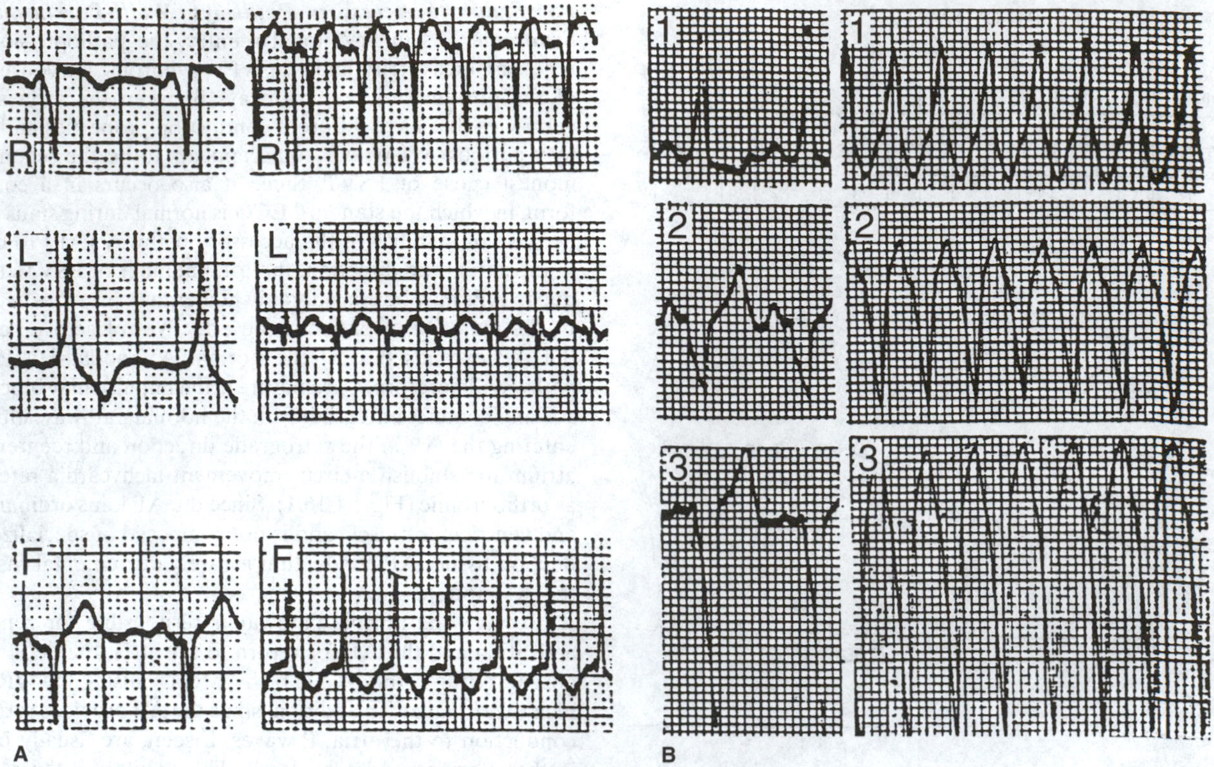

FIGURE 24-16 WPW syndrome with reciprocating tachycardia. *A.* Before and during an "orthodromic" tachycardia. *B.* From another patient before and during an "antidromic" tachycardia.

fibrillation alone in 20 percent, and both in 16 percent.[38] Since the reentrant tachyarrhythmias tend to be more rapid than those in patients with AV nodal reentry, they may be more symptomatic. Light-headedness, near-syncope, and syncope appear to occur more commonly in WPW with PSVT or atrial fibrillation than in AV nodal reentry. A risk of sudden death in patients with WPW has been emphasized, but the magnitude of the risk is unknown, even among those with APs that have short refractory periods. Other factors that appear to influence risk are the presence of multiple bypass tracts and a family history of premature sudden death.[39]

Electrocardiographic Features During normal sinus rhythm, the presence of an AP capable of antegrade conduction (manifest WPW) is recognized by the presence of a short PR interval, followed by slurred initial forces of the QRS complex—the delta wave—resulting from early activation (preexcitation) of the portion of ventricular muscle because specialized conduction has been bypassed. Several algorithms have been developed to identify the location of the AP electrocardiographically.[40,41] Some useful general rules include the following:

1. If the delta wave is positive in lead I and negative in lead V_1, the AP is probably right-sided; the vectors are generally opposite for left-sided tracts.
2. If the delta wave is positive in the inferior leads, the tract is likely to be anterior, and if it is negative in these leads, posterior. If it is negative in aVL, a left lateral AP is likely (Fig. 24-17).

The most common patterns recorded during PSVT due to WPW syndrome are narrow QRS tachycardias at rates ranging from 160 to 240 per minute. Rates may occasionally be faster or somewhat slower. When the tachycardia is antidromic, the QRS complexes are wide and have characteristics similar to fully preexcited impulses during sinus rhythm or PACs (see Fig. 24-16*B*). In atrial fibrillation with WPW syndrome, if the AP has a refractory period longer than the normal pathway, the delta wave will disappear and patterns typical of atrial fibrillation with narrow QRS complexes will be recorded. In contrast, when the refractory period of the AP is shorter, wide QRS complexes dominate the tracing (Fig. 24-18). Multiple bypass tracts are suggested by multiple wide-QRS-complex morphologies during atrial fibrillation with preexcited conduction (Fig. 24-18*B*). A grossly irregular rhythm with wide QRS complexes and a mean ventricular rate in excess of 200 per minute is a clue supporting WPW with atrial fibrillation in the differential diagnosis of a wide-QRS-complex tachycardia. Another form of wide-QRS tachycardia in WPW is orthodromic tachycardia with functional bundle-branch block. When a patient with left lateral bypass tract abruptly develops a wide QRS complex with a left bundle-branch block pattern during orthodromic tachycardia, the diagnosis of SVT with aberrancy is strongly suspected when the cycle length of the tachycardia *lengthens*. Functional left bundle-branch block delays arrival of the circu-

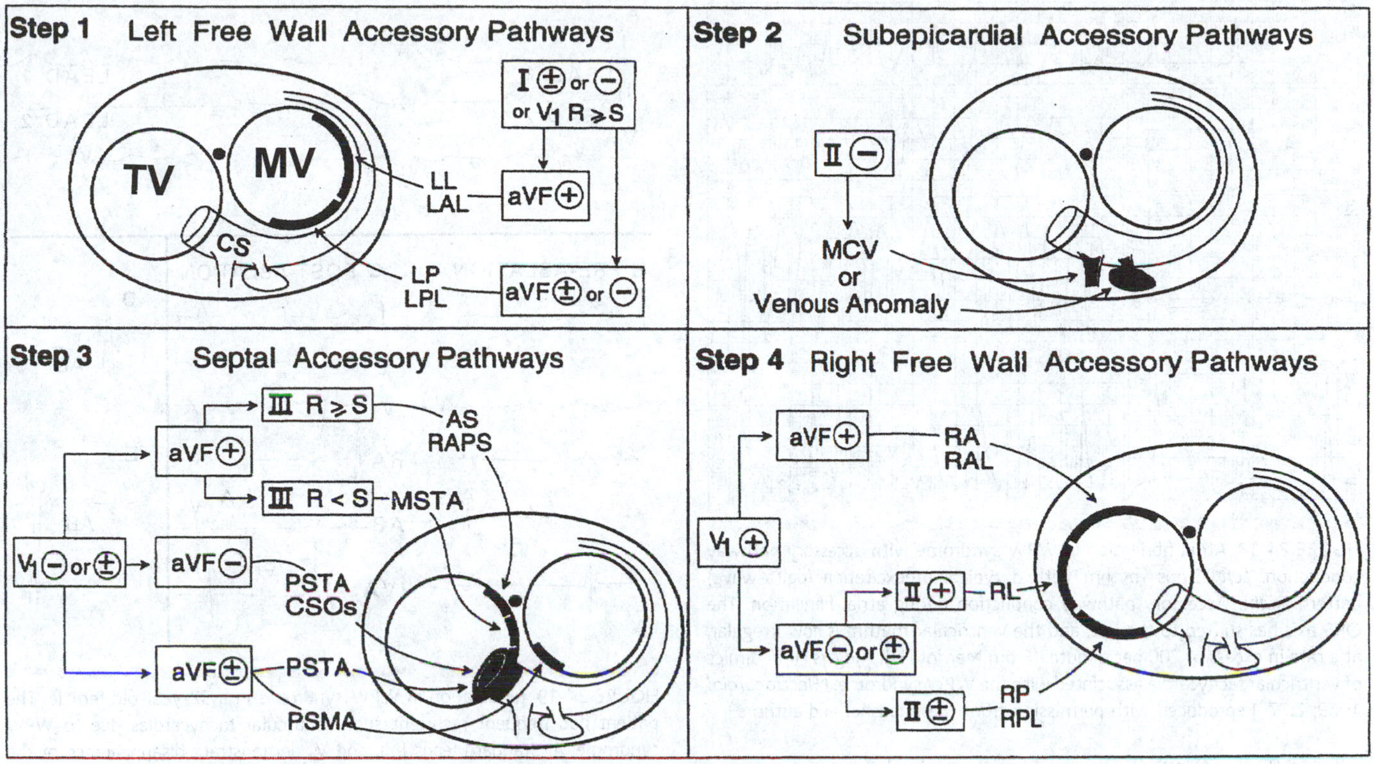

FIGURE 24-17 Localization of accessory pathways in patients with WPW syndrome. The line drawings illustrate the anatomic relationships between the tricuspid (TV) and mitral valves (MV), the coronary sinus (CS), AV conducting system, and accessory pathways. For each accessory pathway location indicated, the combination of QRS vectors most likely to result are shown, based on upright (+) or inverted (−) QRS waveforms. These vectorial guidelines are generally useful but not necessarily precise, since activation patterns from specific sites may vary in individual patients. Nomenclature for accessory pathway location: RA, anterior; RAL, right anterolateral; RL, right lateral; RPL, right posterolateral; RP, right posterior; PSTA, posteroseptal tricuspid annulus; CSOs, coronary sinus ostium; MSTA, mid-septal tricuspid annulus; AS, anteroseptal; RAPS, right anterior paraseptal; MCV, middle cardiac vein (coronary vein); CS, coronary sinus; venous anomaly (coronary sinus diverticulum); PSMA, posteroseptal mitral annulus; LP, left posterior; LPL, left posterolateral; LL, left lateral; LAL, left anterolateral. (From Arruda MS et al.[40] Reprinted with permission from the publisher and authors.)

lating impulse at the distal end of a left-sided AP, thereby lengthening the tachycardia cycle. Under most other conditions, appearance of functional left bundle-branch block correlates with *shortening* of the tachycardia cycle length, because the accelerating tachycardia rate encroaches on the refractory period of the left bundle branch (see also Chap. 23).

Management of PSVT due to WPW Syndrome This form of reentrant SVT is amenable to a broad range of interventions. Careful attention to the details of therapy is required because a subgroup of patients is at risk for potentially lethal arrhythmias due to very rapid conduction across the AP during atrial flutter or fibrillation. This concern influences the pharmacologic approaches to PSVT in the WPW syndrome, since drugs have different effects on APs and the AV node and because reciprocating PSVT may convert to atrial flutter or fibrillation.[42]

Physiologic interventions and vagomimetic drugs can be used safely during acute episodes of reciprocating tachycardia. In addition, adenosine, verapamil diltiazem, propranolol, and membrane-active antiarrhythmic agents, such as procainamide, quinidine, or disopyramide, may be used to convert acute reentrant tachycardias. Verapamil[43,44] and lidocaine[45] may accelerate the ventricular rate during atrial flutter or fibrillation in the WPW syndrome, however, and should be avoided if atrial fibrillation is present or if the patient has previously demonstrated alternation between atrial fibrillation and reciprocating tachycardia. Digoxin must be avoided in patients with WPW because it may shorten the refractory period of the AP[46] as well as atrial muscle. Should this occur in the presence of unrecognized atrial flutter or fibrillation or with the conversion of a reciprocating tachycardia to atrial fibrillation, the patient could develop a life-threatening tachyarrhythmia due to rapid AP conduction.[47] Whenever there is doubt, therapy should be limited to those drugs that will depress conduction in the AP or prolong its refractory period, such as the membrane-active antiarrhythmic agents (e.g., intravenous procainamide), or to agents, such as adenosine, that usually have no effect on an AP. Electrical cardioversion should be used if other means have failed or as initial therapy if the patient has extremely rapid rates causing hemodynamic intolerance of the tachycardia.

The approach to long-term management of patients with WPW syndrome is determined by the physiologic characteristics of the bypass tract and the frequency, duration, and symptoms of arrhythmias. Two primary approaches to therapy are available: drugs and catheter ablation. The latter, using an RF energy

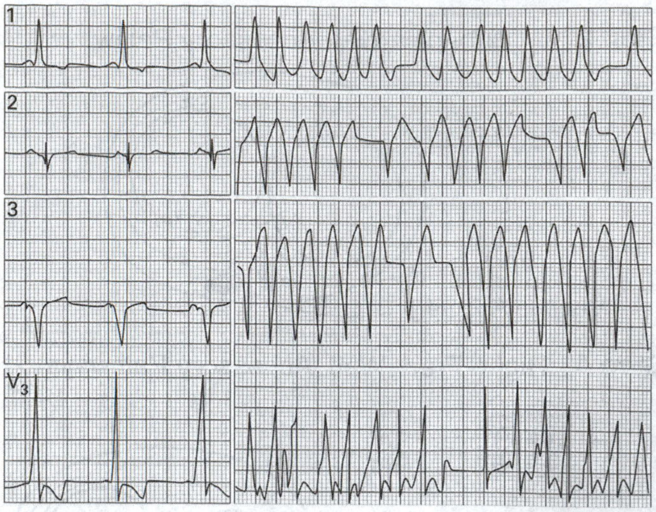

FIGURE 24-18 Atrial fibrillation in WPW syndrome with accessory pathway conduction. *Left.* Sinus rhythm with a typical preexcitation (delta-wave) pattern. *Right.* Accessory pathway conduction during atrial fibrillation. The QRS axis has shifted to the left, and the ventricular rhythm is now irregular, at a rate in excess of 200 per minute. (From Marriott HJL, Rogers HM. Mimics of ventricular tachycardia associated with the WPW syndrome. *J Electrocardiol* 1969; 2:77. Reproduced with permission from the publisher and authors.)

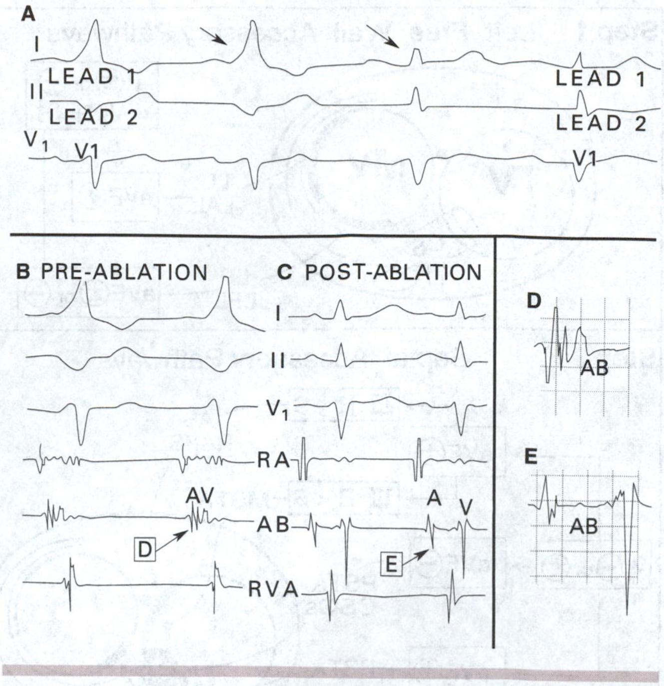

FIGURE 24-19 RF ablation in WPW syndrome in a 52-year-old female. The patient had frequent recurrent supraventricular tachycardias due to WPW syndrome. *A.* Standard leads I, II, and V_1 demonstrate disappearance of the delta wave from one impulse to the next 5 s after beginning the application of RF energy (compare successive QRS complexes indicated by arrows). *B.* Prior to ventricular ablation, the interval between atrial (A) and (V) activation at the site of the ablation catheter is less than 50 ms, and the sharp spike between A and V likely represents activity in the bypass tract. *C.* Immediately after ablation, the AV interval at the site of the ablation catheter is lengthened to 150 ms, and the accessory pathway spike has disappeared. *D, E.* Enlargements from panels B and C, respectively. AB, ablation catheter; RA, right atrium; RVA, right ventricular apex.

source (Fig. 24-19), is the preferred method for treatment of patients with tachycardias symptomatic enough to limit their quality of life (e.g., near-syncope or syncope) or with symptomatic life-threatening arrhythmias in WPW (e.g, atrial fibrillation with short refractory period bypass tract)[34,48] (see Chap. 28). Surgery is a rarely used secondary approach, reserved for the occasional patients requiring treatment and not amenable to catheter ablation or pharmacologic therapy and for some who require surgery for other causes as well.[49] Although intracardiac electrophysiologic studies provide information on drug efficacy and pharmacologic effects on the bypass tract,[50] this invasive procedure is seldom performed for this purpose any longer.[51] Patients who demonstrate a good clinical response to therapy, measured in terms of reduced frequency or rate of tachyarrhythmic episodes, can be managed noninvasively; patients with an intermittent delta wave and no clinical arrhythmia need no therapy. On the other hand, patients who have frequent or poorly tolerated tachyarrhythmias, those who are prone to episodes of atrial flutter or fibrillation[52] (particularly if they develop wide QRS complexes during their tachyarrhythmias, suggesting bypass tract conduction), or those who have a family history of WPW and sudden death[39,53] should be evaluated by electrophysiologic testing. In such patients, catheter ablation using RF energy is the intervention of choice when available in an experienced laboratory and accepted by the patient.[32,48,54] In the event of failure of the technique to interrupt the tract or tracts, surgical interventions may be considered,[55,56] but the threshold for surgical intervention is higher. Among those with symptomatic or life-threatening arrhythmias for whom RF ablation is not available, accepted, or feasible, a clear-cut response to antiarrhythmic therapy is mandated. Among the antiarrhythmic agents, the class IA, IC, and III drugs (see Table 24-5) may be useful. Not all drugs in these categories are approved for this indication in the United States, but efficacy studies are impressive.[57-61] Because of its side-effect profile, the threshold for use of amiodarone has been higher, despite good efficacy[59] (see also Chap. 27). PSVT also occurs in patients with *concealed* WPW syndrome,[35,62] a condition in which the bypass tract is incapable of conducting in the antegrade direction. Thus, there is no delta wave during sinus rhythm, but intact retrograde conduction permits completion of reciprocating tachycardia circuits. The diagnosis is suggested by longer RP intervals on the ECG during tachycardia than occur in AV nodal reentry[35] and can be established by electrophysiologic testing. Management is similar to that for other WPW syndrome patients. However, even though atrial fibrillation may occur, there is no concern about risk of degenerating to ventricular fibrillation. In such patients, the ventricular rate is controlled by normal AV nodal properties, since the AP cannot provide antegrade conduction.

Other Paroxysmal Reentrant SVTs The other reentrant SVTs are far less common than PSVT due to AV node reentry or WPW syndrome. The PSVT due to sinus node reentry[63,64] is difficult to distinguish clinically and by ECG from sinus tachycardia, except for its paroxysmal onset and offset. P-wave morphology is similar to that in sinus tachycardia. Intraatrial reentry[64,65] may be difficult to distinguish from certain forms of automatic ectopic atrial tachycardia. Intraatrial and sinus node reentry are distinguished from PSVT due to AV node reentry or WPW on a standard ECG because P waves precede narrow QRS complexes during these tachycardias.

Atriofascicular and nodoventricular pathways (Mahaim tracts)[66] may cause PSVT with wide QRS complexes having a left bundle-branch block pattern. Intracardiac electrophysiologic studies are usually necessary for specific diagnosis and treatment of these various PSVTs. There is no generally accepted and predictably effective approach to therapy. Intraatrial reentrant tachycardia may be treated with conventional membrane-active antiarrhythmic agents (beta-adrenergic blocking agents, or perhaps Ca^{2+}-entry blockers). Sinus node reentry may respond to digoxin, propranolol, diltiazem, or verapamil. Surgical interventions[67] are only rarely considered for these arrhythmias because of their usually benign nature, but catheter ablation with RF energy has proved to be useful for many (see also Chap. 28).

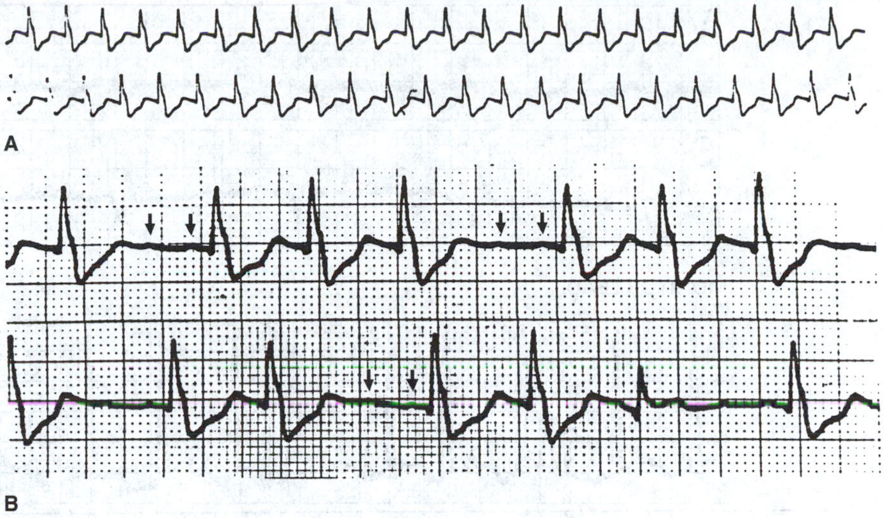

FIGURE 24-20 Ectopic atrial tachycardia. *A.* A 20-s continuous recording demonstrates a regular tachycardia at a ventricular rate of approximately 140 per minute. *B.* During carotid sinus massage, ventricular conduction becomes irregular, and diminutive P waves at twice the basic ventricular rate are evident. Impaired AV conduction with little or no effect on atrial activity is characteristic of the response of an ectopic atrial tachycardia to carotid sinus massage.

ECTOPIC ATRIAL TACHYCARDIAS

These arrhythmias are usually persistent, are commonly referred to as "nonparoxysmal," and may be associated with specific inciting factors. There are experimental and clinical reasons to support the notion that ectopic atrial tachycardias can be due to mechanisms of reentry,[68] automaticity (enhanced spontaneous phase 4 depolarization),[69] or triggered activity.[70] An underlying toxic or metabolic cause is commonly identified as the factor responsible for ectopic atrial tachycardia, but some are persistent or recurrent, likely due to focal atrial disease. When an ectopic atrial rate is in the range of 160 to greater than 200 per minute and associated with 2:1 conduction or variable block in a patient receiving digitalis, a digitalis-toxic rhythm must be suspected strongly. Decompensated chronic lung disease, metabolic abnormalities (including acute alcohol abuse), electrolyte disturbances, and hypoxemia should be considered when digitalis toxicity has been excluded. Various forms of cardiac disease, including acute myocardial infarction, also may cause ectopic atrial tachycardia. Ectopic tachycardias also may originate from atrial suture lines in patients who have previously had complex congenital heart disease surgery.[71] The atrial arrhythmias may appear many years after the surgery.

Electrocardiographic Features P waves are usually normal to small in amplitude and may be difficult to identify when the ventricular rate is rapid (Fig. 24-20). Atrial activity does not slow during carotid sinus massage, but AV conduction is usually impeded, making P waves more evident. When ectopic atrial tachycardia is due to digitalis intoxication or occurs in the presence of hyperkalemia, P waves may be "diminutive" (Fig. 24-21*A*).

Management of Ectopic Atrial Tachycardias Treatment is dictated by identification and reversal of inciting factors, by ablation of a defined focal source when identifiable, and by control of the heart rate when necessary. Temporary pacing is required infrequently. More commonly, the problem is one of a rapid ventricular rate. Attempts to control the ectopic atrial arrhythmias with membrane-active antiarrhythmic drugs have not been generally successful. (Beta-adrenergic blocking agents or Ca^{2+}-entry blocking agents may be successful in controlling the arrhythmia in some patients, but a uniformly beneficial response should not be expected. Electrical cardioversion is not indicated because it is usually unsuccessful.

The mainstay of therapy remains the removal or reversal of inciting factors. If a controllable inciting factor cannot be identified or reversed, antiarrhythmic drugs may be tried. In addition, catheter ablation techniques may have a short-term success rate of as much as 80 percent among those whose arrhythmia has a structural basis.[72] It is not useful for metabolic or toxic causes and is very limited for those having multiple foci of origin.

MULTIFOCAL ATRIAL TACHYCARDIA: CHAOTIC ATRIAL RHYTHM

The diagnosis of multifocal atrial tachycardia, or chaotic atrial rhythm, requires the electrocardiographic identification of P waves having three or more different morphologies, occurring at different cycle lengths (Fig. 24-21*B*). The rhythm, as the name indicates, is usually very irregular, but the rate is not usually excessive (less than 140 per minute).[73] It is most commonly associated with underlying lung disease, metabolic abnormalities, electrolyte disturbances, and, in rare instances, toxic causes, such as digitalis intoxication. Calcium-entry blockers have been tried with some success[74] when given acutely, but there is little success with conventional membrane-active antiarrhythmic ages. Beta-adrenergic blockers have also been suggested,[75] but feasibility of their use may be limited by the nature of the underlying disease (e.g., chronic obstructive pulmonary disease). Removal of inciting factors (e.g., improvement of P_{O_2},

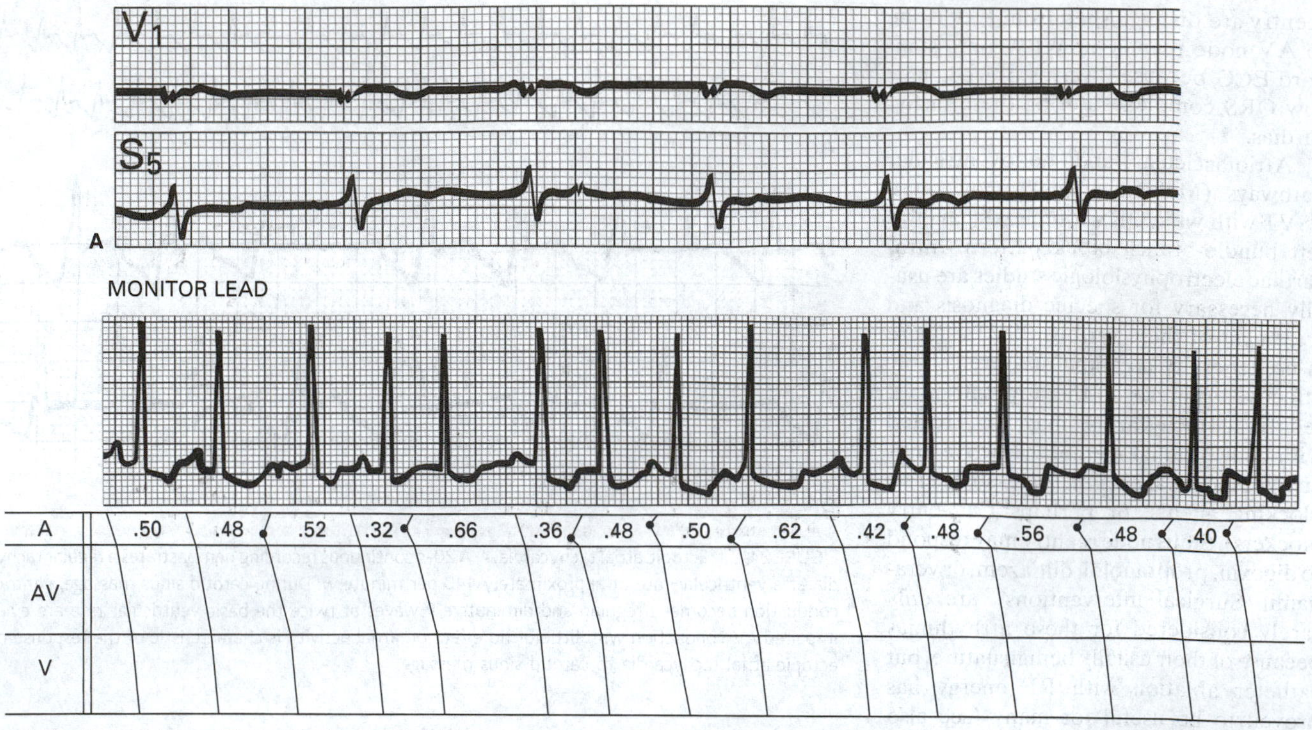

FIGURE 24-21 A. Atrial tachycardia with 2:1 AV block due to digitalis intoxication. Note the diminitive P waves, barely visible even in V_1. *B.* Multifocal (chaotic) atrial tachycardia. Note the constantly changing form of the ectopic P waves and the irregular rhythm at a mean rate of 122 per minute. Three or more distinct P-wave morphologies are required to make the diagnosis.

P_{CO_2}, pH, and/or electrolyte status) has been the most successful approach when the rhythm is associated with pulmonary or metabolic dysfunction, but many patients are forced to tolerate a chronic low-grade tachyarrhythmia because of inefficacy of any approach. There is no role for cardioversion, implantable devices, surgery, or catheter ablation.

ATRIAL FLUTTER

Atrial flutter is a rapid, regular atrial tachyarrhythmia that is less common than the PSVTs or atrial fibrillation. It is observed infrequently in normal individuals[76] but may occur at any age in the presence of underlying atrial abnormalities, such as those secondary to mitral valve disease, congenital heart disease, cardiomyopathies, and, less frequently, coronary artery disease. Subgroups at particularly high risk for developing atrial flutter are children, adolescents, and young adults who have undergone corrective surgery for complex congenital heart diseases, most notably transposition of the great vessels, tetralogy of Fallot, or atrial septal defects.[77]

Atrial flutter has been separated into two types: classic, or type I, and type II.[78] Classic type I flutter is characterized by a single right atrial macroreentrant circuit with defined anatomic and functional boundaries and an obligate pathway through an area of slow conduction, the subeustachian isthmus. This isthmus-dependent conduction pattern in classic type I atrial flutter travels in a counterclockwise rotation up the interatrial septum, down the atrial free wall, and along the crista terminalis, which serves as an anatomic barrier.[79] The other boundaries of this reentrant circuit include the tricuspid valve ring on one side and an area of probable anatomic block in the region extending from the venae cavae to the eustachian valve and ridge on the other side. A clockwise rotation around the same circuit can generate a variant of type I atrial flutter that may occur spontaneously and may also be induced repeatedly during electrophysiologic studies.

The distinction between type I and type II atrial flutter is based upon (1) the ability to entrain and interrupt type I flutter with atrial pacing techniques and (2) a faster atrial rate in type II flutter. Untreated type I flutter usually has atrial rates between 280 and 320 per minute, commonly very close to 300 per minute. Type I, however, may occur infrequently at rates as low as 240 to 250 and as high as 340 per minute. In type II flutter, the atrial rate is commonly at least 340 to 350 per minute and occasionally may be as fast as 450 per minute. The ventricular rate in atrial flutter is usually a defined fraction of the atrial rate, for example, 2:1 conduction in type I flutter generating a characteristic ventricular rate of 150 per minute and 4:1 conduction at 75 per minute. Group beating may occur, often reflecting two levels of block in the AV junction with a Wenckebach phenomenon influencing the impulses conducting below the site of 2:1 block.[80] Clinically, atrial flutter may occur in brief, persistent, or chronic forms, and therapeutic approaches are influenced by the clinical pattern.

Electrocardiographic Features Atrial flutter generates a defined pattern of atrial activity in the ECG. In typical type I atrial flutter with counterclockwise rotation, the classically described sawtooth pattern is identifiable in leads II, III, and aVF (Fig. 24-22). The electrical activity appears continuous in these leads, without a defined isoelectric baseline between flutter waves. In contrast, a discernible isoelectric line may appear in these leads when type I atrial flutter is slower than usual, as may occur in

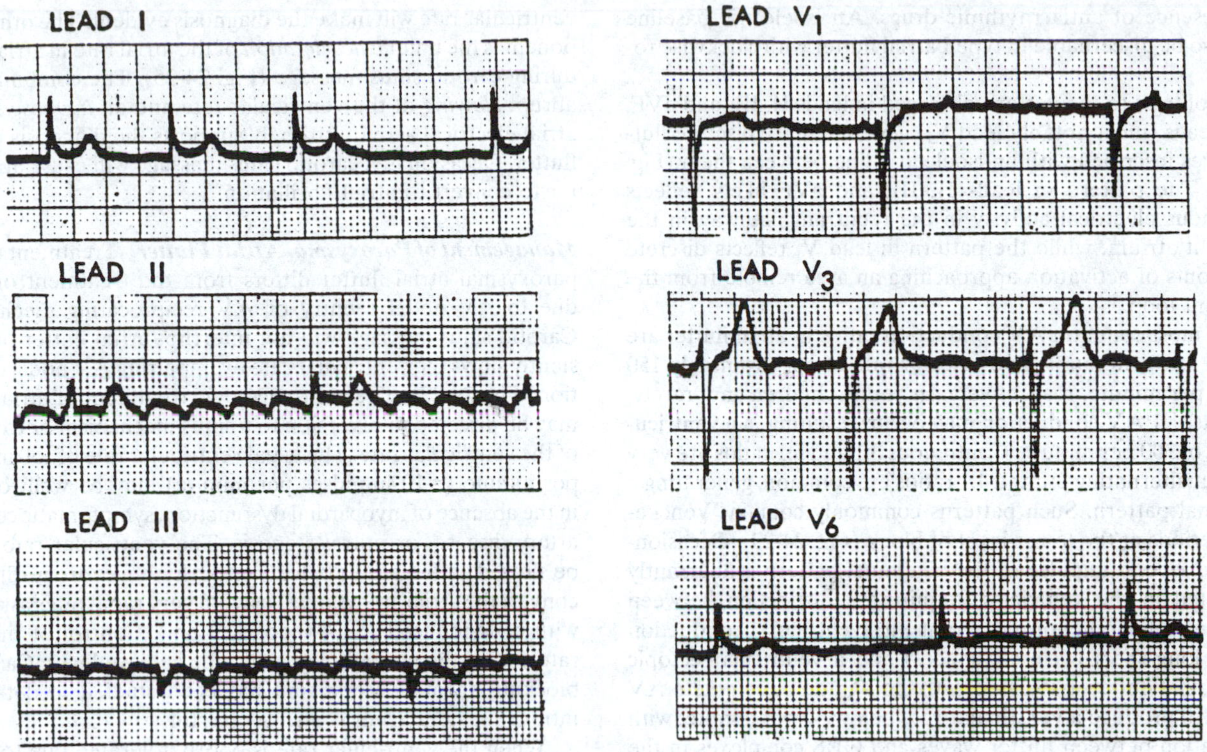

FIGURE 24-22 Atrial flutter. Note the "sawtooth" pattern in leads II and III, discrete atrial waves in V_1, and poorly registered atrial activity in leads I and V_6.

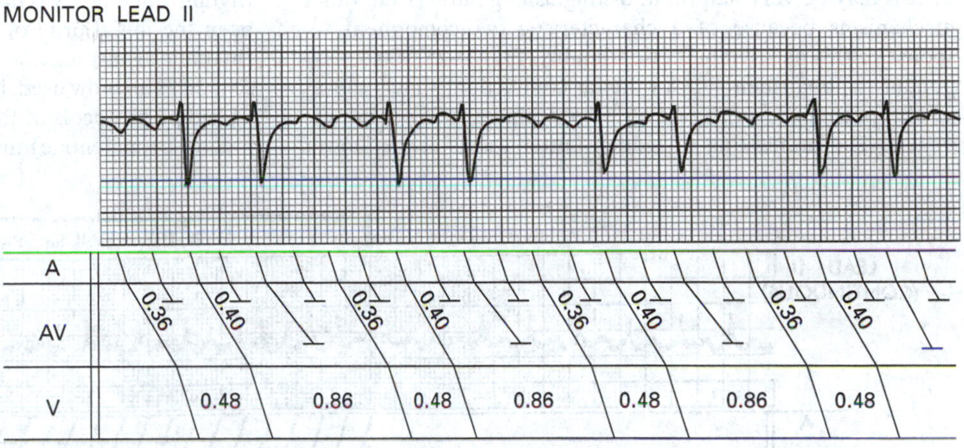

FIGURE 24-23 Atrial flutter with alternating 4:1 and 2:1 conduction. This common cause of bigeminal rhythm is almost always due to 2:1 AV conduction high in the AV junction and 3:2 Wenckebach periods at a lower level, as diagrammed.

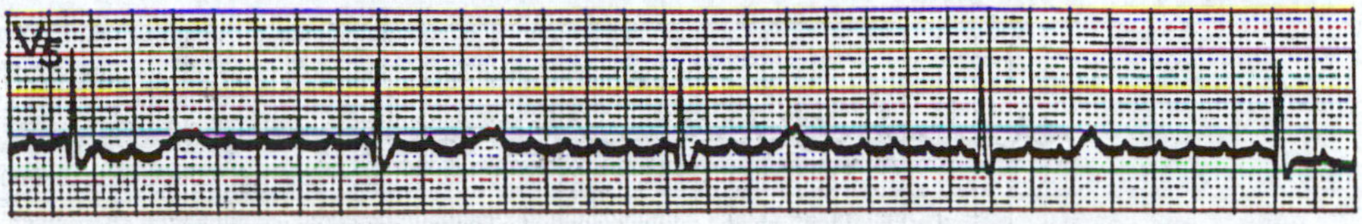

FIGURE 24-24 Atrial flutter (type II) with complete AV block. The atrial rate is 366 per minute, and the ventricular rate is 40 per minute. The ventricular rhythm remains regular, while the relationship between atrial and ventricular complexes varies.

the presence of antiarrhythmic drugs. An isoelectric baseline may also be discernable in type I atrial flutter with clockwise rotation.

In contrast to the pattern observed in leads II, III, and aVF, other leads (most notably lead V_1) generally have discrete flutter waves inscribed with an isoelectric line between them (Fig. 24-22). The pattern in leads II, III, and aVF likely reflects continuous electrical activity in the reentrant pathway in the low right atrium, while the pattern in lead V_1 reflects discrete wavefronts of activation approaching an area remote from the reentrant loop.

The most common AV conduction ratios in atrial flutter are 2:1 and 4:1, generating a ventricular rate of approximately 150 and 75 per minute, respectively. In young children and, rarely, in adults, 1:1 AV conduction may occur, resulting in a ventricular rate of 300 per minute. Continuous 3:1 and 5:1 ratios are very rare, but alternating 2:1 and 4:1 ratios are common, generating a bigeminal pattern. Such patterns commonly contain Wenckebach periods at the lower level of block (Fig. 24-23). Occasionally, the second impulse of the bigeminal pattern is aberrantly conducted in the ventricles, requiring a distinction between Ashman's phenomenon (aberrant intraventricular conduction due to long-short cycle sequences) and a ventricular ectopic beat. Atrial flutter associated with high-grade or complete AV block will produce a ventricular rate below 60 per minute, with dissociation between flutter waves and QRS complexes in the case of complete AV block (Fig. 24-24).

A narrow QRS complex tachycardia at a rate of 150 per minute should always lead to the consideration of atrial flutter. Carotid sinus massage will not interrupt atrial flutter but nonetheless may be very helpful in distinguishing flutter from other mechanisms because of a characteristic two-component response to this parasympathetic stimulus (Fig. 24-25). One component is impairment of AV nodal conduction, which causes an abrupt change from a rate of 150 per minute to 75 per minute or less. The unmasking of hidden flutter waves at the slower ventricular rate will make the diagnosis evident. The other component is the unique *acceleration* of the atrial rate in atrial flutter during carotid sinus massage (Fig. 24-25). The combination of abrupt *slowing* of the ventricular rate and an *increased rate* of atrial electrical activity strongly supports the diagnosis of atrial flutter. Occasionally, carotid sinus massage will cause atrial flutter to convert to atrial fibrillation.

Management of Paroxysmal Atrial Flutter Treatment of acute paroxysmal atrial flutter differs from the treatment of PSVT due to AV nodal reentry or AV reciprocating mechanisms. Carotid sinus massage will not interrupt atrial flutter but transiently slows the ventricular rate by impairing AV nodal conduction (Fig. 24-25). The pharmacologic treatment of atrial flutter may be directed to reversion to a sinus mechanism or to control of the ventricular rate. The usual ventricular rate of 150 impulses per minute (±10 impulses per minute) may be well tolerated in the absence of myocardial dysfunction, symptomatic coronary artery disease, or mitral stenosis. The ventricular rate should be slowed with digitalis before antiarrhythmics are instituted to convert the atrial arrhythmia to avoid very rapid rates associated with drug-induced 1:1 AV conduction.[82] Control of the heart rate during the paroxysm may also be achieved with Ca^{2+}-entry blocking agents.[25] Verapamil has been studied in detail, and intravenous diltiazem is also successful.

When the ventricular rate is poorly tolerated due to effects on hemodynamics or coronary blood flow, electrical cardioversion is used as initial treatment. An attempt using 10 to 50 J may be successful; higher energies are often necessary. Membrane-active antiarrhythmic agents are used to convert flutter to sinus rhythm, but efficacy is unpredictable. Historically, quinidine has been the initial drug of choice, but the other class IA antiarrhythmic agents may be equally effective. Conventional dosing schedules are now used, in contrast to the highly toxic aggressive quinidine protocols of the past. The class IC drugs (e.g., flecainide or propafenone) may also be effective for pharmacologic

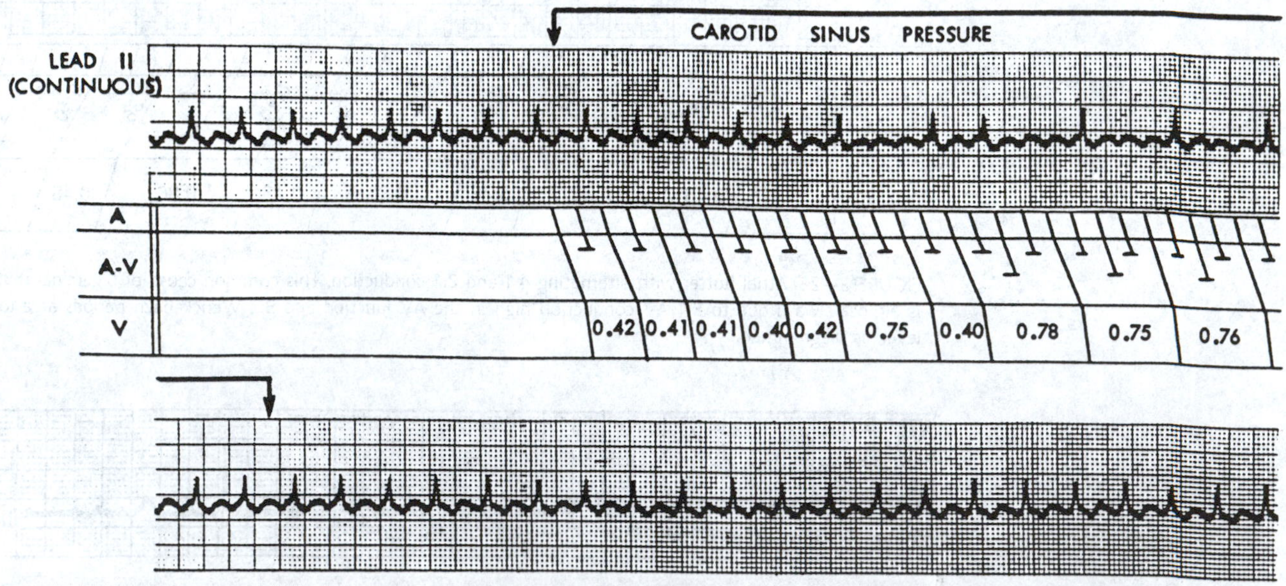

FIGURE 24-25 Atrial flutter and carotid sinus massage. At the beginning of the strip, AV conduction is occurring at the common 2:1 ratio, and flutter waves can be suspected but not proved. However, during carotid sinus massage, the conduction ratio increases to 4:1, and the flutter waves are easily recognized. Note the tendency of the atrial (flutter) rate to increase slightly during the parasympathetic stimulus.

reversion of atrial flutter,[57] although they slow intraatrial conduction without lengthening refractory periods. This drug effect may result in slowing atrial flutter from 300 per minute to less than 240 per minute, allowing 1:1 conduction to the ventricles at rates as high as 220 to 240 per minute. Because of the concomitant rate-dependent effect on ventricular conduction velocity, the slowed atrial rate with 1:1 conduction may generate wide QRS complexes mimicking ventricular tachycardia.[81] Ibutelide, an intravenous drug with class III effects, is also effective for acute treatment of atrial flutter.[86] Its major concern is the short-term risk of torsades de pointes, which necessitates monitoring for several hours after administration. Failing conversion or achieving an acceptable rate with drugs, elective DC cardioversion is usually successful. If cardioversion is contraindicated or fails, an attempt to entrain the atrium with rapid atrial pacing may result in conversion to sinus rhythm[83,84] (see Chap. 31). Occasionally, rapid pacing may convert atrial flutter to atrial fibrillation, which will have a slower ventricular response. Pharmacologic management for recurrences of the paroxysmal form of atrial flutter includes long-term use of antiarrhythmic therapy to prevent the arrhythmia and the use of AV nodal blocking agents to control heart rate during recurrences. For the former, the class IA antiarrhythmic agents, especially quinidine, have been used with variable success. Class IC and class III drugs are potentially useful, but the concern with the mechanism of action of class IC drugs in atrial flutter cited above limits their use. Control of ventricular rate is best achieved with digitalis because of safety and efficacy considerations. Long-term oral use of verapamil for control of rate in recurrent atrial flutter is less predictably effective than intravenous use to slow the rate during a paroxysm.[24] Beta-adrenergic blocking agents have been used, and if the drugs are well tolerated, the dose can be titrated to clinical beta-blocking efficacy by heart rate and blood pressure criteria. Subsequent observations of ventricular rates during recurrences will establish efficacy. There is no known excess incidence of embolic events during paroxysmal atrial flutter or during its reversion. Anticoagulants are not used before, during, or after reversion. In recent years, RF catheter ablation procedures have been used with increasing frequency for patients with atrial flutter, especially for patients with frequent symptomatic episodes of atrial flutter or those resistant to drug therapy. A linear RF ablation lesion across the subeustachian isthmus, between the tricuspid valve annulus and the inferior vena cava, interrupts the reentrant pathway responsible for type I flutter. The procedure has a high probability of permanent clinical success,[85,87] avoiding the need for long-term pharmacologic therapy among these patients.

Management of Persistent Atrial Flutter Atrial flutter may occur in a persistent form secondary to noncardiac factors, such as thyrotoxicosis or pulmonary embolism, although it is most common in the presence of chronic heart disease. Persistent or chronic atrial flutter occurs, but not commonly, in otherwise normal persons. Patients subject to recurrent episodes of persistent atrial flutter can be maintained on long-term antiarrhythmic therapy. However, RF ablation has emerged as the therapy of choice for symptomatic patients in this category.[85] Recurrence of atrial flutter after an RF ablation procedure occurs in approximately 15 percent and is usually due to gaps in the linear lesion across the isthmus, maintaining continuity of conduction in the reentrant pathway.[85,88] These gaps can often be identified and sealed during a repeat RF ablation procedure. If RF ablation fails or is not desired by the patient, therapeutic approaches during recurrences include additional antiarrhythmic agents for reverting atrial flutter and agents that will control the ventricular rate. Acute antiarrhythmic therapy may include intravenous procainamide or ibutilide[86] or orally administered drugs that prolong refractoriness (e.g., sotolol). Electrical reversion, however, may still be required.

Management of Chronic Atrial Flutter Some patients will remain in chronic atrial flutter despite aggressive antiarrhythmic or interventional therapy, and flutter may recur predictably shortly after DC cardioversion. This usually occurs in the setting of advanced heart disease, may occur as the forerunner of chronic atrial fibrillation, and appears to be especially frequent with the variants of flutter, such as type II atrial flutter. It may occur rarely in otherwise normal persons[76] and more commonly in association with other SVTs, such as WPW and AV nodal reentry.[89] If the ventricular rate is adequately controlled and the patient is asymptomatic, chronic atrial flutter need not be treated aggressively. In these cases, there is little justification for the use of complex antiarrhythmic drug regimens with adverse side-effect profiles. Rather, catheter ablation procedures can be used, especially for type I flutter, where the success rate is high. Surgical ablation of atrial flutter is feasible but is used only in rare circumstances, usually in conjunction with surgery being performed for another primary indication.

Control of ventricular rate is the major issue for management. AV nodal blocking agents, such as digoxin, beta-adrenergic blockers, and Ca^{2+}-entry blockers, may be tried. The major problem is the tendency for AV conduction to respond to pharmacologic control in step patterns. The patient who is well controlled with 4:1 conduction at a ventricular rate of 75 per minute may abruptly increase to 150 per minute under conditions of stress, which enhance AV nodal conduction.

In patients with enhanced AV nodal conduction and atrial flutter, it may be difficult to slow the rate below 150 per minute pharmacologically. Verapamil appears to be more effective than digoxin for the AV node with enhanced conduction but is not uniformly effective. Rarely, catheter ablation for AV node modification or interruption, with pacemaker implantation, is used for heart rate control in patients who are resistant to or intolerant of AV nodal blocking drugs and who have failed ablation attempts to interrupt the flutter pathway.

In the past, long-term anticoagulation was not generally recommended for patients with chronic atrial flutter. However, the potential risk of thromboembolism in atrial flutter has been reevaluated,[90,91] and it is now recommended to follow the guidelines of anticoagulation for atrial fibrillation in patients with atrial flutter.[92,93] Although the precise risk of stroke associated with atrial flutter has not been yet established by a large prospective clinical trial, the retrospective observations cited suggest an incidence of stroke similar to that expected in chronic atrial fibrillation. There is transesophageal echocardiographic evidence of atrial clot formation and spontaneous contrast in these patients. Finally, it is clinically difficult to ensure that a patient with atrial flutter will not have occasional periods of atrial fibrillation.

ATRIAL FIBRILLATION

Atrial fibrillation is the commonest among the cardiac rhythm disturbances that require treatment. In cross-sectional popula-

CARDIOVERSION OF ATRIAL FIBRILLATION

Duration	Method	Efficacy
Paroxysmal		
Short-lasting (< 1 hour)	(Spontaneous)	100% [by definition]
	DC Cardioversion	~100% [if necessary]
Long-lasting (> 1; < 48 hours)	(Spontaneous)	< 24 h = >50%; > 24h ~ 25%
	Bolus Therapy [PO, IV]	Added benefit = ~20-30%
	Standard PO Therapy	Uncertain; duration related
	DC Cardioversion	~100%
Persistent 2 Days - Weeks	(Spontaneous)	Rare
	Bolus Therapy [PO, IV]	Benefit higher with disease
	Standard PO Therapy	Low; duration/disease related
	DC Cardioversion	>90% [better with pretreatment]
Chronic Months/Years	(Spontaneous)	-------
	Bolus Therapy [PO, IV]	Low efficacy ; disease-related
	Standard PO Therapy	Usually ineffective
	DC Cardioversion	>70% [may be transient]

FIGURE 24-26 Clinical expression of atrial fibrillation. Atrial fibrillation may occur in brief paroxysms, a more persistent form lasting from days to weeks, or chronically. Approaches to therapy are dictated by these patterns in conjunction with the hemodynamic considerations shown in Fig. 24-27. Methods of management include sedation while awaiting spontaneous conversion, DC cardioversion, bolus antiarrhythmic therapy (oral or intravenous), and standard oral antiarrhythmic therapy. There is a relationship between the efficacy of each therapy and the clinical expression of the arrhythmia. Short-lasting paroxysmal atrial fibrillation (less than 1 h) undergo spontaneous return to sinus rhythm by definition, but DC cardioversion may be necessary based on the hemodynamic response in patients with cardiac diseases such as aortic stenosis or mitral stenosis. Longer-lasting paroxysms of atrial fibrillation or persistent patterns of atrial fibrillation (see the text) may be treated with bolus therapy, standard therapy, or cardioversion, the latter having better efficacy in patients with more advanced disease if they are pretreated with antiarrhythmic agents. Chronic atrial fibrillation will not convert spontaneously but may respond to the various therapies listed. However, long-term maintenance of sinus rhythm is limited among patients in this category, particularly if the heart disease is advanced.

tion studies, there is a large gradient of prevalence across age categories, ranging from less than 0.5 percent in young adults to 1 to 5 percent through the decades from 40 to 70 years and reaching rates in excess of 10 percent in some beyond age 70.[94] The arrhythmia should not be viewed as a single entity for practical clinical purposes. Risk, relevance, and management strategies are heavily influenced by the temporal pattern of the arrhythmia (paroxysmal, persistent, or permanent; Fig. 24-26) and by the clinical setting in which it occurs (Fig. 24-27).

The electrophysiologic mechanism of atrial fibrillation also influences treatment options. The commonest mechanism by far is multiple reentrant atrial wavelet circuits, producing loss of mechanical and electrical synchronization of the atria and variable AV nodal penetration and conduction, which in turn results in an irregular ventricular response. A less common but strategically important mechanism is focal atrial tachycardia originating in muscle fibers in the distal pulmonary veins in the left atrium or the crista terminalis or elsewhere in the right atrium.[20,95] Premature atrial impulses may be an expression of the presence of such sites of focal activity and serve as a guide to ablation therapy. They may also serve as triggers for initiation of the reentrant forms.

The clinical presentations and associations of atrial fibrillation are very broad. At one end of the spectrum is lone atrial fibrillation (absence of any form of structural cardiac abnormality) with arrhythmia symptoms that range from unrecognized to very symptomatic. The other extreme includes patients with advanced structural diseases, such as mitral or aortic stenosis, restrictive cardiomyopathies, or advanced LV dysfunction, in which the onset of atrial fibrillation may cause severe hemodynamic deterioration. Valvular heart disease has received much attention historically. The high prevalence of the arrhythmia in rheumatic mitral valve disease has been emphasized in the past, but it is likely that risk with any cause of mitral valve disease of equivalent severity is just as high. Between these extremes, atrial fibrillation may herald the presence of noncardiac disorders (e.g., thyrotoxicosis), alert to the significance of another cardiac disorder (e.g., WPW syndrome), constitute a transient complicating factor of another cardiac disorder (e.g., acute myocardial infarction or systemic arterial hypertension), or occur during the postoperative period after cardiac surgery.

The hemodynamic consequences of atrial fibrillation are due to two factors: (1) the loss of atrial systole may impair ventricular function in the noncompliant ventricle [e.g., aortic stenosis or left ventricular hypertrophy (LVH)] or the dilated ventricle with systolic dysfunction, and

Atrial Contraction Important	Diastolic Intervals Important
▷ Aortic stenosis	▷ Mitral stenosis
▷ Hypertrophic cardiomyopathy	▷ Coronary artery disease
▷ Hypertension/LV hypertrophy	▷ Dilated cardiomyopathy; CHF
▷ Restrictive cardiomyopathy	▷ Wolf-Parkinson-White syndrome
▷ Dilated cardiomyopathy; CHF	▷ Enhanced A-V nodal conduction

FIGURE 24-27 Hemodynamic factors in atrial fibrillation. Atrial fibrillation creates the potential for two hemodynamic defects: (1) loss of atrial contraction, which provides the presystolic atrial "kick"; and (2) rate-related reduction of the diastolic filling period. Atrial contraction is important to ventricles with reduced compliance and low-output states due to myocardial factors. Diastolic filling time is important in conditions in which a longer diastolic is beneficial to impaired flow states, such as mitral stenosis, coronary atherosclerosis, and some myopathic ventricles.

(2) a rapid ventricular rate will encroach upon the diastolic filling period of the left ventricle and the diastolic flow time of the coronary arteries (see Fig. 24-27). The risk of embolism and stroke is a long-term concern of special importance (see below).

Electrocardiographic Features Atrial fibrillation is characterized electrocardiographically by grossly disorganized atrial electrical activity that is irregular in respect to both rate and rhythm. There is no visually discernible timing pattern to the atrial electrical activity on the surface ECG or to electrogram sequences recorded by catheter electrodes. Specific patterns of AV conduction sequences (ventricular responses) have been proposed as a result of sophisticated analytic techniques;[96] this analysis provides some physiologic insight but does not yet have practical clinical value. Atrial fibrillatory waves are best seen in standard lead V_1 and are usually clearly evident in II, III, and aVF as well. They may be quite large and coarse or almost imperceptible (compare Fig. 24-28*A* and *B*). In the absence of discernible atrial electrical activity, a grossly irregular ventricular rhythm still suggests the presence of atrial fibrillation. Coarse atrial fibrillation is occasionally difficult to distinguish from atrial flutter waves, but the irregular ventricular response, in the absence of a repetitive pattern, is again helpful in making the distinction. In contrast, obvious coarse fibrillatory waves with a regular ventricular response, especially when slow, suggests the coexistence of high-grade AV block with atrial fibrillation.

One of the more challenging exercises in clinical electrocardiography is the distinction between aberrant intraventricular conduction and ventricular ectopy in the presence of atrial fibrillation. Aberrant conduction tends to occur when a long ventricular cycle is followed by a short cycle. This long-short cycle sequence, with the short cycle terminated by an aberrantly conducted beat, is referred to as Ashman's phenomenon.[97] It is important to recognize that *long* and *short* are relative terms in this context and carry no implications of absolute value (compare Figs. 24-29 and 24-30). A series of short cycles, if short enough, may generate runs of consecutively aberrant beats imitating VT (Fig. 24-30). Thus, additional criteria for distinction between aberrancy and ectopy are required. In general, an initial QRS vector similar or identical to that of narrow QRS complexes and a typical right bundle-branch block pattern, in association with a long-short cycle sequence, strongly favor ab-

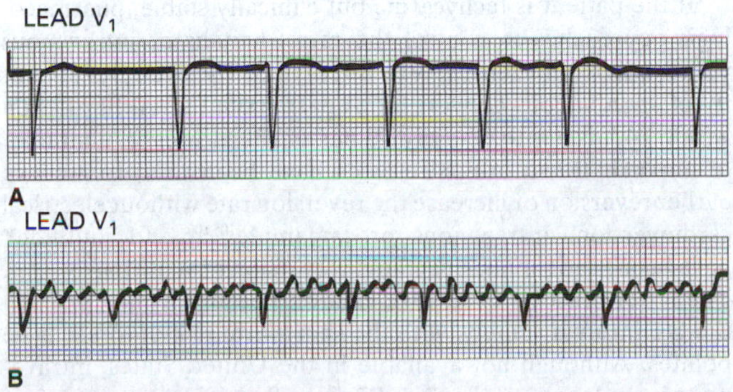

FIGURE 24-28 *A.* Fine atrial fibrillation, leaving virtually no imprint on the baseline ("straight-line" fibrillation). *B.* Coarse atrial fibrillation; the fibrillatory waves are the size of respectable flutter waves but are irregular.

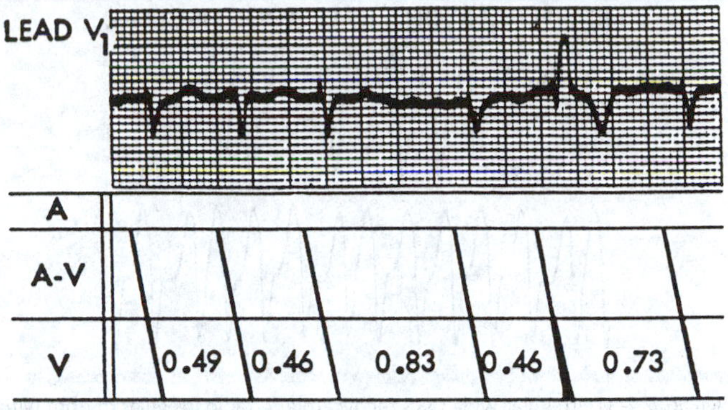

FIGURE 24-29 Ashman's phenomenon. During atrial fibrillation, the impulse ending a short cycle preceded by a relatively long cycle manifests aberrant intraventricular conduction. In this example, the aberrant impulse shows typical right bundle-branch block type aberration in lead V_1, with an rSR pattern and the initial deflection identical to that of the preceding and following normally conducted impulses.

errancy over ectopy.[98] Left bundle-branch block aberrancy also occurs but is far less common. It is more likely when aberrant conduction is persistent (i.e., functional bundle-branch block during a sustained SVT; see Fig. 24-15), while it is unusual in single-cycle aberrancy (Fig. 24-29). Atrial fibrillation alters intraventricular conduction only through the following mechanisms: (1) functional bundle-branch block or aberrancy (Fig. 24-31), (2) loss of delta waves in WPW syndrome with normal pathway conduction during atrial fibrillation, or (3) totally preexcited QRS complexes during atrial fibrillation in WPW syndrome (see Fig. 24-18). The QRS complex during atrial fibrillation will be similar to that recorded during sinus rhythm under all other circumstances. In patients with preexisting bundle-branch block who develop atrial fibrillation with rapid ventricular responses, the distinction from VT may be difficult.

Evaluation and Management of the First Episode of Atrial Fibrillation The first episode of atrial fibrillation requires special considerations. A thorough investigation of the clinical status is needed to determine whether the event is caused by a primary electrical mechanism, underlying structural heart disease, hemodynamic abnormalities, or a systemic disorder that

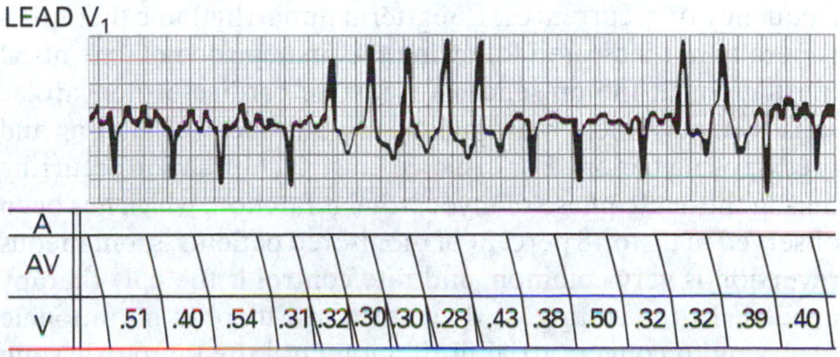

FIGURE 24-30 Atrial fibrillation with repetitive aberrant ventricular conduction. The impulses that end the shortest ventricular cycles (0.28 to 0.32 s) are anomalous, widened complexes. Note that the cycle preceding the onset of the salvos of anomalous beats is *relatively* long in comparison with the anomalous complexes (0.54 and 0.50 s), in accordance with Ashman's phenomenon. Thus, these almost certainly represent a right bundle-branch block type of ventricular aberration rather than ventrcular ectopy.

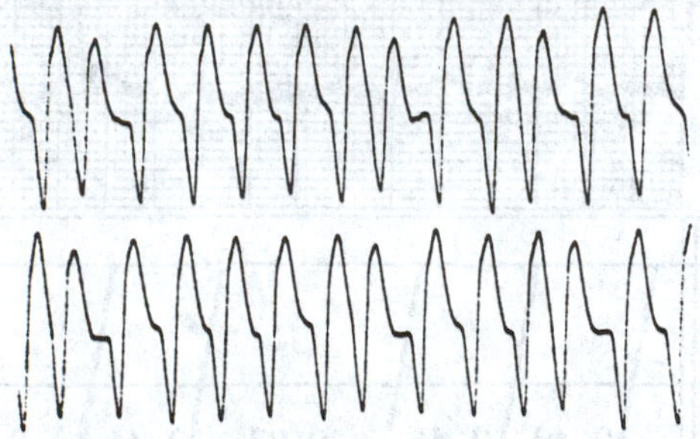

FIGURE 24-31 Irregular wide QRS tachycardia. A rapid irregular rhythm with wide QRS complexes having a left bundle-branch block pattern is recorded. The rhythm is atrial fibrillation with abnormal intraventricular conduction. Irregular, wide QRS tachycardias also occur in WPW syndrome, with atrial fibrillation and conduction down the accessory pathway or in rare cases of irregular ventricular tachycardia.

predisposes to atrial fibrillation. Previously unrecognized mitral or aortic stenosis or regurgitation, hypertension, coronary heart disease, cardiomyopathy, atrial septal defect, pericarditis, or atrial abnormalities secondary to left or right ventricular overload are among cardiac causes that must be excluded. Heart failure may be either a cause or a consequence of atrial fibrillation. Pulmonary emboli and metabolic abnormalities such as thyrotoxicosis also must be considered. The identification of associated factors at the time of the first episode of atrial fibrillation dictate future management. In the absence of an identifiable cause, so-called lone atrial fibrillation, the prognosis is good,[99] especially if it is a single event or intermittently recurrent. Chronic lone atrial fibrillation may indicate a higher risk,[100] although conflicting data[99] question the validity of this conclusion. In a young, healthy individual in whom there is no evidence of structural heart disease, paroxysmal episodes of lone atrial fibrillation may occur under conditions of exogenous precipitating factors, such as excessive cigarette, alcohol, and/or coffee consumption; exposure to so-called "recreational drugs," such as cocaine and amphetamines; stress or fatigue; or upon cessation of extreme exercise.

In the absence of organic heart disease or coexistent WPW syndrome, long-term management after the first episode need include no more than avoidance or removal of precipitating factors and following the patient over time to estimate the frequency of recurrences. Long-term antiarrhythmic therapy is generally not indicated following the first episode of lone atrial fibrillation. In the presence of treatable cardiac or noncardiac causes, management must include attention to precipitating and predisposing factors. For instance, in atrial fibrillation occurring during the acute phase of myocardial infarction, which has been observed in up to 18 percent of monitored patients, spontaneous reversion is very common, and rate control is the only therapy needed. In the setting of thyrotoxicosis, there is no rationale for trying to convert atrial fibrillation until the thyrotoxic state is controlled; in the interim, the ventricular rate may be slowed with propranolol and anticoagulation maintained (see below) until sinus rhythm is restored after the patient is euthyroid. When atrial fibrillation calls attention to previously undiagnosed mitral stenosis, atrial enlargement may limit success of attempts to obtain and maintain sinus rhythm.

Ventricular rate should be controlled, and conversion of atrial fibrillation can await correction of the mitral valve obstruction. In atrial septal defect, atrial fibrillation is generally a sign of advanced hemodynamic deterioration, such as pulmonary hypertension and balanced or reversing shunts; these patients must be evaluated for surgery promptly. In patients with *advanced* heart disease of any etiology and dilated atria, the first episode may herald a chronic fibrillatory state. An attempt to revert the rhythm, either pharmacologically or electrically, the latter usually with a concomitant pharmacologic agent, may be an appropriate option; but the recurrence rate is very high.[101–103] If the patient will benefit from the hemodynamic advantage provided by an atrial contraction, the attempt at reversion is warranted despite the high probability of recurrence. The recent onset of chronic atrial fibrillation has special implications for anticoagulation therapy (see below).

In hemodynamically significant mitral stenosis or aortic stenosis, acute pulmonary edema may complicate the first episode of rapid atrial fibrillation, making immediate control of heart rate or electrical cardioversion mandatory. In mitral stenosis, recurrences can be expected; but even a short time in sinus rhythm can provide hemodynamic benefit and allow institution of therapy that will control the ventricular rate for the next episode. A slower heart rate, with a resultant longer diastolic filling period, may help prevent the recurrence of pulmonary edema. In aortic stenosis, dependence upon the atrial kick for optimal hemodynamic function of the noncompliant hypertrophied left ventricle, rather than encroachment on the diastolic filling period, is the major concern.

Management of Recurrent Episodes of Paroxysmal Atrial Fibrillation Paroxysms of atrial fibrillation lasting less than 48 h in the absence of underlying heart disease are usually managed conservatively. Rest, mild sedation with 5 to 10 mg of diazepam, and Ca^{2+}-entry blockers, beta-adrenergic blockers, or digitalis for control of the ventricular rate constitute an accepted approach. After the first episode, patients who have lone atrial fibrillation can be reassured in respect to the absence of underlying organic heart disease and guided to avoid precipitating factors. In the presence of heart disease, particularly when the hemodynamic circumstances require either the mechanical benefit of atrial systole or a properly controlled ventricular rate for adequate diastolic filling (see Fig. 24-27), immediate reversion to sinus rhythm or slowing of the ventricular rate may be mandatory. The presence of clinical signs of heart failure requires immediate cardioversion to achieve either or both of these goals.

If the patient is tachycardic but clinically stable, pharmacologic approaches to control the rate (digitalis or intravenous verapamil or diltiazem) may be attempted. The overall probability of spontaneous conversion of paroxysmal atrial fibrillation within 24 h is approximately 50 percent.[104] However, a number of antiarrhythmic drug strategies have been used to achieve earlier reversion or increase the reversion rate without electrical cardioversion. Intravenous procainamide[105,106] and ibutilide[86] have been used for pharmacologic reversion of acute paroxysms. The latter must be used with caution because it may prolong the QT interval acutely, with the short-term risk of torsades de pointes. Although not available in the United States, intravenous formulations of the class IC drugs flecainide and propafenone have also been used successfully for treatment of acute atrial fibrillation.[107] Oral bolus therapy using flecainide (300-mg dose) or propafenone (600 mg) in a single dose has been used,[108,109] although it is not clear whether it provides more or simply earlier conversions than in control subjects.[110]

Long-term pharmacologic therapy in the absence of underlying heart disease or in the presence of trivial abnormalities is intended to reduce or eliminate recurrent episodes and to control ventricular rate during recurrences, should they occur. Digitalis, beta-adrenergic blockers, or Ca^{2+}-entry blockers are used for rate control as described for atrial flutter. Digitalis controls ventricular rate at rest, although it appears less effective for limiting effort-induced increases in ventricular rate during atrial fibrillation.[111]

Prevention of episodes of atrial fibrillation may be achieved with class IA, IC, or III antiarrhythmic drugs. If episodes are clinically benign and infrequent, the threshold for such treatment is higher than if they are more frequent and symptomatic. Efficacy is uneven and proarrhythmic or toxic side effects are of concern. During short paroxysms of atrial fibrillation (up to 48 h), anticoagulation is not required prior to reversion; long-term anticoagulation is not necessary for patients subject to brief paroxysmal attacks[112] (see Fig. 24-26; Tables 24-8 and 24-9).

TABLE 24-8 Risk of Stroke and General Approaches to Anticoagulation in Atrial Fibrillation

Age Group, %	Risk Factors[a]	Annual Event Rate if Untreated (95% Confidence Intervals)	Recommendation
<65	Absent	1.0 (0.3–3.1)	Aspirin or no therapy
	Present	4.9 (3.0–8.1)	Warfarin
65–75	Absent	4.3 (2.7–7.1)	Warfarin (aspirin)
	Present	5.7 (3.9–8.3)	Warfarin
>75	Absent	3.5 (1.6–7.7)	Warfarin
	Present	8.1 (4.7–13.9)	Warfarin

[a]Presence of one or more of the following features: previous stroke or transient ischemic attack, hypertension, heart failure (HTN), coronary artery disease (CAD), prosthetic heart valve or hyperthyroidism.

NOTE: Contraindications to warfarin include inability to monitor prothrombin times (target INR 2–3), prior major bleeding event on warfarin, history of major gastrointestinal hemorrhage, history of falls or unstable gait, alcohol abuse or serious liver disease, or uncontrolled hypertension in an elderly patient.

SOURCE: Adapted from American College of Chest Physicians recommendations for anticoagulation for patients with atrial fibrillation. Laupacis A, Albergs G, Dalen J, et al. Antithrombotic therapy in atrial fibrillation, *Chest* 1995; 108:3525–3595; and Atrial Fibrillation Investigators. Risk factors for stroke and efficacy of antithrombotic therapy in atrial fibrillation: Analysis of pooled data from five randomized controlled trials. *Arch Intern Med* 1994; 154:1449–1457. With permission.

Management of Persistent Atrial Fibrillation The decision to intervene in longer episodes of atrial fibrillation is based on the balance between hemodynamic tolerance and the likelihood of being able to control future episodes. Because of the demonstrated effects of "electrical remodeling" of atrial myocytes during persistent atrial fibrillation,[113] which favors persistence of the arrhythmia and resistance to reversion, there is a tendency toward a more aggressive approach to early reversion.[114]

Many patients with organic heart disease have intermittent episodes of persistent atrial fibrillation prior to establishing chronic atrial fibrillation.[115] Among these patients, antiarrhythmic efficacy for control of recurrences is unpredictable. Prediction of the ability to control ventricular rate by AV nodal blocking agents is better but still imperfect. When a patient has had multiple recurrences of persistent atrial fibrillation despite trials of several antiarrhythmic agents and the arrhythmia is well tolerated hemodynamically, many clinicians avoid repeated electrical cardioversions, especially in the presence of advanced heart disease. If elective cardioversion is to be attempted, 3 weeks of anticoagulation should precede the procedure to reduce embolic risk. A more expeditious alternative strategy is to perform a transesophageal echocardiogram to rule out the presence of atrial thrombi.[116] If results are negative, heparin can be started and chemical or electrical cardioversion performed. However, there remains some debate about the efficacy of this strategy.[117]

If cardioversion is not attempted and the patient has recurrent episodes of atrial fibrillation lasting 48 to 72 h, long-term anticoagulant with warfarin is indicated. If the patient is without structural disease, is less than 60 years of age, and has a normal

TABLE 24-9 Anticoagulation of Patients with Atrial Fibrillation

- Indications
  - Rheumatic mitral valve disease with recurrent or chronic atrial fibrillation
  - Dilated cardiomyopathy with recurrent persistent or chronic atrial fibrillation
  - Prosthetic valves
  - Prior to (≥3 weeks) elective cardioversion of persistent or chronic atrial fibrillation
  - Coronary heart disease or hypertensive heart disease with recurrent persistent or chronic atrial fibrillation
  - Atrial fibrillation in thyrotoxicosis (while awaiting long-term control; elective cardioversion)
  - Chronic or persistent lone atrial fibrillation, age ≥60 years
- Controversial, or limited data
  - Coronary or hypertensive heart disease with normal left atrial size, after first episode of paroxysmal atrial fibrillation
  - Elective cardioversion of atrial fibrillation of short duration (2–3 days) with normal left atrial size
  - Chronic or persistent lone atrial fibrillation, age <60 years
- Not indicated
  - Lone atrial fibrillation, paroxysmal (<48 h, age <65)
  - Most clinical settings associated with short paroxysms (minutes to hours)
- Relative contraindications
  - Difficulty controlling prothrombin times
  - Dementia
  - Malignancies, especially associated with bleeding risk
  - Prior major bleeding events
  - Uncontrolled hypertension

echocardiogram and no prior history of embolism, long-term warfarin therapy is unnecessary.

In the presence of advanced or progressive cardiac disease, atrial fibrillation is likely to revert and recur intermittently until the condition evolves into chronic atrial fibrillation. When this occurs, the best therapeutic approach may be control of ventricular rate during recurrences. Membrane-active antiarrhythmic agents are often used in an attempt to limit the number of recurrences, but efficacy is unpredictable, and risk of side effects is high. The flecainide data suggest efficacy,[61,119] especially for patients with good LV function and those free of underlying coronary artery disease.[19] Class III antiarrhythmic drugs, including sotalol,[120] amiodarone,[121] dofetilide,[122] and azemilide,[123] are also effective. The latter two drugs have not yet been approved for use by the U.S. Food and Drug Administration. The long-term benefit of prevention of atrial fibrillation by antiarrhythmic drug therapy versus control of heart rate remains uncertain. A large multicenter study is currently in progress to answer this question.[124]

Management of Chronic (Permanent) Atrial Fibrillation The ventricular rate in chronic atrial fibrillation is usually more predictably controlled than in recurrent episodes of paroxysmal or persistent atrial fibrillation. Pharmacologic or electrical cardioversion in patients with advanced heart disease and atrial enlargement is attempted in the hope of achieving a hemodynamic benefit, but the probability of maintaining sinus rhythm is low.[101–103] Until more data are available, the choice between attempting to restore sinus rhythm and simply controlling heart rate (with anticoagulation) is a matter for individual clinical judgment. Among patients with advanced heart disease who have been electrically cardioverted while taking antiarrhythmic drug therapy, approximately one-third will revert to atrial fibrillation within 1 week and two-thirds within 12 months.[101–103] If the rhythm reverts to chronic atrial fibrillation shortly after cardioversion, the probability of long-term maintenance of sinus rhythm by additional pharmacologic approaches is very low. The ventricular rate is then controlled as outlined above.

Pharmacologic control of ventricular rate may be problematic in recurrent episodes of both persistent and chronic atrial fibrillation. Under both circumstances, catheter modification of the AV junction or complete interruption (catheter ablation) of the AV junction with permanent pacing may provide heart rate control.[125] Other nonpharmacologic strategies for control of atrial fibrillation include surgical procedures designed to establish sinus node control of the ventricular rate and rhythm, implantable device therapy, and catheter ablation procedures. Among the surgical approaches, the "corridor" procedure[126] establishes a pathway from sinus node to AV node, while the MAZE procedure[127] interrupts pathways necessary for maintaining fibrillation and reestablishes both rate control and mechanical function. The MAZE technique has been used both as primary surgery and as an added procedure for patients undergoing cardiac surgery for other reasons.

An implantable atrial defibrillator[128] has been developed for use in patients with chronic recurrent atrial fibrillation. It appears to have only limited applicability as a stand-alone device, but integration of the technology within the platform of conventional implantable cardioverter defibrillators (ICDs)[129] may be useful for patients with paroxysmal atrial fibrillation at risk for life-threatening ventricular arrythmias. Another device strategy being evaluated is the use of dual-site atrial pacing in an attempt to resynchronize atrial depolarization and avoid dispersion of atrial refractoriness.[130]

Catheter ablation techniques for preventing atrial fibrillation (i.e., catheter-based MAZE procedure or ablation of focal triggering sites for atrial fibrillation)[131–132] are currently being evaluated. The ultimate role for these approaches in the management of patients with recurrent or chronic atrial fibrillation remains to be determined.

Anticoagulation of Patients with Atrial Fibrillation Patients with atrial fibrillation have a greater than fivefold increase in risk of stroke compared to control populations without atrial fibrillation.[133–136] In addition, there are specific high-risk subgroups. Among patients with rheumatic heart disease, the risk exceeds by up to 17 times that of a control group.[134,135] Other subgroups at high risk include patients with dilated cardiomyopathy, dilated left atrium of any cause, atrial fibrillation of recent onset, and a history of prior embolism. Patients with atrial fibrillation and LVH are also at increased risk, as are thyrotoxic patients.[137] In one study, the chronic form of lone atrial fibrillation has been reported to be associated with a relative increase in risk of embolic stroke,[138] although other studies have not identified an increased risk. It is generally agreed, however, that patients older than 60 years with lone atrial fibrillation are at risk and should be anticoagulated with warfarin.[139] As a group, the nonrheumatic disease states associated with atrial fibrillation tend to have excess risks in the range of five- to sixfold, according to various studies.[94] Absolute risks differ little among the various rheumatic and nonrheumatic etiologies, however, with event rates in the range of 4 to 6 percent for each, except for lone atrial fibrillation, which has a considerably lower rate.[92,99,138] The risk of embolic events tends to cluster around changes in rhythm, the highest incidence occurring within the first year after onset of chronic atrial fibrillation[134] and a concentrated 1 to 2 percent risk occurring in the first days after restoration of sinus rhythm,[140–142] whether by pharmacologic strategies or DC cardioversion.

The issue of anticoagulation in atrial fibrillation hinges on a balance between efficacy of preventing embolic events and risk of bleeding (see Tables 24-8 and 24-9). Indicators of increased risk of embolic events, in addition to the general presence of structural heart disease, include previous stroke or transient ischemic attack, hypertension, heart failure, prosthetic heart valves, and hyperthyroidism.[137,143] Age and female gender (particularly elderly women) also identify increased risk.[139] Efficacy and risk both relate well to the level of anticoagulation with warfarin. Measured as the now-standard international normalized ratio (INR), benefit is optimal at or above an INR of 2.0, while bleeding risk increases above an INR of 3.5 to 4.0.[143] Until recently, most of the data on efficacy of anticoagulation for reducing incidence of embolic events in atrial fibrillation were from poorly controlled or uncontrolled studies, and there was no consensus based on the available data.[133] The available combination of risk data and retrospective or uncontrolled efficacy data[101,111,133] tended to result in the practice of using long-term anticoagulation for patients with a rheumatic etiology and for those with advanced structural diseases associated with atrial fibrillation (see Table 24-8). Such patients included those with coronary artery disease and a prior embolism, idiopathic dilated cardiomyopathy, and prosthetic cardiac valves. Several recent placebo-controlled studies have now provided clarification of the role and methods for anticoagulation in patients with nonrheumatic atrial fibrillation. In one multicenter randomized trial, the Stroke Prevention in Atrial Fibrillation (SPAF) Study, aspirin, 325 mg/day, and warfarin, with prolongation of prothrombin times to 1.3 to 1.8 times those of the control subjects were each compared to placebo among a population of 1330 patients.[144] During a mean follow-up of 1.3 years, ischemic stroke or systemic embolization occurred at a rate of 6.3 percent per year in the placebo group, compared to 3.6 percent per year in the aspirin-treated group, a 42 percent reduction in the treated group ($p < .02$). Among the patients eligible for warfarin, the event rate in the untreated group was 7.4 percent, compared to 2.3 percent in the treated group, a 67 percent reduction ($p < .01$). Primary embolic events and deaths combined were reduced by 58 percent in the warfarin group and 32 percent in the aspirin group.

Thus, both warfarin and aspirin were effective, but the design of the study prevented comparison of the two treatments. Although both chronic atrial fibrillation and intermittent atrial fibrillation were included in the study, the data reported do not permit a determination of any difference in risk or benefit for the two patterns. In another study, the Canadian Atrial Fibrillation Anticoagulation (CAFA) Study, the placebo group experienced a 5.2 percent embolism/stroke rate compared to 3.5 percent in a warfarin-treated group, a relative reduction of 37 percent with treatment.[145] The differences did not reach statistical significance, since the study was prematurely terminated because of outcome data from other large studies suggesting benefit. Among two other studies, the Copenhagen AFASK Study[146] and the Boston Area Anticoagulation Trial in Atrial Fibrillation,[148] warfarin again demonstrated significant reductions in risk (82 and 87 percent, respectively), while aspirin demonstrated only a 14 percent reduction in the Copenhagen study (nonsignificant),[146] even though it was associated with a 42 percent reduction in the SPAF study.[144] Collectively, these studies demonstrate a significant benefit for reduction of embolism and stroke in nonrheumatic atrial fibrillation patients with the use of warfarin and likely with aspirin as a less effective alternative (see Chap. 89). More recent data have reaffirmed that warfarin is superior to aspirin and provided additional insight into effective warfarin dose ranges.[148] In patients at high risk for embolic events, fixed low-dose warfarin (0.5 to 3.0 mg/day; INR = 1.2 to 1.5) plus aspirin (325 mg/day) was inferior to conventional dose-adjusted warfarin (INR target = 2.0 to 3.0). Indications for anticoagulation prior to elective cardioversion have not undergone the same scrutiny for efficacy as has now been provided for intermittent and chronic atrial fibrillation. Nonetheless, there is enough information available to warrant the routine use of anticoagulation prior to elective cardioversion of recent onset (more than 48 to 72 h), persistent atrial fibrillation or chronic atrial fibrillation, particularly when associated with an enlarged left atrium or other structural diseases regardless of etiology. Anticoagulation with warfarin is started 3 to 4 weeks before elective cardioversion and is maintained for 3 to 4 weeks subsequently. If there is concern about the ability of a patient to recognize a recurrence of atrial fibrillation, it may be warranted to maintain anticoagulation indefinitely, particularly if the patient has advanced structural heart disease.

The risk-benefit data are less clear for anticoagulation prior to elective cardioversion of atrial fibrillation of short duration (less than or equal to 48 h), particularly lone atrial fibrillation or when associated with minimal structural disease and normal atrial dimensions. The potential efficacy of anticoagulation must be weighed against its risk. Patients receiving anticoagulants retain a risk of embolization ranging from 1 to greater than 3 percent per year,[94,102,142–147] depending upon disease states. Furthermore, there is a significant incidence of life-threatening bleeding or major events requiring transfusion among patients on long-term anticoagulation. In one report,[149] the incidence was 4.3 percent per treatment-year. In the SPAF study,[144] however, bleeding risk hovered around 1.5 percent and did not differ among aspirin-treated, warfarin-treated, and placebo groups. Lower warfarin dosing than used previously, titrated to an INR of 2.0 to 3.0,[150] may be one reason for the reduction of bleeding risk with warfarin use. Since the risk of bleeding is increased significantly with an INR of 5.0, the inability to control the prothrombin time, including the inability of the patient to comply with the prescribed dosages, must be considered relative contraindications. The major complication of intracranial bleeding may have an incidence of 1 to 2 percent per treatment-year.[151] Table 24-9 lists indications and relative contraindications for anticoagulation in patients with atrial fibrillation. The physician must balance accepted indications and risks in judging whether to use anticoagulation in individual patients. In most circumstances now, however, one should err on the side of use rather than avoidance if the risk-benefit relationship is not clear, assuming the INR is assiduously maintained between 2.0 and 3.0 in candidates at higher risk for bleeding complications.

ATRIOVENTRICULAR JUNCTIONAL AND ACCELERATED VENTRICULAR RHYTHMS

Rhythm disturbances that originate in the AV junction include premature AV junctional impulses, accelerated junctional rhythms, and AV junctional tachycardias that may be automatic or reentrant. Echo beats and tachycardias that incorporate the atria and AV junction as part of the reentrant pathway in PSVT due to AV nodal reentry or WPW syndrome are discussed elsewhere. Junctional escape rhythms at rates of 40 to 60 per minute during sinus bradycardia or AV block are normal physiologic backup phenomena that are usually hemodynamically stable; failure of normal junctional escape mechanisms may result in significant bradycardias.

The normal inherent rate of AV junctional automatic activity is 40 to 60 per minute, and those of subordinate pacemakers at the fascicular or ventricular level are 20 to 40 per minute. Faster rates from either of these levels are considered "accelerated" for rates up to 100 impulses per minute, at which point they take on the general definition of a tachycardia. Accelerated junctional and ventricular rhythms and most nonparoxysmal AV junctional tachycardias are thought to be due to enhanced automatic activity (phase 4 depolarization).[152,153] Other forms of abnormal automaticity, including triggered activity initiated by afterdepolarizations, may also originate in the AV junction[154,155] (see also Chap. 23).

AV Junctional Premature Beats

AV junctional premature beats occur much less frequently than do premature atrial or ventricular complexes. The timing of P

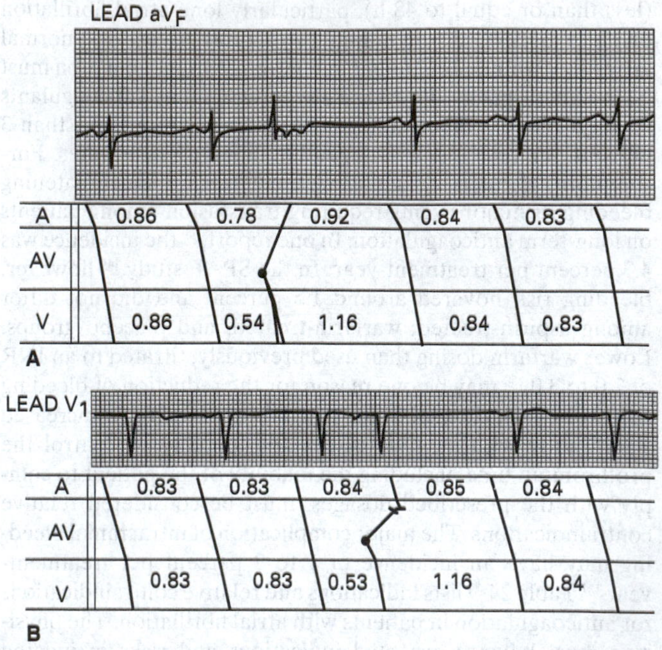

FIGURE 24-32 *A.* AV junctional extrasystole. The retrograde P wave follows the premature QRS complex, which shows some degree of ventricular aberration. *B.* The fourth complex is an AV premature impulse without retroconduction to the atria, leaving the sinus rhythm undisturbed.

waves and QRS complexes is variable, however. The P waves may precede QRS complexes by 0.12 s or less, may be concealed within the QRS complexes, or may appear in the ST segment following the QRS complex (Fig. 24-32). The P waves are usually inverted in leads II, III, and aVF; isoelectric to slightly negative in leads I and V_6; and upright in the right precordial leads. The QRS complexes are narrow except when aberrant intraventricular conduction is present. When the P waves precede the QRS complex, distinction from premature atrial complexes may be difficult, and when aberrant intraventricular conduction is present and the P wave is within or after the QRS complex, the distinction from premature ventricular complexes may be impossible without intracardiac recordings. AV junctional premature beats generally require no treatment; when treated, however, they are approached using the same principles applied to the treatment of premature ventricular complexes (see below).

Accelerated Junctional and Accelerated Ventricular Rhythms

Accelerated rhythms derive from subordinate pacemakers and emerge when the sinus rate is less than the normally suppressed focus. Sinus bradycardia combined with enhanced automaticity of the subordinate site is the common pathophysiology. Ischemia (especially inferior wall myocardial ischemia or infarction), digitalis intoxication, electrolyte disturbances (especially hypokalemia), and hypoxemia may enhance phase 4 depolarization in the AV junction or intraventricular specialized conducting system, accelerating the rate of impulse formation of the subordinate pacemakers located at these sites. Digitalis intoxication, various degrees of AV block, and sinus node depression may accompany AV junctional acceleration, producing complex ECG patterns. In inferior wall ischemia, subordinate pacemaker acceleration is commonly associated with sinus node depression, the latter permitting escape and usurpation of pacemaker function, even with only modest AV junctional acceleration (e.g., 60 to 70 impulses per minute). These rhythms are almost always hemodynamically stable.

The typical electrocardiographic pattern is apparent shortening of the PR interval as the PP intervals prolong, leading to emergence of the subordinate QRS complexes as they assume the pacemaker function (Fig. 24-33). After a variable duration, the PP interval begins to shorten, P waves reappear in front of the QRS complex, and ventricular capture by atrial activity is reestablished. The QRS complexes of accelerated AV junctional rhythm commonly have slightly altered vectors, durations, and morphology, often accompanied by minor changes in the T-wave vectors. Such alterations are due to slight changes in conduction patterns resulting from the altered origin of the propagating wavefront in the ventricles. These changes may be diagnostically useful.

Accelerated AV junctional and ventricular rhythms generally require no specific antiarrhythmic therapy. In ischemia, they are usually self-limiting in duration and of no major consequence hemodynamically; when associated with digitalis intoxication or electrolyte disturbances, they promptly reverse with control of these toxic or metabolic influences. In fact, specific antiarrhythmic drugs might suppress a subordinate pacemaker that is needed to maintain cardiac output in the presence of dysfunction of normal sinus node pacemakers. If a faster ventricular rate or AV sequencing is desirable for hemodynamic benefits, attempts to enhance cardiac rates may be achieved pharmacologically or by pacing. Atropine, 0.6 to 1.2 mg intravenously, may increase sinus rate and allow the sinus to resume its normal pacemaking function if AV conduction is intact. Atropine will have little or no influence on the rate of the accelerated AV junction focus. Temporary atrial or ventricular pacing may be used to support the heart rate if it is slow enough to impair hemodynamics, but pacing is rarely necessary.

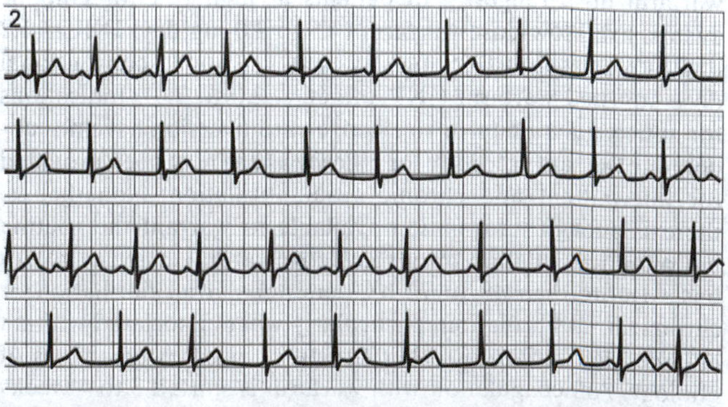

FIGURE 24-33 Accelerated idiojunctional rhythm with isorhythmic AV dissociation. After four sinus beats, the sinus rate slows slightly, enabling an accelerated junctional pacemaker to escape at a rate of 94 per minute. After several seconds, the sinus pacemaker accelerates and recaptures the ventricles. The same sequence is then repeated (the strips are continuous). (From Marriott HJL. *Workshop in Electrocardiography*. Tampa, FL: Tampa Tracings; 1972. Reproduced with permission from the publisher and author.)

AV Junctional Tachycardia

Enhanced AV junctional rhythm may occasionally double its rate abruptly to a true tachycardic range.[156] This phenomenon likely represents an automatic focus firing at the faster rate with 2:1 exit block, which abruptly changes to 1:1 exit. In acute ischemic events, it may be desirable to reduce the rate with antiarrhythmic agents. These incidents are commonly self-limited, however, and will usually cease spontaneously or revert to 2:1 exit block.

Ectopic or persistent nonparoxysmal AV junctional tachycardia may occur intermittently in patients with chronic heart disease and appears to be more frequent and more important in children, particularly after surgical correction of congenital defects.[157,158] The response to treatment is unpredictable, and the rhythm may be resistant to conventional antiarrhythmic drugs. Catheter ablation has been suggested for some patients, however.[158]

An arrhythmia referred to as permanent junctional reciprocating tachycardia (PJRT) is characterized by a long RP–short PR reentry pattern and is due to a very slowly conducting retrograde accessory pathway.[159–161] It is persistent but not truly incessant, occasionally causes tachycardia-induced cardiomyopathy, tends to occur in children, and is difficult to treat pharmacologically. Some success with class IC antiarrhythmic agents has been reported in children,[162] but catheter ablation has become the treatment of choice.

VENTRICULAR ARRHYTHMIAS

Approaches to the evaluation and management of ventricular arrhythmias have changed dramatically in recent years. New insight into risks of ventricular arrhythmias in various clinical settings, clarification of the risk-benefit ratio of antiarrhythmic drug treatment, and the refinement of nonpharmacologic methods of therapy all have developed in parallel in recent years. The equilibrium between the risk implied by an arrhythmia and the proarrhythmic risk of a drug[163–165] was dramatically emphasized by the results of the Cardiac Arrhythmia Suppression Trial (CAST)[21,227] and Survival with Oral D-Sotalol (SWORD)[166] study, which resulted in major changes in indications and methods for treatment of some ventricular arrhythmias.

The *urge* to treat, based upon limited scientific support in the past, has yielded to indications based upon the *need* to treat, modulated by a better definition of the *risk* of treatment. Clinical approaches to the patient with ventricular arrhythmias require a clear analysis of the interrelationships between electrocardiographic forms of arrhythmias, the specific clinical setting in which it occurs, and realistic goals of therapy (see Tables 24-1 and 24-3).

Definitions, Classification of Risk, and End Points of Therapy

Forms of ventricular arrhythmias may be separated into the various patterns of ambient PVCs and of sustained arrhythmias, such as sustained VT or Ventricular fibrillation (VF). The former are present intermittently and identify risk in the presence of structural heart disease. They may also serve a triggering function for hemodynamically significant or life-threatening arrhythmias (VT or VF) under appropriate conditions.

TABLE 24-10 Specific Forms of Ventricular Tachycardia

Duration	ECG Pattern
Salvo (3–5 impulses)	Uniform morphology VT
Nonsustained VT (6 impulses, 29 s)	Polymorphic VT, torsades de pointes
Sustained VT (≥30 s)	Right ventricular outflow pattern
	Bidirectional tachycardia

The conventional definition of VT, three or more consecutive ventricular ectopic impulses at a rate of 120 or greater, is too broad to apply to current evaluation and management strategies. A distinction between bursts of nonsustained VT lasting for up to 30 s and sustained VT lasting 30 s or more (Table 24-10) is more useful for evaluation at the bedside, ambulatory monitoring data, the results of invasive electrophysiologic testing, and responses to therapy. In addition to defining VT by its duration, useful information is contained in the definition of VT from its ECG pattern. Slow, monomorphic patterns of nonsustained VT are less symptomatic and may denote lower risk than faster, polymorphic VT patterns.

Data on the risk predicted by PVCs after convalescence from myocardial infarction have been analyzed relative to both frequency and forms.[167–172] Based upon the frequency in Fig. 24-34, most studies demonstrate increased risk with frequencies of 10 or more ectopic impulses per hour, and one major study demonstrated a sharp increase in risk moving across the range of 1 to 9 impulses per hour.[172] Similarly, in the hierarchy of

HIERARCHY OF FREQUENCIES	HIERARCHY OF FORMS
CLASS 0 – NIL	CLASS A – UNIFORM MORPHOLOGY, UNIFOCAL
CLASS I – RARE < 1 ectopic impulse/hour	CLASS B – MULTIFORM, MULTIFOCAL
CLASS II – INFREQUENT 1 to 9 ectopic impulses/hour	CLASS C – REPETITIVE FORMS • COUPLETS • SALVOS, REPETITIVE RESPONSES (3–5 consecutive inpulses)
CLASS III – INTERMEDIATE 10 to 29 ectopic impulses/hour	CLASS D – NON-SUSTAINED VENTRICULAR TACHYCARDIA (from 6 consecutive ectopic impulses to runs lasting up to 30 seconds)
CLASS IV – FREQUENT ≥ 30 ectopic impulses/hour	CLASS E – SUSTAINED VENTRICULAR TACHYCARDIA (runs of ectopic activity ≥ 30 seconds)

FIGURE 24-34 Classification of ventricular arrhythmias based on hierarchies of frequency and forms. Hierarchical schemes for estimating risk of ventricular arrhythmias have been developed based on frequency and forms of ventricular arrhythmias. In some clinical settings, frequencies in the range of 1 to 9 ectopic impulses per hour become significant, and in most settings of clinically significant heart disease, risk based on frequency plateaus in the range of 10 to 30 ectopic impulses per hour. Among forms of ventricular arrhythmias, the repetitive forms, particularly salvos or nonsustained ventricular tachycardia, indicate higher risk in most clinical settings. (Modified from Myerburg et al.[138] Reproduced with permission from the publisher and authors.)

forms, couplets indicate only a small increase in risk compared to uniform or multiform single PVCs,[172] and salvos indicate a significantly higher risk.[171,172] There are insufficient data to determine whether longer runs (i.e., nonsustained VTs of six consecutive impulses) constitute an even higher risk. Patterns such as bigeminy and trigeminy are simply an expression of frequency and contain no inherent information concerning risk beyond frequency.

For evaluating risk and prescribing therapy, clinical information beyond the pattern of the arrhythmia itself must be considered. Very high frequencies and/or advanced forms usually connote little or no increased risk in the absence of structural heart disease, except for certain polymorphic nonsustained VTs. Risk begins to increase with the presence of structural heart disease and becomes prominent with falling EF.[171,172] A simplified but useful clinically based classification incorporates both form and frequency along with clinical disease information. Bigger[173] suggested classifying ventricular arrhythmias as benign, potentially malignant, and malignant based on these considerations. As an extension of this concept, frequency, forms, severity of cardiac disease, and LV function (EF) can be integrated into a clinical classification of benign (no independent increase in risk), significant (independent increase in risk), and potentially lethal (untreated, can lead to proximate fatality). While these clinically based approaches have not been quantitated, they do provide a conceptual framework for classifying arrhythmias.

Management of PVCs must be further analyzed in regard to specific etiology (e.g., low-risk mitral valve prolapse versus high-risk idiopathic dilated cardiomyopathy), and PVCs in acute or subacute clinical settings must be distinguished from those occurring in chronic settings. Finally, end points of therapy that are based upon suppression of underlying ectopy (i.e., background PVCs) are separated from end points based upon prevention of potentially lethal arrhythmias (i.e., sustained VT or VF; see Table 24-1). *There are no data supporting the notion that PVC suppression itself improves mortality rates, despite the connotation of risk in specific clinical settings. Indications for therapy are based on symptoms, evaluated in the light of the known or suspected risks of therapy.*

Premature Ventricular Contractions

ELECTROCARDIOGRAPHIC RECOGNITION OF PVCS

Ventricular arrhythmias originate in the specialized conducting tissue distal to the bifurcation of the bundle of His or in true ventricular myocardium. Accordingly, they are characterized by a prolonged ventricular depolarization (i.e., wide QRS complex), an alteration in the sequence of ventricular activation (i.e., a change in the QRS vector), and alterations in the timing sequence of consecutive QRS complexes (i.e., prematurity or escape rhythms). None of these criteria is totally sensitive and specific for ectopic impulses of ventricular origin. On occasion, PVCs demonstrate narrow QRS complexes, have a vector very similar to the normal QRS vector, or have timing little changed from the normal sinus sequence. Nonetheless, the majority of impulses originating in the ventricles have QRS complexes of at least 0.12 s and a shift in the QRS vector, and most single PVCs or initiating beats for runs of ventricular ectopic activity are premature. PVCs may fail to conduct to the atria or may demonstrate retrograde atrial activation. In either case, the sinus cycle is usually not interrupted, resulting in a *fully compensatory pause* (Fig. 24-35). The pause is characterized by an interval between the P wave of the sinus impulse immediately before the PVC and the first sinus P wave after the PVC equal to twice the sinus cycle length (Fig. 24-35*A*). If the sinus rate is relatively slow, PVCs may be interpolated between two sinus beats with no alteration of the sinus cycle length (Fig. 24-35*B*). Exceptions to the compensatory pause rule do occur (Fig. 24-36) and occasionally complicate diagnostic criteria. PVCs that presumably originate in the fascicles of the specialized conducting system may have more narrow QRS complexes with only slight alterations in the QRS vector.

PVCs are usually coupled to the preceding sinus beat by a fixed coupling interval. This generalization has exceptions, in that PVCs having different QRS morphologies may have different coupling intervals,[174] and PVCs having the same morphology in a given patient may have different coupling intervals as pathophysiologic conditions change. The pattern of fixed coupling has led to a concept of a physiologic relationship between the sinus beat and the PVC, an argument in favor of reentrant or triggered-activity mechanisms for common PVCs. In contrast, parasystolic rhythms refer to an independent ectopic rhythm, with the focus of origin being protected in the sense that descending impulses cannot enter and reset the parasystolic focus but can create a field of refractoriness around it, limiting the rate and timing of impulses that exit the focus. Thus, the parasystolic

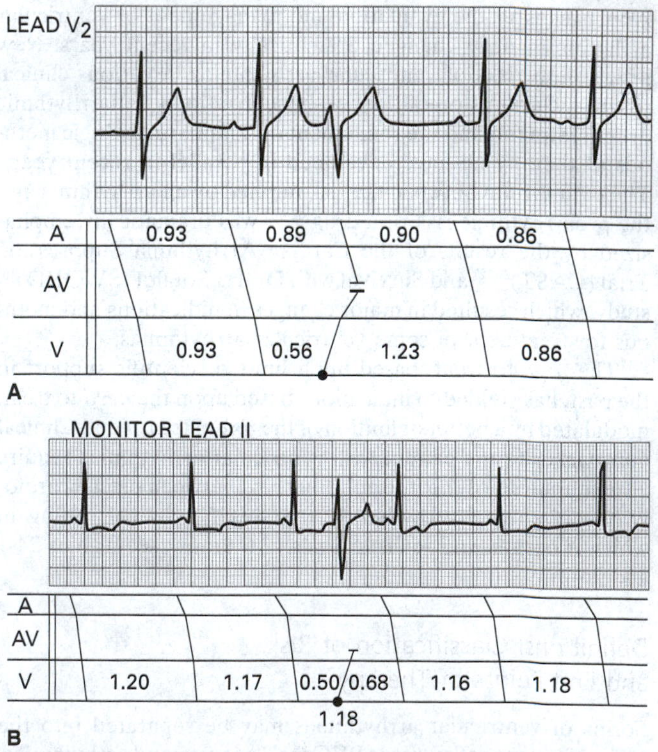

FIGURE 24-35 Ventricular premature contractions. *A*. The third impulse is wide and bizarre, and since the sinus rhythm is undisturbed (next sinus P wave indicated by arrow), the postextrasystolic pause is compensatory. *B*. The fourth impulse is an interpolated ventricular premature contraction; it is sandwiched between two consecutive conducted sinus beats.

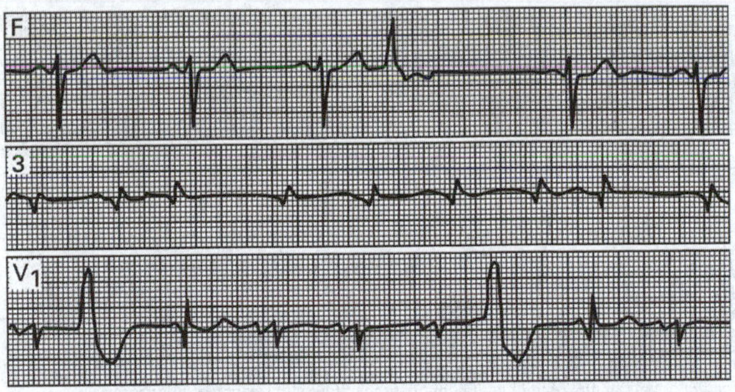

FIGURE 24-36 Exceptions to the rules for compensatory pauses. *Top.* Ventricular extrasystole with less than compensatory pause. Retrograde conduction to the atria (retrograde P wave deforms first part of ST segment) discharges the sinus pacemaker early and thus shortens the postextrasystolic cycle. *Middle.* Atrial premature contraction followed by fully compensatory pause. The third and eighth beats are atrial extrasystoles, but presumably because they suppress the sinus pacemaker, they are followed by compensatory pauses. *Bottom.* Ventricular extrasystoles with less than compensatory pauses. Each postextrasystolic cycle ends in an escape beat and so is slightly less than compensatory.

focus, automatic in nature, can deliver impulses to the myocardium but cannot be reset by impulses originating elsewhere. Accordingly, the ECG reflects the presence of competing pacemakers, the sinus node, and a protected automatic ectopic ventricular focus, creating the classic triad of (1) variable coupling between sinus beats and ectopic QRS complexes, (2) fusion beats, and (3) a fixed common denominator of interectopic intervals between manifest parasystolic extrasystoles (Fig. 24-37). However, classic concepts of parasystole have been altered by the discovery that parasystole may be modulated by relationships between the parasystolic focus and impulses originating in the sinus node. Sinus impulses occurring early in the parasystolic cycle tend to shorten the cycle length of the parasystolic focus, whereas those arriving in the latter half of the cycle tend to lengthen the cycle length of the parasystolic focus.[175] Parasystolic patterns may also occur with atrial extrasystolic activity.

MANAGEMENT OF PREMATURE VENTRICULAR CONTRACTIONS

Management of PVCs in the Absence of Significant Structural Heart Disease PVCs occur in many healthy individuals. In the absence of heart disease, there is little or no increased risk,[176] and the risk-benefit ratio of antiarrhythmic therapy does not support a need for routine treatment. For the patient who complains of disturbing or disabling palpitations due to PVCs, however, the clinician may have to treat for symptom relief (Fig. 24-38). Reassurance and avoidance of potentially aggravating factors (e.g., tobacco, coffee, caffeine-containing soft drinks, environmental stress, or stimulants) should be tried before pharmacologic therapy. For the latter, mild anxiolytic drugs or beta-adrenergic blockers (which may sedate, reduce PVC frequency, and decrease the strength of postextrasystolic impulses causing the perception of palpitations) are preferred. When used for this purpose, low doses of beta-adrenergic blockers are often sufficient. The end point, relief of symptoms, may not necessarily be accompanied by significantly reduced PVC frequency. The frequency of PVCs may be modulated by underlying heart rate,[177] and thus manipulations of sympathetic and parasympathetic balance may be useful. Because of their side-effect profiles, class I antiarrhythmic agents are rarely indicated in this clinical setting, and the class III agent amiodarone is unnecessarily potent. PVCs are often more prominent with pregnancy and premenstrually and increase in frequency with age.[178]

There may be an urge to be more aggressive in the management of patients who have advanced forms of PVCs (e.g., salvos or nonsustained VT) or a high frequency of PVCs (30 or more PVCs per hour) in the absence of structural disease. Kennedy et al.,[176] however, reported no increased risk of death in a cohort of such persons followed for a mean of over 6 years. Some specific forms of nonsustained VT, for example, polymorphic runs, may predict some increase in risk (see below).

The occurrence of PVCs in patients with mitral valve prolapse has gained special attention for three reasons: (1) the high prevalence of mitral valve prolapse, (2) the prevalence of PVCs in patients with mitral valve prolapse, and (3) the very small risk of sustained VT or VF. Annoying palpitations are a common complaint, but the arrhythmia does not require treatment in the vast majority. There are limited data suggesting that the patients at highest risk for serious ventricular arrhythmias can be subgrouped by the presence of nonspecific ST-T wave changes in leads II, III, and aVF[179,180] in conjunction with advanced grades of ventricular arrhythmias and redundancy of the mitral valve echocardiographically.[181] The approach to treatment of patients with benign forms of PVCs in mitral valve prolapse should be no different than that outlined for individuals with no structural abnormalities. Beta-adrenergic blocking agents are often sufficient to control the symptoms, and membrane-active antiarrhythmic drugs should be avoided.

Patients at risk for more serious arrhythmias, as outlined above, may require more aggressive treatment; membrane-active drugs are considered for use in this special situation for patients with salvos or nonsustained VT. The rare mitral valve prolapse patient who has had sustained VT or survived after VF is managed by the approaches generally used for these potentially lethal arrhythmias in other clinical settings (see below).

Management of PVCs in Acute Syndromes PVCs are nearly ubiquitous in acute myocardial infarction, but the threshold for treatment remains unsettled. The original concept of "warning arrhythmias" published by Lown et al.[182] remains an indication for aggressive treatment, even though the predictive value of such warning arrhythmias remains unsubstantiated.[183,184]

The concept of routine treatment of all patients with acute infarctions with lidocaine to prevent PVCs as well as VT or VF[185,186] is no longer applied, having yielded to a threshold for treatment at various frequencies of manifest PVCs. Suppression of PVCs in acute myocardial infarction is usually accomplished with intravenous lidocaine (a bolus of 50 to 100 mg followed by a continuous infusion of 2 to 4 mg/min), with intravenous procainamide as a second choice (100 mg every 5 min to a total dose of 500 to 750 mg, followed by an infusion of 1 to 4 mg/min). Both drugs have significant side effects, especially with improper dosing. Furthermore, these drugs have not been shown to change hospital mortality rates for patients for whom prompt medical attention and electrical defibrillation are avail-

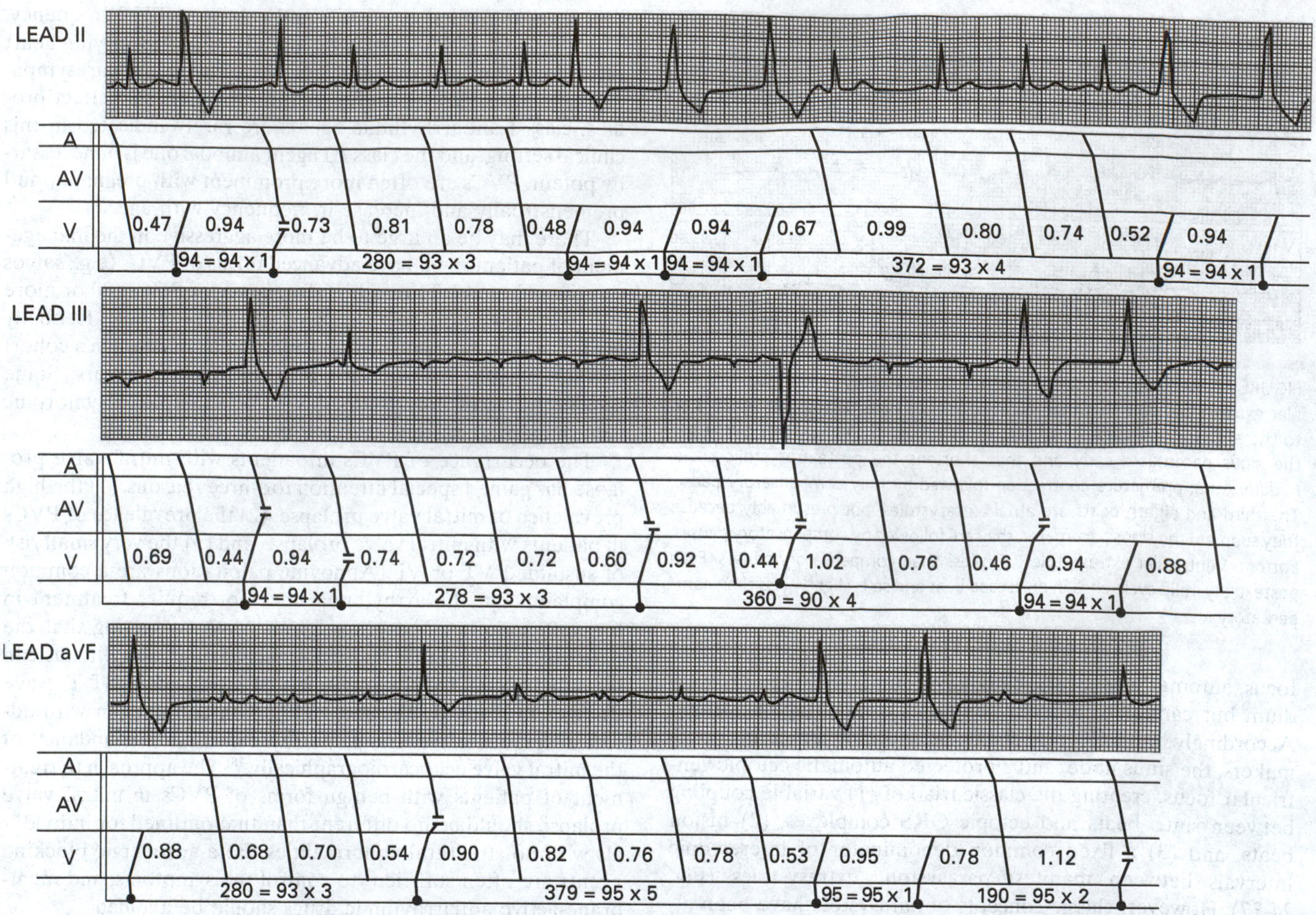

FIGURE 24-37 Ventricular parasystole. The strips are continuous. Note that (1) the interval between an ectopic beat and the preceding sinus beat varies; (2) the interectopic intervals all have a common denominator of 0.90 to 0.95 s; and (3) there are occasional fusion beats (third beat in top strip; fourth beat in second strip; last beat in bottom strip). (From Hurst JW, Myerburg R. *Introduction to Electrocardiography*. New York: McGraw-Hill; 1973. Reproduced with permission from the publisher and authors.)

VENTRICULAR ARRHYTHMIAS - LEVELS OF SYMPTOMS

SYMPTOM-FREE → UNAWARE OF RHYTHM

MINIMAL SYMPTOMS → PALPITATIONS

LIFESTYLE LIMITING → LIGHTHEADEDNESS

HEMODYNAMIC EFFECTS → SYNCOPE

LIFE-THREATENING → CARDIAC ARREST

FIGURE 24-38 Approaches to management of ventricular arrhythmias. Treatment of ventricular arrhythmias is dictated by symptoms and clinical risk. Asymptomatic PVCs in the absence of disease usually need not be treated. Ventricular arrhythmias in the presence of advanced and/or acute disease states commonly indicate high risk, although therapy is not necessarily targeted to the PVCs themselves. A range of considerations of risk versus quality of life exists between these two extremes (see the text for details).

able. Lidocaine levels and binding both increase during the course of acute myocardial infarction,[187] theoretically rendering free drug levels stable. The practice of tapering the lidocaine infusion to avoid toxicity[188] is not appropriate if free drug concentration represents active drug and does not rise (see also Chap. 42).

A number of other acute cardiac states are associated with the emergence of PVCs. For example, PVCs may emerge during and immediately after transient myocardial ischemia and are accompanied by a risk for sustained VT or VF.[189–191] The primary intervention for controlling PVCs in these settings is the reversal of ischemia.[189] On first contact, however, intravenous lidocaine or procainamide should be administered to suppress the arrhythmias. Clinical circumstances characterized by myocardial reperfusion—such as Prinzmetal's angina, thrombolysis in AMI, or balloon deflation during percutaneous transluminal coronary angioplasty (PTCA)—may cause reperfusion-induced arrhythmias. The arrhythmias generated include PVCs and accelerated ventricular rhythms (e.g., postthrombolysis or PTCA) or nonsustained VT (often polymorphic) after reversal of coronary spasm.[191] These arrhythmias are usually transient and self-limiting but may evolve into sustained VT or VF.[190,191] Although there are theoretical and experimental reasons to suspect that Ca^{2+}-mediated electrophysiologic disturbances occur during reperfusion,[192,194] intravenous lidocaine is currently used to treat reperfusion-induced arrhythmias. It is used in the same dose and with the same infusion techniques as in acute myocardial infarction. Severe heart failure and acute pulmonary edema are commonly accompanied by frequent and advanced forms of PVCs;[194,195] as in acute myocardial infarction with low-output states, the PVCs are considered secondary to the hemodynamic abnormality (see Fig. 24-1). The use of antiarrhythmic agents while the hemodynamic status is being stabilized is appropriate but may have only limited success until adequate hemodynamic control is achieved.

Acute and subacute myocarditis and pericarditis are commonly accompanied by PVCs, and sustained VT or VF may occur infrequently,[196] even in the absence of significant myocardial dysfunction. Frequent PVCs and salvos or nonsustained VT are usually treated until the carditis has resolved. In those patients who have not had sustained VT or VF conventional antiarrhythmic agents are given orally and titrated to suppression of the PVCs if possible, or at least to achieve suppression of repetitive forms. Antiarrhythmic therapy is continued for a minimum of 2 months, and then the patient is taken off antiarrhythmic drugs while still being monitored. If advanced forms do not reappear, the drug is not restarted; if they do reappear, treatment is continued for another 2 to 3 months, after which the same procedure is carried out. Myocarditis that has not evolved into a cardiomyopathic state is only rarely followed by frequent or complex forms of PVCs beyond 6 months. Virtually all other acute cardiac syndromes and many acute systemic disorders may be associated with PVCs that will abate with resolution of the initiating abnormality.

Management of Chronic PVCs in the Presence of Cardiac Disease Chronic PVCs carry a different connotation in patients with established heart disease than in those free of disease. Sudden and total death rates are increased in patients who have frequent or repetitive PVCs in the major categories of chronic cardiac disease in the United States, including chronic ischemic heart disease,[168–172] hypertensive heart disease, and the cardiomyopathies.[1,194,195,197,198]

When frequent PVCs and/or salvos or runs of nonsustained VT are accompanied by a reduced EF, both the arrhythmia and the EF contribute to risk, and the rate of sudden death is increased.[200,201] Bigger et al.[201] observed a 2-year mortality rate of 42 percent for postinfarction patients with salvos or nonsustained VT and an EF of less than 30 percent, compared to a 2-year mortality rate of 12 percent for patients with salvos or nonsustained VT and an EF of 50 percent or more. The 2-year rate fell to 7 percent for patients with only single PVCs and an EF of 50 percent or more.

Management of frequent and repetitive forms of chronic PVCs after myocardial infarction has changed dramatically since the results of the CAST study were published.[21,199] Previous studies[200,201] as well as CAST itself[21] had demonstrated that PVC suppression was feasible in these patients, but CAST clearly demonstrated a significant excess risk of sudden cardiovascular death among the treatment groups receiving the two class IC agents (flecainide and encainide) evaluated in the study. CAST II, the continuation of the study with moricizine, the one drug that had not crossed a boundary of significance during CAST I, demonstrated neither benefit nor adverse effect, showing only an early classic proarrhythmic mortality risk, which did not influence long-term outcome.[199] By design, the enrollment in the moricizine arm of CAST I and in CAST II was a population with more advanced disease. Meta-analyses of data derived from previous smaller randomized studies, as well as the subsequent (SWORD) study,[166] testing the effect of antiarrhythmic drugs on mortality rates after myocardial infarction, also suggested an adverse effect of most antiarrhythmic drugs when used in postmyocardial infarction patients.[202] Accordingly, the drugs used in CAST are now contraindicated following myocardial infarction in patients with asymptomatic or mildly symptomatic PVCs, and there is a trend away from the use of any membrane-active antiarrhythmic agent in such patients. Recent large randomized, placebo-controlled trials testing the possible benefit of amiodarone in postmyocardial infarction patients (EMIAT and CAMIAT) demonstrated no benefit on total mortality rates.[203,204] Beta-adrenoceptor blocking agents, however, have a substantial beneficial effect on long-term outcome in the postmyocardial infarction patient[205,206] as well as improving total mortality rates in the subgroups of the amiodarone postmyocardial infarction trials in whom beta-adrenoceptor–blocking agents were used with amiodarone.[207] In addition, beta-adrenoceptor–blocking agents are effective in suppressing repetitive forms of PVCs in many patients.[209]

Beta blockers, therefore, have evolved as the drugs of choice following myocardial infarction in patients with mildly symptomatic PVCs. While no properly randomized study directed to a sudden and total death outcome as a result of PVC suppression using beta-adrenoceptor–blocking agents has been reported, the existing randomized data on mortality rates in patients following myocardial infarction in general demonstrates beneficial effects.[205,206]

In patients with *symptomatic* PVCs (e.g., palpitations or repetitive beats) following myocardial infarction, especially when accompanied by a low EF, management becomes more difficult. Such patients have a higher mortality rate, and it is not known whether the CAST data should be extrapolated to this population. Because of CAST, class IC agents are avoided in these patients, but clinicians may use other antiarrhythmic drugs if they are well tolerated and no adverse effects are observed. However, the threshold for initiation of therapy is generally higher than it was prior to CAST. Even if the EF is depressed, beta-adrenergic blocking agents should be tried initially. If they are effective and well tolerated, they are the preferred treatment. Class III (e.g., sotalol and amiodarone) and perhaps class IA drugs also appear to be safe and may be used if treatment is necessary.

Chronic PVCs are very common in patients with advanced idiopathic dilated cardiomyopathy and in patients with hypertrophic cardiomyopathy, and both groups have a major risk of arrhythmic sudden death. In some reports, more than 90 percent of patients with dilated cardiomyopathy have frequent PVCs, and over 50 percent have salvos or nonsustained VT.[194,195] Efficacy of antiarrhythmic therapy for both suppression of chronic PVCs and prevention of VT and VF is unclear and perhaps is quite limited in these patients. Treatment is controversial. It is not known whether the CAST data can be extrapolated to this group or whether there is any mortality benefit from the use of antiarrhythmic drugs among these patients. When treatment is prescribed, the patient should be hospitalized for initiation of antiarrhythmic therapy because of proarrhythmic risk in cardiomyopathy.[214] Secondary ventricular arrhythmias in patients who have chronic heart failure (see Fig. 24-1) may respond to control of heart failure. In one carefully designed study, treatment with an angiotensin-converting enzyme inhibitor had a very favorable effect on both parameters of heart failure and ventricular ectopy.[215]

When antiarrhythmic drugs are to be used, the selection of a drug or a combination of drugs for high-risk patients with chronic PVCs is complex. The class IA drugs are moderately effective but have a high incidence of allergic reactions (e.g., procainamide) and poorly tolerated side effects (e.g., quinidine causing thrombocytopenia). They may also produce significant further myocardial depression in patients with an already reduced EF (e.g., disopyramide). Moricizine appears to be better tolerated, but all have significant risks of proarrhythmic effects, although many of these events are not life-threatening.[216] Among the class IB agents (e.g., tocainide and mexiletine), efficacy might be good in some patients and the proarrhythmic incidence is lower, but there is a high incidence of uncomfortable side effects. The currently available IC agents (flecainide and propafenone) are very effective for reducing ventricular ectopy and are well tolerated in patients with normal or only minimally depressed LV function. Their use is not indicated for patients with ischemic heart disease because of the adverse outcome observed in CAST[21] and is limited more generally by the fact that the incidence of proarrhythmic effects and myocardial depression is highest in the subgroup at greatest need for the intervention: those with repetitive forms and impaired LV function. It is not yet known, however, whether the higher absolute risk of adverse effects in patients with abnormal LV function is balanced by a benefit in this higher-risk group.[217] Specifically, the long-term effects of the class I agents on death rates in groups of patients other than the lower-risk category enrolled in CAST are unknown at present.

There are differences in adverse proarrhythmic effects among the various drug groups. Class IA drugs are predominantly associated with classical proarrhythmia. Class III drugs have the same pattern of proarrhythmia, perhaps with a lower incidence of torsades de pointes for amiodarone. Sotalol demonstrates a dose-dependent incidence of torsades de pointes, in contrast to the idiosyncratic pattern for the class IA drugs. The common denominator between class IA and class III drugs, which likely contributes to this concordant proarrhythmic pattern, is moderate to marked prolongation of repolarization, as reflected in QT interval prolongation. In contrast, the class IC drugs, which have minimal effect on repolarization, have a low rate of classic proarrhythmia: torsades de pointes. They may, however, worsen clinical arrhythmias or generate a new rapid sinusoidal sustained VT.[219] In addition, the excess death rate in CAST, attributed to proarrhythmia, extended over the entire period of drug exposure rather than being close in time to the start of treatment. A possible explanation for this pattern is a tendency for the class IC drugs to interact with sporadic intercurrent events, such as transient ischemia or LV dysfunction.[22] Such an explanation is consistent with disturbed conduction patterns (depolarization) contributing to proarrhythmia rather than repolarization abnormalities[15] (see also Chap. 27). It is also consistent with the observation in CAST that increased risk of mortality in the flecainide and encainide arms was accompanied by a decreased incidence of nonfatal ischemic events compared to their placebo groups. Combining drug classes has been found to be effective by some, although carefully controlled studies are limited;[220] combinations such as a class IA and a class IB drug may be tried. The class II drugs, beta-adrenergic blocking agents, have been mentioned earlier, and many consider them the first choice of therapy even if the EF is reduced. They may be used in combination with class I drugs in some patients. Class III drugs have been approved only for use in life-threatening arrhythmias, although amiodarone and sotalol are both appropriate for selected patients with symptomatic runs of nonsustained VT and advanced LV dysfunction. The available data on amiodarone is promising for patients with life-threatening arrhythmias,[221,222] but the specific benefit for patients with PVCs and nonsustained VT in the presence of advanced heart disease is unclear. In the Survival Trial of Antiarrhythmic Therapy in Congestive Heart Failure (CHF-STAT) study, which randomized ischemic and nonischemic myopathies and PVCs to amiodarone and placebo, no mortality benefit was observed.[223] Another study, GESICA, which randomized cardiomyopathic patients to the same drug versus placebo, however, showed a survival benefit for the amiodarone-treated group.[224] PVC stratification was not carried out in the latter. In both studies, amiodarone-treated patients with nonischemic cardiomyopathies tended to respond more favorably to the drug than those with ischemic cardiomyopathies. The class IV drugs, Ca^{2+}-entry blockers, have no role in the treatment of chronic PVCs.

With any of these drugs or drug combinations, attention to underlying heart disease and systemic factors is necessary. Treatment for limiting the frequency of episodes of transient ischemia, maximizing LV function, maintaining electrolyte balance, and controlling blood pressure all may act in concert with antiarrhythmic agents to limit the risk of cardiac morbidity

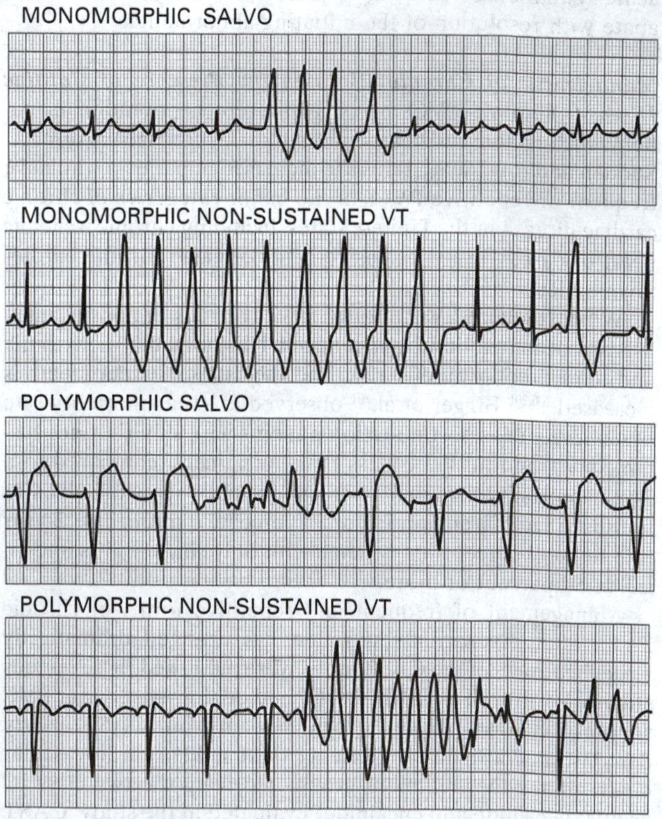

FIGURE 24-39 Nonsustained forms of VT. Runs of repetitive ventricular impulses (rate 100 per minute) lasting less than 30 s are subgrouped into salvos of three to five consecutive impulses and nonsustained VT of six or more impulses in duration. Both forms may be further defined according to morphology as monomorphic or polymorphic.

and mortality in patients with chronic PVCs. The end point of treatment (see Table 24-1) of patients who have structural heart disease and high-risk forms and frequency of chronic PVCs is not at all clear. The pharmacodynamics of PVC suppression differ from those of VT prevention,[225] and quantitative PVC suppression is difficult to achieve.

Suppression of advanced forms of PVCs (e.g., couplets, salvos, and nonsustained VT) is sometimes achieved,[226] even if quantitative PVC suppression fails. General guidelines have included suppression of 70 to 80 percent of total PVCs on a 24-h ambulatory monitor[227] and complete (or nearly complete) suppression of repetitive forms.[228] An ongoing trial, MADIT II, is designed to determine whether mortality rates can be improved by ICDs in postmyocardial infarction patients with PVCs and ejection fractions of 30 percent or less.[229]

Nonsustained Ventricular Tachycardia

Nonsustained runs of VT (salvos of three to five consecutive impulses or nonsustained VT of six impulses to 30 s; Fig. 24-39) are considered indicators of high risk for potentially fatal arrhythmias (sustained VT or VF) in most clinical settings. There are important exceptions, however. Patients who have no organic disease or limited cardiac abnormalities do not appear to have increased risk, although some patients who have very rapid polymorphic VT may be at increased risk. Even in the absence of an increased mortality risk, symptoms such as transient light-headedness, near-syncope, or syncope require therapy (see Fig. 24-38). At the other extreme, cardiomyopathy patients and those who have advanced coronary artery disease with a very low EF are among the highest risk groups. Conceptually, nonsustained VT may be viewed as self-terminating VT or as an intense triggering event in a susceptible myocardium.[1]

Treatment is generally similar to that outlined for other patterns of PVCs, although patients with prior myocardial infarction who have nonsustained VT and low EFs and are inducible into VT in the clinical electrophysiology laboratory are thought to be at higher risk than those with nonsustained VT who have better EFs and are noninducible.[210] In MADIT, ICD therapy demonstrated lower mortality rates than with the best conventional therapy in a randomized study design of such patients (nonsustained VT, EF 35 percent or less, inducible sustained VT, and failed supression of inducibility of VT during programmed stimulation-guided therapy with intravenous procainamide).[211] In the Multicenter Unsustained Tachycardia Trial (MUSTT), a similar group of patients appeared to benefit from ICDs, as opposed to electrophysiologically guided drug therapy.[230]

Repetitive Monomorphic Ventricular Tachycardia

Repetitive monomorphic VT is an uncommon form of repetitive salvos or runs of nonsustained VT, often separated from one another by only a few sinus impulses (Fig. 24-40).[233] Occasionally, this arrhythmia is continuous and fulfills the definition of sustained VT. The tachycardia rate is usually 150 or less per minute but may be greater than 200 per minute in rare cases. The syndrome is more common in women and is usually benign.[233,234] The QRS patterns of the tachycardia on 12-lead ECGs suggest a right ventricular outflow tract origin (left bundle-branch block pattern with an axis between 0° and +90°, or slightly rightward), and the mechanism is likely a form of enhanced automaticity.[235] Treatment is considered only when structural heart disease is also present, when the palpitations are poorly tolerated by the patient, or when the patient has light-headedness, near-syncope, or syncope caused by the arrhythmia. Membrane-active antiarrhythmic drugs should be avoided if possible, and beta-adrenoceptor and Ca^{2+}-entry blocking agents are effective in some. Catheter ablation is an option for the more sustained or symptomatic forms and has a high probability of success[236] (Fig. 24-41).

Sustained Ventricular Tachycardia

Sustained VT may originate in the specialized conducting system distal to the bundle of His, in ventricular myocardium, or by an interaction between the two. By definition, it occurs at a heart rate of 100 per minute or more and lasts for 30 s or more. A ventricular rhythm faster than 40 to 50 impulses per minute but slower than 100 per minute is referred to as an accelerated ventricular rhythm. Runs of VT lasting less than

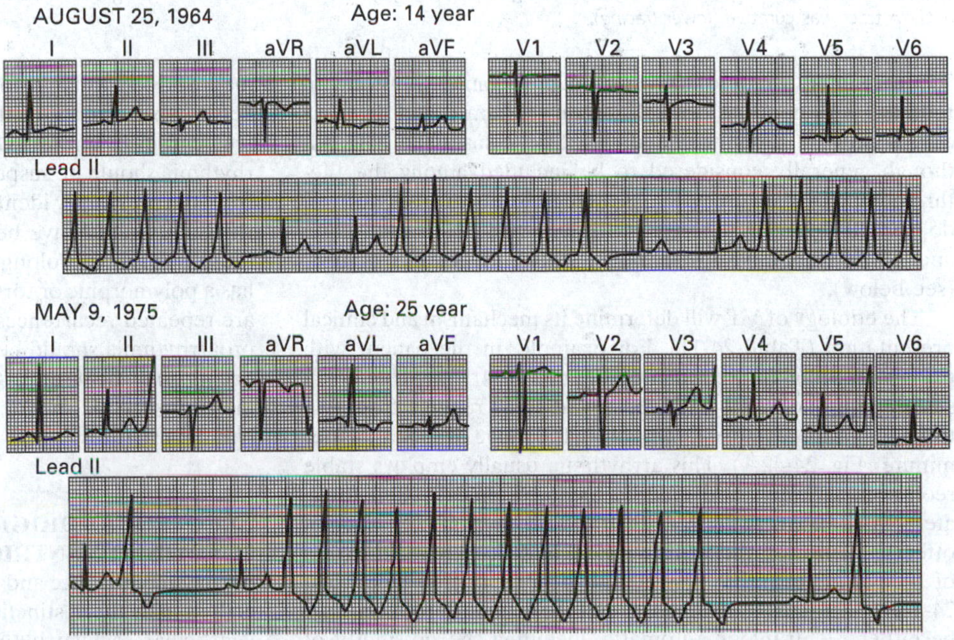

FIGURE 24-40 Repetitive monomorphic ventricular tachycardia. This condition is commonly benign but may be symptomatic in some patients. The most benign form (Gallavardin tachycardia or Parkinson-Papp syndrome) is characterized by runs of nonsustained VT commonly separated by only a few sinus beats. It is occasionally sustained and usually suppresses with exercise. It is commoner in women and has a QRS morphology suggesting a right ventricular outflow tract origin. In this example, an 11-year follow-up shows persistence of the arrhythmia, with no other significant ECG abnormalities, in a patient who has remained asymptomatic without therapy.

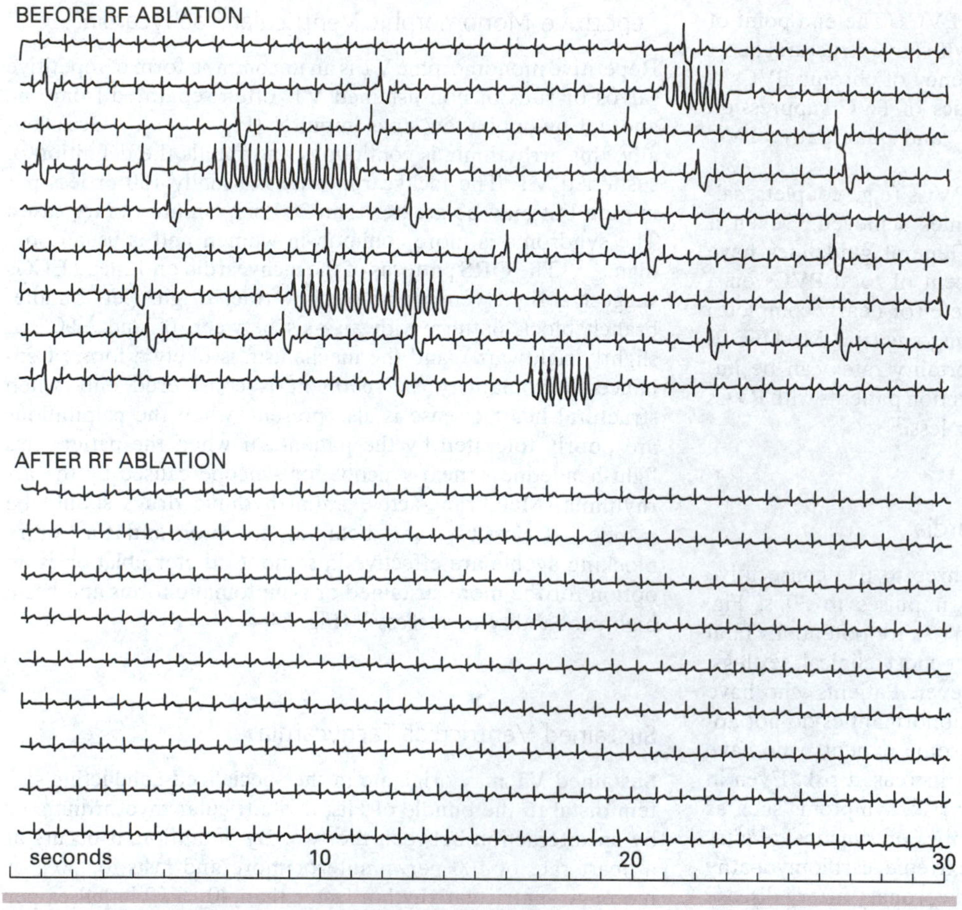

FIGURE 24-41 Symptomatic repetitive monomorphic ventricular tachycardia. In this example, the patient presented with a 6-month history of palpitations, episodic lightheadedness, and a few episodes of syncope. The arrhythmia was observed on ambulatory monitoring (*upper tracing*); RF ablation of a focus in the right ventricular outflow tract was curative (*lower tracing*).

30 s that impair hemodynamics enough to cause symptoms of reduced peripheral or central nervous system blood flow are considered the functional equivalent of a sustained VT. Although generally considered to be included among the life-threatening cardiac arrhythmias, benign forms of sustained VT do exist. They occur in persons without structural heart disease, and a functional basis can be identified in some instances (see below).

The etiology of VT will determine its mechanism and clinical presentation (Table 24-11). For example, in the patient with prior myocardial infarction and a defined ventricular aneurysm, sustained monomorphic VT occurs at rates ranging from 140 to 200 per minute, most commonly in the range of 150 to 180 per minute (Fig. 24-42*A*). This arrhythmia usually employs stable reentrant pathways and may be hemodynamically well tolerated. In contrast, patients with transient myocardial ischemia often have more rapid ventricular tachyarrhythmias (in excess of 200 per minute) that may be polymorphic or sinusoidal (Fig. 24-42*B*). The mechanism is not clearly defined but likely may be either reentrant or automatic, including the possibility of triggered activity. These forms of VT tend to be hemodynamically and electrically unstable, with a higher risk of degenerating to VF than chronic recurrent monomorphic VT. They tend to persist for only short periods of time, in contrast to the sustained mono-morphic VTs, which may persist for hours in some patients. These forms of VT either degenerate to VF, convert to a stable monomorphic VT, or spontaneously revert to sinus rhythm (see also Chap. 23).

Some patients will tolerate sustained monomorphic VT remarkably well, although the risk that sustained VT will degenerate into VF must always be kept in mind. When the hemodynamic status is stable and there is no evidence of myocardial ischemia, acute infarction, or poor central nervous system perfusion, electrical cardioversion can await a therapeutic trial of intravenous drug. With acute myocardial infarction, falling blood pressure, or evidence of ischemia, immediate cardioversion is indicated. In patients who are already receiving antiarrhythmic agents because of prior sustained VT or for treatment of other ventricular arrhythmias, recurrent sustained VT presents a challenging therapeutic problem. If it is known that the patient has not complied with antiarrhythmic regimens, standard intravenous regimens may be tried, but more commonly this is not the case. Plasma concentrations of the prescribed antiarrhythmics should be ordered at the time of presentation, even though the information may not be available for initial management. The distinction between recurrence of the previous VT and proarrhythmic effects caused by antiarrhythmic agents is a major dilemma. Proarrhythmia should be suspected if the VT morphology is different from the previously identified clinical VT morphology, if antiarrhythmic agents have been recently prescribed or changed, if there is marked prolongation of the QT interval, or if the VT has a polymorphic or torsades de pointes configuration. If there are repeated recurrences after cardioversion, the possibility of proarrhythmia should be seriously entertained, and temporary pacing may be useful. Other causes of repeated recurrence include ischemia, heart failure, autonomic surges, or electrolyte disturbances.

ELECTROCARDIOGRAPHIC RECOGNITION OF SUSTAINED VENTRICULAR TACHYCARDIA

Having met the rate and duration criteria for a sustained tachyarrhythmia, the distinction between sustained VT and supraventricular tachyarrhythmias with abnormal intraventricular conduction patterns is based upon a complex set of electrocardiographic criteria. The evaluation of the patient's general clinical status, short of cardiac arrest, is only of limited value for distinguishing very rapid SVT from VT as the cause of hypotension or syncope. Nonetheless, the distinction between SVT and

TABLE 24-11 Causes of Ventricular Tachycardias

Clinical Setting	Common Mechanisms
Structural heart disease	
Chronic ischemic heart disease	Reentry
Acute ischemia and reperfusion	Automatic, triggered activity, reentry
Dilated cardiomyopathy	Reentry (bundle brunch), automatic, triggered activity (EAD, DAD)
Hypertrophic cardiomyopathy	Triggered activity (EAD); reentry (?)
Right ventricular dysplasia	Reentry; triggered activity (?)
Congenital heart defects	Automatic, reentry
Postsurgical correction of congenital heart defects	Reentry
Channel abnormalities	
Congenital long QT syndrome (torsades de pointes)	Triggered activity (EAD)
Brugada's syndrome (mono- or polymorphic VT)	Reentry (?: ventricular refractory period dispersion); triggered activity (?)
Idiopathic	
Right outflow tract VT	Automatic
Left posteroseptal VT	Automatic, reentry
Other, less common locations	Automatic
Drug induced	
Acquire long QT (torsades de pointes)	Triggered activity (EAD)
Digitalis toxicity (bidirectional tachycardia)	Triggered activity (DAD) (?)

ABBREVIATIONS: DAD = delayed after depolarization; EAD = early after depolarization.

VT at the bedside is important because of its clinical and therapeutic implications.

Electrocardiographic criteria derive from atrioventricular timing relationships and from QRS durations, configurations, and axes. The presence of ventriculoatrial dissociation with clearly discernible P waves independent of a regular QRS rhythm is strongly suggestive of VT (Fig. 24-43*A*), as is the presence of P waves associated with alternate QRS complexes (Fig. 24-44). The latter, best identified in lead V_1, is due to 2:1 retrograde block because of the rate of the tachycardia. The presence of a 1:1 relationship between P waves and QRS complexes, with a short RP interval (as in Fig. 24-43*B*), is also considered supportive evidence for VT. A variety of SVTs with aberrant intraventricular conduction may mimic this pattern, however, and therefore it is not conclusive. Finally, in the presence of ventriculoatrial dissociation, a fortuitously timed sinus impulse may fuse with the wide QRS complex due to VT and produce a single cycle of an altered (usually narrowed) QRS complex (Fig. 24-43*C*). Such fusion beats are helpful when present but are not common.

A QRS duration greater than 0.14 s favors VT as the cause of a wide QRS complex tachyarrhythmia. It is nonspecific, however, and is commonly observed in patients with SVT in the presence of a preexisting bundle-branch block. SVT with QRS complexes greater than 0.14 s occurs only rarely as a consequence of aberrant intraventricular conduction when QRS complexes are normal during sinus rhythm. In addition, antidromic tachycardias in WPW syndrome usually have QRS complexes longer than 0.14 s in duration and therefore may mimic VT. The mean QRS axis is also of limited help in distinguishing between SVT with aberration and VT. Abnormal left-axis deviation (−30° or beyond) favors VT but does not exclude SVT with preexisting bundle-branch block or various supraventricular arrhythmias associated with accessory pathways. Some unusual VTs are associated with a left bundle-branch block pattern and right-axis deviation.

QRS configurations have been carefully studied in both VT and SVT with aberrant intraventricular conduction and are of considerable help in distinguishing between the two. Generally, concordantly positive or negative QRS complexes across the precordium from V_1 to V_6 strongly favor VT over aberrant intraventricular conduction (Fig. 24-45). In addition, patterns in specific leads may be helpful. In V_1, a right bundle-branch block configuration that is monophasic (R) or biphasic (qR) suggests VT, while a triphasic pattern (rSR) strongly favors aberrant intraventricular conduction.[237] R-wave amplitude in V_1 during the tachycardia that exceeds that during sinus rhythm favors VT, and an initial R wave during the tachycardia of 30 ms duration or longer also favors VT. In V_1 and V_2, a notched downslope on an S wave suggests VT, as does an interval of 70 ms or more from onset of the QRS to the negative peak of the S wave. In lead V_6, a deep S wave with an R:S ratio below 1 and a qR or QS pattern both favor VT.[238,239] Each of these criteria may be altered or modified in individual cases by the presence of preexisting intraventricular conduction abnormalities.

Several additional features of tachyarrhythmias may be helpful. Polymorphic tachyarrhythmias are almost exclusively ventricular in origin but must be carefully distinguished from atrial fibrillation in patients with WPW syndrome who have multiple bypass tracts.[240] A tachycardia characterized by a wide QRS pattern with a left bundle-branch configuration in the precordial leads and right-axis deviation in the frontal plane leads is also usually ventricular in origin. A regular rhythm with alternating QRS axes (a bidirectional pattern) alteration is likely to be ventricular in origin, while paired group beating with bidirec-

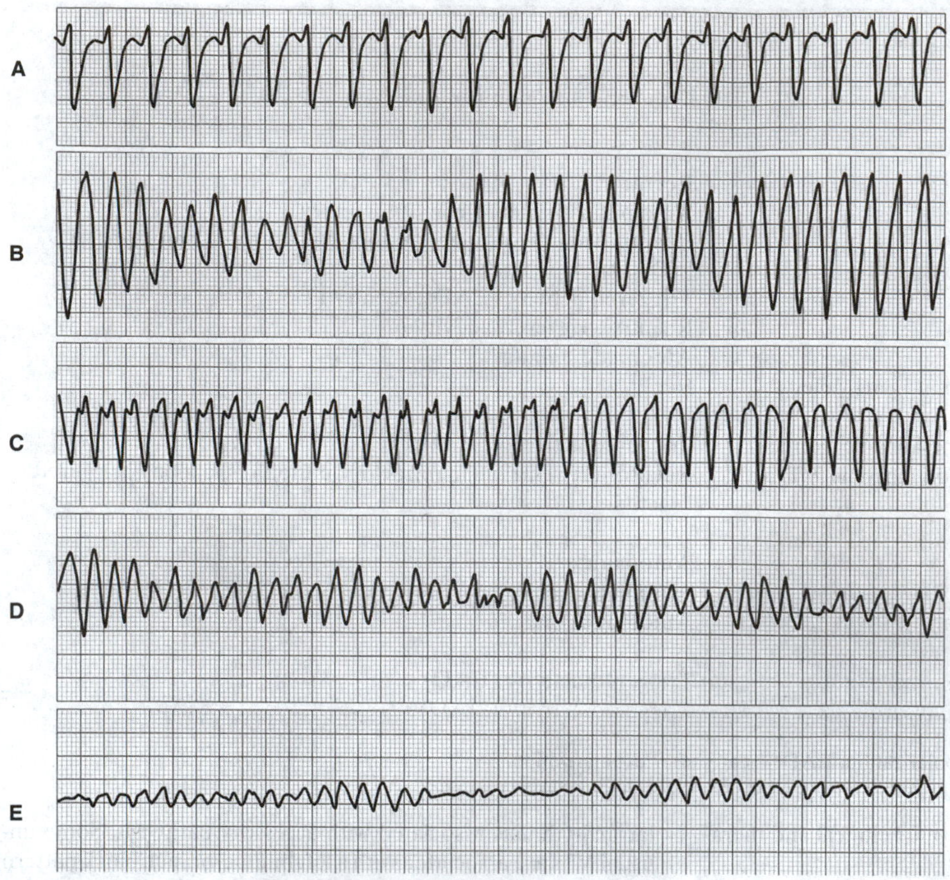

FIGURE 24-42 Different forms of sustained potentially fatal VTs. *A* Sustained monomorphic VT recorded from a patient with a LV aneurysm. *B*. Sustained polymorphic VT in a patient with myocardial ischemia. *C*. Ventricular flutter: a sine wave configuration at a cycle length of 200 to 220 ms. *D*. Coarse VF. *E*. Fine VF. A careful distinction between the different morphologies and rates of tachyarrhyhmia contains important information for prognosis and management.

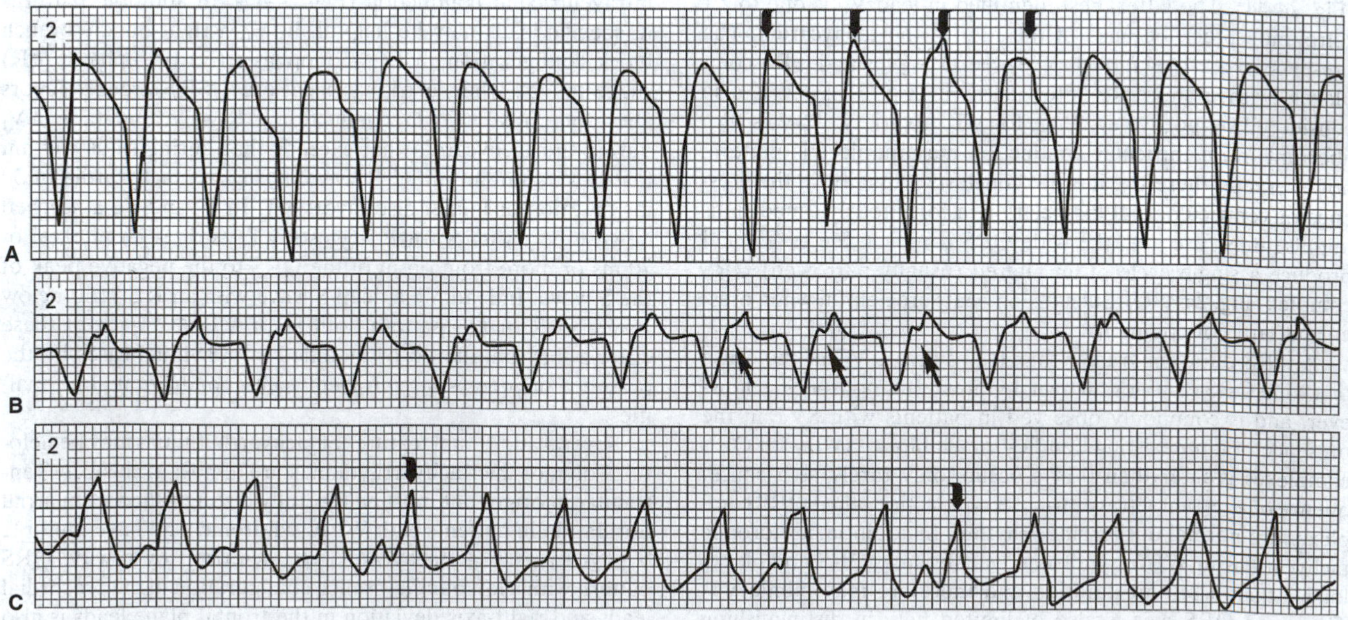

FIGURE 24-43 *A*. Ventricular tachycardia with regular independent P waves (*arrows*). *B*. Ventricular tachycardia with retrograde conduction to the atria (retrograde P waves indicated by *arrows*.) *C*. Ventricular tachycardia with fusion (Dressler's) beats (*arrows*). Note the sinus P wave preceding each fusion beat.

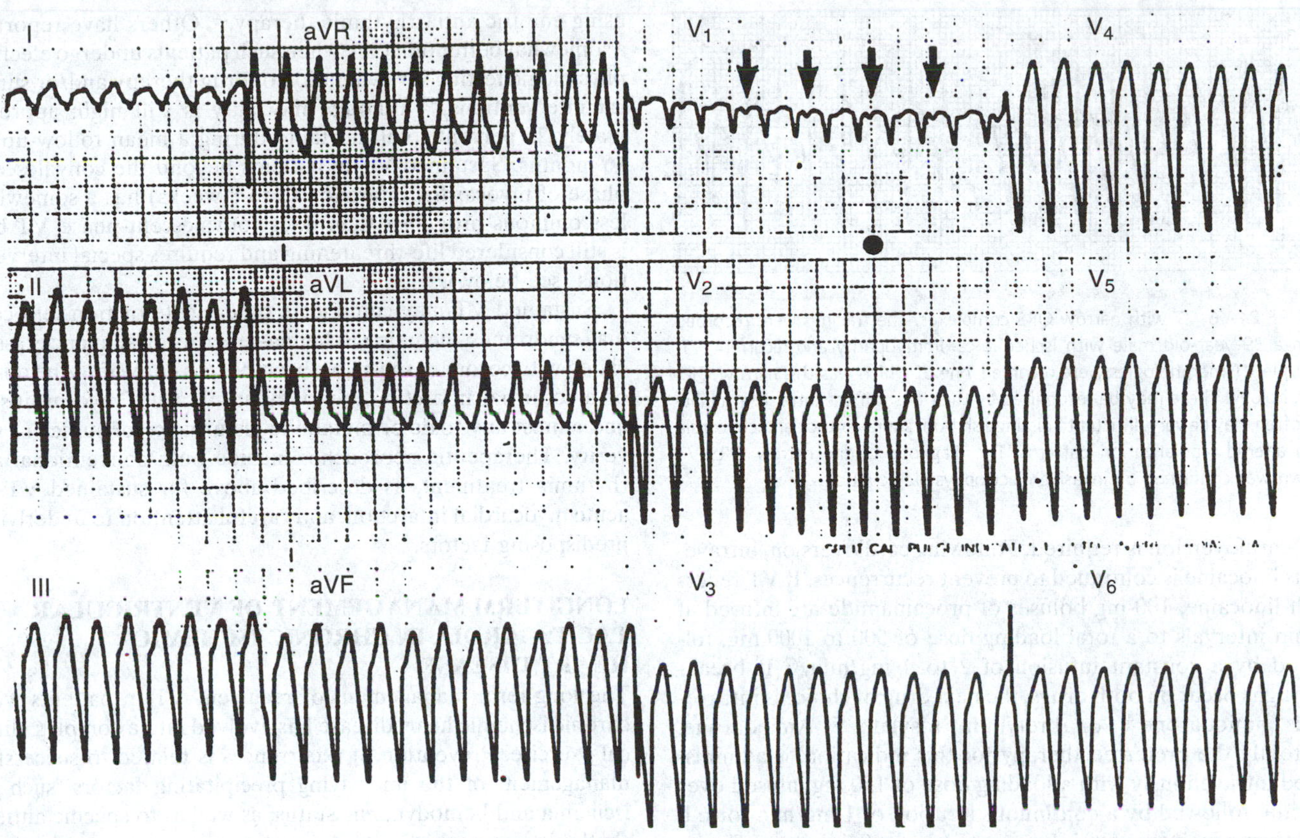

FIGURE 24-44 A rapid wide QRS tachycardia in a 22-year-old female with a history of prior chest wall trauma and a LV aneurysm. VT is suggested by the history and QRS pattern (see the text), but useful confirmatory information is present in the form of 2:1 retrograde conduction, resulting in P waves following alternate QRS complexes, most clearly seen in lead V_1 (*arrows*). In difficult cases, the presence of a 2:1 VA conduction pattern is strongly supportive of VT.

tional alteration is likely to be due to aberrant conduction terminating the shorter cycles. Finally, VTs, presumably originating in proximal bundle branches or fascicles, may inscribe relatively or absolutely narrow QRS complexes Fig. 24-46.

The cycle length of tachyarrhythmias is of little additional value in distinguishing between VTs and SVTs. Although monomorphic VTs associated with coronary heart disease and LV aneurysms tend to have rates below 220 per minute, ventricular arrhythmias due to ischemia and/or reperfusion may be considerably faster, in some instances approaching 250 to 280 per minute (Fig. 24-42*B*). SVTs, particularly those associated with WPW syndrome, may approach similar rates and may be difficult to distinguish from VTs. Antiarrhythmic drugs may also alter electrocardiographic patterns. An example is the slowing of atrial flutter by class IA or class IC antiarrhythmic agents to atrial rates of 240 per minute or less, allowing 1:1 conduction. Particularly for the class IC agents, slowed intraventricular conduction at these rates widens the QRS complexes, resulting in patterns that may be difficult to distinguish from rapid sustained *ventricular* tachyarrhythmias.

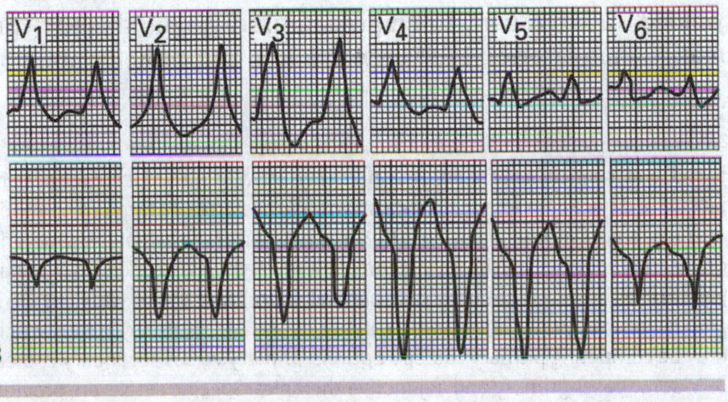

FIGURE 24-45 VT with concordant QRS complexes across precordium. *A*. All upright. *B*. All inverted.

ACUTE MANAGEMENT OF SUSTAINED MONOMORPHIC VENTRICULAR TACHYCARDIA

Sustained monomorphic VT may occur in acute or chronic ischemic heart disease syndromes, in idiopathic dilated or hypertrophic cardiomyopathy, and, less frequently, in inflammatory or infiltrative disease states. It occurs occasionally as a primary electrical disturbance. Management depends upon the clinical setting and the clinical characteristics of the tachycardia.

In acute myocardial infarction, sustained VT occurs most commonly within 24 h of the onset. Although degeneration into VF is uncommon, sustained VT carries that risk and must be treated aggressively. If the patient is clinically stable and the arrhythmia electrically stable, a 75- to 100-mg bolus of intravenous lidocaine, followed by a continuous infusion of 1 to 4 mg/min, may be tried. The infusion dose depends upon the patient's age, size, and general clinical status.[241] In heart failure and low-output states, the dose should be reduced. If the VT does not revert immediately or if the patient is hypotensive, immediate

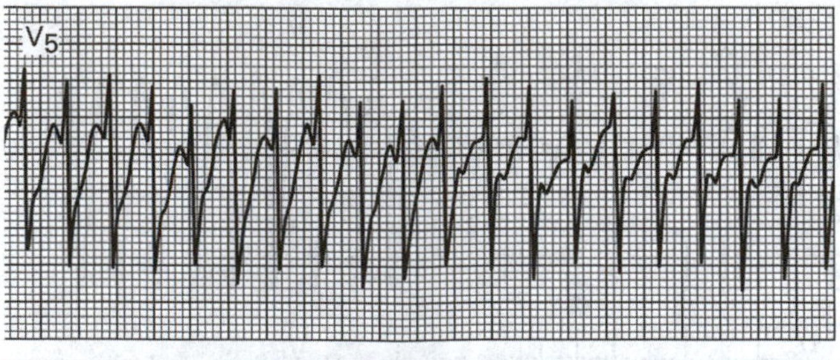

FIGURE 24-46 VT with narrow QRS complexes. The tracings were recorded from a 39-year-old male with ischemic cardiomyopathy and recurrent VT. Multiple VT morphologies were recorded, one of which was this narrow QRS morphology. These may be recognized by their onset if the latter is available but often may be very difficult to distinguish from supraventricular tachycardia with altered repolarization patterns. The diagnosis of the narrow QRS VT shown was confirmed by invasive electrophysiologic studies.

DC cardioversion is required. Following cardioversion, intravenous lidocaine is continued to prevent recurrences. If VT recurs with lidocaine, 100-mg boluses of procainamide are infused at 5-min intervals to a total loading dose of 500 to 1000 mg, followed by a constant infusion of 2 to 4 mg/min.[242] If breakthroughs occur on both drugs, the next drug of choice is intravenous amiodarone[243] or bretylium tosylate.[244] Amiodarone, currently the preferred therapy for this indication, is administered intravenously with a loading dose of 150 mg infused over 10 min, followed by a continuous infusion of 1 mg/min for 6 h and then a maintenance infusion at a rate of 0.5 mg/min. Bretylium, less commonly used than in the past, is administered as a loading dose of 5 mg/kg intravenously infused over 15 min, repeated if necessary, and followed by a 0.5- to 2.0-mg/min infusion. Total dose should not exceed 25 mg/kg per 24 h. Antiarrhythmic therapy may be stopped after 48 to 72 h, since the risk of recurrence is small at that point. Sustained VT during the acute phase of transmural myocardial infarction is due to transient factors and does not predict later recurrent arrhythmias (see also Chap. 42).

A second category of sustained VT related to acute myocardial infarction is that which occurs during the convalescent period.[245] It is unrelated pathophysiologically to the VT that occurs early and has much more serious long-term implications. It is most common in patients with large anterior wall myocardial infarction. Management of the acute event requires intravenous antiarrhythmic drugs and/or cardioversion, using an algorithm similar to that described for acute-phase VT. There is, however, a very high death rate during follow-up of these patients, in part related to the size of the infarct. One report cited an 83 percent death rate during a mean follow-up of 7 months using empiric antiarrhythmic therapy.[246] Others have reported a somewhat better outcome when such patients undergo electrophysiologic testing for evaluation of drug therapy and/or surgical interventions,[247] although mortality is still high: approximately 25 percent total mortality during a mean follow-up of 16 months. Sustained VT in patients beyond the convalescent phase of myocardial infarction (6 to 8 weeks) has a somewhat less ominous prognosis than does convalescent-phase VT but is still considered life-threatening and requires special interventions (see below).[246]

Sustained VT may complicate other acute or transient cardiac syndromes, including ischemia-reperfusion sequences associated with coronary spasm or thrombolysis early after the onset of myocardial infarction, heart failure,[248] acute myocarditis,[196] and almost any toxic or metabolic disturbance of sufficient severity. Therapeutic approaches include both conventional arrhythmia treatment, as described above for sustained VT in acute myocardial infarction, and careful attention to underlying predisposing factors.

LONG-TERM MANAGEMENT OF VENTRICULAR TACHYCARDIA IN CHRONIC ISCHEMIC HEART DISEASE

The long-term management of recurrent VT in patients with chronic ischemic heart disease has evolved into a complex clinical exercise. Prevention of recurrences is related to successful management of the underlying precipitating factors, such as ischemia and hemodynamic status, as well as to specific antiarrhythmic approaches.

Four general approaches to antiarrhythmic therapy are available: (1) antiarrhythmic therapy guided by invasive electrophysiologic testing or by ambulatory monitoring or exercise testing, (2) surgical procedures designed to excise or cryoablate reentrant pathways or automatic foci, (3) catheter ablation procedures, and (4) ICDs (Fig. 24-47). The relative proportion of patients managed by each of these four techniques has changed in recent years, with fewer and more selective surgical approaches, fewer antiarrhythmic drug trials, and broader use of ICD therapy. The use of catheter ablation techniques for VT in chronic ischemic heart disease is largely palliative,[249] often employed as adjunctive therapy with other primary approaches. As technology improves, however, it may develop broader applications (see below).

Pharmacologic Management Invasive electrophysiologic testing to guide pharmacologic therapy in patients with recurrent monomorphic sustained VT due to ischemic heart disease has yielded, in large part, to empiric antiarrhythmic therapy (primarily amiodarone), ICD implantation, and catheter ablation.

FIGURE 24-4724-47 Therapeutic options for patients with ventricular tachyarrhythmias or cardiac arrest in association with coronary artery disease. Six categories of arrhythmias or clinical events are presented, and for each the associated observations during programmed electrical stimulation are provided. Four categories of therapeutic option are shown. Under "Drug Therapy," membrane-active antiarrhythmic drugs include amiodarone unless amiodarone is cited specifically, in which case the other membrane-active antiarrhythmic drugs are not considered therapeutic options. Also included in drug therapy are the beta-adrenergic–blocking agents. The second category is surgical and interventional approaches, which include antiarrhythmic surgery and catheter-based and surgical revascularization procedures. The third category is implantable devices, under which indications and preferred programming modes are presented. Catheter ablation is the final category. For each of the categories of therapy, indications shown on the bottom of the illustration discriminate patients with EFs greater than 35 percent (*blue*) and those with EFs of 35 percent or less (*red*). Therapeutic categories are not mutually exclusive and may be competing primary therapy options, primary versus secondary choices, or in some cases primary and adjunctive therapies. Specific details are provided in the text.

CLINICAL EVENT	LABORATORY-INDUCED ARRHYTHMIA	DRUG THERAPY	SURGERY; ANGIOPLASTY	IMPLANTABLE DEVICE	CATHETER ABLATION
SUSTAINED VT, MONOMORPHIC: Hemodynamically Stable	Single Morphology VT	Membrane-active drugs +++ / +	Anti-arrhythmic; ±Anti-ischemic? ++ / ++	Tiered Therapy	Yes +++ / ++
	Multiple Morphology VTs	Membrane-active [lower success rate] ++ / +	Anti-ischemic, if substrate identified	+ / +++	Very low success rate + / +
	Non-inducible	Amiodarone +++ / ++	+++ / ++	Defibrillation mode + / +++	No - / -
SUSTAINED VT, MONOMORPHIC: Hemodynamically Unstable	Single Morphology VT	Membrane-actives; β-adrenergic blockers ++ / +	Anti-ischemic, if substrate identified	Defibrillation mode [Tiered Therapy?]	No
	Multiple Morphology VTs	Membrane-actives [lower success rate]; β-adrenergic blockers? + / -		++ / +++	
	Non-inducible	Amiodarone + / -	++ / ++	Defibrillation mode +++ / +++	- / -
POLYMORPHIC VENTRICULAR TACHYCARDIA: Reversible Cause not Identified	Sustained VT, Non-sustained VT, Non-inducible	β-adrenergic blockers (selected cases); Amiodarone? + / -	Anti-ischemic, if substrate identified ++ / ++	Defibrillation mode +++ / +++	No - / -
VENTRICULAR FIBRILLATION	Sustained Monomorphic VT	Amiodarone ++ / -	Anti-ischemic, if substrate identified	Defibrillation mode [Tiered Therapy?]	No
	Non-sustained VT Polymorphic VT Non-inducible	Amiodarone; β-adrenergic blockers? (selected cases) ++ / -		++ / +++	
	Non-inducible	Amiodarone + / -	++ / ++	Defibrillation mode +++ / +++	- / -
CARDIAC ARREST Unknown Mechanism [Suspected VT/VF]	Non-sustained VT, Non-inducible	Amiodarone + / -	Anti-ischemic, if substrate identified ++ / ++	Defibrillation mode +++ / +++	No - / -
UNEXPLAINED SYNCOPE: Suspected Ventricular Arrhythmia	Sustained VT	Membrane Actives; Amiodarone ++ / -	Anti-ischemic, if substrate identified	Defibrillation mode [Tiered Therapy?] ++ / +++	Uncertain + / -
	Non-sustained VT; VF; Non-inducible	No - / -	++ / ++	Defibrillation mode +++ / +++	No - / -

+++ = Acceptable as primary therapy or effective adjunctive
++ = Uncertain primary efficacy; useful adjunctive
+ = Adjunctive; selected cases
- = Not recommended

EF >35% (first rating of each pair) / EF ≤35% (second rating of each pair)

At one time the index for the initial treatment strategy for such patients, the initial study free of antiarrhythmic drugs required to demonstrate inducibility of the clinical VT and its characteristics at baseline, is now largely used for risk stratification. Several clinical trials[211,230–232] have demonstrated that inducibility predicts risk along with better outcomes with ICD therapy than with drug therapy in high-risk patients.[230] It is also useful in conjuction with ablation or surgical procedures.

Although there have been controversies about the validity of different protocols for programmed electrical stimulation in patients who have clinical sustained ventricular arrhythmias,[251] up to 95 percent of inducible sustained monomorphic VTs can be induced by right ventricular stimulation, using up to two drive cycle lengths between 600 and 400 ms from two right ventricular locations (apex and outflow tract) with up to three extrastimuli (see also Chap. 26). In at least 80 percent of patients with chronic ischemic heart disease and recurrent monomorphic sustained VT, the clinical tachyarrhythmias can be induced during a baseline study free of antiarrhythmic agents. The subsequent identification of a drug regimen that will prevent reinduction into the same sustained monomorphic VT is associated with a reduction of risk of recurrent VT at 1 year of follow-up. The risk appears to decrease from 30 to 40 percent if VT remains inducible on therapy to 10 to 15 percent if therapy results in noninducibility.[252] The results of acute intravenous testing of a drug should not be extrapolated to long-term oral therapy without retesting on the oral regimen, because intravenous regimens do not predict responses on oral drugs.[253] In addition, a drug capable of preventing induction of a VT previously induced during baseline testing can be identified in only a minority of patients (approximately 20 to 35 percent in various studies). Moreover, the success rate for membrane-active drugs is considerably lower if multiple monomorphic VTs are induced at baseline.[254] Left ventricular EF strongly influences probability of recurrence. Among cardiac arrest survivors, an EF of 30 percent or less predicts a mortality rate approximately twice as high as for patients in the same category with EFs above 30 percent.[255] A similar relationship likely exists for patients who present clinically with sustained VT. Unfortunately, all statements about the potential benefit of therapy guided by programmed electrical stimulation are based upon comparisons of groups who did (responders) or did not (nonresponders) convert from an inducible status to a noninducible status as a result of the therapy. Randomized, placebo-controlled studies of patients who convert to a noninducible status on therapy, with a similar strategy for patients with VT that remains inducible, are still lacking. Such studies would determine whether it is the therapy or simply the ability to change inducibility status that is determining outcome. In one study of patients who had had VT or VF and met criteria for both the invasive electrophysiologic approach (i.e., inducibility at baseline) and the ambulatory monitoring approach (30 or more PVCs per hour), a randomized comparison revealed a significantly lower arrhythmia recurrence rate with therapy guided by the invasive testing technique:[256] 20 percent recurrence rate of symptomatic VT at 24 months with invasive procedures versus 50 percent with noninvasive procedures. The study, however, did not identify a difference in death rate, possibly because of the small number of patients randomized. In another study, a drug or drug combination that did not prevent inducibility during invasive electrophysiologic study but did prolong the cycle length of induced VT by more than 100 ms with stable hemodynamics predicted a favorable mortality outcome, even though the incidence of recurrent VT was not different from that in those who failed to show any measure of a successful response.[257] Patients who have a partial response to a drug regimen (i.e., induced runs of 6 or more but fewer than 15 impulses) also appear to have a lower risk of recurrent VT.[258] Many electrophysiologists currently will accept induced runs of less than 10 impulses on therapy as a satisfactory end point, and almost all will accept less than 6. Any change in therapy established by invasive electrophysiologic testing because of drug intolerance or clinical failure should be evaluated by repeat testing.[252,259]

Finally, a recently reported trial in postmyocardial infarction patients, the MUSTT study, demonstrated that patients who had nonsustained VT on ambulatory monitoring with inducible VT at baseline study and failed antiarrhythmic drug therapy during repeat study had better long-term survival rates if they received ICDs than if they received drug therapy.[250] It is important to note that patients who received ICDs based on failed electrophysiologic testing—considered a high-risk group—did even better than those who had a successful electrophysiologic study on drug therapy.

Noninvasive management strategies for VT require identification of frequent (i.e., 10 to 30 PVCs per hour in various studies) and/or repetitive PVC forms (i.e., salvos or nonsustained VT) at baseline monitoring or VT induced during exercise testing. Reduction of PVC frequency (80 percent or more suppression) and abolition of complex forms has been used as the index of a successful end point. This approach has been reported to be successful in some studies,[226,260] even among patients who have failed to achieve a successful end point by invasive electrophysiologic testing.[260] Unfortunately, the *residual risk* among many patient groups with successful noninvasive or invasive end points is still very high.[261] Thus, because of the *relative* benefit of ICDs in several patient groups compared to empiric amiodarone, many clinicians now prefer implantable devices for both primary and secondary prevention of life-threatening arrhythmias in these high-risk patients.

A large multicenter randomized trial, entitled Electrophysiological Study Versus Electrocardiographic Monitoring (ESVEM), was designed to compare programmed electrical stimulation with ambulatory monitoring techniques for guiding therapy in patients who had sustained VT, had survived cardiac arrest, or had syncope presumed due to a ventricular arrhythmia.[262,263] The data showed no difference between the two methods for prediction of efficacy or mortality benefit, although there was a small trend favoring programmed stimulation during early follow-up in the coronary disease subgroup (see Chap. 30). Failure by both invasive and noninvasive criteria connotes a poor prognosis and requires other considerations for therapy, namely, surgery or implantable devices.

Pharmacologic therapy has an increasingly important role as adjunct therapy in patients who have implanted defibrillators. It is used to reduce VT events requiring ICD therapy, slow tachycardia rates to favor antitachycardia pacing therapy over shocks, and reduce the incidence of atrial tachycardia that can initiate shock therapy unnecessarily (e.g., atrial fibrillation or flutter). A randomized trial has demonstrated that these goals can be achieved.[264]

Surgical Therapy Patients who have recurrent sustained monomorphic VT associated with prior myocardial infarction and inducibility into a hemodynamically stable tachycardia were uniformly considered for antiarrhythmic surgery until recent years. The indication was reinforced by the presence of discrete ventricular aneurysms and bypassable coronary artery lesions. With the development of ICDs capable of flexible antitachycardia pacing programs, many patients who were formerly surgical candidates are now receiving ICDs. However, surgery is still recommended, in the absence of contraindications, for a small number of such patients,[252,265,266] particularly if they require revascularization surgery as well or their tachycardias are not easily pace-terminated during induction studies. Patients without discrete aneurysms who have large dyskinetic areas may have sites of origin of VT mapped in the cardiac electrophysiology laboratory and operating room if they are inducible into stable monomorphic tachycardias. Mapping allows the identification of areas that may be attacked by endocardial resection or surgical cryoablation.[267] Map-guided surgical procedures employing resection, cryoablation, and revascularization have markedly improved the clinical outcome of surgically treated patients.[268] Overall surgical results have also benefited from the preferred use of ICDs in patients previously referred for surgery out of desperation (see Chap. 30). Coronary bypass surgery may be used as primary therapy for patients who have recurrent VT initiated by transient ischemic episodes.[269] It is also a valuable adjunct to antiarrhythmic surgery (see Fig. 24-47).

Catheter Ablation Procedures for Ventricular Tachyarrhythmias The combination of LV endocardial mapping by catheter techniques and RF energy delivery systems provides the capability for catheter ablation therapy of sustained, hemodynamically stable VTs.[249,270,271] While these techniques are currently limited to only a small fraction of patients as primary therapy,[271] they are useful as an adjunct to ICD therapy (Fig. 24-48). Improvements of mapping techniques capable of storage and recall of spatial activation maps[272,273] and improved energy delivery systems will enhance the use of catheter ablation as primary therapy and as more effective ancillary therapy in the future.

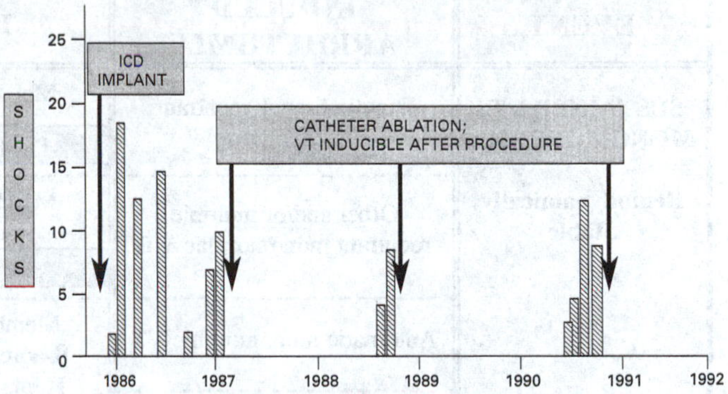

FIGURE 24-48 Catheter ablation for VT as an adjunct to an ICD. A 57-year-old male with recurrent life-threatening episodes of sustained VT who received an ICD had multiple shocks for arrhythmias that were resistant to all antiarrhythmic agents attempted. LV mapping and catheter ablation in a VT reentrant pathway in 1987 provided freedom from recurrent ICD discharges for approximately 19 months, after which the multiple ICD discharges recurred. Additional ablation procedures 18 or more months apart provided relief from the recurrent discharges despite the fact that VT remained inducible. While of limited value as primary therapy for life-threatening ventricular arrhythmias in patients with coronary heart disease or cardiomyopathy because of risk of recurrence (see the text), this procedure can provide benefit as an adjunct to other primary forms of therapy by avoiding frequent discharges and improving the quality of life.

Implantable Defibrillators As a result of the outcomes of several large clinical trials[211,230-232] and advances in technology that resulted in a significant decrease in device size and range of functions, the role of ICD therapy for patients with ventricular tachyarrhythmias has expanded dramatically in recent years (see Fig. 24-47). It is no longer necessary or desirable to test a long sequence of antiarrhythmic drugs in patients with sustained monomorphic VT. For those subgroups among whom ICDs have not been demonstrated to be superior to drug therapy (e.g., those with EFs greater than 40 percent), failure of no more than one or two drugs during electrophysiologic study is generally considered an indication for ICD therapy. Their use is amplified by such enrichments as antitachycardia pacing, allowing effective programmable tiered-therapy algorithms, back-up bradyarrhythmia pacing (including dual-chamber pacing in some devices), and electrogram storage for retrieving and analyzing events.

Patients who present with clinical VT and have inducible, hemodynamically *unstable* VT associated with ischemia before surgery should receive an ICD after revascularization surgery if they remain inducible into VT. The routine use of an ICD after antiarrhythmic surgery, even if successful by postsurgical programmed stimulation study, has been advocated[275] but has gained only limited acceptance. The CABG-Patch trial tested the value of ICDs after revascularization surgery among patients with positive signal-averaged ECGs but no history of clinical VT. The results demonstrated no cumulative survival benefit of this strategy[276] even though there was a suggestion that the devices reduced arrhythmic deaths.[277]

ICDs are indicated for patients with recurrent or unstable VT whose arrhythmias cannot be controlled medically or surgically or who belong to subgroups that have been demonstrated to benefit specifically from device therapy. Antitachycardia pacing capabilities and programmable tiered therapy have expanded the scope of ICD therapy for recurrent sustained VT. The availability of antitachycardia pacing obviates the need for antiarrhythmic surgery in many patients who had been consid-

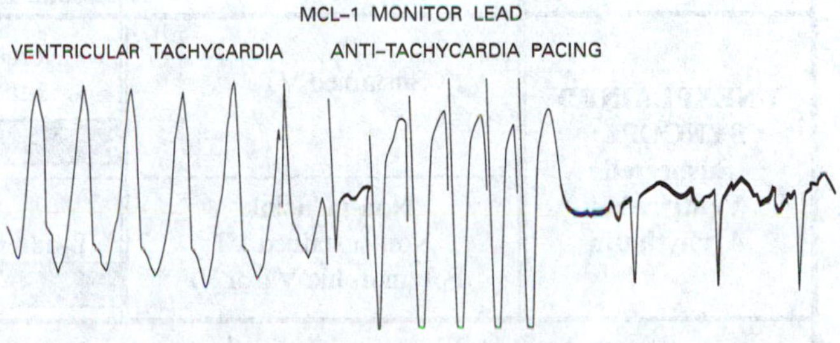

FIGURE 24-49 ICD with antitachycardia pacing. The figure demonstrates the end of a run of induced sustained VT (*left*) followed by antitachycardia pacing that converts the rhythm back to normal sinus (*right*). The device will revert to a defibrillator mode if programmed pacing sequences fail to convert the rhythm.

CLINICAL EVENT	LABORATORY-INDUCED ARRHYTHMIA	DRUG THERAPY	Drug: EF >35%	Drug: EF ≤35%	IMPLANTABLE DEVICE	Device: EF >35%	Device: EF ≤35%	CATHETER ABLATION	Ablation: EF >35%	Ablation: EF ≤35%
SUSTAINED VT, MONOMORPHIC: Hemodynamically Stable	Bundle-branch reentrant tachycardia	Membrane-active drugs	+++	++	Tiered Therapy			Yes	+++	+++
	Other and/or multiple reentrant monomorphic VTs	Membrane-active drugs [unknown efficacy]	++	+		++	+++	Low success rate	++	++
	Automatic monomorphic VT	Membrane-active drugs; β-adrenergic blockers (?); Hemodynamically-active drugs (?)			No	-	-	Uncertain efficacy	+	+
	Non-inducible		+++	++	Defibrillation mode	+	+++	No	-	-
SUSTAINED VT, MONOMORPHIC: Hemodynamically Unstable	Single morphology VT, including bundle-branch reentrant tachycardia	Membrane-active drugs; β-adrenergic blockers (?);	++	+	Defibrillation mode [Tiered Therapy?]			For bundle-branch reentrant tachycardia	++	+
	Multiple Morphology VTs	Membrane-active drugs [lower success rate]; β-adrenergic blockers?	++	-		++	+++	No		
	Non-inducible	Amiodarone	++	-	Defibrillation mode	++	+++		-	-
POLYMORPHIC VENTRICULAR TACHYCARDIA: Reversible Cause not Identified	Sustained VT, Non-sustained VT, Non-inducible	β-adrenergic blockers [selected cases]; Amiodarone (?)	+	-	Defibrillation mode	+++	+++	No	-	-
VENTRICULAR FIBRILLATION	Sustained Monomorphic VT	Amiodarone			Tiered Therapy	+++	+++	For B-BR	++	+
	Non-sustained VT Polymorphic VT Non-inducible		++	-	Defibrillation mode	+++	+++	No	-	-
CARDIAC ARREST Unknown Mechanism [Suspected VT/VF]	Non-sustained VT, Non-inducible	Amiodarone [efficacy unknown]	+	-	Defibrillation mode	+++	+++	No	-	-
UNEXPLAINED SYNCOPE: Suspected Ventricular Arrhythmia	Sustained VT	Membrane-active drugs [uncertain efficacy]	++	-	Tiered therapy or defibrillation mode	++	+++	For B-BR only	+	-
	Non-inducible; Non-sustained VT; Polymorphic VT or VF	Amiodarone; β-adrenergic blockers (?)	++	+	Defibrillation mode	+++	+++	No	-	-

+++ = Acceptable as primary therapy or effective adjunctive
++ = Uncertain primary efficacy; useful adjunctive
+ = Adjunctive; selected cases
- = Not recommended
EF >35%
EF ≤35%

FIGURE 24-50 Therapeutic options for patients with VTs or cardiac arrest due to nonischemic cardiomyopathies. See the legend for Fig. 24-47 for a description of the figure design. The surgical/angioplasty category is excluded for the nonischemic cardiomyopathies. The indications, based upon priorities of therapy, are the same as described for coronary heart disease–related arrhythmias. See the text for further details.

ered surgical candidates on the basis of anatomy and physiology in the past (Fig. 24-49; see also Chap. 30).

LONG-TERM MANAGEMENT OF VENTRICULAR TACHYCARDIA IN NONISCHEMIC HEART DISEASE

Sustained VT in patients with idiopathic dilated cardiomyopathy, dilated cardiomyopathies due to specific etiologies, or hypertrophic cardiomyopathies carries a poor prognosis. Management approaches differ from those used for patients with ischemic heart disease (Fig. 24-50). Invasive electrophysiologic testing, to identify risk or guide therapry is less predictably useful in the small fraction of patients with dilated cardiomyopathy who have clinical sustained monomorphic VT[278,279] than it is in coronary heart disease patients. In a subgroup of these patients, however, sustained VT is due to bundle-branch reentry,[280] which can be cured by catheter ablation of the right bundle branch. Electrophysiologically guided management does not appear useful in idiopathic dilated cardiomyopathy patients who have survived out-of-hospital VF or have clinical nonsustained VT.[281] There is almost no role for surgical therapy in these patients at present, but the ICD is an appropriate means of management. The device appears effective for reverting potentially fatal arrhythmias in patients who have cardiomyopathy,[282] but the long-term outcome may be dominated by LV function. The evaluation of ICD therapy in these patients has been confounded by the observation that, in some (perhaps a substantial fraction) of these patients, sudden death is caused by the bradyarrhythmic asystole–pulseless electrical activity complex, which would not benefit from any form of antiarrhythmic therapy.[283] The availability of ICD with electrogram storage capability should begin to clarify the magnitude of this problem. Ultimately, identification of groups at risk for specific mechanisms will help define the best therapy, but such data are currently lacking.

Sustained VT is also a late consequence and poor prognostic sign in patients with hypertrophic cardiomyopathy.[284–286] In this setting, the use of electrophysiologic testing has been limited because of unvalidated concerns about the ability to cardiovert the severely hypertrophied and obstructed ventricle,[286,287] and there is no uniform opinion regarding the best approach to management of these patients, other than the accepted need for therapy. The recent trend toward ICD therapy, rather than pharmacologic therapy, particularly among higher-risk subgroups, has now received support from multicenter observational data suggesting ICD benefit.[288] Preoperative electrophysiologic testing is generally avoided in patients with severe aortic stenosis who have survived sustained VT or VF.

Less Common Clinical Causes of Sustained Monomorphic Ventricular Tachycardia

CATECHOLAMINE- AND METABOLICALLY MEDIATED VENTRICULAR TACHYCARDIA

In a small number of patients, sustained VT appears to be mediated by catecholamines or other neurophysiologic influences.[289,290] Sustained VT in these patients is commonly induced by physical or emotional stress. Isoproterenol infusions may be used to initiate the VT, which may then be suppressed and subsequently prevented by beta-adrenergic blocking agents

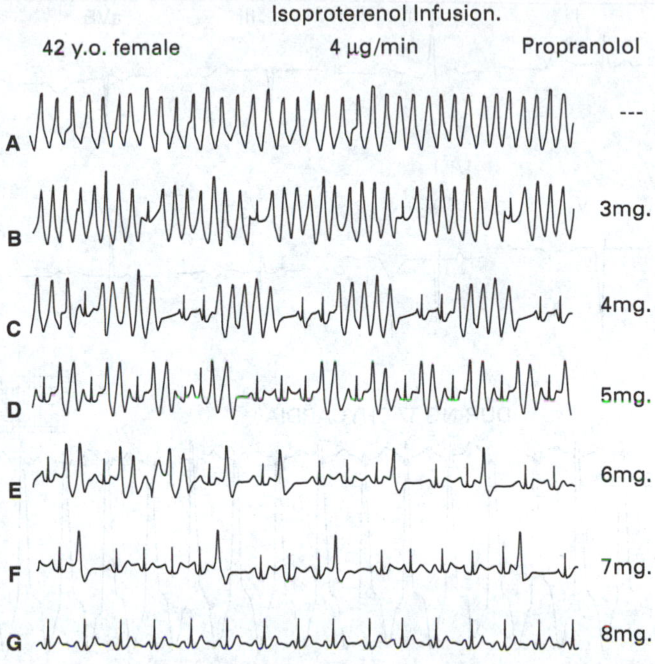

FIGURE 24-51 Catecholamine-mediated VT in an otherwise healthy female. Psychologic stress or isoproterenol infusion could initiate the arrhythmia in this patient. During this sequence, a 4-μg/min isoproterenol infusion initiated the VT (*A*), and the patient was treated with intravenous propranolol. After the first 3 mg of propranolol (*B*), occasional sinus beats interrupted the tachycardia. On a milligram-by-milligram basis up to a total dose of 8 mg of propranolol, there was further suppression of VT to the point of salvos (*C*, *D*, *E*), frequent PVCs (*F*), and complete suppression of ectopic activity (*G*).

(Fig. 24-51). Another small group of patients have sustained VT that may respond to Ca^{2+}-entry blockers.[291–293] This is a heterogeneous group of VTs that includes adenosine-sensitive VT,[291] and an unusual VT with a right bundle-branch block, left-axis deviation QRS pattern originating in the low interventricular septum.[293] Catecholamine-mediated VT may occur in the presence or absence of structural heart disease; when it is responsive to Ca^{2+}-entry blockers, it generally occurs in the absence of structural heart disease.

RIGHT VENTRICULAR DYSPLASIA AND VENTRICULAR ARRHYTHMIAS

Arrhythmogenic right ventricular dysplasia (ARVD) or right ventricular cardiomyopathy (RVCM) may be associated with nonsustained or sustained VT and/or sudden cardiac death. Patients with a stable monomorphic VT without near-syncope may have a better prognosis,[294] but it is clear that sudden death, presumably due to VF, may be the first and only manifestation of the disease.[295]

The term isolated right ventricular cardiomyopathy[295,297] has been used as an alternative for ARVD, and, more recently, the ARVD-RVCM complex[298] is being labeled simply right ventricular dysplasia (RVD). The entity may occur sporadically or in familial clusters, with up to 40 to 50 percnt currently appearing to be familial. A number of loci are identified from linkage analyses studies in affected families,[299,300] but no specific gene abnormalities have been identified to date.

The 12-lead electrocardiographic pattern of the patient with ARVD is helpful. In sinus rhythm, anterior precordial T-wave

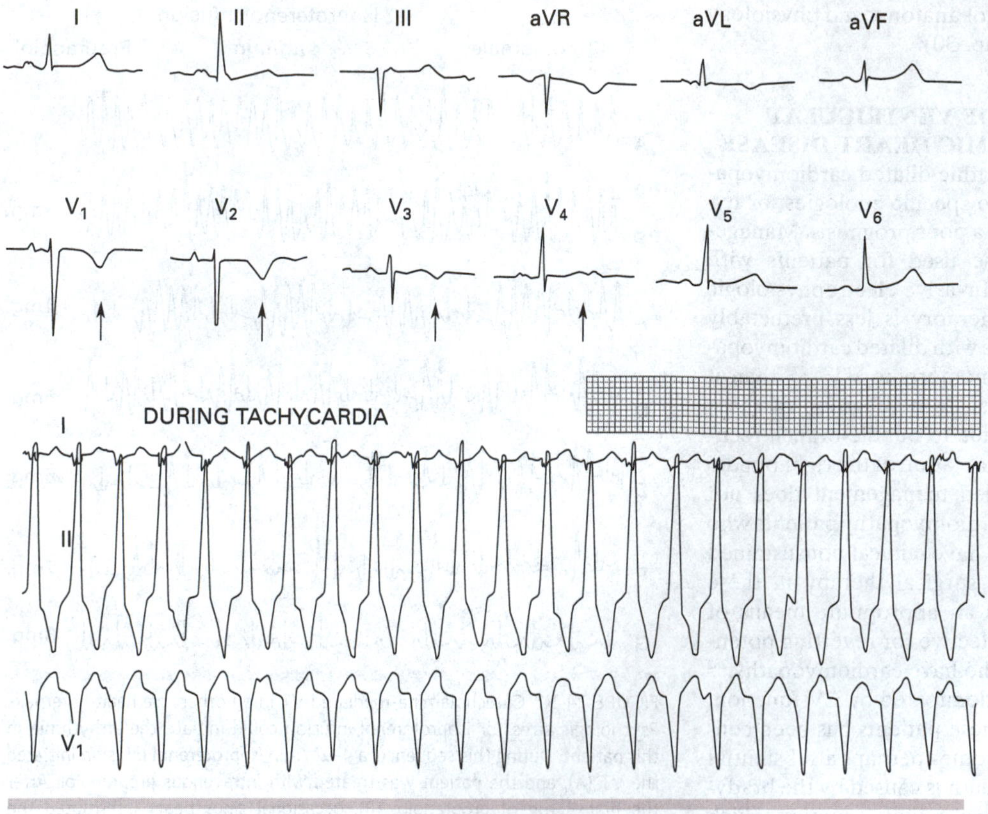

FIGURE 24-52 Right ventricular dysplasia with VT. Episodic wide QRS tachycardia with near-syncope in a 33-year-old man. The left bundle-branch block pattern of the tachycardia suggests a right ventricular origin, and the inverted T waves in V_1 to V_3 are characteristic of right ventricular dysplasia.

inversions are commonly present (Fig. 24-52), sometimes with notching in the early part of the ST segment of V_1 and V_2 as well (epsilon waves). The monomorphic tachycardia has a left bundle-branch block morphology, reflecting its origin from the right ventricle.

At initial presentation, the future course cannot be predicted, and preventive measures should be aggressive. Pharmacologic and surgical approaches have been used for the management of ARVD.[294,296] Amiodarone and class IC drugs have been suggested to be effective for ARVD patients with symptomatic arrhythmias. However, because of its high risk of sudden death and unpredictable response to treatment, there is an increasing trend toward the use of ICD therapy, especially in patients with symptomatic arrhythmias, syncope, and a family history of sudden death in affected family members.

VENTRICULAR TACHYCARDIA AFTER CONGENITAL HEART DISEASE SURGERY

Sustained VT or VF may appear years after repair of complex congenital heart defects,[301] especially tetralogy of Fallot and transposition of the great vessels. The arrhythmias are potentially lethal and must be treated pharmacologically,[302] surgically,[303] or with ICDs in selected cases.

BIDIRECTIONAL VENTRICULAR TACHYCARDIA

Bidirectional ventricular tachycardia (Fig. 24-53) is usually a manifestation of digitalis intoxication and responds to standard measures.

Polymorphic Ventricular Tachycardia, Including Torsades de Pointes

The polymorphic VTs, including the specific variant referred to as torsades de pointes, is a tachycardia pattern with important clinical implications. As a group, the polymorphic tachycardias tend to be more unstable electrically than the monomorphic tachycardias, occur at faster rates, have a higher likelihood of producing transient central nervous system symptoms (syncope or near-syncope) due to reduced cardiac output, and establish a higher risk for spontaneous degeneration to VF. The polymorphic tachycardias generally do not persist as long as the monomorphic tachycardias, either spontaneously reverting to a normal rhythm, degenerating to VF, or triggering a monomorphic tachycardia in susceptible patients.

The specific variant of polymorphic tachycardia characterized by QRS peaks that seem to twist around the baseline (Fig. 24-54) is referred to as torsades de pointes. The orthodox definition of torsades de pointes includes the predisposing electrocardiographic pattern, namely, a prolonged QT interval.[304] The same electrocardiographic pattern, however, may occur in the absence of QT prolongation.[305] Torsades de pointes may occur as a consequence of congenital prolongation of the QT interval or may be associated with acquired QT prolongations due to any of a group of diverse factors (see below). Less specific patterns of polymorphic VT may also occur in a number of other acquired disease settings, often not associated with prolonged QT intervals or with transient prolongations.

CONGENITAL LONG QT INTERVAL SYNDROME

The congenital long QT interval syndrome, which is present persistently from childhood, is characterized by the presence of long QT intervals and/or prominent U waves on the standard 12-lead ECG (Fig. 24-55). The affected patients are prone to episodes of torsades de pointes, which may cause transient light-

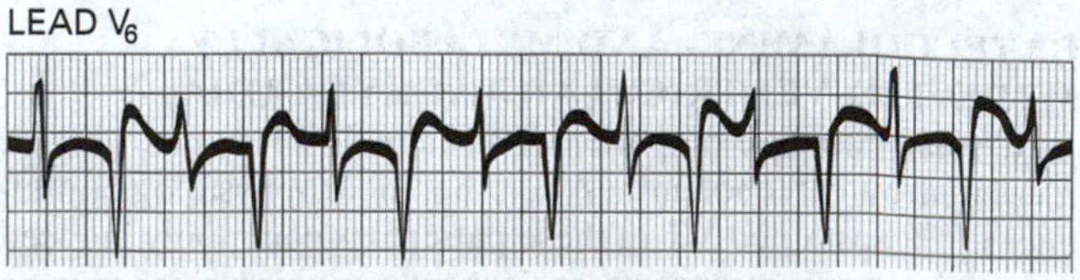

FIGURE 24-53 Bidirectional tachycardia. The tachycardia is regular at a rate of 160, but the vector of the QRS-T complexes alternates.

headedness, syncope, or sudden cardiac death. Arrhythmias may occur at rest, under emotional stress or with exercise (Fig 24-56). The two general patterns of the syndrome are the Romano-Ward syndrome,[306,307] which has an autosomal dominant inheritance pattern, and the much less common Jervell and Lange-Nielsen syndrome,[308] which has an autosomal recessive inheritance pattern and is associated with congenital deafness.

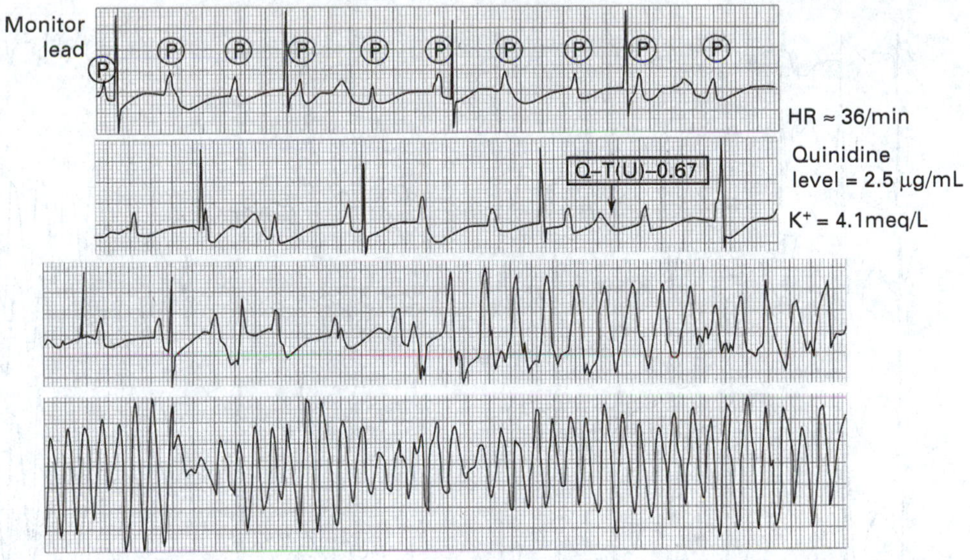

FIGURE 24-54 Torsades de pointes. The patient, a 49-year-old female, has complete heart block and was receiving quinidine sulfate for a ventricular arrhythmia. The rhythm shown in the bottom two strips occurred shortly after institution of therapy. Note the prolonged QT(U) interval (0.67 s) and the onset of classical torsades de pointes.

For many years, congenital long QT interval syndrome has been viewed as a consequence of abnormal patterns of cardiac autonomic neural innervation, based in part upon the fact that the entity could be treated with beta-adrenergic blocking agents or surgical ablation of the left stellate ganglion.[309] Progress in the molecular genetics of the syndrome, however, has clearly demonstrated that inherited defects in membrane ion-channel molecular structure and function underlie the disease. The ion-channel abnormalities constitute the structural basis of the disorder at a molecular level; neurophysiologic, environmental, or transient risk factors (e.g., stress or hypokalemia) may then trigger the arrhythmias.

Multiple specific mutations have been identified at loci on five chromosomes and the specific gene products and their physiologic dysfunctions studied (Fig. 24-57).[311,312,325,326] The first abnormality suggested from linkage analysis was on chromosome 11. An association with the Harvey-*ras* gene was suggested, but subsequent observations demonstrated that the affected locus encodes a component of a potassium channel, I_{KS}, the slowly activating delayed rectifier channel. This channel also appears to be affected in at least one variety of the Jervell and Lange-Nielsen syndrome. Subsequently, two other gene loci have been identified among multiple families. An abnormality has been mapped to a locus on chromosome 7, which encodes HERG,[311] the rapidly activating delayed rectifier channel, I_{KR}, which carries a major repolarizing current. Another locus, SCN5A, on chromosome 3, encodes the human cardiac sodium channel gene.[312] One defective pattern on the latter gene encodes a three-amino acid deletion, which results in failure of the channel to close properly after activation. The depolarizing leak of sodium current competes with and delays repolarization by the normal potassium channels. Drugs that block the sodium channel, such as mexiletine, have been suggested as a possible pharmacologic therapy for this specific variant of the syndrome.[313] A fourth locus for an as yet unidentified genetic abnormality on chromosome 4 has been identified in a single family and may be a unique mutant in that family.[314] Finally, the fifth locus affected is chromosome 21. It encodes

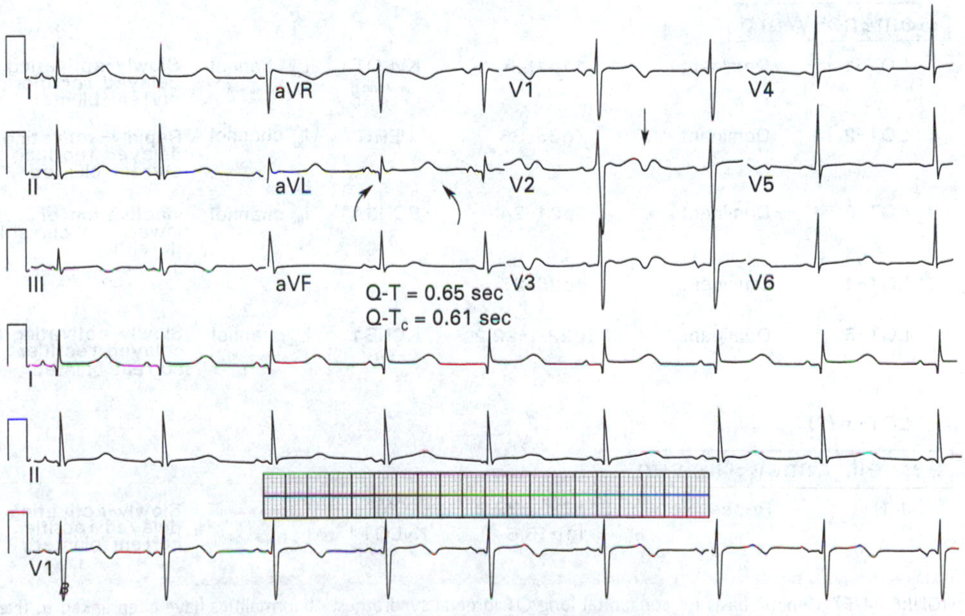

FIGURE 24-55 Congenital long QT interval syndrome. A 12-lead ECG was recorded in a 25-year-old female with congenital deafness and a history of recurrent syncope throughout her life (Jervell and Lange-Nielsen syndrome). Many episodes of syncope occurred during or immediately after exercise and were commonly preceded by palpitations. She had never been treated. The tracing reveals a corrected QT interval of 610 ms with marked notching of the TU waves in the anterior precordial leads.

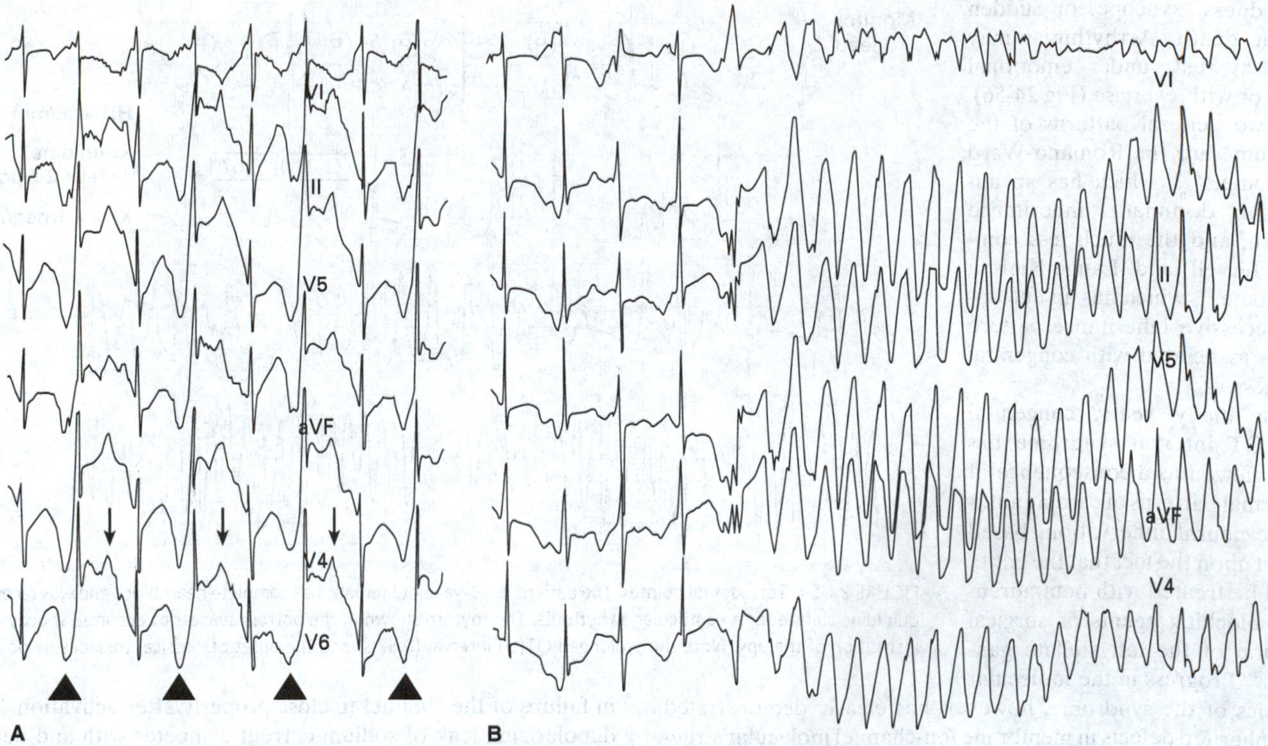

FIGURE 24-56 Congenital long QT interval syndrome. Treadmill stress testing was carried out in the patient shown in Fig. 24-55. *A*. At 4 min and 2 s into a Bruce protocol, ST-T alternans was observed, followed shortly by torsades de pointes (*B*).

GENETICS OF CONGENITAL LONG Q-T SYNDROMES

Syndrome	Inheritance	Chromosome	Gene	Product	Defect
Romano-Ward					
LQT-1	Dominant	11p15.5	KvLQT1 [or KCNQ1]	I_{KS} channel [alpha-subunit]	Slowly-activating delayed rectifier current blunted
LQT-2	Dominant	7q35-36	HERG	I_{KR} channel	Rapidly-activating delayed rectifier current blunted
LQT-3	Dominant	3p21-24	SCN5A	I_{Na} channel	Inactivation of inward Na^+ current defective
LQT-4	Dominant	4q25-27	?	?	?
LQT-5	Dominant	21q22.1-22.2	KCNE1 [minK]	I_{KS} channel [beta-subunit]	Slowly-activating delayed rectifier current blunted
⋮					
LQT-n (?)		?	?	?	?
Jervell, Lange-Nielsen					
JLN	Recessive	21q22.1-22.2 11p15.5	KCNE1 KvLQT1 [or KCNQ1]	I_{KS} [beta-subunit] I_{KS} [alpha-subunit]	Slowly-activating delayed rectifier current blunted

FIGURE 24-57 Genetic basis for congenital long QT interval syndromes. Abnormalities have been linked to five chromosomes among families with the Romano-Ward form of congenital long QT interval syndromes. At present, specific genetic abnormalities and gene products are identified, in part, for four of the five. Multiple mutations or deletions are possible at each locus. The genetic basis for the Jervell and Lange-Nielsen syndrome (autosomal recessive inheritance and associated deafness) includes LQT-1 abnormalities in some families, but other loci are likely as well. The last two columns provide the gene products and defective currents for each of the known loci. See the text for further details.

another subunit of I_{KS} and has a role in both the Romano-Ward and the Jervell and Lange-Nielsen forms of the syndrome. A syndrome of torsades de pointes with normal QT intervals has been described. It may also have a congenital basis, although cases are infrequent and adequate studies have not yet occurred. In addition, some subjects genotypically affected with known long QT interval variants are intermittently or persistently normal phenotypes, at least based on ECGs.

ACQUIRED LONG QT INTERVAL SYNDROME

The commonest causes for acquired long QT interval syndromes are the antiarrhythmic drugs, classically quinidine, but also other class IA agents and class III agents. Prolongation of the QT interval usually precedes the arrhythmia.[275] Bradycardia, hypokalemia, and hypomagnesemia potentiate the risk.[316–318] QT prolongation induced by class IA agents appears to be idiosyncratic, often appearing in a dose-independent manner at the onset of therapy. It occurs among a small subsegment of the population exposed to the drugs, suggesting specific individual susceptibility, but no inheritance pattern has as yet been identified. It is commoner among women because women have longer QT intervals. However, other factors that interact with repolarization may act to generate risk of arrhythmias sporadically, unrelated to initiation of therapy. These factors include hypokalemia, bradycardia, LV dysfunction, and possibly LV hypertrophy. The class III drugs, particularly sotalol, prolong the QT interval in a dose-dependent pattern, consistent with its major pharmacologic effect of blocking the delayed rectifier channel and thus prolonging the QT interval. This fact has implications for monitoring adverse drug effects at the initiation of therapy.

There is a growing list of other drugs that may also block repolarizing currents, prolong the QT interval, and establish susceptibility to torsades de pointes (Table 24-12), including the phenothiazines, certain antibiotics, pentamidine (Nebupent), cocaine, and terfenadine (Seldane) and other antihistamines, among others. The mechanisms of terfenadine-induced torsades de pointes is particularly instructive.[319] In addition to having antihistamine effects, the parent compound blocks the delayed rectifier current, which can result in prolongation of the QT interval. Under normal conditions after oral ingestion, however, the parent compound is converted by a P450 enzyme in the liver to a metabolite that is an effective antihistamine but does not block the delayed rectifier current. Concomitant use of drugs that block specific enzymes in the hepatic P450 enzyme system, [e.g., ketoconazole (Nizoral)], however, allows the parent compound to be absorbed and to circulate, creating the propensity to torsades de pointes in a small group of patients. Sudden deaths have been reported with this combination therapy.[320] Other causes of acquired long QT interval syndrome with torsades de pointes include acute ischemia and reperfusion, acute central nervous system injury, liquid protein diets, and various other drugs.[317,321,322]

ELECTROCARDIOGRAPHIC FEATURES

Torsades de pointes is characterized by sequential beat-to-beat variations in mean QRS axis, causing the QRS complexes to appear to twist about the baseline (see Figs. 24-54 and 24-56). Characteristically, the tachycardia rate varies between 150 and 300 per minute, and the QT interval is prolonged during sinus rhythm. Episodes of tachycardia may be nonsustained or sustained, preceded by a long-short cycle sequence initiated by late PVCs, and may degenerate into VF.

TABLE 24-12 Drugs Associated with Acquired Long QT Syndrome and to Be Avoided in Congenital Long QT Syndrome

Antiarrhythmics
Class IA: quinidine, procainamide, disopyramide
Class III: sotalol, dofetilide, ibutilide, bretylium, N-acetyl procainamide, amiodarone (rare)
Antibiotics
Macrolides: erythromycin, clindamycin, clarithromycin, trimethoprim-sulfamethoxazole, chloroquine, pentamidine, amantadine, halofantrine
Antifungals
Itraconazole, ketoconazole
Psychotropics
Antidepressants: tricyclics (i.e., amitriptyline and desipramine), tetracyclics, fluvoxamine
Haloperidol, droperidol, thiothixene, doxepin, risperidone, phenothiazines
Antihistamines
Astemizole, terfenadine
Others
Cisapride
Glibenclamide
Organophosphate insecticides
Diuretics, with hypokalemia, hypomagnesemia, or hypocalcemia

NOTE: Some drugs cause risk only in combination (e.g., terfenadine and ketoconazole). Some observations are based on limited clinical data from case reports (e.g., clindamycin and newer nonsedating H_1 receptor antagonists); this list is current at the time of writing in an evolving field requiring continuous physician updating.

Torsades de pointes is a classic proarrhythmic manifestation of class IA antiarrhythmic agents. Class IC antiarrhythmic agents may express proarrhythmia in the form of an incessant monomorphic VT that is sinusoidal in pattern and often at rates less than 160 per minute (see also Chap. 23).

MANAGEMENT OF CONGENITAL LONG QT INTERVAL SYNDROME

The clinical expression of arrhythmias in congenital long QT interval syndrome is episodic and transient, ranging from palpitations to syncope to sudden death. Ambient arrhythmias are not usually sustained enough to make acute management a common clinical need. When required, however, intravenous beta-adrenergic blockade, intravenous Mg^{2+}, pacing, and/or lidocaine are appropriate, depending on the genetic variant and pattern of the arrhythmia. A new category of drugs, the K^+-channel openers, may ultimately prove useful as well.

Because of the continuing risk of transition of torsades de pointes to VF in patients with congenital long QT interval syndrome throughout life, careful long-term management is important from the time of diagnosis. A 12-lead ECG should be recorded in anyone with *unexplained* near-syncope, syncope, and/or symptomatic palpitations, especially with repetitive beats. In selected patients, stress testing and ambulatory monitoring may help clarify uncertain findings. Genetic testing should be carried out in selected members of affected families. An important subgroup consists of symptomatic relatives with phenotypically normal ECGs, since ECG expression appears to be intermittent, or even silent, in some.[321,322]

Long-term therapy includes beta-adrenergic blockade and/or left cardiac sympathetic denervation.[309,324] ICD implantation is indicated for patients with arrhythmias resistant to beta-adrenergic blockers or survivors of cardiac arrest due to long QT syndrome. Recurrent syncope without arrhythmia documentation despite beta-adrenergic blocker therapy is also an indication, especially if there is a family history of sudden death. Finally, ICD implantation may be considered for genotypically positive relatives in a family with a strong history of fatal long QT syndrome.

The present information on a variety of genetically controlled ion-channel dysfunctions may lead to new therapeutic approaches in the future. For instance, mexiletine may be a specific therapy for the variant associated with the SCN5A gene on chromosome 3, which encodes the cardiac sodium channel.[313] It is possible that other channel-specific therapies will be identified in the future.

MANAGEMENT OF ACQUIRED LONG QT INTERVAL SYNDROME

Treatment is directed at the underlying cause, or causes, with careful attention to electrolyte and metabolic disturbances and to identifying and reversing or removing iatrogenic factors. Although electrical cardioversion may interrupt torsades de pointes, the arrhythmia frequently recurs as long as the offending influence is present. In addition, many runs are nonsustained. Intravenous magnesium sulfate is often effective, especially when torsades de pointes is due to quinidine. It may be given in a dose of 2 g over 2 min followed by an infusion of 2 to 20 mg/min. Although Mg^{2+} will effectively control the arrhythmia, it will not reduce the duration of the QT interval. That must await clearance of the offending agent.

Overdrive atrial or ventricular pacing to induce rate-related QT shortening may also be required. Acceleration of the underlying heart rate with isoproterenol infusion to shorten the acquired QT interval prolongation may be effective but should be avoided in patients with symptomatic ischemic heart disease, if possible. Lidocaine also may be beneficial, as may other class IB drugs. These drugs tend to shorten the QT interval in normal myocardium. Class IA and class III antiarrhythmic agents should be avoided, since they prolong the QT interval.

THE SYNDROME OF RIGHT BUNDLE-BRANCH BLOCK, ST-SEGMENT ELEVATION, AND LIFE-THREATENING VENTRICULAR ARRHYTHMIAS (BRUGADA'S SYNDROME)

A complex of right bundle-branch block, ST-segment elevation in the anterior precordial leads, and risk of sudden death has been described. The reported patients often have spontaneous and inducible polymorphic VT, sustained or nonsustained, with normal QT intervals. There is no associated structural heart disease described to date, and some patients are aymptomatic. It is commonest in adolescent and young adult males, among whom it appears to confer a high risk of sudden death.[325,329,330] It has been suggested as the basis for so-called "sleep death" in young Asian males.[331] The syndrome is familial, and a mutation on chromosome 3 (SCN5A, the cardiac Na^+-channel) has been identified,[330] and others suggested.[330]

The diagnosis may be difficult because the right bundle-branch block and ST elevations may be subtle and intermittent.[325] They may be unmasked or enhanced by antiarrhythmic drug challenges with procainamide or flecainide[328,329] (Fig. 24-58), although the sensitivity and specificity of such challenges remains unknown. The entity is considered high risk, and ICD therapy has been suggested, even for asymptomatic affected individuals, particularly if there is a history of sudden death in young family members. Unfortunately, there are no prospective studies comparing ICDs to antiarrhythmic drug therapy for this disorder.

Ventricular Fibrillation and Flutter

Ventricular fibrillation is a terminal arrhythmia, uniformly requiring rapid initiation of emergency measures. Ventricular flutter with loss of consciousness and rapid unstable VT are clinical and hemodynamic equivalents of VF and treated identically when accompanied by the clinical picture of cardiac arrest. VF occurs most commonly in the setting of acute ischemic events (unstable angina pectoris or acute myocardial infarction) or unpredictably in advanced chronic ischemic heart disease. In the latter, it may be triggered by transient ischemia and perhaps transient or uncontrolled hemodynamic dysfunction. Moreover, it is the apparent mode of death in 25 to 50 percent of all cardiac fatalities. Among patients with nonischemic cardiomyopathies,[322,333] cardiac arrest is the mode of death in up to 50 percent of all fatalities. In the past, it has been assumed that VF is the mechanism of most of these events, but it is clear now that a substantial proportion of these events are due to bradyarrhythmias and asystole[333] and, it is important to note, to acute hemodynamic dysfunction.

VF may also develop during ischemia caused by coronary artery spasm, some hypoxic states, atrial fibrillation with rapid ventricular responses in WPW syndrome, pacing on the T-wave or asynchronized cardioversion, electrical accidents due to improper grounding of electrical devices, or proarrhythmic effects of antiarrhythmic drugs. A particularly high-risk setting for VF is acute myocardial infarction with right or left bundle-branch block. VF may occur de novo, but among patients with out-of-hospital cardiac arrest, VT commonly precedes the onset of VF (see also Chap. 23).

ELECTROCARDIOGRAPHIC FEATURES

The electrocardiographic pattern of VF is described by gross disorganization without identifiable repetitive waveforms or intervals (see Fig. 24-42*D* and *E*). At the onset VF may be "coarse" in pattern, but over time it loses its amplitude and becomes "fine" (less than 0.2 mV). Successful defibrillation and survival rates are decreased in patients with the fine pattern of VF. In ventricular flutter (see Fig. 24-42*C*), a sine wave configuration is present, having a cycle length in the range of 200 to 240 ms. Rapid polymorphic VTs may be difficult to distinguish from VF electrocardiographically, but maintained consciousness suggests VT rather than VF, the latter defined by loss of effective mechanical function. Hemodynamic findings may be initially stable in ventricular flutter or very rapid polymorphic VT, but hypotension, loss of consciousness, and degeneration to VF are common.

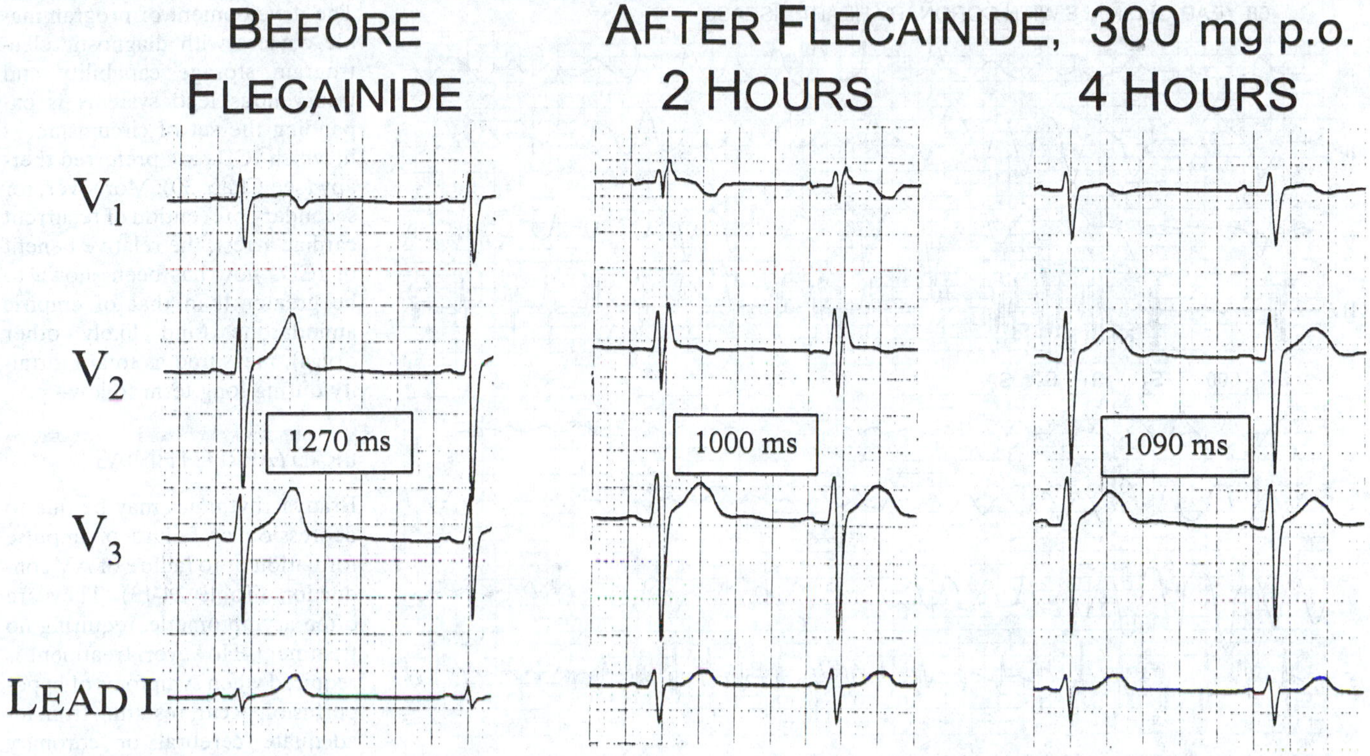

FIGURE 24-58 Syndrome of right bundle-branch block and ST-segment elevation in the anterior precordial leads and risk of sudden cardiac death (Brugada). In this syndrome, the electrocardiographic hallmarks of right bundle-branch block and ST elevation in the anterior leads are not consistently present, but they may be evoked by drug provocation using procainamide or flecainide. The left panel shows strips from leads V_1, V_3, and I, recorded from a 17-year-old male with Brugada's syndrome and a strong Family history of sudden cardiac death in males. The baseline ECG was normal. After a 300-mg oral bolus of flecainide, an ECG recorded 2 h later revealed a ST-segment elevation and a right bundle-branch block pattern in leads V_1 and V_2. After 4 h, this had reverted to baseline. See the text for details.

MANAGEMENT OF VENTRICULAR FLUTTER AND VENTRICULAR FIBRILLATION

There are two major goals of therapy: (1) immediate life support and resuscitation and (2) long-term prevention of recurrences. Basic life support with standard cardiopulmonary resuscitation (Chap. 34) is used until emergency defibrillation at 200 J or more can be carried out (see Chaps. 29A and 29B). After three unsuccessful shocks at energies up to 360 J, 1 mg of epinephrine should be administered by intravenous push and defibrillation attempted again.

Early defibrillation is essential to survival.[334] Resistance of defibrillation may occur due to the patient's size, improper paddle placement, improper use of conducting media, acidosis, hypoxemia, or electrolyte disturbances.[335] Some antiarrhythmic drugs may raise the defibrillation threshold. Energy thresholds for defibrillation may be decreased by administration of bretylium, lidocaine, or epinephrine, the latter especially when the fibrillatory waveform is fine. Immediate steps to improve metabolic and electrolyte disturbances are required, paramount of which is to establish an airway, followed by techniques to support ventilation.[336] In rare instances, "spontaneous" reversion of VF[336] or "medical" defibrillation with bretylium[243] has been reported. A physiologic or pharmacologic increase in catecholamines has been postulated as the underlying mechanism.

After successful defibrillation, careful attention to the total clinical status of the patient and prophylactic antiarrhythmic drugs are required. Intravenous therapy with lidocaine is commonly used initially. For recurrent and resistant cases, intravenous procainamide or amiodarone[337] can be administered intravenously, the latter having replaced bretylium tosylate in order of priority and urgency. In addition to oxygenation and improving the metabolic milieu, aggressive steps to identify and treat or prevent recurrent ischemia or heart failure are necessary, since they may act as pathophysiologic triggers for recurrences.[4,248]

In the in-hospital setting, early recognition and aggressive treatment of VT may prevent VF. In the patient with acute myocardial infarction, early VF (48 h), as with early VT, is not associated with an independent influence on posthospital mortality risk and does not justify long-term antiarrhythmic therapy.[339-341] When VF occurs as a convalescent-phase complication of acute myocardial infarction, however, aggressive long-term antiarrhythmic management is indicated (see above).[342,343] The vast majority of patients who have VT or VF in the convalescent phase after acute myocardial infarction (3 days to 8 weeks) will have inducible ventricular arrhythmias at baseline electrophysiologic study.[247]

Among survivors of out-of-hospital VF not caused by acute myocardial infarction, control of ischemia and heart failure is essential. The clinical context[344,345] is evaluated in terms of the interaction between structural abnormalities (e.g., coronary heart disease, myopathy, hypertrophy, or anatomic electrical abnormalities) and functional states (e.g., ischemia-reperfusion, or systemic factors, including congestive heart failur, metabolic

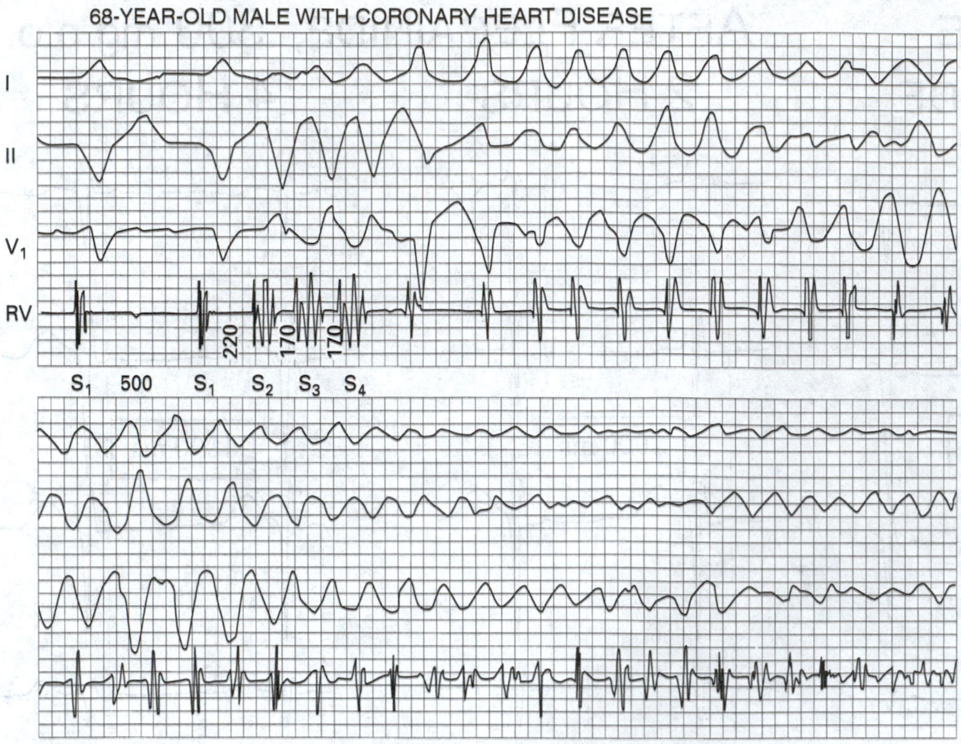

FIGURE 24-59 Programmed electrical stimulation study in a survivor of out-of-hospital cardiac arrest. The patient had ischemic heart disease, and polymorphic VT degenerating to VF was reproducibly induced prior to bypass surgery. After surgery, the tachycardia was no longer inducible.

and electrolyte disturbances, neurophysiologic interactions, and toxic effects). For long-term estimate of the risk of arrhythmic death, invasive electrophysiologic testing of pharmacologic efficacy is one accepted approach.[346] Only about 33 to 40 percent of survivors, however, will be inducible into a reproducibly inducible ventricular tachyarrhythmia at baseline.[345,346] A similar fraction will be inducible into nonsustained VT or VF (Fig. 24-59), and 20 to 30 percent are noninducible. The subgroup whose unexpected VF is related to transient ischemia, in contrast to an underlying structural basis, is less likely to be inducible at baseline.[347] With high-risk forms of arrhythmias on ambulatory monitoring or exercise testing but without inducible arrhythmia at baseline by invasive testing, drug therapy can be guided by suppression of these spontaneous arrhythmias by noninvasive techniques[226,260,261] as long as the EF is greater than 40 percent. For such patients with lower EFs, the use of ICDs is emerging as the preferred treatment.

Usefulness of long-term drug therapy is limited by the fact that no more than 20 to 30 percent of the patients with inducible arrhythmias will have a drug identified that will prevent inducibility. In one randomized study without placebo control (ESVEM), a class III antiarrhythmic agent with beta-blocking effect, sotalol, appeared more effective than other drugs for survivors of VT and VF.[263] Whether amiodarone will have equivalent (or greater) benefit remains to be determined.

Patients who have recurrences despite drug therapy predicted to be effective during testing, those in whom an end point of therapy cannot be established, or those in whom the risk of recurrence remains high because underlying precipitating factors cannot be adequately controlled should receive ICDs.[345]

The development of programmable devices with diagnostic electrogram storage capability and transvenous lead systems is expanding the set of circumstances in which ICDs are preferred therapy (see Chap. 30). Moreover, for secondary prevention of recurrent cardiac arrest, the relative benefit of ICDs now has been shown to be greater than that of empiric amiodarone (and likely other drugs), measured as total mortality during long-term follow-up.

BRADYARRHYTHMIAS

Bradyarrhythmias may be due to depression or failure of impulse formation or to failure of AV conduction (Table 24-13). They are often asymptomatic, requiring no treatment. However, treatment is required when symptoms of hypoperfusion occur, resulting from inadequate cerebral or coronary blood flow, or worsening of congestive heart failure at rest or during exercise. Symptoms are almost always due to inadequate heart rate, although under some circumstances, such as with aortic stenosis or hypertrophic cardiomyopathy, loss of synchronized atrial contraction may contribute to symptoms. Bradyarrhythmias may be due solely to cardiac factors but are often caused or aggravated by noncardiac factors, such as drugs, autonomic imbalance, hypothyroidism, hypothermia, or hyperkalemia.[348] Furthermore, the hypoperfusion associated with bradycardia may be multifactorial, such as may occur in acute inferior wall infarction, in which bradycardia and LV

TABLE 24-13 Classification of Bradyarrhythmias

Failure of Impulse Formation

- Sinus bradycardia
- Sinus pauses, sinus arrest, SA block
- Sick-sinus syndrome
- Carotid sinus hypersensitivity syndrome
- Neurocardiogenic cardioinhibitory syncope

AV Conduction Abnormalities

- First-degree heart block
- Second-degree heart block
  - Type I (Wenckebach)
  - Type II
- Third-degree heart block
  - Paroxysmal
  - Intermittent, transient
  - Chronic: congenital, acquired
- AV dissociation

dysfunction may be additive. In all cases, careful evaluation of both cardiac and noncardiac factors is necessary. If the patient is symptomatic, the first step in management is to increase the heart rate, which is readily accomplished by parasympatholytic drugs (e.g., atropine) or sympathomimetic drugs (e.g., isoproterenol). Underdosing with atropine (e.g., 0.3 mg) may cause a centrally mediated bradycardia and should be avoided. In addition, sympathomimetics must be used cautiously in all patients and avoided in the patient with ischemic symptoms. Temporary external pacing offers a logical alternative.[349,350] Stable, reliable increases in heart rate are afforded by temporary ventricular demand pacing from a pacing catheter positioned in the right ventricular apex. Temporary dual-chamber pacing is required in cases in which synchronized atrial contraction is deemed beneficial, such as bradycardia associated with inferior wall and right ventricular infarction.[351] General circulatory support and elimination of drugs that aggravate bradycardia is the second step in management.

Failure of Impulse Formation

SINUS BRADYCARDIA

Sinus bradycardia ranges from a benign asymptomatic physiologic adjustment in heart rate to a symptomatic expression of sinus node dysfunction. The asymptomatic forms are most often benign and related to physiologic (e.g., training effect) or pathologic (e.g., inferior wall infarction) excesses in vagal tone.[352–356] Drugs that can cause sinus node depression include beta blockers, calcium channel blockers, amiodarone, lithium, cimetidine, and adenosine. Radiographic contrast materials can also cause it in sensitive patients. Although most commonly due to impaired impulse formation, it may also be caused by impaired conduction from the sinus node to atrial muscle (SA block).

Electrocardiographic Features of Sinus Bradycardia and Sinoatrial Block Sinus bradycardia is defined as a rate less than 60 impulses per minute, with the pacemaker impulse originating in the sinus node, resulting in P waves of normal amplitude and vector. It is rarely considered outside of the physiologic range until rates are under 50 per minute. In well-trained athletes and during sleep, rates of 40 per minute or less may occur as a normal variant. Sinus bradycardia may be accompanied by some degree of sinus arrhythmia.

SA block is categorized as first-degree (delayed conduction), second-degree (intermittent), or third-degree (complete) block. Vagal stimulation, digitalis, and ischemia are the most common predisposing factors in this rare conduction disorder. SA block is recognized by the absence of expected P waves and the subsequent QRS complex. First- and third-degree SA blocks cannot be recognized on the standard clinical ECG, but second-degree SA block may be identified because of its intermittent pattern. Characteristically, in SA Wenckebach, the PP and RR intervals will progressively shorten together before a dropped P-QRS complex results in a pause; a recurrent pattern may be identified (Fig. 24-60*B*). SA Wenckebach periods are frequently overlooked or mislabeled as sinus arrhythmia. Intermittent 2:1 block may also be deduced from standard rhythm strips (Fig. 24-61), but persistent 2:1 SA block is indistinguishable from sinus bradycardia.

Management of Sinus Bradyarrhythmias Treatment of patients who have asymptomatic bradycardia is often unnecessary. In the symptomatic patient, elimination of reversible aggravating factors is an essential step in management. When this is ineffective or negative chronotropic agents are essential to overall patient management, permanent pacing may be needed (see Chap. 31). A similar approach is taken for patients with sinus pauses, sinus arrest, or SA exit block, which may be associated with myocardial infarction, myocarditis, sinus node fibrosis, digitalis excess, or excess vagal tone.[357,358] In the patient with symptomatic hypersensitive carotid sinus syndrome,[359,360] medical treatment is usually inadequate. Permanent ventricular or dual-chamber pacing[361] is usually effective but occasionally may not relieve symptoms because of a coexisting vasodepressor reflex.[362]

The complex of neurocardiogenic syncope, or neurally mediated vasodepressor syncope, has combined manifestations of sinus bradycardia and vasodepressor responses. It is revealed by the response to head-up tilt testing and is due to an abnormal reflex, the afferent limb of which originates in the LV wall.[363] The efferent limb is parasympathetic, causing both decreases in peripheral vascular tone, leading to hypotension, and sinus node depression, leading to sinus bradycardia or a junctional escape rhythm. In the majority of patients, the vasodepressor component dominates, limiting the effectiveness of pacing therapy.[364] However, among the subgroup of patients in whom the cardioinhibitory component predominates, cardiac pacing featuring "rate-drop response" or a similar algorithm appears to be effective.[365] Among pharmacologic agents,[366,367] beta-adrenergic blockers have been most useful, presumably by the mechanism of blocking the sympathetically mediated afferent limb of the reflex[367] (see Chap. 32).

SICK-SINUS SYNDROME

Sick-sinus syndrome[368–370] is a general term used to indicate abnormalities of cardiac impulse formation and intraatrial and AV conduction[352,371,372] that may be manifested by various combinations of brady- and tachyarrhythmias.[373] Treatment, therefore, must be individualized to each patient's manifestations of the syndrome.[374] Often the patient is asymptomatic, or the symptoms are mild and nonspecific. Negative chronotropic agents are avoided or discontinued,[370,375] and permanent pacing may be delayed until the patient is more clearly symptomatic.[376,377] Although decisions regarding therapy often can be made from the combination of clinical, ECG, and monitoring data, invasive electrophysiologic studies may assist in decision making in some patients. Quantitative measures of sinus node function, such as sinus node recovery time and perhaps SA conduction time, and of conduction system status, such as HV interval and its response to membrane suppressants, are occasionally helpful. In the clearly symptomatic patient, treatment may include a combination of antiarrhythmic agents and permanent pacing for intrinsic and drug-induced bradycardias. Ironically, the eventual development of atrial fibrillation in patients with sick-sinus syndrome may alleviate symptoms, since heart rate control in atrial fibrillation can be more consistently achieved. Dual-chamber pacing is preferred, to avoid pacemaker syndrome, since 50 to 80 percent of patients with sick-sinus syndrome have preserved ventriculoatrial conduction (see Chap. 31), and DDD pacing with rate-responsive functions is preferred for patients with intermittent or persistent sinus bradyarrhythmias. Among patients with-

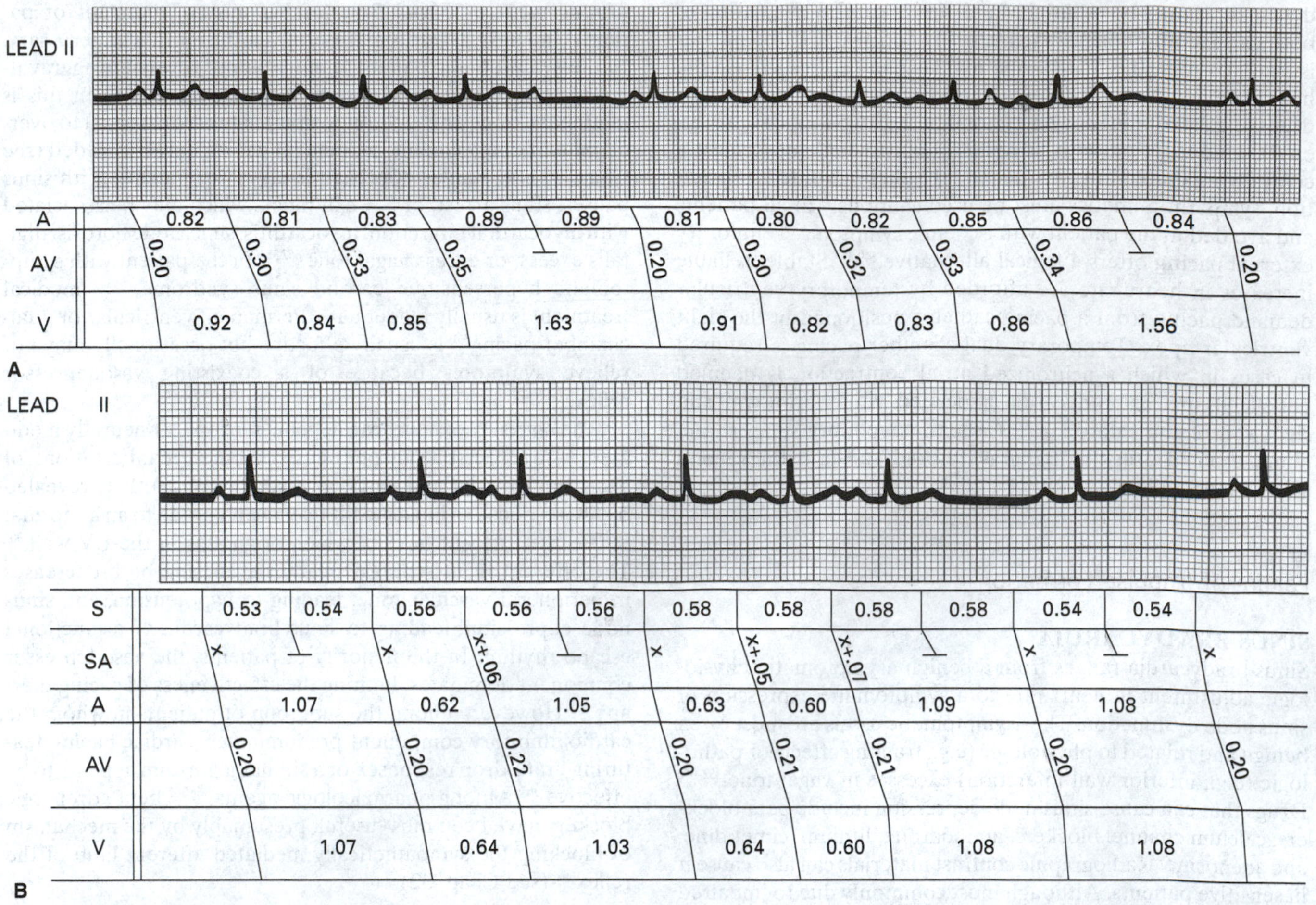

FIGURE 24-60 Wenckebach phenomenon. *A.* A 5:4 and 6:5 AV Wenckebach period. Note that the PR interval progressively lengthens, but by a decreasing increment; therefore, the ventricular cycle tends to shorten (at least for the first two cycles following the dropped beat). *B.* A 3:2 and 4:3 SA Wenckebach period with 2:1 SA block at beginning and end of strip. (From Hurst JW, Myerburg R. *Introduction to Electrocardiography*. New York: McGraw-Hill; 1973. Reproduced with permission from the publisher and authors).

out evidence of AV nodal dysfunction or requiring AV nodal blocking drugs, pacing in the AAI mode, using a single atrial lead, is feasible. This system is less expensive and avoids the risks and complications of a second lead implant (ventricular), which may be important in patients with difficult vascular access. Later development of AV nodal disease is uncommon among these patients, and it usually presents in a slowly progressive pattern.[378–380] DDD pacing with automatic mode-switching function is useful for patients with intermittent tachyarrhythmias, and rate-responsive VVI pacing is preferred for patients with chronic atrial fibrillation.[381]

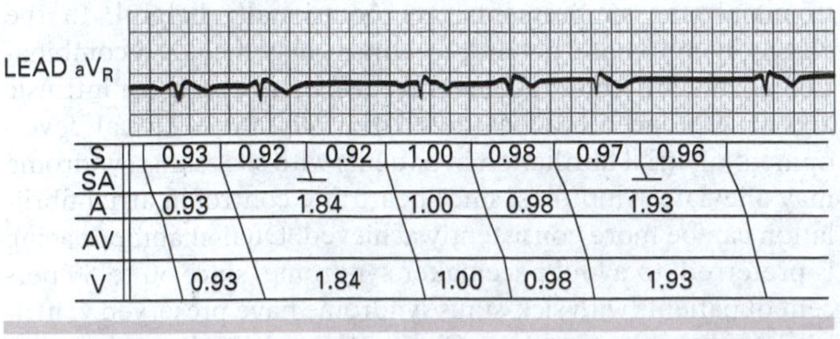

FIGURE 24-61 SA block. In each pause the entire P-QRS-T sequence is missing, and the long cycle is approximately equal to two of the sinus cycles. The pattern is the equivalent of a Möbitz-type II block at the level of the AV junction.

Digitalis is used with caution[375] and, when needed, is easier to titrate once the patient has a permanent pacemaker. When such patients require therapy with antiarrhythmic drugs that slow sinus rates and/or impair AV conduction (e.g., beta blockers or amiodarone), management of drug therapy may be facilitated by pacemaker backup.

It is important to recognize that the risk of development of new-onset atrial fibrillation is high in patients with sick-sinus syndrome, approximately 5.2 percent per year in a retrospective analysis of several studies. The incidence of the arrhythmia and its thromboembolic complications may be reduced by atrial or DDD pacing, compared to VVI or no pacing.[382,383] Anticoagulation should be considered part of the management of patients with sick-sinus syndrome, especially when they have documented atrial fibrillation episodes. Although there is clearly a symptomatic improvement in patients with sick-sinus syndrome by cardiac pacing and a trend toward reduction of incidence of heart failure, it is not yet known whether cardiac pacing improves survival.[382,383]

CAROTID SINUS HYPERSENSITIVITY

The pathophysiology of carotid sinus hypersensitivity is poorly understood. Among the explanations are abnormalities of the

TABLE 24-14 Effect of Maneuvers on Sinus Node and Conducting System Function

Maneuver	Effect on SN	Functional (AV Nodal Block)	Structural (AV Nodal, Hisian, or Infrahisian Disease)
Atropine	↑ Heart rate	Improve AV conduction, decrease block	Worsen AV conduction, increase block
Exercise	↑ Heart rate	Improve AV conduction, decrease block	Worsen AV conduction, increase block
CSM	↓ Heart rate	Worsen AV conduction, increase block	Improve AV conduction, decrease block

ABBREVIATIONS: CSM = carotid sinus massage; SN = sinus node.

neuromuscular structures surrounding the carotid sinus mechanoreceptors, a central defect of the autonomic nervous system, and association with artherosclerotic disease.[384,385] A hypersensitive response to carotid sinus stimulation is defined as asystole due to sinus arrest of more than 3 s, a substantial symptomatic decrease in blood pressure, or both. It is important to evaluate and correlate the patient's symptoms because an abnormal response to carotid sinus pressure may be found in elderly patients or in patients sensitized by digitalis or other drugs, without clinical significance. In patients with associated syncope or near syncope, pacing is indicated.[385–388]

Atrioventricular Conduction Abnormalities

Abnormal prolongation or block of AV node conduction can be due to physiologic, reversible or permanent acquired or congenital causes (Tables 24-14 and 24-15). Although the term *block* is applied generally to most patterns of conduction abnormalities, it is a misnomer when referring to impaired impulse conduction through the AV node or the bundle branches, in which there is an abnormal delay, rather than complete block, of conduction. Delayed conduction may result from normal physiologic variations (e.g., vagal tone) or pathologic influences.[389] Management is determined by assessing the degree of block, symptoms, and clinical setting. Recurrent episodes of the Wenckebach phenomen (type I, second-degree AV block) may be asymptomatic and require no therapy in the well-conditioned individual or athlete. These individuals may have resting heart rates of 40 impulses per minute or less and as low as 30 per minute during sleep, due to sinus bradycardia and/or second-degree AV block. Sinus pauses as long as 2.8 s may occur. All of these phenomena are due to high vagal tone in this setting.[390,391] In contrast, transient second-degree or complete AV block accompanying an acute anterior wall myocardial infarction is usually infranodal, a marker of massive muscle loss and predictive of a high mortality rate, even without symptoms of AV block and despite permanent pacing,[392,393] whether or not symptoms of AV block have occurred.

AV block associated with inferior wall myocardial infarction is much commoner (10 to 15 percent versus 5 percent) than with anterior wall infarction and has a more benign prognosis. It is usually due to AV nodal, rather than infranodal, conduction abnormalities and is commonly vagally mediated rather than structural. Onset is within the first 24 h, and it is almost always transient and commonly reversible with atropine, if treatment is needed at all. This form of AV block is not associated with an adverse long-term prognosis, although in-hospital mortality rates are slightly increased. Temporary pacing is occasionally required, but permanent pacing is very rarely indicated.

ELECTROCARDIOGRAPHIC PATTERNS

First-degree AV block is defined as a PR interval in excess of 0.2 s at normal heart rates. When the QRS complexes are of normal duration and configuration, it is usually due to prolonged conduction at the level of the AV node. If bundle-branch or fascicular block is present, the conduction delay may be at the level of either the AV node or the His-Purkinje system.

Second-degree AV block is characterized by intermittent failure of conduction from atria to ventricles and is further subdivided into type I (Wenckebach phenomenon) and Möbitz type II second-degree block. Type I second-degree AV block is characterized electrocardiographically by progressive lengthening of the PR interval, eventually leading to a nonconducted P wave (Fig. 24-60*A*). This often recurs with regularity, and patterns of "group beating" are recognized. The degree of block can be quantified by the conduction ratio, the ratio of the number of P waves to the number of QRS complexes in each episode or period terminated by the pause. Because the magnitude of PR lengthening typically is less with subsequent RR intervals, the RR intervals themselves progressively shorten before the pause caused by the blocked P wave. Atypical patterns may demonstrate lengthening of RR intervals in later cycles of a Wenckebach period. The greatest decrement between successive RR intervals occurs from the first to the second cycle of a Wenckebach period, and, even with atypical patterns, shortening of the second RR cycle is always present. Wenckebach block may be physiologic in athletes (especially during sleep) or induced by digitalis. It is almost always due to impaired conduction across the AV node and is usually accompanied by a QRS complex of normal duration (see also Chap. 31). A Wenckebach conduction pattern may occur rarely across an area of disease in the His-Purkinje system.

In type II second-degree AV block, appropriately timed P waves fail to conduct, but there is not a pattern of progressive PR lengthening. Isolated P waves may fail to conduct, or fixed patterns (e.g., 2:1 at rates that are expected to conduct 1:1 under normal physiologic conditions) may occur. Infranodal block is the rule, and QRS complexes tend to be widened due to disease in the His bundle or intraventricular conducting system. Type II block is most often associated with organic cardiac disease and is frequently progressive. When the QRS complex is narrow with Möbitz type II block, block in the His bundle is likely (Fig. 24-62); when it is widened, block below the His bundle is the rule. At times, the conduction ratio of P waves to QRS complexes is fixed at 2:1. Only a single PR interval is recorded, and PR lengthening cannot be discerned; therefore, the absolute distinction between type I (2:1 Wenckebach) and type II block cannot be made. A narrow QRS complex and type I block at other times on the tracing suggest that 2:1 block is a manifesta-

TABLE 24-15 Etiologies of AV Block

	Reversible or Transient	Permanent
Physiologic		
Heightened vagal tone (athlete, sleep apnea)	+	−
Neurogenic		
Carotid hypersensitivity syndrome	+	−
Neurocardiogenic syncope	+	−
Congenital		
Congenital heart disease	−	+
Maternal systemic lupus erythematosus	−	+
Coronary artery disease		
Acute myocardial infarction		
Anterior	+	+
Inferior	++	+
Ischemic cardiomyopathy	−	+
Cardiomyopathy	−	+
Infiltrative disease	−	+
Amyloidosis		
Sarcoidosis		
Hemochromatosis		
Infectious disease		
Endocarditis	+	++
Myocarditis		
Lyme disease	+	−
Tuberculosis, rheumatic fever, siphylis	−	+
Viral: measles, mumps, adult varicella	++	+
Chagas disease	−	+
Collagen vascular disease	+	++
Systemic lupus erythematosus		
Rheumatoid arthritis		
Scleroderma		
Others		
Idiopathic fibrosis (Lev's disease)	−	+
Calcific infiltration (Lenegre's disease)	−	+
Drug induced	+	−
Digitalis		
Beta blockers		
Calcium channel blockers		
Amiodarone		
Lithium		
Cimetidine		
Adenosine		
Metabolic	+	−
Hyperkalemia		
Addison's disease		
Hypermagnesemia		
Traumatic	+	+
Surgery		
RF energy, catheter trauma		
Radiation		
Tumors	−	+
Mesothelioma		
Melanoma		
Rhabdomyoma		
Hodgkin's disease		
Neuromuscular disease	−	+
Myotonic muscular dystrophy		
Kearns-Sayer syndrome		
Peroneal muscular atrophy		
Erb's dystrophy		

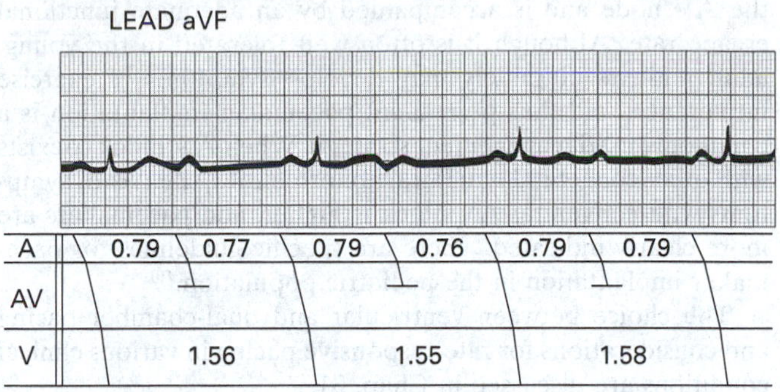

FIGURE 24-62 A form of second-degree AV block. There are two P waves to each QRS 2:1 AV block (alternate sinus impulses are blocked). This pattern can be caused by block in the AV node (Wenckebach), intra-Hisian block, or distal block (see the text).

tion of type I block (Wenckebach–AV nodal) physiology. Wide QRS complexes favor type II block. If the PR interval of conducted beats is 300 ms or longer, conduction block is likely at the level of the AV node; if it is 160 ms or less, Hisian or infra-Hisian block is likely. Evidence of VA conduction, such as retrograde P waves following a PVC favors the His-Purkinje system as the site of block. The response to certain maneuvers can be of help establishing the site of block (see Table 24-14).[415] In the electrophysiology laboratory, recording an HV interval of greater than 80 ms (normal = 45 to 55 ms) identifies high risk for AV block, and a pacemaker is indicated if the patient is symptomatic. If the HV is 100 ms or more, a pacemaker implantation is indicated, even in asymptomatic patients.[410]

Occasionally, the intervals between P waves may vary, with a pattern of shorter PP intervals when a QRS is between the two P waves, and the PP interval is longer when the two P waves are consecutive. This phenomenon is called ventriculophasic sinus arrhythmia and is related to baroreceptor reflexes. High conduction ratios, such as 3:1 and greater, may be diagnosed simply as paroxysmal or high-grade AV block.

In third-degree (complete) AV block, the atrial and ventricular rates are regular but dissociated (Fig. 24-63). At times, the P waves and QRS rates are so similar (isorhythmic dissociation) as to make this judgment difficult. Maneuvers by the patient, such as arm movement, standing up, or marching in place, may increase the sinus rate (P waves) without corresponding changes in the ventricular escape rate, confirming loss of AV conduction. In contrast, the development of 1:1 conduction suggests that the impaired conduction was at the AV nodal level. Morphology of the QRS complexes suggests the escape of junctional (narrow

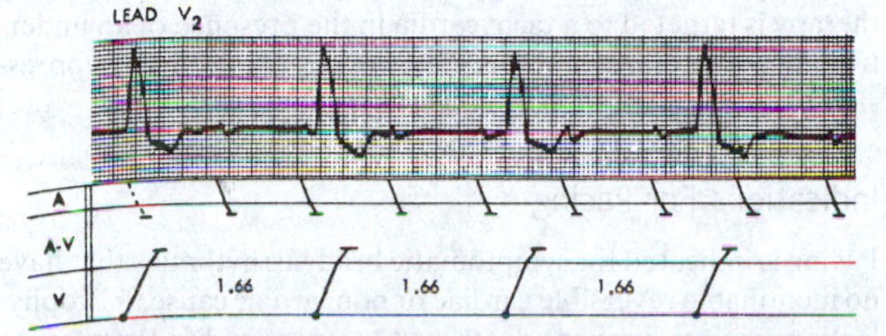

FIGURE 24-63 Complete (third-degree) AV block. There is a regular idioventricular rhythm at rate 36 impulses per minute, and the P waves indicate their independence by changing their relationship to the QRS complexes.

QRS) or ventricular (wide QRS) subordinate pacemakers. Complete AV block may be preceded by years of varying and/or progressive lower grades of block, as well as by bundle-branch and fascicular blocks. It is common to observe long rhythm strips that demonstrate not quite complete AV block. Occasional capture beats interrupt a regular escape rhythm. The conducted P waves are critically timed within a narrow range, usually at a long interval after the preceding escape QRS complex. The clinical implication of this pattern is the same as complete heart block. Transient AV block or sinus pauses on telemetry or ambulatory monitoring are common and occasionally of concern. Occurring at night or without symptoms, sinus pauses of less than 3 s are not uncommon (2.4 percent of patients) and usually represent variations in response to autonomic fluctuations rather than disease. Pauses greater than 3 s are rarer (0.8 percent of patients) and may require further evaluation. Patients with sleep apnea may develop sinus pauses or transient AV block, usually preceded by a decrease in sinus rate, a clue of increased vagal tone. These patients require therapy for the respiratory problem rather than pacemaker implantation.[410]

MANAGEMENT OF ATRIOVENTRICULAR BLOCK

First-Degree Heart Block Isolated first-degree AV block is asymptomatic and is not an indication for temporary or permanent pacing.[410,416,417] However, one possible exception is a subgroup of patients with marked first-degree AV block (greater than 300 ms) associated with LV dysfunction and symptoms of congestive heart failure in whom a shorter AV interval caused by sequential AV pacing results in hemodynamic improvement.[410,414]

Second-Degree Heart Block Möbitz type I AV block, or the Wenckebach phenomenon, is usually associated with an adequate ventricular rate and is rarely symptomatic.[415] It occurs in highly trained athletes[419] and is a normal response to rapid atrial pacing. In most patients who have the Wenckebach phenomenon secondary to AV nodal disease, routine prophylactic pacing is not advised, since it is minimally symptomatic (if at all) and tends not to progress.[369] Rarely, the effective ventricular rate is slow and patients are symptomatic, requiring pacing if vagolytic maneuvers are ineffective. The prognosis in patients who have underlying organic heart disease is determined by the extent of the underlying disease, not the Möbitz type I block.[420] Second-degree heart block is common in the acute phase of inferior wall myocardial infarction and rarely requires temporary pacing in this setting. Reversion is usually prompt—measured in hours to days.

Möbitz type II block is less common but implies more significant disease in the conduction system. The site of block is almost always below the AV node and usually below the bundle of His. Therefore, slower escape rhythms and risk of progression to complete heart block are of concern. It is almost always associated with a defined disease process. Permanent pacing is indicated,[410] except where Möbitz type II block is induced by rapid artificial pacing.[421,422] The purpose of pacing is primarily to protect against symptomatic events, such as syncope, and thus to protect the patient from injuring him- or herself or others. Available data do not suggest that pacemakers will prolong the life of patients with Möbitz type II block. The selection among specific designs of pacing devices is discussed in Chap. 31.

A special circumstance involves 2:1 AV block in which the underlying mechanism and site of block remain obscure. The decision to treat is inferred from the clinical setting. Wide QRS complexes, sudden onset of periods of block, and inadequate escape rates favor type II block, whereas narrow complexes and coincident episodes of typical type I block favor Wenckebach block.

Another variant pattern is multilevel block in the AV junction. This commonly occurs during atrial tachycardias and may be functional, pharmacologic, or pathologic. The pattern of multilevel block during atrial tachycardia may be deceiving. This pattern is a basic 2:1 pattern with Wenckebach conduction patterns of the impulses that conduct through the area of 2:1, and it produces group beating of the ventricles. This may result in relatively slow ventricular rates, but the primary problem is the atrial arrhythmias with physiologic or insignificant pathologic responses at the level of the AV node. His-bundle electrograms may be diagnostic, but such invasive studies are indicated only when needed for a therapeutic decision.[422–425]

Paroxysmal AV Block Runs of consecutive atrial impulses that fail to conduct to the ventricles may last for up to 10 to 20 s and may be associated with syncope. Unless a clearly defined, reversible cause is identified, permanent pacing is required. Bradycardia-dependent AV block, or phase 4 block, usually affects patients with underlying conduction system disease. It is characterized by spontaneous phase 4 depolarization of tissue in the His-Purkinje system. The partially depolarized tissue impairs ventricular conduction of propagating impulses of sinus origin, most commonly affecting the conduction in the left bundle-branch system (bradycardia-dependent left bundle-branch block). Block by this mechanism at a more proximal site in the conducting system may result in complete heart block, not responsive to atropine or isoproterenol, but only to cardiac pacing. A precordial thump may produce a PVC able to depolarize and reset the ventricle including the site of automatic activity, thereby allowing resumption AV conduction down the distal conducting system.[426–429]

Complete AV Block Complete heart block may be acute in onset or slowly progressive and chronic; it may produce abrupt, clinically significant symptoms or may remain asymptomatic and be discovered incidentally. When acute and symptomatic, evaluation and rate support are urgently needed. Pharmacologic intervention with atropine or isoproterenol is usually most readily available.

The latter should be avoided in the presence of ischemic heart disease, and external pacing instituted if needed.[437,438] Reliable rate control is achieved by ventricular or dual-chamber temporary cardiac pacing. Permanent pacing is indicated unless those factors responsible for the heart block are reversible or when transient complete block complicates an acute inferior wall myocardial infarction.[410] Since the advent of thrombolytic therapy and primary angioplasty in acute myocardial infarction, the incidence of complete heart block in myocardial infarction has decreased. However, in acute anterior wall infarction, the prognosis remains grave, even after permanent pacemaker implantation.[395,401,404]

Isolated congenital AV block usually occurs at the level of the AV node and is accompanied by an adequate junctional escape rate. Although it is often well tolerated in the young, adult patients ultimately may develop symptoms of exercise intolerance, and thus permanent pacemaker implantation is a commonly used management strategy. When AV block coexists with other congenital structural abnormalities, the risk of symptoms with congenital AV block is higher, and pacemakers are more clearly indicated. There are specific guidelines for pacemaker implantation in the pediatric population.[410]

The choice between ventricular and dual-chamber pacing and considerations for rate-responsive pacing in various clinical conditions are discussed in Chap. 31.

Atrioventricular Dissociation

AV dissociation is not synonymous with AV block but occurs in conjunction with block as well as in its absence. It implies an abnormality of intrinsic pacemaker activity that may be slowing of normal pacemaker activity (*default*), acceleration of a normally subordinate or latent pacemaker (*usurpation*), AV block, or a combination of these phenomena.

ELECTROCARDIOGRAPHIC FINDINGS

AV dissociation implies that the atria and ventricles each have manifest independent pacemakers. In the setting of AV block, a junctional or ventricular pacemaker emerges as an escape rhythm; if it fails or if the escape is too slow, AV block will become a symptomatic or terminal rhythm. The atria and ventricles may beat independently if a normally subordinate junctional or ventricular pacemaker discharges faster than the sinus or atrial pacemaker and 1:1 retrograde conduction is absent. Since AV block is not necessarily present, ventricular capture by impulses of sinus origin commonly occur as a result of fortuitous timing relationships between sinus node activity and ventricular refractoriness. At times, capture beats and junctional or ventricular beats coincide and generate fusion beats (Fig. 24-64).

MANAGEMENT

Treatment, when needed, is directed toward the underlying cause. It is important to evaluate whether symptoms are present and whether they are due to a rapid or slow rate. Suppression of tachyarrhythmias, such as AV dissociation in VT, is the primary goal when symptoms are related primarily to the tachyarrhythmia and an intact intrinsic or artificial pacemaker is present. Intermittent ventricular ectopy may be an escape phenomenon in an otherwise asymptomatic patient who has an underlying persistent bradycardia. In such cases, rate support with pacing is indicated to relieve bradycardia symptoms, and the escape ventricular ectopy will resolve secondarily. If initial therapy is targeted to a tachycardia in the presence of an underlying bradycardia, symptoms may worsen due to drug suppression of lower intrinsic pacemaker sites.[430]

Indications For Pacing

Pacing is indicated for symptomatic bradyarrhythmias that have no identifiable reversible cardiac or noncardiac cause.[410] Prophylactic pacing to prevent death or the onset of life-threatening symptoms is controversial, since increased risk of death is more likely related to the severity of underlying organic heart disease. The mortality benefits of pacing, though theoretically sound,

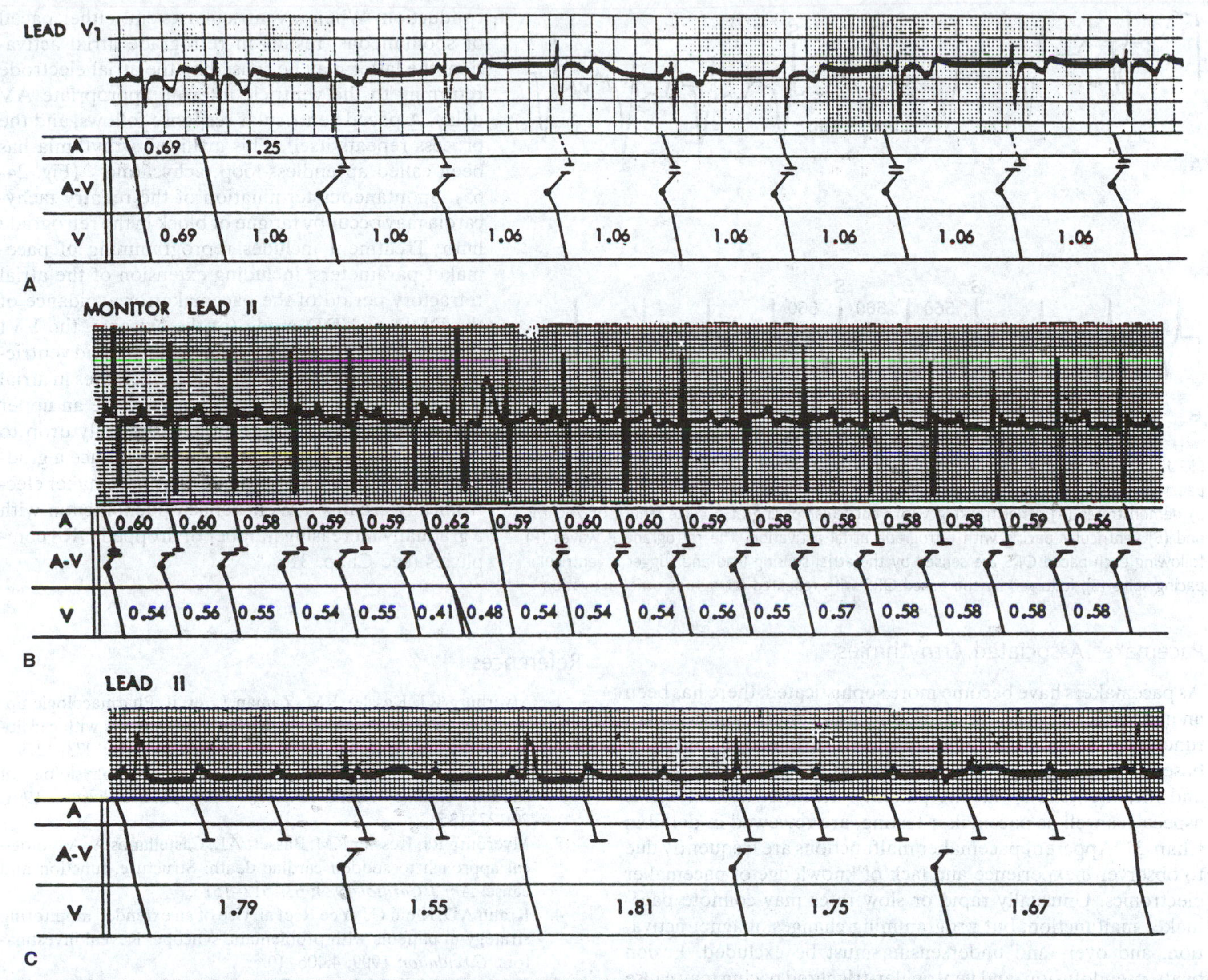

FIGURE 24-64 AV dissociation *A*. Sinus arrhythmia. The bradycardic phase enables the AV node to escape, with resulting dissociation. *B*. AV tachycardia. The tachycardia enables the AV pacemaker to usurp control of the ventricles, with resulting dissociation; the seventh and eighth beats are ventricular captures, the seventh, ending the shorter cycle, showing ventricular aberration. *C*. High-grade AV block permits the AV node to escape (second, fourth, and fifth beats), with resulting dissociation.

often lack rigorous proof of effectiveness. Less controversial is the use of permanent pacing for morbidity benefit, namely, to reduce symptomatic bradyarrhythmic events and their consequences (see also Chap. 31).

Temporary pacing is indicated for AV block associated with acute anterior wall infarction if the heart rate is excessively slow and/or associated with rate-dependent hypotension, and if there is a newly acquired left or right bundle-branch block accompanied by hemiblock.[431] The availability of external pacing techniques[349,350] has tended to relax the sense of urgency for prophylactic pacing catheters in these settings. New left bundle-branch block or preexisting right or left bundle-branch block is managed with less immediate urgency and often does not require pacing. Permanent pacing is often recommended for those with acute anterior wall infarction who have had transient complete heart block.[432] The change in long-term survival, however, is not well documented.[433] Temporary pacing can often be avoided in AV block associated with inferior infarction, since block is often related to ischemia or parasympathetic reflexes, is usually asymptomatic, and reverses with time.[434] If hypotension occurs in inferior infarction that is not due to hypovolemia or right ventricular infarct, temporary pacing for severe sinus bradycardia or higher grades of AV block is often used. Permanent pacing after AV block in inferior infarction is required only very rarely.

Permanent prophylactic pacing in bifascicular block without symptoms of transient AV block is not routinely recommended.[435,436] In patients at high risk for complete heart block (e.g., Kearns-Sayre syndrome) or recurrent neurologic symptoms associated with advanced HV prolongation (e.g., HV longer than 70 to 80 ms), however, prophylactic pacing may be of benefit.[437] Guidelines for permanent cardiac pacemaker implantation have been published[410] and are further discussed in Chap. 31.

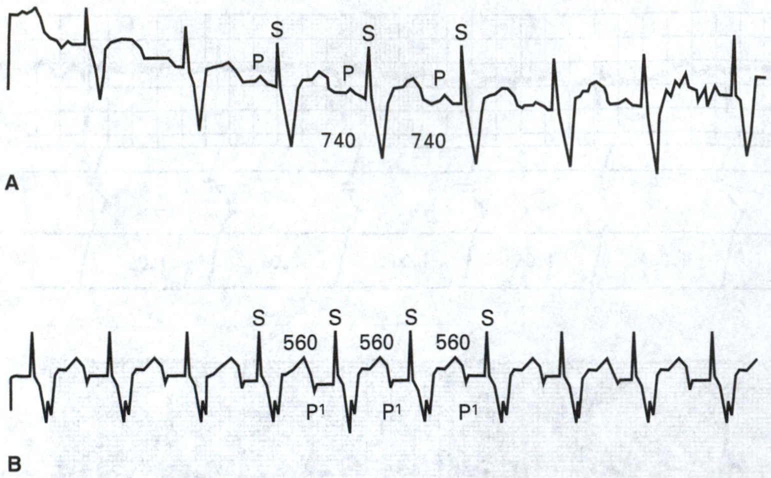

FIGURE 24-65 Pacemaker-mediated (endless-loop) tachycardia. The patient had a DDD pacemaker and presented with episodes of sustained rapid heart action. The tracing (lead II) demonstrates (*A*) atrial tracking with ventricular pacing at a cycle length of 740 ms and (*B*) ventricular pacing with retrograde atrial activation. The retrograde P waves (P) following each paced QRS are sensed by the atrial sensing lead and trigger a ventricular pacing spike (S), followed by the paced QRS with repeated retrograde atrial activation.

Pacemaker-Associated Arrhythmias

As pacemakers have become more sophisticated, there has been an increasing need to identify normal and abnormal pacemaker function and related arrhythmias electrocardiographically. The baseline pacing pattern is dependent on the pacemaker design and the interaction with the patient's intrinsic rhythm. These aspects, as well as pacemaker testing, are reviewed in detail in Chap. 31. Apparent pacemaker malfunctions are frequently due to observer inexperience and lack of knowledge of pacemaker electronics. Unusually rapid or slow rates may connote pacemaker malfunction, but programming changes, magnet activation, and over- and undersensing must be excluded. Fusion beats, pseudofusion, and ventricular-triggered pacing may cause confusion. Fusion beats occur when there is overlap in the timing of paced and normal beats and the morphology of the fused complex is midway between the normal and paced QRS complexes. Ventricular-triggered pacing becomes confusing when a PVC occurs and is thought to be triggered by the pacemaker because of the width of the complex and the presence of a pacemaker artifact. The pacing artifact occurs slightly after the initiation of the PVC, providing a clue to ventricular ectopy. Inappropriate bradycardias may be induced by oversensing by the pacemaker or by normal sensing of extracardiac stimuli, such as myopotentials (skeletal muscle activity) or extracorporeal inhibition by electromagnetic or RF waves. "Cross-talk" can result in arrhythmias, for instance, when the ventricular lead senses atrial activity.

Dual-chamber pacing may lead to a variety of arrhythmias that are actually an undesirable byproduct of normal pacemaker function. Arrhythmias may be initiated by asynchronous ventricular or atrial stimulation (DVI pacemakers), interruption of ventricular sensing during ventricular blanking (all dual-chamber pacemakers), or asynchronous atrial or ventricular stimulation in the magnet mode (all dual-chamber pacemakers). Furthermore, dual-chamber units create an artificial bypass tract that may become operative in the presence of ventriculoatrial conduction. When a ventricular event, either paced or spontaneous, results in retrograde atrial activation, the latter may be sensed by the atrial electrode returning to the ventricle after an appropriate AV delay. A paced ventricular response follows, and the process repeats itself. This artificial arrhythmia has been called an endless-loop tachycardia[438] (Fig. 24-65). Spontaneous termination of the reentry tachycardia may occur by fatigue or block in the retrograde limb. Treatment includes reprogramming of pacemaker parameters, including extension of the atrial refractory period of the pacemaker or avoidance of the DDD or VDD mode (at the extreme, the VVI mode is used). In order to guard against rapid ventricular pacing and response to sudden increases in atrial rate, physiologic pacemakers tend to have an upper rate limit control. Earlier models suddenly drop to 2:1 pacing rates. Recent models often induce a gradual Wenckebach-type response. The pacemaker electronically creates a Wenckebach phenomenon with a gradually increasing number of dropped QRS complexes (see Chap. 31).

References

1. Myerburg RJ, Kessler KM, Zaman L, et al. Pharmacologic approaches to management of arrhythmias in patients with cardiomyopathy and heart failure. *Am Heart J* 1987; 114:1273–1279.
2. Myerburg RJ, Kessler KM, Castellanos A. Pathophysiology of sudden cardiac death. *Pacing Clin Electrophysiol* 1991; 23:127–135.
3. Myerburg RJ, Kessler KM, Bassett AL, Castellanos A. A biological approach to sudden cardiac death: Structure, function and cause. *Am J Cardiol* 1989; 63:1512–1516.
4. Krahn AD, Klein GJ, Yee R, et al. Use of an extended monitoring strategy in patients with problematic syncope: Reveal investigators. *Circulation* 1999; 4:406–10.
5. Ranger S, Talajic M, Lemery R, et al. Amplification of flecainide-induced ventricular conduction slowing by exercise: A potentially significant clinical consequence of use-dependent sodium channel blockade. *Circulation* 1989; 79:1000–1006.
6. Rinne C, Klein GJ, Sharma AD, Yee R. Clinical usefulness of the 12-lead electrocardiogram in the Wolff-Parkinson-White syndrome. *Cardiol Clin* 1987; 5:499–509.
7. Breithardt G, Cain ME, El-Sherif N, et al. Standards for analysis of ventricular late potentials using high-resolution or signal-averaged electrocardiography: A statement by a task force committee of the European Study of Cardiology, the American Heart Association, and the American College of Cardiology. *J Am Coll Cardiol* 1991; 17:999–1006.
8. Kuchar DL, Thorburn CW, Sammel NL. Prediction of serious arrhythmic events after myocardial infarction: Signal-averaged electrocardiogram, Holter monitoring, and radionuclide ventriculography. *J Am Coll Cardiol* 1987; 9:531–538.
9. Kleiger RE, Miller JP, Bigger JT, Moss AJ. Decreased heart rate variability and its association with increased mortality after acute myocardial infarction. *Am J Cardiol* 1987; 59:256–262.
10. Huikuri HV, Valkama JO, Airaksinen KE, et al. Frequency domains measures of heart rate variability before the onset of nonsustained and sustained ventricular tachycardia in patients with coronary artery disease. *Circulation* 1993; 87:1220–1228.
11. La Rovere MT, Specchia G, Mortara A, Schwartz PJ. Baroreflex sensitivity, clinical correlates and cardiovascular mortality among

patients with first myocardial infarction: A prospective study. *Circulation* 1988; 78:816–824.
12. La Rovere MT, Bigger JT Jr, Marcus FI, et al. Baroreflex sensitivity and heart rate variability in prediction of total cardiac mortality after myocardial infarction. *Lancet* 1998; 351:478–484.
13. Gepstein L, Evans S. Electroanatomical mapping of the heart: Basic concepts and implications for the treatment of cardiac arrythmias. *PACE* 1998; 21(part II):638–648.
14. Schilling RJ, Peters NS, Davies DW. Mapping and ablation of ventricular tachycardia with the aid of a non-contact mapping system. *Heart* 1999; 81:570–575.
15. Task Force of the Working Group on Arrhythmias of the European Society of Cardiology. The Sicilian gambit: A new approach to the classification of antiarrhythmic drugs based on their actions on antiarrhythmogenic mechanisms. *Circulation* 1991; 84:1831–1851.
16. Bauernfeind RA, Amat-y-Leon F, Dhingra RC, et al. Chronic nonparoxysmal sinus tachycardia in otherwise healthy persons. *Ann Intern Med* 1979; 91:702–710.
17. Packer DL, Bardy GH, Worley SJ, et al. Tachycardia-induced cardiomyopathy: A reversible form of left ventricular dysfunction. *Am J Cardiol* 1986; 57:563–570.
18. Rodriguez LM, Smeets JL, Xie B, et al. Improvement in left ventricular function by ablation of atrioventricular nodal conduction in selected patients with lone atrial fibrillation. *Am J Cardiol* 1993; 72:1137–1141.
19. Lee RJ, Kalman JM, Fitzpatrick AP, et al. Radiofrequency catheter modification of the sinus node for "inappropriate" sinus tachycardia. *Circulation* 1995; 92:2919–2928.
20. Chen PS, Wu TJ, Ikeda T, et al. Focal source hypothesis of atrial fibrillation. *J Cardiovasc Electrophysiol* 1998; 31(suppl):32–34.
21. Echt DS, Liebson PR, Mitchell B, et al. Mortality and morbidity in patients receiving encainide, flecainide, or placebo: The Cardiac Arrhythmia Suppression Trial. *N Engl J Med* 1991; 324:781–788.
22. Akhtar M, Breithardt G, Camm AJ, et al. CAST and beyond: Implications of the Cardiac Arrhythmia Suppression Trial. *Circulation* 1990; 81:1123–1127.
23. DiMarco JP, Sellers TD, Lerman BB, et al. Diagnostic and therapeutic use of adenosine in patients with supraventricular tachyarrhythmias. *J Am Coll Cardiol* 1985; 6:417–425.
24. Rinkenberger RL, Prystowsky EN, Heger JJ, et al. Effects of intravenous and chronic oral verapamil administration in patients with supraventricular tachyarrhythmias. *Circulation* 1980; 62:996–1010.
25. Waxman HL, Myerburg RJ, Appel R, Sung RJ. Verapamil for control of ventricular rate in paroxysmal supraventricular tachycardia and atrial fibrillation or flutter. A double-blind randomized cross-over study. *Ann Intern Med* 1981; 94:1–6.
26. Stewart RB, Bardy GH, Greene LH. Wide complex tachycardia: Misdiagnosis and outcome after emergent therapy. *Ann Intern Med* 1986; 104:766–771.
27. Rozanski JJ, Zaman L, Castellanos A. Electrophysiologic effects of diltiazem hydrochloride in supraventricular tachycardia. *Am J Cardiol* 1982; 49:621–628.
28. Betriu A, Chaitman BR, Bourassa MG, et al. Beneficial effect of intravenous diltiazem in the acute management of paroxysmal supraventricular tachyarrhythmias. *Circulation* 1983; 67:88–94.
29. Wu D, Denes P, Dhingra R, et al. The effects of propranolol on induction of A-V nodal reentrant paroxysmal tachycardia. *Circulation* 1974; 50:665–677.
30. Wu D, Hung JS, Kuo CT, et al. Effects of quinidine on atrioventricular nodal reentrant paroxysmal tachycardia. *Circulation* 1981; 64:823–831.
31. Lee MA, Morady F, Kadish A, et al. Catheter modification of the atrioventricular junction with radiofrequency energy for control of atrioventricular nodal reentry tachycardia. *Circulation* 1991; 83:827–835.
32. Calkins H, Sousa J, El-Atassi R, et al. Diagnosis and cure of the Wolff-Parkinson-White syndrome or paroxysmal supraventricular tachycardias during a single electrophysiologic test. *N Engl J Med* 1991; 324:1612–1618.
33. Myerburg RJ, Cox MM, Interian A Jr, et al. Cycling of inducibility of paroxysmal supraventricular tachycardia in women and its implications for timing of electrophysiologic procedures. *Am J Cardiol* 1999; 83:1049–1054.
34. Ross DL, Johnson DC, Denniss AR, et al. Curvative surgery for atrioventricular junctional ("A-V nodal") reentrant tachycardia. *J Am Coll Cardiol* 1985; 6:1383–1392.
35. Sung RJ, Castellanos A, Gelband H, Myerburg RJ. Mechanisms of reciprocating tachycardia initiated during sinus rhythm in concealed Wolff-Parkinson-White syndrome. *Circulation* 1976; 54:338–344.
36. Lee SH, Chen SA, Wu TJ, et al. Effects of pregnancy on first onset and symptoms of paroxysmal supraventricular tachycardia. *Am J Cardiol* 1995; 76:675–678.
37. Klein GT, Yee R, Sharma AD. Longitudinal electrophysiologic assessment of asymptomatic patients with the Wolff-Parkinson-White electrocardiographic pattern. *N Engl J Med* 1989; 320: 1229–1233.
38. Wellens HJJ. Wolff-Parkinson-White syndrome: I. Diagnosis, arrhythmias and identification of the high risk patient. *Mod Concepts Cardiovasc Dis* 1983; 52:53–56.
39. Vidaillet HJ Jr, Pressley JC, Henke E, et al. Familial occurrence of accessory A-V pathways (preexcitation syndrome). *N Engl J Med* 1987; 317:65–69.
40. Arruda MS, McClelland JH, Wang X, et al. Development and validation of an ECG algorithm for identifying accessory pathway ablation site in Wolff-Parkinson-White syndrome. *J Cardiovasc Electrophysiol* 1998; 9:2–12.
41. Xie B, Heald SC, Bashir Y, et al. Localization of accessory pathways from the 12-lead electrocardiogram using a new algorithm. *Am J Cardiol* 1994; 74:161–165.
42. Sung RJ, Castellanos A, Mallon SM, et al. Mechanisms of spontaneous alteration between reciprocating tachycardia and atrial flutter-fibrillation in the Wolff-Parkinson-White syndrome. *Circulation* 1977; 56:409–415.
43. Gulamhusein S, Ko P, Carruthers SG, Klein GJ. Acceleration of the ventricular response during atrial fibrillation in the Wolff-Parkinson-White syndrome after verapamil. *Circulation* 1982; 65:348–354.
44. McGovern B, Garan H, Ruskin JN. Precipitation of cardiac arrest by verapamil in patients with Wolff-Parkinson-White syndrome. *Ann Intern Med* 1986; 104:791–794.
45. Akhtar M, Gilbert CJ, Shenasa M. Effect of lidocaine on atrioventricular response via the accessory pathway in patients with Wolff-Parkinson-White syndrome. *Circulation* 1981; 63:435–441.
46. Wellens HJJ, Durrer D. Effect of digitalis on atrioventricular conduction and circus movement tachycardias in patients with Wolff-Parkinson-White syndrome. *Circulation* 1973; 47:1229–1233.
47. Sellers TD, Bashore TM, Gallagher JJ. Digitalis in the preexcitation syndrome: Analysis during atrial fibrillation. *Circulation* 1977; 56:260–267.
48. Jackman WM, Wang X, Friday KJ, et al. Catheter ablation of accessory atrioventricular pathways (Wolff-Parkinson-White syndrome by radiofrequency current. *N Engl J Med* 1991; 324:1605–1611.
49. Guiraudon GM, Guiraudon CM, Klein GJ, et al. Operation for the Wolff-Parkinson-White syndrome in the catheter ablation era. *Ann Thorac Surg* 1994; 57:1084–1088.
50. Josephson ME, Wellens HJJ. Electrophysiologic evaluation of supraventricular tachycardia. *Cardiol Clin* 1997; 15:567–586.
51. Prystowsky EN. Indications for intracardiac electrophysiologic studies in patients with supraventricular tachycardia. *Circulation* 1987; 75(suppl III):III119–III122.

52. Klein GJ, Bashore TM, Sellers TD, et al. Ventricular fibrillation in the Wolff-Parkinson-White syndrome. *N Engl J Med* 1979; 301:1080–1085.
53. Castellanos A, Myerburg RJ. Changing perspectives in the preexcitation syndromes. *N Engl J Med* 1987; 317:109–111.
54. Scheinman MM. Catheter ablation for patients with ventricular preexcitation syndromes. In: Benditt DG, Benson DW, eds. *Cardiac Preexcitation Syndromes*. Boston: Martinus Nijhoff; 1986:493.
55. Cox JL, Cain ME. Surgery for preexcitation syndromes. In: Benditt DG, Benson DW, eds. *Cardiac Preexcitation Syndromes*. Boston: Martinus Nijhoff; 1986:527.
56. Guiraudon GM, Klein GJ, Sharma AD, et al. Surgery for Wolff-Parkinson-White syndrome: Further experience with an epicardial approach. *Circulation* 1986; 74:525–529.
57. Camm J, Hellestrand KJ, Nathan AW, Bexton RS. Clinical usefulness of flecainide acetate in the treatment of paroxysmal supraventricular arrhythmias. *Drugs* 1985; 29:7–13.
58. Prystowsky EN, Klein G, Rinkenberger RL, et al. Clinical efficacy and electrophysiologic effects of encainice in patients with Wolff-Parkinson-White syndrome. *Circulation* 1984; 69:278–287.
59. Fogoros RN, Anderson KP, Winkle RA, et al. Amiodarone: Clinical efficacy and toxicity in 96 patients with recurrent drug refractory arrhythmias. *Circulation* 1983; 68:88–94.
60. Breithardt G, Borggrefe M, Wiebringhaus E, Seipel L. Effect of propafenone in the Wolff-Parkinson-White syndrome: Electrophysiologic findings and long term follow-up. *Am J Cardiol* 1984; 54:29D–39D.
61. Pritchett EL, DaTorre SD, Platt ML, et al. Flecainide acetate treatment of paroxysmal supraventricular tachycardia and paroxysmal atrial fibrillation: Dose-response studies. *J Am Coll Cardiol* 1991; 17:297–303.
62. Neuss H, Schlepper M, Thormann J. Analysis of reentry mechanisms in the three patients with concealed Wolff-Parkinson-White syndrome. *Circulation* 1975; 51:75–81.
63. Wu D, Amat-y-Leon F, Denes P, et al. Demonstration of sustained sinus and atrial reentry as a mechanism of paroxysmal supraventricular tachycardia. *Circulation* 1975; 51:234–243.
64. Wu D, Denes P, Amat-y-Leon F, et al. Clinical electrocardiographic and electrophysiologic observations in patients with paroxysmal supraventricular tachycardia. *Am J Cardiol* 1978; 41:1045–1051.
65. Coumel P, Flammang D, Attuel P, Leclercq JF. Sustained intra-atrial reentrant tachycardia: Electrophysiologic study of 20 cases. *Clin Cardiol* 1979; 2:167–178.
66. Gallagher JJ, Smith WM, Kassell JH, et al. Role of Mahaim fibers in cardiac arrhythmias in man. *Circulation* 1981; 64:176–189.
67. Cox JL. The status of surgery for cardiac arrhythmias. *Circulation* 1985; 71:413–417.
68. Allessie MA, Bonke FIM, Schopman FJG. Circus movement in rabbit atrial muscle as a mechanism of tachycardia: III. The "leading circle" concept: A new model of circus movement in cardiac tissue without the involvement of an anatomical obstacle. *Circ Res* 1977; 41:9–18.
69. Gelband H, Bush HL, Rosen MR, et al. Electrophysiologic properties of isolated preparations of human atrial myocardium. *Circ Res* 1972; 30:290–300.
70. Mary-Rabine L, Hordof AJ, Danilo P Jr, et al. Mechanisms for impulse initiation in isolated human atrial fibers. *Circ Res* 1980; 47:267–277.
71. Lesh MD, Kalman JM, Saxon LA, Dorostkar PC. Electrophysiology of "incisional" reentrant atrial tachycardia complicating surgery for congenital heart disease. *Pacing Clin Electrophysiol* 1997; 20:2107–2111.
72. Poty H, Saoudi N, Haissaguerre M, et al. Radiofrequency catheter ablation of atrial tachycardias. *Am Heart J* 1996; 131:481–489.
73. Shine KI, Kastor JA, Yurchak PM. Multifocal atrial tachycardia: Clinical and electrocardiographic features in 32 patients. *N Engl J Med* 1968; 279:344–349.
74. Salerno DM, Anderson B, Sharkey PJ, Iber C. Intravenous verapamil for treatment of multifocal atrial tachycardia with and without calcium pretreatment. *Ann Intern Med* 1987; 107: 623–628.
75. Wang K, Goldfarb JL, Gobel F, Richman HG. Multifocal atrial tachycardia. *Arch Intern Med* 1977; 137:161–164.
76. Fosmoe RJ, Averill KH, Lamb LE. Electrocardiographic findings in 67,375 asymptomatic subjects: II. Supraventricular arrhythmias. *Am J Cardiol* 1960; 6:84–95.
77. Garson A, Bink-Boelkens M, Hesslein PS, et al. Atrial flutter in the young: A collaborative study of 380 cases. *J Am Coll Cardiol* 1985; 6:871–878.
78. Waldo AL, Henthorn RW, Plumb VJ. Atrial flutter: Recent observations in man. In: Josephson ME, Wellens HJJ, eds. *Tachycardias: Mechanisms, Diagnosis, Treatment*. Philadelphia: Lea & Febiger; 1982:113.
79. Olgin JE, Kalman JM, Lesh MD. Conduction barriers in human atrial flutter: Correlation of electrophysiology and anatomy. *J Cardiovasc Electrophysiol* 1996; 7:1112–1126.
80. Slama R, Leclercq JF, Rosengarten M, et al. Multilevel block in the atrioventricular node during atrial tachycardia and flutter alternating with Wenckebach phenomenon. *Br Heart J* 1979; 42:463–470.
81. el-Harari MB, Adams PC. Atrial flutter with 1:1 atrioventricular conduction caused by propafenone. *Pacing Clin Electrophysiol* 1998; 21:1999–2001.
82. Robertson CE, Miller HC. Extreme tachycardia complicating the use of disopyramide in atrial flutter. *Br Heart J* 1980; 44:602–603.
83. Waldo AL, MacLean WH, Karp RP, et al. Entrainment and interruption of atrial flutter with atrial pacing: Studies in man following open heart surgery. *Circulation* 1977; 56:737–745.
84. Camm J, Ward D, Spurrell R. Response of atrial flutter to overdrive atrial pacing and intravenous disopyramide phosphate, singly and in combination. *Br Heart J* 1980; 44:240–247.
85. Olgin JE, Lesh MD. The laboratory evaluation and role of catheter ablation for patients with atrial flutter. *Cardiol Clin* 1997; 15:677–690.
86. Ellenbogen KA, Stambler BS, Wood MA, et al. Efficacy of intravenous ibutelide for rapid termination of atrial fibrillation and atrial flutter: A dose-response study. *J Am Coll Cardiol* 1996; 28:130–136.
87. Waldo AL, Mackall JA, Biblo LA. Mechanisms and medical management of patients with atrial flutter. *Cardiol Clin* 1997; 15:661–676.
88. Saxon LA, Kalman JM, Olgin JE, et al. Results of radiofrequency catheter ablation for atrial flutter. [review]. *Am J Cardiol* 1996; 77:1014–1016.
89. Benditt DG, Pritchett EL, Gallagher JJ. Spectrum of regular tachycardias with wide QRS complexes in patients with accessory atrioventricular pathways. *Am J Cardiol* 1978; 42:828–838.
90. Wood KA, Eisenberg SJ, Kalman JM, et al. Risk of thromboembolism in chronic atrial flutter. *Am J Cardiol* 1997; 79:1043–1047.
91. Waldo AL. Atrial flutter: Mechanisms, clinical features, and management. In: Zipes DP, Jalife J, eds. *Cardiac Electrophysiology: From Cell to Bedside*, 3d ed. Philadelphia: Saunders; 1999:468.
92. Seidl K, Hauer B, Schwick NG, et al. Risk of thromboembolic events in patients with atrial flutter. *Am J Cardiol* 1998; 82:580–583.
93. Dunn MI. Thrombolism with atrial flutter *Am J Cardiol* 1998; 82:638.
94. Cairns JA, Connolly ST. Nonrheumatic atrial fibrillation: Risk of stroke and role of antithrombotic therapy. *Circulation* 1991; 84:469–481.
95. Hwang C, Karagueuzian HS, Chen PS. Idiopathic paroxysmal atrial fibrillation induced by a focal discharge mechanism in the

left superior pulmonary vein: Possible roles of the ligament of Marshall. *J Cardiovasc Electrophysiol* 1999; 10:636–648.

96. Shrier A, Dubarsky H, Rosengarten M, et al. Prediction of complex atrioventricular conduction rhythms in humans with use of the atrioventricular nodal recovery curve. *Circulation* 1987; 76:1196–1205.
97. Gouaux JL, Ashman R. Auricular fibrillation with aberration simulating ventricular paroxysmal tachycardia. *Am Heart J* 1947; 34:366–373.
98. Marriott HJL, Sandler LA. Criteria, old and new, for differentiating between ectopic ventricular beats and aberrant ventricular conduction in the presence of atrial fibrillation. *Prog Cardiovasc Dis* 1966; 9:18–28.
99. Kopecky SL, Gersh BJ, McGoon MD, et al. The natural history of lone atrial fibrillation: A population-based study over three decades. *N Engl J Med* 1987; 317:669–674.
100. Gajewski J, Singer RB. Mortality in an insured population with atrial fibrillation. *JAMA* 1981; 245:1540–1544.
101. Morris JM, Peter RH, Mcintosh HD. Electrical conversion of atrial fibrillation: Immediate and long-term results and selection of patients. *Ann Intern Med* 1966; 65:216–231.
102. Mancini GBJ, Goldberger AL. Cardioversion of atrial fibrillation: Consideration of embolization, anticoagulation, prophylactic pacemaker and long-term success. *Am Heart J* 1982; 104:617–621.
103. Van Gelder IC, Crijns HJ, Van Gilst WH, et al. Prediction of uneventful cardioversion and maintenance of sinus rhythm from direct-current electrical cardioversion of chronic atrial fibrillation and flutter. *Am J Cardiol* 1991; 68:41–46.
104. Danias PG, Caulfield TA, Weigner MJ, et al. Likelihood of spontaneous conversion of atrial fibrillation to sinus rhythm. *J Am Coll Cardiol* 1998; 31:588–592.
105. Fenster PE, Comess KA, Marsh R, et al. Conversion of atrial fibrillation to sinus rhythm by acute intravenous procainamide infusion. *Am Heart J* 1983; 106:501–504.
106. Prystowsky EN, Benson DW Jr, Fuster V, et al. Management of patients with atrial fibrillation: A statement for health care professionals from the subcommittee on electrocardiography and electrophysiology of the American Heart Association. *Circulation* 1996; 93:1262–1277.
107. Suttorp MJ, Kingma JH, Jessurun ER, et al. The value of class IC antiarrhythmic drugs for acute conversion of paroxysmal atrial fibrillation or flutter to sinus rhythm. *J Am Coll Cardiol* 1990; 16:1722–1727.
108. Capucci A, Villani GQ, Aschieri D, Piepoli M. Safety of oral propafenone in the conversion of recent onset atrial fibrillation to sinus rhythm: A prospective parallel placebo-controlled multicentre study. *Int J Cardiol* 1999; 68:187–196.
109. Capucci A, Lenzi T, Boriani G, et al. Effectiveness of loading oral flecainide for converting recent-onset atrial fibrillation to sinus rhythm in patients without organic heart disease or with only systemic hypertension. *Am J Cardiol* 1992; 70:69–72.
110. Capucci A, Villani GQ, Piepoli MF, Aschieri D. The role of oral 1C antiarrhythmic drugs in terminating atrial fibrillation. *Curr Opin Cardiol* 1999; 14:4–8.
111. Klein HO, Kaplinsky E. Verapamil and digoxin: Their respective effects on atrial fibrillation and their interaction. *Am J Cardiol* 1982; 50:894–902.
112. Dunn M, Alexandre J, DeSilva R, Hildner F. Antithrombotic therapy in atrial fibrillation. *Chest* 1986; 89:68s–73s.
113. Wijffels MCEF, Kirchhof CJHJ, Dorland R, Allessie MA. Atrial fibrillation begets atrial fibrillation: A study in awake chronically instrumented goats. *Circulation* 1995; 92:1954–1968.
114. Allessie MA, Konings K, Kirchhof CJHJ, Wijffels M. Electrophysiologic mechanisms of perpetuation of atrial fibrillation. *Am J Cardiol* 1996; 77:10A–23A.
115. Takahashi N, Seki A, Imataka K, Fuji J. Clinical features of paroxysmal atrial fibrillation: An observation of 94 patients. *Jpn Heart J* 1981; 22:143–149.
116. Leung DY, Davidson PM, Cranney GB, Walsh WF. Thromboembolic risks of left atrial thrombus detected by transesophageal echocardiogram. *Am J Cardiol* 1997; 79:626–629.
117. Manning WJ, Silverman DI. Cardioversion of atrial fibrillation. *N Engl J* Med 1999; 341:1313.
118. Manning WJ, Douglas PS. Transesophageal echocardiography and atrial fibrillation: Added value or expensive toy? *Ann Intern Med* 1998; 128:685–687.
119. Berns E, Rinkenberger RL, Jeang MK, et al. Efficacy and safety of flecainide acetate for atrial tachycardia or fibrillation. *Am J Cardiol* 1987; 59:1337–1341.
120. The d,1 Sotalol Afib/Afl Study Group. Efficacy, safety and dose-response study of d,1 sotalol (Betapace) for prevention of recurrence of atrial fibrillation and atrial flutter [abstract]. *PACE* 1998; 21:812.
121. Deedwania PC, Singh BN, Ellenbogen K, et al. Spontaneous conversion and maintenance of sinus rhythm by amiodarone in patients with heart failure and atrial fibrillation: Observations from the Veterans Affairs Congestive Heart Failure Trial of Antiarrhythmic Therapy (CHF-STAT). *Circulation* 1998; 98:2574–2579.
122. Torp-Pedersen C, Moller M, Bloch-Thomsen PE, et al. Dofetilide in patients with congestive heart failure and left ventricular dysfunction: Danish Investigations of Arrhythmia and Mortality on Dofetilide Study Group. *N Engl J Med* 1999; 341:857–865.
123. Camm AJ, Karam R, Pratt CM. The azimilide post-infarct survival evaluation (ALIVE) trial. *Am J Cardiol* 1998; 81: 35D–39D.
124. Waldo AL. Management of atrial fibrillation: The need for AFFIRMative action. AFFIRM Investigators. Atrial Fibrillation Follow-up Investigation of Rhythm Management. *Am J Cardiol* 1999; 84:698–700.
125. Morady E, Calkins H, Langberg JJ, et al. A prospective randomized comparison of direct current and radiofrequency ablation of the atrioventricular junction. *J Am Coll Cardiol* 1993; 21:102–109.
126. Leitch JM, Klein G, Yee R, Guiraudon G. Sinus node-atrioventricular node isolation: Long-term results with the "corridor" operation for atrial fibrillation. *J Am Coll Cardiol* 1991; 17:970–975.
127. Sundt TM 3d, Camillo CJ, Cox JL. The maze procedure for cure of atrial fibrillation. *Cardiol Clin* 1997; 15:739–748.
128. Timmermans C, Rodriguez LM, Ayers GM, et al. Design and preliminary data of the Metrix Atrioverter Expanded Indication Trial. *J Interv Card Electrophysiol* 2000; 4(suppl 1):197–199.
129. Jung W, Wolpert C, Esmailzadeh B, et al. Clinical experience with implantable atrial and combined atrioventricular defibrillators. *J Interv Card Electrophysiol* 2000; 4(suppl 1):185–195.
130. Fitts SM, Hill MR, Mehra R, et al. Design and implementation of the Dual Site Atrial Pacing to Prevent Atrial Fibrillation (DAPPAF) clinical trial: DAPPAF Phase 1 Investigators. *J Interv Card Electrophysiol* 1998; 2(2):139–144.
131. Swartz JF, Pellersels C, Silvers, J, et al. A catheter-based curative approach to atrial fibrillation in humans [abstr]. *Circulation* 1994; 90(suppl I):I-335.
132. Jais P, Haissaguerre M, Shah DC, et al. A focal source of atrial fibrillation treated by discrete radiofrequency ablation [see comments]. *Circulation* 1997; 95:572–576.
133. Chen PS, Athill CA, Wu TJ, et al. Mechanisms of atrial fibrillation and flutter and implications for management. *Am J Cardiol* 1999; 84(9A):125R–130R.
134. Wolf PA, Dawber TR, Thomas HE. Epidemiologic assessment of chronic atrial fibrillation and risk of stroke: The Framingham study. *Neurology* 1978; 28:973–977.
135. Wolf PA, Kannel WB, McGee DL, et al. Duration of atrial

fibrillation and imminence of stroke: The Framingham study. *Stroke* 1983; 14:664–667.
136. Kannel WB, Abbott RD, Savage DD, McNamara PM. Epidemiologic features of chronic atrial fibrillation. *N Engl J Med* 1982; 306:1018–1022.
137. Staffurth JS, Gibberd MC. Arterial embolism in thyrotoxicosis with atrial fibrillation. *Br Med J* 1977; 2:688–690.
138. Brand FN, Abbott RD, Kannel WB, Wolf PA. Characteristics and prognosis of lone atrial fibrillation. *JAMA* 1985; 254:3449–3453.
139. Wolf PA, Abbott RD, Kannel WB. Atrial fibrillation: A major contributor to stroke in the elderly: The Framingham study. *Arch Intern Med* 1987; 147:1561–1564.
140. Lown B. Electrical reversion of cardiac arrhythmias. *Br Heart J* 1967; 29:469–489.
141. Resenkov L, McDonald I. Complications in 220 patients with cardiac dysrhythmias treated by phased direct current shock and indications for electrocardioversion. *Br Heart J* 1967; 29: 926–936.
142. Bjerkelund CJ, Orning OM. The efficacy of anticoagulant therapy in preventing embolism related to DC electrical conversion of atrial fibrillation. *Am J Cardiol* 1969; 23:208–216.
143. Laupacis A, Albergs G, Dalen J, et al. American College of Chest Physicians recommendations for anticoagulation for patients with atrial fibrillation: Antithrombotic therapy in atrial fibrillation. *Chest* 1995; 108:3525–3595.
144. Stroke Prevention in Atrial Fibrillation Investigators. Stroke prevention in atrial fibrillation study: Final results. *Circulation* 1991; 84:527–539.
145. Connolly SJ, Laupacis A, Gent M, et al. Canadian atrial fibrillation anticoagulation (CAFA) study. *J Am Coll Cardiol* 1991; 18:349–355.
146. Peterson P, Boysen G, Godtfredsen J, et al. Placebo-controlled, randomized trial of warfarin and aspirin for prevention of thromboembolic complications in chronic atrial fibrillation: The Copenhagen AFASAK study. *Lancet* 1989; 1:175–179.
147. Boston Area Anticoagulation Trial in Atrial Fibrillation Investigators. The effect of low-dose warfarin on the risk of stroke in patients with non-rheumatic atrial fibrillation. *N Engl J Med* 1990; 323:1505–1511.
148. Stroke Prevention in Atrial Fibrillation Investigators. Adjusted-dose warfarin versus low-intensity, fixed-dose warfarin plus aspirin for high-risk patients with atrial fibrillation: Stroke Prevention and Atrial Fibrillation III randomized clinical trial. *Lancet* 1996; 348:633–638.
149. Forfar JC. A 7-year analysis of haemorrhage in patients on long-term anticoagulant treatment. *Br Heart J* 1979; 42:128–132.
150. European Atrial Fibrillation Trial Study Group. Optimal oral anticoagulant therapy in patients with nonrheumatic atrial fibrillation and recent cerebral ischemia. *N Engl J Med* 1995;33:5–10.
151. Whisnant JP, Cartlidge NEF, Elveback LR. Carotid and vertebral-basilar transient ischemic attacks: Effect of anticoagulants, hypertension, and cardiac disorders on survival and stroke occurrence—a population study. *Ann Neurol* 1978; 3:107–115.
152. Hoffman BF, Rosen MR. Cellular mechanisms for cardiac arrhythmias. *Circ Res* 1981; 43:1–15.
153. Friedman PL, Stewart JR, Wit AL. Spontaneous and induced cardiac arrhythmias in subendocardial Purkinje fibers surviving extensive myocardial infarction in dogs. *Circ Res* 1973; 33:612–626.
154. Rosen MR, Fisch C, Hoffman BF, et al. Can accelerated atrioventricular junctional escape rhythms be explained by delayed afterdepolarizations? *Am J Cardiol* 1980; 45:1272–1284.
155. Sclarowsky S, Strasberg B, Fuchs J, et al: Multiform accelerated idioventricular rhythm in acute myocardial infarction: Electrocardiographic characteristics and response to verapamil. *Am J Cardiol* 1983; 52:43–47.
156. deSoyza N, Bissett JK, Kane JJ, et al. Association of accelerated idioventricular rhythm and paroxysmal ventricular tachycardia in acute myocardial infarction. *Am J Cardiol* 1974; 34:667–670.
157. Garson A, Gillette PC. Junctional ectopic tachycardia in children: Electrocardiography, electrophysiology and pharmacologic response. *Am J Cardiol* 1979; 44:298–302.
158. Gillette PC, Garson A, Porter J, et al. Junctional automatic ectopic tachycardia: New proposed treatment of transcatheter His bundle ablation. *Am Heart J* 1983; 106:619–623.
159. Green M, Heddle B, Dassen W, et al. Value of QRS alternation in determining the site of origin of narrow QRS supraventricular tachycardia. *Circulation* 1983; 68:368–373.
160. Brugada P, Bar FWHM, Vanagt EJ, et al. Observations in patients showing A-V junctional echoes with a shorter P-R than R-P interval: Distinction between intranodal reentry and reentry using an accessory pathway with a long conduction time. *Am J Cardiol* 1981; 48:611–622.
161. Brugada P, Farre H, Green M, et al. Observations in patients with supraventricular tachycardia having a P-R interval shorter than the R-P interval: Differentiation between atrial tachycardia and reciprocating atrioventricular tachycardia using an accessory pathway with long conduction times. *Am Heart J* 1984; 107:556–570.
162. Perry JC, McQuinn RL, Smith RT, et al. Flecainide acetate for resistant arrhythmias in the young: Efficacy and pharmacokinetics. *J Am Coll Cardiol* 1989; 14:185–191.
163. Velebit V, Podrid P, Lown B, et al. Aggravation and provocation of ventricular arrhythmia by antiarrhythmic drugs. *Circulation* 1982; 65:886–894.
164. Ruskin JN, McGovern B, Garan H, et al. Antiarrhythmic drugs: A possible cause of out-of-hospital cardiac arrest. *N Engl J Med* 1983; 309:1302–1306.
165. Starmer CF, Lastra AA, Nesterenko VV, Grant AO. Proarrhythmic response to sodium channel blockade: Theoretical model and numerical experiments. *Circulation* 1991; 84:1364–1377.
166. Waldo AL, Camm AJ, deRuyter H, et al. Effect of D-sotalol on mortality in patients with left ventricular dysfunction after recent and remote myocardial infarction: The SWORD Investigators, Survival with Oral D-Sotalol. *Lancet* 1996; 348:7–12. Published erratum appears in *Lancet* 1996; 348:416.
167. Myerburg RJ, Kessler KM, Luceri RFM, et al. Classification of ventricular arrhythmias based on parallel hierarchies of frequency and form. *Am J Cardiol* 1984; 54:1355–1358.
168. Moss AJ, Schnitzler R, Green R, DeCamilla J. Ventricular arrhythmias 3 weeks after acute myocardial infarction. *Ann Intern Med* 1971; 75:837–841.
169. Vismara LA, Amsterdam BA, Mason DT. Relation of ventricular arrhythmias in the late-hospital phase of acute myocardial infarction to sudden death after hospital discharge. *Am J Med* 1975; 59:6–12.
170. Ruberman W, Weinblatt E, Goldberg JD, et al. Ventricular premature complexes and sudden death after myocardial infarction. *Circulation* 1981; 64:297–305.
171. Schulze RA, Strauss HW, Pitt B. Sudden death in the year following myocardial infarction: Relationship of ventricular premature contractions in the late hospital phase and left ventricular ejection fraction. *Am J Med* 1977; 62:192–199.
172. Bigger JT, Fleiss JL, Kleiger R, et al. The relationships among ventricular arrhythmias, left ventricular dysfunction, and mortality in the 2 years after myocardial infarction. *Circulation* 1984; 69:250–258.
173. Bigger JT Jr. Current approaches to drug treatment of ventricular arrhythmias. *Am J Cardiol* 1987; 60:10F–20F.
174. Kessler KM, McAuliff D, Chakko S, et al. Multiform ventricular complexes: A transitional arrhythmia form? *Am Heart J* 1989; 118:441–444.
175. Castellanos A, Luceri RM, Moleiro F, et al. Annihilation, entrain-

ment and modulation of ventricular parasystolic rhythms. *Am J Cardiol* 1984; 54:17–322.

176. Kennedy HL, Whitlock JA, Sprague MK, et al. Long-term follow-up of asymptomatic healthy subjects with frequent and complex ventricular ectopy. *N Engl J Med* 1985; 313:193–197.
177. Winkle RA. The relationship between ventricular ectopic beat frequency and heart rate. *Circulation* 1982; 66:439–446.
178. Kostis JB, McCrone K, Moreyra AE, et al. Premature ventricular complexes in the absence of identifiable heart disease. *Circulation* 1981; 63:1351–1356.
179. Campbell RWF, Godman MG, Fiddler GI, et al. Ventricular arrhythmias in the syndrome of balloon deformity of mitral valve: Definition of possible high risk group. *Br Heart J* 1976; 38:1053–1057.
180. Pocock WA, Bosman CK, Chesler E, et al. Sudden death in primary mitral valve prolapse. *Am Heart J* 1984; 107:378–382.
181. Nishimura RA, McGoon MD, Shub C, et al. Echocardiographically documented mitral valve prolapse: Long-term follow-up of 237 patients. *N Engl J Med* 1985; 313:1305–1309.
182. Lown B, Fakhro AM, Hood WB, Thorn GW. The coronary care unit: New perspectives and directions. *JAMA* 1967; 199:156–166.
183. El-Sherif N, Myerburg RJ, Scherlag BJ, et al. Electrocardiographic antecedents of primary ventricular fibrillation: Value of the R-on-T phenomenon in myocardial infarction. *Br Heart J* 1976; 38:415–422.
184. DeSozya N, Meacham D, Murphy ML, et al. Evaluation of warning arrhythmias before paroxysmal ventricular tachycardia during acute myocardial infarction in man. *Circulation* 1979; 60:814–818.
185. Wyman MG, Hammersmith L. Comprehensive treatment plan for the prevention of primary ventricular fibrillation in acute myocardial infarction. *Am J Cardiol* 1974; 33:661–667.
186. Lie KI, Wellens HJJ, Van Capelli FJ. Lidocaine in the prevention of primary ventricular fibrillation: A double-blind randomized study of 212 consecutive patients. *N Engl J Med* 1974; 291:1324–1326.
187. Routledge PA, Stargel WW, Wagner GS, Shand DG. Increased alpha-1-acid glycoprotein and lidocaine distribution in myocardial infarction. *Ann Intern Med* 1980; 293:701–704.
188. LeLorier J, Genon D, Latour Y. Pharmacokinetics of lidocaine after prolonged intravenous infusions in uncomplicated myocardial infarction. *Ann Intern Med* 1977; 87:700–702.
189. Maseri A, Severi S, Marzulio P. Role of coronary arterial spasm in sudden coronary ischemic death. *Ann NY Acad Sci* 1982; 382:204–217.
190. Tzivoni D, Keren A, Granot H, et al. Ventricular fibrillation caused by myocardial reperfusion in Prinzmetal's angina. *Am Heart J* 1983; 105:323–325.
191. Myerburg RJ, Kessler KM, Mallon SM, et al. Life-threatening ventricular arrhythmias in patients with silent myocardial ischemia due to coronary artery spasm. *N Engl J Med* 1992; 326:1451–1455.
192. Kimura S, Bassett AL, Saoudi NC, et al. Cellular electrophysiologic changes and "arrhythmias" during experimental ischemia and reperfusion in isolated cat ventricular myocardium. *J Am Coll Cardiol* 1986; 7:833–841.
193. Furukawa T, Bassett AL, Furukawa N, et al. The ionic mechanism of reperfusion-induced early afterdepolarizations in feline left ventricular hypertrophy. *J Clin Invest* 1993; 91:1521–1531.
194. Maskin CS, Siskin SJ, LeJemtal TH. High prevalence of nonsustained ventricular tachycardia in severe congestive heart failure. *Am Heart J* 1983; 207:896–901.
195. Chakko CS, Gheorghiade M. Ventricular arrhythmias in severe heart failure: Incidence, significance, and effectiveness of antiarrhythmic therapy. *Am Heart J* 1985; 109:497–504.
196. Vignola PA, Aonuma K, Swaye PS, et al. Lymphocytic myocarditis presenting as unexplained ventricular arrhythmias: Diagnosis with endomyocardial biopsy and response to immunosuppression. *J Am Coll Cardiol* 1984; 4:812–819.
197. Meinertz T, Hofmann T, Kasper W, et al. Significance of ventricular arrhythmias in idiopathic dilated cardiomyopathy. *Am J Cardiol* 1984; 53:902–907.
198. Holmes J, Kubo SH, Cody RJ, Kligfield P. Arrhythmias in ischemic and nonischemic dilated cardiomyopathy: Prediction of mortality by ambulatory electrocardiography. *Am J Cardiol* 1985; 55:146–151.
199. The Cardiac Arrhythmia Suppression Trial II Investigators. Effect of the antiarrhythmic agent moricizine in survival after myocardial infarction. *N Engl J Med* 1992; 327:227–233.
200. Bigger JT. Methodology for clinical trials with antiarrhythmic drugs to prevent cardiac deaths: U.S. experience. *Cardiology* 1987; 74(suppl 2):40–56.
201. The Cardiac Arrhythmia Pilot Study (CAPS) Investigators. Effects of encainide, flecainide, imipramine, and moricizine on ventricular arrhythmias during the year after acute myocardial infarction: The CAPS study. *Am J Cardiol* 1988; 61:501–509.
202. Hine LK, Laird NM, Hewitt P, Chalmers TC. Meta-analysis of empirical long-term antiarrhythmic therapy after myocardial infarction. *JAMA* 1989; 262:3037–3040.
203. Julian DG, Camm AJ, Frangin G, et al. Radomised trial of effect of amiodarone on mortality in patients with left-ventricular dysfunction after recent myocardial infarction: EMIAT. *Lancet* 1997; 349:667–674.
204. Cairns JA, Connolly SJ, Roberts R, et al. Randomised trial of outcome after myocardial infarction in patients with frequent or repetitive ventricular premature depolarisations: CAMIAT. *Lancet* 1997; 349:675–682.
205. Beta-Blocker Heart Attack Research Group. A randomized trial of propranolol in patients with acute myocardial infarction: 1. Mortality results. *JAMA* 1982; 247:1707–1714.
206. Pederson TR, Norwegian Multicenter Study Group. Six-year follow-up of the Norwegian multicenter study on timolol after acute myocardial infarction. *N Engl J Med* 1985; 313:1055–1058.
207. Ogunyankin KO, Singh BN. Mortality reduction by antiadrenergic modulation of arrhythmogenic substrate: Significance of combining beta blockers and amiodarone. *Am J Cardiol* 1999; 84:76R–82R.
208. Boutitie F, Boissel JP, Connolly SJ, et al. Amiodarone interaction with beta-blockers: Analysis of the merged EMIAT (European Myocardial Infarct Amiodarone Trial) and CAMIAT (Canadian Amiodarone Myocardial Infarction Trial) databases. *Circulation* 1999; 99:2268–2275.
209. Woosley RL, Kornhauser D, Smith R, et al. Suppression of chronic ventricular arrhythmias with propranolol. *Circulation* 1979; 60:819–827.
210. Gomes JA, Harriman RI, Kaing P, et al. Programmed electrical stimulation in patients with high-grade ventricular ectopy: Electrophysiologic findings and prognosis for survival. *Circulation* 1984; 70:43–51.
211. Moss AM, Hall WJ, Cannom DS, et al. Improved survival with an implanted defibrillator in patients with coronary disease at high risk for ventricular arrhythmia. *N Engl J Med* 1996; 335:1933–1940.
212. Gomes JA, Winters SL, Stewart D, et al. A new noninvasive index to predict sustained ventricular tachycardia and sudden death in the first year after myocardial infarction: Based on signal-averaged electrocardiogram, radionucleotide ejection fraction, and Holter monitoring. *J Am Coll Cardiol* 1987; 10:349–357.
213. Bigger JT, Fleiss JL, Steinman RC, et al. Frequency domain measures of heart period variability and mortality after myocardial infarction. *Circulation* 1992; 85:164–171.
214. Morganroth J, Anderson JL, Gentzkow CD. Classification by type of arrhythmia predicts frequency of adverse cardiac events from flecainide. *J Am Coll Cardiol* 1986; 8:607–615.

215. Webster MWI, Fitzpatrick MA, Nicholis MG, et al. Effect of enalapril on ventricular arrhythmias in congestive heart failure. *Am J Cardiol* 1985; 56:566–569.
216. Myerburg RJ, Kessler KM, Chakko S, et al. Future evaluation of antiarrhythmic therapy. *Am Heart J* 1994; 127:1111–1118.
217. Myerburg RJ, Kessler KM, Castellanos A. Sudden cardiac death: Epidemiology, transient risk, and intervention assessment. *Ann Intern Med* 1993; 119:1187–1197.
218. Minardo JD, Heger JJ, Miles WM, et al. Clinical characteristics of patients with ventricular fibrillation during antiarrhythmic drug therapy. *N Engl J Med* 1988; 319:257–262.
219. Myerburg RJ, Kessler KM, Cox MM, et al. Reversal of proarrhythmic effects of flecainide acetate and encainide hydrochloride by propranolol. *Circulation* 1989; 80:1571–1579.
220. Anderson JL. Rationale of combination antiarrhythmic drug therapy. *Cardiovasc Clin* 1985; 16:307–327.
221. Herre JM, Sauve MJ, Malone P, et al. Long-term results of amiodarone therapy in patients with recurrent sustained ventricular tachycardia or ventricular fibrillation. *J Am Coll Cardiol* 1989; 13:442–449.
222. The CASCADE Investigators. Randomized antiarrhythmic drug therapy in survivors of cardiac arrest (the CASCADE Study). *Am J Cardiol* 1993; 72:280–288.
223. Singh SN, Fletcher RD, Fisher SB, et al. Amiodarone in patients with congestive heart failure and asymptomatic ventricular arrhythmia. *N Engl J Med* 1995; 333:77–82.
224. Doval HC, Nul DR, Grancelli HO, et al. Randomised trial of low-dose amiodarone in severe congestive heart failure. *Lancet* 1994; 344:493–498.
225. Myerburg RJ, Kessler KM, Kiem I, et al. The relationship between plasma levels of procainamide, suppression of premature ventricular contractions, and prevention of recurrent ventricular tachycardia. *Circulation* 1981; 64:280–290.
226. Graboys TB, Lown B, Podrid PJ, DeSilva R. Long-term survival of patients with malignant ventricular arrhythmias treated with antiarrhythmic drugs. *Am J Cardiol* 1982; 50:437–443.
227. Morganroth J, Michelson EL, Horowitz LN, et al. Limitations of routine long-term electrocardiographic monitoring to assess ventricular ectopic frequency. *Circulation* 1978; 58:408–414.
228. Vlay SC, Kallman CH, Reid RP. Prognostic assessment of survivors of ventricular tachycardia and ventricular fibrillation with ambulatory monitoring. *Am J Cardiol* 1984; 54:87–90.
229. Klein H, Auricchio A, Reek S, Geller C. New primary prevention trials of sudden cardiac death in patients with left ventricular dysfunction: SCD-HEFT and MADIT-II. *Am J Cardiol* 1999; 83:91D–97D.
230. Buxton AE, Marchlinski FE, Doherty JU, et al. Repetitive monomorphic ventricular tachycardia: Clinical and electrophysiologic characteristics in patients with and without organ heart disease. *Am J Cardiol* 1984; 54:997–1002.
231. The Antiarrhythmic versus Implantable Defibrillators (AVID) Investigators. A comparison of antiarrhythmic drug therapy with implantable defibrillators in patients resuscitated from near-fatal ventricular arrhythmias. *N Engl J Med* 1997; 337:1576–1583.
232. Connolly SJ, Gent M, Roberts RS, et al. Canadian Implantable Defibrillator Study (CIDS): A randomized trial of the implantable cardioverter defibrillator against amiodarone. *Circulation* 2000; 101:1293–1302.
233. Gallavardin L, Veil P. Deux nouveaux cas d'extrasystolic-ventriculaire avec salves tachycardiques. *Arch Mal Coeur* 1929; 22:738–741.
234. Coumel P, Leclercq JF, Attuel P, et al. Tachycardies ventriculaires en salves: Etude electrophysiologique et therapeutique. *Arch Mal Coeur* 1980; 73:155–164.
235. Rahilly GT, Prystowsky EN, Zipes DP, et al. Clinical and electrophysiologic findings in patients with otherwise normal electrocardiograms. *Am J Cardiol* 1982; 50:459–468.
236. Klein LS, Shih H-T, Hackett FK, et al. Radiofrequency catheter ablation of ventricular tachycardia in patients without structural heart disease. *Circulation* 1992; 85:1666–1674.
237. Marriott HJL. Differential diagnosis of supraventricular and ventricular tachycardia. *Cardiology* 1990; 77:209–220.
238. Wellens HJJ, Bar FRWM, Lie KI. The value of the electrocardiogram in the differential diagnosis of a tachycardia with a widened QRS complex. *Am J Med* 1978; 64:27–33.
239. Wellens HJJ, Bar FRHM, Vanagt EJDM, Brugada P. Medical treatment of ventricular tachycardia: Considerations in the selection of patients for surgical treatment. *Am J Cardiol* 1982; 49:187–193.
240. Colavita PG, Packer DL, Pressley JC, et al. Frequency, diagnoses, and clinical characteristics of patients with multiple atrioventricular pathways. *Am J Cardiol* 1987; 59:601–606.
241. Thompson PD, Melmon KL, Richardson JA, et al. Lidocaine pharmacokinetics in advanced heart failure, liver disease and renal failure in humans. *Ann Intern Med* 1973; 78:499–508.
242. Giardina EG, Heissenbuttel RH, Bigger JT. Intermittent intravenous procainamide to treat ventricular arrhythmias: Correlation of plasma concentration with effect on arrhythmia, electrocardiogram, and blood pressure. *Ann Intern Med* 1973; 78:183–193.
243. Holder DA, Sniderman AD, Fraser G, Fallen EL. Experience with bretylium tosylate by a hospital cardiac arrest team. *Circulation* 1977; 55:541–544.
244. Scheinman MM, Levine JH, Cannom DS, et al. Dose-ranging study of intravenous amiodarone in patients with life-threatening ventricular tachyarrhythmias. *Circulation* 1995; 92:3264–3272.
245. Myerburg RJ, Zaman L, Luceri R, et al. Antiarrhythmic drug therapy after myocardial infarction. In: Kulbertus HE, Wellens HJJ, eds. *The First Year after a Myocardial Infarction.* Mt. Kisco, NY: Futura; 1983:321.
246. Wellens HJJ, Bar FWH, Vanagt EJDM, Brugada P. Medical treatment for ventricular tachycardia: Considerations in the selection of patients for surgical therapy. *Am J Cardiol* 1982; 49:186–193.
247. DiMarco JP, Lerman BB, Kron IL, Sellers TD. Sustained ventricular tachyarrhythmias within 2 months of acute myocardial infarction: Results of medical and surgical therapy in patients resuscitated from the initial episode. *J Am Coll Cardiol* 1985; 6:759–768.
248. Packer M. Sudden unexpected death in patients with congestive heart failure: A second frontier. *Circulation* 1985; 72:681–685.
249. Garan H, Kuchar D, Freeman C, et al. Early assessment of the effect of map-guided transcatheter intracardiac electric shock on sustained ventricular tachycardia secondary to coronary artery disease. *Am J Cardiol* 1988; 61:1018–1023.
250. Buxton AE, Lee KL, Fisher JD, et al. A randomized study of the prevention of sudden death in patients with coronary artery disease, Multicenter Unsustained Tachycardia Trial Investigators. *N Engl J Med* 1999; 341:1882–1890.
251. Wellens HJJ, Brugada P, Stevenson WG. Programmed electrical stimulation of the heart in patients with life-threatening ventricular arrhythmias: What is the significance of induced arrhythmias and what is the correct stimulation protocol? *Circulation* 1985; 72:1–7.
252. Swerdlow CD, Winkle RA, Mason JW. Determinant of survival in patients with ventricular tachycardias. *N Engl J Med* 1983; 308:1436–1442.
253. Interian A Jr, Zaman L, Velez-Robinson E, et al. Paired comparisons of efficacy of intravenous and oral procainamide in patients with inducible sustained ventricular tachyarrhythmias. *J Am Coll Cardiol* 1991; 17:1581–1586.
254. Mitrani RD, Biblo LA, Carlson M, et al. Multiple monomorphic ventricular tachycardia configurations predict failure of antiarrhythmic drug therapy guided by electrophysiologic study. *J Am Coll Cardiol* 1993; 22:1117–1122.
255. Wilbur DJ, Garan H, Finkelstein D, et al. Out-of-hospital cardiac

arrest: Use of electrophysiologic testing in the prediction of long-term outcome. *N Engl J Med* 1988; 318:19–24.

256. Mitchell LB, Duff HJ, Manyari DE, Wyse DG. A randomized clinical trial of the noninvasive and invasive approaches to drug therapy of ventricular tachycardia. *N Engl J Med* 1987; 317:1681–1687.
257. Waller TJ, Kay HR, Spielman SR, et al. Reduction in sudden death and total mortality by antiarrhythmic therapy evaluated by electrophysiologic drug testing: Criteria of efficacy in patients with sustained ventricular tachycardia. *J Am Coll Cardiol* 1987; 10:83–89.
258. Rae AP, Greenspan AM, Spielman SR, et al. Antiarrhythmic drug efficacy for ventricular tachyarrhythmias associated with coronary artery disease as assessed by electrophysiologic studies. *Am J Cardiol* 1985; 55:1494–1499.
259. Myerburg RJ, Kessler KM, Estes D, et al. Long-term survival after pre-hospital cardiac arrest: Analysis of outcome during an 8-year study. *Circulation* 1984; 70:538–546.
260. Kim SG, Seiden SW, Felder SD, et al. Is programmed stimulation of value in predicting the long-term success of antiarrhythmic therapy for ventricular tachycardias? *N Engl J Med* 1986; 315:356–362.
261. Kim SG. The management of patients with life-threatening ventricular tachyarrhythmias: Programmed stimulation or Holter monitoring (either or both)? *Circulation* 1987; 76:1–5.
262. The ESVEM Investigators. Determinants of predicted efficacy of antiarrhythmic drugs in the Electrophysiologic Study Versus Electrocardiographic Monitoring Trial. *Circulation* 1993; 87:323–329.
263. Mason JW, Electrophysiologic Study Versus Electrocardiographic Monitoring Investigators. A comparison of electrophysiologic testing with Holter monitoring to predict antiarrhythmic-drug efficacy for ventricular tachyarrhythmias. *N Engl J Med* 1993; 329:445–451.
264. Pacifico A, Hohnloser SH, Williams JH, et al. Prevention of implantable-defibrillator shocks by treatment with sotalol: D,l-Sotalol Implantable Cardioverter-Defibrillator Study Group. *N Engl J Med* 1999; 340:1855–1862.
265. Weiner I, Mindich B, Pitchon R. Determinant of ventricular tachycardia in patients with ventricular aneurysms: Results of intraoperative epicardial and endocardial mapping. *Circulation* 1982; 65:856–861.
266. Josephson ME, Harken AH, Horowitz LN. Endocardial excision: A new surgical technique for the treatment of recurrent ventricular tachycardia. *Circulation* 1979; 60:1430–1439.
267. Gallagher JJ, Anderson RW, Kasell JH, et al. Cryoablation of drug resistant ventricular tachycardia in a patient with a variant of scleroderma. *Circulation* 1978; 57:190–197.
268. Cox JL. Ventricular tachycardia surgery: A review of the first decade and a suggested contemporary approach. *Semin Thorac Cardiovasc Surg* 1989; 1:97–103.
269. Condini MA, Sommerfeldt I, Eybel CE, et al. Efficacy of coronary bypass grafting in exercise-induced ventricular tachycardia. *J Thorac Cardiovasc Surg* 1981; 81:502–506.
270. Fontaine G, Lechat PH, Cansell A, et al. Advances in the treatment of cardiac arrhythmias in the last decade: Definition and role of ablative techniques. In: Fontaine G, Scheinman MM, eds. *Ablation in Cardiac Arrhythmias.* Mt. Kisco, NY: Futura; 1987:5.
271. Stevenson WG. Ventricular tachycardia after myocardial infarction: From arrhythmia surgery to catheter ablation. *J Cardiovasc Electrophysiol* 1995; 6:942–950.
272. Stevenson WG, Delacretaz E, Friedman PI, Ellison KE. Identification and ablation of macroreentrant ventricular tachycardia with the CARTO electroanatomical mapping system. *Pacing Clin Electrophysiol* 1998; 21:1448–1456.
273. Schilling RJ, Peters NS, Davies DW. Mapping and ablation of ventricular tachycardia with the aid of a non-contact mapping system. *Heart* 1999, 81:570–575.
274. Kleman JM, Castle LW, Kidwell GA, et al. Nonthoracotomy-versus-thoracotomy-implantable defibrillators: Intentions-to-treat comparison of clinical outcomes. *Circulation* 1994; 90:2833–2842.
275. Platia EV, Griffith LSC, Watkins L, et al. Treatment of malignant ventricular arrhythmias with endocardial resection and implantation of the automatic cardioverter-defibrillator. *N Engl J Med* 1986; 314:213–216.
276. Bigger JT Jr. Prophylactic use of implanted cardiac defibrillators in patients at high risk for ventricular arrhythmias after coronary-artery bypass graft surgery: Coronary Artery Bypass Graft (CABG) Patch Trial investigators. *N Engl J Med* 1997; 337:1569–1575.
277. Bigger JT Jr, Whang W, Rottman JN, Mechanisms of death in the CABG Patch Trial: A randomized trial of implantable cardiac defibrillator prophylaxis in patients at high risk of death after coronary artery bypass graft surgery. *Circulation* 1999; 99:1416–1421.
278. Poll DS, Marchinski FE, Buxton AE, Josephson ME. Usefulness of programmed stimulation in idiopathic dilated cardiomyopathy. *Am J Cardiol* 1986; 58:992–997.
279. Rae AP, Spielman SC, Kutalek SP, et al. Electrophysiologic assessment of antiarrhythmic drug efficacy for ventricular tachyarrhythmias associated with dilated cardiomyopathy. *Am J Cardiol* 1987; 59:291–295.
280. Caceres J, Jazayeri M, McKinnie J, et al. Sustained bundle branch reentry mechanism of clinical tachycardia. *Circulation* 1989; 79:256–270.
281. Das SK, Morady F, DiCarlo L, et al. Prognostic usefulness of programmed ventricular stimulation in idiopathic dilated cardiomyopathy without symptomatic ventricular arrhythmias. *Am J Cardiol* 1986; 58:998–1000.
282. Myerburg RJ, Luceri RM, Thurer R, et al. Time to first shock and clinical outcome in patients receiving automatic implantable cardioverter defibrillators. *J Am Coll Cardiol* 1989; 14:508–514.
283. Myerburg RJ, Estes D, Zaman L, et al. Outcome of resuscitation from bradyarrhythmic or asystolic prehospital cardiac arrest. *J Am Coll Cardiol* 1984; 4:1118–1122.
284. Anderson KP. Sudden death, hypertension, hypertrophy. *J Cardiovasc Pharm* 1984; 6:(suppl III):S498–S503.
285. Goodwin JF, Krikler DM. Arrhythmia as a cause of sudden death in hypertrophic cardiomyopathy. *Lancet* 1976; 2:937–940.
286. Kowey PR, Eisenberg R, Engel TR. Sustained arrhythmias in hypertrophic obstructive cardiomyopathy. *N Engl J Med* 1984; 310:1566–1569.
287. Anderson KP, Stinson EB, Derby GC, et al. Vulnerability of patients with obstructive hypertrophic cardiomyopathy to ventricular arrhythmia induction in the operating room. *Am J Cardiol* 1983; 51:811–816.
288. Maron BJ, Shen WK, Link MS, et al. Efficacy of the implantable cardioverter-defibrillator for the prevention of sudden cardiac death in hypertrophic cardiomyopathy. *N Engl J Med* 2000; 342:365–373.
289. Coumel P, Rosengarten MD, Lecieroq JF, Attuel P. Role of sympathetic nervous system in non-ischemic ventricular arrhythmias. *Br Heart J* 1982; 47:137–147.
290. Sung RJ, Shapiro WA, Shen EN, et al. Effects of verapamil on ventricular tachycardias possibly caused by reentry, automaticity, and triggered activity. *J Clin Invest* 1983; 72:350–360.
291. Lerman BB, Belardinelli L, West A, et al. Adenosine-sensitive ventricular tachycardia: Evidence suggesting cyclic AMP-mediated triggered activity. *Circulation* 1986; 74:270–280.
292. Ward DE, Nathan AW, Camm AJ. Fascicular tachycardia sensitive to calcium antagonists. *Eur Heart J* 1984; 5:896–905.

293. Ohe T, Shimomura S, Aihara N, et al. Idiopathic sustained left ventricular tachycardia: Clinical and electrophysiologic characteristics. *Circulation* 1988; 77:560–568.
294. Marcus FI, Fontaine GH, Guiraudon G, et al. Right ventricular dysplasia: A report of 24 adult cases. *Circulation* 1982; 65:384–398.
295. Thiene G, Nava A, Corrado D, et al. Right ventricular cardiomyopathy and sudden death in young people. *N Engl J Med* 1988; 318:129–133.
296. Guiraudon GM, Klein GJ, Guiamhusein SS, et al. Total disconnection of the right ventricular free wall: Surgical treatment of right ventricular tachycardia associated with right ventricular dysplasia. *Circulation* 1983; 67:463–470.
297. Fitchett DH, Sugrue DD, MacArthur CG, Oakley CM. Right ventricular dilated cardiomyopathy. *Br Heart J* 1984; 51:25–29.
298. Fortaine G, Fontaliran F, Rosas Andrade F, et al. The arrhythmogenic right ventricle: Dysplasia versus cardiomyopathy. *Heart Vessels* 1995; 10:227–235.
299. Rampazzo A, Nava A, Miorin M, et al. ARVD4, a new locus for arrhythmogenic right ventricular cardiomyopathy maps to chromosome 2 long arm. *Genomics* 1997; 45:259–262.
300. Ahmad F, Li D, Karibe A, et al. Localization of a gene responsible for arrhythmogenic right ventricular dysplasia to chromosome 3p23. *Circulation* 1998; 98:2791–2795.
301. Dunnigan A, Pritzker MR, Benditt DG, Benson DW. Life-threatening ventricular tachycardias in late survivors of surgically corrected tetralogy of Fallot. *Br Heart J* 1984; 52:198–206.
302. Garson A, Randall DC, Gillette PC, et al. Prevention of sudden death after repair of tetralogy of Fallot: Treatment of ventricular arrhythmias. *J Am Coll Cardiol* 1985; 6:221–227.
303. Harken AH, Horowitz LN, Josephson ME. Surgical correction of recurrent sustained ventricular tachycardia on complete repair of tetralogy of Fallot. *J Thorac Cardiovasc Surg* 1980; 80:779–781.
304. Fontaine G, Frank R, Grosgogeat Y. Torsades de pointes: Definition and management. *Mod Concepts Cardiovasc Dis* 1982; 51:103–108.
305. Leenhardt L, Glaser E, Burguera M, et al. Short-coupled variant of torsade de pointes: A new electrocardiographic entity in the spectrum of idiopathic ventricular tachyarrhythmias. *Circulation* 1994; 89:206–215.
306. Ward OC. A new familial cardiac syndrome in children. *J Irish Med Assoc* 1964; 54:103–106.
307. Romano C. Congenital cardiac arrhythmia. *Lancet* 1965; 1:658–659.
308. Jervell A, Lange-Nielsen F. Congenital deaf mutism, functional heart disease with prolongation of the Q-T interval, and sudden death. *Am Heart J* 1957; 54:59–78.
309. Schwartz PJ, Locati EH, Moss AJ, et al. Left cardiac sympathetic denervation in the therapy of congenital long QT syndrome: A worldwide report. *Circulation* 1991; 84:503–511.
310. Keating MT, Atkinson D, Dunn C, et al. Linkage of a cardiac arrhythmia, the long Q-T syndrome, and the Harvey *ras*-1 gene. *Science* 1991; 252:704–706.
311. Curran ME, Splawski I, Timothy KW, et al. A molecular basis for cardiac arrhythmia: HERG mutations cause long QT syndrome. *Cell* 1995; 80:795–803.
312. Wang Q, Shen J, Splawski I, et al. SCN5A mutations associated with an inherited cardiac arrhythmia, long Q-T syndrome. *Cell* 1995; 80:805–811.
313. Schwartz PJ, Priori SG, Locati EH, et al. Long Q-T syndrome patients with mutations of the SCN5A and HERG genes have differential responses to Na^{+}-channel blockade and to increases in heart rate: Implications for gene-specific therapy. *Circulation* 1995; 92:3381–3386.
314. Schott JJ, Charpentier F, Peltier S, et al. Mapping of a gene for long Q-T syndrome to chromosome 4q25-27. *Am J Hum Genet* 1995; 57:1114–1122.
315. Denes P, Gabster A, Huang SK. Clinical, electrocardiographic and follow-up observations in patients having ventricular fibrillation during Holter monitoring. *Am J Cardiol* 1981; 48:9–27.
316. Krikler DM, Curry PVL. Torsades de pointes, an atypical ventricular tachycardia. *Br Heart J* 1976; 38:117–120.
317. Smith WM, Gallagher JJ. "Les torsades de pointes": An unusual ventricular arrhythmia. *Ann Intern Med* 1980; 93:578–584.
318. Keren A, Tzivoni D, Gavish D, et al. Etiology, warning signs and therapy of torsades de pointes: A study of ten patients. *Circulation* 1981; 64:1167–1174.
319. Monahan BP, Ferguson CL, Killeavy ES, et al. Torsades de pointes occurring in association with terfenadine use. *JAMA* 1990; 264:2788–2790.
320. Woosley RL, Chen Y, Freiman JP, Gillis RA. Mechanism of the cardiotoxic actions of terfenadine. *JAMA* 1993; 269:1532–1536.
321. Ackerman MJ. The long QT syndrome: Ion channel diseases of the heart. *Mayo Clinic Proc* 1998; 73:250–269.
322. Priori S, Barhanin J, Hauer RN, et al. Genetic and molecular basis of cardiac arrhythmias: Impact on clinical management. *Circulation* 1999; 99:518–528.
323. Stratmann HG, Kennedy HL. Torsades de pointes associated with drugs and toxins: Recognition and management. *Am Heart J* 1987; 113:1470–1482.
324. Schwartz PJ, Locati EH, Moss AJ, et al. Left cardiac sympathetic denervation in the therapy of congenital long QT syndrome: A worldwide report. *Circulation* 1991; 84:503–511.
325. Brugada J, Brugada R, Brugada P. Right bundle-branch block and ST-segment elevation in leads V_1 through V_3: A marker for sudden death in patients without demonstrable structural heart disease. *Circulation* 1998; 97:457–460.
326. Splawski I, Tristani-Firouzi M, Lehmann MH, et al. Mutations in the hminK gene cause long QT syndrome and suppress Iks function. *Nature Genet* 1997; 17:338–340.
327. Neyroud N, Tesson F, Denjoy I, et al. A novel mutation in the potassium channel gene KVLQT1 causes the Jervell and Lange-Nielsen cardioauditory syndrome. *Nature Genet* 1997; 15:186–189.
328. Krishnan SC, Josephson ME. ST segment elevation induced by class IC antiarrhythmic agents: Underlying electrophysiologic mechanisms and insights into drug-induced proarrhythmia. *J Cardiovasc Electrophysiol* 1998; 9:1167–1172.
329. Brugada J, Brugada P. Further characterization of the syndrome of right bundle branch block, ST segment elevation, and sudden cardiac death. *J Cardiovasc Electrophysiol* 1997; 8:325–331.
330. Chen Q, Kirsch GE, Zhang D, et al. Genetic basis and molecular mechanism for idiopathic ventricular fibrillation. *Nature* 1998; 392:293–296.
331. Nademanee K, Veerakul G, Nimmannit S, et al. Arrhythmogenic marker for the sudden unexplained death syndrome in Thai men. *Circulation* 1997; 96:2595–2600.
332. Packer M. Sudden unexpected death in patients with congestive heart failure: A second frontier. *Circulation* 1985; 72:681–685.
333. Luu M, Stevenson WG, Stevenson LW, et al. Diverse mechanisms of unexpected cardiac arrest in advanced heart failure. *Circulation* 1991; 80:1675–1680.
334. Cummins RO, Ornato JP, Thies WH, Pepe P. Improving survival from sudden cardiac arrest: The "chain of survival" concept. *Circulation* 1991; 83:1832–1847.
335. Creed JD, Packard JM, Lambrew CT, Lewis AJ. Defibrillation and synchronized cardioversion. In: McIntyre KM, Lewis AJ, eds. *Textbook of Advanced Cardiac Life Support.* Dallas: American Heart Association; 1983:89.
336. Emergency Cardiac Care Committee and Subcommittees, American Heart Association. Guidelines for cardiopulmonary resuscitation and emergency cardiac care. *JAMA* 1992; 268:2172–2275.
337. Kudenchuk PJ, Cobb LA, Copass MK, et al. Amiodarone for resuscitation after out-of-hospital cardiac arrest due to ventricular fibrillation. *N Engl J Med* 1999; 341:871–878.

338. Interian A, Trohman RG, Castellanos A, et al. Spontaneous conversion of ventricular fibrillation in cardiogenic shock for acute myocardial infarction. *Am J Cardiol* 1987; 50:1200–1201.
339. Behar S, Goldbourt U, Reicher-Reiss H, Kaplinsky E. Prognosis of acute myocardial infarction complicated by primary ventricular fibrillation. *Am J Cardiol* 1990; 66:1208–1211.
340. Volpi A, Cavalli A, Franzosi MG, et al. One-year prognosis of primary ventricular fibrillation complicating acute myocardial infarction. *Am J Cardiol* 1989; 63:1174–1178.
341. Nicod P, Gilpin E, Dittrich H, et al. Late clinical outcome in patients with early ventricular fibrillation after myocardial infarction. *J Am Coll Cardiol* 1988; 11:464–470.
342. Lie KI, Leim KL, Schullenberg RM, et al. Early identification of patients developing late in-hospital ventricular fibrillation after discharge from the coronary care unit. *Am J Cardiol* 1978; 41:674–677.
343. Hauer RNW, Lie KI, Liem KL, Durrer D. Long-term prognosis in patients with bundle branch block complicating acute anteroseptal infarction. *Am J Cardiol* 1982; 49:1581–1585.
344. Myerburg RJ, Kessler KM, Castellanos A. Sudden cardiac death: Structure, function and time-dependence of risk. *Circulation* 1992; 85(suppl I):I2–I10.
345. Myerburg RJ, Kessler KM. Management of patients who survive cardiac arrest. *Mod Concepts Cardiovasc Dis* 1986; 55:61–66.
346. Wilber DJ, Garan H, Finkelstein D, et al. Out-of-hospital cardiac arrest: Use of electrophysiologic testing in the prediction of long-term outcome. *N Engl J Med* 1988; 318:19–24.
347. Morady F, DiCarlo L, Winston S, et al. Clinical features and prognosis of patients with out-of-hospital cardiac arrest and a normal electrophysiologic study. *J Am Coll Cardiol* 1984; 4:39–44.
348. Kunis RL, Garfein OB, Pepe AJ, Dwyer EM. Deglutition syncope and atrioventricular block selectively induced by hot food and liquid. *Am J Cardiol* 1985; 55:613.
349. Falk RH, Zoll PM, Zoll RH. Safety and efficiency of non-invasive cardiac pacing: A preliminary report. *N Engl J Med* 1983; 309:1166–1168.
350. Zoll PM, Zoll RH, Falk RH, et al. External non-invasive temporary cardiac pacing: Clinical trials. *Circulation* 1985; 71:937–944.
351. Love JC, Haffajee MD, Gore MD, Alpert JS. Reversibility of hypotension and shock by atrial or atrioventricular sequential pacing in patients with right ventricular infarction. *Am Heart J* 1984; 108:5–13.
352. Kang PS, Gomes JA, Kelen G, El-Sherif N. Role of autonomic regulatory mechanism in sinoatrial conduction and sinus nodal automaticity in sick sinus syndrome. *Circulation* 1981; 64:832–838.
353. Yabek SM, Swensson RE, Jarmakani JM. Electrocardiographic recognition of sinus node dysfunction in children and young adults. *Circulation* 1977; 56:235–239.
354. Mackintosh AF. Sinoatrial disease in young people. *Br Heart J* 1981; 45:62–66.
355. Rasmussen V, Haunso S, Skagen K. Cerebral attacks due to excessive vagal tone in heavily trained persons: A clinical and electrophysiologic study. *Acta Med Scand* 1978; 204:401–405.
356. Bharati S, Nordenberg A, Bauernfeind R, et al. The anatomic substrate for the sick sinus syndrome in adolescents. *Am J Cardiol* 1980; 46:156–172.
357. DeMoulin JC, Kulbertus HE. Histopathological correlates of sinoatrial disease. *Br Heart J* 1978; 40:1384–1389.
358. Thery C, Gosselin B, Lekieffre J, Warrenbourg H. Pathology of the sinoatrial node: Correlation with electrocardiographic findings in 111 patients. *Am Heart J* 1977; 93:735–740.
359. Walter PF, Crawley IS, Dorney ER. Carotid sinus hypersensitivity and syncope. *Am J Cardiol* 1978; 42:396–403.
360. Davies AB, Stephens MR, Davies AG. Carotid sinus hypersensitivity in patients presenting with syncope. *Br Heart J* 1979; 42:583–586.
361. Madigan NP, Fiaker GC, Curtis JJ, et al. Carotid sinus hypersensitivity: Beneficial effects of dual-chamber pacing. *Am J Cardiol* 1984; 53:1034–1040.
362. Wenger TL, Dohrmann ML, Strauss HC, et al. Hypersensitive carotid sinus syndrome manifested as cough syncope. *PACE* 1980; 3:332–339.
363. Sra JS, Anderson AJ, Sheikh SH, et al. Unexplained syncope evaluated by electrophysiologic studies and head-up tilt testing. *Ann Intern Med* 1991; 114:1013–1019.
364. Sra JS, Jazayeri MR, Avitall B, et al. Comparison of cardiac pacing with drug therapy in the treatment of neurocardiogenic (vasovagal) syncope with bradycardia or asystole. *N Engl J Med* 1993; 328:1085–1090.
365. Connolly SJ, Sheldon RS, Roberts RS, Gent M. The North American Vasovagal Pacemaker Study: A randomized trial of permanent pacing for the prevention of vasovagal syncope. *J Am Coll Cardiol* 1999; 3:16–20.
366. Calkins H. Pharmacologic approaches to therapy for vasovagal syncope. *Am J Cardiol* 1999; 84:20Q–25Q.
367. Cox MM, Pearlman BA, Mayor MR, et al. Acute and long-term beta-adrenergic blockade for neurocardiogenic syncope. *J Am Coll Cardiol* 1995; 26:1293–1298.
368. Bigger JT Jr, Reiffel JA. Sick sinus syndrome. *Annu Rev Med* 1979; 30:91–118.
369. Chung EK. Sick sinus syndrome: Current views. *Mod Concepts Cardiovasc Dis* 1980; 49:61–66.
370. Crossen KJ, Cain ME. Assessment and management of sinus node dysfunction. *Mod Concepts Cardiovasc Dis* 1986; 55:43–48.
371. Narula OS. Atrioventricular conduction disturbances in patients with sinus bradycardia. *Circulation* 1971; 44:1096–1110.
372. Jordan JA, Yamaguchi L, Mandel WJ. Studies on the mechanisms of sinus node dysfunction in a sick sinus syndrome. *Circulation* 1978; 57:217–223.
373. Rosenqvist M, Vallin H, Edhag O. Clinical electrophysiologic course of sinus node diseases: Five-year follow-up study. *Am Heart J* 1985; 109:513–522.
374. Benditt DG, Benson DW, Kreitt J, et al. Electrophysiologic effects of theophylline in young patients with symptomatic bradyarrhythmias. *Am J Cardiol* 1983; 52:1223–1229.
375. Gomes JA, Kang PS, El-Sherif N. Effects of digitalis on the human sick sinus node after pharmacologic autonomic blockade. *Am J Cardiol* 1981; 48:783–788.
376. Dhingra RC, Amat-y-Leon F, Wyndham C, et al. Clinical significance of prolonged sinoatrial conduction time. *Circulation* 1977; 55:8–15.
377. Gann D, Tolentino A, Samet P. Electrophysiologic evaluation of elderly patients with sinus bradycardia: A long-term follow-up study. *Ann Intern Med* 1979; 90:24–29.
378. Katritsis D, Camm AJ. AAI pacing mode: When is it indicated and how should it be achieved? *Clin Cardiol* 1993; 16:339–343.
379. Rosenqvist M, Obel IW. Atrial pacing and the risk for AV block: Is there a time for change in attitude? *PACE* 1989; 12:97–101.
380. Brandt J, Anderson H, Fahraeus T, Schuller H. Natural history of sinus node disease treated with atrial pacing in 213 patients: Implications for selection of stimulation mode. *J Am Coll Cardiol* 1992; 20:633–639.
381. Rosenqvist M, Brandt J, Schuller H. Atrial versus ventricular pacing in sinus node disease: A treatment comparison study. *Am Heart J* 1986; 111:292–297.
382. Lamas GA, Estes NM, Schneller S, Flaker GC. Does dual chamber or atrial pacing prevent atrial fibrillation? The need for a randomized controlled trial. *PACE* 1992; 15:1109–1113.
383. Andersen HR, Nielsen JC, Thomsen PEB, et al. Long term follow up of patients from a randomised trial of atrial versus ventricular pacing for sick sinus syndrome. *Lancet* 1994; 344:1523–1528.
384. Kallikazaros I, Stratos C, Tsioufis C, et al. Carotid sinus hypersensitivity in patients undergoing coronary angiography: Relation

with severity of carotid arteriosclerosis and extent of coronary artery disease. *J Cardiovasc Electrophysiol* 1997; 8:1218–1228.

385. Jeffreys M, Wood DA, Lampe F, et al. The heart response to carotid sinus massage in a sample of healthy elderly people. *PACE* 1996; 19:1488–1492.
386. Sugrue DD, Gersh BJ, Holmes DR, et al. Symptomatic "isolated" carotid sinus hypersensitivity: Natural history and results of treatment with anticholinergic drugs or pacemaker. *J Am Coll Cardiol* 1986; 7:158–162.
387. Peretz DI, Gerein AN, Miyagishima RT. Permanent demand pacing for hypersensitive carotid sinus syndrome. *Can Med Assoc J* 1973; 108:1131–1134.
388. Brignole M, Menozzi C, Gianfranchi L, et al. Neurally mediated syncope detected by carotid sinus massage and head-up tilt test in sick sinus syndrome. *Am J Cardiol* 1991; 68:1032–1036.
389. Denes P. Atrioventricular and intraventricular block. *Circulation* 1987; 75(suppl III):III19–III25.
390. Meytes I, Kaplinsky E, Yahini JH, et al. Wenckebach A-V block: A frequent feature following heavy physical training. *Am Heart J* 1975; 90:426–430.
391. Talan DA, Bauernfeind RA, Ashley WW, et al. Twenty-four hour continuous ECG recordings in long-distance runners. *Chest* 1982; 82:19–24.
392. Hindman MC, Wagner GS, JaRo M, et al. The clinical significance of bundle branch block complicating acute myocardial infarction: Indications for temporary and permanent pacemaker insertion. *Circulation* 1978; 58:689–699.
393. Col JJ, Weinberg SL. The incidence and mortality of intraventricular conduction defects in acute myocardial infarction. *Am J Cardiol* 1972; 29:344–350.
394. Ritter WS, Atkins JM, Blomqvist CG, Mullins CB. Permanent pacing in patients with transient trifascicular block during acute myocardial infarction. *Am J Cardiol* 1976; 38:205–208.
395. Ginks WR, Sutton R, Oh W, Leatham A. Long-term prognosis after acute anterior infarction with atrioventricular block. *Br Heart J* 1977; 39:186–189.
396. Domenighetti G, Perret C. Intraventricular conduction disturbances in acute myocardial infarction: Short- and long-term prognosis. *Eur J Cardiol* 1980; 11:51–59.
397. DePasquale NP, Bruno MS. Natural history of combined right bundle branch block and left anterior hemiblock (bilateral bundle branch block). *Am J Med* 1973; 54:297–303.
398. Breithardt G, Cain ME, el-Sherif N, et al. Standards for analysis of ventricular late potentials using high-resolution or signal-averaged electrocardiography: A statement by a task force committee of the European Society of Cardiology, the American Heart Association, and the American College of Cardiology. *J Am Coll Cardiol* 1991; 17:999–1006.
399. Lamas GA, Muller JE, Turi ZG, et al. A simplified method to predict occurrence of complete heart block during acute myocardial infarction. *Am J Cardiol* 1986; 57:1213–1219.
400. Juma Z, Castellanos A, Myerburg RJ. Prognostic significance of the electrocardiogram in patients with coronary heart disease. In: Wellens HJJ, Kulbertus HE, eds. *What's New in Electrocardiography*. The Hague: Martinus Nijhoff; 1981:5.
401. Clemmensen P, Bates ER, Califf RM, et al. Complete atrioventricular block complicating inferior wall acute myocardial infarction treated with reperfusion therapy. *Am J Cardiol* 1991; 67:225–230.
402. Goldberg RJ, Zevallos JC, Yarzebski J, et al. Prognosis of acute myocardial infarction complicated by complete heart block: The Worcester Heart Attack Study. *Am J Cardiol* 1992; 69:1135–1141.
403. Behar S, Zissman E, Zion M, et al. Prognostic significance of second-degree atrioventricular block in inferior wall acute myocardial infarction. *Am J Cardiol* 1993; 72:831–834.
404. Berger PB, Ruocco NA, Ryan TJ, et al. Incidence and prognostic implications of heart block complicating inferior myocardial infarction treated with thrombolytic therapy: Results from TIMI II. *J Am Coll Cardiol* 1992; 20:533–540.
405. Nicod P, Gilpin E, Dittrich H, et al. Long-term outcome in patients with inferior myocardial infarction and complete atrioventricular block. *J Am Coll Cardiol* 1988; 12:589–594.
406. Dubois C, Piérard LA, Smeets JP, et al. Long-term prognostic significance of atrioventricular block in inferior acute myocardial infarction. *Eur Heart J* 1989; 10:816–820.
407. Ector H, Rolies L, De Geest H. Dynamic electrocardiography and ventricular pauses of 3 seconds and more: Etiology and therapeutic implications. *PACE* 1983; 6:548–551.
408. Mymin D, Mathewson FA, Tate RB, Manfreda J. The natural history of primary first-degree atrioventricular heart block. *N Engl J Med* 1986; 315:1183–1187.
409. Barold SS. Indications for permanent cardiac pacing in first-degree AV block: Class I, II, or III? *PACE* 1996; 19:747–751.
410. Gregoratos G, Cheitlin MD, Conill A, et al. ACC/AHA guidelines for implantation of cardiac pacemakers and arrhythmia devices: A report of the American College of Cardiology/American Heart Association Task Force on Practice Guidelines (Committee on Pacemaker Implantation). *J Am Coll Cardiol* 1998; 31:1175–1209.
411. Brecker SJD, Xiao HB, Sparrow J, Gibson DG. Effects of dual chamber pacing with short atrioventricular delay in dilated cardiomyopathy. *Lancet* 1992; 340:1308–1312.
412. Nishimura RA, Hayes DL, Holmes DR, Tajik AJ. Mechanism of hemodynamic improvement by dual-chamber pacing for severe left ventricular dysfunction: An acute Doppler and catheterization hemodynamic study. *J Am Coll Cardiol* 1995; 25:281–288.
413. Hochleitner M, Hortnagl H, Fridrich L, Gschnitzer F. Long-term efficacy of physiologic dual-chamber pacing in the treatment of end-stage idiopathic dilated cardiomyopathy. *Am J Cardiol* 1992; 70:1320–1325.
414. Auricchio A, Sommariva L, Salo RW, et al. Improvement of cardiac function in patients with severe congestive heart failure and coronary artery disease by dual chamber pacing with shortened AV delay. *PACE* 1993; 16:2034–2043.
415. Zipes DP. Current topics: Second degree atrioventricular block. *Circulation* 1979; 60:465–472.
416. Barold SS, Jais P, Shah DC, et al. Exercise-induced second-degree AV block: Is it type I or type II? *J Cardiovasc Electrophysiol* 1997; 8:1084–1086.
417. Mymin D, Mathewson FA, Tate RB, Manfreda J. The natural history of primary first-degree atrioventricular heart block. *N Engl J Med* 1986; 315:1183–1187.
418. Barold SS. Indications for permanent cardiac pacing in first-degree AV block: Class I, II, or III? *PACE* 1996; 19:747–751.
419. Zeppilli P, Feniel R, Sassara M, et al. Wenckebach second degree A-V block in top-ranking athletes: An old problem revisited. *Am Heart J* 1980; 100:281–294.
420. Strasberg B, Amat-y-Leon F, Dhingra RC, et al. Natural history of chronic second degree atrioventricular nodal block. *Circulation* 1981; 63:1043–1049.
421. Damato AN, Varghese PJH, Caracta AR, et al. Functional 2:1 A-V block within the His Purkinje system: Simulation of type II A-V block. *Circulation* 1973; 47:534–542.
422. Woelfel A, Simpson RJ Jr, Foster JR. Functional "type I-like" distal atrioventricular block induced by atrial pacing. *Am J Cardiol* 1984; 54:1363–1364.
423. Zipes DP, Dimarco JP, Gillette PC, et al. Guidelines for clinical intracardiac electrophysiological and catheter ablation procedures: A report of the American College of Cardiology/American Heart Association Task Force on Practice Guidelines (Committee on Clinical Intracardiac Electrophysiologic and Catheter Ab-

lation Procedures), developed in collaboration with the North American Society of Pacing and Electrophysiology. *Circulation* 1995; 92:673–691.

424. Gallastregui J, Hariman RJ. Indications for intracardiac electrophysiologic studies in patients with atrioventricular and intraventricular blocks not associated with acute myocardial infarction. *Circulation* 1987; 75(suppl III):III103–III106.
425. Bhandari AK, Rahimtoola SH. Intracardiac electrophysiologic studies in patients with atrioventricular and intraventricular blocks not associated with acute myocardial infarction. Discussion. *Circulation* 1987; 75(suppl III):III107–III109.
426. Prystowsky EN, Klein GJ. Bundle branch block. In: *Cardiac Arrhythmias: An Integrated Approach for the Clinician.* New York: McGraw-Hill; 1994:47.
427. Josephson ME. Intraventricular conduction disturbances. In: *Clinical Cardiac Electrophysiology: Techniques and Interpretations*, 2d ed. Philadelphia: Lea & Febiger, 1992:117.
428. Edhag O, Herrlin B, Lagergren H. Paroxysmal complete heart block due to bradycardia-dependent "phase 4" fascicular block in a patient with sinus node dysfunction and bifascicular block. *PACE* 1984; 7:839–843.
429. Corrado G, Levi RJ, Nau GJ, Rosenbaum MB. Paroxysmal atrioventricular block related to phase 4 bilateral bundle branch block. *Am J Cardiol* 1974; 33:553–556.
430. Tenczer J, Littmann L, Rohia N, Fenyvesi T. The effects of overdrive pacing and lidocaine on atrioventricular junctional rhythm in man: The role of abnormal automaticity. *Circulation* 1985; 72:480–486.
431. Gunnar RM, Bourdillon PVD, Dixon DW, et al. ACC/AHA guidelines for the early management of patients with acute myocardial infarction. *Circulation* 1990; 82:664–707.
432. Hindman MC, Wagner GS, Jaro M. The clinical significance of bundle branch block complicating acute myocardial infarction: 2. Indications for temporary and permanent pacemaker insertion. *Circulation* 1978; 58:689–699.
433. Watson RDS, Glober DR, Page AJF, et al. The Birmingham trial of permanent pacing in patients with intraventricular conduction disorders after acute myocardial infarction. *Am Heart J* 1984; 108:496–501.
434. Kastor JA. Atrioventricular block. *N Engl J Med* 1975; 292: 462–465.
435. Dhingra RC, Palileo E, Strasberg B, et al. Significance of the HV interval in 517 patients with chronic bifascicular block. *Circulation* 1982; 64:1265–1271.
436. McAnulty JH, Rahimtoola DH, Murphy ES, et al. A prospective study of sudden death in high risk bundle branch block. *N Engl J Med* 1978; 299:209–215.
437. Scheinman MM, Peters RW, Modin G, et al. Prognostic value of infranodal conduction time in patients with chronic bundle branch block. *Circulation* 1977; 56:240–244.
438. Furman S, Fischer JD. Endless loop tachycardia in the A-V universal (DDD) pacemaker. *PACE* 1982; 5:486–489.

C H A P T E R 25

LONG-TERM CONTINUOUS ELECTROCARDIOGRAPHIC RECORDING

R. Joe Noble / Eric N. Prystowsky

Long-term electrocardiographic recording is a method of recording the electrocardiogram (ECG) over extended time periods; the recording is subsequently analyzed for rhythm and ST-segment and T-wave alterations.[1-3] Technological advances in the past few years have provided a diversity of recording, transmitting, and analysis systems.

INDICATIONS

Ambulatory ECG (AECG) recording may be helpful in recognizing, characterizing, and less frequently, quantitating arrhythmias in patients with symptoms potentially related to an arrhythmia; the recording of a rhythm disturbance simultaneous with a patient's symptoms may be the only means of diagnosis, particularly when the symptoms and arrhythmia are relatively infrequent (Fig. 25-1). Importantly, the recording of a normal rhythm when the patient is symptomatic may prove equally valuable in excluding a rhythm disturbance as the cause for the patient's symptoms. Not only is it important to correlate an abnormal rate and rhythm with the symptom complex but, from the ambulatory record, also to determine the precise mechanism of arrhythmia. Some concept of the frequency of the arrhythmia, as demonstrated by the ambulatory record, is clinically helpful, but precise quantitation of the frequency of premature ventricular complexes, for instance, is rarely required.

AECG recordings may be indicated in certain patients to assess risk for future cardiac events—specifically in those patients with idiopathic hypertrophic cardiomyopathy, patients who have survived myocardial infarction with substantial left ventricular (LV) dysfunction, patients with long QT intervals, patients with dilated cardiomyopathy and symptoms consistent with arrhythmia, and in some patients with the Wolff-Parkinson-White syndrome.[4] The value of AECG in predicting risk is compromised by low sensitivity and specificity. Furthermore, since the effect of treatment of any arrhythmia recorded in these conditions is unclear, there is little support for routine AECG recording in risk stratification.[4]

Patients who undergo treatment for complex arrhythmias, such as sustained supraventricular tachyarrhythmias or ventricular tachycardia, may benefit from AECG recordings in order to assess the efficacy of therapy—both suppression of arrhythmia and rate control (Fig. 25-2). Similarly, patients in whom pacemakers have been implanted who have symptoms consistent with pacemaker malfunction or who require evaluation of their rate-responsive physiologic pacing function may require long-term AECG recording.

Heart rate variability and QT dispersion may be measured accurately by long-term AECG recording, which also may be helpful in patients with sleep apnea or those having suffered a previous myocardial infarction in whom further prognostic information is sought. However, the predictive value of the measurement limits it application.[4]

The recording of the pattern on AECG (as opposed to the rhythm) may be helpful in the detection of myocardial ischemia. Long-term AECG recording is indicated for patients suspected of Prinzmetal's variant angina, in whom the simultaneous recording of ST-segment elevation with symptoms should confirm the diagnosis (Fig. 25-3). Long-term recording may be of diagnostic help in patients with symptomatic angina who are unable to undergo exercise testing; preoperative risk stratification would be one indication.

Another potential use of prolonged ECG pattern recording is to correlate symptoms that occur during normal daily activity with ECG evidence of ischemia. In this setting, the demonstration of significant ST segment–T-wave alterations that cannot be reproduced by hyperventilation or by change in position, particularly when reinforced by documentation in the patient's diary of simultaneous symptoms of angina, proves highly suggestive of ischemic heart disease. Particularly in patients in whom exercise testing produces negative results

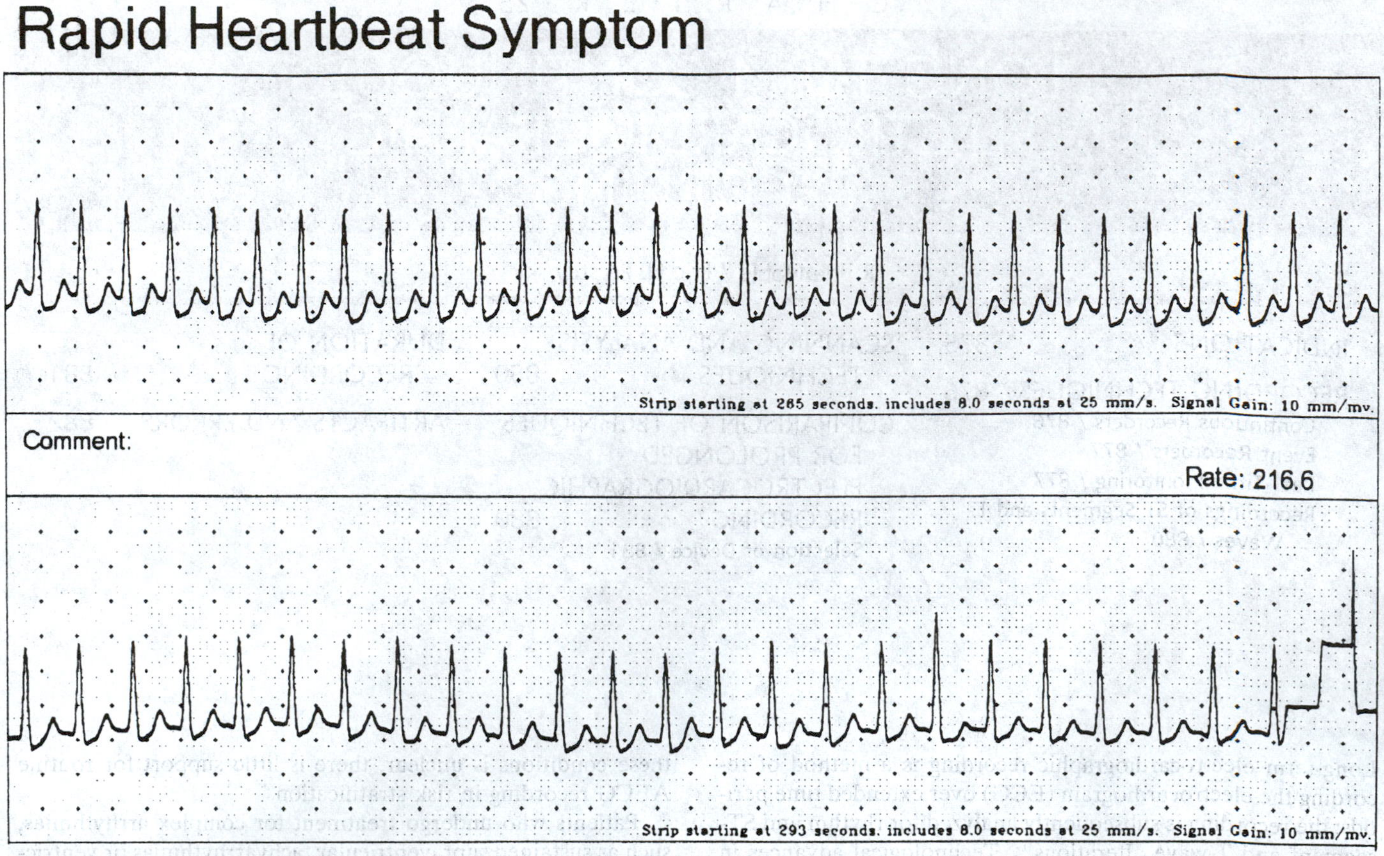

FIGURE 25-1 An episode of rapid paroxysmal supraventricular tachycardia captured with a hand-held event recorder during a typical period of symptoms.

yet symptoms highly suggestive of myocardial ischemia continue with other specific activities, AECG recording provides useful information.

The reader is referred to *Guidelines for Ambulatory Electrocardiography*, published jointly by the American College of Cardiology and the American Heart Association, for a more complete consideration of clinical indications for ambulatory AECG recordings.[4]

RECORDING TECHNIQUES

Three general types of instruments for acquiring data are currently available: continuous recorders, intermittent or event recorders, and instruments for real-time recording and transmission of ECGs (Table 25-1).

Continuous Recorders

The ECG can be recorded continuously on cassette tape or digitally in solid-state memory. The tape recorder is a battery-powered, miniature device with a very slow tape speed that is small enough to be suspended by a strap over the shoulder or around the waist.

All digital recording systems amplify, digitize, and store the ECG in solid-state memory. Two types of digital recorders are available. In the first, each QRS complex is recorded, similar in this sense to the continuous tape recording. "Full disclosure" of the ECG is provided by enhanced storage capacity on a memory card the size of a credit card. With the second, microcomputers and microelectronic circuits sample the cardiac rhythm in real time as it is being recorded, convert the analog signal into a digital signal, and analyze the data in terms of maximal and minimal rates, RR intervals, and changes in RR intervals. Within minutes of the instrument's disconnection from the patient, the information can be retrieved in the form of a histogram covering the entire recording period, and a printout of selected segments in real time can be obtained. This instrument is different from those used to make continuous tape or digital recordings in that the actual ECG has not been recorded on tape; only the histogram has been stored. Selected brief segments of the patient's ECG, e.g., 6- to 10-s intervals, also can be stored, however. Microcomputers that can analyze electronic data over prolonged periods, even several days, have been developed.

The lead systems on recorders vary from one manufacturer to another. Meticulous attention must be paid to placing the electrodes on the patient's chest, since poor electrode contact will produce technically inadequate recordings.

Event Recorders

An alternative method records not continuously but only when the patient senses symptoms or an event. Of the numerous event recorders available, there are two basic types, which are differentiated on the basis of memory.

In the *postevent recorder*, without memory, the unit may continuously monitor the ECG via attached leads. The patient wears the recorder continuously, activating it when symptoms appear; this device does not record the ECG until it is activated. Alternatively, the patient may carry a miniature solid-state recorder (sufficiently small to fit into a pocket or purse) with which the rhythm can be recorded whenever the symptoms appear simply by placing the unit on the precordium. Some newer devices are the size of a credit card, to be carried in a wallet or worn as a necklace or wristwatch. The recorded data are stored in memory until the patient submits the information either directly or transtelephonically to an ECG receiver, where it is recorded. When a tape is employed, the tape is then erased, and subsequent data can be recorded and transmitted to facilitate the recording of rhythm or pattern during several symptomatic episodes. When digital acquisition devices are used, a prolonged, continuous event can be recorded and stored or the device can be programmed to acquire multiple events.

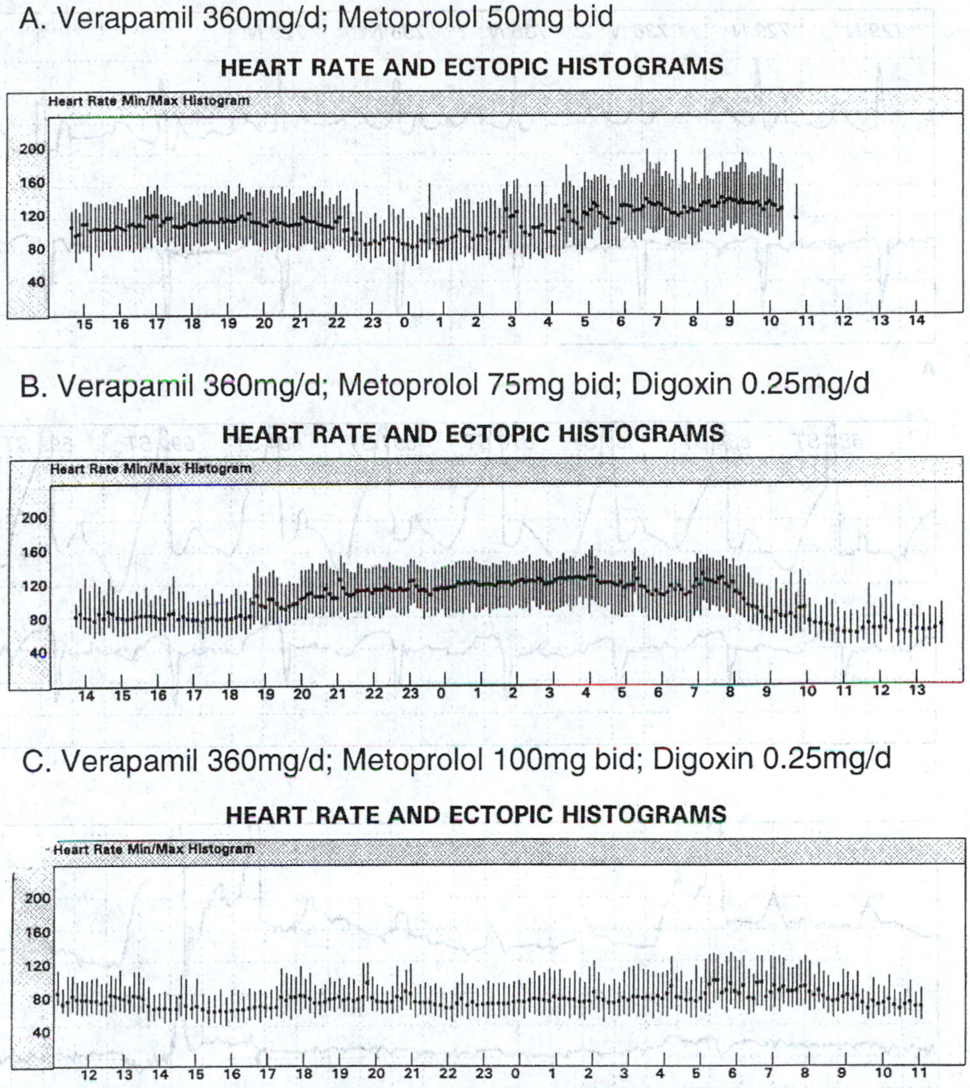

FIGURE 25-2 Histograms of serial 24-h AECG to evaluate rate control in a patient with atrial fibrillation. In *A* and *B* the overall ventricular rate during the monitoring period was too fast. Adequate rate control is shown in *C*. (With permission from *American Journal of Cardiology* from manuscript, Prystowsky, EN. "Management of atrial fibrillation: Therapeutic options and clinical decisions," in press.)

With a *preevent recorder*, employing a memory loop, the rhythm is monitored continuously via leads either at the extremities or over the precordium, connected to a recorder typically worn on a belt. Patients activate the unit when they experience symptoms so that an abnormal rhythm or an ECG synchronous with the symptoms can be recorded. The loop recorder is capable of recording information several seconds or minutes before or after a recognized event; the number of events that can be recorded and the allotment of recording time prior to and after activation of the unit are programmable.

A miniaturized *event recorder* has been developed that can be implanted subcutaneously to be mechanically activated by the patient to record an ECG when the patient suffers serious symptoms (such as syncope) at widely spaced intervals.[5,6] Incorporating a memory loop, the preevent ECG is recorded, and the resulting recording is transmitted by telemetry to a receiver for analysis.

Event recording is also provided by some newer-generation DDD pacemakers and implantable cardioverter defibrillators (Fig. 25-4). These instruments automatically recognize abnormal rhythms, such as tachycardia, and provide, via telemetric transmission, either actual ECG records or an analysis of the number, rate, and duration of recognized arrhythmias.

Real-Time Monitoring

As another variation, the device that acquires data can transmit the ECG information directly and transtelephonically, in real time, without recording the data in the unit. With such a device, for instance, the patient can transmit his or her ECG daily or even multiple times each day, with or without symptoms, at some distance from the medical institution to the recording station.

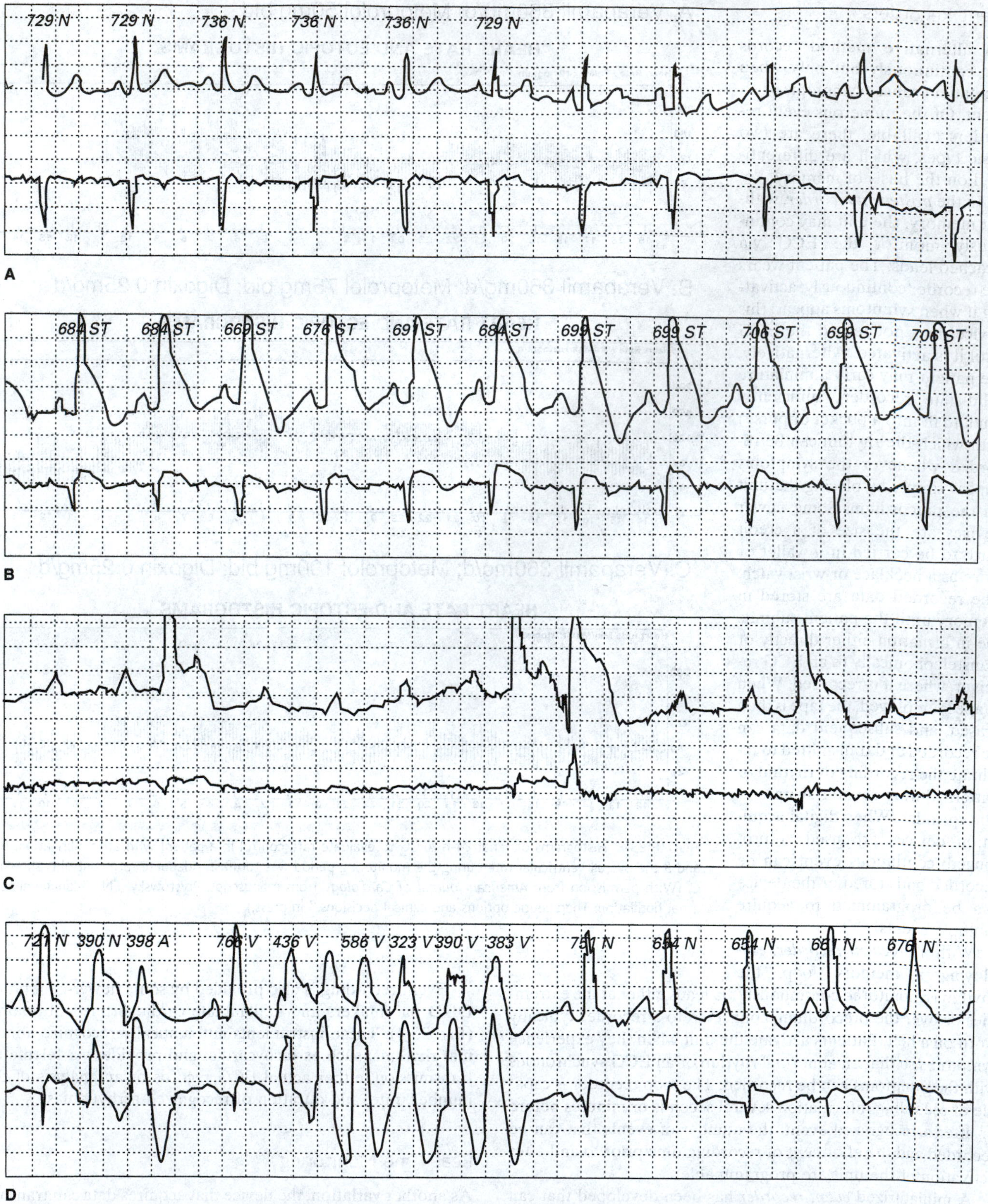

FIGURE 25-3 AECG recording in Prinzmetal's variant angina. *A.* Control. Lead II (*top*), precordial lead (*bottom*). *B.* Marked ST-segment elevation (resembling monophasic action potential), associated with mild angina. *C.* High-grade atrioventricular block and continued ST-segment elevation, associated with near syncope. *D.* Nonsustained ventricular tachycardia with continued ST-segment elevation associated with palpitations and light-headedness.

TABLE 25-1 Types of Electrocardiographic Recording Instruments

Type	Recording	Scanning	Transmitting
	HOLTER		
Analog	All ECG complexes "Full Disclosure"	Technician with computer assistance, templating, area determination and superimposition	None
Digital—continuous recording	All ECG complexes "Full Disclosure"	Technician with computer assistance, templating, area determination and superimposition	Transtelephonic
Digital—real-time analysis	Computer analysis of ECG and selected ECG printouts	Real time by microprocessor with retrospective technician editing	None
	EVENT RECORDER		
"Postevent," nonlooping, without memory			
Hand-held (including credit card size) wristwatch–type	ECG, selected by patient activation	Direct visualization	Transtelephonic
Automatic electronic sensor, in DDD pacemaker	ECG, when activated automatically by sensor	Direct visualization of analysis or ECG	Direct telemetry
"Preevent," looping, with memory monitor worn with attached electrodes	ECG, selected by patient activation, with memory of preevent	Direct visualization	Transtelephonic
Subcutaneous, implanted digital recorder	ECG, selected by patient activation with memory of preevent	Direct visualization	Direct telemetry
Automatic electronic sensor, in ICD or pacemaker	ECG, when activated by firing of ICD or recognized by sensor in pacemaker, with memory	Direct visualization of analysis or ECG	Direct telemetry
	REAL TIME		
Real-time transtelephonic monitoring	ECG at central monitoring station—no recording at device	Direct visualization	Transtelephonic

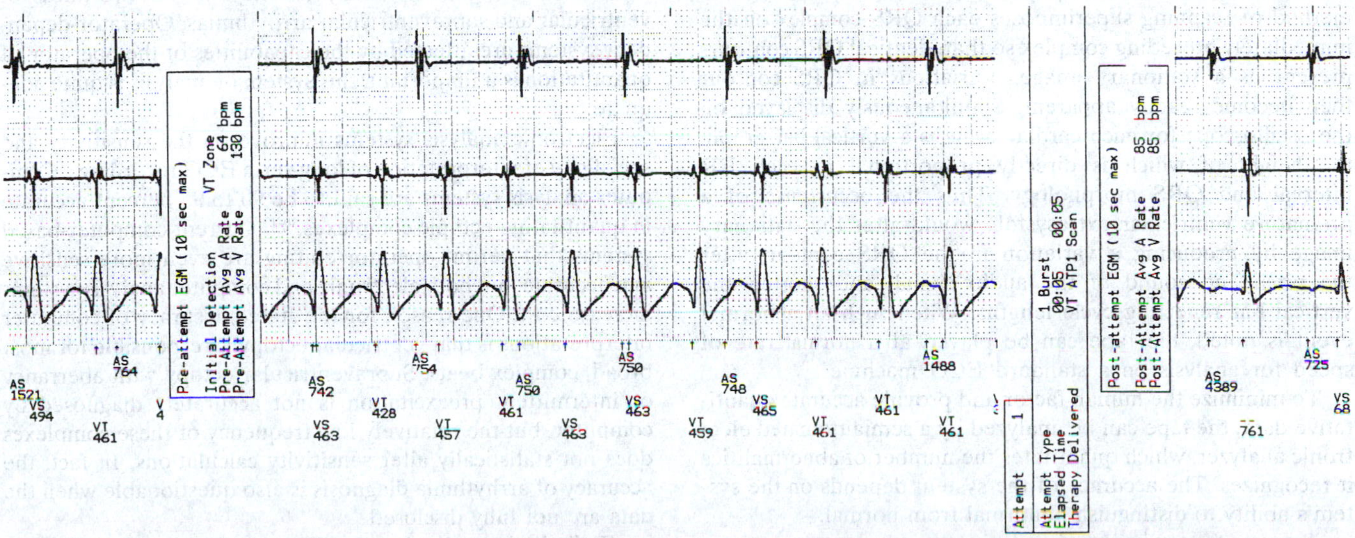

FIGURE 25-4 Intracardiac electrograms from a dual-chamber implantable cardioverter defibrillator (ICD) for an episode of ventricular tachycardia. The simultaneous tracings are the atrial electrocardiogram, ventricular electrocardiogram, anda far-field electrocardiogram. Note atrioventricular dissociation during ventricular tachycardia (*left* and *center*) and normal sinus rhythm after termination of ventricular tachycardia by antitachycardia pacing (*right*).

Recordings of ST Segments and T Waves

For several reasons, both technical and physiologic, long-term ECG recording devices do not provide the same degree of reliability in interpretation of the pattern of the ST segment and T wave as in the detection of rhythm disturbances.[7–8] Technical limitations include certain characteristics of the patient's ECG; normal sinus rhythm, an isoelectric ST segment, and absence of broad Q waves, intraventricular conduction delays, and LV hypertrophy are prerequisites. The patient cannot be treated with digitalis and some other drugs that alter ST-segment–T-wave morphology. Electrode preparation and placement must be meticulous. AECG recordings of ST-segment–T-wave morphology should be performed only by physicians and institutions trained and experienced in these techniques. With these considerations, however, newer-generation digital recording systems and those with improved low-frequency characteristics more accurately reproduce ST-T segments; some new systems either directly record or derive full 12-lead ECGs.

Even more important than these technical considerations, however, are certain physiologic limitations. For instance, standing, hyperventilation, eating, anxiety, use of drugs, and change in heart rate or autonomic tone are all daily events that may result in depression of the ST segment or inversion of the T wave to simulate ischemic changes. Striking ST-segment elevation has been recorded during prolonged recording in patients without organic heart disease.[9]

SCANNING AND ANALYSIS TECHNIQUES

The recording can be analyzed by scanning the tape or digital record at high speed, by printing it out directly, or—as in the case of microcomputers—by processing during the recording and printing out the analysis at the end of sampling.

Scanning techniques include technician-dependent analysis, in which a technician interprets the cardiac rhythm as it is played back at high speed on an oscilloscope at 30 to 240 times the speed of the actual event. One commonly used method of scanning superimposes each QRS complex on the immediately preceding complex so that identical QRS contours present as a stationary image. Variations in QRS contour then become readily apparent. Simultaneously displayed on the oscilloscope for each cardiac cycle is a vertical bar graph, the height of which is directly proportional to each RR interval and QRS morphology. Thus the occurrence of a premature ventricular extrasystole would alter the stationary image by producing a variation in the QRS contour, alter the pitch and sound of the audio signal, and shorten the vertical bar reflecting cycle lengths. When such an abnormal event is noted, the tape can be played at a normal rate of speed for analysis on a standard ECG machine.

To minimize the human factor and provide accurate quantitative data, the tape can be analyzed by a semiautomated electronic analyzer, which quantitates the number of abnormalities it recognizes. The accuracy of the system depends on the system's ability to distinguish abnormal from normal.

A computer can be interfaced with the scanner to quantitate the data even more accurately. The playback analysis can occur at up to 240 times the normal rate. Electronic analyzers and computers, as well as the scanner, can be programmed to recognize the patient's own QRS complex template and then to recognize any deviation from normal. The computer program can provide summaries of heart rates, heart rate variability, frequency of premature atrial or ventricular extrasystoles, coupling intervals, runs of tachycardia or other arrhythmias, and variations in QRS, ST, QT, or T-wave pattern during any time period. Hard copies can be printed out for verification. When arrhythmias or pattern changes are detected, an automatic ECG printout can be triggered by the event marker or by the computer.

Scanning services are available and generally can provide reasonably accurate analysis at less cost than can small institutions or offices with smaller volumes of long-term ECG recordings. Recorders can be purchased, leased, or rented.

An alternative to scanning is the direct printout of the entire record. Prolonged ECG records are compressed to reduce the amount of paper that the physician must examine; when brief events are recorded, compression is not necessary. By writing out the entire ECG directly, the need for a trained technician and scanners may be obviated.

Since microcomputers assess the ECG in real time, as it is recorded, there is no need for a scanner or expert technician when the results are printed out. The physician evaluates the trend chart or any recorded rhythm strip.

As noted in Table 25-1, all the event recordings, the real-time recording, as well as some of the continuous recordings can be transmitted transtelephonically to receivers for analysis and interpretation. These recordings of implanted pacemakers or defibrillators are available by telemetry.

COMPARISON OF TECHNIQUES FOR PROLONGED ELECTROCARDIOGRAPHIC RECORDING

Operator-dependent high-speed audiovisual analysis of the tape, without direct printout or electronic analysis, recognizes serious rhythm disturbances. On the other hand, the operator can fail to recognize as many as one-third to two-thirds of ventricular and supraventricular arrhythmias. Operator-dependent systems are affected by the capabilities of the operator. If quantitation is unimportant, this system of analysis is quite adequate.

Electronic analysis systems improve on the sensitivity and specificity of interpretation of long-term ECG recordings. Computer analysis systems are said to be 90 to 95 percent accurate in quantitating ectopic complexes.[10–12] Current computer-based systems that permit operator editing are even more sensitive and accurate, but both electronic and computer analysis systems increase cost. One reason for the stated accuracy of computer interpretations is that ventricular ectopy is responsible for most broad, complex beats. Supraventricular ectopy with aberrancy or intermittent preexcitation is not accurately diagnosed by computer, but the relatively low frequency of these complexes does not statistically alter sensitivity calculations. In fact, the accuracy of arrhythmia diagnosis is also questionable when the data are not fully disclosed.

"Full disclosure"—i.e., hard-copy printout of the entire record—provides a visual analysis of the record to identify complex disturbances such as ventricular tachycardia or prolonged asystolic intervals. In addition, it is often useful to have hard-copy ECG data available (as opposed to those derived from analysis of the ECG data) with which to compare subsequent records. The direct printout does not quantitate the actual number of events. Assuming care in interpretation, the direct printout may be more sensitive than high-speed operator-dependent and semiautomated systems with operator editing in identifying pairs or triplets of consecutive ectopic complexes.

An event recorder does not require a scanner or an experienced technician; however, the continuously recording event recorder itself is more expensive than a continuously recording tape recorder. The postevent recorder, without memory, which the patient applies only when symptoms appear, is less expensive. Both types of event recorders provide an ECG record more quickly than a system that requires scanning,[13] but neither creates a long-term record of the ECG during asymptomatic intervals. The automatic event recorders incorporated in pacemakers and implantable defibrillators are limited by the accuracy and sensitivity of the algorithm used to detect abnormalities yet enhanced by analysis of intracardiac signals. Any event recorder clearly allows correlation between the patient's symptoms and the rhythm. The only technique currently available to record rhythm events leading up to and following infrequently occurring symptoms is the memory-loop event recorder.

When more rapid identification of a rhythm abnormality in an outpatient is essential, as in the patient with a potentially dangerous rhythm disturbance, real-time transmitters permit frequent and even automatic transtelephonic transmission of the ambulatory record to a hospital or clinic telemetry receiver. The monitor technician can then quickly identify a serious rhythm abnormality and arrange for the patient's proper management.

Those microcomputers which analyze the rhythm in real time, simultaneous with the recording, should prove at least as accurate as other high-speed playback analysis systems. More important, longer periods can be monitored than are practical for other systems. The cost of the analysis is independent of the duration of recording, so patient cost should be less for prolonged periods of monitoring. Finally, the analysis of the entire recording and the actual printout of the specific ECG segment are available within minutes of the recording. On the other hand, only limited segments of actual ECG records are generally available, and the accuracy of abnormal rhythm or pattern recognition remains dependent on the computer algorithm; this recognition is far from perfect, since many problems in the computer analysis of complex rhythm disturbances remain unsolved.

When the ECG pattern is monitored for ischemia, newer-generation methodologies—either digital or with enhanced low-frequency recording—are required. Whichever system is employed, the ultimate accuracy of ECG interpretation depends on the technician and overreading physician; scanners and computers cannot differentiate complex patterns (supraventricular arrhythmias with aberrancy as opposed to ventricular arrhythmias or preexcitation) or even artifacts. The clinical application of the data is solely the function of the responsible physician. No data-acquisition system or scanner, no computer, and no technician can substitute for the well-trained physician in determining the significance of any recorded data and their clinical utility.

Selection of Device

The ultimate selection of a long-term ECG recording system depends on individual patient needs. If a precise count of ectopy is required, a continuous recorder with computer-based analysis is essential. These devices are also very useful to evaluate ventricular rate control in atrial fibrillation (see Fig. 25-2). On the other hand, if the purpose of the recording is to detect ventricular tachycardia or asystole, an event recorder, a microcomputer, or direct printout of the entire record would be an excellent choice. Either a microcomputer or an event recorder provides an opportunity to monitor over prolonged periods of time, and either is of benefit to the patient whose rhythm disturbance occurs infrequently. When the goal is to correlate the patient's rhythm or ECG pattern with symptoms that are very infrequent (at weekly intervals or less), the patient-applied and patient-activated event recorder is the optimal choice. However, if the patient's symptoms are of such brief duration (seconds) or severe (frank syncope) to preclude capture by such a unit, then a loop event recorder is required. This and the direct printout are less expensive for an individual physician's or small clinic's use, and both are more cost-effective than prolonged ambulatory (Holter) recordings, whether indicated for assessment of palpitations[14,15] or such serious symptoms as syncope[15] (see Fig. 25-1). The implantable event recorder with memory may prove optimal for those patients with syncopal events so widely spaced (months) as to render other devices impractical.[6]

Except with large scanning services, it is impractical for an individual physician to have available all the monitoring techniques for each individual patient's needs. Hence the physician's selection of a system is based on his or her own patient population, the frequency of using this test, the availability of dependable scanning services, and the associated cost analysis. The physician would do well to realize that any or all of the systems described herein are available alone or in combination. The more detailed and precisely quantitated the final report, generally the more expensive are the equipment and personnel required. All systems recognize marked tachycardia or bradycardia and, qualitatively at least, detect ectopy. For clinical purposes, this amount of information is usually sufficient. The practicing physician does not really require precise quantitation, since the therapeutic and prognostic significance of such quantitation is not yet known. In short, technology exceeds clinical assimilation of the results at the present time.

DURATION OF RECORDING

Arrhythmias are often evanescent, occurring only rarely. In such patients, 24-h ECG recordings are unlikely to detect the abnormal rhythm. Even when arrhythmias are frequent, marked variation in the frequency and complexity of the rhythm disturbance is expected, with variations occurring during and between days. Spontaneous reduction in the frequency of ventricular ectopy of 50 to 90 percent is common.[16,17] For screening purposes, 24-h ECG tape recording seems an optimal compromise between the practical limits of recording and the point of diminishing return.[18–20]

If a reduction in total number of premature ventricular complexes is the goal of antiarrhythmic therapy, then more than one control 24-h ECG recording and several recordings while the patient is receiving therapy are required to prove efficacy.[18,19]

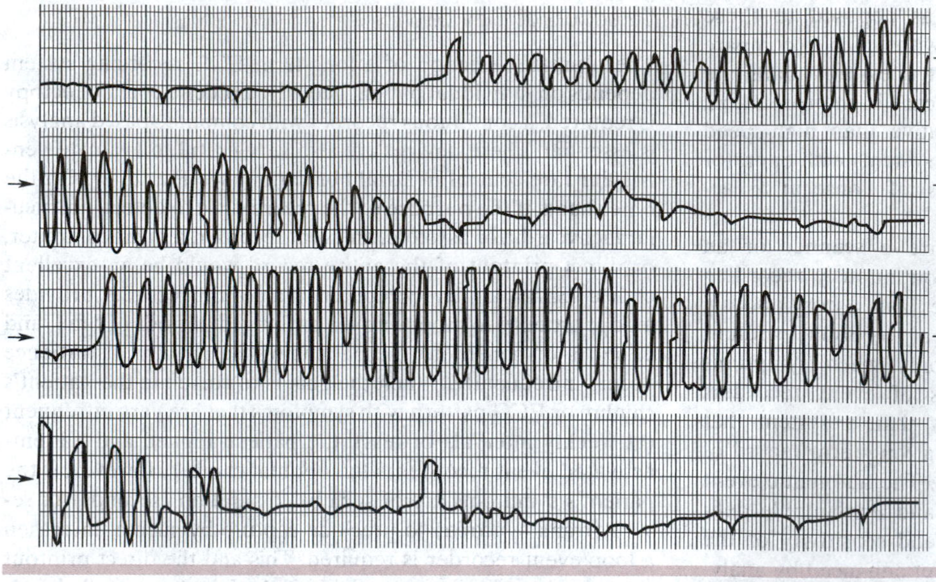

FIGURE 25-5 Artifact recorded on monitor. A loose electrode was responsible for the artifactual tracing mimicking ventricular flutter/fibrillation recorded by the monitor.

The total number of premature ventricular complexes must be reduced by about 80 percent.[16,17,21,22] On the other hand, since it has not yet been demonstrated that reducing the total number of premature ventricular complexes necessarily implies the elimination of more dire ventricular rhythm disturbances or sudden death, this is often not the physician's goal. Instead, simply preventing sustained, symptomatic ventricular tachycardia may be the therapeutic goal,[23] in which case multiple 24-h recordings are less essential.

The frequency and degree of ST-segment depression also vary chronologically.[24-26] Forty-eight hours is probably the optimal duration for monitoring ST-segment changes.[27] When comparing a 48-h recording prior to and following therapy, the frequency of ST-segment deviation must be reduced by 75 percent to infer a therapeutic efficacy.[28]

The ideal duration of recording varies from patient to patient, depending on the physician's goals. If the objective is to correlate the cardiac rhythm or pattern with a symptom such as syncope, palpitations, or chest pain, then the monitoring period must be extended sufficiently to incorporate a symptomatic period, whether these intervals occur with a frequency of hours or months. The actual recording period, however, may be only seconds.

ARTIFACTS AND ERRORS

Artifacts registered during prolonged ECG recording have mimicked virtually every variety of supraventricular and ventricular bradycardia and tachycardia and have led to misdiagnosis[29,30] and inappropriate and unnecessary treatment.[31]

Most of these artifacts are identical to those plaguing the standard 12-lead ECG but are simply detected more frequently due to the length of the recording; however, many are unique to extended recording by virtue of the magnetic tape recorder.

Probably the most common artifact is that resulting from a

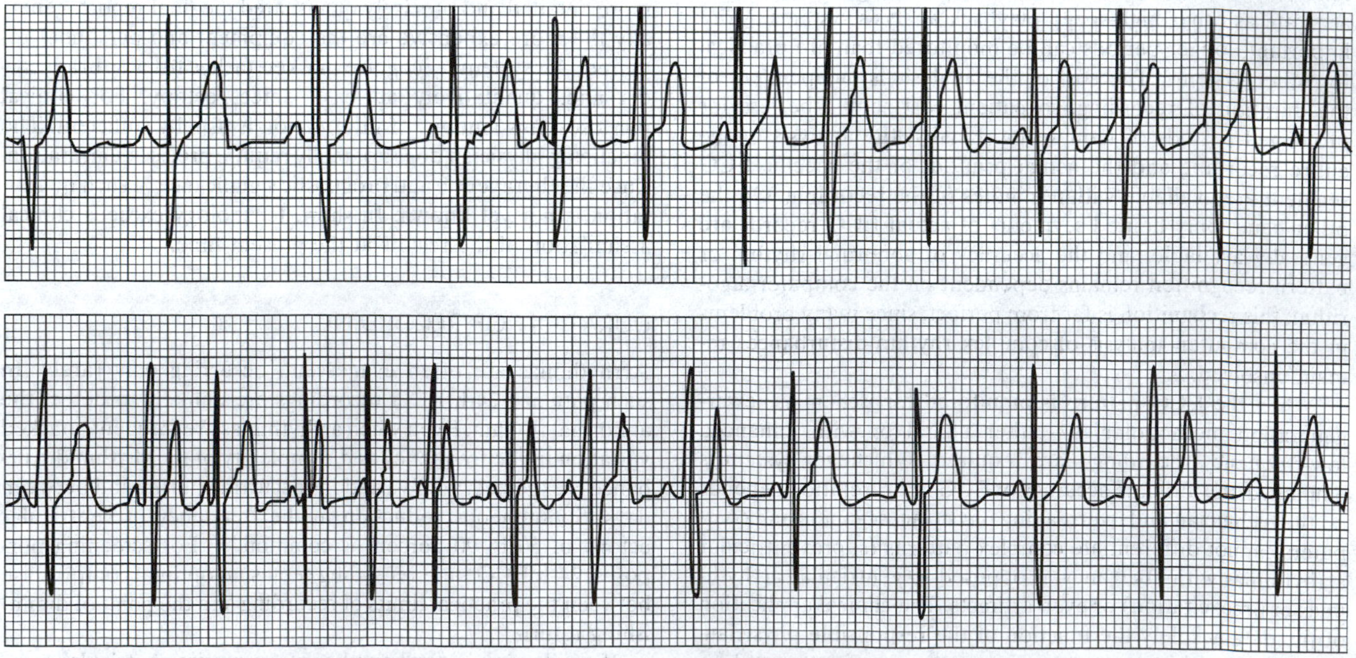

FIGURE 25-6 Deceleration of tape during recording. Supraventricular tachycardia is simulated toward the end of the top and beginning of the second trace as the tape, which transiently slowed as a result of battery failure during recording, was played back on recording paper at proper speed. Note the foreshortening of the duration of the P wave, PR interval, QRS complex, and QT interval.

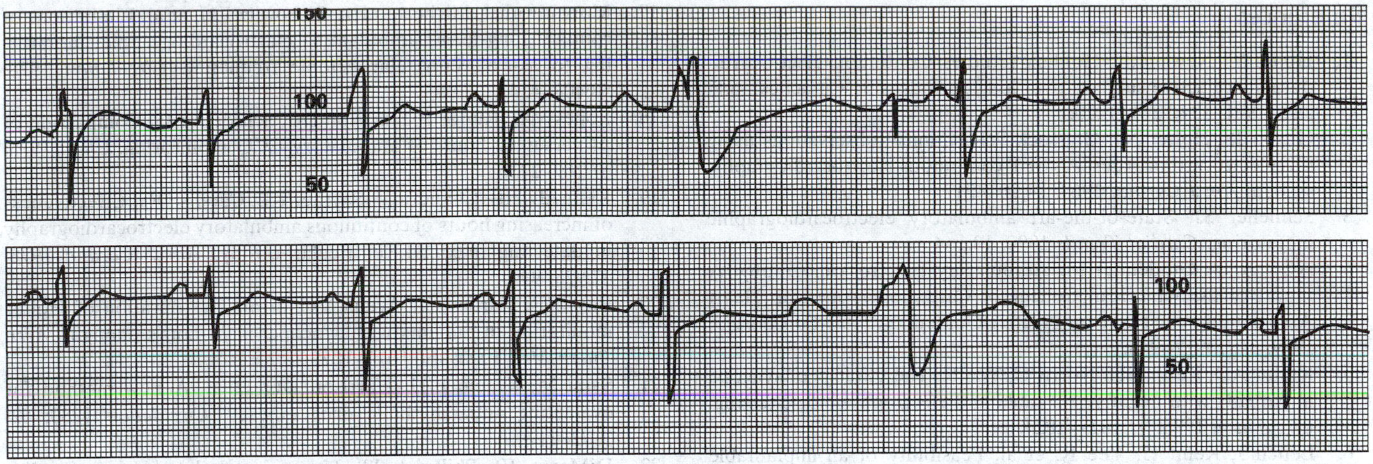

FIGURE 25-7 Deceleration of tape during playback. Slowing or sticking of the tape during playback spreads out the P wave, PR interval, and QRS complex to resemble sinus deceleration or transient atrioventricular or intraventricular conduction delay (fifth complex in top trace; sixth complex in bottom trace).

loose electrode (Fig. 25-5) or mechanical "stimulation" of the electrode. Failure of either the battery or the motor of the recorder generally results in a slowing of the tape speed as the ECG is recorded. When played back, the heart rate will appear fast; i.e., it will mimic a tachycardia (Fig. 25-6). The interpreter may be alerted to the artifact by the concomitant shortening of all ECG intervals (PR, QRS, QT, and RR) and decrease in QRS voltage. Conversely, transient slowing or sticking of the tape during playback will suggest bradycardia or atrioventricular (AV) or intraventricular conduction disturbances (Fig. 25-7). Recording an ECG on a previously used tape that is incompletely erased results in the simultaneous registration of two ECGs and potentially the misinterpretation of a "parasystolic" ectopic rhythm (Fig. 25-8). Digital recording in solid-state memory eliminates these various mechanical failures of tape recordings.

The technician and/or physician who interprets prolonged ECG recordings must have a working knowledge of these and other potential artifacts in order to interpret the records properly.

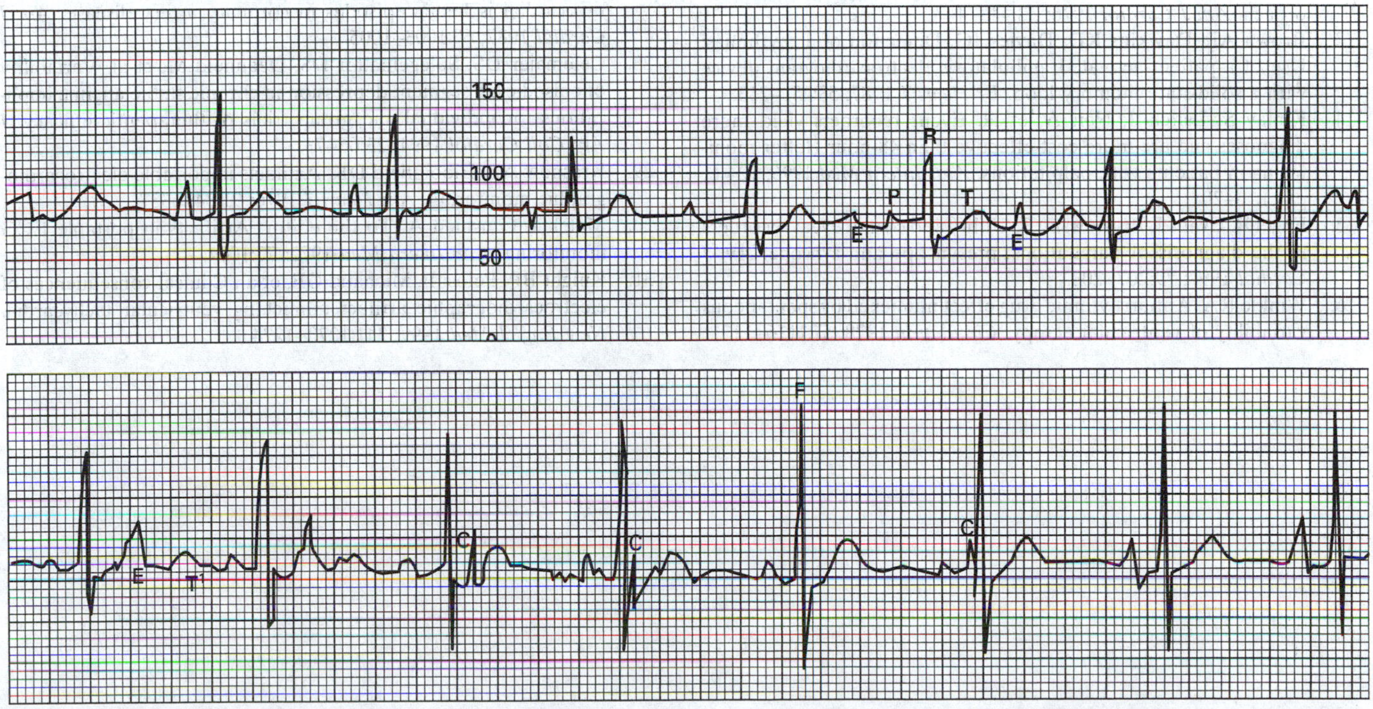

FIGURE 25-8 Incomplete erasure of tape. Two independent ventricular rhythms are identified: a larger QRS, labeled *R*, whose P wave and T wave are also labeled, and a smaller QRS, considered "ectopic" and labeled *E*; its T wave is labeled *T*. The sequence could be recorded with a piggyback heart transplant or in Siamese twins. Alternatively, ectopic complex E may be misinterpreted to represent a parasystolic rhythm even fusing with complex R at F. The very short coupling intervals (C) preclude this possibility and indicate that the ECG record of one patient is superimposed on that of another.

References

1. Holter NJ. New method for heart studies: Continuous electrocardiography of active subjects over long periods is now practical. *Science* 1961; 134:1214–1220.
2. Gilson JS, Holter NJ, Glassock WR. Clinical observations using this electrocardiocorder: AVSEP continuous electrocardiographic system. *Am J Cardiol* 1964; 14:204–217.
3. Schneller SJ. State-of-the-art ambulatory electrocardiographic monitoring. *Cardiol Trends* 1990; 10:1–4.
4. ACC/AHA Guidelines for Ambulatory Electrocardiography: A report of the American College of Cardiology/American Heart Association Task Force on Practice Guidelines. *J Am Coll Cardiol* 1999; 34:(3)917–948.
5. Krahn AD, Kelin GH, Norris C, Yee R. The etiology of syncope in patients with negative tilt table and electrophysiologic testing. *Circulation* 1995; 92:1819–1824.
6. Leitch J, Kelin G, Yee R, et al. Feasibility of an implantable arrhythmia monitor. *Pacing Clin Electrophysiol* 1992; 15:2232–2235.
7. Hinkle LE Jr, Meyer J, Stevens M, Carver ST. Recordings of the ECG of active men. *Circulation* 1967; 36:752–765.
8. Crawford MH, Mendoza CA, O'Rourke RA, et al. Limitations of continuous ambulatory electrocardiogram monitoring for detecting coronary artery disease. *Ann Intern Med* 1978; 89:1–5.
9. Golding B, Wolf E. Tzivoni D, Stern S. Transient S-T elevation detected by 24-hour ECG monitoring during normal daily activity. *Am Heart J* 1973; 86:501–507.
10. Stein IM, Plunkett J, Troy M. Comparison of techniques for examining long-term ECG recordings. *Med Instrum* 1980; 14: 69–72.
11. Fitzgerald JW, Spitz AL, Winkle RA, Harrison DC. Quantitation of ambulatory electrocardiograms (abstract). *Circulation* 1977; 56(suppl 3):178.
12. Knoebel SB, Lovelace DE, Rasmussen S, Wash SE. Computer detection of premature ventricular complexes: A modified approach. *Am J Cardiol* 1976; 38:440–447.
13. Brown AP, Dawkins KD, Davies JG. Detection of arrhythmias: Use of a patient-activated ambulatory electrocardiogram device with a solid-state memory loop. *Br Heart J* 1987; 58:251–253.
14. Kinlay S, Leitch J, Neil A, et al. Event recorders yield more diagnoses and are more cost-effective than 48-hour Holter monitoring in patients with palpitations. *Ann Intern Med* 1996; 124 (1 pt 1):16–20.
15. Fogel R, Evans J, Prystowsky E. Utility and cost of event recorders in the diagnosis of palpitations, presyncope and syncope. *Am J Cardiol* 1997; 79:207–208.
16. Winkle RA. Antiarrhythmic drug effect mimicked by spontaneous variability of ventricular ectopy. *Circulation* 1978; 57:1116–1121.
17. Morganroth J, Michelson EL, Horowitz LN, et al. Limitations of routine long-term ambulatory electrocardiographic monitoring to assess ventricular ectopic frequency. *Circulation* 1978; 58:408–414.
18. Lopes MG, Runge P, Harrison DC, Schroeder JS. Comparison of 24 versus 12 hours of ambulatory ECG monitoring. *Chest* 1975; 67:269–273.
19. Kennedy HL, Chandra V, Sayther KL, Caralis DG. Effectiveness of increasing hours of continuous ambulatory electrocardiography in detecting maximal ventricular ectopy. *Am J Cardiol* 1978; 42:925–930.
20. Bass EB, Curtiss EI, Arena VC, et al. The duration of Holter monitoring in patients with syncope: is 24 hours enough? *Arch Intern Med* 1990; 150:1073–1078.
21. Sami M, Kraemer H, Harrison DC, et al. A new method for evaluating antiarrhythmic drug efficacy. *Circulation* 1980; 62: 1172–1179.
22. DiMarco JP, Philbrick JT. Uses of ambulatory electrocardiographic (Holter) monitoring. *Ann Intern Med* 1990; 113:53–68.
23. Winkle RA, Alderman EL, Fitzgerald JW, Harrison DC. Treatment of recurrent symptomatic ventricular tachycardia. *Ann Intern Med* 1976; 85:1–7.
24. Nabel EG, Barry J, Rocco MB, et al. Variability of transient myocardial ischemia in ambulatory patients with coronary artery disease. *Circulation* 1988; 78:60–67.
25. Nademanee K, Christenson PD, Intarachot V, et al. Variability of indexes for myocardial ischemia: A comparison of exercise treadmill test, ambulatory electrocardiographic monitoring and symptoms of myocardial ischemia. *J Am Coll Cardiol* 1989; 13:574–579.
26. Celemajer DS, Spiegelhalter DJ, Deanfield M, et al. Variability of episodic ST segment depression in chronic stable angina; implications for individual and group trials of therapeutic efficacy. *J Am Coll Cardiol* 1994; 23:66–73.
27. Tzivoni D, Gavish A, Benhorin J, et al. Day-to-day variability of myocardial ischemic episodes in coronary artery disease. *Am J Cardiol* 1987; 60:1003–1005.
28. Celemajer DS, Spiegelhalter DS, Deanfield M, et al. Variability of episodic ST segment depression in chronic stable angina: implications for individual and group trials of therapeutic efficacy. *J Am Coll Cardiol* 1994; 23:66–73.
29. Krasnow AZ, Bloomfield DK. Artifacts in portable electrocardiographic monitoring. *Am Heart J* 1976; 91:349–357.
30. Malek J, Glushien A. To the editor: Artifacts in portable ECG monitoring. *Ann Intern Med* 1972; 77:1004.
31. Knight BP, Pelosi F, Michaud GF, et al. Clinical consequences of electrocardiographic artifact mimicking ventricular tachycardia. *New Engl J Med* 1999; 341:1270–1274.

CHAPTER 26

TECHNIQUES OF ELECTROPHYSIOLOGIC EVALUATION

Masood Akhtar

The recording of intracavitary electrocardiographic signals and various forms of pacing programs have experienced enormous growth during the past 3 decades. Recordings of intracardiac signals from the region of the His bundle, initially made by Scherlag et al.,[1] were rapidly applied to clinical problems including atrioventricular (AV) blocks and supraventricular and ventricular tachyarrhythmias.[1–10] Such recordings were then complemented by pacing to unmask sinus node dysfunction and AV conduction abnormalities as well as to initiate supraventricular tachycardias (SVTs).[3-8] Intracardiac electrophysiologic studies (EPSs) have since found utility in a variety of cardiac arrhythmias, including sinus node dysfunction, intraventricular and AV conduction disturbances, SVTs, ventricular tachycardias (VTs), preexcitation syndromes, and ventricular fibrillation (VF). Such studies are now also employed as a prelude to correction of various arrhythmias and conduction defects. This chapter addresses recording and pacing techniques and their clinical utility.[9,10]

TECHNIQUES OF INTRACARDIAC ELECTROPHYSIOLOGIC STUDIES

The exact type of electric signal recordings, specific equipment used, and pacing protocol depend upon the nature of the clinical problem, the type of electrophysiologic assessment, and the anticipated course of action. Routine cardiac EPSs are performed while patients are in a nonsedated postabsorptive state.[11] Although some degree of sedation is advisable in apprehensive patients, the use of drugs that may alter the properties of the cardiac conduction system should be avoided. Antiarrhythmic drugs are usually stopped prior to these studies. In selected cases, antiarrhythmic drugs may be continued if a clinical event occurred while the patient was on a specific agent. Customarily, other cardioactive drugs that are necessary for nonarrhythmic cardiovascular problems such as hypertension, angina, and heart failure are continued.

The typical electrode catheters used for both recording and cardiac stimulation are multipolar (sizes varying from 4 to 8 F). Catheters can be inserted via peripheral veins such as the antecubital or femoral veins and, at times, the subclavian or internal jugular veins. When a catheter is intended to be left in place for several days, subclavian and internal jugular veins are preferable. After using local anesthesia, a guide wire is inserted percutaneously through a needle, and a sheath is advanced over the guide wire. A catheter is then guided fluoroscopically through the sheath to position in the appropriate cardiac chamber. For most electrophysiologic testing, the catheter is placed in the high right atrium, at the His bundle, or at the right bundle branch region across the tricuspid valve and right ventricular apex or outflow. For accessory pathways or AV junctional tachycardias, a catheter is placed in the region of the coronary sinus. Heparinization is recommended at approximately 1000 units per hour. For EPSs, good contact between the electrodes and the walls of the various chambers is critical. For His bundle and right bundle branch recording, the catheter is introduced via the femoral vein, advanced across the tricuspid valve, and gradually withdrawn until an appropriate recording from the right bundle and/or the His bundle is obtained (Fig. 26-1). A coronary sinus catheter can be placed via an arm, internal jugular, or subclavian vein. If necessary, coronary sinus catheterization can also be accomplished via a femoral approach. Right atrial catheter placement can be done via any of the larger peripheral veins. For a routine study, left-

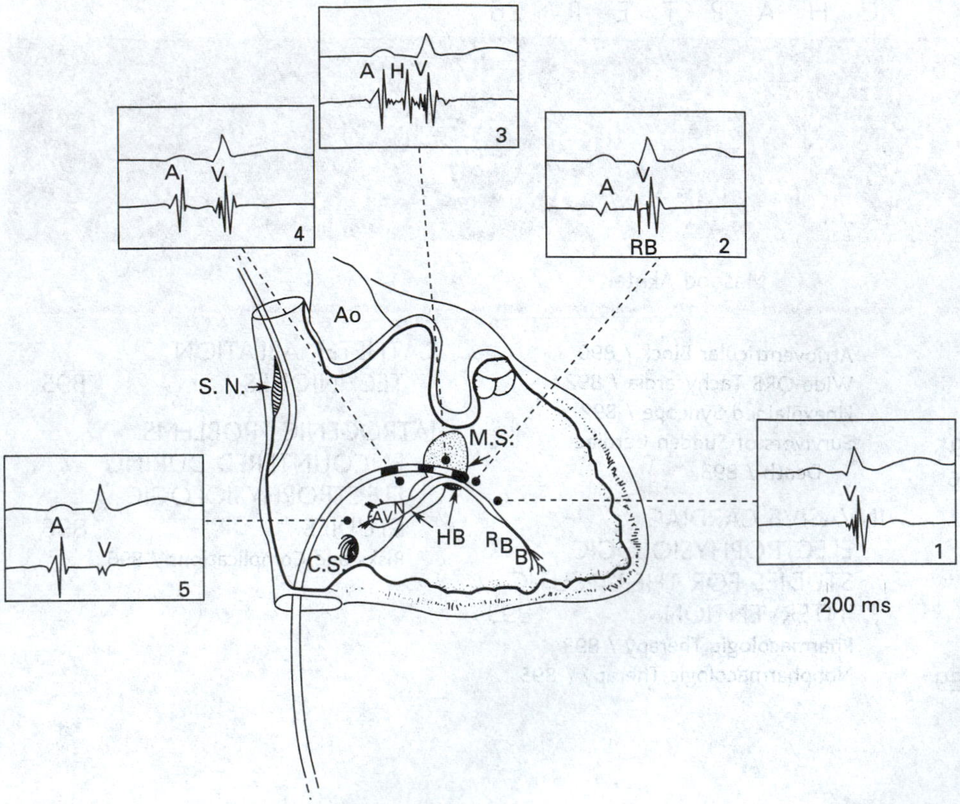

FIGURE 26-1 Intracardiac recordings from the specialized conduction system in the atrioventricular (AV) junction. The recording of various electrograms along the right side of the interventricular septum with gradual withdrawal of the catheter across the tricuspid valve is shown. The intracardiac recordings are labeled. Numbers 1 through 5 refer to intracardiac location of catheters along with corresponding electrogram. CS = coronary sinus; SN = sinus node; Ao = aorta; MS = membranous septum; AVN = atrioventricular node; HB = His bundle; RBB = right bundle branch; A = atrial deflection; H and RB = His and right bundle potentials; V = ventricular deflection. (From Gallagher and Damato.[52] Reproduced with permission from the publisher and authors.)

sided heart catheterization is seldom necessary. In patients with VT and/or left-sided accessory pathways, however, this is performed for diagnostic or therapeutic purposes. Continuous heparinization is desirable for left heart catheterization to avoid thromboembolic complications.

Electrophysiologic Recordings

Once the electrode catheters are placed appropriately, the connections are made via a junction box and isolation units to prevent excess current in the event of random electrical surges. All of the electrograms are displayed simultaneously on a multichannel oscilloscopic recorder. In addition to the intracardiac signals, several unfiltered surface electrocardiographic leads (i.e., X, Y, and Z or leads I, II, or aV_F and V_1) are recorded. To reduce the noise generated with the low-frequency signals, the usual filtering frequency for intracardiac signals is between 30 and 40 Hz for the high-pass and 500 Hz for the low-pass filters. Although appropriately placed electrode catheters will record desired signals at any filtering frequency, filter settings between 30 to 40 and 500 Hz are best suited for sharp intracardiac signals such as those from the His bundle and accessory pathways (Fig. 26-2). Undesirable low-frequency signals can be reduced by a high-pass filter setting of more than 50 to 100 Hz. On the other hand, 60-cycle interference can be eliminated with a low-pass filter setting at 50 Hz. Alteration in the high-bandpass filter for surface electrocardiography can markedly alter the scalar electrocardiographic morphology. Amplification is frequently necessary to identify desirable signals from the specialized conduction system. This can lead to superimposition of the larger myocardial signals on various electrocardiographic tracings. In most recording equipment, however, limiting filters allow the adjustment of amplitude limits.

The main value of intracardiac/electrocardiographic tracings is timing of electric events and to determine the direction of impulse propagation. To acquire true local electrical activity, a bipolar electrogram with an interelectrode distance of less than 1 cm is desirable. When unipolar electrograms are obtained, a rapid intrinsic deflection will identify a point of local activation. For routine intracardiac electrocardiographic studies, unipolar electrograms provide relatively limited advantage over bipolar signals, and therefore the latter are more often utilized. The foregoing description relates to the routine diagnostic invasive EPSs. In other clinical situations, different types of diagnostic methods are employed. For example, during intraoperative mapping, direct placement of electrodes over the epicardium or endocardium is necessary to get appropriate signals for identifying the precise origin and route of impulse propagation.[12] These electrodes can be in the form of either handheld probes or plaques that can be placed or sutured over the myocardium. Socks and balloons incorporating several electrodes can also be used for epicardial and endocardial mapping techniques, respectively.[13,14] All electrical signals can be recorded on either a disk or frequency-modulated tape for permanent storage.

More recently, several other types of mapping and recording equipment have emerged to locate the origin of cardiac arrhythmias more accurately. Two of the systems likely to find clinical utility in the mapping of arrhythmic origins are (1) nonfluoroscopic electromagnetic endocardial mapping ([CARTO, Biosense (Cordis Webster) Marlton, NJ] and (2) noncontact mapping (EnSite, Endocardial Solutions, Saint Paul, MN).

1. The CARTO system consists of a magnetic field generator locator pad placed under the patient table, a sensor-mounted

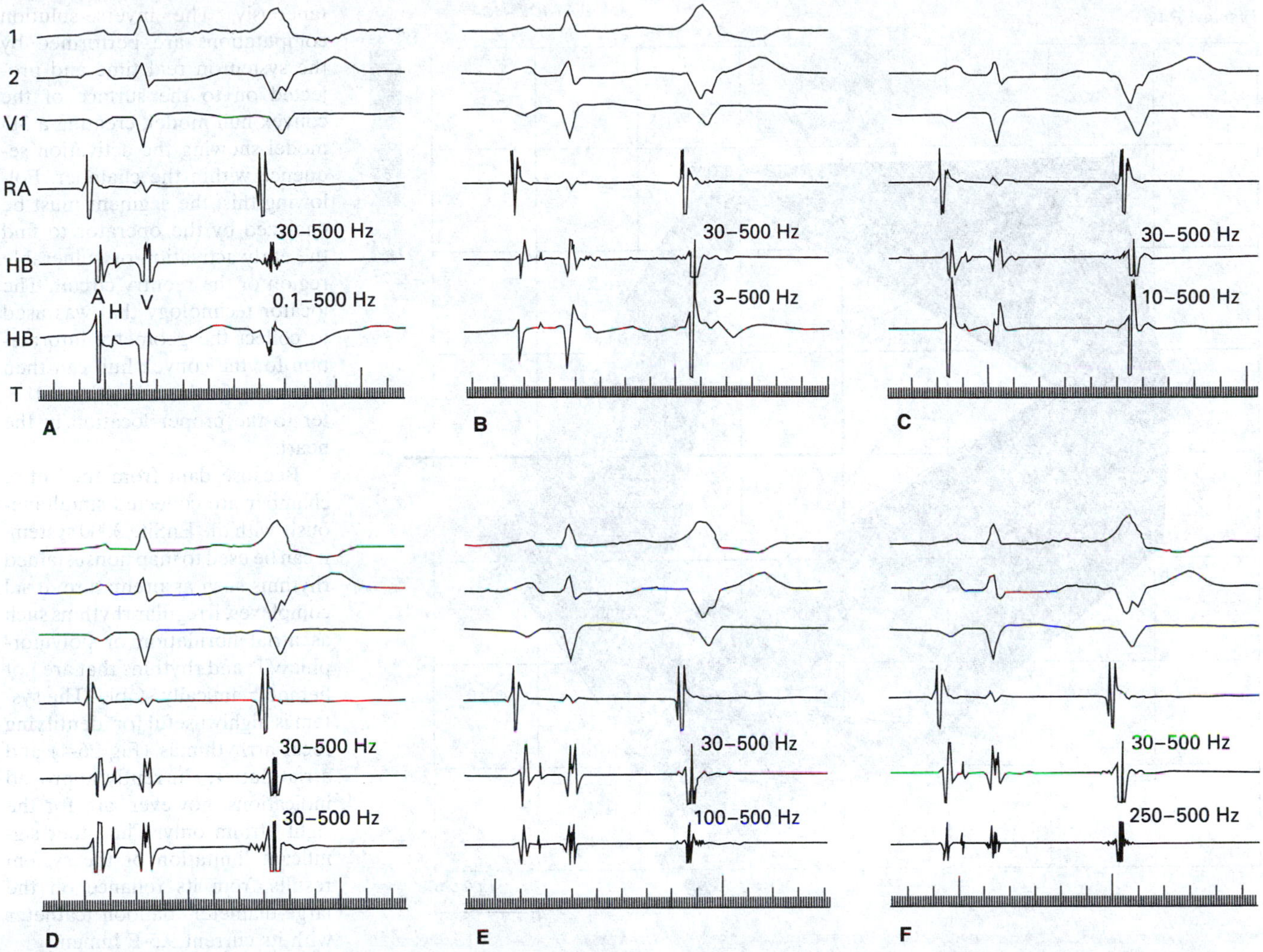

FIGURE 26-2 Effects of various filtering frequencies on the morphologic appearance of intracardiac electrograms *A* through *F*. The tracings from top to bottom are electrocardiographic leads I, II, V_1, right atrial (RA), two His bundle (HB) electrograms, and time (T) line. Similar abbreviations are used in subsequent figures and tracings. In each panel, the first beat is of sinus origin and is followed by a spontaneous ventricular premature beat. The top HB, RA, and RV are filtered at 30 to 500 Hz (i.e., the usual filtering frequencies). The bottom HB tracing shows the effect of various filtering frequencies on the appearance. The low-frequency signals are mostly eliminated at high-bandpass filter frequency settings above 10 Hz (*C*). The low-bandpass filter settings above 500 Hz generally do not have a significant effect on the intracardiac electrogram appearance. It should be pointed out that the high-bandpass setting reduces the overall magnitude of the electrogram, necessitating an increase in amplification. It should also be noted that, at all frequencies depicted, the HB deflection can be clearly identified. (From Akhtar.[11] Reproduced with permission from the publisher and authors.)

catheter and a reference catheter placed intracardially, a mapping system and a graphic computer.[15] The catheter tip allows orientation in relation to the reference signal. The accuracy of catheter tip position is within a millimeter of arrhythmia location in this low magnetic field. By moving the sensor sequentially, one can generate a three-dimensional (3D) activation map. By color coding, both the earliest and the latest directions of electrical activation can be recorded. Once the initial fluoroscopy-guided placement of reference catheter and other catheters is satisfactory, several points are acquired. A 3D map is generated, and sensor-mounted catheters are manipulated further without the help of fluoroscopy.

Aside from creation of an accurate map guiding the origin and activation sequence, the CARTO system is also helpful in separating micro from macro reentry circuits. For example, in atrial flutter, by virtue of its large circuit, the impulse propagation along the entire route can be outlined. The atrial tachycardia, on the other hand, can be distinguished by its radial spread from an atrial focus. A typical map generated during this technique is shown in Fig. 26-3, Plate 75.

2. Noncontact mapping using the Endocardial Solutions EnSite 3000 system.[16] The Endocardial Solutions EnSite 3000 is a new endocardial mapping system that takes a different approach to such mapping (Fig. 26-4, Plate 76). Like the CARTO system, the EnSite 3000 system also makes use of an amplifier and computer system with custom software. The EnSite catheter uses a balloon design with a 64-electrode array arranged over the outside of the balloon. This balloon is positioned in the center of the chamber and does not come in

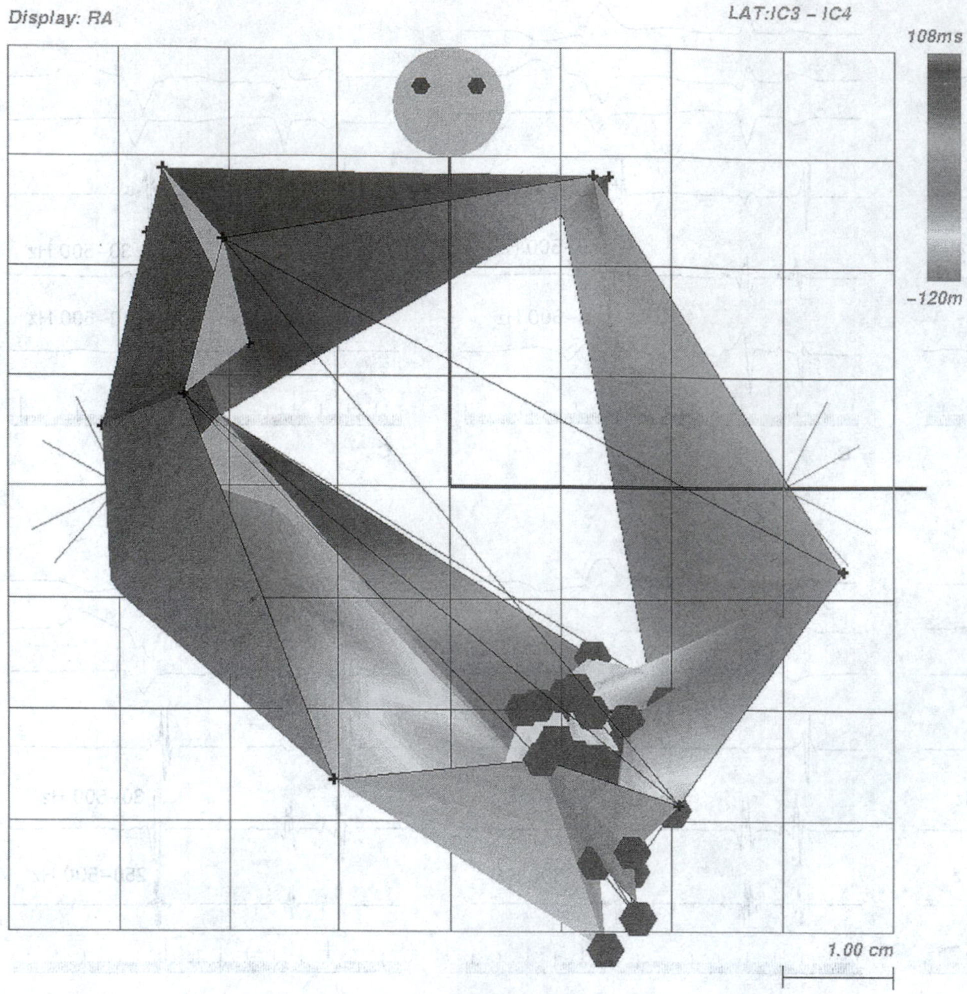

FIGURE 26-3 (Plate 75) Anterior-posterior view of the right atrium during typical, inferior vena cava (IVC)-tricuspid valve annulus isthmus-dependent atrial flutter using the Biosense CARTO system. The *red* shows the earliest activation with respect to the timing reference (typically the proximal coronary sinus recording), and the *blue* and the *violet* represent areas of late activation. The *gray* areas are where early activation meets late activation, a characteristic of reentrant tachycardias. The *brown* hexagons mark the location of radiofrequency lesions positioned on the isthmus to ablate the atrial flutter. RA = right atria.

contact with the walls of the chamber being mapped. Using data from the 64-electrode array catheter, the computer uses sophisticated algorithms to compute an *inverse solution* to determine the activation sequence on the endocardial surface. Data from all points in the chamber are acquired simultaneously.

To create a map, the balloon catheter is positioned in the chamber and deployed. A conventional (roving) deflectable catheter is also positioned in the chamber and used to collect geometry information. A 5-kHz signal is emitted from the tip electrode of the conventional catheter, and the computer analyzes this signal to determine the position of the roving catheter relative to the position of the balloon. The roving catheter is moved throughout the chamber, and the location information is collected by the system. Using this information, the computer creates a model, called a *convex hull*, of the chamber during diastole. After the chamber geometry is determined, mapping can begin. The arrhythmia is induced, and data are acquired. The data acquisition process is performed automatically by the system, and all data for the entire chamber are acquired simultaneously. The inverse-solution computations are performed by the system in real time and projected on to the surface of the convex-hull model, creating a 3D model showing the activation sequence within the chamber. Following this, the segment must be analyzed by the operator to find the early activation or vulnerable region of the reentry circuit. The locator technology that was used to collect the geometry information for the convex hull can then be used to guide an ablation catheter to the proper location in the heart.

Because data from the entire chamber are collected simultaneously with the EnSite 3000 system, it can be used to map nonsustained rhythms such as premature atrial complexes, irregular rhythms such as atrial fibrillation or polymorphic VT, and rhythms that are not hemodynamically stable. The system is highly useful for identifying focal arrhythmias (Fig 26-4) and atrial flutter. Currently approved indications, however, are for the right atrium only. The other significant limitation of the system results from its reliance on the large-diameter balloon catheter with its current 9.5-F lumen.

These mapping systems, both of which are relatively new, provide electrophysiologists with new tools for diagnosing and treating what are often complex arrhythmias. They make use of state-of-the-art technology to accomplish their objectives and improve the state of the art in arrhythmia management. Because these technologies are so new, further enhancements can be expected that will further the usefulness of advanced mapping techniques in the practice of electrophysiology.

Programmed Electrical Stimulation

After satisfactory placement of the electrode catheters, patches, or other forms of recording equipment, baseline recordings are made and programmed stimulation is initiated. The usual site of pacing is the right atrium or left atrium via the coronary sinus. For ventricular stimulation, the pacing sites are the right ventricular apex, outflow tract, and rarely some other right ventricular site. A variety of pacing programs can be utilized, depending upon the nature of the underlying arrhythmic problem under investigation. At least two formats of pacing protocol are common. The first is incremental pacing, which is pacing at a constant cycle length with gradual shortening until the occurrence of a desirable event, such as induction of a tachycardia or production of AV block. Otherwise the incremental atrial pacing is continued until the onset of AV nodal Wenckebach's phenomenon: a physiologic response at faster pacing rates. Fixed-cycle-length ventricular pacing is also used for the induction of supraventricular tachyarrhythmias and study of ventriculoatrial conduction. Bursts of pacing at a constant cycle length are occasionally used to induce SVT, VT, or VF or for study of sinus node function and integrity of subsidiary pacemakers.

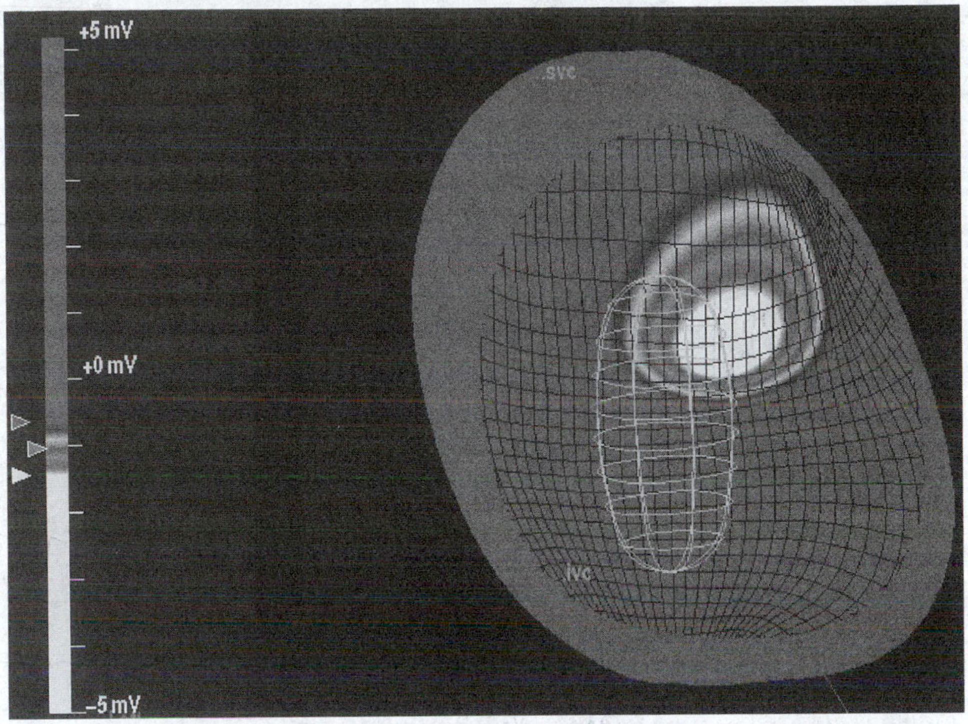

FIGURE 26-4 (Plate 76) Activation of the right atrium during focal atrial tachycardia, mapped with the Endocardial Solutions EnSite 3000 system. The *white* represents tissue that is fully activated, and *purple* is tissue that is not yet activated. SVC = superior vena cava; IVC = inferior vena cava.

The second pacing format is premature (or extra) stimulation from atrial or ventricular sites. For the study of a physiologic phenomenon, refractory periods, and conduction characteristics, a single extra stimulus is usually applied after a series of beats with a constant cycle length (Fig. 26-5). The scanning is initiated late during electrical diastole, and the coupling interval is progressively decreased until the atrial and/or ventricular muscle is refractory. For induction of SVTs, single, two, or more extra stimuli are delivered (Fig. 26-6). For the induction of VT, up to three ventricular extra stimuli are employed. The sensitivity of pacing protocols seems to be directly related to the number of extra stimuli utilized.[17] This occurs, however, at the expense of specificity when polymorphic VT/VF can be induced at very short coupling intervals by using multiple extra stimuli. Regardless of the pacing protocol, the induction of sustained monomorphic VT constitutes a specific response and is seldom induced in patients not prone to such arrhythmias clinically. In contrast, the induction of polymorphic VT/VF with three extra stimuli at short coupling intervals can be nonspecific and does not provide a reliable guide for serial testing. Both polymorphic VT and VF can be avoided to a great extent at short coupling intervals (<200 ms) and the induction of latency between the stimulus artifact and the local ventricular electrograms is avoided.[18]

During routine EPSs, a variety of electrophysiologic parameters are measured, including sinus node function and intraatrial, AV nodal, and His-Purkinje system conduction. Initiation of SVT and VT is attempted to determine the mechanisms, the site of origin (by pacing and mapping techniques), and the potential of overdrive termination as a therapy option. After baseline studies, intravenous drugs are frequently administered to facilitate either induction of tachycardias, aggravation of sinus node function, or production of AV block (Fig. 26-7), or to determine drug efficacy.[17] At the completion of testing, the catheters are withdrawn, and gentle pressure is applied at the area of catheter insertion. Unless arterial catheterization is performed, patients are usually allowed to ambulate after 4 to 6 h. The role of EPSs in patient management has evolved over the past decades from a purely diagnostic method to a frequently applied therapeutic tool. A brief outline of the value of clinical EPSs in various arrhythmia settings is outlined separately under diagnostic and therapeutic categories.

INVASIVE ELECTROPHYSIOLOGIC STUDIES FOR DIAGNOSIS

Sinus Node Dysfunction[3,4]

EPSs are generally performed to detect suspected sinus node dysfunction in patients with dizziness, presyncope, syncope, etc., in whom the diagnosis cannot be made noninvasively. The most frequently performed test is that of sinus node suppression by using overdrive atrial pacing. After pacing at several basic cycle lengths for a period of approximately 30 s or longer, the pacing is interrupted. The resultant escape interval, which is called *sinus node recovery time*, is measured. By deducting the predominant sinus cycle length from this interval, one can obtain the so-called corrected sinus node recovery time. In one study, sinus node recovery time in patients with sinus node disease averaged 3087 ms,[3] and averaged 1073 ms in normal individuals. In another series,[6] the value for corrected sinus node recovery time was less than 525 ms in normal individuals and exceeded those values in patients with overt sinus node dysfunction. Direct sinus node recordings have been obtained by amplification of recording from catheters placed in close proximity to the sinus node,[20,21] where both the sinus node automaticity and sinoatrial conduction can be determined more accurately.

In the vast majority of patients with true sinus node disease, sinoatrial conduction abnormalities are the predominant reason for sinus node dysfunction. The sinoatrial conduction time in

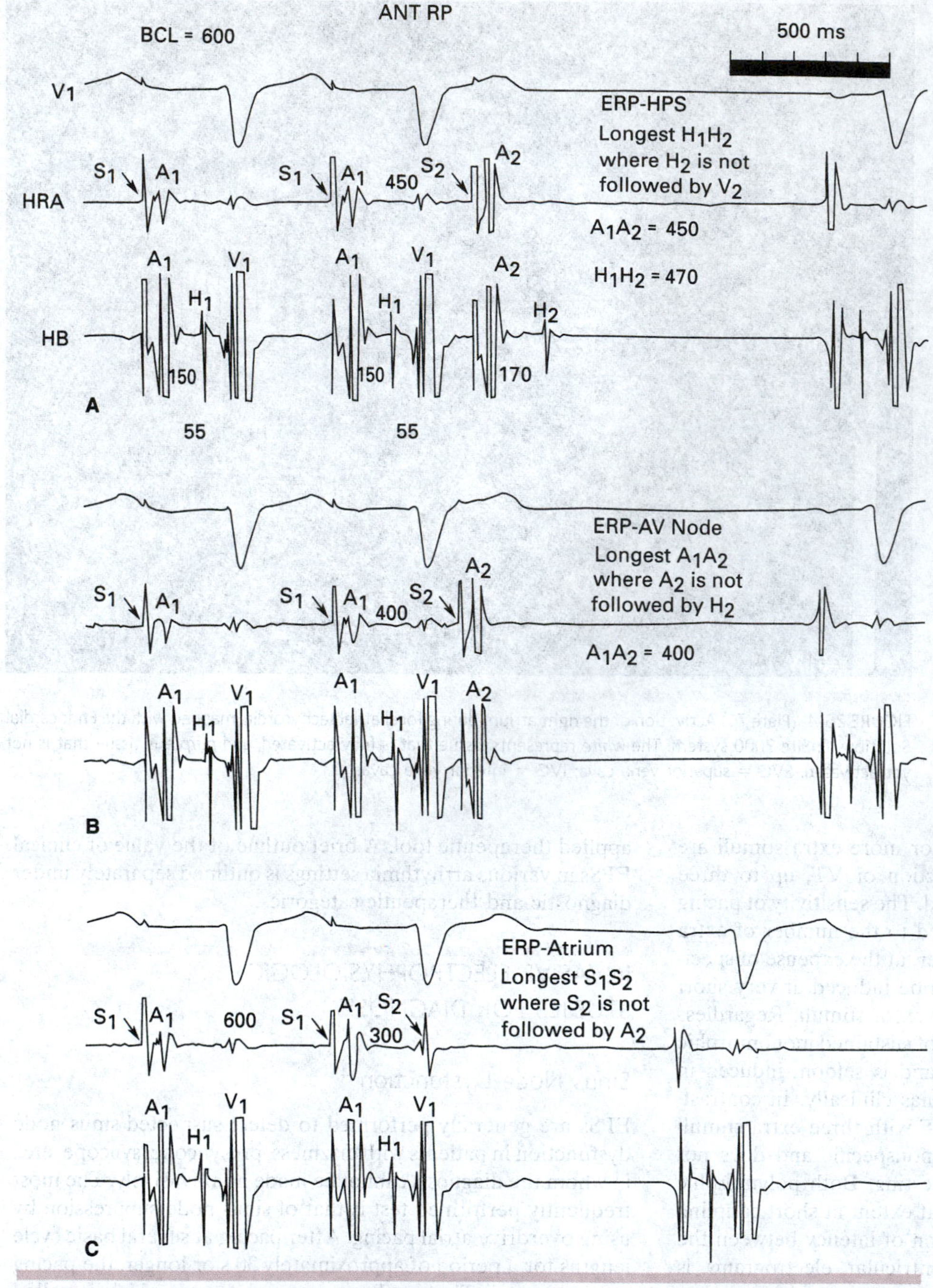

FIGURE 26-5 Determination of cardiac refractory periods during atrial pacing (*A* through *C*). During a basic cycle-length pacing at 600 ms (S_1S_1 or A_1A_1), atrial premature stimulation (S_2 or A_2) at progressively shorter coupling intervals (S_1S_2 or A_1A_2) is depicted. The definition of the effective refractory period (ERP) of the His-Purkinje system (HPS), atrioventricular node, and atrium are labeled. ANT RP = antegrade refractory period. (From Akhtar.[11] Reproduced with permission from the publisher and authors.)

the absence of obvious sinus node disease is less than 100 ms. The sensitivity of sinus node recovery time for the detection of sinus node dysfunction is 54 percent, whereas that of sinoatrial conduction time is 51 percent, with a combined sensitivity of the two tests of around 64 percent. Poor sensitivity of such testing relates in part to the fact that, in previous studies, documented episodes of sinus bradycardia or sinus arrest due to neurocardiogenic mechanisms may have been included as examples of sinus node dysfunction.[22] The specificity of the two tests combined is approximately 88 percent. It is important to test the AV conduction in patients with sinus node dysfunction, since the former is also frequently abnormal. In patients with bradycardia/tachycardia syndrome, tachycardias are frequent, particularly those arising in the atrium, and testing may also be necessary for the proper diagnosis and therapy of the concomitant tachyarrhythmia.

Atrioventricular Block

In asymptomatic patients with first-degree AV block (prolonged PR interval), electrophysiologic assessment is unnecessary, regardless of the QRS morphology of the conducted beats. In asymptomatic individuals with second-degree AV block, electrophysiologic assessment is used to find the site of the block (Fig. 26-8). Patients with intra-Hisian or infra-Hisian block tend to have a more unpredictable course, and permanent pacing is desirable.[23] On the other hand, asymptomatic patients with AV nodal block generally do not require permanent pacing. Even though the intranodal block usually presents as Wenckebach's phenomenon or Mobitz type I, it is not uncommon to see Wenckebach phenomena within the His-Purkinje system or within the His bundle. There is no difference in prognosis regardless of how the infra- or intra-Hisian second-degree block manifests itself, i.e., type I versus type II (Fig. 26-8). On occasion, intranodal blocks are preceded by no discernible change in PR interval and from a surface electrocardiogram may appear as forms of Mobitz type II. The absolute length of the PR interval is usually quite diagnostic in that it is markedly prolonged (i.e., >300 ms), and there is a PR shortening exceeding 100 ms following the block beat (Fig. 26-8). In symptomatic patients with second-degree AV block, the role of EPS is limited because permanent pacing is the appropriate intervention. On the other hand, if the patient's symptoms cannot be explained on the basis of AV block and may be related to another arrhythmia, such as VT, EPSs should be considered. In patients with third-degree or complete AV

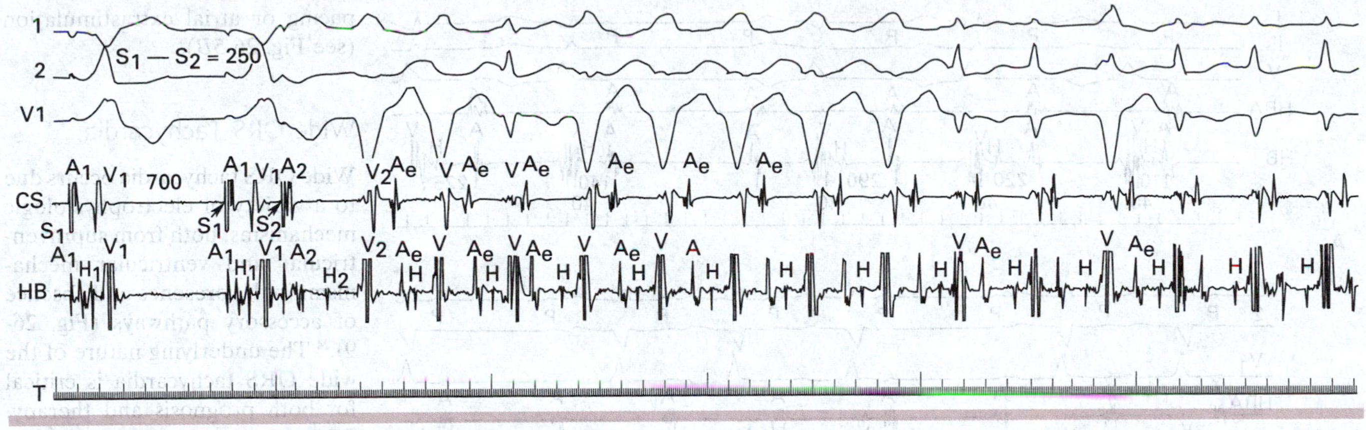

FIGURE 26-6 Induction of supraventricular tachycardia (SVT) in Wolff-Parkinson-White syndrome. The tracings are labeled. Atrial pacing from coronary sinus (CS) is done at a 700-ms basic cycle. During the basic drive pacing, left free wall accessory pathway conduction to the ventricle produces ventricular preexcitation. A single premature beat (S_2) blocks in the accessory pathway (AP) and conducts over the normal pathway with a left bundle branch block morphology, and the SVT is initiated. Note the intermittent normalization of the QRS complex during this SVT. (From Jazayeri et al.[53] Reproduced with permission from the publisher and authors.)

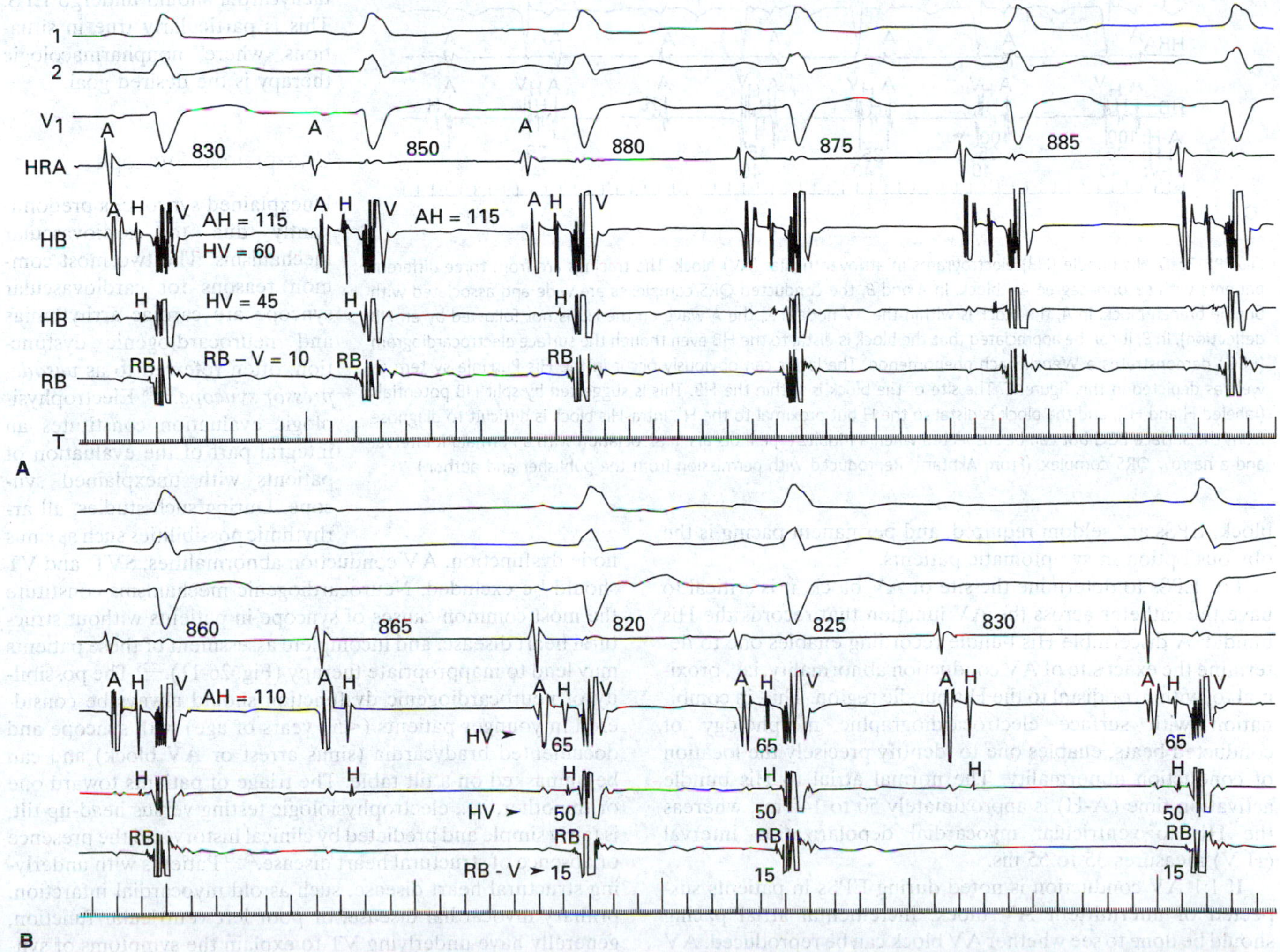

FIGURE 26-7 Atrioventricular (AV) block in the His-Purkinje system (HPS). *A*. Control. A 1:1 AV conduction is depicted in a patient with unexplained syncope. Following 150 mg of intravenous procainamide (*B*), a second-degree AV block in the HPS is noted (i.e., His bundle potential is not followed by a QRS complex), an abnormal response to a small dose of procainamide suggesting AV block in the HPS as a potential cause of syncope.

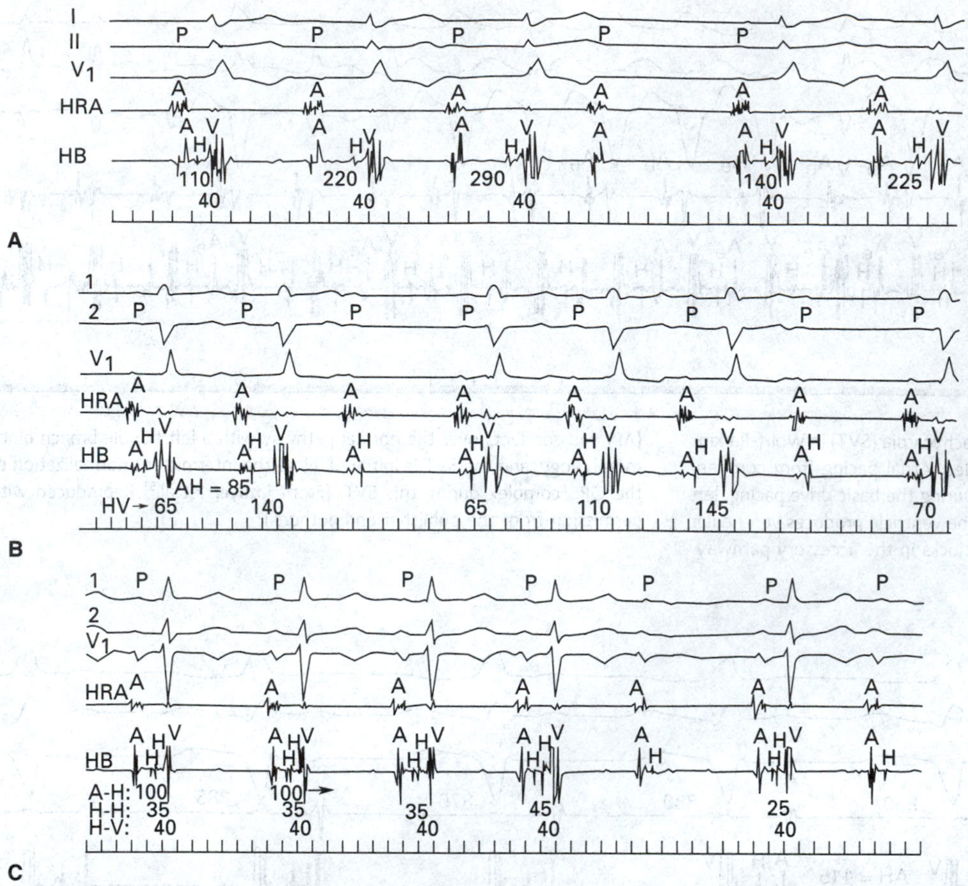

FIGURE 26-8 His bundle (HB) electrograms in atrioventricular (AV) block. The tracings are from three different patients with second-degree AV block. In *A* and *B*, the conducted QRS complexes are wide and associated with bundle branch block. In *A*, the block is within the AV node (i.e., the A wave on the HB is not followed by an HB deflection). In *B*, it can be appreciated that the block is distal to the HB even though the surface electrocardiogram (ECG) demonstrates a Wenckebach phenomenon. The latter can obviously occur in the His-Purkinje system as well, as depicted in this figure. *C*. The site of the block is within the HB. This is suggested by split HB potentials (labeled H and H′), and the block is distal to the H but proximal to the H′. Intra-His block is difficult to diagnose from the surface ECG but can be suspected when a Mobitz type II occurs in association with a normal PR interval and a narrow QRS complex. (From Akhtar.[11] Reproduced with permission from the publisher and author.)

block, EPSs are seldom required, and permanent pacing is the obvious option in symptomatic patients.

For EPSs to determine the site of AV block, it is critical to have the catheter across the AV junction that records the His bundle. A discernible His bundle recording enables one to determine the exact site of AV conduction abnormality, i.e., proximal to, within, or distal to the His bundle region. This, in combination with surface electrocardiographic morphology of conducted beats, enables one to identify precisely the location of conduction abnormality. The normal atrial to His bundle activation time (A-H) is approximately 50 to 140 ms, whereas the His to ventricular myocardial depolarization interval (H-V) measures 35 to 55 ms.

If 1:1 AV conduction is noted during EPSs in patients suspected of intermittent AV block, incremental atrial pacing should be done to see whether AV block can be reproduced. AV block in the His-Purkinje system is abnormal during incremental atrial pacing but is a physiologic response during atrial extrastimulation (see Fig. 26-5*A*) or with abrupt acceleration of atrial pacing rate. First- and second-degree blocks in the AV node are considered physiologic responses during incremental atrial pacing or atrial extrastimulation (see Fig. 26-5*B*).

Wide QRS Tachycardia

Wide QRS tachycardia occurs due to a variety of electrophysiologic mechanisms, both from supraventricular and ventricular mechanisms in the presence and absence of accessory pathways (Fig. 26-9).[24] The underlying nature of the wide QRS tachycardia is critical for both prognosis and therapy. EPSs have proven invaluable in distinguishing the various etiologies (Fig. 26-10). With few exceptions, when the nature of the arrhythmic problem is not known and the direction of therapy is not clear, patients with wide QRS tachycardia should undergo EPS. This is particularly true in situations where nonpharmacologic therapy is the desired goal.

Unexplained Syncope

Unexplained syncope is predominantly due to cardiovascular mechanisms. The two most common reasons for cardiovascular syncope are cardiac arrhythmias and neurocardiogenic dysfunction, often referred to as *vasodepressor syncope*.[23–28] Electrophysiologic evaluation constitutes an integral part of the evaluation of patients with unexplained syncope. During such studies, all arrhythmic possibilities such as sinus node dysfunction, AV conduction abnormalities, SVT, and VT should be excluded. Neurocardiogenic mechanisms constitute the most common causes of syncope in patients without structural heart disease, and incomplete assessment of these patients may lead to inappropriate therapy (Fig. 26-11).[22,25] The possibility of neurocardiogenic dysfunction should always be considered in younger patients (<50 years of age) with syncope and documented bradycardia (sinus arrest or AV block) and can be unmasked on a tilt table. The triage of patients toward one or the other, i.e., electrophysiologic testing versus head-up tilt, is fairly simple and predicted by clinical history and the presence or absence of structural heart disease.[25–30] Patients with underlying structural heart disease, such as old myocardial infarction, primary myocardial disease, or poor left ventricular function, generally have underlying VT to explain the symptoms of syncope (Fig. 26-12). When arrhythmias occur in patients without overt structural heart disease, sinus node dysfunction, AV block (particularly intra-Hisian block), or SVTs are likely. Less frequently, VT can occur in the absence of an overt structural heart disease.

Survivors of Sudden Cardiac Death

In most patients with documented episodes of cardiac arrest from the onset, VF can be documented. Patients dying suddenly generally have underlying structural heart disease (usually coronary artery disease or primary myocardial disease) and are prone to VT/VF due to electrical instability. It seems prudent to investigate both the nature and extent of organic heart disease and also to assess vulnerability to recurrent VT/VF. At present, EPS is considered a routine part of the overall patient assessment in this group of individuals.[31,32]

EPSs in survivors of VT/VF are desirable for a variety of reasons. Some are listed here:

1. Not infrequently, the underlying VT leading to cardiac arrest is bundle branch reentry or BBR (Fig. 26-13). Almost 40 percent of patients with monomorphic VT in association with idiopathic dilated cardiomyopathy and valvular heart disease have BBR as the underlying mechanism. This arrhythmia is preferably managed with bundle branch ablation, which is curative, rather than with an implantable cardioverter defibrillator (ICD) alone.

2. Several VT morphologies or other types of tachycardia may be induced in addition to VT. Lack of awareness of such arrhythmias may complicate patient management. For example, the presence of rapid SVT may require separate attention to prevent unnecessary ICD shocks.

3. In some cases, supraventricular arrhythmia may trigger VT/VF. This may happen in patients with severe coronary artery disease, congestive heart failure, Wolff-Parkinson-White syndrome, etc. Elimination of the underlying causes is a more rational therapeutic approach in such cases.

4. Patients with VT/VF often have underlying sick sinus syndrome or AV block, which can be further aggravated with antiarrhythmic drugs and may require permanent pacing. Assessment for this eventuality can be done during the conduct of an EPS and may help selection of a particular device. Because of the increasing flexibility of these devices this need for EPS may be less relevant in the future.

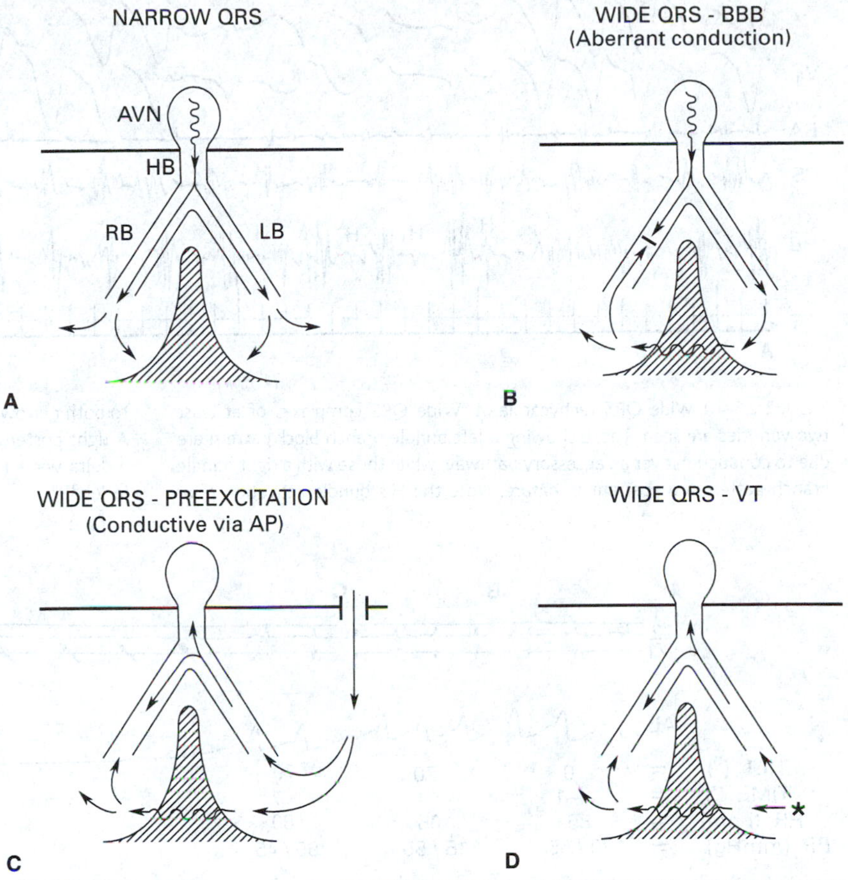

FIGURE 26-9 Wide QRS tachycardia. Routes of impulse propagation during a wide QRS tachycardia in various settings are depicted. It should be noted that only in *A* and *B* is His bundle activation expected to precede ventricular activation. This helps the delineation from other causes of wide QRS tachycardia shown in *C* and *D*.

INVASIVE CARDIAC ELECTROPHYSIOLOGIC STUDIES FOR THERAPEUTIC INTERVENTION

Because of the episodic nature of most cardiac arrhythmias, the efficacy of any therapeutic intervention is difficult to assess unless the arrhythmia in question can be replicated. Diagnostic EPS provides that opportunity, and it seems logical to use the same tool to assess therapeutic interventions.[34-36] This method to assess efficacy can be applied for both pharmacologic and nonpharmacologic therapy.

Pharmacologic Therapy

It is arguable whether the assessment of pharmacologic intervention is essential in patients with relatively benign cardiac arrhythmias. The clinical course can be observed to determine whether control has been achieved. With life-threatening tachycardias, such as VT/VF, or with severe manifestations of cardiac arrhythmias, such as syncope or presyncope, it is desirable to assess efficacy of pharmacologic intervention (Fig. 26-14).[35,36] The technique of drug testing has been developed whereby the elimination of inducibility of a given tachycardia is assessed following a drug administration. Both the drug efficacy or inefficacy can be evaluated by this method. When drug therapy does eliminate induction of a previously inducible tachycardia, the addition of isoproterenol will frequently demonstrate reversal of therapeutic drug effect.[37,38] This is helpful in considering additional beta-blocker therapy. The latter can be accomplished with ease in patients with good left ventricular function, whereas the addition of beta blockers may pose a problem in patients with VT and poor left ventricular function. Failure of serial drug testing is associated with a significant recurrence rate and a strong indication for nonpharmacologic intervention.

Some controversy has arisen regarding the value of EPS for prediction of drug efficacy in comparison to ambulatory monitoring.[39] However, because of the infrequency of spontane-

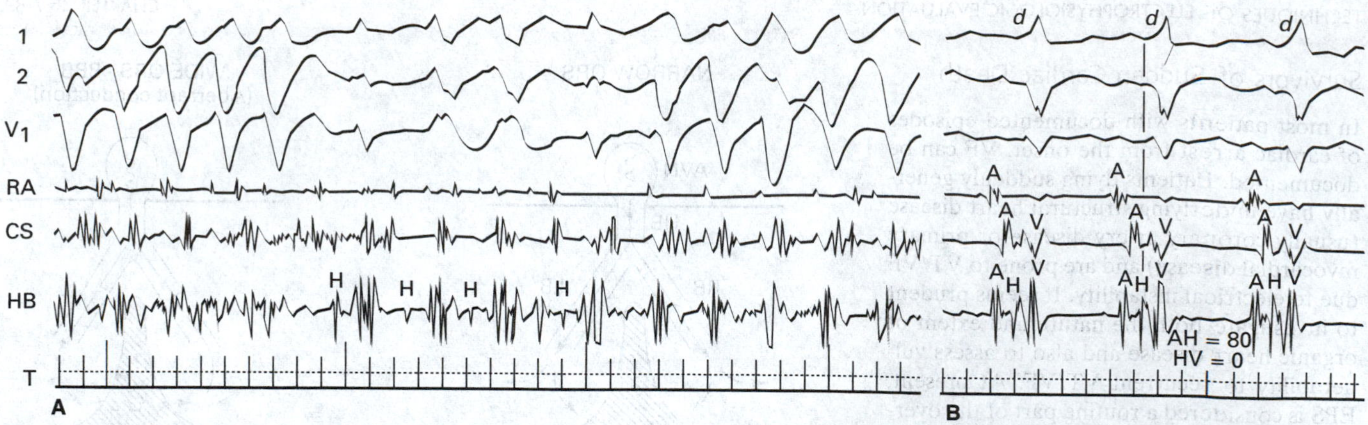

FIGURE 26-10 Wide QRS tachycardia. *A*. Wide QRS complexes of at least two varieties are seen. Those showing a left bundle branch block pattern are due to conduction over an accessory pathway, while those with a right bundle branch pattern are aberrant in nature. Note the His bundle activation prior to both narrow and aberrant complexes but not before preexcited complexes. A right posteroseptal preexcitation can be appreciated in *B*, with a short PR, a delta wave (*d*), an His to ventricle (HV) of zero, and negative delta wave in lead V_1.

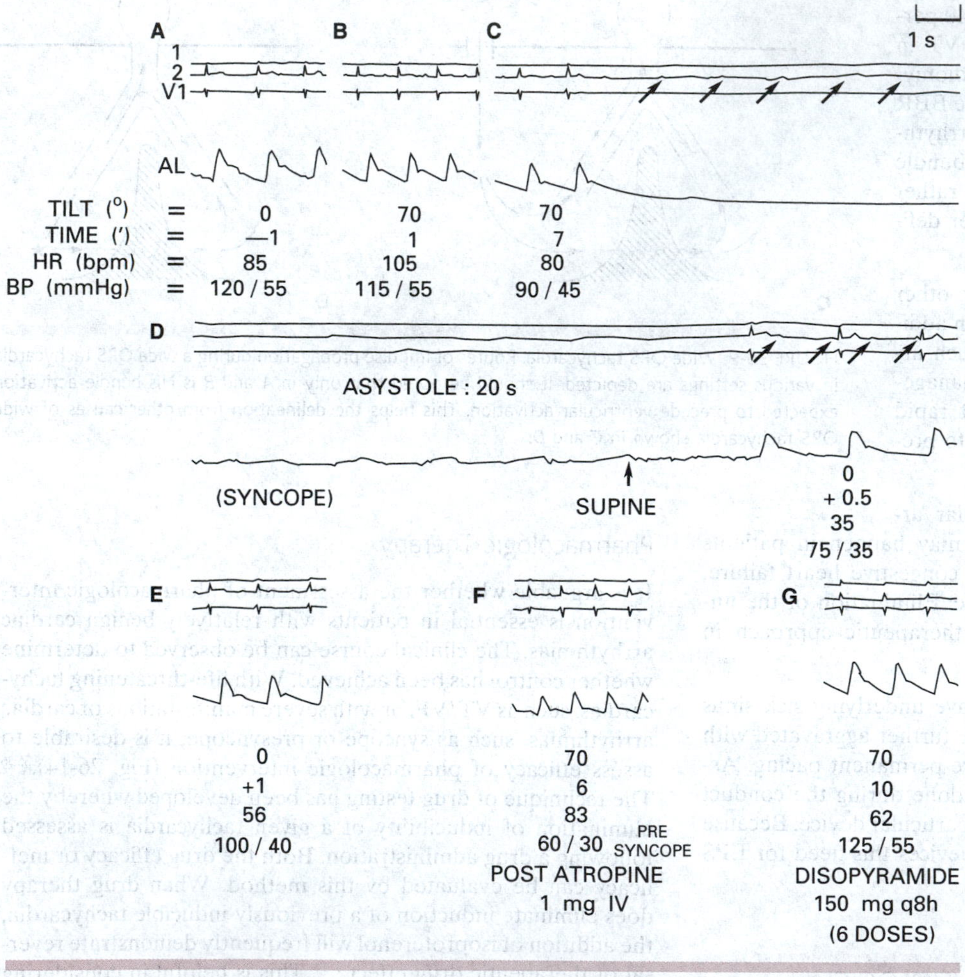

FIGURE 26-11 Asystole in neurocardiogenic syncope. Note the normal heart rate (HR) and blood pressure (BP) in supine position. At the beginning of head-up tilt at 70° (*B*), some degree of tachycardia is noted. Seven minutes after the onset of tilt (*C*), an episode of atrioventricular block occurs and is followed by sinus arrest and a total asystole of 20 s. Syncopal episodes follow. Presyncope is still present when asystole is prevented by atropine (*F*). Findings in *C* might tempt one to prescribe permanent pacing, an inappropriate choice of therapy. In this patient with neurocardiogenic syncope, disopyramide (*G*) prevented hypotension and syncope without the need for a permanent pacemaker. This patient has remained asymptomatic on this therapy for more than 6 years now. (From Sra et al.[22] Reproduced with permission from the publisher and authors.)

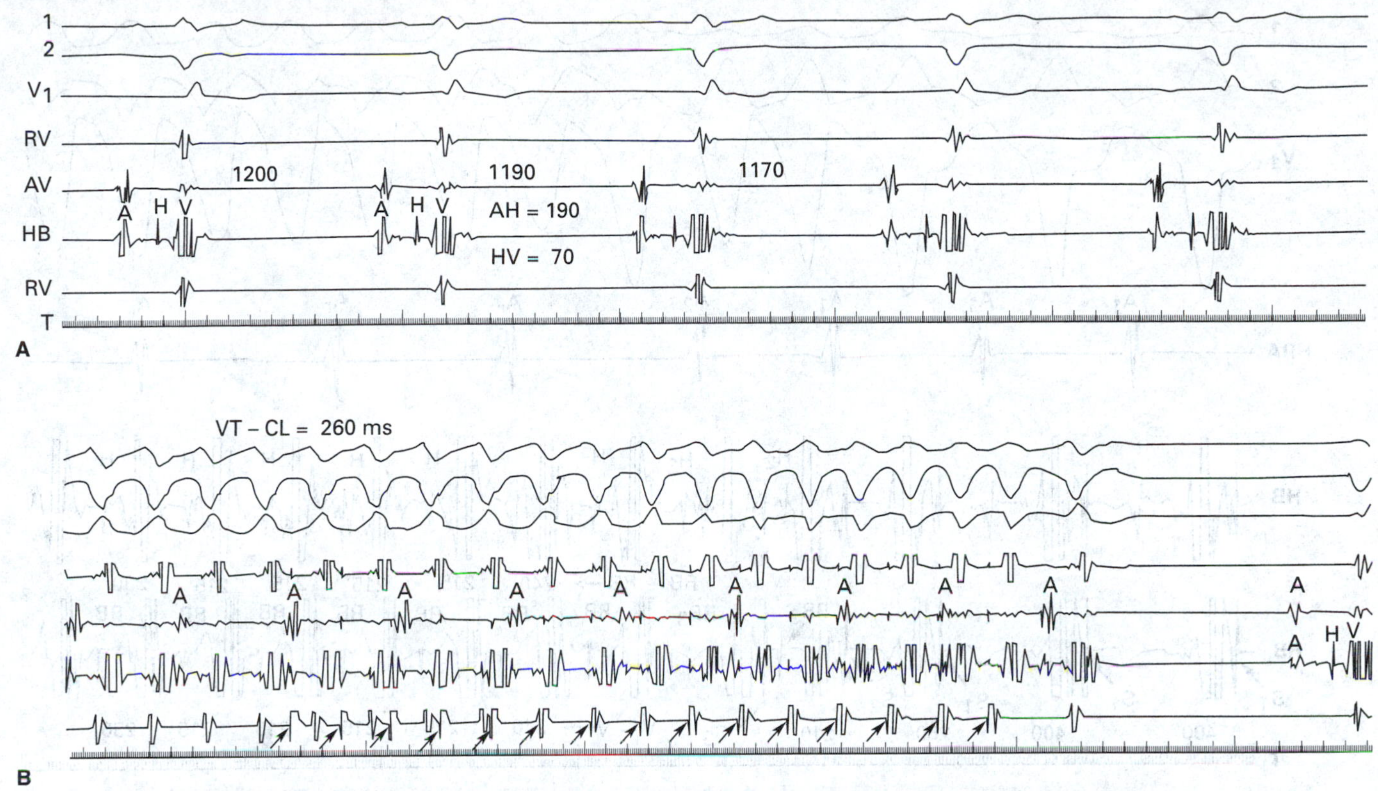

FIGURE 26-12 Arrhythmic causes of syncope. *A.* Sinus rhythm in a patient with unexplained syncope. Sinus bradycardia, bifascicular block, and a long PR interval from surface electrocardiogram suggest possible bradycardia etiology. In this patient, however, ventricular tachycardia (*B*) was inducible with ventricular extrastimulation and was the actual cause of syncope. Control of ventricular tachycardia (VT) without a pacemaker was sufficient to prevent syncope in this patient. Termination of tachycardia and restoration of sinus rhythm are shown in *B*.

ous VT/VF in most patients with life-threatening ventricular arrhythmias, ambulatory monitoring is an impractical approach. At present, serial drug studies with multiple oral antiarrhythmic agents are seldom carried out for SVT or VT.

Nonpharmacologic Therapy

Nonpharmacologic intervention has become an integral part of patient management in cardiac arrhythmias. With documented cardiac arrest from VF, implantation of an automatic ICD is fairly common, and electrophysiologic assessment before such therapy is routine.[40] Both preoperative and postimplant electrophysiologic evaluation can be done through permanent leads of an ICD through a wand and programmer. Pacing, antitachycardia function, low-energy cardioversion, and cardiac defibrillation can all be programmed with newer devices. When problems are encountered following discharge of a patient with an ICD, electrophysiologic reassessment via ICD is frequently necessary, both for reprogramming and for the detection of any unexplained events. For assessment of certain other electrophysiologic parameters (e.g., AV conduction and mechanism of SVTs), however, transvenous catheterization may be necessary.

Patients with coronary artery disease and mappable VT are also candidates for VT surgery when it cannot be managed with ICD, antiarrhythmic drugs and for catheter ablation.[41–43] Preoperative EPS assessment for this possibility is important. Surgery for VT in the form of endocardial resection or cryoablation can be performed very effectively and relatively safely in patients with a left ventricular ejection fraction greater than 20 percent. This curative procedure provides effective control in approximately 75 percent of the patients who have monomorphic VT that can be appropriately mapped, and it may be considered when other forms of therapies are ineffective.

Surgery for SVT has gone through a significant evolution. The introduction of catheter ablative techniques has made it rare for patients to undergo surgery for Wolff-Parkinson-White syndrome and/or AV nodal reentrant tachycardia. Some individuals with resistant atrial fibrillation and flutter and those who fail catheter ablative therapy may still be considered candidates for such a procedure, but this is now becoming exceedingly less frequent.

CATHETER ABLATION TECHNIQUES[44–48]

The realization that the origin of VT and SVT can be effectively mapped has made the catheter ablative technique a rational approach. The radiofrequency form of energy delivered through a catheter has permitted controlled trauma to cardiac tissue to abolish or modify reentrant circuits. This is true for both SVT and VT. Unifocal atrial tachycardia, AV nodal reentry of all varieties, and accessory pathways including atriofascicular fibers can be cured in over 90 percent of patients with radiofrequency catheter ablation. Among the VTs, BBR tachycardia seen in association with dilated cardiomyopathy (both ischemic and nonischemic) and valvular disease is an ideal substrate for catheter ablation. Patients with monomorphic VT associated with

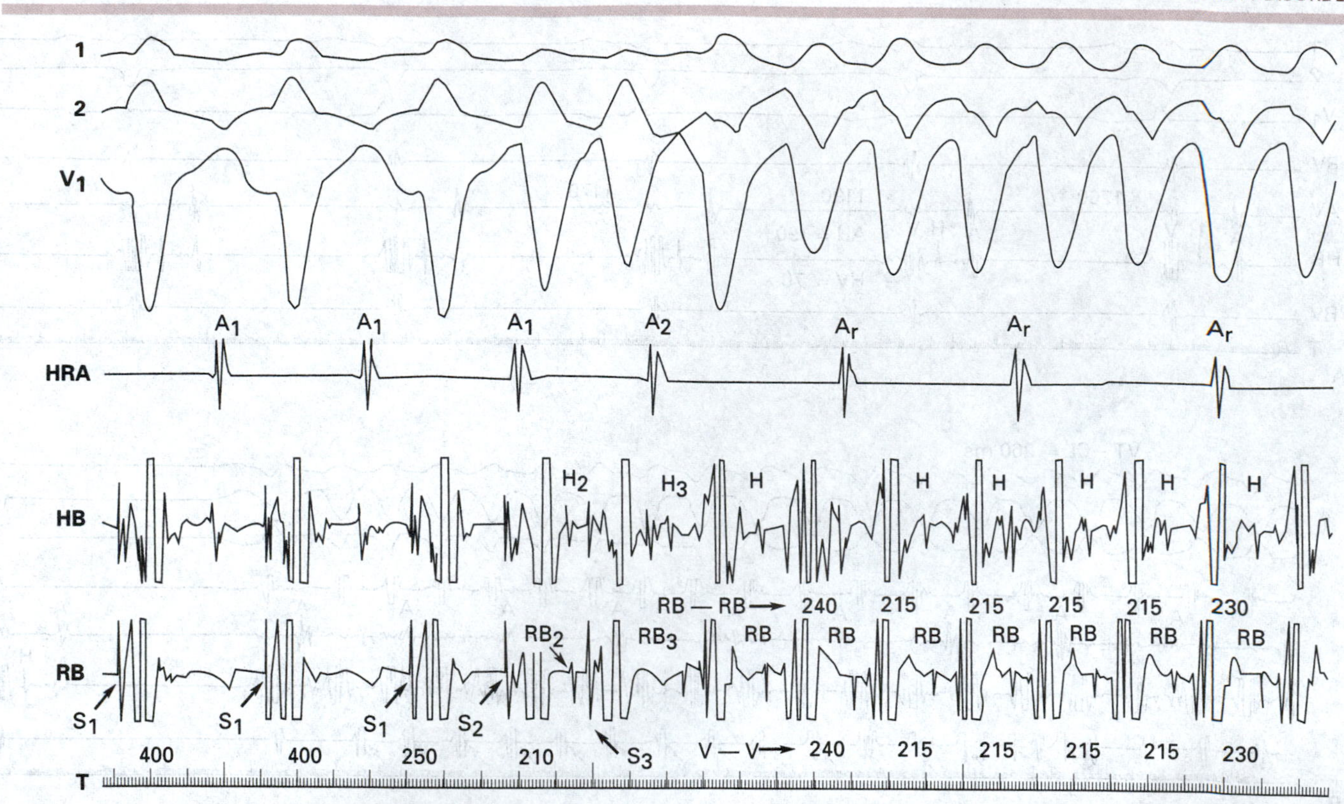

FIGURE 26-13 Induction of sustained ventricular tachycardia due to bundle branch reentry (BBR). The surface electrocardiogram and intracardiac tracings are labeled. Basic cycle length (S_1S_1) is 400 ms during ventricular pacing. Sustained BBR is induced with two extra stimuli (S_2S_3). Note that the His bundle and right bundle (RB) deflections precede the QRS, suggesting supraventricular tachycardia with aberrant conduction. However, there is 2:1 ventricular atrial (VA) block, indicating the ventricular nature of this tachycardia. Without His bundle/right bundle (HB/RB) recordings, the diagnosis can be difficult and, consequently, the likelihood of inappropriate therapy will be high. RB-RB and V-V (ventricular) intervals are labeled. (From Jazayeri et al.[54] Reproduced with permission from the publisher and authors.)

myocardial scarring or other substrates can also be considered candidates, particularly when they are not suitable for VT surgery and have failed drug therapy. Additionally, in patients with incessant VT or frequency VT with inadequate control despite ICD therapy, VT ablation should be considered. By using the electromagnetic mapping, the scarred area can be mapped during sinus rhythm and ablation of this substrate can effectively eliminate VT. Noncontact mapping techniques outlined earlier are likely to further help improve ablation success rate with unifocal or possibly multifocal tachycardias.

IATROGENIC PROBLEMS ENCOUNTERED DURING ELECTROPHYSIOLOGIC STUDIES

Mechanical irritation from catheters during placement and even when not being manipulated can cause a variety of arrhythmias and conduction disturbances.[49] These include induction of atrial, junctional, and ventricular ectopic beats and right bundle branch block and thus AV block in the His-Purkinje system in patients with preexisting left bundle branch block during right ventricular catheterization.[47] Obviously, AV block in the His-Purkinje system can occur in patients with preexisting right bundle branch block during left ventricular catheterization. Ventricular stimulation can also occur from physical movement of the ventricular catheter coincident with atrial contraction, producing electrocardiographic patterns of ventricular preexcitation. Recognition of all these iatrogenic patterns is important for avoiding misinterpretation of electrophysiologic phenomena and the significance of findings in the laboratory.

Certain types of arrhythmias must be avoided at all costs, such as atrial and VF. Atrial fibrillation will obviously not permit study of any other form of SVT, and VF will require prompt cardioversion, making it difficult to continue the EPS. If atrial fibrillation must be initiated for diagnostic purposes (i.e., to assess ventricular response over the accessory pathway in Wolff-Parkinson-White syndrome), it should be done at the end of the study. Patients with a prior history of atrial fibrillation are more prone to the occurrence of sustained atrial fibrillation in the laboratory. Frequently, this will occur during initial placement of catheters, and excessive manipulation of catheters in the atria should therefore be avoided. Catheter trauma resulting in abolition of accessory pathway conduction or reentrant pathway may make the curative ablation difficult or impossible.

Risks and Complications

The complication rate is relatively low when only right heart catheterization is done, with almost negligible mortality.[50,51] Other complications include deep venous thrombosis, pulmonary embolism, infection at catheter sites, systemic infection,

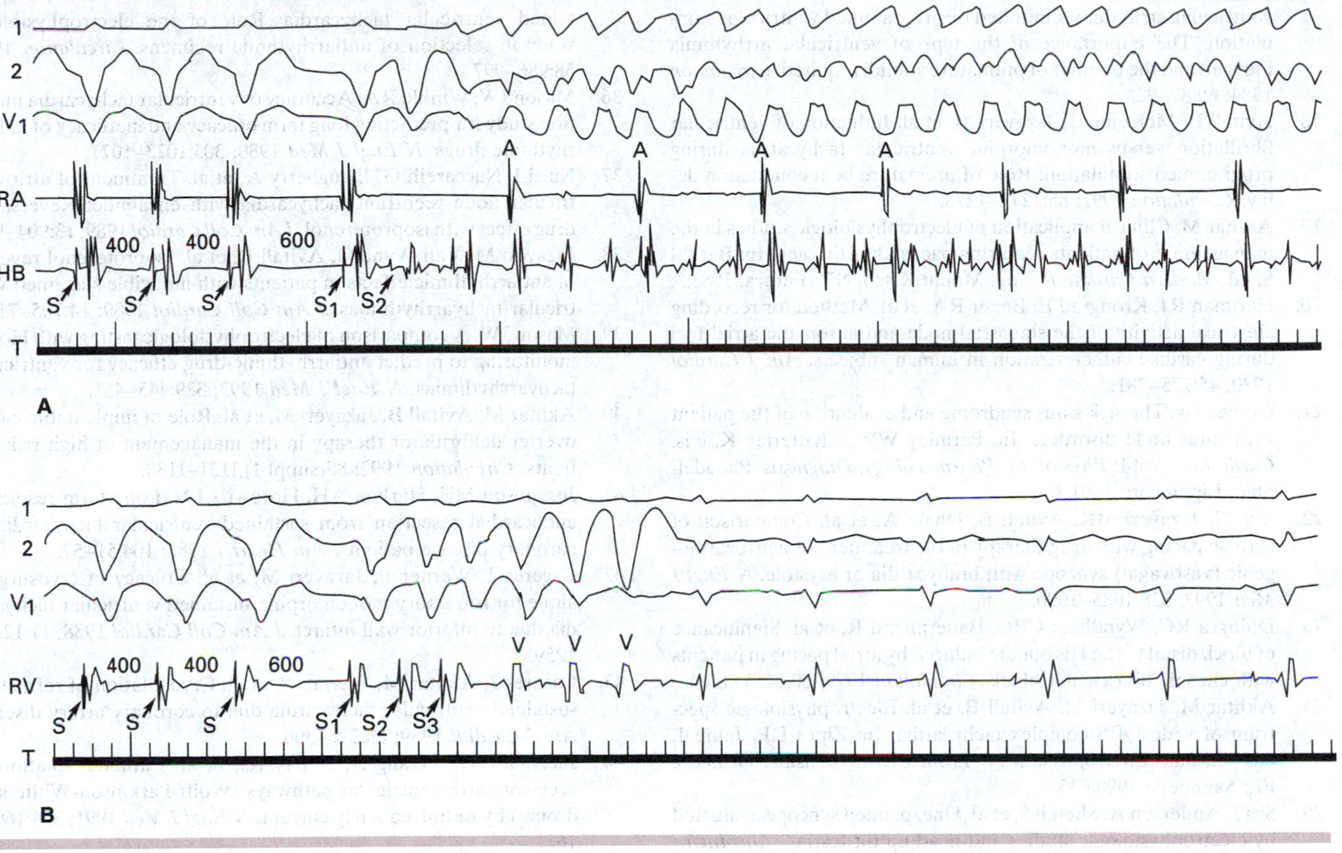

FIGURE 26-14 *A*. Control. *B*. Post procainamide (PA) + mexiletine. Initiation of sustained monomorphic ventricular tachycardia (VT) of myocardial origin is shown in *A*. After oral procainamide and mexiletine, the sustained VT could not be induced despite using a more aggressive pacing protocol.

pneumothorax, and perforation of a cardiac chamber or coronary sinus. Potentially lethal arrhythmias such as rapid VT or VF are common in the laboratory. These are not necessarily counted as complications, however, but are often expected and anticipated. Nonetheless, their common occurrence makes the electrophysiology laboratory a place for only highly trained personnel equipped to handle such problems.

References

1. Scherlag BJ, Lau SH, Helfant RH, et al. Catheter technique for recording His bundle activity in man. *Circulation* 1969; 39:13–18.
2. Goldreyer BN, Bigger JT. Spontaneous and induced reentrant tachycardia. *Ann Intern Med* 1969; 70:87–98.
3. Mandel WJ, Hayakawa H, Danzig R, Marcus HS. Evaluation of sinoatrial node function in man by overdrive suppression. *Circulation* 1971; 44:59–66.
4. Narula OS, Samet P, Javier RP. Significance of the sinus node recovery time. *Circulation* 1972; 45:140–158.
5. Damato AN, Lau SH, Helfant RH, et al. A study of heart block in man using His bundle recordings. *Circulation* 1969; 39:297–305.
6. Narula OS, Scherlag BJ, Samet P, Javier RP. Atrioventricular block: Localization and classification by His bundle recordings. *Am J Med* 1971; 50:146–165.
7. Goldreyer BN, Damato AN. The essential role of atrioventricular conduction delay in the initiation of paroxysmal supraventricular tachycardia. *Circulation* 1971; 43:679–687.
8. Wellens HJJ, Schuilenberg RM, Durrer D. Electrical stimulation of the heart in patients with the Wolff-Parkinson-White syndrome type A. *Circulation* 1971; 43:99–114.
9. Mason JW, Winkel RA. Electrode catheter arrhythmia induction in the selection and assessment of antiarrhythmic drug therapy for recurrent ventricular tachycardia. *Circulation* 1978; 58:971–985.
10. Ruskin JN, DiMarco JP, Garan H. Out of hospital cardiac arrest: Electrophysiologic observations in selection of long-term antiarrhythmic therapy. *N Engl J Med* 1980; 303:607–613.
11. Akhtar M. Invasive cardiac electrophysiologic studies: An introduction. In: Parmley WW, Chatterjee K, eds. *Cardiology*, vol 1: *Physiology, Pharmacology, Diagnosis*. Philadelphia: Lippincott; 1991:1.
12. Josephson ME, Harken PH, Horowitz LN. Endocardial excision: A new surgical technique for the treatment of recurrent ventricular tachycardia. *Circulation* 1979; 60:1430–1439.
13. Fann JI, Loeb JM, LoCicero III J, et al. Endocardial activation mapping and endocardial pace-mapping using a balloon apparatus. *Am J Cardiol* 1985; 55:1076.
14. Mickleborough LL, Harris L, Downar E, et al. A new intraoperative approach for endocardial mapping of ventricular tachycardia. *J Thorac Cardiovasc Surg* 1988; 95:271.
15. Gepstein L, Hayam G, Ben-Haim SA. A novel method for nonfluoroscopic catheter-based electroanatomical mapping of the heart. *Circulation* 1997; 95:1611–1622.
16. Schilling RJ, Peters NS, Davies DW. A non-contact catheter for simultaneous endocardial mapping in the human left ventricle: Comparison of contact and reconstructed electrograms during sinus rhythm. *Circulation* 1998; 98:887–898.
17. Brugada P, Green M, Abdollah H, Wellens HJ. Significance of

ventricular arrhythmias initiated by programmed ventricular stimulation: The importance of the type of ventricular arrhythmia induced and the number of premature stimuli required. *Circulation* 1984; 69:87–92.
18. Avitall B, McKinnie J, Jazayeri M, et al. Induction of ventricular fibrillation versus monomorphic ventricular tachycardia during programmed stimulation: Role of premature beat conduction delay. *Circulation* 1992; 85:1271–1278.
19. Akhtar M. Clinical application of electrophysiologic studies in the management of patients requiring pacemaker therapy. In: Barold S, ed. *Modern Cardiac Pacing*. Mount Kisco, NY: Futura; 1985:3.
20. Hariman RJ, Krongrad E, Boxer RA, et al. Method for recording electrical activity of the sinoatrial node and automatic atrial foci during cardiac catheterization in human subjects. *Am J Cardiol* 1980; 45:775–781.
21. Gomes JA. The sick sinus syndrome and evaluation of the patient with sinus node disorders. In: Parmley WW, Chatterjee K, eds. *Cardiology*, vol 1: *Physiology, Pharmacology, Diagnosis*. Philadelphia: Lippincott; 1991:1.
22. Sra JS, Jazayeri MR, Avitall B, Dhala A, et al. Comparison of cardiac pacing with drug therapy in the treatment of neurocardiogenic (vasovagal) syncope with bradycardia or asystole. *N Engl J Med* 1993; 328:1085–1090.
23. Dhingra RC, Wyndham CRC, Bauernfiend R, et al. Significance of block distal to the His bundle induced by atrial pacing in patients with chronic bifascicular block. *Circulation* 1979; 60:1455–1464.
24. Akhtar M, Jazayeri M, Avitall B, et al. Electrophysiologic spectrum of wide QRS complex tachycardia. In: Zipes DP, Jalife J, eds. *Cardiac Electrophysiology: From Cell to Bedside*. Orlando, FL: Saunders; 1990:635.
25. Sra J, Anderson A, Sheikh S, et al. Unexplained syncope evaluated by electrophysiologic studies and head-up tilt testing. *Ann Intern Med* 1991; 114:1013–1019.
26. DiMarco JP, Garan H, Ruskin JN. Cardiac electrophysiologic techniques in recurrent syncope of unknown cause. *Ann Intern Med* 1981; 95:542–548.
27. Akhtar M, Shenasa M, Denker S, et al. Role of cardiac electrophysiologic studies in patients with unexplained recurrent syncope. *Pacing Clin Electrophysiol* 1983; 6:192–201.
28. Morady F, Scheinman MM. The role and limitations of electrophysiologic testing in patients with unexplained syncope. *Int J Cardiol* 1983; 4:229–234.
29. Teichman SL, Felder DS, Matos JA, et al. The value of electrophysiologic studies in syncope of undetermined origin: Report of 150 cases. *Am Heart J* 1985; 110:469–479.
30. Moazez F, Peter T, Simonson J, et al. Syncope of unknown origin: Clinical noninvasive and electrophysiologic determinants of arrhythmia induction and symptom recurrence during long-term follow-up. *Am Heart J* 1991; 121:81–88.
31. Akhtar M, Garan H, Lehmann MH, Troup PJ. Sudden cardiac death: Management of high-risk patients. *Ann Intern Med* 1991; 114:499–512.
32. Ruskin JN, DiMarco JP, Garan H. Out-of-hospital cardiac arrest: Electrophysiologic observations and selection of long-term antiarrhythmic therapy. *N Engl J Med* 1980; 303:607–612.
33. Morady F, Scheinman MM, Hess DS, et al. Electrophysiologic testing in the management of survivors of out-of-hospital arrest. *Am J Cardiol* 1983; 51:85–89.
34. Wu D, Wyndham CR, Denes P, et al. Chronic electrophysiological study in patients with recurrent paroxysmal tachycardia: A new method for developing successful oral antiarrhythmic therapy. In: Kulbertus HE, ed. *Reentrant Arrhythmias*. Baltimore: University Park Press; 1976:294.
35. Horowitz LN, Josephson ME, Farshidi A, et al. Recurrent sustained ventricular tachycardia: Role of the electrophysiologic study in selection of antiarrhythmic regimens. *Circulation* 1978; 58:986–997.
36. Mason JW, Winkle RA. Accuracy of ventricular tachycardia induction study for predicting long term efficacy and inefficacy of antiarrhythmic drugs. *N Engl J Med* 1980; 303:1073–1077.
37. Niazi I, Naccarelli G, Dougherty A, et al. Treatment of atrioventricular node reentrant tachycardia with encainide: Reversal of drug effect with isoproterenol. *J Am Coll Cardiol* 1989; 13:904–910.
38. Jazayeri M, Van Wyhe G, Avitall B, et al. Isoproterenol reversal of antiarrhythmic effects in patients with inducible sustained ventricular tachyarrhythmias. *J Am Coll Cardiol* 1989; 14:705–711.
39. Mason JW. A comparison of electrophysiologic testing with Holter monitoring to predict antiarrhythmic-drug efficacy for ventricular tachyarrhythmias. *N Engl J Med* 1993; 329:445–451.
40. Akhtar M, Avitall B, Jazayeri M, et al. Role of implantable cardioverter defibrillator therapy in the management of high risk patients. *Circulation* 1992; 85(suppl I):I131–I139.
41. Josephson ME, Harken AH, Horowitz LN. Long-term results of endocardial resection from sustained ventricular tachycardia in coronary disease patients. *Am Heart J* 1982; 104:51–57.
42. Caceres J, Werner P, Jazayeri M, et al. Efficacy of cryosurgery alone for refractory monomorphic sustained ventricular tachycardia due to inferior wall infarct. *J Am Coll Cardiol* 1988; 11:1254–1259.
43. Caceres J, Akhtar M, Werner P, et al. Cryoablation of refractory sustained ventricular tachycardia due to coronary artery disease. *Am J Cardiol* 1989; 63:296–300.
44. Jackman WM, Wang X, Friday KJ, et al. Catheter ablation of accessory atrioventricular pathways (Wolff-Parkinson-White syndrome) by radiofrequency current. *N Engl J Med* 1991; 324:1605–1611.
45. Calkins H, Sousa J, El-Atassi R, et al. Diagnosis and cure of the Wolff-Parkinson-White syndrome or paroxysmal supraventricular tachycardias during a single electrophysiologic test. *N Engl J Med* 1991; 324:1612–1618.
46. Jazayeri M, Hempe SL, Sra JS, et al. Selective transcatheter ablation of the fast and slow pathways using radiofrequency energy in patients with atrioventricular nodal reentrant tachycardia. *Circulation* 1992; 85:1318–1328.
47. Saoudi N, Atallah G, Kirkorian G, Touboul P. Catheter ablation of the atrial myocardium in human type I atrial flutter. *Circulation* 1990; 81:762–771.
48. Klein LS, Shih HT, Hackett FK, et al. Radiofrequency catheter ablation of ventricular tachycardia in patients without structural heart disease. *Circulation* 1992; 85:1666–1674.
49. Akhtar M, Damato AN, Gilbert-Leeds CJ, et al. Induction of iatrogenic electrocardiographic patterns during electrophysiologic studies. *Circulation* 1977; 56:60–65.
50. Di Marco JP, Garan H, Ruskin JN. Complications in patients undergoing cardiac electrophysiologic procedures. *Ann Intern Med* 1982; 97:490–493.
51. Horowitz L. Risks and complications of clinical cardiac electrophysiologic studies: A prospective analysis of 1000 consecutive patients. *J Am Coll Cardiol* 1987; 9:1261–1268.
52. Gallagher JJ, Damato AN. Technique of recording His bundle activity in man. In: Grossman W, ed. *Cardiac Catheterization and Angiography*. Philadelphia: Lea and Febiger; 1980:283.
53. Jazayeri M, Caceres J, Tchou P, et al. Electrophysiologic characteristics of sudden QRS axis deviation during orthodromic tachycardia. *J Clin Invest* 1989; 83:952–959.
54. Jazayeri M, Sra J, Akhtar M. Wide QRS complexes: Electrophysiologic basis of a common electrocardiographic diagnosis. *J Cardiovasc Electrophysiol* 1992; 3:36–39.

CHAPTER 27

ANTIARRHYTHMIC DRUGS

Raymond L. Woosley

Antiarrhythmic drugs have been developed with the expectation that they would extend and improve life for many patients with cardiovascular disease and those with a history of life-threatening arrhythmias. Their usefulness, however, has been, limited by ineffectiveness and/or toxicity. In mortality trials, benefit has not been clearly demonstrated, and worsened mortality rates have been observed with several drugs. Care must be taken, therefore, in deciding on the mode of treatment or in fact whether to treat at all. Many antiarrhythmic agents are available today, and more are under development. So many are needed because no agent is completely effective for all patients, and every agent has the potential for inducing serious adverse effects. Drug selection is often empiric. In fact, the side-effect profiles of the available drugs are very different and are often the determining factor in drug selection. Known side effects may completely eliminate the use of certain classes of drugs for a specific patient. Because of the narrow margin between effective and potentially toxic dosages, it is essential that physicians be thoroughly familiar with the clinical pharmacology, dosage, and adverse effects of any of these agents.

The use of antiarrhythmic drugs has been dramatically altered by the findings of the Cardiac Arrhythmia Suppression Trial (CAST).[1] This landmark study was designed to test the hypothesis that suppression of asymptomatic ventricular arrhythmias in patients with recent myocardial infarction would reduce mortality rates due to cardiac arrest and/or arrhythmic sudden death. Prior to the CAST, antiarrhythmic drugs were prescribed for these patients to suppress asymptomatic arrhythmias and thus improve mortality rates. Based on the results of a feasibility and planning trial, the Cardiac Arrhythmia Pilot Study (CAPS), the CAST evaluated encainide, flecainide, and moricizine. These drugs were chosen because they were all tolerated and had reasonable ability to suppress symptomatic ventricular arrhythmias. In April 1989, the CAST was interrupted by the Data Safety and Monitoring Committee, and encainide and flecainide were removed because they had been found to increase mortality rates two- to threefold. The CAST II continued to evaluate the remaining drug, moricizine. However, the CAST II was also terminated prematurely in August 1991 when it became apparent that moricizine was producing a similar trend toward harm, and there was no reasonable chance that a beneficial effect on the mortality rate could be detected.[2] These results shocked the medical community but have influenced thinking in this and many other areas of medicine. Hine et al.[3] reported a meta-analysis of the CAST and similar studies with sodium channel–blocking antiarrhythmic drugs and found overall support for the conclusion of the CAST. The CAST has also led to recommendations by the U.S. Food and Drug Administration (FDA) for more restrictive labeling for all sodium channel–blocking antiarrhythmic drugs. In 1991, these drugs were given class labeling with indications for the treatment of documented ventricular arrhythmias that, in the judgment of the physician, are life threatening. Exceptions among the sodium channel–blocking drugs are quinidine, propafenone, and flecainide, which have an additional indication for supraventricular arrhythmias.

Because of discouraging results with sodium channel–blocking drugs, drugs that prolong the action potential (often termed class III) have been studied. Developers had been encouraged, since one drug with this action, amiodarone, may improve, or at least not worsen, mortality rates in patients with cardiac disease.[4,5] Dofetilide, ibutilide, and the *d*-isomer of sotalol all prolong the action potential duration and were developed in the hope that they would have the efficacy of amiodarone but lack its propensity to cause serious side effects. However, the first of these drugs to be evaluated in a mortality trial, *d*-sotalol, was found to increase mortality rates after myocardial infarction.[6] Development of *d*-sotalol was halted, but the other two have been marketed with restrictions placed on their indications and/or clinical use. Clearly, antiarrhythmic drugs are the most complex drugs in clinical use today and require care in their use.

CLASSIFICATION OF ANTIARRHYTHMIC DRUGS

Antiarrhythmic drugs are often classified according to their electrophysiologic effects.[7] The scheme most often employed

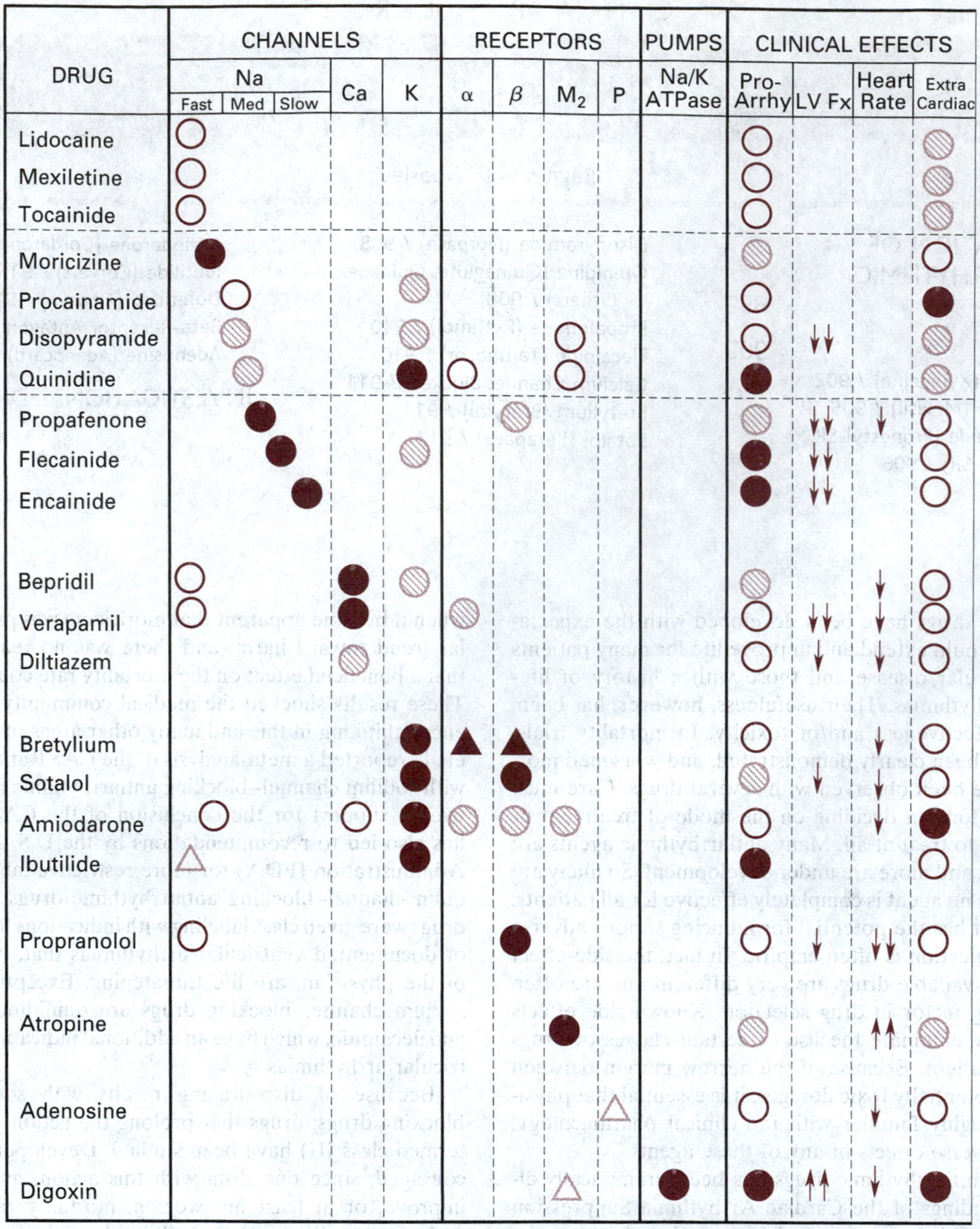
DRUG
CHANNELS
Na
Fast
Med
Slow
Ca
K
RECEPTORS
α
β
M2
P
PUMPS
Na/K ATPase
CLINICAL EFFECTS
Pro-Arrhy
LV Fx
Heart Rate
Extra Cardiac
Lidocaine
Mexiletine
Tocainide
Moricizine
Procainamide
Disopyramide
Quinidine
Propafenone
Flecainide
Encainide
Bepridil
Verapamil
Diltiazem
Bretylium
Sotalol
Amiodarone
Ibutilide
Propranolol
Atropine
Adenosine
Digoxin

FIGURE 27-1 Summary of the potentially most important actions of drugs on membrane channels, receptors, and ionic pumps in the heart. Listed are drugs used to modify cardiac rhythm. Most are marketed as antiarrhythmic agents. The drugs (rows) are ordered in a fashion similar to the columns so that generally the darker symbols for their predominant action or actions form a diagonal. Drugs with multiple actions (e.g., amiodarone) depart strikingly from the diagonal trend. The actions of drugs on the sodium, calcium, and potassium channels are indicated. Sodium channel blockade is subdivided into three groups of actions characterized by fast (300 ms), medium (med; 300–1500 ms), and slow (greater than or equal to 1500 ms) time constants for recovery from block. This parameter is a measure of "use dependence" and predicts the likelihood that a drug will decrease conduction velocity of normal sodium-dependent tissues in the heart and perhaps the propensity of a drug for causing bundle-branch block or proarrhythmia. Drug interactions with receptors alpha, beta, M_2, and P (alpha- and beta-adrenergic, muscarinic subtype, and A_1 purinergic) and drug effects on the sodium-potassium pump (Na/K ATPase) are indicated. Symbols indicate the type of actions at receptors or channels (Antagonist relative potency: ○ low; ● moderate; ● high; △, agonist; ▲, agonist/antagonist). Filled triangles for bretylium indicate its biphasic action to initially stimulate alpha and beta receptors by release of norepinephrine, followed by blocking of norepinephrine release and indirect antagonism of these receptors. (Adapted from the Task Force of the Working Group on Arrhythmias of the European Society of Cardiology,[9] with permission.)

was originally proposed by Vaughan Williams as a classification of drug actions that should be antiarrhythmic, not a classification of drugs.[7] This is a subtle but important distinction that is made for the following reasons:

- Most antiarrhythmic drugs have multiple actions; hence, their pharmacology is more complex than indicated by a simple drug classification scheme.
- The actions of a given drug differ in different cardiac tissues.
- Many antiarrhythmic agents have pharmacologically active metabolites whose activity may be quite different from and in a class other than that of the parent compound.
- The relative amounts of these metabolites produced are genetically determined for several of these drugs and often vary extensively within the population.

Drugs having class I action possess "local anesthetic," or "membrane-stabilizing," activity. Their predominant action is to block the fast inward sodium channel. This produces a decrease in the maximum depolarization rate, $\dot{V}_{max}$, of the action potential (phase 0) and slows intracardiac conduction. These agents have been further subclassified as belonging to class IA, IB, or IC on the basis of their effects on specific aspects of intracardiac conduction and refractoriness.[8] Drugs having class IA action include quinidine, procainamide, and disopyramide. These agents also produce measurable increases in ventricular refractoriness and prolongation of the QT interval. Lidocaine, mexiletine, and tocainide have actions belonging to class IB. Their potency for blocking sodium channels is only moderate, and in isolated tissues they shorten the action potential duration (APD) and refractoriness. They generally exert little effect on PR, QRS, or QT intervals. Drugs with class IC actions are the more potent agents: flecainide and propafenone. Because these are potent sodium channel inhibitors, slowing conduction velocity while having little effect on repolarization, they increase the PR and QRS intervals but cause little change in QT.

Class II action refers to beta-adrenergic antagonism, possessed by agents such as propranolol, timolol, and metoprolol. While these drugs are effective for treatment of supraventricular arrhythmias and tachyarrhythmias secondary to excessive sympathetic activity, they are not very effective in the treatment of severe arrhythmias, such as recurrent ventricular tachycardia. Although the mechanism is unknown, they are the only antiarrhythmic drugs found clearly effective in preventing sudden cardiac death in patients with prior myocardial infarction.

Drugs whose predominant effect is to prolong the duration of the cardiac action potential and refractoriness have class III action. These drugs include amiodarone, sotalol, bretylium, ibutilide, dofetilide, and *N*-acetylprocainamide (NAPA), the major metabolite of procainamide.

Class IV action is calcium channel antagonism. Antiarrhythmic drugs with this action include verapamil, bepridil, diltiazem, and nifedipine.

Because of the many limitations of the Vaughan Williams classification of antiarrhythmic drugs, a new approach has been proposed,[9] termed the Sicilian gambit. This classification system is based on the differential effects of antiarrhythmic drugs on (1) channels, (2) receptors, and (3) transmembrane pumps. The grouping is based primarily on the predominant action of drugs but also considers the other ancillary actions that may be clinically relevant. As shown in Fig. 27-1, because of the sequence of drugs listed, the symbols for these primary actions are generally aligned diagonally. For example, in this system quinidine is a sodium channel antagonist with potassium channel- and alpha-blocking activity. This provides a more complete and accurate description of the pharmacologic actions of the drugs than simply designating it class IA. When combined with an understanding of the electrophysiologic role of these actions, one can predict the effects likely to occur in vivo. In this case one would expect conduction slowing, increased APD (and refractoriness), and vasodilation to result from these three actions of quinidine.

The Sicilian gambit also creates a framework in which newly discovered actions of drugs can be readily added. It emphasizes the multiple actions of drugs and the subtle differences and similarities that exist, and is more complete. At present, our understanding of the pharmacology of these drugs has progressed to the point that oversimplification can be misleading. The increased detail of the new system reflects the current state of our knowledge at a level necessary for optimal use of these drugs.

Due to the low efficacy of any one agent, the treatment of acute or chronic ventricular arrhythmias frequently necessitates the use of multiple drugs, sequentially or in combination. One may produce increased sodium channel blockade and, it is hoped, increase drug efficacy by using combinations of drugs with different kinetics of interaction with the sodium channel. Basic to these considerations is an understanding of the regulation of sodium channel function. Hodgkin and Huxley[10] proposed that sodium channels exist in three distinct states: open, closed, and inactivated. According to the modulated receptor theory of cardiac sodium channel regulation proposed by Hille and by Hondeghem and Katzung,[11] sodium channels in each of these states have differing affinities for a given local anesthetic drug (Fig. 27-2).

The theory also provides a potential explanation for the phenomenon of "frequency," or "use," dependence. Use dependence is the increase in conduction block observed at an increasing rate of stimulation in response to sodium channel–blocking antiarrhythmic agents. Since an increase in the rate of stimulation increases the number of sodium channels in the open and inactivated states, antiarrhythmic agents having

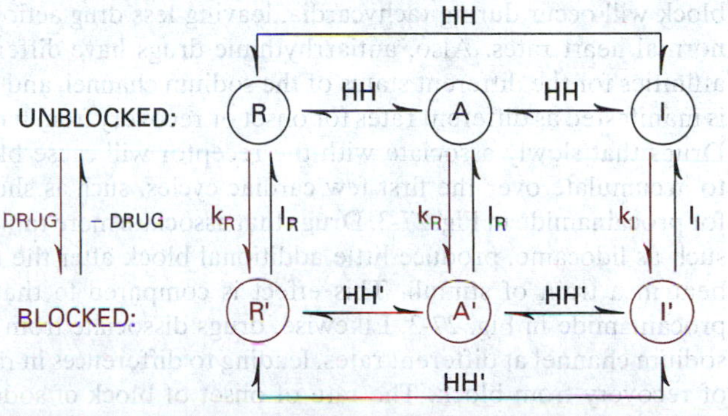

FIGURE 27-2 Diagram of the modulated receptor mechanism for antiarrhythmic drug action. The three fractions of the sodium channel population proposed by Hodgkin and Huxley are represented in the upper part of the figure in the drug-free condition and in the lower part of the figure blocked by an antiarrhythmic agent (R', A', and I', respectively). HH, standard Hodgkin-Huxley rate constants; HH', HH with voltage dependence altered by drug binding; k_R, k_A, and k_I, association rate constants; l_R, l_A, and l_I, dissociation rate constants for the respective channel fractions. (From Hondeghem and Katzung,[11] reproduced with permission from the authors and the American Heart Association.)

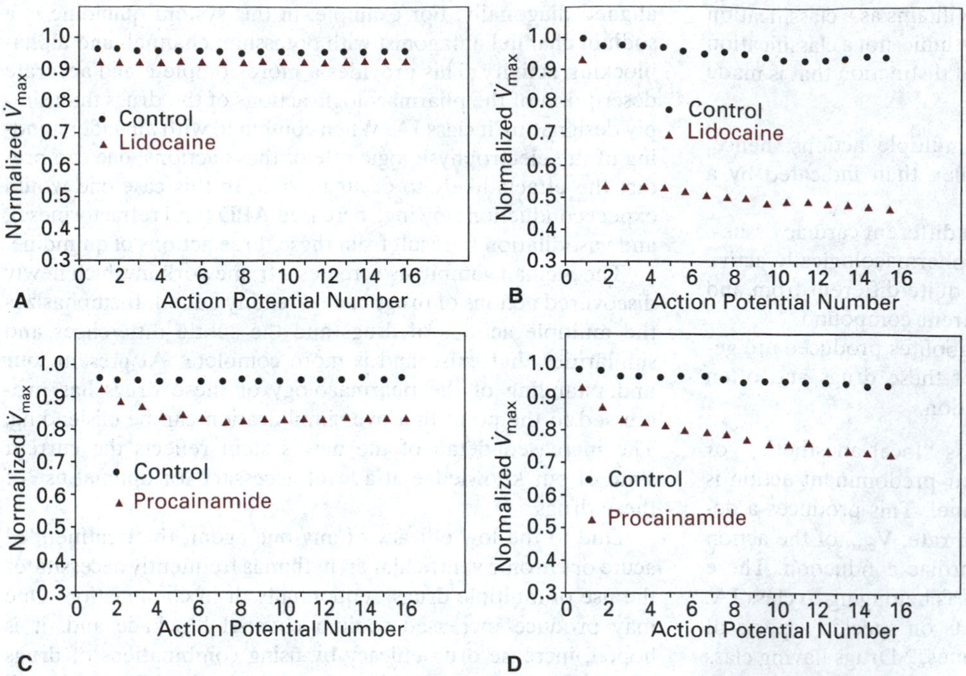

FIGURE 27-3 Rate- (interval-)dependent depression of $\dot{V}_{max}$ by lidocaine and procainamide. Following a 20-s rest period, a train of 16 action potentials was elicited using interstimulus intervals (ISIs) of 1 s or 200 ms in the presence (triangles) or absence (circles) of lidocaine or procainamide. For the duration of the train, $\dot{V}_{max}$ was relatively constant when measured at either ISI in the absence of drug. *A.* In the presence of lidocaine (22 μM), stimulation at an ISI of 1 s produced no use-dependent block. *B.* However, stimulation at 200 ms produced a 50 percent reduction in $\dot{V}_{max}$ from baseline, which was first observed for the second action potential and was constant thereafter. *C.* A different pattern is seen in the presence of 276 μM procainamide, which produced a significant depression of $\dot{V}_{max}$ at an ISI of 1 s. *D.* This depression was more pronounced when the ISI was shortened to 200 ms. Unlike the case for lidocaine, the use-dependent depression of $\dot{V}_{max}$ due to procainamide required multiple action potentials to approach steady-state values. (From Ehring BR, Moyer JW, Hondeghem LM. Quantitative structure activity studies of antiarrhythmic properties in a series of lidocaine and procainamide derivatives. *J Pharmacol Exp Ther* 1989; 244:479–492. Reproduced with permission from the publisher and authors.)

greater affinity for activated (open) or inactivated channels (as opposed to rested channels) would have a greater opportunity to bind to the receptor and slow conduction. Therefore, greater block will occur during tachycardia, leaving less drug action at normal heart rates. Also, antiarrhythmic drugs have different affinities for the different states of the sodium channel, and this is manifested as different rates for onset or recovery from block. Drugs that slowly associate with the receptor will cause block to accumulate over the first few cardiac cycles, such as shown for procainamide in Fig. 27-3. Drugs that associate more rapidly, such as lidocaine, produce little additional block after the first beat in a train of stimuli. This effect is compared to that of procainamide in Fig. 27-3. Likewise, drugs dissociate from the sodium channel at different rates, leading to differences in rates of recovery from block. The rate of onset of block of sodium channels has been proposed as a means of subclassifying antiarrhythmic drugs.[12] This is the electrophysiologic correlate of the subclassification of sodium channel blockers proposed by Harrison that was based on differences in clinical effects of the drugs.[8]

This chapter reviews the clinical pharmacology and applications of the currently available antiarrhythmic drugs, excluding digoxin, beta-receptor antagonists, and calcium channel blockers, which are addressed in other chapters. The drugs reappear in the same order as listed in Fig. 27-1, an updated revision of the Sicilian gambit classification. The pharmacokinetics, usual dosages, and ranges of plasma concentration for the major drugs are listed in Tables 27-1 and 27-2.

DRUGS

Lidocaine (Xylocaine)

CLINICAL APPLICATIONS

Lidocaine, introduced as a local anesthetic, was first used as an antiarrhythmic agent in the 1950s for the treatment of arrhythmias arising during cardiac catheterization.[13] It is still the most widely used intravenous antiarrhythmic drug. Since extensive first-pass metabolism makes it unsatisfactory for oral use, congeners such as mexiletine were developed that would possess similar sodium channel–blocking actions and be active when taken orally.

Lidocaine is very often the drug of first choice for the acute suppression of ventricular arrhythmias. Although such therapy does not reduce total mortality rates, it is effective in decreasing the incidence of primary ventricular fibrillation in patients with documented acute myocardial infarction.[14,15] Because of the complex pharmacokinetics of lidocaine, a monitored environment is desirable to permit evaluation of the patient's response and detection of toxicity.

Lidocaine has little effect on atrial tissue in vitro,[16] consistent with the clinical observation that it has no value in treating supraventricular tachyarrhythmias. Although lidocaine has been used to decrease the ventricular response during atrial fibrillation in patients whose atrioventricular (AV) conduction follows an accessory pathway,[17] some workers have reported accelerated conduction,[18] and other drugs, such as procainamide, are preferred in this situation.

MECHANISM OF ACTION

In concentrations similar to those attained during clinical use, lidocaine reduces $\dot{V}_{max}$ and produces shortening or no change in APD and the effective refractory period of normal Purkinje fibers. This contrasts with quinidine and procainamide, which additionally block potassium channels and produce lengthening of APD.[19,20] Lidocaine has little effect on the electrophysiology of the normal conduction system, but in patients with conduction system abnormalities, it has produced variable effects. Some studies have failed to detect significant changes in conduction,[21,22] while others have found slowing of ventricular rate or potentiation of infranodal block in patients with conduction

TABLE 27-1 Pharmacokinetics of Antiarrhythmic Drugs

Agent	Inactivation or Elimination,[a] %	Protein Binding, %	V_D, L/kg	Elimination Half-life, h	Bioavailability, %	Apparent Oral Clearance, mL/min
Quinidine	Hepatic, 50–90 Renal, 10–30	80–90	2.5	3–19	70	200–400
Procainamide	Hepatic, 40–70[b] Renal, 30–60	15	2	2–4	100	400–700
Disopyramide	Hepatic, 20–30 Renal, 40–50	20–50	0.6	6–8	80–90	90
Lidocaine	Hepatic, 90	40–70	1.1	1.5–4	35[c]	700–1000[c]
Tocainide	Hepatic, 30–40 Renal, 40	10	1.5–3	8–20	90	150–200
Mexiletine	Hepatic, 85–90[b] Renal, 10–15	70	5.5–9.5	8–20	90	400–700
Flecainide	Hepatic, 70[b] Renal, 30	40	7–10	7–26	90–95	200–800
Propafenone	Hepatic, 99[b]	90	3–4	2–24[b]	10–50[b]	800–5000[b]
Amiodarone	Hepatic, 99	95	20–200	13–103 days	20–80	6500–11,000
Bretylium	Renal, 90	Low	3–4	4–16	25[c]	1300
Ibutilide	Hepatic, 93	40	11	2–12		
Dofetilide	Renal, 80	60–70	3	10	>90	—

[a]Renal elimination of unchanged drug.
[b]Dependent on metabolic phenotype (see text).
[c]Not recommended for oral administration.

TABLE 27-2 Dosage and Plasma Concentration Ranges for Antiarrhythmic Agents[a]

Agent	Usual Initial Dosage[b]	Modification of Dosage in Disease[c]	Dosage Range	Maximum Single Dose	Therapeutic Range,[d] μg/mL
Quinidine (sulfate)	200 mg q 6 h	None	800–2400 mg/day	600	0.7–5.5
Procainamide (sustained release)	500 mg q 6 h	↓ CHF ↓ RI	2000–6000 mg/day	1500	4–8
Disopyramide	100 mg q 6 h	↓ CHF ↓ HI ↓ RI	300–1200 mg/day	300	2–5
Lidocaine	See text	↓ CHF ↓ HI	1–4 mg/min IV	—	1.5–5
Tocainide	400 mg q 8 h	↓ HI ↓ RI	1200–2400 mg/day	800	4–10
Mexiletine	200 mg q 8 h	↓ CHF ↓ HI?	600–1200 mg/day	400	0.7–2
Flecainide	50–100 mg q 12 h	↓ CHF ↓ RI ↓ HI?	200–400 mg/day	200	0.2–1
Propafenone	150 mg q 8 h	See text	300–900 mg/day	300	0.5–3?
Amiodarone	600–1400 mg/day (load)	None	200–600 mg/day	600	1–2
Bretylium	See text	↓ RI	1–4 mg/min IV	—	—
Ibutilide	1 mg, repeat after 10 min	—	0.01 mg/kg–1 mg × 2	1 mg	—
Dofetilide	500 mcg bid	↓ RI	125–1000 mcg/d	500 mcg	0.001–0.003

[a]These are general guidelines only. Dosage should be determined for each patient based on clinical presentation, disease states, clinical response, and tolerance to the drug.
[b]Dosage usually recommended in absence of significant cardiac, renal, or hepatic failure.
[c]CHF, congestive heart failure; HI, hepatic insufficiency; RI, renal insufficiency. See text for details.
[d]The range of therapeutic plasma concentrations is a statistical range that should be considered only a guideline to therapy.

system defects.[23,24] Variability in dosage and pharmacokinetics may explain some of these discrepancies.

CLINICAL PHARMACOLOGY

Orally administered lidocaine is well absorbed, but it has poor oral bioavailability because it undergoes extensive first-pass hepatic metabolism. Lidocaine clearance is well approximated by measurement of liver blood flow.[25,26] The two desethyl metabolites, which are excreted by the kidneys, have less antiarrhythmic potency than the parent drug and may contribute to the production of central nervous system side effects occurring with lidocaine.[27,28] Following intravenous administration, lidocaine's biphasic disposition is well represented by a two-compartment pharmacokinetic model.[29] Since antiarrhythmic activity is correlated with lidocaine's concentration in the central compartment and the half-life of distribution out of this compartment is rapid (8 min), regimens employing a series of multiple loading doses and a maintenance infusion should be used to achieve and then maintain a therapeutic concentration in plasma and myocardial tissue.

Regardless of the initial regimen employed, during prolonged constant infusion the lidocaine concentration eventually reaches steady state, dependent only on the drug infusion rate and clearance of lidocaine. The time required to reach steady-state conditions is approximately 8 to 10 h in normal individuals and up to 20 to 24 h in some patients with heart failure and/or liver disease. This is longer than often anticipated because of the failure to recognize the relatively long elimination half-life (1.5 to 2 h in normal subjects and longer in patients with heart failure or hepatic disease).

DOSAGE AND ADMINISTRATION

The primary use of lidocaine is for acute rapid suppression of highly symptomatic ventricular arrhythmias. Single intravenous boluses will achieve only transient therapeutic effects because the drug is rapidly distributed out of the plasma and myocardium; therefore, multiple loading doses should be used in order to achieve more sustained therapeutic plasma levels of lidocaine rapidly. Based on pharmacokinetic models validated in clinical studies, several regimens have been designed to maintain a relatively constant therapeutic level. For a stable patient, a total loading dose of lidocaine should be approximately 3 to 4 mg/kg body weight administered over 20 to 30 min. After injection of an initial dose of 1 mg/kg over 2 min, a series of three loading boluses can be administered slowly (approximately 50 mg each over 2 min) 8 to 10 min apart, while the patient is continuously observed for the development of side effects. Loading should be stopped should the transient, usually mild, central nervous system side effects persist or serious unwanted effects occur.

Another effective and well-tolerated loading regimen was suggested by Wyman et al.[30] For a 75-kg person, an initial bolus of 75 mg is recommended, followed by 50 mg every 5 min repeated three times to a total dose of 225 mg. This regimen usually achieves and maintains plasma concentrations within usual therapeutic guidelines (1.5 to 5 μg/mL). A priming dose of 75 mg followed by a loading infusion of 150 mg over 18 min has also been used successfully.[31] At the time of initiation of the loading regimen, a maintenance infusion, designed to replace ongoing losses due to drug elimination, should be started. This may be calculated as the product of the desired plasma concentration (about 3 μg/mL) and the expected clearance. This calculation usually yields a dosage in the range of 20 to 60 μg/kg of body weight per minute.

Even in normal individuals, there is great variability in the peak plasma concentration and, consequently, in the calculated size of the central compartment for lidocaine. Therefore, during loading, the patient's electrocardiogram (ECG), blood pressure, and mental status should be monitored; the process should be stopped at the first sign of lidocaine excess. When symptomatic arrhythmias persist in the presence of documented adequate dosage, defined by side effects or plasma concentration in excess of 5 to 7 μg/mL, another agent should be used.

If the maintenance infusion has reached steady state but the concentration is below the level needed to prevent recurrence and the arrhythmia reappears while side effects are absent, the appropriate actions are as follows: (1) obtain a plasma sample for measurement of lidocaine concentration for future reference, (2) administer a small bolus of lidocaine (25 to 50 mg over 2 min), and (3) increase the maintenance infusion rate proportionally. The plasma concentration can be used to estimate clearance for calculation of the final maintenance infusion (i.e., maintenance dosage = clearance × desired plasma concentration, and clearance = infusion rate ÷ plasma concentration measured at steady state). Little therapeutic effect is evident at lidocaine plasma concentrations below 1.5 μg/mL, while the risk of toxicity increases above 5 μg/mL. In some patients, however, concentrations in the range of 5 to 9 μg/mL may be required for arrhythmia suppression and can safely be achieved with cautious drug administration.[32]

Once steady-state conditions have been achieved, simply terminating a lidocaine infusion will result in a gradual decline in plasma levels over the next 8 to 10 h as elimination occurs. Not only is there no reason to taper lidocaine infusions, but it may be dangerous if oral antiarrhythmic therapy is initiated too early, since unpredictable additive effects may occur between lidocaine and newly started oral therapy. If a patient has reached steady-state equilibrium, it is possible to estimate when the plasma lidocaine concentration will fall below usually therapeutic levels. The plasma lidocaine concentration should be determined at the time the infusion is terminated, and the number of half-lives needed for that level to reach approximately 1.5 μg/mL can be estimated. The half-life of lidocaine for an individual patient can be estimated from the following equation: $t_{1/2}$ = plasma concentration × V_D × 0.693/infusion rate, where V_D is the final volume of distribution.

The measured plasma concentration and the infusion rate are known components of the equation. V_D is usually 1.1 L/kg but may be reduced by 50 percent or more in patients with heart failure.

MODIFICATION OF DOSAGE IN DISEASE STATES

Initial loading regimens require no adjustment in patients with renal or liver disease[29]; however, maintenance infusions must be decreased in liver disease and heart failure to compensate for decreased clearance. Since clearance alone is altered in liver disease, with little change in the volume of distribution, the half-life of elimination is prolonged greatly (as much as 5 h), and steady-state conditions may not be achieved until 20 to 25 h following the institution of an intravenous infusion. Despite the fact that lidocaine metabolites are excreted by the kidneys, renal disease has not been reported to exert any significant effect on lidocaine dosing regimens. With mechanical ventilation, there is often a decrease in cardiac output and hepatic blood flow, and a decrease in lidocaine dosage may be required.[33] Patients with congestive heart failure achieve lidocaine levels that are almost double those in normal individuals given the same dose.[29] Since the central volume of distribution is generally halved in heart failure, loading doses should be reduced by 50 percent; since clearance is also approximately halved, maintenance doses should be reduced proportionately from an infusion rate of 30 μg/kg body weight per minute used for usual patients to about half that figure. The time required to achieve steady-state conditions following the institution of a maintenance infusion is still 8 to 10 h in many patients with heart failure because of concomitant changes in V_D and clearance, resulting in a half-life similar to that seen in patients without heart failure.

In summary, general recommendations for initial lidocaine dosage selection should be adjusted for each patient based on clinical presentation, clinical response, and the results of plasma level monitoring. Some patients with congestive heart failure may experience toxicity when given an infusion as low as 0.5 mg/mL; thus, blood level monitoring is essential for proper dosage adjustment. In postmyocardial infarction patients receiving lidocaine infusions for more than 24 h, plasma lidocaine levels can increase, and the elimination phase half-life can increase up to 50 percent.[34] This increase is due, in part, to changes occurring in protein binding of lidocaine during the first few days of therapy. Assays for plasma lidocaine measure the sum of both protein-bound and free lidocaine as total lidocaine and thus do not give a true picture of the amount of free drug available. An increase in plasma lidocaine occurring at this time often reflects an elevation in plasma levels of alpha-1-acid glycoprotein (AAG), to which it binds,[35] and does not always indicate an increase in free, active drug. In this case, the lidocaine dosage should not be reduced to compensate for the higher total plasma concentration as long as the patient displays no adverse effects. Subsequent decreases in AAG concentrations will result in an apparent decrease in plasma lidocaine, which may reflect a drop in only that fraction bound to AAG.

ADVERSE REACTIONS

Central nervous system symptoms are the most frequent side effects of lidocaine administration. A rapid bolus can induce tinnitus or seizures. With more gradual attainment of excessive levels, drowsiness, dysarthria, confusion, hallucinations, and dysesthesia may occur. Excessive lidocaine can also cause coma, which should be a consideration in patients after cardiac arrest. Lidocaine can depress cardiac function, which decreases its clearance, and produces an even greater increase in lidocaine concentrations. Advanced degrees of sinus node dysfunction have been reported in isolated instances.[36,37] In patients with known conduction abnormalities below the AV node, lidocaine should be administered cautiously, if at all, unless a temporary pacemaker is readily available.

DRUG INTERACTIONS

An additive or synergistic depression of myocardial function or conduction may occur when using lidocaine combined with other antiarrhythmic agents,[38] especially during conversion from lidocaine to another antiarrhythmic agent. A pharmacokinetic drug interaction between propranolol and lidocaine has been described experimentally and in humans in which beta-adrenergic blockade caused decreases in cardiac output and liver blood flow, with a resultant decreased lidocaine clearance.[39] Cimetidine has been reported to decrease lidocaine's volume of distribution, decrease splanchnic (and hence liver) blood flow, and inhibit the enzymes responsible for lidocaine metabolism. This may raise lidocaine plasma concentrations, and both loading and maintenance dosages may require downward adjustment in patients receiving cimetidine.[40]

Mexiletine (Mexitil)

CLINICAL APPLICATIONS

Mexiletine is used in the treatment of ventricular arrhythmias and has, on occasion, been effective in treating arrhythmias that were refractory to other agents. Success rates vary between 6 and 60 percent, and more than half of the studies suggest limited efficacy (less than 20 percent).[41] Mexiletine does not prolong the QT interval and therefore can be useful for patients with a history of drug-induced torsades de pointes or long-QT syndrome when quinidine, sotalol, procainamide, or disopyramide are contraindicated. While the rate of response to mexiletine when used alone is low, it has been combined successfully with quinidine,[42] propranolol,[43] or procainamide.[44] This mode of therapy takes advantage of the additive, and perhaps synergistic, antiarrhythmic response produced by the combination of these agents. Since lower than usual dosages of both agents can be used, dosage-related adverse effects are reduced concomitantly. Mexiletine exerts minimal effects on both hemodynamics and myocardial contractility, even in patients with severe congestive heart failure.[45]

MECHANISM OF ACTION

Mexiletine is an orally active lidocaine congener with class IB sodium channel–blocking activity and structural similarity to tocainide. It was originally developed as an anorexiant and anticonvulsant agent, and its antiarrhythmic properties were only later recognized. Mexiletine blocks fast sodium channels, decreasing V_{max} and shortening the repolarization phase of ventricular myocardium.[46]

CLINICAL PHARMACOLOGY

The systemic bioavailability of mexiletine approximates 90 percent,[47] with a large volume of distribution (5.5 to 9.5 L/kg), reflecting extensive tissue uptake. About 1 percent of total body content of mexiletine is in the plasma compartment, with approximately 70 percent of this bound to serum proteins. Mexiletine has little first-pass metabolism but is eliminated primarily by hepatic metabolism, with only 10 to 15 percent being excreted unchanged in the urine. Its half-life of elimination is between 8 and 20 h (9 and 12 h for healthy subjects), with the time needed to reach steady state ranging between 1 and 3 days.[48] Mexiletine undergoes extensive hepatic metabolism by cytochrome P450 2D6 (CYP2D6),[49,50] and, consequently, clearance is extremely variable (see below).[51]

DOSAGE AND ADMINISTRATION

Mexiletine therapy should be initiated with a low dosage, which is increased at 2- to 3-day intervals until efficacy or intolerable side effects, such as tremor or other central nervous system symptoms, develop. With normal renal function, the recommended initial oral mexiletine dosage is 200 mg every 8 h. As with most drugs having extensive liver metabolism, clearance will be widely variable within the population. This is especially true for mexiletine because CYP2D6, responsible for its metabolism, is absent in 7 percent of the Caucasian population. Also, consideration of dosage adjustment to compensate for the action of agents (discussed below) that induce or inhibit hepatic mexiletine metabolism is required.

MODIFICATION OF DOSAGE IN DISEASE STATES

Patients with renal failure who also inherit a deficiency of hepatic CYP2D6 are likely to have extremely slow elimination for mexiletine,[52] and for this reason, all renal failure patients should be given low initial doses. Elimination half-life and clearance may be prolonged by overt congestive heart failure[53] and hepatic failure,[54] and dosage reduction is required.

ADVERSE REACTIONS

Adverse reactions to mexiletine are dose-related and neurologic and include tremor, visual blurring, dizziness, dysphoria, and nausea. Thrombocytopenia has been reported to occur infrequently with mexiletine therapy,[55,56] and a positive antinuclear antibody test result occurs rarely. Severe bradycardia and abnormal prolongation of sinus node recovery time have been reported in patients with the sick-sinus syndrome,[57] and, at high concentrations, worsening of heart block has been reported.[58] Oral mexiletine does not depress ventricular function or induce increased heart failure,[59] although intravenous mexiletine, which is not available in the United States, has been noted to increase congestive heart failure.[60]

DRUG INTERACTIONS

The hepatic metabolism of mexiletine can be increased by phenobarbital, phenytoin (Dilantin), or rifampicin, which reduce the half-life of mexiletine, possibly changing an effective dose to an ineffective one.[41,48,61] Conversely, if treatment with an inducing agent is stopped, an effective dose may become toxic.

In one study, mexiletine decreased the clearance and increased the plasma concentrations of theophylline.[62] Quinidine inhibits the CYP2D6 enzyme primarily responsible for the metabolic clearance of mexiletine, and plasma concentration of mexiletine may increase in those individuals who express the enzyme (93 percent of Caucasians).

Procainamide (Pronestyl-SR, Procan-SR)

CLINICAL APPLICATIONS

Procainamide, like quinidine, is effective against both supraventricular and ventricular arrhythmias.[63] Although the two drugs have similar electrophysiologic effects, they are clinically different, and one agent may be effective for a patient when the other is not. Procainamide is useful in acute management of patients with reentrant supraventricular tachycardia and atrial fibrillation and flutter associated with Wolff-Parkinson-White syndrome.[64]

Although lidocaine is more often used, procainamide is also used intravenously to suppress ventricular arrhythmias occurring immediatiely following myocardial infarction or to convert sustained ventricular tachycardia. Since it takes approximately 20 min to administer a loading dose of procainamide safely, its use is limited to those situations where adequate time is available. Its advantage over lidocaine is the potential for conversion to oral therapy using the same agent. Lidocaine is usually used, however, because the initial loading dose can be given within a 2- to 5-min period.

The active metabolite of procainamide, *N*-acetylprocainamide (acecainide or NAPA), produces class III antiarrhythmic activity in some patients, although not always those who respond to procainamide.[65] This is most likely due to the very different electrophysiologic actions of procainamide and NAPA.[66] NAPA was investigated as an antiarrhythmic drug and was shown to be effective in the treatment of ventricular arrhythmias, but since its use was limited by a narrow therapeutic index, development was halted.[65]

The development of procainamide as an antiarrhythmic agent resulted from a systematic search for a useful congener of procaine, whose use was precluded by adverse reactions.[67] Since procainamide is an effective agent but is not without adverse effects, it has served as a prototype for development of several of the newer antiarrhythmic agents.

MECHANISM OF ACTION

Like other agents demonstrating class I activity, procainamide slows conduction and decreases automaticity and excitability of atrial and ventricular myocardium and Purkinje fibers.[68] Because of its effect on potassium channels, it also prolongs APD and refractoriness. Compared to quinidine, procainamide has very little vagolytic activity and does not prolong the QT interval to as great an extent.[63] NAPA has predominantly class III antiarrhythmic activity; it prolongs APD and refractoriness in both atrial and ventricular myocardium and prolongs the QT interval.[69,70] It has little or no effect on $\dot{V}_{max}$ in either Purkinje fibers or ventricular cells and does not alter His-Purkinje conduction velocity because of its very low potency as a sodium channel antagonist.

CLINICAL PHARMACOLOGY

Procainamide is rapidly absorbed and 100 percent orally bioavailable. About 15 percent of procainamide is bound to serum proteins. Its short half-life of elimination, 2 to 4 h in patients with normal renal function, necessitates dosing every 3 to 6 h. Dosing every 6, 8, or 12 h is possible with sustained-release preparations, and the frequency depends upon the formulation. The varied formulations and their very different dosing requirements often create confusion and can lead to dangerous mistakes in dosing.

Slightly more than half of the general population are phenotypically rapid acetylators of procainamide and quickly convert it to NAPA, a metabolite with very pure class III antiarrhythmic action.[65] As would be expected, however, the response to one agent does not predict response to the other. When each is given as the sole agent, the usually effective plasma concentration is 4 to 8 μg/mL for procainamide and 7 to 15 μg/mL for NAPA.[65] During oral procainamide therapy, both agents are present in variable amounts, and there is no way to determine readily the contribution of NAPA to arrhythmia suppression under these conditions. Consequently, the utility of measuring plasma levels of procainamide during chronic therapy is limited because of this variable hepatic conversion to NAPA. Monitoring plasma concentrations for determination of compliance or prevention of toxicity is feasible and recommended (see below).

DOSAGE AND ADMINISTRATION

Procainamide is available for either intravenous or oral use. With normal renal and cardiac function, the initial recommended oral maintenance dose is 50 mg/kg per day. Frequent administration is required for oral procainamide, which is inconvenient and makes compliance difficult. Sustained-release forms of procainamide are available, which permits dosing every 6, 8, or 12 h, depending upon the formulation. During chronic therapy, levels of NAPA may accumulate to effective or toxic levels in some individuals, resulting in achievement of maximum pharmacologic effect long after the time procainamide has reached steady state.[65,71] Therefore, the elimination half-life of 2 to 4 h for procainamide may be misleading as a predictor of time to the occurrence of stable pharmacologic action. Thus, dosage should be initiated at conservative levels, and the patient should be monitored carefully until both procainamide and its metabolite have reached steady state. Patients with ventricular tachycardia may need higher dosages[65] for prevention of arrhythmia induction by programmed stimulation,[72] although such dosages often lead to adverse effects. Since the electrophysiologic effects of procainamide and NAPA are quite different, monitoring of patients receiving procainamide should at some point include measurement of plasma concentrations of both agents to determine their relative concentrations. Patients who are rapid acetylators or who have impaired renal function usually have plasma concentrations of NAPA higher than those of procainamide at steady state. These individuals should be monitored for excessive accumulation of NAPA during dose titration to maintain plasma levels of NAPA below 20 μg/mL. The practice of using the sum of the plasma concentration of procainamide and NAPA is not recommended.

When administered intravenously, procainamide can be given as a constant 25-min loading infusion of 275 μg/min per kilogram of body weight or by a series of doses (100 mg delivered over 3 min) given every 5 min, up to a total dose of 1 g.[73,74] If the loading infusion is well tolerated with no hypotension and less than 25 percent QRS or QT widening, a maintenance intravenous infusion of 20 to 60 μg/kg per minute can then be given. Larger and more rapid loading infusions of 1 g over 15 to 20 min have been given in the electrophysiology laboratory to prevent induction of ventricular tachycardia by programmed ventricular stimulation. A second loading infusion of 0.5 to 1 g has been given in some instances where an initial loading infusion was well tolerated but ineffective. These large dosages are accompanied by a higher incidence of hypotension and conduction disturbance and often result in attainment of unacceptably high plasma concentration.

MODIFICATION OF DOSAGE IN DISEASE STATES

With renal dysfunction or a low cardiac output, both procainamide and NAPA in usual doses may accumulate to potentially toxic levels, and the dose should be reduced.[75] Increased plasma levels of procainamide and/or NAPA may occur with congestive heart failure because of decreased urinary excretion and hydrolysis of procainamide.[76] On the other hand, one study of procainamide pharmacokinetics following a single intravenous bolus revealed no difference in volume of distribution, clearance, elimination half-life, unbound drug fraction, and peak procainamide concentrations between patients with congestive heart failure and normal individuals.[77] Although intravenous procainamide does depress myocardial contractility and lower blood pressure, worsening of heart failure is uncommon during oral therapy when the usual dosages and plasma concentrations are maintained.

ADVERSE REACTIONS

Side effects associated with long-term procainamide therapy limit its usefulness. Up to 40 percent of patients discontinue therapy in the first 6 months due to adverse reactions. The potential exists for arrhythmia aggravation, including the development of torsades de pointes due to procainamide or, more often, NAPA.[78] Therefore, just as with all agents possessing class IA activity, procainamide should not be used in patients with a long-QT syndrome, a history of torsades de pointes, or hypokalemia.[79] In order to reduce the occurrence of proarrhythmia, potassium levels should be maintained above 4 meq/L when taking procainamide. Heart block and sinus node dysfunction can occur in patients with preexisting conduction system abnormalities.[80]

Between 15 and 20 percent of patients receiving chronic oral procainamide therapy develop a lupus-like syndrome, which is often difficult to recognize but regresses with discontinuation of treatment. The syndrome usually begins insidiously as mild arthralgia but progresses to frank arthritis, fever, malar erythematous rash, and pleural and/or pericardial effusions, with serum antibodies against nucleoprotein (histone) appearing as antinuclear antibodies with a "smooth" or "diffuse" pattern. These symptoms abate if procainamide is discontinued and generally resolve at a rate proportional to their duration.

Almost all patients treated chronically develop detectable antinuclear antibodies, but only 15 to 20 percent develop symptoms of the lupus syndrome. Therefore, it is unnecessary to discontinue therapy solely because of the positive antinuclear antibody titer. The patient should be fully informed of the symptoms, which should be reported, so that therapy can be discontinued at the earliest symptoms or signs of the lupus syndrome. Continuing procainamide after the development of the early symptoms of the lupus syndrome is dangerous because of the above-noted possibility of pleural effusion and potentially lethal pericardial tamponade.[81]

More recently, procainamide therapy has been associated with the development of agranulocytosis. It has been suggested, but not proven, that the sustained-release form of the drug may be especially capable of inducing this toxicity.[82] The manufacturer recommends that a white blood count be obtained every 2 weeks for the first 3 months.

DRUG INTERACTIONS

Unlike quinidine, procainamide does not cause an increase in digoxin levels. There are few reports of interactions between procainamide and other drugs. Its clearance is reduced between 30 and 50 percent by cimetidine, which blocks the renal tubular secretion of procainamide.[83,84] A similar competition has been found between procainamide and its predominant metabolite, NAPA.[85] Ranitidine affects procainamide pharmacokinetics by reducing both its renal clearance and its absorption, the former by 14 to 23 percent and the latter by 10 to 24 percent, depending on the dose.[86]

Disopyramide (Norpace)

CLINICAL APPLICATIONS

Disopyramide is effective against a broad range of supraventricular and ventricular arrhythmias, its antiarrhythmic profile being similar to that of quinidine and procainamide. Disopyramide, in contrast to quinidine and procainamide, is better suited for long-term therapy, having relatively little associated chronic toxicity. While newer than quinidine or procainamide, disopyramide is still one of the older antiarrhythmic agents, having been in use in the United States since 1977. Its negative inotropic and anticholinergic actions occur frequently and limit its usefulness.

MECHANISMS OF ACTION

The class IA antiarrhythmic effects of disopyramide are predominantly those associated with sodium and potassium channel blockade. Its effects are similar to those of quinidine and procainamide on automaticity, conduction, and refractoriness in atrial and ventricular tissue.[87]

CLINICAL PHARMACOLOGY

The oral bioavailability of disopyramide is 80 to 90 percent.[88] Its half-life of elimination, usually 6 to 8 h, is lengthened to as much as 15 h in cardiac patients.[89] About half of the compound is eliminated by the kidneys unchanged, and the remainder as an active metabolite resulting from hepatic *N*-dealkylation.[90] Protein binding of disopyramide is complex, with between 20 and 50 percent of disopyramide being bound to plasma proteins. For most drugs, the percentage bound to plasma protein is a constant over the usual range of therapeutic concentrations. The saturation of disopyramide-binding sites on plasma proteins at usual doses means that there are disproportionate increases in levels of free drug in plasma compared to the magnitude of dosage increment.[91]

DOSAGE AND ADMINISTRATION

Loading doses are not recommended with disopyramide. The usually effective dosage for disopyramide is 100 to 400 mg three to four times daily, to a maximal dose of 800 mg/day. Therapy should be very carefully titrated, beginning with low doses and allowing ample time for achievement of steady-state equilibrium.

While rapid fluctuations in plasma concentration are undesirable, they are difficult to avoid because of disopyramide's saturable protein binding. The controlled-release form of disopyramide may be useful in reducing adverse effects by decreasing fluctuations in the concentration of free disopyramide in plasma.[92] Because of saturable protein binding,[16] the generally accepted therapeutic range for total disopyramide in plasma, 2 to 5 μg/mL, should not be strictly relied on. While monitoring the plasma concentrations of free disopyramide has been recommended,[93] the range of concentrations associated with arrhythmia suppression has not been clearly delineated and overlaps with that causing adverse effects.

MODIFICATION OF DOSAGE IN DISEASE STATES

The patient's response to disopyramide should be monitored especially closely following acute myocardial infarction because both the absorption and elimination of disopyramide are decreased at this time.[94] In fact, in view of the negative inotropic actions of disopyramide and changes in levels of binding proteins in plasma following a myocardial infarction, other antiarrhythmic agents should be considered first.

Disopyramide is contraindicated in patients with uncompensated heart failure because it can worsen failure.[95] The initial dosage of disopyramide should be reduced to 50 to 100 mg every 12 h in patients with renal insufficiency[96] or decreased hepatic function.[97]

ADVERSE REACTIONS

The predominant side effects of disopyramide include new or worsened congestive heart failure and symptoms resulting from dose-related anticholinergic actions, including urinary retention, constipation, dry mouth, and esophageal reflux. Because of this anticholinergic action, patients with obstructive uropathy or glaucoma should not receive this agent.[98] For some patients, the anticholinergic side effects can be prevented or alleviated by concomitant use of cholinesterase inhibitors, such as physostigmine and neostigmine, without reduction in antiarrhythmic efficacy.[99] As with all agents that prolong repolarization, disopyramide should not be used in patients with long-QT syndrome, hypokalemia, or a history of torsades de pointes[100] because of the potential for arrhythmia aggravation. Direct actions of disopyramide on the sinus node can lead to excessive bradycardia in patients with sinus nodal dysfunction,[101] and this may contribute to development of torsades de pointes in patients with hypokalemia.[102]

DRUG INTERACTIONS

Disopyramide does not increase digoxin levels,[103] and the effects of warfarin are not potentiated by disopyramide.[104] Phenytoin, rifampicin, and phenobarbital induce hepatic metabolism of disopyramide, thus increasing its elimination and potentially leading to loss of antiarrhythmic effect.[105] Significant depression of myocardial contractility may result from the combined administration of disopyramide with beta-adrenergic or calcium channel antagonists and should be avoided in patients with impairment of ventricular function.[106]

Quinidine (Quinaglute, Quinadex, Others)

CLINICAL APPLICATIONS

Quinidine has been used successfully for a variety of supraventricular and ventricular arrhythmias, including conversion of atrial fibrillation or flutter,[107,108] supraventricular tachycardia,[107,108] ventricular extrasystoles,[109] and ventricular tachycardia and fibrillation.[110,111] Digitalis is used in the treatment of atrial fibrillation, atrial flutter, and other arrhythmias. This important drug is discussed in Chap. 23.

A grouped analysis of six small placebo-controlled trials in patients with atrial fibrillation showed a statistically significant increase in mortality rate for the patients treated with quinidine.[112] Because of the similar negative effects on mortality rate seen in the CAST and CAST II, one must assume that the results of this meta-analysis are valid until a definitive prospective study is available.

MECHANISM OF ACTION

Quinidine has multiple actions, but the action thought by many to be primarily responsible for its efficacy is block of the rapid inward sodium channel. This results in a decrease in $\dot{V}_{max}$ of the action potential upstroke and slowed conduction, more marked in the His-Purkinje system than in the atria. The effects of quinidine on sodium channels are greatest at increased heart rate and less negative membrane potential; that is, they are pH-, rate-, and voltage-dependent. Dose-related changes in the ECG are increases in PR, QRS, and QT_c intervals, which reflect the multiple actions of quinidine.[113]

CLINICAL PHARMACOLOGY

The effective dosage of quinidine varies among individuals because of several factors. Although quinidine sulfate is usually administered every 6 h, there are wide interindividual differences in its elimination half-life, which varies from 3 to 19 h.[114] Plasma protein binding also varies widely, ranging from 50 to 95 percent.[114] Oral bioavailability is approximately 70 percent, and clearance after oral administration ranges from 200 to 400 mL/min. Quinidine is inactivated or eliminated by both hepatic metabolism (50 to 90 percent) and renal elimination (10 to 30 percent). Several potentially active metabolites are formed in amounts that vary among individuals,[115] but for most, their clinical role has not been determined. One of the metabolites of quinidine, 3-hydroxyquinidine, has been shown to possess antiarrhythmic activity when given to humans.[115] Experimental data indicate some contribution by metabolites of quinidine to its antiarrhythmic action.[116,117,118]

DOSAGE AND ADMINISTRATION

Quinidine therapy (as the sulfate) is usually initiated with an oral dosage of 200 mg every 6 h, and the dosage is carefully titrated every 3 or more days. Elderly patients often require lower dosages of quinidine because of both reduced clearance and volume of distribution. Quinidine is available commercially in at least three different forms: quinidine sulfate, gluconate, and polygalacturonate. Since the quinidine content varies among these at 83, 62, and 60 percent, respectively, the need for dosage adjustment should be considered if one form is substituted for another. The usually effective dosage of quinidine sulfate ranges from 800 to 2400 mg/day, with the maximum recommended single dose being 600 mg. Because the half-life varies from 3 to 19 h, one should wait 4 days between dosage increases to prevent unexpected drug accumulation. The range of therapeutic plasma concentrations measured using assays that differentiate quinidine from its metabolites is 0.7 to 5.5 μg/mL.[119,120] Rapid escalation in quinidine dosage has been used to convert atrial fibrillation, but this therapy is no longer recommended because of unnecessary toxicity.

Intravenous therapy with quinidine is usually avoided if alternatives are feasible. Vasodilation and hypotension result from quinidine-induced alpha-adrenergic blockade. If quinidine is given intravenously (as quinidine gluconate), the patient should be carefully monitored and the infusion rate should be no greater than 16 mg/min. This should be discontinued if hypotension is observed or the QRS is prolonged by more than 30 percent.

MODIFICATION OF DOSAGE IN DISEASE STATES

No adjustment in initial dosage is usually needed for patients with renal or hepatic disease,[121,122] although, due to decreased protein binding in patients with hepatic failure, lower than usual total plasma concentration can produce toxicity.[123] Slower dose titration is advisable to permit attainment of steady state and complete accumulation of active metabolites; however, because the usual range of effective dosages is wide, dosage for these patients is not markedly different. Patients with rapid quinidine elimination may require higher dosages (up to 600 mg every 6 h). This is often due to induction of hepatic metabolism caused by other drugs.

Patients with congenital long-QT syndrome, hypokalemia, or a history of torsades de pointes[124] should not be given quinidine because of their increased risk for this form of proarrhythmic event. For patients with congestive heart failure, problems associated with use of quinidine are proarrhythmia and digitalis (either digitoxin or digoxin) toxicity. Prudent use of quinidine in individuals taking digitalis requires the following: (1) that titration begin at a reduced dosage, (2) that dosage of any cardiac glycoside being administered concomitantly be reduced, and (3) that plasma electrolyte levels, especially potassium levels, be maintained above 4 meq/L.

Although quinidine does possess some direct negative inotropic effects, they are usually counteracted by its vasodilatory effect; therefore, oral quinidine is well tolerated hemodynamically when given at dosages producing usual plasma concentrations, even in patients with reduced ventricular function.[125] In a study of over 650 patients, 35 percent of whom had congestive heart failure, quinidine therapy resulted in no induction or worsening of congestive heart failure.[126] On the other hand, a significant problem for patients with congestive heart failure receiving quinidine therapy is proarrhythmia, with quinidine-induced torsades de pointes being potentiated in the setting of bradycardia and low serum levels of magnesium or potassium.[102,127]

ADVERSE REACTIONS

Marked prolongation of the QT interval has been seen in some patients receiving low or usual dosages of quinidine, and the risk of torsades de pointes is markedly increased. This arrhythmia may be responsible for quinidine syncope, which occurs in as many as 5 to 10 percent of patients within the first days of quinidine treatment, and for quinidine-induced sudden death.[128] Torsades de pointes usually occurs in patients (more often females than males) with low serum concentrations of quinidine, hypokalemia, poor ventricular function, and bradycardia.[128,129] In a study by Drici et al., dihydrotestosterone reduced the sensitivity to the effects of quinidine on the QT interval in animals.[130] This study[130] and a subsequent study by Benton et al.[131] in which women were shown to be more sensitive to the effects of quinidine on the QT interval, provide evidence that sex hormones have direct effects on cardiac tissue that may be responsible for the difference in the incidence of torsades de pointes in men and women.[129]

For patients who develop torsades de pointes, treatment with pacing or isoproterenol is very effective. Magnesium sulfate injection is often recommended as initial therapy for torsades de pointes, although controlled trials are not available. These measures should also include correction of hypokalemia. Clinically, it is essential to distinguish torsades de pointes from polymorphic ventricular tachycardia occurring in the setting of a normal QT interval, because the latter should be treated with local anesthetic antiarrhythmic drugs and may be worsened by the above-mentioned treatment for torsades de pointes.

Since quinidine acts via alpha-adrenergic blockade to produce vasodilatation,[132] hypotension may occur, especially in patients concomitantly receiving nitrates or other vasodilators.

Other adverse effects include a high incidence of diarrhea and vomiting, tinnitus at high plasma levels, rare thrombocytopenia,[133] and, in unusual cases, conduction block in patients with existing conduction system disease.[126] In patients treated with quinidine for atrial flutter without prior AV nodal blockade by digitalis, there have been reports of sudden increases in AV conduction and rapid ventricular rates.[132] This results from a slight reduction of the flutter rate and enhanced AV nodal conduction due to the anticholinergic effects of quinidine. This permits 1:1 conduction through the AV node, often at 200 to 250 beats per minute. This may be of particular concern for patients receiving other drugs that increase conduction time through the AV node, such as beta-adrenergic agonists.

DRUG INTERACTIONS

Quinidine metabolism is inhibited by cimetidine[134] and induced by phenytoin, phenobarbital,[135] and rifampicin,[133] with the latter agents leading to reduced, often subtherapeutic, quinidine concentrations. Clinical digoxin toxicity has been described in 20 to 40 percent of patients receiving quinidine and digoxin concurrently.[134] The magnitude of this interaction is dependent on quinidine dosage, and in some patients it may not appear until the dosage is increased to higher levels.[136,137] The rise in digoxin levels appears with the first dose of quinidine; therefore, it is suggested that digoxin dosage be halved when quinidine therapy is initiated. A similar interaction has been reported for quinidine and digitoxin.

Quinidine is a potent inhibitor of the hepatic cytochrome P450 (CYP) specific for debrisoquine metabolism (CYP2D6),[138,139] although it is not metabolized by this specific P450 isozyme.[140,141] Thus, it may interfere with the biotransformation and actions of pharmacologic agents dependent on this cytochrome for their metabolism, which include propafenone, mexiletine, flecainide, metoprolol, timolol, sparteine, and bufuralol.[142] Quinidine worsens neuromuscular blockade in patients with myasthenia gravis[143] and may prolong the effects of succinylcholine.[144]

Propafenone (Rythmol)

CLINICAL APPLICATIONS

Propafenone was developed in Germany, where it has been marketed since 1977. It is similar to other antiarrhythmic agents in overall efficacy and tolerance by patients. It has a role in the treatment of many types of arrhythmias, including supraventricular arrhythmias.[145]

CLINICAL PHARMACOLOGY

Propafenone has been described as having class IC antiarrhythmic activity because of its potent ability to slow conduction velocity with little change in APD.[146,147] It has a marked structural similarity to propranolol, and studies have shown that propafenone can accumulate during continued administration to levels capable of producing clinically significant beta-adrenergic inhibition.[148]

Propafenone, like mexiletine and flecainide, is eliminated by a metabolic pathway that has a polymorphic pattern of inheritance. Patients deficient in CYP2D6 activity have very slow elimination of propafenone and fail to form measurable quantities of the potentially active metabolite, 5-hydroxypropafenone.[149] The accumulation of high concentrations of propafenone leads to significant beta-receptor antagonism at both low and high dosages in poor metabolizers but only at high dosages in extensive metabolizers of propafenone.[150] Although metabolic phenotype does not seem to dramatically influence the antiarrhythmic response to propafenone in many patients,[149] it clearly influences the degree of beta blockade occurring during therapy.

DOSAGE AND ADMINISTRATION

Effective dosages range from 300 to 900 mg/day in two to four divided dosages. In order to prevent unexpected accumulation of pharmacologic action, propafenone dosage should not be changed more frequently than every 3 days; there is slow elimination of the parent drug in poor metabolizers, and there is slow accumulation of the metabolite or metabolites in extensive metabolizers.

Patients with reduced ventricular function, especially those receiving propafenone, should be carefully monitored for deterioration in ventricular function, which may result from beta-adrenergic receptor antagonism and/or the direct negative inotropic effect.[151]

MODIFICATION OF DOSAGE IN DISEASE STATES

Dosage recommendations for patients with cardiac, renal, or hepatic dysfunction are not yet available.

DRUG INTERACTIONS

It is very likely that there will be drug interactions between propafenone and other agents that utilize or inhibit cytochrome CYP2D6 for their metabolism. Such an interaction has been documented already between propafenone and metoprolol[152] and should be expected with timolol, many antidepressants, many neuroleptics, and perhaps other agents. Quinidine, which inhibits this cytochrome, inhibits the formation of 5-hydroxypropafenone in extensive metabolizers[153]; however, the clinical consequence of such inhibition is unknown and difficult to predict. One would expect greater beta blockade to occur after combining quinidine with propafenone therapy because of the resulting higher propafenone concentrations.

Flecainide (Tambocor)

CLINICAL APPLICATIONS

Flecainide is very effective in suppressing a variety of ventricular and supraventricular tachycardias.[154,155] The finding of increased mortality rates when flecainide is given to patients with ischemic heart disease has led to restricted usage (see above); however, there has been no evidence to indicate that this increase in mortality rate is seen when flecainide is given to treat supraventricular arrhythmias in patients without known coronary artery disease.[156] Overall, the antiarrhythmic response to flecainide in patients with symptomatic life-threatening ventricular arrhythmias is not markedly better than with older agents, such as quinidine or procainamide.[154,157] Although it is far better tolerated than older agents, the negative inotropic actions of flecainide restrict its use to patients having moderately well-preserved ventricular function. Likewise, its potential to increase mortality rates in patients with ischemic heart disease limits its usefulness.

MECHANISM OF ACTION

Flecainide has sodium channel–blocking activity and is considered to have class IC actions. It has also been found to block the delayed rectifier potassium channel in feline ventricular myocytes, and this action may be clinically relevant.[158]

Flecainide slows intraventricular conduction velocity more than it prolongs effective refractory periods.[159] It prolongs AH and HV intervals and measurably increases PR and QRS intervals on the surface ECG at therapeutic doses. The QT_c interval is slightly increased, primarily due to prolongation of the QRS, but its ability to block the delayed rectifier potassium channel may contribute to QT changes.

CLINICAL PHARMACOLOGY

The systemic bioavailability of oral flecainide is 90 to 95 percent,[160] and flecainide is predominantly metabolized in the liver to compounds that are not pharmacologically active at the concentrations usually found in plasma.[154] Flecainide, like many other antiarrhythmic agents, is metabolized by CYP2D6.[161] Because flecainide is also eliminated by the kidneys to a considerable extent, the enzyme deficiency has little effect on the pharmacokinetics of flecainide. If, however, those patients without the enzyme develop renal insufficiency or if renal patients are given a drug that blocks the metabolism of flecainide, extremely high plasma concentrations are likely to occur.[162] A potential advantage of flecainide is its very slow elimination, with half-life ranging from 7 to 23 h in normal individuals and tending to be even longer (14 to 26 h) in patients with cardiac disease, even in the absence of heart failure.[160,163]

DOSAGE AND ADMINISTRATION

The usual dosage of flecainide for ventricular arrhythmias is 100 to 150 mg every 12 h in patients without cardiac or renal failure. A total daily dosage of more than 400 mg may sometimes be used under close medical monitoring (see below). Patients with supraventricular tachycardia are recommended to receive 50 mg every 12 h as a starting dose. The range of therapeutic plasma concentrations of flecainide is reported to be between 200 and 1000 ng/mL, although adverse effects may occur in some patients at concentrations within this range,[164,165] and many patients tolerate concentrations well above this range. To reduce the incidence of adverse effects, flecainide therapy should start with a low dosage that is maintained until steady state has been reached (at least 4 days) and altered relative to clinical response.

MODIFICATION OF DOSAGE IN DISEASE STATES

With cardiac failure, the usual initial dose is 50 to 100 mg every 12 h. Since 7 percent of Caucasian patients with renal failure will not have the CYP2D6 enzyme and because flecainide is usually eliminated by both metabolism and renal excretion, all patients with renal failure should be given very low dosages and titrated very carefully. Plasma concentration monitoring will be essential in patients with renal disease or cardiac or hepatic dysfunction. Any significant reduction in ejection fraction should be expected to lengthen elimination half-life and hence the time needed to attain steady-state equilibrium, while reductions in clearance may occur in renal or hepatic dysfunction and lead to higher plasma concentrations at steady state.

ADVERSE REACTIONS

Although aggravation of arrhythmias seen in the early days of the evaluation of flecainide was often due to excessive initial doses and frequent dose increments, flecainide has a potential to induce proarrhythmic events, even when prescribed as recommended. This is especially true in patients with severe heart disease and if flecainide is given in higher dosages.[166] Because of its negative inotropic effects at dosages necessary to suppress arrhythmias, flecainide produces a measurable decrease in left ventricular function in most patients.[167,168] The increased mortality rate seen in the CAST seemed to be confined to patients with structural heart disease.[156] A retrospective study of five multiple-dose efficacy trials showed that, of patients with a history of congestive heart failure, oral flecainide precipitated heart failure in 15 percent. A dose-related depression of myocardial performance was found after rapid (1 to 2 mg/kg) intravenous injections.[169]

Other side effects of flecainide include depression of sinus node activity in patients with preexisting sinus node dysfunction[170] and prolongation of QRS and PR intervals on the surface ECG. If below 25 percent, these effects do not necessarily indicate excessive dosage.

Flecainide increases pacing thresholds by as much as 200 percent and should therefore be used with caution in patients dependent upon pacemakers.[171,172] Since it also increases the threshold for electrical defibrillation, patients with implanted devices should be evaluated carefully.[173]

DRUG INTERACTIONS

Cimetidine reduces flecainide clearance and prolongs flecainide elimination half-life.[174] Studies in normal volunteers have demonstrated an increase in the plasma concentrations of digoxin and propranolol when flecainide is coadministered.[175,176] Not unexpectedly, propranolol and flecainide have been found to have additive negative inotropic effects. An interaction with amiodarone, resulting in elevation of plasma flecainide concentration and necessitating reduction of flecainide dosage, has been described.[177]

Calcium Channel Blockers

Some calcium channel blockers are also used as antiarrhythmic agents.[178,179] Verapamil and diltiazem are useful in the management of supraventricular tachycardia, where they are administered to slow the ventricular rate in patients with atrial fibrillation or flutter and to treat and prevent AV nodal reentrant tachycardia. Intravenous diltiazem is useful for the temporary control of rapid ventricular rate during atrial fibrillation and flutter. In controlled clinical trials, conversion to sinus rhythm occurred with diltiazem and placebo with equal frequency.

Bretylium (Bretylol)

CLINICAL APPLICATIONS

Bretylium is effective for acute therapy of ventricular tachycardia and/or ventricular fibrillation. Because of its sympatholytic activity, bretylium tosylate was first evaluated in the 1950s for the treatment of hypertension; however, a very high incidence of orthostatic hypotension and unreliable oral absorption led to its disfavor for chronic therapy. After its antiarrhythmic activity was discovered in animals,[180] it was eventually marketed in the United States as intravenous therapy for life-threatening ventricular arrhythmias. Bretylium is usually employed only after patients have not responded to lidocaine.

MECHANISM OF ACTION

In addition to the indirect electrophysiologic changes caused by a biphasic action on postganglionic autonomic neurons, bretylium has a direct class III action that causes an increase in APD and refractoriness in ventricular muscle and Purkinje fibers.[181] When clinically relevant concentrations of bretylium are studied in normal tissues, no changes are seen in $\dot{V}_{max}$, maximum diastolic potential, or conduction velocity. Studies have found that bretylium reduces the degree of dispersion of repolarization across the boundary between normal and ischemic tissue by acting predominantly on normal tissue.[182] Transient increases in membrane potential and conduction velocity are seen early after bretylium administration and are presumed to be due to the local release of catecholamines.

When initially administered, bretylium causes the release of norepinephrine from postganglionic adrenergic neurons.[183] Bretylium is transported into the neuron by the norepinephrine pump, and extensive accumulation in the neuron is then associated with a blockade of further release or uptake of norepinephrine by the neuron. The blockade of uptake of circulating or infused catecholamines leads to supersensitivity that is functionally similar to a denervated state.

CLINICAL PHARMACOLOGY

Bretylium is poorly absorbed after oral administration, with average bioavailability of approximately 25 percent, and is available only for parenteral administration. It is eliminated almost entirely unchanged in the urine, and clearance correlates well with creatinine clearance.[184]

DOSAGE AND ADMINISTRATION

The usual intravenous dosage for bretylium is 5 mg/kg given at a rate dependent upon the clinical setting.[185] During cardiac emergencies, it should be given by rapid injection into a central intravenous line. In less acute situations, giving a loading infusion of the same dose, but over 10 to 20 min, will reduce the incidence of nausea and vomiting. The loading dose should be repeated after 20 min if the arrhythmia is still present. A total loading dose of 20 mg/kg may be required, and dosages up to 9 g in 24 h have been given without serious adverse effects. Maintenance infusions of 1 to 4 mg/min should be given, depending upon body size and renal function. Heart rhythm and blood pressure should be monitored carefully, especially during the first few hours of bretylium therapy.

MODIFICATION OF DOSAGE IN DISEASE STATES

In patients with renal insufficiency, bretylium clearance is reduced and half-life prolonged; therefore, the maintenance infusion for bretylium should be reduced to the lowest effective dosage. There are few data to guide dosage adjustment in cardiac or hepatic impairment, but it is unlikely that the dosage should be altered in these patients.

ADVERSE REACTIONS

When bretylium is given by rapid intravenous injection, many patients experience nausea and vomiting. The release of norepinephrine by bretylium has the potential to cause increased blood pressure, but severe hypertension has not been described. Increased frequency of ventricular arrhythmias is often seen at this time and can lead to the need for more frequent cardioversion. The reduction in peripheral vascular resistance can cause symptomatic hypotension in volume-depleted patients, but this can be readily corrected if recognized, although hypotension could prove dangerous in patients with fixed valvular obstruction. Bradycardia has been reported in some patients with abnormalities of the conduction system when given large intravenous dosages of bretylium.

In stable patients, either initial or subsequent doses of bretylium can cause a transient increase in heart rate, blood pressure, contractility, peripheral vascular resistance, and arrhythmia frequency, followed by a fall in standing blood pressure and peripheral vascular resistance.[186] Orthostatic hypotension is almost uniformly seen in patients receiving bretylium and sometimes lasts for days after discontinuation of therapy. Dosages that are well below those required for antiarrhythmic efficacy are capable of causing orthostatic hypotension. When hypotension develops during bretylium therapy, it should be corrected with intravenous volume expansion to enable adequate doses of bretylium for suppression of arrhythmias.

DRUG INTERACTIONS

Other than those with tricyclic antidepressants, no drug interactions have been reported. One would expect, however, that there might be competition for renal tubular secretion with procainamide, NAPA, cimetidine, and other organic bases.

Sotalol (Betapace)

CLINICAL APPLICATIONS

Sotalol has been used for up to 20 years in many countries for angina and hypertension, and it was in this setting that its value as an antiarrhythmic agent was first observed. Sotalol is unlike other beta-adrenergic antagonists in that it prolongs the action potential, producing a dose-related increase in refractoriness of cardiac tissues.[187] This unique combination of properties makes sotalol effective in a variety of supraventricular and ventricular arrhythmias. It has been found to be effective in patients with sustained ventricular tachycardia evaluated by programmed ventricular stimulation. In a controlled comparison to procainamide, sotalol was effective in 30 percent of patients with inducible sustained ventricular tachycardia, whereas only 20 percent responded to procainamide ($p < .2$).[188] This is consistent with the response rate for sotalol (31 percent) in the Electrophysiology Study Versus ECG Monitoring (ESVEM) trial sponsored by the National Institutes of Health, which compared therapy guided by programmed electrical stimulation to therapy guided by ambulatory monitoring.[189] In this study, a mean of only 12 percent of patients responded to the other antiarrhythmic drugs evaluated.

MECHANISM OF ACTION

Sotalol has two main actions, each of which can contribute to its antiarrhythmic efficacy.[190] The drug was originally synthesized for its actions as a beta-adrenergic receptor antagonist. Unlike other beta-receptor antagonists, it markedly prolongs refractoriness in atrial and ventricular tissues, a class III antiarrhythmic action. These actions slow heart rate, decrease AV nodal conduction, and increase refractoriness of atrial, ventricular, AV nodal, and AV accessory pathways in both the anterograde and retrograde directions.[191] When given in dosages between 160 and 640 mg/day, there are increases of 40 to 100 ms in the QT interval and 10 to 40 ms in QT_c.[192]

CLINICAL PHARMACOLOGY

Oral bioavailability of sotalol is greater than 90 percent, and peak concentrations are seen 2.5 to 4 h after a dose. It is not bound to plasma proteins and is eliminated by the kidneys unchanged, with an elimination half-life of approximately 12 h. Because of the relatively long half-life and twice daily dosing regimen, it is recommended that testing for efficacy be conducted near the end of the dosing interval at steady state. The age of the patient per se does not influence the pharmacokinetics of sotalol other than that due to the natural decline in renal function that occurs with age.

DOSAGE AND ADMINISTRATION

Sotalol is available only in the oral form in the United States. The recommended initial dose of sotalol is 80 mg every 12 h. In patients with relatively normal renal function, steady state is reached in 2 to 3 days. If evaluation at this dosage indicates a lack of response without evidence of excessive effects on repolarization (QT below 500 ms), the dosage may be increased to 160 mg twice daily and, if necessary, to 240 mg twice daily. Some patients with life-threatening arrhythmias have required dosages of 640 mg/day. Accelerated titration regimens have been used with close monitoring without apparent increase in the frequency of adverse events.[193]

MODIFICATION OF DOSAGE IN DISEASE STATES

Because sotalol is mainly eliminated unchanged in the urine, the dosage must be adjusted for altered renal function. For patients with a creatinine clearance greater than 60 mL/min, the usual dosing interval is every 12 h. If the creatinine clearance (CL_{CR}) is between 30 and 60 mL/min, the recommended interval between doses is 24 h. For patients with CL_{CR} between 10 and 30 mL/min, the interval should be every 36 to 48 h or the usual dose halved and given every 24 h. The dosage for patients with CL_{CR} below 10 mL/min should be individualized. Because of the increased risk of proarrhythmia and congestive heart failure, patients with reduced cardiac output should be given lower doses and monitored carefully.

ADVERSE REACTIONS

A major concern with sotalol treatment has been the occurrence of torsades de pointes. Reports of this syndrome have predominantly been cases of suicidal overdoses or in patients who were receiving concomitant diuretics and inadequate potassium replacement. Clearly, hypokalemia and bradycardia are predisposing factors for the development of this arrhythmia during sotalol therapy, as they are with quinidine, disopyramide, and procainamide. The manufacturer observed an overall incidence of torsades de pointes of 2 percent, broken down to 4 percent of patients with sustained ventricular tachycardia and 1.5 percent of patients with supraventricular arrhythmias. It is more common in females and patients with congestive heart failure and those with a history of sustained ventricular tachycardia (7 percent). The incidence of torsades de pointes should be minimized by careful screening and consideration of predisposing factors, such as gender, bradycardia, baseline prolongation of the QT interval, and electrolyte disturbances, (especially hypokalemia); careful dose escalation beginning at 160 mg/day; and limiting the maximum QT-interval prolongation to less than 550 ms.

The incidence of new or worsened congestive heart failure is only about 3 percent. This may be attenuated because of the increased inotropy produced by its action to prolong repolarization. Other side effects typical of beta blockers are to be expected, including bronchospasm in asthmatic patients, masking the signs and symptoms of hypoglycemia in diabetic patients, and catecholamine hypersensitivity withdrawal syndrome.

DRUG INTERACTIONS

Concomitant use of sotalol with agents that prolong repolarization has the potential to increase the likelihood of torsades de pointes. No pharmacokinetic interactions have been seen with sotalol and/or warfarin, digoxin, cholestyramine, or hydrochlorothiazide. Because of the beta-blocking actions of sotalol, it is likely that there would be increased pharmacologic effect if the drug is combined with amiodarone, calcium channel blockers, antihypertensive agents, or antiarrhythmic agents.

Amiodarone (Cordarone)

CLINICAL APPLICATIONS

Although amiodarone has been reported to have efficacy in a wide range of arrhythmias, the FDA has recommended it only for life-threatening ventricular arrhythmias refractory to other available forms of therapy. Nevertheless, there are now numerous trials in the literature describing the efficacy of amiodarone in the conversion and slowing of atrial fibrillation, AV nodal reentrant tachycardia, and tachycardias associated with the Wolff-Parkinson-White syndrome.[194,195] The reasons for the limited labeling of amiodarone are (1) the documented potentially lethal complications of chronic amiodarone therapy, (2) the complications associated with its variable onset of action, and (3) multiple dangerous drug interactions.

After the results of CAST, antiarrhythmic drugs have been examined for their effects on mortality rate. After several small or uncontrolled trials seemed to indicate that amiodarone could have a beneficial effect on mortality rate,[4,196] adequate trials were undertaken. The Veteran's Administration trial, Congestive Heart Failure Survival Trial of Antiarrhythmic Therapy (CHF STAT),[5] examined the effects of amiodarone on total mortality rate in patients with a history of congestive heart failure, more than 10 premature ventricular contractions per hour on ambulatory monitoring, and an ejection fraction below 40 percent. The study found no difference in the placebo- and amiodarone-treated arms. Two other major trials have evaluated amiodarone in patients with recent myocardial infarction. The Canadian Myocardial Infarction Amiodarone Trial (CAMIAT)[197] and the European Myocardial Infarction Amiodarone Trial (EMIAT)[198] were recently completed. The results of these trials are mixed, in that neither found amiodarone to reduce overall mortality rate, but the Canadian trial reported a reduced incidence of ventricular fibrillation or arrhythmic death among survivors of myocardial infarction with ventricular ectopy. It is important to note that there was no increase in mortality rate, as has been seen with other antiarrhythmic drugs. In recent years, there have been attempts to perform meta-analyses of the many trials with amiodarone.[199,200] They have generally confirmed a modest reduction in mortality rate in cardiac patients. One study concluded that the benefit could be extended to patients with congestive heart failure,[200] but another did not.[199] The NIH-sponsored Antiarrhythmics versus Implanted Devices (AVID) trial found that the devices were superior to amiodarone in reducing mortality rates in patients who had been resuscitated from sudden death or who had sustained ventricular tachycardia.

In 1993, an intravenous formulation of amiodarone became available in the United States. Although it had been used extensively in most countries for many years, controlled trials only became available in recent years. Three completed controlled trials demonstrated the value of amiodarone in patients with recurrent life-threatening ventricular tachycardia or fibrillation. A comparison of three dosages found that the recurrence of arrhythmia decreased with increasing dosages of 125, 500, and 1000 mg per 24 h.[201] Hypotension was the major side effect seen, but it occurred equally in all groups, about 26 percent. The second study in a similar group of patients was a comparison of bretylium to two doses of amiodarone.[202] The arrhythmia event rate for the first 48 h of therapy was equivalent for the high dose of amiodarone and bretylium, and both were more effective than the low dose of amiodarone. Hypotension was common in all groups but significantly higher in the bretylium group. Amiodarone was approved for intravenous therapy of ventricular arrhythmia by the FDA in 1998. Although not yet approved in labeling, a recent study found intravenous amiodarone effective for prevention of postoperative atrial fibrillation.[203]

MECHANISM OF ACTION

Amiodarone is an iodinated benzofuran that has structural similarity to thyroxine and procainamide and was originally developed as an antianginal agent. It was incidentally noted to suppress a wide variety of ventricular and supraventricular arrhythmias. This efficacy has been assumed to be due to its prolongation of refractoriness and APD in myocardial tissue (Vaughan Williams class III antiarrhythmic activity), although amiodarone has been found to have many diverse pharmacologic actions (see Table 27-1); the action or actions responsible for its high degree of antiarrhythmic efficacy remain unidentified.

In intracellular recordings of rabbit cardiac myocytes, amiodarone prolongs APD and increases refractoriness of both atrial and ventricular myocardium, Purkinje fibers, and sinus and AV nodal tissues. Amiodarone decreases phase 3 depolarization of myocardial cells, blocks sodium channels that are in the inactivated state, and slows phase 4 depolarization of the sinus node as well as conduction through the AV node.[204,205] The electrophysiologic actions of the major metabolite of amiodarone, desethylamiodarone (DEA), differ from those of amiodarone, with the metabolite having greater effects on sodium channels and, hence, upon conduction.[206] Intracoronary injection of amiodarone has shown little cardiac effect compared to the ability of DEA to prolong cardiac refractoriness.[207]

Electrophysiologic changes in humans depend on the route of administration and the duration of therapy. Following acute intravenous amiodarone administration, prolongation of the AH interval and an increase in the refractory periods of the AV node and bypass tracts are seen, but this may be due to the presence of the solubilizing agent polysorbate 80 (Tween 80) in the intravenous formulation. No acute changes occur in either sinus rate or atrial or ventricular refractoriness, which are prolonged during chronic oral therapy. Chronic amiodarone therapy also prolongs the AH and HV intervals and the PR and QT intervals of the surface ECG. Data conflict on the time course of these changes and how they may relate to antiarrhythmic efficacy.

Changes in APD and refractoriness are seen in hypothyroidism that are similar to changes resulting from oral amiodarone therapy.[208] Since these changes can be prevented in animals by coadministration of thyroid hormone with amiodarone,[209] some have concluded that the antiarrhythmic efficacy of amiodarone is due to production of "cardiac hypothyroidism." This is supported by the observation that the major metabolite of amiodarone causes noncompetitive inhibition of thyroid hormone binding to nuclear receptors.[210] On the other hand, amiodarone also causes noncompetitive blockade of alpha and beta receptors[211] and muscarinic receptors,[212] and both calcium and sodium channel blockade, any combination of which may contribute to its antiarrhythmic efficacy.

CLINICAL PHARMACOLOGY

Amiodarone is a highly lipid-soluble compound with extremely variable and complex pharmacokinetics. It is slowly absorbed from the gastrointestinal tract, and bioavailability varies over a fourfold range.[213] Amiodarone is extensively metabolized to DEA, and little, if any, is excreted unchanged in the urine. Concentrations of DEA in plasma vary from 0.4 to 2.0 times that of amiodarone during chronic therapy.[214] This metabolite has antiarrhythmic potency equal to or greater than amiodarone in in vitro and animal models.[215] Amiodarone is rapidly concentrated in some tissues, including myocardium, but accumulates more slowly in others, such as adipose tissue. It redistributes out of myocardial tissue while still accumulating in adipose and other tissues.[214,216] Until all tissues are saturated, rapid redistribution out of the myocardium may be responsible for early recurrence of arrhythmias after discontinuation of therapy or rapid reduction of dosage. Because of drug accumulation in tissues, the volume of distribution for amiodarone is very large, 20 to 200 L/kg.[216] After intravenous administration, the measured half-life in plasma is from 4.8 to 68.2 h,[217] with tissue uptake being the primary factor responsible for the decline in plasma concentration. As tissues become saturated, however, the decline in plasma levels is slow, reflecting mainly elimination and slow redistribution of the drug out of adipose and muscle tissues. This leads to slow and extremely variable elimination from plasma, with half-lives ranging from 13 to 103 days at steady state.[216] It is also possible that amiodarone inhibits its own elimination after chronic therapy, contributing to the differences between half-life early in therapy to that after prolonged therapy.

DOSAGE AND ADMINISTRATION

Without a loading-dose regimen, amiodarone requires several weeks to months before producing its antiarrhythmic action. Large intravenous dosages or oral loading dosages can hasten the onset of therapeutic effects. From small prospective studies, loading dosages have varied from 600 to 1400 mg/day for 2 to

21 days.[218] Recent large clinical trials have utilized a lower loading dose, of 600 to 800 mg daily for 14 days.[5,219] Because of relatively rapid redistribution out of myocardial tissue, the dosage should be tapered over a period of several weeks. The usual maintenance dose varies from 200 to 600 mg/day, and because of the severe nature of adverse reactions, the lowest effective dosage should be prescribed. Patients with supraventricular arrhythmias may respond to lower dosages than those with ventricular arrhythmias, but there are many exceptions. Because of the variable pharmacokinetics and oral bioavailability, such generalizations may be unreliable. Some patients with extensive absorption (approximately 80 to 90 percent bioavailability) of even low doses may have the same drug exposure as a person with limited bioavailability given a high dose.

For intravenous administration, the manufacturer recommends a three-phase infusion over the first 24 h: 150 mg over 10 min, followed by 360 mg over the next 6 h, followed by 0.5 mg/min. The drug can be continued at this rate, but monitoring of plasma concentrations is recommended. An additional 150 mg can be infused over 10 min for those patients who continue to have recurrent ventricular tachycardia or fibrillation or whose arrhythmia recurs during downward titration of the infusion. Concentrations of drug greater than 3 mg/mL should be infused through a central catheter to prevent phlebitis. Also, the surfactant properties of the drug alter the size of a drop of infusate, and pumps that count drops will give approximately 30 percent less drug than intended.

Amiodarone concentrations are usually between 1 and 2 μg/mL during effective oral therapy.[220,221] Similar concentrations of DEA accumulate during therapy and, although this is unproven, are likely to contribute to antiarrhythmic efficacy. Because of extensive overlap between the range of concentrations required for arrhythmia suppression and those associated with toxicity, monitoring of plasma concentrations is of limited value. Clearly, levels of amiodarone above 3 to 4 μg/mL for prolonged periods of time are associated with a higher incidence of adverse effects.[222]

MODIFICATION OF DOSAGE IN DISEASE STATES

Long-term oral therapy with amiodarone appears to be well tolerated hemodynamically in patients with congestive heart failure. In the CHF STAT study, discussed above, amiodarone failed to prolong life for congestive heart failure patients with arrhythmias but was associated with improved ventricular function as measured by radionuclide ejection fraction.[5]

ADVERSE REACTIONS

Intravenous amiodarone at dosages greater than 5 mg/kg decreases cardiac contractility and peripheral vascular resistance, producing severe hypotension in some instances. Some of this effect, like the electrophysiologic effects described earlier, may be due to the effects of polysorbate 80 or benzyl alcohol, since oral administration at usual dosages improves myocardial contractility.

The safety of amiodarone is controversial. The early reports found it to be very well tolerated and described it as the "ideal antiarrhythmic drug." Some studies continue to find that it is relatively safe and effective, even in the treatment of arrhythmias in children.[223] The early experience with amiodarone in the United States, with a very high incidence of intolerable and sometimes lethal reactions, may have been the result of high dosages required for control of life-threatening arrhythmias. In less urgent conditions, lower dosages are given and are much better tolerated. Determination of the incidence of adverse reactions is difficult because of highly variable dosages and durations of treatment.[204,224]

The most serious adverse reaction is lethal interstitial pneumonitis,[204,225] which may be more common in patients with preexisting lung disease. Monitoring is essential, since the pneumonitis is reversible if detected early. A chest x-ray every 3 months may be useful, but serial pulmonary function tests are of little value for follow-up. Hyper- or hypothyroidism is seen in about 4 percent of patients treated chronically.[208] Accumulation of corneal microdeposits is almost uniform during long-term therapy and in many cases can progress to the point of interfering with vision.[226] Some Caucasian patients develop a slate-gray or bluish discoloration of sun-exposed areas of the skin.[227] Many also complain of photosensitivity, which can sometimes be prevented or alleviated with sunscreens and garments. Thirty percent or more of patients have abnormally elevated serum hepatic enzyme levels, and progression to jaundice and cirrhosis has been reported.[228,229] Serial laboratory tests to screen for amiodarone toxicity can be costly and generally are of limited value; however, it is wise to obtain a reliable assessment of baseline test results, including complete blood count, blood chemistry, tests of thyroid and pulmonary function, a slit-lamp examination, and measurement of blood levels of other drugs whenever possible.

DRUG INTERACTIONS

Amiodarone interferes with the clearance of many drugs. This may involve the formation of a metabolically inactive cytochrome P450 Fe(II)–metabolite complex, which has been described in animals treated with amiodarone,[230] and may explain the reduced metabolism and unexpected accumulation of warfarin,[231] quinidine, procainamide, disopyramide, mexiletine, and propafenone[232] and the resulting bleeding, heart block, or torsades de pointes. It does not, however, explain interaction with drugs eliminated predominantly by the kidneys, such as digoxin.[233] The elimination of other drugs may be impaired by amiodarone, and the lowest effective dosage should be sought.

Ibutilide (Corvert)

CLINICAL APPLICATIONS

Ibutilide was given FDA approval for the rapid conversion of recent-onset atrial fibrillation or flutter in 1995.[234,235] It has completed testing in other arrhythmias or in patients with atrial fibrillation or flutter of long duration (greater than 90 days). It should not be given to patients who have hypokalemia, hypomagnesemia, or QT_c prolongation at baseline greater than 440 ms. In placebo-controlled studies summarized in the manufacturer's labeling, the placebo conversion rate for atrial fibrillation or flutter was approximately 2 percent. Ibutilide terminated the arrhythmia in approximately 44 percent of patients treated with 1 mg followed by either 0.5 or 1 mg. Approximately 20 percent of patients responded to the first infusion, and approximately 25 percent of those not responding to the first infusion responded to the second infusion. Response usually occurred at 20 to 30 min, ranging from 5 to 88 min after infusion. The response in patients with atrial fibrillation and atrial flutter was not significantly different in the early trials performed. However, in patients with postoperative arrhythmias, there was a greater response in patients with atrial flutter, with an overall conversion rate of 57 percent compared to 15 percent with placebo.[236] Ibutilide may have value in conversion of atrial fibrillation in patients with Wolff-Parkinson-White syndrome.[236]

MECHANISM OF ACTION

Ibutilide is a remarkably potent methanesulfonamide analog of sotalol that has class III action to prolong cardiac refractoriness and action potential duration.

The mechanism of action of ibutilide is unclear. The manufacturer's data indicate that the class III action of the drug is due to an increase in inward sodium current, as observed in guinea pig ventricular myocytes at 10^{-7}-*M* concentrations. They observed that higher concentrations (10^{-5} *M*) increase an outward potassium current to shorten action potential duration.[237] Other investigators reported that, as has been seen with dofetilide, sotalol, and other methanesulfonamides, 10^{-8} *M* concentrations of ibutilide block the rapid component of the delayed rectifier potassium current, I_{KR}, in mouse and human cardiac cells.[238]

CLINICAL PHARMACOLOGY

Ibutilide is available only for intravenous administration. When given over 10 min, it distributes rapidly in a multiexponential fashion, with the relevant component having a half-life from 2 to 12 h (mean 6 h). The plasma concentration and pharmacokinetics are highly variable, and dosing is recommended on the basis of weight. The drug is mainly eliminated by oxidative hepatic metabolism, and systemic clearance is rapid (about 29 mL/min per kilogram). Since formal drug interaction studies have not been performed, it is not possible to anticipate which enzymes are likely responsible for its elimination.

DOSAGE AND ADMINISTRATION

Ibutilide is given undiluted or diluted in saline as an infusion over 10 min. The recommended dose for a patient over 60 kg is 1 mg and for a patient under 60 kg, 0.01 mg/kg. For patients whose arrhythmias have not converted by 10 min after completion of the first dose, a second dose of equal size may be administered. Since conversion of the arrhythmias is usually associated with peak levels, slower infusion rates are not likely to be as effective.

It is essential that patients receiving ibutilide be treated in a carefully monitored environment during and at least 4 h subsequent to treatment. The FDA-approved labeling recommends that skilled personnel, facilities, and medication for defibrillation or resuscitation be readily available.

MODIFICATION OF DOSAGE IN DISEASE STATES

Although specific studies with heart failure and renal or hepatic disease have not been conducted, current information does not indicate that any dosage adjustments should be necessary in these conditions. Patients with severe left ventricular dysfunction, however, have a higher risk of developing ventricular arrhythmias, including torsades de pointes. Since the duration of drug effect is determined by distribution, it is very possible that patients with severe congestive heart failure will have decreased volumes of distribution and hence an exaggerated and prolonged duration of effect.

ADVERSE REACTIONS

The most serious adverse reaction to ibutilide is torsades de pointes. There were, however, only 586 patients participating in trials before marketing, and patients with a QT_c greater than 440 ms or potassium concentrations less than 4 meq/L were excluded. In spite of these precautions, the incidence of sustained polymorphic ventricular tachycardia requiring cardioversion was 1.7 percent. Another 2.7 percent developed nonsustained polymorphic ventricular tachycardia, 4.9 percent had nonsustained monomorphic ventricular tachycardia, 1.5 percent had AV block, and 1.9 percent had bundle-branch block. The risk of polymorphic ventricular tachycardia was highest in patients who were female and/or who had evidence of reduced ventricular performance. The incidence of these adverse effects may well be higher in general clinical use, where electrolyte disorders and concomitant therapies may be more common. Bradycardia and multiple episodes of sinus arrest have been reported.[236,239] A single case of acute renal failure has been reported with ibutilide.[240]

DRUG INTERACTIONS

No specific drug interaction studies have been performed. Concomitant beta-receptor or calcium channel antagonists do not apparently interact, although data are limited. The manufacturer's labeling warns against combining ibutilide with other drugs that prolong the QT interval. During the development of ibutilide, such drugs were discontinued for at least five half-lives prior to administration of ibutilide and were not allowed until at least 4 h after administration.

Dofetilide (Tikosyn)

CLINICAL APPLICATIONS

Dofetilide was approved and marketed in 2000 for oral therapy of atrial fibrillation and flutter. In controlled trials of approximately 1000 patients, about 30 percent of patients with atrial fibrillation given a dosage of 500 μg bid converted to normal sinus rhythm, compared to 6 percent in the control group treated with sotalol and 1 percent of patients given placebo. Prevention of recurrence was demonstrated, with 62 to 71 percent remaining in sinus rhythm after 6 months, compared to 59 percent for sotalol and 26 to 37 percent for placebo (personal communication, S. Singh, Washington, DC). A large mortality trial (the Danish Investigators of Arrhythmia and Mortality on Dofetilide trial, or DIAMOND) in 1518 patients with reduced ejection fraction and symptoms of heart failure examined the effects of dofetilide on mortality rate and atrial fibrillation. A decrease in the incidence of hospitalization for heart failure was observed. Although the antiarrhythmic efficacy of dofetilide was confirmed in the lower incidence of atrial fibrillation, a positive effect on mortality rate was not observed. However, because of the previously observed increases in mortality rate with sodium channel blockers (CAST[1,241] and CAST II[2]) and with *d*-sotalol (SWORD[6]), the lack of harm in the DIAMOND trial with dofetilide[242] was interpreted as a positive indication of the safety of the drug. A caveat to this safety was the potentially important role of extensive screening and monitoring for potential harm. Even with these efforts, 3.3 percent of patients in this trial developed torsades de pointes. Because of the risk of torsades de pointes, the manufacturer will require physicians to receive special training prior to prescribing dofetilide, and the FDA has required that labeling include a warning that therapy should be initiated in the hospital, with continuous ECG monitoring for at least 3 days.

MECHANISM OF ACTION

Dofetilide is one of the most potent I_{KR} blockers of the rapid component of the delayed rectifier potassium current (I_{KR}) ever synthesized. Perhaps an additional advantage is the twofold greater ability to prolong action potential duration in atrial compared to ventricular tissue.[243] It does not depress cardiac function at usual dosages, even in patients with reduced ejection fraction.

CLINICAL PHARMACOLOGY

Dofetilide is well absorbed after oral administration and is partially metabolized by cytochrome P450 3A4[244] to inactive metabolites and excreted predominantly in urine. In most patients, the elimination half-life ranges from 8 to 10 h but is prolonged, and clearance is reduced in patients with renal failure. Dofetilide is susceptible to several drug interactions because it is metabolized by CYP3A4 (see below). It is very likely that these interactions increase the risk of torsades de pointes.

DOSAGE AND ADMINISTRATION

The recommended dosage of dofetilide is 500 μg bid. Lower dosages are recommended for patients who develop excessive QT_c prolongation on 500 μg bid. In the largest clinical trial, excessive was defined as greater than 550 ms or greater than 20 percent longer than baseline.

MODIFICATION OF DOSAGE IN DISEASE STATES

Dosage should be reduced in patients with renal disease (250 mg bid for creatinine clearance 60 to 40 mL/min and 250 mg daily for creatinine clearance 40 to 20 mL/min). Data are not available for adjustment of dosage in patients with liver disease. It is not clear whether the greater risk of torsades de pointes in women is influenced by a pharmacokinetic difference between sexes.

ADVERSE DRUG REACTIONS

The major adverse effect of dofetilide is torsades de pointes. The overall incidence during clinical development was 0.9 percent. In the DIAMOND trial, 3.3 percent of patients with a history of heart failure developed torsades de pointes.

DRUG INTERACTIONS

Concomitant administration of dofetilide with verapamil, ketoconazole, or cimetidine (but not ranitidine) results in increased plasma concentrations of dofetilide, especially in patients with reduced renal function.[245] Because it is known to be a substrate for CYP3A4, there may be other important interactions with erythromycin, other macrolides, or antifungals. No interactions have been seen between dofetilide and digoxin or warfarin.

Beta-Receptor Antagonists

See Chap. 40 for a discussion of beta-receptor antagonists.

Adenosine (Adenocard)

CLINICAL APPLICATIONS

Adenosine is very effective for the acute conversion of paroxysmal supraventricular tachycardia (PSVT) due to reentry involving the AV node. Sixty percent of patients respond at a dose of 6 mg, and an additional 32 percent respond when given a higher dose, of 12 mg. Because of the fleeting and relatively selective action of adenosine on the AV node, some have suggested that it be used as a diagnostic tool in patients with narrow- and wide-complex tachycardia.[246] However, it is preferable, when possible, to make the correct diagnosis before giving any drugs, because of their risk of adverse effects.

MECHANISM OF ACTION

Adenosine is a nucleoside formed in the body by serial dephosphorylation of adenosine triphosphate (ATP), from cyclic adenosine monophosphate, or from hydrolysis of *S*-adenosylhomocysteine. It is formed both intra- and extracellularly, and its actions are rapidly terminated by active transport into cells followed by metabolism. The actions of adenosine are highly dependent on the rate and route of administration. A rapid intravenous injection into a central venous line is thought to activate carotid body chemoreceptors and usually produces an initial increase in blood pressure of 10 to 15 mmHg, followed by a small and transient decrease. These reflexes are attenuated during surgery, and in this setting adenosine decreases peripheral vascular resistance, increases cardiac output, and increases heart rate moderately. Bolus injections also produce biphasic effects on heart rate. Approximately 20 s after injection, sinus bradycardia occurs for 10 to 15 s, followed by sinus tachycardia thought to be due to chemoreceptor activation. Activation of the carotid chemoreceptors stimulates respiration and causes secondary activation of pulmonary stretch receptors. Adenosine has a direct effect of slowing AV nodal conduction, which can result in transient AV block. Although adenosine has no direct effect on the His-Purkinje system, it does attenuate the effects of catecholamine stimulation and, in patients with heart block, can block acceleration of the ventricular escape rate by isoproterenol. Adenosine usually has no effect on anterograde or retrograde accessory pathway conduction. Pathways that demonstrate decremental conduction often respond to adenosine, probably because they are partially depolarized and can be hyperpolarized by adenosine. Slow injections into a peripheral line often produce no clinical benefit or changes in blood pressure or heart rate.

The development of synthetic agonists and antagonists of adenosine receptors has made possible the subclassification of A_1 and A_2 receptor subtypes. The A_1 receptors are present in myocardial cells and mediate the negative inotropic, dromotropic, and chronotropic actions of adenosine. The A_2 receptors are present in the endothelium and vascular smooth muscle cells and cause coronary vasodilatation when activated.

The efficacy of adenosine in PVST is most likely due to the following actions in atrial myocardium and the AV node: (1) hyperpolarization of sinoatrial nodal cells and slowing of rate of firing, (2) shortening of the action potential of atrial cells, and (3) depression of conduction velocity in the AV node. These actions are due to activation of A_1 adenosine-receptor subtypes, which leads to activation of cyclic AMP-independent, acetylcholine/adenosine-regulated potassium current, $IK_{ACh,Ado}$.

CLINICAL PHARMACOLOGY

After intravenous injection, adenosine is rapidly transported into red blood cells and endothelial cells. A half-life of elimination has ranged from 1.5 to 10 s. The drug is rapidly metabolized in the plasma and in cells to form inosine and adenosine monophosphate. Maximal pharmacologic effects are seen within 30 s after injection into a peripheral intravenous line but occur within 10 to 20 s when given into a central line.

DOSAGE AND ADMINISTRATION

Adenosine should be injected intravenously into a proximal tubing site and flushed quickly with saline solution. For adults, the initial dose is 6 mg injected over 1 to 2 s. If the arrhythmia persists, a 12-mg dose can be injected 1 to 2 min later. This can be repeated, but doses larger than 12 mg are not recommended by the manufacturer. A dosage regimen based on body weight has been proposed, with an initial dose of 50 μg/kg incremented by 50 μg/kg until the PSVT is terminated or side effects become intolerable.[246] Higher doses may be required for patients who have received caffeine or theophylline because of their antagonistic effects at A_1 receptors. Lower doses are recommended if the patients are receiving dipyridamole or carbamazepine.

MODIFICATION OF DOSAGE IN DISEASE STATES

Although the pharmacokinetics of adenosine are unlikely to be altered in patients with renal or hepatic disease, these patients often have electrolyte imbalances that could alter the clinical response. Although patients with congestive heart failure have not been reported to respond abnormally, cardiac transplant patients appear to require one-third to one-fifth of the usual dose because of denervation hypersensitivity.[247]

ADVERSE REACTIONS

Adenosine is contraindicated in patients with sick-sinus syndrome or second- or third-degree heart block unless the patient has a functioning artificial pacemaker. Because of the rapid clearance of adenosine, side effects such as facial flushing, dyspnea, or chest pressure last less than 60 s. Although intrapulmonary administration of adenosine has precipitated bronchospasm in asthmatic patients, this has not been reported with intravenous administration. Other less frequent side effects include nausea, lightheadedness, headache, sweating, palpitations, hypotension, and blurred vision. Intravenous theophylline, which has been recommended to reverse the effects of adenosine, should be prepared and ready for injection in high-risk patients.

DRUG INTERACTIONS

Several proven interactions can increase or decrease the activity of adenosine. Dipyridamole pretreatment increases the potency of adenosine, probably because it blocks cellular uptake of adenosine.[248] On the other hand, caffeine and theophylline antagonize the actions of adenosine.[249] The manufacturer cautions that carbamazepine may potentiate the actions of adenosine.

INVESTIGATIONAL DRUGS

Only a few new antiarrhythmic agents are currently under development in the United States. Several of these are analogs of amiodarone, such as ATI-2001,[250] dronedarone,[251] and SR-33589.[252] Some impetus for the development of these agents lies in the hope that they will have the efficacy of amiodarone without complex pharmacokinetics and/or its toxicity.[250–252]

Azimilide is another drug with class III action that was initially believed to be a highly selective blocker of the slow component of the delayed rectifier (I_{KS}), but recent studies suggest that azimilide also blocks I_{KR}. It is unclear whether the effects on I_{KS} contribute any novel aspects to its actions or safety. I_{KS} blockade is thought to be desirable because the effect is resistant to antagonism by isoproterenol. Other drugs, such as ambasilide, are also in clinical development, and chromanol 293B is in preclinical testing.

A new class of serotonergic antagonist drugs is being developed. Stimulation of 5-HT_4 receptors increases atrial chronotropic and inotropic responses. Whether other electrophysiologic effects are produced is unknown. In humans and swine, 5-HT_4 receptors are present only in atrium. In porcine atrial tissue, RS-100302 prolonged the effective refractory period and minimally slowed conduction velocity. The drug produced no electrophysiologic effects on ventricular tissue. It terminated pacing-induced atrial flutter in six of eight animals and atrial fibrillation in eight of nine animals, and prevented reinduction of sustained tachycardia in all animals. The electrophysiologic profile of RS-100302 suggests that it may have atrial antiarrhythmic potential without producing ventricular proarrhythmic effects.

References

1. CAST investigators. Preliminary report: Effect of encainide and flecainide on mortality in a randomized trial of arrhythmia suppression after myocardial infarction. *N Eng J Med* 1989; 321:406–412.
2. CAST-II investigators. Effect of the antiarrhythmic agent moricizine on survival after myocardial infarction. *N Eng J Med* 1992; 327:227–233.
3. Hine LK, Laird NM, Hewitt P, Chalmers TC. Meta-analysis of empirical long-term antiarrhythmic therapy after myocardial infarction. *JAMA* 1989; 262:3037–3040.
4. Pfisterer ME, Kiowski W, Brunner H, et al. Long-term benefit of 1-year amiodarone treatment for persistent complex ventricular arrhythmias after myocardial infarction. *Circulation* 1993; 87:309–311.
5. Singh SN, Fletcher RD, Fisher SG, et al. Amiodarone in patients with congestive heart failure and asymptomatic ventricular arrhythmia: Survival Trial of Antiarrhythmic Therapy in Congestive Heart Failure. *N Engl J Med* 1995; 333:77–82.
6. Waldo AL, Camm AJ, deRuyter H, et al. Effect of D-sotalol on mortality in patients with left ventricular dysfunction after recent and remote myocardial infarction. The SWORD Investigators. Survival With Oral D-Sotalol. *Lancet* 1996; 348:7–12.
7. Vaughan Williams EM. A classification of antiarrhythmic actions reassessed after a decade of new drugs. *J Clin Pharmacol* 1984; 24:129–147.
8. Harrison DC. Antiarrhythmic drug classification: New science and practical applications. *Am J Cardiol* 1985; 56:185–187.
9. Task Force of the Working Group on Arrhythmias of the European Society of Cardiology. The Sicilian gambit: A new approach to the classification of antiarrhythmic drugs based on their actions on arrhythmogenic mechanisms. *Circulation* 1991; 84:1831–1851.
10. Hodgkin AL, Huxley AF. A quantitative description of membrane current and its application to conduction and excitation in nerve. *J Physiol* 1952; 117:500–544.
11. Hondeghem LM, Katzung BG. Test of a model of antiarrhythmic drug action: Effects of quinidine and lidocaine on myocardial conduction. *Circulation* 1980; 61:1217–1224.
12. Campbell TJ. Kinetics of onset of rate-dependent effects of class I antiarrhythmic drugs are important in determining their effects

on refractoriness in guinea-pig ventricle, and provide a theoretical basis for their subclassification. *Cardiovasc Res* 1983; 17:344–352.
13. Southworth JL, McKusick VA, Pierce EC II, Rawson FL Jr. Ventricular fibrillation precipitated by cardiac catheterization. *JAMA* 1950; 143:717–720.
14. Lie KI, Wellens HJ, van Capelle FJ, Durrer D: Lidocaine in the prevention of primary ventricular fibrillation: A double-blind, randomized study of 212 consecutive patients. *N Eng J Med* 1974; 291:1324–1326.
15. MacMahon S, Collins R, Peto R, et al. Effects of prophylactic lidocaine in suspected acute myocardial infarction. *JAMA* 1988; 260:1910–1916.
16. Pedersen LE, Bonde J, Graudal NA, et al. Quantitative and qualitative binding characteristics of disopyramide in serum from patients with decreased renal and hepatic function. *Br J Clin Pharmacol* 1987; 23:41–46.
17. Josephson ME, Kastor JA, Kitchen JG III. Lidocaine in Wolff-Parkinson-White syndrome with atrial fibrillation. *Ann Intern Med* 1976; 84:44–45.
18. Akhtar M, Gilbert CJ, Shenasa M. Effect of lidocaine on atrioventricular response via the accessory pathway in patients with Wolff-Parkinson-White syndrome. *Circulation* 1981; 63:435–441.
19. Davis LD, Temte JV. Electrophysiological actions of lidocaine on canine ventricular muscle and Purkinje fibers. *Circ Res* 1969; 24:639–655.
20. Bigger JT Jr, Mandel WJ. Effect of lidocaine on the electrophysiological properties of ventricular muscle and Purkinje fibers. *J Clin Invest* 1970; 49:63–77.
21. Kunkel F, Rowland M, Scheinman MM. The electrophysiologic effects of lidocaine in patients with intraventricular conduction defects. *Circulation* 1974; 49:894–899.
22. Bekheit S, Murtagh JG, Morton P, Fletcher E. Effect of lidocaine on conducting system of human heart. *Br Heart J* 1973; 35:305–311.
23. Gupta PK, Lichstein E, Chadda KD. Lidocaine-induced heart block in patients with bundle branch block. *Am J Cardiol* 1974; 33:487–492.
24. Aravindakshan V, Kuo C-S, Gettes LS. Effect of lidocaine on escape rate in patients with complete atrioventricular block: A. Distal His block. *Am J Cardiol* 1977; 40:177–183.
25. Stenson RE, Constantino RT, Harrison DC. Interrelationships of hepatic blood flow, cardiac output, and blood levels of lidocaine in man. *Circulation* 1971; 43:205–211.
26. Zito RA, Reid PR. Lidocaine kinetics predicted by indocyanine green clearance. *N Engl J Med* 1978; 298:1160–1163.
27. Blumer J, Strong JM, Atkinson AJ Jr. The convulsant potency of lidocaine and its *N*-dealkylated metabolites. *J Pharmacol Exp Ther* 1973; 186:31–36.
28. Narang PK, Crouthamel WG, Carliner NH, Fisher ML. Lidocaine and its active metabolites. *Clin Pharmacol Ther* 1978; 24:654–662.
29. Thomson PD, Melmon KL, Richardson JA, et al. Lidocaine pharmacokinetics in advanced heart failure, liver disease and renal failure in humans. *Ann Intern Med* 1973; 78:499–508.
30. Wyman MG, Slaughter RL, Farolino DA, et al. Multiple bolus technique for lidocaine administration in acute ischemic heart disease: II. Treatment of refractory ventricular arrhythmias and the pharmacokinetic significance of severe left ventricular failure. *J Am Coll Cardiol* 1983; 2:764–769.
31. Stargel WW, Shand DG, Routledge PA, et al. Clinical comparison of rapid infusion and multiple injection methods for lidocaine loading. *Am Heart J* 1981; 102:872–876.
32. Alderman EL, Kerber RE, Harrison DC. Evaluation of lidocaine resistance in man using intermittent large-dose infusion techniques. *Am J Cardiol* 1974; 34:342–349.
33. Richard C, Berdeaux A, Delion F, et al. Effect of mechanical ventilation on hepatic drug pharmacokinetics. *Chest* 1986; 90:837–841.
34. LeLorier J, Grenon D, Latour Y, et al. Pharmacokinetics of lidocaine after prolonged intravenous infusions in uncomplicated myocardial infarction. *Ann Intern Med* 1977; 87:700–702.
35. Routledge PA, Shand DG, Barchowsky A, et al. Relationship between alpha 1-acid glycoprotein and lidocaine disposition in myocardial infarction. *Clin Pharmacol Ther* 1981; 30:154–157.
36. Cheng TO, Wadhwa K. Sinus standstill following intravenous lidocaine administration. *JAMA* 1973; 223:790–792.
37. Marriott HJL, Phillips K. Profound hypotension and bradycardia after a single bolus of lidocaine. *J Electrocardiol* 1974; 7:79–82.
38. Cote P, Harrison DC, Basile J, Schroeder JS. Hemodynamic interaction of procainamide and lidocaine after experimental myocardial infarction. *Am J Cardiol* 1973; 32:937–942.
39. Ochs HR, Carstens G, Greenblatt DJ. Reduction in lidocaine clearance during continuous infusion and by coadministration of propranolol. *N Engl J Med* 1980; 303:373–377.
40. Feeley J, Wilkinson GR, McAllister CB, Wood AJJ. Increased toxicity and reduced clearance of lidocaine by cimetidine. *Ann Intern Med* 1982; 96:592–593.
41. Campbell RWF. Mexiletine. *N Engl J Med* 1987; 316:29–34.
42. Duff HJ, Kolodgie FD, Roden DM, Woosley RL. Electropharmacologic synergism with mexiletine and quinidine. *J Cardiovasc Pharmacol* 1986; 8:840–846.
43. Leahey EB Jr, Heissenbuttel RH, Giardina E-GV, Bigger, JT Jr. Combined mexiletine and propranolol treatment of refractory ventricular arrhythmia. *Br Med J* 1980; 281:357–358.
44. Ruskin JN, DiMarco JP, Garan H. Out-of-hospital cardiac arrest: Electrophysiologic observations and selection of long-term antiarrhythmic therapy. *N Engl J Med* 1980; 303:607–613.
45. Stein J, Podrid P, Lown B. Effects of oral mexiletine on left and right ventricular function. *Am J Cardiol* 1984; 54:575–578.
46. Yamaguchi I, Singh BN, Mandel WJ. Electrophysiological effects of mexiletine on isolated rabbit atria and canine ventricular muscle Purkinje fiber. *Cardiovasc Res* 1979; 13:288–296.
47. Prescott LF, Clements JA, Pottage A. Absorption, distribution, and elimination of mexiletine. *Postgrad Med J* 1977; 53(suppl 1):50–55.
48. Woosley RL, Wang T, Stone W, et al. Pharmacology, electrophysiology, and pharmacokinetics of mexiletine. *Am Heart J* 1984; 107:1058–1065.
49. Brown JE, Shand DG. Therapeutic drug monitoring of antiarrhythmic agents. *Clin Pharmacokinet* 1982; 7:125–148.
50. Beckett AH, Chidomere EC. The distribution, metabolism and excretion of mexiletine in man. *Postgrad Med J* 1977; 53(suppl 1):60–66.
51. Campbell NPS, Kelley JG, Adgey AAJ, Shanks RG. The clinical pharmacology of mexiletine. *Br J Clin Pharmacol* 1978; 6: 103–108.
52. el Allaf D, Henrard L, Crochelet L, et al. Pharmacokinetics of mexiletine in renal insufficiency. *Br J Clin Pharmacol* 1982; 14:431–435.
53. Leahey EB Jr, Giardina E-GV, Bigger JT Jr. Effect of ventricular failure on steady state kinetics of mexiletine. *Clin Res* 1980; 26:239A.
54. Pentikainen PJ, Hietakorpi S, Halinen MO, Lampinen LM. Cirrhosis of the liver markedly impairs the elimination of mexiletine. *Eur J Clin Pharmacol* 1986; 30:83–88.
55. Fasola GP, D'Osualdo F, de Pangher V, Barducci E. Thrombocytopenia and mexiletine. *Ann Intern Med* 1984; 100:162.
56. Girmann G, Pees H, Scheurlen PG. Pseudothrombocytopenia and mexiletine. *Ann Intern Med* 1984; 100:767.
57. Roos JC, Paalman ACA, Dunning AJ. Electrophysiological effects of mexiletine in man. *Br Heart J* 1976; 38.1262–1271.
58. Campbell RWF, Dolder MA, Prescott LF, et al. Comparison of procainamide and mexiletine in prevention of ventricular arrhythmias after acute myocardial infarction. *Lancet* 1975; 1:1257–1259.

59. Stein J, Podrid PJ, Lampert S, et al. Long-term mexiletine for ventricular arrhythmia. *Am Heart J* 1984; 107:1091–1098.
60. Saunamaki KI. Hemodynamic effects of a new anti-arrhythmic agent mexiletine (Ko 1173) in ischaemic heart disease. *Cardiovasc Res* 1975; 9:788–792.
61. Pentikainen PJ, Koivula IH, Hiltunen HA. Effect of rifampicin treatment on the kinetics of mexiletine. *Eur J Clin Pharmacol* 1982; 23:261–266.
62. Bigger JT Jr. The interaction of mexiletine with other cardiovascular drugs. *Am Heart J* 1984; 107:1079–1085.
63. Hoffman BF, Rosen MR, Wit AL. Electrophysiology and pharmacology of cardiac arrhythmias: VII. Cardiac effects of quinidine and procaine amide. *Am Heart J* 1975; 90:117–122.
64. Wellens HJ, Braat S, Brugada P, et al. Use of procainamide in patients with the Wolff-Parkinson-White syndrome to disclose a short refractory period of the accessory pathway. *Am J Cardiol* 1982; 50:1087–1089.
65. Roden DM, Reele SB, Higgins SB, et al. Antiarrhythmic efficacy, pharmacokinetics and safety of *N*-acetylprocainamide in human subjects: Comparison with procainamide. *Am J Cardiol* 1980; 46:463–468.
66. Jaillon P, Winkle RA. Electrophysiologic comparative study of procainamide and *N*-acetylprocainamide in anesthetized dogs: Concentration-response relationships. *Circulation* 1979; 60:1385–1394.
67. Mark LC, Kayden HJ, Steele JM, et al. The physiologic disposition and cardiac effects of procaine amide. *J Pharmacol Exp Ther* 1951; 102:5–15.
68. Komeichi K, Tohse N, Nakaya H, et al. Effects of *N*-acetylprocainamide and sotalol on ion currents in isolated guinea-pig ventricular myocytes. *Eur J Pharmacol* 1990; 187:313–322.
69. Dangman KH, Hoffman BF. In vivo and in vitro antiarrhythmic and arrhythmogenic effects of *N*-acetyl procainamide. *J Pharmacol Exp Ther* 1981; 217:851–862.
70. Jaillon P, Rubenson D, Peters F, et al. Electrophysiologic effects of *N*-acetylprocainamide in human beings. *Am J Cardiol* 1981; 47:1134–1140.
71. Funck-Brentano C, Lineberry MD, Light RT, et al. Pharmacokinetic and pharmacodynamic interaction on *N*-acetyl procainamide and procainamide in man. *J Cardiovasc Pharmacol* 1989; 14:364–373.
72. Myerburg RJ, Kessler KM, Kiem I, et al. Relationship between plasma levels of procainamide, suppression of premature ventricular complexes and prevention of recurrent ventricular tachycardia. *Circulation* 1981; 64:280–290.
73. Giardina E-GV, Heissenbuttel RH, Bigger JT Jr. Intermittent intravenous procainamide to treat ventricular arrhythmias: Correlation of plasma concentration with effect on arrhythmia, electrocardiogram and blood pressure. *Ann Intern Med* 1973; 78:183–193.
74. Lima JJ, Goldfarb AL, Conti DR, et al. Safety and efficacy of procainamide infusions. *Am J Cardiol* 1979; 43:98–105.
75. Karlsson, E. Clinical pharmacokinetics of procainamide. *Clin Pharmacokinet* 1978; 3:97–107.
76. du Souich P, Erill S. Metabolism of procainamide in patients with chronic heart failure, chronic respiratory failure and chronic renal failure. *Eur J Clin Pharmacol* 1978; 14:21–27.
77. Kessler KM, Kayden DS, Estes DM, et al. Procainamide pharmacokinetics in patients with acute myocardial infarction or congestive heart failure. *J Am Coll Cardiol* 1986; 7:1131–1139.
78. Olshansky B, Martins J, Hunt S. *N*-acetyl procainamide causing torsades de pointes. *Am J Cardiol* 1982; 50:1439–1441.
79. Brachmann J, Scherlag BJ, Rosenshtraukh LV, Lazzara R. Bradycardia-dependent triggered activity: Relevance to drug-induced multiform ventricular tachycardia. *Circulation* 1983; 68:846–856.
80. Wyse DG, McAnulty JH, Rahimtoola SH. Influence of plasma drug level and the presence of conduction disease on the electrophysiologic effects of procainamide. *Am J Cardiol* 1979; 43:619–626.
81. Kosowsky BD, Taylor J, Lown B, Ritchie RF. Long-term use of procaine amide following acute myocardial infarction. *Circulation* 1973; 47:1204–1210.
82. Ellrodt AG, Murata GH, Riedinger MS, et al. Severe neutropenia associated with sustained-release procainamide. *Ann Intern Med* 1984; 100:197–201.
83. Somogyi A, McLean A, Heinzow B. Cimetidine-procainamide pharmacokinetic interaction in man: Evidence of competition for tubular secretion of basic drugs. *Eur J Clin Pharmacol* 1983; 25:339–345.
84. Christian CD Jr, Meredith CG, Speeg KV Jr. Cimetidine inhibits renal procainamide clearance. *Clin Pharmacol Ther* 1984; 36:221–227.
85. Funck-Brentano C, Jared LL, Roden DM, Woosley RL. Interaction of procainamide and *N*-acetylprocainamide in man. *Circulation* 1987; 76(Suppl):IV–520.
86. Somogyi A, Bochner F. Dose and concentration dependent effect of ranitidine on procainamide disposition and renal clearance in man. *Br J Clin Pharmacol* 1984; 18:175–181.
87. Mirro MJ, Watanabe AM, Bailey JC. Electrophysiological effects of disopyramide and quinidine on guinea pig atria and canine Purkinje fibers. *Circ Res* 1980; 46:660–668.
88. Dubetz DK, Brown NN, Hooper WD, et al. Disopyramide pharmacokinetics and bioavailability. *Br J Clin Pharmacol* 1978; 6:279–281.
89. Rangno RE, Warnica W, Ogilvie RI, et al. Correlation of disopyramide pharmacokinetics with efficacy in ventricular tachyarrhythmia. *J Int Med Res* 1976; 4(suppl 1):54–58.
90. Hinderling PH, Garrett ER. Pharmacodynamics of the antiarrhythmic disopyramide in healthy humans: Correlation of the kinetics of the drug and its effect. *J Pharmacokinet Biopharm* 1976; 4:231–242.
91. Meffin PJ, Robert EW, Winkle RA, et al. The role of concentration-dependent plasma protein binding in disopyramide disposition. *J Pharmacokinet Biopharm* 1979; 7:29–46.
92. Davies RF, Siddoway LA, Shaw L, et al. Immediate- versus controlled-release disopyramide: Importance of saturable binding. *Clin Pharmacol Ther* 1993; 54:16–22.
93. Edvardsson N, Olsson SB. Clinical value of plasma concentrations of antiarrhythmic drugs. *Eur Heart J* 1987; 8(suppl A):83–89.
94. Kumana CR, Rambihar VS, Tanser PH, et al. A placebo-controlled study to determine the efficacy of oral disopyramide phosphate for the prophylaxis of ventricular dysrhythmias after acute myocardial infarction. *Br J Clin Pharmacol* 1982; 14:519–527.
95. Podrid PJ, Schoenberger A, Lown B. Congestive heart failure caused by oral disopyramide. *N Engl J Med* 1980; 302:614–617.
96. Johnston A, Henry JA, Warrington SJ, Hamer NAJ. Pharmacokinetics of oral disopyramide phosphate in patients with renal impairment. *Br J Clin Pharmacol* 1980; 10:245–248.
97. Bonde J, Gradual NA, Pedersen LE, et al. Kinetics of disopyramide in decreased hepatic function. *Eur J Clin Pharmacol* 1986; 31:73–77.
98. Mokler CM, Hillman RA. Nature of the anticholinergic action of some antiarrhythmic drugs. *Pharmacol Res Commun* 1972; 4:171–178.
99. Teichman SL, Ferrick A, Kim SG, et al. Disopyramide-pyridostigmine interaction: Selective reversal of anticholinergic symptoms with preservation of antiarrhythmic effect. *J Am Coll Cardiol* 1987; 10:633–641.
100. Schweitzer P, Mark H. Torsades de pointes caused by disopyramide and hypokalemia. *Mt Sinai J Med* 1982; 49:110–114.
101. LaBarre A, Strauss HC, Scheinman MM, et al. Electrophysiologic effects of disopyramide phosphate on sinus node function in patients with sinus node dysfunction. *Circulation* 1979; 59:226–235.

102. Roden DM, Hoffman BF. Action potential prolongation and induction of abnormal automaticity by low quinidine concentrations in canine Purkinje fibers: Relationship to potassium and cycle length. *Circ Res* 1985; 56:857–867.
103. Risler T, Burk M, Peters U, et al. On the interaction between digoxin and disopyramide. *Clin Pharmacol Ther* 1983; 34: 176–180.
104. Sylven C, Anderson P. Evidence that disopyramide does not interact with warfarin. *Br Med J* 1983; 286:1181.
105. Kessler JM, Keys PW, Stattford RW. Disopyramide and phenytoin interaction. *Clin Pharm* 1982; 1:263–264.
106. Cumming AD, Robertson C. Interaction between disopyramide and practolol. *Br Med J* 1979; 2:1264.
107. Sodermark T, Edhag O, Sjogren A, et al. Effect of quinidine on maintaining sinus rhythm after conversion of atrial fibrillation or flutter: A multicenter study from Stockholm. *Br Heart J* 1975; 37:486–492.
108. Levi GF, Proto C. Combined treatment of atrial fibrillation with quinidine and beta-blockers. *Br Heart J* 1972; 34:911–914.
109. Bloomfield SS, Romhilt DW, Chou T-C, Fowler NO. Natural history of cardiac arrhythmias and their prevention with quinidine in patients with acute coronary insufficiency. *Circulation* 1973; 47:967–973.
110. Carliner NH, Crouthamel WG, Fisher ML, et al. Quinidine therapy in hospitalized patients with ventricular arrhythmias. *Am Heart J* 1979; 98:708–715.
111. Winkle RA, Gradman AH, Fitzgerald JW. Antiarrhythmic drug effect assessed from ventricular arrhythmia reduction in the ambulatory electrocardiogram and treadmill test: Comparison of propranolol, procainamide and quinidine. *Am J Cardiol* 1978; 42:473–480.
112. Coplen SE, Antman EM, Berlin JA, et al. Efficacy and safety of quinidine therapy for maintenance of sinus rhythm after cardioversion: A meta-analysis of randomized control trials. *Circulation* 1990; 82:1106–1114.
113. Denes P, Gabster A, Huang SK. Clinical, electrocardiographic and follow-up observations in patients having ventricular fibrillation during Holter monitoring: Role of quinidine therapy. *Am J Cardiol* 1981; 48:9–16.
114. Sokolow M, Edgar AL. Blood quinidine concentrations as a guide in the treatment of cardiac arrhythmias. *Circulation* 1950; 1:576–592.
115. Vozeh S, Oti-Amoako K, Uematsu T, Follath F. Antiarrhythmic activity of two quinidine metabolites in experimental reperfusion arrythmia: Relative potency and pharmacodynamic interaction with the parent drug. *J Pharmacol Exp Ther* 1987; 43:297–301.
116. Vozeh S, Bindschedler M, Huy-Riem HA, et al. Pharmacodynamics of 3-hydroxyquinidine alone and in combination with quinidine in healthy persons. *Am J Cardiol* 1987; 59:681–684.
117. Kavanagh KM, Wyse DG, Mitchell LB, et al. Contribution of quinidine metabolites to electrophysiologic responses in human subjects. *Clin Pharmacol Ther* 1989; 46:352–358.
118. Thompson KA, Blair IA, Woosley RL, Roden DM. Comparative in vitro electrophysiology of quinidine, its major metabolites and dihydroxyquinidine. *J Pharmacol Exp Ther* 1987; 241:84–90.
119. Drayer DE, Lorenzo B, Reidenberg MM. Liquid chromatography and fluorescence spectroscopy compared with a homogeneous enzyme immunoassay technique for determining quinidine in serum. *Clin Chem* 1981; 27:308–310.
120. Lehmann CR, Boran KJ, Pierson WP, et al. Quinidine assays: Enzyme immunoassay versus high performance liquid chromatography. *Ther Drug Monit* 1986; 8:336–339.
121. Drayer DE, Lowenthal DT, Restivo KM, et al. Steady-state serum levels of quinidine and active metabolites in cardiac patients with varying degrees of renal function. *Clin Pharmacol Ther* 1978; 24:31–39.
122. Kessler KM, Humphries WC, Black M, Spann JF. Quinidine pharmacokinetics in patients with cirrhosis or receiving propranolol. *Am Heart J* 1978; 96:627–635.
123. Ochs HR, Greenblatt DJ, Woo E. Clinical pharmacokinetics of quinidine. *Clin Pharmacokinet* 1980; 5:150–168.
124. Kay GN, Plumb VJ, Arciniegas JG, et al. Torsades de pointes: The long-short initiating sequence and other clinical features: Observations in 32 patients. *J Am Coll Cardiol* 1983; 2:806–817.
125. Gottlieb SS, Weinberg M. Hemodynamic and neurohormonal effects of quinidine in patients with severe left ventricular dysfunction secondary to coronary artery disease or idiopathic dilated cardiomyopathy. *Am J Cardiol* 1991; 67:728–731.
126. Cohen IS, Jick H, Cohen SI. Adverse reactions to quinidine in hospitalized patients: Findings based on data from the Boston Collaborative Drug Surveillance Programs. *Prog Cardiovasc Dis* 1977; 20:151–163.
127. Dargie HJ, Cleland JGF, Leckie BJ, et al. Relation of arrhythmias and electrolyte abnormalities to survival in patients with severe chronic heart failure. *Circulation* 1987; 75(suppl IV):IV-98–IV-107.
128. Roden DM, Woosley RL, Primm RK. Incidence and clinical features of the quinidine-associated long-QT syndrome: Implications for patient care. *Am Heart J* 1986; 111:1088–1093.
129. Makkar RR, Fromm BS, Steinman RT, et al. Female gender as a risk factor for torsades de pointes associated with cardiovascular drugs. *JAMA* 1993; 270:2590–2597.
130. Drici MD, Burklow TR, Haridasse V, et al. Sex hormones prolong the QT interval and down-regulate potassium channel expression in the rabbit heart. *Circulation* 1996; 94:1471–1474.
131. Benton RE, Sale M, Flockhart DA, Woosley RL. Greater quinidine induced QT_c interval prolongation in women. *Clin Pharm Ther* 2000; 67:413–418.
132. Schmid PG, Nelson LD, Mark AL, et al. Inhibition of adrenergic vasoconstriction by quinidine. *J Pharmacol Exp Ther* 1974; 188:124–134.
133. Nair MR, Duvernoy WF, Leichtman DA. Severe leukopenia and thrombocytopenia secondary to quinidine. *Clin Cardiol* 1981; 4:247–257.
134. Polish LB, Branch RA, Fitzgerald GA. Digitoxin-quinidine interaction: Potentiation during administration of cimetidine. *South Med J* 1981; 74:633–634.
135. Data JL, Wilkinson GR, Nies AS. Interaction of quinidine with anticonvulsant drugs. *N Engl J Med* 1976; 294:699–702.
136. Leahey EB Jr, Reiffel JA, Drusin RE, et al. Interactions between quinidine and digoxin. *JAMA* 1978; 240:533–534.
137. Bussey HI. The influence of quinidine and other agents on digitalis glycosides. *Am Heart J* 1982; 104:289–302.
138. Brinn R, Brosen K, Gram LF, et al. Spartine oxidation is practically abolished in quinidine-treated patients. *Br J Clin Pharmacol* 1986; 22:194–197.
139. Spiers CJ, Murray S, Boobis AR, et al. Quinidine and the identification of drugs whose elimination is impaired in subjects classified as poor metabolizers of debrisoquine. *Br J Clin Pharmacol* 1986; 22:739–743.
140. Guengerich FP, Muller-Enoch D, Blair IA. Oxidation of quinidine by human liver cytochrome P-450. *Mol Pharmacol* 1986; 30:287–295.
141. Mikus G, Ha HR, Vozeh S, et al. Pharmacokinetics and metabolism of quinidine in extensive and poor metabolizers of spartine. *Eur J Clin Pharmacol* 1986; 31:69–72.
142. Brosen K, Gram LF, Haghfelt T, Bertilsson L. Extensive metabolizers of debrisoquin become poor metabolizers during quinidine treatment. *Pharmacol Toxicol* 1987; 60:312–314.
143. Kornfeld P, Horowitz SH, Genkins G, Papatestas AE. Myasthenia gravis unmasked by antiarrhythmic agents. *Mt Sinai J Med* 1976; 43:10–14.
144. Grogono AW. Anesthesia for atrial fibrillation: Effect of quinidine on muscle relaxation. *Lancet* 1963; 2:1039–1040.

145. Connolly SJ, Mulji AS, Hoffert DL, et al. Randomized placebo-controlled trial of propafenone for treatment of atrial tachyarrhythmias after cardiac surgery. *J Am Coll Cardiol* 1987; 10:1145–1148.
146. von Philipsborn G, Gries J, Hofmann HP, et al. Pharmacological studies on propafenone and its main metabolite 5-hydroxypropafenone. *Arzneimittelforschung* 1984; 34:1489–1497.
147. Valenzuela C, Delgado C, Tamargo J. Electrophysiological effects of 5-hydroxypropafenone on guinea pig ventricular muscle fibers. *J Cardiovasc Pharmacol* 1987; 10:523–529.
148. McLeod AA, Stiles GL, Shand DG. Demonstration of beta adrenoceptor blockade by propafenone hydrochloride: Clinical pharmacologic, radioligand binding, and adenylate cyclase activation studies. *J Pharmacol Exp Ther* 1984; 228:461–466.
149. Siddoway LA, Thompson KA, McAllister CB, et al. Polymorphism of propafenone metabolism and disposition in man: Clinical and pharmacokinetic consequences. *Circulation* 1987; 75:785–791.
150. Lee JT, Kroemer HK, Silberstein DJ, et al. The role of genetically determined polymorphic drug metabolism in the beta-block produced by propafenone. *N Engl J Med* 1990; 322:1764–1768.
151. Baker BJ, Dinh H, Kroskey D, et al. Effect of propafenone on left ventricular ejection fraction. *Am J Cardiol* 1984; 54 (suppl):20D–22D.
152. Wagner F, Kalusche D, Trenk D, et al. Drug interaction between propafenone and metoprolol. *Br J Clin Pharmacol* 1987; 24:213–220.
153. Funck-Brentano C, Kroemer HK, Pavlou H, et al. Genetically-determined interaction between propafenone and low dose quinidine: Role of active metabolites in modulating net drug effect. *Br J Clin Pharmacol* 1989; 27:435–444.
154. Roden DM, Woosley RL. Flecainide. *N Engl J Med* 1986; 315:36–41.
155. Hellestrand KJ, Nathan AW, Bexton RS, et al. Cardiac electrophysiologic effects of flecainide acetate for paroxysmal reentrant junctional tachycardias. *Am J Cardiol* 1983; 51:770–776.
156. Pritchett EL, Wilkinson WE. Mortality in patients treated with flecainide and encainide for supraventricular arrhythmias. *Am J Cardiol* 1991; 67:976–980.
157. The Flecainide-Quinidine Research Group. Flecainide versus quinidine for treatment of chronic ventricular arrhythmias: A multicenter clinical trial. *Circulation* 1983; 67:1117–1123.
158. Follmer CH, Colatsky TJ. Block of delayed rectifier potassium current, I_K, by flecainide and E-4031 in cat ventricular myocytes. *Circulation* 1990; 82:289–293.
159. Estes NAM III, Garan H, Ruskin JN. Electrophysiological properties of flecainide acetate. *Am J Cardiol* 1984; 53(suppl):26B–29B.
160. Conard GJ, Ober RE. Metabolism of flecainide. *Am J Cardiol* 1984; 53(suppl):41B–51B.
161. Haefeli WE, Bargetzi MJ, Follath F, et al. Potent inhibition of cytochrome p450IID6 (debrisoquin 4-hydroxylase) by flecainide in vitro and in vivo. *J Cardiovasc Pharmacol* 1990; 15:776–779.
162. Johnston A, Warrington S, Turner P. Flecainide pharmacokinetics in healthy volunteers: The influence of urinary pH. *Br J Clin Pharmacol* 1985; 20:333–338.
163. Franciosa JA, Wilen M, Weeks CE, et al. Pharmacokinetics and hemodynamic effects of flecainide in patients with chronic low output heart failure. *J Am Coll Cardiol* 1983; 1:699.
164. Winkelman BR, Leinberger H. Life-threatening flecainide toxicity: A pharmacodynamic approach. *Ann Intern Med* 1987; 106:807–814.
165. Salerno DM, Granrud GA, Sharkey P, et al. Pharmacodynamics and side effects of flecainide acetate. *Clin Pharmacol Ther* 1986; 40:101–107.
166. Morganroth J, Horowitz LN. Flecainide: Its proarrhythmic effect and expected changes on the surface electrocardiogram. *Am J Cardiol* 1984; 53(suppl):89B–94B.
167. Josephson MA, Kaul S, Hopkins J, et al. Hemodynamic effects of intravenous flecainide relative to the level of ventricular function in patients with coronary artery disease. *Am Heart J* 1985; 109:41–45.
168. Muhiddin KA, Turner P, Blackett A. Effect of flecainide on cardiac output. *Clin Pharmacol Ther* 1985; 37:260–263.
169. Josephson MA, Ikeda N, Singh BN. Effects of flecainide on ventricular function: Clinical and experimental correlations. *Am J Cardiol* 1984; 53:95B–100B.
170. Vik-Mo H, Ohm O-J, Lund-Johansen P. Electrophysiological effects of flecainide acetate in patients with sinus nodal dysfunction. *Am J Cardiol* 1982; 50:1090–1094.
171. Hellestrand KJ, Nathan AW, Bexton RS, Camm AJ. Electrophysiologic effects of flecainide acetate on sinus node function, anomalous atrioventricular connections and pacemaker thresholds. *Am J Cardiol* 1984; 53(suppl):30B–38B.
172. Hellestrand KJ, Burnett PJ, Milne JR, et al. The effect of the antiarrhythmic agent flecainide on acute and chronic pacing thresholds. *PACE* 1983; 6:892–899.
173. Hernandez R, Mann DE, Breckinridge S, et al. Effects of flecainide on defibrillation thresholds in the anesthetized dog. *J Am Coll Cardiol* 1989; 14:777–781.
174. Tjandra-Maga TB, van Hecken A, van Melle P, et al. Altered pharmacokinetics of oral flecainide by cimetidine. *Br J Clin Pharmacol* 1986; 22:108–110.
175. Weeks CE, Conard GJ, Kvam DC, et al. The effect of flecainide acetate, a new antiarrhythmic, on plasma digoxin levels. *J Clin Pharmacol* 1986; 26:27–31.
176. Lewis GP, Holtzman JL. Interaction of flecainide with digoxin and propranolol. *Am J Cardiol* 1984; 53(suppl):52B–57B.
177. Shea P, Lal R, Kim SS, et al. Flecainide and amiodarone interaction. *J Am Coll Cardiol* 1986; 7:1127–1130.
178. Rowland E. Antiarrhythmic drugs: Class IV. *Eur Heart J* 1987; 8(suppl A):61–63.
179. Singh BN, Nademanee K, Baky SH. Calcium antagonists: Clinical use in the treatment of arrhythmias. *Drugs* 1983; 25:125–153.
180. Bacaner MB. Treatment of ventricular fibrillation and other acute arrhythmias with bretylium tosylate. *Am J Cardiol* 1968; 21:530–543.
181. Bigger JT Jr, Jaffe CC. The effect of bretylium tosylate on the electrophysiologic properties of ventricular muscle and Purkinje fibers. *Am J Cardiol* 1971; 27:82–92.
182. Cardinale R, Sasyniuk, BI. Electrophysiological effects of bretylium tosylate on subendocardial Purkinje fibers from infarcted canine hearts. *J Pharmacol Exp Ther* 1978; 204:159–174.
183. Nishimura M, Watanabe Y. Membrane action and catecholamine release action of bretylium tosylate in normoxic and hypoxic canine Purkinje fibers. *J Am Coll Cardiol* 1983; 2:287–295.
184. Narang PK, Adir J, Josselson J, Yacobi A. Pharmacokinetics of bretylium in man after intravenous administration. *J Pharmacokinet Biopharm* 1980; 8:363–372.
185. Chow MSS, Kluger J, DiPersio DM, et al. Antifibrillatory effects of lidocaine and bretylium immediately postcardiopulmonary resuscitation. *Am Heart J* 1985; 110:938–943.
186. Duff HJ, Roden DM, Yacobi A, et al. Bretylium: Relations between plasma concentrations and pharmacologic actions in high-frequency ventricular arrhythmias. *Am J Cardiol* 1985; 55:395–401.
187. Singh BN, Nademanee K. Sotalol: A beta-blocker with unique antiarrhythmic properties. *Am Heart J* 1987; 114:121–139.
188. Singh BN, Kehoe R, Woosley RL, et al. Multicenter trial of sotalol compared with procainamide in the suppression of inducible ventricular tachycardia: A double-blind, randomized parallel evaluation. Sotalol Multicenter Study Group. *Am Heart J* 1995; 129:87–97.

189. Mason JW, ESVEM Investigators. A comparison of seven antiarrhythmic drugs in patients with ventricular tachyarrhythmias. *N Engl J Med* 1993; 329:452–458.
190. Wang T, Bergstrand RH, Thompson KA, et al. Concentration-dependent pharmacologic properties of sotalol. *Am J Cardiol* 1986; 57:1160–1165.
191. Kopleman HA, Woosley RL, Lee JT et al. Electrophysiologic effects of intravenous and oral sotalol for sustained ventricular tachycardia secondary to coronary artery disease. *Am J Cardiol* 1988; 61:1006–1011.
192. Hohnloser SH, Woosley RL. Sotalol. *N Engl J Med* 1994; 331:31–38.
193. Barbey JT, Sale ME, Woosley RL, et al. Pharmacokinetic, pharmacodynamic, and safety evaluation of an accelerated dose titration regimen of sotalol in healthy middle-aged subjects. *Clin Pharmacol Ther* 1999; 66:91–99.
194. Graboys TB, Podrid PJ, Lown B. Efficacy of amiodarone for refractory supraventricular tachyarrhythmias. *Am Heart J* 1983; 106:870–876.
195. Horowitz LN, Spielman SR, Greenspan AM, et al. Use of amiodarone in the treatment of persistent and paroxysmal atrial fibrillation resistant to quinidine therapy. *J Am Coll Cardiol* 1985; 6:1402–1407.
196. Peters RW, Fisher ML. Use of amiodarone. *Choices Cardiol* 1994; 8:57–60.
197. Cairns JA, Connolly SJ, Roberts R, et al. Randomized trial of outcome after myocardial infarction in patients with frequent or repetitive ventricular premature depolarizations: CAMIAT. *Lancet* 1997; 349:675–682.
198. Julian DG, Camm AJ, Frangin G, et al. Randomized trial of effect of amiodarone on mortality in patients with left-ventricular dysfunction after recent myocardial infarction: EMIAT. *Lancet* 1997; 349:667–674.
199. Connolly SJ. Meta-analysis of antiarrhythmic drug trials. *Am J Cardiol* 1999; 84:90R–93R.
200. Piepoli M, Villani GQ, Ponikowski P, et al. Overview and meta-analysis of randomised trials of amiodarone in chronic heart failure. *Int J Cardiol* 1998; 66:1–10.
201. Scheinman MM, Levine JH, Cannom DS, et al. Dose-ranging study of intravenous amiodarone in patients with life-threatening ventricular tachyarrhythmias. *Circulation* 1995; 92:3264–3272.
202. Kowey PR, Levine JH, Herre JM, et al. Randomized, double-blind comparison of intravenous amiodarone and bretylium in the treatment of patients with recurrent, hemodynamically destabilizing ventricular tachycardia or fibrillation. *Circulation* 1995; 92:3255–3263.
203. Guarnieri T, Nolan S, Gottlieb SO, et al. Intravenous amiodarone for the prevention of atrial fibrillation after open heart surgery: The amiodarone reduction in coronary heart (ARCH) trial. *J Am Coll Cardiol* 1999; 34:343–347.
204. Mason JW. Amiodarone. *N Engl J Med* 1987; 316:455–466.
205. Mason JW, Hondeghem LM, Katzung BG. Amiodarone blocks inactivated cardiac sodium channels. *Pflugers Arch* 1983; 396:79–81.
206. Talajic M, DeRoode MR, Nattel S. Comparative electrophysiologic effects of intravenous amiodarone and desmethylamiodarone in dogs: Evidence for clinically relevant activity of the metabolite. *Circulation* 1987; 75:265–271.
207. Nanas JN, Mason JW. Pharmacokinetics and regional electrophysiological effects of intracoronary amiodarone administration. *Circulation* 1995; 91:451–461.
208. Albert SG, Alves LE, Rose EP. Thyroid dysfunction during chronic amiodarone therapy. *J Am Coll Cardiol* 1987; 9:175–183.
209. Singh BN, Nademanee K. Amiodarone and thyroid function: Clinical implications during antiarrhythmic therapy. *Am Heart J* 1983; 106:857–869.
210. Latham KR, Sellitti DF, Goldstein RE. Interaction of amiodarone and desethylamiodarone with solubilized nuclear thyroid hormone receptors. *J Am Coll Cardiol* 1987; 9:872–876.
211. Charlier R, Deltour G, Baudine A, Chaillet F. Pharmacology of amiodarone, and anti-anginal drug with a new biological profile. *Arzneimittelforschung* 1968; 18:1408–1417.
212. Cohen-Armon M, Schreiber G, Sokolovsky M. Interaction of the antiarrhythmic drug amiodarone with the muscarinic receptor in rat heart and brain. *J Cardiovasc Pharmacol* 1984; 6:1148–1155.
213. Pourbaix S, Berger Y, Desager J-P, et al. Absolute bioavailability of amiodarone in normal subjects. *Clin Pharmacol Ther* 1985; 37:118–123.
214. Adams PC, Holt DW, Storey GC, et al. Amiodarone and its desethyl metabolite: Tissue distribution and morphologic changes during long-term therapy. *Circulation* 1985; 72:1064–1075.
215. Nattel S, Davies M, Quantz M. The antiarrhythmic efficacy of amiodarone and desethylamiodarone, alone and in combination, in dogs with acute myocardial infarction. *Circulation* 1988; 77:200–208.
216. Holt DW, Tucker GT, Jackson PR, McKenna WJ. Amiodarone pharmacokinetics. *Br J Clin Pract* 1986; 44(suppl):109–114.
217. Plomp TA, van Rossum JM, Robles de Medina EO, et al. Pharmacokinetics and body distribution of amiodarone in man. *Arzneimittelforschung* 1984; 34:513–520.
218. Siddoway LA, McAllister CB, Wilkinson GR, et al. Amiodarone dosing: A proposal based on its pharmacokinetics. *Am Heart J* 1983; 106:951–956.
219. Cairns JA, Connolly SJ, Gent M, Roberts R. Post-myocardial infarction mortality in patients with ventricular premature depolarizations. *Circulation* 1991; 84:550–557.
220. Escoubet B, Coumel P, Poirier J-M, et al. Suppression of arrhythmias within hours after a single oral dose of amiodarone and relation to plasma and myocardial concentrations. *Am J Cardiol* 1985; 55:696–702.
221. Mostow ND, Vrobel TR, Noon D, Rakita L. Rapid suppression of complex ventricular arrhythmias with high-dose oral amiodarone. *Circulation* 1986; 73:1231–1238.
222. Greenberg ML, Lerman BB, Shipe JR, et al. Relation between amiodarone and desethylamiodarone plasma concentrations and electrophysiological effects, efficacy and toxicity. *J Am Coll Cardiol* 1987; 9:1148–1155.
223. Coumel P, Fidelle J. Amiodarone in the treatment of cardiac arrhythmias in children: One hundred thirty-five cases. *Am Heart J* 1980; 100:1063–1069.
224. Mason JW, Amiodarone Toxicity Study Group. Toxicity of amiodarone. *Circulation* 1985; 72(suppl):III-272.
225. Veltri EP, Reid PR. Amiodarone pulmonary toxicity: Early changes in pulmonary function tests during amiodarone rechallenge. *J Am Coll Cardiol* 1985; 6:802–805.
226. Orlando RG, Dangel ME, Schaal SF. Clinical experience and grading of amiodarone keratopathy. *Ophthalmology* 1984; 91:1184–1187.
227. Zachary CB, Slater DN, Holt DW, et al. The pathogenesis of amiodarone-induced pigmentation and photosensitivity. *Br J Dermatol* 1984; 110:451–456.
228. Simon JB, Manley PN, Brien JF, Armstrong PW. Amiodarone hepatotoxicity simulating alcoholic liver disease. *N Engl J Med* 1984; 311:167–172.
229. Rigas B, Rosenfeld LE, Barwick KW, et al. Amiodarone hepatotoxicity: A clinicopathologic study of five patients. *Ann Intern Med* 1986; 104:348–351.
230. Larrey D, Tinel M, Letteron P, et al. Formation of an inactive cytochrome P-450 Fe(II)-metabolite complex after administration of amiodarone in rats, mice and hamsters. *Biochem Pharmacol* 1986; 35:2213–2220.
231. Almog S, Shafran N, Halkin H, et al. Mechanism of warfarin potentiation by amiodarone: Dose- and concentration-dependent

inhibition of warfarin elimination. *Eur J Clin Pharmacol* 1985; 28:257–261.

232. Marcus FI. Drug interactions with amiodarone. *Am Heart J* 1983; 106:924–930.

233. Fenster PE, White NW Jr, Hanson CD. Pharmacokinetic evaluation of the digoxin-amiodarone interaction. *J Am Coll Cardiol* 1985; 5:108–112.

234. Stambler BS, Wood MA, Ellenbogen KA. Comparative efficacy of intravenous ibutilide versus procainamide for enhancing termination of atrial flutter by atrial overdrive pacing. *Am J Cardiol* 1996; 77:960–966.

235. Guo GB, Ellenbogen KA, Wood MA, Stambler BS. Conversion of atrial flutter by ibutilide is associated with increased atrial cycle length variability. *J Am Coll Cardiol* 1996; 27:1083–1089.

236. Vanderlugt JT, Mattioni T, Denker S, et al. Efficacy and safety of ibutilide fumarate for the conversion of atrial arrhythmias after cardiac surgery. *Circulation* 1999; 100:369–375.

237. Lee KS. Ibutilide, a new compound with potent class III antiarrhythmic activity, activates a slow inward Na^+ current in guinea pig ventricular cells. *J Pharmacol Exp Ther* 1992; 262:99–108.

238. Yang T, Snyders DJ, Roden DM. Ibutilide, a methanesulfonanilide antiarrhythmic, is a potent blocker of the rapidly activating delayed rectifier K^+ current (I_{Kr}) in AT-1 cells: Concentration-, time-, voltage-, and use-dependent effects. *Circulation* 1995; 91:1799–1806.

239. Amin NB, Borzak S, Housholder S, Tisdale JE. Sinus bradycardia and multiple episodes of sinus arrest following administration of ibutilide. *Heart* 1998; 79:628–629.

240. Franz MR, Geppert A, Kain R, et al. Acute renal failure after ibutilide. *Lancet* 1999; 353:467.

241. Akiyama T, Pawitan Y, Greenberg H, et al. Increased risk of death and cardiac arrest from encainide and flecainide in patients after non-Q-wave acute myocardial infarction in the Cardiac Arrhythmia Suppression Trial. *Am J Cardiol* 1991; 68:1551–1555.

242. Torp-Pedersen C, Moller M, Bloch-Thomsen PE, et al. Dofetilide in patients with congestive heart failure and left ventricular dysfunction. Danish Investigations of Arrhythmia and Mortality on Dofetilide Study Group. *N Engl J Med* 1999; 341:857–865.

243. Baskin EP, Lynch JJ Jr. Differential atrial versus ventricular activities of class III potassium channel blockers. *J Pharmacol Exp Ther* 1998; 285:135–142.

244. Walker DK, Alabaster CT, Congrave GS, et al. Significance of metabolism in the disposition and action of the antidysrhythmic drug, dofetilide: In vitro studies and correlation with in vivo data. *Drug Metab Dispos* 1996; 24:447–455.

245. Abel S, Nichols DJ, Brearley CJ, Eve MD. Effect of cimetidine and ranitidine on pharmacokinetics and pharmacodynamics of a single dose of dofetilide. *Br J Clin Pharmacol* 2000; 49:64–71.

246. Lerman BB, Belardinelli L. Cardiac electrophysiology of adenosine: Basic and clinical concepts. *Circulation* 1991; 83:1499–1509.

247. Ellenbogen KA, Thames MD, DiMarco JP, et al. Electrophysiologic effects of adenosine in the transplanted human heart: Evidence for supersensitivity. *Circulation* 1990; 81:821–828.

248. Lerman BB, Wesley RC, Belardinelli L. Electrophysiologic effects of dipyridamole on atrioventricular nodal conduction and supraventricular tachycardia: Role of endogenous adenosine. *Circulation* 1989; 80:1536–1543.

249. DiMarco JP, Sellers TD, Lerman BB, et al. Diagnostic and therapeutic use of adenosine in patients with supraventricular tachyarrhythmias. *J Am Coll Cardiol* 1985; 6:417–425.

250. Raatikainen MJ, Napolitano CA, Druzgala P, Dennis DM. Electrophysiological effects of a novel, short-acting and potent ester derivative of amiodarone, ATI-2001, in guinea pig isolated heart. *J Pharmacol Exp Ther* 1996; 277:1454–1463.

251. Verduyn SC, Vos MA, Leunissen HDM, et al. Evaluation of the acute electrophysiologic effects of intravenous dronedarone, an amiodarone-like agent, with special emphasis on ventricular repolarization and acquired torsades de pointes arrhythmias. *J Cardiovasc Pharmacol* 1999; 33:212–222.

252. Manning AS, Bruyninckx C, Ramboux J, Chatelain P. SR 33589, a new amiodarone-like agent: Effect on ischemia- and reperfusion-induced arrhythmias in anesthetized rats. *J Cardiovasc Pharmacol* 1995; 26:453–461.

CHAPTER 28

TREATMENT OF CARDIAC ARRHYTHMIAS WITH CATHETER-ABLATIVE TECHNIQUES

Eugen C. Palma / Melvin M. Scheinman

Over the past several years, various techniques have been introduced using catheter ablative procedures for patients with cardiac arrhythmias. Particularly impressive are some of the newer techniques using radiofrequency energy sources for patients with supraventricular arrhythmias. This chapter reviews the techniques, results, and clinical indications for these procedures.

TECHNIQUES

Ablation of the Atrioventricular Junction

The technique of catheter ablation of the atrioventricular (AV) junction was first developed in canines[1] and subsequently applied for control of drug-refractory atrial arrhythmias in patients.[2,3] Multipolar electrode catheters are inserted by vein and positioned just across the tricuspid valve and against the apex of the right ventricle (Fig. 28-1). The catheter across the tricuspid valve is manipulated to allow recording of the largest unipolar His bundle potential[2] (Fig. 28-2). Radiofrequency energy of 350 to 500 kHz is applied between the distal electrode and a large back patch. After persistent AV block is observed, a permanent cardiac pacemaker is inserted (Fig. 28-3).

AV Nodal Modification for Patients with Atrial Fibrillation

A more recent innovation has been the use of AV nodal modification for achieving rate control in patients with atrial fibrillation.[4–6] This technique involves placement of radiofrequency lesions over the posterior or midseptum in order to achieve the desired reduction in rate during atrial fibrillation. The procedure entails a 16 percent risk of inducing complete AV block, which usually occurs within the first 72 h after the ablation.[6] In addition, a late recurrence of rapid rate has been reported in approximately 10 percent of patients.[6] The available data over a 19-month follow-up period suggest that the bulk of suitably selected patients with atrial fibrillation and rapid rate resistant to drug therapy will respond to AV nodal modification. However, this technique is of no value for the relief of symptoms related to the irregular rhythm per se.

Ablation of Accessory Pathways

Patients with accessory extranodal pathways often experience reentrant arrhythmias, with the circuit of the tachycardia involving antegrade conduction over the normal AV nodal conduction system and retrograde conduction over the accessory pathway.[7] Surgical techniques have in the past proved very effective and safe in the interruption of these pathways.[8] More recently, a number of catheter techniques have been introduced for catheter ablation of these pathways. Fisher et al.[9] were the first to use this technique for ablation of left free wall accessory pathways via the coronary sinus. Accessory AV pathways occur anywhere along the cardiac annulus or in the septum. The majority of pathways are found traversing the left AV groove. These pathways are currently approached by inserting a steerable multipolar electrode catheter into the femoral artery with retrograde catheterization of the left ventricle.[10] The catheter is then placed under the mitral annulus in the putative site of the accessory pathway (Fig. 28-4). An alternative technique involves use of transseptal catheterization with placement of

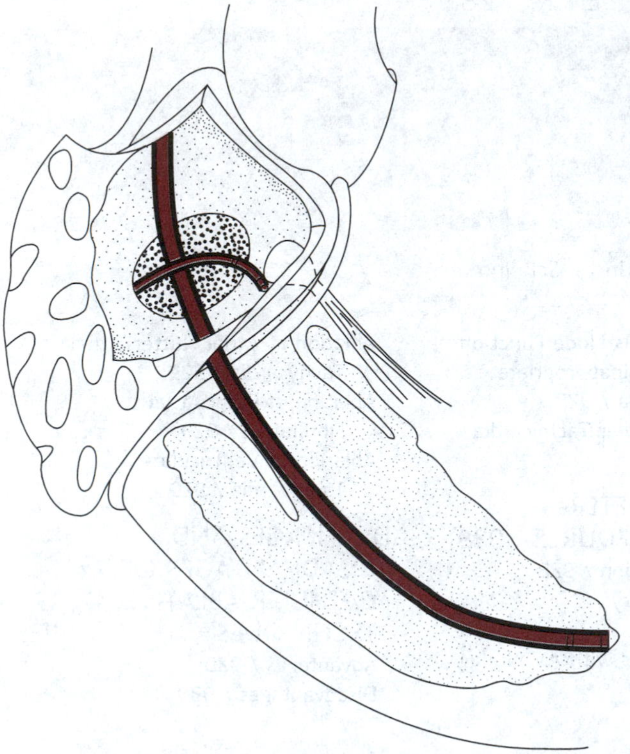

FIGURE 28-1 Catheter positions for patients undergoing AV junctional ablation. One catheter is placed over the region of the AV node, while a second catheter is placed against the apex of the right ventricle.

the catheter along the atrial margin of the mitral annulus.[11] One or more applications of radiofrequency energy are used to ablate the pathways. In contrast, most septal and all right free wall pathways are approached by right-sided catheterization.

Modification of the AV Node in AV Nodal Reentrant Tachycardia

Patients with AV nodal reentrant tachycardia are thought to have two pathways within or in close proximity to the AV node. These pathways show fast and slow conducting properties and have different refractory periods. Techniques have been introduced that allow for selective ablation of either pathway. The fast pathway is approached by withdrawing the catheter to a more proximal location while recording the His bundle potential, which is associated with a large-amplitude atrial electrogram and a very small or absent His deflection.[12] Application of radiofrequency energy to this area results in abrupt prolongation of the PR interval, since ablation of the fast pathway forces conduction to occur over the slow pathway. An alternative technique for ablation of the slow pathway was introduced by Roman et al.,[13] where the radiofrequency energy is applied posteriorly between the os of the coronary sinus and the septal leaflet of the tricuspid valve. Successful application of the latter technique does not result in a change in the PR interval. The approach described for slow-pathway ablation may be accomplished successfully either by using anatomic landmarks or searching for specific so-called slow-pathway potentials. This technique has proved to be more effective and safer than attempts at fast-pathway ablation.

Ablation of Atrial Flutter/Atrial Tachycardia

Very effective techniques have been introduced recently for ablation of atrial flutter. Patients with a "typical" flutter pattern have a reentrant circuit localized to the right atrium. The critical slow zone appears to reside in the isthmus between the inferior vena cava and the tricuspid annulus.[14] A catheter is used to apply serial lesions, creating a line of block across the isthmus, with initial results suggesting success in 85 to 90 percent of patients.[15]

Patients with atrial tachycardia may be treated with catheter-

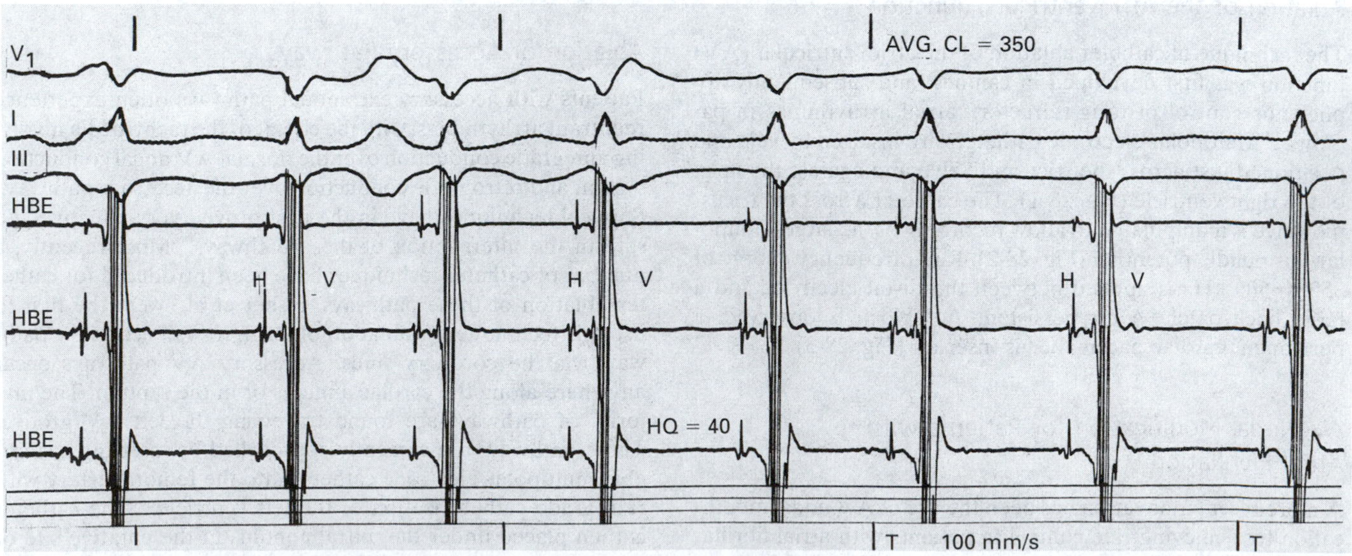

FIGURE 28-2 Atrial fibrillation with rapid ventricular response prior to ablation.

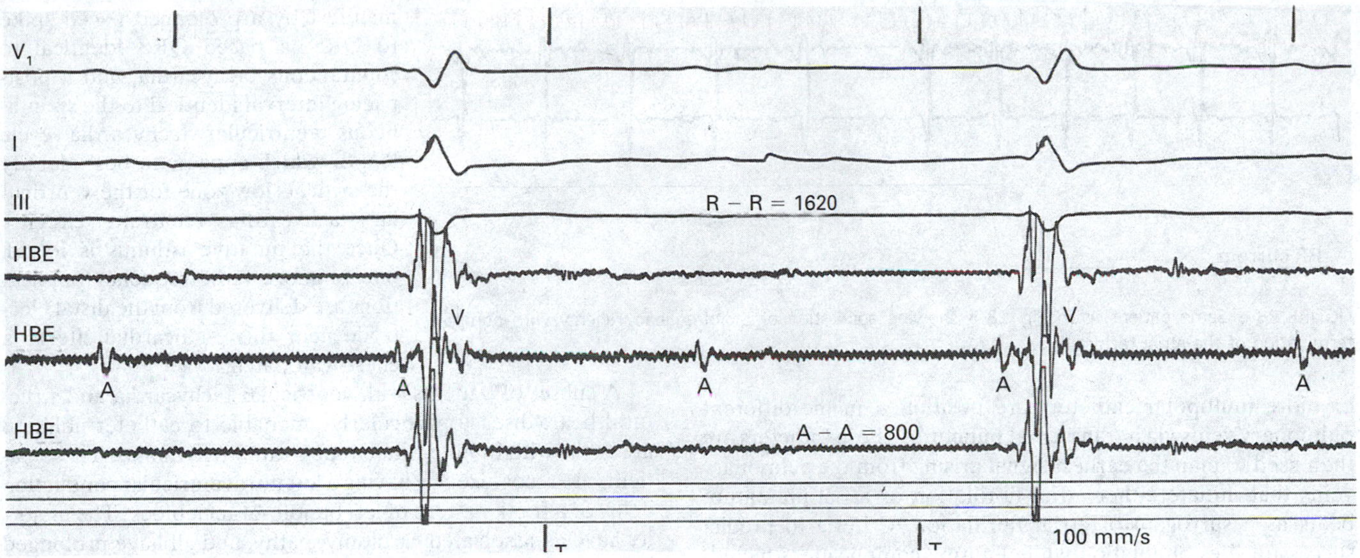

FIGURE 28-3 After completion of the ablation, complete AV block is achieved.

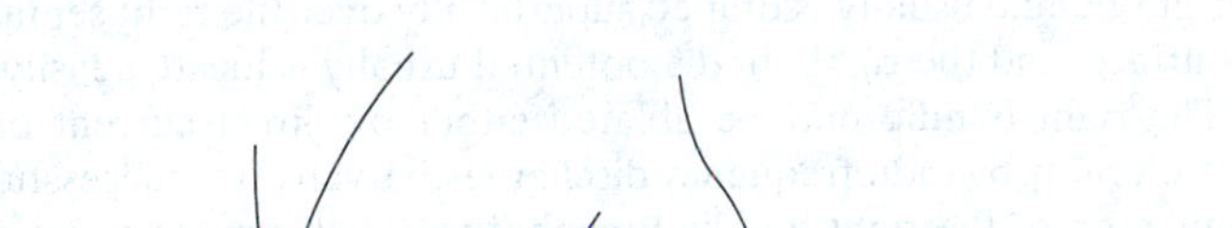

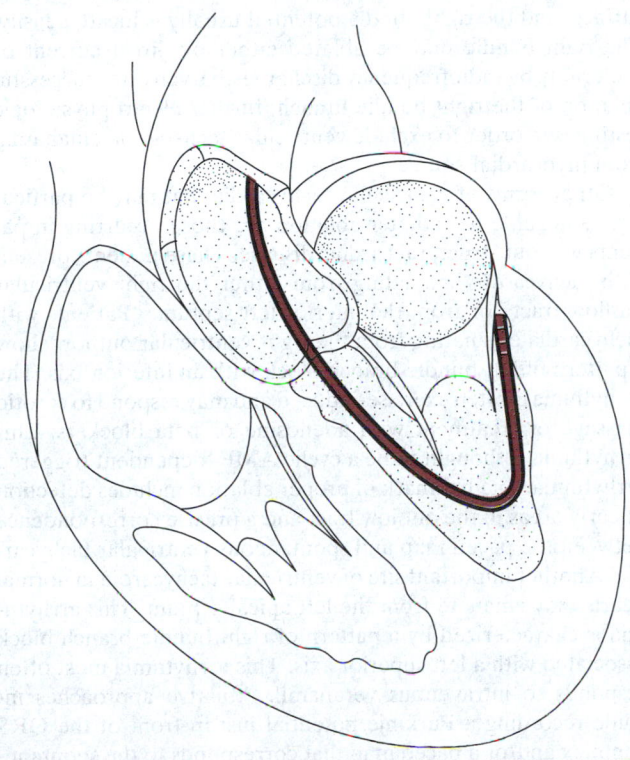

FIGURE 28-4 Schema depicting retrograde aortic technique for ablation of a left free wall accessory pathway. The catheter is passed across the aortic valve and placed under the mitral annulus.

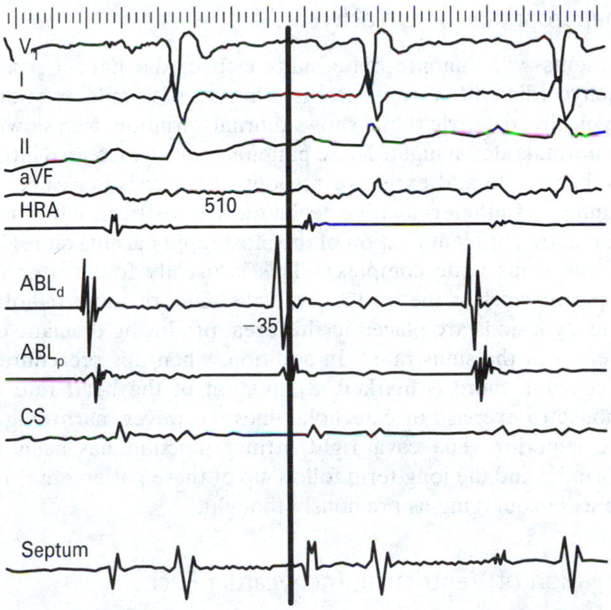

FIGURE 28-5 Simultaneous surface V_1, I, II, and intracardiac recordings from the high right atrium (HRA), distal (ABL_d), and proximal (ABL_p) electrodes from the ablating catheter, coronary sinus (CS), and low right atrial septum (Septum) in a patient with atrial tachycardia. The earliest atrial electrogram was 35 ms prior to inscription of the surface P waves.

ablative techniques.[16] The catheter is manipulated to find the earliest endocardial atrial potential relative to the surface P wave (Fig. 28-5). Foci of atrial tachycardia are localized along the crista terminalis or atrial appendage in the right atrium. Left atrial foci occur around the superior pulmonary veins or left atrial appendage.[17] Once the earliest site is located, radiofrequency energy is applied to ablate the atrial focus (Fig. 28-6).

Ablation of Focal Atrial Fibrillation

Recently, a subset of patients with atrial fibrillation has been discovered to have the initiation of atrial fibrillation arise from foci located in the pulmonary veins.[18,19] The successful ablation of these initiating foci has been encouraging as a possible cure for this subset of atrial fibrillation. However, while the initial results have been encouraging, further study on the efficacy and short- and long-term complications of this procedure is still needed. In order to map the site of these initiating foci, one

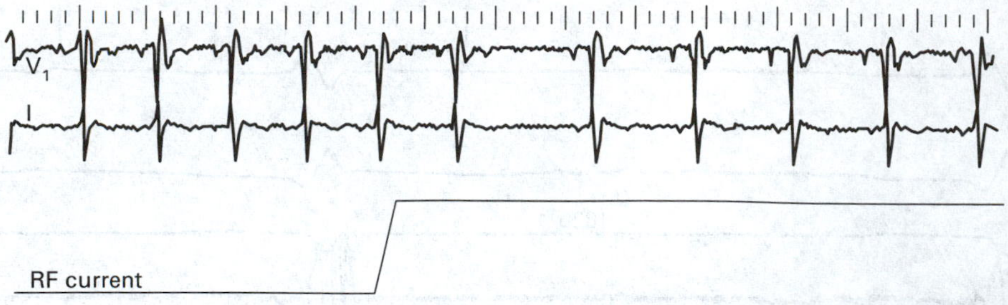

FIGURE 28-6 Same patient as in Fig. 28-5 showing application of radiofrequency energy with abrupt termination of the atrial tachycardia.

or more multipolar catheters are positioned in the different pulmonary veins via a transseptal puncture. These catheters are then used to map the earliest signal arising from the pulmonary veins that initiate either atrial fibrillation or atrial premature beats as a surrogate of atrial fibrillation. Criteria to predict successful sites of ablation while limiting complications including that of pulmonary vein stenosis are still being developed.

Modification of Sinus Node Function in Patients with Inappropriate Sinus Tachycardia

Patients with inappropriate sinus tachycardia have a resting tachycardia with abrupt increases in rate with mild exertion.[20] Typically, the arrhythmia shows diurnal variation, with slowing to normal rates at night. These patients have an increased intrinsic heart rate and excessive response to exercise or catecholamines.[20] Catheter-ablative techniques have been introduced that allow for identification of the most rapid pacemaker region of the sinus node complex.[21] This is usually found over the superior crest of the crista terminalis. One or more radiofrequency lesions are placed in this area, producing dramatic decreases in the sinus rate.[22] In addition, when this procedure is successful, there is marked attenuation of the heart rate response to exercise or catecholamines. However, narrowing of the superior vena cava–right atrium junction has been reported,[23] and the long-term follow-up of these patients may not be as encouraging as previously thought.

Ablation of Ventricular Tachycardia Foci

One of the most demanding of the catheter-ablative techniques is attempted ablation of foci initiating ventricular tachycardia. For this procedure, multipolar electrode catheters are inserted into the right ventricle, coronary sinus, and left ventricle. Ventricular tachycardia is induced by using standard stimulation protocols, and the catheters are manipulated within the ventricles to determine the earliest ventricular endocardial electrogram (during ventricular tachycardia) in relation to at least three reference orthogonal surface leads.[24] Ventricular overdrive pacing is used in an attempt to entrain the tachycardia and to prove that the earliest endocardial potentials precede (rather than follow) the tachycardia complex. In addition, the putative focus of ventricular tachycardia is paced in an effort to determine whether the paced complexes are identical or similar to the induced tachycardia.[25] The latter procedure is known as *pace mapping*. For patients with ventricular tachycardia due to coronary artery disease, concealed entrainment is manifest by a prolonged paced spike to QRS, a paced QRS identical to spontaneous tachycardia, and a postpacing interval identical to the spontaneous ventricular tachycardia cycle length, which appears to best identify the critical slow zone for the ventricular tachycardia reentrant circuit.[26] Once the putative isthmus is found, one or more radiofrequency applications are delivered from the distal electrode near this endocardial site to a chest-wall patch.

A subset of patients with ventricular tachycardia and structural heart disease particularly amenable to catheter ablation are those with bundle-branch reentrant arrhythmias. These patients are recognized by having a left intraventricular conduction delay or a frank pattern of left bundle-branch block. The majority have an associated cardiomyopathy, and all have prolonged infranodal conduction. In these patients, the tachycardic mechanism involves bundle-to-bundle conduction.[27] Catheter cure may be achieved by ablation of the right bundle branch. The right bundle usually is draped superficially over the right septal surface, and the right bundle potential usually is located easily. The right bundle may be ablated either by direct current or preferably by radiofrequency discharges.[27] Even after successful ablation of the right bundle branch, further electrophysiologic testing is in order to exclude ventricular tachycardia emanating from myocardial sources.

Other forms of ventricular tachycardia that may be particularly amenable to catheter ablation are those occurring in patients without structural cardiac disease. These patients present with tachycardia emanating from either the right ventricular outflow tract[28] or from the inferior left septum.[29] Patients with tachycardia emanating from the right ventricular outflow show a pattern of left bundle-branch block with an inferior axis. The arrhythmia is often exercise-induced and may respond to carotid massage or treatment with adenosine or beta blockers. This arrhythmia is thought to be a cyclic AMP–dependent triggered arrhythmia. The hallmark of proper ablation includes detection of early areas in the outflow tract and a precise correspondence between the paced map and spontaneous ventricular tachycardia. Another important site of ventricular tachycardia in normal hearts may emanate from the left apical septum. This arrhythmia is characterized by a pattern of right bundle-branch block associated with a left superior axis. This arrhythmia most often responds to intravenous verapamil. Ablative approaches include recording a Purkinje potential just in front of the QRS complex and/or a paced map that corresponds to the spontaneous tachycardia.

RESULTS OF CATHETER-ABLATIVE PROCEDURES

AV Junctional Ablation

In 1998, the largest prospective study in the United States relating to the various ablative procedures was gathered from the voluntary ablation registry of NASPE[30] (Tables 28-1 and 28-2). At present, AV junctional ablation is performed using radiofre-

TABLE 28-1 Results of Catheter Ablation from NASPE Voluntary Registry, 1998

	AVJ Ablation	Accessory Pathway Ablation LFW	RFW	Septal	AVNRT	Atrial Flutter	Atrial Tachycardia	IAST
Total performed	629	418	83	186	1197	477	227	42
Percent success	98.2	93.8	96.4	84.0	96.1	85.8	72.7	71.4
Significant complications, number (%)	6 (0.9)	26 (6.2)	3 (3.6)	6 (11.1)	27 (2.20)	13 (2.54)	7 (2.99)	2 (4.65)

ABBREVIATIONS: LFW, left free wall; RFW, right free wall; AVNRT, atrioventricular node reentrant tachycardia; IAST, inappropriate sinus node tachycardia.
SOURCE: Unpublished data from NASPE Voluntary Registry, 1998.

quency energy application, with a success rate of 98.2 percent and very infrequent complications. The most serious complication is postprocedure death, which occurred in 1 of 629 patients undergoing ablation. The death was due to loss of pacemaker capture after the procedure.

Ablation of Accessory Pathways

In the NASPE voluntary registry,[30] ablation of accessory pathways was attempted in 654 patients. The overall rate of successful ablation for left-sided pathways was 94 percent, as compared with a success rate of 96 percent for right free wall and 84 percent for septal accessory pathways. Significant complications, including 4 procedure-related deaths, occurred in 1.8 percent of patients. The major complications reported were hematoma/bleeding (12 patients), cardiac tamponade (7 patients), inadvertent heart block (5 patients), and damage to the coronary arteries, including a patient who required angioplasty.

Ablation for Patients with AV Node Reentry

The largest reported series of patients undergoing catheter treatment of AV node reentry again comes from the NASPE voluntary registry,[30] which included 1197 patients who underwent ablation of a slow pathway. The success rate was 96 percent in these patients, with the development of inadvertent AV block in only 4 patients (0.33 percent).

Ablation of Atrial Flutter/Atrial Tachycardia

A total of 477 patients underwent attempted flutter ablation in the NASPE registry. The reported success rate for flutter was 85 percent and for atrial tachycardia (227 patients) 72 percent. Reported complications included development of complete AV block (3 patients) and cardiac tamponade (3 patients).

TABLE 28-2 Results of Catheter Ablation for Ventricular Tachycardia from NASPE Voluntary Registry, 1998

	VT with CAD	VT with Cardiomyopathy	VT with Structurally Normal Heart
Total performed	53	42	119
Success (%)	58.5	61.9	84.9

ABBREVIATIONS: VT, ventricular tachycardia.
SOURCE: Unpublished data from NASPE Voluntary Registry, 1998.

Ablation of Focal Atrial Fibrillation

To date, in the published series of patients who have undergone ablation of focal atrial fibrillation, no recurrence of atrial fibrillation has been reported in 62 and 86 percent of patients in 8- and 6-month follow-up periods.[18,19] Reported complications[19,32] have included cerebral transient ischemic attacks (2 patients), hemothorax (1 patient), hemopericardium (1 patient), and pulmonary vein stenosis (5 patients).

Ablation of Ventricular Tachycardia

Successful ablation was more frequent in those with ventricular tachycardia associated with no structural heart disease (85 percent), including those with right ventricular outflow tract tachycardia or left septal tachycardia, compared with ablation for ventricular tachycardia associated with coronary artery disease (58 percent) or idiopathic cardiomyopathy (62 percent).[30] Major complications included a post-procedural death from presumed respiratory failure and cardiac tamponade, pulmonary edema, systemic emboli, AV block, and femoral artery thrombosis.

ADVANTAGES AND DISADVANTAGES OF CATHETER-ABLATIVE TECHNIQUES

Advantages

The use of catheter-ablative techniques has greatly affected our approach to the management of patients with supraventricular tachycardia. Catheter ablation of the AV junction has replaced the need for surgical ablation of the His bundle for patients with atrial arrhythmias refractory to drug therapy. Furthermore, use of catheter procedures allows cure of patients with reentrant supraventricular arrhythmias. The initial reports suggest a cure rate of 90 to 100 percent with minimal serious adverse effects.[31] For selected patients with ventricular tachycardia, catheter-ablative procedures may obviate the need for surgical intervention. This is particularly true for patients with bundle-branch reentry or for those with right ventricular outflow tract or left septal tachycardias.

Disadvantages

The chief disadvantage of AV junctional ablation is the need for chronic cardiac pacing after successful ablation. Another serious adverse effect is the reported 2 to 4 percent incidence of polymorphous ventricular tachycardia occurring in the post-ablative period.[33] This arrhythmia is more common in patients with severe myocardial disease, bradycardia, and electrolyte abnormalities, and may be prevented by temporarily pacing the heart at relatively fast rates immediately after ablation. The chief complication reported for patients undergoing AV modification procedures for AV nodal reentry is the risk of complete AV block. Attempted ablation of the slow AV nodal pathway promises to diminish or obviate this risk.

The risks of catheter ablation of accessory pathways appears to be related to the pathway site. Reported complications for left free wall pathways include the risk of systemic embolization, tamponade, or damage to the left circumflex coronary artery. Ablation of septal pathways carries the risk of causing inadvertent complete AV block. Fortunately, the risk of significant complications appears to be on the order of approximately 2 percent.

Major complications have been reported in the use of catheter-ablation treatment of ventricular tachycardia. Such complications include the risk of cerebrovascular accidents, damage to the aortic valve, or tamponade.

CONCLUSION

The introduction of catheter-ablative techniques has completely revolutionized our approach to the management of patients with supraventricular tachycardia. These techniques have evolved to the point where curative ablative procedures are recommended as the treatment of choice for all symptomatic patients with tachycardias mediated by accessory pathways or with atrial flutter and for most patients with symptomatic AV nodal reentrant tachycardia. Complete AV junctional ablation is the procedure of choice for those with drug-refractory atrial arrhythmias, whereas selected patients with ventricular arrhythmias may benefit from catheter-ablative techniques; however, the vast majority of these patients are best managed by drugs, devices, or surgical therapy.

References

1. Gonzalez R, Scheinman M, Margaretten W, Rubinstein M. Closed-chest electrode-catheter technique for His bundle ablation in dogs. *Am J Physiol* 1981; 241:H283–H287.
2. Scheinman MM, Morady F, Hess DS, Gonzalez R. Catheter-induced ablation of the atrioventricular junction to control refractory supraventricular arrhythmias. *JAMA* 1982; 248:851–855.
3. Gallagher JJ, Svenson RH, Kasell JH, et al. Catheter technique for closed-chest ablation of the atrioventricular conduction system: A therapeutic alternative for the treatment of refractory supraventricular tachycardia. *N Engl J Med* 1982; 306:194–200.
4. Williamson BD, Man KC, Daoud E, et al. Radiofrequency catheter modification of atrioventricular conduction to control the ventricular rate during atrial fibrillation. *N Engl J Med* 1994; 331:910–917.
5. Della Bella P, Carbucicchio C, Tondo C, Riva S. Modulation of atrioventricular conduction by ablation of the "slow" atrioventricular node pathway in patients with drug-refractory atrial fibrillation or flutter. *J Am Coll Cardiol* 1995; 25:39–46.
6. Morady F, Hasse C, Strickberger A, et al. Long-term follow-up after radiofrequency modification of the atrioventricular node in patients with atrial fibrillation. *J Am Coll Cardiol* 1997; 27:113–121.
7. Gallagher JJ, Gilbert M, Swenson RH, et al. Wolff-Parkinson-White syndrome: The problem, evaluation, and surgical correction. *Circulation* 1975; 51:767–785.
8. Gallagher JJ, Sealy WC, Cox JL, Kasell JH. Results of surgery for preexcitation in 200 consecutive cases. In: Levy S, Scheinman MM, eds. *Cardiac Arrhythmias: From Diagnosis to Therapy*. Mt. Kisco, NY: Futura; 1984:323–340.
9. Fisher JD, Brodman R, Kim SG, et al. Attempted nonsurgical electrical ablation of accessory pathways via the coronary sinus in the Wolff-Parkinson-White syndrome. *J Am Coll Cardiol* 1984; 4:685–694.
10. Jackman WM, Wang XH, Friday KJ, et al. Catheter ablation of accessory atrioventricular pathways (Wolff-Parkinson-White syndrome) by radiofrequency current. *N Engl J Med* 1991; 324:1605–1611.
11. Lesh MD, Van Hare GF, Scheinman MM, et al. Comparison of the retrograde and transseptal methods for ablation of left free wall accessory pathways. *J Am Coll Cardiol* 1993; 22:542–549.
12. Lee MA, Morady F, Kadish A, et al. Catheter modification of the atrioventricular junction with radiofrequency energy for control of atrioventricular nodal reentry tachycardia. *Circulation* 1991; 83:827–835.
13. Roman CA, Wang X, Friday KJ, et al. Catheter technique for selective ablation of slow pathway in AV nodal reentrant tachycardia (abstract). *PACE* 1990; 13:498.
14. Olgin JE, Kalman JM, Fitzpatrick AP, Lesh MD. Role of right atrial endocardial structures as barriers to conduction during human type I atrial flutter: Activation and entrainment mapping guided by intracardiac echocardiography. *Circulation* 1995; 92:1839–1848.
15. Saxon LA, Kalman JM, Olgin JE, et al. Results of catheter ablation for atrial flutter. *Am J Cardiol* 1995; 26:431–438.
16. Tracy CM, Swartz JF, Fletcher RD, et al. Radiofrequency catheter ablation of ectopic atrial tachycardia using paced activation sequence mapping. *J Am Coll Cardiol* 1993; 21:910–917.
17. Tang CW, Scheinman MM, Van Hare GF, et al. Use of P wave configuration during atrial tachycardia to predict site of origin. *J Am Coll Cardiol* 1995; 26:1315–1324.
18. Haissaguerre M, Jais P, Shah D, et al. Spontaneous initiation of atrial fibrillation by ectopic beats originating in the pulmonary veins. *N Engl J Med* 1998; 339:659–666.
19. Chen SA, Hsieh M, Tai C, et al. Initiation of atrial fibrillation by ectopic beats originating from the pulmonary veins. *Circulation* 1999; 100:1879–1886.
20. Morillo CA, Klein GJ, Thakur RK, et al. Mechanism of inappropriate sinus tachycardia: Role of sympathovagal balance. *Circulation* 1994; 90:873–877.
21. Kalman JM, Lee RJ, Fisher WG, et al. Radiofrequency catheter modification of sinus pacemaker function guided by intracardiac echocardiography. *Circulation* 1995; 92:3070–3081.
22. Lee RJ, Kalman JM, Fitzpatrick AP, et al. Radiofrequency catheter modification of the sinus node for "inappropriate" sinus tachycardia. *Circulation* 1995; 92:2919–2928.
23. Man KC, Knight B, Tse HF, et al. Radiofrequency catheter ablation of inappropriate sinus node tachycardia guided by activation mapping. *J Am Coll Cardiol* 2000; 35(2):451–457.
24. Marchlinski FE, Almendrah JM, Cassidy DM, et al. Localization of endocardial site for catheter ablation of ventricular tachycardia. In: Fontaine G, Scheinman MM, eds. *Ablation in Cardiac Arrhythmias*. Mount Kisco, NY: Futura; 1987:289–302.
25. Josephson ME, Waxman HL, Cain ME, et al. Ventricular activation during ventricular endocardial pacing: II. Role of pace mapping to localize origin of ventricular tachycardia. *Am J Cardiol* 1982; 50:11–22.

26. Stevenson WG, Weiss JN, Weiner I, et al. Resetting of ventricular tachycardia: Implications for localizing the area of slow conduction. *J Am Coll Cardiol* 1988; 11:522.
27. Tchou P, Jazayeri M, Denker S, et al. Transcatheter electrical ablation of right bundle branch: A method of treating macroreentrant ventricular tachycardia attributed to bundle branch reentry. *Circulation* 1988; 78:246–257.
28. Klein LS, Shih H-T, Hackett FK, et al. Radiofrequency catheter ablation of ventricular tachycardia in patients without structural heart disease. *Circulation* 1992; 85:1666.
29. Coggins DL, Lee RJ, Sweeney J, et al. Radiofrequency catheter ablation as a cure for idiopathic tachycardia of both left and right ventricular origin. *J Am Coll Cardiol* 1994; 23:1333–1341.
30. Scheinman MM. NASPE Ablation Registry on catheter ablation for 1998 (unpublished data).
31. Calkins H, Sousa J, el-Atassi R, et al. Diagnosis and cure of the Wolff-Parkinson-White syndrome or paroxysmal supraventricular tachycardias during a single electrophysiologic test. *N Engl J Med* 1991; 324:1612–1618.
32. Haïssaguerre M, Jaïs P, Shah DC, et al. Electrophysiological end points for catheter ablation of atrial fibrillation initiated from multiple pulmonary venous foci. *Circulation* 2000; 101:1409–1417.
33. Geelen P, Brugada J, Andries E, et al. Ventricular fibrillation and sudden death after radiofrequency catheter ablation of the atrioventricular junction. *Pacing Clin Electrophysiol* 1997; 20 (2 pt 1):343–348.

CHAPTER 29A

PRINCIPLES OF EXTERNAL AND INTERNAL CARDIOVERSION AND DEFIBRILLATION

Bernard Lown / Regis A. DeSilva

The application of electrical current is standard treatment for termination of atrial and ventricular tachyarrhythmias in emergency situations and when these conditions are refractory to pharmacologic treatment.[1] *Cardioversion* is the discharge of electrical energy synchronized on the R wave, while *defibrillation* refers to unsynchronized discharge. Cardioversion is, by definition, a synchronized direct-current discharge; thus this term does not apply to ventricular defibrillation or to the pharmacologic reversal of arrhythmias. The standard unit of measurement is the joule (J), and 1 J equals 1 watt-second. As there may be a wide discrepancy between the stored energy level indicated on the defibrillator and the actual delivered energy, the device should be periodically checked across a standardized resistance for reliability. The electrophysiologic basis for cardioversion is probably the closure of the "excitable gap" in a reentrant electrical circuit. Abolition of the circuit for the arrhythmia may be accomplished with energy levels as low as 1 to 5 J, and this might account for the success in terminating reentrant arrhythmias such as atrial flutter and ventricular tachycardia. Defibrillation requires much higher energy levels, which may be due to the necessity for depolarizing a large number of multiple asynchronous reentrant circuits. Energy requirements for cardioversion and defibrillation may be affected by such factors as the duration of the arrhythmia, electrolyte imbalance, underlying metabolic states, and the use of antiarrhythmic drugs such as amiodarone.

PROCEDURE

Elective cardioversion should preferably be done early in the morning in the fasting state. In urgent cases, meals should be withheld for as long as possible. Serum levels for electrolytes, digoxin, blood urea nitrogen, and creatinine should be obtained and hypokalemia corrected before cardioversion is attempted. Digitalis glycosides should be withheld only on the day of cardioversion, but if digitalis toxicity is suspected, the procedure is postponed until the problem is resolved. An intravenous line is inserted, vital signs and the electrocardiogram (ECG) are monitored, and equipment for cardiopulmonary resuscitation (CPR) is made available. General anesthesia is administered via a face mask or intravenous diazepam or midazolam is used for sedation.

Synchronization with the tallest R wave on the ECG prevents accidental triggering of ventricular fibrillation (VF); (see Fig. 29B-1) resynchronization should be checked after each discharge, as the device may revert to the default setting for defibrillation. Improper synchronization may occur when there is bundle-branch block with a tall R wave, when the T wave is highly peaked, and with artifactual spikes from a malfunctioning pacemaker. Electrodes are placed in either an anterolateral or an anteroposterior position. The anterior electrode is placed parasternally over the right second and third intercostal spaces. The lateral electrode is positioned over the cardiac apex. If a flat posterior electrode is available, it is placed at the tip of the angle of the left scapula. Current flow in either configuration is along the long axis of the heart, encompasses the bulk of cardiac tissue and minimizes travel through high-impedance bony tissue. Electrode paste, with firm pressure on the paddles, should be used to provide adequate electrical contact and reduce transthoracic impedance. Bridging of the electrodes by conductive paste should be avoided, as this will reduce the amount of energy delivered to the heart. Pregelled adhesive electrodes may also be used in the positions described above. Prior to discharge, cardiopulmonary resuscitation (CPR) should be stopped and an "All clear" signal should be given to avoid the accidental shocking of attendants. Defibrillator waveforms are discussed in Chap. 29B.

Energy titration reduces both energy use and complications. The initial setting may be as low as 10 J, as this may be successful for atrial flutter and stable ventricular tachycardia. Energy output is increased progressively to 25, 50, 100, 200, and 360 J. Lead II of the ECG is monitored to determine whether normal sinus rhythm (NSR) has been reestablished. If serious ventricular arrhythmias emerge after a discharge, especially if digitalis toxicity is suspected, the procedure is discontinued. Alternatively, xylocaine may be administered prophylactically before the next discharge and cardioversion cautiously continued. Following cardioversion, a proper airway is maintained and adequate ventilation delivered until recovery from anesthesia occurs. Vital signs and cardiac rhythm are monitored for at least 24 h to detect the late emergence of malignant ventricular arrhythmias or recurrence of the underlying arrhythmia.

TREATMENT OF SPECIFIC ARRHYTHMIAS

Atrial Fibrillation

Approximately 50 percent of patients admitted to hospital for atrial fibrillation (AF) will revert spontaneously to normal sinus rhythm (NSR) within 48 h.[2] Cardioversion is the treatment of choice if spontaneous or pharmacologic reversion to NSR does not occur, if the patient is symptomatic with chest pain during myocardial infarction, or during rapid ventricular rates in preexcitation syndrome when VF may supervene. Normal rhythm following cardioversion obviates the need for long-term anticoagulation. There is also a decrease in fatigue, increase in exercise capacity, and improvement in cerebral blood flow. Both physical and electrical remodeling occurring with AF may be reversed following cardioversion, with changes in right and left atrial volumes.[3,4] Treatment with sotalol, quinidine, disopyramide, or verapamil for at least 48 h before cardioversion may prevent early recurrence. Success of cardioversion in maintaining NSR is dependent on factors such as the duration of arrhythmia, the size of the left atrium, underlying conduction system disease, presence of valvular heart disease, and the patient's age. Overall, the success rate is over 90 percent using 200 J or less and the mean energy level required is 87 J (see also Chap. 29B). The use of atropine to abolish high vagal tone facilitates reversion to NSR.[5] Infusion of ibutelide promotes reversion to NSR experimentally. The use of high-energy cardioversion with 720 J has also been described for refractory AF.[6] Recurrence of arrhythmia is predicted by a left atrial size of 45 mm or greater and a less than 10 percent increase in the *a* wave on Doppler echocardiography following cardioversion.[7]

Higher energy levels may be required to terminate AF in congestive heart failure. Treatment of heart failure before cardioversion will increase the success rate. Acute myocardial infarction is not a contraindication to cardioversion and, in fact, prompt reversion will help prevent infarct extension by decreasing heart rate and reducing oxygen consumption. In patients with conduction system disease, emergence of atrial ectopic activity, severe sinus bradycardia, sinus arrest, junctional rhythm, or multifocal atrial tachycardia may follow cardioversion, with gradual restoration of NSR. In such cases, atropine or isoproterenol treatment may be required. If conduction system disease is suspected (e.g., a slow ventricular response in the absence of drug treatment), a temporary pacemaker is inserted prior to cardioversion, as asystole may result following the shock. Energy titration, as described earlier, anticipates this complication, and if pacing is not available, cardioversion should be abandoned if the first few discharges evoke severe bradyarrhythmia.

Cardioversion may not benefit patients with severe mitral valve disease who have "giant" scarred atria, those with mitral valve replacement, and patients with chronic recurrent paroxysmal atrial tachyarrhythmias. Although successful low-energy internal cardioversion can be performed and implantable devices are available for long-term treatment of AF, these methods are rarely indicated and seldom justified.

Thromboembolism is a major risk of atrial fibrillation resulting from stasis and inadequate emptying of the left atrial appendage and low transmitral flow velocity. Anticoagulation reduces the incidence of emboli and is recommended in the absence of contraindications.[8,9] Warfarin is started a minimum of 3 weeks before cardioversion to maintain a prothrombin time of 1.3 to 1.5 times the control value, or an International Normalized Ratio (INR) of 2.0–3.0. Treatment is maintained for 4 weeks after cardioversion because delayed embolism may occur. Such embolism may result if there is delayed resumption of atrial activity due to "stunning" after successful cardioversion of AF. Doppler echocardiography is useful in documenting the presence of atrial contraction, as the absence of an atrial *a* wave suggests electromechanical dissociation.[7] Anticoagulation beyond 4 weeks may be indicated in the presence of recurrent bouts of AF, prosthetic valves, or cardiomyopathy or if there is a history of previous embolization or stroke.

In cases where AF is known to be of acute onset (i.e., <24 h) or in emergency situations, cardioversion may be performed without long-term anticoagulation. Heparin is started and simultaneous treatment with warfarin may be necessary, as AF may recur or embolization may occur later due to delayed resumption of atrial contraction. In elective cases, the absence of thrombus documented by transesophageal echocardiography (TEE) is not an adequate reason to withhold anticoagulation as it does not protect the patient from the risk of thromboembolism.[10–13] Because of differences in sophistication of the equipment used for TEE, patient selection, and conflicting data, absence of intraatrial clot by TEE cannot be recommended as the standard for decision making prior to cardioversion.[12] Late embolic complications result from one of three possible mechanisms: delayed resumption of atrial mechanical activity due to stunning of the atria, formation of clots after cardioversion during sinus rhythm, or relapse of AF. In 98 percent of cases, embolization occurs within 10 days of cardioversion.[14] If warfarin is contraindicated, aspirin may be utilized, but there is no persuasive evidence that such treatment protects against embolism during or following cardioversion.

Atrial Flutter

If drug treatment with an agent such propafenone or sotalol is unsuccessful, cardioversion is the treatment of choice for this arrhythmia. In many cases, the arrhythmia does not recur and maintenance of drug treatment may be unnecessary. The arrhythmia is often benign unless there is 1:1 atrioventricular conduction, when syncope may occur. Low-energy shocks easily revert atrial flutter to sinus rhythm. The mean energy level generally required is 25 J, and in 95 percent of cases 50 J or less suffices. Anticoagulation should be administered before and after cardioversion, as for AF, because of the risk of embolism.

Supraventricular Tachycardia

Because this arrhythmia is often responsive to vagal maneuvers and/or to several antiarrhythmic drugs, cardioversion is only rarely necessary for reversion. If such treatment fails, cardioversion with energy levels between 100 and 360 J is required. In paroxysmal atrial tachycardia with block due to digitalis intoxication, cardioversion is extremely hazardous, as VF and death may result. When digitalis toxicity is suspected, energy titration is cautiously attempted, with xylocaine pretreatment for ventricular arrhythmia if necessary. If low-energy discharges provoke high grades of arrhythmia or atrioventricular block, cardioversion is discontinued.

Ventricular Tachycardia

When a chest thump and intravenous xylocaine or procainamide fail to terminate ventricular tachycardia (VT), cardioversion should be performed promptly. Unless the arrhythmia is clinically unstable, sedation is administered. Energy titration is performed in stable VT and as little of 1 to 5 J may succeed; in 90 percent of cases, 10 J or less is successful in terminating the arrhythmia. Only rarely is more than 100 J necessary. When VT is rapid and the QRS complex and T wave indistinguishable, or if the patient becomes syncopal due to hemodynamic deterioration, an unsynchronized discharge of 100 J is delivered immediately. If this attempt fails, discharges of 200, 300, and 360 J should be administered consecutively until sinus rhythm is restored. Polymorphic VT and torsades de pointes, which are not self-terminating or responsive to drugs, may be similarly treated.

Ventricular Fibrillation

Unsynchronized discharge is the treatment of choice for VF and is performed using a standard defibrillator or an automatic external defibrillator (AED). This setting is also used for "blind defibrillation" in an unmonitored patient in cardiac arrest; the electrode positions are similar to those used for cardioversion. The procedure for defibrillation is delivery of an initial shock of 200 J following institution of CPR, followed by a second 200- or 300-J shock and a third 360-J shock if VF persists. If these attempts fail, 0.5 to 1.0 mg of intravenous epinephrine is given and defibrillation at 360 J is attempted again. There is no clear evidence that there is a relationship between body weight and energy requirements for defibrillation. For children, 1 to 2 J/kg is recommended; in small children and infants, a little as 10 J might suffice.

A variety of lightweight AEDs using either damped sinusoidal or monophasic truncated exponential waveforms, with varying types of hardware and software, are now available.[15–17] These devices include features such as strip-chart recorders, screen displays, and voice-synthesizer messages for the operator and devices to record the ECG and the voices of the operators. These defibrillators are equipped with computerized algorithms that recognize VF or rapid VT, permitting automatic or semiautomatic firing of the device within 8 to 10 s. These devices are intended for use in the field, where highly trained personnel are not available and therapeutic options are limited. Adhesive defibrillator pads are attached to the patient's chest in the position suggested for standard defibrillation. Resuscitative maneuvers are stopped and radio transmitters and receivers not operated during initial signal recording so as to prevent interference. Signal recognition may take up to 15 s before the defibrillator discharges; prior to this the device will automatically announce the imminent delivery of a shock by providing a printed message, a visual alarm, or a voice statement so that the attendants are not accidentally shocked. Following delivery of the first shock, CPR is not reinstituted so that the device can accomplish signal analysis and deliver additional shocks if necessary. Following successful termination of ventricular fibrillation, the airway is kept clear of secretions and vomitus, adequate ventilation with supplemental oxygen is continued, and the patient is monitored in an appropriate setting for further management. If defibrillation occurs outside of a medical facility, the patient is intubated if necessary, hemodynamically stabilized, and transported to a hospital as soon as possible.

The major determinant of success or failure of defibrillation relates to the time elapsed between the onset of cardiac arrest and defibrillation. Failure to terminate VF may be due to operator error or due to irreversibility of the underlying condition. In refractory VF, correction of hypoxia, acid-base imbalance, and electrolyte derangements as well as administration of isoproterenol (to convert fine-grain fibrillation to coarse-grain fibrillation) all render successful defibrillation more likely. If this approach is unsuccessful, rapid serial delivery of two or three 360-J shocks may succeed owing to reduction in transthoracic impedance following consecutive shocks. Rarely, fine-grain fibrillation may appear as asystole on a monitor and defibrillation should be attempted. In this setting, automatic defibrillators may fail to trigger a discharge. Current-based defibrillation (rather than an energy-based system) delivering approximately 30 to 40 A per shock has been advocated to increase success rates.[17–19] Automatic measurement of transthoracic impedance (ranging from 70 to 80 ohms in adults) before delivery of the shock avoids delivery of high currents in patients with low chest impedance and low currents in those with high impedance. Thus, success rates for defibrillation may be increased and cardiac damage minimized. If all defibrillation attempts fail to revive the patient, a rapid and thorough assessment of the resuscitative and defibrillation procedures is necessary to check for errors, such as improper electrode placement and the use of inappropriate energy levels. With AEDs, it is essential to check for proper contact of the defibrillator pads and for proper signal analysis. If, however, no errors are detected and if the patient is unresponsive, a decision about terminating resuscitation is warranted, as severe brain damage occurs with prolonged resuscitation.

COMPLICATIONS

Morphologic and functional cardiac damage may follow the use of high-energy shocks. Creatine kinase elevation following electrical discharge is transient, derives from skeletal muscle, and usually does not mask the diagnosis of acute myocardial infarction. Intracellular potassium is released from electrical trauma and may contribute to the intractability of ventricular fibrillation. Hyperkalemia may result from repeated high-energy shocks. The occurrence of postcardioversion ventricular arrhythmias is related to the presence of hypokalemia, digitalis toxicity, severe heart disease, improper synchronization, and the repeated use of high-energy discharges. Asystole and cardiac arrest are rare and occur when there is severe conduction system disease. When VF occurs several hours after cardioversion, it may be due to toxicity from digoxin, quinidine, or other antiarrhythmic agents.

Pulmonary edema following cardioversion occurs most often in the presence of mitral or aortic valvular disease or left ventricular dysfunction. It may also relate to electrically induced alterations in myocardial function, fluid overload, delayed return of atrial function, and pulmonary embolism. The risk of systemic embolization has already been discussed. Unexplained hypotension, possibly due to vasodilation, sometimes occurs after cardioversion; fluid replacement will usually correct this problem.

In the presence of implanted cardioverter-defibrillators (ICD) and pacemakers, defibrillator electrodes should be placed at least 12 cm from the generator before discharge to prevent temporary or permanent malfunction. Additionally, the metal generator may absorb electrical energy and reduce the effectiveness of the discharge. Following cardioversion or defibrillation, pacing thresholds may increase due to myocardial burns caused by transmission of electrical energy to the paced site. Because the pacing threshold may increase gradually over weeks with subsequent loss of capture by the pacemaker, serial threshold measurements should be checked not only immediately following discharge but also for 2 months afterward.

Cardioversion has been safely performed during pregnancy and fetal death has not been reported as a direct consequence of treatment. Nonetheless, fetal monitoring with an obstetrician in consultation is appropriate in this situation. Despite the possible complications described with the use of electrical energy, cardioversion and defibrillation have been performed for several decades now with a high degree of safety.

The implantable atrial defibrillator is discussed in Chap. 29B.

References

1. Lown B. Electrical reversion of cardiac arrhythmias. *Br Heart J* 1967; 29:469–489.
2. Dell'Orfano JT, Patel H, Wolbrette DL, et al. Acute treatment of atrial fibrillation: Spontaneous conversion rates and cost of care. *Am J Cardiol* 1999; 83:788–790.
3. Yu WC, Tai CT, Hsieh MH, et al. Reversal of atrial electrical remodeling following cardioversion of long-standing atrial fibrillation in man. *Cardiovasc Res* 1999; 42:470–476.
4. Gosselink AT, Crijns HJ, Hamer HP. Changes in left and right atrial size after cradioversion of atrial fibrillation: Role of mitral valve disease. *J Am Coll Cardiol* 1993; 22:1666–1672.
5. Sutton AGC, Khurana C, Hall JA, et al. The use of atropine for facilitation of direct current cardioversion from atrial fibrillation—Results of a pilot study. *Clin Cardiol* 1999; 22:712–714.
6. Saliba W, Juratli SW, Chung MK, et al. Higher energy synchronized external direct current cardioversion for refractory atrial fibrillation. *J Am Coll Cardiol* 1999; 34:2031–2034.
7. Dethy M, Chassat C, Roy D, et al. Doppler echocardiographic predictors of recurrence of atrial fibrillation. *Am J Cardiol* 1988; 62:723–726.
8. DeSilva RA, Graboys TB, Podrid PJ, et al. Cardioversion and defibrillation. *Am Heart J* 1980; 100:881–895.
9. Laupacis A, Albers G, Dalen J, et al. Antithrombotic therapy in atrial fibrillation. *Chest* 1998; 114(suppl 5):579S–589S.
10. Black IW, Fatkin D, Sagar KB et al. Exclusion of atrial thrombus by transesophageal echocardiography does not preclude embolism after cardioversion of atrial fibrillation: A multicenter study. *Circulation* 1994; 89:2509–2513.
11. Fatkin D, Kuchar DL. Transesophageal echocardiography before and during direct current cardioversion of atrial fibrillation: Evidence for "atrial stunning" as a mechanism of thromboembolic complications. *J Am Coll Cardiol* 1994; 23:307–316.
12. Stöllberger C, Chnupa P, Kronik G, et al. Transesophageal echocardiography to assess embolic risk in patients with atrial fibrillation. *Ann Intern Med* 1998; 630–638.
13. Silverman DI, Manning WJ. Role of echocardiography in patients undergoing elective cardioversion of atrial fibrillation. *Circulation* 1998; 98:479–486.
14. Berger M, Schweitzer P. Timing of thromboembolic events after electrical cardioversion of atrial fibrillation or flutter: A retrospective analysis *Am J Cardiol* 1998; 82:1545–1547.
15. Kerber RE, Becker LB, Bourland JD, et al. Automatic external defibrillators for public access: Recommendations for specifying and reporting arrhythmia analysis algorithm performance, incorporating new waveforms, and enhancing safety. *Circulation* 1997; 95:1677–1682.
16. Weisfeldt ML, Kerber RE, McGoldrick P, et al. *American Heart Association Report on the Public Access Defibrillation Conference,* December 8–10, 1994. *Circulation* 1995; 92:2740–2747.
17. Cummins RO, ed. *Advanced Cardiac Life Support* (manual). Dallas: American Heart Association; 1997:4-11–4-22.
18. Kerber RE, Martins JB, Kienzle MG, et al. Energy, current and success in defibrillation and cardioversion: Clinical studies using an automated impedance-based method of energy adjustment. *Circulation* 1988; 77:1038–1046.
19. Lerman BB, DiMarco JP, Haines DE. Current-based versus energy-based ventricular defibrillation: A prospective study. *J Am Coll Cardiol* 1988; 12:1259–1264.

CHAPTER 29B

CLINICAL APPLICATION OF EXTERNAL AND INTERNAL CARDIOVERSION AND DEFIBRILLATION

Carl Timmermans / Luz-Maria Rodriguez / Hein J. J. Wellens

Electricity was first applied to the heart in 1775 when Abildgaard used electric current both to stun and to revive animals.[1] The first successful human ventricular defibrillation was reported by Beck in 1947.[2] Cardioversion of atrial fibrillation to sinus rhythm by a synchronized direct current shock was introduced by Lown in 1962[3] (see Chap. 29A). Nowadays, the application of electric current is a standard treatment for termination of atrial and ventricular tachyarrhythmias. *Cardioversion* refers to the discharge of electrical energy synchronized on the R wave, whereas *defibrillation* refers to an unsynchronized discharge. Further progress in the electrical treatment of tachyarrhythmias was made when external defibrillation paddles or skin patches were replaced by internal defibrillation electrodes (or patches) and when biphasic, instead of monophasic sinusoidal, defibrillator waveforms were used (see also Chap. 29A).

EXTERNAL CARDIOVERSION AND DEFIBRILLATION

Technique

After the procedure has been explained to the patient, a physical examination should be performed prior to elective external cardioversion. Patients should be cardioverted in a fasting state. The serum potassium level should be normal. Knowledge of renal function is helpful in guiding the dosage of adjunctive medication. If there is clinical or electrocardiographic suspicion of digitalis toxicity, the procedure needs to be postponed. The use of anticoagulation is discussed in the section "Treatment of Specific Arrhythmias," below. The patient should have a reliable intravenous access, and dentures should be removed. A short-acting anesthetic or sedative agent (preferably with amnesic effects, e.g., midazolam) is administrated by a qualified physician. The cardioversion should be carried out in an area with facilities for an eventual cardiopulmonary resuscitation. A 12-lead electrocardiogram is recorded before and after the procedure, and during the cardioversion, a rhythm strip is obtained, or at least the patient's rhythm should be shown on a monitor screen. Synchronization of shock delivery with the R wave of the QRS complex is essential during cardioversion. Although properly synchronized shocks rarely, if ever, induce ventricular fibrillation, unsynchronized shocks may be delivered in the ventricular vulnerable period of the preceding beat (near the apex of the T wave) and result in ventricular fibrillation (Fig. 29B-1). The appropriateness of synchronization of each shock delivery always should be verified because a large or tall T wave or P wave, artifacts, or noise can be misidentified as the R wave. Improper synchronization also may occur when the QRS complex has a right bundle-branch block configuration with a tall secondary R wave.

The two standard electrode positions are the anterolateral and anteroposterior positions. In the anterolateral position, the anterior electrode is placed parasternally over the right second and third intercostal spaces, and the lateral electrode is placed just below the fourth intercostal space in the midaxillary line. In the anteroposterior position, the anterior electrode is placed as previously mentioned, and the posterior electrode is positioned just below the left scapula. In case of failure to terminate the arrhythmia, shock delivery can be repeated using the other electrode location. Some authors do not recommend the anterolateral position for cardioversion of atrial fibrillation because this position probably does not provide optimal current flow through the atria.[4]

Successful defibrillation and cardioversion requires sufficient flow of electric current through the appropriate chambers of the heart. Current flow is determined by the shock strength and the transthoracic impedance. Most available defibrillators have a maximum energy setting of 360 J, representing the maximal

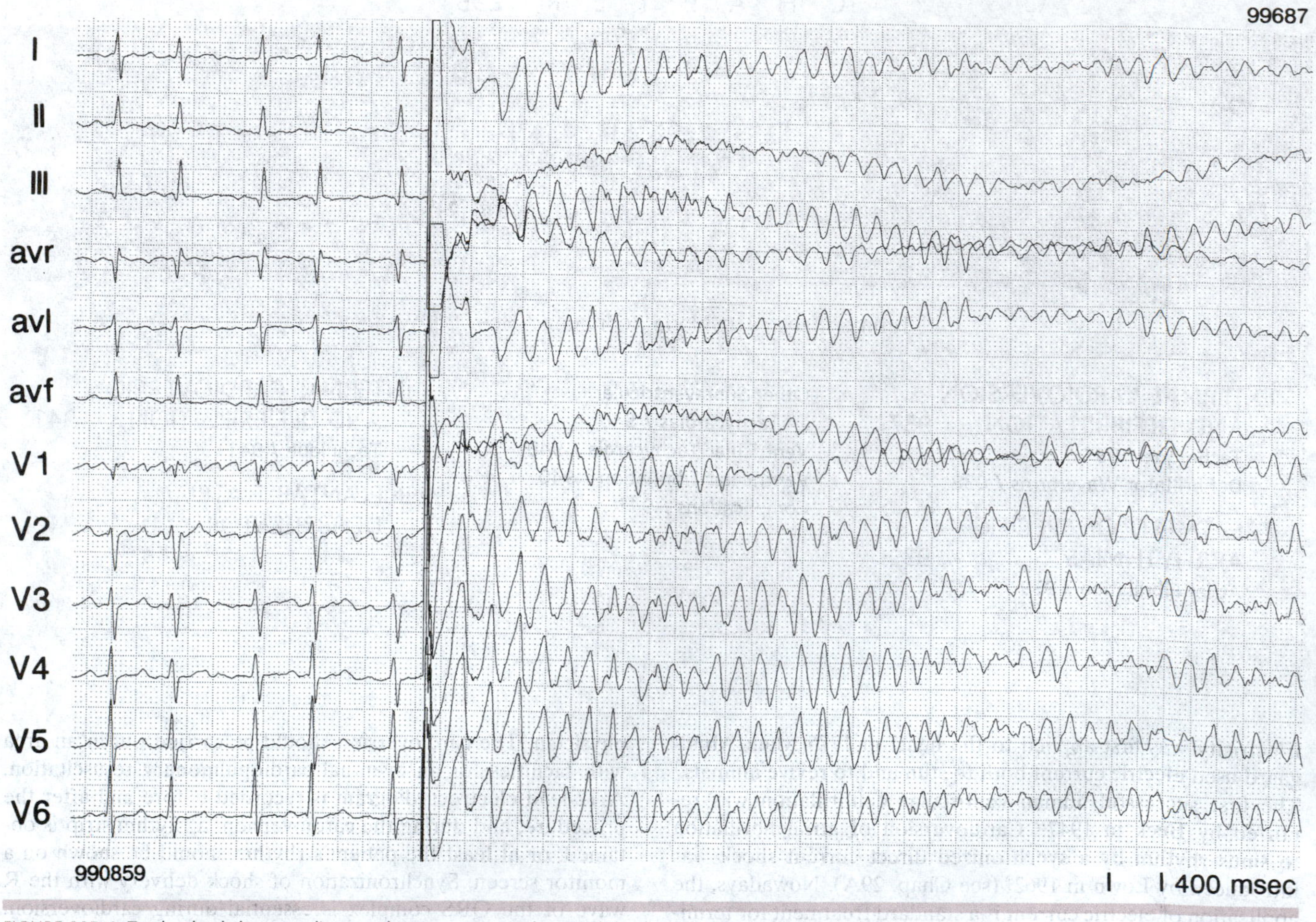

FIGURE 29B-1 Twelve-lead electrocardiogram showing an unsynchronized shock producing ventricular fibrillation in a patient who underwent internal cardioversion of atrial fibrillation.

amount of energy delivered through a 50-Ω resistance. It was determined that the transthoracic impedance in adults of a first shock of 100 J or more varies between 25 and 150 Ω, with an average of 75 Ω.[5] If the impedance is high, low-energy shocks will fail to terminate the arrhythmia. Several authors reported on the different factors that influence transthoracic impedance, including the electrode size, the distance between the electrodes, the couplant medium and pressure between the electrode and the chest wall, the phase of respiration, a recent sternotomy, and previous shocks.[4,6] Optimal electrode size seems to be 8 to 12 cm in diameter for adults. This electrode size also should be used for children weighing more than 10 kg. Wide separation of the electrodes must be maintained especially if the coupling medium is a paste or gel. In women, the lateral electrode should be placed lateral to or under the breast. Although self-adhesive disposable electrode pads have advantages in certain circumstances with high-risk cardiac patients, their slightly higher impedance makes their use not optimal in patients predisposed to a high transthoracic impedance. Firm electrode pressure with the patient in full expiration reduces transthoracic impedance and enhances the likelihood of shock success. A sternotomy reduces transthoracic impedance for at least 1 month after the procedure. Finally, impedance also lowers after repeated shock delivery.

Prior to each shock delivery, attendants should be warned in order to avoid their accidental shocking. Following cardioversion, a proper airway is maintained, and adequate ventilation is delivered until recovery from anesthesia occurs.

Defibrillator Waveforms

Alternating current was first used for ventricular defibrillation. It is a sine wave that oscillates between positive and negative polarity with a well-defined frequency (Fig. 29B-2*A*). Because of significant side effects and technical constraints, alternating current was replaced by a single-capacitor discharge or direct-current defibrillation.[7] A single-capacitor discharge generates a high-voltage peaked wave with an exponential decay (undamped exponential waveform,[3,7] see Fig. 29B-2*B*). Rounding of this initial peak using an inductor (damped capacitor discharge) gave rise to the until now most frequently used monophasic damped sinusoidal waveform for external defibrillation and cardioversion (Fig. 29B-3). Depending on the defibrillator characteristics and the impedance of the patient, the monophasic sinusoidal waveform does not oscillate between the baseline (critically damped capacitor discharge; Edmark waveform, see Fig. 29-3*A*) or has one or more terminal negative components (underdamped capacitor discharge; Lown or Gurvich waveform).[7] Less frequently, a defibrillator uses an undamped capacitor discharge with a long time constant that is then truncated

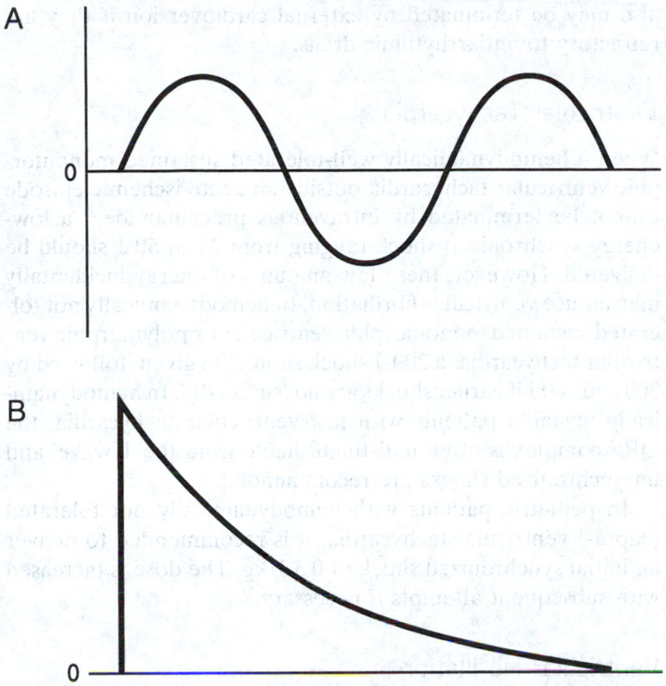

FIGURE 29B-2 *A.* Alternating current. *B.* Direct current.

so that it resembles a square or trapezoidal wave (monophasic truncated exponential waveform,[7] see Fig. 29-3*B*). Only limited clinical information is available on the effectiveness of this waveform.[8]

Due to the development of an implantable cardioverter defibrillator, biphasic waveforms have been examined in several experimental and clinical studies over the last two decades. A biphasic truncated waveform, which consists of both a positive and a negative phase (see Fig. 29-3*C*), may offer several technical advantages over a monophasic sinusoidal waveform and seems to allow external defibrillation at lower energy levels. These lower amounts of energy, together with removal of the inductor, makes an external defibrillator using a biphasic waveform small, light, cheap, and easy to maintain. In a multicenter study it was demonstrated that 115- to 130-J biphasic truncated transthoracic shocks defibrillate ventricular fibrillation as well as 200-J monophasic damped sine-wave transthoracic shocks.[9] However, in this study, the 115- or 130-J biphasic shocks appeared to be not as successful as the 360-J monophasic shocks.

Recently, low-energy impedance-compensating biphasic waveforms have been evaluated for the treatment of ventricular as well as atrial arrhythmias. These defibrillators automatically adjust the duration of the waveform for the transthoracic impedance of the patient during shock delivery.[10]

TREATMENT OF SPECIFIC ARRHYTHMIAS

Atrial Fibrillation

Because cardioversion of atrial fibrillation is a safe and effective method to restore sinus rhythm, the procedure should be attempted at least once in every patient with chronic atrial fibrillation. Furthermore, due to the proarrhythmogenic effect of antiarrhythmic drugs, cardioversion also may be preferred to the intravenous administration of these drugs in patients with symptomatic, long-standing paroxysmal atrial fibrillation. Overt congestive heart failure and hyperthyroidism should be controlled as much as possible before cardioversion. Acute myocardial infarction is not a contraindication to cardioversion; prompt restoration of sinus rhythm would help prevent infarct extension by decreasing the heart rate and reducing oxygen consumption. If atrioventricular conduction disturbances are suspected (e.g., a slow ventricular response in the absence of antiarrhythmic drug treatment), cardioversion should be avoided because asystole may result or should be performed after the insertion of a temporary transvenous pacing catheter.

The immediate success rate of external cardioversion varies between 70 and 94 percent.[3,11] This variation in outcome may be due to the use of different definitions for a successful cardioversion, other patient characteristics, and pretreatment with antiarrhythmic drugs. The probability of a successful cardioversion depends mainly on the duration of the atrial fibrillation episode.[3,11] Other factors such as the transthoracic impedance,[5] left atrial size, and the patient's age[12] are also important for acute success. The maintenance of sinus rhythm after cardioversion is less favorable. In a metaanalysis performed by Coplen et al.,[13] only 45, 33, and 25 percent of the patients who were not taking antiarrhythmic drugs remained in sinus rhythm at 3, 6, and 12

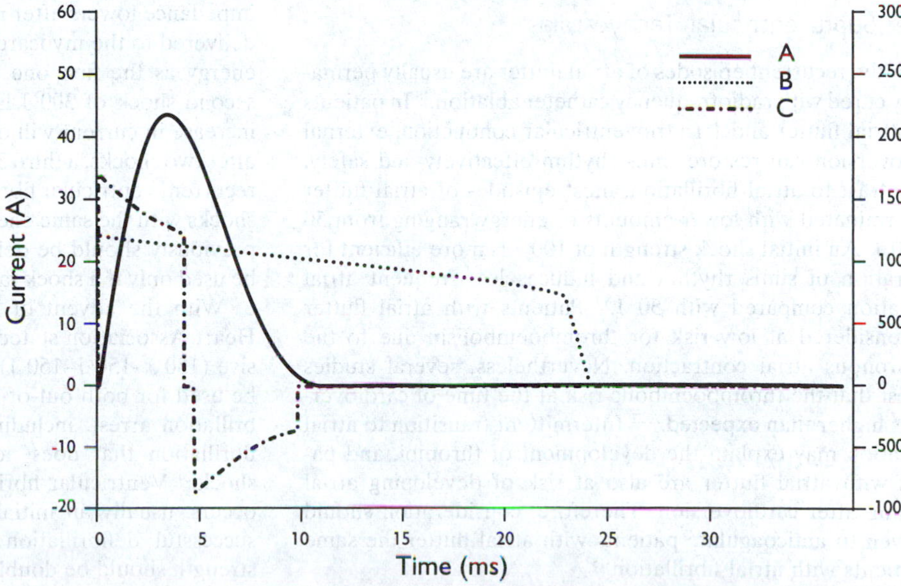

FIGURE 29B-3 Clinically used transthoracic defibrillator waveforms. *A.* Monophasic sinusoidal waveform. *B.* Monophasic truncated exponential waveform. *C.* Biphasic truncated waveform.

months after cardioversion, respectively. Although the administration of antiarrhythmic drugs prolongs to a certain extent the arrhythmia-free period after external cardioversion, use of these drugs is not without risk. Several clinical variables including etiology and duration of atrial fibrillation, age, and echocardiographic variables such as size and function of the left atrium and left atrial appendix are considered to have a certain predictive value for the recurrence of the arrhythmia.

The initial shock strength should be 100 J, followed by a second 200-J shock and a third 360-J shock if atrial fibrillation persists. In patients in whom 360 J fails to restore sinus rhythm, a second 360-J shock may be delivered again. Shocks lower than 200 J are particularly likely to be effective when the duration of atrial fibrillation is shorter than 24 h or when the patient does not have structural heart disease or is not receiving antiarrhythmic drugs.[14]

Patients undergoing electrical cardioversion are at risk for thromboembolic complications. Two mechanisms may be responsible: (1) dislodgment of a preexisting atrial thrombus after resumption of mechanical atrial activity and (2) left atrial appendage stunning or impaired function immediate after cardioversion. It is recommended for patients with atrial fibrillation of unknown or long duration that anticoagulation should be given for 3 weeks before elective cardioversion to maintain an international normalized ratio (INR) of 2.0 to 3.0. Anticoagulation should be continued for 4 weeks after successful cardioversion. It is usual clinical practice not to give anticoagulation to patients certain to have had the onset of atrial fibrillation within the preceding 24 to 48 h.[15] The absence of a thrombus documented by transesophageal echocardiography is not an adequate reason to withhold anticoagulation because it does not protect the patient from the risk for thromboembolism.[16] Even if short-term anticoagulation is combined with transesophageal echocardiography, this approach has not yet proved to be safer than the prophylactic anticoagulation 3 weeks before cardioversion.[17] In any case, the short-term anticoagulation needs to be extended to 4 weeks after cardioversion.

Other Supraventricular Tachycardias

Presently, recurrent episodes of atrial flutter are usually permanently cured with radiofrequency catheter ablation.[18] In patients with atrial flutter and 1:1 atrioventricular conduction, external cardioversion can restore sinus rhythm effectively and safely. In contrast to atrial fibrillation, most episodes of atrial flutter are terminated with lower amounts of energy ranging from 50 to 100 J. An initial shock strength of 100 J is more efficient for restoration of sinus rhythm and induces less frequent atrial fibrillation compared with 50 J.[19] Patients with atrial flutter are considered at low risk for thromboembolism due to the synchronous atrial contraction. Nevertheless, several studies suggest that the thromboembolic risk at the time of cardioversion is higher than expected.[20,21] Intermittent transition to atrial fibrillation may explain the development of thrombi, and patients with atrial flutter are also at risk of developing atrial stunning after cardioversion. Therefore, consideration should be given to anticoagulate patients with atrial flutter the same as patients with atrial fibrillation.[15]

Other supraventricular tachycardias rarely require external cardioversion unless they produce hypotension, heart failure, or myocardial ischemia (see also Chap. 29A). These arrhythmias also may be terminated by external cardioversion if they are refractory to antiarrhythmic drugs.

Ventricular Tachycardia

When a hemodynamically well-tolerated sustained monomorphic ventricular tachycardia outside an acute ischemic episode cannot be terminated by intravenous procainamide,[22] a low-energy synchronized shock ranging from 25 to 50 J should be delivered. However, these low amounts of energy incidentally may induce ventricular fibrillation. In hemodynamically not tolerated sustained monomorphic ventricular or polymorphic ventricular tachycardia, a 200-J shock should be given, followed by 300 and 360 J if earlier shocks are not successful. In hemodynamically unstable patients with fast ventricular tachycardia, the QRS complex is often indistinguishable from the T wave, and unsynchronized shocks are recommended.

In pediatric patients with hemodynamically not tolerated (supra-) ventricular tachycardia, it is recommended to deliver an initial synchronized shock of 0.5 J/kg. The dose is increased with subsequent attempts if necessary.[23]

Ventricular Fibrillation

Ventricular fibrillation is best explained as a re-entrant mechanism where the waves initially follow certain routes and thereafter degenerate into smaller reentry circuits. This pattern of ventricular activation causes loss of coordinated myocyte contraction and results in loss of mechanical function of the ventricles, leading to death. The arrhythmia is eminently treatable with an unsynchronized discharge of electrical energy. The recommended first shock strength for defibrillation is 200 J. If the first shock fails to defibrillate, a second 200- or 300-J shock should be delivered. The following arguments favor the administration of a second shock of 200 J. First, every defibrillation attempt with a selected amount of energy has a certain probability to terminate ventricular fibrillation. For repeated shocks, the probability should be additive. Second, since transthoracic impedance lowers after repeated shocks, higher current will be delivered to the myocardium using a second shock of the same energy as the first one. The argument favoring the use of a second shock of 300 J is that a greater and more predictable increase in current will occur. If ventricular fibrillation persists after two shocks, a third 360-J shock should be given.[23] In case of recurrent ventricular fibrillation after a successful defibrillation, shocks with the same energy level as those which were effective previously should be delivered. Higher shock energies should be used only if a shock fails to terminate ventricular fibrillation.

With the advent of biphasic defibrillators, the American Heart Association stated that low-energy (150-J), nonprogressive (150 J–150 J–150 J) biphasic waveform defibrillators may be used for both out-of-hospital and in-hospital ventricular fibrillation arrest, including persistent or recurrent ventricular fibrillation that does not respond to the initial low-energy shock.[24] Ventricular fibrillation is uncommon in children; if it occurs, usually an initial shock strength of 2 J/kg is used. If successful defibrillation has not been obtained, the shock strength should be doubled and repeated. If defibrillation fails, a second shock of 4 J/kg needs to be delivered.[23]

Ventricular fibrillation is the most common cardiac mechanism for sudden death. In the chain-of-survival concept, early defibrillation is a key link to improve survival.[25] Technological improvements in automated external defibrillators, developed almost 20 years ago, made possible the use of defibrillation by non(para)medics. Self-adhesive pads attached to the patient on the standard electrode positions recommended for conventional external defibrillation are used for recording the electrogram and for eventual defibrillation. The automated external defibrillators are fitted with accurate arrhythmia analysis algorithms that recognize ventricular fibrillation or rapid ventricular tachycardia when presented with approximately 8 s of cardiac rhythm, permitting defibrillation within 8 to 10 s either automatically or by advising a rescuer to press a button that delivers a shock. A potential clinical advantage of automated external defibrillators using the conventional monophasic waveform over newer devices equipped with biphasic waveforms for treatment of patients in out-of-hospital arrest awaits proper clinical trials.[24]

Complications

The overall incidence of complications with external cardioversion and defibrillation is low. No myocardial injury occurs following the delivery of even high-energy shocks, as detected by the release of the cardiac isotype of troponin I, a highly specific marker of myocardial lesions.[26] After cardioversion, ST-segment elevation and negative T-waves occasionally may occur. The ST-segment changes usually persist several minutes after shock delivery, whereas the T-wave changes usually last longer. These electrocardiographic changes are related to the amount of energy delivered, but their exact mechanism is unknown. It has been postulated that postshock transient enhanced permeability of the cellular membrane occurs, allowing ionic exchange that leads to membrane depolarization (electroporation).[27] The electroporation is macroscopically manifested as ST-segment changes.

The occurrence of serious ventricular arrhythmias is related to the presence of hypokalemia, digitalis toxicity, severity of heart disease, improper synchronization, and the repeated use of high levels of energy. Asystole and cardiac arrest are rare and occur when there are severe conduction disturbances. Postshock bradycardia may be due to an underlying sick sinus syndrome, the use of antiarrhythmic drugs, or the presence of myocardial ischemia. The risk of embolization after cardioversion of atrial arrhythmias is prevented by adequate anticoagulation.

Damage to the electric circuitry of pacemakers or to the electrode-myocardial interface may occur following cardioversion or defibrillation.[28] Defibrillation electrodes should be placed as far from the pacemaker as possible, preferably in the anteroposterior position. Because pacing thresholds may increase gradually over weeks with subsequent loss of capture by the device, serial pacing threshold measurements for 2 months are recommended. Pulmonary edema, occurring minutes to hours after cardioversion, is a rare complication. It may be due to delayed return of left atrial function, left ventricular dysfunction, and possibly neurohumoral mechanisms.[29] Unexplained hypotension sometimes occurs after cardioversion, and fluid treatment will correct this problem. External cardioversion and defibrillation cause first-degree skin burns, which are related to the amount of energy used.[30] Rarely, fractures of vertebrae or long bones following cardioversion or defibrillation may occur.

INTERNAL CARDIOVERSION AND DEFIBRILLATION

Initially, the intracardiac delivery of energy was used for the development of implantable cardioverter defibrillators. Chapter 30 is dedicated to the use of these devices for the treatment of ventricular tachyarrhythmia. Only recently, internal cardioversion was introduced as a new treatment modality for patients with atrial fibrillation. The gradual replacement of external defibrillation paddles or skin patches by defibrillation electrodes resulted in effective intracardiac cardioversion of atrial fibrillation using only a small fraction of the energy required for external cardioversion. An esophageal electrode–cutaneous patch configuration allowed the cardioversion of patients with atrial fibrillation with an amount of energy three to four times lower than the energy required for conventional external cardioversion.[31] An early attempt to obtain lower atrial defibrillation thresholds using a single right atrial electrode in combination with a cutaneous patch was disappointing.[32] However, a randomized comparison of this technique with conventional external cardioversion demonstrated a higher immediate success rate of internal cardioversion compared with external cardioversion.[33] In the first study where both defibrillation electrodes were located in the right side of the heart, none of the patients with atrial fibrillation were cardioverted successfully.[34] Only after experimental studies in sheep was it recognized that the optimal lead configuration for internal defibrillation of atrial fibrillation required electrodes encircling as much of the fibrillating atrium as possible.[35] In that study, four right atrial electrode positions (superior vena cava, right atrial appendage, and middle and low right atrium) and three left atrial positions (coronary sinus, left pulmonary artery, and left axillary subcutaneous patch) were evaluated. Additionally, the efficacy of monophasic and biphasic waveforms was compared. It was shown that a 3/3-ms biphasic shock delivered between the right atrium and the coronary sinus had the lowest defibrillation threshold (1.3 ± 0.4 J). The remarkably low amount of energy to convert atrial fibrillation in animals prompted several centers to investigate the use of intracardiac shocks in patients with atrial fibrillation.

Technique

Similar to external cardioversion, evaluation of patients undergoing elective internal cardioversion of atrial fibrillation includes a clinical history, a physical examination, routine laboratory and thyroid function tests, and a 12-lead electrocardiogram. The same oral anticoagulation recommendations should be used as discussed previously for external cardioversion, except that the anticoagulant needs to be interrupted before the procedure to perform a safe venous puncture. Patients are cardioverted in a fasting state, and whenever needed, conscious sedation is provided. Although several techniques are used for internal cardioversion, the following is the most frequently used. Three temporary catheters are inserted in the venous system and positioned under fluoroscopic guidance. Two large-surface-area catheters are used for shock delivery, and a third quadripolar catheter is used for R-wave synchronization and temporary ventricular postshock pacing. In case no ventricular catheter is inserted, the surface electrocardiogram is used for R-wave synchronization. Improperly synchronized shocks, also of low energy, induce ventricular fibrillation (see Fig. 29B-1). The first

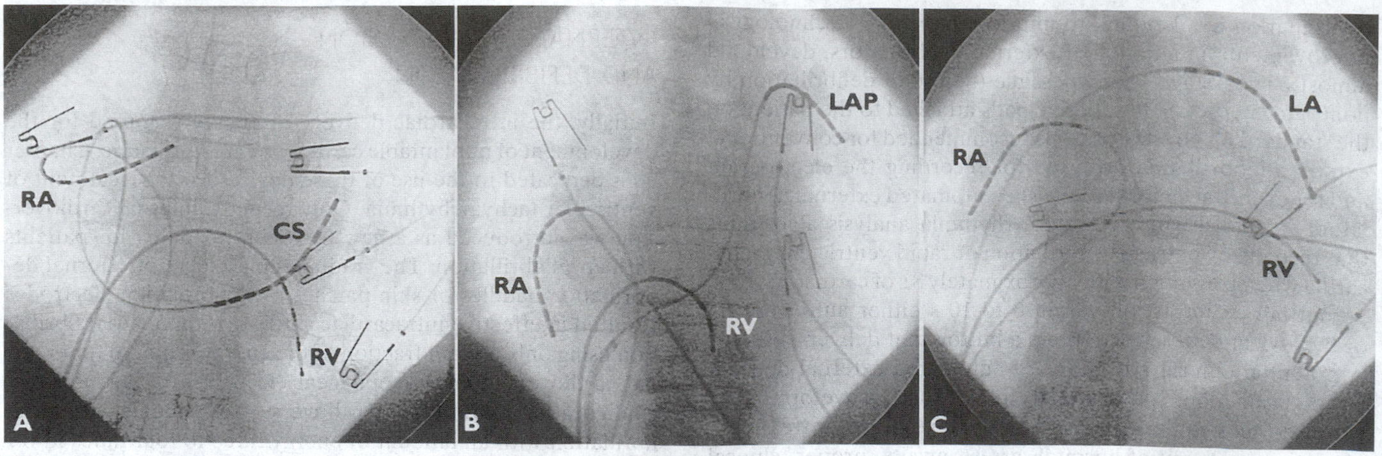

FIGURE 29B-4 Three temporary catheters are inserted in the venous system for internal cardioversion of atrial fibrillation. Most frequently, two large-surface-area catheters for shock delivery are positioned in the right atrium and the distal coronary sinus (*A*). If the catheter cannot be inserted in the coronary sinus, alternative positions are the left pulmonary artery (*B*) or the left atrium through a patent foramen ovale (*C*). A third catheter, used for R-wave synchronization and temporary ventricular postshock pacing, is positioned in the right ventricular apex.

defibrillation catheter is advanced in the distal coronary sinus, and the second preferably is positioned in the right atrium appendix or, otherwise, in the lateral wall of the right atrium (Fig. 29B-4*A*). The defibrillation catheters are connected to an external defibrillator delivering biphasic shocks. The quadripolar catheter is placed in the apex of the right ventricle and is also connected to an external pacemaker. The right atrial and right ventricular catheters usually are introduced via a femoral approach. The coronary sinus catheter can be inserted through a femoral, subclavian, jugular, or brachial vein. Alternative positions for the defibrillation catheters are the left pulmonary artery (see Fig. 29B-4*B*) or the left atrium through a patent foramen ovale (see Fig. 29B-4*C*).

Internal cardioversion of atrial fibrillation has several clinical applications such as the treatment of patients resistant to external cardioversion or in whom general anesthesia is contraindicated or hazardous, the conversion to sinus rhythm of inadvertently induced atrial fibrillation during an electrophysiologic study, and the evaluation of patients with recurrent symptomatic atrial fibrillation, resistant to antiarrhythmic drugs, for treatment with an implantable atrial defibrillator. A comparison of the reported success rates and energy requirements for catheter-based restoration of sinus rhythm is not only difficult because of the variable use of a preestablished energy limit for termination of the procedure but also because of the heterogeneous populations treated, the evaluation of several technological improvements of the defibrillation system, and the differences in lead configurations.

Between December of 1995 and February of 1999, 120 patients (89 men, mean age 59 ± 12 years) with a mixture of heart disease seen in the general population with atrial fibrillation underwent 141 internal cardioversions in our hospital. Most of the patients were taking antiarrhythmic drugs at the time of the procedure. The left atrial size ranged from 42 to 70 (53 ± 6) mm and the left ventricular ejection fraction from 21 to 72 (55 ± 12) percent. Atrial fibrillation was induced in 16 patients, and in the other 125 patients the average duration of the treated spontaneous episode was 306 ± 564 (0.1–3650) days. In all procedures, a right atrium to coronary sinus defibrillation vector was used. Shocks were delivered using a 0.5-J start, a 0.5-J step-up protocol until 3 J, followed by 1.0-J steps until cardioversion of atrial fibrillation occurred. All 141 atrial fibrillation episodes were cardioverted successfully with a mean energy of 5.6 ± 4.7 (0.4–35) J. In patients with long-standing atrial fibrillation, the atrial defibrillation threshold is higher than in patients with induced or paroxysmal atrial fibrillation. Although internal cardioversion has a higher acute efficacy in restoring sinus rhythm as compared with external cardioversion, the long-term outcome seems to be independent of the method of cardioversion.

An intriguing phenomenon after internal and external cardioversion of atrial fibrillation is the immediate reinitiation of the arrhythmia occurring within minutes of successful shock delivery (Fig. 29B-5). Because the intracardiac electrograms following an internal cardioversion are frequently monitored, immediate resumption of atrial fibrillation is detected more often as compared with external cardioversion.[36] Complications of internal cardioversion are rare and, if they occur, are related to the invasive nature of the procedure, improper synchronization, and inadequate anticoagulation.

IMPLANTABLE ATRIAL DEFIBRILLATOR

Antiarrhythmic drugs and external defibrillation are presently the primary modes of treatment of patients with atrial fibrillation. Due to the limited efficacy and safety of antiarrhythmic drugs and the repeated hospitalizations for external cardioversion requiring anesthesia, several non-pharmacologic options have been developed, especially for patients with recurrent atrial fibrillation. One of them, the implantable atrial defibrillator, only recently has been evaluated clinically. At present, a stand-alone atrial defibrillator and an atrioventricular cardioverter-defibrillator with dual-chamber pacemaker facilities are available. Because these devices are intended for use outside the hospital, ventricular tachyarrhythmia induced by atrial shocks, especially from a stand-alone atrial defibrillator, could have disastrous consequences. Prior experimental animal studies[37] resulted in programming the atrial shock synchronized to a QRS complex that occurs at least 500 ms after the preceding

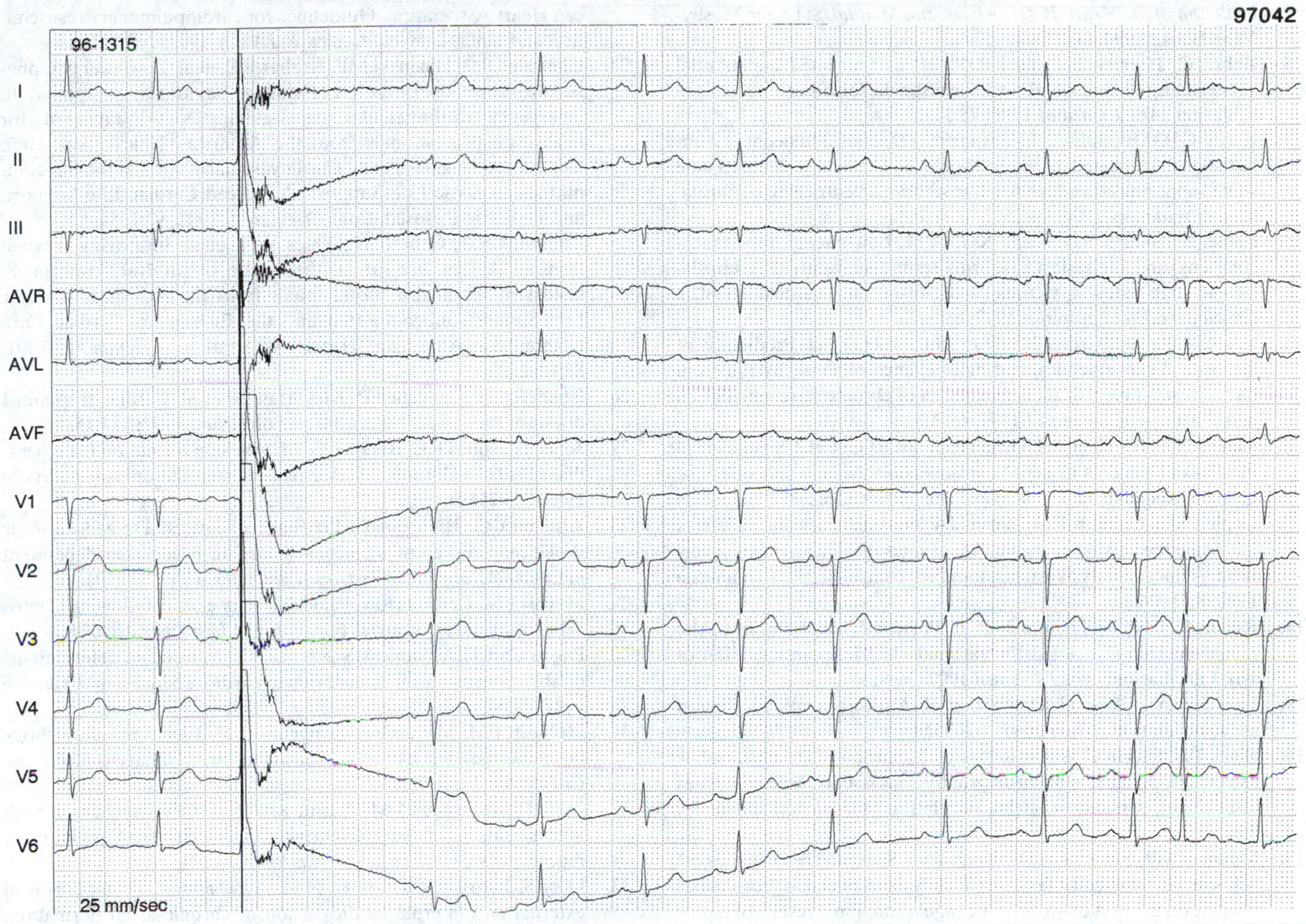

FIGURE 29B-5 Twelve-lead electrocardiogram recorded during internal cardioversion of atrial fibrillation. A 1-J biphasic shock, synchronized to the R wave, terminated atrial fibrillation. Note that after eight sinus beats, an atrial premature beat reinitiated atrial fibrillation. (From Timmermans C et al: Immediate reinitiation of atrial fibrillation following internal atrial defibrillation. *J Cardiovasc Electrophysiol* 1998; 9:122. Reproduced with permission from the publisher.)

QRS complex, in the absence of a long-short sequence, to avoid the potential ventricular proarrhythmia risk in a stand-alone atrial defibrillator.

In selected patients with recurrent atrial fibrillation, a stand-alone atrial defibrillator was able to restore sinus rhythm promptly and safely with low amounts of energy.[38] Ambulatory therapy with the stand-alone atrial defibrillator is feasible because the device can terminate most of the episodes of atrial fibrillation in the patient's ambient setting without induction of ventricular proarrhythmia. Interestingly, in the majority of patients, atrial fibrillation can be treated with the device without sedation. The need for sedation is related to the number of shocks delivered to treat an atrial fibrillation episode.[39] A clinical study for the evaluation of a dual-chamber cardioverter-defibrillator for termination of spontaneous atrial fibrillation episodes in patients without indication for implantation of a ventricular defibrillator is presently ongoing. Whether an implantable atrial defibrillator modifies the natural history of atrial fibrillation, improves quality of life, and is cost-effective needs to be defined.

References

1. Driscol TE, Ratnoff OD, Nygaard OF. The remarkable Dr. Abildgaard and countershock: The bicentennial of his electrical experiments on animals. *Ann Intern Med* 1975; 83:878.
2. Beck CS, Pritchard WH, Feil HS. Ventricular fibrillation of long duration abolished by electrical shock. *JAMA* 1947; 135:985.
3. Lown B. Electrical reversion of cardiac arrhythmias. *Br Heart J* 1967; 29:469.
4. Ewy GA. Optimal technique for electrical cardioversion of atrial fibrillation. *Circulation* 1992; 86:1645.
5. Kerber RE, Martins JB, Kienzle MG, et al. Energy, current, and success in defibrillation and cardioversion: Clinical studies using an automated impedance-based method of energy adjustment. *Circulation* 1988; 77:1038.
6. Kerber RE, Grayzel J, Hoyt R, et al. Transthoracic resistance in human defibrillation: Influence of body weight, chest size, serial shocks, paddle size and paddle contact pressure. *Circulation* 1981; 63:676.
7. Jones JL. Waveforms for implantable cardioverter defibrillators (ICDs) and transchest defibrillation. In: Tacker WA Jr, ed. *Defi-*

brillation of the Heart: ICDs, AEDs, and Manual. St Louis: Mosby-Year Book; 1994:46.

8. Behr JC, Hartley LL, York DK, et al. Truncated exponential versus damped sinusoidal waveform shocks for transthoracic defibrillation. *Am J Cardiol* 1996; 78:1242.
9. Bardy GH, Marchlinski FE, Sharma AD, et al. Multicenter comparison of truncated biphasic shocks and standard damped sine wave monophasic shocks for transthoracic ventricular defibrillation. *Circulation* 1996; 94:2507.
10. Poole JE, White RD, Kanz KG, et al. Low-energy impedance-compensating biphasic waveforms terminate ventricular fibrillation at high rates in victims of out-of-hospital cardiac arrest. *J Cardiovasc Electrophysiol* 1997; 8:1373.
11. Van Gelder IC, Crijns HJ, Van Gilst WH, et al. Prediction of uneventful cardioversion and maintenance of sinus rhythm from direct-current electrical cardioversion of chronic atrial fibrillation and flutter. *Am J Cardiol* 1991; 68:41.
12. Van Gelder IC, Crijns HJGM, Tieleman RG, et al. Chronic atrial fibrillation: Success of serial cardioversion therapy and safety of oral anticoagulation. *Arch Intern Med* 1996; 156:2585.
13. Coplen SE, Antman EM, Berlin JA, et al. Efficacy and safety of quinidine therapy for maintenance of sinus rhythm after cardioversion: A meta-analysis of randomized control trials. *Circulation* 1990; 82:1106.
14. Ricard P, Lévy S, Trigano J, et al. Prospective assessment of the minimum energy needed for external electrical cardioversion of atrial fibrillation. *Am J Cardiol* 1997; 79:815.
15. Laupacis A, Albers G, Dalen J, et al. Antithrombotic therapy in atrial fibrillation. *Chest* 1995; 108:352S.
16. Black IW, Fatkin D, Sagar KB, et al. Exclusion of atrial thrombus by transesophageal echocardiography does not preclude embolism after cardioversion of atrial fibrillation. *Circulation* 1994; 89: 2509.
17. Manning WJ, Silverman DI, Keighley CS, et al. Transesophageal echocardiographically facilitated early cardioversion from atrial fibrillation using short-term anticoagulation: Final results of a prospective 4.5-year study. *J Am Coll Cardiol* 1995; 25:1354.
18. Nabar A, Rodiguez LM, Timmermans C, et al. Isoproterenol to evaluate resumption of conduction after right atrial isthmus ablation in type I atrial flutter. *Circulation* 1999; 99:3286.
19. Pinski SL, Sgarbossa EB, Ching E, et al. A comparison of 50-J versus 100-J shocks for direct-current cardioversion of atrial flutter. *Am Heart J* 1999; 137:439.
20. Irani WN, Grayburn PA, Afridi I. Prevalence of thrombus, spontaneous echo contrast, and atrial stunning in patients undergoing cardioversion of atrial flutter: A prospective study using transesophageal echocardiography. *Circulation* 1997; 95:962.
21. Lanzarotti CJ, Olshansky B. Thromboembolism in chronic atrial flutter: Is the risk underestimated? *J Am Coll Cardiol* 1997; 30:1506.
22. Gorgels AP, van den Dool A, Hofs A, et al. Comparison of procainamide and lidocaine in terminating sustained monomorphic ventricular tachycardia. *Am J Cardiol* 1996; 78:43.
23. Emergency Cardiac Care Committee and Subcommittees, American Heart Association. Guidelines for cardiopulmonary resuscitation and emergency cardiac care. *JAMA* 1992; 268:2171.
24. Cummins RO, Hazinski MF, Kerber RE, et al. Low-energy biphasic waveform defibrillation: Evidence-based review applied to emergency cardiovascular care guidelines. A statement for healthcare professionals from the American Heart Association Committee on Emergency Cardiovascular Care and the Subcommittees on Basic Life Support, Advanced Cardiac Life Support, and Pediatric Resuscitation. *Circulation* 1998; 97:1654.
25. Cummins RO, Ornato JP, Thies WH, et al. Improving survival from sudden cardiac arrest: the "chain of survival" concept: A statement for health professionals from the Advanced Cardiac Life Support Subcommittee and the Emergency Cardiac Care Committee, American Heart Association. *Circulation* 1991; 83:1832.
26. Bonnefoy E, Chevalier P, Kirkorian G, et al. Cardiac troponin I does not increase after cardioversion. *Chest* 1997; 111:15.
27. Jones JL, Jones RE, Balasky G. Microlesion formation in myocardial cells by high-intensity electric field stimulation. *Am J Physiol* 1987; 253:H480.
28. Altamura G, Bianconi L, Lo Bianco F, et al. Transthoracic dc shock may represent a serious hazard in pacemaker dependent patients. *Pacing Clin Electrophysiol* 1995; 18(pt. II):194.
29. Mayosi BM, Commerford PJ. Pulmonary edema following electrical cardioversion of atrial fibrillation. *Chest* 1996; 109:278.
30. Pagan-Carlo LA, Stone MS, Kerber RE. Nature and determinants of skin "burns" after transthoracic cardioversion. *Am J Cardiol* 1997; 79:689.
31. McNally EM, Meyer EC, Langendorf R. Elective countershock in unanesthetized patients with use of an esophageal electrode. *Circulation* 1966; 33:124.
32. Jain SC, Bhatnagar VM, Azami Ru, et al. Elective countershock in atrial fibrillation with an intracardiac electrode: A preliminary report. *J Assoc Physicians India* 1970; 18:821.
33. Lévy S, Lauribe P, Dolla E, et al. A randomized comparison of external and internal cardioversion of chronic atrial fibrillation. *Circulation* 1992; 86:1415.
34. Nathan AW, Bexton RS, Spurrell RAJ, et al. Internal transvenous low energy cardioversion for the treatment of cardiac arrhythmias. *Br Heart J* 1984; 52:377.
35. Cooper RAS, Alferness CA, Smith WA, et al. Internal cardioversion of atrial fibrillation in sheep. *Circulation* 1993; 87:1673.
36. Timmermans C, Rodriguez LM, Smeets JLRM, et al. Immediate reinitiation of atrial fibrillation following internal atrial defibrillation. *J Cardiovasc Electrophysiol* 1998; 9:122.
37. Ayers GM, Alferness CA, Ilina M, et al. Ventricular proarrhythmic effects of ventricular cycle length and shock strength in a sheep model of transvenous atrial defibrillation. *Circulation* 1994; 89:413.
38. Wellens HJJ, Lau CP, Lüderitz B, et al. Atrioverter: an implantable device for the treatment of atrial fibrillation. *Circulation* 1998; 98:1651.
39. Timmermans C, Nabar A, Rodriguez LM, et al. Use of sedation during cardioversion with the implantable atrial defibrillator. *Circulation* 1999; 100:1499.

CHAPTER 30

THE IMPLANTABLE CARDIOVERTER DEFIBRILLATOR

Peter A. O'Callaghan / Jeremy N. Ruskin

HISTORICAL PERSPECTIVE

Sudden and unexpected cardiac death (SCD) is estimated to claim 300,000 lives annually in the United States.[1] Despite a significant reduction in total cardiac mortality rates in recent years, the proportion of deaths that are sudden has remained unchanged. In-field electrocardiogram monitoring has demonstrated that the principal cause of SCD in victims of out-of-hospital cardiac arrest is ventricular fibrillation (VF).[2] In more than 80 percent of cases, sudden death is caused by the abrupt onset of ventricular tachycardia (VT) that progresses to VF.[3] Since self-termination of VF is exceedingly rare, the single most important factor determining survival is the time between event onset and first defibrillation attempt.[4] Overall mortality rates associated with out-of-hospital cardiac arrest are unacceptably high, mainly because of the delay in providing effective therapy.[5] In Seattle, Washington, only 10 percent of all out-of-hospital SCD victims are discharged from the hospital neurologically intact, despite good emergency medical response times, prompt cardiopulmonary resuscitation, and the use of automatic external defibrillators.[6]

As originally conceived by Mirowski, the implantable cardioverter defibrillator (ICD) was designed to circumvent the delay in providing definitive therapy to ambulatory individuals with life-threatening ventricular tachyarrhythmias.[7] The internal defibrillator responds by delivering an internal electrical shock within 10 to 20 s of arrhythmia onset, a time frame in which the potential for arrhythmia reversal approaches 100 percent. The first experimental model was successfully tested in 1969 in a dog.[8] After 10 years of research and development, Mirowski and coworkers implanted the first ICD in a human at the Johns Hopkins University Medical Center in 1980.[9] In the original article, the authors state, "It is intended to protect patients at particularly high risk of sudden death whenever and wherever they are stricken by these lethal arrhythmias . . . the only purpose of this device is to achieve defibrillation automatically, before the victim of a lethal arrhythmia can be reached by a cardiac resuscitation team." In 1985, the ICD received approval from the U.S. Food and Drug Administration for market release. Since then, the indications for ICD implantation have greatly expanded, and the number of devices implanted annually has steadily increased, reaching 50,000 new implants worldwide in 1999.

FUNCTIONAL CHARACTERISTICS

The ICD system consists of two basic components: a pulse generator and a lead electrode or electrodes for arrhythmia detection and for therapy delivery. In addition to internal defibrillation, ICDs also provide pacing (antitachycardia and antibradycardia), synchronized cardioversion, telemetry, and diagnostics (event electrograms and history logs). The pulse generator is essentially a self-powered computer within a hermetically sealed titanium can.[10] Lithium vanadium oxide batteries and defibrillator capacitors occupy the bulk of the space. The operational circuitry—including resistors, capacitors, transformers, and microprocessors—occupies the remaining space and is separated into low-power circuit components (sensing and pacing) and high-power circuit components (defibrillation). A header made of epoxy provides an electrical interface between the internal circuitry and the lead electrode as well as electrical insulation from the surrounding tissues. Since the 1990s, designs have focused on a progressive increase in device functions combined with a gradual reduction in pulse generator size.

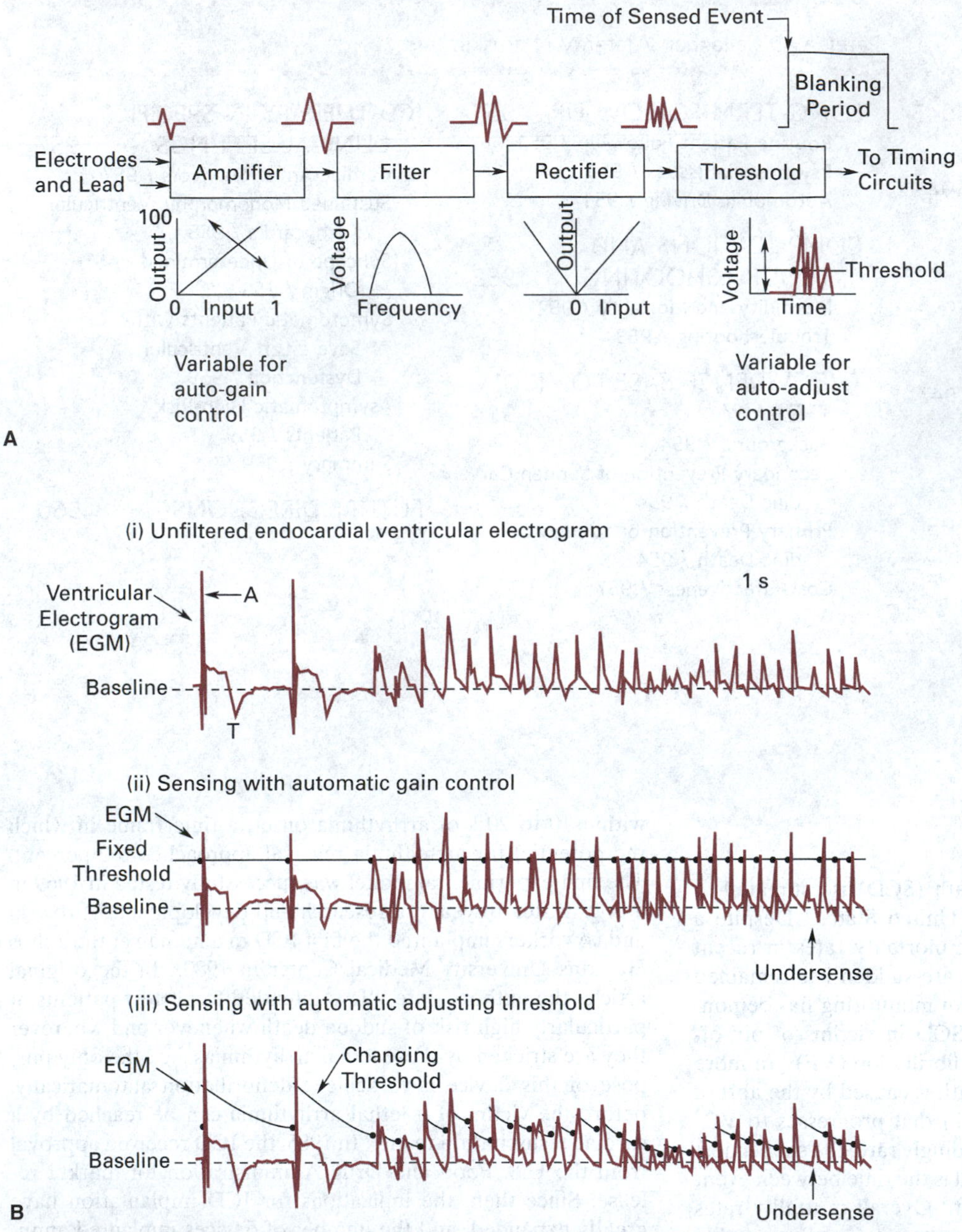

FIGURE 30-1 Sensing of electrogram signals by implantable cardioverter-defibrillators. *A*. A functional block diagram for an ICD sense amplifier consists of an amplifier that may be fixed or have automatic gain control, a band-pass filter to reject low-frequency T waves and high-frequency noise, a rectifier to eliminate polarity dependency, and a threshold detector that may be fixed or autoadjusting. The net result is a single pulse for each ventricular depolarization that is used by timing circuits to determine a series of cycle lengths. The effects of each block on a biphasic electrogram are shown above the blocks, and each functional operation is shown below each block. *B*. Sinus rhythm and ventricular fibrillation signals are shown for the raw electrogram in panel *i*, for automatic gain control in panel *ii*, and for automatic adjusting threshold in panel *iii*. With automatic gain control, the small electrograms are amplified compared to panel *i*, and sensing is shown by the dots where the signal crosses the fixed threshold. With automatic adjusting threshold, the electrograms are the same as in panel *i*, and the threshold varies according to the amplitude of the electrogram; sensing is again shown by the dots where the signal crosses the variable threshold. (From Olson,[11] with permission.)

Sensing Ventricular Depolarizations

Reliable sensing of ventricular depolarizations is essential for proper functioning of the ICD. Sensing electrodes transmit raw (unfiltered) electrograms to the sense amplifier of the ICD. The sense amplifer amplifies, filters, and rectifies the incoming signals. It then compares them to a sensing threshold and produces a set of RR intervals for the detection algorithm to use (Fig. 30-1*A*). Intracardiac electrogram amplitude can vary markedly among rhythms, such as sinus rhythm, VT, and VF, or even during the same rhythm (e.g., VF). Fixed gain and sensitivity, as used in pacemaker technology, would result in either undersensing or oversensing, depending on the settings chosen. Therefore, all ICDs utilize some form of automatically adjusting signal amplifier (Fig. 30-1*B*). Automatic gain control automatically and continuously varies the gain so that the amplitude of the processed signal is constant. Autoadjusting sensitivity threshold sets the sensitivity to a proportion of the amplitude of the last sensed event, and the sensitivity then gradually increases until the next event is sensed. Sensed events are then analyzed using a detection algorithm. The range of all possible ventricular cycle lengths is divided into rate zones that do not overlap, including a VF zone, VT zones (between 0 and 3 programmable), a normal rate zone, and a bradycardia zone.

Ventricular Fibrillation Detection

Devices employ rate criteria as the sole method of detecting VF. An

X/Y detector triggers when *X* out of the previous *Y* sensed intervals (typical setting 8/12 intervals) are shorter than the VF detection interval. This approach is very good at ignoring the effect of a small number of undersensed events due to small-amplitude signals during VF. The utilization of rate detection in an *X/Y* detection algorithm results in maximal sensitivity at the expense of specificity. Any tachycardia with a cycle length less than the tachycardia detection interval will be detected as VF by the device, and VF therapy will be initiated. At the end of capacitor charging and prior to the delivery of therapy, a reconfirmation algorithm must be fulfilled (noncommitted device). This prevents inappropriate shock therapy for self-terminating events, such as nonsustained VT.

Ventricular Tachycardia Detection

ICDs have multiple programmable tachyarrhythmia detection zones. Although rate is the principal detection criterion, the VT detection algorithm is different from that in the VF zone. In contrast to VF detection, most VT detection algorithms require a programmable number of consecutive intervals shorter than the VT detection interval. An interval longer than the detection interval (e.g., due to RR variability in atrial fibrillation) would reset the counters.

In certain patients, both ventricular and supraventricular tachycardias (e.g., sinus tachycardia, atrial fibrillation, or atrial flutter) may result in ventricular rates within the VT zone or zones. Up to 25 percent of ICD discharges are inappropriate when rate is employed as the sole criterion for VT therapy.[12] These inappropriate discharges are poorly tolerated by patients and constitute a major clinical problem.

To increase specificity, optional VT detection enhancements are programmable. This approach should be limited to tachycardia rates that are hemodynamically tolerated by the patient. Detection enhancements include sudden onset, rate stability, and electrogram morphologic (QRS width) criteria. These programmable options are not available in the VF zone, where maximal sensitivity is required. The onset criterion is intended to distinguish sinus tachycardia with a gradual rate increase from VT characterized by a sudden rate increase (e.g., greater than 9 percent shortening in cycle length at onset of episode). The rate stability criterion is used to differentiate sustained monomorphic VT with a small variation in cycle length (e.g., less than 40 ms) from atrial fibrillation with large cycle length variability. The electrogram morphologic criterion measures the width of the intracardiac electrogram to differentiate ventricular from supraventricular tachycardias with normal conduction. Although programming these options improves specificity, it does so at the risk of prolonging detection times and of failure to detect an episode of VT. "Sustained-rate duration" is a programmable maximum period of time (e.g., 30 to 120 s) during which therapy is inhibited if the programmed enhancement criteria are not met. At the end of this period, if the tachycardia rate persists above the VT cutoff rate, therapy will be delivered. As a safety feature, sustained-rate duration is nearly always programmed "on" whenever enhancement criteria are employed. In one study, programming stability and onset criteria plus sustained-rate duration significantly reduced inappropriate therapies to 13 percent, compared to 28 percent in patients using a rate criterion only.[13] Addition of an electrogram morphologic criterion can reduce inappropriate detection even further.[14] However, optimal programming of ICD width criterion requires testing during exercise as well as at rest.[15]

The lack of specificity of VT detection despite optional VT detection enhancements is a significant limitation of single-chamber ICDs. Dual-chamber pacemaker-defibrillators, requiring an additional atrial lead, provide not only the hemodynamic benefits of dual-chamber pacing but also dual-chamber detection algorithms.[16] Detection algorithms in these devices employ a stepwise analysis of rate, stability, atrioventricular (AV) association, and onset (ventricular acceleration, atrial acceleration, or nonaccelerated).[17] Again, these programmable options are not available in the VF zone, where maximal sensitivity is required. Preliminary clinical experience is mixed. In one study, all episodes (122) of VT and VF were correctly diagnosed, and 51 of 53 episodes of supraventricular tachyarrhythmias were correctly diagnosed. Only 2 episodes of atrial fibrillation with rapid regular ventricular rates were incorrectly diagnosed as VT.[18] However, a nonrandomized study comparing a dual-chamber ICD with an optimally programmed single-chamber device found that the number of inappropriate therapies for atrial fibrillation was not decreased.[19]

Ventricular Fibrillation Therapy

ICDs employ electrical defibrillation as the sole therapy option for the treatment of VF. In contrast to cardiac pacing, which requires depolarization during diastole of a small number of cells located very close to the electrode, defibrillation requires depolarization of the majority of ventricular myocardial cells, many of which are relatively refractory and can be up to 10 cm away. Successful defibrillation may require voltages up to 100 times greater than the voltage of the ICD battery (approximately 6.4 V). A capacitor is used to store charge immediately prior to therapy delivery. This energy is then delivered between the high-voltage electrodes and depolarizes the intervening myocardium, thereby restoring baseline rhythm (Fig. 30-2). Reversing electrode polarity during capacitor discharge (biphasic waveform) lowers defibrillation energy requirements and was one of the main factors that facilitated the introduction of smaller, lower-energy pectoral devices.[20,21]

The time interval between VF onset and delivery of defibrillation energy is usually 10 to 15 s, with capacitor charge time accounting for most of the delay. During this time, the subject may experience presyncope or syncope with restoration of consciousness after successful defibrillation and restoration of cardiac output. One study of ICD recipients found that 16 percent of patients who received device therapy experienced syncope. In comparison, 65 percent of these patients had experienced syncope during tachyarrhythmia prior to device implantation.[22]

Ventricular Tachycardia Therapy

In contrast to VF therapy, treatment options in the VT zone or zones include antitachycardia pacing (ATP), cardioversion, and defibrillation. Therapy progresses through a programmable sequence of responses (tiered therapy) until the episode is terminated. Most sustained monomorphic VTs, particularly in patients with coronary artery disease, are due to reentry and can be terminated by a critical pacing sequence.[23] Pacing at faster rates increases the probability of VT termination but also increases the risk of tachycardia acceleration. ATP, with backup

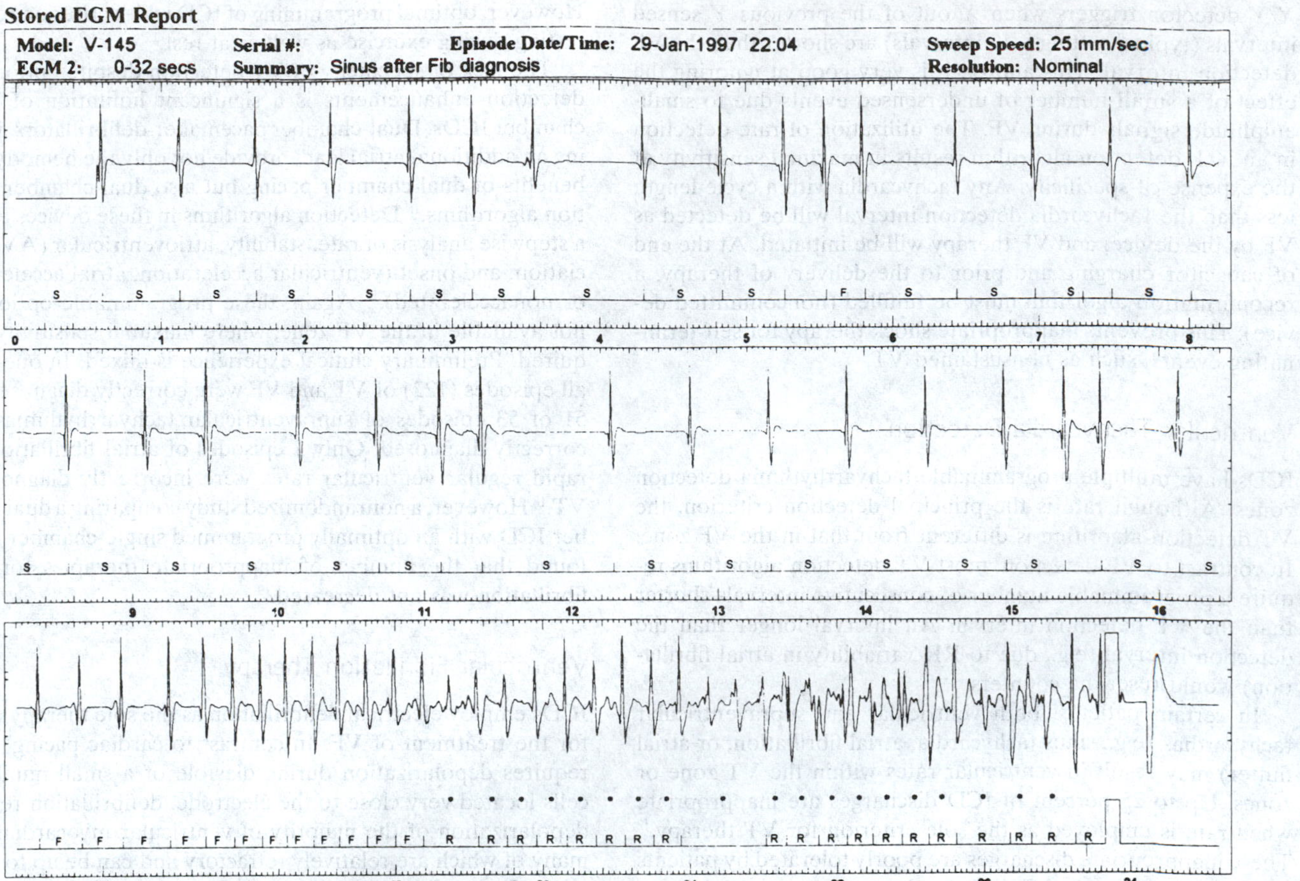

FIGURE 30-2 Stored electrogram of successful defibrillation of ventricular fibrillation. The recording is a continuous 32-s strip consisting of a waveform channel and a status channel. Sinus rhythm (S) with ectopy is seen in the first and second panels. At the start of the third panel, before the 17-s mark, the rhythm morphology changes and the cycle length shortens, consistent with a spontaneous episode of VF. The device begins to classify these intervals as fibrillation (F). Just after the 19-s mark, the detection criterion is met. Device charging (*) and reconfirmation (R) of the arrhythmia begin as recorded in the status channel. Immediately before the 24-s mark, a high-voltage shock is delivered, denoted by a full-scale positive rectangular marker in both the waveform and status channels. This restores sinus rhythm (S). Sinus redetection is denoted by an arrow in the status channel and a negative deflection in the marker channel. Total duration of VF is approximately 8 s. Information regarding the device, date and time of the episode, screen sweep speed, the electrogram number and duration, and the reason the event was stored is located in the oblong box at the top of the page. (Courtesy of Ventritex, Inc.)

defibrillation if acceleration occurs, is an attractive, well-tolerated treatment that avoids high-energy shock therapy, which is painful and diminishes battery life (Fig. 30-3). The most common form of ATP is adaptive-burst pacing, which delivers a train of stimuli at a fixed percentage of the tachycardia cycle length. Repeated and more aggressive pacing trains can be administered, resulting in either termination of the tachycardia or progression to the next treatment modality (cardioversion or defibrillation). ATP is extremely effective, with over 90 percent successful termination of spontaneous VTs.[24,25] Gross et al. reported that the addition of ATP to ICD therapy significantly reduced the cumulative occurrence of first ICD shock from 36 to 28 percent at a mean follow-up of 2 years.[26]

Cardioversion, in contrast to defibrillation, is a synchronized shock, usually of low energy. Compared to high-energy defibrillation, low-energy cardioversion reduces the time to therapy and conserves battery life. Efficacy rates and acceleration rates are similar for these two treatment modalities.[27]

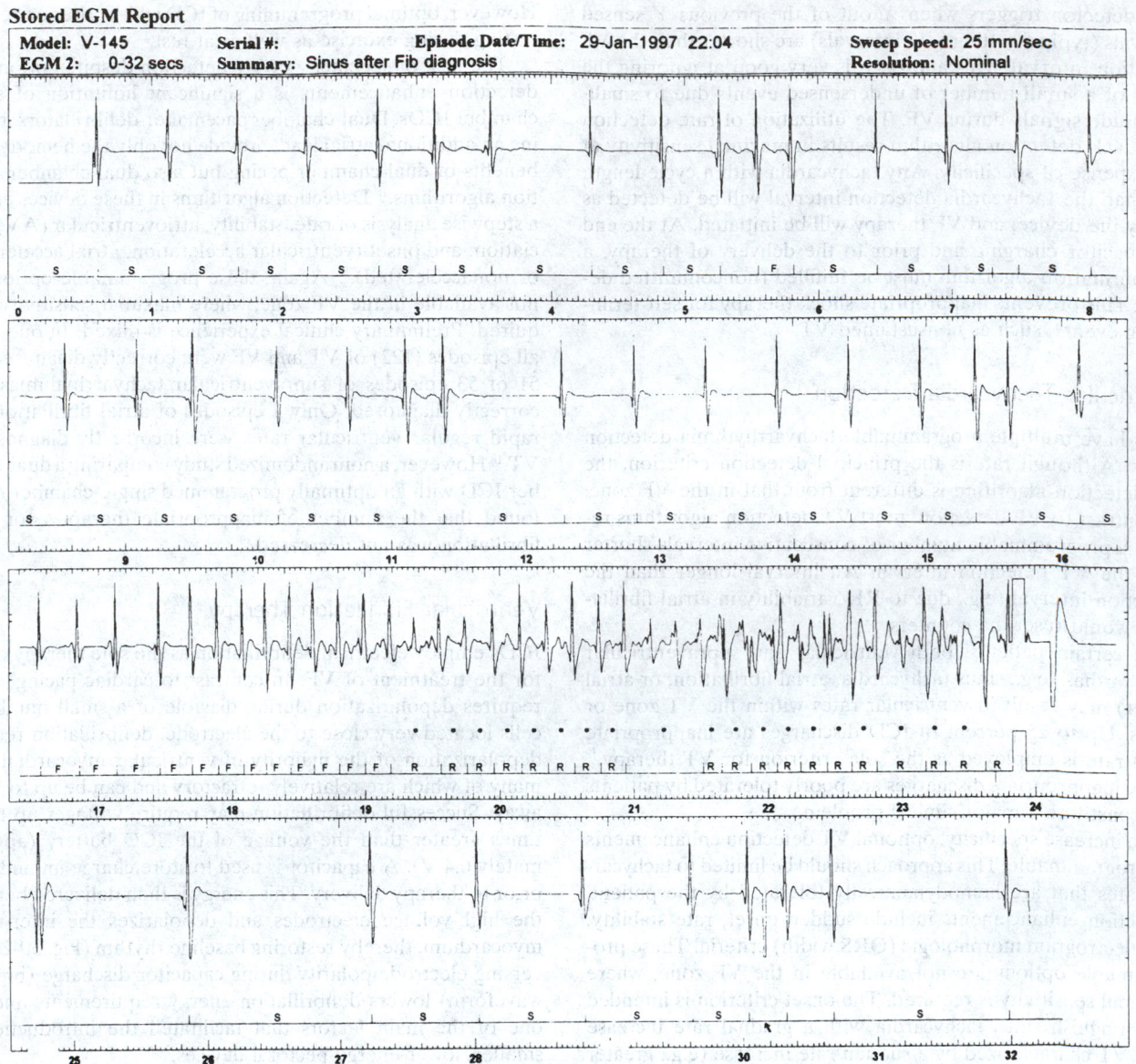

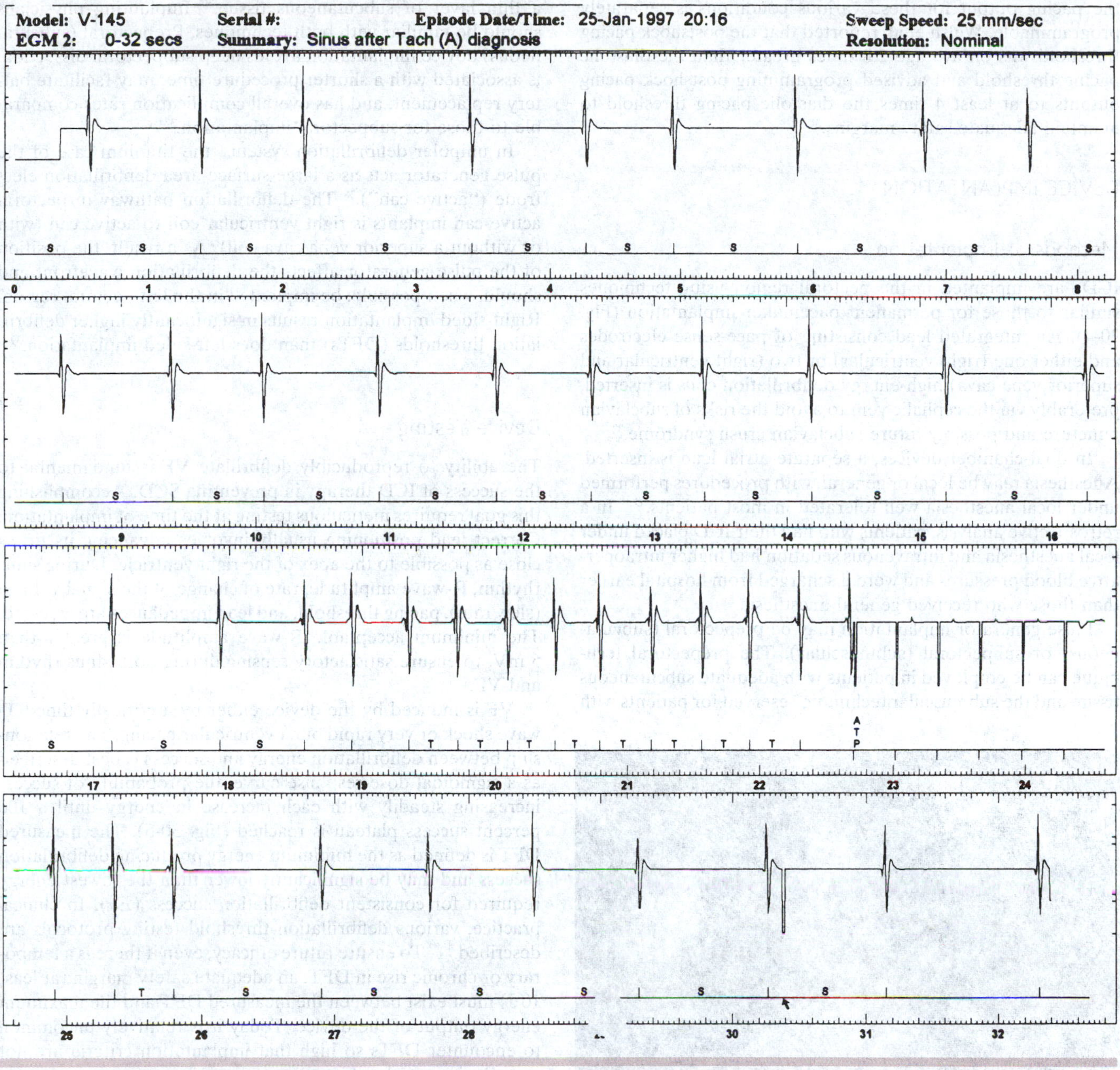

FIGURE 30-3 Stored electrogram of successful antitachycardia pacing of VT. The recording is a continuous 32-s strip consisting of a waveform channel and a status channel. Baseline rhythm, seen in the first and second panels, is atrial fibrillation with a relatively slow ventricular rate, which is annotated as sinus (S) because it falls within the normal rate zone. In the third panel, after the 19-s mark the electrogram morphology changes, the rhythm becomes regular, and the cycle length shortens, consistent with a spontaneous episode of VT. The device begins to classify these intervals as VT (T). Just before the 23-s mark, the detection criterion is met, and antitachycardia pacing (ATP) therapy is delivered. This terminates the tachycardia and restores baseline rhythm. Redetection of baseline rhythm is denoted by an arrow in the status channel and a negative deflection in the marker channel. Successful ATP in this patient avoided high-energy shock delivery. (Courtesy of Ventritex, Inc.)

Bradycardia Pacing

Bradycardia ventricular demand pacing is a standard feature of all single-chamber ICDs. Dual-chamber pacemaker-defibrillators provide not only improved diagnostic specificity but also the benefits of dual-chamber pacing, rate-responsiveness, and mode switching. In contrast to single-chamber devices, dual-chamber ICDs have reasonable longevity despite continuous pacing. Approximately 20 percent of ICD recipients need antibradycardia pacing, and most of them would benefit from a dual-chamber device.[28] If one includes patients with poor ejection fraction and patients who would benefit from dual-chamber sensing, it is possible that up to 50 percent of ICD recipients may benefit from implantation of a dual-chamber ICD.[29,30]

Pacing thresholds during VT and after defibrillation are frequently higher than those needed for bradycardia pacing, and the pacing output for these various conditions is separately programmable. Welsh et al. reported that the postshock pacing threshold was on average 2.8 times greater than the diastolic pacing threshold and advised programming postshock pacing outputs to at least 4 times the diastolic pacing threshold to maintain adequate safety margins.[31]

DEVICE IMPLANTATION

Methods of Implantation

ICDs are implanted in the pectoral region using techniques similar to those for permanent pacemaker implantation (Fig. 30-4). An integrated lead consisting of pace-sense electrodes and either one (right ventricular) or two (right ventricular and superior vena cava) high-energy defibrillation coils is inserted, preferably via the cephalic vein to avoid the risks of subclavian puncture and possibly future subclavian crush syndrome.[32]

In dual-chamber devices, a separate atrial lead is inserted. Anesthesia may be local or general, with procedures performed under local anesthesia well tolerated in most patients.[33,34] In a retrospective analysis, patients who had their ICD placed under local anesthesia and intravenous sedation had higher intraoperative blood pressures and were discharged from hospital earlier than those who received general anesthesia.[35]

Pulse generator implantation may be prepectoral (subcutaneous) or subpectoral (submuscular). The prepectoral technique can be employed in patients with adequate subcutaneous tissue and the submuscular technique reserved for patients with a thin layer of subcutaneous tissue.[36] Implanting physicians should be familiar with both techniques. Prepectoral (subcutaneous) device implantation avoids deep subpectoral dissection, is associated with a shorter procedure time, may facilitate battery replacement, and has overall complication rates comparable to those for subpectoral implantation.[37]

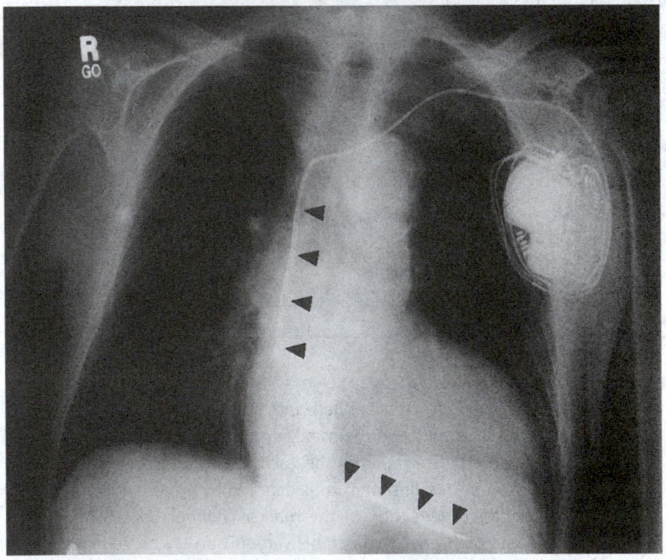

FIGURE 30-4 Posteroanterior chest x-ray of pectoral ICD device. A single integrated lead is inserted via the cephalic vein and positioned at the right ventricular apex. This is attached to a pulse generator implanted in the left pectoral region. ICDs are implanted using techniques similar to permanent pacemaker implantation. The integrated lead consists of right ventricular and superior vena cava defibrillation coils (*arrows*) and a tip electrode. In addition to the defibrillation coils, the titanium case of the pulse generator acts as a large-surface-area defibrillation electrode (active can). The defibrillation pathway in this patient is right ventricular coil to both superior vena cava coil and active can.

In unipolar defibrillation systems, the titanium case of the pulse generator acts as a large-surface-area defibrillation electrode ("active can").[38] The defibrillation pathway in pectoral active-can implants is right ventricular coil to active can (with or without a superior vena cava coil). As a result, the position of the pulse generator affects the defibrillation wavefront and should, when possible, be implanted in the left pectoral region. Right-sided implantation results in significantly higher defibrillation thresholds (DFTs) than does left-sided implantation.[39]

Device Testing

The ability to reproducibly defibrillate VF is fundamental to the success of ICD therapy in preventing SCD. Accomplishing this goal requires meticulous testing at the time of implantation. Correct lead positioning usually involves advancing its tip as close as possible to the apex of the right ventricle. During sinus rhythm, R-wave amplitude, rate of change of the signal voltage (slew rate), pacing threshold, and lead impedances are assessed. The minimum acceptable R-wave amplitude is greater than 5 mV, to ensure satisfactory sensing during both sinus rhythm and VF.

VF is induced by the device either by a critically timed T-wave shock or very rapid burst ventricular pacing. The relationship between defibrillation energy and success is best described as a sigmoidal dose-response curve, the probability of success increasing steadily with each increase in energy until a 100 percent success plateau is reached (Fig. 30-5). The measured DFT is defined as the minimum energy producing defibrillation success and may be significantly lower than the lowest energy required for consistent defibrillation success (E_{99}). In clinical practice, various defibrillation threshold testing protocols are described.[41,42] To ensure future efficacy, even if there is a temporary or chronic rise in DFT, an adequate safety margin (at least 10 J) must exist between the measured DFT and the maximum energy output of the device. Today it is relatively uncommon to encounter DFTs so high that implantation criteria are not met. Boriani et al. achieved a safety margin of greater than or equal to 10 J and successfully implanted a single-lead unipolar system with a maximum energy output of only 29 J in 54 of 55 patients (98 percent).[43] If high DFTs are encountered at implantation, repeat testing can be performed after repositioning the lead (usually by attempting to get as close to the right ventricular apex as possible); changing the lead polarity, pulse duration, or waveform; adding additional defibrillation electrodes; or changing to a higher-energy-output device. In addition, in unipolar systems, a pneumothorax can greatly increase the high voltage impedance, resulting in high DFTs.[44] Finally, the role of antiarrhythmic drugs should be considered. When high DFTs are found at the time of implantation in patients who have been taking chronic oral amiodarone, we recommend completing the procedure and repeating DFT testing after a 4-week drug-washout period.

Predischarge Testing and Programming

Prior to discharge, the pace-sense characteristics of the ICD system are assessed in all patients and posteroanterior and lateral chest x-rays are reviewed to rule out lead dislodgment. Modern ICD systems employ integrated lead technology that combine both pace-sense and defibrillation functions. Changes in lead position that can potentially result in failure to detect or terminate VF invariably result in a change in pace-sense variables relative to implant values.[45] It is our practice to reserve predischarge arrhythmia induction testing for select patients with marginal implant characteristics or in whom routine testing raises the possibility of a device malfunction.

The characteristics of induced VT correlate poorly with those of subsequent spontaneous VT episodes due to the frequent induction of faster, "nonclinical" VTs.[46] Fortunately, empirically programmed ATP successfully terminates VT in over 90 percent of cases.[47] In addition, even in VF survivors, the most common tachyarrhythmia recorded during follow-up is monomorphic VT.[48] Therefore, in the majority of ICD recipients, empiric programming of a VT zone should be considered prior to discharge.

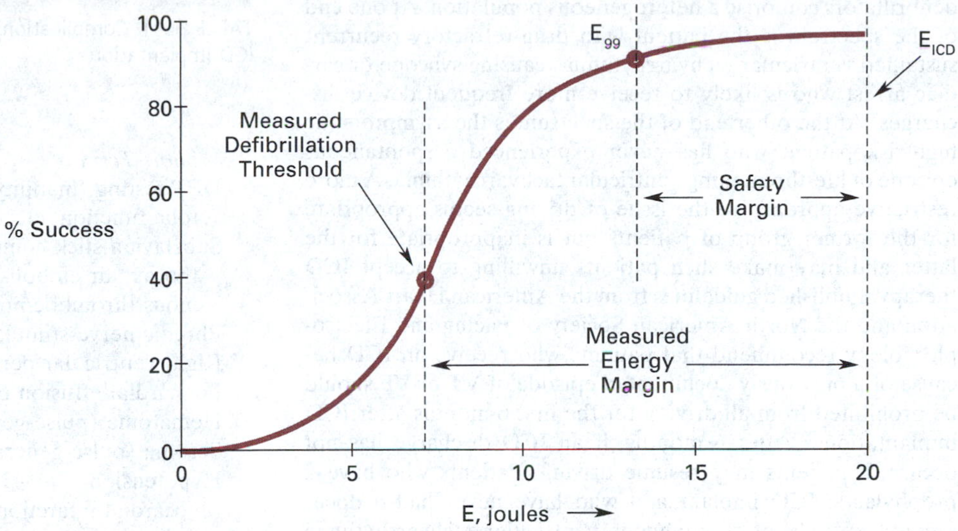

FIGURE 30-5 Percent probability for successful defibrillation versus shock energy. The measured ICD energy margin is the energy difference between the lowest conversion success [defibrillation threshold (DFT)] and the programmed ICD energy: energy margin = E_{ICD} − DFT. The ICD safety margin is the energy difference between the lowest energy required for consistent defibrillation success (E_{99}) and the programmed ICD energy: safety margin = E_{ICD} − E_{99}. (Adapted from Singer and Lang,[40] with permission.)

LONG-TERM FOLLOW-UP

Routine Patient Follow-up

Patients are reviewed routinely every 3 months to assess the pace-sense and impedance characteristics of the ICD system, to assess the charge times, and to diagnose the cause of any delivered therapy. Radiographs of the ICD system are obtained annually. Fortunately, careful regular follow-up will identify the majority of asymptomatic problems. If routine assessment reveals a significant alteration in the pace-sense or impedance characteristics of the system and if no defibrillation shock was recently administered, DFTs are rechecked noninvasively under intravenous sedation to confirm an adequate defibrillation safety margin. Tokano et al. performed serial DFT testing in 31 patients who received biphasic defibrillation systems. After 2 years' follow-up 5 patients, (15 percent) had an increase in defibrillation energy requirements of 10 J or more, and 1 patient (3 percent) required surgical revision of the system.[49]

All patients with an ICD should be considered for pulse generator replacement when there is evidence of battery depletion, since late shocks occurring many years after primary implantation appear to define a continuing need for this therapy in many patients.[50] At the time of elective pulse generator replacement, the pace-sense characteristics of the ICD system are reassessed, and VF is induced in order to confirm satisfactory sensing and ability to defibrillate VF with a safety margin of 10 J or more. Occasionally, a patient's defibrillation energy requirements may be unexpectedly elevated at the time of generator replacement, and appropriate revision of the system or implantation of a new integrated lead is required.

Psychosocial Issues

The ICD is generally well tolerated in the vast majority of patients for whom it is recommended. Quality of life declines in the first 6 months postimplantation but by 12 months has returned to preimplant levels.[51] Depression, anxiety, and reduced sexual function may occur after device implantation. Factors that adversely affect quality of life include frequent or inappropriate shocks, device malfunction, or product recall.[52,53] Since shock delivery has a major impact on quality of life, it is appropriate to consider measures such as concomitant drug therapy, empiric programming of ATP for VT, and use of detection enhancement algorithms to minimize the risk of both appropriate and inappropriate shock delivery during long-term follow-up.[13,14,26] In a prospective, multicenter trial of ICD patients randomized to receive either sotalol or placebo, sotalol significantly reduced the mean annual number of shocks (1.4 shocks) compared to placebo (3.9 shocks) and significantly prolonged the time interval to first shock.[54]

Automobile Driving

A major concern among ICD patients is driving restrictions. Because of the risk of an arrhythmia recurrence or the delivery of high-energy shocks, restrictions on driving should be considered and discussed with all patients prior to device implantation. The period for greatest risk of ICD discharge is within the first 6 months after implantation. Patients receiving implantable defibrillators comprise a heterogeneous population. At one end of the spectrum is the patient with drug-refractory recurrent sustained ventricular tachyarrhythmias causing syncope or cardiac arrest who is likely to receive more frequent device discharges. At the other end of the spectrum is the asymptomatic high-risk patient who has never experienced a spontaneous episode of life-threatening ventricular tachyarrhythmia. A more restrictive approach to the issue of driving seems appropriate for the former group of patients but is inappropriate for the latter and may make such patients unwilling to accept ICD therapy. Published guidelines from the American Heart Association and the North American Society of Pacing and Electrophysiology recommend that patients who receive an ICD because of a previously documented episode of VT or VF should be prohibited from all driving for the first 6 months after ICD implantation.[55] After 6 months, if an ICD discharge has not occurred, patients may resume driving. Patients who have a prophylactic ICD implant and who have never had a documented episode of spontaneous ventricular tachyarrhythmia should not be prohibited from noncommercial driving. The recommendations make no distinction between patients whose primary treatment is antiarrhythmic drug therapy rather than ICD therapy.

COMPLICATIONS AND TROUBLESHOOTING

Morbidity and Mortality

ICD therapy is associated with well-known risks (Table 30-1) that must be weighed against the potential benefits of automatic ventricular tachyarrhythmia therapy. The last 10 years have seen a simplification of device implantation from nonthoracotomy transvenous abdominal implantation to single-lead pectoral implantation. A multicenter study of 473 patients implanted with a pectoral unipolar device reported successful device implantation in 98 percent of patients; in 7 percent of patients, implant criteria either were not met or were not fully assessed. No patient died within 24 h of the procedure, and the 1-month (perioperative) mortality rate was 0.9 percent.[57] Patients were followed for a mean of 6 months. Twenty-nine patients (6 percent) has serious procedure- or device-related complications requiring surgical intervention. A study of over 3000 patients who had nonthoracotomy ICD systems implanted in either an abdominal, a prepectoral, or a subpectoral position found that the 1-year cumulative complication-free survival rate was 88 percent and did not differ significantly among the three groups.[58] However, the complication rate depends on the definitions used and the duration of follow-up. If one includes mild device-related complications (e.g., inappropriate therapy delivery), approximately 50 percent of patients experience an adverse event within the first year of ICD implantation.[59] This needs to be considered when recommending device implantation in high-risk asymptomatic patients.

Lead-related problems, such as dislodgment, insulation defects, or conductor fracture, which can result in failure to sense, failure to pace, and either inappropriate defibrillation shocks or inability to defibrillate VF, remain a significant problem despite the enormous advances in lead technology. A comparison of abdominal versus pectoral implants followed for a mean of 4 months postimplantation found that pectoral devices were associated with significantly fewer severe lead-related events, the majority of which were dislodgments (5 versus 11 percent).[60]

TABLE 30-1 Complications Associated with Pectoral ICD Implantation

PROCEDURE-RELATED
Short-Term
DFT testing (inability to defibrillate, worsening systolic function, electromechanical dissociation)
Subclavian stick complications (pneumothorax, hemothorax, air embolism, subclavian artery puncture)
Venous thromboembolism
Phrenic nerve stimulation
Right ventricular perforation
Pericardial effusion or tamponade
Hematoma (pulse-generator pocket)
Seroma (pulse-generator pocket)
Hypotension
Myocardial infarction
Cerebrovascular accident
Proarrhythmia (atrial fibrillation, increased frequency of ventricular tachyarrhythmia: "electrical storm")
Long-Term
Infection
Erosion
Migration
Venous thromboembolism
Endocarditis
Shoulder-related problems
SYSTEM-RELATED
Lead dislodgment (Gross-, microdislodgment, Twiddler's syndrome)
Lead conductor fracture
Lead insulation defect
Lead perforation (+/− diaphragmatic pacing)
Loose set screw
Exit block (high pacing threshold)
Inappropriate shock delivery
Premature battery depletion
Device recall

SOURCE: Modified from O'Callaghan and Ruskin,[56] with permission.

One of the most devastating complications is infection of the ICD system. Pectoral devices avoid the infection risks associated with tunneling to the abdomen or placement of a subcutaneous patch. Of 950 patients who had a transvenous system implanted, the infection rate was 0.6 percent, compared to 1.9 percent in patients who had a transvenous system plus a subcutaneous patch.[61] Infection resembles that observed with permanent pacemaker implantation. Direct intraoperative contamination is the source of most infections. However, due to the low virulence of some organisms (e.g., *Staphylococcus epidermis*), infections may not become obvious for some considerable time after implantation. In general, explantation of the entire ICD system is required. After a regimen of intense antibiotic therapy and if all clinical evidence of infection is resolved, reimplantation at a different site may be performed, but the risk of reinfection is higher than following a primary implant.

Troubleshooting

The differentiation of appropriate from inappropriate device function in a patient who has received an ICD discharge is a challenging problem. The initial step toward management is device interrogation to determine whether the ICD therapy was appropriate or inappropriate. ICDs have advanced from devices providing basic diagnostic data, such as event counts or RR intervals only, to sophisticated electrocardiographic monitoring units. Analysis of stored intracardiac electrograms recorded

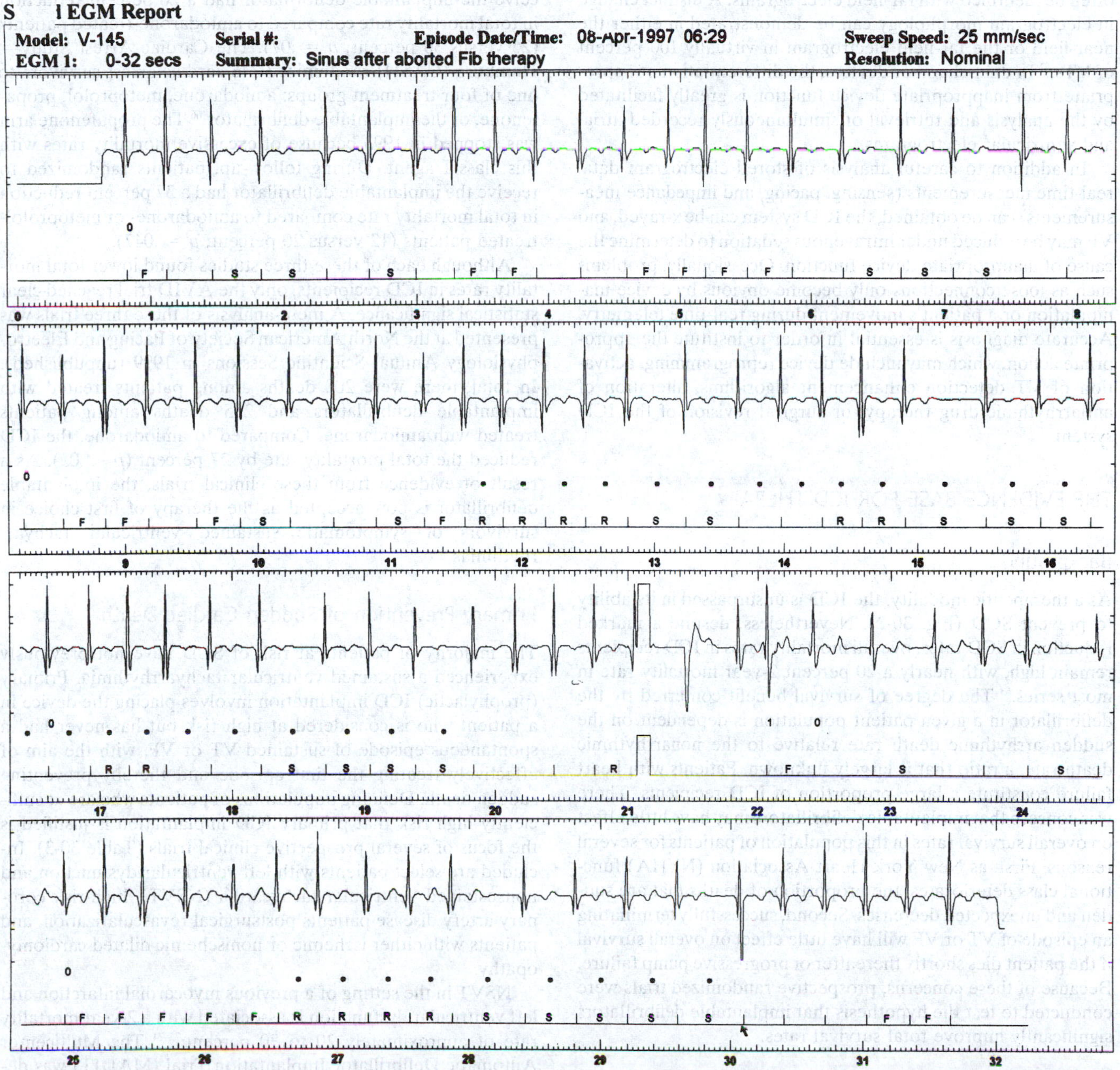

FIGURE 30-6 Stored electrogram of inappropriate shock delivery due to atrial fibrillation. The recording is a continuous 32-s strip consisting of a waveform channel and a status channel. Atrial fibrillation is seen throughout the recording. In the first panel, the ICD classifies the shorter intervals as fibrillation (F). In the second panel, before the 12-s mark the detection criterion for VF is met. Device charging (*) and reconfirmation (R) of the arrhythmia begin as recorded in the status channel. In the third panel, a high-voltage shock is delivered inappropriately at the 21-s mark, denoted by a full-scale positive rectangular marker in both the waveform and status channels. Atrial fibrillation persists, and the detection criterion for VF is met a second time, in panel 4 before the 27-s mark. During device charging, the ventricular rate slows, and redetection of "sinus rhythm" (normal rate zone) aborts shock therapy. Sinus redetection is denoted by an arrow in the status channel and a negative deflection in the marker channel. Information regarding the device, date and time of the episode, screen sweep speed, the electrogram number and duration, and the reason the event was stored is located in the oblong box at the top of the page. (Courtesy of Mary Guy RN, ICD Clinic, Massachusetts General Hospital. From O'Callaghan and Ruskin,[56] with permission.)

during the time interval preceding and following ICD therapy, in addition to marker channels that annotate each sensed event, results in a confident diagnosis of the causes of most ICD therapies (Fig. 30-6). In general, changes in electrogram morphology compared to sinus rhythm are consistent with ventricular tachyarrhythmias, while an identical electrogram morphology is consistent with supraventricular arrhythmias. Atrial activity can often be identified with far-field electrograms. A distinct change in electrogram morphology can be demonstrated in either the near-field or the far-field electrogram in virtually 100 percent of VTs.[62] In dual-chamber devices, the differentiation of appropriate from inappropriate device function is greatly facilitated by the analysis and retrieval of simultaneously recorded atrial and ventricular electrograms.

In addition to careful analysis of stored electrogram data, real-time measurements (sensing, pacing, and impedance measurements) can be obtained, the ICD system can be x-rayed, and VF may be induced under intravenous sedation to determine the cause of inappropriate device function. Occasionally, problems such as loose connections only become obvious by device manipulation or a patient's movement during real-time telemetry. Accurate diagnosis is essential in order to institute the appropriate action, which may include device reprogramming, activation of VT detection enhancement algorithms, alteration of antiarrhythmic drug therapy, or surgical revision of the ICD system.

THE EVIDENCE BASE FOR ICD THERAPY

Background

As a therapeutic modality, the ICD is unsurpassed in its ability to prevent SCD (Fig. 30-2). Nevertheless, despite a marked reduction in SCD rates, overall mortality rates in ICD recipients remain high, with nearly a 20 percent 2-year mortality rate in most series.[63] The degree of survival benefit conferred by the defibrillator in a given patient population is dependent on the sudden arrhythmic death rate relative to the nonarrhythmic death rate, a ratio that is largely unknown. Patients with heart failure constitute a large proportion of ICD recipients. There was concern that implantable defibrillators may have little effect on overall survival rates in this population of patients for several reasons. First, as New York Heart Association (NYHA) functional class deteriorates, the proportion of deaths that are sudden and unexpected decreases. Second, successfully terminating an episode of VT or VF will have little effect on overall survival if the patient dies shortly thereafter of progressive pump failure. Because of these concerns, prospective randomized trials were conducted to test the hypothesis that implantable defibrillators significantly improve total survival rates.

Secondary Prevention of Sudden Cardiac Death

The results of three large prospective ICD trials comparing implantable defibrillators to antiarrhythmic drug therapy (mainly amiodarone) in patients with life-threatening ventricular tachyarrhythmias have consistently shown that the implantable defibrillator improves overall survival (Table 30-2). In the Antiarrhythmic Versus Implantable Defibrillator (AVID) trial of over 1000 patients, implantable defibrillators resulted in a 31 percent reduction in total mortality rate at 3 years compared to the antiarrhythmic drug therapy group (25 versus 36 percent; $p < .02$; Fig. 30-7).[64] The Canadian Implantable Defibrillator Study (CIDS) randomized over 600 patients presenting with sustained ventricular tachyarrhythmias to treatment with either the implantable defibrillator or amiodarone.[65] After 3 years' follow-up, patients randomized to receive the implantable defibrillator had a 20 percent reduction in total mortality rate compared to amiodarone-treated patients (25 versus 30 percent; $p = .07$). The Cardiac Arrest Study—Hamburg (CASH) randomized 346 cardiac arrest survivors to one of four treatment groups: amiodarone, metoprolol, propafenone, or the implantable defibrillator.[66] The propafenone arm was stopped in 1993 because of excessive mortality rates with this class I agent. During follow-up, patients randomized to receive the implantable defibrillator had a 37 percent reduction in total mortality rate compared to amiodarone- or metoprolol-treated patients (12 versus 20 percent; $p = .047$).

Although each of these three studies found lower total mortality rates in ICD recipients, only the AVID trial reached clear statistical significance. A meta-analysis of these three trials was presented at the North American Society of Pacing and Electrophysiology Annual Scientific Sessions in 1999 (unpublished). In total, there were 200 deaths among patients treated with implantable defibrillators and 255 deaths among patients treated with amiodarone. Compared to amiodarone, the ICD reduced the total mortality rate by 27 percent ($p < .05$). As a result of evidence from these clinical trials, the implantable defibrillator is now accepted as the therapy of first choice in survivors of symptomatic sustained ventricular tachyarrhythmias.

Primary Prevention of Sudden Cardiac Death

The majority of patients at risk of SCD have not previously experienced a sustained ventricular tachyarrhythmia. Primary (prophylactic) ICD implantation involves placing the device in a patient who is considered at high risk but has never had a spontaneous episode of sustained VT or VF, with the aim of effectively treating the first episode and thereby preventing sudden death. Defining populations of patients who are at sufficiently high risk that primary ICD implantation is justified is the focus of several prospective clinical trials (Table 30-3). Included are select patients with left ventricular dysfunction and nonsustained ventricular tachycardia (NSVT), high-risk coronary artery disease patients postsurgical revascularization, and patients with either ischemic or nonischemic dilated cardiomyopathy.

NSVT in the setting of a previous myocardial infarction and left ventricular dysfunction is associated with a 2-year mortality rate of approximately 20 to 30 percent.[72–74] The Multicenter Automatic Defibrillator Implantation Trial (MADIT) was designed to determine whether prophylactic ICD implantation in patients with prior myocardial infarction, left ventricular ejection fraction (LVEF) less than or equal to 35 percent, NSVT, and inducible, nonsuppressible VT or VF would improve survival rates compared to conventional medical therapy.[67] Amiodarone was used in 74 percent of the conventional therapy group 1 month after randomization, but by the end of the study only 45 percent of the conventional group were still taking amiodarone. Total mortality rates in the ICD group were sig-

TABLE 30-2 Multicenter Secondary Prevention ICD Trials

Trial	Study Population	Treatment Groups	Sample Size	Primary End Point	Study Period	Outcome
AVID[64] (Antiarrhythmics versus Implantable Defibrillators)	(1) Cardiac arrest survivors or (2) VT with either syncope or hypotension + EF < 40%	ICD vs amiodarone or guided sotalol therapy	1016 patients	Total mortality rate	1993–1997	31% reduction in total mortality rate at 3 years with ICD ($p < .02$)
CIDS[65] (Canadian Implantable Defibrillator Study)	(1) Cardiac arrest survivors or (2) syncopal VT or (3) symptomatic VT + EF < 35% or (4) SUO + documented spontaneous or induced VT	ICD vs amiodarone	~ 600 patients	Total mortality rate	1990–1997	20% reduction in total mortality rate at 3 years with ICD ($p < .07$, NS)
CASH[66] (Cardiac Arrest Study—Hamburg)	Cardiac arrest survivors and inducible VT or VF	ICD vs amiodarone vs metoprolol vs propafenone[a]	346 patients	Total mortality rate	1987–1995	37% reduction in total mortality rate with ICD compared to amiodarone or metoprolol (one-sided $p = .047$)

[a]Propafenone limb terminated in 1993 due to excessive mortality rate.
ABBREVIATIONS: SUO = syncope of undetermined origin; NS = non-significant.

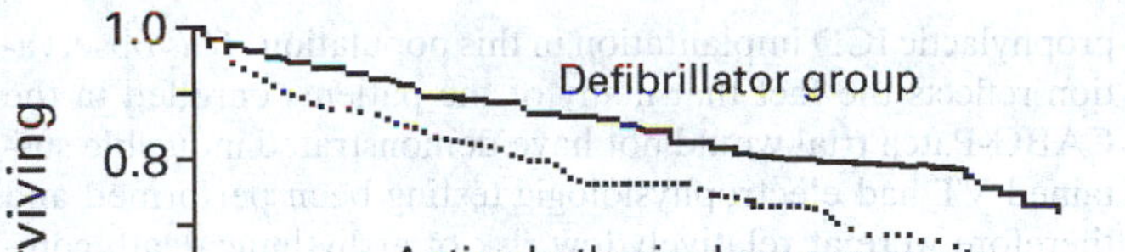

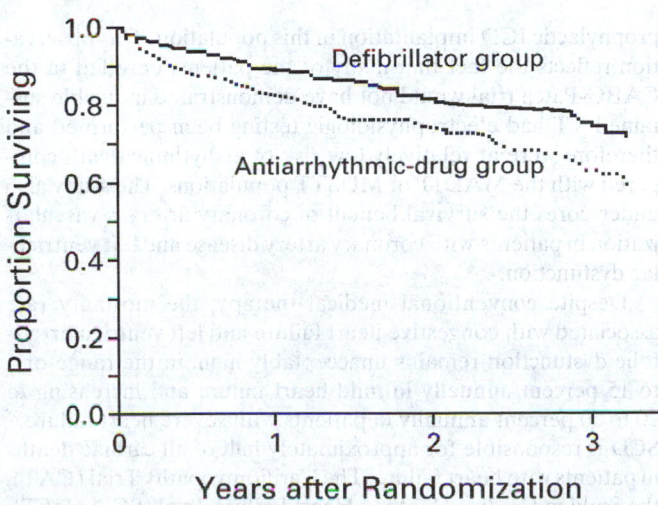

FIGURE 30-7 The Antiarrhythmic Versus Implantable Defibrillator (AVID) Trial. Overall survival in the defibrillator group and the antiarrhythmic drug group up to 3 years after randomization in the AVID trial. Survival was better among patients treated with the implantable defibrillator ($p < .02$). (From the AVID Investigators,[64] with permission.)

nificantly less than in the conventional treatment group. The Multicenter UnSustained Tachycardia Trial (MUSTT) was designed to determine whether electrophysiologically guided antiarrhythmic therapy would reduce the risk of sudden death among patients with coronary artery disease, LVEF less than or equal to 40 percent, NSVT, and inducible VT or VF compared to no antiarrhythmic therapy.[68] Patients randomized to antiarrhythmic therapy (ICD or electrophysiologically guided drug therapy) had a significantly reduced arrhythmic mortality rate compared to the conservative treatment group. It is noteworthy that the improvement in outcome was entirely due to the ICD patients; electrophysiologically guided drug therapy (mostly class I agents) did not improve and may have worsened outcome. Although not a primary end point of the trial, Kaplan-Meier estimates of overall mortality rate show significantly fewer deaths in ICD patients than in either of the other two groups (Fig. 30-8). Therefore, the results of the MADIT and MUSTT trials confirm that, in patients with coronary artery disease, depressed LVEF, NSVT, and inducible sustained ventricular tachyarrhythmias who have never had a spontaneous episode of sustained VT or VF, the ICD is effective in significantly reducing the risk of SCD and prolonging overall survival.

The Coronary Artery Bypass Graft (CABG) Patch trial randomized patients with LVEF less than 36 percent and a positive signal-averaged electrocardiogram who were undergoing coronary artery bypass surgery to a prophylactic ICD or no specific antiarrhythmic therapy.[69] There was no survival benefit from

TABLE 30-3 Multicenter Primary Prevention ICD Trials

Trial	Study Population	Treatment Groups	Sample Size	Primary End Point	Study Period	Outcome
MADIT[67] (Multicenter Automatic Defibrillator Implantation Trial)	Prior MI with LVEF <35%, NSVT, and inducible nonsuppressible VT or VF	ICD vs conventional medical therapy	196 patients	Total mortality rate	1990–1996	Total mortality rate in ICD group significantly less than in conventional group (16 vs 39%, $p < .01$)
MUSTT[68] (Multicenter Unsustained Tachycardia Trial)	CAD with LVEF <40%, NSVT and inducible VT or VF	Antiarrhythmic therapy (ICD or EP-guided antiarrhythmic drug) vs no antiarrhythmic therapy	704 patients	Cardiac arrest or death from arrhythmia	1990–1998	5-year incidence of cardiac arrest or death from arrhythmia significantly less among "antiarrhythmic therapy" than among "no antiarrhythmic therapy" patients (25 vs 32% $p = .04$)
CABG-Patch[69] (Coronary Artery Bypass Graft Patch Trial)	CABG with LVEF <36% and positive SAECG	ICD + CABG vs CABG only	900 patients	Total mortality rate	1990–1997	At 4-year follow-up, total actuarial mortality rate in ICD group no different than for control group (27 vs 24%, $p = .7$)
CAT[70] (Cardiomyopathy Trial)	Dilated cardiomyopathy with LVEF <30% and no symptomatic ventricular arrhythmias	ICD vs control group	~720 patients	Total mortality rate	1991–present	No possible benefit from ICD determined at interim analysis (1997)
SCD-HeFT[71] (Sudden Cardiac Death in Heart Failure Trial)	Ischemic or dilated cardiomyopathy with congestive heart failure (NYHA II–III) and LVEF <35%	ICD vs amiodarone vs conventional group	~2500 patients	Total mortality rate	1996–present	Ongoing
MADIT-II[71] (Second Multicenter Automatic Defibrillator Implantation Trial)	Prior myocardial infarction with LVEF <30%	ICD vs conventional group	~1200	Total mortality rate	1998–present	Ongoing

ABBREVIATIONS: CABG = coronary artery bypass graft; CAD = coronary artery disease; EP = electrophysiologic; MI = myocardial infarction; Rx = treatment; SAECG = signal-averaged electrocardiogram.

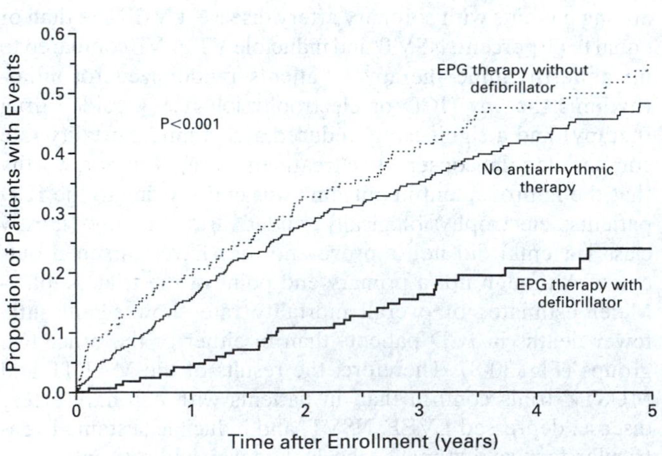

FIGURE 30-8 The Multicenter Unsustained Tachycardia Trial (MUSTT). Kaplan-Meier estimates of overall mortality rate according to whether the patients received treatment with electrophysiologically guided (EPG) therapy without defibrillator (i.e., antiarrhythmic drug therapy), no antiarrhythmic therapy, or electrophysiologically guided therapy with a defibrillator. Mortality rates were significantly less in the ICD-treated patients than in the other two groups. (From Buxton et al.,[68] with permission.)

prophylactic ICD implantation in this population. This observation reflects the fact that many of the patients enrolled in the CABG-Patch trial would not have demonstrated inducible sustained VT had electrophysiologic testing been performed and therefore were at relatively low risk of arrhythmic death compared with the MADIT or MUSTT populations. The study also underscores the survival benefit of coronary artery revascularization in patients with coronary artery disease and left ventricular dysfunction.

Despite conventional medical therapy, the mortality rate associated with congestive heart failure and left ventricular systolic dysfunction remains unacceptably high, in the range of 5 to 15 percent annually in mild heart failure and increasing to 20 to 50 percent annually in patients with severe heart failure.[75] SCD is responsible for approximately half of all cardiac deaths in patients with heart failure. The Cardiomyopathy Trial (CAT), the Sudden Cardiac Death in Heart Failure Trial (SCD-HeFT), and the second Multicenter Automatic Defibrillator Implantation Trial (MADIT-II) will address the issue of whether the ICD improves survival in a population of cardiomyopathy patients irregardless of the presence or absence of arrhythmia markers (inducibility, NSVT, etc.).[70,71] Preliminary results from the CAT trial suggest that the ICD does not improve overall survival, however our future approach to the management of heart failure patients awaits the results of SCD-HeFT and MADIT-II.

The results of negative ICD trials (CABG-Patch and CAT) emphasize the fact that ICDs prolong survival in a population of patients only if that population has a sufficiently high incidence of life-threatening ventricular tachyarrhythmias and a sufficiently low incidence of death from all other causes. The real challenge over the next few years will be developing means of accurately identifying patients at sufficiently high risk of life-threatening ventricular tachyarrhythmias and sufficiently low risk of death from all other causes in whom ICD therapy is both efficacious and cost effective.[76]

Cost-Effectiveness

The cost of ICD therapy compared to alternative therapies will be the focus of much study and discussion in the next few years. In addition to hardware costs (approximately $20,000 to $25,000), there are implantation costs, hospital admission charges, and the cost of routine follow-up and pulse generator replacement. Treatment strategy is central to the issue of overall costs. In the early 1990s, management of patients with life-threatening ventricular tachyarrhythmia consisted of serial antiarrhythmic drug testing, with ICD therapy reserved for those patients whose arrhythmias were not adequately suppressed. This strategy was characterized by long hospitalizations and frequent progression to late ICD implantation, resulting in substantial costs. In recent years, the strategy of ICD implantation as first-line therapy and the progression from thoracotomy and abdominal implantation to transvenous pectoral implantation has significantly reduced the length of hospital stay and substantially lowered the initial cost of ICD therapy.[77,78]

Long-term costs need to be compared with outcome measures, including total mortality rate and quality of life, in order to assess cost effectiveness. In the AVID trial, the average length of additional life associated with ICD therapy was 2.7 months. The estimated cost per life-year saved was $127,000.[79] In the MADIT trial, the average length of additional life associated with ICD therapy was 10.3 months, and the estimated cost per life-year saved was $27,000.[80] The cost analysis of MADIT, in contrast to AVID, compares favorably with other cardiac interventions. The difference is most likely due to differences in patients' selection. The MADIT patients, all of whom had inducible nonsuppressible ventricular tachyarrhythmias (NSVTs) on electrophysiologic testing, were at higher risk of death than were the AVID patients, as evidenced by the poorer prognosis in the conventional arm of MADIT compared to that in the antiarrhythmic-drug arm of AVID. These results emphasize the fact that the patients' selection largely determines the cost effectiveness of ICD therapy. The most cost-effective use of the ICD is in patients at high risk of death due to ventricular tachyarrhythmia and at low risk of death from all other causes. More accurate risk stratification is necessary to ensure that ICD therapy is applied in an optimally efficient and cost-effective manner.

ICD THERAPY IN SPECIFIC CLINICAL SETTINGS

The American College of Cardiology (ACC) and the American Heart Association (AHA) advise ICD therapy in cardiac arrest survivors, in patients with spontaneous sustained ventricular tachycardia, in select patients with syncope of undetermined origin, and in select patients with coronary artery disease, left ventricular dysfunction, and NSVT (Table 30-4).[81] In these clinical circumstances, the implantable defibrillator is now regarded as the treatment of first choice. The role of antiarrhythmic therapy in these patients is mainly limited to adjunctive therapy in ICD recipients who have other tachyarrhythmias (e.g., atrial fibrillation) or who are receiving frequent shocks and require suppressive drug therapy. Future drug trials in patients with ICDs may result in the development of new, safer antiarrhythmic drugs.

Cardiac Arrest Survivors

Aborted SCD is, in the majority of cases, caused by life-threatening ventricular tachyarrhythmias (VF and hypotensive VT). Structural heart disease is almost invariably present, which in adult populations is most frequently coronary artery disease.[82] Survivors of cardiac arrest, in the absence of an acute myocardial infarction (first 48 h), are at high risk of future recurrence. Data from the 1970s, which today reflect the natural history of this condition, show a 36 percent 1-year mortality rate in patients who were successfully resuscitated, hospitalized, and discharged home following an out-of-hospital VF arrest.[83]

The role of ischemia in the pathogenesis of SCD is not clearly defined. Only a small proportion of cardiac arrest survivors have clinical evidence of an acute myocardial infarction. Nonetheless, since the majority of cardiac arrest survivors have evidence of significant chronic coronary atherosclerosis, transient ischemia is suspected as the major trigger factor for life-threatening ventricular tachyarrhythmias. Cardiac catheterization identifies those survivors of SCD who have critical obstructive coronary artery disease. It is our practice to revascularize these patients whenever feasible. Cardiac arrest occurring in the setting of acute clinical ischemia or within 48 h of an acute myocardial infarction is, with rare exception, treated in the conventional manner without electrophysiologic workup or ICD implantation. In addition, select patients with significant multivessel coronary artery disease, reversible ischemia on functional assessment, and no obvious arrhythmic substrate (no prior Q-wave infarction, preserved left ventricular function, and negative signal-averaged ECG) usually require revascularization rather than ICD implantation. In this group, we perform an electrophysiologic study following revascularization, and those with no inducible arrhythmias are considered to be a low-risk group, whose treatment usually consists of beta blockade.[84] These two groups (patients with acute clinical ischemia and patients with significant multivessel coronary artery disease, reversible ischemia, and no obvious arrhythmic substrate) account for only a minority of cardiac arrest survivors. The majority of cardiac arrest survivors have an obvious arrhythmic substrate [prior Q-wave infarction, depressed LVEF, positive signal-averaged ECG, or inducible sustained monomorphic VT (SMVT)], and, in addition to revascularization, we advise ICD implantation.

Until now, it has been assumed that ventricular tachyarrhythmias due to a transient or reversible disorder are adequately treated by correcting the underlying cause; this is supported by the current ACC-AHA guidelines. Recent analysis of the AVID trial registry of screened nonrandomized patients has reported that the overall mortality rate in these patients is as great as in

TABLE 30-4 ACC-AHA Guidelines for ICD Implantation[81]

CLASS I: ICD INDICATED

1. Cardiac arrest due to VT or VF not due to a transient or reversible cause
2. Spontaneous sustained VT
3. Syncope of undetermined origin with clinically relevant, hemodynamically significant sustained VT or VF induced at electrophysiologic study when drug therapy is ineffective, not tolerated, or not preferred
4. Nonsustained VT with coronary artery disease, prior myocardial infarction, left ventricular dysfunction, and inducible VF or sustained VT at electrophysiologic study that is not suppressible by a class I antiarrhythmic drug

CLASS II: ICD MAY BE INDICATED

1. Cardiac arrest presumed to be due to VF when electrophysiologic testing is precluded by other medical conditions
2. Severe symptoms attributable to ventricular tachyarrhythmias while awaiting cardiac transplantation
3. Familial or inherited conditions with a high risk for life-threatening ventricular tachyarrhythmias, such as long-QT syndrome or hypertrophic cardiomyopathy
4. Nonsustained VT with coronary artery disease, prior myocardial infarction, left ventricular dysfunction, and inducible sustained VT or VF at electrophysiologic study
5. Recurrent syncope of undetermined etiology in the presence of ventricular dysfunction and inducible ventricular arrhythmias at electrophysiologic study when other causes of syncope have been excluded

CLASS III: ICD CONTRAINDICATED

1. Syncope of undetermined cause in a patient without inducible ventricular tachyarrhythmias
2. Incessant VT or VF
3. VF or VT resulting from arrhythmias amenable to surgical or catheter ablation, for example, atrial arrhythmias associated with Wolf-Parkinson-White syndrome, right ventricular outflow tract VT, idiopathic left ventricular tachycardia, or fascicular VT
4. Ventricular tachyarrhythmias due to a transient or reversible disorder, for example, acute myocardial infarction, electrolyte imbalance, drugs, or trauma
5. Significant psychiatric illnesses that may be aggravated by device implantation or preclude systematic follow-up
6. Terminal illness with projected life expectancy ≤6 months
7. Patients with coronary artery disease, left ventricular dysfunction, and prolonged QRS duration in the absence of spontaneous or inducible sustained or nonsustained VT who are undergoing coronary bypass surgery
8. NYHA class IV drug-refractory congestive heart failure in patients who are not candidates for cardiac transplantation

SOURCE: Gregoratos et al.,[81] with permission.

patients with prior cardiac arrest.[85] Determining whether this high mortality rate is due to sudden arrhythmic death or progressive pump failure requires further study and may significantly affect our management of these patients.

Sustained Monomorphic Ventricular Tachycardia

In patients with SMVT that has resulted in a cardiac arrest or syncope, the ICD is usually employed as first-line therapy. In patients with SMVT that is tolerated hemodynamically, other potential therapeutic options include empiric amiodarone therapy, electrophysiologically guided antiarrhythmic drug therapy, transcatheter radiofrequency ablation, and arrhythmia surgery. Empiric amiodarone therapy is associated with high rates of drug discontinuation due to adverse side effects. "Guided" drug therapy using either invasive electrophysiologic study or noninvasive Holter monitoring has failed to adequately protect against arrhythmia recurrence and has largely been abandoned. Catheter ablation, the treatment of choice in patients with VT and structurally normal hearts, is usually only employed as adjunctive therapy in patients with underlying structural heart disease, typically in patients with implanted devices. Catheter ablation is suitable in only about 10 percent of patients with spontaneous sustained ventricular tachycardia.[86] Arrhythmia surgery is the only therapy with SCD rates similar to those for ICD therapy.[87,88] Although this approach can be curative, perioperative mortality rates are much higher than those associated with ICD implantation, ranging from 9 to 15 percent. Combined aneurysmectomy and intraoperative map-guided subendocardial resection yields a low rate of arrhythmia recurrence and is only indicated in highly selected patients who have a discrete left ventricular aneurysm.

In summary, compared to the other available treatments, ICD therapy is widely applicable, well tolerated, and associated with good short-term and long-term results. Today it is the preferred mode of therapy in the vast majority of patients with structural heart disease and SMVT. The various therapeutic options available should be considered as complementary rather than competing therapies. In managing individual patients, more than one therapy or even all therapies may be employed over a period of time.

Syncope of Undetermined Origin

Syncope is a common, usually benign condition. However, when associated with structural heart disease and inducible VT at electrophysiologic study, it carries a high risk of SCD. One representative study reported a sudden death rate of 48 percent at 3 years in patients with syncope of undetermined origin and inducible sustained VT, compared to 9 percent in patients with negative electrophysiologic study results.[89] The risk of death in patients presenting with syncope plus inducible ventricular tachyarrhythmia on electrophysiologic study is similar to that in patients presenting with documented spontaneous VT or VF.[90] The ACC-AHA guidelines recommend ICD therapy in patients with syncope of undetermined origin, structural heart disease, and inducible hypotensive ventricular tachycardia.[81] However, follow-up of small series of such patients have reported a high total mortality rate despite ICD therapy.[91] Whether ICD therapy truly reduces the total mortality rate in this group can only be answered by a prospective, randomized trial. The CIDS trial randomized patients with syncope of undetermined origin and documented or induced sustained VT.[65] Analysis of this subgroup should help resolve this issue.

Patients with idiopathic dilated cardiomyopathy who present with syncope have a high mortality rate, and, in contrast to coronary artery disease patients, the role of electrophysiologic study is ill defined. According to the ACC-AHA guidelines, ICD therapy is contraindicated in patients with syncope of undetermined origin and no inducible ventricular tachyarrhythmia. Knight et al. reported on 14 consecutive patients with nonischemic cardiomyopathy, unexplained syncope, and a negative electrophysiologic test result who underwent defibrillator implantation.[92] Fifty percent of patients received appropriate shocks during 2 years' follow-up, supporting the use of ICD therapy in these patients. Prospective studies are needed to identify which patients with dilated cardiomyopathy and undetermined syncope may benefit from ICD implantation. Meanwhile, these patients need careful clinical assessment, and select patients may benefit from implantable event loop-recording devices.

Symptomatic Patients with Severe Left Ventricular Dysfunction

Patients with poor left ventricular function who have experienced a spontaneous episode of life-threatening ventricular tachyarrhythmia are a high risk of both SCD and death due to progressive pump failure. Successfully terminating an episode of VT or VF will have little effect on overall survival if the patient dies shortly thereafter of pump failure. In the past, this observation raised the concern that implantable defibrillators may have little effect on overall survival in this patient population. It is somewhat surprising that subgroup analysis of both the AVID and CIDS trials has found that patients with a LVEF less than or equal to 35 percent derive the greatest survival benefit from defibrillator therapy.[93,94] Patients with an LVEF greater than 35 percent had similar survival benefit up to 3 years postrandomization with either empiric amiodarone or device therapy, probably due to a lower arrhythmia recurrence rate. Bocker et al. also assessed the potential benefit of ICD therapy in 603 patients with and without heart failure and concluded that patients with NYHA functional class I to III heart failure benefited in terms of overall survival from ICD implantation.[95] ICD therapy is contraindicated in patients with NYHA class IV heart failure unless they have experienced an episode of life-threatening ventricular tachyarrhythmia and are awaiting cardiac transplantation.

Patients awaiting heart transplantation who have experienced a spontaneous episode of life-threatening ventricular tachyarrhythmia deserve special consideration. Not only are they at risk of sudden tachyarrhythmic death, but they also are at high risk of sudden death due to bradyarrhythmias or electromechanical dissociation and of death due to progressive pump failure.[96] Nevertheless, it has been reported that cardiac transplant candidates who have experienced a spontaneous episode of life-threatening ventricular tachyarrhythmia can be effectively protected against sudden arrhythmic death despite having a high incidence of appropriate shocks early after implantation.[97]

Asymptomatic High-Risk Patients

Since the prognosis associated with a first cardiac arrest is very poor, an effective primary prevention strategy is required to identify and effectively treat patients at high risk of sudden death who have not yet experienced a spontaneous episode of life-threatening ventricular tachyarrhythmia (hypotensive VT or VF). The results of the MADIT and MUSTT trials confirm that, in a clearly defined high-risk group of patients with coronary artery disease, depressed left ventricular function, NSVT, and inducible sustained ventricular tachyarrhythmias, the ICD is effective in significantly reducing the risk of SCD and prolonging overall survival. In clinical practice, however, patients with coronary artery disease, depressed left ventricular function, and NSVT are common, and there is at present no consensus as to which patients should proceed to invasive electrophysiologic study and possible ICD implantation. In addition, the cost effectiveness of screening large numbers of these patients has not been assessed. We do not recommend routine screening of patients with left ventricular dysfunction to detect the presence of NSVT. However, in selected patients with severe left ventricular dysfunction due to who are brought to our attention because of recurrent NSVT, we recommend electrophysiologic testing and, if MADIT or MUSTT criteria are met, ICD implantation.

Primary prevention in many patients with cardiomyopathy is limited by our inability to accurately identify those at risk of SCD. The issue of whether the ICD improves survival in cardiomyopathy patients irregardless of the presence or absence of arrhythmia markers (e.g., inducibility, NSVT, etc.) is at present being addressed by SCD-HeFT and MADIT-II trials (Table 30-3). The ability of noninvasive markers to predict overall mortality rates and arrhythmic events in over 200 patients with idiopathic dilated cardiomyopathy over a 5-year follow-up period is currently being undertaken and should help identify patients who may benefit most from ICD therapy.[98]

Patients awaiting heart transplantation who have never experienced a spontaneous episode of life-threatening ventricular tachyarrhythmia deserve special consideration. Although ICD therapy is contraindicated in patients with NYHA class IV heart failure, due to a high incidence of nontachyarrhythmic deaths, it has been argued that ICD should be implanted in all NYHA class III patients as a "bridge" to transplantation. To date, no prospective randomized trial has been conducted to assess the benefit of such a strategy.

Summary

The ICD is now accepted as first-line therapy in the management of most patients who have experienced a spontaneous episode of life-threatening ventricular tachyarrhythmia. Much work needs to be done to accurately identify those patients at high risk of arrhythmic death who are at relatively low risk of death from all other causes and who would benefit from prophylactic ICD therapy. Prospective randomized trials have identified specific subgroups of patients who benefit from ICD therapy (MADIT and MUSTT patients), but a clear strategy regarding the screening and the investigation of such patients is required.

FUTURE DIRECTIONS

Implantable cardioverter-defibrillator technology is evolving rapidly. Nonetheless, ICD devices are far from ideal, and many advances can be anticipated in the years ahead.[99] Advances in battery and capacitor technology, improved lead systems, and more efficient defibrillation waveforms will hopefully enable the ICD of the future to more closely approach the size of today's permanent pacemakers. Increased battery longevity is required to reduce the morbidity associated with pulse-generator replacements and to improve the cost-effectiveness of ICD therapy. Integrated arrhythmia management systems incorporating sophisticated dual-chamber pacing, dual-chamber cardioversion, and dual-chamber defibrillation will be employed in patients with paroxysmal supraventricular and ventricular tachyarrhythmias. The incorporation of a reliable hemodynamic sensor to differentiate hemodynamically stable from hypotensive tachyarrhythmias would help identify the most appropriate therapy for each arrhythmia.

More important than technological advances in the next few years will be a clearer understanding of the role of ICD therapy in the primary prevention of SCD. Careful selection of patients to reduce overall mortality rates as well as SCD will ensure that both patients and society benefit.

References

1. Gillum RF. Sudden coronary death in the United States. *Circulation* 1989; 79:756–765.
2. Kerber RE, Jensen SR, Gascho JA, et al. Determinants of defibrillation: A prospective analysis of 183 patients. *Am J Cardiol* 1983; 52:739–745.
3. DeLuna AB, Coumel P, Leclercq JF. Ambulatory sudden cardiac death: Mechanisms of production of fatal arrhythmias on the basis of 157 cases. *Am Heart J* 1989; 117:151–159.
4. Pionkowski RS, Thompson BM, Gruchow HW, et al. Resuscitation time in ventricular fibrillation: A prognosis indicator. *Ann Emerg Med* 1983; 12:733–738.
5. Weaver WD, Cobb LA, Hallstrom AP, et al. Factors influencing survival after out-of-hospital cardiac arrest. *J Am Coll Cardiol* 1986; 7:752–757.
6. Poole JE, Bardy GH. Sudden cardiac death. In: Zipes DP, Jalife J, eds. *Cardiac Electrophysiology: From Cell to Bedside*, 2d ed. Philadelphia: Saunders; 1995:812.
7. Mirowski M. The automatic implantable cardioverter/defibrillator: An overview. *J Am Coll Cardiol* 1985; 6:461–466.
8. Mirowski M, Mower MM, Staewen WS, et al. Standby automatic defibrillator: An approach to prevention of sudden cardiac death. *Arch Intern Med* 1970; 126:158–161.
9. Mirowski M, Reid PR, Mower MM, et al. Termination of malignant ventricular arrhythmias with an implanted automatic defibrillator in human beings. *N Engl J Med* 1980; 303:322–324.
10. Nelson RS. The pulse generator. In: Kroll MW, Lehmann MH, eds. *Implantable Cardioverter Defibrillator Therapy: The Engineering-Clinical Interface*. Norwell, MA: Kluwer Academic; 1996:241.
11. Olson WH. Tachyarrhythmia sensing and detection. In: Singer I, ed. *Implantable Cardioverter Defibrillator*. New York: Futura; 1994:71.
12. Marchlinski FE, Callans DJ, Gottlieb CD, et al. Benefit and lessons learned from stored electrogram information in implantable defibrillators. *J Cardiovasc Electrophysiol* 1995; 6:832–851.
13. Weber M, Bocker D, Bansch D, et al. Efficacy and safety of the initial use of stability and onset criteria in implantable cardioverter defibrillators. *J Cardiovasc Electrophysiol* 1999; 10:145–153.
14. Barold HS, Newby KH, Tomassoni G, et al. Prospective evaluation of new and old criteria to discriminate between supraventricular and ventricular tachycardia in implantable defibrillators. *Pacing Clin Electrophysiol* 1998; 21:1347–1355.
15. Duru F, Schonbeck M, Luscher TF. The potential for inappropriate ventricular tachycardia confirmation using the intracardiac electrogram (EGM) width criterion. *Pacing Clin Electrophysiol* 1999; 22:1039–1046.
16. Nair M, Saoudi N, Kroiss D, et al. Automatic arrhythmia identification using analysis of the atrioventricular association: Application to a new generation of implantable defibrillators. *Circulation* 1997; 95:967–973.
17. Korte T, Jung W, Wolpert C, et al. A new classification algorithm for discrimination of ventricular from supraventricular tachycardia in a dual chamber implantable cardioverter defibrillator. *J Cardiovasc Electrophysiol* 1998; 9:70–73.
18. Lavergne T, Daubert JC, Chauvin M, et al. Preliminary clinical experience with the first dual chamber pacemaker defibrillator. *Pacing Clin Electrophysiol* 1997; 20:182–188.
19. Kuhlkamp V, Dornberger V, Mewis C, et al. Clinical experience with the new detection algorithms for atrial fibrillation of a defibrillator with dual chamber sensing and pacing. *J Cardiovasc Electrophysiol* 1999; 10:905–915.
20. Neuzner J, Pitschner HF, Huth C, et al. Effects of biphasic waveform pulse on endocardial defibrillation efficacy in humans. *Pacing Clin Electrophysiol* 1994; 17:207–212.
21. Block M, Hammel D, Bocker D, et al. A prospective randomized cross-over comparison of mono- and biphasic defibrillation using nonthoracotomy lead configurations in humans. *J Cardiovasc Electrophysiol* 1994; 5:581–590.
22. Olatidoye AG, Verroneau J, Kluger J. Mechanisms of syncope in implantable cardioverter-defibrillator recipients who receive device therapies. *Am J Cardiol* 1998; 82:1372–1376.
23. Almendral J, Arenal A, Villacastin JP, et al. The importance of antitachycardia pacing for patients presenting with ventricular tachycardia. *Pacing Clin Electrophysiol* 1993; 16:535–539.
24. The PCD Investigator Group. Clinical outcome of patients with malignant ventricular tachyarrhythmias and a multiprogrammable implantable cardioverter-defibrillator implanted with or without thoracotomy: An international multicenter study. *J Am Coll Cardiol* 1994; 23:1521–1530.
25. Porterfield JG, Porterfield LM, Smith BA, et al. Conversion rates of induced versus spontaneous ventricular tachycardia by a third generation cardioverter defibrillator. *Pacing Clin Electrophysiol* 1993; 16:170–178.
26. Gross JN, Sackstein RD, Song SL, et al. The antitachycardia pacing ICD: Impact on patient selection and outcome. *Pacing Clin Electrophysiol* 1993; 16:165–169.
27. Brady GH, Poole JE, Kudenchuk PJ, et al. A prospective randomized repeat-crossover comparison of antitachycardia pacing with low-energy cardioversion. *Circulation* 1993; 87:1889–1896.
28. Geelen P, Lorga A, Chauvin M, et al. The value of DDD pacing in patients with an implantable cardioverter defibrillator. *Pacing Clin Electrophysiol* 1997; 20:177–181.
29. Best PJ, Hayes DL, Stanton MS. The potential usage of dual chamber pacing in patients with implantable cardioverter defibrillators. *Pacing Clin Electrophysiol* 1999; 22:79–85.
30. Higgins SL, Williams SK, Pak JP, et al. Indications for implantation

of a dual-chamber pacemaker combined with an implantable cardioverter-defibrillator. *Am J Cardiol* 1998; 81:1360–1362.
31. Welsh PJ, Joglar JA, Hamdan MH, et al. The effect of biphasic defibrillation on the immediate pacing threshold of a dedicated bipolar, steroid-eluting lead. *Pacing Clin Electrophysiol* 1999; 22:1229–1233.
32. Roelke M, O'Nunain SS, Osswald S, et al. Subclavian crush syndrome complicating transvenous cardioverter defibrillator systems. *Pacing Clin Electrophysiol* 1995; 18:973–979.
33. Van Rugge FP, Savalle LH, Schalij MJ. Subcutaneous single-incision implantation of cardioverter-defibrillators under local anesthesia by electrophysiologists in the electrophysiology laboratory. *Am J Cardiol* 1998; 81:302–305.
34. Lipscomb KJ, Linker NJ, Fitzpatrick AP. Subpectoral implantation of a cardioverter defibrillator under local anaesthesia. *Heart* 1998; 79:253–255.
35. Pinosky ML, Reeves ST, Fishman RL, et al. Intravenous sedation for placement of automatic implantable cardioverter-defibrillators. *J Cardiothorac Anesth* 1996; 10:764–766.
36. Manolis AS, Chiladakis J, Vassilikos V, et al. Pectoral cardioverter defibrillators: Comparison of prepectoral and submuscular implantation techniques. *Pacing Clin Electrophysiol* 1999; 22:469–478.
37. Gold MR, Peters RW, Johnson JW, et al. Complications associated with pectoral cardioverter-defibrillator implantation: Comparison of subcutaneous and submuscular approaches. *J Am Coll Cardiol* 1996; 28:1278–1282.
38. Bardy GH, Johnson G, Poole JE, et al. A simplified, single-lead unipolar transvenous cardioversion-defibrillation system. *Circulation* 1993; 88:543–547.
39. Friedman PA, Rasmussen MJ, Grice S, et al. Defibrillation thresholds are increased by right-sided implantation of totally transvenous implantable cardioverter defibrillators. *Pacing Clin Electrophysiol* 1999; 22:1186–1192.
40. Singer I, Lang D. Defibrillation threshold: Clinical utility and therapeutic implications. *Pacing Clin Electrophysiol* 1992; 15:932–949.
41. Lang JL, KenKnight BH. Implant support devices. In: Singer I, ed. *Implantable Cardioverter Defibrillator*. New York: Futura; 1994:223.
42. Singer I, Lang D. The defibrillation threshold. In: Kroll MW, Lehmann MH, eds. *Implantable Cardioverter Defibrillator Therapy: The Engineering-Clinical Interface*. Norwell, MA: Kluwer Academic, 1996:89.
43. Boriani G, Frabetti L, Biffi M, et al. Clinical experience with downsized lower energy output implantable cardioverter defibrillators. *Int J Cardiol* 1998; 66:261–266.
44. Luria D, Stanton MS, Eldar M, et al. Pneumothorax: An unusual cause of ICD defibrillation failure. *Pacing Clin Electrophysiol* 1998; 21:474–475.
45. Weiss DN, Zilo P, Luceri RM, et al. Predischarge arrhythmia induction testing of implantable defibrillators may be unnecessary in selected cases. *Am J Cardiol* 1997; 80:1562–1565.
46. Monahan KM, Hadjis T, Hallett N, et al. Relation of induced to spontaneous ventricular tachycardia from analysis of stored far-field implantable defibrillator electrograms. *Am J Cardiol* 1999; 83:349–353.
47. Schaumann A, von zur Muhlen F, Herse B, et al. Empirical versus tested antitachycardia pacing in implantable cardioverter defibrillators: A prospective study including 200 patients. *Circulation* 1998; 97:66–74.
48. Ruppel R, Schluter CA, Boczor S, et al. Ventricular tachycardia during follow-up in patients resuscitated from ventricular fibrillation: Experience from stored electrograms of implantable cardioverter-defibrillators. *J Am Coll Cardiol* 1998; 32:1724–1730.
49. Tokanao T, Pelosi F, Flemming M, et al. Long-term evaluation of the ventricular defibrillation energy requirement. *J Cardiovasc Electrophysiol* 1998; 9:916–920.
50. Grimm W, Marchlinski FE. Shock occurrence in patients with an implantable cardioverter-defibrillator without spontaneous shocks before first generator replacement for battery depletion. *Am J Cardiol* 1994; 73:969–970.
51. May CD, Smith PR, Murdock CJ, et al. The impact of the implantable cardioverter defibrillator on quality-of-life. *Pacing Clin Electrophysiol* 1995; 18:1411–1418.
52. Sneed NV, Finch NJ, Leman RB. The impact of device recall on patients and family members of patients with automatic implantable cardioverter defibrillators. *Heart Lung* 1994; 23:317–322.
53. Heller SS, Ormont MA, Lidagoster L, et al. Psychosocial outcome after ICD implantation: A current perspective. *Pacing Clin Electrophysiol* 1998; 21:1207–1215.
54. Pacifico A, Hohnloser SH, Williams JH, et al. Prevention of implantable-defibrillator shocks by treatment with sotalol. *N Engl J Med* 1999; 340:1855–1862.
55. Epstein AE, Miles WM, Benditt DG, et al. Personal and public safety issues related to arrhythmias that may affect consciousness: Implications for regulation and physician recommendations, a medical/scientific statement from the American Heart Association and the North American Society of Pacing and Electrophysiology. *Circulation* 1996; 94:1147–1166.
56. O'Callaghan PA, Ruskin JN, The current status of implantable cardioverter defibrillators. *Curr Probl Cardiol* 1997; 22: 645–708.
57. Bardy GH, Yee R, Jung W. Multicenter experience with a pectoral unipolar implantable cardioverter-defibrillator. *J Am Coll Cardiol* 1996; 28:400–410.
58. Pacifico A, Johnson JW, Stanton MS, et al. Comparison of results in two implantable defibrillators. *Am J Cardiol* 1998; 82: 875–880.
59. Rosenqvist M, Beyer T, Block M, et al. Adverse events with transvenous implantable cardioverter-defibrillators: A prospective multicenter study. *Circulation* 1998; 98:663–670.
60. Hoffman E, Steinbeck G. Experience with pectoral versus abdominal implantation of a small defibrillator: A multicenter comparison in 778 patients, European Jewel Investigators. *Eur Heart J* 1998; 19:1085–1098.
61. Smith PN, Vidaillet HJ, Hayes JJ, et al. Infections with nonthoracotomy implantable cardioverter defibrillators: Can these be prevented? *Pacing Clin Electrophysiol* 1998; 21:42–55.
62. Callans DJ, Hook BG, Marchlinski FE. Use of bipolar recordings from patch-patch and rate sensing leads to distinguish rhythms in patients with implantable cardioverter-defibrillators. *Pacing Clin Electrophysiol* 1991; 14:1917–1922.
63. Block M, Breithardt G. Long-term follow-up and clinical results of implantable cardioverter-defibrillators. In: Zipes DP, Jalife J, eds. *Cardiac Electrophysiology: From Cell to Bedside*, 2d ed. Philadelphia: Saunders; 1995:1412.
64. The Antiarrhythmics versus Implantable Defibrillators (AVID) Investigators. A comparison of antiarrhythmic-drug therapy with implantable defibrillators in patients resuscitated from near-fatal ventricular arrhythmias. *N Engl J Med* 1997; 337:1576–1583.
65. Connolly SJ, Gent M, Roberts RS, et al. Canadian Implantable Defibrillator Study (CIDS): A randomized trial of the implantable cardioverter defibrillator against amiodarone. *Circulation* 2000; 101:1297–1302.
66. Kuck HK. Cardiac Arrest Study—Hamburg (CASH), 1999. Located on internet at http://www.acc.org/lectures/trials.cash.hmtl.
67. Moss AJ, Hall WJ, Cannom DS, et al. Improved survival with an implanted defibrillator in patients with coronary artery disease at high risk for ventricular arrhythmia. *N Engl J Med* 1996; 335:1933–1940.
68. Buxton AE, Lee KL, Fisher JD, et al. A randomized study of the prevention of sudden death in patients with coronary artery disease. *N Engl J Med* 1999; 341:1882–1890.
69. Bigger JT, for the Coronary Artery Bypass Graft (CABG) Patch Trial Investigators. Prophylactic use of implanted cardiac defibril-

lators in patients at high risk for ventricular arrhythmias after coronary artery bypass graft surgery. *N Engl J Med* 1997; 337:1568–1575.
70. The German Dilated Cardiomyopathy Study Investigators. Prospective studies assessing prophylactic therapy in high risk patients: The German Dilated Cardiomyopathy Study (GDCMS), study design. *Pacing Clin Electrophysiol* 1992; 15:697–700.
71. Klein H, Auricchio A, Reek S, et al. New primary prevention trials of sudden cardiac death in patients with left ventricular dysfunction: SCD-HeFT and MADIT-II. *Am J Cardiol* 1999; 83:91D–97D.
72. Bigger JT, Fleiss JL, Kleiger R, et al. The relationships among ventricular arrhythmias, left ventricular dysfunction, and mortality in the 2 years after myocardial infarction. *Circulation* 1984; 69:250–258.
73. Waldo AL, Camm AJ, deRuyter H, et al. Effect of d-sotalol on mortality in patients with left ventricular dysfunction after recent and remote myocardial infarction. *Lancet* 1996; 348:7–12.
74. Pfeffer MA, Braunwald E, Moye LA, et al. Effect of captopril on mortality and morbidity in patients with left ventricular dysfunction after myocardial infarction: Results of the Survival and Ventricular Enlargement Trial. *N Engl J Med* 1992; 327:669–677.
75. Uretsky BF, Sheahan RG. Primary prevention of sudden cardiac death in heart failure: Will the solution be shocking? *J Am Coll Cardiol* 1997; 30:1589–1597.
76. Fogoros RN. The impact of the implantable defibrillator on mortality: The axiom of overall implantable cardioverter-defibrillator survival. *Am J Cardiol* 1996; 78:57–61.
77. Gold MR, Froman D, Kavesh NG, et al. A comparison of pectoral and abdominal transvenous defibrillator implantation: Analysis of costs and outcomes. *J Intervent Cardiac Electrophysiol* 1998; 2:345–349.
78. Cardinal DS, Connelly DT, Steinhaus DM, et al. Cost savings with nonthoracotomy implantable cardioverter-defibrillators. *Am J Cardiol* 1996; 78:1255–1259.
79. Garratt CJ. A new evidence base for implantable defibrillator therapy. *Eur Heart J* 1998; 19:189–191.
80. Mushlin AI, Hall WJ, Zwanziger J, et al. The cost-effectiveness of automatic implantable cardiac defibrillators: Results from MADIT. *Circulation* 1998; 97:2129–2135.
81. Gregoratos G, Cheitlin MD, Epstein AE, et al. ACC/AHA guidelines for implantation of cardiac pacemakers and antiarrhythmic devices: A report of the American College of Cardiology/American Heart Association Task Force on Practice Guidelines (Committee on Pacemaker Implantation). *J Am Coll Cardiol* 1998; 31:1175–1209.
82. Engelstein ED, Zipes DP. Sudden cardiac death. In: Alexander RW, Schlant RC, Fuster V, eds. *Hurst's The Heart*, 9th ed. New York: McGraw-Hill; 1998:1081.
83. Cobb LA, Baum RS, Alvarez H, et al. Resuscitation from out-of-hospital ventricular fibrillation: Four years follow-up. *Circulation* 1975; 52:223–228.
84. Kelly P, Ruskin JN, Vlahakes GJ, et al. Surgical coronary revascularization in survivors of prehospital cardiac arrest: Its effect on inducible ventricular arrhythmias and long-term survival. *J Am Coll Cardiol* 1990; 15:267–273.
85. Anderson JL, Hallstrom AP, Epstein AE, et al. Design and results of the antiarrhythmics vs implantable defibrillators (AVID) registry, the AVID investigators. *Circulation* 1999; 99:1692–1699.
86. Kim YH, Sosa-Suarez G, Trouton TG, et al. Treatment of ventricular tachycardia by transcatheter radiofrequency ablation in patients with ischemic heart disease. *Circulation* 1994; 89:1094–1102.
87. Hargrove WC, Josephson ME, Marchlinski FE, et al. Surgical decisions in the management of sudden cardiac death and malignant ventricular arrhythmias. *J Thorac Cardiovasc Surg* 1989; 97:923–928.
88. Geha AS, Elefteriades JA, Hsu J, et al. Strategies in the surgical treatment of malignant ventricular arrhythmias. *Ann Surg* 1992; 216:309–316.
89. Bass EB, Elson JJ, Fogoros RN, et al. Long-term prognosis of patients undergoing electrophysiologic studies for syncope of unknown origin. *Am J Cardiol* 1988; 62:1186–1191.
90. Olshansky B, Hahn EA, Hartz VL, et al. Clinical significance of syncope in the electrophysiologic study versus electrocardiographic monitoring (ESVEM) trial, the ESVEM Investigators. *Am Heart J* 1999; 137:878–886.
91. Mittal S, Iwai S, Stein KM, et al. Significance and outcome of inducible VT in patients with coronary artery disease and syncope [abstr]. *Circulation* 1998; 98:I-787.
92. Knight BP, Goyal R, Pelosi F, et al. Outcome of patients with nonischemic dilated cardiomyopathy and unexplained syncope treated with an implantable defibrillator. *J Am Coll Cardiol* 1999; 33:1971–1973.
93. Domanski MJ, Saksena S, Hallstrom A. Benefit with implantable cardioverter-defibrillators in patients with malignant ventricular arrhythmias and varying degrees of left ventricular dysfunction [abstr]. *Circulation* 1998; 98:I-191.
94. Krahn AD, Klein GJ, Yee R, et al. The effect of ejection fraction on the relative benefit of the implantable defibrillator in the Canadian Implantable Defibrillator Study [abstr]. *Circulation* 1998; 98:I-93.
95. Bocker D, Bansch D, Heinecke A, et al. Potential benefit from implantable cardioverter-defibrillator therapy in patients with and without heart failure. *Circulation* 1998; 98:1636–1643.
96. DEFIBRILAT Study Group. Actuarial risk of sudden death while awaiting cardiac transplantation in patients with atherosclerotic heart disease. *Am J Cardiol* 1991; 68:545–546.
97. Lorga-Filho A, Geelan P, Vanderheyden M, et al. Early benefit of implantable cardioverter defibrillator therapy in patients waiting for cardiac transplantation. *Pacing Clin Electrophysiol* 1998; 21:1747–1750.
98. Grimm W, Glaveris C, Hoffmann, C et al. Noninvasive arrhythmia risk stratification in idiopathic dilated cardiomyopathy: Design and first results of the Marburg Cardiomyopathy Study. *Pacing Clin Electrophysiol* 1998; 21:2551–2556.
99. Morris MM, KenKnight BH, Warren JA, et al. A preview of implantable cardioverter defibrillator systems in the next millennium: An integrated cardiac rhythm management approach. *Am J Cardiol* 1999; 83:48D–54D.

CHAPTER 31

CARDIAC PACEMAKERS

Raul D. Mitrani / Robert J. Myerburg / Agustin Castellanos

The concept for bradycardia pacemakers originated in the 1950s. Over the past 4 decades, cardiac pacing has undergone tremendous growth, while the pacer units themselves have been downsized. Current units are capable of fully programmable dual-chamber pacing, rate response to activity and metabolic changes, have telemetry of pacer function, incorporate algorithms to respond to changes in intrinsic rhythms, and can store a history of patients' arrhythmic events. Besides providing bradycardia support, pacers are an integral part of patients' comprehensive arrhythmia and hemodynamic management strategies. A number of current and comprehensive reviews are available,[1–3] and the reader is referred to these for more detailed discussion of selected topics.

The basic pacemaker system consists of a pulse generator connected to one or two leads attached to the heart. Almost all pacemakers use a lithium-iodide battery. Pacing is accomplished by sending current pulses through the lead to a distal electrode (cathode), which initiates depolarization of the myocardium. Current returning through the anode completes the electrical circuit.

CODES FOR CARDIAC PACING

Pacemakers are coded by a specific abbreviation according to the type of pacemaker and mode of pacing. In common usage, the first three or four letters are used, but a total of five letters have been defined by the North American Society of Pacing and Electrophysiology (NASPE) and the British Pacing and Electrophysiology Group (BPEG) (Table 31-1).[4]

The first three letters refer to the type of pacemaker or

TABLE 31-1 The NASPE/BPEG Pacemaker Code

Chamber Paced	Chamber Sensed	Response to Sensed Event	Programmability/Rate Response
O (none)	O	O	O
A (atrium)	A	I (inhibit)	R (rate responsive)
V (ventricle)	V	T (triggered)	P (simple programmable)
D (dual)	D	D (I + T)	M (multiprogrammable)
S (single chamber, A or V)	S		C (communicating)

NOTE: In current terminology, only rate responsiveness (*R*) is indicated by the fourth position. All current pacers have full programmability; therefore, the letters *P*, *M*, and *C* are no longer used.

pacing mode that is being employed. The first letter refers to the chamber(s) being paced and the second letter refers to the chamber(s) being sensed. The letter A indicates atrial pacing or sensing, and V refers to ventricular pacing or sensing. If A and V are both being paced and/or sensed, the designation D, dual-chamber pacing or sensing, is used. The third letter refers to the response to a sensed event. The pacemaker can either inhibit (I) pacing output from one or both of its leads, or it can trigger (T) pacing at a programmable interval after the sensed event. The detailed description and indications for different pacing modes will be described.

The fourth letter designation represents either the type of programmability or whether the pacemaker is capable of providing rate-responsive pacing. Lastly, the fifth letter represents cardiac devices that are capable of treating atrial or ventricular tachyarrhythmias. In common usage, only the rate responsiveness of the pacemaker is noted in the fourth letter designation, and the fifth letter designation is only used for atrial pacers with antitachycardia function.

TEMPORARY PACING

Temporary pacing is a modality required to provide patients with heart rate support when they experience intermittent or persistent hemodynamically relevant bradyarrhythmias or to provide standby pacing for patients at increased risk for sudden and complete heart block. Occasionally, temporary pacing is used to control sustained atrial or ventricular tachyarrhythmias. The end point for temporary pacing is either resolution of a temporary indication for pacing or implantation of a permanent pacemaker for a continuing indication. The clinician must decide whether to insert a temporary transvenous pacemaker versus relying on a noninvasive external unit.[5]

Indications

Indications for pacer implant can be divided according to whether there is consensus opinion as to the appropriateness of the indication (Table 31-2). The indications for temporary pacing are listed in Table 31-3. In general, indications for temporary pacing may include patients who are at high risk for developing complete heart block, such as is the case in patients with acute myocardial infarctions and alternating bundle branch blocks. Other indications for temporary pacing include those indications for permanent pacing when patients are symptomatic and cannot wait for the permanent pacemaker. In general, it would be advisable to place the permanent pacemaker as soon as possible to avoid the risks of temporary pacemaker placement.

Temporary pacing is also indicated when a patient has bradycardia causing symptomatic or hemodynamic compromise. Temporary pacing at rates of 80 to 100 beats per minute can be used to prevent bradycardia-dependent ventricular arrhythmias or those associated with a long QT interval and torsade de pointes. Temporary atrial pacing is occasionally used in patients to restore atrioventricular (AV) synchrony in patients with temporary sinus arrest who have intact AV conduction. Toxic drug effects, such as digitalis toxicity, or metabolic abnormalities, such as hyperkalemia, may produce a temporary symptomatic bradycardia requiring temporary pacing.[6]

Lyme disease is a specific cause of carditis that has been associated with various degrees of AV block in some patients.[6,7] In the presence of high-degree or complete AV block (see Chap. 23), the escape rhythm consists of a slow wide QRS or there may be a systole. Temporary cardiac pacing is necessary in the more advanced cases, but implantation of a permanent pacemaker is generally not necessary for patients with Lyme disease since the AV block almost always resolves.

Occasionally, temporary pacing is used for management of tachyarrhythmias for overdrive pacing of atrial or ventricular arrhythmias. The most common clinical setting is generally in the postoperative period after major cardiac surgery, when atrial flutter may be pace terminated into sinus rhythm.[8]

Temporary Pacing in Acute Myocardial Infarction

The use of temporary pacing in acute myocardial infarction can be accomplished by transcutaneous systems in those patients

TABLE 31-2 Consensus for Appropriateness of Pacer Implant Indication

Class I	Conditions for which there is general agreement that permanent pacemakers should be implanted.
Class IIa	Conditions for which permanent pacemakers are frequently used but there is divergence of opinion with respect to the necessity of their insertion. Weight of evidence/opinion is in favor of pacemaker use.
Class IIb	Conditions for which permanent pacemakers are frequently used but there is divergence of opinion with respect to the necessity of their insertion. Weight of evidence/opinion is in favor of pacemaker use.
Class III	Conditions for which there is general agreement that devices are unnecessary.

TABLE 31-3 Indications for Temporary (Transvenous) Pacing

Symptomatic sinus nodal dysfunction/bradyarrhythmias
Drug or electrolyte induced
Symptomatic high-degree or third-degree AV block
Acquired or congenital heart block with symptoms
Postoperative after cardiac surgery
After radiofrequency ablation of the AV junction
Acute myocardial infarction
Class I indications
Asystole
New bifascicular block with first-degree AV block
Alternating bundle branch block
Symptomatic bradycardia with hypotension from any etiology unresponsive to drug therapy
Mobitz type II second-degree AV block
Class IIa indications
New or indeterminate RBBB with LAHB or LPHB or first-degree AV block
New or indeterminate LBBB
Recurrent sinus pauses not responsive to atropine
Incessant VT, for atrial or ventricular overdrive pacing
Class IIb indications
Bifascicular block of indeterminate age
New or age-indeterminate isolated RBBB
Bradycardia-dependent tachyarrhythmias/long QT syndrome with torsades de pointes

NOTE: See Table 31-2 for definition of class I or class II indications.
ABBREVIATIONS: AV = atrioventricular; LAHB = left anterior hemiblock; LBBB = left bundle branch block; LPHB = left posterior hemiblock; RBBB = right bundle branch block.
SOURCE: Adapted from Ryan et al.[9] Reproduced with permission from the publisher and authors.

without active need for pacing and in those patients at low to moderate risk for developing complete heart block. Because transcutaneous systems are uncomfortable during active pacing for prolonged periods of time, transvenous pacing may be placed in patients requiring active pacing or in those patients at increased risk for developing complete heart block (Table 31-3).[9]

In patients with inferior infarction, any conduction disturbance is likely to be proximal to the His bundle. Therefore, patients with inferior infarction require temporary cardiac pacing only if there are symptoms (angina, hypotension, etc.) associated with the bradycardia or for persistent rates less than 40 beats per minute.

Although patients with inferior myocardial infarction are less likely to require temporary pacing compared with patients with anterior infarction, the recent guidelines on the use of temporary pacing in patients with acute infarction do not differentiate between anterior and inferior infarction.[9] Temporary pacing is indicated in the presence of high-degree (Mobitz type II second-degree AV block) or complete AV block because of the likelihood that these patients will be hemodynamically unstable with their bradyarrhythmia. Any symptomatic bradycardia with hypotension is also an indication for temporary pacing. Additionally, the presence of new bifascicular block generally places patients at increased risk for complete AV block, especially with associated first-degree AV block; therefore, temporary pacing would be reasonable. It is unclear whether patients with new left bundle branch block with normal PR interval or new right bundle branch block (with normal axis) require temporary pacing.

Selected patients with right ventricular infarction or other patients who require AV synchrony may require dual-chamber AV pacing. However, most patients who need temporary transvenous pacing receive a single ventricular lead because of its ease of use.

Techniques for Temporary Pacing

Techniques and clinical competence required to implant temporary pacemakers have been described elsewhere.[1,10,11] Catheters are generally placed into the right heart by percutaneous sheaths placed into the internal jugular, subclavian, brachial, or femoral vein. For temporary VVI pacing, the catheter is advanced under fluoroscopic guidance into the right ventricle. If fluoroscopy is not available, the pacing catheter can be advanced into the right ventricle by using intracardiac electrograms to position the lead.

Alternatively, transcutaneous pacing is a common method for noninvasively pacing patients who require a prophylactic temporary backup pacer or require emergent pacing.[5,12] It can be activated quickly in situations in which emergency ventricular pacing is required. The unit incorporates two large pads placed in an anterior and posterior position. The main drawback is the high energy requirements (50 to 100 mA at 20 to 40 ms), which cause skeletal muscle stimulation and pain; therefore, this should not be used for extended periods in awake patients.

INDICATIONS FOR PERMANENT PACING

The indications for permanent pacemakers can be divided into three classifications (Table 31-2) and are listed in Table 31-4 according to the most recent indications published by a joint task force by the American College of Cardiology and American Heart Association in 1998.[13] These recommendations serve as guidelines, and there are other clinical factors that may affect the decision to implant a pacer. Many indications for pacemaker implantation are predicated by the presence of symptoms. However, many symptoms such as fatigue or subtle symptoms of congestive heart failure may be recognized only in retrospect, after placement of a permanent pacemaker.

Pacing in Acquired Atrioventricular Block

It is generally agreed that complete heart block, permanent or intermittent, at any anatomic level associated with symptoms such as dizziness, lightheadedness, syncope, congestive heart failure, or confusion is an indication for a permanent pacemaker. In the absence of symptoms, pacing is indicated for patients with third-degree AV block, especially with awake heart rates of less than 40 beats per minute or pauses of longer than 3 s.

In the presence of bifascicular or trifascicular block, intermittent third-degree or type II second-degree AV block usually indicates the need for a permanent pacemaker. When patients with these conduction patterns present with syncope, a pacemaker is usually required. However, an electrophysiology study may be useful to rule out other causes of syncope (e.g., ventricular tachycardia) particularly if structural heart disease is present.

TABLE 31-4 Indications for Permanent Pacemaker

	Class I	Class II	Class III
Acquired AV block	Third-degree AV block with: Bradycardia and symptoms due to AV block Requirement of drugs that result in symptomatic bradycardia After catheter ablation of the AV junction or after postoperative AV block not expected to resolve Neuromuscular diseases with AV block Escape rhythm <40 bpm or asystole >3 s in awake symptom-free patients Second-degree AV block, permanent or intermittent, with symptomatic bradycardia	*Class IIa* Asymptomatic complete AV block with average awake ventricular rate >40 bpm Asymptomatic type II second-degree AV block (permanent or intermittent) Asymptomatic type I second-degree AV block at or below the bundle of His (documented by electrophysiologic studies) First degree AV block with symptoms suggestive of pacemaker syndrome and documented alleviation of symptoms with temporary pacing *Class IIb* Marked first-degree AV block in patients with congestive heart failure	Asymptomatic first-degree AV block Asymptomatic type I second-degree AV block above the level of the bundle of His AV block expected to resolve
After myocardial infarction	Persistent second- or third-degree AV block in the His-Purkinje system or Transient advanced infranodal AV block and associated BBB Symptomatic second- or third-degree AV block at any level	*Class IIb* Persistent advanced AV block at the AV node level	Transient AV conduction disturbances without intraventricular conduction defects or with isolated left anterior fascicular block Acquired left anterior fascicular block Persistent first-degree AV block in the presence of old or age-indeterminate BBB
Bifascicular or trifascicular block	Intermittent complete heart block associated with symptoms Type II second-degree AV block	*Class IIa* Bifascicular or trifascicular block with syncope not proven to be due to AV block but other causes of syncope not identifiable HV interval >100 ms or pacing-induced infra-His block	Fascicular block without AV block or symptoms Fascicular block with first-degree AV block without symptoms
Sinus node dysfunction	Sinus node dysfunction with documented symptomatic bradycardia (in some patients, this will occur as a result of long-term essential drug therapy of a type and dose for which there is no acceptable alternative) Symptomatic chronotropic incompetence	*Class IIa* Sinus node dysfunction, occurring spontaneously or as a result of necessary drug therapy, with heart rates <40 bpm without clear association between significant symptoms and bradycardia *Class IIb* In minimally symptomatic patients, chronic heart rate <30 bpm while awake	Sinus node dysfunction in asymptomatic patients, including those in whom substantial sinus bradycardia is a consequence of long-term drug treatment Sinus node dysfunction in patients in whom symptoms suggestive of bradycardia are clearly documented not to be associated with a slow heart rate Sinus node dysfunction with symptomatic bradycardia due to nonessential drug therapy
Hypersensitive carotid sinus and neurocardiac syndromes	Recurrent syncope associated with clear, spontaneous events provoked by carotid sinus stimulation; minimal carotid sinus pressure induces asystole of >3 s duration in the absence of any medication that depresses the sinus node or AV conduction	*Class IIa* Recurrent syncope without clear, provocative events and with a hypersensitive cardioinhibitory response *Class IIb* Syncope with associated bradycardia reproduced by head-up tilt (with or without provocative maneuvers or isoproterenol)	A hyperactive cardioinhibitory response to carotid sinus stimulation in the absence of symptoms Vague symptoms (dizziness or light-headedness) with a hyperactive cardioinhibitory response to carotid sinus stimulation Recurrent syncope, light-headedness or dizziness in the absence of a cardioinhibitory response

SOURCE: Adapted from Gregoratos et al.,[13] with permission.
See Table 31-2 for definition of classes I, II, and III indications.
ABBREVIATIONS: AV = atrioventricular; BBB = bundle branch blocks; bpm = beats per minute.

Additionally, during electrophysiology study, permanent pacing may be indicated if there is a markedly prolonged HV interval (>100 ms)[14] or nonphysiologic pacing or drug-induced infra-His block.[15]

Second-degree AV block associated with symptomatic bradycardia is an indication for pacing. In asymptomatic patients with second-degree AV block, type II, cardiac pacing may be required if the level of block is infranodal, because the progression to complete heart block is common.[16] Although type I second-degree AV block is usually located at the AV nodal level, there are patients with bundle branch block or intraventricular conduction delays in whom type I second-degree AV block is located at an infranodal level. These patients should be approached similar to patients with second-degree type II AV block, since the risk of progression to complete heart block remains high. Lastly, with 2:1 AV block, the level of block may be difficult to determine. In the presence of a bundle branch block or intraventricular conduction delay and 2:1 AV block, the level of block is usually infranodal and therefore may be an indication for pacing.

In asymptomatic and otherwise healthy patients, the presence of intermittent second-degree, type I AV block may be due to enhanced vagal tone.[17,18] In asymptomatic elderly patients with daytime type I second-degree AV block and structural heart disease, however, there is some divergence of opinion as to whether permanent pacing should[19–21] or should not[13,18] be considered. Many patients may become symptomatic during clinical follow-up.[18,19]

Due to the benign prognosis first-degree AV block is not considered an indication for permanent pacing.[13,22] However, with marked first-degree AV block (PR > 0.30 s), inappropriately timed atrial systole that occurs after ventricular systole can lead to symptoms similar to having retrograde ventriculoatrial conduction. This may be of hemodynamic consequence in some patients, particularly with left ventricular systolic or diastolic dysfunction.[23,24] Additionally, because there is not an appropriately timed ventricular systole occurring at the end of atrial systole, end-diastolic mitral regurgitation develops, which may be of clinical significance in patients with left ventricular systolic dysfunction.[25] Therefore, dual-chamber pacing may be indicated in select patients with marked first-degree AV block in whom hemodynamic improvement can be demonstrated by temporary pacing to resynchronize the atrium and ventricles.[13]

Of note, patients with neuromuscular diseases with AV block should be considered for DDD pacing, since progression of conduction system disease is not uncommon.[26–28]

Pacing in Congenital Atrioventricular Block

Congenital heart block is usually due to AV nodal block. Patients tend to be asymptomatic and typically have narrow QRS complex rhythms. However, congenital AV block is associated with serious and possible fatal complications, including syncope and sudden death.[29–32] In one study,[30] a mean daytime heart rate less than 50 beats per minute was associated with sudden death or need for pacemaker. Exercise testing is useful to assess heart rate response at rest and exercise.[30] Other indicators of poor outcome include prolonged QT interval (corrected for heart rate), cardiomegaly, atrial enlargement, decreased left ventricular systolic function, mean ventricular rates lower than median for age, periods of junctional exit block, and mitral regurgitation.[30–32]

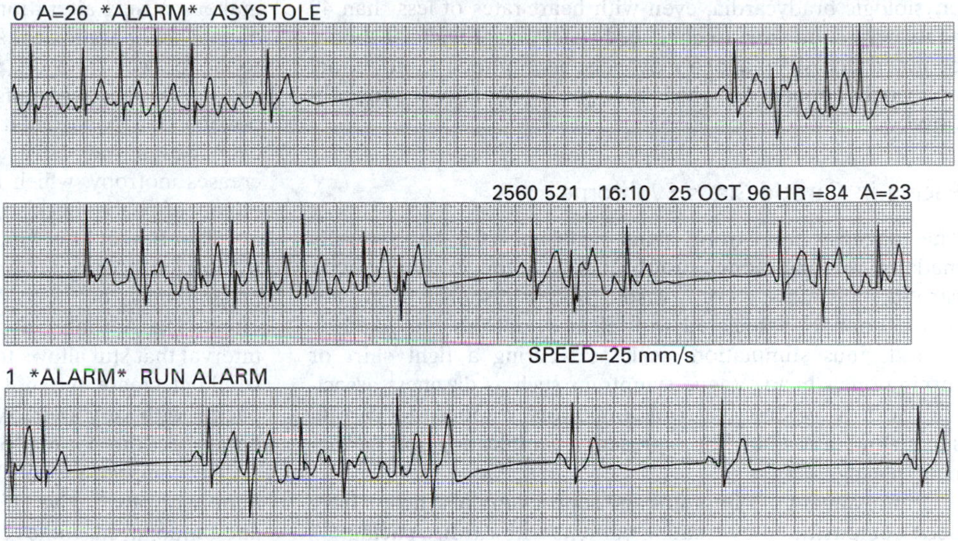

FIGURE 31-1 This is a continuous electrocardiographic tracing from a patient with sick sinus syndrome who complained of palpitations and near-syncope. The patient was mostly symptomatic from the pauses following abrupt termination of his atrial fibrillation. Note the frequent abrupt terminations, followed by pauses up to 6 s before resumption of atrial fibrillation.

Therefore, cardiac pacing is indicated in all symptomatic patients with congenital AV block. Furthermore, cardiac pacing is now recommended even for symptom-free adults. In the largest series published to date, there was reported a 5 percent mortality risk in adults older than 15 years with congenital AV block in the absence of heart disease. Eight of 102 patients whose cases were followed for 7 to 30 years had fatal Stokes-Adams attacks.[31] Syncope, mitral regurgitation, and/or heart failure occurred in 30 percent of this cohort.[31,32]

Pacing in Sinus Nodal Dysfunction

Sinus nodal dysfunction has become the most common indication for pacing in the United States. Pacing therapy has been demonstrated to be superior to medical therapy with theophylline for patients with sinus nodal dysfunction.[33] The guidelines (Table 31-4) stress the importance of correlating symptoms with bradyarrhythmias. Often, it is difficult to correlate ECG findings with symptoms. Furthermore, symptoms may be nebulous. For instance, the presence of fatigue and dyspnea may be due to a bradyarrhythmia but may also be due to lack of conditioning or other cardiac dysfunction.

The presence of the tachycardia/bradycardia syndrome is especially common in patients with paroxysmal atrial arrhythmias (Fig. 31-1). The bradyarrhythmia often occurs at the termination of tachycardia and can lead to pauses of several seconds. Drugs used to suppress tachyarrhythmias may lead to symptomatic bradycardia, in which case a bradycardia pacemaker would be required.

Patients with asymptomatic bradyarrhythmias should be evaluated carefully prior to placing a pacemaker. In general, an absolute heart rate of less than 30 beats per minute is an indication for pacer placement, even in the absence of symptoms. An exercise test can demonstrate intact sinus nodal function in patients with otherwise asymptomatic bradyarrhythmias who do not require pacing therapy. Athletes commonly have physiologic bradycardia, even with heart rates of less than 40 beats per minute, due to enhanced vagal tone. Finally, it should be noted that sleep apnea may cause asymptomatic, nocturnal bradyarrhythmias,[34] in which case pacing therapy is not indicated.

Pacing in Carotid Sinus Syndrome

The diagnosis for carotid sinus syndrome (CSS) is typically made by demonstrating asystolic pauses of longer than 3 s with carotid sinus massage or a vasodepressor response of greater than 50 mmHg associated with clear symptoms provoked by carotid sinus stimulation, such as wearing a tight shirt or turning one's head. Vague symptoms such as dizziness associated with a hyperactive cardioinhibitory response to carotid sinus stimulation do not represent an indication for permanent pacing.

Improvement of symptoms and suppression of syncope have been demonstrated by treating patients with cardiac pacing,[35–38] particularly dual-chamber pacing.[36–38] Single-chamber atrial pacing is contraindicated because of the increased risk of transient AV block. Some studies suggest that hemodynamic evaluation of patients may enable them to be stratified into groups among whom VVI pacing would be sufficient. However, DDD pacing is probably better in most patients with CSS, because of the presence of vasodepressor and cardioinhibitory reflexes.

Cardiac Pacing in Neurocardiogenic Syncope

The role of pacing for neurocardiogenic syncope is controversial. Because these are younger patients who generally respond to medication, pacing is not required in most patients.[39] Cardiac pacing has been shown to prevent the bradycardia and AV block associated with neurocardiogenic syncope, but patients still typically experience hypotension, vasodilatation, and other associated symptoms.[39–41] The Vasovagal Pacemaker Study demonstrated a role for pacing in patients with vasovagal syncope refractory to standard medical therapy.[42] Therefore, patients with refractory neurocardiogenic syncope may benefit from pacing, especially if they have a predominant cardioinhibitory component.[43]

Pacing in Hypertrophic Cardiomyopathy

In patients with hypertrophic cardiomyopathy (HCM) and left ventricular outflow tract (LVOT) gradients, DDD pacing with a programmed short AV interval has been proposed as therapy to reduce LVOT gradient and improve symptoms.[44–47] This concept is based on early studies where it was shown that DDD pacing with short AV interval decreased the LVOT gradient by a mean of 35 mmHg,[44] and there was improvement of symptoms associated with HCM. An observational study involving 84 patients whose cases were followed for a mean of 2.3 years showed improvement of symptoms in nearly all patients, and there was reduction in the left ventricular wall thickness by more than 4 mm in a subgroup of patients.[47] However, 15 percent of the patients required AV junction ablation to allow ventricular preexcitation by the pacer.

The mechanism by which DDD pacing reduces LVOT gradient remains controversial. With ventricular pacing at short AV interval, the right ventricular apex is preexcited by the pacemaker, causing alteration of the left ventricular activation sequence and paradoxical septal motion. This causes the septum to move away from the posterior left ventricular wall in early systole, thereby widening the LVOT during systole. It is also possible that ventricular pacing alters myocardial perfusion, decreases mitral valve systolic anterior motion, and/or decreases inotropy, which may also contribute to the beneficial effects of pacing in this disorder.

Therefore, if DDD pacing is used as therapy for obstructive hypertrophic cardiomyopathy, placement of pacing lead and programming of the AV interval are crucial for a beneficial effect. The AV interval should be programmed to the longest interval that still allows for left ventricular preexcitation, which would decrease but not eliminate the deleterious effects of pacing with very short AV intervals.[46] Echocardiography may help select the optimal pacing AV interval.

The long-term clinical effectiveness of DDD pacing in patients with obstructive HCM remains controversial. Some recent and randomized studies cast some doubt as to the clinical effectiveness of pacing for objectively improving functional capacity, quality of life, and LVOT gradient.[46,48,49] One small randomized study failed to demonstrate improvement in exercise response to DDD pacing.[48] Another study in patients with symptomatic obstructive HCM showed that when patients were randomized to backup AAI pacing versus DDD pacing with short AV interval, there was no difference in subjective improvement.[49] LVOT gradient was reduced by 40 percent in 57 percent of patients and remained unchanged in the other 43 percent of patients. Only 12 percent of patients (all older than age 65) showed improvement in functional capacity after 12 months in the study. Therefore, based on this randomized double-blind study, pacing could not be routinely recommended for drug-refractory patients with obstructive HCM but, rather, may be considered for select patients with medically refractory obstructive HCM as an alternative to surgical myectomy.[50]

Patients with hypertensive cardiac hypertrophy with cavity obliteration may also show clinical improvement with DDD pacing.[51] In contrast to obstructive HCM, patients with nonobstructive symptomatic HCM experience limited symptomatic improvement and no objective evidence of hemodynamic benefit with DDD pacing and short AV interval.[52]

Pacing in Dilated Cardiomyopathy and Congestive Heart Failure

Initial reports suggested that patients with congestive heart failure and dilated cardiomyopathy may benefit from dual-chamber pacing by altering and optimizing timing of left atrial to left ventricular activation or improving left ventricular contractile function. There was initial enthusiasm that pacing with a short AV interval may improve hemodynamic function[24,25] and that the patients with first-degree AV block derived the most benefit.[25] An acute hemodynamic study demonstrated that pacing with a short AV interval could eliminate presystolic mitral regurgitation in patients with first-degree AV block, restore normal AV relationships, and improve hemodynamic function.[25] Subsequent studies showed that standard DDD pacing does not improve hemodynamic function in patients with physiologic PR intervals.[53,54] On this basis, DDD pacing is possibly indicated in patients with dilated cardiomyopathy or marked first-degree AV block and where acute hemodynamic studies demonstrate improvement by dual-chamber pacing.[13]

Whereas pacing the ventricles with short AV interval may have limited benefit, the ability to pace the ventricles in a more synchronous manner to improve mechanical efficiency has also been studied. Ventricular pacing typically is achieved by pacing through a lead placed in the right ventricular apex, which may not produce the most efficient ventricular mechanical function. Pacing through the His-Purkinje system in theory may provide more physiologic ventricular activation patterns but is currently not readily available.[54a] Pacing from the right ventricular septum or outflow track may enable earlier left ventricular activation and, hence, more simultaneous contraction. However the results of hemodynamic improvement using right ventricular outflow tract pacing has shown a trend for improvement in some studies,[55,56] whereas other studies[57–59] show no benefit at all compared with right ventricular apical (RVA) pacing.

It has been proposed that left ventricular or biventricular pacing may optimize hemodynamic function in patients with dilated congestive cardiomyopathy, particularly those patients with intraventricular conduction delay. Left ventricular pacing can be accomplished by either an epicardial lead or a transvenous lead through the coronary sinus venous system. An acute hemodynamic study[58] was performed on patients with severe heart failure, intraventricular conduction delay (usually left bundle branch block), and increased capillary wedge pressure. These patients had measurement of hemodynamic parameters during either right ventricular pacing or biventricular pacing, which was compared with AAI pacing (control values). These results showed improvement of cardiac index and decrease in capillary wedge pressure with either right ventricular pacing or biventricular pacing compared with AAI pacing. Furthermore, biventricular pacing showed more hemodynamic benefit compared with right ventricular pacing. Another study on patients with congestive heart failure and wide QRS duration showed that epicardial left ventricular pacing, with or without concurrent right ventricular pacing, improved hemodynamic function at optimized AV intervals compared with control values.[60] Therefore, left ventricular pacing may evolve as a therapeutic pacing technique in patients with congestive dilated cardiomyopathy and intraventricular conduction delay.

PACEMAKER HARDWARE

Implant and Explant

Nearly all pacemakers are implanted through a transvenous approach by either cardiologists or surgeons. The choice of using an operating room or a catheterization laboratory for the implant procedure probably plays little role in procedural-related complications, but a cardiac catheterization laboratory involves lower hospital costs.[61,62]

A full description of the surgical procedure has been reviewed elsewhere.[1,63] Venous access for lead placement generally is through a subclavian venipuncture or a cephalic vein cutdown. The use of subclavian venipuncture is technically easier, and this vein can almost always accommodate two leads. With the subclavian venipuncture, there exists the risk of subclavian artery puncture, pneumothorax, or air embolus. Furthermore, pacing leads placed medially incur an additional long-term risk of being "crushed" by the clavicle and first rib leading to lead insulation breaks or fractures (Fig. 31-2). Lateral puncture of the subclavian or axillary vein using intravenous contrast may allow for safe lateral subclavian venous puncture.[64] A cephalic vein cutdown[65] may also avoid some of the risks associated with subclavian vein puncture; however, this vein is not always accessible and cannot always accommodate two pacing leads.

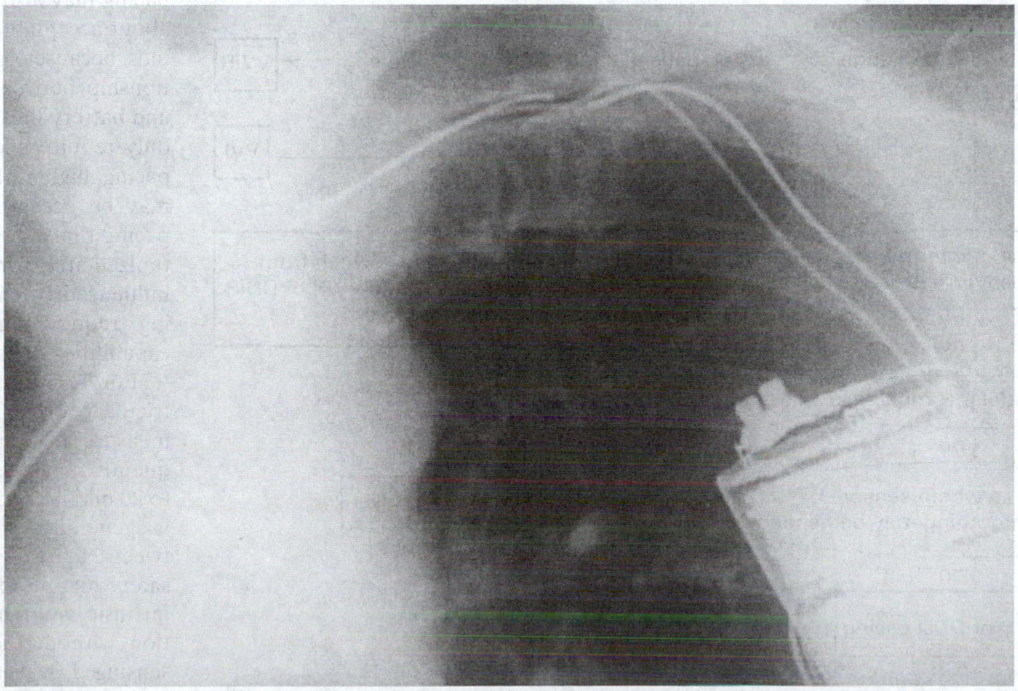

FIGURE 31-2 Close-up of a chest x-ray of a patient with a dual-chamber pacemaker. Note complete fracture of both leads at the costoclavicular junction, causing complete pacemaker malfunction.

Explanations of pacemaker generators are routinely performed during pacemaker generator changes. However, removal of pacemaker leads can be difficult due to fibrosis between chronically implanted leads and surrounding cardiac, valvular, and vascular structures. Traditional methods for extraction of chronically implanted leads involve specialized extraction sheaths that are glided over implanted leads to tear and peel away the encapsulating tissue.[66] Recently, a technique using ultraviolet excimer laser light has been introduced to facilitate lead extraction by allowing advancement of sheaths over pacer leads without excessive mechanical tearing of fibrotic tissues.[67,68] Compared with mechanical extraction, laser-assisted extraction demonstrated a greater success rate in lead removal (94 percent versus 64 percent) and less time to remove leads,[67] with no difference in complications.

Hardware

The pacemaker system consists of a pulse generator and the pacing lead(s). Pacemaker system selection should be primarily based on the medical and surgical requirements of the patient. It is unusual that one pacemaker system would be most optimal and cost effective for all patients. An algorithm for choosing a pacemaker system and pacing mode is presented in Fig. 31-3.

Pacemaker leads can be unipolar or bipolar (Figs. 31-4 and 31-5). Unipolar leads use a distal electrode in the catheter as the cathode and the shell of the pacemaker generator as the anode. Therefore, the myocardium and adjacent tissue complete the circuit. A bipolar lead consist of two separate conductors and electrodes within the lead. Since the electrodes for sensing in a bipolar lead are much closer together, bipolar signals are sharper with less extraneous noise (Fig. 31-6).

Unipolar leads are simpler to design, smaller in diameter and, because of their simplicity, probably less likely to fail.[69] Because of their small size, it is easier to pass two unipolar leads through a cephalic venous approach. However, there are several disadvantages to unipolar lead systems. Because the unipolar lead uses body tissue to complete the circuit, there is the possibility of causing muscle stimulation. Most pacemakers avoid this by placing the stimulating surface of the pacemaker anterior such that it interfaces with subcutaneous tissue and not the pectoralis muscle. Unipolar sensing is far more likely to pick up extracardiac signals, including myopotentials (Fig. 31-6), far-field sensing of remote cardiac potentials, and electromagnetic interference. Finally, unipolar pacing is generally contraindicated in patients with a concomitant implantable defibrillator. Therefore, most leads implanted today are bipolar.

Leads are attached to the heart by active or passive fixation. Active fixation involves the use of some type of exposed or retractable screw within the lead system that fixes the lead to the heart (Fig. 31-5). Passive fixation involves the use of tines, which are short protuberances that extend proximal to the distal electrode and interact with myocardial tissue to hold the lead in place. Active fixation leads are used more in the atrium and allow fixation of the leads almost anywhere within the right atrium or ventricle. The use of either type of lead probably has little effect on complication rate or lead dislodgment rate when used by experienced operators.

Lead Placement and Acute Threshold Testing

Atrial and ventricular leads are placed into the appropriate chambers after ensuring adequate pacing and sensing thresholds (Table 31-5). The basic premise in obtaining acute pacing and sensing thresholds during implant is that these thresholds may degenerate over time, and adequate safety margins need to be obtained to ensure safe long-term pacing and sensing. Furthermore, one should be aware of the type of unit implanted, its capabilities for pacing outputs, programmed sensitivities, and pacing modality (bipolar versus unipolar). The indication for pacing may also affect decisions about acceptable pacing thresholds, because of the inverse relationship between current drain and battery life. In patients who only require occasional backup pacing, higher pacing thresholds may be acceptable. Therefore, pacing thresholds should be optimized at the time of implant as influenced by the patient's pacing requirements and pacing capabilities of the pacemaker.

For sensing functions, ventricular electrograms should measure at least 5 mV and frequently measure in excess of 10 to 20 mV. Ventricular sensitivity is generally programmed between 2 to 3 mV so that adequate safety margin exists for sensing intrinsic ventricular depolarization without the risk of oversensing T waves or other artifacts. Atrial electrograms are lower in amplitude than ventric-

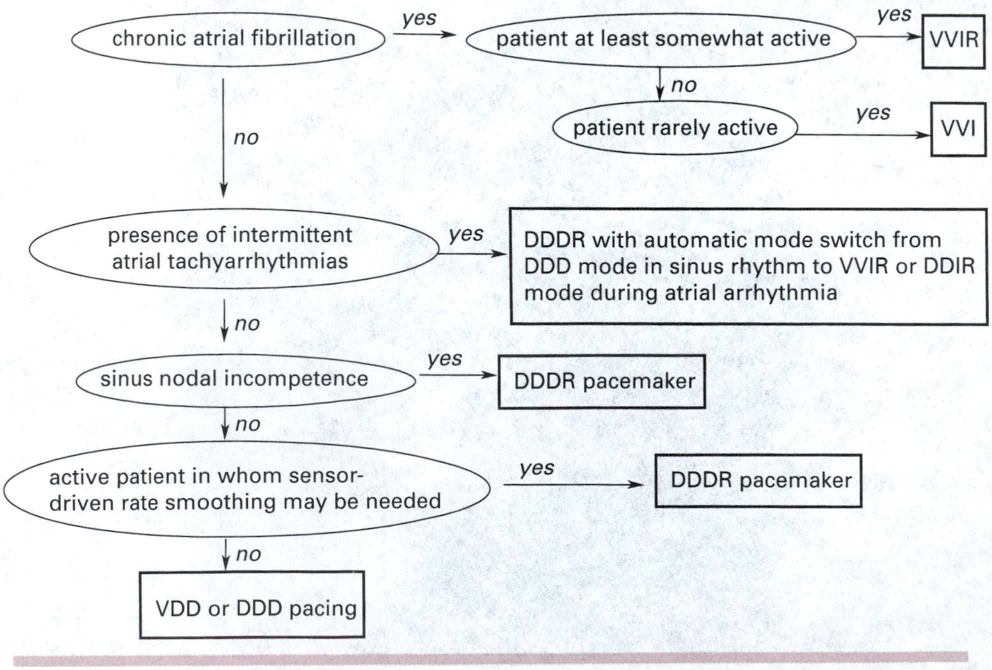

FIGURE 31-3 An algorithm for choosing a pacemaker model and pacemaker mode in patients with intermittent or fixed atrioventricular block. See the text for details.

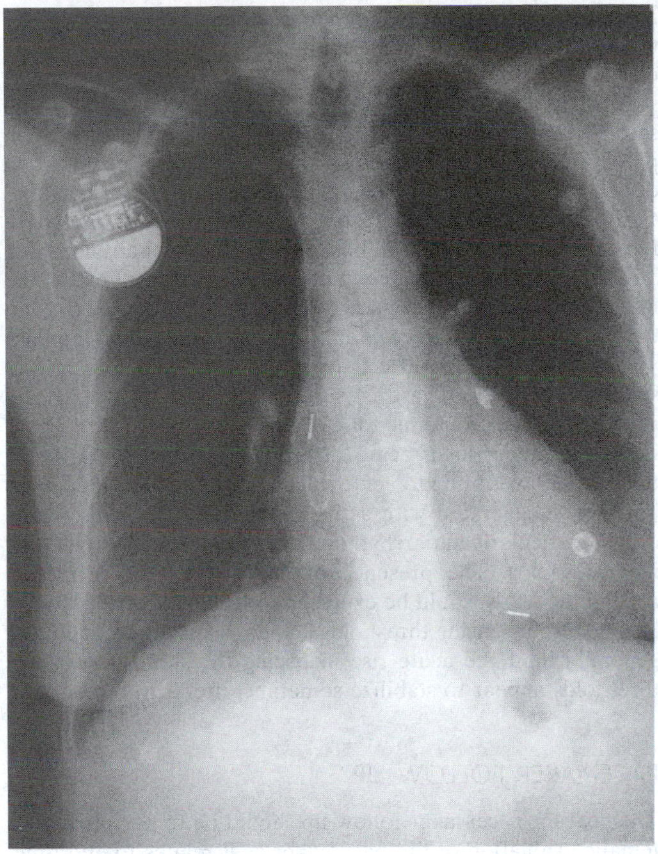
A

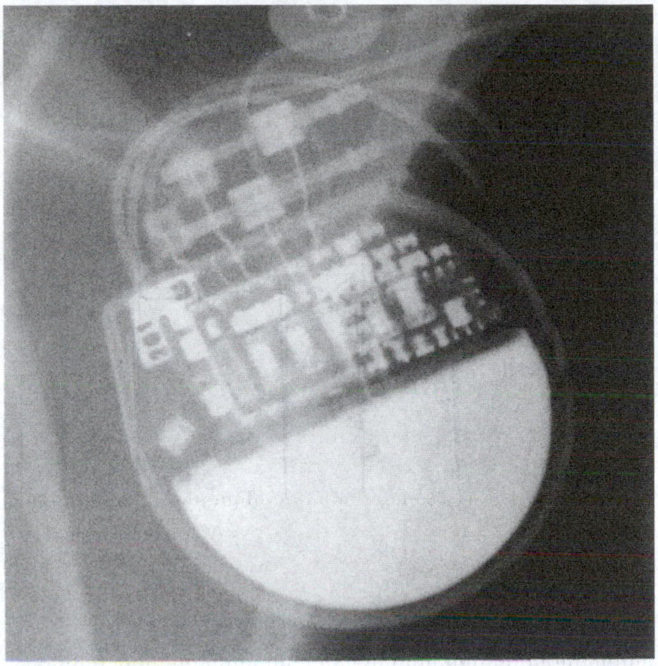
B

FIGURE 31-4 *A*. Chest x-ray of a patient with a dual-chamber unipolar pacemaker. The leads are placed in the right atrial appendage and in the right ventricular apex, respectively. Note only one electrode at the distal tip of each lead. *B*. Close inspection of the pacemaker generator shows that the ventricular lead has pulled out of the header with very minimal contact between the ventricular electrodes and the metal contacts in the pacemaker header. This caused intermittent failure to sense and pace in this patient.

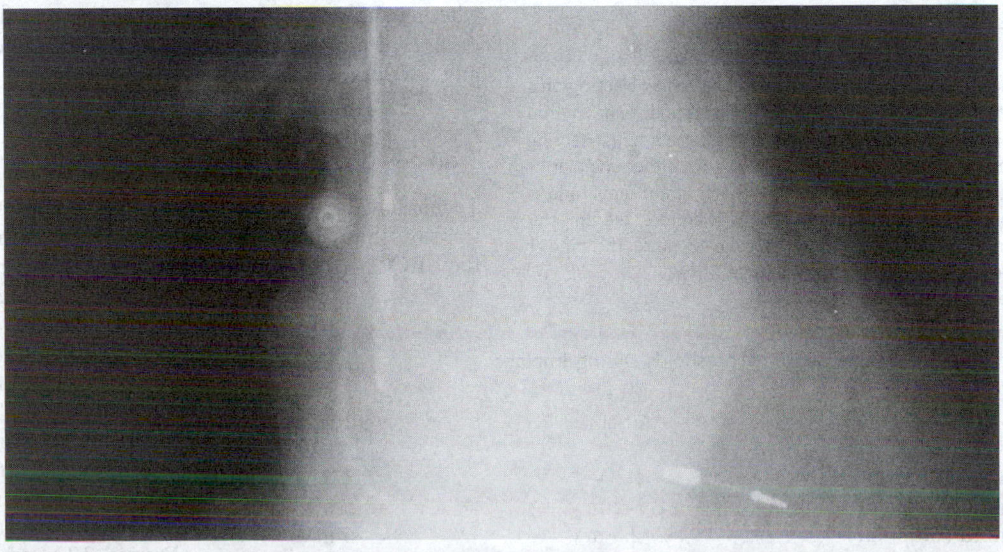

FIGURE 31-5 Chest x-ray from a patient with a bipolar dual-chamber pacing system. The atrial lead is attached to the right atrial appendage by active fixation (screw-in lead), and the screw is visible on the chest x-ray. The ventricular lead is attached to the ventricle by passive fixation.

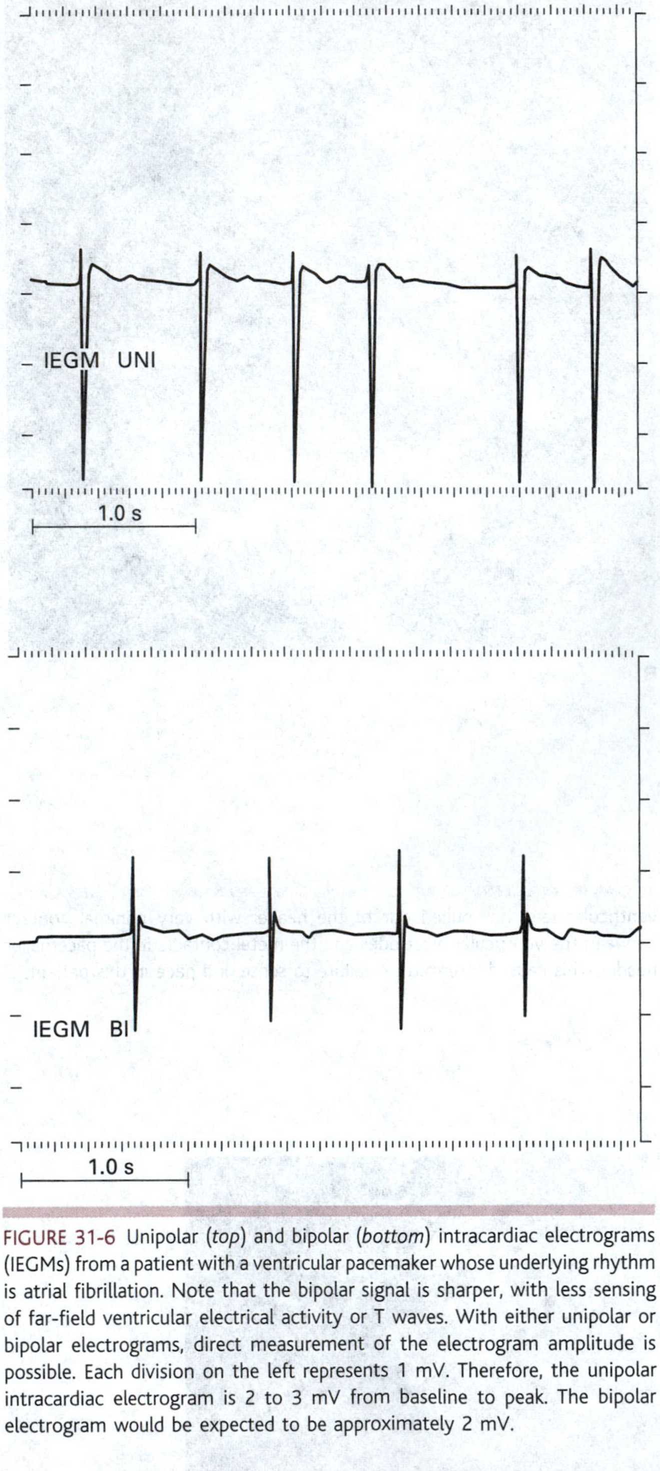

FIGURE 31-6 Unipolar (*top*) and bipolar (*bottom*) intracardiac electrograms (IEGMs) from a patient with a ventricular pacemaker whose underlying rhythm is atrial fibrillation. Note that the bipolar signal is sharper, with less sensing of far-field ventricular electrical activity or T waves. With either unipolar or bipolar electrograms, direct measurement of the electrogram amplitude is possible. Each division on the left represents 1 mV. Therefore, the unipolar intracardiac electrogram is 2 to 3 mV from baseline to peak. The bipolar electrogram would be expected to be approximately 2 mV.

ular electrograms; however, a minimum atrial electrogram of 1 to 2 mV should be obtained. In unipolar systems, a larger atrial electrogram is important because of the increased risk of oversensing myopotentials or other artifactual signals if the atrial sensitivity is programmed to less than 1 mV. In patients with paroxysmal atrial fibrillation or flutter, the atrial electrogram during tachycardia might be smaller than during sinus rhythm. Conversely, in patients with marked sinus bradycardia where it is expected that there will be nearly 100 percent atrial pacing, atrial sensing thresholds may not be as important. Finally, the minimum programmed sensitivity available by the pacer (0.15 to 0.5 mV) may influence acceptable sensing thresholds at implant.

Many factors may affect atrial or ventricular pacing and sensing thresholds. There is variation to these thresholds depending on the autonomic tone or the electrolyte status. There is an expected rise in acute thresholds within 1 to 4 weeks following implant due to acute inflammation, which appears to be more exaggerated with active fixation lead systems. Many drugs, particularly antiarrhythmic medications, may affect pacing thresholds. The presence of new myocardial infarction around the leads would be expected to lead to deterioration of pacing and/or sensing thresholds. Leads that are steroid eluting generally limit the acute rise in pacing threshold. Long-term thresholds appear to stabilize sometime after 3 to 6 months.[70]

PACEMAKER FOLLOW-UP

The goal for pacemaker follow-up should be to perform a systematic evaluation of the pacemaker as it relates to and functions with the patient and his or her individual needs. These goals are outlined in Table 31-6. Complete guidelines for pacemaker follow-up have been described.[71]

In the first several months after pacer implant, several evaluations of pacer function may be required in order to optimize pacing outputs, rate responsiveness, and other features. There is a stable period of pacer function starting 6 to 12 months following implant until the expected time for battery depletion. Therefore, direct evaluations of pacer function may be performed once or twice per year during this time, depending on whether the patient is pacer dependent and depending on the pacer type and whether any of the pacer components are under any advisory warnings.

Transtelephonic Monitoring

Technology is available for simple devices used by patients to transmit their ECG by telephone to a receiving station so that their ECG rhythm may be analyzed to detect normal or abnormal pacemaker function.[71,72] In this way, a spontaneous pacing rhythm can be assessed for normal or abnormal pacing function. More importantly, by applying a magnet to the pacemaker and observing the *magnet rate* during the transtelephonic monitoring (TTM), the battery status can be assessed. During TTM, changes in pacing rate or loss of output could always be detected. Ventricular oversens-

TABLE 31-5 Acceptable Pacing and Sensing Thresholds During Implant

	Atrial	Ventricular
Pacing threshold at 0.5 ms	<1.2 V	<1.0 V
Sensing threshold (bipolar)	>1.5–2 mV	>5 mV
Sensing threshold (unipolar)	>2–2.5 mV	>5 mV
Impedance*	300–1400 ohm	300–1400 ohm

*New high-impedance leads result in less current drain and improved longevity.

TABLE 31-6 Goals of Pacemaker Follow-up

TTM or Direct	Direct or indirect measurement of battery voltage and anticipate need for replacement
TTM	Evaluation of pacing and sensing during normal pacer function and during application of magnet
Direct	Lead function: sensing, pacing thresholds, and impedance measurement; telemetry of lead during various arm/chest positions to expose any subtle lead insulation defects
Direct	Optimization of pacing outputs and parameters based on results of pacing tests, patient clinical condition, and medications
Direct	Evaluation of diagnostic information stored in pacemakers and integrate information with overall patient management strategy
Direct	Patient education

ABBREVIATIONS: TTM = transtelephonic monitoring; Direct = direct evaluation of pacemaker using specific programmer.

ing or atrial pace/sense problems can sometimes be detected during TTM.[72]

Follow-up using TTM should be used to supplement and not replace direct evaluation of pacer function. The frequency of follow-up should be individualized according to the type of pacemaker, whether the patient is pacemaker dependent, age of pulse generator and expected longevity, presence of any pacemaker component under advisory or warning, and patient clinical factors. As depletion of pacer battery occurs, TTM may be used as often as every month to appropriately determine the timing for pacer replacement.

Components for Direct Evaluation of Pacemaker Systems

CHECKING PACING THRESHOLDS AND PROGRAMMING PACING OUTPUTS

Pacemakers should always be programmed for maximal safety particularly in patients who are pacemaker dependent. To understand how to program pacemakers safely and efficiently, some basic principles are reviewed.

Current Drain Ultimately, the longevity of the battery will be a function of the current drain versus battery capacity. There is nominal current drain for operating pacemaker circuitry, which varies according to the pacer type; however, most current drain results from pacing output. The current delivered per pacing pulse is a function of the voltage divided by the lead impedance ($I = V/R$)—Ohm's law. Therefore, it is desirable to be able to implant leads with low pacing voltage thresholds. Additionally, leads designed to have high impedance appear to decrease long-term current drain.[73]

Strength-Duration Curve The strength-duration curve (Fig. 31-7) relates voltage and pulse width. This curve is dynamic during the first 2 to 3 months following implant. With an acute rise in threshold, the curve is expected to shift upward two to four times and then subsequently shift back downward at a level greater than the initially obtained values. At pulse widths less than 0.2 ms, the curve is steep; at pulse widths exceeding 1.0 ms, the curve is flat. With this kind of relationship, programming pulse widths greater than 1 ms generally does not add safety margin to the pacing output but does substantially increase battery current drain. Similarly, programming pacing pulse widths less than 0.2 to 0.3 ms may not allow sufficient safety margin at even high voltage amplitudes.

Total Energy Expenditure of the Pacemaker This is defined as energy = $(\text{voltage})^2$ multiplied by pulse width divided by impedance. According to this relationship, the energy expenditure has an exponential relationship to voltage output but has a linear relationship to pulse width. Therefore, it is preferable to reduce voltage output rather than pulse width to conserve battery life.

Calculating Pacing Threshold At implant, it is standard to fix the pulse width at 0.5 ms and reduce the voltage until the lowest voltage that maintains consistent pacing—which is the pacing threshold (Fig. 31-8). One can fix the pulse width at any value, however (usually between 0.3 and 1.0 ms), and calculate a voltage threshold. Similarly, one can fix the voltage at a certain value and reduce the pulse width to the lowest value that maintains consistent pacing, which would also define the pacing threshold. Either method is acceptable to define a pacing threshold.

Safety Margin The safety margin for pacing outputs can be calculated by multiples of either the pulse width or the voltage threshold. For example, if the voltage threshold at 0.5 ms is

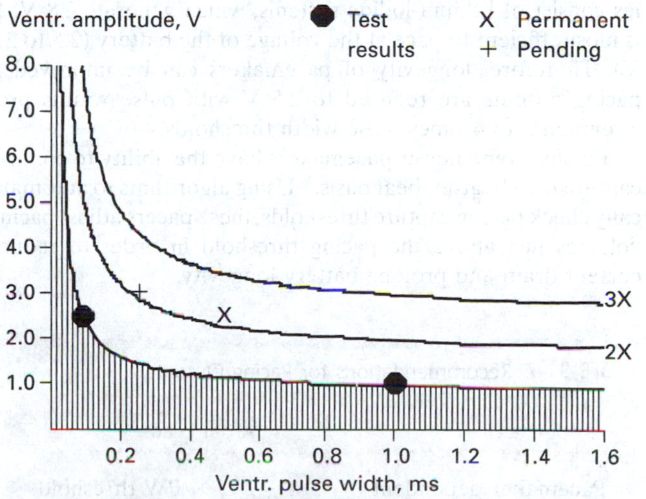

FIGURE 31-7 A sample of a strength-duration curve. The voltage threshold at 2.5 V was 0.1 ms, and the pulse-width threshold at 1.0 ms was 1.0 V. Sample curves are shown providing for two and three times the safety margin for programming voltage and pulse width. Ventr. = ventricular.

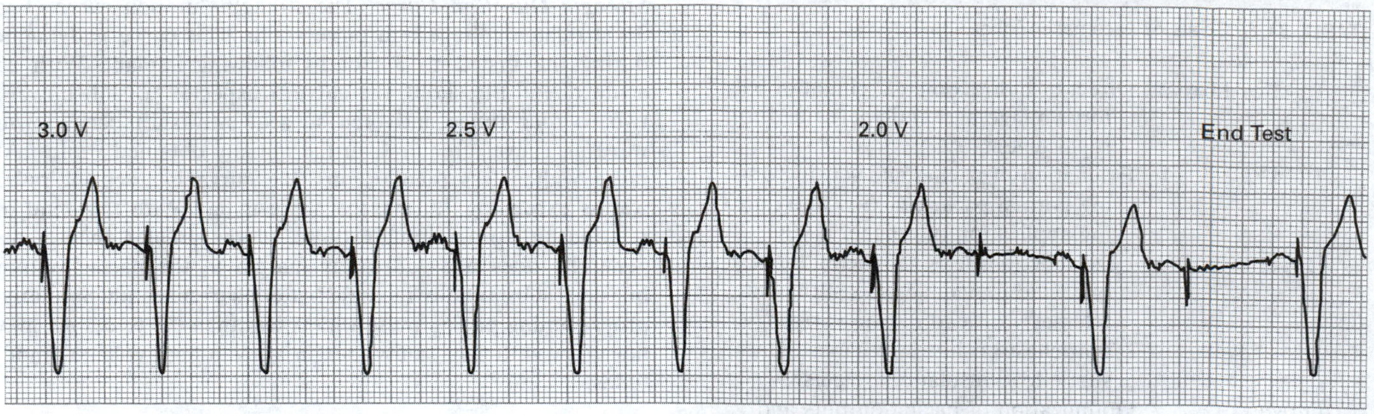

FIGURE 31-8 Ventricular pacing threshold in a patient can be calculated by holding the pulse width constant and automatically decreasing the voltage in 0.5-V decrements every four complexes. As shown, ventricular pacing was maintained at 2.5 V but was inconsistent at 2.0 V. Therefore, the voltage threshold in this patient was 2.5 V at 0.5 ms.

1.5 V, then a pacing output of 0.5 ms and 3.0 V would yield an energy safety margin of fourfold, given the relationship between energy and voltage. Similarly, if the pulse width threshold at 3.0 V is 0.15 ms, then a pacing output of 3.0 V and 0.6 ms would provide an energy safety margin of fourfold.

Acute Pacing Outputs Because the extent of the acute rise in pacing thresholds may be difficult to predict, it is better to program high pacing outputs at implant and during the first 6 to 24 weeks after implant. A greater safety margin may be desired in patients who are pacemaker dependent. Typically, greater safety margins are also desired in ventricular leads rather than atrial leads. Steroid-eluting leads generally result in blunting of the acute rise in threshold,[74] which may allow for lower pacing outputs early after implant.

Chronic Pacing Outputs In the time frame of 2 to 6 months, the pacing thresholds stabilize. Therefore, chronic pacing outputs may be programmed (Table 31-7). Almost all pacing batteries consist of lithium-iodide systems, which generate 2.8 V. It is most efficient to pace at the voltage of the battery (2.5 to 2.8 V). Therefore, longevity of pacemakers can be improved if pacing outputs are reduced to 2.5 V with pulse widths programmed 2 to 4 times pulse-width thresholds.

Finally, some newer pacemakers have the ability to confirm capture on a beat-by-beat basis.[75] Using algorithms to automatically check pacing capture thresholds, these pacers adjust pacing voltages just above the pacing threshold in order to reduce current drain and prolong battery longevity.

TABLE 31-7 Recommendations for Pacing Outputs

	Atrial Leads	Ventricular Leads
Pacemaker dependent	2–3 × PW threshold 1.5–1.8 × V threshold	4 × PW threshold 2 × V threshold
Not pacemaker dependent	2 × PW threshold 1.5 × V threshold	2–3 × PW threshold 1.5–1.8 × V threshold

ABBREVIATIONS: PW = pulse width; V = voltage.

OTHER FEATURES

Sensing Sensing of atrial and ventricular intracardiac electrograms can be evaluated by different algorithms. To test atrial sensing, the pacemaker needs to be programmed temporarily at a programmed atrial rate less than the intrinsic sinus rate. To test ventricular sensing, the pacer can be temporarily reprogrammed to the VVI mode if the programmed rate is less than the intrinsic heart rate. Alternatively, with intact AV conduction, the AV delay can be increased to allow AV conduction and thereby allow for ventricular sensing in the DDD mode. Increasing the programmed sensitivity until the intrinsic P or R wave is no longer sensed (Fig. 31-9) is another method to test sensing threshold. Telemetry of atrial or ventricular electrograms allows for direct measurement of the electrogram amplitude (Fig. 31-6). Lastly, some pacemakers have algorithms whereby the pacemaker automatically measures atrial and ventricular electrograms.

Lead Function Lead function is assessed by checking pacing and sensing function and by measuring impedance. Although there is a wide variability of normal lead impedances, chronic lead impedances should not widely vary between outpatient follow-up visits. A fractured lead exhibits a markedly elevated lead impedance. Insulation breaks manifest by reduced lead impedances. Lead fractures or insulation breaks often are intermittent problems. Therefore, normal lead impedances and pacing and sensing thresholds do not rule out these problems. The leads can be stressed by having the patient change position and do various provocative arm movements to facilitate diagnosis of lead-related problems that are not otherwise observed.

Battery Function Almost all pacemakers use lithium-iodide batteries, which have an initial battery voltage of 2.8 V. Battery voltages can be directly measured and, at a certain level (elective replacement index, ERI), the pace-

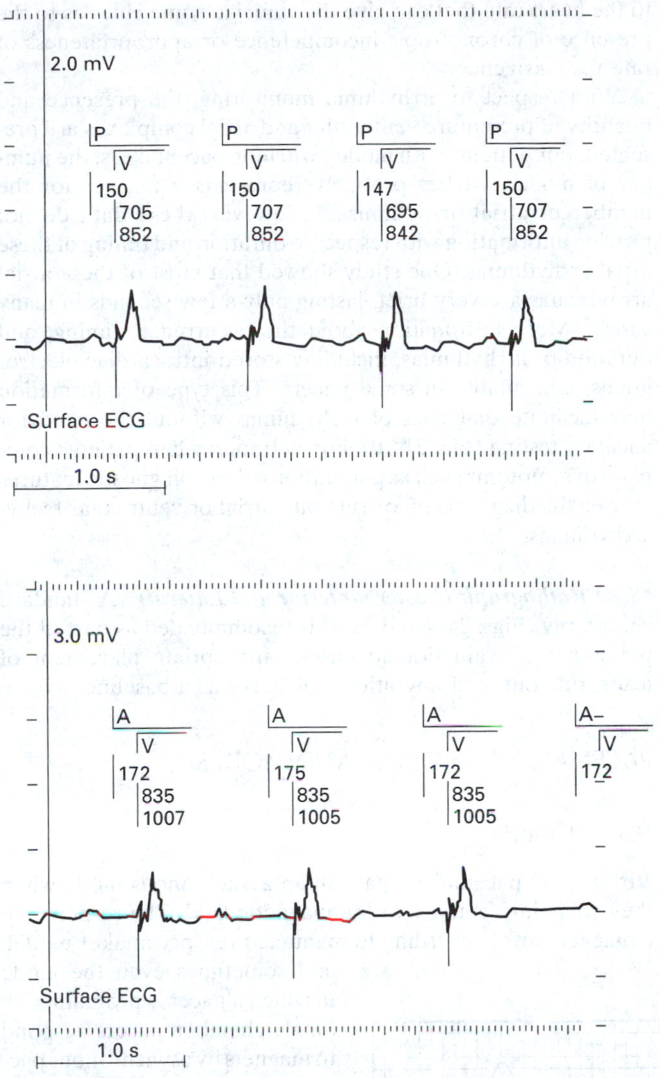

FIGURE 31-9 *Top*. P-wave synchronous ventricular pacing, with marker channels "P" indicating sensed P waves and "V" indicating paced ventricular complex. At 2 mV, there was appropriate P-wave sensing. *Bottom*. "A" indicates that the pacemaker is pacing the atrium. At the programmed sensitivity of 3 mV, there was undersensing of the P wave and therefore atrial pacing occurred. Hence, the sensed P-wave amplitude is between 2 and 3 mV.

maker unit requires elective generator change. At a lower battery voltage (end of life, EOL), there is potential loss of pacemaker function; therefore, immediate generator change is mandated.

Battery function can also be assessed without formal interrogation. Many pacemakers reset to a VVI mode at a preset pacing rate, or the pacing rate decreases to less than the programmed lower rate of the pacemaker when battery function reaches the ERI or EOL stage. Additionally, the magnet mode causes asynchronous pacing at a preset *magnet* rate for each particular pacemaker model. This magnet rate varies according to whether the battery status is adequate or not.

Rate Responsiveness Rate-responsive pacemakers require periodic adjustments of the rate-responsive features to optimize clinical responsiveness. The programmable variables include a rate-responsive upper pacing rate, which may be a separate programmable variable than the upper tracking rate. A rate-response slope may be programmed to determine the pacing rate at a certain activity level. Some pacemakers store data with respect to the use of rate responsiveness over a certain period. Otherwise, one can simply have the patient walk briskly for 2 to 3 min and assess the heart rate to determine whether it is appropriate given the patient's age and clinical status. Some pacemakers offer algorithms whereby the physician chooses the appropriate heart rate for "brisk walking," and the pacemaker automatically calculates the optimal rate-responsive programming.

Pacer Diagnostic Function Modern pacemakers have increased memory capabilities to store diagnostic information. The basic diagnostic feature displays counts or percentages of pacing versus sensing in the atrial and ventricular chambers. If a patient has complete heart block but has intact sinus nodal function, it would be expected that there be 100 percent ventricular pacing with predominant atrial sensing. The breakdown of pacing and sensing in each chamber can be stratified according

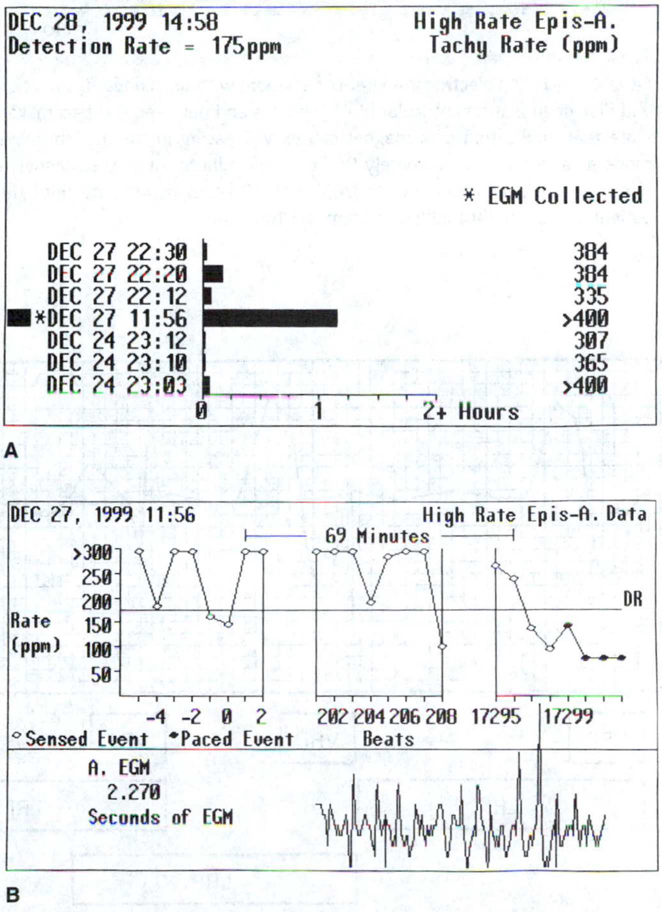

FIGURE 31-10 *A*. Shown are rate histograms demonstrating seven episodes of atrial fibrillation lasting from a few minutes to an episode lasting over an hour. *B*. This graphic demonstrates the beat-to-beat rate just before onset of the atrial tachyarrhythmia, after 200 beats, and just after termination of the arrhythmia, 69 min later. A snapshot of the stored intraatrial electrograms (A-EGMs) confirms atrial fibrillation as the mechanism. DEC, December; Tachy, tachycardia.

to the heart rate that can give the clinician some clues as to the presence of chronotropic incompetence or appropriateness of rate responsiveness.

With respect to arrhythmia monitoring, the presence and quantity of premature ventricular and atrial complexes are presented. For patients with mode-switching pacemakers, the number of mode switches probably represents a marker for the number of atrial arrhythmias.[76] However, these data do not provide information with respect to duration and timing of these atrial arrhythmias. One study showed that most of these atrial arrhythmias are very brief, lasting only a few seconds in many cases.[77] More information about the occurrence, timing, and duration of arrhythmias, including stored intracardiac electrograms, is available in some pacers. This type of information may facilitate diagnosis of arrhythmias without the need for ancillary testing (Fig. 31-10). Furthermore, when patients complain of symptoms such as palpitations, these diagnostic features may enablediagnosis of, or rule out, atrial or ventricular tachyarrhythmias.

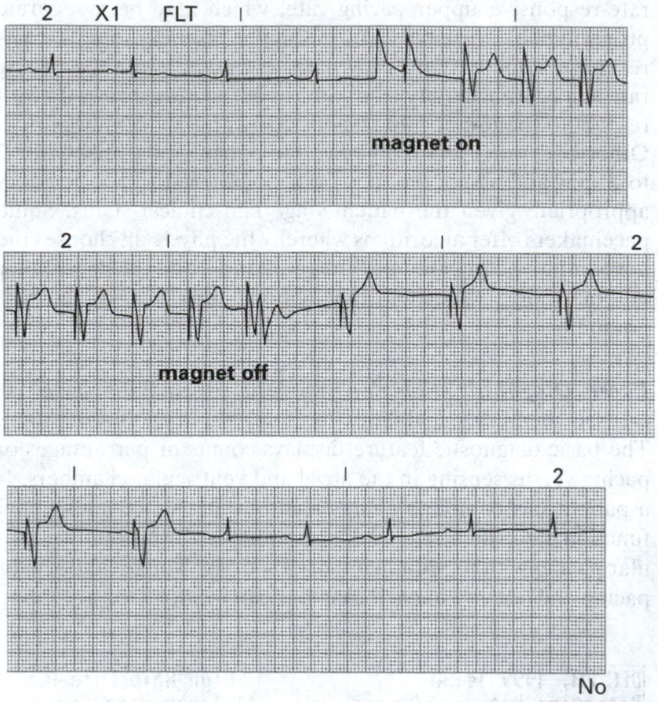

FIGURE 31-11 An electrocardiogram of a patient with sinus nodal dysfunction and first-degree atrioventricular block who has an implanted VVI pacemaker. Note that application of a magnet causes VVI pacing in the asynchronous mode at a rate of approximately 95 beats per minute. After the magnet is removed, the pacemaker reverts to VVI at 50 beats per minute until the patient's sinus rhythm inhibits pacemaker function.

Chest Radiograph (Posteroanterior and Lateral) A standard chest x-ray (Figs. 34-4 and 34-5) is recommended as part of the predischarge evaluation to ensure appropriate placement of leads, rule out lead migration, and serve as a baseline.

PACEMAKER FUNCTION AND MODES

Magnet Mode

Virtually all pacemakers pace in an asynchronous mode when they come into contact with a magnetic field. The response to a magnet varies according to manufacturer, pacemaker model, and sometimes even the mode in which a pacer is programmed. Single-chamber pacers respond to magnets by asynchronous pacing at either the programmed rate or a special magnet rate (Fig. 31-11). This allows a simple noninvasive method to assess pacing at the bedside, office, or by TTM. In patients who are pacemaker dependent and experiencing oversensing thereby inhibiting pacemaker output, a magnet is a convenient short-term method to ensure pacing. Furthermore, pacemakers usually have one magnet rate for a battery that is intact and another one for a battery that is at ERI or at EOL. If these rates are known, applying a magnet to a pacemaker is an easy noninvasive method to assess battery status.

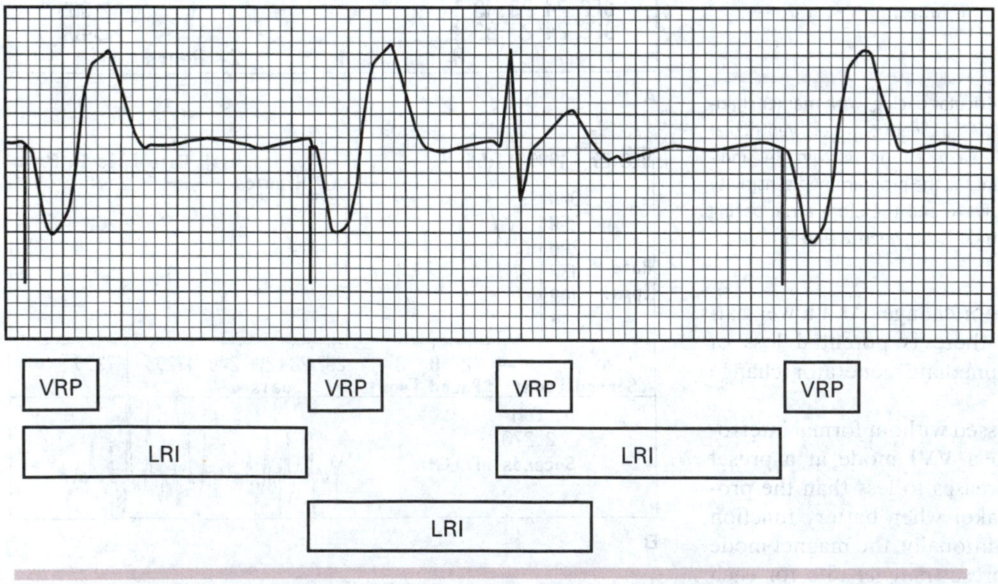

FIGURE 31-12 Schematic diagram of the pacemaker timing cycles during VVI pacing. After a ventricular paced or ventricular sensed event, the pacemaker begins a ventricular refractory period (VRP). This is a programmable value usually between 250 and 400 ms. During this time, a sensed ventricular event will not initiate a new timing interval and will not reset the pacemaker. The lower rate interval (LRI) of the pacemaker corresponds to the programmed lower rate. If this interval expires and there is no sensed ventricular event following the end of the ventricular refractory period, the pacemaker stimulates the ventricle (second and fourth complex) and the VRP and LRI begin anew. If there is an intrinsic ventricular depolarization between the end of the VRP and during the LRI, then ventricular output is inhibited and the VRP and LRI begin anew.

VVI Mode

In the VVI mode, a pacemaker operates as shown in Fig.

31-12. The lower rate is converted to an interval (milliseconds). After a paced or sensed ventricular event, a programmable refractory period prevents inappropriate sensing of T waves. After the pacemaker ventricular refractory period, there is an interval extending to the escape interval during which time the pacemaker senses a ventricular event, if one occurs before the end of the interval; otherwise, there is ventricular pacing output.

Hysteresis is a programmable function in which the ventricular escape interval is longer after a sensed ventricular event than after a paced ventricular event. This feature can be used in patients with sinus rhythm so that VVI pacing would not initiate until the sinus rate drops below the hysteresis rate, which is lower than the pacemaker rate (Fig. 31-13).

AAI Pacing

AAIR is an excellent mode of pacing in patients with sinus node dysfunction and normal AV nodal and His-Purkinje function.[78,79] The timing sequences are the same for AAI as for VVI pacing. Atrial sensitivities are programmed at lower values (increased sensitivity) to sense intrinsic P waves safely. This frequently leads to oversensing of far-field ventricular electrograms, which can be avoided by programming a longer refractory period.

Patients with sinus nodal dysfunction may develop AV block, which may be a source of concern when using AAI pacing. However, with careful selection of patients,[78,79] including normal PR intervals, absence of bundle branch block, and AV Wenckebach occurring at atrial pacing rates of more than 120 beats per minute, the risk of development of second- or third-degree AV block is less than 0.6 percent per year.

DDD Pacing

DDD pacing is the most common pacing mode for dual-chamber pacemakers. The timing sequences for DDD pacing are described in Fig. 31-14. This mode is used for patients with AV node and/or sinus node dysfunction.

DDD PACING IN PATIENTS WITH SINUS NODE DYSFUNCTION

Patients with sinus node dysfunction may have intermittent or chronic sinus bradycardia requiring intermittent or continuous atrial pacing. If patients have intact AV conduction, the pacemaker functions as an AAI pacer. Due to medications that slow AV conduction and/or intrinsic AV nodal or His-Purkinje disease, however, patients with DDD pacemakers frequently demonstrate fused ventricular complexes originating from ventricular stimulation and through the AV conduction system. The degree of fusion of the ventricular complex between pacing from a right ventricular lead and conduction down the AV nodal–His-Purkinje system depends in large part on the difference between the programmed AV interval and the intrinsic AV conduction time.

For ventricular output to be inhibited in patients with DDD pacemakers, the pacemaker AV interval must be longer than the conduction time between the sensed or paced atrial complex to the right ventricular lead. A very long AV interval (more than 0.25 s) may decrease the benefit of AV synchrony when AV pacing does occur. It is not uncommon that pacemakers sense the ventricular electrogram late during ventricular depolarization especially with right ventricular conduction delay or right bundle branch block. Pacemaker *pseudofusion* occurs when there is ventricular pacing within the QRS complex (Fig. 31-15).

PATIENTS WITH ATRIOVENTRICULAR BLOCK AND NORMAL SINUS NODE FUNCTION

In the DDD mode, if the lower rate of the pacer is programmed at a sufficiently low value to permit atrial tracking, the pacemaker stimulates the ventricle synchronous with intrinsic P waves. If a patient does not require atrial pacing, it may be reasonable to implant a dual-chamber pacer with a single tripolar or quadripolar lead that allows atrial sensing and ventricular pacing and sensing (Fig. 31-16). These VDD pacing systems allow for ease of implant and for bipolar atrial sensing. Atrial sensing may not be as reliable compared to a fixed atrial lead, which may lead to occasional atrial undersensing.[80,81] In a recent prospective comparison between single-lead VDD systems to DDD leads, however, there were lower P-wave amplitudes in the group with VDD systems, but no significant clinical differences with respect to atrial undersensing.[82]

DDD versus VVI Pacing

Multiple retrospective and observational studies[83–91] and a few prospective studies[92–94] demonstrate hemodynamic, clinical, and

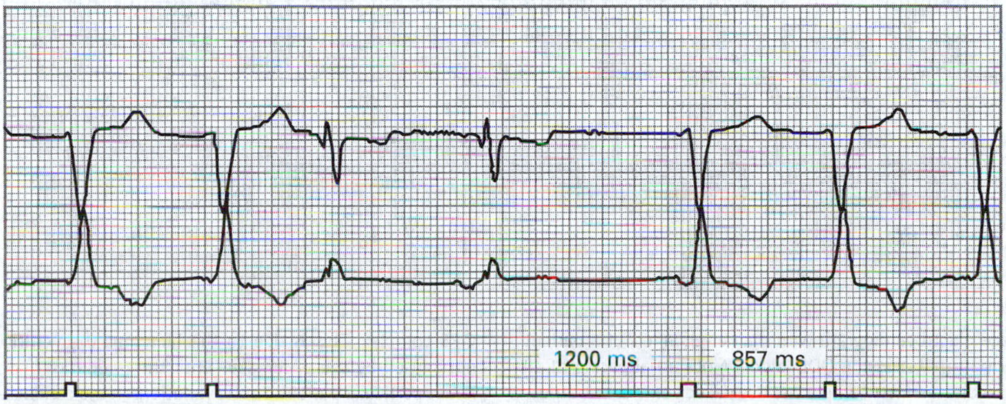

FIGURE 31-13 A patient with atrial fibrillation and the VVI pacemaker with lower rate of 70 pulses per minute (857 ms) and hysteresis rate of 50 beats per minute (1200 ms). The square pulses in the bottom line represent pacing output. This tracing (two leads recorded simultaneously) represents normal hysteresis function. See the text for discussion.

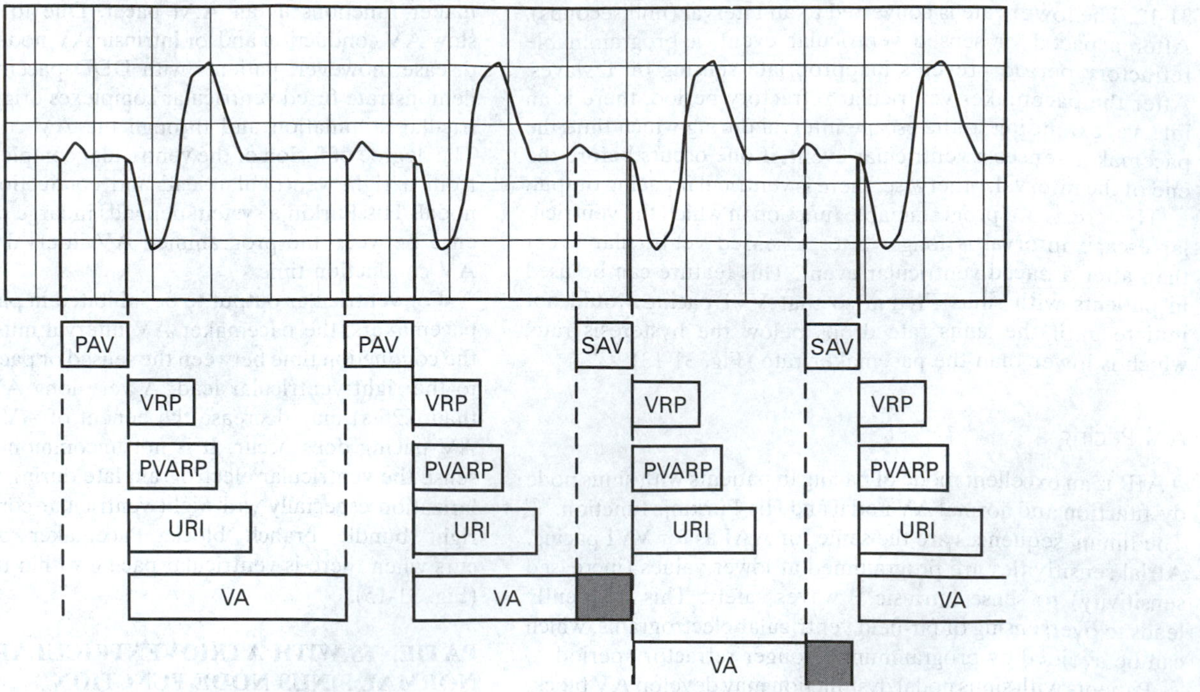

FIGURE 31-14 Schematic diagram of DDD pacing with selected timing cycles and refractory periods. After a paced atrial complex, the paced atrioventricular interval (PAV) begins. If there is no ventricular depolarization before this interval expires, the pacemaker response is to output a ventricular impulse. After a paced ventricular output, several refractory periods and timing cycles are initiated. The ventricular refractory period (VRP) is the time during which a ventricular event will not reset the timing intervals. The postventricular refractory period (PVARP) represents the time during which an atrial event will not be sensed or will not reset the timing intervals. The upper rate interval represents the shortest interval (maximum rate) that a pacemaker will ventricular pace corresponding to the programmed upper tracking rate. The ventricular-atrial escape interval (VA) represents the time during which, if there is no sensed atrial electrogram, atrial pacing occurs. The programmed lower rate corresponds to the AV interval and the VA interval. During the first two complexes, there were no sensed atrial complexes; therefore, the VA interval expired and atrial pacing occurred. During the third and fourth complexes, there were sensed atrial electrograms following the PVARP and before the VA interval expired (shaded area in the VA bar). Note that atrial sensing usually occurs after the start of the P wave, representing the atrial conduction time to the atrial electrodes. The programmed AV interval following a sensed atrial complex (SAV) may be programmed at a value lower than the PAV to obtain equivalent PR intervals.

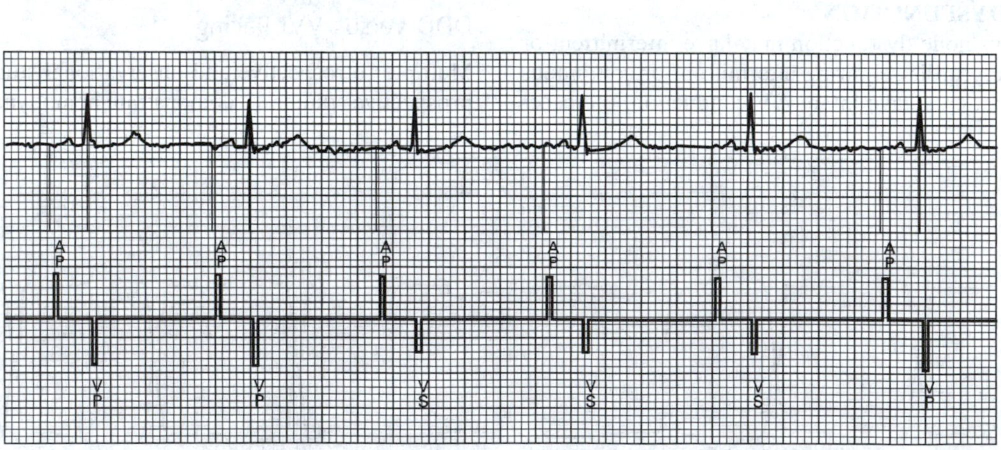

FIGURE 31-15 Surface electrocardiogram with marker channels of a patient with a dual-chamber pacemaker in the DDD mode. Note atrial pacing of all complexes. The first, second, and last complexes have paced ventricular outputs in the middle of the QRS complex. Compared to the third, fourth, and fifth complexes, which do not have these ventricular pacing spikes, there is no change in the QRS complex. This is consistent with "pseudofusion" of the QRS complex. This is due to the fact that the ventricular depolarization is not sensed by the pacemaker until the middle or end of the QRS complex in this particular patient. Subtle variations in the conducted PR interval account for the fact that some of the complexes have a paced ventricular complex and some do not.

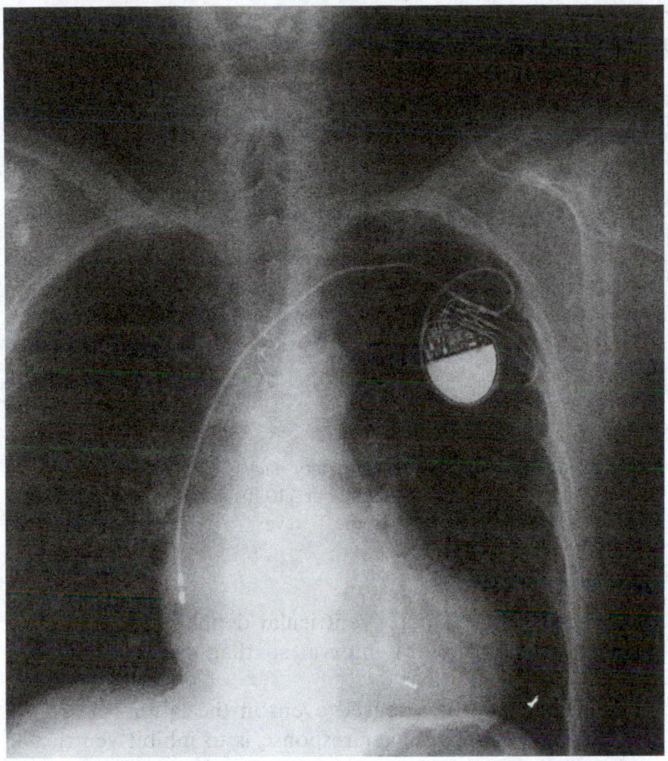

FIGURE 31-16 Chest x-ray showing a single lead in the heart. Note the bipolar electrodes in the atrium and the single electrode in the ventricle. This pacemaker system is capable of VDD pacing. Therefore, it senses atrial depolarizations and can pace or sense in the ventricle.

quality-of-life benefits of dual-chamber or atrial-based pacing versus ventricular pacing. Therefore, it appears prudent to implant DDD pacers in most patients with intact atrial function but not all patients.

In patients with congestive heart failure due to left ventricular systolic dysfunction, the dependence of cardiac output to AV synchrony appears to decrease secondarily to the already increased left ventricular filling pressures. Patients with fixed stroke volume (i.e., left ventricular systolic dysfunction) may depend almost exclusively on heart rate for cardiac output[83] and, therefore, may have limited benefit from AV synchrony. However, any improvement in cardiac output with restoration of AV synchrony may be clinically significant. Additionally, clinical conditions such as left ventricular hypertrophy or diastolic dysfunction generally are dependent on adequate preload to maintain cardiac output. Restoration of AV synchrony appears to be particularly significant for these patients.

Patients with Sick Sinus Syndrome

In patients with sick sinus syndrome, dual-chamber pacing has been shown to be superior to VVI pacing.[92,93,95–97] Many studies have demonstrated that atrial-based pacing (DDD) is associated with decreased clinical events, including atrial fibrillation, congestive heart failure, stroke, and death,[88–98] mainly but not exclusively in patients with sick sinus syndrome. Several mechanisms by which atrial-based pacing is beneficial in patients with sick sinus syndrome may not apply to the subset of patients with AV block. Patients with sick sinus syndrome are more likely to have intact VA conduction compared with patients with high-degree or complete AV block. VVI pacing in patients with retrograde VA conduction causes atrial contractions against closed AV valves, leading to atrial distension and transient increases in pulmonary capillary wedge and jugular venous pressures. Increased atrial distension may predispose individuals to atrial fibrillation. This is apt to be more evident in the patients with sick sinus syndrome who already have paroxysmal atrial fibrillation or are at risk for such arrhythmias. Sympathetic activity is elevated during VVI versus dual-chamber pacing, which contributes to increased morbidity and possible mortality.[99] Even in the absence of retrograde conduction, VVI pacing with VA dissociation leads to atrial systoles throughout the cardiac cycle, which can also lead to a similar deleterious effect on atrial size and function. Therefore, dual-chamber pacing appears to reduce the incidence of atrial fibrillation and embolic complications.[88,90,93]

Andersen and colleagues published short- and long-term reports on a randomized study comparing single- and dual-chamber pacing in patients with sick sinus syndrome.[92,93] In their long-term study, they reported a reduction of embolic events, atrial fibrillation, and mortality with use of atrial-based pacing. Additionally, they found progressive benefit from atrial pacing compared with ventricular pacing, which resulted in overall improvement of survival based on total mortality and death from cardiovascular causes. Additionally, many studies have shown that maintenance of AV synchrony improves quality of life particularly at rest.[86,87] In fact, many patients who have VVI pacers may not recognize the extent of their symptoms until they have an upgrade to a DDD system.

Atrioventricular Block

In patients with AV block, the advantage of dual-chamber pacing has been demonstrated by some authors[98,100] but not by others.[91,94] In a retrospective study from the Mayo Clinic[91] on an elderly population, long-term survival was not affected by the mode of pacing. Lamas et al.[94] published a series on 407 elderly patients (older than age 65) who were randomized to have a dual-chamber pacer programmed to either VVI[R] or DDD[R] modes. These authors concluded that the main quality-of-life benefits associated with DDDR pacing were noted in the group of patients with sick sinus syndrome, and there were no quality-of-life benefits noted in the patients with pacers implanted for AV block.[94]

Therefore, there now appear to be adequate data supporting the use of atrial-based pacing (AAI, DDI, and DDD) in patients with sick sinus syndrome. The benefit of dual-chamber versus ventricular pacing in patients with advanced or complete AV block appears to be controversial. In patients with intact sinus node function and AV block, however, it is prudent to at least implant a single-lead VDD system, if not a complete dual-chamber pacing system, to restore AV synchrony in order to restore physiologic pacing.

PACING TIMING INTERVALS AND UPPER RATE BEHAVIOR

Atrioventricular Interval

The AV interval is divided into three zones. The first 20 to 40 ms of this interval is the atrial blanking period. The ventricular

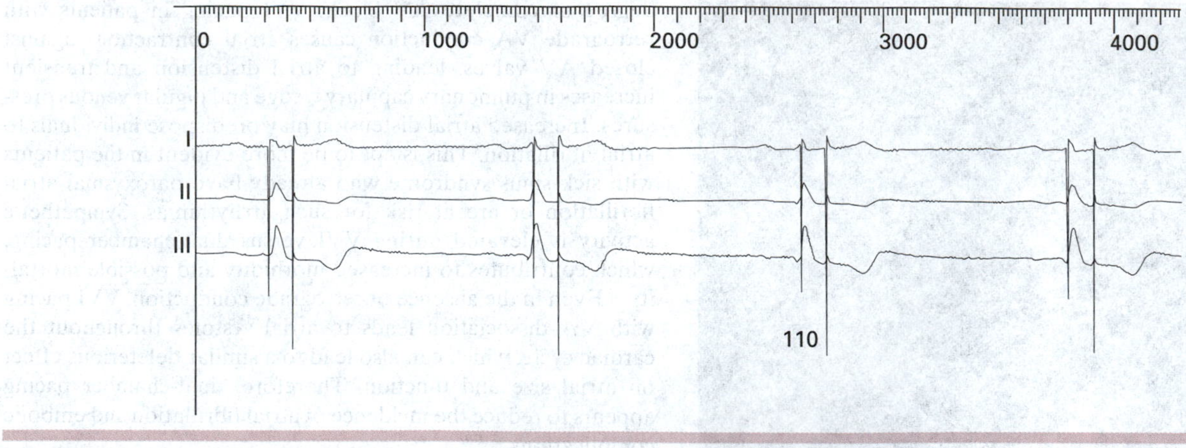

FIGURE 31-17 Surface leads I, II, and III are shown at paper speed of 50 mm/s. Note that there is complete undersensing of the P wave. The pacemaker therefore tends to pace at the lower rate interval, which corresponds with an intrinsic QRS complex. This QRS complex is sensed within the ventricular safety period, triggering ventricular safety pacing. For this particular pacemaker, ventricular safety pacing occurs at 110 ms after atrial pacing in order to avoid ventricular pacing during the T wave.

channel is blanked during this period to prevent inappropriate sensing of atrial output (crosstalk). Crosstalk is a greater problem in unipolar than in bipolar systems. The next part of the AV interval occurs from the end of the blanking period to approximately 100 to 120 ms after the atrial pacing output. If a ventricular sensed event occurred at this point, it would be nonphysiologic because of the short elapsed AV interval. The pacemaker responds with a ventricular output at a short AV interval (100 to 120 ms), which is a safety feature [ventricular safety pacing (Fig. 31-17)]. Ventricular safety pacing is a feature that ensures ventricular pacing in case the sensed event was not a ventricular depolarization; instead, pacing occurs at a short interval so that the pacing output falls before the T wave.

Finally, if there is a sensed event in the latter part of the AV interval, the pacemaker response is to inhibit ventricular pacing output.

Upper Rate Behavior

The total atrial refractory period (TARP) consists of the AV interval and the postventricular atrial refractory period (PVARP). The TARP is a programmable value that can be calculated in milliseconds. Ventricular tracking of atrial events cannot exceed a frequency shorter than the TARP. By dividing 60,000 by the TARP, a rate can be calculated that is the upper rate at which a pacemaker can track atrial events at a 1:1 ratio. At atrial rates exceeding this value, every other atrial event will fall within the pacemaker refractory period (PVARP) and there will be 2:1 pacemaker AV block. Therefore, the rate corresponding to the TARP corresponds to the pacemaker 2:1 rate.

The upper tracking rate is a separate programmable value. The upper tracking rate is generally programmed at a rate less than that corresponding to the TARP. This leads to pacemaker Wenckebach behavior when the patient's atrial rate exceeds the programmed upper rate (Fig. 31-18). The Wenckebach interval is defined as the difference between

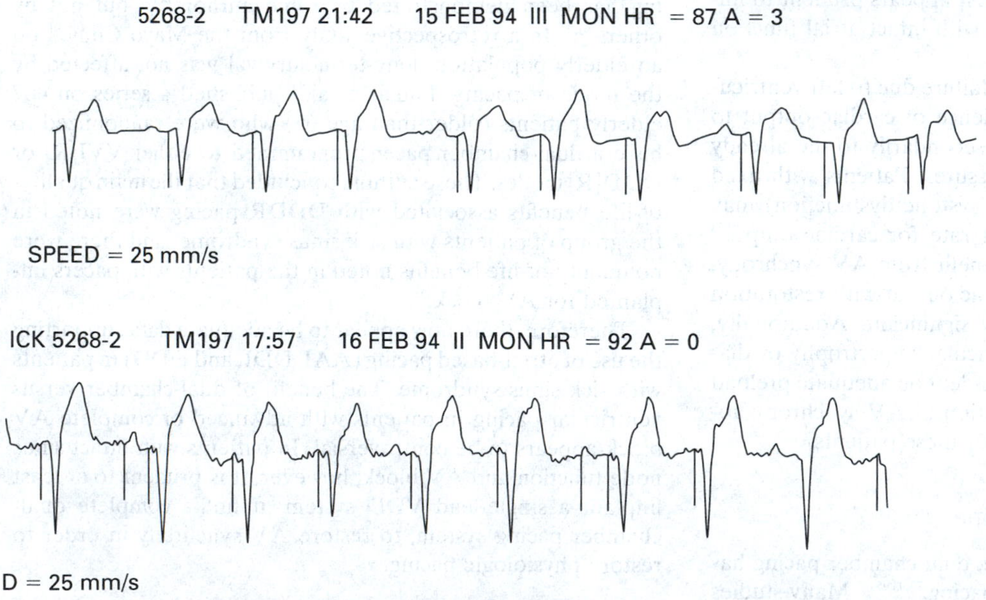

FIGURE 31-18 *Top.* Sinus tachycardia in a patient with atrioventricular block and a DDD pacemaker with a programmed upper rate of 100 beats per minute, which is less than the intrinsic sinus rate. Note that the interval between the sensed P wave and the paced ventricular complex lengthens progressively, until there is a P wave (within the T wave) following the first, fourth, and seventh paced ventricular complexes without subsequent ventricular pacing, consistent with pacemaker Wenckebach. *Bottom.* The pacemaker is programmed in the DDDR mode with upper rate of 100 beats per minute. The presence of rate response, during activity, acts to smooth the upper rate, preventing the longer pauses during pacemaker Wenckebach.

the programmed upper rate and the rate corresponding to the TARP.

Therefore, when a patient has a sinus or other atrial tachycardia, the pacemaker can track the P waves in a 1:1 fashion up to either the upper programmed rate of the pacer or to the pacemaker 2:1 rate, which ever is lower. If the 2:1 pacemaker rate is lower, there may be deleterious hemodynamic consequences for an exercising patient in whom the ventricular response would abruptly drop by nearly half. For this reason, a Wenckebach interval is preferred by programming the TARP to a sufficiently short interval or the upper rate of the pacemaker to a rate that is less than the 2:1 AV block rate.

Various strategies are available for active patients with DDD pacemakers who require physiologic upper rates. Many pacemakers offer autoadjusting AV intervals that shorten with increasing rates. By shortening the AV interval, the TARP decreases, which allows greater upper tracking rates before reaching the rate of 2:1 AV block. Another strategy involves sensor-driven rate smoothing.[101] The rate-responsive features are activated, and, in fact, a separate upper sensor-driven rate, different than the upper atrial tracking rate, may be programmed. This enables maintenance of increased ventricular pacing rates driven by the sensor when the pacer would otherwise respond with AV Wenckebach or 2:1 AV block.

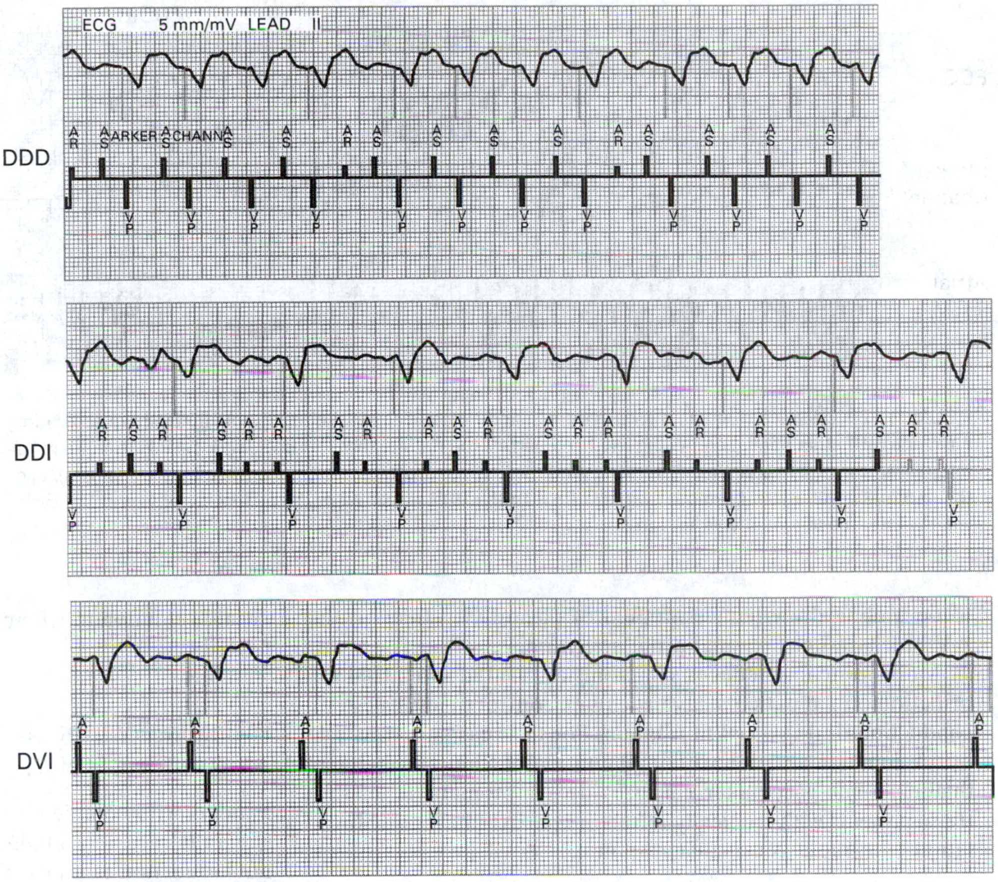

FIGURE 31-19 Tracings of a patient with a dual-chamber pacemaker who has underlying atrial fibrillation. Electrocardiograms and corresponding marker channels are shown for pacing modes DDD, DDI, and DVI, respectively. Note that during DDD the pacemaker rhythm is an irregularly irregular paced ventricular rhythm at, but not exceeding, the upper rate of the pacemaker. In the DDI mode, there is no tracking of the atrial fibrillation; therefore, it functions effectively as a VVI pacemaker so long as the patient is in atrial fibrillation. In the last tracing, the mode is DVI; therefore, there is no sensing of atrial electrograms, which accounts for the AV sequential pacing pattern. This mode is generally not used when the DDI mode is available. AR = sensed atrial electrogram in the pacemaker refractory period; AS = sensed atrial electrogram; VP = ventricular paced complex.

USE OF PACEMAKERS IN DIFFERENT CLINICAL SITUATIONS

Paroxysmal Atrial Fibrillation, Flutter, and Other Tachyarrhythmias

DDD pacing is problematic in the presence of atrial tachyarrhythmias. During atrial fibrillation, there are so many sensed atrial events occurring at rapid rates that a DDD pacemaker responds with an attempt to track these electrograms up to but not exceeding the upper rate (Figs. 31-19 and 31-20). The ECG hallmark is an irregularly irregular ventricular paced rhythm at a mean rate just below the upper rate. Of course, if the patient has intrinsic AV conduction, the patient's ventricular rate is not controlled by the pacemaker but rather by the intrinsic AV nodal conduction.

There are various strategies for preventing inappropriate upper tracking behavior during atrial tachyarrhythmias. In a patient with intact AV conduction and paroxysmal atrial tachyarrhythmias, DDI or DDIR modes would be appropriate (Fig. 31-19). In this mode of pacing, there is no tracking of atrial events. If there is a sinus or other atrial sensed electrogram, the pacer will inhibit atrial pacing output. Ventricular pacing occurs only at the lower rate interval. For patients with sick sinus syndrome, the clinical problem necessitating a pacemaker is the bradycardia resulting from intrinsic sinus node dysfunction or the bradyarrhythmias resulting from therapy to suppress the tachyarrhythmias. Therefore, DDIR is a very effective pacing mode for patients with sick sinus syndrome who have intrinsic AV conduction.

At the initiation of atrial fibrillation or other atrial tachyarrhythmia, many pacers can automatically switch pacer modes from DDD[R] to VVI[R] or DDI[R] (Fig. 31-20). The automatic mode switch may occur at the upper rate of the pacemaker or at a separate programmable mode switch rate. It may occur with single or multiple sequential premature atrial complexes, depending on the pacemaker model. Mode switching appears

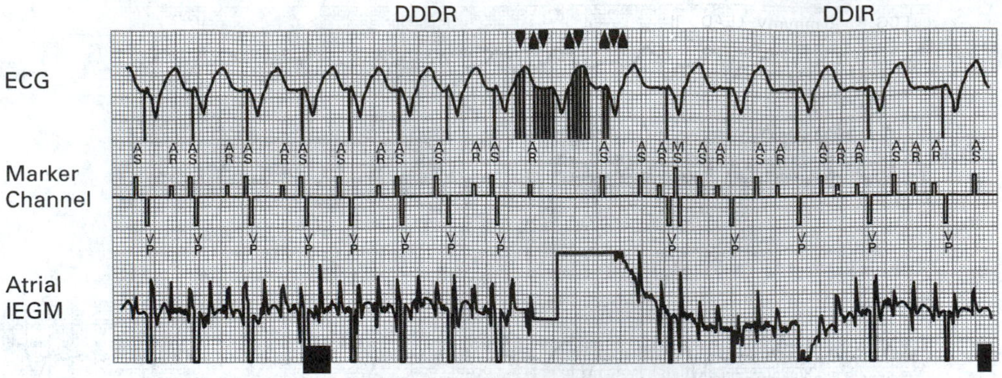

FIGURE 31-20 Electrocardiogram, marker channels, and intracardiac atrial electrograms (IEGMs) are shown for a patient with atrial fibrillation. At the left-hand part of the tracing, there is upper track pacing at an irregular rate due to the atrial fibrillation. Automatic mode switch was programmed on (indicated by the triangles), and the pacemaker automatically mode switched (MS) to the DDIR mode. Note the prolonging of ventricular cycle lengths after mode switch was activated.

to be a clinically effective method of pacing in patients with AV block and paroxysmal atrial arrhythmias.[102–104]

Mode switching reduces symptoms associated with atrial fibrillation only if patients have adequate control of intrinsic AV conduction during atrial fibrillation. For this reason, a strategy of AV junction ablation with implantation of a mode-switching dual-chamber pacemaker can provide symptomatic relief for those patients with medically refractory paroxysmal atrial fibrillation with rapid ventricular response.[103,104]

Prevention of Atrial Fibrillation by Pacing

The initiation and maintenance of atrial fibrillation involve several pathophysiologic mechanisms, the most dominant of which is multiple reentrant pathways (see Chaps. 23 and 24). Pacing therapy may reduce dispersion of refractoriness in the atrium, a feature in reentry, or eliminate pause-dependent initiation of arrhythmias. As discussed above atrial-based pacing (AAI or DDD) reduces the incidence of atrial fibrillation compared with VVI pacing in those patients who require pacing; it is unknown, however, whether atrial pacing in itself may reduce the occurrence of atrial fibrillation. In patients with sick sinus syndrome who require bradycardia pacing support, it has been suggested[105–107] that standard atrial pacing reduces the frequency of atrial fibrillation. These studies examined the arrhythmia-free interval before and after atrial pacing. In another study of patients who had atrial fibrillation without sinus nodal dysfunction, however, DDD pacers were implanted 3 months prior to planned AV junction ablation, and these pacers were programmed to DDD pacing at 70 beats per minute or to backup DDI pacing at 30 beats per minute.[108] The patients who were actively paced did not have fewer episodes of atrial fibrillation. Therefore, pacing in itself may not reduce the occurrence of atrial fibrillation but may be helpful in the management of those patients who have sinus nodal dysfunction.

It has been reported that dual-site atrial pacing may reduce the occurrence of episodes of atrial fibrillation.[106,107] One lead is placed in the right atrium and a second lead is placed in the coronary sinus ostium or inside the coronary sinus to advance left atrial depolarization. In theory, synchronization of the atria may reduce dispersion of refractoriness and thereby reduce the occurrence of atrial fibrillation.

Pacing in Chronic Atrial Fibrillation or Other Atrial Tachyarrhythmia

Patients with persistent atrial tachyarrhythmias and high-degree or complete AV block generally require a VVIR pacemaker unless their functional status is limited, in which case a VVI pacemaker would suffice. DDD[R] may be implanted in select patients with persistent atrial fibrillation in whom cardioversion to sinus rhythm is expected.

Pacing in Complete or Intermittent Third-Degree Atrioventricular Block

Patients with complete or intermittent third-degree AV block generally receive a DDD pacemaker (Fig. 31-3). If their sinus nodal function is intact, the ventricles are paced synchronous with the P wave after a programmed AV delay. Because some of these patients would not require atrial pacing, some manufacturers offer a single tripolar or quadripolar lead that utilizes a bipole in the atrial cavity for atrial sensing, and the distal electrode(s) are attached to the right ventricle for ventricular pacing and sensing (Fig. 31-16). This mode of pacing, VDD, facilitates implant, since only one lead is required.

Pacing in Carotid Sinus Syndrome and Vasovagal Syncope

Patients with one of the neurally mediated syncope syndromes generally have intact sinus and AV nodal function. Because of combined vasodepressor and cardioinhibitory responses, patients usually require dual-chamber pacing when a pacer is implanted. Additionally, these patients benefit from an interventional pacing rate (80 to 100 pulses per minute) during their vasovagal episodes and only require backup pacing at rates of 40 to 50 pulses per minute during other times. Therefore, one algorithm is to use dual-chamber hysteresis so that when a patient's heart rate drops to the lower rate, pacing is initiated at the interventional rate. This algorithm has limitations, since a patient's heart rate needs to exceed the interventional pacing before inhibiting the pacer. Some pacemakers now offer *rate-drop response* pacing, which involves interventional pacing (80 to 110 pulses per minute with gradual decline in paced rate at 1 to 5 minutes) that is triggered by a steep drop in a patient's intrinsic heart rate. Based on the North American Vasovagal Pacing Study, there was a reduction in syncope from 70 percent in the control group to 22 percent in patients who had pacers implanted with the rate-drop response feature.[42]

Pacing in Cardiac Transplant Patients

After orthotopic cardiac transplant, there is a high incidence of chronotropic incompetence resulting in slow junctional rhythm, sinus arrest, or sinus bradycardia. Bradycardia tends to resolve spontaneously in most patients, but 6 to 21 percent of patients may require permanent pacing.[109] Although symptomatic bradycardia is generally an early finding after transplantation, up to 5 percent of patients following transplant may have symptomatic bradycardia as a late finding.[110] During the implant, the atrial lead is positioned in the donor atrium. A DDDR or AAIR pacer is placed, depending on whether AV conduction is intact.[111]

HEMODYNAMICS OF CARDIAC PACING

In theory, a pacemaker optimizes and maintains AV synchrony and optimizes ventricular activation and heart rate to enable cardiac output to meet the metabolic needs of the patient, whether he or she is resting, sleeping, or exercising. There are many variables involved in determining cardiac output through an effect on stroke volume, such as the autonomic tone, physical condition of the patient, left ventricular diastolic and systolic function, and peripheral vascular resistance. As seen in Table 31-8, many variables in pacing systems can affect cardiac hemodynamic function.

Atrioventricular Interval

The role of the AV interval and the optimal AV interval for improving hemodynamic function has been studied.[112–114] For most patients, the optimal AV interval corresponds to the physiologic range (i.e., an AV interval of approximately 150 ± 50 ms). In clinical practice, however, most patients' quality of life is not significantly different between AV intervals that are *optimized by noninvasive assessment* versus AV intervals that are *suboptimal*.[114]

There are other considerations when programming AV intervals. With AV sequential pacing, the start of the P wave corresponds to the start of the AV interval while, with P-wave synchronous ventricular pacing, the start of the P wave begins approximately 20 to 70 ms prior to the start of the AV interval, depending on the conduction time from the sinus node to the atrial electrodes. The optimal AV interval for P-wave synchronous ventricular pacing would be shorter than the optimal AV interval for AV sequential pacing.[112] Therefore, to achieve similar hemodynamic effects from ventricular pacing following a sensed or paced P wave, the sensed AV interval should be programmed approximately 40 to 50 ms shorter than the paced AV interval. Additionally, left ventricular cardiac function is more dependent on left atrial to left ventricular relationships rather than right atrial to right ventricular AV interval. For this reason, there is much variability between patients with respect to programming AV intervals.

TABLE 31-8 Effects of Cardiac Pacing Variables on Hemodynamic Function

Feature	Effects
AV synchrony	Improves hemodynamic function in patients with diastolic dysfunction
	Required for most patients with one of the neurally mediated syncope syndromes
	Prevents AV valve regurgitation that is observed with ventricular contraction against open AV valves
	Prevents increase in pulmonary venous or central venous pressure seen when atria contract against closed AV valves
AV interval	Short AV interval in patients with hypertrophic cardiomyopathy
	Shorter AV interval after sensed P wave than during AV sequential pacing to have equivalent PR intervals
	In patients with dilated cardiomyopathy, physiologic AV interval may be preferable to markedly prolonged PR interval
Rate responsiveness	Useful in patients with chronotropic incompetence
	Useful as a rate-smoothing feature during upper tracking rate behavior in DDD patients to prevent deleterious effects of pacemaker AV Wenckebach or 2:1 AV block
Pacing site	Right ventricular apex is preferred in patients with hypertrophic cardiomyopathy to have left ventricular apical preexcitation preceding septal activation
	Multisite ventricular pacing is under study in patients with congestive heart failure, dilated cardiomyopathy, and intraventricular conduction delay

ABBREVIATIONS: AV = atrioventricular.

Pacemaker Syndrome

The pacemaker syndrome is a constellation of signs and symptoms representing adverse reaction to VVI pacing.[115–117] Most of the symptoms relate to loss of AV synchrony and also to retrograde conduction. These include orthostatic hypotension, near syncope, fatigue, exercise intolerance, malaise, weakness, cough, awareness of heartbeat, chest fullness, neck fullness, headache, chest pain, and other symptoms that may be nonspecific. On exam, these patients may have intermittent or persistent cannon A waves and possible liver pulsation. ECG demonstrates VVI pacing present at the time of the symptoms.

The basis for pacemaker syndrome is not only loss of AV synchrony but also the presence of ventricular-atrial conduction. Atrial contraction against closed AV valves leads to increases in jugular and pulmonary venous pressure causing cough and malaise in patients with intact cardiac function and congestive heart failure in other patients with structural heart disease. Distended atria can lead to reflex vasodepressor effects mediated by the autonomic nervous system and diuresis mediated by elevated levels of atrial natriuretic peptide.[118,119] Therefore, if patients have decreased cardiac output and arterial pressure secondary to VVI pacing, autonomic and humoral reflexes can lead to further hypotension and hemodynamic deterioration.

DDI pacing may produce pacemaker syndrome if the sinus rate exceeds the lower rate. DDD pacing can lead to pacemaker syndrome in select patients with severe intraatrial conduction delay who experience inappropriate timing between left atrial systole and left ventricular contraction.[120] This may necessitate the addition of a coronary sinus pacing lead to advance left atrial systole.[121]

The management of pacemaker syndrome usually requires restoration of AV synchrony. In many patients, an upgrade to a dual-chamber pacer is indicated. In some patients with intact sinus and AV conduction, lowering the pacing rate in VVI mode and using the hysteresis mode may promote sinus rhythm, lessening the symptoms associated with pacemaker syndrome. Using the VVIR mode by itself will not prevent or reduce symptoms from the pacemaker syndrome. Many patients may experience mild symptoms of the pacemaker syndrome and not recognize the symptoms until after an upgrade to a dual-chamber pacemaker.[122] Most patients prefer DDD pacing to VVI pacing[117,122,123] in various clinical and hemodynamic studies.

RATE-RESPONSIVE PACEMAKERS

The ability of a pacemaker to increase the lower rate in response to a physical or physiologic stimulus is termed *rate-responsive, rate-adaptive,* or *sensor-driven* pacing. The letter R in the fourth position of the NASPE/BPEG pacing code indicates rate-responsive pacing. Sensor systems that respond to parameters or activities that correlate with physiologic need for increased cardiac pacing rate provide input to the pacer, which increases the pacer lower rate. Numerous sensors have been developed with the goal of providing sensor input into the pacemaker, which can be then used to provide rate-adaptive pacing.[124–133]

Hemodynamic Evaluation of Rate-Adaptive Pacing

Cardiac output is a function of ventricular rate and stroke volume, modified by variables such as AV synchrony, ventricular preload, ventricular afterload, and autonomic state. In normal individuals at rest, pacing-induced increase in ventricular rate usually results in a transient increase in cardiac output followed by decrease in stroke volume, returning cardiac output toward normal. When there is a physiologic need for increased cardiac output, however, such as during exercise, stroke volume is maintained during increased ventricular pacing rate.

The role of the atrium and the need for AV synchrony remain less certain during faster rates compared with heart rates under 100 beats per minute. In patients with AV and ventricular-atrial block, pacing in the VDD mode compared with VVI pacing matched to the atrial rate (without AV synchrony) appears to provide similar cardiac output.[134,135] Multiple studies have shown that the change in work capacity correlates with ventricular rate during exercise whether the ventricular rate is triggered by spontaneous atrial activity or by a pacemaker sensor. Therefore, AV synchrony may be less important in patients during exercise who achieve or require heart rates in excess of 120 beats per minute. Nevertheless, VVIR pacing is not a substitute for DDD pacing.

If a patient has a VVI pacemaker and ventriculoatrial conduction, or a DDD pacing programmed with long AV intervals such that the P wave is closer to the preceding R wave, deleterious hemodynamic consequences may result. In this circumstance, there would be a decrease in cardiac output, since the atrium would consistently pace against closed AV valves, producing increases in the pulmonary and jugular venous pressures. This would also produce symptoms of the pacemaker syndrome. Dual-chamber pacemakers currently available often have options of rate-adaptive AV intervals. This provides the advantage of maintaining normal AV relationships during exercise and prevent retrograde atrial contraction.

RATE-ADAPTIVE SENSORS

Multiple rate adaptive sensors are available or under development.[124–133] Actively based sensors are used most commonly. These are piezoelectric crystal systems that are very sensitive to detection of vibration induced by up-down motion (activity) or acceleration, particularly (forward-backward motion).

The drawback of activity-based pacers is that they do not provide feedback that is proportional to physiologic need. For instance, climbing up stairs requires more work than going down stairs; however, going down stairs is usually faster and would activate the sensor more than climbing up stairs. This leads to faster-paced rates while going down stairs. Similarly, other activity with little body vibrations may produce ineffective rate adaptation from the pacemaker. Therefore, true physiologic sensors are desirable for rate-responsive pacing. The role of physiologic sensors is to provide some measurable index of activity, exercise, or catecholamine state that can provide a more accurate input to the pacemaker for rate-adaptive pacing. The QT interval is affected by heart rate but also independently by catecholamines. Therefore, pacers can measure the interval from the ventricular stimulus to the end of the sensed T wave and modulate heart rate based on this measurement. The drawback of this technique is that the patient has to be ventricular paced in order to measure the QT, or stimulus-T, interval.

Since there exists a close relationship between respiratory rate or minute ventilation and heart rate, various sensors incorporate measurements of respiratory effort. These systems are based on measurement of transthoracic impedance between the pacemaker lead and the pulse generator. The impedance increases with inspirations and decreases with expiration; the amplitude of the impedance change is proportional to the tidal volume. Minute ventilation is the product of the tidal volume and respiratory rate. Thus, minute ventilation can provide an accurate physiologic estimate of metabolic needs. One of the disadvantages of this system is that energy is required to measure impedance, which increases current drain from the pacemaker.

A number of other sensor systems are available or under development. Many use physiologic parameters, such as pH, oxygen saturation, stroke volume, or temperature. The premise behind all of these are that the measured parameters can provide an accurate measure of a patient's metabolic needs, which can be used to guide rate responsiveness. There are various benefits and drawbacks to the different methods.

DUAL SENSORS

Some sensors systems provide the advantage of more physiologic pacing during steady state but have a slow response time during initiation of exercise. Other sensors, particularly activity sensors, have fast response times at initiation of activity but may not produce physiologic responses during peak or steady-state activity. Pacers with dual sensors can provide patients with rapid responses during the start of exercise to augment the heart rate and a more physiologic sensor (QT, minute ventilation) to provide more proportional heart rate response during steady state.[136,137] The benefit of dual sensors has not been conclusively demonstrated in long-term randomized studies, and, in fact, one acute exercise study demonstrated no clinical advantage of dual sensor over single-sensor rate-responsive pacing.[138]

Programming Rate-Adaptive Parameters

The parameters for programming rate responsiveness include the lower and upper activity rates, which may be separate from the upper tracking rate. A treadmill test may be required to optimize pacemaker programming. In practice, it is often sufficient to have the patient walk for a few minutes and program the rate-responsive features to achieve what would be expected to be a physiologic pacing rate for that patient. Different pacers have different algorithms that can automate the adjustments of the rate responsiveness. In most patients, it is difficult to demonstrate clinical effectiveness of automatic rate-response optimization versus fixed rate-responsive programming in the office or clinic.[139]

PACEMAKER COMPLICATIONS

Pacemaker complications can occur at the time of implantation[66,140] or, less likely, can occur late after implantation (Table 31-9). Overall, early complications have been reported in the range of 3 to 11 percent,[1,66,140,141] depending on the definition of complication, duration, and intensity of follow-up.

TABLE 31-9 Complications Related to Pacemakers

Early complications, related to implant	
Pneumothorax	0.5–1.9%
Large hematoma	0.5–1.7%
Cardiac perforation	0.2–1.2%
Lead dislodgment, atrial	1.6–3.8%
Lead dislodgment, ventricular	0.5–1.4%
Venous thrombosis	2–5%
Other complications	
Wound dehiscence	
Infection	
Pain	
High thresholds	
Loose setscrew	
Lead failure	
Pacemaker failure	
Diaphragmatic stimulation	
Skin erosion	
Pacemaker syndrome	

Complications of Pacemaker Implant

Cardiac perforation is a potentially serious and often unrecognized complication of pacemaker lead insertion. This may be recognized at the time of lead insertion by fluoroscopic position of the lead, a paced QRS complex having right bundle branch block pattern, diaphragmatic stimulation, or hypotension resulting from cardiac tamponade. In the absence of anticoagulation, perforation usually does not lead to tamponade if the lead is withdrawn and repositioned. After implantation, cardiac perforation may be recognized by pericardial pain, friction rub, increasing ventricular pacing threshold, diaphragmatic stimulation, or pericardial effusion. The presence of these signs is not diagnostic of cardiac perforation, and echocardiograms should be performed to examine the lead position. If perforation is suspected, and the patient is hemodynamically stable, clinical observation is often the prudent course.

Other implant-related complications include subclavian arterial puncture, pneumothorax, hemothorax, and air embolus. Rarely, a lead may be introduced into the left ventricle through an inadvertent subclavian arterial puncture or through an unrecognized atrial or ventricular septal defect.[142,143]

Complications of venous leads include venous occlusion with resulting superior vena cava syndrome or thrombosis of the subclavian vein with ipsilateral arm edema.[144–147] Acute thrombosis may be treated with heparin and warfarin and managed conservatively if the patient responds to anticoagulation. Invasive and surgical interventions, including venoplasty and stent placement, have been described.[144,147] Most occlusions, partial or complete, may occur over time and tend to be asymptomatic because of the formation of venous collaterals.[148]

Infections related to pacemaker implantation are rare. The use of prophylactic antibiotics and irrigation of the pacemaker pocket with antibiotic solution may help prevent infection, especially from local flora.[149,150] Early infections may be caused by *Staphylococcus aureus* and can be aggressive. Late infections are commonly related to *Staphylococcus epidermidis* and may have a more indolent course. Occasionally, pacemaker infections are misdiagnosed as pacemaker allergy. Other signs of infection include local inflammation and abscess formation, erosion of the pacer, and fever with positive blood culture without an identifiable focus of infection. Transesophageal echocardiography may help determine whether vegetations are present on the pacemaker lead.[151,152] If the pacemaker is infected, removal of the pacemaker leads and generator is usually required.[153]

Mechanical Complications

During implant, the leads are connected to the pulse generator by a setscrew mechanism. If the setscrew is loose (Fig. 31-4), then pacemaker malfunction may occur, manifested by increased impedance and intermittent or complete failure to capture.

The pacemaker leads are subject to long-term complications. The insulation of the leads may break, leading to problems with oversensing (due to electrical noise), undersensing, and failure to capture (due to current leak). This problem often manifests intermittently and may be difficult to detect during a routine pacer check. The patient may complain of pectoral muscle stimulation due to current leak around an insulation break.[154] An abnormally low impedance with demonstrable lead malfunction is diagnostic for insulation break. Subtle insulation breaks may be detected by having the patient perform provocative maneuvers while monitoring an ECG (and marker channels) and or measuring impedances.

Leads may also fracture over time (Fig. 31-2). Early lead fractures lead to increased impedances associated with failure to capture, oversensing, and undersensing. Some leads use retention wires to preform an atrial lead so that it is more likely to attach and remain within the atrial appendage. Fracture of a retention wire does not cause any pacemaker malfunction, but it can lead to serious complications, including cardiac perforation and death, when it penetrates through the insulation into the atrial cavity.[155]

Twiddler's syndrome is a term applied to patients who intentionally or unintentionally manipulate their pulse generator, causing twisting of the entire pacemaker system. This leads to lead dislodgment or fracture. This may also result from an excessively large pacemaker pocket allowing rotation of the pacemaker.

Electromagnetic Interference of Pacemaker Function

In general, electromagnetic interference (EMI) can originate from a variety of sources that have the potential to affect pacemaker function adversely. In Table 31-10 are listed some of the more common sources of EMI with potential pacemaker effects.

Unipolar pacemakers are usually more susceptible to EMI interference than are bipolar pacemakers because the sensing circuit encompasses a larger area compared with bipolar sensing. Factors that affect EMI interference have to do with the source of the interference and the proximity to the pacemaker generator. Many of these sources are located in a hospital environment or specialized places such as construction sites. Magnetic resonance imaging scans are contraindicated in patients with pacemakers, although there are case reports of patients with pacers undergoing MRI scans without adverse events.[156] Sources of EMI at home and the office usually do not pose a problem for patients. There is concern, however, that electronic article surveillance devices, found commonly in retail establishments, can interfere with pacemaker function,[157,158] if patients linger by these devices.

The effects of EMI vary according to its source and the type of pacemaker. Inhibition of pacing output can potentially be life threatening for patients who are pacemaker dependent. If the EMI is interpreted as atrial events by the pacemaker, then inappropriate ventricular pacing may occur in patients with DDD pacemakers, since these pacemakers attempt to *track* these events, which are interpreted as atrial. EMI often causes electrical noise that causes the pacemaker to function in a *noise reversion mode*. The actual function of this mode differs among the different pacemakers, but this mode involves switching to an asynchronous pacing mode. After elimination of this interference, pacers generally revert to the previously programmed mode; however, it is possible for EMI to cause pacemakers to revert to a backup pacing mode. Backup pacing in some models is unipolar VVI pacing at a preset rate.

Occasionally, EMI causes permanent damage to the pulse generator. Therapeutic radiation can damage the complementary metal oxide semiconductors (CMOS) that are part of most modern pacemakers. Generally, doses in excess of 5000 rad, but as little as 1000 rad, may induce pacemaker circuitry damage, which in turn can cause pacemaker failure or even induce a runaway pacemaker. If the pacemaker cannot be shielded from the field of radiation, then consideration should be given to reimplanting the pacemaker at a distant site.

In studies[159,160] examining interactions between pacemakers and cellular telephones, it was noted that digital telephones may cause intermittent pacemaker dysfunction. These adverse effects observed included pacemaker inhibition, inappropriate ventricular tracking (in VDD or DDD pacemakers), or resetting the pacemaker to a backup asynchronous mode. Factors associated with interference include unipolar pacing systems, digital cellular phones, increased output by the cellular phone, and close proximity of the cellular phone to the pacer. Because of the diversity of cellular phones and pacemakers that have different shielding capabilities against electromagnetic interference, it is difficult to draw firm conclusions on the use of digital cellular telephones.[159] No consistent problems have been detected with analog telephones. It is advisable that patients use cellular telephones that are analog or to keep digital cellular (with power outputs greater than 3 W) phones 20 cm away from their pacemaker generator.

TABLE 31-10 Sources of Electromagnetic Interference and Potential Effects

	Possible Pacemaker Response		
Type of Interference	Damage to Pacemaker	Total Inhibition	Rate Increase
Magnetic resonance imaging	Y	N	Y
Cellular phones (digital)	N	Y	Y
Electrocautery	U	Y	Y
Defibrillation (external or internal)	U	N	N
Extracorporeal shock-wave lithotripsy	U	Y	U
Therapeutic radiation	Y	N	N
Radiofrequency ablation	U	Y	U
Electroshock therapy	U	U	U

ABBREVIATIONS: N = no; Y = yes; U = unlikely, but possible.

PACEMAKER MALFUNCTION

Pacemaker malfunction can be categorized as loss of capture, abnormal pacing rate, undersensing, oversensing, or other erratic behavior. The approach to diagnosing pacemaker malfunction is to inspect the ECG carefully, interrogate the pacemaker; check pacing and sensing thresholds, lead impedances, and battery voltage/magnet rate; and perform a chest x-ray. Many instances of pacemaker malfunction actually represent normal function of the pacemaker (Table 31-11). Usually, causes of pacer malfunction may

TABLE 31-11 Suspected Malfunction Occurring During Normal Pacer Function

Observation	Suspected Problem	Possible Normal Pacer Function
Pacing artifacts delivered in the middle of normal QRS complexes	Pacemaker undersensing	Pseudofusion
Unexplained pauses after sensed but not paced complexes	Pacemaker oversensing	Hysteresis
Pacer rate less than lower rate, which occurs at night	Pacemaker oversensing at night	Different sleep rate/lower rate
Rapid pacing rates	Pacemaker oversensing of EMI in atrial channel or other atrial events causing upper rate tracking	Scanning hysteresis/rate drop response causing an increased "intervention" pacing rate for vasovagal episodes
	Pacemaker-mediated tachycardia	Activation of rate-response sensors Upper rate tracking of unsuspected atrial tachyarrhythmia or sinus tachycardia
DDD pacer operating in VVI mode	Malfunction of pacer	Pacer reset due to EMI or low battery Pacer that mode switched due to atrial tachyarrhythmia

ABBREVIATION: EMI = electromagnetic interference.

be diagnosed noninvasively, but, occasionally, surgery is required to diagnose problems.

Abnormal Pacing Rates

Abnormal pacing rates can be due to normal or abnormal pacing function (Table 31-11). Failure of the pacemaker to output is usually due to oversensing. Occasionally, there is pacemaker output that is not visible because of bipolar pacing producing very low amplitude pacing artifacts (artifacts from digital ECG recording are commonly difficult to visualize). Conversely, absence of pacing stimuli may be due to interruption of current flow from a lead fracture, insulation break, or a loose setscrew.

Abnormally fast pacing rates usually are due to normal pacing function. They may be in response to rate-adaptive sensors. In DDD pacemakers, upper rate pacing may be due to sinus tachycardia, atrial tachyarrhythmias, or pacemaker-mediated tachycardia (Table 31-12). In either case, the pacemaker function is normal and is responding either to a rapid atrial rate or to retrograde atrial activity. Rarely, very rapid ventricular pacing ("runaway pacemakers") can cause life-threatening problems requiring disconnection of the pacemaker. Occasionally, abnormal pacing rates can be due to an unstable lead position where the lead is swinging between heart chambers.

Loss of Capture

The loss of pacemaker capture occurs when there is a visible pacing stimulus and no atrial or ventricular depolarization. This may be intermittent or persistent. Most problems occur at the pacemaker lead/tissue interface. For instance, lead dislodgment can cause obvious failure to capture. An increase in the pacing threshold above the pacing output can occur as part of the rise above initial threshold within a few weeks following lead placement (Fig. 31-21) or because of drug therapy, electrolytes, myocardial infarction, or ischemia. Fracture of the lead, insulation breaks, and loose setscrews are mechanical problems that can cause failure to capture. Lastly, battery depletion may cause the pacing output to decline sufficiently such that pacing failure occurs.

Loss of capture requires a check of pacing threshold and of pacing lead impedance and a chest x-ray. For instance, if the problem is an elevated pacing threshold, pacing outputs must be increased. Abnormal lead impedances may confirm a lead failure and the need for lead replacement.

TABLE 31-12 Causes of Upper Rate Behavior in DDD Pacemakers (and Atrioventricular Block)

	ECG Characteristics	Response to Magnet
Sinus tachycardia	1:1 Atrioventricular pacing, pacemaker Wenckebach or 2:1 block depending on the PVARP, upper rate, and sinus rate	No change in paced rhythm after magnet removed
Atrial fibrillation	Irregularly irregular paced ventricular rhythm up to but not exceeding the upper rate	No change in paced rhythm after magnet removed
Pacemaker-mediated tachycardia	Regular paced ventricular rhythm equal to or less than upper rate	Termination of tachycardia

ABBREVIATION: PVARP = postventricular atrial refractory period.

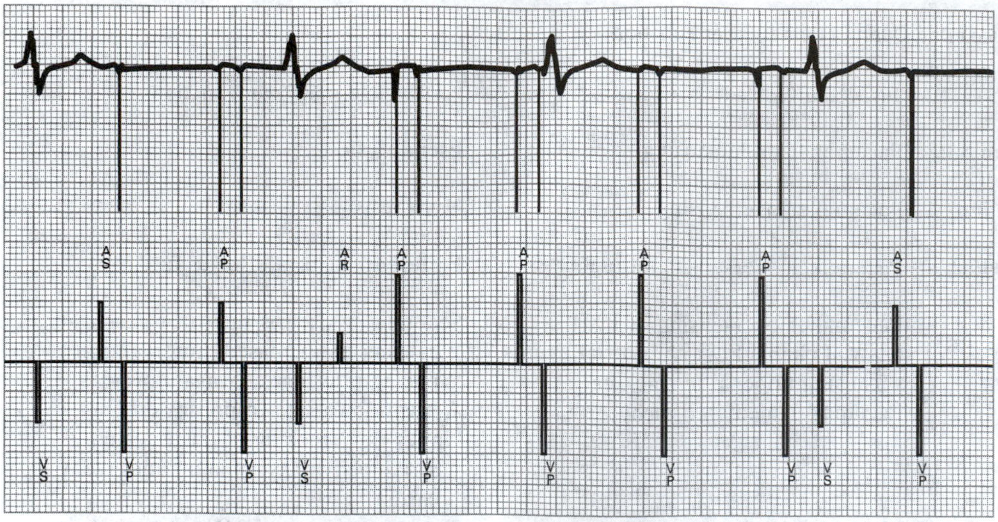

FIGURE 31-21 Electrocardiogram marker channels of a patient with a dual-chamber pacemaker. Note that the atrial pacing outputs (APs) are capturing the atrium, and there is appropriate P-wave sensing (AS or AR). However, none of the ventricular outputs are capturing the ventricle. This is a tracing of a patient who had a pacemaker placed 3 weeks prior to acquisition of this ECG, and the pacing threshold had exceeded the tracing output.

Oversensing

This problem leads to abnormal pacing rates with pacemaker pauses. Generally, unipolar lead systems are more susceptible to oversensing. The sources for oversensing can be intracardiac, extracardiac, or due to EMI. Analysis of ECG, especially with pacemaker interrogation and pacemaker marker channels, may help to determine the cause. If the oversensing is regular, analysis of the pauses may suggest T-wave or P-wave oversensing. T-wave oversensing usually can be eliminated by decreasing the sensitivity (increasing the millivoltage required to sense electrical activity) or increasing the ventricular refractory period.

Oversensing due to lead fracture, insulation break, or other electrode problems will usually be random and erratic (Fig. 31-22). With early lead problems, the malfunction is intermittent and may be exacerbated by certain body positions or motions. In later stages, the combination of oversensing, undersensing, and failure to capture is almost always diagnostic of a lead-related problem. Programming to an asynchronous mode may temporarily control this problem while awaiting a lead replacement, which should be carried out as promptly as possible.

Crosstalk inhibition is a phenomena usually seen in unipolar pacers. It is due to ventricular sensing of atrial output. This is currently a rare problem because of blanking periods and ventricular safety pacing.

Myopotential oversensing is usually a problem in unipolar but not bipolar systems. These skeletal myopotentials generate interference, which tends to correspond to certain activity. The optimal solution is reprogramming the sensitivity to a level high enough to avoid myopotential sensing while preserving adequate safety margin to sense intrinsic cardiac depolarizations.

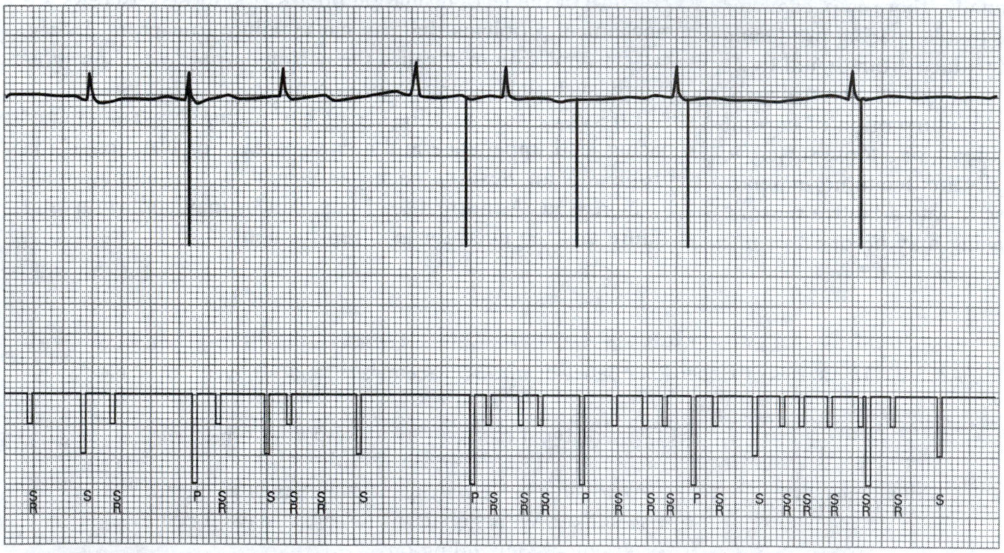

FIGURE 31-22 Electrocardiogram and marker channels are shown for a patient with a ventricular lead impedance break. Note that based on the ECG there is failure to sense, as manifested by the second and fourth pacing outputs coming very shortly after the QRS complex. There is failure to capture, demonstrated by the second and third pacing outputs, which should capture the ventricle. There is also evidence of oversensing, as demonstrated by the long pause between the fourth and fifth pacing outputs during a diastolic period that exceeds the interval between the previous two pacing outputs. In general, when there is evidence of oversensing, undersensing, and failure to capture, then the likely etiology is either a lead insulation break, lead fracture, or other mechanical problem. The marker channels confirm the above ECG findings. There are sensed ventricular events (S or SR) that do not correspond to surface QRS complexes, consistent with oversensing. Additionally, the erratic pattern of sensed ventricular events is consistent with electrical noise. There are also lack-of-sense markers corresponding to QRS complexes; finally, there are ventricular pace markers (P) that fail to capture the ventricle.

Undersensing

An inadequate intracardiac signal can lead to undersensing (Fig. 31-17). The intracardiac electrograms can deteriorate due to inflammation or scar formation at the tissue lead interface. Additionally, certain drugs, electrolyte abnormalities, infarction, ischemia, lead fracture, or insulation breaks can lead to undersensing. Cardioversion or defibrillation can also cause attenuation of intracardiac electrograms. Usually, undersensing is a greater problem in the atrium than in the ventricle. The optimal solution is to program an enhanced sensitivity (decrease sensing level). With bipolar systems, the programmed sensitivity can usually be reduced to 0.18 mV in the atrium, without oversensing of myopotentials or other extraneous signals.

Other etiologies for undersensing occur when intrinsic atrial or ventricular complexes fall within one of the programmed refractory periods. Undersensing can also result from a pacer that was inadvertently programmed to an asynchronous mode (occasionally occurring with battery depletion or pacemaker generator reset).

References

1. Furman S, Hayes DL, Holmes DR. *A Practice of Cardiac Pacing,* 3d ed. Mount Kisco, NY: Futura; 1993.
2. Mitrani RD, Simmons JD, Interian A Jr, et al. Cardiac pacemakers: Current and future status. *Curr Probl Cardiol* 1999; 6: 341–420.
3. Ellenberger KA, Kay GN, Wilkoff BL, eds. *Clinical Cardiac Pacing*. Philadelphia: WB Saunders; 1995.
4. Bernstein AD, Camm AJ, Fletcher R, et al. The NASPE/BPEG generic pacemaker code for antibradyarrhythmia and adaptive rate pacing and antitachyarrhythmia devices. *PACE* 1987; 10:794–799.
5. Zoll PM, Zoll RH, Falk RH, et al. External noninvasive temporary cardiac pacing: Clinical trials. *Circulation* 1985; 71:937–944.
6. McAllister HF, Klementowicz PT, Andrews C, et al. Lyme carditis: An important cause of reversible heart block. *Ann Intern Med* 1989; 110:339.
7. Rubin DA, Sorbera C, Baum S, et al. Acute reversible diffuse conduction system disease due to Lyme disease. *PACE* 1990; 13:1367–1373.
8. Waldo AL, MacLean WA, Karp RB, et al. Continuous rapid atrial pacing to control recurrent or sustained supraventricular tachycardias following open heart surgery. *Circulation* 1976; 54:245–250.
9. Ryan TJ, Anderson JL, Antman EM, et al. ACC/AHA guidelines for the management of patients with acute myocardial infarction. *J Am Coll Cardiol* 1996; 28:1328–1428.
10. Francis GS (lead author) and the ACP/ACC/AHA Task Force on Clinical Privileges in Cardiology. Clinical competence in insertion of a temporary transvenous ventricular pacemaker. *J Am Coll Cardiol* 1994; 23:1254–1257.
11. Hauser RG, Vicari RM. Temporary pacing: Indications, modes and techniques. *Med Clin North Am* 1986; 70:813–827.
12. Trigano JA, Birkui PJ, Mujica J. Noninvasive transcutaneous cardiac pacing: Modern instrumentation and new perspectives. *PACE* 1992; 15:1937.
13. Gregoratos G, Cheitlin MD, Conill A, et al. ACC/AHA guidelines for implantation of cardiac pacemakers and antiarrhythmia devices. *J Am Coll Cardiol* 1998; 31:1175–1209.
14. Scheinman MM, Peters RW, Sauve MJ, et al. Value of HQ interval in patients with bundle branch block and the role of prophylactic permanent pacing. *Am J Cardiol* 1982; 50:1316–1322.
15. Dhingra RC, Wyndham C, Bauernfeind R, et al. Significance of block distal to the His-bundle induced by atrial pacing in patients with chronic bifascicular block. *Circulation* 1979; 60:1455–1464.
16. Dhingra RC, Denes P, Wu D, et al. The significance of second degree AV block and bundle branch block. *Circulation* 1974; 49:638–646.
17. Zipes D. Second degree AV block. *Circulation* 1979; 60:465–472.
18. Strasberg B, Amat-Y-Leon F, Dhingra RC, et al. Natural history of chronic second-degree AV block. *Circulation* 1981; 63:1043–1049.
19. Connelly DT, Steinhaus DM. Mobitz type I atrioventricular block: An indication for permanent pacing? *PACE* 1996; 19: 261–264.
20. Shaw DB, Kekwick CA, Veale D, et al. Survival in second degree AV block. *Br Heart J* 1985; 53:587–593.
21. Clarke M, Sutton R, Ward D, et al. Recommendations for pacemaker prescription for symptomatic bradycardia: Report of a working party of the British Pacing and Electrophysiology Group. *Br Heart J* 1991; 66:185–191.
22. Mymin D, Mathewson FA, Tate RB, Manfreda J. The natural history of primary first degree AV heart block. *N Engl J Med* 1986; 315:1183–1187.
23. Barold SS. Indications for permanent cardiac pacing in first-degree AV block: Class I, II, or III? *PACE* 1996; 19:747–751.
24. Brecker SJD, Xiao HB, Sparrow J, Gibson DG. Effects of dual chamber pacing with short atrioventricular delay in dilated cardiomyopathy. *Lancet* 1992; 340:1308–1312.
25. Nishimura RA, Hayes DL, Holmes DR, Tajik AJ. Mechanism of hemodynamic improvement by dual-chamber pacing for severe left ventricular dysfunction: An acute Doppler and catheterization hemodynamic study. *J Am Coll Cardiol* 1995; 25:281–288.
26. Hiromasa S, Ikeda T, Kubota K, et al. Myotonic dystrophy: Ambulatory electrocardiogram, electrophysiologic study, and echocardiographic evaluation. *Am Heart J* 1987; 113:1482–1488.
27. Stevenson WG, Perloff JK, Weiss JN, Anderson TL. Facioscapulohumeral muscular dystrophy: Evidence for selective, genetic electrophysiologic cardiac involvement. *J Am Coll Cardiol* 1990; 15:292–299.
28. Charles R, Holt S, Ka JM, et al. Myocardial ultrastructure and the development of AV block in Kearns-Sayre syndrome. *Circulation* 1981; 63:214–219.
29. Dewey RC, Capeless MA, Levy AM. Use of ambulatory electrocardiographic monitoring to identify high risk patients with congenital complete heart block. *N Engl J Med* 1987; 316:835.
30. Reybrouck T, Van den Eynde BB, Cumoulin M, Van der Hauwaert LG. Cardiorespiratory response to exercise in congenital complete AV block. *Am J Cardiol* 1989; 64:896.
31. Michaelsson M, Jonzon A, Riesenfeld T. Isolated congenital complete atrioventricular block in adult life: A prospective study. *Circulation* 1995; 92:442–449.
32. Michaelsson M, Riesenfeld T, Jonzon A. Natural history of congenital complete atrioventricular block. *PACE* 1997; 20:2098–2101.
33. Alboni P, Menozzi C, Brignole M, et al. Effects of permanent pacemaker and oral theophylline in sick sinus syndrome: The THEOPACE study—A randomized controlled trial. *Circulation* 1997; 9:260–266.
34. Stegman SS, Burroughs JM, Henthorn RW. Asymptomatic bradyarrhythmias as a marker for sleep apnea: Appropriate recognition and treatment may reduce the need for pacemaker therapy. *PACE* 1996; 19:899–904.
35. Sugrue DD, Gersh BJ, Holmes DR, et al. Symptomatic "isolated" carotid sinus hypersensitivity: Natural history and results of treatment with anticholinergic drugs or pacemaker. *J Am Coll Cardiol* 1986; 7:158–162.
36. Brignole M, Sartore B, Barra M, et al. Ventricular and dual-chamber pacing for treatment of carotid sinus syndrome. *PACE* 1989; 12:582–590.
37. Brignole M, Menozzi C, Lolli G, et al. Pacing for carotid sinus syndrome and sick sinus syndrome. *PACE* 1990; 13:2071–2075.
38. Brignole M, Menozzi C, Lolli G, et al. Validation of a method for choice of pacing mode in carotid sinus syndrome with or without sinus bradycardia. *PACE* 1991; 14:196–203.
39. El-Bedawi KM, Wahbha MMAE, Hainsworth R. Cardiac pacing

does not improve orthostatic tolerance in patients with vasovagal syncope. *Clin Autonom Res* 1994; 4:233–237.
40. Maloney JD, Jaeger FJ, Rizo-Patron C, Zhu DW. The role of pacing for the management of neurally mediated syncope: Carotid sinus syndrome and vasovagal syncope. *Am Heart J* 1994; 127:1030–1037.
41. Sra JS, Jazayeri MR, Avitall B, et al. Comparison of cardiac pacing with drug therapy in the treatment of neurocardiogenic (vasovagal) syncope with bradycardia or asystole. *N Engl J Med* 1993; 328:1085–1090.
42. Connolly SJ, Sheldon R, Roberts RS, Bent M, on behalf of the Vasovagal Pacemaker Study Investigators. The North American Vasovagal Pacemaker Study: A randomized trial of permanent cardiac pacing for the prevention of vasovagal syncope. *J Am Coll Cardiol* 1999; 33:16–20.
43. Shah CP, Thakur RK, Xie B, Pathak P. Dual chamber pacing for neurally mediated syncope with a prominent cardioinhibitory component. *PACE* 1999; 22:999–1003.
44. Fananapazir L, Cannon RO, Tripodi D, Panza JA. Impact of dual-chamber permanent pacing in patients with obstructive hypertrophic cardiomyopathy with symptoms refractory to verapamil and beta-adrenergic blocker therapy. *Circulation* 1992; 85:2149–2161.
45. Jeanrenaud X, Goy JJ, Kappenberger L. Effects of dual-chamber pacing in hypertrophic obstructive cardiomyopathy. *Lancet* 1992; 339:1318–1323.
46. Nishimura RA, Hayes DL, Ilstrup DM, et al. Effect of dual-chamber pacing on systolic and diastolic function in patients with hypertrophic cardiomyopathy: Acute Doppler echocardiographic and catheterization hemodynamic study. *J Am Coll Cardiol* 1996; 27:421–430.
47. Fananapazir L, Epstein ND, Curiel RV, et al. Long term results of dual-chamber (DDD) pacing in obstructive hypertrophic cardiomyopathy: Evidence for progressive symptomatic and hemodynamic improvement and reduction of left ventricular hypertrophy. *Circulation* 1994; 90:2731–2742.
48. Nishimura RA, Trusty JM, Hayes DL, et al. Dual-chamber pacing for hypertrophic obstructive cardiomyopathy: A randomized, double blind crossover trial. *J Am Coll Cardiol* 1997; 29:435–441.
49. Maron BJ, Nishimura RA, McKenna WJ, et al. Assessment of permanent dual-chamber pacing as a treatment for drug refractory symptomatic patients with obstructive hypertrophic cardiomyopathy: A randomized, double-blind, crossover study (M-PATHY). *Circulation* 1999; 99:2927–2933.
50. Ommen SR, Nishimura RA, Squires RW, et al. Comparison of dual-chamber pacing versus septal myectomy for the treatment of patients with hypertrophic obstructive cardiomyopathy. *J Am Coll Cardiol* 1999; 34:191–196.
51. Kass DA, Chen CH, Talbot MW, et al. Ventricular pacing with premature excitation for treatment of hypertensive-cardiac hypertrophy with cavity obliteration. *Circulation* 1999; 100:807–812.
52. Cannon RO, Tripodi D, Dilsizian V, et al. Results of permanent dual-chamber pacing in symptomatic nonobstructive hypertrophic cardiomyopathy. *Am J Cardiol* 1994; 73:571–576.
53. Gold MR, Feliciano Z, Gottlieb SS, Fisher ML. Dual-chamber pacing with a short atrioventricular delay in congestive heart failure: A randomized study. *J Am Coll Cardiol* 1995; 26:967–973.
54. Shinbane JS, Chu E, DeMarco T, et al. Evaluation of acute dual-chamber pacing with a range of atrioventricular delays on cardiac performance in refractory heart failure. *J Am Coll Cardiol* 1997; 30:1295–1300.
54a. Deshmulch P, Casavant DA, Romanyshyn M, Anderson K. Permanent, direct His-bundle pacing. A novel approach to cardiac pacing in patients with normal His-Purkinje activation. *Circulation* 2000; 101:869–877.
55. Buckingham TA, Candinas R, Schläpfer J, et al. Acute hemodynamic effects of atrioventricular pacing at differing sites in the right ventricle individually and simultaneously. *PACE* 1997; 20:909–915.
56. DeCock CC, Meyer A, Kamp O, Visser CA. Hemodynamic benefits of right ventricular outflow tract pacing: Comparison with right ventricular apex pacing. *PACE* 1998; 21:536–541.
57. Blanc JJ, Etienne Y, Gilard M, et al. Evaluation of different ventricular pacing sites in patients with severe heart failure: Results of an acute hemodynamic study. *Circulation* 1997; 96:3273–3277.
58. Leclercq C, Cazeau S, Le Breton H, et al. Acute hemodynamic effects of biventricular DDD pacing in patients with end-stage heart failure. *J Am Coll Cardiol* 1998; 32:1825–1831.
59. Victor F, Leclerq C, Mabo P, et al. Optimal right ventricular pacing site in chronically implanted patients. *J Am Coll Cardiol* 1999; 33:311–316.
60. Auricchio A, Stellbrink C, Block M, et al. Effect of pacing chamber and atrioventricular delay on acute systolic function of paced patients with congestive heart failure. *Circulation* 1999; 99:2993–3001.
61. Stamato NJ, O'Toole MF, Enger EL. Permanent pacemaker implantation in the cardiac catheterization laboratory versus the operating room: An analysis of hospital charges and complications. *PACE* 1992; 15:2236–2239.
62. Yamamura KH, Kloostrman EM, Alba J, et al. Analysis of charges and complications of permanent pacemaker implantation in the cardiac catheterization laboratory versus operating room. *PACE* 1999; 22:1820–1824.
63. Smyth NPD. Pacemaker implantation: Surgical techniques. *Cardiovasc Clin* 1983; 14:31–44.
64. Higano ST, Hayes DL, Spittell PC. Facilitation of the subclavian-introducer technique with contrast venography. *PACE* 1990; 13:681–684.
65. Parsonnet V, Roelke M. The cephalic vein cutdown versus subclavian puncture for pacemaker/ICD lead implantation. *PACE* 1999; 22:695–697.
66. Smith HJ, Fearnot NE, Byrd CL, et al. Five-years experience with intravascular lead extraction. *PACE* 1994; 17:2016–2020.
67. Wilkoff BL, Byrd CL, Love CJ, et al. Pacemaker lead extraction with the laser sheath: Results of the pacing lead extraction with the excimer sheath (PLEXES) trial. *J Am Coll Cardiol* 1999; 33:1671–1676.
68. Epstein LM, Byrd CL, Wilkoff BL, et al. Initial experience with larger laser sheaths for the removal of transvenous pacemaker and implantable defibrillator leads. *Circulation* 1999; 100: 516–525.
69. Moller M, Arnsbo P. Appraisal of pacing lead performance from the Danish pacemaker register. *PACE* 1996; 19:1327–1336.
70. Gumbrielle TP, Bourke JP, Sinkovic M, et al. Long-term thresholds of nonsteroidal permanent pacing leads: A 5-year study. *PACE* 1996; 19:829–835.
71. Bernstein AD, Irwin ME, Parsonnet V, et al. Report of the NASPE Policy conference on antibradycardia pacemaker follow-up: Effectiveness, needs and resources. *PACE* 1994; 17(pt 1):1714–1729.
72. Sweesy W, Erickson SL, Crago JA, et al. Analysis of the effectiveness of in office and transtelephonic follow-up in terms of pacemaker system complications. *PACE* 1994; 17:2001.
73. Ellenbogen KA, Wood MA, Gilligan DM, et al. Steroid eluting high impedance pacing leads decrease short and long-term current drain: Results from a multicenter clinical trial—CapSure Z investigators. *PACE* 1999; 22:39–48.
74. Mond HG, Stokes KB. The steroid eluting electrode: A 10-year experience. *PACE* 1996; 19:1016–1020.
75. Clarke M, Liu B, Schuller H, et al. Automatic adjustment of pacemaker stimulation output correlated with continuously monitored capture thresholds: A multicenter study. *PACE* 1998; 21:1567–1575.
76. Ricci R, Puglisi A, Azzolini P, et al. Reliability of a new algorithm

for automatic mode switching from DDDR to DDIR pacing in sinus node disease patients with chronotropic incompetence and recurrent paroxysmal atrial fibrillation. *PACE* 1996; 19(pt 2): 1719–1723.

77. Mitrani RD, Pollack W, Interian A, et al. Pacemaker diagnostic information can be used to follow episodes of atrial tachyarrhythmia in patients. *Arch Mal Coeur* 1998; spec 3:209.
78. Brandt J, Anderson H, Fahraens T, Schuller H. Natural history of sinus node disease treated with atrial pacing in 213 patients: Implications for selection of stimulation mode. *J Am Coll Cardiol* 1992; 20:633.
79. Andersen HR, Nielsen JC, Thomsen PEB, et al. Atrioventricular conduction during long-term follow-up of patients with sick sinus syndrome. *Circulation* 1998; 98:1315–1321.
80. Crick JCP. European multicenter prospective follow-up study of 1002 implants of a single lead VDD pacing system. *PACE* 1991; 14:1724–1744.
81. Naegeli B, Osswald S, Pfisterer M, Burkart F. VDDR pacing: Short- and long-term stability of atrial sensing with a single lead system. *PACE* 1996; 19(pt 1):455–464.
82. Wiegand UKH, Bode F, Schneider R, et al. Atrial sensing and AV synchrony in single lead VDD pacemakers: A prospective comparison to DDD devices with bipolar atrial leads. *J Cardiovasc Electrophysiol* 1999; 10:513–520.
83. Oldroyd KG, Rae A, Carter R, et al. Double blind crossover comparison of the effects of dual chamber pacing (DDD) and ventricular adaptive (VV1R) pacing on neuroendocrine variables, exercise performance and symptoms in complete heart block. *Br Heart J* 1991; 65:188–193.
84. Karlof I. Hemodynamic effect of atrial triggered versus fixed rate pacing at rest and during exercise in complete heart block. *Acta Med Scand* 1975; 197:195–206.
85. Alpert MA, Curtis JJ, Sanfelippo W, et al. Comparative survival following permanent ventricular and dual chamber pacing for patients with chronic symptomatic sinus node dysfunction with and without congestive heart failure. *Am Heart J* 1987; 13: 958–965.
86. Lukl J, Doupal V, Heinc P. Quality-of-life during DDD and dual sensor VV1R pacing. *PACE* 1994; 17:1844.
87. Lau CP, Tai YT, Lee PWE, et al. Quality-of-life in DDR pacing: AV synchrony or rate adaptation? *PACE* 1994; 17:1838.
88. Rosenqvist NI, Brandi J, Schuller H. Atrial versus ventricular pacing in sinus node disease: A treatment comparison study. *Am Heart J* 1986; 111:292–297.
89. Feuer N, Shandling AH, Messenger JC, et al. Influence of cardiac pacing mode on the long-term development of atrial fibrillation. *Am J Cardiol* 1989; 64:1376–1379.
90. Hesselson AB, Parsormet V, Bernstein AD, Bonavita GJ. Deleterious effects of long-term single-chamber ventricular pacing in patients with sick sinus syndrome: The hidden benefits of dual-chamber pacing. *J Am Coll Cardiol* 1992; 19:1542–1549.
91. Jahangir A, Shen WK, Neubauer SA, et al. Relation between mode of pacing and long-term survival in the very elderly. *J Am Coll Cardiol* 1999; 33:1208–1216.
92. Andersen HR, Thuesen L, Bagger JP, et al. Prospective randomised trial of atrial versus ventricular pacing in sick-sinus syndrome. *Lancet* 1994; 344:1523–1528.
93. Andersen HR, Nielsen JC, Thomsen PEB, et al. Long-term follow up of patients from a randomised trial of atrial versus ventricular pacing for sick-sinus syndrome. *Lancet* 1997; 350:1210–1216.
94. Lamas GA, Orav EJ, Stambler BS, et al. Quality of life and clinical outcomes in elderly patients treated with ventricular pacing as compared with dual-chamber pacing. *N Engl J Med* 1998; 338:1097–1104.
95. Sasaki Y, Furihata A, Suyama K, et al. Comparison between ventricular inhibited pacing and physiologic pacing in sick sinus syndrome. *Am J Cardiol* 1991; 67:771–774.
96. Sgarbossa EB, Pinski SL, Maloney JD, et al. The role of pacing modalities in long-term survival in the sick sinus syndrome. *Ann Intern Med* 1993; 119:359–365.
97. Sgarbossa EB, Pinski SL, Maloney JD, et al. Chronic atrial fibrillation and stroke in paced patients with sick sinus syndrome: Relevence of clinical characteristics and pacing modalities. *Circulation* 1993; 88:1045–1053.
98. Linde-Edelstam C, Gullberg B, Nordlander R, et al. Longevity in patients with high degree AV block paced in the atrial synchronous or the fixed rate ventricular inhibited mode. *PACE* 1992; 14:304–313.
99. Taylor JA, Morillo CA, Eckberg DL, Ellenbogen KA. Higher sympathetic nerve activity during ventricular (VVI) than during dual-chamber (DDD) pacing. *J Am Coll Cardiol* 1996; 28:1753–1758.
100. Alpert MA, Curtiss JJ, Sanfellippo JF, et al. Comparative survival after permanent ventricular and dual-chamber pacing for patients with chronic high degree AV block with and without preexistent congestive heart failure. *J Am Coll Cardiol* 1986; 7:925–932.
101. Higano ST, Hayes DL, Eisinger G. Sensor driven rate smoothing in a DDDR pacemaker. *PACE* 1989; 12:922–929.
102. Kamalvand K, Kotsakis TK, Bucknall C, Sulke N. Is mode switching beneficial? A randomized study in patients with paroxysmal atrial tachyarrhythmias. *J Am Coll Cardiol* 1997; 30:496–504.
103. Brignole M, Gianfranchi L, Menozzi C, et al. Assessment of atrioventricular junction ablation and DDDR mode-switching pacemaker versus pharmacological treatment in patients with severely symptomatic paroxysmal atrial fibrillation: A randomized controlled study. *Circulation* 1997; 96:2617–2624.
104. Marshall HJ, Harris ZI, Griffith MJ, et al. Prospective randomized study of ablation and pacing versus medical therapy for paroxysmal atrial fibrillation: Effects of pacing mode and mode-switch algorithm. *Circulation* 1999; 99:1587–1592.
105. Stabile G, Senatore G, DeSimone A, et al. Determinants of efficacy of atrial pacing in preventing atrial fibrillation recurrences. *J Cardiovasc Electrophysiol* 1999; 10:2–9.
106. Saksena S, Praiash A, Hill M, et al. Prevention of recurrent atrial fibrillation with chronic dual-site right atrial pacing. *J Am Coll Cardiol* 1996; 28:687–694.
107. Delfaut P, Saksena S, Prakash A, Krol RB. Long-term outcome of patients with drug-refractory atrial flutter and fibrillation after single- and dual-site right atrial pacing for arrhythmia prevention. *J Am Coll Cardiol* 1998; 32:1900–1908.
108. Gillis AM, Wyse G, Connolly SJ, et al. Atrial pacing periablation for prevention of paroxysmal atrial fibrillation. *Circulation* 1999; 99:2553–2558.
109. Melton IC, Gilligan DM, Wood MA, Ellenbogen KA. Optimal cardiac pacing after heart transplantation. *PACE* 1999; 22:1510–1527.
110. Weinfeld MS, Kartashov A, Piana R, et al. Bradycardia: A late complication following cardiac transplantation. *Am J Cardiol* 1996; 78:969–971.
111. Woodard DA, Conti JB, Mills RM Jr, et al. Permanent atrial pacing in cardiac transplant patients. *PACE* 1997; 20(pt 1):2398–2404.
112. Janosik DL, Pearson AC, Buckingham TA, et al. The hemodynamic benefit of differential atrioventricular delay intervals for sensed and paced atrial events during physiologic pacing. *J Am Coll Cardiol* 1989; 14:499–507.
113. Pearson AC, Janosik DL, Redd RR, et al. Doppler echocardiographic assessment of the effect of varying atrioventricular delay and pacemaker mode on left ventricular filling. *Am Heart J* 1988; 115:611–621.
114. Frielingsdor J, Deseo T, Gerber AE, Bertel O. A comparison of quality-of-life in patients with dual-chamber pacemakers and individually programmed atrioventricular delays. *PACE* 1996; 19:1147–1154.
115. Furman S. Pacemaker syndrome. *PACE* 1994; 17:14.
116. Schuller N, Brandt J. The pacemaker syndrome: Old and new causes. *Clin Cardiol* 1991; 14:336–340.

117. Travill CM, Sutton R. Pacemaker syndrome: An iatrogenic condition. *Br Heart J* 1992; 68:163.
118. Clemo HF, Buamgarten CM, Stambler BS, et al. Atrial natriuretic factor: Implications of cardiac pacing and electrophysiology. *PACE* 1994; 17:70.
119. Noll B, Irrappe J, Goke B, et al. Influence of pacing mode and rate on peripheral levels of atrial natriutetic peptide (ANP). *PACE* 1989; 12:1763–1769.
120. Grant SCD, Bennet DH. Atrial latency in a dual chamber pacing system causing inappropriate sequence of cardiac chamber activation. *PACE* 1992; 15:116.
121. Daubert C, Mabo P, Berder V, et al. Atrial tachyarrhythmias associated with high degree interatrial conduction block: Prevention by permanent atrial resynchronisation. *Eur J Pacing Electrophysiol* 1994; 3:35.
122. Sulke N, Drisas A, Bostock J, et al. "Subclinical" pacemaker syndrome: A randomized study of symptom free patients with ventricular demand (VV1) pacemakers upgraded to dual-chamber devices. *Br Heart J* 1992; 67:57.
123. Sulke N, Chambers J, Dritsas A, Sowton E. A randomized double-blind crossover comparison of four rate-responsive pacing models. *J Am Coll Cardiol* 1991; 17:696.
124. Bloomfield P, Macareavey D, Kerr F, et al. Long-term follow-up of patients with the QT rate adaptive pacemaker. *PACE* 1989; 12:1114.
125. Alt E, Hirgstetter C, Heinz M, et al. Rate control of physiologic pacemakers by central venous blood temparature. *Circulation* 1986; 73:1206–1212.
126. Benditt DG, Mianulli M, Fetter J, et al. Single chamber cardiac pacing with activity initiated chronotropic response: Evaluation by cardiopulmonary exercise testing. *Circulation* 1987; 75: 184–189.
127. Benditt DG, Milstein S, Buetikofer J, et al. Sensor-triggered, rate variable cardiac pacing: Current technologies and clinical implications. *Ann Intern Med* 1987; 107:714–724.
128. Bennett T, Sharma A, Sutton R. Development of a rate adaptive pacemaker based on the maximum rate-of-rise of right ventricular pressure (RV dP/dt max). *PACE* 1992; 15:219–234.
129. Lau DP, Antoniou A, Ward DE, et al. Initial clinical experience with a minute ventilation sensing rate modulated pacemaker: Improvements in exercise capacity and symptomatology. *PACE* 1988; 11:1815–1822.
130. Lau CO, Tai Y, Fong P. Clinical experience with an activity sensing DDDR pacemaker using an accelerometer sensor. *PACE* 1992; 15:334–343.
131. Ruiter J, Heemels J, Kee D, et al. Adaptive rate pacing controlled by the right ventricular preejection interval: Clinical experience with a physiological pacing system. *PACE* 1992; 15:886–894.
132. Windecker S, Bubien RS, Halperin L, et al. Two-year experience with rate-modulated pacing controlled by mixed venous oxygen. *PACE* 1998; 21:1396–1404.
133. Cl'ementy J. Dual chamber rate responsive pacing system driven by contractility: Final assessment after 1 year follow-up—The European PEA Clinical Investigation Group. *PACE* 1998; 21:2192–2197.
134. Wirtzfeld A, Schmidt G, Himmeier FC, et al. Physiological pacing: Present status and future developments. *PACE* 1987; 12:749–751.
135. Nordlander R, Hedman A, Pehrsson SK. Rate responsive pacing and exercise capacity: A comment. *PACE* 1989; 12:749–751.
136. Celiker A, Alehan D, Tokel NK, et al. Experience with dual-sensor rate-responsive pacemakers in children. *Eur Heart J* 1996; 17:1251–1255.
137. Leung SK, Lau CP, Tng MO. Cardiac output is a sensitive indicator of difference in exercise performance between single and dual sensor pacemakers. *PACE* 1998; 21:35–41.
138. Sulke N, Tan K, Kamalvand K, et al. Dual sensor VVIR mode pacing: Is it worth it? *PACE* 1996; 19:1560–1567.
139. Schubert A, Van Langen H, Michels K, Meinertz T. A prospective randomized comparison between fixed rate response programming and automatic rate response optimization in activity-triggered DDDR pacemakers: Thera Pacemaker Study. *Cardiology* 1998; 89:25–28.
140. Kiviniemi MS, Pirnes MA, Eranen JK, et al. Complications related to permanent pacemaker therapy. *PACE* 1999; 22:711–720.
141. Chauhan A, Grace AA, Newell SA, et al. Early complications after dual chamber versus single chamber pacemaker implantation. *PACE* 1994; 17:2012–2015.
142. Mazzetti H, Cussaut A, Tentori C, et al. Transarterial permanent pacing of the left ventricle. *PACE* 1990; 13:588–592.
143. Winner SJ, Boon NA. Transvenous pacemaker electrodes placed unintentionally in the left ventricle: Three cases. *Postgrad Med J* 1989; 65:98–102.
144. Spittell PC, Vlietstra RE, Hayes DL, et al. Venous obstruction due to permanent transvenous pacemaker electrodes: Treatment with percutaneous transluminal balloon venoplasty. *PACE* 1990; 13:2714.
145. Spittell PC, Hayes DL. Venous complications after insertion of a transvenous pacemaker. *Mayo Clin Proc* 1992; 67:258–265.
146. Mazzetti H, Dussaut A, Tentori C, et al. Superior vena cava occlusion and/or syndrome related to pacemaker leads. *Am Heart J* 1993; 125:831.
147. Lindsay HS, Chennells PM, Perrins EJ. Successful treatment by balloon venoplasty and stent insertion of obstruction of the superior vena cava by an endocardial pacemaker lead. *Br Heart J* 1994; 71:363–365.
148. Kataoka H. Ten-year follow-up of a patient with pacemaker induced superior vena cava syndrome. *PACE* 1997; 20:1734–1735.
149. Da Costa A, Kirkorian G, Cucherat M, et al. Antibiotic prophylaxis for permanent pacemaker implantation: A meta-analysis. *Circulation* 1998; 97:1796–1801.
150. Da Costa A, Lelievre H, Kirkorian G, et al. Role of the preaxillary flora in pacemaker infections: A prospective study. *Circulation* 1998; 97:1791–1795.
151. Vilacosta I, Zamorano J, Camino A, et al. Infected transvenous permanent pacemakers: Role of transesophageal echocardiography. *Am Heart J* 1993; 125:904–906.
152. Vilacosta I, Sarria C, San Roman JA, et al. Usefulness of transesophageal echocardiography for diagnosis of infected tranvenous permanent pacemakers. *Circulation* 1994; 89:2684–2687.
153. Smith HJ, Fernot NE, Byrd CL, et al. Five-years experience with intravascular lead extraction. *PACE* 1994; 17:2016.
154. Chauvin M, Brecheumacher C. Muscle stimulation caused by a pacemaker current leakage: The role of the insulation failure of a polyurethane coating. *J Electrophysiol* 1987; 1:326–329.
155. Parsonnet V, Roelke M, Bernstein AD. Reduced frequency of retention wire fractures suggests that elective explantation of affected atrial leads is no longer indicated. *PACE* 2000; 23:380–383.
156. Gimbel JR, Johnson D, Levine PA, Wilkoff BL. Safe performance of magnetic resonance imaging on five patients with permanent cardiac pacemakers. *PACE* 1996; 19:913–919.
157. Food and Drug Administration: Important information on anti-theft and metal detector systems and pacemakers, ICDs, and spinal cord stimulators. *DHHS* September 28, 1998.
158. McIvor ME, Redding J, Floden E, Sheppard RC. Study of pacemaker and ICD triggering by electronic article surveillance devices (SPICED-TEAS). *PACE* 1998; 21:1847–1861.
159. Naegeli B, Osswald S, Deola Ni Burkart F. Intermittent pacemaker dysfunction caused by digital mobile telephones. *J Am Coll Cardiol* 1996; 27:1471–1477.
160. Hayes DL, Wang PJ, Reynolds DW, et al. Interference with cardiac pacemakers by cellular telephones. *N Engl J Med* 1997; 336:1473–1479.

PART FIVE

SYNCOPE, SUDDEN DEATH, AND CARDIOPULMONARY RESUSCITATION

C H A P T E R 32

DIAGNOSIS AND MANAGEMENT OF SYNCOPE

Harisios Boudoulas / Steven D. Nelson / Stephen F. Schaal / Richard P. Lewis

Syncope is a sudden and transient loss of consciousness. The occurrence of syncope in the general population, as reflected in the 26-year surveillance of the Framingham Study, is 3.0 percent in men and 3.5 percent in women in the general population. As a general rule, the incidence of syncope increases with age.[1]

As an initial presentation, syncope denotes a diversity of disorders ranging from a benign episode to sudden death. Studies in recent years have documented the multiple causes and the widely divergent mortality risks associated with an episode of syncope. On the basis of these studies, patients with a transient episode of altered consciousness (presyncope) and those with complete loss of consciousness (syncope) can be classified into three broad categories[2] (Table 32-1): *cardiac syncope, noncardiac syncope,* and *syncope of undetermined cause.* The relative incidence of these categories varies with the clinical site from which the patients are selected. In the emergency room, noncardiac syncope is most common. For patients admitted to the hospital, cardiac syncope is the most common diagnosis.[3]

Clearly, the highest mortality occurs among those with cardiac syncope. Among all patients with syncope associated with cardiac disease, sudden death is extremely high.

NONCARDIAC SYNCOPE (Table 32-2)

Sudden transient loss or impairment of consciousness occurs under a wide variety of circumstances. The pathophysiologic mechanisms, diagnostic features, and therapy for these disorders are discussed below.

Neurocardiogenic Syncope

The syndrome of neurocardiogenic syncope, the common faint (also referred to as neurally mediated hypotension, vasovagal syncope, and vasodepressor syncope), is one of the most common causes of syncope. This disorder is considered to be an abnormality in the complex neurocardiovascular interactions responsible for maintaining systemic and cerebral perfusion (Fig. 32-1).[4–10]

PATHOPHYSIOLOGY

The pathophysiology of neurocardiogenic syncope is quite complex and incompletely understood. Under normal circumstances, upright posture causes venous pooling and a transient decrease in arterial pressure, resulting in an unloading of baroreceptors. Reflex augmentation of sympathetic activity and parasympathetic withdrawal result in peripheral arterial vasoconstriction, venoconstriction, and an increase in heart rate and contractility. These adaptive mechanisms serve to maintain normal systemic and cerebral perfusion. Neuroendocrine systems (e.g., renin-angiotensin and vasopressin) may be important modulators of homeostasis during prolonged periods of orthostatic stress.[11]

Individuals susceptible to neurocardiogenic syncope are unable to maintain the adaptive neurocardiovascular responses to upright posture for prolonged periods. These patients tend to have a modest reduction in central blood volume, which is aggravated by upright posture. Increases in circulating catecholamines and cardiac adrenergic tone in response to orthostatic stress result in increased myocardial contractility.[12] Studies in animal models suggest that, under these conditions, cardiopulmonary mechanoreceptors are activated, resulting in increased neural traffic across afferent C fibers leading to the central nervous system vasomotor center; this in turn results in reflex paradoxical vasodilation (vasodepressor response) and bradycardia (cardioinhibitory response).[13] The final result is hypotension, cerebral hypoperfusion, cerebral hypoxia, and syncope. This paradoxical reflex is believed to be a variant of the Bezold-Jarisch reflex and has also been documented during nitrate therapy for acute myocardial ischemia, and during acute hemor-

TABLE 32-1 Classification of Syncope

I. Noncardiac	III. Undetermined cause
II. Cardiac	

rhagic syndromes.[14,15] In addition, vasomotor center activation is believed to cause several of the prodromal symptoms of diaphoresis, nausea, vomiting, and dyspnea that frequently accompany neurocardiogenic syncope. Recent evidence from patients with denervated hearts (i.e., cardiac transplantation patients) and those with neurocardiogenic syncope raises the possibility that other neurohumoral mechanisms, primarily involving the peripheral circulation, may play an important role.[16]

The mechanism of paradoxical vasodilation observed during neurocardiogenic syncope is incompletely understood. Clinical studies have shown that serum epinephrine concentrations surge prior to the syncopal event with resultant intense β_2 activation, which may cause inappropriate vasodilation and syncope. Withdrawal of peripheral sympathetic neural activity at the time of neurocardiogenic syncope has also been demonstrated by direct recordings of sympathetic neural activity.[17]

The paradoxical bradycardia (cardioinhibitory response) during neurocardiogenic syncope is due to a surge in cardiac parasympathetic tone and usually lags vasodilation by several seconds.[18] The cardioinhibitory response is highly variable, ranging from a relative bradycardia with heart rates in the 40 to 60 beats per minute range to profound periods of asystole. Variable degrees of atrioventricular (AV) block and junctional escape rhythms are observed as well. *Bradycardia aggravates but is not the principal cause of hypotension during neurocardiogenic syncope.* Maintaining heart rate with atropine or cardiac pacing will often reduce, but not prevent, symptomatic hypotension

TABLE 32-2 Classification of Noncardiac Syncope

Neurocardiogenic
Orthostatic
Cerebrovascular
Seizure disorders
Carotid sinus hypersensitivity
Situational
Cough
Swallowing
Valsalva
Micturition
Defecation
Diver's
Postprandial
Metabolic, drugs
Hypoxia
Hypoglycemia
Hyperventilation, panic attacks
Ethanol, other drugs
Other forms of syncope or conditions mimicking syncope
Vertigo
Migraine
Psychiatric

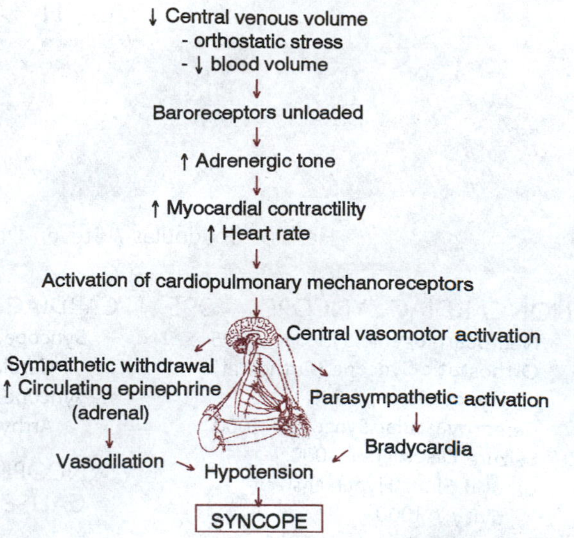

FIGURE 32-1 Presumed mechanisms of neurocardiogenic syncope. Schematic presentation. ↑ = increase; ↓ = decrease.

during neurocardiogenic syncope. Elderly patients with neurocardiogenic syncope are likely to have a predominant vasodepressor response without a significant cardioinhibitory component.

CLINICAL CHARACTERISTICS

Predisposition to neurocardiogenic syncope occurs under a wide variety of clinical circumstances. Indeed, the neurocardiogenic reaction per se may be the ultimate cause of most types of syncope. Neurocardiogenic syncope is often noted in individuals receiving sympathetic blocking agents and vasodilator drugs for hypertension, in elderly individuals receiving tranquilizers, in patients with acute or chronic anemia, and in those with transient reductions in blood volume, such as occur following a brisk diuresis or blood donation. Neurocardiogenic syncope complicates acute febrile infections and occurs with prolonged recumbency in chronic illness. Normal individuals at prolonged bed rest have a propensity for fainting, particularly when they arise abruptly from a sitting or recumbent position. Neurocardiogenic syncope is probably the most frequent cause of cardiovascular collapse during dental manipulations (dental syncope).[19] Neurocardiogenic syncope has been noted to follow strenuous exercise and may also occur during rapid acceleration in air flight, particularly when centrifugal force is applied in the head-to-foot position. Neurocardiogenic syncope of an unusual type may occur in pregnancy, being precipitated when the patient is supine and reversed when the patient assumes a lateral decubitus or upright posture (see Chap. 82).

The identification of aggravating factors (*triggers*) is important not only for the diagnosis but also for the prevention of syncope. Situations that decrease central venous volume or increase cardiovascular adrenergic tone are particularly important in the aggravation of neurocardiogenic syncope. The postprandial state, exertion in warm environments, prolonged upright posture, sodium restriction or diuretic use, and emotional or stressful situations are but a few important triggers to consider. Evidence suggests a relationship between chronic fatigue syndrome and neurocardiogenic syncope.[20]

The classic syncopal spell is often preceded by a constellation of prodromal symptoms occurring several seconds prior to the syncopal event. The prodrome may include symptoms of nausea, headache, diaphoresis, dizziness, chest pain, palpitations, dyspnea, and paresthesia. These symptoms may also persist for several minutes to several hours after the syncopal episode has resolved. Patients with sudden loss of consciousness may not report prodromal symptoms. Usually the spell occurs when the patient is upright and is less likely while seated. *Syncope while supine should prompt the search for etiologies other than neurocardiogenic syncope.*

During the syncopal episode, patients typically appear pale and diaphoretic, with a slow, diminished pulse. Occasionally, seizure-like activity may occur during asystolic periods. The syncopal spell classically resolves spontaneously once the patient is in the supine position but may recur if the patient stands or sits upright soon after the initial spell. The observations of a bystander are particularly helpful. *If the patient experiences a prolonged period of confusion after the syncopal event or is incontinent, etiologies other than neurocardiogenic syncope should be considered.*

Natural History The frequency and clinical significance of neurocardiogenic syncope are highly variable. Neurocardiogenic syncope may occur as a single isolated event or as a cluster of spells over weeks to months, or it may be a recurrent lifetime problem. The overall prognosis in patients with neurocardiogenic syncope is quite favorable compared with arrhythmic or left ventricular outflow obstructive forms of cardiac syncope. A very small subset of patients has been described as having *malignant* neurocardiogenic syncope.[21,22] This form of syncope is characterized by profound periods of asystole with sudden loss of consciousness, potentially leading to severe trauma and a theoretically increased risk of ischemia-mediated ventricular tachyarrhythmias. This risk is greatest in patients with underlying structural heart disease.

DIAGNOSTIC EVALUATION

Head-up tilt (HUT) testing has become a useful diagnostic study for the identification of patients with neurocardiogenic syncope.[23–25] The sensitivity, specificity, and reproducibility of HUT testing depend on the patient population studied and the HUT protocol employed.[23–30] HUT at an angle of 60° to 90° for a time period of 20 to 60 min has been found to yield a sensitivity ranging from 20 to 74 percent. Longer durations of HUT (45 to 60 min) lead to improved sensitivity without a significant increase in false-positive responses. Recent studies suggest that the optimal HUT angle should be between 60° and 80°. Tilt angles less than 45° sacrifice sensitivity, whereas angles greater than 80° can result in more false-positive results.[24] An average of 63 percent of patients studied with HUT after a negative electrophysiologic study were found to have a positive HUT response, suggesting that a significant proportion of patients with unexplained syncope have neurocardiogenic syncope. Isoproterenol infusion during HUT testing has been shown to improve sensitivity.[23] Low-dose isoproterenol infusion ($<2\ \mu g/min$) has been shown to nearly double the number of positive responses compared with baseline (short-duration HUT), with an acceptable specificity of 93 percent and reproducibility of 83 percent.[28] High doses of isoproterenol, especially at HUT angles of greater than 80°, markedly increase the incidence of false-positive responses.[29] High-dose intravenous isoproterenol, intravenous adenosine, and sublingual nitroglycerin during HUT have all been shown to increase sensitivity with some reduction in specificity and significant reduction in the time required to perform the test.[31–33]

MANAGEMENT

The management of recurrent neurocardiogenic syncope is challenging and sometimes unsatisfactory. The choice of therapy should be based on an understanding of the neurocardiovascular cascade that eventually culminates in neurocardiogenic syncope. First-line therapy includes counseling the patient to avoid dehydration, prolonged periods of standing motionless, and situations known to trigger syncope. Increased salt intake may be beneficial, if not contraindicated. Patients should be educated to recognize premonitory symptoms and, if they are present, to assume a recumbent position and cough in order to maintain cerebral perfusion. Data suggest that tilt training may improve outcome.[34]

The severity and frequency of recurrence of neurocardiogenic syncope are highly variable. As a result, its pharmacologic management must be highly individualized. Patients with infrequent, near-syncopal spells may respond to general measures alone. Frequent syncopal spells, especially if trauma occurs, usually necessitate pharmacologic interventions.

Therapeutic options include volume expansion, beta-adrenergic receptor blockade, anticholinergic agents, serotonin reuptake inhibitors, methylxanthines, alpha-agonists, and dual-chamber cardiac pacing. A stepped approach to pharmacologic therapy is advisable, starting with low initial doses, as these patients seem to be more prone to adverse reactions than the general population. The dose can be gradually titrated until the frequency and severity of spells are diminished. If one class of drug is ineffective, a combination of drugs, each acting on different limbs responsible for the neurocardiogenic syncope, may be beneficial. Several centers report the use of HUT testing to predict the clinical outcome of therapy. This approach has been questioned by two placebo-controlled trials that showed no significant difference in HUT response during treatment with active drug versus placebo.[35,36]

Volume Expansion A significant proportion of patients with neurocardiogenic syncope have evidence of mild reduction in central plasma volume, and plasma volume expansion can prevent recurrence. Simple measures such as liberalizing salt and fluid intake may suffice.[37] Custom-fitted, counterpressure support garments that extend from the ankle to the waist may be of benefit in highly motivated individuals. In some instances, fludrocortisone acetate may be helpful in augmenting salt retention and volume expansion. The initial dose is 0.1 mg daily; this may be increased by increments of 0.1 mg every 5 to 7 days. The maintenance dose varies from 0.1 to 1.0 mg daily.[38] Potential side effects include recumbent hypertension, marked fluid retention, congestive heart failure, and hypokalemia.

Beta Blockers Increased adrenergic stimulation with resultant activation of cardiac mechanoreceptors is believed to be an important mechanism in the pathophysiologic cascade that culminates in neurocardiogenic syncope. The negative inotropic effect of beta blockers may theoretically prevent activation of the ventricular mechanoreceptors or block the peripheral vasodilator effects of beta-adrenergic receptor stimulation. Oral metoprolol has been shown to prevent symptom recurrence in patients with neurocardiogenic syncope. In addition, intravenous metoprolol can blunt the hypotension and bradycardia during HUT testing. Recent studies suggest that patients who require isoproterenol infusion during tilt to elicit neurocardiogenic syncope are more likely to respond to beta blockers than are patients who are tilt positive without isoproterenol provocation.

Anticholinergic Agents During neurocardiogenic syncope, certain subsets of patients experience profound bradycardia that can aggravate the hypotension associated with vasodilation. This subset is believed to have a sudden surge in vagal activity because the bradyarrhythmia, but not the vasodilation, can be prevented by intravenous atropine. The profound bradyarrhythmias are primarily observed in the young and presumably healthy age group. Despite the unimpressive response of neurocardiogenic syncope to atropine, certain other anticholinergic drugs may be of benefit, if tolerated. The anticholenergic activity of propantheline bromide may be an effective treatment.[39]

Transdermal scopolamine has been shown to be a useful preventive agent in certain subsets of patients with recurrent neurocardiogenic syncope. Its mechanism of action is poorly understood but is probably related to its peripheral anticholinergic actions, as well as a depressant effect on the central nervous system transmission to the autonomic nervous system. These central actions of scopolamine are believed to be important for the prevention of the nausea of motion sickness, which may incidentally involve neuropathways common to the vasovagal pathways.[40]

The class 1A antiarrhythmic drug, disopyramide, has known anticholinergic and negative inotropic properties. These properties, which are considered undesirable effects of disopyramide in the therapy of tachyarrhythmias, may prevent the activation of cardiopulmonary mechanoreceptors and the neurogenic reflex observed in neurocardiogenic syncope. Disopyramide has been shown to prevent tilt-induced syncope and to prevent spontaneous syncopal spells. Disopyramide, however, must be used with caution because of its potential for proarrhythmia. In addition, the noncardiovascular anticholinergic side effects of disopyramide may be intolerable for some patients.

Serotonin Reuptake Inhibitors Serotonin may be an important mediator of inappropriate vasodilation and bradycardia in animal models of hemorrhagic shock. Blockade of serotonin receptors with methysergide can block this event. Nonrandomized studies suggest that the serotonin reuptake inhibitors fluoxetine hydrochloride (Prozac) and sertraline hydrochloride (Zoloft) may both be beneficial in the prevention of neurocardiogenic syncope after 4 to 6 weeks of therapy in approximately 55 percent of patients with severe, recurrent neurocardiogenic syncope.[41] A randomized, double-blinded, placebo-controlled trial showed that paroxetine hydrochloride-treated patients had an 18 percent incidence of recurrence versus a 53 percent recurrence rate in the placebo group.[42]

Methylxanthines Theophylline appears to reduce the frequency of neurocardiogenic syncope in patients who can tolerate this durg. Two separate clinical studies have shown that theophylline can prevent recurrences in greater than 70 percent of patients.[43] Even low doses of theophylline (6 to 12 mg/kg per day) appear to have benefit in those patients who cannot tolerate higher doses. Unfortunately, side effects such as nervousness, anxiety, and gastrointestinal abnormalities limit the usefulness of theophylline in this setting. Methylxanthines, such as theophylline, appear to have three different pharmacologic effects that may be beneficial therapeutically. In low concentrations, methylxanthines are potent adenosine receptor antagonists. At *therapeutic* serum concentrations, theophylline acts as a phosphodiesterase inhibitor and as a calcium transport inhibitor, both of which may be important in maintaining peripheral vascular tone.

Alpha-Agonists Nonrandomized studies in a small number of patients have suggested that alpha-agonists may prevent neurocardiogenic syncope due to a patent vasoconstrictor effect that may reduce venous pooling and concomitant reflex arteriolar vasodilation. However, two double-blinded, randomized placebo-controlled trials have yielded mixed results. Etilefrine was no better than placebo in the prevention of syncope. In contrast, the alpha-agonist medodrine reduced the incidence of HUT-induced syncope and improved quality of life compared with placebo control.[44,45]

Cardiac Pacing Similar to the use of anticholinergics, pacing is valuable in preventing the component of hypotension that is due to bradycardia; however, peripheral vasodilation may still occur despite heart rate control as noted. *Cardiac pacing should be reserved for those patients who have documented episodes of prolonged bradycardia associated with the syncopal spell.* Pacing may be especially beneficial in those rare patients with malignant neurocardiogenic syncope due to cardiac asystole.[46,47] These patients typically require pharmacologic therapy in addition to cardiac pacing to prevent the vasodepressor component. Dual-chamber pacing with rate-drop response is the preferred mode of pacing. The North American Vasovagal Pacemaker Study was the first randomized trial to confirm the effectiveness of pacing in patients with frequent syncope, positive head-up tilt, and relative bradycardia.[48]

Orthostatic Syncope (Orthostatic Hypotension)

Orthostatic hypotension is a disorder in which assumption of the upright posture is associated with a fall in arterial pressure associated with light-headedness, blurring of vision, and a sense of weakness and unsteadiness.[2,49–55] Hypotension is progressive over a period of seconds to minutes, depending on the degree of loss in reflex adaptation. If the fall in perfusion pressure to the brain is profound, syncope occurs. If the individual assumes the recumbent posture, arterial pressure rapidly normalizes and consciousness is restored.

From the diagnostic viewpoint, orthostatic hypotension is conveniently classified under three major causes:[2] *venous pooling and/or blood volume depletion, pharmacologic agents,* and *neurogenic causes* (Table 32-3). In certain cases, circulating endogenous vasodilators may result in orthostatic hypotension and syncope.

TABLE 32-3 Causes of Orthostatic Syncope

Venous pooling or volume depletion
Prolonged bed rest
Prolonged standing
Pregnancy
Venous varicosities
Blood loss
Dehydration
Pharmacologic agents
Antihypertensive
Sympathetic blocking agents
Calcium channel blockers
Converting enzyme inhibitors
Nitrates
Diuretics
Antidepressants, antipsychotic
Phenothiazides
Tranquilizers
Antiparkinsonian
Central nervous system depressants
Neurogenic
Diabetes mellitus
Alcoholic neuropathy
Spinal cord disease
Amyloidosis
Multiple sclerosis
Multiple cerebral infarcts
Parkinsonism
Tabes dorsalis
Syringomyelia
Idiopathic orthostatic hypotension
Shy-Drager syndrome (multiple system atrophy)
Circulating endogenous vasodilators
Hyperbradykinism
Mastocytosis
Carcinoid syndrome

VENOUS POOLING AND/OR BLOOD VOLUME DEPLETION

Excessive venous pooling accounts for the postural hypotension accompanying sustained bed rest, prolonged standing, pregnancy, and marked venous varicosities. Tall, asthenic individuals with poorly developed musculature are particularly prone to this form of postural hypotension. Deconditioning of normal autonomic reflex vasoconstriction may contribute to the orthostatic hypotension associated with prolonged bed rest and following extended periods of weightlessness in astronauts.[2] Blood volume depletion accounts for the orthostatic hypotension associated with dehydration, excessive diuresis, anemia, hemorrhage, excessive gastrointestinal fluid loss, third-space sequestration, prolonged fever, renal dialysis, excessive perspiration, adrenal insufficiency, pheochromocytoma, and diabetes insipidus.[56-60]

PHARMACOLOGIC AGENTS

Pharmacologically induced postural hypotension is a side effect in the administration of several classes of drugs, including antihypertensives, sympathetic blocking agents, diuretics, nitrates, calcium channel blockers, converting enzyme inhibitors, antidepressants, phenothiazines, tranquilizers, antipsychotic drugs, antiparkinsonian drugs, and central nervous system depressants.

NEUROGENIC CAUSES

Neurogenic postural hypotension has been observed in a wide variety of diseases affecting the autonomic nervous system. Specific entities include diabetes mellitus, alcoholic neuropathy, spinal cord injury, idiopathic orthostatic hypotension, and Shy-Drager syndrome (Table 32-3).[57-62] Administration of adrenergic blocking drugs and vasodilators may accentuate the predisposition to orthostatic hypotension in patients with primary neurogenic postural hypotension.

In the idiopathic form of orthostatic hypotension, postural hypotension is accompanied by relatively fixed heart rate, heat intolerance, anhidrosis, nocturnal polyuria, urinary and anal sphincter dysfunction, and impotency.[59,60] In the Shy-Drager syndrome, orthostatic hypotension is accompanied by multiple central nervous system manifestations and is referred to as *multiple system atrophy*.[57,61]

The central nervous system manifestations in multiple system atrophy may be indistinguishable from those of idiopathic Parkinson's disease and may precede or follow the onset of orthostatic hypotension. The prognosis appears to be worse in patients with multiple system atrophy than in those with idiopathic orthostatic hypotension, with death often resulting from general debilitation and its complications. Severe supine hypertension may complicate the presence of orthostatic hypotension.

When the total or central blood volume is depleted in the presence of an intact autonomic nervous system, pallor, coldness of the extremities, tachycardia, and sweating are evident. Relative bradycardia may occur at the time of syncope, and the clinical presentation may be identical to that of neurocardiogenic syncope. When orthostatic hypotension is due to loss or severe impairment of autonomic reflexes, the syncope is associated with little or no change in heart rate, and there is an absence of the pallor, sweating, and other manifestations observed in patients with intact autonomic reflexes.

THERAPY

Effective therapy in postural hypotension is closely linked to an accurate diagnosis. Primary emphasis must be based on treatable causes, in particular, pharmacologically induced postural hypotension, blood volume loss, venous pooling, and reversible disease entities. A summary of treatment modalities currently applied among patients with chronic orthostatic hypotension is presented in Table 32-4.[2] The wide variety of recommended approaches reflects the frequently disappointing therapeutic response to each of these modalities. Commonly, multiple maneuvers are necessary to achieve optimum control of postural hypotension. Of singular importance is the need to have the patient avoid experiences, such as dehydration, that accentuate postural hypotension and to restrict the use of pharmacologic agents that induce blood volume depletion, vasodilation, and sympathetic blockade. *Patients should be instructed about simple adaptive maneuvers, including slow rising from a recumbent or sitting position, flexing of the calf muscles during assumption of the*

TABLE 32-4 Treatment of Chronic Orthostatic Hypotension

- Evaluation for reversible and accentuating disease entities
- Specific modalities for irreversible orthostatic hypotension
  - Mechanical measures
    - Head-up position of bed
    - Lower body compression garment
    - Slow motion and calf muscle flexing on arising
  - Volume expansion
    - High-salt diet
    - Fludrocortisone acetate
  - Pharmacologic agents
    - Sympathomimetics
    - Vasoconstrictors

upright posture, and avoidance of prolonged immobility during standing.[63,64] Erythropoietin administration to expand red blood cell mass and blood volume has been used to maintain pressure in the upright posture in certain cases of orthostatic hypotension.[65]

Cerebrovascular Syncope

In patients with extensive occlusive disease of the origins of the brachiocephalic vessels, such as pulseless disease (e.g., aortic arch syndrome and Takayasu's arteritis), syncope is not uncommon.[2,66] With lesser degrees of cerebral occlusive disease, as with atherosclerotic narrowing, transient lowering of arterial pressure such as that immediately following assumption of the upright posture may be followed by vague symptoms suggesting impaired cerebral blood flow. In patients with cerebrovascular occlusive disease, a transient decrease in cardiac output and arterial pressure may provoke syncope at levels of arterial pressure that would otherwise be tolerated (see below, "Multifactorial Syncope").

Impairment or loss of consciousness in relation to changing positions of the head, particularly hyperextension and lateral rotation, has been attributed to mechanical narrowing of the vertebral arteries by skeletal deformities of the cervical spine. Such symptoms have been observed in patients with Klippel-Feil deformity, cervical spondylosis, and severe cervical osteoarthritis. Altered consciousness is often preceded by vestibular symptoms. When vertigo is a predominant symptom, the syndrome of benign postural vertigo must be considered.

Among patients with major occlusive disease of the carotid-vertebrobasilar arterial system, manual compression of the carotid artery as a test for carotid sinus hypersensitivity may induce syncope, at times associated with focal neurologic signs. The occurrence of syncope under such circumstances may be misdiagnosed as carotid sinus syndrome. The occurrence of a cerebrovascular accident following manual compression of the carotid sinus has been reported in patients with carotid disease, and *carotid sinus massage should be avoided in patients with symptomatic or suspected occlusive carotid vascular disease.*

Syncope in the *subclavian steal syndrome* is caused by major occlusive disease of the subclavian artery proximal to the origin of the vertebral artery. During upper extremity exercise, blood flow is shunted retrograde, by the circle of Willis, to the distal subclavian artery. The consequent decrease in cerebral circulation induces cerebral ischemia.[2,66] This syndrome is suggested by the findings of diminished brachial arterial pressure on the affected side, a bruit that is maximal over the supraclavicular area adjacent to the origin of the vertebral artery, and the induction of symptoms by exercise of the involved extremity.

Although focal neurologic symptoms and signs are the usual neurologic manifestations of cerebral emboli, transient loss of consciousness can be a primary presenting symptom. *Syncopal episodes are more likely to occur when atherosclerotic occlusive disease involves the vertebrobasilar system, with compromised perfusion to the medullary arousal center.* In vertebrobasilar vascular insufficiency, syncope or presyncope is nearly always preceded by symptoms of vertigo, diplopia, dysarthria, and ataxia. The episodes are generally attributed to microemboli arising from an atherosclerotic plaque, although vasospasm or postural hypotension may contribute (see Chap. 89).

THERAPY

The treatment of recurrent syncope in cerebrovascular disease is predicated on an accurate diagnosis. In this regard, it is essential to segregate the potential contribution of cardiac and vascular factors and their interplay. Anticoagulants and/or platelet antiaggregant agents are recommended for the prevention of embolic disease from the heart or central vessels (see Chap. 44). Surgical endarterectomy should be considered in carotid arterial occlusive disease.

Seizure Disorders

The various forms of syncope from the loss of consciousness during a generalized convulsive seizure are often differentiated on the basis of history alone.[67,68] Grand mal epilepsy as a cause of sudden loss of consciousness is suggested by the dramatic nature of the onset of the attack, which is often preceded by an aura. Other observations that aid in distinguishing epilepsy are the absence of hypotension and cardiac arrhythmia (other than sinus tachycardia); the presence of sustained tonic-clonic convulsive movements with upturning of the eyes; prolonged unconsciousness; urinary incontinence; and postictal drowsiness, headache, and confusion. While any of these findings occasionally occur in episodes of syncope, the frequent association of these several events generally allows differentiation of epilepsy as its cause. In fact, it is common for patients with true syncope to be incorrectly diagnosed as having a seizure disorder. Akinetic seizures and absence (petite mal) seizures may be difficult to differentiate from syncope. The occurrence in childhood, a past history of recurrent episodes, and the absence of pallor in witnessed episodes are helpful diagnostic findings. *Temporal lobe seizures are the most likely form of epilepsy to masquerade as syncope.*

An abnormal electroencephalogram (EEG) between episodes of altered consciousness can aid in distinguishing a seizure disorder when clinical observations are not definitive, and in some instances continuous EEG and electrocardiogram (ECG) monitoring are required.

Carotid Sinus Hypersensitivity

Compression of the carotid sinus in normal persons is often associated with transient slowing of the heart rate and mild hypotension. In some patients, such stimulation is followed by a profound slowing of heart rate and/or a marked diminution of arterial pressure. This disorder is referred to as *carotid sinus hypersensitivity*.

There are three forms of carotid sinus syncope, as originally described by Weiss and Baker:[69] cardioinhibitory, vasodepressor, and mixed type.

CARDIOINHIBITORY TYPE

The cardioinhibitory type of carotid sinus syncope which is the most common, is associated with slowing of the heart rate secondary to marked sinus bradycardia, sinoatrial block, and/or high-degree AV block. Syncope in this instance is related to the prolonged asystole rather than to a fall in peripheral vascular resistance.

VASODEPRESSOR TYPE

The vasodepressor type of carotid sinus syncope is that form of the syndrome in which syncope occurs as a result of a primary decrease in arterial pressure in the absence of profound bradycardia. Presyncopal signs, such as nausea, sweating, and pallor, are usually not observed, and the fall in arterial pressure may be precipitous.

MIXED FORM

In the mixed form of carotid sinus syncope with bradycardia and hypotension, the vasodepressor component may not be evident until after atropine blockade or during cardiac pacing. Under such circumstances, carotid sinus massage uncovers the hypotension in the absence of bradycardia.

Carotid sinus syncope and presyncope are commonly found in elderly patients in whom symptoms of light-headedness and impaired consciousness may be initiated by relatively minor stimulation of the carotid sinus.[2] Carotid sinus hypersensitivity in the elderly is often associated with generalized atherosclerosis.

Manual carotid sinus compression in elderly persons enjoins caution whenever this maneuver is attempted. Digital carotid massage should first be attempted with a very gentle and brief (2 to 4 s) compression, always when the patient is supine and with monitoring of the heart rate and blood pressure.[70–73] *The presence of carotid artery bruits is a relative contraindication to carotid massage.*

Carotid sinus syncope has been observed in patients with neoplasms, inflammatory masses, and lymph nodes in the neck adjacent to the carotid sinus.[74] Carotid sinus syncope is well established as a complication of carotid body and parotid tumors. In certain patients, carotid sinus hypersensitivity may be documented only when carotid sinus massage is performed in the upright position or during HUT studies with careful attention to the blood pressure response.

THERAPY

Thorough patient education concerning avoidance of carotid sinus pressure may be effective in preventing syncopal episodes. Anticholinergic and sympathomimetic agents may be tried, but inadequacy of drug therapy and the occurrence of side effects usually necessitate pacemaker therapy. AV sequential pacing appears to minimize the hypotensive effect of cardiac pacing and, hence, is the preferred form of pacemaker therapy in the mixed form of carotid sinus syncope. It is important that pacemaker effectiveness be verified objectively through observation of the effect of carotid sinus stimulation on cardiac rhythm and arterial pressure following pacemaker insertion.

Situational Syncope

The term *situational syncope* has been applied to a group of syndromes that is defined by the circumstances that precipitate the event. In the past, the syncope in these disorders has been attributed mainly to mechanical factors. Recent observations suggest that, at least in part, neurocardiogenic factors contribute to the syncope.[75]

COUGH SYNCOPE

Also called laryngeal vertigo, tussive syncope, and posttussive syncope, cough syncope is associated with loss of consciousness following a paroxysm of vigorous coughing. It is often seen in robust men and children but rarely in women. Cerebral blood flow is impaired by the marked increase in cerebrospinal fluid pressure during coughing, which increases cerebrovascular resistance. There is also a *concussive effect* transmitted via the cerebrospinal fluid. Reflex-induced sinus bradycardia, sinus arrest, and AV block have been observed in patients with cough syncope.[76]

In the treatment of cough syncope, the patient should be informed of the deleterious effects of vigorous coughing. Cessation of smoking and initiation of bronchodilator and anti-inflammatory therapy for associated bronchitis are mandatory for the prevention of cough-induced syncope.

SWALLOWING, OR DEGLUTITION, SYNCOPE

Deglutition syncope has been reported in association with tumor, diverticulum, achalasia, stricture, and spasm of the esophagus. In some patients, no abnormality can be identified radiologically or endoscopically. Syncope is usually associated with sinus bradycardia, sinus arrest, or high-degree AV block.[77]

Similar mechanisms have been implicated in syncope following distension of the viscera, glossopharyngeal neuralgia, fainting associated with irritation of the pleura or peritoneum, and cardiac asystole associated with esophagoscopy or bronchoscopy.[78]

VALSALVA SYNCOPE

Valsalva syncope is related to prolonged increases in intrathoracic pressure that may be observed during a sustained Valsalva maneuver. With prolonged exhalation against a closed glottis, there is a progressive fall in venous return, arterial pressure, and cardiac output.[2] These hemodynamic changes may be sufficient to impair cerebral circulation. An episode of Valsalva syncope may be the first indication of the presence of a disorder predisposing an individual to syncope (e.g., cerebrovascular occlusive disease or sick sinus syndrome). Instruction to the patient regarding avoidance of sustained Valsalva maneuvers is essential in preventing recurring episodes.

MICTURITION SYNCOPE

Micturition syncope is often seen in adult men with nocturia. During or immediately following voiding, there is a loss of consciousness, often without premonitory symptoms. The ingestion of large quantities of alcoholic beverages before retiring is common.[2,79] A similar type of syncope may be observed following drainage of the distended bladder or after removal of large quantities of ascitic fluid. The loss of consciousness in these circumstances may be related to bradycardia and a sudden reflex decrease in peripheral arterial resistance induced by the precipitous fall of intraabdominal volume. The loss of consciousness of typical micturition syncope is precipitated by such factors as the Valsalva maneuver in the upright posture and the peripheral vasodilation associated with a warm bed and recent alcohol consumption.

DEFECATION SYNCOPE

Defecation syncope occurs most commonly in the elderly, usually after arising from bed at night or during manual disimpaction of the rectum.[2,80] It has been attributed to sudden decompression of the rectum. Valsalva-related syncope could also explain some instances of this form of syncope. Many patients with defecation syncope have underlying gastrointestinal or cardiovascular disease.

DIVER'S SYNCOPE

Diver's syncope is an unusual and poorly understood form of loss of consciousness or even sudden death that may occur in underwater diving. In some instances diver's syncope may represent a form of neurocardiogenic syncope. Hypoxia and bradycardia of the diving reflex may be contributing factors.

POSTPRANDIAL SYNCOPE

Hypotension postprandially may result in presyncope and/or syncope and is most common in the elderly. The mechanisms of postprandial hypotension and syncope are not fully understood. Possible contributing factors include inadequate sympathetic nervous system compensation for meal-induced splanchnic blood pooling, impairments in baroreflex function, inadequate postprandial increase in cardiac output, impairment of peripheral vasoconstriction, and release of gastrointestinal peptides.[81,82]

TREATMENT

Therapy of situational syncope should be individualized and should be addressed to the specific circumstance associated with it. Episodes of syncope may be prevented by anticholinergic drugs such as atropine if they are administered prior to a procedure. Other measures include avoidance of vasodilators before meals and/or resting in a supine position after meals for patients with postprandial hypotension and sitting while urinating for men with micturition syncope. Octreotide, a somatostatin analog, has been shown to be effective in patients with postprandial hypotension, but it is expensive and must be given parenterally.[81,82]

Metabolic Syncope

HYPOXIA-RELATED SYNCOPE

Hypoxia may induce syncope that is related directly to a lack of oxygen or to an episode of neurocardiogenic syncope initiated during a period of oxygen lack. In the presence of cardiovascular disease, pulmonary insufficiency, and anemia, symptoms of hypoxia occur at lesser levels of oxygen deprivation. The impairment of consciousness due to hypoxia is accompanied by sinus tachycardia, while arterial pressure is usually normal. Short-term exposure to moderate altitude may be related to otherwise unexplained syncope in healthy, young adults. The environmental setting in which impaired consciousness due to hypoxia occurs usually leaves little difficulty in its differentiation from other forms of syncope.

HYPOGLYCEMIA-RELATED SYNCOPE

This form of syncope may be associated with weakness, sweating, a sensation of hunger, confusion, and altered consciousness. The symptoms are unrelated to posture and usually respond promptly to food ingestion or intravenous glucose administration. Impaired consciousness is usually associated with sinus tachycardia and is rarely accompanied by hypotension. In contrast to syncope of circulatory origin, it is gradual in onset. Hypoglycemia has been implicated as a possible factor that may trigger neurocardiogenic syncope.

HYPERVENTILATION, PANIC ATTACKS, AND SYNCOPE

In normal persons, anxiety is accompanied by varying degrees of hyperventilation. In the hyperventilation syndrome or in a panic episode, anxiety is associated with an inordinate degree of hyperventilation. Symptoms of hypocapnia and alkalosis may dominate the clinical picture. During the episode, the patient may complain of a tightness in the chest and a feeling of suffocation. These symptoms may be followed by confusion, a sense of unreality, bewilderment, light-headedness, and a feeling of panic. Symptoms of palpitation, precordial oppression, and dyspnea may suggest an acute cardiac or pulmonary catastrophe. Digital and circumoral paresthesias may develop and, in severe cases, may be accompanied by carpopedal spasm, which is probably related to alkalosis-induced decreases in serum ionized calcium. The symptoms may be protracted and persist while the subject is sitting or recumbent. During hyperventilation, there is slight hypotension but no profound fall in arterial pressure, while the heart rate is rapid. Although mentation is impaired, complete loss of consciousness rarely occurs. Typical neurocardiogenic syncope may be superimposed, making identification of the syndrome more difficult. *The induction of a typical episode by voluntary hyperventilation is helpful in distinguishing this syndrome and aids in educating the patient regarding the prevention and control of attacks.*

Other Forms of Syncope or Conditions Mimicking Syncope

MIGRAINE-RELATED SYNCOPE

Symptoms suggesting syncope are unusual in ordinary types of migraine. In rare instances in which the basilar arterial system is involved (as opposed to the more usually affected carotid system), the premonitory aura of migraine terminates in a period of unconsciousness of several minutes' duration. The unconsciousness is slow in onset and may be preceded by a dreamlike state. When the patient awakens, there is severe headache, typically in the occipital area. This form of migraine usually afflicts young women and has a strong menstrual association. The symptoms in syncopal migraine may suggest hyperventilation and/or hysterical syncope.

HYSTERICAL SYNCOPE

Altered consciousness of circulatory origin may be mimicked by hysteria. Hysterical episodes occur most frequently in young adults, often with severe emotional illness, and generally in the presence of an audience.[83] The individual slumps gently, even gracefully, to the floor or in a convenient chair or sofa, typically without injury or awkwardness. The patient may be motionless or may exhibit symbolic restrictive movements. Episodes are of varying duration and may last an hour or more. Although the patient is unresponsive to verbal stimulation, there is evidence, such as eyelid movement, that consciousness is well preserved, and no abnormalities in pulse, arterial pressure, or skin color are evident.

CARDIAC SYNCOPE

Either severe obstruction of cardiac output or disturbances of cardiac rhythm can produce syncope of cardiac origin.[2,84–95] Obstructive lesions and arrhythmias frequently coexist; indeed, one abnormality may accentuate the other. Common disorders associated with cardiac syncope are listed in Table 32-5.

Syncope Related to Obstruction of Cardiac Output

Obstruction to cardiac output sufficient to cause syncope may occur on the left or right side of the heart. Syncope, particularly that occurring with effort, is a major symptom of aortic stenosis and is often the initial presentation. The mechanisms are unclear, but studies suggest a reflex fall in peripheral vascular resistance as the usual cause. Failure of cardiac output to increase adequately during exercise, while peripheral resistance decreases, may play a role (see also Chap. 56). Transient arrhythmias can also induce syncope in aortic stenosis. Syncope associated with effort (often occurring immediately after effort) is observed in patients with hypertrophic cardiomyopathy as well. Nonexertional syncope related to acute decreases in preload or afterload, to inotropic stimulation, or to transient arrhythmias may also occur in hypertrophic cardiomyopathy (see also Chap. 67). Left-sided heart prosthetic valve malfunction can produce transient and at times profound obstruction to blood flow with syncope (see Chap. 60). A left atrial myxoma may obstruct left ventricular filling, leading to low cardiac output and syncope. The obstruction of left ventricular inflow in atrial myxoma may be posturally induced (see also Chap. 77). Mitral stenosis can produce cardiac syncope but usually does so only when tachycardia or other arrhythmias supervene (see also Chap. 57).

Primary pulmonary hypertension and pulmonary hypertension secondary to congenital heart disease may both be complicated by syncope, particularly effort-related syncope. In these conditions, limitation of right ventricular outflow markedly inhibits the cardiac output during increased peripheral demand. The fall in peripheral resistance in the presence of an inability to increase cardiac output may result in profound hypotension. A reflex fall in peripheral resistance similar to that which occurs with aortic stenosis may play a role. In a young patient without a cardiac murmur who presents with syncope during or shortly after exertion, primary pulmonary hypertension should be considered (see also Chap. 52). In pulmonary stenosis and pulmonary embolism, similar mechanisms may account for syncope. Pulmonary embolism as a cause of syncope should also be suspected in paraplegic patients.[96] In tetralogy of Fallot, the magnitude of flow through the right-to-left shunt increases when systemic resistance falls with effort, since the right ventricular outflow obstruction is usually fixed. This shunting results in marked arterial hypoxia, which may precipitate a syncopal episode (see also Chap. 63).

Cardiac tamponade, which affects both the right side and the left side of the heart, can produce syncope, but this is extremely rare. The likelihood of syncope is increased by concomitant arrhythmias.

TABLE 32-5 Common Disorders Associated with Cardiac Syncope

Left-sided heart
Aortic stenosis
Hypertrophic cardiomyopathy
Prosthetic valve malfunction
Mitral stenosis
Left atrial myxoma (rare)
Right-sided heart
Eisenmenger syndrome
Tetralogy of Fallot
Pulmonary embolism
Pulmonary stenosis
Primary pulmonary hypertension
Cardiac tamponade
Cardiac arrhythmia
Sinoatrial disease
Atrioventricular block
Supraventricular tachycardia
Ventricular tachycardia/fibrillation
Pacemaker related

Syncope Related to Cardiac Arrhythmia

Arrhythmias are a common cause of syncope and must be considered in any patient, particularly when cardiac disease is present. Either extreme of ventricular rate—bradycardia or tachycardia—can depress cardiac output to the point of critical hypotension with cerebral hypoperfusion and syncope. As noted earlier for other forms of syncope, a neurocardiogenic reaction may be precipitated by the hemodynamic effects of arrhythmias (see also Chaps. 23 and 24). The most common arrhythmias producing syncope or presyncope are profound sinus bradycardia, sinoatrial exit block or sinus pause, high-grade AV block, supraventricular tachycardia and ventricular tachycardia/fibrillation. Although arrhythmias occur in the absence of demonstrable underlying cardiac disease, they are usually secondary to such disorders as ischemic heart disease, cardiomyopathy, valvular heart disease (including mitral valve prolapse), and primary conduction system disease.

Primary degenerative disease of the sinus node and the specialized conduction tissue is the most common cause of sinoatrial disease (*sick sinus syndrome;* see Chap. 24). The sick sinus syndrome may be manifested by persistent or episodic sinus bradycardia or sinoatrial exit block, often with impaired junctional escape rhythm. The presence of alternating sinus bradycardia or sinoatrial block with paroxysmal supraventricular tachycardia of diverse types is quite common and is referred to as the *bradycardia-tachycardia syndrome. Syncope often occurs with asystole or bradycardia at the termination of tachycardia, when overdrive suppression of the sinoatrial or junctional pacemakers is present.*[2] A high incidence of associated AV and intraventricular conduction defects occurs in the sick sinus syndrome. AV block, impaired junctional escape rhythm, or ventricular arrhythmias may actually be responsible for syncope in the setting of sick sinus syndrome.

High-grade AV block may be due to disease of either the AV node or the His-Purkinje system. Block of the AV node is usually associated with a functional junctional pacemaker and a normal QRS complex, whereas AV block due to disease of the His-Purkinje system is usually associated with a wide complex idioventricular escape rhythm, which may be quite slow. Bifascicular block associated with a prolonged PR interval is associated with a substantial risk of developing high-grade AV block and syncope. Progression to high-grade AV block in patients with bifascicular block and a normal PR interval is less common. Ventricular tachycardia can cause syncope in patients with AV block or other bradycardic rhythms (see Chap. 24).

Sinus bradycardia, AV block, or cardiac asystole may be mediated by reflex vagal mechanisms and have been observed in a variety of disease states or during diagnostic procedures. Ventricular asystole (usually sinus arrest, although AV block can occasionally be noted) is most commonly due to neurocardiogenic syncope. Transient sinus bradycardia or AV block can also occur in apparently healthy young individuals; certain of these patients may have mitral valve prolapse.[93] Paroxysmal supraventricular tachycardias usually do not produce syncope in young individuals. Syncope, however, may occur in individuals who have accessory AV pathways due to the Wolff-Parkinson-White (WPW) syndrome, wherein supraventricular tachycardia is associated with a very rapid ventricular response. Studies have shown, though, that syncope during supraventricular tachycardia may be related to vasomotor factors and not be due solely to heart rate (Fig. 32-2).[97,98] AV node reentry, atrial fibrillation, or atrial flutter may be associated with a rapid ventricular rate in the setting of baseline short PR interval, or tachycardia occurring during or after exercise may cause syncope. Patients with cardiac disease, particularly obstructive outflow disorders, and older individuals may more commonly have hypotension significant enough to cause cerebral hypoperfusion and syncope.

Paroxysmal ventricular tachycardia may produce syncope at any age. The tachycardia is usually a manifestation of cardiac disease in which there are structural abnormalities and/or ischemia. Ventricular tachycardia is the most common arrhythmic cause of syncope in most series. In some patients, ventricular and supraventricular tachycardia may coexist (see Chap. 24).

Syncope may occur with ventricular tachycardia in the setting of the long QT syndrome. The long QT interval syndrome may be congenital or acquired (see Chaps. 11 and 24). The recognition of the long QT syndromes depends on demonstration of QT prolongation and of recurrent syncope, which is almost always due to ventricular arrhythmia. The ventricular arrhythmia is usually torsades de pointes. Ventricular tachycardia in the long QT syndromes is often triggered by exercise or stress reaction. A pause preceding the onset of tachycardia is common since the early after-depolarizations thought responsible for torsades are bradycardia dependent.[94,99]

It is particularly important to recognize the polymorphic ventricular tachycardia associated with acquired long QT syndromes, because it is a potentially life-threatening side effect of many drugs and metabolic abnormalities. The most frequent causes of acquired long QT syndromes are antiarrhythmic drugs and electrolyte disorders (hypokalemia and hypomagnesemia).

A variety of other drugs may produce arrhythmias or arrhythmia aggravation, resulting in syncope or presyncope. Beta-blocking drugs, calcium-channel-blocking agents, sotalol, and amiodarone are some of the more common agents that may cause significant sinus bradycardia or AV block. Digitalis may occasionally cause sinoatrial exit block or AV block, particularly in patients with sinoatrial or AV node disease. Supraventricular and ventricular tachycardias can be a result of digitalis therapy, particularly in patients with organic heart disease and hypokalemia. Theophylline and beta agonists, used for therapy of chronic obstructive pulmonary disease, may precipitate ventricular or supraventricular arrhythmias. Therapy with diuretics often causes hypokalemia and hypomagnesemia, which predispose individuals to supraventricular and ventricular arrhythmias. Both caffeine and alcohol may precipitate either atrial or ventricular tachycardia.

In patients with an artificial ventricular pacemaker, syncope may be secondary to pacemaker malfunction or to the pacemaker syndrome (see Chap. 31). Dual-chamber pacemakers can produce pacemaker-mediated tachycardias when there is retrograde conduction of the ventricular impulse to the atria. Improvements in technology have reduced the incidence of this complication.[100,101]

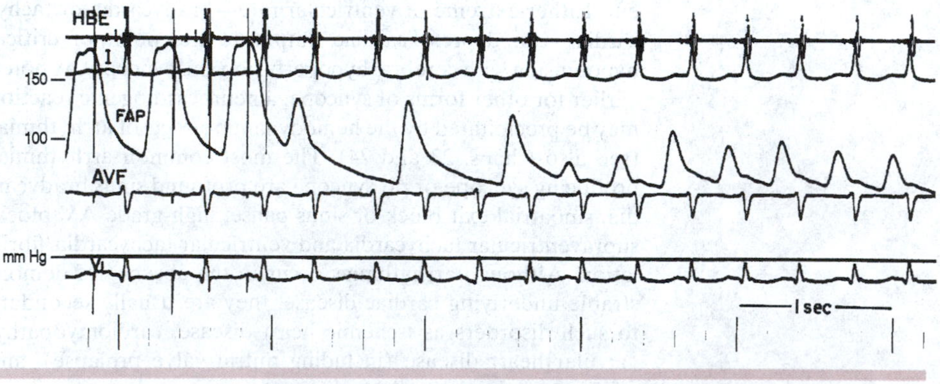

FIGURE 32-2 Atrial premature depolarization induced supraventricular tachycardia in a patient with tachycardia and syncope. Tachycardia rate was 170 beats per minute but associated with moderate hypotension in supine state. HBE = His bundle electrocardiogram; FAP = femoral artery pressure; AVF = scalar electrocardiographic lead. (From Schaal SF et al.[165] Reproduced with permission from the publisher and authors.)

DIAGNOSTIC EVALUATION OF SYNCOPE ASSOCIATED WITH CARDIAC DISEASE

While the history and physical examination often establish the diagnosis of obstructive cardiac syncope, laboratory studies are usually required for the determination of the severity of the disorder. Cardiac catheterization is required when corrective cardiac surgery is contemplated.

By far, the most challenging diagnostic evaluation occurs when arrhythmic cardiac syncope is suspected. Such patients often have evidence of underlying cardiovascular disease, which, when present, portends a poor prognosis. Thus, diagnostic studies directed to the nature and severity of the underlying cardiac disease must be pursued in addition to the arrhythmia evaluation.[102]

The various diagnostic tests used for the evaluation of arrhythmic syncope are listed in Fig. 32-3. Because of the transient nature of most arrhythmias, the routine ECG is generally of limited value. It is, however, very useful in identifying patients with abnormalities that may predispose individuals to syncope, such as prior infarction, WPW pattern, and AV or bundle branch block.

The technique of signal-averaged ECG for detecting late potentials can be used as a noninvasive screening test for detecting a high-risk subset of patients prone to lethal ventricular arrhythmias. The accuracy of the signal-averaged ECG in predicting the induction of sustained monomorphic ventricular tachycardia in high-risk patients with coronary artery disease who undergo electrophysiologic studies is good. The signal-averaged ECG may be helpful in some instances of other myocardial disease such as right ventricular dysplasia.[103–107]

Exercise testing can directly provoke arrhythmias in patients with a history suggesting exercise-induced arrhythmias. It should be performed when exertional arrhythmias are suspected but not documented by ambulatory monitoring or when ischemia is suspected (see also Chap. 14).[108,109] Continuous ECG monitoring is a widely used screening test for suspected arrhythmic syncope. It has low yield in unselected patients. *It is important to recognize that one 24-h monitoring period may not be sufficient for detecting transient rhythm disturbances. The diagnostic yield, moreover, increases only slightly with more prolonged monitoring* (see also Chap. 25).[108–110]

When ambulatory monitoring does not document an arrhythmia, a patient-activated electrocardiographic device (event recorder) may prove efficacious. This type of monitoring is effective in documenting infrequent arrhythmia. It should not be used in patients with suspected life-threatening arrhythmias.[111–113] Extended monitoring with an implantable loop recorder has been demonstrated to provide diagnostic ability in approximately two-thirds of patients with syncope of undetermined cause.[114,115]

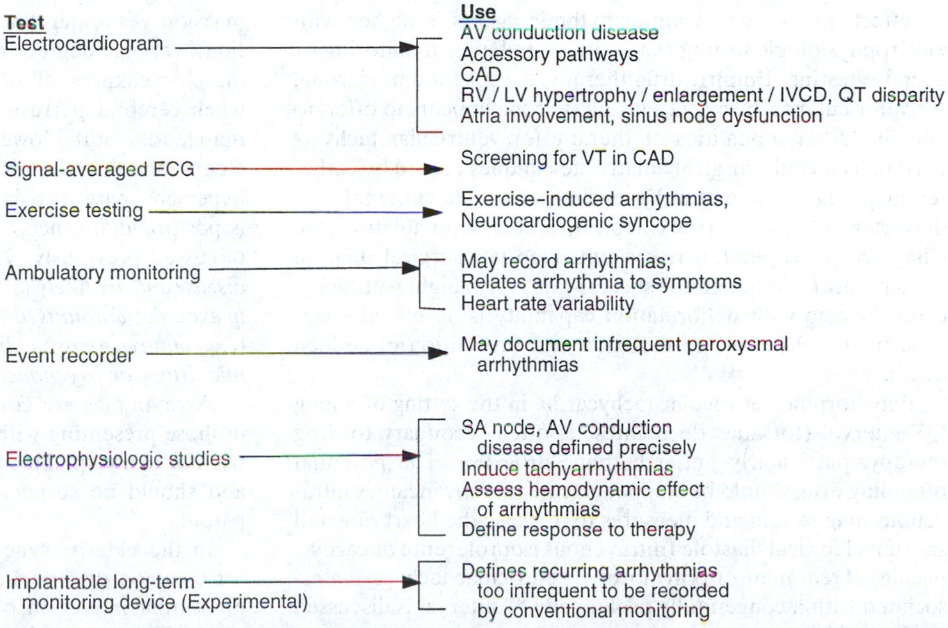

Test
Use
Electrocardiogram
AV conduction disease
Accessory pathways
CAD
RV / LV hypertrophy / enlargement / IVCD, QT disparity
Atria involvement, sinus node dysfunction
Signal-averaged ECG
Screening for VT in CAD
Exercise testing
Exercise-induced arrhythmias,
Neurocardiogenic syncope
Ambulatory monitoring
May record arrhythmias;
Relates arrhythmia to symptoms
Heart rate variability
Event recorder
May document infrequent paroxysmal arrhythmias
Electrophysiologic studies
SA node, AV conduction disease defined precisely
Induce tachyarrhythmias
Assess hemodynamic effect of arrhythmias
Define response to therapy
Implantable long-term monitoring device (Experimental)
Defines recurring arrhythmias too infrequent to be recorded by conventional monitoring

FIGURE 32-3 Diagnostic tests that can be used for the evaluation of arrhythmic syncope. AV = atrioventricular; CAD = coronary artery disease; RV/LV = right ventricular/left ventricular; IVCD = intraventricular conduction defect; VT = ventricular tachycardia; SA = sinoatrial.

When noninvasive testing is inconclusive for the diagnosis of suspected arrhythmic syncope, an electrophysiologic study should be performed on high-risk patients (i.e., those with underlying heart disease, suspicious arrhythmia by ECG monitoring, or recurrent syncope). Patients without identifiable heart disease are less likely to have the cause of syncope identified by electrophysiologic study. The cause of syncope most commonly identified by electrophysiologic study is ventricular tachycardia.

Electrophysiologic studies are useful in stratifying risk among symptomatic patients with bundle branch block or patients with bifascicular block. Patients with normal electrophysiologic study results have a favorable prognosis even without treatment. Patients undergoing permanent pacing on the basis of electrophysiologic testing also have a favorable prognosis, with a low rate of symptom recurrence.[116–121]

The prognosis in patients with syncope due to supraventricular tachycardia is usually good, since therapeutic approaches are available (i.e., drugs and radiofrequency ablation). The prognosis in patients with inducible ventricular tachycardia is less favorable but is improved when specific therapy can be demonstrated to inhibit the inducibility of ventricular tachycardia or with the use of an implantable cardioverter-defibrillator.

TREATMENT OF CARDIAC SYNCOPE

Obstructive Heart Disease For patients with syncope caused by obstructive heart disease, cardiac surgery is often the treatment of choice.[2] Patients with hypertrophic cardiomyopathy and syncope may respond well to pharmacologic therapy. Recent studies have suggested that an AV sequential pacemaker might control symptoms in certain patients with hypertrophic cardiomyopathy.[122–130] In rare cases with severe obstruction and persistent symptoms, surgery must be considered (see Chap. 67). Among all patients with obstructive heart disease and recurrent syncope, the diagnosis of fixed pulmonary hypertension is most difficult to treat because effective therapeutic options are limited (see Chap. 52).

Arrhythmic Syncope A detailed discussion of therapy for cardiac arrhythmias is presented in Chap. 24. Some general principles of arrhythmia management as they apply to patients with syncope are summarized here. Treatment of arrhythmic syncope requires accurate definition of the arrhythmia associated with syncope or presyncope.

The bradycardic rhythm disturbances responsible for syncope, primarily AV and sinoatrial pauses or exit block, usually require the implantation of a pacemaker. Patients receiving drugs that cause or contribute to the bradyarrhythmia, however, may benefit from withdrawal or substitution of the offending agent. Patients with bradycardia-tachycardia syndrome usually require pacemaker therapy, because the antiarrhythmic agents required for control of the tachycardia will often further suppress sinoatrial function.

Implicit in the approach to the tachycardias causing syncope is the accurate diagnosis of a specific tachycardia. The definition of the tachycardia and the response to antiarrhythmic therapy are often best achieved in the electrophysiologic laboratory. Patients with syncope due to supraventricular tachycardia associated with an accessory pathway are most often approached with catheter ablation of the accessory pathway.[131,132] Catheter ablation is also a successful mode of therapy in patients with AV nodal reentry supraventricular tachycardia or other supraventricular tachycardias associated with a rapid heart rate (see Chap. 28).

Therapy of paroxysmal ventricular tachycardia responsible for syncope is best guided by pharmacologic testing in the electrophysiologic laboratory.[133–139] Predictive accuracy of therapeutic effectiveness due to antiarrhythmic agents is higher with electrophysiologic testing than with ambulatory monitoring or exercise testing. Empiric drug therapy, except for amiodarone, for ventricular tachycardia causing syncope appears to offer no benefit. Other modalities of therapy for ventricular tachyarrhythmias include surgical ablative techniques guided by catheter mapping, antitachycardia pacing, automatic internal cardioverter-defibrillator (see Chap. 30), and catheter ablation (see Chap. 28). The operative risk is quite high with surgical ablation of tachycardia, although the success rate is also high. Antitachycardia pacing with defibrillation capability is an effective approach to tachycardia termination and prevention of sudden death.

Polymorphic ventricular tachycardia in the setting of a long QT interval (torsades de pointes) is often secondary to drug therapy, particularly antiarrhythmic drug use. The potential offending drug should be stopped. Acute therapy includes intravenous magnesium and measures to increase the heart rate and shorten electrical diastole (intravenous isoproterenol or cardiac pacing). Treatment of polymorphic ventricular tachycardia associated with a congenitally prolonged QT interval is discussed in Chap. 24.

Pacemaker-induced hypotension and syncope are rectified by changing from ventricular pacing to AV sequential pacing when hypotension due to loss of atrial transport or neurocardiogenic response is responsible for symptoms. Identification of pacemaker-mediated tachycardia usually requires only pacemaker programming changes. Pacemaker malfunction or myopotential inhibition requires a change in programming or replacement of the defective part of the system.

SYNCOPE OF UNDETERMINED CAUSE

Despite careful diagnostic evaluation, the cause of syncope often cannot be defined. Unexplained syncope probably has a broad spectrum of etiologies. The varying mortality rate among patients with syncope of undetermined cause probably reflects the varying incidence of undetected cardiac syncope. A certain number of these patients probably have experienced syncope of multiple causes.

SPECIAL PROBLEMS IN SYNCOPE

Syncope in the Elderly

Elderly persons are particularly prone to develop syncope or presyncope. The aging process can result in diminished cerebral oxygen delivery by a variety of physiologic mechanisms, including decreased cerebral blood flow from low cardiac output, cerebral vascular disease, decreased hemoglobin, and lower arterial P_{O_2}. In addition, cerebral arteriolar sclerosis may be present and may necessitate a normal arterial perfusion pressure. Thus, many older patients have only marginal cerebral oxygen delivery at rest.[140–143] Physiologic defenses against a fall in blood pressure may also be impaired as discussed previously.

The aged may also suffer from multiple sensory deficits (e.g., in vision, vestibular function, and peripheral sensory nerve function), variable degrees of dementia, bradykinesis, arthritis, and muscle weakness, all of which enhance the likelihood of a fall when cerebral perfusion is marginal. *Drop* attacks, in which muscle tone in the lower extremities is lost, are frequent in the elderly and must be distinguished from syncope. Carotid sinus hypersensitivity also is relatively common in the elderly, as is postprandial syncope; these entities should be evaluated as discussed previously. *The elderly frequently have multisystem disease and are likely to be taking several medications, sometimes in excessive amounts, that may aggravate the tendency to syncope (e.g., antihypertensive drugs, diuretics, vasodilators, antiarrhythmic drugs, or psychoactive drugs).*

Arrhythmias are common in elderly individuals, especially in those presenting with syncope. Syncope is a significant contributor to unexplained automobile accidents among the elderly and should be suspected when external causes are not apparent.[144–146]

In the elderly, syncope may be the presenting complaint for common disorders such as pneumonia, viral illness, acute myocardial infarction, or occult hemorrhage. Thus, the management of syncope in the aged often requires initial management of underlying diseases, with subsequent evaluation to determine whether such therapy controls syncope.

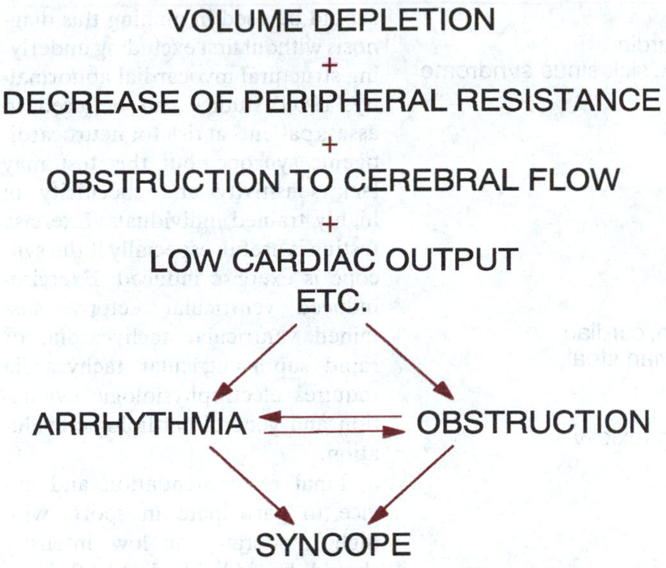

FIGURE 32-4 Frequently, multiple factors must be present simultaneously or in sequence for syncope to occur as a result of an arrhythmia or obstruction to cardiac output. (From Boudoulas H and Lewis RP.[159] Reproduced with permission from the publisher and authors.)

Multifactorial Syncope

In many instances, syncope requires that a constellation of events occur, either simultaneously or in sequence. Without the full complex, the patient may note only light-headedness or perhaps no definable symptoms. A carefully recorded history is required to elucidate such complex presentations.

Transient abnormalities such as fever, fatigue, hypoglycemia, or drug ingestion may increase the likelihood of syncope. Coexisting diseases may decrease the patient's physiologic defenses for maintaining adequate cerebral perfusion to sustain consciousness. A cardiac arrhythmia that ordinarily would not produce syncope may become a contributory factor when other predisposing factors are present (Fig. 32-4). With respect to combined causes of syncope, it is notable that, in the original description of Adams-Stokes syncope, the patients exhibited a permanently slow pulse rate accompanied by aortic stenosis.

The development of the neurocardiogenic reaction may determine whether a given stimulus initiates syncope. This relationship has been shown in such diverse causes of syncope as aortic stenosis, vasodilator drug therapy, volume loss, pulmonary embolism, tachyarrhythmias, pacemaker syndrome, postprandial state in the elderly, and after exercise. A common pathophysiologic mechanism that may trigger neurocardiogenic syncope is diminished venous return to the right side of the heart.

Syncope and Sudden Death

Sudden death is common among those with known cardiac syncope (both obstructive and arrhythmic), but occasionally sudden death may also occur in presumptive noncardiac syncope and syncope of unknown cause. It would appear therefore that, in some patients, syncope is a harbinger of sudden death. Patients with advanced heart failure and syncope are at especially high risk for sudden death regardless of the etiology.[147–149] Syncope is also associated with a high mortality rate in patients with hypertrophic cardiomyopathy. It is not always clear to what extent the occurrence of syncope per se is a risk factor for sudden death or whether the risk is more related to the underlying disease.

Recurrent Syncope

In up to one-third of all patients with syncope, it is a recurring event. For most patients, the persistence of syncope increases morbidity from trauma but does not increase mortality. Such recurrences most often reflect a lack of effective therapy and/or a failure to establish the correct diagnosis.

Unexplained syncope in patients with negative initial diagnostic studies has a broad spectrum of etiologies, the most common of which is bradycardia. An implantable long-term monitoring device is useful for establishing a diagnosis when symptoms are recurrent but too infrequent for conventional monitoring techniques.[114,115,150] Recurrent syncope is particularly common in a subset of patients with mitral valve prolapse in whom dysautonomia, arrhythmia, and hypovolemia all play a role.[93] In certain patients with unexplained recurrent syncope, especially in individuals with multiple physical symptoms, screening for psychiatric disorder may be necessary. In patients with recurrent syncope, advice regarding the avoidance of certain activities, such as working with dangerous equipment, is needed and, in some cases in which public safety is involved, a change in jobs is required (e.g., pilots or bus drivers).

Exercise and Syncope

Individuals with a history of syncope associated with activity and who participate in physical activities or competitive athletics

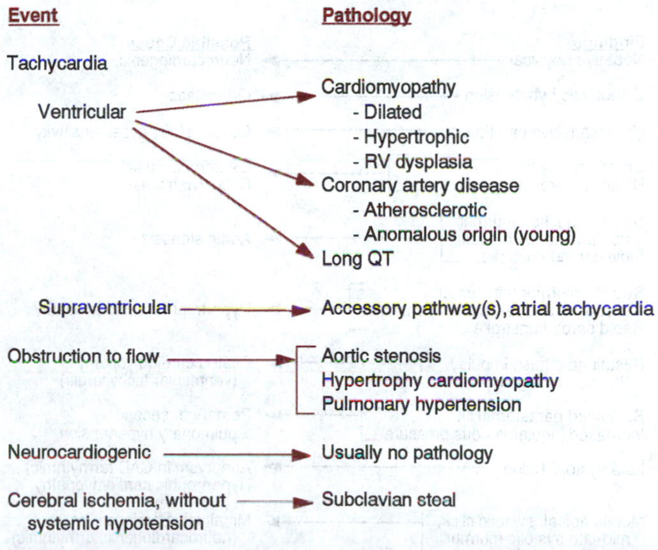

FIGURE 32-5 Exercise-induced syncope. Events and underlying pathology. RV = right ventricular.

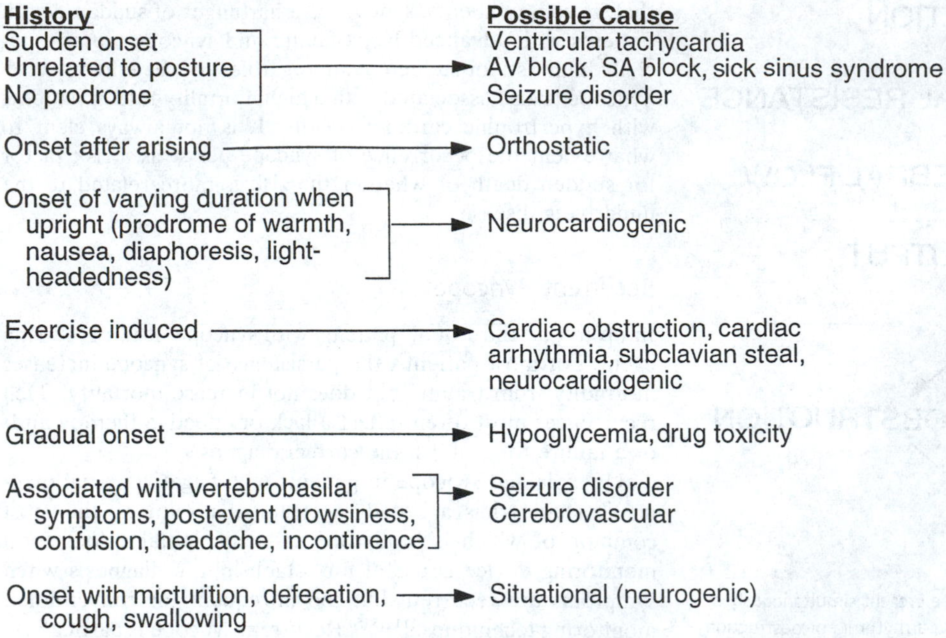

FIGURE 32-6 Differential diagnosis of syncope based on history. AV = atrioventricular; SA = sinoatrial.

constitute a special problem. Since exercise syncope may be a manifestation of serious underlying cardiac disease, complete evaluation is indicated to define the cause of syncope prior to recommendation for participation in sports. *Identification of myocardial abnormalities by physical examination and echocardiogram is paramount to the prevention of potential sudden cardiac death.*[151–158]

Syncope may occur during or immediately after exercise. The most common causes of exercise-induced syncope are shown in Fig. 32-5. Neurocardiogenic syncope is not uncommon in highly trained individuals with high resting vagal tone, but caution should be used in making this diagnosis without first excluding underlying structural myocardial abnormality. HUT studies can be used to assess patients at risk for neurocardiogenic syncope, but this test may lack sensitivity and specificity in highly trained individuals. Exercise testing is useful, especially if the syncope is exercise induced. Exercise-induced ventricular ectopy, sustained ventricular tachycardia, or rapid supraventricular tachycardia requires electrophysiologic evaluation and general cardiologic evaluation.

Final recommendation and advice to participate in sports with high, moderate, or low intensity should be individualized. Recommendations should be balanced between restricting activity unduly and reducing chance of death or injury from the participation in sports.

DIAGNOSTIC EVALUATION OF SYNCOPE: AN OVERVIEW

In the initial approach to the diagnosis of syncope, it is essential to distinguish the underlying cause in terms of the three basic categories outlined in Table 32-1. This differentiation is accomplished in a majority of patients by a history (Fig. 32-6), physical examination (Fig. 32-7), and ECG (Fig. 32-8) and is supplemented by routine laboratory studies, including echocardiography (Fig. 32-9). Further, Figs. 32-5 and 32-10 provide a useful framework for initiating a diagnostic evaluation of syncope based on age and in situations when syncope is induced with physical activities.[159–164]

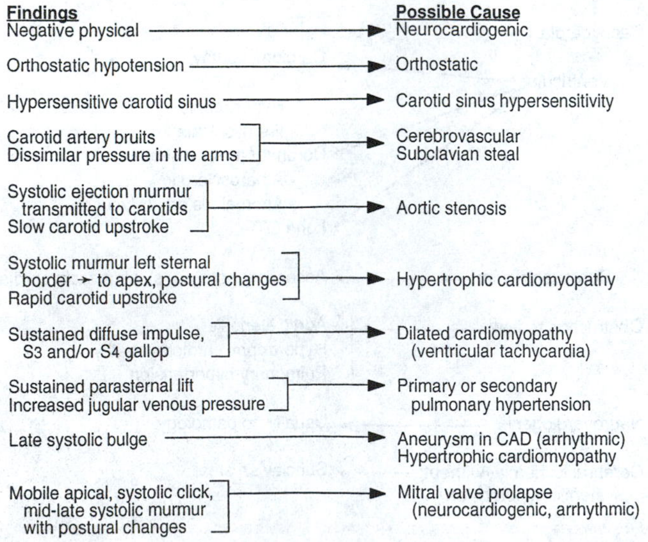

FIGURE 32-7 Differential diagnosis of syncope based on physical examination. CAD = coronary artery disease.

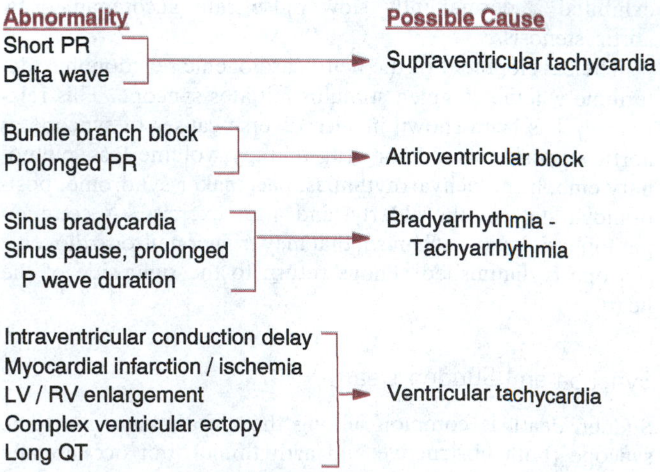

FIGURE 32-8 Differential diagnosis of syncope based on the electrocardiogram. LV/RV = left ventricular/right ventricular.

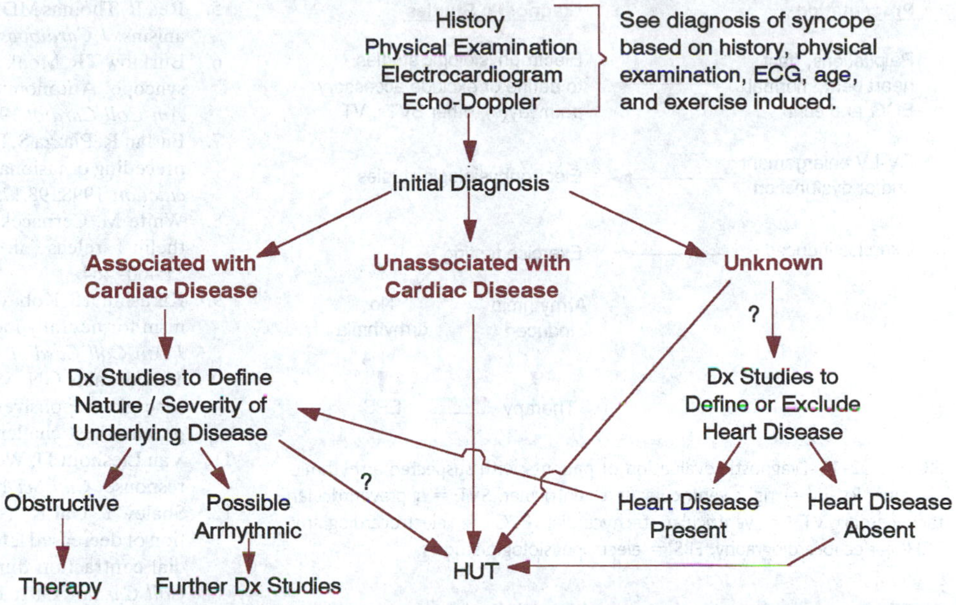

FIGURE 32-9 Basic schema for diagnostic evaluation of syncope. ECG = electrocardiogram; Dx = diagnostic; HUT = head-up tilt.

Children, Adolescent, Young Adults

Neurocardiogenic (common)
Cardiac
- Supraventricular tachycardia
  - Accessory AV pathway(s)
- Ventricular tachycardia
  - Idiopathic long QT
  - Cardiomyopathy
  - Right ventricular dysplasia
  - Congenital heart disease
  - Post corrective surgery
- AV block
  - Congenital
  - Postcorrective surgery

Seizure disorders

Middle Age

Neurocardiogenic
Orthostatic
Cardiac
- Arrhythmic
- Obstruction

Seizure disorders
Pharmacologic agents

Elderly

Cardiac
- Arrhythmic
- Obstructive

Orthostatic
Neurocardiogenic
Drug induced
Cerebrovascular
Carotid sinus hypersensitivity
Seizure disorders
Combined causes

FIGURE 32-10 Common causes of syncope by age. AV = atrioventricular.

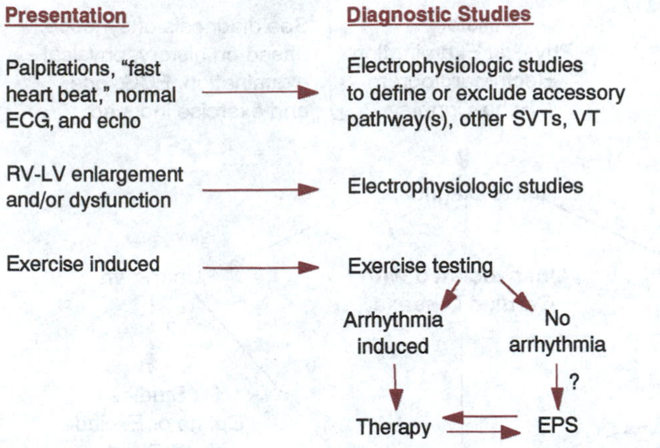

FIGURE 32-11 Diagnostic evaluation of patients with suspected arrhythmic syncope. RV-LV = right ventricular/left ventricular; SVT = supraventricular tachycardia; VT = ventricular tachycardia; ECG = electrocardiogram; ECHO = echocardiography; EPS = electrophysiologic studies.

The extent of evaluation should initially be predicated on the estimation of mortality and morbidity risk, which is high in cardiac syncope or syncope associated with cardiac disease and low in syncope without structural heart disease. Although cost effectiveness in diagnostic testing should be practiced, the need for an assiduous search should not be dismissed when lethal disease is suspected.

Complete evaluation of syncope is required for the elderly and for patients with suspected arrhythmic syncope (Fig. 32-11). When patients in such a selected group undergo a thorough evaluation, including an electrophysiologic study, an arrhythmic basis for syncope can be found in the majority of patients. *Negative results are often as important as actual identification of an arrhythmia, since the negative evaluation usually denotes a favorable long-term prognosis.* Long-term follow-up suggests that both morbidity and mortality risks can be reduced by therapy guided by electrophysiologic study results. Unfortunately, no controlled studies exist (or are likely to be done) to establish these benefits conclusively.

The diagnostic evaluation of patients with syncope of unknown cause presents a perplexing problem, particularly when syncope occurs repeatedly and because it may be a harbinger of sudden death. As the understanding of the mechanisms and the breadth of causes of syncope improves (particularly the role of multiple causes), it is reasonable to suspect that the incidence of patients with syncope of unknown cause will be further diminished in the future. In certain cases, devices with extended monitoring capabilities can be used.

References

1. Savage DD, Corwin L, McGee DL, et al. Epidemiologic features of isolated syncope: The Framingham Study. *Stroke* 1985; 16: 626–629.
2. Boudoulas H, Weissler AM, Lewis RP, et al. The clinical diagnosis of syncope. *Curr Probl Cardiol* 1982; 7:6–40.
3. Kapoor WN, Karpf M, Wieland S, et al. A prospective evaluation and follow-up of patients with syncope. *N Engl J Med* 1983; 309:197–204.
4. Abbond F. Neurocardiogenic syncope. *N Engl J Med* 1993; 328: 1117–1120.
5. Rea R, Thomas MD. Neural control and vasovagal syncope mechanisms. *J Cardiovasc Electrophysiol* 1993; 4:587–595.
6. Burklow TR, Moak JP, Bailey JJ, et al. Neurally mediated cardiac syncope: Autonomic modulation after normal saline infusion. *J Am Coll Cardiol* 1999; 33:2059–2066.
7. Furlan R, Piazza S, Dell'Orto S, et al. Cardiac autonomic patterns preceding occasional vasovagal reactions in healthy humans. *Circulation* 1998; 98:1756–1761.
8. White M, Cernacek P, Courtemanche M, et al. Impaired endothelin-1 release in tilt-induced syncope. *Am J Cardiol* 1998; 81:460–464.
9. Kikushima S, Kobayashi Y, Nakagawa H, et al. Triggering mechanism for neurally mediated syncope induced by head-up tilt test. *J Am Coll Cardiol* 1999; 33:350–357.
10. Theodorakis GN, Markianos M, Livanis EG, et al. Central serotonergic responsiveness in neurocardiogenic syncope: A clomipramine test challenge. *Circulation* 1998; 98:2724–2730.
11. Van Lieshout JJ, Wouter W, Karemaker JM, et al. The vasovagal response. *Clin Sci* 1991; 81:575–586.
12. Shalev Y, Gal R, Tchou p, et al. Echocardiographic demonstration of decreased left ventricular dimension and vigorous myocardial contraction during syncope induced by head-up tilt. *J Am Coll Cardiol* 1991; 18:748–751.
13. Thoren P. Role of cardiac vagal C-fibers in cardiovascular control. *Rev Physiol Biochem Pharmacol* 1979; 86:1–94.
14. Mark A. The Bezold-Jaisch reflex revisited: Clinical implications of inhibitory reflexes originating in the heart. *J Am Coll Cardiol* 1983; 1:90–102.
15. Rosoff MH, Cohen MV. Profound bradycardia after amyl nitrate in patients with a tendency to vasovagal episodes. *Br Heart J* 1986; 55:97–100.
16. Fitzpatrick AP, Banner N, Cheng A, et al. Vasovagal reactions may occur after orthotopic heart transplantation. *J Am Coll Cardiol* 1993; 21:1132–1137.
17. Sra JS, Murthy V, Natale A, et al. Circulatory and catecholamine changes during head-up tilt testing in neurocardiogenic (vasovagal) syncope. *Am J Cardiol* 1994; 73:33–37.
18. Chen MY, Goldenberg IF, Milstein S, et al. Cardiac electrophysiologic and hemodynamic correlates of neurally-mediated syncope. *Am J Cardiol* 1989; 63:66–72.
19. Boorin MR. Anxiety: Its manifestation and role in the dental patient. *Dent Clin North Am* 1995; 39:523–539.
20. Bou-Holagah I, Rowe PC, Kan J, et al. The relationship between neurally mediated hypotension and the chronic fatigue syndrome. *JAMA* 1995; 274:961–967.
21. Milstein S, Buetikofer J, Lesser J, et al. Cardiac asystole: A manifestation of neurally-mediated hypotension-bradycardia. *J Am Coll Cardiol* 1989; 14:1626–1632.
22. Folino AF, Buja GF, Martini B, et al. Prolonged cardiac arrest and complete AV block during upright tilt test in young patients with syncope of unknown origin: Prognostic and therapeutic implications. *Eur Heart J* 1992; 13:1416–1421.
23. Almquist A, Goldenberg IF, Milstein S, et al. Provocation of bradycardia and hypotension by isoproterenol and upright posture in patients with unexplained syncope. *N Engl J Med* 1989; 320:346–351.
24. Fitzpatrick AP, Theodorakis G, Vardas P, et al. Methodology of head-up tilt testing in patients with unexplained syncope. *J Am Coll Cardiol* 1991; 17:125–130.
25. Bloomfield D, Maurer M, Bigger JT. Effects of age on outcome of tilt-table testing. *Am J Cardiol* 1999; 83:1055–1058.
26. Sneddon JF, Slade A, Seo H, et al. Assessment of the diagnostic value of head-up tilt testing in the evaluation of syncope in hypertrophic cardiomyopathy. *Am J Cardiol* 1994; 73:601–604.
27. Kenny RA, Bayliss J, Ingram A, et al. Head-up tilt: A useful test for investigating unexplained syncope. *Lancet* 1986; 1:1352–1355.

28. Morello CA, Klein GJ, Zandri S, et al. Diagnostic accuracy of a low-dose isoproterenol head-up tilt protocol. *Am Heart J* 1995; 129:901–906.
29. Natale A, Akhtar M, Jazayeri M, et al. Provocation of hypotension during head-up tilt testing in subjects with no history of syncope or presyncope. *Circulation* 1995; 92:54–58.
30. Sheldon R, Rose S, Flanagan P, et al. Risk factors for syncope recurrence after a positive tilt-table test in patients with syncope. *Circulation* 1996; 93:973–981.
31. Shen WK, Jahangir A, Beinborn D, et al. Utility of a single-stage isoproterenol tilt table test in adults: A randomized comparison with passive head-up tilt. *J Am Coll Cardiol* 1999; 33:985–990.
32. Zeng C, Zhu Z, Hu W, et al. Value of sublingual isosorbide dinitrate before isoproterenol tilt test for diagnosis of neurally mediated syncope. *Am J Cardiol* 1999; 83:1059–1063.
33. Mittal S, Stein KM, Markowitz SM, et al. Induction of neurally mediated syncope with adenosine. *Circulation* 1999; 99:1318–1324.
34. Di Girolamo E, Di Iorio C, Leonzio L, et al. Usefulness of a tilt training program for the prevention of refractory neurocardiogenic syncope in adolescents: A controlled study. *Circulation* 1999; 100:1798–1801.
35. Morillo CA, Leitch JW, Yee R, et al. A placebo-controlled trial of intravenous and oral disopyramide for prevention of neurally mediated syncope induced by head-up tilt. *J Am Coll Cardiol* 1993; 22:1843–1848.
36. Moya A, Permanyer-Miralda G, Sagrista-Sauleda J, et al. Limitations of head-up tilt test for evaluating the efficacy of therapeutic interventions in patients with vasovagal syncope: Results of a controlled study of etilefrine versus placebo. *J Am Coll Cardiol* 1995; 25:65–69.
37. Younoszai AK, Franklin WH, Chan DP, et al. Oral fluid therapy: A promising treatment for vasodepressor syncope. *Arch Pediatr Adolesc Med* 1998; 152:165–168.
38. Schatz IJ. Management of orthostatic hypotension. In: Schatz IJ, ed. *Orthostatic Hypotension.* Philadelphia: FA Davis; 1986:98.
39. Yu SC, Sung RJ. Clinical efficacy of propantheline bromide in neurocardiogenic syncope: Pharmacodynamic implications. *Cardiovasc Drugs Ther* 1997; 10:687–692.
40. Kosinski D, Grubb BP, Temesy-Armos P. Pathophysiological aspects of neurocardiogenic syncope: Current concepts and new perspectives. *PACE* 1995; 18:716–724.
41. Grubb BP, Samoil D, Kosinski D, et al. Use of sertraline hydrochloride in the treatment of refractory neurocardiogenic syncope in children and adolescents. *J Am Coll Cardiol* 1994; 24: 490–495.
42. Di Girolamo E, Di Lorio C, Sabatini P, et al. Effects of paroxetine hydrochloride, a selective serotonin reuptake inhibitor, on refractory vasovagal syncope: A randomized, double-blind, placebo-controlled study. *J Am Coll Cardiol* 1999; 33:1227–1230.
43. Nelson SD, Stanley M, Love CJ, et al. The autonomic and hemodynamic effects of oral theophylline in patients with vasodepressor syncope. *Arch Intern Med* 1991; 151:2425–2429.
44. Ward CR, Gray JC, Gilroy JJ, et al. Midodrine: A role in the management of neurocardiogenic syncope. *Heart* 1998; 79:45–49.
45. Raviele A, Brignole M, Sutton R, et al. Effect of etilefrine in preventing syncopal recurrence in patients with vasovagal syncope: A double-blind, randomized, placebo-controlled trial—The Vasovagal Syncope International Study. *Circulation* 1999; 99: 1452–1457.
46. Sheldon R, Koshman ML, Wilson W, et al. Effect of dual-chamber pacing with automatic rate-drop sensing on recurrent neurally medicated syncope. *Am J Cardiol* 1998; 81:158–162.
47. Ammirati F, Colivicchi F, Toscano S, et al. DDD pacing with rate drop response function versus DDI with rate hysteresis pacing for cardioinhibitory vasovagal syncope. *Pacing Clin Electrophysiol* 1998; 21:2178–2181.
48. Connolly SJ, Sheldon R, Roberts RS, et al. The North American Vasovagal Pacemaker Study (VPS): A randomized trial of permanent cardiac pacing for the prevention of vasovagal syncope. *J Am Coll Cardiol* 1999; 33:16–20.
49. Schatz IJ. Orthostatic hypotension: Functional and neurogenic causes. *Arch Intern Med* 1984; 144:773–777.
50. Ziegler MG. Postural hypotension. *Annu Rev Med* 1980; 31: 239–245.
51. Levine BD, Giller CA, Lane LD, et al. Cerebral versus systemic hemodynamics during graded orthostatic stress in humans. *Circulation* 1994; 90:298–306.
52. Jacob G, Shannon JR, Costa F, et al. Abnormal norepinephrine clearance and adrenergic receptor sensitivity in idiopathic orthostatic intolerance. *Circulation* 1999; 99:1706–1712.
53. Jacob G, Shannon JR, Black B, et al. Effects of volume loading and pressor agents in idiopathic orthostatic tachycarda. *Circulation* 1997; 96:575–580.
54. Furlan R, Jacob G, Snell M, et al. Chronic orthostatic intolerance: A disorder with discordant cardiac and vascular sympathetic control. *Circulation* 1998; 98:2154–2159.
55. Masaki KH, Schatz IJ, Burchfiel CM, et al. Orthostatic hypotension predicts mortality in elderly men: The Honolulu Heart Program. *Circulation* 1998; 98:2290–2295.
56. Leier CV, Boudoulas H. *Cardiorenal Disorders and Diseases,* 2d ed. New York: Futura; 1992.
57. Shy GM, Drager GA. A neurologic syndrome associated with orthostatic hypotension. *Arch Neurol* 1960; 2:511–527.
58. Kontos HA, Richardson DW, Norvell JE. Norepinephrine depletion in idiopathic orthostatic hypotension. *Ann Intern Med* 1975; 82:336–341.
59. Ziegler MG, Lake CR, Kopin IJ. The sympathetic-nervous-system defect in primary orthostatic hypotension. *N Engl J Med* 1977; 296:293–297.
60. Kopin IJ, Polinsky RJ, Oliver JA, et al. Urinary catecholamine metabolites distinguish different types of sympathetic neuronal dysfunction in patients with orthostatic hypotension. *J Clin Endocrinol Metab* 1983; 57:632–637.
61. Khurana RK, Nelson E, Azzarelli B, et al. Shy-Drager syndrome: Diagnosis and treatment of cholinergic dysfunction. *Neurology* 1980; 30:805–809.
62. Cryer PE, Silverberg AB, Santiago JV, et al. Plasma catecholamines in diabetes: The syndromes of hypoadrenergic and hyperadrenergic postural hypotension. *Am J Med* 1978; 64:407–416.
63. Henry R, Rowe J, O'Mahony D. Haemodynamic analysis of efficacy of compression hosiery in elderly fallers with orthostatic hypotension. *Lancet* 1999; 354:45–46.
64. Ector H, Reybrouck T, Heidbuchel H, et al. Tilt training: A new treatment for recurrent neurocardiogenic syncope and severe orthostatic intolerance. *Pacing Clin Electrophysiol* 1998; 21: 193–196.
65. Hoeldtke RD, Streeten DHP, Phil D. Treatment of orthostatic hypotension with erythropoietin. *N Engl J Med* 1993; 329: 611–615.
66. Bousser MG, Dubois B, Castaigne P. Transient loss of consciousness in ischemic cerebral events: A study of 557 ischemic strokes and transient ischemic attacks. *Ann Intern Med* 1980; 132: 300–307.
67. Benbadis SR, Wolgamuth BR, Goren H, et al. Value of tongue biting in the diagnosis of seizures. *Arch Intern Med* 1995; 155:2346–2349.
68. Delanty N, Vaughan CJ, French JA. Medical causes of seizures. *Lancet* 1998; 352:383–390.
69. Weiss S, Baker JP. The carotid sinus reflex in health and disease: Its role in the causation of fainting and convulsions. *Medicine (Baltimore)* 1933; 12:297–354.
70. Graux P, Carlioz R, Guyomar Y, et al. Characteristics and influence of different clinical forms on the development and prog-

nosis of carotid sinus syndrome. *Arch Mal Coeur* 1995; 88:999–1006.
71. El-Sayed H, Hainsworth R. Relationship between plasma volume, carotic baroreceptor sensitivity and orthostatic tolerance. *Clin Sci* 1995; 88:463–470.
72. Nishizaki M, Arita M, Sakurada H, et al. Long-term follow-up of the reproducibility of carotid sinus hypersensitivity in patients with carotid sinus syndrome. *Jpn Circ J* 1995; 59:33–39.
73. Tea SH, Mansourati J, L'Heveder G, et al. New insights into the pathophysiology of carotid sinus syndrome. *Circulation* 1996; 93:1411–1416.
74. Cicogna R, Bonomi FG, Curnis A, et al. Peripharyngeal space lesions syncope-syndrome: A newly proposed reflexogenic cardiovascular syndrome. *Eur Heart J* 1993; 14:1476–1483.
75. Sumiyoshi M, Nakata Y, Mineda Y, et al. Response to head-up tilt testing in patients with situational syncope. *Am J Cardiol* 1998; 82:1117–1118.
76. Mattle HP, Nirkko AC, Baumgartner RW, et al. Transient cerebral circulatory arrest coincides with fainting in cough syncope. *Neurology* 1995; 45:498–501.
77. Bortolotti M, Cirignotta F, Labo G. Atrioventricular block induced by swallowing in a patient with diffuse esophageal spasm. *JAMA* 1982; 248:2297–2299.
78. Ferrante L, Artico M, Nardacci B, et al. Glossopharyngeal neuralgia with cardiac syncope. *Neurosurgery* 1995; 36:58–63.
79. Godec CJ, Cass AS. Micturition syncope. *J Urol* 1981; 126: 551–556.
80. Kapoor WN, Peterson J, Karpf M. Defecation syncope: A symptom with multiple etiologies. *Arch Intern Med* 1986; 146:2377–2382.
81. Jansen RW, Connelly CM, Kelley-Gagnon M, et al. Postprandial hypotension in elderly patients with unexplained syncope. *Arch Intern Med* 1995; 155:945–952.
82. Jansen RWMM, Lipsitz LA. Postprandial hypotension: Epidemiology, pathophysiology, and clinical management. *Ann Intern Med* 1995; 122:286–295.
83. Kapoor WN, Fortunato M, Hanusa BH, et al. Psychiatric illnesses in patients with syncope. *Am J Med* 1995; 99:505–512.
84. Aminoff MJ, Scheimman MM, Griffin JC, et al. Electrocerebral accompaniments of syncope associated with malignant ventricular arrhythmias. *Ann Intern Med* 1988; 108:791–796.
85. Constantin L, Martins JB, Fincham RW, et al. Bradycardia and syncope as manifestations of partial epilepsy. *J Am Coll Cardiol* 1990; 15:900–905.
86. Grech ED, Ramsdale DR. Exertional syncope in aortic stenosis: Evidence to support inappropriate left ventricular baroreceptor response. *Am Heart J* 1991; 121:603–606.
87. Schwartz LS, Goldfisher J, Sprague GJ, et al. Syncope and sudden death in aortic stenosis. *Am J Cardiol* 1969; 23:647–658.
88. Nienaber CA, Hiller S, Speilmann RP, et al. Syncope in hypertrophic cardiomyopathy: Multivariate analysis of prognostic determinants. *J Am Coll Cardiol* 1990; 15:948–955.
89. Dressler W. Effort syncope as an early manifestation of primary pulmonary hypertension. *Am J Med Sci* 1952; 223: 131–143.
90. Scarpa WJ. The sick sinus syndrome. *Am Heart J* 1983; 92: 648–651.
91. Talwar KK, Edvardsson N, Varnauskas E. Paroxysmal vagally mediated AV block with recurrent syncope. *Clin Cardiol* 1985; 8:337–340.
92. Beder SD, Cohen MH, Riemenschneider TA. Occult arrhythmias as the etiology of unexplained syncope in children with structurally normal hearts. *Am Heart J* 1985; 109:309–313.
93. Boudoulas H, Wooley CF. Mitral Valve: *Floppy Mitral Valve, Mitral Valve Prolapse, Mitral Valvular Regurgitation*, 2d ed. Armonk, NY: Futura Publishing Company; 2000.
94. Moss AJ, Schwartz PJ, Crampton RS, et al. The long QT syndrome: Prospective longitudinal study of 328 families. *Circulation* 1991; 84:1136–1144.
95. Menozzi C, Brignole M, Alboni P, et al. The natural course of untreated sick sinus syndrome and identification of the variables predictive of unfavorable outcome. *Am J Cardiol* 1998; 82:1205–1209.
96. Chen SY, Wang YH, Hwang JJ, et al. Pulmonary embolism presenting as syncope in paraplegia: A case report. *Arch Phys Med Rehabil* 1995; 76:387–390.
97. Brignole M, Gianfranchi L, Menozzi C, et al. Role of autonomic reflexes in syncope associated with paroxysmal atrial fibrillation. *J Am Coll Cardiol* 1993; 22:1123–1129.
98. Leitch JW, Klein GJ, Yee R, et al. Syncope associated with supraventricular tachycardia. *Circulation* 1992; 85:1064–1071.
99. Zareba W, Moss AJ, Schwartz PJ, et al. Influence of the genotype on the clinical course of the long-QT syndrome. *N Engl J Med* 1998; 339:960–965.
100. Ausubel K, Boal BH, Furmen S. Pacemaker syndrome: Definition and evaluation. *Cardiol Clin* 1985; 3:587–589.
101. Lamas GA, Orav EJ, Stambler BS, et al. Quality of life and clinical outcomes in elderly patients treated with ventricular pacing as compared with dual-chamber pacing. *N Engl J Med* 1998; 338:1097–1104.
102. Oh JH, Hanusa BH, Kapoor WN. Do symptoms predict cardiac arrhythmias and mortality in patients with syncope? *Arch Intern Med* 1999; 159:375–380.
103. Corrado D, Basso C, Thiene G, et al. Spectrum of clinicopathologic manifestations of arrhythmogenic right ventricular cardiomyopathy/dysplasia: A multicenter study. *J Am Coll Cardiol* 1997; 30:1512–1520.
104. Winters SL, Stewart D, Gomes JA. Signal averaging of the surface QRS complex predicts inducibility of ventricular tachycardia in patients with syncope of unknown origin: A prospective study. *J Am Coll Cardiol* 1987; 10:775–781.
105. Nalos PC, Gang ES, Mandel WJ, et al. The signal averaged electrocardiogram as a screening test for inducibility of sustained ventricular tachycardia in high risk patients: A prospective study. *J Am Coll Cardiol* 1987; 9:539–548.
106. Cain ME, Anderson JL, Arnsdorf MF, et al. ACC Expert Consensus Document: Signal-averaged electrocardiography. *J Am Coll Cardiol* 1996; 27:238–249.
107. Steinberg JS, Prystowsky E, Freedman RA, et al. Use of the signal-averaged electrocardiogram for predicting inducible ventricular tachycardia in patients with unexplained syncope: Relation to clinical variables in a multivariate analysis. *J Am Coll Cardiol* 1994; 23:99–106.
108. Boudoulas H, Schaal SF, Lewis RP, et al. Superiority of 24-hour outpatient monitoring over multi-stage exercise testing for the evaluation of syncope. *J Electrocardiol* 1979; 12:103–108.
109. Boudoulas H, Geleris P, Schaal SF, et al. Comparison between electrophysiologic studies and ambulatory monitoring in patients with syncope. *J Electrocardiol* 1983; 16:91–96.
110. Dewey RC, Capeless MA, Levy AM. Use of ambulatory electrocardiographic monitoring to identify high-risk patients with congenital complete heart block. *N Engl J Med* 1987; 316: 835–839.
111. Linzer M, Prystowsky EN, Brunetti LL, et al. Recurrent syncope of unknown origin diagnosed by ambulatory continuous loop ECG recording. *Am Heart J* 1988; 116:1632–1634.
112. Fetter JG, Stanton MS, Benditt DG, et al. Transtelephonic monitoring and transmission of stored arrhythmia detection and therapy data from an implantable cardioverter defibrillator. *Pacing Clin Electrophysiol* 1995; 18:1531–1539.
113. Kinlay S, Leitch JW, Neil A, et al. Cardiac event recorders yield more diagnoses and are more cost-effective than 48-hour Holter monitoring in patients with palpitations. *Ann Intern Med* 1996; 124:16–20.

114. Krahn AD, Klein GJ, Yee R, et al. Use of an extended monitoring strategy in patients with problematic syncope. *Circulation* 1999; 99:406–410.
115. Zimetbaum PJ, Kim KY, Josephson ME, et al. Diagnostic yield and optimal duration of continuous-loop event monitoring for the diagnosis of palpitations. *Ann Intern Med* 1998; 128:890–895.
116. Kushner JA, Kou WH, Kadish AM, et al. Natural history of patients with unexplained syncope and a nondiagnostic electrophysiologic study. *J Am Coll Cardiol* 1989; 74:391–396.
117. Boudoulas H, Schaal SF, Lewis RP. Electrophysiologic risk factors in syncope. *J Electrocardiol* 1978; 11:339–342.
118. Englund A, Bergfeldt L, Rehnqvist N, et al. Diagnostic value of programmed ventricular stimulation in patients with bifascicular block: A prospective study of patients with and without syncope. *J Am Coll Cardiol* 1995; 26:1508–1515.
119. Bellinder G, Nordlander R, Pehrsson SK, et al. Atrial pacing in the management of sick sinus syndrome: Long-term observation for conduction disturbances and supraventricular tachyarrhythmias. *Eur Heart J* 1986; 7:105–109.
120. Moss AJ, Liu JE, Gottlieb S, et al. Efficacy of permanent pacing in the management of high-risk patients with long QT syndrome. *Circulation* 1991; 84:1524–1529.
121. Link MS, Kim KMS, Homoud MK, et al. Long-term outcome of patients with syncope associated with coronary artery disease and a nondiagnostic electrophysiologic evaluation. *Am J Cardiol* 1999; 83:1334–1337.
122. Nishimura RA, Giuliani ER, Brandenburg RO, et al. Hypertrophic cardiomyopathy. In: Giuliani ER, Gersh BJ, McGoon MD, eds. *Mayo Clinic Practice of Cardiology,* 3d ed. St. Louis: CV Mosby; 1996:689.
123. Henein MY, O'Sullivan CA, Ramzy IS, et al. Electromechanical left ventricular behavior after nonsurgical septal reduction in patients with hypertrophic obstructive cardiomyopathy. *J Am Coll Cardiol* 1999; 34:1117–1122.
124. Ommen SR, Nishimura RA, Squires RW, et al. Comparison of dual-chamber pacing versus septal myectomy for the treatment of patients with hypertrophic obstructive cardiomyopathy. *J Am Coll Cardiol* 1999; 34:191–196.
125. Fananapazir L. Advances in molecular genetics and management of hypertrophic cardiomyopathy. *JAMA* 1999; 281:1746–1747.
126. Henein MY, O'Sullivan C, Sutton GC, et al. Stress-induced left ventricular outflow tract obstruction: A potential cause of dyspnea in the elderly. *J Am Coll Cardiol* 1997; 30:1301–1307.
127. Spirito P, Maton BJ. Perspectives on the role of new treatment strategies in hypertrophic obstructive cardiomyopathy. *J Am Coll Cardiol* 1999; 33:1071–1075.
128. Kappenberger L, Linde C, McKenna DW, et al. Pacing in hypertrophic obstructive cardiomyopathy: A randomized crossover study. *Eur Heart J* 1997; 18:1249–1256.
129. Suda K, Kohl T, Kovalchin JP, et al. Echocardiographic predictors of poor outcome in infants with hypertrophic cardiomyopathy. *Am J Cardiol* 1997; 80:595–600.
130. Knight C, Kurbaan AS, Seggewiss H, et al. Nonsurgical septal reduction for hypertrophic obstructive cardiomyopathy: Outcome in the first series of patients. *Circulation* 1997; 95:2075–2081.
131. Jackman WM, Xunzhang W, Friday K, et al. Catheter ablation of accessory atrioventricular pathways (Wolff-Parkinson-White syndrome) by radio-frequency current. *N Engl J Med* 1991; 324:1605–1611.
132. Calkins H, Sousa J, El-Atassi R, et al. Diagnosis and cure of the Wolff-White-Parkinson syndrome or paroxysmal supraventricular tachycardia during a single electrophysiologic test. *N Engl J Med* 1991; 324:1612–1618.
133. Weiner DA, Levine SR, Klein MD. Ventricular arrhythmias during exercise testing: Mechanism, response to coronary bypass surgery and prognostic significance. *Am J Cardiol* 1984; 53:1553–1559.
134. Mirowski M, Reid PR, Mower MM, et al. Termination of malignant ventricular arrhythmias with an implanted automatic defibrillator in human beings. *N Engl J Med* 1980; 330:322–324.
135. Jung W, Anderson M, Camm AJ, et al. Recommendations for driving of patients with implantable cardioverter defibrillators. *Eur Heart J* 1997; 18:1210–1219.
136. Olatidoye AG, Verroneau J, Kluger J. Mechanisms of syncope in implantable cardioverter-defibrillator recipients who receive device therapies. *Am J Cardiol* 1998; 82:1372–1376.
137. Mittal S, Iwai S, Stein KM, et al. Long-term outcome of patients with unexplained syncope treated with an electrophysiologic-guided approach in the implantable cardioverter-defibrillator era. *J Am Coll Cardiol* 1999; 34:1082–1089.
138. Knight BP, Goyal R, Pelosi F, et al. Outcome of patients with nonischemic dilated cardiomyopathy and unexplained syncope treated with an implantable defibrillator. *J Am Coll Cardiol* 1999; 33:1964–1970.
139. De Divitiis M, Galderisi M, Santangelo L, et al. Impact of heart rate and atrioventricular delay on left ventricular diastolic filling in patients with dual-chamber pacing for sick sinus syndrome or atrioventricular block. *Am J Cardiol* 1998; 82:816–820.
140. Lipsitz LA. Syncope in the elderly. *Ann Intern Med* 1983; 99:92–105.
141. Jonsson PV, Lipsitz LA, Kelley M, et al. Hypotensive responses to common daily activities in institutionalized elderly. *Arch Intern Med* 1990; 150:1518–1524.
142. Lipsitz LA, Nyquist RP Jr, Wei JY, et al. Postprandial reduction in blood pressure in the elderly. *N Engl J Med* 1983; 309: 81–83.
143. O'Mahony D. Pathophysiology of carotid sinus hypersensitivity in elderly patients. *Lancet* 1995; 346:950–952.
144. Rehm CG, Ross SE. Syncope as etiology of road crashes involving elderly drivers. *Am Surg* 1995; 61:1006–1008.
145. Rehm CG, Ross SE. Elderly drivers involved in road crashes: A profile. *Am Surg* 1995; 61:435–437.
146. Lurie KG, Iskos D, Sakaguchi S, et al. Resumption of motor vehicle operation in vasovagal fainters. *Am J Cardiol* 1999; 83:604–606.
147. Bondar RL, Kassam MS, Stein F, et al. Simultaneous cerebrovascular and cardiovascular responses during presyncope. *Stroke* 1995; 26:1794–1800.
148. Middlekauff HR, Stevenson WG, Stevenson LW, et al. Syncope in advanced heart failure: High risk of sudden death regardless of origin of syncope. *J Am Coll Cardiol* 1993; 21:110–116.
149. Kapoor WN, Hanusa BH. Is syncope a risk factor for poor outcomes? Comparison of patients with and without syncope. *Am J Med* 1996; 100:646–655.
150. Lascault G, Barnay C, Cazeau S, et al. Etude preliminaire d'un stimulateur double chambre a fonction diagnostique. *Arch Mal Coeur* 1995; 88:451–457.
151. Leenhardt A, Lucet V, Denjoy I, et al. Catecholaminergic polymorphic ventricular tachycardia in children: A 7-year follow-up of 21 patients. *Circulation* 1995; 91:1512–1519.
152. Salim MA, DiSessa TG. QT interval response to exercise in children with syncope. *Am J Cardiol* 1994; 73:976–978.
153. Noh CI, Song JY, Kim HS, et al. Ventricular tachycardia and exercise related syncope in children with structurally normal hearts: Emphasis on repolarization abnormality. *Br Heart J* 1995; 73:544–547.
154. Sinkovec M, Rakovec P, Zorman D, et al. Exertional syncope in a patient with aortic stenosis and right coronary artery disease. *Eur Heart J* 1995; 16:276–278.
155. Williams CC, Bernhardt DT. Syncope in athletes. *Sports Med* 1995; 19:223–234.
156. Thomson HL, Atherton JJ, Khafagi FA, et al. Failure of reflex venoconstriction during exercise in patients with vasovagal syncope. *Circulation* 1996; 93:953–959.

157. Balaji S, Oslizlok PC, Allen MC, et al. Neurocardiogenic syncope in children with a normal heart. *J Am Coll Cardiol* 1994; 23:779–785.
158. Liberthson RR. Sudden death from cardiac causes in children and young adults. *N Engl J Med* 1996; 334:1039–1044.
159. Boudoulas H, Lewis RP. Cardiac syncope: Diagnosis, mechanism, and management. In: Hurst JW, ed. *The Heart,* 6th ed. New York: McGraw-Hill; 1986:321.
160. Calkins H, Shyr Y, Frumin H, et al. The value of the clinical history in the differentiation of syncope due to ventricular tachycardia, atrioventricular block, and neurocardiogenic syncope. *Am J Med* 1995; 98:365–373.
161. Kapoor WN. Workup and management of patients with syncope. *Med Clin North Am* 1995; 79:1153–1170.
162. Gilman JK. Syncope in the emergency department. *Emerg Med Clin North Am* 1995; 13:955–971.
163. Kroenke K, Lucas CA, Rosenberg ML, et al. Causes of persistent dizziness: A prospective study of 100 patients in ambulatory care. *Ann Intern Med* 1992; 117:898–904.
164. Krahn AD, Klein GJ, Norris C, et al. The etiology of syncope in patients with negative tilt table and electrophysiological testing. *Circulation* 1995; 92:1819–1824.
165. Schaal SF, Nelson SD, Boudoulas H, Lewis RP. Syncope. *Curr Probl Cardiol* 1992; 14:211–264.

C H A P T E R 33

SUDDEN CARDIAC DEATH

Duane S. Pinto / Mark E. Josephson

DEFINITION OF SUDDEN CARDIAC DEATH

Sudden cardiac death describes the unexpected natural death due to a cardiac cause within a short time period from the onset of symptoms in a person without any prior condition that would appear fatal. It is most often due to a sustained ventricular tachyarrhythmia. Disparities in definitions have led to differences in the classification of deaths and have influenced the outcomes of studies looking at the incidence of sudden cardiac death.[1–11] The definition of sudden cardiac death should include the time interval from onset of the symptoms leading to collapse and then to death, the unexpected nature of the event, and the specific cause of death. Although many cardiovascular disorders increase the risk of sudden cardiac death, the presence or absence of preexisting cardiovascular disease is not necessary. More recent definitions have focused on time intervals of 1 h or less, which normally identify sudden cardiac death populations having a high proportion (up to 91 percent) of arrhythmic death.[12,13] The information necessary to establish a diagnosis of sudden cardiac death is often not available. For instance, up to 40 percent of sudden deaths are not witnessed, making a determination of the time of onset of symptoms to loss of consciousness impossible.[14–16] Prodromal symptoms such as palpitations, chest pain, and dyspnea may suggest a cardiovascular etiology such as arrhythmia, ischemia, or congestive heart failure but are not specific.[11,17]

Advances in emergency medical services, technological advances such as automatic external defibrillators, and community-based interventions have resulted in a contradiction in terms. Biologic death is an absolute and irreversible event, while patients can survive a cardiac arrest that would lead to sudden cardiac death if left untreated. Processes such as malignant arrhythmias, pump failure, and coronary ischemia that initiate the cascade of events leading to cardiovascular collapse can be modified, and the episode of sudden cardiac death can be averted. Ultimately, though, the distinction between sudden cardiac death, nonsudden cardiac death, and noncardiac death is relevant more from a historical perspective, and total mortality rate is a more definitive end point in assessing the efficacy of an intervention aimed at improving survival.

EPIDEMIOLOGY

Incidence

Sudden cardiac death accounts for approximately 300,000 to 400,000 deaths yearly in the United States, depending on the definition used (Table 33-1).[1–11] When its definition is restricted to death less than 2 h from onset of symptoms, 12 percent of all natural deaths were sudden, and 88 percent of those were due to cardiac disease. In autopsy-based studies, a cardiac etiology of

TABLE 33-1 Incidence of Sudden Cardiac Death in Selected Regional Population Studies

Study	Patient Population	Definition of Sudden Cardiac Death	SCD (CHD Deaths)	Annual Incidence of SCD (per 1000 population)	Known CHD, %	Proportion of CHD Deaths, %	Comments
Framingham,[1–3] 1948–1974	5128 M + F 30–62 years; no prior CHD	<1 h	M: 160 (350) F: 73 (196)	*Age:* *45–54* *55–64* *65–74* M: 1.1 2.7 2.6 F: 0.3 0.4 1.2	M: 50 F: 36	M: 46 F: 35	18% M (24% F) had SCD as first symptom of CHD
Tecumseh,[4] 1959–1965	M + F ≥30 years	<1 h		2.0	40	46	
Baltimore,[5,6] 1964–1965	M + F 40–64 years	<24 h, witnessed	661 (1098)	*<2 h* *2–24 h* M: 2.02 1.14 F: 0.39 0.34	51	60	
Allegheny,[7] 1970–1981	White M 35–44 years	<24 h, OOH, no disability	433		43	78	50% decline in CHD mortality, 77% due to decrease in SCD mortality
Worcester,[8] 1975–1988	M + F ≥25 years	OOH + ER		*1975* *1978* *1981* *1984* 2.65 1.74 1.70 1.48			
Minnesota,[9] 1970–1980	M + F 30–74 years	OOH + ER		*Year:* *1970* *1980* M: 3.11 2.44 F: 0.96 0.7	M: 26[a] F: 16	M: 67 F: 60	
40 U.S. states,[10] 1980–1985	M + F 35–74 years	OOH + ER	223,864 (399,324)	M: 1.91[b] F: 0.57	56	M: 60 F: 50	
Denmark,[11] 1982	M + F ≥25 years	<24 h	166	*Age:* *25–50* *50–69* *≥70* M: 1.1 2.7 2.6 F: 0.3 0.4 1.2	75	13% of all deaths (1309)	19% had no prodrome or known heart disease

[a]Acute myocardial infarction only.
[b]White population only.
ABBREVIATIONS: CHD = coronary heart disease; ER = emergency room; F = female; M = male; OOH = out-of-hospital; SCD = sudden cardiac death.

sudden death has been reported in 60 to 70 percent of sudden death victims.[15,16] Sudden cardiac death is the most common and often the first manifestation of coronary heart disease (CHD) and is responsible for half the deaths from cardiovascular disease, which remains the main cause of death in this country. In the Framingham Study,[1–3] a 26-year survey of 5128 subjects (age 30 to 62) without evidence of cardiac disease at entry, 13 percent of all natural deaths were sudden, accounting for 50 percent of the deaths from CHD. Fifty percent of sudden cardiac deaths in men and 64 percent in women occurred in people without known CHD. The proportion of sudden cardiac death was lower (20 to 34 percent) in patients with known CHD. Sudden cardiac death was the first symptom of CHD in 10 percent of all coronary events in men and 8 percent of those in women.

The overall annual incidence of sudden cardiac death in the United States is probably best estimated with data derived from the National Center for Health Statistics.[10] This data base from 40 states represents 71 percent of the U.S. population. Based on a combination of the place of death (out of hospital or emergency room) and diagnosis of CHD as an estimate of sudden cardiac death, the sudden cardiac death incidence in 1985 was 1.9 in men and 0.6 in women, resulting in 223,864 deaths of a total of 399,324 deaths from ischemic heart disease. Sudden cardiac death rates in developed countries outside the United States are comparable to those inside the United States. Using methods similar to those of the National Center for Health Statistics study,[10] the World Health Organization reported an annual incidence of sudden cardiac death of 1.9 in men and 0.6 in women, again accounting for nearly half the deaths from CHD in a surveillance study of 3.5 million men and women aged 20 to 64 years.[17] Sudden cardiac death rates in developing countries are considerably lower, paralleling the rates of ischemic heart disease as a whole (Fig. 33-1). In the United States, several populations-based studies have documented a decline (15 to 19 percent) in the incidence of sudden cardiac deaths caused by CHD since the early 1980s.[7,18]

Influence of Age, Race, and Gender

AGE

The incidence of sudden cardiac death increases with age in men and women as well as whites and nonwhites because of the higher prevalence of ischemic heart disease at older ages (Fig. 33-2).[3] Among sudden natural deaths, the proportion of cardiac causes increases with advancing age. Among patients with CHD, however, the proportion of coronary deaths that are sudden decreases with age.[1,3]

RACIAL DIFFERENCES

An analysis of cardiac death rates from 40 U.S. states between 1980 and 1985 showed that the rate of sudden coronary death is higher in blacks than in whites (men, 66 versus 61 percent; women, 56 versus 50 percent).[10] The annual age-adjusted incidence of sudden cardiac death in a cohort of 860 white and 117 black cardiac arrest victims in Seattle between 1984 and 1986 was also higher in blacks than in whites: 3.4 percent versus 1.6 percent per 1000 population (p <.001).[19] A similar difference was reported in an analysis of 6451 cardiac arrest victims in Chicago.[20] Not only was the sudden cardiac death rate higher, but the overall survival was also lower in blacks than in whites (10.2 percent versus 16.7 percent, p <.07, in Seattle, and 0.8 percent versus 2.6 percent, p <.001, in Chicago). In both studies, blacks were less likely to receive bystander cardiopulmonary resuscitation (CPR); however, differences in outcome could not be accounted for by differences in emergency medical team response time or administration of advanced cardiac life support. Possible explanations for these findings include limitations in access to preventive care, prehospital delays in patient activation of emergency medical services, and denial or self-treatment of prodromal symptoms. Blacks are also prescribed diuretics more often than whites, leading to an increased risk of hypokalemia and possibly sudden cardiac death.[2] These issues warrant further investigation.

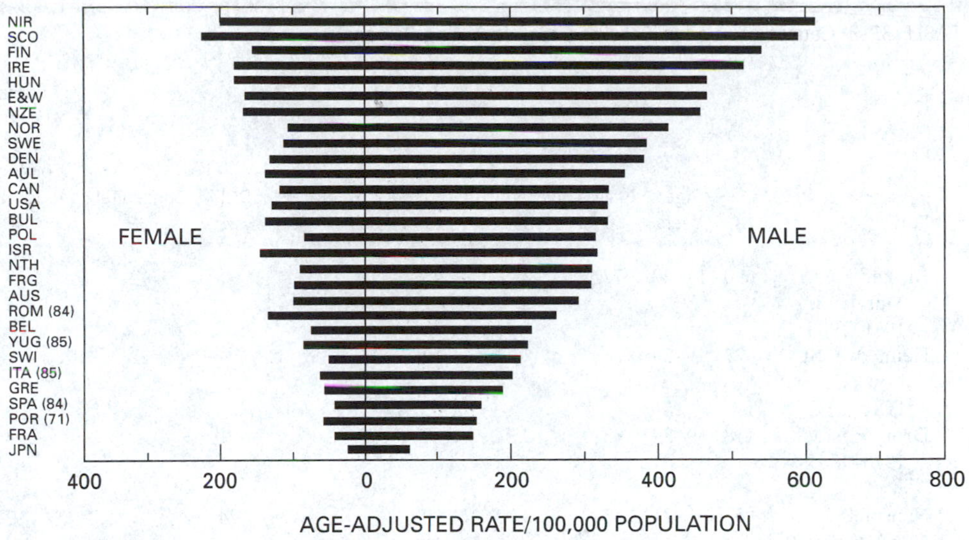

FIGURE 33-1 Sudden cardiac death rates by gender and country, ages 35 to 74 years, compiled from death certificates by the World Health Organization, Geneva, 1986. (From Manolio TA, Furberg CD. Epidemiology of sudden cardiac death. In: Akhtar M, Myerburg RJ, Ruskin JN, eds. *Sudden Cardiac Death*. Baltimore: Williams & Wilkins; 1994:3. Reproduced with permission from the publisher and authors.)

GENDER

Sudden cardiac death has a much higher incidence in men than in women, reflecting gender differences in the incidence of CHD.[1–3] Between 70 and 89 percent of sudden cardiac deaths occur in men, and the annual incidence of sudden cardiac death in men is overall three to four times higher than in women. As is the case with coronary disease, however, this disparity decreases with advancing age, with a male–female ratio for sudden cardiac death of 7:1 in 45- to 64-year-olds and 2:1 in 65- to 74-year-olds.

A higher percentage (64 percent) of sudden cardiac death in women than in men (50 percent) occurs in patients without prior evidence of coronary heart disease.[3] Among survivors of cardiac arrest, women are more likely than men to have other forms of structural heart disease (valvular heart disease, 13 percent versus 5 percent; idiopathic dilated cardiomyopathy, 19 percent versus 10 percent) or a "normal" heart (10 percent versus 3 percent).[21]

SUDDEN CARDIAC DEATH IN THE YOUNG

Sudden cardiac death accounts for 19 percent of sudden deaths in children between 1 and 13 years of age and 30 percent between 14 and 21 years.[22] The overall incidence is low, 600 cases per year, compared with approximately 300,000 per year in the adult population. Structural cardiac abnormalities can be identified in over 90 percent of young victims of sudden cardiac death (Table 33-2).[22–34] About 40 percent of sudden cardiac deaths in the pediatric population occur in patients with surgically treated congenital cardiac abnormalities; in the majority of young victims, however, sudden cardiac death is often the first manifestation of underlying cardiac disease in otherwise healthy-appearing individuals.[35] The most common underlying pathologic conditions in people who die of sudden cardiac death in the first three decades of life are myocarditis, hypertrophic cardiomyopathy, congenital coronary artery anomalies, atherosclerotic coronary heart disease, conduction system abnormali-

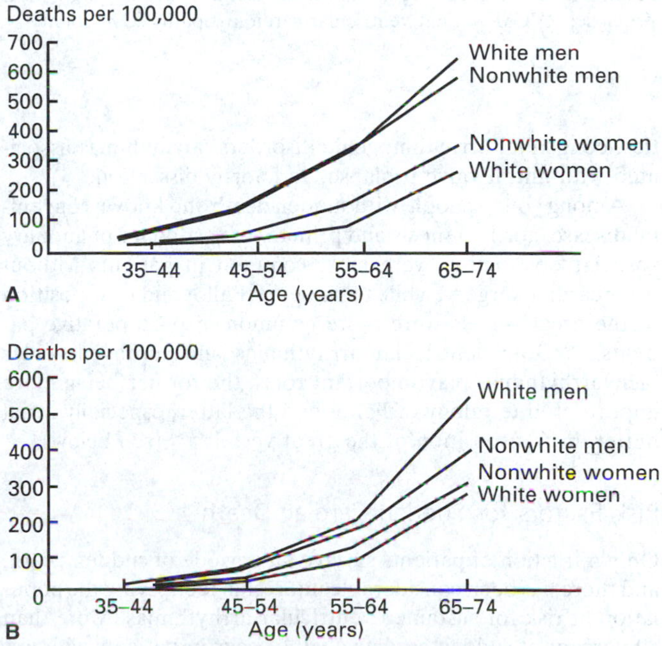

FIGURE 33-2 Plots of mortality rates (deaths per 100,000) for ischemic heart disease occurring (*A*) out of hospital or in emergency room (an estimate for sudden cardiac death rate) and (*B*) in the hospital, by age, gender, and race in 40 states during 1985. (From the National Center for Health Statistics. Reproduced from Gillum,[10] with permission.)

TABLE 33-2 Causes of Sudden Cardiac Death in Young Persons

Study	n	Age, Years	Male, %	Myocarditis, %	CHD, %	HCM, %	RVCM, %	DCM, %	Congenital, %	Primary Arrhythmia or Conduction Abnormality, %	MVP, %	Preceding Symptoms	Exertion Related, %
Burke,[24] Maryland, 1981–1988	690	14–40	77	5	48	10			2	3			5
Kennedy,[25] St. Louis C., 1981–1982	27	1–29			19	11			22				8
Drory,[26] Israel, 1976–1985	118	9–39	83	25	58	13				4		Dizziness, chest pain, syncope (54%)	23
Neuspiel,[22] Allegheny C., 1972–1980	51	1–21	58	27	10			24		12		Prior heart disease (41%)	22
Topaz,[28] St. Paul, 1960–1983	50	7–35	58	24	4	12			6		24	Family history (16%)	16
Thiene,[31] Northern Italy, 1979–1993	163	18–35		7	35	6	12	5	5	10	10		
Keeling,[33] Oxford, UK, 1965–1984	42	2–20		14	2	12		7	64				
Shen,[34] Olmstead C., 1960–1984	31	20–40	65	10	46	5	8		10	5			3

ABBREVIATIONS: CHD = coronary heart disease; DCM = dilated cardiomyopathy; HCM = hypertrophic cardiomyopathy; MVP = mitral valve prolapse; RVCM = right ventricular cardiomyopathy; C = county.

ties, congenital arrhythmogenic disorders, arrhythmias associated with mitral valve prolapse, and aortic dissection.

Among young people with sudden death and known congenital disease, aortic stenosis and primary or secondary pulmonary vascular obstruction were most common in patients without prior cardiac surgery, while tetralogy of Fallot and transposition of the great vessels were more common in postoperative patients.[35,36] Both ventricular arrhythmias and supraventricular tachyarrhythmias play important roles, the former being more important in tetralogy of Fallot and the latter, especially atrial flutter, in transposition of the great vessels[37–39] (see below).

Risk Factors for Sudden Cardiac Death

Only a fraction of patients survive an episode of sudden death, and there has been considerable interest in identifying the population at risk for sustained ventricular arrhythmias. More than 80 percent of sudden cardiac deaths occur in patients with underlying coronary disease, and the risk factors for sudden cardiac death largely reflect those for CHD (see Chap. 35). Left ventricular dysfunction and CHD confer the highest risk for sudden cardiac death.[40] In the Framingham Study, a multivariate model based on risk factors such as age, systolic blood pressure, left ventricular hypertrophy, intraventricular block or nonspecific abnormalities on the electrocardiogram (ECG), elevated serum cholesterol level, glucose intolerance, decreased vital capacity, smoking, relative weight, and heart rate found that 53 percent of men and 42 percent of women who were at risk for sudden death were in the upper decile of this analysis (Fig. 33-3).[1–3]

Despite the fact that numerous population-based studies have shown a strong relationship between risk factors for CHD and sudden cardiac death, none of them has identified a single set of risk factors that are specific for sudden cardiac death (Table 33-3).[1,2,40–43] The inability to determine a profile based on coronary risk factors that is specific for sudden cardiac death reflects the fact that these factors are manifestations of chronic disease processes that create the structural basis for sustained arrhythmia. These structural abnormalities may be necessary but are not sufficient to cause an episode of sudden cardiac death. Triggers such as acute ischemia, alterations in hemodynamic status, electrolyte abnormalities, transient drug or toxin effects, or circadian variations in vasoconstriction, plaque stability, and thrombosis may precipitate an event.[44–46] A challenge for the future will be to identify these triggers so that patients at risk for malignant arrhythmias can be targeted for intervention.

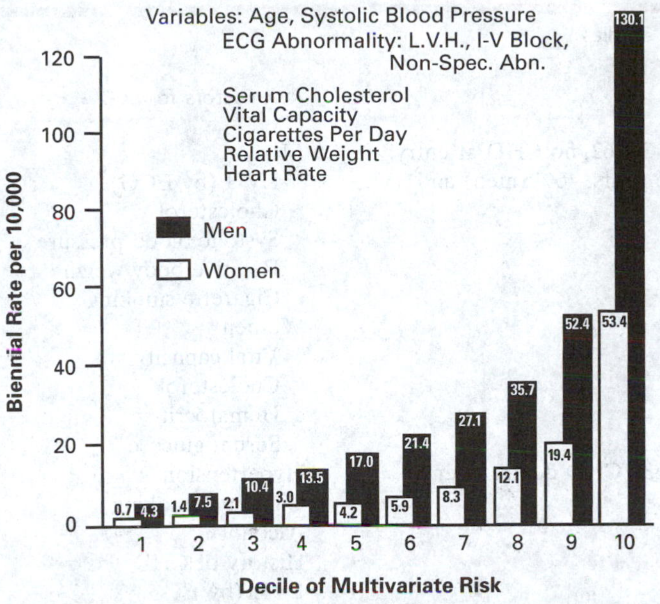

FIGURE 33-3 Risk of sudden cardiac death by decile of multivariate risk: 26-year follow-up, the Framingham Study. ECG, electrocardiographic; I-V, intraventricular; LVH, left ventricular hypertrophy; Non-Spec. Abn., nonspecific abnormality. (Reproduced from Kannel and Schatzkin,[2] with permission.)

LIFESTYLE FACTORS

Observations suggest that changes in lifestyle factors can be of potential importance in protecting patients with CHD from dying suddenly.[1,2,47–57]

Alcohol Individuals who consume high amounts of alcohol (more than 5 drinks per day) have increased risks of ventricular arrhythmia and sudden cardiac death. The relationship is less clear for drinkers of light to moderate amounts. A recent prospective analysis of 21,537 males in the Physicians Health Study demonstrated a decreased risk of sudden cardiac death. Men who consumed light to moderate amounts of alcohol (2 to 6 drinks per week) had a significantly reduced risk of sudden cardiac death compared with those who rarely or never consumed alcohol.[47,48]

Cigarette Smoking Smoking is one of the few coronary risk factors that has been associated with a disproportionate number of sudden deaths as compared to coronary deaths. Smoking has been shown to induce physiologic changes that predispose to sudden cardiac death, such as increases in platelet adhesiveness, decreases in ventricular fibrillation threshold, acceleration of heart rate, increases in blood pressure, induction of coronary spasm, decreases in oxygen-carrying capacity of the circulation by accumulation of carboxyhemoglobin and impairment of myoglobin utilization, and short-term nicotine-induced catecholamine release.[49] A postmortem study linked smoking and the presence of acute coronary thrombus. Fresh thrombus was found in 59 of 113 men who died suddenly, and cigarette smoking was a risk factor in 75 percent of these men, compared with 41 percent of the men with stable plaques ($p < .001$).[50] In the Framingham Study, the annual incidence of sudden cardiac deaths increased from 13 per 1000 in nonsmokers to 31 per 1000 in those smoking more than 20 cigarettes per day.[1,2,49] People who stopped smoking had a prompt reduction in CHD mortality rate compared with those who continued to smoke, irrespective of the duration of previous smoking habits.[51]

Stress and Socioeconomic Status There are many reports linking stress, particularly emotional stress, to sudden cardiac death.[52–54] For instance, in the hours following the Northridge earthquake in California in 1994, there was a more than fourfold increase in sudden cardiac death in patients with known or unknown CHD, illustrating the role of emotional stress as trigger for sudden cardiac death in this population.[55] Based on the difference of average and actual daily sudden cardiac death rates in that period, it was estimated that as many as 40 percent of sudden cardiac deaths are precipitated by emotional stress.

Socioeconomic factors, presumably associated with higher levels of stress, can also contribute to sudden cardiac death. For instance, a more than threefold increase of sudden cardiac death following myocardial infarction was reported in men with low levels of education and complex ventricular ectopy compared with better-educated men with the same arrhythmias.[56] In a study of sudden cardiac death in women, those who died suddenly were less often married, had fewer children, and had greater educational discrepancies with their spouses than did age-matched controls in the same neighborhood.[57]

Physical Activity There is increasing evidence that regular physical activity may help prevent CHD and its complications.[2,58–62] On the other hand, the value of vigorous exercise in patients with known CHD is controversial, and several clinical and autopsy-based studies have reported triggering of sudden cardiac death and acute myocardial infarction by vigorous exercise.[63–66] Emergency medical records show that in adults, 11 to 17 percent of cardiac arrest victims collapsed during or immediately after exertion, although the amount of exertion is rarely quantified.[59] The increased risk of cardiac arrest due to ventricular fibrillation during or after exercise is also evident from cardiac rehabilitation programs and exercise stress testing in patients with heart disease. These studies are of selected patients with known heart disease who are already at risk for sudden death, but in these situations, cardiac arrests rates of 1 in 12,000 to 15,000 (rehabilitation) and 1 per 2000 (stress testing) have been reported. This rate is at least six times higher than the general incidence of sudden cardiac death for patients known to have heart disease.[59] Because of immediate and successful defibrillation in most cases, these reported cases of cardiac arrest have rarely been fatal. These observations, however, do support the concept that vigorous physical activity can trigger cardiac arrest due to ventricular fibrillation. On the other hand, there is increasing experimental evidence that regular exercise may prevent ischemia-induced ventricular fibrillation and death.[60,65] Thus, it appears that regular participation in moderate-intensity activities is associated with reduced rates of cardiovascular morbidity and mortality, while the risks of sudden cardiac death and myocardial infarction are transiently increased during acute bouts of high-intensity activity.

SUDDEN CARDIAC DEATH IN COMPETITIVE ATHLETES Sudden cardiac death in competitive athletes is an extremely rare event. Between 10 and 25 sports-related sudden deaths from cardiac causes occur annually in the United States.[23] The annual incidence of sudden cardiac death during exercise is 1 per 200,000

TABLE 33-3 Risk Factors for Sudden Cardiac Death in Population-Based Studies

Study	Study Population	Risk Factors for SCD
Kannel et al.[1,2] (Framingham Study)	5128 men and women, age 30–62, no CHD at entry: 546 CHD deaths over 26 years, 46% (men) and 35% (women) SCD	Men LVH (by ECG) Cholesterol Systolic blood pressure Relative body weight Cigarette smoking Women Vital capacity Cholesterol Hematocrit Serum glucose
Hinkle et al.[40]	269,755 men, age 20–65: 1839 CHD deaths over 5 years, 60% SCD	Hypertension Cigarette smoking Alcohol History of CHD LVH (by ECG) Enlarged heart (CXR) CHF PVCs
Demirovic[41] (Yugoslavia Cardiovascular Disease study)	6614 men, age 35–62, no CHD at entry: 143 CHD deaths over 15 years, 75% SCD	Age Blood pressure Cigarette smoking
Beaglehole et al.,[42] Aukland, New Zealand	300 cases of SCD, age <70	Cigarette smoking Low-level HDL
Kagan et al.,[43] Hawaii	7591 middle-aged Japanese men living in Hawaii	Blood pressure Cholesterol Cigarette smoking Positive family history LVH (by ECG)

ABBREVIATIONS: CHD = coronary heart disease; CHF = congestive heart failure; CXR = chest x-ray; HDL = high-density lipoproteins; LVH = left ventricular hypertrophy; PVC = premature ventricular contraction; SCD = sudden cardiac death.

in competitive high school athletes[29] and 1 per 250,000 among unscreened young runners.[67] Collapse usually occurs during or shortly after exercise, either in training or during competition. Although, unfortunately, sudden cardiac death is often the first manifestation of their disease, the majority of sudden cardiac deaths in athletes occur in persons with underlying cardiac disease.[24,68–70] Age has been shown to be the most useful variable in predicting the underlying cardiac disease (Fig. 33-4). In athletes below 35 years of age, the vast majority of sudden cardiac deaths arise from a variety of congenital cardiovascular diseases, most commonly hypertrophic cardiomyopathy (36 percent) and congenital coronary artery anomalies (19 percent).[69] Arrhythmogenic right ventricular dysplasia, myocarditis, arrhythmias associated with mitral valve prolapse, the Wolff-Parkinson-White syndrome, and aortic dissection are much less common. Coronary artery disease was present in 10 percent, compared with 80 percent in those older than 35 years.[68] Arrhythmogenic right ventricular dysplasia was the most common finding in a cohort from northern Italy, accounting for 22 percent.[71] Hypertrophic cardiomyopathy accounted for only 2 percent of sudden cardiac deaths in this population.[72]

Screening programs for identifying relatively rare cardiac abnormalities in a large population of asymptomatic athletes are often costly and inefficient.[73] Guidelines for such screening have therefore been published. They are based mainly on detailed personal and family history, physical examination, and ECG, with echocardiography and other noninvasive tests reserved for those with any positive finding during the initial evaluation.[74] Guidelines have also been published outlining which athletes with cardiac arrhythmias can participate in competitive athletics[74] (see also Chap. 85).

MECHANISM OF SUDDEN CARDIAC DEATH

Relationship between Structure and Function in Sudden Cardiac Death

A vast majority of patients who have experienced sudden cardiac death have cardiac structural abnormalities. In the adult population, these consist predominantly of coronary heart disease, cardiomyopathies, valvular heart disease, and abnormalities of the conduction system. These structural changes provide the substrate for ventricular tachyarrhythmias that are the cause of sudden cardiac death in most cases. It is important to recognize the role of triggering factors, such as fluctuations in the

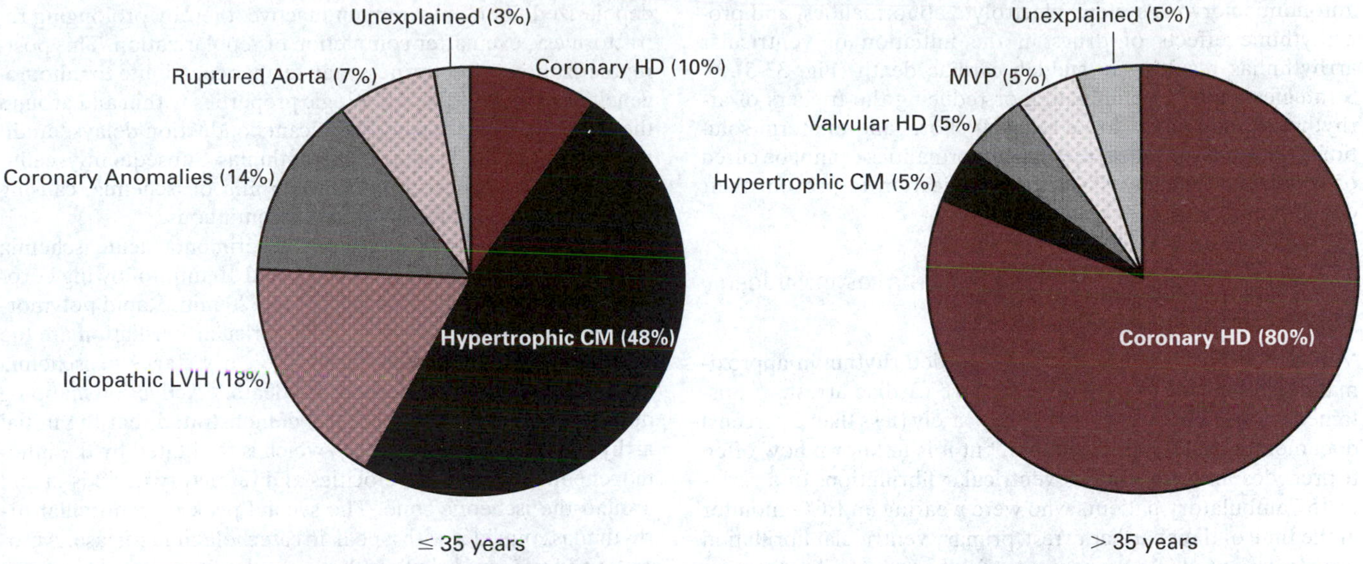

FIGURE 33-4 Causes of sudden cardiac death in competitive athletes by age group. There is evidence of structural heart disease in nearly all athletes who die suddenly of cardiac causes. In athletes younger than 35 years, hypertrophic cardiomyopathy is more prevalent, while, in those older than 35 years, coronary heart disease is the most frequent cause. CM, cardiomyopathy; HD, heart disease; LVH, left ventricular hypertrophy; MVP, mitral valve prolapse. (Reproduced from Maron et al.,[69] with permission.)

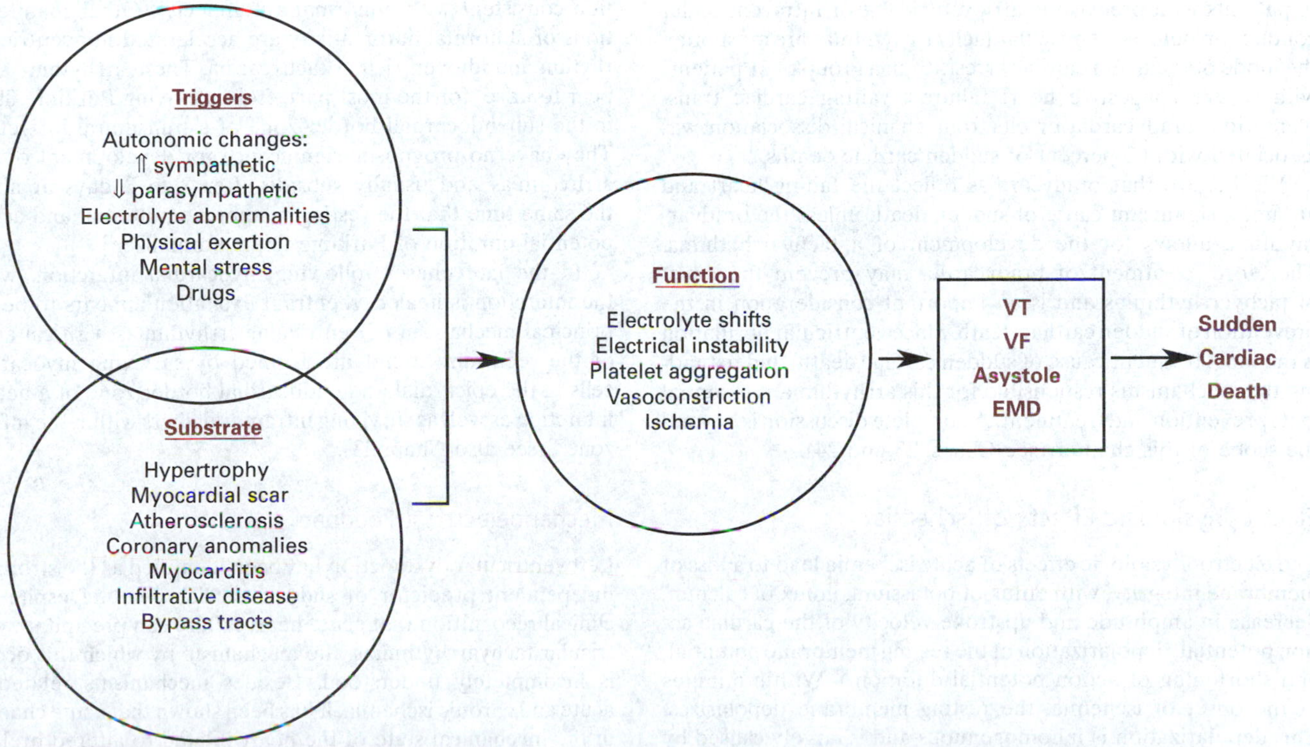

FIGURE 33-5 Interaction between structural cardiac abnormalities, functional changes, and triggering factors in the pathophysiology of sudden cardiac death. The role of triggering factors, such as changes in autonomic tone or reflexes, is increasingly being recognized. EMD, electromechanical dissociation; VF, ventricular fibrillation; VT, ventricular tachycardia.

autonomic nervous system, electrolyte abnormalities, and proarrhythmic effects of drugs in the initiation of ventricular arrhythmias resulting in sudden cardiac death (Fig. 33-5).[75,76] Strategies aimed at eliminating or reducing the triggers of arrhythmias may prove to be efficient short- and midterm solutions, since many of the structural abnormalities cannot be cured or require long-term risk-factor modification to prevent their development.

Tachyarrhythmias versus Bradyarrhythmias in Sudden Cardiac Death

Ventricular fibrillation is the first recorded rhythm in approximately 70 percent of patients who have cardiac arrest.[77,78] Sustained ventricular tachycardia is only rarely (less than 2 percent) documented as the initial rhythm, but it is unknown how often it precedes and precipitates ventricular fibrillation. In a series of 157 ambulatory patients who were wearing an ECG monitor at the time of their cardiac arrest, primary ventricular fibrillation was documented in 8 percent, ventricular tachycardia degenerating into ventricular fibrillation in 62 percent, and torsades de pointes in 13 percent.[79]

Electromechanical dissociation and asystole are found in about 30 percent of patients experiencing cardiac arrest, and this finding is usually related to the time interval from collapse to first monitoring of the rhythm, suggesting that it is a later manifestation of cardiac arrest.[77,78] The incidence of bradycardia as the first documented rhythm varies according to the population studied. In patients who have died suddenly while wearing an ambulatory ECG monitor, bradyarrhythmias as the initial rhythm were documented in 17 percent (26 of 231), but even in patients with preexisting atrioventricular or intraventricular conduction defects, ventricular tachyarrhythmias are most often the mode of recurrent cardiac arrest.[79,80] In a group of 21 patients with severe congestive heart failure awaiting cardiac transplantation, bradycardia or electromechanical dissociation was associated with 62 percent of sudden cardiac deaths.[81]

We believe that bradycardias reflect the failing heart and are not a significant cause of sudden death unless the bradyarrhythmia allows for the development of a tachyarrhythmia. Therefore, treatment of bradycardia may prevent the onset of tachyarrhythmias and is an important consideration in the prevention of sudden cardiac death. Since ventricular fibrillation is the most frequent cause of sudden cardiac death, understanding the mechanisms responsible for this arrhythmia is essential in its prevention and treatment. A complete discussion is beyond the scope of this chapter (see Chaps. 23 and 24).

Electrophysiologic Effects of Ischemia

The electrophysiologic effects of acute ischemia lead to a loss of membrane integrity, with efflux of potassium, influx of calcium, decrease in amplitude and upstroke velocity of the cardiac action potential, depolarization of the resting membrane potential, and shortening of action potential duration.[82] Within minutes of the onset of ischemia, the resting membrane depolarizes. This depolarization is inhomogenuous and is largely caused by local abnormalities in extracellular potassium levels and acidosis. Refractory periods in the ischemic zone and action potential duration shorten. Despite shortening of the action potential duration, fast sodium and slow calcium channels in partially depolarized fibers may remain inactive, thereby prolonging refractoriness, even after completion of repolarization. This postrepolarization refractoriness may further contribute to inhomogeneities in the electrophysiologic properties within and around the ischemic zone, causing significant conduction delays, unidirectional block, and reentrant arrhythmias. Subsequently, cellular uncoupling occurs after 20 to 25 min of ischemia, causing conduction to become slow and discontinuous.[83]

Ventricular arrhythmias during experimental acute ischemia occur in two peaks, one between 2 and 10 min following coronary occlusion and the second at 15 to 20 min. Rapid polymorphic ventricular tachycardias and ventricular fibrillation are the characteristic arrhythmias during the early stages of ischemia and are the cause of sudden cardiac death.[84] Activation mapping during ventricular fibrillation has demonstrated that the initial arrhythmias are due to reentry, which is facilitated by the inhomogeneous conduction velocities and refractory periods in and around the ischemic zone. The second peak of ventricular arrhythmias coincides with a peak in catecholamine release. Automatic and triggered rhythms have also been implicated in these arrhythmias. Ventricular arrhythmias can be a sign of reperfusion after thrombolysis, percutaneous revascularization, or spontaneous reperfusion. In addition, it appears that the rate, time, and degree of reperfusion influence the incidence, rate, and duration of these arrhythmias. More work is needed to further define these relationships.[85]

In the subacute phase of myocardial infarction (within the first 3 days), sudden cardiac death may occur due to ventricular fibrillation initiated by early, frequent premature ventricular complexes (PVCs). Such PVCs have been shown, in experimental models, to be predominantly due to abnormal impulse initiation consistent with abnormal automaticity. Other manifestations of abnormal automaticity are accelerated idioventricular rhythm and idioventricular tachycardia. These arrhythmias appear to arise, for the most part, from surviving Purkinje fibers in the subendocardial border zone of a transmural infarction. They have no prognostic significance for development of late arrhythmias and usually subside after 2 to 3 days at about the same time that the resting membrane potential and action potential duration of Purkinje fibers normalize.[82]

In the late phases following myocardial infarction, when the infarction is healed, reentrant excitation appears to be the principal mechanism of ventricular arrhythmias. Critical areas of the reentrant circuit are formed by surviving myocardial cells in the epicardial and endocardial border zone of a healed infarction as well as surviving intramural fibers within the infarct zone[84] (see also Chap. 23).

Mechanoelectrical Feedback

Left ventricular dysfunction has been identified as the strongest independent predictor of sudden cardiac death. Despite the clinical recognition that acute heart failure can precipitate ventricular tachyarrhythmias, the mechanism by which this occurs is incompletely understood. Besides mechanisms related to acute and chronic ischemia, it has been shown that acute changes in the mechanical state of the heart related to altered preload and contractility can have direct electrophysiologic effects that may precipitate arrhythmias; this relationship is usually referred to as mechanoelectrical feedback.[86] An increase in both left ventricular preload and contractility has been shown to shorten action potential duration in the canine ventricle.[86] An increase in right ventricular pressure has been shown to shorten action potential duration in humans.[87] The cellular mechanism by which this occurs is unknown, but there is some evidence that these changes might be mediated by fluctuation of intracellular calcium levels.[86]

Role of the Autonomic Nervous System in the Genesis of Arrhythmias

There is increasing evidence that cardiac abnormalities associated with a high risk of sudden cardiac death are accompanied by changes in autonomic innervation of the heart. Myocardial infarction, for instance, has been shown to cause regional cardiac sympathetic and parasympathetic denervation.[88] The denervated areas show supersensitivity to catecholamine infusion, with disproportionate shortening of action potential duration and refractoriness.[89] This autonomic heterogeneity may predispose to arrhythmia development by creating dispersion of refractoriness and/or conduction.

Sensitivity to sympathetic activation favors the onset of life-threatening cardiac arrhythmias, while vagal activation has been shown to have a protective effect in the presence of tonic sympathetic stimulation.[90] This is thought to be due, at least in part, to the antiadrenergic effects of vagal stimulation via reduction of norepinephrine release and inhibition of adenylate cyclase via inhibitory G proteins. Because it is difficult to study the effects of vagal activity on ventricular electrophysiologic properties directly, the behavior of the sinus node has been used as a surrogate by measuring indices of heart rate variability (reflecting primarily tonic vagal activity) and evaluating baroreflex sensitivity (a measure of reflex vagal activity). In dogs, decreased baroreflex sensitivity is associated with an increased susceptibility to ventricular fibrillation and sudden cardiac death provoked by ischemia in a chronic (4-week) infarct model.[65] Myocardial infarction reduced baroreflex sensitivity 4 weeks after myocardial infarction in 73 percent of animals studied compared to control animals. A transient (less than 3 months) decrease in baroreflex sensitivity following myocardial infarction has also been demonstrated in humans.[91] The prognostic value of baroreflex sensitivity in humans has been suggested in several studies.[92,93]

CARDIAC DISEASES ASSOCIATED WITH SUDDEN CARDIAC DEATH

Table 33-4 summarizes cardiac abnormalities associated with sudden death.

Ischemic Heart Disease

CORONARY ATHEROSCLEROSIS

In survivors of cardiac arrest, CHD is present in 40 to 86 percent of patients, depending on age and gender of the population.[94] There is ample evidence to support the concept that the electrical instability caused by acute ischemia is more important than infarction in the pathogenesis of sudden cardiac death. Although the majority of patients who suffer sudden cardiac death have severe multivessel coronary disease, fewer than half of the patients resuscitated from ventricular fibrillation evolve evidence of myocardial infarction by elevated cardiac enzymes, and less than 20 percent have Q-wave myocardial infarction.[77] Holter monitoring at the time of arrest has infrequently shown evidence of ischemic ECG changes before the event.[95–97] In postmortem examinations and in catheterization studies, there was a significant (75 to 85 percent) stenosis in at least two major coronary arteries in as many as 76 percent of patients. Detailed pathologic studies have confirmed the presence of acute coronary arterial lesions (plaque fissure, plaque hemorrhage, and thrombosis) in up to 95 percent of patients dying suddenly, but only a fraction had total occlusion.[50,66,98–100] Thus, the important observation is that sudden cardiac death can occur in the absence of infarction but is usually in the presence of diffuse coronary disease.[101]

Coronary collateralization may play an important role in the presentation of coronary artery disease as sudden cardiac death. Studies looking at occluded arteries demonstrated that minimally stenosed coronary arteries were a weaker stimulus for development of collaterals than were high-grade lesions.[102] This mitigating effect of coronary collateralization is further supported by a study of exercise testing in 894 healthy men followed for a mean of 12.7 years. In this study, the initial coronary event was acute myocardial infarction or sudden cardiac death in 73 percent of those with a normal stress test result, as opposed to 20 percent of those with an abnormal stress test result.[103] It has been hypothesized that chronic ischemia may be a stimulus for development of coronary collaterals, which in turn could have a protective effect during acute coronary occlusion. It should be noted that patients with silent ischemia during exercise testing have the same likelihood of developing an acute myocardial infarction or sudden cardiac death as do symptomatic patients.[104]

Since coronary artery disease is the major substrate of sudden cardiac death, risk stratification following myocardial infarction is an important step in the prevention of sudden cardiac death. Few variables, mainly, frequent PVCs (more than 10 per hour), nonsustained ventricular tachycardia, reduced left ventricular ejection fraction (less than 40 percent), and use of digitalis are independent risk factors for sudden versus nonsudden cardiac death following myocardial infarction.[105–109] The incidence of sudden cardiac death in the first 2 years after myocardial infarction ranged from 11 to 18 percent in these studies. Patients with both nonsustained ventricular tachycardia and left ventricular dysfunction have the worst prognosis.[109]

The variables identified to predict sudden cardiac death following myocardial infarction in these studies are better in selecting a low-risk population for sudden cardiac death than in predicting who will go on to die suddenly. In the absence of frequent PVCs and with a normal left ventricular ejection fraction following myocardial infarction, the risk of sudden cardiac death is low (less than 2 percent in the first year).[110] Even when all clinical risk factors for sudden cardiac death are present following myocardial infarction, the reported risk varies between 10 and 40 percent and generally does not warrant prophylactic antiarrhythmic therapy. It is hoped that risk-stratification models incorporating other methods (e.g., heart rate variability, baroreflex sensitivity, nonlinear dynamics, T-wave alternans, and imaging of the cardiac autonomic innervation) of assessing such triggers of sudden cardiac death as autonomic fluctuations and electrical instability will enhance their positive predictive value (see also Chap. 42).

TABLE 33-4 Cardiac Abnormalities Associated with Sudden Cardiac Death

Ischemic Heart Disease	
Coronary atherosclerosis	Coronary artery spasm
Acute myocardial infarction	Coronary artery dissection
Chronic ischemic cardiomyopathy	Coronary arteritis
Anomalous origin of coronary arteries	Small vessel disease
Hypoplastic coronary artery	
Nonischemic Heart Disease	
Cardiomyopathies	Drug-induced and other toxic agents
Idiopathic dilated cardiomyopathy	Antiarrhythmic drugs (class Ia, Ic, and III)
Hypertrophic cardiomyopathy	Erythromycin
Hypertensive cardiomyopathy	Clarithromycin
Right ventricular cardiomyopathy	Astemizole
Infiltrative and inflammatory heart disease	Terfenadine
Sarcoidosis	Pentamidine
Amyloidosis	Ketoconazole
Hemochromatosis	Trimethoprim-sulfamethoxazole
Myocarditis	Psychotropic drugs (tricyclic antidepressants, haloperidol, phenothiazines, chloral hydrate)
Valvular heart disease	Probucol
Aortic stenosis	Cisapride
Aortic regurgitation	Cocaine
Mitral valve prolapse	Chloroquine
Infective endocarditis	Alcohol
Congenital heart disease	Phosphodiesterase inhibitors
Tetralogy of Fallot	Organophosphates
Transposition of the great vessels (post–Mustard-Senning)	Electrolyte abnormalities
Ebstein's anomaly	Hypokalemia
Pulmonary vascular obstructive disease	Hypomagnesemia
Congenital aortic stenosis	Hypocalcemia
Primary electrical abnormalities	Anorexia nervosa and bulimia
Long-QT syndrome	Liquid protein dieting
Wolff-Parkinson-White syndrome	Diuretics
Congenital heart block	
Idiopathic ventricular tachycardia	
Idiopathic ventricular fibrillation	
Syndrome of right bundle-branch block, ST elevation, and sudden death (Brugada syndrome)	
Nocturnal death in Southeast Asian men	

NONATHEROSCLEROTIC DISEASE OF THE CORONARY ARTERIES

Several nonatherosclerotic diseases of the coronary arteries are associated with increased risk of sudden cardiac death precipitated by cardiac ischemia. Congenital coronary artery anomalies, found in approximately 1 percent of all patients undergoing angiography and in 0.3 percent of patients undergoing autopsy, have been complicated by sudden cardiac death, often exercise-related, in up to about 30 percent of patients.[111] Origin of the left main coronary artery from the right aortic sinus or origin of the right coronary artery from the left coronary sinus were most frequently the cause. It has been postulated that acute ischemia is due to compression of the anomalous coronary artery between the pulmonary artery and aorta during exercise-induced expansion of these vessels and to diminished coronary flow reserve due to the slitlike orifice and acute takeoff angle of the anomalous vessel.[111]

Life-threatening ventricular arrhythmias and sudden cardiac death have been described in patients with coronary artery spasm (Prinzmetal's angina or variant angina). In a series of 81 patients with coronary artery spasm, 13 patients (16 percent) had at least one episode of cardiac arrest due to ventricular fibrillation.[112,113] Significant arrhythmias during attacks of variant angina were documented in 41 percent of these patients and appeared to be associated with a higher risk of sudden cardiac death. Calcium channel blockers are effective in many patients in preventing coronary spasm and appear also to protect from malignant ventricular arrhythmias if the attacks can be completely abolished.[112,113]

Sudden cardiac death has been described as a rare complication of coronary artery dissection in Marfan's syndrome, after labor and delivery, secondary to trauma or coronary catheterization, as a consequence of syphilitic aortitis, or as an extension of aortic dissection. Myocardial bridges have been reported in association with sudden cardiac death during exercise, but they are also an incidental finding at autopsy in up to 25 percent of patients dying of other causes.[114] Coronary arteritis and subsequent infarction have been reported in Kawasaki's disease, giant-cell arteritis, Beçhet's disease, systemic lupus erythematosus, and Churg-Strauss syndrome.[115–120]

Cardiomyopathies

IDIOPATHIC DILATED CARDIOMYOPATHY

Idiopathic dilated cardiomyopathy is the substrate for approximately 10 percent of sudden cardiac deaths in the adult population. The mortality rate for idiopathic dilated cardiomyopathy is high, reaching 10 to 50 percent annually, and seems most closely tied to the severity of pump dysfunction.[121] Mortality rates are higher among patients with advanced heart failure, but the proportion of sudden cardiac deaths is not increased.[122] In an overview of 14 studies including 1432 patients with idiopathic dilated cardiomyopathy, the mean mortality rate after a follow-up of 4 years was 42 percent, with 28 percent of deaths classified as sudden.[121] Sudden cardiac death in idiopathic dilated cardiomyopathy is usually attributed to both polymorphic and monomorphic ventricular tachyarrhythmias occurring in the setting of a high frequency of complex ventricular ectopy.[123] The terminal event may, however, also be asystole or electromechanical dissociation, especially in patients with advanced left ventricular dysfunction.[81] Factors potentially contributing to the generation of arrhythmias in idiopathic dilated cardiomyopathy are mechanoelectrical feedback, electrolyte depletion due to chronic diuretic therapy, excessive activation of the sympathetic nervous and renin-angiotensin systems, and proarrhythmic effects of antiarrhythmic drugs.[124]

Risk stratification of patients with idiopathic dilated cardiomyopathy is difficult because there are few clinical predictors specific for sudden cardiac death.[125] The only clinical variable that identifies patients with a higher risk of sudden cardiac death is unexplained syncope, and these patients should undergo further evaluation.[121,126] A recent study looked at patients with implantable defibrillators, nonischemic dilated cardiomyopathy, and unexplained syncope with negative electrophysiologic test results. Fifty percent of the patients received appropriate shocks for ventricular arrhythmias within a mean of 10 ± 14 months from implantation.[127] Patients with idiopathic dilated cardiomyopathy have a very high incidence of ventricular ectopy, with simple PVCs, complex PVCs, and nonsustained ventricular tachycardia present in 94 percent, 76 percent, and 40 percent, respectively, thus limiting their prognostic value by a low specificity.[123] The prognostic value of intraventricular conduction delays on ECG, which are associated with decreased survival rates, is, again, not specific for sudden cardiac death, and late potentials recorded by signal-averaged ECGs can be detected only in a minority of patients with idiopathic dilated cardiomyopathy.[128] It is clear that induction of polymorphic ventricular tachycardia or fibrillation during electrophysiologic testing is nonspecific and that the absence of inducible ventricular tachyarrhythmias in this population does not accurately predict a low risk for sudden cardiac death[129] (see Chap. 66). In up to 40 percent of patients with nonischemic dilated cardiomyopathy, inducible monomorphic ventricular tachycardia can be due to a macro-reentry circuit, such as bundle-branch reentry, that is readily amenable to catheter ablation.[130]

HYPERTROPHIC CARDIOMYOPATHY

The incidence of sudden cardiac death in patients with hypertrophic cardiomyopathy (HCM) is 2 to 4 percent per year in adults and 4 to 6 percent per year in children and adolescents.[131] A review of 78 patients with HCM who died suddenly or survived a cardiac arrest episode showed that 71 percent were younger than 30 years of age, 54 percent were without functional limitation, and 61 percent were performing sedentary or minimal physical activity at the time of cardiac arrest.[132] The mechanism of sudden cardiac death in HCM is not clear. Primary arrhythmias, hemodynamic events with diminished stroke volume, and/or ischemia have been implicated.[131,133] It must be emphasized that atrial arrhythmias can lead to ischemia and hemodynamic compromise leading to sudden death in these patients. Assessment of autonomic function in patients with HCM revealed abnormal responses of heart rate and blood pressure to exercise in two-thirds, which was associated with a more malignant clinical course, suggesting that autonomic imbalance may be important in the genesis of sudden cardiac death in these patients.[134]

There are few predictors of sudden cardiac death in patients with HCM. A clinical history of spontaneous, sustained monomorphic VT or sudden death in family members indicates a worse prognosis, as does onset of symptoms in childhood.[132] Hemodynamic and echocardiographic variables such as left ventricular wall thickness or the presence of outflow tract obstruction are not useful in identifying patients at high risk for sudden cardiac death. Ambulatory ECG monitoring has been reported to be of some value in identifying patients with HCM at risk for sudden cardiac death.[135] The prognostic value of electrophysiologic study in the absence of spontaneous, sustained ventricular tachycardia is limited, and in fact the study itself may be dangerous. Sustained ventricular tachyarrhythmias, predominantly rapid polymorphic ventricular tachycardia, have been induced in 27 to 43 percent of patients with HCM at electrophysiologic study, but their prognostic significance is controversial.[135] The predictive value of asymptomatic nonsustained ventricular tachycardia is also limited.[136] Paced electrogram fractionation in hypertrophic cardiomyopathy may be helpful in determining which patients are at risk for ventricular fibrillation.[137] The absence of inducible, sustained monomorphic ventricular tachyarrhythmias, absence of nonsustained ventricular tachycardia on ambulatory ECG, and no history of "impaired consciousness" (i.e., cardiac arrest or syncope) identified a subset (22 percent) of patients with HCM with a low (less than 1 percent) risk for sudden cardiac death.[136] A large number of mutations in genes coding for the β-myosin heavy chain, cardiac troponin T, cardiac troponin I, α-tropomyosin, myosin-binding protein C, and myosin light chains 1 and 2 in patients with HCM have been identified. Genotype-phenotype correlation studies have shown that mutations carry prognostic significance. Some mutations of the β-myosin heavy chain are associated with a benign prognosis, while other mutations are associated with a high incidence of sudden cardiac death. Mutations in cardiac troponin T are associated with a mild degree of hypertrophy but a high incidence of sudden cardiac death[139,140] (see Chaps. 62 and 67). As with most genetic disorders, the phenotypic expression of the same genetic abnormality is highly variable.

HYPERTENSIVE CARDIOMYOPATHY

Left ventricular hypertrophy has been identified as one of the strongest blood pressure–independent risk factors for sudden death, acute myocardial infarction, congestive heart failure, and other cardiovascular disease and deaths.[141–143] Hypertensive patients with left ventricular hypertrophy have a significantly greater prevalence of PVCs and complex ventricular arrhythmias than do patients without left ventricular hypertrophy or normotensive patients. In the Framingham Study, ECG evidence of left ventricular hypertrophy doubled the risk of sudden cardiac death. Echocardiographic studies showed an incremental risk for cardiovascular deaths of 1.73 in men and 2.12 in women for each 50 g increment in the index of left ventricular mass.[144] A possible mechanism for the increased mortality rate in patients with left ventricular hypertrophy is ventricular tachyarrhythmia.[141] Decreased coronary blood flow, flow reserve, and endothelial dysfunction may all be factors favoring the development of transient ischemia,[142] and long-term, repeated transient ischemic episodes could lead to interstitial fibrosis, which may underlie the arrhythmias in this population.[145] Other potential contributing factors to the increased risk of sudden cardiac death in hypertensive cardiomyopathy are the electrolyte disturbances associated with diuretic therapy of hypertension.[146,147] It remains to be shown that the reduction of hypertrophy or concomitant ventricular ectopy confers a clinical benefit that exceeds the one from the reduction of arterial pressure alone[143,148] (see also Chap. 51).

ARRHYTHMOGENIC RIGHT VENTRICULAR DYSPLASIA

Arrhythmogenic right ventricular dysplasia (ARVD) is predominantly right ventricular cardiomyopathy characterized by fatty or fibrofatty replacement of myocardium. It is a rare cause of sudden cardiac death except in a few endemic regions.[31] Recurrent ventricular tachycardia with multiple left bundle-branch block morphologies typifies this disorder. It is a familial disorder in approximately 30 percent of cases, with an autosomal dominant mode of inheritance. The gene defect has been localized to chromosomes 1, 3, and 14.[149–152] In the fibrofatty variety, patchy myocarditis, programmed cell death, and/or congenital abnormalities of development appear to lead to myocardial atrophy and repair by fibrofatty replacement, which may become the basis for reentrant ventricular arrhythmia. The left ventricle and ventricular septum can be involved in 50 to 67 percent of cases, especially later in the course of the disease, and such involvement confers a poor prognosis.[153,154]

The electrocardiographic manifestations in sinus rhythm include T-wave inversion in V_1–V_3 or complete or incomplete right bundle-branch block. Intraventricular conduction delay may produce a terminal notch on the QRS complex called an epsilon wave in approximately 50 percent of patients. The ventricular ectopy is usually of a left bundle-branch pattern, with a QRS axis between −90° and +110°, and generally arises from one of three sites of fatty degeneration. Called the triangle of dysplasia, these sites are the right ventricular outflow and inflow tract and apex. Any patient with frequent premature beats of a left bundle-branch morphology and left-axis deviation should be evaluated for this disorder.

In patients with ARVD, particularly at early stages of the disease, ventricular tachycardia is often precipitated by exercise, and its induction is usually found to be catecholamine sensitive at electrophysiologic study.[31,155] The course and prognosis of ARVD are highly variable and difficult to predict. The annual incidence of sudden cardiac death in ARVD has been estimated to be about 2 percent despite various treatments[156,157] (see Chap. 24).

Valvular Heart Disease

The risk of sudden cardiac death in asymptomatic patients with aortic stenosis or regurgitation appears to be low.[158,159] In contrast, in the presurgical era, sudden cardiac death was one of the three most common types of death in symptomatic patients with aortic stenosis, the other two being bacterial endocarditis and congestive heart failure.[160] There appears to be an increased risk of sudden cardiac death following aortic valve replacement for aortic stenosis or regurgitation.[161,162] In 831 patients receiving a Björk-Shiley prosthesis in the aortic (341 patients), mitral (345 patients), or double-valve (145 patients) position, the incidence of sudden cardiac death in the subgroups was 1.8 percent, 3.5 percent, and 4 percent, respectively, over a follow-up period of 7 years.[162] Malignant tachyarrhythmias have been suggested as the cause of sudden cardiac death in such patients, since the presence of PVCs is more frequent in patients who die suddenly than in those who die of other causes. Transient complete heart block is relatively common following both aortic (17.6 percent) and mitral (13 percent) valve replacement, pointing to bradyarrhythmias as the potential precipitating factor for sudden cardiac death[163] (see also Chap. 56).

MITRAL VALVE PROLAPSE

Whether or not mitral valve prolapse (MVP) is a cause of sudden cardiac death is controversial. The prevalence of MVP is so high (4 to 5 percent of the general population and up to 17 percent of young women) that its presence may just be a coincidental finding in victims of sudden cardiac death and not causally related.[164,165] The overall 8-year probability of survival in a group of 237 asymptomatic or minimally symptomatic patients with echocardiographically documented MVP who were prospectively followed was not significantly different from that for a matched control population.[165] On the other hand, MVP may not always be benign. MVP is the only structural cardiac disease found in a significant number of victims of sudden cardiac death, especially in the young female population.[28,166] Of course, they may have had a primary electrical disease unrelated to mitral valve prolapse.[167] Patients with MVP associated with mitral regurgitation and left ventricular dysfunction are clearly at higher risk for such complications as infective endocarditis, cerebroembolic events, and sudden cardiac death.[168,169] Some victims of sudden cardiac death with MVP, mild mitral regurgitation, and normal left ventricular function have been treated with antiarrhythmic agents, raising the possibility of proarrhythmia as the cause of death.

Ambulatory electrocardiography in patients with mitral valve prolapse who experienced sudden cardiac death suggests that, based on the increased incidence of complex ventricular ectopy, the cause of sudden cardiac death in patients with MVP is a ventricular tachyarrhythmia.[167] A prolonged QTc interval and changes in autonomic tone have also been related to sudden cardiac death in patients with MVP.[170] Several risk factors for sudden cardiac death have been identified in asymptomatic or mildly symptomatic MVP patients without significant mitral regurgitation, including mitral valve annular circumference, thickness of the anterior and posterior mitral valve leaflets, presence and extent of endocardial plaque, and presence or absence of redundant mitral valve leaflets on M-mode echocardiography[165,170] (see Chap. 58).

Inflammatory and Infiltrative Myocardial Disease

Any inflammatory disease can cause sudden cardiac death due to either ventricular tachyarrhythmias or complete heart block. Histologic findings suggestive of myocarditis have been reported in 10 to 44 percent of young victims of sudden cardiac death (Table 33-2).[23] In adults, the diagnosis of myocarditis is made much less frequently, perhaps because of concurrent structural heart disease or because the late manifestations of the disease are indistinguishable from idiopathic dilated cardiomyopathy (see Chap. 69). In South America, however, myocarditis due to specific pathogens, such as Chagas' disease, is the most frequent cause of cardiomyopathy and related sudden cardiac death.[171] Patients with infective endocarditis may also be at risk for sudden cardiac death due to coronary emboli from valvular vegetations. More often, sudden cardiac death is caused by acute hemodynamic deterioration due to valvular failure. Intramyocardial abscesses can also precipitate ventricular tachycardia and lead to sudden cardiac death.

Infiltrative cardiomyopathies, such as primary or secondary amyloidosis, hemochromatosis, or sarcoidosis, have been associated with predominantly cardiac conduction defects but also ventricular tachyarrhythmias and sudden cardiac death. Ventricular tachycardia is sometimes the mode of presentation of sarcoidosis, can usually be reproduced by programmed electrical stimulation, and is associated with a high rate of recurrent arrhythmia and sudden cardiac death[172] (see also Chap. 68).

Congenital Heart Disease

An increased risk of sudden cardiac death due to an arrhythmia has been found predominantly in four congenital conditions: tetralogy of Fallot, transposition of the great vessels, aortic stenosis, and pulmonary vascular obstruction.[35] Patients who have undergone reparative surgery for tetralogy of Fallot have a reported risk of sudden cardiac death of 6 percent before age 20.[37,173,174] A QRS duration of 180 ms or more was found to be the most sensitive predictor of sudden cardiac death and ventricular tachyarrhythmias in 178 adults after repair of tetralogy of Fallot and correlated with other parameters of right ventricular volume overload.[174] Transposition of the great vessels (post–Mustard-Senning) is associated with a 2 to 8 percent rate of late sudden cardiac death, which is due in some cases to sinus node dysfunction and in others to ventricular tachyarrhythmias[38,39] (see Chap. 63). Sudden cardiac death is often (45 to 60 percent) the mode of death in patients with primary or secondary pulmonary hypertension (see Chap. 52). Death is often precipitated by general anesthesia, dehydration, exertion, or pregnancy. Any process that decreases systemic vascular resistance increases right-to-left shunting and decreases pulmonary flow. The resultant peripheral desaturation may trigger lethal arrhythmias and sudden cardiac death.[175] The sudden cardiac death risk in congenital aortic stenosis is estimated to be 1 percent and occurs predominantly in symptomatic patients with severe left ventricular hypertrophy. Ebstein's anomaly is frequently (up to 25 percent) associated with the presence of accessory pathways and the Wolff-Parkinson-White syndrome, which carries a small risk of sudden cardiac death (see below). Congenital heart block without associated structural heart disease occurs in 1 of 20,000 infants, and a moderate decrease in heart rate is usually well tolerated. A maternal risk factor is systemic lupus erythematosus. As previously noted, patients with severe bradycardia, however, have a tendency to develop ventricular arrhythmias. Pacemaker therapy has virtually eliminated the risk of sudden cardiac death in this population.[175]

Primary Electrical Abnormalities

LONG-QT SYNDROME

Sudden cardiac death is one of the hallmarks of the idiopathic long-QT syndrome (LQTS), a group of genetically distinct disorders each resulting from a mutation in one of six genes encoding cardiac ion channels or auxiliary ion-channel subunits.[176–178,341] The prolonged QT interval reflects abnormal prolongation of repolarization. Other characteristics of this disorder, in addition to prolonged (greater than 460 ms) QT interval, include abnormal T-wave contours, relative sinus bradycardia, a family history of early sudden death, a propensity for recurrent syncope, and sudden cardiac death due to polymorphic ventricular tachycardia (torsades de pointes) and ventricular fibrillation. Over 90 percent of the congenital forms of LQTS have been linked to six specific chromosomal defects, resulting in a genetically based classification (LQTS 1 through 6) with important functional and prognostic implications.[178]

The six defects have been mapped to chromosome *11p15.5* (LQTS1), chromosome *7q35-36* (LQTS2), chromosome *3p21-24* (LQTS3), chromosome *4q25-27* (LQT4), and chromosome *21* (LQTS5 and LQTS6). Several mutations have been identified in each gene, and this locus heterogeneity appears to be important prognostically. Defects in outward currents (potassium) or impaired inactivation of inward currents (sodium) can cause abnormal prolongation of the action potential repolarization, enhancing the propensity to develop early afterdepolarizations that may initiate arrhythmias[178] (see Chaps. 23 and 24). Recent data suggest that reentry due to transventricular heterogeneity is responsible for sustaining the arrhythmia.[179]

Five of these genes have been identified as encoding ion-channel proteins (LQTS1, LQTS2, LQTS3, LQTS5, and LQTS6). Four of them (LQTS1, LQTS2, LQTS5, and LQTS6) encode potassium channels. The gene products of LQTS1 and LQTS5 combine to form the slow delayed-rectifier potassium current, I_{K_S}. LQTS1, also referred to as KVLQT1, encodes the alpha subunit of the channel, and LQTS5, or KCNE1, encodes the beta subunit, called minK. Similarly, the products of LQTS2, known as HERG, and LQTS6, or KCNE2, combine to form the rapid delayed-rectifier potassium current, I_{K_R}. LQTS3, or SCN5A, encodes the cardiac sodium channel. The protein encoded by LQTS4 remains unknown.[180–183] Mutations in KVLQT1 account for approximately 50 percent of all cases of the LQTS. The congenital LQTS associated with deafness, or Jervell-Lange-Nielsen syndrome, appears to be caused by homozygous mutations of the KVLQT1 gene.[184]

Carriers of the LQT gene have been reported to have a 5 percent incidence of aborted sudden cardiac death and a 63 percent incidence of recurrent syncope.[177] The mean age at presentation was 24 years, and the annual incidences of sudden cardiac death and recurrent syncope were 1.3 percent and 8.6 percent, respectively, in a series of 196 patients enrolled in an international registry.[176] Multivariate analysis in the registry population identified female gender, congenital deafness, history of syncope, and a documented episode of torsades de pointes or ventricular fibrillation as independent risk factors for postenrollment syncope or sudden cardiac death.[176] Exercise-related cardiac events dominate the clinical picture of LQTS1 patients, and auditory stimuli tend to be a trigger for arrhythmic events in LQTS2 patients.[185] Echocardiographic studies have also been reported to reveal specific wall motion abnormalities associated with an increased risk (relative risk 2.75) of syncope and sudden cardiac death.[186] Genetic typing in the future may facilitate risk stratification, providing valuable information not only about the underlying abnormality but also about the expected severity of the disease and preferred therapy.[178]

WOLFF-PARKINSON-WHITE SYNDROME

The risk of sudden cardiac death in patients with Wolff-Parkinson-White syndrome is less than 1 per 1000 patient-years of follow-up.[187] Although a rare event, it is an important one to consider, since it usually occurs in otherwise healthy individuals and, in the era of catheter ablation of accessory pathways, is a curable cause of sudden cardiac death.[188] Almost all survivors of sudden cardiac death with Wolff-Parkinson-White syndrome have had symptomatic arrhythmias prior to the event, but up to 10 percent had sudden cardiac death as their first manifestation of the disease.[189–193] The mechanism of sudden cardiac death in most patients with this syndrome is presumably the development of atrial fibrillation with rapid ventricular rates due to conduction over an accessory pathway and subsequent degeneration into ventricular fibrillation. Sudden cardiac death survivors tend to have a higher prevalence of atrial fibrillation, multiple bypass tracts, and Atrioventricular Nodal Reentrant Tachycardia (AVNRT). There are no good predictors during sinus rhythm for the development of sudden death in these patients. Spontaneous or exercise-induced intermittent loss of preexitation is helpful in identifying patients who will have a slower ventricular response in atrial fibrillation. Loss of preexitation due to enhanced conduction through the atrioventricular node or other causes of antegrade block in the accessory pathway must be excluded for this finding to be reliable. The best predictor for development of ventricular fibrillation during atrial fibrillation is the spontaneous occurrence of a rapid ventricular response over the accessory pathway, with the shortest interval between preexcited ventricular beats (i.e., those conducted over the accessory pathway) being less than 220 ms.[188–192] Although this short RR interval is a highly sensitive marker, identifying virtually 100 percent of patients at high risk for ventricular fibrillation, its specificity is low, since this finding is present in approximately 20 percent of asymptomatic patients with Wolff-Parkinson-White syndrome[189] and 50 percent of those with mild to moderate symptoms due to atrioventricular reentrant tachycardia.[190] In symptomatic patients, an electrophysiologic study offers the opportunity to assess conduction properties of the accessory pathways, the propensity to develop tachyarrhythmias, and the possibility of curing the patient with catheter ablation at minimal risk. There is no proof that refractory period measurements predict sudden death in asymptomatic or symptomatic patients.

IDIOPATHIC VENTRICULAR TACHYCARDIA

Several distinct clinical or electrophysiologic patterns in patients with idiopathic monomorphic ventricular tachycardia have been described. Sudden cardiac death rarely occurs in these populations.[194] They include a reentrant form, known as verapamil-sensitive ventricular tachycardia or idiopathic left ventricular tachycardia, typically located in the region of the left posterior fascicle, an automatic form that may originate from either ventricle and paroxysmal or repetitive forms that originate from the right ventricular outflow tract. Eighty percent of cases of idiopathic ventricular tachycardias originate from the right ventricular outflow tract and typically have a left bundle-branch block with inferior axis pattern. These arrhythmias are sensitive to vagal maneuvers, such as administration of adenosine, and can be provoked by isoproterenol.[195] Ventricular tachycardia originating from the left ventricular outflow tract is uncommon. The reentrant form generally arises from the left inferior septum posteriorly and has a right bundle-branch block pattern with left-axis deviation but can arise more apically, in which case the axis is right and superior. Calcium channel blockers are effective in suppressing this arrhythmia, and vagal maneuvers, β-blockers, and lidocaine are usually ineffective.

In contrast, several types of idiopathic polymorphic ventricular tachycardias have been described and are associated with an unfavorable prognosis. These arrhythmias include idiopathic ventricular fibrillation (see below), torsades de pointes with a short coupling interval, and catecholaminergic polymorphic ventricular tachycardia. They can occur in sporadic or familial forms and are frequently but not uniformly associated with catecholamine release during physical or emotional stress. Patients with catecholaminergic polymorphous ventricular tachycardia have a favorable response to β-blocker therapy, while those with idiopathic ventricular fibrillation and short-coupled torsades de pointes may not.[196]

Idiopathic Ventricular Fibrillation Although the list of potential causes of sudden cardiac death continues to grow, a definite cause of sudden cardiac death cannot be established in approximately 1 percent of patients dying suddenly or after successful resuscitation from cardiac arrest.[197] These instances of sudden cardiac death without evident cause are presumed to be due to idiopathic ventricular fibrillation. The incidence of idiopathic ventricular fibrillation is higher in selected populations, such as younger patients (up to 14 percent in patients below 40 years of age) who had sudden cardiac death[198] or female survivors of sudden cardiac death unrelated to myocardial infarction (10 percent).[21] The risk of recurrent ventricular fibrillation in this young and otherwise healthy patient population ranges between 22 and 37 percent at 2 to 4 years.[197,199,200] In survivors of cardiac arrest due to idiopathic ventricular fibrillation, the diagnosis is made by exclusion if extensive cardiac workup (including physical examination, laboratory tests for acute myocardial infarction and electrolyte abnormalities, ECG, exercise test, echocardiographic study, cardiac catheterization, and electrophysiologic study to exclude significant conduction system abnormalities or accessory pathways) reveals no abnormality that is thought to account for the ventricular fibrillation episode. In a review of 54 published cases of presumed idiopathic ventricular fibrillation, patients were younger (mean age 36 ± 16 years) than those who had sudden cardiac death associated with structural heart disease, and there was a relatively higher proportion of women.[197] Noninvasive evaluation, including exercise testing and ambulatory ECG monitoring, may help confirm the diagnosis of idiopathic ventricular fibrillation in selected patients in whom rapid, nonsustained runs of polymorphic ventricular tachycardia can be documented. Unfortunately, such markers are present in fewer than half the patients with this disorder.[197,201] The prognostic role of electrophysiologic evaluation in these patients is controversial: sustained rapid polymorphic ventricular tachycardia or ventricular fibrillation is inducible in 38 to 75 percent of patients studied[197,200–202]; however, these arrhythmias are generally considered a nonspecific finding,[203,204] and noninducibility of ventricular fibrillation in this patient population did not predict a more favorable outcome.[200]

The syndrome of sudden cardiac death associated with right bundle-branch block and persistent ST-segment elevation in ECG leads V_1–V_3 in patients without demonstrable structural heart disease is known as the Brugada syndrome.[205] Symptomatic patients and those in whom ventricular tachycardia or ventricular fibrillation are inducible at the time of electrophysiologic study have a high incidence of sudden death.[206,207] This syndrome is genetically determined, and three mutations of the gene for the sodium channel SCN5A have been found in chromosome 3. These mutations are distinct from those identified in the LQTS and in right ventricular dysplasia.[208]

A sudden unexpected nocturnal death syndrome is described in young, apparently healthy males from Southeast Asia.[209] This syndrome is known among Asian-Pacific populations and has several names. The Thai describe it as *Lai Tai* (death during sleep). In the Philippines, it is known as *Bangungut* (to rise and moan in sleep followed by death) and as *Pokkuri* (unexpected sudden death at night) by the Japanese.[210] A majority of these patients have been found to have the electrocardiographic manifestations of the Brugada syndrome.[211,212]

In any case, it should be kept in mind that the diagnosis of "idiopathic" ventricular fibrillation is made by exclusion and therefore depends on the sensitivity of the diagnostic tests used. With the development and validation of new diagnostic tools, many forms of "idiopathic" sudden cardiac death in "structurally normal" hearts may have to be reclassified.

Drugs and Other Toxic Agents

PROARRHYTHMIA

The apparent paradox that antiarrhythmic agents can cause arrhythmias has been recognized since the introduction of quinidine in 1918.[213] The results of the Cardiac Arrhythmia Suppression Trial (CAST) showed an increased mortality rate in postinfarction patients treated with encainide, flecainide, and moricizine compared with placebo, despite effective antiarrhythmic efficacy as documented by the suppression of PVCs.[214] Besides antiarrhythmic drugs, many other agents with diverse actions have been implicated in the induction of tachyarrhythmias.[215] Among commonly used drugs associated with the risk of producing ventricular arrhythmias leading to sudden cardiac death are erythromycin, terfenadine, hismanal, pentamidine, and certain psychotropic drugs, such as tricyclic antidepressants and chlorpromazine, which generally affect repolarization. Phosphodiesterase inhibitors and other positive inotropic agents that increase intracellular calcium loading have also been shown to be proarrhythmic and to increase the risk of sudden cardiac death, despite their beneficial effects on hemodynamic parameters.[216] Suggested proarrhythmia mechanisms of classes Ia and III antiarrhythmic drugs—as well as psychotropic drugs, erythromycin, and pentamidine—include increased prolongation of refractoriness (QT interval of the ECG) and development of early afterdepolarizations[217] (Table 33-4). The initiation of the arrhythmia is often triggered by bradycardia or a characteristic "long-short" coupling interval that initiates a pause-dependent prolongation of the QT interval. The ventricular tachycardia in this setting has commonly a typical torsades de pointes morphology. This form of proarrhythmia may be facilitated by electrolyte abnormalities such as hypokalemia or hypomagnesemia. It is usually an early event during drug therapy (within 3 days), and concomitant therapy with digitalis and diuretic agents may predispose patients to this complication.[218] Since it is not possible to predict who will develop proarrhythmic effects, initiation of antiarrhythmic therapy in a telemetry unit is recommended (see Chaps. 23, 24, and 27).

A second mechanism of proarrhythmia, observed predominantly with class IC antiarrhythmic drugs such as flecainide and propafenone, appears to be associated with acute ischemic events and occurs more frequently in patients with ischemic cardiomyopathy.[219] It is believed that the antiarrhythmic drug exacerbates ischemia-induced myocardial conduction delays in an heterogeneous fashion and promotes reentrant ventricular tachycardias.[219]

COCAINE AND ALCOHOL

The increasingly widespread use of cocaine in the United States has led to the realization that this drug can precipitate life-threatening cardiac events, including sudden cardiac death. In a series of 41 survivors of cardiac arrest due to ventricular fibrillation in patients 18 to 35 years of age, one-third had ingested alcohol or drugs (cocaine, heroin, or tricyclic agents).[220] The combination of alcohol and cocaine is especially dangerous due to the generation of a unique metabolite, cocaethylene, that has enhanced cardiotoxicity.[221] Cocaine causes coronary vasoconstriction, increases cardiac sympathetic effects, and precipitates cardiac arrhythmias irrespective of the amount ingested, prior use, or whether there is an underlying cardiac abnormality.[222] The combination of increased oxygen demand due to sympathetic stimulation and diminished coronary flow due to vasoconstriction may precipitate ischemia-induced arrhythmias and sudden cardiac death (see Chap. 71).

ELECTROLYTE ABNORMALITIES

Hypokalemia is often found in patients during and following resuscitation from a cardiac arrest. Although it is often a secondary phenomenon due to catecholamine-induced potassium shift into the cells, primary hypokalemia can also be arrhythmogenic. There is an almost linear inverse relationship between serum potassium concentration and the probability of ventricular tachycardia in patients with acute myocardial infarction.[223] A decrease in the extracellular potassium level hypopolarizes the resting membrane potential, shortens the plateau duration, prolongs the phase of rapid repolarization in ventricular fibers, and causes an increase in pacemaker activity in Purkinje cells, triggering ventricular arrhythmias.[224] These changes in repolarization may increase the dispersion of the recovery of excitability and facilitate reentrant ventricular arrhythmias.[224] Many of the electrophysiologic effects of hypokalemia are similar to those caused by digitalis and catecholamine stimulation, explaining the high risk of ventricular arrhythmias when a combination of these factors is present.

An association between magnesium deficiency and sudden cardiac death has been reported in humans, especially as a cofactor in drug-induced torsades de pointes.[225] Hypomagnesemia in humans is generally associated with congestive heart failure, digitalis use, chronic diuretic use, hypokalemia, and hypocalcemia, making it difficult to establish whether the hypomagnesemia alone caused the sudden cardiac death. Acute administration of magnesium has been successfully used in the treatment of drug-induced torsades de pointes, although hypomagnesemia is not usually documented in this situation.

Changes in intracellular concentration of calcium may also be arrhythmogenic.[224] An increase in intracellular calcium concentration causes oscillatory release of calcium from the sarcoplasmic reticulum and gives rise to delayed afterdepolarizations, which may lead subsequently to ventricular arrhythmias due to triggered activity. Increases in intracellular calcium are believed to play a significant role in arrhythmias associated with digitalis glycosides, catecholamine-induced ventricular tachycardia, reperfusion arrhythmias, and the proarrhythmic effect seen with phosphodiesterase inhibitors and other positive inotropic agents.

Several studies in patients with hypertension who received treatment with diuretics suggested an increased risk of sudden cardiac death due to therapy with non–potassium-sparing diuretics.[226] Drug-induced potassium or magnesium depletion leading to cardiac arrhythmias has been suggested as the underlying mechanism (see also Chap. 23).

Electrolyte abnormalities are thought to be the cause of sudden cardiac death in patients with severe eating disorders, such as anorexia nervosa and bulimia, or patients who are on liquid protein diets. Sudden cardiac death due to ventricular tachycardia related to prolongation of the QT interval has been reported in a few patients with anorexia nervosa and bulimia.[227] It is thought to account partially for the high fatality rate of this eating disorder.

CLINICAL PRESENTATION AND MANAGEMENT OF THE PATIENT WITH CARDIAC ARREST

Out-of-Hospital Cardiac Arrest

Cardiac arrest is characterized by abrupt loss of consciousness that would uniformly lead to death in the absence of an acute intervention, although spontaneous reversions rarely occur. About 75 percent of cardiac arrests occur at home, and about two-thirds are witnessed.[14,228,229] Individuals who live alone and women appear more likely to have unwitnessed deaths.[230] The average age of cardiac arrest victims is around 65 years, and 70 to 80 percent are men.[229]

As discussed above, the most common mechanisms of cardiac arrest are ventricular tachyarrhythmias, followed by bradyarrhythmias, or asystole. The most important determinant of successful resuscitation is the time interval from cardiovascular collapse to initial intervention. Since most patients are found in ventricular fibrillation, the time to successful defibrillation is a key element in the acute management of the cardiac arrest victim (see also Chap. 34). The importance of early intervention is reflected in the "chain of survival" concept of emergency cardiac care systems: early access, early CPR, early defibrillation, and early advanced cardiac life support.[231] This concept has led to the development of tiered medical emergency systems in most urban areas. Following activation of the emergency call (911) system, the first response consists of the nearest emergency medical technicians or fire departments who are trained to provide basic CPR and defibrillation. The second response is by paramedics who are trained in advanced cardiac life support, including endotracheal intubation, intravenous medications, and additional defibrillation if necessary.

Initiation of bystander CPR by people trained in basic cardiac life support is another important element of early intervention and improves the chances of successful resuscitation. In an overview of 17 controlled studies of survival from out-of-hospital cardiac arrest, bystander CPR was associated with a greater than twofold odds ratio of survival (28 ± 16 percent of 5565 patients receiving bystander CPR versus 12 ± 11 percent of 8329 patients who did not).[231] The association between early CPR and improved survival appears to be related to the beneficial effects of CPR on ventricular fibrillation. The earlier CPR is performed, the greater the proportion of patients who are found in ventricular fibrillation as opposed to bradycardia or asystole.[78] Further, successful defibrillation is more likely when early CPR is performed. Community-based CPR training programs, such as those implemented in Seattle and Minneapolis, resulted in training of 20 to 25 percent of the adult population and have led to a higher likelihood of bystander CPR being administered in out-of-hospital cardiac arrest. The percentage of patients receiving bystander CPR varies in the communities studied between 8 and 54 percent, with an average around 30 percent.[229] A more efficient approach is targeted CPR training for persons who have an increased likelihood of having to perform CPR. It has been suggested that learning CPR be a mandatory course in high school, much like learning how to drive a car.[232]

In order to improve the time to initial defibrillation, early defibrillation by nonmedical personnel has been advocated. The widespread use of automatic external defibrillators has the potential to improve significantly the availability of early defibrillation.[231,233] These are relatively simple and inexpensive devices that have an automatic detection and treatment algorithm for ventricular tachyarrhythmias, but whether widespread use of these devices will translate into improved overall mortality rates and quality of life remains to be determined. The addition of interposed abdominal compression to standard CPR techniques has been reported to improve the outcome, particularly in patients found in asystole or electromechanical dissociation.[234]

Although duration of arrest is the most important determinant of successful ventricular defibrillation, other factors should be kept in mind. It has been estimated that in humans only about 4 percent of the transthoracic current actually traverses the heart, the rest being shunted by the thoracic cage and lungs.[235] The transthoracic impedance is inversely proportional to the size of defibrillator patches and the force applied on the paddles. It also depends on the location of the paddles and the paddle-skin coupling material, and it decreases with the number of shocks applied.[236] To improve defibrillation efficacy, especially in individuals with large chests and expected high transthoracic impedance, the operator should use a gel, cream, or saline-soaked gauze between the paddles and the skin and press firmly on the largest hand-held paddles available; several successive shocks may be necessary.[237] Recent experimental evidence suggests that ischemia-triggered release of endogenous adenosine may have deleterious effects on the success of defibrillation.[238] Development of specific adenosine antagonists and their administration during CPR in patients found in ventricular fibrillation might further improve defibrillation success.

SURVIVAL AND PROGNOSIS AFTER CARDIAC ARREST

Survival to hospital discharge after cardiac arrest varies from 1.4 to 28 percent.[77,78,229,239,240] Marked differences in survival rates following out-of-hospital cardiac arrest have been reported in different communities, being lowest in large cities such as New York (1.4 percent) and Chicago (4 percent)[196] and highest (28 percent) in Seattle, an urban community where many of the early intervention concepts have been pioneered.[241] The in-hospital mortality rate following successful resuscitation outside the hospital remains high, in the range of 30 to 50 percent[77,78,242] (Fig. 33-6). The most important factors associated with increased in-hospital mortality rates after out-of-hospital cardiac arrest are cardiogenic shock after defibrillation, age 60 years or greater, requirement of four or more shocks for defibrillation, absence of an acute myocardial infarction, and coma on admission to the hospital.[77,242]

Survival depends largely on the initial recorded rhythm.[77,78,229,239,240] Some 40 to 60 percent of patients who are found in ventricular fibrillation are successfully resuscitated, but only about one-fourth of patients survive to be discharged from the hospital. The outcome is much better in the small (less than 7 percent) group of patients in whom ventricular tachycardia is the initial documented rhythm: 88 percent survive to the hospital and 76 percent are discharged alive. Bradycardias and electromechanical dissociation as the presenting rhythms are associated with the worst prognosis, and very few (less than 5 percent) of these patients survive to discharge from the hospital.[78] Other factors associated with improved survival are a low "comorbidity index," reflecting chronic conditions such as history of heart failure, diabetes, hypertension, and gastrointestinal disorders as well as recent symptoms prior to the event.[243]

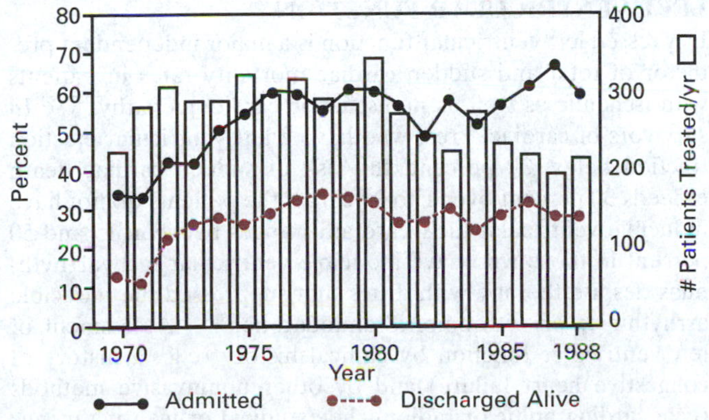

FIGURE 33-6 Percentage of out-of-hospital cardiac arrest victims admitted to the hospital by emergency medical service personnel and subsequently discharged alive during the period from 1970 to 1988. (From Cobb LA et al. Community-based interventions for sudden cardiac death: Impact, limitations, and changes. *Circulation* 1992; 85:I98–I102. Reproduced with permission from the publisher and authors.)

An important consideration in the treatment of the cardiac arrest victim is the appropriateness of CPR and the use of life-sustaining therapies in patients with a low likelihood of survival, such as chronically ill people found in asystole or electromechanical dissociation. Their chances of surviving until hospital discharge are less than 1 percent. Further, many older people prefer to die suddenly rather than experience chronic suffering.[244] Advance directives, when available, and consultation with family members and personal physicians might aid in the difficult decision process of when to administer supportive care rather than aggressive management.

MANAGEMENT OF CARDIAC ARREST SURVIVORS AND RISK STRATIFICATION FOR SUDDEN CARDIAC DEATH

Establishing the Underlying Cardiac Pathology

The initial management following successful resuscitation from cardiac arrest consists of allowing a period of hemodynamic and respiratory stabilization, after which every effort should be made to establish the cause of cardiac arrest and likelihood of recurrence. For this, the underlying cardiac disease should first be determined. History and physical examination may provide the first clues. Myocardial infarction must be excluded by serial enzyme and electrocardiographic studies. Echocardiographic studies can determine left ventricular function, regional wall motion abnormalities, valvular heart disease, or cardiomyopathies. Stress-imaging studies can demonstrate inducible ischemia. Cardiac catheterization is often recommended to evaluate the coronary anatomy and right and left ventricular hemodynamic parameters. Other tests, such as radionuclide studies, magnetic resonance imaging, or cardiac biopsy, may be necessary in selected patients. As discussed above, an underlying cardiac disease can be found in nearly all patients.

PRIMARY VERSUS SECONDARY CARDIAC ARREST One of the important questions following cardiac arrest is whether it was primarily due to acute circulatory or respiratory failure or to an arrhythmia. Although all these events are usually present during the arrest, it is important to distinguish whether the arrhythmia preceded or followed the hemodynamic collapse. While several clinical and historical clues help to answer this question (Table 33-5), the distinction sometimes cannot be made with certainty. Separating primary from secondary cardiac arrest has important prognostic and therapeutic consequences. In 142 survivors of cardiac arrest with coronary artery disease, the 1-year survival rate was 89 percent, 80 percent, and 71 percent in the patients classified as having had cardiac arrest secondary to acute myocardial infarction (44 percent of patients), secondary to an ischemic event (34 percent), or due to a primary arrhythmic event (22 percent), respectively.[96] Patients who present with cardiac arrest secondary (and within 48 h) to an acute transmural myocardial infarction have a prognosis similar to that of those who have an acute myocardial infarction without an arrhythmia.[77] Specific antiarrhythmic therapy is therefore usually not recommended if cardiac arrest occurs during or within 2 days of an acute Q-wave myocardial infarction. In

TABLE 33-5 Differences in Clinical Status Immediately before Death in Patients Dying Primarily of Arrhythmia versus Circulatory Failure

Clinical Status Immediately before Death	Arrhythmic Deaths $n = 82$	Circulatory Failure Deaths $n = 59$
Comatose	0/82 (0%)	56/59 (95%)
Standing or actively moving	39/82 (48%)	0/59 (0%)
Terminal arrhythmia		
Ventricular fibrillation	15/18 (83%)	3/9 (33%)
Asystole	3/18 (17%)	6/9 (67%)
Duration of terminal illness		
<1 h	53/82 (65%)	4/59 (7%)
>24 h	17/82 (21%)	48/59 (81%)
Nature of terminal illness		
Acute cardiac events	80/82 (98%)	8/59 (14%)
Noncardiac events	1/82 (1%)	51/59 (86%)

SOURCE: Modified with permission from Hinkle et al.[13]

contrast, if the arrhythmia is the primary event and myocardial infarction developed secondary to the acute hemodynamic deterioration during the arrhythmia, then antiarrhythmic therapy with a drug or device is recommended unless a transient or reversible cause is identified.[96]

Every effort should be made to exclude potentially reversible causes of sudden cardiac death (Table 33-6), including transient ischemic episodes in patients who are candidates for complete revascularization and in whom the onset of the arrhythmia is clearly preceded by ischemic ECG changes or symptoms.

Other reversible etiologies for cardiac arrest include transient severe electrolyte disturbances and proarrhythmic effects of antiarrhythmic drugs and other pharmacologic agents. It can be difficult to establish a causal relationship between the proarrhythmic agent and the malignant ventricular arrhythmia, as opposed to its being a coincidental finding. A pathologic prolongation of the QT_c interval preceding initiation of the arrhythmia and return of the QT_c interval to normal following discontinuation of the presumed proarrhythmic agent is strongly suggestive of a cause-effect relationship. Occasionally, especially when type IA agents are implicated in the cardiac arrest event, electrophysiologic evaluation, with programmed stimulation after washout and following reexposure to these agents, is necessary to confirm proarrhythmia as the sole cause of the episode of cardiac arrest. Another setting in which a reversible etiology for cardiac arrest is often present is in the hemodynamically unstable patient in the early postoperative period following cardiac surgery. Infusion of positive inotropic agents, electrolyte imbalances, and hypoxia are often precipitating factors.

TABLE 33-6 Potentially Reversible Causes of Cardiac Arrest Due to Ventricular Fibrillation

Myocardial ischemia	Electrolyte abnormalities
Prinzmetal's angina	Hypoxia
Proarrhythmia	Acute congestive heart failure
Antiarrhythmic agents	
Other drugs	

Risk Stratification for Sudden Cardiac Death

Several clinical, noninvasive, and invasive strategies can aid in the risk stratification of patients for sudden cardiac death. The underlying cardiac disease largely determines the choice of appropriate testing.

CLINICAL HISTORY

Four independent prognostic variables for sudden cardiac death related to clinical history were identified in a study of 200 patients who suffered from ventricular fibrillation or sustained ventricular tachycardia following myocardial infarction: (1) cardiac arrest at the time of the first documented episode of arrhythmia, (2) New York Heart Association (NYHA) class III or IV, (3) ventricular fibrillation or ventricular tachycardia occurring early after myocardial infarction (3 days to 2 months), and (4) history of multiple previous myocardial infarctions.[245] Risk stratification for sudden cardiac death using these four variables can identify subgroups with a sudden cardiac death incidence ranging from 0 to 28 percent. It is noteworthy that patients with hemodynamically tolerated ventricular tachycardia occurring more than 2 months after myocardial infarction, a subgroup that constituted 40 percent of the study population, were reported to have a 0 percent incidence of sudden cardiac death at 26 months. Syncope in patients with a left ventricular ejection fraction below 30 percent is associated with increased risk of sudden cardiac death (about 50 percent at 3 years) irrespective of finding an arrhythmic cause.[246]

LEFT VENTRICULAR FUNCTION

Depressed left ventricular function is a major independent predictor of total and sudden cardiac mortality rates in patients with ischemic as well as nonischemic cardiomyopathy.[247–250] In survivors of cardiac arrest who have a left ventricular ejection fraction below 30 percent, the risk of sudden cardiac death exceeds 30 percent over 1 to 3 years if the patients do not have inducible ventricular tachycardia; it ranges between 15 and 50 percent in those who have inducible ventricular tachyarrhythmias despite therapy with drugs that suppressed the inducible arrhythmias or with empiric amiodarone.[251–253] Assessment of left ventricular function by clinical history (e.g., a history of congestive heart failure) and by other noninvasive methods (echocardiographic or radionuclide studies) or invasive means (angiography) is therefore essential in the evaluation of a patient at risk for sudden cardiac death.[248] Unfortunately, detection of severe left ventricular dysfunction serves to predict the total cardiac mortality rate but does not distinguish patients who will die suddenly from those who will die of progressive congestive heart failure.[124,248,249]

ELECTROCARDIOGRAPHIC ABNORMALITIES

In survivors of out-of-hospital cardiac arrest, the presence of atrioventricular block or intraventricular conduction defects on ambulatory ECG (72 h) is associated with a higher recurrence rate of cardiac arrest (10 of 14 patients versus 1 of 28 patients without).[78] Other ECG parameters that have been reported to be associated independently with an increased risk of sudden cardiac death are prolongation of the QT interval (in the absence of inherited or acquired long-QT syndrome),[254] increased dispersion of the QT interval,[255,256] and an increase in resting heart rate above 90, particularly in men without a history of coronary artery disease.[257]

Detection of nonsustained ventricular arrhythmias by ambulatory ECG monitoring has been reported to be of value in the risk stratification of patients for sudden cardiac death.[247,258–261] The incidence of sudden cardiac death in the 2 years following myocardial infarction in 766 patients enrolled in the Multicenter Post-Infarction Research Group increased with the frequency of PVCs detected during 24-h ECG monitoring from 3 percent for less than 1 per hour to 14 percent for more than 30 per hour; similarly, patients with nonsustained ventricular tachycardia runs had a higher (17 percent) incidence of sudden cardiac death than did those with single PVCs (6 percent).[247] The prognostic value of ambulatory ECG monitoring in patients with congestive heart failure is limited by the high incidence of these arrhythmias (up to 88 percent) in this population, resulting in a low specificity of this parameter.[262]

BAROREFLEX SENSITIVITY

Reduced baroreflex sensitivity, reflecting mainly an impairment in the vagal efferent component of the baroreceptor reflex, may help to predict cardiovascular mortality rates and arrhythmic events, particularly in patients following myocardial infarction.[91–93] In two prospective studies including a total of 200 patients following myocardial infarction, baroreflex sensitivity was significantly reduced in the 14 patients with sudden cardiac death or life-threatening arrhythmias compared to those without (less than 3 ms/mmHg versus 8 ms/mmHg).[95,263] The prognostic significance of baroreflex sensitivity was not diminished in patients with reduced left ventricular function and carried the highest relative risk for arrhythmic events, superior to that of other prognostic variables, including left ventricular function.

HEART RATE VARIABILITY

Another noninvasive measure of sympathovagal balance is heart rate variability, beat-to-beat variations of RR intervals and their mathematically derived parameter. Several measures of heart rate variability have been reported to be associated with an increased risk of sudden and total cardiac death following myocardial infarction, underscoring the importance of the autonomic nervous system in the evolution of life-threatening arrhythmias.[261,264–266] In a study of 808 survivors of myocardial infarction, heart rate variability of less than 50 ms carried a 5.3 relative risk of death compared with the group with a heart rate variability of greater than 100 ms.[264] In a prospective study of 6693 nonselected and consecutive patients who underwent 24-h ambulatory ECG monitoring, those with a heart rate variability of less than 25 ms had a fourfold higher risk of sudden cardiac death than did patients with higher variability.[266] The sensitivity, specificity, positive predictive value, and relative risk in the prediction of arrhythmic events following myocardial infarction have been reported to be 60, 94, 55, and 10.4 for reduced heart rate variability [standard deviation of RR intervals (SDNN), less than 50 ms] and 80, 91, 44, and 23.1, respectively, for decreased baroreflex sensitivity (less than 3.0 ms/mmHg).[267] A prospective international study is in progress to assess the prognostic significance of diminished baroreflex sensitivity and heart rate variability 20 days after myocardial infarction in a large population.[268]

NONLINEAR DYNAMICS

According to the chaos theory, apparently irregular events such as ventricular ectopy are nonrandomly distributed in time, and their clustering can be quantified by fractal geometric analysis.[269] Fractal clustering of ventricular ectopy has been associated with sudden cardiac death in patients with mitral regurgitation and has also been demonstrated in other patients with life-threatening ventricular arrhythmias. The physiologic correlate for a low fractal dimension appears to be transient increases in cardiac sympathetic tone.[270]

T-WAVE ALTERNANS

Macroscopic T-wave changes with an alternating pattern have been observed in patients with long-QT syndrome prior to onset of ventricular fibrillation as well as in the setting of mechanical alternans, as is sometimes present during cardiac tamponade. Recent studies have indicated that T-wave alternans that is discernible only by computer-averaging techniques may be a more ubiquitous phenomenon that can identify patients at risk for ventricular arrhythmias.[271] Techniques for computer-assisted analysis of T-wave alternans are being developed and may provide a quantitative, noninvasive method for assessing susceptibility to ventricular fibrillation. T-wave alternans assessed by computer analysis has been shown to predict arrhythmia-free survival over 20 months, with a nearly 90 percent sensitivity and specificity in a small cohort of 66 patients[272] (see Chaps. 23 and 24). The positive predictive accuracy of this test appears to be similar to that of others with a very high negative predictive value.

LATE POTENTIALS

Late potentials, microvolt waveforms extending the duration of a filtered QRS complex detected by signal-averaging electrocardiography (SAECG), have been shown to be helpful in the risk stratification of patients following myocardial infarction. The prognostic significance of late potentials has been demonstrated in several studies, which reported a 17 to 29 percent incidence of sudden cardiac death, ventricular fibrillation, or sustained ventricular tachycardia in patients with an abnormal SAECG, in contrast to 0.8 to 3.5 percent in those without.[273] Although the negative predictive value of a normal SAECG is good, the application of SAECG in risk stratification for sudden cardiac death is limited by a low positive predictive value in patients following myocardial infarction as well as by its low sensitivity in patients with nonischemic cardiomyopathies[130,274,275] (see also Chap. 23). The sensitivity, specificity, and positive predictive value of SAECG are all improved when used in patients with known left ventricular dysfunction after myocardial infarction and/or nonsustained ventricular tachycardia.[275]

ELECTROPHYSIOLOGIC STUDIES

Electrophysiologic studies have advanced our understanding of life-threatening ventricular arrhythmias and facilitated the development of new therapies for their prevention and treatment. Induction of sustained monomorphic ventricular tachycardia is the generally accepted end point for programmed stimulation, while induction of nonsustained ventricular arrhythmias, polymorphic ventricular tachycardia, or ventricular fibrillation may be a nonspecific finding, depending on the aggressiveness of the stimulation protocol.[204,276] Information obtained during the electrophysiologic study—such as ventricular tachycardia rate, morphology, origin, mechanism, and hemodynamic stability—is crucial to determining whether the patient is a candidate for serial drug testing, catheter ablation therapy, surgical therapy, or an implantable defibrillator. In patients who present with sustained monomorphic ventricular tachycardia, ventricular tachycardia is reproducibly inducible in the vast majority, especially in those with coronary artery disease.[276] Electrophysiologic testing is also useful in patients with structural heart disease presenting with unexplained syncope. Ventricular tachycardia is the most common abnormal finding in these patients, but demonstration of His-Purkinje conduction disease or hemodynamically unstable supraventricular tachycardia can also be important. In patients with CHD, reduced left ventricular function, and documented nonsustained ventricular tachycardia, electrophysiologic studies can help select patients who would benefit from antiarrhythmic therapy. In survivors of cardiac arrest due to ventricular fibrillation, the prognostic value of electrophysiologic testing is less clear. Since sustained ventricular tachycardia or ventricular fibrillation is inducible in fewer than half the patients, suppression of induction of ventricular fibrillation by antiarrhythmic therapy is an unreliable end point, and even patients with no inducible ventricular arrhythmias remain at a high risk for recurrent cardiac arrest.[277,278] Nevertheless, in survivors of cardiac arrest, electrophysiologic study may reveal the mechanism of arrest, have prognostic significance, and help select an appropriate therapy.[279,280] The routine use of electrophysiologic testing following myocardial infarction and in patients with nonischemic cardiomyopathy is controversial, and the appropriate end points are unclear[277,281] (see Chap. 26).

TREATMENT OPTIONS FOR PATIENTS AT RISK FOR SUDDEN CARDIAC DEATH

General Considerations

There are few direct and randomized comparisons of various treatment strategies to prevent sudden cardiac death. Since reduction of sudden cardiac death rates does not necessarily parallel a reduction in total mortality rate, reduction in total mortality rate is a more appropriate end point in assessing antiarrhythmic efficacy. Patient selection affects the outcome of different treatment strategies. For example, in patients at low risk of sudden cardiac death, proarrhythmia or procedural mortality rates may outweigh the benefits achieved with an antiarrhythmic intervention. On the other hand, in patients at high risk for recurrent cardiac arrest, the risk-benefit profile of antiarrhythmic treatment strategies may be more favorable. Selection of therapy is further limited by the patient's baseline characteristics. For instance, only patients with inducible sustained ventricular arrhythmias are good candidates for electrophysiologically guided antiarrhythmic drug therapy, and radiofrequency ablation of ventricular tachycardia is an option only in patients with hemodynamically stable monomorphic ventricular tachycardia or bundle-branch reentry. In an era of limited health care resources, the cost-effectiveness of different treatment strategies is another element to be considered in choosing therapy. Last but not least, quality of life is an important aspect in the selection of the most appropriate therapy.

Pharmacologic Therapy

BETA BLOCKERS

Of all the therapies currently available for the prevention of sudden cardiac death, none is more established or more effective in patients with coronary heart disease than beta blockers.[282,283] Although beta blockers are less effective in suppressing spontaneous or induced ventricular ectopy when compared with other membrane-active antiarrhythmic agents, both nonselective beta blockers (timolol and propranolol) and cardioselective agents (e.g., metoprolol) have been shown in placebo-controlled, randomized trials to reduce total mortality rates by 20 to 36 percent, in large part because of a reduction of sudden cardiac death.[283–286] The benefits of beta blockade are additive to those of standard treatment for congestive heart failure. The Metoprolol CR/XL Randomized Intervention Trial in Congestive Heart Failure (MERIT-HF) trial demonstrated a 34 percent decrease in the mortality rate due to all causes, a 38 percent decrease in the cardiovascular mortality rate, and a 41 percent decrease in sudden death in 3991 patients who were randomized to beta blockers or placebo while being treated with standard medical therapy, including angiotensin-converting enzyme (ACE) inhibition, digitalis, and diuretics.[287]

In a review of 19,000 post–myocardial infarction patients who were randomized to beta blockers or placebo, active treatment was associated with a decrease in total mortality rate of 20 percent, of sudden cardiac death rate of 30 percent, and of reinfarction of 35 to 40 percent.[288] Beta blockers are effective in the setting of ventricular arrhythmias provoked by a high sympathetic tone, as in patients with congenital long-QT syndrome,[176] arrhythmogenic right ventricular dysplasia,[157] or congestive heart failure.[289] It is important to note that the beneficial effects of beta blockers on cardiac mortality rate are most pronounced in patients who are at higher risk for sudden cardiac death, such as patients with congestive heart failure, atrial and ventricular arrhythmias post–myocardial infarction, and diabetes[282] (see also Chaps. 23 and 42).

ANGIOTENSIN-CONVERTING ENZYME INHIBITORS

Vasodilator therapy is an effective treatment in patients with congestive heart failure and has been shown to reduce mortality rates by up to 40 percent in the first year.[290–292] The effect of ACE inhibitors on sudden cardiac death in established heart failure is less clear. In studies of patients with class I through IV congestive heart failure treated with ACE inhibitors or placebo, approximately 20 percent of patients died suddenly, without a significant difference in the sudden death mortality rate.[290–292] The situation is somewhat different in patients without heart failure in the post–myocardial infarction setting. Several trials have demonstrated a significant reduction in overall deaths in post–myocardial infarction patients (ejection fraction less than 35 percent) with or without mild heart failure. These studies have demonstrated a significant or trend toward a significant decrease in sudden cardiac death.[293–296] A recent metaanalysis analyzed 15 trials that included 15,104 post–myocardial infarction patients treated with ACE inhibitors. There were 900 sudden cardiac deaths in these studies, and a significant or trend toward significant reduction in sudden cardiac death in all of the larger (n >500) trials.[297]

CLASS I ANTIARRHYTHMIC DRUGS

The role of antiarrhythmic drug therapy in the prevention of sudden cardiac death has changed considerably since placebo-controlled trials such as Cardiac Arrhythmia Suppression Trial (CAST) demonstrated that suppression of spontaneous nonsustained ventricular arrhythmias with certain drugs does not necessarily result in improved survival rates.[214] In CAST, type IC antiarrhythmic drugs, such as encainide, flecainide, and moricizine, were associated with excess deaths from arrhythmias in asymptomatic post-infarction patients with frequent ventricular ectopy despite effective suppression of spontaneous ventricular ectopy[214] (Table 33-7). These results were interpreted as being due to an excessive proarrhythmic effect, which outweighed the lower mortality risk of these patients. Whether the risk-benefit ratio between pro- and antiarrhythmic effect of antiarrhythmic drugs is different in other patient populations or with other antiarrhythmic drugs is not clear, since there are very few placebo-controlled, randomized trials with total mortality rate as an end point.

There is no evidence that other class I antiarrhythmic drugs can prolong survival in any patient group studied, and they may even be harmful. Results of a meta-analysis of empiric long-term antiarrhythmic therapy after myocardial infarction with mostly class I antiarrhythmic agents (mexiletine, phenytoin, tocainide, flecainide, encainide, procainamide, aprindine, imipramine, and moricizine) showed either no beneficial effects or detrimental effects on mortality rate despite effective reduction of PVCs.[298,299] A meta-analysis of lidocaine in acute myocardial infarction suggested an increase in in-hospital mortality rate despite a reduction in the prevalence of ventricular fibrillation.[300] Empiric use of these drugs in patients with sustained ventricular arrhythmias has been associated with a very high rate of sudden cardiac death, between 30 and 70 percent at 2 years.[301] In a randomized trial between electrophysiologically guided conventional (i.e., class I drugs) therapy versus empiric amiodarone in survivors of cardiac arrest (CASCADE), overall survival rates were lower in the conventional arm (78, 62, and 32 percent at 2, 4, and 6 years, respectively).[302] The propafenone arm was stopped early in the Cardiac Arrest Study—Hamburg (CASH) because of excess mortality rates in cardiac arrest survivors compared with amiodarone, beta blockers, and implantable defibrillators[303] (see also Chap. 24).

SOTALOL

Sotalol, in the currently marketed form of a racemic mixture of the d- and l-stereoisomers, is a potent class III antiarrhythmic agent with nonselective beta-blocking effects.[304] Sotalol has been reported to suppress inducible ventricular tachycardia in 30 to 40 percent of patients who present with sustained ventricular arrhythmias. In a randomized trial of sotalol and other antiarrhythmic agents in patients with sustained ventricular tachycardia, the arrhythmia recurrence rate (21 percent at 1 year) and the arrhythmic death rate (12 percent at 4 years) was half of that achieved with class I agents.[305] However, since most patients receiving sotalol had failed other antiarrhythmic agents, the results were biased in favor of sotalol. The beta-blocking effect of sotalol seems to be essential for its benefit. The Survivor With Oral d-Sotalol (SWORD) trial of the d-isomer (class III antiarrhythmic effect only, devoid of beta-blocking effect) in patients with prior myocardial infarction was associated with increased mortality rates[306] (Table 33-7). The most serious side effect encountered with sotalol is proarrhythmia (mostly torsades de pointes), which has been reported to occur in up to 8 percent of treated patients.[303] In survivors of cardiac arrest, sotalol therapy was less effective than implantable cardioverter defibrillators.[307]

AMIODARONE

Amiodarone is widely considered the most effective antiarrhythmic agent for therapy of supraventricular and ventricular arrhythmias. It is a class III antiarrhythmic agent with additional class I, II, and IV properties and has unusual pharmacokinetics with a delayed onset of action and an elimination half-life of up to 53 days after chronic therapy[308] (see Chap. 27). In contrast to that of other antiarrhythmic agents, the long-term clinical efficacy of amiodarone is poorly predicted by the results of electrophysiologic evaluation.[252,253] Uncontrolled trials in patients with sustained ventricular tachycardia or ventricular fibrillation demonstrated a relatively low incidence of sudden cardiac death in patients treated with amiodarone, despite a high recurrence rate of ventricular arrhythmias. The sudden cardiac death rates at 1, 3, and 5 years in two series of 462 and 589 patients with mostly sustained ventricular arrhythmias were 9 percent, 15 to 16 percent, and 21 to 22 percent, respectively, whereas the arrhythmia recurrence rates were approximately 20 percent, 30 percent, and 40 percent during the same time period.[252,253] Again, the most important predictor of sudden cardiac death in patients treated with amiodarone for sustained ventricular tachycardia or ventricular fibrillation is left ventricular ejection fraction. In a series of 122 such patients with mostly coronary artery disease, the actuarial probability of sudden cardiac death at 5 years was 5 percent when the ejection fraction was greater than or equal to 40 percent and 49 percent when the ejection fraction was less than 40 percent.[309]

Amiodarone has been shown to reduce significantly sudden cardiac death rates following myocardial infarction in several placebo-controlled randomized studies, but its effects on the total mortality rate are inconsistent.[310] The Basel Antiarrhythmic Study of Infarct Survival (BASIS), a prospective randomized trial of empiric amiodarone, ambulatory ECG-guided conventional antiarrhythmic therapy, or placebo in 312 patients with complex ventricular ectopy following myocardial infarction showed that amiodarone significantly reduced the total mortality rate at 1 year from 13 percent in the placebo group to 5 percent in amiodarone-treated patients (p <.05).[311] On the other hand, amiodarone therapy did not reduce the total mortality rate compared with placebo in nearly 2700 post–myocardial infarction patients enrolled in the Canadian Amiodarone Myocardial Infarction Arrhythmia Trial (CAMIAT)[312] and the European Myocardial Infarction Amiodarone Trial (EMIAT),[313] despite a 50 percent risk reduction in the arrhythmic mortality rate (Table 33-7).

In patients with congestive heart failure who are at high risk for sudden cardiac death, prophylactic therapy with amiodarone was shown to decrease the mortality rate (by 28 percent) in the Argentinean Grupo de Estudio de la Sobrevida en la Insufficiencia Cardiaca en Argentina (GESICA) trial[314] but not in the Survival Trial of Antiarrhythmic Therapy in Congestive Heart

TABLE 33-7 Trials for Primary Prevention of Sudden Cardiac Death

	N	CAD	Low EF	PVCs	NSVT	Therapy	Follow-up, Months	Findings	Comments
Coronary Artery Disease									
Class IC									
CAST (1989)	1498	+	+	+	–	Encainide or flecainide vs. placebo	10	7.7% mortality (treatment) vs. 3.0% (placebo)	Terminated prematurely due to excess mortality in treatment group
Amiodarone BASIS (1990)	312	+	–	+	–	Amio vs. mexiletine or quinidine vs. no therapy	72	5% mortality (amio) vs. 10% (class I) vs. 13% (placebo)	Amio improved survival, non-significant trend with Holter-guided PVC suppression
EMIAT (1997)	1486	+	+	–	–	Amio vs. placebo	21	7.2% mortality (both groups), 35% RR in arrhythmic death	Amio reduced arrhythmic death rate without affecting total survival
CAMIAT (1997)	1202	+	–	+	–	Amio vs. placebo	21	3.3% VF/SCD (amio) vs. 6.0% (placebo), RR 21.2%	Prophylactic amio improved survival for frequent or repetitive PVCs
ICD									
MADIT (1996)	196	+	+	+	+	ICD vs. conventional therapy	27	15.7% mortality (ICD) vs. 38.6% (placebo), RR 46%	Terminated prematurely because of significant ICD benefit
CABG-Patch (1997)	900	+	+	–	–	ICD vs. no ICD	36	No difference in all-cause mortality	All patients had abnormal SAECG; no benefit of prophylactic ICD
MUSTT (1999)	704	+	+	+	+	EP-guided or ICD vs. no therapy	60	25% mortality (EP-guided or ICD) vs. 32% (no therapy)	EP-guided therapy with ICDs, but not with antiarrhythmic drugs, reduced the risk of SCD in high-risk patients with CAD
Sotalol									
Julian et al. (1982)	1456	+	–	–	–	*d,l*-sotalol vs. placebo	12	7.3% mortality (sotalol) vs. 8.9% (placebo), RR 18%	*d,l*-sotalol may reduce mortality by up to 25%
SWORD (1996)	3121	+	+	–	–	*d*-sotalol vs. placebo	5	5.0% mortality (sotalol) vs. 3.1% (placebo)	Trial terminated due to excess mortality in the treatment group
CHF Amiodarone Trials									
GESICA (1994)	516	~1/3	–	–	–	Amio vs. standard therapy	24	33.5% mortality (amio) vs. 41.4% (control)	Amio improved survival in symptomatic heart failure
CHF-STAT (1995)	674	~2/3	+	–	–	Amio vs. placebo	45	30.6% mortality (amio) vs. 29.2% (placebo)	No survival benefit with amio; trend to improved survival in DCM

Abbreviations: + = inclusion criterion; – = not inclusion criterion; amio = amiodarone; CAD = coronary artery disease; CHF = congestive heart failure; DCM = dilated cardiomyopathy; EF = ejection fraction; ICD = implantable cardioverter-defibrillator; NSVT = nonsustained ventricular tachycardia; PVCs = premature ventricular contractions; RR = risk reduction; SCD = sudden cardiac death; VF = ventricular fibrillation. See text for clinical trial abbreviations.

Source: Modified with permission from Welch PJ, Page RL, Hamdan MH. Management of ventricular arrhythmias: A trial-based approach. *J Am Coll Cardiol* 1999; 34:621–630. Julian DG, Prescott RJ, Jackson FS. Controlled trial of sotalol for one year after myocardial infarction. *Lancet* 1982; 1:1142–1147.

Failure (STAT-CHF).[315] Comparison of the two patient populations and subgroup analysis suggested that prophylactic amiodarone may be more beneficial in patients with nonischemic cardiomyopathy, found in greater number in the GESICA study (Table 33-7). The consequence of these amiodarone trials is that this drug can be used safely in patients with left ventricular dysfunction, and, in contrast to some class I agents, it does not increase mortality rates. Therefore, amiodarone is the drug of choice when antiarrhythmic drug treatment is indicated in patients with left ventricular dysfunction.

In patients who survived cardiac arrest not associated with myocardial infarction, empiric amiodarone therapy has been shown to be superior to electrophysiologically guided conventional therapy.[302] Rates for survival free of cardiac death, resuscitated cardiac arrest, and defibrillator shocks associated with syncope at 1, 3, and 5 years was 91 percent, 76 percent, and 63 percent, respectively, in the amiodarone-treated patients, compared with 77 percent, 56 percent, and 46 percent in the conventionally treated patients. The efficacy of amiodarone in reducing total mortality rates in patients with ventricular fibrillation or hemodynamically unstable ventricular tachycardia compared to implantable cardioverter-defibrillator (ICD) treatment has been evaluated prospectively in the randomized Amiodarone versus Implantable Defibrillator (AVID) study, which reported a survival benefit in the patients randomized to ICD therapy.[307] Prospective, randomized trials addressed a similar question in cardiac arrest survivors in the Canadian Implantable Defibrillator Study (CIDS)[316,317] and CASH[303,318] (see below).

Intravenous Amiodarone Intravenous amiodarone in the United States remains a powerful parenteral drug for the acute treatment of patients with life-threatening ventricular arrhythmias.[319] The efficacy of intravenous amiodarone in patients with recurrent, hemodynamically unstable ventricular tachycardia refractory to lidocaine, procainamide, and bretylium is approximately 40 percent in prospective studies, and about 80 percent of the arrhythmias are suppressed within the first 48 h. A loading dose of 5 mg/kg over the first 30 min and a total dose of 1000 mg in the first 24 h is recommended. Additional boluses of 150 mg may be necessary for arrhythmia control.[320] Compared with bretylium, intravenous amiodarone was at least as effective and caused significantly less hypotension than did bretylium in 302 patients with recurrent or incessant ventricular arrhythmias refractory to lidocaine and procainamide[321] (see also Chaps. 24 and 27).

The use of intravenous amiodarone in out-of-hospital cardiac arrest was recently studied. Intravenous amiodarone was compared to placebo in 504 patients suffering out-of-hospital cardiac arrest that was refractory to three or more precordial shocks. Patients receiving 300 mg of intravenous amiodarone had an improved rate of survival to admission to the hospital as compared to placebo. Whether use of intravenous amiodarone confers a survival benefit remains to be determined.[322]

Device Therapy

AUTOMATIC IMPLANTABLE CARDIOVERTER-DEFIBRILLATOR

The ICD was initially developed to recognize ventricular fibrillation or rapid ventricular tachycardia and terminate it automatically by delivering one or more high-energy shocks.[323] Newer-generation defibrillators have the additional ability to deliver low-energy cardioversion, antitachycardia pacing for ventricular tachycardia, and antibradycardia pacing. In addition, the extended storage capabilities of new defibrillator systems permit retrospective analysis of the stored electrograms during arrhythmia detection, allowing more accurate conclusions about the type of arrhythmia recognized by the device (supraventricular or ventricular), their mode of initiation, and effects of additional antiarrhythmic therapy.

The first generation of epicardial defibrillators required a thoracotomy to place the sensing and defibrillator leads epicardially, and the generator size mandated implantation of the device in an abdominal pocket. The development of biphasic waveforms, "active cans" (the generator case itself serves as a defibrillator electrode), and more efficient capacitors has made it possible to reduce the size of the defibrillators, which can now be implanted subpectorally with a transvenous endocardial lead system that integrates both pace-sense and high-voltage defibrillation abilities. Endocardial placement has reduced the perioperative mortality rate associated with defibrillator implants from 4 to 5 to less than 1.0 percent.[324]

ICDs are very effective in terminating ventricular tachyarrhythmias. In a large data base of 2834 epicardial and endocardial defibrillators implanted in 2807 patients between 1989 and 1993, 98.8 percent of 7470 ventricular fibrillation episodes were detected, and 97.9 percent of 42,132 ventricular tachycardia episodes were successfully terminated by the device.[324] The long-term outcome of patients with implantable defibrillators is also favorable, considering that virtually all patients receiving such devices are at high risk for sudden cardiac death, since they had either cardiac arrest or recurrent ventricular tachycardia refractory to medical therapy prior to implantation of the device. Defibrillator therapy has been shown to effectively reduce the annual incidence of sudden cardiac death in patients with severe underlying cardiac disease (less than 5 percent)[325,326] as well as in patients without significant structural heart disease (0 percent).[327] Despite effective reduction of the mortality rate from sudden cardiac death, however, long-term survival in patients with severely depressed left ventricular function is still poor despite defibrillatory therapy, and the overall cardiac mortality rate does not appear to be reduced in direct proportion to the reduction in sudden cardiac death.[328]

To investigate the potential benefit of ICD therapy compared with antiarrhythmic drug treatment in secondary prevention, the AVID, CASH, and CIDS studies randomized patients with documented sustained ventricular arrhythmia to one of these two treatment strategies. AVID and CIDS enrolled patients with ventricular fibrillation or poorly tolerated ventricular tachycardia and left ventricular dysfunction. In the AVID trial, which enrolled 1016 such patients, the ICD group had 38 and 25 percent reductions in the overall mortality rate at 1 and 3 years, respectively, compared to the group of patients taking amiodarone or sotalol.[307] CIDS enrolled 659 patients. Preliminary results after 1 year of follow-up were recently reported, and a 20 percent reduction in mortality rate with ICD was demonstrated.[317] CASH enrolled patients with cardiac arrest secondary to a ventricular arrhythmia regardless of the underlying disease or ventricular function. The final results have not yet been published, although a 2-year 39 percent reduction of the mortality rate due to all causes in the ICD arm compared with the drug arm (metoprolol or amiodarone) has been reported by the investigators.[318] These studies show that, compared to the best currently available antiarrhythmic drug therapy, ICDs improve survival rates in patients with a history of ventricular fibrillation or ventricular tachycardia (Table 33-7).

Several studies looking at the primary prevention or prophylactic use of defibrillators in high-risk populations have been completed (Table 33-7). The Multicenter Automatic Defibrillator Implantation Trial (MADIT)[329] demonstrated a survival benefit of defibrillator therapy compared with conventional therapy in patients who are post–myocardial infarction with nonsustained ventricular tachycardia, left ventricular dysfunction, and inducible sustained ventricular tachycardia that was not suppressed by procainamide. It has led to the approval of prophylactic implantation of defibrillators in this narrowly defined patient population. The Multicenter Unsustained Tachycardia Trial (MUSTT) was a randomized, controlled trial to test the hypothesis that electrophysiologically guided antiarrhythmic therapy would reduce the risk of sudden death among patients with coronary artery disease, a left ventricular ejection fraction of 40 percent or less, and asymptomatic, nonsustained ventricular tachycardia. Patients in whom sustained ventricular tachyarrhythmias were induced by programmed stimulation were assigned to receive either antiarrhythmic therapy, including drugs and implantable defibrillators, as indicated by the results of electrophysiologic testing, or no antiarrhythmic therapy. Electrophysiologically guided antiarrhythmic therapy with implantable defibrillators, but not with antiarrhythmic drugs, reduced the risk of sudden death in high-risk patients with coronary disease[330] (Fig. 33-7). The Coronary Artery Bypass Graft (CABG) Patch trial enrolled patients with coronary artery disease scheduled for elective coronary artery bypass grafting (CABG) who also had a left ventricular ejection fraction of less than 30 percent and an abnormal SAECG. Nine hundred patients were randomized to receive either an ICD at the time of CABG or usual care and followed for a mean of 32 months. This study found no significant difference in the primary end point of total mortality at 30 days and a mean of 32 months.[331] The findings were not surprising in view of the known benefit of revascularization in preventing sudden cardiac death (see below) and the poor positive predictive value of the SAECG (Table 33-7).

The number of patients who could benefit from an ICD implant is increasingly larger due to the lower mortality and morbidity rates associated with the implantation of newer endocardial devices, which can be implanted with techniques similar to those of bradycardia pacemaker insertion. ICDs can effectively protect against both tachycardic and bradycardic sudden cardiac death regardless of the underlying heart disease or various triggers of arrhythmias. Since their mode of action is therapeutic rather than preventive, ICD therapy might effectively be combined with other antiarrhythmic strategies, such as drugs or catheter ablation, to prevent frequent recurrences of tachyarrhythmias. Despite the undisputed efficacy of implantable defibrillators in preventing sudden cardiac death, there are several major questions that remain to be answered: (1) Which patients will benefit most from defibrillator therapy?, (2) Do ICDs improve quality of life?, (3) Are ICDs cost-effective compared with antiarrhythmic drug therapy?, and (4) Will adjunctive antiarrhythmic drug therapy add to the efficacy of ICDs? (see also Chap. 30).

PERMANENT PACEMAKER

Permanent pacing appears to have a beneficial effect on survival in patients with congenital long-QT syndrome.[332,333] The beneficial effects of permanent pacing may be related to prevention of bradycardia and pauses, potentially contributing to a more homogeneous repolarization, as well as rate-dependent shortening of the QT_c interval in patients with mutation in the sodium channel gene (*SCN5A*)[178] (see Chap. 24). This is an unreliable approach and is unlikely to be used in the future due to the development of small, dual-chambered ICDs.

Patients with obstructive hypertrophic cardiomyopathy are at increased risk for sudden cardiac death may also benefit from pacemaker implantation. In a series of 84 patients with this condition who had severe, drug-refractory symptoms and a history of syncope in half the patients, only two sudden cardiac deaths occurred during the 2.5-year follow-up period after pacemaker implantation.[334] This approximately 1 percent annual mortality rate compares favorably with the annual incidence of sudden cardiac death in hypertrophic cardiomyopathy of 2 to 4 percent

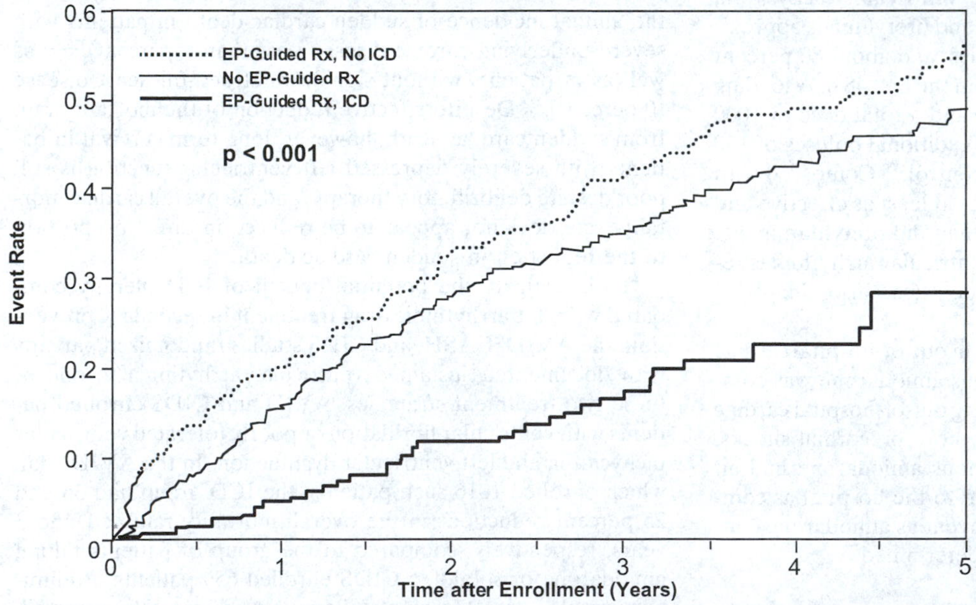

FIGURE 33-7 Kaplan-Meier estimates of the rates of overall mortality in a randomized trial of electrophysiologically guided (EPG) therapy versus no antiarrhythmic therapy (MUSTT Trial). The p value refers to two comparisons: between the patients in the group assigned to EPG therapy who received treatment with a defibrillator (solid dark line) and those who did not receive such treatment (dotted line), and between the patients assigned to electrophysiologically guided therapy who received treatment with a defibrillator and those assigned to no antiarrhythmic therapy (thin solid line). (Reproduced from Buxton et al.,[330] with permission.)

per year in adults and 4 to 6 percent per year in children and adolescents[134] demonstrated in previous studies. Most studies have shown a decrease in left ventricular outflow tract gradient, however, pacing may have deleterious effects on other hemodynamic parameters, and there are no controlled trials demonstrating improved survival[334,335] (see Chap. 67).

Role of Surgery

REVASCULARIZATION

There is a reduced prevalence of sudden cardiac death after CABG.[336,337] Among the 13,476 patients in the Coronary Artery Surgical Study (CASS) registry, all of whom had significant coronary artery disease, operable vessels, and no significant valvular disease, the mean incidence of sudden cardiac death during the 4.6-year average follow-up was 5.2 percent in patients treated medically and 1.8 percent in those treated surgically.[336] The beneficial effect of CABG was even more pronounced in the subgroup of patients with reduced left ventricular ejection fraction and multivessel disease, where the survival rate free from sudden cardiac death at 5 years was 91 percent for the surgical group versus 69 percent in the medical group. CABG also seems to be beneficial in patients with cardiac arrest prior to hospitalization. In an uncontrolled study of 265 survivors of cardiac arrest, 32 percent underwent CABG and 68 percent were treated medically.[338] After adjusting for differences in baseline variables between the two treatment groups, the use of CABG was associated with a significant risk reduction in recurrent cardiac arrest (risk ratio 0.48, confidence interval 0.24 to 0.97). The protective effect of CABG against recurrent cardiac arrest appears to be best in patients with reversible ischemia as the major pathophysiologic factor in sudden cardiac death. These patients are characterized by critical coronary artery disease, significant regions of myocardium at risk for ischemia, and no inducible monomorphic ventricular arrhythmias at electrophysiologic study.[251,338] Despite the encouraging results of CABG in survivors of cardiac arrest, it should be noted that only a minority of these patients are candidates for operative revascularization and that monomorphic ventricular tachycardia, which is often associated with ventricular scars from healed myocardial infarctions, is usually not controlled by myocardial revascularization alone.[339]

ANTIARRHYTHMIA SURGERY

Electrophysiologically guided subendocardial resection and cryoablation are potentially curative surgical options in patients with recurrent monomorphic ventricular tachycardia in whom areas of slow conduction around myocardial scars are critical for sustaining ventricular tachycardia. Long-term follow-up of this operative technique has yielded a clinical success rate of nearly 90 percent in eliminating the presenting ventricular tachycardia in patients who survive surgery. The technique is limited, however, by the high surgical mortality rate of 10 to 15 percent.[340] These data, gathered in the 1980s, may exaggerate the operative risk, since current myocardial preservation is improved. We believe that the use of this therapy should be revisited. The best candidates for electrophysiologically guided subendocardial resection are patients who require coronary revascularization and have a well-defined left ventricular aneurysm.

Another surgical technique aimed at reducing sudden cardiac death rates in high-risk patients is left cardiac sympathetic denervation in the therapy of congenital long-QT syndrome.[341] The goal of this surgery is selective partial sympathetic denervation of the heart. In a review of 85 long-QT patients who continued to have recurrent syncope and cardiac arrest despite beta-blocker therapy and subsequently underwent left sympathectomy, the cardiac event rate was reduced from 22 ± 32 to 1 ± 3 per patient, and the number of patients with cardiac events decreased from 99 to 45 percent.[341] The rate of sudden cardiac death over a follow-up period of nearly 6 years was 8 percent (see also Chap. 24). This therapy, which, when successful, is almost always associated with development of Horner's syndrome, has fallen out of favor as a result of the evolution of ICD therapy.

CATHETER ABLATION THERAPY

Catheter ablation of arrhythmias has emerged as a curative approach for many supraventricular arrhythmias and a few specific forms of ventricular tachycardias.[188] The role of catheter ablation in the prevention of sudden cardiac death is less well established, but this therapy form has been successfully employed in selected cases. Rarely, supraventricular tachycardias with a rapid ventricular response may degenerate into fatal ventricular tachyarrhythmias and cardiac arrest.[342] Radiofrequency catheter ablation can eliminate the risk of a rapid ventricular response by abolishing conduction over an accessory pathway in patients with Wolff-Parkinson-White syndrome, or it can slow or completely block conduction over the atrioventricular node in patients with atrial arrhythmias and rapid, medically uncontrolled atrioventricular conduction.

Radiofrequency catheter ablation can potentially prevent sudden cardiac death in patients with documented and inducible bundle-branch reentrant ventricular tachycardia as the only mechanism of cardiac arrest.[343] The role of catheter ablation in other forms of ventricular tachycardia is less well established. Catheter ablation of ventricular tachycardia in patients with structural heart disease is currently feasible in only a small subset of patients who present with a hemodynamically relatively well-tolerated monomorphic ventricular tachycardia.[344] Although the acute success rate in eliminating the index arrhythmia in a few specialized centers is near 60 percent, these patients often have extensive coronary heart disease, and other ventricular tachycardia morphologies recur frequently during follow-up, necessitating additional therapies.[345] Improved mapping techniques of the ventricular tachycardia circuit, better catheters, and perhaps other energy sources may help improve the efficacy of catheter ablation for ventricular tachycardia and potentially expand its role in the prevention of sudden cardiac death (see also Chap. 28).

SUMMARY

Sudden cardiac death affects more than 300,000 individuals in the United States annually and accounts for half the mortality rate due to coronary heart disease. The vast majority of people who have experienced sudden cardiac death have underlying structural heart disease, which in the adult population is most frequently coronary heart disease, but a variety of other cardiac disorders can cause sudden cardiac death as well. Ventricular tachycardia and fibrillation and, less often, bradycardia and asystole are responsible for sudden cardiac death. Enhanced sympathetic tone appears to be important in triggering or predisposing to sudden cardiac death. Long-term survival following a cardiac arrest episode is still poor (less than 30 percent). The time delay to defibrillation and/or bystander administration of CPR directly influences survival. ICDs appear to be the most effective therapeutic option for treating survivors of cardiac arrest. Beta blockers and ACE inhibitors are helpful in the prevention of sudden cardiac death, in part through a reduction in the incidence of myocardial infarction. Proof for the use of other prophylactic medications, including antiarrhythmics, to prevent sudden cardiac death is inadequate. The most important factor limiting our ability to alter the incidence of sudden cardiac death is our inability to identify with acceptable sensitivity and specificity a large percentage of the individuals who experience sudden cardiac death. Short-term efforts to improve the survival of sudden cardiac death victims should be directed toward delivering CPR and electrical therapy as soon as possible after the onset of an arrest.[232] Long-term goals should be focused on the prevention of sudden cardiac death and encompass basically four interrelated, stepwise objectives:[232] (1) more accurate and specific identification of the patients at risk, (2) identification and characterization of mechanisms responsible for ventricular tachycardia–ventricular fibrillation, and bradycardia-asystole, (3) identification of interventions that prevent these arrhythmias, and (4) testing of these interventions in the individuals at risk.

References

1. Kannel WB, Thomas HE Jr. Sudden coronary death: The Framingham Study. *Ann NY Acad Sci* 1982; 382:3–20.
2. Kannel WB, Schatzkin A. Sudden death: Lessons from subsets in population studies. *J Am Coll Cardiol* 1985; 5(suppl B):141B–149B.
3. Kannel WB, Cupples LA, D'Agostino RB. Sudden death risk in overt coronary heart disease: The Framingham Study. *Am Heart J* 1987; 113:799–804.
4. Chiang BN, Perlman LV, Fulton M, et al. Predisposing factors in sudden cardiac death in Tecumseh, Michigan. *Circulation* 1970; 41:31–37.
5. Kuller LH, Lilienfeld A, Fischer R. Epidemiological study of sudden and unexpected deaths due to arteriosclerotic heart disease. *Circulation* 1966; 34:1056–1068.
6. Kuller LH, Lilienfeld A, Fischer R. An epidemiological study of sudden and unexpected death in adults. *Medicine* 1967; 46:341–361.
7. Kuller LH, Perper JA, Dai WS, et al. Sudden death and the decline in coronary heart disease mortality. *J Chronic Dis* 1986; 39:1001–1019.
8. Goldberg RJ, Gore JM, Alpert JS, et al. Incidence and acute fatality rates of acute myocardial infarction (1975–1988): The Worcester Heart Attack Study. *Am Heart J* 1988; 115:761–767.
9. Gillum RF, Folsom A, Luepker RV, et al. Sudden death and acute myocardial infarction in a metropolitan area, 1970–1980: The Minnesota Heart Survey. *N Engl J Med* 1983; 309:1353–1358.
10. Gillum RF. Sudden coronary death in the United States: 1980–1985. *Circulation* 1989; 79:756–765.
11. Madsen JK. Ischemic heart disease and prodromes of sudden death. *Br Heart J* 1985; 54:27–32.
12. Goldstein S. The necessity of a uniform definition of sudden coronary death: Witnessed death within 1 hour of the onset of acute symptoms. *Am Heart J* 1982; 103:156–159.
13. Hinkle LE, Thaler HT. Clinical classification of cardiac deaths. *Circulation* 1982; 65:457–464.
14. de Vreede-Swagemakers JJ, Gorgels AP, Dubois-Arbouw WI, et al. Out-of-hospital cardiac arrest in the 1990's: A population-based study in the Maastricht area on incidence, characteristics and survival. *J Am Coll Cardiol* 1997; 30:1500–1505.
15. Leach IH, Blundell JW, Rowley JM, et al. Acute ischemic lesions in death due to ischemic heart disease: An autopsy study of 333 cases of out-of-hospital death. *Eur Heart J* 1995; 16:1181–1185.
16. Matoba R, Shikata I, Iwai K, et al. An epidemiologic and histopathological study of sudden cardiac death in Osaka Medical Examiner's office. *Jpn Circ J* 1989; 53:1581–1588.
17. Myocardial Infarction Community Registers. *Public Health in Europe 5*. Copenhagen: Regional Office for Europe, World Health Organization; 1976.
18. Goldberg RJ. Declining out-of-hospital sudden coronary death rates: Additional pieces of the epidemiologic puzzle. *Circulation* 1989; 79:1369–1373.
19. Cowie MR, Fahrenbuch CE, Cobb LA, et al. Out-of-hospital cardiac arrest: Racial differences in outcome in Seattle. *Am J Public Health* 1993; 83:955–959.
20. Becker LB, Han BH, Meyer PM, et al. Racial differences in the incidence of cardiac arrest and subsequent survival. *N Engl J Med* 1993; 329:600–606.
21. Albert CM, McGovern BA, Newell JB, et al. Sex differences in cardiac arrest survivors. *Circulation* 1996; 93:1170–1176.
22. Neuspiel DR, Kuller LH. Sudden and unexpected natural death in childhood and adolescence. *JAMA* 1985; 254:1321–1325.
23. Liberthson RR. Sudden death from cardiac causes in children and young adults. *N Engl J Med* 1996; 334:1039–1044.
24. Burke AP, Farb A, Virmani R, et al. Sports-related sudden cardiac death in young adults. *Am Heart J* 1991; 121:568–575.
25. Kennedy HL, Whitlock JA, Buckingham TA, et al. Long-term follow-up of asymptomatic healthy subjects with frequent and complex ventricular ectopy. *N Engl J Med* 1985; 312:193–197.
26. Drory Y, Turetz Y, Hiss Y, et al. Sudden unexpected deaths in persons less than 40 years of age. *Am J Cardiol* 1991; 68:1388–1392.
27. Driscoll DJ, Edwards WD. Sudden unexpected death in children and adolescents. *J Am Coll Cardiol* 1985; 5(suppl 6):118B–121B.
28. Topaz O, Edwards JE. Pathologic features of sudden death in children, adolescents and young adults. *Chest* 1985; 87:476–482.
29. Maron BJ, Gohman TE, Aeppli D. Prevalence of sudden cardiac death during competitive sports activities in Minnesota high school athletes. *J Am Coll Cardiol* 1998; 32:1881–1884.
30. Kramer MR, Drory Y, Lev B. Sudden death in young Israeli soldiers: Analysis of 83 cases. *Isr J Med Sci* 1989; 25:620–624.
31. Thiene G, Nava A, Corrado D, et al. Right ventricular cardiomyopathy and sudden death in young people. *N Engl J Med* 1988; 318:129–133.
32. Molander N. Sudden natural death in later childhood and adolescence. *Arch Dis Child* 1982; 57:572–576.
33. Keeling JW, Knowles SAS. Sudden death in childhood and adolescence. *J Pathol* 1989; 159:221–224.
34. Shen WK, Edwards WD, Hammill SC, et al. Sudden unexpected nontraumatic death in 54 young adults: A 30-year population-based study. *Am J Cardiol* 1995; 76:148–152.
35. Garson A Jr, McNamara DG. Sudden death in a pediatric cardiology population, 1958–1983: Relation to prior arrhythmias. *J Am Coll Cardiol* 1985; 5(Suppl 6):134B–137B.
36. Lambert EC, Menon VA, Wagner HR, et al. Sudden unexpected death from cardiovascular disease in children: A cooperative international study. *Am J Cardiol* 1974; 34:89–96.
37. Chandar JS, Wolff GS, Garson A Jr, et al. Ventricular arrhythmias in postoperative tetralogy of Fallot. *Am J Cardiol* 1990; 65:655–661.
38. Hayes CJ, Gersony WM: Arrhythmias after the Mustard operation for transposition of the great arteries: A long-term study. *J Am Coll Cardiol* 1986; 7:133–137.

39. Duster MC, Bink-Boelkens MT, Wampler D, et al. Long-term follow-up of dysrhythmias following the Mustard procedure. *Am Heart J* 1985; 109:1323–1326.
40. Hinkle LE. Short-term risk factors for sudden death. *Ann NY Acad Sci* 1982; 382:22–37.
41. Demirovic J. Risk factors in the incidence of sudden cardiac death and possibilities for its prevention. Doctoral thesis. Belgrade, Yugoslavia: University of Belgrade Press; 1985.
42. Beaglehole R, Stewart AW, Bonita R, et al. Myocardial infarction and sudden death in Auckland. *NZ Med J* 1984; 97:715–718.
43. Kagan A, Yano K, Reed DM, et al. Predictors of sudden cardiac death among Hawaiian-Japanese men. *Am J Epidemiol* 1989; 130:268–277.
44. Lavery CE, Mittleman MA, Cohen MC, et al. Nonuniform night-time distribution of acute cardiac events: A possible effect of sleep states. *Circulation* 1997; 9:3321–3327.
45. Willich SN, Maclure M, Mittleman M, et al. Sudden cardiac death: Support for a role of triggering in causation. *Circulation* 1993; 87:1442–1450.
46. Mittleman MA, Siscovick DS. Physical exertion as a trigger of myocardial infarction and sudden cardiac death. *Cardiol Clin* 1996; 14:263–270.
47. Albert CM, Manson JE, Cook NR, et al. Moderate alcohol consumption and the risk of sudden cardiac death among U.S. male physicians. *Circulation* 1999; 100:944–950
48. de Vreede-Swagemakers JJ, Gorgels AP, Weijenberg MP, et al. Risk indicators for out-of-hospital cardiac arrest in patients with coronary artery disease. *J Clin Epidemiol* 1999; 52:601–607.
49. Kannel WB. Update on the role of cigarette smoking in coronary heart disease. *Am Heart J* 1981; 101:319–328.
50. Burke AP, Farb A, Malcom GT, Liang YH, et al. Coronary risk factors and plaque morphology in men with coronary disease who died suddenly. *N Engl J Med* 1997; 336:1276–1282.
51. Hallstrom AP, Cobb LA, Ray R. Smoking as a risk factor for recurrence of sudden cardiac arrest. *N Engl J Med* 1986; 314:271–274.
52. Lampert R, Jain D, Burg MM, et al. Destabilizing effects of mental stress on ventricular arrhythmias in patients with implantable cardioverter-defibrillators. *Circulation* 2000; 101: 158–164.
53. Lown B. Sudden cardiac death: Biobehavioral perspective. *Circulation* 1987; 76(1, part 2):I186–I196.
54. Engel GL. Sudden and rapid death during psychologic stress: Folklore or folk wisdom? *Ann Intern Med* 1971; 74:771–782.
55. Leor J, Poole WK, Kloner RA. Sudden cardiac death triggered by an earthquake. *N Engl J Med* 1996; 334:413–419.
56. Weinblatt E, Ruberman W, Goldberg JD, et al. Relation of education to sudden death after myocardial infarction. *N Engl J Med* 1978; 299:60–65.
57. Talbott E, Kuller LH, Petre K, et al. Biologic and psychosocial risk factors of sudden death from coronary disease in white women. *Am J Cardiol* 1977; 39:858–864.
58. Lakka TA, Venalainen JM, Rauramaa R, et al. Relation of leisure-time physical activity and cardiorespiratory fitness to the risk of acute myocardial infarction in men. *N Engl J Med* 1994; 330:1549–1554.
59. Cobb LA, Weaver WD. Exercise: A risk factor for sudden death in patients with coronary heart disease. *J Am Coll Cardiol* 1986; 7:215–219.
60. Lemaitre RN, Siscovick DS, Raghunathan TE, et al. Leisure-time physical activity and the risk of primary cardiac arrest. *Arch Intern Med* 1999; 159:686–690.
61. Williams PT. Physical activity and public health. *JAMA* 1995; 274:533–534.
62. Brownell KD, Bachorik PS, Ayerle RS. Changes in plasma lipid and lipoprotein levels in men and women after a program of moderate exercise. *Circulation* 1982; 65:477–484.
63. Mittleman MA, Maclure M, Toffer GH, et al. Triggering of acute myocardial infarction by heavy physical exertion: Protection against triggering by regular exertion. *N Engl J Med* 1993; 329:1677–1683.
64. Thompson PD, Stern MP, Williams P, et al. Deaths during jogging or running: A study of 18 cases. *JAMA* 1979; 242:1265–1267.
65. Mittleman MA, Siscovick DS. Physical exertion as a trigger of myocardial infarction and sudden cardiac death. *Cardiol Clin* 1996; 14:263–270.
66. Burke AP, Farb A, Malcom GT, et al. Plaque rupture and sudden death related to exertion in men with coronary artery disease. *JAMA* 1999; 281:921–926.
67. Koplan JP. Cardiovascular deaths while running. *JAMA* 1979; 242:2578–2579.
68. Maron BJ, Shirani J, Poliac LC, et al. Sudden death in young competitive athletes. Clinical, demographic, and pathological profiles. *JAMA* 1996; 276:199–204.
69. Maron BJ, Roberts WC, McAllister HA, et al. Sudden death in young athletes. *Circulation* 1980; 62:218–229.
70. Jensen-Urstad M. Sudden death and physical activity in athletes and nonathletes. *Scand J Med Sci Sports* 1995; 5:279–284.
71. Corrado D, Thiene G, Nava A, et al. Sudden death in young competitive athletes: Clinicopathologic correlations in 22 cases. *Am J Med* 1990; 89:588–596.
72. Corrado D, Basso C, Schiavon M, et al. Screening for hypertrophic cardiomyopathy in young athletes. *N Engl J Med* 1998; 339:364–369.
73. Maron BJ, Bodison S, Wesley Y, et al. Results of screening a large population of intercollegiate athletes for cardiovascular disease. *J Am Coll Cardiol* 1987; 10:1214–1222.
74. Maron BJ, Mitchell JH. 26th Bethesda Conference: Recommendations for determining eligibility for competition in athletes with cardiovascular abnormalities. *J Am Coll Cardiol* 1994; 24: 848–899.
75. Myerburg RJ, Kessler KM, Bassett AL, et al. A biological approach to sudden cardiac death: Structure, function and cause. *Am J Cardiol* 1989; 63:1512–1516.
76. Willich SN, Maclure M, Mittleman M, et al. Sudden cardiac death: Support for a role of triggering in causation. *Circulation* 1993; 87:1442–1450.
77. Green HL. Sudden arrhythmic cardiac death: Mechanisms, resuscitation and classification: The Seattle perspective. *Am J Cardiol* 1990; 65:4B–12B.
78. Myerburg RJ, Conde CA, Sung RJ, et al. Clinical, electrophysiologic, and hemodynamic profile of patients resuscitated from prehospital cardiac arrest. *Am J Med* 1980; 68:568–576.
79. Bayes de Luna A, Coumel P, Leclercq JF. Ambulatory sudden cardiac death: Mechanisms of production of fatal arrhythmia. *Am Heart J* 1989; 117:151–159.
80. Nikolic G, Bishop RL, Singh JB. Sudden death during Holter monitoring. *Circulation* 1982; 66:218–225.
81. Luu M, Stevenson WG, Stevenson LW, et al. Diverse mechanisms of unexpected cardiac arrest in advanced heart failure. *Circulation* 1989; 80:1675–1680.
82. Janse MJ, Wit AL. Electrophysiologic mechanisms of ventricular arrhythmias resulting from myocardial ischemia and infarction. *Physiol Rev* 1989; 69:1049–1154.
83. Dillon SM, Allessie MA, Ursell PC, et al. Influence of anisotropic tissue structure on reentrant circuits in the epicardial border zone of subacute canine infarcts. *Circ Res* 1988; 63:182–206.
84. Pogwizd SM, Corr PB. Mechanisms underlying the development of ventricular fibrillation during early myocardial ischemia. *Circ Res* 1990; 66:672–695.
85. Balke CW, Kaplinsky E, Michelson EL, et al. Reperfusion ventricular tachyarrhythmias: Correlation with antecedent coronary artery occlusion tachyarrhythmias and duration of myocardial ischemia. *Am Heart J* 1981; 101:449–456.

86. Lerman BB, Burkhoff D, Yue DT, et al. Mechanoelectrical feedback: Independent role of preload and contractility in modulation of canine ventricular excitability. *J Clin Invest* 1985; 76:1843–1850.
87. Levine JH, Guarnieri T, Kadish AH, et al. Changes in myocardial repolarization in patients undergoing balloon valvuloplasty for congenital pulmonary stenosis: Evidence for contraction-excitation feedback in humans. *Circulation* 1988; 77:70–77.
88. Barber MJ, Mueller TM, Henry DP, et al. Transmural myocardial infarction in the dog produces sympathectomy in noninfarcted myocardium. *Circulation* 1983; 67:787–796.
89. Inoue H, Zipes DP. Results of sympathetic denervation in the canine heart: Supersensitivity that may be arrhythmogenic. *Circulation* 1987; 75:877–887.
90. Takahashi N, Zipes DP. Vagal modulation of adrenergic effects on canine sinus and atrioventricular nodes. *Am J Physiol* 1983; 244:H775–H781.
91. Schwartz PJ, Zaza A, Pala M, et al. Baroreflex sensitivity and its evolution during the first year after myocardial infarction. *J Am Coll Cardiol* 1988; 12:629–636.
92. La Rovere MT, Specchia G, Mortara A, et al. Baroreflex sensitivity, clinical correlates and cardiovascular mortality among patients with a first myocardial infarction: A prospective study. *Circulation* 1988; 78:816–824.
93. Farrell TG, Odemuyiwa O, Bashir Y, et al. Prognostic value of baroreflex sensitivity after acute myocardial infarction. *Br Heart J* 1992; 66:129–137.
94. Goldstein S, Landis J, Leighton R, et al. Characteristics of the resuscitated out-of-hospital cardiac arrest victim with coronary heart disease. *Circulation* 1981; 64:977–984.
95. Bigger JT Jr. Patients with malignant or potentially malignant ventricular arrhythmias: Opportunities and limitations of drug therapy in prevention of sudden death. *J Am Coll Cardiol* 1985; 5:23B–26B.
96. Kempf FC Jr, Josephson ME. Cardiac arrest recorded on ambulatory electrocardiograms. *Am J Cardiol* 1984; 53:1577–1582.
97. Myerburg RJ, Kessler KM, Bassett AL, et al. A biological approach to sudden cardiac death: Structure, function and cause. *Am J Cardiol* 1989; 63:1512–1516.
98. Margolis JR, Hirshfeld JW Jr, McNeer JF, et al. Sudden death due to coronary artery disease: A clinical, hemodynamic, and angiographic profile. *Circulation* 1975; 52(6 suppl):III180–III188.
99. Davies MJ. Anatomic features in victims of sudden coronary death: Coronary artery pathology. *Circulation* 1992; 85(1 suppl):I19–I24.
100. Roberts WC, Kragel AH, Gertz D, et al. Coronary arteries in unstable pectoris, acute myocardial infarction and sudden coronary death. *Am Heart J* 1994; 127:1588–1593.
101. Kuller LH, Perper JA, Dai WS, et al. Sudden death and the decline in coronary heart disease mortality. *J Chronic Dis* 1986; 39:1001–1019.
102. Ambrose JA, Tannenbaum MA, Alexopoulos D, et al. Angiographic progression of coronary artery disease in the development of myocardial infarction. *J Am Coll Cardiol* 1988; 12:56–62.
103. McHenry PL, O'Donnell J, Morris SN, et al. The abnormal exercise electrocardiogram in apparently healthy men: A predictor of angina pectoris as an initial coronary event during long-term follow-up. *Circulation* 1984; 70:547–551.
104. Weiner DA, Ryan TJ, McCabe CH, et al. Risk of developing an acute myocardial infarction or sudden death in patients with exercise-induced silent myocardial ischemia: A report from the Coronary Artery Surgery Study (CASS) registry. *Am J Cardiol* 1988; 62:1155–1158.
105. Goldstein S, Friedman L, Hutchinson R, Aspirin Myocardial Infarction Study Group. Timing, mechanism and clinical setting of witnessed deaths in postmyocardial infarction patients. *J Am Coll Cardiol* 1984; 3:1111–1117.
106. Marcus FI, Cobb LA, Edwards JE, Multicenter Post-infarction Research Group. Mechanism of death and prevalence of myocardial ischemic symptoms in the terminal event after acute myocardial infarction. *Am J Cardiol* 1988; 61:8–15.
107. Holmes DR Jr, Davis K, Gersh BJ, Participants in the Coronary Artery Surgery Study (CASS). Risk factor profiles of patients with sudden cardiac death and death from other cardiac causes: A report from the Coronary Artery Surgery Study (CASS). *J Am Coll Cardiol* 1989; 13:524–530.
108. Muharji J, Rude RE, Poole WK, et al. Risk factors for sudden death after acute myocardial infarction: Two year follow-up. *Am J Cardiol* 1984; 54:31–36.
109. Bigger JT Jr, Fleiss JL, Rolnitzky LM. Prevalence, characteristics and significance of ventricular tachycardia detected by 24-hour continuous electrocardiographic recordings in the late hospital phase of acute myocardial infarction. *Am J Cardiol* 1986; 58:1151–1160.
110. Middlekauff HR, Stevenson WG, Tilliseh JH. Prevention of sudden death in survivors of myocardial infarction: A decision analysis approach. *Am Heart J* 1992; 123:475–480.
111. Taylor AJ, Rogan KM, Virmani R. Sudden cardiac death associated with isolated congenital coronary artery anomalies. *J Am Coll Cardiol* 1992; 20:640–647.
112. MacAlpin RN. Cardiac arrest and sudden unexpected death in variant angina: Complications of coronary spasm that can occur in the absence of severe organic coronary stenosis. *Am Heart J* 1993; 125:1011–1017.
113. Myerburg RJ, Kessler KM, Mallon SM, et al. Life threatening ventricular tachycardia in patients with silent myocardial ischemia due to coronary artery spasm. *N Engl J Med* 1992; 326:1451–1455.
114. Roberts WC, Dicicco BS, Waller BF, et al. Origin of the left main from the right coronary artery or from the right aortic sinus with intramyocardial tunneling to the left side of the heart via the ventricular septum: The case against clinical significance of myocardial bridge or coronary tunnel. *Am Heart J* 1982; 104:303–305.
115. Corrado D, Thiene G, Cocco P, et al. Non-atherosclerotic coronary artery disease and sudden death in the young. *Br Heart J* 1992; 68:601–607.
116. Hunsaker JC III, O'Connor WN, Lie JT. Spontaneous coronary arterial dissection and isolated eosinophilic coronary arteritis: Sudden cardiac death in a patient with a limited variant of Churg-Strauss syndrome. *Mayo Clin Proc* 1992; 67:761–766.
117. Goldeli O, Ural D, Komsuoglu B, et al. Abnormal QT dispersion in Behçet's disease. *Int J Cardiol* 1997; 61:55–59.
118. Tanaka N, Naoe S, Masuda H, et al. Pathological study of sequelae of Kawasaki disease (MCLS): With special reference to the heart and coronary arterial lesions. *Acta Pathol Jpn* 1986; 36:1513–1527.
119. Cohle SD, Titus JL, Espinola A, et al. Sudden unexpected death due to coronary giant cell arteritis. *Arch Pathol Lab Med* 1982; 106:171–172.
120. Mandell BF. Cardiovascular involvement in systemic lupus erythematosus. *Semin Arthritis Rheum* 1987; 17:126–141.
121. Tamburro P, Wilber D. Sudden death in idiopathic dilated cardiomyopathy. *Am Heart J* 1992; 124:1035–1045.
122. Packer M. Lack of correlation between ventricular arrhythmias and sudden death in patients with chronic heart failure. *Circulation* 1992; 85(1 suppl):I50–I56.
123. Larsen L, Markham J, Haffajee CI. Sudden death in idiopathic dilated cardiomyopathy: Role of ventricular arrhythmias. *Pacing Clin Electrophysiol* 1993; 16:1051–1059.
124. Tomaselli GF, Beukelmann DJ, Calkins HG, et al. Sudden cardiac death in heart failure: The role of abnormal repolarization. *Circulation* 1994; 90:2534–2539.
125. Hofmann T, Meinertz T, Kasper W, et al. Mode of death in idiopathic dilated cardiomyopathy: A multivariate analysis of prognostic determinants. *Am Heart J* 1988; 116:1455–1463.

126. Josephson ME. Should ICDs be implanted in all patients with dilated cardiomyopathy and unexplained syncope? *J Am Coll Cardiol* 1999; 33:1971–1973.
127. Knight BP, Goyal R, Pelosi F, et al. Outcome of patients with nonischemic dilated cardiomyopathy and unexplained syncope treated with an implantable defibrillator. *J Am Coll Cardiol* 1999; 33:1964–1970.
128. Middlekauff HR, Stevenson WG, Woo MA, et al. Comparison of frequency of late potentials in idiopathic dilated cardiomyopathy and ischemic cardiomyopathy with advanced congestive heart failure and their usefulness in predicting sudden death. *Am J Cardiol* 1990; 66:1113–1117.
129. Naccarelli GV, Prystowsky EN, Jackman WM, et al. Role of electrophysiologic testing in managing patients who have ventricular tachycardia unrelated to coronary artery disease. *Am J Cardiol* 1982; 50:165–171.
130. Caceres J, Jazayeri M, McKinnie J, et al. Sustained bundle branch reentry as a mechanism of clinical tachycardia. *Circulation* 1989; 79:256–270.
131. McKenna WJ, Camm AJ. Sudden death in hypertrophic cardiomyopathy. *Circulation* 1989; 80:1489–1492.
132. Maron BJ, Roberts WC, Epstein SE. Sudden death in hypertrophic cardiomyopathy: A profile of 78 patients. *Circulation* 1992; 65:1388–1394.
133. Dilsizian V, Bonow RO, Epstein SE, et al. Myocardial ischemia detected by thallium scintigraphy is frequently related to cardiac arrest and syncope in young patients with hypertrophic cardiomyopathy. *J Am Coll Cardiol* 1993; 22:796–804.
134. Counihan PJ, Fei L, Bashir Y, et al. Assessment of heart rate variability in hypertrophic cardiomyopathy: Association with clinical and prognostic features. *Circulation* 1993; 88:1682–1690.
135. Fananapazir L, Chang AC, Epstein SE, et al. Prognostic determinants in hypertrophic cardiomyopathy: Prospective evaluation of a therapeutic strategy based on clinical, Holter, hemodynamic, and electrophysiologic findings. *Circulation* 1992; 86:730–740.
136. Spirito P, Rapezzi C, Autore C, et al. Prognosis of asymptomatic patients with hypertrophic cardiomyopathy and nonsustained ventricular tachycardia. *Circulation* 1994; 90:2743–2747.
137. Saumarez RC, Heald S, Gill J, et al. Primary ventricular fibrillation is associated with increased paced right ventricular electrogram fractionation. *Circulation* 1995; 92:2565–2571.
138. Fananapazir L, Tracy CM, Leon MB, et al. Electrophysiologic abnormalities in patients with hypertrophic cardiomyopathy: A consecutive analysis of 155 patients. *Circulation* 1989; 80:1259–1268.
139. Marian AJ, Roberts R. Molecular genetic basis of hypertrophic cardiomyopathy: Genetic markers for sudden cardiac death. *J Cardiovasc Electrophysiol* 1998; 9:88–99.
140. Moolman JC, Corfield VA, Posen B, et al. Sudden death due to troponin T mutations. *J Am Coll Cardiol* 1997; 29:549–555.
141. Zehender M, Faber T, Koscheck U, et al. Ventricular tachyarrhythmias, myocardial ischemia, and sudden cardiac death in patients with hypertensive heart disease. *Clin Cardiol* 1995; 18:377–383.
142. Frohlich ED. State of the art lecture: Risk mechanisms in hypertensive heart disease. *Hypertension* 1999; 34:782–789.
143. Messerli FH. Hypertension and sudden cardiac death. *Am J Hypertens* 1999; 12:181S–188S.
144. Levy D, Garrison RJ, Savage DD, et al. Prognostic implications of echocardiographically determined left ventricular mass in the Framingham Heart Study. *N Engl J Med* 1990; 322:1561–1566.
145. Tanaka M, Fujiwara H, Onodera T. Quantitative analysis of myocardial fibrosis in normals, hypertensive hearts and hypertrophic cardiomyopathy. *Br Heart J* 1986; 55:575–581.
146. Siscovick DS, Raghunathan TE, Psaty BM, et al. Diuretic therapy for hypertension and the risk of primary cardiac arrest. *N Engl J Med* 1994; 330:1852–1857.
147. Hoes AW, Grobbee DE, Lubsen J, et al. Diuretics, beta-blockers, and the risk for sudden cardiac death in hypertensive patients. *Ann Intern Med* 1995; 123:481–487.
148. O'Kelly BF, Massie BM, Tubau JF, Szlachcic J. Coronary morbidity and mortality, preexisting silent coronary artery disease and mild hypertension. *Ann Intern Med* 1989; 110:1017–1026.
149. Ahmad F, Li D, Karibe A, Gonzalez O, et al. Localization of a gene responsible for arrhythmogenic right ventricular dysplasia to chromosome 3p23. *Circulation* 1998; 98:2791–2795.
150. Rampazzo A, Nava A, Danieli G, et al. The gene for arrhythmogenic right ventricular cardiomyopathy maps to chromosome 14q23-q24. *Hum Mol Genet* 1994; 3:959–962.
151. Severini GM, Krajinovic M, Pinamonti B, et al. A new locus for arrhythmogenic right ventricular dysplasia on the long arm of chromosome 14. *Genomics* 1996; 31:193–200.
152. Rampazzo A, Nava A, Erne P, et al. A new locus for arrhythmogenic right ventricular cardiomyopathy (ARVD2) maps to chromosome 1q42-q43. *Hum Mol Genet* 1995; 4:2151–2154.
153. Zipes DP, Wellens HJ. Sudden cardiac death. *Circulation* 1998; 98:2334–2351.
154. Corrado D, Basso C, Thiene G, et al. Spectrum of clinicopathologic manifestations of arrhythmogenic right ventricular cardiomyopathy/dysplasia: A multicenter study. *J Am Coll Cardiol* 1997; 30:1512–1520.
155. Haissaguerre M, Le Metayer P, D'Ivernois C, et al. Distinctive response of arrhythmogenic right ventricular disease to high dose isoproterenol. *PACE* 1990; 13:2119–2126.
156. Marcus FI, Fontaine GH, Frank R, et al. Long term follow-up in patients with arrhythmogenic right ventricular disease. *Eur Heart J* 1989; 10(suppl D):68–73.
157. Lemery R, Brugada P, Janssen J, et al. Nonischemic sustained ventricular tachycardia: Clinical outcome in 12 patients with arrhythmogenic right ventricular dysplasia. *J Am Coll Cardiol* 1989; 14:96–105.
158. Pellikka PA, Nishimura RA, Bailey KR, et al. The natural history of adults with asymptomatic, hemodynamically significant aortic stenosis. *J Am Coll Cardiol* 1990; 15:1012–1017.
159. Bonow RO, Lakatos E, Maron BJ, et al. Serial long-term assessment of the natural history of asymptomatic patients with chronic regurgitation and normal left ventricular systolic function. *Circulation* 1991; 84:1625–1635.
160. Braunwald E. On the natural history of severe aortic stenosis. *J Am Coll Cardiol* 1990; 15:1018–1020.
161. Foppl M, Hoffmann A, Amann FW, et al. Sudden cardiac death after aortic valve surgery. *Clin Cardiol* 1989; 12:202–207.
162. Alvarez L, Escudero C, Figuera D, et al. Late sudden cardiac death in the follow-up of patients having a heart valve prosthesis. *J Thorac Cardiovasc Surg* 1992; 104:502–510.
163. Keefe DL, Griffin JC, Harrison DC, et al. Atrioventricular conduction abnormalities in patients undergoing isolated aortic or mitral valve replacement. *PACE* 1985; 8:393–398.
164. Farb A, Tang AL, Atkinson JB, et al. Comparison of cardiac findings in patients with mitral prolapse who die suddenly to those who have congestive heart failure from mitral regurgitation and to those with fatal noncardiac conditions. *Am J Cardiol* 1992; 70:234–239.
165. Nishimura RA, McGoon MD, Shub C, et al. Echocardiography documented mitral valve prolapse: Long term follow-up of 238 patients. *N Engl J Med* 1985; 313:1305–1309.
166. Vohra J, Sathe S, Warren R, et al. Malignant ventricular arrhythmias in patients with mitral valve prolapse and mild mitral regurgitation. *PACE* 1993; 16:387–393.
167. Martini B, Basso C, Thiene G. Sudden death in mitral valve prolapse with Holter monitoring–documented ventricular fibrillation: Evidence of coexisting arrhythmogenic right ventricular cardiomyopathy. *Int J Cardiol* 1995; 49:274–278.
168. Marks AR, Choong CY, Sanfilippo AJ, et al. Identification of

high-risk and low-risk subgroups of patients with mitral-valve prolapse. *N Engl J Med* 1989; 320:1031–1036.
169. Devereux RB. Diagnosis and prognosis of mitral valve prolapse. *N Engl J Med* 1989; 320:1077–1079.
170. Puddu PE, Pasternac A, Tubau JF, et al. QT interval prolongation and increased plasma catecholamine levels in patients with mitral valve prolapse. *Am Heart J* 1983; 105:422–428.
171. Ramos SG, Matturi L, Rossi L, et al. Lesions of mediastinal paraganglia in chronic chagasic cardiomyopathy: Cause of sudden death? *Am Heart J* 1996; 131:417–420.
172. Winters SL, Cohen M, Greenberg S, et al. Sustained ventricular tachycardia associated with sarcoidosis: Assessment of the underlying cardiac anatomy and the prospective utility of programmed ventricular stimulation, drug therapy and implantable antitachycardia device. *J Am Coll Cardiol* 1991; 18:937–943.
173. Cullen S, Celermajer DS, Franklin RCG, et al. Prognostic significance of ventricular arrhythmias after repair of tetralogy of Fallot: A 12-year prospective study. *J Am Coll Cardiol* 1994; 23:1151–1155.
174. Gatzoulis MA, Till JA, Somerville J, et al. Mechanoelectrical interaction in tetralogy of Fallot: QRS prolongation relates to right ventricular size and predicts malignant ventricular arrhythmias and sudden death. *Circulation* 1995; 92:231–237.
175. Moss AJ, Adams FH. Sudden cardiac death. In: Moss AJ, Adams FH, eds, *Heart Disease in Infants, Children and Adolescents Including the Fetus and Young Adult,* 5th ed: Vol II. Baltimore: Williams & Wilkins; 1995:1610.
176. Moss AJ, Schwartz PJ, Crampton RS, et al. The long QT syndrome: A prospective international study. *Circulation* 1985; 71:17–24.
177. Vincent GM, Timothy KW, Leppert M, et al. The spectrum of symptoms and QT intervals in carriers of the gene for the long-QT syndrome. *N Engl J Med* 1992; 327:846–852.
178. Roden DM, Lazzara R, Rosen M, et al. Multiple mechanisms in the long QT syndrome: Current knowledge, gaps, and future directions. The SADS Foundation Task Force on LQTS. *Circulation* 1996; 94:1996–2012.
179. Antzelevitch C, Shimizu W, Yan GX, et al. The M cell: Its contribution to the ECG and to normal and abnormal electrical function of the heart. *J Cardiovasc Electrophysiol* 1999; 10:1124–1152.
180. Wang Q, Chen Q, Li H, et al. Molecular genetics of long QT syndrome from genes to patients. *Curr Opin Cardiol* 1997; 12:310–320.
181. Towbin JA. New revelations about the long-QT syndrome. *N Engl J Med* 1995; 333:384–385.
182. Ackerman MJ. The long QT syndrome: Ion channel diseases of the heart. *Mayo Clin Proc* 1998; 73:250–269.
183. Abbott GW, Sesti F, Splawski I, et al. MiRP1 forms I_{Kr} potassium channels with HERG and is associated with cardiac arrhythmia. *Cell* 1999; 97:175–187.
184. Splawski I, Timothy KW, Vincent GM, et al. Molecular basis of the long-QT syndrome associated with deafness. *N Engl J Med* 1997; 336:1562–1567.
185. Wilde AA, Jongbloed RJ, Doevendans PA, et al. Auditory stimuli as a trigger for arrhythmic events differentiate HERG-related (LQTS2) patients from KVLQT1-related patients (LQTS1). *J Am Coll Cardiol* 1999; 33:327–332.
186. Nador F, Beria G, De Ferrari GM, et al. Unsuspected echocardiographic abnormality in the long QT syndrome: Diagnostic, prognostic and pathogenetic implications. *Circulation* 1991; 84:1530–1542.
187. Munger TM, Packer DL, Hammill SC, et al. A population study of the natural history of Wolff-Parkinson-White syndrome in Olmsted County, Minnesota, 1953–1989. *Circulation* 1993; 87:866–873.
188. Jackman WM, Wang XZ, Friday KJ, et al. Catheter ablation of accessory atrioventricular pathways (Wolff-Parkinson-White syndrome) by radiofrequency current. *N Engl J Med* 1991; 324:1605–1611.
189. Leitch JW, Klein GJ, Yee R, et al. Prognostic value of electrophysiologic testing in asymptomatic patients with Wolff-Parkinson-White pattern. *Circulation* 1990; 82:1718–1723.
190. Zardini M, Yee R, Thakur RK, et al. Risk of sudden arrhythmic death in the Wolff-Parkinson-White syndrome: Current perspectives. *Pacing Clin Electrophysiol* 1994; 17:966–975.
191. Klein GJ, Bashore TM, Sellers TD, et al. Ventricular fibrillation in the Wolff-Parkinson-White syndrome. *N Engl J Med* 1979; 301:1080–1085.
192. Chen SA, Chiang CE, Tai CT, et al. Longitudinal clinical and electrophysiological assessment of patients with symptomatic Wolff-Parkinson-White syndrome and atrioventricular node reentrant tachycardia. *Circulation* 1996; 93:2023–2032.
193. Bromberg BI, Lindsay BD, Cain ME, et al. Impact of clinical history and electrophysiologic characterization of accessory pathways on management strategies to reduce sudden death among children with Wolff-Parkinson-White syndrome. *J Am Coll Cardiol* 1996; 27:690–695.
194. Lemery R, Brugada P, Bella PD, et al. Nonischemic ventricular tachycardia: Clinical course and long-term follow-up in patients without clinically overt heart disease. *Circulation* 1989; 79: 990–999.
195. Lerman BB, Stein KM, Markowitz SM. Adenosine-sensitive ventricular tachycardia: A conceptual approach. *J Cardiovasc Electrophysiol* 1996; 7:559–569.
196. Leenhardt A, Glaser E, Burguera M, et al. Short-coupled variant of torsades de pointes: A new electrocardiographic entity in the spectrum of tachyarrhythmias. *Circulation* 1994; 89:206–215.
197. Viskin S, Belhassen B. Idiopathic ventricular fibrillation. *Am Heart J* 1990; 120:661–671.
198. Morady F, Scheinman MM, Hess DS, et al. Clinical characteristics and results of electrophysiologic testing in young adults with ventricular tachycardia or ventricular fibrillation. *Am Heart J* 1983; 106:1306–1314.
199. Siebels J, Schneider MAE, Geiger M, et al. Unexpected recurrences in survivors of cardiac arrest without organic heart disease [abstr]. *Eur Heart J* 1991; 12(suppl):86.
200. Wever EF, Hauer RN, Oomen A, et al. Unfavorable outcome in patients with primary electrical disease who survived an episode of ventricular fibrillation. *Circulation* 1993; 88:1021–1029.
201. Wellens HJ, Lemery R, Smeets JL, et al. Sudden death without overt heart disease. *Circulation* 1992; 85(suppl I):I92–I97.
202. Aizawa Y, Naitoh N, Washizuka T, et al. Electrophysiological findings in idiopathic recurrent ventricular fibrillation: Special reference to mode of induction, drug testing, and long-term outcomes. *PACE* 1996; 19:929–939.
203. Brugada P, Abdollah H, Heddle B, et al. Results of a ventricular stimulation protocol using a maximum of 4 premature extrastimuli in patients without documented or sustained ventricular arrhythmias. *Am J Cardiol* 1983; 52:1214–1218.
204. DiCarlo LA Jr, Morady F, Schwartz AB, et al. Clinical significance of ventricular fibrillation-flutter induced by programmed ventricular stimulation. *Am Heart J* 1985; 109:959–963.
205. Brugada P, Brugada J. Right bundle branch block, persistent ST segment elevation and sudden cardiac death, a distinct clinical and electrocardiographic syndrome. *J Am Coll Cardiol* 1992; 20:1391–1396.
206. Atarashi H, Ogawa S, Harumi K, et al. Characteristics of patients with right bundle branch block and ST-segment elevation in right precordial leads. Idiopathic Ventricular Fibrillation Investigators. *Am J Cardiol* 1996; 78:581–583.
207. Brugada J, Brugada R, Brugada P. Right bundle-branch block and ST-segment elevation in leads V1 through V3: A marker for sudden death in patients without demonstrable structural heart disease. *Circulation* 1998; 97:457–460.

208. Chen Q, Kirsch GE, Zhang D, et al. Genetic basis and molecular mechanism for idiopathic ventricular fibrillation. *Nature* 1998; 392:293–296.
209. Kirschner RH, Eckner FA, Baron RC. The cardiac pathology of sudden, unexplained nocturnal death in Southeast Asian refugees. *JAMA* 1986; 256:2700–2705.
210. Gotoh K. A histopathological study of the conduction system in so-called "Pokkuri disease" (sudden unexpected cardiac death of unknown origin in Japan). *Jpn Circ J* 1976; 40:753–768.
211. Nademanee K, Veerakul G, Nimmannit S, et al. Arrhythmogenic marker for the sudden unexplained death syndrome in Thai men. *Circulation* 1997; 96:2595–2600.
212. Corrado D, Nava A, Buja G, et al. Familial cardiomyopathy underlies syndrome of right bundle branch block, ST segment elevation and sudden death. *J Am Coll Cardiol* 1996; 27:443–448.
213. Frey W. Weitere Erfahrungen mit Chinidin bei absoluter Herzunregelmä bigkeit. *Wien Klin Wochenschr* 1918; 55:849–853.
214. Echt DS, Liebson PR, Mitchell B, et al. Mortality and morbidity in patients receiving encainide, flecainide, or placebo: The Cardiac Arrhythmia Suppression Trial. *N Engl J Med* 1991; 324:781–778.
215. Podrid PJ. Aggravation of arrhythmia: A complication of antiarrhythmic drugs. *J Cardiovasc Electrophysiol* 1993; 4:311–319.
216. Packer M, Medina N, Yushak M. Hemodynamic and clinical limitations of long term inotropic therapy with amrinone in patients with severe congestive heart failure. *Circulation* 1984; 70:1038–1047.
217. Patterson E, Szabo B, Scherlag BJ, et al. Arrhythmogenic effects of antiarrhythmic drugs. In: Zipes DP, Jalife J, eds. *Cardiac Electrophysiology: From Cell to Bedside*. Philadelphia: Saunders; 1995:496.
218. Minardo JD, Heger JJ, Miles WM, et al. Clinical characteristics of patients with ventricular fibrillation during antiarrhythmic drug therapy. *N Engl J Med* 1988; 319:257–262.
219. Nattel S, Pederson DH, Zipes DP. Alteration in regional myocardial distribution and arrhythmogenic effects of aprindine produced by coronary artery occlusion in the dog. *Cardiovasc Res* 1981; 15:80–85.
220. Raymond JR, van den Berg EK Jr, Knapp MJ. Nontraumatic prehospital death in young adults. *Arch Intern Med* 1988; 148:303–308.
221. Hearn WL, Flynn DD, Hine GW, et al. Cocaethylene: A unique cocaine metabolite displays high affinity for the dopamine transporter. *J Neurochem* 1991; 56:698–701.
222. Isner JM, Estes M III, Thompson PD, et al. Acute events temporally related to cocaine abuse. *N Engl J Med* 1986; 315:1438–1443.
223. Nordrehaug JE, Johanessen KA, van der Lippe G. Serum potassium concentrations as a risk factor of ventricular arrhythmias early in acute myocardial infarction. *Circulation* 1985; 71:645–649.
224. Gettes LS. Electrolyte abnormalities underlying lethal ventricular arrhythmias. *Circulation* 1992; 85(suppl I):I70–I76.
225. Eisenberg MJ. Magnesium deficiency and sudden death. *Am Heart J* 1992; 124:544–549.
226. Hoes AW, Grobbe DE, Peet TM, et al. Do non-potassium-sparing diuretics increase the risk of sudden cardiac death in hypertensive patients? Recent evidence. *Drugs* 1994; 47:711–733.
227. Isner JM, Roberts WC, Heymsfield SB, et al. Anorexia nervosa and sudden death. *Ann Intern Med* 1985; 102:49–52.
228. Litwin PE, Eisenberg MS, Hallstrom AP, et al. The location of collapse and its effect on survival from cardiac arrest. *Ann Emerg Med* 1987; 16:787–791.
229. Eisenberg MS, Horwood BT, Cummins RO, et al. Cardiac arrest and resuscitation: A tale of 29 cities. *Ann Emerg Med* 1990; 19:179–186.
230. Kuller LH, Perper JA, Cooper MC. Sudden and unexpected death due to atherosclerotic heart disease. *Mod Trends Cardiol* 1974; 3:292–332.
231. Cummins RO, Ornato JP, Thies WH, et al. Improving survival from sudden cardiac arrest: The "chain of survival" concept. *Circulation* 1991; 83:1832–1847.
232. Zipes DP. Sudden cardiac death: Future approaches. *Circulation* 1992; 85(suppl I):I160–I166.
233. Weaver WD, Cobb LA, Fahrenbruch CE, et al. Use of the automatic external defibrillator in the management of out-of-hospital cardiac arrest. *N Engl J Med* 1988; 319:661–666.
234. Sack JB, Kesselbrenner MB, Jarrad A. Interposed abdominal compression CPR and resuscitation outcome during asystole and electromechanical dissociation. *Circulation* 1992; 86:1692–1700.
235. Lerman BB, Deale OC. Relation between transcardiac and transthoracic current during defibrillation in humans. *Circ Res* 1990; 67:1420–1426.
236. Kerber RE, Grayzel J, Hoyt R, et al. Transthoracic resistance in human defibrillation: Influence of body weight, chest size, serial shocks, paddle size and paddle contact pressure. *Circulation* 1981; 63:676–682.
237. Emergency Cardiac Care Committee and Subcommittees, American Heart Association. Guidelines for cardiopulmonary resuscitation and emergency cardiac care. *JAMA* 1992; 268: 2172–2295.
238. Lerman BB, Engelstein ED. Metabolic determinants of defibrillation: Role of adenosine. *Circulation* 1995; 91:838–844.
239. Becker LB, Ostrander MP, Barrett J, et al. Outcome of CPR in a large metropolitan area: Where are the survivors? *Ann Emerg Med* 1991; 20:355–361.
240. Lombardi G, Gallagher EJ, Gennis P. Outcome of out-of-hospital cardiac arrest in New York City: The pre-hospital arrest survival evaluation (PHASE) study. *JAMA* 1994; 271:678–683.
241. Cobb LA, Hallstrom AP. Community-based cardiopulmonary resuscitation: What have we learned? *Ann NY Acad Sci* 1982; 382:330–342.
242. Dickey W, Adgey J. Mortality within hospital after resuscitation from ventricular fibrillation outside hospital. *Br Heart J* 1992; 67:334–338.
243. Hallstrom AP, Cobb LA, Yu BH. Influence of comorbidity on the outcome of patients treated for ventricular fibrillation. *Circulation* 1996; 93:2019–2022.
244. Longstreth WT, Cobb LA, Fahrenbruch CE, et al. Does age affect outcomes of out-of-hospital cardiopulmonary resuscitation? *JAMA* 1990; 264:2109–2110.
245. Brugada P, Talajic M, Smeets J, et al. The value of the clinical history to assess prognosis of patients with ventricular tachycardia or ventricular fibrillation after myocardial infarction. *Eur Heart J* 1989; 10:747–752.
246. Middlekauff HR, Stevenson WG, Saxon LA. Prognosis after syncope: Impact of left ventricular function. *Am Heart J* 1993; 125:121–127.
247. Bigger JT, Fleiss JL, Kleiger R, Multicenter Post-Infarction Research Group. The relationship among ventricular arrhythmias, left ventricular dysfunction, and mortality in the 2 years after myocardial infarction. *Circulation* 1984; 69:250–258.
248. Greenberg H, McMaster P, Dwyer EM Jr, Multicenter Post-infarction Research Group. Left ventricular dysfunction after acute myocardial infarction: Results of a prospective multicenter study. *J Am Coll Cardiol* 1984; 4:867–874.
249. Wilson JR, Schwartz J, Sutton M, et al. Prognosis in severe heart failure: Relation to hemodynamic measurements and ventricular ectopic activity. *J Am Coll Cardiol* 1983; 2:403–410.
250. Stevenson WG, Stevenson LW, Middlekauf HR, et al. Sudden death prevention in patients with advanced ventricular dysfunction. *Circulation* 1993; 88:2953–2961.
251. Wilber DJ, Garan H, Finkelstein D, et al. Out-of-hospital cardiac arrest: Use of electrophysiologic testing in the prediction of long-term outcome. *N Engl J Med* 1988; 318:19–24.
252. Herre JM, Sauve MJ, Malone P, et al. Long term results of amiodarone therapy in patients with recurrent sustained ventricu-

lar tachycardia or ventricular fibrillation. *J Am Coll Cardiol* 1989; 13:442–449.

253. Weinberg BA, Miles WM, Klein LS, et al. Five-year follow-up of 589 patients treated with amiodarone. *Am Heart J* 1993; 125:109–120.
254. Algra A, Tijssen JG, Roelandt JR, et al. QT_c prolongation measured by standard 12-lead electrocardiography is an independent risk factor for sudden death due to cardiac arrest. *Circulation* 1991; 83:1888–1894.
255. Day CP, McComb JM, Campbell RWF. QT dispersion, an indication of arrhythmia risk in patients with long QT intervals. *Br Heart J* 1990; 63:342–344.
256. Barr CS, Naas A, Freeman M, et al. QT dispersion and sudden unexpected death in chronic heart failure. *Lancet* 1994; 343: 327–329.
257. Shaper AG, Wannamethee G, Macfarlane PW, et al. Heart rate in ischemic heart disease and sudden cardiac death in middle-aged British men. *Br Heart J* 1993; 70:49–55.
258. Holmes J, Kubo SH, Cody RJ, et al. Arrhythmias in ischemic and nonischemic dilated cardiomyopathy: Prediction of mortality by ambulatory electrocardiography. *Am J Cardiol* 1985; 55: 146–151.
259. Gomes JA, Winters SL, Stewart D, et al. A new noninvasive index to predict ventricular tachycardia and sudden death in the first year after myocardial infarction: Based on signal averaged electrocardiogram, radionuclide ejection fraction and Holter monitoring. *J Am Coll Cardiol* 1987; 10:349–357.
260. Kuchar DL, Thornburn CW, Sammel NL. Prediction of serious arrhythmic events after myocardial infarction: Signal averaged electrocardiogram, Holter monitoring and radionuclide ventriculography. *J Am Coll Cardiol* 1987; 9:531–538.
261. Farrell TG, Bashir Y, Cripps T, et al. Risk stratification for arrhythmic events in post-infarction patients based on heart rate variability, ambulatory electrocardiographic variables and the signal-averaged electrocardiogram. *J Am Coll Cardiol* 1991; 18:687–697.
262. Chakko CS, Cheorghiade M. Ventricular arrhythmias in severe heart failure: Incidence, significance, and effectiveness of antiarrhythmic therapy. *Am Heart J* 1985; 109:497–504.
263. Hull SS Jr, Vanoli E, Adamson PB, et al. Exercise training confers anticipatory protection from sudden death during myocardial ischemia. *Circulation* 1994; 89:548–552.
264. Kleiger RE, Miller JP, Bigger JT, Multicenter Post-Infarction Research Group. Decreased heart rate variability and its association with increased mortality after acute myocardial infarction. *Am J Cardiol* 1987; 59:256–262.
265. Bigger JT Jr, Fleiss JL, Steinman RC, et al. Frequency domain measures of heart period variability and mortality after myocardial infarction. *Circulation* 1992; 85:164–171.
266. Algra A, Tijssen JG, Roelandt JR, et al. Heart rate variability from 24 hour electrocardiography and the 2-year risk for sudden death. *Circulation* 1993; 88:180–185.
267. Barron HV, Lesh MD. Autonomic nervous system and sudden cardiac death. *J Am Coll Cardiol* 1996; 27:1053–1060.
268. Schwartz PJ, La Rovere MT, Vanoli E. Autonomic nervous system and sudden cardiac death: Experimental basis and clinical observations for post-myocardial infarction risk stratification. *Circulation* 1992; 85(suppl I):I77–I91.
269. Stein KM, Borer JS, Hochreiter C, et al. Fractal clustering of ventricular ectopy and sudden death in mitral regurgitation. *J Electrocardiol* 1992; 25:S178–S181.
270. Stein KM, Karagounis LA, Anderson JL, et al. Fractal clustering of ventricular ectopy correlates with sympathetic tone preceding ectopic beats. *Circulation* 1995; 91:722–727.
271. Rosenbaum DS, He B, Cohen RJ. New approaches for evaluating cardiac electrical activity: Repolarization alternans and body surface imaging. In: Zipes DP, Jalife J, eds. *Cardiac Electrophysiology: From Cell to Bedside*. Philadelphia: Saunders; 1995: 1187.
272. Rosenbaum DS, Jackson LE, Smith JM, et al. Electrical alternans and vulnerability to ventricular arrhythmias. *N Engl J Med* 1994; 330:235–241.
273. Simson MB. Noninvasive identification of patients at high risk for sudden cardiac death: Signal-averaged electrocardiography. *Circulation* 1992; 85(suppl I):I145–I151.
274. Mancini DM, Wong SL, Simson MB. Prognostic value of an abnormal signal-averaged electrocardiogram in patients with nonischemic congestive cardiomyopathy. *Circulation* 1993; 87:1083–1092.
275. Gomes JA, Winters SL, Stewart D, et al. A new noninvasive index to predict sustained ventricular tachycardia and sudden death in the first year after myocardial infarction: Based on signal-averaged electrocardiogram, radionuclide ejection fraction and Holter monitoring. *J Am Coll Cardiol* 1987; 10:349–357.
276. Ruskin JN. Role of invasive electrophysiologic testing in the evaluation of and treatment of patients at high risk for sudden cardiac death. *Circulation* 1992; 85(suppl I):I152–I159.
277. Andresen D, Steinbeck G, Bruggeman T, et al. Prognosis of patients with sustained ventricular tachycardia and of survivors of cardiac arrest not inducible by programmed stimulation. *Am J Cardiol* 1992; 70:1250–1254.
278. Poole JE, Mathisen TL, Kudenchuck PJ, et al. Long-term outcome in patients who survived out-of-hospital ventricular fibrillation and who undergo electrophysiologic studies: Evaluation by electrophysiologic subgroups. *J Am Coll Cardiol* 1990; 16:657–665.
279. Benditt DG, Benson DW Jr, Klein GJ, et al. Prevention of recurrent sudden cardiac arrest: Role of provocative electropharmacologic testing. *J Am Coll Cardiol* 1983; 2:418–425.
280. Waller TJ, Kay HR, Spielman SR, et al. Reduction in sudden death and total mortality by antiarrhythmic therapy evaluated by electrophysiologic drug testing: Criteria of efficacy in patients with sustained ventricular tachyarrhythmia. *J Am Coll Cardiol* 1987; 10:83–89.
281. Bourke JP, Richards DAB, Ross DL, et al. Routine programmed electrical stimulation in survivors of acute myocardial infarction for prediction of spontaneous ventricular tachyarrhythmias during follow-up: Results, optimal stimulation protocol and cost-effective screening. *J Am Coll Cardiol* 1991; 18:780–788.
282. Kendall MJ, Lynch KP, Hjalmarson A, et al. Beta-blockers and sudden cardiac death. *Ann Intern Med* 1995; 123:358–367.
283. Yusuf S, Peto R, Lewis J, et al. β-Blockade during and after myocardial infarction: An overview of the randomized trials. *Prog Cardiovasc Dis* 1985; 27:335–371.
284. Beta Blocker Heart Attack Research Group. A randomized trial of propranolol in patients with acute myocardial infarction: I. Mortality results. *JAMA* 1982; 247:1707–1714.
285. Schwartz PJ, Motolese M, Pollavini G, et al. Prevention of sudden cardiac death after a first myocardial infarction by pharmacological or surgical antiadrenergic interventions. *J Cardiovasc Electrophysiol* 1992; 3:2–16.
286. Norwegian Multicenter Study Group. Timolol-induced reduction in mortality and reinfarction in patients surviving myocardial infarction. *N Engl J Med* 1981; 304:801–807.
287. Goldstein S, Hjalmarson A. The mortality effect of metoprolol CR/XL in patients with heart failure: Results of the MERIT-HF trial. *Clin Cardiol* 1999; 22(suppl V):V30–V35.
288. Singh BN. Advantages of beta-blockers versus antiarrhythmic agents and calcium-antagonists in secondary prevention after myocardial infarction. *Am J Cardiol* 1990; 66:9C–20C.
289. Furberg C, Hawkins C, Lichstein E. Effect of propranolol in postinfarction patients with mechanical or electrical complications. *Circulation* 1984; 69:761–765.
290. CONSENSUS Trial Study Group. Effects of enalapril on mortal-

ity in severe congestive heart failure: Results of the Cooperative North Scandinavian Enalapril Survival Study (CONSENSUS). *N Engl J Med* 1987; 316:1429–1435.
291. SOLVD Investigators. Effect of enalapril on survival in patients with reduced left ventricular ejection fractions and congestive heart failure. *N Engl J Med* 1991; 325:293–302.
292. SOLVD Investigators. Effect of enalapril mortality and the development of heart failure in asymptomatic patients with reduced left ventricular ejection fractions. *N Engl J Med* 1992; 327:685–691.
293. Pfeffer MA, Braunwald E, Moye LA, et al. Effect of captopril on mortality and morbidity in patients with left ventricular dysfunction after myocardial infarction. *N Engl J Med* 1992; 327:669–677.
294. Ambrosioni E, Borghi C, Magnani B, et al. The effect of the angiotensin converting enzyme inhibitor zofenopril on mortality and morbidity after anterior myocardial infarction. *N Engl J Med* 1995; 332:80–85.
295. Kober L, Torp-Pedersen C, Carlsen JE, et al. A clinical trial of the angiotensin-converting enzyme inhibitor trandolapril in patients with left ventricular dysfunction after myocardial infarction. *N Engl J Med* 1995; 333:1670–1676.
296. Cohn JN, Johnson G, Ziesche S, et al. A comparison of enalapril with hydralazine-isosorbide dinitrate in the treatment of chronic congestive heart failure. *N Engl J Med* 1991; 325:303–310.
297. Domanski MJ, Exner DV, Borkowf CB, et al. Effect of angiotensin converting enzyme inhibition on sudden cardiac death in patients following acute myocardial infarction: A meta-analysis of randomized clinical trials. *J Am Coll Cardiol* 1999; 33:598–604.
298. Hine L, Laird N, Hewitt P, et al. Meta-analysis of empirical long-term antiarrhythmic therapy after myocardial infarction. *JAMA* 1989; 262:3037–3040.
299. Teo KK, Yusuf S, Furberg CD. Effects of prophylactic antiarrhythmic drug therapy in acute myocardial infarction. *JAMA* 1993; 270:1589–1595.
300. Hine LK, Laird N, Hewitt P, et al. Meta-analysis evidence against prophylactic use of lidocaine in acute myocardial infarction. *Arch Intern Med* 1989; 149:2694–2698.
301. Moosvi AR, Goldstein S, Medendorp SV, et al. Effect of empiric antiarrhythmic therapy in resuscitated out-of-hospital cardiac arrest: Victims with coronary artery disease. *Am J Cardiol* 1990; 65:1192–1197.
302. CASCADE Investigators. Randomized antiarrhythmic drug therapy in survivors of cardiac arrest (the CASCADE study). *Am J Cardiol* 1993; 72:280–287.
303. Siebels J, Kuck KH. Implantable cardioverter defibrillator compared with antiarrhythmic drug treatment in cardiac arrest survivors [The Cardiac Arrest Study—Hamburg (CASH)]. *Am Heart J* 1994; 127:1139–1144.
304. Hohnloser SH, Woosley RL. Drug therapy: Sotalol. *N Engl J Med* 1994; 331:31–38.
305. Mason JW. A comparison of electrophysiologic study to electrocardiographic monitoring for prediction of antiarrhythmic drug efficacy in patients with ventricular tachyarrhythmias. *N Engl J Med* 1993; 329:445–451.
306. Waldo AL, Camm AJ, deRuyter H, et al. Effect of *d*-sotalol on mortality in patients with left ventricular dysfunction after recent and remote myocardial infarction: The SWORD Investigators. (Survival with Oral *d*-Sotalol). *Lancet* 1996; 348:7–12.
307. Antiarrhythmics versus Implantable Defibrillators (AVID) Investigators. A comparison of antiarrhythmic-drug therapy with implantable defibrillators in patients resuscitated from near-fatal ventricular arrhythmias. *N Engl J Med* 1997; 337:1576–1583.
308. Zipes DP, Prystowsky EN, Heger JJ. Amiodarone: Electrophysiologic actions, pharmacokinetics and clinical effects. *J Am Coll Cardiol* 1984; 3:1059–1071.
309. Olson PJ, Woelfel A, Simpson RJ Jr, et al. Stratification of sudden death risk in patients receiving long-term amiodarone treatment for sustained ventricular tachycardia or ventricular fibrillation. *Am J Cardiol* 1993; 71:823–826.
310. Nademanee K, Singh BN, Stevenson WG, et al. Amiodarone and post MI patients. *Circulation* 1993; 88:764–774.
311. Burkart F, Pfisterer M, Kioski W, et al. Effect of antiarrhythmic therapy on mortality in survivors of myocardial infarction with asymptomatic complex ventricular arrhythmias: Basel Antiarrhythmic Study of Infarct Survival (BASIS). *J Am Coll Cardiol* 1990; 16:1711–1718.
312. Cairns JA, Connolly SJ, Roberts R, et al. Randomized trial of outcome after myocardial infarction in patients with frequent or repetitive ventricular premature depolarizations: CAMIAT. Canadian Amiodarone Myocardial Infarction Trial Investigators. *Lancet* 1997; 349:675–682.
313. Julian DJ, Camm AJ, Frangin G, et al. Randomized trial of effect of amiodarone on mortality in patients with left-ventricular dysfunction after recent myocardial infarction. EMIAT, European Myocardial Infarction Amiodarone Trial Investigators. *Lancet* 1997; 349:667–674.
314. Doval HC, Nul DR, Grancelli HO, et al. Randomized trial of low-dose amiodarone in severe congestive heart failure: Grupo de Estudio de la Sobrevida en la Insuficiencia Cardiaca en Argentina (GESICA). *Lancet* 1994; 344:493–498.
315. Singh SN, Fletcher RD, Fisher SG, et al. Amiodarone in patients with congestive heart failure and asymptomatic ventricular arrhythmia: Survival Trial of Antiarrhythmic Therapy in Congestive Heart Failure. *N Engl J Med* 1995; 13:333:77–82.
316. Connolly SJ, Gent M, Roberts RS, et al. Canadian Implantation Defibrillator Study (CIDS): Study design and organization. *Am J Cardiol* 1993; 72:103F–108F.
317. Connolly SJ, on behalf of the CIDS Investigators. The CIDS study: Final results. Oral presentation at the Annual Session of the American College of Cardiology meeting, Atlanta, March 29–April 1, 1998.
318. Kuck KH, on behalf of the CASH Investigators. The CASH study: Final results. Oral presentation at the Annual Session of the American College of Cardiology, Atlanta, March 29–April 1, 1998.
319. Scheinman MM. Parenteral antiarrhythmic drug therapy in ventricular tachycardia/ventricular fibrillation: Evolving role of class III agents—Focus on amiodarone. *J Cardiovasc Electrophysiol* 1995; 6:914–919.
320. Levine JH, Massumi A, Scheinman MM, et al. Intravenous amiodarone for recurrent sustained hypotensive ventricular tachyarrhythmias. *J Am Coll Cardiol* 1996; 27:67–75.
321. Kowey PR, Levine JH, Herre JM, et al. Randomized, double-blind comparison of intravenous amiodarone and bretylium in the treatment of patients with recurrent, hemodynamically destabilizing ventricular tachycardia or fibrillation. *Circulation* 1995; 92:3255–3263.
322. Kudenchuk PJ, Cobb LA, Copass MK, et al. Amiodarone for resuscitation after out-of-hospital cardiac arrest due to ventricular fibrillation. *N Engl J Med* 1999; 341:871–878.
323. Mirowski M, Reid PR, Mower MM, et al. Termination of malignant ventricular arrhythmias with an implanted automatic defibrillator in human beings. *N Engl J Med* 1980; 303:322–324.
324. Zipes DP, Roberts D, for the Pacemaker-Cardioverter-Defibrillator Investigators. Results of the International Study of the implantable pacemaker cardioverter-defibrillator: A comparison of epicardial and endocardial lead systems. *Circulation* 1995; 92:59–62.
325. Fogoros RN, Elson JJ, Bonnet CA, et al. Efficacy of the automatic implantable cardioverter-defibrillator in prolonging survival in patients with severe underlying cardiac disease. *J Am Coll Cardiol* 1990; 16:381–386.

326. Winkle RA, Mead RH, Ruder MA, et al. Long-term outcome with the automatic implantable cardioverter-defibrillator. *J Am Coll Cardiol* 1989; 13:1353–1361.
327. Meissner MD, Lehmann MH, Steinman RT, et al. Ventricular fibrillation in patients without significant structural heart disease: A multicenter experience with implantable cardioverter defibrillator therapy. *J Am Coll Cardiol* 1993; 21:1406–1412.
328. Powell AC, Fuchs T, Finkelstein DM, et al. Influence of implantable cardioverter defibrillators on the long term prognosis of survivors of out of hospital cardiac arrest. *Circulation* 1993; 88:1083–1092.
329. Moss AJ, Hall WJ, Cannom DS, et al. Improved survival with an implanted defibrillator in patients with coronary disease at high risk for ventricular arrhythmia. Multicenter Automatic Defibrillator Implantation Trial Investigators. *N Engl J Med* 1996; 335:1933–1940.
330. Buxton AE, Lee KL, Fisher JD, et al. A randomized study of the prevention of sudden death in patients with coronary artery disease. Multicenter Unsustained Tachycardia Trial Investigators. *N Engl J Med* 1999; 341:1882–1890.
331. Bigger JT Jr. Prophylactic use of implanted cardiac defibrillators in patients at high risk for ventricular arrhythmias after coronary-artery bypass graft surgery. Coronary Artery Bypass Graft (CABG) Patch Trial Investigators. *N Engl J Med* 1997; 337:1569–1575.
332. Moss AJ, Liu JE, Gottlieb S, et al. Efficacy of permanent pacing in the management of high-risk patients with long QT syndrome. *Circulation* 1991; 84:1524–1529.
333. Eldar M, Griffin JC, VanHare GF, et al. Combined use of beta-adrenergic blocking agents and long-term cardiac pacing for patients with long QT syndrome. *J Am Coll Cardiol* 1992; 20:830–837.
334. Fananapazir L, Epstein ND, Curiel RV, et al. Long-term results of dual chamber (DDD) pacing in obstructive hypertrophic cardiomyopathy: Evidence for progressive symptomatic and hemodynamic improvement and reduction of left ventricular hypertrophy. *Circulation* 1994; 90:2731–2742.
335. Nishimura RA, Hayes DL, Ilstrup DM, et al. Effect of dual-chamber pacing on systolic and diastolic function in patients with hypertrophic cardiomyopathy: Acute Doppler echocardiographic and catheterization hemodynamic study. *J Am Coll Cardiol* 1996; 27:421–430.
336. Holmes DR Jr, Davis KB, Mock MB, et al. The effect of medical and surgical treatment in patients with coronary artery disease: A report from the Coronary Artery Surgery Study. *Circulation* 1986; 73:1254–1263.
337. Varnauskas E, European Coronary Surgery Study Group. Survival, myocardial infarction and employment status in a prospective randomized study of coronary bypass surgery. *Circulation* 1985; 72(suppl V):V90–V101.
338. Every NR, Fahrenbruch CE, Hallstrom AP, et al. Influence of coronary bypass surgery on subsequent outcome of patients resuscitated from out of hospital cardiac arrest. *J Am Coll Cardiol* 1992; 19:1435–1439.
339. Kelly P, Ruskin JN, Vlahakes GJ, et al. Surgical coronary revascularization in survivors of prehospital cardiac arrest: Its effect on inducible ventricular arrhythmias and long-term survival. *J Am Coll Cardiol* 1990; 15:267–273.
340. Hargrove WC, Josephson ME, Marchlinski FE, et al. Surgical decisions in the management of sudden cardiac death and malignant ventricular arrhythmias: Subendocardial resection, the automatic internal defibrillator, or both. *J Thorac Cardiovasc Surg* 1989; 97:923–928.
341. Schwartz PJ, Locati EH, Moss AJ. Left cardiac sympathetic denervation in the therapy of congenital long QT syndrome: A world-wide report. *Circulation* 1991; 84:503–511.
342. Wang YS, Scheinmann MM, Chien WW, et al. Patients with supraventricular tachycardia presenting with aborted sudden death: Incidence, mechanism and long-term follow-up. *J Am Coll Cardiol* 1991; 18:1711–1719.
343. Langberg JJ, Desai J, Dullet N, et al. Treatment of macroreentrant ventricular tachycardia with radiofrequency ablation of the right bundle branch. *Am J Cardiol* 1989; 63:1010–1013.
344. Stevenson WG, Khan H, Sager P, et al. Identification of reentry circuit sites during catheter mapping and radiofrequency ablation of ventricular tachycardia late after myocardial infarction. *Circulation* 1993; 88:1647–1670.
345. Gonska BD, Cao K, Schaumann A, et al. Catheter ablation of ventricular tachycardia in 136 patients with coronary artery disease: Results and long-term follow-up. *J Am Coll Cardiol* 1994; 24:1506–1514.

CHAPTER 34

CARDIOPULMONARY RESUSCITATION AND THE SUBSEQUENT MANAGEMENT OF THE PATIENT

Nisha Chandra-Strobos / Myron L. Weisfeldt

INTRODUCTION: HISTORICAL ISSUES

Since biblical times, humans have attempted to restore life to the dead or nearly dead individual. The modern era of resuscitation began in the 1930s, when Wiggers pioneered the study of the mechanisms and treatment of ventricular fibrillation.[1] Major developments occurred in 1954, when Elam and colleagues showed that mouth-to-mouth or mouth-to-nose resuscitation was superior to the Schafer prone method of resuscitation in terms of efficacy of ventilation.[2,3] The importance of the circulation of blood was also recognized, and direct or internal cardiac massage became an accepted technique as early as 1916. Largely due to its complication rates and limited practical usefulness, it was replaced by noninvasive techniques of resuscitation.[4,5] In 1960, Kouwenhoven and coworkers developed the present technique of external chest compression in the supine position and coupled this with artificial respiration.[6] This technique of cardiopulmonary resuscitation (CPR) gained rapid popularity and was shown to be effective.[7] Only recently has the importance of prompt defibrillation taken a primary position in resuscitation efforts. Studies in large populations have confirmed that survival from prehospital cardiac arrest is dependent upon both prompt CPR and prompt defibrillation.

MECHANISMS OF MOVEMENT OF BLOOD DURING CARDIOPULMONARY RESUSCITATION

The original hypothesis suggested that blood flow to the periphery during external chest compression resulted from direct compression of the heart between the sternum and the vertebral column.[6] According to this concept, chest compression ("systole"), similar to internal cardiac massage, resulted in blood being squeezed from both ventricles into the great arteries as the pulmonary and aortic valves opened.

Retrograde flow of blood was prevented by closure of the mitral and tricuspid valves. During the release phase of chest compression ("diastole"), the ventricles recoiled to their original shape and filled by a suction effect, while elevated arterial pressure was thought to close both the pulmonic and aortic valves.

This widely held concept is not, however, consistent with a number of observations in animal models[8] and humans[9]; these suggest a correlation between the rise in intrathoracic pressure during chest compression and the apparent magnitude of carotid flow and pressure. The importance of fluctuations in intrathoracic pressure as a means for generating blood flow is further supported by the observations of Criley et al. that, by the continuous and early initiation of coughing, patients in ventricular fibrillation can maintain consciousness as long as cough is continued.[10] The critical ingredient of the cough is clearly a rise in intrathoracic pressure, probably with no cardiac compression. Criley's observations strongly suggest that following cardiac arrest, a rise in intrathoracic pressure is a potent mechanism for the movement of blood to the brain in humans.[10]

EXPERIMENTAL OBSERVATIONS

For brain blood flow to occur during CPR, a carotid arterial-to-jugular pressure gradient must be present during chest compression. In large animals, chest compression during CPR results in an essentially equal rise in central venous, right atrial, pulmonary artery, aortic, esophageal, and lateral pleural space pressures with no transcardiac gradient being developed (Fig. 34-1).[11]

In large animals, aortic pressure is transmitted directly to the carotid arteries, but retrograde transmission of intrathoracic venous pressure into the jugular veins is prevented by valves at the thoracic inlet. Thus, during chest compression ("systole"), a peripheral arteriovenous pressure gradient appears, and blood flow occurs consequent to this gradient. During compression, there is no pressure gradient across the heart; therefore, the heart cannot be the pump responsible for generating blood flow during CPR. In fact, the heart functions merely as a passive conduit. When chest compression is released ("diastole"), intrathoracic pressures fall toward zero, and venous flow into the right side of the heart and lungs occurs.

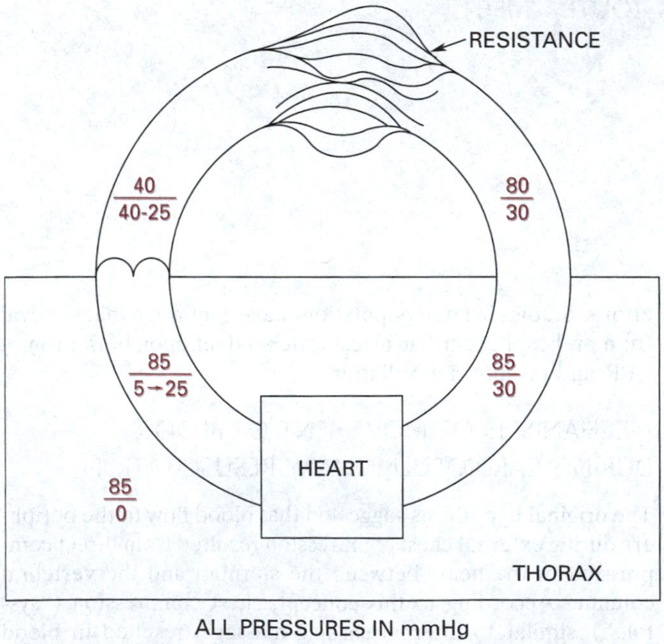

FIGURE 34-1 Representative pressures recorded during conventional cardiopulmonary resuscitation with forward carotid flow. Pressures are those recorded during compression. Intrathoracic pressures were indexed from esophageal pressures. There is no significant pressure gradient across the heart. The extrathoracic arterial pressure is similar to the intrathoracic aortic pressure. The extrathoracic venous pressure is markedly lower than the intrathoracic venous (right atrial) pressure. There is an extrathoracic arteriovenous pressure gradient that results in forward flow.

During diastole, a modest gradient also develops between the intrathoracic aorta and the right atrium and determines myocardial flow. Limited retrograde flow occurs into the aorta from extrathoracic arteries, raising aortic diastolic pressure and increasing coronary flow. The rise in intrathoracic pressure during chest compression is likely a consequence of airway collapse, which occurs at the level of the small bronchioles and results in air trapping. With the release of chest compression, this airway collapse is relieved.[12]

Unlike the hemodynamic pattern described above, in some animals intrathoracic vascular pressures during vigorous chest compression are much higher than pleural pressure.[13] In such animals, the rise in vascular pressures probably results from compression of the heart during chest compression, and the classic mechanism of direct cardiac compression is probably operating in these animals. Even during cardiac compression, however, venous valves at the thoracic inlet remain essential for establishing a peripheral arteriovenous pressure gradient, which facilitates peripheral flow. It is likely that flow produced by the two mechanisms operating simultaneously can occur, and in such situations the resultant flow is additive.

The position of the mitral valve during chest compression came to be regarded as a marker for the mechanism of blood flow during CPR, with mitral valve closure suggesting direct cardiac compression.[14] Some investigators, using transesophageal echocardiography, have demonstrated mitral valve closure during CPR in humans.[15] Others have reported that the mitral valve remains open during chest compression.[16] Animal studies have demonstrated that mitral valve closure or position cannot be used to identify the primary mechanism for blood flow during CPR.[17]

Studies of the perfusion of vital organs indicate that during CPR (irrespective of the primary mechanism for blood flow), cerebral flow is dependent on the gradient between the carotid artery and the intracranial pressure during systole, with myocardial flow being dependent on the gradient between the aorta and right atrium during diastole.[18]

OBSERVATIONS IN HUMANS

Unfortunately, at this point we can draw no final conclusion as to the frequency or importance of the two mechanisms (cardiac compression or generalized increase in intrathoracic pressure) during conventional cardiopulmonary resuscitation in humans. Published studies, however, suggest that manipulation of intrathoracic pressure is probably the dominant mechanism.[19] In a number of patients, comparable arterial and right atrial pressures have been observed as well as the presence of a pressure gradient at the thoracic inlet upon withdrawing an intravascular catheter from the superior vena cava to the extrathoracic internal jugular vein.[11,20,21] This hemodynamic pattern favors the concept of forward flow of blood through manipulation of intrathoracic pressure. This concept is further strengthened by the observation that maneuvers designed to increase intrathoracic pressure during chest compression—such as prolonged compression or vest CPR—are rewarded by a significant increase in peripheral arterial pressure. Recent studies have also shown increased peripheral arterial pressures in man during CPR with the use of an inspiratory airflow resistance valve. Inspiratory resistance is designed to reduce "diastolic" intrathoracic pressure (during the release phase of chest compression) and thereby increase net intrathoracic pressure fluctuations.[23] Perhaps the strongest evidence supporting the theory of manipulation of intrathoracic pressure as a mechanism for blood flow in humans is found in the documented efficacy of "cough CPR."[10] In some patients, who are usually thin-chested, with cardiomegaly, extremely high arterial pressures are generated with conventional CPR. In a few of these patients, central venous pressure was found to be lower than arterial pressure. This hemodynamic picture suggests cardiac compression. In other patients, however, this higher arterial pressure may reflect higher generalized intrathoracic pressure during chest compression. This may be a result of functional airway obstruction due to airway collapse, pulmonary congestion, and/or bronchospasm.[12] In the majority of the patients in whom radial artery pressure has been measured during CPR, the arterial pressure has been relatively low and similar to that seen in the dog during conventional CPR.[19,20]

In human beings (and also in animals), it is not essential to think about the mechanisms of blood flow during CPR in an exclusive fashion. As the force of chest compression changes or as chest wall anatomy and chest compliance change during prolonged resuscitation, the dominant mechanism for blood flow (during resuscitation) may also change.

Building on these concepts, several experimental maneuvers and techniques have been developed to increase arterial pressure during chest compression. Following clinical evaluation, some are now being considered for limited clinical use. Some of these techniques require special equipment, whereas others can be performed by unequipped health care providers.

EXPERIMENTAL AND ALTERNATIVE TECHNIQUES OF CARDIOPULMONARY RESUSCITATION

"High-impulse CPR" requires no special equipment and has been shown to improve vascular pressures.[13] It incorporates high-force, rapid down-thrust chest compression. However, clinical experience with this technique is limited.

Interposed abdominal compression (IAC) CPR can be performed by three unequipped health care providers. In this technique, the upper abdomen is compressed when the chest is released. The mechanism of benefit with IAC CPR in humans is unclear but may relate to improved venous return, decreased arterial runoff, or greater rise in intrathoracic pressure (with the diaphragm pushed up before chest compression). This technique increases carotid flow and improves survival in animals. Human clinical trials during in-hospital IAC CPR have also shown improved survival as compared with conventional CPR.[24] Based on these results, the 2000 American Heart Association (AHA) Guidelines for CPR suggest that IAC CPR be considered an alternative to conventional in-hospital CPR (class 2A recommendation).[25] The clinical value of this technique in the prehospital arrest patient, however, remains unproven.

Recently, the technique of phased chest and abdominal compression-decompression has also undergone animal and clinical testing. This technique is a mechanized IAC CPR in which the rescuer uses a special chest-abdomen manual compression device (the Lifestick Resuscitator); the chest and abdomen are thus compressed alternately. Its originators suggest that this technique, although similar to IAC CPR, is safer and more effective. Clinical studies are presently ongoing.[26]

The technique of perithoracic high-pressure vest inflation without airway manipulation (vest CPR) requires special equipment and allows cyclic increments in intrathoracic pressure to 100 to 150 mmHg during external chest compression. It has been shown to significantly increase cerebral and myocardial blood flow during CPR in animals. This technique employs a special computer-controlled pneumatic vest device positioned around the chest. Initial human data confirm higher vascular pressures during vest CPR as compared with conventional resuscitation.[22] Survival studies are lacking. A multicenter randomized survival trial was terminated prior to target patient enrollment. Data suggests that this technique may be of value as an alternative to standard CPR for short-term hemodynamic support.[26]

Active compression-decompression CPR (ACD CPR) requires a special suction-cup plunger-type device that can be readily deployed by first responders. It incorporates a negative pressure "pull" on the thorax during the release phase of chest compression and slightly improves vascular pressures and air exchange during CPR.[27] The mechanism of benefit from this technique of resuscitation may relate to improved venous return and/or increased intrathoracic pressure during chest compression as a consequence of changes in the bony thorax. Except for one 500-patient French study, all other recent, large, in-hospital and out-of-hospital studies in cardiac arrest patients have shown no survival benefit of ACD CPR.[28,29] It may, however, be of some value in improving short-term resuscitation outcomes. Lurie et al. have reported on the hemodynamic benefits of an inspiratory impedance valve attached to the endotracheal tube during resuscitation. Preliminary human data suggests that this device, coupled with ACD CPR, increases coronary perfusion pressures and improves end-tidal CO_2.[23] Larger clinical studies are necessary before the clinical usefulness of this technique is assessed.

In cardiac arrest in animals, aortic infusion during CPR (via catheters placed retrograde) has been shown to improve coronary flow and survival. However, human experience with this technique is limited. Emergency cardiopulmonary bypass and hypothermia during cardiac arrest is also undergoing clinical evaluation following promising animal studies. The initial clinical experience is favorable and a multicenter trial is ongoing. In summary, recent data suggest that several experimental CPR techniques may offer short-term survival benefit—i.e., survival to hospital admission—but the data on long-term improved outcome as compared to conventional CPR is less compelling for all strategies studied.

Although such experimental techniques lend themselves to limited clinical use, their study has resulted in a better understanding of physiology, which, in turn, allows several aspects of conventional external chest compression to be manipulated in order to optimize vital-organ perfusion pressures.[30] First, greater sternal force augments myocardial and cerebral perfusion but can also result in greater tissue injury. Second, adequate duration of compression during each chest compression–release cycle is critical for maintaining maximal myocardial and cerebral blood flow during resuscitation. At higher rates of chest compression, more time per minute is spent in chest compression. Based on these data, changes in the AHA recommendations regarding chest compression rate have evolved. The 2000 standards recommend that chest compressions be performed at a rate of approximately 100/min.[25]

DIAGNOSIS AND IDENTIFICATION OF CARDIAC ARREST

Cardiac arrest is defined as the sudden cessation of effective cardiac pumping function as a result of either ventricular asystole (electrical or mechanical) or ventricular fibrillation. Rapid diagnosis and treatment are essential because (1) more than a few minutes of total cardiac arrest result in permanent cerebral anoxic damage and (2) the success of resuscitative measures is related to the rapidity with which they are instituted following arrest. Based on these and other observations, the concept of early activation of emergency medical systems (EMS) has evolved for victims of out-of-hospital cardiac arrest[25] (see also Chap. 36).

Preliminary Patient Evaluation and Triage

Cardiac arrest should be considered in the differential diagnosis of sudden collapse in any patient. It can be clinically confirmed by pulseless major vessels and absent heart sounds.

Although respirations (agonal respirations) may continue for a minute or two, the patient with cardiac arrest rapidly becomes cyanotic and unconscious.

Once the diagnosis of cardiac arrest is made and no trauma is suspected, the unconscious patient should be positioned supine on a firm surface and the airway opened using the head tilt–chin lift technique or alternative strategies, as described below (in the discussion of ventilation during CPR). The patient should immediately receive rescue breathing either with a bag–valve mask device or with mouth-to-mouth breathing. Simple airway barrier devices, which are easily deployed, can be used to minimize direct patient contact and are preceived as being more hygienic during mouth-to-mouth resuscitation. Following airway opening and rescue breathing, chest compressions should be promptly initiated at approximately 100/min. Recent animal data suggests that ventilation can be deferred for several minutes in witnessed cardiac arrest without changing survival if chest compressions are initiated promptly. In addition, a recent study that randomized patients receiving dispatcher-assisted CPR to ventilation or no ventilation failed to demonstrate any benefit of early ventilation.[31] These and other data have raised several questions regarding the need and benefit for early ventilation in patients in cardiac arrest. Nevertheless, the AHA continues to recommend early ventilation for all patients.[25]

If available, an electrocardiogram (ECG) can confirm the diagnosis and identify asystole, ventricular fibrillation, or electromechanical dissociation as the mechanism of arrest. However, cardiopulmonary resuscitation (CPR) should be initiated immediately, as described above, once the clinical diagnosis is made without delaying to obtain this information. If a defibrillator but not an ECG is immediately available, a 200-J countershock should be administered without delay. Prehospital CPR studies in several patients have confirmed that, early in cardiac arrest, the mechanism of arrest is usually ventricular fibrillation and that survival is critically dependent on the time to defibrillation.[32] Most hospitals and paramedics are now equipped with defibrillators with "quick look" paddles that simultaneously allow the ECG rhythm to be analyzed. On the basis of the rhythm, an etiology for the arrest can then be explored in a more focused way and appropriate therapy initiated. A recent debate has emerged prompted by animal data from Niemann et al. showing that animals receiving CPR prior to early defibrillation did better than those in whom no CPR preceded defibrillation.[33] This observation is further supported by recent data from Cobb et al. showing that 90 s of "high-quality" CPR prior to defibrillation improved outcome in patients receiving bystander CPR.[34] The current recommendation is that if defibrillation is delayed, CPR should be performed immediately. However, if a defibrillator is available, the value of "predefibrillation CPR" is unclear. Clearly, if defibrillation fails to restore circulation, CPR should be performed immediately. Also, if collapse time without CPR is known to be more than 2 to 4 min, 90 s of initial CPR will likely be of value.

AUTOMATIC EXTERNAL DEFIBRILLATORS

Given the value of early defibrillation, automatic external defibrillators (AEDs) were developed for use by first (minimally trained) professional responders, and were shown to dramatically improve survival after prehospital arrest.[35,36] AEDs have an approximately 90 percent sensitivity and specificity for successfully recognized ventricular fibrillation. They are designed for use by first responders or persons with little medical training (e.g., fire fighters, EMS technicians). These devices have varying degrees of automation and can deliver several successive defibrillatory shocks via two self-adhesive electrodes placed by the user directly on the left anterior and left lateral chest. Most manual physician- or paramedic-operated waveform defibrillators deliver monophasic shocks. In recent years commercially available AEDs deliver a biphasic waveform shock. Recent research has focused on the relative efficacy of these two waveforms. Data suggests that biphasic-waveform defibrillation using shocks <200 J are safe and as effective as (if not more so) higher-energy monophasic shocks. Also, animal data suggests less postshock myocardial dysfunction following biphasic-waveform defibrillation. Various modifications of the biphasic waveform (sawtooth pattern, etc.) are being evaluated. Current recommendations do not clearly rank one defibrillatory waveform over the other; both are acceptable.

AEDs have been successfully used by nontraditional health care professionals (airline crews, police, and security guards) with dramatic improvement in patient survival. This program has been termed *public-access defibrillation.* All such AED defibrillation programs have been under strict physician-guided training and supervision. Perhaps the most compelling results of this strategy of emergency care were reported recently by White et al. in Rochester, Minnesota, where police-initiated AED defibrillation and resuscitation resulted in a survival to hospital discharge of approximately 50 percent (Fig. 34-2).[31] The value of training the on-site nontraditional health care provider was further tested and ratified when Valenzuela et al. trained casino security guards and demonstrated significant increases in resuscitation rates. They have demonstrated the compelling benefit of early defibrillation (Fig. 34-3).[37] Some authors have questioned the cost effectiveness of deploying first responder AEDs. A treatment should be considered economically attractive if it is associated with an incremental cost effectiveness ratio of less than twice the average annual income per life year (i.e., approximately $50,000 per life year). Modeling studies and clinical trials have demonstrated that the cost effectiveness of first responder AED programs is well within the cost of programs deemed to be clinically appropriate, if achieved by a low intensity intervention such as police or lay responder defibrillation (estimated cost $29,000 to $46,700 per year). Available data suggests that time to defibrillation is not cost-effectively reduced by adding to existing EMS systems.[38] In a dramatic move to test the value of early AED deployment, several AEDs have been prominently positioned at O'Hare Airport and have been successfully used by airport patrons. Recent state and federal legislation that endorses early AED deployment by trained supervised persons and indemnifies users, trainers, and other owners of AEDs has paved the way to evaluate public-access defibrillation.

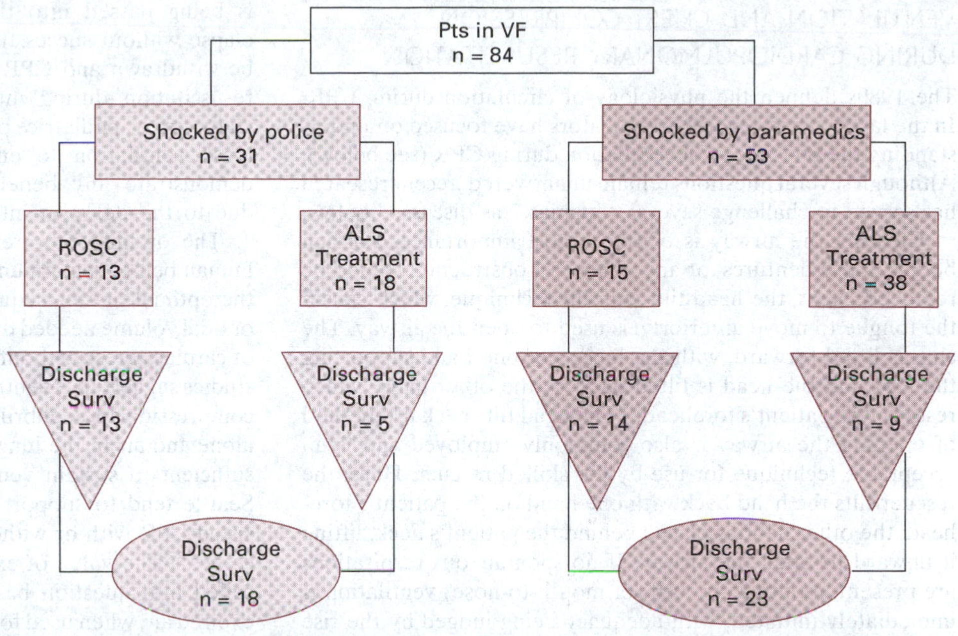

FIGURE 34-2 Police and paramedical treatment groups and patient outcome. VF = ventricular fibrillation; ROSC = restoration of spontaneous circulation; ALS = advanced life support. (From White et al.,[35] with permission.)

The use of AEDs by nontraditional health care professionals and possibly by trained lay persons is currently the focus of intense research. It is highly recommended that all first-responder EMS units be equipped with AEDs. Several agencies have developed training programs that incorporate AEDs and basic CPR training. However, the duration of training needed to correctly teach the use of an AED is likely much less than that currently used by most training agencies (i.e., only 3 or less hours appear to be needed).

RESPIRATORY ARREST

Respiratory arrest is the cessation of effective respiratory effort. It can result from airway obstruction (due to a foreign body or other causes), drowning, smoke inhalation, drug overdose, head trauma, cerebrovascular accident, or suffocation. When respiratory arrest occurs suddenly (as with foreign-body obstruction), the patient rapidly becomes cyanotic, though a palpable pulse with blood pressure, consciousness, and ineffective respiratory efforts may be maintained for several minutes. Opening the airway and/or rescue breathing may be all that is necessary to resuscitate such a patient.

The Heimlich maneuver is recommended for relieving foreign-body airway obstruction. It is implemented by standing behind the victim and delivering a series of sharp thrusts to the upper abdomen with a closed fist.[39] Abdominal thrusts can also be used directly in the unconscious, supine patient by the trained health care provider to help dislodge a foreign body mechanically. The Heimlich maneuver can also be self-administered by placing the fist between the navel and the xiphoid process and delivering a series of quick upward thrusts. If incorrectly administered, this maneuver can lead to visceral damage.[40] When properly used, however, the technique is both safe and effective.

Manual removal of a foreign body in the unconscious victim should be done only by trained health care providers. This can be achieved by opening the victim's mouth and attempting to dislodge any obvious foreign body with a finger. As a single method, back blows may not be as effective as the Heimlich maneuver in adults.

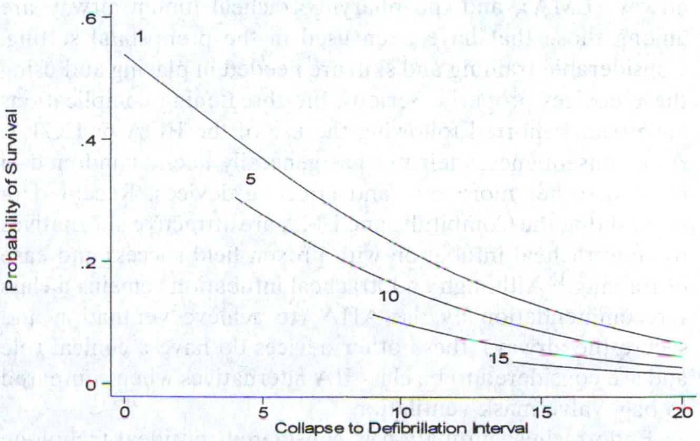

FIGURE 34-3 Relationship of collapse to CPR and defibrillation to survival: simplified model. Graphical representation of simplified (includes collapse to CPR and collapse to defibrillation only) predictive model of survival after witnessed out-of-hospital cardiac arrest due to VF. Each curve represents change in probability of survival as delay (minutes) to defibrillation increases for a given collapse-to-CPR interval (minutes). (From Valenzuela et al.,[37] with permission.)

VENTILATION AND CHEST COMPRESSION DURING CARDIOPULMONARY RESUSCITATION

The 1980s defined the physiology of circulation during CPR. In the last 5 years, several investigators have focused on understanding the physiology of ventilation during CPR (see below). Although several questions remain unanswered, recent research has served to challenge several "dogmas," as discussed below.

Clearing the airway is of the utmost importance. Foreign bodies, loose dentures, or any other oral obstruction should be removed. Next, the head tilt–chin lift technique, which causes the tongue to move anteriorly, is used to open the airway. The chin is lifted forward, with the fingers of one hand supporting the jaw, and the head is tilted back by the other hand, which rests on the patient's forehead.[35] The head tilt–neck lift method of opening the airway is also commonly employed and is an acceptable technique for use by the skilled rescuer. Here, the rescuer tilts the head back with one hand on the patient's forehead; the other hand is placed behind the patient's neck, lifting it upward to open the airway. If no spontaneous respirations are present, mouth-to-mouth (or mouth-to-nose) ventilation is immediately initiated, with adequacy being judged by the rise and fall of the patient's chest with each breath. To minimize gastric distention, it is necessary to deliver slow (2-s) ventilatory breaths.

Equipped rescuers will use a barrier device or a bag–valve mask technique of ventilation together with a small plastic oral "airway," which moves the tongue anteriorly. Adequate ventilation is difficult with the bag–valve mask technique, since a single rescuer often has difficulty maintaining an adequate seal on the face, and rapid bag deflation commonly results in gastric distention and aspiration. Slow (2-s) ventilation must be employed if the bag-mask technique is used.

Several invasive airway adjuncts have also been developed for use by nonphysician health care providers in prehospital situations, and several newer devices have been shown to be superior to the bag–valve mask technique of ventilation.[41] The esophageal obturator airway (EOA), esophageal gastric tube airway (EGTA), the Combitube, the laryngeal tracheal mask airway (LMA), and the pharyngotracheal lumen airway are among those that have been used in the prehospital setting. Considerable training and skill are needed in placing and using these devices properly. Serious, life-threatening complications have been reported following the use of the EOA or EGTA. As a consequence, their use has generally been abandoned in favor of other more safe and effective devices. Recent data suggest that the Combitube and LMA are attractive alternatives to endotracheal intubation with proven field success and ease of training.[42] Although endotracheal intubation remains a class I recommendation by the AHA (to achieve ventilation and secure the airway), these other devices do have a clinical role and are considered to be class IIA alternatives when compared to bag–valve mask ventilation.

Endotracheal intubation is considered the ideal technique for ensuring adequate ventilation during CPR. Whenever possible, a nasogastric tube should be inserted following intubation to drain the stomach and thus decrease the chances of aspiration. Intubation can be rapidly implemented, but much valuable time can be wasted by repeated unskilled attempts at intubation. If this technique is used, CPR should be discontinued for no more than 20 to 30 s while the tube is being passed into the airway. If more than 20 to 30 s elapse without successful intubation, the laryngoscope should be withdrawn and CPR reinstituted. The concern of delaying resuscitation during intubation was supported by a recent study in a pediatric population that compared bag–valve mask ventilation to endotracheal intubation and failed to demonstrate any benefit of endotracheal intubation, likely due to the delay in intubating patients.

The optimal requirements for ventilation during CPR in human beings remain unknown. No study has clearly identified the optimal timing, sequence in relation to chest compression, or tidal volume needed during CPR. During the first few minutes of cardiac arrest without prior hypoxia, as noted above, animal studies suggest that ventilation is less important relative to chest compression and defibrillation. Airflow from chest compression alone and air in the lungs at the time of arrest may be initially sufficient to sustain ventilation.[43,44] Recent human data from Seattle tend to support this observation, since dispatcher-assisted CPR with or without ventilation resulted in similar outcomes.[31] The value of expired air ventilation has further been called into question based on animal studies that show that expired air, when used for ventilation, actually worsens outcome in a ventricular fibrillation cardiac arrest model. The value of immediate expired air ventilation for victims of witnessed cardiac arrest has thus clearly been called into question. There are few data on the value (or lack thereof) of ventilation in the victim of an unwitnessed arrest. Based on these data, the new AHA guidelines for resuscitation recommend 100 chest compressions per minute with a 15:2 compression-ventilation ratio (for both single and two rescuer CPR) and ventilation with two breaths slowly delivered over 2 s with a tidal volume sufficient to achieve obvious chest rise (10 to 12 mL/kg) or if a bag-valve mask is used, 400 to 600 mL per breath.

In addition to these recommendations, it is critical, in performing chest compression, to use sufficient force to depress the sternum by approximately 2 in. (5 to 6 cm). As this is usually difficult to gauge, sufficient chest compression force should be used to generate a palpable femoral or carotid arterial pulse.

Airway, breathing, chest compression (ABC) is the specific sequence used to initiate CPR in the United States, with survival rates as high as 35 percent in cities with advanced EMS systems[32,36] (see Chap. 36). ABC is also used in many other countries. However, in the Netherlands, CAB (chest compression first followed by airway opening and breathing) is the common technique for CPR implementation, with resuscitation outcomes similar to those reported for ABC in the United States. Despite its proven efficacy, the recently perceived risk of infectious disease transmission during CPR has reduced the willingness of both lay and medical personnel to initiate mouth-to-mouth ventilation and CPR in unknown victims of cardiac arrest. In an effort to respond to these concerns and encourage the lay administration of CPR, some cities have mandated the public availability and use of barrier devices during mouth-to-mouth ventilation. The effectiveness of such barrier devices is, however, unknown. To overcome this limitation, potential rescuers who are reluctant to initiate CPR because of the perceived risk of infection should be encouraged to activate the EMS system immediately, open the victim's airway, and then initiate and continue chest compressions only until paramedics arrive (i.e., C–A). The paramedics can then initiate ventilation with the necessary protective equipment. It is important to note that a randomized comparison with CAB (chest compression, airway, breathing) or CAD (chest compression, airway opening, defibrillation) has never been done.

DEFINITIVE THERAPY

The AHA's *2000 Guidelines for Cardiopulmonary Resuscitation and Emergency Cardiac Care* adopted a new classification for therapeutic recommendations.[25] This classification allows a relative therapeutic value to be assigned to a given strategy of treatment based on scientific data. It is as follows:

1. Class I: Definitely helpful
2. Class IIA: Acceptable, probably helpful
3. Class IIB: Acceptable, possibly helpful, probably not harmful
4. Class III: Not indicated, may be harmful
5. Indeterminate: clinical data too preliminary or insufficient to allow classification into the other four categories

During cardiac arrest, the ECG will usually show rapid ventricular tachycardia or fibrillation, asystole, or heart block—or it may be near normal.

Ventricular Tachycardia or Fibrillation

With ventricular fibrillation, an attempt at electrical defibrillation should be made as quickly as possible. Successful defibrillation is accomplished by the passage of adequate electrical current (amperes) through the heart (see also Chap. 32). Current flow is dependent on the energy chosen (joules) and the transthoracic impedance (ohms), or resistance to current flow. Factors that affect transthoracic impedance include the energy selected, electrode size, skin-paddle coupling material, the number and time interval of previous shocks, the distance between the electrodes (size of the chest), phase of ventilation, and paddle electrode pressure.[45] Human transthoracic impedance ranges from 15 to 150 ohms, with the average adult impedance being 70 to 80 ohms. If transthoracic impedance is high, low-energy shocks are ineffective in generating enough current to achieve successful defibrillation. Transthoracic impedance can be reduced by firm pressure on hand-held electrode paddles and a gel/cream or saline-soaked gauze pads between the electrode and the skin.[45] In addition, proper electrode/paddle placement is essential; one electrode should be placed to the right of the upper sternum below the clavicle and the other to the left of the nipple, with the center of the electrode in the midaxillary line. An acceptable alternative is one electrode anteriorly over the left precordium and the other posteriorly behind the heart in the right infrascapular location. The latter positioning is best achieved by using preadhesive rather than hand-held electrodes. In female patients with large breasts, the electrodes are best placed to the right of the upper sternum and either under or lateral to the left breast. Direct current is employed during defibrillation. The paddles, coated with low-resistance gel, are applied firmly to the chest and then for monophasic defibrillations discharged with 200 J, which is repeated at 200 to 300 J if the first shock is unsuccessful. The current AHA standards suggest that a third 360-J shock should be delivered if ventricular fibrillation persists.[25] These three shocks should be delivered in rapid succession. Prospective studies by Adgey and others have shown 85 to 90 percent successful defibrillation using only 200 J in patients weighing up to 90 kg.[46,47] Some advocate higher-energy defibrillation, but few currently use more than 400 J.[48] High-energy defibrillation likely causes more cardiac injury, and increases postshock myocardial dysfunction; there is no clear evidence that it increases the frequency of successful resuscitation.[49] As mentioned above, several defibrillators have biphasic defibrillatory shock-wave forms. Most conventional manual defibrillators use the monophasic exponential wave form, whereas several AEDs deliver a biphasic defibrillatory shock wave at lower energy levels with equal if not greater success.

When the ECG shows fine fibrillation waves, defibrillation efforts are often unsuccessful. Although commonly practiced, the early use of epinephrine in such situations is not supported by improved survival in clinical trials. Nevertheless, it is suggested that the administration of epinephrine (5 to 10 mL of 1:10,000) intravenously (IV) may result in a more vigorous and coarse fibrillation that is more responsive to defibrillation. This effect is possibly due to improved coronary flow following epinephrine administration (see below), although recent data raise the question of epinephrine-induced deleterious myocardial effects, especially at higher doses.[50] If defibrillation fails, it is likely that marked acidosis or hypoxemia is present. Emphasis should be on modest hyperventilation with supplemental oxygen to correct both hypoxemia and metabolic acidosis.[51] Sodium bicarbonate might then be administered (1 meq/kg) to aid in the management of acidosis, and defibrillation should be repeated with 360 J. By using instantaneous Fourier transformation analysis, Brown et al. have demonstrated that the coarseness of the waveform of ventricular fibrillation may be highly predictive of subsequent survival and appears to correlate with coronary flow.[52] Preliminary human data to confirm these observations are limited.

In a recent study, the value of intravenous amiodarone in shock-refractory ventricular fibrillation/ventricular tachycardia (VF/VT) was tested in patients who had experienced prehospital cardiac arrest. Athough it improved survival to hospital admission, there was no difference in survival to hospital discharge between those who did and did not receive amiodarone.[53] Although often given, there are few data to support the use of lidocaine, bretylium, procainamide, or magnesium in such patients—i.e., those with shock refractory VF/FT (class of recommendation indeterminate).[54–56] Based on these data, it appears that amiodarone may be of some short-term benefit in patients with recurrent VT/VF. Amiodarone is usually dosed as a bolus of 150 to 300 mg over 10 min, 1.0 to 2.0 mg/min for 6 h, then 0.5 to 1.0 mg/min for 6 to 24 h. For recurrent VF in the setting of ischemia, intravenous propranolol or other intravenous beta blockers or amiodarone may be effective.[54] Beta blockers seem particularly helpful in the setting of primary ventricular fibrillation complicating acute myocardial infarction.[54] In fact, the early benefit of amiodarone has been ascribed by some to its beta blocking properties.

Hyperkalemia is a readily treated condition that can cause atrioventricular (AV) block, impaired intraatrial and intraventricular conduction, and occasionally ventricular fibrillation or, less commonly, asystole. It can be recognized by the development of tall, peaked T waves with a normal QT interval and sine wave–like ventricular tachycardia. Life-threatening hyperkalemia responds most readily to calcium infusion; 10 to 30 mL of 10% calcium gluconate is infused intravenously over 1 to 5 min under constant ECG monitoring. Calcium counteracts the adverse effects of potassium on the neuromuscular membranes but does not alter plasma potassium. Its effect, though immediate, is transient. Hyperkalemia should subsequently be treated by glucose-insulin or ion-exchange resins (Chap. 31). Sodium bicarbonate is also used as an agent to lower potassium.

With VT in an alert and responsive patient, cough may reverse the arrhythmia without defibrillation, and repeated cough may maintain the conscious state as a result of the rise in intrathoracic pressure.[10,57] It is an appropriate strategy for immediate use pending more definitive drug or electrical intervention. It is commonly used in the cath lab. The efficacy of the precordial thump (precordial chest blows) has been variably reported in patients with VT. A thump is generally ineffective for terminating prehospital VF. Hence, it should never be used in the patient with VT and a pulse unless a defibrillator is immediately available.

Asystole or Heart Block

For patients with prehospital cardiac arrest, asystole has been shown to be an ominous rhythm with a very low likelihood of successful resuscitation.[32] On the other hand, asystole due to vagal stimulation is the commonest cause of cardiac arrest associated with anesthesia induction and surgical procedures. Asystole also occurs as a result of heart block or sinus node disease (see Chap. 34). Atropine (0.5 mg) given intravenously and repeated in 5 min can be used acutely to prevent or reverse severe bradycardia in many of these settings.

If asystole is witnessed or of short duration, vigorous blows to the precordium may sometimes restart the heart. Rhythmic chest blows may maintain limited perfusion and can be continued if needed while palpating the femoral or carotid pulse until other treatment is available. If the chest blow fails, CPR should be initiated and intravenous epinephrine (5 to 10 mL of 1:10,000) administered. Possible treatable causes of asystole—such as acidosis, hypoxemia, hyper- or hypokalemia, and hypothermia—should be considered and treated appropriately if suspected. If an overdose of calcium channel blocker is suspected, calcium chloride, 1 g given as an intravenous bolus, may be very effective (class IIA recommendation). Resuscitation measures may result in the return of a slow ventricular rhythm, which can subsequently be supported with atropine (1 to 2 mg IV) until a temporary pacemaker is placed. Temporary pacing is the optimal treatment for true asystole or profound bradycardia. Obviously, considerable skill and training are required for temporary transvenous pacemaker placement (see Chap. 31). Transcutaneous pacing has been developed as a noninvasive and simple technique that can be implemented rapidly. It uses external surface electrodes with a high-voltage pacing source. Higher voltages are required to overcome transthoracic resistance, but they are painful and are therefore used mainly on unconscious patients. The energy delivered to the heart by this technique is variable, as is its efficacy. Recently, pacing sources with longer pacing stimulus duration have been developed and may offer less painful and more effective pacing. Prehospital studies of transcutaneous pacing for asystole have not confirmed an improvement in survival.[58] It may, however, be of some benefit for patients early in asystole (class IIB intervention). Clinical evidence does not support its routine use in all patients with asystole.

In rare instances, very fine VF may result in an almost straight line on a single-lead ECG and thus be mistaken for asystole. In such cases, where the diagnosis of asystole is in question, it is suggested that a perpendicular ECG lead be viewed. Rotation of "quick look" ECG paddles by 90 degrees easily achieves this. If ventricular fibrillation is present, the perpendicular ECG lead will demonstrate a typical fibrillation pattern; whereas in true asystole, a straight line will be seen in all ECG leads. If VF is diagnosed, the initial treatment should be according to the outline above—i.e, three successive countershocks. There is little value in defibrillating true asystole.

Electromechanical Dissociation

In *electromechanical dissociation* (EMD), there is evidence of organized electrical activity on the ECG at a reasonable rate, but failure of effective perfusion (no pulse or blood pressure). The most treatable causes of this condition are hypovolemia due to severe hemorrhage, pericardial tamponade, tension pneumothorax, hypoxia, hypothermia, acidosis, hyperkalemia, and massive pulmonary embolism. Signs of these problems should be sought and definitive therapy undertaken with fluids and/or blood replacement, pericardiocentesis, placement of a pleural needle or tube, endotracheal intubation, and other maneuvers as deemed necessary. These conditions should also be strongly considered if CPR results in no palpable pulse or evidence of perfusion. Unfortunately, many patients with electromechanical dissociation have primary myocardial failure. Following diagnosis, ventilation should be optimized and epinephrine administered. Calcium chloride has been used for EMD, but prospective studies have not shown it to improve survival.[59] In acute myocardial infarction, sudden electromechanical dissociation is a sign of myocardial rupture. In such cases, pericardiocentesis and surgical repair can rarely result in survival.

ESTABLISHMENT OF AN INTRAVENOUS ROUTE

While external chest compression and artificial ventilation are continued, a plastic catheter should be inserted into a large peripheral vein. Drug administration during CPR should be preferentially accomplished only from a source above the diaphragm, since there is little cephalad flow from veins below the diaphragm. If a peripheral vein cannot be cannulated, a cutdown should be attempted or a central venous line placed by a percutaneous route. If CPR is properly performed, drugs administered through a peripheral line will often reach the arterial circulation within 15 to 30 s.[51] Recent data suggest that a 20-mL fluid bolus significantly improves peripheral drug delivery to the central compartment. Larger amounts of fluids should be used if drugs are given via a femoral line. Intracardiac injections are unnecessary except when there is no intravenous access. If an intravenous route is unavailable, epinephrine (1 to 2 mg in 10 mL of sterile distilled water) and lidocaine (50 to 100 mg in 10 mL of sterile distilled water) can be administered by way of the endotracheal tube into the bronchial tree. The drug should be injected through a long catheter passed beyond the tip of the endotracheal tube. Cardiac compression should be withheld, and several insufflations with an Ambu bag should immediately follow drug administration to aid drug absorption through aerosolization.

MAJOR DRUGS USED DURING CARDIOPULMONARY RESUSCITATION

Drugs that are used for the treatment of various arrhythmias are mentioned above. Catecholamines are used in cardiac arrest to (1) increase arterial and coronary perfusion during and following CPR, (2) stimulate spontaneous contraction during asystole, (3) make fine VF more responsive to defibrillation, and (4) act as an inotropic agent.

Epinephrine was among the earliest pressors evaluated during resuscitation. It is effective in achieving several of these goals, although recent data have highlighted its possible deleterious effects on postresuscitation left ventricular function. Both animal and clinical studies have extensively evaluated the hemodynamic effects of epinephrine during resuscitation. Animal studies show that during conventional CPR, cerebral and myocardial perfusion pressures are low. Epinephrine increases brain and heart flow by two mechanisms: (1) It prevents carotid artery collapse and raises arterial pressure during both chest compression and the release phase of chest compression (i.e., "systole" and "diastole," respectively). This results in higher carotid arterial systolic and aortic diastolic pressures, which, in turn, are reflected in higher cerebral perfusion and myocardial perfusion pressures and flow. (2) It preferentially reduces blood flow to the external carotid, renal, and splanchnic beds, thereby redirecting flow toward the brain and heart.[60,61]

Arterial collapse at the thoracic inlet has been shown to be the critical limiting factor for cerebral perfusion pressure and flow during prolonged CPR. Arterial collapse results from high extravascular intrathoracic pressures, low intravascular volumes, and loss of arterial tone. Collapse results in a precipitous fall in carotid arterial and hence cerebral perfusion pressure. Epinephrine during CPR can not only reverse arterial collapse but also prevent it from developing. With the administration of epinephrine during conventional manual CPR in the dog, cerebral blood flow can be maintained at approximately 15 percent and myocardial flow at approximately 5 percent of prearrest values for 20 min.

These data strongly support the early and frequent use of epinephrine during CPR in an effort to optimize the perfusion of vital organs. The recommended dose of epinephrine (1 mg IV every 3 to 5 min) is comparable to a 0.007 to 0.014 mg/kg dose in a 70-kg person. This dose has been questioned, since animal studies using higher doses of epinephrine have shown improved blood flow to vital organs and improved survival.[61] Other studies of higher doses of epinephrine, however, have shown increased myocardial oxygen demand despite this improved blood flow.[62] Higher than recommended doses of epinephrine have been reported to increase arterial pressure and coronary perfusion pressure in a small number of human studies. These studies spawned an intense interest in the use of higher doses of epinephrine during CPR. Results from several prospective randomized out-of-hospital clinical trials of more than 2400 adult cardiac arrest victims, however, have shown no statistically significant improvement in survival to hospital admission or discharge or improved neurologic survival when higher doses of epinephrine (0.1 to 0.2 mg/kg) were compared with standard doses.[63,64] On the other hand, these trials did not demonstrate any obvious deleterious effect of the higher doses of epinephrine.

Recent retrospective studies suggest that higher cumulative doses of epinephrine are associated with worse hemodynamic and neurologic outcome event when duration of cardiac arrest are accounted for. Hence, most experts would use 1 mg IV uniformly. Higher doses worsen postresuscitation myocardial dysfunction, hence its use is not routinely recommended.[25] The recommended dose is 0.5 to 1 mg IV, and this dose should be repeated at approximately 3- to 5-min intervals unless effective cardiac activity is restored. If an intravenous route is not available, epinephrine can be administered down the endotracheal tube; 10 mL of a 1:10,000 solution should be used, and this can also be repeated every 3 to 5 min.

The benefits of epinephrine are principally due to the alpha vasoconstriction induced by this agent. The inotropic effects of the drug may not be helpful, since these effects increase myocardial oxygen demand, even during ventricular fibrillation, when supply or blood flow is limited.[62] Consequently, there is some interest in using a pure vasoconstrictor during CPR rather than epinephrine. Animal studies of vital organ perfusion and human survival studies comparing epinephrine and phenylepinephrine (a pure alpha vasoconstrictor) have yielded similar results. Vasopressin has recently been evaluated as an alternative pressor agent, with promising results.[64a] Animal studies have demonstrated it to be as effective as pressor but with less resultant myocardial dysfunction as compared to epinephrine. Initial human data has been encouraging. However, a large prospective randomized out-of-hospital study of vasopressin versus epinephrine failed to confirm any survival benefit of this agent.[64b] It may be considered an alternative pressor to epinephrine for patients in shock-refractory VF (class IIB).

Norepinephrine is a potent vasoconstrictor and generally produces a rise in blood pressure; it is also an inotropic agent. Its disadvantage is renal and mesenteric vasoconstriction, and it should not be used in the initial phase of resuscitation. This agent is most useful where severe hypotension is present but where the chronotropic effects of epinephrine are not desirable (as in acute myocardial infarction or severe ischemia). This agent should be administered cautiously, since severe tissue injury results from extravasation around an intravenous site. A large prehospital trial failed to identify any differences in survival following treatments with norepinephrine, high-dose epinephrine, or standard epinephrine.[63]

Similarly, dopamine (a chemical precursor of norepinephrine) and dobutamine (a synthetic catecholamine) are preferred for use as inotropic agents because of their lesser chronotropic effect. Recent animal data suggests that dobutamine may be particularly effective in reducing postresuscitation left ventricular dysfunction. Isoproterenol (a synthetic catecholamine) is a pure adrenergic agonist and effective vasodilator. Therefore, its use during CPR is contraindicated since it can significantly decrease vital organ perfusion pressures. In patients with a palpable pulse, however, it is useful for treatment of bradycardia due to heart block or asystole until a temporary pacemaker is placed (see also Chap. 31).

Sodium Bicarbonate

The recent AHA recommendations deemphasize the role of sodium bicarbonate and suggest that much less sodium bicarbonate should be used than previously advocated for acid-base control during cardiac arrest. As with other types of metabolic acidosis, if adequate alveolar ventilation is achieved, the metabolic acidosis of arrest is partially corrected through P_{CO_2} excretion.[51] Recent clinical trials failed to demonstrate improved outcome from cardiac arrest with buffer therapy.[65] Rather, several deleterious effects of bicarbonate administration including respiratory acidosis, hypernatremia, and hyperosmolality have been reported. Ideally, sodium bicarbonate should be given according to the results of measurement of arterial blood pH, P_{CO_2} determination, and calculation of the base deficit. Bicarbonate should be used, if at all, only after more established interventions such as defibrillation, ventilation with endotracheal intubation, and pharmacologic therapies (epinephrine and antiarrhythmic drugs) have been tried.[25] If needed, 1 meq/kg of sodium bicarbonate should be administered; then no more than half this dose may be repeated every 15 min. Excessive use of sodium bicarbonate can result in metabolic alkalosis, hypernatremia, and hyperosmolality. Some benefit of the usual bicarbonate solution (7.2 percent) may occur as a result of the hyperosmolality of the solution temporarily drawing fluid into the intravascular compartment.

On the other hand, bicarbonate may be most useful during the immediate postresuscitation period, when a profound metabolic acidosis occurs. In most instances during CPR, its use should be considered as a class IIB recommendation.[30]

Calcium Chloride

Calcium chloride (5 to 7 mg/kg) enhances the contractile state of the heart and is indicated in treating severe hypotension due to an overdose of calcium channel blocker or hyperkalemia. It is no longer recommended for use in asystole or electromechanical dissociation.

TERMINATION OF CARDIOPULMONARY RESUSCITATION

Despite resuscitative efforts, the patient in cardiac arrest may not regain spontaneous circulation. The decision to end (or even initiate) CPR should be based on a physician's assessment of the patient's prior advance directives (if known) and the cerebral, cardiovascular, and general status of the patient.[66,67] Recent prospective and retrospective data confirm that survival is unlikely in patients who have no return of spontaneous circulation after 30 min of ACLS care.[68] Recent studies have demonstrated that continued in-hospital CPR efforts (in patients failing prehospital advanced cardiac life support) are not only expensive but also unsuccessful.[69] Persistent deep unconsciousness and absence of respiration, reflex response, or pupillary reaction suggest cerebral death, and resuscitative efforts are usually unproductive. These guidelines, however, should be altered in patients with hypothermia, barbiturate overdose, and perhaps following electrocution, where recovery has been seen even after hours of resuscitation.[70]

POSTARREST CARE

Patients who have been successfully resuscitated usually require monitoring in an intensive care setting. These patients are prone to develop cardiac arrhythmias, hemodynamic and ventilatory instability, and ischemic encephalopathy. Ventilatory support with a respirator may well be necessary initially. Serial arterial blood-gas determinations should be made to identify hypoxemia and assess the rapidly changing acid-base status. Commonly, hyperventilation was employed postresuscitation to not only treat acidosis but also help reduce CNS edema. Recent studies raise the possibility of worsening cerebral ischemia with low P_{CO_2} levels after brain ischemia. Based on these observations, normal ventilation is preferred in the comatose postresuscitation patient.

Several therapeutic strategies have been employed in animal models to help reduce hypoxic encephalopathy after cardiac arrest. None (including emergency cardiopulmonary bypass, which is currently undergoing clinical testing) have clearly been shown to be beneficial in humans.

The treatment of encephalopathy after cardiac arrest involves the prevention of further hypoxia and hypotension. For cerebral edema after cardiac arrest, methylprednisolone (60 to 100 mg) or dexamethasone sodium phosphate (12 to 20 mg IV every 6 h) has been recommended, but there is no conclusive evidence that these agents are beneficial. High-dose barbiturates or lidoflazine have also been shown to reduce postarrest brain injury in animal studies; the value of this therapy in human beings is negligible. In animals, mild to moderate hypothermia appears to be neuroprotective following an ischemic event. Clinical data are limited but suggestive of benefit. Trials are ongoing. The prognosis of the patient with anoxic encephalopathy is related to the depth and continued duration of cerebral dysfunction (see also Chap. 89). Failure to exhibit neurologic improvement 24–72 h following resuscitation is usually an ominous sign. Clinical and laboratory evaluations (electroencephalography, sensory evoked potentials) are often employed to help define prognosis and thus guide further care in such individuals.

Other potential life-threatening problems in the postarrest period include acute renal failure, bowel infarction, infection, adult respiratory distress syndrome, and sepsis. Patients regaining consciousness may have postarrest amnesia or may develop psychotic behavior.

OUTCOME OF RESUSCITATION

In their initial study, Kouwenhoven and colleagues reported a 24 percent successful resuscitation and discharge rate from the hospital. Recent studies have shown that with a paramedical response system, a near 40 percent successful out-of-hospital resuscitation rate can be achieved.[32,71] Many of these patients die in hospital, however, with the dominant cause of death being anoxic encephalopathy. Recent data suggest that somatosensory evoked potentials may be useful and highly predictive in identifying patients who are likely to have irreversible brain injury.[72] The critical factors for successful out-of-hospital resuscitation include approximately 7 min total duration of CPR, approximately 4 min from collapse to the initiation of CPR, and approximately 10 min to successful delivery of the first countershock.

It is important to point out, however, that the quality of life for patients surviving to hospital discharge is often quite good, with most discharged patients being able to return to gainful employment.

CHAIN OF SURVIVAL

The concept of a "chain of survival" has been adopted by several agencies and underscores the importance of an integrated public education and health care system if outcome from prehospital cardiac arrest is to be optimized.[25] Early access (to EMS systems), early CPR (to include bystander CPR), early defibrillation (to include the use of AEDs), and early *advanced cardiac life support* (ACLS) care are the major links in the chain, and any one weak link weakens the whole chain of survival.

This is best exemplified in two recent publications that reported on prehospital cardiac arrest outcomes in New York and Chicago, where survival rates were only 1 to 2 percent. Despite a mature EMS system and considerable public training in CPR, delayed defibrillation—due to traffic, elevators, and other factors—contributed significantly to the poor outcome in these studies.[73,74] Other cities, where prompt defibrillation has been possible, have reported a 20 to 30 percent survival rate.[75] To overcome this tragic limitation, AEDs were developed and have been shown to facilitate prompt defibrillation and thereby improve survival (Fig. 34-3). Hence, the American Heart Association and American College of Cardiology have jointly recommended that all professional first-responder units (especially in rural areas where long transport times are common) be equipped with AEDs.

If mortality from out-of-hospital arrest is to be reduced, public education programs to increase awareness of the warning signs of a heart attack and teach CPR are critical (Fig. 34-3). Despite many years of public education, the incidence of bystander CPR nationwide remains low.[73,74] This may have several explanations, including a lack of training in high-risk populations, poor performance or lack of retention despite training, unnecessarily complex training programs, or a fear of communicable disease during mouth-to-mouth resuscitation. This last issue has become particularly significant in the 1990s. Individuals should be reassured that the likelihood of disease transmission is minimal, 70 percent of arrest victims collapse at home, and if an individual is still unwilling to do mouth-to-mouth CPR, he or she should be taught to at least activate EMS ("call") and start chest compressions ("pump"). Ventilation ("blow") could then be started by suitably equipped trained EMS rescuers. Present data indicate that a refocusing of basic life support (BLS) training programs is essential, with efforts being targeted at simplification of training, with specific education and training penetration into high-risk patient groups (older patients and minority groups). The CPR message must be kept simple (for example, "call-pump-blow"). These goals must be achieved if the first two links in the chain of survival (early access and early CPR) are to be strengthened. Universal 911 would facilitate early and easy access and should be encouraged in all communities. Minimal standards of performance and excellence for EMS systems should be established and monitored. Dispatcher-assisted CPR teaches CPR on the telephone to the person who is calling to report the arrest (while professional help is in transit) and has been shown to be effective. The Seattle–King County EMS system is proof that such efforts directly improve outcome (Fig. 34-3).[75] On the other hand, the Chicago–New York experience is a chilling reminder of the consequence of one weak link in the chain of survival. The outcome from prehospital arrest can be improved only if each community strives to optimize its own chain of survival.

References

1. Wiggers CJ. The physiologic basis for cardiac resuscitation from ventricular fibrillation method of serial defibrillation. *Am Heart J* 1940; 20:413–422.
2. Comroe JH. Retrospectroscope: In comes the good air. *Am Rev Respir Dis* 1979; 119:803–809.
3. Elam JO, Brown ES, Elder JD. Artificial respiration by mouth-to-mask method. *N Engl J Med* 1954; 250:749–754.
4. Sanders AB, Kern KB, Ewy GA. Open chest massage for resuscitation from cardiac arrest. *Resuscitation* 1988; 16:153–154.
5. Eldor J, Frankel DZN, Davidson JT. Open chest cardiac massage: A review. *Resuscitation* 1988; 16:155–162.
6. Kouwenhoven WB, Jude JR, Knickerbocker GG. Closed chest cardiac massage. *JAMA* 1960; 173:1064–1067.
7. Jude JR, Kouwenhoven WB, Knickerbocker GG. Cardiac arrest: Report of application of external cardiac massage on 118 patients. *JAMA* 1961; 178:1063–1071.
8. Weale FE, Rothwell-Jackson RL. The efficiency of cardiac massage. *Lancet* 1962; 1:990–992.
9. MacKenzie GJ, Taylor SH, McDonald AH, Donald KW. Hemodynamic effects of external cardiac compression. *Lancet* 1964; 1:1342–1345.
10. Criley JM, Blaufuss AN, Kissel GL. Cough-induced cardiac compression. *JAMA* 1976; 236:1246–1250.
11. Rudikoff MT, Maughan WL, Effron M, et al. Mechanisms of flow during cardiopulmonary resuscitation. *Circulation* 1980; 61:345–351.
12. Halperin H, Brower R, Weisfeldt ML, et al. Air trapping in the lungs during cardiopulmonary resuscitation in dogs: A mechanism for generating changes in intrathoracic pressure. *Circ Res* 1989; 65:946–954.
13. Maier GW, Tyson GS, Olsen CO, et al. The physiology of external cardiac massage: High impulse cardiopulmonary resuscitation. *Circulation* 1984; 70:86–101.
14. Feneley MP, Maier GW, Gaynor JW, et al. Sequence of mitral valve motion and transmitral blood flow during manual cardiopulmonary resuscitation in dogs. *Circulation* 1987; 76:363–375.
15. Deshmukh HG, Weil MH, Gudipati CV, et al. Mechanism of blood flow generated by precordial compression during CPR: I. Studies on closed chest precordial compression. *Chest* 1989; 95:1092–1099.
16. Werner JA, Greene HL, Janko CL, Cobb LA. Visualization of cardiac valve motion in man during external chest compression using two-dimensional echocardiography: Implications regarding the mechanism of blood flow. *Circulation* 1981; 63:1417–1421.
17. Halperin HR, Weiss JL, Guerci AD, et al. Cyclic elevation of intrathoracic pressure can close the mitral valve during cardiac arrest in dogs. *Circulation* 1988; 78:754–760.
18. Koehler RC, Chandra N, Guerci AD, et al. Augmentation of cerebral perfusion by simultaneous chest compression and lung inflation with abdominal binding following cardiac arrest in dogs. *Circulation* 1983; 67:266–275.
19. Swenson RD, Weaver WD, Nisaken RA, et al. Hemodynamics in humans during conventional and experimental methods of cardiopulmonary resuscitation. *Circulation* 1988; 78:630–639.
20. Chandra NC, Tsitlik JE, Halperin HR, et al. Observations of hemodynamics during cardiopulmonary resuscitation. *Crit Care Med* 1990; 18:929–934.
21. Paradis N, Martin G, Goetting M, et al. Simultaneous aortic, jugular bulb, and right atrial pressures during cardiopulmonary

resuscitation in humans: Insights into mechanisms. *Circulation* 1989; 80:361–368.

22. Halperin HR, Tsitlik JE, Gelfand N, et al. A preliminary study of cardiopulmonary resuscitation with circumferential compression of the chest with use of a pneumatic vest. *N Engl J Med* 1993; 329:762–768.
23. Plaisance P, Lurie KG, Payen D. Inspiratory impedance during ACD-CPR. *Circulation* 2000; 101:989–994.
24. Sack J, Kesselbrenner M, Bergman D. Survival from in-hospital arrest with interposed abdominal counterpulsation during cardiopulmonary resuscitation. *JAMA* 1992; 276:379–385.
25. Guidelines 2000 for cardiopulmonary resuscitation and emergency cardiovascular care international consensus on science. *Circulation* 2000 (in press).
26. Tang W, Weil MH, Schock, et al. Phased chest and abdominal compression-decompression. *Circulation* 1997; 95:1335–1340.
27. Cohen TJ, Tucker KJ, Lurie KG, et al. Active compression-decompression resuscitation: A new method of cardiopulmonary resuscitation. *JAMA* 1992; 267:2916–2923.
28. Stiell IG, Hébert PC, Wells GA, et al. The Ontario trial of active compression-decompression cardiopulmonary resuscitation for in-hospital and prehospital cardiac arrest. *JAMA* 1996; 275:1417–1423.
29. Gueugniaud P, Mols P, Goldstein P, et al. A comparison of repeated high doses and repeated standard doses of epinephrine for cardiac arrest outside the hospital. *N Engl J Med* 1998; 339:1595–1601.
30. Halperin HR, Tsitlik JE, Guerci AD, et al. Determinants of blood flow to vital organs during cardiopulmonary resuscitation in dogs. *Circulation* 1986; 73:539–551.
31. Hallstrom A, Cobb L, Johnson E, Copass M. Cardiopulmonary resuscitation by chest compression alone or with mouth to mouth ventilation. *NEJM* 2000; 342:1546–1553.
32. Eisenberg MS, Horwood BT, Cummins RO, et al. Cardiac arrest after resuscitation: A tale of 29 cities. *Ann Emerg Med* 1990; 19:179–186.
33. Niemann JT, Cairns CB, Sharma J, Lewis RJ. Treatment of prolonged ventricular fibrillation: Immediate countershock versus high dose epinephrine and CPR preceding countershock. *Circulation* 1992; 85(1):281–287.
34. Cobb LA, Fahrenbruch CE, Walsh TR. Influence of cardiopulmonary resuscitation prior to defibrillation in patients with out-of-hospital ventricular fibrillation. *JAMA* 1999; 281:1182–1188.
35. White RD, Asplin BR, Bugliosi TF, Hankins DG. High release survival from out-of-hospital ventricular fibrillation with rapid defibrillation by both police and paramedics. *Acad Emerg Med* 1996; 3:422.
36. Weaver WD, Hill D, Fahrenbruch CE, et al. Use of the automatic external defibrillation in the management of out-of-hospital cardiac arrest. *N Engl J Med* 1988; 319:661–666.
37. Valenzuela TD, Roe DJ, Cretin S, et al. Estimating effectiveness of cardiac arrest interventions. A logistic regression survival model. *Circulation* 1997; 96:3308–3313.
38. Nichol G, Hallstrom A, Ornato JP, et al. Potential cost-effectiveness of public access defibrillation in the United States. *Circulation* 1998; 97(13):1315–1320.
39. Heimlich HJ. A life saving maneuver to prevent from choking. *JAMA* 1975; 234:398–401.
40. Visintine RE, Baick CH. Ruptured stomach after Heimlich maneuver. *JAMA* 1975; 234:415.
41. Pepe PE, Zacharich BS, Chandra NC. Update on invasive airway techniques in resuscitation. *Ann Emerg Med* 1993; 22:393–403.
42. Rumball CJ, MacDonald D. The PTL, Combitube, Laryngeal Mask, and Oral Airway. A randomized prehospital comparative study of ventilatory device effectiveness and cost-effectiveness in 470 cases of cardiorespiratory arrest. *Prehospital Emergency Care* 1997; 1:1–10.
43. Chandra NC, Gruben KG, Tsitlik JE, et al. Observations of ventilation during resuscitation of a canine model. *Circulation* 1994; 90:3070–3075.
44. Locke CJ, Berg RA, Sanders AB, et al. Bystander cardiopulmonary resuscitation: Concerns about mouth to mouth contact. *Arch Intern Med* 1995; 155:938–943.
45. Sirna SJ, Fergusson DW, Charbonnier F, Kerber RE. Electrical cardioversion in humans: Factors affecting transthoracic impedance. *Am J Cardiol* 1988; 62:1048–1052.
46. Adgey AAJ, Patton JN, Campbell NPS, Webb SW. Ventricular defibrillation: Appropriate energy levels. *Circulation* 1979; 60: 219–223.
47. Gascho JA, Crampton RS, Cherwek ML, et al. Determinants of ventricular defibrillation in adults. *Circulation* 1979; 60:231–240.
48. Tacker WA, Ewy GA. Emergency defibrillation dose, recommendation and rationale. *Circulation* 1979; 60:223–225.
49. Weaver WD, Cobb LA, Copass MK, Hallstrom AP. Ventricular defibrillation: A comparative trial using 175-J and 320-J shocks. *N Engl J Med* 1982; 307:1101–1106.
50. Tang W, Weil MH, Sun S, et al. Epinephrine increases the severity of postresuscitation myocardial dysfunction. *Circulation* 1995; 92:3089–3093.
51. Bishop RL, Weisfeldt ML. Sodium bicarbonate administration during cardiac arrest: Effect of arterial pH, P_{CO_2} and osmolality. *JAMA* 1976; 235:506–509.
52. Brown CG, Dzwoncyk R, Martin DR. Physiologic measurement of the ventricular fibrillation ECG signal: Estimating the duration of ventricular fibrillation. *Circulation* 1993; 22:70–74.
53. Kudenchuk PJ, Cobb LA, Copass MK, et al. Amiodarone for resuscitation after out-of-hospital cardiac arrest due to ventricular fibrillation. *N Engl J Med* 1999; 341:871–878.
54. Levine JH, Massumi A, Scheinman MM, et al. Intravenous amiodarone for recurrent sustained hypotensive ventricular tachyarrhythmias. *Circulation J Am Coll Cardiol* 1996; 27:67–75.
55. Kowey PR, Levine JH, Herre JM, et al. Randomized, double-blind comparison of intravenous amiodarone and bretylium in the treatment of patients with recurrent, hemodynamically destabilizing ventricular tachycardia and fibrillation. *Circulation* 1995; 92:3255–3263.
56. Haynes RE, Copass MK, Chinn TL, Cobb LA. Comparison of bretylium tosylate and lidocaine in management of out-of-hospital ventricular fibrillation: A randomized clinical trial. *Am J Cardiol* 1981; 48:353–356.
57. Wei JY, Greene HL, Weisfeldt ML. Cough-facilitated conversion of ventricular tachycardia. *Am J Cardiol* 1980; 45:174–176.
58. Cummins RO, Grave JR, Larsen MP, et al. Out-of-hospital transcutaneous pacing by emergency medical technicians in patients with asystolic cardiac arrest. *N Engl J Med* 1993; 328:1377–1382.
59. Stueven HA, Thompson BM, Aprahamian C, Tonsfeldt DJ. Calcium chloride: Reassessment of use in asystole. *Ann Emerg Med* 1984; 13:820–822.
60. Michael JR, Guerci AD, Koehler RC, et al. Mechanisms by which epinephrine augments cerebral and myocardial perfusion during cardiopulmonary resuscitation in dogs. *Circulation* 1984; 69: 822–835.
61. Brown CG, Wermn HA, Davis EA, et al. The effects of graded doses of epinephrine on regional myocardial blood flow during cardiopulmonary resuscitation in swine. *Circulation* 1987; 75: 491–497.
62. Ditchey RV, Lindenfeld J. Failure of epinephrine to improve the balance between myocardial oxygen supply and demand during closed chest resuscitation in dogs. *Circulation* 1988; 78: 382–389.
63. Callaham M, Madsen CD, Barton CW, et al. A randomized clinical trial of high-dose epinephrine and norepinephrine vs standard dose epinephrine in prehospital cardiac arrest. *JAMA* 1992; 268:2667–2672.

64. Brown CG, Martin DR, Pepe PE, et al. A comparison of standard-dose and high-dose epinephrine in cardiac arrest outside the hospital. *N Engl J Med* 1992; 327:1051–1055.

64a. Lindner KH, Prengel AW, Brinkmann A, et al. Vasopressin administration in refractory cardiac arrest. *Ann Intern Med* 1996; 124:1061–1064.

64b. Stiell et al. Randomized, double blind controlled study of vasopressin vs epinephrine adult cardiac arrest. *Lancet* (in press).

65. Dybvik T, Strand T, Steen PA. Buffer therapy during out-of-hospital cardiopulmonary resuscitation. *Resuscitation* 1995; 29:89–95.

66. Luce JM, Raffin TA. Withholding and withdrawal of life support from critically ill patients. *Chest* 1988; 94:621–626.

67. Niemann JT. Cardiopulmonary resuscitation. *N Engl J Med* 1992; 327:1075–1080.

68. Pepe PE, Brown CG, Bonnin MJ, et al. Prospective validation criteria for on-scene termination of resuscitation after out-of hospital cardiac arrest. *Ann Emerg Med* 1993; 22:884–885 (abstract).

69. Gray WA, Capone RJ, Most AS: Unsuccessful emergency medical resuscitation—Are continued efforts in the emergency department justified? *N Engl J Med* 1991; 325:1393–1398.

70. Ravitch MM, Lane R, Safar P, et al. Lightning stroke: Report of a case with recovery after cardiac massage and prolonged artificial respiration. *N Engl J Med* 1961; 264:36–38.

71. Eisenberg MS, Hallstrom A, Bergner L. Long-term survival after out-of-hospital cardiac arrest. *N Engl J Med* 1982; 306:1340–1343.

72. Berek K, Lechleitner P, Luef G, et al. Early determination of neurological outcome after prehospital cardiopulmonary resuscitation. *Stroke* 1995; 26:543–549.

73. Lombardi G, Gallagher J, Gennis P. Outcome of out-of-hospital cardiac arrest in New York City: The pre-hospital arrest survival evaluation (PHASE) study. *JAMA* 1994; 271:678–683.

74. Becker LB, Ostrander MP, Barrett J, Kondos GT. Outcome of CPR in a large metropolitan area—Where are the survivors? *Ann Emerg Med* 1991; 20:355–361.

75. Cummins RO. From concept to standard-of-care? Review of the clinical experience with automated external defibrillators. *Ann Emerg Med* 1989; 12:1269–1275.

PART SIX

CORONARY HEART DISEASE

CHAPTER 35

ATHEROGENESIS AND ITS DETERMINANTS

Erling Falk / Valentin Fuster

INTRODUCTION

Despite steady progress in treatment of cardiovascular diseases, people are still dying of these diseases, although at later ages.[1] In the United States as well as in many other countries, cardiovascular diseases remain by far the number 1 cause of death for both men and women of all ethnic backgrounds and, no less important, cause the greatest disability. By the year 2020, coronary heart disease (CHD) and stroke will hold first and fourth places, respectively, in the World Health Organization's list of leading causes of disability.[2] A worldwide epidemic of cardiovascular diseases is evolving, and atherosclerosis, often with thrombosis superimposed, is by far the most frequent underlying cause.

It has been known for decades that the earliest lesions of atherosclerosis, fatty streaks, are present in the aorta from early childhood, but today we know that atherosclerosis begins already during fetal development, particularly in fetuses of hypercholesterolemic mothers.[3] Therefore, literally, a life-long effort is needed to prevent this disease and its dreadful consequences. Although a genetic predisposition to atherosclerosis may be present, the vast majority of atherosclerosis-related diseases, including CHD, are acquired; that is, the clinical manifestations of atherosclerosis, which usually appear in later life, are largely preventable. This fact is the major challenge to the world of cardiology at the turn of the millennium.

Definition

Atherosclerosis is a complex inflammatory-fibroproliferative response to retention of plasma-derived atherogenic lipoproteins in the arterial intima.[4,5] Literally, both softening (*athére* is Greek for gruel or porridge) and hardening (*skleros* is Greek for hard) need to be present to qualify for the diagnosis atherosclerosis; that is, *atherosclerosis* is not synonymous with *arteriosclerosis*. The latter term is broader, covering all diseases leading to arterial hardening, including native atherosclerosis, restenosis after angioplasty, and transplant vascular disease. These conditions all share some pathologic processes, but the mix of lipid accumulation, smooth muscle proliferation, and immune activation differs markedly.[6] It is important to recognize this distinction between atherosclerosis and arteriosclerosis, particularly when dealing with animal models of arterial diseases, because it is the lipid-related atheromatous component that is dangerous in human atherosclerosis, not the smooth muscle cell–related sclerotic component. The lipid-related component destabilizes plaques and thus is responsible for the great majority of all the life-threatening complications of human atherosclerosis: plaque disruption with superimposed thrombosis.[7]

Susceptibility to Atherosclerosis

Some individuals are more susceptible to atherosclerosis than others (e.g., males compared with females), and the same applies to different arterial segments within an individual. Atherosclerosis is a focal intimal disease of large and medium-sized systemic arteries, including the aorta, iliofemoral, coronary, carotid (bifurcation) and, to a lesser extent, intracranial arteries. Secondary changes may occur in the underlying media and adventitia, particularly in the more advanced stages of the disease. For unknown reasons, some arteries (such as the internal mammary arteries) are highly resistant to atherosclerosis. Although the epicardial coronary arteries appear to be the most susceptible arteries in the body, intramyocardial arteries are highly resistant to atherosclerosis.

ATHEROGENESIS IN SUSCEPTIBLE MICE

To reproduce in animals a vascular disease resembling human atherosclerosis, atherogenic lipoprotein concentrations need to be above a certain level. Normal wild-type mice do not develop hypercholesterolemia and are thus fundamentally resistant to atherosclerosis, even when fed a high-fat high-cholesterol diet that induces the disease in other species, such as rabbits, pigs, birds, and nonhuman primates. By inactivating and/or overexpressing selected genes, however, hypercholesterolemic atherosclerosis-prone mice have been created, for example, mice deficient in apolipoprotein E (apoE$^{-/-}$)[8,9] or low-density lipoprotein receptor (LDLR$^{-/-}$),[10] or both,[11] double knockouts deficient in both the LDLR and apobec-1 protein,[12] and LDLR$^{-/-}$ mice expressing human apolipoprotein B 100 (apoB100).[13] Among mammals, research using the mouse has several unique advantages, including the extensive knowledge of, and the ability to manipulate, the murine genome. Over the past decade, remarkable progress has been made in our knowledge of vascular biology through the use of genetically engineered mice, and mice are being increasingly used as a model for the study of atherosclerosis and its risk factors.[14–16]

The most commonly used genetically altered murine models for studies of atherosclerosis are mice deficient in apoE and/or LDLR. ApoE is a ligand for receptors that clear chylomicron and very low-density lipoprotein remnant particles. Consequently, apoE$^{-/-}$ mice develop severe hypercholesterolemia and atherosclerosis spontaneously on a normal chow diet, in contrast to LDLR$^{-/-}$ mice, which only do so when fed a high-fat high-cholesterol diet.[17] The atherosclerotic lesions that develop in these atherosclerosis-prone mice are morphologically quite similar to those in humans, which is why the mouse has become the most common experimental animal model for atherosclerosis research. Therefore, a more detailed description of atherogenesis in these mice is appropriate.

Endothelial Dysfunction

Endothelial function is generally similar in blood vessels from normal mice compared with blood vessels from other species.[18] For example, acetylcholine (the classic endothelium-dependent agonist) relaxes the mouse aorta as well as the carotid, coronary, mesenteric, and pulmonary arteries.[18] The relaxation observed in response to acetylcholine in murine blood vessels is endothelium dependent and, thus, similar to that observed in many other species, including humans.[18] In hypercholesterolemic atherosclerosis-prone mice, endothelium-dependent relaxation is impaired, i.e., endothelial dysfunction is present,[19–22] consistent with studies of atherosclerosis in other experimental animals and in humans.[18]

Transfer of the human apolipoprotein A1 (apoA1) gene tends to normalize the impaired endothelial function in these mice,[22] apparently without preventing subendothelial lipid deposition, endothelial activation [vascular cell adhesion molecule 1 (VCAM-1 expression)] or monocyte adherence to the activated endothelium.[23] Nevertheless, lesion formation is dramatically reduced.[24,25] The atheroprotective effect of the mouse's own native apoA1 has been more difficult to prove,[26–28] but clear protective effect has been documented.[29]

Lesion-Prone Areas

In aortas of normocholesterolemic mice, VCAM-1 and intercellular adhesion molecule 1 (ICAM-1), but not E-selection, are expressed by endothelial cells in regions predisposed to atherosclerotic lesion formation.[30] The complex hemodynamics in these lesion-prone areas may also increase the local transendothelial passage of lipoproteins and promote their retention and modification in the subendothelial space.[31] Oxidative modified LDL (oxLDL) has many proinflammatory properties which may explain the local upregulation of these inducible endothelial cell adhesion molecules, even before lesion formation, in hypercholesterolemic atherosclerosis-prone animals.[30]

Injuring Lipoprotein Retention

The first event in the birth of a plaque is the transendothelial passage of atherogenic lipoproteins into the subendothelial space, where they are retained and modified.[4,5,32] In normal mice, the subendothelial space contains an acellular matrix of branching filaments (presumed to be mainly proteoglycans) and numerous collagen fibrils without any visible lipid deposition[4]—normal mice do not spontaneously form an arterial intima.[33] The retention of lipoproteins in the subendothelial space provides a microenvironment where lipoprotein modification and aggregation can occur.[4] Modification, e.g., oxidation, of the retained lipoprotein makes it more atherogenic.[34,35] OxLDL is proinflammatory, cytotoxic, and recognized by the macrophage scavenger receptor promoting intracellular lipid accumulation and foam cell formation. In vitro studies suggest that lipoprotein retention involves interactions between apoB and matrix proteoglycans[36,37] and appears to be an important if not the key step in lesion development.

The concentration of a particular macromolecule within the subendothelial matrix depends on its plasma concentration, molecular size, permeability (the arterial endothelium is permeable to all plasma proteins), degree of retention (trapping) and rate of degradation within intima, and efflux from intima as well as on the location along the arterial tree.[38,39]

Inflammatory/Immune Response

One of the earliest detectable cellular responses in atherogenesis is the focal recruitment of circulating monocytes and, to a lesser extent, T cells into the arterial intima is.[40] The persistence of this cellular response seems to underlie disease progression (Fig. 35-1).[41] A few B cells may also be present,[42] but granulocytes are rare in atherosclerosis. Atherosclerotic lesions develop initially beneath an intact but activated endothelium at lesion-prone sites, preferentially affecting the outer walls of bifurcations and the inner wall of curvatures. The local factors responsible for the focal development of lesions are not well understood, but hemodynamic shear stress, the frictional force acting on the endothelial cell surface as a result of blood flow, is weaker in the susceptible lesion-prone areas.[31,43] Hemodynamic shear stress is an important determinant of endothelial function and phenotype. High shear stress (>15 dyne/cm^2) induces endothelial quiescence and an atheroprotective gene expression profile, whereas low shear stress (<4 dyne/cm^2), which is prevalent at atherosclerosis-prone sites, stimulates an atherogenic phenotype.[31,43] The endothelium mediates the transendothelial trafficking of leukocytes into the intima by expressing specific and inducible adhesion molecules such as VCAM-1 and ICAM-1. These adhesion molecules are upregulated at lesion-prone sites in apoE$^{-/-}$ mice prior to lesion formation and thus probably play an important role in the recruitment of mononuclear cells during atherogenesis.[40] Sites of predilection for lesion development include the aortic root, the lesser curvature of the aortic arch, the principal branches of the aorta (in particular, the coronary arteries and the brachiocephalic trunk), the carotid bifurcations, the aortic bifurcation, the iliac arteries, and the pulmonary arteries. Adhesion of monocytes to the endothelial surface was seen already at 6 weeks, macrophage foam cell lesions (fatty streaks) developed as early as 8 weeks, and, as lesions continued to progress, smooth muscle cells appeared and advanced atherosclerotic plaques were present after 15 weeks. The latter consisted of a fibrous cap containing smooth muscle cells surrounded by connective tissue matrix that covered a necrotic core with numerous foamy macrophages. Thus, the apoE$^{-/-}$ mouse contains the entire spectrum of lesions observed during atherogenesis and was the first mouse model to develop lesions similar to those in humans.[44]

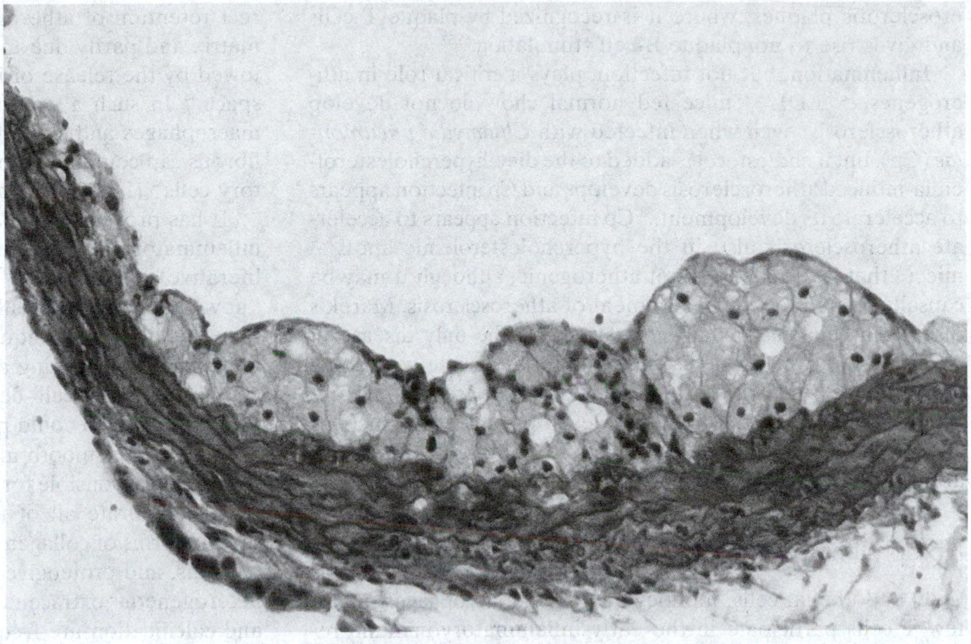

FIGURE 35-1 (Plate 77) An early atherosclerotic lesion (fatty streak) in the aortic root of a 3-month-old apolipoprotein E$^{-/-}$ mouse fed a high-fat Western-type diet for 6 weeks. The lesion consists of lipid-laden monocyte-derived macrophage foam cells and a few lymphocytes (T cells) beneath an intact endothelium. Elastin trichrome stain.

Leukocyte adhesion to the endothelium alone however, is, not enough to get monocytes and T cells into the intima. They have to pass through the endothelium and, for that, one or more chemokines (chemotactic cytokines) are needed.[45,46] The proinflammatory chemokine monocyte chemoattractant protein 1 (MCP-1) attracts potently both monocytes and T cells, but not neutrophils, eosinophils, and B cells, and plays a fundamental role in the recruitment of these cells.[47] Endothelial cells, smooth muscle cells, and macrophages all contribute to overexpression of MCP-1 in atherosclerosis. Thus, once within the intima, monocytes recruit themselves by secreting MCP-1.[45,48–50] MCP-1 appears to be uniquely essential for monocyte recruitment in several inflammatory diseases,[51] including atherosclerosis.[49,50] Additionally, MCP-1 may induce tissue factor expression in plaque cells and thus increase the risk of atherosclerosis-mediated luminal thrombosis.[52] A prime candidate for upregulation of MCP-1 in the vessel wall is minimally oxidized LDL, linking hypercholesterolemia to fatty-streak formation, plaque progression, and tissue factor expression.[53]

Once within intima and activated, macrophages may secrete a variety of potent cytokines that profoundly influence local cellular accumulation and function. Macrophages can both initiate the oxidation of LDL and take up oxLDL by specific scavenger receptors. Lesion size is reduced in atherosclerosis-prone mice lacking the macrophage-expressed oxygenating enzyme 12/15-lipoxygenase[54] and scavenger receptors, suggesting that lipoprotein oxidation and uptake are key events in atherogenesis.[35]

The humoral and cellular immune system modulates the development of atherosclerosis.[35,55] Plaque T cells and their products [e.g., interferon-γ (IFN-γ)] appear to promote atherosclerosis, whereas nonplaque B cells and their products (e.g., antibodies) are atheroprotective.[56,57] Hyperimmunization with oxLDL, resulting in high antibody titers, and polyclonal immunoglobulin therapy protect against atherosclerosis, whereas splenectomy (removal of a B cell–enriched immune organ) promotes atherosclerosis in apoE$^{-/-}$ mice.[57] In contrast, all proatherogenic activities of the immune system discovered until now have been associated with inflammatory responses elicited by macrophages and T cells within plaques.[57] Neither B nor T cells, however, are required for the development and growth of plaques, documented in apoE$^{-/-}$ × RAG mice lacking lymphocytes.[58,59] A variety of antigens are formed in developing plaques with immune activation and subsequent modulation, mediated by both cellular and humoral events, of the ongoing atherosclerotic process.[55] Further evidence of immune activation is the upregulated expression of the immune mediator CD40 and its ligand CD154 by all cell types present in advanced atherosclerotic lesions.[60] The interaction of CD40 with CD154 mediates both humoral and cellular immune responses, and blocking this interaction reduces lesion formation in atherosclerosis-prone mice.[61,62]

There are a number of candidate antigens in the lesion that could be responsible for immune activation, including modified LDL,[35] heat-shock proteins,[63–65] β_2-glycoprotein I,[66] and microbial antigens. Of these, the most extensive data support an important role for oxLDL, which is abundantly present in atherosclerotic plaques, where it is recognized by plaque T cells and gives rise to nonplaque B-cell stimulation.[55,57]

Inflammation, but not infection, plays a critical role in atherogenesis.[67] $LDL^{-/-}$ mice fed normal chow do not develop atherosclerosis, even when infected with *Chlamydia pneumoniae* (Cp), but if cholesterol is added to the diet, hypercholesterolemia-induced atherosclerosis develops and Cp infection appears to accelerate its development.[68] Cp infection appears to accelerate atherosclerosis also in the hypercholesterolemic $apoE^{-/-}$ mice;[69] that is, Cp alone is not atherogenic, although it may be causally related to the development of atherosclerosis. Marek's disease in chickens (avian herpesvirus) is the only disease in which an infection alone causes an arterial disease with some morphologic similarities to human atherosclerosis, but full-blown human-like atherosclerosis develops only if the chickens concomitantly are fed a cholesterol-rich diet.[70] This infectious arterial disease in birds is preventable by vaccination.[71]

Fibroproliferative Response

Only endothelial cells, monocyte-derived macrophages, and a few T cells participate in the early inflammatory/immune response, giving rise to early atherosclerotic lesions (fatty streaks) (Fig. 35-1, Plate 77). In disease progression, this pure inflammatory/immune response is accompanied by a fibroproliferative response in which the vascular smooth muscle cell plays a dominant role.[72] Smooth muscle cells are not normally present in the mouse intima, but they are, of course, present in the adjacent tunica media, from which they migrate into intima to become the matrix-synthesizing cell in the developing atherosclerotic plaque.[72] Macrophages and T cells continue to be present throughout plaque development and probably promote rather than retard progression.

Lipids begin to accumulate extracellularly, partly due to direct retention of atherogenic lipoproteins in the extracellular matrix and partly due to foam cell necrosis and apoptosis followed by the release of intracellular lipids to the extracellular space.[44] In such a way, a *necrotic* lipid-rich core with foamy macrophages and cholesterol crystals may form, covered by a fibrous cap containing both smooth muscle cells and inflammatory cells[44] (Fig. 35-2, Plate 78).

It has proved much easier to prevent and regress the early inflammatory/immune response than the subsequent fibroproliferative response,[58,59,72–76] and, consequently, much more is known about the molecular mechanisms controlling the former than the latter. All plaque cells, including smooth muscle cells, are capable of forming a large number of growth factors and cytokines, and T cell–derived IFN-γ and responses mediated by CD40 ligation could play important roles in lesion progression.[56,60–62] The smooth muscle cell is the principal connective-tissue cell responsible for healing and repair of the arterial wall. It can elaborate all of the proteins of the matrix, including several forms of collagen (e.g., types I, III, and IV), elastic fiber proteins, and proteoglycans, which together create a complex, heterogeneous extracellular matrix.[72] Cartilaginous metaplasia[77] and calcification are frequently seen in advanced lesions, and both intimal calcification[78] and medial[79] calcification have been studied in atherosclerosis-prone mice.

In normal arteries and in arteries with early atherosclerosis, vasa vasorum are confined to adventitia, but neovascularization of plaques may occur with disease progression. In $apoE^{-/-}$ mice, the incidence of neovascularization is generally low but appears to increase in more advanced and thicker lesions. Thus, thin-walled capillary-like vessels (i.e., neovascularization) have been identified in 15 (13 percent) of 114 advanced aortic lesions from cholesterol-fed $apoE^{-/-}$ mice aged 36 to 60 weeks.[80]

Fibrinogen is not required for, and does not appear to influence, the development and progression of advanced lesions in mice, documented in double gene knockout mice lacking both apoE and fibrinogen.[75] On the other hand, the loss of a key fibrinolytic factor — plasminogen — greatly accelerates lesion formation in $apoE^{-/-}$ mice.[81] Plasminogen deficiency may accelerate atherosclerosis by influencing processes in the vessel wall unrelated to fibrin(ogen) and impaired fibrinolysis.

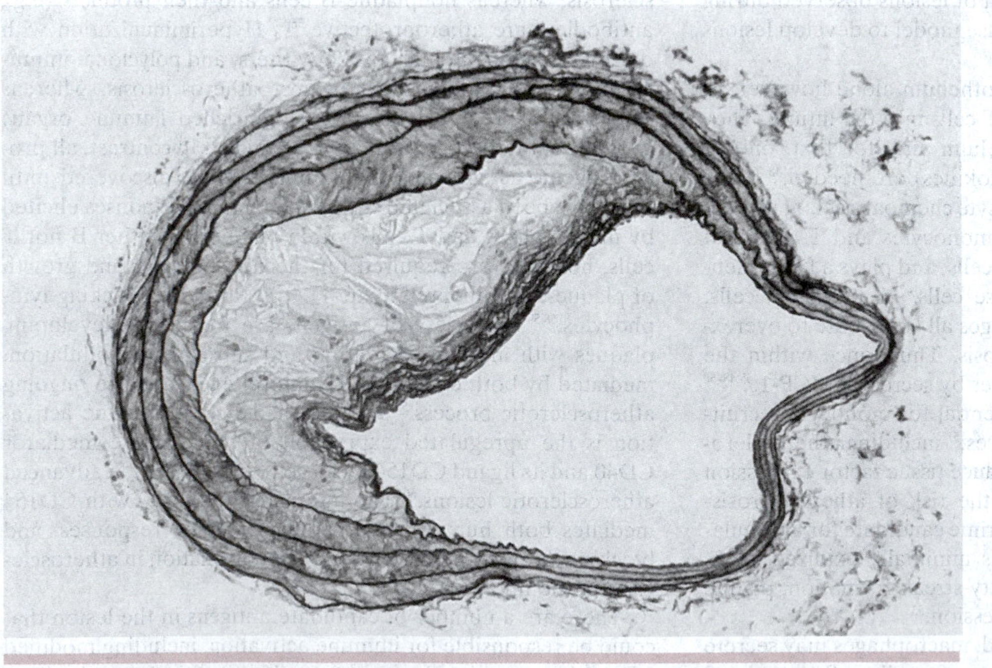

FIGURE 35-2 (Plate 78) An advanced atherosclerotic plaque in the brachiocephalic trunk of a 6-month-old apolipoprotein $E^{-/-}$ mouse fed normal chow. The plaque appears vulnerable morphologically, consisting of a lipid-rich core with cholesterol crystals covered by a thin fibrous cap. Orcein, staining elastic tissue black.

PLATELET-VESSEL WALL INTERACTION

Before the creation of gene-manipulated atherosclerosis-prone mice, Paigen and colleagues evaluated the potential contribution of platelets to the development of atherosclerosis by comparing the severity of atherosclerosis in susceptible C57BL/6 mice carrying either a normal or a variant phenotype for platelet function.[82] Five genetically distinct mutants with increased bleeding times and abnormal dense granules were studied, and three of these mutants (light ear, maroon, and ruby eye) developed less atherosclerosis than the controls on the atherogenic diet.[82] The result indicates that some particular component of platelet function affects atherosclerosis. Other defects than those in platelets are, however, present in these mice, which precludes any firm conclusion regarding the significance of the platelet–vessel wall interaction in atherogenesis in these mice.

Platelets may contribute to atherogenesis in at least two different ways: mural thrombi may form on denuded plaques and subsequently be incorporated into developing lesions, and/or they may serve as a source of platelet-derived growth factors and stimulate smooth muscle cell proliferation. Although the endothelium is intact, but activated, early during atherogenesis in both humans and atherosclerosis-prone mice, endothelial denudation or frank plaque rupture with subsequent thrombus formation contribute significantly to plaque development in humans. Spontaneous endothelial denudation with subsequent platelet adhesion (monolayer) or thrombus formation (aggregation) have not been described in mice.

Plaque Disruption and Thrombosis

Although we have learned a lot about atherogenesis by studying the initiation and development of lesions in atherosclerosis-prone mice, nothing has been learned about atherosclerosis-mediated thrombogenesis—the final pathogenetic chain of events precipitating life-threatening heart attacks in humans. Plaque rupture with superimposed thrombosis, which is a rather common feature of human atherosclerosis, is extremely rare in mice and all other animal models of atherosclerosis.[83] This shortcoming is probably the most significant distinction between human atherosclerosis and human-like atherosclerosis in mice.[75]

A variety of proteinases, mostly released by infiltrating macrophages, have been implicated in plaque rupture in humans, but the actual enzymatic culprits have not yet been conclusively identified.[84] Of the many proteinases present in plaques, members of the matrix metalloproteinase (MMP) family, cysteine proteinases (e.g., elastolytic cathepsins S and K), and serine proteinases [mostly plasminogen and its activators: urokinase-type plasminogen activator (u-PA) and tissue-type plasminogen activator (t-PA)] have received much attention.[84] Atherosclerotic plaques in apo$E^{-/-}$ mice contain a lot of macrophages, both superficially in plaque and at their base, many of which express MMPs, including MMP-3, MMP-9, MMP-12, and MMP-13.[85,86] However, although macrophages at the base of plaques often infiltrate and destroy the internal elastic membrane, media, and adjacent adventitia, which may give rise to aneurysm formation, the plaque surface almost always remains intact without disruption and/or thrombosis. Not a single case of plaque disruption with superimposed thrombosis in mice has been reported. We have performed a meticulous search for ruptured and thrombosed plaques in middle-aged apo$E^{-/-}$ mice (age, >1 year), some of which had died spontaneously of natural causes. Although we have studied several hundred mice, each of which contained many rupture-prone plaques, only two ruptured plaques were identified, one with superimposed thrombosis (Fig. 35-3, Plate 79).

Remodeling

Consistent with what is observed in human atherosclerosis, arteries in apo$E^{-/-}$ mice remodel in response to plaque growth with no correlation between lesion mass and lumen loss.[87] In the ascending aorta, a normal lumen is preserved due to compensatory vascular enlargement during plaque growth, in contrast to the external carotid arteries, where stenotic lesions tend to develop associated with adventitial inflammation and medial atrophy.[87] Vascular remodeling with preservation of the aortic lumen despite marked intimal thickening has also been described in apo$E^{-/-}$ × $LDLR^{-/-}$ mice.[88]

Vascular Protection

Preventing or retarding atherosclerosis is more than just controlling lipid and other major risk factors. Atherosclerosis is a lipid-driven disease, but not all mice or all arteries within the same mouse are equally susceptible to atherosclerosis;[83] that is, hypercholesterolemia does not necessarily lead to advanced atherosclerosis. The final result depends critically on the participation of many processes not directly related to lipid, and the inhibition of just one necessary step in the pathogenetic chain

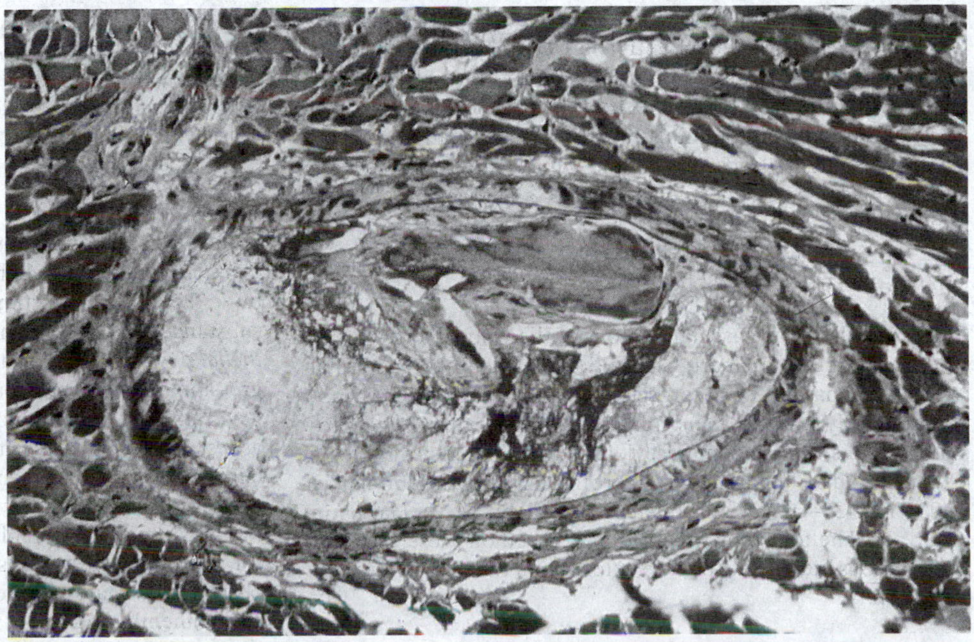

FIGURE 35-3 (Plate 79) Ruptured coronary plaque with occlusive thrombosis superimposed (natural death of a 21-month-old apolipoprotein $E^{-/-}$ mouse). Spontaneous plaque rupture and/or luminal thrombosis are extremely rare in animal models of atherosclerosis. Elastin trichrome stain.

of events is enough to prevent or retard plaque development. To date, most interventions have targeted the initial step in atherogenesis—hypercholesterolemia—but it may prove to be as, or even more, effective to target subsequent but necessary steps for lesion development in the vessel wall.

TARGETING MONOCYTE/MACROPHAGE FUNCTIONS

Some monocyte/macrophage functions are crucial in the initiation and progression of lesions, documented by reduced lesion development in hypercholesterolemic atherosclerosis-prone mice lacking ICAM-1,[89] macrophage-colony stimulating factor,[90–92] MCP-1,[49,50] MCP-1 receptor CCR2 on monocytes,[53,93] macrophage-expressed 12/15-lipoxygenase,[54] or macrophage scavenger receptors,[94–96] or mice treated with an antibody against the M-CSF receptor c-fms.[73] In contrast, macrophage overexpression of MCP-1 accelerates atherosclerosis.[48]

TARGETING OTHER EVENTS NOT MEDIATED BY LOW-DENSITY LIPOPROTEIN

Interventions, in addition to the monocyte/macrophage-related just described, that have proved to *slow the development of lesions* in atherosclerosis-prone mice, and not mediated by LDL lowering, include apoA1 overexpression;[24,25,29,76,97] apoA1 Milano injection;[98] inactivation IFN-γ receptor;[56] immunization with oxLDL[99,100] or native LDL;[100] antioxidant treatment with high-dose vitamin E[101] (compared with lower dosing),[102] (co)antioxidants H212/43,[103] DPPD,[104] or licorice;[105] treatment with estrogen,[106] L-arginine,[107] the angiotensin-converting enzyme inhibitor captopril,[108] the angiotensin-II receptor antagonist losartan,[109] (cf. Makaritsis et al.[110]), or normal human polyspecific immunoglobulins;[111] inhibition or blocking of endothelin ET_A receptor[20] or interleukin-1 receptor;[112] CD40 ligation;[61,62] angiogenesis (advanced lesions only);[113] and cellular receptor for advanced glycation end products (in diabetic mice);[114] dietary soy protein;[115] and iron-deficient diet.[116]

Interventions that have proved to *accelerate the development of atherosclerosis* independently of LDL cholesterol include probucol (paradoxically and in contrast to other antioxidants such as vitamin E),[117–119] Cp infection,[68,69] cytomegalovirus infection,[120] interleukin 12 administration,[121] immunization with β_2-glycoprotein I,[122,123] absence of the tumor-suppressor protein p53,[124] plasminogen deficiency,[81] and angiotensin II injection.[125]

HUMAN ATHEROSCLEROSIS

The Committee on Vascular Lesions of the Council on Arteriosclerosis, American Heart Association, has defined the normal arterial intima and its atherosclerosis-prone regions,[126] asymptomatic early lesions,[127] and advanced and potentially symptomatic lesions.[128] Based on these definitions, a practical histologic classification of human atherosclerotic lesions was published in 1995 (Fig. 35-4),[129] which is summarized by M. J. Davies in Chap. 36. The following description is based on these excellent publications but differs to some extent from the 1995 AHA classification.

Endothelial Dysfunction

Atherogenic stimuli may give rise to nonadaptive changes in endothelial structure and function, such as enhanced permeabil-

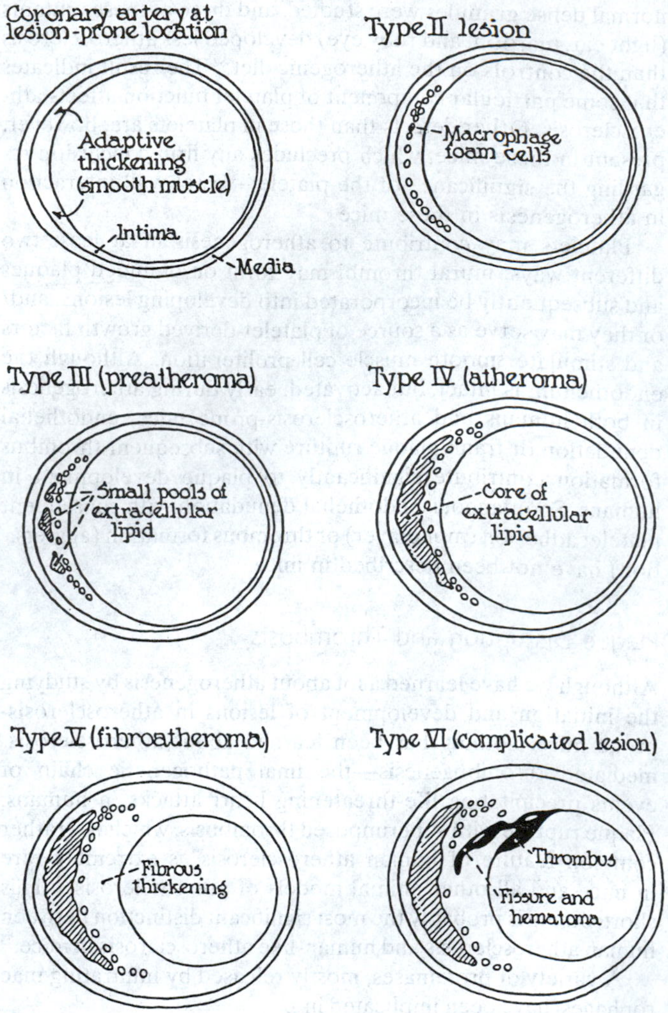

FIGURE 35-4 The 1995 American Heart Association classification of atherosclerotic lesions. The type I (initial) lesion, which consists of small, isolated groups of macrophages containing lipid droplets, is not shown in this figure. (Adapted from Stary et al.[128] Reproduced with permission from the publisher and authors.)

ity to plasma lipoproteins, hyperadhesiveness for blood leukocytes, and functional imbalances in local pro- and antithrombotic factors, growth stimulators and inhibitors, and vasoactive substances.[129] These manifestations, collectively termed *endothelial dysfunction*, play an important role in the initiation, progression, and clinical complications of atherosclerosis.[129] It is generally assumed, but not proved, that endothelial dysfunction as just defined equates with endothelial dysfunction as identified clinically as an impairment in endothelium-dependent vasodilation, largely mediated by the endogenous vasodilator nitric oxide and usually reversible. The mere presence of risk factors for ischemic heart disease, such as hypercholesterolemia, hypertension, cigarette smoking, diabetes mellitus, hyperhomocyst(e)inemia, and aging, is associated with endothelial dysfunction as defined clinically, even in the microcirculation and in arteries, such as the brachial artery, that are resistant to atherosclerosis.[130,131] Thus, clinically defined endothelial dysfunction is related to atherosclerosis but not necessarily causally.

Atherosclerosis-Prone Areas

The normal human intima is covered by endothelial cells and contains, in contrast to intima of many laboratory animals (including mice), smooth muscle cells, isolated macrophages, occasional mast cells, and extracellular matrix.[127] The latter constitutes up to 60 percent of the volume and contains proteoglycans (predominantly chondroitin and dermatan sulfates), collagens (predominantly types I and III), elastin, and other components such as fibronectin, laminin, and plasma proteins.[127] Apparently, all plasma proteins are present in lesion-free intima in concentrations related directly to the protein's plasma concentration and inversely to its molecular weight. In the normal artery, LDL is present in intima but is usually not detectable in media.[126]

Regardless of atherogenic stimuli, nonobstructive intimal thickenings are present at constant locations in everyone from birth, particularly at bifurcations, and progress with time. Such adaptive intimal thickenings develop in response to mechanical forces such as pressure, circumferential stretch or tension, and shear stress.[126] Low shear stress and, probably more importantly, oscillatory flow and flow reversal may promote both adaptive intimal thickening and subsequent influx and accumulation of atherogenic lipoproteins.[31] Reduced wall shear stress (dilatation) and increased wall tensile stress (hypertension) promote adaptive intimal thickening, which tends to normalize shear and tension.[126] Eccentric intimal thickening is frequently seen near bifurcations and branch points where shear and tensile stresses are not uniformly distributed, and diffuse thickening may develop in relatively straight arterial segments with evenly distributed stresses.[126] Evidence suggests that the shape of a vessel, rather than the flow patterns, may determine the degree of adaptive intimal thickening and ultimately constitute a risk factor for development of symptomatic lesions.[132]

In human arteries, there is no need for migration of smooth muscle cells into the intima from the media to initiate plaque formation, in contrast to many laboratory animals, where the intima does not normally contain smooth muscle cells. Under the influence of atherogenic stimuli, adaptive intimal thickenings appear to be good soil for the development of atherosclerosis.[133] The smooth muscle cells present early in preexisting intimal thickenings and later show "clonality" in superimposed atherosclerotic lesions, suggesting clonal expansion during lesion development.[134] Although advanced lesions are not confined to regions with adaptive intimal thickenings, particularly not in hyperlipidemia-induced atherosclerosis in animals, lesions form earlier and more rapidly in these atherosclerosis-prone areas than elsewhere.[33] In humans, the topographic distribution of eccentric intimal thickening and of advanced atherosclerotic lesions is similar in the coronary arteries, the carotid bifurcation, the parasellar carotid artery, and the aorta.[126,132,135]

Fatty Streaks

The early lesions of atherosclerosis develop under an intact but activated and dysfunctioning endothelium, particularly in atherosclerosis-prone areas with preexisting intimal thickening. Inflammation and immune responses play an important role in atherogenesis from its very beginning.[67,136,137] Hypercholesterolemia is associated with increased endothelial permeability, increased transcytosis and intimal retention of lipoproteins, and endothelial activation with focal expression of VCAM-1 leading to monocyte and T-lymphocyte recruitment. Within intima, the monocyte-derived macrophages engulf the blood-derived LDLs, probably via their scavenger receptors after oxidative modification, and become lipid-filled foam cells. These inflammatory cells constitute by far the major part of the early fatty-streak lesion, with a ratio of approximately 1:10 to 1:50 between T cells and macrophages, and they probably play a significant role in the progression of fatty streaks to mature atherosclerotic plaques.[137] The presence of activated macrophages and T cells strongly suggests that an immunologic reaction has taken place in the atherosclerotic plaque. The antigens that elicit this response are not yet known, and both autoantigens (e.g., against oxidized LDL) and microorganisms (e.g., Cp) have been proposed to play a role.[137]

Although immunoglobulins are found in abundance in lesions, B cells are noticeably absent from human plaque. Similarly, although plasma cells have been noted in inflammatory infiltrates in the adventitia surrounding atherosclerotic arteries, few if any such cells have been seen in the plaque itself.[35]

Accumulations of lipid-filled foam cells within intima may be visible to the naked eye as yellow dots or streaks—fatty streaks. Microscopically, fatty streaks are highly cellular inflammatory lesions consisting of macrophage foam cells (intracellular lipid) and T lymphocytes (immune reaction). Extracellular lipid is hardly identifiable microscopically and B lymphocytes and polymorphonuclear neutrophil (PMN) are not seen. Fatty streaks do not protrude into the lumen, and they are therefore asymptomatic.

The fate of fatty streaks remains controversial. It has been known for decades that aortic fatty streaks are present in infants all over the world, irrespective of ethnicity or prevalence of ischemic heart disease in the population.[138] Recently, it was shown that fatty streaks are present already in arteries of human fetuses,[139,140] but, associated with the low blood cholesterol in late pregnancy and early childhood, fetal aortic fatty streaks may regress, just to progress again later during childhood.[3] In laboratory animals, fatty streaks are the most readily produced lesions and regress completely when serum cholesterol is reduced. It is generally assumed that fatty streaks can progress to more advanced lesions because they occur at the same anatomic sites and because transitional stages have been observed.[127] A smaller subgroup of fatty streaks, those superimposed on preexisting intimal thickenings, appear to be particularly prone to progress to advanced symptomatic lesions, but the mode of progression and the factors controlling it are not clear.[127] For example, aortic fatty streaks are universally present in all populations around the world early in life, even in populations at low risk for symptomatic atherosclerosis later in life, such as the South African Bantu.[138] Females have more aortic fatty streaks than males early in life even though males develop more advanced lesions than females later in life.[138,141] Blacks have more aortic fatty streaks than whites early in life, but the latter have more advanced lesions than the former later in life.[138,141] The thoracic aorta has more fatty streaks than the abdominal aorta early in life, but the opposite applies for advanced lesions later in life.[138] These contrasting relations seen in the human aorta between asymptomatic fatty streaks in young persons and advanced and potentially symptomatic lesions in adults may put into question the relevance of results obtained in short-term animal experiments in which only the development of foam cell lesions (fatty streaks) in aorta are studied.

Advanced Plaques

Advanced lesions may cause luminal narrowing and produce symptoms. In contrast to mice and many other laboratory animals, smooth muscle cells are already present within the human intima early during atherogenesis, beneath developing fatty streaks.[127] When lipids begin to accumulate extracellulary, then atherogenesis has passed beyond the fatty-streak stage. Oxidatively modified LDL is present in atherosclerotic plaques but not in the normal intima.[35,67] Two different processes are responsible for the extracellular accumulation of lipids: blood-derived atherogenic lipoprotein particles may be trapped and retained directly within the proteoglycan-rich extracelluar matrix, and/or lipid may be released from macrophage foam cells following their death. Macrophages both proliferate and die within atherosclerotic plaques, and the balance probably depends on whether the lesion is progressing, quiescent, or regressing.

Progression beyond the fatty-streak stage is not only associated with lipid accumulation; also, connective tissue, produced by smooth muscle cells, accumulates, giving rise to very heterogeneous atherosclerotic lesions. Some plaques are lipid rich, whereas others are lipid poor, and morphologically dissimilar plaques may evolve next to each other.[6] The endothelium is intact early during atherogenesis, but denuded areas, often related to superficial foam cell infiltration (inflammation), with adherent platelets are later seen over mature plaques.[142,143] Then, growth factors released from adherent platelets and microthrombi may stimulate the smooth muscle cells within the plaques to produce more connective tissue matrix.[72] Because of a leaky endothelium, not only lipoproteins but also many other blood-derived components, including albumin and fibrinogen, are present in evolving lesions.[144]

Neovascularization, often expressing leukocyte adhesion molecules such as VCAM-1 and ICAM-1 and associated with inflammatory cell infiltration, is frequently present at the base of advanced plaques, and it has been suggested that these "new" vessels could play an active role in the recruitment of leukocytes into plaques and thus contribute to the progression of the disease.[145] Extravasated erythrocytes are also frequently seen in these neovascularized areas.

VULNERABLE PLAQUES

A subset of the advanced lesions is particularly dangerous—the vulnerable plaques—because they are at high risk of becoming complicated by luminal thrombosis (Fig. 35-5, Plate 80). Disruption of vulnerable plaques with superimposed thrombosis is the most frequent cause of the acute coronary syndromes of unstable angina, myocardial infarction, and sudden coronary death.[7,146,147]

The risk of plaque disruption depends more on plaque type than on plaque size: lipid-rich and soft plaques are more vulnerable and prone to rupture than are collagen-rich and hard plaques.[7] Furthermore, plaques are highly thrombogenic after disruption, because of a high content of tissue factor.[148] Pathoanatomic studies have identified three major determinants of a plaque's vulnerability to rupture (Fig. 35-6): (1) the size of the lipid-rich core, (2) inflammation with plaque degradation, and (3) lack of smooth muscle cells with impaired healing.

Lipid accumulation, macrophage infiltration, and lack of smooth muscle cells destabilize plaques, making them vulnerable to rupture. In contrast, smooth muscle cell–mediated healing and repair processes stabilize plaques, protecting them against disruption.[136] Plaque size or stenosis severity tell nothing about a plaque's vulnerability.[149] Many vulnerable plaques are invisible angiographically due to their small size and compensatory vascular remodeling.

Lipid Accumulation The atheromatous core of a plaque is avascular, hypocellular, lipid rich, soft like gruel, and totally devoid of supporting collagen.[7] The size of such a soft core is, of course, critical for the stability of a plaque. At autopsy, Gertz and Roberts found much larger atheromatous cores in coronary plaques with disrupted (compared with intact) surface,[150] and Davies and coworkers found a strong relation between core size and plaque rupture in aorta.[151] Recent studies using immunohistochemical and tunnel staining techniques have identified macrophage-specific antigens and apoptotic nuclear fragments within the gruel, indicating that lipid and other cell constituents released from dead macrophage foam cells could contribute significantly to the formation and growth of the atheromatous core, which is why it also has been referred to as the "graveyard of dead macrophages," emphasizing the inflammatory origin of this destabilizing core.[152–154]

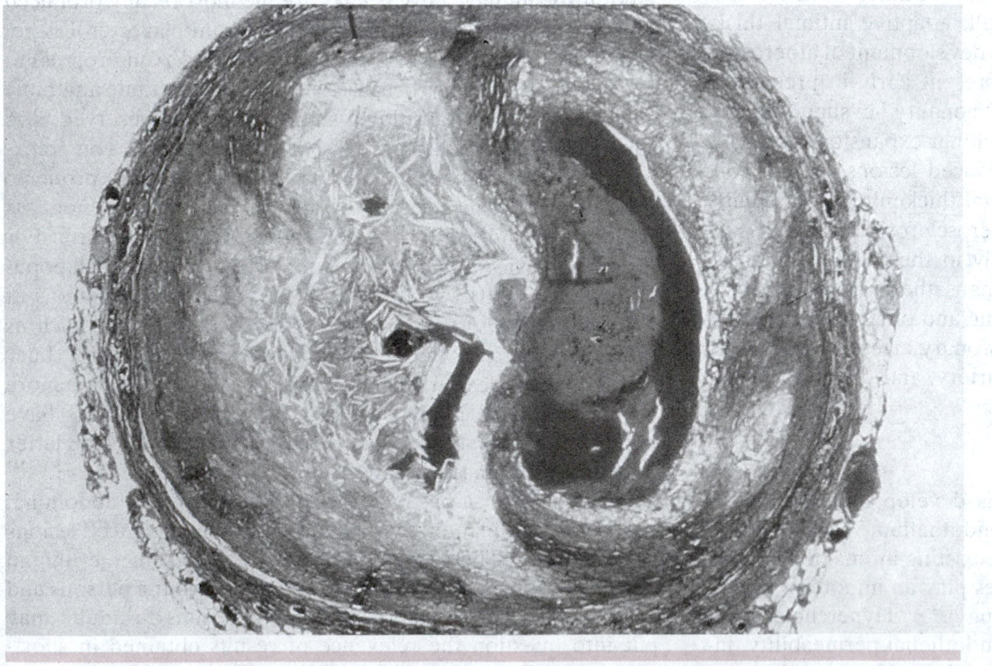

FIGURE 35-5 (Plate 80) Cross-sectioned coronary artery, containing a vulnerable plaque (large lipid-rich core covered by a thin fibrous cap) with ruptured surface and a nonocclusive luminal thrombosis superimposed. Trichrome stain.

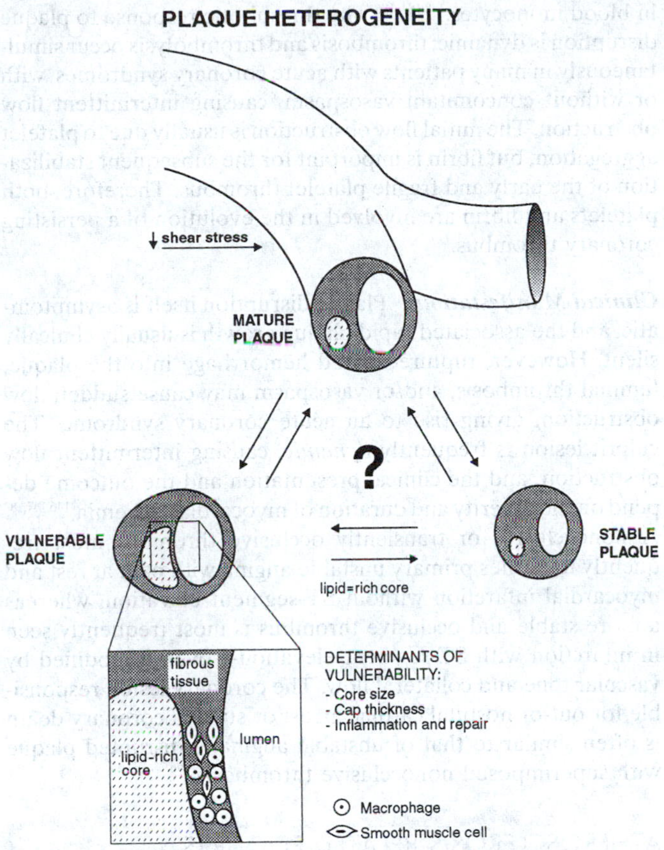

FIGURE 35-6 Advanced atherosclerotic plaques are extremely heterogeneous in composition. A subset of the advanced plaques are vulnerable (i.e., rupture-prone) with high risk of becoming complicated by luminal thrombosis. The relation between vulnerable and stable plaques is not well defined. (Adapted from Ravn and Falk.[412] Reproduced with permission from the publisher and authors.)

Plaque Degradation Disrupted fibrous caps are usually heavily infiltrated by macrophage foam cells,[7,155] and recent observations have revealed that such rupture-related macrophages are activated, indicating ongoing inflammation at the site of plaque disruption.[156] Van der Wal and colleagues identified superficial macrophage infiltration in plaques beneath all 20 coronary thrombi examined, whether or not the underlying plaque was disrupted or just eroded,[156] although a more recent study of coronary thrombi responsible for sudden coronary death could not confirm that observation.[157] Evaluated by immunohistochemical technique, van der Wal and coworkers found that macrophages and adjacent T lymphocytes (smooth muscle cells were usually lacking at rupture sites) were activated, indicating ongoing disease activity.[156] Further evidence of immune activation is the upregulated expression of CD40 receptor and its ligand by all cell types present in advanced atherosclerotic lesions.[60] Comparable results were obtained by the same group in a study of atherectomy specimens showing an inverse relation between the extent of inflammatory activity in plaque tissues of culprit lesions and the clinical stability of the ischemic syndrome.[158] There was considerable overlap between groups, however, indicating that not all patients with clinically stable angina have histologically stable plaques.[158] These observations confirmed the findings of a previous study of atherectomy specimens from culprit lesions responsible for stable angina, unstable rest angina, or non-Q-wave infarction.[159] Culprit lesions responsible for the acute coronary syndromes contained significantly more macrophages than did lesions responsible for stable angina pectoris (14 versus 3 percent of plaque tissue occupied by macrophages).[159]

Macrophages are capable of degrading extracellular matrix by phagocytosis or by secreting proteolytic enzymes such as members of the MMP family (collagenases, gelatinases, and stromeolysins), cysteine proteinases (e.g., elastolytic cathepsins S and K), and serine proteinases (mostly plasminogen and its activators, u-PA and t-PA), which may weaken the fibrous cap, predisposing it to rupture.[83,160] All these proteinases have been identified in human plaques and have been implicated in plaque rupture, but the actual enzymatic culprits have not yet been conclusively identified.[83] The MMPs are secreted in a latent zymogen form requiring extracellular activation, after which they are capable of degrading virtually all components of the extracellular matrix. The MMPs and their cosecreted tissue inhibitors or metalloproteinases, TIMP-1 and TIMP-2, are critical for cell migration, tumor invasion and metastasis, and vascular remodeling. Collagen confers stability to plaques, and human monocyte-derived macrophages grown in culture are indeed capable of degrading the old and mature collagen present in advanced aortic plaques.[161] Simultaneously, they express MMP-1 (interstitial collagenase) and induce MMP-2 (gelatinolytic) activity in the culture medium.[161] Besides macrophages, a wide variety of cells may produce MMPs. Activated mast cells may secrete powerful proteolytic enzymes such as tryptase and chymase that can activate pro-MMPs secreted by other cells (e.g., macrophages), and mast cells are actually present in shoulder regions of mature plaques and at sites of disruption, although at very low density.[162] Neutrophils are also capable of destroying tissue by secreting proteolytic enzymes but are rare in intact plaques.[137,156]

Several infectious agents have been suggested to play an active role in the development of cardiovascular diseases, particularly Cp but also herpesviruses (including cytomegalovirus) and *Helicobacter pylori*.[163–165] *Chlamydia* has been identified in atherosclerotic plaques;[166] it contains lipopolysaccharide and heat-shock protein 60, which are well-known strong inducers of many enzymes including MMPs.[167] Nonspecific but sensitive blood markers of inflammation (acute-phase reactants such as C-reactive protein and serum amyloid A) have been identified as strong risk factors for future cardiovascular events in apparently healthy men[168] and women,[169] in patients with stable[170] and unstable angina,[171–173] and after myocardial infarction.[174]

Impaired Healing Obviously, the thickness and collagen content of the fibrous cap is very important for its strength and stability: the thinner the cap is, the weaker it is and the more vulnerable is the plaque to rupture.[175] Ruptured aortic caps contain fewer smooth muscle cells and less collagen than intact caps,[151,176] and smooth muscle cells are usually missing at the actual site of disruption.[156,162]

Collagen is responsible for the mechanical strength of the fibrous cap and is synthesized by intimal smooth muscle cells. It is important to realize that smooth muscle cell proliferation and matrix synthesis may, in fact, be good in protecting plaques against disruption, whereas local loss of smooth muscle cells or impaired smooth muscle cell function may be bad, leading to gradual plaque destabilization due to impaired healing and repair.[136] It is unknown why smooth muscle cells are lacking at sites of disruption, but apoptotic cell death could play an important role.[153,154]

Complicated Plaques

We use the term *complicated plaques* when referring to advanced lesions complicated by luminal thrombosis and/or plaque hemorrhage. Such an acute plaque event causes rapid progression of the lesion[177] and is probably the most important mechanism responsible for the unpredictable, sudden, and rapid progression of coronary lesions observed by serial angiographic examination. As just described, plaque disruption with superimposed thrombosis is the most frequent cause of a life-threatening acute myocardial infarction.

PLAQUE DISRUPTION

Vulnerable plaques rupture frequently. Autopsy data indicate that 9 percent of healthy persons harbor disrupted plaques (without superimposed thrombosis) in their coronary arteries, increasing to 22 percent in persons with diabetes or hypertension.[178] In fatal coronary artery disease, more than one disrupted plaque, with or without superimposed thrombosis, is usually present in the coronary arteries.[155,179]

The plaque surface is disrupted most often where the cap is thinnest and most heavily infiltrated by macrophages and therefore weakest, namely, at the cap's shoulders.[7,180] The weak shoulder regions, however, are also points where biomechanical and hemodynamic forces acting on plaques appear to be concentrated.[180,181] Thus, plaque disruption is probably the result of a dynamic interaction between *intrinsic* plaque changes (vulnerability) and *extrinsic* forces imposed on the plaque (triggers); the former predispose a plaque to rupture, whereas the latter may precipitate it. As the presence of a vulnerable plaque is a prerequisite for plaque disruption, plaque vulnerability is probably more important than rupture triggers in determining the risk of a future heart attack. If no vulnerable plaques are present in the coronary arteries, there is no rupture-prone substrate for a potential trigger to function on. Furthermore, the fact that exercise stress testing in individuals with advanced coronary artery disease rarely triggers an acute coronary event suggests that plaque vulnerability ultimately plays a more important role in plaque rupture than does physiologic stress or other potential triggers.

LUMINAL THROMBOSIS

The most feared consequence of coronary plaque disruption is thrombotic occlusion of the artery. About 75 percent of thrombi responsible for acute coronary syndromes are precipitated by plaque disruption whereby the highly thrombogenic gruel is exposed to the flowing blood.[155,182,183] In the remaining 25 percent, superficial plaque erosion without frank disruption (i.e., no deep injury) is usually present.[2] Most disrupted plaques are resealed by a small mural thrombus, and only sometimes does a major luminal thrombus evolve. There are three major determinants of the thrombotic response to plaque disruption/erosion: (1) the local thrombogenic substrate, (2) the local flow disturbances, and (3) the systemic thrombotic propensity.

Inflammatory cells might also play an important role in the thrombotic response to plaque disruption/erosion via tissue factor expressed locally in plaque macrophages and systemically in blood monocytes.[148,184–186] The thrombotic response to plaque disruption is dynamic; thrombosis and thrombolysis occur simultaneously in many patients with acute coronary syndromes, with or without concomitant vasospasm, causing intermittent flow obstruction. The initial flow obstruction is usually due to platelet aggregation, but fibrin is important for the subsequent stabilization of the early and fragile platelet thrombus. Therefore, both platelets and fibrin are involved in the evolution of a persisting coronary thrombus.[187]

Clinical Manifestations Plaque disruption itself is asymptomatic, and the associated rapid plaque growth is usually clinically silent. However, rupture-related hemorrhage into the plaque, luminal thrombosis, and/or vasospasm may cause sudden flow obstruction, giving rise to an acute coronary syndrome. The culprit lesion is frequently *dynamic*, causing intermittent flow obstruction, and the clinical presentation and the outcome depend on the severity and duration of myocardial ischemia.[146,147,187] A nonocclusive or transiently occlusive thrombus most frequently underlies primary unstable angina with pain at rest and myocardial infarction without ST-segment elevation, whereas a more stable and occlusive thrombus is most frequently seen in infarction with ST-segment elevation—overall modified by vascular tone and collateral flow. The coronary lesion responsible for out-of-hospital cardiac arrest or sudden coronary death is often similar to that of unstable angina: a disrupted plaque with superimposed nonocclusive thrombosis.[179]

ATHEROSCLEROSIS-RELATED FEATURES

Patients with CHD generally have many atherosclerotic plaques in their coronary arteries, which vary considerably in their composition. Although coronary angiography may show only one or a few stenotic lesions, many more plaques are observed on intravascular ultrasound examination in living patients and at autopsy in deceased patients.[188,189] Only a minority of plaques protrude into and compromise the lumen because of compensatory abluminal vascular enlargement (remodeling) during plaque growth.[190] Thus, the lumen may remain normal despite buildup of large volumes of atherosclerotic plaque in the vessel wall. For all practical purposes, diagnostically as well as therapeutically, coronary atherosclerosis is a diffuse disease with superimposed focal luminal narrowing.

Arterial Remodeling and Luminal Narrowing

Vascular remodeling is the ability of the vessel wall to reorganize its cellular and extracellular components in response to a chronic stimulus.[191] In human atherosclerosis, there is ample evidence for active remodeling during the early stages of disease prior to significant lumenal stenosis. It was originally assumed that atherogenesis was always associated with more or less compensatory enlargement of coronary arteries during plaque growth,[190] but recent studies suggest that remodeling is bidirectional.[192] Plaques responsible for acute coronary syndromes are usually relatively large and associated with compensatory enlargement, which tends to preserve a normal lumen despite the presence of significant, and potentially dangerous, vessel wall disease. In contrast, plaques responsible for stable angina are usually smaller but, nevertheless, may cause more severe luminal narrowing because of concomitant local shrinkage of the artery.[193] The reason for these different modes of remodeling is unknown, but processes in adventitia could play a critical role.

Stenosis as Predictor

The vulnerability and thrombogenicity of atherosclerotic plaques rather than their obstructive capability (stenosis severity), together with the status of the collateral circulation, have emerged as the most important determinants for the occurrence, type, and outcome of acute coronary events.[7,146,147] Thus, coronary angiography is not a good method to identify high-risk thrombosis-prone lesions, partly because the size of a plaque and its vulnerability correlate poorly, if at all,[149] and partly because vascular remodeling tends to preserve the lumen better with the larger but vulnerable plaques (compensatory enlargement) than with the smaller and stable plaques (shrinkage).[193]

The great majority of heart attacks and ischemic strokes originate from atherosclerotic lesions that, prior to the acute events, only were mild-to-moderately stenotic; i.e., they were hemodynamically insignificant and probably asymptomatic (Fig. 35-7). Although the risk for occlusion, or myocardial infarction or stroke, increases with stenosis severity, the great majority of coronary occlusions (71 percent) in the Coronary Artery Surgery Study and myocardial infarctions (86 percent) in pooled studies originated from lesions that caused less than 70 to 80 percent angiographic stenosis prior to the acute events.[7] The reason is that stenotic lesions are markers of plaque burden, and lower-risk nonstenotic lesions will always by far outnumber the higher-risk stenotic ones and altogether increase the risk for an acute event much more than the few stenotic lesions at higher individual risk. And the same holds for ischemic stroke. Asymptomatic plaques at the carotid bifurcation, contralateral to symptomatic lesions, were evaluated and followed in the European Carotid Surgery Trial ($n = 2240$).[194] Only 13 (19 percent) of 67 new strokes were judged to have originated from initially asymptomatic lesions that at baseline caused more than 70 percent angiographic stenosis (Fig. 35-7). The reason: lower-risk nonstenotic carotid plaques ($n = 2113$) outnumbered by far the stenotic ones ($n = 127$) at higher risk.

Vasoconstriction

Plaque disruption and vasospasm often coexist, and the former most likely gives rise to the latter.[7] Abnormal coronary vasoreactivity is common in acute coronary syndromes but *spasm* is usually confined to the culprit lesion, suggesting that it is caused by locally released vasoactive substances.[195] The plaque, particularly macrophages in disrupted plaques responsible for unstable angina, may contain potent vasoconstrictors such as endothelin 1,[196,197] and superimposed thrombosis may also contain or generate vasoconstrictors such as thrombin and platelet-derived serotonin and thromboxane A_2.[147]

Coronary Calcification

Focal calcification in atherosclerotic plaques is very common and increases with age, both in men and women. Both lipid-rich and collagen-rich components may calcify, and the process may be active and controlled, resembling calcification in bone, rather than being passive and *dystrophic*.[198,199] Coronary calcification in adults is almost always atherosclerosis related and

Coronary stenosis: progression to occlusion

Serial angiography in 298 patients*

Stenosis at baseline	Segments n	Occlusion, 5-year %	n	
< 5%	2161	.7	15	
5 - 49%	430	2	10	51
50 - 80%	258	10	26	
81 - 95%	89	24	21	
All	2938		72	

*Alderman EL et al. *J Am Coll Cardiol* 1993; 22:1141-54

Coronary stenosis: progression to MI

Serial angiography in 239 patients#

Stenosis prior to MI	Segments n	Culprit for MI %	n	
0%	2674	0.3	8	
25%	287	3.5	10	
50%	123	4.1	5	29
75%	76	7.9	6	
90 - 99%	115	8.7	10	
All	3275		39	

#Nobuyoshi M et al. *J Am Coll Cardiol* 1991; 18:904-10

Carotid stenosis: progression to stroke

Angiography in 2240 patients¶

Stenosis at baseline	n	Ipsilateral stroke %, 3 y	n, 4.5 y	
0 - 29%	1270	1.8	28	54
30 - 69%	843	2.1	26	
70 - 99%	127	5.7	13	
All	2240		67	

¶European Carotid Surgery Trial. *Lancet* 1995; 345:209-12

FIGURE 35-7 Most coronary occlusions (*top*, 51/72 = 71 percent), myocardial infarctions (*middle*, 29/39 = 74 percent), and ischemic strokes of carotid origin (*bottom*, 54/67 = 81 percent) are caused by acute thrombosis superimposed on atherosclerotic lesions that, prior to the acute events, were asymptomatic and only mildly to moderately stenotic. Overall, nonstenotic atherosclerotic lesions by far outnumber the stenotic ones at higher individual risk, which is why most acute clinical events originate from nonstenotic lesions at relative low individual risk. MI = myocardial infarction.

intimal.[200] Medical calcification (Mönckeberg's calcinosis) is rare in coronary arteries, even in diabetic persons where it frequently occurs in other arteries, particularly the muscular arteries of the legs.[201] Both autopsy and clinical data indicate that coronary calcification is a marker for, and correlates closely with, the overall atherosclerotic plaque burden,[202–204] but calcification of a plaque does not correlate with its flow-limiting capacity (degree of stenosis) [202,203] or its risk of sudden occlusion (vulnerability). If anything, heavily calcified plaques appear to be more stable than noncalcified plaques.[203,205–207] The vascular remodeling phenomenon is the likely explanation for the poor correlation of plaque calcification with lumen narrowing and/or stenosis severity.[202]

It is possible to detect and quantify coronary artery calcification noninvasively by electron-beam (or *ultrafast*) computed tomography (EBCT). Plaque calcification detected by EBCT is not necessarily an end-stage irreversible phenomenon; recent data suggest that it may regress with lipid-lowering therapy.[208] Taking age, sex, and clinical presentation into account, coronary calcification may noninvasively identify patients, rather than plaques, at increased risk, because the overall plaque burden, of which coronary calcification is a marker, rather than the severity of individual plaques/stenoses, predicts future coronary events in both symptomatic and asymptomatic adults. The more plaques there are, the greater is the likelihood of one of them being vulnerable and prone to thrombose.

FACTORS INFLUENCING ATHEROGENESIS

Atherosclerosis is the result of multiple and complex gene-environment interactions. Genetic factors alone may cause symptomatic atherosclerosis (e.g., homozygous LDLR deficiency), but it is rare. Most frequently, the genetic background determines an individual's response to proatherogenic factors and the susceptibility of the vessel wall to atherogenic stimuli, but environmental factors may markedly influence the speed of disease progression (plaque development) and, thus, determine whether CHD develops. In high-risk societies, epidemiologic studies with autopsy follow-up have revealed a large individual variation in the extent of atherosclerosis (plaque burden) in apparently homogeneous subgroups.[209] The three factors that most consistently have been shown to correlate with the extent of atherosclerotic lesions per se at autopsy in men (high total cholesterol, low HDL cholesterol, and high blood pressure) explain together only about 25 percent of the individual variation.[209] Thus, a large part of the individual variation in the development of atherosclerosis remains unexplained. Only sparse and inconclusive data are available for women.

Several major and independent risk factors for the clinical manifestations of atherosclerosis have been identified, including elevated serum total (and LDL) cholesterol, low serum HDL cholesterol, cigarette smoking, elevated blood pressure, diabetes mellitus, and advancing age.[210] If left untreated, any of these major risk factors has the potential to produce clinical disease. Nevertheless, in principle, only a single absolutely necessary and truly independent etiologic agent for atherosclerosis exists, and it is a high level of serum LDL cholesterol (or its surrogate, serum total cholesterol).[210–212] A strongly positive relation exists between serum cholesterol levels and CHD worldwide, and atherosclerotic events are rare in populations with total cholesterol less than 4 mmol/L (150 mg/dL), even in the presence of other major risk factors.[212–214] At higher cholesterol levels, smoking, hypertension, low HDL cholesterol, and diabetes mellitus promote development of coronary atherosclerosis and predispose individuals to CHD, but these statistically independent risk factors can not by themselves cause atherosclerosis.[211] In affluent societies, however, many patients with CHD have serum cholesterol levels within or below the average range for these high-risk populations, and there is considerable overlap (about 80 percent) in the distribution of cholesterol values among men with and without CHD.[215] Known risk factors for CHD, of which serum cholesterol concentration is just one, explain only half of the variance in the occurrence of the disease.[216] Although it is said that as many as 50 percent of CHD patients lack major cardiovascular risk factors,[217] recently published data indicate that very few, less than 5 to 10 percent, of young adult and middle-aged men and women in the United States lack major risk factors, defined as serum cholesterol level less than 5.17 mmol/L (<200 mg/dL), blood pressure less than or equal to 120/80 mmHg, no smoking, and no diabetes. In this small low-risk subgroup, long-term mortality is much lower and longevity is much greater.[218] Both human and experimental studies strongly indicate that a certain serum cholesterol level (~4 mmol/L; 150 mg/dL) needs to be present to initiate and drive the disease in the vessel wall: atherosclerosis.[210,216] Below that level, CHD is rare, regardless of other risk factors.

Except for LDL cholesterol, very little is known about the specific relation of cardiovascular risk factors to atherosclerosis. The matter is complicated by the fact that symptomatic human plaques develop over decades and are extremely heterogeneous. Even plaques developed next to each other in the same coronary artery and thus exposed to the same systemic risk factors may look very dissimilar. If a particular risk factor plays a pathogenetic role in arterial occlusive disease, it could, in principle, do so by (1) accelerating the atherosclerotic process itself (plaque burden), (2) destabilizing established plaques (vulnerability, erosin, and rupture), and/or (3) promoting thrombosis on plaques via local (plaque thrombogenicity) and/or systemic factors. With these different pathways in mind, the role of the major risk factors in atherogenesis will be discussed.

Lipoproteins

Elevated serum total (and LDL) cholesterol and low serum HDL cholesterol are major independent risk factors for CHD.[210] Epidemiologic observations, angiographic studies, and lipid-lowering trials, as well as experimental studies, confirm the importance of LDL as a cause of atherosclerosis in both men and women with or without symptoms of CHD.[211,214] An elevated LDL-cholesterol level appears to be the primary CHD risk factor, and the higher the total and LDL cholesterol levels are, the greater is the risk of an atherosclerotic event.[210,211] A strongly positive relation exists between serum cholesterol levels and CHD worldwide,[212–214] and no threshold has been identified below which a lower blood cholesterol is not associated with a lower risk of CHD; the lower the cholesterol, the lower the risk of CHD, even in Chinese populations who, by Western standards, have a low cholesterol concentration.[219] Normal laboratory animals with low cholesterol levels do not develop atherosclerosis.

A low level of HDL cholesterol is a potent individual predictor for CHD in populations in which average cholesterol levels are relatively high, but it may not hold as a predictor in populations in which mean levels of serum total (and LDL) cholesterol are low.[211] In this regard, low HDL cholesterol resembles the other independent major risk factors (smoking, hypertension, and diabetes): it appears to promote coronary atherosclerosis when a high LDL level is present, but not when it is absent.[211] Thus, low HDL cholesterol and nonlipid risk factors aggravate the effect of LDL cholesterol, especially when total and LDL cholesterol are only moderately elevated; 5 to 6.5 mmol/L (190 to 250 mg/dL) and 3 to 4.5 mmol/L (115 to 175 mg/dL), respectively.[214]

Atherosclerosis is due to influx, retention, and modification of atherogenic lipoproteins in the intima, including LDL, intermediate-density lipoproteins (IDLs), and small species of very low density lipoproteins (VLDLs). The degree to which lipoproteins cause atherosclerosis depends in part on their size, explaining why large VLDLs and chylomicrons, which are too large to enter the artery wall, are not atherogenic.[214] The smallest lipoproteins, HDLs, enter the artery wall quite easily but also leave the artery wall easily and do not cause atherosclerosis. In fact, HDL probably affords protection by facilitating the removal of cholesterol from the vessel wall (reverse cholesterol transport).[214] Cholesterol and triglycerides are lipid components of all these various lipoproteins, and measurements of cholesterol or triglycerides therefore do not accurately reflect the particular lipoproteins that cause atherosclerosis. ApoB is a protein common to LDLs, IDLs, VLDLs, and chylomicrons. Since the latter are not present in plasma in the fasting state, almost all apoB is in atherogenic lipoproteins, which is why a fasting plasma apoB level is a good marker of cardiovascular risk.[214]

The relationship of triglycerides to atherosclerosis has been a source of confusion, partly because not all triglyceride-rich lipoproteins are atherogenic (smaller VLDLs versus larger VLDLs and chylomicrons) and partly because VLDLs and HDLs are metabolically closely linked (HDL-cholesterol concentrations are usually low when triglyceride concentrations are high).[214] Severe hypertriglyceridemia due to chylomicrons and large forms of VLDL is not atherogenic (but may cause pancreatitis), in contrast to less severe hypertriglyceridemia due to small VLDLs and IDLs (VLDLs normally carry most of the plasma triglyceride). Recent data have more clearly identified hypertriglyceridemia as a risk factor for CHD.[214] The strong inverse association between plasma HDL cholesterol and CHD is a consistent observation, but exactly how this relationship comes about is not entirely understood. HDL cholesterol may, as already described, be a reciprocal measure of atherogenic lipoproteins such as small VLDLs, it may protect the vessel wall by inhibiting LDL oxidation, and/or it may promote the removal of cholesterol from the vessel wall (reverse cholesterol transport).[214] Experimental studies suggest that HDL and its major protein component, apoA1, indeed have an innate atheroprotective effect.[76,220-222]

Prospective epidemiologic studies with autopsy follow-up have shown that serum total cholesterol measured during life correlates with the amount of atherosclerosis (plaque burden) in all arterial segments studied (aorta and coronary and cerebral arteries) in men (only one small study included females).[209] In the only study in which HDL cholesterol was measured, it correlated inversely with coronary atherosclerosis.[209] Recent data from the Bogalusa Heart Study, a long-term epidemiologic study of cardiovascular risk factors in children and young adults, revealed that antemortem risk factors relate strongly to atherosclerosis in autopsied children and young adults.[223,224] LDL cholesterol, triglycerides, body mass index, and elevated blood pressure correlated positively with both fatty streaks and more advanced lesions in coronary arteries; no significant correlation was found with HDL cholesterol.[223]

In the multicenter Pathobiological Determinants of Atherosclerosis in Youth (PDAY) study, HDL cholesterol and non-HDL cholesterol in blood obtained postmortem correlated negatively and positively, respectively, with the extent of atherosclerosis in autopsied persons ($n = 715$).[225] Neither apoA1 nor apoB measures were as strongly or consistently correlated with extent of lesions as the corresponding lipid measure (HDL cholesterol and non-HDL cholesterol, respectively).[225] Including all available risk factors (sex, age, race, smoking status, hypertension, and the lipid measures) in a predictive model, only up to 25 percent of the variation in raised lesions were explained, and HDL cholesterol and non-HDL cholesterol alone increased the explanatory capability by only 2.5 percent. Thus, the larger part of the individual variation in the development of atherosclerosis remains unexplained.

High plasma concentrations of lipoprotein(a) [Lp(a)] identifies persons at increased risk of ischemic heart disease (IHD), but whether Lp(a) is causally related to occlusive arterial disease is unknown. Lp(a) predominantly localizes in atherosclerotic plaques,[39,226] but neither Lp(a) concentration nor its size correlated strongly or consistently with the extent of atherosclerosis in autopsied persons in the PDAY study.[225] It was therefore concluded that Lp(a), which contains apo(a) (which bears significant homology to plasminogen), probably acts by interfering with the thrombotic complications to atherosclerosis rather than promoting atherosclerosis itself.

Regarding plaque composition, recent studies of sudden coronary deaths indicate that elevated total cholesterol and reduced HDL cholesterol, but particularly a high total-to-HDL ratio, predispose men and postmenopausal women to the development of vulnerable rupture-prone plaques with superimposed thrombosis.[227,228]

Smoking

Cigarette smoking is a major, and the single most modifiable, risk factor for atherosclerosis-related clinical events, both in high-risk[211,229] and low-risk[230-232] populations. As many as 30 percent of all CHD deaths in the United States each year are attributable to cigarette smoking, and smoking is the predominant cause of peripheral arterial disease and abdominal aortic aneurysm, it is a major risk factor for ischemic stroke, and it increases the risk of many other chronic diseases.[229] Evaluated statistically by multivariate analysis, smoking contributes to CHD risk independently of other risk factors, but this does not mean that smoking is an independent cause of CHD. Cigarette smoking is pathogenetically a cholesterol-dependent risk factor and acts synergistically with other risk factors, substantially increasing the risk of CHD.[211,229] Smoking is only weakly, if at all, atherogenic, and smoking alone does not cause a high incidence of CHD, exemplified by low CHD rates in populations in which cigarette smoking is heavy but total cholesterol levels are uniformly low (<4 mmol/L; 150 mg/dL).[212] A dose-related and potentially reversible impairment of endothelium-dependent vasodilation was found in healthy young adults who smoked cigarettes,[233] and smoking also contributes to coronary artery spasm.[234]

Cigarette smoking is a strong predictor of myocardial infarction but not for uncomplicated angina pectoris.[211,235,236] This could mean that smoking does not cause coronary atherosclerosis per se but rather increases the risk for thrombotic events in those who already have reached a certain level of coronary atherosclerosis. Support for this view comes from prospective epidemiologic studies with autopsy follow-up: smokers do not have significantly more extensive coronary atherosclerosis, evaluated grossly as intimal surface covered by plaques, than nonsmokers.[209,237-241] This finding is supported by the more recent PDAY study, in which the extent of coronary atherosclerosis did not correlate significantly with serum thiocyanate (a marker of exposure to smoke, measured post mortem)[141] but, evaluated microscopically, established plaques appeared to be more rapidly progressing and thus reaching an advanced stage of the disease earlier.[242] A coronary thrombus is more freqently found in smokers than in nonsmokers dying suddenly of CHD,[227,228] and preliminary data suggest that smoking may increase the thrombogenicity of plaques by upregulating tissue factor expression.[243] In contrast to coronary atherosclerosis, aortic atherosclerosis and particularly abdominal aortic aneurysm are strongly related to smoking.[141,209,237,238,240,241]

A strong synergistic interaction exists between hypercholesterolemia and smoking in the genesis of myocardial infarction: the former promotes coronary atherosclerosis and the latter, in turn, precipitates myocardial infarction.[211] The specific mechanisms by which cigarette smoking precipitates myocardial infarction are not known but are most likely related to thrombosis on coronary plaques mediated by local factors (plaque thrombogenicity) and/or systemic smoking-dependent factors.[244,245] Some of the evidence for smoking being thrombogenic rather than atherogenic are[244,245] (1) smoking is a strong risk factor for thrombus-mediated events (myocardial infarction and sudden death), but not for symptoms caused by atherosclerosis alone (angina pectoris); (2) angiographically, smoking is associated with rapid coronary occlusion (thrombosis) rather than slow nonocclusive plaque progression (atherosclerosis); (3) after thrombolysis for myocardial infarction, less residual vessel wall disease persists (atherosclerosis) in smokers than in nonsmokers;[246-248] (4) smoking is associated with a systemic hyperthrombotic state (systemic thrombin generation, activated platelets, and high fibrinogen);[249,250] (5) pathoanatomically, smoking is strongly related to coronary thrombosis and only weakly to the underlying atherosclerosis; and (6) smoking cessation rapidly and markedly reduces risk for myocardial infarction, indicating that the responsible process is rapidly reversible.[244,251] Finally, also in experimental animals is smoking more thrombogenic than atherogenic; it promotes platelet-dependent cyclic flow variation after arterial injury,[252] but forced cigarette smoking does not induce coronary atherosclerosis in nonhuman primates.[253]

In the United States, about 43 percent of nonsmoking children and 37 percent of nonsmoking adults are exposed to environmental tobacco smoke, and passive smoking appears to be associated with a small increase in the risk of CHD.[254] Thus, the public health consequences of passive smoking with regard to CHD may be important.[254]

Hypertension

Systemic arterial hypertension is a major independent risk factor for CHD, although it pathogenetically appears to be a cholesterol-dependent accelerator of atherosclerosis.[212,213] When hypertension is defined as a systolic blood pressure of 140 mmHg or greater, a diastolic blood pressure of 90 mmHg or greater, or both, it is associated with a relative risk of 1.5 (Seven Countries Study)[255] to 2.0 (Framingham Study)[256] for death from CHD, in both high-risk (United States and Northern Europe) and low-risk populations (Japan and Mediterranean Southern Europe).[255]

It is generally assumed that hypertension accelerates atherosclerosis directly by way of increased blood pressure, but it has been suggested that associated hormonal changes, including generation of angiotensin II by systemic and/or local renin-angiotensin systems, could also play a pathogenetic role.[67] However, the original observation of an association between the insertion (I)/deletion (D) polymorphism of the angiotensin-converting enzyme (ACE) gene, which explains as much as 30 to 40 percent of the total variation in serum ACE activity,[257] and myocardial infarction was not confirmed in the two largest studies to date,[258,259] and increased serum ACE activity has never been shown to be a risk factor for CHD.[257] The recently published Heart Outcomes Prevention Evaluation trial may shed new light on that question.[260]

Hypertension and hypercholesterolemia interact strongly in promotion of coronary atherosclerosis.[211] Hypertension does not induce atherosclerosis in normal laboratory animals with low cholesterol levels; it is not in itself atherogenic. In populations where total cholesterol is less than 4 mmol/L (150 mg/dL), atherosclerotic events are rare, even in people with hypertension.[212] That the blood pressure needs to be above a certain level to accelerate atherosclerosis is best illustrated by the following examples: (1) atherosclerosis does not develop in veins unless exposed to higher-than-normal pressure (e.g., veins used as coronary bypass grafts), (2) atherosclerosis does not develop to any significant degree in pulmonary arteries unless pulmonary hypertension is present, (3) more atherosclerosis is present in high-pressure arteries proximal to congenital aortic coarctation than in downstream low-pressure arteries, and (4) much less atherosclerosis develops in coronary arteries originating anomalously from the low-pressure pulmonary trunk than from the high-pressure aorta[261,262] (Fig. 35-8, Plate 81). Furthermore, in the International Atherosclerosis Project ($n > 20,000$), much more coronary and aortic atherosclerosis was found at autopsy in hypertensive compared with normotensive individuals—a relation already present from a young age.[263] But much more conclusive, prospective epidemiologic studies with autopsy follow-up revealed that blood pressure measured during life was a powerful and consistent predictor for the extent of raised atherosclerotic lesions per se: the higher the pressure during life, the more severe atherosclerosis post mortem in aorta and coronary and cerebral arteries[218,237-241]—an association that is present already in children and young adults.[223] Thus, hypertension and atherosclerosis are related, probably causally. Also, the PDAY study has provided evidence for the association between hypertension and the development of atherosclerotic lesions.[264,265]

The principal components of blood pressure consist of a steady component (mean arterial pressure) and a pulsatile com-

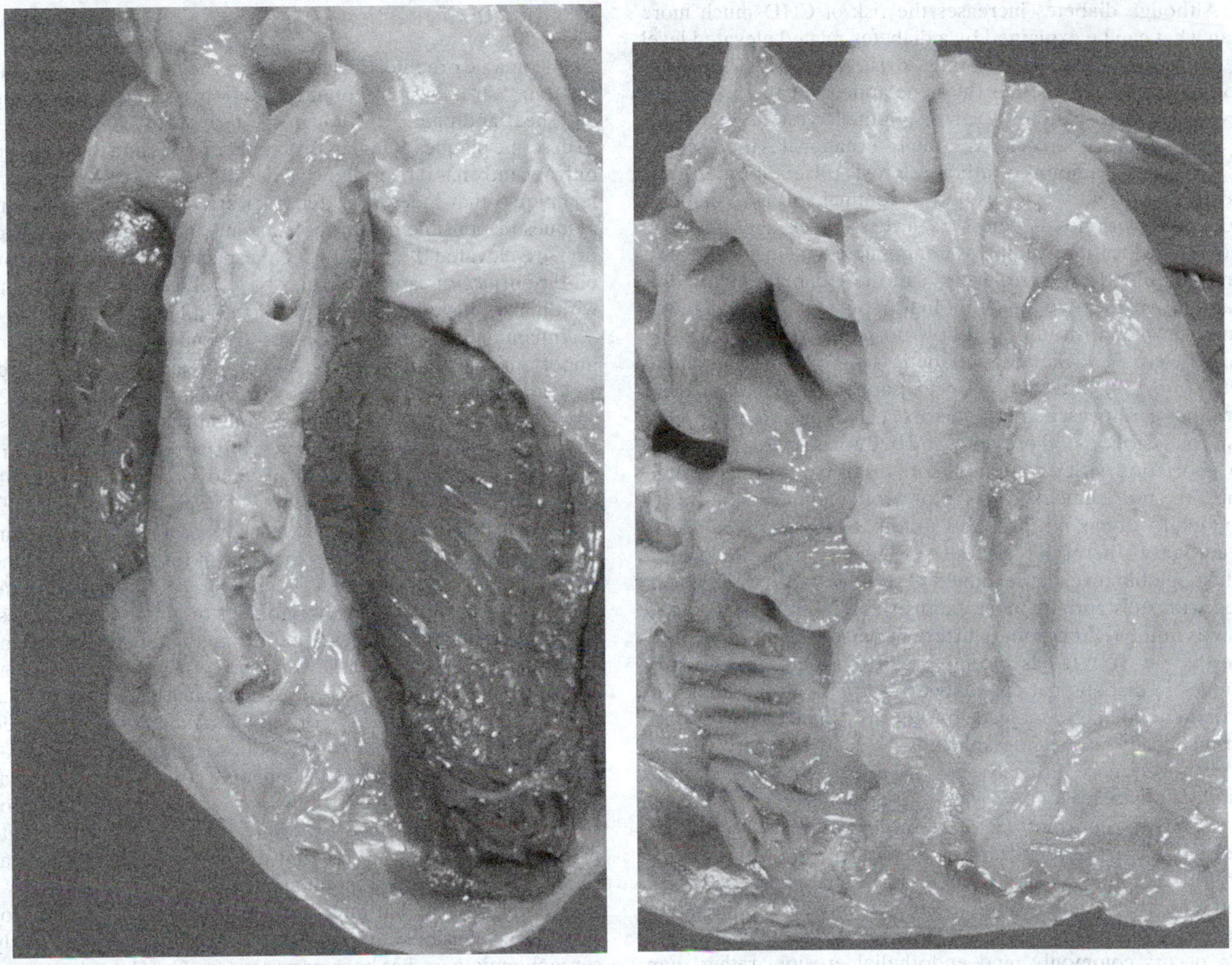

FIGURE 35-8 (Plate 81) Experiment of nature, illustrating the pathogenetic role of blood pressure in atherogenesis. The left anterior descending coronary artery (LAD) is departing normally and thus exposed to systemic blood pressure; the LAD is severely atherosclerotic, stiff, and calcified (*A*). In contrast, the right coronary artery (RC) is originating anomalously from the lower-pressure pulmonary trunk; the RC is elastic and compliant without atherosclerosis (*B*).

ponent (pulse pressure). As large-artery stiffness increases in middle-aged and elderly subjects, systolic pressure rises and diastolic pressure falls (isolated systolic hypertension), with a resulting increase in pulse pressure.[266] Recent data from the Framingham Heart Study indicate that pulse pressure is superior to both systolic and diastolic blood pressures in predicting CHD risk, and age-related large-artery stiffening may thus constitute an important component of CHD risk in the elderly.[266]

Diabetes

Yet another pathogenetically cholesterol-dependent, but statistically independent, major cardiovascular risk factor is non-insulin-dependent diabetes mellitus (NIDDM).[211] NIDDM and hypercholesterolemia interact strongly in the genesis of CHD.[211] In populations where total cholesterol is less than 4 mmol/L (150 mg/dL), atherosclerotic events are rare, even in diabetics.[212] Diabetes is, however, a powerful and gender-dependent risk factor in North America and Europe, increasing the risk of CHD three- to sevenfold in women compared with two- to threefold in men.[267] In fact, as recently expressed in a Scientific Statement from the American Heart Association, "diabetes *is* a cardiovascular disease."[268] Also, the precursor to type 2 diabetes, insulin resistance with impaired glucose tolerance, carries a strongly increased risk for cardiovascular disease, but the individual roles of insulin resistance itself, hyperinsulinemia, hyperglycemia (and advanced glycation end products),[113] hemostatic abnormalities (platelets, coagulation, and fibrinolysis), and conventional risk factors such as dyslipidemia (high triglycerides, low HDL, and small dense LDL particles) and hypertension are not clear. Not only hyperglycemia but also glucose levels in the nondiabetic range are associated with an increased risk of atherosclerosis-related diseases.[269–272] Thus, the mechanisms by which diabetes promotes atherosclerosis and/or its clinical manifestations are poorly understood.

Although diabetes increases the risk of CHD much more than what can be explained by a diabetes-related elevated level of conventional risk factors (e.g., dyslipidemia and hypertension), it is unclear whether the same applies for the underlying vessel wall disease: atherosclerosis. In the largest autopsy study of diabetes and atherosclerosis, the International Atherosclerosis Project, the amount of atherosclerosis (plaque burden) was greater in coronary arteries and abdominal aortas in diabetes (compared with nondiabetes), regardless of sex, age, race, and geographic location, but it was not possible to adjust for cholesterol and blood pressure levels.[263] In the Honolulu Heart Program, a prospective epidemiologic study among Japanese-American men with autopsy follow-up, more extensive coronary atherosclerosis was found in diabetics (n = 83) than in nondiabetics (n = 159), but the difference disappeared after adjustment for other cardiovascular risk factors such as age, smoking, cholesterol, systolic blood pressure, and body mass index. There was no association with duration of diabetes or type of treatment.[273] Thus, the more adverse risk factor profile among diabetics accounted for some, but probably not all, of the observed excess of coronary atherosclerosis. In the PDAY study, however, glycohemoglobin levels exceeding 8 percent (n = 10) were associated with substantially more extensive fatty streaks and raised lesions in the right coronary artery in persons 25 to 34 years of age (n = 648).[274] It has recently been reported that coronary plaques in diabetic patients appear morphologically similar to those in nondiabetic subjects, but there is some evidence, both pathologically and angiographically, that the coronary arteries are involved more diffusely and that disease may extend more distally in diabetes.[275]

If diabetes does not accelerate atherosclerosis, it could increase the risk of atherosclerosis-mediated events by promoting thrombotic complications. Diabetes is associated with increased platelet activity and elevated plasma fibrinogen and plasminogen activator inhibitor 1 (PAI-1) levels.[276] Endothelial dysfunction occurs commonly, and endothelial erosion, rather than plaque rupture, appears to be the dominant mechanism underlying coronary thrombosis in patients with diabetes.[182]

Diabetes predisposes individuals to medial artery calcification (MAC, Mönckeberg's calcinosis), especially of the muscular arteries of the legs, but is practically never seen in the coronary arteries of adults.[202] MAC is a nonobstructive condition (apparently independent of and unrelated to atherosclerosis) leading to reduced arterial compliance. MAC is a strong independent predictor of future cardiovascular events in patients with type 2 diabetes, supporting the hypothesis that reduced arterial elasticity (arterial stiffening) could play a role in arterial occlusion in diabetes.[277–279]

There are no well-controlled studies conclusively demonstrating that intensive blood-glucose control will reduce atherosclerotic events in patients with diabetes.[275] Only a relatively small and nonsignificant reduction was seen in the U.K. Prospective Diabetes Study (type 2 diabetes), contrasting a substantial and highly significant reduction in microvascular complications.[280] On the other hand, lipid-lowering with a statin appears to benefit all people at risk, including diabetics and those with only *impaired fasting glucose*, defined as a fasting glucose level of 6.0 to 6.9 mmol/L.[281] Intensive insulin treatment in type 2 diabetes has been shown to have survival benefits after acute myocardial infarction.[282]

Inflammation/Infection

The Roman Cornelius Celsus, living in the first century, gave us the four "cardinal signs" of inflammation: redness and swelling, with heat and pain.[283] Although the term "hot" has been used to describe plaques at high risk of rapid progression to occlusion, only recently has it been shown clinically, using a catheter-based technique, that indeed the temperature of high-risk coronary plaques responsible for unstable angina and myocardial infarction are elevated 0.7°C and 1.5°C, respectively,[284] and hot spots on the surface of carotid plaques have been shown to correlate with macrophage infiltration, i.e., local inflammation.[285]

Inflammation, but not necessarily chronic infection, plays an important role in the initiation and progression of atherosclerosis,[67] and systemic blood markers of inflammation such as C-reactive protein, serum amyloid A, and fibrinogen (acute-phase reactants) have emerged as powerful predictors of coronary events[286,287] in asymptomatic men[168] and women,[169] in patients with stable[170] and unstable angina,[171–173] and after infarction.[174] These sensitive but nonspecific markers of low-grade systemic inflammation are produced in the liver in response to cytokine stimulation (e.g., interleukins 1 and 6),[288,289] but it is unclear whether the proinflammatory cytokines originate from the vessel wall itself (macrophages?), reflecting the quantity (burden) or quality (activity) of atherosclerosis, or from nonvascular sources, reflecting inflammatory states such as chronic infections. Other novel markers of vascular inflammation include the soluble forms of leukocyte adhesion molecules, such as sICAM-1,[290,291] which may reflect ongoing atherosclerosis. Proinflammatory cytokines, regardless of their sources, and the processes they mediate may accelerate atherogenesis and/or its manifestations, but it still remains unknown whether inflammation per se represents a modifiable risk factor.[292]

The hypothesis that infection is causally related to atherosclerosis is plausible but unproven. Most evidence, particularly seroepidemiologic, has been presented for Cp, *Helicobacter pylori* (Hp), and certain herpesviruses [particularly cytomegalovirus (CMV)].[163,164,293–295] Recent observational,[296–300] interventional,[301,302] and pathoanatomic[303–306] evidence have, however, weakened the case for a possible causal role of Cp in occlusive vascular disease, and the evidence for Hp is still questionable.[307,308] CMV may play a greater role in restenosis after angioplasty and transplant vascular disease than in atherosclerosis.[164,308] If infection plays a pathogenetic role, vaccination and/or antimicrobial agents might offer protection.

It has been extremely difficult, if not impossible, to culture infectious agents from atherosclerotic lesions, but this does not preclude their involvement in lesion formation.[164] CMV genomic DNA and antigens are commonly found in the human arterial tree, both in plaque and in plaque-free vessel walls (90 versus > 50 percent, i.e., considerable overlap),[164,309] in contrast to Cp DNA and antigens that appear to be confined to diseased vessel walls (up to 73 percent of coronary plaques were defined Cp positive by immunohistochemistry).[166,167] Hp has not been detected in vessel walls.

To date, more than 20 inflammation-associated cell adhesion molecules and almost 50 proinflammatory cytokines have been described,[45] and a significant number of these have already been shown to be present in human atherosclerotic plaques.[310–318] Acute-phase reactants are also frequently present in advanced lesions, including fibrinogen,[144,319] C-reactive protein,[320,321] and serum amyloid A (expressed in lesions).[322] The relation, if any, of local inflammation in plaques to systemic markers of inflammation such as C-reactive protein has not yet been reported. No inflammatory markers of cardiovascular risk have been related with any histopathologic changes at the plaque level, and no published evidence suggests that atherosclerotic lesions containing infectious agent–related products differ histologically from those without signs of plaque infection.[323]

Hemostatic Factors

Several systemic hemostatic factors, including fibrinogen, factor VII, PAI-1, t-PA, and platelets, have been identified as determinants of future CHD events.[324–326] Thrombin generation and platelet activation play a causal role in atherosclerosis-mediated luminal thrombosis and, most likely, also in the slow progression of atherosclerotic lesions. Platelets can adhere to denuded areas and release their granules, which contain cytokines and growth factors that, together with thrombin, may contribute to activation, migration, and proliferation of cells and thus promote plaque development.[67] Local generation of plasmin may itself, but most likely via activation of latent MMPs, digest the extracellular matrix, which is essential for cell migration. If unopposed, matrix degradation may ultimately culminate in plaque disruption.[324]

The mere presence of a positive relation between abnormal hemostasis and CHD does not indicate whether the former is a cause of, related to, or a consequence of, the latter. The most powerful and most consistent predictor of CHD among the hemostatic factors—fibrinogen—is strongly related to smoking, diabetes, and C-reactive protein (an acute-phase reactant like fibrinogen), all of which are strong, consistent, and independent predictors of CHD.[326] To answer the question about causality and, if present, its strength, studying CHD risk in persons with congenital abnormalities in coagulation, fibrinolysis and platelet function provides important information. Although conflicting results have been published,[327,328] gene polymorphisms associated with different plasma levels of fibrinogen ($G_{-455}\rightarrow A$),[329,330] prothrombin (G20210A),[331] factor V (G1691A, Leiden),[331] factor VII (e.g., G10976A, R353Q),[331–333] factor VIII,[330] t-PA (I/D),[334] and PAI-1 (4G/5G)[330,335] appear not to be, or at best weakly, causally related to atherosclerosis or arterial thrombosis, even though many of these abnormalities are causally related to venous thrombosis.[330] On the other hand, polymorphisms of the platelet fibrinogen (PIA1/A2, glycoprotein IIIa)[331,336,337] and collagen (C3550T, glycoprotein Ib; 807T/873A, glycoprotein Ia/IIa)[338] receptor genes appear, at least under certain circumstances, to be causally related to coronary thrombosis and myocardial infarction, rather than to coronary atherosclerosis, emphasizing the primary role of platelets in arterial thrombosis. Prothrombotic genetic risk factors appear to be particularly important in precipitating myocardial infarction in young persons without severe atherosclerosis, and there is a strong adverse interaction with smoking.[331] It is possible to prevent arterial occlusion and, if it occurs, accelerate reperfusion and prevent reocclusion by targeting hemostatic factors (antiplatelet agents, anticoagulants, and fibrinolytic agents), but it has never been proven that such treatments also prevent or retard the slow progression of atherosclerosis not mediated by luminal thrombosis.

Homocyst(e)ine

Numerous retrospective case-control studies have identified mild-to-moderate homocyst(e)inemia as a strong and independent risk factor for CHD, stroke, and peripheral vascular disease,[339–342] and a clear association between plasma homocyst(e)ine (Hcy) and the anatomic extent of carotid, coronary, aortic, and peripheral vascular diseases has been demonstrated in several studies,[343,344] including at least one in a low-risk population.[345] Many prospective studies, but not all,[346–348] have, however, failed to demonstrate such an association, and it has been suggested that elevated Hcy could be a marker, or a consequence, rather than a cause of cardiovascular disease.[349–351] An argument against Hcy being causally related to CHD is the fact that the homozygous form of the thermolabile methylene-tetrahydrofolate reductase (MTHFR) gene, although leading to elevated Hcy levels in those with low folate levels, has not consistently been associated with an increased CHD risk.[351] If Hcy is a causative factor, the mechanisms by which homocysteine causes occlusive vascular disease remain to be identified.[343]

Using high nonphysiologic concentrations in vitro, potential proatherogenic effects of Hcy have been identified, such as endothelial toxicity[352,353] and promotion of smooth muscle cell growth and collagen production.[354,355] In vivo, hyperhomocyst(e)inemia is associated with endothelial dysfunction,[356] but there is no experimental evidence from animal studies indicating that mildly to moderately elevated Hcy is a cause of atherosclerosis.[343,350,357] Also in humans is elevated Hcy associated with endothelial dysfunction,[358,359] probably mediated by increased oxidant stress because antioxidant vitamin C normalizes the impaired endothelium-dependent vasodilation seen with hyperhomocyst(e)inemia and the associated metabolic changes.[360]

Elevated Hcy appears to be more closely linked to thrombus-mediated coronary events (myocardial infarction) than to coronary atherosclerosis as seen on angiography,[361] and elevated Hcy is also linked to venous thrombosis.[351,362,363] Prothrombotic effects of Hcy have been described, such as downregulation of thrombomodulin on endothelial cells[364] and upregulation of tissue factor on both endothelial cells[365] and macrophages.[366] In homocystinuria, an inborn error of Hcy metabolism associated with extremely high plasma Hcy (usually >100 μmol/L), the few published autopsy reports confirm that both arterial and venous thrombosis are frequent and occur at an early age but apparently often without concomitant atherosclerosis.[367]

Alcohol

Generally, men and women who consume one to three drinks a day live longer than nondrinkers, due to reduced risk of CHD.[368] It also holds for low-risk Chinese people.[369] The inverse association between moderate alcohol intake and CHD is documented in over 40 prospective studies in diverse populations,[368] suggesting that mild to moderate alcohol intake is associated with a 10 to 40 percent lower risk of CHD than with no alcohol intake. The five largest cohort studies, with nearly 30,000 heart disease events, showed a consistent 20 percent reduction in CHD mortality among people who drank about 1 U of alcohol a day compared with nondrinkers.[370] This reduction is generally attributed to the beneficial effects of alcohol on lipids and hemostatic factors.[368] Moderate alcohol intake is strongly and consistently associated with higher concentrations of HDL cholesterol and apoA1 and lower concentrations of fibrinogen and is weakly associated with increased triglyceride concentration.[368] It was calculated that such changes, believed to be causally related to CHD, overall may reduce the CHD risk by 25 percent. Alcohol also inhibits platelet aggregation, which may substantially reduce the risk of CHD[371] and may promote fibrinolysis.[372,373] The effect of moderate alcohol intake on blood pressure is likely to be minor, but heavy intake (more than four drinks a day) is associated with hypertension[368] and increased risk of hemorrhagic stroke.[374–376] Several large cross-sectional studies have reported strong positive associations between alcohol and increased insulin sensitivity,[368] and moderate drinking seems to be associated with extraordinary benefit in patients with late-onset diabetes, possibly due to their greater baseline risk of CHD.[377]

With regard to wine, beer, and spirits, no consistent evidence has emerged that any one beverage confers a greater health benefit than another, indicating that a substantial portion of the benefit is mediated by ethanol.[377] Some studies suggest, however, that wine offers additional benefits.[378–381] A possible special effect associated with wine drinking could be due to specific nonalcoholic compounds in wine, particularly in red wine (e.g., antioxidant polyphenols).[382–384] Alternatively, it could be due to confounding lifestyle factors associated with wine intake.[385] Moderate wine drinking seems to be associated with a healthier lifestyle in California (less smoking and more education)[386] and Britain (less smoking and obesity),[387] a healthier diet in Denmark (higher intake of fruit, vegetables, and fish),[385] and better subjective health in Finland.[388]

The health benefit associated with regular and moderate alcohol intake may not extend to populations with irregular drinking patterns and/or substantial higher consumptions. For example, in Central and Eastern Europe and the former Soviet Union, a growing body of epidemiologic research indicates a positive rather than negative association between alcohol consumption and cardiovascular deaths, especially sudden cardiac deaths.[389] In binge drinkers, atheroprotective changes in HDL are not seen, and irregular heavy drinking appears to be associated with an increased risk of rebound thrombosis, occurring after cessation of drinking, and sudden death due to ventricular fibrillation.[389–392]

In France, the CHD mortality rate is much lower that in Britain (1:4 in men and 1:6 in women, 1992 data) and other high-risk countries, despite similar average values of major CHD risk factors (except fewer female smokers in France). Low-dose alcohol consumption, in particular wine drinking, has been suggested as the most likely explanation for this lower-than-expected CHD mortality rate in France, called the *French paradox*.[371,393,394] However, a novel *time lag* hypothesis has recently been suggested to explain this paradox.[395] Animal fat consumption and serum cholesterol concentration were lower in France than in Britain up to 1970, and only in recent years have these major determinants of CHD been similar in the two countries. For a chronic disease like atherosclerosis that evolves over decades, it seems more appropriate to compare current mortality data with levels of risk factors in the past (30 year ago) rather than recent levels. If so done, the French paradox apparently disappears.[395] The same argument holds for cigarette smoking and lung cancer where the time lag between exposure and clinical disease is well recognized; current disease correlates better with smoking habits decades ago than with recent habits.[395] Many countries with high wine consumption are also those in which saturated fat consumption used to be low but increased in recent years (France, Italy, Spain, and Switzerland, for example). The low mortality from CHD reflects the earlier low levels of saturated fat consumption, for which wine may simply be an indirect marker.[395]

Sex

The major cardiovascular risk factors are similar for both sexes, but men develop CHD 10 to 15 years earlier than women.[396] By age 60 in the United States, only 1 in 17 women has had a coronary event, as compared with 1 in 5 men. After age 60, however, CHD becomes the leading cause of death among women as well as among men, and as many women as men eventually die of the disease.[396] Diabetes mellitus is a particularly strong risk factor among women, nearly eliminating the normal protection offered by female sex. The striking influence of sex on CHD risk is cholesterol dependent, because neither men nor women develop CHD unless total cholesterol is greater than 4 mmol/L (150 mg/dL), and the higher the level is, the greater is the chance of an event, and the earlier the event occurs irrespective of sex.[212]

Estrogen may be the most obvious factor responsible for the protection against CHD conferred by the premenopausal state. With menopause, LDL levels begin to increase, whereas HDL levels stop climbing or decrease slightly.[397] This leads to a worsening of the LDL-to-HDL ratio. Although estrogen replacement therapy overall restores the deteriorated lipid profile,[397] estrogen may have beneficial effects that go beyond changes in serum lipids. In particular, estrogen may have direct atheroprotective effects on the vessel wall (estrogen receptors are present in vascular cells), suggested by the improvement of endothelial function seen with estrogen administration.[398] In nonhuman primates[399,400] and rabbits,[401] estrogen reduced diet-induced atherosclerosis, probably via an endothelium-dependent mechanism.[402]

Premature menopause (before age 45) due to oophorectomy or occurring naturally is known to lead to an increased CHD risk.[214] However, a simple hysterectomy with the ovaries and, consequently, estrogen production left intact also appears to increase the risk, and it has been suggested that this could be due to the loss of menstruation.[403] Iron is a powerful oxidant that mediates lipid peroxidation, which may explain the positive association between total body iron stores and cardiovascular risk found in epidemiologic studies. The *iron hypothesis*, suggesting that iron stores and CHD are causally related, has recently been revived by the finding of an increased CHD risk in heterozygous carriers of a common hemochromatosis gene mutation.[404,405]

In the International Atherosclerosis Project (IAP, 1960–1964), white men were unusually susceptible to atherosclerosis as compared with other sex-race subgroups, and sex differences in extent of aortic, coronary, and cerebral atherosclerosis were striking among whites but minimal among blacks.[209,406] In contrast, in the PDAY study initiated much later (1985) and involving young adults only (15 to 34 years of age), white men were no longer the most susceptible subgroup when evaluated by the same method as that used in the IAP (intimal surface grossly covered by plaques); there were no obvious sex differences, and blacks of both sexes appeared to be at least as susceptible to atherosclerosis as were white men.[407] When evaluated microscopically, however, coronary lesions appeared to progress faster in males than in females, evidenced by the presence of much more advanced plaque in 30- to 34-year-old men compared with age-matched women.[407] Regarding rapid thrombus-mediated plaque progression, the underlying mechanism appears to be in part sex dependent: plaque erosion (versus rupture) is more frequent in females than in males.[182,183,228]

Aging

Age is a powerful risk factor for CHD. The development of atherosclerosis increases markedly with age up to an age of about 65, regardless of sex and ethnic background.[141,223] Although atherosclerosis and the incidence of stable angina (caused by atherosclerosis alone) seem to increase less markedly beyond age 65,[408] most new-onset heart attacks (atherosclerosis plus thrombosis) occur after age 65, especially among women,[409] and the CHD mortality rate increases almost exponentially with age among elderly persons.[408] The reason for this paradox (more dangerous but not more extensive atherosclerosis with aging) is unknown but could be due to age-related changes superimposed on preexisting atherosclerosis and, of course, an increase in case fatality rates among the elderly. For example, increased pulse pressure and systolic blood pressure caused by age-related arterial stiffening are powerful predictors for myocardial infarction and coronary death, [266] and treatment of systolic hypertension even in very old patients reduces risk for both stroke and CHD.[410]

Although age is a strong and independent risk factor for CHD, the independent contribution of age to CHD risk is cholesterol dependent. In populations in which average serum total cholesterol levels are less than 4 mmol/L (150 mg/dL), atherosclerotic events are rare even among older persons.[213] Atherosclerotic events are also rare among North Americans and Europeans with that low cholesterol level, but only about 5 percent of persons older than 40 years of age have a total cholesterol level less than 4 mmol/L in these populations.[212] The mean serum total cholesterol of umbilical blood of newborns is approximately 1.9 mmol/L (75 mg/dL), but within 2 weeks of life that value rises to a mean of 4 mmol/L (150 mg/dL) and remains at that level until approximately age 20 years, when it gradually starts to rise. The average serum total cholesterol level in the United States in persons 20 to 74 years of age is 5.5 mmol/L (215 mg/dL).[411] Men have higher levels earlier in life, and women have higher levels in later life.[212]

CONCLUSION

Atherosclerosis is a complex and multifactorial disease, which means that many avenues for intervention can be applied. A certain blood-cholesterol level is necessary to initiate and drive the disease, but cholesterol alone is rarely enough for the development of symptomatic atherosclerotic lesions. Although many cardiovascular risk factors, such as smoking and hypertension, are not atherogenic on their own, they accelerate the development of occlusive arterial disease, and clinically it may be more rewarding to treat accelerators of the disease rather than its initiator, hypercholesterolemia. Maximum benefit, of course, is achieved by treating both. Experimental studies have clearly documented that the inhibition of just one necessary step in the atherogenetic chain of events in the vessel wall (e.g., macrophage recruitment) may markedly prevent or retard the development of mature plaques responsible for clinical disease.

References

1. Fuster V. Epidemic of cardiovascular disease and stroke: The three main challenges. *Circulation* 1999; 99:1132–1137.
2. Murray CJ, Lopez AD. Mortality by cause for eight regions of the world: Global Burden of Disease Study. *Lancet* 1997; 349:1269–1276.
3. Napoli C, Glass CK, Witztum JL, et al. Influence of maternal hypercholesterolaemia during pregnancy on progression of early atherosclerotic lesions in childhood: Fate of Early Lesions in Children (FELIC) study. *Lancet* 1999; 354:1234–1241.
4. Tamminen M, Mottino G, Qiao JH, et al. Ultrastructure of early lipid accumulation in apoE-deficient mice. *Arterioscler Thromb Vasc Biol* 1999; 19:847–853.
5. Williams KJ, Tabas I. The response-to-retention hypothesis of atherogenesis reinforced. *Curr Opin Lipidol* 1998; 9:471–474.
6. Davies MJ. *Atlas of Coronary Artery Disease*. Philadelphia: Lippincott-Raven; 1998.
7. Falk E, Shah PK, Fuster V. Coronary plaque disruption. *Circulation* 1995; 92:657–671.
8. Plump AS, Smith JD, Hayek T, et al. Severe hypercholesterolemia and atherosclerosis in apolipoprotein E–deficient mice created by homologous recombination in ES cells. *Cell* 1992; 71: 343–353.
9. Zhang SH, Reddick RL, Piedrahita JA, Maeda N. Spontaneous hypercholesterolemia and arterial lesions in mice lacking apolipoprotein E. *Science* 1992; 258:468–471.
10. Ishibashi S, Goldstein JL, Brown MS, et al. Massive xanthomatosis and atherosclerosis in cholesterol-fed low density lipoprotein receptor–negative mice. *J Clin Invest* 1994; 93:1885–1893.
11. Ishibashi S, Perrey S, Chen Z, et al. Role of the low density lipoprotein (LDL) receptor pathway in the metabolism of chylomicron remnants: A quantitative study in knockout mice lacking the LDL receptor, apolipoprotein E, or both. *J Biol Chem* 1996; 271:22,422–22,427.
12. Powell-Braxton L, Veniant M, Latvala RD, et al. A mouse model of human familial hypercholesterolemia: Markedly elevated low density lipoprotein cholesterol levels and severe atherosclerosis on a low-fat chow diet. *Nat Med* 1998; 4:934–938 [published erratum appears in *Nat Med* 1998; 4:1200].
13. Sanan DA, Newland DL, Tao R, et al. Low density lipoprotein receptor–negative mice expressing human apolipoprotein B-100 develop complex atherosclerotic lesions on a chow diet: No accentuation by apolipoprotein(a). *Proc Natl Acad Sci USA* 1998; 95:4544–4549.
14. Breslow JL, Plump A, Dannerman M, et al. New mouse models of lipoprotein disorders and atherosclerosis. In: Fuster V, Ross R, Topol EJ, eds. *Atherosclerosis and Coronary Artery Disease*, vol 1. Philadelphia: Lippincott-Raven; 1996:363–378.
15. Smith JD, Breslow JL. The emergence of mouse models of atherosclerosis and their relevance to clinical research. *J Intern Med* 1997; 242:99–109.
16. Carmeliet P, Moons L, Collen D. Mouse models of angiogenesis, arterial stenosis, atherosclerosis and hemostasis. *Cardiovasc Res* 1998; 39:8–33.
17. Lichtman AH, Clinton SK, Iiyama K, et al. Hyperlipidemia and atherosclerotic lesion development in LDL receptor–deficient

mice fed defined semipurified diets with and without cholate. *Arterioscler Thromb Vasc Biol* 1999; 19:1938–1944.
18. Faraci FM, Sigmund CD. Vascular biology in genetically altered mice: Smaller vessels, bigger insight. *Circ Res* 1999; 85:1214–1225.
19. Bonthu S, Heistad DD, Chappell DA, et al. Atherosclerosis, vascular remodeling, and impairment of endothelium-dependent relaxation in genetically altered hyperlipidemic mice. *Arterioscler Thromb Vasc Biol* 1997; 17:2333–2340.
20. Barton M, Haudenschild CC, d'Uscio LV, et al. Endothelin ETA receptor blockade restores NO-mediated endothelial function and inhibits atherosclerosis in apolipoprotein E–deficient mice. *Proc Natl Acad Sci USA* 1998; 95:14,367–14,372.
21. Lamping KG, Nuno DW, Chappell DA, Faraci FM. Agonist-specific impairment of coronary vascular function in genetically altered, hyperlipidemic mice. *Am J Physiol* 1999; 276(4 pt 2): R1023–R1029.
22. Deckert V, Lizard G, Duverger N, et al. Impairment of endothelium-dependent arterial relaxation by high-fat feeding in ApoE-deficient mice: Toward normalization by human ApoA-I expression. *Circulation* 1999; 100:1230–1235.
23. Dansky HM, Charlton SA, Barlow CB, et al. Apo A-I inhibits foam cell formation in Apo E-deficient mice after monocyte adherence to endothelium. *J Clin Invest* 1999; 104:31–39.
24. Plump AS, Scott CJ, Breslow JL. Human apolipoprotein A-I gene expression increases high density lipoprotein and suppresses atherosclerosis in the apolipoprotein E–deficient mouse. *Proc Natl Acad Sci USA* 1994; 91:9607–9611.
25. Paszty C, Maeda N, Verstuyft J, Rubin EM. Apolipoprotein AI transgene corrects apolipoprotein E deficiency–induced atherosclerosis in mice. *J Clin Invest* 1994; 94:899–903.
26. Zhang SH, Reddick RL, Avdievich E, et al. Paradoxical enhancement of atherosclerosis by probucol treatment in apolipoprotein E–deficient mice. *J Clin Invest* 1997; 99:2858–2866.
27. Hughes SD, Verstuyft J, Rubin EM. HDL deficiency in genetically engineered mice requires elevated LDL to accelerate atherogenesis. *Arterioscler Thromb Vasc Biol* 1997; 17:1725–1729.
28. Voyiaziakis E, Goldberg IJ, Plump AS, et al. ApoA-I deficiency causes both hypertriglyceridemia and increased atherosclerosis in human apoB transgenic mice. *J Lipid Res* 1998; 39:313–321.
29. Boisvert WA, Black AS, Curtiss LK. ApoA1 reduces free cholesterol accumulation in atherosclerotic lesions of apoE-deficient mice transplanted with apoE-expressing macrophages. *Arterioscler Thromb Vasc Biol* 1999; 19:525–530.
30. Iiyama K, Hajra L, Iiyama M, Li H, et al. Patterns of vascular cell adhesion molecule-1 and intercellular adhesion molecule-1 expression in rabbit and mouse atherosclerotic lesions and at sites predisposed to lesion formation. *Circ Res* 1999; 85:199–207.
31. Traub O, Berk BC. Laminar shear stress: Mechanisms by which endothelial cells transduce an atheroprotective force. *Arterioscler Thromb Vasc Biol* 1998; 18:677–685.
32. Tabas I. Nonoxidative modifications of lipoproteins in atherogenesis. *Annu Rev Nutr* 1999; 19:123–139.
33. Schwartz SM. The intima: A new soil (editorial). *Circ Res* 1999; 85:877–879.
34. Palinski W, Ord VA, Plump AS, et al. ApoE-deficient mice are a model of lipoprotein oxidation in atherogenesis: Demonstration of oxidation-specific epitopes in lesions and high titers of autoantibodies to malondialdehyde-lysine in serum. *Arterioscler Thromb* 1994; 14:605–616.
35. Witztum JL, Palinski W. Are immunological mechanisms relevant for the development of atherosclerosis? (editorial). *Clin Immunopathol* 1999; 90:153–156.
36. Camejo G, Hurt-Camejo E, Wiklund O, Bondjers G. Association of apo B lipoproteins with arterial proteoglycans: Pathological significance and molecular basis. *Atherosclerosis* 1998; 139: 205–222.
37. Kovanen PT, Pentikainen MO. Decorin links low-density lipoproteins (LDL) to collagen: A novel mechanism for retention of LDL in the atherosclerotic plaque. *Trends Cardiovasc Med* 1999; 9:86–91.
38. Nielsen LB. Transfer of low density lipoprotein into the arterial wall and risk of atherosclerosis. *Atherosclerosis* 1996; 123:1–15.
39. Nielsen LB. Atherogenecity of lipoprotein(a) and oxidized low density lipoprotein: Insight from in vivo studies of arterial wall influx, degradation and efflux. *Atherosclerosis* 1999; 143:229–243.
40. Nakashima Y, Raines EW, Plump AS, et al. Upregulation of VCAM-1 and ICAM-1 at atherosclerosis-prone sites on the endothelium in the apoE-deficient mouse. *Arterioscler Thromb Vasc Biol* 1998; 18:842–851.
41. Patel SS, Thiagarajan R, Willerson JT, Yeh ET. Inhibition of alpha$_4$ integrin and ICAM-1 markedly attenuate macrophage homing to atherosclerotic plaques in ApoE-deficient mice. *Circulation* 1998; 97:75–81.
42. Zhou X, Hansson GK. Detection of B cells and proinflammatory cytokines in atherosclerotic plaques of hypercholesterolaemic apolipoprotein E knockout mice. *Scand J Immunol* 1999; 50: 25–30.
43. Malek AM, Alper SL, Izumo S. Hemodynamic shear stress and its role in atherosclerosis. *JAMA* 1999; 282:2035–2042.
44. Nakashima Y, Plump AS, Raines EW, et al. ApoE-deficient mice develop lesions of all phases of atherosclerosis throughout the arterial tree. *Arterioscler Thromb* 1994; 14:133–140.
45. Reckless J, Rubin EM, Verstuyft JB, et al. Monocyte chemoattractant protein-1 but not tumor necrosis factor-alpha is correlated with monocyte infiltration in mouse lipid lesions. *Circulation* 1999; 99:2310–2316.
46. Reape TJ, Groot PHE. Chemokines and atherosclerosis. *Atherosclerosis* 1999; 147:213–225.
47. Rollins BJ. Chemokines (review). *Blood* 1997; 90:909–928.
48. Aiello RJ, Bourassa PA, Lindsey S, et al. Monocyte chemoattractant protein-1 accelerates atherosclerosis in apolipoprotein E–deficient mice. *Arterioscler Thromb Vasc Biol* 1999; 19:1518–1525.
49. Gu L, Okada Y, Clinton SK, et al. Absence of monocyte chemoattractant protein-1 reduces atherosclerosis in low density lipoprotein receptor–deficient mice. *Mol Cell* 1998; 2:275–281.
50. Gosling J, Slaymaker S, Gu L, Tseng S, et al. MCP-1 deficiency reduces susceptibility to atherosclerosis in mice that overexpress human apolipoprotein B. *J Clin Invest* 1999; 103:773–778.
51. Lu B, Rutledge BJ, Gu L, et al. Abnormalities in monocyte recruitment and cytokine expression in monocyte chemoattractant protein 1–deficient mice. *J Exp Med* 1998; 187:601–608.
52. Schecter AD, Rollins BJ, Zhang YJ, et al. Tissue factor is induced by monocyte chemoattractant protein-1 in human aortic smooth muscle and THP-1 cells. *J Biol Chem* 1997; 272:28,568–28,573.
53. Boring L, Gosling J, Cleary M, Charo IF. Decreased lesion formation in CCR2$^{-/-}$ mice reveals a role for chemokines in the initiation of atherosclerosis. *Nature* 1998; 394:894–897.
54. Cyrus T, Witztum JL, Rader DJ, et al. Disruption of the 12/15-lipoxygenase gene diminishes atherosclerosis in apo E-deficient mice. *J Clin Invest* 1999; 103:1597–1604.
55. Zhou X, Paulsson G, Stemme S, Hansson GK. Hypercholesterolemia is associated with a T helper (Th) 1/Th2 switch of the autoimmune response in atherosclerotic apo E-knockout mice. *J Clin Invest* 1998; 101:1717–1725.
56. Gupta S, Pablo AM, Jiang XC, et al. IFN-gamma potentiates atherosclerosis in ApoE knock-out mice. *J Clin Invest* 1997; 99:2752–2761.
57. Caligiuri G. The immune response in atherosclerosis and acute coronary syndromes. Thesis, Karolinska Institute, Stockholm, 1999.
58. Daugherty A, Puré E, Delfel-Butteiger D, et al. The effects of total lymphocyte deficiency on the extent of atherosclerosis in apolipoprotein E$^{-/-}$ mice. *J Clin Invest* 1997; 100:1575–1580.

59. Dansky HM, Charlton SA, Harper MM, Smith JD. T and B lymphocytes play a minor role in atherosclerotic plaque formation in the apolipoprotein E–deficient mouse. *Proc Natl Acad Sci USA* 1997; 94:4642–4646.
60. Mach F, Schonbeck U, Bonnefoy JY, et al. Activation of monocyte/macrophage functions related to acute atheroma complication by ligation of CD40: Induction of collagenase, stromelysin, and tissue factor. *Circulation* 1997; 96:396–399.
61. Mach F, Schonbeck U, Sukhova GK, et al. Reduction of atherosclerosis in mice by inhibition of CD40 signalling. *Nature* 1998; 394:200–203.
62. Lutgens E, Gorelik L, Daemen MJ, et al. Requirement for CD154 in the progression of atherosclerosis. *Nat Med* 1999; 5:1313–1316.
63. Wick G, Schett G, Amberger A, et al. Is atherosclerosis an immunologically mediated disease? *Immunol Today* 1995; 16:27–33.
64. Xu Q, Kiechl S, Mayr M, et al. Association of serum antibodies to heat-shock protein 65 with carotid atherosclerosis: Clinical significance determined in a follow-up study. *Circulation* 1999; 100:1169–1174.
65. Mayr M, Metzler B, Kiechl S, et al. Endothelial cytotoxicity mediated by serum antibodies to heat shock proteins of *Escherichia coli* and *Chlamydia pneumoniae*: Immune reactions to heat shock proteins as a possible link between infection and atherosclerosis. *Circulation* 1999; 99:1560–1566.
66. George J, Harats D, Gilburd B, et al. Immunolocalization of beta$_2$-glycoprotein I (apolipoprotein H) to human atherosclerotic plaques: Potential implications for lesion progression. *Circulation* 1999; 99:2227–2230.
67. Ross R. Atherosclerosis: An inflammatory disease. *N Engl J Med* 1999; 340:115–126.
68. Hu H, Pierce GN, Zhong G. The atherogenic effects of chlamydia are dependent on serum cholesterol and specific to *Chlamydia pneumoniae. J Clin Invest* 1999; 103:747–753.
69. Moazed TC, Campbell LA, Rosenfeld ME, et al. *Chlamydia pneumoniae* infection accelerates the progression of atherosclerosis in apolipoprotein E–deficient mice. *J Infect Dis* 1999; 180: 238–241.
70. Fabricant CG, Fabricant J, Litrenta MM, et al. Virus-induced atherosclerosis. *J Exp Med* 1978; 148:335–340.
71. Fabricant C, Fabricant J, Minick CR, et al. Herpes virus induced atherosclerosis in chickens. *Fed Proc* 1983; 42:2476–2479.
72. Ross R. The biology of atherosclerosis. In: Topol EJ, ed. *Comprehensive Cardiovascular Medicine*. Philadelphia: Lippincott-Raven; 1998:13.
73. Murayama T, Yokode M, Kataoka H, et al. Intraperitoneal administration of anti–c-fms monoclonal antibody prevents initial events of atherogenesis but does not reduce the size of advanced lesions in apolipoprotein E–deficient mice. *Circulation* 1999; 99:1740–1746.
74. Hasty AH, Linton MF, Brandt SJ, et al. Retroviral gene therapy in ApoE-deficient mice: ApoE expression in the artery wall reduces early foam cell lesion formation. *Circulation* 1999; 99:2571–2576.
75. Xiao Q, Danton MJ, Witte DP, et al. Fibrinogen deficiency is compatible with the development of atherosclerosis in mice. *J Clin Invest* 1998; 101:1184–1194.
76. Tangirala RK, Tsukamoto K, Chun SH, et al. Regression of atherosclerosis induced by liver-directed gene transfer of apolipoprotein A-I in mice. *Circulation* 1999; 100:1816–1822.
77. Tse J, Martin-McNaulty B, Halks-Miller M, et al. Accelerated atherosclerosis and premature calcified cartilaginous metaplasia in the aorta of diabetic male Apo E knockout mice can be prevented by chronic treatment with 17 beta-estradiol. *Atherosclerosis* 1999; 144:303–313.
78. Qiao JH, Xie PZ, Fishbein MC, et al. Pathology of atheromatous lesions in inbred and genetically engineered mice: Genetic determination of arterial calcification. *Arterioscler Thromb* 1994; 14: 1480–1497.
79. Towler DA, Bidder M, Latifi T, et al. Diet-induced diabetes activates an osteogenic gene regulatory program in the aortas of low density lipoprotein receptor–deficient mice. *J Biol Chem* 1998; 273:30,427–30,434.
80. Moulton KS, Heller E, Konerding MA, et al. Angiogenesis inhibitors endostatin or TNP-470 reduce intimal neovascularization and plaque growth in apolipoprotein E–deficient mice. *Circulation* 1999; 99:1726–1732.
81. Xiao Q, Danton MJ, Witte DP, et al. Plasminogen deficiency accelerates vessel wall disease in mice predisposed to atherosclerosis. *Proc Natl Acad Sci USA* 1997; 94:10,335–10,340.
82. Paigen B, Holmes PA, Novak EK, Swank RT. Analysis of atherosclerosis susceptibility in mice with genetic defects in platelet function. *Arteriosclerosis* 1990; 10:648–652.
83. Dansky HM, Charlton SA, Sikes JL, et al. Genetic background determines the extent of atherosclerosis in ApoE-deficient mice. *Arterioscler Thromb Vasc Biol* 1999; 19:1960–1968.
84. Parks WC. Who are the proteolytic culprits in vascular disease? *J Clin Invest* 1999; 104:1167–1168.
85. Carmeliet P, Moons L, Lijnen R, et al. Urokinase-generated plasmin activates matrix metalloproteinases during aneurysm formation. *Nat Genet* 1997; 17:439–444.
86. Jeng AY, Chou M, Sawyer WK, et al. Enhanced expression of matrix metalloproteinase-3, -12, and -13 mRNAs in the aortas of apolipoprotein E–deficient mice with advanced atherosclerosis. *Ann NY Acad Sci* 1999; 878:555–558.
87. Seo HS, Lombardi DM, Polinsky P, et al. Peripheral vascular stenosis in apolipoprotein E–deficient mice: Potential roles of lipid deposition, medial atrophy, and adventitial inflammation. *Arterioscler Thromb Vasc Biol* 1997; 17:3593–3601.
88. Bonthu S, Heistad DD, Chappell DA, et al. Atherosclerosis, vascular remodeling, and impairment of endothelium-dependent relaxation in genetically altered hyperlipidemic mice. *Arterioscler Thromb Vasc Biol* 1997; 17:2333–2340.
89. Bourdillon MC, et al. ICAM-1 deficiency reduces atherosclerotic lesions in double knockout mice (apoE$^{-/-}$/ICAM-1$^{-/-}$) fed a fat or a chow diet. In: 71st EAS Congress; 1999:94.
90. Smith JD, Trogan E, Ginsberg M, et al. Decreased atherosclerosis in mice deficient in both macrophage colony-stimulating factor (op) and apolipoprotein E. *Proc Natl Acad Sci USA* 1995; 92: 8264–8268.
91. Qiao JH, Tripathi J, Mishra NK, et al. Role of macrophage colony-stimulating factor in atherosclerosis: Studies of osteopetrotic mice. *Am J Pathol* 1997; 150:1687–1699.
92. Rajavashisth T, Qiao JH, Tripathi S, et al. Heterozygous osteopetrotic (op) mutation reduces atherosclerosis in LDL receptor–deficient mice. *J Clin Invest* 101:2702–2710.
93. Dawson TC, Kuziel WA, Osahar TA, Maeda N. Absence of CC chemokine receptor-2 reduces atherosclerosis in apolipoprotein E–deficient mice. *Atherosclerosis* 1999; 143:205–211.
94. Suzuki H, Kurihara Y, Takeya M, et al. A role for macrophage scavenger receptors in atherosclerosis and susceptibility to infection. *Nature* 1997; 386:292–296.
95. Sakaguchi H, Takeya M, Suzuki H, et al. Role of macrophage scavenger receptors in diet-induced atherosclerosis in mice. *Lab Invest* 1998; 78:423–434.
96. Febbraio M, Podrez EA, Smith JD, et al. Targeted disruption of the class B scavenger receptor CD36 protects against atherosclerotic lesion development in mice. *J Clin Invest* 2000; 105:1049–1056.
97. Benoit P, Emmanuel F, Caillaud JM, et al. Somatic gene transfer of human ApoA-I inhibits atherosclerosis progression in mouse models. *Circulation* 1999; 99:105–110.
98. Shah PK, Nilsson J, Kaul S, et al. Effects of recombinant apolipoprotein A-I (Milano) on aortic atherosclerosis in apolipoprotein E–deficient mice. *Circulation* 1998; 97:780–785.
99. George J, Afek A, Gilburd B, et al. Hyperimmunization of apo-

E-deficient mice with homologous malondialdehyde low-density lipoprotein suppresses early atherogenesis. *Atherosclerosis* 1998; 138:147–152.

100. Freigang S, Horkko S, Miller E, et al. Immunization of LDL receptor–deficient mice with homologous malondialdehyde-modified and native LDL reduces progression of atherosclerosis by mechanisms other than induction of high titers of antibodies to oxidative neoepitopes. *Arterioscler Thromb Vasc Biol* 1998; 18:1972–1982.
101. Pratico D, Tangirala RK, Rader DJ, et al. Vitamin E suppresses isoprostane generation in vivo and reduces atherosclerosis in ApoE-deficient mice. *Nat Med* 1998; 4:1189–1192.
102. Shaish A, George J, Gilburd B, et al. Dietary beta-carotene and alpha-tocopherol combination does not inhibit atherogenesis in an ApoE-deficient mouse model. *Arterioscler Thromb Vasc Biol* 1999; 19:1470–1475.
103. Witting PK, Pettersson K, Ostlund-Lindqvist AM, et al. Inhibition by a coantioxidant of aortic lipoprotein lipid peroxidation and atherosclerosis in apolipoprotein E and low density lipoprotein receptor gene double knockout mice. *FASEB J* 1999; 13:667–675.
104. Tangirala RK, Casanada F, Miller E, et al. Effect of the antioxidant N,N′-diphenyl 1,4-phenylenediamine (DPPD) on atherosclerosis in apoE-deficient mice. *Arterioscler Thromb Vasc Biol* 1995; 15:1625–1630.
105. Fuhrman B, Buch S, Vaya J, et al. Licorice extract and its major polyphenol glabridin protect low-density lipoprotein against lipid peroxidation: In vitro and ex vivo studies in humans and in atherosclerotic apolipoprotein E–deficient mice. *Am J Clin Nutr* 1997; 66:267–275.
106. Elhage R, Arnal JF, Pieraggi MT, et al. 17 beta-Estradiol prevents fatty streak formation in apolipoprotein E–deficient mice. *Arterioscler Thromb Vasc Biol* 1997; 17:2679–2684.
107. Aji W, Ravalli S, Szabolcs M, et al. L-Arginine prevents xanthoma development and inhibits atherosclerosis in LDL receptor knockout mice. *Circulation* 1997; 95:430–437.
108. Hayek T, Attias J, Smith J, et al. Antiatherosclerotic and antioxidative effects of captopril in apolipoprotein E–deficient mice. *J Cardiovasc Pharmacol* 1998; 31:540–544.
109. Keidar S, Attias J, Smith J, et al. The angiotensin-II receptor antagonist, losartan, inhibits LDL lipid peroxidation and atherosclerosis in apolipoprotein E–deficient mice. *Biochem Biophys Res Commun* 1997; 236:622–625.
110. Makaritsis KP, Gavras H, Du Y, et al. Alpha$_1$-adrenergic plus angiotensin receptor blockade reduces atherosclerosis in apolipoprotein E–deficient mice. *Hypertension* 1998; 32:1044–1048.
111. Nicoletti A, Kaveri S, Caligiuri G, et al. Immunoglobulin treatment reduces atherosclerosis in apoE knockout mice. *J Clin Invest* 1998; 102:910–918.
112. Elhage R, Maret A, Pieraggi MT, et al. Differential effects of interleukin-1 receptor antagonist and tumor necrosis factor binding protein on fatty-streak formation in apolipoprotein E–deficient mice. *Circulation* 1998; 97:242–244.
113. Moulton KS, Heller E, Konerding MA, et al. Angiogenesis inhibitors endostatin or TNP-470 reduce intimal neovascularization and plaque growth in apolipoprotein E–deficient mice. *Circulation* 1999; 99:1726–1732.
114. Schmidt AM, Yan SD, Wautier JL, Stern D. Activation of receptor for advanced glycation end products: A mechanism for chronic vascular dysfunction in diabetic vasculopathy and atherosclerosis. *Circ Res* 1999; 84:489–497.
115. Ni W, Tsuda Y, Sakono M, Imaizumi K. Dietary soy protein isolate, compared with casein, reduces atherosclerotic lesion area in apolipoprotein E–deficient mice. *J Nutr* 1998; 128:1884–1889.
116. Lee TS, Shiao MS, Pan CC, Chau LY. Iron-deficient diet reduces atherosclerotic lesions in apoE-deficient mice. *Circulation* 1999; 99:1222–1229.
117. Zhang SH, Reddick RL, Avdievich E, et al. Paradoxical enhancement of atherosclerosis by probucol treatment in apolipoprotein E–deficient mice. *J Clin Invest* 1997; 99:2858–2866.
118. Bird DA, Tangirala RK, Fruebis J, et al. Effect of probucol on LDL oxidation and atherosclerosis in LDL receptor–deficient mice. *J Lipid Res* 1998; 39:1079–1090.
119. Moghadasian MH, McManus BM, Godin DV, et al. Proatherogenic and antiatherogenic effects of probucol and phytosterols in apolipoprotein E–deficient mice: Possible mechanisms of action. *Circulation* 1999; 99:1733–1739.
120. Hsich E, Johnson TM, Zhou YF, et al. Cytomegalovirus infection increases development of atherosclerosis in apoE knockout mice (abstr). *FASEB J* 1999; 13:A692.
121. Lee TS, Yen HC, Pan CC, Chau LY. The role of interleukin 12 in the development of atherosclerosis in ApoE-deficient mice. *Arterioscler Thromb Vasc Biol* 1999; 19:734–742.
122. George J, Afek A, Gilburd B, et al. Induction of early atherosclerosis in LDL-receptor-deficient mice immunized with beta$_2$-glycoprotein I. *Circulation* 1998; 98:1108–1115.
123. Afek A, George J, Shoenfeld Y, et al. Enhancement of atherosclerosis in beta-2-glycoprotein I–immunized apolipoprotein E–deficient mice. *Pathobiology* 1999; 67:19–25.
124. Guevara NV, Kim HS, Antonova EI, Chan L. The absence of p53 accelerates atherosclerosis by increasing cell proliferation in vivo. *Nat Med* 1999; 5:335–339.
125. Keidar S, Attias J, Heinrich R, et al. Angiotensin II atherogenicity in apolipoprotein E deficient mice is associated with increased cellular cholesterol biosynthesis. *Atherosclerosis* 1999; 146: 249–257.
126. Stary HC, Blankenhorn DH, Chandler AB, et al. A definition of the intima of human arteries and of its atherosclerosis-prone regions: A report from the Committee on Vascular Lesions of the Council on Arteriosclerosis, American Heart Association. *Circulation* 1992; 85:391–405.
127. Stary HC, Chandler AB, Glagov S, et al. A definition of initial, fatty streak, and intermediate lesions of atherosclerosis: A report from the Committee on Vascular Lesions of the Council on Arteriosclerosis, American Heart Association. *Circulation* 1994; 89:2462–2478.
128. Stary HC, Chandler AB, Dinsmore RE, et al. A definition of advanced types of atherosclerotic lesions and a histological classification of atherosclerosis: A report from the Committee on Vascular Lesions of the Council on Arteriosclerosis, American Heart Association. *Circulation* 1995; 92:1355–1374.
129. DiCorleto PE, Gimbrone MA. Vascular Endothelium. In: Fuster V, Ross R, Topol EJ, eds. *Atherosclerosis and Coronary Artery Disease*, vol 1. Philadelphia: Lippincott-Raven; 1996:387.
130. Biegelsen ES, Loscalzo J. Endothelial function and atherosclerosis. *Coron Artery Dis* 1999; 10:241–256.
131. Reddy KG, Nair RN, Sheehan HM, Hodgson JM. Evidence that selective endothelial dysfunction may occur in the absence of angiographic or ultrasound atherosclerosis in patients with risk factors for atherosclerosis. *Am Coll Cardiol* 1994; 23:833–843.
132. Weninger WJ, Muller GB, Reiter C, et al. Intimal hyperplasia of the infant parasellar carotid artery: A potential developmental factor in atherosclerosis and SIDS. *Circ Res* 1999; 85:970–975.
133. Schwartz SM, De Blois D, O'Brien ER. The intima: Soil for atherosclerosis and restenosis. *Circ Res* 1995; 77:445–465.
134. Chung IM, Schwartz SM, Murry CE. Clonal architecture of normal and atherosclerotic aorta: Implications for atherogenesis and vascular development. *Am J Pathol* 1998; 152:913–923.
135. Ikari Y, McManus BM, Kenyon J, Schwartz SM. Neonatal intima formation in the human coronary artery. *Arterioscler Thromb Vasc Biol* 1999; 19:2036–2040.
136. Libby P. Molecular bases of the acute coronary syndromes. *Circulation* 1995; 91:2844–2850.
137. Hansson GK. Immune responses in atherosclerosis. In: GK Hans-

son, P Libby, eds: *Immune Functions of the Vessel Wall*. Harwood Academic; 1996.
138. McGill HC Jr. George Lyman Duff memorial lecture: Persistent problems in the pathogenesis of atherosclerosis. *Arteriosclerosis* 1984; 4:443–451.
139. Napoli C, D'Armiento FP, Mancini FP, et al. Fatty streak formation occurs in human fetal aortas and is greatly enhanced by maternal hypercholesterolemia: Intimal accumulation of low density lipoprotein and its oxidation precede monocyte recruitment into early atherosclerotic lesions. *J Clin Invest* 1997; 100:2680–2690.
140. Napoli C, Witztum JL, De Nigris F, et al. Intracranial arteries of human fetuses are more resistant to hypercholesterolemia-induced fatty streak formation than extracranial arteries. *Circulation* 1999; 99:2003–2010.
141. McGill HC Jr, McMahan CA, Malcom GT, et al. Effects of serum lipoproteins and smoking on atherosclerosis in young men and women. The PDAY Research Group: Pathobiological Determinants of Atherosclerosis in Youth. *Arterioscler Thromb Vasc Biol* 1997; 17:95–106.
142. Davies MJ, Woolf N. Atherosclerosis: What is it and why does it occur? *Br Heart J* 1993; 69(suppl):S3–S11.
143. Burrig K-F. The endothelium of advanced arteriosclerotic plaques in humans. *Arterioscler Thromb* 1991; 11:1678–1689.
144. Falk E, Fernández-Ortiz A. Role of thrombosis in atherosclerosis and its complications. *Am J Cardiol* 1995; 75:5B–11B.
145. O'Brien KD, McDonald TO, Chait A, et al. Neovascular expression of E-selectin, intercellular adhesion molecule-1, and vascular cell adhesion molecule-1 in human atherosclerosis and their relation to intimal leukocyte content. *Circulation* 1996; 93:672–682.
146. Fuster V, Badimon L, Badimon J, Chesebro JH. The pathogenesis of coronary artery disease and the acute coronary syndromes. *N Eng J Med* 1992; 326:242–250 and 310–318.
147. Fuster V, Fayad ZA, Badimon JJ. Acute coronary syndromes: Biology. *Lancet* 1999; 353(suppl II):5–9.
148. Toschi V, Gallo R, Lettino M, et al. Tissue factor modulates the thrombogenicity of human atherosclerotic plaque. *Circulation* 1997; 95:594–599.
149. Mann JM, Davies MJ. Vulnerable plaque: Relation of characteristics to degree of stenosis in human coronary arteries. *Circulation* 1996; 94:928–931.
150. Gertz SD, Roberts WC. Hemodynamic shear force in rupture of coronary arterial atherosclerotic plaques. *Am J Cardiol* 1990; 66:1368–1372.
151. Davies MJ, Richardson PD, Woolf N, et al. Risk of thrombosis in human atherosclerotic plaques: Role of extracellular lipid, macrophage, and smooth muscle cell content. *Br Heart J* 1993; 69:377–381.
152. Ball RY, Stowers EC, Burton JH, et al. Evidence that the death of macrophage foam cells contributes to the lipid core of atheroma. *Atherosclerosis* 1995; 114:45–54.
153. Geng Y-J, Libby P. Evidence for apoptosis in advanced human atheroma. *Am J Pathol* 1995; 147: 251–266.
154. Björkerud S, Björkerud B. Apoptosis is abundant in human atherosclerotic lesions, especially in inflammatory cells (macrophages and T cells), and may contribute to the accumulation of gruel and plaque instability. *Am J Pathol* 1996; 149:367–380.
155. Falk E. Plaque rupture with severe pre-existing stenosis precipitating coronary thrombosis: Characteristics of coronary atherosclerotic plaques underlying fatal occlusive thrombi. *Br Heart J* 1983; 50:127–134.
156. Van der Wal AC, Becker AE, Van der Loos CM, Das PK. Site of intimal rupture or erosion of thrombosed coronary atherosclerotic plaques is characterized by an inflammatory process irrespective of the dominant plaque morphology. *Circulation* 1994; 89:36–44.
157. Farb A, Burke AP, Tang AL, et al. Coronary plaque erosion without rupture into a lipid core: A frequent cause of coronary thrombosis in sudden coronary death. *Circulation* 1996; 93:1354–1363.
158. Van der Wal AC, Becker AE, Koch KT, et al. Clinically stable angina pectoris is not necessarily associated with histologically stable atherosclerotic plaques. *Heart* 1996; 76:312–316.
159. Moreno PR, Falk E, Palacios IF, et al. Macrophage infiltration in acute coronary syndromes: Implications for plaque rupture. *Circulation* 1994; 90:775–778.
160. Galis ZS, Sukhova GK, Lark MW, Libby P. Increased expression of matrix-metalloproteinases and matrix degrading activity in vulnerable regions of human atherosclerotic plaques. *J Clin Invest* 1994; 94:2493–2503.
161. Shah PK, Falk E, Badimon JJ, et al. Human monocyte-derived macrophages induce collagen breakdown in fibrous caps of atherosclerotic plaques: Potential role of matrix-degrading metalloproteinases and implications for plaque rupture. *Circulation* 1995; 92:1565–1569.
162. Kovanen PT, Kaartinen M, Paavonen T. Infiltrates of activated mast cells at the site of coronary atheromatous erosion or rupture in myocardial infarction. *Circulation* 1995; 92:1084–1088.
163. Danesh J, Collins R, Peto R. Chronic infections and coronary heart disease: Is there a link? (review). *Lancet* 1997; 350:430–436.
164. Libby P, Egan D, Skarlatos S. Roles of infectious agents in atherosclerosis and restenosis: An assessment of the evidence and need for future research. *Circulation* 1997; 96:4095–4103.
165. Kol A, Libby P. The mechanisms by which infectious agents may contribute to atherosclerosis and its clinical manifestations. *Trends Cardiovasc Med* 1998; 8:191–199.
166. Muhlestein JB, Hammond EH, Carlquist JF, et al. Increased incidence of *Chlamydia* species within the coronary arteries of patients with symptomatic atherosclerotic versus other forms of cardiovascular disease. *J Am Coll Cardiol* 1996; 27:1555–1561.
167. Kol A, Sukhova GK, Lichtman AH, Libby P. Chlamydial heat shock protein 60 localizes in human atheroma and regulates macrophage tumor necrosis factor-α and matrix metalloproteinase expression. *Circulation* 1998; 98:300–307.
168. Ridker PM, Cushman M, Stampfer MJ, et al. Inflammation, aspirin and the risk of cardiovascular disease in apparently healthy men. *N Engl J Med* 1997; 336:973–979.
169. Ridker PM, Buring JE, Shih J, et al. Prospective study of C-reactive protein and the risk of future cardiovascular events among apparently healthy women. *Circulation* 1998; 98:731–733.
170. Thompson SG, Kienast J, Pyke SD, et al. Hemostatic factors and the risk of myocardial infarction or sudden death in patients with angina pectoris. *N Engl J Med* 1995; 332:635–641.
171. Liuzzo G, Biasucci LM, Galimore R, et al. The prognostic value of C-reactive protein and serum amyloid A protein in severe unstable angina. *N Engl J Med* 1994; 331:417–424.
172. Toss H, Lindahl B, Siegbahn A, Wallentin L. Prognostic influence of increased fibrinogen and C-reactive protein levels in unstable coronary artery disease. *Circulation* 1997; 96:4204–4210.
173. Morrow DA, Rifai N, Antman EM, et al. C-reactive protein is a potent predictor of mortality independently of and in combination with troponin T in acute coronary syndromes: A TIMI 11A substudy. *J Am Coll Cardiol* 1998; 31:1460–1465.
174. Ridker PM, Rifai N, Pfeffer MA, et al. Inflammation, pravastatin, and the risk of coronary events after myocardial infarction in patients with average cholesterol levels. *Circulation* 1998; 98: 839–844.
175. Loree HM, Kamm RD, Stringfellow RG, Lee RT. Effects of fibrous cap thickness on peak circumferential stress in model atherosclerotic vessels. *Circulation Res* 1992; 71:850–858.
176. Burleigh MC, Briggs AD, Lendon CL, et al. Collagen types I and III, collagen content, GAGs and mechanical strength of human atherosclerotic plaque caps: Span-wise variations. *Atherosclerosis* 1992; 96:71–81.

177. Mann J, Davies MJ. Mechanisms of progression in native coronary artery disease: Role of healed plaque disruption. *Heart* 1999; 82:265–268.
178. Davies MJ, Bland JM, Hangartner JRW, et al. Factors influencing the presence or absence of acute coronary artery thrombi in sudden ischaemic death. *Eur Heart J* 1989; 10:203–208.
179. Davies MJ, Thomas A. Thrombosis and acute coronary-artery lesions in sudden cardiac ischemic death. *N Engl J Med* 1984; 310:1137–1140.
180. Richardson PD, Davies MJ, Born GVR. Influence of plaque configuration and stress distribution on fissuring of coronary atherosclerotic plaques. *Lancet* 1989; 2:941–944.
181. Cheng GC, Loree HM, Kamm RD, et al. Distribution of circumferential stress in ruptured and stable atherosclerotic lesions: A structural analysis with histopathological correlation. *Circulation* 1993; 87:1179–1187.
182. Davies MJ. The composition of coronary-artery plaques (editorial). *N Engl J Med* 1997; 336:1312–1314.
183. Arbustini E, Dal Bello B, Morbini P, et al. Plaque erosion is a major substrate for coronary thrombosis in acute myocardial infarction. *Heart* 1999; 82:269–272.
184. Jude B, Agraou B, McFadden EP, et al. Evidence for time-dependent activation of monocytes in the systemic circulation in unstable angina, but not in acute myocardial infarction or in stable angina. *Circulation* 1994; 90:1662–1668.
185. Badimon JJ, Lettino M, Toschi V, et al. Local inhibition of tissue factor reduces the thrombogenicity of disrupted human atherosclerotic plaques: Effects of tissue factor pathway inhibitor on plaque thrombogenicity under flow conditions. *Circulation* 1999; 99:1780–1787.
186. Mallat Z, Hugel B, Ohan J, et al. Shed membrane microparticles with procoagulant potential in human atherosclerotic plaques: A role for apoptosis in plaque thrombogenicity. *Circulation* 1999; 99:348–353.
187. Falk E, Fuster V, Shah PK. Interrelationship between atherosclerosis and thrombosis. In: Verstraete M, Fuster V, Topol EJ, eds. *Cardiovascular Thrombosis: Thrombocardiology and Thromboneurology*. Philadelphia: Lippincott-Raven; 1998:45.
188. Ge J, Erbel R, Gerber T, et al. Intravascular ultrasound imaging of angiographically normal coronary arteries: A prospective study in vivo. *Br Heart J* 1994; 71:572–578.
189. Roberts WC. Diffuse extent of coronary atherosclerosis in fatal coronary artery disease. *Am J Cardiol* 1990; 65:2F–6F.
190. Glagov S, Weisenberg E, Zarins CK, et al. Compensatory enlargement of human atherosclerotic coronary arteries. *N Engl J Med* 1987; 316:1371–1375.
191. Gibbons GH, Dzau VJ. The emerging concept of vascular remodeling. *N Engl J Med* 1994; 330:1431–1438.
192. Mintz GS, Kent KM, Pichard AD, et al. Contribution of inadequate arterial remodeling to the development of focal coronary artery stenoses: An intravascular ultrasound study. *Circulation* 1997; 95:1791–1798.
193. Smits PC, Pasterkamp G, Quarles van Ufford MA, et al. Coronary artery disease: Arterial remodelling and clinical presentation. *Heart* 1999; 82:461–464.
194. European Carotid Surgery Trialists Collaborative Group. Risk of stroke in the distribution of an asymptomatic carotid artery. *Lancet* 1995; 345:209–212.
195. Bogaty P, Hackett D, Davies G, Maseri A. Vasoreactivity of the culprit lesion in unstable angina. *Circulation* 1994; 90:5–11.
196. Lerman A, Edwards BS, Hallett JW, et al. Circulating and tissue endothelin immunoreactivity in advanced atherosclerosis. *N Engl J Med* 1991; 325:997–1001.
197. Zeiher AM, Goebel H, Schachinger V, Ihling C. Tissue endothelin-1 immunoreactivity in the active coronary atherosclerotic plaque: A clue to the mechanism of increased vasoreactivity of the culprit lesion in unstable angina. *Circulation* 1995; 91:941–947.
198. Donley GE, Fitzpatrick LA. Noncollagenous matrix proteins controlling mineralization: Possible role in pathologic calcification of vascular tissue. *Trends Cardiovasc Med* 1998; 8:199–206.
199. Wexler L, Brundage B, Crouse J, et al. Coronary artery calcification: Pathophysiology, epidemiology, imaging methods, and clinical implications—A statement for health professionals from the American Heart Association Writing Group. *Circulation* 1996; 94:1175–1192.
200. Blankenhorn DH. Coronary arterial calcification: A review. *Am J Med Sci* 1961; 242:41–49.
201. Lachman AS, Spray TL, Kerwin DM, et al. Medial calcinosis of Monckeberg: A review of the problem and a description of a patient with involvement of peripheral, visceral and coronary arteries. *Am J Med* 1977; 63:615–622.
202. Sangiorgi G, Rumberger JA, Severson A, et al. Arterial calcification and not lumen stenosis is highly correlated with atherosclerotic plaque burden in humans: A histologic study of 723 coronary artery segments using nondecalcifying methodology. *J Am Coll Cardiol* 1998; 31:126–133.
203. Mintz GS, Pichard AD, Popma JJ, et al. Determinants and correlates of target lesion calcium in coronary artery disease: A clinical, angiographic and intravascular ultrasound study. *J Am Coll Cardiol* 1997; 29:268–274.
204. Baumgart D, Schmermund A, Goerge G, et al. Comparison of electron beam computed tomography with intracoronary ultrasound and coronary angiography for detection of coronary atherosclerosis. *J Am Coll Cardiol* 1997; 30:57–64.
205. Hodgson JM, Reddy KG, Suneja R, et al. Intracoronary ultrasound imaging: Correlation of plaque morphology with angiography, clinical syndrome and procedural results in patients undergoing coronary angioplasty. *J Am Coll Cardiol* 1993; 21:35–44.
206. Rasheed Q, Nair R, Sheehan H, Hodgson JM. Correlation of intracoronary ultrasound plaque characteristics in atherosclerotic coronary artery disease patients with clinical variables. *Am J Cardiol* 1994; 73:753–758.
207. Gertz SD, Roberts WC. Hemodynamic shear force in rupture of coronary arterial atherosclerotic plaques. *Am J Cardiol* 1990; 66:1368–1372.
208. Callister TQ, Raggi P, Cooil B, et al. Effect of HMG-CoA reductase inhibitors on coronary artery disease as assessed by electron-beam computed tomography. *N Engl J Med* 1998; 339:1972–1978.
209. Solberg LA, Strong JP. Risk factors and atherosclerotic lesions: A review of autopsy studies. *Arteriosclerosis* 1983; 3:187–198.
210. Grundy SM, Pasternak R, Greenland P, et al. Assessment of cardiovascular risk by use of multiple-risk-factor assessment equations: A statement for healthcare professionals from the American Heart Association and the American College of Cardiology. *Circulation* 1999; 100:1481–1492.
211. Grundy SM, Wilhelmsen L, Rose G, et al. Coronary heart disease in high-risk populations: Lessons from Finland. *Eur Heart J* 1990; 11:462–471.
212. Roberts WC. Preventing and arresting coronary atherosclerosis. *Am Heart J* 1995; 130:580–600.
213. Keys A. *Seven Countries: A Multivariate Analysis of Death and Coronary Heart Disease*. Cambridge: Harvard University Press; 1980.
214. Wood D, Backer GD, Faergeman O, et al. Prevention of coronary heart disease in clinical practice: Recommendations of the Second Joint Task Force of European and Other Societies on Coronary Prevention. *Eur Heart J* 1998; 19:1434–1503.
215. Kannel WB. Range of serum cholesterol values in the population developing coronary artery disease. *Am J Cardiol* 1995; 76(suppl C):69C–77C.
216. Walker ARP. Cholesterol: How low is low enough? *BMJ* 1999; 318:538.
217. Epstein SE, Zhou YF, Zhu J. Infection and atherosclerosis: Emerging mechanistic paradigms. *Circulation* 1999; 100:e20–e28.

218. Stamler J, Stamler R, Neaton JD, et al. Low risk-factor profile and long-term cardiovascular and noncardiovascular mortality and life expectancy: Findings for 5 large cohorts of young adult and middle-aged men and women. *JAMA* 1999; 282:2012–2018.
219. Chen Z, Peto R, Collins R, et al. Serum cholesterol concentration and coronary heart disease in population with low cholesterol concentrations. *BMJ* 1991; 303:276–282.
220. Badimon JJ, Badimon L, Galvez A, et al. High density lipoprotein plasma fractions inhibit aortic fatty streaks in cholesterol-fed rabbits. *Lab Invest* 1989; 60:455–461.
221. Badimon JJ, Badimon L, Fuster V. Regression of atherosclerotic lesions by high density lipoprotein plasma fraction in the cholesterol-fed rabbit. *J Clin Invest* 1990; 85:1234–1241.
222. Dansky HM, Fisher EA. High-density lipoprotein and plaque regression: The good cholesterol gets even better (editorial). *Circulation* 1999; 100:1762–1763.
223. Berenson GS, Srinivasan SR, Bao W, et al. Association between multiple cardiovascular risk factors and atherosclerosis in children and young adults: The Bogalusa Heart Study. *N Engl J Med* 1998; 338:1650–1656.
224. Berenson GS, Srinivasan SR. Prevention of atherosclerosis in childhood (comment). *Lancet* 1999; 354:1223–1224.
225. Rainwater DL, McMahan CA, Malcom GT, et al. Lipid and apolipoprotein predictors of atherosclerosis in youth: Apolipoprotein concentrations do not materially improve prediction of arterial lesions in PDAY subjects. The PDAY Research Group. *Arterioscler Thromb Vasc Biol* 1999; 19:753–761.
226. Scanu AM. Atherothrombogenicity of lipoprotein(a): The debate. *Am J Cardiol* 1998; 82:26Q–33Q.
227. Burke AP, Farb A, Malcom GT, et al. Coronary risk factors and plaque morphology in men with coronary disease who died suddenly. *N Engl J Med* 1997; 336:1276–1282.
228. Burke AP, Farb A, Malcom GT, et al. Effect of risk factors on the mechanism of acute thrombosis and sudden coronary death in women. *Circulation* 1998; 97:2110–2116.
229. Ockene IS, Miller NH. Cigarette smoking, cardiovascular disease, and stroke: A statement for healthcare professionals from the American Heart Association. American Heart Association Task Force on Risk Reduction. *Circulation* 1997; 96:3243–3247.
230. Chen Z-M, Xu Z, Collins R, et al. Early health effects of the emerging tobacco epidemic in China: A 16-year prospective study. *JAMA* 1997; 278:1500–1504.
231. Lam TH, He Y, Li LS, et al. Mortality attributable to cigarette smoking in China. *JAMA* 1997; 278:1505–1508.
232. Jee SH, Suh I, Kim IS, Appel LJ. Smoking and atherosclerotic cardiovascular disease in men with low levels of serum cholesterol: The Korea Medical Insurance Corporation Study. *JAMA* 1999; 282:2149–2155.
233. Celermajer DS, Sorensen KE, Georgakopoulos D, et al. Cigarette smoking is associated with dose-related and potentially reversible impairment of endothelium-dependent dilation in healthy young adults. *Circulation* 1993; 88:2149–2155.
234. Yoshimura M, Yasue H, Nakayama M, et al. Genetic risk factors for coronary artery spasm: Significance of endothelial nitric oxide synthase gene $T^{-786}{\rightarrow}C$ and missense Glu^{298}Asp variants (abstr). *Circulation* 1999; 100(suppl I):I-819.
235. Kannel WB, Higgins M. Smoking and hypertension as predictors of cardiovascular risk in population studies. *J Hypertens* 1990; 8(suppl):S3–S8.
236. Wilhelmsen L. Coronary heart disease: Epidemiology of smoking and intervention studies of smoking. *Am Heart J* 1988; 115: 242–249.
237. Solberg LA, Strong JP, Holme I, et al. Stenoses in the coronary arteries: Relation to atherosclerotic lesions, coronary heart disease, and risk factors—The Oslo Study. *Lab Invest* 1985; 53: 648–655.
238. Reed DM, MacLean CJ, Hayashi T. Predictors of atherosclerosis in the Honolulu Heart Program: I. Biologic, dietary, and lifestyle characteristics. *Am J Epidemiol* 1987; 126:214–225.
239. Reed DM, Resch JA, Hayashi T, et al. A prospective study of cerebral artery atherosclerosis. *Stroke* 1988; 19:820–825.
240. Reed DM, Strong JP, Resch J, Hayashi T. Serum lipids and lipoproteins as predictors of atherosclerosis: An autopsy study. *Arteriosclerosis* 1989; 9:560–564.
241. Reed D, Marcus E, Hayashi T. Smoking as a predictor of atherosclerosis in the Honolulu heart program. *Adv Exp Med Biol* 1990; 273:17–25.
242. Zieske AW, Takei H, Fallon KB, Strong JP. Smoking and atherosclerosis in youth. *Atherosclerosis* 1999; 144:403–408.
243. Moreno PR, Leon MN, Vyalkov VA, et al. Coronary plaque composition and tissue factor in cigarette smokers (abstr). *Circulation* 1998; 98(suppl I):I-145.
244. Bøttcher M, Falk E. Pathology of the coronary arteries in smokers and nonsmokers. *J Cardiovasc Risk* 1999; 6:299–302.
245. Seltzer CC. The negative association in women between cigarette smoking and uncomplicated angina pectoris in the Framingham Heart Study data. *J Clin Epidemiol* 1991; 44:871–876.
246. Grines CL, Topol EJ, O'Neill WW, et al. Effect of cigarette smoking on outcome after thrombolytic therapy for myocardial infarction. *Circulation* 1995; 91:298–303.
247. Barbash GI, Reiner J, White HD, et al. Evaluation of paradoxic beneficial effects of smoking in patients receiving thrombolytic therapy for acute myocardial infarction: Mechanism of the "smoker's paradox" from the GUSTO-I trial, with angiographic insights. Global Utilization of Streptokinase and Tissue-Plasminogen Activator for Occluded Coronary Arteries. *J Am Coll Cardiol* 1995; 26:1222–1229.
248. Lundergan CF, Reiner JS, McCarthy WF, et al. Clinical predictors of early infarct-related artery patency following thrombolytic therapy: Importance of body weight, smoking history, infarct-related artery and choice of thrombolytic regimen—The GUSTO-I experience. Global Utilization of Streptokinase and t-PA for Occluded Coronary Arteries. *J Am Coll Cardiol* 1998; 32:641–647.
249. Roald HE, Orvim U, Bakken IJ, et al. Modulation of thrombotic responses in moderately stenosed arteries by cigarette smoking and aspirin ingestion. *Arterioscler Thromb* 1994; 14:617–621.
250. Hung J, Lam JY, Lacoste L, Letchacovski G. Cigarette smoking acutely increases platelet thrombus formation in patients with coronary artery disease taking aspirin. *Circulation* 1995; 92:2432–2436.
251. Nyboe J, Jensen G, Appleyard M, Schnohr P. Smoking and the risk of first acute myocardial infarction. *Am Heart J* 1991; 122:438–447.
252. Folts JD, Bonebrake FC. The effects of cigarette smoke and nicotine on platelet thrombus formation in stenosed dog coronary arteries: Inhibition with phentolamine. *Circulation* 1982; 65: 465–470.
253. Rogers WR, Carey KD, McMahan A, et al. Cigarette smoking, dietary hyperlipidemia, and experimental atherosclerosis in the baboon. *Exp Mol Pathol* 1988; 48:135–151.
254. He J, Vupputuri S, Allen K, et al. Passive smoking and the risk of coronary heart disease: A meta-analysis of epidemiologic studies. *N Engl J Med* 1999; 340:920–926.
255. Van den Hoogen PCW, Feskens EJM, Nagelkerke NJD, et al. The relation between blood pressure and mortality due to coronary heart disease among men in different parts of the world. *N Engl J Med* 2000; 342:1–8.
256. Kannel WB. Blood pressure as a cardiovascular risk factor: Prevention and treatment. *JAMA* 1996; 275:1571–1576.
257. Agerholm-Larsen B, Tybjærg-Hansen A, Schnohr P, Nordestgaard BG. ACE gene polymorphism explains 30–40% of variability in serum ACE activity in both women and men in the popula-

tion at large: The Copenhagen City Heart Study (letter). *Atherosclerosis* 1999; 147:425–427.
258. Lindpaintner K, Pfeffer MA, Kreutz R, et al. A prospective evaluation of an angiotensin-converting-enzyme gene polymorphism and the risk of ischemic heart disease. *N Engl J Med* 1995; 332:706–711.
259. Agerholm-Larsen B, Nordestgaard BG, Steffensen R, et al. ACE gene polymorphism: Ischemic heart disease and longevity in 10150 individuals—A case-referent and retrospective cohort study based on the Copenhagen City Heart Study. *Circulation* 1997; 95:2358–2367.
260. Yusuf S, Sleight P, Pogue J, et al. Effects of an angiotensin-converting-enzyme inhibitor, ramipril, on cardiovascular events in high-risk patients. The Heart Outcomes Prevention Evaluation Study Investigators. *N Engl J Med* 2000; 342:145–153.
261. Roberts WC. Frequency of systemic hypertension in various cardiovascular diseases. *Am J Cardiol* 1987; 60:1E–8E.
262. Falk E. Cardiac causes of death in hypertension. *Scand J Clin Lab Invest* 1989; 49(suppl 196):33–41.
263. Robertson WB, Strong JP. Atherosclerosis in persons with hypertension and diabetes mellitus. *Lab Invest* 1968; 18:538–551.
264. McGill HC Jr, Strong JP, Tracy RE, et al. Relation of a postmortem renal index of hypertension to atherosclerosis in youth. The Pathobiological Determinants of Atherosclerosis in Youth (PDAY) Research Group. *Arterioscler Thromb Vasc Biol* 1995; 15:2222–2228.
265. McGill HC Jr, McMahan CA, Tracy RE, et al. Relation of a postmortem renal index of hypertension to atherosclerosis and coronary artery size in young men and women. Pathobiological Determinants of Atherosclerosis in Youth (PDAY) Research Group. *Arterioscler Thromb Vasc Biol* 1998; 18:1108–1118.
266. Franklin SS, Khan SA, Wong ND, et al. Is pulse pressure useful in predicting risk for coronary heart disease? The Framingham Heart Study. *Circulation* 1999; 100:354–360.
267. Mosca L, Grundy SM, Judelson D, et al. Guide to preventive cardiology for women: AHA/ACC Scientific Statement Consensus Panel statement. *Circulation* 1999; 99:2480–2484.
268. Grundy SM, Benjamin IJ, Burke GL, et al. Diabetes and cardiovascular disease: A statement for healthcare professionals from the American Heart Association. *Circulation* 1999; 100:1134–1146.
269. Gerstein HC, Yusuf S. Dysglycaemia and risk of cardiovascular disease. *Lancet* 1996; 347:949–950.
270. Gerstein HC, Pais P, Pogue J, Yusuf S. Relationship of glucose and insulin levels to the risk of myocardial infarction: A case-control study. *J Am Coll Cardiol* 1999; 33:612–619.
271. Laakso M. Hyperglycemia and cardiovascular disease in type 2 diabetes. *Diabetes* 1999; 48:937–942.
272. Coutinho M, Gerstein HC, Wang Y, Yusuf S. The relationship between glucose and incident cardiovascular events: A metaregression analysis of published data from 20 studies of 95,783 individuals followed for 12.4 years. *Diabetes Care* 1999; 22: 233–240.
273. Burchfiel CM, Reed DM, Marcus EB, et al. Association of diabetes mellitus with coronary atherosclerosis and myocardial lesions: An autopsy study from the Honolulu Heart Program. *Am J Epidemiol* 1993; 137:1328–1340.
274. McGill HC Jr, McMahan CA, Malcom GT, et al. Relation of glycohemoglobin and adiposity to atherosclerosis in youth. Pathobiological Determinants of Atherosclerosis in Youth (PDAY) Research Group. *Arterioscler Thromb Vasc Biol* 1995; 15: 431–440.
275. American Diabetes Association. Consensus development conference on the diagnosis of coronary heart disease in people with diabetes: 10–11 February 1998, Miami, Florida. *Diabetes Care* 1998; 21:1551–1559.
276. Marso SP, Mak K-H, Topol EJ. Diabetes mellitus: Biological determinants of atherosclerosis and restenosis. *Semin Intervent Cardiol* 1999; 4:129–143.
277. Lehto S, Niskanen L, Suhonen M, et al. Medial artery calcification: A neglected harbinger of cardiovascular complications in non-insulin-dependent diabetes mellitus. *Arterioscler Thromb Vasc Biol* 1996; 16:978–983.
278. Niskanen L, Siitonen O, Suhonen M, Uusitupa MI. Medial artery calcification predicts cardiovascular mortality in patients with NIDDM. *Diabetes Care* 1994; 17:1252–1256.
279. Salomaa V, Riley W, Kark JD, et al. Non-insulin-dependent diabetes mellitus and fasting glucose and insulin concentrations are associated with arterial stiffness indexes: The ARIC Study. Atherosclerosis Risk in Communities Study. *Circulation* 1995; 91:1432–1443.
280. UK Prospective Diabetes Study (UKPDS) Group. Intensive blood-glucose control with sulphonylureas or insulin compared with conventional treatment and risk of complications in patients with type 2 diabetes (UKPDS 33). *Lancet* 1998; 352:837–853 [published erratum appears in *Lancet* 1999; 354:602].
281. Haffner SM, Alexander CM, Cook TJ, et al. Reduced coronary events in simvastatin-treated patients with coronary heart disease and diabetes or impaired fasting glucose levels: Subgroup analyses in the Scandinavian Simvastatin Survival Study. *Arch Intern Med* 1999; 159:2661–2667.
282. Malmberg K. Prospective randomised study of intensive insulin treatment on long term survival after acute myocardial infarction in patients with diabetes mellitus. DIGAMI (Diabetes Mellitus, Insulin Glucose Infusion in Acute Myocardial Infarction) Study Group. *BMJ* 1997; 314:1512–1515.
283. Anderson WAD, Kissane JM, eds. *Pathology*, 7th ed. St Louis: CV Mosby; 1977:25.
284. Stefanadis C, Diamantopoulos L, Vlachopoulos C, et al. Thermal heterogeneity within human atherosclerotic coronary arteries detected in vivo: A new method of detection by application of a special thermography catheter. *Circulation* 1999; 99:1965–1971.
285. Casscells W, Hathorn B, David M, et al. Thermal detection of cellular infiltrates in living atherosclerotic plaques: Possible implications for plaque rupture and thrombosis. *Lancet* 1996; 347: 1447–1451.
286. Danesh J, Collins R, Appleby P, Peto R. Association of fibrinogen, C-reactive protein, albumin, or leukocyte count with coronary heart disease: Meta-analyses of prospective studies. *JAMA* 1998; 279:1477–1482.
287. Lagrand WK, Visser CA, Hermens WT, et al. C-reactive protein as a cardiovascular risk factor: More than an epiphenomenon? *Circulation* 1999; 100:96–102.
288. Biasucci LM, Vitelli A, Liuzzo G, et al. Elevated levels of interleukin-6 in unstable angina. *Circulation* 1996; 94:874–877.
289. Ikonomidis I, Andreotti F, Economou E, et al. Increased proinflammatory cytokines in patients with chronic stable angina and their reduction by aspirin. *Circulation* 1999; 100:793–798.
290. Hwang SJ, Ballantyne CM, Sharrett AR, et al. Circulating adhesion molecules VCAM-1, ICAM-1, and E-selectin in carotid atherosclerosis and incident coronary heart disease cases. The Atherosclerosis Risk in Communities (ARIC) study. *Circulation* 1997; 96:4219–4225.
291. Ridker PM, Hennekens CH, Roitman-Johnson B, et al. Plasma concentration of soluble intercellular adhesion molecule 1 and risks of future myocardial infarction in apparently healthy men. *Lancet* 1998; 351:88–92.
292. Libby P, Ridker PM. Novel inflammatory markers of coronary risk: Theory versus practice (editorial). *Circulation* 1999; 100: 1148–1150.
293. International Symposium on Infection and Atherosclerosis. *Am Heart J* 1999; 138(5 pt 2, suppl):S417–S560.
294. Meier CR, Derby LE, Jick SS, et al. Antibiotics and risk of

subsequent first-time acute myocardial infarction. *JAMA* 1999; 281:427–431.

295. Danesh J, Youngman L, Clark S, et al. *Helicobacter pylori* infection and early onset myocardial infarction: Case-control and sibling pairs study. *BMJ* 1999; 319:1157–1162.
296. Ridker PM, Kundsin RB, Stampfer MJ, et al. Prospective study of *Chlamydia pneumoniae* IgG seropositivity and risks of future myocardial infarction. *Circulation* 1999; 99:1161–1164.
297. Ridker PM, Hennekens CH, Buring JE, et al. Baseline IgG antibody titers to *Chlamydia pneumoniae, Helicobacter pylori,* herpes simplex virus, and cytomegalovirus and the risk for cardiovascular disease in women. *Ann Intern Med* 1999; 131:573–577.
298. Nieto FJ, Folsom AR, Sorlie PD, et al. *Chlamydia pneumoniae* infection and incident coronary heart disease: The Atherosclerosis Risk in Communities Study. *Am J Epidemiol* 1999; 150: 149–156.
299. Kaehler J et al. Antibodies to *Chlamydia pneumoniae* in unstable angina: Results from the CAPTURE trial (abstr). *Circulation* 1999(suppl).
300. Danesh J, Wong Y, Ward M, Muir J. Chronic infection with *Helicobacter pylori, Chlamydia pneumoniae,* or cytomegalovirus: Population based study of coronary heart disease. *Heart* 1999; 81:245–247.
301. Anderson JL, Muhlestein JB, Carlquist J, et al. Randomized secondary prevention trial of azithromycin in patients with coronary artery disease and serological evidence for *Chlamydia pneumoniae* infection: The Azithromycin in Coronary Artery Disease—Elimination of Myocardial Infection with *Chlamydia* (ACADEMIC) study. *Circulation* 1999; 99:1540–1547.
302. Jackson LA, Smith NL, Heckbert SR, et al. Lack of association between first myocardial infarction and past use of erythromycin, tetracycline, or doxycycline. *Emerg Infect Dis* 1999; 5: 281–284.
303. Weiss SM, Roblin PM, Gaydos CA, et al. Failure to detect *Chlamydia pneumoniae* in coronary atheromas of patients undergoing atherectomy. *J Infect Dis* 1996; 173:957–962.
304. Paterson DL, Hall J, Rasmussen SJ, Timms P. Failure to detect *Chlamydia pneumoniae* in atherosclerotic plaques of Australian patients. *Pathology* 1998; 30:169–172.
305. Jantos CA, Nesseler A, Waas W, et al. Low prevalence of *Chlamydia pneumoniae* in atherectomy specimens from patients with coronary heart disease. *Clin Infect Dis* 1999; 28:988–992.
306. Meijer A, Van der Vliet JA, Roholl PJ, et al. *Chlamydia pneumoniae* in abdominal aortic aneurysms: Abundance of membrane components in the absence of heat shock protein 60 and DNA. *Arterioscler Thromb Vasc Biol* 1999; 19:2680–2686.
307. Koenig W, Rothenbacher D, Hoffmeister A, et al. Infection with *Helicobacter pylori* is not a major independent risk factor for stable coronary heart disease: Lack of a role of cytotoxin-associated protein A–positive strains and absence of a systemic inflammatory response. *Circulation* 1999; 100:2326–2331.
308. Epstein SE, Zhu J. Lack of association of infectious agents with risk of future myocardial infarction and stroke: Definitive evidence disproving the infection/coronary artery disease hypothesis (editorial). *Circulation* 1999; 100:1366–1368.
309. Hendrix MG, Salimans MM, Van Boven CP, Bruggeman CA. High prevalence of latently present cytomegalovirus in arterial walls of patients suffering from grade III atherosclerosis. *Am J Pathol* 1990; 136:23–28.
310. Hansson GK, Libby P. The role of lymphocyte. In: Fuster V, Ross R, Topol EJ, eds. *Atherosclerosis and Coronary Artery Disease.* Philadelphia: Lippincott-Raven; 1996:557–568.
311. Duplaa C, Couffinhal T, Labat L, et al. Monocyte/macrophage recruitment and expression of endothelial adhesion proteins in human atherosclerotic lesions. *Atherosclerosis* 1996; 121: 253–266.
312. Thorne SA, Abbot SE, Stevens CR, et al. Modified low density lipoprotein and cytokines mediate monocyte adhesion to smooth muscle cells. *Atherosclerosis* 1996; 127:167–176.
313. Moyer CF, Sajuthi D, Tulli H, Williams JK. Synthesis of IL-1 alpha and IL-1 beta by arterial cells in atherosclerosis. *Am J Pathol* 1991; 138:951–960.
314. Rus HG, Niculescu F, Vlaicu R. Tumor necrosis factor-alpha in human arterial wall with atherosclerosis. *Atherosclerosis* 1991; 89:247–254.
315. Endres M, Laufs U, Merz H, Kaps M. Focal expression of intercellular adhesion molecule-1 in the human carotid bifurcation. *Stroke* 1997; 28:77–82.
316. Lawn RM, Pearle AD, Kunz LL, et al. Feedback mechanism of focal vascular lesion formation in transgenic apolipoprotein(a) mice. *J Biol Chem* 1996; 271:31,367–31,371.
317. Tipping PG, Hancock WW. Production of tumor necrosis factor and interleukin-1 by macrophages from human atheromatous plaques. *Am J Pathol* 1993; 142:1721–1728.
318. Reape TJ, Groot PHE. Chemokines and atherosclerosis. *Atherosclerosis* 1999; 147:213–225.
319. Rabbani LE, Loscalzo J. Recent observations on the role of hemostatic determinants in the development of the atherothrombotic plaque. *Atherosclerosis* 1994; 105:1–7.
320. Reynolds GD, Vance RP. C-reactive protein immunohistochemical localization in normal and atherosclerotic human aortas. *Arch Pathol Lab Med* 1987; 111:265–269.
321. Hatanaka K, Li XA, Masuda K, et al. Immunohistochemical localization of C-reactive protein-binding sites in human atherosclerotic aortic lesions by a modified streptavidin-biotin–staining method. *Pathol Int* 1995; 45:635–641.
322. Meek RL, Urieli-Shoval S, Benditt EP. Expression of apolipoprotein serum amyloid A mRNA in human atherosclerotic lesions and cultured vascular cells: Implications for serum amyloid A function. *Proc Natl Acad Sci USA* 1994; 91:3186–3190.
323. Kol A, Libby P. The mechanisms by which infectious agents may contribute to atherosclerosis and its clinical manifestations. *Trends Cardiovasc Med* 1998; 8:191–199.
324. Fuster V, Gotto AM, Libby P, et al. Task Force 1: Pathogenesis of coronary disease—The biologic role of risk factors. *J Am Coll Cardiol* 1996; 27:964–976.
325. Meade TW, Miller GJ, Rosenberg ED. Characteristics associated with the risk of arterial thrombosis. In: Verstraete M, Fuster V, Topol EJ, eds. *Cardiovascular Thrombosis: Thrombocardiology and Thromboneurology*. Philadelphia: Lippincott-Raven; 1998: 77.
326. Maresca G, Blasio AD, Marchioli R, Minno GD. Measuring plasma fibrinogen to predict stroke and myocardial infarction: An Update. *Arterioscler Thromb Vasc Biol* 1999; 19:1368–1377.
327. Iacoviello L, Di Castelnuovo A, De Knijff P, et al. Polymorphisms in the coagulation factor VII gene and the risk of myocardial infarction. *N Engl J Med* 1998; 338:79–85.
328. Doggen CJM, Cats VM, Bertina RM, Rosendaal FR. Interaction of coagulation defects and cardiovascular risk factors: Increased risk of myocardial infarction associated with factor V Leiden or prothrombin 20210A. *Circulation* 1998; 97:1037–1041.
329. Tybjærg-Hansen A, Agerholm-Larsen B, Humphries SE, et al. A common mutation (G−455→A) in the β-fibrinogen promoter is an independent predictor of plasma fibrinogen, but not of ischemic heart disease. *J Clin Invest* 1997; 99:3034–3039.
330. DeLoughery TG. Coagulation abnormalities and cardiovascular disease. *Curr Opin Lipidol* 1999; 10:443–448.
331. Ardissino D, Mannucci PM, Merlini PA, et al. Prothrombotic genetic risk factors in young survivors of myocardial infarction. *Blood* 1999; 94:46–51.
332. Doggen CJ, Manger CV, Bertina RM, et al. A genetic propensity to high factor VII is not associated with the risk of myocardial infarction in men. *Thromb Haemost* 1998; 80:281–285.
333. Tamaki S, Iwai N, Nakamura Y, et al. Variation of the factor

VII gene and ischemic heart disease in Japanese subjects. *Coron Artery Dis* 1999; 10:601–606.
334. Steeds R, Adams M, Smith P, et al. Distribution of tissue plasminogen activator insertion/deletion polymorphism in myocardial infarction and control subjects. *Thromb Haemost* 1998; 79: 980–984.
335. Ridker PM, Hennekens CH, Lindpaintner K, et al. Arterial and venous thrombosis is not associated with the 4G/5G polymorphism in the promotor of the plasminogen activator inhibitor gene in a large cohort of US men. *Circulation* 1997; 95:59–62.
336. Walter DH, Schachinger V, Elsner M, et al. Platelet glycoprotein IIIa polymorphisms and risk of coronary stent thrombosis. *Lancet* 1997; 350:1217–1219.
337. Goldschmidt-Clermont PJ, Coleman LD, Pham YM, et al. Higher prevalence of GPIIIa PlA2 polymorphism in siblings of patients with premature coronary heart disease. *Arch Pathol Lab Med* 1999; 123:1223–1229.
338. Moshfegh K, Wueillemin WA, Redondo M, et al. Association of two silent polymorphisms of platelet glycoprotein Ia/IIa receptor with risk of myocardial infarction: A case-control study. *Lancet* 1999; 353:351–354.
339. Boushey CJ, Beresford SA, Omenn GS, Motulsky AG. A quantitative assessment of plasma homocysteine as a risk factor for vascular disease: Probable benefits of increasing folic acid intakes. *JAMA* 1995; 274:1049–1057.
340. Robinson K, Arheart K, Refsum H, et al. Low circulating folate and vitamin B_6 concentrations: Risk factors for stroke, peripheral vascular disease, and coronary artery disease. European COMAC Group. *Circulation* 1998; 97:437–443.
341. Refsum H, Ueland PM, Nygard O, Vollset SE. Homocysteine and cardiovascular disease. *Annu Rev Med* 1998; 49:31–62.
342. Malinow MR, Bostom AG, Krauss RM. Homocyst(e)ine, diet, and cardiovascular diseases: A statement for healthcare professionals from the Nutrition Committee, American Heart Association. *Circulation* 1999; 99:178–182.
343. Hankey GJ, Eikelboom JW. Homocysteine and vascular disease. *Lancet* 1999; 354:407–413.
344. McQuillan BM, Beilby JP, Nidorf M, et al. Hyperhomocysteinemia but not the C677T mutation of methylenetetrahydrofolate reductase is an independent risk determinant of carotid wall thickening. The Perth Carotid Ultrasound Disease Assessment Study. *Circulation* 1999; 99:2383–2388.
345. Chao C-L, Tsai H-H, Lee C-M, et al. The graded effect of hyperhomocysteinemia on the severity and extent of coronary atherosclerosis. *Atherosclerosis* 1999; 147:379–380.
346. Stampfer MJ, Malinow MR, Willett WC, et al. A prospective study of plasma homocyst(e)ine and risk of myocardial infarction in US physicians. *JAMA* 1992; 268:877–881.
347. Arnesen E, Refsum H, Bonaa KH, et al. Serum total homocysteine and coronary heart disease. *Int J Epidemiol* 1995; 24:704–709.
348. Ridker PM, Manson JE, Buring JE, et al. Homocysteine and risk of cardiovascular disease among postmenopausal women. *JAMA* 1999; 281:1817–1821.
349. Evans RW, Shaten BJ, Hempel JD, et al. Homocyst(e)ine and risk of cardiovascular disease in the Multiple Risk Factor Intervention Trial. *Arterioscler Thromb Vasc Biol* 1997; 17:1947–1953.
350. Kuller LH, Evans RW. Homocysteine, vitamins, and cardiovascular disease (editorial). *Circulation* 1998; 98:196–199.
351. Cattaneo M. Hyperhomocysteinemia, atherosclerosis and thrombosis. *Thromb Haemost* 1999; 81:165–176.
352. Wall RT, Harlan JM, Harker LA, Striker GE. Homocysteine-induced endothelial cell injury in vitro: A model for the study of vascular injury. *Thromb Res* 1980; 18:113–121.
353. Upchurch GR Jr, Welch GN, Fabian AJ, et al. Homocyst(e)ine decreases bioavailable nitric oxide by a mechanism involving glutathione peroxidase. *J Biol Chem* 1997; 272:17,012–17,017.
354. Tsai JC, Perrella MA, Yoshizumi M, et al. Promotion of vascular smooth muscle cell growth by homocysteine: A link to atherosclerosis. *Proc Natl Acad Sci USA* 1994; 91:6369–6373.
355. Majors A, Ehrhart LA, Pezacka EH. Homocysteine as a risk factor for vascular disease: Enhanced collagen production and accumulation by smooth muscle cells. *Arterioscler Thromb Vasc Biol* 1997; 17:2074–2081.
356. Lentz SR, Sobey CG, Piegors DJ, et al. Vascular dysfunction in monkeys with diet-induced hyperhomocyst(e)inemia. *J Clin Invest* 1996; 98:24–29.
357. Pasceri V, Willerson JT. Homocysteine and coronary heart disease: A review of the current evidence. *Semin Intervent Cardiol* 1999; 4:121–128.
358. Celermajer DS, Sorensen K, Ryalls M, et al. Impaired endothelial function occurs in the systemic arteries of children with homozygous homocystinuria but not in their heterozygous parents. *J Am Coll Cardiol* 1993; 22:854–858.
359. Chambers JC, Obeid OA, Kooner JS. Physiological increments in plasma homocysteine induce vascular endothelial dysfunction in normal human subjects. *Arterioscler Thromb Vasc Biol* 1999; 19:2922–2927.
360. Kanani PM, Sinkey CA, Browning RL, et al. Role of oxidant stress in endothelial dysfunction produced by experimental hyperhomocyst(e)inemia in humans. *Circulation* 1999; 100:1161–1168.
361. Nygard O, Nordrehaug JE, Refsum H, et al. Plasma homocysteine levels and mortality in patients with coronary artery disease. *N Engl J Med* 1997; 337:230–236.
362. Ray JG. Meta-analysis of hyperhomocysteinemia as a risk factor for venous thromboembolic disease. *Arch Intern Med* 1998; 158:2101–2106.
363. Ridker PM, Hennekens CH, Selhub J, et al. Interrelation of hyperhomocyst(e)inemia, factor V Leiden, and risk of future venous thromboembolism. *Circulation* 1997; 95:1777–1782.
364. Lentz SR, Sadler JE. Inhibition of thrombomodulin surface expression and protein C activation by the thrombogenic agent homocysteine. *J Clin Invest* 1991; 88:1906–1914.
365. Fryer RH, Wilson BD, Gubler DB, et al. Homocysteine, a risk factor for premature vascular disease and thrombosis, induces tissue factor activity in endothelial cells. *Arterioscler Thromb* 1993; 13:1327–1333.
366. Durand P, Lussier-Cacan S, Blache D. Acute methionine load-induced hyperhomocysteinemia enhances platelet aggregation, thromboxane biosynthesis, and macrophage-derived tissue factor activity in rats. *FASEB J* 1997; 11:1157–1168.
367. Rubba P, Mercuri M, Faccenda F, et al. Premature carotid atherosclerosis: Does it occur in both familial hypercholesterolemia and homocystinuria? Ultrasound assessment of arterial intima-media thickness and blood flow velocity. *Stroke* 1994; 25:943–950.
368. Rimm EB, Williams P, Fosher K, et al. Moderate alcohol intake and lower risk of coronary heart disease: Meta-analysis of effects on lipids and haemostatic factors. *BMJ* 1999; 319:1523–1528.
369. Yuan J-M, Ross RK, Gao Y-T, et al. Follow up study of moderate alcohol intake and mortality among middle aged men in Shanghai, China. *BMJ* 1997; 314:18–23.
370. Law M, Wald N. Why heart disease mortality is low in France: The time lag explanation. *BMJ* 1999; 318:1471–1476.
371. Renaud S, De Lorgeril M. Wine, alcohol, platelets, and the French paradox for coronary heart disease. *Lancet* 1992; 339:1523–1526.
372. Ridker PM, Vaughan DE, Stampfer MJ, et al. Association of moderate alcohol consumption and plasma concentration of endogenous tissue-type plasminogen activator. *JAMA* 1994; 272: 929–933.
373. Lee AJ, Flanagan PA, Rumley A, et al. Relationship between alcohol intake and tissue plasminogen activator antigen and other haemostatic factors in the general population. *Fibrinolysis* 1995; 8:49–54.

374. Iso H, Kitamura A, Shimamoto T, et al. Alcohol intake and the risk of cardiovascular disease in middle-aged Japanese men. *Stroke* 1995; 26:767–773.
375. Hommel M. Alcohol for stroke prevention? *N Engl J Med* 1999; 341:1605–1606.
376. Lee AJ, Flanagan PA, Rumley A, et al. Relationship between alcohol intake and tissue plasminogen activator antigen and other haemostatic factors in the general population. *Fibrinolysis* 1995; 8:49–54.
377. Valmadrid CT, Klein R, Moss SE, et al. Alcohol intake and the risk of coronary heart disease mortality in persons with older-onset diabetes mellitus. *JAMA* 1999; 282:239–246.
378. Rimm EB, Klatsky A, Stampfer MJ. Review of moderate alcohol consumption and reduced risk of coronary heart disease: Is the effect due to beer, wine, or spirits? *BMJ* 1996; 312:731–736.
379. Klatsky AL, Armstrong MA. Alcoholic beverage choice and risk of coronary artery disease mortality: Do red wine drinkers fare best? *Am J Cardiol* 1993; 71:467–469.
380. Grønbæk M, Deis A, Sørensen TIA, et al. Mortality associated with moderate intakes of wine, beer, or spirits. *BMJ* 1995; 310:1165–1169.
381. Truelsen T, Grønbæk M, Schnohr P, Boysen G. Intake of beer, wine, and spirits and risk of stroke: The Copenhagen City Heart Study. *Stroke* 1998; 29:2467–2472.
382. Folts JD. Antithrombotic potential of grape juice and red wine for preventing heart attacks. *Pharm Biol* 1998; 36:1–7.
383. Stein JH, Keevil JG, Aeschlimann S, Folts JD. Purple grape juice improves endothelial function and reduces the susceptibility of LDL cholesterol to oxidation in patients with coronary artery disease. *Circulation* 1999; 100;1050–1055.
384. Wollny T, Aiello L, Di Tommaso D, et al. Modulation of haemostatic function and prevention of experimental thrombosis by red wine in rats: A role for increased nitric oxide production. *Br J Pharmacol* 1999; 127:747–755.
385. Tjønneland A, Grønbæk M, Stripp C, Overvad K. Wine intake and diet in a random sample of 48763 Danish men and women. *Am J Clin Nutr* 1999; 69:49–54.
386. Klatsky AL, Armstrong MA, Klipp H. Correlates of alcoholic beverage preference: Traits of persons who choose wine, liquor or beer. *Br J Addict* 1990; 85:1279–1289.
387. Wannamethee SG, Shaper AG. Type of alcoholic drink and risk of major coronary heart disease events and all-cause mortality. *Am J Public Health* 1999; 89:685–690.
388. Poikolainen K, Vartiainen E. Wine and good subjective health. *Am J Epidemiol* 1999; 150:47–50.
389. McKee M, Britton A. The positive relationship between alcohol and heart disease in Eastern Europe: Potential physiological mechanisms. *J R Soc Med* 1998; 91:402–407.
390. Kauhanen J, Kaplan GA, Goldberg DE, Salonen JT. Beer binging and mortality: Results from the Kuopio ischaemic heart disease risk factor study, a prospective population based study. *BMJ* 1997; 315:846–851.
391. Iso H, Kitamura A, Shimamoto T, et al. Alcohol intake and the risk of cardiovascular disease in middle-aged Japanese men. *Stroke* 1995; 26:767–773.
392. Albert CM, Manson JE, Cook NR, et al. Moderate alcohol consumption and the risk of sudden cardiac death among US male physicians. *Circulation* 1999; 100:944–950.
393. Simini B, Serge Renaud. Serge Renaud: From French paradox to Cretan miracle. *Lancet* 2000; 355:48.
394. Criqui MH, Ringel BL. Does diet or alcohol explain the French paradox? *Lancet* 1994; 344:1719–1723.
395. Law M, Wald N. Why heart disease mortality is low in France: The time lag explanation. *BMJ* 1999; 318:1471–1476.
396. Grundy SM, Balady GJ, Criqui MH, et al. Primary prevention of coronary heart disease: Guidance from Framingham—A statement for healthcare professionals from the AHA Task Force on Risk Reduction, American Heart Association. *Circulation* 1998; 97:1876–1887.
397. Walsh BW, Schiff I, Rosner B, et al. Effects of postmenopausal estrogen replacement on the concentrations and metabolism of plasma lipoproteins. *N Engl J Med* 1991; 325:1196–1204.
398. Bush DE, Jones CE, Bass KM, et al. Estrogen replacement reverses endothelial dysfunction in postmenopausal women. *Am J Med* 1998; 104:552–558.
399. Adams MR, Kaplan JR, Manuck SB, et al. Inhibition of coronary artery atherosclerosis by 17-beta estradiol in ovariectomized monkeys: Lack of an effect of added progesterone. *Arteriosclerosis* 1990; 10:1051–1057.
400. Kushwaha RS, Lewis DS, Carey KD, McGill HC Jr. Effects of estrogen and progesterone on plasma lipoproteins and experimental atherosclerosis in the baboon (*Papio* sp.). *Arterioscler Thromb* 1991; 11:23–31.
401. Haarbo J, Leth-Espensen P, Stender S, Christiansen C. Estrogen monotherapy and combined estrogen-progestogen replacement therapy attenuate aortic accumulation of cholesterol in ovariectomized cholesterol-fed rabbits. *J Clin Invest* 1991; 87:1274–1279.
402. Holm P, Andersen HL, Andersen MR, et al. The direct antiatherogenic effect of estrogen is present, absent, or reversed, depending on the state of the arterial endothelium: A time course study in cholesterol-clamped rabbits. *Circulation* 1999; 100:1727–1733.
403. Ornstein DL, Zacharski LR. Coronary artery disease in men and women. *N Engl J Med* 1999; 341:1933–1934.
404. Roest M, Van der Schouw YT, De Valk B, et al. Heterozygosity for a hereditary hemochromatosis gene is associated with cardiovascular death in women. *Circulation* 1999; 100:1268–1273.
405. Tuomainen TP, Kontula K, Nyyssonen K, et al. Increased risk of acute myocardial infarction in carriers of the hemochromatosis gene Cys282Tyr mutation: A prospective cohort study in men in eastern Finland. *Circulation* 1999; 100:1274–1279.
406. Strong JP, Restrepo C, Guzman M. Coronary and aortic atherosclerosis in New Orleans: II. Comparison of lesions by age, sex, and race. *Lab Invest* 1978; 39:364–369.
407. Wissler RW, Strong JP. Risk factors and progression of atherosclerosis in youth. PDAY Research Group: Pathological Determinants of Atherosclerosis in Youth. *Am J Pathol* 1998; 153:1023–1033.
408. Maseri A. *Ischemic Heart Disease*. New York: Churchill Livingstone; 1995.
409. Denke MA, Grundy SM. Hypercholesterolemia in elderly persons: Resolving the treatment dilemma. *Ann Intern Med* 1990; 112:780–792.
410. SHEP Cooperative Research Group. Prevention of stroke by antihypertensive drug treatment in older persons with isolated systolic hypertension: Final results of the Systolic Hypertension in the Elderly Program (SHEP). *JAMA* 1991; 265:3255–3264.
411. Sempos CT, Cleeman JI, Carroll MD, et al. Prevalence of high blood cholesterol among US adults: An update based on guidelines from the second report of the National Cholesterol Education Program Adult Treatment Panel. *JAMA* 1993; 269:3009–3014.
412. Ravn HB, Falk E. Histopathology of plaque rupture. *Cardiol Clin* 1999 May; 17(2):263–270.

CHAPTER 36

PATHOLOGY OF CORONARY ATHEROSCLEROSIS

Michael J. Davies

THE PROCESS OF ATHEROSCLEROSIS

Atherosclerosis is an intimal disease of systemic arteries that range in size from the aorta to the epicardial coronary arteries. Atherosclerosis is characterized by discrete intimal plaques, although at an advanced stage the lesions may coalesce. Each plaque has variable combinations of extracellular lipid, lipid contained within cells that have foamy cytoplasm, and connective tissue matrix proteins, such as collagen, produced by smooth muscle cells. The majority of the foam cells are macrophages derived from monocytes, which enter the plaque from the arterial lumen.

Lipid is a fundamental component of the atherosclerotic plaque, which is essentially an inflammatory/repair response in the vessel wall invoked by lipid.[1] Lesions that consist entirely of proliferating smooth muscle cells, such as the response to endothelial denudation in animal models, are a repair response to mechanical injury and are not strictly atherosclerosis. Intimal thickening that consists solely of connective tissue and smooth muscle cells is also an adaptive response of the vessel wall to flow and occurs at branching points in human coronary arteries from a young age.[2,3] While this diffuse intimal thickening without a lipid component is not atherosclerosis as such, it does occur commonly in subjects who have atherosclerotic disease and plaques. Such intimal thickening can be measured by ultrasound in the carotid arteries in vivo and has been used as a surrogate marker for the detection of risk and in evaluating lipid-lowering therapy.[4]

Morphologic Forms of Atherosclerotic Plaques

The intimal surface of an opened human coronary artery reveals several types of plaque. Some are flat yellow dots or lines (fatty streaks), and others are raised above the surface as oval humps, which range in color from white to yellow (raised fibrolipid plaques).

Observations made on human necropsies allow a developmental sequence to be proposed for plaques based on cohorts of individuals dying at different ages from noncardiac disease.[2] In children from 5 to 10 years of age, fatty streaks often are present in the coronary arteries, suggesting that they are the initial point in a sequence of plaque development.[5] Raised plaques appear later in life and, by 20 years of age, are present in areas such as the proximal left anterior descending coronary artery, where fatty streaks are most prevalent in earlier life.[5] *By middle age, most subjects will have coronary plaques of all types, suggesting that plaque initiation continues throughout life.*

Plaque Evolution

The American Heart Association has recommended a nomenclature for the types of plaques and has suggested ways in which they may evolve.[6] The initial lesion (type I) develops when monocytes adhere to the endothelial surface and migrate from the lumen of an artery to accumulate in the intima. The type II lesion is the fatty streak that consists of a focal accumulation of lipid-filled foam cells largely of monocyte origin immediately beneath the intact endothelium. The type III lesion contains in addition small pools of extracellular lipid. While type I to type III plaques are the precursors of more advanced lesions, they do not cause clinical symptoms.

Type IV is characterized by two additional features. Smooth muscle cells appear within the lesion beneath the endothelium, and the pools of extracellular lipid coalesce to form a lipid core. Type V shows significant connective tissue deposition and the formation of a fibrous capsule containing the lipid core. The

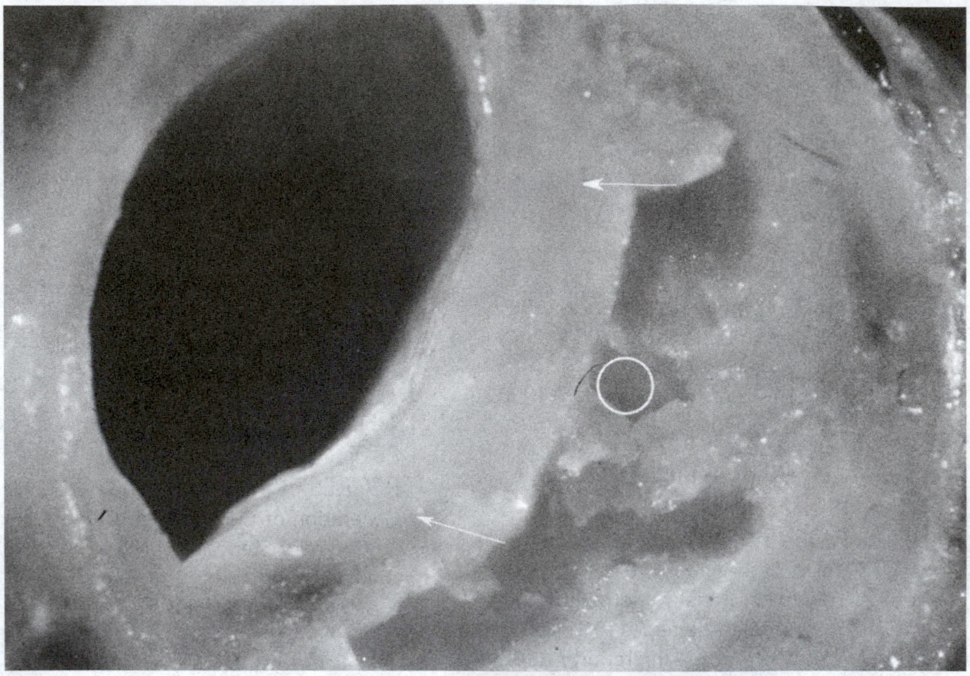

FIGURE 36-1 Human coronary artery in which there is a large lipid-rich plaque with a core (○) and a thick cap (*arrows*). This lesion would be designated as a type Va plaque.

portion of this capsule separating the core from the lumen is the plaque cap.

Plaques with a lipid core and a fibrous cap are designated as type Va (Figs. 36-1 and 36-2). *Type VI plaques are those complicated by thrombosis, which predominantly develops in type Va plaques.* Some plaques have heavy calcification (type Vb). Yet another form of advanced plaque (type Vc) is almost entirely composed of collagen and smooth muscle cells.

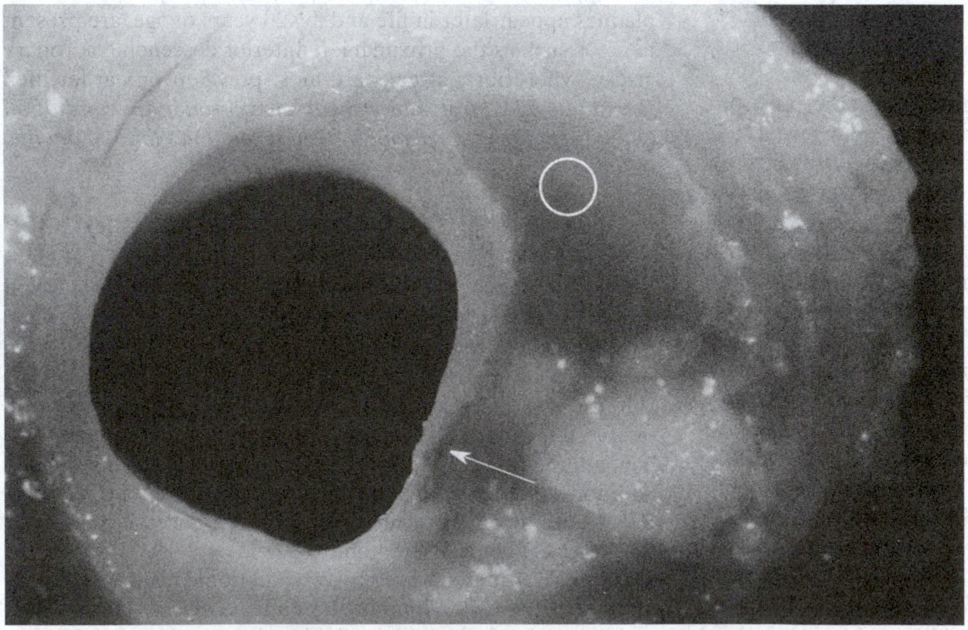

FIGURE 36-2 Human coronary artery in which there is a large lipid-rich plaque with a core (○), but in contrast to Fig. 36-1, the cap (*arrow*) is thin. This lesion is also a type Va plaque.

In general, the plaques found in subjects with ischemic heart disease show the complete spectrum of possible morphologies. There are, however, individuals who show a more uniform pattern. Virtually all the plaques may contain very large amounts of extracellular lipid, or virtually all the plaques consist of connective tissue with a rich connective mucin content and a minimal lipid component. Such variations from individual to individual may depend on the profile of risk factors. Smoking and elevated homocysteine levels may produce lesions that have different characteristics than those associated with high plasma lipids.[7,8] The great majority of descriptive work on plaques is based on the hyperlipidemic white male, and there is evidence emerging that women may have a somewhat different plaque morphology. In familial hypercholesterolemia and diabetes, diffuse intimal involvement with many foam cells rather than the formation of discrete plaques occurs.

Basic Mechanisms in Plaque Formation

FOAM CELL FORMATION

In experimental models and human disease, the first morphologic phenomenon observed in plaque formation is adhesion of monocytes to an intact endothelial surface.[1,9] This adhesion is followed by monocyte migration into the intima. In the intima, monocytes are activated, converted to macrophages, and may divide. Lipid uptake by macrophages then leads to the formation of the foam cell. These observations have created a paradox in that although plasma low-density lipoprotein (LDL) freely enters the intima, it should not be taken up by macrophages, which lack the appropriate receptor. The apparent paradox can now be explained in the context of the chemical changes that LDL undergoes as it is modified by the cells in the arterial wall. The first minor modifications of the LDL molecule occur close to the endothelial surface.[10] This initial change produces a proinflammatory molecule called *minimally modified low-density lipoprotein* (MMLDL) that contributes to the endothelial expression of molecules mediating monocyte adhesion, such as *vascular cell adhesion molecule* (VCAM).[11] Other inflammatory mediators such as *intercellular adhesion molecule* (ICAM), *monocyte chemotactic protein* (MCP-1),[12] and *macrophage colony-stimulating factor* (MCSF)[13] are also induced (see also Chaps. 6 and 36). These factors act in concert to cause monocyte migration and to allow the incoming monocytes to establish themselves and divide in the intima. Further changes in the LDL molecule lead to an oxidized form (oxidized LDL) that is recognized by the *macrophage scavenger receptor.* The scavenger receptor does not downregulate, as does the receptor for native LDL, and the cell becomes laden with lipid because of continued unregulated uptake. The macrophage foam cells that result produce a range of inflammatory cytokines including *tumor necrosis factor alpha* (TNF-α)[14] and metalloproteinases as well as the procoagulant *tissue factor.*[15] This sequence of lipid oxidation and lipid uptake by macrophages forms a credible explanation for the formation of foam cells, and oxidized LDL has been shown within macrophages in both human and rabbit atherosclerosis[16] (see also Chap. 35).

Transgenic models of atherosclerosis show the importance of these inflammatory mediators. Apoliprotein B knockout mice, for example, show a very marked susceptibility to form plaques when given lipid diets. Animals in whom in addition MCP-1 or its receptor or MCSF or VCAM or the scavenger receptors are knocked out show a profound attenuation of atherosclerotic lesions. MCP-1 is suggested by these models to be a major component of monocyte recruitment in plaques.[17,18]

LIPID CORE FORMATION

Lipid cores are potential spaces in the connective tissue matrix of the intima that are filled with cellular debris and cholesterol. Active plaques contain numerous macrophages clustered at the edge of the core, with the expression of a range of metalloproteinases that likely are engaged in the active destruction of the collagen matrix. Some extracellular lipid may be derived directly from LDL bound to proteoglycans within the intima,[19] but much of the cholesterol and esters in the lipid core is released from the cytoplasm of dying foam cells. Macrophages may be killed by lipid peroxides formed by LDL oxidation, but there is now evidence that cell death is by apoptosis.[20] Deprivation of growth factors such as MCSF-1 may induce apoptosis, particularly in association with the TNF-α present in large amounts in cellular plaques. Tissue factor (TF) expression by macrophages within the core makes this area of the plaque highly thrombogenic if it is exposed to the arterial lumen.[21]

SMOOTH MUSCLE PROLIFERATION AND CAP FORMATION

The caps of plaques with a lipid core consist of a lattice of collagen within which are lacunae containing smooth muscle cells that produce the connective tissue matrix. Intimal smooth muscle cells have the tendancy to die by apoptosis, and many caps of plaques become relatively acellular. Smooth muscle cell migration and proliferation, as well as collagen deposition, are driven by growth factors produced by virtually every cell type, including smooth muscle cells themselves.[22] Platelets, fibrin, and thrombin also can stimulate smooth muscle cell proliferation if deposited on the vessel wall, and there is increasing recognition that fibrinogen passes into the intima and can be converted to fibrin. Such fibrin is usually removed by plasminogen activation. Any residual fibrin-thrombin complexes are potent stimulators of smooth muscle cell proliferation. The plaque cap is now recognized as a dynamic structure in which there is deposition of collagen[23] balanced by degradation of the connective tissue matrix by a range of proteases. Numerous cytokines control this balance.

IMMUNE MECHANISMS IN PLAQUE FORMATION

Plaques contain T-lymphocytes,[24] the function of which may be, in part, to modify smooth muscle cell proliferation via the production of interferon-γ. CD40L-positive lymphocytes are present in plaques and react with CD40-positive macrophages to cause activation, cytokine expression, tissue factor expression, and metalloproteinase production. In experimental models, blockade of CD40L attenuates plaque formation.[25] A significant proportion of lymphocytes within plaques are potentially cytotoxic producing perforins and granzymes and may contribute to death of smooth muscle cells and macrophages. B-lymphocytes are absent from the plaque itself but are present, often in large numbers, in the adjacent adventitia. Oxidized LDL is strongly antigenic, and the B-lymphocytes produce autoantibodies that can be measured in the plasma and may provide a marker of the activity or extent of the atherosclerotic process.[26]

A significant proportion of subjects with coronary atherosclerosis show colonization of the plaques by the intracellular bacterium *Chlamydia pneumoniae.* The frequency of such direct infection of the plaque is high, as shown by immunofluorescence studies when 40 to 50 percent of individuals with atherosclerosis have some positive plaques. Studies by polymerase chain reaction (PCR) for the detection of chlamydial DNA are less frequently positive. The current perception is that chlamydia reach the plaque by entering a monocyte in the lung or upper respiratory tract and then enter the bloodstream and migrate into the plaque. The higher frequency of immunohistochemical positivity than PCR positivity may suggest that the organism grows only for a limited time, but the capular antigens persist within macrophages. Chlamydia within macrophages in the plaque potentially would upregulate inflammatory activity and enhance plaque progression. Chlamydial heat-shock protein upregulates TNF-α production.[27,28] Antibiotic therapy may or may not turn out to be effective in slowing plaque progression.[29,30]

PLAQUE VASCULARIZATION

The normal media is avascular, but once intimal thickening occurs, new vessels grow in from the adventitia and reach the base of the plaque. Neovascularization may be visible on angiography in life.[31] The vessels that lie close to the base of the core are thin-walled, and extravasation of red cells is very common. When the core contains platelets, however, a direct continuity with the lumen is found via a cap tear (see below). Transmedial vessels strongly express adhesion molecules such as VCAM and may be another route by which monocytes enter the plaque.[32] Transgenic mouse models show that inhibition of new vessel formation will attenuate plaque formation.[33]

ENDOTHELIAL STATUS OVER PLAQUES

In early plaque formation (types I–III), the endothelial surface is intact, and there is no exposure of the subendothelial connective tissue matrix and therefore no adhesion of platelets to the vessel wall. The endothelium is structurally intact, although this does not mean that it is functionally normal. Once later plaque formation has occurred (types IV–V), however, small foci of endothelial loss do occur, and this denudation injury exposes connective tissue, allowing the formation of a monolayer of platelets adherent to the vessel wall. Associated with denudation injury is evidence of increased endothelial cell turnover. The thrombi that form are ultramicroscopic but do indicate endothelial instability in the atherosclerotic artery. Observational studies show that endothelial cell loss is associated with the proximity to macrophages.[34,35] Macrophages may induce endothelial cell apoptosis as well as producing a range of proteolytic enzymes that cut loose the endothelial cell from its attachment to the vessel wall.[36]

CLINICAL SYMPTOMS AND PLAQUE TYPES

The presence of advanced plaques of types IV and Va allows clinical symptoms to develop. Atherosclerosis is a biphasic disease; in the first stage, advanced plaques are generated, but the patient is asymptomatic; in the second stage, symptoms develop. Plaques are ubiquitous in Western populations, but not everyone develops ischemic heart disease.

Large-scale epidemiologic studies—including the International Geographic Survey,[37] the Pathological Determinants of Atherosclerosis in Youth (PDAY) study,[4] and the Bogalusa Heart Study[38]—have produced consistent information: *In all geographic populations, the mean number of coronary plaques present in a large number of autopsied patients who die from all causes predicts the incidence of ischemic heart disease in that population.* The risk factors for large numbers of subjects developing ischemic heart disease depend on how many advanced plaques are present. Smokers will, on average, have more plaques than nonsmokers. Similar data exist for hyperlipidemia, hypertension, and diabetes (see Chap. 38). Thus risk factors operate in part by increasing the number of plaques that potentially can progress to cause symptoms. Such epidemiologic studies, however, do not mean that an individual cannot die of a single, strategically placed plaque.

The majority of types IV and Va advanced plaques are clinically silent and angiographically invisible because they do not encroach on the lumen of a coronary artery. Two mechanisms are responsible for this phenomenon. First, the media behind an atherosclerotic plaque undergoes thinning and atrophy, which allows the plaque to bulge outward rather than inward. Second, *the development of an intimal plaque causes remodeling of the arterial wall, increasing the external diameter and allowing the plaque to be accommodated without altering the lumen dimensions.*[39] Intravascular ultrasound confirms that coronary angiography is very insensitive for the detection of plaques[40] (see also Chap. 47).

Plaque Heterogeneity

Common to all type Va plaques is the presence of a fibromuscular cap, but even so, there is considerable heterogeneity (see Figs. 36-1 and 36-2). The cap may be relatively thick and uniform, or it may vary in thickness with interspersed thin areas. Thick caps have high numbers of smooth muscle cells, whereas relatively thin caps often have fewer smooth muscle cells and contain appreciable numbers of macrophages. The lipid core may occupy over 70 percent of the overall volume of the plaque or as little as 10 percent. Core margins may be surrounded by macrophages, or there may be no macrophages. *Plaque heterogeneity therefore involves both the micromorphology of the lesion (core size, cap thickness) and the degree of inflammatory activity.* A plaque in inflammatory terms can be "hot" or "burnt out." There is no readily discernible relation between plaque size and any of the variables that contribute to plaque heterogeneity.

Mechanisms of Induction of Symptoms

Three major mechanisms lead to clinical symptoms (see also Chap. 35). First, thrombosis leads to acute decreases in flow in a coronary artery. Second, a plaque grows without the clinically apparent involvement of thrombosis to the point that the lumen size is reduced to a degree that causes flow limitation during exercise.

Finally, in subjects with coronary atherosclerosis, coronary vasomotor tonal responses are abnormal. This disordered control of tone, which reflects in part endothelial dysfunction (see also Chaps. 6 and 36) may take the form of local spasm at the site of an eccentric plaque in which there is a residual segment of normal vessel wall, or vasospasm may be a more generalized phenomenon.

Acute Ischemic Syndromes

The major factor initiating acute ischemia in the crescendo form of unstable angina, acute myocardial infarction, and a high proportion of sudden ischemic deaths is a thrombus of sufficient size to protrude into the arterial lumen. This assertion does not imply that thrombosis is the only factor, but necropsy studies, angiography, and angioscopy, as well as the success of fibrinolytic therapy in restoring arterial patency in infarct-related arteries, all indicate a dominant role for thrombosis.

FACTORS INDUCING PLAQUE THROMBOSIS

Postmortem study of human coronary thrombi causing death has shown the involvement of two distinct processes.[41]

Endothelial Erosion The endothelial surface over many plaques of types IV and Va has been shown to develop small foci of endothelial cell loss[34,35] that expose the subendothelial connective tissue and lead to local ultramicroscopic areas of platelet adhesion (Fig. 36-3). The extension of this process to cause large areas of endothelial denudation over a plaque leads to much larger thrombi capable of causing symptoms. The characteristics of these thrombi are that they are adherent to the luminal surface of the plaque, which is otherwise intact, and there is no intraplaque thrombosis (Fig. 36-4).

Plaque Disruption Major coronary thrombi are also caused by plaque disruption (also known as *plaque cracking, fissuring, rupture,* or *ulceration*). In disruption, the cap of a plaque with a lipid-rich core will tear; blood from the lumen of the artery then enters the lipid core, where the presence of tissue factor and collagen induces platelet adhesion, aggregation, and activation.[41] Thrombus formation within the core itself expands and distorts the plaque, whereas the torn cap may project into the lumen (Fig. 36-5). Necropsy study of disrupted coronary and aortic plaques compared with intact plaques in the same individuals shows that plaques with a large lipid core occupying more than 50 percent of overall plaque volume and having a high macrophage density, a thin cap, and low smooth muscle cell density are the most vulnerable to rupture.[42] Of interest, core size and cap thickness, which are two major determinants of plaque vulnerability, are not statistically related, and neither is related to absolute plaque size or to the degree of stenosis.

Plaque disruption is responsible for at least 80 percent of major coronary thrombi causing sudden death or myocardial infarction in white males.[42] In contrast, the frequencies of disruption and erosion are almost equal in women with coronary thrombi.[43,44]

Postdisruption Events

The events that follow an episode of plaque cap disruption are dynamic and occur in stages (Fig. 36-6). Progression can be halted at any stage. The initial stage, in the past, often has been referred to as *plaque* or *intimal hemorrhage, intraplaque hematoma,* and *hemorrhagic dissection.* These names imply that the intraplaque component is predominantly composed of red blood cells. A large component of platelets and fibrin is also present, justifying the name *intraplaque thrombus.*[42] Within the area of the torn cap at the interface with the lumen, the thrombus composition is predominantly densely packed fibrin. From this transition zone, mural thrombus may project out into the lumen without totally preventing antegrade flow. In the final stage, thrombus is predominantly made up of a loose network of fibrin-containing enmeshed red blood cells and totally occludes the arterial lumen.

Plaque disruption is a stimulus to the formation of thrombosis within the lumen. Many factors control whether or not thrombosis occurs. The magnitude of the tear varies. At one extreme it may be a narrow fissure running from the lumen to the core; at the other extreme the whole cap may be lost with extrusion of core material

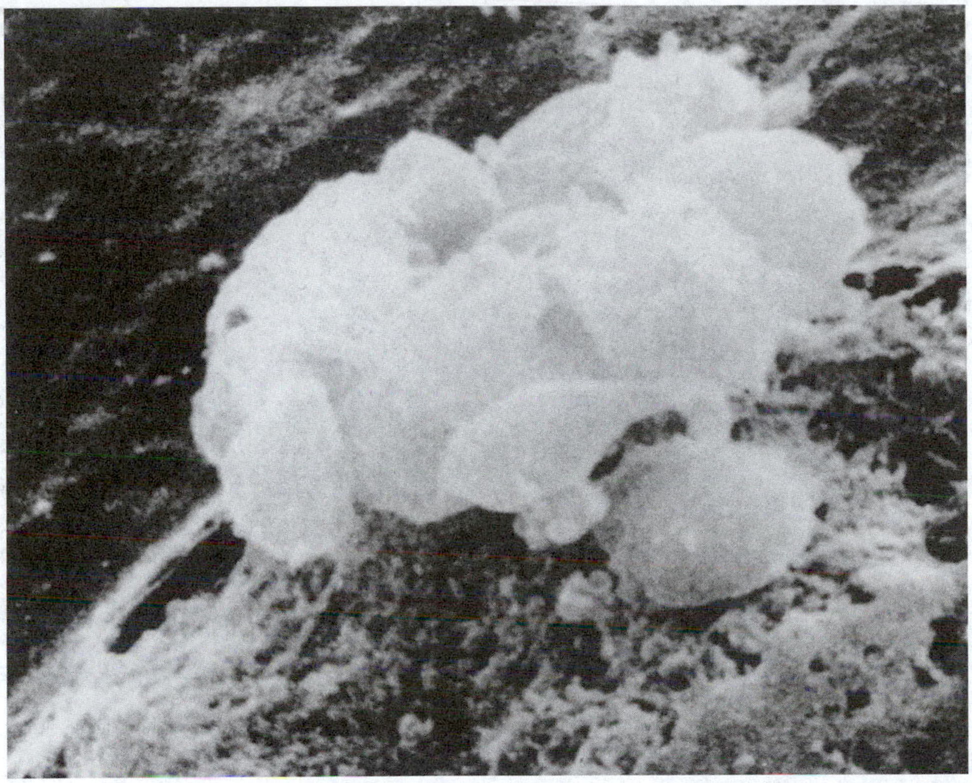

FIGURE 36-3 Scanning electron micrograph of human coronary artery. A single endothelial cell has undergone denudation. Over the exposed subendothelial tissue, a small clump of platelets has formed. No platelets adhere to adjacent intact endothelial cells.

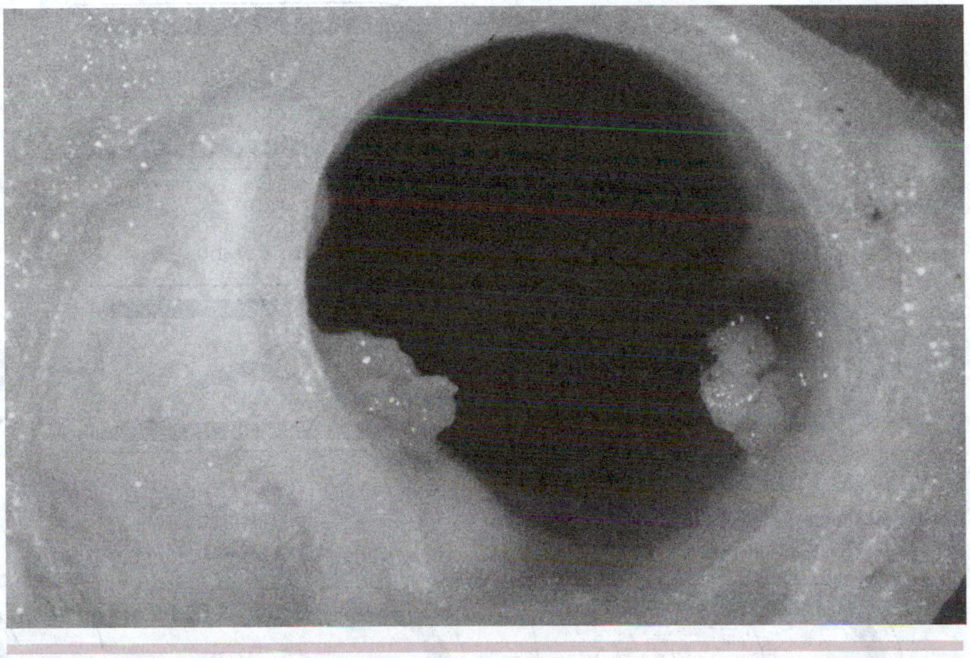

FIGURE 36-4 Two small thrombi due to endothelial erosion over a plaque. The thrombi are stuck onto the surface of the plaque—there is no intraplaque component of thrombus.

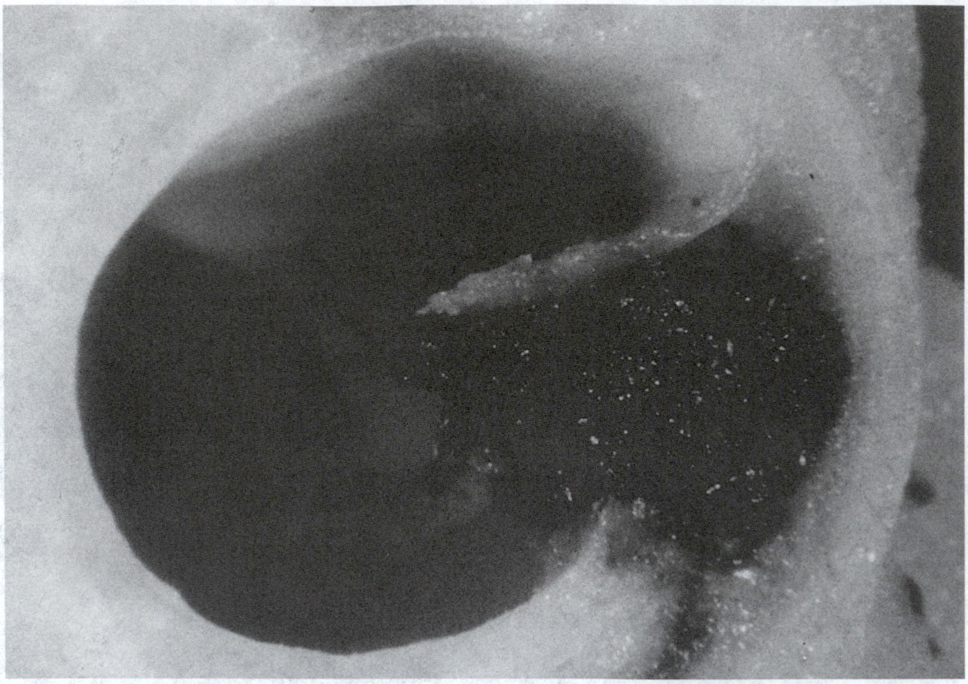

FIGURE 36-5 Plaque disruption in which the torn cap of a plaque projects into the lumen. The original site of the lipid core is filled with thrombus, which protrudes into but does not occlude the lumen.

into the lumen. Another important factor is the local blood flow. Reduction of flow, either due to spasm or because of a large expansion of the plaque by thrombus within the core, increases the likelihood of major thrombosis within the lumen. The systemic balance of prothrombotic and natural fibrinolytic mechanisms is another factor influencing whether or not major intraluminal thrombi follow the stimulus of an episode of plaque disruption.

Plaque Healing

Plaque disruption is followed by a healing response. Natural fibrinolysis will remove a variable amount of the thrombus, which is followed by smooth muscle cell proliferation and deposition of new collagen. This healing process is analogous to that which follows angioplasty. The end stage of an episode of plaque disruption can

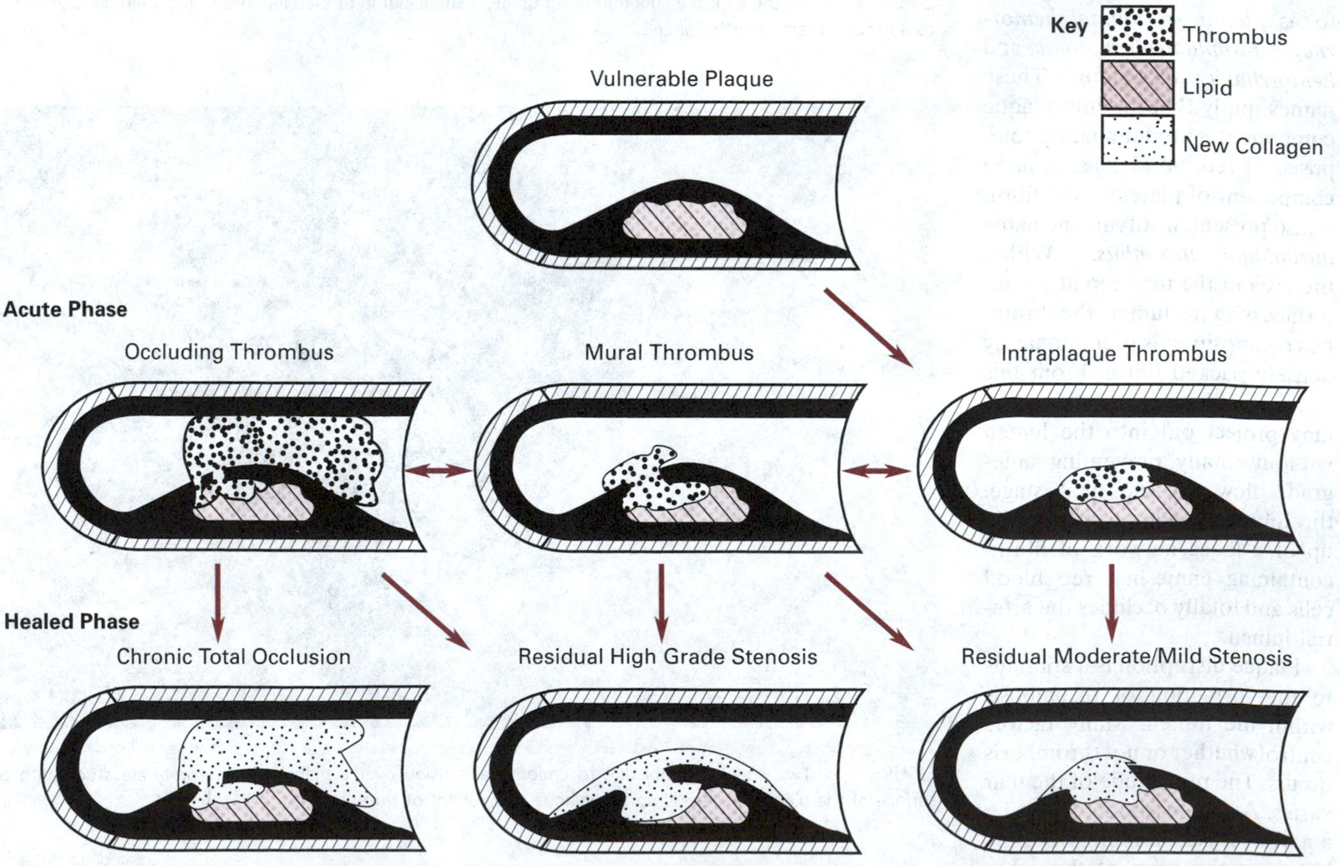

FIGURE 36-6 Diagram of the dynamic state of the acute thrombotic response with different stages—intraplaque, mural nonocclusive, and occlusive thrombus. The end result, after healing by smooth muscle cell proliferation, ranges from chronic total occlusion to a mild increase in stenosis.

range from a trivial increase in plaque size through more significant increases in size resulting in an increase in stenosis severity to chronic total occlusion (see Fig. 36-6).

Mechanism of Intimal Tears

Reconstruction of human atherosclerotic plaques that have undergone disruption shows that the majority have a large core of extracellular cholesterol occupying over 50 percent of the plaque by volume. Computer models of plaques using finite-element analysis have been used to show the distribution of circumferential wall stress in systole.[45,46] Normally, systolic circumferential stress is evenly distributed. Lipid cores are soft and cannot sustain stress, which has to be distributed elsewhere. The displaced stress is redistributed to the plaque cap. Focal points of maximal stress may be up to 10 times greater than that experienced by the rest of the arterial wall. Studies of coronary plaques show that the site of tearing coincides with the calculated point of maximal stress.[46] Concentration of stress on the plaque cap is also particularly enhanced in thin caps of plaques, causing minimal stenosis.[47] All these studies emphasize the concept that plaques with lipid cores and thin caps are mechanically inefficient, with stresses impinging excessively on the cap.

Another important aspect of plaque disruption is the innate mechanical strength of the cap tissue. Mechanical testing in vitro of cap tissue shows that a reduction in collagen and glycosoaminoglycans and an increase in the number of lipid-filled macrophages interact to reduce the amount of stress needed to fracture the tissue even after correction for the cross-sectional area of the test sample.[48] Collagen types and elastin content do not alter absolute tissue strength. These results lead to consideration of whether or not the cap is undergoing active destruction by proteases. Macrophages have the capacity when activated by the cytokines TNF-α and interleukin 1 (IL-1) to secrete inactive *metalloproteinases* (MMP). These connective tissue–degrading enzymes include interstitial collagenase (MMP1), gelatinase B (MMP9), stromelysins 1, 2, and 3 (MMP3, -10, and -11), and a membrane type (MTMPP). When activated by plasmin or by inactivation of intrinsic inhibitors in the tissue, these metalloproteinases can degrade the connective tissue matrix. Macrophages in plaques also produce cathepsins K and S, which will degrade elastin.[49] Both metalloproteinase mRNA and protein have been found in large amounts in the cap and core area,[30,50,51] but their activity may be neutralized by tissue inhibitors (TIMPS). Sections of plaques laid on a gelatin substrate in vitro, however, show that lysis occurs in focal areas, indicating that active degradation of collagen is occurring.[51] Evidence of enhanced collagen destruction in lipid-rich plaques also has been shown by the presence of collagen breakdown products identified by specific immunohistochemistry.[52] *Plaque cap tears therefore can be seen as resulting from a destructive process initiated by macrophages that gains ascendancy over the repair process of collagen deposition by smooth muscle cells.*

DETAILED PATHOLOGY OF CLINICAL SYNDROMES IN ISCHEMIC HEART DISEASE

Unstable Angina

Intermittent ischemia occurring at rest is the hallmark of unstable angina and is related to "dynamic" stenosis; i.e., the obstruction to flow varies rather than being fixed (see Chap. 41). Two main mechanisms, mural thrombosis at the site of a culprit plaque and varying vasomotor tone, have been proposed. Neither process is exclusive, and both may operate contemporaneously.

Angiographic studies in unstable angina of the crescendo form, in which there is a clear risk of subsequent acute infarction, emphasize the presence of eccentric stenoses with ragged outlines, designated as type II, and of intraluminal filling defects.[53] Necropsy studies (Fig. 36-7) confirm that these angiographic appearances are due to nonocclusive thrombi developing over a disrupted plaque. *A major cause of unstable angina therefore is a culprit plaque over which thrombus is arrested at an intermediate stage in which it is neither occlusive nor resolved sufficiently to allow the plaque to reseal and heal.*

Necropsy studies of unstable angina are biased toward the worst-case scenario. To an extent, this limitation can be over-

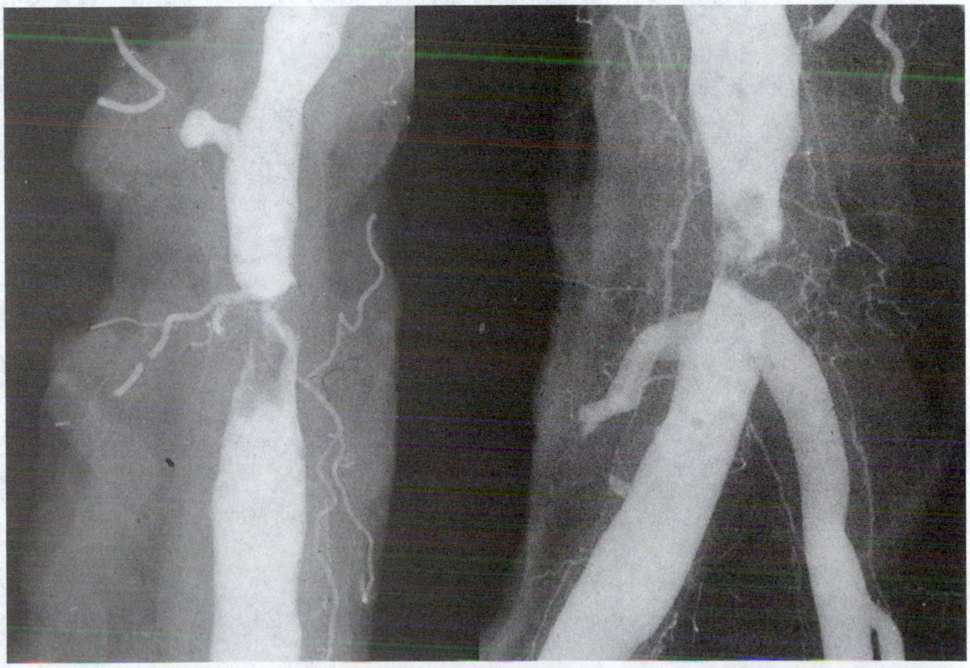

FIGURE 36-7 Postmortem angiograms of two patients who died suddenly after a prodrome of intermittent resting chest pain. Both had disrupted plaques. The angiograms show the typical eccentric stenoses with ragged edges. Both have related intraluminal thrombi—proximal in one (*left*) and distal in the other (*right*).

come by studies of plaque material retrieved by atherectomy of the culprit lesion. Such studies confirm that macrophage infiltration is a feature of unstable plaques.[54] A number of atherectomy studies have shown that thrombotic material is recovered from a far higher proportion of plaques causing unstable as compared with stable angina but that this correlation is not 100 percent.[55,56] A far smaller proportion of apparently stable plaques also shows thrombotic material. Haft et al.,[57] for example, found thrombus in atherectomy material in 49 of 57 patients with unstable angina (86 percent) and in 7 of 24 patients with stable angina (29 percent). Atherectomy removes a random portion of the plaque, and this may explain the absence of thrombus in some patients with unstable angina. Timing is also important. Atherectomy samples that show accelerated growth with storiform smooth muscle cell proliferation[58] can be explained by the sample's having been taken after healing is initiated.[59] Angioscopy is probably more sensitive than angiography in identifying plaque thrombosis. A recent study[60] shows 70 of 95 (73.7 percent) patients with unstable angina had plaque thrombus. Four of 27 patients (14.8 percent) who had only exercise-related pain showed thrombus.

Pathologic studies show that platelet emboli into the distal myocardium lead to small foci of acute myocardial necrosis in subjects dying suddenly after unstable angina.[61,62] These small platelet emboli within the myocardium show intense expression of the type IIb/IIIa receptor (Fig. 36-8).

The arterial pathology of unstable angina differs from that of acute myocardial infarction only in that the artery remains open and some antegrade flow is retained, whereas in the latter antegrade flow ceases for at least a period of time, usually some hours. Unstable angina of the crescendo type, non-Q-wave or nontransmural infarction, and transmural infarction are different points in a continuous spectrum. It is therefore not surprising that sensitive methods of detecting myocardial necrosis, such as measuring plasma troponin-T levels, can be used to detect subjects with the clinical diagnosis of unstable angina who are at high risk of death or further infarction.[63]

The essence of the arterial pathology of unstable angina is that the process of thrombosis is arrested at the point of exposed mural thrombus. This arrest represents a balance between many active forces and does not imply that the thrombotic surface has become inert. The risk of thrombotic occlusion developing at the site remains increased for at least 6 to 12 weeks, and systemic hypercoagulative activity is also elevated for several months. Residual thrombotic material continues to be highly thrombogenic until it is completely replaced by smooth muscle cells and new connective tissue.[64]

Vasomotor Tonal Abnormalities in Unstable Angina

There is now abundant evidence in humans and in animals that atherosclerotic arteries have inappropriate vasoconstrictor responses. Vasoconstriction, which has been induced both by exercise and intracoronary infusion of acetylcholine, is caused by a failure of normal vasodilatory responses due, at least in part, to diminished nitric oxide release by the endothelium (see Chaps. 6 and 36).

Some cases of unstable angina have localized dynamic vasoconstriction, either at a site of eccentric stenosis or in a segment with minimal or no angiographic narrowing.[65,66] It is uncertain why one such lesion should acquire vasomotor excitability. Increased endothelin-1 production within plaques may be a contributing factor.[67] In one case, small amounts of thrombus, too small to be detected angiographically, were found on the endothelial surface at surgery.[68] The local release of vasoactive substances by platelets is one possible cause of spasm, and this possibility is supported by experimental models of coronary injury in pigs.[69] Another postulated cause is related to the heavy adventitial inflammation; mast cells may release pharmacologically active substances that act directly on adventitial nerve tissue.[70] The Prinzmetal variant form of angina frequently occurs in arteries that have some angiographic evidence of atherosclerosis but without an element of high-grade fixed stenosis[71] (see also Chap. 41). The greater frequency of unstable angina with either normal or mildly diseased arteries on angiography in women suggests they have a larger vasospastic component than males with acute ischemic events.[72]

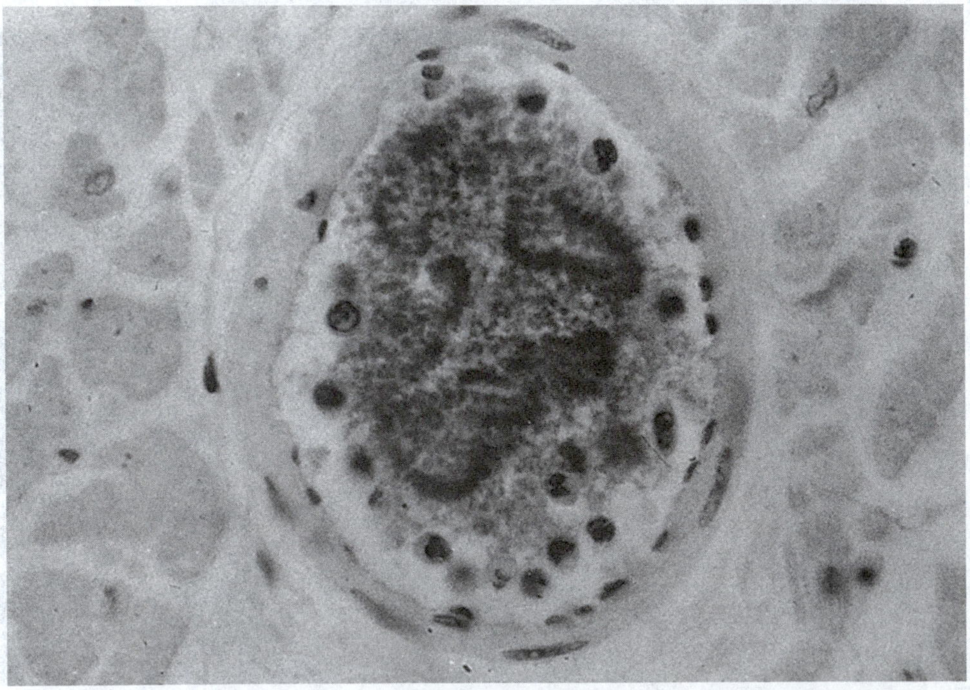

FIGURE 36-8 An intramyocardial artery distal to a disrupted plaque in a major epicardial artery is occluded by a mass of platelets and white blood cells. The platelets are expressing the type IIb/IIIa receptor (immunohistochemical staining with type IIb/IIIa antibody).

Acute Myocardial Infarction

The blood supply of the mammalian myocardium is regional; each major branch of the coronary arteries supplies a specific segment of myocardium. There is considerable interspecies variation in the degree of innate crossflow between adjacent epicardial arteries; humans and pigs share the property of having little natural collateral development.

In experimental animal models, the only way to produce regional infarction is to occlude the coronary artery supplying a given area. Clinical studies of regional myocardial infarction in humans confirm the importance of occlusion of the subtending ("infarct-related") artery. Angiography during the early hours of infarction shows the subtending artery to the region to be occluded.[73] The frequency with which occlusion is detected after a myocardial infarction diminishes with the passage of time; as antegrade flow returns (because of spontaneous lysis of thrombus), filling defects are seen within the lumen over a type II stenosis. Fibrinolytic therapy increases the speed with which the subtending artery reopens. These data suggest that a dynamic thrombotic process is occurring. Necropsy studies show a higher frequency of total thrombotic occlusion than equivalent angiographic studies of survivors of acute infarction. These findings suggest that persistent occlusion has an adverse influence on survival, probably by being linked to larger infarct size.[74]

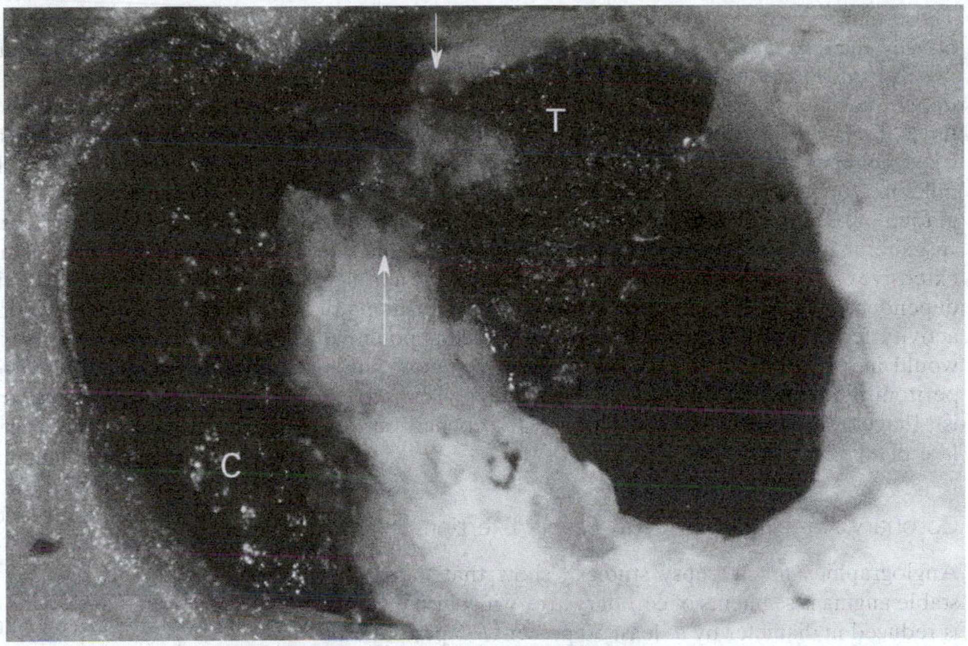

FIGURE 36-9 Plaque disruption related to an acute regional infarct. There is a mass of thrombus within the lipid core (*C*), which is continuous with thrombus (*T*) in the lumen via a discrete fissure (*arrows*) in the cap. The thrombus is not occlusive, presumably due to natural lysis.

Reconstruction of the microanatomy of occlusive coronary thrombi shows the majority to be due to plaque rupture in which there is both an intraplaque and an intraluminal component (Fig. 36-9). The thrombus found at autopsy varies in suggesting that it is formed by an intermittent process taking place over some days. The intraplaque component of the thrombus consists predominantly of platelets; the thrombus within the fissure site is formed of densely packed fibrin. Much of the intraluminal thrombus, particularly that distal to the fissured plaque, is "venous" in type, suggesting that it has formed in a static column of blood. At least part of the intraluminal thrombus thus may be a late phenomenon. In vivo radiolabeling studies in subjects who subsequently died of acute infarction show that both fibrinogen and platelets given after the onset of the infarction can be incorporated into the coronary thrombus. Detailed studies, however, showed that the thrombus within the fissured plaque is not labeled, i.e., predates infarction, whereas a proportion of thrombus in the lumen is labeled, i.e., postdates infarction.[75]

INTERRELATION OF INFARCT MORPHOLOGY AND ARTERIAL THROMBI

Human regional infarcts may be formed of transmural necrosis of uniform age. Such infarcts are closely analogous to experimental infarction in the dog and represent the consequences of thrombus occurring suddenly and progressing to occlusion over a very short time in a vessel in which there was minimal or no preexisting stenosis. There may be preexisting high-grade stenosis, however, that has invoked collateral formation. In such arteries, thrombosis may occur without causing any infarction. Thrombosis may be mural and associated with distal embolization of platelet masses or intermittently occlusive prior to the final occlusive episode. Antegrade flow may or may not be restored spontaneously within a period of hours. These more complex developmental patterns of thrombosis are associated with regional infarcts that are built up by the coalescence of small, often microscopic areas of necrosis of different ages. Retention of areas of viable myocardium mixed with necrotic areas is common. Infarcts that are regional but confined to the subendocardial zone (nontransmural) are almost always of this type. In humans, nontransmural infarction, as compared with transmural infarction, has a higher frequency of previously established collateral flow and/or restoration of antegrade flow over the culprit plaque.[76,77] The sinister complications of infarct expansion, infarct rupture, and cardiogenic shock are virtually confined to transmural infarcts and are associated withpersistent total occlusion of long segments of coronary artery.

Coronary Syndromes and Markers of Inflammation

Atherosclerosis is an inflammatory response to modified lipids[78] within focal areas of the intima. All plaques at some point in their evolution have such an inflammatory response,[79] but this may burn out or progress to cause plaque disruption or endothelial erosion with resulting thrombosis and the potential to cause acute coronary syndromes.

A wide range of markers of inflammatory activity including C-reactive protein,[80] fibrinogen, neoptenin, and soluble intercellular adhesion molecule (ICAM) on a population basis give an indication of the risk of acute ischemic events in the future.

These markers are not elevated to a degree that is strikingly outside the normal range, but, for example, if a population is divided into quartiles of the level of C-reactive protein, the upper quartile has a risk of myocardial infarction around three times the lowest quartile.[81] Such data can be interpreted in two ways, neither being exclusive of the other. The level of systemic inflammatory activity may be a measure of the total active plaque burden in the aorta and carotid and coronary arteries. In general, subjects with severe aortic disease have the most extensive coronary plaque formation. Alternatively, a non-lipid-dependent mechanism may be elevating overall inflammatory activity feeding back on the plaques. Such factors potentially would include *Helicobacter* and chlamydial infection, chronic peritonitis, rheumatoid arthritis, etc. Experimental evidence exists that elevation of systemic mediators will secondarily upregulate plaque inflammation.[82]

Coronary Artery Pathology in Stable Exertional Angina

Angiographic and necropsy studies[83] show that the basis of stable angina is segments of coronary artery in which the lumen is reduced in diameter by at least 50 percent (75 percent cross-sectional area) compared with the adjacent normal artery. Such stenoses are potentially flow-limiting on exertion. The number of arteries involved and the number of stenotic segments vary widely from case to case, with autopsy studies inevitably showing the more severe end of the spectrum. The morphology of lesions causing chronic high-grade stenosis can best be appreciated in coronary arteries that have been fixed after autopsy by perfusion with formalin at systolic pressures. In such preparations, the lumen is nearly circular in outline, indicating that the slitlike lumen shape shown in many pathology studies is an artifact. Segments of high-grade stenosis may be eccentric; i.e., there is an arc of vessel wall that has retained its normal media opposite the plaque[84] (see Fig. 36-2). Alterations in vascular tone in this residual segment of normal media may alter the cross-sectional area of the lumen. Stenoses may be concentric, however, surrounding the lumen and limiting variation in lumen size.

Many patients with stable angina but without a clinical history of infarction are found at autopsy to have a healed regional infarct. Arteries that supply such regions may be totally occluded by fibrous tissue, have high-grade stenosis due to complex type Vb plaques, or have many new, small vascular channels contained within the original lumen. This last appearance is pathognomonic of recanalization by organization of previous occlusive thrombus. In subjects with stable angina, such recanalized segments also may be present and unrelated to old scars, illustrating the fact that thrombotic occlusion is not inevitably followed by infarction. In one autopsy study of 54 men with stable angina who died within 6 h of the onset of symptoms, 38 patients had microscopic evidence of previous healed myocardial infarction; of these, 33 (87 percent) had one or more arterial segments in which the lumen was multichanneled. In the 16 patients who did not have microscopic evidence of an old infarction, 10 (62.5 percent) had one or more arterial segments that were multichanneled.[83]

CORONARY ANASTOMOSES (COLLATERALS)

Anastomotic flow is impossible to demonstrate in life or at necropsy without angiography. Anastomoses occur at several different levels. Local adventitial vessels open and provide very localized anastomoses at sites of short segments of high-grade or total chronic occlusion. While such periarterial vessels may show up strikingly in angiograms, the caliber of individual vessels is small, and useful flow may not be achieved. Similar-sized vessels develop within the arterial lumen, passing through an old organized thrombus. Larger anastomoses develop between adjacent arteries on the epicardial surface. These may be as much as 1000 μm in diameter and are probably preexisting smaller arteries altered by flow-induced pressure differentials between different coronary beds. These anastomoses at the epicardial surface are probably the most important functionally and develop a characteristic corkscrew configuration in angiograms. In areas of nontransmural scarring within the myocardium, a plexus of large subendocardial vessels appears that has a structure resembling that of venous sinusoids. In very diffusely scarred ventricles, these channels fill throughout the ventricle from injection into one coronary artery.

MECHANISMS OF PROGRESSION AND REGRESSION

Any morphologic explanation of disease progression must take into account a number of clinical observations.[85–89] Sequential clinical angiographic studies show that progression is phasic and unpredictable in any particular arterial segment. High-grade lesions do not necessarily appear at sites where lower-grade lesions were present previously. New lesions causing luminal stenosis over 50 percent in diameter can appear between two angiographic examinations in apparently normal segments of artery. The sites of future acute occlusions causing infarction cannot be predicted. The progression of separate lesions in an individual is unrelated, and the progression of lesions in "normal" segments is often greater than in areas recognized to have an irregular outline. Thus individual plaques can enter an accelerated growth phase that is unrelated to their degree of stenosis. Despite this unpredictable behavior, high-grade stenoses (>70 percent by diameter) do tend to progress, particularly if the segment is long. Chronic total occlusions follow such high-grade lesions three times more frequently than in the case of less severe lesions[89] but frequently do not invoke infarction because of collateral development. Sequential coronary angiograms show that increases in the overall extent of disease also predict the risk of acute ischemic events in the future.[90,91]

Episodes of plaque disruption were regarded initially as events that inevitably caused thrombosis within the arterial lumen and therefore usually were manifest as episodes of acute myocardial ischemia. Several pathology studies have altered this concept. In a significant proportion of patients who had coronary atherosclerosis but who died of noncardiac causes such as accidents, small, recent plaque disruptions were found at autopsy. Up to 16 percent of such individuals who have diabetes and/or hypertension have these lesions.[92] In three studies of patients who died of acute myocardial ischemia, many were found at necropsy to have had two or three separate areas of disruption, although one was usually larger and regarded as the culprit lesion causing death.[93–95] Such data suggest that *episodes of plaque disruption are a characteristic feature of the progression of atherosclerosis and that many are clinically silent.*

An episode of plaque disruption heals by smooth muscle proliferation, replacing residual thrombus. The repair process is identical to that which follows plaque disruption produced by angioplasty. The final outcome of an episode of plaque disruption can range from chronic total occlusion at one extreme to a mild increase in stenosis at the other extreme (see Fig. 36-6).

Generation of Chronic High-Grade Coronary Stenosis

The simplest model of the generation of significant coronary stenosis is that the plaque simply grows by the process of atherosclerosis (lipid accumulation–collagen formation) in a linear fashion until the lumen is narrowed to a degree that limits flow. Sequential angiography, however, often shows that high-grade stenotic lesions appear within a year at sites that were normal previously by angiography.

As plaques grow slowly, the artery wall remodels to accommodate the lesion, compromising lumen size. The external cross-sectional area of a coronary artery may increase by up to 80 percent of its normal size. Such compensatory dilatation is often sufficient to allow relatively large plaques not to encroach on the lumen and be angiographically invisible. At points of high-grade coronary stenosis, the degree of remodeling is often minimal (inadequate remodeling) or even shows a reduction in the artery size (negative remodeling). Thus stenosis arises both from an increase in plaque size and from the degree of remodeling.[96,97] Failure of remodeling may reflect the rate of plaque growth. Reconstruction of segments of high-grade stenosis in pathology studies show at least 70 percent of lesions to have healed disruption that would have triggered accelerated smooth muscle proliferation and a sudden increase in the rate of plaque growth.[59]

Lipid Lowering and Atherosclerosis

Lipid-lowering trials have shown consistently that disease progression can be slowed but that the degree of reduction in narrowing of established stenoses is minimal. Trials designed to study the risk of acute events after lipid lowering by drugs, however, have demonstrated a 30 percent drop in acute ischemic events and a fall in all-cause mortality. The effect becomes apparent after 18 months of therapy (see also Chap. 38).

Acute coronary syndromes largely are due to thrombosis developing on plaques that are vulnerable, i.e., have an increased risk of causing thrombus compared with other plaques in that individual that remain inert for years. The determinants of vulnerability are a large lipid core, a thin cap, endothelial loss, and reduced smooth muscle cell content. All these characteristics reflect a high density and activity of macrophages, i.e., active inflammation. The degree of risk for any individual of developing an acute event depends on the absolute numbers of vulnerable, highly active inflammatory plaques.

Lipid lowering in experimental models of atherosclerosis shows a very consistent message in that plaque morphology is significantly altered, although the reduction in size is small.[99] The number of macrophages falls, cytokine activity falls, metalloproteinase activity falls, smooth muscle density rises, and the plaque becomes more solid due to collagen deposition.[100,101] Such changes would reduce plaque vulnerability to thrombosis. In human subjects, while lipid lowering has systemic effects and improves endothelial function, the time course of benefit is consistent with the induction of quantitative changes in plaques reducing vulnerability. The equal benefit observed in males and females would suggest that both erosion and disruption risks are reduced.

References

1. Ross R. The pathogenesis of atherosclerosis: A perspective for the 1990s. *Nature* 1993; 362:801–809.
2. Stary HC. Evolution and progression of atherosclerotic lesions in coronary arteries of children and young adults. *Arteriosclerosis* 1989; 9:1–19.
3. Glagov S, Bassiouny HS, Giddens DP, Zarins CK. Intimal thickening: Morphogenesis, functional significance and detection. *J Vasc Invest* 1995; 1:2–14.
4. Adams M, Nakagomi A, Keech A, et al. Carotid intima-media thickness is only weakly correlated with the extent and severity of coronary artery disease. *Circulation* 1995; 92:2127–2134.
5. Wissler RW. An overview of the quantitative influence of several risk factors on progression of atherosclerosis in young people in the United States. *Am J Med Sci* 1995; 310:S29–S36.
6. Stary HC, Chandler AB, Dinsmore RE, et al. A definition of advanced types of atherosclerotic lesions and a histological classification of atherosclerosis: A report from the Committee on Vascular Lesions of the Council on Atherosclerosis, American Heart Association. *Circulation* 1995; 92:1355–1374.
7. Burke A, Farb A, Malcom G, et al. Coronary risk factors and plaque morphology in men with coronary disease who died suddenly. *N Engl J Med* 1997; 336:1276–1282.
8. Boston A, Selhub J. Homocysteine and arterioclerosis: Subclinical and clinical disease associations. *Circulation* 1999; 99:2361–2363.
9. Faggiotto A, Ross R, Harker L. Studies of hypercholesterolemia in the non-human primate: I. Changes that lead to fatty streak formation. *Arteriosclerosis* 1984; 4:323–340.
10. Steinberg D, Witztum JL. Lipoproteins and atherogenesis. *JAMA* 1990; 264:3047–3052.
11. O'Brien KD, Allen MD, McDonald TO, et al. Vascular cell adhesion molecule-1 is expressed in human coronary atherosclerotic plaques: Implications for the mode of progression of advanced coronary atherosclerosis. *J Clin Invest* 1993; 92:945–951.
12. Nelken NA, Coughlin SR, Gordon D, Wilcox JN. Monocyte chemoattractant protein-1 in human atheromatous plaques. *J Clin Invest* 1991; 88:1121–1127.
13. Rosenfeld ME, Yla-Herttuala S, Lipton BA, et al. Macrophage colony-stimulation factor mRNA and protein in atherosclerotic lesions of rabbits and man. *Am J Pathol* 1992; 140:291–300.
14. Rayment NB, Moss E, Faulkner L, et al. Synthesis of TNFα and TGFβ mRNA in the different microenvironments within atheromatous plaques. *Cardiovasc Res* 1996; 32:1123–1130.
15. Annex BH, Denning SM, Channon KM, et al. Differential expression of tissue factor protein in directional atherectomy specimens from patients with stable and unstable coronary syndrome. *Circulation* 1995; 91:619–622.
16. Witztum JL, Berliner JA. Oxidized phospholipids and isoprostanes in atherosclerosis. *Curr Opin Lipidiol* 1998; 9:441–448.
17. Gu L, Okada Y, Clinton S, et al. Absence of monocyte chemoattractant protein-1 reduces atherosclerosis in low density lipoprotein receptor-deficient mice. *Mol Cell* 1998; 2:275–281.
18. Reckless J, Rubin E, Verstuyft J, et al. Monocyte chemoattractant protein-1 but not tumor necrosis factor-alpha is correlated with monocyte infiltration in mouse lipid lesions. *Circulation* 1999; 99:2310–2316.

19. Guyton JR, Klemp KF. Development of the atherosclerotic core region: Chemical and ultrastructural analysis of microdissected atherosclerotic lesions from human aorta. *Arterioscler Thromb* 1994; 14:1305–1314.
20. Ball RY, Stower EC, Burton JH, Cary NR. Evidence that the death of macrophage foam cells contributes to the lipid core of atheroma. *Atherosclerosis* 1995; 114:45–54.
21. Badimon J, Lettino M, Toschi V, et al. Local inhibition of tissue factor reduces the thrombogenicity of disrupted human atherosclerotic plaques: Effects of tissue factor pathway inhibitor on plaque thrombogenicity under flow conditions. *Circulation* 1999; 99:1780–1787.
22. Raines EW, Ross R. Smooth muscle cells and the pathogenesis of the lesions of atherosclerosis. *Br Heart J* 1993; 69:S30–S37.
23. Libby P. Molecular bases of the acute coronary syndromes. *Circulation* 1995; 91:2844–2850.
24. Libby P, Hansson GK. Involvement of the immune system in human atherogenesis: Current knowledge and unanswered questions. *Lab Invest* 1991; 64:5–15.
25. Mach F, Schonbeck U, Sukhova G, et al. Reduction of atherosclerosis in mice by inhibition of CD40 signalling. *Nature* 1998; 394:200–203.
26. Salonen JT, Yla-Herttuala S Yamamoto R, et al. Auto-antibody against oxidised LDL and progression of carotid atherosclerosis. *Lancet* 1992; 339:883–887.
27. Kol A, Bourcier T, Lichtman A, Libby P. Chlamydial and human heat shock protein 60s activate human vascular endothelium, smooth muscle cells, and macrophages. *J Clin Invest* 1999; 103:571–577.
28. Kol A, Sukhova G, Lichtman A, Libby P. Chlamydial heat shock protein 60 localizes in human atheroma and regulates macrophage tumor necrosis factor-alpha and matrix metalloproteinase expression. *Circulation* 1998; 98:300–307.
29. Thomas M, Wong Y, Thomas D, et al. Relation between direct detection of *Chlamydia pneumoniae* DNA in human coronary arteries at postmortem examination and histological severity (Stary grading) of associated atherosclerotic plaque. *Circulation* 1999; 99:2733–2736.
30. Anderson J, Muhlestein J, Carlquist J, et al. Randomized secondary prevention trial of azithromycin in patients with coronary artery disease and serological evidence of *Chlaymdia pneumoniae* infection. The Azithromycin in Coronary Artery Disease: Elimination of Myocardial Infarction with Chlamydia (ACADEMIC) study. *Circulation* 1999; 99:1540–1547.
31. Barger AC III, Beeuwkes R. Rupture of coronary vasa vasorum as a trigger of acute myocardial infarction. *Am J Cardiol* 1990; 66:41G–43G.
32. O'Brien KD, McDonald TO, Chait A, et al. Neovascular expression of E-selectin, intercellular adhesion molecule-1, and vascular cell adhesion molecule-1 in human atherosclerosis and their relation to intimal leukocyte content. *Circulation* 1996; 93:672–682.
33. Moulton K, Heller E, Konerding M, et al. Angiogenesis inhibitors endostatin or TNP-470 reduce intimal neovascularization and plaque growth in apolipoprotein E–deficient mice. *Circulation* 1999; 99:1726–1732.
34. Davies MJ, Woolf N, Rowles PM, Pepper J. Morphology of the endothelium over atherosclerotic plaques in human coronary arteries. *Br Heart J* 1988; 60:459–464.
35. Burrig KF. The endothelium of advanced arteriosclerotic plaques in humans. *Arterioscler Thromb* 1991; 11:1678–1689.
36. Yang JJ, Kettritz R, Falk RJ, et al. Apoptosis of endothelial cells induced by the neutrophil serine proteases proteinase 3 and elastase. *Am J Pathol* 1996; 149:1617–1626.
37. McGill HC. *The Geographic Pathology of Atherosclerosis*. Baltimore: Williams & Wilkins; 1968:38.
38. Tracy RE, Newman WP, Wattigney WA, Berenson GS. Risk factors and atherosclerosis in youth: Autopsy findings of the Bogalusa Heart Study. *Am J Med Sci* 1995; 310:S37–S41.
39. Glagov S, Weisenberd E, Zarins CK, et al. Compensatory enlargement of human atherosclerotic coronary arteries. *N Engl J Med* 1987; 316:1371–1375.
40. Tuzcu EM, Hobbs RE, Rincon G, et al. Occult and frequent transmission of atherosclerotic coronary disease with cardiac transplantation: Insights from intravascular ultrasound. *Circulation* 1995; 91:1706–1713.
41. Davies M. Stability and instability: Two faces of coronary atherosclerosis. The Paul Dudley White Lecture 1995. *Circulation* 1996; 94:2013–2020.
42. Davies MJ, Richardson PD, Woolf N, et al. Risk of thrombosis in human atherosclerotic plaques: Role of extracellular lipid, macrophage, and smooth muscle cell content. *Br Heart J* 1993; 69:377–381.
43. Farb A, Burke AP, Tang AL, et al. Coronary plaque erosion without rupture into a lipid core: A frequent cause of coronary thrombosis in sudden coronary death. *Circulation* 1996; 93:1354–1363.
44. Arbustini E, Bello B, Morbini P, et al. Plaque erosion is a major substrate for coronary thrombosis in acute myocardial infarction. *Heart* 1999; 82:1–4.
45. Richardson PD, Davies MJ, Born GVR. Influence of plaque configuration and stress distribution on fissuring of coronary atherosclerotic plaques. *Lancet* 1989; 2:941–944.
46. Cheng GC, Loree HM, Kamm RD, et al. Distribution of circumferential stress in ruptured and stable atherosclerotic lesions: A structural analysis with histopathological correlation. *Circulation* 1993; 87:1179–1187.
47. Loree HM, Kamm RD, Stringfellow RG, Lee RT. Effects of fibrous cap thickness on peak circumferential stress in model atherosclerotic vessels. *Circ Res* 1992; 71:850–858.
48. Lendon CL, Davies MJ, Born GVR, Richardson PD. Atherosclerotic plaque caps are locally weakened when macrophages density is increased. *Atherosclerosis* 1991; 87:87–90.
49. Sukhova G, Shi G, Simon D, et al. Expression of the elastolytic cathepsins S and K in human atheroma and regulation of their production in smooth muscle cells. *J Clin Invest* 1998; 102: 576–583.
50. Henney AM, Wakeley PR, Davies MJ, et al. Localization of stromelysin gene expression in atherosclerotic plaques by in situ hybridization. *Proc Natl Acad Sci USA* 1991; 88:8154–8158.
51. Galis ZS, Sukhova GK, Lark MW, Libby P. Increased expression of matrix metalloproteinases and matrix degrading activity in vulnerable regions of human atherosclerotic plaques. *J Clin Invest* 1994; 94:2493–2503.
52. Sukhova G, Schonbeck U, Rabkin E, et al. Evidence for increased collagenolysis by interstitial collagenases-1 and -3 in vulnerable human atheromatous plaques. *Circulation* 1999; 99:2503–2509.
53. Ambrose JA, Winters SL, Arora RR. Angiographic evolution of coronary artery morphology in unstable angina. *J Am Coll Cardiol* 1986; 7:472–478.
54. Moreno PR, Falk E, Palacios IF, et al. Macrophage infiltration in acute coronary syndromes: Implications for plaque rupture. *Circulation* 1994; 90:775–778.
55. Escaned J, van Suylen RJ MacLeod DC, et al. Histologic characteristics of tissue excised during directional coronary atherectomy in stable and unstable angina pectoris. *Am J Cardiol* 1993; 71:1442–1447.
56. Rosenschein U, Ellis SG, Haudenschild CC, et al. Comparison of histopathologic coronary lesions obtained from directional atherectomy in stable angina versus acute coronary syndromes. *Am J Cardiol* 1994; 73:508–510.
57. Haft JI, Christou CP, Goldstein JE, Carnes RE. Atherectomy and complex coronary lesions. In: Ambrose JA, ed. *Complex*

Coronary Lesions in Acute Coronary Syndromes. Armonk, NY: Futura; 1996:73.
58. Flugelman MY, Virmani R, Correa R, et al. Smooth muscle cell abundance and fibroblast growth factors in coronary lesions of patients with nonfatal unstable angina: A clue to the mechanism of transformation from the stable to the unstable clinical state. *Circulation* 1993; 88:2493–2500.
59. Mann J, Davies MJ. Mechanisms of progression in native coronary artery disease: Role of healed plaque disruption. *Heart* 1999; 82:265–268.
60. White CJ, Ramee SR, Collins TJ, et al. Coronary thrombi increase PTCA risk: Angioscopy as a clinical tool. *Circulation* 1996; 93:253–258.
61. Davies MJ, Thomas AC, Knapman PA, Hangartner R. Intramyocardial platelet aggregation in patients with unstable angina suffering sudden ischemic cardiac death. *Circulation* 1986; 73: 418–427.
62. Falk E. Unstable angina with fatal outcome: Dynamic coronary thrombosis leading to infarction and/or sudden death. *Circulation* 1985; 71:699–708.
63. Lindahl B, Venge P, Wallentin L, FRISC Study Group. Relation between troponin T and the risk of subsequent cardiac events in unstable coronary artery disease. *Circulation* 1996; 93:1651–1657.
64. Badimon L, Chesebro JH, Badimon JJ. Thrombus formation on ruptured atherosclerotic plaques and rethrombosis on evolving thrombi. *Circulation* 1992; 86:III74–III85.
65. Reddy KG, Nair RN, Sheehan HM, Hodgson JM. Evidence that selective endothelial dysfunction may occur in the absence of angiographic or ultrasound atherosclerosis in patients with risk factors for atherosclerosis. *J Am Coll Cardiol* 1994; 23:833–843.
66. Yamagishi M, Miyatake K, Tamai J, et al. Intravascular ultrasound detection of atherosclerosis at the site of focal vasospasm in angiographically normal or minimally narrowed coronary segments. *J Am Coll Cardiol* 1994; 23:352–357.
67. Zeiher AM, Goebel H, Schachinger V, Ihling C. Tissue endothelin-1 immunoreactivity in the active coronary atherosclerotic plaque: A clue to the mechanism of increased vasoreactivity of the culprit lesion in unstable angina. *Circulation* 1995; 91:941–947.
68. Brown B, Bolson EL, Dodge HT. Dynamic mechanisms in human coronary stenosis. *Circulation* 1984; 70:917–922.
69. Lam JY, Chesebro JH, Steele PM, et al. Is vasospasm related to platelet deposition: Relationship in a porcine preparation of arterial injury in vivo. *Circulation* 1987; 76:243–248.
70. Kohchi K, Takebayashi S, Hiroki T, Nobuyoshi M. Significance of adventitial inflammation of the coronary artery in patients with unstable angina: Results at autopsy. *Circulation* 1995; 71:709–716.
71. Roberts WC, Curry RC, Isner JM. Sudden death in Prinzmetal's angina with coronary spasm documented by arteriography: Analysis of three necropsy cases. *Am J Cardiol* 1982; 50:203–210.
72. Hochman J, Tamis J, Thompson T, et al. Sex, clinical presentation, and outcome in patients with acute coronary syndromes. *N Engl J Med* 1999; 341:226–232.
73. Stadius ML, Maynard C, Fritz JK. Coronary anatomy and left ventricular function in the first 12 hours of acute myocardial infarction: The Western Washington Randomized Intracoronary Streptokinase Trial. *Circulation* 1985; 72:292–301.
74. Davies MJ, Woolf N, Robertson WB. Pathology of acute myocardial infarction with particular reference to occlusive coronary thrombi. *Br Heart J* 1976; 38:659–664.
75. Fulton WFM. Pathological concepts in acute coronary thrombosis: Relevance to treatment. *Br Heart J* 1993; 70:403–408.
76. DeWood MA, Sifter WF, Simpson CS. Coronary arteriographic findings soon after non-Q-wave myocardial infarction. *N Engl J Med* 1986; 315:417–423.
77. Piek JJ, Becker AE. Collateral blood supply to the myocardium at risk in human myocardial infarction: A quantitative post-mortem assessment. *J Am Coll Cardiol* 1988; 11:1290–1296.
78. Ross R. Atherosclerosis: An inflammatory disease. *N Engl J Med* 1999; 340:115–126.
79. van der Wal A, Becker A, Koch K, et al. Clinically stable angina pectoris is not necessarily associated with histological stable atherosclerotic plaques. *Heart* 1996; 76:312–316.
80. Lagrand W, Visser C, Hermens W, et al. C-reactive protein as a cardiovascular risk factor: More than an epiphenomenon? *Circulation* 1999; 100:96–102.
81. Ridker PM, Cushman M, Stampfer MJ, et al. Inflammation, aspirin and the risk of cardiovascular disease in apparently healthy men. *N Engl J Med* 1997; 336:973–979.
82. Libby P, Egan D, Skarlatos S. Roles of infectious agents in atherosclerosis and restenosis: An assessment of the evidence and need for future research. *Circulation* 1997; 96:4095–4103.
83. Hangartner JRW, Charleston AJ, Davies MJ, Thomas AC. Morphological characteristics of clinically significant coronary artery stenosis in stable angina. *Br Heart J* 1986; 56:501–508.
84. Waller BF. The eccentric coronary atherosclerotic plaque: Morphologic observations and clinical relevance. *Clin Cardiol* 1989; 12:14–20.
85. Moise A, Lesperance J, Theroux P, et al. Clinical and angiographic predictors of new total coronary occlusion in coronary artery disease: Analysis of 313 non-operated patients. *Am J Cardiol* 1984; 54:1176–1181.
86. Ambrose JA, Tannenbaum MA, Alexopoulos D, et al. Angiographic progression of coronary artery disease and the development of myocardial infarction. *J Am Coll Cardiol* 1988; 12:56–62.
87. Little WC, Constantinescu M, Applegate RJ. Can coronary angiography predict the site of a subsequent myocardial infarction in patients with mild-to-moderate artery disease? *Circulation* 1988; 78:1157–1166.
88. Giroud D, Li JM, Urban P, et al. Relation of the site of acute myocardial infarction to the most severe coronary arterial stenosis at prior angiography. *Am J Cardiol* 1992; 69:729–732.
89. Petursson KK, Jonmundsson EH, Brekkan A, Hardarson T. Angiographic predictors of new coronary occlusions. 1995; 129: 515–520.
90. Waters D, Craven TE, Lesperance J. Prognostic significance of progression of coronary atherosclerosis. *Circulation* 1993; 87: 1067–1075.
91. Azen SP, Mack WJ, Cashin Hemphill L, et al. Progression of coronary artery disease predicts clinical coronary events: Long-term follow-up from the cholesterol lowering atherosclerosis study. *Circulation* 1996; 93:34–41.
92. Davies MJ, Bland JM, Hangartner JWR, et al. Factors influencing the presence or absence of acute coronary artery thrombi in sudden ischaemic death. *Eur Heart J* 1989; 10:203–208.
93. Davies MJ, Thomas AC. Thrombosis and acute coronary artery lesions in sudden cardiac ischaemic death. *N Engl J Med* 1984; 310:1137–1140.
94. Falk E. Plaque rupture with severe pre-existing stenosis precipitating coronary thrombosis: Characteristics of coronary atherosclerotic plaque underlying fatal occlusive thrombi. *Br Heart J* 1983; 50:127–131.
95. Frink RJ. Chronic ulcerated plaques: New insights into the pathogenesis of acute coronary disease. *J Invas Cardiol* 1994; 6:173–185.
96. Varnava A. Coronary artery remodelling. *Heart* 1998; 79:109–110.
97. Smits P, Bos L, Quarles van Ufford M, et al. Shrinkage of human coronary arteries is an important determinant of *de novo* atherosclerotic luminal stenosis: An in vivo intravascular ultrasound study. *Heart* 1998; 79:143–147.
98. Small DM, Bond MG, Waugh D, et al. Physicochemical and histological changes in the arterial wall of non-human primates

during progression and regression of atherosclerosis. *J Clin Invest* 1984; 73:1590–1605.

99. Kaplan JR, Manuck SB, Adams MR, et al. Plaque changes and arterial enlargement in atherosclerotic monkeys after manipulation of diet and social environment. *Arterioscler Thromb* 1993; 13:254–263.
100. Shiomi M, Ito T, Tsukada T, et al. Reduction of serum cholesterol levels alters lesional composition of atherosclerotic plaques: Effect of pravastatin sodium on atherosclerosis in mature WHHL rabbits. *Arterioscler Thromb Vasc Biol* 1995; 15:1938–1944.
101. Aikawa M, Rabkin E, Okada Y, et al. Lipid lowering by diet reduces matrix metalloproteinase activity and increases collagen content of rabbit atheroma: A potential mechanism of lesions stabilization (see Comments). *Circulation* 1998; 97:2433–2444.

CHAPTER 37

CORONARY BLOOD FLOW AND MYOCARDIAL ISCHEMIA

Attilio Maseri / Gaetano Antonio Lanza / Tommaso Sanna / Stefano Rigattieri

REGULATION OF CORONARY BLOOD FLOW

The task of the coronary circulation is to supply the myocardium with oxygen and substrates and remove metabolic waste products. Contractile cardiac function relies on aerobic metabolism and, as basal oxygen extraction is about 60 percent,[1] an adequate increase of coronary blood flow is required to meet increased myocardial oxygen consumption (M_{VO_2}).

During strenuous exercise coronary blood flow can increase about five times.[2] The maximal increase in coronary flow above resting levels is defined *coronary flow reserve* and is expressed as the ratio between the flow during maximal vasodilatation and basal flow.[3] Low M_{VO_2} at rest requires a low coronary flow; therefore it is associated with a larger coronary flow reserve than a high resting M_{VO_2}.

Vascular resistance in the coronary circulation is distributed into several functional compartments arranged in series. It is mainly determined by M_{VO_2} and modulated by neural stimuli, local vasoactive autacoids, and circulating vasoactive substances. The transmural distribution of resistance across the ventricular wall is largely determined by extravascular tissue compressive forces.

A brief description of determinants of M_{VO_2}, of the functional anatomy of the coronary circulation, and of the distribution of coronary vascular resistance is useful for a better understanding of the regulation of myocardial blood flow (see also Chap. 40).

Determinants of Myocardial Oxygen Consumption

Mechanical work performed by the myocardium is the most important determinant of M_{VO_2}, as the latter decreases to only 15 to 20 percent in the nonbeating heart. Heart rate, myocardial wall tension, and myocardial inotropic state are the major determinants of metabolic activity and therefore of M_{VO_2}.[4]

Heart rate is by far the major determinant of M_{VO_2}: when the heart rate doubles, myocardial oxygen uptake also approximately doubles. Myocardial tension developed during systole is directly proportional to aortic pressure (afterload), myocardial fiber length and ventricular volume (preload).* Myocardial oxygen uptake approximately doubles as mean aortic pressure is increased from 75 to 175 mmHg at constant heart rate and stroke volume. Finally, myocardial inotropic state determines ventricular performance independent of both preload and afterload. M_{VO_2} increases by about 30 percent when *dp/dt*† is doubled by extrasystolic potentiation or by norepinephrine at constant heart rate, aortic pressure, and cardiac output.

Direct measurement of M_{VO_2} requires determination of coronary blood flow and arteriovenous difference of blood oxygen content. Therefore, a number of noninvasive, indirect indices were proposed. Of these, the rate-pressure product (heart rate × systolic blood pressure) is the simplest one and is well correlated with direct measures of M_{VO_2} in a variety of physiologic and experimental conditions.

Functional Compartments of the Coronary Circulation

About 75 percent of total vascular resistance occurs in the arterial system, which can be divided into three functional com-

* According to Laplace's law, wall tension = (pressure × radius)/2 × wall thickness.

† *dp/dt* indicates the rate of pressure development in the left ventricle.

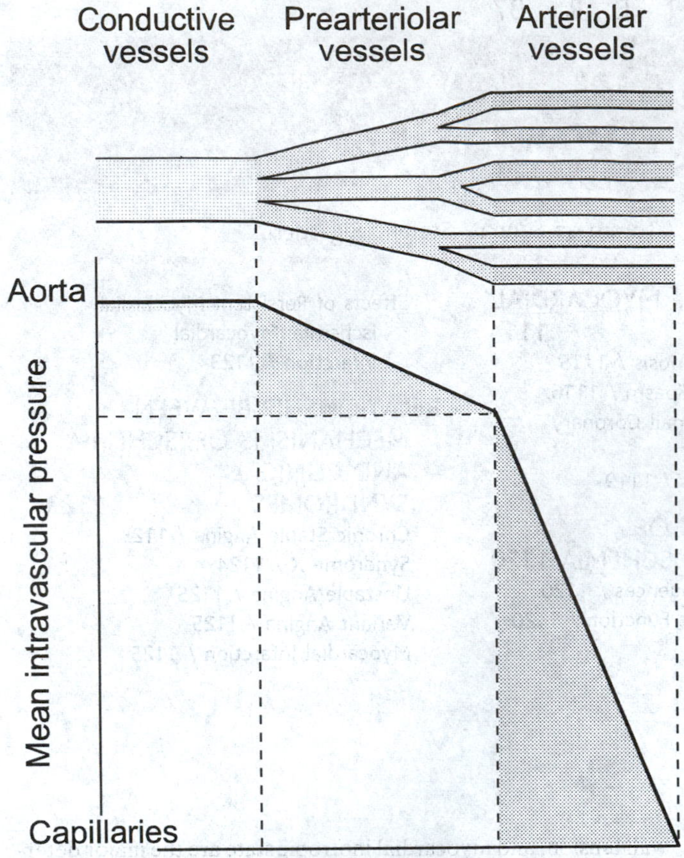

FIGURE 37-1 Schematic illustration of the subdivision of coronary arterial system into conductive, prearteriolar, and arteriolar vessels. Resistance to flow is negligible in conductive vessels (epicardial arteries) and maximal in arterioles, which are under the control of myocardial metabolic activity. Prearteriolar vessels offer an appreciable resistance to flow, but, unlike arterioles, are not under direct metabolic vasodilator control. Their specific function is to maintain pressure at the origin of arterioles within a narrow range when aortic pressure and coronary flow vary. The arterioles are the major site of metabolic regulation of flow. (From Maseri[46] by permission.)

partments arranged in series: conductive vessels, prearteriolar vessels, and arteriolar vessels (Fig. 37-1).

1. The proximal compartment is represented by the large epicardial coronary arteries; these vessels have conductive function and do not contribute significantly to vascular resistance, as the pressure drop along their length is negligible. During systole, their blood content increases by about 25 percent as a result of anterograde flow from the aorta and retrograde flow from squeezed intramyocardial vessels. The elastic energy accumulated in the vessel wall during systole is transformed into blood kinetic energy at the beginning of diastole. About 60 percent of the wall thickness of conductive vessels is represented by the muscular media, which is responsible for myogenic autoregulation of the vascular lumen in response to changes in aortic pressure and for modulation of coronary tone in response to flow-mediated endothelium-dependent vasodilators, circulating vasoactive substances, and neural stimuli. Conversely, the caliber of large conduit arteries is totally unaffected by myocardial metabolites because of their extramural position.
2. The intermediate compartment is represented by prearterioles, which are resistive vessels connecting epicardial conduit arteries to the arterioles. The proximal and distal ends of prearterioles cannot be defined anatomically, but their diameter is in the range of 100 to 500 μm. They contribute to about 30 percent of total coronary flow resistance, but their vasomotor control mechanisms are much more like those of epicardial arteries than those of arterioles because they are largely unaffected by myocardial metabolic vasodilators. The main function of prearterioles is to maintain the driving pressure at the origin of arterioles within an optimal range. This regulatory function is mediated by myogenic autoregulation and flow-dependent vasodilatation in response to shear stress. Prearteriolar resistance is also modulated by neural stimuli and by local autacoids.
3. The distal arterial compartment is represented by the arterioles, which are the main site of metabolic regulation of coronary blood flow. They are smaller than 100 μm in diameter and are responsible for about 40 percent of coronary flow resistance. Also, their tone can be modulated by neural stimuli and local autacoids. At the arteriolar site, the effects of constrictor stimuli strong enough to induce ischemia are directly opposed by locally released myocardial vasodilator metabolites.

In an integrated response model,[5] an increase in metabolic demand of the myocardium initially causes arteriolar vasodilatation (metabolic domain) which is followed by a transient decrease in pressure at their origin, with consequent myogenic regulation (myogenic domain) as well as by an increase in flow, leading to flow-mediated, endothelium-dependent vasodilatation in proximal vessels (flow-sensitive domain). Arterioles branch into metaarteriolar and capillary vessels, which provide a regional microdistribution of flow that, under physiologic conditions, exhibits spatial and temporal heterogeneity. Such physiologic heterogeneity may have pathophysiologic consequences, as coronary hypoperfusion severe enough to cause ischemia was shown to produce a nonuniform maximal dilation of microvessels and a variable response to adenosine in adjacent myocardial regions.[6]

Diffusion of oxygen and substrates to myocardial cells takes place at the capillary level. On average, there is one capillary for each myocardial fiber, but their density is about 20 percent higher in the subendocardial layers.

The venous side of the coronary circulation has so far received little attention, although it contributes a detectable fraction of total coronary flow resistance and can influence capillary recruitment and blood volume content in the ventricular wall, increasing diastolic fiber length and therefore myocardial oxygen consumption ("garden hose" effect).

Physiologic Control Of Myocardial Perfusion

The in-series distribution of resistance as well as total vascular resistance are largely determined by changes of coronary vasomotor tone, while the transmural distribution of perfusion across the left ventricular wall is largely determined by extravascular compressive forces.

EXTRAVASCULAR MECHANICAL FORCES

At variance with all other organs, the heart generates its own perfusion pressure, and extravascular forces squeeze the vessels closed when extravascular pressure is higher than intravascular distending pressure.[7]

During systole, intramyocardial left ventricular pressure is sufficiently high to prevent systolic flow across the whole wall (perhaps with the exception of the outermost layers) and to squeeze intramyocardial blood forward out of the capillaries, venules, and veins toward the coronary sinus and backward from subendocardial and midwall layers toward epicardial arteries.[8] The extravascular compressive forces are highest in the subendocardium and decrease linearly toward the subepicardium. As intramyocardial tissue pressure is higher in subendocardial layers,[9] subendocardial vessels are squeezed more than subepicardial ones, so they take a longer time to refill and resume their caliber during diastole,[10] particularly when perfusion pressure is low (e.g., distal to flow-limiting coronary stenosis or in the presence of aortic stenosis) (Fig. 37-2). When poststenotic pressure is reduced, subendocardial perfusion is further impaired by tachycardia, which shortens the duration of diastole,[11] and by increased left ventricular diastolic pressure, which increases extravascular compressive forces in subendocardial layers. The higher extravascular resistance, together with a higher basal M_{VO_2}, determines a greater susceptibility to ischemia in subendocardial layers.

REGULATION OF CORONARY VASOMOTOR TONE

The mechanisms of contraction and relaxation of vascular smooth muscle cells are influenced by several factors and are not the same in the different compartments of the coronary circulation. Vasomotor tone is mainly determined by M_{VO_2} in arteriolar vessels (metabolic vasodilatation) and by perfusion pressure and flow-mediated vasodilatation in prearterioles and in large arteries (myogenic and endothelial control); it is also influenced by neurogenic stimuli, local autacoids, and circulating vasoactive substances in all vascular compartments.

Metabolic Regulation Arteriolar vasomotor tone is under metabolic control, as arterioles are directly exposed to the effects of the myocardial metabolites, which diffuse into the interstitial space. When M_{VO_2} increases, vasodilator metabolites released from myocardial cells diffuse into the arteriolar wall, causing smooth muscle cell relaxation. The resulting arteriolar vasodilatation causes flow to increase, so that vasodilator metabolites are washed out and flow is reset at a higher level.

Adenosine is a major component of myocardial metabolic regulation of flow.[12] According to a "microhypoxia" model, adenosine production reflects adenosine triphosphate (ATP) degradation resulting from a local myocardial imbalance between oxygen supply and demand. ATP dephosphorylation first results in the formation of adenosine monophosphate (AMP), and then, by 5′-nucleotidase action, in adenosine production. Adenosine, diffusing into the interstitial space and arteriolar wall, can stimulate alpha$_2$-receptors of smooth muscle cells, inducing adenylate-cyclase activation, cyclic-AMP synthesis, and consequent smooth muscle cell relaxation.

However, adenosine is unlikely to be the only component of metabolic vasodilatation[13] and of reactive hyperemia following

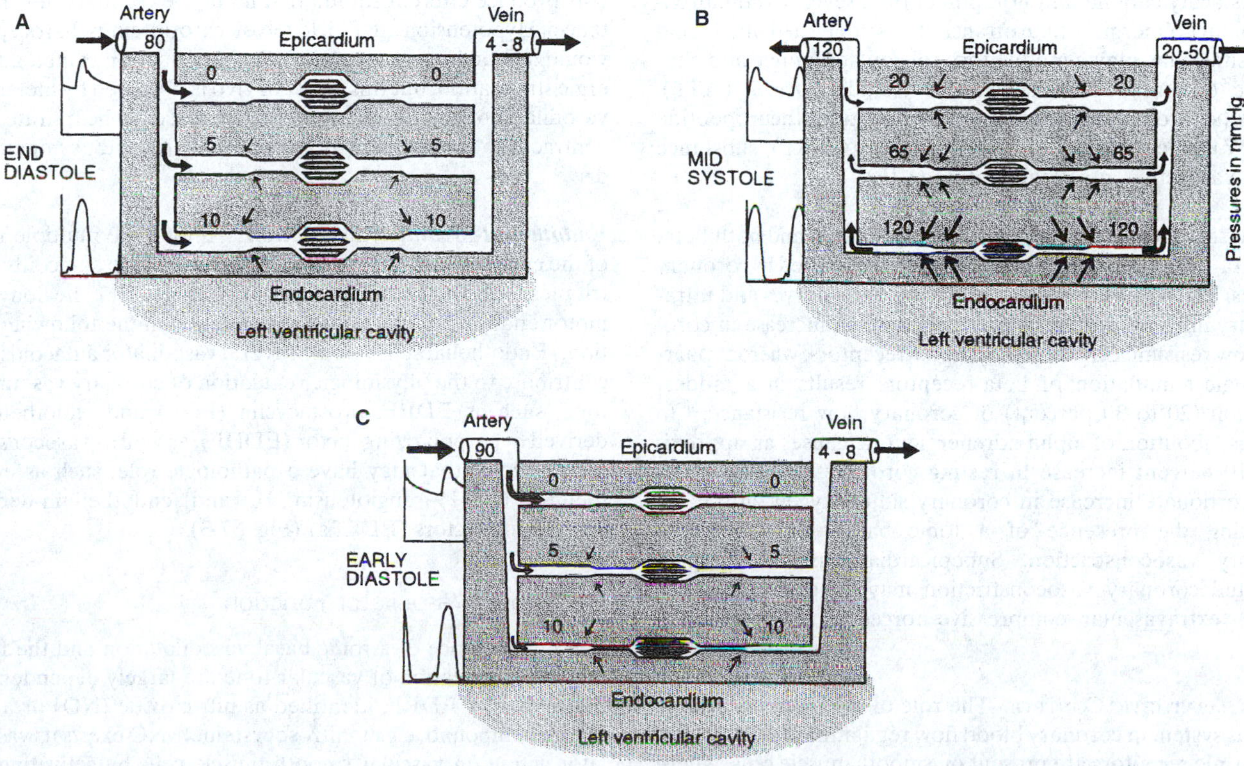

FIGURE 37-2 Changes in interstitial and intravascular pressure and vessel caliber across the left ventricular free wall during the cardiac cycle. During systole, interstitial tissue pressure is greater in subendocardial than in subepicardial layers; therefore subendocardial vessels are squeezed more than subepicardial ones at the end of systole and take longer to resume their full diastolic dimension. In the presence of a low perfusion pressure, subendocardial flow is also impaired by reduced diastolic time, during tachycardia, and by elevated left ventricular diastolic pressure. (From Maseri,[46] modified from Hoffman et al.,[10] by permission.)

release of coronary occlusion.[14] Oxygen tension, pH, potassium, osmotic pressure[15] and ATP-sensitive potassium channels[16] also contribute to metabolic regulation of flow.

Myogenic Regulation When metabolic requirements do not vary, the heart, like other organs, exhibits an intrinsic tendency to maintain blood flow constant despite changes in arterial perfusion pressure. Pressure-flow curves in experimental models show that flow remains nearly constant over a range of perfusion pressure from 60 to 120 mmHg, partly resulting from myogenic control. Myogenic control of vasomotor tone tends to keep the vessel wall tension constant in response to changes in vascular distending pressure: myogenic tone increases when pressure increases and decreases when pressure decreases.

The role of myogenic control of vasomotor tone cannot be easily separated from the effects of stretch-induced release of endothelium-derived relaxing factor (EDRF, see below) and of metabolic regulation. However, myogenic activity has been demonstrated in coronary vessels 40 to 200 μm in diameter[17] and the responses of vascular tone to changes in transmural pressure is not affected by endothelial denudation, confirming that myogenic activity is an intrinsic property of vascular smooth muscle cells.

Neural Regulation Coronary vessels are innervated both by sympathetic and parasympathetic efferents of the autonomic nervous system.[18] Nerve endings are mainly located at the adventitial-medial border of vessels and their density is greater in prearterioles and arterioles than in epicardial coronary arteries. Besides acetylcholine and norepinephrine, several "nonadrenergic noncholinergic" neurotransmitters identified in axonal varicosities may play a modulatory role on adrenergic and cholinergic output.[19] These substances include purines (ATP), amines (serotonin and dopamine), and peptides [neuropeptide Y (NPY), calcitonin gene-related peptide (CGRP), substance P, and vasoactive intestinal peptide (VIP)].

Sympathetic Control Both $alpha_1$ and $alpha_2$ and both $beta_1$ and $beta_2$ adrenergic receptors have been identified in coronary arteries. Electrical stimulation of sympathetic nerves and intracoronary infusion of norepinephrine cause an increase in coronary flow resistance mediated by alpha-receptors, whereas pharmacologic stimulation of beta-receptors results in a modest reduction (20 to 30 percent) of coronary flow resistance.[20] In humans, abolition of alpha-adrenergic tone causes an approximate 10 percent increase in resting coronary blood flow and a proportionate increase in coronary sinus oxygen saturation, indicating the presence of a tonic basal, alpha-mediated coronary vasoconstriction. Subepicardial alpha-adrenergic–mediated coronary vasoconstriction may counterbalance the greater extravascular compressive forces in subendocardial layers.[21]

Parasympathetic Control The role of the parasympathetic nervous system in coronary blood flow regulation is still unclear. Muscarinic receptors are present on smooth muscle cells, where they trigger contraction; on sympathetic nerve varicosities, where acetylcholine inhibits norepinephrine release; and on the endothelium, where their activation induces EDRF release.[22] However, the extent to which acetylcholine released at the site of vagal nerve endings in the adventitia reaches endothelial receptors is unknown. The variable effect of cholinergic stimulation may depend on the balance among its different sites of action. VIP co-released with acetylcholine exerts a significant vasodilator effect.[23]

Purinergic Control Two types of purinergic receptors have been identified: P_1, which is most sensitive to adenosine and mediates smooth muscle cell relaxation both directly and by endothelial release of EDRF, and P_2, which is most sensitive to ATP and mediates endothelial release of EDRF but also direct vasoconstriction. ATP was found to be released from nerve terminals together with norepinephrine. However, the role of purine release by nerve endings in the regulation of coronary blood flow and coronary vasomotion is not well defined.

Peptides NPY is released with norepinephrine during sympathetic nerve stimulation[24] and its infusion was shown to cause severe myocardial ischemia by microvascular constriction in patients with normal coronary arteries (see below). Both CGRP and substance P are also found in cardiac nerves; their intracoronary infusion causes EDRF release and dose-dependent dilation of epicardial coronary arteries with a maximum effect similar to that produced by nitrates.

Reflex Control Coronary vasomotor tone is also under the influence of cardiac reflexes; afferent stimuli arising outside the heart (from chemoreceptors in the carotid bodies and from mechanoreceptors in the carotid sinus, aortic arch and lungs) may produce efferent stimuli that influence coronary flow resistance. Hypotension at the level of carotid sinus baroceptors would tend to increase coronary flow resistance by alpha-adrenergic stimulation, but this effect in vivo is obscured by metabolic vasodilatation in response to the increase in heart rate and contractility consequent to enhanced cardiac sympathetic drive.

Endothelial-Mediated Regulation Among the multiple roles of the endothelium, the production of vasoactive autacoids contributes to the regulation of coronary blood flow. (The nonvasomotor endothelial functions are presented in the following section.) Endothelial cells release several vasodilator autacoids that contribute to the physiologic regulation of coronary vasomotor tone, such as EDRF, prostacyclin (PGI_2) and endothelium-derived hyperpolarizing factor (EDHF), as well as vasoconstrictor autacoids that may have a pathologic role, such as endothelin-1 (ET-1), angiotensin II, and endothelium-derived contracting factors (EDCFs) (Fig. 37-3).

Physiologic Vasodilator Function

The maintenance of a tonic basal vasodilatation and the flow-mediated regulation of vascular tone are largely dependent on the release of EDRF, identified as nitric oxide (NO) or a NO carrier compound, e.g., L-nitrosocysteine.[25] NO exerts its vasodilator action on vascular smooth muscle cells by activating the enzyme guanylate cyclase, which leads to cyclic-GMP production. EDRF is released in response to a large number of agonists acting on endothelial receptors, including neurotransmitters (acetylcholine and norepinephrine), substances released by platelets (serotonin, adenosine diphosphate) or formed during coagulation of the blood (thrombin), and autacoids formed in the vessel wall, such as histamine, bradykinin, and endothelin. Moreover, EDRF is released also in response to pulsatile stretch and flow shear stress.

EDRF has a 5-s half-life and is continuously released, tonically reducing basal vasomotor tone as the infusion of its inhibitor NG-monomethyl-L-arginine (LNMMA) reduces forearm blood flow and coronary diameter in humans[26,27] and causes blood pressure increase in animals.

Flow-mediated vasodilatation in large arteries and in prearteriolar vessels reduces wall shear stress when flow increases. Fluid shear stress and viscous drag, through endothelial mechanotransduction, cause EDRF release as well as transcriptional changes, with protein synthesis and vascular remodeling.[28]

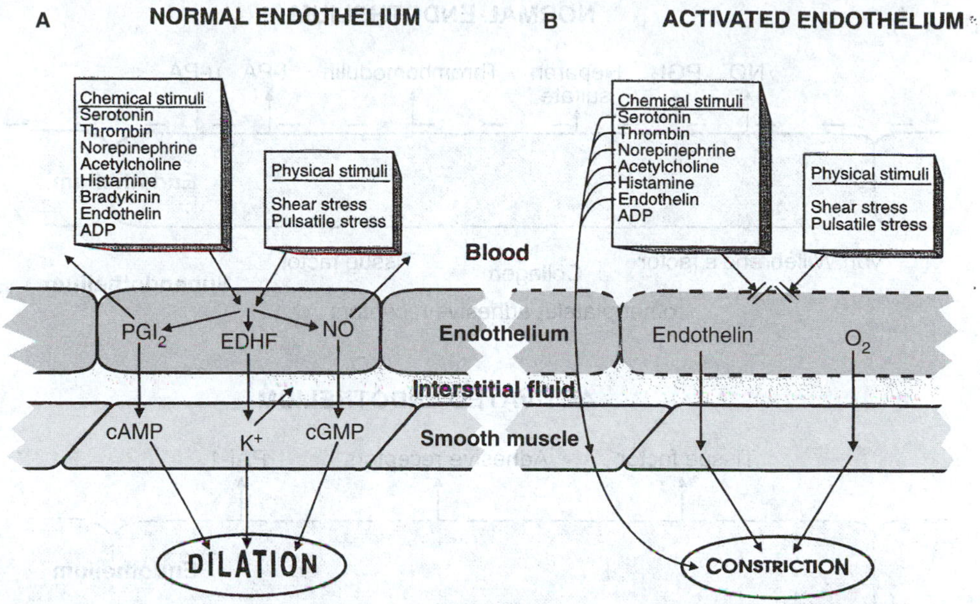

FIGURE 37-3 Vasoactive functions of the endothelium. *A.* Normal endothelium produces a variety of vasodilator substances. *B.* Activated endothelium causes loss of vasodilator functions and produces vasoconstrictor substances. ADP, adenosine diphosphate; PGI_2, prostacyclin; EDHF, endothelium-derived hyperpolarizing factor; NO, nitric oxide; cAMP, cyclic adenosine-monophosphate; K^+, potassium ions; cGMP, cyclic guanosine-monophosphate; O_2^-, superoxide anion. (From Maseri[46] by permission.)

Coronary vascular resistance is also modulated by PGI_2 and by EDHF. PGI_2 is synthesized from arachidonic acid, has a 10-s half-life, and is released in response to pulsatile pressure, bradykinin, thrombin, serotonin, and platelet-derived growth factor (PDGF). It contributes to resting conduit and resistance vessel tone and to flow-mediated vasodilatation.[29] EDHF is most likely a short-lived metabolite of arachidonic acid,[30] thought to open ligand-gated potassium channels, and is released in response to several stimuli, including shear stress, pulsatile flow, acetylcholine, substance P, bradykinin, and CGRP.

Pathologic Vasoconstrictor Function

Vasoconstrictor autacoids are released by endothelial cells in several pathologic conditions (hypertension, diabetes, atherosclerosis, and acute inflammation), but their physiologic role is uncertain.

ET-1, a 21–amino acid peptide released abluminally by endothelial cells, is the most powerful vasoconstrictor known.[31] Despite its short plasmatic half-life (about 5 min), it exerts a prolonged action, interacting with two major types of receptors (ET_A and ET_B) and activating the membrane phospholipase C. Its release is reduced by NO and stimulated by thrombin, angiotensin II, catecholamines, interleukin-1β, transforming growth factor beta, and by hypoxia and ischemia.[32] ET-1 was shown to exert a potent vasoconstrictor effect on small coronary vessels; in dogs, intracoronary infusion of ET-1 causes severe reduction in coronary flow without constriction of angiographically detectable arteries (see below). Under physiologic conditions, there seems to be no significant role for ET-1–mediated regulation of coronary blood flow, as myocardial perfusion is not affected by ET-1 antagonists.

Other endothelial constrictor substances include angiotensin II (produced through a local angiotensin-converting enzyme) and EDCFs, including prostaglandin H_2 and oxygen-derived free radicals.[33]

Blood/Vessel Wall Interface

In addition to its vasomotor function, the endothelium plays a major role in the homeostasis of the vessel wall and in the control of the blood/vessel wall interface. The latter is of fundamental importance, as coronary thrombosis is a major pathogenetic mechanism of acute coronary syndromes.

HOMEOSTASIS OF THE VESSEL WALL

Endothelial cells produce several constituents of the basement membrane and of the intercellular intimal matrix. They also synthesize growth factors for smooth muscle cells as well as heparan sulfates and NO, which inhibit cellular growth and migration.[34,35] The integrity of the endothelium is essential for preventing the diffusion of atherogenic components into the arterial wall. The response of smooth muscle cells to trophic stimuli produced by the endothelium depends on their phenotype:[36] cells in the proliferative phenotype respond with increased protein synthesis and proliferation to growth factors and to constrictor stimuli, whereas cells in the mature contractile phenotype respond with contraction.

CONTROL OF BLOOD/VESSEL WALL INTERFACE

The endothelium plays a key role in preserving blood fluidity and in preventing thrombosis (Fig. 37-4*A*). This overall function is performed by different mechanisms. The glycocalyx of endothelial cells, represented by proteoglycans such as heparan sulfate, forms an electronegative barrier, which prevents adhesion of platelets and circulating cells. NO production also prevents platelet adhesion, and PGI_2 opposes platelet aggregation.[37]

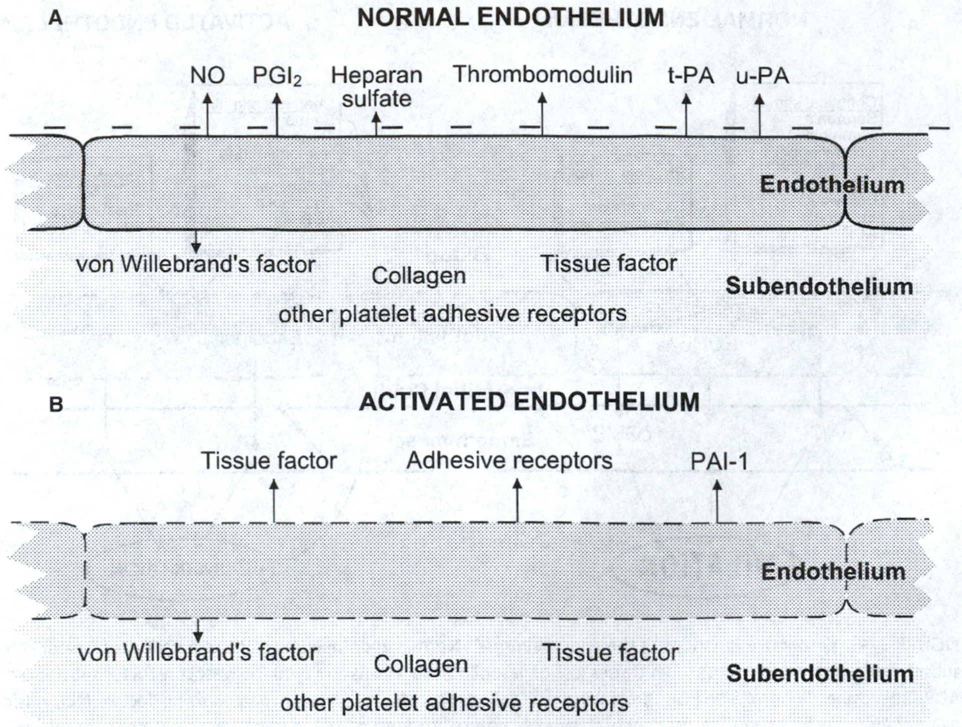

FIGURE 37-4 Anticoagulant role of normal endothelium (*A*) and procoagulant role of activated endothelium (*B*). The anticoagulant properties are due to electronegative charges, to the production of nitric oxide (NO) (which antagonizes platelet adhesion), prostacyclin (PGI_2) (which antagonizes platelet aggregation), heparan sulfate (which catalyzes binding of antithrombin III to thrombin), thrombomodulin (which activates protein C), and tissue and urokinase plasminogen activators (t-PA and u-PA) (which activate plasminogen). Activation of the endothelium causes the loss of anticoagulant functions, the expression of adhesive receptors for leukocytes and platelets and the production of tissue factor and of plasminogen activator inhibitors (PAI-1). (From Maseri[46] by permission.)

Moreover, endothelial cells produce and bind anticoagulants such as heparan sulfate, which catalyzes the inactivation of thrombin by plasma antithrombin III, and thrombomodulin, which binds thrombin and protein C, leading, ultimately, to factor V and VIII inactivation. Finally, endothelial cells are involved in fibrinolysis by the secretion of two plasminogen activators, a urokinase type (u-PA) and a tissue type (t-PA).

ALTERATIONS OF ENDOTHELIAL FUNCTION

Chronic Endothelial Dysfunction Patients with coronary atherosclerosis and also individuals with cardiovascular risk factors (such as hypertension, diabetes, hypercholesterolemia, hyperomocysteinemia, and smoking) show a reduced or abolished vasodilator response to acetylcholine.[33] However, acetylcholine is also a direct powerful constrictor of vascular smooth muscle cells; therefore it is impossible to establish whether an abnormal vasomotor response to acetylcholine is due to defective endothelial EDRF production or to enhanced smooth muscle vasoconstrictor response. The latter possibility is suggested by the preserved dilator effect to substance P in atherosclerotic vessels.[38] It is also unknown to what extent an abnormal response to acetylcholine implies alterations of the endothelial antithrombotic properties. As many patients with extensive coronary atherosclerosis may remain totally free from ischemic events for months and years, it would seem reasonable to consider the possibility that, in some patients and under some circumstances, coronary atherosclerosis may be associated with the development of compensatory, protective factors.

Acute Inflammatory Activation Increasing evidence suggests that inflammatory activation of the endothelium may play a role in the pathogenesis of some acute ischemic syndromes, determining a rapid switch of its functional properties from vasodilator to vasoconstrictor and from anticoagulant to procoagulant.[39,40] Also, in the absence of detectable histologic changes such as erosion or fissure, endothelial activation by inflammatory cytokines abolishes EDRF and PGI_2 release and stimulates ET-1 release, induces the expression of tissue factor and of adhesive receptors for platelets and leukocytes on the luminal surface, causes the production of plasminogen activator inhibitors (PAI-1), and inhibits that of plasminogen activators (u-PA, t-PA) and of heparan sulfate (Fig. 37-4*B*). In addition, cytokines may also activate metalloproteases, with consequent endothelial erosions and lysis of the plaque caps.[41,42] The causes of such inflammatory processes may be multiple, acute, and chronic, infectious or noninfectious,[43] and be variably modulated by the individual inflammatory and immune responses.[44,45]

Therefore, acute activation of the endothelium and of the vascular wall is one of the possible mechanisms that set the stage for local thrombosis and vasoconstriction in presence of a very variable severity of the chronic atherosclerotic background.

MECHANISMS OF MYOCARDIAL ISCHEMIA

Myocardial ischemia develops when coronary blood flow becomes inadequate to meet myocardial oxygen and metabolic substrate requirements for maintaining adequate cardiac function. Myocardial ischemia can result from (1) an increase of myocardial workload, and hence oxygen demand, in the presence of a flow-limiting coronary artery stenosis or (2) a reduction of coronary blood flow caused by epicardial or microvascular coronary artery constriction or by acute thrombosis. These mechanisms may act in combination in some patient as well as in different ischemic episodes in a same patient (Fig. 37-5).[46]

In clinical practice, coronary stenoses are often considered the only or main cause of myocardial ischemia, because they are the most obvious and readily plausible culprits. Indeed, acute thrombosis can be recognized until thrombi are lysed or become incorporated into the atherosclerotic plaques. The detection of coronary spasm and of dynamic stenosis is even more elusive, because they are very transient and usually require repetition of angiography following nitrates or provocative tests. Finally, microvascular constriction may only be indirectly inferred by slow distal flow dye progression at angiography or by special diagnostic studies (see also Chap. 40).

The clinical presentation of anginal syndromes can provide useful clues about the role of these distinct pathogenetic mechanisms in precipitating myocardial ischemia.

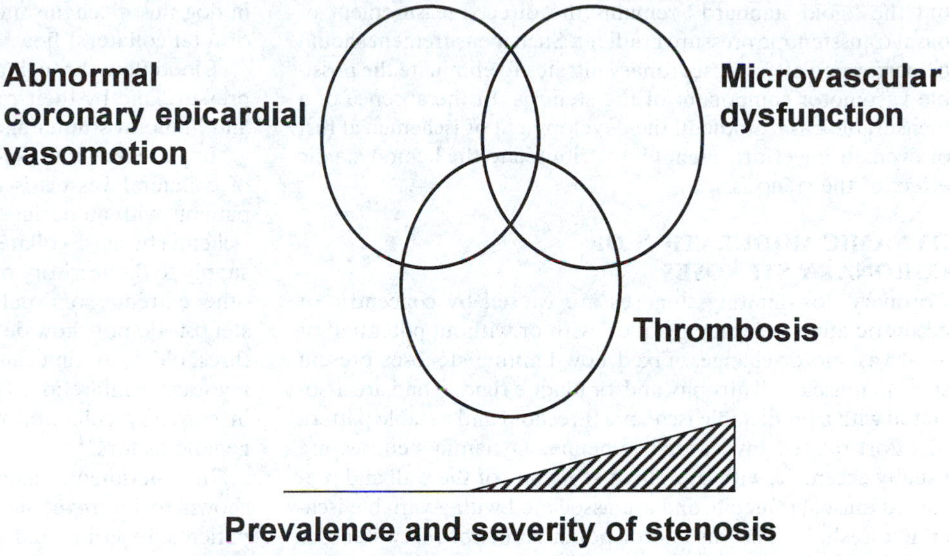

FIGURE 37-5 Pathophysiologic components of myocardial ischemia. The different clinical ischemic syndromes may result from fixed obstruction to coronary blood flow caused by atherosclerotic plaques, from coronary vasoconstriction of epicardial or of microvascular vessels and from coronary thrombosis. (Modified from Maseri A, Crea F, Lanza GA. Coronary vasoconstriction: Where do we stand in 1999? An important, multifaceted, but elusive role. *Cardiologia* 1999; 44:115, by permission.)

Flow-Limiting Stenosis

EFFECTS OF FLOW-LIMITING STENOSIS ON BLOOD FLOW

The presence of epicardial coronary artery stenosis, caused by atherosclerotic plaques, is by far the most frequent angiographic finding in any cardiac ischemic syndrome. However, a stenosis becomes flow-limiting only when it determines a measurable transstenotic pressure gradient at rest. The transstenotic pressure gradient increases with increase in flow, more than doubling when blood flow doubles.

A basal gradient at rest may not cause myocardial ischemia, as flow is maintained by compensatory distal arteriolar dilatation. In turn, compensatory arteriolar dilatation implies a local reduction of coronary flow reserve. The greater the basal transstenotic pressure gradient, the greater the reduction of coronary flow reserve and the lower the level of cardiac work at which myocardial ischemia appears during effort (*ischemic threshold*).

Experimental studies in dogs showed that the acute reduction of coronary diameter by more than 50 percent causes a measurable basal transstenotic pressure gradient.[47] Further decreases in diameter cause an exponential increase of transstenotic pressure gradient and reduction of maximal coronary blood flow (Fig. 37-6). A sudden 85 to 90 percent reduction of an epicardial coronary artery diameter is required to exhaust compensatory arteriolar dilatation and cause myocardial ischemia at rest. The decrease of poststenotic pressure may be reduced by the gradual development of collateral blood flow (see ahead).

In presence of a decreased poststenotic pressure, ischemia initially occurs in subendocardial layers, because the subendocardium is more vulnerable to ischemia than the subepicardium (see above).

The general relationship between severity of coronary stenosis as assessed on coronary angiography and impairment of coronary flow reserve has been confirmed in patients.[48,49] However, the angiographic judgment of the hemodynamic consequences of coronary stenoses is difficult because (1) quantitative angiography does not allow an accurate three-dimensional measurement of severe stenoses; (2) the lumen reduction is estimated with reference to the coronary segment proximal to the stenosis, which may be restricted by atheroma or, conversely, enlarged because of vascular remodeling; (3) the stenosis resistance is linearly related to the length of the stenosis and to the flow turbulence caused by the stenosis irregularities.

Several invasive and noninvasive methods have been proposed to assess the hemodynamic effects of coronary stenoses,[50]

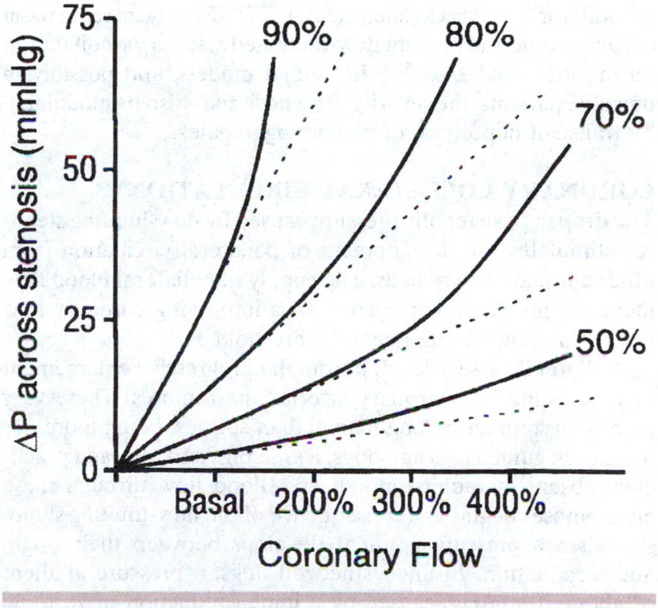

FIGURE 37-6 Schematic illustration of the relationship between coronary blood flow and transstenotic pressure gradient. This relationship becomes curvilinear because of energy losses caused by blood flow turbulence across the stenosis (*solid lines*). Poststenotic pressure decreases progressively with the increase of stenosis severity and, for a given stenosis, it decreases markedly with increasing flow. In the absence of collateral flow, an 80 percent diameter stenosis causes a drop in poststenotic pressure of about 12 mmHg, which would increase to about 30 mmHg when flow doubles. (From Maseri,[46] modified from Klocke,[47] by permission.)

but the "gold standard" remains the direct measurement of basal transstenotic pressure gradient. Such measurement should be performed after intracoronary nitrates to eliminate the possible vasomotor component of the stenosis. In the absence of a measurable basal gradient, the development of ischemia, at rest or even during effort, cannot be attributed to the hemodynamic effect of the stenosis.

DYNAMIC MODULATION OF CORONARY STENOSES

Coronary flow-limiting stenoses are caused by concentric or eccentric atherosclerotic plaques, with or without potential for local vasomotor changes. Fixed flow-limiting stenoses present smooth muscle cell atrophy and/or plaque rigidity and are associated with a predictable ischemic threshold and a stable pattern of effort-related myocardial ischemia. Dynamic stenoses are usually eccentric, with compliant segments of the wall and preserved muscular media, and are associated with a variable ischemic threshold. The vasomotor potential of coronary stenoses can also be assessed directly at angiography by intracoronary infusion of vasodilator and/or vasoconstrictor substances.[51,52]

Vasoconstriction at the site of stenoses may result from (1) neural vasoconstrictor stimuli, (2) impairment of vasodilator mechanisms, (3) increased response of dysfunctional vascular smooth muscle cells to vasoconstrictor stimuli, or (4) variable combination of these mechanisms. For example, exercise and cold pressor test cause vasodilatation in normal vessels but vasoconstriction at the site of stenoses.[53,54] Vasoconstrictor autacoids, produced locally by the endothelium (endothelin)[55,56] in the adventitia (histamine, leukotrienes) or released by activated platelets (thromboxane A_2, serotonin), are also powerful potential constrictor stimuli. Defective production and/or release of vasodilator substances (in particular, EDRF) may increase basal coronary tone and prevent flow-mediated arterial vasodilatation during increased M_{VO_2}.[57–59] In animal models, and possibly in unstable patients, the severity of stenosis may also be modulated by transient deposition of platelet aggregates.

CORONARY COLLATERAL CIRCULATION

The drop in poststenotic pressure caused by flow-limiting stenoses stimulates the development of collateral circulation from other coronary artery beds. The supply of collateral blood flow increases poststenotic pressure, thus improving coronary flow reserve and increasing ischemic threshold.

Collateral vessels develop from the progressive enlargement of preexisting intercoronary arterial anastomoses. These vary greatly in number among mammalian species, being more numerous in guinea pigs and dogs, less in pigs and rats, and practically absent in rabbits and sheep. Blood flow through these anastomoses begins as a consequence of the flow-limiting stenosis, when a pressure gradient develops between their origin and termination. In unanesthetized dogs, a pressure gradient of about 10 mmHg, caused by a lumen reduction of 70 to 80 percent, has been shown to elicit the development of collateral flow.[46]

Preexisting anastomoses progressively transform into mature collaterals over a period of 3 to 6 months by initial widening and remodeling, subsequent proliferation of endothelial and smooth muscle cells, and development of a smooth muscle coat, leading to vessels with a final diameter of 20 to 200 μm. Collateral blood flow may also develop by vessel neoformation, but in dog this mechanism contributes only by less than 5 percent of total collateral flow.[46]

Blood flow through collaterals is determined by the driving pressure and by their resistance, which is influenced by neural and humoral stimuli and by local vasoactive autacoids.[60–63]

In patients with flow-limiting stenoses, the number and size of collateral vessels is quite variable. At one extreme, some patients with an occluded coronary artery do not have signs of ischemia because collateral circulation provides adequate blood supply to the territory of the occluded coronary branch. At the other extreme, some patients with severe flow-limiting coronary stenosis do not show detectable improvement of their ischemic threshold over time and, when the vessel occludes, develop myocardial infarction. The causes of these individual differences in coronary collateral circulation are likely to be related to genetic factors.[64]

In experimental animals, no intervention was convincingly shown to improve the development of collateral vessels. In patients, heparin[65] and fibroblastic growth factor 1 (FGF-1)[66,67] have been suggested to promote collateral growth, but the data are still uncertain.

CORONARY STEAL DISTAL TO FLOW-LIMITING STENOSIS

In the presence of flow-limiting stenoses, myocardial ischemia may develop as a result of a diversion of blood flow from a myocardial region with a very severe impairment of coronary flow reserve, determining an almost maximal arteriolar dilatation in basal conditions, toward a myocardial region with sufficiently preserved coronary flow reserve.

Such a coronary diversion may occur (1) from the subendocardium, as a result of vasodilatation of subepicardial vessels, which increases subepicardial flow but causes a further critical drop of poststenotic pressure (*transmural coronary steal*)[46,68] or (2) from collateralized territories when the parent coronary artery supplying the collaterals presents a flow-limiting stenosis proximal to their origin. In this case, arteriolar dilatation in the territory of the stenosed parent artery increases flow thus causing a further drop of perfusion pressure at the origin of collaterals, which reduces collateral flow (*lateral coronary steal*).[69] In both instances the vasodilatation responsible for the blood flow steal can be induced by vasodilator drugs or an increase in M_{VO_2}.

Coronary Artery Spasm

Epicardial coronary artery spasm is the pathogenetic mechanism of variant angina, but it can play a role in some patients who present with acute coronary syndromes (see also Chap. 40).

CORONARY SPASM IN VARIANT ANGINA

In patients who present with a variant form of angina (see below), myocardial ischemia is caused by an occlusive epicardial coronary spasm.[46] Usually, spasm develops at the site of subcritical or critical stenoses, but it may also occur in angiographically normal coronary arteries, the so-called variant of the variant form of angina. Occlusive spasm causes transmural ischemia with ST-segment elevation, but when spasm is subocclusive, it may cause subendocardial ischemia and ST-segment depression.[70]

In patients with variant angina, spasm tends to recur in the same arterial segment and can be precipitated by sympathetic and parasympathetic stimuli and by a variety of triggers, such as ergonovine, histamine, dopamine, acetylcholine, and serotonin, acting on different receptors, as well as by an increase in arterial pH to 7.65 to 7.70.[71–76] Collectively, these findings suggest a local smooth muscle hyperreactivity to a wide variety of constrictor stimuli. Such hyperreactivity may be caused by a variety of postreceptoral intracellular abnormalities.[46,60] The postmortem findings at the site of coronary spasm are not specific, but fibromuscular hyperplasia was observed in some cases. The animal model of coronary spasm developed in minipigs[77] is unlikely to adequately reflect the mechanisms of vasospastic angina occurring in patients.

CORONARY SPASM IN ACUTE CORONARY SYNDROMES

Although occlusive spasm is typically observed in patients with variant angina, it may also represent a pathogenetic component of other, more common acute coronary syndromes, including unstable angina,[78] unheralded myocardial infarction,[79,80] resuscitated sudden cardiac death,[81] and postcoronary bypass graft angina.[82] In fact, there appears to be a higher prevalence of coronary spasm in patients with acute coronary syndromes (20 to 38 percent) than in patients with stable angina (<6 percent).[46] Coronary spasm has been found to occur more frequently in Asian patients than in Caucasian patients with a recent acute myocardial infarction[80] (Fig. 37-7).

The differences in clinical presentation between variant angina and other ischemic syndromes suggest possible different underlying pathogenetic mechanisms. In unstable plaques, the degree of constriction produced by thromboxane A_2, serotonin, and thrombin could be greatly amplified geometrically at the site of fresh mural thrombi and, in some patients, a local smooth muscle coronary hyperreactivity may contribute to the transition from a nonocclusive platelet-fibrin mural thrombus to an occlusive red thrombus.[46]

Dysfunction of Small Coronary Vessels

The possibility that an impairment of coronary blood flow could occur at the level of distal rather than proximal coronary vessels, has received little consideration until recently, as epicardial coronary artery stenoses, spasm, and thrombosis provide readily available, plausible mechanisms for ischemia. However, several animal and clinical studies indicated that ischemia can be also caused by small coronary vessel constriction.[83,84]

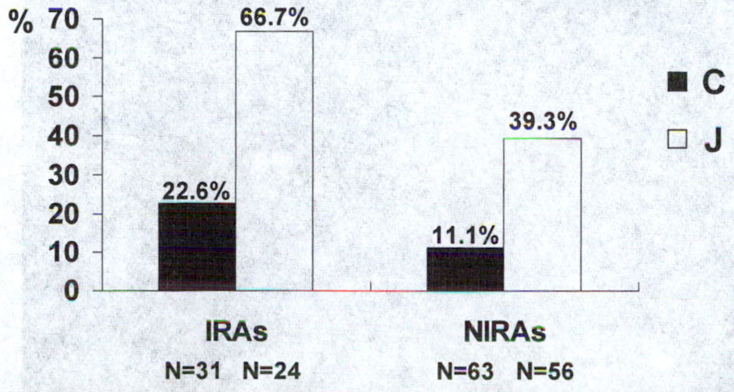

FIGURE 37-7 Induction of coronary spasm by intracoronary acetylcholine injection in infarct-related arteries (IRAs) and non-infarct-related arteries (NIRAs) of Japanese (J) and Italian (C) patients with a recent acute myocardial infarction. Japanese patients had about a threefold higher prevalence of spastic response in both IRAs and NIRAs. The spastic response was more frequent in IRAs than in NIRAs in Japanese, but not in Italian Caucasian, patients. (Modified from Pristipino et al.[80] by permission.)

PHARMACOLOGIC STUDIES IN HUMANS

In patients with angiographically normal coronary arteries, the intracoronary infusion of neuropeptide Y and that of high doses of acetylcholine was found to induce myocardial ischemia without changes of large epicardial vessels but with extremely slow dye progression or diffuse constriction of distal branches, respectively, indicating microvascular constriction.[46,85] In patients with coronary stenoses, the intracoronary infusion of serotonin caused myocardial ischemia with only small changes in stenosis lumen but with diffuse constriction of distal branches and reduced filling of collateral vessels. In dogs, endothelin infusion caused marked ischemia without detectable changes of epicardial vessels, suggesting powerful microvascular constriction.[46,85]

CLINICAL CLUES TO MICROVASCULAR DYSFUNCTION

In some patients in whom myocardial ischemic episodes cannot be blamed on fixed or dynamic epicardial coronary stenoses, constriction of small coronary vessels could account for the development of myocardial ischemia (see also Chap. 40).

Patients with occlusion of a single epicardial coronary artery and no other stenoses may present very wide variations in the ischemic threshold during daily life and exercise testing, which cannot be attributed to dynamic modulation of stenoses or spasm and are most likely caused by vasomotor changes in small distal coronary vessels.[86]

Patients with single-vessel disease following successful percutaneous coronary angioplasty (PTCA) may continue to present with angina, ST-segment depression on exercise testing, and perfusion defects on stress myocardial scintigraphy;[87] in such patients, a dysfunction of small coronary vessels has been confirmed by intracoronary Doppler blood flow measurements and myocardial positron emission tomography (PET) following administration of vasodilator stimuli.[88,89] Microvascular dysfunction is most likely responsible for the reduced coronary dilator response of nonstenosed coronary arteries in patients with coronary disease[90,91] and also in patients with risk factors but no flow-limiting coronary stenoses.[92,93]

Patients with syndrome X who present with angina pectoris, positive exercise testing but angiographically normal coronary arteries and no evidence of epicardial spasm[94] may suffer from some form of microvascular dysfunction. Such a possibility is suggested by stress-induced myocardial perfusion defects on radionuclide studies,[95,96] transient ischemic ST-segment changes during effort test, and reproduction of typical anginal pain with or without ST-segment ischemic changes, by dipyridamole.

However, an ischemic origin of this syndrome is widely questioned because, in the vast majority of studies, no myocardial lactate production or left ventricular dysfunction can be detected during angina and transient ischemic ST-segment changes.[97,98] This apparent paradox could be explained by a patchily distributed coronary microvascular dysfunction, causing dispersed small foci of ischemia. A patchily distributed small vessel constriction may not cause detectable contractile abnormalities or lactate production but rather electrocardiographic

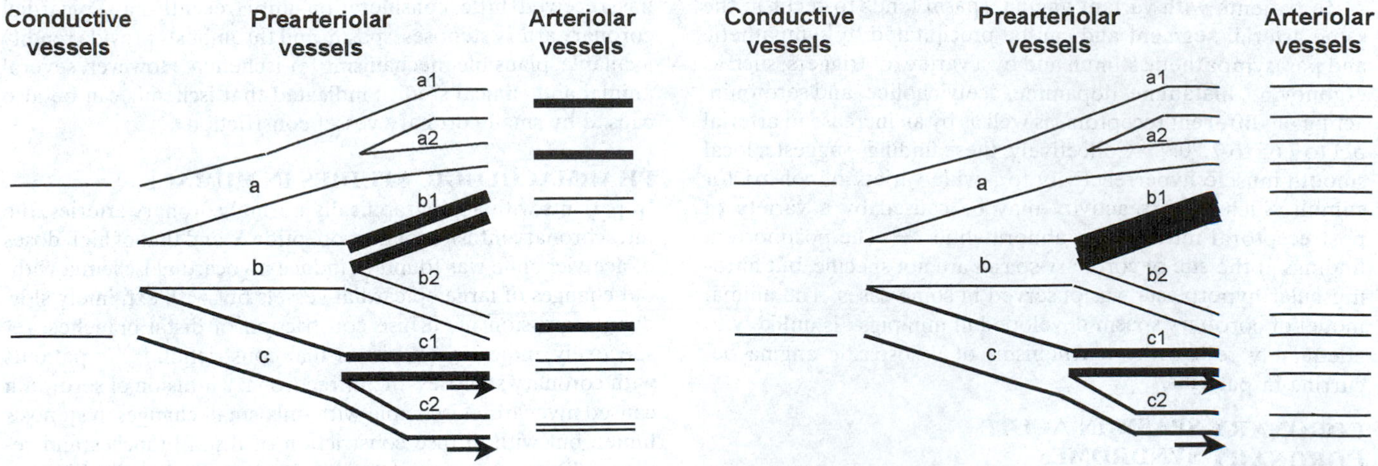

FIGURE 37-8 Model of patchily distributed prearteriolar vasoconstriction in syndrome X. A patchily distributed prearteriolar constriction may be present in basal conditions (b1,c1,c2) (*left panel*). As flow increases during metabolic or pharmacologic arteriolar dilation, the pressure drop through constricted prearterioles increases and perfusion pressure at the origin of distal arterioles decreases, thus resulting in small focal areas of myocardial ischemia (*right panel*). Blood flow steal may also occur from the territory supplied by the most constricted prearterioles toward the region supplied by less constricted prearteriolar vessels (c1,c2). At the end of severely constricted prearterioles, distending pressure may become lower than the critical closing pressure, thus resulting in prearteriolar occlusion (b1). Compensatory myocardial release of adenosine in response to blood flow reduction distal to constricted prearterioles may be sufficient to maintain adequate flow, thus avoiding ischemia, but it may cause angina, particularly when associated with enhanced pain sensitivity. (Modified from Maseri A, Crea F, Kaski JC, et al. Mechanisms of angina pectoris in syndrome X. *J Am Coll Cardiol* 1991; 17:499, by permission.)

(ECG) changes and myocardial perfusion defects when sufficiently confluent.[46,85] This possibility is suggested by observations in animal models, in which ischemia was caused by impaired coronary microcirculation by microspheres[46] or endothelin-1 infusion.[99]

Recent data showing intracardiac production of lipid peroxidation products, which are sensitive markers of ischemia-reperfusion injury,[100] during angina and ischemic ST changes following atrial pacing in syndrome-X patients strongly support the microvascular ischemic origin of the syndrome.[101,102] The occurrence of myocardial ischemia sufficiently confluent and extensive to be detected by phosphorus nuclear magnetic resonance has been reported in 20 percent of syndrome-X patients during the hand-grip stress test.[103]

SITE OF MICROVASCULAR DYSFUNCTION

Theoretically, myocardial ischemia caused by microvascular dysfunction may result from abnormal constriction or failure of adequate dilatation of arteriolar or prearteriolar vessels. Arteriolar constriction as a cause of myocardial ischemia would require constrictor stimuli sufficiently strong to overcome the dilator effect of ischemic metabolites on the arterioles them-

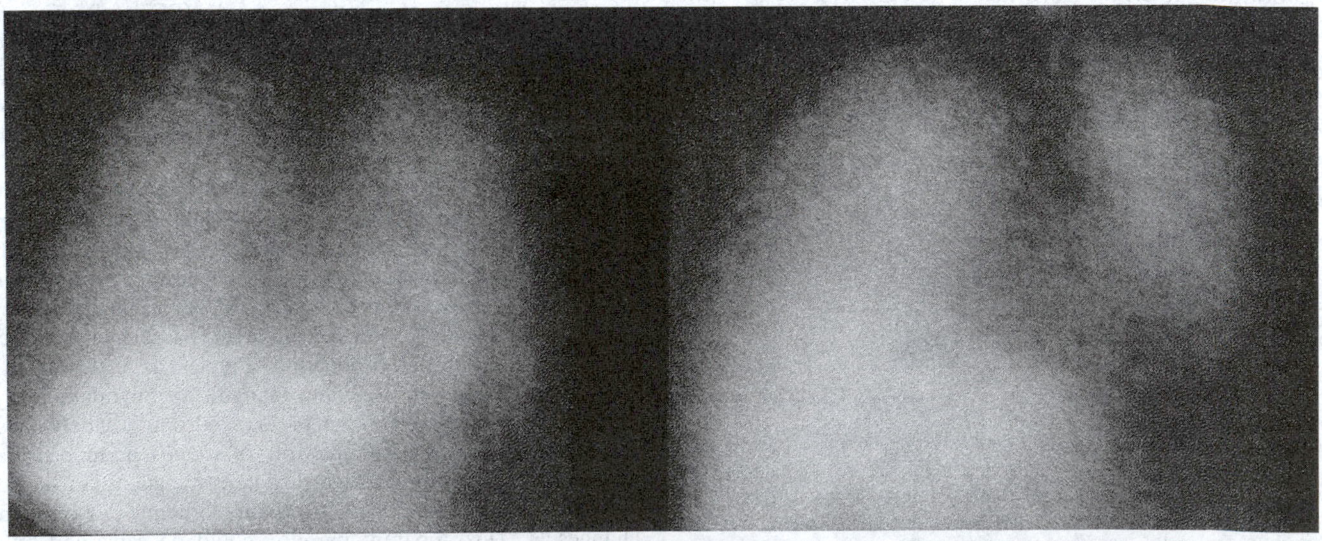

FIGURE 37-9 Typical cardiac scintigrams obtained 3 h after the injection of one-half of the same dose of ^{123}I metaiodobenzylguanidine (MIBG) in a healthy subject (*left panel*) and the other one-half in a patient with syndrome X (*right panel*). Cardiac MIBG uptake was normal in the control subject and totally absent in the syndrome X patient, in contrast with his normal lung and liver MIBG uptake. The total absence of cardiac MIBG uptake was confirmed in follow-up studies at 1 and 12 months, consistent with a persistent impairment of cardiac sympathetic function. (From Lanza et al.[114] by permission.)

selves.[46,85] The prearteriolar vessels appear to be a more likely site of microvascular alterations responsible for myocardial ischemia. An increased, patchily distributed prearteriolar vasoconstriction was proposed as a causal mechanism of syndrome X[46,85] (Fig. 37-8).

MECHANISMS OF MICROVASCULAR DYSFUNCTION

In patients with coronary stenoses, the causes of small coronary vessel dysfunction are commonly attributed to atherosclerosis, although such dysfunction may also be related to neurohumoral stimuli[104] or to vascular abnormalities (e.g., perivascular fibrosis, medial hypertrophy) associated with systemic diseases, such as hypertension or diabetes.[105,106] Small vessel dysfunction in these patients is also frequently attributed to EDRF deficiency on the basis of an abnormal vasomotor response to acetylcholine, but a reduced vasodilator response or a vasoconstrictor response to acetylcholine[107,108] could also be caused by an increased constrictor effect of the drug on smooth muscle cells.

In patients with syndrome X, the mechanisms responsible for microvascular dysfunction can be multiple and not necessarily the same in all patients. They may include (1) structural abnormalities, such as fibrosis and medial hypertrophy;[46] (2) impaired endothelial and nonendothelial vasodilator function;[109] (3) enhanced constrictor response of smooth muscle cells, possibly related to an increased membrane Na^+-H^+ exchanger activity;[110,111] (4) increased release of local vasoconstrictor autacoids—e.g., endothelin 1[112,113] or angiotensin;[46] and (5) abnormal neural stimuli. Evidence of abnormal cardiac sympathetic function was documented by ^{123}I-metaiodobenzylguanidine (MIBG) scintigraphy, which showed total absence of cardiac MIBG uptake in 42 percent of patients and regional defects, matching thallium perfusion defects, in another 33 percent of cases[114] (Fig. 37-9).

Each of these putative mechanisms of microvascular dysfunction may involve a very variable number of prearteriolar vessels. Therefore there may be a spectrum of vascular involvement ranging from very sparse foci of microvascular dysfunction to confluent alteration of all small coronary vessels in large vascular territories.

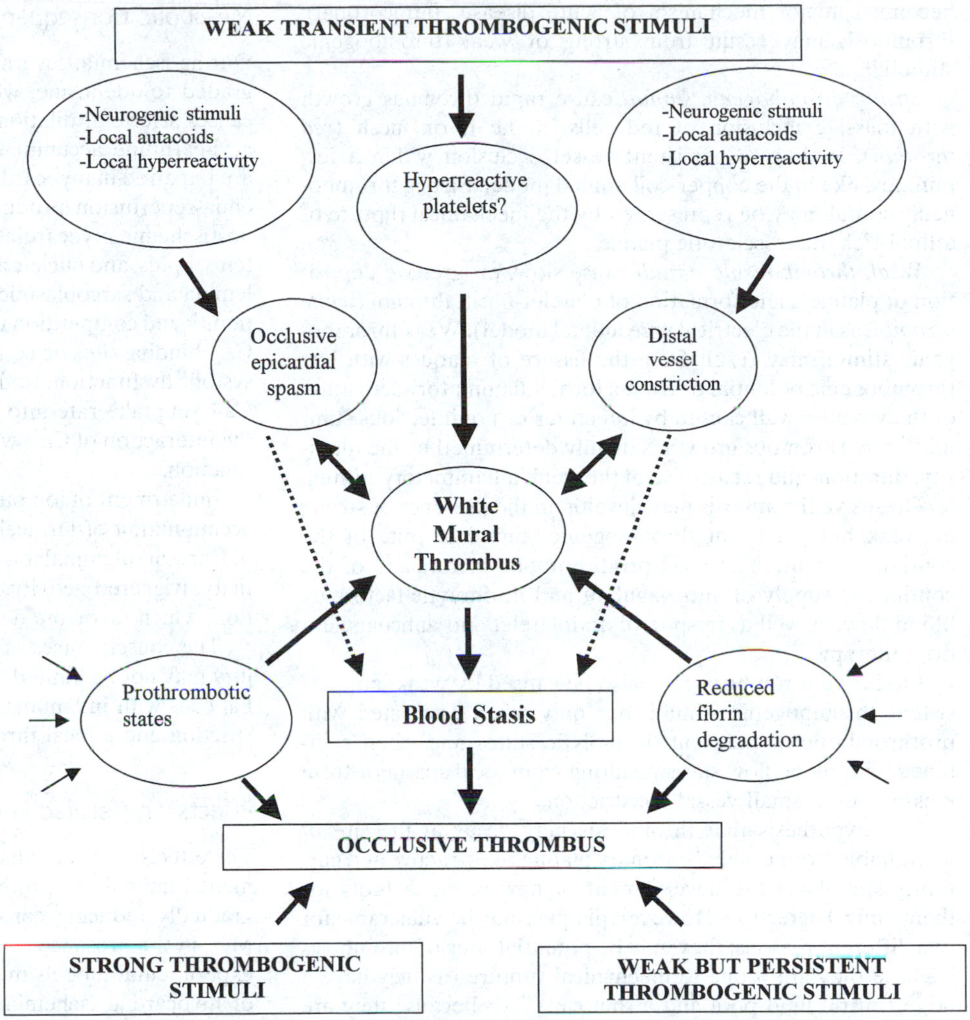

FIGURE 37-10 Vicious circles leading to the formation and growth of an occlusive coronary thrombus. An occlusive red thrombus can form rapidly within minutes at the site of highly thrombogenic injury (for example, the rupture of a strongly thrombogenic plaque). An occlusive platelet thrombus can form gradually at the site of a weak but very persistent thrombogenic stimuli (for example, a persisting inflammatory process). A mural thrombus resulting from a weakly thrombogenic plaque fissure or from a transient local inflammatory process may evolve into occlusive thrombosis only in the presence of prothrombotic states or of blood flow stasis induced by local or distal coronary constriction. The components of these vicious circles and their gain may have a variable importance and prevalence in different groups of patients. Prothrombotic states may result from any acquired or genetic alteration that leads to enhanced platelet reactivity or thrombin activity or to reduced fibrinolysis. (From Maseri[115] by permission.)

Acute Thrombosis

Intraluminal thrombi are the most common finding in patients with acute coronary syndromes. Most thrombi are composed of platelets and fibrin in variable proportions and often develop at the site of non-flow-limiting coronary stenoses. Thrombosis may reduce or interrupt blood flow by itself or in combination with local or distal vasoconstriction (triggered by thromboxane, serotonin, and thrombin)[115] (Fig. 37-10). Fresh thrombi may have a different fate. They may (1) grow to occlude the artery; (2) lyse completely; or (3) become organized and contribute to plaque growth.

MECHANISMS OF ACUTE THROMBOSIS

Thrombus formation is the first physiologic self-limiting step of vascular injury repair—but, under some circumstances, it may become a major mechanism of acute disease. Intracoronary thrombosis may result from strong or weak thrombogenic stimuli.[115]

Strong thrombogenic stimuli cause rapid thrombus growth with massive inclusion of red cells in the fibrin mesh (*red thrombi*), leading to persistent vessel occlusion within a few minutes, like in the copper-coil animal model. Strong thrombogenic stimuli may be represented by the mechanical rupture of a lipid-rich atherosclerotic plaque.

Weak thrombogenic stimuli cause slow, progressive deposition of platelets and formation of platelet-fibrin thrombi (*white thrombi*, as in the electrical wire animal model). Weak thrombogenic stimuli may result from the fissure of plaques with low thrombogenic potential or from a local inflammatory activation of the vascular wall caused by infectious or noninfectious stimuli.[40,116–118] Thrombus growth is mainly determined by the intensity, duration, and recurrence of the weak inflammatory stimuli.

Occlusive thrombosis may develop in the presence of strong or weak but persistent thrombogenic stimuli in spite of the continuous dilution of local prothrombotic factors and of the continuous supply of anticoagulant and fibrinolytic factors by blood flow, as well as in spite of antiplatelet and anticoagulant drug therapy.

Occlusive thrombosis may also be caused by weak, nonpersistent thrombogenic stimuli, but only when associated with prothrombotic or deficient fibrinolytic states and when combined with blood flow stasis resulting from local spasm or from massive distal small vessel constriction.

The hypothesis that thrombosis may occur at the site of identifiable "vulnerable" coronary plaques is attractive and currently stimulates the development of new research tools for their clinical detection. However, plaques may be vulnerable for two different reasons: they may be potential sites of thrombosis because they are prone to mechanical rupture (as they have a large central lipid pool and a thin cap)[119] or because they are the site of inflammatory processes.[45] Plaque vulnerability may last days, weeks, or months.

The different mechanisms responsible for coronary thrombosis or contributing to it and acute coronary occlusion may not have the same prevalence in different geographic, ethnic, age, and sex groups; yet they may influence the individual response to antiplatelet, antithrombotic, and acute reperfusion strategies.

CONSEQUENCES OF MYOCARDIAL ISCHEMIA

Myocardial ischemia causes myocardial cells to switch from aerobic to anaerobic metabolism with a progressive depletion of high-energy phosphate stores and impairment of mechanical and electrical function. When prolonged or repetitive, ischemia also modifies cell gene expression, which may contribute to postischemic cell dysfunction.

The most obvious clinical manifestation of myocardial ischemia is anginal pain, but most ischemic episodes are clinically silent. The consequences of myocardial ischemia vary according to its severity, extension, duration, mode of onset, and recurrence and may result in global impairment of contractile function and life-threatening arrhythmias as well as in preconditioning, stunning, hibernation, or myocardial infarction, which occurs when severe ischemia persists for longer than 30 min.

Metabolic Consequences

During ischemia, several metabolic changes occur. ATP is degraded to adenosine, which, diffusing out of cardiomyocytes, causes arteriolar dilation and anginal pain. Free fatty acids and acyl-carnitine accumulate and protein synthesis and turnover are impaired in myocardial cells. Furthermore, myocardial ischemia-reperfusion produces free radicals, which contribute to postischemic myocardial cell dysfunction by reacting with proteins, lipids, and nucleic acids. Impaired Ca^{2+} release from sarcolemma and sarcoplasmic reticulum, cross-bridge cycling inhibition,[120] and competition of H^+ accumulating during ischemia for Ca^{2+} binding sites on contractile proteins thus also contribute to systolic dysfunction. Reduced ATP availability and a decreasing Ca^{2+} reuptake rate into sarcoplasmatic reticulum also prolong the interaction of Ca^{2+} with myofilaments, causing diastolic dysfunction.

Impairment of ion pumps causes loss of intracellular K^+ and accumulation of intracellular Na^+, Ca^{2+}, and H_2O. Alterations of transsarcolemmal ion gradients may cause increased automaticity, triggered activity, and abnormalities of impulse conduction, which favor the development of reentry circuits.[121]

The consequences of ischemia and ischemia-reperfusion injury may not be limited to the myocytes but extend to endothelial cells with inflammatory changes,[122–124] resulting in vasoconstriction and a local thrombogenic tendency.

Effects on Cardiac Function

The effects of myocardial ischemia have been studied in experimental animals by producing a sudden coronary occlusion, by gradually reducing coronary flow at rest, and by increasing M_{VO_2} in the presence of a flow-limiting coronary stenosis. Such experimental models mimic, at least in part, the consequences of myocardial ischemia observed in variant angina, unstable angina, and effort angina, respectively (see ahead).

EFFECTS OF SUDDEN CORONARY OCCLUSION

Occlusion of a major coronary artery is followed within a few seconds by a typical sequence of events that includes a reduction in the velocity of ventricular relaxation and contraction, ST-segment elevation, increased end-diastolic pressure with dyssynchrony (delayed onset of contraction in ischemic myocardial segments), hypokinesis (reduced contractility), akinesis (cessation of contraction), and dyskinesis (paradoxical expansion of affected segment during systole). The sequence of hemodynamic and electrocardiographic events observed in experimental animals is similar to that observed in patients during episodes of occlusive epicardial coronary artery spasm (Fig. 37-11) or during coronary angioplasty balloon occlusion in patients.[46] It is typically characterized by the following sequence of events: a decrease in peak relaxation $-dp/dt$, a decrease of peak contraction dp/dt, an increase in diastolic pressures, and a fall in systolic and in pulse pressure. In patients with variant angina and coronary occlusive spasm, pain, when present, usually appears only several seconds or minutes later.

EFFECTS OF GRADED REDUCTION OF CORONARY FLOW AT REST

In anesthetized dogs, a 25 percent reduction of basal coronary blood flow through a major coronary branch is associated with increased myocardial extraction of oxygen and with decreased oxygen consumption.[46] Further reductions of flow are followed by a decrease in the rate of left ventricular relaxation and contraction, then by ST-segment depression, elevation of end-diastolic pressure, decreased stroke volume, and, finally, by elevation of the ST segment, which develops when flow is reduced to about 70 percent and myocardial ischemia becomes transmural. Local contractile function in subendocardial layers begins to fall slightly when regional subendocardial flow is reduced by 10 to 20 percent and becomes marked as flow decreases by 50 to 80 percent. Segments with a flow reduction greater than 80 percent show paradoxical movement, with bulging of the left ventricular wall[46] (Fig. 37-12).

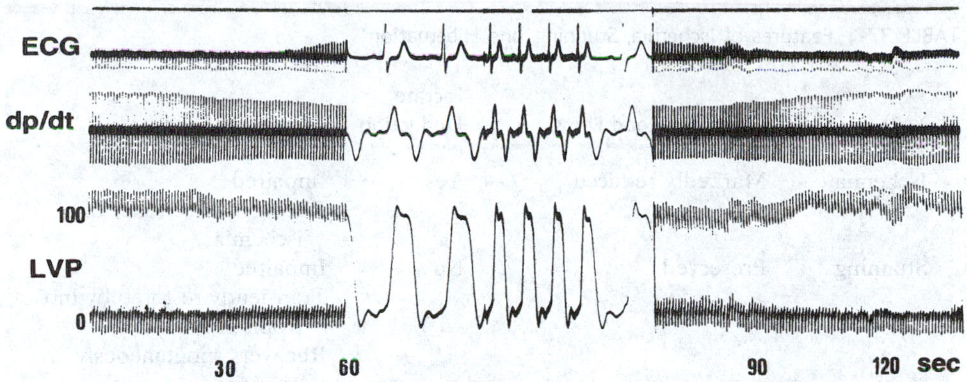

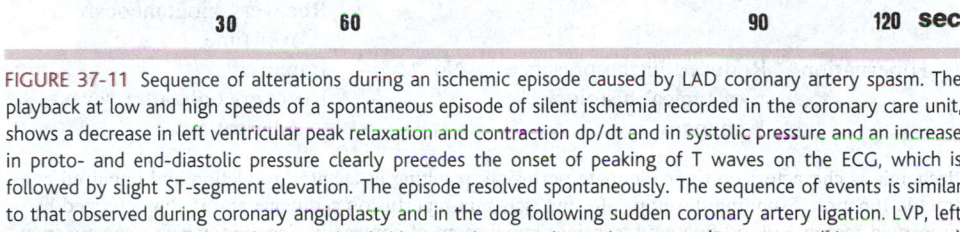

FIGURE 37-11 Sequence of alterations during an ischemic episode caused by LAD coronary artery spasm. The playback at low and high speeds of a spontaneous episode of silent ischemia recorded in the coronary care unit, shows a decrease in left ventricular peak relaxation and contraction dp/dt and in systolic pressure and an increase in proto- and end-diastolic pressure clearly precedes the onset of peaking of T waves on the ECG, which is followed by slight ST-segment elevation. The episode resolved spontaneously. The sequence of events is similar to that observed during coronary angioplasty and in the dog following sudden coronary artery ligation. LVP, left ventricular pressure; dp/dt, left ventricular dp/dt; ECG, electrocardiographic tracing. (From Maseri[46] by permission.)

EFFECT OF INCREASED WORKLOAD IN THE PRESENCE OF A FLOW-LIMITING STENOSIS

When exercise reduces mean transmural blood flow by 30 percent in chronically instrumented dogs with coronary artery stenosis, a mild reduction of systolic thickening is observed, whereas in the normally perfused wall, thickening increases by 20 percent.[46] During exercise, severe regional dysfunction develops when mean flow is about 80 percent lower than in nonischemic myocardial segments. Thus a severe reduction of coronary blood flow is necessary to produce detectable effects on global ventricular contractile function.[46]

At variance with the late occurrence of pain following sudden coronary occlusion by spasm, anginal pain may precede electrocardiographic changes in about one-third of the cases during effort-induced ischemia.[46]

PRECONDITIONING

The term *preconditioning* was originally used with reference to the ability of short periods of ischemia to limit infarct size after subsequent prolonged coronary occlusion in animals. However, it is now used also to include a protective effect of transient ischemia on myocardial suffering induced by subsequent ischemic episodes. An early ischemic preconditioning after an ischemic episode was reported during the initial 2 h (early preconditioning), but a later protection was also reported beginning 24 h after the preconditioning stimulus and extending to 48 h (delayed preconditioning).[125] Findings compatible with early ischemic preconditioning were reported following balloon occlusion during coronary angioplasty, in preinfarction angina, in coronary artery bypass surgery, and in exercise-induced ischemia (warmup phenomenon).[46] In experimental settings, ischemic preconditioning was also shown to reduce ventricular tachyarrhythmias appearing in the ischemic or reperfusion phase of ischemic episodes, and a reduction of ischemia-related ventricular arrhythmias following episodes of transmural myocardial ischemia was reported in patients with vasospastic angina.[126] Preconditioning could partly explain the more favorable prognosis of patients in whom acute myocardial infarction is preceded by unstable angina.[127,128]

The bases of preconditioning are not completely understood. Extrapolation of experimental results to patients should be cautious. Early preconditioning is thought to derive from phosphorylation of a sarcolemmal protein, possibly the ATP-sensitive K^+ channel, resulting from G protein–coupled receptor activation of protein kinase C. Late preconditioning may be mediated by activation of genes encoding for protective proteins such as heat-shock proteins and growth factors (see also Table 37-1).

STUNNING

The term *stunning* defines a prolonged but reversible contractile dysfunction observed after an episode of transient myocardial

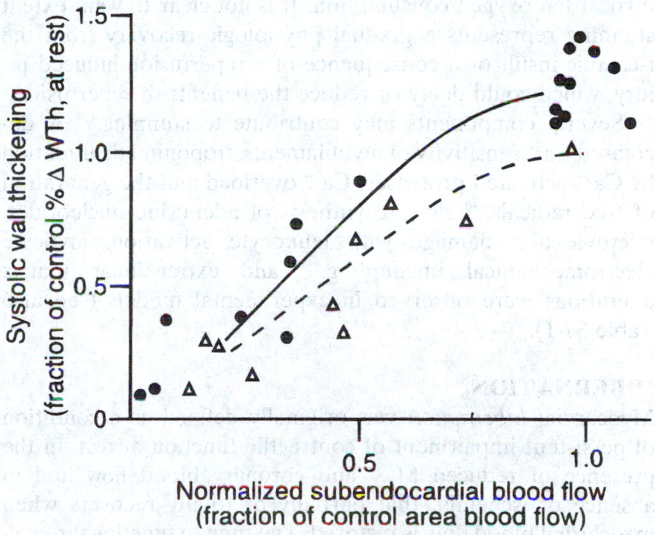

FIGURE 37-12 Effect of decrease of subendocardial blood flow on systolic segment shortening. In conscious dogs the percentage decrease of subendocardial segment shortening is small until blood flow is reduced by 20 percent. Systolic bulging (segment lengthening) develops only when flow is reduced by more than 80 percent. (From Maseri,[46] modified from Gallagher et al.,[148] by permission.)

TABLE 37-1 Features of Ischemia, Stunning, and Hibernation[a]

	Coronary Blood Flow	Lactate Production	Contractile Function
Ischemia	Markedly reduced	Yes	Impaired Recovers after relief of ischemia
Stunning	Preserved	No	Impaired Transiently restored by inotropic stimulation Recovers spontaneously over time
Hibernation	Reduced in the presence of typical histologic changes	No	Impaired Recovers only after revascularization

[a]Ischemia is characterized by inadequate perfusion, resulting in lactate production and impaired contractile function. Stunning develops after an ischemia-reperfusion sequence and is characterized by preserved regional blood flow and transient impairment of contractile function, which recovers spontaneously over time. Hibernation may develop after repeated episodes of ischemia-reperfusion, and is characterized by myocardial histologic changes, absence of contraction, reduced M_{VO_2}, reduced regional blood flow but no lactate production. Contractile function recovers following revascularization over a period of weeks and months.

ischemia. It has been observed in animals following sudden coronary occlusion lasting 10 to 15 minutes or after repeated shorter periods of occlusion as well as in patients after positive exercise tests, in ischemic peri-infarction regions, and following extracorporeal circulation. The spontaneous recovery of cardiac contractile function may take hours or days, depending on the severity and duration of ischemia, but contraction can be transiently restored by inotropic stimuli such as after extrasystolic potentiation or beta-adrenergic drugs. In stunned myocardium, the delayed recovery of contractile function is associated with a normal average myocardial perfusion in the presence of reduced myocardial oxygen consumption. It is not clear to what extent stunning represents a gradual physiologic recovery from the ischemic insult or a consequence of a reperfusion-induced injury, which could delay or reduce the benefits of reperfusion.

Several components may contribute to stunning.[129] A decreased Ca^{2+} sensitivity of myofilaments, troponin I degradation by Ca^{2+}-activated proteases, Ca^{2+} overload and the generation of free radicals,[130] slow resynthesis of adenosine nucleotides, microvascular damage with leukocyte activation, myocyte electromechanical uncoupling,[131] and extracellular matrix alterations were observed in experimental models (see also Table 37-1).

HIBERNATION

Myocardial *hibernation* was originally defined as a condition of persistent impairment of contractile function at rest, in the presence of reduced M_{VO_2} and coronary blood flow and in absence of ischemia, that partially or totally recovers when myocardial blood flow is restored. The time to functional recovery of hibernated myocardium after revascularization varies from 10 days to 6 months and is related to the severity of structural changes of cardiomyocytes and interstitium.

Hibernation is characterized[132] by progressive loss of sarcomeres, sarcoplasmatic reticulum, and T tubules in cardiomyocytes with glycogen replacement. Mitochondria appear small and scattered and nuclei distorted, with uniformly dispersed heterochromatin. Hibernated myocardial cells have normal ATP, total adenine nucleotides, and phosphocreatine content and exhibit normal glucose uptake and no lactate production. Several of these characteristics suggest that hibernation may be the result of a dedifferentiation process related to changes in gene expression, as hibernated cardiomyocytes show many features of neonatal cardiomyocytes.[132]

Hibernation is caused by a severe reduction of coronary flow reserve, as a result of which any increase in M_{VO_2} and any further reduction in coronary blood flow (e.g., by vasoconstriction or platelet aggregation) results in repeated episodes of myocardial ischemia-reperfusion (see also Table 37-1).

CLINICAL MANIFESTATIONS OF MYOCARDIAL ISCHEMIA

Chest Pain The most obvious clinical manifestation of myocardial ischemia, irrespective of its multiple causal mechanisms, is angina pectoris. However, myocardial ischemia may occur without angina and angina may occur without detectable signs of myocardial ischemia. Typically anginal pain is retrosternal in location, with a crushing, squeezing, or burning character. It may radiate to the throat, neck, ulnar side of the left and/or right arm, interscapular region, epigastrium, and the jaw and teeth. The intensity of the discomfort can vary greatly, from a mild feeling of retrosternal fullness or tingling in only one dermatome to a diffuse, unbearable pain. These features are totally unrelated to the actual cause of ischemia and are not completely specific for ischemia, as they may also be caused by cardiac nonischemic causes and by extracardiac causes.

Myocardial ischemia, with or without angina, may occasionally present with other symptoms, including dyspnea (when ischemia is extensive with transient impairment of left ventricular function or ischemia of papillary muscles with mitral regurgitation), palpitations, syncope, or cardiac arrest (when ischemia is associated with arrhythmias).

Anginal pain originates from the stimulation of polymodal receptors (more abundant around small coronary vessels) by chemical mediators produced during ischemia.[46] The best studied of such mediators is adenosine. The algogenic effects of adenosine were studied by its intracoronary infusion and are mediated by $alpha_1$ receptors, while its vasodilator effects are mediated by $alpha_2$ receptors.[133]

Comparison of pain location during selective intracoronary infusion of adenosine in the right and left coronary arteries has shown that, in nearly 70 percent of patients, afferent stimuli from different myocardial regions cannot be discriminated, thus suggesting that they converge on the same neurons of the dorsal roots of spinal cord.[134] In contrast, in the remaining 30 percent of patients, anginal pain during infusion of adenosine in the separate coronary beds caused a different location of pain. The possibility that a different location of pain in the same person reflects a different location of myocardial ischemia has been confirmed in patients undergoing PTCA and with a second myocardial infarction.[135,136] Moreover, convergence of afferent painful stimuli from different visceral organs and somatic dermatomes on the same ascending neurons can cause noncardiac pain to have features indistinguishable from angina. The central transmission of painful stimuli is strongly modulated at the spinal cord level by a "gating" system regulated by descending and afferent stimuli. After modulation at the spinal cord level, afferent stimuli reach thalamic centers and are finally projected to the cortex, where their processing and decoding occur.

Painless Ischemia The total lack of pain represents one extreme of the spectrum of the possible clinical presentations of myocardial ischemia. Painless ischemia can only be diagnosed by techniques capable of detecting ischemia and depends entirely on their sensitivity and specificity. Continuous ECG recording reveals that about 70 percent of episodes of transient myocardial ischemia do not cause chest pain or any other symptom.[46] The percentage of episodes of silent ischemia is similar in chronic stable angina, unstable angina, variant angina, and microvascular angina. Thus, the presence or absence of pain is totally unrelated to the actual cause of transient ischemia. Furthermore, myocardial infarction (MI) may be totally silent in about 20 percent of the cases.

The reasons why myocardial ischemia does not elicit pain in the majority of cases are multiple.[134] Although angina is less likely to accompany myocardial ischemia when it is brief, there is no strict relationship between duration and extension of ischemia and development of chest pain also in the same patient.

The gating system at the spinal cord and possibly at the thalamic level, together with the cortical decoding of afferent stimuli, probably play a major role in determining the perception of pain. Moreover, personality, emotional status, and previous experience of pain may modulate such perception.

Arrhythmias Arrhythmias are major potential consequences of acute ischemia, as they are responsible for most of the deaths observed during the early phases of acute MI as well as in variant angina, and thus for sudden death in the community.

During ischemia, increased automaticity, triggered activity, conduction delay and reentry may cause the development of ventricular tachycardia and ventricular fibrillation. Moreover, altered impulse formation and conduction defects may cause asystole and atrioventricular block.

The arrhythmic response to ischemic insult of individual patients is unpredictable but is influenced by the cardiac anatomic background (left ventricular hypertrophy, previous infarction), sympathetic activity (as suggested also by experimental studies on cardiac sympathetic denervation) and nervous autonomic imbalance.

Fatal ventricular arrhythmias are exceptional during mild transient ischemic episodes, but they may develop after the onset or soon after the termination of episodes of severe subendocardial ischemia and in transmural ischemia caused by occlusive spasm or by occlusive thrombosis. Reperfusion arrhythmias, although particularly common in anesthetized animals, are less frequently observed both in patients with variant angina and during myocardial reperfusion in acute MI.[46]

Effects of Persistent Myocardial Ischemia: Myocardial Infarction

In dogs, focal cell necrosis begins about 20 min following coronary flow interruption. Such foci become confluent in subendocardial layers by 40 min, reaching subepicardial layers with a progressive wavefront at about 3 to 4 h. By this time, necrosis has developed, on average, to about 90 percent of its final extension, which is reached after 6 h.

In patients, the extension of myocardial necrosis depends not only on the area perfused by the occluded vessel, the level of myocardial oxygen consumption, and the presence of collaterals but also on the intermittence of coronary occlusion. Actually, MI is a dynamic process with intermittence of occlusion occurring in about two-thirds of the cases during the initial 6 h.[46] Therefore it is reasonable to undertake reperfusion strategies in all patients irrespective of actual delay from the onset of symptoms as long as ECG shows persistent massive ischemia without completed necrosis. The impairment of global myocardial function depends on the extension of myocardial necrosis. When infarction involves more than 15 percent of the left ventricle, ejection fraction decreases and left ventricular end-systolic volume and pressure increase. When it involves more than 25 percent of the left ventricle, signs of heart failure develop; when it involves more than 40 percent, cardiogenic shock occurs. The development of primary ventricular fibrillation is independent of infarct size but strongly influenced by high adrenergic tone.

RELATIONSHIP BETWEEN MECHANISMS OF ISCHEMIA AND CLINICAL SYNDROMES

The mechanisms responsible for the development of ischemia do not influence the location and radiation of anginal pain but may determine specific clinical patterns of anginal episodes that, at least in typical cases, provide useful clues for personalized patient management. Therefore a carefully collected clinical history is the fundamental first step in the assessment of the pathogenetic mechanisms of MI and for the selection of the appropriate sequence of diagnostic tests.

Chronic Stable Angina

Some patients presenting with chronic stable angina report that anginal pain develops predictably only and every time they exceed a rather fixed level of exertion that they learn to recognize and avoid. The pain disappears within 1 to 2 min after the interruption of the effort or after sublingual nitrates. In these patients, the fixed anginal threshold suggests that myocardial ischemia is caused exclusively by an excessive increase in oxygen demand in the presence of a fixed coronary stenosis (*fixed-threshold effort angina*) (see Chap. 40).

On careful questioning, however, the majority of patients with chronic stable angina report that they have "good and bad days" and a variable threshold for angina, which sometimes develops unpredictably for efforts usually well tolerated and occasionally also at rest (*mixed angina*). A variable ischemic threshold, with "good days" during which patients have a good

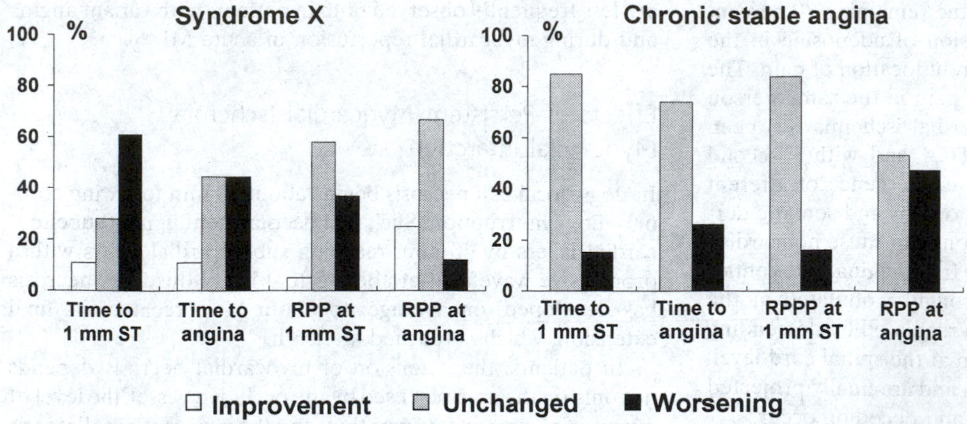

FIGURE 37-13 Acute effects of nitrates on exercise testing in syndrome X. The administration of isosorbide dinitrate (ISDN, 5 mg sublingual) significantly improved exercise test variables in patients with chronic stable angina and documented coronary artery disease (*right panel*). In contrast, ISDN caused a worsening of exercise variables in a significant number of patients with syndrome X (*left panel*). ST, ST segment; RPP, rate pressure product. (Modified from Lanza GA, Manzoli A, Bia E, et al. Acute effects of nitrates on exercise testing in patients with syndrome X: Clinical and pathophysiological implications. *Circulation* 1994; 90:2695, by permission.)

effort tolerance, is suggestive of a strong modulation of residual flow reserve by changes in vasomotor tone at the level of a potential flow-limiting stenosis or in distal vessels; therefore it represents an indication for vasodilator therapy. This indication is supported by a significant increase of effort tolerance on exercise testing following sublingual nitrates. Conversely, a low effort tolerance, persisting after sublingual nitrates, represents a mandatory indication for drugs that reduce M_{VO_2} and for coronary angiography with a view to revascularization procedures.

Syndrome X

Patients with a chronic stable pattern of mixed angina, "ischemic" ST-segment depression, and/or myocardial perfusion defects during stress test, but angiographically normal coronary arteries are classified as having syndrome X.[94] In these patients, angina also predominantly occurs on exertion, typically with a variable ischemic threshold and occasionally at rest, but very seldom at night. Although the location and radiation of pain are often indistinguishable from those of patients with flow-limiting stenosis, some distinct features raise the suspicion of syndrome X: (1) patients usually report persistence of angina for several minutes after the interruption of exertion, and many report attacks lasting over 30 min; (2) they have a poor response to sublingual nitrates, which were also shown to worsen exercise tolerance, in sharp contrast with their established beneficial effect in patients with flow-limiting stenosis (Fig. 37-13); (3) they show a variable individual response to prophylactic long-acting nitrates, calcium antagonists, and beta blockers,[137] possibly because of differences in the underlying causes of microvascular dysfunction; (4) they develop their typical pain (often with transient ischemic ECG changes) during dipyridamole test but without development of left ventricular contractile abnormalities; (5) they often have an enhanced response to painful stimuli,[138] which contributes to explain the paradox of severe angina in the absence of detectable myocardial contractile dysfunction (Fig. 37-14); and (6) Holter monitoring demonstrates that some episodes of chest pain and ST-segment depression are not associated with tachycardia, and it may show episodes of transient ST-segment depression in patients with a negative exercise test, suggestive of possible episodic occurrence of microvascular constriction.[139]

The diagnosis of syndrome X is confirmed by (1) the evidence of a cardiac origin of pain because of its consistent association with transient ischemic ECG changes and/or myocardial perfusion defects during exercise test or by diagnostic ECG changes on Holter monitoring;[140] (2) normal coronary angiogram; and (3) the exclusion of epicardial coronary spasm

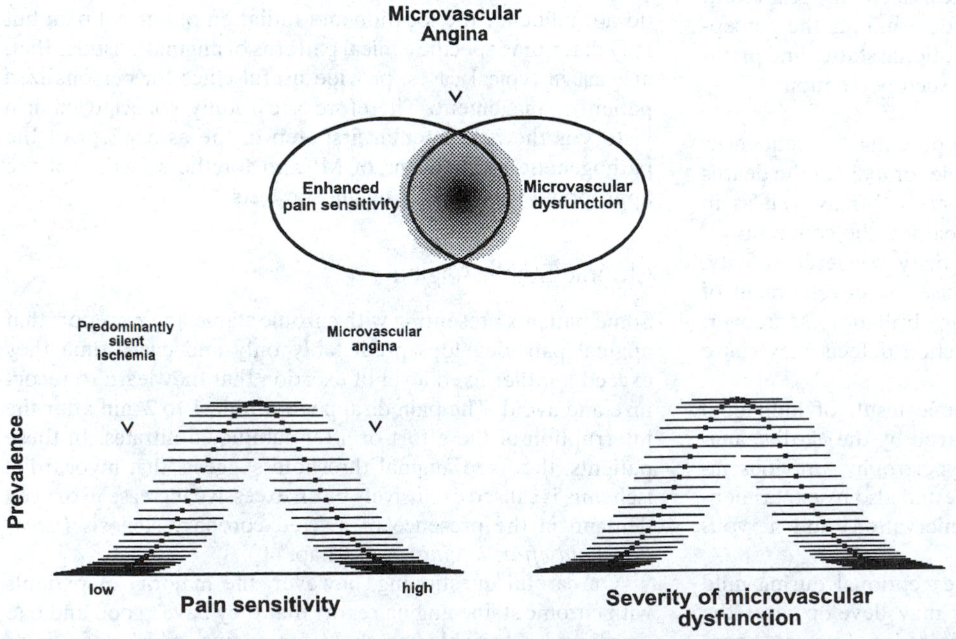

FIGURE 37-14 Main pathogenetic mechanisms of syndrome X. Syndrome X likely results from a variable combination of two components: a coronary microvascular dysfunction and an increased pain sensitivity, both of which may have a bell-shaped prevalence in the population. (From Maseri[46] by permission.)

on the basis of distinct clinical history, absence of transient episodes of ST-segment elevation, and failure to induce coronary spasm by provocative tests (see also Chap. 40).

Unstable Angina

The characteristic clinical feature of unstable angina is the sudden appearance and/or worsening of angina, with more frequent and prolonged attacks occurring at rest or on efforts that were previously well tolerated. In patients with a de novo angina and those with known ischemic heart disease (in the absence of anemia, fever, hyperthyroidism and tachyarrhythmias), this pattern of presentation suggests a transient, recurring impairment of myocardial perfusion by thrombosis and vasoconstriction. The crescendo, waxing, waning, and persistence of anginal attacks over a period of days and weeks suggests stimuli causing thrombosis and vasoconstriction. A sudden reduction of the ischemic threshold on exertion suggests a rapid development or increased severity of a flow-limiting stenosis by organized thrombus. Many patients continue to present recurrent instability and/or to develop MI in the initial weeks and months following hospital discharge. Unstable patients are also at an increased risk of restenosis following PTCA. The waxing and persistance of instability and restenosis following PTCA are correlated with elevated blood levels of systemic markers of inflammation—for example C-reactive protein[140] and interleukin 6[141]—consistent with the hypothesis that inflammatory cytokines may be an important component of instability.

In the first few days after onset, the presentation of unstable angina may be clinically indistinguishable from that of an acute onset of variant angina, unless repeated short episodes of transient ST-segment elevation are detected on the ECG. The absence of detectable systemic inflammatory markers is a distinctive feature of variant angina as opposed to unstable angina[142] (see also Chap. 41).

Variant Angina

The clinical diagnosis of variant angina can only be suspected when sufficient time has elapsed from the onset of symptoms to allow the emergence of a distinctive pattern of angina. The following features suggest the clinical diagnosis of variant angina: (1) a report of pain occurring predominantly at rest, without apparent cause, more often at night, in the early morning hours or at the same time of the day, usually with preserved effort tolerance (many patients with variant angina report with amazement that they have anginal attacks without apparent cause and yet can perform considerable efforts without symptoms); (2) anginal episodes are usually of short duration (2 to 5 min) and respond to sublingual nitrates within 1 to 2 min (at variance with syndrome X); (3) anginal episodes may occur in clusters of two to three in the early morning hours and then be absent throughout the day; (4) anginal episodes may be associated with syncope caused by ventricular tachycardia/ventricular fibrillation[81] or by complete atrioventricular block; (5) the exercise stress test is usually negative but in some patients it may cause ST-segment elevation during or after the test; the exercise test becomes negative after sublingual nitrate administration.

The clinical suspicion elicited by these features is supported by the demonstration of ST-segment elevation, usually a typical "lesion wave," during angina. The demonstration of ST-segment elevation can be obtained by chance with a standard 12-lead ECG, by Holter monitoring, or soon after or during the exercise stress test. The diagnosis is confirmed by the angiographic demonstration of spasm occurring spontaneously or following provocative tests. Among these, ergonovine and hyperventilation have a 100 percent specificity but a low sensitivity, whereas acetylcholine seems to have a greater sensitivity but a lower specificity.

The occlusive spasm typically occurs at the site of coronary stenosis, but it may also occur in angiographically normal coronaries, in particular in Asian patients.[143] The diagnosis of variant angina is a mandatory indication for calcium antagonists and nitrates, as beta blockers are totally ineffective.

Myocardial Infarction

In some patients MI develops totally unheralded with the single first episode of uninterrupted anginal pain that brings them to hospital. In others, the final persistent episode of pain is preceded by a typical history of unstable angina. In an intermediate group, the final episode of persistent pain is preceded by one or two isolated anginal attacks, compatible with a hyperacute presentation of preinfarction unstable angina. During the initial 6 h from the onset of symptoms in unselected patients with acute MI, the infarct-related artery recanalizes spontaneously in 40 percent of the cases and exhibits occasional, transient reperfusion in about 70 percent. Spontaneous and early reperfusion seems to be more frequent in patients in whom MI is preceded by unstable angina[144] (see also Chap. 42).

Thus in some patients, coronary occlusion appears to develop like lightning out of a blue sky and to be persistent and uninterrupted, compatible with the fissure of a strongly thrombogenic plaque, with a persistent coronary inflammatory stimulus or with persistent spasm or distal coronary vessel constriction. In some patients with a history of preinfarction unstable angina, the coronary occlusion is transient and very occasional before the final episode; in others, the final coronary occlusion exhibits spontaneous, transient, or persistent recanalization, consistent with waxing, waning, and recurrence of weak inflammatory thrombogenic stimuli.

The presence of systemically detectable inflammatory markers in about 70 percent of patients with Braunwald class IIIB unstable angina and the much higher recurrence of instability among the 50 percent of patients in whom the elevation persists at discharge and at 3 months[145] may represent an objective marker of inflammatory thrombogenic triggers. This possibility is supported by the elevation of such markers at the time of hospital admission in nearly all patients in whom MI was preceded by unstable angina but in less than 50 percent of those in whom MI was totally unheralded.[146] The absence of inflammatory markers also allows an objective distinction of variant angina,[142] which sometimes has a clinical presentation indistinguishable from that of the more common form of unstable angina.

Different pathogenetic components of coronary occlusion are also suggested by the earlier recanalization in response to t-PA observed in patients with preinfarction angina as compared to those with a totally unheralded MI.[127]

The prodromal symptoms of MI also provide clues about its pathogenetic mechanisms. In some patients, MI occurs without any apparent cause; in others, a history of severe psychological distress[147] or of flu-like symptoms can be elicited on careful questioning. These prodromal symptoms may be associated with a different mode of presentation of acute MI and might provide clues of distinct pathogenetic mechanisms, which may not have the same prevalence in different age, sex, geographic, and ethnic groups.

Understanding the precise mechanisms of acute coronary occlusion would allow more effective coronary reperfusion strategies to be reserved to those patients who are unlikely to respond to simpler ones. The alternative is to treat indiscriminately all patients with the newest, most efficacious, but possibly also more complex and expensive coronary reperfusion strategies. The subgroups of patients that benefit from antiplatelet drugs, anticoagulants, beta blockers, statins, and ACE inhibitors should be identified. Again, the alternative is to prescribe indiscriminately all these treatments to each patient, with the consequent burden of polytherapy, risk of low compliance, and high cost.

References

1. Porenta G, Cherry S, Czernin J, et al. Noninvasive determination of myocardial blood flow, oxygen consumption and efficiency in normal humans by carbon-11 acetate positron emission tomography imaging. *Eur J Nucl Med* 1999; 26:1465.
2. Pitkanen OP, Nuutila P, Raitakari OT, et al. Coronary flow reserve in young men with familial combined hyperlipidemia. *Circulation* 1999; 99:1678.
3. Vassalli G, Hess OM. Measurement of coronary flow reserve and its role in patient care. *Basic Res Cardiol* 1998; 93:339.
4. Braunwald E. Myocardial oxygen consumption: The quest for its determinants and some clinical fallout. *J Am Coll Cardiol* 1999; 34:1365.
5. Kuo L, Davis MJ, Chilian WM. Longitudinal gradients for endothelium-dependent and independent vascular responses in the coronary microcirculation. *Circulation* 1995; 92:518.
6. Coggins DL, Flynn AE, Austin RE, et al. Nonuniform loss of regional flow reserve during myocardial ischemia in dogs. *Circ Res* 1990; 67:253.
7. Beyar R, Sideman S. Dynamic interaction between myocardial contraction and coronary flow. *Adv Exp Med Biol* 1997; 430:123.
8. Spaan JAE. Mechanical determinants of myocardial perfusion. *Basic Res Cardiol* 1995; 90:89.
9. Armour JA, Randall WC. Canine left ventricular intramyocardial pressures. *Am J Physiol* 1995; 220:1833.
10. Hoffman JIE, Baer RW, Hanley FL, et al. Regulation of transmural myocardial blood flow. *J Biochem Eng* 1985; 107:2.
11. Merkus D, Kajiya F, Vink H, et al. Prolonged diastolic time fraction protects myocardial perfusion when coronary blood flow is reduced. *Circulation* 1999; 100:75.
12. Berne RM. Cardiac nucleotides in hypoxia: Possible role in regulation of coronary blood flow. *Am J Physiol* 1963; 204:317.
13. Yada T, Richmond KN, Van Bibber R, et al. Role of adenosine in local metabolic coronary vasodilation. *Am J Physiol* 1999; 276:H1425.
14. DeFily DV, Chilian WM. Coronary microcirculation: Autoregulation and metabolic control. *Basic Res Cardiol* 1995; 90:112.
15. Ishizaka H, Kuo L. Endothelial ATP-sensitive potassium channels mediate coronary microvascular dilation to hyperosmolarity. *Am J Physiol* 1997; 273:H104.
16. Dellsperger KC. Potassium channels and the coronary circulation. *Clin Exp Pharmacol Physiol* 1996; 23:1096.
17. Miller FJ Jr, Dellsperger KC, Gutterman DD. Myogenic constriction of human coronary arterioles. *Am J Physiol* 1997; 273:H257.
18. Feigl EO. Neural control of coronary blood flow. *J Vasc Res* 1998; 35:85.
19. Saetrum Opgaard O, Gulbenkian S, Edvinsson L. Innervation and effects of vasoactive substances in the coronary circulation. *Eur Heart J* 1997; 18:1556.
20. Saetrum Opgaard O, Edvinsson L. Mechanical properties and effects of sympathetic co-transmitters on human coronary arteries and veins. *Basic Res Cardiol* 1997; 92:168.
21. Baumgart D, Heusch G. Neuronal control of coronary blood flow. *Basic Res Cardiol* 1995; 90:142.
22. Saetrum Opgaard O, Edvinsson L. Effect of parasympathetic and sensory transmitters on human epicardial coronary arteries and veins. *Pharmacol Toxicol* 1996; 78:273.
23. Feliciano L, Henning RJ. Vagal nerve stimulation during muscarinic and beta-adrenergic blockade causes significant coronary artery dilation. *J Auton Nerv Syst* 1998; 68:78.
24. Tanaka E, Mori H, Chujo M, et al. Coronary vasoconstrictive effects of neuropeptide Y and their modulation by the ATP-sensitive potassium channel in anesthetized dogs. *J Am Coll Cardiol* 1997; 29:1380.
25. Fleming I, Busse R. NO: the primary EDRF. *J Mol Cell Cardiol* 1999; 31:5.
26. Tousoulis D, Crake T, Tentolouris C, et al. Effects of inhibition of nitric oxide synthesis in proximal and distal segments in patients with normal arteries and in patients with coronary artery disease. *J Am Coll Cardiol* 1995; 25(suppl):117A.
27. Tousoulis D, Tentolouris C, Crake T, et al. Basal and flow-mediated nitric oxide production by atheromatous coronary arteries. *J Am Coll Cardiol* 1997; 29:1256.
28. Bassenge E. Control of coronary blood flow by autacoids. *Basic Res Cardiol* 1995; 90:112.
29. Duffy SJ, Castle SF, Harper RW, et al. Contribution of vasodilator prostanoids and nitric oxide to resting flow, metabolic vasodilation, and flow-mediated dilation in human coronary circulation. *Circulation* 1999; 100:1951.
30. Campbell WB, Gebremedhin D, Pratt PF, et al. Identification of epoxyeicosatrienoic acids as endothelium-derived hyperpolarizing factors. *Circ Res* 1996; 78:415.
31. Masaki T. Possible role of endothelin in endothelial regulation of vascular tone. *Annu Rev Pharmacol Toxicol* 1995; 35:235.
32. Lüscher TF, Oemar BS, Boulanger CM, et al. Molecular and cellular biology of endothelin and its receptors. In: *Molecular Reviews*. London: Chapman & Hall; 1996:96.
33. Mombouli JV, Vanhoutte PM. Endothelial dysfunction: From physiology to therapy. *J Mol Cell Cardiol* 1999; 31:61.
34. Ruschitzka FT, Noll G, Luscher TF. The endothelium in coronary artery disease. *Cardiology* 1997; 88:3.
35. Luscher TF. Endothelial control of vascular tone and growth. *Clin Exp Hypertens A* 1990; 12:897.
36. Li S, Sims S, Jiao Y, et al. Evidence from a novel human cell clone that adult vascular smooth muscle cells can convert reversibly between noncontractile and contractile phenotypes. *Circ Res* 1999; 85:338.
37. Bombeli T, Mueller M, Haeberli A. Anticoagulant properties of the vascular endothelium. *Thromb Haemost* 1997; 77:408.
38. Crossman DC, Larkin SW, Dashwood MR, et al. Responses of atherosclerotic human coronary arteries in vivo to the endothelium-dependent vasodilator substance P. *Circulation* 1991; 84:2001.
39. Vallance P, Collier J, Bhagat K. Infection, inflammation, and infarction: Does acute endothelial dysfunction provide a link? *Lancet* 1997; 349:1391.
40. Kinlay S, Selwyn AP, Libby P, et al. Inflammation, the endothelium, and the acute coronary syndromes. *J Cardiovasc Pharmacol* 1998; 32:S62.
41. Libby P. Molecular bases of the acute coronary syndromes. *Circulation* 1995; 91:2844.

42. Maseri A, Sanna T. The role of plaque fissures in unstable angina: Fact or fiction? *Eur Heart J* 1998; 19(suppl K):K2.
43. Maseri A. Antibiotics for acute coronary syndromes: Are we ready for megatrials? *Eur Heart J* 1999; 20:89.
44. Caligiuri G, Liuzzo G, Biasucci LM, et al. Immune system activation follows inflammation in unstable angina: Pathogenetic implications. *J Am Coll Cardiol* 1998; 32:1295.
45. Liuzzo G, Kopecky SI, Frye RL, et al. Perturbation of the T-cell repertoire in patients with unstable angina. *Circulation* 1999; 100:2135.
46. Maseri A. *Ischemic Heart Disease.* New York: Churchill Livingstone; 1995.
47. Klocke FJ. Measurements of coronary blood flow and degree of stenosis: Current clinical implications and continuing uncertainties. *J Am Coll Cardiol* 1983; 1:31.
48. Di Carli M, Czernin J, Hoh CK, et al. Relation among stenosis severity, myocardial blood flow, and flow reserve in patients with coronary artery disease. *Circulation* 1995; 91:1944.
49. Beanlands RSB, Muzik O, Melon P, et al. Noninvasive quantification of regional myocardial flow reserve in patients with coronary atherosclerosis using nitrogen-13 ammonia positron emission tomography: Determination of extent of altered vascular reactivity. *J Am Coll Cardiol* 1995; 26:1465.
50. Rutishauser W. The Denolin Lecture 1998. Towards measurement of coronary blood flow in patients and its alteration by interventions. *Eur Heart J* 1999; 20:1076.
51. Tousoulis D, Davies GJ, Toutouzas PC. Vasomotion of coronary arteries: From nitrates to nitric oxide. *Cardiovasc Drugs Ther* 1999; 13:295.
52. Tousoulis D, Crake T, Kaski JC, et al. Enhanced vasomotor responses of complex coronary stenoses to acetylcholine in stable angina pectoris. *Am J Cardiol* 1995; 75:725.
53. Dubois-Rande JL, Dupouy P, Aptecar E, et al. Comparison of the effects of exercise and cold pressor test on the vasomotor response of normal and atherosclerotic coronary arteries and their relation to the flow-mediated mechanism. *Am J Cardiol* 1995; 76:467.
54. Julius BK, Vassalli G, Mandinov L, et al. Alpha-adrenoceptor blockade prevents exercise-induced vasoconstriction of stenotic coronary arteries. *J Am Coll Cardiol* 1999; 33:1499.
55. Petronio AS, Amoroso G, Limbruno U, et al. Endothelin-1 release from atherosclerotic plaque after percutaneous transluminal coronary angioplasty in stable angina pectoris and single-vessel coronary artery disease. *Am J Cardiol* 1999; 84:1085.
56. Lerman A, Holmes DR Jr, Bell MR, et al. Endothelin in coronary endothelial dysfunction and early atherosclerosis in humans. *Circulation* 1995; 92:2426.
57. Yokoyama I, Momomura S, Ohtake T, et al. Improvement of impaired myocardial vasodilatation due to diffuse coronary atherosclerosis in hypercholesterolemics after lipid-lowering therapy. *Circulation* 1999; 100:117.
58. Nishikawa Y, Ogawa S. Importance of nitric oxide in the coronary artery at rest and during pacing in humans. *J Am Coll Cardiol* 1997; 29:85-92.
59. Schachinger V, Zeiher AM. Quantitative assessment of coronary vasoreactivity in humans in vivo: Importance of baseline vasomotor tone in atherosclerosis. *Circulation* 1995; 92:2087.
60. Traverse JH, Judd D, Bache RJ. Dose-dependent effect of endothelin-1 on blood flow to normal and collateral-dependent myocardium. *Circulation* 1996; 93:558.
61. Lamping KG. Response of native and stimulated collateral vessels to serotonin. *Am J Physiol* 1997; 272(5 pt 2):H2409.
62. Klassen CL, Traverse JH, Bache RJ. Nitroglycerin dilates coronary collateral vessels during exercise after blockade of endogenous NO production. *Am J Physiol* 1999; 277(3 pt 2): H918–H23.
63. Altman JD, Klassen CL, Bache RJ. Cyclooxygenase blockade limits blood flow to collateral-dependent myocardium during exercise. *Cardiovasc Res* 1995; 30:697.
64. Schultz A, Lavie L, Hochberg I, et al. Interindividual heterogeneity in the hypoxic regulation of VEGF: Significance for the development of the coronary artery collateral circulation. *Circulation* 1999; 100:547.
65. Fujita M, Kihara Y, Hasegawa K, et al. Heparin potentiates collateral growth but not growth of intramyocardial endarteries in dogs with repeated coronary occlusion. *Int J Cardiol* 1999; 70:165.
66. Schumacher B, Pecher P, von Specht BU, et al. Induction of neoangiogenesis in ischemic myocardium by human growth factors: First clinical results of a new treatment of coronary heart disease. *Circulation* 1998; 97:645.
67. Sellke FW, Laham RJ, Edelman ER, et al. Therapeutic angiogenesis with basic fibroblast growth factor: Technique and early results. *Ann Thorac Surg* 1998; 65:1540.
68. Hamasaki S, Arima S, Fukumoto N, et al. Tanaka H. Mechanisms of limited maximum coronary flow in severe single-vessel coronary artery disease in humans due to vertical steal. *Am J Cardiol* 1997; 80:1597.
69. Holmvang G, Fry S, Skopicki HA, Abraham SA, et al. Relation between coronary "steal" and contractile function at rest in collateral-dependent myocardium of humans with ischemic heart disease. *Circulation* 1999; 99:2510.
70. Lanza GA, Maseri A. Diagnosis and treatment of coronary artery spasm. *Cardiol Rev* 1996; 1:1.
71. Lanza GA, Pedrotti P, Pasceri V, et al. Autonomic changes associated with spontaneous coronary spasm in patients with variant angina. *J Am Coll Cardiol* 1996; 28:1249.
72. Yamakado T, Kasai A, Masuda T, et al. Exercise-induced coronary spasm: Comparison of treadmill and bicycle exercise in patients with vasospastic angina. *Coron Artery Dis* 1996; 7:819.
73. Song JK, Lee SJ, Kang DH, et al. Ergonovine echocardiography as a screening test for diagnosis of vasospastic angina before coronary angiography. *J Am Coll Cardiol* 1996; 27:1156.
74. Kugiyama K, Murohara T, Yasue H, et al. Increased constrictor response to acetylcholine of the isolated coronary arteries from patients with variant angina. *Int J Cardiol* 1995; 52:223.
75. Ishida T, Hirata K, Sakoda T, et al. 5-HT1D beta receptor mediates the supersensitivity of isolated coronary artery to serotonin in variant angina. *Chest* 1998; 113:243.
76. Nakao K, Ohgushi M, Yoshimura M, et al. Hyperventilation as a specific test for diagnosis of coronary artery spasm. *Am J Cardiol* 1997; 80:545.
77. Katsumata N, Shimokawa H, Seto M, et al. Enhanced myosin light chain phosphorylations as a central mechanism for coronary artery spasm in a swine model with interleukin-1 beta. *Circulation* 1997; 96:4357.
78. Maseri A, Crea F, Lanza GA. Coronary vasoconstriction: Where do we stand in 1999: An important, multifaceted but elusive role. *Cardiologia* 1999; 44:115.
79. Mongiardo R, Finocchiaro ML, Beltrame J, et al. Low incidence of serotonin-induced occlusive coronary artery spasm in patients with recent myocardial infarction. *Am J Cardiol* 1996; 78:84.
80. Pristipino C, Beltrame JF, Finocchiaro ML, et al. Major racial differences in coronary constrictor response between Japanese and Caucasians with recent myocardial infarction. *Circulation* 2000; 101:1102.
81. Chevalier P, Dacosta A, Defaye P, et al. Arrhythmic cardiac arrest due to isolated coronary artery spasm: Long-term outcome of seven resuscitated patients. *J Am Coll Cardiol* 1998; 31:57.
82. Caputo M, Nicolini F, Franciosi G, et al. Coronary artery spasm after coronary artery bypass grafting. *Eur J Cardiothorac Surg* 1999; 15:545.
83. DeFily DV, Nishikawa Y, Chilian WM. Endothelin antagonists block alpha$_1$-adrenergic constriction of coronary arterioles. *Am J Physiol* 1999; 276(3 pt 2):H1028.

84. Miao L, Nunez BD, Susulic V, et al. Cocaine-induced microvascular vasoconstriction but differential systemic haemodynamic responses in Yucatan versus Yorkshire varieties of swine. *Br J Pharmacol* 1996; 117:559.
85. Cianflone D, Lanza GA, Maseri A. Microvascular angina in patients with normal coronary arteries and with other ischaemic syndromes. *Eur Heart J* 1995; 16(suppl I):96.
86. Pupita G, Maseri A, Kaski JC, et al. Myocardial ischemia caused by distal coronary-artery constriction in stable angina pectoris. *N Engl J Med* 1990; 323:514.
87. Versaci F, Tomai F, Nudi F, et al. Differences of regional coronary flow reserve assessed by adenosine thallium-201 scintigraphy early and six months after successful percutaneous transluminal coronary angioplasty or stent implantation. *Am J Cardiol* 1996; 78:1097.
88. Kern MJ, Puri S, Bach RG, et al. Abnormal coronary flow velocity reserve after coronary artery stenting in patients: Role of relative coronary reserve to assess potential mechanisms. *Circulation* 1999; 100:2491.
89. Kosa I, Blasini R, Schneider-Eicke J, et al. Early recovery of coronary flow reserve after stent implantation as assessed by positron emission tomography. *J Am Coll Cardiol* 1999; 34:1036.
90. Gregorini L, Marco J, Kozakova M, et al. Alpha-adrenergic blockade improves recovery of myocardial perfusion and function after coronary stenting in patients with acute myocardial infarction. *Circulation* 1999; 99:482.
91. Kramer CM, Rogers WJ, Theobald TM, et al. Remote noninfarcted region dysfunction soon after first anterior myocardial infarction: A magnetic resonance tagging study. *Circulation* 1996; 94:660.
92. Zeiher AM, Krause T, Schächinger V, et al. Impaired endothelium-dependent vasodilation of coronary resistance vessels is associated with exercise-induced myocardial ischemia. *Circulation* 1995; 91:2345.
93. Yokoyama I, Ohtake T, Momomura S, et al. Reduced coronary flow reserve in hypercholesterolemic patients without overt coronary stenosis. *Circulation* 1996; 94:3232.
94. Kaski JC. Cardiac syndrome X and microvascular angina. In Kaski JC, ed. *Chest Pain with Normal Coronary Angiograms*. Dordrecht: Kluwer Academic Publishers; 1999:1.
95. Kao CH, Wang SJ, Ting CT, Chen YT. Tc-99m sestamibi myocardial SPECT in syndrome X. *Clin Nucl Med* 1996; 21:280.
96. Rosano GM, Peters NS, Kaski JC, et al. Abnormal uptake and washout of thallium-201 in patients with syndrome X and normal-appearing scans. *Am J Cardiol* 1995; 75:400.
97. Panza JA, Laurienzo JM, Curiel RV, et al. Investigation of the mechanism of chest pain in patients with angiographically normal coronary arteries using transesophageal dobutamine stress echocardiography. *J Am Coll Cardiol* 1997; 29:293.
98. Rosano GMC, Kaski JC, Arie S, et al. Failure to demonstrate myocardial ischaemia in patients with angina and normal coronary arteries: Evaluation by continuous coronary sinus pH monitoring and lactate metabolism. *Eur Heart J* 1996; 17:1175.
99. Watanabe S, Buffington CW, Moresea G. Comparison of myocardial ischemia induced by endothelin vs mechanical stenosis in pigs. *Am J Physiol* 1995; 268(3 pt 2):H1276.
100. Rigattieri S, Buffon A, Ramazzotti V, et al. Oxidative stress in ischemia-reperfusion injury: Assessment by three independent biochemical markers. *Ital Heart J* 2000; 1:68.
101. Buffon A, Santini SA, Rigattieri S, et al. Transient intracardiac lipid peroxidation induced by atrial pacing in syndrome X: A definitive demonstration of an ischemic mechanism? *Circulation* 1997; 96:I-270.
102. Crea F, Buffon A, Gaspardone A, et al. Alternative mechanisms for myocardial ischemia in syndrome X—New diagnostic markers. In Kaski JC, ed. *Chest Pain with Normal Coronary Angiograms. Pathogenesis, Diagnosis and Management*. Boston: Kluwer Academic Publishers; 1999:123.
103. Buchthal SD, den Hollander JA, Merz NB, et al. Abnormal myocardial phosphorus-31 nuclear magnetic resonance spectroscopy in women with chest pain but normal coronary angiograms. *N Engl J Med* 2000; 342:829.
104. Baumgart D, Haude M, Gorge G, et al. Augmented alpha-adrenergic constriction of atherosclerotic human coronary arteries. *Circulation* 1999; 99:2090.
105. Virdis A, Ghiadoni L, Lucarini A, et al. Presence of cardiovascular structural changes in essential hypertensive patients with coronary microvascular disease and effects of long-term treatment. *Am J Hypertens* 1996; 9(4 pt 1):361.
106. Kawaguchi M, Techigawara M, Ishihata T, et al. A comparison of ultrastructural changes on endomyocardial biopsy specimens obtained from patients with diabetes mellitus with and without hypertension. *Heart Vessels* 1997; 12:267.
107. Zeiher AM, Krause T, Schachinger V, et al. Impaired endothelium-dependent vasodilation of coronary resistance vessels is associated with exercise-induced myocardial ischemia. *Circulation* 1995; 91:2345.
108. Quyyumi AA, Dakak N, Andrews NP, et al. Contribution of nitric oxide to metabolic coronary vasodilation in the human heart. *Circulation* 1995; 92:320.
109. Chauhan A, Mullins PA, Taylor G, et al. Both endothelium-dependent and endothelium-independent function is impaired in patients with angina pectoris and normal coronary angiograms. *Eur Heart J* 1997; 18:60.
110. Koren W, Koldanov R, Peleg E, et al. Enhanced red cell sodium-hydrogen exchange in microvascular angina. *Eur Heart J* 1997; 18:1296–1299.
111. Gaspardone A, Ferri C, Crea F, et al. Enhanced activity of sodium-lithium countertransport in patients with cardiac syndrome X: A potential link between cardiac and metabolic syndrome X. *J Am Coll Cardiol* 1998; 32:2031–2034.
112. Kaski JC, Elliot PM, Salomone O, et al. Concentration of circulating plasma endothelin in patients with angina and normal coronary arteries. *Br Heart J* 1995; 74:620.
113. Lanza GA, Luscher TF, Pasceri V, et al. Effects of atrial pacing on arterial and coronary sinus endothelin-1 levels in syndrome X. *Am J Cardiol* 1999; 84:1187.
114. Lanza GA, Giordano A, Pristipino C, et al. Abnormal cardiac adrenergic nerve function in patients with syndrome X detected by [^{123}I]metaiodobenzylguanidine myocardial scintigraphy. *Circulation* 1997; 96:821.
115. Maseri A. From syndromes to specific disease mechanisms: The search for the causes of myocardial infarction. *Ital Heart J* 2000; 1:20.
116. Dechend R, Maass M, Gieffers J, et al. *Chlamydia pneumoniae* infection of vascular smooth muscle and endothelial cells activates NF-kappaB and induces tissue factor and PAI-1 expression: A potential link to accelerated arteriosclerosis. *Circulation* 1999; 100:1369.
117. Mayr M, Metzler B, Kiechl S, et al. Endothelial cytotoxicity mediated by serum antibodies to heat shock proteins of *Escherichia coli* and *Chlamydia pneumoniae*: Immune reactions to heat shock proteins as a possible link between infection and atherosclerosis. *Circulation* 1999; 99:1560.
118. Ikeda U, Takahashi M, Shimada K. Monocyte-endothelial cell interaction in atherogenesis and thrombosis. *Clin Cardiol* 1998; 21:11.
119. Gutstein DE, Fuster V. Pathophysiology and clinical significance of atherosclerotic plaque rupture. *Cardiovasc Res* 1999; 41:323.
120. Shah AM, Mebazaa A, Yang ZK, et al. Inhibition of myocardial crossbridge cycling by hypoxic endothelial cells: A potential mechanism for matching oxygen supply and demand. *Circ Res* 1997; 80:688.

121. Ehlert FA, Goldberger JJ. Cellular and pathophysiological mechanisms of ventricular arrhythmias in acute ischemia and infarction. *PACE* 1997; 20:967.
122. Niessen HW, Lagrand WK, Visser CA, et al. Upregulation of ICAM-1 on cardiomyocytes in jeopardized human myocardium during infarction. *Cardiovasc Res* 1999; 41:603.
123. Kaikita K, Ogawa H, Yasue H, et al. Increased plasma soluble intercellular adhesion molecule-1 levels in patients with acute myocardial infarction. *Jpn Circ J* 1997; 61:741.
124. Siminiak T, Dye JF, Egdell RM, et al. The release of soluble adhesion molecules ICAM-1 and E-selectin after acute myocardial infarction and following coronary angioplasty. *Int J Cardiol* 1997; 61:113.
125. Tomai F, Crea F, Chiariello L, et al. Ischemic preconditioning in humans: Models, mediators and clinical relevance. *Circulation* 1999; 100:559.
126. Pasceri V, Lanza GA, Patti G, et al. Preconditioning by transient myocardial ischemia confers protection against ischemia-induced ventricular arrhythmias in variant angina. *Circulation* 1996; 94:1850.
127. Andreotti F, Pasceri V, Hackett DR, et al. Preinfarction angina as a predictor of more rapid coronary thrombolysis in patients with acute myocardial infarction. *N Engl J Med* 1996; 334:7.
128. Braunwald E. Acute myocardial infarction—The value of being prepared. *N Engl J Med* 1996; 334:51.
129. Baker AJ. Cellular and extracellular mechanisms causing myocardial stunning. *J Am Coll Cardiol* 1999; 34:603.
130. Bolli R. Causative role of oxyradicals in myocardial stunning: A proven hypothesis: A brief review of the evidence demonstrating a major role of reactive oxygen species in several forms of postischemic dysfunction. *Basic Res Cardiol* 1998; 93:156.
131. Murphy AM, Kogler H, Georgakapoulos D, et al. Transgenic mouse model of stunned myocardium. *Science* 2000; 287:488.
132. Vanoverschelde J-L J, Wijns W, Borgers M, et al. Chronic myocardial hibernation in humans. From bedside to bench. *Circulation* 1997; 95:1961.
133. Crea F, Gaspardone A. New look to an old symptom: Angina pectoris. *Circulation* 1997; 96:3766.
134. Crea F, Gaspardone A, Kaski JC, et al. Relationship between stimulation site of cardiac afferent nerves by adenosine and location of cardiac pain: Results of a study in patients with stable angina. *J Am Coll Cardiol* 1992; 20:1498.
135. Pasceri V, Patti G, Maseri A. Changing features of anginal pain after PTCA suggest a stenosis on a different artery rather than restenosis. *Circulation* 1997; 96:3278.
136. Pasceri V, Cianflone D, Finocchiaro ML, et al. Relation between myocardial infarction site and pain location in acute Q-wave myocardial infarction. *Am J Cardiol* 1995; 75:224.
137. Lanza GA, Colonna G, Pasceri V, et al. A. Atenolol-vs-amlodipine-vs-isosorbide-5-mononitrate on anginal symptoms in syndrome X. *Am J Cardiol* 1999; 84:854.
138. Pasceri V, Lanza GA, Buffon A, et al. Role of abnormal pain sensitivity and behavioral factors in determining chest pain in syndrome X. *J Am Coll Cardiol* 1998; 31:62.
139. Lanza GA, Manzoli A, Pasceri V, et al. Ischemic-like ST-segment changes during Holter monitoring in patients with angina pectoris and normal coronary arteries but negative exercise testing. *Am J Cardiol* 1997; 79:1.
140. Liuzzo G, Biasucci LM, Gallimore et al. The prognostic value of C-reactive protein and serum amyloid, a protein in severe unstable angina. *N Engl J Med* 1994; 331:417.
141. Biasucci LM, Vitelli A, Liuzzo G, et al. Elevated levels of interleukin-6 in unstable angina. *Circulation* 1996; 94:874.
142. Liuzzo G, Biasucci LM, Rebuzzi AG, et al. Plasma protein acute-phase response in unstable angina is not induced by ischemic injury. *Circulation* 1996; 94:2373.
143. Beltrame JF, Sasayama S, Maseri A. Racial heterogeneity in coronary artery vasomotor reactivity: Differences between Japanese and Caucasian patients. *J Am Coll Cardiol* 1999; 33:1442.
144. Masahatu I, Ikaru U, Hironobu T, et al. Implications of prodromal angina pectoris in anterior wall acute myocardial infarction: Acute angiographic findings and long-term prognosis. *J Am Coll Cardiol* 1997; 30:970.
145. Biasucci LM, Liuzzo G, Grillo RL, et al. Elevated levels of C-reactive protein at discharge in patients with unstable angina predict recurrent instability. *Circulation* 1999; 99:885.
146. Liuzzo G, Biasucci LM, Gallimore R, et al. Enhanced inflammatory response in patients with pre-infarction angina. *J Am Coll Cardiol* 1999; 15:1696.
147. Pignalberi C, Patti G, Chimenti C, et al. Role of different determinants of psychological distress in acute coronary syndromes. *J Am Coll Cardiol* 1998; 32:613.

CHAPTER 38

DYSLIPIDEMIA, OTHER RISK FACTORS, AND THE PREVENTION OF CORONARY HEART DISEASE

David J. Maron / Paul M. Ridker / Thomas A. Pearson / Scott M. Grundy

Identification and management of risk factors are essential for preventing coronary heart disease (CHD) in asymptomatic individuals (*primary prevention*) and for preventing recurrent events in patients with established disease (*secondary prevention*). *Risk factor management should be conceived as prevention or treatment of the atherosclerotic disease process itself and, as such, should be included as an integral part of any management plan for the many acute or chronic manifestations of this disease.* The intensity of risk factor intervention should correspond to the patient's level of risk.[1] The presence of unmodifiable risk factors may necessitate more intense management of modifiable risk factors. The 27th Bethesda Conference proposed a classification scheme according to the strength of evidence that risk factor intervention favorably affects outcome.[1] This chapter is organized to reflect that classification scheme (Table 38-1) and reviews risk assessment for primary prevention, reviews CHD risk factors, discusses the efficacy and cost-effectiveness of managing risk factors, and provides practical recommendations for preventive cardiology practice.

RISK ASSESSMENT IN PRIMARY PREVENTION

As detailed in this chapter, the efficacy of secondary prevention of CHD using a variety of therapies has been well established. Therefore, an individual with established CHD or other atherosclerotic disease should be considered at highest risk for a CHD event and deserves the most aggressive evidence-based risk-reduction therapy. The therapeutic success achieved in secondary prevention of CHD has generated enthusiasm for extending this success to primary prevention in clinical practice. The essential issues for primary prevention are the selection of patients and selection of appropriate interventions. The first step in patient selection is to estimate a patient's risk. The key parameter for risk assessment for medical intervention is the *absolute risk*, i.e., the probability of developing CHD over a finite period.

Categories of Absolute Risk

For the sake of simplicity, absolute risk can be divided into three categories: high, intermediate, and low.[2] Patients at high

TABLE 38-1 Cardiovascular Risk Factors: The Evidence Supporting Their Association with Disease, the Usefulness of Measuring Them, and Their Responsiveness to Intervention

	Evidence for Association with CVD			Response to	
Risk Factor	Epidemiologic	Clinical Trials	Clinical Measurement Useful?	Nonpharmacologic Therapy	Pharmacologic Therapy
Category I (risk factors for which interventions have been proved to lower CVD risk)					
LDL cholesterol	+++	+++	+++	++	+++
HDL cholesterol	+++	++	+++	++	++
Atherogenic diet	+++	++	++	+++	−
Cigarette smoking	+++	++	+++	+++	+++
Hypertension	+++	+++ (stroke)	+++	++	+++
Left ventricular hypertrophy	+++	+	++	−	++
Thrombogenic factors	+++ (fibrinogen)	+++ (aspirin, warfarin)	+ (fibrinogen)	+	+++ (aspirin, warfarin)
Category II (risk factors for which interventions are likely to lower CVD risk)					
Diabetes mellitus	+++	+	+++	++	+++
Physical inactivity	+++	++	++	++	−
Triglycerides; small dense LDL	++	+	+++	++	+++
Obesity	+++	−	+++	++	+
Category III (risk factors associated with increased CVD risk that, if modified, might lower risk)					
Psychosocial factors	++	+	+++	+	−
Lipoprotein(a)	+	+	+	−	+
Homocysteine	++	−	+	+	++
Inflammation makers	++	+	+	−	+
No alcohol consumption	+++	−	++	++	−
Oxidative stress	++	−	−	+	++
Postmenopausal status (women)	+++	−	+++	−	+++
Category IV (risk factors associated with increased CVD risk but which cannot be modified)					
Age	+++	−	+++	−	−
Male gender	+++	−	+++	−	−
Low socioeconomic status	+++	−	+++	−	−
Family history of early-onset CVD	+++	−	+++	−	−

ABBREVIATIONS: CVD = cardiovascular disease; HDL = high-density lipoprotein; LDL = low-density lipoprotein: +, weak, somewhat consistent evidence; ++, moderately strong, rather consistent evidence; +++, very strong, consistent evidence; − evidence poor or nonexistent.
SOURCE: Modified from Fuster V, Pearson TA,[1] with permission.

risk deserve aggressive risk-reduction therapy. Those at intermediate risk also deserve medical intervention to the extent that therapy is effective, safe, and cost-effective. Finally, low-risk patients can be encouraged by their physicians to follow public health recommendations for primary prevention of CHD.

Each category of absolute risk can be examined in quantitative terms (Table 38-2). Patients at high risk are those whose absolute risk for CHD equals that of patients who already manifest clinical CHD.[2,3] Evidence from clinical trials of cholesterol-lowering therapy indicates that patients with a prior history of myocardial infarction (MI) have a 10-year risk for recurrent nonfatal or fatal MI of about 26 percent.[3–5] Patients with stable angina pectoris have a 10-year risk for acute MI of about 20 percent.[6,7] Thus, it is reasonable to say that *patients without manifest CHD who have a 10-year risk for MI of greater than 20 percent are at high risk.* These patients also can be said to have a *CHD risk equivalent.*[3] In accord, *intermediate-risk patients have a 10-year risk for MI of 10 to 20 percent.* Assignment of risk category is first made by measurements of standard risk factors.[2] In some patients, however, estimates of absolute risk may require adjustment on the basis of other kinds of risk factors or the presence of subclinical coronary artery disease.[2] *Low-risk patients are those whose 10-year risk for MI is less than 10 percent.*

TABLE 38-2 Risk Categories

Risk Category	10-Year Absolute Risk for Myocardial Infarction (%) (Nonfatal + Fatal)
High	>20
Intermediate	10–20
Low	<10

Identification of High-Risk Patients (Coronary Heart Disease Risk Equivalents)

NONCORONARY FORMS OF CLINICAL ATHEROSCLEROTIC DISEASE

Patients in this group include those with peripheral arterial disease, abdominal aortic aneurysm, and symptomatic carotid artery disease. The absolute risk for MI in patients with noncoronary forms of atherosclerotic disease equals that for recurrent MI in patients with established CHD.[8]

TYPE 2 DIABETES

Patients with type 2 diabetes who do not manifest CHD still appear to carry a risk for major coronary events equivalent to that of nondiabetic patients with established CHD.[9] Moreover, many patients with type 2 diabetes have had a silent MI, and many other asymptomatic patients have silent ischemia. This has led the American Diabetes Association to designate type 2 diabetes as a CHD risk equivalent.[10]

HIGH-RISK PATIENTS WITH MULTIPLE RISK FACTORS

The category of CHD risk equivalents has been extended to include asymptomatic patients who have multiple risk factors (other than diabetes).[11] A modified version of the Framingham score sheet is presented in Table 38-3. Framingham scores are used to estimate the absolute risk for the development of CHD over the next decade.[12] Table 38-4 shows absolute risk for *hard CHD* (nonfatal and fatal MI) and excludes *soft CHD* (stable and unstable angina). *Hard* CHD seems a better end point for defining CHD risk equivalency because risk-reduction therapy is aimed primarily at reducing risk for MI. When absolute 10-year risk for hard CHD exceeds 20 percent, a CHD risk equivalent is identified.

HIGH-RISK PATIENTS IDENTIFIED BY MAJOR RISK FACTORS PLUS SUBCLINICAL ATHEROSCLEROSIS

Many patients will be found to be at intermediate risk by Framingham scoring (Tables 38-3 and 38-4), i.e., absolute 10-year risk will be 10 to 20 percent.[13] Some of these patients undoubtedly will be at higher risk because of advanced subclinical coronary atherosclerosis. If the latter could be identified by noninvasive methods, risk could be raised to a level of CHD risk equivalent. The potential utility of noninvasive testing for this purpose has recently been reviewed in the American Heart Association's Prevention V Conference.[2] In the past, noninvasive testing in asymptomatic patients has been contentious. Many investigators are concerned that asymptomatic patients with advanced subclinical atherosclerosis will be labeled as having CHD; if so, patients receiving this label might be referred inappropriately for invasive procedures. *Only if noninvasive techniques are used for risk assessment (prognosis) and not for diagnosis can noninvasive testing be justified for asymptomatic patients.* The goal of such testing thus is to identify persons who will benefit from aggressive medical therapy for risk reduction, not for case finding for invasive intervention. Some authorities question whether the scientific evidence supporting this testing is sufficient to justify its recommendation.[14] Still others doubt that it is cost-effective. Various techniques for noninvasive testing and their utility in risk assessment are reviewed briefly below.

Exercise Treadmill Testing Exercise treadmill testing identifies patients whose coronary atherosclerosis has advanced sufficiently to produce myocardial ischemia with exercise (see also Chap. 14). A considerable body of data exists on risk prognostication on men of ages 45 to 70 years.[15] Exercise testing has reduced predictive value when the pretest probability for CHD is low. In middle-aged men, the combination of standard risk

TABLE 38-3 Scoring for Global Risk Assessment (Adjusted Framingham Scoring Points for Risk Factors)

	Risk Points	
Risk Factor	Men	Women
Age		
<34	−1	−9
35–39	0	−4
40–44	1	0
45–49	2	3
50–54	3	6
55–59	4	7
60–64	5	8
65–69	6	9
70–74	7	10
Total cholesterol (mg/dL)		
<160	−3	−2
169–199	0	0
200–239	1	1
240–279	2	2
≥280	3	3
Blood pressure (mmHg)		
<120	0	−3
120–129	0	0
130–139	1	1
140–159	2	2
>160	3	3
Smoker		
No	0	0
Yes	2	2
HDL cholesterol (mg/dL)		
<35	2	5
35–44	1	2
45–49	0	1
50–59	−1	0
≥60	−2	−3
Plasma glucose (mg/dL)		
<110	0	0
110–126	1	2
>126	2	4

Adding up the Points

Age________ Cholesterol________
Diabetes________ HDL cholesterol________
Smoker________ Blood pressure________
Total________

Adjusting Framingham Age Points for Coronary Calcium Scores

Percentile of Calcium Score[a]	Point Adjustment[b]
0–24th	−2
25–49th	−1
50–74th	+1
75–89th	+2
>90th	+3

[a]For percentile of calcium score, see Table 38-5.
[b]The adjustment shown should be substituted for the age score of a given patient, whether men or women.

TABLE 38-4 Absolute Risk Estimates for Hard Coronary Heart Disease (CHD) According to Framingham Points[a]

Framingham Risk Points	Absolute 10-Year Risk (%) Hard CHD Men	Women
1	2	1
2	3	2
3	4	2
4	5	2
5	6	2
6	7	2
7	9	3
8	13	3
9	16	3
10	20	4
11	25	7
12	30	8
13	35	11
14	45	13
15		15
16		18
17		20

[a]Hard CHD = nonfatal and fatal myocardial infarction.
[b]See Table 38-3.

factors and an abnormal exercise ECG denotes a high risk for developing clinical CHD. Risk for angina pectoris is 12-fold elevated above that of men with a normal test result.[15] Risk for MI is elevated fourfold. These extremely high risk ratios are sufficient to elevate an intermediate-risk category to the level of CHD risk equivalent.

Electron-Beam Computerized Tomography Electron-beam computerized tomography (EBCT) can be used to identify coronary calcification, which is a close correlate of coronary atherosclerosis.[16–19] As shown by EBCT, coronary calcium increases progressively with advancing age in parallel with coronary atherosclerosis (Table 38-5).[20] The finding of a certain degree of coronary calcium by EBCT (Table 38-5) may provide a means to improve on the risk estimate denoted by age in the Framingham algorithm (Tables 38-3 and 38-4). Patients at apparently intermediate risk with a high calcium score may be reclassified as having a CHD risk equivalent (see also Chap. 17).

Carotid B-mode Ultrasonography Carotid B-mode ultrasonography, which measures the intimal-medial thickness (IMT) of carotid arteries, provides an independent approximation of coronary atherosclerosis.[2] The extent of carotid atherosclerosis correlates with coronary atherosclerosis.[21–23] Recent reports indicate that carotid IMT carries independent predictive power for development of CHD.[24,25] Like coronary calcium scores, IMT scores could be used to replace age as a risk factor in the Framingham algorithm.[3,26] A high IMT score thus could elevate some apparently intermediate-risk patients to the level of CHD risk equivalent.

INFLAMMATORY MARKERS

Inflammatory markers also may improve risk prognostication in apparently intermediate-risk patients. For example, high-sensitivity C-reactive protein has been reported to carry independent predictive power.[27,28] An elevated concentration of circulating inflammatory markers might point to the presence of unstable coronary lesions. If this is confirmed, abnormalities in inflammatory markers could be used to raise a finding of intermediate risk by conventional risk factors to a CHD risk equivalent.

TABLE 38-5 Calcium Score Nomogram for 9728 Consecutive Subjects (the Number of Patients in Each Group Is in Parentheses)

Men (5433) Age	35–39 (479)	40–44 (859)	45–49 (1066)	50–54 (1085)	55–59 (853)	60–64 (613)	65–70 (478)
Calcium Scores							
25th percentile	0	0	0	0	3	14	28
50th percentile	0	0	3	16	41	118	151
75th percentile	2	11	44	101	187	434	569
90th percentile	21	64	176	320	502	804	1178
Women (4297) Age	**35–39 (288)**	**40–44 (589)**	**45–49 (822)**	**50–54 (903)**	**55–59 (693)**	**60–64 (515)**	**65–70 (485)**
Calcium Scores							
25th percentile	0	0	0	0	0	0	0
50th percentile	0	0	0	0	0	4	24
75th percentile	0	0	0	10	33	87	123
90th percentile	4	9	23	66	140	310	362

Source: From Raggi et al.,[20] with permission.

UNDERLYING AND PROVISIONAL RISK FACTORS

Finally, should *underlying risk factors*—e.g., obesity, physical inactivity, diet, genetic factors, and socioeconomic status—and *provisionally atherogenic risk factors*—e.g., elevated concentrations of triglycerides, lipoprotein(a), [Lp(a)], small dense low-density lipoprotein (LDL) particles, homocysteine, and coagulation factors—be used to adjust the risk of patients found to be at intermediate risk by Framingham scoring? The best approach may be to attempt to modify these factors directly through appropriate therapy, but not to use them in risk assessment. Nevertheless, this question is contentious and its answer unresolved.

RISK ASSESSMENT IN ELDERLY PATIENTS

The predictive power of conventional risk factors declines in older patients, and age becomes the predominant risk factor. Thus, the reliability of the Framingham algorithm is suspect in people over age 65. For this reason, measures of myocardial ischemia, coronary plaque burden, or markers of inflammation could be especially useful in differentiating between high-risk and intermediate-risk elderly patients. The demonstration that aggressive medical therapy significantly reduces risk for CHD in the older population increases the need to define absolute risk in this population more accurately.

Intermediate-Risk and Low-Risk Patients

For patients found to be at intermediate risk by Framingham scoring, additional noninvasive evaluation for subclinical atherosclerotic disease may be considered to define their risk status further (see above). Patients at intermediate risk by the Framingham algorithm deserve medical intervention. Primary prevention is for the long run. Even though these patients are not at high absolute risk for the short term, their risk mounts over time. In view of the proven effectiveness of risk-reduction therapies, there is a growing debate over whom among intermediate-risk patients should receive drug therapy for risk reduction. The issue revolves around efficacy, safety, and cost-effectiveness of drug therapies. Advances in pharmacologic therapy promise to improve safety and to reduce costs; therefore, in the future, it should be possible to extend the benefits of risk-reducing drugs to more patients. In addition, advances in nondrug therapies may also make these options more attractive to many patients.

An important question is how to manage patients with a single categorical risk factor but who are otherwise at low risk. A fundamental principle of primary prevention is that *all categorical risk factors must be treated, regardless of absolute risk.*[29] For example, cigarette smoking can cause cancer and cardiovascular disease even in the absence of other risk factors. Hypertension alone can cause stroke, heart failure, and kidney failure. Therefore, patients with categorical risk factors must not be ignored even if they are found to have a low absolute risk by Framingham scoring (Tables 38-3 and 38-4).

RISK FACTORS FOR WHICH INTERVENTIONS HAVE PROVED TO LOWER RISK OF CORONARY HEART DISEASE

Dyslipidemia

LOW-DENSITY LIPOPROTEIN CHOLESTEROL

Evidence of several types supports the concept that LDL is the primary atherogenic factor, and controlled clinical trials show that lowering LDL reduces the risk for CHD. Accordingly, the National Cholesterol Education Program (NCEP)[8] has identified LDL cholesterol as the primary target of lipid-lowering therapy. Five decades of research on the role of LDL in the pathogenesis of CHD represents one of the major advances in modern medicine and public health.[30] This evidence is summarized briefly.

Low-Density Lipoprotein as the Primary Atherogenic Agent Many studies in laboratory animals indicate that raising serum levels of LDL and related lipoproteins will initiate and sustain atherogenesis.[31] Moreover, humans with genetic forms of severely elevated LDL exhibit premature atherosclerotic disease.[32] Both of these examples demonstrate that elevated LDL alone, without the need for other CHD risk factors, is independently atherogenic. For many years, it was believed that the major action of LDL was merely to deposit its cholesterol within the arterial wall. More recently, LDL has been found to be a proinflammatory agent:[33] it sets into motion the chronic inflammatory response that is the hallmark of the atherosclerotic lesion. Elevated LDL appears to be involved with all stages of atherogenesis: endothelial dysfunction, plaque formation and growth, plaque instability and disruption, and thrombosis. Elevated LDL-cholesterol levels in the plasma lead to increased retention of LDL particles in the arterial wall, their oxidation, and the secretion of various inflammatory mediators and chemoattractants[35] (see Chap. 35). One sequela of this is the disruption of endothelial cell function by oxidized LDL,[35] with subsequent loss of production of nitric oxide. Treatment of elevated LDL-cholesterol levels has been shown to reestablish normal coronary vasodilatory response to acetylcholine.[36,37] LDL is also a potent mitogen for smooth muscle cells.

The primacy of LDL as a pathogenic agent is supported by epidemiologic data of several types. In different populations, the risk for CHD is positively correlated with the serum total cholesterol level;[38] the total cholesterol level in turn is highly correlated with LDL-cholesterol levels.[8] The association between serum cholesterol levels and CHD risk is curvilinear (or long-linear).[38] Risk rises exponentially at higher cholesterol levels. In populations that have very low total (and LDL) cholesterol, risk for CHD likewise is low, even when other CHD risk factors (cigarette smoking, hypertension, and diabetes) are common.[32] This latter observation strongly suggests that an elevated LDL cholesterol is the *primary* risk factor.

Primary and Secondary Prevention There is a long history of clinical trials of cholesterol-lowering therapy that have included dietary and drug trials.[30] One trial also induced cholesterol lowering by intestinal surgery.[39] Some trials have included patients with established CHD (secondary prevention), and others recruited patients without CHD (primary prevention). The aggregate results of early trials, both primary and secondary prevention, demonstrated that cholesterol-lowering therapy (or lipoprotein modification) reduces risk for CHD.[40] However, earlier trials failed to show that cholesterol reduction decreased total mortality.[40,41] This latter deficiency left many clinicians skeptical of the benefits of cholesterol-lowering therapy.

The introduction of HMG-CoA reductase inhibitors (statins), which are powerful LDL-lowering drugs, made possible a more effective test of the cholesterol hypothesis.[42,43] Since 1993, five major trials with statins have been published: three secondary prevention[4,5,44] and two primary prevention trials.[45,46] The results of these studies are summarized in Table 38-6. All trials showed a marked reduction in major coronary events. Three found a reduction in total mortality.[5,44,45] No increases in noncardiovascular mortality occurred in any of the trials. These trials documented convincingly that cholesterol-lowering therapy is both safe and effective for reducing CHD risk.

In this same time period, a series of angiographic trials was

TABLE 38-6 Clinical Outcome Studies Using Statins

Study n (% Women)	Intervention	Baseline LDL (mg/dL)	% LDL Reduction	On-trial LDL (mg/dL)[a]	% Reduction in Total Mortality	% Reduction in Coronary Events	% Reduction in CABG and PTCA
Secondary prevention trials							
4S 4444 (19)	Simvastatin 20–40 mg/day	188	35	120	30 ($p = .003$)	34 ($p < .0001$)	37 ($p < .0001$)
CARE 4159 (14)	Pravastatin 40 mg/day	139	32	95	9 (NS)	24 ($p = .003$)	27 ($p < .001$)
LIPID 9014 (17)	Pravastatin 40 mg/day	150	25	113	22 ($p < .0001$)	24 ($p < .0001$)	22[b] ($p < .001$)
Primary prevention trials							
WOSCOPS 6595 (0)	Pravastatin 40 mg/day	192	26	142	22 ($p = .051$)	31 ($p < .001$)	37 ($p = .009$)
AFCAPS/TexCAPS 6605 (15)	Lovastatin 20–40 mg/day	150	25	113	0 (NS)	37 ($p < .001$)	33 ($p = .001$)

[a]On-trial LDL-C values are calculated from published data.
[b]Results for CABG; the need for PTCA was reduced by 19% ($p = .024$).
ABBREVIATIONS: 4S = Scandinavian Simvastatin Survival Study; CARE = Cholesterol and Recurrent Events trial; LIPID = Long-Term Intervention with Pravastatin in Ischaemic Disease Trial; WOSCOPS = West of Scotland Coronary Prevention Study; AFCAPS/TexCAPS = Air Force/Texas Coronary Atherosclerosis Prevention Study.
SOURCE: From Maron et al.,[298] with permission.

performed to determine whether reducing LDL-cholesterol levels would decrease progression or promote regression of coronary atherosclerotic lesions. These trials typically employed aggressive cholesterol-lowering therapy, often with combined drug regimens. Indeed, most studies revealed that marked reductions of LDL levels will slow progression, and in some cases promote regression, of coronary lesions.[47,48] Although measurable angiographic changes in lesion size were small, the incidence of major coronary events was reduced strikingly. This observation engendered the concept that LDL reduction *stabilizes* coronary lesions rather than causing them to shrink markedly. Seemingly, LDL lowering modifies lesion structure and composition more than it changes lesion size. Consequently, short-term cholesterol-lowering therapy appears to reduce the likelihood of coronary plaque rupture and thrombosis.

Practice Recommendations for Low-Density Lipoprotein Lowering LDL lowering can be accomplished with nondrug and drug therapies. *The importance of nondrug therapies must not be minimized.* Chief among them are reducing intake of cholesterol-raising fatty acids (saturated and *trans* fatty acids) and dietary cholesterol.[8] The major sources of dietary saturated fatty acids are dairy fats (e.g., milk, butter, cream, cheese, and ice cream) and animal fats [e.g., fatty cuts of meat (especially hamburger), fatty processed meats, lard and tallow]. *Trans* fatty acids are present in shortening, hard margarine, and processed foods containing these forms of fat. Rich sources of dietary cholesterol are eggs, dairy fats, and other animal products. Current intake of cholesterol-raising fatty acids in the United States is in the range of 15 percent of total calories. For patients on cholesterol-lowering therapy, this should be reduced to less than 7 percent. Dietary cholesterol should be lowered to less than 200 mg/day. Achieving a desirable body weight will reduce LDL-cholesterol levels in most overweight patients and will decrease risk for CHD in several other ways.[49]

There is growing interest in obtaining further risk reduction by use of dietary adjuncts. A daily intake of 3 g/day of plant stanols will reduce LDL-cholesterol concentrations 10 to 15 percent beyond that which can be achieved by reducing cholesterol-raising fatty acids and cholesterol in the diet.[50] High-intakes of dietary fiber will produce another 3 to 5 percent decrease in LDL levels.[51] Unsaturated fatty acids (monounsaturated, *n*-6 polyunsaturated, and *n*-3 polyunsaturated fatty acids) will lower LDL and may reduce global risk for CHD via several other mechanisms.[52]

Statins head the list of cholesterol-lowering drugs. Table 38-7 compares the efficacy of the currently available statins in patients without hypertriglyceridemia. Most patients tolerate statins with few side effects. Occasional patients will have a mild rise in liver transaminases, but this change is currently not believed to be an indication of hepatotoxicity. Rare patients will exhibit signs and symptoms of myopathy. This side effect is more likely to occur in patients who have chronic renal failure or liver disease or who are on drugs that utilize or inhibit the cytochrome P450 3A4 pathway. For every doubling of the dose of a statin, the LDL-cholesterol level will fall by about 6 percent; a more efficacious way to enhance LDL lowering is to combine statins with bile acid sequestrants. For patients with borderline elevated triglycerides (200 to 400 mg/dL) and high LDL, niacin or a statin is an acceptable first-line drug. When triglycerides exceed 400 mg/dL, a fibrate or niacin is usually the most appropriate first-line agent.

Goals of Therapy Lowering Low-Density Lipoprotein For patients with established CHD, the NCEP recommends an LDL-cholesterol goal of ≤100 mg/dL.[8] This recommendation is based on the combined data from epidemiologic studies, angiographic trials, and end-point trials. New clinical trials have been initiated to define the optimal LDL-cholesterol goal for secondary prevention. However, the NCEP contends that multiple lines of evidence already converge to support an LDL-cholesterol target of ≤100 mg/dL.[53] The American Heart Association recom-

TABLE 38-7 Comparative Efficacy of the Six Currently Available Statins on Lipids and Lipoproteins in Patients Without Hypertriglyceridemia

Statin Drug (mg)						Change in Lipid and Lipoprotein Levels (%)			
Atorvastatin	Simvastatin	Lovastatin	Pravastatin	Fluvastatin	Cerivastatin	Total	LDL	HDL	Triglycerides
—	10	20	20	40	0.2	−22	−27	+4–8	−10–15
10	20	40	40	80	0.4	−27	−34	+4–8	−10–20
20	40	80	—	—	—	−32	−41	+4–8	−15–25
40	80	—	—	—	—	−37	−48	+4–8	−20–30
80	—	—	—	—	—	−42	−55	+4–8	−25–35

NOTE: For the purpose of illustration, the lipid and lipoprotein responses are based on short-term clinical trials and are approximations of what might be observed in clinical practice.
ABBREVIATIONS: HDL = high-density lipoprotein; LDL = low-density lipoprotein.
SOURCE: From Maron et al.,[298] with permission.

mends starting cholesterol-lowering drugs immediately in all CHD patients when the LDL-cholesterol level is >130 mg/dL.[54] Whether to initiate cholesterol-lowering drugs in patients whose baseline LDL-cholesterol is in the range of 100 to 129 mg/dL is unsettled. Without question, these patients should receive maximal nondrug therapy, possibly including dietary adjuncts (see above). Such therapy alone will often achieve the LDL-cholesterol goal of ≤100 mg/dL.

For patients with noncoronary forms of atherosclerotic disease, the NCEP also recommends an LDL-cholesterol goal of ≤100 mg/dL.[8] This is because other atherosclerotic disease constitutes a CHD risk equivalent. Patients with CHD risk equivalents should have the same goal for LDL cholesterol as patients with known CHD, i.e., ≤100 mg/dL.

For patients at intermediate risk (Table 38-2), a reasonable LDL-cholesterol goal is <130 mg/dL. The last NCEP report essentially made such a recommendation, although the method for establishing CHD risk was not with the Framingham algorithm (Tables 38-3 and 38-4). Rather it recommended counting categorical risk factors (Table 38-8), which is less precise for estimating absolute risk. Most men over age 65 who are not found to be at high risk can be considered to be at intermediate risk; their LDL-cholesterol goal should be <130 mg/dL. Women under age 55 generally are at lower risk than men of equivalent age and should be evaluated by Framingham scoring for risk stratification. The strategy for achieving an LDL-cholesterol level <130 mg/dL should be initiated with nondrug therapy, but some patients undoubtedly will require LDL-lowering drugs.

Finally, for patients who are at low risk (Table 38-2), the LDL-cholesterol goal is <160 mg/dL. This target can be considered to be a minimal goal, but it must be recognized that the desirable LDL in primary prevention is <130 mg/dL.[8] Most low-risk patients, however, are not candidates for cholesterol-lowering drugs unless their LDL-cholesterol levels are very high, e.g., >190 mg/dL. In low-risk patients whose baseline LDL-cholesterol concentration is in the range of 160 to 189 mg/dL, clinical judgment is required whether to start cholesterol-lowering drugs.[8] Most patients whose LDL is in this range should achieve an LDL-cholesterol level of < 160 mg/dL with maximal nondrug therapy including dietary adjuncts.

Cost-Effectiveness of Drug Therapy for Lowering Low-Density Lipoprotein Cost-effectiveness analysis is used to consider both the effectiveness of an intervention and its cost and is commonly expressed as a ratio of cost in dollars per quality-adjusted years of life gained[1] (see also Chap. 94). The validity of the assumptions used to determine direct and indirect cost is critical to computing an accurate ratio. By convention, less than $20,000 per year of life saved is considered highly cost-effective, $20,000 to $40,000 is relatively cost-effective, and greater than $60,000 is considered expensive. Studies of the cost-effectiveness of cholesterol lowering have demonstrated the importance of effective therapies in patients at highest risk. Studies of LDL-cholesterol reduction with statins have demonstrated cost-effectiveness in CHD patients. Estimates of cost per year of life range from $22,900 in asymptomatic 55- to 64-

TABLE 38-8 National Cholesterol Education Program Risk Categories for Primary Prevention

Intermediate-to-high risk

Two or more major risk factors in the presence of LDL cholesterol ≥160 mg/dL[a]

- Cigarette smoking
- Hypertension (blood pressure >140/90 mmHg) or on treatment for hypertension
- Low HDL cholesterol (<35 mg/dL)
- Age (men >45 years; women >55 years or post-menopausal)
- Family history of premature coronary heart disease
- Diabetes mellitus

Low risk

Zero to one risk factor in the presence of LDL cholesterol ≥160 mg/dL

[a]Subtract one risk factor if HDL cholesterol >60 mg/dL.
ABBREVIATIONS: HDL = high-density lipoprotein; LDL = low-density lipoprotein.
SOURCE: From National Cholesterol Education Program,[8] with permission.

year-old men with total cholesterol <250 mg/dL to actual cost savings in hypercholesterolemic, male CHD patients 45 to 54 years old.[55] In a direct cost analysis of the Scandinavian Simvastatin Survival Study, cost of simvastatin therapy ranged from $3800 for 70-year-old men with a cholesterol level of 309 mg/dL to $27,400 for 35-year-old women with a cholesterol level of 213 mg/dL.[56] When indirect costs were considered, the results ranged from a savings in the youngest patient to a cost of $13,300 per year of life gained in older patients. In contrast, the use of less effective agents, such as bile acid-binding resins, in low-risk, asymptomatic patients does not appear to be cost-effective.[57]

ATHEROGENIC DYSLIPIDEMIA: HYPERTRIGLYCERIDEMIA, LOW HIGH-DENSITY LIPOPROTEIN, AND SMALL DENSE LOW-DENSITY LIPOPROTEIN

Although high LDL is the primary lipid risk factor, other lipid parameters increase the risk of CHD in persons with or without an elevated LDL cholesterol. Specifically, the combination of *elevated concentrations of triglycerides, small dense LDL and low levels of high-density lipoprotein (HDL) is referred to as atherogenic dyslipidemia.*[58] This is a complex dyslipidemia that usually results from a generalized metabolic derangement. Although an elevated LDL cholesterol deserves primary emphasis for management, atherogenic dyslipidemia is assuming increasing importance as a contributor to CHD because of the growing prevalence of obesity in the United States and worldwide.[58] Most patients with atherogenic dyslipidemia have a generalized metabolic disorder called *insulin resistance.* This syndrome is described later in this chapter.

Relation of Atherogenic Dyslipidemia to Coronary Heart Disease A long-standing debate is whether the individual components of atherogenic dyslipidemia are independent risk factors. This question has been difficult to resolve because each of the three lipid components is highly correlated with the other two. Nevertheless, there is growing evidence for independent atherogenicity of each component. For triglycerides, *recent meta-analyses of multiple prospective studies strongly suggest that elevated serum triglycerides are an independent risk factor for CHD.*[59,60] *Other prospective studies show that a low HDL-cholesterol level is an independent risk factor.*[61,62] Two important mechanisms by which HDL is thought to play a protective role against atherosclerosis are reverse cholesterol transport and inhibition of LDL oxidation. *A lesser body of data also suggests that small, dense LDL particles are more atherogenic than normal-sized LDL.*[63] Atherogenic dyslipidemia is commonly accompanied by the other atherogenic risk factors of the metabolic syndrome[58] (see the section "Insulin Resistance Syndrome" below).

Primary and Secondary Prevention Among Subjects with Atherogenic Dyslipidemia No controlled clinical trials have been conducted to address specifically whether modifying atherogenic dyslipidemia will reduce risk for CHD. Indirect evidence comes from post hoc analyses of large clinical trials and from trials using drugs that modify atherogenic dyslipidemia. The latter drugs include nicotinic acid and the fibric acids. These drugs have only small effects on LDL levels, and most changes occur in the components of atherogenic dyslipidemia. The results of clinical trials[64–69] in which nicotinic acid or a fibric acid was used are shown in Table 38-9. None of these trials except for the Veterans Affairs High-Density Lipoprotein Cholesterol Intervention Trial (VA-HIT)[69] specifically targeted patients with atherogenic dyslipidemia. Nevertheless, most of the trials either showed a significant reduction in coronary events by drug therapy or a trend toward a reduction. In the Helsinki Heart Study,[65] the Stockholm Ischemic Heart Disease Study,[67] and the Bezafibrate Infarction Prevention Study,[68] the most favorable results were observed in patients with elevated triglycerides, an indicator of atherogenic dyslipidemia. These trials generally did not reveal a reduction in total mortality, nor were they statistically powered to do so. Nonetheless, taken as a whole, these trials are strongly suggestive that modification of atherogenic dyslipidemia by drug therapy will reduce the risk for CHD. This likelihood is enhanced by the findings of angiographic trials that fibrates slow progression of coronary atherosclerosis.[65,70]

It must be noted that statins also modify atherogenic dyslipidemia by reducing remnants of triglyceride-rich lipoproteins, reducing concentrations of small dense LDL, and by raising HDL-cholesterol levels modestly. Thus, some of the risk reduc-

TABLE 38-9 Clinical Trials with Drugs That Modify Atherogenic Dyslipidemia

Name of Clinical Trial	Type of Trial	Drug	Number of Patients	Coronary Events on Drug Therapy
WHO Trial[64]	Primary prevention	Clofibrate	15,745[a]	20% (p = .05)
Helsinki Heart Study[65]	Primary prevention	Gemfibrozil	4061[b]	−34% (p <.02)
Coronary Drug Project[66]	Secondary prevention	Nicotinic Acid	1119[c] (2789)[d]	−22% (p <.05)
Coronary Drug Project[66]	Secondary prevention	Clofibrate	1103[c] (2789)[d]	−5% (NS)
Stockholm Study[67]	Secondary prevention	Clofibrate + nicotinic acid	555[b]	−36% (p <.01)
BIP[68]	Secondary prevention	Bezafibrate	3122[b]	−9.4% (p = .26)
VA-HIT[69]	Secondary prevention	Gemfibrozil	2531[b]	−22% (p <.006)

[a]Three groups of patients. Patients divided between two high-cholesterol groups and one low-cholesterol group. Comparison was between two high-cholesterol groups.
[b]Patients divided between drug and control groups (open label design).
[c]Number of patients on drug therapy.
[d]Number of patients on placebo therapy.

tion from the statin trials could be related to favorable modification of the component of atherogenic dyslipidemia as well as to lowering of LDL-cholesterol levels.

Practice Recommendations for Atherogenic Dyslipidemia First-line treatment of atherogenic dyslipidemia is weight control and physical activity. Most patients with atherogenic dyslipidemia are either overweight [body mass index (BMI), 25 to 29 kg/m^2] or obese (BMI $\geq$30 kg/m^2).[49] Weight reduction in these patients often will improve the lipoprotein abnormalities associated with this form of dyslipidemia.[49] Introduction of regular physical activity will further correct the lipoprotein pattern. Not only will weight control and regular exercise improve atherogenic dyslipidemia, it also will mitigate the other components of the metabolic syndrome.[71] The increasing prevalence of obesity and physical inactivity in the United States has caused a corresponding increase in the metabolic syndrome among Americans. This unfortunate trend threatens to reverse the advances made in reducing morbidity and mortality from cardiovascular disease over the past two decades. It also poses a challenge to physicians to modify their practice to place more emphasis on lifestyle changes.

Both fibric acids and nicotinic acid will improve the lipoprotein pattern in patients with atherogenic dyslipidemia. Fibric acids have been shown to activate nuclear receptors (PPAR alpha) that favorably modify regulators of lipoprotein metabolism in the liver.[72] The mechanism of action of nicotinic acid is not known, but its effects are similar to those of fibric acids, except that nicotinic acid is more effective for raising HDL-cholesterol levels.[73] Unfortunately, nicotinic acid has several side effects that prevent its use in high doses in many patients. Nonetheless, the drug is usually well tolerated in moderate doses (1.0 to 1.5 g/day).

The primary goal of lipid therapy in patients with atherogenic dyslipidemia is to reduce LDL-cholesterol concentration to the targets recommended for primary and secondary prevention. In many patients, statin therapy will be required to achieve the LDL target. If abnormalities persist after reaching the LDL goal, renewed efforts at weight control and increased physical activity may be indicated. If these measures are not successful, a second lipid-lowering drug may be added to modify these other lipoproteins. Either a fibric acid or nicotinic acid can be employed as the second agent to achieve the secondary NCEP goals of HDL > 35 mg/dL and triglycerides < 200 mg/dL. The combination of fibrates with a high dose of a statin should be avoided because of the increased risk of myopathy.

Some investigators believe that an appropriate target of therapy in patients with atherogenic dyslipidemia is non-HDL cholesterol.[74,75] This fraction includes cholesterol in LDL and in remnants of triglyceride-rich lipoproteins. If non-HDL cholesterol is taken as a target of therapy, the goals of therapy are 30 mg/dL higher than the LDL-cholesterol goals for secondary and primary prevention. An alternate target is the serum triglyceride level. Although clinical trials are suggestive of benefit, there is no universal agreement among authorities that additional risk reduction is achieved by targeting atherogenic dyslipidemia beyond LDL cholesterol.

LIPOPROTEIN(a)

Lp(a) consists of an LDL particle linked via a disulfide bond to an apolipoprotein(a) [apo(a)] polypeptide chain. Because of homology between apo(a) and plasminogen, Lp(a) has been hypothesized to serve as a competitive inhibitor for plasminogen binding and thus may inhibit endogenous fibrinolysis.[76] Lp(a) is largely genetically determined, and distributions differ between men and women, as well as between races.

Several retrospective case-control studies support the view that Lp(a) is an independent risk factor for thromboembolic disease. However, results of the major prospective studies evaluating baseline Lp(a) concentration and future risks of MI and stroke have been inconsistent.[77–83] One possibility to explain these divergent results may relate to the fact that Lp(a) appears to be a greater marker of risk among patients with hypercholesterolemia[78,84] or among younger individuals only.[85] Another possibility is that electrophoretically detected Lp(a) may be a better marker than actual plasma level.[86,87]

Primary and Secondary Prevention Although nicotinic acid and estrogen appear to reduce Lp(a) levels in some patients, no clinical trials have been conducted to test whether reducing plasma levels results in reduced risk.

Practice Recommendations It is not yet clear whether Lp(a) provides information independent of the conventional lipid profile, and no recommendation for screening can be made. If elevated levels prove clearly to increase risk among hypercholesterolemic individuals, it may be prudent to lower LDL-cholesterol levels even more aggressively in such individuals than current guidelines dictate. Knowledge of Lp(a) levels may also be useful in the selection of LDL-lowering drugs (e.g., niacin) and may identify a possible treatable cause in the occasional patient with CHD and none of the major risk factors. Unfortunately, many commercial assays for plasma Lp(a) are poorly standardized.[88]

Atherogenic Diet

An atherogenic diet and a lack of physical activity are considered leading preventable causes of death, second only to tobacco use.[89] Considerable epidemiologic data indicate that populations with diets high in cholesterol and animal fats have high rates of CHD.[90,91] Conversely, those populations consuming large amounts of calories as vegetables, cereals, and fish have lower rates of CHD.[90] Countries that increased their animal fat consumption during the 1970s and 1980s increased their CHD mortality rates, while those that decreased their annual fat consumption showed CHD mortality reductions.[92] Similarly, populations consuming larger amounts of sodium in their diet have higher average blood pressures.[93] Caloric imbalance, in part due to excess calorie consumption, is related to a rising prevalence of obesity. On an individual basis, recent clinical trials of modified diets have demonstrated reductions in angiographic progression[94] and in recurrence of clinical disease.[95]

It has been assumed that the harmful effects of the *Western* diet have been mediated by saturated fats, dietary cholesterol, and sodium, via their effects on traditional risk factors such as LDL cholesterol, body weight, diabetes, and blood pressure. A portion of the effect of a Western diet appears to be attributable to these factors. However, there is evidence for mechanisms other than the traditional risk factors. The Western Electric Study adjusted for these factors and continued to find an independent risk associated with dietary cholesterol.[96] The Lyon

Diet Heart Study compared a Mediterranean-type diet high in alpha-linolenic acid with a Western diet and showed a 65 percent reduction in recurrent coronary events despite no demonstrable change in any of the traditional risk factors.[95] Mechanisms suggested as explanatory of these benefits include antioxidant, anti-inflammatory, and antiplatelet effects. This apparent independent benefit of a diet low in saturated fat, cholesterol, and sodium, and high in monounsaturated fats, fruits, vegetables, and fish provides the rationale for inclusion of *atherogenic diet* as a separate, modifiable risk factor.

PRIMARY PREVENTION
Reduction in the dietary consumption of animal fat, cholesterol, and sodium should be the mainstay of population-wide coronary disease prevention. Population-wide cholesterol reductions observed in the United States from 1979 to 1991 are attributed solely to changes in dietary consumption patterns.[97] Two older clinical trials of long-term inpatients demonstrated reductions in coronary endpoints of 34 to 50 percent among patients on low saturated fat and cholesterol diets.[98,99] Therefore, *dietary interventions should be the initial step in the treatment of dyslipidemia, hypertension, diabetes, and obesity.*

SECONDARY PREVENTION
Studies of low-fat diets, such as the STARS Trial[100] and the Lifestyle Heart Study[94] have used angiographic end points and shown a marked reduction in LDL cholesterol and a reduction in new or progressive coronary stenoses. However, these studies are too small to test for clinical end-point reduction. The Oslo Diet-Heart Study demonstrated a significant reduction in reinfarction rates with a low saturated fat diet as well as a smoking cessation program.[101] As noted, the Lyon Diet Heart Study, with a Mediterranean-type diet enriched in alpha-linolenic acid, demonstrated a 65 percent reduction in recurrent cardiac events and death over a 4-year period of follow-up.[95] *The magnitude of benefit was similar to or greater than those shown in numerous trials of lipid-lowering drugs.*

COST-EFFECTIVENESS
Dietary interventions might be targeted at the general population or at high-risk groups such as coronary disease patients. Population-wide interventions to alter eating behaviors intend to make relatively small changes in dietary habits in a large number of people. Studies from Finland[102] and the United States[103] suggest that population-wide education programs can reduce LDL-cholesterol levels 3 to 4 percent at a cost of $4 to $10 per person per year. Using a model to project benefits of such programs, Goldman et al. predicted that the Finnish program would cost $10,000 per year of life saved, whereas the U.S. program would actually be cost saving.[104] The cost-effectiveness of such a population-wide intervention was compared with a more individualized dietary intervention in a study of Norwegian men.[105] The population-wide approach cost approximately $20 per year of life saved versus $20,000 per year of life saved for the program of individual counseling. *Both approaches are considered highly cost-effective and favorable to drug treatment in that study.*

PRACTICE RECOMMENDATIONS
The current dietary recommendations emphasize a well-balanced diet low in saturated fat, cholesterol, and sodium, while rich in fruits and vegetables.[102] Very low fat diets are poorly complied with and have little long-term safety and efficacy data to support them.[106] A diet with less than 30 percent of calories from fat is generally recommended, but with caloric content compatible with maintenance of ideal body weight. For patients with vascular disease or hyperlipidemia, less than 7 percent of calories from saturated fat and less than 200 mg of dietary cholesterol per day are suggested. Monounsaturated fats and omega-3 fatty acids from fish may be a beneficial source of calories, as compared with carbohydrates.[107] Consultation with a registered dietitian or other nutrition specialist can be recommended as part of a risk-modification program in high-risk patients.

Cigarette Smoking

Strong dose-responsive relationships between cigarette smoking and CHD have been observed in both sexes, in the young and in the elderly, and in all racial groups.[108] Cigarette smoking increases risk two- to threefold and interacts with other risk factors to multiply risk. There is no evidence that filters or other modifications of the cigarette reduce risk.[109] Pipe smoking and cigar smoking, when not inhaled, as well as oral tobacco use, whether chewing tobacco or snuff, carry rather small risks but are related to later resumption of cigarette smoking. Clearly, cigarette smoking remains a leading preventable cause of mortality, much of it due to cardiovascular disease.

Whereas active cigarette smoking has long been established as a cardiovascular risk factor, exposure to environmental tobacco smoke, or passive smoking, has increasingly been recognized as a modifiable risk factor.[110,111] In a recent meta-analysis of 18 epidemiologic studies, exposure to tobacco smoke by nonsmokers was consistently associated with a 20 to 30 percent increase in risk.[112] This is in addition to an increased risk for respiratory tract cancers and other smoking-related diseases.

Pathophysiologic studies have identified a panoply of mechanisms through which cigarette smoking may cause CHD. Smokers have increased levels of oxidation products, including oxidized LDL.[113] Cigarette smoking also lowers the cardioprotective levels of HDL. These effects, along with direct effects of carbon monoxide and nicotine, produce endothelial damage. Possibly through these mechanisms, smokers have increased vascular reactivity.[113,114] The reduced capacity of the blood to carry oxygen also lowers the threshold for myocardial ischemia and increases the risk of coronary spasm. Cigarette smoking is also related to increased levels of fibrinogen and increased platelet aggregability.[115]

PRIMARY PREVENTION
Cessation of smoking is associated with a precipitous fall in CHD events. *In a previous smoker, the relative risk declines nearly to that of a nonsmoker in a year or less.*[116] It is estimated that a 35-year-old who quits smoking extends survival by 3 to 5 years,[117] with much of the improved life expectancy caused by a reduction in CHD deaths.

SECONDARY PREVENTION
The risk of a recurrent event in a patient surviving an MI is strikingly reduced by smoking cessation. Compared with a patient who continues to smoke, the risk of recurrence can be reduced by 50 percent.[118,119] *The benefits of achieving complete*

abstinence from smoking for a patient with CHD compare favorably with the health benefits of any intervention in modern cardiology.

COST-EFFECTIVENESS

Interventions to achieve smoking cessation are among the most cost-effective in either primary or secondary prevention, with or without the use of nicotine replacement therapy.[120,121] Physician counseling of middle-aged patients without vascular disease is estimated to cost only $1000 to $1400 per year in men and $1700 to $3000 per year in women.[122] The use of nicotine gum by these patients increased the cost to up to $9000 per year in men and $13,500 per year in women.[123] In contrast, counseling to achieve smoking cessation in MI patients is exceptionally cost-effective, costing only $250 per year of life saved.[124]

PRACTICE RECOMMENDATIONS

Nothing less than complete cessation of smoking and other tobacco use should be acceptable in patients with cardiovascular disease. Moreover, the home and work environments to which patients return should be smoke free, both to encourage cessation and to reduce the risk from passive smoking. Cardiovascular specialists often have unique and time-limited opportunities to influence the behaviors of patients. After an acute event, the patient and their family members may be especially receptive to a smoking cessation intervention.

Smoking Cessation Clinical Practice Guidelines were first published by the Agency for Health Care Policy and Research in 1996 and form the basis for a successful smoking cessation program.[125] Those guidelines emphasize that tobacco use status be documented in every patient and that every smoker should be offered one or more of three effective treatment interventions. Even a brief intervention may be effective and should, at a minimum, be provided to every patient who uses tobacco (Table 38-10). Three elements of a treatment program found to be effective include social support, skills training/problem solving, and nicotine replacement. More intense efforts by the care provider to achieve complete cessation will generally result in a greater success rate. The huge reduction in risk resulting from smoking cessation in the cardiovascular disease patient provides a strong rationale for sustained and intense efforts to be expended.

Addiction to tobacco is a major barrier to cessation, and a number of pharmacologic agents can be recommended as an adjunct to a concurrent behavioral intervention on the basis of clinical trials demonstrating significantly increased rates of smoking cessation.[126] Bupropion SR, nicotine gum, nicotine inhaler, nicotine nasal spray, and nicotine patch are all first-line drugs to prevent nicotine withdrawal; clonidine is reserved for second-line therapy. Safety of the use of these agents in coronary disease patients was initially a concern, but several studies have now established the lack of association between the use of nicotine replacement agents and further cardiac events.[127–129]

TABLE 38-10 Strategies for Successful Cessation of Cigarette Smoking: The Four A's

Ask	Systematically identify all tobacco users at every visit (e.g., include tobacco as a vital sign). Determine exposure to environmental tobacco smoke at home or at work. Identify patients with nicotine addiction.
Advise	Provide a clear, strong, and personalized message, urging every tobacco user to quit. Review benefits of quitting and risk of continuing. Assess patient's willingness to quit.
Assist	Have the patient develop a quit plan, including setting a quit date, identifying sources of support for cessation for family and friends, removing tobacco and other cues from the home and work environment. Provide counseling, information materials and other behavioral interventions. Recommend use of pharmacotherapy including bupropion SR, nicotine gum, nicotine inhaler, nicotine nasal spray or nicotine patch.
Arrange	Provide a reminder on the quit date. See the patient shortly after the quit date to assess success. If unsuccessful, identify barriers and solutions to their removal

SOURCE: From Fiore M et al.[125] and Pearson TA.[299]

Hypertension

(See also Chap. 51.) Several major prospective epidemiologic studies have found that both systolic and diastolic hypertension have a strong, positive, continuous, and graded relationship to CHD without evidence of a threshold risk level of blood pressure.[130–132] Among populations in different countries, the relative risk for CHD imposed by a given increase in blood pressure is similar, but the absolute risk at a given blood pressure value varies substantially.[133] This may be due to widely varying baseline risk among populations. Hypertension clusters with insulin resistance, hyperinsulinemia, glucose intolerance, dyslipidemia, left ventricular hypertrophy, and obesity, and occurs in isolation in less than 20 percent of individuals.[134] The potential mechanisms by which hypertension may cause coronary events include impaired endothelial function, increased endothelial permeability to lipoproteins, increased adherence of leukocytes, increased oxidative stress, hemodynamic stress that may trigger acute plaque rupture, and increased myocardial wall stress and oxygen demand. A widened pulse pressure, an indicator of arterial stiffness, is gaining an evidence base as another blood pressure measurement that predicts CHD.[135]

PRIMARY PREVENTION

A meta-analysis of 17 randomized trials of antihypertensive drugs in over 47,000 men and women with mild to moderate hypertension found that stroke was reduced by 38 percent and CHD was reduced by 16 percent.[131] The mean difference in diastolic blood pressure over 5 years between treatment and control groups was 5 to 6 mmHg. An important subset in whom events were reduced was elderly subjects with isolated systolic hypertension (systolic blood pressure ≥160 mmHg; diastolic blood pressure ≤90 mmHg).

For a prolonged 5- to 6-mmHg difference, observational studies predict a reduction of 35 to 40 percent in stroke risk and 20 to 25 percent in CHD risk. Although clinical trials indicate that antihypertensive therapy achieves the reduction in stroke expected from observational studies, the reduction in CHD is not as great as expected. Potential explanations for this are (1) the shortfall was due to chance, (2) the duration of observation was too short and the full benefit was not seen, (3) the treatment benefits were partially offset by metabolic side effects of medications, (4) excessive reduction in diastolic blood pressure led to excess CHD events, or (5) metabolic disturbances associated with hypertension that potentiate CHD were not corrected by the antihypertensive therapy used in the studies (see the section "Insulin Resistance Syndrome," below). Most of these trials were based on high-dose diuretic therapy, with or without beta blockers, leading some experts to propose that adverse metabolic consequences of high-dose diuretics were responsible for the less than expected benefits of antihypertensive treatment. Nevertheless, diuretics and beta blockers are the only classes of antihypertensives extensively tested to date that have been shown to reduce CHD morbidity and mortality in primary prevention. The efficacy of newer antihypertensives in reducing initial coronary events is currently being tested.[136] Blood pressure can be lowered by weight loss, exercise, salt restriction, and avoidance of alcohol,[132] but the long-term utility of these measures to prevent CHD in hypertensives has not been tested in randomized controlled studies.

SECONDARY PREVENTION

Clinical trials to test the effect of blood pressure lowering per se in CHD patients have not been performed.

COST-EFFECTIVENESS

Treatment of hypertension for primary prevention is highly cost-effective, with an estimated cost per year of life saved of about $23,000 (in 1993 dollars) for moderate to severe hypertension and twice as much for mild hypertension.[1] Estimates (in 1993 dollars) vary depending on the choice of medication, ranging from $14,000 per year of life saved for propranolol, to $20,000 for hydrochlorothiazide, and up to $90,000 for newer medications. The cost-effectiveness of blood pressure lowering for secondary prevention is unknown.

PRACTICE RECOMMENDATIONS

The Joint National Committee on Detection, Evaluation, and Treatment of High Blood Pressure recommends a treatment goal of <140/90 mmHg.[132] A goal of <130/85 is appropriate for patients with diabetes, renal insufficiency, or CHF.[132,137] Please refer to Chap. 51 for a complete discussion of the treatment of hypertension.

Left Ventricular Hypertrophy

Left ventricular hypertrophy (LVH), defined either by electrocardiography or echocardiography, is a potent independent risk factor for CHD, roughly doubling the risk of cardiovascular death in both men and women.[138] LVH is the adaptive response of the heart to chronic pressure or volume overload (see Chap. 67). In addition to hypertension, LVH is associated with obesity, salt intake, advanced age, and heredity.[139] Progressive LVH may lead to decreased left ventricular compliance, decreased coronary reserve, ventricular ectopy, and impaired systolic function. The Framingham Heart Study observed that ECG evidence of LVH regression was associated with a reduction in cardiovascular disease morbidity and mortality.[140] Another observational, prospective evaluation of LVH using echocardiography indicated an improved prognosis among patients with a reduction of left ventricular mass on antihypertensive therapy.[141] Most antihypertensive drugs can reduce LVH (except direct vasodilators, e.g., hydralazine and minoxidil),[132] although not all drugs are equally effective in this regard despite their equipotent blood pressure-lowering capabilities. An analysis of several comparative studies and some meta-analyses, including only double-blind, randomized, controlled clinical studies with parallel group design, indicates that angiotensin-converting enzyme (ACE) inhibitors reduced left ventricular mass by 12 percent, calcium channel blockers by 11 percent, beta blockers by 5 percent, and diuretics by 8 percent.[142] A study of the effect of monotherapy with six antihypertensive agents on reduction of left ventricular mass revealed that captopril, hydrochlorothiazide, and atenolol reduced left ventricular mass and that diltiazem, clonidine, and prazosin did not.[143] The impact of new antihypertensive agents such as angiotensin II-receptor antagonists is still uncertain. Randomized clinical trials have not yet tested whether regression of LVH lowers CHD risk, but the observational data merit its classification as a risk factor that should be modified.[132]

Thrombogenic Factors

See the section "Antiplatelet and Anticoagulant Therapy," below.

RISK FACTORS FOR WHICH INTERVENTIONS ARE LIKELY TO LOWER RISK OF CORONARY HEART DISEASE

Insulin Resistance Syndrome: The Basis of Multiple Risk Factors

Reaven[144,145] has hypothesized that *resistance to insulin-stimulated glucose uptake and compensatory hyperinsulinemia are the common metabolic bases for a cluster of coronary risk factors, particularly hypertension, diabetes, hypertriglyceridemia, low HDL, predominance of small dense LDL, and a prothrombotic state* with elevated levels of plasma fibrinogen, plasminogen activator inhibitor 1 (PAI-1), and factor VII.[146] This clustering has been called the *insulin resistance syndrome* or the *metabolic syndrome.* Interestingly, hypertensive individuals, both treated and untreated, obese and nonobese, are hyperinsulinemic compared with a matched group of normotensive individuals. Also, patients with atherogenic dyslipidemia have an increased frequency of hypertension. Hypertriglyceridemia or low HDL, major components of the syndrome, can be considered as *markers* for the presence of the metabolic syndrome. Obesity, particularly when located abdominally, exacerbates insulin resistance, and weight loss improves insulin sensitivity. Insulin sensitivity is associated with endothelial nitric oxide production in healthy persons, providing a clue as to how insulin resistance may promote CHD directly.[147] Furthermore, hyperinsulinemia has been found in a prospective study to be an independent risk factor for CHD in nondiabetic men after adjusting for body weight, blood pressure, and dyslipidemia.[148]

Some experts believe the primary mechanism for insulin resistance is lipid overload in skeletal muscle, liver, and pancreatic beta cells. This overload of tissues with lipid may derive both from an excess of adipose tissue (obesity) and physical inactivity. In skeletal muscle, lipid overload impairs glucose uptake and promotes hyperglycemia.[149] In the liver, lipid overload contributes to atherogenic dyslipidemia. And in pancreatic beta cells, excess lipid overstimulates the secretion of insulin, producing hyperinsulinemia.[150] In a significant portion of the population, the adverse consequences of an overload of tissues with lipid are accentuated by an underlying genetic susceptibility to insulin resistance.[146]

A comprehensive lifestyle approach is required to address the cluster of risk factors related to insulin resistance. Weight loss and physical activity are clear goals because they counteract insulin resistance. Although a low-fat diet is clearly beneficial for hypercholesterolemia, it might be detrimental in insulin-resistant, hypertriglyceridemic patients.[145]

Diabetes Mellitus

(See Chap. 78 for a complete discussion about diabetes and CHD.) Diabetes mellitus is an independent risk factor for CHD, increasing risk by two to four times for men and women, respectively.[9,71] CHD is the leading cause of death among diabetics, and approximately 25 percent of MI survivors have diabetes.[8,71] *Diabetic patients without a history of MI have as high a risk of coronary mortality as nondiabetic patients with a history of MI.*[9] Once patients with type 2 diabetes suffer a myocardial infarction, their prognosis for survival is much worse than that for CHD patients without diabetes.[151,152]

Diabetes abolishes the usual protection from CHD afforded a premenopausal woman.[71] Diabetic women have twice the risk of recurrent MI compared with diabetic men.[153] The greater risk of CHD in diabetic women compared to diabetic men may be explained in part by the greater adverse effect of diabetes on lipoproteins in women.[154] Potential mechanisms by which diabetes may cause atherosclerosis include low HDL, high triglycerides/increased lipoprotein remnant particles, increased small dense LDL, elevated Lp(a) concentration, enhanced lipoprotein oxidation, glycation of LDL, increased fibrinogen, increased platelet aggregability, increased PAI-1, impaired fibrinolysis, increased von Willebrand factor, hyperinsulinemia, and impaired endothelial function. Most patients with type 2 diabetes have multiple risk factors. High-risk populations in the United States include whites, blacks, Hispanics, and South Asians.

PRIMARY AND SECONDARY PREVENTION

Despite overwhelming observational data that diabetes increases the risk of CHD, few data are available to determine whether glycemic control reduces risk. The University Group Diabetes Program was the first large-scale randomized clinical trial to study cardiovascular end points in patients with type 2 diabetes, and treatment with sulfonylurea therapy was associated with *increased* cardiovascular mortality.[155] The Diabetes Control and Complications Trial studied the effect of intensive insulin therapy in patients with type 1 diabetes.[156] Intensive therapy reduced microvascular end points, but the study was not of sufficient size to examine CHD end points. The United Kingdom Prospective Diabetes Study (UKPDS) examined the impact of intensive glycemic control with sulfonylureas or insulin compared with conventional therapy on the risk of complications in patients with type 2 diabetes.[157] The treatment goal in the intensive therapy group was a fasting glucose of <108 mg/dL. In the conventional treatment group, drugs were added to diet only if there were hyperglycemic symptoms or if the fasting glucose was >270 mg/dL. After a 10-year follow-up, there was a significant reduction in microvascular end points but not in macrovascular end points. There was no evidence that intensive treatment with sulfonylureas or insulin had an adverse effect on macrovascular disease.

COST-EFFECTIVENESS

The cost-effectiveness of treating diabetes for primary and secondary prevention of CHD has not been established.

PRACTICE RECOMMENDATIONS

Weight loss and exercise are key therapeutic interventions because they improve the constellation of metabolic abnormalities that accompany diabetes. Although the optimal proportion of dietary fat and carbohydrate is controversial, calorie restriction for obesity and avoidance of sugar and saturated fat are definitely recommended. *Beta blockers should not be withheld from diabetic patients following MI unless strong contraindications exist, because diabetic MI survivors have fewer deaths if treated with a beta blocker.*[158] Although there is no consistent evidence to support intensive glycemic control as a strategy to reduce macrovascular end points, aggressive lipid management in patients with diabetes lowers CHD risk. The NCEP and American Diabetes Association guidelines recommend a more aggressive LDL goal (<100 mg/dL) in primary prevention of CHD in diabetics.[8,71] The American Heart Association (AHA) recommends near-normal fasting glucose and hemoglobin A_{1c} (HgA_{1c}) ≤1 percent above normal as treatment goals for patients with diabetes.[71]

Physical Inactivity

Physical inactivity is an independent risk factor for CHD[159] *and roughly doubles the risk.* There is a dose-response relation between the amount of exercise performed weekly, from 700 to 2000 kcal of energy, and death from cardiovascular disease and all causes.[159] Data linking sedentary lifestyle with CHD derive from numerous lines of evidence, including animal studies, observational studies, and clinical trials. Moderate-intensity exercise reduces coronary atherosclerosis and widens coronary arteries in monkeys fed an atherogenic diet compared with monkeys fed the same diet but forced to be sedentary. Physical activity slows progression of angiographically defined coronary atherosclerosis in humans.[160] Over 50 observational studies, primarily of men, have established that physical fitness, on-the-job physical activity, and leisure-time physical activity reduce the risk of CHD.[161] These studies of physical activity are subject to important potential biases, including self-selection and unmeasured confounding variables. The risk of MI and sudden cardiac death is greatest during exercise, but the overall risk of MI and sudden cardiac death is reduced among those who exercise regularly.[162] The greatest potential for reduced mortality is in sedentary individuals who become moderately active.[159] Moderate-intensity activity, as opposed to high-intensity activity, produces most of the beneficial effects of physical activity on cardiovascular mortality. A recent prospective study of more than 72,000 apparently healthy female nurses indicated that brisk walking and vigorous exercise are associated with substantial and similar reductions in coronary events.[163] In addition to decreasing myocardial oxygen demand and increasing myocardial efficiency and electrical stability, other potential mechanisms of benefit include increasing HDL, lowering triglycerides, reducing blood pressure, reducing obesity, improving insulin sensitivity, decreasing platelet aggregation, and increasing fibrinolysis.[161]

PRIMARY PREVENTION

A randomized, controlled trial of physical activity for primary prevention of CHD is not likely to be conducted because of cost and compliance issues.

SECONDARY PREVENTION

(See Chap. 50 on cardiac rehabilitation.) Meta-analyses of randomized trials of cardiac rehabilitation with exercise in over 4000 MI survivors demonstrated a 20 to 25 percent reduction in cardiovascular mortality, although there were no significant differences in nonfatal reinfarction.[164,165] Most of the studies combined exercise training with other risk factor modification. The small number of trials with exercise as the only intervention does not permit definitive conclusions. The benefit of physical activity in female CHD patients is uncertain.

COST-EFFECTIVENESS

The cost-effectiveness of physical activity for primary prevention is not established. Given the low monetary cost of physical activity and its numerous favorable effects on other risk factors, exercise for primary prevention is likely to be highly cost-effective. The cost-effectiveness of cardiac rehabilitation has been estimated (in 1993 dollars) at less than $8000 per quality-adjusted year of life gained.[8]

PRACTICE RECOMMENDATIONS

The American College of Sports Medicine and the Centers for Disease Control and Prevention recommend that every adult should accumulate 30 min or more of moderate-intensity physical activity on most, preferably all, days.[166] Only about 20 percent of U.S. adults meet this goal. The AHA recommends a minimal goal of 30 min of moderate-intensity activity three to four times a week for individuals with and without CHD.[167,168] Large-scale studies indicate that high-intensity physical activity is *not* required to achieve a mortality benefit, and that 200 calories expended daily in moderate-intensity physical activity will confer the majority of CHD risk reduction that exercise can provide. To accomplish this requires about 30 min of brisk walking; however, intermittent activity also provides substantial benefit.[167] Therefore, the minimal goal of 30 min can be accumulated in short bouts of typical daily activities like walking, climbing stairs, housework, and gardening. Exercise testing should be recommended to apparently healthy men over 40 and women over 50 who are sedentary, as well as to younger adults with coronary risk factors, before starting a *vigorous* physical activity program (intensity $>$ 60 percent individual maximum oxygen consumption).[169] For secondary prevention, exercise testing is recommended to guide exercise prescription, and high-risk patients should exercise in a medically supervised setting.[167] Structured exercise programs, whether on site or at home, help compliance with an exercise prescription[170] (see also Chap. 50).

Obesity

Obesity is defined by the AHA as a major risk factor for CHD.[171] Obesity promotes insulin resistance, hyperinsulinemia, type 2 diabetes, hypertension, hypertriglyceridemia, low HDL cholesterol, small dense LDL, prothrombotic factors, and LVH.[132] It is associated with an increase in cardiovascular and all-cause mortality.[132,172]

Body mass index (BMI) has been adopted widely as a measure of adiposity. BMI is calculated as weight (kg)/height squared (m^2) and estimated as [weight (pounds)/height (inches)^2] $\times$ 704.5 *Overweight* is defined as a BMI of 25 to 29.9, and *obesity* is defined as BMI $\geq$ 30. The number of overweight and obese adults in the United States has increased since 1960. Nearly one-third of adults in the United States are overweight, and an additional one-fifth meet the definition of obese.[172] BMI correlates with total body fat content. Abdominal obesity adds to the health risks of obesity, and waist circumference correlates positively with abdominal fat content. In adults with a BMI between 25 and 35, increased relative risk is indicated in men with a waist circumference of $>$102 cm ($>$40 inches) and in women of $>$88 cm ($>$35 inches).[132]

In univariate analysis, many observational studies have found obesity strongly and positively correlated with the risk of CHD. In multivariate analysis, when controlling statistically for risk factors such as hypertension, diabetes, and dyslipidemia, obesity is usually not found to be an independent risk factor. This reflects that many of the adverse consequences of obesity are mediated through resultant metabolic risk factors acting as pathogenetic links in the causal pathway. Nevertheless, some large prospective observational studies of long duration indicate that obesity is independently related to coronary and cardiovascular mortality in men and women.[173–175] In general, the greater the degree of overweight, the higher is the risk of coronary mortality. Weight loss improves insulin sensitivity and glucose disposal, reduces HbA_{1c} in patients with type 2 diabetes, reduces blood pressure and triglycerides, produces a modest reduction in LDL, and increases HDL cholesterol.[132]

PRIMARY AND SECONDARY PREVENTION

Although weight loss leads to a number of favorable short-term changes in metabolism, it is unknown whether long-term weight loss results in reduced CHD events. No primary or secondary prevention trials of weight loss have been conducted.

COST-EFFECTIVENESS

The cost-effectiveness of weight loss is unknown. Given the favorable effect of weight loss on other risk factors, it may prove to be highly cost-effective.

PRACTICE RECOMMENDATIONS

BMI should be listed as a vital sign, used to assess overweight and obesity, and used to monitor changes in body weight. Tracking body weight alone can be used to determine the efficacy of weight-loss therapy. National Institutes of Health guidelines recommend that waist circumference be measured in patients with a BMI between 25 and 35 because of its incremental predictive power.[132] Treatment of overweight (BMI, 25 to 29.9) is recommended only when patients have two or more risk factors, increased waist circumference, or CHD or a CHD risk equivalent. Treatment should focus on diet and exercise to prevent weight gain and to produce moderate weight loss over years. The initial goal of weight-loss therapy is to reduce body weight by approximately 10 percent from baseline in 6 months. For patients with BMI in the range of 27 to 35, a decrease of 300 to 500 kcal/day will result in this degree of weight loss. Lost weight is usually regained unless a program consisting of dietary therapy, physical activity, and behavior therapy is continued indefinitely.

Smoking cessation is associated with weight gain, on average 4.5 to 7 lb. The health hazards of smoking exceed the risks of moderate obesity; therefore, cigarette smokers should be given the clear message that smoking cessation is of the highest priority even if it results in weight gain. Weight-loss drugs approved by the Food and Drug Administration for long-term use may be useful as an adjunct to diet and physical activity for patients with a BMI ≥ 30 and for patients with a BMI ≥ 27 with CHD or obesity-related risk factors. CHD end-point trials with weight-loss drugs, however, have not been conducted. Fenfluramine and dexfenfluramine have been withdrawn from the market because of associated valvular heart disease.

Postmenopausal Status

CHD is relatively uncommon in premenopausal women. There is a dramatic rise in CHD incidence in women after age 55, coinciding with increasing age and a decline in endogenous estrogen levels. Early menopause (natural or surgical) is associated with increased CHD risk.[176] These observations are consistent with the notion that estrogen deficiency permits or promotes CHD and that estrogen reduces risk. Numerous observational studies show that postmenopausal users of estrogen replacement therapy (ERT) have a 50 percent lower risk of initial CHD events compared with nonusers.[176] Because of their observational design, these studies have been subject to selection bias and uncontrolled or unknown confounding variables. In most of these studies, ERT has been unopposed by concomitant progestin therapy. Proposed mechanisms by which estrogen may confer benefit include raising HDL; lowering LDL, small dense LDL, Lp(a), and fibrinogen levels; inhibiting LDL oxidation; and enhancing endothelium-dependent and endothelium-independent coronary vasodilation.

Unopposed ERT increases the risk of endometrial carcinoma, but the addition of a progestin erases that risk.[176] Estrogen with or without progestin may increase slightly the risk of breast cancer, particularly among older women who have taken hormones for 5 or more years.[176,177] For women aged 65 to 74 years, the absolute risk of dying of CHD over the next 10 years is 15 times that of dying of endometrial cancer and 6 times that of dying of breast cancer.[178] The Postmenopausal Estrogen/Progestin Interventions Trial assessed differences between placebo, unopposed estrogen, and three estrogen/progestin combinations over 3 years on selected CHD risk factors in healthy postmenopausal women.[179] Compared with placebo, estrogen alone or in combination with a progestin raised HDL cholesterol and lowered fibrinogen levels. The best regimen for raising HDL cholesterol was unopposed estrogen, but in women with an intact uterus this caused a high rate of atypical or adenomatous endometrial hyperplasia.

PRIMARY AND SECONDARY PREVENTION

The Heart and Estrogen/Progestin Replacement Study (HERS) investigated the impact of estrogen plus progestin on the risk of CHD in 2763 postmenopausal women with established coronary disease and an intact uterus.[180] Subjects were randomly assigned 0.625 mg of conjugated equine estrogens plus 2.5 mg of medroxyprogesterone daily or a placebo with a mean follow-up of 4 years. There was no difference in the primary end point of nonfatal MI or CHD death. The lack of an overall effect occurred despite a net 11 percent lower LDL level and 10 percent higher HDL level in the hormone treatment group. Although there was no difference overall between groups, there was a statistically significant time trend, with more CHD events in the hormone group in year 1 and fewer events in years 4 and 5. More women in the hormone group suffered venous thromboembolic events and gallbladder disease. Other large randomized trials of hormone replacement therapy for primary and secondary prevention are currently in progress.

COST-EFFECTIVENESS

The cost-effectiveness of ERT for prevention of CHD is undefined.

PRACTICE RECOMMENDATIONS

On the basis of HERS, we recommend that postmenopausal women with CHD who have not been on ERT should not be started routinely on hormone therapy for the purpose of preventing CHD events. Those with CHD who have been on ERT for at least 2 years without a CHD event should not have hormone therapy discontinued. For postmenopausal women without known CHD, clinical trial evidence is still lacking and the decision whether to treat must be individualized according to other health risks. Oral estrogen therapy is contraindicated in women with hypertriglyceridemia (e.g., serum triglycerides >400 mg/dL).

RISK FACTORS FOR WHICH INTERVENTIONS MIGHT LOWER RISK OF CORONARY HEART DISEASE

Psychosocial Factors

The role of personality, environment, social support, social contact, stress and lack of control at work, and depression have all been associated with increased risk for CHD. See Chap. 80 for a discussion of these topics.

Acute emotional reactions have been implicated as triggers of acute coronary syndromes. In the absence of atherosclerosis, mental stress causes vasodilation or no change in the diameter of epicardial coronary arteries. In the presence of atherosclerosis, mental stress induces silent myocardial ischemia[181] and coronary vasoconstriction.[182] An episode of anger is capable of triggering acute MI.[183] There was a fivefold increase in the number of sudden cardiac deaths related to atherosclerosis on the day of one of the strongest earthquakes ever recorded in North America.[184] Most of these deaths did not occur in association with heavy physical exertion and were presumably related to major emotional stress. In most cases, the length of time between the earthquake and sudden death was less than 1 h. A mechanism by which acute emotional stress could trigger coronary events is release of catecholamines, leading to an increase in heart rate, blood pressure, myocardial oxygen demand, vasoconstriction, platelet aggregability, and coagulation with an inhibition of fibrinolysis. These factors could contribute to the rupture of a vulnerable plaque, with subsequent thrombosis, or to the precipitation of ventricular arrhythmias.

PRACTICE RECOMMENDATIONS

Optimal comprehensive secondary prevention should include attempts to identify and treat depression and anxiety in patients with CHD. Group support and stress management can be provided in formal cardiac rehabilitation programs.

Total Plasma Homocysteine Level

Total plasma homocysteine level reflects the sum of homocysteine and homocysteinyl moieties of oxidized disulfides, homocystine, and cysteine-homocysteine. Together, these amino acid derivatives appear to have direct toxic effects on the vascular endothelium and can result in the oxidation of LDL, both important steps in atherogenesis. Although there are genetic determinants of total homocysteine level (see Chap. 62), the most important factor affecting plasma concentration is dietary intake of folate and vitamins B_6 and B_{12}.[185] Of note, folate fortification exists in the United States, and less than 1 percent of the population has low levels of folic acid.[186]

A series of cross-sectional and case-control studies strongly supports an independent association between total plasma homocysteine level and atherosclerotic risk.[187] In addition, prospective studies have found increased risk of MI[188–193] and stroke[194] among patients with moderate hyperhomocysteinemia. However, not all large-scale studies are positive.[195–197] When pooled, these data suggest that as much as 10 percent of the population risk of CHD may be attributable to homocysteine level.[187]

PRIMARY AND SECONDARY PREVENTION

Although folate and vitamins B_6 and B_{12} reduce homocysteine concentration,[198] no randomized trial data are yet available to indicate that reducing plasma levels reduces risk.

PRACTICE RECOMMENDATIONS

Measurement of homocysteine may be useful in patients with CHD in the absence of major risk factors or with a history of recurrent arterial thromboses.

Oxidative Stress

Oxidative modification of LDL has been hypothesized to play a major role in the initiation and progression of atherosclerosis.[34] Because naturally occurring antioxidants such as vitamins E, C, and beta-carotene may slow this process, there has been substantial interest in these compounds as agents for both primary and secondary prevention. A series of observational epidemiologic studies supports the hypothesis that increased dietary intake of antioxidants is associated with reduced cardiovascular risk, with the strongest evidence for vitamin E.[199–202] Unfortunately, it is impossible to conclude from observational studies that a given vitamin supplement is responsible for observed vascular risk reduction, since individuals who take vitamins are also likely to employ other preventive lifestyle and dietary measures. This issue can only be resolved through large-scale, randomized clinical trials.

PRIMARY PREVENTION

In the Alpha-Tocopherol, Beta-Carotene Cancer Prevention Study, which enrolled 29,133 male smokers,[203] there was no evidence that vitamin E (given as 50 mg of alpha-tocopherol daily) reduced the subsequent risk of CHD or stroke, and a small increase in rates of cerebral hemorrhage was reported. In the same trial, beta-carotene was associated with a small increase in lung cancer and deaths due to CHD. In the Carotene and Retinol Efficacy Trial conducted among 18,314 smokers, former smokers, and asbestos-exposed workers,[204] the combined use of 30 mg/day of beta-carotene plus 25,000 IU of retinol was associated with a small but statistically significant increase in lung cancer and all-cause mortality, as well as a nonsignificant increase in cardiovascular mortality. In constrast, among 22,071 men participating in the Physicians' Health Study who were randomly allocated to 50 mg of beta-carotene on alternate days for a period of 12 years, supplementation resulted in no evidence of benefit or harm in terms of the incidence of cardiovascular disease or cancer.[205]

SECONDARY PREVENTION

In the Cambridge Heart Antioxidant Study,[206] higher doses of vitamin E were found to reduce rates of nonfatal MI substantially among a group of patients with known CHD. Specifically, in this high-risk secondary prevention trial, the use of 400 to 800 IU of alpha-tocopherol daily over an average period of only 17 months was associated with a statistically significant 47 percent risk reduction in cardiovascular death and nonfatal infarction. By contrast, in the large-scale Heart Outcomes Prevention Evaluation (HOPE) trial, these effects were not confirmed, as no overall benefit was observed among those randomly allocated to vitamin E.[207]

PRACTICE RECOMMENDATIONS

Based on these randomized trial data, it is impossible to make recommendations for or against supplementation with vitamin C to prevent CHD, although beta-carotene and vitamin E appear to carry no benefit. Given observational evidence suggesting benefit for diets rich in fruits and vegetables, however, it is prudent to continue such diets that contain several hundred micronutrients that may have chemopreventive properties.

No Alcohol Consumption

Heavy alcohol intake is associated with increased risks of death from several causes and is a major public health concern. However, cross-sectional, case-control, and prospective cohort studies indicate that mild to moderate alcohol consumption is associated with reduced rates of CHD compared with abstainers.[208–210] These studies suggest a J-shaped relationship between level of alcohol consumption and total mortality such that a protective effect is apparent at low levels of consumption (one to two beverages daily), whereas there is substantial hazard among heavy consumers.[211] In large part, this dose-dependent balance reflects summation of three effects: (1) a positive association between alcohol use and cancer; (2) a U-shaped relationship between alcohol use and total cardiovascular disease due to increased risks of cardiomyopathy, sudden death, and hemorrhagic stroke among heavy drinkers; and (3) a well-established L-shaped protective effect for coronary disease.[211,212]

Several mechanisms are important in the cardioprotective effect of moderate alcohol use. Alcohol intake increases total HDL-cholesterol levels as well as HDL2 and HDL3 subfractions.[213-216] Alcohol consumption also has potentially beneficial effects on fibrinolytic function[217,218] and on platelet aggregation.[219,220]

PRIMARY AND SECONDARY PREVENTION

There have been no randomized trials of alcohol use for primary or secondary prevention.

PRACTICE RECOMMENDATIONS

How best to advise patients concerning the potential use of alcohol for cardiovascular protection is a complex process, because of this agent's potential for abuse.[221] Abstinence is advised for patients who are pregnant or who have hepatic disorders, pancreatic disease, congestive heart failure, idiopathic cardiomyopathy, or degenerative neurologic conditions. On the other hand, the recommendation to drink moderately (one drink per day for women and two drinks for men) may be safe when made on a case-by-case basis in the absence of a history of abuse or medical contraindication.[221] Whether specific beverage type matters in terms of cardiovascular protection is uncertain. Evidence indicating benefits for white wine, red wine, beer, and liquor suggest that alcohol content rather than type is the more important predictor of cardiovascular risk reduction.[209,210]

UNMODIFIABLE RISK FACTORS

Age and Sex as Risk Factors for Atherosclerotic Disease

The incidence and prevalence of CHD increase sharply with age, so that age might be considered one of the most potent cardiovascular risk factors. Atherosclerotic involvement of the coronary arteries is well established in men by young adulthood, as shown in Korean War and Vietnam War casualties.[222,223] CHD incidence rates in men are similar to those in women 10 years older.[224] Approximately 52 percent of women and 46 percent of men will eventually die of atherosclerotic disease.[225] The increased risk for men and older persons should trigger more intense management of modifiable risk factors. Persons at very advanced age (e.g., 75+ years) should have the risks and benefits of preventive cardiology interventions weighed on an individual basis.

Socioeconomic Status: An Unmodifiable Coronary Risk Factor?

At any one point in time, markedly different CHD rates may be observed between socioeconomic subgroups of the population, as defined by occupation, education, income, or other measures. As a group becomes affluent, its members use their new wealth to purchase high-fat and high-salt foods, tobacco products, and automobiles. Less affluent groups lag behind this development, achieving access to these deleterious behaviors later. Affluent groups then learn about and adopt healthful lifestyles, reducing deleterious behaviors. Again, less affluent and less educated groups lag behind, eventually exceeding the rates of CHD in those educated groups whose CHD rates have begun to fall.

Currently, persons with low socioeconomic status are at high risk for CHD. A number of mechanisms may explain this.[226] First, risk factors for atherosclerosis, such as smoking, hypertension, obesity, and sedentary lifestyle, are higher in persons with low socioeconomic status. Second, some of these risk factors, as well as psychosocial responses to stressors, may increase exposure to CHD triggers in these groups. Finally, these groups may have less access to care.

Family History of Early-Onset CHD

Over 35 case-control and prospective studies have consistently identified an association between CHD and a history of first-degree relatives with early-onset CHD.[227] This risk generally persists even after adjustment for other risk factors. The family history most predictive of coronary disease is that of a first-degree relative developing CHD at an early age. Although CHD in a male relative with onset at age 55 or less or a female relative with onset at age 65 or less is defined as a positive family history, the larger the number of relatives with early-onset CHD or the younger the age of CHD onset in the relative, the stronger is the predictive value.[228,229]

Although considered a nonmodifiable risk factor, a positive family history should result in the careful screening of individual risk factors known to aggregate in families. Such familial aggregations may represent monogenic factors with known phenotypic expressions and inheritance patterns, polygenic factors with less clear modes of expression and inheritance, or shared environments. In early-CHD families, Williams et al.[229] estimate that only 10 percent of families will not have a concordant risk factor, most of which are amenable to intervention. Thus, family members of patients with CHD at a young age represent fruitful targets for risk factor assessment. *However, risk factor screening often does not extend beyond the coronary patient. A strong recommendation that siblings and children of early-CHD patients be screened for CHD risk factors should be delivered to each patient and their family members.*

OTHER PHARMACOLOGIC THERAPY

Antiplatelet and Anticoagulant Therapy

See also Chap. 44.

PRIMARY PREVENTION

Several prevention trials of aspirin have been completed in healthy men. The largest of these, the Physicians' Health Study, enrolled 22,071 apparently healthy male physicians aged 40 to 84 years of age and randomized them to 325 mg aspirin on alternate days or to placebo.[230] Among those given active aspirin, a highly statistically significant 44 percent reduction in nonfatal MI was observed. In this study, aspirin had little effect on the clinical characteristics of MI[231] or on the rate of development of angina pectoris.[232] When the Physicians' Health Study data are combined with those of a similar trial among British men,[233] an overall 32 percent reduction in risk of first nonfatal MI appears to be associated with chronic aspirin prophylaxis.[234] These trials have also demonstrated the efficacy of low-dose aspirin in the prevention of MI among patients with stable angina pectoris.[235] In the Thrombosis Prevention Trial, low-dose aspirin (75 mg daily) and low-dose warfarin (target INR = 1.5) were both effective, although combination therapy as compared with monotherapy remains controversial.[236]

SECONDARY PREVENTION

At least 25 trials have been completed in the study of antiplatelet therapy for secondary prevention.[237] Overall, among patients with known clinical manifestations of atherosclerotic disease, antiplatelet therapy is associated with a 32 percent reduction in subsequent MI, 27 percent reduction in subsequent nonfatal stroke, and 15 percent reduction in vascular mortality.[238] Although thienopyridines such as clopidogrel also appear effective, evidence that these agents are superior to aspirin alone is marginal.[239]

Few studies of anticoagulant therapy in the secondary prevention of coronary disease are available. In the Dutch Sixty Plus Study,[240] patients over 60 years of age who had been taking anticoagulants following infarction were randomly assigned to continue or discontinue warfarin. Patients continuing anticoagulant therapy had a 26 percent lower mortality rate and a 51 percent lower reinfarction rate.

The utility of warfarin initiated soon after infarction has also been demonstrated.[241] In a trial of 1214 patients with acute or subacute MI, the randomized use of warfarin with a target INR between 2.8 and 4.8 was associated with a 24 percent reduction in mortality, a 34 percent reduction in nonfatal reinfarction, and a 55 percent reduction in stroke over a mean period of 37 months. These reductions were achieved with acceptably low bleeding rates for those assigned to warfarin.

COST-EFFECTIVENESS

For primary prevention, aspirin is likely to be extremely cost-effective because of its low cost and high efficacy for preventing MI. Following MI, both aspirin and anticoagulant therapy have been shown to be cost saving.[21]

PRACTICE RECOMMENDATIONS

The United States Preventive Services Task Force has recommended that low-dose aspirin be considered in men age 40 and over who are at high risk for MI and lack contraindications.[242] Although observational data generally support the use of aspirin in women,[243] the risk-to-benefit ratio in women may differ from that of men, since the average age at first infarction is higher. For secondary prevention, 80 to 325 mg of aspirin daily is recommended, with treatment continued indefinitely. If aspirin is contraindicated, clopidogrel and then warfarin are recommended for secondary prevention, with an INR goal of 2 to 3.5.[137,167]

Fibrinogen

Plasma fibrinogen level has been shown in several studies to predict the future risk of MI and stroke.[244–248] When pooled, these studies indicate that individuals with fibrinogen concentrations in the upper third of the control distribution have a relative risk of future cardiovascular disease 2.0 to 2.5 times that of individuals with lower levels.[249] High fibrinogen levels result in increased whole blood viscosity and may play a direct role in atherogenesis and platelet aggregation. While fibrinogen levels increase with smoking, age, oral contraceptive use, and diabetes, fibrinogen is poorly correlated with dyslipidemia and therefore may provide additional risk information beyond lipid and lipoprotein measurement.

HIGH-SENSITIVITY C-REACTIVE PROTEIN

C-reactive protein (CRP) is a hepatically derived marker of low-grade systemic inflammation that largely reflects circulating cytokine function. When measured with high-sensitivity assays, CRP can be detected within the normal range and used for cardiovascular risk prediction. To date, several large-scale prospective studies have shown the inflammatory marker high-sensitivity CRP (hs-CRP) to be a potent predictor of future myocardial infarction, stroke, and peripheral vascular occlusion among apparently healthy men and women,[27,250–252] as well as among high-risk smokers[253] and the elderly[254] (see Fig. 38-1). Levels of hs-CRP are also elevated among those with acute coronary syndromes at high risk for recurrent events[255,256] and among post-MI patients at high risk for recurrent instability.[257] These effects are independent of other risk factors and appear to add to the predictive value of lipid screening in terms of risk prediction.[28] Thus, as a clinical marker reflecting the presence of an enhanced systemic inflammatory response, hs-CRP appears to have utility in the detection of high-risk patients for plaque instability.

PRIMARY AND SECONDARY PREVENTION

Exercise frequency and body mass both correlate with hs-CRP levels,[258,259] and randomized trial data indicate that lipid reduction with pravastatin lowers hs-CRP in an LDL-independent manner.[260] Further, the effectiveness of low-dose aspirin in reducing risk of first MI appears related to hs-CRP level.[250] However, no data are yet available which indicate that reducing plasma levels of hs-CRP reduces vascular risk.

PRACTICE RECOMMENDATIONS

Practice guidelines for hs-CRP screening are in development. As hs-CRP levels appear to add to the predictive value of lipid screening[28] and pedict risk even among those with low levels of LDL cholesterol, knowledge of hs-CRP may be of use as an adjunct to lipid profiling on a population basis. A standardized commercial assay for hs-CRP has recently been approved by the Food and Drug Administration for use in cardiovascular risk assessment.[261]

Endogenous Fibrinolysis: Tissue Plasminogen Activator, PAI-1, and *D*-Dimer

The activity of the endogenous fibrinolytic system reflects a balance between plasma concentration of tissue-type plasminogen activator (tPA) and its primary inhibitor, PAI-1. Prospective studies of initially healthy individuals[262,263] as well as patients with known CHD[264] indicate that elevated antigen levels of both enzymes are associated with increased risk of future MI. Further, prospective data also indicate that tPA antigen level is a potent marker of risk for stroke.[265]

Because both tPA and PAI-1 contribute to the net fibrinolytic balance, it has been hypothesized that individuals at risk for future vascular occlusive events suffer from a net inhibition of fibrinolytic function, a finding supported in at least one prospective study.[266] Other data, however, indicate that elevations of *D*-dimer are also associated with increased risk of future MI[267] and peripheral vascular disease.[268,269] Since plasma *D*-dimer levels increase with fibrinogen turnover, these data raise the possibility that the endogenous fibrinolytic system is activated among individuals at risk.

Evidence is not available to support fibrinogen reduction as a measure to prevent CHD, although smoking cessation, physical activity, and hormone replacement therapy[179,270] all favorably affect fibrinogen levels. Other fibrinogen-reducing agents, such as bezafibrate, are also under investigation in ongoing clinical trials.[271] Many factors affect endogenous fibrinolytic activity, including obesity, estrogen status, and exercise. In addition, pharmacologic interventions may soon be available that can favorably shift fibrinolytic function in an attempt to reduce vascular risk. To date, aspirin therapy, alcohol use, and ACE inhibitors have all shown promise in this regard.[272]

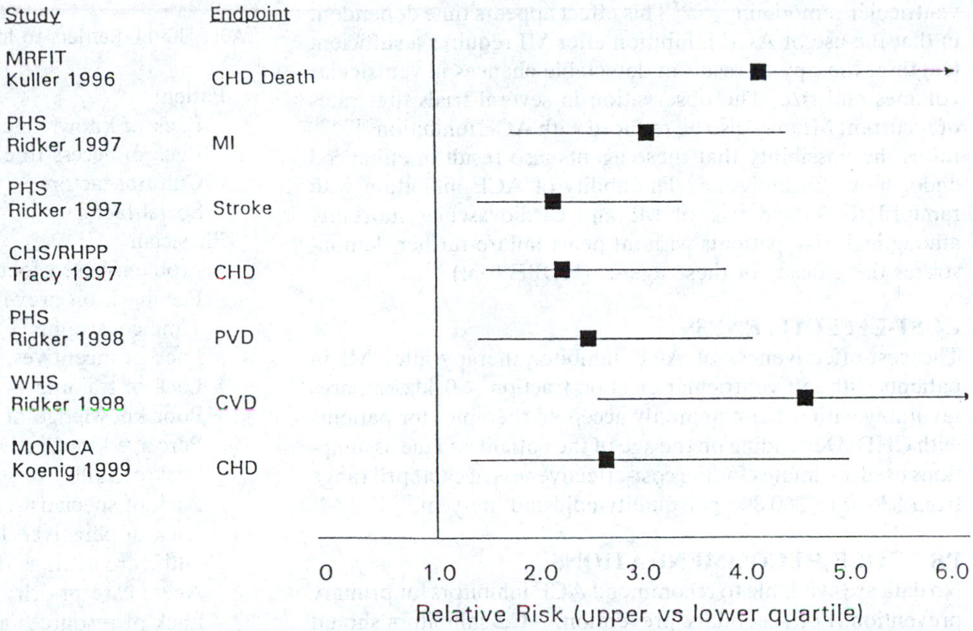

FIGURE 38-1 Prospective studies of high-sensitivity C-reactive protein as a risk factor for future cardiovascular disease in populations free of clinical disease. ABBREVIATIONS: MRFIT = Multiple Risk Factor Intervention Trial; PHS = Physicians' Health Study; CHS/RHPP = Cardiovascular Health Study/Rural Health Promotion Project; WHS = Women's Health Study; MONICA = Monitoring of Trends and Determinants of Cardiovascular Disease; CHD = coronary heart disease; MI = myocardial infarction; PVD = peripheral vascular disease. (From Ridker and Haughie,[300] with permission.)

Beta-Adrenergic Blocking Agents

Beta-adrenergic blocking agents reduce heart rate, systemic blood pressure, and ventricular contractility, all factors that decrease myocardial oxygen consumption (see Chap. 3). Beta blockers further have antiarrhythmic properties and appear to increase thresholds for ventricular fibrillation.[273]

PRIMARY PREVENTION

Little clinical trial data are available that directly test beta-blocking agents in the primary prevention of MI. The use of this class of agents in the treatment of hypertension, however, has been shown to be efficacious for CHD prevention,[274] and beta blockers have few long-term side effects.

SECONDARY PREVENTION

The utility of beta-blocking agents in the acute, subacute, and chronic phases following MI has been demonstrated in many clinical trials. Overview analyses indicate that therapy with beta blockers reduces mortality approximately 20 percent compared with placebo.[275,276] The mortality effect of long-term beta blockade results primarily from prevention of sudden death (pooled relative risk = 0.68), presumably due to a reduction in the incidence and complexity of ventricular arrhythmias. Beta blockers have also proven effective in reducing rates of nonfatal reinfarction (pooled relative risk = 0.74), an effect more likely to result from chronic reductions in heart rate, contractility, and vascular stress.

COST-EFFECTIVENESS

Estimates of the cost of beta blockers after MI range from $3600 per year of life saved when used in high-risk patients to $23,400 per year of life saved when used in low-risk patients.[277] This is cost-effective as compared with other accepted CHD interventions.

PRACTICE RECOMMENDATIONS

For primary prevention, beta blockers are recommended as first-line therapy for hypertension.[132] For secondary prevention, beta blockers are recommended in post-MI patients with arrhythmias, left ventricular dysfunction, and inducible ischemia.[167] Although specific studies of beta-blocker cessation are not available, it is commonly recommended that beta-blocker therapy be continued indefinitely as long as side effects are not present.[273]

Angiotensin-Converting Enzyme Inhibitors

PRIMARY PREVENTION

Although ACE inhibitors are used widely as first-line therapy for hypertension, no data on primary prevention with this class of drugs are available. A large-scale trial is in progress.[136]

SECONDARY PREVENTION

ACE inhibitors reduce mortality in patients with congestive heart failure and reduced left ventricular ejection fraction.[278–280] More recently, this class of agents has been recognized as important adjunctive therapy following acute MI.[281] The primary rationale for using these agents in this setting is based on the experimental observation that ACE inhibition slows the process of ventricular remodeling.[282,283] This effect appears time dependent in that the use of ACE inhibition after MI requires a sufficient length of therapy to result in detectable changes in ventricular volumes and size. The observation in several trials that rates of recurrent MI may also be reduced with ACE inhibition[281,284,285] raises the possibility that these agents also result in enhanced endogenous fibrinolysis.[286] The ability of ACE inhibition with ramipril to reduce risk of MI and cardiovascular mortality among high-risk patients without heart failure further demonstrates the efficacy of these agents (HOPE trial).[207]

COST-EFFECTIVENESS

The cost-effectiveness of ACE inhibitor therapy after MI in patients with left ventricular ejection fraction < 0.40 compares favorably with other commonly accepted therapies for patients with CHD. Depending on the age of the patient and the assumptions used, estimates for the cost-effectiveness of captopril range from $3600 to $60,800 per quality-adjusted life-year.[287]

PRACTICE RECOMMENDATIONS

No data are available to recommend ACE inhibitors for primary prevention. For secondary prevention, ACE inhibitors should be prescribed to patients with congestive heart failure and reduced left ventricular function unless contraindicated. The results of the recent HOPE trial suggest it is reasonable to prescribe ramipril for patients with CHD or CHD risk equivalent and normal left ventricular function.[207] We await the results of ongoing trials to learn whether other ACE inhibitors will confer a similar benefit for patients with normal left ventricular function.

THE PRACTICE OF PREVENTIVE CARDIOLOGY

The evidence for a causal role of risk factors in the etiology of CHD and the feasibility and efficacy of risk factor modification in lowering CHD risk is some of the most convincing in all of medicine. Despite this, there are both qualitative and quantitative gaps in our treatment of coronary risk factors, even in patients at highest risk. Qualitative gaps entail the lack of any risk factor detection and management in many patients. Among patients with established coronary disease, only 40 to 60 percent receive beta blockers, only 60 percent of patients with reduced left ventricular ejection fractions receive ACE inhibitors, and only 70 to 90 percent take aspirin.[288,289] Likewise, many of those patients receiving treatment are not being treated to the goals as set by various guidelines or as documented as efficacious in randomized clinical trials. For example, in a recent study of 4888 patients receiving treatment for lipid disorders, only 17 percent of CHD patients reached their LDL-cholesterol goal of ≤100 mg/dL, and only 37 percent of high-risk (2+ risk factors), non-CHD patients reached their goal of <130 mg/dL.[290] Thus, preventive cardiology strategies backed by strong evidence for efficacy and cost-effectiveness are simply not being applied sufficiently widely, constituting a missed opportunity to reduce costs and improve prognosis.

Barriers to Implementation of Preventive Cardiology Services

A number of barriers to the implementation of preventive services can be identified at the patient, physician, health care setting, and community/society levels (Table 38-11).[291,292] The improved implementation of proven interventions therefore requires a variety of strategies targeted at patients, healthcare providers, inpatient care settings, ambulatory care settings, and health systems.

TABLE 38-11 Barriers to Implementation of Preventive Services

Patient
Lack of knowledge and motivation
Lack of access to care
Cultural factors
Social factors
Physician
Problem-based focus
Feedback on prevention is negative or neutral
Time constraints
Lack of incentives, including reimbursement
Lack of training
Poor knowledge of benefits
Perceived ineffectiveness
Lack of skills
Lack of specialist-generalist communication
Lack of perceived legitimacy
Health care settings (hospitals, practices, etc.)
Acute care priority
Lack of resources and facilities
Lack of systems for preventive services
Time and economic constraints
Poor communication between specialty and primary care providers
Lack of policies and standards
Community/society
Lack of policies and standards
Lack of reimbursement

SOURCE: From Pearson TA et al.,[292] with permission.

Strategies to Improve Preventive Cardiology Services

IMPROVING PATIENT COMPLIANCE

While there is a pervasive tendency to blame the patient, health care providers can take a number of actions to improve their patients' compliance with the treatment regimen.[293,294] These include (1) encouragement to engage in prevention and treatment behaviors essential to adherence with a regimen, such as acceptance and understanding of the need to control risk factors, (2) establishment of specific behavioral or physiological goals, (3) skills training of patients for adopting and maintaining the recommended behaviors, (4) recommending self-monitoring of progress toward the goals, and (5) helping patients anticipate and resolve problems that keep the goals from being realized. This will require regular communication between providers and patients about the goals and actions agreed upon.[293]

IMPROVING PERFORMANCE BY HEALTH CARE PROVIDERS

Providers must foster effective communication with both their patients and other health professionals on the preventive cardiology team.[293] Strategies to improve this communication include

TABLE 38-12 American Heart Association Guide to Comprehensive Risk Reduction for Patients with Coronary and Other Vascular Disease

Risk Intervention	Recommendations
Smoking Goal complete cessation	Strongly encourage patient and family to stop smoking. Provide counseling, nicotine replacement, and formal cessation programs as appropriate.
BP control Goal <140/90 mmHg or <130/85 mmHg if heart failure, renal insufficiency or diabetes.	Initiate lifestyle modification—weight control, physical activity, alcohol moderation, and moderate sodium restriction—in all patients with blood pressure ≥130 mmHg systolic or 85 mmHg diastolic. Add blood pressure medication, individualized to other patient requirements and characteristics (i.e., age, race, need for drugs with specific benefits) **if** blood pressure is not less than 140 mmHg systolic or 90 mmHg diastolic **or** if blood pressure is not <130 mmHg systolic or 85 mmHg diastolic for individuals with heart failure, renal insufficiency, or diabetes.
Lipid management Primary goal LDL <100 mg/dL Secondary goals HDL >35 mg/dL; TG <200 mg/dL	Start AHA Step II Diet in all patients: ≤30% fat, <7% saturated fat, <200 mg/ day cholesterol and promote physical activity. Assess fasting lipid profile. In post-MI patients, lipid profile may take 4 to 6 weeks to stabilize. Add drug therapy according to the following guide:

LDL <100 mg/dL	LDL 100 to 130 mg/dL	LDL > 130 mg/dL	HDL <35 mg/dL
No drug therapy	Consider adding drug therapy to diet, as follows:	Add drug therapy to diet, as follows:	Emphasize weight management and physical activity. Advise smoking cessation. If needed to achieve LDL goals, consider niacin, statin, fibrates.

↘ Suggested drug therapy ↙

TG <200 mg/dL	TG 200 to 400 mg/dL	TG >400 mg/dL
Statin Resin Niacin	Statin Niacin	Consider combined drug therapy (niacin, fibrates, statin)

If LDL goal not achieved, consider combination drug therapy.

Risk Intervention	Recommendations
Physical activity Minimum goal 30 min 3 to 4 times per week	Assess risk, preferably with exercise test, to guide prescription. Encourage minimum of 30 to 60 min of activity 3 or 4 times weekly (walking, jogging, cycling, or other aerobic activity) supplemented by an increase in daily lifestyle activities (e.g., walking breaks at work, gardening, household work). Maximum benefit 5 to 6 h a week. Advise medically supervised programs for moderate- to high-risk patients.
Weight management Goal BMI 21–25 kg/m^2	Measure patient's weight and height, BMI, and waist-to-hip ratio at each visit as part of routine evaluation. Start weight management and physical activity as appropriate. Desirable BMI range: 21–25 kg/m^2. Desirable waist circumference <40 inches in men and <36 inches in women.
Diabetes management Near normal fasting plasma glucose and near normal HbA_{1c}(<7)	Appropriate hypoglycemic therapy to achieve near normal fasting plasma glucose as indicated by HbA_{1c}. Treatment of other risks (e.g., physical activity, weight management, blood pressure) and for cholesterol management see recommendations above.
Antiplatelet agents/ anticoagulants	Start aspirin 80 to 325 mg/day if not contraindicated. Consider clopidogrel as an alternative if aspirin contraindicated. Manage warfarin to international normalized ratio = 2 to 3.5 post-MI patients not able to take aspirin.
ACE inhibitors post-MI	Start early post-MI in stable high-risk patients [anterior MI, previous MI, Killip class II (S_3 gallop, rales, radiographic CHF)]. Continue indefinitely for all with LV dysfunction (ejection fraction ≤40%) or symptoms of failure. Use as needed to manage blood pressure or symptoms in all other patients.
Beta blockers	Start in high-risk post-MI patients (arrhythmia, LV dysfunction, inducible ischemia) at 5 to 28 days. Continue 6 months minimum. Observe usual contraindications. Use as needed to manage angina, rhythm, or blood pressure in all other patients.
Estrogens	Estrogen replacement: individualize consistent with other health risks.

ABBREVIATIONS: ACE = angiotensin-converting enzyme; AHA = American Heart Association; BMI = body mass index; HDL = high-density lipoprotein; LDL = low-density lipoprotein; LV = left ventricular; MI = myocardial infarction; TG = triglycerides; CHF = congestive heart failure.

SOURCE: Adapted from Gibbons et al.,[137] and Smith et al.,[167] with permission.

TABLE 38-13 American Heart Association Guide to Primary Prevention of Cardiovascular Diseases

Risk Intervention	Recommendations
Smoking Goal complete cessation	Ask about smoking status as part of routine evaluation. Reinforce nonsmoking status. Strongly encourage patient and family to stop smoking. Provide counseling, nicotine replacement, and formal cessation programs as appropriate.
Blood pressure control Goal <140/90 mmHg or <130/85 mmHg if heart failure, renal insufficiency or diabetes	Measure blood pressure in all adults at least every 2 years. Promote lifestyle modification: weight control, physical activity, moderation in alcohol intake, and moderate sodium restriction. If blood pressure ≥140/90 mmHg after 6 months of lifestyle modification or if initial blood pressure >160/100 mmHg or >130/85 mmHg with heart failure, renal insufficiency or diabetes, add blood pressure medication. Individualize therapy to patient's age, race, need for drugs with specific benefits, etc.
Cholesterol management Primary goal LDL <160 mg/dL if 0–1 risk factors or LDL <130 mg/dL if ≥2 risk factors Secondary goals HDL >35 mg/dL; TG <200 mg/dL	Ask about dietary habits as part of routine evaluation. Measure total and HDL cholesterol in all adults ≥20 years and assess positive and negative risk factors at least every 5 years. For all persons: promote AHA Step I diet (≤30% fat, <10% saturated fat, <300 mg/day cholesterol), weight control, and physical activity. Measure LDL if total cholesteral ≥240 mg/dL or ≥200 mg/dL with ≥2 risk factors or if HDL <35 mg/dL. If LDL ≥160 mg/dL with 0–1 risk factors; or ≥130 mg/dL on 2 occasions with ≥2 risk factors; then Start Step II diet (≤30% fat, <7% saturated fat, <200 mg/dL cholesterol) and weight control. Rule out secondary causes of high LDL (LFTs, TFTs, UA). If LDL ≥160 mg/dL plus 2 risk factors; or ≥190 mg/dL; or ≥220 mg/dL in men <35 y; or in pre-menopausal women; then consider adding drug therapy to diet therapy for LDL levels > those listed above that persist despite Step II diet. Risk factors: age (men ≥45 years, women ≥55 years or postmenopausal), hypertension, diabetes, smoking, HDL <35 mg/dL, family history of CHD in first-degree relatives (in male relatives <55 years, female relatives <65 years). HDL ≥60 mg/dL, subtract 1 risk factor from the number of positive risk factors.

Suggested drug therapy for high LDL levels (≥160 mg/dL) (drug selection priority modified according to TG level)

TG <200 mg/dL	TG 200–400 mg/dL	TG >400 mg/dL
Statin Resin Niacin	Statin Niacin	Consider combined drug therapy (niacin, fibrates, statin)

HDL <35 mg/dL: Emphasize weight management and physical activity, avoidance of cigarette smoking. Niacin raises HDL. Consider niacin if patient has ≥2 risk factors and high LDL (except patients with diabetes).

If LDL goal not achieved, consider combination drug therapy.

Risk Intervention	Recommendations
Physical activity Goal Exercise regularly 3–4 times per week for 30–60 min	Ask about physical activity status and exercise habits as part of routine evaluation. Encourage 30 min of vigorous-intensity dynamic exercise 3 to 4 times per week as well as increased physical activity in daily life style activities (e.g., walking breaks at work, gardening, household work). Advise medically supervised programs for those with low functional capacity and/or comorbidities.
Weight management Goal BMI 21–25 kg/m^2	Measure patient's weight and height, BMI, and waist-to-hip ratio at each visit as part of routine evaluation. Start weight management and physical activity as appropriate. Desirable BMI range: 21–25 kg/m^2. Desirable waist circumference <40 inches in men and <36 inches in women.
Diabetes management: Near normal fasting plasma glucose and near normal HbA_{1c}(<7)	Appropriate hypoglycemic therapy to achieve near normal fasting plasma glucose as indicated by HbA_{1c}. Treatment of other risks (e.g., physical activity, weight management, blood pressure and for cholesterol management see recommendations for patients with coronary disease on other side.)
Estrogens	Consider estrogen replacement in all postmenopausal women, especially those with multiple CHD risk factors. Individualize recommendation consistent with other health risks.

ABBREVIATIONS: BMI = body mass index (704.5); CHD = coronary heart disease; HDL = high-density lipoprotein; LDL = low-density lipoprotein; LFT = liver function test; TFT = thyroid function test; TG = triglycerides; UA = uric acid.

SOURCE: Adapted from Grundy et al.,[168] with permission.

verbal and written instructions, negotiation of goals and a plan with the patient, and anticipation of barriers to successful attainment of goals. There also must be documentation and monitoring of progress toward goals, with assessment of patient compliance at each visit and reminder systems (e.g., listing smoking status as a vital sign) to assure that risk factors are identified and attended to. One barrier to physician action in this area is a perceived lack of legitimacy by cardiovascular specialists for involvement in risk factor management. *Professional societies counter this problem by strongly recommending that risk factor management be part of the optimal care of patients at high risk for cardiovascular disease and therefore be the responsibility of all health care providers.*[1]

IMPROVING THE INPATIENT CARE SETTING

The admission to an inpatient unit provides an enormous opportunity for risk behavior change that should not be missed, for several reasons. First, the opportunity to reduce short-term risk in patients following infarction or revascularization has not been extensively studied, but several interventions such as antiplatelet therapy, ACE inhibitors, beta blockers, and even lipid management appear to provide benefit within days or weeks. Second, the patient and family are aroused to the risk of disability and death, and their receptivity to behavior-change messages is likely highest at this time. Finally, the message communicated to the patient and their primary care provider is that behavior change is an important, integral part of their postcoronary care, along with revascularization and pharmacotherapy.

The inpatient setting can be reorganized to provide efficient risk factor assessment and management. The joint AHA/American College of Cardiology (ACC) guidelines for comprehensive risk reduction for patients with coronary and other vascular disease provide a convenient list of risk factor goals and modification strategies (Table 38-12).[167] These can be transcribed onto a simple checklist or more elaborate care protocols. The cardiovascular specialist should confirm the diagnosis of prevalent risk factors, set goals for treatment, and integrate a treatment plan into the overall regimen of care. However, the physician is often not the best person to carry out the plan, due in part to time constraints, acute care focus, and short hospital length of stay. A better model is the multidisciplinary team approach, with nurses, nutritionists, and exercise physiologists assigned specific tasks for the patient's care. A strategy with proven effectiveness is the nurse case-manager approach, with a nurse initiating care in the hospital and following the patient to the ambulatory care setting. In one randomized trial of this approach, smoking cessation, LDL-cholesterol levels, and aerobic capacity all improved in patients assigned to a system of nurse case management, as compared with usual care.[295]

IMPROVING THE AMBULATORY CARE SETTING

The AHA guidelines for primary prevention of cardiovascular diseases (Table 38-13) and for comprehensive risk reduction for patients with coronary and other vascular disease (Table 38-12) provide clear risk factor goals and risk-reduction strategies.[168] The office or clinic should strive to develop an environment supportive of risk factor management, including staff trained in behavior-modification skills, follow-up protocols, and tracking systems and reminders. A clear assignment of tasks and responsibilities is important, with defined roles for the physician, nurse, nutritionist, and even receptionist.

A number of specialty units might be convenient platforms for risk factor management. Cardiac rehabilitation has been documented, in meta-analyses of randomized clinical trials, to reduce coronary disease recurrence and death significantly, especially when the service includes risk factor modification.[164] The patients' extended exposure (after 12 weeks or longer) to a supportive environment provides the opportunity for behavior change, monitoring, and reinforcement. Likewise, a nurse case-manager program with extension to the ambulatory care setting provides long-term continuity and support for meaningful behavior change.[295]

IMPROVING THE HEALTH SYSTEM

Supportive of this are a large number of guidelines from professional societies, expert bodies, and governmental agencies that support preventive cardiology practices. The joint AHA/ACC guidelines in risk reduction[167] are coordinated with more extensive guidelines for individual risk factors, including hyperlipidemia,[8] hypertension,[132] smoking,[296] cardiac rehabilitation,[297] and obesity.[49] These provide clear recommendations for health care providers as to the goals and scenarios required for optimal risk reduction. Increasingly, these guidelines are being used in quality assurance programs that use provision of preventive services and attainment of risk factor goals as quality-of-care indicators. The use of preventive cardiology services as such quality indicators has motivated health care systems to implement the reorganization and reallocation of resources that have been shown to be effective in improving preventive cardiology care.

References

1. Fuster V, Pearson TA. 27th Bethesda Conference: Matching the intensity of risk factor management. *J Am Coll Cardiol* 1996; 27:957.
2. Smith SC, Greenland P, Grundy SM. Beyond secondary prevention: Identifying the high-risk patient for primary prevention. Executive Summary: American Heart Association Prevention Conference. *Circulation* 2000; 101:111.
3. Grundy SM. Primary prevention of coronary heart disease: Integrating risk assessment. *Circulation* 1999; 100:988.
4. Sacks FM, Pfeffer MA, Moye LA, et al. The effect of pravastatin on coronary events after myocardial infarction in patients with average cholesterol levels. Cholesterol and Recurrent Events Trial Investigators. *N Engl J Med* 1996; 335:1001.
5. Lipid Study Group. Prevention of cardiovascular events and death with pravastatin in patients with coronary heart disease and a broad range of initial cholesterol levels. The Long-Term Intervention with Pravastatin in Ischaemic Disease (LIPID) Study Group. *N Engl J Med* 1998; 339:1349.
6. Cleland JG. Can improved quality of care reduce the costs of managing angina pectoris? *Eur Heart J* 1996; 17:29.
7. Juul-Moller S, Edvardsson N, Jahnmatz B, et al. Double-blind trial of aspirin in primary prevention of myocardial infarction. *Lancet* 1992; 340:1421.
8. National Cholesterol Education Program. Second report of the Expert Panel on Detection, Evaluation, and Treatment of High Blood Cholesterol in Adults (Adults Treatment Panel II). *Circulation* 1994; 89:1333.
9. Haffner SM, Lehto S, Ronnemaa T, et al. Mortality from coronary heart disease in subjects with type 2 diabetes and in nondiabetic subjects with and without prior myocardial infarction. *N Engl J Med* 1998; 339:229.
10. American Diabetes Association. Management of dyslipidemia in

adults with diabetes. American Diabetes Association: Clinical recommendations. *Diabetes Care* 1999; 22:S56.
11. Wood D, De Backer G, Faergeman O, et al. Prevention of coronary heart disease in clinical practice: Recommendations of the Second Joint Task Force of European and Other Societies on Coronary Prevention. *Atherosclerosis* 1998; 140:199.
12. Grundy SM, Pasternak R, Greenland P, et al. Assessment of cardiovascular risk by use of multiple-risk-factor assessment. *Circulation* 1999; 100:1481.
13. Wilson PW, D'Agostino RB, Levy D, et al. Prediction of coronary heart disease using risk factor categories. *Circulation* 1998; 97:1837.
14. Pitt B, Rubenfire M. Risk stratification for the detection of preclinical coronary artery disease. *Circulation* 1999; 99:2610.
15. Froelicher VF, Follansbee WP, Labovitz, AJ, et al. Special application: Screening apparently healthy individuals. In: Froelicher VF, Follansbee WP, Labovitz AJ, Myers J, eds. *Exercise and the Heart.* Boston: Mosby; 1993:208–229.
16. Rumberger JA, Schwartz RS, Simons DB, et al. Relation of coronary calcium determined by electron beam computed tomography and lumen narrowing determined by autopsy. *Am J Cardiol* 1994; 73:1169.
17. Rumberger JA, Simons DB, Fitzpatrick LA, et al. Coronary artery calcium area by electron-beam computed tomography and coronary atherosclerotic plaque area: A histopathologic correlative study. *Circulation* 1995; 92:2157.
18. Budoff MJ, Georgiou D, Brody A, et al. Ultrafast computed tomography as a diagnostic modality in the detection of coronary artery disease: A multicenter study. *Circulation* 1996; 93:898.
19. Guerci AD, Spadaro, LA, Popma JJ, et al. Relation of coronary calcium score by electron beam computed tomography to arteriographic findings in asymptomatic and symptomatic adults. *Am J Cardiol* 1997; 79:128.
20. Raggi P, Callister TQ, Cooil B, et al. Identification of patients at increased risk of first unheralded acute myocardial infarction by electron-beam computed tomography. *Circulation* 2000; 101:850.
21. Cairns JA, Markham BA. Economics and efficacy in choosing oral anticoagulants or aspirin after myocardial infarction. *JAMA* 1995; 273:965.
22. Crouse JR, Craven TE, Hagaman AP. Association of coronary disease with segment-specific intimal-medial thickening of the extracranial carotid artery. *Circulation* 1995; 92:1141.
23. Visona A, Pesavento R, Lusiani L, et al. Intimal medial thickening of common carotid artery as indicator of coronary artery disease. *Angiology* 1996; 47:61.
24. Hodis HN, Mack WJ, LaBree L, et al. The role of carotid arterial intima-media thickness in predicting clinical coronary events. *Ann Intern Med* 1998; 128:262.
25. O'Leary DH, Polak JF, Kronmal RA, et al. Carotid-artery intima and media thickness as a risk factor for myocardial infarction and stroke in older adults: Cardiovascular Health Study Collaborative Research Group. *N Engl J Med* 1999; 340:14.
26. Grundy SM. Age as a risk factor: You are as old as your arteries. *Am J Cardiol* 1999; 83:1455.
27. Ridker PM, Buring JE, Shih J, et al. Prospective study of C-reactive protein and the risk of future cardiovascular events among apparently healthy women. *Circulation* 1998; 98:731.
28. Ridker PM, Glynn RJ, Hennekens CH. C-reactive protein adds to the predictive value of total and HDL cholesterol in determining risk of first myocardial infarction. *Circulation* 1998; 97:2007.
29. Grundy SM, Balady GJ, Criqui MJ, et al. Primary prevention of coronary heart disease: Guidance from Framingham—A statement for healthcare professionals from the AHA Task Force on Risk Reduction. American Heart Association. *Circulation* 1998; 97:1876.
30. Grundy SM. Cholesterol-lowering clinical trials: A historical perspective. In: Grundy SM, ed. *Cholesterol Lowering Therapy: Evaluation of Clinical Trial Evidence.* New York: Marcel Dekker; 1999:1.
31. Babiak J, Rudel LL. Lipoproteins and atherosclerosis. *Baillieres Clin Endocrinol Metab* 1987; 1:515.
32. Goldstein JL, Kita T, Brown MS. Defective lipoprotein receptors and atherosclerosis: Lessons from an animal counterpart of familial hypercholesterolemia. *N Engl J Med* 1983; 309:288.
33. Navab M, Berliner JA, Watson AD, et al. The Yin and Yang of oxidation in the development of the fatty streak: A review based on the 1994 George Lyman Duff Memorial Lecture. *Arterioscler Thromb Vasc Biol* 1996; 16:831.
34. Steinberg D, Parthasarathy S, Carew TE, et al. Beyond cholesterol: Modifications of low-density lipoprotein that increase its atherogenicity. *N Engl J Med* 1989; 320:915.
35. Flavahan NA. Atherosclerosis or lipoprotein-induced endothelial dysfunction: Potential mechanisms underlying reduction in EDRF/nitric oxide activity. *Circulation* 1992; 85:1927.
36. Treasure CB, Klein JL, Weintraub WS, et al. Beneficial effects of cholesterol-lowering therapy on the coronary endothelium in patients with coronary artery disease. *N Engl J Med* 1995; 332:481.
37. Anderson TJ, Meredith IT, Yeung AC, et al. The effect of cholesterol-lowering and antioxidant therapy on endothelium-dependent coronary vasomotion. *N Engl J Med* 1995; 332:488.
38. Law MR, Wald, NJ, Thompson SG. By how much and how quickly does reduction in serum cholesterol concentration lower risk of ischaemic heart disease? *BMJ* 1994; 308:367.
39. Buchwald H. Program on the surgical control of hyperlipidemias (POSCH) trial: A pivotal 25-year study. In Grundy SM, ed. *Cholesterol Lowering Therapy: Evaluation of Clinical Trial Evidence.* New York: Marcel Dekker; 1999:117.
40. Gordon DJ. Cholesterol lowering and total mortality. In: Rifkind BM, ed. *Lowering Cholesterol in High Risk Individuals and Populations.* New York: Marcel Dekker; 1995:33.
41. Gordon DJ. Cholesterol and mortality: What can meta-analysis tell us? In: Gallo LL, ed. *Cardiovascular Disease,* 2nd ed. New York: Plenum; 1995:333.
42. Endo AL. The discovery and development of HMG-CoA reductase inhibitors. *J Lipid Res* 1992; 33:1569.
43. Grundy SM. HMG-CoA reductase inhibitors for treatment of hypercholesterolemia. *N Engl J Med* 1988; 319:24.
44. Scandinavian Simvastatin Survival Study. Randomised trial of cholesterol lowering in 4444 patients with coronary heart disease: The Scandinavian Simvastatin Survival Study. *Lancet* 1994; 344:1383.
45. Shepherd J, Cobbe SM, Ford l, et al. Prevention of coronary heart disease with pravastatin in men with hypercholesterolemia. West of Scotland Coronary Prevention Study Group. *N Engl J Med* 1995; 333:1301.
46. Downs JR, Clearfield M, Weis S, et al. Primary prevention of acute coronary events with lovastatin in men and women with average cholesterol levels: Results of AFCAPS/TexCAPS. Air Force/Texas Coronary Atherosclerosis Prevention Study. *JAMA* 1998; 279:1615.
47. Brown BG, Zhao XQ, Sacco DE, et al. Lipid lowering and plaque regression: New insights into prevention of plaque disruption and clinical events in coronary disease. *Circulation* 1993; 87:1781.
48. Holmes CL, Schulzer M, Mancini GBJ. Angiographic results of lipid-lowering trials: A systematic review and meta-analysis. In: Grundy SM, ed. *Cholesterol-Lowering Therapy: Evaluation of Clinical Trial Evidence.* New York: Marcel Dekker; 1999:191.
49. National Heart, Lung, and Blood Institute (NHLBI). *Clinical Guidelines on the Identification, Evaluation, and Treatment of Overweight and Obesity in Adults: The Evidence Report.* Bethesda; MD: National Institutes of Health, NHLBI; 1998.
50. Cater NB, Grundy SM. Lowering serum cholesterol with plant sterols and stanols: Historical perspectives. In: Nguyen TT, ed. *Postgraduate Medicine Special Report: New Developments in Di-*

etary Management of High Cholesterol. New York: McGraw-Hill; 1998:6.

51. Van Horn L. Fiber, lipids, and coronary heart disease: A statement for healthcare professionals from the Nutrition Committee, American Heart Association. *Circulation* 1997; 95:2701.
52. Grundy SM. The optimal ratio of fat-to-carbohydrate in the diet. *Annu Rev Nutr* 1999; 19:325.
53. Lee TH, Cleeman JI, Grundy SM, et al. Clinical goals and performance measures for cholesterol management in secondary prevention of coronary heart disease. *JAMA* 2000; 283:294.
54. Grundy SM, Balady GJ, Criqui MH, et al. When to start cholesterol-lowering therapy in patients with coronary heart disease: A statement for healthcare professionals from the American Heart Association Task Force on Risk Reduction. *Circulation* 1997; 95:1683.
55. Goldman L, Weinstein MC, Goldman PA, et al. Cost-effectiveness of HMG-CoA reductase inhibition for primary and secondary prevention of coronary heart disease. *JAMA* 1991; 265:1145.
56. Johannesson M, Jonsson B, Kjekshus J, et al. Cost effectiveness of simvastatin treatment to lower cholesterol levels in patients with coronary heart disease. Scandinavian Simvastatin Survival Study Group. *N Engl J Med* 1997; 336:332.
57. Cohen DJ, Goldman L, Weinstein C. The cost-effectiveness of programs to lower serum cholesterol. In: Rifkind BM, ed. *Lowering Cholesterol in High-Risk Individuals and Populations.* New York: Marcel Dekker; 1995:311.
58. Grundy SM. Hypertriglyceridemia, atherogenic dyslipidemia, and the metabolic syndrome. *Am J Cardiol* 1998; 81:18B.
59. Hokanson JE, Austin MA. Plasma triglyceride level is a risk factor for cardiovascular disease independent of high-density lipoprotein cholesterol level: A meta-analysis of population-based prospective studies. *J Cardiovasc Risk* 1996; 3:213.
60. Assmann G, Schulte H, Funke H, et al. The emergence of triglycerides as a significant independent risk factor in coronary artery disease. *Eur Heart J* 1998; 19:M8.
61. Miller NE. High-density lipoprotein: A major risk factor for coronary atherosclerosis. *Baillieres Clin Endocrinol Metab* 1987; 1:603.
62. Vega GL, Grundy SM. Hypoalphalipoproteinemia (low high density lipoprotein) as a risk factor for coronary heart disease. *Curr Opin Lipidol* 1996; 7:209.
63. Austin MA, King MC, Vranizan KM, et al. Atherogenic lipoprotein phenotype: A proposed genetic marker for coronary heart disease risk. *Circulation* 1990; 82:495.
64. Report from the Committee of Principal Investigators. A co-operative trial in the primary prevention of ischaemic heart disease using clofibrate: Report from the Committee of Principal Investigators. *Br Heart J* 1978; 40:1069.
65. Frick MH, Elo O, Haapa K, et al. Helsinki Heart Study: Primary-prevention trial with gemfibrozil in middle-aged men with dyslipidemia—Safety of treatment, changes in risk factors, and incidence of coronary heart disease. *N Engl J Med* 1987; 317:1237.
66. Coronary Drug Project Research Group. Clofibrate and niacin in coronary heart disease. *JAMA* 1975; 231:360.
67. Carlson LA, Rosenhamer G. Reduction of mortality in the Stockholm Ischaemic Heart Disease Secondary Prevention Study by combined treatment with clofibrate and nicotinic acid. *Acta Med Scand* 1988; 223:405.
68. Goldbourt U, Brunner D, Behar S, et al. Baseline characteristics of patients participating in the Bezafibrate Infarction Prevention (BIP) Study. *Eur Heart J* 1998; 19:H42.
69. Rubins HB, Robins SJ, Collins D, et al. Gemfibrozil for the secondary prevention of coronary heart disease in men with low levels of high-density lipoprotein cholesterol. Veterans Affairs High-Density Lipoprotein Cholesterol Intervention Trial Study Group. *N Engl J Med* 1999; 341:410.
70. Ericsson CG, Hamsten A, Nilsson J, et al. Angiographic assessment of effects of bezafibrate on progression of coronary artery disease in young male postinfarction patients. *Lancet* 1996; 347:849.
71. Grundy SM, Benjamin IJ, Burke GL, et al. Diabetes and cardiovascular disease: A statement for healthcare professionals from the American Heart Association. *Circulation* 1999; 100:1134.
72. Staels B, Dallongeville J, Auwerx J, et al. Mechanism of action of fibrates on lipid and lipoprotein metabolism. *Circulation* 1998; 98:2088.
73. Vega GL, Grundy SM. Lipoprotein responses to treatment with lovastatin, gemfibrozil, and nicotinic acid in normolipidemic patients with hypoalphalipoproteinemia. *Arch Intern Med* 1994; 154:73.
74. Garg A, Grundy SML. Management of dyslipidemia in NIDDM. *Diabetes Care* 1990; 13:153.
75. Frost PH, Havel RJ. Rationale for use of non-high-density lipoprotein cholesterol rather than low-density lipoprotein cholesterol as a tool for lipoprotein cholesterol screening and assessment of risk and therapy. *Am J Cardiol* 1998; 81:26B.
76. Scanu AM. Lipoprotein(a): A genetic risk factor for premature coronary heart disease. *JAMA* 1992; 267:3326.
77. Ridker PM, Hennekens CH, Stampfer MJ. A prospective study of lipoprotein(a) and the risk of myocardial infarction. *JAMA* 1993; 270:2195.
78. Schaefer EJ, Lamon-Fava S, Jenner JL, et al. Lipoprotein(a) levels and risk of coronary heart disease in men. The Lipid Research Clinics Coronary Primary Prevention Trial. *JAMA* 1994; 27:999.
79. Cremer P, Nagel D, Labrot B, et al. Lipoprotein Lp(a) as predictor of myocardial infarction in comparison to fibrinogen, LDL cholesterol and other risk factors: Results from the prospective Gottingen Risk Incidence and Prevalence Study (GRIPS). *Eur J Clin Invest* 1994; 24:444.
80. Wald NJ, Law M, Watt HC, et al. Apolipoproteins and ischaemic heart disease: Implications for screening. *Lancet* 1994; 343:75.
81. Ridker PM, Stampfer MJ, Hennekens CH. Plasma concentration of lipoprotein(a) and the risk of future stroke. *JAMA* 1995; 273:1269.
82. Cantin BF, Gagnon S, Moorjani JP, et al. Is lipoprotein(a) an independent risk factor for ischemic heart disease in men? The Quebec Cardiovascular Study. *J Am Coll Cardiol* 1998; 31:519.
83. Wild SH, Fortmann SP, Marcovina SM. A prospective case-control study of lipoprotein(a) levels and apo(a) size and risk of coronary heart disease in Stanford Five-City Project participants. *Arterioscler Thromb Vasc Biol* 1997; 17:239.
84. Maher VM, Brown BG, Marcovina SM, et al. Effects of lowering elevated LDL cholesterol on the cardiovascular risk of lipoprotein(a). *JAMA* 1995; 274:1771.
85. Orth-Gomer K, Mittleman MA, Schenck-Gustafsson K, et al. Lipoprotein(a) as a determinant of coronary heart disease in young women. *Circulation* 1997; 95:329.
86. Bostom AG, Gagnon DR, Cupples LA, et al. A prospective investigation of elevated lipoprotein(a) detected by electrophoresis and cardiovascular disease in women. The Framingham Heart Study. *Circulation* 1994; 90:1688.
87. Nguyen TT, Ellefson RD, Hodge DO, et al. Predictive value of electrophoretically detected lipoprotein(a) for coronary heart disease and cerebrovascular disease in community-based cohort of 9936 men and women. *Circulation* 1997; 96:1390.
88. Tate JR, Rifai N, Berg K, et al. International Federation of Clinical Chemistry standardization project for the measurement of lipoprotein(a): Phase I Evaluation of the analytical performance of lipoprotein(a) assay systems and commercial calibrators. *Clin Chem* 1998; 44:1629.
89. McGinnis JM, Foege W. Actual causes of death in the United States. *JAMA* 1993; 270:2207.
90. Kesteloot H, Joossens JV. Nutrition and international patterns of disease. In: Marmot M, Elliott P, eds. *Coronary Heart Disease*

Epidemiology: From Etiology to Public Health. Oxford: Oxford University Press; 1993:152.
91. Keys A. *Seven Countries: A Multivariate Analysis of Death and Coronary Heart Disease.* Cambridge: Harvard University Press; 1980.
92. Epstein FH. The relationship of lifestyle to international trends in CHD. *Int J Epidemiol* 1989; 18(3 suppl):S203.
93. INTERSALT Cooperative Research Group. Intersalt: An international study of electrolyte excretion and blood. *BMJ* 1988; 297:319.
94. Ornish D, Brown SE, Scherwitz LW, et al. Can lifestyle changes reverse coronary heart disease? The Lifestyle Heart. *Lancet* 1990; 336:129.
95. De Lorgeril M, Salen P, Martin JL, et al. Mediterranean diet, traditional risk factors, and the rate of cardiovascular complications after myocardial infarction: Final report of the Lyon Diet Heart Study. *Circulation* 1999; 99:779.
96. Shekelle RB, Stamler J. Dietary cholesterol and ischaemic heart disease. *Lancet* 1989; 1:1177.
97. Johnson CL, Rifkind BM, Sempos CT, et al. Declining serum total cholesterol levels among US adults. The National Health and Nutrition Examination Surveys. *JAMA* 1993; 269:3002.
98. Dayton S, Pearce MC, Hashimoto S. A controlled trial of a diet high in unsaturated fat in preventing complications of atherosclerosis. *Circulation* 1969; 39:1.
99. Turpeinen O. Effect of cholesterol-lowering diet on mortality from coronary heart disease. *Circulation* 1979; 59:1.
100. Watts GF, Lewis B, Brunt JN, et al. Effects on coronary artery disease of lipid-lowering diet, or diet plus cholestyramine, in the St Thomas' Atherosclerosis Regression Study (STARS). *Lancet* 1992; 339:563.
101. Leren P. The Oslo diet-heart study: Eleven-year report. *Circulation* 1970; 42:935.
102. Puska P, Salonen JT, Nissinen A, et al. Change in risk factors for coronary heart disease during 10 years of a community intervention programme (North Karelia Project). *BMJ* 1983; 287:1840.
103. Farquhar JW, Fortmann SP, Flora JA, et al. Effects of communitywide education on cardiovascular disease risk factors. *JAMA* 1990; 264:359.
104. Goldman L, Gordon DJ, Rifkind BM, et al. Cost and health implication of cholesterol lowering. *Circulation* 1992; 85:1960.
105. Kristiansen IS, Eggen AE, Thelle DS. Cost effectiveness of incremental programmes for lowering serum cholesterol concentration: Is individual intervention worth while? *BMJ* 1991; 302:119.
106. Lichtenstein AH, Van Horn L. Very low fat diets. *Circulation* 1998; 98:935.
107. Kris-Etherton PM. AHA Science Advisory: Monounsaturated fatty acids and risk of cardiovascular disease. American Heart Association, Nutrition Committee. *Circulation* 1999; 100:1253.
108. US Department of Health and Human Services. *The Health Consequences of Smoking: Cardiovascular Disease—A Report of the Surgeon General.* Washington, DC: Office of Smoking and Health, US Government Printing Office; 1983.
109. Castelli WP, Garrison RJ, Dawber TR, et al. The filter cigarette and coronary heart disease: The Framingham story. *Lancet* 1981; 2:109.
110. Fielding JE, Phenow KJ. Health effects of involuntary smoking. *N Engl J Med* 1988; 319:1452.
111. Glantz SA, Parmley WW. Passive smoking and heart disease: Mechanisms and risk. *JAMA* 1995; 273:1047.
112. He J, Vupputuri S, Allen K, et al. Passive smoking and the risk of coronary heart disease: A meta-analysis of epidemiologic studies. *N Engl J Med* 1999; 340:920.
113. Frei B, Forte TM, Ames BN, et al. Gas phase oxidants of cigarette smoke induce lipid peroxidation and changes in lipoprotein properties in human blood plasma: Protective effects of ascorbic acid. *Biochem J* 1991; 277:133.
114. Celermajer DS, Sorensen KE, Georgakopoulos D, et al. Cigarette smoking is associated with dose-related and potentially reversible improvement of endothelium-dependent dilation in healthy young adults. *Circulation* 1993; 88:2149.
115. Rival J, Riddle JM, Stein PD. Effects of chronic smoking on platelet function. *Thromb Res* 1987; 45:75.
116. Gordon T, Kannel WB, McGee D, et al. Death and coronary attacks in men after giving up cigarette smoking: A report from the Framingham Study. *Lancet* 1974; 2:1345.
117. Tsevat J, Weinstein MC, Williams LW, et al. Expected gains in life expectancy from various coronary heart disease risk factor modifications *Circulation* 1991; 83:1194.
118. Wilhelmsson C, Vedin JA, Elmfeldt D, et al. Smoking and myocardial infarction. *Lancet* 1975; 1:415.
119. Hermanson B, Omenn GS, Kronmal RA, et al. Beneficial six-year outcome of smoking cessation in older men and women with coronary artery disease: Results from the CASS Registry. *N Engl J Med* 1988; 319:1365.
120. Tsevat J. Impact and cost-effectiveness of smoking interventions. *Am J Med* 1992; 93:43S.
121. Goldman L, Garber AM, Grover SA, et al. 27th Bethesda Conference: Matching the intensity of risk factor management. *J Am Coll Cardiol* 1996; 27:1020.
122. Cummings SR, Rubin SM, Oster G. The cost-effectiveness of counseling smokers to quit. *JAMA* 1989; 261:75.
123. Oster G, Huse DM, Delea TE, et al. Cost-effectiveness of nicotine gum as an adjunct to physician's advice. *JAMA* 1986; 256:1315.
124. Krumholz HM, Cohen BJ, Tsevat J, et al. Cost-effectiveness of a smoking cessation program after myocardial infarction. *J Am Coll Cardiol* 1993; 22:1697.
125. Fiore M, Bailey W, Cohen S, et al. *Smoking Cessation: Clinical Practice Guidelines No. 18.* Washington, DC: Agency for Healthcare Policy and Research, Public Health Service, US Department of Health and Human Services; 1996.
126. Hughes JR, Goldstein MG, Hurt RD, et al. Recent advances in the pharmacotherapy of smoking. *JAMA* 1999; 281:72.
127. Benowitz NL. The role of nicotine in smoking-related cardiovascular disease. *Prev Med* 1997; 26:412.
128. Blann AD, Steele C, McCollum CN. The influence of smoking and of oral and transdermal nicotine on blood. *Thromb Haemost* 1997; 78:1093.
129. Lucini D, Bertocchi F, Malliani A, et al. Autonomic effects of nicotine patch administration in habitual cigarette smokers: A double-blind, placebo-controlled study using spectral analysis of RR interval and systolic arterial pressure variabilities. *J Cardiovas-Pharmacol* 1998; 31:714.
130. MacMahon S, Peto R, Cutler J, et al. Blood pressure, stroke, and coronary heart disease: Part 1. Prolonged differences in blood pressure: Prospective observational studies corrected for the regression dilution bias. *Lancet* 1990; 335:765.
131. Collins R, MacMahon S. Blood pressure, antihypertensive drug treatment and the risks of stroke and of coronary heart disease. *Br Med Bull* 1994; 50:272.
132. Joint National Committee on Prevention, Evaluation, and Treatment of High Blood Pressure. *The Sixth Report of the Joint National Committee on Prevention, Detection, Evaluation, and Treatment of High Blood Pressure.* Bethesda, MD: National Institutes of Health; National Heart, Lung, and Blood Institute; 1997.
133. Van den Hoogen PCW, Feskens EJM, Jaglekerke NJD. The relation between blood pressure and mortality due to coronary heart disease among men in different parts of the world. *N Engl J Med* 2000; 342:1.
134. Kannel WB. Blood pressure as a cardiovascular risk factor: Prevention and treatment. *JAMA* 1996; 275:1571.
135. Franklin SS, Khan SA, Wong ND, et al. Is pulse pressure useful in predicting risk for coronary heart disease? The Framingham Heart Study. *Circulation* 1999; 100:354.

136. Davis BR, Cutler JA, Gordon DJ, et al. Rationale and design for the antihypertensive and lipid lowering treatment. *Am J Hypertens* 1996; 9:342.
137. Gibbons RJ, Chatterjee K, Daley J, et al. ACC/AHA/ACP-ASIM guidelines for the management of patients with chronic stable angina: A report of the American College of Cardiology/American Heart Association Task Force on Practice Guidelines (Committee on Management of Patients with Chronic Stable Angina). *J Am Coll Cardiol* 1999; 33:2092.
138. Levy D, Garrison RJ, Savage DD, et al. Prognostic implications of echocardiographically determined left ventricular mass in the Framingham Heart Study. *N Engl J Med* 1990; 322:1561.
139. Harjai KJ. Potential new cardiovascular risk factors: Left ventricular hypertrophy. *Ann Intern Med* 1999; 131:376.
140. Levy D, Salomon M, D'Agostino RB, et al. Prognostic implications of baseline electrocardiographic features and their serial changes in subjects with left ventricular hypertrophy. *Circulation* 1994; 90:1786.
141. Verdecchia P, Schillaci G, Borgioni C, et al. Prognostic significance of serial changes in left ventricular mass in essential hypertension. *Circulation* 1998; 97:48.
142. Schlaich MP, Schmieder RE. Left ventricular hypertrophy and its regression: Pathophysiology and therapeutic approach—Focus on treatment by antihypertensive agents. *Am J Hypertens* 1998; 11:1394.
143. Gottdiener JS, Reda DJ, Massie BM, et al. Effect of single-drug therapy on reduction of left ventricular mass in mild to moderate hypertension: comparison of six antihypertensive agents. The Department of Veterans Affairs Cooperative Study Group on Antihypertensive Agents. *Circulation* 1997; 95:2007.
144. Reaven GM. Banting Lecture 1988: Role of insulin resistance in human disease. *Diabetes* 1988; 37:1595.
145. Reaven GM. Syndrome X: 6 years later. *J Intern Med* 1994; 736:13.
146. Reaven GM. Insulin resistance and its consequences: Non-insulin-dependent diabetes mellitus and coronary heart disease. In: LeFoith, Taylor Sl, Olefsky JM, eds. *Diabetes Mellitus.* Philadelphia: Lippincott-Raven; 1996:509.
147. Petrie JR, Ueda S, Webb DJ, et al. Endothelial nitric oxide production and insulin sensitivity: A physiological link with implications for pathogenesis of cardiovascular disease. *Circulation* 1996; 93:1331.
148. Despres JP, Lamarche B, Mauriege P, et al. Hyperinsulinemia as an independent risk factor for ischemic heart disease. *N Engl J Med* 1996; 334:952.
149. Boden G. Fatty acids and insulin resistance. *Diabetes Care* 1996; 19:394.
150. Dobbins RL, Chester MW, Daniels MB, et al. Circulating fatty acids are essential for efficient glucose-stimulated insulin secretion after prolonged fasting in humans. *Diabetes* 1998; 47:1613.
151. Stone PH, Muller JE, Hartwell T, et al. The effect of diabetes mellitus on prognosis and serial left ventricular function after acute myocardial infarction: Contribution of both coronary disease and diastolic left ventricular dysfunction to the adverse prognosis. The MILIS Study Group. *J Am Coll Cardiol* 1989; 14:49.
152. Smith JW, Marcus FI, Serokman R. Prognosis of patients with diabetes mellitus after acute myocardial infarction. *Am J Cardiol* 1984; 54:718.
153. Abbott RD, Donahue RP, Kannel WB, et al. The impact of diabetes on survival following myocardial infarction in men vs women: The Framingham Study. *JAMA* 1988; 260:3456.
154. Walden CE, Knopp RH, Wahl PW, et al. Sex differences in the effect of diabetes mellitus on lipoprotein triglyceride and cholesterol concentrations. *N Engl J Med* 1984; 311:953.
155. Meinert Cl, Knatterud GL, Prout TE, et al. A study of the effects of hypoglycemic agents on vascular complications in patients with adult-onset diabetes: II. Mortality results. *Diabetes* 1970; 19:789.
156. Diabetes Control and Complications Trial Reseach Group. The effect of intensive treatment of diabetes on the development and progression of long-term complications in insulin-dependent diabetes mellitus. The Diabetes Control and Complications Trial Research Group. *N Engl J Med* 1993; 329:977.
157. UK Prospective Diabetes Study Group. Intensive blood-glucose control with sulphonylureas or insulin compared with conventional treatment and risk of complications in patients with type 2 diabetes (UKPDS 33). *Lancet* 1998; 352:837.
158. Gundersen T, Kjekshus J. Timolol treatment after myocardial infarction in diabetic patients. *Diabetes Care* 1983; 6:285.
159. Fletcher GF, Balady G, Blair SN, et al. Statement on exercise: Benefits and recommendations for physical activity. *Circulation* 1996; 94:857.
160. Hambrecht R, Niebauer J, Marburger C, et al. Various intensities of leisure time physical activity in patients with coronary artery disease: Effects on cardiorespiratory fitness and progression of coronary atherosclerotic lesions. *J Am Coll Cardiol* 1993; 22:468.
161. Haskell WL. Sedentary lifestyle as a risk factor for coronary heart disease. In: Pearson TA, ed. *Primer in Preventive Cardiology.* Dallas: American Heart Association; 1994:173.
162. Siscovick DS, Weiss NS, Fletcher RH, et al. The incidence of primary cardiac arrest during vigorous exercise. *N Engl J Med* 1984; 311:874.
163. Manson JE, Hu FB, Rich-Edwards JW, et al. A prospective study of walking as compared with vigorous exercise in the prevention of coronary heart disease in women. *N Engl J Med* 1999; 341:650.
164. Oldridge NB, Guyatt GH, Fischer ME, et al. Cardiac rehabilitation after myocardial infarction: Combined experience of randomized clinical trials. *JAMA* 1988; 260:945.
165. O'Connor GT, Buring JE, Yusuf S, et al. An overview of randomized trials of rehabilitation with exercise after myocardial infarction. *Circulation* 1989; 80:234.
166. Pate RR, Pratt M, Blair SN, et al. Physical activity and public health: A recommendation from the Centers for Disease Control and Prevention and the American College of Sports Medicine. *JAMA* 1995; 273:402.
167. Smith SC Jr, Blair SN, Criqui MH, et al. AHA consensus panel statement: Preventing heart attack and death in patients with coronary disease. The Secondary Prevention Panel. *Circulation* 1995; 92:2.
168. Grundy SM, Balady GJ, Criqui MH, et al. Guide to primary prevention of cardiovascular disease: A statement for healthcare professionals from the Task Force on Risk Reduction. American Heart Association Science Advisory and Coordinating Committee. *Circulation* 1997; 95:2329.
169. Fletcher GF, Balady G, Froelicher VF, et al. Exercise standards: A statement for healthcare professionals from the American Heart Association. Writing Group. *Circulation* 1995; 91:580.
170. King AC, Haskell WL, Taylor CB. Group- vs home-based exercise training in healthy older men and women. *JAMA* 1991; 266:1535.
171. Eckel RH, Krauss RM. American Heart Association call to action: Obesity as a major risk factor. *Circulation* 1998; 97:2099.
172. Calle EE, Thun MJ, Petrilli JM, et al. Body-mass index and mortality in a prospective cohort of U.S. adults. *N Engl J Med* 1999; 341:1097.
173. Hubert HB, Feinleib M, McNamara PM, et al. Obesity as an independent risk factor for cardiovascular disease: A 26-year follow-up of participants in the Framingham Heart Study. *Circulation* 1983; 67:968.
174. Manson JE, Willett WC, Stampfer MJ, et al. Body weight and mortality among women. *N Engl J Med* 1995; 333:677.
175. Jousilahti P, Tuomilehto J, Vartiainen E, et al. Body weight, cardiovascular risk factors, and coronary mortality. *Circulation* 1996; 93:1372.
176. Belchetz PE. Hormonal treatment of postmenopausal women. *N Engl J Med* 1994; 330:1062.

177. Colditz GA, Hankinson SE, Hunter DJ, et al. The use of estrogens and progestins and the risk of breast cancer in postmenopausal women. *N Engl J Med* 1995; 332:1589.
178. Goldman L, Tosteso AN. Uncertainty about postmenopausal estrogen: Time for action, not debate. *N Engl J Med* 1991; 325:800.
179. Writing Group for the PEPI Trial. Effects of estrogen or estrogen/progestin regimens on heart disease risk factors in postmenopausal women: The Postmenopausal Estrogen/Progestin Interventions (PEPI) Trial. The Writing Group for the PEPI Trial. *JAMA* 1995; 273:199.
180. Hulley SD, Grady D, Bush T, et al. Randomized trial of estrogen plus progestin for secondary prevention of coronary heart disease in postmenopausal women. Heart and Estrogen/progestin Replacement Study (HERS) Research Group. *JAMA* 1998; 280:605.
181. Rozanski A, Bairey CN, Krantz DS, et al. Mental stress and the induction of silent myocardial ischemia in patients with coronary artery disease. *N Engl J Med* 1988; 318:1005.
182. Yeung AC, Vekshtein VI, Krantz DS, et al. The effect of atherosclerosis on the vasomotor response of coronary arteries. *N Engl J Med* 1991; 325:1551.
183. Mittleman MA, Maclure M, Sherwood JB, et al. Triggering of acute myocardial infarction onset by episodes of anger. *Circulation* 1995; 92:1720.
184. Leor J, Poole WK, Kloner RA. Sudden cardiac death triggered by an earthquake. *N Engl J Med* 1996; 334:413.
185. Selhub J, Jacques PF, Wilson PW, et al. Vitamin status and intake as primary determinants of homocysteinemia in an elderly population. *JAMA* 1993; 270:2693.
186. Jacques PF, Selhub J, Bostom AG, et al. The effect of folic acid fortification on plasma folate and total homocysteine concentrations. *N Engl J Med* 1999; 340:1449.
187. Boushey CJ, Beresford SA, Omenn GS, et al. A quantitative assessment of plasma homocysteine as a risk factor for vascular disease: Probable benefits of increasing folic acid intakes. *JAMA* 1995; 274:1049.
188. Stampfer MJ, Malinow MR, Willett WC, et al. A prospective study of plasma homocyst(e)ine and risk of myocardial infarction in US physicians. *JAMA* 1992; 268:877.
189. Arnesen E, Refsum H, Bonaa KH, et al. Serum total homocysteine and coronary heart disease. *Int J Epidemiol* 1995; 24:704.
190. Wald NJ, Watt HC, Law MR, et al. Homocysteine and ischemic heart disease: Results of a prospective study with implications regarding prevention. *Arch Intern Med* 1998; 158:862.
191. Bostom AG, Silbershatz H, Rosenberg IH, et al. Nonfasting plasma total homocysteine levels and all-cause and cardiovascular disease mortality in elderly Framingham men and women. *Arch Intern Med* 1999; 159:1077.
192. Ridker PM, Manson JE, Buring JE, et al. Homocysteine and risk of cardiovascular disease among postmenopausal women. *JAMA* 1999; 281:1817.
193. Nygard O, Nordrehaug JE, Refsum H, et al. Plasma homocysteine levels and mortality in patients with coronary artery disease. *N Engl J Med* 1997; 337:230.
194. Perry IJ, Refsum H, Morris RW, et al. Prospective study of serum total homocysteine concentration and risk of stroke in middle-aged British men. *Lancet* 1995; 346:1395.
195. Evans RW, Shaten BJ, Hempel JD, et al. Homocyst(e)ine and risk of cardiovascular disease in the Multiple Risk Factor intervention Trial. *Arterioscler Thromb Vasc Biol* 1997; 17:1947.
196. Alfthan G, Pekkanen J, Jauhiainen M, et al. Relation of serum homocysteine and lipoprotein(a) concentrations to atherosclerotic disease in a prospective Finnish population based study. *Arterioscler Thromb Vasc Biol* 1994; 106:9.
197. Folsom AR, Nieto FJ, McGovern PG, et al. Prospective study of coronary heart disease incidence in relation to fasting total homocysteine, related genetic polymorphisms, and B vitamins: The Atherosclerosis Risk in Communities (ARIC) Study. *Circulation* 1998; 98:204.
198. Malinow MR, Duell PB, Hess DL, et al. Reduction of plasma homocyst(e)ine levels by breakfast cereal fortified with folic acid in patients with coronary heart disease. *N Engl J Med* 1998; 338:1009.
199. Stampfer MJ, Hennekens CH, Manson JE, et al. Vitamin E consumption and the risk of coronary disease in women. *N Engl J Med* 1993; 328:1444.
200. Rimm EB, Stampfer A, Ascherio E, et al. Vitamin E consumption and the risk of coronary heart disease in men. *Engl J Med* 1993; 328:1450.
201. Greenberg ER, Baron JA, Karagas MR, et al. Mortality associated with low plasma concentration of beta carotene and the effect of oral supplementation. *JAMA* 1996; 275:699.
202. Jha P, Flather M, Lonn E, et al. The antioxidant vitamins and cardiovascular disease: A critical review of epidemiologic and clinical trial data. *Ann Intern Med* 1995; 123:860.
203. The Alpha-Tocopherol, Beta Carotene Cancer Prevention Study Group. The effect of vitamin E and beta carotene on the incidence of lung cancer and other cancers in male smokers. *N Engl J Med* 1994; 330:1029.
204. Omenn GS, Goodman GE, Thornquist MD, et al. Effects of a combination of beta carotene and vitamin A on lung cancer and cardiovascular disease. *N Engl J Med* 1996; 334:1150.
205. Hennekens CH, Buring JE, Manson JE, et al. Lack of effect of long-term supplementation with beta carotene on the incidence of malignant neoplasms and cardiovascular disease. *N Engl J Med* 1996; 334:1145.
206. Stephens NG, Parsons A, Schofield PM, et al. Randomised controlled trial of vitamin E in patients with coronary disease. *Lancet* 1996; 347:781.
207. Yusuf S, Sleight P, Pgue J, et al. Effects of an angiotensin-converting enzyme inhibitor, ramipril, on cardiovascular events in high-risk patients. The Heart Outcomes Prevention Evaluation Study Investigators. *N Engl J Med* 2000; 342:145.
208. Moore RD, Pearson TA. Moderate alcohol consumption and coronary artery disease: A review. *Medicine Baltimore* 1986; 65:242.
209. Stampfer MJ, Colditz GA, Willett WC, et al. A prospective study of moderate alcohol consumption and the risk of coronary disease and stroke in women. *N Engl J Med* 1988; 319:267.
210. Rimm EB, Giovannucci El, Willett WC, et al. Prospective study of alcohol consumption and risk of coronary disease in men. *Lancet* 1991; 338:464.
211. Gaziano JM. Alcohol and coronary heart disease. *Biol Effects Low Level Exposure (Newsl)* 1995; 4:1.
212. Maclure M. Demonstration of deductive meta-analysis: Ethanol intake and risk of myocardial infarction. *Epidemiol Rev* 1993; 15:328.
213. Langer RD, Criqui MH, Reed DM. Lipoproteins and blood pressure as biological pathways for effect of moderate alcohol consumption on coronary heart disease. *Circulation* 1992; 85:910.
214. Suh I, Shaten BJ, Cutler JA, et al. Alcohol use and mortality from coronary heart disease: The role of high-density lipoprotein cholesterol. The Multiple Risk Factor Intervention Trial Research Group. *Ann Intern Med* 1992; 116:881.
215. Haskell WL, Camargo C Jr, Williams PT, et al. The effect of cessation and resumption of moderate alcohol intake on serum high-density-lipoprotein subfractions. A controlled study. *N Engl J Med* 1984; 310:805.
216. Gaziano JM, Buring JE, Breslow JL, et al. Moderate alcohol intake, increased levels of high-density lipoprotein and its subfractions, and decreased risk of myocardial infarction. *N Engl J Med* 1993; 329:1829.
217. Ridker PM, Vaughan DE, Stampfer MJ, et al. Association of moderate alcohol consumption and plasma concentration of endogenous tissue-type plasminogen activator. *JAMA* 1994; 272:929.
218. Hendriks HF, Veenstra J, Velthuis-te Wierik EJ, et al. Effect of moderate dose of alcohol with evening meal on fibrinolytic factors. *BMJ* 1994; 308:1003.

219. Deykin D, Janson P, McMahon L. Ethanol potentiation of aspirin-induced prolongation of the bleeding time. *N Engl J Med* 1982; 306:852.
220. Elmer O, Goransson G, Zoucas E. Impairment of primary hemostasis and platelet function after alcohol ingestion in man. *Haemostasis* 1984; 14:223.
221. Pearson TA, Terry P. What to advise patients about drinking alcohol: The clinician's conundrum. *JAMA* 1994; 272:967.
222. Enos WFJ, Beyer JC, Holmes RH. Pathogenesis of coronary disease in American soldiers killed in Korea. *JAMA* 1955;58:912.
223. McNamara JJ, Molot MA, Stemple JF, et al. Coronary artery disease in combat casualties in Vietnam. *JAMA* 1971; 216:1185.
224. Castelli WP. Epidemiology of coronary heart disease: The Framingham Study. *Am J Med* 1984; 76:4.
225. Thom TJ. Cardiovascular disease mortality among United States women. In: Eaker ED, ed. *Coronary Heart Disease in Women.* New York: Haymarket Doyma; 1987.
226. Kaplan GA, Keil JE. Socioeconomic factors and cardiovascular disease: A review of the literature. *Circulation* 1993; 88:1973.
227. Hopkins PN, Williams RR. Human genetics and coronary heart disease: A public health perspective. *Annu Rev Nutr* 1989; 9:303.
228. Rissanen AM. Familial aggregation of coronary heart disease in a high incidence area. *Br Heart J* 1979; 42:294.
229. Williams RR, Hopkins PN, Wu LL, et al. Evaluating family history to prevent early coronary heart disease. In: Person TA, ed. *Primer in Preventive Cardiology.* Dallas: American Heart Association; 1994:93.
230. Steering Committee of the Physicians' Health Study Research Group. Final report on the aspirin component of the ongoing Physicians' Health Study. *N Engl J Med* 1989; 321:129.
231. Ridker PM, Manson JE, Buring JE, et al. Clinical characteristics of nonfatal myocardial infarction among individuals on prophylactic low-dose aspirin therapy. *Circulation* 1991; 84:708.
232. Manson JE, Grobbee DE, Stampfer MJ, et al. Aspirin in the primary prevention of angina pectoris in a randomized trial. *Am J Med* 1990; 89:772.
233. Peto R, Gray R, Collins K, et al. Randomised trial of prophylactic daily aspirin in British male doctors. *BMJ* 1988; 296:313.
234. Hennekens CH, Peto R, Hutchison GB, et al. An overview of the British and American aspirin studies [Letter]. *N Engl J Med* 1988; 318:923.
235. Ridker PM, Manson JE, Gaziano JM, et al. Low-dose aspirin therapy for chronic stable angina: A randomized, placebo-controlled clinical trial. *Ann Intern Med* 1991; 114:835.
236. Medical Research Council's General Practice Research Framework. Thrombosis prevention trial: Randomised trial of low-intensity oral anticoagulation with warfarin and low-dose aspirin in the primary prevention of ischaemic heart disease in men at increased risk. The Medical Research Council's General Practice Research Framework. *Lancet* 1998; 351:233.
237. Hennekens CH, Buring JE, Sandercock P, et al. Aspirin and other antiplatelet agents in the secondary and primary prevention of cardiovascular disease. *Circulation* 1989; 80:749.
238. Antiplatelet Trialists' Collaboration. Collaborative overview of randomised trials of antiplatelet therapy: Prevention of death, myocardial infarction, and stroke by prolonged antiplatelet therapy in various categories of patients. Antiplatelet Trialists' Collaboration. *BMJ* 1994; 308:81.
239. CAPRIE Steering Committee. A randomized, blinded, trial of clopidogrel versus aspirin in patients at risk of ischaemic events (CAPRIE). *Lancet* 1996; 348:1329.
240. Sixty Plus Reinfarction Study Research Group. A double-blind trial to assess long-term oral anticoagulant therapy in elderly patients after myocardial infarction: Report of the Sixty Plus Reinfarction Study Research Group. Lancet 1980; 2:989.
241. Smith P, Amesen H, Holme I. The effect of warfarin on mortality and reinfarction after myocardial infarction. *N Engl J Med* 1990; 323:147.
242. US Preventive Services Task Force. Aspirin prophylaxis. In: *Guide to Clinical Preventive Services: Report of the US Preventive Services Task Force.* Baltimore: Williams and Wilkins; 1989.
243. Manson JE, Stampfer MJ, Colditz GA, et al. A prospective study of aspirin use and primary prevention of cardiovascular disease in women. *JAMA* 1991; 266:521.
244. Meade TW, Mellows S, Brozovic M, et al. Haemostatic function and ischaemic heart disease: Principal results of the Northwick Park Heart Study. *Lancet* 1986; 2:533.
245. Wilhelmsen L, Svardsudd K, Korsan-Bengtsen K, et al. Fibrinogen as a risk factor for stroke and myocardial infarction. *N Engl J Med* 1984; 311:501.
246. Kannel WB, Wolf PA, Castelli WP, et al. Fibrinogen and risk of cardiovascular disease: The Framingham Study. *JAMA* 1987; 258:1183.
247. Thompson SG, Kienast J, Pyke SD, et al. Hemostatic factors and the risk of myocardial infarction or sudden death in patients with angina pectoris. European Concerted Action on Thrombosis and Disabilities Angina Pectoris Study Group. *N Engl J Med* 1995; 332:635.
248. Ma J, Hennekens CH, Ridker PM, et al. A prospective study of fibrinogen and risk of myocardial infarction in the Physicians' Health Study. *J Am Coll Cardiol* 1999; 33:1347.
249. Ernst E, Resch KL. Fibrinogen as a cardiovascular risk factor: A meta-analysis and review of the literature. *Ann Intern Med* 1993; 118:956.
250. Ridker PM, Cushman M, Stampfer MJ, et al. Inflammation, aspirin, and the risk of cardiovascular disease in apparently healthy men. *N Engl J Med* 1997; 336:973.
251. Koenig W, Sund M, Frohlich M, et al. C-Reactive protein, a sensitive marker of inflammation, predicts future risk of coronary heart disease in initially healthy middle-aged men: Results from the MONICA (Monitoring Trends and Determinants in Cardiovascular Disease) Augsburg Cohort Study, 1984 to 1992. *Circulation* 1999; 99:237.
252. Ridker PM, Cushman M, Stampfer MJ, et al. Plasma concentration of C-reactive protein and risk of developing peripheral vascular disease. *Circulation* 1998; 97:425.
253. Kuller LH, Tracy RP, Shaten J, et al. Relation of C-reactive protein and coronary heart disease in the MRFIT nested case-control study. Multiple Risk Factor Intervention Trial. *Am J Epidemiol* 1996; 144:537.
254. Tracy RP, Lemaitre RN, Psaty BM, et al. Relationship of C-reactive protein to risk of cardiovascular disease in the elderly: Results from the Cardiovascular Health Study and the Rural Health Promotion Project. *Arterioscler Thromb Vasc Biol* 1997; 17:1121.
255. Liuzzo G, Biasucci LM, Gallimore JR, et al. The prognostic value of C-reactive protein and serum amyloid A protein in severe unstable angina. *N Engl J Med* 1994; 331:417.
256. Morrow DA, Rifai N, Antman EM, et al. C-reactive protein is a potent predictor of mortality independently of and in combination with troponin T in acute coronary syndromes: A TIMI 11A substudy. Thrombolysis in Myocardial Infarction. *J Am Coll Cardiol* 1998; 31:1460.
257. Ridker PM, Rifai N, Pfeffer MA, et al. Inflammation, pravastatin, and the risk of coronary events after myocardial infarction in patients with average cholesterol levels. Cholesterol and Recurrent Events (CARE) Investigators. *Circulation* 1998; 98:839.
258. Smith JK, Dykes R, Douglas JE, et al. Long-term exercise and atherogenic activity of blood mononuclear cells in persons at risk of developing ischemic heart disease. *JAMA* 1999; 281:1722.
259. Visser M, Bouter LM, McQuillen GM, et al. Elevated C-reactive protein levels in overweight and obese adults. *JAMA* 1999; 282:2131.
260. Ridker PM, Rifai N, Pfeffer MA, et al. Long-term effects of pravastatin on plasma concentration of C-reactive protein. The

Cholesterol and Recurrent Events (CARE) Investigators. *Circulation* 1999; 100:230.
261. Rifai N, Tracy RP, Ridker PM. Clinical efficacy of an automated high-sensitivity C-reactive protein assay. *Clin Chem* 1999; 45: 2136.
262. Ridker PM, Vaughan DE, Stampfer JE, et al. Endogenous tissue-type plasminogen activator and risk of myocardial infarction. *Lancet* 1993; 341:1165.
263. Thogersen AM, Jansson JH, Boman K, et al. High plasminogen activator inhibitor and tissue plasminogen activator levels in plasma precede a first acute myocardial infarction in both men and women: Evidence for the fibrinolytic system as an independent primary risk factor. *Circulation* 1998; 98:2241.
264. Thompson SG, Kienast J, Pyke SD, et al. Hemostatic factors and the risk of myocardial infarction or sudden death in patients with angina pectoris. European Concerted Action on Thrombosis and Disabilities Angina Pectoris Study Group. *N Engl J Med* 1995; 332:635.
265. Ridker PM, Hennekens CH, Stampfer MJ, et al. Prospective study of endogenous tissue plasminogen activator and risk of stroke. *Lancet* 1994; 343:940.
266. Meade TW, Ruddock V, Stirling Y, et al. Fibrinolytic activity, clotting factors, and long-term incidence of ischaemic heart disease in the Northwick Park Heart Study. *Lancet* 1993; 342:1076.
267. Ridker PM, Hennekens CH, Cerskus A, et al. Plasma concentration of cross-linked fibrin degradation product (*D*-dimer). *Circulation* 1994; 90:2236.
268. Fowkes FG, Lowe GD, Housley E, et al. Cross-linked fibrin degradation products, progression of peripheral arterial disease, and risk of coronary heart disease. *Lancet* 1993; 342:84.
269. Lowe GD, Yamell JW, Sweetnam PM, et al. Fibrin *D*-dimer, tissue plasminogen activator, plasminogen activator inhibitor, and the risk of major ischaemic heart disease in the Caerphilly Study. *Thromb Haemost* 1998; 79:129.
270. Nabulsi AA, Folsom AR, White A, et al. Association of hormone-replacement therapy with various cardiovascular risk factors in postmenopausal women. *N Engl J Med* 1993; 328:1069.
271. Goldbourt U, Behar S, Reicher-Reiss H, et al. Rationale and design of a secondary prevention trial of increasing serum HDL cholesterol and reducing triglycerides after myocardial infarction in patients with clinically manifest atherosclerotic heart disease (the Bezafibrate Infarction Prevention Study). *Am J Cardiol* 1993; 71:909.
272. Vaughan DE, Rouleau JL, Ridker PM, et al. Effects of ramipril on plasma fibrinolytic balance in patients with acute anterior myocardial infarction. HEART Study Investigators. *Circulation* 1997; 96:442.
273. Stone PH, Sacks FM. *Strategies for secondary prevention.* In: Manson JE, ed. Primary Prevention of Myocardial Infarction. London: Oxford University Press: 1996.
274. Wikstrand J, Warnold I, Olsson G, et al. Primary prevention with metoprolol in patients with hypertension: Mortality. *JAMA* 1988; 259:1976.
275. Yusuf S, Peto R, Lewis J, et al. Beta blockade during and after myocardial infarction: An overview of the randomized trials. *Prog Cardiovasc Dis* 1985; 27:335.
276. Lau J, Antman EM, Jimenez-Silva J, et al. Cumulative meta-analysis of therapeutic trials for myocardial infarction. *N Engl J Med* 1992; 327:248.
277. Goldman L, Sia ST, Cook EF, et al. Costs and effectiveness of routine therapy with long-term beta-adrenergic antagonists after acute myocardial infarction. *N Engl J Med* 1988; 319:152.
278. Consensus Clinical Trial Study Group. Effects of enalapril on mortality in severe congestive heart failure. *N Engl J Med* 1987; 316:1429.
279. SOLVD Investigators. Effect of enalapril on survival in patients with reduced left ventricular ejection fractions and congestive heart failure. The SOLVD Investigators. *N Engl J Med* 1991; 325:293.
280. SOLVD Investigators. Effect of enalapril on mortality and the development of heart failure in asymptomatic patients with reduced left ventricular ejection fractions. The SOLVD Investigators. *N Engl J Med* 1992; 327:685.
281. Pfeffer JM, Fischer TA, Pfeffer MA. Angiotensin-converting enzyme inhibition and ventricular remodeling after myocardial infarction. *Annu Rev Physiol* 1995; 57:805.
282. Pfeffer MA, Lamas GA, Vaughan DE, et al. Effect of captopril on progressive ventricular dilatation after anterior myocardial infarction. *N Engl J Med* 1988; 319:80.
283. Sharpe N, Murphy J, Smith H, et al. Treatment of patients with symptomless left ventricular dysfunction after myocardial infarction. *Lancet* 1988; 1:255.
284. Pfeffer MA, Braunwald E, Moye LA, et al. Effect of captopril on mortality and morbidity in patients with left ventricular dysfunction after myocardial infarction: Results of the survival and ventricular enlargement trial. The SAVE Investigators. *N Engl J Med* 1992; 327:669.
285. Yusuf S, Pepine CJ, Garces C, et al. Effect of enalapril on myocardial infarction and unstable angina in patients with low ejection fractions. *Lancet* 1992; 340:1173.
286. Ridker PM, Gaboury CL, Conlin PR, et al. Stimulation of plasminogen activator inhibitor in vivo by infusion of angiotensin II. Evidence of a potential interaction between the renin-angiotensin system and fibrinolytic function. *Circulation* 1993; 87:1969.
287. Tsevat J, Duke D, Goldman L, et al. Cost-effectiveness of captopril therapy after myocardial infarction. *J Am Coll Cardiol* 1995; 26:914.
288. Vogel RA. Risk factor intervention and coronary artery disease: Clinical strategies. *Coron Artery Dis* 1995; 6:466.
289. Pearson TA. The American College of Cardiology: Evaluation of Preventive Therapeutics (ACCEPT) Study. 2000 (in preparation).
290. Pearson TA. The Lipid Treatment Assessment Project (L-TAP): A multicenter survey to evaluate the percentages of dyslipidemic patients receiving lipid-lowering therapy and achieving low-density lipoprotein cholesterol goals. *Arch Intern Med* 2000; 160:459.
291. Kottke TE, Blackburn H, Brekke ML, et al. The systematic practice of preventive cardiology. *Am J Cardiol* 1987; 59:690.
292. Pearson TA, McBride PE, Miller NH, et al. 27th Bethesda Conference: Matching the intensity of risk factor management. *J Am Coll Cardiol* 1996; 27:1039.
293. Houston-Miller N, Hill M, Kottke T, et al. The multilevel compliance challenge: Recommendations for a call to action. *Circulation* 1997; 95:1085.
294. Levine DM. Behavioral and psychosocial factors, progress and strategies. In: Pearson TA, ed. *Primer in Preventive Cardiology.* Dallas: American Heart Association; 1994:214.
295. DeBusk RF, Miller NH, Superko HR, et al. A case-management system for coronary risk factor modification after acute myocardial infarction. *Ann Intern Med* 1994; 120:721.
296. US Department of Health and Human Services. *Treating Tobacco Use and Dependence: A Clinical Practice Guideline.* Washington, DC: US Department of Health and Human Services; 2000.
297. Wenger NK, Froelicher ES, Smith LK. *Cardiac Rehabilitation as Secondary Prevention.* Bethesda, MD: National Heart, Lung, and Blood Institute; 1995.
298. Maron DJ, Fazio S, Linton MF. Current perspectives on statins. *Circulation* 2000; 101:207.
299. Pearson TA. Smoking cessation: Clinical evaluation and management of the cigarette smoker. In: Kelly WN, ed. *Textbook of Internal Medicine.* Philadelphia: Lippincott; 1992:1870.
300. Ridker PM, Haughie P. Prospective studies of C-reactive protein as a risk factor for cardiovascular disease. *J Investig Med* 1998; 46:391.

CHAPTER 39

NONATHEROSCLEROTIC CORONARY HEART DISEASE

Bruce F. Waller

Although atherosclerotic disease of the coronary arteries is the most common cause of luminal narrowing and coronary heart disease, there are multiple nonatherosclerotic (congenital and acquired) causes of severe luminal narrowing and subsequent clinical coronary events (angina pectoris, acute myocardial infarction, and sudden death) (Table 39-1).

Various nonatherosclerotic coronary artery diseases can reduce or interrupt coronary arterial blood flow by various mechanisms: (1) fixed luminal obstructions (internal narrowing), (2) encroachment of the lumen by disease of the arterial wall or adjacent tissues (external narrowing), or (3) both.[1] Reduction in coronary arterial blood flow also may result from dynamic changes in the walls of an otherwise normal artery (spasm) or from a disproportion of myocardial oxygen supply and demand. In view of current trends toward rapid coronary artery reperfusion to salvage jeopardized myocardium during evolving acute myocardial infarction, the various nonatherosclerotic etiologies of coronary artery disease must be kept in mind.

FREQUENCY OF NONATHEROSCLEROTIC CORONARY NARROWING PRODUCING FATAL MYOCARDIAL INFARCTION

Approximately 4 to 7 percent of all patients with acute myocardial infarction and nearly 4 times this percentage for patients under age 35 do not have atherosclerotic coronary artery disease (CAD) as demonstrated by coronary arteriography, at necropsy, or both.[1–5] In view of the fact that coronary angiography simply represents an image of one lumen, the specificity for etiology of the coronary luminal narrowing is extremely low. Review of necropsy studies[1,3,4] suggests that approximately 95 percent of patients with fatal acute myocardial infarction have at least one major epicardial coronary artery with severe luminal narrowing or total occlusion (Fig. 39-1). The remaining 5 percent of patients apparently have normal major epicardial coronary arteries. Of the 95 percent of patients with severe coronary

TABLE 39-1 Nonatherosclerotic Causes of Coronary Artery Disease (Coronary Heart Disease)

- Congenital anomalies
  - Anomalous origin from the aorta
  - Right-from-left sinus of Valsalva
  - Left-from-right sinus of Valsalva
  - Single coronary artery
  - Atresia of coronary ostium
  - High-takeoff coronary ostium
  - Ostial ridges
  - Anomalous origin from the pulmonary trunk
  - Fistula
  - Myocardial bridges (tunneled epicardial artery)
- Embolus
  - Natural
  - Thrombus
  - Tumor
  - Calcium
  - Vegetation (infective, noninfective)
  - Iatrogenic
  - Cardiac surgery
  - Cardiac catheterization
  - Coronary angioplasty
  - Prosthetic valves
  - Paradoxical
- Dissection
  - Coronary artery
  - Aortic
- Spasm
- Trauma
  - Nonpenetrating
  - Penetrating
  - Surgery
  - Catheterization
- Arteritis
  - Takayasu's disease
  - Polyarteritis nodosa
  - Systemic lupus erythematosus
  - Kawasaki's syndrome (mucocutaneous lymph node syndrome)
  - Syphilis
  - Other infections (infective endocarditis, *Salmonella*, parasites)
  - Buerger's disease
  - Giant-cell arteritis
- Metabolic disorders
  - Mucopolysaccharidoses (Hurler, Hunter)
  - Homocystinuria
  - Fabry's disease
  - Amyloid
- Intimal proliferation
  - Irradiation therapy
  - Cardiac transplantation
  - Fibromuscular hyperplasia (methysergide therapy)
  - Ostial cannulation
  - Transluminal balloon angioplasty
  - Idiopathic infantile arterial calcification (juvenile internal sclerosis)
  - Cocaine
- External compression
  - Aortic aneurysm
  - Tumor metastases
  - Muscle bridges
- Thrombosis without underlying atherosclerotic plaque
  - Polycythemia
  - Thrombocytosis
  - Hypercoagulability
- Substance abuse
  - Cocaine
  - Amphetamines
- Myocardial oxygen demand-supply disproportion
  - Aortic stenosis
  - Systemic hypotension
  - Carbon monoxide poisoning
  - Increased myocardial function (thyrotoxicosis)
- Intramural coronary artery disease (small vessel disease)
  - Hypertrophic cardiomyopathy
  - Amyloid
  - Cardiac transplantation
  - Neuromuscular
  - Diabetes mellitus
- Normal coronary arteries

SOURCES: Adapted from Waller,[1] Alpert and Braunwald,[2] Cheitlin et al.,[4] and Baim and Harrison.[5]

artery luminal narrowing, 95 percent have typical atherosclerotic plaque, with a superimposed thrombus in 85 percent of these.

The remaining 5 percent of the patients with severe coronary artery luminal narrowing have a host of etiologies (see Table 39-1), including coronary arteritis, trauma, systemic metabolic disorders, intimal fibrous proliferation, and coronary emboli. Medical centers with large populations of cardiac transplant patients will exceed the 5 percent nonatherosclerotic approximation owing to the high frequency of intimal fibrous proliferation in the coronary arteries late after transplantation. Of the 5 percent of patients seen at necropsy after fatal acute myocardial infarction with normal or nearly normal epicardial coronary arteries, perhaps 50 to 60 percent represent clinical coronary spasm, but the remaining 40 to 50 percent represent a combination of congenital coronary artery anomalies, spontaneous recanalization, and mismatches of coronary supply and myocardial demand (see also Chap. 35).

CONGENITAL CORONARY ARTERY ANOMALIES

Variation in the origin, course, or distribution of the epicardial coronary arteries is found in 1 to 2 percent of the population[1,6–14]

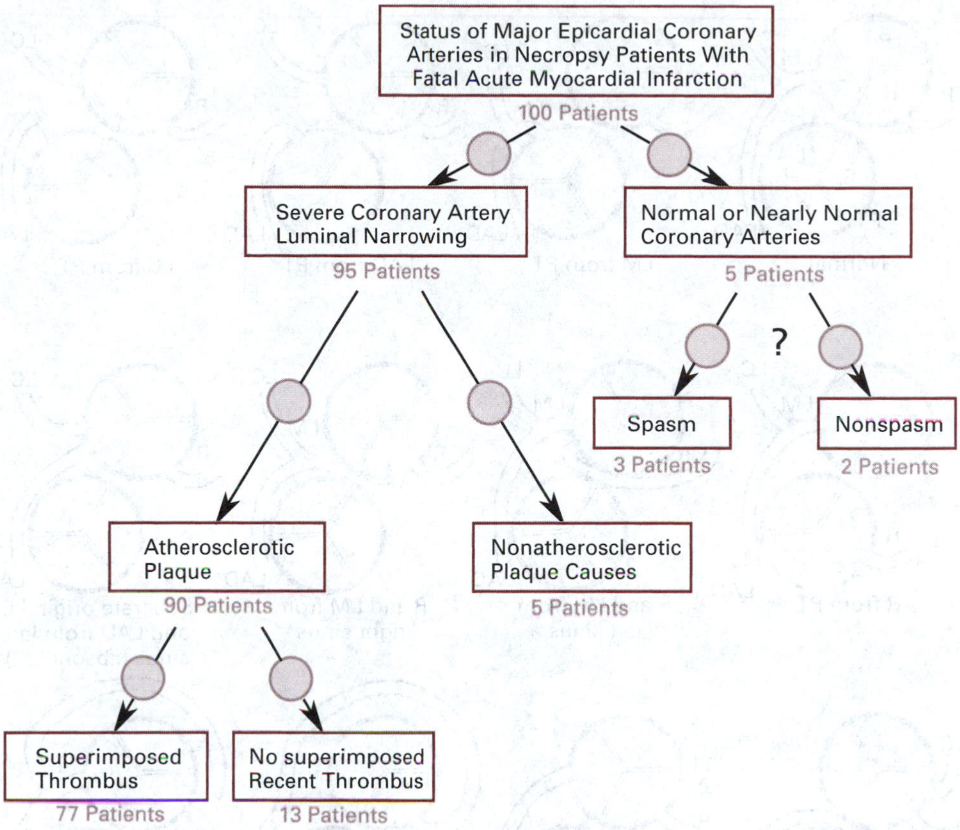

FIGURE 39-1 Diagram displaying the approximate breakdown of status of major epicardial coronary arteries in necropsy patients with fatal acute myocardial infarction. (From Waller.[10] Reproduced with permission from the publisher, editor, and author.)

TABLE 39-2 Certain Coronary Arterial Anomalies Associated with Clinical Coronary Events or Coronary Artery Narrowing

Anomalous origin of one or more coronary arteries from the aorta	High-takeoff coronary ostia
Origin of both right (R) and left (L) from same sinus of Valsalva	Ostial narrowing
R + LM (left main) from right sinus	Syphilis
R + LM (left main) from left sinus	Takayasu's disease (pulseless disease)
Single coronary artery	Fibromuscular hyperplasia (drug-induced)
Arising from right sinus	Aortic valve surgery
Arising from left sinus	Fibrous ridges
Arising from posterior sinus	Protruding masses
Anomalous origin of one or more coronary arteries from pulmonary trunk (PT)	Calcific nodules
Origin of R from PT	Supravalvular aortic stenosis
Origin of LM from PT	Aortic dissection
Origin of left anterior descending from PT	Adhesion of aortic cusp to sinus wall
Origin of left circumflex from PT	Embolism
Coronary artery atresia	Fibroelastosis
Atresia of R	Coronary artery fistula
Atresia of LM	Myocardial bridges

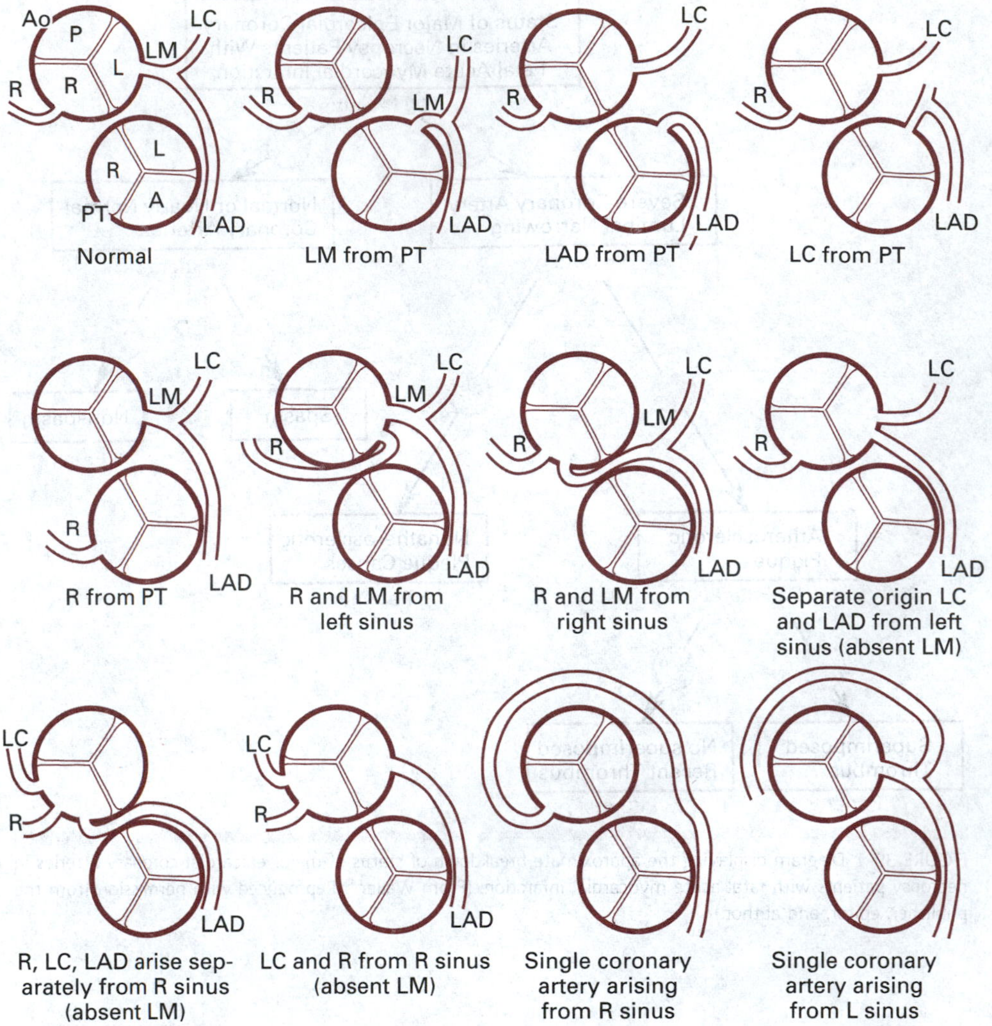

FIGURE 39-2 Diagram showing various congenital coronary artery anomalies that have been associated with clinical symptomatic heart disease. A, anterior cusp; Ao, aorta; L, left cusp; LAD, left anterior descending; LC, left circumflex; LM, left main; P, posterior cusp; PT, pulmonary trunk; R, right cusp or right coronary artery.

(Table 39-2 and Fig. 39-2). Certain types of these anomalies—including ostial lesions, passage of a major artery between the walls of the pulmonary trunk, a major coronary artery originating from the pulmonary trunk, or perhaps myocardial bridges—may produce ischemia with subsequent myocardial infarction[8] (see also Chaps. 15 and 63).

Origin of Both Right and Left Coronary Arteries from the Same Sinus of Valsalva

When either the right or left coronary artery arises from the left or right sinus of Valsalva, respectively, the anomalous vessel transverses the base of the heart in a course anterior to the pulmonary trunk, posterior to the aorta, or between the aorta and the pulmonary trunk (Figs. 39-3 and 39-4). At least 43 cases have been reported with necropsy where the origin of the left main coronary artery is from the right sinus with passage between the aorta and pulmonary trunk.[7] In 79 percent of these patients,[3,4] death was related to the anomaly with sudden death or an acute myocardial infarction. At necropsy, 5 of 26 patients younger than 20 years old had myocardial infarcts.[7] When the right coronary artery originates from the left sinus of Valsalva and passes between the aorta and the pulmonary trunk, symptoms of myocardial ischemia, infarction, or sudden death may occur.[7] Of 12 patients with this anomaly,[9] 3 died suddenly, and 2 had angina or syncope. At necropsy, transmural ventricular scars (healed infarction) were seen in 2.

The mechanism of ischemia, infarction, and/or sudden death in this coronary anomaly appears related to the shape of the coronary ostium of the anomalous vessel (Fig. 39-4). Normally, the coronary ostia are round to oval in shape, but in this anomaly, the coronary artery has an acute angle of takeoff that makes the ostium slitlike in shape. With increased cardiac output, the aorta dilates with stretching of the aortic wall so that this slitlike ostium may become severely narrowed (see Figs. 39-3 and 39-4). Similar mechanisms of coronary ischemia with exercise and aortic dilatation occur in case of the presence of a very acute angle of takeoff of the left main coronary artery (see Fig. 39-5) or of valvelike ridges at the ostia (see Fig. 39-6). It is unlikely that there is "compression" of the anomalous coronary artery by the aorta and pulmonary trunk in view of the marked differences in diastolic pressures. At best, there would be an anterior shift of the anomalous vessel rather than a viselike compression.

Single Coronary Artery

Origin of the entire coronary circulation from a single aortic ostium has been termed *single coronary artery*. This anomaly is rare in the absence of other associated anomalies of the heart. One or more branches of the single artery may cross the base of the heart in a fashion described above and thus may be exposed to the risks of ischemia owing to acute angulation.[5] Angina pectoris and myocardial lactate production have been demonstrated in patients with single coronary arteries in whom coronary atherosclerosis or an anomalous coronary artery passage was absent[13] (see also Chap. 63).

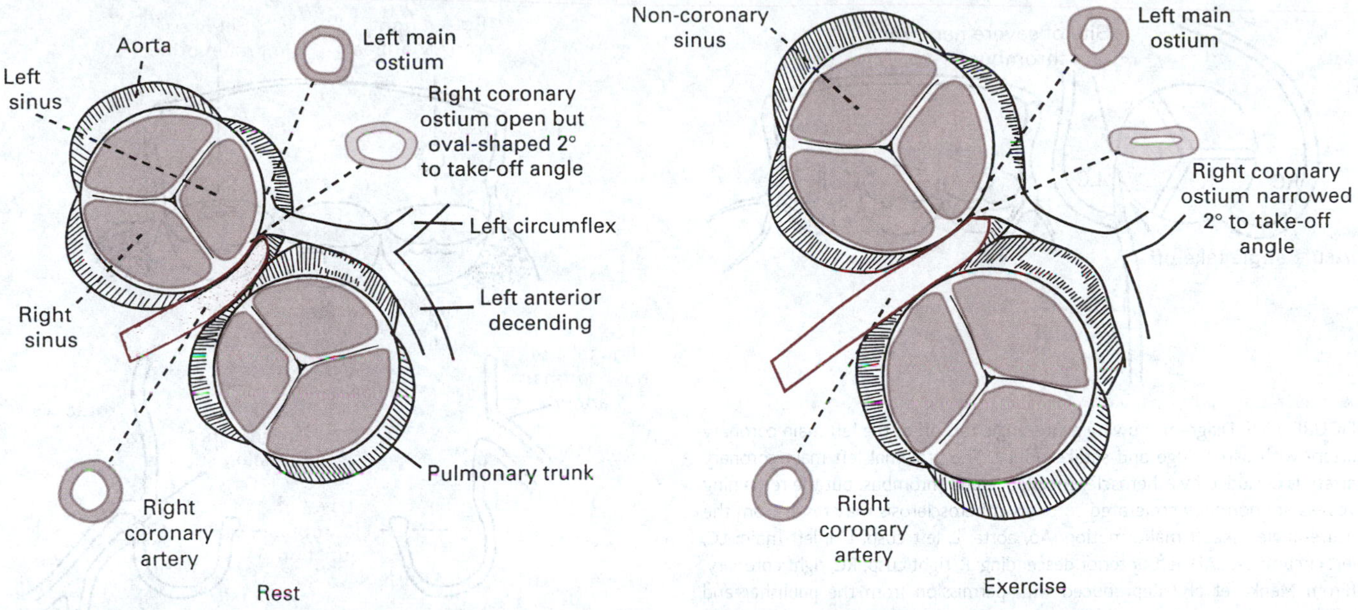

FIGURE 39-3 Diagram showing the proposed mechanism of myocardial ischemia produced by anomalous origin of the right coronary artery from the left sinus of Valsalva. With exercise, the aorta and pulmonary trunk dilate, thereby reducing the already narrowed coronary ostium of the anomalous right coronary. (From Waller.[10] Reproduced with permission from the publisher, editor, and author.)

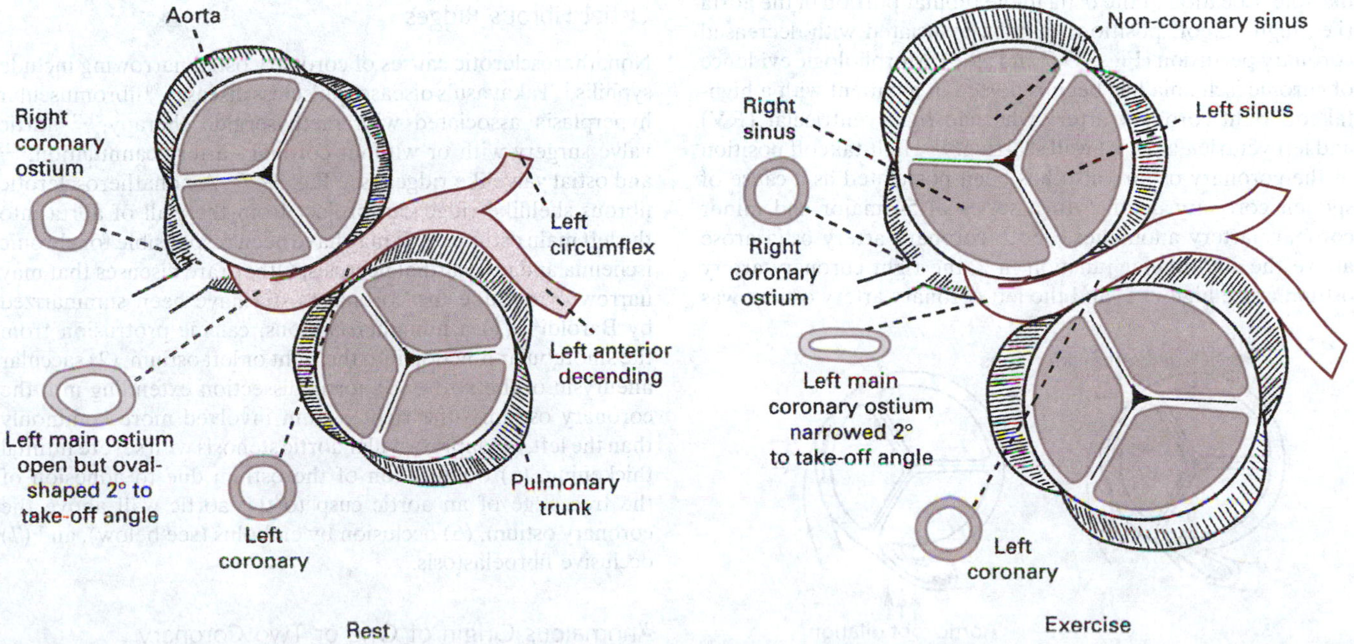

FIGURE 39-4 Diagram showing the proposed mechanism of myocardial ischemia produced by anomalous origin of the left coronary artery from the right sinus of Valsalva. With exercise, the aorta and pulmonary trunk dilate, thereby reducing the already narrowed coronary ostium of the anomalous left coronary. (From Waller.[10] Reproduced with permission from the publisher, editor, and author.)

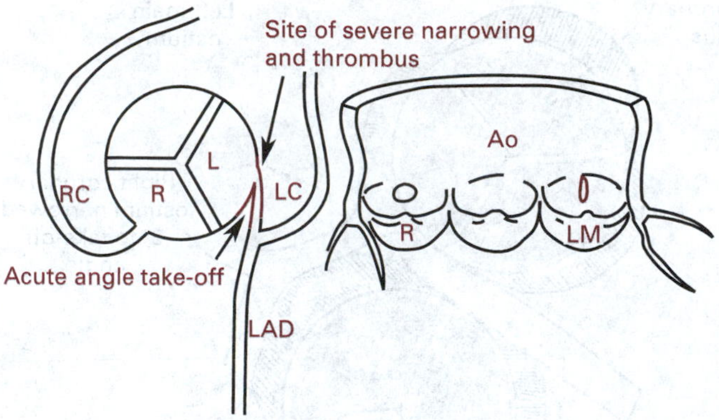

FIGURE 39-5 Diagram showing acute-angle takeoff of the left main coronary artery with ostial ridge and slitlike orifice. The proximal left main coronary artery is occluded by atherosclerotic plaque and thrombus, but the remaining vessels are normal. Accelerated coronary atherosclerosis may result from the acute-angle takeoff malformation. Ao, aorta; L, left cusp; LM, left main; LC, left circumflex; LAD, left anterior descending; R, right cusp; RC, right coronary. (From Menke et al.[11] Reproduced with permission from the publisher and author.)

Coronary Artery Atresia

Atresia of one of the two main coronary ostia may be associated with myocardial ischemia and infarction in infancy or childhood.[5] The involved vessel becomes dependent on collateral coronary blood flow from the contralateral coronary artery.

High-Takeoff Coronary Ostia

Normally, the coronary ostia are located within the sinuses of Valsalva, which optimizes coronary arterial blood flow in diastole. Location of the ostia in the tubular portion of the aorta (i.e., high-takeoff position) may be associated with decreased coronary perfusion (Figs. 39-7 and 39-8). Morphologic evidence of chronic ischemia has been reported in a patient with a high-takeoff right coronary artery who had right ventricular (RV) and left ventricular (LV) wall scarring.[14,15] High-takeoff position of the coronary ostium also has been postulated as a cause of sudden coronary death.[16] In a series of 54 major and minor coronary artery anomalies,[17] both coronary artery ostia arose above the sinotubular junction in 2, the right coronary artery ostium arose high in 5, and the left coronary artery ostium was in a high-takeoff position in 3. In 2 cases of high origin of the right coronary artery ostium, ischemia and death were attributed to the ostial lesion in 1.[18]

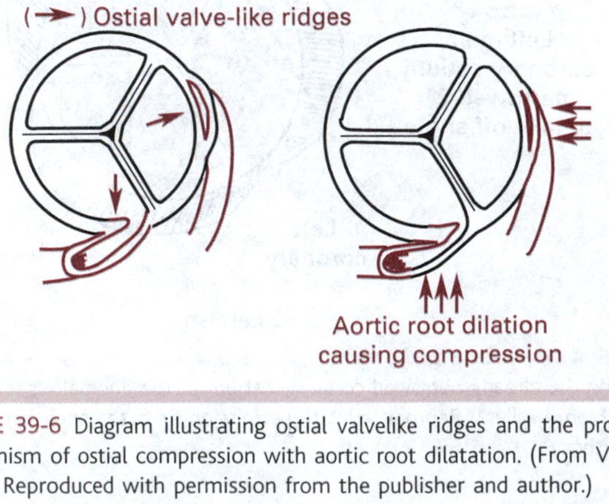

FIGURE 39-6 Diagram illustrating ostial valvelike ridges and the proposed mechanism of ostial compression with aortic root dilatation. (From Virmani et al.[12] Reproduced with permission from the publisher and author.)

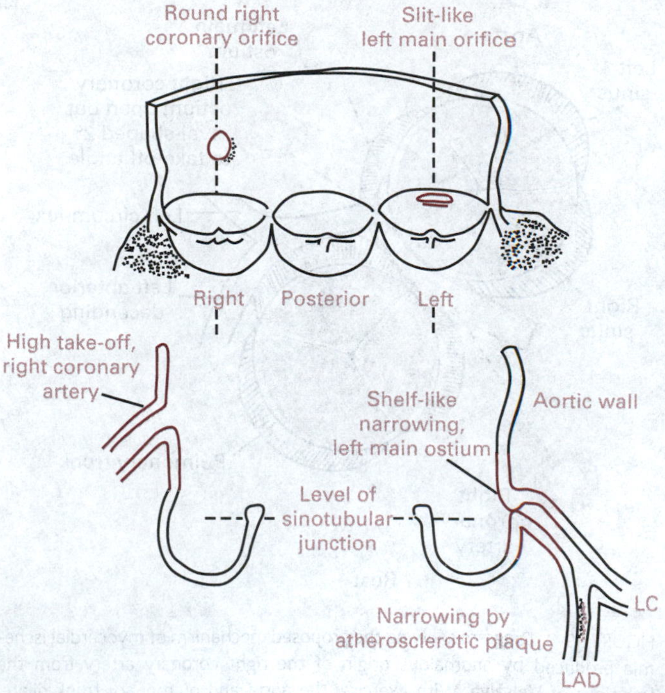

FIGURE 39-7 Diagram showing high-takeoff position of the right coronary artery and the nonatherosclerotic fibrous ridge occluding the left main coronary ostium. LAD, left anterior descending; LC, left circumflex. (From Foster et al.[14] Reproduced with permission from the publisher and author.)

Ostial Fibrous Ridges

Nonatherosclerotic causes of coronary ostial narrowing include syphilis,[19] Takayasu's disease (pulseless disease),[20] fibromuscular hyperplasia associated with methysergide therapy,[21,22] aortic valve surgery with or without coronary artery cannulation,[14,23] and ostial valvelike ridges (see Fig. 39-7). A nonatherosclerotic fibrous shelflike ridge can project from the wall of aorta into the left main ostium.[14,15] It may have been responsible for chronic ischemia and myocardial necrosis. Other rare diseases that may narrow or occlude the coronary ostia have been summarized by Baroldi[24]: (1) a nonatheromatous, calcific protrusion from the sinotubular junction into the right or left ostium, (2) saccular aneurysm of the aorta, (3) aortic dissection extending into the coronary ostium—the right ostium involved more commonly than the left, (4) supravalvular aortic stenosis with severe intimal thickening, (5) obliteration of the ostium due to adhesion of the free edge of an aortic cusp to the aortic wall above the coronary ostium, (6) occlusion by embolus (see below), and (7) occlusive fibroelastosis.

Anomalous Origin of One or Two Coronary Arteries from the Pulmonary Trunk

Anomalous origin of a coronary artery from the pulmonary trunk (Figs. 39-9 and 39-10) may be responsible for myocardial ischemia and infarction in infants and children. In more than

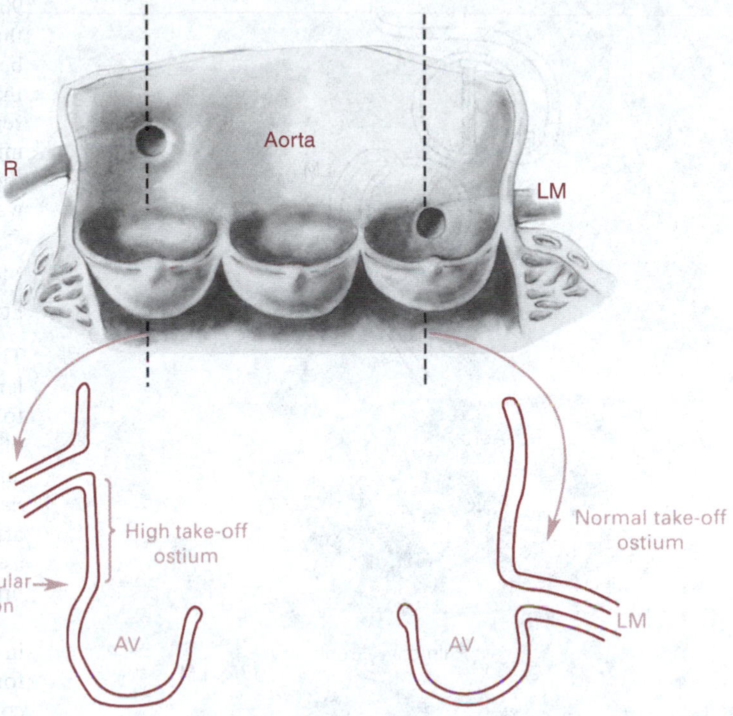

FIGURE 39-8 Diagram showing origin of right coronary ostium above the sinotubular junction "high-takeoff position." AV, aortic valve; L, left cusp; LM, left main; R, right cusp or right coronary artery.

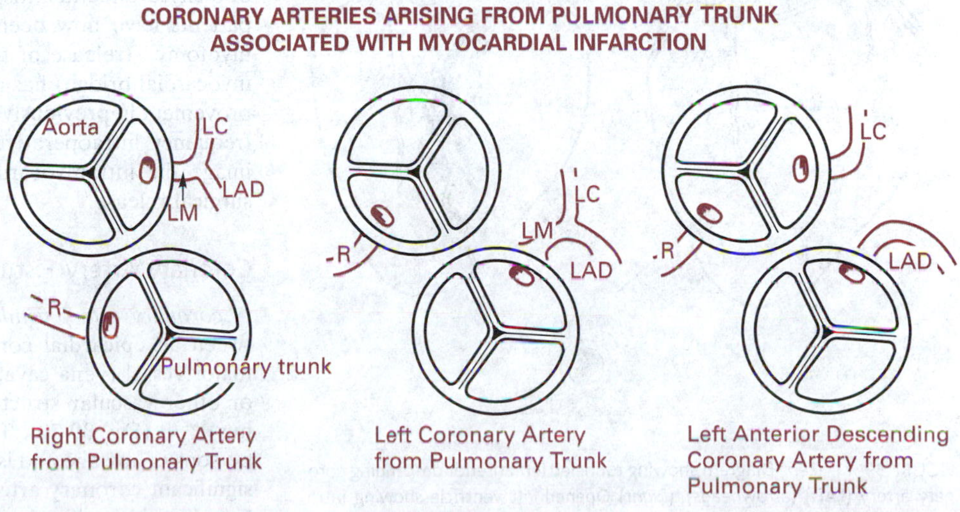

FIGURE 39-9 Anomalous origin of one or two major epicardial coronary arteries from the pulmonary trunk. For abbreviations, see Fig. 39-2. (From Waller.[1] Reproduced with permission from the publisher, editor, and author.)

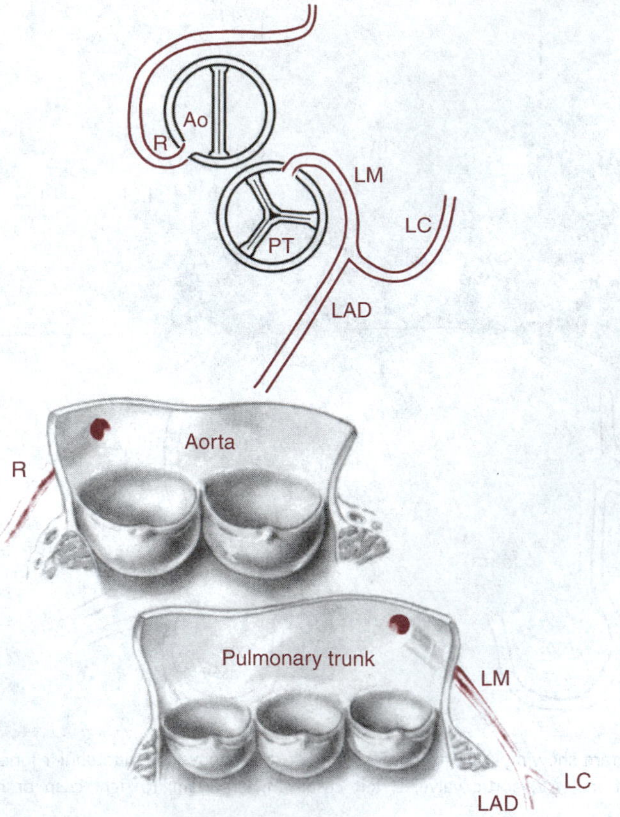

FIGURE 39-10 Anomalous origin of the main (LM) coronary artery from the pulmonary trunk causing acute myocardial infarction in an infant. Of interest is that both the anomalous LM and normal right coronary arteries arise in high-takeoff positions from the pulmonary trunk and aorta (Ao), respectively. LAD, left anterior descending; LC, left circumflex.

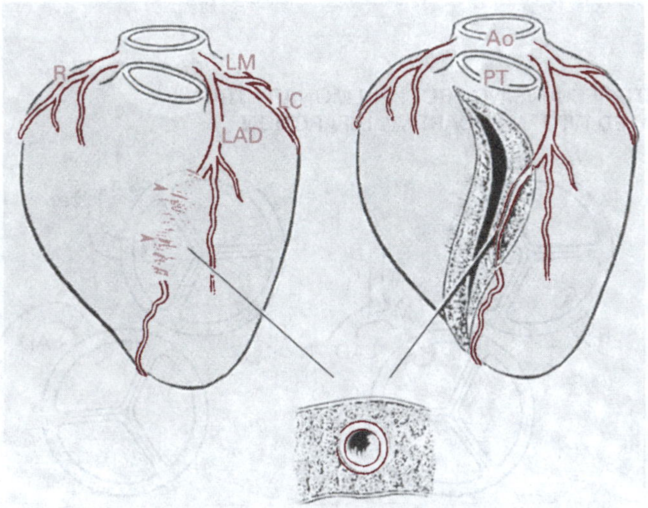

FIGURE 39-11 (*Left*) Diagram showing tunneled left anterior descending coronary artery (LAD) (*arrowheads*). (*Right*) Opened left ventricle showing intramyocardial segment. (*Below*) Transverse section of LV wall showing tunneled coronary artery surrounded by myocardium. (From Waller.[1] Reproduced with permission from the publisher, editor, and author.)

90 percent of cases,[5,7] the left main artery is the anomalous one; thus the anteroseptal and anterolateral LV myocardium may be at jeopardy for injury. Asymptomatic older patients with this coronary artery anomaly are usually found when they present with an abnormal electrocardiogram (ECG), a systolic murmur, or sudden death.[7] The murmur and abnormal ECG are the result of papillary muscle and/or anteroseptal myocardial wall damage (see Chap. 42).

Myocardial Bridges (Tunneled Epicardial Coronary Artery)

The coronary arteries may dip into the myocardium for varying lengths and then reappear on the heart's surface (Figs. 39-11 to 39-18). The muscle overlying the intramyocardial segment of the epicardial coronary artery is termed a *myocardial bridge*, and the artery coursing within the myocardium is called a *tunneled artery*[25–63] (see Figs. 39-11 to 39-13). Tunneled coronary arteries have long been recognized anatomically,[25] but suggested associations between myocardial ischemia and myocardial bridges have heightened their clinical relevance.[26,27]

Tunneled coronary arteries have been presumed congenital in origin.[28] At least three factors have been postulated to account for differences between the high frequency of tunneled major coronary arteries observed at necropsy (5–86 percent[29,30,57]) and the lower frequency of tunneled coronary arteries observed angiographically (0.5–12 percent[26,31,32,58–60]) or associated with symptoms of myocardial ischemia (18 percent[32]): (1) length of the tunneled coronary segment, (2) degree of systolic compression, and (3) heart rate. Longer tunneled segments of coronary arteries,[27] more severe systolic diameter narrowing of the tunneled segment,[27] and tachycardia[33] may contribute to the production of myocardial ischemia with myocardial bridging (see Figs. 39-17 and 39-18). The length of coronary tunneling may not always be an important factor in causing myocardial ischemia, since three patients with left main intramyocardial tunneling of greater than 40 mm have been described without evidence of myocardial ischemia[34,35] (Fig. 39-19).

Treatment of symptomatic, clinically recognized myocardial bridges has involved beta and calcium-channel blockers (control of tachycardia and antispasmodic effects) and surgery. Several patients have now been reported[61–63] in which "supraarterial myotomy" (release of the myocardial bridge, excision of the myocardial bridge) has resulted in relief of symptoms and improvement in previously abnormal nuclear imaging tests. High-frequency intraoperative echocardiography has been used to image the intramyocardial coronary artery before and after surgical release.[61]

Coronary Artery Fistula

A *coronary artery fistula* is an abnormal communication between an epicardial coronary artery and a cardiac chamber, major vessel (vena cava, pulmonary veins, pulmonary artery), or other vascular structure (mediastinal vessels, coronary sinus)[5,64–113] (Fig. 39-20). This infrequent abnormality can affect persons of any age and is the most important hemodynamically significant coronary artery anomaly.[5,64–113] Many are small and found incidentally during coronary arteriography, whereas others are identified as the cause of a continuous murmur, myocardial ischemia and angina, acute myocardial infarction, sudden death, coronary steal, congestive heart failure, endocarditis, stroke, arrhythmias, coronary aneurysm formation (rupture, emboli), or superior vena cava syndrome.[64–76] Of over 33,000 patients undergoing coronary arteriography,[34] coronary artery fistula occurred in 0.1 percent,[76] whether due to congenital[77–85] or acquired causes[76–113] (Table 39-3). Fistulas from the right coronary artery are more common than from the left,[64–113] and over 90 percent of the fistulas drain into the venous circulation.[64–113] Most fistulas are single communications, but multiple fistulas have been identified.[106] The natural history of coronary artery fistulas is variable, with long periods of stability in some and sudden onset or gradual progression of symptoms in others. Spontaneous closure is uncommon.[106–108] Surgical repair of the fistula is recommended for symptomatic patients and for those asymptomatic patients at risk for future complications (coronary steals, aneurysms, large shunts).[109–112] Transcatheter embolization of fistulas has been reported.[113] Direct connection between a major epicardial coronary artery and a cardiac chamber or major vessel (vena cava, coronary sinus, pulmonary artery) is the most common hemodynamically significant coronary artery anomaly[5] (see Fig. 39-19). Myocardial ischemia has been documented in some patients with coronary artery fistulas who have no evidence of coronary atherosclerosis.[5]

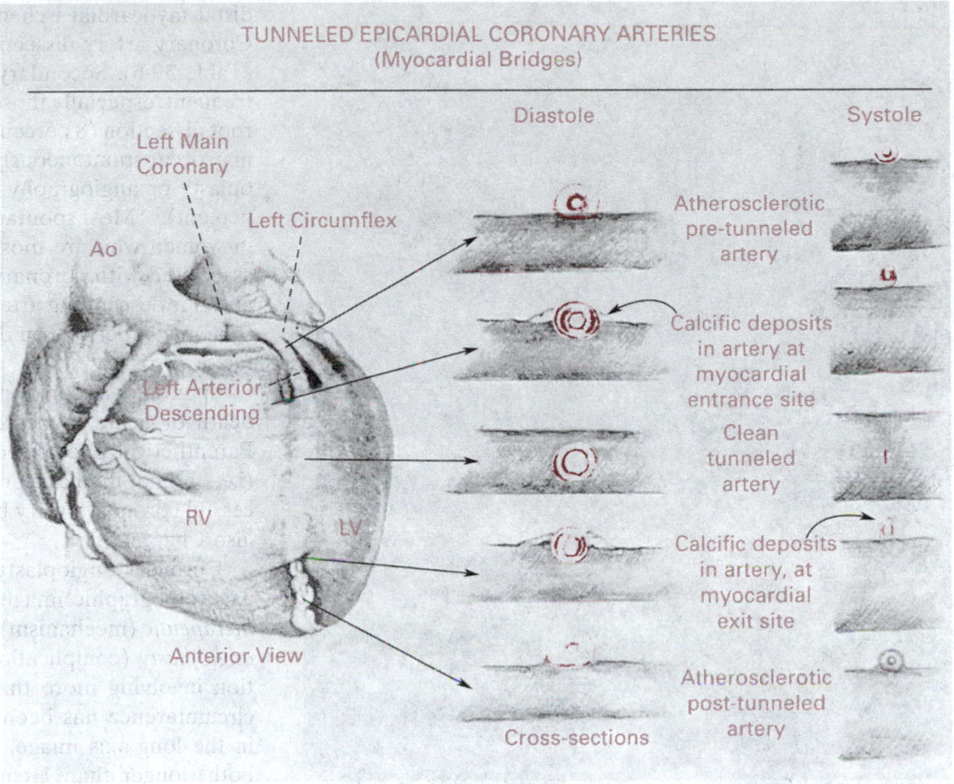

FIGURE 39-12 Diagram showing segments of tunneled and nontunneled epicardial coronary artery with changes during ventricular systole and diastole. Ao, aorta; LV, left ventricle; RV, right ventricle. (From Waller.[10] Reproduced with permission from the publisher, editor, and author.)

CORONARY ANEURYSMS

Aneurysm formation of the coronary arteries may result from congenital or acquired conditions. Congenital coronary artery aneurysms are found most commonly in the right coronary artery.[114] Abnormal flow patterns within the aneurysm may lead to thrombus formation with subsequent vessel occlusion, distal thromboembolization, and myocardial infarction.[115] In general, angina pectoris or acute myocardial infarction present in patients younger than 20 years of age should prompt suspicion of a congenital coronary artery anomaly or a congenital coronary artery aneurysm.[114] Coronary artery aneurysms are found in about 1.5 percent of patients studied at necropsy or by coronary arteriography.[37] Coronary artery aneurysms, which may be multiple, can be congenital or the result of atherosclerosis, trauma, angioplasty, atherectomy, laser procedures, arteritis (including syphilis), mycotic emboli, mucocutaneous lymph node syndrome (Kawasaki's disease), systemic lupus erythematosus,[116] or dissection (spontaneous or secondary) (Table 39-4). Atherosclerosis-induced aneurysms are thought to result from primary thinning and/or destruction of the media and may represent up to 50 percent of the causes (see Table 39-4). Angioplasty, atherectomy, vasculitis, and arteritis also may damage the arterial wall (media) and lead to coronary aneurysms.

CORONARY ARTERY EMBOLI

Coronary arterial emboli (Figs. 39-21 to 39-25) are clinically suspected in patients who develop severe chest pain with acute myocardial infarction in the presence of a prosthetic left-sided valve, active infective endocarditis, native left-sided valve stenosis, atrial fibrillation, LV aneurysm, dilated cardiomyopathy (see Fig. 39-22), known cardiac tumor, or during cardiac catheterization or cardiac surgery. Coronary emboli can be due to natural, iatrogenic, or "paradoxical" causes (Table 39-5; see also Figs. 39-21 to 39-25).[117–138] Coronary embolism most often involves the left anterior descending coronary artery.[36]

Coronary embolism is suspected as the cause of acute myocardial infarction when, at necropsy, the zone of necrosis is large but discrete (since there was little time to develop effective collaterals). Embolic coronary artery lesions can resolve completely and spontaneously and provide an explanation for angiographically normal coronary arteries several months following an acute myocardial infarction.[36]

The consequences of coronary embolism depend on two major factors (see Fig. 39-25): the size of the embolus and the size of the lumen of the artery in which it becomes impacted.[139,140] The smaller the embolus, the greater is the chance that it will travel distally to a small coronary arterial segment and the less is the likelihood of myocardial infarction or fatal arrhythmia.[139]

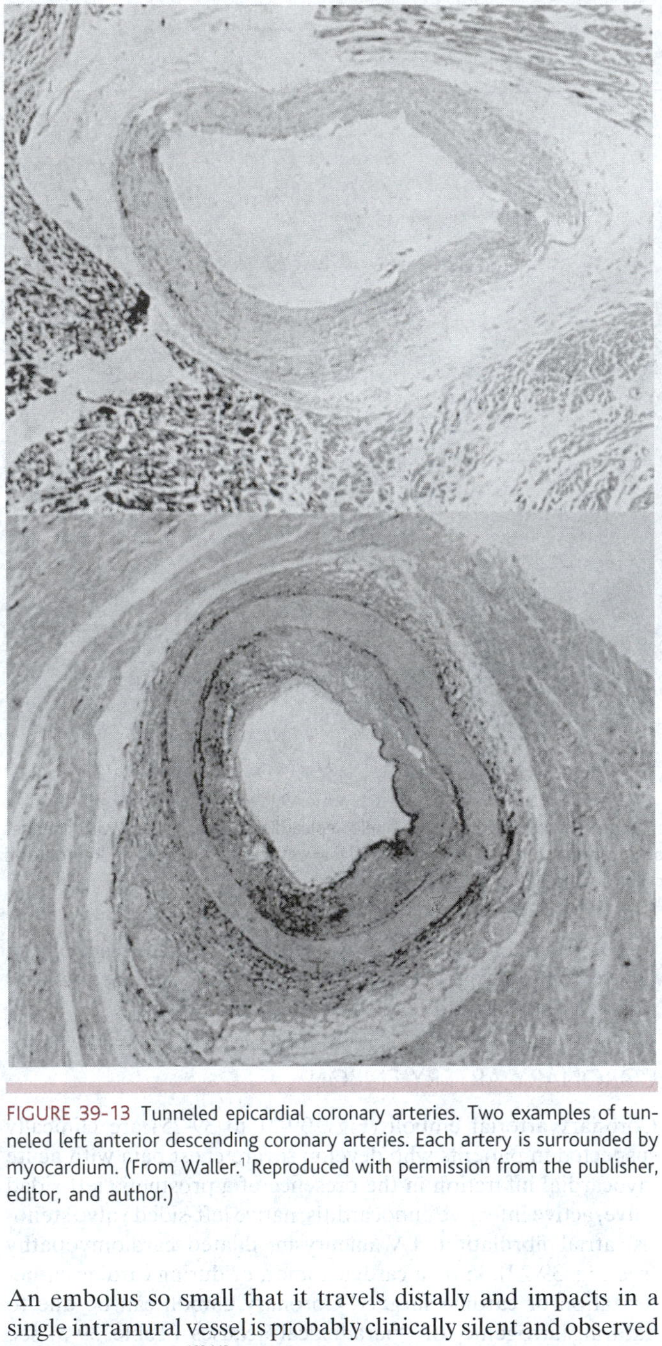

FIGURE 39-13 Tunneled epicardial coronary arteries. Two examples of tunneled left anterior descending coronary arteries. Each artery is surrounded by myocardium. (From Waller.[1] Reproduced with permission from the publisher, editor, and author.)

An embolus so small that it travels distally and impacts in a single intramural vessel is probably clinically silent and observed only at necropsy.[139,140] The status of the coronary lumen before the embolus appears also determines the subsequent myocardial consequences. An embolus to a previously normal coronary artery is likely to migrate distally and result in localized myocardial infarction because of absence of collaterals. An embolus traveling to a previously diseased coronary artery is more likely to impact proximally. Emboli to the left main coronary arteries are rare but usually fatal[140] (see Fig. 39-24).

CORONARY ARTERY DISSECTION

Separation of the media by hemorrhage with or without an associated intimal tear is termed *coronary artery dissection*. The medial separation forces the intimal-medial layer (wall of the true channel) toward the true coronary lumen and produces distal myocardial ischemia/infarction (Figs. 39-26 and 39-27). Coronary artery dissections may be primary or secondary[141–168] (Table 39-6). Secondary coronary artery dissections are more frequent, especially those associated as an extension from aortic root dissection (8 percent).[5] Primary coronary artery dissections may occur spontaneously or as a consequence of coronary angioplasty or angiography, cardiac surgery, or chest trauma (0.3 percent).[158] Most spontaneous coronary artery dissections occur in women who are most commonly postpartum; they may be associated with coronary artery wall eosinophils.[141–165] The left anterior descending artery is the one most frequently involved. Systemic hypertension does not appear to provide a significant factor of risk.[114]

Spontaneous coronary artery dissection may result in sudden death or acute myocardial infarction and subsequent death. Parenthetically, localized and limited coronary artery dissection (i.e., intimal-medial tear) appears necessary for a clinically successful coronary artery balloon angioplasty procedure[143,144] (see also Chap. 45).

Coronary angioplasty dissections viewed in short- or long-axis tomographic images help distinguish dissections that are *therapeutic* (mechanism) from those which are *complications of angioplasty* (complications).[168] In the short-axis image, dissection involving more than 50 percent of the coronary medial circumference has been considered a complication. Similarly, in the long-axis image, dissections (antegrade, retrograde, or both) longer than 1 cm in length also have been defined as a complication of angioplasty (Fig. 39-28). A combination of dissection greater than 50 percent of the short-axis circumference and greater than 1 cm antegrade or retrograde of long-axis length may result in "intussusception" of intimal-medial tissue. Spiral dissections ("the ugly") are among the most serious dissection injuries after balloon angioplasty (Fig. 39-29). The spiral dissection as reviewed angiographically appears to alternate from side to side, extending antegrade and retrograde (see Fig. 39-29*A*), or it has an unaltered dissection course but appears alternating from limited angiographic views (see Fig. 39-29*B*).

CORONARY ARTERY SPASM

Coronary artery luminal narrowing produced by spasm has been associated with angina pectoris, acute myocardial infarction, and sudden death[141,169–195] (see also Chap. 41). Despite the extensive clinical information about coronary artery spasm, relatively few necropsy data are available.[169–181] Smooth muscle cells in the coronary artery wall may contract in response to various neurologic and pharmacologic stimuli and temporarily reduce the vessel lumen. Specific pathogenesis of this disorder is unknown.[180] Enhanced α-adrenergic tone[191] and various vasoactive substances—such as histamine, catecholamines, prostaglandins, and thromboxane[189–192]—are presently thought to be relevant factors. Necropsy findings have been reviewed in 13 previously reported patients and in 3 new patients[141,180,195] (Figs. 39-30 and 39-31).

Most of the 13 previous patients with clinical evidence of spasm had significant fixed coronary luminal narrowing due to atherosclerotic plaque, although coronary angiograms during life did not recognize these lesions found at necropsy.[141,195] In one of the original patients described by Prinzmetal et al.,[169] both major epicardial coronary arteries were "markedly sclerotic," and the "posterior coronary artery" was 80 percent narrowed. Of the subsequent 12 necropsy patients, 10 had at least one major artery severely narrowed by atherosclerotic plaque at necropsy.[169–181] The 3 necropsy patients with clinical spasm[141,180] all had severe luminal coronary narrowing by atherosclerotic plaque at least in the artery in which spasm had been demonstrated during life (see Figs. 39-30 and 39-31). In general, histologic sections of the left anterior descending artery at the site of spasm disclosed luminal concentric plaque that had a predominance of smooth muscle cells, suggesting that the lesion may have been responsive to pharmacologic and neurologic stimuli compared with "garden variety" fibrotic and calcified atherosclerotic plaque (see Fig. 39-31). In a patient with normal angiograms and documented myocardial infarction, "intimal ridges" were observed on postmortem angiography; these were interpreted as evidence of spasm.[194] Similar ridges have been noted at necropsy in a patient with coronary artery spasm.[195] Histology of the ridges disclosed typical atherosclerotic plaque,[196] suggesting that varying degrees of dynamic muscular contraction may be superimposed on fixed atherosclerotic lesions, presumably related to the amount of smooth muscle present.[141] Coronary artery smooth muscle depletion ("medial attenuation"), which accompanies advanced degrees of luminal narrowing by atherosclerotic plaque, suggests diminished potential for coronary wall spasm.[196] It has been suggested recently that medial "contraction" bands may represent a morphologic-histologic marker for arteries that have spasm during life[197] (see also Chap. 41).

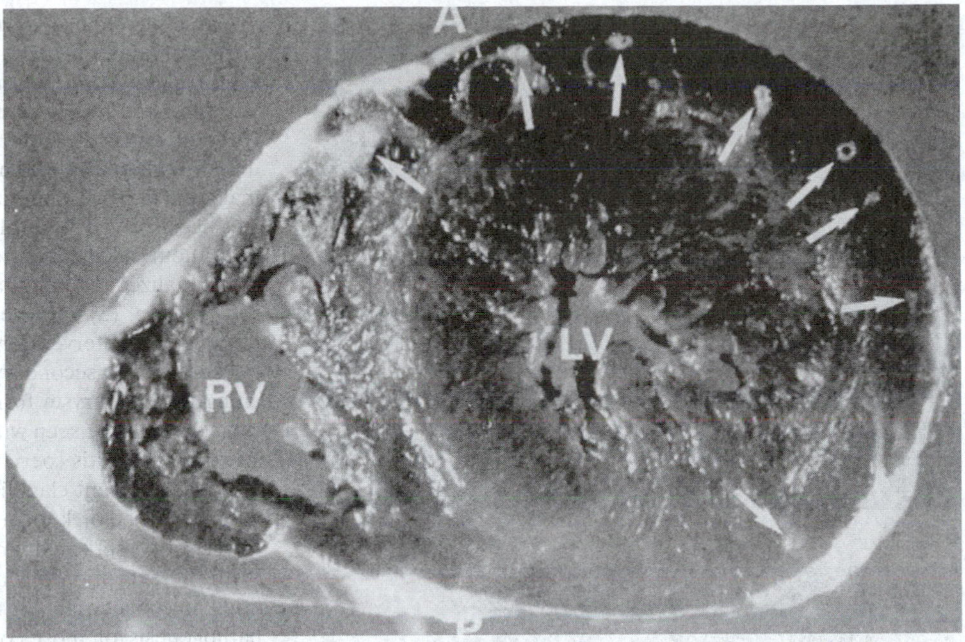

FIGURE 39-14 Transverse section of ventricular myocardium showing the "arcade" of tunneled epicardial coronary arteries (*arrows*). A, anterior; LV, left ventricle; RV, right ventricle; P, posterior. (From Waller.[1] Reproduced with permission from the publisher, editor, and author.)

Eccentric atherosclerotic plaques have a segment of disease-free wall with preserved media that presumably has the potential for spasm.[198] In patients with clinical coronary spasm, unstable and stable angina pectoris, and episodes of silent myocardial ischemia, where 448 segments were narrowed by more than 75 percent in cross-sectional area by plaques, 15 percent of these segments had a variable arc of disease-free wall with normal media.[199] Other studies have found a similar 15 to 20 percent of the coronary wall normal in 70 percent of patients studied.[200–205] This disease-free coronary segment represents a site of "vasospastic potential" and could convert a hemodynamically insignificant lesion of less than 50 percent cross-sectional area into a hemodynamically significant one of more than 75 percent narrowing.

Three newly recognized associations and/or causes of coronary artery spasm include general anesthesia,[184] "allergic angina" (histamine-induced),[185] and postpartum bromocriptine use.[186] Acute ST-segment elevation has been noted following induction of general anesthesia in some patients with angiographically normal coronary arteries.[184] In postpartum women receiving bromocriptine in the presence of pregnancy-induced hypertension, acute myocardial infarction has occurred.[186] Coronary spasm also occurs with balloon angioplasty and coronary interventional procedures,[187] catheter-related angiography, and neurofibromatosis.[188]

Endothelial cell dysfunction has been proposed to explain coronary vasospasm.[189] In response to increases in shear stress, platelet products, and other agonists, normal endothelial cells release endothelium-derived relaxing factor (nitric oxide), resulting in vasodilation.[189] When endothelium is damaged, as occurs with hypertension, elevated cholesterol, smoking, or use of cocaine, endothelial nitric oxide is reduced or lost. Thus, when platelets aggregate at such sites with release of vasospastic substances such as serotonin (5HT) and thromboxane A_2, arterial smooth muscle cells contract, causing spasm.[190]

CORONARY ARTERY TRAUMA

Coronary artery trauma may produce myocardial ischemia and/or acute myocardial infarction. Traumatic injury may result from a nonpenetrating blunt chest wall injury such as a steering-wheel impact, penetration trauma such as a laceration from a stab wound or bullet, coronary artery bypass surgery as from inadvertent ligation, laceration, or intimal dissection, or after coronary angiography or angioplasty resulting in dissection, rupture, or embolus. Nonpenetrating trauma may produce coronary artery injury and subsequent myocardial infarction due to coronary artery dissection, contusion and thrombosis, fistula formation, and/or coronary artery aneurysm formation.[5] Extensive coronary artery dissections occur more commonly as the result of catheter or cannula injury in normal or nearly normal

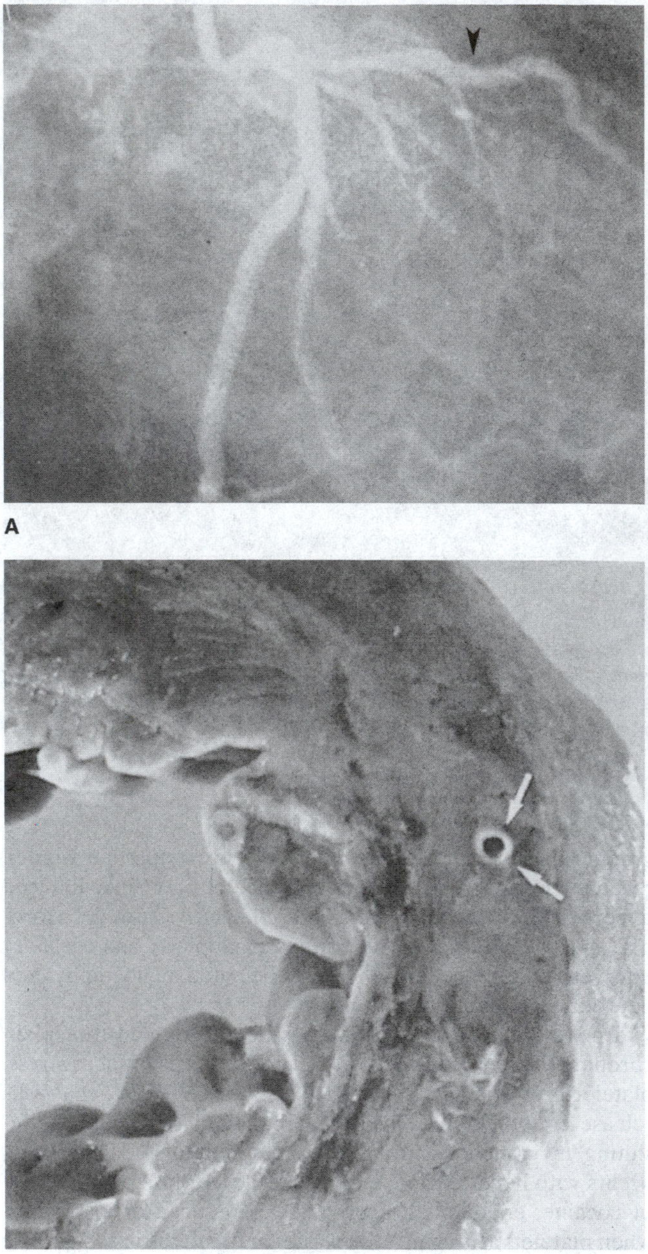

A

B

FIGURE 39-15 Tunneled epicardial coronary artery. *A.* Coronary angiogram showing tunneled segment of epicardial coronary artery. *B.* Corresponding segment of tunneled left circumflex coronary artery (*arrow*). (From Waller.[1] Reproduced with permission from the publisher, editor, and author.)

arteries as opposed to coronary arteries with severe atherosclerotic plaque (see also Chap. 79).

CORONARY ARTERY ARTERITIS (VASCULITIS)

Epicardial coronary artery arteritis (vasculitis) is a rare event but has been reported in several conditions (Table 39-7). The resulting coronary artery injury may lead to myocardial ischemia/infarction with or without associated coronary artery thrombosis. This type of coronary artery damage has been classified by route(s) of entry[24]: *direct extension* from adjacent organ or tissue infections, e.g., epicardial or myocardial abscess from aortic valve endocarditis, pericardial infections such as tuberculosis; *hematogenous spread* through the coronary lumen or vasa vasorum; and *unknown* route of entry. In the direct extension route of entry the adventitial layer of the artery is involved initially, whereas in the hematogenous route the coronary intimal layer is involved initially. Evidence of coronary artery arteritis has included[24] the following: (1) focal arterial necrosis with or without calcification, (2) acute coronary artery thrombosis or recanalized thrombus associated with underlying atherosclerotic plaque, (3) rupture of the vessel wall unassociated with trauma or an interventional procedure, (4) coronary artery wall thickening with secondary luminal narrowing, or (5) wall thickening with aneurysm formation.[204] Specific coronary artery lesions also may be seen with systemic diseases such as tuberculosis or polyarteritis (periarteritis).

A more recent classification of coronary artery vasculitides has been based on known and unknown causes and involvement of size of vessel (medium-sized, small-sized)[205,206] (Table 39-8). With the exception of infectious angiitis resulting from syphilitic, mycobacterial, or rickettsial infection, the causes and pathogenesis of most coronary artery vasculitides are either unknown or incompletely understood.[207] Vasculitic syndromes may be caused by deposition of immune complexes in the vessel walls.[209–214] The specific antigen has been identified in only a few cases, such as hepatitis B. Circulating immune complexes associated with hepatitis B infection may cause more than one type of vasculitic syndrome,[205] producing periarteritis nodosa in arteries of muscles and hypersensitivity angiitis in venules while eliciting the production of anti-immunoglobulin antibodies, leading to cryoglobulinemia. Thus a classification of vasculitides *based solely* on immunologic studies is incomplete[205] (see also Chap. 76).

General Concepts

The earliest vasculitic syndrome was named *periarteritis nodosa*[215] because of the nodules along the course of small arteries.[205] Because the inflammatory changes are not only periarterial, *polyarteritis* may be a better term.[216] Periarteritis nodosa has become a "wastebasket designation" of any vasculitis whose cause is unknown.[205] The term *necrotizing angiitis*[217] has been used to designate arterial and venous lesions; there are five types[217,218]: (1) hypersensitivity angiitis, (2) allergic granulomatous angiitis, (3) rheumatoid arteritis, (4) periarteritis nodosa, and (5) temporal arteritis. The term *hypersensitivity angiitis* has been considered synonymous with small-vessel vasculitis and is used to imply that the angiitis is due to an allergic response to proteins, drugs, vaccines, or infections.[205] Allergic *granulomatous angiitis* (Churg-Strauss syndrome) is a variant of polyarteritis characterized by necrotizing vasculitis with extravascular granulomas and eosinophilia associated with asthma or allergic rhinitis.[205,219–221] *Rheumatic arteritis*[222] describes vascular lesions in rheumatic diseases with both rheumatic and necrotizing vascular lesions. *Temporal arteritis* (giant-cell arteritis) involves large and small extracranial arteries, including the coronary arteries, and blindness may be a serious complication.[205,223–228] Despite its limitations, this classification[217,218] remains a basis for the diagnosis of vasculitides. The classification of coronary vasculitis is closely tied to that of vasculitides in general[205] and

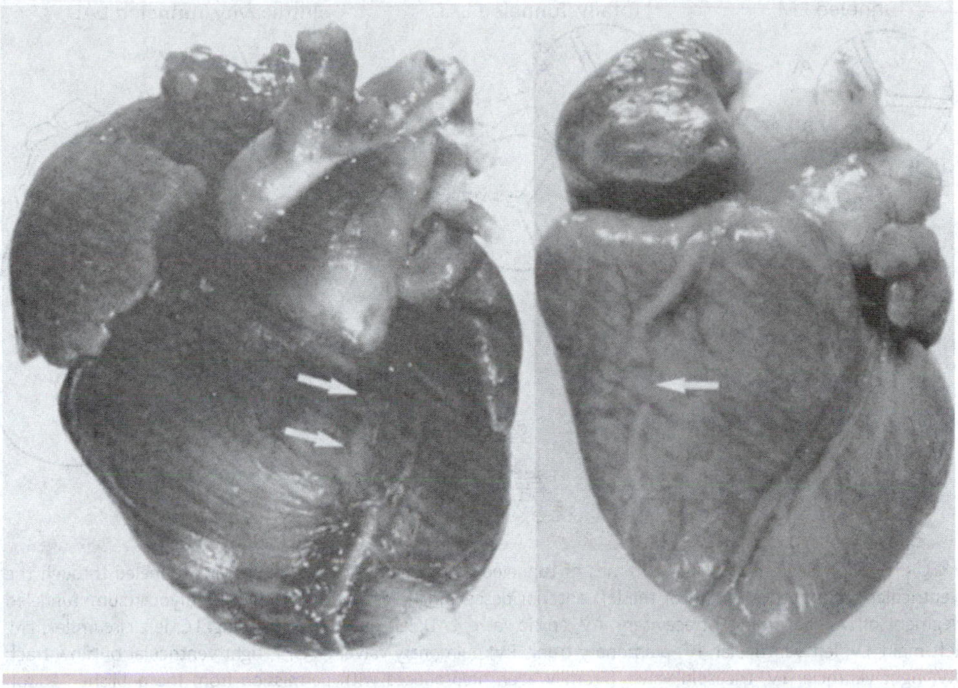

FIGURE 39-16 Tunneled left anterior epicardial coronary arteries from two newborn infants. (*Left*) Tunneled left anterior descending. (*Right*) Tunneled marginal branch of right coronary artery. (From Waller.[1] Reproduced with permission from the publisher, editor, and author.)

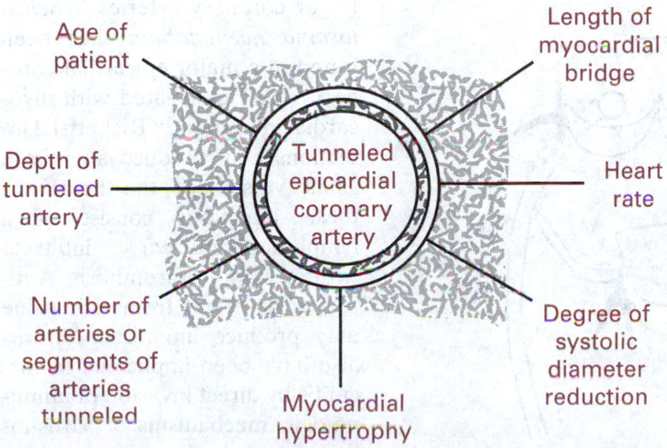

FIGURE 39-17 Diagram showing some of the clinical and anatomic factors in a tunneled epicardial coronary artery. (From Waller.[1] Reproduced with permission from the publisher, editor, and author.)

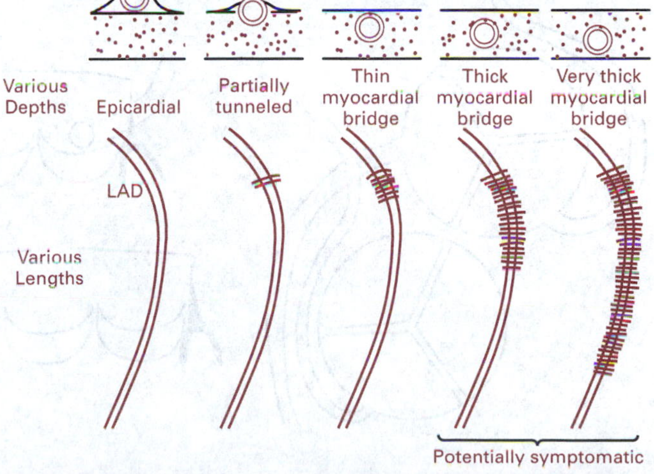

FIGURE 39-18 Diagram showing morphologic variations in tunneling (length of tunneled segment, depth of tunneled segment). (From Waller.[1] Reproduced with permission from the publisher, editor, and author.)

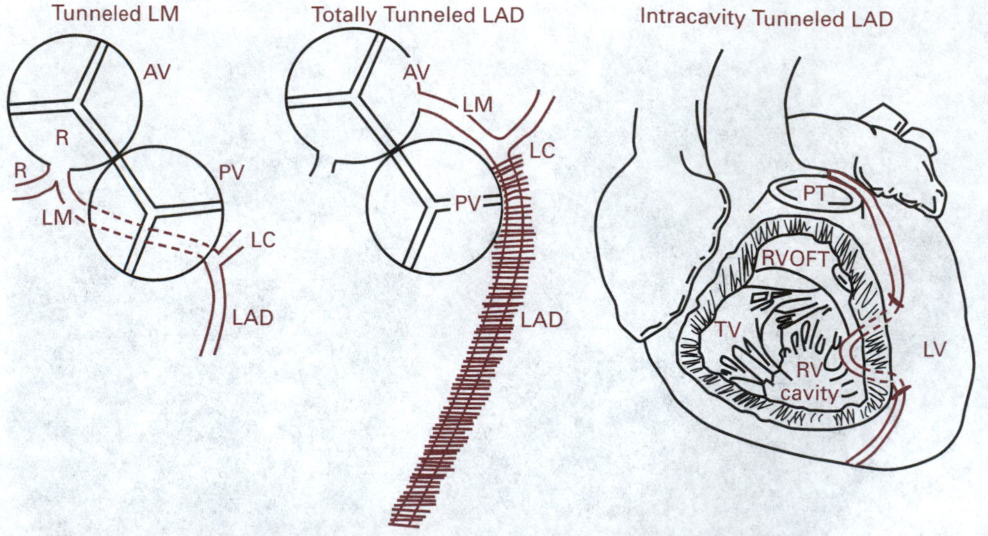

FIGURE 39-19 Diagram showing extremes of tunneled coronary arteries: left main (LM) tunneled through the ventricular septum, total length of the left anterior descending (LAD) located within the myocardium, tunneled segment of LAD becoming intracavitary. AV, aortic valve; LAD, left anterior descending; LC, left circumflex; LM, left main; LV, left ventricular; PT, pulmonary trunk; PV, pulmonary valve; RVOFT, right ventricular outflow tract; RV, right ventricle; TV, tricuspid valve. (From Waller.[1] Reproduced with permission from the publisher, editor, and author.)

relates to the predominant type and size of vessels affected[229,230] (see Table 39-8 and Chap. 79).

Infectious Angiitis

Various microorganisms may cause vasculitis in vessels of any size and involve the vessel by extension of the acute or chronic infective process from an adjacent tissue or organ[24] or from the lumen by hematogenous spread (see Table 39-8). The inflammatory response produces variable reactions including suppurative inflammation (bacteria),[231] proliferative response (typhoid[232]), hemorrhagic response (anthrax), and histiocytic and granulomatous response (leprosy, syphilis, tuberculosis).[4,205] The most important angiitic infections affecting the coronary arteries include syphilis, tuberculosis, and syphilitic arteritis. All three stages of syphilis show arteritic features. The most important vascular lesion of tertiary syphilis, coronary ostial stenosis, seen in up to 4 percent of patients,[5,233–236] can occur independent of aortic involvement.[205,235] Syphilitic arteritis is characterized by a chronic inflammation with adventitial fibrosis and patchy destruction of media with a lymphoplasmacytic infiltrate. Gummas can be found in 20 percent of patients,[237] but spirochetes are detected rarely.[205] The first 3 to 4 mm of the left and right coronary arteries may be involved with an obliterative arteritis[114]; angina and acute myocardial infarction may result from syphilitic involvement.[236]

TUBERCULOUS ARTERITIS

Tuberculous coronary arteritis occurs mainly in patients with pericardial and myocardial tuberculosis.[238,239] Granuloma may involve the adventitia, intima, or entire wall[24,239] and result from several infectious angiitic agents. Endocarditis and septicemia are the most common underlying causes of infectious angiitis and mycotic aneurysm formation.[205,240] Any type of gram-positive or gram-negative organism may be involved. Myocarditis with abscesses and pericarditis frequently accompany infectious coronary angiitis. Mucormycosis, aspergillosis, and *Candida* (Fig. 39-32) are examples of fungi and systemic yeast infections associated with coronary angiitis. Malarial parasites and parasitized red blood cells also may plug larger coronary arteries.[241] *Schistosoma haematobium* has been found in a major epicardial coronary artery associated with myocardial infarction.[242] Rickettsial infections may produce angiitis in small vessels of the heart[205,243]; these infections consist of a lymphomononuclear infiltrate with or without thrombosis. A direct toxic effect from rickettsiae may produce angiitis.[244] Viruses also have been implicated in vasculitis by direct invasion of immunologic mechanisms.[205] Virus-induced vasculitides in humans are represented by polyarteritis associated with hepatitis B antigenemia[205,245,246] and herpes zoster.[205]

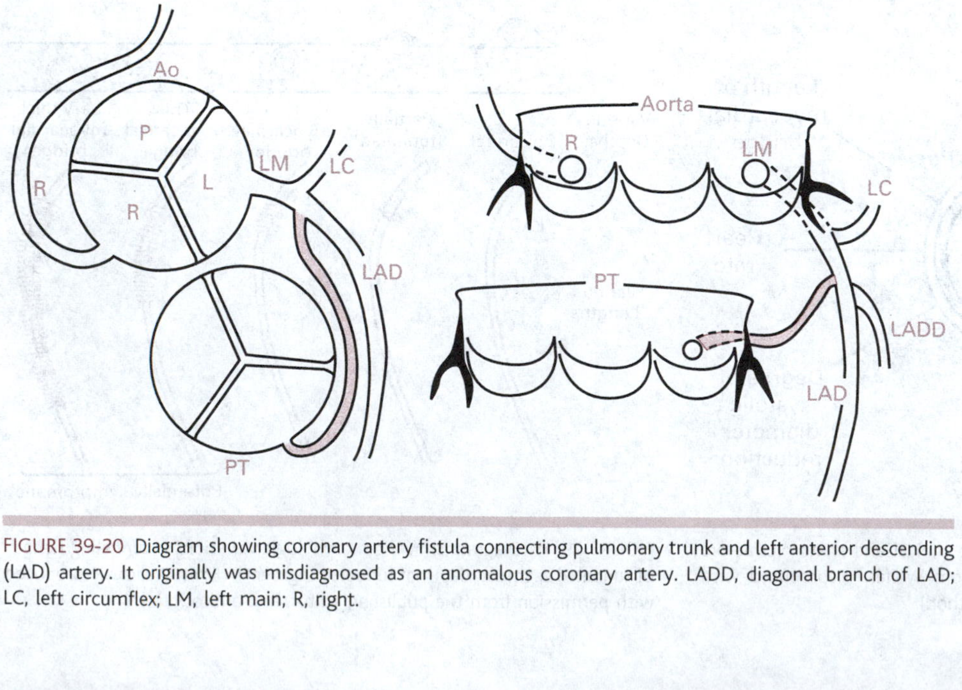

FIGURE 39-20 Diagram showing coronary artery fistula connecting pulmonary trunk and left anterior descending (LAD) artery. It originally was misdiagnosed as an anomalous coronary artery. LADD, diagonal branch of LAD; LC, left circumflex; LM, left main; R, right.

TABLE 39-3 Causes and Associations of Coronary Artery Fistula

I. Congenital[77–85]
   1. Embryonic
   2. Multiple; systemic hemangioma

II. Acquired
   1. Closed-chest ablation of accessory pathway[86]
   2. Percutaneous coronary balloon angioplasty[87–89]
   3. Hypertrophic cardiomyopathy[90]
   4. Right/left ventricular septal myectomy[101]
   5. Penetrating and nonpenetrating trauma[102–104]
   6. Acute myocardial infarction[91,93]
   7. Dilated cardiomyopathy[94]
   8. Mitral valve surgery[95]
   9. "Sign" of mural thrombus[96]
   10. Tumor[100]
   11. Permanent pacemaker placement[99]
   12. Cardiac transplant[92]
   13. Endomyocardial biopsy[97,98]
   14. Coronary artery bypass grafting[105]

Noninfectious Angiitis

Various noninfectious causes of angiitis involve large to medium-sized (predominately medium-sized and small) blood vessels[205] (see Table 39-8).

TAKAYASU'S ARTERITIS

Takayasu's disease (pulseless disease) is one of the coronary vasculitides associated with aortitis; others are temporal arteritides and rheumatic disease (see also Chaps. 88 and 90). Takayasu's disease is a chronic, occlusive inflammatory disease of unknown etiology[205,247–256] with a worldwide distribution and greater incidence in young to middle-aged female Asians.[249–250] Involvement of the coronary arteries occurs in 15 to 25 percent of patients and may be the lethal complication[248,250–255,257] (Fig. 39-33), commonly involving the coronary ostium[248,257,258–263] with segmental involvement of distal coronary arteries.[252–255,264] Rarely, diffuse coronary arteritis is produced by Takayasu's disease.[265]

TABLE 39-4 Causes of Coronary Arterial Aneurysms

- Atherosclerosis (destruction of coronary media)
- Trauma
- Angioplasty
- Atherectomy
- Laser
- Arteritis (including syphilis, lupus erythematosus)
- Mycotic emboli
- Mucocutaneous lymph node syndrome (Kawasaki's disease)
- Congenital
- Dissection
- Neoplasm
- Connective tissue disorders (Ehlers-Danlos, Marfan's)

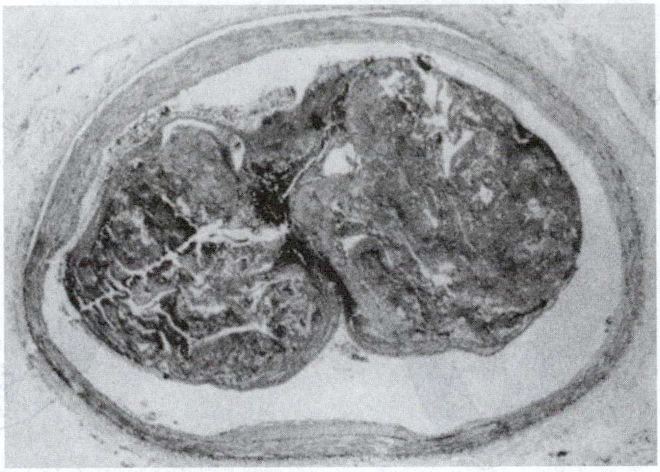

FIGURE 39-21 Coronary artery embolus. Fibrin-platelet thrombus occluding the left anterior descending coronary artery. The source of the embolus was not established, but the patient recently underwent cardiac surgery. (From Waller.[1] Reproduced with permission from the publisher, editor, and author.)

GRANULOMATOUS GIANT-CELL ARTERITIS (TEMPORAL ARTERITIS)

Granulomatous giant-cell arteritis may occur independently or, more commonly, may be associated with temporal arteritis in 10 to 15 percent of patients.[205,226–228,266–277] Histologically proven giant-cell coronary arteritis is rare, and cases leading to fatal myocardial infarction are even rarer[205,266,269–272,274] (Fig. 39-34). The arterial wall lesion is a granulomatous inflammation with giant cells found along degenerative internal elastic membrane.[274] The intima becomes greatly thickened, and ultimately, the vessel is converted into a fibrous cord. Luminal thrombosis also may have been present in 16 patients with temporal arteritis reported by Harrison[275]; only 1 case involved the epicardial coronary arteries. Giant-cell arteritis of the intramural (intramyocardial) coronary arteries (Fig. 39-35) also may occur in association with temporal arteritis and giant-cell arteries[266] (see also Chaps. 76, 88, and 90).

Rheumatic Arteritis

Rheumatic diseases commonly affect the aorta and are morphologically indistinguishable from granulomatous aortitis.[205,276–293] Coronary arteritis at necropsy has been detected in up to 20 percent of patients with rheumatoid arthritis, usually involving small intramural vessels.[276–297] The small-vessel arteritis also may involve conduction system vessels leading to various forms of heart block.[291–293] Rheumatoid coronary vasculitis producing myocardial infarction is rare.[282–285,296,297] Histologically, extraaortic rheumatoid vasculitis (coronary artery vasculitis) is usually a polyarteritis type of necrotizing angiitis[205,281,286–290] and not a giant-cell arteritis (Fig. 39-36). Small myocardial vessels also may be severely narrowed in ankylosing spondylosis. Occlusion of the left main ostium has been described.[293]

Buerger's Disease

Thromboangiitis obliterans (Buerger's disease), which is very rare[205,298–307] (Fig. 39-37), is a nonatherosclerotic, occlusive, inflammatory vascular disease of unknown cause occurring mainly

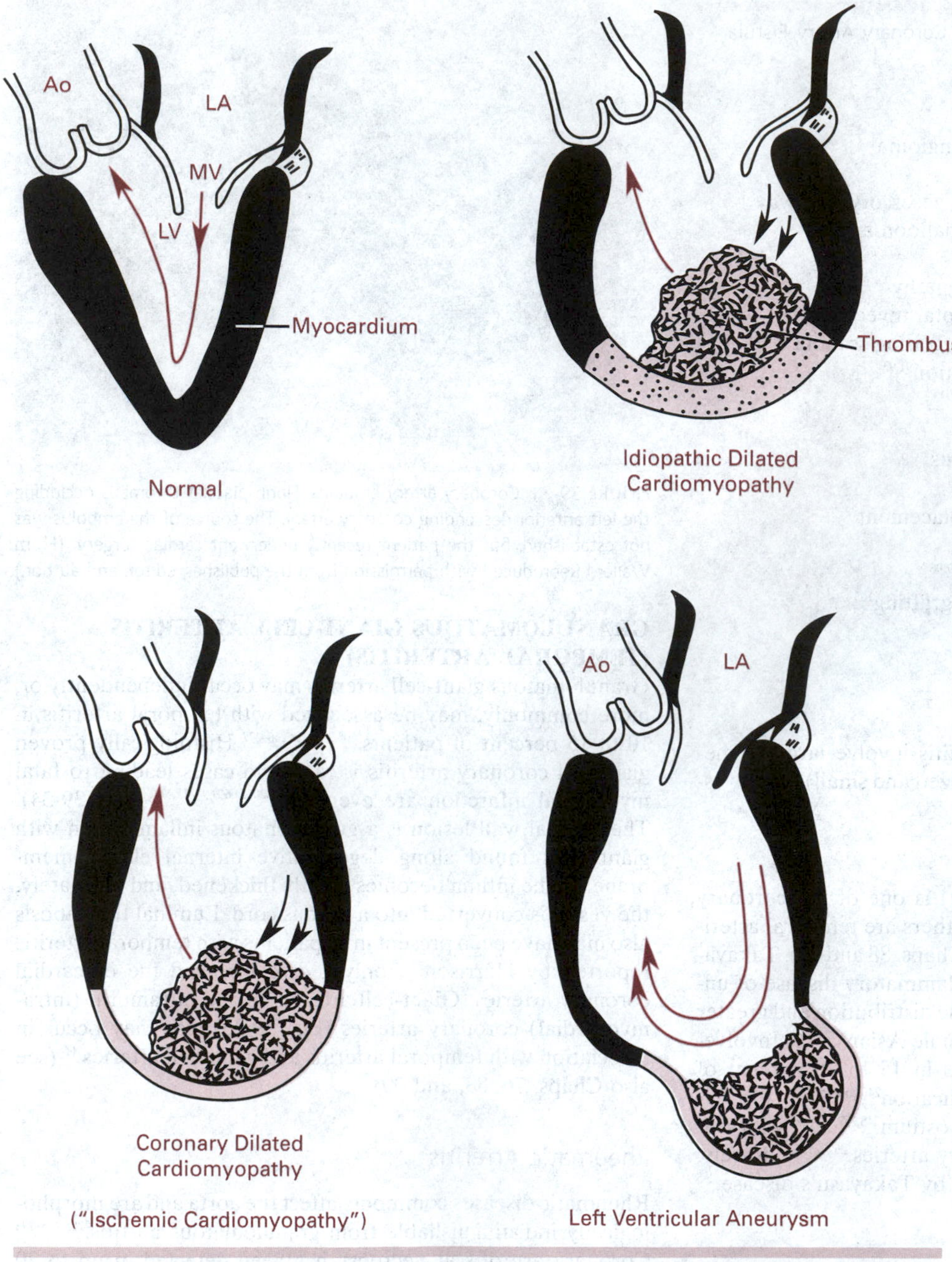

FIGURE 39-22 Diagram showing factors associated with emboli from LV thrombus in three conditions: (1) idiopathic dilated cardiomyopathy (IDC), (2) coronary dilated cardiomyopathy (CDC), and (3) LV aneurysm. Thrombus protruding into the LV cavity (IDC, CDC) is more likely to embolize than thrombus protected within the sac of an LV aneurysm. Underlying myocardial contraction is more likely to propel thrombus out the LV outflow tract than paradoxical motion of LV aneurysm. Ao, aorta; LA, left atrium; MV, mitral valve. (From Cabin and Roberts.[138] Reproduced with permission from the publisher, editor, and author.)

in young males who are heavy smokers of cigarettes[205] (see also Chap. 90). In a few patients, the coronary arteries have shown focal polymorphonuclear infiltrates, histiocytes, and giant cells with or without coronary artery thrombosis.[304] Coronary involvement is rare,[304] although coronary thrombosis may be seen.[308] Buerger's disease involving a saphenous vein bypass graft also has been documented.[309]

Polyarteritis (Necrotizing) Angiitis

CLASSIC POLYARTERITIS NODOSA

Classic polyarteritis nodosa is a chronic systemic disease manifest by infarction or hemorrhage in various target organs as the result of necrotizing vasculitis.[215] Male patients are affected twice as often as female, with a mean age of 45 years.[205,310–314] It is probably the most common cause of coronary angiitis with both epicardial and intramural coronary arteries being affected[24,310–320] (Fig. 39-38). In a review of 66 necropsy cases,[315] 41 (62 percent) had involvement of the epicardial coronary arteries, including 25 (61 percent) with involvement of both the epicardial and intramural coronary arteries, whereas 16 (39 percent) had only involvement of the intramural arteries. Frequently, various stages of acute disease and healing are seen in the same arterial segment. The acute phase has an acute cellular reaction with destruction of the media and internal elastic membrane.[316] The healing stage results in fibrous internal proliferation. Coronary arteries may dilate to form small berry-like aneurysms (becoming occluded by thrombus), rupture, or produce fatal myocardial infarction,[315,317–320] pericardial tamponade, or sudden death (see also Chap. 76).

INFANTILE POLYARTERITIS

Polyarteritis nodosa occurring in infants under 2 years of age (infantile polyarteritis) differs from the clinical pathologic features of classic polyarteritis nodosa.[205,321–324] Infantile disease involves a higher frequency (79 percent) of coronary vasculitis and aneurysmal disease of the coronary arteries with sparing of vessels in other locations[205,321–324] (Fig. 39-39). Kawasaki's disease may involve children up to 8 or 10 years of age[205] rather than being confined to patients under age 2 as in infantile polyarteritis.[325]

TABLE 39-5 Etiology of Coronary Artery Emboli

Natural	Iatrogenic
Vegetation	Cardiac surgery (ostial cannulization, prosthetic valve, patch repair)
Active infective endocarditis (native valve)	Cardiac catheterization and angiography (catheter thrombus, catheter fragments)
Active infective endocarditis (prosthetic valve)	Coronary angioplasty, other interventions, catheter balloon valvuloplasty and thrombolysis
Mural endocarditis	Prosthetic valves (thrombus, vegetation, occluders, leaflets, cloth covering, struts)
Noninfective (marantic) endocarditis	Cardioversion (left atrial thrombus, left ventricular thrombus)
Calcific deposit	Cardiac resuscitation (thrombus)
Aortic valve stenosis	Trauma—blunt penetrating, nonpenetrating, foreign body (bullet)
Mitral valve stenosis	"Paradoxical"
Intracardiac thrombus	Congenital heart disease (atrial septal defect, ventricular septal defect)
Left ventricle (myocardial infarction, cardiomyopathy, fibroelastosis with mural thrombus, ventricular aneurysm)	Probe patent foramen ovale defect (thrombophlebitis, right atrial catheters)
Left atrium—appendage (low-cardiac-output states)	Pulmonary hypertension (acquired atrial septal defect)
Left atrium—body (mitral stenosis, native or prosthetic)	Interatrial flap valve (fossa ovale aneurysm)
Pulmonary veins (mitral stenosis)	
Intracardiac tumor	
Primary (myxoma)	
Secondary (extension from pulmonary veins, lymphatic extension, direct extension)	
Coronary artery	
Plaque rupture (cholesterol)	
Thrombus dislodgment	

SOURCE: Waller.[1] Reproduced with permission from the author, editor, and publisher.

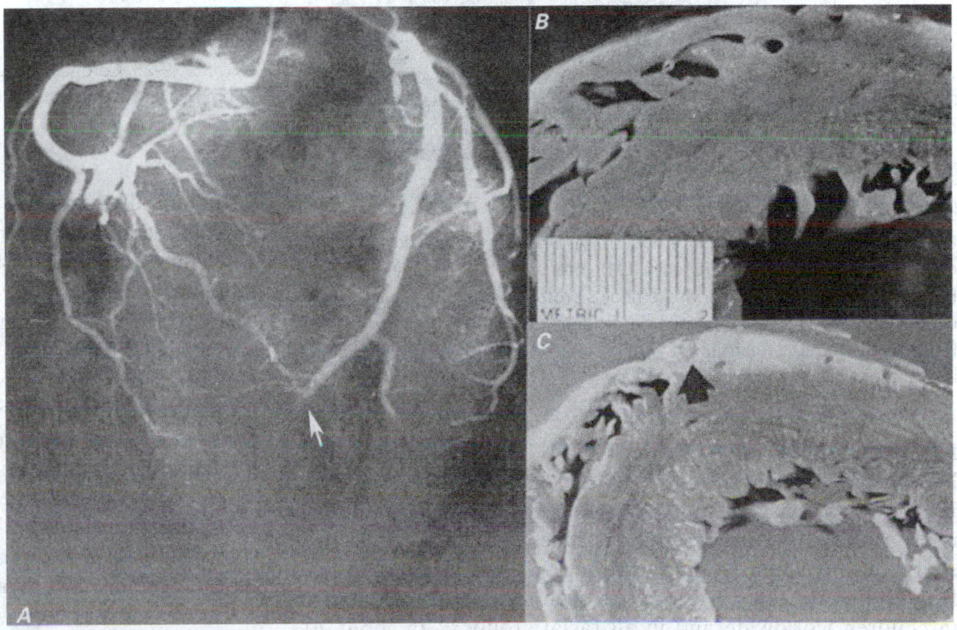

FIGURE 39-23 Coronary artery embolus. *A*. Postmortem coronary angiogram showing normal epicardial coronary arteries except for sudden cutoff of the distal third of the left anterior coronary artery (*arrow*). *B*. Portion of anterior left ventricle and proximal left anterior descending coronary artery showing normal artery. *C*. Site (*arrow*) of embolic occlusion of the left anterior descending coronary artery. The remaining distal left anterior descending, right, left circumflex, and left main coronary arteries were normal. (From Waller.[1] Reproduced with permission from the publisher, editor, and author.)

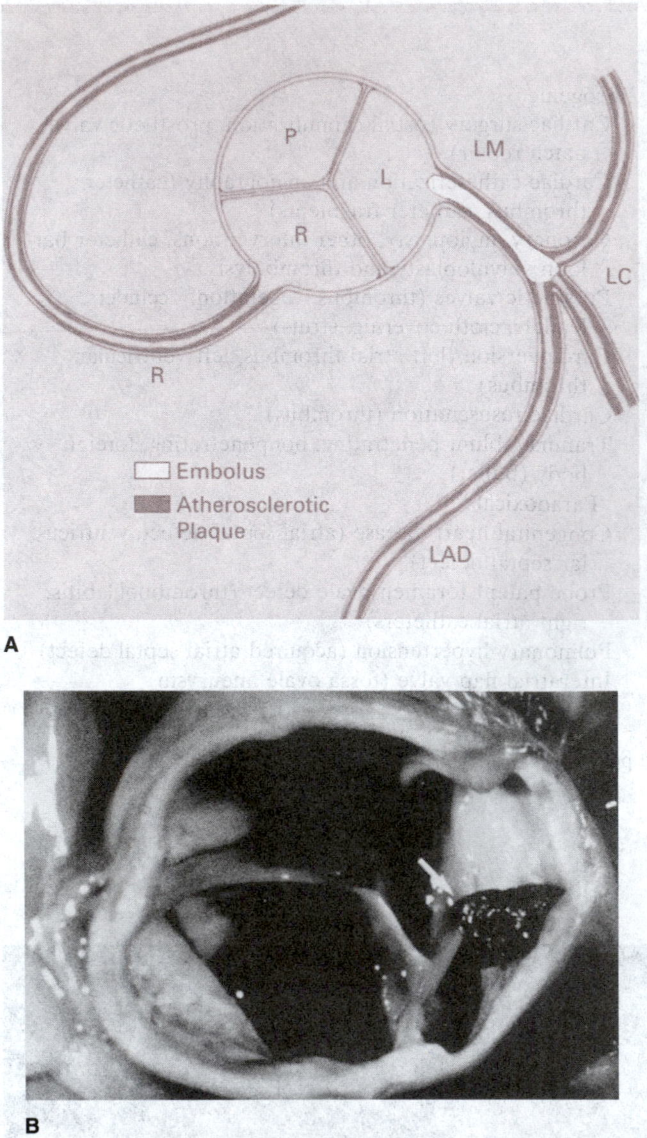

FIGURE 39-24 Coronary artery embolism. *A*. Diagram showing location and extent of occlusion of the left main (LM) coronary artery by an embolus. *B*. Photograph of aortic root showing embolus protruding from the LM coronary ostium (*arrow*). LAD, left anterior descending; LC, left circumflex; R, right. (From Waller et al.[140] Reproduced with permission from the publisher, editor, and author.)

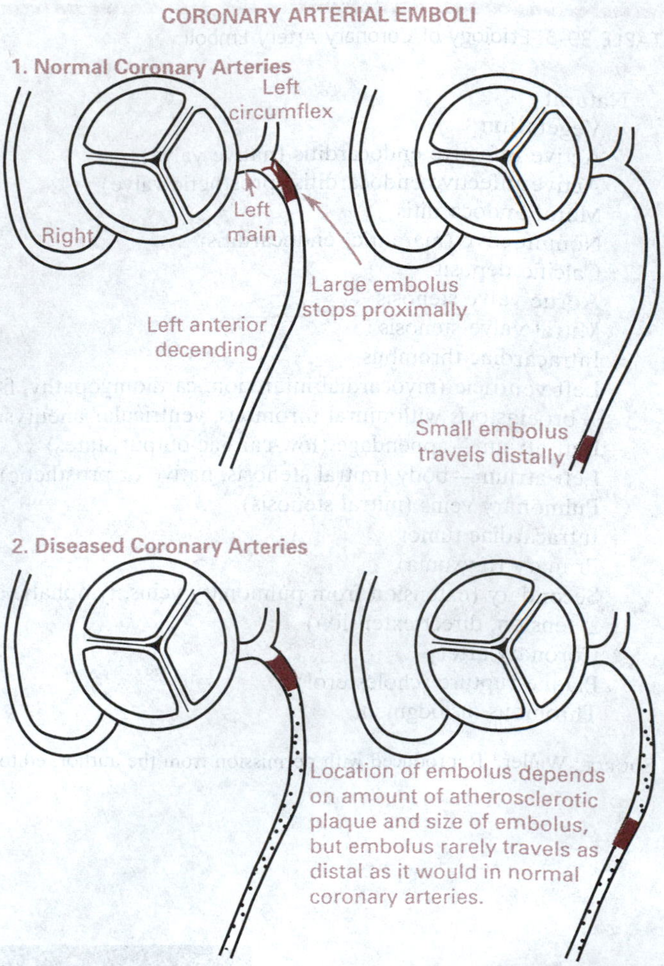

FIGURE 39-25 Coronary emboli in normal and diseased coronary arteries. (From Waller.[1] Reproduced with permission from the publisher, editor, and author.)

KAWASAKI'S DISEASE (MUCOCUTANEOUS LYMPH NODE SYNDROME)

Kawasaki's disease, or mucocutaneous lymph node syndrome, is an acute febrile exanthematous illness of children first described in the Japanese literature in 1967 and reported in the English literature in 1974.[326] It has been reported subsequently in children worldwide and in all racial groups.[327] In about 20 percent of children with the acute illness, a vasculitis of the coronary vasa vasorum leads to coronary arterial aneurysm formation, thrombosis, acute myocardial infarction, and sudden death.[326–339] Estimates of death from acute infarction or ventricular fibrillation range from 1 to 2 percent.[332–334] Late presentation with myocardial infarction secondary to dislodged aneurysmal thrombosis also may occur[332,333,335,337] (Figs. 39-40 and 39-41). Pathologically, the acute phase shows a necrotizing angiitis involving media and adventitial layers. Some children have survived into adulthood, with coronary artery aneurysms identified later in life[339] (see Figs. 39-40 and 39-41). The differential diagnosis of coronary artery aneurysms in adults includes previously undiagnosed Kawasaki's disease presumably occurring during childhood. Coronary arteriography results in 1100 children aged 4 months to 13 years identified 262 (24 percent) patients with the disease. In these, coronary occlusion was present in 76 percent, segmental stenosis in 5.7 percent, localized stenosis in 23.7 percent, aneurysms in 35.5 percent, and dilatation in 27.5 percent.[338] The incidence of both occlusion and segmental stenosis was lowest in the group studied shortly after onset of the illness, whereas the prevalence of coronary aneurysm was highest in this early group.

Allergic Granulomatosis and Angiitis: Wegener's Granulomatosis and Churg-Strauss Syndrome

Wegener's granulomatosis is a necrotizing vasculitis of unknown cause classically involving the upper and lower respiratory tracts and the kidneys.[205,342–355] Cardiovascular involvement in Wegener's granulomatosis was described in one of three cases reported in 1936.[345] About 30 additional necropsy cases have been described subsequently, 14 of these (48 percent) showed small-vessel necrotizing coronary vasculitis[205,353,354] (Fig. 39-42). Fibrinoid necrosis of the small and medium-sized coronary arteries[342] and occlusion of larger epicardial coronary arteries with myocardial infarction[343] have been reported. In a large clinical series of patients with Wegener's granulomatosis, 12 percent had cardiac involvement largely manifest by pericarditis and coronary arteritis.[355] Some patients with this disease develop unusual cardiac complications such as pericardial tamponade and later constrictive pericarditis, high-grade atrioventricular block, and atrial tachycardia resistant to usual treatment measures. In this series,[355] all patients improved with cyclophosphamide therapy.

Churg-Strauss syndrome (allergic granulomatosis and angiitis) is a variant of polyarteritis nodosa[205,219] occurring in patients with asthma or an allergy history.[219–221,356] It is characterized by necrotizing angiitis with extravascular granulomas and eosinophilia. The heart is commonly involved with this disease, with granulomatous vasculitis of the coronary arteries (see Fig. 39-42). Granulomatous myocarditis may occur with or without the coronary angiitis[357] (see also Chap. 76).

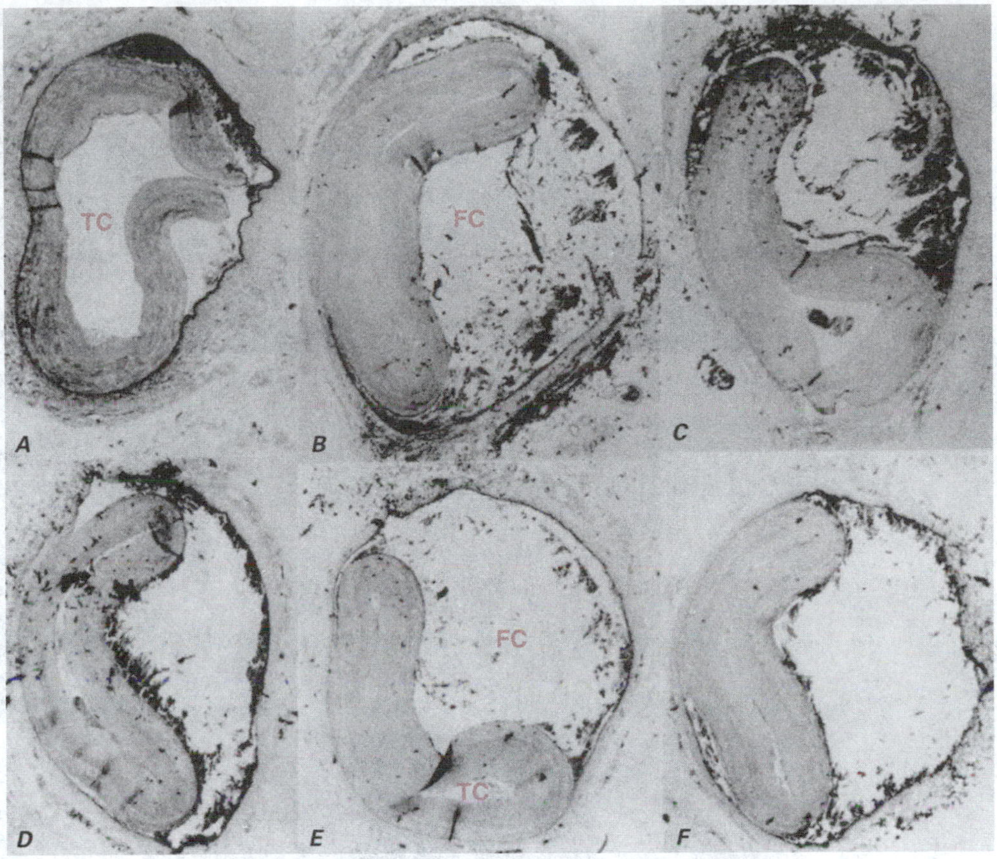

FIGURE 39-26 Coronary artery dissection. Serial cross section (*A-F*) showing dissection of the left anterior descending coronary artery. The true channel (TC) is severely compromised by external compression from the false channel (FC) ("dissection channel"). (From Waller.[1] Reproduced with permission from the publisher, editor, and author.)

Collagen Vascular Disease Vasculitis

Collagen vascular diseases generally involve arthritis, myositis, carditis, dermatitis, and inflammatory vascular changes to varying degrees.[358] They include systemic lupus erythematosus, rheumatoid vasculitis, systemic sclerosis, and polymyositis. Rheumatoid vasculitis was discussed earlier. One of the most common conditions with coronary artery vasculitis is systemic lupus erythematosus (Fig. 39-43). Several young patients with this disease and absent coronary atherosclerosis have suffered acute myocardial infarction[359–362] (see also Chap. 76). At necropsy, the coronary arteries in these patients have shown internal fibrous proliferation, possibly representing healed arteritis. Necrotizing vasculitis frequently leads to fatal coronary thrombosis and myocardial infarction,[205,360] rarely associated with thrombotic occlusion of all three major arteries.[360] Smaller intramural coronary arteries are also involved frequently with fibrinoid necrosis and subsequent fibrosis.[114] Recently, myocardial infarction has been seen with a proximal right coronary artery aneurysm at necropsy. It was postulated that the coronary artery aneurysm represented a sequela of systemic lupus erythematosus arteritis similar to Kawasaki's disease.[362] Necrotizing vasculitis occurs less commonly in other entities of collagen vascular disease such as dermatopolymyositis,[363] systemic sclerosis,[364] Behçet's syndrome,[365] and Cogan's syndrome.[205,366]

Hypersensitivity Angiitis (Allergic Vasculitis)

Hypersensitivity angiitis describes a miscellaneous group of necrotizing vasculitides that involve both epicardial and intramural coronary arteries.[205] This includes drug-induced vasculitis,[367] which, when generalized, may involve the heart. Histologically, drug-induced vasculitis cannot be separated from primary vasculitis or from hypersensitivity angiitis associated with a known underlying disease or malignancy such as serum sickness, mixed cryoglobulinemia, Schönlein-Henoch purpura, etc.[205] (see Table 39-8). A correct diagnosis cannot be made without clinical information about drug use. Organ-transplantation arteritis[205,368] is also in this category, representing a form of immune-mediated vascular injury (see Chap. 32).

METABOLIC DISORDERS

Specific metabolic substances may accumulate in the walls of large and small coronary arteries as a result of inborn errors of metabolism. The deposition of this material may severely narrow the coronary artery lumen and produce acute myocar-

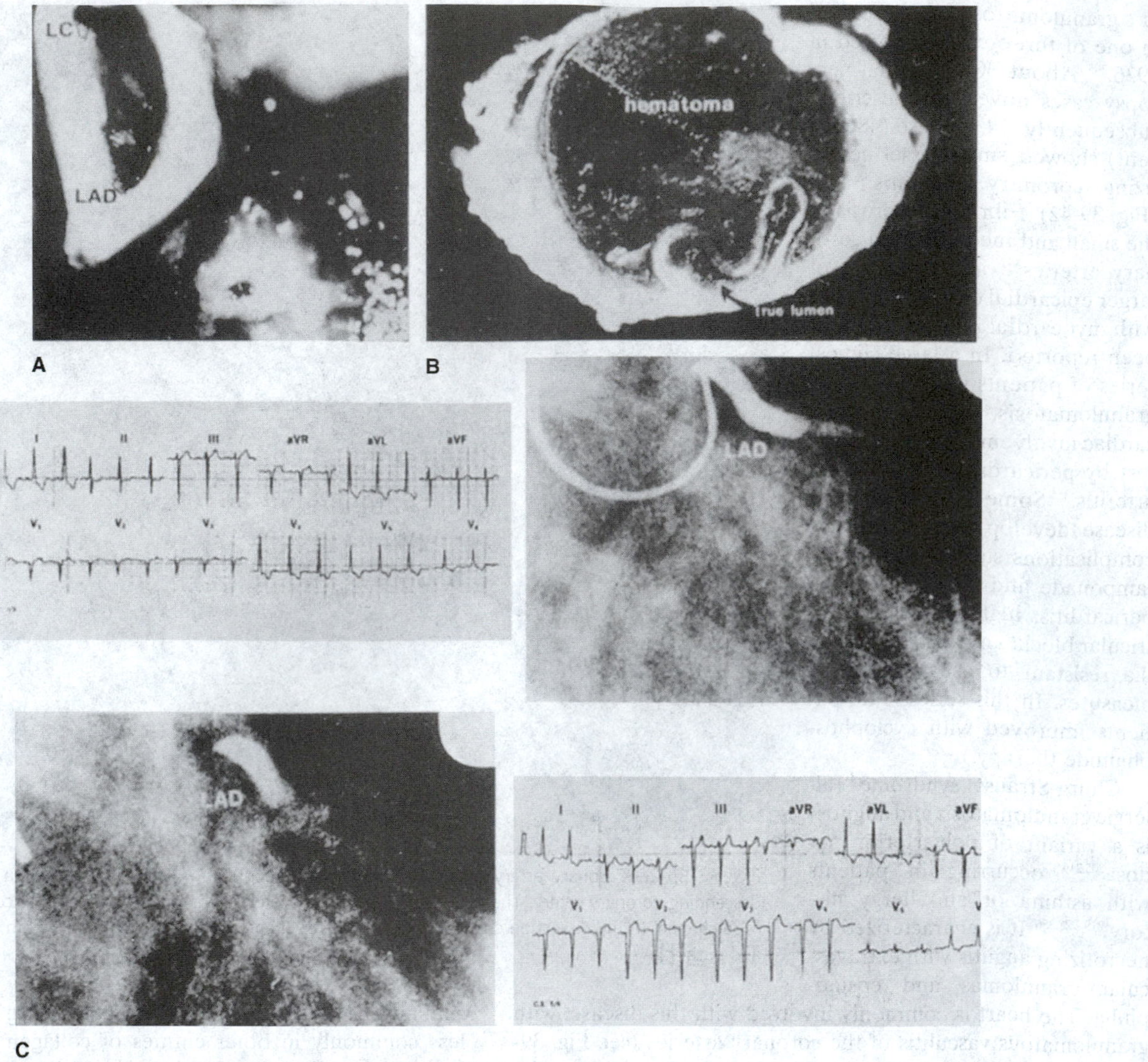

FIGURE 39-27 Coronary artery dissection. Occlusion of the left anterior descending (LAD) artery due to dissection. *A.* The LAD and left circumflex (LC) are seen through the left main artery. *B.* Cross section shows hematoma in false channel severely narrows native (true channel) unobstructed lumen. *C.* Sequential electrocardiographic and angiographic findings. (From Isner and Donaldson.[141] Reproduced with permission from the publisher, editor, and author.)

dial infarction.[5] Inherited inborn errors of metabolism that are known to affect major epicardial coronary arteries include Hunter's and Hurler's diseases (mucopolysaccharidoses).[293,369–371] The involvement of the coronary arteries in these disorders may be so severe as to totally occlude the vessel and to produce myocardial ischemia/infarction. Other disorders of metabolism such as primary oxalosis,[372] Fabry's disease,[114] Sandhoff's disease (gangliosidoses),[373] and homocystinuria may affect smaller coronary vessels by severe intimal proliferation[374] (see also Chap. 62).

INTIMAL PROLIFERATION

Fibrous hyperplasia and smooth muscle proliferation in the coronary arteries may narrow the lumen severely and produce myocardial ischemia/infarction. The process may be associated with mediastinal irradiation,[375] fibromuscular hyperplasia of the renal arteries,[5] use of methysergide,[22,376] ostial cannulation during cardiac surgery, aortic valve replacement,[23] and unknown causes.[377,378–380] Up to 50 percent of patients undergoing cardiac transplantation develop significant narrowing of epicardial coronary arteries or total occlusion by intimal fibrous proliferation within 3 to 5 years after transplantation.[381] Myocardial infarction and sudden death may result from this "chronic rejection" process. Fibrosis of the intramural vessels also may occur. Intimal damage from immunologic rejection is believed to be the basis for the accelerated intimal fibrous hyperplasia involving the coronary arteries (see also Chap. 22). A morphologic assessment of 61 human cardiac allografts of short- and long-term survival has been provided.[382] Allographs were divided into two groups: fibrous lesions confined to the proximal region of epicardial arteries and those with diffuse necrotizing vasculitis of the entire system. Disease in the proximal region begins as concentric fibrous thickening. Diffuse disease (necrotizing vasculitis) invariably was associated with acute myocardial rejection with severe intimal lesions of large and small epicardial and intramu-

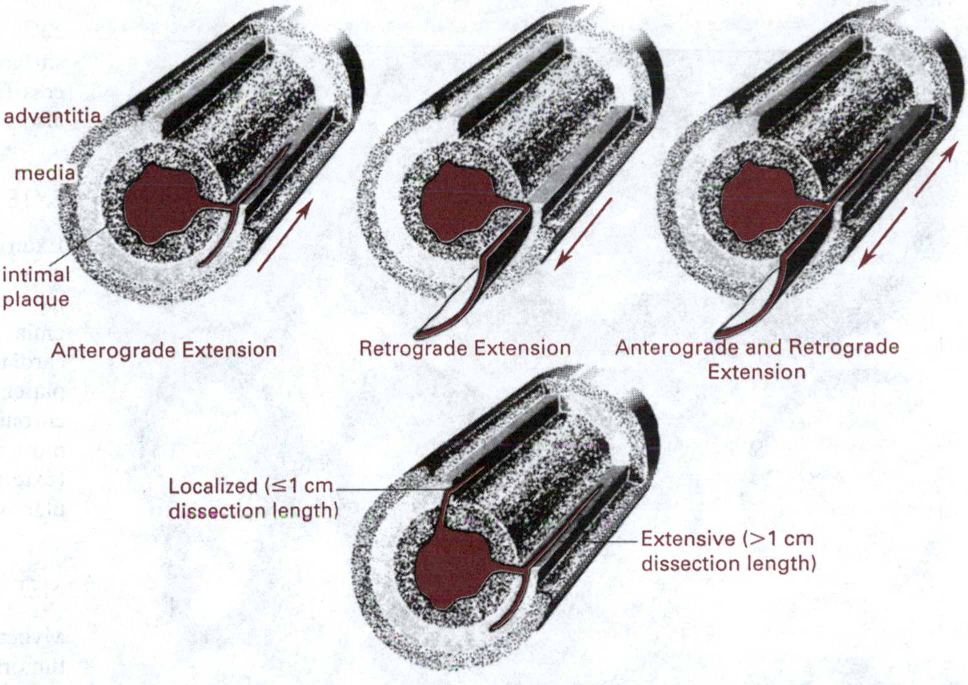

FIGURE 39-28 Diagram showing morphologic definition of coronary artery dissections in balloon angioplasty (long-axis plane): localized (mechanism) (1 cm in total dissection length) and extension (complications) (≥1 cm in total length). (From Waller et al.[168] Reproduced with permission from the author, editor, and publisher.)

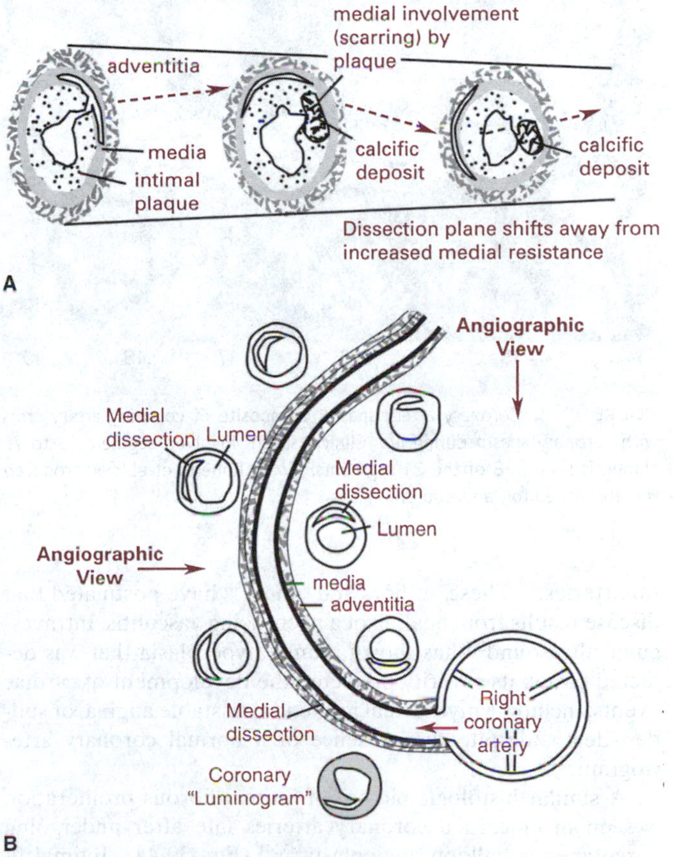

FIGURE 39-29 Diagram showing pathologic change accounting for angiographic appearance of coronary artery "spiral" dissection. *A.* Alteration in course of dissection. *B.* Angiographic appearance of unaltered course of dissection. (From Waller et al.[168] Reproduced with permission from the author, editor, and publisher.)

TABLE 39-6 Causes of Coronary Artery Dissections[141–168]

- I. Spontaneous
  - A. Post- or peripartum[142,146,148,156,160,161,163,164,166,167]
  - B. With or without eosinophilia[142,156,161,163]
  - C. Idiopathic[145,150–152,154,158,159,162,163,165]
  - D. Systemic hypertension[155]
  - E. Coronary spasm
  - F. Aortic root dissection[163] (hypertension, medial degeneration)
  - G. Arteritis[162]
  - H. Fibromuscular hyperplasia
- II. Trauma
  - A. Post- or peripartum[146,148,160,164,167]
  - B. Blunt chest[157] (penetrating, nonpenetrating)
  - C. Coronary angiography[153]
  - D. Coronary interventions[147,168] (angioplasty, atherectomy, laser, stenting, rotablade)
  - E. Cardiac surgery (coronary bypass, coronary ostial cannulation, endarterectomy)
  - F. Aortic root dissection[149] (surgery, nonpenetrating, penetrating)

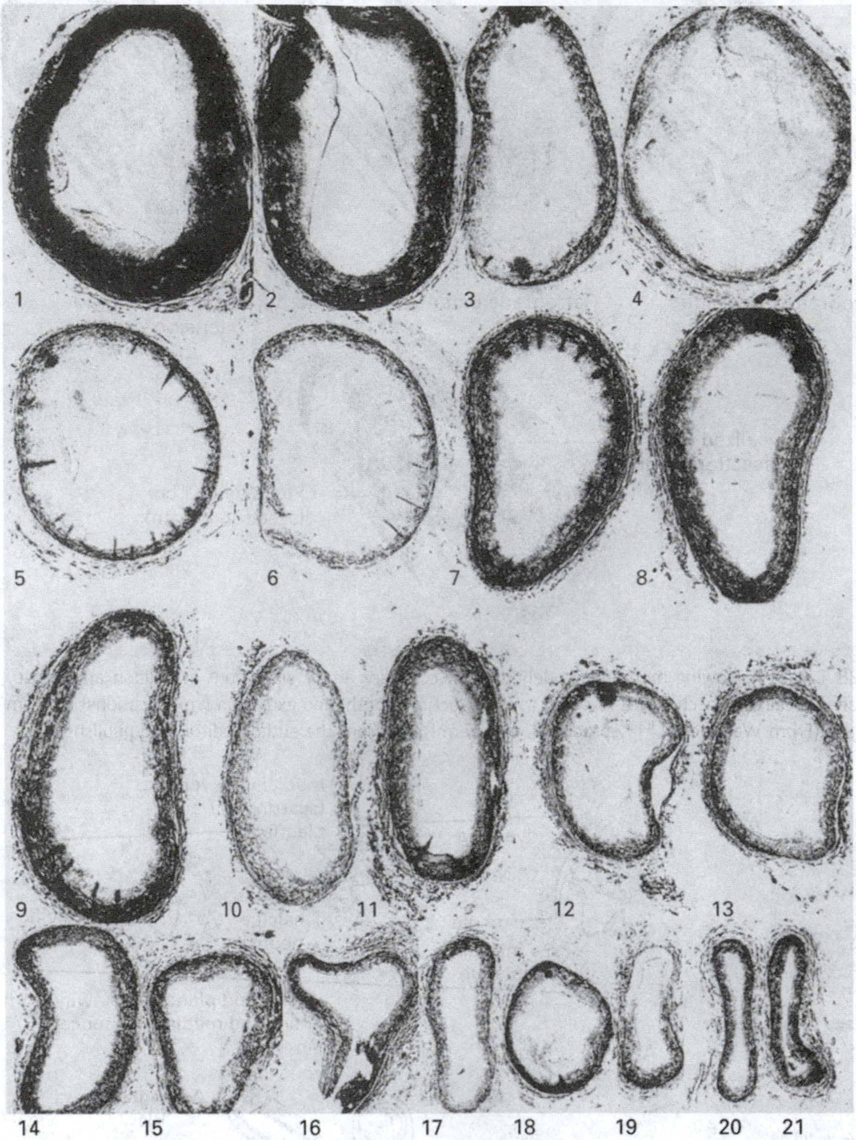

FIGURE 39-30 Coronary artery spasm. Composite of coronary artery cross sections of a patient with coronary spasm during life. Clinical spasm involved segments 3 to 7. Severe atherosclerotic plaque is seen in 8 of the 21 segments. (From Roberts et al.[180] Reproduced with permission from the author, editor, and publisher.)

ral arteries.[382] These authors and others[383] have postulated that disease results from healing of a necrotizing vasculitis. Intravascular ultrasound[384] has shown intimal hyperplasia that was detected easily; its severity predicted the development of cardiac events, including myocardial infarction, unstable angina, or sudden death, despite the presence of a normal coronary arteriogram.

A similar histologic picture of intimal fibrous proliferation is seen in epicardial coronary arteries late after undergoing percutaneous balloon angioplasty[143,144] (Fig. 39-44). Intimal fibrous proliferation of the left main coronary artery has been reported late after balloon angioplasty of a lesion in the proximal left anterior descending coronary artery.[385] This may be due to intimal reaction from balloon rubbing of the intimal surface and/or extension of the fibrous process from the angioplasty dilation site (see also Chap. 45).

EXTERNAL COMPRESSION

External compression of the epicardial coronary arteries may result in severe luminal narrowing and progressive myocardial ischemia. External compression of a major epicardial coronary artery has been reported in patients with sinus of Valsalva aneurysms, chronic aortic dissection,[386] and epicardial tumor metastases.[387,388] Myocardial bridging (external muscle compression during ventricular systole) was reviewed earlier.

METASTATIC IMPLANTS

Myocardial metastatic lesions from various tumors—including carcinomas, sarcomas, and lymphomas—may mimic a healed myocardial infarct at necropsy (Fig. 39-45). The discrete location or locations of these metastatic deposits generally are unrelated to specific coronary arterial supply zones, and the lesions usually are surrounded by normal myocardium. These two gross observations suggest the lesions are metastatic tumor implants rather than healed myocardial infarcts (see also Chap. 77).

RADIATION-INDUCED CAD

Intimal proliferation of epicardial coronary arteries involving the ostium, main segment, or both is well known and increasingly reported.[375,389–400] "Accelerated" or "premature" coronary atherosclerosis has been noted in young individuals undergoing previous mediastinal irradiation for various types of malignancies.[401–404] Internal proliferation following mediastinal radiation 5 to 10 years earlier is described as "intimal thickening *without* medial abnormalities." The intimal lesions (ostial or main segment of artery) consists of fibrous tissue *without* extra cellular lipid deposits.[375,399] Coronary ostial stenosis has an incidence of 0.13 to 2.7 percent of patients undergoing mediastinal irradiation treatment.[375,399] A few patients have developed acute myocardial infarction or unstable angina as a result of the radiation-induced lesions treated by myocardial revascularization[394,398] or angioplasty[398] (see also Chap. 71).

Because of their fibrous nature, many radiation-induced lesions do not provide the best substrate for dilation techniques.[143,144,385] Chemotherapy-induced myocardial infarction in a young man without coronary disease has been reported.[405] Cardiac invasion by tumor, hypercoagulable states, and coronary artery spasm are possible etiologies.[405] Vascular toxicity, including myocardial infarction, has been reported following antineoplastic regimens containing *Vinca* alkaloids.[405]

CORONARY ARTERY THROMBOSIS WITHOUT UNDERLYING ATHEROSCLEROTIC PLAQUE (THROMBOSIS IN SITU)

Thrombotic occlusion of the coronary system unassociated with underlying atherosclerotic plaque may be seen with several hematologic diseases: thrombocytopenic purpura,[35] leukemia,[406] polycythemia vera,[407] sickle cell anemia,[114] and primary thrombocytosis.[408] Occasionally, acute myocardial infarction may be the initial manifestation of these hematologic disorders. A main factor responsible for the myocardial ischemia in these conditions is blockage of small intramural coronary vessels by platelet aggregates.[409] These platelet aggregates initially may form in the major coronary arteries and then embolize distally.

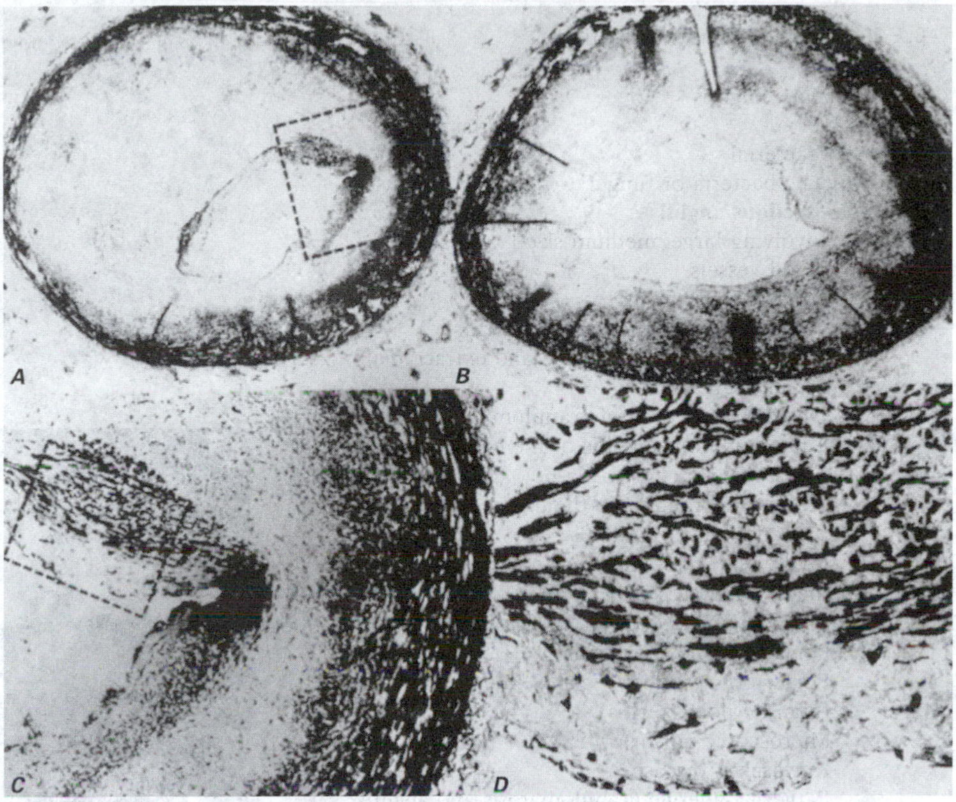

FIGURE 39-31 Coronary artery spasm. *A*, *B*. Histologic sections of the left anterior descending coronary artery at the approximate site of spasm showing severe luminal narrowing. *C*, *D*. Higher magnifications of the internal plaque showing the predominance of smooth muscle cells. (From Roberts et al.[180] Reproduced with permission from the author, editor, and publisher.)

SUBSTANCE ABUSE

Cocaine abuse is now a major health hazard; more than 22 million Americans have tried cocaine at least once, and 5 million are current users.[410] Recent reports have documented that cocaine abuse can result in myocardial ischemia and infarction in the absence of CAD,[410–420] and cocaine-induced coronary artery vasoconstriction has been reported in patients following the intranasal administration of cocaine[415,421–424] (see also Chap. 71).

Several instances of coronary artery thrombosis and spasm have been reported in patients who abuse cocaine. Acute coronary thrombosis in association with cardiac events—including angina, acute myocardial infarction, and sudden death—has been reported.[410,413,422–424] In some instances, there is underlying atherosclerotic plaque; in others, the coronary arteries are normal. Coronary thrombosis occurring in coronary arteries free of atherosclerotic plaque suggests the role of cocaine-induced spasm, massive norepinephrine release in the heart, or possible primary thrombogenicity of cocaine or its metabolites.[421] Coronary spasm has been associated with cocaine use and has been postulated as a mechanism of myocardial infarction in cocaine users with clean coronary arteries.[410,425–431] In such cases, fibrointimal proliferation with coronary narrowing was attributed

TABLE 39-7 Some Conditions Associated with Coronary Artery Arteritis (Vasculitis)

Tuberculosis[24,238,239]
Polyarteritis nodosa[24,205,310–324]
Giant-cell arteritis[205,226–228,266–277]
Systemic lupus erythematosus[205,358–362]
Buerger's disease (thromboangiitis obliterans)[205,303–307]
Wegener's granulomatosis[205,342–355]
Salmonella[4,340]
Leprosy[4]
Mucocutaneous lymph node syndrome[326–339]
Takayasu's disease[208,247–265]
Typhus[232]
Infective endocarditis[341]
Rheumatic diseases[205,276–297]
Ankylosing spondylitis[293]
Syphilis[5,114,205,233–237]
Malaria[241]
Schistosoma haematobium[242]
Rickettsial infections[205,242–244]
Viruses[205,245,246]

SOURCE: Waller.[1] Reproduced with permission from the author, editor, and publisher.

TABLE 39-8 Classification of Vasculitides

1. **Infectious angiitis**
   - Syphilitic
   - Mycobacterial
   - Pyogenic bacteria or fungal
   - Rickettsial
   - Viral
   - Whipple bacillus
2. **Noninfectious angiitis**
   - A. Involving large, medium-sized, and small blood vessels
     - Takayasu's arteritis
     - Granulomatous (giant-cell) arteritis
     - Cranial (temporal) arteritis and extracranial giant-cell arteritis
     - Disseminated visceral granulomatous angiitis
     - Granulomatous angiitis of the central nervous system
     - Arteritis of rheumatic-rheumatoid disease and spondyloarthropathies
   - B. Involving predominantly medium-sized and small blood vessels
     - Thromboangiitis obliterans (Buerger's disease)
     - Polyarteritis (periarteritis)
     - Polyarteritis nodosa
     - Infantile polyarteritis
     - Microscopic polyarteritis
     - Kawasaki's disease
     - Pathergic-allergic granulomatosis and angiitis
     - Wegener's granulomatosis
     - Churg-Strauss syndrome
     - Necrotizing sarcoid granulomatosis
     - Vasculitis of collagen vascular disease:
     - Rheumatic fever
     - Relapsing polychondritis
     - Rheumatoid arthritis
     - Systemic sclerosis
     - Seronegative arthropathies
     - Sjögren's syndrome
     - Systemic lupus erythematosus
     - Behçet's syndrome
     - Cogan's syndrome
     - Dermatomyositis/polymyositis
   - C. Involving predominantly small blood vessels
     - Hypersensitivity angiitis (synonym: leukocytoclastic or allergic vasculitis)
     - Serum sickness
     - Mixed cryoglobulinemia
     - Schönlein-Henoch purpura
     - Drug-induced angiitis
     - Hypocomplementemia
     - Inflammatory bowel disease
     - Malignancy-associated vasculitis
     - Primary biliary cirrhosis
     - Retroperitoneal fibrosis
     - Goodpasture's syndrome

SOURCE: Lie.[205] Reproduced with permission from the author, editor, and publisher.

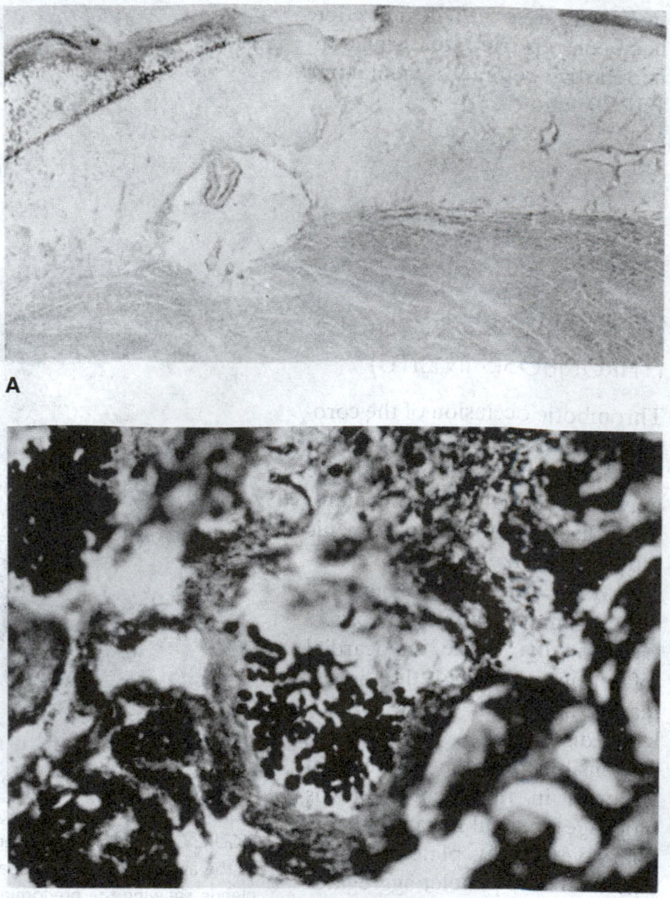

FIGURE 39-32 Coronary arteritis. *A*. Extensive yeast (*Candida*) pericarditis, which involves the adventitial layer of a branch of a major subepicardial coronary artery. *B*. Close-up shows the budding yeast organisms (GMS stain). (From Waller.[1] Reproduced with permission from the author, editor, and publisher.)

to underlying coronary artery spasm that caused focal vessel endothelial injury, platelet adherence, and aggregation. Platelets liberate platelet-derived growth factor (PDGF), which can induce intimal proliferative lesions. In patients with underlying coronary plaque, cocaine-induced spasm also may produce endothelial disruption at the surface of the plaque and promote platelet aggregation and further vasoconstriction from the release of platelet prostaglandins[432] (see also Chap. 71).

Recently, two drugs have been the center of debate over their potential for abuse versus use as psychotherapeutic agents and their complication in induction of arrhythmias.[433] Use of MDMA ("Ecstasy," 3,4-methylenedioxymethamphetamine) and MDEA ("Eve," 3,4-methylenedioxymethamphetamine) has been associated with five sudden deaths.[433] In three of these, "Eve" and "Ecstasy" may have induced fatal arrhythmias.

MYOCARDIAL OXYGEN DEMAND-SUPPLY DISPROPORTION

In this category are disease states in which there is failure to deliver adequate oxygen to the myocardium over a prolonged

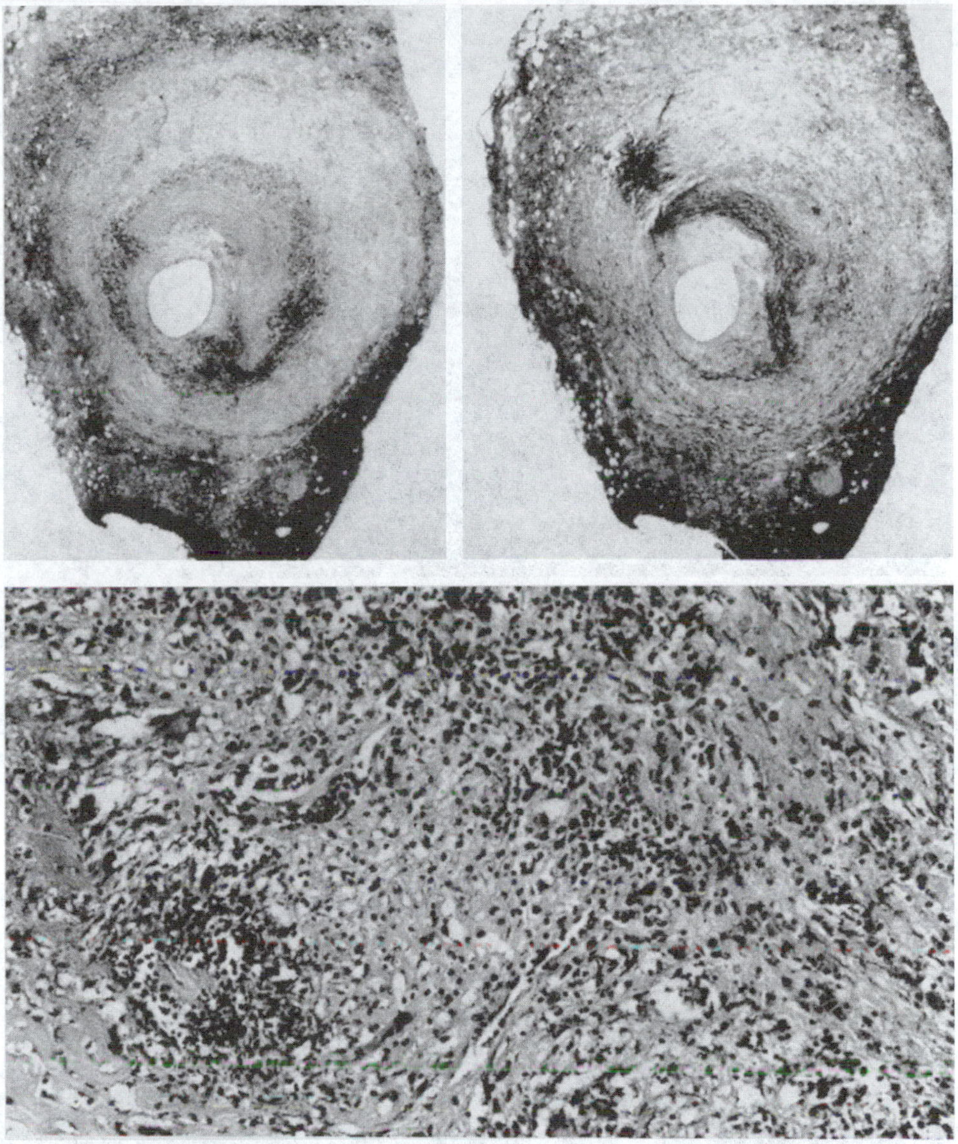

FIGURE 39-33 (*Top*) Matching hematoxylin-eosin (*left*) and elastic (*right*) stained sections of coronary artery in Takayasu's arteritis. Note transmural fibrosis and inflammatory infiltrate in media of artery (×16). (*Bottom*) Close-up view of lymphoplasmacytic infiltrate with giant cells in media of coronary artery (×160). (From Lie.[205] Reproduced with permission from the author, editor, and publisher.)

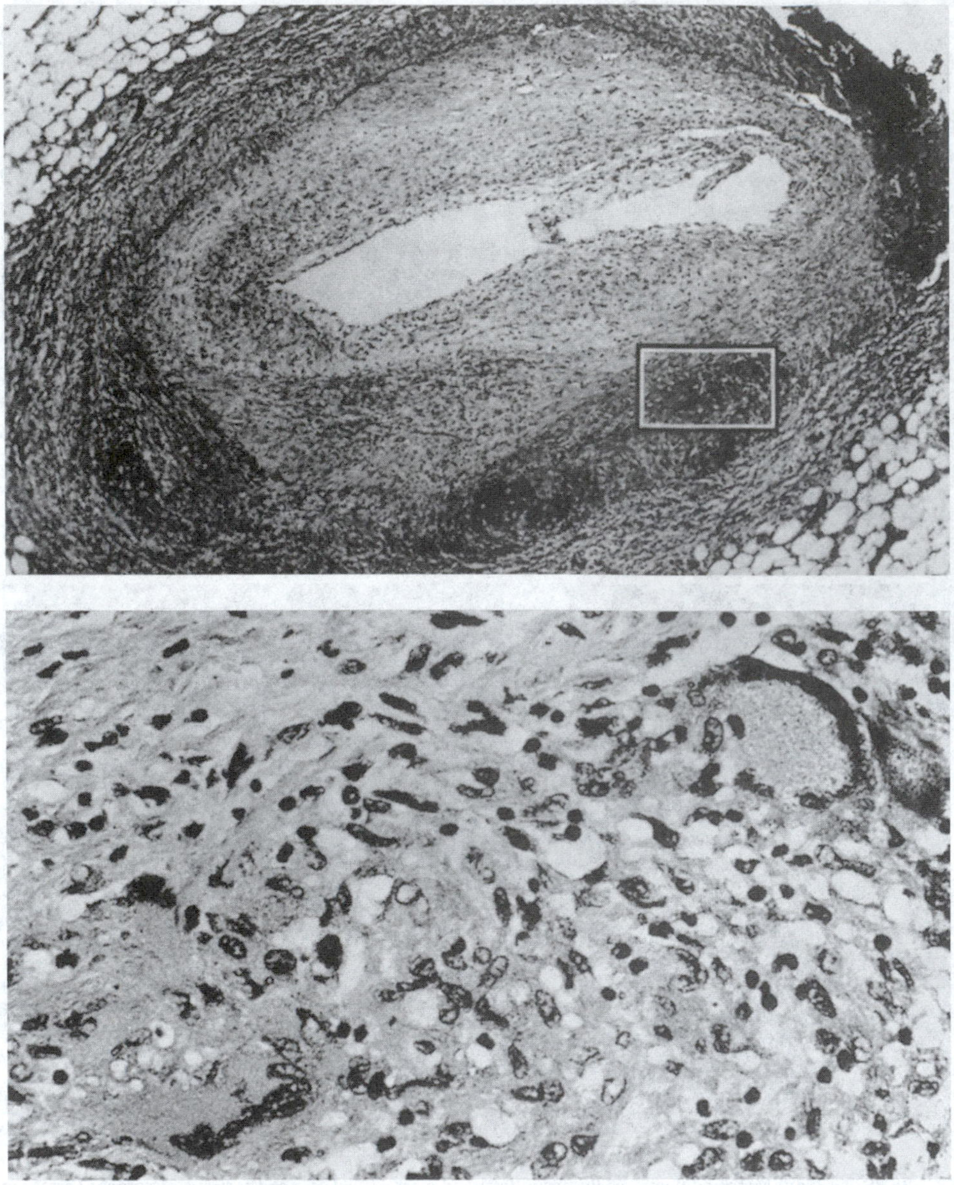

FIGURE 39-34 (*Top*) Low-power view of granulomatous coronary arteritis associated with giant-cell aortitis (hematoxylin-eosin, ×40). (*Bottom*) Close-up view of boxed area (hematoxylin-eosin, ×400). (From Lie.[205] Reproduced with permission from the author, editor, and publisher.)

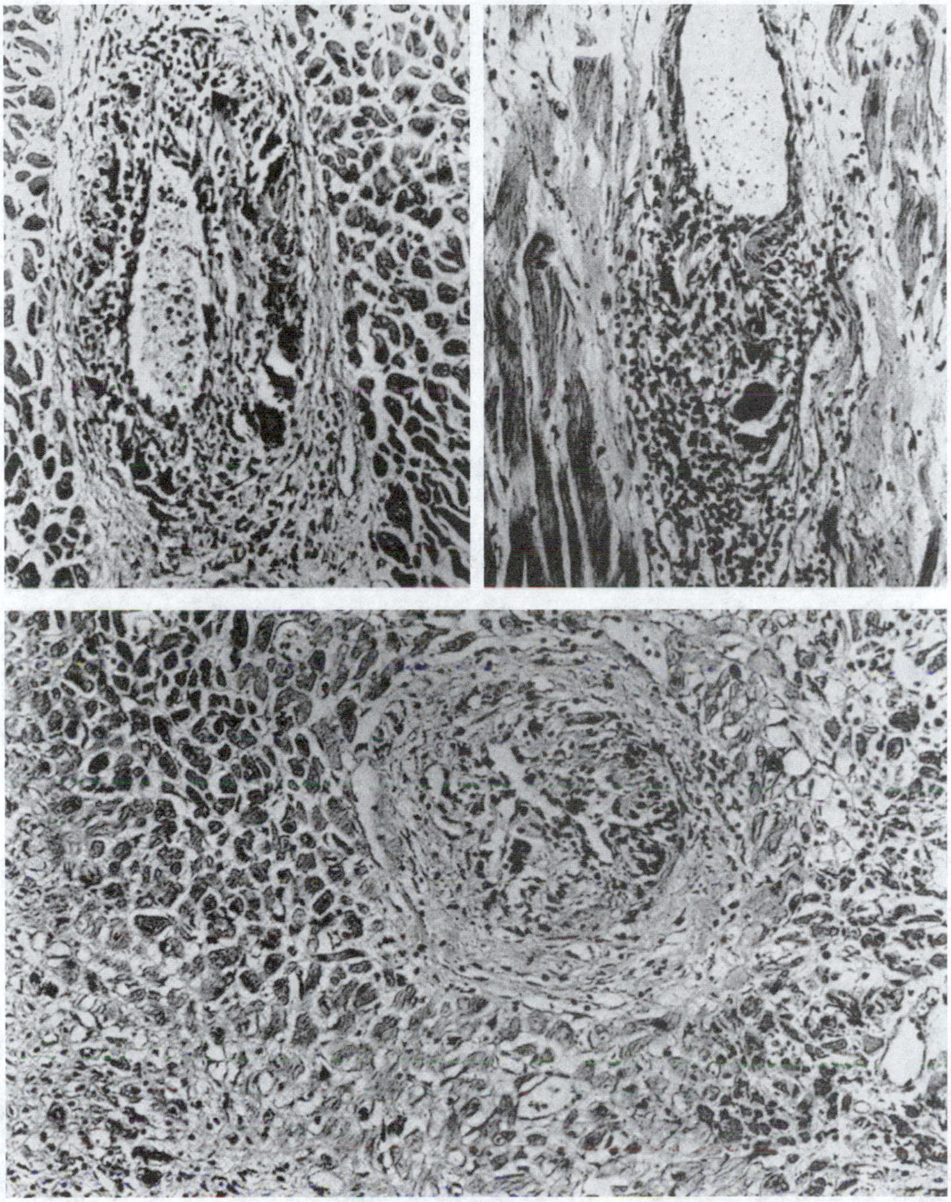

FIGURE 39-35 (*Top left and right*) Giant-cell arteritis of intramural coronary arteries associated with temporal arteritis and giant cell arteritis (hematoxylin-eosin, ×160). (*Bottom*) Granulomatous coronary arteritis in disseminated visceral giant-cell angiitis (hematoxylin-eosin, ×160). (From Lie.[205] Reproduced with permission from the author, editor, and publisher.)

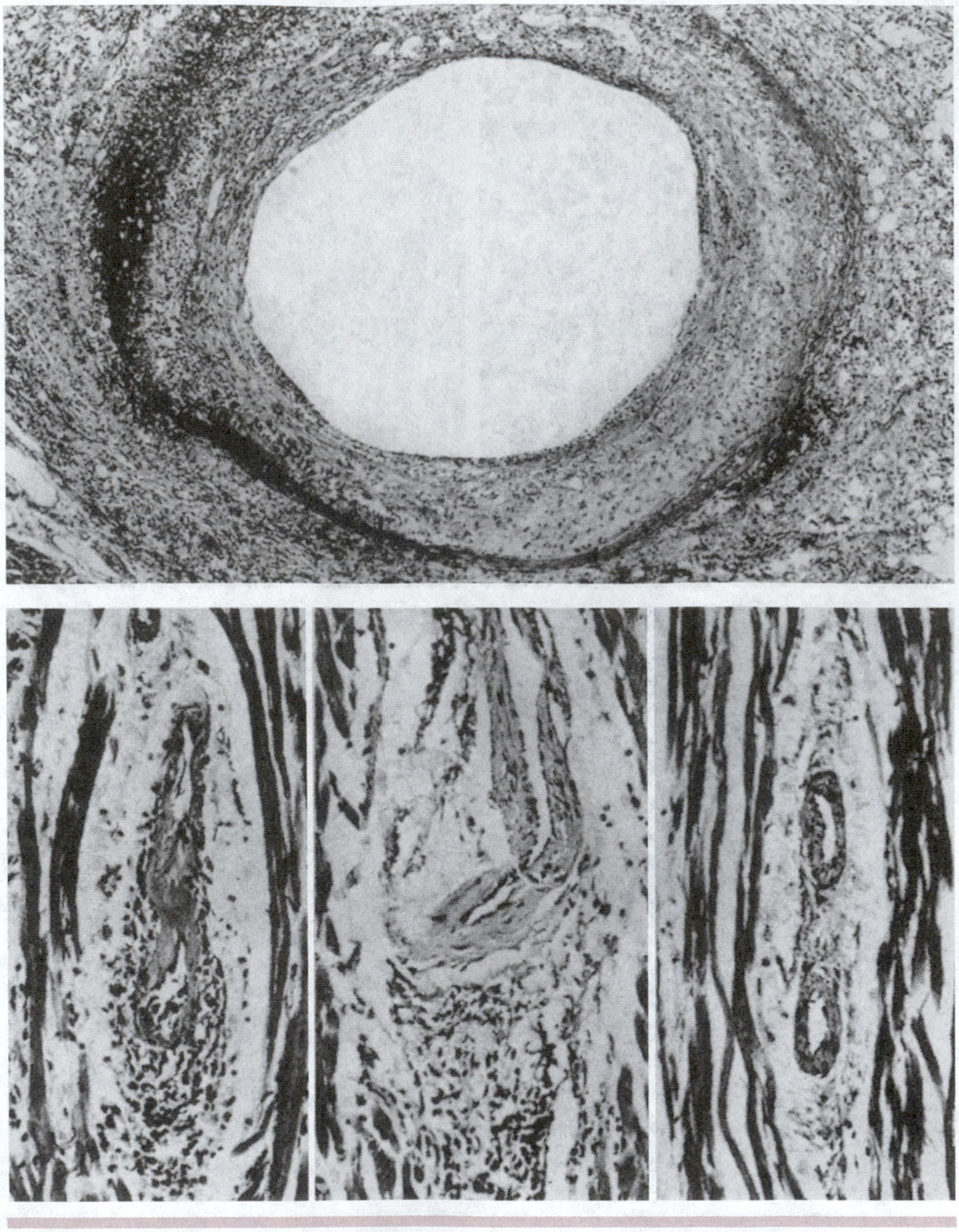

FIGURE 39-36 (*Top*) Polyarteritis-type necrotizing angiitis of epicardial coronary artery in rheumatoid arthritis (hematoxylin-eosin, ×160). (*Bottom*) Variations of small-vessel coronary artery arteritis in rheumatic fever (hematoxylin-eosin, ×160). (From Lie.[205] Reproduced with permission from the author, editor, and publisher.)

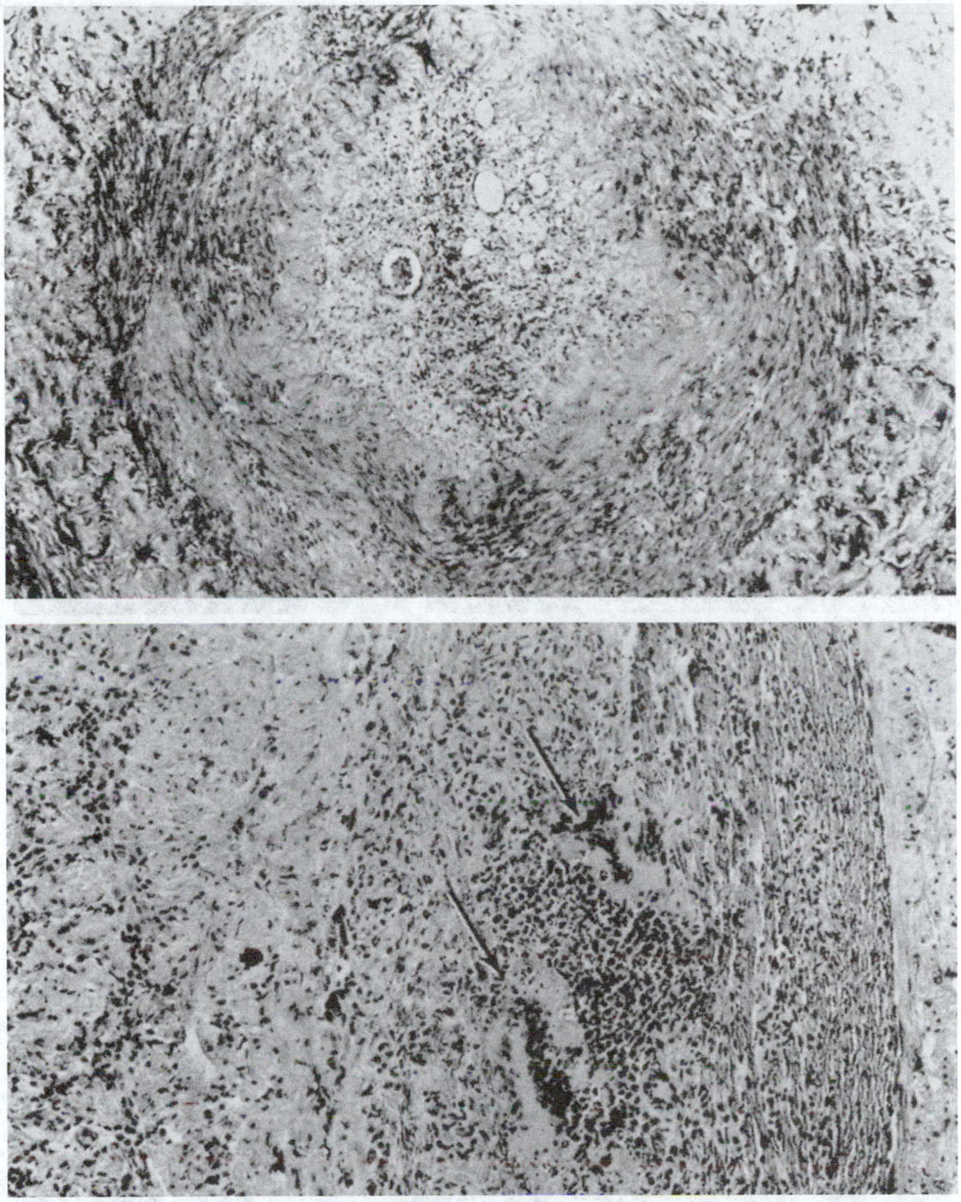

FIGURE 39-37 (*Top*) Subacute stage of Buerger's disease of coronary artery with organizing thrombus (hematoxylin-eosin, ×160). (*Bottom*) Involvement of coronary vein in Buerger's disease with typical intraluminal microabscesses and giant cells (*arrows*) (hematoxylin-eosin, ×160). (From Lie.[205] Reproduced with permission from the author, editor, and publisher.)

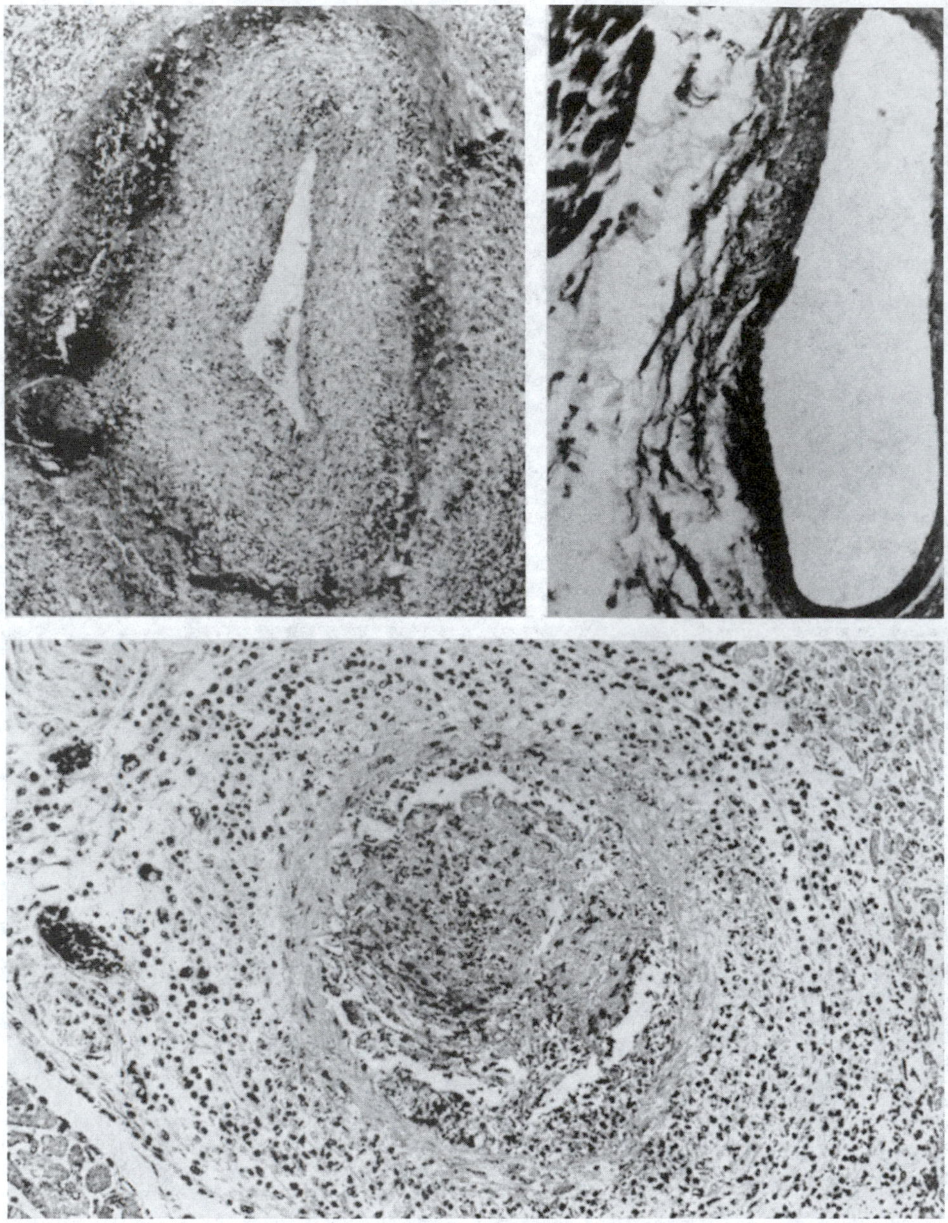

FIGURE 39-38 (*Top*) Necrotizing angiitis (*left*) and histologically normal (*right*) segments of epicardial coronary arteries in classic polyarteritis nodosa (hematoxylin-eosin, ×16). (*Bottom*) Necrotizing angiitis with fibrinoid necrosis of intramural coronary artery (hematoxylin-eosin, ×160). (From Lie.[205] Reproduced with permission from the author, editor, and publisher.)

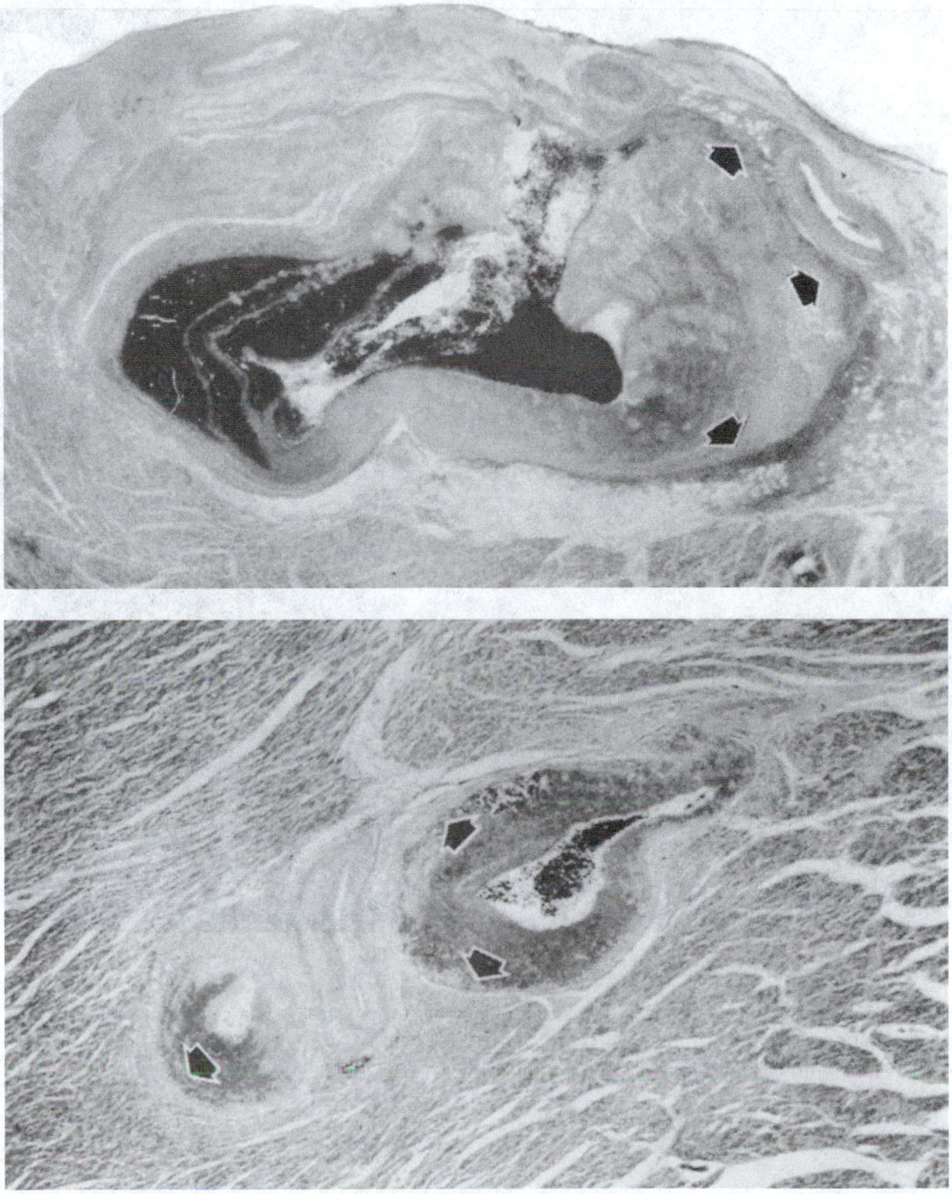

FIGURE 39-39 Necrotizing angiitis with aneurysmal disruption of epicardial (*arrows, top*) and intramural (*arrows, bottom*) coronary arteries in infantile polyarteritis nodosa (hematoxylin-eosin, ×160). (From Lie.[205] Reproduced with permission from the author, editor, and publisher.)

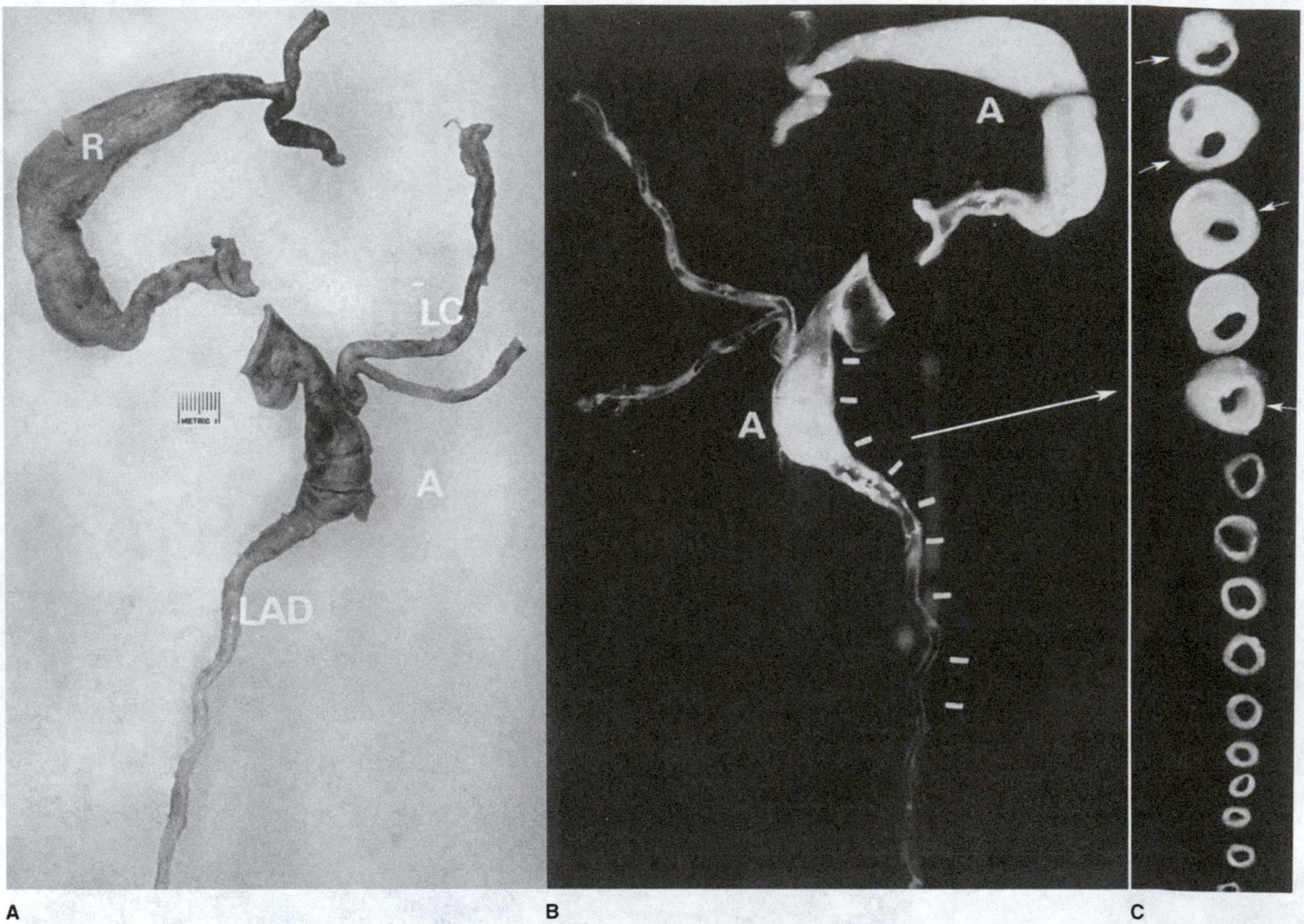

FIGURE 39-40 *A*. Epicardial coronary artery aneurysm involving the proximal left anterior descending (LAD) and right coronary artery (A) from an adult with probable Kawasaki's disease as a child. LC, left circumflex. *B*. Radiograph of coronary arterial tree in *A* showing calcific deposits. Cross section of the aneurysm (*A*) is shown in *C*. Arrows indicate calcific deposits.

period or increased myocardial wall tension requiring increased oxygen supply. The classic example of the first situation is carbon monoxide poisoning,[4] which has been associated with extensive nontransmural infarction in the presence of normal epicardial coronary arteries. Prolonged shock from any cause also can result in extensive nontransmural necrosis and frequently is associated with transmural necrosis of the papillary muscles. One example of increased myocardial wall tension requiring increased coronary oxygen supply is aortic valve stenosis[4] (see Chap. 56). In the face of increased oxygen demand with increased muscle mass, coronary blood supply may be limited by poor perfusion resulting from the lower coronary arterial pressure. In addition, poor perfusion results from the high coronary arterial resistance caused by increased wall pressure on the intramural coronary arteries and the high LV end-diastolic pressure from a stiff ventricle, with further limitation of the time in diastole for coronary blood flow occasioned by tachycardia.[4] Excessive myocardial oxygen demand exceeding supply and resulting in myocardial ischemia/infarction also may be seen in thyrotoxicosis,[434] which reflects increased metabolic rates and the adverse affects of tachycardia.

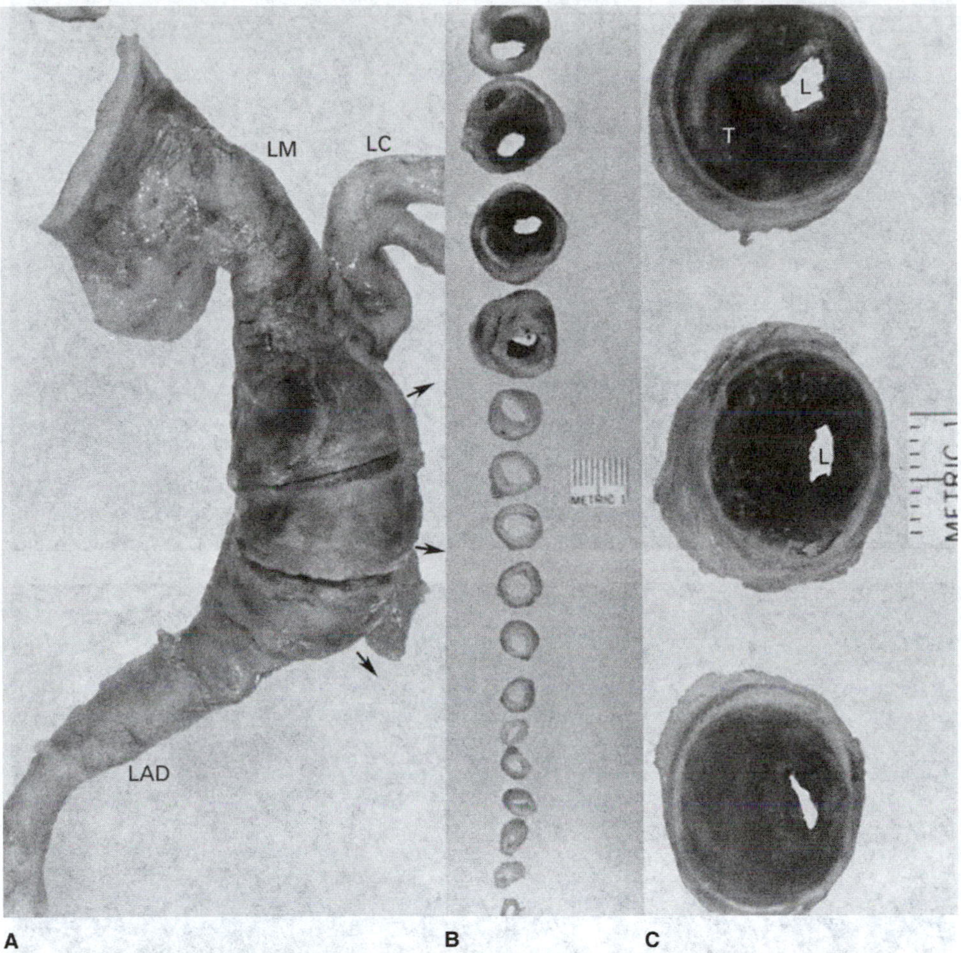

FIGURE 39-41 *A.* Close-up of left anterior descending (LAD) coronary aneurysm from Fig. 39-40 with cross sections displayed in *B.* Note the intraaneurysmal thrombus. *C.* Close-up of three transverse sections of coronary aneurysm shown in *A* and *B.* LM, left main; LC, left circumflex.

INTRAMURAL CAD (SMALL-VESSEL DISEASE)

Acute myocardial infarction may result from abnormally thickened or totally occluded intramural coronary arteries in the presence of normal extramural (epicardial) coronary arteries. A few of the conditions in this category include (1) hypertrophic cardiomyopathy, (2) diabetes mellitus, (3) amyloid heart disease,[434] (4) neuromuscular disorders (Friedreich's ataxia, progressive muscular dystrophy), (5) cardiac transplantation, (6) rheumatoid arthritis, (7) collagen-vascular disorders (scleroderma, systemic lupus erythematosus), (8) metabolic abnormalities (mucopolysaccharidoses, gangliosidoses), and (9) polyarteritis nodosa.[435–439]

Histologic abnormalities of small-vessel coronary arteries have been reported in individuals who have died from toxic oil syndrome involving rapeseed oil adulterated with aniline.[440] Many of those who later died had scleroderma-like illnesses. Dense fibrosis of the sinus node, resembling scleroderma, was found with cystic degeneration of the sinus node (resembling lupus erythematosus) and fibromuscular dysplasia of small coronary vessels.

NORMAL EPICARDIAL CORONARY ARTERIES

There have been relatively few necropsy reports of patients with acute myocardial infarction who had angiographically normal coronary arteries and normal coronary arteries at necropsy.[3,4,434,441,442] Of 100 consecutive necropsy cases of acute myocardial infarction,[3] 7 percent had infarcts without evidence of coronary luminal narrowing. In 10 patients with a typical picture of acute myocardial infarction who died within 25 days of onset of symptoms, the coronary arterial systems showed minimal or no luminal narrowing by atherosclerosis. No thrombotic material was observed in the coronary arteries despite the fact that the acute myocardial infarction was 2 days old in 5 patients and 3 to 4 days old in 3. Possible explanations for this have included coronary artery spasm, coronary artery disease in vessels too small to be visualized angiographically, or coronary artery thrombosis or embolus with subsequent clot lysis. Myocardial infarction in postpartum women with normal epicardial coronary arteries has included two additional causes for possible spasm in these patients: bromocriptine used for suppression of lactation[186,443–451] and antiphospholipid syndrome with elevated anticardiolipin antibody levels, false-positive syphilis serology, and a history of deep venous thrombosis.[452]

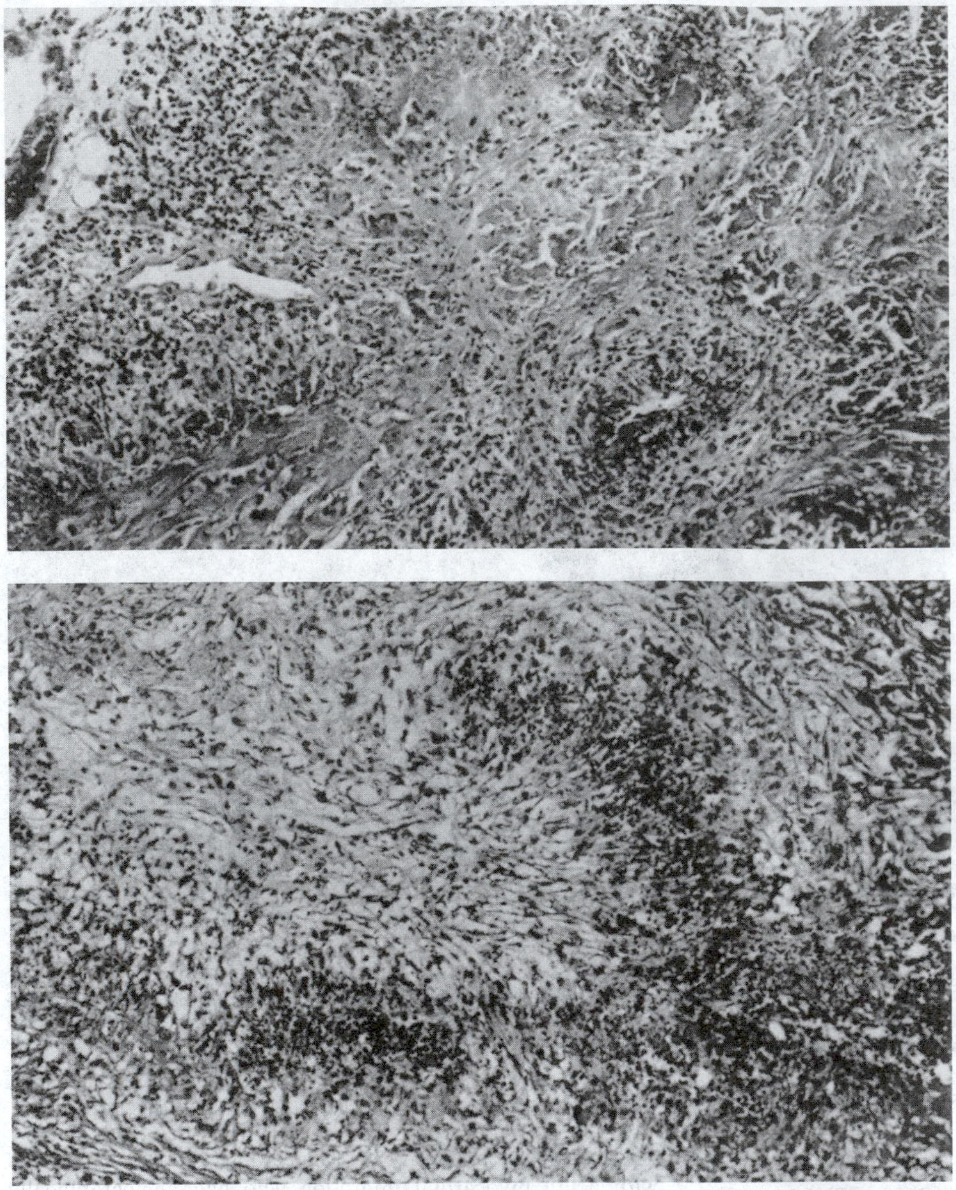

FIGURE 39-42 Granulomatous necrotizing angiitis of coronary arteries in Wegener's granulomatosis (*top*) and Churg-Strauss syndrome (*bottom*) (hematoxylin-eosin, ×160). (From Lie.[205] Reproduced with permission from the author, editor, and publisher.)

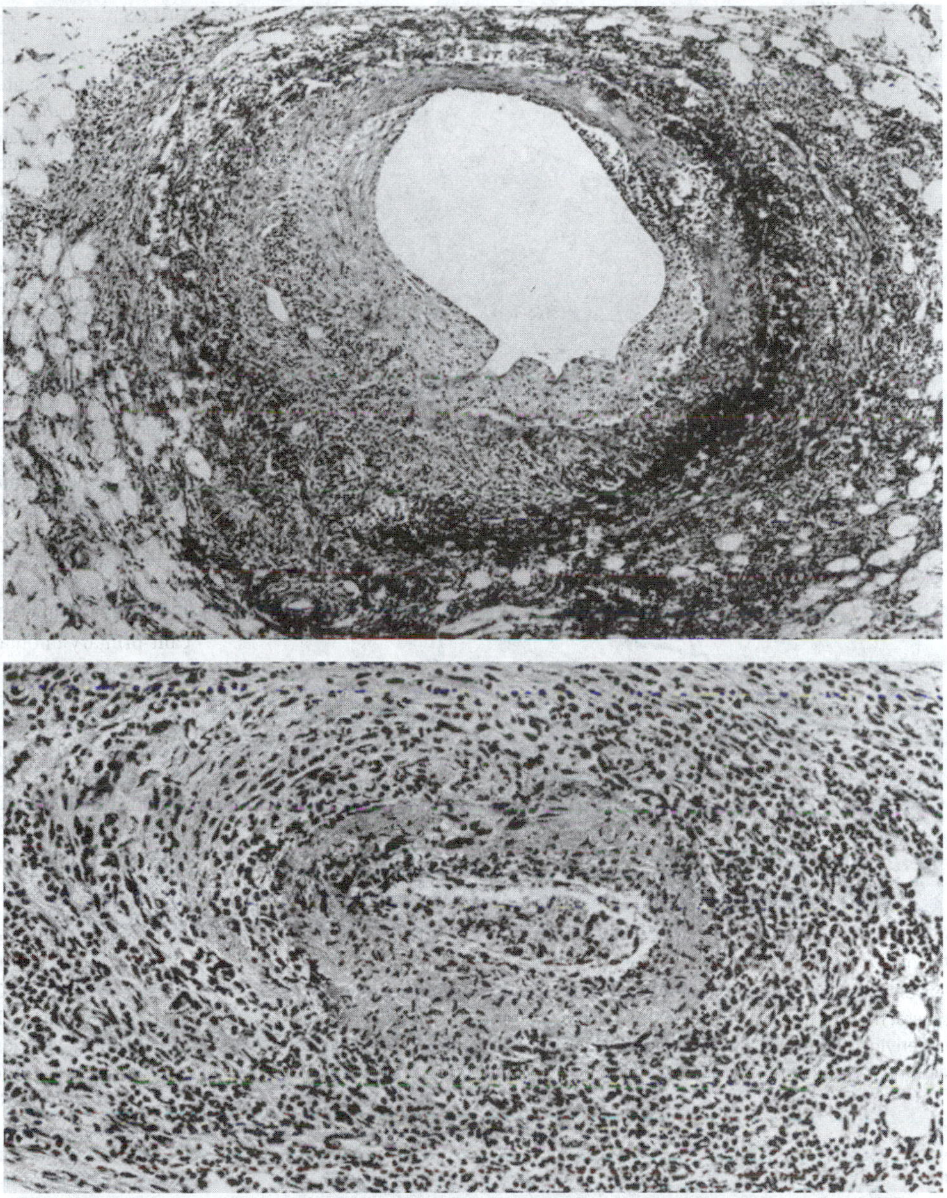

FIGURE 39-43 Necrotizing angiitis of epicardial (*top*) and intramural (*bottom*) coronary arteries in systemic lupus erythematosus (hematoxylin-eosin, ×160).

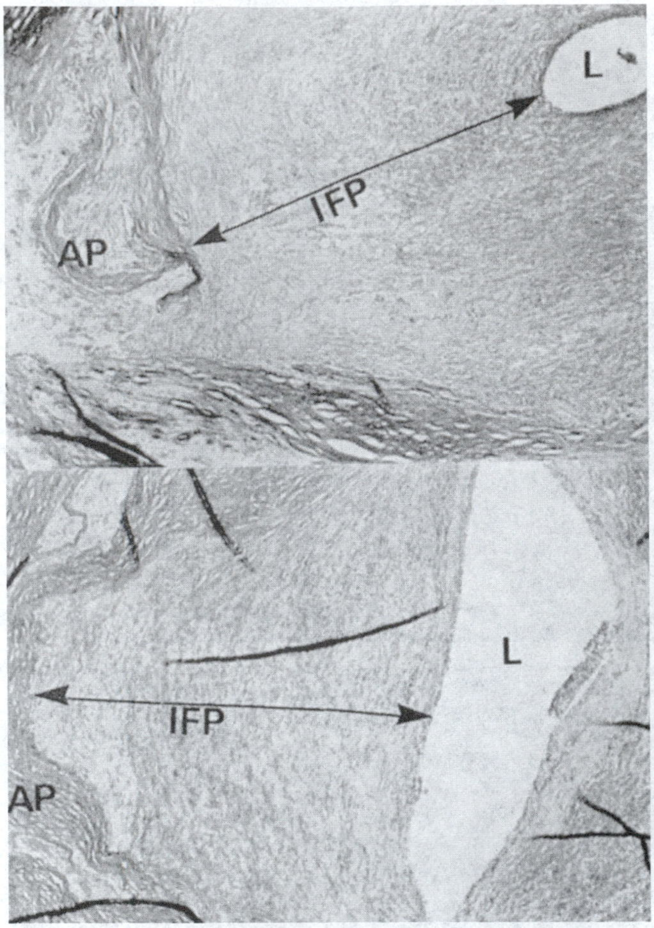

FIGURE 39-44 Intimal fibrous proliferation. Severe luminal narrowing of the left anterior descending coronary artery by intimal fibrous proliferation (IFP) several months after percutaneous balloon angioplasty. The IFP superimposes underlying atherosclerotic plaque (AP). L, lumen. (From Waller.[1] Reproduced with permission from the author, editor, and publisher.)

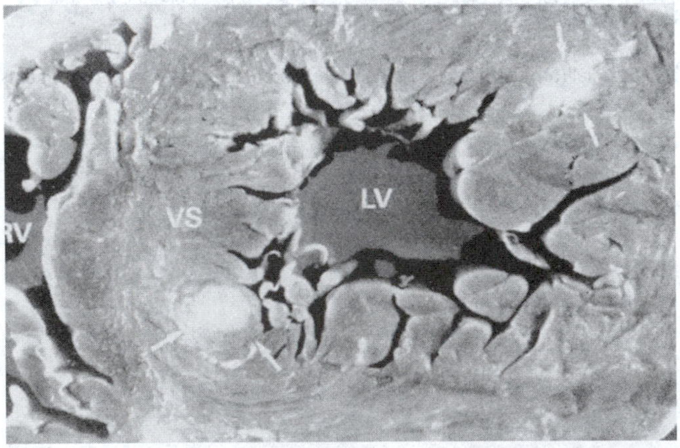

FIGURE 39-45 Metastatic deposits mimicking myocardial infarction. Transverse section of cardiac ventricle showing two discrete myocardial metastatic deposits of lymphoma. These whitish deposits may be mistakenly interpreted as healed myocardial infarctions in a patient with clean epicardial coronary arteries. LV, left ventricle; RV, right ventricle; VS, ventricular septum. (From Waller.[1] Reproduced with permission from the author, editor, and publisher.)

References

1. Waller BF. Atherosclerotic and nonatherosclerotic coronary artery factors in acute myocardial infarction. In: Pepine CJ, ed. *Acute Myocardial Infarction*. Philadelphia: Davis; 1989:29–104.
2. Alpert JS, Braunwald E. Acute myocardial infarction: Pathological, pathophysiological and clinical manifestations. In: Braunwald E, ed. *Heart Disease: A Textbook of Cardiovascular Medicine*. Philadelphia: Saunders; 1984:1262–1300.
3. Eliot RS, Baroldi G. Necropsy studies in myocardial infarction with minimal or no coronary luminal reduction due to atherosclerosis. *Circulation* 1974; 49:1127–1131.
4. Cheitlin MD, McAllister HA, deCastro CM. Myocardial infarction without atherosclerosis. *JAMA* 1975; 231:951–959.
5. Baim DS, Harrison DC. Nonatherosclerotic coronary heart disease (including coronary artery spasm). In: Hurst JW et al, eds. *The Heart*, 5th ed. New York: McGraw-Hill; 1982:1158–1170.
6. Engel HJ, Torres C, Page HL. Major variations in anatomical origin of the coronary arteries: Angiographic observations in 4250 patients without associated congenital heart disease. *Cathet Cardiovasc Diag* 1975; 1:157–161.
7. Roberts WC. Major anomalies of coronary arterial origin seen in adulthood. *Am Heart J* 1986; 111:941–963.
8. Levin DC, Fellows KE, Abrams HL. Hemodynamically significant primary anomalies of the coronary arteries: Angiographic aspects. *Circulation* 1978; 58:25–34.
9. Roberts WC, Siegel RJ, Zipes DP. Origin of the right coronary artery from the left sinus of Valsalva and its functional consequences: Analysis of 10 necropsy patients. *Am J Cardiol* 1982; 49:863–868.
10. Waller BF. Exercise related sudden death in young (age <30 years) and old (age >30 years) conditioned athletes. In: Wenger NK, ed. *Exercise and the Heart*, 2d ed. Philadelphia: Davis; 1985:9–73.
11. Menke DM, Jordan MD, Sut CH, et al. Isolated and severe left main coronary atherosclerosis and thrombosis: A complication of acute angle takeoff of the left main coronary artery. *Am Heart J* 1986; 112:1319–1320.
12. Virmani R, Chun PKC, Goldstein RE, et al. Acute takeoffs of the coronary arteries along the aortic wall and congenital coronary ostial valve-like ridges: Association with sudden death. *J Am Coll Cardiol* 1984; 3:766–771.
13. Joswig BF, Warren SE, Vieweg WV, Hagan AD. Transmural myocardial infarction in the absence of coronary arterial luminal narrowing in a young man with single coronary arterial anomaly. *Cathet Cardiovasc Diag* 1978; 4:297–301.
14. Foster L, Waller BF, Pless JE. Hypoplastic coronary arteries and high takeoff position of the right coronary artery. *Chest* 1985; 88:299–301.
15. Foster L, Waller BF. Nonatherosclerotic fibrous ridges: A previously unrecognized cause of ostial left main stenosis. *J Indiana Med Assoc* 1983; 76:682–683.
16. Vlodaver Z, Amplatz K, Burchell HB, Edwards JE. *Coronary Heart Disease: Clinical, Angiographic and Pathologic Profiles*. New York: Springer-Verlag; 1976.
17. Alexander RW, Griffith GC. Anomalies of the coronary arteries and their clinical significance. *Circulation* 1956; 14:800–805.
18. Burth HC. Hoher und trichterformiger Ursprung der Herz Kanzarterien. *Beitr Pathol Anal* 1963; 128:139–148.
19. Holt S. Syphilitic ostial occlusion. *Br Heart J* 1977; 39:469–470.
20. Young JA, Sengupta A, Khaja FU. Coronary arterial stenosis, angina pectoris and atypical coarctation of the aorta due to nonspecific arteritis: Treatment, with aortocoronary bypass graft. *Am J Cardiol* 1973; 32:356–361.
21. Rozavi M. Unusual forms of coronary artery disease. In: D Vedt, ed. *Cleveland Clinic Cardiovascular Consultations*. Philadelphia: Davis; 1975:25.

22. Hudgson P, Foster JB, Walton JN. Methysergide and coronary artery disease. *Am Heart J* 1967; 74:854–855.
23. Yates JD, Kirsh MM, Sodeman TM, et al. Coronary ostial stenosis: A complication of aortic valve replacement. *Circulation* 1974; 49:530–534.
24. Baroldi G. Diseases of the coronary arteries. In: Silver MD, ed. *Cardiovascular Pathology*. New York: Churchhill-Livingstone; 1983:341.
25. Reyman HC. Disertatis de vasis cordis propiis. *Bibl Anat* 1737; 2:366–373.
26. Noble J, Bourassa MG, Petitclerc R, Dyrda I. Myocardial bridging and milking effect of the left anterior descending coronary artery: Normal variant or obstruction? *Am J Cardiol* 1976; 37:993–999.
27. Faruqui AM, Maloy WC, Felner JM, et al. Symptomatic myocardial bridging of the coronary artery. *Am J Cardiol* 1978; 41:1305–1310.
28. Visscher DW, Mildes BM, Waller BF. Tunneled ("bridged") left anterior descending coronary artery in a newborn without clinical or morphological evidence of myocardial ischemia. *Cath Cardiovasc Diag* 1983; 9:493–498.
29. Edwards JC, Burnsides C, Swarm RL, Lansing AJ. Arteriosclerosis and extramural portions of coronary arteries in the human heart. *Circulation* 1956; 13:235–241.
30. Polacek P. Relation of myocardial bridges and loops in the coronary arteries to coronary occlusions. *Am Heart J* 1961; 61:44–52.
31. Levin DC, Fellows KE, Abrams HL. Hemodynamically significant primary anomalies of the coronary arteries: Angiographic aspects. *Circulation* 1978; 58:25–34.
32. Kramer JR, Kitazume H, Proudin WI, Sones IM. Clinical significance of isolated coronary bridges: Benign and frequent condition involving the left anterior descending artery. *Am Heart J* 1982; 103:283–288.
33. Ishimori T, Raizner AE, Chahine RA, et al. Myocardial bridges in man: Clinical correlations and angiographic accentuation with nitroglycerin. *Cathet Cardiovas Diag* 1977; 3:59–65.
34. Roberts WC, Dicicco BS, Waller BF, et al. Origin of the left main from the right coronary artery or from the right aortic sinus with intramyocardial tunneling to the left side of the heart via the ventricular septum: The case against clinical significance of myocardial bridge or coronary tunnel. *Am Heart J* 1982; 104: 303–305.
35. Schulte MA, Waller BF, Hull MT, Pless JE. Origin of the left anterior descending artery from the right aortic sinus with intramyocardial tunneling to the left side of the heart via the ventricular septum: A case against clinical and morphologic significance of myocardial bridging. *Am Heart J* 1985; 110:499–501.
36. Angelini P, Trivellato M, Donis J, Leachman RD. Myocardial bridges: A review. *Prog Cardiovasc Dis* 1983; 26:75–88.
37. Isner JM, Donaldson RF. Coronary angiographic and morphologic correlation. *Cardiol Clin* 1984; 2:571–592.
38. Nakajima K, Taki J, Bunko H, et al. Demonstration of therapeutic effect in a patient with myocardial bridge by exercise-myocardial SPECT imaging. *Clin Nucl Med* 1985; 10:116–117.
39. Kramer JR, Kitazume H, Krauthamer D, et al. The prevalence of myocardial bridging and septal squeeze in patients with significant aortic stenosis. *Cleve Q* 1984; 51:35–38.
40. Carvalho VB, Macruz R, Decort LV, et al. Hemodynamic determinants of coronary constriction in human myocardial bridges. *Am Heart J* 1984; 108:73–80.
41. Kitazume H, Kramer JR, Krauthamer D, et al. Myocardial bridges in obstructive hypertrophic cardiomyopathy. *Am Heart J* 1983; 106:131–135.
42. Pichard AD, Casanegra P, Marchant E, Rodriguez JA. Abnormal regional myocardial flow in myocardial bridging of the left anterior descending coronary artery. *Am J Cardiol* 1981; 47:978–982.
43. Chee TP, Jensen DP, Padnick MB, et al. Myocardial bridging of the left anterior descending coronary artery resulting in subendocardial infarction. *Arch Intern Med* 1981; 141:1703–1704.
44. Traube C, Rafii S, Greenfield DH, et al. Progression of the milking effect of the coronary artery. *Chest* 1981; 79:475–476.
45. Greenspan M, Iskandrian AS, Catherwood E, et al. Myocardial bridging of the left anterior descending artery: Evaluation using exercise thallium-201 myocardial scintigraphy. *Cathet Cardiovasc Diagn* 1980; 6:173–180.
46. Kuhn FE, Reagan K, Mohler ER III, et al. Evidence for endothelial dysfunction and enhanced vasoconstriction in myocardial bridges. *Am Heart J* 1991; 122:1764–1766.
47. Voelker W, Euchner U, Dittmann H, Karsch KR. Long-term clinical course of patients with angina and angiographically normal coronary arteries. *Clin Cardiol* 1991; 14:307–311.
48. Feld H, Guadanino V, Hollander G, et al. Exercise-induced ventricular tachycardia in association with a myocardial bridge. *Chest* 1991; 1295–1296.
49. Furniss SS, Williams DO, McGregor CG. Systolic coronary occlusion due to myocardial bridging: A rare cause of ischemia. *Int J Cardiol* 1990; 26:116–117.
50. Somanath HS, Reddy KN, Gupta SK, et al. Myocardial bridge (MB): An angiographic curiosity? *Ind Heart J* 1989; 41:296–300.
51. Vasan RS, Bahl VK, Rajani M. Myocardial infarction associated with a myocardial bridge. *Int J Cardiol* 1989; 25:240–241.
52. Theron HD, Kleynhans PH, Marx JD, Jordaan PJ. Myocardial bridging as a cause of myocardial infarction: A case report. *S Afr Med J* 1988; 74:243–244.
53. Bennett JM, Bomerus P. Thallium-201 scintigraphy perfusion defect with dipyridamole in a patient with a myocardial bridge. *Clin Cardiol* 1988; 11:268–270.
54. Kracoff OH, Ovsyshcher I, Gueron M. Malignant course of a benign anomaly: Myocardial bridging. *Chest* 1987; 92:1113–1115.
55. Bestetti RB, Finzi LA, Amaral FT, et al. Myocardial bridging of coronary arteries associated with an impending acute myocardial infarction. *Clin Cardiol* 1987; 10:129–131.
56. Bestetti RB, Costa RS, Zucolotto S, Oliveira JS. Fatal outcome associated with autopsy proven myocardial bridging of the left anterior descending coronary artery. *Eur Heart J* 1989; 10: 573–576.
57. Ferreira AG Jr, Trotter SE, Konig B Jr, et al. Myocardial bridges: Morphological and functional aspects. *Br Heart J* 1991; 66: 364–367.
58. Irvin RG. The angiographic prevalence of myocardial bridging in man. *Chest* 1982; 81:198–202.
59. Channer KS, Bukis E, Hartnell G, Rees JR. Myocardial bridging of the coronary arteries. *Clin Radiol* 1989; 40:355–359.
60. Wymore P, Yedlicka JW, Garcia-Medina V, et al. The incidence of myocardial bridges in heart transplants. *Cardiovasc Int Radiol* 1989; 12:202–206.
61. Watanabe G, Ohhira M, Takemura H, et al. Surgical treatment for myocardial bridge using intraoperative echocardiography. *J Cardiovasc Surg* 1989; 30:1009–1012.
62. Betriu A, Tubau J, Sanz G, et al. Relief of angina by periarterial muscle resection of myocardial bridges. *Am Heart J* 1980; 100: 223–226.
63. Pey J, de Dios RM, Epeldegui A. Myocardial bridging and hypertrophic cardiomyopathy: Relief of ischemia by surgery. *Int J Cardiol* 1985; 8:327–330.
64. Gupta NC, Beauvais J. Physiologic assessment of coronary artery fistula. *Clin Nucl Med* 1991; 16:40–42.
65. Theman TE, Crosby DR. Coronary artery steal secondary to coronary arteriovenous fistula. *Can J Surg* 1981; 24:231–233, 236.
66. Nakashima M, Takashima S, Hashimoto K, Shiraishi M. Association of stroke and myocardial infarction in children. *Neuropediatrics* 1982; 13:47–49.
67. Macri R, Capulzini A, Fazzini L, et al. Congenital coronary artery

fistula: Report of five patients, diagnostic problems and principles of management. *Thorac Cardiovasc Surg* 1982; 30:167–171.
68. Sethia B, Pollock JC. Coronary artery fistula following rupture of aneurysm of the sinus node artery into the right atrium. *Thorac Cardiovasc Surg* 1985; 33:191–192.
69. Zalman F, Andia AM, Wu KT, et al. Atherosclerotic coronary artery aneurysm progressing to coronary artery fistula: Presentation as myocardial infarction with continuous murmur. *Am Heart J* 1987; 114:427–429.
70. Fyfe DA, Edwards WD, Driscoll DJ. Myocardial ischemia in patients with pulmonary atresia and intact ventricular septum. *J Am Coll Cardiol* 1986; 8:402–406.
71. Lau G. Sudden death arising from a congenital coronary artery fistula. *Forens Sci Int* 1995; 73:125–130.
72. Takahashi M, Sekiguchi H, Fujikawa H, et al. Multiple saccular aneurysm formation in a patient with bilateral coronary artery fistula: A case report and review of the literature. *Cardiology* 1995; 86:174–176.
73. Takahashi M, Sekiguchi H, Fujikawa H, et al. Multicystic aneurysmal dilatation of bilateral coronary artery fistula. *Cathet Cardiol Diagn* 1994; 31:290–292.
74. Cason BA, Gordon HJ. Coronary steal caused by a coronary artery fistula. *J Cardiothorac Vasc Anesth* 1992; 6:65–67.
75. Rein AJ, Yatsiv I, Simcha A. Intracardiac causes of superior vena cava obstruction. *Eur J Pediatr* 1988; 148:98–100.
76. Vavuranakis M, Bush CA, Boudoulas H. Coronary artery fistulas in adults: Incidence, angiographic characteristics, natural history. *Cathet Cardiovasc Diagn* 1995; 35:116–120.
77. Aydogan U, Onursal E, Cantez T, et al. Giant congenital coronary artery fistula to left superior vena cava and right atrium with compression of left pulmonary vein simulating cor triatriatum: Diagnostic value of magnetic resonance imaging. *Eur J Cardiovasc Surg* 1994; 8:97–99.
78. Vigneswaran WT, Pollock JC. Pulmonary atresia with ventricular septal defect and coronary artery fistula: A late presentation. *Br Heart J* 1988; 59:387–388.
79. Shizukuda Y, Yonekura S, Tsuchihashi K, et al. A case of a right coronary artery to left ventricle fistula observed over twenty years. *Jpn J Med* 1989; 28:510–514.
80. Wilde P, Watt I. Congenital coronary artery fistulae: Six new cases with a collective review. *Clin Radiol* 1980; 31:301–311.
81. Mori K, Onoe T, Ooka T. Three main coronary arteries to pulmonary artery fistula. *Jpn Circ J* 1981; 45:209–212.
82. Schneeweiss A, Rath S, Neufeld HN. Bilateral congenital coronary artery fistula. *Thorax* 1981; 36:697–698.
83. Adams P, Morris L, Ross I. Congenital left coronary artery–right ventricular fistula. *Austr Pediatr J* 1983; 19:47–50.
84. Nakashima T, Tsuji T, Miyanaga H, et al. A case of blue rubber bleb nevus syndrome with coronary artery fistula to left ventricle. *Gastroenterol Jpn* 1983; 18:255–259.
85. Liu PR, Leong KH, Lee PC, Chen YT. Congenital coronary artery–cardiac chamber fistulae: A study of fourteen cases. *Chung Hua i Hsueh Tsa Chih* 1994; 54:160–165.
86. Mabo P, Le Breton H, De Place C, Daubert C. Asymptomatic pseudoaneurysm of the left ventricle and coronary artery fistula after closed-chest ablation of an accessory pathway. *Am Heart J* 1992; 124:1637–1639.
87. Bata IR, MacDonald RG, O'Neill BJ. Coronary artery fistula as a complication of percutaneous transluminal coronary angioplasty. *Can J Cardiol* 1993; 9:331–335.
88. Iannone LA, Iannone DP. Iatrogenic left coronary artery fistula-to-left ventricle following PTCA: A previously unreported complication with nonsurgical management. *Am Heart J* 1990; 120:1215–1217.
89. Cheng TO. Coronary artery fistula related to dilatation of totally occluded vessel. *Clin Cardiol* 1994; 17:166.
90. Geist M, Rozenman Y, Hasin Y, Gotsman MS. Coronary artery–pulmonary artery fistula associated with hypertrophic cardiomyopathy. *Clin Cardiol* 1994; 17:93–94.
91. Shirai K, Ogawa M, Kawaguchi H, et al. Acute myocardial infarction due to thrombus formation in congenital coronary artery fistula. *Eur Heart J* 1994; 15:577–579.
92. Uchida N, Baudet E, Roques X, et al. Surgical experience of coronary artery–right ventricular fistula in a heart transplant patient. *Eur J Cardiothorac Surg* 1995; 9:106–108.
93. Uy R, Sharma B, Franciosa JA. Acquired coronary artery fistula to the left ventricle after acute myocardial infarction. *Am J Cardiol* 1986; 58:557–558.
94. Doi YL, Takata J, Hamashige N, et al. Congenital coronary arteriovenous fistula associated with dilated cardiomyopathy. *Chest* 1987; 91:464–466.
95. Lee RT, Mudge GH, Colucci WS. Coronary artery fistula after mitral valve surgery. *Am Heart J* 1988; 115:1128–1130.
96. Lucca MJ, Tomlinson GC. Acquired coronary artery fistula: A sign of mural thrombus. *Cathet Cardiovasc Diagn* 1988; 15:273–276.
97. Sandhu JS, Uretsky BF, Zerbe TR, et al. Coronary artery fistula in the heart transplant patient: A potential complication of endomyocardial biopsy. *Circulation* 1989; 79:350–356.
98. Henzlova MJ, Nath H, Bucy RP, et al. Coronary artery to right ventricle fistula in heart transplant recipients: A complication of endomyocardial biopsy. *J Am Coll Cardiol* 1989; 14:258–261.
99. Saeian K, Vellinga T, Troup P, Wetherbee J. Coronary artery fistula formation secondary to permanent pacemaker placement. *Chest* 1991; 99:780–781.
100. Sherman D, Smith C, Marboe C, et al. Right atrial angiosarcoma causing a coronary artery fistula: Diagnosis by transesophageal echocardiography. *Am Heart J* 1993; 126:254–256.
101. Gildein HP, Kleinert S, Layangool T, Wilkinson JL. Acquired coronary artery fistula in children after ventricular septal myectomy of the right or left ventricular outflow tract. *Am Heart J* 1995; 130:1124–1126.
102. Lowe JE, Adams DH, Cummings RG, et al. The natural history and recommended management of patients with traumatic coronary artery fistulas. *Ann Thorac Surg* 1983; 36:295–305.
103. Haas GE, Parr GV, Trout RG, Hargrove WC III. Traumatic coronary artery fistula. *J Trauma* 1986; 26:854–857.
104. Kwan T, Salciccioli L, Elsakr A, et al. Coronary artery fistula coexisting with a ventricular septal defect due to a penetrating gunshot wound. *Cathet Cardiovasc Diagn* 1995; 34:235–239.
105. Tami LF. Coronary artery-right ventricular fistula after coronary artery bypass grafting. *Clin Cardiol* 1993; 16:155–157.
106. Sapin P, Frantz E, Jain A, et al. Coronary artery fistula: An abnormality affecting all age groups. *Medicine* 1990; 69:101–113.
107. Hackett D, Hallidie-Smith KA. Spontaneous closure of coronary artery fistula. *Br Heart J* 1984; 52:477–479.
108. Griffiths SP, Ellis K, Hordof AJ, et al. Spontaneous complete closure of a congenital coronary artery fistula. *J Am Coll Cardiol* 1983; 2:1169–1173.
109. John S, Perianayagam WJ, Muralidharan S, et al. Surgical treatment of congenital coronary artery fistula. *Thorax* 1981; 36:350–354.
110. Rim RS, Yang YJ, Chiu IS, et al. Surgical management of congenital coronary artery fistula. *J Formos Med Assoc* 1985; 84:683–692.
111. Wellens F, Deuvaert F, Leclerc JL, Primo G. Coronary artery fistula: An absolute surgical indication. *Acta Chir Belg* 1984; 84:339–344.
112. Kostis JB, Burns JJ, Moreyra AE, Pichard AD. Recurrent coronary artery fistula. *Clin Cardiol* 1984; 7:307–313.
113. Reidy JF, Anjos RT, Qureshi SA, et al. Transcatheter embolization in the treatment of coronary artery fistulas. *J Am Coll Cardiol* 1991; 18:187–192.
114. Wenger NK. Nonatherosclerotic causes of myocardial ischemia

and necrosis. In: Hurst JW et al, eds. *The Heart*, 4th ed. New York: McGraw-Hill; 1978:1345–1362.
115. Glickel SZ, Maggs PR, Ellis FH. Coronary artery aneurysm. *Ann Thorac Surg* 1978; 25:372–376.
116. Sumino H, Kanda T, Sasaki T, et al. Myocardial infarction secondary to coronary aneurysm in systemic lupus erythematosus: An autopsy case. *Angiology* 1995; 46:527–530.
117. Teja K, Crampton RS. Intramural coronary arteritis from cholesterol emboli: A rare case of unstable angina preceding sudden death. *Am Heart J* 1985; 110:168–170.
118. Choy DS, Stertzer S, Loubeau JM, et al. Embolization and vessel wall perforation in argon laser recanalization. *Lasers Surg Med* 1985; 5:297–308.
119. Arvan S. Mural thrombi in coronary artery disease: Recent advances in pathogenesis, diagnosis, and approaches to treatment. *Arch Intern Med* 1984; 144:113–116.
120. Charles RG, Epstein EJ. Diagnosis of coronary embolism: A review. *J R Soc Med* 1983; 76:863–869.
121. Hartman RB, Harrison EE, Pupello DF, et al. Characteristics of left ventricular thrombus resulting in perioperative embolism: A complication of coronary artery bypass grafting. *J Thorac Cardiovasc Surg* 1983; 86:706–709.
122. Rath S, Har-Zahav Y, Battler A, et al. Coronary arterial embolus from left atrial myxoma. *Am J Cardiol* 1984; 54:1392–1393.
123. Tubbs RR, Picha GC, Levin HS, et al. Cotton emboli of the coronary arteries. *Hum Pathol* 1980; 11:76–80.
124. Keon WJ, Heggtveit HA, Leduc J. Perioperative myocardial infarction caused by atheroembolism. *J Thorac Cardiovasc Surg* 1982; 84:849–855.
125. Charles RG, Epstein EJ, Holt S, Coulshed N. Coronary embolism in valvular heart disease. *Q J Med* 1982; 51:147–161.
126. Camann WR, Sacks GM, Schools AG, et al. Nearly fatal cardiovascular collapse during total hip replacement: Probable coronary arterial embolism. *Anesth Analg* 1991; 72:245–248.
127. Wiegand V, Tebbe U, Helmchen U, Kreuzer H. Coronary arterial embolism due to valvular debris after percutaneous valvuloplasty of calcific mitral stenosis. *Clin Cardiol* 1988; 11:793–796.
128. Goulah RD, Rose MR, Strober M, Haft JI. Coronary dissection following chest trauma with systemic emboli. *Chest* 1988; 93:887–888.
129. Mercereau D, Klinke WP. Paradoxical coronary embolism associated with an unusual interatrial flap valve. *Can J Cardiol* 1988; 4:140–143.
130. Saenz CB, Harrell RR, Sawyer JA, Hood WP. Acute percutaneous transluminal coronary angioplasty complicated by embolism to a coronary artery remote from the site of infarction. *Cathet Cardiovasc Diagn* 1987; 13:266–268.
131. Lifschultz BD, Donoghue ER, Leestma JE, Boade WA. Embolization of cotton pledgets following insertion of porcine cardiac valve bioprostheses. *J Foren Sci* 1987; 32:1796–1800.
132. Johnson D, Gonzalez-Lavin L. Myocardial infarction secondary to calcific embolization: An unusual complication of bioprosthetic valve degeneration. *Ann Thorac Surg* 1986; 42:102–103.
133. Cina SJ, Raso DS, Crymes LW, Upshur JK. Fatal suture embolism to the left anterior descending coronary artery: A case report and review of the literature. *Am J Forens Med Pathol* 1994; 15:142–145.
134. Saber RS, Edwards WD, Bailey KR, et al. Coronary embolization after balloon angioplasty or thrombolytic therapy: An autopsy study of 32 cases. *J Am Coll Cardiol* 1993; 22:1283–1288.
135. Hopkins HR, Pecirep DP. Bullet embolization to a coronary artery. *Ann Thorac Surg* 1993; 56:370–372.
136. Nagaoka H, Funakoshi N, Innami R, et al. Left ventricular aneurysm, normal coronary arteries and embolization in a patient with systemic lupus erythematosus. *Chest* 1993; 103: 287–288.
137. Yutani C, Imakita M, Ueda-Ishibashi H, et al. Coronary artery embolism with special reference to invasive procedures as the source. *Mod Pathol* 1992; 5:244–249.
138. Cabin HS, Roberts WC. Left ventricular aneurysm, intraaneurysmal thrombus and systemic embolus in coronary heart disease. *Chest* 1980; 77:586–590.
139. Roberts WC. Coronary embolism: A review of causes, consequences and diagnostic considerations. *Cardiovasc Med* 1978; 3:699–709.
140. Waller BF, Dixon DS, Kem RW, Roberts WC. Embolus to the left main coronary artery. *Am J Cardiol* 1982; 50:658–660.
141. Isner JM, Donaldson RF. Coronary angiographic and morphologic correlation. In: Waller BF, ed. *Cardiac Morphology*. Philadelphia: Saunders; 1984:571–592.
142. Rabinowitz M, Virmani R, McAllister HA. Spontaneous coronary artery dissection and eosinophilic infiltration: A cause-and-effect relationship? *Am J Med* 1982; 72:923–928.
143. Waller BR. Pathology of transluminal balloon angioplasty used in the treatment of coronary heart disease. *Hum Pathol* 1987; 18:476–484.
144. Waller BF. Crackers, breakers, stretchers, drillers, scrapers, shavers, burners, welders and melters: The future of atherosclerotic coronary artery disease? A clinical-morphologic assessment. *J Am Coll Cardiol* 1989; 13:969–987.
145. Antoniucci D, Magi Diligenti L. Spontaneous dissection of the three major coronary arteries. *Eur Heart J* 1990; 11:1130–1134.
146. Mather PJ, Hansen CL, Goldman B, et al. Postpartum multivessel coronary dissection. *J Heart Lung Transplant* 1994; 13:533–537.
147. Wasserman L, Wolf P, Podolin R, Bloor CM. Dissecting aneurysm of a coronary artery due to percutaneous transluminal balloon angioplasty. *Am J Cardiovasc Pathol* 1990; 3:271–274.
148. Ehya H, Weitzner S. Postpartum dissecting aneurysm of coronary arteries in a patient with sarcoidosis. *South Med J* 1980; 73:87–88.
149. Lantos G, Sos TA, Sniderman KW, et al. Dissecting hematoma of the thoracic aorta extending into a coronary artery: Angiographic demonstration. *Radiology* 1980; 135:329–330.
150. Molloy PJ, Ablett MB, Anderson KR. Left main stem coronary artery dissection. *Br Heart J* 1980; 43:705–708.
151. Shin P, Minamino T, Onishi S, Kitamura H. Dissecting aneurysms of the coronary arteries. *Acta Pathol Jpn* 1982; 32:713–724.
152. van der Bel-Kahn J. Recurrent primary coronary artery dissecting aneurysm. *Am J Clin Pathol* 1982; 78:394–398.
153. Morise AP, Hardin NJ, Bovill EG, Gundel WD. Coronary artery dissection secondary to coronary arteriography: Presentation of three cases and review of the literature. *Cathet Cardiovasc Diagn* 1981; 7:283–296.
154. Gibson WG, Reimer KA. Multiple coronary artery dissections in old age: A unique case. *Arch Pathol Lab Med* 1980; 104:419–421.
155. Paidipaty BB, Husain M, Puri VK. Right coronary artery occlusion after acute proximal dissection. *Crit Care Med* 1983; 11:574–575.
156. Virmani R, Forman MB, Robinowitz M, McAllister HA. Coronary artery dissections. *Cardiol Clin* 1984; 2:633–646.
157. Boland J, Limet R, Trotteur G, et al. Left main coronary dissection after mild chest trauma: Favorable evolution with fibrinolytic and surgical therapies. *Chest* 1988; 93:213–214.
158. Nishikawa H, Nakanishi S, Nishiyama S, et al. Primary coronary artery dissection: Its incidence, mode of the onset and prognostic evaluation. *J Cardiol* 1988; 18:307–317.
159. Wisecarver J, Jones J, Goaley T, McManus B. Spontaneous coronary artery dissection: The challenge of detection, the enigma of cause. *Am J Forens Med Pathol* 1989; 10:60–62.
160. Movsesian MA, Wray RB. Postpartum myocardial infarction. *Br Heart J* 1989; 62:154–156.
161. Burkey D, Love J, Fanning J, Lambrew C. Multiple spontaneous coronary artery dissections in a middle aged woman: Support for an underlying eosinophilic arteritis predisposing to intimal disruption. *Cathet Cardiovasc Diagn* 1993; 30:303–305.

162. Siegel RJ, Koponen M. Spontaneous coronary artery dissection causing sudden death: Mechanical arterial failure or primary vasculitis. *Arch Pathol Lab Med* 1994; 118:196–198.
163. Bateman AC, Gallagher PJ, Vincenti AC. Sudden death from coronary artery dissection. *J Clin Pathol* 1995; 48:781–784.
164. Sage MD, Koelmeyer TD, Smeeton WM. Fatal postpartum coronary artery dissection: A light- and electron-microscope study. *Am J Forens Med Pathol* 1986; 7:107–111.
165. Thayer JO, Healy RW, Maggs PR. Spontaneous coronary artery dissection. *Ann Thorac Surg* 1987; 44:97–102.
166. Emori T, Goto Y, Maeda T, et al. Multiple coronary artery dissections diagnosed in vivo in a pregnant woman. *Chest* 1993; 104:289–290.
167. Shaver PJ, Carrig TF, Baker WP. Postpartum coronary artery dissection. *Br Heart J* 1978; 40:83–86.
168. Waller BF, Orr CM, Pinkerton CA, et al. Coronary balloon angioplasty dissections: The good, the bad, and the ugly. *J Am Coll Cardiol* 1992; 20:701–706.
169. Prinzmetal M, Kennamer R, Merliss R, Wada T. Angina pectoris: I. A variant form of angina pectoris. Preliminary report. *Am J Med* 1959; 27:375–388.
170. Peretz DI. Variant angina pectoris of Prinzmetal. *Can Med Assoc J* 1961; 85:1101–1102.
171. Gianelly R, Mugler F, Harrison DC. Prinzmetal's variant of angina pectoris with only slight coronary atherosclerosis. *Calif Med* 1968; 108:129–132.
172. Silvermann ME, Flamm MD. Variant angina pectoris: Anatomic findings and prognostic implications. *Ann Intern Med* 1971; 75:339–343.
173. Dhurandhar RW, Watt DL, Silver MD, et al. Prinzmetal's variant form of angina with arteriographic evidence of coronary arterial spasm. *Am J Cardiol* 1972; 30:902–905.
174. Cosby RS, Giddins JA, See JR, Mayo M. Variant angina: Case reports and critique. *Am J Med* 1972; 53:739–742.
175. Cheng TO, Bashour T, Kelser GA, et al. Variant angina of Prinzmetal with normal coronary arteriograms: A variant of the variant. *Circulation* 1973; 47:476–485.
176. Donsky MS, Harris MD, Curry GC, et al. Variant angina pectoris: A clinical and coronary arteriographic spectrum. *Am Heart J* 1975; 89:571–578.
177. Wiener L, Kasparian H, Duca PR, et al. Spectrum of coronary arterial spasm: Clinical, angiographic and myocardial metabolic experience in 29 cases. *Am J Cardiol* 1976; 38:945–955.
178. Bharati S, Dhingra RC, Lev M, et al. Conduction system in a patient with Prinzmetal's angina and transient atrioventricular block. *Am J Cardiol* 1977; 39:120–125.
179. Maseri A, L'Abbate A, Baroldi G, et al. Coronary vasospasm as a possible cause of myocardial infarction: A conclusion derived from the study of "preinfarction" angina. *New Engl J Med* 1978; 299:1271–1277.
180. Roberts WC, Curry RC, Isner JM, et al. Sudden death in Prinzmetal's angina with coronary spasm documented by angiography: Analysis of 3 necropsy patients. *Am J Cardiol* 1982; 50:203–210.
181. Brown BF. Coronary vasospasm: Observations linking the clinical spectrum of ischemic heart disease to the dynamic pathology of coronary, atherosclerosis. *Arch Intern Med* 1981; 141:716–722.
182. Conti CR. Large vessel coronary vasospasm: Diagnosis, natural history and treatment. *Am J Cardiol* 1985; 55:41B–49B.
183. Lambert CR, Pepine CJ. Coronary artery spasm and acute myocardial infarction. *Cardiovasc Clin* 1989; 20:131–140.
184. Zainea M, Duvernoy WF, Chauhan A, et al. Acute myocardial infarction in angiographically normal coronary arteries following induction of general anesthesia. *Arch Intern Med* 1994; 154:2495–2498.
185. Kounis NG, Zavras GM. Histamine induced coronary artery spasm: The concept of allergic angina. *Br J Clin Pract* 1991; 45:121–128.
186. Ruch A, Duhring JL. Postpartum myocardial infarction in a patient receiving bromocriptine. *Obstet Gynecol* 1989; 74: 448–451.
187. Fischell TA. Coronary artery spasm after percutaneous transluminal coronary angioplasty: Pathophysiology and clinical consequences. *Cathet Cardiovasc Diagn* 1990; 19:1–3.
188. Halper J, Factor SM. Coronary lesions in neurofibromatosis associated with vasospasm and myocardial infarction. *Am Heart J* 1984; 108:420–422.
189. Shepherd JT, Katusic ZS, Vedernikov Y, Vanhoutte PM. Mechanisms of coronary vasospasm: Role of endothelium. *J Mol Cell Cardiol* 1991; 23(suppl 1):125–131.
190. Kalsner S. Coronary artery spasm: Multiple causes and multiple roles in heart disease. *Biochem Pharmacol* 1995; 49:859–871.
191. Hillis LD, Braunwald E. Coronary artery spasm. *New Engl J Med* 1978; 299:695–702.
192. Ginsburg R, Birstow MR, Harrison DC, Stinson EB. Studies with isolated human coronary arteries: Some general observations, potential mediators of spasm, role of calcium antagonists. *Chest* 1980; 78:180–186.
193. Maseri A, Severi S, De Nes M, et al. "Variant" angina: One aspect of a continuous spectrum of vasospastic myocardial ischemia. *Am J Cardiol* 1978; 42:1019–1035.
194. El-Maraghi NRH , Sealey BJ. Recurrent myocardial infarction in a young man with coronary arterial spasm, demonstrated at autopsy. *Circulation* 1980; 61:199–207.
195. Isner JM, Donaldson RF, Katsas GC. Spasm at autopsy: A prospective study (abstract). *Circulation* 1983; 68:III-1028.
196. Isner JM, Fortin AH, Fortin RV. Depletion of smooth muscle from the media of atherosclerotic coronary arteries: A potential factor in the pathogenesis of myocardial ischemia and the variable response to anti-anginal therapy (abstract). *Clin Res* 1983; 31: 193A.
197. Factor SM, Cho S. Smooth muscle contraction bands in the media of coronary arteries: A postmortem marker of antemortem coronary spasm? *J Am Coll Cardiol* 1985; 6:1329–1337.
198. Waller BF. The eccentric coronary atherosclerotic plaque: Morphologic observations and clinical relevance. *Clin Cardiol* 1988; 12:14–20.
199. Hangartner JRW, Charleston AJ, Davies MJ, Thomas AC. Morphologic characteristics of clinically significant coronary artery stenosis in stable angina. *Br Heart J* 1986; 56:501–508.
200. Quyyumi AA, Al-Rufaii HK, Olsen EGJ, Fox KM. Coronary anatomy in patients with various manifestations of three vessel coronary artery disease. *Br Heart J* 1985; 54:362–366.
201. Hort W, Moosdorf R, Kalbfleisch H, et al. Postmortale Untersuchungen uber Lokalisation und Form der starksten Stenosen in den Koronararterien und ihre Beziehung zu den Risikofaktoren. *Z Kardiol* 1977; 66:333–340.
202. Freudenberg H, Lichtlen PR. Das Normale Wandsegment bei Koronarstenosen—ein postmortale Studie. *Z Kardiol* 1981; 70:863–869.
203. Saner HE, Gobel FL, Salomonowitz E, et al. The disease-free wall in coronary atherosclerosis: Its relation to degree of obstruction. *J Am Coll Cardiol* 1985; 6:1096–1099.
204. Manion WC. Infectious angiitis. In: Orbison JL, Smith DE, eds. *The Peripheral Blood Vessels*. Baltimore: Williams & Wilkins; 1963:221.
205. Lie JT. Coronary vasculitis: A review in the current scheme of classification of vasculitis. *Arch Pathol Lab Med* 1987; 111:224–233.
206. Parillo JE, Fauci AS. Coronary vasculitis. In: Ansell BM, Simkin PA, eds. *The Heart and Rheumatic Disease*. Woburn, MA: Butterworth; 1984:213–233.
207. Manion WC. Infectious angiitis. In: Orbison JL, Smith DE, eds. *The Peripheral Blood Vessels*. Baltimore: Williams and Wilkins; 1963:221–231.

208. DeShazo RD. The spectrum of systemic vasculitis. A classification to aid diagnosis. *Postgrad Med* 1975; 58:78–82.
209. Paronetto F. Systemic nonsuppurative necrotizing angiitis. In: Miescher PA, Muller-Eberhard HJ, eds. *Textbook of Immunopathology*, 2d ed. New York: Grune & Stratton; 1976:1012–1024.
210. Christian CL, Sergent JS. Vasculitis syndromes: Clinical and experimental models. *Am J Med* 1976; 61:385–392.
211. Conn DL, McDuffie FC, Holley KE, Schroeter AL. Immunologic mechanisms in systemic vasculitis. *Mayo Clin Proc* 1976; 51:511–518.
212. Fauci AS, Haynes BF, Katz P. The spectrum of vasculitis: Clinical, pathogenic, immunologic, and therapeutic considerations. *Ann Intern Med* 1978; 89:660–676.
213. Soter NA, Austen KF. Pathogenetic mechanisms in necrotizing vasculitides. *Clin Rheum Dis* 1980; 6:233–253.
214. McCluskey RT, Fienberg R. Vasculitis in primary vasculitides, granulomatoses, and connective tissue diseases. *Hum Pathol* 1983; 14:305–315.
215. Kussmaul A, Maier R. Uber eine bisher nicht beschriebene eigenthumliche Arterienerkrankung (periarteritis nodosa), die mit Morbus Brightii und rapid fortschreitender allgemeiner Muskellahmung einhergeht. *Dtsch Arch Klin Med* 1866; 1:484–518.
216. Dickson WE. Polyarteritis acuta nodosa and periarteritis nodosa. *J Pathol Bacteriol* 1908; 12:31–57.
217. Zeek PM. Periarteritis nodosa: A critical review. *Am J Clin Pathol* 1952; 22:777–790.
218. Zeek PM. Periarteritis and other forms of necrotizing angiitis. *New Engl J Med* 1953; 248:764–772.
219. Churg J, Strauss L. Allergic granulomatosis, allergic angiitis, and periarteritis nodosa. *Am J Pathol* 1951; 27:277–294.
220. Churg J. Allergic granulomatosis and granulomatous vascular syndromes. *Ann Allergy* 1963; 21:619–628.
221. Lanham JG, Elkon KB, Pusey CD, Hughes GF. Systemic vasculitis with asthma and eosinophilia: A clinical approach to the Churg-Strauss syndrome. *Medicine* 1984; 63:65–81.
222. Von Glahn WC, Pappenheimer AM. Specific lesions of peripheral blood vessels in rheumatism. *Am J Pathol* 1926; 2:235–250.
223. Huthinson J. Diseases of the arteries: On a peculiar form of thrombotic arteritis of the aged which is sometimes productive of gangrene. *Arch Surg Lond* 1890; 1:323–329.
224. Horton BT, Magath TB, Brown GE. An underscribed form of arteritis of the temporal vessels. *Mayo Clin Proc* 1932; 7:700–701.
225. Horton BT, Magath TB, Brown GE. Arteritis of the temporal vessels. *Arch Intern Med* 1934; 53:400–410.
226. Cooke WT, Cloake PC, Govan AD, Colbeck JC. Temporal arteritis: A generalized vascular disease. *Q J Med* 1946; 15:47–75.
227. Hamilton CR, Shelley WM, Tumulty PA. Giant cell arteritis: Including temporal arteritis and polymyalgia rheumatica. *Medicine* 1971; 50:1–27.
228. Ostberg G. On arteritis: With special reference to polymyalgia arteritica. *Acta Pathol Microbiol Immunol Scand A* 1973; 237:1–59.
229. Somer T. Thrombo-embolic and vascular complications in vasculitis syndromes. *Eur Heart J* 1993; 14(suppl K):24–29.
230. Kawai S, Fukuda Y, Okada R. Atherosclerosis of the coronary arteries in collagen disease and allied disorders with special reference to vasculitis as a preceding lesion of coronary atherosclerosis. *Jpn Circ J* 1982; 46:1208–1221.
231. Karsner HT. *Acute Inflammations of Arteries*. Springfield, IL: Charles C Thomas; 1947.
232. Allen AC, Spitz S. A comparative study of the pathology of scrub typhus (Tsutsugamushi disease) and other rickettsial diseases. *Am J Pathol* 1945; 21:603–682.
233. Moritz AR. Syphilitic coronary arteritis. *Arch Pathol Lab Med* 1931; 11:44–59.
234. Bruenn HG. Syphilitic disease of the coronary arteries. *Am Heart J* 1934; 9:421–436.
235. Scharfman WB, Wallach JB, Angrist A. Myocardial infarction due to syphilitic coronary ostial stenosis. *Am Heart J* 1950; 40:603–613.
236. Holt S. Syphilitic ostial occlusion. *Br Heart J* 1977; 39:469–470.
237. Heggtveit HA. Syphilitic aortitis: A clinicopathologic study of 100 cases, 1950 to 1960. *Circulation* 1964; 29:346–355.
238. Rose AG. Cardiac tuberculosis. A study of 19 patients. *Arch Pathol Lab Med* 1987; 111:422–426.
239. Gouley BA, Bellet S, McMillan TM. Tuberculosis of the myocardium: Report of six cases with observations on involvement of coronary arteries. *Arch Intern Med* 1933; 51:244–263.
240. Manion WC. Infectious angiitis. In: Orbison JL, Smith DE, eds. *The Peripheral Blood Vessels*. Baltimore: Williams & Wilkins; 1963; 221–231.
241. Merkel WC. Plasmodium falciparum malaria: The coronary and myocardial lesions observed in autopsy in two cases of acute fulminating *P. falciparum* infection. *Arch Pathol* 1946; 41: 290–298.
242. Gazayerli M. Unusual site of a schistosome worm in the circumflex branch of the left coronary artery. *J Egypt Med Assoc* 1939; 22:34–39.
243. Allen AC, Spitz S. A comparative study of the pathology of scrub typhus (Tsutsugamuschi's disease) and other rickettsial diseases. *Am J Pathol* 1945; 21:603–681.
244. Moe JB, Mosher DF, Kenyon RH, et al. Functional and morphological changes during experimental Rocky Mountain spotted fever in guinea pigs. *Lab Invest* 1976; 35:235–245.
245. Sergent JS. Vasculitides associated with viral infections. *Clin Rheum Dis* 1980; 6:339–350.
246. Sergent JS, Lockshin MD, Christian CL, Gocke DJ. Vasculitis with hepatitis B antigenemia: Long-term observations in nine patients. *Medicine* 1976; 55:1–18.
247. Heibel RH, O'Toole JD, Curtiss EI, et al. Coronary arteritis in systemic lupus erythematosus. *Chest* 1976; 69:700–703.
248. Cipriano PR, Silverman JF, Perlroth MG, et al. Coronary arterial narrowing in Takayasu's aortitis. *Am J Cardiol* 1977; 39:744–750.
249. Judge RD, Currier RD, Gracie WA, Figley MM. Takayasu's arteritis and the aortic arch syndrome. *Am J Med* 1962; 32: 379–392.
250. Strachan RW. The natural history of Takayasu's arteriopathy. *Q J Med* 1964; 33:57–69.
251. Ueda H. Clinical and pathological studies of aortitis syndrome: Committee report. *Jpn Heart J* 1968; 9:76–87.
252. Hachiya J. Current concepts of Takayasu's arteritis. *Semin Roentgenol* 1970; 5:245–259.
253. Lupi-Herrera E, Sanchez-Torres G, Marcus-Hamer J, et al. Takayasu's arteritis: Clinical study of 107 cases. *Am Heart J* 1977; 93:94–103.
254. Ischikawa K. Natural history and classification of occlusive thromboarteriopathy (Takayasu's disease). *Circulation* 1978; 57:27–35.
255. Rose AG, Sinclair-Smith CC. Takayasu's arteritis: A study of 16 cases. *Arch Pathol Lab Med* 1980; 104:231–237.
256. Hall S, Barr W, Lie JT, et al. Takayasu arteritis: A study of 32 North American patients. *Medicine* 1985; 64:89–99.
257. Aufderheide AC, Henke BW, Parker EH. Granulomatous coronary arteritis (Takayasu's disease). *Arch Pathol Lab Med* 1981; 105:647–649.
258. Hashimoto Y, Numano F, Maruyama Y, et al. Thallium 201 stress scintigraphy in Takayasu arteritis. *Am J Cardiol* 1991; 67:879–882.
259. Kinare SG. Cardiac lesions in nonspecific aortoarteritis: An autopsy study. *Ind Heart J* 1994; 46:65–69.
260. Takei M, Sasaki Y, Suyama K, et al. Surgically treated case of complete obstruction of the left main coronary artery caused by Takayasu's arteritis. *Am Heart J* 1993; 126:458–459.
261. Tanaka M, Abe T, Takeuchi E, et al. Revascularization for coronary ostial stenosis in Takayasu's disease with calcified aorta. *Ann Thorac Surg* 1992; 53:894–895.

262. Nakano S, Shimazaki Y, Keneko M, et al. Transaortic patch angioplasty for left coronary ostial stenosis in a patient with Takayasu's aortitis. *Ann Thorac Surg* 1992; 53:694–696.
263. Aufderheide AC, Henke BW, Parker EH. Granulomatous coronary arteritis. *Arch Pathol Lab Med* 1981; 105:647–649.
264. Rosen H, Gaton E. Takayasu's arteritis of coronary arteries. *Arch Pathol Lab Med* 1972; 94:225–229.
265. Case 46-1967. Case records of the Massachusetts General Hospital: Weekly clinicopathological exercise. *New Engl J Med* 1967; 277:1025–1033.
266. Lie JT, Failoni DD, Davis DC. Temporal arteritis with giant cell aortitis, coronary arteritis, and myocardial infarction. *Arch Pathol Lab Med* 1986; 110:857–860.
267. Klein RG, Hunder GG, Stanson AW, Sheps SG. Large vessel involvement in giant cell (temporal) arteritis. *Ann Intern Med* 1975; 83:806–812.
268. Harris M. Dissecting aneurysm of the aorta due to giant cell arteritis. *Br Heart J* 1968; 30:840–844.
269. Morrison AN, Abitbol M. Granulomatous arteritis with myocardial infarction: A case report with autopsy findings. *Ann Intern Med* 1955; 42:691–700.
270. Crompton MR. The visual changes in temporal (giant cell) arteritis: Report of a case with autopsy findings. *Brain* 1959; 82:377–390.
271. Martin JF, Kittas C, Triger DR. Giant cell arteritis of coronary arteries causing myocardial infarction. *Br Heart J* 1980; 43: 487–489.
272. Save-Soderbergh J, Malmvall BE, Andersson R, Bengtsson RA. Giant cell arteritis as a cause of death: Report of nine cases. *JAMA* 1985; 255:493–496.
273. Lie JT. Disseminated visceral giant cell arteritis: Histopathologic description and differentiation from other granulomatous vasculitides. *Am J Clin Pathol* 1978; 69:299–305.
274. Ainsworth RW, Gresham GA, Balmforth GV. Pathologic changes in temporal arteries removed from unselected cadavers. *J Clin Pathol* 1961; 14:115–119.
275. Harrison CV. Giant-cell or temporal arteritis: A review. *J Clin Pathol* 1948; 1:197–211.
276. Paulley JW. Coronary ischemia and occlusion in giant cell (temporal) arteritis. *Acta Med Scand* 1980; 208:257–263.
277. Zvaifler NJ, Weintraub AM. Aortitis and aortic insufficiency in chronic rheumatic disorders: A reappraisal. *Arthritis Rheum* 1963; 6:241–245.
278. Heggtveit HA, Hennigar GR, Morrione TG. Panaortitis. *Am J Pathol* 1963; 42:151–172.
279. Reimer KA, Rodgers RF, Oyasu R. Rheumatoid arthritis with rheumatoid heart disease and granulomatous aortitis. *JAMA* 1976; 235:2510–2512.
280. Sokoloff L. Cardiac involvement in rheumatoid arthritis and allied disorders: current concepts. *Mod Concepts Cardiovasc Dis* 1964; 33:847–850.
281. Lie JT. Rheumatoid arthritis and heart disease. *Prim Cardiol* 1982; 8:137–152.
282. Swezey RL. Myocardial infarction due to rheumatoid arthritis. *JAMA* 1967; 199:855–857.
283. Karten I. Arteritis, myocardial infarction, and rheumatoid arthritis. *JAMA* 1969; 210:1717–1720.
284. Voyles WF, Searles RP, Bankhurst AD. Myocardial infarction caused by rheumatoid vasculitis. *Arthritis Rheum* 1980; 23:860–883.
285. Morris PB, Imber MJ, Heinsimer JA, et al. Rheumatoid arthritis and coronary arteritis. *Am J Cardiol* 1986; 57:689–690.
286. Pagel W. Polyarteritis nodosa and the rheumatic diseases. *J Clin Pathol* 1951; 4:137.
287. Cruickshank B. The arteritis of rheumatoid arthritis. *Ann Rheum Dis* 1954; 13:136–145.
288. Schmid FR, Cooper NS, Ziff M, McEwen C. Arteritis in rheumatoid arthritis. *Am J Med* 1961; 30:56–83.
289. Glass D, Soter NA, Schur PH. Rheumatoid vasculitis. *Arthritis Rheum* 1976; 19:950–952.
290. Scott DG, Bacon PA, Tribe CR. Systemic rheumatoid vasculitis: A clinical and laboratory study of 50 cases. *Medicine* 1981; 60:288–297.
291. James TN. De Subitaneis Mortibus: XXIII. Rheumatoid arthritis and ankylosing spondylitis. *Circulation* 1977; 55:669–677.
292. Hoffman FG, Leight L. Complete atrioventricular block associated with rheumatoid disease. *Am J Cardiol* 1965; 16:585–592.
293. Grismer JT, Anderson WR, Weiss L. Chronic occlusive rheumatic coronary vasculitis and myocardial dysfunction. *Am J Cardiol* 1976; 20:739–745.
294. Kawai S, Okada R, Sugimoto H, et al. An autopsied case of a two month old infant with granulomatous pancarditis having severe vasculitis and valvulitis. *Jpn Circ J* 1983; 47:1325–1330.
295. Bely M, Apathy A, Beke Martos E. Cardiac changes in rheumatoid arthritis. Acta Morphol Hung 1992; 40:149–186.
296. Voyles WF, Searles RP, Bankhurst AD. Myocardial infarction caused by rheumatoid vasculitis. *Arthritis Rheum* 1980; 23:860–863.
297. Fujita M, Abe M, Itoh T, et al. Nonarthritic rheumatoid valvulitis with coronary arteritis causing myocardial infarction. *Virchows Arch* 1992; 420:109–112.
298. Buerger L. Thromboangiitis obliterans: A study of the vascular lesions leading to presenile spontaneous gangrene. *Am J Med Sci* 1908; 136:567–580.
299. McKusick VA, Harris WS, Otteson OE, et al. Buerger's disease: A distinct clinical and pathologic entity. *JAMA* 1962; 181:5–12.
300. Wessler S. Buerger's disease revisited. *Surg Clin North Am* 1969; 49:703–713.
301. Williams G. Recent views on Buerger's disease. *J Clin Pathol* 1969; 22:573–578.
302. Vink M. Symposium on Buerger's disease. *J Cardiovasc Surg* 1973; 14:1–51.
303. Gilkes R, Dow J. Aortic involvement in Buerger's disease. *Br J Med* 1973; 46:110–114.
304. Saphir O. Thromboangiitis obliterans of the coronary arteries and its relation to arteriosclerosis. *Am Heart J* 1936; 12:521–535.
305. Gore I, Burrows S. A reconsideration of the pathogenesis of Buerger's disease. *Am J Clin Pathol* 1958; 29:319–330.
306. Ohno H, Matsuda Y, Takashiba K, et al. Acute myocardial infarction in Buerger's disease. *Am J Cardiol* 1986; 57:690–691.
307. Mautner GC, Mautner SL, Lin F, et al. Amounts of coronary arterial luminal narrowing and composition of the material causing the narrowing in Buerger's disease. *Am J Cardiol* 1993; 71:486–490.
308. Averbuck SH, Silbert S. Thromboangiitis obliterans: Cause of death. *Arch Intern Med* 1934; 54:436–465.
309. Lie JT. Thromboangiitis obliterans (Buerger's disease) in a saphenous vein arterial graft. *Hum Pathol* 1999 (in press).
310. Fronert PP, Sheps SG. Long-term follow-up study of polyarteritis nodosa. *Am J Med* 1967; 43:8–14.
311. Sack M, Cassidy JT, Bole GG. Prognostic factors in polyarteritis. *J Rheumatol* 1975; 2:411–420.
312. Leib ES, Restivo C, Paulus HE. Immunosuppressive and corticosteroid therapy of polyarteritis nodosa. *Am J Med* 1979; 67:941–947.
313. Cohen RD, Conn DL, Ilstrup DM. Clinical features, prognosis, and response to treatment in polyarteritis. *Mayo Clin Proc* 1980; 55:146–155.
314. Scott DG, Becon PA, Elliott PJ, et al. Systemic vasculitis in a district general hospital 1972–1980: Clinical and laboratory classification and prognosis in 80 cases. *Q J Med* 1982; 51:292–311.
315. Holsinger DR, Osmondson PJ, Edwards JE. The heart in polyarteritis nodosa. *Circulation* 1962; 25:610–617.
316. Arkin A. A clinical and pathological study of periarteritis nodosa. *Am J Pathol* 1930; 6:401–426.

317. Sinclair W, Nitsch E. Polyarteritis nodosa of the coronary arteries: Report of a case with rupture of an aneurysm and intrapericardial hemorrhage. *Am Heart J* 1949; 38:898–904.
318. Przybojewski JZ. Polyarteritis nodosa in the adult: Report of a case with repeated myocardial infarction and a review of cardiac involvement. *S Afr Med J* 1981; 60:512–518.
319. Swalwell CI, Reddy SK, Rao VJ. Sudden death due to unsuspected coronary vasculitis. *Am J Forens Med Pathol* 1991; 12:306–312.
320. Sugihara N, Genda A, Shimizu M, et al. Intramural coronary angiitis of periarteritis nodosa proved by endomyocardial biopsy. *Am Heart J* 1990; 119:1414–1416.
321. Ettinger RE, Nelson AM, Buske EC, Lie JT. Polyarteritis nodosa in childhood: A clinical pathologic study. *Arthritis Rheum* 1979; 22:820–825.
322. Petty RE, Maligilavy DB, Cassidy JT, Sullivan DB. Polyarteritis in childhood: A clinical description of eight cases. *Arthritis Rheum* 1977; 20:392–394.
323. Roberts FB, Fetterman GH. Polyarteritis nodosa in infancy. *J Pediatr* 1963; 63:519–529.
324. Munro-Faure H. Necrotizing arteritis of the coronary vessels in infancy: Case report and review of the literature. *Pediatrics* 1959; 23:914–926.
325. Tanaka N, Naoe S, Masuda H, Ueno T. Pathological study of sequelae of Kawasaki disease (MCLS): With special reference to the heart and coronary arterial lesions. *Acta Pathol Japan* 1986; 36:1513–1527.
326. Kawasaki T, Kosaki F, Okawa S, et al. A new infantile acute febrile mucocutaneous lymph node syndrome (MLNS) prevailing in Japan. *Pediatrics* 1974; 54:271–276.
327. Melish ME. Kawasaki syndrome (the mucocutaneous lymph node syndrome). *Annu Rev Med* 1982; 33:569–585.
328. Tanaka N. Kawasaki disease (acute febrile infantile mucocutaneous lymph node syndrome) in Japan: Relationship with infantile polyarteritis nodosa. *Pathol Microbiol* 1975; 43:204–218.
329. Langing BH, Larson EJ. Are infantile periarteritis nodosa with coronary artery involvement and fatal mucocutaneous lymph node syndrome the same? Comparison of 20 patients from North America with patients from Hawaii and Japan. *Pediatrics* 1977; 59:651–662.
330. Amano S, Hozama F, Hamashima Y. Pathology of Kawasaki disease: I. Pathology and morphology of the vascular changes. *Jpn Circ J* 1979; 43:633–643.
331. Amano S, Hozama F, Hamashima Y. Pathology of Kawasaki disease: II. Distribution and incidence of the vascular lesions. *Jpn Circ J* 1979; 43:741–748.
332. Fukushige J, Nihill MR, McNamara DG. Spectrum of cardiovascular lesions in mucocutaneous lymph node syndrome. *Am J Cardiol* 1980; 45:98–107.
333. Kitamura S, Kawashima Y, Fujita T, et al. Aortocoronary bypass grafting in a child with coronary artery obstruction due to mucocutaneous lymph node syndrome: Report of a case. *Circulation* 1976; 53:1035–1040.
334. Kato H, Koike S, Yamamoto M, et al. Coronary aneurysms in infants and young children with acute febrile mucocutaneous lymph node syndrome. *J Pediatr* 1975; 86:892–898.
335. Tanimoto T, Kamiya T, Misawa H, et al. An autopsied case of an elementary school boy with sudden death four years after Kawasaki disease: On the problem of present method of cardiac mass screening of school children. *Jpn Circ J* 1981; 45:1438–1442.
336. Kitamura S, Kawachi K, Harima R, et al. Surgery for coronary heart disease due to mucocutaneous lymph node syndrome: Report of 6 patients. *Am J Cardiol* 1983; 51:444–448.
337. Quam JP, Edwards WD, Bambara JF, Luzier TL. Sudden death in an adolescent four years after recovery from mucocutaneous lymph node syndrome. *J Forens Sci* 1986; 31:1135–1141.
338. Suzuki A, Kamiya T, Kuwahara N, et al. Coronary arterial lesions of Kawasaki disease: Cardiac catheterization findings of 1100 cases. *Pediatr Cardiol* 1986; 7:3–9.
339. Sakai Y, Takayanagi K, Inoue T, et al. Coronary artery aneurysms and congestive heart failure: Possible long term course of Kawasaki disease in an adult. A case report. *Angiology* 1988; 39:625–630.
340. Hennigar GR, Thabet R, Bundy WE, Sutton LE. Salmonellosis complicated by pancarditis: Report of a case with autopsy findings. *J Pediatr* 1953; 43:524–531.
341. Saphir O, Katz LN, Gore I. The myocardium in subacute bacterial endocarditis. *Circulation* 1950; 1:1155–1167.
342. Parrillo JE, Fauci AS. Necrotizing vasculitis, coronary angiitis and the cardiologist. *Am Heart J* 1980; 99:547–554.
343. Gatenby PA, Lytton DG, Bulteau VG, et al. Myocardial infarction in Wegener's granulomatosis. *Aust NZ J Med* 1976; 6:336–340.
344. Klinger H. Grenzformen der periarteritis nodosa. *Frankfurt Z Pathol* 1931; 42:455–480.
345. Wegener F. Uber generalisierte, septische Gefasserkrankugen. *Verh Dtsch Ges Pathol* 1936; 29:202–210.
346. Wegener F. Uber eine eigenartige rhinogene Granulomatose mit besonderer Beteiligung des Arteriensystems und der Nieren. *Beitr Pathol Anat* 1939; 102:36–68.
347. Fahey J, Leonard E, Churg J, Godman G. Wegener's granulomatosis. *Am J Med* 1954; 17:168–179.
348. Godman G, Churg J. Wegener's granulomatosis: Pathology and review of the literature. *Arch Pathol Lab Med* 1954; 58:533–553.
349. Fienberg R. Pathergic granulomatosis. *Am J Med* 1955; 19: 829–831.
350. Walton EW. Giant cell granuloma of the respiratory tract (Wegener's granulomatosis). *Br Med J* 1958; 2:265–270.
351. Fauci AS, Wolff SM. Wegener's granulomatosis: Studies in 18 patients and a review of the literature. *Medicine* 1973; 52:535–561.
352. Pambakian H, Tighe JR. Breast involvement in Wegener's granulomatosis. *J Clin Pathol* 1971; 24:343–347.
353. Forstot JZ, Overlie PA, Neufeld GK, et al. Cardiac complications of Wegener granulomatosis: A case report of complete heart block and review of the literature. *Semin Arthritis Rheum* 1980; 10:148–154.
354. Allen DC, Doherty CC, O'Reilly DP. Pathology of the heart and the cardiac conduction system in Wegener's granulomatosis. *Br Heart J* 1964; 52:674–678.
355. Schiavone WA, Ahmad M, Ockner SA. Unusual cardiac complications of Wegener's granulomatosis. *Chest* 1985; 88:745–748.
356. Lie JT. Classification of vasculitis and a reappraisal of allergic granulomatosis and angiitis. *Mt Sinai J Med* 1986; 53:429–439.
357. Cupps TR, Fauci AS. *The Vasculitides.* Philadelphia: Saunders; 1981:211.
358. Rich AR. Hypersensitivity in disease, with special reference to periarteritis nodosa, rheumatic fever, disseminated lupus erythematosus, and rheumatoid arthritis. *Harvey Lect* 1947; 42:106–147.
359. Meller J, Conde CA, Deppisch LM, et al. Myocardial infarction due to coronary atherosclerosis in three young adults with systemic lupus erythematosus. *Am J Cardiol* 1975; 35:309–314.
360. Bonfiglio TA, Botti RE, Hagstrom JWC. Coronary arteritis, occlusion and myocardial infarction due to lupus erythematosus. *Am Heart J* 1972; 83:153–158.
361. Benisch BM, Pervez N. Coronary artery vasculitis and myocardial infarction with systemic lupus erythematosus. *N Y State J Med* 1974; 74:873–874.
362. Sumino H, Kanda T, Sasaki T, et al. Myocardial infarction secondary to coronary aneurysm in systemic lupus erythematosus: An autopsy case. *Angiology* 1995; 46:527–530.
363. Denbow CE, Lie JT, Tancredi RG, Bunch TW. Cardiac involvement in polymyositis: A clinicopathologic study of 20 autopsied patients. *Arthritis Rheum* 1979; 22:1088–1092.

364. Follansbee WP. The cardiovascular manifestations of systemic sclerosis. *Curr Probl Cardiol* 1986; 11:245–297.
365. Schimizu T, Ehrlich GE, Inaba G, Hayashi K. Behçet disease. *Semin Arthritis Rheum* 1979; 8:223–260.
366. Haynes BF, Kaiser-Kupfer MI, Mason P, Fauci AS. Cogan syndrome: Studies in 13 patients, long term follow-up and a review of the literature. *Medicine* 1980; 59:426–441.
367. Mullick FG, McAllister HA, Wagner BM, Fenoglio JJ Jr. Drug related vasculitis: Clinicopathologic correlation in 30 patients. *Hum Pathol* 1979; 10:313–325.
368. Uys CJ, Rose AG. Pathologic findings in long term cardiac transplants. *Arch Pathol Lab Med* 1984; 108:112–116.
369. Brosius FC, Roberts WC. Coronary artery disease in the Hurler syndrome. *Am J Cardiol* 1981; 47:649–653.
370. Renteria VG, Ferrans VJ, Roberts WC. The heart in the Hurler syndrome: Gross histologic and ultrastructural observations in five necropsy cases. *Am J Cardiol* 1976; 38:487–501.
371. Lindsay S. The cardiovascular system in gargoylism. *Br Heart J* 1950; 12:17–32.
372. Stauffer M. Oxalosis: Report of a case with a review of the literature and discussion on pathogenesis. *New Engl J Med* 1960; 263:386–390.
373. Blieden LC, Desnick RJ, Carter JB, et al. Cardiac involvement in Sandhoff's disease: An inborn error of glycosphingolipid metabolism. *Am J Cardiol* 1974; 34:83–88.
374. Blieden LC, Moller JH. Cardiac involvement in inherited disorders of metabolism. *Prog Cardiovasc Dis* 1974; 16:615–631.
375. Brosius FC III, Waller BF, Roberts WC. Radiation heart disease: Analysis of 16 young (aged 15 to 33 years) necropsy patients who received over 3500 rads to the heart. *Am J Med* 1981; 70:519–530.
376. Brill IC, Brodeur MTH, Oyama AA. Myocardial infarction in two sisters less than 20 years old. *JAMA* 1971; 217:1345–1348.
377. Trimble AS, Bigelow WG, Wigle ED. Coronary ostial stenosis: A late complication of coronary perfusion in open-heart surgery. *J Thorac Cardiovasc Surg* 1969; 57:792–795.
378. Lie JT, Berg KK. Isolated fibromuscular dysplasia of the coronary arteries with spontaneous dissection and myocardial infarction. *Hum Pathol* 1987; 18:654–656.
379. Przybojewski JZ, Rossouw J. Severe isolated left mainstem coronary artery stenosis: A case report. *S Afr Med J* 1986; 69:133–136.
380. Dominguez FE, Tate LG, Robinson MJ. Familial fibromuscular dysplasia presenting as sudden death. *Am J Cardiovasc Pathol* 1988; 2:269–272.
381. Billingham M. Personal communication, 1988.
382. Johnson DE, Gao SZ, Schroeder JS, et al. The spectrum of coronary artery pathologic findings in human cardiac allografts. *J Heart Transplant* 1989; 8:349–359.
383. Gravanis MB. Allograft heart accelerated atherosclerosis: Evidence for cell mediated immunity in pathogenesis. *Mod Pathol* 1989; 2:495–505.
384. Mehra MR, Ventura HO, Stapleton DD, et al. Presence of severe intimal thickening by intravascular ultrasonography predicts cardiac events in cardiac allograft vasculopathy. *J Heart Lung Transpl* 1995; 14:632–639.
385. Waller BF, Pinkerton CA, Foster LN. Morphologic evidence of accelerated left main coronary artery stenosis: A late complication of percutaneous transluminal angioplasty of the proximal left anterior descending coronary artery. *J Am Coll Cardiol* 1987; 9:1019–1023.
386. Giritsky AS, Ricci MT, Reitz BA, Shumway NE. Extrinsic coronary artery obstruction by chronic aortic dissection. *Ann Thorac Surg* 1981; 32:289–293.
387. Gardia-Rinaldi R, Von Koch L, Howell JP. Aneurysm of the sinus of Valsalva producing obstruction of the left main coronary artery. *J Thorac Cardiovascular Surg* 1976; 72:123–126.
388. Kopelson G, Herwig KJ. The etiologies of coronary artery disease in cancer patients. *Int J Radiat Oncol Biol Phys* 1978; 4:895–906.
389. Applefeld MM, Wiernik PH. Cardiac disease after radiation therapy for Hodgkin's disease: Analysis of 48 patients. *Am J Cardiol* 1983; 51:1679–1681.
390. SebagMontefiore D, Hope Stone H. Radiation induced coronary heart disease. *Br Heart J* 1993; 69:481–482.
391. Radwaner BA, Geringer R, Goldmann AM, et al. Left main coronary artery stenosis following mediastinal irradiation. *Am J Med* 1987; 82:1017–1020.
392. Schulman HE, Korr KS, Myers TJ. Left internal thoracic artery graft occlusion following mediastinal radiation therapy. *Chest* 1994; 105:1881–1882.
393. Benoff LJ, Schweitzer P. Radiation therapy induced cardiac injury. *Am Heart J* 1995; 129:1193–1196.
394. Reber D, Birnbaum DE, Tollenaere P. Heart diseases following mediastinal irradiation: Surgical management. *Eur J Cardiothorac Surg* 1995; 9:202–205.
395. Raviprasad GS, Salem BI, Gowda S, Leidenfrost R. Radiation induced mitral and tricuspid regurgitation with severe ostial coronary artery disease: A case report with successful surgical treatment. *Cathet Cardiovasc Diagn* 1995; 35:146–148.
396. Simon EB, Ling J, Mendizabal RC, Midwall J. Radiation induced coronary artery disease. *Am Heart J* 1984; 108:1032–1034.
397. Chen MF, Yang CY, Wu CC, et al. Heart diseases following radiotherapy. *J Formos Med Assoc* 1991; 90:398–402.
398. Handler CEE, Livesey S, Lawton PA. Coronary ostial stenosis after radiotherapy: Angioplasty or coronary artery surgery? *Br Heart J* 1989; 61:208–211.
399. Grollier G, Commeau P, Mercier V, et al. Post radiotherapeutic left main coronary ostial stenosis: Clinical and histological study. *Eur Heart J* 1988; 9:567–570.
400. Tenet W, Missri J, Hager D. Radiation induced stenosis of the left main coronary artery. *Cathet Cardiovasc Diagn* 1986; 12:169–171.
401. McEniery PT, Dorosti K, Schiavone WA, et al. Clinical and angiographic features of coronary artery disease after chest irradiation. *Am J Cardiol* 1987; 60:1020–1024.
402. Mittal B, Deutsch M, Thompson M, Dameshek HL. Radiation induced accelerated coronary arteriosclerosis. *Am J Med* 1986; 81:183–184.
403. Om A, Ellahham S, Vetrovec GW. Radiation induced coronary artery disease. *Am Heart J* 1992; 124:1598–1602.
404. Orzan F, Brusca A, Conte MR, et al. Severe coronary artery disease after radiation therapy of the chest and mediastinum: Clinical presentation and treatment. *Br Heart J* 1993; 69:496–500.
405. House KW, Simon SR, Pugh RP. Chemotherapy induced myocardial infarction in a young man with Hodgkin's disease. *Clin Cardiol* 1992; 15:122–125.
406. Fomina LG. A case of myocardial infarct in acute leukemia. *Sov Med* 1960; 24:141–143.
407. Wirth L. Myocardial infarction as the initial manifestation of polycythemia vera. *Milit Med* 1960; 125:544–548.
408. Spach MS, Howell DA, Harris JS. Myocardial infarction and multiple thrombosis in a child with primary thrombocytosis. *Pediatrics* 1963; 31:268–276.
409. James TN. Pathology of the small coronary arteries. *Am J Cardiol* 1963; 20:679–691.
410. Isner JM, Estes NAM III, Thompson PD, et al. Acute cardiac events temporally related to cocaine abuse. *New Engl J Med* 1968; 315:1438–1443.
411. Simpson RW, Edwards WD. Pathogenesis of cocaine-induced ischemic heart disease. *Arch Pathol Lab Med* 1986; 110:479–484.
412. Zimmerman FH, Gustafson GM, Kemp HG. Recurrent myocardial infarction associated with cocaine abuse in a young man with normal coronary arteries: Evidence for coronary artery spasm culminating in thrombosis. *J Am Coll Cardiol* 1987; 9:964–968.
413. Smith HWB, Liberman HA, Brody SL, et al. Acute myocardial infarction temporally related to cocaine use: Clinical angiographic

and pathophysiologic observations. *Ann Intern Med* 1987; 107:13–18.

414. Patel R, Haider B, Ahmed S, Regan TJ. Cocaine-related myocardial infarction: High prevalence of occlusive coronary thrombi without significant obstructive atherosclerosis (abstract). *Circulation* 1988; 78(suppl II):II-436.
415. Lange RA, Cigarroa RG, Yancy CW, et al. Cocaine-induced coronary artery vasoconstriction. *New Engl J Med* 1989; 321: 1557–1562.
416. Waller BF. Cocaine and the heart. *Indiana Med* 1988; 81:956–959.
417. Inoue H, Zipes DP. Cocaine induced supersensitivity and arrhythmogenesis. *J Am Coll Cardiol* 1988; 11:867–874.
418. Pallasch TJ, McCarty FM, Jastak JT. Cocaine and sudden cardiac death. *J Oral Maxillofac Surg* 1989; 47:1188–1191.
419. Perreault CL, Hauge NL, Morgan KG, et al. Negative inotropic and relaxant effects of cocaine on myopathic human ventricular myocardium and epicardial coronary arteries in vitro. *Cardiovasc Res* 1993; 27:262–268.
420. Virmani R, Robinowitz M, Smialek JE, Smyth DF. Cardiovascular effects of cocaine: An autopsy study of 40 patients. *Am Heart J* 1988; 115:1068–1076.
421. Lam D, Goldschlager N. Myocardial injury associated with polysubstance abuse. *Am Heart J* 1988; 115:675–680.
422. Rod JL, Zucker RD. Acute myocardial infarction shortly after cocaine inhalation. *Am J Cardiol* 1987; 59:161.
423. Kossowsky WA, Lyon AF. Cocaine and myocardial infarction: A probable connection. *Chest* 1984; 86:729–731.
424. Hollander JE, Hoffman RS. Cocaine-induced myocardial infarction: An analysis and review of the literature. *J Emerg Med* 1992; 10:169–177.
425. Miller GW. The cocaine habit. *Am Fam Physician* 1985; 31:173–176.
426. Wetli CV, Wright RK. Death caused by recreational cocaine use. *JAMA* 1979; 241:2519–2522.
427. Benchimol A, Bartall H, Desser KB. Acceleration of ventricular rhythm and cocaine abuse. *Ann Intern Med* 1978; 88:519–520.
428. Nanji AA, Filipenko JD. Asystole and ventricular fibrillation associated with cocaine intoxication. *Chest* 1984; 85:132–133.
429. Schachne JS, Roberts BH, Thompson PD. Coronary artery spasm and myocardial infarction associated with cocaine use. *New Engl J Med* 1984; 310:1665–1666.
430. Howard RE, Hueter DC, Davis GJ. Acute myocardial infarction following cocaine abuse in a young woman with normal coronary arteries. *JAMA* 1985; 254:95–96.
431. Simpson RW, Edwards WD. Pathogenesis of cocaine-induced ischemic heart disease: Autopsy finding in a 21-year-old man. *Arch Pathol Lab Med* 1986; 110:479–484.
432. Virmani R, Robinowitz M, Smialek JE, Smyth DF. Cardiovascular effects of cocaine: An autopsy study of 40 patients. *Am Heart J* 1988; 115:1068–1076.
433. Dowling GP, McDonough ET, Bost RO. Eve and ecstasy: A report of five deaths associated with the use of MDEA and MDMA. *J Am Coll Cardiol* 1987; 257:1615–1617.
434. Barbour DJ, Roberts WC. Frequency of acute and healed myocardial infarcts in fatal cardiac amyloidosis. *Am J Cardiol* 1988; 62:1134–1135.
435. Nichols GR, Davis GJ, Lefkowitz JB. Sudden death due to fibromuscular dysplasia of the sinoatrial nodal artery. *J Ky Med Assoc* 1989; 87:504–505.
436. James TN. Morphologic characteristics and functional significance of focal fibromuscular dysplasia of small coronary arteries. *Am J Cardiol* 1990; 65:12G–22G.
437. Mosseri M, Yarom R, Gotsman MS, Hasin Y. Histologic evidence for small vessel coronary artery disease in patients with angina pectoris and patent large coronary arteries. *Circulation* 1986; 74:964–972.
438. Oberai B, Adams CW, High OB. Myocardial and renal arteriolar thickening in cigarette smokers. *Atherosclerosis* 1984; 52:185–190.
439. Arey JB, Segal R. Fibromuscular dysplasia of intramyocardial coronary arteries. *Pediatr Pathol* 1987; 7:97–103.
440. James TN, Posada de la Paz M, Abaitua Borda I, et al. Histologic abnormalities of large and small coronary arteries, neural structures, and the conduction system of the heart found in postmortem studies of individuals dying from the toxic oil syndrome. *Am Heart J* 1991; 121:803–815.
441. Friedberg CK, Horn H. Acute myocardial infarction not due to coronary artery occlusion. *JAMA* 1939; 112:1675–1679.
442. Baroldi G, Scomazzoni X. *Coronary Circulation in the Normal and Pathologic Heart.* Washington: American Registry of Pathology, Armed Forces Institute of Washington, DC, U.S. Government Printing Office; 1967:1–80.
443. Department of Health and Human Services, Food and Drug Administration Docket No. 94N-0304. Notice of Hearing on Proposal to Withdraw Approval of the Indication for Prevention of Physiological Lactation: Bromocriptine. Rockville MD: Center for Drug Evaluation and Research; 1999:1–12.
444. Iffy L, Ten Hove W, Frisoli G. Acute myocardial infarction in the puerperium in patients receiving bromocriptine. *Am J Obstet Gynecol* 1986; 155:371–373.
445. Hara M, Takakura T, Nanimatsu K, et al. Acute myocardial infarction probably induced by the oral administration of Bromocriptine: A case report. *J Cardiol* 1989; 19:609–614.
446. Eichman FM. Recurrent myocardial infarction in a post partum patient receiving bromocriptine. *Clin Cardiol* 1992; 15:781–783.
447. Larrazet F, Spaulding C, Lobreau HJ, et al. Possible bromocriptine-induced myocardial infarction. *Ann Intern Med* 1993; 118:197–200.
448. Rosenkranz S, Deutsch HI, Erdmann E: 33 jährige Patientin met postpatalem Myohardinforkt. *Der Internist* 1997; 38:602–605.
449. Oakley C. Coronary artery disease. In: Oakley C, ed. *Heart Disease in Pregnancy.* London: British Medical Journal Publishing Group; 1997:237–247.
450. Pop C, Metz D, Matei M, et al. Infarctus du myocarde du postpartum induit par le Parlodel. *Arch Des Mal du Cour* 1998; 91:1171–1174.
451. Sandoz Pharmaceuticals Parlodel Pachage inserts. In: *Physicians Desk Reference*, 42d to 53d eds. Oradell, NJ: Medical Economics Company; 1988–1999.
452. Thorp JM, Chescheir NC, Fann B. Postpartum myocardial infarction in a patient with antiphospholipid syndrome. *Am J Perinatol* 1994; 11:1–3.

CHAPTER 40

DIAGNOSIS AND MANAGEMENT OF PATIENTS WITH CHRONIC ISCHEMIC HEART DISEASE

Robert A. O'Rourke / Robert C. Schlant / John S. Douglas, Jr.

Ischemic heart disease remains a major public health problem.[1] Chronic stable angina is the first indicator of ischemic heart disease in about 50 percent of patients. The reported annual incidence of angina is 213 per 100,000 population over the age of 30. The number of patients with stable angina in the United States approximates 16.5 million people, not including individuals who do not seek medical attention for their chest pain or who are shown to have a noncardiac cause of chest discomfort. Angina pectoris is a clinical syndrome that consists of discomfort or pain in the chest, jaw, shoulder, back, or arm. Typically it is precipitated or aggravated by exertion or emotional stress and relieved by nitroglycerin. Angina usually occurs in patients with coronary artery disease (CAD) affecting one or more large epicardial arteries. Angina often is present in individuals with valvular heart disease, hypertrophic cardiomyopathy, and uncontrolled hypertension, however. It also occurs in patients with normal coronary arteries and myocardial ischemia due to coronary artery spasm or endothelial dysfunction. The symptom of angina is often observed in patients with noncardiac disorders affecting the esophagus, chest wall, or lungs.

HISTORICAL PERSPECTIVE

In 1768, William Herberden presented his classic description of angina pectoris in a lecture before the Royal College of Physicians; it was published in 1772.[2] This classic description was published again with minor changes in a chapter entitled "Pectoris Dolor" in his *Commentaries on the History and Cure of Diseases,* which was translated from the Latin and published by his son, also named William Herberden, in 1802.[3] The following quotation is from the original lecture:

> There is a disorder of the breast, marked with strong and peculiar symptoms, considerable for the kind of danger belonging to it, and extremely rare, of which I do not recollect any mention among medical authors. The seat of it, and sense of strangling and anxiety, with which it is attended, may make it not improperly be called angina pectoris. Those who are afflicted with it are seized, while they are walking, and more particularly when they walk soon after eating, with a painful and most disagreeable sensation in the breast, which seems as if it would take their life away, if it were to increase or to continue: the moment they stand still all this uneasiness vanishes. In all other respects the patients are at the beginning of this disorder perfectly well, and in particular have no shortness of breath, from which it is totally different.
>
> After it has continued some months, it will not cease so instantaneous upon standing still; and it will come on, not only when the persons are walking, but when they are lying down, and oblige them to rise up from their beds every night for many months together; and in one or two very inveterate cases it has been brought on by the motion of a horse or a carriage, and even by swallowing, coughing, going to stool or speaking, or by any disturbance of mind. I have heard once and only one person, say that he had known it to attack him when he was up and standing still or sitting.
>
> . . . but all the rest, whom I have seen, who are at least twenty, were men, and almost all above 50 years old, and most of them with a short neck, and inclining to be fat. When a fit of this sort comes on by walking, its duration is very short, as it goes off almost immediately upon stopping. If it comes on in the night, it will last an hour or two; and I have met one, in whom it once continued for several days, during all which time the patient seemed to be in imminent danger of death.
>
> But the natural tendency of this illness be to kill the patients suddenly, yet unless it have a power of preserving a person from all other ails, it will easily be believed that some of those, who are afflicted with it, may die in a different manner, since this disorder will last, as I have known it more than once, near twenty years, and most usually attacks only those who are above fifty years of age. I have accordingly observed one, who sunk under a lingering illness of a different nature.
>
> The os sterni is usually pointed to as the seat of this malady, but it seems sometimes as if it was under the lower part of it, and at other times under the middle or upper part, but always inclining more to the left side, and sometimes there is with it a pain about the middle of the left arm. What the particular mischief is, which is referred to these different parts of the sternum, it is not easy to guess, and I have had no opportunity of knowing with certainty. It may be a strong cramp, or an ulcer, or possibly both.

The syndrome of angina pectoris was described as rare in textbooks of medicine in 1866 (Austin Flint) and 1892 (William Osler). Paul Dudley White wrote: "[angina pectoris] was uncommon in my early professional years. But when the automobile came in the 1920s and the population at large became more prosperous and over nourished, the current epidemic of coronary heart disease, as shown mainly by the symptom angina pectoris, began and incidentally involved younger and younger men."[4] In the United States, the peak mortality rate from coronary heart disease (CHD) occurred about 1962 to 1965; since then, it has been decreasing steadily.[5]

ETIOLOGY AND CLASSIFICATION

Coronary atherosclerosis is the cause of angina pectoris in most patients (see Chaps. 35 to 38). Many nonatherosclerotic causes of CAD (Tables 39-1 and 39-2) also can produce angina pectoris or myocardial infarction. Other conditions particularly associated with angina pectoris include congenital coronary artery abnormalities (see Chap. 64), aortic stenoses (see Chap. 56) mitral stenoses with resulting severe right ventricular hypertension (see Chap. 52), hypertrophic cardiomyopathy (see Chap. 67), and systemic arterial hypertension[6] (see Chap. 51).

Disorders in which angina occurs less frequently include aortic regurgitation (see Chap. 56), idiopathic dilated cardiomyopathy (see Chap. 66), and luetic heart disease. Mitral valve prolapse (see Chap. 58) rarely causes true angina pectoris. Certain conditions may alter the balance between myocardial oxygen supply-demand and precipitate or aggravate angina pectoris, including severe anemia, tachycardia, fever, hyperthyroidism, and Paget's disease of bone.

The Canadian Cardiovascular Society Grading Scale (see Table 10-2) is commonly used to classify the severity of angina pectoris, with the most severe symptoms occurring at rest and the least severe only with excessive exercise.

DIAGNOSIS

History and Physical Examination

The first step is to obtain a detailed description of the symptom complex in order to characterize the chest pain or discomfort. Five descriptors typically are considered: (1) location, (2) quality, (3) duration of the discomfort, (4) inciting factors, and (5) factors relieving the pain.[1]

After a description of the chest discomfort is obtained, the physician makes an integrated assessment of various components. The most commonly used classification scheme for chest pain divides patients into three groups: *typical angina, atypical angina,* or *noncardiac chest pain*[7,8] (Table 40-1).

Angina is further labeled as *stable* when its characteristics are usually unchanged for 60 days or *unstable* (see Chap. 41). The presence of unstable angina predicts a much higher short-term risk of an acute coronary event. *Unstable angina* is defined as angina that presents in one of three major ways: *rest angina, severe new-onset angina,* or *prior angina increasing in severity* (see Chap. 41). Recently, the acute coronary syndromes of unstable angina and nonST-segment elevation myocardial infarction have been linked together by their similar presentation and treatment.[8a]

Usually, the discomfort of chronic stable angina pectoris is precipitated by physical activity, emotions, eating, or cold

TABLE 40-1 Clinical Classification of Angina

Typical angina (definite)
1. Substernal chest discomfort with a characteristic quality and duration that is
2. provoked by exertion or emotional stress and
3. relieved by rest or NTG.
Atypical angina (probable)
Meets two of the above characteristics.
Noncardiac chest pain
Meets one or none of the typical anginal characteristics.

SOURCE: Modified from Diamond et al.[7]

weather. Certain patients are able to describe accurately the extent and type of exercise at which they reproducibly experience their chest pain (see Chap. 10). Many patients with angina will develop chest discomfort if they walk up a hill after a large meal with a cold wind blowing in their face. Emotions, particularly anger, excitation, and frustration, often precipitate angina in patients with CAD. Cigarette smoking induces chest discomfort or lowers the exertion threshold for angina in some patients. A history of cocaine use should be sought because it can precipitate myocardial ischemia with or without infarction by coronary vasoconstriction.[9]

When stable angina pectoris develops, it often increases to a plateau over 10 to 30 s and usually disappears within minutes if the exertion is discontinued. Occasionally, the angina will disappear despite continued physical activity, so-called walk-through angina. Most patients have discomfort that lasts only several minutes or up to 10 to 15 min, and rarely, up to 30 min (see Chap. 10).

The discomfort of angina is most often located substernally or just to the left of the sternum. Some patients, when describing the discomfort, clench their fist over their upper sternum (Levine's sign), a sign of high diagnostic accuracy. Less often, angina is located over the precordium. The discomfort is rarely localized only to the apex of the heart. Nevertheless, angina can be located anywhere from the epigastrium to the neck, and rarely it may be located only in the neck, throat, arm, or back.

The pain often radiates down the arms or to the neck, jaw, teeth, shoulders, or back. Radiation to the left side is more common, but both sides can be involved. The radiation, characteristically down the ulnar aspect of the arm, often is described as numbness. Increased heat or humidity also may lower the exertional threshold at which angina occurs.

Disorders that increase myocardial oxygen requirement ($M\dot{V}_{O_2}$) may exacerbate the occurrence of angina pectoris and sometimes may be associated with angina in the absence of moderate or severe CAD stenosis on coronary arteriography.

Patients with stable angina may have many episodes of myocardial ischemia that are asymptomatic or silent. Also, myocardial ischemia may result in symptoms from either systolic or diastolic left ventricular (LV) dysfunction without the chest discomfort characteristic of angina pectoris. Like chest discomfort due to angina, *angina equivalent* symptoms usually are associated with exertion and are relieved by rest and nitroglycerin. *Exertional dyspnea* likely is due to reduced diastolic LV compliance resulting from myocardial ischemia. *Exertional fatigue* or exhaustion probably results from an acute decrease in cardiac output due to diminished systolic LV function and/or associated mitral regurgitation from transient papillary muscle dysfunction.

In general, when myocardial ischemia is produced, an *ischemic cascade* occurs. Regional diastolic and systolic dysfunction precede global diastolic and then systolic dysfunction, which in turn often occurs prior to changes in the electrocardiogram (ECG) and before the symptoms of angina pectoris (Fig. 40-1). Noninvasive testing often is useful in detecting ischemia (see below). The detection of LV diastolic dysfunction by Doppler mitral valve recording or by diastolic filling curves using radionuclide ventriculography has many limitations (see Chaps. 13 and 16). Although diaphoresis and alterations in blood pressure and heart rate may occur, the physical examination is often normal. An examination performed during an episode of pain, however, can be useful. A fourth (most common) or third heart sound, a mitral regurgitant systolic murmur, reversed splitting of the S_2, bibasilar pulmonary rates, or palpable ectopic cardiac impulses that disappear when the pain subsides are all predictive of CAD (see Chap. 10). Carotid sinus pressure often terminates angina chest pain. Evidence of noncoronary atherosclerotic disease such as a carotid bruit, diminished pedal pulse, or abdominal aneurysm increases the likelihood of CAD. An elevated

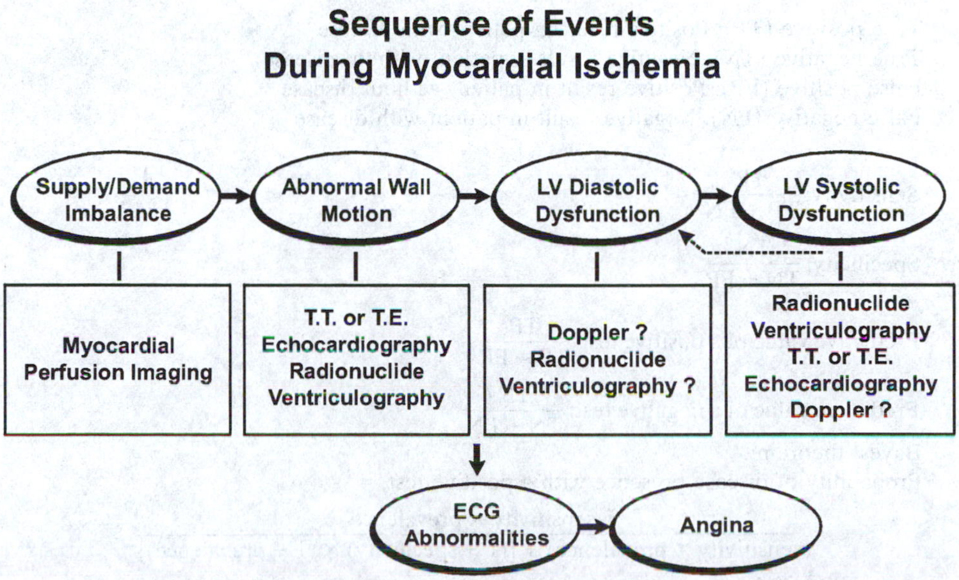

FIGURE 40-1 Sequence of events in the ischemic cascade plus noninvasive tests for detecting its presence. T.T., transthoracic; T.E., transesophageal.

TABLE 40-2 Pretest Likelihood of CAD in Symptomatic Patients According to Age and Sex* (Combined Diamond/Forrester and CASS Data)[7–10]

	Nonanginal Chest Pain		Atypical Angina		Typical Angina	
Age, years	Men	Women	Men	Women	Men	Women
30–39	4	2	34	12	76	26
40–49	13	3	51	22	87	55
50–59	20	7	65	31	93	73
60–69	27	14	72	51	94	86

*Each value represents the percent with significant CAD on catheterization.
Source: Modified from Gibbons et al.[1]

blood pressure, xanthomas, and retinal exudates point to the presence of CAD risk factors[6] (see Chap. 10).

Clinical Assessment of the Likelihood of CAD

The clinicopathologic study performed by Diamond and Forrester[10] demonstrated that it is possible to predict the probability of CAD after the history and the physical examination. By combining data from several angiographic studies performed before 1980, they showed that simple clinical observations of pain type, age, and sex were powerful predictors of the probability of CAD.

The utility of the Diamond and Forrester approach was confirmed subsequently in prospective studies at Duke and Stanford.[11–13] In both men and women referred for cardiac catheterization or for cardiac stress testing, the initial clinical characteristics most helpful in predicting CAD were determined. In these studies, age, sex, and pain type were the most powerful predictors (Table 40-2). Smoking, Q waves, or ST-segment–T-wavechanges on ECG, hyperlipidemia, and diabetes further strengthened the predictive abilities of these models.[1,13]

Special Tests for Diagnosis

Most special tests in patients with suspected stable angina are performed either to establish the diagnosis and/or to determine the risk for coronary events.[1] In general, men with a history of classic angina pectoris have a higher probability of having significant CAD on coronary arteriography than do women. Table 40-2 indicates the likelihood for each gender by age and characteristics of the chest discomfort. It also indicates why women have more false-positive responses to ECG exercise testing than do men (see Chap. 14). Terms useful in the evaluation and selection of diagnostic tests for CAD are listed in Table 40-3. Bayes' theorem states that the pretest prevalence of disease influences the posttest likelihood of significant CAD (see Chap. 14). Figure 40-2 illustrates the impact of Bayes' theorem when evaluating several diagnostic tests for CAD. More accurate data on the sensitivity and specificity of noninvasive testing for diagnosis of CAD are provided in Chaps. 13, 14, 16, and 17.

If an exercise ECG test was performed by a 55-year-old woman with atypical chest pain and a pretest likelihood for coronary disease of 0.46, a positive ECG stress test response would indicate her posttest likelihood to be 0.86. If she had a positive thallium scan, her likelihood of disease would increase to 0.98; however, if her thallium scan were negative, the probability of disease would decrease to 0.63.

On the other hand, diagnostic tests should only be performed when necessary to answer a specific clinical question. Thus a diagnostic test may be of limited additional diagnostic value in patients with either a very high (>0.90) or a very low (<0.10) pretest risk for CAD.[1]

TABLE 40-3 Glossary of Terms

True positive (TP): Positive result in patient with disease
True negative (TN): Negative result in patient without disease
False positive (FP): Positive result in patient without disease
False negative (FN): Negative result in patient with disease

Sensitivity: $\frac{TP}{TP + FN}$

Specificity: $\frac{TN}{TN + FP}$

Predictive value of a positive test: $\frac{TP}{TP + FP}$

Predictive value of a negative test: $\frac{TN}{TN + FN}$

Bayes' theorem:
Probability of disease presence with a positive test =

$$\frac{\text{sensitivity} \times \text{prevalence}}{(\text{sensitivity} \times \text{prevalence}) + [(1 - \text{specificity}) \times (1 - \text{prevalence})]}$$

Probability of disease presence with a negative test =

$$\frac{(1 - \text{sensitivity}) \times \text{prevalence}}{[(1 - \text{sensitivity}) \times \text{prevalence}] + [\text{specificity} \times (1 - \text{prevalence})]}$$

ELECTROCARDIOGRAM AND CHEST ROENTGENOGRAM

A resting 12-lead ECG should be recorded in all patients with symptoms suggestive of angina; however, it will be normal in up to 50 percent of patients with chronic stable angina. ECG evidence of LV hypertrophy or ST-segment–T-wave changes consistent with myocardial ischemia favor the diagnosis of angina pectoris. Evidence of prior Q-wave myocardial infarction (MI) on the ECG makes CAD very likely. Patients with a completely normal resting ECG rarely have significant LV systolic dysfunction.

The presence of arrhythmias (e.g., atrial fibrillation or ventricular tachyarrhythmias) on the ECG in patients with chest pain also increases the probability of underlying CAD; however, these arrhythmias frequently are caused by other types of cardiac disease. Various degrees of atrioventricular (AV) block occur in patients with chronic CAD but have a very low specificity for the diagnosis. Left anterior fascicular block, right bundle-branch block (RBBB), and left bundle-branch block (LBBB) often are present in patients with CAD and frequently indicate multivessel CAD. However, these findings also lack specificity for the diagnosis of chronic stable angina.

An ECG obtained during chest pain is abnormal in about 50 percent of patients with angina and a normal resting ECG. Sinus tachycardia is frequent; bradyarrhythmias are less common. ST-segment elevation or depression establishes a high likelihood of angina and indicates ischemia at a low workload, suggesting an unfavorable prognosis. Many high-risk patients with severe episodes of angina need no further noninvasive testing. Coronary arteriography usually defines the severity of CAD and determines the necessity and feasibility of myocardial revascularization. In patients with ST-segment–T-wave depression or inversion on the resting ECG, pseudonormalization of these abnormalities during pain is another indicator that CAD is likely.[14] The occurrence of tachyarrhythmias, AV block, left anterior fascicular block, or bundle-branch block during chest pain also increases the probability of CHD and often leads to coronary arteriography.

The *chest roentgenogram* often is normal in patients with stable angina pectoris. Its usefulness as a routine test is *not* well established. It is more likely to be abnormal in patients with previous or acute MI, those with a noncoronary artery cause of chest pain, and those with noncardiac chest pain.

Coronary artery calcification increases the likelihood of symptomatic CAD. *Fluoroscopically detectable* coronary calcification is correlated with major vessel occlusion in 94 percent of patients with chest pain[15]; however, the sensitivity of the test is less than 40 percent.

Electron beam computed tomography (EBCT) (see Chap. 17) is being used with increased frequency. However, the specificity of a positive result may be as low as 49 percent, and the predictive accuracy is less than 70 percent. The role of EBCT in CAD diagnosis and risk stratification has been controversial.[16] A recent report of an ACC/AHA expert consensus writing group does not recommend EBCT for routine screening of asymptomatic patients for CAD or for its use in most patients with chest pain.[17] It also is of little use in detecting vulnerable plaques.[17a]

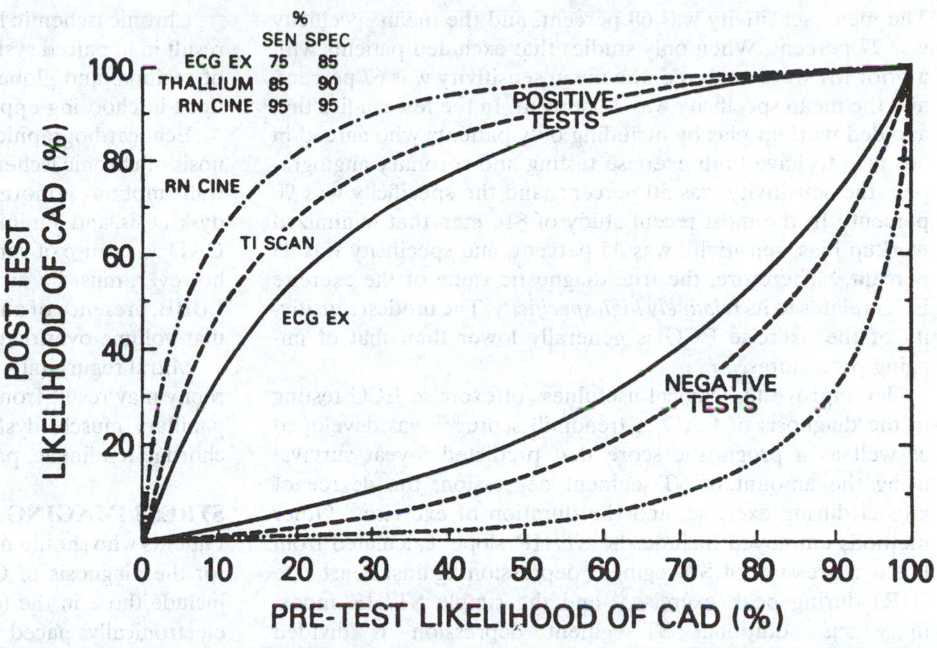

FIGURE 40-2 Probability of CAD. Comparison of ECG exercise testing (ECG Ex), thallium perfusion imaging (Tl Scan), and radionuclide cineangiography (RN CINE). Sensitivity (SEN) and specificity (SPEC) values are approximations derived from published series. (From Epstein et al. *Am J Cardiol* 1980; 46:491. Reproduced with permission from the publisher and authors.)

EXERCISE ECG STRESS TESTING

Exercise ECG stress testing is a well-established procedure that has been in widespread clinical use for many decades.[18] Although usually a safe procedure, both MI and death occur at a rate of up to 1 per 2500 tests[19] (see Chap. 14). Absolute contraindications include acute MI within 2 days, cardiac arrhythmias causing symptoms or hemodynamic compromise, symptomatic and severe aortic stenoses, symptomatic heart failure, acute pulmonary embolus or infarction, acute myocarditis or pericarditis, and acute aortic dissection.

For optimizing the information obtained, the protocol should be tailored to the individual patient, with exercise lasting at least 6 min.[20] Exercise capacity should be reported in estimated metabolic equivalents (METs) of exercise (1 MET is the standard basal oxygen uptake of 3.5 ml/kg/min) as well as in minutes.

The ECG, heart rate, and blood pressure should be monitored carefully and recorded during each stage of exercise, as well as during ST-segment abnormalities and chest pain, as detailed in Chap. 14.

Interpretation of the exercise ECG should include symptomatic response, exercise capacity, hemodynamic response, and ECG changes. The most important ECG abnormalities are ST-segment depression and ST-segment elevation (in leads without diagnostic Q waves) of greater than 1 mm for at least 60 to 80 ms after the end of the QRS complex. Although exercise testing often is terminated when subjects reach a standard percentage (often 85 percent of age-predicted maximum heart rate), there is a *great variability* in maximum heart rate among individuals. Many stress testing laboratories still utilize approaches that are not up to date.

A meta-analysis of 147 published reports describing 24,074 patients who underwent both coronary angiography and exercise testing found wide variation in sensitivity and specificity.[17]

The mean sensitivity was 68 percent, and the mean specificity was 77 percent. When only studies that excluded patients with a prior MI were analyzed, the mean sensitivity was 67 percent, and the mean specificity was 72 percent. In the few studies that avoided workup bias by including only patients who agreed in advance to have both exercise testing and coronary angiography, the sensitivity was 50 percent, and the specificity was 90 percent.[1] In the most recent study of 814 men that minimized workup bias, sensitivity was 45 percent, and specificity was 85 percent.[21] Therefore, the true diagnostic value of the exercise ECG relates to its *relatively high specificity*. The modest sensitivity of the exercise ECG is generally lower than that of imaging procedures.

To improve the clinical usefulness of exercise ECG testing in the diagnosis of CAD, a treadmill score[20,22] was developed as well as a prognostic score that predicted 5-year survival using the amount of ST-segment depression, the degree of angina during exercise, and the duration of exercise.[23] Other methods employed include the ST/HR slope, calculated from linear regression of ST-segment depression against heart rate (HR) during peak exercise,[24] and the simple ST/HR index, in which additional ST-segment depression is divided by the overall change in heart rate throughout the exercise period.[25] The cost-effectiveness of these techniques remains unknown.

Diagnostic testing is most valuable when the pretest probability of obstructive CAD is intermediate. In these conditions, the test result has the largest effect on the posttest probability of disease and thus on clinical decisions. Intermediate probability has been defined arbitrarily as between 10 and 90 percent; this definition has been used in several reports, including the ACC/AHA Exercise Test Guidelines.[18]

Special issues in ECG exercise testing include the effect of digoxin on ST–T wave changes, the usefulness of withholding beta-blocking drugs when possible, changes in ST-segment depression in patients with LBBB or RBBB, changes in the exercise ECG in patients with LV hypertrophy on ECG with or without repolarization abnormalities, and the usefulness of ECG testing in patients with resting ST-segment depression; these are discussed in great detail in Chap. 14 and ref. 18.

Exercise induced ST-depression usually occurs with LBBB and does not necessarily indicate ischemia.[26] However, in RBBB, ST-segment depression in the left chest leads (V_{5-6}) or inferior leads (II, aV_F) during exercise has the same significance as it does when the resting ECG is normal.

The difficulties of using exercise testing for diagnosing obstructive CAD in women have led to speculation that initial stress imaging may be preferable to standard ECG stress testing. There are insufficient data, however, to justify replacing standard exercise testing with stress imaging when evaluating women for CAD, and *women with a completely normal resting ECG* do not have a greater incidence of false-positive tests than men.[1]

REST ECHOCARDIOGRAPHY

Echocardiography can be useful for establishing a diagnosis of CAD and in defining the consequences of CAD in selected patients with chronic chest pain presumed to be chronic stable angina[1] (see Chap. 13). However, most patients undergoing a diagnostic evaluation for angina do not need a resting echocardiogram.[1]

Chronic ischemic heart disease, with or without angina, can result in impaired systolic LV function. The extent and severity of regional and global abnormalities are important considerations in choosing appropriate medical or surgical therapy.[25]

Echocardiographic findings that may help establish the diagnosis of chronic ischemic heart disease include regional systolic wall motion abnormalities, such as hypokinesis, akinesis, dyskinesis, and diminished segmental wall thickening.[27] Chronic CAD as a cause of ventricular septal wall motion abnormalities, however, must be distinguished from other conditions such as LBBB, presence of an intraventricular pacemaker, right ventricular volume overload, or prior cardiac surgery.[27]

Mitral regurgitation demonstrated by Doppler echocardiography may result from global LV systolic dysfunction, regional papillary muscle dysfunction, scarring and shortening of the chordae tendineae, papillary muscle rupture, or other causes.[27]

STRESS IMAGING FOR DIAGNOSIS

Patients who should undergo cardiac stress testing with imaging for the diagnosis of CAD as opposed to exercise ECG alone include those in the following categories: (1) complete LBBB, electronically paced ventricular rhythm, preexcitation syndromes, and other similar ECG conduction abnormalities, (2) patients who have greater than 1 mm of resting ST-segment depression, including those with LV hypertrophy or those taking drugs such as digitalis, (3) patients who are unable to exercise to a level high enough to give meaningful results on routine stress ECG (pharmacologic stress imaging should be considered), and (4) patients with angina who have undergone prior revascularization, in whom localization of ischemia, establishing the functional significance of lesions, and demonstrating myocardial viability are important considerations. In our experience, false-positive ECG tests often occur in patients with hypertension, no evidence of LV hypertrophy on the ECG, but LV hypertrophy by echocardiography. Stress imaging is utilized in most patients with a history of hypertension even when the resting ECG is normal.

Several methods can be used to induce stress, including (1) exercise (treadmill or bicycle) and (2) pharmacologic techniques (dobutamine or vasodilator drugs). When the patient can exercise to an appropriate level of cardiovascular stress for 6 to 12 min, exercise stress testing generally is preferred to pharmacologic stress.[1]

Myocardial Perfusion Imaging In patients with suspected or known chronic stable angina, the largest accumulated experience in myocardial perfusion imaging (MPI) has been with the isotope thallium-201; however, the available evidence suggests that the newer isotopes technetium-99m (^{99m}Tc) sestamibi and ^{99m}Tc tetrofosmin provide similar diagnostic accuracy (see Chap. 16). Thus, for the most part, these isotopes can be used interchangeably, with a similar diagnostic accuracy for CAD.[27]

MPI may use either planar or single-photon-emission computed tomography (SPECT), visual analyses, or quantitative techniques (see Chap. 16). Quantification using horizontal or circumferential profiles may improve the test's sensitivity, especially in patients with single-vessel disease. For the less commonly used thallium-201 planar scintigraphy, average reported values of sensitivity and specificity (uncorrected for posttest referral bias) have been in the range of 83 and 88 percent, respectively, for visual analysis and 90 and 80 percent, respectively, for quantitative analyses.[28] Thallium-201 SPECT generally is more sensitive than planar imaging for diagnosing CAD, localizing hypoperfused vascular segments, identifying left anterior descending and left circumflex coronary artery stenoses, and accurately predicting multivessel CAD. The average sensitivity and specificity of exercise thallium-201 SPECT imaging (uncorrected for referral bias) are in the range of 89 and 76 percent, respectively, for qualitative analyses and 90 and 70 percent, respectively, for quantitative analyses.[28]

Pharmacologic stress uses dipyridamole or adenosine-induced coronary vasodilatation as an adjunct to thallium-201 myocardial perfusion imaging.[29] Dipyridamole planar scintigraphy has a high sensitivity (90 percent average) and acceptable specificity (70 percent average) for the detection of CAD. Dipyridamole SPECT with thallium-201 or ^{99m}Tc sestamibi is as accurate as planar imaging, and results of myocardial perfusion imaging during adenosine infusion are similar to those obtained with dipyridamole and exercise imaging[30] (see Chap. 16). Evidence of CAD is demonstrated by redistribution defects comparing stress and resting scintigrams (ischemia), fixed defects at rest (scar), and LV dilatation or lung uptake of isotope during stress[28] (see Chap. 16).

Stress Echocardiography Stress echocardiography is based on the assessment of myocardial thickening during stress compared with baseline (see Chap. 13). Echocardiographic findings suggestive of myocardial ischemia include (1) decrease in wall motion in one or more LV segments with stress, (2) diminution in systolic wall thickening in one or more segments during stress, and (3) compensatory hyperkinesis in complementary (nonischemic) wall segments.[27] The use of digital acquisition and storage, as well as side-by-side display of cine loops of LV images acquired at rest and at different levels of stress, has improved efficiency and accuracy in interpretation of stress echocardiograms.[27]

In 36 studies including 3210 patients, the reported overall sensitivities (uncorrected for referral bias) ranged from 70 to 97 percent. The average overall sensitivity was 85 percent for exercise echocardiography and 82 percent for dobutamine stress

TABLE 40-4 Comparative Advantages of Stress Echocardiography and Stress Radionuclide Perfusion Imaging in Diagnosis of CAD

Advantages of stress echocardiography
1. Higher specificity
2. Versatility. More extensive evaluations of cardiac anatomy and function
3. Greater convenience/efficacy/availability
4. Lower cost

Advantages of stress perfusion imaging
1. Higher technical success rate
2. Higher sensitivity, especially for single-vessel coronary disease involving the left circumflex
3. Better accuracy in evaluating possible ischemia when multiple resting LV wall motion abnormalities are present
4. More extensive published data base, especially in evaluation of prognosis

SOURCE: From Gibbons et al.[1]

TABLE 40-5 Invasive Testing: Coronary Angiography (Recommendations for Coronary Angiography to Establish a Diagnosis in Patients with Suspected Angina, Including Those with Known CAD Who Have a Significant Change in Anginal Symptoms)

Class I
1. Patients with known or possible angina pectoris who have survived sudden cardiac death

Class IIa
1. Patients with an uncertain diagnosis after noninvasive testing in whom the benefit of a more certain diagnosis outweighs the risk and cost of coronary angiography
2. Patients who cannot undergo noninvasive testing due to disability, illness, or morbid obesity
3. Patients with an occupational requirement for a definitive diagnosis
4. Patients who by virtue of young age at onset of symptoms, noninvasive imaging, or other clinical parameters are suspected of having a nonatherosclerotic cause of myocardial ischemia (coronary artery anomaly, Kawasaki disease, primary coronary artery dissection, radiation-induced vasculoplasty)
5. Patients in whom coronary artery spasm is suspected and provocative testing may be necessary
6. Patients with a high pretest probability of left main or 3-vessel CAD

Class IIb
1. Patients with recurrent hospitalization for chest pain in whom a definite diagnosis is judged necessary
2. Patients with an overriding desire for a definitive diagnosis and a greater than low probability of CAD

Class III
1. Patients with significant comorbidity in whom the risk of coronary arteriography outweighs the benefits of the procedure
2. Patients with an overriding personal desire for a definitive diagnosis and a low probability of CAD

Class I: Conditions for which there is evidence and/or general agreement that a given procedure or treatment is useful and effective.
Class II: Conditions for which there is conflicting evidence and/or a divergence of opinion about the usefulness/efficacy of a procedure or treatment.
IIa: Weight of evidence/opinion is in favor of usefulness/efficacy.
IIb: Usefulness/efficacy is less well established by evidence/opinion.
Class III: Conditions for which there is evidence and/or general agreement that the procedure/treatment is not useful and in some cases may be harmful.

SOURCE: From Gibbons et al.[1]

echocardiography.[24] The reported sensitivity of exercise echocardiography for multivessel disease was higher (approximately 90 percent) than the sensitivity for single-vessel disease (approximately 79 percent). In this series of studies, specificity averaged approximately 86 percent for exercise echocardiography and 85 percent for dobutamine echocardiography.[27]

Pharmacologic stress echocardiography is best accomplished using dobutamine because it enhances myocardial contractile performance and wall motion, both of which can be evaluated directly by echocardiography (see Chap. 13). In 36 studies, average sensitivity and specificity (uncorrected for referral bias) of dobutamine stress echocardiography in the detection of CAD were 82 and 85 percent, respectively.[27]

Additional information concerning the sensitivity of exercise imaging in patients receiving beta blockers, the need for pharmacologic stress imaging in patients with LBBB, and the accuracy of myocardial perfusion and echocardiographic imaging in selected patient subgroups is included in Chaps. 13, 14, and 16.

Echocardiographic and MPI have complementary roles, and both add value to routine stress ECG under appropriate circumstances, as outlined earlier. The choice of which test to perform depends importantly on issues of local expertise, available facilities, and considerations of cost-effectiveness. A summary of the comparative advantages of stress myocardial perfusion imaging and stress echocardiography is provided in Table 40-4.

Coronary Angiography for Diagnosis Direct referral for diagnostic coronary angiography in patients with chest pain, possibly due to myocardial ischemia, is appropriate when noninvasive tests are contraindicated or likely to be inadequate due to illness, disability, or physical characteristics.[1] Many patients with obesity, chronic obstructive pulmonary disease, bronchospasm, and heart failure are likely to have suboptimal imaging tests; diagnostic coronary angiography will provide accuracy diagnostic information with minimal risk.

Patients with noninvasive tests that are abnormal but not clearly diagnostic often require clarification of an uncertain diagnosis by coronary angiography. In certain cases, a second noninvasive test (imaging modality) may be recommended for a patient with a low likelihood of CAD but an intermediate risk treadmill result. Coronary angiography is likely to be most appropriate for a patient with a high-risk treadmill outcome.[1]

In individuals with symptoms consistent with but not diagnostic of stable angina, coronary angiography may be a necessity when the patient's occupation or activity could constitute a risk to themselves or others (e.g., pilots, firefighters, professional athletes).[1] When typical or atypical symptoms suggest stable angina and there is high clinical probability of severe CAD, direct referral for coronary angiography may be indicated and cost-effective.[31] In diabetic patients, the diagnosis of chronic stable angina can be particularly difficult because of the absence of characteristic symptoms of myocardial ischemia due to the autonomic and sensory neuropathy (see also Chap. 78). Thus a lower threshold for coronary angiography is appropriate. Special groups for the consideration of coronary angiography include women, who more often have atypical chest discomfort, and the elderly, in whom symptoms are common, noninvasive testing may be difficult, and comorbid conditions that mimic angina pectoris are frequent.[1] Coronary angiography is useful in patients in whom coronary artery spasm is suspected, in younger patients with signs or symptoms of myocardial ischemia possibly due to coronary anomalies, in patients with a history of cocaine use, and in patients experiencing sudden death or ventricular arrhythmias.[1,32] The ACC/AHA recommendations concerning the value of coronary angiography are listed in Table 40-5. Coronary angiographic findings in patients with chronic stable angina are depicted in Fig. 40-3.[32]

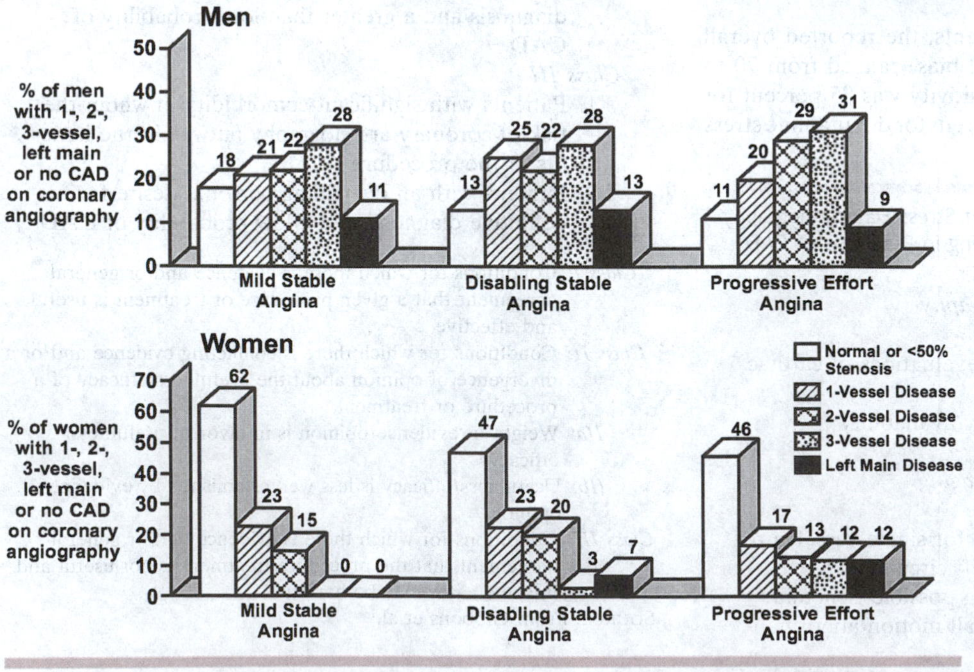

FIGURE 40-3 Prevalence of zero- to three-vessel CAD or coronary angiography in men and women related to severity of angina. (Modified from Douglas JS Jr, Hurst JW. Limitations of symptoms in the recognition of coronary atherosclerotic heart disease. In: Hurst JW, ed. *Update I: The Heart*. New York: McGraw-Hill; 1979:3. Reproduced with permission from the publisher and authors.)

DIFFERENTIAL DIAGNOSIS

Table 40-6 lists the differential diagnoses of angina pectoris. Usually, the distinction is clear if an accurate history is obtained and a complete, accurate physical examination is performed (see Chap. 10).

Patients with hypertensive or valvular heart disease may have chest pain that is located at the apex rather than substernally and that is often associated with hyperesthesia of the left breast or precordium.[6] Many patients with no functional heart disease have pain over the LV apex that often occurs at rest. Chest wall pain, cervical arthritis, and subdeltoid bursitis can occur with exertion and are relieved by rest. Importantly, patients frequently have more than one type of chest pain.[1]

TABLE 40-6 Differential Diagnosis of Angina Pectoris

- Cardiovascular
  - Myocardial ischemia
    - Coronary atherosclerosis
    - Coronary vasospasm
    - Congenital coronary artery disease
      - Anomalous origin
      - Aberrant coronary artery
      - Coronary arteriovenous fistula
    - Kawasaki's disease
    - Small vessel disease
    - Microvascular angina (syndrome X)
    - Systemic arterial hypertension
    - Hypertrophic cardiomyopathy
    - Idiopathic dilated cardiomyopathy
    - Aortic valve disease
    - Coronary artery dissection (Marfan's syndrome)
    - Pulmonary hypertension
    - Right ventricular hypertension
    - Chronic obstructive pulmonary disease
    - Syphilitic aortitis coronary ostial disease
    - Collagen vascular disease
      - Periarteritis nodosa
      - Systemic lupus erythematosus
      - Rheumatoid arthritis
    - Cardiac amyloid
    - Cardiac tumors
    - Hereditary connective tissue disorders
      - Pseudoxanthoma elasticum
      - Cystic medial necrosis
      - Homocystinuria
      - Gargoylism
    - Severe anemia, hypoxia
    - High-dose x-irradiation
    - Withdrawal from chronic nitroglycerin exposure
  - Nonmyocardial ischemia
    - Aortic dissection
    - Discrete thoracic aortic aneurysm
    - Mitral valve prolapse
    - Tachycardia, bradycardia
    - Palpitations
    - Pericarditis
- Thoracic-respiratory
  - Pulmonary embolism, infarction
  - Pneumothorax
  - Pneumomediastinum (mediastinal emphysema)
  - Pleuritis
  - Epidemic pleurodynia (Bornholm's disease)
  - Mediastinitis
  - Intrathoracic malignancy
  - Café Coronary
- Gastrointestinal
  - Gastroesophageal reflux, esophagitis
  - Esophageal spasm
  - Esophageal rupture (Mallory-Weiss syndrome; Boehaave's syndrome)
  - Esophageal impaction
  - Hiatal hernia
  - Cholecystitis, gallstones
  - Gastritis
  - Peptic ulcer disease
  - Pancreatitis
  - Splenic infarction
  - Splenic flexure syndrome
- Neuromuscular/skeletal
  - Chest wall pain
  - Costochondritis (Tietze's syndrome)
  - Cervical or thoracic degenerative arthritis, nerve compression, radiculopathy
    - Cervical vertebral disk
    - Intercostal neuralgia
  - Thoracic outlet (scalenus anticus) syndrome
  - Shoulder arthropathies
    - Shoulder hand syndrome
  - Fibromyalgia (myofascial pain syndrome; fibromyositis)
    - Pectoral, intercostal, seratus anterior
    - Precordial catch syndrome
  - Cardiac causalgia
  - Bursitis
  - Superficial thrombophlebitis of thoracic veins (Mondor's syndrome)
  - Xiphoidalgia
  - Diaphragmatic flutter
- Neurocutaneous
  - Herpes zoster
- Breast
  - Pendulous breast syndrome
  - Brassiere syndrome
- Psychologic
  - Anxiety
  - Hyperventilation
  - Panic attacks
  - Depression
  - Self-gain
  - Munchausen syndrome

PATHOPHYSIOLOGY

In patients with stable angina pectoris due to atherosclerotic CAD, the correlation between the severity or extent of atherosclerosis and the magnitude of angina symptoms is poor. Also, no definite relation exists between the location of the chest discomfort and the site of the myocardial ischemia. Women have angina as the initial manifestation of CAD more often than men, who often present with acute MI. The pathology of coronary atherosclerosis is discussed in detail in Chap. 36. The nonatherosclerotic causes of CHD are discussed in Chap. 39.

A disparity between the supply of coronary blood flow (CBF) and the metabolic demands of the myocardium ($M\dot{V}_{O_2}$) is the primary factor in ischemic heart disease. This imbalance may result in clinical manifestations of ischemia when myocardial demand exceeds the capacity of the coronary arteries to deliver an adequate supply of oxygen. In normal hearts there is an excess CBF reserve so that ischemia does not occur even with very vigorous exercise.[34]

Arteriosclerotic disease in either the epicardial coronary arteries or in the coronary microvasculature may cause an imbalance between supply and demand at even modest levels of exercise. An understanding of the determinants of CBF and myocardial metabolic demand is important in the management of chronic ischemic heart disease.[6]

Myocardial Oxygen Demand

The major relevant determinants of $M\dot{V}_{O_2}$ are heart rate, contractility, and systolic wall stress (Fig. 40-4). A detailed discussion of the major and minor determinants of myocardial oxygen demand is presented in Chaps. 3 and 37. Heart rate is one of the most important determinants of $M\dot{V}_{O_2}$ and can be altered easily by medical therapy in most patients.[35]

Myocardial contractility, partially reflected in the isovolumic rate of change of LV pressure (*dP/dt*), is a major determinant of $M\dot{V}_{O_2}$ but not usually a primary factor for therapeutic inter-

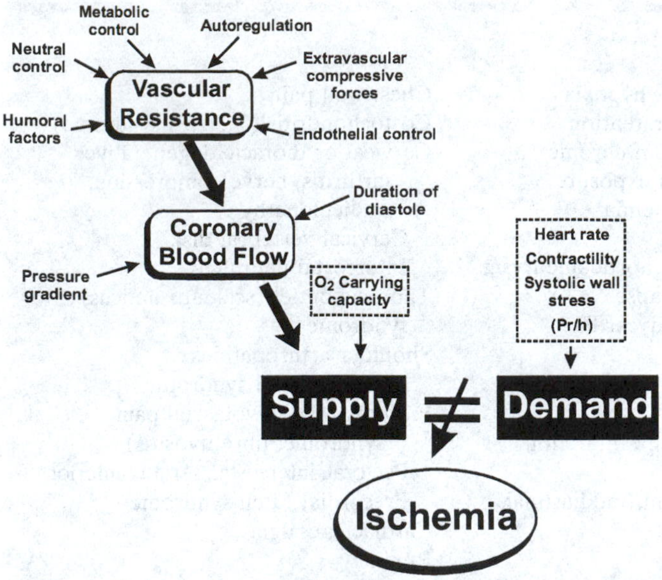

FIGURE 40-4 Factors controlling myocardial oxygen demand. *P*, systolic pressure; *r*, radius; *h*, wall thickness. (Modified from Ardehali A, Ports TA. Myocardial oxygen supply and demand. *Chest* 1990; 98:699–705. Reproduced with permission from the publisher and authors.)

vention. However, LV systolic wall stress is an important consideration in the medical treatment of angina pectoris.

Systolic wall stress is directly related to the LV systolic pressure (P) and radius (r) and inversely related to wall thickness (h). Thus, reducing systolic pressure afterload (i.e., treating hypertension) can decrease $M\dot{V}_{O_2}$. Decreasing preload by venodilation, and thus reducing LV size and oxygen consumption, is an important mechanism for the efficacy of nitrate therapy in angina pectoris. Positive inotropic agents actually may decrease $M\dot{V}_{O_2}$ in patients with an enlarged left ventricle if the results of a diminished LV radius outweigh those of increasing contractility.

Myocardial Oxygen Supply

Oxygen supply to the myocardium depends on the oxygen-carrying capacity of the blood and on CBF (see Fig. 40-4). Although a decrease in oxygen-carrying capacity may contribute to the development or exacerbation of myocardial ischemia in severe anemia, myocardial ischemia related to oxygen supply usually results from inadequate CBF.

The arteriolar resistance vessels are normally the primary regulators of CBF because the epicardial arteries are low-resistance conduits. Narrowing of the large coronary arteries transiently by vasospasm or permanently by obstructive lesions may increase the coronary resistance sufficiently to reduce CBF.

In the past decade, the pathophysiologic role of the coronary microvasculature has been recognized,[36,37] either concomitantly with atherosclerotic narrowing of the large-conduit arteries or predominantly in anginal syndromes with normal epicardial arteries (syndrome X).[38,39]

The determinants of CBF are relatively complex and include (1) metabolic control, (2) autoregulation, (3) extravascular compressive forces, (4) duration of diastole, (5) humoral agents composed of both circulating hormones and autocrine and paracrine factors produced within the arterial wall and in particular by the endothelium, (6) neural control, and (7) the difference between aortic diastolic pressure and right atrial pressure[6] (see Fig. 40-4).

CBF is relatively constant, being autoregulated during perfusion pressures between 60 and 160 mmHg.[40] Below a perfusion pressure of 60 mmHg, vasodilator reserve disappears, and blood flow is directly related to perfusion pressure. Experimentally, loss of vasodilator reserve occurs distal to lesions with an 85 percent decrease in diameter.[41] A decrease in CBF, likely due to vasoconstriction and loss of vasodilator reserve, has been observed despite an increase in blood pressure during cold pressor stimulation in patients with significant CAD.[42]

Extravascular compressive forces, including intrapericardial, intramyocardial, and intraventricular pressures, are important in the control of CBF and account for 30 to 50 percent of the vascular resistance.[6] Since intramyocardial and intraventricular pressures are maximal during systole and are exerted maximally on the subendocardium, LV subendocardial blood flow decreases during systole. Thus subendocardial blood flow is most vulnerable whenever total blood flow is decreased or $M\dot{V}_{O_2}$ is increased and blood flow is limited. Because of the systolic compressive forces, the subendocardium is also critically dependent on the duration of diastole for its blood flow (see Chap. 37).

CBF is regulated by systemic hormones and by neural control mechanisms similar to other vascular beds. Angiotensin II is a coronary vasoconstrictor; beta-adrenergic agonists dilate and alpha-adrenergic agonists constrict coronary arteries, although there are some regional differences in distribution of receptors in vessels of different sizes.[6] Importantly, the integrated vasomotor response to the various vasoactive stimuli affecting a coronary artery or arteriole appears greatly influenced by the functional state of the endothelium (see Chaps. 6 and 37).

Endothelial Function and Coronary Vasomotor Control

The phenomenon of endothelial-dependent relaxation[43] and the identification of endothelial-derived relaxing factor as nitric oxide[44] are discussed in detail in Chap. 6. The defect in endothelial-dependent dilatation in atherosclerotic epicardial coronary arteries that vasoconstrict in response to stimuli that normally cause vasodilation, such as acetylcholine, exercise, or cold pressure testing, is discussed in Chap. 37, as is the role of dysfunctional endothelium in both the stable and unstable coronary artery syndromes.

The majority view is that endothelium-dependent vasodilator mechanisms are predominant in nondiseased epicardial coronary arteries. Thus interventions such as exercise,[45] mental stress,[46] cold pressure testing,[47] or even pacing-induced tachycardia,[48] which normally induce increases in $M\dot{V}_{O_2}$ and flow, are associated with epicardial dilatation that is at least partially endothelial-dependent. The presence of even nonocclusive, early atherosclerosis appears to attenuate this vasodilator mechanism and results in prevailing constrictor forces.[6]

The local infusion of the alpha-adrenergic agonist phenylephrine does not constrict normal coronary arteries of patients with intact endothelial-dependent dilatation.[49] However, vasoconstriction occurs in even minimally diseased coronary arteries at low concentrations of phenylephrine. Thus in CAD there appears to be both loss of endothelial-dependent dilatation and an enhanced vasoconstrictor sensitivity to catecholamines. This disordered vasomotor control is an important contributor to the variability in anginal threshold commonly observed in many patients.[50]

Moderate vasoconstriction of a minimal stenosis may have little hemodynamic importance, whereas the same degree of vasoconstriction of a higher-grade stenosis may markedly decrease blood flow and induce ischemia.

The Microvasculature and Coronary Ischemia

The recognition of the likely importance of the coronary microvascular resistance vessels in the pathogenesis of angina pectoris resulted from studies of patients with angina-like chest pain and angiographically normal epicardial coronary arteries.[51–55]

The coronary etiology of the chest pain is supported by the frequent but not universal evidence of ischemia in these patients during exercise testing[56]; many were found to have abnormal vasodilator reserve.[56] Specifically, in patients with angina and angiographically normal coronary arteries, endothelial-dependent vasodilatation of the resistance arteries, as reflected in the responses of CBF to infusion of the endothelial-dependent vasodilator acetylcholine, was diminished relative to controls.[58]

In contrast, the flow responses to the non-endothelial-dependent dilators, isosorbide dinitrate and papaverine were no different between patients and controls, suggesting that the intrinsic vasodilator capacity of the resistance arteries was not defective. Similar defects in endothelial-dependent increases in CBF have been observed in LV hypertrophy associated with hypertension, another condition that may be associated with angina pectoris with angiographically normal epicardial coronary arteries.[58]

The histopathology of biopsy specimens from patients with normal epicardial coronaries but with anginal syndromes has demonstrated capillary narrowing with swollen endothelium encroaching on the lumen as well as decreased capillary density. Thus the coronary microvasculature can develop dysfunction of vasomotor control mechanisms and of endothelial-dependent vasodilation that may become clinically significant in the setting of increased demand or $M\dot{V}_{O_2}$. In this situation, the loss of vasodilator reserve and/or the actual constriction of resistance arterioles may induce ischemia and chest pain.[6]

Spectrum of Pathophysiologic Mechanisms Associated with the Stable Coronary Ischemia Syndromes

Symptomatic myocardial ischemia due primarily to microvascular abnormalities in the control of coronary vascular tone partially explains the characteristics of stable angina syndromes. Angina pectoris or anginal equivalents, with a *relatively constant* threshold for inducing ischemic symptoms due to a fixed stenoses of an epicardial coronary artery, also in part determine the spectrum of angina symptoms. Most patients have a somewhat variable threshold for inducing angina from day to day or even at different times of the day.

Interestingly, the same activity that causes chest discomfort in the early morning may not do so in the afternoon or evening. Yet the patient may have a consistent level of exercise for inducing ischemia on protocol exercise testing because of the augmented $M\dot{V}_{O_2}$ that is due to increases in heart rate, contractility, and blood pressure and the associated increment in systolic wall stress. This is explained by the presence of both flow-limiting epicardial coronary stenosis and associated episodic vasoconstriction.

Maseri et al.[50] have termed have termed this phenomenon *mixed angina*. Myocardial ischemia is induced by both an increase in $M\dot{V}_{O_2}$ and a decrease in CBF. The site(s) of vasoconstriction may be at an epicardial stenoses, in the microvasculature, or at both locations.[61] The concept of a *variable flow reserve* that interacts with differing metabolic demands to produce intermittent ischemia is depicted in Fig. 40-5*A* and *B*.

In the stable anginal syndromes, the predominant vasoconstrictors are likely neural and hormonal, whereas in the unstable (acute) coronary syndromes, platelet and coagulation products as well as inflammatory mediators are important contributors (see Chap. 41). Patients with predominantly vasoconstrictor pathophysiology in an epicardial vessel have been classified as having *vasospastic angina* or *Prinzmetal's variant angina* (see Chap. 41).

Cellular Bases for the Clinical Manifestations of Ischemia

The cellular effects of myocardial ischemia are discussed in detail in Chaps. 36 and 37. The rapid decreases in systolic function and diastolic compliance that are associated with creatine phosphate depletion and ionic shifts will increase LV end-

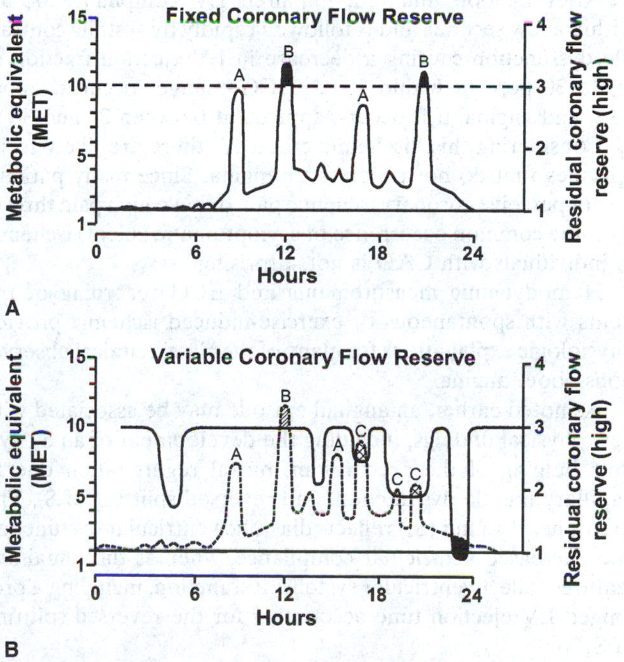

FIGURE 40-5 Concept of variable coronary flow reserve in the presence of variable atherosclerotic obstruction. *A*. Episodes not associated with ischemia. *B*. Ischemic episode occurring at levels of exercise exceeding threshold of residual coronary flow reserve. *C*. Ischemic episodes occurring at lower levels of exercise when residual coronary flow is reduced. *D*. Ischemic episodes occurring at rest in the presence of maximal reduction in residual coronary flow reserve. --, residual coronary flow reserve; - - -, variable atherosclerotic obstruction as measured by MED. (Modified from Cohn PF. Mechanisms of myocardial ischemia. *Am J Cardiol* 1992; 70:14G–18G; and Maseri A. Role of coronary artery spasm in symptomatic and silent myocardial ischemia. *J Am Coll Cardiol* 1987; 9:249–262. Reproduced with permission from the authors and publishers.)

diastolic pressure. Elevated pulmonary vascular pressures often stimulate mechanoreceptors and mediate the dyspnea response. Dyspnea may be associated with angina or may be present as an anginal equivalent in patients who do not develop chest discomfort.

The metabolic abnormalities due to ischemia cause cellular depolarization and the flow of electric currents between normal and ischemic areas that are reflected on the ECG.[6] ST-segment depression reflecting subendocardial underperfusion is the most common ECG manifestation of ischemia in chronic stable angina during ambulatory recordings or exercise testing.[62] The ST-segment depression observed during exercise testing or ambulatory ECG recordings is not commonly associated with complex or life-threatening ventricular arrhythmias; exercise-induced ventricular ectopic activity is not a reliable predictor of cardiac events in asymptomatic persons.[63]

The Coronary Ischemia Cascade

Studies in which hemodynamic and ECG recordings have been performed during spontaneous episodes of ischemia, either in unstable patients or during balloon inflation at angioplasty, have provided insights into the sequential responses evoked at the onset of ischemia and are consistent with those described in animals undergoing acute coronary artery ligation[64] (see Fig. 40-1).

After balloon inflation, impaired LV compliance occurs within a few seconds and is followed rapidly by systolic contractile dysfunction causing a decrease in LV ejection fraction of up to 30 percent within 10 s.[64] ECG changes occur at about 20 s, and angina, if it occurs, appears at between 25 and 30 s.

Considering this "ischemic cascade," there are likely to be episodes that do not progress to angina. Since many patients do not perceive coronary ischemic pain or have high pain thresholds, the common occurrence of asymptomatic (silent) ischemia in individuals with CAD is not surprising.

Hemodynamic measurements and ECG recording of patients with spontaneous or exercise-induced ischemia provide physiologic explanations for many of the classic clinical observations about angina.

As noted earlier, an anginal episode may be associated with new physical findings, including the development of an S_4, systolic bulging of the precordium, mitral regurgitation due to papillary muscle dysfunction, and reversed splitting of S_2. The fourth heart sound (S_4) reflects diastolic ventricular dysfunction and decreased ventricular compliance, whereas the remaining features reflect ventricular systolic dysfunction, including a prolonged LV ejection time accounting for the reversed splitting of S_2.

In addition, the crescendo-decrescendo nature of anginal pain is reflected in the crescendo-decrescendo pattern of the development and resolution of ischemic ST-segment changes and elevations in LV filling pressure recorded during exercise-induced angina.

Circadian Rhythm of Coronary Ischemia

The prevalence of MI, unstable angina, variant angina, and silent ischemia is greatest in the morning during the first few hours after awakening, and the threshold for precipitating anginal attacks in patients with stable angina also appears to be lowest in the morning.[65,66] Patients often develop ST-segment depression and angina at lower thresholds during exercise testing in the morning than later in the day. Studies with ambulatory ECG recordings have confirmed that the incidence of both painful and painless episodes of ST-segment depression is highest in the morning[66] and, in particular, in the first few hours after awakening (Fig. 40-6).

The diurnal variation in ischemic threshold is attributed to the endogenous rhythms of catecholamine secretion and to the sensitivity to coronary vasoconstrictors, both of which appear to peak in the morning. The increase in sympathetic nervous system activity is associated with increases in heart rate, blood pressure, contractility, and $M\dot{V}O_2$. The lowered morning anginal threshold and the higher morning systolic blood pressure have *important therapeutic implications.* A decrease in the frequency of ischemia can be achieved by blunting the morning surge of beta-adrenergic stimulation by the administration of beta blockers. The control of hypertension by the *early morning use of antihypertensive drugs* is also important. In patients with recurrent morning angina, the use of nitroglycerin (TNG) soon after awakening may prevent angina in many instances.

Mechanisms of Anginal Pain

Angina pain is a useful warning system, but it is often too insensitive. Pain stimuli arise within the myocardium and most likely stimulate free nerve endings in or near small coronary vessels. Impulses travel in afferent unmyelinated or small myelinated cardiac sympathetic nerves through the upper five thoracic sympathetic ganglia to dorsal horn cells and through the spinothalamic tract of the thalamus and then to the cortex.[67]

Integration and modification of these impulses occur at several levels, including the cerebral cortex. This modulation also

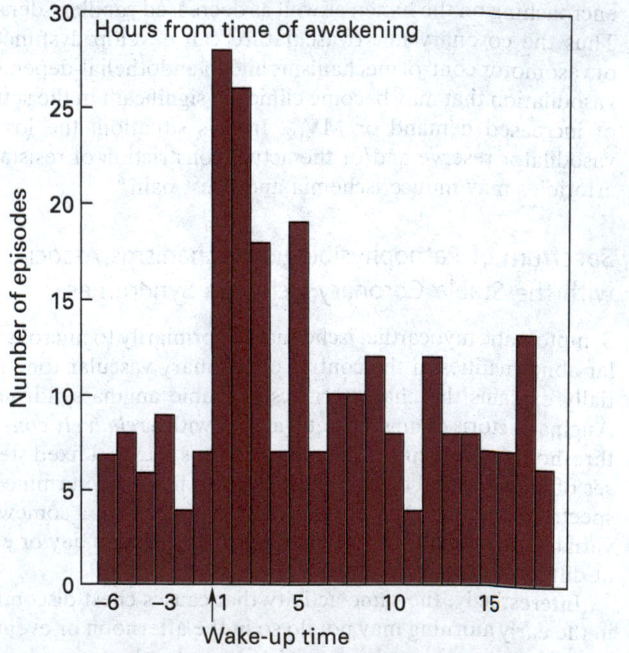

FIGURE 40-6 When the frequency of episodes is displayed hourly from the time of awakening, the peak activity occurs in the first and second hour after arising. (From Rocco et al.[67] Reproduced with permission from the authors and publishers.)

may contribute importantly to the variability in anginal threshold. At the cortical level, psychosocial and cultural factors may alter the perception of pain. The radiation patterns of angina are determined by the levels of the thoracic spinal cord that share the sensory inputs from the heart and from somatic structures.

The nature of the stimuli causing angina has been difficult to delineate. The causes are probably chemical, and several molecules, including kinins, serotonin, hydrogen ions, and inflammatory mediators, have been proposed. By contrast, adenosine, which is increased during ischemia, has been shown to cause anginal-type pain during intravenous infusion in normal volunteers.[68] The precise mechanisms causing angina pain are yet to be defined.

ASYMPTOMATIC (SILENT) ISCHEMIA IN STABLE CAD

The presence of unrecognized myocardial infarction due to the absence of pain was mentioned by Herrick in 1912.[69] The frequent presence of extensive CAD and MI at autopsies of apparently asymptomatic persons was recognized later.[70] Direct evidence of asymptomatic (silent) ischemia during ECG exercise testing and during ambulatory ECG recording stimulated interest in this clinical entity.[71]

Prevalence of Silent Ischemia

Asymptomatic ischemic episodes may be present in patients with any of the ischemic coronary syndromes, including unstable angina and silent ischemia after MI; they may be observed in patients who are totally asymptomatic or who have chest discomfort with some episodes of ischemia but not with others.[72] The prevalence of silent ischemic episodes approaches 40 percent in patients with chronic stable angina or in those with a history of instability.[73] The incidence of asymptomatic ischemia occurring in individuals with extensive CAD has been estimated at 5 percent.[74] ST-segment depression of 60 s or more on ambulatory recordings is uncommon in patients with no evidence of CAD.[75,76]

A prospective study of 68-year-old men with a 9.9 and a 6.6 percent prevalence of a history of angina pectoris or MI, respectively, demonstrated ST-segment depression on ambulatory ECG recordings. In 25 percent[77]; 92 percent of the "ischemic" episodes were asymptomatic, but ST-segment depression was associated with an increased risk of coronary events.

The true prevalence of silent ischemia is difficult to determine and obviously will depend on age and the presence and extent of CAD. In the presence of CAD, however, it is apparent that episodes of asymptomatic ischemia are often more common than are painful episodes.[78]

Pathophysiology of Silent Ischemia

An obvious possible explanation for painful as opposed to asymptomatic ischemia is that the ischemia, and thus the noxious stimulus, is more severe in the former. The correlation between the duration and severity of an ischemic episode and the development of anginal pain in chronic stable angina, however, is only fair.[79] Symptomatic episodes last slightly longer and have a slightly higher frequency of severe ST-segment depression than do painless ones, but there is considerable overlap. In several clinical studies, the intensity of the ischemic stimulus did not appear to account for the variability in the perception of pain in chronic ischemic heart disease.[80]

An alternative reason for lack of pain with myocardial ischemia is neurologic.[81] Neuropathy with defective sensory efferent nerves definitely occurs in some patients and is particularly prevalent in diabetics. Modification of pain stimuli in the central nervous system (CNS) may contribute importantly to the variable expression of ischemic pain. This modulation may occur in spinal centers because transcutaneous nerve,[81] esophageal,[82] and dorsal column stimulation[83] can increase anginal threshold. Modulation of pain-mediating efferent messages also may occur at supraspinal centers. Psychological or cultural factors also may affect pain perception. Subsets of patients with predominantly painless ischemic episodes tend to have a higher threshold and tolerance for painful stimuli than those who experience pain.[84–86] Thus processing of pain signals in the CNS likely contributes to the variability of anginal threshold or to the absence of pain.

Diabetic patients have a relatively high incidence of painless MI and definite silent ischemic episodes as documented by exercise testing and ambulatory ECG recordings (also Chap. 78).[87–90]

Causes and Functional Consequences of Asymptomatic Ischemia

Ischemia caused by the increased $M\dot{V}_{O_2}$ associated with exercise testing often is silent.[91] Ambulatory ECG recordings have provided insights into potential mechanisms of many episodes of painless or painful ischemia during daily living. The heart rate at the onset of ischemia is generally lower with ambulatory ECG recordings than with exercise testing.[92] These observations suggest that coronary vasoconstriction likely contributes to many episodes of silent ischemia.

Clinical Implications of Silent Ischemia

Asymptomatic silent ischemia is a common component of both acute and chronic coronary artery syndromes. Thus it may have the same clinical importance as symptomatic ischemia.[93] The important indicators of risk are the extent and severity of ischemia, regardless of how it is detected or manifested, and whether the disease is in a stable or unstable phase. Whether ECG monitoring for silent ischemia and changing therapy to decrease or eliminate it diminish morbidity and mortality in a cost-effective manner is unproven.[76]

Evidence of high-risk ischemia detected by exercise ECG testing, with or without myocardial imaging, and implications for treatment are discussed later. Therapeutically, it is appropriate to treat high-risk ischemia whether or not it is associated with pain. Persistent severe ischemia despite medical therapy should lead to consideration of myocardial revascularization.

The role of ambulatory ECG recordings *alone* without stress testing to detect asymptomatic ischemia in routine patient care is *minimal,* and ACC/AHA practice guidelines on this topic have been published recently.[76]

Treatment of Silent Ischemia

Most medical or interventional strategies that reduce symptomatic ischemia also will reduce asymptomatic ischemia.[94–96] The available data from early clinical trials of the treatment of asymptomatic (silent) ischemia in stable CAD have been summarized recently.[94–96] Nitroglycerin (TNG) is highly effective, and beta blockers appear to be somewhat more effective than calcium antagonists. Calcium antagonists may be most effective in preventing ischemia occurring at lower heart rates because coronary artery vasoconstriction may be a predominant factor in this situation. In patients with ischemic CAD, the total ischemic burden, and not just symptoms, may be the appropriate therapeutic target.

RISK STRATIFICATION OF PATIENTS WITH CHRONIC ISCHEMIC HEART DISEASE

The prognosis for the patient with chronic CHD is usually related to four patient factors.[1] *LV performance* is the strongest predictor of long-term survival in patients with CHD, and the ejection fraction (EF) is the most often used measure of the presence and the degree of LV dysfunction. The second predictive factor is the *anatomic extent and severity* of atherosclerotic involvement of the coronary arteries. The number of stenosed coronary arteries is the most common measure of this factor. The third patient factor affecting prognosis is evidence of a *recent coronary plaque rupture* indicating a much higher short-term risk for cardiac death or nonfatal MI. Worsening clinical symptoms with unstable features are an important clinical marker of a complicated plaque (see Chap. 41). The fourth prognostic factor is *general health and noncoronary comorbidity*.

History and Physical Examination for Prognosis

Useful information relative to *risk stratification* can be obtained from the history. This includes demographics such as age and gender, as well as a medical history focusing on hypertension, diabetes, hypercholesterolemia, smoking, peripheral vascular disease, and previous MI.

The physical examination can be useful in risk stratification by defining the presence or absence of signs that may alter the probability of *severe* CAD.[1] Useful physical findings include those suggesting vascular disease (abnormal fundi, decreased peripheral pulses, bruits), long-standing hypertension (high blood pressure, abnormal fundi), aortic valve stenoses or hypertrophic obstructive cardiomyopathy (systolic murmur, abnormal carotid arterial pulse, abnormal LV impulse), left-sided heart failure (third heart sounds, displaced LV impulse, bibasilar rales), and right-sided heart failure (elevated jugular venous pressure, hepatomegaly, ascites, peripheral edema).[1] Hubbard et al.[97] identified five clinical markers that independently predicted severe three-vessel and left main CAD, including age, typical angina, diabetes, male gender, and prior MI, which were used to develop a five-point cardiac risk score.

ECG and Chest Roentgenogram for Prognosis

Patients with chronic stable angina who have abnormalities on resting ECG are at greater risk than those with normal ECGs.[98] Evidence of one or more prior MIs on ECG indicates a greater risk for cardiac events. The presence of Q waves in multiple ECG leads, often accompanied by an R wave in lead V_1 (posterior infarction), commonly is associated with a markedly reduced left ventricular ejection fraction (LVEF), an important factor in the natural history of patients with CAD.[99] Persistent ST-segment–T-wave inversions, particularly in V_1 to V_3, are associated with an increased prevalence of future coronary events and a poor prognosis.[99]

On the chest roentgenogram the presence of cardiomegaly, a LV aneurysm or pulmonary venous congestion is associated with a poorer long-term prognosis than occurs in patients with a normal chest x-ray.

The presence of calcium in the coronary arteries on chest x-ray or fluoroscopy in patients with symptomatic CAD suggests an increased risk of cardiac events. Although the presence and amount of coronary artery calcification by electron beam computed tomography correlate to some extent with the severity of CAD, there is considerable patient variation.[16] Also, placques vulnerable to rupture with resulting acute coronary syndromes rarely contain much calcium.

Noninvasive Testing for Prognosis

ASSESSMENT OF LV FUNCTION

LV global systolic function and volumes are important predictors of prognosis in patients with cardiac disease.[1] In patients with chronic CHD, LVEF measured at rest by either echocardiography (usually qualitative and less reliable) or radionuclide ventriculography (RVG) is predictive of long-term prognosis. As LVEF decreases, subsequent mortality increases; a resting ejection fraction of greater than 35 percent is associated with an annual mortality rate of more than 3 percent per year.[1]

Radionuclide LVEF may be measured at rest using a gamma camera, a ^{99m}Tc tracer, and first-pass or gated equilibrium blood pool angiography (RVG) or by gated SPECT perfusion imaging using a technetium-based isotope[27] (see Chap. 16). LV diastolic function also can be estimated from RVG diastolic filling curves. LV systolic function can be measured by quantitative two-dimensional echocardiography (see Chap. 13), and LV diastolic function can be assessed by transmitral valve Doppler recording.[13]

In patients with chronic stable angina and a history of previous MI, segmental wall motion abnormalities are apparent not only in the zone(s) of prior infarction but also in areas with ischemic "stunning" or "hibernation" of myocardium that are nonfunctional but still viable.[100] In patients with CHD, the presence, severity, and mechanism of mitral regurgitation can be detected reliably using transthoracic and transesophageal two-dimensional imaging and Doppler echocardiographic techniques (see Chap. 13).

Echocardiography is the definitive test for detecting intracardiac thrombi.[27] LV thrombi are most common in stable angina pectoris patients who have significant LV wall motion abnormalities. In patients with anterior and apical infarctions, the presence of LV thrombi denotes an increased risk of both embolism and death (see Chap. 41).

ECG EXERCISE TESTING

Unless cardiac catheterization is clearly indicated, symptomatic patients with suspected or known CAD usually should undergo exercise testing to assess the risk of future cardiac events, unless they have confounding features on their resting ECG or are unable to exercise[1] (see Chap. 14). Also, demonstration of exercise-induced ischemia is desirable for most patients who are being evaluated for revascularization.

Several studies have shown that risk assessment in patients with a normal ECG who are not taking digoxin and who are physically capable *usually* should start with the exercise test[1,102] (see Chap. 14). In contrast, a stress-imaging technique should be used for patients with ECG evidence of LV hypertrophy, widespread resting ST-segment depression (>1 mm), complete LBBB, ventricular paced rhythm, or preexcitation.[17] The primary evidence that ECG exercise testing can be used to estimate prognosis and assist in management decisions consists of seven observational studies.[1,18] One of the strongest and most consistent prognostic markers is the *maximum exercise capacity*.[103,104]

A second group of *prognostic markers* relates to exercise-induced ischemia (see Chap. 14). ST-segment depression and ST-segment elevation (in leads without pathologic Q waves and not in aV_R) best summarize the prognostic information related to ischemia. Other variables are less powerful, including angina, the number of leads with ST-segment depression, and the configuration of the ST-segment depression and the duration of ST-segment deviation into the recovery phase.

The *Duke treadmill score* combines this information and provides a way to calculate risk.[103,105] The Duke treadmill score equals the exercise time in minutes minus five times the peak ST-segment deviation during or after exercise (in millimeters) minus four times the angina index (which has a value of 0 if there is no angina, 1 if angina occurs, and 2 if angina is the reason for stopping the test). Among outpatients with suspected CAD, two-thirds of patients with scores indicating low risk had a 4-year survival of 99 percent (average annual mortality of 0.25 percent), and the 4 percent who had scores indicating high risk had a 4-year survival of 79 percent (average annual mortality rate of 5 percent) (Table 40-7). Recent studies indicate that this approach is equally applicable in men and women.[106]

STRESS IMAGING FOR PROGNOSIS

Stress-imaging studies using radionuclide MPI techniques or two-dimensional echocardiography at rest and during stress are beneficial for risk stratification and determining the most effective treatment strategy for patients with chronic stable angina.[1] Whenever feasible, treadmill or bicycle exercise should be used as the most desirable forms of stress because exercise provides the most information concerning patient's symptoms, cardiovascular function, and hemodynamic response during usual activity (see Chap. 16). The inability to perform a bicycle or exercise treadmill test has been shown to be a serious and negative prognostic factor for patients with chronic CAD.[1]

In patients unable to exercise adequately, various types of pharmacologic stress (as discussed under diagnosis) are commonly used for *risk stratification*. The type of pharmacologic stress selected will depend on specific patient factors, including the patient's heart rate and blood pressure, evidence of bronchospastic disease, the presence of LBBB or a pacemaker, and the likelihood of ventricular arrhythmias. Pharmacologic agents often are used to increase workload or to cause an increase in overall CBF.[107,108]

MPI has played a major role in the risk stratification of patients with CAD.[27] Either planar (less common) or SPECT imaging using thallium-201 or ^{99m}Tc perfusion tracers, with images obtained at stress and during rest, provides important information concerning the severity of functionally significant CAD (see Chap. 16).

Stress echocardiography has been used more recently for detecting the presence and amount of ischemia in patients with chronic stable angina. Accordingly, the amount of prognostic data obtained with this approach is less extensive. The presence or absence of inducible myocardial wall motion abnormalities, however, has useful predictive value in patients undergoing exercise or pharmacologic stress echocardiography.[27,109–112] A negative stress echocardiographic study denotes a low cardiovascular event rate during follow-up.

MYOCARDIAL PERFUSION IMAGING FOR PROGNOSIS

Normal poststress thallium scan results are highly predictive of a benign prognosis even in patients with known CAD.[1] An analysis of 16 studies involving 3594 patients followed for an average of 29 months indicated a rate per year of cardiac death and MI of 0.9 percent, little different from that of the general population.[113,114] In a recent prospective study of 5183 consecutive patients undergoing myocardial perfusion imaging during stress and later at rest, patients with normal scans were at low risk (<0.5 percent per year) for the composite end point of cardiac death and MI during 642 ± 226 days of mean follow-up[115] (see Chap. 16).

The number, extent, and site of abnormalities on stress MPI reflect the location and severity of functionally significant coronary artery stenoses (see Chap. 16). Lung uptake of thallium-201 on postexercise or pharmacologic stress images is an indicator of stress-induced global LV dysfunction and is associated with pulmonary venous hypertension in the presence of multivessel CAD.[115] Transient poststress ischemic LV dilatation also correlates with severe two- or three-vessel CAD (see Chap. 16). SPECT may be more accurate than planar imaging for determining the size of defects, for detecting particularly left circumflex CAD, and for localizing abnormalities in the distribution of individual coronary arteries. More false-positive results are likely to result from photon attenuation during SPECT imaging, however.

The determination of both myocardial perfusion and LV function at rest may help determine the extent and severity of CAD.[1] This combined information can be obtained by performing two separate exercise tests (e.g., stress MPI and stress RVG), or by combining the studies after a single exercise test (first-pass RVG) with ^{99m}Tc-based agents followed by MPI, or

TABLE 40-7 Survival According to Risk Groups Based on Duke Treadmill Scores

Risk Group (Score)	Percentage of Total	Four-Year Survival	Annual Mortality (percent)
Low (≥ +5)	62	0.99	0.25
Moderate (−10 to +4)	34	0.95	1.25
High (< −10)	4	0.79	5.0

SOURCE: From Gibbons et al.[1]

by perfusion imaging using ECG gating. The use of ECG gated ^{99m}Tc sestamibi SPECT imaging at rest and with exercise or pharmacologic stress provides important prognostic information concerning LVEF and the extent of reversible ischemia (see Chap. 16).

Pharmacologic stress perfusion imaging for risk stratification is preferable to *exercise perfusion* imaging in patients with LBBB.[116] Recently, 245 patients with LBBB underwent SPECT imaging with thallium-201 (n = 173) or ^{99m}Tc sestamibi (n = 72) during dipyridamole (n = 153) or adenosine (n = 92) stress.[134] The 3-year survival was 57 percent in the high-risk group compared with 87 percent in the low-risk group (p = 0.001).

STRESS ECHOCARDIOGRAPHY FOR PROGNOSIS

Stress echocardiography is both sensitive and specific for detecting inducible myocardial ischemia in patients with chronic stable angina.[27] Compared with standard exercise treadmill testing, stress echocardiography provides additional clinical value for detecting and localizing myocardial ischemia. Several studies indicate that patients at low, intermediate, and high risk for cardiac events can be stratified by the presence or absence of inducible wall motion abnormalities on stress echocardiography testing.[109–112] The presence of ischemia on the exercise echocardiogram is independent and additive to clinical and exercise data in predicting cardiac events in both men and women.[117,118]

The prognosis is not benign in patients with a positive stress echocardiographic study, and morbid or fatal cardiovascular events are more likely. The overall event rates, however, are rather variable, and the cost-effectiveness of using routine stress echocardiographic testing to establish prognosis is uncertain.[1]

Coronary Angiography for Prognosis

The availability of powerful but expensive therapeutic strategies to reduce the long-term morbidity and mortality of CAD dictate that the patients most likely to benefit because of increased risk be determined. The assessment of cardiac risk and the need for further testing usually begin with simple, repeatable, and inexpensive assessments of history and physical examination that lead to noninvasive or invasive testing depending on outcome. Clinical risk factors generally are additive, and a crude estimate of 1-year mortality can be obtained from these variables. Methods for the accurate identification of vulnerable plaques, however, are lacking. Magnetic resonance imaging (MRI) offers significant promise in this regard.[1]

Risk stratification of patients with chronic stable angina by stress testing with exercise or pharmacologic agents has been shown to permit identification of groups of patients with low, intermediate, or high risk for subsequent cardiac events[1,27,28] (see Chap. 18).

The randomized trials of coronary artery bypass grafting (CABG) demonstrated that patients randomized to initial CABG had a lower mortality than those assigned to medical therapy only if they were at substantial risk (annual mortality > 3 percent).[119,120] Coronary angiography is appropriate for patients whose mortality risk is in this range. Noninvasive test findings that identify high-risk patients are listed in Table 40-8. Patients identified as at high risk generally are referred for coronary arteriography independent of their symptomatic status. The ACC/AHA guidelines for risk stratification using coronary angiography in patients with stable angina are listed in Table 40-9.

TABLE 40-8 Noninvasive Risk Stratification

High risk (greater than 3% annual mortality rate)
1. Severe resting left ventricular dysfunction (LVEF < 35%)
2. High-risk treadmill score (score ≤ −11)
3. Severe exercise left ventricular dysfunction (exercise LVEF < 35%)
4. Stress-induced large perfusion defect (particularly if anterior)
5. Stress-induced multiple perfusion defects of moderate size
6. Large, fixed perfusion defect with LV dilatation or increased lung uptake (thallium-201)
7. Stress-induced moderate perfusion defect with LV dilatation or increased lung uptake (thallium-201)
8. Echocardiographic wall motion abnormality (involving greater than two segments) developing at low dose of dobutamine (≤10 mg/kg/min) or at a low heart rate (<120 beats/min)
9. Stress echocardiographic evidence of extensive ischemia

Intermediate risk (1% < 3% annual mortality rate)
1. Mild/moderate resting left ventricular dysfunction (LVEF = 35%–49%)
2. Intermediate-risk treadmill score* (−11 < score < 5)
3. Stress-induced moderate perfusion defect without LV dilatation or increased lung intake (thallium-201)
4. Limited stress echocardiographic ischemia with a wall motion abnormality only at higher doses of dobutamine involving less than or equal to two segments

Low risk (less than 1% annual mortality rate)
1. Low-risk treadmill score (score ≥ 5)
2. Normal or small myocardial perfusion defect at rest or with stress
3. Normal stress echocardiographic wall motion or no change of limited resting wall motion abnormalities during stress

*Duke treadmill score; see text.
SOURCE: From Gibbons et al.[1]

TREATMENT OF CHRONIC STABLE ANGINA

There are two major purposes in the treatment of stable angina. The first is to prevent MI and death and thereby *increase the quantity of life*. The second is to reduce symptoms of angina and the frequency and severity of ischemia, which should *improve the quality of life*. Therapy directed toward preventing death has the highest priority. The choice of therapy often depends on the clinical response to initial medical therapy, although some patients (and many physicians) prefer coronary revascularization in situations where either may be successful.

TABLE 40-9 Recommendations for Coronary Angiography for Risk Stratification in Patients With Chronic Stable Angina

Class I
1. Patients with disabling [Canadian Cardiovascular Society (CCS) classes III and IV] chronic stable angina despite medical therapy
2. Patients with high-risk criteria on noninvasive testing regardless of anginal severity
3. Patients with angina who have survived sudden cardiac death or serious ventricular arrhythmia
4. Patients with angina and symptoms and signs of congestive heart failure
5. Patients with clinical characteristics that indicate a high likelihood of severe CAD

Class IIa
1. Patients with significant LV dysfunction (ejection fraction < 45%), CCS class I or II angina, and demonstrable ischemia but less than high-risk criteria on noninvasive testing
2. Patients with inadequate prognostic information after noninvasive testing

Class IIb
1. Patients with disabling CCS class I or II angina, preserved LV function (ejection fraction > 45%), and less than high-risk criteria on noninvasive testing

Class III
1. Patients with disabling CCS classes I or II angina who respond to medical therapy and have no evidence of ischemia on noninvasive testing
2. Patients who prefer to avoid revascularization

NOTE: See classes I–III as described at bottom of Table 40-5.
SOURCE: From Gibbons et al.[1]

It must be stressed that the pharmacologic treatment of chronic CAD has greatly improved and may even be superior to revascularization therapy for many patients.[120a] Patient education, cost-effectiveness, and patient preference are important components in this decision-making process.

Pharmacotherapy to Prevent MI

ANTIPLATELET AGENTS

Aspirin exerts an antithrombotic effect by inhibiting cyclooxygenase and synthesis of platelet thromboxane A_2. In the Physicians' Health Study, aspirin given on alternative days to asymptomatic individuals was associated with a decreased incidence of MI.[121] In the Swedish Angina Pectoris Aspirin Trial (SAPAT), in patients with stable angina, the addition of 75 mg aspirin to sotalol resulted in a 34 percent reduction in primary outcome events of MI and sudden death and a 32 percent decrease in secondary vascular events.[122]

Ticlopidine is a thienopyridine derivative that inhibits platelet aggregation induced by adenosine diphosphate and low concentrations of thrombin, collagen, thromboxane A_2, and platelet-activating factor.[123] It has *not* been shown to decrease adverse cardiovascular events and may induce neutropenia and often thrombotic thrombocytopenia purpura (TTP).

Clopidogrel, also a thienopyridine derivative, is chemically related to ticlopidine, but it appears to possess a greater antithrombotic effect than ticlopidine. In a randomized trial that compared clopidogrel with aspirin in patients with previous MIs, stroke, or peripheral vascular disease, clopidogrel was slightly more effective than aspirin in decreasing the combined risk of MI, vascular death, or ischemic stroke.[124] Aspirin, 75 to 325 mg per day, should be used routinely in all patients with acute and chronic ischemic heart disease with and without clinical symptoms in the absence of contraindications. In those unable to take aspirin, clopidogrel may be used instead. Warfarin is the third choice.

ANTITHROMBOTIC THERAPY

Disturbed fibrinolytic function after exercise appears to be associated with an increased risk of subsequent cardiovascular death in patients with chronic stable angina, providing the rationale for long-term antithrombotic therapy. In small placebo-controlled trials among patients with chronic stable angina, daily subcutaneous administration of low-molecular-weight heparin deceased the fibrinogen level and improved the exercise time to ST-segment depression.[125] The clinical experience of such therapy, however, is extremely limited. The efficacy of newer antiplatelet and antithrombotic agents such as glycoprotein IIb/IIa inhibitors and recombinant hirudin in the management of patients with chronic stable angina has not been established. Low-intensity oral anticoagulation with warfarin decreased the risk of ischemic events in a randomized trial of patients with risk factors for atherosclerosis but without symptoms of angina.[126]

LIPID-LOWERING AGENTS

Recent clinical studies have conveniently demonstrated that low-density lipoprotein (LDL)–lowering agents can decrease the risk of adverse ischemic events in patients with established CAD (see Chap. 38). In the Scandinavian Simvastatin Survival Study (4S),[127] treatment with an HMG-CoA reductase inhibitor in patients with documented CAD (including stable angina) and a baseline total cholesterol concentration between 212 and 308 mg/dL was associated with 30 to 35 percent reduction in both mortality rate and major coronary events. In the Cholesterol And Recurrent Events (CARE) study,[128] in men and women with previous MI and total cholesterol levels of less than 240 mg/dL and LDL-cholesterol levels of 115 to 174 mg/dL, treatment with a HMG-CoA reductase inhibitor (statin) was associated with a 24 percent reduction in risk for nonfatal MI. Thus lipid-lowering therapy should be recommended even in the presence of mild to moderate elevations of LDL-cholesterol in patients with chronic stable angina. Ongoing studies[128a,128b] suggest that a reduction of LDL-cholesterol below 100 mg/dL will further reduce cardiac events (see Chap. 38).

Antianginal and Anti-ischemic Therapy

Antianginal and anti-ischemic drug therapy consists of beta-adrenoreceptor blocking agents (beta blockers), calcium antagonists, and nitrates. Drug interactions are described in Chap. 81. There is a tendency for physicians to give *lower doses* of antianginal medications than those proven to be effective in clinical trials and after higher doses or combined therapy are neglected in patients who could be "angina-free," if treated more appropriately; this is particularly true with beta-blocker therapy. For example, the usual dose for angina is 50 to 200 mg of metoprolol twice daily.

BETA BLOCKERS

The decrease in heart rate, contractility, arterial pressure, and usually LV wall stress with beta blockers is associated with decreased $\dot{M}V_{O_2}$. A reduction in heart rate also increases diastolic coronary artery perfusion time, which may enhance LV perfusion. Although beta blockers have the potential to increase coronary vascular resistance by the formation of cyclic AMP, the clinical relevance of this pharmacodynamic effect remains to be demonstrated.

All beta blockers without intrinsic sympathetic activity appear to be equally effective in angina pectoris. In patients with chronic stable exertional angina, these agents decrease the heart rate–blood pressure product during exercise, and the onset of angina or the ischemic threshold during exercise is delayed or avoided.[1] When treating stable angina, it is essential that the dose of beta blockers be adjusted to lower the resting heart rate to 55 to 60 beats per minute. In patients with more severe angina, the heart rate can be reduced to less than 50 beats per minute if there are no symptoms associated with bradycardia and AV block does not develop (see Chap. 81). In patients with exertional angina, beta blockers attenuate the increase in heart rate during exercise, which ideally should not exceed 75 percent of the heart rate response associated with the onset of ischemia. It is often useful for the patient to perform exercise (sit-ups, running in place) before and after the institution of beta-blocker therapy. If the heart rate increase with exercise is not significantly reduced by therapy, the dose of the beta blocker is inadequate. Beta blockers are definitely effective in reducing exercise-induced angina. Three controlled studies comparing beta blockers with calcium antagonists[129–132] report equal efficacy in the treatment of chronic stable angina.

In patients with postinfarction stable angina and those who require antianginal therapy after revascularization, treatment with beta blockers appears to be effective in controlling symptomatic and asymptomatic ischemic episodes. Beta blockers are still the anti-ischemic drugs of choice in elderly patients with stable angina.[1]

Beta blockers frequently are combined with nitrates for treating chronic stable angina. This combination of therapy appeared to be more effective in several studies than nitrates or beta blockers alone.[133–135] Beta blockers also may be combined with calcium antagonists. For combination therapy, slow-released dihydropyridine derivatives or new-generation long-acting dihydropyridine derivatives are the calcium antagonists of choice.[1]

In the International Multicenter Angina Exercise (IMAGE) study,[132] both metoprolol and nifedipine were effective as monotherapy in increasing exercise time, although metoprolol was more effective than nifedipine. The combination therapy also increased the exercise time to ischemia compared with either drug alone. The absolute contraindications to the use of beta blockers are severe bradycardia, preexisting high-degree AV block, sick sinus syndrome, and severe, unstable LV failure (see Chap. 81). Asthma and bronchospastic disease, severe depression, and peripheral vascular disease are relative contraindications (see Chap. 81). Fatigue, inability to perform exercise, lethargy, insomnia, nightmares, worsening claudication, and impotence are frequently experienced side effects. Most patients with chronic CAD and diabetes can be treated with beta blockers (see Chap. 78).

CALCIUM ANTAGONISTS

These agents, also considered in Chap. 81, reduce the transmembrane flux of calcium by the calcium channels. There are three types of voltage-dependent calcium channels: L type, T type, and N type.

All calcium antagonists exert a negative inotropic effect, depending on dosage. In smooth muscle, calcium ions also regulate the contractile mechanism, and calcium antagonists reduce smooth muscle tension in the peripheral vascular bed, thus causing vasodilation. All the calcium antagonists cause dilatation of the epicardial conduit vessels and the arterial resistance vessels, the former being the primary mechanism for the beneficial effect of calcium antagonists for relieving vasospastic angina. Calcium antagonists also decrease $\dot{M}V_{O_2}$ demand primarily by reducing the systemic vascular resistance and arterial pressure. The negative inotropic effect of calcium antagonists also decreases the $\dot{M}V_{O_2}$.

Randomized clinical trials comparing calcium antagonists and beta blockers have demonstrated that calcium antagonists are equally effective as beta blockers in relieving angina and improving exercise time to onset of angina or ischemia.[1] The calcium antagonists are effective in reducing the incidence of angina in patients with vasospastic angina.[136,137]

In a *retrospective case-controlled study* reported in patients with hypertension, treatment with immediate-acting nifedipine, diltiazem, and verapamil was associated with an increased risk of MI of 31 to 61 percent.[138] Although a subsequent meta-analysis of immediate-release and short-acting nifedipine in patients with MI and unstable angina reported a dose-related influence on excess mortality,[139] further analysis of the published reports failed to confirm an increased risk of adverse cardiac events with calcium antagonists.[140,141] Importantly, long-acting calcium antagonists, including slow-release and long-acting dihydropyridine and nondihydropyridine derivatives, are effective in relieving symptoms in patients with chronic stable angina. They should be used in combination with beta blockers when initial treatment with beta blockers is not successful or as a substitute for beta blockers when initial treatment leads to unacceptable side effects. Many patients with two- or three-vessel CAD are asymptomatic on combined beta blocker and calcium antagonist therapy. Some have further improvement on triple therapy (combined beta blocker, calcium antagonist, and long-acting nitrates). Further information concerning the potential side effects of the calcium antagonists is given elsewhere (see Chap. 81).

NITROGLYCERIN AND NITRATES

Nitrates are endothelium-independent vasodilators that produce beneficial effects by both reducing the $\dot{M}V_{O_2}$ and improving CBF perfusion. The decreased $\dot{M}V_{O_2}$ results from the reduction of LV volume and arterial pressure primarily due to reduced preload. Nitroglycerin also exerts antithrombotic and antiplatelet effects in patients with stable angina.[1]

Nitrates dilate large epicardial arteries and collateral vessels. The vasodilating effect on epicardial coronary arteries with or without atherosclerotic CAD is beneficial in relieving coronary vasospasm in patients with vasospastic angina.

In patients with exertional stable angina, nitrates improve exercise tolerance, time to onset of angina, and time to ST-segment depression during treadmill exercise testing. In combination with beta blockers or calcium antagonists, nitrates produce greater antianginal and anti-ischemic effects in patients with stable angina.[142–145]

The interaction between nitrates and sildenafil (Viagra) is discussed in detail elsewhere.[146] The coadministration of nitrates and sildenafil significantly increases the risk of potentially life-threatening hypotension (see Chap. 81).

The major problem with long-term use of nitroglycerin and long-acting nitrates is development of nitrate tolerance.[147] Tolerance develops not only to antianginal and hemodynamic effects but also to platelet antiaggregatory effects.[148] The mechanism for development of nitrate tolerance remains unclear. For practical purposes, the administration or nitrates with an adequate nitrate-free interval (8–12 h) appears to be the most effective method of preventing nitrate tolerance. Unfortunately, this means that patients with unpredictable episodes of myocardial ischemia should not be treated with nitrate therapy alone because for part of each 24 h they will be "unprotected."

The primary consideration in the choice of pharmacologic agents for treatment of angina should be to *improve prognosis*. Aspirin and lipid-lowering therapies have been shown to reduce the risk of death and nonfatal myocardial infarction in both primary and secondary prevention trials. Beta blockers also reduce cardiac events when used as secondary prevention in postinfarction patients and reduce mortality and morbidity among patients with hypertension. Nitrates have not been shown to reduce mortality with acute infarction or in patients with chronic CAD.

Recommended drug therapy using calcium antagonists versus beta blockers in patients with angina-associated conditions are listed in Table 40-10.

Treatment of Risk Factors

The recommendations of the AHA for the treatment of risk factors are detailed in Chap. 38. *The risk factors to which interventions have been shown to reduce the incidence of CAD events include* (1) cigarette smoking, (2) LDL-cholesterol, (3) systemic hypertension, (4) LV hypertrophy, and (5) thrombogenic factors (see Chap. 38).

The causal role of *LDL-cholesterol* in the pathogenesis of atherosclerotic CAD has been enhanced by recent randomized, controlled clinical trials of lipid-lowering therapy. Several primary and secondary prevention trials have shown that LDL-cholesterol lowering is associated with a reduced risk of CAD (see Chap. 38). Angiographic trials provide firm evidence linking cholesterol reduction to favorable trends in coronary anatomy.

Data from numerous observational studies indicate a continuous and graded relation between blood pressure and cardiovascular disease risk.[149,150] Hypertension predisposes patients to coronary events both as a result of the direct vascular injury caused by increases in blood pressure and by its effects on the myocardium, including increased wall stress and $\dot{M}V_{O_2}$.

CAD, diabetes, LV hypertrophy, heart failure, retinopathy, and nephropathy are indicators of increased cardiovascular disease risk in hypertensive patients. The target of therapy is a reduction in blood pressure to less than 130 mmHg systolic and less than 85 mmHg diastolic in patients with CAD and coexisting diabetes, heart failure, or renal failure.[149]

Treatment of *hypertension* begins with nonpharmacologic means. When lifestyle modifications and dietary alterations adequately reduce blood pressure, pharmacologic intervention may be unnecessary (see Chaps. 38 and 51).

When pharmacologic treatment is necessary (usually the case), beta blockers or calcium antagonists may be especially useful in patients with hypertension and angina pectoris; however, short-acting calcium antagonists should not be used.[151]

Epidemiologic studies have implicated *LV hypertrophy* as a risk factor for development of MI, congestive heart failure, and sudden death.[152] LV hypertrophy also has been shown to predict a poorer prognosis in patients with definite CAD.[153] In the Framingham Heart Study,[154] the subjects who demonstrated ECG evidence of LV hypertrophy regression on follow-up were at a substantially reduced risk for cardiovascular events.

Coronary artery thrombosis is a trigger of acute MI. Aspirin has been documented to reduce the risk for CHD in both primary and secondary prevention settings.[1] Elevated plasma fibrinogen levels predict CAD risk in prospective observational studies[155] (see Chap. 38).

Risk factors for which interventions are likely to reduce the incidence of coronary disease events include diabetes mellitus, high-density lipoprotein (HDL)–cholesterol, obesity, physical inactivity, and postmenopausal status (see Chap. 38).

Diabetes mellitus, which is defined as a fasting blood sugar level of more than 126 mg/dL,[156] is present in a significant minority of adult Americans. Data supporting an important role of diabetes mellitus as a risk factor for cardiovascular disease comes from a number of observational settings. This is true for both type I and type II diabetes. Atherosclerosis accounts for 80 percent of all diabetic mortality,[157,158] with CAD alone responsible for 75 percent of total atherosclerotic deaths (see Chaps. 38 and 78). The goal is to maintain a blood glucose HbA_1c level of less than 7 percent and a blood glucose level of less than 140 mg/dL. In diabetic patients with hypertension, microalbuminuria, or decreased LV systolic function, angiotensin converting enzyme (ACE) inhibitors appear indicated. This may apply to most diabetics with CAD.[158a]

Observational studies and clinical trials have demonstrated a strong inverse association between *HDL-cholesterol* and CAD risk (see Chap. 38). This inverse relation is observed in both men and women and among asymptomatic persons as well as patients with established CAD.[1] The National Cholesterol Adult Treatment Panel II has defined a low HDL-cholesterol level as less than 35 mg/dL.[159]

Obesity is a common condition associated with increased risk for CHD and mortality (see Chap. 38). New AHA guidelines for weight control have been published recently.[160]

Multiple randomized, controlled trials comparing exercise training with a "no exercise" control group have demonstrated a statistically significant improvement in exercise tolerance for the exercise group versus the control group.[1] The threshold for ischemia is likely to increase with exercise training because training reduces the heart rate–blood pressure product at a given submaximal exercise workload[1] (see Chap. 38).

When hormone production decreases in the perimenopausal period over several years, the risk of CAD rises in postmenopausal women. By age 75, the risk of atherosclerotic cardiovascular disease among men and women is equal.[1] The first published randomized trial of estrogen plus progestin therapy in postmenopausal women with known CAD did not show any reduction in cardiovascular events over 4 years of follow-up[161] despite an 11 percent lower LDL-cholesterol level and a 10 percent higher HDL-cholesterol level in those women receiving hormone replacement. Other randomized trials of hormone-

TABLE 40-10 Recommended Drug Therapy (Calcium Antagonist versus Beta Blocker) in Patients with Angina and Associated Conditions

Condition	Recommended Treatment and Alternative	Avoid
Medical conditions		
Systemic hypertension	Beta blockers (calcium antagonists)	
Migraine or vascular headaches	Beta blockers (verapamil or diltiazem)	
Asthma or chronic obstructive pulmonary disease with bronchospasm	Verapamil or diltiazem	Beta blockers
Hyperthyroidism	Beta blockers	
Raynaud's syndrome	Long-acting slow-release calcium antagonists	Beta blockers
Insulin-dependent diabetes mellitus	Beta blockers (particularly if prior myocardial infarction) or long-acting slow-release calcium antagonists	
Non-insulin-dependent diabetes mellitus	Beta blockers or long-acting slow-release calcium antagonists	
Depression	Long-acting slow-release calcium antagonists	Beta blockers
Mild peripheral vascular disease	Beta blockers or calcium antagonists	
Severe peripheral vascular disease with rest ischemia	Calcium antagonists	Beta blockers
Cardiac arrhythmias and conduction abnormalities		
Sinus bradycardia	Long-acting slow-release calcium antagonists that do not decrease heart rate	Beta blockers, diltiazem, verapamil
Sinus tachycardia (not due to heart failure)	Beta blockers	
Supraventricular tachycardia	Verapamil, diltiazem, or beta blockers	
Atrioventricular block	Long-acting slow-release calcium antagonists that do not slow AV conduction	Beta blockers, verapamil, diltiazem
Rapid artrial fibrillation (with digitalis)	Verapamil, diltiazem, or beta blockers	
Ventricular arrhythmias	Beta blockers	
Left ventricular dysfunction		
Congestive heart failure		
Mild (LVEF ≥ 40%)	Beta blockers	
Moderate to Severe (LVEF < 40%)	Amlodipine or felodipine (nitrates)	Verapamil, diltiazem
Left-sided valvular heart disease		
Mild aortic stenosis	Beta blockers	
Aortic insufficiency	Long-acting slow-release dihydropyridines	
Mitral regurgitation	Long-acting slow-release dihydropyridines	
Mitral stenosis	Beta blockers	
Hypertrophic cardiomyopathy	Beta blockers, nondihydropyridine calcium antagonist	Nitrates, dihydropyridine, calcium antagonists

SOURCE: From Gibbons et al.[1]

replacement therapy in primary and secondary prevention of CAD in postmenopausal women are in progress.

Risk factors for which interventions may reduce the incidence of coronary disease events include psychosocial factors, triglycerides, lipoprotein (a), homocysteine, oxidative stress, and consumption of alcohol (see Chap. 38).

Triglyceride levels are predictive of CHD in a variety of observational studies and clinical settings.[162] However, much of the association of triglycerides with CHD risk is related to other factors, including diabetes, obesity, hypertension, high LDL-cholesterol, and low HDL-cholesterol[163] (see Chap. 38).

Lipoprotein(a) is a lipoprotein particle that has been linked to CHD risk in observational studies. Elevated lipoprotein(a) levels are largely genetically determined and found in 15 to 20 percent of patients with premature CHD.[164,165] Increased *homocysteine* levels are associated with increased risk of CAD, peripheral arterial disease, and carotid disease.[166,167] Elevated homocysteine levels can occur as a result of inborn errors of metabolism such as homocysteinuria, and homocysteine levels also can be increased by deficiencies of vitamin B_6, vitamin B_{12}, and folate, which commonly occur in older patients[167] (see Chap. 38).

Extensive laboratory data indicate that oxidation of LDL-cholesterol promotes and accelerates the atherosclerosis process.[168] Observational studies have documented an association between dietary intake of antioxidant vitamins (vitamin C, vitamin E, and β-carotene) and reduced risk for CHD[169] (see Chap. 38).

Observational studies have shown repeatedly an inverse relation of *moderate alcohol intake* to the risk of CHD events.[170]

However, excessive alcohol intake can promote many other medical problems that outweigh its beneficial effects on CHD risk.

Risk factors associated with increased risk but that cannot be modified or when modified are unlikely to change the incidence of CHD events include age, male gender, and a positive family history of premature CHD. The latter is defined as definite MI or sudden death before age 55 in a father or other male first-degree relative or before age 65 in a mother or other female first-degree relative[1] (see Chap. 38).

MYOCARDIAL REVASCULARIZATION

There are currently two well-established revascularization approaches to treatment of chronic stable angina caused by coronary atherosclerosis. One is CABG surgery, in which segments of autologous arteries or veins are used to reroute blood around relatively stenotic segments of the proximal coronary artery. The other is percutaneous coronary interventions (PCIs) using catheter-borne or laser techniques to open usually short areas of stenoses from within the coronary artery. These techniques are described in greater detail in Chaps. 45 and 48. Revascularization is also potentially feasible with transthoracic (laser) myocardial revascularization in patients in whom neither CABG nor PCI is feasible (see Chap. 48). The recommendations of the ACC/AHA/ACP-ASIM for revascularization with PCIs or CABG in patients with stable angina are listed in Table 40-11.

Patients with stable angina pectoris may be appropriate candidates for revascularization either by CABG surgery or PCIs. In general, this is an individual decision to be made by the patient with knowledge of the advantages or disadvantages either of medical therapy alone or revascularization with either CABG or PCIs.

There are two general indications for revascularization procedures: the presence of symptoms that are not acceptable to the patient either because of (1) restriction of physical activity and lifestyle as a result of limitations or side effects from medications or (2) the presence of findings that indicate clearly that the patient would have a better prognosis for revascularization than with medical therapy. Considerations regarding revascularization are based on an assessment of the grade or class of angina experienced by the patient, the presence and severity of myocardial ischemia on noninvasive testing, the degree of LV function, and the distribution and severity of coronary artery stenoses.

A recent meta-analysis of three major large multicenter randomized trials of initial surgery versus medical management (performed in the 1970s) as well as other smaller trials has confirmed the surgical benefits achieved by surgery at 10 postoperative years for patients with three-vessel disease, two-vessel disease, or even one-vessel disease that included a severe stenoses of the proximal left anterior descending coronary artery[119] (see Chap. 48).

The advantages of PCIs for the treatment of CAD include a low level of procedure-related morbidity, a low procedure-related mortality rate in properly selected patients, a short hospital stay, early return to activity, and the feasibility of multiple procedures. However, PCIs are not feasible in all patients; they are accompanied by a significant incidence of restenoses, and there is an occasional need for emergency CABG surgery (see Chap. 45).

Three randomized studies have compared PCIs with medical management alone for the treatment of chronic stable angina.[171–173] All these randomized studies of PCIs versus medical management have involved patients at a low risk of mortality even with medical management and did not assess patients with moderate to severe CAD (see Chap. 45). Multiple trials have compared the strategy of an initial PCI with initial CABG surgery for treatment of multivessel CAD (see Chaps. 45 and 48). The results of all these trials have shown that early and late survival rates have been equivalent for the PCI and CABG surgery groups. In the Bypass Angioplasty Revascularization Intervention (BARI) trial, the subgroups of patients with treated diabetics had a significantly better survival rate with CABG surgery.[174] This was true, however, on post hoc analysis of the clinical variables, including diabetes, which was not a prerandomization blocking variable.

The randomized studies of invasive therapy for chronic angina have all excluded patients who developed recurrent angina after previous CABG surgery. Few existing data define outcomes for risk-stratified groups of patients who develop recurrent angina after bypass surgery. Those which do indicate that patients with ischemia produced by late atherosclerotic stenoses in vein grafts are at a higher risk with medical management alone than those with ischemia produced by native-vessel disease.

FOLLOW-UP OF PATIENTS WITH CHRONIC STABLE ANGINA

Published evidence of the efficacy of specific strategies for the follow-up of patients with chronic stable angina on patient outcome are nonexistent. The ACC/AHA/ACP-ASIM guidelines[1] for monitoring of symptoms and antianginal therapy during patient follow-up are as follows:

For the patient with successfully treated chronic stable angina, a follow-up evaluation every 4 to 12 months is appropriate. During the first year of therapy, evaluations every 4 to 6 months are recommended. After the first year of therapy, annual evaluations are recommended if the patient is stable and reliable enough to return for evaluation when anginal symptoms become worse or other symptoms occur.[1] At the time of follow-up, a general assessment of the patient's functional and health status and quality of life may reveal additional issues that affect angina. Symptoms that have worsened should follow reevaluation as outlined above. A detailed history of the patient's daily activity is critical because angina symptoms may remain stable only because stressful activities have been eliminated.

A careful history of the characteristics of the patient's angina including provoking and alleviating factors must be repeated at each visit. Detailed questions should be asked about common drug side effects. The patient's adherence to the treatment program must be assessed.

The physical examination should be determined by the patient's history. Every patient should have weight, blood pressure, and pulse noted. The jugular venous pressure, carotid pulse magnitude and upstroke, and presence or absence of carotid bruits should be noted. Pulmonary examination with special attention to rales, rhonchi, wheezing, and decreased breath sounds is required. A cardiac examination should note the presence of fourth and third heart sounds, a new or changed systolic

TABLE 40-11 Revascularization for Chronic Stable Angina (Recommendations for Revascularization with PTCA or Other Catheter-Based Techniques and CABG in Patients with Stable Angina)

Class I

1. CABG for patients with significant left main coronary disease.
2. CABG for patients with three-vessel disease. The survival benefit is greater in patients with abnormal LV function (ejection fraction < 50%).
3. CABG for patients with two-vessel disease with significant proximal left anterior descending CAD and either abnormal LV function (ejection fraction < 50%) or demonstrable ischemia on noninvasive testing.
4. PCI for patients with two- or three-vessel disease with significant proximal left anterior descending CAD, who have anatomy suitable for catheter-based therapy, normal LV function and who do not have treated diabetes.
5. PCI or CABG for patients with one- or two-vessel disease CAD without significant proximal left anterior descending CAD, but with a large area of viable myocardium and high risk criteria on noninvasive testing.
6. CABG for patients with one- or two-vessel disease CAD without significant proximal left anterior descending CAD who have survived sudden cardiac death or sustained ventricular tachycardia.
7. In patients with prior PCI, CABG, or PCI for recurrent stenosis associated with a large area of viable myocardium or high-risk criteria on noninvasive testing.
8. PTCA or CABG for patients who have not been treated successfully by medical therapy and can undergo revascularization with acceptable risk.

Class IIa

1. Repeat CABG for patients with multiple saphenous vein graft stenoses, especially when there is significant stenosis of a graft supplying the LAD. It may be appropriate to use PTCA for focal saphenous vein graft lesions or multiple stenoses in poor candidates for reoperative surgery.
2. Use of PCI or CABG for patients with one- or two-vessel disease CAD without significant proximal LAD disease but with a moderate area of viable myocardium and demonstrable ischemia on noninvasive testing.
3. Use of PCI or CABG for patients with one-vessel disease with significant proximal LAD disease.

Class IIb

1. Compared with CABG, PCI for patients with two- or three-vessel disease with significant proximal left anterior descending CAD, who have anatomy suitable for catheter-based therapy, and who have treated diabetes or abnormal LV function.
2. Use of PCI for patients with significant left main coronary disease who are not candidates for CABG.
3. PCI for patients with one- or two-vessel disease CAD without significant proximal left anterior descending CAD, who have survived sudden cardiac death or sustained ventricular tachycardia.

Class III

1. Use of PCI or CABG for patients with one- or two-vessel CAD without significant proximal left anterior descending CAD, who have mild symptoms that are unlikely due to myocardial ischemia or who have not received an adequate trial of medical therapy and
   a. Have only a small area of viable myocardium or
   b. Have no demonstrable ischemia on noninvasive testing
2. Use of PCI or CABG for patients with borderline coronary stenoses (50% to 60% diameter in locations other than the left main coronary artery) and no demonstrable ischemia on noninvasive testing.
3. Use of PCI or CABG for patients with insignificant coronary stenosis (<50% diameter).
4. Use of PCI in patients with significant left main coronary disease who are candidates for CABG.

NOTE: PTCA is used in these recommendations to indicate PTCA or other catheter-based techniques, such as stents, atherectomy, and laser therapy. See classes I–III as described at the bottom of Table 40-5.

murmur, the location of the LV impulse, and any change from previous examinations. Clearly, the vascular examination should identify any change in peripheral pulses and new bruits; the abdominal examination should identify hepatomegaly and the presence of any pulsatile mass suggesting abdominal aortic aneurysm. The presence of new or worsening peripheral edema should be noted.

The American Diabetes Association recommends that patients not known to have diabetes should have a *fasting blood glucose* measured every 3 years and an annual measurement of glycosylated hemoglobin for individuals with established diabetes. Fasting blood work 6 to 8 weeks after initiating lipid-lowering drug therapy should include liver function testing and assessment of the cholesterol profile. This should be repeated every 8 to 12 weeks during the first year of therapy and at 4- to 6-month intervals thereafter.

An ECG should be repeated when medications affecting cardiac conduction are initiated or changed. A repeat ECG is indicated for a change in the anginal pattern, symptoms or finding suggestive of an arrhythmia or conduction abnormality, and near or frank syncope. There is no clear evidence showing that routine, periodic ECGs are useful in the absence of a change in history or physical examination.

In the absence of a change in clinical status, low-risk patients with an estimated annual mortality rate of less than 1 percent over each year of the interval do not require repeat stress testing

TABLE 40-12 Recommendations for Echocardiography, Treadmill Exercise Testing, Stress Imaging Studies, and Coronary Angiography during Patient Follow-Up

Class I

1. Chest x-ray for patients with evidence of new or worsening congestive heart failure.
2. Assessment of LV ejection fraction and segmental wall motion in patients with new or worsening congestive heart failure or evidence of intervening MI by history or ECG.
3. Echocardiography for evidence of new or worsening valvular heart disease.
4. Treadmill exercise test for patients without prior revascularization who have a significant change in clinical status, are able to exercise, and do not have any of the ECG abnormalities listed below in number 5.
5. Stress imaging procedures for patients without prior revascularization who have a significant change in clinical status and are unable to exercise or have one of the following ECG abnormalities:
   a. Preexcitation (Wolff-Parkinson-White) syndrome.
   b. Electronically paced ventricular rhythm.
   c. More than 1 mm of rest ST-segment depression.
   d. Complete left bundle-branch block.
6. Stress imaging procedures for patients who have a significant change in clinical status and required a stress imaging procedure on their initial evaluation because of equivocal or intermediate-risk treadmill results.
7. Stress imaging procedures for patients with prior revascularization who have a significant change in clinical status.
8. Coronary angiography in patients with marked limitation of ordinary activity. (CCS class III despite maximal medical therapy).

Class IIb

Annual treadmill exercise testing in patients who have no change to clinical status, can exercise, have none of the ECG abnormalities listed in number 5 above, and have an estimated annual mortality of >1%.

Class III

1. Echocardiography or radionuclide imaging for assessment of LV ejection fraction and segmental wall motion in patients with a normal ECG, no history of MI, and no evidence of congestive heart failure.
2. Repeat treadmill exercise testing in <3 years in patients who have no change in clinical status and an estimated annual mortality ≤1% on their initial evaluation as demonstrated by one of the following:
   a. Low-risk Duke treadmill score (without imaging).
   b. Low-risk Duke treadmill score with negative imaging.
   c. Normal LV function and a normal coronary angiogram.
   d. Normal LV function and insignificant CAD.
3. Stress imaging procedures for patients who have no change in clinical status and a normal rest ECG, are not taking digoxin, are able to exercise, and did not require a stress imaging procedure on their initial evaluation because of equivocal or intermediate-risk treadmill results.
4. Repeat coronary angiography in patients with no change in clinical status, no change on repeat exercise testing or stress imaging, and insignificant CAD on initial evaluation.

NOTE: See classes I–III as described at the bottom of Table 40-5.

for 3 years after the initial evaluation.[1] These include those with low-risk Duke treadmill scores either without imaging or with negative imaging, those with normal LV function and normal coronary angiograms, and those with normal LV function and insignificant CAD. *Annual follow-up for noninvasive testing in the absence of a change in symptoms* has not been studied adequately; it may be useful in high-risk patients with an estimated annual mortality rate of greater than 5 percent. Follow-up testing should be performed in a stable high-risk patient only if the initial decision not to proceed with revascularization may change if the patient's estimated risk worsens. Patients with an immediate-risk (>1 and <3 percent) annual mortality rate are more problematic because of limited data. They may need testing at an interval of 1 to 3 years depending on the individual circumstances. The ACC/AHA/ACP-ASIM recommendations for echocardiography, treadmill exercise testing, stress imaging studies and coronary angiography during patient follow-up are also listed in Table 40-12.

MANAGEMENT OF SPECIAL CATEGORIES

Systemic Arterial Hypertension

Patients with systemic arterial hypertension (SAH) often have angina pectoris. In most patients, significant coronary atherosclerosis of the epicardial blood vessels is present, but some patients with SAH may have angina pectoris or even fatal MI without significant obstruction of the large epicardial vessels. A major mistake is to send a patient for noninvasive testing when his or her hypertension has not been treated. In some patients there may be a marked increase in $M\dot{V}_{O_2}$ that exceeds the CBF reserve, whereas others may have microvascular angina (syndrome X).

In many patients, treatment of the hypertension with a beta blocker, calcium antagonist, or angiotension-converting enzyme inhibitor also will decrease $M\dot{V}_{O_2}$ and prevent the development of angina pectoris. In general, efforts should be made to control the blood pressure both at rest and during exercise. It is now know that many patients with an elevated systolic and/or diastolic blood pressure above the normal variation during exercise will develop severe fixed SAH. Efforts should be made to control the blood pressure both at rest and during exertion.

Chronic Obstructive Pulmonary Disease/Asthma

Beta blockers should be avoided in the subset of patients who have true bronchospastic lung disease, and the use of nitrates and calcium antagonists is preferred. Since many of these patients receive medications for their pulmonary disease that may increase their heart rate or even produce supraventricular tachycardia, it is preferable to use a heart rate–slowing calcium antagonist such as diltiazem or verapamil. Many patients with a history of only asthma or mild chronic obstructive pulmonary disease may be able to tolerate small doses of cardioselective beta blockers with careful monitoring.

Elderly Patients

In general, elderly patients tolerate calcium antagonists better than beta blockers. The presence of sinus tachycardia or atrial fibrillation is a relative contraindication to the selection of dihydropyridines such as nifedipine or amlodipine. In such patients, diltiazem or verapamil or even a beta blocker is preferable. On the other hand, beta blockers, verapamil, and diltiazem can exacerbate AV block, and verapamil produces constipation in many elderly patients. Also, some elderly patients develop postural hypotension from short-acting nitrates.

Peripheral Vascular Disease

Patients with peripheral vascular disease may have a worsening of their symptoms when treated with a nonselective beta blocker, permitting unopposed alpha-induced vasoconstriction. Alternatively, the worsening symptoms may be due to a decrease in arterial perfusion pressure. In general, it is preferable to treat patients with chronic stable angina who have peripheral vascular disease with nitrates and a calcium antagonist.

Diabetes Mellitus

Patients with chronic stable angina who have diabetes mellitus and hypoglycemic episodes due to insulin probably should be treated with nitrates and calcium antagonists (see Chap. 78). If it is necessary to use a beta blocker, a cardioselective agent should be chosen, since it is less likely to impair the recognition of and recovery from insulin-induced hypoglycemia. In most diabetics, cardioselective beta blockers are well tolerated. The BARI-II Diabetes Study is evaluating the efficacy at *early* myocardial revascularization in diabetes with CAD.

Chronic Renal Disease

While beta blockers and calcium antagonists normally can be used effectively in patients with chronic angina and chronic renal insufficiency, careful monitoring may be necessary because many beta blockers and calcium antagonists (see Chap. 84) are excreted primarily by the kidneys.

CHRONIC MANIFESTATIONS OF CHRONIC ISCHEMIC HEART DISEASE

Heart Failure

Patients with severe CAD that produces a loss of 20 percent or more of the myocardium or that results in a ventricular septal defect or significant mitral regurgitation may cause important LV failure. While there may be significant hypertrophy of the remaining myocytes and interstitium (see Chap. 20), the ventricle is unable to compensate completely, and heart failure often results with a decreased stroke volume and elevated diastolic filling pressures. A syndrome of heart failure may result that is clinically predominant and often more incapacitating than any symptom of angina pectoris (see Chap. 66).

Patients with severe LV dysfunction due to CAD have a poor prognosis. Usually it reflects permanent, irreversible loss of myocytes. In some patients severe chronic CAD is associated with persistently impaired LV function at rest due to reduced CBF that can be partially or completely restored to normal either by improving blood flow (more common) or by reducing oxygen demand. This concept of "hibernating" myocardium is important because there can be significant improvement following good LV revascularization. While this does not occur routinely, it must be considered before concluding that the LVEF of an individual patient is too low to consider revascularization surgery or that the etiology of the heart failure is not CHD. MPI imaging techniques, magnetic resonance imaging (MRI), dobutamine echocardiography, and positron-emission tomography (PET) are useful in detecting myocardial viability (see Chap. 19).

The treatment of patients with heart failure due to CHD is the same as for most patients with combined systolic and diastolic LV failure and includes diuretics, an ACE inhibitor, digitalis, beta blockers, and spironolactone (see Chap. 28).

Cardiac transplantation is also frequently performed for severe heart failure due to CAD (see Chap. 22). A patient with heart failure who has a large LV aneurysm may benefit from aneurysmectomy if there is sufficient remaining functioning LV tissue. Similarly, heart failure due to severe mitral regurgitation sometimes can be improved significantly by corrective mitral valve surgery, which is often combined with myocardial revascularization. The operative mortality for this procedure can be high; in patients with severe functional mitral regurgitation, mitral valve repair with a reduced annular size can improve patient symptoms considerably (see Chap. 48).

Cardiac Arrhythmias, Conduction Disturbances

Chronic ischemic heart diseases causes many cardiac arrhythmias. The basic management is discussed in Chap. 24. In general, beta blockers should be employed whenever there is no strong contraindication, and type IC antiarrhythmic agents should be avoided unless the patient is symptomatic. In patients with atrial fibrillation, the ventricular response rate should be controlled with digoxin.

Patients with chronic atrial fibrillation also should be maintained on warfarin (INR = 2–3) unless there is a contraindication, in which case aspirin (80–325 mg/day) should be used. Patients in heart failure who have atrial fibrillation may benefit from an effective atrial contraction restored by electrical cardioversion. Unfortunately, large percentages revert to atrial fibrillation in the next few months. Nonetheless, cardioversion sometimes can improve overall function significantly even though for a short time. Patients with recurrent symptomatic ventricular tachycardia or ventricular fibrillation can be treated with an implantable cardioverter-defibrillator. The use of these devices is discussed in Chap. 29.

Embolic Disease

Patients with ischemic disease are likely to have systemic emboli, particularly patients with a history of systemic embolus, chronic atrial fibrillation, ventricular aneurysm, a large dyskinetic or hypokinetic area of myocardium, or a severely depressed LVEF. Such patients should be considered for chronic, long-term, low-dose warfarin therapy (INR = 2–3).

CHEST PAIN WITH NORMAL CORONARY ARTERIES

The combination of chest pain with many of the features of angina pectoris, although frequently atypical, and normal epicardial coronary arteries at cardiac catheterization has been known since the entity was first described in the 1960s. The early studies identified many of the features of what was subsequently characterized as a syndrome: female predominance, the frequent presence of ischemic ST-segment changes on the exercise ECG, inconsistent relationship between ECG changes and metabolic or hemodynamic evidence of ischemia, and pain that could be very severe, prolonged, variable in location, precipitated by unusual events, and unresponsive to usual anti-ischemic therapy.

The term *syndrome X* was applied to this diagnostic combination in 1973[175]; it is usually used to describe patients with the common features of angina-like pain and normal epicardial coronaries, but the term is also used to categorize groups that undoubtedly are pathophysiologically heterogeneous.[176–178] The continued use of this term is unfortunate and has been discouraged,[179] especially since there is a *metabolic syndrome X*, characterized by insulin resistance, hyperinsulinemia, and diabetes, that is associated with abnormal lipids, hypertension, and abdominal obesity[179] (see Chap. 78). A more specific term such as *angina with normal coronary arteriography* is preferable.

References

1. Gibbons RJ, Chatterjee K, Daley J, et al. ACC/AHA/ACP-ASIM guidelines for the management of patients with chronic stable angina: A report of the ACC/AHA Task Force on Practice Guidelines (Committee on the Management of Patients with Chronic Stable Angina). *J Am Coll Cardiol* 1999; 33:2097–2197.
2. Herberden W. Some account of disorder of the breast. *Med Trans R Coll Phys (Lond)* 1772; 2:59–67.
3. Herberden W. *Commentaries on the History and Care of Disease*. London: T Payne; 1802.
4. White PD. Angina pectoris: Historical background. In: Paul O, ed. *Angina Pectoris*. New York: Medcom Press; 1974:1.
5. Fuster V. Epidemic of cardiovascular disease and stroke: The three main challenges. In: *American Heart Association 71st Scientific Sessions*. Dallas, Texas: American Heart Association; 1999.
6. Schlant RC, Alexander RW. Diagnosis and management of patients with chronic ischemic disease. In: Alexander RW, Schlant RC, Fuster V, et al, eds. *Hurst's the Heart*, 9th ed. New York: McGraw-Hill; 1998:1275.
7. Diamond GA, Staniloff HM, Forrester JS, et al. Computer-assisted diagnosis in the noninvasive evaluation of patients with suspected coronary disease. *J Am Coll Cardiol* 1983; 1:444–455.
8. Chaitman BR, Bourassa MG, Davis K, et al. Angiographic prevalence of high-risk coronary artery disease in patient subsets (CASS). *Circulation* 1981; 64:360–367.

8a. O'Rourke RA, Hochman JS, Cohen MC, et al. New approaches to diagnosis and management of unstable angina and nonST-segment elevation myocardial infarction. 2000 (in press).

9. Lange RA, Cigarroa RG, Yancy CWJ, et al. Cocaine-induced coronary-artery vasoconstriction. *N Engl J Med* 1989; 321:1557–1562.
10. Diamond GA, Forrester JS. Analysis of probability as an aid in the clinical diagnosis of coronary-artery disease. *N Engl J Med* 1979; 300:1350–1358.
11. Pryor DB, Harrell FE, Lee KL, et al. Estimating the likelihood of significant coronary artery disease. *Am J Med* 1983; 75:771–790.
12. Sox HC, Hickam DH, Marton KL, et al. Using the patient's history to estimate the probability of coronary artery disease. *N Engl J Med* 1979; 300:1350S.
13. Pryor DB, Shaw L, McCants CB, et al. Value of the history and physical in identifying patients at increased risk for coronary artery disease. *Ann Intern Med* 1993; 18:81–90.
14. Castellanos A, Kessler KM, Myerburg RJ. The resting electrocardiogram. In: Alexander RW, Schlant RC, Fuster V, et al, eds. *Hurst's The Heart*, 9th ed. New York: McGraw-Hill; 1998:351.
15. Margolis JR, Chen JT, Kong Y, et al. The diagnostic and prognostic significance of coronary artery calcification: A report of 800 cases. *Radiology* 1980; 137:609–616.
16. Wexler L, Brundage B, Crouse J, et al. Coronary artery calcification, pathophysiology, epidemiology, imaging methods and clinical implications. *Circulation* 1996; 94:1175–1192.
17. O'Rourke R, Brundage B, Froelicher V, et al. American College of Cardiology/American Heart Association consensus document on electron beam computed tomography for the diagnosis of coronary artery disease (Committee on Electron Beam Computer Tomography). *Circulation* 2000; 20:(July 4, 2001).

17a. DeTrano RC, Duherty TM, Davies MJ, et al. Predicting coronary events with coronary calcium: Pathophysiologic and clinical problems. *Curr Probl Card* 2000; 25:369–404.

18. Gibbons RJ, Balady GJ, Beasley JW, et al. AHA guidelines for exercise testing. *J Am Coll Cardiol* 1997; 30:260–315.
19. Stuart RJ, Ellestad MH. National survey of exercise stress testing facilities. *Chest* 1980; 77:94–97.
20. Myers J, Froelicher VF. Optimizing the exercise test for pharmacological investigations. *Circulation* 1990; 82:1839–1846.
21. Froelicher VF, Lehmann KG, Thomas R, et al. The electrocardiographic exercise test in a population with reduced workup bias: Diagnostic performance, computerized interpretation, and multivariable prediction. Veterans Affairs Cooperative Study in Health Services 016 (QUEXTA) Study Group, Quantitative Exercise Testing and Angiography. *Ann Intern Med* 1998; 128:965–974.
22. Veragari J, Hakki AH, Heo J, Iskandrian AS. Merits and limitations of quantitative treadmill exercise score. *Am Heart J* 1987; 114:819–826.
23. Mark DB, Shaw L, Harrell FE, et al. Prognostic value of a treadmill exercise score in outpatients with suspected coronary artery disease. *N Engl J Med* 1991; 325:849–853.

24. Kligfield P, Ameisen O, Okin PM. Heart rate adjustment of ST segment depression for improved detection of coronary artery disease. *Circulation* 1989; 79:245–255.
25. Lachterman B, Lehmann KG, Detrano R, et al. Comparison of the ST/heart rate index to standard ST criteria for analysis of the exercise electrocardiogram. *Circulation* 1990; 82:44–50.
26. Whinnery JE, Froelicher VF, Stuart AJ. The electrocardiographic response to maximal treadmill exercise in asymptomatic men with left bundle branch block. *Am Heart J* 1977; 94:316–324.
27. Cheitlin MD, Alpert JS, Armstrong WF, et al. ACC/AHA guidelines for the clinical application of echocardiography: A report of the American College of Cardiology/American Heart Association Task Force on Practice Guidelines (Committee on Clinical Application of Echocardiography), developed in collaboration with the American Society of Echocardiography. *Circulation* 1997; 95:1686–1744.
28. Ritchie JL, Bateman TM, Bonow RO, et al. Guidelines for clinical use of cardiac radionuclide imaging: Report of the American College of Cardiology/American Heart Association Task Force on Assessment of Diagnostic and Therapeutic Cardiovascular Procedures (Committee on Radionuclide Imaging), developed in collaboration with the American Society of Nuclear Cardiology. *J Am Coll Cardiol* 1995; 25:521–547.
29. Verani MS. Pharmacologic stress myocardial perfusion imaging. *Curr Probl Cardiol* 1993; 18:481–525.
30. Nishimura S, Mahmarian JJ, Boyce TM, Verani MS. Equivalence between adenosine and exercise thallium-201 myocardial tomography: A mulitcenter, prospective, crossover trial. *J Am Coll Cardiol* 1992; 20:265–275.
31. Patterson RE, Eisner RL, Horowitz SF. Comparison of cost effectiveness and utility of exercise ECG, single photon emission tomography and coronary angiography for diagnosis of coronary artery disease. *Circulation* 1995; 91:54–65.
32. Spaulding CM, Joly LM, Rosenberg A, et al. Immediate coronary angiography in survivors of out-of-hospital cardiac arrest. *N Engl J Med* 1997; 336:1629–1633.
33. Douglas JS Jr, Hurst JW. Limitations of symptoms in the recognition of coronary atherosclerotic heart disease. In: Hurst JW, ed. *Update I: The Heart.* New York: McGraw-Hill; 1979:3.
34. Barnard RJ, Duncan HW, Livesay JJ, Buckberg GD. Coronary vasodilator reserve and flow distribution during near-maximal exercise in dogs. *J Appl Physiol Respir Environ Exerc Physiol* 1977; 43:988–992.
35. Boerth RC, Covell JW, Pool PE, Ross J Jr. Increased myocardial oxygen consumption and contractile state associated with increase in heart rate in dogs. *Circ Res* 1969; 24:725–734.
36. Pupita G, Maseri A, Kaski JC, et al. Myocardial ischemia caused by distal coronary artery constriction in stable angina pectoris. *N Engl J Med* 1990; 323:514–520.
37. McGorisk GM, Treasure CB. Endothelial dysfunction in coronary heart disease. *Curr Opin Cardiol* 1996; 11:341–350.
38. Egashira K, Inou T, Hirooka Y, et al. Evidence of impaired endothelium-dependent coronary vasodilatation in patients with angina pectoris and normal coronary angiograms. *N Engl J Med* 1993; 328:1659–1664.
39. Cannon RO III, Camici PG, Epstein SE. Pathophysiological dilemma of syndrome X. *Circulation* 1992; 85:883–892.
40. Dole WP. Autoregulation of the coronary circulation. *Prog Cardiovasc Dis* 1987; 29:369–387.
41. Gould KL, Lipscomb K, Calvert C. Compensatory changes of the distal coronary vascular bed during progressive coronary constriction. *Circulation* 1975; 51:1085–1094.
42. Mudge GH Jr, Grossman W, Mills RM Jr, et al. Reflex increase in coronary vascular resistance in patients with ischemic heart disease. *N Engl J Med* 1976; 295:1333–1337.
43. Furchgott RF, Zawadzski JV. The obligatory role of endothelial cells in the relaxation of arterial smooth muscle by acetylcholine. *Nature* 1980; 288:373–376.
44. Palmer RMJ, Ferrige AG, Moncada S. Nitric oxide release accounts for the biological activity of endothelium-derived relaxing factor. *Nature* 1987; 327:524–526.
45. Bortone AS, Hess OM, Eberli FR. Abnormal coronary vasomotion during exercise in patients with normal coronary arteries and reduced coronary flow reserve. *Circulation* 1991; 83:26–37.
46. Yeung AC, Vekshtein VI, Krantz DS, et al. The effect of atherosclerosis on the vasomotor response of coronary arteries to mental stress. *N Engl J Med* 1991; 325:1551–1556.
47. Nabel EG, Ganz P, Gordon JB, et al. Dilation of normal and constriction of atherosclerotic coronary arteries caused by the cold pressor testing. *Circulation* 1988; 77:43–52.
48. Nabel EG, Ganz P, Gordon JB, et al. Paradoxical narrowing of atherosclerotic coronary arteries induced by increases in heart rate. *Circulation* 1990; 81:850–859.
49. Vita JA, Treasure CB, Yeung AC, et al. Patients with evidence of coronary endothelial dysfunction as assessed by acetylcholine infusion demonstrate marked increase in sensitivity to constrictor effects of catecholamines. *Circulation* 1992; 85:1390–1397.
50. Maseri A, Chierchia S, Kaski JC. Mixed angina pectoris. *Am J Cardiol* 1985; 56:30E-33E.
51. Maseri A, Crea F, Kaski JC. Mechanisms of angina pectoris in syndrome X. *J Am Coll Cardiol* 1991; 17:499–506.
52. Cannon RO III, Camici PG, Epstein SE. Pathophysiological dilemma of syndrome X. *Circulation* 1992; 85:883–892.
53. Fuh MM-T, Jeng C-Y, Young MM, et al. Insulin resistance, glucose intolerance, and hyperinsulinemia in patients with microvascular angina. *Metabolism* 1993; 42:1090–1092.
54. Quyyumi AA, Cannon RO III, Panza JA, et al. Endothelial dysfunction in patients with chest pain and normal coronary arteries. *Circulation* 1992; 86:1864–1871.
55. Opherk D, Schuler G, Wetterauer K, et al. Four-year follow-up study in patients with angina pectoris and normal coronary arteriograms ("syndromes X"). *Circulation* 1989; 80:1610–1616.
56. Legrand V, Hodgson JM, Bates ER, et al. Abnormal coronary flow reserve and abnormal radionuclide exercise test results in patients with normal coronary angiograms. *J Am Coll Cardiol* 1985; 6:1245–1253.
57. Cannon RO III, Watson RM, Rosing DR, Epstein SE. Angina caused by reduced vasodilator reserve of the small coronary arteries. *J Am Coll Cardiol* 1983; 1:1359–1373.
58. Egashira K, Inou T, Hirooka Y, et al. Evidence of impaired endothelium-dependent coronary vasodilatation in patients with angina pectoris and normal coronary angiograms. *N Engl J Med* 1993; 328:1659–1664.
59. Treasure CB, Klein JL, Vita JA, et al. Hypertension and left ventricular hypertrophy are associated with impaired endothelium-mediated relaxation in human coronary resistance vessels. *Circulation* 1993; 87:86–93.
60. Mosseri M, Schaper J, Admon D, et al. Coronary capillaries in patients with congestive cardiomyopathy or angina pectoris with patent main coronary arteries: Ultrastructural morphometry of endomyocardial biopsy samples. *Circulation* 1991; 48:203–210.
61. Maseri A, Crea F, Kaski JC, Davies G. Mechanisms and significance of cardiac ischemic pain. *Prog Cardiovasc Dis* 1992; 35:1–18.
62. Deanfield JE. Characteristics of silent and symptomatic ischemia in chronic stable angina: Comparison with unstable and vasospastic angina. In: Singh BM, ed. *Silent Myocardial Ischemia and Angina: Prevalence, Prognostic and Therapeutic Significance.* New York: Pergamon Press; 1988:104–111.
63. Nair CK, Aronow MH, Sketch R, et al. Diagnostic and prognostic significance of exercise-induced premature ventricular complexes in men and women: A four-year follow-up. *J Am Coll Cardiol* 1983; 1:1201–1206.

64. Sigwart U, Grbic M, Payot J, et al. Ischemic events during coronary artery balloon occlusion. In: Rutishauser W, Roskamm H, eds. *Silent Myocardial Ischemia*. Berlin: Springer–Verlag; 1984:29.
65. Muller JE, Stone PH, Turi ZG, et al. Circadian variation in the frequency of onset of acute myocardial infarction. *N Engl J Med* 1985; 313:1315–1322.
66. Rocco MB, Barry J, Campbell S, et al. Circadian variation of transient myocardial ischemia in patients with coronary artery disease. *Circulation* 1987; 75:395–400.
67. Rosen SD, Paulesu E, Frith CD, et al. Central nervous pathways mediating angina pectoris. *Lancet* 1994; 344:147–150.
68. Sylven C, Beerman B, Jonzon B. Angina pectoris-like pain provoked by intravenous adenosine in healthy volunteers. *Br Med J* 1986; 293:227–230.
69. Herrick JB. Clinical features of sudden obstruction of the coronary arteries. *JAMA* 1912; 59:2015–2020.
70. Roseman MD. Painless myocardial infarction: A review of the literature and analysis of 220 cases. *Ann Intern Med* 1954; 41:1–8.
71. Froelicher VF, Yanowitz FG, Thompson AJ. The correlation of coronary angiography and the electrocardiographic response to maximal treadmill testing in 76 asymptomatic men. *Circulation* 1973; 48:597–604.
72. Cohn PF. Asymptomatic coronary artery disease: Pathophysiology, diagnosis, management. *Mod Concepts Cardiovasc Dis* 1981; 50:55–60.
73. Serneri GGN, Doddi M, Arata L, et al. Silent ischemia in unstable angina is related to an altered cardiac norepinephrine handling. *Circulation* 1993; 87:1928–1937.
74. Cohn PF. Prevalence of silent myocardial ischemia. In: Cohn PF, ed. *Silent Myocardial Ischemia and Infarction*. New York: Marcel Dekker; 1986:71–80.
75. Deanfield JE, Ribiero P, Oakley K, et al. Analysis of ST-segment changes in normal subjects: Implications for ambulatory monitoring in angina pectoris. *Am J Cardiol* 1984; 54:1321–1325.
76. Crawford NH, Bernstein SJ, DiMarco J, et al. ACC/AHA guidelines for ambulatory electrocardiography. *Circulation* 1999; 34: 912–948.
77. Hedblad B, Juul-Moller S, Svensson K, et al. Increased mortality in men with ST segment depression during 24 h ambulatory long-term ECG recording: Results from prospective population study "Men born in 1914," from Malmo, Sweden. *Eur Heart J* 1989; 10:149–158.
78. Pepine CJ, Coy K, Lambert C. Silent myocardial ischemia during daily activities in asymptomatic patients with positive treadmill tests. In: Singh B, ed. *Silent Myocardial Ischemia and Angina*. New York: Pergamon Press; 1988:93–103.
79. Deanfield JE, Maseri A, Selwyn AP, et al. Myocardial ischaemia during daily life in patients with stable angina: Its relation to symptoms and heart rate changes. *Lancet* 1983; 3:753–758.
80. Cannon RO III, Watson RM, Rosing DR, Epstein SE. Angina caused by reduced vasodilator reserve of the small coronary arteries. *J Am Coll Cardiol* 1983; 1:1359–1373.
81. Mannheimer C, Carlsson CA, Vedin A, Wilhelmsson C. Transcutaneous electrical nerve stimulation (TENS) in angina pectoris. *Pain* 1986; 26:291–300.
82. Davies HA, Page Z, Rush EM, et al. Esophageal stimulation lowers exertional angina threshold. *Lancet* 1985; 1:1011–1014.
83. Pepine CJ, Coy K, Lambert C. Silent myocardial ischemia during daily activities in asymptomatic patients with positive treadmill tests. In: Singh B, ed. *Silent Myocardial Ischemia and Angina*. New York: Pergamon Press; 1988:93.
84. Droste C, Roskamm H. Experimental pain measurements in patients with asymptomatic myocardial ischemia. *J Am Coll Cardiol* 1983; 1:940–945.
85. Glazier JJ, Chierchia S, Brown MJ, Maseri A. Importance of generalized defective perception of painful stimuli as a cause of silent myocardial ischemia in chronic stable angina pectoris. *Am J Cardiol* 1986; 58:667–672.
86. Falcone C, Sconocchia R, Guasti L, et al. Dental pain threshold and angina pectoris in patients with coronary artery disease. *J Am Coll Cardiol* 1988; 12:348–352.
87. Bradley RF, Partamian JO. Coronary heart disease in the diabetic patient. *Med Clin North Am* 1993; 78:1093–1104.
88. Fearman I, Faccio E, Melei J. Autonomic neuropathy and painless myocardial infarction in diabetic patients: Histology evidence of their relationships. *Diabetes* 1977; 26:1147–1158.
89. Nesto RW, Phillips RT, Kett KG. Angina and exertional myocardial ischemia in diabetic and nondiabetic patients: Assessment by exercise thallium scintigraphy. *Ann Intern Med* 1988; 108:170–175.
90. Chiariello M, Indolfi C, Cotecchia MR. Asymptomatic transient ST changes during ambulatory ECG monitoring in diabetic patients. *Am Heart J* 1985; 110:529–534.
91. Coy KM, Imperi GA, Lambert CR, Pepine CJ. Silent myocardial ischemia during daily activities in asymptomatic men with positive exercise test responses. *Am J Cardiol* 1987; 59:45–49.
92. Deanfield JE, Kensett M, Wilson RA, et al. Silent myocardial ischaemia due to mental stress. *Lancet* 1984; 2:1001–1005.
93. Bertolet BD, Hill JA, Pepine CJ. Treatment strategies for daily life silent myocardial ischemia: A correlation with potential pathogenic mechanisms. *Prog Cardiovasc Dis* 1992; 35:97–118.
94. Rogers WJ, Bourassa MG, Andrews TC, et al. Asymptomatic Cardiac Ischemia Pilot (ACIP) Study: Outcome at 1 year for patients with asymptomatic cardiac ischemia randomized to medical therapy or revascularization. *J Am Coll Cardiol* 1995; 26:594–605.
95. Pepine CJ, Sharaf B, Andrews TC, et al. Relation between clinical, angiographic and ischemic findings at baseline and ischemia-related adverse outcomes at 1 year in Asymptomatic Cardiac Ischemia Pilot Study. *J Am Coll Cardiol* 1997; 29:1483–1489.
96. Davies RF, Goldberg AD, Forman S, et al. Asymptomatic Cardiac Ischemia Pilot (ACIP) study two-year follow-up: Outcomes of patients randomized to initial strategies of medical therapy versus revascularization. *Circulation* 1997; 95:2037–2043.
97. Hubbard BL, Gibbons RJ, Lapeyre AC, et al. Identification of severe coronary artery disease using simple clinical parameters. *Arch Intern Med* 1992; 152(2):309–312.
98. Hammermeister KE, DeRouen TA, Dodge HT. Variables predictive of survival in patients with coronary disease: Selection by univariate and multivariate analyses from the clinical, electrocardiographic, exercise, arteriographic, and quantitative angiographic evaluations. *Circulation* 1979; 59(3):421–430.
99. Califf RM, Mark DB, Harrell FE, et al. Importance of clinical measures of ischemia in the prognosis of patients with documented coronary artery disease. *Circulation* 1988; 11(1):20–26.
100. Oh JK, Gibbons RJ, Christian TF, et al. Correlation of regional wall motion abnormalities determined by technetium-99m sestamibi imaging in patients treated with reperfusion therapy during acute myocardial infarction. *Am Heart J* 1996; 131:32–37.
101. Guidelines for percutaneous transluminal coronary angioplasty: A report of the American College of Cardiology/American Heart Association Task Force on Assessment of Diagnostic and Therapeutic Cardiovascular Procedures (Committee on Percutaneous Transluminal Coronary Angioplasty). *J Am Coll Cardiol* 1993; 22(7):2033–2054.
102. Christian TF, Miller TD, Bailey KR, Gibbons RJ. Exercise tomographic thallium-201 imaging in patients with severe coronary artery disease and normal electrocardiograms. *Ann Intern Med* 1994; 121(11):825–832.
103. Mark DB, Hlatky MA, Harrell FE, et al. Exercise treadmill score for predicting prognosis in coronary artery disease. *Ann Intern Med* 1987; 106(6):793–800.
104. Morrow K, Morris CK, Froelicher VF, et al. Prediction of cardio-

vascular death in men undergoing noninvasive evaluation for coronary artery disease. *Ann Intern Med* 1993; 118(9):689–695.
105. Mark DB, Shaw L, Harrell FE, et al. Prognostic value of a treadmill exercise score in outpatients with suspected coronary artery disease. *N Engl J Med* 1991; 325:849–853.
106. Alexander KP, Shaw LJ, Shaw LK, et al. Value of exercise treadmill testing in women. *J Am Coll Cardiol* 1998; 32(6):1657–1664.
107. Beleslin BD, Ostojic M, Stepanovic J, et al. Stress echocardiography in the detection of myocardial ischemia: Head-to-head comparison of exercise, dobutamine, and dipyridamole tests. *Circulation* 1994; 90:1168–1176.
108. Dagianti A, Penco M, Agati L, et al. Stress echocardiography: Comparison of exercise, dipyridamole and dobutamine in detecting and predicting the extent of coronary artery disease [published erratum appears in *J Am Coll Cardiol* 1995; 26:114]. *J Am Coll Cardiol* 1995; 26(1):18–25.
109. Williams MJ, Odabashian J, Lauer MS, et al. Prognostic value of dobutamine echocardiography in patients with left ventricular dysfunction. *J Am Coll Cardiol* 1996; 27:132–139.
110. Afridi I, Quinones MA, Zoghbi WA, Cheirif J. Dobutamine stress echocardiography: Sensitivity, specificity, and predictive value for future cardiac events. *Am Heart J* 1994; 127:1510–1515.
111. Kamaran M, Teague SM, Finkelhor RS, et al. Prognostic value of dobutamine stress echocardiography in patients referred because of suspected coronary artery disease. *Am J Cardiol* 1995; 76:887–891.
112. Marcovitz PA, Shayna V, Horn RA, et al. Value of dobutamine stress echocardiography in determining the prognosis of patients with known or suspected coronary artery disease. *Am J Cardiol* 1996; 78:404–408.
113. Brown KA, Prognostic value of thallium-201 myocardial perfusion imaging: A diagnostic tool comes of age. *Circulation* 1991; 83:363–381.
114. National Center for Health Statistics. *Vital Statistics of the United States, 1979,* Vol II: Mortality, Part A (U.S. Department of Health and Human Services publication PHS84–1101). Washington: US Government Printing Office; 1984.
115. Hachamovitch R, Berman DS, Shaw LJ, et al. Incremental prognostic value of myocardial perfusion single photon emission computed tomography for the prediction of cardiac death: Differential stratification for risk of cardiac death and myocardial infarction [published erratum appears in *Circulation* 1999; 98(2):190]. *Circulation* 1998; 97(6):533–543.
116. Wagdy HM, Hodge D, Christian TF, et al. Prognostic value of vasodilator myocardial perfusion imaging in patients with left bundle-branch-block. *Circulation* 1998; 97(16):1563–1570.
117. Marwick T, D'Hondt AM, Baudhuin T, et al. Optimal use of dobutamine stress for the detection and evaluation of coronary artery disease: Combination with echocardiography or scintigraphy, or both? *J Am Coll Cardiol* 1993; 22(1):159–167.
118. Marwick TH. Use of exercise echocardiography for the prognostic assessment of patients with stable chronic coronary artery disease. *Eur Heart J* 1997; 18(suppl D):D97–D101.
119. Yusuf S, Zucker D, Peduzzi P, et al. Effect of coronary artery bypass graft surgery on survival: Overview of 10-year results from randomized trials by the Coronary Artery Bypass Graft Surgery Trialists Collaboration [published erratum appears in *Lancet* 1994; 344 (8934):1446]. *Lancet* 1994; 344(8922):563–570.
120. Emond M, Mock MB, Davis KB, et al. Long-term survival of medically treated patients in the Coronary Artery Surgery Study (CASS) registry. *Circulation* 1994; 90(6):2645–2657.
120a. O'Rourke R, Boden W, Weintraub W, et al. Medical therapy versus percutaneous coronary intervention: Implications of the Avert Study and the Courage Trial. *Curr Prac Med* 1999; vol 2, 11:225–227.
121. Final report on the aspirin component of the ongoing Physicians' Health Study. Steering Committee of the Physicians' Health Study Research Group. *N Engl J Med* 1989; 321:129–135.
122. Juul-Moller S, Edvardsson N, Jahnmatz B, et al. Double-blind trial of aspirin in primary prevention of myocardial infarction in patients with stable chronic angina pectoris: The Swedish Angina Pectoris Aspirin Trial (SAPAT) group. *Lancet* 1992; 340(8833):1421–1425.
123. McTavish D, Faulds D, Goa KL. Ticlopidine: An updated review of its pharmacology and therapeutic use in platelet-dependent disorders. *Drugs* 1990; 40(2):238–259.
124. CAPRIE Steering Committee. A randomized, blinded trial of clopidogrel versus aspirin in patients at risk of ischemic events (CAPRIE). *Lancet* 1996; 348(9038):1329–1339.
125. Melandri G, Semprini F, Cervi V, et al. Benefit of adding low molecular weight heparin to the conventional treatment of stable angina pectoris: A double-blind, randomized, placebo-controlled trial. *Circulation* 1993; 88(6):2517–2523.
126. Thrombosis prevention trial: Randomised trial of low-intensity oral anticoagulation with warfarin and low-dose aspirin in the primary prevention of ischaemic heart disease in men at increased risk. The Medical Research Council's General Practice Research Framework. *Lancet* 1998; 351:233–241.
127. Randomized trial of cholesterol lowering in 4444 patients with coronary heart disease: The Scandinavian Simvastatin Survival Study (4S). *Lancet* 1994; 344:1383–1389.
128. Sacks FM, Pfeffer MA, Moye LA, et al. The effect of pravastatin on coronary events after myocardial infarction in patients with average cholesterol levels: Cholesterol and Recurrent Events Trial investigators. *N Engl J Med* 1996; 335(14):1001–1009.
128a. Pedersen T, Olsson A, Faergeman O, et al. Lipoprotein changes and reduction in the incidence of major coronary heart disease events in the Scandinavian Simvastatin Survival Study (4S). *Circulation* 1998; 97:1453–1460.
128b. Gould A, Rossouw J, Santanello N, et al. Cholesterol reduction yields clinical benefit impact of Statin Trials. *Circulation* 1998; 86:946–952.
129. Wallace WA, Wellington KL, Chess MA, Liang CS. Comparison of nifedipine gastrointestinal therapeutic system and atenolol on antianginal efficacies and exercise hemodynamic responses in stable angina pectoris. *Am J Cardiol* 1994; 73(1):23–28.
130. de Vries RJ, van den Heuvel AF, Lok DJ, et al. Nifedipine gastrointestinal therapeutic system versus atenolol in stable angina pectoris: The Netherlands Working Group on Cardiovascular Research (WCN). *Int J Cardiol* 1996; 57:143–150.
131. Fox KM, Mulcahy D, Findlay I, et al. The Total Ischaemic Burden European Trial (TIBET): Effects of atenolol, nifedipine SR and their combination on the exercise test and the total ischaemic burden in 608 patients with stable angina. The TIBET Study Group. *Eur Heart J* 1996; 17(1):96–103.
132. Savonitto S, Ardissiono D, Egstrup K, et al. Combination therapy with metoprolol and nifedipine versus monotherapy in patients with stable angina pectoris: Results of the International Multicenter Angina Exercise (IMAGE) study. *J Am Coll Cardiol* 1996; 27(2):311–316.
133. van de Ven LL, Vermeulen A, Tana JG, et al. Which drug to choose for stable angina pectoris: A comparative study between bisoprolol and nitrates. *Int J Cardiol* 1995; 47(3):217–223.
134. Waysbort J, Meshulam N, Brunner D. Isosorbide-5-mononitrate and atenolol in the treatment of stable exertional angina. *Cardiology* 1991; 79(suppl 2):19–26.
135. Krepp HP. Evaluation of the antianginal and anti-ischemic efficacy of slow release isosorbide-5-mononitrate capsules, bupra-

nolol and their combination, in patients with chronic stable angina pectoris. *Cardiology* 1991; 79(suppl 2):14–18.
136. Pepine CJ, Feldman RL, Whittle J, et al. Effect of diltiazem in patients with variant angina: A randomized double-blind trial. *Am Heart J* 1981; 101(6):719–725.
137. Antman E, Muller J, Goldberg S, et al. Nifedipine therapy for coronary-artery spasm: Experience in 127 patients. *N Engl J Med* 1980; 302(23):1269–1273.
138. Psaty BM, Heckbert SR, Koepsell TD, et al. The risk of myocardial infarction associated with antihypertensive drug therapies. *JAMA* 1995; 274(8):620–625.
139. Furberg CD, Psaty BM, Meyer JV. Nifedipine: Dose-related increase in mortality in patients with coronary heart disease. *Circulation* 1995; 92(5):1326–1331.
140. Opie LH, Messerli FH. Nifedipine and mortality: Grave defects in the dossier. *Circulation* 1995; 92(5):1068–1073.
141. Ad Hoc Subcommittee of the Liaison Committee of the World Health Organisation and the International Society of Hypertension. Effects of calcium antagonists on the risks of coronary heart disease, cancer and bleeding. *J Hypertens* 1997; 15:105–115.
142. Schneider W, Maul FD, Bussmann WD, et al. Comparison of the antianginal efficacy of isosorbide dinitrate (ISDN) 40 mg and verapamil 120 mg three times daily in the acute trial and following two-week treatment. *Eur Heart J* 1998; 9:149–158.
143. Ankier SI, Fay L, Warrington SJ, Woodings DF. A multicentre open comparison of isosorbide-5-mononitrate and nifedipine given prophylactically to general practice patients with chronic stable angina pectoris. *J Int Med Res* 1989; 17(2):172–178.
144. Emanuelsson H, Ake H, Kristi M, Arina R. Effects of diltiazem and isosorbide-5-mononitrate, alone and in combination, on patients with stable angina pectoris. *Eur J Clin Pharmacol* 1989; 36:561–566.
145. Akhras F, Jackson G. Efficacy of nifedipine and isosorbide mononitrate in combination with atenolol in stable angina. *Lancet* 1991; 338(8774):1036–1039.
146. Cheitlin MD, Hutter AM Jr, Brindis RG, et al. ACC/AHA expert consensus documents: Use of sildenafil (Viagra) in patients with cardiovascular disease. *J Am Coll Cardiol* 1999; 33:273–282.
147. Fung HL, Bauer JA. Mechanisms of nitrate tolerance. *Cardiovasc Drugs Ther* 1994; 8(3):489–499.
148. Chirkov YY, Chirkova LP, Horowitz JD. Nitroglycerin tolerance at the platelet level in patients with angina pectoris. *Am J Cardiol* 1997; 80(2):128–131.
149. The sixth report of the Joint National Committee on prevention, detection, evaluation, and treatment of high blood pressure. *Arch Intern Med* 1997; 157(21):2413–2446.
150. Stamler J, Neaton J, Wentworth DN. Blood pressure (systolic and diastolic) and risk of fatal coronary heart disease. *Hypertension* 1989; 13(suppl 5):I2–I12.
151. Alderman MH, Cohen H, Roque R, Madhavan S. Effect of long-acting and short-acting calcium antagonist on cardiovascular outcomes in hypertensive patients. *Lancet* 1997; 349(9052):594–598.
152. Kannel WB, Gordon T, Castelli WP, Margolis JR. Electrocardiographic left ventricular hypertrophy and risk of coronary heart disease: The Framingham Study. *Ann Intern Med* 1970; 72(6):813–822.
153. Ghali JK, Liao Y, Simmons B, et al. The prognostic role of left ventricular hypertrophy in patients with or without coronary artery disease. *Ann Intern Med* 1992; 117(10):831–836.
154. Levy D, Salomon M, D'Agostino RB, et al. Prognostic implications of baseline electrocardiographic features and their serial changes in subjects with left ventricular hypertrophy. *Circulation* 1994; 90(4):1786–1793.
155. Ernst E, Resch KL. Fibrinogen as a cardiovascular risk factor: A meta-analysis and review of the literature. *Ann Intern Med* 1993; 118(12):956–963.
156. American Diabetes Association. Clinical practice recommendations 1998: Screening for type 2 diabetes. *Diabetes Care* 1998; 21(suppl 1):1–98.
157. The effect of intensive treatment of diabetes on the development and progression of long-term complications in insulin-dependent diabetes mellitus: The Diabetes Control and Complications Trial Research Group. *N Engl J Med* 1993; 329:977–986.
158. Getz GS. Report on the workshop on diabetes and mechanisms of atherogenesis, September 17 and 18, 1992, Bethesda, Maryland. *Arterioscler Thromb* 1993; 13:459–464.
158a. Heart Outcomes Prevention Evaluation Study Investigators. Effects of ramipril on cardiovascular outcomes in people with diabetes mellitus: Results of the HOPE study and MICRO-HOPE sub-study. *Lancet* 2000; 355:253–259.
159. National Cholesterol Education Program. Second report of the expert panel on detection, evaluation, and treatment of high blood cholesterol in adults (adult treatment panel II). *Circulation* 1994; 89(3):1333–1445.
160. Eckel RH. Obesity and heart disease: A statement for healthcare professionals from the Nutrition Committee, American Heart Association. *Circulation* 1997; 96(9):3248–3250.
161. Hulley S, Grady D, Bush T, et al. Randomized trial of estrogen plus progestin for secondary prevention of coronary heart disease in postmenopausal women: Heart and Estrogen/Progestin Replacement Study (HERS) research group. *JAMA* 1998; 280(7):605–613.
162. Jeppesen J, Hein HO, Suadicani P, Gyntelberg F. Triglyceride concentration and ischemic heart disease: An eight-year follow-up in the Copenhagen male study [published erratum appears in *Circulation* 1999; 98(2):190]. *Circulation* 1998; 97(11):1029–1036.
163. Reaven GM. Insulin resistance and compensatory hyperinsulinemia: Role in hypertension, dyslipidemia, and coronary heart disease. *Am Heart J* 1991; 121(4 pt 2):1283–1288.
164. Coronary Heart Disease. Triglyceride, high-density lipoprotein, and coronary heart disease. *JAMA* 1993; 269:505–510.
165. Genest JJ, Jenner JL, McNamara JR, et al. Prevalence of lipoprotein (a) [Lp(a)] excess in coronary artery disease. *Am J Cardiol* 1991; 67(13):1039–1045.
166. Clarke R, Daly L, Robinson K, et al. Hyperhomocysteinemia: An independent risk factor for vascular disease. *N Engl J Med* 1991; 324(17):1149–1155.
167. Stampfer MJ, Malinow MR, Willett WC, et al. A prospective study of plasma homocysteine and risk of myocardial infarction in US physicians. *JAMA* 1992; 268(7):877–881.
168. Berliner JA, Navab M, Fogelman AM, et al. Atherosclerosis: Basic mechanisms. Oxidation, inflammation, and genetics. *Circulation* 1995; 91(9):2488–2496.
169. Nyyssonen K, Parviainen MT, Salonen R, et al. Vitamin C deficiency and risk of myocardial infarction: Prospective population study of men from eastern Finland. *Br Med J* 1997; 314(7081):634–638.
170. Gaziano JM, Buring JE, Breslow JL, et al. Moderate alcohol intake, increased levels of high-density lipoprotein and its subfractions, and decreased risk of myocardial infarction. *N Engl J Med* 1993; 329(25):1829–1834.
171. Parisi AF, Folland ED, Hartigan P. A comparison of angioplasty with medical therapy in the treatment of single-vessel coronary artery disease: Veterans Affairs ACME Investigators. *N Engl J Med* 1992; 326(1):10–16.
172. Coronary angioplasty versus medical therapy for angina: The second Randomised Intervention Treatment of Angina (RITA-2) trial. RITA-2 trial participants. *Lancet* 1997; 350(9076):461–468.
173. Pitt B, Waters D, Brown WV, et al. Aggressive lipid-lowering

therapy compared with angioplasty in stable coronary artery disease: Atorvastatin versus Revascularization Treatment Investigators. *N Engl J Med* 1999; 341(2):70–76.

174. Comparison of coronary bypass surgery with angioplasty in patients with multivessel disease: The Bypass Angioplasty Revascularization Investigation (BARI) investigators [published erratum appears in *N Engl J Med* 1997; 336(2):147]. *N Engl J Med* 1996; 335(4):217–225.

175. Kemp HG. Left ventricular function in patients with the anginal syndrome and normal coronary arteriograms. *Am J Cardiol* 1973; 32(3):375–376.

176. Kemp HG, Elliott WC, Gorlin R. The anginal syndrome with normal coronary arteriography. *Trans Assoc Am Physicians* 1967; 80:59–70.

177. Cannon RO III, Canici PG, Epstein SE. Pathophysiological dilemma of syndrome X. *Circulation* 1992; 85:883–892.

178. Pupita G, Maseri A, Kaski JC, et al. Myocardial ischemia caused by distal coronary artery constriction in stable angina pectoris. *N Engl J Med* 1990; 323(8):514–520.

179. Kaplan MN. Syndromes X: Two too many. *J Am Coll Cardiol* 1992; 69:1643–1644.

CHAPTER 41

DIAGNOSIS AND MANAGEMENT OF PATIENTS WITH UNSTABLE ANGINA

David D. Waters

Unstable angina is an acute coronary syndrome that does not involve myocardial necrosis. It is characterized clinically by new-onset or worsening angina. The usual underlying pathophysiologic mechanism involves the rupture or erosion of an atherosclerotic plaque with thrombus formation that severely obstructs the coronary artery lumen. In 1996, 1,367,000 patients were hospitalized with this diagnosis in the United States.[1]

Important advances in the management of unstable angina have occurred in the last decade. Serum markers such as C-reactive protein and the troponins facilitate more accurate risk stratification. New therapies, specifically low-molecular-weight heparins and platelet glycoprotein (GP) IIb/IIIa receptor antagonists, have improved outcomes in high-risk patients. The introduction of coronary stents has reduced the incidence of acute vessel closure and restenosis. The exact indications for these newer therapies have not been defined completely across different strata of risk in patients with unstable angina. Physicians therefore must continue to integrate the results of new trials into their practice and exercise finely tuned judgment in the management of these patients. Unstable angina and the closely related condition non–ST-segment elevation myocardial infarction (NSTEMI) are very common manifestations of coronary artery disease.[1]

DEFINITION AND CLASSIFICATION

The term *unstable angina* has superseded older labels such as *preinfarction angina, acute coronary insufficiency,* and *intermediate coronary syndrome*. Unstable angina can be defined conveniently as new-onset or worsening angina within the previous 60 days or postinfarction angina (after the first 24 h from the onset of infarction).

Several systems have been proposed for classifying unstable angina. Distinguishing *primary* from *secondary* unstable angina is of clinical value. Acute worsening of a coronary stenosis (as described below) causes primary unstable angina by limiting coronary blood flow. Secondary unstable angina arises as a consequence of increased myocardial oxygen demand superimposed on severe underlying coronary disease. The major determinants of myocardial oxygen demand are heart rate, inotropic state, and the loading conditions of the left ventricle, primarily afterload. Thus, conditions with the potential to provoke secondary unstable angina include tachyarrhythmia, fever, hypoxia, anemia, hypertensive crisis, and thyrotoxicosis. Secondary unstable angina should resolve after successful treatment of the precipitating condition. Various classifications have been proposed for primary unstable angina, based on the presenting symptoms.[2-4] In 1973, Gazes and associates[2] defined three subgroups: (1) initial onset of progressive, crescendo angina and pain at rest in a patient previously free from symptoms, (2) the same presentation occurring suddenly in a patient with previously stable angina, and (3) episodes of prolonged pain at rest, lasting more than 15 min, not related to obvious precipitating factors.

The classification proposed by Braunwald (Table 41-1) includes three levels of severity and three clinical circumstances, yielding nine categories in all.[4] The presence or absence of electrocardiographic (ECG) changes and the intensity of medical therapy also were considered. A higher clinical category was more commonly associated with intracoronary thrombus and complex lesions in one study.[5] The components of the Braunwald classification have been shown to correlate with clinical outcomes. Specifically, a 48-h pain-free interval and the absence of ECG changes are associated with decreased risk, while postinfarction unstable angina and the need for maximal medical therapy carry a higher risk.[6,7] The Braunwald classification sometimes is used to categorize patients for research purposes, but no system is widely used in clinical practice. Braunwald has proposed a pictographic system to display the pathophysiologic components that contribute to unstable angina in a specific patient (Fig. 41-1).[8]

TABLE 41-1 Braunwald Classification of Unstable Angina

Severity	
Class I	New-onset, severe, or accelerated angina (angina of less than 2 months' duration, severe or occurring more than three times/day, or angina that is distinctly more frequent and precipitated by distinctly less exertion; no rest pain within 2 months)
Class II	Angina at rest, subacute (angina at rest within the preceding month but not within the preceding 48 h)
Class III	Angina at rest, acute (angina at rest within the preceding 48 h)
Clinical Circumstances	
Class A	Secondary unstable angina (a clearly identified condition extrinsic to the coronary vascular bed that has intensified myocardial ischemia, e.g., anemia, hypotension, tachyarrhythmia)
Class B	Primary unstable angina
Class C	Postinfarction unstable angina (within 2 weeks of a documented myocardial infarction)
Intensity of Treatment	
1.	Absence of treatment or minimal treatment
2.	Standard therapy for chronic stable angina (conventional doses of oral beta blockers, nitrates, and calcium channel blockers)
3.	Maximal therapy (maximally tolerated doses of all three categories of oral therapy and intravenous nitroglycerin)

SOURCE: Adapted from Braunwald,[4] with permission.

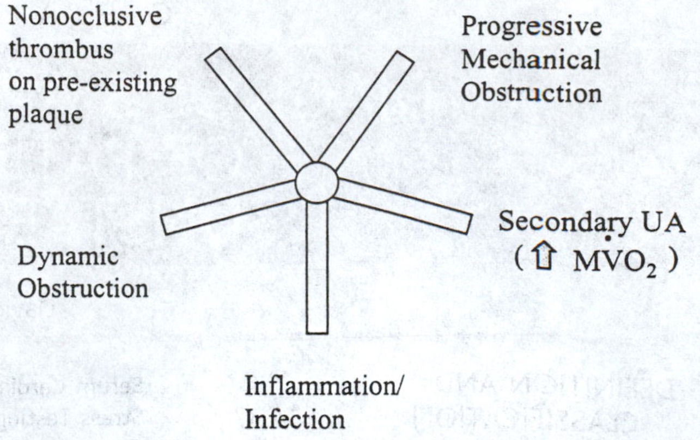

FIGURE 41-1 Framework for considering the pathophysiologic components that contribute to unstable angina in a specific patient. Varying contributions are possible from each of the five arms. Some patients will have predominantly one cause, while in others two or more mechanisms will contribute significantly. (From Braunwald,[8] with permission.)

The recognition of three specific forms of primary unstable angina is worthwhile because the pathophysiology, prognosis, and management of those forms are different. Variant, or Prinzmetal's, angina (discussed later in this chapter) is caused by coronary spasm and usually can be controlled with calcium channel blockers. Unstable angina within 6 months after coronary angioplasty almost invariably is caused by restenosis. Since the underlying mechanism is cellular proliferation instead of plaque rupture, antithrombotic drugs are not needed and intravenous nitroglycerin provides effective treatment.[9] Unstable angina in a patient with previous coronary bypass surgery often involves advanced atherosclerosis of venous bypass grafts and a lower likelihood of long-term symptomatic relief compared with other patients with unstable angina.[10,11] As is discussed below, patients with unstable angina should be classified according to their level of short-term risk. High-, intermediate-, and low-risk categories have been established on the basis of clinical and ECG data available at the time of the first assessment.[12]

PATHOPHYSIOLOGY

Progression of coronary atherosclerotic plaque can be divided into five phases and different lesions (Fig. 41-2).[13] Disruption of a type IV or type VA lesion exposes the underlying thrombogenic substrate, leading to the formation of a thrombus. This acute type VI lesion can heal without producing symptoms. However, when the thrombus totally or subtotally occludes the lumen, an acute coronary syndrome may result. The factors that contribute to the development of an acute coronary syndrome (Table 41-2) also represent potential targets for therapy.

Plaque Disruption

The mechanisms involved in plaque disruption and the transformation of coronary atherosclerosis from a stable phase to an

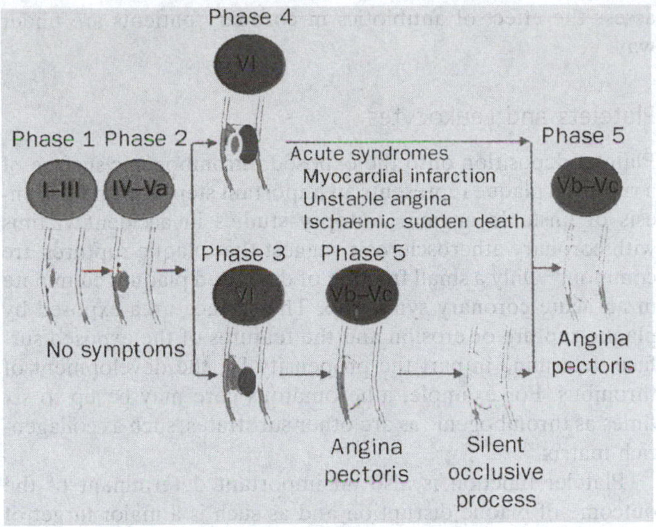

FIGURE 41-2 Phases of coronary lesion morphology and progression, with correlation to clinical syndromes. Unstable angina is caused by phase 2, type IV and type Va, lesions that are disrupted and progress to phases 3 and 4, type VI. (From Fuster et al.,[13] with permission.)

unstable phase have been studied intensively in recent years. Mechanical factors contribute to plaque disruption: A thin fibrous cap is more prone to rupture than is a thick one, and plaque rupture occurs commonly at the shoulders, where the plaque joins the adjacent vessel wall.[14] A lipid pool within a plaque influences the biomechanical properties of the plaque and increases the risk of rupture; conversely, fibrosis and calcification appear to decrease the risk of rupture.[14,15]

Plaque erosion, as well as plaque rupture, can initiate an acute coronary syndrome.[16] Erosion usually occurs centrally through a thinning cap as opposed to taking place at the plaque shoulders. Plaque erosion appears to be more common in women smokers, and plaque rupture in hyperlipidemic men.[17,18] In a study of women who died from sudden coronary death, plaque erosion was common in the premenopausal age group and plaque rupture was common in older women with hyperlipidemia.[18] Diabetes and hypertension were most common in women with healed infarcts. Macrophages and T cells invariably are found in close proximity to sites of plaque rupture but are not prominent features of plaque erosion.

TABLE 41-2 Factors That Modulate the Development of Acute Coronary Syndromes

Coronary factors
Location of the culprit coronary lesion
Stenosis length, contour, and severity
Extent of plaque rupture or erosion
Inflammatory substrate
Endothelial function
Degree of coronary vasoconstriction
Extent of collaterals
Thrombotic factors
Platelet aggregability and reactivity
Leukocyte activation
Intrinsic clotting factors
Plaque tissue factor levels
Level of fibrinolytic activity
Blood viscosity
Systemic factors
Heart rate and blood pressure
Catecholamine levels (smoking, cocaine, stress)
Cholesterol levels, including Lp(a)

Inflammation

In addition to biomechanical factors, inflammation appears to play a key role in plaque disruption. Macrophages and T lymphocytes accumulate in atherosclerotic plaques because of the expression of adhesion molecules on monocytes, endothelial cells, and leukocytes.[19,20] Once within the plaque, these cells release growth and chemotactic factors and are involved in the local oxidation of low-density lipoprotein (LDL) cholesterol and other products. These processes stimulate smooth muscle cell proliferation and the production of foam cells.

T lymphocytes produce interferon-gamma (INF-gamma), a cytokine that markedly inhibits the production of collagen by smooth muscle cells in vulnerable regions of the plaque cap.[21] INF-gamma also inhibits the proliferation of smooth muscle cells. In addition to impaired synthesis of collagen, accelerated degradation of collagen and other components of the matrix contributes to weakening of the fibrous cap. The matrix metalloproteinases, a family of enzymes that includes collagenases and gelatinases, are released by foam cells and are able to degrade the collagen that provides strength to the fibrous cap.[21] Tissue inhibitors of metalloproteinases (TIMPs) normally are expressed by vascular smooth muscle cells; however, in the critical areas of the fibrous cap, foam cells predominate and smooth muscle cells are sparse. Under the influence of cytokines, smooth muscle cells produce a different form of gelatinase, with no increase in the production of TIMPs.

Elevated peripheral blood levels of specific matrix metalloproteinases have been reported in patients with acute coronary syndromes.[22] Furthermore, atherectomy specimens from patients with unstable angina, but not stable angina, exhibit active synthesis of a specific gelatinase.[23] Nuclear factor-κB (NF-κB) also has been found in the peripheral blood of patients with unstable angina but not stable angina.[24] NF-κB resides inactive in the cytoplasm of lymphocytes, monocytes, endothelial cells, and smooth muscle cells, where after stimulation it transcriptionally activates interleukins, interferon, tumor necrosis factor-alpha, and adhesion molecules. It is thus a specific marker of inflammation.

In a detailed study of 20 culprit lesions, macrophages and T lymphocytes were found to be clustered at the immediate site of plaque rupture.[25] These cells and nearby smooth muscle cells expressed high levels of the same human leukocyte antigen (HLA)-DR transplantation antigen, indicating both activation and "cross-talk" among the cells. Mast cells also have been found in culprit lesions of unstable angina patients but not stable angina patients.[26] These mast cells stained positively for TNF-alpha and were in proximity to macrophages containing matrix metalloproteinase and gelatinase. Taken together, these findings indicate that an inflammatory stimulus unleashes a biochemical storm within the susceptible plaque, leading to rupture of the fibrous cap.

C-reactive protein (CRP) is a nonspecific acute-phase reactant. Increased serum levels of CRP[27,28] were reported to be elevated in most patients with unstable angina and myocardial infarction but not in those with stable angina. The short-term prognosis was worse in unstable angina patients with elevated levels.[28] In a larger study of stable and unstable angina patients undergoing coronary arteriography,[29] CRP levels averaged slightly higher than normal in both groups, and an elevated CRP level was a strong predictor of coronary events over the subsequent 2 years. The cytokine interleukin-6, which is the main producer of CRP in the liver, is elevated in unstable angina but not in stable angina.[30] Interleukin-6 and interleukin-1 receptor antagonist levels were higher on admission in unstable angina patients who were destined to have a complicated course than in unstable angina patients without complications in a recent study.[31]

Infection

The stimulus that initiates the acute inflammatory process in unstable angina has not been identified. Atherosclerosis itself, as defined by the "response to injury" hypothesis, is a chronic, low-grade inflammatory condition.[32] Considerable controversy exists about whether infectious agents play a role either in atherogenesis or in the transformation of stable to unstable coronary disease.[33,34]

Chlamydia pneumoniae, cytomegalovirus, and *Helicobacter pylori* have been identified within human atherosclerotic lesions.[33] Mechanisms by which chlamydia may contribute to atherogenesis or plaque disruption have been identified: Chlamydia heat shock protein and human heat shock protein are located together within macrophages, where they stimulate TNF-alpha and matrix metalloproteinase production.[35] Also, antibodies against chlamydia heat shock proteins could cross-react against heat shock proteins produced by endothelium, resulting in endothelial damage and accelerated atherosclerosis.[36]

Antibodies to chlamydia, cytomegalovirus, and *Helicobacter* are found more often in patients with atherosclerosis than in controls.[33,34] However, these associations do not prove causality. Antibodies to these agents are found in a high proportion of the population, particularly in members of the lower socioeconomic classes.[37] In prospective studies, antibodies to cytomegalovirus or *Helicobacter* did not predict future cardiovascular events, although total mortality was higher in subjects with antibodies to *Helicobacter.*[37,38]

If infection contributes to the initiation of acute coronary syndromes, appropriate antibiotic treatment should reduce coronary events in infected individuals. In a small study of postinfarction patients, adverse cardiovascular events during follow-up increased with increasing antibody titers to chlamydia.[39] Patients with high titers were randomized to azithromycin or placebo, and events were reduced significantly in the antibiotic-treated group. However, in another small trial of azithromycin in coronary patients with a seropositive reaction to chlamydia, no reduction in events was seen despite a significant reduction in the levels of inflammatory markers.[40] In the ROXIS pilot study, patients with unstable angina or non-Q-wave infarction were randomized to either roxithromycin or placebo for 1 month, with a total follow-up of 6 months.[41] The drug reduced end point events significantly. Larger, more definitive trials to assess the effect of antibiotics in coronary patients are under way.

Platelets and Leukocytes

Platelet deposition onto the exposed, thrombogenic surface of a ruptured plaque represents an important step in the pathogenesis of unstable angina. Autopsy studies in accident victims with coronary atherosclerosis suggest that plaque ruptures are common.[42] Only a small fraction of disrupted plaques culminate in an acute coronary syndrome. The surface area exposed by plaque rupture or erosion and the features of the exposed surface determine in part the propensity for the development of thrombus. For example, atheromatous core may be up to six times as thrombogenic as are other substrates, such as collagen-rich matrix.[43]

Platelet function is also an important determinant of the outcome of plaque disruption and as such is a major target of therapy. Patients with stable coronary or peripheral vascular disease already have increased platelet reactivity compared with normal controls.[44,45] Healthy endothelium releases nitric oxide, which inhibits platelet aggregation. This protective mechanism is attenuated in patients with atherosclerosis.[46]

In unstable angina, platelets are activated and generate thromboxane and prostaglandin metabolites.[47] Severe or persistent unstable angina is associated with the highest thromboxane output, and stabilization of unstable angina is accompanied by a return to normal levels.[48,49] Not only is the release of nitric oxide by the endothelium attenuated, the platelets themselves exhibit impaired nitric oxide production in patients with unstable angina.[50]

P-selectin is a membrane glycoprotein found both in the alpha granules of platelets and in endothelial cells. P-selectin mediates both platelet-leukocyte and endothelial cell–leukocyte adhesive interactions. Plasma P-selectin levels increase significantly in unstable angina and myocardial infarction but not in stable angina.[51] Neutrophils also are activated in unstable angina, and neutrophil-platelet adhesion is increased.[52] Neutrophil and monocyte adhesion molecules have been reported to increase in unstable angina,[20] particularly when measured in the coronary sinus soon after an episode of rest angina.[53]

Activated platelets and activated leukocytes thus interact in the acute phase of unstable angina to facilitate platelet-thrombus deposition. The interaction involves not only cellular elements but also the coagulation cascade.

Thrombosis and Fibrinolysis

Activated platelets and leukocytes interact to stimulate the coagulation system. Monocytes release tissue factor, a small glycoprotein that initiates the extrinsic clotting cascade, leading to an increase in thrombin generation.[54,55] Transient increases in thrombin-antithrombin III and prothrombin fragment 1+2 can be demonstrated in the hour after an ischemic attack in most patients with unstable angina.[56] This finding indicates that intermittent thrombus deposition, stimulated by all the mechanisms discussed above, causes transient coronary flow reductions and thus the symptoms of ischemia at rest.

Tissue factor is also present in the lipid-rich core of atherosclerotic plaque and may be one of the major determinants of the thrombogenicity of plaques when they rupture.[57] When tissue factor is specifically inhibited, platelet and fibrin deposition onto the ruptured plaque is reduced.[58] Tissue factor content is higher in unstable than in stable angina culprit lesions and correlates with areas of macrophages and smooth muscle cells.[59] Unstable angina patients with high circulating levels of tissue factor have unfavorable outcomes.[60] This finding implies that tissue factor plays a key role in the evolution of the unstable plaque.

Overactivity of other components of the coagulation system has been reported in unstable angina, including levels of factor XII, bradykinin precursor, and fibrinogen.[61] Lower tissue-type plasminogen activator (TPA) and plasminogen activator inhibitor-1 (PAI-1) levels indicate that impairment of the fibrinolytic system also is present in unstable angina.[61]

Vasoconstriction

Culprit lesions in unstable angina exhibit a heightened response to vasoconstrictor stimuli.[62] This response is not present in other coronary segments and also is not seen in the culprit lesions of patients with stable angina. One explanation for this is that endothelin levels are higher in culprit lesions in unstable angina patients as a result of the inflammatory component of those patients' condition.[63] However, under experimental conditions, the degree of vasoconstriction varies directly with the amount of platelet deposition.[64] The process of platelet aggregation and thrombus formation releases potent vasoconstrictors such as thromboxane A_2 and serotonin. Vasoconstriction, or the absence of appropriate vasodilation, probably contributes significantly to the development of ischemic episodes in patients with unstable angina and represents a potential target for therapy.

Evolution of the Culprit Lesion

The angiographic aspects of the culprit lesion have been defined before, during, and after an episode of unstable angina. If a patient with unstable angina has previously had a coronary angiogram, the culprit lesion usually can be documented to have progressed markedly since that time.[65] Lesions that progress to cause acute coronary events are usually not severely stenotic; in fact, two-thirds of them are less than 50 percent in diameter stenosis and thus would not be targets for revascularization.[66] Angiographic features of a lesion that predict that it will precipitate an acute coronary event include greater asymmetry, greater length, and a steeper outflow angle.[67]

At the time of an episode of unstable angina, the culprit lesion is likely to be asymmetric or eccentric, with a narrow base or neck, compared with control lesions.[68] These angiographic features reflect the underlying pathology: plaque disruption with thrombus. Obvious thrombus is visible at angiography in a minority of unstable angina patients. However, coronary angioscopy reveals plaque rupture with overlying thrombus in most culprit lesions.[69,70]

During the months after an episode of unstable angina, the culprit lesion is far more likely to progress and precipitate another coronary event than are other lesions in the same patient or lesions in stable patients.[71,72] Lesions with irregular borders, overhanging edges, or obvious thrombus at angiography are more likely to precipitate another event in the ensuing months than smooth lesions are. Whether more aggressive treatment with antiplatelet or antithrombotic drugs can modify the evolution of such complex lesions is not known.

DIAGNOSIS

A patient with unstable angina seeks medical attention because he or she has recognized either that new symptoms have appeared or that a previously stable pattern of symptoms has become unstable. The diagnostic difficulty usually lies in determining whether the chest pain is due to myocardial ischemia. Patients with suspected unstable angina must be evaluated rapidly and efficiently. A prompt and accurate diagnosis permits the timely initiation of appropriate therapy, which is important because complications are clustered in the early phases of acute coronary syndromes and because appropriate treatment reduces the rate of complications.

Patients with chest pain lasting for longer than 20 min, hemodynamic instability, or recent syncope or presyncope should be referred to a hospital emergency department.[1] Other patients with suspected unstable angina may be seen initially either in an emergency department or in an outpatient facility where a 12-lead ECG can be obtained quickly.

Initial Evaluation

The initial assessment should be directed toward determining whether the symptoms are caused by myocardial ischemia and, if so, the level of risk. If chest pain and ST-segment elevation >1 mm in two contiguous leads are present, reperfusion with thrombolytic therapy or primary angioplasty should be considered without delay. In the absence of these findings, the patient's clinical features should indicate whether the probability that symptoms are due to myocardial ischemia is high, intermediate, or low (Table 41-3). In a patient known to have coronary disease, typical symptoms are highly likely to be caused by myocardial ischemia, particularly if the patient confirms that the symptoms are identical to previous episodes with objective documentation. However, even if chest pain has some typical features, it is unlikely to be related to myocardial ischemia in a young individual who is known not to have risk factors for coronary disease. In one prospective multicenter study, older age, male sex, and the presence of chest or left arm pain or pressure as the presenting symptom all increased the likelihood that a patient was experiencing acute myocardial ischemia.[73]

When unstable angina is suspected in a patient younger than age 50, it is particularly important to ask about cocaine use regardless of social class or ethnicity.[1] As is discussed in Chap. 71, cocaine can cause coronary vasospasm and thrombosis in addition to its direct effects on heart rate and arterial pressure and has been implicated as a cause of acute coronary syndromes. Unstable angina may be more difficult to diagnose than is stable angina because of the absence of some of the distinguishing features. The characteristic relation between stable angina and physical exertion or other stressful activities is a key diagnostic feature of stable angina that is lacking in unstable angina. Unstable angina may be poorly relieved by nitroglycerin, whereas this is rarely true for stable angina. The duration of an episode of chest discomfort is usually longer and more variable in unstable angina than in stable angina.

The sensation of myocardial ischemia usually is located in the retrosternal area but may be felt only in the epigastrium,

TABLE 41-3 Likelihood That Unstable Angina Symptoms Are Caused by Myocardial Ischemia

HIGH LIKELIHOOD
Any of the following features:
Known coronary disease
Definite angina in men age 60 years or older or women 70 years or older
Hemodynamic or ECG changes during pain
Variant angina
ST elevation or depression of at least 1 mm
Marked symmetric T-wave inversion in multiple precordial leads
INTERMEDIATE LIKELIHOOD
Absence of high-likelihood features and any of the following:
Definite angina in men younger than age 60 or women younger than 70 years
Probable angina in men 60 years or older or women 70 years or older
Probably not angina in diabetics or in nondiabetics with two or more other risk factors[a]
Extracardiac vascular disease
ST depression of 0.05 to 1 mm
T-wave inversion of at least 1 mm in leads with dominant R waves
LOW LIKELIHOOD
Absence of high- or intermediate-likelihood features but may have:
Chest pain, probably not angina
One risk factor but not diabetes
T waves flat or inverted <1 mm in leads with dominant R waves
Normal ECG

[a]Risk factors include diabetes, smoking, hypertension, and hypercholesterolemia.
SOURCE: Adapted from Braunwald et al.,[12] with permission.

back, arms, or jaw. The description may include adjectives such as *burning, squeezing, pressurelike,* or *heavy* but rarely includes *sharp, jabbing,* or *knifelike*. The physician should be cautioned that atypical features do not completely rule out the possibility of unstable angina. For example, in one study of patients presenting to the emergency department, acute ischemia ultimately was found to be present in 22 percent of patients who used the terms *sharp* and *stabbing* to describe their symptoms and 7 percent of patients whose pain was reproduced on palpation.[74]

Nausea, sweating, or shortness of breath may accompany episodes of unstable angina. In elderly or diabetic patients, these symptoms may be the only indication that myocardial ischemia is present. Elderly and diabetic patients also have a greater likelihood of having multivessel disease. Women who present with unstable angina are more likely to have diabetes, hypertension, hyperlipidemia, and heart failure and to be older than men; they are less likely to be smokers and to have had a previous infarction or a previous coronary revascularization (Table 41-4).[75] At coronary angiography, they are less likely to have significant coronary lesions.[75] In a recent large series of unstable angina patients, female sex had an independent protective effect against death or myocardial infarction within the first 30 days, with an odds ratio of 0.65 (95 percent confidence interval of 0.49 to 0.87).[75]

On physical examination, transient signs of left ventricular dysfunction such as basilar rales or a ventricular gallop may accompany or follow shortly after an episode of unstable angina. More ominous signs of severe transient left ventricular dysfunction, such as hypotension and peripheral hypoperfusion, fortunately are not encountered commonly. Physical examination may reveal precipitating causes of or contributing factors to unstable angina, such as pneumonia and uncontrolled hypertension.

The Electrocardiogram

An ECG must be obtained as part of the initial evaluation of a patient with suspected unstable angina. The diagnostic yield is enhanced greatly if a tracing also can be recorded during an episode of chest pain. A normal ECG during chest pain does not rule out unstable angina as a likely diagnosis; however, it does indicate that an ischemic area, if present, is not extensive or severe enough to induce ECG changes and thus is a favorable prognostic sign.

Transient ST depression of at least 1 mm (Fig. 41-3) that appears during chest pain and disappears after relief represents objective evidence of transient myocardial ischemia. When ST depression is a persistent feature of ECGs recorded with or without chest pain, the finding is less specific. A common ECG pattern in patients with unstable angina is a persistently negative T wave over the involved territory (Fig. 41-4). This usually indicates that a severe stenosis is present in the corresponding coronary artery.[76] Myocardial stunning distal to the culprit lesion probably accounts for this ECG abnormality.[77] Deeply negative T waves occasionally are seen across all the precordial leads and point to a proximal, severe left anterior descending (LAD) coronary artery stenosis as the culprit lesion.[78]

In unstable angina patients, the ECG may show Q waves from an old infarct or a left bundle branch block resulting from extensive prior left ventricular damage. Patients with such findings are at increased risk because they are less likely than other patients to be able to tolerate an additional insult to the myocardium.[79,80] Myocardial ischemia is less likely to induce ST-segment changes in a territory that has Q waves, and when it does, the change usually consists of ST elevation.

ECG abnormalities may appear or evolve in the absence of new symptoms in patients with acute coronary syndromes. For example, the development of significant Q waves may be the first indicator that the diagnosis is myocardial infarction, not unstable angina. T-wave abnormalities may appear, worsen, or resolve. It is therefore worthwhile to obtain serial ECGs during the first 48 h as well as during episodes of chest pain. Continuous 12-lead ECG monitoring can be performed using new multiprocessor-controlled, programmable devices. The limited clinical experience with this technology suggests that it can detect episodes of ST depression when the presenting ECG is normal and that this information has prognostic as well as diagnostic value.[81] Continuous vector cardiography ST-segment monitoring has been used by investigators who have reached the same conclusion.[82]

TABLE 41-4 Clinical Features in Men and Women Presenting with Unstable Angina

	Men	Women	*p* value
Number of patients	2801	1690	
Age (median, 25th, 75th percentile)	64 (54, 71)	68 (60, 75)	<.001
Hypertension	45%	57%	<.001
Diabetes	17%	23%	<.001
Current or former smoker	74%	38%	<.001
Hypercholesterolemia	39%	47%	<.001
Prior myocardial infarction	38%	27%	<.001
Prior angina	82%	82%	.54
Prior congestive heart failure	6.1%	10.2%	<.001
Prior bypass surgery	16.6%	9.2%	<.001
Heart rate (median, 25th, 75th percentile)	71 (62, 83)	76 (67, 86)	<.001
Systolic blood pressure (mmHg)	138 (120, 150)	140 (125, 160)	<.001
Killip class 2–4 on presentation	9.6%	12.5%	<.001

SOURCE: Adapted from Hochman et al.,[75] with permission.

Serum Cardiac Markers

In the traditional paradigm, elevated serum levels of cardiac enzymes or the MB isoenzyme of creatine kinase (CK) could be used to distinguish between unstable angina and acute myocardial infarction. The diagnosis of unstable angina could be retained when minor elevations in CK or CK-MB were detected by serial sampling, but it was recognized that this was a negative prognostic sign.[83]

The widespread availability of other serum cardiac markers, particularly the troponins, has enriched this paradigm. One-fifth to one-quarter of patients with unstable angina will have elevated levels of troponin T or troponin I on admission or soon thereafter, and most of them will have normal levels of CK-MB. Several large studies have demonstrated that elevations of either troponin T or troponin I are independent predictors of adverse events in populations with either unstable angina alone or unstable angina and non-Q-wave infarction.[80,82,84–88] The troponin complex in cardiac and skeletal muscle consists of three subunits, which have been termed T, I, and C. The amino acid sequence of troponins T and I but not troponin C differ in cardiac muscle versus skeletal muscle. Immunoassays based on monoclonal antibodies have been developed to detect cardiac troponin T and cardiac troponin I. The sensitivity and specificity of these two markers appear to be roughly equal when used in populations with a high prevalence of acute coronary syndromes.[88] However, troponin I theoretically could be more specific because it is less likely to be generated by skeletal muscle disease or injury.[88] A rapid bedside assay for cardiac troponin T has

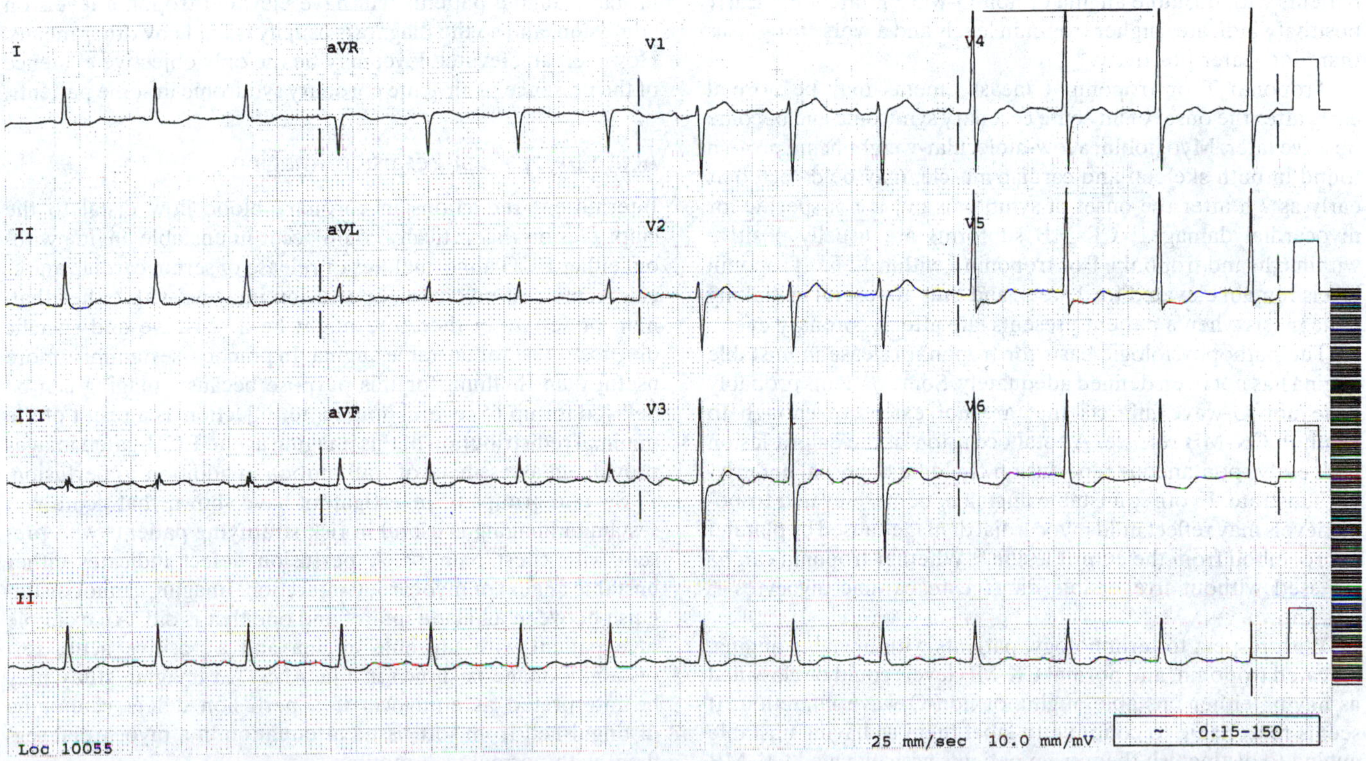

FIGURE 41-3 Electrocardiogram recorded during an episode of chest pain at rest in a patient with unstable angina. ST depression >1 mm is present in leads V_4 to V_6. This abnormality was not present on the baseline tracing. The chest pain and ST depression disappeared promptly after the administration of sublingual nitroglycerin.

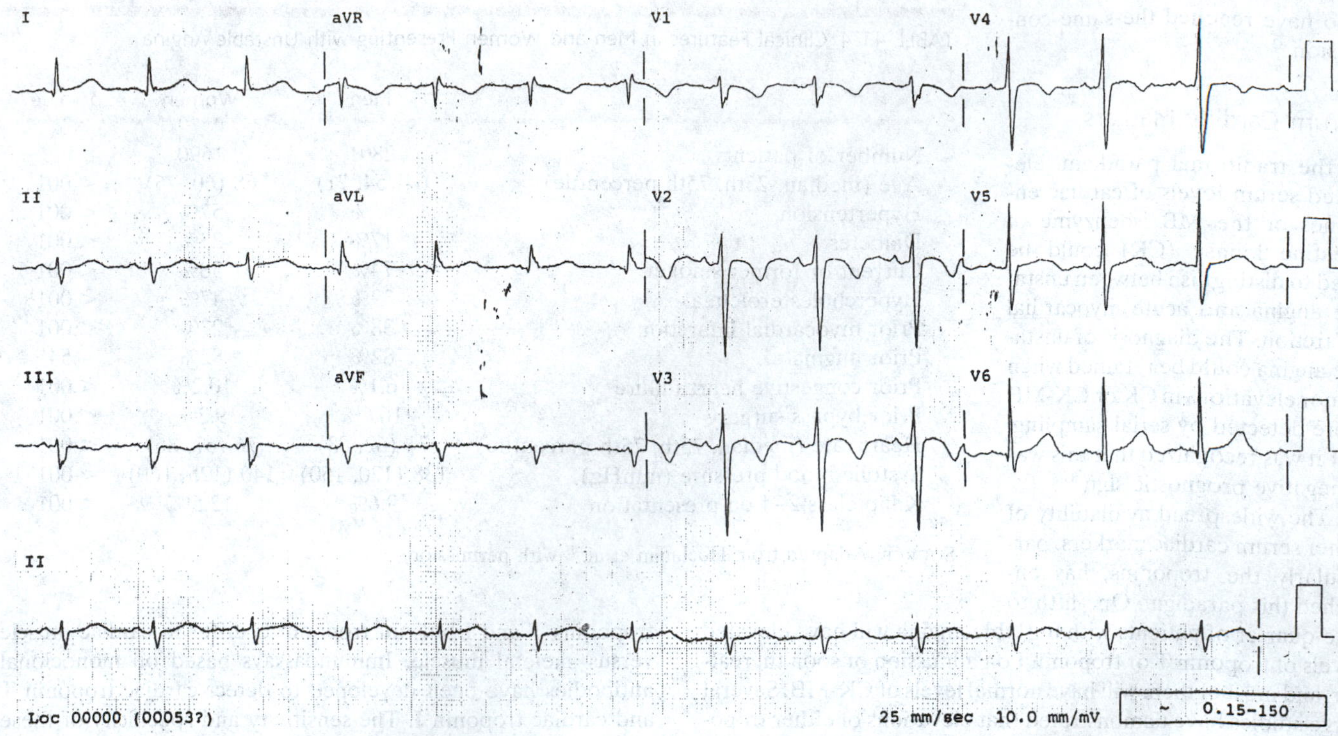

FIGURE 41-4 Electrocardiogram recorded from a patient hospitalized with unstable angina during a pain-free interval. The negative T waves in V_1 to V_4 had been upright on a previous tracing. The culprit lesion was located in the left anterior descending coronary artery.

been developed,[89] and a positive result of this test has been shown to be predictive of in-hospital adverse events among patients with unstable angina or non-Q-wave infarction.[90] Early positivity indicates higher troponin levels and a worse prognosis than does later positivity.[90]

Troponin T or troponin I measurements may be normal early after the onset of an acute coronary syndrome and become positive later. Myoglobin, a low-molecular-weight heme protein found in both skeletal and cardiac muscle, may be detected as early as 2 h after the onset of symptoms but is not specific for myocardial damage.[91] CK-MB subforms are usually positive within 6 h, and troponin T or troponin I within 12 h.[91] Troponin levels remain elevated for 1 week and thus are useful in making a diagnosis when a patient presents late after a coronary event.

The pathophysiologic basis for troponin release in unstable angina has not been defined adequately. Some patients probably have non-Q-wave infarcts that are not extensive enough to result in CK-MB release. A total occlusion of the culprit lesion with early spontaneous reperfusion could be the usual underlying substrate. In other unstable angina patients, elevated troponin levels may reflect mild myocardial damage caused by platelet microemboli from the culprit lesion.[92] Whether troponin can be released without irreversible damage to cardiac myocytes is not known.

With respect to terminology, patients with unstable angina, elevated troponin, and normal CK-MB levels could be classified as having either unstable angina or non-Q-wave infarction. It seems reasonable to continue to label them as having unstable angina to distinguish them from patients with elevated CK-MB levels. These patients should, however, be treated as high risk compared with unstable angina patients with normal troponin levels.

Cardiac troponins are less useful for the diagnosis of unstable angina than they are for risk stratification. Only a minority of unstable angina patients will have elevated troponin levels on admission, and so the diagnosis usually is made by other means. However, an elevated level may be the only objective evidence of the presence of an acute coronary syndrome in some patients.

Acute Myocardial Perfusion Imaging

Intermittent reductions in coronary blood flow distal to the culprit lesion theoretically could occur in unstable angina without either ECG abnormalities or release of serum cardiac markers. Acute rest myocardial perfusion imaging with either thallium or sestamibi therefore might be a sensitive and specific diagnostic test for unstable angina. In practice, sestamibi is more useful than thallium for this purpose because imaging can be delayed for up to several hours after injection as a result of the minimal redistribution of this imaging agent. ECG-gated images provide an assessment of wall motion in addition to perfusion.

Several groups of investigators have shown that acute rest sestamibi imaging is useful in risk stratifying patients who present with chest pain.[93–96] A perfusion defect indicates either unstable angina or myocardial infarction. Imaging cannot distinguish between an acute infarct and one that is old. An example of a patient with unstable angina and a positive acute rest sestamibi image is shown in Fig. 41-5. An imaging study may be interpreted as equivocal if a perfusion defect cannot be distinguished from soft tissue attenuation in a myocardial segment with normal wall motion.

The sensitivity and specificity of acute rest imaging are very high if sestamibi is injected during an episode of chest pain, but sensitivity decreases if the injection is done within the ensuing hours.[97] The negative predictive value of a normal perfusion study is extremely high when the injection is done during symptoms. However, acute rest imaging will miss a few patients with acute coronary syndromes (less than 5 percent with experienced readers) and so patient management decisions cannot be made solely on the basis of one test result.

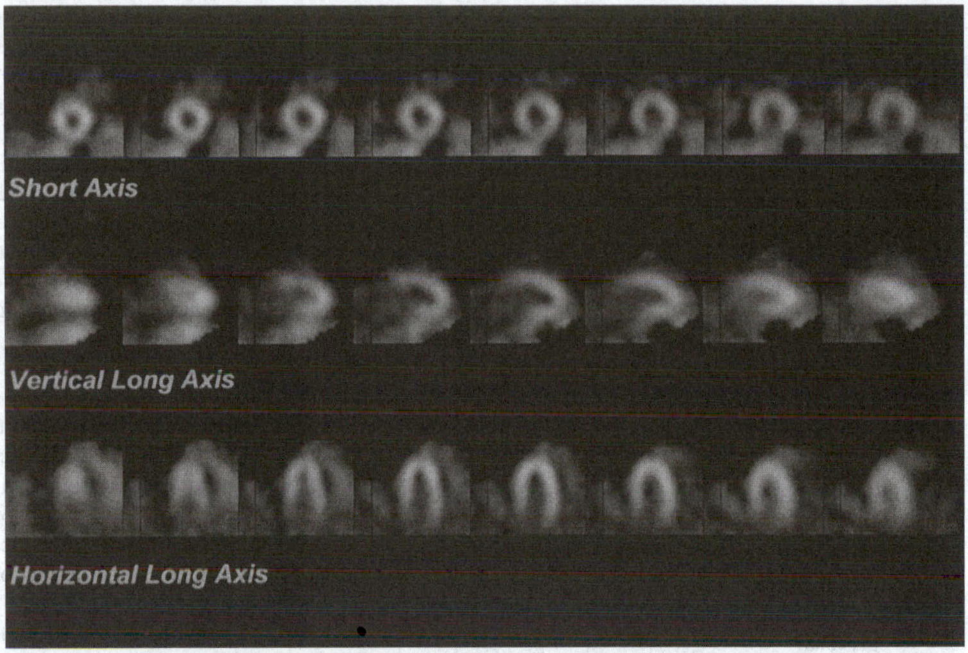

FIGURE 41-5 An acute sestamibi imaging study from a patient with unstable angina. The patient was injected after an episode of angina at rest. The short axis and vertical long axis views reveal a posterior and inferior perfusion defect. This defect could be due to previous or acute infarction or to acute ischemia. However, gated single-photon emission computed tomography (SPECT) imaging demonstrated normal wall motion, suggesting ischemia rather than infarction. (Courtesy of Dr. Gary Heller, University of Connecticut School of Medicine.)

Chest Pain Units

The evaluation of patients with chest pain who may have unstable angina or myocardial infarction is often fraught with uncertainty. Hospitalizing all such patients for an extensive workup when the probability that active coronary disease accounts for their symptoms is neither cost-effective nor necessary. However, missing the diagnosis of unstable angina may result in unnecessary myocardial infarction or death. The chest pain unit has been developed as a solution to this problem.

Most chest pain units are in or adjacent to the emergency department and employ a set of criteria designed to select low-risk patients.[98–100] These criteria usually include chest pain that may indicate myocardial ischemia but with a normal or unchanged ECG and a normal first set of cardiac enzymes.[100] In a study of over 10,000 patients presenting to emergency departments with chest pain, the likelihood of a major cardiovascular event declined over time, with 41 percent occurring within 12 h and 62 percent within 24 h.[101] Events could be predicted by a set of simple clinical measures available at baseline and updated at 12 h.[101] This information provides a rationale for the design of chest pain units.

In most units, CK-MB is measured at 3- to 4-h intervals for 9 to 12 h, sometimes with other serum markers. Patients receive an aspirin, an intravenous line, ECG monitoring, and 12-lead ECGs during chest pain and at specific intervals. If no evidence of active coronary disease is detected at the end of this observation period, a stress test may be performed for diagnostic and prognostic purposes.

Chest pain units have been reported to reduce the rate of missed infarctions from approximately 5 percent to 0.5 percent of patients, as estimated from return visits within 72 h.[100] Missed diagnoses of unstable angina probably are reduced as well, although this rate is difficult to measure. Hospitalizations, hospital days, and total costs are reduced because approximately 75 percent of patients are discharged directly from the unit.[99,100]

Although most chest pain units accept only patients at low risk for an acute coronary event, a randomized trial has demonstrated that patients with unstable angina who are judged to be at intermediate risk also can be managed in this environment.[102] Nearly half the patients randomized to the chest pain unit strategy completed the observation period, had a negative stress test, and were discharged home, to be evaluated further as outpatients. The rate of serious complications, mainly myocardial infarction, was not significantly different at 30 days and 6 months between the two groups.

RISK STRATIFICATION

The evaluation of a patient with unstable angina requires not only the establishment of the diagnosis but also an assessment of the short-term risk. This risk assessment determines the appropriate intensity of therapy. At the low end of the risk scale, a patient may be discharged home with aspirin and a beta blocker, to be followed as an outpatient. At the opposite end of the scale, a patient may be hospitalized in a coronary care unit, be treated with multiple drugs, and undergo coronary arteriography urgently as a prelude to revascularization.

Clinical Features

The 1994 report of the Agency for Health Care Policy and Research (Table 41-5) categorized unstable angina patients into low-, intermediate-, and high-risk groups on the basis of the data available at the time of the first assessment.[12] High-risk patients have ongoing chest pain that lasts longer than 20 min, reversible ST changes of at least 1 mm, or signs of serious left ventricular dysfunction. Low-risk patients have worsening angina without rest pain, are not older than age 65, and have a normal or unchanged ECG without evidence of a previous infarct.

The risk assessment should be updated during hospitalization because patients frequently change categories. Continuing angina with ST changes despite medical therapy is an ominous

TABLE 41-5 Short-Term Risk of Death or Myocardial Infarction in Patients Presenting with Symptoms Suggesting Unstable Angina

HIGH RISK

At least one of the following features must be present:
- Prolonged, ongoing (>20 min) rest pain
- Pulmonary edema
- Angina with new or worsening mitral regurgitation murmurs
- Rest angina with dynamic ST changes of at least 1 mm
- Angina with S_3 or rales
- Angina with hypotension

INTERMEDIATE RISK

No high-risk features but must have any of the following:
- Rest angina now resolved but not low likelihood of coronary disease
- Rest angina (>20 min or relieved with rest or nitroglycerin)
- Angina with dynamic T-wave changes
- Nocturnal angina
- New onset Canadian Cardiovascular Society class III or IV angina in past 2 weeks but not low likelihood of coronary disease
- Q waves or ST depression of at least 1 mm in multiple leads
- Age >65 years

LOW RISK

No high- or intermediate-risk features but may have any of the following:
- Increased angina frequency, severity, or duration
- Angina provoked at a lower threshold
- New-onset angina within 2 weeks to 2 months
- Normal or unchanged ECG

SOURCE: Adapted from Braunwald et al.,[12] with permission.

sign that should precipitate urgent coronary arteriography with a view to revascularization, because the risk of myocardial infarction is high. Most episodes of myocardial ischemia are silent, and some investigators have reported that episodes of ST depression detected by Holter monitoring are a better predictor of an unfavorable outcome.[103]

Serum Cardiac Markers

Troponin measurements should be used in the risk stratification of patients with unstable angina to supplement the assessment from clinical features and the results of the ECG. Elevated troponin levels strongly predict coronary events over the short term. The odds ratio for cardiac death or myocardial infarction within 30 days for an elevated troponin T was 2.7 (95 percent confidence interval of 2.1 to 3.4), based on 12 studies including a total of 2847 unstable angina patients.[88] The odds ratio for an elevated troponin I was 4.2 (95 percent confidence interval of 2.7 to 6.4), based on 9 studies of 1901 unstable angina patients.[88] The sensitivity and specificity of troponin T and troponin I are not significantly different.[88]

A major advantage of troponin measurements is that troponins contribute to risk independently of most of the other major predictors. For example, in one large study, elevated troponin T, age, hypertension, number of antianginal drugs, and ECG changes at baseline predicted cardiac death or myocardial infarction in a multivariate analysis.[84] In that study, the amount of troponin T elevation was also a predictor, with risk increasing for each quintile of troponin T elevation. The combination of troponin T elevation and ST depression identified a group at particularly high risk.

Measuring troponin not just at baseline but also at 8 and 16 h after admission has been shown to add useful prognostic information.[104] Elevated troponin levels predict an adverse outcome not just in unstable angina patients but also in the broader population of patients with chest pain presenting to emergency departments.[105] Evidence from a trial of a low-molecular-weight heparin suggests that elevated troponin may be a marker that identifies patients who will benefit from antithrombotic therapy.[106]

High levels of the inflammatory markers CRP, serum amyloid A, and interleukin-6 are associated with a poorer prognosis in unstable angina patients.[28,31,107] Markers of activation of the coagulation system also have been reported to predict risk, including fibrinopeptide A[108] and fibrinogen.[109] The early rise in von Willebrand factor was an independent predictor of events within 30 days in one study.[110] However, in practice, the only serum marker that should be measured routinely for risk stratification in unstable angina is troponin T or I.

Stress Testing

Stress testing often is used as a risk assessment tool in patients with unstable angina. Low-risk and some intermediate-risk patients whose symptoms stabilize with medical therapy undergo stress testing for advanced risk stratification. Those with high-risk findings (Fig. 41-6) such as reversible perfusion defects or ST depression at low exercise levels undergo coronary arteriography, and those with negative or low-risk results are managed medically. This approach has been validated by studies in unstable angina patients demonstrating that these abnormalities correlate with a higher event rate during follow-up.[111–114] For example, in one study, 60 percent of patients with a reversible perfusion defect compared with 12 percent of those with a normal exercise sestamibi scan experienced cardiac death, nonfatal infarction, or rehospitalization for unstable angina during a 12-month follow-up.[114] Patients with low exercise tolerance, exercise-induced ST depression, and larger perfusion defects are more likely to have three-vessel coronary disease than are patients without these high-risk findings.[115]

Patients who complete a stay in a chest pain unit without objective evidence of myocardial ischemia can safely undergo stress testing for diagnostic and prognostic purposes.[116] In one study, 71 percent of chest pain unit patients completed stage 1 of a Bruce protocol without evidence of myocardial ischemia, and their rate of infarction or coronary revascularization over the next 6 months was only 2 percent.[116]

In patients who are unable to exercise, dipyridamole or dobutamine can be used as the stress and sestamibi imaging or echocardiography can be used as the method of assessment. Stress testing is not needed in patients whose clinical features already put them at high risk. Patients with continuing angina despite medical therapy. ST depression, or hemodynamic impairment during spontaneous attacks of rest angina or elevated troponin levels should proceed directly to coronary arteriography.

Coronary Angiography

Risk in coronary patients traditionally has been assessed according to the number of vessels with at least 50 percent diameter stenosis and the presence and severity of left ventricular dysfunction. Older studies indicate that these variables are important predictors of outcome in unstable angina.[117–119] However, their prognostic impact is probably less than it is in stable coronary disease because the risk of short-term events in unstable angina is dominated by features of the culprit lesion, such as whether it induces ST depression or troponin release. Culprit lesions are far more likely to progress and initiate other coronary events in the months after an episode of unstable angina than are other coronary lesions in the same patients.[71,72]

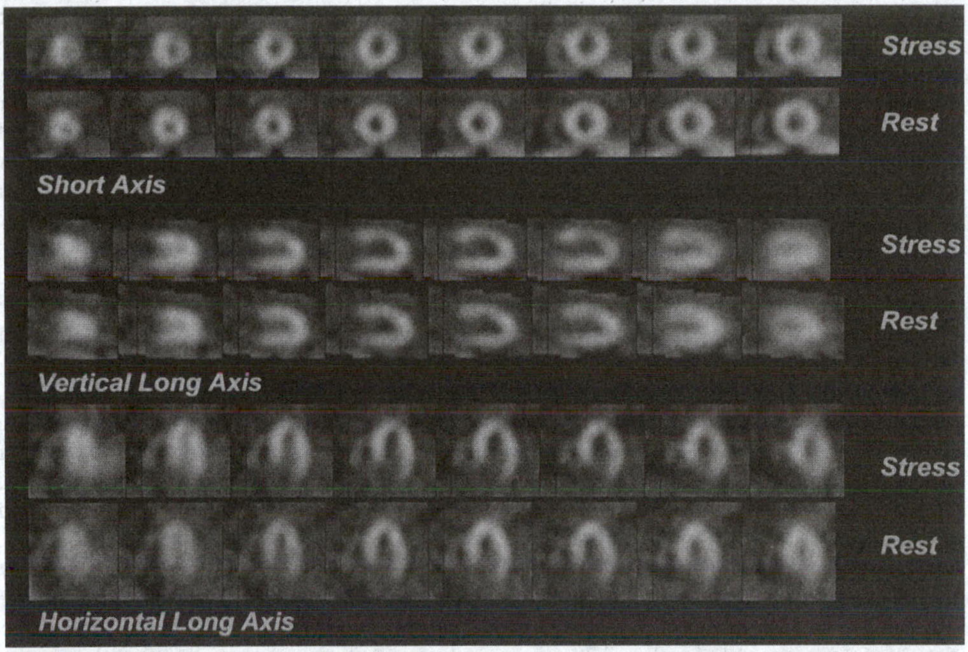

FIGURE 41-6 Stress and rest sestamibi images from a patient with unstable angina. A reversible perfusion defect is present in the anterior wall, best seen in the vertical long axis view. (Courtesy of Dr. Gary Heller, University of Connecticut School of Medicine.)

Among patients with unstable angina who undergo coronary arteriography, approximately one-quarter will have one-vessel, one-quarter two-vessel, and one-quarter three-vessel involvement; 10 percent will have significant left main stenosis; and the other 15 percent will have narrowings of less than 50 percent or normal vessels on angiography. Patients with left main stenosis of at least 50 percent or three-vessel disease with left ventricular dysfunction will obtain a survival benefit from coronary bypass surgery.[120,121] Although noninvasive testing is sensitive and specific enough to detect many of these patients, the only certain method for diagnosing these conditions is angiography.

At the other extreme, patients without significant lesions at angiography benefit from a reorientation of their management. Noncardiac causes of chest pain should be considered, as well as other potential diagnoses, such as syndrome X and variant angina. Antithrombotic and antiplatelet drugs often can be discontinued, and the need for antianginal medication can be reassessed. The unstable angina patients who are most likely to have no significant lesions at angiography tend to be women with no ST-segment abnormalities on ECG.[122] Nevertheless, the finding of no significant lesions at angiography is usually a surprise. These patients have a low coronary event rate during follow-up even though their symptoms often persist.[122]

Risk Stratification with Combinations of Predictors

In clinical practice, several variables usually are integrated into a global assessment of risk. The combination of ST-segment abnormalities and elevated troponin levels has been shown to be useful. In one study that used these two indicators, the risk of death or infarction within 30 days was 25.8 percent, 3.1 percent, and 1.7 percent in high-, intermediate-, and low-risk groups, respectively.[24] In a Thrombin Inhibition in Myocardial Ischemia (TRIM) substudy, the composite end point of death, myocardial infarction, or refractory angina within 30 days was predicted by ST depression, inverted T waves in at least five leads, elevated troponin or myoglobin levels, female sex, and age of 65 or higher.[123] Death or infarction occurred in 14 percent, 6 percent, and 3 percent of high-, intermediate-, and low-risk groups, respectively.

In summary, the short-term outcome of unstable angina can be predicted by a variety of methods (Table 41-5). Risk assessment should be updated during hospitalization as new information becomes available so that high-risk patients are not undertreated and low-risk patients are not overtreated. The most important predictors are the clinical presentation (Table 41-3), ST depression during attacks, elevated troponin levels, and continuing episodes in spite of medical therapy.

PROGNOSIS

Prognosis in patients with unstable angina can be viewed as a composite of the prognosis expected from the extent of coronary disease and left ventricular function overlaid with the short-term risk associated with the culprit lesion and the unstable state. The short-term risk is related almost entirely to myocardial infarction and its complications and to recurrences of unstable angina. Risk is highest in the hours, days, and first month after the onset of symptoms. The incremental risk associated with the unstable state dissipates completely by 1 year.[71,72] For example, 11 percent of unstable angina patients in one series experienced a myocardial infarction between hospital discharge and 1 year but the subsequent annual infarction rate was less than 2 percent.[124]

Published data on the prognosis in unstable angina are influenced by patient selection and treatment and can be quite misleading. The inclusion and exclusion criteria for clinical trials may bias the prognosis by eliminating low-risk or high-risk patients. If younger patients with atypical symptoms and no objective evidence of myocardial ischemia are included in large numbers, the prognosis of the cohort under study will tend to be better. By contrast, if ECG changes or elevated troponin levels are required, the prognosis will tend to be worse. The prognosis has improved dramatically over the past two decades with the introduction of increasingly more sophisticated medical therapy and revascularization techniques. As recently as the early 1980s, aspirin was not used routinely in the treatment of unstable angina. Results from that era are therefore below current expectations.

In a compilation of 10 representative series with a total of nearly 2000 unstable angina patients, excluding those with new-onset or postinfarction angina, the mortality was 4 percent in the hospital and 10 percent at 1 year.[125] Survival without infarction was 89 percent at 1 month and 79 percent at 1 year. Among 4488 unstable angina patients in GUSTO-IIb, the mortality rate was 2.4 percent at 30 days, 5 percent at 6 months, and 7 percent at 1 year.[126] The infarction rate was 4.8 percent at 30 days and 6.2 percent at 6 months. Recurrent ischemia had a major impact on these rates; for example, the 30-day infarction rate increased from 2.3 percent to 7.2 percent to 21.7 percent in patients with no ischemia, ischemia, and refractory ischemia, respectively. These outcomes are representative of the results of modern therapy in the late 1990s.

TREATMENT

The goals of treatment in unstable angina are to control symptoms and prevent myocardial infarction. Nitroglycerin, beta blockers, and to a lesser extent calcium channel blockers reduce the risk of recurrent ischemic attacks. Revascularization eliminates ischemia entirely in patients with favorable anatomy, and in some subgroups, coronary bypass surgery has been shown to prolong life. The risk of myocardial infarction is reduced by antiplatelet and antithrombotic therapy.

Nitroglycerin and Nitrate Therapy

In patients with unstable angina, sublingual nitroglycerin usually relieves attacks promptly, although it may be somewhat less efficacious than it is in stable angina patients. Patients with unstable angina often are treated with an infusion of intravenous nitroglycerin to prevent further attacks. A common starting dose is 10 μg/min. The dose can be increased in increments of 10 μg/min until symptoms are controlled or unwanted side effects develop. The most common adverse effects are headache, nausea, dizziness, hypotension, and reflex tachycardia.

The evidence that intravenous nitroglycerin prevents ischemic attacks in unstable angina patients is sparse (Table 41-6). In two studies of 35 and 40 patients, respectively, intravenous nitroglycerin reduced the number of angina episodes during treatment compared with a pretreatment period.[127,128] However, a placebo control group was not included in the design of either study. No studies of sufficient power have examined whether intravenous nitroglycerin or other nitrate preparations reduce the risk of infarction in unstable angina.

Nitroglycerin acts through several mechanisms that could provide benefit in patients with unstable angina. As a venodilator at low doses and an arteriolar dilator at higher doses, it reduces preload and afterload and thus myocardial oxygen consumption. The drug directly dilates coronary stenoses and thus increases oxygen delivery to the ischemic region.[129] Nitroglycerin increases collateral flow and favorably redistributes regional coronary flow. Because of its preferential effect on capacitance vessels as opposed to resistance vessels, it does not have the potential to induce coronary steal, unlike other vasodilators.[130]

Nitroglycerin and longer-acting nitrates act by releasing nitric oxide in vascular smooth muscle through an enzymatic process.[130] Sulfhydryl-donating compounds are necessary for this activity, and their rapid depletion during chronic therapy with nitroglycerin or other nitrate preparations rapidly leads to tolerance to the hemodynamic effects of the drug.[131] In stable patients, intermittent nitrate therapy is recommended to circumvent nitrate tolerance; however, some studies have shown that a rebound increase in ischemic episodes occurs during nitrate-free intervals.[132] Rebound myocardial ischemia after abrupt interruption of intravenous nitroglycerin infusion also has been reported in unstable angina patients.[133]

A second strategy for avoiding nitrate tolerance involves the concomitant administration of a sulfhydryl donor such as captopril or *N*-acetylcysteine. Although this approach is not employed in patients with unstable angina, a randomized trial in 200 patients demonstrated that the combination of transdermal nitroglycerin and *N*-acetylcysteine reduced the incidence of death, myocardial infarction, and refractory angina requiring hospitalization over 4 months compared with placebo or transdermal nitroglycerin alone.[134] Combined therapy caused intolerable headache in one-third of patients, limiting its clinical utility.

Considerable data can be marshaled to support the argument that the antiplatelet effects of nitroglycerin explain that drug's efficacy in treating unstable angina. Early studies demonstrated that nitroglycerin inhibits platelet aggregation.[135] Nitroglycerin and other nitrates activate cyclic guanosine monophosphate (GMP) in platelets. Cyclic GMP modulates the availability of intracellular platelet calcium and thus influences the response of platelets to receptor-mediated activation.[135]

At therapeutic doses, nitroglycerin reduces platelet aggregability to adenosine diphosphate and thrombin in unstable angina patients.[136] The drug also has been shown to reduce platelet thrombin deposition in an experimental model that simulates plaque rupture.[137] Platelet aggregation induced by thrombin and platelet thrombin deposition appear to be reduced by nitroglycerin even after tolerance to the hemodynamic effects of the drug has developed.[138] Intravenous nitroglycerin usually is replaced with transdermal nitroglycerin or an oral nitrate preparation after an angina-free interval of 1 or 2 days. In unstable angina patients who undergo coronary angiography and angioplasty, intravenous nitroglycerin usually is discontinued 12 to 24 h after the procedure. The doses of transdermal or oral nitrates that are prescribed for patients with unstable angina are similar to those used in stable angina patients. In most cases, they are lower than the doses found to be effective in preventing angina in clinical studies.

TABLE 41-6 Clinical Trials of Anti-Ischemic Therapy in Unstable Angina

Author[a]	Year	Active Treatment	Comparison Group	No. Patients	Duration of Study	End Point	Primary Results	Comments
Kaplan et al.[127]	1983	IV Nitroglycerin (NTG)	None	35	In hospital	Rest angina episodes	90% decrease in episodes	No control group
Curman et al.[128]	1983	IV NTG	Oral/topical nitrates	40	In hospital	Rest angina episodes	Fewer episodes in both groups	No difference between groups
Muller et al.[143]	1984	Nifedipine	Propranolol, oral nitrates	126	14 days	Angina relief	Equal angina relief in both groups	MI rate 9/63 in both groups
Gottlieb et al.[144]	1986	Propranolol	Placebo	82	4 weeks	Angina recurrence	Propranolol superior	Nitrates plus nifedipine in both groups
Théroux et al.[145]	1985	Diltiazem	Propranolol	100	5.1 months	Angina in hospital death/MI during follow-up (FU)	Equal angina relief in both groups	Equal rates of death/MI during FU
Andre-Fouet et al.[146]	1983	Diltiazem	Propranolol	70	In hospital	Angina	Equal angina relief in both groups	Diltiazem superior in variant angina patients
HINT[147]	1986	Nifedipine Metoprolol	Placebo	515	48 h	Recurrent angina death/MI	MI rate higher with nifedipine compared with metoprolol	Angina relief when nifedipine added to metoprolol
Gerstenblith et al.[150]	1982	Nifedipine	Placebo	138	4 months	Death/MI/coronary artery bypass grafting (CABG)	Nifedipine better than placebo	Nifedipine benefit in variant angina patients

[a]Several small studies are not included (see references 152, 153, 158, and 159).

Beta Blockers

Ischemia occurs when myocardial oxygen demand exceeds the delivery of oxygenated blood to a territory of myocardium distal to the culprit lesion. The major determinants of myocardial oxygen consumption are heart rate, myocardial inotropic state, and left ventricular afterload. Treatment strategies to prevent episodes of unstable angina can be divided into those which increase regional blood flow and those which reduce myocardial oxygen demand.

Beta blockers are the most useful category of drug in reducing myocardial oxygen demand, primarily by slowing heart rate but also by decreasing myocardial contractility and afterload. Heart rate and arterial pressure often increase during episodes of rest angina.[139,140] This unwanted response can be limited by beta-adrenergic blockade.

Beta blockers attenuate the coronary vasodilating effect of beta-adrenergic stimulation and allow alpha-adrenergic vasoconstriction to predominate. In patients with Prinzmetal's variant angina, beta blockers may increase the frequency or duration of attacks,[141,142] presumably through this mechanism. However, in patients with unstable angina, the potentially harmful effect of beta blockers on coronary blood flow does not appear to be clinically relevant.

Although it is widely accepted that beta blockers are useful in controlling ischemic episodes in patients with unstable angina, the data to support this claim are mainly inferential or have been derived from small trials without placebo-treated controls (Table 41-6). These trials date from the early 1980s, an era when patients were not treated routinely with aspirin and heparin.

Muller and coworkers randomly allocated 126 patients with unstable angina to propranolol plus isosorbide dinitrate or to nifedipine for 14 days.[143] The principal end point—the absence of recurrent chest pain for at least 48 h—was attained with equal frequency in the two groups; however, the propranolol and nitrate combination was more effective in patients not previously taking a beta blocker, and nifedipine was more effective in patients who had been receiving beta blockers before admission. The incidence of myocardial infarction during the 14-day treatment period was 14 percent (9 of 63) in both groups. Four patients in the nifedipine group died, compared with none in the group treated with propranolol.

Gottlieb and associates randomized 81 unstable angina patients either to propranolol at a dose of at least 160 mg/day or to placebo.[144] Baseline therapy in all patients included long-acting nitrates and nifedipine 80 mg/day. The cumulative probability of experiencing recurrent angina was significantly lower in the propranolol group. Myocardial infarction during the 4 weeks of the trial occurred in 6 of 42 propranolol-treated patients and 3 of 39 controls, a difference that was not statistically significant.

Théroux and colleagues randomized 100 patients with unstable angina to propranolol 240 mg/day or diltiazem 360 mg/day.[145] Transient ST-segment changes during an episode of chest pain were a requirement for study entry, and patients with Prinzmetal's variant angina or those already being treated with a beta blocker were excluded. Both drugs significantly reduced the frequency of angina episodes during hospitalization, and their antianginal efficacy was approximately equivalent. After 5.1 months of follow-up, 2 of 50 patients in each treatment group had died; 4 propranolol-treated and 5 diltiazem-treated patients experienced myocardial infarction. Similar results were found with respect to angina relief in a randomized comparison of propranolol and diltiazem in 70 unstable angina patients.[146]

The largest trial of a beta blocker in unstable angina was the Holland Interuniversity Nifedipine/Metoprolol Trial (HINT).[147] The 338 patients not receiving a beta blocker on admission were randomized to nifedipine 60 mg/day, metoprolol 200 mg/day, both drugs, or double placebo therapy. The rate of recurrent ischemia or myocardial infarction within 48 h, the main end point of HINT, was reached by 37 percent of placebo patients, 47 percent of nifedipine patients, 28 percent of metoprolol patients, and 30 percent of patients receiving combination therapy. Metoprolol was significantly better than nifedipine with respect to this end point. The trend in favor of metoprolol compared with placebo was not statistically significant.

Taken together, these trials indicate that beta blockers effectively reduce symptoms in unstable angina patients who are not already taking one of these drugs on admission. Whether or not a beta blocker also reduces the risk of myocardial infarction is uncertain. The trials in unstable angina are much too small to answer this question and are confounded by the use of nifedipine in the comparison groups. Five old randomized trials involving approximately 4700 patients with "threatened myocardial infarction" assessed the effect of acute intravenous beta blockade followed by oral treatment for 1 week.[148] Most patients in these studies had prolonged chest pain without ECG evidence of infarction on admission. A 13 percent reduction in the risk of infarction, from 32 percent to 29 percent, was reported in an overview of these trials, a difference of borderline statistical significance ($p < .04$). Neither antiplatelet nor antithrombotic therapy was used in these trials, and so their relevance to patients treated with current therapy is uncertain.

During chronic therapy, a long-acting beta blocker is preferable to a short-acting one because it can be given once per day. However, in the context of unstable angina, it is reasonable to try to achieve beta blockade within hours, not days. Therefore, beta blockade sometimes is initiated with intravenous boluses titrated to reduce heart rate. Early heart rate control is particularly important in high-risk patients and those with tachycardia or a high arterial pressure on admission. A reasonable target heart rate in unstable angina patients is 50 to 60 beats per minute at rest. The main contraindications to beta blockers in unstable angina are reactive airway disease, sinus node dysfunction or atrioventricular block, and severe heart failure. Most patients with chronic obstructive pulmonary disease will tolerate a beta blocker; a $beta_1$-selective agent (for example, metoprolol or atenolol) is theoretically less likely to provoke bronchoconstriction. In some patients with conduction system disease, permanent pacing may be indicated in part so that chronic beta blocker therapy can be given. Mild heart failure that is stable is not a contraindication to beta blockers in patients with unstable angina. Diltiazem or verapamil should be considered when a beta blocker cannot be used.

Calcium Channel Blockers

Calcium channel blockers increase coronary blood flow both globally and to the ischemic zone. Diltiazem and verapamil both slow heart rate, reduce afterload, and reduce myocardial contractility; they thus reduce myocardial oxygen demand. Most dihydropyridine calcium channel blockers induce a reflex increase in heart rate in the absence of beta blockade, a feature that is likely to mitigate any benefit in regard to myocardial ischemia. Dihydropyridine calcium channel blockers sometimes worsen myocardial ischemia and produce other "proischemic" complications in a minority of patients.[149]

The calcium channel blocker that has been used most often among the limited number of studies of unstable angina is the short-acting formulation of nifedipine. The rapid absorption and short half-life of this preparation produce frequent abrupt changes in arterial pressure and heart rate. Whether the poor results seen with nifedipine in trials of unstable angina and postinfarction patients would have been different with a long-acting formulation is open to debate.

As was noted above, in the study of Muller and colleagues[143] comparing propranolol and nifedipine in 126 unstable angina patients, nifedipine was more effective in controlling angina in patients who were already taking a beta blocker on admission but was less effective in other patients. The infarction rate during 14 days of treatment was 14 percent in both the propranolol and nifedipine treatment groups.

HINT was terminated prematurely because of a significantly higher rate of infarction in nifedipine-treated patients.[147] Among patients not already receiving a beta blocker on admission, recurrent ischemia or infarction within 48 h, the primary end point, occurred more often with nifedipine than it did with propranolol. However, among the 177 patients pretreated with a beta blocker, nifedipine was superior to placebo, with a relative risk for the primary end point of 0.68 (95 percent confidence interval of 0.47 to 0.97).

Gerstenblith and coinvestigators randomized 138 unstable angina patients taking propranolol and long-acting nitrates to nifedipine 80 mg/day or to placebo.[150] The primary end point of the trial—death, infarction, or coronary bypass surgery within 4 months—was reached by 43 of 70 placebo patients and 30 of 68 nifedipine-treated patients ($p = .03$). Nifedipine was particularly beneficial ($p = .02$) in the 52 patients with transient ST elevation during attacks, who presumably had coronary spasm, with little difference seen between the groups for the remainder of the study patients.

The potential of nifedipine at a dose of 80 mg/day to prevent "threatened myocardial infarction" was assessed in a double-blind, placebo-controlled trial of 105 patients.[151] Entry criteria included chest pain lasting longer than 45 min and ECG ST-segment changes, and treatment was initiated a mean of 4.6 h after the onset of pain. The incidence of progression to infarction of 75 percent in both groups was not altered by nifedipine. A further 66 patients with documented infarction on admission also were randomized to the same treatments in another part of the trial. At the end of the 14-day treatment period, mortality among the entire 171 patients was higher in the nifedipine group: 7.9 percent versus 0 percent ($p = .018$).

Taken together, these trials provide fairly strong evidence that nifedipine is harmful when used in unstable angina patients who are not receiving beta blockers but that it may be helpful in controlling angina in patients with an adequate level of beta blockade. Even when the addition of nifedipine does control angina in patients whose unstable angina was previously refractory, the risk of infarction or death over the next few months in the absence of revascularization remains very high.[152] Long-acting formulations of nifedipine and newer dihydropyridines such as amlodipine have not been evaluated in unstable angina trials.

As was mentioned above, two trials compared diltiazem to propranolol in a total of 170 patients with unstable angina.[145,146] The two drugs were equally effective in controlling angina and were associated with equal rates of myocardial infarction. In two small series in which intravenous diltiazem was compared with an intravenous nitrate for the control of myocardial ischemic episodes, diltiazem was reported to be superior.[153,154]

Verapamil has not been studied in large numbers of patients with unstable angina. In two small, placebo-controlled trials, the frequency of ischemic episodes was reduced significantly.[155,156] Long-term follow-up of these patients showed continued control of symptoms but a high incidence of infarction and death.[157] Verapamil and propranolol were compared in two small clinical trials.[158,159] Both drugs reduced the frequency of ischemic episodes, with verapamil being somewhat superior to propranolol. Both diltiazem and verapamil are effective in preventing ischemic episodes caused by coronary spasm, a condition that was present in some of the patients in these trials.

Diltiazem and verapamil are reasonable choices for treating unstable angina patients for whom beta blockers are contraindicated. The scant evidence discussed above suggests that both drugs reduce the frequency of attacks in unstable angina, but there is no evidence that they prevent infarction. The combination of diltiazem or verapamil with a beta blocker is not commonly used in unstable angina because the effects of these calcium channel blockers on heart rate and myocardial contractility are additive to the effects of beta blockers.

Antianginal Therapy

An oral beta blocker at a dose that reduces heart rate and an intravenous nitroglycerin infusion are a reasonable treatment to control symptoms in a high-risk or intermediate-risk unstable angina patient. Low-risk and some intermediate-risk patients can be treated with oral or transdermal nitrates and beta blockers. A patient who develops unstable angina while taking two or three antianginal drugs should be treated with intravenous nitroglycerin, but the symptoms will be harder to control compared with an unstable angina patient who previously took no antianginal drugs.

In most patients hospitalized with unstable angina, symptoms do not recur after the institution of antianginal therapy. Patients with refractory unstable angina have a much higher risk of developing myocardial infarction than do patients whose angina is controlled with drugs. Patients who are labeled as refractory often become asymptomatic when medical therapy is intensified; for example, in one study an increase in medical therapy relieved symptoms in 83 percent of patients transferred because their unstable angina was refractory.[160] Intraaortic balloon counterpulsation prevents myocardial ischemia effectively in patients whose unstable angina is truly refractory.[161] This mechanical approach improves myocardial blood flow and reduces myocardial oxygen demand by collapsing the resistance to left ventricular ejection in early systole. Intraaortic balloon counterpulsation is needed for the control of symptoms in less than 1 percent of patients with unstable angina, but it also is used in high-risk patients at the time of coronary angioplasty to provide a margin of safety. Intraaortic balloon counterpulsation causes lower limb ischemia in approximately 10 percent of cases, but this complication almost always resolves after removal of the device.

Aspirin

Aspirin inhibits cyclooxygenase activity in all body cells. This inhibition is irreversible for the life span of a platelet, normally a median of 8 days. As a consequence, the platelet is unable to produce thromboxane A_2, the platelet-specific prostaglandin that induces platelet aggregation. Aspirin also may influence the pathophysiology of unstable angina through other mechanisms. For example, aspirin inhibits prostacyclin production by the endothelium but also has been shown to block cyclooxygenase-dependent endothelium-derived vasoconstriction.[162]

Four trials have demonstrated conclusively that aspirin reduces the risk of myocardial infarction in patients with unstable angina (Table 41-7).[163–166] In the Veterans Administration study, 1338 men hospitalized with crescendo angina, prolonged pain, or pain at rest were randomized to aspirin 324 mg/day or placebo within 7 days.[163] The study duration was 12 weeks, and the primary end point was death or acute myocardial infarction. The principal outcome was reduced from 10.1 percent to 5.0 percent (p = .0005). In the Canadian multicenter trial, 555 unstable angina patients were randomized to aspirin 325 mg four times per day or placebo within 8 days of admission and were followed on therapy for a mean of 18 months.[164] The risk reduction for cardiac death or nonfatal myocardial infarction was identical to that in the Veterans Administration study at 51 percent, from 17.0 percent to 8.6 percent (p = .008). Sulfinpyrazone also was tested in this trial but showed no benefit.

Théroux and associates randomized 479 unstable angina patients to aspirin 325 mg twice daily or placebo at hospital admission, a mean of 8 h after the last episode of pain, with a mean follow-up of 6 days.[165] Patients also were randomized to intravenous heparin in a factorial design. Aspirin reduced the risk of death or myocardial infarction from 6.3 percent to 2.6 percent, a 63 percent decrease (p = .04). The Research Group on Instability in Coronary Artery Disease (RISC) randomized 796 men with unstable angina or non-Q-wave infarction within 4 weeks to aspirin 75 mg/day or placebo.[166] An additional 115 men were excluded per the protocol because their predischarge exercise tests revealed no evidence of myocardial ischemia. Aspirin reduced the risk of death and nonfatal infarction in both unstable angina and non-Q-wave infarction categories. At 5 days, the reduction was from 5.8 percent to 2.55 percent (p = .033), and at 30 days it was from 17.1 percent to 6.5 percent (p = .0001).

The results of these trials are remarkably consistent, and the risk reduction with aspirin for the prevention of death or nonfatal infarction is relatively large: from one-half to two-thirds. These findings attest to the central role platelets play in the pathophysiology of unstable angina. These studies show that the benefit from aspirin begins with the onset of unstable angina and extends for more than 1 year. Other trials have demonstrated that aspirin reduces the risk of infarction in stable coronary patients, and so the drug should be continued for life after an episode of unstable angina. The dose of aspirin used in these trials ranged from 75 to 1300 mg/day. Gastrointestinal side effects increase with increasing dose levels. A dose of 325 mg acutely and a dose of 81 mg during chronic treatment are sufficient to inhibit the platelet cyclooxygenase pathway maximally.

Women were excluded from two of the four trials[163,166] and represented one-quarter to one-third of the patients in the other two studies.[164,165] However, it seems reasonable to assume that the benefit of aspirin extends to women with unstable angina, particularly since aspirin has been shown to reduce coronary events across the broad spectrum of patients with atherosclerosis.

The Antiplatelet Trialists' Collaboration meta-analysis of 145 trials with more than 100,000 patients randomized to antiplatelet therapy or placebo showed consistent benefit in cere-

TABLE 41-7 Clinical Trials of Aspirin in Unstable Angina

Author	Year	No. Patients	Dose	Duration of Follow-Up	Death/MI Rate in Aspirin Group, %	Death/MI Rate in Control Group, %	*p* value	Relative Risk	Comments
Lewis et al.[163]	1983	1266	324 mg/day	12 weeks	5.0	10.1	.0005	0.49	Men only
Cairns et al.[164]	1985	555	325 mg qid	18 months	8.6	17.0	.008	0.49	Not intention to treat
Théroux et al.[165]	1988	239	325 mg bid	6 days	3.3	11.9	.01	0.29	Treatment begun at 8 h
RISC[166]	1990	796	75 mg/day	3 months	6.5	17.1	.001	0.36	Men only, non-Q-wave MI included

brovascular disease and stable and unstable coronary disease.[167] Almost all the antiplatelet therapy in these trials consisted of aspirin. Few treatments show a cost/benefit ratio that is superior to that of aspirin in the treatment of unstable angina.

Angiotensin-converting enzyme (ACE) inhibitors promote the release of prostaglandins, and inhibition of prostaglandin synthesis with aspirin or other nonsteroidal anti-inflammatory drugs attenuates the acute vasodilatory effect of ACE inhibition. In the SOLVED trial,[168] the CONSENSUS II trial,[169] and the GUSTO-1 trial,[170] a negative interaction between aspirin and ACE inhibitors was reported. However, in a data base of 11,576 patients with coronary disease, 5-year adjusted mortality was lower in ACE inhibitor–treated patients who also took aspirin than it was in those who did not in the presence or absence of heart failure.[171] On the basis of the information that is currently available, it appears reasonable not to withhold aspirin from coronary patients who are receiving ACE inhibitors in the absence of severe heart failure.

Ticlopidine and Clopidogrel

Ticlopidine and clopidogrel are thienopyridines, and their mechanism of action differs from that of aspirin (Fig. 41-7). Both drugs inhibit adenosine diphosphate (ADP)-mediated platelet activation.[172] Because they act independently of the arachidonic acid pathway, the antiplatelet activities of aspirin and either ticlopidine or clopidogrel are synergistic. Ticlopidine induces neutropenia in 1 to 3 percent of patients and also rarely causes severe adverse dermatologic effects. The drug also is limited by its slow onset of action: 3 to 4 days for the inhibition of platelet aggregation to exceed 50 percent and up to 2 weeks for the effect to plateau. The effect of ticlopidine also persists after treatment has been discontinued.

Ticlopidine 250 mg twice per day was compared to conventional antianginal therapy without aspirin in a randomized but open-label trial in 652 unstable angina patients.[173] Over a 6-month follow-up period, the rate of fatal or nonfatal infarction was 7.3 percent in the ticlopidine group and 13.6 percent in controls, a 46 percent reduction ($p = .009$). However, the benefit of treatment developed only after 2 weeks; this is consistent with the known delayed onset of action of the drug. On the basis of this trial, ticlopidine has been considered as an alternative in unstable angina patients who cannot tolerate aspirin. Ticlopidine has been widely used with aspirin to prevent thrombotic complications in the weeks after coronary stenting, based on clinical trial evidence that it is superior to aspirin alone in this situation.[174] However, ticlopidine is rapidly being supplanted by clopidogrel for this indication because of the better safety profile of clopidogrel.

Clopidogrel is more potent than ticlopidine in inhibiting ADP-induced platelet aggregation in vitro and has a more rapid onset of action. Within 2 h of oral administration, antiplatelet activity can be detected, and the effect on platelet aggregation becomes maximal between 4 and 7 days. The usual dose is 75 mg once daily. The utility of clopidogrel in treating unstable angina is being assessed in a randomized clinical trial. In the Clopidogrel versus Aspirin in Patients at Risk of Ischemic Events (CAPRIE) trial, clopidogrel reduced the combined end point of ischemic stroke, myocardial infarction, and vascular

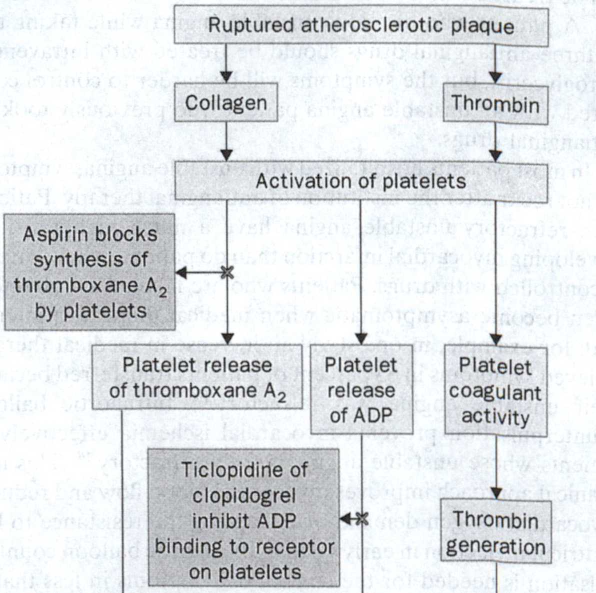

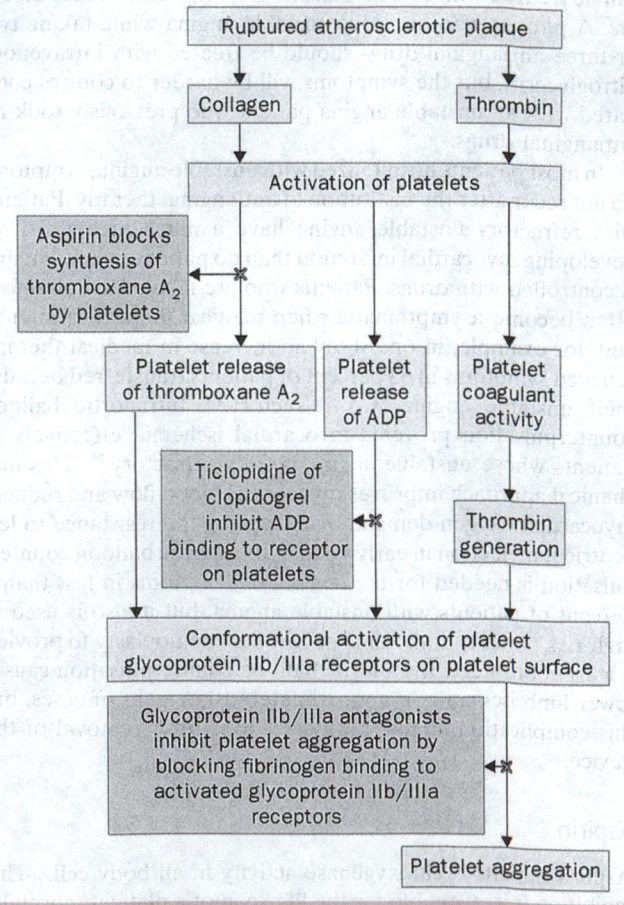

FIGURE 41-7 Sites of action of platelet inhibitors. (From Hirsh and Weitz,[219] with permission.)

death by 8.7 percent ($p = .043$) for up to 3 years compared with aspirin in 19,185 patients with vascular disease.[175] Patients with peripheral arterial disease appeared to benefit more than did patients with previous infarction or stroke. The risk of gastrointestinal hemorrhage severe enough to stop the drug was higher with clopidogrel than it was with aspirin but was still less than 1 percent. Clopidogrel is not associated with the increased potential for neutropenia seen with ticlopidine. For these reasons, clopidogrel is preferred over ticlopidine in patients with unstable angina who do not tolerate aspirin.

Platelet Glycoprotein IIb/IIIa Receptor Inhibitors

Platelet membranes contain glycoprotein receptors, many of which are integrins.[176] Integrins are heterodimeric molecules composed of alpha and beta subunits. These subunits are combined in unique patterns to form receptors specific for various ligands. The $\alpha_{IIb}\beta_3$ integrin, or platelet IIb/IIIa receptor (Fig. 41-8), changes from its resting state to its active state when the platelet is activated by agonists or other platelets and serves as a receptor for fibrinogen and von Willebrand factor.[176] Fibrinogen binding is central to platelet aggregation and thrombus formation in the arterial circulation.

Blockade of the platelet GP IIb/IIIa receptor is a theoretically attractive concept. Unlike aspirin and clopidogrel, which do not block thrombin-induced platelet aggregation, GP IIb/IIIa inhibitors block aggregation in response to all potential agonists (Fig. 41-7). Different receptors, GP Ib and GP IV, mediate platelet adhesion to the subendothelial matrix. Thus, hemorrhage should not be a major problem even with complete blockade of GP IIb/IIIa receptors.[176]

The first GP IIb/IIIa blocker to be approved and widely used clinically is abciximab, the Fab fragment of a monoclonal antibody to the $\alpha_{IIb}\beta_3$ integrin. Other GP IIb/IIIa inhibitors are either peptides or smaller molecules. Eptifibatide is the peptide GP IIb/IIIa inhibitor that has been approved for use in the United States. Tirofiban, lamifiban, fradafiban, xemilofiban, orbofiban, sibrafiban, roxifiban, lotrafiban, and lefradiban are all small-molecule GP IIb/IIIa inhibitors. Only tirofiban has been approved for use in the United States, but several of the other drugs are in the later stages of clinical development. All the currently approved drugs must be administered by parenteral infusion, but the last six compounds on the above list of small-molecule GP IIb/IIIa inhibitors will be for oral use.

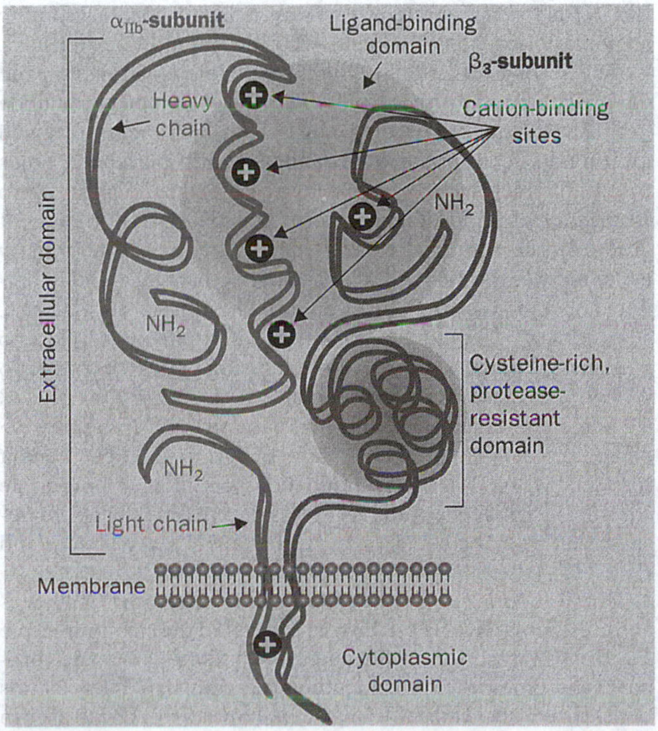

FIGURE 41-8 Schematic representation of the $\alpha_{IIb}\beta_3$ integrin, or the platelet IIb/IIIa receptor. (From Topol et al.,[176] with permission.)

Coronary Intervention Trials with GP IIb/IIIa Inhibitors

Platelet GP IIb/IIIa inhibitors have been evaluated mainly in patients with acute coronary syndromes (including unstable angina and NSTEMI patients), patients undergoing coronary angioplasty, and patients in both categories (Fig. 41-9). The Evaluation of c7E3 Fab for Prevention of Ischemic Complications (EPIC) trial enrolled 2099 patients considered at high risk for coronary angioplasty, including patients with unstable angina.[177] All these patients were treated with aspirin and heparin, and randomization was to placebo, a weight-adjusted abciximab bolus, or a bolus followed by an infusion of abciximab for 12 h. The primary end point was a composite of death, myocardial infarction, urgent repeat revascularization, or stent or balloon pump placement within 30 days after randomization. The event rate was 12.8 percent in the placebo group, 11.4 percent with bolus abciximab, and 8.3 percent in the bolus plus infusion group ($p = .008$ versus placebo). Benefit was most pronounced in unstable angina patients, with a 71 percent decrease in the primary end point and a 94 percent decrease in death or myocardial infarction (11.1 percent placebo versus 0.6 percent bolus plus infusion group, $p < .0001$). The benefit of abciximab in the EPIC patients persisted to 6 months[178] and 3 years.[179]

The Evaluation in PTCA to Improve Long-Term Outcome with abciximab GP IIb/IIIa blockade (EPILOG) trial compared a bolus plus 12-h infusion of abciximab to placebo in all but high-risk patients undergoing coronary angioplasty.[180] EPILOG is thus complementary to EPIC. Nearly half the EPILOG patients had unstable angina as their diagnosis, but patients with ECG changes within the 24 h preceding randomization were excluded. Randomization was to placebo plus standard-dose heparin and to abciximab with low-dose or standard-dose heparin. EPILOG was stopped after 2792 of the planned 4800 patients were enrolled because the composite end point of death, infarction, or urgent revascularization at 30 days was 11.7 percent in the placebo group and 5.2 percent and 5.4 percent in the abciximab groups ($p < .0001$). The clinical benefit of abciximab in EPILOG was maintained to 1 year.[181] Among unstable angina patients, the end point of death, myocardial infarction, or urgent intervention at 1 year was reached by 16.8 percent in the placebo group and 9.0 percent in the abciximab groups. Taken together, EPIC and EPILOG firmly established that abciximab reduces the rate of coronary events across a broad range of patients undergoing coronary angioplasty, including those with unstable angina.

The c7E3 Fab Antiplatelet Therapy in Unstable Refractory Angina (CAPTURE) trial differed from EPIC and EPILOG in that it evaluated pretreatment with abciximab before coronary

Trial	Agent	No	Placebo (%)	IIb/IIIa (%)
Percutaneous coronary intervention trials				
EPIC	Abciximab	2099	10·1	7·0
IMPACT-II	Eptifibatide	4010	8·4	7·1
EPILOG	Abciximab	2792	9·1	4·0
CAPTURE	Abciximab	1265	9·0	4·8
RESTORE	Tirofiban	2139	6·3	5·1
EPISTENT	Abciximab	2399	10·2	5·2
Unstable angina/non-Q-wave MI trials				
PRISM	Tirofiban	3231	7·0	5·7
PRISM Plus	Tirofiban	1570	11·9	8·7
PARAGON	Lamifiban	2282	11·7	11·3
PURSUIT	Eptifibatide	10 948	15·7	14·2
Overall		**32 735**	**11·1**	**9·0**

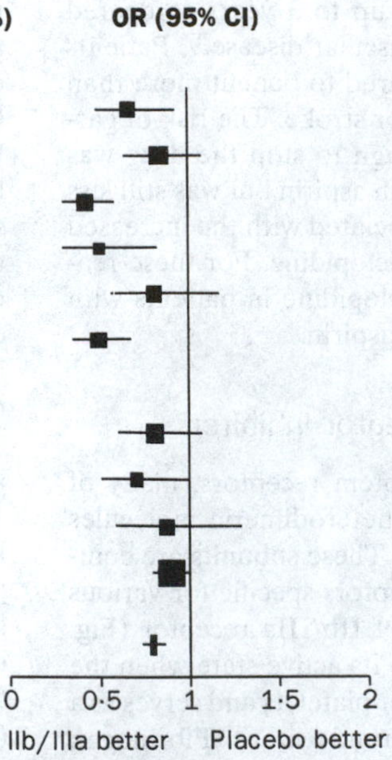

FIGURE 41-9 Randomized, placebo-controlled trials of platelet GP IIb/IIIa inhibitors during percutaneous coronary interventions and trials of unstable angina and non-Q-wave infarction. The event rates are for death or nonfatal myocardial infarction at 30 days. The graphic depicts odds ratio and 95 percent confidence intervals, with the size of the box being proportional to the sample size of the trial. (From Topol et al.,[176] with permission.)

angioplasty among high-risk unstable angina patients.[182] To qualify, patients had to have chest pain with ischemic ECG changes within 48 h despite intravenous heparin and intravenous glyceryl trinitrate. All these patients also received aspirin and heparin. Placebo or abciximab bolus plus infusion was begun 18 to 24 h before angioplasty and continued until 1 h after the procedure. After the enrollment of 1265 patients, the trial was stopped prematurely. The primary end point—death, myocardial infarction, or urgent intervention within 30 days—was reached by 15.9 percent of placebo patients and 11.3 percent of abciximab patients (p =.012). Clinical benefit developed before the angioplasty procedure (Fig. 41-10): The infarction rate during this short interval was 2.6 percent among placebo-treated patients and 0.6 percent among abciximab-treated patients (p = .029). In contrast to the EPIC and EPILOG trials, the

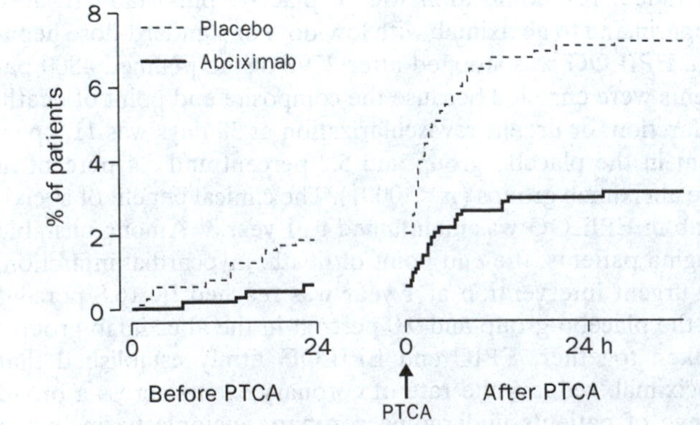

FIGURE 41-10 Reduction in the incidence of myocardial infarction with abciximab in the CAPTURE trial.[182] The benefit of abciximab was present both in the first 24 h before angioplasty (p = .029) and during and for the 24 h after angioplasty (p = .021). (From CAPTURE investigators,[182] with permission.)

benefit of abciximab treatment in CAPTURE was attenuated by 6 months.

Abciximab and coronary stenting were assessed in a wide spectrum of patients undergoing angioplasty in the Evaluation of Platelet IIb/IIIa Inhibitor for Stenting (EPISTENT) trial.[183] Slightly more than one-third of the 2399 EPISTENT patients had unstable angina within 48 h. Randomization was to stenting plus placebo, stenting plus abciximab (bolus plus 12-h infusion), or balloon angioplasty plus abciximab. The primary end point—a composite of death, myocardial infarction, or the need for urgent revascularization within 30 days—occurred at a rate of 10.8 percent in the stent/placebo group, 5.3 percent in the stent/abciximab group (odds ratio 0.48, 95 percent confidence interval 0.33 to 0.69), and 6.9 percent in the balloon/abciximab group (odds ratio 0.63, 95 percent confidence interval 0.45 to 0.88). By 6 months, death or myocardial infarction had occurred in 11.4 percent of the stent/placebo group, 5.6 percent of the stent/abciximab group (odds ratio 0.47, 95 percent confidence interval 0.33 to 0.68, $p < .001$), and 7.8 percent of the balloon/abciximab group (odds ratio 0.67, 95 percent confidence interval 0.49 to 0.92, p = .01).[184] EPISTENT demonstrated that the benefit of abciximab during angioplasty extends to patients who receive elective stents.

The Second Integrilin to Minimize Platelet Aggregation and Coronary Thrombosis (IMPACT-II) trial evaluated eptifibatide in 4010 patients undergoing angioplasty.[185] Patients received aspirin and heparin and were randomized to placebo, a bolus of eptifibatide followed by a lower-dose infusion for 20 to 24 h, or a bolus plus a higher-dose infusion. In each treatment group, 38 percent of patients had unstable angina. The primary end point was the 30-day composite of death, myocardial infarction, unplanned revascularization, or stenting for abrupt closure. The primary end point occurred in 11.4 percent of placebo patients, 9.2 percent of lower-dose infusion patients (odds ratio 0.79, 95 percent confidence interval 0.61 to 1.01, p = .063), and 9.9 percent of higher-dose infusion patients (odds ratio 0.86, 95 percent confidence interval 0.67 to 1.10, p = .22). The benefit seen in IMPACT-II with eptifibatide was thus of borderline statistical significance and was less impressive than the results seen with abciximab in EPIC, EPILOG, CAPTURE, and EPISTENT (Fig. 41-9).

The Randomized Efficacy Study of Tirofiban for Outcomes and Restenosis (RESTORE) trial evaluated the small-molecule GP IIb/IIIa inhibitor tirofiban in 2139 patients with acute coronary syndromes who were undergoing angioplasty.[186] Two-thirds of the patients had unstable angina. All were treated with aspirin and heparin. Tirofiban or placebo was begun after the lesion was crossed with the guidewire and was continued for 36 h, longer than in the other trials, because of the rapid reversibility of platelet inhibition with tirofiban. The primary end point was a composite similar but not identical to the preceding trials: death, infarction, repeat target lesion angioplasty, coronary bypass surgery, or coronary stenting by 30 days. Although a statistically significant reduction in events was seen with tirofiban at day 2 and day 5 after the procedure, by 30 days (the primary end point), the rate was 12.2 percent in the placebo group and 10.3 percent in the tirofiban group, a 16 percent relative reduction ($p = .16$).

Taken together, these trials indicate that platelet GP IIb/IIIa inhibition at the time of angioplasty reduces ischemic complications. The benefit with respect to the primary end point of the trials was less with eptifibatide and tirofiban (15 to 20 percent) than with abciximab (30 to 60 percent); however, the 95 percent confidence intervals overlap, and the drugs have not been compared directly in the same trial. If variability in efficacy does exist, potential explanations might be that abciximab gradually dissociates from the GP IIb/IIIa receptor over 36 h after the drug is discontinued, that abciximab also blocks the $\alpha_v\beta_3$ vitronectin receptor, or that the dose of eptifibatide selected for IMPACT-II was too low. The risk of hemorrhage during angioplasty with GP IIb/IIIa inhibitors can be reduced by early sheath removal, meticulous care of arterial puncture sites, and lower, weight-adjusted doses of heparin than were used traditionally.

Acute Coronary Syndrome Trials with GP IIb/IIIa Inhibitors

In addition to the six large trials discussed above in which GP IIb/IIIa inhibitors were tested during coronary angioplasty, four large trials have assessed the value of these drugs in patients with unstable angina or non-Q-wave myocardial infarction (also known as NSTEMI). Whereas abciximab was the drug used most frequently in the angioplasty trials, eptifibatide and the small-molecule GP IIb/IIIa inhibitors predominated in the acute coronary syndrome trials (Fig. 41-9).

The Platelet Receptor Inhibition in Ischemic Syndrome Management (PRISM) study enrolled 3232 patients with an acute coronary syndrome including chest pain within 24 h.[187] One-quarter of these patients had non-Q-wave infarction, and the remainder had unstable angina with ECG abnormalities. With aspirin as baseline therapy, patients were randomized according to a double-blind protocol either to a weight-adjusted bolus plus infusion of tirofiban or to a bolus and infusion of heparin to maintain the activated partial thromboplastin time at twice the control value. Treatment continued for 48 h, and the primary end point was a composite of death, myocardial infarction, or refractory ischemia during this period. The end point was reached by 5.6 percent of heparin-treated patients and 3.8 percent of tirofiban-treated patients (odds ratio 0.67, 95 percent confidence interval 0.48 to 0.92, $p = .01$). By 30 days, the primary end point with the addition of readmission for unstable angina was 17.1 percent in the heparin group and 15.9 percent in the tirofiban group, a difference that was not statistically significant. However, mortality at 30 days was lower in the tirofiban group at 2.3 percent compared with 3.6 percent ($p = .02$).

The Platelet Receptor Inhibition in Ischemic Syndrome Management in Patients Limited by Unstable Signs and Symptoms (PRISM-PLUS) study enrolled 1915 unstable angina and non-Q-wave infarction patients with prolonged or repetitive chest pains within 12 h and ECG changes.[188] Study treatment was continued for 72 h, and coronary angioplasty was done in 475 of the patients between 48 and 72 h. Randomization was to tirofiban, heparin, or tirofiban plus heparin, with all patients receiving aspirin unless it was contraindicated. The tirofiban bolus and infusion doses were one-third lower in patients treated with heparin than they were in those treated with tirofiban alone. The study was stopped prematurely for the group receiving tirofiban alone because of excess mortality at 7 days: 4.6 percent versus 1.1 percent among patients receiving heparin alone ($p = .012$). This early increase in mortality was explained by the investigators as most likely being due to chance, since no such increase was seen in PRISM. The frequency of the primary end point at 7 days—a composite of death, myocardial infarction, or refractory ischemia—was 17.9 percent in the heparin group and 12.9 percent in the heparin plus tirofiban group (odds ratio 0.68, 95 percent confidence interval 0.53 to 0.88, $p = .004$). This advantage persisted to 30 days and to 6 months. Death or myocardial infarction occurred within 7 days in 8.3 percent of the heparin-only patients and 4.9 percent of the heparin and tirofiban group ($p = .006$). This absolute difference of 3.6 percent narrowed slightly to 3.0 percent by 6 months, when the rates of death and infarction were 15.3 percent and 12.3 percent ($p = .06$). In the subset of patients who underwent angioplasty between 48 and 72 h, the risk of death, infarction, refractory ischemia, or rehospitalization for unstable angina over the next 30 days was reduced from 15.3 percent to 8.8 percent with combination therapy compared with heparin alone (odds ratio 0.55, 95 percent confidence interval 0.32 to 0.94). The benefit of combination therapy over heparin alone was of roughly equal magnitude in patients with unstable angina or non-Q-wave infarction.

The findings of PRISM and PRISM-PLUS are somewhat contradictory. PRISM indicates that tirofiban may be superior to heparin as acute therapy for unstable angina in patients taking aspirin. PRISM-PLUS suggests that the combination of aspirin, heparin, and tirofiban is superior to aspirin and heparin. The benefit of tirofiban added to aspirin and heparin among angioplasty patients in PRISM-PLUS was of greater magnitude and lasted longer than the benefit seen with this combination of treatment in RESTORE. However, the results of RESTORE are more credible because the number of patients was much larger: 2139 compared with 475 angioplasty patients in PRISM-PLUS. Pretreatment and selection biases might have influenced the angioplasty subgroup in PRISM-PLUS.

The Platelet glycoprotein IIb/IIIa in Unstable Angina Receptor Suppression Using Integrilin Therapy (PURSUIT) trial enrolled 10,948 patients with unstable angina or non-Q-wave infarction to eptifibatide or placebo.[189] Baseline therapy consisted of aspirin and heparin. Study drug treatment lasted for 3 days, with an additional day if coronary intervention was done near 72 h. The primary end point, a composite of death or nonfatal myocardial infarction at 30 days, was 15.7 percent in the placebo group and 14.2 percent in the eptifibatide group ($p = .04$). The treatment effect occurred consistently across most subgroups except for women, who had a statistically nonsignificant 10 percent higher event rate with eptifibatide. The absolute risk reduction of 1.5 percent was less than the 3.2 percent absolute risk reduction seen in PRISM-PLUS (Fig. 41-9). The Platelet IIb/IIIa Antagonism for the Reduction of Acute coronary syndrome events in a Global Organization Network (PARAGON) trial tested lamifiban, a small-molecule GP IIb/IIIa inhibitor that has not yet been approved for use in the United States.[190] Low-dose lamifiban and high-dose lamifiban, with and without heparin, were compared to a placebo plus heparin group. All patients received aspirin. A total of 2282 patients with unstable angina and ECG changes were enrolled. The primary end point of death or myocardial infarction at 30 days occurred at a rate of 11.7 percent in the placebo group, 10.6 percent in the low-dose lamifiban group, and 12.0 percent in the high-dose lamifiban group. These differences were not statistically significant. At 6 months, the composite event rate was 13.7 percent for the low-dose lamifiban group compared with 17.9 percent for controls ($p = .027$). The high-dose lamifiban plus heparin group experienced more intermediate or major bleeding than did controls: 12.1 percent compared with 5.5 percent ($p = .002$).

The oral small-molecule GP IIb/IIIa inhibitors have failed to reduce coronary events in three large, recently completed trials.[191,192,192a] In the Sibrafiban versus Aspirin to Yield Maximum Protection from Ischemic Heart Events Post-acute Coronary Syndromes (SYMPHONY) study,[191] 9233 patients who had stabilized after an acute coronary syndrome were randomly assigned to aspirin, low-dose sibrafiban, or high-dose sibrafiban. The primary end point was a composite of death, nonfatal infarction, or severe recurrent ischemia at 90 days. Sibrafiban showed no additional benefit over aspirin, and was associated with more dose-related bleeding.

In the Evaluation of Oral Xemilofiban in Controlling Thrombotic Events (EXCITE) trial,[192] 7232 patients were randomized to placebo or oral xemilofiban beginning just before coronary angioplasty and continuing for 182 days. This trial was not limited to patients with unstable angina. The primary end point (a composite of death, nonfatal infarction, or urgent revascularization) was not reduced by active treatment. The Orbofiban in Patients with Unstable Coronary Syndromes–Thrombolysis in Myocardial Infarction 16 (OPUS-TIMI 16) trial[192a] enrolled 10,302 unstable angina patients to either of two doses of orbofiban or placebo. The trial was halted early because of excess mortality in one of the active treatment groups. The composite end point was not reduced by either dose of orbofiban at either 30 days or 10 months. The reason for the early increase in mortality is unclear, but may be related to intermittent platelet activation with the oral GP IIb/IIIa platelet inhibitors.

Guidelines for the Use of GP IIb/IIIa Inhibitors

Although GP IIb/IIIa inhibitors have firmly established their usefulness in a wide spectrum of patients undergoing coronary angioplasty, their value in unstable angina patients who are not undergoing intervention is incompletely defined. GP IIb/IIIa inhibitors have not been compared to clopidogrel or to low-molecular-weight heparins or studied in patients taking these drugs as background therapy.

The current high cost of these drugs makes it tempting to limit their use to high-risk patients. In a subgroup analysis from the CAPTURE study,[193] patients with troponin T elevations at study entry had a high event rate and derived a large benefit from abciximab therapy (odds ratio for death or myocardial infarction 0.32, 95 percent confidence interval 0.14 to 0.62, $p = .002$). Patients without elevated troponin T levels experienced a low event rate and did not benefit from abciximab.

Current guidelines recommend that eptifibatide or tirofiban be added to aspirin and heparin in the treatment of patients with some high-risk features or with refractory ischemia.[1] These drugs should be continued during coronary angioplasty and for 12 to 24 h after the procedure for tirofiban and for 24 to 72 h after the procedure for eptifibatide.[1] Abciximab also can be used in patients with unstable angina in whom angioplasty is planned within the following 24 h.[1] However, when abciximab is administered before diagnostic coronary angiography, the prolonged platelet inhibition it induces may force a delay in the urgent coronary bypass surgery that is needed for some patients. When aspirin and unfractionated heparin are used with GP IIb/IIIa inhibitors, the dose of heparin should be conservative during coronary procedures, and heparin should be discontinued after the procedure if it is uncomplicated.[1]

Heparin

Heparin binds with antithrombin to form a complex that inactivates thrombin and activated factors X, XII, XI, and IX.[194] The principal inhibitory effect of heparin on coagulation probably occurs through the inhibition of thrombin-induced activation of factor V and factor VIII. Fibrin binds thrombin and protects it from inactivation by the heparin-antithrombin complex. Platelets inhibit the anticoagulant effect of heparin by binding factor Xa and protecting it from inactivation.

The pharmacokinetics of heparin are complex, and the dose-response relationship is nonlinear. Heparin therapy is monitored to maintain the activated partial thromboplastin time (APTT) ratio within 1.5 to 2.5 times normal. The anticoagulant response to a standard dose of heparin varies widely among patients so that even when a weight-based nomogram is used in a clinical study, the APTT falls outside the therapeutic range more than one-third of the time.[195] Results in routine clinical practice are probably much worse. Pooled analyses of randomized trials have revealed an average incidence of major bleeding of 6.8 percent in continuous-infusion groups and 14.2 percent in intermittent-infusion groups (odds ratio 0.42, $p = .01$).[196]

Heparin was used to treat patients with unstable angina before that diagnostic term was used commonly,[2] but good clinical trial data in support of its use did not emerge until the 1980s (Table 41-8). In a randomized, double-blind, placebo-controlled trial of 214 patients with unstable angina, myocardial infarction developed during 7 days of treatment in 9 (17 percent) of 54 patients taking placebo, 8 (13 percent) of 60 taking atenolol, 1 (2 percent) of 51 receiving heparin, and 2 (4 percent) of 49 on combined therapy.[197] The improved prognosis of heparin-treated patients was maintained during follow-up, and all five deaths occurred among patients who did not receive heparin. The impact of this trial was attenuated by a design problem in that 186 additional patients were withdrawn after randomization because of incorrect recruitment.

Théroux and colleagues randomized 479 patients with unstable angina to aspirin, heparin, combination therapy, or double placebo a mean of 8 h after the last episode of chest pain, with a mean follow-up of 6 days.[165] The results of this trial with respect to aspirin were discussed earlier in this chapter. The incidence of death or nonfatal myocardial infarction was reduced dramatically with heparin from 14 of 118 patients in the placebo group to 3 of 240 in the heparin groups (11.9 percent versus 1.25 percent, $p < .001$). Heparin also reduced the fre-

TABLE 41-8 Clinical Trials of Unfractionated Heparin in Unstable Angina

Author	Year	No. Patients	Background Therapy	Duration of Follow-Up	MI Rate with Heparin, %	MI Rate in Controls, %	*p* Value	Relative Risk	Comments
Telford and Wilson[197]	1981	214	Also randomized to atenolol	In hospital	3	14.9	.024	0.20	No background aspirin therapy
RISC[166]	1990	796	Also randomized to aspirin	5 days of heparin	3.4[a]	4.9[a]	NS[b]	0.70	No significant benefit at 3 months; men only
Théroux et al.[198]	1993	484	Aspirin	6 days	0.8	3.7	.035	0.22	Treatment begun a mean of 8 h after last chest pain
Holdwright et al.[199]	1994	285	Aspirin	30 days	27.2[a]	30.5[a]	NS	0.89	Very high event rate
Gurfinkel et al.[200]	1995	143	Aspirin	In hospital	6.0	9.5	NS	0.60	Treatment begun a mean of 6 h after last chest pain
Cohen et al.[202]	1994	214	Aspirin	12 weeks	6.0	8.3	NS	0.69	Heparin followed by coumadin

[a]Includes death as well as myocardial infarction in the end point.
[b]NS = not significant.

quency of refractory angina 60 percent. The combination of heparin and aspirin was not superior to aspirin alone in the prevention of death or nonfatal infarction. In an extension of the trial, heparin and aspirin were compared directly in a total of 484 patients.[198] Death or myocardial infarction occurred in 3.7 percent of aspirin-treated patients and 0.8 percent of heparin-treated patients ($p = .035$).

Aspirin and heparin also were tested in a factorial design in the RISC trial.[166] RISC enrolled 796 men with unstable angina or non-Q-wave infarction. As was discussed above, aspirin exhibited a marked protective effect in this study. The effect of heparin on the event rate was not statistically significant, although a trend in its favor was seen during the 5 days in which it was administered. In two smaller trials comparing aspirin to aspirin plus heparin, no difference was seen between the treatment groups.[199,200] The Antithrombotic Therapy in Acute Coronary Syndromes (ATACS) trial randomized 69 patients in a pilot study and 214 patients in the main trial to aspirin alone or to aspirin plus heparin followed by warfarin.[201,202] The composite end point of recurrent angina with ECG changes, myocardial infarction, or death within 12 weeks was reduced in the main trial by combination therapy from 27 percent to 10.5 percent ($p = .004$). A meta-analysis of these trials concluded that the addition of heparin to aspirin in the treatment of unstable angina reduces the rate of myocardial infarction approximately one-third.[203]

The way in which heparin is administered may influence its efficacy in treating unstable angina. In a trial of unstable angina patients who were refractory to medical therapy, heparin significantly decreased the frequency of angina attacks and the number of episodes of silent myocardial ischemia when it was administered as a bolus followed by an infusion but not when it was given as a bolus every 6 h.[204] In another study of refractory unstable angina patients done by the same investigators, both subcutaneous heparin and heparin given as a bolus and an infusion profoundly reduced the frequency of myocardial ischemic episodes.[205]

Discontinuation of heparin in unstable angina patients can results in a reactivation of refractory ischemic episodes within hours.[206] Aspirin or warfarin may block this phenomenon. Rebound has been described with other thrombin inhibitors, but the mechanism has not been defined. However, it has been shown that thrombin generation increases and tissue factor pathway inhibitor levels decrease within 24 h of heparin cessation.[207] Gradual weaning from heparin, as opposed to abrupt cessation, results in less thrombin generation.[207] Mild thrombocytopenia occurs in 10 to 20 percent of patients treated with unfractionated heparin.[208] In 2 to 10 percent of patients, a more severe form of thrombocytopenia develops. This antibody-mediated response occurs within 5 to 10 days after the initiation of treatment and is associated with thromboembolic sequelae in 30 to 80 percent of cases.[208] Other adverse effects of heparin include osteoporosis, skin necrosis, alopecia, hypersensitivity reactions, and hypoaldosteronism.[196]

Low-Molecular-Weight Heparins

Unfractionated heparin consists of a heterogeneous mixture of polysaccharide chains ranging in molecular weight from approximately 3000 to 30,000. Low-molecular-weight heparins (LMWHs) are fragments of unfractionated heparin produced by enzymatic or chemical depolymerization processes that yield chains with average molecular weights of approximately 5000.[209] The main difference between the two types of heparin is that unfractionated heparin has equivalent activity against factor Xa and thrombin while LMWHs have greater activity against factor Xa.[209] The reason for this difference is that long heparin chains such as those present predominantly in regular heparin are required to bind both antithrombin and thrombin (Fig. 41-11).

Both types of heparin interfere with thrombin-induced platelet activation by inhibiting the thrombin–glycoprotein Ib interaction, but standard heparin is more potent than LMWHs in this regard.[210] However, a disadvantage of regular heparin is that it inhibits activation of the protein C anticoagulant pathway more than a LMWH does.[211]

Compared with unfractionated heparin, LMWHs produce a more predictable anticoagulant response because of their better bioavailability, longer half-life, and dose-independent clearance.[209] The plasma half-life of a LMWH after subcutaneous injection ranges from 3 to 6 h, and so once- or twice-daily administration is feasible. In contrast to unfractionated heparin, monitoring is not required with the use of LMWHs, with the possible exception of plasma antifactor Xa levels in patients with renal insufficiency.[209] LMWH caused less bleeding than unfractionated heparin did in laboratory animal experiments

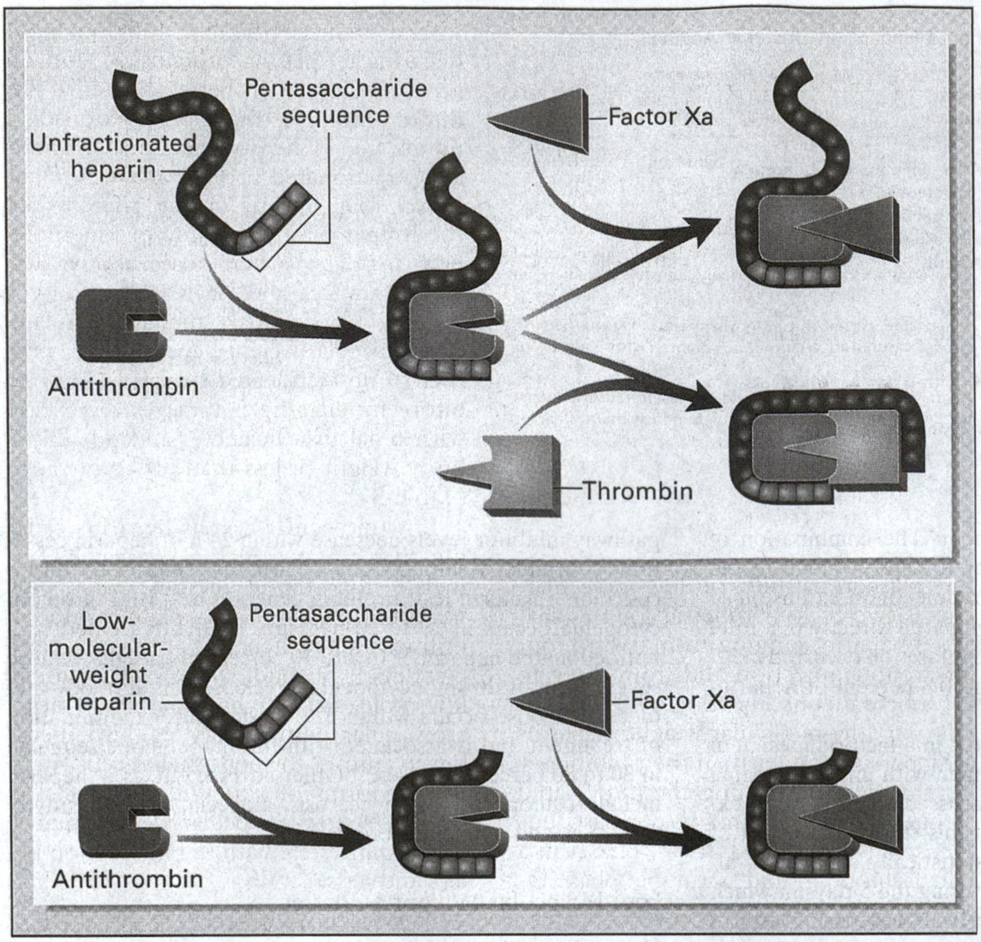

FIGURE 41-11 Binding of unfractionated heparin (*top*) and low-molecular-weight heparin (*bottom*) to antithrombin. When bound to either form of heparin, antithrombin undergoes a conformational change that accelerates its interaction inactivating factor Xa. In contrast, formation of the heparin-antithrombin-thrombin complex (*top panel, bottom right*) requires the long saccharide chain of unfractionated heparin. (From Weitz,[209] with permission.)

and in some clinical trials.[209] The main disadvantage of LMWHs is that they are far more expensive than unfractionated heparin.

LMWHs are somewhat more effective than standard heparin in preventing deep vein thrombosis after general or orthopedic surgery, according to meta-analyses of clinical trials.[195] Thrombus size by venography and a small trial in patients with established venous thrombosis showed better outcomes with LMWHs compared with unfractionated heparin.[195] In light of these encouraging findings and the obvious practical advantages of LMWHs, trials of LMWHs for unstable angina were anticipated with enthusiasm.

The first of these trials, a small open-label trial, showed that LMWHs plus aspirin reduced the risk of myocardial infarction better than did standard heparin plus aspirin or aspirin alone.[200] In a more definitive trial, the Fragmin during Instability in Coronary Artery Disease (FRISC) study, 1506 patients with unstable angina or non-Q-wave myocardial infarction were randomly assigned to a weight-adjusted dose of the LMWH dalteparin twice daily or to placebo.[212] After 6 days, the dose was changed to 7500 IU once daily and was continued for 35 to 45 days. All patients without contraindications took aspirin. The primary end point—the rate of death or myocardial infarction during the first 6 days—was reduced with dalteparin (odds ratio 0.37, 95 percent confidence interval 0.20 to 0.68). The benefit of treatment persisted to 40 days but was attenuated, mainly because of an increase in events among smokers in the active treatment group after the dose was reduced from twice daily to once daily. The results of FRISC demonstrated that LMWH is superior to placebo in aspirin-treated patients with unstable angina, but a more important issue is how LMWH compares with intravenous unfractionated heparin.

The Fragmin in Unstable Coronary Artery Disease (FRIC) study was the first trial to address this question. In the open-label, acute phase of FRIC, 1482 patients with unstable angina or non-Q-wave infarction were randomized to either dalteparin, administered as in FRISC, or dose-adjusted intravenous standard heparin for 6 days.[213] All the patients received aspirin. The primary end point—a composite of death, myocardial infarction, or recurrence of angina—was 9.3 percent in the dalteparin group and 7.6 percent in the standard heparin group. Although this difference is not statistically significant, fewer deaths occurred in the unfractionated heparin group (3 versus 11, $p = .05$). After 6 days, most of the patients continued to the double-blind phase of the trial, in which they were treated from days 6 to 45 with dalteparin 7500 IU subcutaneously once daily or with placebo. During this period, the composite end point was 12.3 percent in both groups. The authors concluded that dalteparin at this dose during the month after hospital discharge provided no additional benefit over aspirin but speculated that twice-daily treatment might.

Thus, in the Fragmin and Fast Revascularisation during Instability in Coronary artery disease (FRISC II) trial, 2267 patients with unstable angina or non-Q-wave infarction were randomly assigned to subcutaneous dalteparin twice daily or to placebo for 3 months after at least 5 days of treatment with open-label dalteparin.[214] Half the patients had ST depression at study entry, and more than half had troponin T elevations. After 30 days, the rate of death or nonfatal infarction was 3.1 percent with dalteparin and 5.9 percent with placebo (odds ratio 0.53, 95 percent confidence interval 0.35 to 0.80). However, by 3 months this difference had shrunk to 6.7 percent versus 8.0 percent, which was not statistically significant. In the subgroup with elevated troponin T levels at baseline, dalteparin reduced the relative risk of death or infarction to 3 months by 30 percent and the absolute risk by 2.7 percent ($p = .07$). In troponin-negative patients, treatment beyond 5 days with dalteparin showed no benefit.

The Efficacy and Safety of Subcutaneous Enoxaparin in

Non-Q-Wave Coronary Events (ESSENCE) study randomly assigned 3171 patients with unstable angina or non-Q-wave infarction to enoxaparin 1 mg/kg subcutaneously twice daily or to continuous unfractionated heparin for a period of 2 to 8 days.[215] All the patients received aspirin. The primary end point—a composite or death, myocardial infarction, or recurrent angina at 14 days—was 16.6 percent with enoxaparin and 19.8 percent with regular heparin ($p = .019$). This difference persisted to 30 days, and the need for revascularization to this point also was reduced significantly with enoxaparin. An economic substudy indicated that total medical costs to 1 month were lower in enoxaparin-treated patients because the added cost of the drug was more than compensated for by savings from reduced events.[216]

The Thrombolysis in Myocardial Infarction (TIMI) 11B trial randomly assigned 3910 patients with unstable angina or non-Q-wave infarction to enoxaparin or standard heparin for 3 to 8 days, with 60 percent of the population continuing treatment with enoxaparin or placebo for 43 days.[217] Enoxaparin reduced events compared with unfractionated heparin during the acute phase of the trial (odds ratio 0.83, 95 percent confidence interval 0.69 to 1.00, $p = .048$). No additional benefit or loss of benefit was seen with continued therapy. In another trial, 3468 patients with unstable coronary disease were allocated randomly to unfractionated heparin or to 6 days or 14 days of treatment with the LMWH nadroparin.[218] No benefit of the LMWH was seen in this study; in fact, at 3 months the composite end point of death, infarction, or refractory ischemia occurred in 22.2 percent of unfractionated heparin patients, 22.3 percent of those in the 6-day LMWH group, and 26.2 percent of those in the 14-day treatment group ($p = .03$).

In summary, trials of LMWH in unstable angina and non-Q-wave infarction have yielded conflicting results (Table 41-9). Two trials, ESSENCE and TIMI 11B, demonstrated that enoxaparin is superior to unfractionated heparin for the first few days of therapy. The only acute comparison between dalteparin and standard heparin, FRIC, had inadequate statistical power to detect a difference between treatments. Theoretically, enoxaparin may be superior to dalteparin because of its higher anti-factor Xa to anti-factor IIa ratio. The early benefit of LMWH treatment appears to dissipate over the ensuing months, and continuing therapy was not beneficial in most trials. However, in FRISC II, treatment from 5 days to 3 months with dalteparin produced an impressive reduction in death or infarction at 1 month, with gradual loss of that benefit thereafter.

Heparin is recommended for the acute treatment of all unstable angina patients except those determined to be at low risk.[1] Unfractionated heparin should be started with an intravenous bolus of 60 to 70 units/kg followed by a constant infusion of approximately 16 units/kg per hour, adjusted to maintain the APTT at 1.5 to 2.5 times control, or to 50 to 70 s.[1] Subcutaneous administration of enoxaparin or dalteparin may be used instead of unfractionated heparin.[1] The dose of enoxaparin is 1 mg/kg twice daily, and the dose of dalteparin is 120 IU/kg (maximum of 10,000 IU) twice daily. Either standard heparin or an LMWH should be continued for 2 to 5 days, until the patient has been stabilized for 24 h, or until revascularization is performed.[1] The dose of unfractionated heparin should be conservative during coronary angioplasty when aspirin and GP IIb/IIIa inhibitors are being administered concomitantly, and heparin should be discontinued after an uncomplicated procedure.[1] Scant information is available on the combined use of LMWHs and GP IIb/IIIa inhibitors, particularly during coronary interventions; however, this combination is probably acceptable.[1]

Hirudin and Other Direct Thrombin Inhibitors

Hirudin is a 65-amino-acid polypeptide that was isolated from the salivary glands of the medicinal leech and now is produced through recombinant DNA technology.[219] Recombinant hirudin

TABLE 41-9 Major Clinical Trials of Low-Molecular-Weight Heparins (LMWH) in Patients with Unstable Angina or Non-Q-Wave Infarction

Trial	LMWH	No. Patients	Duration of Follow-Up	Death/MI Rate in LMWH Group, %	Death/MI Rate in Control Group[a], %	Relative Risk (RR) (95% Confidence Interval)	Comments
FRISC-I[212]	Dalteparin	1506	6 days	1.8	4.8	0.37 (0.20–0.68)	At 40 days, death/MI reduced from 10.7% to 8.0%; RR 0.75 (0.54–1.03)
FRIC[213]	Dalteparin	1482	6 days	3.9	3.6	1.07 (0.63–1.80)	From days 6–45, death/MI reduced from 4.7% to 4.3%; RR 0.92 (0.54–1.57)
FRISC-II[214]	Dalteparin	2267	3 months	6.7	8.0	0.81 (0.60–1.10)	At 30 days, death/MI reduced from 5.9% to 3.1%; RR 0.53 (0.35–0.80)
ESSENCE[215]	Enoxaparin	3171	14 days	4.9	6.1	0.80 (p – .13)	Death/MI/recurrent angina reduced from 19.8% to 16.6%; RR 0.80 (0.67–0.96)
TIMI-11B[217]	Enoxaparin	3910	8 days	4.6	5.9	0.77 (0.58–1.02)	Death/MI/urgent revascularization reduced from 14.5% to 12.4%; RR 0.83 (0.69–1.0)
FRAXIS[218]	Nadroparin	3468	90 days	8.8[b]	7.9[b]	1.10 ($p = .46$)	No benefit for any end point at any time point

[a]Control group treated with unfractionated heparin in all trials except FRISC-I.
[b]Includes mortality only.

binds tightly to thrombin without requiring a cofactor, forming a slowly reversible complex. Hirudin has been shown to be more effective than heparin or LMWH in the prevention of venous thrombosis in patients undergoing total hip replacement[220] and has been approved for use in patients with heparin-induced thrombocytopenia.[219]

Hirudin and standard heparin were compared in 8011 patients with acute chest pain without ST elevation and in 4131 patients with ST elevation in the Global Use of Strategies to Open Occluded Coronary Arteries (GUSTO) IIb study.[221] No differences in drug efficacy were seen between patients with and without ST elevation. A trend toward early benefit was seen with hirudin, with a 1.3 percent rate of death or myocardial infarction at 24 h compared with 2.1 percent in the heparin group ($p = .001$). However, by 30 days, the difference between the treatments for the primary end point of the trial was 8.9 percent versus 9.8 percent ($p = .06$).

The Organization to Assess Strategies for Ischemic Syndrome (OASIS-2) compared a slightly higher dose of hirudin to unfractionated heparin in 10,141 patients with unstable angina or suspected infarction without ST elevation.[222] Hirudin reduced the composite end point of cardiovascular death or myocardial infarction during the 3 days of treatment (odds ratio 0.76, 95 percent confidence interval 0.59 to 0.99), with statistically borderline benefit persisting to 7 days ($p = .077$). Major bleeding was more common with hirudin than it was with heparin.

Bivalirudin, a hirudin analog, was compared with heparin during coronary angioplasty in patients with unstable angina or postinfarction angina.[223] Bivalirudin caused less bleeding than heparin did and produced better results in the subgroup with postinfarction angina but did not significantly reduce the primary end point of the trial. Other direct thrombin inhibitors, such as argatroban and inogratran, have been investigated in acute coronary syndromes with disappointing results.[219] For example, inogratran was less effective than standard heparin in a trial involving 1209 patients with unstable coronary disease.[224]

Despite the encouraging early benefit compared with unfractionated heparin seen in GUSTO IIb and OASIS-2, hirudin is not currently recommended for use in patients with unstable angina.

Anticoagulation

Markers of ongoing thrombin generation remain elevated for months in some patients with unstable angina, and such markers have been correlated with increased risk.[108,225] In a small trial comparing aspirin to aspirin plus warfarin in unstable angina, the combination reduced progression of the culprit lesion compared with aspirin alone.[226] Additionally, the combined-therapy group showed a trend toward fewer infarctions during the 10 weeks of the study. For these reasons, the combination of aspirin to block platelets and oral anticoagulants to suppress activation of the coagulation system has attracted interest for its potential to reduce events in the long term after an episode of unstable angina.

In the ATACS study, 214 unstable angina patients who were not previously taking aspirin were randomized to aspirin alone or to aspirin plus intravenous heparin followed by coumadin for 12 weeks.[202] The combination therapy significantly reduced ischemic events at 12 weeks, but most of the difference occurred early, during treatment with heparin, and the difference during coumadin therapy was not statistically significant.

The OASIS investigators conducted two pilot studies of anticoagulation in patients with unstable angina or non-Q-wave infarction.[227] In the first, aspirin plus a fixed low dose of warfarin, 3 mg/day, was compared with aspirin alone in 309 patients. The composite end point of death, infarction, or refractory angina during the 6 months of treatment was actually lower—3.9 percent versus 6.5 percent—in the group without warfarin, but the difference did not attain statistical significance. Major bleeding occurred in four warfarin plus aspirin and no aspirin-only patients, and minor bleeding was more common in warfarin patients. In the second phase of the pilot study, warfarin was given at a higher, adjusted dose to maintain the International Normalized Ratio (INR) between 2.0 and 2.5. Although only 197 patients were enrolled in this phase, the reduction in the composite rate of cardiovascular death, myocardial infarction, or refractory angina with warfarin was impressive (odds ratio 0.42) and approached statistical significance ($p = .08$). Long-term anticoagulation is being evaluated in a substudy of OASIS-2.

Thrombolytic Therapy

Myocardial infarction and unstable angina share a common pathophysiologic substrate: plaque rupture or erosion with overlying thrombosis. Thrombolysis effectively reopens occluded culprit arteries and reduces mortality in patients with acute infarction. It was therefore thought that thrombolytic therapy might prove useful in treating unstable angina.

A meta-analysis of nine small, randomized controlled clinical trials of thrombolysis in unstable angina, with heparin as background therapy, revealed an increased risk of myocardial infarction with active treatment (odds ratio 2.38, 95 percent confidence interval 1.15 to 4.94).[228] The failure of thrombolytic therapy for unstable angina and non-Q-wave infarction was confirmed in the TIMI-IIIB trial.[229] Among the 1473 patients randomized to intravenous tissue plasminogen activator or to placebo, the rate of fatal or nonfatal myocardial infarction at 6 weeks was 7.4 percent with thrombolysis and 4.9 percent with placebo ($p = .04$). In patients not receiving heparin initially, the event rate was 15.2 percent with TPA and 0 percent with placebo ($p = .01$). In another trial, urokinase was given at the time of coronary angioplasty in unstable angina patients to prevent ischemic events.[230] However, both acute closure and clinical end points were more common with the thrombolytic agent than with placebo.

The reason why thrombolytic therapy does not reduce events in unstable angina is not known. However, thrombolysis stimulates ongoing thrombin formation and also activates platelets.[228] These mechanisms are likely to be more important in patients with unstable angina than in patients with Q-wave-infarction. Thrombolytic therapy should be avoided in patients with unstable angina.

Coronary Revascularization

Coronary bypass surgery and coronary angioplasty frequently are performed in patients with unstable angina; however, the precise indications for revascularization, the choice of procedure, and its timing are controversial. Randomized trials comparing revascularization to medical therapy in patients with unstable angina were first performed more than 20 years ago. The results of all but the most recent trials are not applicable to current clinical decision making because major advances in medical and interventional practices have vastly improved the outcomes with both types of therapy. Randomized trials in this area are difficult to perform and interpret because of small sample sizes, frequent crossovers from medical to interventional treatment, and exclusion criteria that tend to eliminate the high-risk patients who might benefit the most from coronary revascularization.

An overview of the 10-year results from the clinical trials comparing coronary bypass surgery with medical treatment for stable angina indicate that patients with left main coronary artery stenosis or three-vessel disease obtain the greatest benefit from surgery.[121] In low-risk groups such as patients with single-vessel involvement, no survival advantage can be demonstrated with bypass surgery. These conclusions also may be relevant to patients with unstable angina.

In the Veterans Administration Cooperative Study of Unstable Angina, 468 men age less than 70 years were randomized to medical or surgical therapy.[231–233] Those with left main coronary stenosis, previous bypass surgery, recent infarction, or ejection fractions less than 30 percent were excluded. Surgery consisted of saphenous venous bypasses only, a mean of 2.7 per patient, and 30-day surgical mortality was 4.1 percent.[231] By 2 years, one-third of the patients assigned to medical therapy had crossed over to surgery. Overall mortality at 5 years was 19 percent in medically assigned patients and 16 percent in bypass patients, a difference that was not statistically significant.[232] The rates of myocardial infarction also were not significantly different between the groups. High-risk subsets appeared to benefit from surgery; for example, 5-year mortality among patients with three-vessel disease was 11 percent in the bypass surgery group and 24 percent in the medical group ($p = .02$). For patients with three-vessel disease and left ventricular dysfunction, the mortality advantage for surgery is even greater: 29 percent compared with 9 percent ($p < .05$). Surgery appeared to nullify partially the increased risk associated with lower ejection fractions. By 10 years, mortality was 38 percent in the medical group and 39 percent in the surgical group.[233] The relationship between a low ejection fraction and a survival benefit from surgery persisted (Fig. 41-12).

A common feature of the VA trial and trials in stable angina is that bypass surgery provides the greatest survival benefit to patients with the most advanced coronary disease and left ventricular dysfunction. Many patients with unstable angina are limited by exertional angina when they attempt to resume normal activities after the acute episode. Coronary bypass surgery effectively eliminates angina in 80 to 90 percent of cases. The long-term results of coronary bypass surgery for unstable angina have been good. In a compilation of more than 6000 patients from 14 reports from 1978 to 1988, operative mortality was less than 4 percent and 5-year survival was nearly 90 percent despite previous infarction in half the population, three-vessel disease in more than half, and left main stenosis in one-fifth.[234] Since that time, operative techniques have improved dramatically and the population of unstable angina patients undergoing bypass surgery has become older and sicker. These two factors have tended to cancel each other out, and so outcome statistics have remained relatively stable.

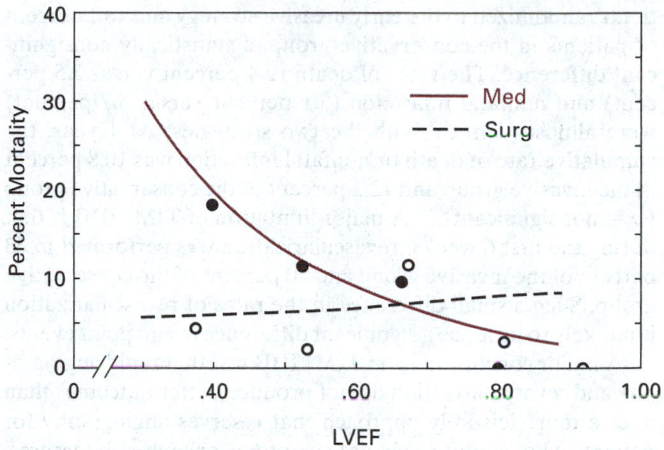

FIGURE 41-12 Mortality at 2 years according to baseline ejection fraction in the Veterans Administration Cooperative Study of Unstable Angina.[231] Although no overall mortality difference between the groups was seen, a relation between ejection fraction and outcome was evident. Survival was poor in medically treated patients with low ejection fractions. In surgically treated patients, survival was independent of ejection fraction. (From Luchi et al.,[231] with permission.)

In its early phases of development, coronary angioplasty was applied to patients with unstable angina. The initial results were not as good as they were in patients with stable coronary disease. Advances in catheter technology have led to improved outcomes in all patient categories, with a narrowing of the gap between unstable and stable patients. The widespread use of coronary stents and GP IIb/IIIa inhibitors has further reduced the risk of coronary angioplasty in patients with unstable coronary disease.

Recent trials of coronary revascularization in unstable angina have compared an "aggressive" approach with a "conservative" approach. The aggressive approach involves early coronary angiography with revascularization by either coronary angioplasty or bypass surgery, depending on the coronary anatomy. Usually, patients with one or two severe narrowings are treated with angioplasty and those with more extensive disease undergo bypass surgery. The conservative approach limits coronary arteriography, usually to patients who require revascularization to control persistent symptoms and to those with very high-risk features.

In the TIMI IIIB trial, 1473 patients with unstable angina or non-Q-wave infarction were randomized within 24 h of chest pain to an early invasive or a conservative strategy.[229] The invasive group underwent coronary arteriography within 18 to 48 h after randomization, followed by a revascularization procedure when possible. Coronary arteriography was done in the conservative group for recurrent chest pain at rest with ischemic ECG changes, episodes of ST depression on ambulatory ECG monitoring, high-risk features on a stress test at the time of hospital discharge, severe angina after discharge, or hospitalization for a recurrence of unstable angina. Two-thirds of the patients had unstable angina, and the remainder had non-Q-wave infarction. Patients also were randomized in a factorial design to TPA or placebo, as was described above. The primary end point of the trial—death, myocardial infarction, or a failed symptom-limited exercise test within 6 weeks—occurred in 16.2 percent of patients randomized to the early invasive strategy and 18.1 percent of patients in the conservative group, a statistically nonsignificant difference. The rates of death (2.4 percent versus 2.5 percent) and nonfatal infarction (5.1 percent versus 5.7 percent) were almost identical with the two strategies. At 1 year, the cumulative rate of death or nonfatal infarction was 10.8 percent in the invasive group and 12.2 percent in the conservative group (p = not significant).[235] A major limitation of TIMI IIIB is that during the first 6 weeks, revascularization was performed in 63 percent of the invasive group and 50 percent of the conservative group. Such a small difference in the rates of revascularization is unlikely to produce a significant difference in end point events.

A major conclusion from TIMI IIIB was that rapid angiography and revascularization do not produce better outcomes than does a more leisurely approach that reserves angiography for patients who exhibit recurrent symptoms or high-risk features.

The Veterans Affairs Non-Q-Wave Infarction Strategies in Hospital (VANQWISH) trial[236] included no patients with unstable angina, but its results may be relevant to all acute coronary syndromes. The 920 patients were assigned randomly to an invasive approach or a conservative approach. The composite end point of death or nonfatal infarction occurred more frequently in the invasive group during the first year: At hospital discharge, the difference was 7.8 percent versus 3.3 percent ($p = .004$); at 1 month, 10.4 percent versus 5.7 percent ($p = .012$); and at 1 year, 24 percent versus 18 percent ($p = .05$). By the end of the 23-month follow-up, the difference between the treatment groups had narrowed and was no longer statistically significant. VANQWISH has been criticized because revascularization was actually performed in only 44 percent of the patients assigned to the invasive strategy but in 33 percent of patients in the conservative group. Additionally, in the invasive patients who underwent bypass surgery, the mortality rate within 1 month of surgery was 11.6 percent, higher than the norm for this type of patient.

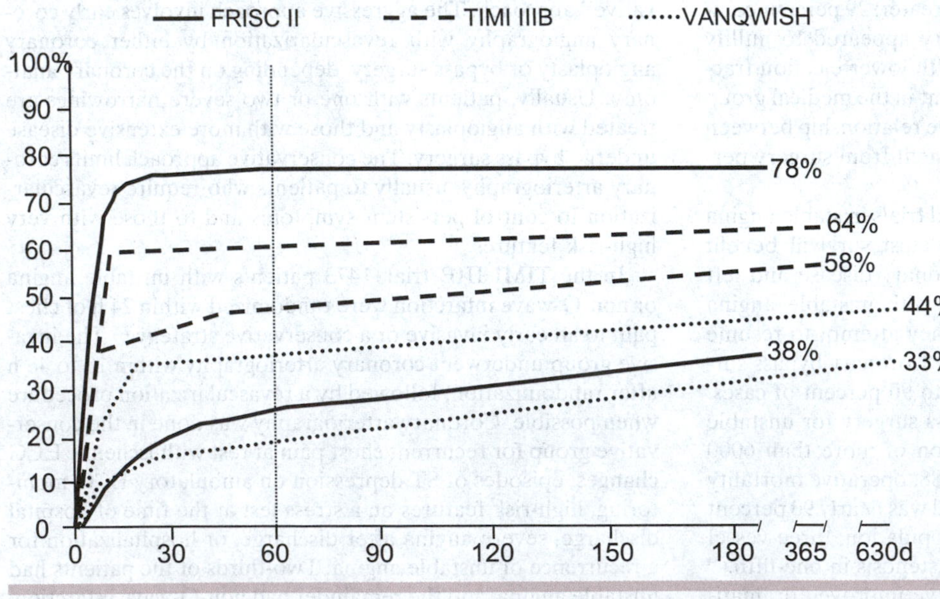

FIGURE 41-13 Proportion of patients in the invasive and noninvasive treatment groups of TIMI IIIB,[229] VANQWISH,[236] and FRISC II[237] who underwent revascularization during the first year. The differences between invasive and noninvasive groups are small in TIMI IIIB and VANQWISH and large in FRISC II. This factor may partially explain why revascularization was shown to be beneficial in FRISC II but not in the other two trials. (Courtesy of Dr. Lars Wallentin, for the FRISC II investigators, with permission.)

In the FRISC II study described above, 2457 patients with unstable coronary disease were randomized in a 2 by 2 factorial design to dalteparin or to placebo and to an invasive or noninvasive treatment strategy.[237] More than half the patients had elevated troponin T levels, and nearly half had ischemic ECG changes; one or the other of these criteria was necessary for entry into the trial. In the invasive arm, coronary angiography was performed within a few days of admission and revascularization was done shortly thereafter if feasible. An important difference between FRISC II and TIMI IIIB or VANQWISH is that most of the invasive patients underwent revascularization and most of the noninvasive patients did not, allowing a true comparison between the two approaches (Fig. 41-13). In the invasive group, the mean time from enrollment to angioplasty was 4 days and the mean time to bypass surgery was 7 days. By 10 days, 71 percent of the invasive patients and only 9 percent of the noninvasive patients had undergone revascularization. At 6 months, these rates were 77 percent and 37 percent, respectively. The mortality rate within 30 days among invasive patients who had bypass surgery was only 2.1 percent.

The primary end point of FRISC II—death or nonfatal infarction at 6 months—occurred in 9.4 percent of invasive patients and 12.1 percent of patients in the noninvasive group (odds ratio 0.78, 95 percent confidence interval 0.62 to 0.98, $p = .031$). During the first 2 weeks, the rate of death or infarction was higher in the invasive group than in the noninvasive group as a result of events associated with the procedures, but the curves crossed at 4 weeks (Fig. 41-14). Patients in the invasive group had a reduction in angina of about 50 percent compared with the noninvasive group during the first 6 months of follow-up ($p < .001$) and also were significantly less likely to be readmitted to the hospital. Dalteparin was effective in reducing events in the entire study and in the noninvasive group but had little effect in the invasive group (9.1 percent dalteparin versus 9.7 percent placebo event rates). The event rate during the first 2 months was lowest in the dalteparin/noninvasive group. FRISC II clearly demonstrated that revascularization improves outcomes for unstable angina patients with ischemic ST changes or elevated troponin levels if the procedures can be done with a low rate of complications. With modern antiplatelet and antithrombotic therapy, revascularization does not need to be done urgently, within the first day or two after admission, but should be done within the first week or two. The early benefit seen with antiplatelet or antithrombotic drugs tended to dissipate within the first month or two in some of the clinical trials of these drugs.

Survey data indicate that unstable angina patients who undergo revascularization outside clinical trial settings may not obtain benefit from the procedure. In the OASIS prospective registry

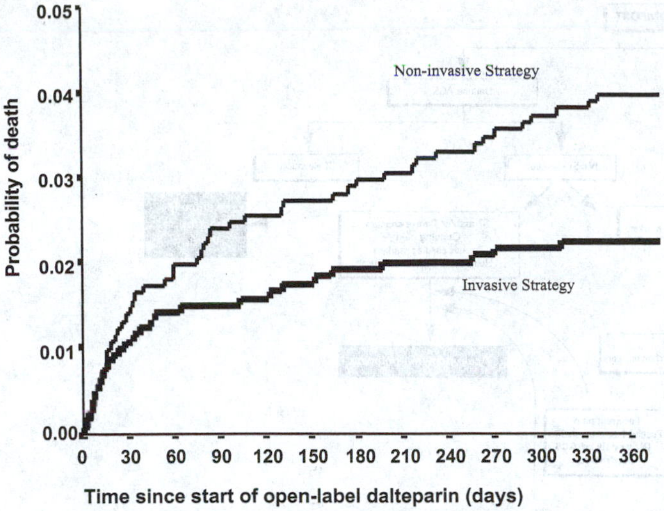

FIGURE 41-14 Incidence of death or myocardial infarction in patients randomized to the invasive and noninvasive strategies in the FRISC II trial.[237] At 6 months (the primary end point of the study), outcome was better in the invasive group ($p = .031$). This benefit persisted to 1 year. (Courtesy of Lars Wallentin, for the FRISC II investigators,[237] with permission.)

of 8000 unstable angina patients treated in 95 hospitals in six countries, revascularization was performed in 49 percent of patients in the United States and Brazil, 34 percent of patients in Canada and Australia, and 17 percent of patients in Hungary and Poland.[238] The 6-month rates of death or myocardial infarction did not differ among patients in the three groups, although angina during follow-up was eliminated more effectively in countries with more intervention. Across the six countries, low-risk unstable angina patients benefited from being treated in a hospital with catheterization facilities, but the outcome of high-risk patients was significantly worse.

An Integrated Approach to Treatment

The treatment of unstable angina should be individualized to take into account the specific features of the disease and the particular circumstances of the patient. Nevertheless, the algorithms that have been developed recently provide a useful framework (Fig. 41-15). It should be remembered that unstable angina is an acute episode related to one active culprit lesion but that the patient has diffuse atherosclerosis. Coronary disease is a chronic condition that usually causes recurrent events that are spread out over many years. Thus, smoking cessation, cholesterol lowering, and control of hypertension and diabetes may be at least as important in the long term as are the specific treatment decisions related to the acute event. An episode of unstable angina may be viewed as an opportunity to improve the patient's profile with respect to secondary prevention.

VARIANT ANGINA

In 1959, Prinzmetal and associates described a syndrome characterized by angina at rest with transient ST-segment elevation.[239] Exercise tolerance usually was well preserved, and the attacks were cyclical in nature, often occurring in the early morning hours. The attacks did not last longer than ordinary anginal episodes, and the ST-segment elevation disappeared rapidly as the chest pain receded. Ventricular arrhythmias and atrioventricular block sometimes occurred at the height of an attack, and both myocardial infarction and sudden death were common complications (see also Chap. 40).

With the advent of coronary angiography, it soon became apparent that the syndrome was caused by coronary spasm, usually focal and often at the site of a coronary stenosis.[240] The underlying coronary lesion can vary from a subtotal occlusion to a very mild stenosis, and in some cases the coronary arteries are angiographically normal. Coronary spasm occurs in more than one artery in some patients,[241] and the site of spasm can fluctuate from one vessel to another.[242]

Pathophysiology

A large number of etiologic explanations for variant angina have been proposed or rejected. Evidence of parasympathetic nervous system overactivity[243] and reduced sympathetic activity[244] has been presented; however, coronary spasm has been demonstrated in the transplanted, denervated heart,[245] making central neural mechanism unlikely. The frequency of attacks of variant angina is not reduced by alpha-adrenergic blockade,[246] blockade of serotonin receptors,[247] inhibition of thromboxane A_2 production,[248] or the administration of prostacyclin.[249] Magnesium deficiency,[250] hyperinsulinemia,[251] and vitamin E deficiency[252] have been reported to be present in patients with variant angina. Vitamin C attenuates the abnormal coronary vasoconstriction in patients with variant angina, purportedly by inhibiting oxygen free radical generation[253] (see also Chap. 37).

Whether nitric oxide activity at sites of coronary spasm is normal or abnormal is controversial.[254,255] A mutation of the endothelial nitric oxide synthetase (eNOS) gene recently was reported to be significantly more common in patients with coronary spasm than in controls.[256] Depressed endothelial nitric oxide production could predispose patients with this defect to coronary spasm.

Coronary spasm usually is localized to the site of an atherosclerotic lesion. Even variant angina patients with no evident narrowing at angiography invariably will have atherosclerosis demonstrable by intracoronary ultrasound at the site of focal spasm.[257] Asian patients with variant angina appear to have generalized coronary artery hyperactivity, whereas in white patients the abnormality is focal.[258]

The pathophysiologic consequences of coronary spasm are well understood. Severe spasm rapidly induces transmural ischemia, resulting in segmental dyskinesis and ST-segment elevation. If the ischemic zone is large, cardiac output and systemic arterial pressure decrease. The risk of serious ventricular arrhythmias increases with the severity and extent of ischemia. Prolonged spasm can induce intracoronary thrombosis, which may persist to cause myocardial infarction.[259]

Clinical Features

Variant angina is uncommon, and the presenting symptoms are usually not remarkable enough to be distinguished immediately from those of unstable angina. Angina at rest occurs with a cyclical pattern, often with attacks occurring in the early morning hours. Exertional angina coexists in slightly more than half these patients, but with an extremely variable ischemic thresh-

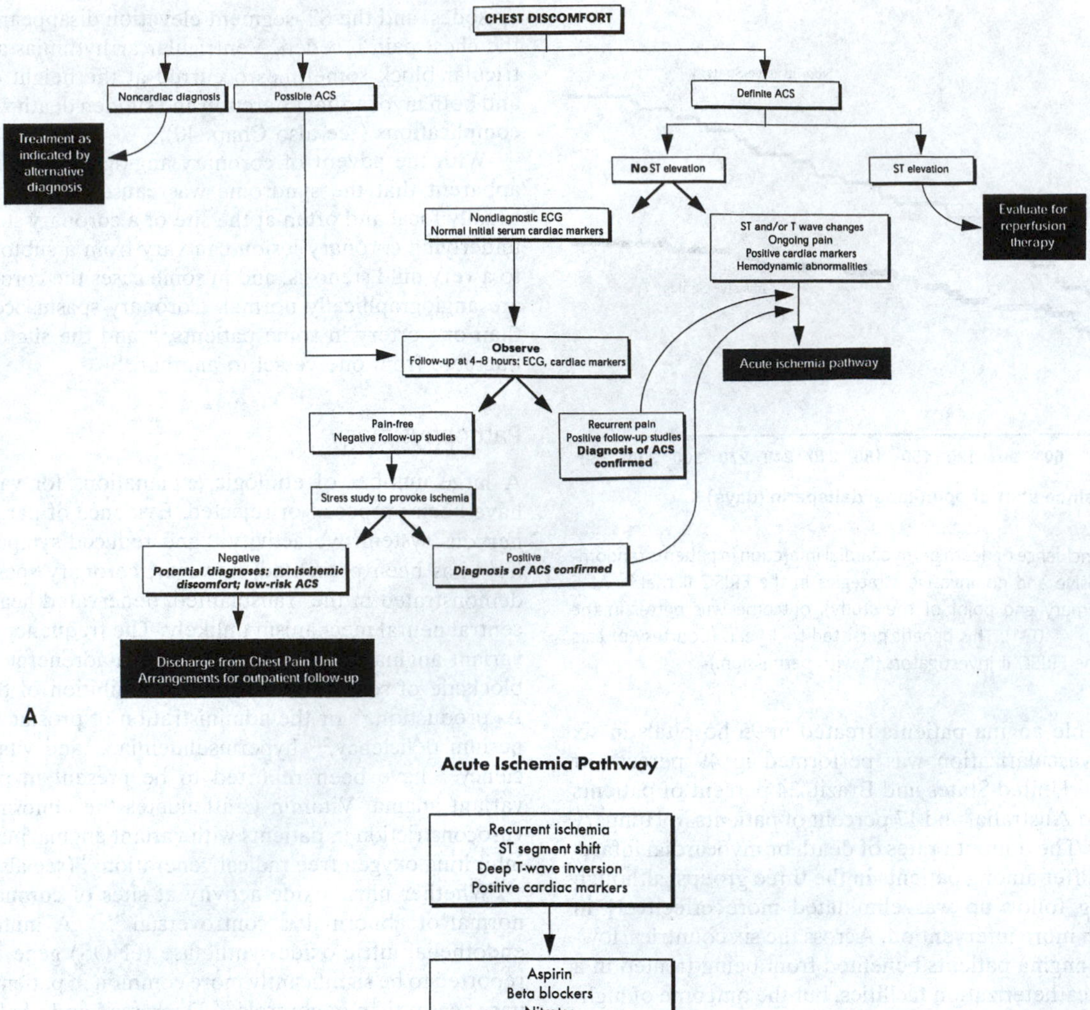

FIGURE 41-15 Algorithm for managing patients with chest discomfort suggestive of unstable angina (*panel A*). The acute ischemic pathway (*panel B*) includes patients with documented unstable angina. This generalized guideline must be adapted to each patient's specific circumstances. (Adapted from the ACC/AHA guidelines for the management of patients with unstable angina,[1] with permission.)

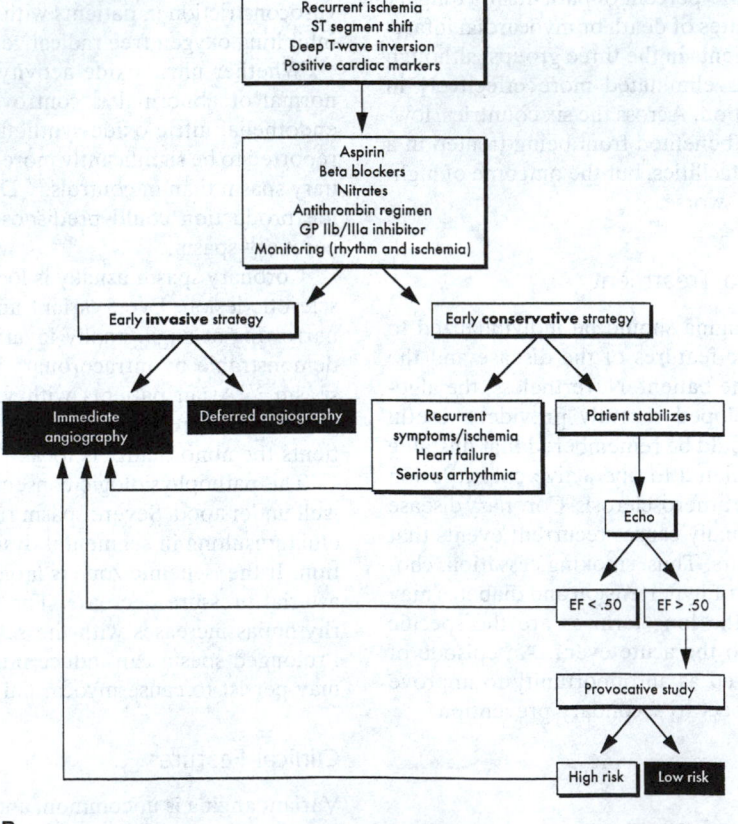

old.[260] Variant angina can appear during the recovery phase of myocardial infarction[261] or soon after coronary bypass surgery[262] or angioplasty.[263]

Most patients with variant angina are heavy cigarette smokers, but their age, sex, and risk factor profiles are otherwise similar to those of other coronary patients.[264] Those with angiographically normal coronary arteries tend to be younger and more often are women. One-quarter of variant angina patients have a history of migraine headaches, and one-quarter have symptoms of Raynaud's phenomenon.[265] Thus, in some cases variant angina may be part of a more generalized vasospastic diathesis. Syncope, presumably caused by ischemia-induced ventricular arrhythmia or atrioventricular block, during rest angina is a useful clue to the diagnosis. Rare cases of life-threatening ventricular arrhythmias caused by silent myocardial ischemia resulting from coronary spasm have been reported.[266,267]

Cocaine causes coronary vasoconstriction and can precipitate coronary spasm, sometimes with myocardial infarction. This topic is discussed in Chap. 71.

Physical examination of variant angina patients between attacks reveals no abnormalities. Routine laboratory tests, including cardiac enzymes, are normal.

Diagnostic Procedures

Variant angina can be diagnosed most easily by recording an ECG during an episode of rest angina. The ST-segment elevation that occurs during an attack disappears promptly after the administration of nitroglycerin. Coronary spasm can induce ST elevation, ST depression, or pseudonormalization of abnormally negative T waves (Fig. 41-16). When variant angina is suspected, ambulatory ECG monitoring or an event monitor sometimes can be useful to confirm the diagnosis. Exercise testing will provoke angina with ST elevation in approximately one-third of variant angina patients during an active phase of the disease.[268] This response to an exercise test often leads to the diagnosis of variant angina when it was not previously suspected. Provocative testing has been used to confirm the diagnosis of variant angina when a spontaneous attack cannot be documented. The cold pressor response, exercise, and hyperventilation are physiologic stimuli for coronary spasm, but each has a sensitivity that is too low to be useful clinically.[268] The pharmacologic agents ergonovine and acetylcholine provoke coronary spasm with a sensitivity of approximately 90 percent in patients with variant angina.[268,269] Intracoronary acetylcholine is probably the preferred method, but a temporary pacemaker must be placed before right coronary (or dominant left coronary) injections are done because of the high incidence of bradyarrhythmias and conduction disturbances from cholinergic effects in the atrioventricular node.

All patients with variant angina should undergo coronary angiography unless an absolute contraindication is present. Coronary angiography is the only certain method to distinguish between patients who have severe organic multivessel disease and those who have only mild narrowings or angiographically normal arteries.

Treatment

Variant angina is difficult to treat because attacks occur unpredictably and frequently without an obvious precipitating factor.

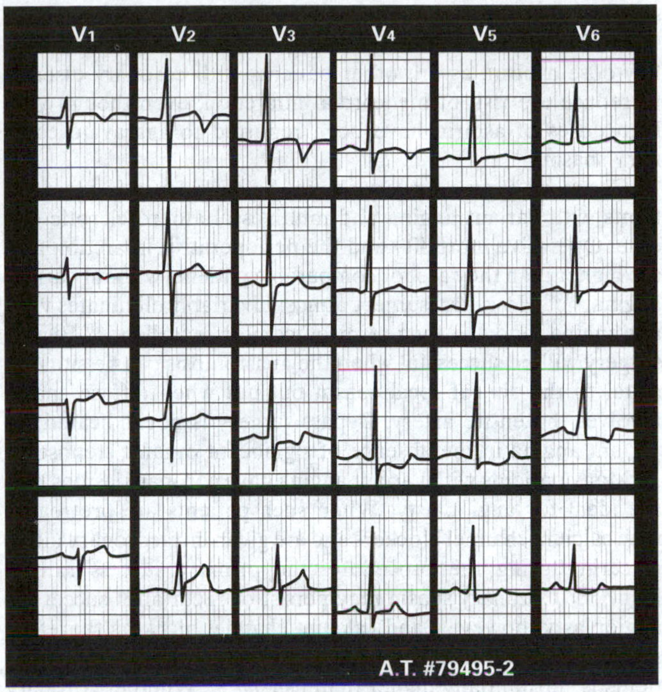

FIGURE 41-16 Electrocardiogram (leads V_1 to V_6) from a patient with active variant angina. Negative T waves are present in the control tracing (*top*). The other three tracings were recorded during separate episodes of rest angina and show pseudonormalization of T waves, ST depression, and ST elevation, respectively.

For the patient's well-being, the goal of therapy therefore should be the elimination of all attacks. Spontaneous remission is a common outcome,[270] but myocardial infarction is a common complication within the first 3 months of diagnosis, particularly in patients with underlying multivessel disease.[271] Nitroglycerin relieves variant angina attacks within minutes and should be used promptly. Long-acting nitrates are effective in preventing variant angina attacks, but the development of nitrate tolerance limits their utility. Beta-adrenergic blockers should not be used in variant angina patients because of their propensity to increase the frequency and duration of attacks.[141,142]

Calcium channel blockers are very effective in preventing attacks of variant angina.[272–275] More than half the patients treated with one of these drugs become completely asymptomatic. The response is better at higher doses, for example, long-acting nifedipine 80 mg/day, diltiazem 360 mg/day, verapamil 480 mg/day, or amlodipine 20 mg/day. The efficacy of these drugs in preventing variant angina is roughly equal. Patients with an incomplete response to one drug often become angina-free on a combination of nifedipine and either diltiazem or verapamil. Evidence from uncontrolled studies suggests that treatment with calcium channel blockers reduces the risk of myocardial infarction.[271,276]

Approximately 20 percent of variant angina patients will not respond to treatment with two calcium channel blockers plus a long-acting nitrate. Although not approved in the United States for this indication, amiodarone,[277] guanethidine,[278] and clonidine[278] have been reported to be effective in some of these refractory patients. Therapy for ventricular arrhythmias and conduction disturbances that complicate attacks in some cases should be directed toward the elimination of all episodes of spasm.[267] Patients with variant angina should be treated with low-dose aspirin, as are other patients with coronary disease, to reduce the risk of myocardial infarction, even though very high doses of aspirin have been reported to aggravate coronary spasm.[279]

Coronary bypass surgery should be considered in most patients with variant angina and multivessel atherosclerotic disease. Operative mortality and the perioperative infarction rate are higher than they are for comparable patients without variant angina.[280,281] However, surgery almost invariably eliminates variant angina, and the long-term outcome is excellent.[280] Bypass surgery will be successful when the anastomosis can be situated distal to the site of focal spasm but not when diffuse spasm involves the entire artery. Bypass surgery is not indicated for variant angina in the absence of significant organic stenoses.

Many patients with variant angina have coronary lesions that are ideal for angioplasty. When such patients are pretreated with calcium channel blockers and are given intracoronary nitroglycerin during the procedure, the primary success rate is high.[263,282] Coronary spasm may persist or recur after successful angioplasty, however, and calcium channel blockers therefore should be continued. The restenosis rate in variant angina patients is substantially higher than usual.[263,283] Whether coronary stenting improves outcomes for variant angina patients is not known. Coronary angioplasty is not indicated for patients with coronary spasm who have normal or nearly normal arteries on coronary angiography.

Prognosis

The long-term prognosis of variant angina has been reported for several large series of patients from different countries.[271,276,280,284] The extent and severity of the underlying coronary disease appear to be the most important factors influencing the outcome (Fig. 41-17). Survival without infarction at 1 year in a consecutive series of 217 patients was 93 percent for those without stenoses of 70 percent or more, 86 percent for patients with single-vessel disease, and 65 percent for those with multivessel disease.[271] At 5 years, the corresponding figures were 83 percent, 74 percent, and 44 percent, respectively. Other variables that correlate with a poor outcome include the presence of abnormal left ventricular function, ventricular arrhythmias during attacks, multivessel spasm, and the absence of treatment with calcium channel blockers. The majority of these patients will become angina-free within months or years.[270] Variant angina will recur in rare cases after a long asymptomatic interval. More commonly, patients will develop other manifestations of coronary disease. Some evidence indicates that recurrent coronary spasm accelerates the progression of coronary atherosclerosis, with a histologic pattern of neointimal hyperplasia that resembles restenosis.[285,286]

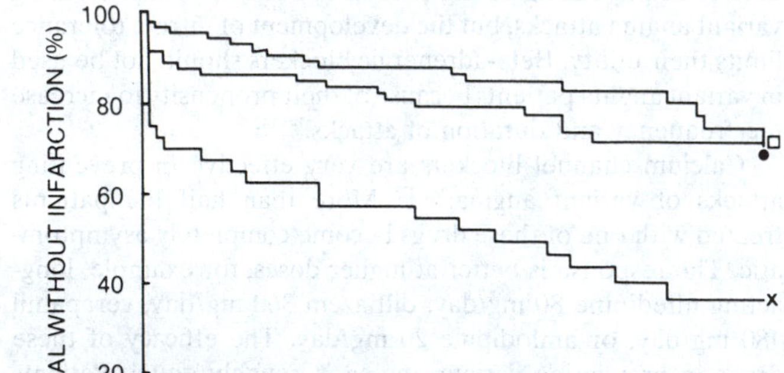

• < 70%	87	76	70	67	52	41	31	18
□ 1 VD	81	67	63	55	49	36	20	7
x 2-3 VD	40	26	22	22	18	13	9	5

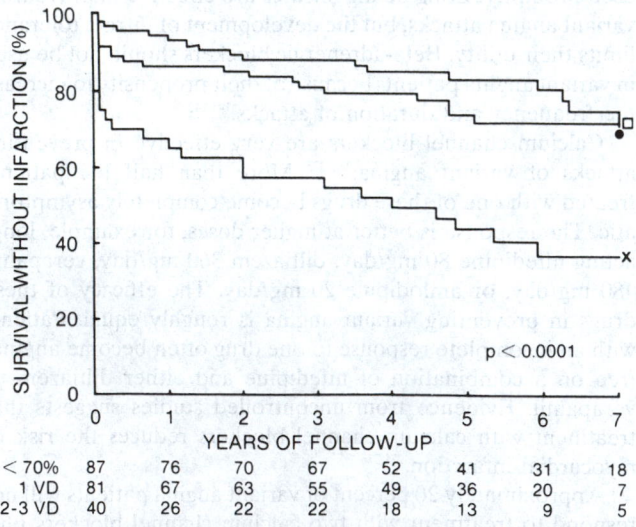

FIGURE 41-17 Survival without myocardial infarction in variant angina patients with no stenoses of 70 percent or more (●), those with one-vessel disease (□), and those with multivessel disease (x). The outcome in the latter group of patients is much worse than that in the other two groups. Events are clustered in the early follow-up period. (From Walling et al.,[271] with permission.)

References

1. Braunwald E, Antman EM, Beasley JW, et al. ACC/AHA guidelines for the management of patients with unstable angina and non–ST-segment elevation myocardial infarction. A report of the American College of Cardiology/American Heart Association Task Force on Practice Guidelines (Committee on the Management of Patients With Unstable Angina). *J Am Coll Cardiol* 2000; September.
2. Gazes PC, Mobley EM, Faris HM, et al. Preinfarctional (unstable) angina—a prospective study—ten year follow-up. *Circulation* 1973; 48:331–337.
3. Rizik DG, Healy S, Margulis A, et al. A new clinical classification for hospital prognosis of unstable angina. *Am J Cardiol* 1995; 75:993–997.
4. Braunwald E. Unstable angina: A classification. *Circulation* 1989; 80:410–414.
5. Ahmed WH, Bittl JA, Braunwald E. Relation between clinical presentation and angiographic findings in unstable angina pectoris, and comparison with that in stable angina. *Am J Cardiol* 1993; 72:544–550.
6. Van Miltenburg-van Zijl AJM, Simoons ML, Veerhoek RJ, Bossuyt PMM. Incidence and follow-up of Braunwald subgroups in unstable angina pectoris. *J Am Coll Cardiol* 1995; 25:1286–1292.
7. Lindenfeld J, Morrison DA. Toward a stable clinical classification of unstable angina. *J Am Coll Cardiol* 1995; 25:1293–1294.
8. Braunwald E. Unstable angina: An etiologic approach to management. *Circulation* 1998; 98:2219–2222.
9. Doucet S, Malekianpour M, Théroux P, et al. Randomized trial comparing intravenous nitroglycerin and heparin for treatment of unstable angina secondary to restenosis after coronary artery angioplasty. *Circulation* 2000; 101:955–961.
10. Waters DD, Walling A, Roy D, Théroux P. Previous coronary artery bypass grafting as an adverse prognostic factor in unstable angina pectoris. *Am J Cardiol* 1986; 58:465–469.
11. Chen L, Théroux P, Lespérance J, et al. Angiographic features of vein grafts versus ungrafted coronary arteries in patients with unstable angina and previous bypass surgery. *J Am Coll Cardiol* 1996; 28:1493–1499.
12. Braunwald E, Jones RH, Mark DB, et al. Diagnosing and managing unstable angina. *Circulation* 1994; 90:613–622.
13. Fuster V, Fayal ZA, Badimon JJ. Acute coronary syndromes: Biology. *Lancet* 1999; 353(suppl II):5–9.
14. Davies MJ, Richardson PD, Woolf N, et al. Risk of thrombosis in human atherosclerotic plaques: Role of extracellular lipid, macrophages, and smooth muscle content. *Br Heart J* 1993; 69:377–381.

15. Davies MJ. Stability and instability: Two faces of coronary atherosclerosis. *Circulation* 1996; 94:2013–2020.
16. Farb A, Burke AP, Tang AL, et al. Coronary plaque erosion without rupture into a lipid core: A frequent cause or coronary thrombosis in sudden coronary death. *Circulation* 1996; 93:1354–1363.
17. Burke AP, Farb A, Malcom GT, et al. Coronary risk factors and plaque morphology in men with coronary disease who die suddenly. *N Engl J Med* 1997; 336:1276–1282.
18. Burke AP, Farb A, Malcom GT, et al. Effect of risk factors on the mechanism of acute thrombosis and sudden coronary death in women. *Circulation* 1998; 97:2110–2116.
19. Sato T, Takebayashi S, Kohehi K. Increased subendothelial infiltration of the coronary arteries with monocytes/macrophages in patients with unstable angina. *Atherosclerosis* 1995; 68:191–197.
20. Mazzone A, De Servi S, Ricevuti G, et al. Increased expression of neutrophil and monocyte adhesion molecules in unstable coronary artery disease. *Circulation* 1993; 88:358–363.
21. Libby P. Molecular basis of acute coronary syndromes. *Circulation* 1995; 91:2844–2850.
22. Kai H, Ikeda H, Yasukawa H, et al. Peripheral blood levels of matrix metalloproteinases-2 and -9 are elevated in patients with acute coronary syndromes. *J Am Coll Cardiol* 1998; 32:368–372.
23. Brown DL, Hibbs MS, Kearney M, et al. Identification of 92-kD gelatinase in human coronary atherosclerotic lesions: Association of active enzyme synthesis with unstable angina. *Circulation* 1995; 91:2125–2131.
24. Ritchie ME. Nuclear factor-κB is selectively and markedly activated in humans with unstable angina pectoris. *Circulation* 1998; 98:1707–1713.
25. Van der Wall AC, Becer AE, van der Loos CM, Das PK. Site of intimal rupture or erosion of thrombosed coronary atherosclerotic plaques is characterized by an inflammatory process irrespective of dominant plaque morphology. *Circulation* 1994; 89:36–44.
26. Kaartinen M, van der Wal AC, van der Loos CM, et al. Mast cell infiltration in acute coronary syndromes: Implications for plaque rupture. *J Am Coll Cardiol* 1998; 32:606–612.
27. Berk BC, Weintraub WS, Alexander RW. Elevation of C-reactive protein in "active" coronary artery disease. *Am J Cardiol* 1990; 65:168–172.
28. Liuzzo G, Biasucci LM, Gallimore JR, et al. The prognostic value of C-reactive protein and serum amyloid A protein in severe unstable angina. *N Engl J Med* 1994; 331:417–424.
29. Haverkate F, Thompson SG, Pyke SDM, et al., for the European Concerted Action on Thrombosis and Disabilities Angina Pectoris Study Group. Production of C-reactive protein and risk of coronary events in stable and unstable angina. *Lancet* 1997; 349:462–466.
30. Biasucci LM, Vitelli A, Liuzzo G, et al. Elevated levels of interleukin-6 in unstable angina. *Circulation* 1996; 94:874–877.
31. Biasucci LM, Liuzzo G, Fantuzzi G, et al. Increasing levels of interleukin (IL)-1Ra and IL-6 during the first 2 days of hospitalization in unstable angina are associated with increased risk of in-hospital coronary events. *Circulation* 1999; 99:2079–2084.
32. Ross R. Atherosclerosis—an inflammatory disease. *N Engl J Med* 1999; 340:115–126.
33. Libby P, Egan D, Skarlatos S. Roles of infectious agents in atherosclerosis and restenosis: An assessment of the evidence and need for future research. *Circulation* 1997; 96:4095–4103.
34. Ridker PM. Inflammation, infection and cardiovascular risk: How good is the evidence? *Circulation* 1998; 97:1671–1674.
35. Kol A, Sukhova GK, Lichtman AH, Libby P. Chlamydial heat shock protein 60 localizes in human atheroma and regulates macrophage tumor necrosis factor-α and matrix metalloproteinase expression. *Circulation* 1998; 98:300–307.
36. Mayr M, Metzler B, Kiechl S, et al. Endothelial cytotoxicity mediated by serum antibodies to heat shock proteins of *Escherichia coli* and *Chlamydia pneumoniae:* Immune reactions to heat shock proteins as a possible link between infection and atherosclerosis. *Circulation* 1999; 99:1560–1566.
37. Strachan DP, Mendall MA, Carrington D, et al. Relation of *Helicobacter pylori* infection to 13-year mortality and incident ischemic heart disease in the Caerphilly Prospective Heart Disease Study. *Circulation* 1998; 98:1286–1290.
38. Ridker PM, Hennekens CH, Stampfer MJ, Wang F. Prospective study of herpes simplex virus, cytomegalovirus, and the risk of future myocardial infarction and stroke. *Circulation* 1998; 98:2796–2799.
39. Gupta S, Leatham EW, Carrington D, et al. Elevated *Chlamydia pneumoniae* antibodies, cardiovascular events, and azithromycin in male survivors of myocardial infarction. *Circulation* 1997; 96:404–407.
40. Anderson JL, Muhlestein JB, Carlquist J, et al. Randomized secondary prevention trial of azithromycin in patients with coronary artery disease and serological evidence for *Chlamydia pneumoniae* infection: The Azithromycin in Coronary Artery Disease: Elimination of Myocardial Infection with Chlamydia (ACADEMIC) Study. *Circulation* 1999; 99:1540–1547.
41. Gurfinkel E, Bozovich G, Daroca A, et al., for the ROXIS Study Group. Randomized trial of roxithromycin in non-Q-wave coronary syndromes: ROXIS pilot study. *Lancet* 1997; 350:404–407.
42. Davies M, Bland J, Hangartner J, et al. Factors influencing the presence or absence of acute coronary artery thrombi in sudden ischemic death. *Eur Heart J* 1989; 10:203–208.
43. Fernàndez-Ortiz A, Badimon JJ, Falk E, et al. Characterization of the relative thrombogenicity of atherosclerotic plaque components: Implications for consequences of plaque rupture. *J Am Coll Cardiol* 1994; 23:1562–1569.
44. Furman MI, Benoit SE, Barnard MR, et al. Increased platelet reactivity and circulating monocyte-platelet aggregates in patients with stable coronary artery disease. *J Am Coll Cardiol* 1998; 31:352–358.
45. Davi G, Gresele P, Violi F, et al. Diabetes mellitus, hypercholesterolemia, and hypertension but not vascular disease per se are associated with persistent platelet activation in vivo: Evidence derived from the study of peripheral arterial disease. *Circulation* 1997; 96:69–75.
46. Diodati JG, Dakak N, Gilligan DM, Quyyumi AA. Effect of atherosclerosis on endothelium-dependent inhibition of platelet activation in humans. *Circulation* 1998; 98:17–24.
47. Fitzgerald DJ, Roy L, Catella F, Fitzgerald A. Platelet activation in unstable coronary disease. *N Engl J Med* 1986; 315:983–989.
48. Grande P, Grauholt AM, Madsen JK. Unstable angina pectoris: Platelet behavior and prognosis in progressive angina and intermediate coronary syndrome. *Circulation* 1990; 81(suppl I):I-16–I-19.
49. Hamm CW, Lorenz RL, Bleifeld W, et al. Biochemical evidence of platelet activation in patients with persistent unstable angina. *J Am Coll Cardiol* 1987; 10:998–1004.
50. Freedman JE, Ting B, Hankin B, et al. Impaired platelet production of nitric oxide predicts presence of acute coronary syndromes. *Circulation* 1998; 98:1481–1486.
51. Ikeda H, Takajo Y, Ichiki K, et al. Increased soluble form of P-selectin in patients with unstable angina. *Circulation* 1995; 92:1693–1696.
52. Ott I, Neumann FJ, Gawaz M, et al. Increased neutrophil-platelet adhesion in patients with unstable angina. *Circulation* 1996; 94:1239–1246.
53. De Servi S, Mazzone A, Ricevuti G, et al. Clinical and angiographic correlates of leukocyte activation in unstable angina. *J Am Coll Cardiol* 1995; 26:1146–1150.

54. Neri Seneri GG, Abbate R, Gori AM, et al. Transient intermittent lymphocyte activation is responsible for the instability of angina. *Circulation* 1992; 86:790–797.
55. Jude B, Agraou B, McFadden EP, et al. Evidence for time-dependent activation of monocytes in the systemic circulation in unstable angina but not in acute myocardial infarction or in stable angina. *Circulation* 1994; 90:1662–1668.
56. Biasucci L, Liuzzo G, Caligiuri G, et al. Temporal relation between ischemic episodes and activation of the coagulation system in unstable angina. *Circulation* 1996; 93:2121–2127.
57. Toschi V, Gallo R, Lettino M, et al. Tissue factor modulates the thrombogenicity of human atherosclerotic plaques. *Circulation* 1997; 95:594–599.
58. Badimon JJ, Lettino M, Toschi V, et al. Local inhibition of tissue factor reduces the thrombogenicity of disrupted human atherosclerotic plaques: Effects of tissue factor pathway inhibitor on plaque thrombogenicity under flow conditions. *Circulation* 1999; 99:1780–1787.
59. Moreno PR, Bernardi VH, López-Cuéllar J, et al. Macrophages, smooth muscle cells, and tissue factor in unstable angina: Implications for cell-mediated thrombogenicity in acute coronary syndromes. *Circulation* 1996; 94:3090–3097.
60. Soejima H, Ogawa H, Yasue H, et al. Heightened tissue factor associated with tissue factor pathway inhibitor and prognosis in patients with unstable angina. *Circulation* 1999; 99:2908–2913.
61. Hoffmeister HM, Jur M, Wendal HP, et al. Alterations of coagulation and fibrinolytic and kallikrein-kinin systems in the acute and postacute phases in patients with unstable angina pectoris. *Circulation* 1995; 91:2520–2527.
62. Bogaty P, Hackett D, Davies G, Maseri A. Vasoreactivity of the culprit lesion in unstable angina. *Circulation* 1994; 90:5–11.
63. Zeiher A, Goebel H, Schächinger V, Ihling C. Tissue endothelin-1 immunoreactivity in the active coronary atherosclerotic plaque: A clue to the mechanism of increased vasoreactivity of the culprit lesion in unstable angina. *Circulation* 1995; 91:941–947.
64. Lam JYT, Chesebro JH, Steele PM, et al. Is vasospasm related to platelet deposition? In vivo relationship in a pig model of arterial injury. *Circulation* 1987; 75:243–248.
65. Moise A, Théroux P, Taeymans Y, et al. Unstable angina and progression of coronary atherosclerosis. *N Engl J Med* 1983; 309:685–689.
66. Falk E, Shah PK, Fuster V. Coronary plaque disruption. *Circulation* 1995; 92:657–671.
67. Ledru F, Théroux P, Lespérance J, et al. Geometric features of coronary artery lesions favoring acute occlusion and myocardial infarction: A quantitative angiographic study. *J Am Coll Cardiol* 1999; 33:1353–1361.
68. Ambrose JA, Winters SL, Stern A, et al. Angiographic morphology and the pathogenesis of unstable angina pectoris. *J Am Coll Cardiol* 1985; 5:609–616.
69. Sherman CT, Litvack F, Grundfest W, et al. Coronary angioscopy in patients with unstable angina pectoris. *N Engl J Med* 1986; 315:913–919.
70. De Feyter PJ, Ozaki Y, Baptista J, et al. Ischemia-related lesion characteristics in patients with stable or unstable angina: A study with intracoronary angioscopy and ultrasound. *Circulation* 1995; 92:1408–1413.
71. Chen L, Chester MR, Redwood S, et al. Angiographic stenosis progression and coronary events in patients with "stabilized" unstable angina. *Circulation* 1995; 91:2319–2324.
72. Chen L, Chester MR, Crook R, Kaski JC. Differential progression of complex culprit stenoses in patients with stable and unstable angina pectoris. *J Am Coll Cardiol* 1996; 28:597–603.
73. Pozen MW, D'Agostino RB, Selker HP, et al. A predictive instrument to improve coronary-care-unit admission practices in acute ischemic heart disease: A prospective multicenter clinical trial. *N Engl J Med* 1984; 310:1273–1278.
74. Lee TH, Cook EF, Weisberg M, et al. Acute chest pain in the emergency room: Identification and examination of low-risk patients. *Arch Intern Med* 1985; 145:65–69.
75. Hochman J, Tamis JE, Thompson TD, et al., for the Global Use of Strategies to Open Occluded Coronary Arteries in Acute Coronary Syndromes IIb investigators. Sex, clinical presentation and outcomes in patients with acute coronary syndromes. *N Engl J Med* 1999; 341:226–232.
76. Haines DE, Raabe DS, Gundel WD, Wackers FJT. Anatomic and prognostic significance of new T-wave inversion in unstable angina. *Am J Cardiol* 1983; 52:14–18.
77. Renkin J, Wijns W, Ladha Z, Col J. Reversal of segmental hypokinesis by coronary angioplasty in patients with unstable angina, persistent T wave inversion, and left anterior descending coronary artery stenosis: Additional evidence for myocardial stunning in humans. *Circulation* 1990; 82:913–921.
78. De Zwaan C, Bär FW, Janssen JHA, et al. Angiographic and clinical characteristics of patients with unstable angina showing an ECG pattern indicating critical narrowing of the proximal LAD coronary artery. *Am Heart J* 1989; 117:657–664.
79. Cannon CP, McCabe CH, Stone PH, et al., for the TIMI III Registry ECG Ancillary Study investigators. The electrocardiogram predicts one-year outcome of patients with unstable angina and non-Q wave myocardial infarction: Results of the TIMI III Registry ECG Ancillary Study. *J Am Coll Cardiol* 1997; 30: 133–140.
80. Ohman EM, Armstrong PW, Christenson RH, et al., for the GUSTO-IIa investigators. Cardiac troponin T levels for risk stratification in acute myocardial ischemia. *N Engl J Med* 1996; 335:1333–1341.
81. Patel DJ, Knight CJ, Holdwright DR, et al. Long-term prognosis in unstable angina: The importance of early risk stratification using continuous ST segment monitoring. *Eur Heart J* 1998; 19:240–249.
82. Nørgaard BL, Andersen K, Dellborg M, et al., for the TRIM study group. Admission risk assessment by cardiac troponin T in unstable coronary artery disease: Additional prognostic information from continuous ST segment monitoring. *J Am Coll Cardiol* 1999; 33:1519–1527.
83. Armstrong PW, Chiong MA, Parker JO. The spectrum of unstable angina: Prognostic role of serum creatine kinase determination. *Am J Cardiol* 1982; 49:1849–1852.
84. Lindahl B, Venge P, Wallentin L, for the FRISC Study Group. Relation between troponin T and the risk of subsequent cardiac events in unstable coronary artery disease. *Circulation* 1996; 93:1651–1657.
85. Antman EM, Tanasijevic MJ, Thompson B, et al. Cardiac specific troponin I levels to predict the risk of mortality in patients with acute coronary syndromes. *N Engl J Med* 1996; 335:1342–1349.
86. Lüscher MS, Thygesen K, Ravkilde J, Heickendorff L, for the TRIM Study Group. Applicability of cardiac troponin T and I for early risk stratification in unstable coronary artery disease. *Circulation* 1997; 96:2578–2585.
87. Galvani M, Ottani F, Ferrini D, et al. Prognostic influence of elevated values of cardiac troponin I in patients with unstable angina. *Circulation* 1997; 95:2053–2059.
88. Olatidoye AG, Wu AHB, Feng YJ, Waters D. Prognostic role of troponin T versus troponin I in unstable angina pectoris for cardiac events with meta-analysis comparing published studies. *Am J Cardiol* 1998; 81:1405–1410.
89. Muller-Bardorff M, Freitag H, Scheffold T, et al. Development and characterization of a rapid assay for bedside determinations of cardiac troponin T. *Circulation* 1995; 92:2869–2875.
90. Antman EM, Sacks DB, Rifai N, et al. Time to positivity of

a rapid bedside assay for cardiac-specific troponin T predicts prognosis in acute coronary syndromes: A Thrombolysis in Myocardial Infarction (TIMI) 11A substudy. *J Am Coll Cardiol* 1998; 31:326–330.

91. Zimmerman J, Fromm R, Meyer D, et al. Diagnostic marker cooperative study for the diagnosis of myocardial infarction. *Circulation* 1999; 99:1671–1677.
92. Davies MJ, Thomas AC, Knapman PA, Hangartner JR. Intramyocardial platelet aggregation in patients with unstable angina suffering sudden ischemic cardiac death. *Circulation* 1985; 73: 418–427.
93. Bilodeau L, Théroux P, Gregoire J, et al. Technetium-99m sestamibi tomography in patients with spontaneous chest pain: Correlations with clinical, electrocardiographic and angiographic findings. *J Am Coll Cardiol* 1991; 18:1684–1691.
94. Hilton TC, Thompson RC, Williams HJ, et al. Technetium-99m sestamibi myocardial perfusion imaging in the emergency room evaluation of chest pain. *J Am Coll Cardiol* 1994; 23:1016–1022.
95. Varetto T, Cantalupi D, Altieri A, Orlandi C. Emergency room technetium-99m sestamibi imaging to rule out acute myocardial ischemic events in patients with nondiagnostic electrocardiograms. *J Am Coll Cardiol* 1993; 22:1804–1808.
96. Kontos MC, Jesse RL, Schmidt KL, et al. Value of actue rest sestamibi perfusion imaging for evaluation of patients admitted to the emergency department with chest pain. *J Am Coll Cardiol* 1997; 30:976–982.
97. Azar RR, Fram DB, Fossati AT, et al. How long do Tc-99m-sestamibi myocardial perfusion defects last after resolution of acute ischemia? An angioplasty model (abstract). *Circulation* 1997; 96:(suppl I):I-309.
98. Gaspoz J, Lee TH, Weinstein MC, et al. Cost effectiveness of a new short-stay unit to "rule out" acute myocardial infarction in low risk patients. *J Am Coll Cardiol* 1994; 24:1249–1259.
99. Gomez MA, Anderson JL, Karagounis LA, et al., for the ROMIO Study Group. An emergency department-based protocol for rapidly ruling out myocardial ischemia reduces hospital time and expense: Results of a randomized study (ROMIO). *J Am Coll Cardiol* 1996; 28:25–33.
100. Graff LG, Dallara J, Ross MA, et al. Impact on the care of the emergency department chest pain patient from the Chest Pain Evaluation Registry (CHEPER) Study. *Am J Cardiol* 1997; 80:563–568.
101. Goldman L, Cook EF, Johnson PA, et al. Prediction of the need for intensive care in patients who come to emergency departments with acute chest pain. *N Engl J Med* 1996; 334:1498–1504.
102. Farkouh ME, Smars PA, Reeder GS, et al., for the Chest Pain Evaluation in the Emergency Room (CHEER) Investigators. A clinical trial of a chest-pain observation unit for patients with unstable angina. *N Engl J Med* 1998; 339:1882–1888.
103. Bugiardini R, Borghi A, Pozzati A, et al. Relation of severity of symptoms to transient myocardial ischemia and prognosis in unstable angina. *J Am Coll Cardiol* 1995; 25:597–604.
104. Newby LK, Christenson RH, Ohman EM, et al., for the GUSTO-IIa Investigators. Value of serial troponin T measures for early and late risk stratification in patients with acute coronary syndromes. *Circulation* 1998; 98:1853–1859.
105. Polanczyk CA, Lee TH, Cook EF, et al. Cardiac troponin I as a predictor of major cardiac events in emergency department patients with acute chest pain. *J Am Coll Cardiol* 1998; 32:8–14.
106. Lindahl B, Venge P, Wallentin L, for the Fragmin in Unstable Coronary Artery Disease (FRISC) Study Group. Troponin T identifies patients with unstable coronary artery disease who benefit from long-term antithrombotic protection. *J Am Coll Cardiol* 1997; 29:43–48.
107. Morrow DA, Rifai N, Antman EM, et al. C-reactive protein is a potent predictor of mortality independently of and in combination with troponin T in acute coronary syndromes: A TIMI 11A substudy: Thrombolysis in Myocardial Infarction. *J Am Coll Cardiol* 1998; 31:1460–1465.
108. Ardissino D, Merlini PA, Gamba G, et al. Thrombin activity and early outcome in unstable angina pectoris. *Circulation* 1996; 93:1634–1639.
109. Becker RC, Cannon CP, Bovill EG, et al., for the TIMI III investigators. Prognostic value of plasma fibrinogen concentration in patients with unstable angina and non-Q-wave myocardial infarction (TIMI IIIB Trial). *Am J Cardiol* 1996; 78:142–147.
110. Montalescot G, Philippe F, Ankri A, et al., for the French investigators in the ESSENCE trial. Early increase of von Willebrand factor predicts adverse outcome in unstable coronary artery disease: Beneficial effects of enoxaparin. *Circulation* 1998; 98:294–299.
111. Swahn E, Areskog M, Berglund U, et al. Predictive importance of clinical findings and a predischarge exercise test in patients with suspected unstable coronary artery disease. *Am J Cardiol* 1987; 59:208–214.
112. Wilcox I, Freedman SB, Allman KC, et al. Prognostic significance of a predischarge exercise test in risk stratification after unstable angina pectoris. *J Am Coll Cardiol* 1991; 18:677–683.
113. Brown KA. Prognostic value of thallium-201 myocardial perfusion imaging in patients with unstable angina who respond to medical treatment. *J Am Coll Cardiol* 1991; 17:1053–1057.
114. Stratmann HG, Younis LT, Wittry MD, et al. Exercise technetium-99m myocardial tomography for risk stratification of men with medically treated unstable angina pectoris. *Am J Cardiol* 1995; 76:236–240.
115. Freeman MR, Chisholm RJ, Armstrong PW. Usefulness of exercise electrocardiography and thallium scintigraphy in unstable angina pectoris in predicting the extent and severity of coronary artery disease. *Am J Cardiol* 1988; 62:1164–1170.
116. Polanczyk CA, Johnson PA, Hartley LH, et al. Clinical correlates and prognostic significance of early negative exercise tolerance test in patients with acute chest pain seen in the hospital emergency department. *Am J Cardiol* 1998; 81:288–292.
117. Alison HW, Russell RO, Mantle JA, et al. Coronary anatomy and arteriography in patients with unstable angina pectoris. *Am J Cardiol* 1978; 41:204–209.
118. Ouyang P, Brinker JA, Mellits ED, et al. Variables predictive of successful medical therapy in patients with unstable angina: Selection by multivariate analysis from clinical, electrocardiographic, and angiographic evaluations. *Circulation* 1984; 70: 367–376.
119. Russell RO, Moraski RE, Kouchoukos N, et al. Unstable angina pectoris: National cooperative study group to compare medical and surgical therapy: II. In-hospital experience and initial follow-up results in patients with one, two and three vessel disease. *Am J Cardiol* 1978; 42:839–848.
120. Luchi RJ, Scott SM, Dupree RH, and the principal investigators and their associates of Veterans Administration Cooperative Study No. 28. Comparison of medical and surgical therapy for unstable angina pectoris. *N Engl J Med* 1987; 316:977–984.
121. Yusuf S, Zucker D, Peduzzi P, et al. Effect of coronary artery bypass graft surgery on survival: Overview of 10-year results from randomised trials by the Coronary Artery Bypass Graft Surgery Trialists Collaboration. *Lancet* 1994; 344:563–570.
122. Diver DJ, Bier JD, Ferreira PE, et al., for the TIMI-IIIA Investigators. Clinical and arteriographic characterization of patients with unstable angina without critical coronary arterial narrowing (from the TIMI-IIIA Trial). *Am J Cardiol* 1994; 74:531–537.
123. Holmvang L, Lüscher MS, Clemmensen P, et al., and the TRIM study group. Very early risk stratification using combined ECG and biochemical assessment in patients with unstable coronary artery disease (a Thrombin Inhibition in Myocardial Ischemia [TRIM] substudy). *Circulation* 1998; 98:2004–2009.

124. Van Domburg RT, van Miltenburg-van Zihl AJ, Veerhoek RJ, Simoons ML. Unstable angina: Good long-term outcome after complicated early course. *J Am Coll Cardiol* 1988; 31:1534–1539.
125. Betriu A, Heras M, Cohen M, Fuster V. Unstable angina: Outcome according to clinical presentation. *J Am Coll Cardiol* 1992; 19:1659–1663.
126. Armstrong PW, Fu Y, Chang WC, et al., for the GUSTO-IIb investigators. Acute coronary syndromes in the GUSTO-IIb trial: Prognostic insights and impact of recurrent ischemia. *Circulation* 1998; 98:1860–1868.
127. Kaplan K, Davison R, Parker M, et al. Intravenous nitroglycerin for the treatment of angina at rest unresponsive to standard nitrate therapy. *Am J Cardiol* 1983; 51:694–698.
128. Curman GD, Heinsimer JA, Lozner EC, Fung HL. Intravenous nitroglycerin in the treatment of spontaneous angina pectoris: A prospective, randomized trial. *Circulation* 1983; 67:276–282.
129. Brown BG, Bolson E, Petersen RB, et al. The mechanisms of nitroglycerin action: Stenosis vasodilatation as a major component of the drug response. *Circulation* 1981; 64:1089–1097.
130. Harrison DG, Bates JN. The nitrovasodilators: New ideas about old drugs. *Circulation* 1993; 87:1461–1467.
131. Abrams J. Tolerance to organic nitrates. *Circulation* 1986; 74:1181–1185.
132. Pepine CJ, Lopez LM, Bell DM, et al., for the TIDES-II investigators. Effects of intermittent transdermal nitroglycerin on occurrence of ischemia after patch removal: Results of the Second Transdermal Intermittent Dosing Evaluation Study (TIDES-II). *J Am Coll Cardiol* 1997; 30:955–961.
133. Figueras J, Lidon R, Cortadellas J. Rebound myocardial ischemia following abrupt interruption of intravenous nitroglycerin infusion in patients with unstable angina at rest. *Eur Heart J* 1991; 12:405–411.
134. Ardissino D, Merlini PA, Savonitto S, et al. Effect of transdermal nitroglycerin or N-acetylcysteine, or both, in the long-term treatment of unstable angina pectoris. *J Am Coll Cardiol* 1997; 29:941–947.
135. Stamler JS, Loscalzo J. The antiplatelet effects of organic nitrates and related nitroso compounds in vitro and in vivo and their relevance to cardiovascular disorders. *J Am Coll Cardiol* 1991; 18:1529–1536.
136. Diodati J, Théroux P, Latour JG, et al. Effects of nitroglycerin at therapeutic doses on platelet aggregation in unstable angina pectoris and acute myocardial infarction. *Am J Cardiol* 1990; 66:683–688.
137. Johnstone MT, Lam JYT, Lacoste L, et al. Methylene blue inhibits the antithrombotic effect of nitroglycerin. *J Am Coll Cardiol* 1993; 21:255–259.
138. Hébert D, Xiang JX, Lam JYT. Persistent inhibition of platelets during continuous nitroglycerin therapy despite hemodynamic tolerance. *Circulation* 1997; 95:1308–1311.
139. Cannom DS, Harrison DC, Schroeder JS. Hemodynamic observations in patients with unstable angina pectoris. *Am J Cardiol* 1974; 33:17–22.
140. Figueras J, Cinca J. Acute arterial hypertension during spontaneous angina in patients with fixed coronary stenosis and exertional angina: An associated rather than a triggering phenomenon. *Circulation* 1981; 64:60–68.
141. Robertson RM, Wood AJJ, Vaughn WK, Robertson D. Exacerbation of vasotonic angina by propranolol. *Circulation* 1982; 65:281–285.
142. Tilmant PY, Lablanche JM, Thieuleux FA, et al. Detrimental effect of propranolol in patients with coronary arterial spasm countered by combination with diltiazem. *Am J Cardiol* 1983; 52:230–233.
143. Muller JE, Turi ZG, Pearle DL, et al. Nifedipine and conventional therapy for unstable angina pectoris: A randomized, double-blind comparison. *Circulation* 1984; 69:728–739.
144. Gottlieb SO, Weisfeldt ML, Ouyang P, et al. Effect of the addition of propranolol to therapy with nifedipine for unstable angina pectoris: A randomized, double-blind, placebo-controlled trial. *Circulation* 1986; 73:331–337.
145. Théroux P, Taeymans Y, Morissette D, et al. A randomized study comparing propranolol and diltiazem in the treatment of unstable angina. *J Am Coll Cardiol* 1985; 5:717–722.
146. Andre-Fouet X, Usdin JP, Gayet C, et al. Comparison of short-term efficacy of diltiazem and propranolol in unstable angina at rest—A randomized trial in 70 patients. *Eur Heart J* 1983; 4:691–698.
147. Report of the Holland Interuniversity Nifedipine/Metoprolol Trial (HINT) Research Group. Early treatment of unstable angina in the coronary care unit: A randomised, double blind, placebo controlled comparison of recurrent ischaemia in patients treated with nifedipine or metoprolol or both. *Br Heart J* 1986; 56:400–413.
148. Yusuf S, Wittes J, Friedman L. Overview of results of randomized clinical trials in heart disease: II. Unstable angina, heart failure, primary prevention with aspirin, and risk factor modification. *JAMA* 1988; 260:2259–2263.
149. Waters D. Proischemic complications of dihydropyridine calcium channel blockers. *Circulation* 1991; 84:2598–2600.
150. Gerstenblith G, Ouyang P, Achuff SC, et al. Nifedipine in unstable angina: A double-blind, randomized trial. *N Engl J Med* 1982; 306:885–889.
151. Muller JE, Morrison J, Stone PH, et al. Nifedipine therapy for patients with threatened and acute myocardial infarction: A randomized, double-blind, placebo-controlled comparison. *Circulation* 1984; 69:740–747.
152. Blaustein AS, Heller GV, Kolman BS. Adjunctive nifedipine therapy in high-risk, medically refractory, unstable angina pectoris. *Am J Cardiol* 1983; 52:950–954.
153. Fang ZY, Picart N, Abramowicz M, et al. Intravenous diltiazem versus nitroglycerin for silent and symptomatic myocardial ischemia in unstable angina pectoris. *Am J Cardiol* 1991; 68: 42C–46C.
154. Göbel EJAM, Hautvast RWM, van Gilst WH, et al. Randomized, double-blind trial of intravenous diltiazem versus glyceryl trinitrate for unstable angina pectoris. *Lancet* 1995; 346:1653–1657.
155. Parodi O, Maseri A, Simonetti I. Management of unstable angina by verapamil: A double-blind crossover study in CCU. *Br Heart J* 1979; 41:167–174.
156. Mehta J, Pepine CJ, Day M, et al. Short-term efficacy of oral verapamil in rest angina: A double-blind controlled trial in CCU patients. *Am J Med* 1981; 71:977–982.
157. Scheidt S, Frishman WH, Packer M, et al. Long-term effectiveness of verapamil in stable and unstable pectoris: One-year follow-up of patients treated in placebo-controlled double blind randomized clinical trials. *Am J Cardiol* 1982; 50:1185–1190.
158. Parodi O, Simonetti I, Michelassi C, et al. Comparison of verapamil and propranolol therapy for angina pectoris at rest: A randomized, multiple-crossover, controlled trial in the coronary care unit. *Am J Cardiol* 1986; 57:899–906.
159. Capucci A, Bassein L, Bracchetti D, et al. Propranolol v. verapamil in the treatment of unstable angina: A double-blind crossover study. *Eur Heart J* 1983; 4:148–154.
160. Grambow DW, Topol EJ. Effect of maximal medical therapy on refractoriness of unstable angina pectoris. *Am J Cardiol* 1992; 70:577–581.
161. Levine FH, Gold HK, Leinbach RC, et al. Management of acute myocardial ischemia with intraaortic balloon pumping and coronary bypass surgery. *Circulation* 1978; 58:(suppl I): I-69–I-72.
162. Husain S, Andrews NP, Mulcahy D, et al. Aspirin improves

endothelial dysfunction in atherosclerosis. *Circulation* 1998; 97: 716–720.

163. Lewis HD, Davis JW, Archibald DG, et al. Protective effects of aspirin against acute myocardial infarction and death in men with unstable angina. *N Engl J Med* 1983; 309:396–403.
164. Cairns JA, Gent M, Singer J, et al. Aspirin, sulfinpyrazone, or both in unstable angina: Results of a Canadian multicenter trial. *N Engl J Med* 1985; 313:1369–1375.
165. Théroux P, Ouimet H, McCans J, et al. Aspirin, heparin, or both to treat unstable angina. *N Engl J Med* 1988; 319:1105–1111.
166. RISC Group. Risk of myocardial infarction and death during treatment with low dose aspirin and intravenous heparin in men with unstable coronary disease. *Lancet* 1990; 336:827–830.
167. Antiplatelet Trialists' Collaboration. Collaborative overview of randomized trials of antiplatelet therapy: 1. Prevention of death, myocardial infarction, and stroke by prolonged antiplatelet therapy in various categories of patients. *Br Heart J* 1994; 308:81–106.
168. Al-Khadra AS, Salem DN, Rand WM, et al. Antiplatelet agents and survival: A cohort analysis from the Studies on Left Ventricular Dysfunction (SOLVD) trial. *J Am Coll Cardiol* 1998; 31:419–425.
169. Nguyen KN, Aursnes I, Kjekshus J. Interaction between enalapril and aspirin on mortality after myocardial infarction: Subgroup analysis of the Cooperative New Scandinavian Enalapril Survival Study II (Consensus II). *Am J Cardiol* 1997; 79:115–119.
170. Peterson JG, Laur MS, Young JB, et al. Evidence for an adverse interaction between ACE inhibitors and aspirin following myocardial infarction: The GUSTO-1 Trial (abstract). *J Am Coll Cardiol* 1998; 31:96A.
171. Leor J, Reicher-Reiss H, Goldbourt U, et al. Aspirin and mortality in patients treated with angiotensin-converting enzyme inhibitors: A cohort study of 11,575 patients with coronary artery disease. *J Am Coll Cardiol* 1999; 33:1920–1925.
172. Quinn MJ, Fitzgerald DJ. Ticlopidine and clopidogrel. *Circulation* 1999; 100:1667–1672.
173. Balsano F, Rizzon P, Violi F, et al., and the Studio della Ticlopidina nell'Angina Instabile Group. Antiplatelet treatment with ticlopidine in unstable angina: A controlled multicenter clinical trial. *Circulation* 1990; 82:17–26.
174. Leon MB, Baim DS, Popma JJ, et al., for the Stent Anticoagulant Restenosis Study Investigators. A clinical trial comparing three antithrombotic-drug regimens after coronary-artery stenting. *N Engl J Med* 1998; 339:1665–1671.
175. CAPRIE Steering Committee. A randomized, blinded trial of clopidogrel versus aspirin in patients at risk of ischemic events (CAPRIE). *Lancet* 1996; 348:1329–1339.
176. Topol EJ, Byzova TV, Plow EF. Platelet IIb-IIIa blockers. *Lancet* 1999; 353:227–231.
177. The EPIC Investigators. Use of a monoclonal antibody directed against the platelet glycoprotein IIb/IIIa receptor in high-risk coronary angioplasty. *N Engl J Med* 1994; 330:956–961.
178. Topol EJ, Califf RM, Weisman HS, et al., on behalf of the EPIC Investigators. Randomized trial of coronary intervention with antibody against platelet IIb/IIIa integrin for reduction of clinical restenosis: Results at six months. *Lancet* 1994; 343:881–886.
179. Topol EJ, Ferguson JJ, Weisman HS, et al., on behalf of the EPIC Investigators. Long-term protection from myocardial ischemic events in a randomized trial of brief integrin β_3 blockade with percutaneous coronary intervention. *JAMA* 1997; 278: 479–484.
180. The EPILOG Investigators. Platelet glycoprotein IIb/IIIa blockade and low-dose heparin during percutaneous coronary revascularization. *N Engl J Med* 1997; 336:1689–1696.
181. Lincoff AM, Tcheng JE, Califf RM, et al., for the EPILOG Investigators. Sustained suppression of ischemic complications of coronary intervention by platelet IIb/IIIa blockade with abciximab: One-year outcome in the EPILOG Trial. *Circulation* 1999; 99:1951–1958.
182. CAPTURE investigators. Randomised placebo-controlled trial of abciximab before and during coronary intervention in refractory unstable angina: The CAPTURE study. *Lancet* 1997; 349: 1429–1435.
183. EPISTENT investigators. Randomised placebo-controlled and balloon-angioplasty-controlled trial to assess safety of coronary stenting with use of platelet glycoprotein-IIb/IIIa blockade. *Lancet* 1998; 352:87–92.
184. Lincoff AM, Califf RM, Moliterno DJ, et al., for the Evaluation of Platelet IIb/IIIa Inhibition in Stenting investigators. Complementary clinical benefits of coronary-artery stenting and blockade of platelet glycoprotein IIb/IIIa receptors. *N Engl J Med* 1999; 341:319–327.
185. The IMPACT-II investigators. Randomised placebo-controlled trial of effect of eptifibatide on complications of percutaneous coronary intervention: IMPACT-II. *Lancet* 1997; 349:1422–1428.
186. The RESTORE investigators. Effects of platelet glycoprotein IIb/IIIa blockade with tirofiban on adverse cardiac events in patients with unstable angina or acute myocardial infarction undergoing coronary angioplasty. *Circulation* 1997; 96:1445–1453.
187. The Platelet Receptor Inhibition in Ischemic Syndrome Management (PRISM) Study investigators. A comparison of aspirin plus tirofiban with aspirin plus heparin for unstable angina. *N Engl J Med* 1998; 338:1498–1505.
188. The Platelet Receptor Inhibition in Ischemic Syndrome Management in Patients Limited by Unstable Signs and Symptoms (PRISM-PLUS) Study investigators. Inhibition of the platelet glycoprotein IIb/IIIa receptor with tirofiban in unstable angina and non-Q-wave myocardial infarction. *N Engl J Med* 1998; 338:1488–1497.
189. The PURSUIT investigators. Inhibition of the platelet glycoprotein IIb/IIIa with eptifibatide in patients with acute coronary syndromes without persistent ST-segment elevation. *N Engl J Med* 1998; 339:436–443.
190. The PARAGON investigators. International, randomized, controlled trial of lamifiban (a platelet glycoprotein IIb/IIIa inhibitor), heparin, or both in unstable angina. *Circulation* 1998; 97:2386–2395.
191. The SYMPHONY investigators. Comparison of sibrafiban with aspirin for prevention of cardiovascular events after acute coronary syndromes: A randomized trial. *Lancet* 2000; 355:337–345.
192. O'Neill WW, Serruys P, Knudtson M, et al., for the EXCITE investigators. Long-term treatment with a platelet glycoprotein-receptor antagonist after percutaneous coronary revascularization. *N Engl J Med* 2000; 342:1316–1324.
192a. Ferguson JJ. Meeting highlights. Highlights of the 48th Scientific Sessions of the American College of Cardiology. *Circulation* 1999; 100:570–575.
193. Hamm CW, Heeschen C, Goldmann B, et al., for the c7E3 Fab Antiplatelet Therapy in Unstable Refractory Angina (CAPTURE) Study investigators. Benefit of abciximab in patients with refractory unstable angina in relation to serum troponin T levels. *N Engl J Med* 1999; 340:1623–1629.
194. Hirsh J. Heparin. *N Engl J Med* 1991; 321:1565–1573.
195. Waters D, Azar RR. Low-molecular-weight heparins for unstable angina: A better mousetrap? *Circulation* 1997; 96:3–5.
196. Hirsh J, Fuster V. Guide to anticoagulant therapy: I. Heparin. *Circulation* 1994; 89:1449–1468.
197. Telford AM, Wilson C. Trial of heparin versus atenolol in prevention of myocardial infarction in intermediate coronary syndrome. *Lancet* 1981; 1:1225–1228.
198. Théroux P, Waters D, Qui S, et al. Aspirin versus heparin to

prevent myocardial infarction during the acute phase of unstable angina. *Circulation* 1993; 88:2045–2048.
199. Holdwright D, Patel D, Cunningham D, et al. Comparison of the effect of heparin and aspirin versus aspirin alone on transient myocardial ischemia and in-hospital prognosis in patients with unstable angina. *J Am Coll Cardiol* 1994; 24:39–45.
200. Gurfinkel EP, Manos EJ, Mejafl RI, et al. Low molecular weight heparin versus regular heparin or aspirin in the treatment of unstable angina and silent ischemia. *J Am Coll Cardiol* 1995; 26:313–318.
201. Cohen M, Adams PC, Hawkins L, et al. Usefulness of antithrombotic therapy in rest angina pectoris or non-Q-wave myocardial infarction in preventing death and myocardial infarction (a pilot study from the Antithrombotic Therapy in Acute Coronary Syndromes Study Group). *Am J Cardiol* 1990; 66:1287–1292.
202. Cohen M, Adams PC, Parry G, et al., and the Antithrombotic Therapy in Acute Coronary Syndromes Research Group. Combination antithrombotic therapy in unstable rest angina and non-Q-wave infarction in nonprior aspirin users: Primary end points analysis from the ATACS trial. *Circulation* 1994; 89:81–88.
203. Oler A, Whooley MA, Oler J, Grady D. Adding heparin to aspirin reduces the incidence of myocardial infarction and death in patients with unstable angina. *JAMA* 1996; 276:811–815.
204. Neri Serneri GG, Gensini GF, Poggesi L, et al. Effect of heparin, aspirin, or alteplase in reduction of myocardial ischemia in refractory unstable angina. *Lancet* 1990; 335:615–618.
205. Neri Serneri GG, Modesti PA, Gensini GF, et al., for the Studio Epoorine Sottocutanea nell'Angina Instobile (SESAIP) Refrattorie Group. Randomised comparison of subcutaneous heparin, intravenous heparin, and aspirin in unstable angina. *Lancet* 1995; 345:1201–1204.
206. Théroux P, Waters D, Lam J, et al. Reactivation of unstable angina after discontinuation of heparin. *N Engl J Med* 1992; 327:141–145.
207. Becker RC, Spencer FA, Li Y, et al. Thrombin generation after the abrupt cessation of intravenous unfractionated heparin among patients with acute coronary syndromes: Potential mechanisms for heightened prothrombotic potential. *J Am Coll Cardiol* 1999; 34:1028–1035.
208. Brieger DB, Mak KH, Kotte-Marchant K, Topol EJ. Heparin-induced thrombocytopenia. *J Am Coll Cardiol* 1998; 31:1449–1459.
209. Weitz JI. Low-molecular-weight heparins. *N Engl J Med* 1997; 337:688–698.
210. De Candia E, De Cristofaro R, Landolfi R. Thrombin-induced platelet activation is inhibited by high- and low-molecular-weight heparin. *Circulation* 1999; 99:3308–3314.
211. De Cristofaro R, De Candia E, Landolfi R. Effect of high- and low-molecular-weight heparins on thrombin-thrombomodulin interaction and protein C activation. *Circulation* 1998; 98:1297–1301.
212. Fragmin during Instability in Coronary Artery Disease (FRISC) study group. Low-molecular-weight heparin during instability in coronary artery disease. *Lancet* 1996, 347:561–568.
213. Klein W, Buchwald A, Hillis SE, et al., for the FRIC Investigators. Comparison of low-molecular-weight heparin with unfractionated heparin acutely and with placebo for 6 weeks in the management of unstable coronary artery disease: Fragmin in Unstable Coronary Artery Disease Study (FRIC). *Circulation* 1997; 96:61–68.
214. Fragmin and Fast Revascularisation during Instability in Coronary artery disease (FRISC II) investigators. Long-term low-molecular-mass heparin in unstable coronary-artery disease: FRISC II prospective randomised multicentre study. *Lancet* 1999; 354:701–707.
215. Cohen M, Demers C, Gurfinkel EP, et al., for the Efficacy and Safety of Subcutaneous Enoxaparin in Non-Q-Wave Coronary Events study group. *N Engl J Med* 1997; 337:447–452.
216. Mark DB, Cowper PA, Berkowitz SD, et al. Economic assessment of low-molecular-weight heparin (enoxaparin) versus unfractionated heparin in acute coronary syndrome patients: Results from the ESSENCE randomized trial. *Circulation* 1998; 97:1702–1707.
217. Antman E, McCabe CH, Gurfinkel EP, et al. Enoxaparin prevents death and cardiac ischemic events in unstable angina/non-Q-wave myocardial infarction: Results of the Thrombolysis in Myocardial Infarction (TIMI) 11B study. *Circulation* 1999; 100:1593–1601.
218. Leizorovicz A. Preliminary results from the FRAX.I.S study: Oral presentation, hotline session: European Society of Cardiology Scientific Sessions, Vienna, 1998.
219. Hirsh J, Weitz JI. New antithrombotic agents. *Lancet* 1999; 353:1431–1436.
220. Eriksson BI, Wille-Jørgensen P, Kälebo P, et al. A comparison of recombinant hirudin with a low-molecular-weight heparin to prevent thromboembolic complications after total hip replacement. *N Engl J Med* 1997; 337:1329–1335.
221. The Global Use of Strategies to Open Occluded Coronary Arteries (GUSTO) IIb investigators. A comparison of recombinant hirudin with heparin for the treatment of acute coronary syndrome. *N Engl J Med* 1996; 335:775–782.
222. Organization to Assess Strategies for Ischemic Syndrome (OASIS-2) investigators. Effect of recombinant hirudin (lepirudin) compared with heparin on death, myocardial infarction, refractory angina, and revascularisation procedures in patients with acute myocardial ischaemia without ST elevation: A randomised trial. *Lancet* 1999; 353:429–438.
223. Bittl JA, Strony J, Brinker HA, et al., for the Hirulog Angioplasty Study investigators. Treatment with bivalirudin (Hirulog) as compared with heparin during coronary angioplasty for unstable or postinfarction angina. *N Engl J Med* 1995; 333:764–769.
224. TRIM Study Group. A low molecular weight, selective thrombin inhibitor, inogatran *vs* heparin, in unstable coronary artery disease in 1209 patients: A double-blind, randomized, dose-finding study. *Eur Heart J* 1997; 18:1416–1425.
225. Merlini PA, Bauer KA, Oltrona L, et al. Persistent activation of coagulation mechanism in unstable angina and myocardial infarction. *Circulation* 1994; 90:61–68.
226. Williams MJA, Morison IM, Parker JH, Stewart RAH. Progression of the culprit lesion in unstable coronary artery disease with warfarin and aspirin versus aspirin alone: Preliminary study. *J Am Coll Cardiol* 1997; 30:364–369.
227. Anand SS, Yusuf S, Pogue J, et al., for the OASIS Pilot Study investigators. Long-term oral anticoagulation therapy in patients with unstable angina or suspected non-Q-wave myocardial infarction: Organization to Assess Strategies for Ischemic Syndromes (OASIS) Pilot Study results. *Circulation* 1998; 98:1064–1070.
228. Waters D, Lam JYT. Is thrombolytic therapy striking out in unstable angina? *Circulation* 1992; 86:1642–1644.
229. The TIMI IIIB investigators. Effects of tissue plasminogen activator and a comparison of early invasive and conservative strategies in unstable angina and non-Q wave infarction: Results of the TIMI IIIB Trial. *Circulation* 1994; 89:1545–1556.
230. Ambrose JA, Almeida OD, Sharma SK, et al., for the TAUSA Investigators. Adjunctive thrombolytic therapy during angioplasty for ischemic rest angina: Results of the TAUSA trial. *Circulation* 1994; 90:69–77.
231. Luchi RJ, Scott SM, Deupree RH, and the principal investigators and their associates of the Veterans Administration Cooperative Study No. 28. Comparison of medical and surgical treatment for

unstable angina pectoris: Results of a Veterans Administration cooperative study. *N Engl J Med* 1987; 316:977–984.

232. Parisi AF, Khuri S, Deupree RH, et al. Medical compared with surgical management of unstable angina: 5-year mortality and morbidity in the Veterans Administration Study. *Circulation* 1989; 80:1176–1189.
233. Scott SM, Deupree RH, Sharma GVRK, Luchi RJ, associates of the VA cooperative study of unstable angina. VA study of unstable angina: 10-year results showing duration of surgical advantage for patients with impaired ejection fraction. *Circulation* 1994; 90:(part 2):II-120–II-123.
234. Kaiser GC, Schaff HV, Killip T. Myocardial revascularization for unstable angina pectoris. *Circulation* 1989; 79:(suppl I): I-60–I-67.
235. Anderson HV, Cannon CP, Stone PH, et al., for the TIMI IIIB Investigators. One-year results of the Thrombolysis in Myocardial Infarction (TIMI) IIIB clinical trial: A randomized comparison of tissue-type plasminogen activator versus placebo and early invasive versus early conservative strategies in unstable angina and non-Q wave myocardial infarction. *J Am Coll Cardiol* 1995; 26:1643–1650.
236. Boden WE, O'Rourke RA, Crawford MH, et al., for the Veterans Affairs Non-Q-Wave Infarction Strategies in Hospital (VANQWISH) Trial investigators. Outcomes in patients with acute non-Q-wave myocardial infarction randomly assigned to an invasive as compared with a conservative management strategy. *N Engl J Med* 1998; 338:1785–1792.
237. Fragmin and Fast Revascularization during Instability in Coronary artery disease (FRISC II) investigators. Invasive compared with non-invasive treatment in unstable coronary-artery disease: FRISC II prospective randomised multicentre study. *Lancet* 1999; 354:708–715.
238. Yusuf S, Flather M, Pogue J, et al., for the OASIS (Organization to Assess Strategies for Ischemic Syndromes) Registry investigators. Variations between countries in invasive cardiac procedures and outcomes in patients with suspected unstable angina or myocardial infarction without initial ST elevation. *Lancet* 1998; 352:507–514.
239. Prinzmetal M, Kennemer R, Merliss R, et al. Angina pectoris: I. A variant form of angina pectoris. *Am J Med* 1959; 27:375–388.
240. MacAlpin RN, Kattus AA, Alvaro AB. Angina pectoris at rest with preservation of exercise capacity: Prinzmetal's variant angina. *Circulation* 1973; 47:946–958.
241. Onaka H, Hirota Y, Shimada S, et al. Clinical observations of spontaneous angina attacks and multivessel spasm in variant angina pectoris with normal coronary arteries: Evaluation by 24-hour 12-lead electrocardiography with computer analysis. *J Am Coll Cardiol* 1996; 27:38–44.
242. Ozaki Y, Keane D, Serruys PW. Fluctuation of spastic location in patients with vasospastic angina: A quantitative angiographic study. *J Am Coll Cardiol* 1995; 26:1606–1614.
243. Yasue H, Horio Y, Nakamura N, et al. Induction of coronary artery spasm with acetylcholine in patients with variant angina: Possible role of the parasympathetic nervous system in the pathogenesis of coronary artery spasm. *Circulation* 1986; 74:955–963.
244. Sakata K, Yoshida H, Hoshino T, Kurata C. Sympathetic nerve activity in the spasm-induced coronary artery region is associated with disease activity of vasospastic angina. *J Am Coll Cardiol* 1996; 28:460–464.
245. Kushwaha S, Mitchell AG, Yacoub MH. Coronary artery spasm after cardiac transplantation. *Am J Cardiol* 1990; 65:1515–1518.
246. Chierchia S, Davies G, Berkenboom G, et al. α-Adrenergic receptors and coronary spasm: An elusive link. *Circulation* 1984; 69:8–14.
247. Freedman SB, Chierchia S, Rodriguez-Plaza L, et al. Ergonovine-induced myocardial ischemia: No role for serotonergic receptors? *Circulation* 1984; 70:178–183.
248. Robertson RM, Robertson D, Roberts LJ, et al. Thromboxane A_2 in vasotonic angina pectoris: Evidence from direct measurement and inhibitor trials. *N Engl J Med* 1981; 304:998–1003.
249. Chierchia S, Patrono C, Crea F, et al. Effect of intravenous prostacyclin in variant angina. *Circulation* 1982; 65:470–477.
250. Satake K, Lee JD, Shimizu H, et al. Relation between severity of magnesium deficiency and frequency of anginal attacks in men with variant angina. *J Am Coll Cardiol* 1996; 28:897–902.
251. Shimabukuro M, Shinzato T, Higa S, et al. Enhanced insulin response relates to acetylcholine-induced vasoconstriction in vasospastic angina. *J Am Coll Cardiol* 1995; 25:356–361.
252. Miwa K, Miyagi Y, Igawa A, et al. Vitamin E deficiency in variant angina. *Circulation* 1996; 94:14–18.
253. Kugiyama K, Motoyama T, Hirashima O, et al. Vitamin C attenuates abnormal vasomotor reactivity in spasm coronary arteries in patients with coronary spastic angina. *J Am Coll Cardiol* 1998; 32:103–109.
254. Kugiyama K, Yasue H, Okumura K, et al. Nitric oxide activity is deficient in spasm arteries of patients with coronary spastic angina. *Circulation* 1996; 94:266–272.
255. Egashira K, Katsuda Y, Mohri M, et al. Basal release of endothelium-derived nitric oxide at site of spasm in patients with variant angina. *J Am Coll Cardiol* 1996; 27:1444–1449.
256. Nakayama M, Yasue H, Yoshimura M, et al. $T^{-786} \rightarrow C$ mutation in the 5′-flanking region of the endothelial nitric oxide synthase gene is associated with coronary spasm. *Circulation* 1999; 99:2864–2870.
257. Yamagishi M, Miyatake K, Tamai J, et al. Intravascular ultrasound detection of atherosclerosis at the site of focal vasospasm in angiographically normal or minimally narrowed coronary segments. *J Am Coll Cardiol* 1994; 23:352–357.
258. Beltrame JF, Sasayama S, Maseri A. Racial heterogeneity in coronary artery vasomotor reactivity: Differences between Japanese and Caucasian patients. *J Am Coll Cardiol* 1999; 33:1442–1452.
259. Maseri A, Severi S, De Nes M, et al. "Variant" angina: One aspect of a continuous spectrum of vasospastic myocardial ischemia. *Am J Cardiol* 1978; 42:1019–1035.
260. Waters DD, Szlachcic J, Bourassa MG, et al. Exercise testing in patients with variant angina: Results, correlation with clinical and angiographic features and prognostic significance. *Circulation* 1982; 65:265–274.
261. Koiwaya Y, Torii S, Takeshita A, et al. Postinfarction angina caused by coronary arterial spasm. *Circulation* 1982; 65:275–280.
262. Waters D, Théroux P, Crittin J, et al. Previously undiagnosed variant angina as a cause of chest pain after coronary artery bypass surgery. *Circulation* 1980; 61:1159–1164.
263. David PR, Waters DD, Scholl JM, et al. Percutaneous transluminal coronary angioplasty in patients with variant angina. *Circulation* 1982; 66:695–702.
264. Scholl JM, Benacerraf A, Ducimetiere P, et al. Comparison of risk factors in vasospastic angina without significant fixed coronary narrowing and no vasospastic angina. *Am J Cardiol* 1986; 57:199–202.
265. Miller D, Waters DD, Warnica W, et al. Is variant angina the coronary manifestation of a generalized vasospastic disorder? *N Engl J Med* 1981; 304:763–766.
266. Myerburg RJ, Kessler KM, Mallon SM, et al. Life-threatening ventricular arrhythmias in patients with silent myocardial ischemia due to coronary artery spasm. *N Engl J Med* 1992; 326:1451–1455.
267. Chevalier P, Dacosta A, Defaye P, et al. Arrhythmic cardiac arrest due to isolated coronary artery spasm: Long-term out-

come of seven resuscitated patients. *J Am Coll Cardiol* 1998; 31:57–61.

268. Waters DD, Szlachcic J, Bonan R, et al. Comparative sensitivity of exercise, cold pressor and ergonovine testing in provoking attacks of variant angina in patients with active disease. *Circulation* 1983; 67:310–315.
269. Okumura K, Yasue H, Matsuyama K, et al. Sensitivity and specificity of intracoronary injection of acetylcholine for the induction of coronary artery spasm. *J Am Coll Cardiol* 1988; 12:883–888.
270. Waters DD, Bouchard A, Théroux P. Spontaneous remission is a frequent outcome of variant angina. *J Am Coll Cardiol* 1983; 2:195–199.
271. Walling A, Waters DD, Miller DD, et al. Long-term prognosis of patients with variant angina. *Circulation* 1987; 76:990–997.
272. Morikami Y, Yasue H. Efficacy of slow-release nifedipine on myocardial ischemia episodes in variant angina pectoris. *Am J Cardiol* 1991; 68:580–584.
273. Pepine CJ, Feldman RL, Whittle J, et al. Effect of diltiazem in patients with variant angina: A randomized double-blind trial. *Am Heart J* 1981; 101:719–725.
274. Johnson SM, Mauritson DR, Willerson JT, Hillis LD. A controlled clinical trial of verapamil for Prinzmetal's variant angina. *N Engl J Med* 1981; 304:862–866.
275. Chahine RA, Feldman RL, Giles TD, et al. Randomized placebo-controlled trial of amlodipine in vasospastic angina. *J Am Coll Cardiol* 1993; 21:1365–1370.
276. Yasue H, Takizawa A, Nagao M, et al. Long-term prognosis for patients with variant angina and influential factors. *Circulation* 1988; 78:1–9.
277. Rutitzky B, Girotti AL, Rosenbaum MB. Efficacy of chronic amiodarone therapy in patients with variant angina pectoris and inhibition of ergonovine coronary constriction. *Am Heart J* 1982; 103:38–43.
278. Frenneaux M, Kaski JC, Brown M, Maseri A. Refractory variant angina relieved by guanethidine and clonidine. *Am J Cardiol* 1988; 62:832–833.
279. Miwa K, Kambara H, Kawai C. Exercise-induced angina provoked by aspirin administration in patients with variant angina. *Am J Cardiol* 1981; 47:1210–1214.
280. Mark DB, Califf RM, Morris KG, et al. Clinical characteristics and long-term survival of patients with variant angina. *Circulation* 1984; 69:880–888.
281. Shubrooks SJ Jr, Bete JM, Hutter AM Jr, et al. Variant angina pectoris: Clinical and anatomic spectrum and results of coronary bypass surgery. *Am J Cardiol* 1975; 36:142–147.
282. Bertrand ME, Lablanche JM, Thieuleux FA, et al. Comparative results of percutaneous transluminal coronary angioplasty in patients with dynamic versus fixed coronary stenosis. *J Am Coll Cardiol* 1986; 8:504–508.
283. Bertrand ME, Lablanche JM, Thieuleux FA, et al. Relation of restenosis after percutaneous transluminal coronary angioplasty to vasomotion of the dilated coronary arterial segment. *Am J Cardiol* 1989; 63:277–281.
284. Severi S, Davies G, Maseri A, et al. Long-term prognosis of "variant" angina with medical treatment. *Am J Cardiol* 1980; 46:226–232.
285. Ozaki Y, Keane D, Serruys PW. Progression and regression of coronary stenosis in the long-term follow-up of vasospastic angina. *Circulation* 1995; 92:2446–2456.
286. Suzuki H, Kawai S, Aizawa T, et al. Histologic evaluation of coronary plaque in patients with variant angina: Relationship between vasospasm and neointimal hyperplasia in primary coronary lesions. *J Am Coll Cardiol* 1999; 33:198–205.

CHAPTER 42

DIAGNOSIS AND MANAGEMENT OF PATIENTS WITH ACUTE MYOCARDIAL INFARCTION

R. Wayne Alexander / Craig M. Pratt / Thomas J. Ryan / Robert Roberts

BACKGROUND AND INTRODUCTION*

Progress in the understanding of the pathogenesis of acute myocardial infarction (AMI) and of its treatment epitomizes scientific, evidence-based medicine at its best. Although myocardial infarction has long been a clinically recognized entity resulting from coronary artery atherosclerosis, its relative importance is a modern phenomenon. Its appearance as a modern epidemic reflects increasing longevity, permitting manifestation of chronic "degenerative" diseases such as atherosclerosis; the adoption of high-fat diets based on meats, permitted by increasing affluence; and decreased exercise, made possible by the increased mechanization of society. Osler devoted only a few pages in his textbook, published in 1892, to the discussion of AMI.[3]

* The ACC/AHA Guidelines for the Management of Patients With Acute Myocardial Infarction, 1996 version, have been updated in 1999. The 1999 update did not reprint the whole document. Reference to the Guidelines in this chapter will refer to the 1999 citation[1] but may also refer to data in the 1996 document.[2]

The modern era can be said to have begun with the autopsy studies of Herrick, who concluded in 1912 that the clinical syndrome of myocardial infarction results from acute thrombotic occlusion of a coronary artery, with resulting downstream necrosis.[4] This conclusion was generally accepted for 60 years, and the term *coronary thrombosis* was not uncommonly used as the equivalent of *heart attack* or, more formally, *acute myocardial infarction.* The conventional wisdom was challenged in 1972, when it was suggested that coronary artery thrombus may be the result rather than the cause of acute infarction, since autopsy studies—which were frequently performed several days after the acute event—did not uniformly show thrombus.[5] In retrospect, these findings can be explained by spontaneous lysis of a thrombus that had been occlusive for a sufficient amount of time to cause tissue necrosis. Definitive proof of the central role of thrombus formation in the pathogenesis of myocardial infarction came from angiographic studies performed during the first hours of the acute event,[6,7] a diagnostic strategy that had previously been thought to be contraindicated.[8]

The unequivocal demonstration of the role of the thrombus in AMI quickly led to the systematic testing of thrombolytic strategies to abort myocardial infarctions.[9-11] Analysis of data from several small trials of thrombolytic therapy with streptokinase suggested improved mortality in treated patients as early as 1982.[12] These early efforts were followed by a large number of major multicenter clinical trials on the treatment of AMI; these demonstrated in a rigorous fashion the efficacy of beta-adrenergic receptor blockers,[13] streptokinase versus no thrombolytic therapy,[14] and recombinant tissue plasminogen activator versus streptokinase[15] in reducing mortality. These and other major trials are discussed in detail further on. The major point to be made here is that large, adequately powered, randomized studies in the treatment of myocardial infarction have helped set a new standard and approach to the goal of enhancing the evidence-based practice of medicine while moving away from one based on previous practice patterns and intuitive extrapolations from pathophysiologic principles. Key to the success of these very large trials has been the generalizability achieved mostly by the use of broad-entry criteria that facilitated the rapid enrollment of suitable patients and provided robust statistical power to the studies.

The availability of data from well-designed clinical trials has permitted the development, by panels of experts, of evidence-based practice guidelines for the treatment of myocardial infarction.[1,16] Furthermore, the confidence with which recommendations can be made for any particular diagnostic or therapeutic approach can be graded on the basis of judgments as to the strength of the supporting evidence. Thus, a committee convened by the American College of Cardiology/American Heart Association (ACC/AHA) Task Force on Practice Guidelines was charged with revising the ACC/AHA statement, "Guidelines for the Early Management of Patients with Acute Myocardial Infarction," published in 1990.[16] The results of the deliberations of this committee, "Guidelines for the Management of Patients with Acute Myocardial Infarction," were published in late 1996[2] and have been updated.[1] The evidence and expert opinion supporting use of a therapy, intervention, or diagnostic procedure were weighed and expressed in ACC/AHA format as follows:

Class I: Conditions for which there is evidence and/or general agreement that a given procedure or treatment is beneficial, useful, and effective.

Class II: Conditions for which there is conflicting evidence and/or a divergence of opinion about the usefulness/efficacy of a procedure or treatment.

Class IIa: Weight of evidence/opinion is in favor of usefulness/efficacy.

Class IIb: Usefulness/efficacy is less well established by evidence/opinion.

Class III: Conditions for which there is evidence and/or general agreement that a procedure/treatment is not useful/effective and in some cases may be harmful.[1] In general, recommendations in this chapter are associated with a class I, II, or III designation to guide the reader in weighing diagnostic and therapeutic options.

The pathophysiologic bases and consequences of coronary artery disease and myocardial infarction are discussed elsewhere: natural history and prognosis (Chap. 1); pathogenesis of atherosclerosis (Chap. 35); pathology of coronary atherosclerosis (Chap. 36); risk factors and prevention (Chap. 38); nonatherosclerotic causes of coronary heart disease (spontaneous coronary artery dissection, aortic dissection, thrombosis associated with the use of birth-control pills, emboli, congenital coronary anomalies, metabolic abnormalities, blunt chest trauma, vasculitis, and drug abuse, especially cocaine) (Chap. 39); pathophysiology of myocardial ischemia (Chap. 37); pathophysiology of coronary artery disease as related to myocardial ischemic syndromes (Chap. 35); and thrombogenesis and antithrombotic therapy (Chap. 44).

The following are important general facts about myocardial infarction:

1. Approximately 800,000 people in the United States experience AMI annually; of these, about 213,000 die. Of those who die, approximately one-half do so within 1 h of the onset of symptoms, before reaching a hospital.[1,17,18]
2. The majority of early deaths are the result of ventricular arrhythmias that can be readily aborted by defibrillation, either during prehospital care or in coronary care units (CCU) in the hospital.
3. The major cause of myocardial infarction is atherosclerotic disease of the epicardial coronary arteries, as noted. Although luminal narrowing resulting in hemodynamically significant obstruction of blood flow is the major cause of symptoms of coronary ischemia (Chap. 40), the majority of myocardial infarctions occur as a result of the disruption of arterial lesions that are not hemodynamically significant (<60 percent). This breakdown of the structural integrity of the arterial intima occurs because of weakening induced by proteolytic degradation of matrix proteins by products released from inflammatory leukocytes[19] and results in the exposure of blood to thrombogenic intimal material, causing obstructive clot formation. Local vasospasm may contribute to the obstruction. *These observations have led to the concept that the biological state of atherosclerotic lesions and not the extent of stenosis is the major determinant of whether or not plaque rupture and myocardial infarction occur.*
4. Myocardial infarction, or ischemia, is a segmental process limited to the distribution of the affected artery. Impaired contractility usually occurs within seconds of the cessation of blood flow. The process usually begins in the endocardium and spreads toward the epicardium. If flow is restored before cell death occurs, prolonged contractile impairment (stunning) may occur.
5. Episodes of ischemia preceding coronary occlusion enhance the survivability of myocardial cells (*ischemic preconditioning*).
6. Irreversible cardiac injury occurs if occlusion is complete for at least 15 to 20 min. Irreversible injury occurs maximally in the area at risk when occlusion is sustained for 4 to 6 h, but most of the damage occurs in the first 2 to 3 h. Thus, restoration of flow within the first 4 to 6 h is associated with salvage of the myocardium, but the salvage is exponentially greater if restoration occurs in 1 to 2 h.
7. Restoration of blood flow by thrombolysis results in myocardial salvage and improved mortality. The extent of the benefit is dependent upon restoration of near-normal blood flow *(open-artery hypothesis)* and is inversely related to the time between the onset of occlusion (symptoms) and the restoration of blood flow.
8. The percentage of tissue at risk that undergoes necrosis

(infarct size) depends on existing collateral flow, which is highly variable and difficult to predict.

9. The major predictor of long-term outcome is infarct size, which is inversely related to the ejection fraction.
10. Q-wave infarction (usually presenting as ST-segment elevation) is a distinct clinical entity, as compared with non-Q-wave infarction (usually presenting with ST-segment depression). There are differential features in their clinical courses. (Q-wave infarction, untreated, has a relatively high in-hospital mortality rate that is favorably influenced by thrombolysis, whereas non-Q-wave infarction has a lower in-hospital mortality and complication rate with a prolonged vulnerability to reinfarction. Thrombolysis may worsen the clinical outcome.) Although there is no close anatomic correlation between the presence and absence of Q waves and transmural and nontransmural myocardial infarction, the distinct clinical outcomes of patients presenting with ST-segment elevation and ST-segment depression have made this electrocardiographic feature a major initial decision point in assigning therapeutic strategies to patients presenting with symptoms compatible with AMI.
11. Because of their salutary effects on thrombus formation and ventricular arrhythmias, aspirin and beta-adrenergic blockers, respectively, have proved to be effective for secondary prevention in patients who have had a myocardial infarction. Aspirin has also been shown to be modestly effective for primary prevention in middle-aged males.
12. Lipid lowering and smoking cessation have both been shown to be effective in the primary and secondary prevention of myocardial infarction. The enormous progress that has been made in understanding the pathogenesis and treatment of myocardial infarction has resulted in substantial improvements in outcomes in recent years. Indeed, the "natural history" of treated patients has improved dramatically. The mortality rate in the pre-CCU era has been estimated to have been about 30 percent.[20] The mortality rate dropped dramatically, to about 15 percent, in the CCU era, which embraced the use of hemodynamic monitoring, defibrillation, and the use of beta blockers. The increased use of thrombolytics, coronary interventions, aspirin, and angiotensin-converting enzyme inhibitors has decreased the mortality of patients treated for the conventional ST-elevated AMI to 6 to 7 percent.[15,21] This, of course, cannot be claimed for patients in the Medicare population where it is generally accepted that patients over the age of 70 have a mortality rate that approximates 20 percent when admitted for the management of AMI. The major challenge, however, is to bring the principles and lessons learned from the efforts of the past decade to everyday clinical practice.

CLINICAL ASPECTS

Predisposing Characteristics and Circumstances

The standard risk factors for the development of coronary artery disease (dyslipidemia, family history, age, male gender, cigarette smoking, diabetes mellitus, and hypertension) are well established and are discussed in Chap. 38. *Careful consideration of the probabilities of the presence of coronary artery disease is centrally important in the initial assessment and evaluation of testing results of any patient with chest pain.* The experienced clinician will calibrate his or her responses even within the context of algorithmic approaches to the evaluation of chest pain. For example, the 35-year-old male with atypical chest pain whose father died of coronary disease at less than age 50 and whose mother had a coronary bypass at age 55 would be viewed with a higher index of suspicion than he would be if both his parents and grandparents were alive and well. This higher level of concern might translate into ordering diagnostic modalities with a higher level of sensitivity and specificity for detecting coronary artery disease in the former as opposed to the latter case.

As discussed in Chaps. 35, 36, and 38, atherosclerosis generally, and including the disease in the coronary arteries, is a chronic inflammation representing the response of the arterial wall to the stress imposed by various risk factors. AMI has commonly been shown to occur as a result of the disruption of a coronary artery plaque at a site of a high density of inflammatory cells.[21] Thus, AMI can be thought of as resulting from the acute exacerbation of a chronic inflammatory response. There is increasing clinical evidence supporting this view. Thus, unstable angina, a frequent antecedent of myocardial infarction,[22] has been shown to be associated with elevated plasma levels of the acute-phase reactant C-reactive protein.[23,24] Observations from the Physicians' Health Study, which showed that subjects with the highest levels of C-reactive protein have an increased long-term risk of cardiac events, is also supportive of the concept that inflammatory responses are important in the pathogenesis of AMI.[25] *Thus, events precipitating myocardial infarctions can be viewed as exacerbating the arterial inflammatory response and/or increasing the physical forces impinging on a coronary artery lesion weakened by inflammation, which leads to rupture.*

Precipitating Events

There is little direct, but intriguing indirect, evidence that external factors might exacerbate the arterial inflammatory response. An association has been noted between AMI and antecedent mild respiratory syndromes.[25] It is possible that an infection, by activating systemic responses, could stimulate or activate previously quiescent atherosclerotic lesions. A more specific relation between AMI and an infectious agent has been posited in the case of *Chlamydia pneumoniae*.[26–28] Increased antibody titers to *C. pneumoniae* in subsets of patients have been associated with increased risk for acute infarction, and acute infarction–associated increases in circulating immune complexes, followed by a subsequent increase in antibody titers, have been observed.[29] Evidence exists for the presence of chlamydiae in atherosclerotic coronary artery lesions.[30] Thus, it is possible that *C. pneumoniae* infection contributes to the inflammatory responses in atherosclerosis and that acute reinfection activates the inflammatory response, leading to myocardial infarction. This area requires further investigation.

There is considerable evidence associating AMI with emotional or environmental stresses. It is likely that the majority of these stresses involve activation of the sympathetic nervous system, with increases in locally released and circulating catecholamines. Increased sympathetic drive increases cardiac oxygen consumption by increasing contractility and rate. Sympathetic stimulation will also increase shear forces and stress on vascular atherosclerotic lesions by augmenting contraction and torque and elevating blood pressure. Superimposition of these forces on a vessel weakened by inflammation can lead to plaque rupture. Enhanced circulating catecholamine levels can increase the propensity for thrombus formation by activating platelets. Such a scenario likely explains the association (in about 4 to 7 percent of patients) between acute increases in physical exertion and the development of myocardial infarction, especially among those who do not exercise regularly.[31,32] Similarly, episodes of anger increase the risk of precipitating myocardial infarction in susceptible persons.[33] Distressing or changing life events reportedly occur with increased frequency in the months preceding a myocardial infarction.[34–36] Another well-controlled study, however, found no correlation between the occurrence of acute infarction and the presence of unusual life events for up to 4 weeks prior to the event.[31]

It is apparent that any acute stressful event or intervention can precipitate AMI in a patient with "active," susceptible coronary atherosclerotic lesions. Anesthesia and surgery are well known to enhance the risk of myocardial infarction, and cardiac events are the leading cause of perioperative morbidity.[37] Perioperatively, stress can be induced by tachycardia and hypotension,[38] anemia,[39] and hypothermia.[40] A study of patients with coronary disease undergoing noncardiac surgery has shown that the usual perioperative hypothermia was associated with a relative risk of cardiac events of 2.2, as contrasted to a similar group in whom normothermia was maintained.[41] The salutary effects of maintaining normothermia were thought to be due to the prevention of cardiac stress imposed by activation of the sympathetic nervous system. By extension, many of the stressful events—such as pulmonary emboli, stroke, hypoxia, allergic responses, blood loss, etc.—that have been associated with the precipitation of AMI can likely be related to the effects of adrenergic stimulation by an excess of catecholamines.

Myocardial infarction can occur because of low perfusion pressure in shock of any etiology and can arise in severe aortic stenosis even in the absence of coronary artery disease because of excessive oxygen demands in a very hypertrophic ventricle with, for example, marked tachycardia. Other nonatherosclerotic causes of myocardial infarction, including trauma, embolism, and dissection, are discussed in Chap. 39. Vasospasm in the absence of angiographically demonstrable coronary artery disease has been reported to have caused AMI in several patients during general anesthesia.[42] Also, it is likely that vasospasm plays a central role in cocaine-induced myocardial infarction.[43]

Personality Types

It has been claimed that so-called coronary-prone individuals exhibit certain personality traits, such as being a compulsive hard worker, being deadline-driven, and being excessively competitive. Categorizing people with such traits as "type A" and thus as being at increased risk for myocardial infarction was formerly widely discussed.[44] This concept is not widely accepted now,[45] and the psychological contributions to heart disease are generally considered to be more complex (see Chap. 80).

Circadian and Seasonal Variation

Results of the Multicenter Investigation of Limitation of Infarct Size (MILIS) study showed a marked circadian periodicity in the occurrence of myocardial infarction, with a peak prevalence between 6 A.M. and noon. The circadian rhythm was present whether the onset of the infarction was marked subjectively by the appearance of pain or objectively by plasma MB-CK (creatine kinase) levels. There was a threefold increase in the frequency of infarction at peak (9 A.M.) periods as compared with trough (11 P.M.) periods.[46] As a corollary, sudden death attributed to ischemic heart disease has a similar circadian periodicity. Available data suggest that the rhythms both for the occurrence of myocardial infarction and for deaths from ischemic events are actually bimodal. These rhythms are characterized not only by the morning peak but also by a secondary, less pronounced late-afternoon or early-evening peak (6 to 8 P.M.).[47] The mechanisms underlying this temporal distribution of ischemic events are not completely understood but are probably related to diurnal variations in thrombotic tendencies and to sympathetic nervous system activity. There is both an enhanced platelet aggregability[48] and a trough in intrinsic fibrinolytic activity during the morning hours.[49] A similar circadian variation is observed for cerebral infarction,[50] which further implicates an increased propensity for thrombosis in the morning hours. The blunting of the morning peak of myocardial infarction by both aspirin and beta-adrenergic blockers emphasizes the contributions of both the sympathetic nervous system and the coagulation pathways to the circadian rhythm of cardiovascular events.[51]

Other endogenous daily rhythms may be causally related. Ambulatory ST-segment changes in patients with coronary artery disease have demonstrated a close correlation between basal heart rate (which is higher in the morning) and the frequency of ischemic ST-segment changes.[52] These observations may be mechanistically related to the morning increase in tone noted in coronary artery segments with dysfunctional endothelium-dependent dilation in patients with chronic stable angina (see Chaps. 6 and 40).[53] Circadian variations in blood pressure[54] and plasma catecholamine levels[55] that parallel those of ischemic events have been observed. The morning increase in sympathetic activity not only increases the metabolic demand but may also cause coronary vasoconstriction that is unopposed by normal endothelial vasodilator mechanisms, as implied earlier.

There also appear to be exogenous rhythms that influence the development of AMI. In a working population, there is an increased risk for infarction on Mondays.[56] Seasonal variations have also been commented upon, with increases in the winter months of January through March.[57]

Symptoms

Prodromal symptoms antedating AMI are common and occur in at least 60 percent of patients.[58] Since at least 8 to 10 percent of AMIs are painless (not necessarily silent) and many ischemic episodes are silent,[59] it is apparent that the great majority of patients capable of sensing cardiac pain during periods of unstable angina do so in the hours, days, or sometimes weeks prior to the acute event. Most of these symptoms are anginal or angina-like, especially when assessed retrospectively in the context of the character of the pain of the acute infarct. The antecedent symptoms may also be anginal equivalents, such as paroxysmal dyspnea (see Chap. 40). The clinical features of unstable angina are discussed in Chap. 41. If one considers the general feeling of malaise and fatigue that many patients report having experienced prior to acute infarction, it is apparent that it is relatively unusual for the episode to be totally unheralded—a conclusion that is consistent with general clinical experience.

The classic symptoms of AMI involve chest discomfort that is commonly retrosternal or precordial in location and is described as pressure, aching, burning, crushing, squeezing, heavy, swelling, or bursting in quality.[60,61] Typically it has all the features of prolonged angina pectoris that was so eloquently phrased by William Heberden in his original description to the assembly of the Royal College of Physicians in 1772;

> There is a disorder of the breast marked with strong and peculiar symptoms considerable for the kind of danger belonging to it, and not extremely rare, which deserves to be mentioned more at length. The seed of it, and sense of strangling, and anxiety with which it is attended, may make it not improperly be called angina pectoris. They who are afflicted with it, are seized while they are walking (more especially if it be uphill, and soon after eating) with a painful and most disagreeable sensation in the breast, which seems as if it would extinguish life, if it were to increase or to continue; but the moment they stand still, all this uneasiness vanishes.

The location of chest pain is usually of little help in differentiating ischemia/infarction from other causes of chest pain,[62] but severe chest pain (as opposed to vague discomfort) and the presence of associated symptoms (dyspnea, nausea, diaphoresis, etc.) are more commonly associated with AMI.[63] The discomfort often radiates over the anterior chest and frequently into the left arm or both arms (particularly the medial aspect), and/or into the neck or jaw. In unusual instances, the pain may be in the back, particularly between the scapulae. There may be skip areas with retrosternal pain—associated with jaw, antecubital fossa, or wrist pain—or no pain between the two sites. Moreover, the pain may appear only in the referral area. The duration of the pain of infarction is prolonged, lasting conventionally longer than 15 min. While the intensity of the pain is usually steady following an initial crescendo, there is occasionally some waxing and waning. Sudden relief of pain may accompany reperfusion. Associated symptoms may include dyspnea, diaphoresis, nausea, and vomiting. Marked apprehension is common. Occasionally, presenting symptoms include syncope, acute confusion, agitation, stroke, or palpitations.

Approximately 23 percent of myocardial infarctions go unrecognized by patients because of the absence of symptoms or the lack of recognition of the significance of symptoms.[64] The common symptoms in this latter instance are nonclassic or atypical pain, dyspnea, nausea, vomiting, and/or epigastric pain. A myocardial infarction may also masquerade as the development or worsening of congestive heart failure, the appearance of an arrhythmia, an overwhelming sense of apprehension, profound weakness, acute indigestion, pericarditis, embolic stroke, or peripheral embolus.[65] Presentation with painless myocardial infarction is more common in the elderly (age >65 years) than it is in the nonelderly, and this subgroup has an increased frequency of congestive heart failure as the initial presenting symptom.[66]

Physical Findings

GENERAL EXAMINATION

Features of the physical examination during AMI have been the subject of several reviews.[67,68] The patient is frequently sitting up because of a sense of suffocation or a feeling of shortness of breath. Most patients with cardiac pain or myocardial infarction have some sense of impending doom that is reflected in their facial expression. They may have a grayish appearance or one of panic or exhaustion. Diaphoresis is frequent. In severe cases, patients may be quite anxious, with an ashen or pale face beaded with perspiration. The patient should be examined in both the supine and left lateral decubitus position. The major findings pertaining to the heart appear on palpation of the precordium in the left lateral position. It is important to rapidly ascertain the vital signs and the nature, character, and rhythm of the arterial pulse; to observe the jugular venous pulse; to check the peripheral pulses; to palpate the precordium; and to auscultate the chest and precordium. Examination of the extremities should include subjective assessment of the temperature and color of the feet. The presence of very cool feet, especially with acrocyanosis in the setting of tachycardia, suggests low cardiac output.

The heart rate and rhythm are important indicators of cardiac function in the initial hours of myocardial infarction. *A normal rate usually indicates that the patient is not experiencing significant hemodynamic compromise.* In patients with inferior myocardial infarction, heart rates in the 50s and 60s are common in the initial hours. Up to 60 percent of these patients initially have bradycardia, but the rate gradually increases over the next few hours. The bradycardia, which may be associated with secondary hypotension, results from the stimulation of myocardial receptors with vagal afferents. *Persistent sinus tachycardia beyond the initial 12 to 24 h is predictive of a high mortality rate.* The pulse may be low in volume, reflecting decreased stroke volume. The blood pressure is usually normal but may be increased secondary to anxiety, or it may be decreased from cardiac failure. Blood pressure frequently normalizes temporarily with AMI in patients with hypertension. All peripheral pulses should be examined to observe their presence, and their status should be noted both to exclude current occlusion and to provide a baseline in case of future embolic events. The carotid pulse is most useful in assessing systolic upstroke time and stroke volume, which are decreased in the patient with a low output state.

The rhythm of the pulse is important because of the frequency of ectopic atrial and, in particular, ventricular beats in AMI. Observation of the jugular venous pulse is useful in determining whether ectopic beats are atrial or ventricular. A large A wave, indicating that the right atrium is contracting against a closed atrioventricular (AV) valve, suggests that the ectopic beat is ventricular. The respiratory rate is usually within the normal range. However, patients who are extremely anxious often exhibit hyperventilation, and those with pulmonary edema and cardiac failure have an increased respiratory rate associated with shallow inspirations. Abnormal breathing patterns, such as Cheyne-Stokes respirations, are rare unless the patient is in cardiogenic shock.

Examination of the jugular venous pulse is important with AMI, especially in patients with an inferior infarction, because insights can be gained into possible involvement of the right ventricle. The right ventricle is commonly involved with inferior infarction, but right-sided failure is seen only with major right ventricular involvement. It may be manifest by an elevated jugular venous pressure. In addition, in many patients with right ventricular infarction or ischemia, there is also a prominent A wave because of the decreased compliance of the right ventricle.[69] Kussmaul's sign, or an increase in the venous pressure on inspiration, may also be seen in right ventricular infarction/ischemia because of decreased right ventricular compliance. Generally, right ventricular failure commonly reflects left ventricular failure, with secondary elevation in pulmonary and right ventricular pressures. This circumstance usually occurs with large anterior or anterolateral infarction.

EXAMINATION OF THE LUNGS

Basilar rales are frequently detected in AMI. Cardiac failure diagnosed on the basis of mild signs of pulmonary congestion occurs in 30 to 40 percent of patients with otherwise uncomplicated myocardial infarction. A clinical classification proposed by Killip provides some uniformity in terms of describing cardiac failure and pulmonary congestion.[69a] Class I patients do not have any pulmonary rales or a third heart sound. Class II patients have rales of a mild-to-moderate degree, involving less than 50 percent of the lung fields, and may or may not have an S_3 gallop. Class III patients have rales more than halfway up the lung fields and an S_3 gallop. Class IV patients are those in cardiogenic shock.

CARDIAC EXAMINATION

Palpation of the precordium may reveal evidence of regional wall motion abnormalities. Palpation should be performed with the patient initially lying in the supine position; this is often adequate to ascertain whether there is a localized normal apical impulse and also permits assessment for dyskinetic impulses (see Chap. 10). Frequently, one may not feel any precordial impulse with the patient in the supine position because of the decreased intensity of contraction and/or body habitus. With the patient in the left lateral decubitus position, one may palpate a diffuse rather than a localized apical impulse, akinesis, or a paradoxical bulging during late systole; in some patients, there is a palpable atrial contraction corresponding to an audible S_4 gallop due to the decreased compliance of the left ventricle. One or more of these features of decreased contractility or lusitrophy and dysynergy are frequently present in the early hours of AMI, particularly with extensive damage.

The first and second heart sounds are often very soft because of decreased contractility. The first heart sound may also be diminished because of a prolonged PR interval. If there is tachycardia, a shortened PR interval may result in a somewhat accentuated first heart sound. The second heart sound is usually normal; however, with extensive damage, there may be a single second sound. Rarely, paradoxical splitting may reflect severe left ventricular dysfunction. A fourth heart sound is often audible in patients with AMI. A third heart sound is heard in probably only about 15 to 20 percent of AMI patients. A pericardial friction rub can be heard anytime between 24 to 72 h after the onset of myocardial infarction and, since its presence is often transient, frequently repeated auscultation is the best means of detection. The murmur of papillary muscle dysfunction is relatively common early in the course of infarction. This crescendo-decrescendo midsystolic murmur often reflects ischemia of the papillary muscles or the myocardial attachment rather than irreversible injury to these structures. This murmur usually disappears after the first 12 to 24 h if it is soft; however, if the murmur is moderate to loud in intensity, it may persist much longer, possibly throughout the patient's life. Mitral regurgitation is most commonly due to ischemia of the posteromedial papillary muscle (see also Chap. 10). Other findings on physical examination, such as the murmur of papillary muscle rupture or a ruptured ventricular septum, are described in appropriate sections under "Complications."

Diagnosis of Acute Myocardial Infarction

DIFFERENTIAL DIAGNOSIS

Myocardial infarction has typically been diagnosed on the basis of the triad of chest pain, electrocardiographic changes, and elevated plasma enzyme activity. Although AMI occurs without chest pain (20 to 25 percent of cases), chest pain remains the most common symptom and is usually responsible for the patient's seeking medical help. The differential diagnosis of prolonged chest pain is presented in Table 42-1. Chest pain, however, is not specific to cardiac disease, and it is often impossible on the basis of history alone to distinguish ischemia or infarction from other causes of chest pain. The differential diagnosis of chest pain is discussed in Chap. 40. Of patients presenting to the emergency department with chest pain, only about 14 percent are subsequently documented to have AMI.[70–73] Most patients at risk for myocardial infarction will be admitted to evaluate their chest pain unless definite noncardiac causes of chest pain—such as chest wall pain, hyperventilation, pleurisy, gastrointestinal pain, and so on—that are not imminently dangerous can be identified. In the CCU, only about 20 percent of patients admitted with chest pain have AMI.

ELECTROCARDIOGRAPHIC DIAGNOSIS

The electrocardiogram (ECG) is sensitive for detecting myocardial ischemia and infarction but is frequently not powerful enough for differentiating ischemia from necrosis (see Chap.

TABLE 42-1 Differential Diagnosis of Prolonged Chest Pain

AMI
Aortic dissection
Pericarditis
Atypical anginal pain associated with hypertrophic cardiomyopathy
Esophageal, other upper gastrointestinal, or biliary tract disease
Pulmonary disease
Pleurisy: infectious, malignant, or immune disease-related
Embolus with or without infarction
Pneumothorax
Hyperventilation syndrome
Chest wall
Skeletal
Neuropathic
Psychogenic

11).[70,71,74] Serial ECGs during AMI will show some evolutionary changes in the majority of patients.[75] An ECG obtained during cardiac ischemic pain frequently but not always exhibits changes in repolarization. The absence of electrocardiographic changes during pain provides evidence but not proof that the pain is not ischemic in nature. The early electrocardiographic changes of T-wave inversion or ST-segment depression may reflect ischemia or infarction. ST-segment elevation is more specific for AMI and reflects the epicardial injury–associated total occlusion of an epicardial coronary artery. The hallmark of AMI is the development of abnormal Q waves,[76,77] which appear on the average 8 to 12 h from the onset of symptoms but may not develop for 24 to 48 h. Abnormal Q waves usually reflect tissue death and the development of an electrical dead zone. Since abnormal Q waves do not develop immediately, they are not very helpful for initial diagnostic management and therapeutic triage except to signify the presence or absence of prior myocardial infarction. The diagnostic serial electrocardiographic changes consist of ST-segment elevation with the development of T-wave inversion and the evolution of abnormal Q waves (Fig. 42-1).[78] The appearance of abnormal Q waves is very specific to AMI; however, they are present in less than 50 percent of patients with documented AMI.[79] Most of the other patients who have AMI will have electrocardiographic changes restricted to T-wave inversion or ST-segment depression or no change at all. These patients represent the group with non-Q-wave infarction.[80]

The traditional concept that myocardial infarctions can be classified as transmural or nontransmural on the basis of the presence or absence of Q waves is misleading, since autopsy studies have demonstrated convincingly that pathologic Q waves may be associated with nontransmural infarction and may be absent with transmural infarction.[81–83] These misnomers have been replaced by the terms *Q-wave infarction* and *non-Q-wave infarction for transmural and nontransmural infarction*, respectively.[84] The evolution of a non-Q-wave infarction is characterized by a lack of development of an abnormal Q wave and by the appearance of reversible ST-T-wave changes with ST depression that usually returns to normal over a few days, but is occasionally permanent. Differentiation between these two types of infarctions has become entrenched, since there are major differences in their pathogenesis, clinical manifestations, treatment, and prognosis (Table 42-2). The initiating events in the pathogenesis of Q-wave and non-Q-wave infarction are thought to be identical, namely, coronary occlusion induced by a thrombus superimposed on a plaque together with vasoconstriction (see Chap. 36). There is considerable evidence, however, to indicate that in non-Q-wave infarction, early spontaneous reperfusion occurs, the mechanism of which remains uncertain. In contrast, in Q-wave infarction, the coronary occlusion is sustained at least for a long enough period to result in extensive necrosis.

One explanation for early spontaneous reperfusion is the lack of sustained vasoconstriction, which may contribute to occlusion.[85] The evidence supporting the existence of early spontaneous reperfusion in non-Q-wave infarction is as follows:

1. Coronary angiographic studies performed in the early hours after onset show that only about 20 to 30 percent of patients have complete coronary occlusion of infarct-related vessels; however, for Q-wave infarction, it is about 80 to 90 percent.
2. Infarct size is routinely much less than observed with Q-wave infarction, which is consistent with salvage by early reperfusion.
3. Peak plasma CK levels are reached on an average of 12 to 13 h after onset of symptoms, indicating early washout of the enzyme, as opposed to about 27 h after Q-wave infarction.
4. Reperfusion-induced contraction necrosis is extremely common, as it is in patients who undergo early reperfusion induced by thrombolytic therapy.[86]
5. Acute mortality rates are around 2 to 3 percent, compared with 10 percent for Q-wave infarction.
6. The complications are minimal compared with those after a Q-wave infarction.
7. Finally, the long-term prognosis is characterized by recurrent episodes of reinfarction, so that after about 2 years, survival is the same as that after Q-wave infarction.[80,87–90]

Traditional teaching has held that AMI could not be diagnosed electrocardiographically in the presence of a left bundle branch block because of the unpredictability of the depolarization and repolarization patterns. It has been suggested that marked ST-segment deviation, beyond what could be anticipated from the conduction abnormality, could be useful in the diagnosis of AMI in the setting of a left bundle branch block.[91]

The resting ECG is insensitive for detecting the presence of atherosclerotic coronary heart disease; it is normal in 50 percent of patients with angiographically significant coronary obstruction.[92] Nevertheless, an abnormally wide Q wave on a resting ECG has been the standard criterion for the diagnosis of a myocardial infarction for over 60 years.[93]

The electrocardiographic criteria for the diagnosis of AMI as outlined in the MILIS study are the presence, in the setting of chest pain, of any one of the following: (1) new or presumably new Q waves (at least 30 ms wide and 0.20 mV deep) in at least two leads from any of the following: (a) leads II, III, or aV_F; (b) leads V_1 through V_6; or (c) leads I and aV_L; (2) new or presumably new ST-T- segment elevation or depression ($\geq$0.10 mV measured 0.02 s after the J point in two contiguous leads of the previously mentioned lead combination); or (3) a complete left bundle branch block in the appropriate clinical setting. An evaluation of these criteria in 1809 enzyme-confirmed infarctions found that 21 percent of the patients with an infarction had none of these changes.[94] Conversely, over 90 percent of patients who had ST-segment elevation of 0.1 mV, as described previously, were confirmed to have AMI. If the patients also had ST-segment depression in the so-called reciprocal leads, the infarction rate was 3 percent higher. Patients with a left branch bundle block or ST-segment depression without other abnormalities had a lower rate of infarction (46 and 52 to 56 percent, respectively) than those with ST-segment elevation. Furthermore, the presence of abnormal Q waves on the resting ECG accurately predicts the presence and location of left ventricular contraction abnormalities. In a study of 64 patients with abnormal Q waves on the ECG, all patients with abnormal Q waves in the anterior leads and 30 of 33 with abnormal Q waves in the inferior leads demonstrated contraction abnormalities in the corresponding left ventricular segments.[95] The evolution of a Q-wave myocardial infarction can be separated electrocardiographically into four phases: (1) hyperacute, (2) acute, (3) subacute, and (4) chronic stabilized (Fig. 42-1; see Chap. 11).

In the hyperacute phase (Fig. 42-1), the earliest electrocardiographic manifestation of an acute infarction is usually a straightening of the normal upward concavity of the ST-T segment.[96] With further evolution, the straightened ST-T segment becomes elevated. The ST-T segment usually slopes upward, since the portion of the ST-T segment nearest the T wave is more elevated than the proximal portion. Also, the amplitude of the T wave is usually increased. Occasionally, the ST-T segment may be markedly elevated and yet retain its upward concavity. ST-T depressions in leads oriented toward the presumably noninfarcted myocardium were traditionally termed *reciprocal changes*. Studies have indicated that such ST-T depressions usually reflect more extensive infarction. In the subacute phase, the abnormal Q wave representing myocardial necrosis begins to appear, but the T-wave vector still points toward the infarct zone (Fig. 42-1). In the fully evolved phase, the ST-T segment begins to diminish in amplitude and becomes coved or convex upward. It blends into the now symmetrically inverted T waves (see Fig. 42-1). The abnormal Q waves (>0.03 s in duration and more than 25 percent of the R-wave

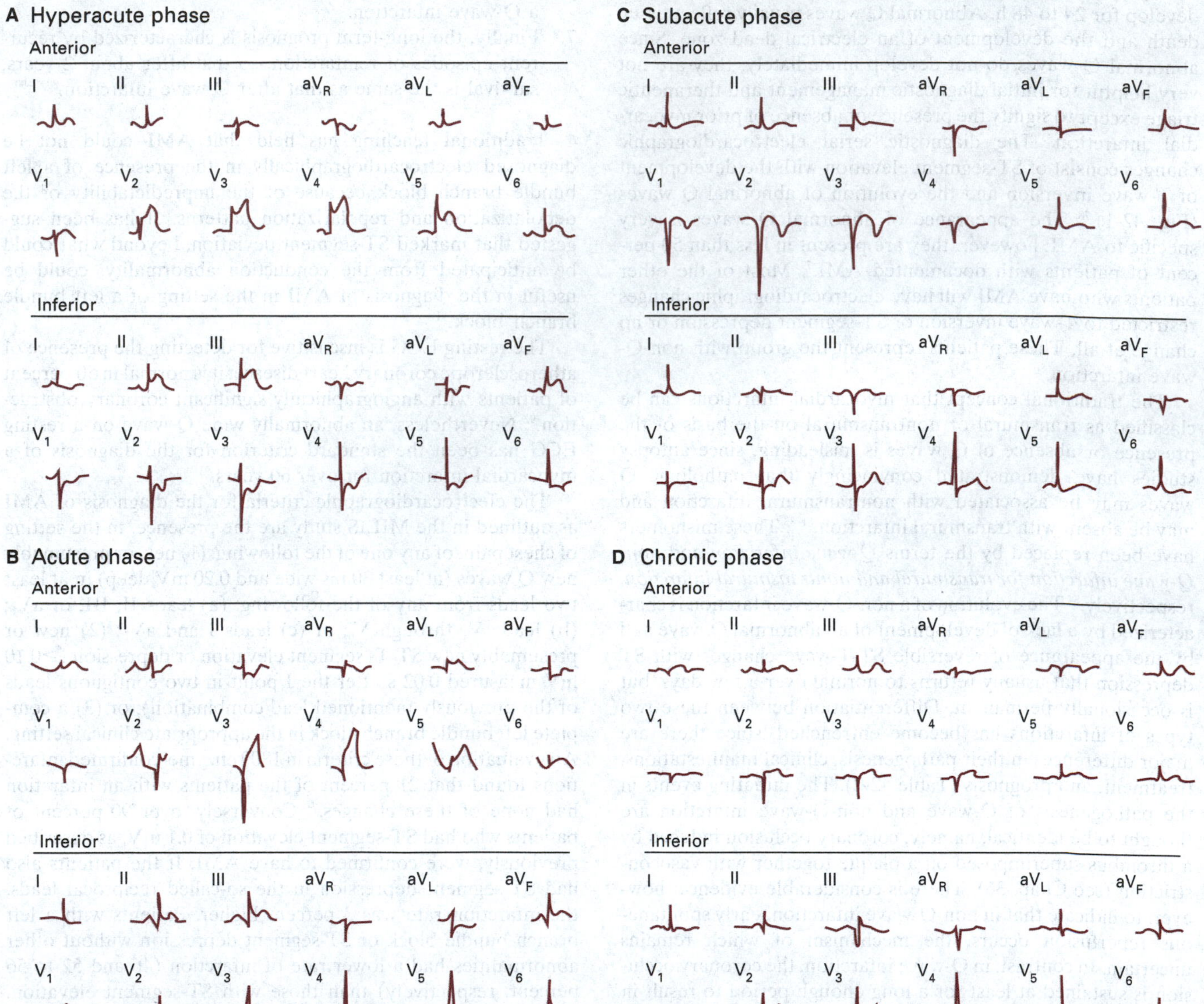

FIGURE 42-1 Electrocardiographic evolution of acute anterior and inferior myocardial infarction. *A*. Hyperacute phase. There is marked ST-segment elevation in V_2 to V_5 in the anterior infarction and in II, III, and aV_F in the inferior infarction. In the inferior infarction, there are reciprocal changes or posterior involvement as reflected in the ST-segment depression in the precordial leads. There are no QRS changes in either case. *B*. Acute phase. Q waves indicating myocardial necrosis develop during this phase. There is some persistent ST-segment elevation and the T-wave vector generally points toward the infarct zone. *C*. Subacute phase. QRS changes are well developed and ST-segment elevation is still present. The T vector, or, more precisely, the terminal portion of the T vector, begins to point away from the infarct zone. *D*. Chronic phase. Minimal or no ST-segment elevation is present, and the T wave is directed away from the infarct zone. (From Wagner et al.,[78] with permission.)

TABLE 42-2 Differences between Patients with Q-Wave and Non-Q-Wave Myocardial Infarction

Characteristic	Q-Wave	Non-Q-Wave
Prevalence	47%	53%
Incidence of coronary occlusion	80–90%	15–25%
ST-T segment elevation	80%	25%
ST-T segment depression	20%	75%
Postinfarction angina	15–25%	30–40%
Incidence of early reinfarction	5–8%	15–25%
1-Month mortality	10–15%	3–5%
2-Year mortality	30%	30%
Infarct size	Moderate to large	Usually small
Residual ischemia	10–20%	40–50%
Acute complication	Common	Uncommon
Therapy		
Thrombolysis	Indicated	Not indicated
Beta-adrenergic blockers	Indicated	Retrospective analysis not definitive
Calcium channel blockers		
Nifedepine	Possibly detrimental	Not determined
Diltiazem	Not indicated	Recommended
Verapamil	Beneficial	Possibly beneficial but not established

amplitude) appear during this stage. During the chronic phase (Fig. 42-1), there is generally resolution of the ST- and T-wave changes, with the only residual change being an abnormal Q wave. Although the ST-T segments again become isoelectric, they are frequently horizontal, with a sharp-angled ST-T junction, rather than exhibiting the normal concavity. Occasionally, in small inferior infarctions, even the abnormal Q waves resolve.

Posterior myocardial infarction occurs in the posterior left ventricular wall. An isolated true posterior infarction is quite uncommon, since such an infarction is usually associated with an inferior or lateral infarction. Since there are no electrocardiographic leads oriented toward the posterior left ventricular wall, the electrocardiographic changes of a true posterior infarction are seen as mirror-image representations in leads V_1 to V_3. Schamroth described the criteria for a true posterior infarction as follows: R waves of 0.04 s in lead V_1 and in contiguous right precordial leads with upright T waves, and, in the acute phase, ST-segment depression and an R/S ratio ≥1 in leads V_1 and V_2.[96] Usually, there are associated changes of an inferior or lateral infarction. As the infarction evolves, the ST-segment depression decreases and the upright T-wave amplitude increases. It is helpful to turn the ECG upside down and look at it from the back while holding it to a strong light. The changes in leads V_1 and V_2, which might be overlooked on a direct glance, are seen as abnormal Q waves, ST-segment elevation, and T-wave inversion when viewed from this perspective.

Similarly, electrocardiographic diagnosis of right ventricular infarction offers special challenges. Since right ventricular infarction generally occurs in the presence of inferior left ventricular infarction, the resulting ST-segment elevation is usually overwhelmed in the conventional precordial leads overlying the right ventricle (V_2 and V_3) by the ST-segment elevation in the opposing left ventricular myocardium on the inferior surface. The right ventricular electrical forces might be manifest in this setting as a diminution of the usual reciprocal ST-segment depression seen in the right precordial leads in inferior infarction. If the injury to the inferior wall is minimal, ST-segment elevation will occasionally be seen in V_2 through V_4 in the presence of right ventricular infarction.[97] Otherwise, ST-segment elevation must be sought in the right chest leads, V_1, and V_{3R} through V_{6R}. ST-segment elevation in these leads provides reasonably strong evidence for the presence of right ventricular infarction.[98] A postmortem study has shown that a 25 percent or greater involvement of the right ventricle was necessary to produce ST-T-segment elevation.[99] Atrial infarction is usually reflected in PR-segment elevation or depression and P-wave abnormalities and is frequently associated with supraventricular arrhythmias, as discussed later.[100]

The phenomenon of "ischemia at a distance" reflects the occurrence, in AMI with ST-segment elevation, of ST-segment depression in other, frequently reciprocal leads. It remains uncertain whether these changes represent true reciprocal changes or subendocardial ischemia in the area, but the presence of the finding is associated with a less favorable prognosis than its absence.[101,102]

Criteria for electrocardiographic diagnosis of AMI in various areas of the heart are discussed more fully in Chap. 11. In view of a lack of sensitivity and specificity of the chest pain history or of the ECG, confirmation of the diagnosis of AMI is based on elevated plasma levels of cardiac-specific isoenzymes.

PLASMA DIAGNOSTIC MARKERS

Tissue Distribution of MB-CK, Troponin T, Troponin I, and Myoglobin Myocardial necrosis is associated with the release of a variety of macromolecules, including enzymes, myoglobin, and contractile proteins that have been evaluated as potential diagnostic markers for AMI. The use of CK and MB-CK has become routine and is highly sensitive, specific, and cost-effective for diagnosing myocardial infarction.[103] The use of total CK alone without MB-CK yields a similar sensitivity, but specificity is markedly lower, in the range of 70 percent.[104] The use of total CK as a diagnostic marker for myocardial infarction is discouraged. CK consists of two monomers, each having a molecular weight of 43,000. The isoenzymes of CK are formed by the association of two M monomers (MM-CK), which predominate in muscle (hence the name); or of two B monomers (BB-CK), which predominate in the brain and internal visceral organs; and a hybrid form (MB-CK), found in the heart, composed of one M subunit and one B subunit. The isoenzymes MM, MB, and BB are located in the cytoplasm of the cell. There are separate genes for each of the monomers, which have been isolated, cloned, and sequenced.[105,106] About 5 percent of cellular MM-CK activity is associated with the M line of the sarcomere in both heart and skeletal muscle and a significant amount is in the Z line in heart muscle.

Fifteen percent of the CK in the myocardium is in the form of MB-CK, which provides for its sensitivity and specificity as a diagnostic marker of AMI. Several investigators have found small amounts of MB-CK in normal adult skeletal muscle,[107,108] whereas others have failed to detect any cytosolic CK other than MM-CK.[109,110] MB-CK is alleged to increase (1 to 5 percent) in skeletal muscle following injury such as chronic exercise,[111,112] inflammation,[113] trauma,[114] and electrical injury.[115] In hereditary muscle diseases, such as Duchenne muscular dystrophy (DMD), there is also increased MB-CK in the range of 1 to 5 percent. During the first 6 weeks of life in utero, only BB-CK is synthesized, while at about the eighth week, M-CK synthesis is induced and rapidly supplants the B-CK in skeletal and cardiac muscle, such that by about the twelfth week, MM-CK predominates.[116,117] It is believed that in DMD, the retained expression of the B-CK reflects the abnormal development of these muscles. It is postulated that in the case of the reaction to muscle injury, undifferentiated skeletal muscle cells differentiate to form mature skeletal myocytes and thus repeat the developmental program of fetal skeletal muscle, but the expression of B-CK is transient.[118] In the adult human heart, 15 percent of total CK activity is MB-CK and the remainder is MM-CK. Myoglobin, with a molecular weight of 17,000, is ubiquitously distributed throughout cardiac and skeletal muscles.[119]

Two new diagnostic cardiac markers have been introduced: troponin T and troponin I,[120] which are part of the sarcomere complex. Troponin T has a molecular weight of 38,000, and troponin I, 23,000. There are three genes for each of the troponins that encode for slow and fast skeletal and cardiac muscle.[121] Cardiac troponin I has 31 amino acids, which are not present in the skeletal forms. The recognition site of the antibody used in the assay is in the cardiac-specific region, which makes the test very specific as a marker for myocardial injury,[122] and since normal plasma levels of troponin I are near 0, it is also very sensitive. Furthermore, studies indicate that cardiac troponin I is not upregulated in skeletal muscle with hypertrophy or injury and the skeletal form is not upregulated in the heart with hypertrophy or injury.[123] Cardiac troponin T has 11 amino acids not present in the skeletal forms, which has permitted the development of a specific diagnostic test.[121] Troponin T has similar sensitivity to troponin I but the first generation assay had less specificity, while the second generation assay appears to have similar specificity to that of troponin I.[121]

Temporal Profiles of MB-CK, Myoglobin, Troponin I, and Troponin T Released into Plasma Plasma MB-CK activity following myocardial infarction is significantly elevated, such that reliable diagnostic sensitivity (>90 percent) is reached within 12 to 16 h of the onset of symptoms. Maximal levels[124] of MB-CK are reached between 14 and 36 h, with a return to normal levels occurring after 48 to 72 h (Fig. 42-2). In patients with minimal cardiac injury, such as occurs in non-Q-wave infarction or following effective early reperfusion, plasma MB-CK activity reaches maximal activity at about 12 to 15 h. In contrast, after Q-wave infarction with reperfusion, it reaches maximal activity at an average of 28 h. The plasma temporal profiles of troponin I and troponin T are very similar to those of total CK and MB-CK. Troponin I and troponin T are released into the plasma so that reliable diagnostic sensitivity (>90 percent) is reached by 12 to 16 h and maximal activity is reached by 24 to 36 h. The levels return to normal within 10 to 12 days.[124] Plasma myoglobin is increased within 2 h of the onset of symptoms and remains increased for at least 7 to 12 h.[119]

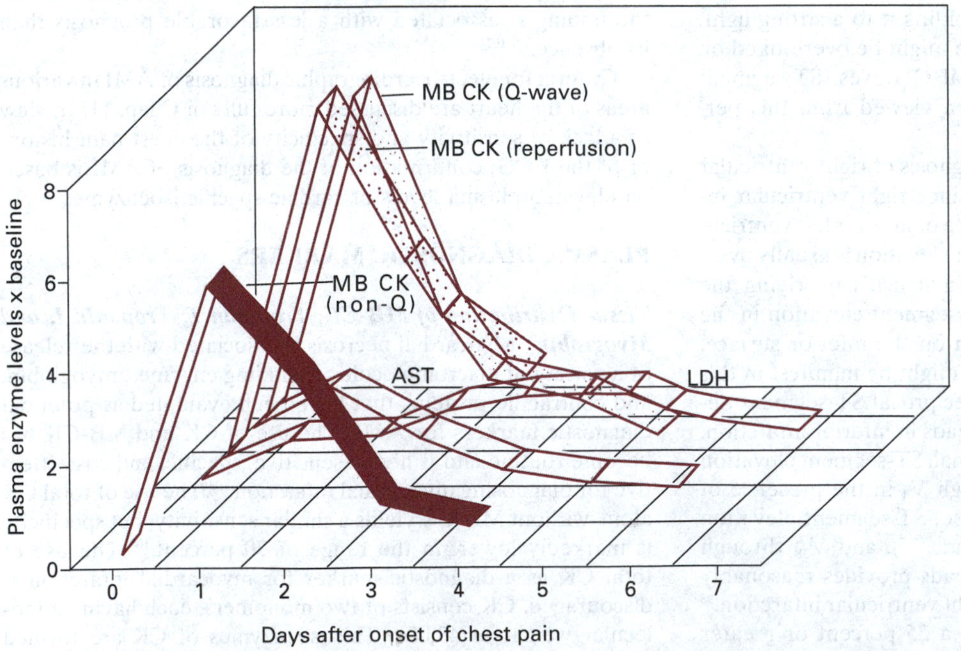

FIGURE 42-2 Typical plasma profiles for the MB isoenzyme of creatine kinase (MB-CK), aspartate amino transferase (AST), and lactate dehydrogenase (LDH) activities following onset of acute myocardial infarction.

Early Diagnosis (6 to 10 h of Onset): MB-CK Subforms and Myoglobin In the United States, over 5 million patients with chest pain go annually to the emergency department, but only about 10 percent with chest pain will subsequently be shown to have myocardial infarction.[124] About 50 percent of patients will have cardiac ischemia, 10 percent will have nonischemic cardiac pain, and about 30 percent will have pain of noncardiac origin.[124] It is important to have an early diagnosis to determine the initial therapeutic regimen and whether hospital admission is needed. In the United States, it is estimated that over $12 billion per year[125] is spent unnecessarily to exclude myocardial infarction in patients admitted to the hospital with chest pain without infarction. Thus, early, rapid diagnosis is required to triage patients, reduce costs, and select appropriate therapy in spite of the difficulty in distinguishing cardiac ischemia from infarction based on the patient's history, physical examination, and the ECG, as noted. This difficulty is emphasized by the observation that over 50 percent of AMI patients in the United States[126] have nonspecific ST-segment changes (non-Q-wave infarction) rather than ST-segment elevation (Q-wave infarction). The only specific electrocardiographic finding on admission for myocardial infarction is the recent development of ST-segment elevation or left bundle branch block. It is estimated that less than 50 percent of patients with AMI will have a diagnostic ECG, which represents only 5 percent of the total patients presenting with chest pain; thus, there is a need for an early objective marker (within 6 h of onset).[71] The ideal diagnostic test should have an assay performance time that is brief, and the marker must have a highly reliable negative predictive value, since only 10 percent of patients will have infarction, as noted. While a false-positive range of 5 to 10 percent is acceptable, a desirable false-negative range is 1 to 2 percent. Assessment of the plasma profile of the markers shows only two plausible candidates, namely, MB-CK subforms and myoglobin.

It was recognized for some time that MM and MB-CK, though present in tissue in single forms, exhibit different forms upon release into the circulation, as detected by electrophoresis.[127] In 1982, it was shown that upon release into the circulation, MM-CK is converted into three forms: MM-3, MM-2, and MM-1, and MB-CK is converted into MB-2 and MB-1, due to the proteolytic activity of carboxypeptidase-N, an enzyme present in the blood of all vertebrates.[128,129] Carboxypeptidase-N cleaves the terminal amino acid, lysine, from the M subunit of the MB-CK, which is positively charged, leaving the remaining molecule more negatively charged (MB-1). The more negative form (MB-1), upon electrophoresis, separates from the parent tissue form (MB-2), giving rise to the two forms of MB-CK in plasma. A new technique utilizing 1400 V, which provides separation of the MB subforms within about 6 min,[130] is coupled with automated densitometric quantification; this produces a value for MB-2 activity, the plasma ratio of MB-2 to MB-1, and total MB-CK activity.[131] The current assay for the MB-CK subforms is completely automated and requires about 25 min. In the plasma, the MB-CK subforms are in equilibrium, with a ratio of MB-2 to MB-1 of 1 to 1. Normally, the baseline plasma MB-CK activity is in the range of 2 to 4 IU/L, or a protein concentration of 3 to 5 ng/L. Thus, for a reliable diagnosis of myocardial infarction based on total MB-CK activity, one requires an increase above 9 IU/L, or, for protein, above 7 ng/L. When infarction occurs, MB-2, the tissue form, is initially released into the circulation in minute amounts so that total plasma MB-CK activity remains within the normal range, but the ratio of MB-2 to MB-1 changes markedly and provides the basis for an early diagnosis of myocardial infarction. In a large, blinded, prospective study involving 1110 patients presenting consecutively with chest pain, it was shown that MB-CK subforms reliably diagnosed myocardial infarction within 6 h of onset of symptoms.[131]

The introduction of troponins T and I necessitated the need to provide comparative diagnostic sensitivity and specificity for all of the markers. A large, multicenter, prospective, double-blind study, the Diagnostic Marker Cooperative Study (DMCS), was performed, comprising 1004 patients admitted consecutively with chest pain.[124] A serial analysis of all markers (MB-CK activity, MB-CK mass, MB-CK subforms, myoglobin, and cardiac troponin T and I) was performed on a sample taken on admission, at 1 h, every 2 h for up to 6 h from onset, and subsequently every 4 h for up to 24 h. Every effort was made to obtain the time of onset of symptoms. In keeping with previous observations, only 11 percent of the patients with chest pain were subsequently documented to have infarction (n = 118), of whom less than 47 percent had a diagnostic ECG (43 percent had ST-segment elevation and 4 percent had a left bundle branch block), with the remainder having nonspecific ST-T changes (non-Q-wave infarction). Cardiac ischemia accounted for 51 percent and nonischemic cardiac pain for another 9 percent, while in 29 percent the pain was of noncardiac origin. The diagnostic sensitivity and specificity of each of the markers are indicated in Table 42-3. MB-CK subforms afforded a sensitivity and specificity of 91 percent for the diagnosis of infarction within 6 h of the onset of symptoms. Myoglobin had a sensitivity of 83 percent during the same interval. The negative predictive value of MB-CK subforms within the initial 6 h of onset was 97 percent and that of myoglobin was 95 percent. Thus, if a patient has a negative MB-CK subform test at 6 h after the onset of symptoms, one can reliably conclude that the patient does not have infarction. During the same interval of 6 h from onset, the total MB-CK (activity or mass assay) and troponins T and I afforded a sensitivity of only 65 percent. A major observation from this study—with significant diagnostic, therapeutic, and cost-saving implications—is the finding that MB-CK subforms correctly diagnosed 92 percent of the patients with myocardial infarction within 60 min of arriving in the emergency department. This was based on the results of the sample collected on admission to the emergency department and on a second sample collected 1 h later (Table 42-4). For the same two samples, however, myoglobin had a sensitivity of 83 percent. The mean time required to make the diagnosis of myocardial infarction using MB-CK subforms was 1.2 h ± 20 min from arrival in the emergency department, and a similar time was required to exclude those without infarction. It is evident from the data in Table 42-3 that total MB-CK, troponin T, and troponin I have high sensitivity and specificity for the diagnosis of myocardial infarction 12 to 16 h from the onset of symptoms. It is noteworthy that the sensitivity of myoglobin decreases after about 7 or 8 h because of rapid renal clearance and thus may not be reliable after 10 to 12 h, particularly in patients with minimal injury.

Sampling Intervals and the Diagnosis of Infarction In patients presenting within the first 10 h of the onset of myocardial infarction, the appropriate marker is either MB-CK subforms or myoglobin, since other markers lack the necessary sensitivity. It is recommended that a blood sample be taken immediately on admission, 1 h later, then every 2 h until 6 h from the onset of symptoms, and then, if positive, every 6 h for 24 to 48 h. The MB-CK subform assay provides a diagnosis based on the first two samples (initial and 1 h) in more than 90 percent of the patients with infarction. Once a sample is positive, one can sample every 6 h for 24 to 48 h. If the sample shows normal values for the MB-CK subforms, one must sample until 6 h from the onset of symptoms to reliably exclude infarction, at

TABLE 42-3 Diagnostic Sensitivity and Specificity of Markers for Myocardial Infarction Based on Time from Onset of Chest Pain

	Early Diagnosis		Late Diagnosis				
Time, hours	2	4	6	10	14	18	22
MARKER							
MB-CK subforms							
Sensitivity (%)	21.1	46.4	91.5	96.2	90.6	80.9	53.1
Specificity (%)	90.5	88.9	89.0	90.2	90.0	89.9	92.2
Myoglobin							
Sensitivity (%)	26.3	42.9	78.7	86.5	62.3	57.5	42.9
Specificity (%)	87.3	89.4	89.4	90.2	88.3	88.8	91.3
Troponin T							
Sensitivity (%)	10.5	35.7	61.7	86.5	84.9	78.7	85.7
Specificity (%)	98.4	98.3	96.1	96.4	96.1	95.7	94.6
Troponin I							
Sensitivity (%)	15.8	35.7	57.5	92.3	90.6	95.7	89.8
Specificity (%)	96.8	94.2	94.3	94.6	92.2	93.4	94.2
Total MB-CK activity							
Sensitivity (%)	21.1	40.7	74.5	96.2	98.1	97.9	89.8
Specificity (%)	100.0	98.8	97.5	97.5	96.1	96.9	96.2
Total MB-CK mass							
Sensitivity (%)	15.8	39.3	66.0	90.4	90.5	95.7	95.7
Specificity (%)	99.2	98.8	100.0	99.6	98.9	99.6	99.1

which time sampling can be discontinued. Sampling for 24 to 48 h in patients with positive MB-CK subforms is optional, but it is recommended for the following reasons: to obtain maximal total plasma MB-CK activity as a rough index of the extent of damage; to follow the decline in MB-CK subform activity as a baseline for subsequent procedures often performed, such as cardiac catheterization or percutaneous transluminal coronary angioplasty (PTCA); and to facilitate detection of early reinfarction, which accounts for 30 to 40 percent of in-hospital deaths in patients recovering from AMI. If the myoglobin is analyzed, a similar sampling algorithm is followed except that the interval required to exclude or include infarction with myoglobin may be longer, since with MB-CK subforms, 90 percent of patients with AMI are diagnosed within 60 min (two samples), whereas only 80 percent over the same interval will be diagnosed with myoglobin. Patients presenting 10 to 12 h or later after the onset of symptoms should have a sample taken on admission; if this is positive, it should be repeated every 6 h for 24 to 48 h. Total MB-CK, troponin T, or troponin I in this time frame will provide the desired diagnostic sensitivity and specificity. Normal total plasma MB-CK activity or protein concentrations at 12 to 16 h from the onset of symptoms excludes infarction with 95 to 100 percent reliability, as does a normal troponin T or I. Plasma myoglobin is not a reliable marker 8 to 10 h after the onset of symptoms. The upper level of normal for MB-2 is ≥2.6 IU/L, with a ratio of MB-2 to MB-1 of ≥1.7. The upper limit of normal for myoglobin is 85 ng/mL. The upper limit of total MB-CK activity is 9 IU/L, and for protein (mass) assays, 7 ng/mL. The upper limit of normal for troponin T is 0.1 ng/mL and for troponin I 1.5 ng/mL. The following guidelines are suggested as enzymatic criteria for the diagnosis of myocardial infarction (Table 42-5).

If there is a serial elevation in plasma MB-CK levels followed by a decrease to baseline, with a change of 25 percent or more between the two values or plasma MB-CK activity increases 50 percent or more between two samples separated by at least 4 h and not more than 12 h:

1. Preferably, the diagnosis is made on the basis of no fewer than two samples in a 24-h period, separated by at least 4 h.
2. If only a single sample is present, the diagnosis must be made on the basis of an elevation above normal by at least twofold.

TABLE 42-4 Diagnostic Sensitivity of Myoglobin and MB-CK Subforms on Admission and 1 h Later

Markers	Sample on Admission (%)	Sample 1 h Later (%)
MB-CK subform	67	91
Myoglobin	63	78

TABLE 42-5 Enzymatic Criteria for Diagnosis of Myocardial Infarction

Serial increase, then decrease of plasma MB-CK, with a change >25% between any two values
MB-CK >10–13 U/L or >5% total CK activity
Increase in MB-CK activity >50% between any two samples, separated by at least 4 h
If only a single sample available, MB-CK elevation > twofold
Beyond 72 h, an elevation of troponin T or I or LDH-1 > LDH-2

3. In patients admitted beyond 72 h from the onset of infarction, troponin T or I is preferred, since MB-CK levels may have returned to normal. The preceding criteria for MB-CK have not been evaluated for troponin T or I but would probably serve as guidelines until further information is available. These principles are incorporated into the protocols for triaging patients in the emergency department, as illustrated in Fig. 42-3.

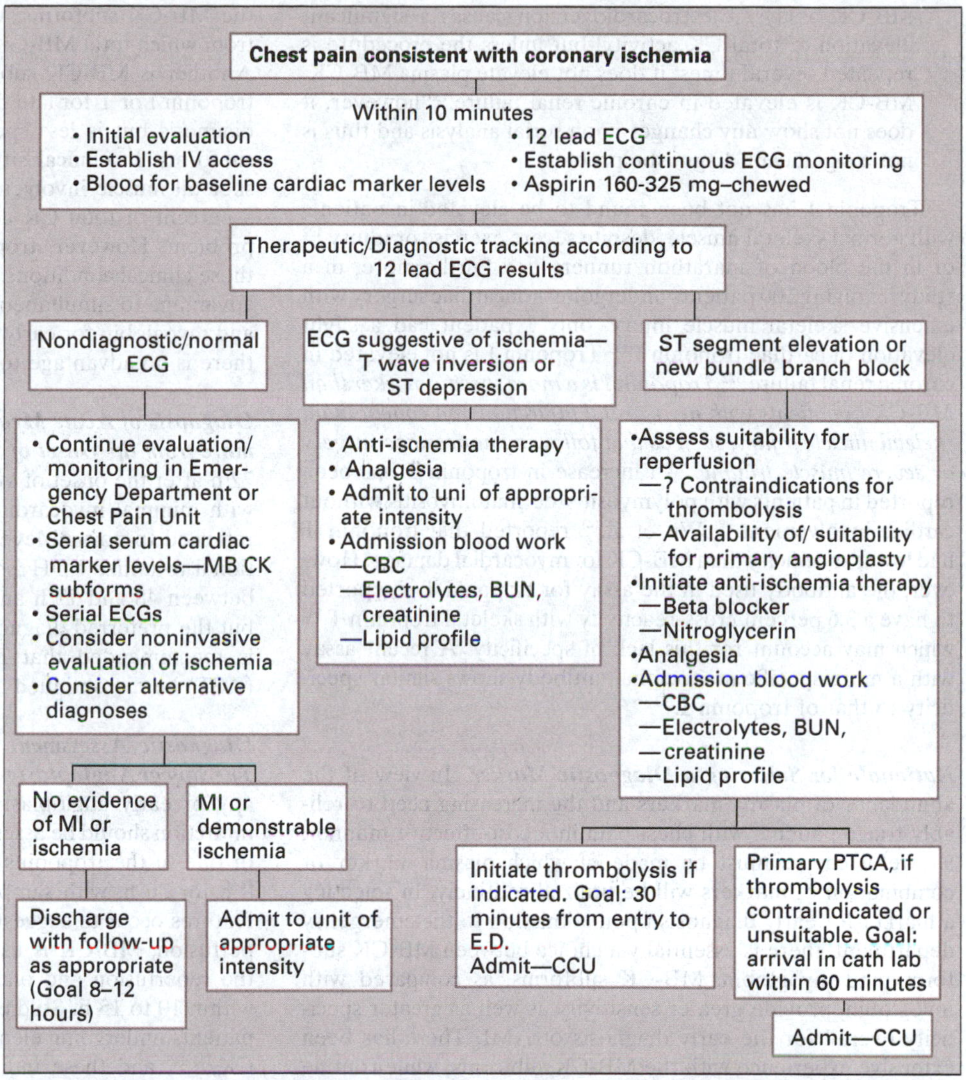

FIGURE 42-3 Algorithm for the initial assessment and evaluation of the patient with acute chest pain in the emergency department. The emergency department should be organized to facilitate the rapid triage of chest pain patients so that the initial evaluation, the obtainment of a 12-lead ECG, and the establishment of intravenous access and continuous monitoring are accomplished within 10 min. The path in the decision tree is determined by the results of the 12-lead ECG. The presence of ST-segment elevation diagnostic of acute myocardial infarction or of presumptively new bundle branch block suggestive of this diagnosis should lead to the immediate consideration of the suitability of the patient for reperfusion therapy, which, if indicated, should be initiated within 30 min of the patient's arrival. The primary PTCA option is applicable only in those settings in which it is immediately available and can be performed by highly qualified interventional cardiologists. In general, patients should not be transferred for angioplasty if thrombolysis is an option, especially if significant delays will be incurred. Thrombolysis is not indicated in patients with only ST-segment depression.

Limitations to Myoglobin, MB-CK, and Troponins I and T Elevated plasma MB-CK as a diagnostic marker for myocardial infarction is associated with a very low incidence of false-negative results if samples are collected frequently and appropriately within 48 to 72 h of the onset of symptoms. However, false-positive results do occur, since trace amounts of MB-CK can be released from tissues other than the heart. Skeletal muscle injury may induce the synthesis of MB-CK and has been documented after crush injury,[114] electrical injury,[115] dermatomyositis and polymyositis,[113] and DMD,[132] as well as in professional athletes and marathon runners.[111,112] If one suspects that elevated plasma MB-CK activity is due to skeletal rather than cardiac muscle, the following should be considered:

1. The appropriate clinical setting, namely, skeletal muscle disease or trauma.
2. An atypical time course for the increase and decrease in plasma MB-CK activity, particularly if prolonged, as one might see in inflammatory disorders.
3. If MB-CK accounts for less than 5 percent of the total CK activity, then a skeletal muscle source should be suspected. Since tissues that contain MB-CK (other than the myocardium), such as skeletal muscle, contain only trace amounts (1 to 2 percent), elevated plasma MB-CK indicative of myocardial infarction should exceed 5 percent of total activity. At the time of peak plasma CK resulting from myocardial infarction, MB-CK levels usually make up 10 to 15 percent of the total activity.
4. A marked elevation of total CK activity of 20- to 30-fold suggests that the cause is more likely to be skeletal muscle injury. Hypothyroidism is associated with elevated levels of both total CK and MB-CK due to diminished clearance.[133] Occasionally, one sees what is referred to as macro CK-1, a complex of CK and macroglobulins, which migrates in the position of MB-CK upon electrophoresis[134,135] and results in a false-positive diagnosis of AMI. Macro CK-1 is common in elderly women and in patients who are chronically ill, with an overall stated incidence of 1.6 percent in hospitalized patients.[135] This is not a problem for assays utilizing MB-CK monoclonal antibody, as is currently the case for most

MB-CK assays. Electrocardioversion causes a significant elevation of total CK activity, but unless the procedure is repeated several times, it does not elevate plasma MB-CK. MB-CK is elevated in chronic renal failure;[136] however, it does not show any changes upon serial analysis and thus is not a significant diagnostic problem.

Troponin I has not been found to be elevated in patients with normal skeletal muscle, despite severe exercise or injury,[122] or in the blood of marathon runners.[137,138] Furthermore, in a study involving 100 patients undergoing noncardiac surgery with extensive skeletal muscle injury, only 1 patient had a slight elevation of cardiac troponin I.[139] Troponin I is not elevated in chronic renal failure.[122] *Troponin I is a more specific marker than MB-CK in patients with myocardial infarction and concomitant skeletal muscle injury, such as that following noncardiac surgery or severe muscle trauma.* An increase in troponin T has been reported in patients with polymyositis/dermatomyositis without cardiac involvement.[140] Wu et al.[141] reported that troponin T had lower specificity than MB-CK for myocardial damage. However, the antibody used in the assay for troponin T is reported to have a 3.6 percent cross-reactivity with skeletal troponin T,[142] which may account for this lack of specificity. A recent assay with a more specific monoclonal antibody shows similar specificity to that of troponin I.[121]

Rationale for Selecting a Diagnostic Marker In view of the abundance of plasma markers and the increasing need to reliably triage patients with chest pain in a cost-effective manner, a careful choice must be made of which plasma marker or combination of markers will be utilized routinely. In selecting a marker for early diagnosis upon admission to the emergency department, there is essentially a choice between MB-CK subforms and myoglobin. MB-CK subforms, as compared with myoglobin, provide greater sensitivity as well as greater specificity overall for the early diagnosis of AMI. There has been extensive experience with the MB-CK subforms, while routine use of myoglobin for the diagnosis of infarction is minimal. Nevertheless, if patients with trauma are avoided, the specificity of myoglobin is quite acceptable, and it is the next best alternative for an early diagnosis, as indicated in Tables 42-3 and 42-4. Both assays are automated and simple to perform, requiring only about 25 min, and are identical in cost. For the diagnosis of patients presenting 10 h or later after the onset of symptoms, total MB-CK, which has been the standard for more than two decades, is extremely sensitive and specific. However, cardiac troponin I or cardiac troponin T, since they are not normally present in the blood and do not appear to be present in skeletal muscle, provide greater specificity than MB-CK in those clinical conditions in which there is concommitant skeletal muscle injury. It is also claimed that troponin I and T may provide increased sensitivity over that of MB-CK since they are not normally present in the blood; however, further studies are required before the claim of greater sensitivity can be accepted. The time required to assay each of these latter three markers is about 25 min, with identical costs. The choice of marker or markers used routinely may depend in part on the various tests with which the laboratory personnel are acquainted. However, there is no reason, based on diagnostic sensitivity and specificity, to assay all of these markers; in addition, the cost would be prohibitive. A single assay for both early and late diagnosis is the MB-CK subforms, which provide an early diagnosis and from which total MB-CK can be derived for the late diagnosis. Another is MB-CK subforms for early diagnosis, plus either troponin I or T for late diagnosis. Myoglobin provides an early diagnosis but is less specific and less sensitive than MB-CK subforms. In clinical situations where there is concommitant skeletal muscle involvement, MB-CK, if elevated, is less than 5 percent of total CK activity and is usually not a diagnostic problem. However, troponin I or T is more appropriate in those clinical conditions. The data from the DMCS indicate no advantage to simultaneously analyzing both MB-CK subforms and myoglobin for early diagnosis; similarly, for late diagnosis, there is no advantage to analyzing multiple markers.

Diagnosis of Acute Myocardial Infarction in Patients 48 h or more from the Onset of Symptoms In patients admitted 48 to 72 h after the onset of symptoms, particularly when associated with minimal myocardial damage, plasma MB-CK may have returned to normal levels. In this situation, it has been traditional to utilize LDH isoenzymes, since LDH-1 activity peaks between 48 and 72 h and remains elevated for 10 to 14 days, but the preferred diagnostic marker is now troponin I or T. It is recommended that LDH, LDH isoenzymes, and SGOT (AST) be discontinued as diagnostic markers for AMI.

Diagnostic Assessment of Patients Undergoing Fibrinolytic Therapy or Angioplasty Patients who receive fibrinolytic therapy or early angioplasty (within 4 to 6 h) for treatment of infarction should be assessed hourly for plasma MB-CK activity or one of the troponins for the first 4 to 6 h, then every 6 to 8 h for 36 h, with sampling reinitiated if chest pain or other features occur to suggest reinfarction. Following successful reperfusion, MB-CK is usually elevated within 30 to 60 min of the reperfusion and plasma activity reaches maximum levels within 10 to 15 h. Studies have shown that 15 to 20 percent of patients undergoing elective PTCA have elevated plasma MB-CK,[143–145] and these individuals have a worse prognosis over the subsequent 6 months.[146] It remains controversial whether routine sampling for MB-CK should be performed after elective PTCA, since changes in treatment based on increased MB-CK have not been assessed. In patients with triple-vessel disease or where complications are more likely, routine sampling with MB-CK subforms is recommended for 6 h; it should be discontinued if the results are normal. If they are positive, sampling should continue for at least 24 h, and the patient should be treated as having had myocardial damage. It is now recognized that increased plasma levels of MB-CK reflect cardiac cell death, and it is likely though not proven that cardiac troponin I and T do so also.

Diagnosis of Early Reinfarction Diagnosis of early reinfarction (within 24 to 48 h) is difficult, since it represents an elevation superimposed on an already elevated plasma marker.[147,148] However, if MB-CK has returned to normal, then the diagnosis is relatively easy, since one sees a secondary increase in plasma MB-CK activity. Detection of early reinfarction with a secondary elevation in plasma MB-CK in patients who undergo successful thrombolysis is more appropriate, since MB-CK activity usually peaks within the first 10 to 15 h and returns to normal by 36 to 48 h. A secondary elevation of MB-CK activity 36 to 48 h after the onset of symptoms provides for a sensitive and specific diagnosis of reinfarction. In the latter situation, reinfarction is defined as an increase of 50 percent or more in the plasma MB-CK activity above the preceding baseline (mean of the two preceding samples) in at least two samples separated by a minimum of 4 h within a 24-h interval, with an absolute value of ±9 IU/L or 7 ng/L in at least one sample.[149] If the MB-CK activity is on the downslope from the antecedent infarction, a 25-percent increase is considered diagnostic; however, this is always less reliable than a secondary elevation after the return of MB-CK activity to baseline. These criteria were found to be reliable in three large clinical trials.[80,134,150] Confirmation of reinfarction occurring early, however, is more appropriately diagnosed using the MB-CK subforms. The MB-2 is near normal by 18 to 24 h and usually peaks at 10 to 12 h, so a well-defined downslope is apparent after 12 to 16 h. The other markers, cardiac troponin T and troponin I, since they remain elevated for 10 to 14 days, and, thus, because of the background, lack the necessary sensitivity. Myoglobin, since it returns to normal early after onset, is also a sensitive marker, but because of venipuncture or other minor skeletal muscle trauma commonly occurring in the hospital setting, makes it nonspecific.

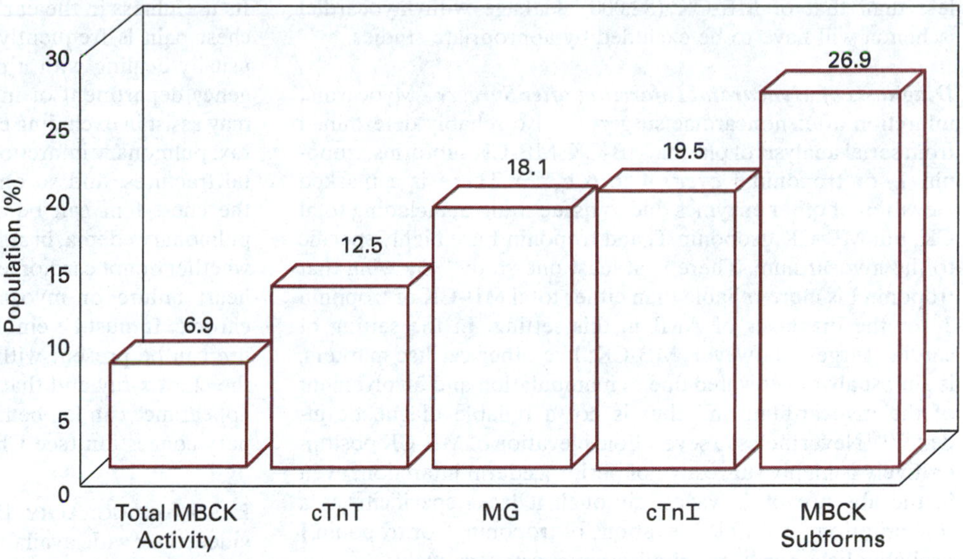

FIGURE 42-4 The above analysis is based on a prospective, multicenter, double-blind study involving the consecutive enrollment of 995 patients presenting to the emergency department. Diagnostic sensitivity and specificity for myocardial infarction of all markers (MB-CK subforms, myoglobin, total MB-CK—activity and mass, troponin T, and troponin I) were assessed serially every 1 to 2 h for 24 h. There were 119 (12.5 percent) patients with infarction and 203 (21 percent) with unstable angina. MB-CK subforms were most sensitive and specific (91 and 89 percent) within 6 h of onset versus myoglobin (MG) (78 and 89 percent). For late diagnosis, total MB-CK activity (derived from subforms) was the most sensitive and specific (96 and 98 percent) at 10 h from onset, followed by troponin I (cTnI) (96 and 93 percent), but not until 18 h, and troponin T (cTnT) (87 and 93 percent) at 10 h. In unstable angina, MB-CK subforms were increased in 29.5 percent, myoglobin in 23.7 percent, troponin I in 19.7 percent, and troponin T in 14.8 percent. (Data from Roberts et al.[154])

Prognostic Role for Biochemical Markers in Assessment of Unstable Angina Several studies have shown that patients presenting with the clinical diagnosis of unstable angina and minor elevations in MB-CK, troponin T, or troponin I have a more adverse outcome with respect to clinical events such as death, myocardial infarction, or the need for revascularization. In the GUSTO IIA trial,[151] of 835 patients with unstable angina, 36 percent had elevated troponin T and experienced increased mortality and other clinical events. Similarly, in the TIMI III trial,[152] of 1404 patients with non-Q-wave infarction and unstable angina, 41 percent had elevated troponin I and experienced increased mortality and other clinical events. In a study involving 593 patients with unstable angina, those with elevated MB-CK had increased mortality and other clinical events.[153]

It is now recommended that patients with unstable angina be assessed with one or more of these markers; however, treatment based on these indications and its long-term outcome have not been assessed. In the DMCS study,[154] there were 178 patients with unstable angina (rest pain of increased frequency or severity); the results of the various markers are shown in Fig. 42-4.[154] This is the only study in which the sensitivity of all of the markers has been compared. There is a dilemma with respect to the interpretation of elevated plasma markers in patients with unstable angina. Does this mean that these proteins are released due to ischemia (reversible injury) or that, in fact, limited infarction has occurred? Data[155] indicate release of CK reflects irreversible injury. In a series of conscious animal studies, it was shown that 20 min of coronary artery occlusion is consistently associated with increased plasma CK activity and, on light and electron microscopy, myocardial necrosis. In contrast, animals undergoing 10 min of coronary occlusion who exhibited severe ischemia—as shown by ST-segment elevation, depletion of myocardial glycogen, and cell swelling—had no increase in plasma CK. In the group of animals undergoing 15 min of coronary occlusion, only 30 percent had increased plasma CK activity, and each of these also showed microinfarction of the myocardium as detected by light and electron microscopy.[155] This finding—coupled with the observation that patients with proven obstructive coronary disease during exercise-induced ischemia, as documented by thallium scintigraphy, exhibited no increase in plasma MB-CK or MB-CK subforms—provides the basis for interpreting elevated plasma MB-CK levels as reflective of irreversible injury.[156] Fibrinolytic therapy has been shown to be detrimental[157] in unstable angina; however, in non-Q-wave infarction, when given on an average of 9 h from onset, it showed no beneficial or detrimental effect. Early fibrinolytic, antithrombin, or antiplatelet therapy in patients with positive MB-CK subforms but ST-segment depression has yet to be evaluated. Similar studies have not been performed to determine whether increased troponin I or troponin T reflects cell death, although, since they are structural sarcomeric proteins, it is highly likely that their release does reflect cell necrosis. Since the molecular weight of troponin I is 23,000, however, and that of troponin T is 39,000, both of which are significantly less than that of MB-CK (82,000), leakage with myocardial ischemia will have to be excluded by appropriate studies.

Diagnosis of Myocardial Infarction after Surgery Myocardial infarction after noncardiac surgery is also reliably determined from serial analysis of plasma MB-CK, MB-CK subforms, troponin T, or troponin I every 4 to 6 h.[104,158] There is a marked elevation of other enzymes due to tissue trauma, including total CK, but MB-CK, troponin T, and troponin I are highly specific to the myocardium. There is at least one study[139] showing that troponin I is more reliable than either total MB-CK or troponin T for the diagnosis of AMI in this setting. In the setting of cardiac surgery, however, MB-CK, like other cardiac markers, is almost always elevated due to manipulation and involvement of the myocardium and thus is not a reliable diagnostic index.[159,160] Nevertheless a severalfold elevation of MB-CK postoperatively is highly suggestive of periprocedural infarction, even in the absence of Q-waves, although it lacks specificity as a sole criterion. Multifold elevations of troponin T or troponin I probably have the same implications postoperatively.

Diagnosis of Previous Infarction Determining whether a patient has had a remote infarction to account for the subsequent development of cardiac failure or other clinical conditions can be difficult. Until recently, the only reliable means of diagnosis was the presence of Q waves on the ECG. Since less than 50 percent of infarctions develop Q waves and since a significant percentage of these Q waves disappear with time, the ECG can be nonspecific and unreliable in diagnosing remote infarction.[161,162] Thallium-201 (^{201}Tl) perfusion scanning has been shown to be extremely reliable, sensitive, and specific in diagnosing remote infarction.[163]

Other Biochemical Alterations The stress of myocardial infarction elicits numerous hormonal and metabolic responses. For example, both catecholamines and growth hormones are elevated. It is noteworthy, however, that serum cholesterol and lipoprotein fractions are relatively unchanged in the initial 1 to 2 days but decrease significantly over subsequent days and weeks. In establishing the baseline levels of these values for guiding future therapeutic interventions, measurements should be performed on admission or should be delayed for 6 to 8 weeks.[164,165] It should also be recognized that if myocardial infarction is occurring in individuals who have hypertension or for any reason are on medications such as diuretics, there may be significant electrolyte abnormalities that need to be treated, particularly in view of the increased propensity for arrhythmias, as with hypokalemia or alkalosis. The other abnormality seen on occasion is that of an increase in blood glucose following myocardial infarction, which, in some cases, particularly in patients with mild or moderate diabetes, may be associated with the development of significant ketoacidosis.[166,167] Not infrequently, it has also been shown that in the early days following myocardial infarction, the glucose tolerance curve is abnormal. It returns to normal after a few weeks. The white blood cell count is usually mildly to moderately elevated in 3 to 5 days.

Noninvasive Imaging in Acute Myocardial Infarction CHEST ROENTGENOGRAM The chest roentgenogram (x-ray) provides important information in the evaluation of chest pain and contributes to an integrative assessment of the clinical situation. Its usefulness in the early stages of evaluation of a patient with chest pain is frequently compromised by the fact that one is usually dealing with a portable study performed in the emergency department or in the CCU. Nonetheless, the chest film may assist in excluding causes of chest pain such as pneumothorax, pulmonary infarction with effusion, aortic dissection, skeletal fractures, and so on. In the patient with acute infarction, the chest film can be useful in establishing the presence of pulmonary edema, in assessing heart size to assist in determining whether or not cardiomegaly is present, and in deciding whether heart failure or myocardial or valvular disease is acute or chronic. It must be emphasized that severe left ventricular failure can be present without manifesting pulmonary edema on the chest x-ray and that, conversely, improvement in the x-ray appearance can lag behind hemodynamic resolution of pulmonary congestion (see Chap. 12).

ECHOCARDIOGRAPHY Because of the quality of the images provided, their wide availability, and the portability of these modalities, two-dimensional and Doppler echocardiography have become very useful tools in the assessment of the patient with suspected AMI[168–170] (see also Chap. 13). Echocardiography is particularly valuable in assessing the patient with a nondiagnostic ECG. The presence of a regional wall motion abnormality provides strong supportive evidence of acute coronary ischemia and is generally present in transmural or Q-wave myocardial infarction.[171–174] Wall motion abnormalities are less common in non-Q-wave infarction but are still present in the majority of cases. Nonetheless, small infarctions can be missed, and a wall motion abnormality may not necessarily be acute.[175] Echocardiography also provides an assessment of ventricular function; it is useful in predicting the prognosis[176] and in diagnosing right ventricular infarction.[177] It can also provide information concerning alternative diagnoses such as aortic dissection and, coupled with Doppler, can provide information on such complications as ruptured chordae tendineae with mitral regurgitation and ventricular septal defect[178] (see Chap. 13). It is useful in detecting ventricular thrombus and pericardial fluid. Thus, echocardiography is extremely useful in the initial assessment of AMI. General guidelines on its clinical use, including those for myocardial infarction, have been published.[179]

MAGNETIC RESONANCE IMAGING Magnetic resonance imaging (MRI) offers great promise in assessing AMI (see Chap. 18A). Its major limitation is logistic, in that it requires transporting patients to the imaging facility—a major concern in the case of the acutely ill. It is potentially useful in the assessment of infarct size and viable myocardium and the extent of the ischemic insult as well as in estimating perfusion to ischemic and nonischemic areas.[180–182] Currently, MRI does not have a defined role in the routine management of AMI.

COMPUTED TOMOGRAPHY Computed tomography (CT) is a powerful tool for cardiac imaging that gives high-resolution structural information (see Chap. 17). Ventricular thickness and dimensions can be assessed.[183] Also, CT is highly sensitive for detecting a left ventricular thrombus.[184] It has the same logistic limitations as MRI in the management of AMI. It does not have a routine role in the management of infarction. Whether electron-beam CT, with its very rapid acquisition times, can

TABLE 42-6 Uses of Radionuclide Testing in Acute Myocardial Infarction

Diagnosis			Risk Assessment		
Indication	Test	Class	Indication	Test	Class
1. Right ventricular infarction	Rest RNA	IIa	1. Residual ischemia	Stress (exercise/pharmacological) thallium with redistribution	I
	^{99m}Tc pyrophosphate	IIa		Stress (exercise/pharmacological) sestamibi with redistribution	
2. Infarction not diagnosed by standard means—early presentation with successful reperfusion	Rest myocardial perfusion imaging	IIb	2. Myocardial infarct size	Tomographic thallium	IIa
	^{99m}Tc pyrophosphate	IIb		Tomographic sestamibi	IIa
3. Infarction not diagnosed by standard means—late presentation	^{99m}Tc pyrophosphate	IIa	3. Hibernating myocardium	Early, late thallium	IIa
4. Routine diagnosis	Any technique	III	4. Ventricular function	RNA	I

ABBREVIATIONS: RNA = radionuclide angiography; ^{99m}Tc = technetium 99m.
SOURCE: The ACC/AHA task force,[185] with permission.

have a role in routine management requires further investigation (see Chap. 17).

RADIONUCLIDE SCINTIGRAPHY The radionuclide techniques available for the diagnosis of AMI are discussed in detail in Chap. 16, and are summarized in Table 42-6.[185] Guidelines for the use of cardiac radionuclide scanning have been published and suggest that the indications for its use in the diagnosis of acute infarction are limited to the unusual case in which history, electrocardiographic changes, and plasma markers are unreliable or unavailable.[185] There is no class I indication in the acute setting, and routine diagnostic use is not indicated (class III).[1,185] Radionuclide scintigraphy may have a diagnostic role in certain patients with right ventricular infarction by showing localized contractile abnormalities[186] or ^{99m}Tc pyrophosphate uptake (class IIa).[185]

ASSESSMENT OF INFARCT SIZE BY IMAGING Infarct size can be assessed by echocardiography (see Chap. 13), computerized tomography (see Chap. 17), magnetic resonance imaging (see Chap. 18A), positron emission tomography (see Chap. 19), or radionuclide scintigraphy (Table 42-6[185]) (see Chap. 16). ^{99m}Tc sestamibi with tomographic imaging has been used to quantitate infarct size,[187,188] and shown to be inversely related to the patient's outcome.[189,190] Thallium 201 can also be used to measure infarct size.[185]

PREHOSPITAL CARE

Recommendations[1]:

Class I

1. Availability of 911 access
2. Availability of an emergency medical services (EMS) system staffed by persons trained to treat cardiac arrest with defibrillation, if indicated, and to triage patients with ischemic-type chest discomfort

Class IIa

1. Availability of a first-responder defibrillation program in a tiered response system
2. Education from health care providers to patients/families about the signs and symptoms of AMI, about accessing EMS, and about medications

Class IIb

1. Use of 12-lead telemetry
2. Prehospital thrombolysis in special circumstances (e.g., transport time is greater than 90 min)

As mentioned previously, modern in-hospital care of the AMI patient has resulted in a substantial reduction in mortality. Some 40 to 65 percent of deaths from AMI, however, occur within an hour of the onset of symptoms and prior to arrival at a hospital.[191,192] Most of these deaths are attributable to ventricular fibrillation (VF).[193] To achieve a further substantial decrease in the mortality rate, it will be necessary to reduce the incidence of deaths outside the hospital.[194] Since, as noted, the earlier thrombolytic therapy can be initiated in eligible patients, the better the outcome, it is also essential to bring patients with chest pain into the medical care system as soon as possible because of the need to shorten the time between the onset of symptoms and the initiation of thrombolytic therapy. To that end, in the United States, the National Heart, Lung and Blood Institute of the National Institutes of Health has instituted the National Heart Attack Alert Program as a coordinated plan to extend the ACC/AHA guidelines promoting rapid identification and treatment of patients with AMI.[195,196]

Recognition and Management

A further reduction in the mortality rate will require the combined efforts of the patient, bystanders, minimally trained "first responders" who are capable of applying defibrillation therapy, and/or paramedics as well as the patient's physician. It has been established that a prolonged delay time in responding to a patient's symptoms is the rate-limiting step in defining the prehospital phase of myocardial infarction. Mean delay time in such response is almost 3 h.[197] Most of this time is consumed in decision making, while failing to recognize or acknowledge the seriousness of the problem.[198] Additional components of the delay between the onset of symptoms and the initiation of definitive therapy involve prehospital evaluation, treatment, and transport time and the time involved with the diagnosis and initiation of treatment in the hospital. The National Registry of Myocardial Infarction found, in a review of 48,128 patients with confirmed AMI, that the average duration of the prehospital phase, defined as onset of chest pain to hospital presentation, was 5.1 h.

STRATEGIES TO REDUCE DELAY

Patient-specific issues for decreasing the delay in seeking assistance primarily involve education. The patient must perceive the symptoms, recognize their possible significance, and conclude that medical help is appropriate. For some patients, the decision time is prolonged because of a lack of knowledge. It is interesting, however, that the length of time patients take to get help is not dependent on educational level, occupation, socioeconomic class, or past history of cardiac disease. In fact, patients with a past history of myocardial infarction or angina have an unexpectedly long decision time,[199] a situation that must be viewed, at least in part, as a failure by physicians to educate patients with established coronary artery disease as to the appropriate response to a change in or reappearance of their symptoms. In other cases, the decision time is prolonged by denial or by "diagnostic trials" with household remedies, patent medications, or previously prescribed drugs. It has been noted that only 10 percent of patients arriving at the hospital within 1 h of the onset of pain utilized nonprescription medications, while 41 percent of those arriving after 12 h did so.[191] The remainder of the delay time is consumed by "human factors," including the time a patient takes to modify existing social obligations and to prepare for going to the hospital. There is evidence that public education can reduce the time required for decision making.[198] It follows that effective efforts by the physician and his or her staff in educating patients with coronary artery disease will have similar effects in inducing appropriate responses to ischemic coronary symptoms. Prodromal symptoms occur in about two-thirds of patients with AMI, as discussed previously, and patients must be taught to recognize them.[194] Patients and their families must be given a specific plan of action after the recognition of symptoms that includes medications to be taken (nitroglycerin and possibly aspirin), mode of transportation to the hospital, and the location of the nearest hospital that offers emergency cardiac care. It is desirable that coronary patients have a copy of their resting ECG with them. They should be instructed not to delay by attempting to contact their physician and should be shown how to use the EMS system and how to contact it (911 in the United States). As opposed to personal transportation, utilizing EMS is desirable, because it permits the earliest possible access to expertise in defibrillation and resuscitation and facilitates evaluation in the field to prepare the hospital to receive the patient, as discussed later. The use of the EMS usually decreases the delay in initiating definitive care.[195] Since the capabilities of the EMS vary by locale, the physician must be familiar with the system in the patient's home area.

Instructions concerning medications to be taken at the onset of symptoms should be individualized. In general, patients are instructed to take nitroglycerin immediately at the onset of angina or a recognized anginal equivalent. If pain is not relieved, another nitroglycerin dose is taken at 5 min and a third at 10 min. If there is no relief by the third dose of nitroglycerin, the patient should be transported to the appropriate emergency facility. The physician should decide whether to incorporate the chewing of an aspirin tablet into this regimen when the decision is made to proceed to the hospital.

Bystanders and family members can play an important role in both shortening patient delay time and responding to an arrest. It has been shown that a spouse's presence accelerated the hospital arrival time.[193] Furthermore, if basic life support is initiated by a bystander within 4 min of cardiac arrest and if defibrillation is accomplished within 8 min, 40 percent of patients will survive and be discharged from the hospital.[200]

EMERGENCY MEDICAL SERVICES

Many communities in the United States are served by a two-tier ambulance service consisting of basic and advanced life support units. Since these are usually more basic support units, the response time of these units is shorter and should ideally be less than 5 min.[1,201] The first responders may be any of a variety of public service employees who are trained in CPR and defibrillation and have been taught to have a sense of urgency in order to identify and treat the AMI patient rapidly. Automatic external defibrillators are safe and effective and can be used by even minimally trained first responders to analyze rhythms and deliver defibrillatory shocks to convert VF.[1,202-206] Incorporation of automatic external defibrillators into emergency medical systems is highly desirable.[1] Minimally, it has been recommended that every ambulance transporting victims of cardiac arrest be equipped with a conventional defibrillator.[204]

The goal of any emergency medical system should be to include individuals who are trained in advanced life support techniques—including the use of antiarrhythmics as well as the administration of intravenous fluids and analgesics—and who can reach the patient as soon as possible in a vehicle equipped as a CCU. Undirected EMS technicians can spend excessive amounts of time evaluating a patient with chest pain and actually delay the ultimate initiation of appropriate therapy.[1] The time elapsed between receiving a 911 call and the actual arrival in the hospital has been assessed, and, at over 46 min, was substantially longer than estimates (under 26 min) taken from the paramedics involved.[198] Most of this field time was consumed by the paramedic on-scene time, which was not prolonged by acquisition of a 12-lead ECG. It has been demonstrated that, by the use of a standardized protocol (Table 42-7[1]), evaluation of the patient with chest pain by experienced emergency medical technicians, acquisition of a 12-lead ECG, and initiation of therapy can be accomplished within 20 min.[1] The protocol should facilitate determination of the likelihood of AMI and the presence of comorbid conditions in which thrombolytic therapy would be dangerous. It should also identify those suspected AMI patients who are at high risk. Patients in this category include those with sinus tachycardia, hypotension, or pulmonary edema or those with signs of shock. It is ideal to be able to record 12-lead ECGs in the field to be transmitted to the hospital physician. The availability of these data facilitates establishing the diagnosis and allows for accelerating preparations to administer thrombolytic therapy.[207-209]

TABLE 42-7 Chest Pain Checklist for Use by EMT/Paramedic for Diagnosis of Acute Myocardial Infarction and Thrombolytic Therapy Screening

Check each finding below. If all [yes] boxes are checked and ECG indicates ST elevation or new BBB, reperfusion therapy with thrombolysis or primary PTCA may be indicated. Thrombolysis is generally not indicated unless all [No] boxes are checked and BP ≤180/110 mmHg.

	Yes	*No*
Ongoing chest discomfort (≥20 min and <12 h)	☐	—
Oriented, can cooperate	☐	—
Age >35 y (>40 if female)	☐	—
History of stroke or TIA	—	☐
Known bleeding disorder	—	☐
Active internal bleeding in past 2 weeks	—	☐
Surgery or trauma in past 2 weeks	—	☐
Terminal illness	—	☐
Jaundice, hepatitis, kidney failure	—	☐
Use of anticoagulants	—	☐
Systolic/diastolic blood pressure		
Right arm: —/—		
Left arm: —/—		
	Yes	*No*
ECG done	☐	—
*High-risk profile**	*Yes*	*No*
Heart rate ≥100 bpm	☐	—
BP ≤100 mmHg	☐	—
Pulmonary edema (rales greater than one half-way up)	☐	—
Shock	☐	—
Pain began — AM/PM		
Arrival time — AM/PM		
Begin transport — AM/PM		
Hospital arrival — AM/PM		

*Transport to hospital capable of angiography and revascularization if needed.

ABBREVIATIONS: EMT = emergency medical technician; ECG = electrocardiogram; BBB = bundle branch block; PTCA = percutaneous transluminal coronary angioplasty; BP = blood pressure; TIA = transient ischemic attack. Adapted from the Seattle/King County EMS Medical Record.

SOURCE: Ryan et al.,[1] with permission.

PREHOSPITAL THROMBOLYSIS

As mentioned previously, there is unequivocal evidence that the earlier thrombolysis is administered to the AMI patient with ST-segment elevation, the more efficacious is the outcome;[14,210,211] in particular, the most favorable results are achieved when therapy is initiated within the first 1 to 2 h after the symptoms appear. It seems logical, therefore, that if thrombolysis could be initiated in appropriate patients during the prehospital phase by general practitioners or by EMS technicians guided by protocol, the 12-lead ECG, and communication with the emergency department physician, outcomes would be improved. Prehospital thrombolysis has been evaluated in several trials.[207,212-214] A meta-analysis of all of the trials showed a modest (17 percent) improvement in outcome, although none of the trials demonstrated significant improvement individually.[212] Prehospital thrombolysis, however, is fraught with a number of difficulties, beginning with the fact that only a small portion of chest pain patients (5 to 10 percent) have an AMI and are eligible to be treated with thrombolytics.[207,209,215,216] Thus, correctly selecting patients for thrombolytic therapy and avoiding its administration when not indicated or when contraindicated is difficult and has significant legal, medical, and economic implications. Because of these difficulties, prehospital thrombolysis should be emphasized primarily in those circumstances in which it can be administered 60 to 90 min before reaching the hospital (because of a long transport time) or when a physician is in the ambulance.[1] Generally, emphasis should be placed on rapid screening and diagnosis in the field to facilitate hospital triage and thrombolytic administration within 30 min of the patient's arrival.

EVALUATION AND MANAGEMENT OF PATIENTS WITH CHEST PAIN IN THE EMERGENCY DEPARTMENT

Recommendation:[1]

Class I

1. Emergency department AMI protocol that yields a targeted clinical examination, a 12-lead ECG within 10 min, and administration of thrombolytic therapy, as appropriate, within 30 min.

Background

In general, the goals of the emergency department with respect to patients with chest pain are to rapidly identify those patients with AMI with both typical and atypical presentations so that appropriate therapy can be initiated; to recognize those patients with acute coronary syndromes (unstable angina) but without myocardial infarction and who, thus, are at high risk; and to assess accurately those patients at low risk who are candidates for noninvasive evaluation and early discharge.[217]

As mentioned previously, the earlier reperfusion therapy is initiated in the subset of patients with diagnostic ST-segment elevation, the more favorable the clinical results (Fig. 42-5).[210]

An important objective, obviously, should be a triage system that minimizes the number of patients at high risk (AMI or unstable angina) who are inadvertently discharged from the emergency department while also minimizing the admission to high-intensity CCUs of low-risk patients without myocardial infarction—a goal of increasing urgency in this era of intense pressures for cost containment. Of patients admitted to a CCU, for example, less than 20 percent will have AMI, as noted.[218,219] In contrast, even in the current era of an enhanced appreciation for atypical presentations, an increased potential for litigation, and a decreased threshold for admission to exclude myocardial infarction, the missed diagnosis rate has still been about 4 percent,[131] a percentage that appears not to have changed substantially since the 1980s.[220–222]

The reasons for misdiagnosis of acute coronary syndromes in the emergency department have been studied extensively and have been reviewed.[217] The misinterpretation of ECGs has been reported to occur in approximately 20 to 40 percent of missed AMIs.[222–224] Equally disturbing are the reports, which are

Presentation features	Percent of patients dead: Fibrinolytic	Percent of patients dead: Control	Stratified statistics: O − E	Stratified statistics: Variance
ECG				
BBB	18.7%	23.6%	−24.5	83.3
ST elev, anterior	13.2%	16.9%	−122.0	420.6
ST elev, inferior	7.5%	8.4%	−27.1	237.4
ST elev, other	10.6%	13.4%	−42.1	159.6
ST depression	15.2%	13.8%	12.9	108.7
Other abnormality	5.2%	5.8%	−9.6	103.2
Normal	3.0%	2.3%	3.4	12.9
Hours from onset				
0–1	9.5%	13.0%	−29.3	83.3
2–3	8.2%	10.7%	−100.2	354.8
4–6	9.7%	11.5%	−78.5	387.6
7–12	11.1%	12.7%	−51.5	336.7
13–24	10.0%	10.5%	−11.1	212.6
Age (years)				
< 55	3.4%	4.6%	−45.9	155.6
55–64	7.2%	8.9%	−86.3	360.0
65–74	13.5%	16.1%	−113.7	533.0
75 +	24.3%	25.3%	−12.6	266.6
Gender				
Male	8.2%	10.1%	−208.1	928.0
Female	14.1%	16.0%	−62.2	436.8
Systolic BP (mmHg)				
< 100	28.9%	35.1%	−38.7	132.2
100–149	9.6%	11.5%	−168.9	850.0
150–174	7.2%	8.7%	−59.2	290.0
175 +	7.2%	8.2%	−10.8	74.1
Heart rate				
< 80	7.2%	8.5%	−83.2	464.9
80–99	9.2%	11.3%	−65.8	287.2
100 +	17.4%	20.7%	−51.7	238.6
Prior MI				
Yes	12.5%	14.1%	−43.7	322.4
No	8.9%	10.9%	−288.5	1001.9
Diabetes				
Yes	13.6%	17.3%	−41.4	145.7
No	8.7%	10.2%	−142.6	830.4
ALL PATIENTS	2820/29315 9.6%	3357/29285 11.5%	−269.5	1377.4

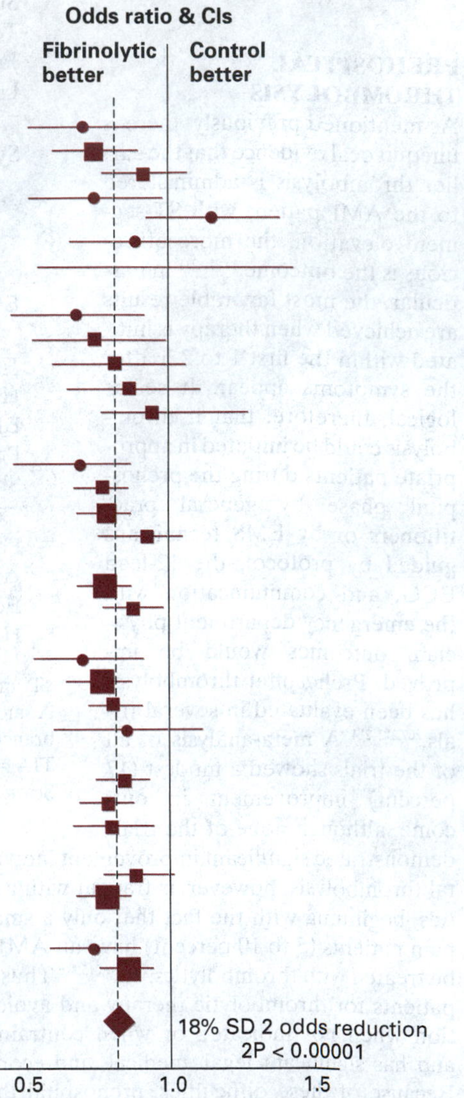

FIGURE 42-5 Proportional effects of fibrinolytic therapy on mortality during days 0 to 35 subdivided by presentation features. "Observed minus expected" (O-E) number of events among fibrinolytic-allocated patients (and its variance) is given for subdivisions of presentation features, stratified by trial. This is used to calculate odds ratios (ORs) of death among patients allocated to fibrinolytic therapy to that among those allocated control. The ORs (squares with areas proportional to the amount of "statistical information" contributed by the trials) are plotted with their 99 percent confidence intervals (CIs) (horizontal lines). Squares to the left of the solid vertical line indicate benefit (significant at $2p < 0.01$ only where the entire CI is to left of vertical line). Overall result and 95 percent CI represented by diamond, with overall proportion reduction in the odds of death and statistical significance given alongside. (From Fibrinolytic Therapy Trialists' Collaborative Group,[210] with permission.)

indictments of training or focus, that patients are discharged even though the physician has recognized ischemic symptoms or electrocardiographic changes.[220,223,224] A major contributing problem is that even experienced clinicians are imprecise in their clinical judgment as to the presence or absence of myocardial infarction in a given patient. Sensitivities of 80 to 90 percent and specificities of approximately 70 to 80 percent in diagnostic precision in determining the presence or absence of AMI based on clinical impressions have been reported.[70,222,225] The diagnostic problem, however, is not limited to the diagnosis of myocardial infarction but also applies to whether unstable angina is present (see also Chap. 41). Patients who are admitted to the hospital with chest pain and only transient ST-segment changes and without aggressive therapy have a 22 percent incidence of death and myocardial infarction after a 28-month follow-up,[226] a figure not dissimilar to that for patients with an initial confirmed infarction. These similarities in outcome of unstable angina and myocardial infarction are not surprising, since the fundamental underlying pathophysiologic mechanisms—disruption of the atherosclerotic plaque and thrombus formation, with or without vasospasm—are likely to be identical, the major difference being the extent of luminal compromise by the thrombus. Thus, the clinical focus should not be simply to "rule out" AMI, but, taking a proactive approach, to "rule in" either acute infarction or unstable angina in an expeditious manner.[217] Once these urgent conditions have been excluded or ascertained to be of low probability, the next level of concern is determining the presence of other acute cardiovascular or cardiopulmonary conditions, such as aortic dissection, pulmonary embolus, and pericarditis. The focus, subsequently, in a hierarchical fashion, is to establish whether or not stable coronary artery disease is present, to identify cardiovascular risk factors, and to consider noncardiac diagnoses, which, in nonurgent cases, can be evaluated further on an outpatient basis.

It has been suggested[217] that management of chest pain in the emergency department can be optimized by having the appropriate clinical focus, developing effective risk stratification approaches, and implementing systematic algorithmic protocols. There has been a great deal of interest in the development of actual or virtual chest pain units to facilitate the expeditious triage and management of patients with chest pain, as discussed later.

Initial Approach, Detection, and Assessment of Risk

Recommendations:[1]

Class I

1. Supplemental oxygen, intravenous access, and continuous electrocardiographic monitoring should be established in all patients with acute ischemic-type chest discomfort.
2. A 12-lead ECG should be obtained and interpreted within 10 min of arrival in the emergency department in all patients with suspected acute ischemic-type chest discomfort.

A major goal of the emergency department in dealing with patients with chest pain is the establishment of a routine approach that leads to a rapid (10 min) preliminary evaluation, acquisition of a 12-lead ECG, and establishment of intravenous access and continuous electrocardiographic monitoring (Fig. 42-3). The initial physical examination and assessment of the history are guided by the differential diagnosis of chest pain, with the goal of establishing whether or not myocardial ischemia is a likely or possible diagnosis. Blood is drawn for baseline cardiac marker levels, and if coronary ischemia is suspected and there are no contraindications, the patient is given aspirin of 160 to 325 mg to chew and swallow. Also, the patient with suspected coronary ischemia is given sublingual nitroglycerine unless the systolic blood pressure is less than 90 mmHg. This should be avoided with severe bradycardia or tachycardia. Because of the potentially catastrophic implications, the history of chest pain alone usually dictates entry into the system for evaluation. In general, the only patients with chest pain who are not systematically evaluated for myocardial ischemia would be those in whom a clear noncardiac cause, such as chest wall tenderness, can be demonstrated unequivocally to be the etiology of the presenting symptoms. Continuous ECG monitoring is essential because of the propensity for the development of sudden and potentially lethal ventricular arrhythmias in any patient with an acute coronary ischemic syndrome. Intravenous access is essential for therapeutic interventions under such circumstances as well as for more general purposes. Additionally, paroxysmal changes in the ST segment may be recognizable on the monitor. The differential diagnosis of chest pain and the clinical recognition of AMI were discussed previously. The causes of chest pain that are not the result of acute pathologic changes compromising the structural integrity of the large coronary arteries are listed in Table 42-8.

As a general rule, and as previously mentioned, one should begin the evaluation of the patient with chest pain with the assumption that one is dealing with myocardial ischemia until

TABLE 42-8 Causes of Chest Pain Other Than Acute Coronary Artery Syndromes

- Cardiovascular
  - Aortic dissection
  - Aortic stenosis
  - Pericarditis
  - Mitral valve prolapse
  - Microvascular angina
    - Hypertrophic cardiomyopathy
    - Syndrome X
  - Pulmonary embolus
  - Arrhythmia/palpitations
- Noncardiovascular
  - Pleurisy
  - Pneumonia
  - Pneumothorax
  - Costochondritis
  - Gastrointestinal
    - Esophageal spasm/reflux
    - Acid peptic disease
    - Cholecystitis
    - Gastritis
- Psychiatric
  - Panic attack
  - Cardiac neurosis
  - Depression
  - Malingering

proven otherwise. The three most serious and urgent alternative diagnoses that need to be considered specifically during the initial evaluation are aortic dissection, acute pulmonary embolus, and acute pneumothorax. Acute pericarditis and myopericarditis need to be considered as well.

Although relatively uncommon, aortic dissection must be considered and ruled in or out during the initial evaluation of the patient with chest pain, since specific intervention can decrease its high mortality. Furthermore, and not unexpectedly, administration of thrombolytic agents in the presence of aortic dissection is associated with high mortality.[227-229] Suspicion of dissection should be heightened especially in hypertensive patients or in those with marfanoid habitus (see also Chaps. 62 and 88). Most patients with aortic dissection who have mistakenly received thrombolytic therapy did not meet the ECG criteria of ST-segment elevation that is usually required.[228] Aortic dissection is usually associated with sudden onset of a severe, tearing pain that may migrate and is frequently felt in the back at some point. Differential blood pressures in the arms may be noted, and pulse differences in the carotids or arms may be observed. An echocardiogram and, in particular, transesophageal echocardiography can be very efficacious in the diagnosis of aortic dissection (see Chaps. 13 and 88).

Pulmonary embolus can be life-threatening and should be suspected in anyone with a sudden onset of shortness of breath and chest pressure or pain, especially if there is a history of being sedentary or immobilized and/or of deep venous thrombosis. There may be a pleural rub, and the chest roentgenogram is usually normal, although arterial hypoxia may be present (see Chap. 53). Similarly, pneumothorax may be associated with persistent chest pain, hypoxemia, and evidence of hypoventilation on physical examination.

Acute pericarditis may mimic AMI in that the pain can be substernal and persistent. Frequently, however, there will be a positional component as well as characteristics of pleurisy, with accentuation by deep breathing. Furthermore, the diffuse ST-segment elevation may lead to a misdiagnosis of myocardial infarction. The key differentiating features in pericarditis include PR depression, the diffuse nature of ST-segment elevation in most leads, and the absence of reciprocal changes (see Chaps. 11 and 72). The presence of a pericardial rub is a key diagnostic finding. Echocardiography, by demonstrating a pericardial effusion in the case of pericarditis or a wall motion abnormality in the case of acute ischemia, can be helpful in making the appropriate diagnosis. Hemorrhagic pericardial effusions have been reported in patients given thrombolytic therapy in the setting of acute pericarditis.[227,228]

Although usually not urgent, it should be kept in mind that esophageal disorders, as assessed retrospectively by motility studies, are very common in patients presenting with chest pain in whom cardiac ischemia is ruled out[230-233] (see also Chap. 40). In fact, among all patients presenting with chest pain, gastroesophageal disease has been observed to be the most common etiology (42 percent), whereas ischemic heart disease was present in 31 percent and chest wall syndromes were responsible in 28 percent.[234] Because of the high frequency of gastrointestinal disease in patients with chest pain, "GI cocktails" or antacids have been used as a diagnostic tool to guide triage and disposition. Only 25 percent of patients with esophageal pain, however, have been reported to obtain pain relief with antacids.[235] Furthermore, coincidental, spontaneous relief of ischemic chest pain at the time of administration of the GI cocktail could be misleading. Similarly, administration of nitroglycerin as a diagnostic strategy for ischemic disease could be misleading, because it can relieve esophageal spasm. Moreover, it has been found that pain relief after nitroglycerin did not predict unstable angina or AMI in the chest pain patient.[236] The use of these "response-to-treatment" strategies as major decision points in the evaluation of chest pain has been discouraged.[217] This reservation, however, applies primarily to those patients without diagnostic ECG changes, and does not preclude giving sublingual nitroglycerin to patients with chest pain and ST-segment elevation as a test of vasospasm or Prinzmetal's angina.

DETECTION

The 12-Lead Electrocardiogram as a Guide to Management Strategy The results of the 12-lead ECG guide the next level of decision making for the patient with chest pain thought to be compatible with myocardial ischemia (Fig. 42-3). The ECG interpretation is assigned to one of three categories: (1) ST-segment elevation in two or more leads or a presumptively new bundle branch block implicating acute coronary occlusion, usually thrombotic; (2) ST-segment depression and/or T-wave inversion implying subtotal occlusion or non-Q infarction; and (3) normal or nondiagnostic. The group with ST- segment elevation or a left bundle branch block is particularly important to define, as it is this group that has been shown to benefit from thrombolytic therapy. ST-segment elevation has a 46 percent sensitivity and a 91 percent specificity for the diagnosis of AMI.[94] There is no indication as yet of the benefit of thrombolytic therapy or primary angioplasty in those patients without ST-segment elevation or bundle branch block, however, appropriately focused randomized trials are lacking.

As discussed previously, the initial ECG is diagnostic in less than 50 percent of patients with AMI,[237,238] and the measurement of serum markers of myocardial damage plays a major role in diagnosis. Measurement of MB-CK is the benchmark laboratory test, and the specificity and sensitivity of samples taken 2 h apart during serial sampling have been reported to be 91 and 94 percent, respectively.[239] The limitations of conventional MB-CK measurements and the role of myoglobin and the troponins have been discussed. The rapid high-voltage method to separate MB-CK-1 and MB-CK-2 and to determine the ratio of the isoforms was described and may be particularly relevant to the initial evaluation in the emergency department, since it quickly provides information that not only facilitates establishing the appropriate diagnosis but also contributes to assigning a risk category to a patient.

RISK STRATIFICATION

Stratifying risk in the patient with AMI is an essential part of the management strategy during all phases of care. It permits not only the more precise calibration of treatment and diagnostic approaches with the level of risk but also, increasingly, facilitates the appropriate utilization of hospital resources. Traditional approaches to initial risk assessment have involved combinations of ECG changes and clinical manifestations. The ECG serves as a basis for initial risk assessment. ST-segment elevation or a new left bundle branch block in the patient with chest pain defines a high-risk group, and in those with elevated ST segments, the mortality correlates positively with the number of leads with the ST changes.[240] The presence of ST-segment depression or T-wave inversion also defines a high-risk group. In patients with unstable angina or non-Q-wave myocardial infarction, ST-segment depression on the initial ECG of at least 1 mm in two leads during pain predicted major clinical events in the subsequent 3 months.[241] A nondiagnostic or normal ECG is associated with low risk. For example, the incidence of myocardial infarction has been reported to be 10, 8, and 41 percent in patients who, at admission, had a normal, a nonspecific, or an abnormal ECG, respectively.[242] The incidence of complications paralleled the infarction rate—a predictable conclusion corroborated by other studies.[243,244] *High risk has been associated with age, ST-segment elevation or depression, T-wave inversions, and Q waves, as well as prolonged chest pain, especially if it radiates to cardiac referral areas.*[70,222,245–247]

Quantitative assessments of risk have been developed to guide the management of patients with chest pain in the emergency department.[244] *Predictors of an increased risk of complications included ECG evidence of ST-segment elevation or Q waves in two or more leads that are not known to have been present previously; ST-segment depression or T-wave inversions consistent with myocardial ischemia and not known to be present previously; pain worse than prior angina or the same as that experienced with prior myocardial infarction; systolic blood pressure of less than 100 mmHg; or rales bilaterally above the bases.* On the basis of these predictors, patients could be divided into four risk groups.[244] Furthermore, the risk could be updated if a complication occurred. This general approach can guide decisions concerning the level of intensity of the unit to which a patient is admitted and the length of observation required.

Blood levels of cardiac markers are prognostically important, as noted. In particular, increased levels of any of the markers—CKMB or the subforms or troponins (I and T), but not myoglobin (×1)—at presentation appear to be strong predictors of risk in patients with acute ischemic syndromes[151,152] (see Chap. 41).

INITIAL MANAGEMENT

As discussed, one frequently does not have a definitive diagnosis of AMI in the patient with chest pain in the emergency department, although this situation may ultimately be improved by the wider availability of the very rapid assays of blood cardiac markers, as discussed earlier. Nevertheless, the initial general treatment of the acute coronary syndromes is the same.

Routine General Measures OXYGEN ADMINISTRATION Recommendations for oxygen administration:[1]

Class I

1. Overt pulmonary congestion
2. Arterial oxygen desaturation (Sa_{O_2} less than 90 percent)

Class IIa

1. Routine administration of oxygen to all patients with uncomplicated myocardial infarction during the first 2 to 3 h

Class IIb

2. Routine administration of supplemental oxygen to patients with uncomplicated myocardial infarction beyond 3 to 6 h

Hypoxemia is not uncommon in patients with AMI, even with an uncomplicated course, and presumably because of ventilation-perfusion mismatch.[248] Oxygen administration has been reported to decrease ST-segment elevation in anterior myocardial infarction.[249] Thus, oxygen administration for up to several days has previously been routine. There is concern with this practice, however, since oxygen may increase vascular resistance, and there may not necessarily be increased delivery to tissues. Because of these concerns and because of the expense of prolonged oxygen administration, there appears to be little justification for extending its use in uncomplicated myocardial infarction with an (Sa_{O_2} of greater than 90 percent beyond 2 to 3 h.[1] Justification of its use in uncomplicated infarction can be based on its potential for limiting of ischemic injury and on the fact that nitroglycerin can induce ventilation-perfusion abnormalities due to its pulmonary vasodilator activity, thus contributing to hypoxia.

Oxygen administration should be continued in patients with pulmonary congestion and desaturation. In patients with complicated myocardial infarction, nasal oxygen or oxygen by face mask may be insufficient to maintain saturation, and positive-pressure breathing or intubation and mechanical ventilation may have to be considered. If necessary, they should be initiated promptly.

ANALGESIA The alleviation of pain and anxiety remains an essential element in the care of the patient with AMI. The pain and accompanying anxiety contribute to excessive activity of the autonomic nervous system and to restlessness. These factors, in turn, increase the metabolic demands of the myocardium. Physician reassurance from the beginning is an essential part of treatment and should be provided with compassion, patience, and confidence. Optimal care of the patient with AMI requires a team of experienced individuals who can help alleviate anxiety by their air of competence and caring.

It is a common clinical observation that reperfusion in AMI is associated with rapid relief of pain, suggesting that the pain is due to ongoing ischemia of the viable myocardium rather than to the effects of tissue necrosis. Thus, the approach to pain consists of the dual strategy of relieving ischemia and attacking the pain directly. Anti-ischemic therapy consists of reperfusion, beta blockers (if appropriate), nitrates, and oxygen administration, as discussed. Narcotics not only relieve pain directly but also indirectly by diminishing the sympathetic nervous system's drive and catecholamine secretion, which will increase blood pressure and drive cardiac chronotrophic and inotrophic responses to increase oxygen consumption and ischemia. The increased sympathetic drive will also enhance the propensity for serious ventricular arrhythmias. Morphine, in most instances, is the drug of choice, since it is well tolerated and offers analgesia without significant cardiac depression.[250] It also relieves anxiety and the feeling of doom commonly described. Morphine sulfate can be given at doses of 2 to 4 mg every 15 min until adequate relief has been obtained, which, in some patients, may require 25 to 30 mg.[251] The peak effect of intravenous morphine occurs within 15 to 20 min, thus requiring titration. Morphine has frequently been given in inadequate doses because of fear of respiratory depression or hypotension. Respiratory depression is less common in patients with myocardial infarction than it is in patients generally, because of the anxiety and respiratory drive from hypoxia, and can be treated with intravenous naloxone should it occur.[1] Hypotension related to morphine is usually orthostatic and volume-dependent and is less common in supine patients.[252] In patients with severe ongoing pain, it may be prudent to avoid concomitant administration of substantial doses of morphine and vasodilators, such as nitroglycerin. In patients with an acute inferior myocardial infarction with bradycardia with or without hypotension, the vagolytic narcotic meperidine may be substituted for the parasympathomimetic morphine. If the patient's anxiety is not controlled by the administration of narcotics, mild sedation with a benzodiazepine is appropriate. Diazepam in doses of 5 mg orally every 8 to 12 h or alprazolam in doses of 0.25 mg every 8 h are most often used.

NITROGLYCERIN Recommendations for intravenous nitroglycerin[1]:

Class I

1. For the first 24 to 48 h in patients with AMI and congestive heart failure, large anterior infarction, persistent ischemia, or hypertension
2. Continued use (beyond 48 h) in patients with recurrent angina or persistent pulmonary congestion

Class IIa

1. None

Class IIb

1. For the first 24 to 48 h in all patients with AMI who do not have hypotension, bradycardia, or tachycardia
2. Continued use (beyond 48 h), perhaps in an oral or topical form, in patients with large or complicated infarction

Class III

1. Patients with systolic pressure less than 90 mmHg or severe bradycardia (less than 50 beats per minute)

Nitroglycerin has become very widely used in the treatment of AMI. It is an anti-ischemic agent not only by virtue of its actions to decrease preload and afterload, and thus to decrease oxygen demand, but also because of its vasodilator actions on epicardial coronary arteries and coronary collaterals. Consequently, and especially in patients with good collaterals, nitroglycerin is likely to increase flow into the ischemic regions.[253,254] Apart from relieving ischemia and pain, intravenous nitroglycerin, in early studies, appeared to reduce the likelihood of developing cardiac failure, infarct extension, or cardiac death. Both clinical data[255,256] and animal studies suggest that the early administration of nitroglycerin limits the extent of myocardial damage and favorably affects survival.[257] Long-term nitrates after reperfusion in animals favorably affect ventricular remodeling.[258]

Small, early trials before the widespread use of reperfusion suggested that the early administration of intravenous nitroglycerin was associated with improved morbidity and mortality. A meta-analysis of these trials suggested that the use of nitrates reduced the odds of mortality after AMI by greater than 30 percent.[259] The efficacy of nitrates in improving short-term mortality after AMI was tested prospectively in the GISSI-3 trial.[260] At 6 weeks, there was no significant difference between the nitrate and control groups. The power to distinguish between the two, however, was diminished, because about one-half of the control group received nitrates during the first 2 days at the discretion of the attending physician. The angiotensin-converting enzyme (ACE) inhibitor lisinopril was tested in a similar fashion in GISSI-3. Mortality was decreased slightly at 6 weeks. The combined use of nitrates and lisinopril was associated with decreased mortality at both 6 weeks and 6 months compared with the no-nitrate group or with the group that received lisinopril alone. There was no significant difference noted at 35 days in comparison with the control group in another large trial, International Study of Infarct Survival (ISIS-4), which evaluated the effects of nitrates on mortality after myocardial infarction.[261] This trial was also compromised by the high frequency of discretionary nitrate use in the control group. A meta-analysis of all randomized, controlled trials involving the use of nitrates in AMI show a small, statistically significant reduction in mortality (about 5 percent).

The weight of the evidence does not justify the routine, long-term use of nitrates in uncomplicated AMI. The use of intravenous nitroglycerin early after acute infarction is justified because of its ease of titration, rapid onset, and ability to be quickly withdrawn in case of complications. Long-term use of nitrates is appropriate in the case of recurrent ischemia, large infarction, congestive heart failure, or hypertension.

COMPLICATIONS AND LIMITATIONS The most serious complication of nitroglycerin is hypotension. The fall in blood pressure may cause reflex tachycardia, and, together with decreased perfusion pressure, may cause or worsen angina. Thus, nitroglycerin should be avoided with a systolic pressure of less than 90 mmHg. Caution should be exercised in the case of inferior wall infarction because of the possibility of right ventricular involvement. Nitroglycerin should be used only with extreme caution if at all in right ventricular infarction, because the right ventricle in this circumstance becomes extremely dependent upon preload, which can be diminished by the venodilating properties of the drug.[262] Similarly, nitroglycerin should be avoided in patients with severe bradycardia (heart rate less than 50 beats per minute), as hypotension may result.[263] If hypotension and bradycardia develop, nitroglycerin should be stopped, legs elevated, fluid administered, and atropine given if needed. Headache is a common side effect of nitrate administration.

Nitrate tolerance is common (see Chap. 81). With intravenous nitroglycerin, this may be recognized only as a diminution of clinical effect after 24 to 48 h. An increase in dose may be required.

DOSAGE OF NITROGLYCERIN Long-acting nitrates should generally not be used as initial therapy in AMI. Intravenous nitroglycerin is preferable, as noted, because of rapidity of onset, ease of titration, and ease of removal in case of complications. Dose titration can be assessed by frequent determinations of blood pressure and heart rate. Invasive monitoring is not essential but is probably prudent if high doses are required or if there is hemodynamic instability or uncertainty about the adequacy of ventricular preload.

Treatment should be initiated with a bolus injection of 12.5 to 25 μg and should be followed by infusion by pump of 10 to 20 μg/min, with increases of 5 to 10 μg every 5 to 10 min while assessing hemodynamic and clinical responses.[1] Control of symptoms is a major end point; in the case of high left ventricular filling pressure, a decrease of 10 to 30 percent in pulmonary artery wedge pressure is the objective. Limitations of nitroglycerin dosing are a decrease in mean arterial pressure of 10 percent in normotensive patients or a decrease of 30 percent in hypertensive patients, but not below a systolic pressure of 90 mmHg, or an increase in heart rate of 10 beats per minute not to exceed 110 beats per minute.

Doses of nitroglycerin greater than 200 μg/min are associated with an increased risk of hypotension. The development of such high requirements may indicate tolerance, and alternative drugs such as ACE inhibitors or nitroprusside should be considered. If tolerance is the issue, responsiveness should return after a 12- to 18-h period off of nitroglycerin.

ASPIRIN Recommendations for aspirin therapy[1]:

Class I

1. A dose of 160 to 325 mg should be given on day 1 of AMI and continued indefinitely on a daily basis thereafter.

Class IIb

1. Other antiplatelet agents such as dipyridamol, ticlopidine, or clopidogrel may be instituted if a true aspirin allergy is present or if the patient is unresponsive to aspirin.

Aspirin has become a standard part of the armamentarium for treating not only AMI but also atherosclerotic vascular disease generally. A 23 percent reduction in mortality at 35 days in patients treated with aspirin during the early stages of AMI was observed in the Second International Study of Infarct Survival (ISIS-2).[211] The reduction in mortality due to aspirin in combination with streptokinase was 42 percent. In a summary of a large number of clinical trials, aspirin has been shown to reduce the incidence of vascular events in patients with AMI at 1 month; a prior history of MI (2 years); a history of transient cerebral ischemia or stroke; and unstable angina.[264]

Aspirin irreversibly inhibits platelet cyclooxygenase, an enzyme that causes formation of thromboxane A_2, a mediator of platelet aggregation.[265] Its antithrombotic and side effects are discussed in detail in Chap. 44. Aspirin should be avoided in cases of true hypersensitivity. In the case of a history of bleeding from acid peptic disease, aspirin rectal suppositories can be used. Ticlopidine or clopidogrel, which are antiplatelet drugs acting as adenosine diphosphate receptor antagonists and can be used in acute infarction in patients in whom aspirin is contraindicated. Their actions do not develop immediately. They are discussed in Chap. 44. Clopidogrel is safer than ticlopidine and was shown to be more effective than aspirin in the CAPRIE (Clopidogrel versus Aspirin in Patients at Risk of Ischemic Events) trial.[266]

Aspirin is an effective antithrombotic at doses as low as 80 mg, but the rapid, acute effect probably requires 160 mg, which is absorbed and is thus clinically effective more quickly if the tablet is chewed rather than swallowed whole. *Thus the patient suspected of having a coronary ischemic syndrome should receive, early in the course, 160 to 325 mg of non-enteric-coated aspirin, which is chewed.*

Management after Triage into Electrocardiographic Subgroups

As discussed earlier, the initial ECG, as a first approximation, permits the assignment of patients with chest pain into subgroups that are distinguishable in terms of therapeutic responsiveness and risk. Thus, those with either ST-segment elevation and presumptively new bundle branch block or those with ST-segment depression and/or T-wave inversion are in high-risk groups, whereas those with either normal ECGs or nonspecific changes are in a low risk category. Furthermore, the high-risk groups can be subdivided into those (ST-segment elevation or new bundle branch block) who have a favorable therapeutic response to thrombolytics and those who do not (ST-segment depression and/or T-wave inversion). *It must be kept in mind that these initial categorizations do not necessarily define ultimate outcome. Thus, patients with no ST-segment elevation at presentation may, in fact, have unstable angina and ultimately have no infarction or may progress to have either a Q-wave or a non-Q-wave infarction. Similarly, those presenting with ST-segment elevation may have a non-Q-wave infarction, although the majority of these will develop Q waves.* This potential for variable outcomes provides the underlying rationale for close monitoring and continuous reassessment of clinical course, risk, and therapeutic strategies during the period of observation and for monitoring both in the emergency department and subsequently in other hospital units.

APPROACH TO THE PATIENT WITH ST-SEGMENT ELEVATION

The approach to the patient with chest pain and ST-segment elevation is guided heavily by the evidence that this subgroup has a high frequency of epicardial coronary artery occlusion by a thrombus that can be halted by prompt reperfusion.[267,268] Furthermore, multiple clinical trials of thrombolytic therapy have shown clinical benefit, but only in those with ST-segment elevation (Fig. 42-5).[210] This efficacy, however, has been shown in men, women, and diabetics and is manifest regardless of any history of previous myocardial infarction, existing heart rate, or recorded blood pressure (if less than 175 mmHg).[210] The greatest benefit is seen in patients with anterior myocardial infarction (and inferior infarction with right ventricular involvement), those with signs of a large infarction (systolic blood pressure less 100 mmHg or heart rate greater than 100 beats per minute), and in those with diabetes. Thus, the evaluation and management of the patient with ischemic chest pain and ST-segment elevation is focused on the rapid assessment of suitability for and delivery of reperfusion therapy. The approach to these patients is summarized in Fig. 42-6.[1]

During the initial evaluation, the patient will have had aspirin given, blood drawn, intravenous access established, a 12-lead ECG showing ST-segment elevation in at least two adjacent leads, nasal oxygen administered, appropriate analgesia, and continuous electrocardiographic monitoring initiated. The appropriate next steps are to administer a beta-adrenergic blocker, if not contraindicated, and to initiate evaluation for reperfusion therapy. Based on the data from nine major clinical trials of thrombolytic therapy summarized by the Fibrinolytic Therapy Trialists Collaborative Group, thrombolytic therapy is efficacious in AMI (although linearly decreasing with the passage of time) for up to 12 h after the onset of symptoms.[210] There was a statistically uncertain benefit from 13 to 18 h. Thus, the 12-h point was chosen as defining the time frame in which the risk-benefit ratio is clearly favorable for administering thrombolytic therapy (Fig. 42-5).

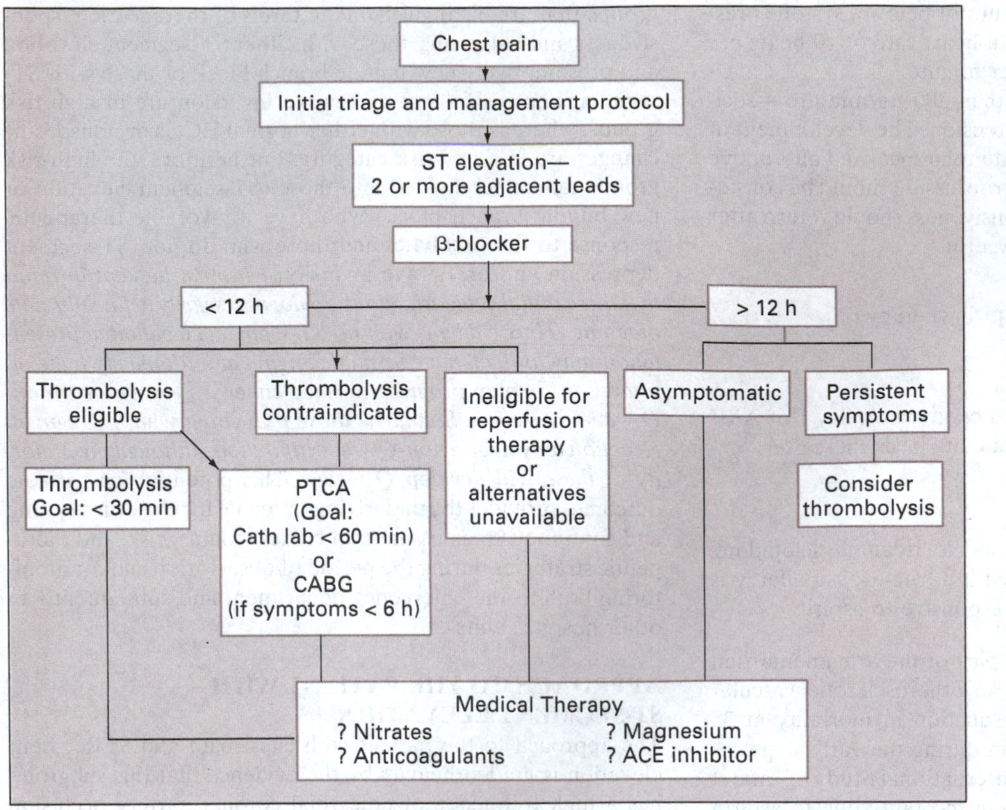

FIGURE 42-6 Evaluation of patients with ST-segment elevation. Algorithm for initial decision making in regard to reperfusion therapy in patients with suspected acute myocardial infarction and ST-segment elevation. Whether or not to administer thrombolytics or to perform primary PTCA is determined by the time from onset of symptoms. For patients in whom more than 12 h have elapsed since the onset of symptoms, reperfusion should be considered only if there are persistent or recurrent symptoms associated with ST-segment elevation. For patients with ST-segment elevation and duration of symptoms between 7 and 12 h, the decision to proceed with a reperfusion strategy requires careful clinical judgment in weighing the risk/benefit issues, as discussed in the text. (Modified from Ryan et al.,[1] with permission.)

Beta-Adrenergic Receptor Blockers Recommendations for early therapy[1]:

Class I

1. Patients without a contraindication to beta-adrenoceptor blocker therapy who can be treated within 12 h of onset of infarction, irrespective of administration of concomitant thrombolytic therapy or performance of primary angioplasty
2. Patients with continuing or recurrent ischemic pain
3. Patients with tachyarrhythmias, such as atrial fibrillation with a rapid ventricular response
4. Non-ST elevation myocardial infarction

Class IIb

1. Patients with moderate left ventricular failure (the presence of bibasilar rales without evidence of low cardiac output) or other relative contraindications to beta-adrenoceptor blocker therapy, provided they can be monitored closely

Class III

1. Patients with severe left ventricular failure

Beta-adrenergic receptor blockers interfere with the positive inotropic and chronotropic effects of catecholamines, thus reducing afterload (blood pressure) and therefore myocardial oxygen consumption. In the myocardial ischemic syndromes, these drugs should decrease ischemia and catecholamine-induced arrhythmias and should potentially reduce infarct size, in part by prolonging diastole and by improving subendocardial perfusion. Most of these theoretical advantages have, in fact, been borne out in clinical trials. The pharmacology of beta-adrenergic blockers is discussed in Chap. 81.

Many studies have demonstrated the clinical efficacy of beta blockers in the treatment of AMI. Analysis of pooled data from 28 trials revealed an average reduction of mortality of 28 percent at 1 week, and the majority of the benefit was seen in the first 48 h.[269] The Beta-Blocker Heart Attack Trial demonstrated that the benefits on mortality persisted and were about 20 percent after 2.5 years.[13] In the First International Study of Infarct Survival, patients were enrolled within the first 12 h from the onset of symptoms and atenolol, 5 to 10 mg, was immediately given intravenously and followed by oral atenolol, 100 mg daily.[13] Seven-day mortality was reduced by 14 percent. In the Metoprolol in Acute Myocardial Infarction (MIAMI) trial, metoprolol, 15 mg, was given intravenously in three divided doses early in the course and followed by 50 mg orally every 6 h for 48 h and then by 100 mg twice daily.[270] Mortality relative to placebo was reduced 12 percent at 15 days. In both of these trials, benefit was seen after 1 day and was sustained. Beta blockers have also enhanced therapeutic efficacy when given adjunctively with thrombolytic therapy. In the Thrombolysis in Myocardial Infarction phase II (TIMI-II) trial of conservative versus invasive strategies after treatment with recombinant tissue-type plasminogen activator (rt-PA), a subgroup was selected to receive either early intravenous followed by daily oral metoprolol or to begin oral metoprolol on day 6 after AMI.[271] The beta-blocker regimen was metoprolol, 15 mg, intravenously, followed by 50 mg orally twice daily for 1 day and 100 mg twice daily subsequently. The alternative protocol involved beginning the oral metoprolol regimen on day 6. The immediate intravenous metoprolol regimen was associated with a 45 percent reduction in nonfatal reinfarction and a 27 percent reduction in recurrent ischemic events in comparison with the group beginning beta-blocker therapy on day 6. Thus, available data strongly support the use of beta blockers early in the course of acute Q-wave myocardial infarction in the absence of contraindications. As discussed later, the data supporting the use of beta blockers in non-Q-wave myocardial infarction are less compelling. The effects of beta blockers in Q-wave MI are summarized in Table 42-9. While metoprolol and atenolol are the only beta blockers approved for use by the Federal Drug Administration in the United States in AMI, it is generally thought that therapeutic efficacy is a class effect of beta blockers lacking intrinsic sympathomimetic activity.

The relative contraindications to beta-blocker therapy are as follows:[1] (1) heart rate less than 60 beats per minute; (2) systolic blood pressure less than 100 mmHg; (3) moderate or severe left ventricular failure; (4) signs of peripheral hypoperfusion; (5) PR interval greater than 240 ms; (6) second- or third-degree AV block; (7) severe chronic pulmonary disease; (8) history of asthma; (9) severe peripheral vascular disease; and (10) insulin-dependent diabetes mellitus. Since these contraindications are relative and not absolute, the clinician has the option of assessing the effects of beta blockade with the short-acting intravenous beta blocker esmolol, which has an onset of action within 5 to 10 min and a half-life of about 30 min. If the beta blockade is tolerated by the patient, long-acting oral beta-blocking drugs can then be used with increased confidence.

Thrombolysis Recommendations[1]:

Class I

1. ST elevation (greater than 0.1 mV in two or more contiguous leads at any time during the observation period); time to therapy 12 h or less since the onset of continuous chest pain discomfort, causing hospital presentation; and age less than 75 years
2. Bundle branch block (obscuring ST-segment analysis and history suggesting AMI)

Comment
Treatment benefit is present regardless of gender, presence of diabetes, blood pressure (if <180 mmHg systolic), heart rate or history of previous myocardial infarction.[210] *Benefit is greater in the setting of anterior myocardial infarction, diabetes, low blood pressure (<100 mmHg systolic) or high heart rate (>100 beats per minute). The earlier therapy begins, the better the outcome with the greatest benefit decidedly occurring when therapy is given within the first 3 h; proven benefit occurs, however, up to at least within 12 h of onset of symptoms. Benefit is less with inferior AMI, except for the subgroup with associated right ventricular infarction (ST-elevation in V_{4R}) or anterior-segment depression indicative of a posterior current of injury as often occurs with occlusion of a large circumflex coronary artery.*

Class IIa

1. ST elevation (as earlier), age 75 years or older

TABLE 42-9 Effects of Beta Blockade in Q-Wave AMI

Reduces ventricular ectopy, atrial fibrillation, and nonfatal cardiac arrest
Reduces frequency of progression of threatened infarction to completed infarction
Reduces recurrent ischemia and infarction during first 6 weeks after initial event

Comment
Persons above age 75 benefit from thrombolytic therapy, but because of the high overall mortality rate, the relative benefit is reduced.[210]

Class IIb

1. ST elevation (as earlier), time to therapy (as previously) greater than 12 to 24 h
2. Blood pressure on presentation >180 mmHg systolic and/or >110 mmHg diastolic associated with a high-risk myocardial infarction

The potential for a therapeutic benefit of thrombolysis when the blood pressure is markedly elevated must be carefully considered against the increased risk of intracranial hemorrhage under these circumstances. Lowering the blood pressure pharmacologically before administering thrombolytics has been recommended but is of unproven benefit. If available, coronary artery bypass grafting or primary PTCA should be considered.[1]

Class III

1. ST-segment elevation, time to therapy >24 h, ischemic pain resolved
2. ST-segment depression only

Comment
In the absence of ST elevation, there is no evidence for benefit in patients with normal electrocardiographic or nonspecific changes. Using current thrombolytic regimens, there is some suggestion of harm (including increased bleeding risk) for patients with ST-segment depression only.[157,210] *When marked ST-segment depression is confined to leads V1-V4, there is a likelihood that this reflects a posterior current of injury and suggests a circumflex artery occlusion for which thrombolytic therapy would be considered appropriate. The prospective analysis of the late assessment of thrombolytic efficacy (LATE) trial*[272] *also casts some uncertainties about withholding thrombolytic therapy from this heterogenous group of patients.*

Indications for Thrombolytic Therapy Reperfusion therapy should be given immediate consideration in all patients presenting with AMI. Patients with ST-segment elevation in two or more contiguous leads or a bundle branch block masking ST-segment changes occurring within 12 h of symptoms are candidates for thrombolytic therapy.[210,273] In the ISIS-2 trial,[274] patients with bundle branch block had a mortality of 28 percent when treated with a placebo versus 19.8 percent when treated with streptokinase and aspirin. A similar beneficial effect was noted in ISIS-3.[275] Patients of unknown age with bundle branch block and with the clinical features of AMI are candidates for thrombolytic therapy.[273] *Patients with ongoing symptoms suggestive of myocardial ischemia should be repeatedly evaluated by 12-lead ECGs as frequently as every 10 to 15 min in order to identify ST-segment elevation as soon as possible.* Conversely, ST-segment elevation in the absence of suggestive symptoms should raise such possibilities as early repolarization, pericarditis, and previous infarction with aneurysm formation. Elderly patients should not be excluded from thrombolytic therapy primarily because of their age or because of the increased risk of bleeding. In patients over 75 years of age enrolled in the GISSI-2 trial, there were 4.2 fewer deaths per 100 patients in those treated with streptokinase than there were in the control group;[276] while in ISIS-2, there were 3.3 fewer deaths per 100 patients in those patients over 70 years of age who were treated.[211] The results of ISIS-3,[275] GUSTO-I,[15] and GUSTO-III[277] showed benefit regardless of age or site of infarction.

Large, placebo-controlled clinical trials have consistently demonstrated reduced mortality in patients receiving thrombolytic therapy within 6 h of the onset of an AMI.[278] In comparison with conventional medical therapy, thrombolytic therapy reduces the 35-day mortality by 21 percent. It is estimated that 34 lives per 1000 patients treated are saved when thrombolysis is used within the first hour of symptom onset, compared to 16 lives saved per 1000 treated when thrombolytics are given 7 to 12 h after the onset of symptoms.[1] The true benefit of thrombolytic therapy between 6 and 12 h has been somewhat unresolved; however, the ACC/AHA guidelines[1] have indicated acceptance that there may be a definite benefit between 6 and 12 h and have, therefore, recommended that the time limit for therapy be up to 12 h from the onset of symptoms. The EMERAS trial[279] showed an insignificant (14 percent) improvement in survival using streptokinase between 6 and 12 h after an infarction, while the LATE trial[280] observed a significant improvement (22 percent) in patients treated with rt-PA up to 12 h after infarction. Results of pooling the data from the LATE, EMERAS, and ISIS trials indicate a statistically significant improvement in survival with the use of thrombolytics up to 12 h after the onset of symptoms. Thus, the benefit of thrombolytics given between 6 and 12 h postinfarction is greater in patients classified with high-risk infarction, such as those with severe heart failure. In patients with anterior infarction, left bundle branch block, or severe hypotension, thrombolytic therapy should be given even if the precise time of onset of symptoms is unknown. Conversely, the young patient with inferior infarction having ST-T-segment elevation might not benefit greatly from thrombolytic therapy after 6 h from the onset of symptoms.

In contrast, patients with ST-segment depression, T-wave inversion, or no ECG changes have not been shown to benefit from thrombolytic therapy, as noted earlier.[281] A major problem in patients with nonspecific ST depresson or T-wave inversion is that less than 20 percent will have infarction as opposed to ST-segment elevation, in which case 90 to 95 percent will have infarction. To properly assess thrombolytic therapy in this group of patients without ST-segment elevation, one would need to have some objective marker other than the ECG to triage for infarction upon admission, which, until recently, was not possible (see previous discussion of MB-CK subforms). In the TIMI-III trial, the importance of differentiating non-Q-wave infarction from unstable angina was demonstrated, in that patients with unstable angina receiving rt-PA experienced an increased incidence of reinfarction and death compared with conventional therapy, and the trial had to be discontinued.[157] However, the mean time of initiating thrombolytic therapy in patients with non-Q-wave infarction was 9 h from the onset of symptoms and was probably too late to have a significant beneficial effect (see "Management of Non-Q-Wave Myocardial Infarction" later). An appropriate trial in which non-Q-wave infarction is diagnosed upon presentation to the emergency department within 20 to 30 min, as with MB-CK subforms or myoglobin, and is followed by thrombolytic therapy or PTCA is yet to be performed. This would be an important trial, since about 50 percent of infarctions in the United States are now non-Q-wave infarctions.[126]

Contraindications to Thrombolytic Therapy The major contraindication to thrombolytic therapy is a cerebrovascular accident (CVA) within the preceding 3 months. A hemorrhagic CVA in the past is an absolute contraindication, whereas a nonhemorrhagic CVA in the more distant past with complete or nearly complete recovery is only a relative contraindication.[282] Patients who have undergone recent (within 2 weeks) major surgery or vaginal delivery are not candidates for thrombolytic therapy, and neither are those with active internal bleeding or bleeding from a peptic ulcer. Puncture of a noncompressible vessel within the previous 10 days makes thrombolytic therapy inadvisable. Other absolute contraindications to thrombolytic therapy include suspected aortic dissection, recent head trauma or known intracranial neoplasm, and pregnancy. Previous exposure to streptokinase or anistreplase (APSAC) requires the use of rt-PA in subsequent attempts at thrombolysis. Systemic arterial hypertension and cardiopulmonary resuscitation should no longer be regarded as absolute contraindications to thrombolytic therapy. The ISIS-2 trial found that, among patients with a systolic blood pressure greater than 175 mmHg, the mortality rate was lower in those receiving streptokinase than it was in control subjects (5.7 versus 8.7 percent).[274] Some practitioners consider a recorded blood pressure greater than 200/120 an absolute contraindication. A history of severe chronic hypertension with diastolic blood pressure greater than 100 mmHg, with or without drug therapy, is a relative contraindication. Most clinicians proceed with thrombolytic therapy in a high-risk patient if elevated blood pressure normalizes promptly, with the easing of pain and anxiety through the use of narcotics and more direct therapy, including nitroglycerin and beta blockers. Califf et al. noted that patients who had brief (<10 min), nontraumatic cardiopulmonary resuscitation had no evidence of tamponade or hemothorax with thrombolytic therapy.[283] Prior administration of cardiopulmonary resuscitation should be considered a relative contraindication, since the risk of further bleeding in the chest may not outweigh the benefit. Other relative contraindications include trauma or surgery less than 2 weeks previously, active peptic ulcer disease, and bleeding diathesis or current use of anticoagulants. The absolute and relative contraindications for thrombolytic therapy are summarized in Table 42-10.

Choice of Thrombolytic Agent Four thrombolytic agents have been approved in the United States: streptokinase (SK), rt-PA, APSAC, and reteplase (r-PA). Each has been shown to limit infarct size, preserve ventricular function, and improve survival rates. These drugs and their pharmacologic properties are discussed in detail in Chap. 44.

In angiographic studies,[284,285] rt-PA and r-PA recanalized the coronary artery at 90 min in about 70 to 75 percent of patients, compared with 55 to 60 percent of those receiving SK or APSAC. Patency determined at 24 to 36 h is essentially the same for all four agents. The time course for this "catch-up" phenomenon in vessel patency, as defined by the GUSTO angiographic substudy, occurs within the first 3 h after administration of the lytic agent.[15] The ISIS-3 trial reported a 30-day mortality rate, which was the same for all three agents (10.5 percent for SK, 10.6 percent for APSAC, and 10.3 percent for rt-PA).[275] Conversely, the GUSTO trial found a 30-day mortality rate of 6.3 percent for the accelerated rt-PA regimen, which was significantly less than the 7.2 percent mortality with SK and subcutaneous heparin and less than the 7.4 percent mortality with SK and intravenous heparin[286] (Table 42-11). This absolute reduction of 1 percent reflects a 14 percent reduction in the risk of death, compared with that of SK or APSAC. A major difference why GUSTO I demonstrated an advantage for rt-PA and GISSI-2 or ISIS-3 did not was the manner in which heparin was used in GUSTO I. In GUSTO III,[277] rt-PA and r-PA exhibited similar beneficial results and a similar incidence of side effects. The 1-year follow-up on the GUSTO-I patients[287] showed that the 1 percent lower mortality rate compared with SK was maintained, which provided further evidence that rt-PA is more effective than SK.

TABLE 42-10 Absolute and Relative Contraindications to Thrombolytic Therapy

Absolute Contraindications	Relative Contraindications
Active internal bleeding	History of nonhemorrhagic cerebrovascular accident in distant past with complete recovery
Intracranial neoplasm or recent head trauma	Prolonged, traumatic CPR
Suspected aortic dissection	Recent trauma or surgery >2 weeks previously
Pregnancy	Active peptic ulcer disease
History of hemorrhagic cerebrovascular accident or recent nonhemorrhagic cerebrovascular accident	History of severe hypertension with diastolic blood pressure >100
Recorded blood pressure >200/120	Bleeding diathesis or concurrent use of anticoagulants
Trauma or surgery that is a potential bleeding source within previous 2 weeks	Previous treatment with SK or APSAC if being considered (does not apply to rt-PA)
Allergy to SK or APSAC if being considered	

ABBREVIATIONS: CPR = cardiopulmonary resuscitation; SK = streptokinase; APSAC = anistreplase; rt-PA = recombinant tissue plasminogen activator.

r-PA is a modified recombinant form of rt-PA with a longer half-life (15 min) and can be given as 2 boluses 30 min apart (see Chap. 44). In the initial open-phase trials (Reteplase Angiographic Phase II International Dose-Finding Trial: RAPID I and RAPID II),[288,289] patency was compared to that of rt-PA. In RAPID I, 60-min patency with r-PA was 78 percent, versus 66 percent for rt-PA, and TIMI-III flow was 51 percent, versus 33 percent for rt-PA. At 90 min after administration, patency was 85 percent for r-PA and 77 percent for rt-PA, with TIMI-III flow being 63 percent for r-PA and 49 percent for rt-PA. These results suggested slightly better patency rates with r-PA than with rt-PA. In the International Joint Efficacy Comparison of Thrombolytics (INJECT) trial of 6000 patients, r-PA was compared with SK.[290] The mortality and the incidence of complications for r-PA was identical to SK. This was followed by the GUSTO-III trial,[291] which compared r-PA with rt-PA, and showed that mortality and bleeding complications were similar. At 30 days, the mortality rate in the r-PA group was 7.43 percent; with rt-PA, it was 7.22 percent. The rate of hemorrhagic strokes was very similar: 0.91 percent for r-PA, versus 0.88 percent for rt-PA. The overall stroke rate was 1.67 for r-PA versus 1.83 for rt-PA. The rate of bleeding events was virtually identical between the two treatments. There remains some lack of clarity, since there were 10,000 patients in the r-PA limb and 5000 in the rt-PA limb, and the confidence limits were somewhat wide, leaving the interpretation open to some extent. Utilizing 95 percent confidence intervals, interpretation may be that rt-PA is 1.1 percent better than r-PA or that r-PA is 0.7 percent better than rt-PA. For this reason, there is still some uncertainty as to whether these drugs are truly equivalent.[291] Nevertheless, the generally accepted conclusion is that the two drugs have similar efficacy and safety.

Bolus administration of a thrombolytic agent, in addition to being more convenient, can be given with the assurance that the patient has received the full dose of the thrombolytic agent, which is not always the case in an infusion that will require 3 h or longer. Two new agents that can be given by bolus have reported results showing similar efficacy to alteplase: one is lanatoplase and the other TNK-tpa. Both agents were found to have comparable rates of intracranial hemorrhage in preliminary trials (0.9-1.1 percent) and are awaiting approval for use by the FDA.

The selection of a thrombolytic agent must be based on its adverse effects as well as upon its efficacy. The major risk with any thrombolytic agent is its propensity for causing bleeding, with the most devastating bleeding being a hemorrhagic stroke. In the GUSTO trial, the frequency of hemorrhagic stroke was 0.49 percent for SK and subcutaneous heparin, 0.54 percent for SK and intravenous heparin, 0.72 percent for rt-PA, and 0.94 percent for combined SK and rt-PA. There was a small but significant excess of hemorrhagic strokes for rt-PA and for the combined rt-PA and SK strategy ($p < 0.001$) compared with the SK arms. The combined end point of death or nonfatal hemorrhagic stroke was, however, significantly reduced in the rt-PA group, compared with the SK groups (6.6 versus 7.5 percent; $p = 0.004$).[286] One reason to choose rt-PA over SK is the 14 percent decreased risk of mortality. Nevertheless, a 10-fold greater cost of rt-PA must be considered. Choosing between rt-PA and r-PA, since both are equally effective and cost the same, may depend on choosing between monitoring an intrave-

TABLE 42-11 30-Day Mortality Rates from the GUSTO Trial

Regimen	Mortality, %
SK and subcutaneous heparin	7.2
SK and intravenous heparin	7.4
Accelerated rt-PA and intravenous heparin	6.3[a]
Combination rt-PA and SK with intravenous heparin	7.0

[a]14% reduction in mortality rate was achieved with the accelerated rt-PA regimen versus the SK strategies ($p = 0.001$).

ABBREVIATIONS: SK = streptokinase; rt-PA = recombinant tissue plasminogen activator.

nous infusion of rt-PA versus 2 bolus injections of r-PA separated by 30 min.

Another thrombolytic agent, TNK-tPA, is in the process of clinical evaluation (see Chap. 44). It has a short half-life of about 17 min and can be given as a single bolus. It is highly fibrin-specific and somewhat resistant to plasminogen activator inhibitor.[292] The phase II trial Assessment of the Safety and Efficacy of a New Thrombolytic (ASSENT-1)[293,294] was performed on 3235 patients, and the results were comparable to that of rt-PA in GUSTO-I and III. In the ASSENT-2 trial[293] the 30-day mortality was 6.17 versus 6.15 percent for rt-PA, and the bleeding rates were also similar. Another thrombolytic agent undergoing clinical trials is that of lanoteplase (see Chap. 44). Preliminary results showed no difference in 30-day mortality, which was 6.6 percent and 6.7 percent with alteplase and lanoteplase, respectively.[295]

Dose and Administration of Thrombolytic Agents Streptokinase is given in a dose of 1.5 million U intravenously over 30 to 60 min. Since antibodies develop and may persist for several years, a subsequent need for thrombolytic therapy, as for early or late reocclusion, would require the use of rt-PA or r-PA. If the patient has had a streptococcal infection within 3 to 6 months, the use of rt-PA is preferable. Although APSAC is identical to SK as a thrombolytic agent, it can be given as a rapid infusion of 30 U over 5 to 10 min. Its therapeutic half-life is similar to that of SK, which is about 90 min. In contrast, the half-life of rt-PA is about 5 min. The FDA-approved dose of rt-PA is an initial bolus of 15 mg, followed by an infusion of 50 mg or 0.75 mg per kilogram of body weight over the next 30 min, and an infusion of 35 mg or 0.50 mg per kilogram of body weight over the subsequent 60 min, for a total of up to 100 mg given over 90 min. Reteplase is given as an initial bolus of 15 megaunits (MU), followed by a second bolus of 15 MU in 30 min.

Overall Strategy for Reperfusion of Patients with Acute Myocardial Infarction The criteria for initiating thrombolytic therapy are as follows (Table 42-12):

1. Patients presenting with chest pain suggestive of myocardial ischemia, having ST-T-segment elevation greater than 1 mm in two contiguous limb leads or greater than 2 mm in two contiguous precordial leads or new left bundle branch block and who are within 6 h of the onset of symptoms should receive thrombolytic therapy if there are no contraindications. In patients presenting between 6 and 12 h of the onset of symptoms, one must weigh more heavily the risk versus the benefit. Patients presenting after 12 h are no longer routinely considered for thrombolytic therapy.
2. Contraindications for thrombolytic therapy are absolute or relative, as discussed earlier (Table 42-10).

TABLE 42-12 Criteria for Initiating Thrombolytic Therapy

Chest pain consistent with angina
ECG changes
ST ↑ ≥ 1 mm, ≥2 contiguous limb leads
ST ↑ ≥ 2 mm, ≥2 contiguous precordial leads
New left bundle branch block
Absence of contraindications

3. In patients receiving rt-PA or r-PA, it is recommended that heparin be given as a bolus at the initiation of infusion (60 U/kg) and then an additional maintenance dose of 12 U/kg/h (with a maximum of 4000 U bolus and a 1000 U/h infusion for patients weighing >70 kg), adjusted to maintain a partial thromboplastin time (PTT) at 1.5 to 2.0 times control (50 to 70 s) for 48 h. Continuation of heparin infusion beyond 48 h should be considered in patients at high risk for systemic or venous thromboembolism. In patients treated with nonselective thrombolytic agents (streptokinase, anistreplase, or urokinase), heparin should be given intravenously for those who are at high risk for systemic emboli (large or anterior myocardial infarction, atrial fibrillation, previous embolus or known left ventricular thrombus). It is recommended that heparin be withheld for 6 h and that aPPT testing begin at that time. Heparin should be started when aPPT returns to 2 times control (approximately 70 s), then infused to keep aPPT 1.5 to 2.0 times control (initial infusion rate approximately 1000 U/h). After 48 h, a change to subcutaneous heparin or warfarin or aspirin alone should be considered.
4. Patients allergic to SK or APSAC who require thrombolytic therapy should receive rt-PA or r-PA. Patients who received SK or APSAC and who again require thrombolytic therapy should receive rt-PA or r-PA.
5. Patients presenting with ST-T-segment depression and chest pain are not candidates for thrombolytic therapy. These patients need to be triaged, as indicated in Fig. 42-3, as to whether their pain is of cardiac or noncardiac origin. If the former, those with either unstable angina (see Chap. 41) or non-ST-elevated infarction should be treated with intravenous unfractionated heparin or low-molecular-weight heparin subcutaneously. In all patients not treated with thrombolytic therapy who do not have a contraindication to heparin, subcutaneous unfractionated heparin (e.g., 7500 U bid) or low-molecular-weight heparin (e.g., Enoxoparin) 1 mg/kg bid should be used. In patients who are at high risk for systemic emboli, intravenous heparin is preferred.
6. As discussed subsequently and in detail in Chapter 46, PTCA as a primary procedure is an alternative to thrombolytic therapy only if performed in a timely fashion by individuals skilled in the procedure and supported by experienced personnel in high volume centers (class I). The individual must perform 75 such PTCA procedures per year, and the center a minimum of 200 PTCAs per year. PTCA is indicated in patients with a contraindication to thrombolytic therapy because of a severe bleeding diathesis or in those who are in cardiogenic shock (class IIa).
7. Elective angioplasty should be reserved for patients who develop ischemia or reinfarction or in whom thrombolytic therapy appears ineffective. In patients in whom angioplasty cannot be performed and who develop recurrent ischemia with possible infarction, the possibility of readministering a thrombolytic agent should be considered; rt-PA may be given in a full dose if the patient has not received it for 24 to 48 h.

Percutaneous Transluminal Coronary Angioplasty as a Primary Therapy for Acute Myocardial Infarction Recommendations[1]:

Class I

1. "As an alternative to thrombolytic therapy in patients with AMI and ST segment elevation or new or presumed new LBBB who can undergo angioplasty of the infarct artery within 12 hours of onset of symptoms or >12 hours if ischemic symptoms persist, if performed in a *timely fashion* by persons skilled in the procedure** and supported by experienced personnel in an appropriate laboratory environment.*"***[1]
2. "In patients who are within 36 hours of an acute ST-elevation/Q-wave or new LBBB MI who develop cardiogenic shock, are <75 years of age, and revascularization can be performed within 18 hours of onset of shock."[1]

Class IIa

1. "As a reperfusion strategy in candidates for reperfusion who have a contraindication to thrombolytic therapy."[1]

Class IIb

1. "In patients with AMI who do not present with ST elevation but who have reduced [less than TIMI (Thrombolysis in Myocardial Infarction) grade 2] flow of the infarct-related artery and when angioplasty can be performed within 12 hours of onset of symptoms."[1]

Class III

"This category applies to patients with AMI who

1. Undergo elective angioplasty of a non-infarct related artery at the time of AMI
2. Are beyond 12 hours after onset of symptoms and have no evidence of myocardial ischemia
3. Have received fibrinolytic therapy and have no symptoms of myocardial ischemia"[1]

Comment
There is serious concern that a routine policy of primary PTCA for patients with AMI will result in unacceptable delays in achieving reperfusion in a substantial number of cases and less than optimal outcomes if performed by less experienced operators. Strict performance criteria must be mandated for primary angioplasty programs so that such delay in revascularization and performance by low-volume operators and centers do not occur. Interventional cardiologists and centers must operate within a specified "corridor of outcomes" to include (1) balloon dilatation within 90 (±30) min of admission and diagnosis of AMI; (2) a documented clinical success rate with TIMI-2 through 3 flow attained in >90 percent of patients without emergency coronary artery bypass graft, stroke, or death; (3) emergency coronary artery bypass graft rate <5 percent among all patients undergoing the procedure; (4) actual performance of angioplasty in a high percentage of patients (85 percent) brought to the laboratory; and (5) mortality rate <10 percent. Otherwise, the focus of treatment should be the early use of thrombolytic therapy.

* Performance standard: balloon inflation within 90 (±30) min of admission.

** Persons who perform >75 PTCA procedures per year.[296]

*** Centers that perform >200 PTCA procedures per year and have cardiac surgical capability.[296]

ANGIOPLASTY AS PRIMARY OR ADJUNCTIVE THERAPY TO THROMBOLYSIS Detailed discussions of PTCA and its indications appear in Chap. 45. Comprehensive discussions of PTCA in the treatment of acute MI are presented in Chapter 46. Direct angioplasty has been compared with thrombolytic therapy in a meta-analysis of 10 randomized trials involving 2606 patients.[297] In 1290 patients treated with primary PTCA, the mortality rate at 30 days was 4.4 percent compared to 6.5 percent in 1316 patients treated with thrombolytic therapy. Pooled rates of nonfatal reinfarction or death were also lower in the PTCA as opposed to the thrombolysis groups. The incidence of stroke was also lower with PTCA than it was with thrombolysis. These authors concluded that "primary PTCA appears to be superior to thrombolytic therapy for treatment of patients with AMI, with the proviso that success rates for PTCA are as good as those achieved in these trials. Data evaluating longer-term outcome, operator expertise, and time delays before treatment are needed before primary PTCA can be recommended universally as the preferred treatment."[297] Registry data (Second National Registry of Myocardial Infarction) of 4939 patients with acute AMI (ST-segment elevation) who received primary PTCA and 24,705 who received alteplase showed similar in-hospital mortality (5.2 percent and 5.4 percent, respectively) in the absence of shock.[298] These results also add some caution against the general embracement of primary PTCA over thrombolysis in the treatment of ST-segment elevation myocardial infarction.

In the case of cardiogenic shock in AMI (ST-segment elevation/new left bundle branch block) primary angioplasty, if rapidly available, offers benefit over thrombolysis as part of a strategy of emergency revascularization.[299] In the Should We Emergently Revascularize Occluded Coronaries for Cardiogenic Shock (SHOCK) Trial, a strategy of emergency revascularization was compared with initial medical stabilization and delayed revascularization based on clinical indicators. The 30-day mortality showed a favorable but not significant ($p = 0.11$) trend for emergency revascularization over initial medical restabilization in the case of mortality at 30 days (46.7 versus 56.0 percent, respectively). The mortality at 6 months, however, was significantly lower ($p = 0.027$) for the emergently revascularized group (53.5 percent) compared to the initially medical stabilized group (65.7 percent). Patients <75 years old had a more favorable outcome with emergency revascularization than did older patients (>75) with a 15.4 percent reduction in 30-day mortality (56.8 versus 41.4 percent, $p < 0.01$). Patients in the emergency revascularization group who were >75 years old fared worse than they did in the medical stabilization group. PTCA was the revascularization procedure in 60 percent, and coronary artery bypass grafting was used in 40 percent of patients with similar outcomes.

Thus, there is increasing evidence of the efficacy of PTCA as an alternative to thrombolysis in the treatment of ST-segment elevation/new left bundle branch block myocardial infarction. It is the method of choice in cardiogenic shock and in the presence of contraindications for thrombolytic therapy. There is increasing concensus that, in high-volume centers with skilled, experienced operators, PTCA is the procedure of choice if it can be performed in a timely manner (generally within the first 2 h). Indeed a report showed a 53 percent reduction in 30-day mortality in patients having PTCA within the first 2 h of pain in comparison to those more than 2 h into their pain.[1,300] Because of the logistic issues involved (including transfer from a community hospital to an interventional center) in obtaining PTCA within an appropriate time frame, the approach of combining a low-dose thrombolytic (to obtain early patency) with PTCA outside of the 2-h time is being explored.[1] These and other issues including the use of stents are discussed in detail in Chapter 45.

Several caveats must be considered before embracing PTCA as the therapy of choice for AMI generally. Only about 20 percent of hospitals in the United States have cardiac catheterization laboratories and relatively few can perform PTCA on an emergency basis. In many cases the time delay involved in transferring a patient to a hospital capable of performing emergency PTCA may outweigh any benefit.[1] *The excellent results for emergency PTCA described earlier were achieved by highly experienced and enthusiastic investigators in hospitals that have devoted extraordinary support and personnel to achieving opening of the coronary artery within 60 to 90 min of arrival.*[1,301,302] Available data suggesting that emergency PTCA may be comparable to thrombolysis in many community settings were alluded to previously.

Heparin as Conjunctive or Adjunctive Therapy Recommendations for heparin administration post-MI[1]:

Class I

1. Patients undergoing percutaneous revascularization.

Class IIa

1. Administer intravenously in patients undergoing reperfusion therapy with rt-PA (alteplase) or r-PA (reteplase).
2. Administer subcutaneously unfractionated heparin (7500 U BID) or low-molecular-weight heparin (enoxaparin 1 mg/kg bid) in all patients not treated with thrombolytic therapy who do not have a contraindication to heparin. Intravenous heparin is acceptable as an alternative and is preferred in patients who have a large or anterior myocardial infarction, atrial fibrillation, a known left ventricular thrombus, or a previous embolus and thus are at high risk for systemic emboli.
3. Administer intravenously in patients treated with nonselective thrombolytic agents (streptokinase or anistreplase) who are at high risk for systemic emboli (anterior or large infarction, history of embolus, atrial fibrillation, or demonstrable left ventricular thrombus).

It is recommended that heparin not be started immediately but that an activated partial thromboplastin time (aPTT) be drawn at 4 h and that heparin be started when the aPTT returns to less than twice control (about 70 s).

Lysis of a thrombus by any thrombolytic agent induces a surface that is perhaps the most thrombogenic known.[285,303] Furthermore, lysis with either rt-PA or SK has been shown to be associated with marked elevation of plasma levels of thrombin, which return to normal after 24 h.[304] Since aspirin has no effect on thrombin-induced platelet aggregation,[305] the use of heparin during the initial 24 to 48 h was assumed to be critical to prevent rethrombosis and reocclusion.

The necessity of heparin for maintaining coronary patency induced by rt-PA was established in the HART trial.[284] In this trial, 208 patients received rt-PA within 4 h of the onset of their infarction. Simultaneously, 50 percent of these patients received heparin administered as a bolus, followed by an intravenous

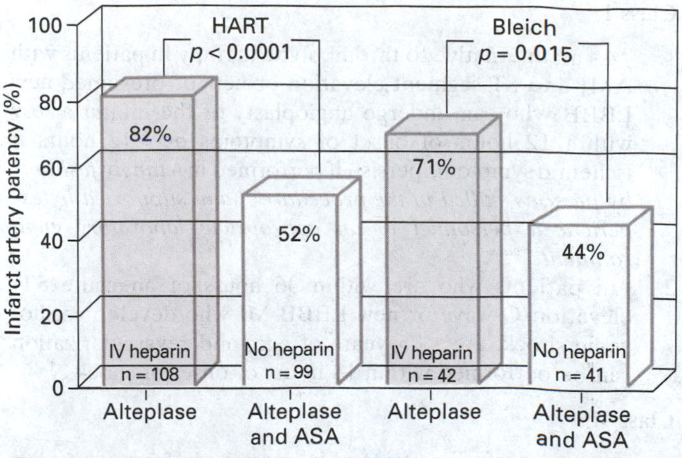

FIGURE 42-7 Influence of effective anticoagulation on early patency rates with rt-PA. Patency assessed angiographically at an average of 18 to 81 h is significantly greater in patients treated with intravenous heparin.

infusion, while the remainder received only oral aspirin in a dose of 81 mg/day. Coronary angiographic studies performed at 18 to 81 h showed a patency of 82 percent in the group receiving heparin and 52 percent in the group receiving aspirin (Fig. 42-7). Stratifying the group on the basis of PTT established an excellent correlation between patency and PTT (Fig. 42-8). In patients with aPTT of <45 s, the patency was only 45 percent; patency was 83 percent or greater in patients with aPTT >45 s.[306] The findings of HART were confirmed by Bleich et al.,[307] who showed that rt-PA given with heparin had a patency of >90 percent; without heparin, the patency rate was 44 percent (Fig. 42-7). In the National Heart Foundation of Australia Study,[308] all patients received rt-PA, followed by intravenous heparin for 24 h. They were then randomized to continue heparin for 72 h or were switched to antiplatelet agents. The study found the patency rate at 72 h to be the same for both groups.

Heparin appears to act by preventing early reocclusion, at least after rt-PA.[309,310] The adjunctive heparin therapy in both GISSI-2 and ISIS-3 was administered by the subcutaneous route (12 h after thrombolytic therapy in GISSI-2 and 4 h afterward in ISIS-3). Such a heparin regimen seems to be suboptimal adjunctive therapy for rt-PA and is believed to be the main

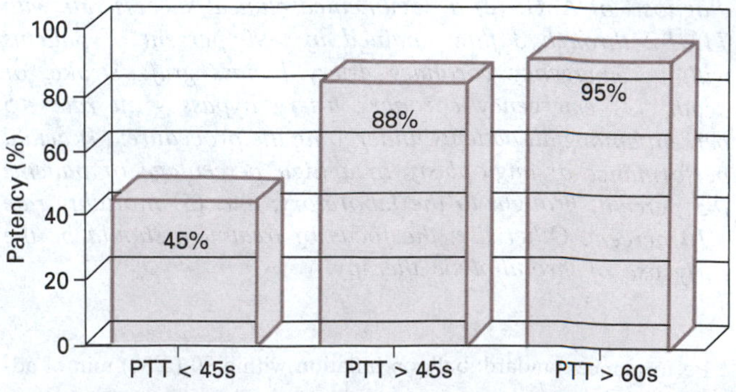

FIGURE 42-8 Retrospective analysis of the HART trial showing the relationship between increased PTT and coronary artery patency (n = 94). This illustrates the importance of heparin.

reason why rt-PA was not shown to be superior over SK in GISSI-2 and ISIS-3. A subcutaneous heparin dose of 12,500 U twice a day used in the megatrials failed to provide therapeutic anticoagulation for at least 24 h in various cohort analytic studies.[311,312] The administration of SK without adjunctive heparin has not been properly tested. However, the ISIS data raise the possibility that it may not be necessary in the early hours, since the marked increase, after SK administration, in plasma levels of fibrinogen breakdown products, which inhibit platelet aggregation, may prevent rethrombosis and reocclusion.[273] In contrast, these platelet-inhibiting breakdown products are not present in high concentrations with the fibrin-selective agents, rt-PA and r-PA. The results of the SCATI trial argue for the existence of a beneficial effect of heparin even in patients treated with SK.[313] In the SCATI trial, patients receiving SK with subcutaneous heparin had a mortality rate of 4.5 percent, while those receiving SK without heparin had a mortality rate of 8.8 percent.[313] The combined data from these studies suggest that heparin is not necessary to achieve reperfusion but is essential in the first 24 h to maintain patency rates with rt-PA. While heparin may be beneficial when SK is used, subcutaneous administration of heparin appears adequate in this circumstance.[273] At present, heparin is recommended in a bolus of 5000 U intravenously followed by an infusion of 1000 to 1200 U/h to keep the PTT at 1.5 to 2.0 times normal. It is recommended that the PTT not be measured until 4 h after heparin therapy is initiated, because it has not yet reached a steady state. If the PTT has increased more than twofold over normal, the same dose of heparin should be continued; if PTT exhibits less than a twofold increase, the infusion rate of heparin should be increased. Initiation of heparin is recommended either during or following completion of thrombolytic therapy, as discussed earlier, and should be maintained in uncomplicated cases for 24 to 48 h.

The use of heparin has also been recommended conjunctively in patients with AMI who are not being treated with the drug for other reasons, i.e., postthrombolysis or postprimary PTCA. Currently, the American Association of Chest Physicians' guidelines recommend heparin 7500 U twice daily subcutaneously as prophylaxis against deep venous thrombosis.[264] Given the enhanced risk of stroke after AMI in patients with atrial arrhythmias, those with large and especially anterior and apical infarction, and those with history of previous stroke,[314] the ACC/AHA guidelines have incorporated this recommendation for broader prophylaxis against systemic embolization.[1] In high-risk patients, the intravenous route is probably preferable. Heparin therapy should be continued for 48 h and judgment should be made at that point about continuation based on individual patient characteristics. Heparin therapy, including precautions concerning the monitoring of platelet counts because of the risk of heparin-induced thrombocytopenia, is discussed in Chap. 44.

Low-molecular-weight heparins are cleavage products of heparin with a mean molecular weight of ~5000 which have higher anti-Xa activity and less antithrombin activity. Low-molecular-weight heparin preparations are widely used in non-ST-segment elevation acute coronary syndromes (unstable angina, non-Q-wave myocardial infarction) as discussed subsequently in Chapter 41. Low-molecular-weight heparins are being evaluated as adjunctive therapy for thrombolysis.[1] Their use has a class IIa recommendation in all patients with ST-segment elevation AMI who have not been treated with thrombolytics and who do not have a contraindication to heparin.[1] High-risk patients for systemic embolization should be treated with heparin, as noted.

Early Coronary Angiography in Patients with ST-Segment Elevation Not Undergoing Primary Percutaneous Transluminal Coronary Angioplasty Recommendations[1]:

Class I

1. None

Class IIa

1. In the presence of cardiogenic shock or persistent hemodynamic instability

Class IIb

1. In the presence of evolving large or anterior infarction and evidence that thrombolysis has not resulted in arterial patency and if adjuvant PTCA is planned

Class III

1. Routine use of angiography and subsequent PTCA within 24 h of administration of thrombolytic agents

Routine immediate or delayed angioplasty is not recommended as a standard mode of therapy following thrombolysis. The TIMI-IIA and TIMI-IIB trials,[315] the TAMI study,[310] The European Cooperative Study Group trial,[316] and the SWIFT trial[317] all showed no reduction in the incidence of coronary reocclusion or hospital mortality rates and no evidence of improved ventricular function with routine immediate or delayed angioplasty compared with elective angioplasty in the case of manifest ischemia following thrombolytic therapy. The TIMI-II trial found that angioplasty either performed routinely at 18 to 48 h when anatomically appropriate or in response to induced or spontaneous ischemia did not improve survival or reduce the reinfarction rate at either 6 weeks or 1 year,[318] and neither did it reduce the need for surgery (Fig. 42-9). At present, the

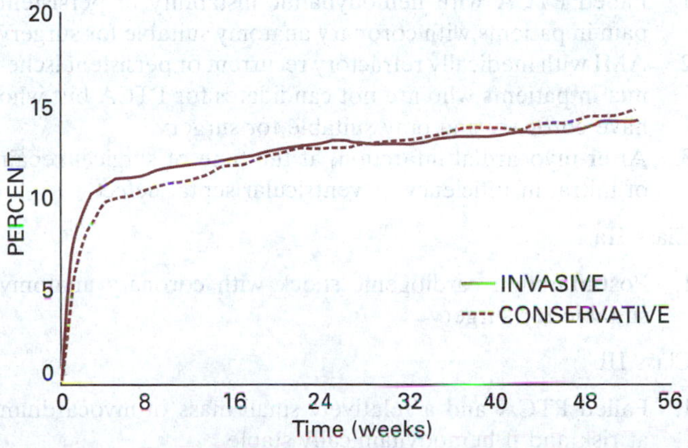

FIGURE 42-9 Kaplan Meier curves for death and infarction in patients assigned to the invasive or conservative strategies in TIMI-2. Routine cardiac catheterization after thrombolytic therapy and revascularization with PTCA or bypass grafting (when anatomically appropriate) was not a superior strategy to catheterization and revascularization when there is development of spontaneous ischemia or ischemia induced by exercise testing. (Reproduced with permission. Williams DO, Braunwald E, Knatterud G, et al.: One-year results of the thrombolysis in myocardial infarction investigation (TIMI) phase II trial. *Circulation* 1992; 85:533–542.[318] Copyright 1992 American Heart Association.)

most widely accepted recommendation is to perform cardiac catheterization for possible angioplasty or bypass surgery in patients who develop angina or manifest evidence of myocardial ischemia during submaximal exercise testing or who develop hemodynamic or ischemic instability. Thus, if intervening with PTCA generally offers no demonstrable benefit after thrombolysis, there is little apparent reason to perform early coronary angiography routinely.

Rescue angioplasty to open occluded arteries after presumptive failed thrombolysis has been advocated and, in fact, studies indicate that TIMI grade 3 flow can be achieved in a high percentage of these patients.[319] In the reported TIMI-IV trial, however, it was found that although a strategy of rescue angioplasty could restore flow that is superior to that of thrombolysis alone, the incidence of adverse events for the strategy as a whole was the same as for not undertaking PTCA (35 percent adverse event rate whether or not PTCA was performed for an occluded artery). Both rates tended to be higher than the incidence in patients with patent arteries (23 percent, $p = 0.07$).[320] *Thus, rescue angioplasty as a routine strategy for failed or presumptively failed thrombolysis cannot be recommended.* This issue is discussed further in Chapter 46.

Patients with cardiogenic shock have a very high mortality (>70 percent) with or without thrombolysis. As noted previously, the results of the reported SHOCK Trial now provide data to suggest that emergency revascularization results in a 41.4 percent survival rate at 30 days.[299] All of these patients received intraaortic balloon assist whether they received revascularization urgently or whether they had initial medical stabilization. These data suggest that other means of metabolically manipulating the myocardial cell may be required for further advances in the management of this lethal complication of AMI.

Emergency or Urgent Coronary Artery Bypass Surgery Recommendations[1]:

Class I

1. Failed PTCA with hemodynamic instability or persistent pain in patients with coronary anatomy suitable for surgery
2. AMI with medically refractory recurrent or persistent ischemia in patients who are not candidates for PTCA but who have coronary anatomy suitable for surgery
3. After myocardial infarction, at the time of surgical repair of mitral insufficiency or ventricular septal defect

Class IIa

1. Postinfarction cardiogenic shock with coronary anatomy suitable for surgery

Class IIb

1. Failed PTCA and a relatively small mass of myocardium at risk and if hemodynamically stable

Class III

1. When the anticipated operative mortality rate exceeds or equals the mortality rate associated with appropriate medical therapy coronary artery bypass grafting in cardiogenic shock in patients in whom other strategies have failed or where they have not been indicated has been associated with mortality rates from about 10 to 40 percent.[321–323] These results are generally better than those associated with PTCA. Thus, AMI patients with multivessel coronary artery disease or cardiogenic shock who have had unsuccessful thrombolysis and/or PTCA and are within 4 to 6 h of the onset of symptoms should be considered for emergency coronary artery bypass grafting.[1]

Arrhythmias Early in the Course of Acute Myocardial Infarction BRADYCARDIA Bradyarrhythmias are relatively common (30 to 40 percent) early in the course of AMI, especially in inferior infarction, or after reperfusion of the right coronary artery, because of the activation of vagal afferents that ultimately result in enhanced parasympathetic tone.[1] Atropine, because of its anticholinergic effects, can be very useful in this situation, since it enhances the discharge rate of the sinus node and facilitates AV conduction,[324] as well as reversing the peripheral effects of excessive cholinergic activity such as vasodilation with associated hypotension. Parasympathomimetic effects with bradycardia, hypotension, and nausea and vomiting are also produced by morphine and can be reversed by atropine. Atropine should be used sparingly and appropriately in AMI, however, because of the protective effect of vagal stimulation against VF.[325]

THE USE OF ATROPINE Recommendations[1]:

Class I

1. Sinus bradycardia with evidence of low cardiac output and hypoperfusion peripherally or frequent ventricular premature complexes at the onset of symptoms of AMI
2. Acute inferior infarction with type I second- or third-degree AV block associated with symptoms of hypotension, ischemic discomfort, or ventricular arrhythmias
3. Sustained bradycardia and hypotension after administration of nitroglycerin
4. Morphine-induced nausea and vomiting
5. Ventricular asystole

Class IIa

1. In patients with inferior infarction and type I second- or third-degree block at the AV-nodal level (narrow QRS complex or known preexisting bundle branch block) who are symptomatic from the low output and/or vagal predominance

Class IIb

1. Vagal symptoms and sinus bradycardia associated with the administration of morphine
2. Patients with inferior infarction who are asymptomatic with type I second-degree heart block or third-degree block at the AV node
3. Second- or third-degree AV block of uncertain mechanism and unavailability of pacing

Class III

1. Asymptomatic sinus bradycardia and a rate of greater than 40 beats per minute with no signs of hypoperfusion or frequent ventricular premature contractions
2. Type II and third-degree AV block and third-degree AV block with new, wide QRS complex (i.e., block below the AV junction)

SINUS BRADYCARDIA, ATRIOVENTRICULAR BLOCK, OR VENTRICULAR ASYSTOLE Atropine is indicated for the treatment of type I second-degree AV block, especially with complicating inferior myocardial infarction, and is useful at times in third-degree AV block at the AV node in restoring AV conduction or for increasing the junctional response rate.[1] By increasing the sinus node rate or by improving AV conduction, atropine may improve signs or symptoms of congestive heart failure, hypotension, or frequent, complex ventricular arrhythmias associated with AV block or sinus bradycardia; thus, pacemaker insertion may be avoided.[1] Treatment of sinus bradycardia or first- or second-degree AV block is generally not indicated in the absence of hemodynamic compromise,[1] and atropine should seldom be used in the treatment of type II AV block (location of block below the AV node). Symptomatic bradycardia that is unresponsive to atropine should be treated with pacing.

Atropine should be administered intravenously at a dosage of 0.5 to 1.0 mg and repeated as necessary to achieve an adequate heart rate every 3 to 5 min, up to a total maximum dose of 2.5 mg, which gives complete vagal blockade.[1] Atropine may also be efficacious in ventricular asystole and should be given intravenously at a dosage of 1.0 mg every 3 to 5 min during cardiopulmonary resuscitation up to a maximum of 2.5 mg if asystole persists.

At doses of 0.5 mg or less, atropine may produce, paradoxically, bradycardia and suppression of AV nodal conduction due to a central or peripheral parasympathomimetic effect.[326] Atropine dosage should be titrated carefully, because tachycardia can be induced and ischemia can be worsened. Thus, atropine should be given in 0.5-mg increments, as noted, to achieve an adequate heart rate of 50 to 60 beats per minute.

HEART BLOCK Heart block develops in about 10 percent of patients with AMI and is associated with an increased mortality during hospitalization, but it does not predict long-term mortality in those who survive to be discharged.[327–329] Intraventricular conduction delay or bundle branch block is also associated with increased in-hospital mortality.[210] The increase in mortality associated with heart block reflects the extent of myocardial damage, not heart block per se. Thus, a heart block in the setting of anterior myocardial infarction reflects extensive infarction and concomitant destruction of the conduction system and is associated with relatively high mortality. In contrast, heart block with inferior myocardial infarction may primarily reflect ischemia of the AV node rather than extensive tissue damage and is associated with a more favorable prognosis. Because of the overwhelming effect of the extent of myocardial damage on prognosis, pacing has not been shown to lessen mortality associated with AV block or bundle branch block.[328,330] It is likely, however, that pacing will benefit subgroups of these patients with severe slowing of ventricular rates but without extensive myocardial damage[330,331] by preventing hypotension, ischemia, and ventricular escape arrhythmias associated with the appearance of a heart block. In AMI, the risk of developing heart block is augmented by the presence of any evidence of conduction system abnormality including first-degree AV block, Mobitz type I or II AV block, left anterior or posterior hemiblock, or a left or right bundle branch block.[1]

TEMPORARY PACING EARLY IN THE COURSE OF ACUTE MYOCARDIAL INFARCTION The "Guidelines for the Management of Patients with Acute Myocardial Infarction"[1] place increased emphasis on transcutaneous pacing in view of the availability of new systems that provide standby status for pacing in AMI patients who do not necessitate immediate pacing and are at intermediate risk for developing heart block. These systems use a single pair of multifunctional electrodes, permitting electrocardiographic monitoring, transcutaneous pacing, and defibrillation.[332] Transcutaneous pacing does not entail the risk and complications of transvenous pacing and, because invasive procedures may thus be avoided or delayed, is well suited for use in the patient who has undergone thrombolysis. Percutaneous pacing is painful; if prolonged pacing is required, the patient should be switched to transvenous systems.

Placement* of Transcutaneous Patches and Active (Demand)† Transcutaneous Pacing Recommendations[1,333]:

Class I

1. Sinus bradycardia (rate less than 50 beats per minute) with symptoms of hypotension (systolic blood pressure less than 80 mmHg) unresponsive to drug therapy†
2. Mobitz type II second-degree AV block†
3. Third-degree heart block†
4. Bilateral bundle branch block (alternating left and right bundle branch block or right bundle branch block with alternating left anterior and posterior fascicular block—irrespective of time of onset)*
5. Newly acquired or age-indeterminant left bundle branch block, right bundle branch block, and anterior or posterior fascicular block*
6. Right bundle branch block or left bundle branch block and first-degree AV block*

Class IIa

1. Stable bradycardia (systolic blood pressure greater than 90 mmHg, no hemodynamic compromise, or compromise responsive to initial drug therapy)*
2. Newly acquired or age-indeterminant right bundle branch block*

Class IIb

1. Newly acquired or age-indeterminant first-degree AV block*

Class III

1. Uncomplicated AMI without evidence of conduction system disease

As noted, transcutaneous pacing is intended to be temporary; if prolonged pacing is required, transvenous pacing should be instituted (discussed later). In addition, patients with a high probability of requiring pacing should have it instituted early on.[1] Technical aspects of transcutaneous pacing have been reviewed.[334]

VENTRICULAR ECTOPY, TACHYCARDIA, AND FIBRILLATION Recommendations[1]:

* Put pacing system in place.
† Activate system.

Class I

1. Ventricular fibrillation should be treated with an unsynchronized electric shock starting with an energy of 200 J. If the initial shock is unsuccessful, a second shock of 200 to 300 J should be administered, and, if required, a third shock of 360 J should be given.
2. Polymorphic ventricular tachycardia (VT) lasting more than 30 s or causing hemodynamic collapse should be treated with an unsynchronized shock, initially of 200 J, and, if necessary, with a second shock of 200 to 300 J, to be followed by a shock of 360 J if the arrhythmia persists.
3. Sustained monomorphic VT associated with hypotension, with blood pressure of less than 90 mmHg, pulmonary edema, or angina should be treated with a synchronized electric shock of 100 J initially, to be followed by high-energy shocks if required.
4. Monomorphic VT that is sustained but not associated with hypotension, angina, or pulmonary edema should be treated with one of the regimens as follows:
   a. Lidocaine bolus from 1.0 to 1.5 mg/kg intravenously with supplemental boluses of 0.5 to 0.75 mg/kg every 5 to 10 min, up to a maximum loading dose of 3 mg/kg as needed. This loading regimen is followed by an infusion of 2 to 4 mg/min (30 to 50 mg/kg/min).
   b. Procainamide at a loading infusion rate of 20 to 30 mg/min to a maximum of 12 to 17 mg/kg total, which may be followed by infusion of 1 to 4 mg/min.
   c. Amiodarone infused initially at 150 mg over 10 min, followed by a constant infusion of 1.0 mg/min for 6 h, and then at a rate of 0.5 mg/min.
   d. Synchronized electrical cardioversion with an initial starting level of 50 J after anesthesia is induced briefly.

Note that drug metabolism can vary depending upon age, body size, and liver and renal function, and that doses may need to be adjusted accordingly.

Class IIa

1. Antiarrhythmic drug infusions may be utilized after an episode of ventricular tachycardia or fibrillation but should be discontinued after 6 to 24 h, when the need for further management of the arrhythmia is reassessed.
2. Metabolic abnormalities of electrolytes and acid-base balances should be corrected as prophylaxis against recurrence when the initial ventricular arrhythmia has been treated.

Class IIb

1. Polymorphic VT, which is refractory to drug treatment, should be managed by focusing on relieving the presumptive underlying ischemia with beta blockers, intraaortic balloon pumping, and/or emergency revascularization. Amiodarone infusion, as noted earlier, may also be useful.

Class III

1. Treatment of isolated ventricular premature beats, couplets, runs of accelerated idioventricular rhythm, and nonsustained VT.
2. Use of antiarrhythmic drugs prophylactically during administration of thrombolytic agents.

Ventricular rhythm abnormalities are common during the early phases of AMI, with an incidence of VF within the first 4 h, so-called primary VF, of 3 to 5 percent, which declines rapidly thereafter.[335] Primary VF is thought to be the result of micro reentry mechanisms in the infarct zone.[1] Postulated triggering mechanisms include hypokalemia, hypomagnesemia, enhanced adrenergic tone, acidosis, increased intracellular calcium, increased free fatty acids, and reperfusion-induced production of free radicals.[336–338] Although the relative contribution of each of these factors to early VT/VF and the effects of their specific treatment are not known,[1] epidemiologic evidence suggests that there has been a decrease in the incidence of primary VF,[339] which may be related generally to more aggressive treatment strategies, including the use of beta blockers. Primary VF is associated with increased in-hospital mortality but not with increased long-term mortality for patients who survive and are discharged.[340]

Post-AMI VT occurs in about 15 percent of patients and is also most commonly manifest during the relatively early period.[335] Ventricular tachycardia is classified according to its electrocardiographic morphology (monomorphic or polymorphic) and by its duration and consequences: sustained (lasting more than 30 s and/or causing hemodynamic compromise earlier, which requires intervention) and nonsustained (not resulting in hemodynamic compromise and lasting less than 30 s).[1] Short runs (5 beats or less) of nonsustained VT are common in the early post-myocardial infarction period and do not require specific treatment.

Because primary VF is one of the major contributors to mortality in the first 24 to 48 h after AMI, a great deal of attention has been paid to attempting to define characteristics of ventricular premature beats that predict VT/VF in order to provide prophylaxis. The hierarchical classification of ventricular arrhythmias according to propensity to cause VT/VF—for example, early coupled R-on-T premature beats as opposed to late-cycle, coupled beats—has fallen out of favor because of the realization that the late-cycle premature beats were equally likely to induce VT/VF.[341]

Accelerated idioventricular rhythm normally occurs frequently during the first hours of AMI,[1] and occurs after thrombolysis as a reperfusion arrhythmia. In neither case is it a premonitory rhythm for VT/VF.[342–344] *Accelerated idioventricular rhythm should ordinarily be observed and not treated specifically.*[1] It has been suggested, however, that if accelerated idioventricular rhythm speeds up to a rate of about 120 beats per minute, it should be considered an automatic rhythm for which suppression with lidocaine should be considered.[341]

Formerly, it was common practice, in order to prevent VT/VF, to treat prophylactically with lidocaine either all patients with AMI or, selectively, those with patterns of premature ventricular contractions thought to predict VT/VF. This approach is no longer common practice, because meta-analysis of trials of lidocaine prophylaxis, although confirming a substantial reduction in primary VF, showed evidence of increased mortality, probably because of episodes of profound bradycardia and asystole.[345] Thus, *routine use of prophylactic lidocaine in AMI in the presence or absence of thrombolysis is not recommended.*

Two prophylactic approaches to the prevention of VT/VF, however, are recommended.[1] Routine administration of beta blockers, as described previously, has been shown to reduce the incidence of VT/VF. Also, since evidence suggests that hypokalemia is a risk factor for VT/VF,[337,338] it is recommended that serum potassium levels be kept above 4.0 meq/L by supplementation as necessary. Although the supporting evidence is less compelling, it is also considered to be good clinical practice to maintain serum magnesium levels above 2.0 meq/L in AMI patients.[1]

TREATMENT OF VENTRICULAR TACHYCARDIA/FIBRILLATION Electrical cardioversion of VT that is hemodynamically compromising should be performed immediately.[335] Rapid polymorphic VT should be considered the equivalent of VF and cardioverted with an unsynchronized shock of 200 J; monomorphic VT at a rate of greater than 150 beats per minute can be treated initially with a synchronized discharge of 100 J.[1,333] Urgent cardioversion for VT with rates of under 150 beats per minute is usually not needed. Ventricular tachycardia that is tolerated hemodynamically can be approached initially with trials of lidocaine, procainamide, or amiodarone, as outlined earlier, with attention being paid to need for dose modifications based on age and renal and hepatic function.

Ventricular fibrillation should initially be treated with an unsynchronized shock of 200 J, then incrementally with 200 to 300 J, and finally with 360 J as needed.[333] There are no definitive data concerning appropriate adjunctive therapy for fibrillation that is difficult to cardiovert.[1] The Advanced Cardiac Life Support (ACLS) protocol recommends the following hierarchical approach, as needed, to adjunctive therapy of resistant VF:[333] (1) epinephrine (1 mg intravenously); (2) lidocaine (1.5 mg/kg intravenously); and (3) bretylium (5 to 10 mg/kg intravenously). Intravenous amiodarone (150 mg intravenously bolus) may also be used.[1] In the case of resistant or recurrent VT/VF, electrolyte imbalances should be sought and corrected and ongoing ischemia suspected. Beta-adrenergic blockers should be used in recurrent VT or primary VF to decrease both sympathetic input to the heart and ischemia.[1] Intravenous amiodarone should be used in these life-threatening ventricular tachyarrhythmias.[346] *If ongoing ischemia is involved, intraaortic balloon pumping or emergency revascularization should be considered.*

APPROACH TO THE PATIENT WITH ISCHEMIC-TYPE CHEST PAIN AND WITHOUT ST-SEGMENT ELEVATION

As discussed previously, the initial criterion differentiating patients with symptoms compatible with AMI for therapeutic purposes is the presence or absence of ST-segment elevation. This distinction is important, because in the absence of ST-segment elevation, there is no therapeutic benefit to thrombolysis in the AMI patient (Fig. 42-5). Patients without ST-segment elevation are less likely to develop Q waves on the ECG, although about one-half of those who present with ST-segment elevation as well will not develop Q waves, especially if thrombolysis is utilized.[347,348] AMI in which Q waves do not develop is categorized as non-Q-wave myocardial infarction (NQWMI), and most patients (90 percent) present with ST-segment depression.[80,131] NQWMI currently accounts for about 50 percent of all AMIs.[87,126]

An important development over the last several years has been the understanding and acknowledgment that the coronary ischemic syndromes (unstable angina, NQWMI, ST-elevation myocardial infarction) represent a continuum that has come to be referred to as *acute coronary syndrome*. ST-segment elevation AMI is clinically distinct, as described. It is apparent that at the time of initial presentation, the clinician does not know whether the patient with chest pain that is compatible with coronary ischemia and with either ST-segment depression and/or T-wave changes or no ECG changes has unstable angina, NQWMI, or another condition. In the case of ST-segment depression and a compatible history, the initial approach in the emergency department is unchanged but the treatment and, especially, the use of drugs interferring with thrombus formation has changed dramatically.

NQWMI, like infarction with Q-waves, is precipitated by plaque disruption.[349,350] Total coronary occlusion demonstrated angiographically is much less common than in Q-wave myocardial infarction.[349] When total occlusion is present, it probably occurs in a well-collateralized vessel.[349,351] These observations—considered together with early data showing that NQWMIs involved loss of a smaller mass of myocardium than did Q-wave myocardial infarctions[352,353]—are consistent with the concept that either NQWMI is associated with less than total compromise of blood flow to a region of myocardium or that early reperfusion occurs. The evidence that early reperfusion is relatively common in NQWMI was reviewed previously. Because of the residual noninfarcted myocardium at risk distal to a disrupted plaque, moreover, patients with NQWMI have a high propensity for recurrent ischemia, infarction, and death[89] and present an opportunity for secondary prevention (Fig. 42-10). Nondiagnostic ECGs (ST-segment depression, T-wave inversion) on admission and NQWMI are more common in the elderly and in those with a history of prior AMI.[208,351] Generally, the incidence of NQWMI may be increasing in concert with the aging population and with the increased use of thrombolytic therapy, beta blockers, and aspirin.[1]

No therapeutic benefit of thrombolytic therapy was detected in patients with ST-segment depression in the first GISSI study and, in fact, mortality was slightly higher in the SK-treated group.[14] Patients with less strikingly abnormal ECGs had a lower mortality rate (8 percent) than the control group with ST-segment depression (16.2 percent) but, similarly, there was no benefit to thrombolytic therapy. The ISIS-2 trial illustrated the same principles.[211] ST-segment depression was associated with relatively high mortality and was not decreased by thrombolytic therapy. The mortality rate was relatively low in patients with only T-wave abnormalities (5 percent) and normal ECGs (1 to 2 percent). In the TIMI-IIIB trial of rt-PA in NQWMI and unstable angina, no benefit was observed with thrombolysis as compared with aspirin and heparin.[157] Data from this trial do indicate that patients with NWQMI or unstable angina who have elevated troponin I on admission have an increased risk of nonfatal myocardial infarction or death in the ensuing 6 weeks. Two important conclusions can be derived from the available data: *(1) thrombolysis cannot be recommended in AMI patients without ST-segment elevation, and (2) in the NQWMI group and based on the admission ECG, there is a graded, decremental spectrum of risk ranging from ST-segment depression to T-wave inversion to normal.* The latter data are consistent with increasingly compelling evidence that the presenting ECG permits risk stratification across the range of the acute coronary syndromes increasing from normal ECG (lowest risk) in ascending order as: T-wave inversion; ST-segment depression; ST-segment elevation; ST-segment elevation and depression.[354]

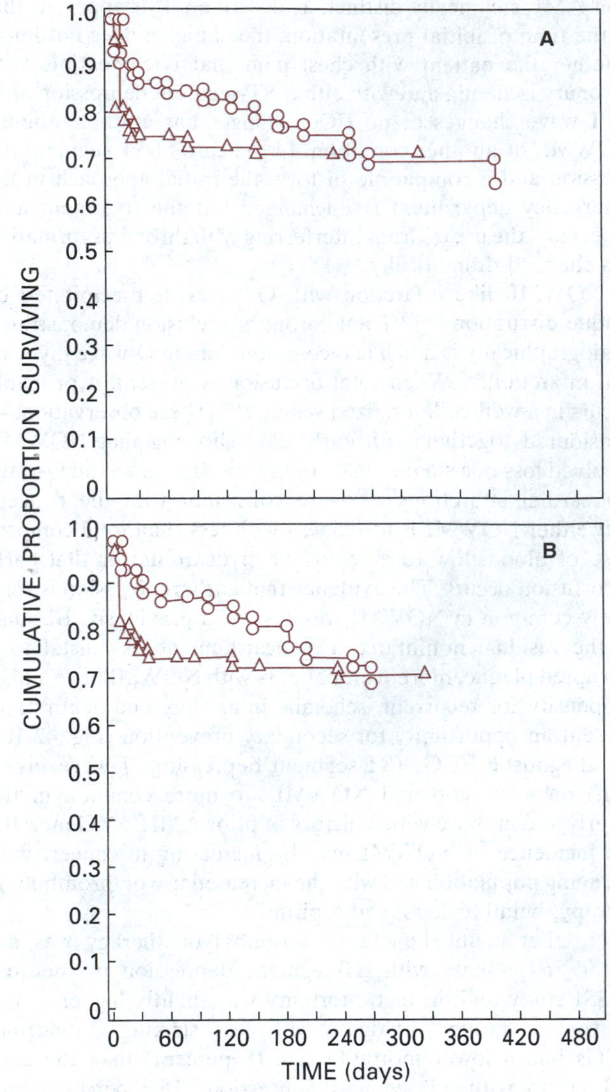

FIGURE 42-10 Comparison of the survival of patients with Q-wave infarction (triangles) to that of patients with non-Q-wave infarction with (circles). Early mortality was higher after Q-wave infarction than it was after non-Q-wave infarction and no recurrence (*A*), but survival was identical for patients with Q-wave infarction and those with non-Q-wave infarction and an early recurrent infarction (*B*). Long-term mortality rates are similar in Q-wave infarction and non-Q-wave infarction with or without early recurrence.

Management of Non-Q-Wave Myocardial Infarction MEDICAL MANAGEMENT Recommendations[1]:

Glycoprotein IIb/IIIa Inhibitors

Class IIa

1. For non-ST-segment elevation myocardial infarction patients with high-risk features and/or recurrent, difficult to control ischemia and who do not have contraindications of risk of bleeding

Beta-Adrenergic Blockers

Class I

1. Non-ST-segment elevation myocardial infarction

Heparin

Class IIa

1. Low-molecular-weight heparin subcutaneously or intravenous unfractionated heparin in NQWMI

Early Coronary Angiography and/or Interventional Therapy

Class I

1. In cases of recurrent (stuttering) or persistent symptoms of ischemia, whether spontaneous or induced, in presence or absence of associated ECG changes

Calcium Channel Blockers

Class I

1. None

Class IIa

1. Verapamil or diltiazem may be given to patients in whom beta-adrenergic blockers are ineffective or contraindicated (i.e., bronchospastic disease) for relief of ongoing ischemia or control of a rapid ventricular response with atrial fibrillation after AMI in the absence of congestive heart failure, left ventricular dysfunction, or AV block.

Class IIb

1. In infarction without ST-segment elevation, diltiazem may be given to patients without left ventricular dysfunction, pulmonary congestion, or congestive heart failure. They may be added to standard therapy after the first 24 h and continued for 1 year.

Class III

1. Nifedipine (short-acting) is generally contraindicated in the routine treatment of AMI because of its negative inotropic effects and the reflex sympathetic activation, tachycardia, and hypotension associated with its use.
2. Diltiazem and verapamil are contraindicated in AMI with associated left ventricular dysfunction or congestive heart failure.

Although the situation may change with the increasing availability of very rapid assays for CK isoforms, it is important to remember that, at present, during the initial evaluation in the emergency department, the NQWMI patient—who by definition does not have diagnostic ST-segment elevation—cannot be distinguished from the patient with unstable angina and no myocardial necrosis. Thus, patients are admitted to the CCU or, if judged to be at relatively low risk, to a unit with continuous electrocardiographic monitoring but of less intensity, and *the initial pharmacologic approach, other than avoiding thrombolytic therapy, is identical* (Fig. 42-3). Serial ECGs and cardiac marker measurements should be performed and, in the case of recurrent pain with the development of ST-segment elevation, thrombolysis or primary PTCA should be performed. If the patient has recurrent, stuttering symptoms, angiography should be performed.

ANTITHROMBOTIC THERAPY **Drugs Blocking the Glycoprotein IIb/IIIa Receptor** The glycoprotein IIb/IIIa receptor is found in the membrane of platelets.[355] When platelets are activated by a variety of stimuli, including thrombin, collagen, adenosine diphosphate, and epinephrine, the glycoprotein IIb/IIIa receptor changes confirmation to be receptive to one end of the fibrinogen dimer. Occupancy of a glycoprotein IIb/IIIa receptor by the other end of the dimer provides the basis for platelet aggregation. Thus, the glycoprotein IIb/IIIa receptor is considered the final common pathway of platelet aggregation.[356] Multiple therapeutic agents have now been developed to block the receptor.

1. Abciximab is a chimeric Fab fragment of a monoclonal antibody to the glycoprotein IIb/IIIa receptor. Although multiple clinical trials have documented the reduction in the composite of death and nonfatal myocardial infarction with abciximab in the setting of percutaneous interventions,[357–360] only one trial has been completed in the setting of non-ST elevation acute coronary syndrome.[357]
2. Eptifibatide is a cyclical heptapeptide, which binds to the receptor with a short half-life.[361]
3. Tirofiban is a small nonpeptide compound that also has a short half-life. It has been evaluated in over 5000 patients in 2 randomized trials of non-ST elevation acute coronary syndrome.[362,363]

The role of antiplatelet therapy in patients with non-Q-wave infarction is evolving. More than 30,000 patients with an acute coronary syndrome without ST-segment elevation (unstable angina and NQWMI) (see Chap 41) have now been randomly assigned into trials comparing glycoprotein IIb/IIIa inhibitors with a placebo in addition to treatment with aspirin and heparin. A direct comparison of the various IIb/IIIa inhibitors is not available and, thus, no specific choice of agent can be made at this time. The three agents available for clinical practice are described earlier. Only one trial[357] has been performed in patients with unstable angina and non-Q-wave infarction using abciximab. Eptifibatide[361] has been evaluated in a trial of 11,000 patients with non-ST elevation, 45 percent of whom had enzymes positive for myocardial necrosis. Tirofiban has been evaluated in 5147 patients in 2 randomized trials[362,363] of non-ST elevation. Again, about 45 percent of the patients in these trials had positive enzymes for infarction. An overview of these trials shows a reduction in the composite end point of death and myocardial infarction and the need for revascularization and procedures.[364] There was no reduction in mortality and, when treatment was discontinued, no further beneficial or detrimental effects were observed. Thus, intravenous glycoprotein IIb/IIIa inhibitors are being accepted increasingly as treatment in NQWMI to stabilize the patients in the acute phase and have a IIa recommendation for patients at high risk and with refractory ischemia.[1] Unfortunately, none of the trials have assessed the effect of this therapy in NQWMI alone. It remains to be determined whether these agents will be effective for *routine* use in patients with NQWMI. Since these agents can only be given intravenously, they can only be given for stabilization of the acute phase.

Low-Molecular-Weight Heparin Low molecular weight heparins are antithrombotics that have higher anti-X_a activity than antithrombin (II_a) activity (see Chap 44). Clinically, there is usually only modest prolongation of the activated partial thromboplastin time (aPTT). The role of low-molecular-weight heparin has been extensively explored in patients with acute coronary syndrome, which include a significant proportion of patients with NQWMI (see also Chap. 41). In the FRISC trial of NQWMI and unstable angina, 746 patients received 7500 IU daily of dalteparin versus 760 patients who received a placebo which included aspirin.[364a] At the six-day evaluation there was a 63 percent reduction in death and nonfatal MI in the dalteparin group, but this difference had disappeared by 40 days. In the FRIC Study, dalteparin was given subcutaneously twice a day and was compared with intravenous heparin in patients with unstable angina and NQWMI, during the acute phase of the first 6 days and thereafter.[365] There was no difference in the composite end points either at 6 days or at 45 days. In the ESSENCE trial (Efficacy and Safety of Subcutaneous Exoxiparin in Non-Q-wave Coronary Events),[365a] the study compared the effectiveness of exoxiparin in unstable angina and NQWMI with that of dalteparin. This was a large multicenter double-blind trial where 3171 patients received either twice daily subcutaneous injections of enoxiparin (1 mg/kg) or continuous intravenous infusions of unfractionated heparin (UFH) during the acute period of 2 to 8 days after hospitalization. The primary end point was a composite of death or myocardial infarction or recurrent angina 14 days after hospitalization. In the enoxiparin group, the end point rate was 16.6 versus 19.8 percent for the UFH group. Patients treated with enoxiparin required less revascularization procedures which continued up until 30 days. A cost-effectiveness analysis showed that, despite a small increase in drug cost ($75 per patient), the lower rate of cardiac catheterization and revascularization procedures led to a savings of $1072 per patient if enoxiparin was used instead of UFH. There is considerable difference among the low-molecular-weight heparins, and enoxiparin is claimed to have a high anti-factor X_a ratio than that of dalteparin. In another trial,[366] two different doses of enoxiparin were compared in patients with unstable angina and non-Q-wave infarction and the dose of 1 mg/kg every 12 h had a hemorrhage incidence of only 1.9 percent compared to 6.5 percent in doses of 1.25 mg/kg. TIMI 11B[367] enrolled 4020 patients with unstable angina and NQWMI and compared two strategies, UFH or enoxiparin. The analysis showed that at 48 h there were significantly fewer events in the enoxiparin group with a 24 percent reduction in relative risk compared to the group receiving UFH. This beneficial effect was maintained through day 43. Thus, it was concluded that enoxiparin is superior to UFH in the treatment of patients with unstable angina and NQWMI. One concern with all of these studies is there is no separation between NQWMI and unstable angina. *Nevertheless, there does appear to be a role for low-molecular-weight heparin in non-Q-wave infarction, and at the present time studies suggest that enoxiparin is superior to that of other preparations.*

There has been no prospective trial assessing aspirin in NQWMI, but retrospective analysis showed significant benefit.[368] It seems prudent to recommend aspirin (160 to 325 mg/day) for NQWMI (Class I).

BETA BLOCKERS IN NON-ST-SEGMENT ELEVATION MYOCARDIAL INFARCTION No prospective studies of beta blockers have been performed solely in patients with NQWMI, but retrospective analyses of trials performed prospectively, involving both Q-wave infarction and NQWMI, generally show no effect of beta blockers on the reinfarction rate in patients recovering from NQWMI.[89,369,370] Beta blockers may be given to relieve pain or arrhythmia, as discussed previously for Q-wave myocardial infarction. The general benefit of beta blockers in the acute coronary syndromes has led to their being recommended (Class I) for use in NQWMI.[1]

CALCIUM CHANNEL BLOCKERS The calcium channel blocker diltiazem (immediate-release form) has been shown to be effective in reducing reinfarction in the Diltiazem Reinfarction Study (DRS) (NQWMI)[80] and in the Multicenter Diltiazem Postinfarction Trial (MDIPIT) (Q-wave myocardial infarction and NQWMI)[371] in patients with preserved left ventricular function and with no evidence of congestive heart failure. The DRS study was performed during hospitalization only (14 days); diltiazem was given in the initial 24 to 48 h after NQWMI and was shown to reduce the reinfarction rate by 47 percent, as compared with conventional therapy over a 2-week period. In the long-term prospective, randomized, blinded MDIPIT study, no overall benefit of diltiazem over conventional therapy was observed. In MDIPIT, 20 percent of patients upon entry had pulmonary congestion or clinical cardiac failure, and diltiazem was associated with increased mortality in this subgroup. In the remaining 80 percent of patients, there was a 27 percent reduction in reinfarction and death in the group receiving diltiazem. Most of this benefit was in the prospective NQWMI substudy of 640 patients in whom diltiazem reduced reinfarction and death by 40 percent at the end of 1 year and 34 percent at the end of 4.5 years in patients without evidence of pulmonary congestion.[372] Analysis in the NQWMI subgroup for either end point alone (reinfarction or death) did not show a statistically significant benefit of diltiazem over the placebo. A meta-analysis of the heart-rate-lowering calcium channel blockers (diltiazem and verapamil) in 3 randomized, blinded clinical trials involving 5670 patients, with a mean follow-up of 550 days, showed a clinical event rate of 20 percent in the placebo group and 18 percent in the calcium channel blocker group ($p < 0.01$).[373] Verapamil has been studied somewhat less extensively than has diltiazem in the treatment of AMI; but when it is used within 2 weeks, a 16.7 percent reduction in death or myocardial infarction has been observed.[374] Verapamil has adverse effects on patients with heart failure or bradyarrhythmias when used within the first 24 to 48 h after AMI.[375,376] Most of the data on the use of calcium channel blockers in AMI were collected before the widespread use of aspirin, low-molecular-weight heparin, and platelet GIIb/IIIa inhibitors, and their precise role in the current management of AMI is somewhat ill defined. Currently in the treatment of non-ST-segment elevation AMI, diltiazem has a Class IIa recommendation only in patients in whom beta blockers are ineffective or contraindicated for relief of ongoing ischemia or control of a rapid ventricular response in atrial fibrillation.[1] The role of sustained-release diltiazem and aspirin is being studied in AMI after thrombolysis in the Incomplete Infarction Trial of European Research Collaborators Evaluating Prognosis Post-Thrombolysis (INTERCEPT).[377]

EARLY INVASIVE/INTERVENTIONAL STRATEGY: EARLY CORONARY ANGIOGRAPHY AND/OR INTERVENTIONAL THERAPY Recommendations[1]:

Class I

1. Patients with recurrent (stuttering) epidoses of spontaneous or induced ischemia or evidence of shock, pulmonary congestion, or left ventricular dysfunction and hypotension

A prospective observational trial (VANQUISH) was performed comparing PTCA with conventional therapy in patients with NQWMI. The mortality was less in patients receiving medical therapy. A contrary view was presented by FRISC II.[378] In addition to the randomization to low-molecular-weight heparins, patients were assigned within 48 h to invasive or noninvasive early management. The invasive strategy consisted of early coronary angiography within 2 to 7 days, whereas the noninvasive strategy consisted of exercise testing with referrals to coronary angiography if the test was positive. At 6 months, the rate of death or myocardial infarction in the invasive group was 9.5 versus 12 percent in the noninvasive group ($p = 0.045$). In this study, men particularly benefited with a difference of 9.1 versus 13.9 percent for the conservative strategy. Further studies will have to be performed to determine whether the invasive strategy is preferred over conservative therapy. This must also be considered in light of the new medical therapy of glycoprotein IIb/IIIa inhibitors and low-molecular-weight heparins being evaluated. Currently, early angiography and/or interventional therapy is indicated (Class I) in non-ST segment elevation myocardial infarction only with spontaneous or induced ischemia.[1]

PROTOCOLS, CLINICAL PATHWAYS, AND CHEST PAIN EVALUATION UNITS

There are increasing pressures, driven by both economic and clinical imperatives, to improve the management of patients with chest pain. The goal of controlling costs has contributed to the need to triage patients with chest pain accurately to levels of care that are appropriate to need and to facilitate evaluation and treatment in the shortest time that is commensurate with good medical care. For example, low-risk patients with normal ECGs frequently do not have to be admitted to the hospital, much less to the intensive care unit (ICU), and can have a total time in the health care facility of hours rather than of days. The medical necessity of achieving rapid, accurate diagnoses has been discussed earlier. These two driving forces have led to the development of predictive algorithms to guide triage decisions.[70,225] For example, one analysis provided evidence that patients with chest pain with ECG changes of ischemia or infarction were, depending on age, the only subgroup with a probability of AMI high enough (21 percent or moderate) to justify admission to the CCU as opposed to an intermediate care unit of reduced intensity.[379] While these algorithms have been shown to be effective in, for instance, reducing ICU admissions without compromising clinical care,[225,245] they have not been widely adopted for a variety of reasons, including the fact that most experienced clinicians are comfortable with their decision making in triaging patients with chest pain.[217]

The continuing need to improve the process of chest pain management has led to the development of clinical pathways, protocols, and practice guidelines that differ from predictive instruments in that they provide structure to the decision-making process rather than influence decision making.[217,380] A chest pain evaluation unit, which may either be a defined area, frequently near the emergency department, or a virtual entity embracing a team approach to chest pain evaluation and management, is frequently central to the strategy to systematize the approach to the patient with chest pain.

In general, the approach is to triage the patient to evaluation and management pathways according to risk based on electrocardiographic findings, history, and symptoms. For example, and at the opposite end of the clinical spectrum, the patient with ST-segment elevation would receive thrombolytic therapy within 30 min of arrival and be rapidly admitted to the CCU, whereas the low-risk patient with a normal ECG would be evaluated in a unit of low intensity and acuity and would be discharged within a matter of hours. There is a great deal of interest in the use of imaging modalities such as nuclear scanning with sestamibi or stress echocardiography to guide decision making in cases of intermediate or low probability for AMI during the initial evaluation period.[217] While the results using the systematized approach of a chest pain evaluation unit appear promising, further assessment is needed in large-scale trials to test both clinical value and cost-effectiveness before a specific strategy can be recommended. The general strategy of systematizing the approach to the patient with chest pain, however, is strongly encouraged.

MANAGEMENT AFTER HOSPITAL ADMISSION

General Approach

Recommendations[1]:

Class I

1. Selection of electrocardiographic monitoring leads based on infarct location and rhythm to maximize diagnostic utility
2. Bed rest with bedside commode privileges for initial 12 h in hemodynamically stable patients who are free of ischemic-type chest discomfort
3. Avoidance of the Valsalva maneuver and straining
4. Optimization of pain relief

Class IIb

1. Routine use of anxiolytics

Class III

1. Prolonged bed rest (more than 12 to 24 h) in stable patients without complications

The general issues involved in the management of the patient with suspected or manifest AMI in the intensive or moderate care unit are to provide for adequate monitoring for the detection of arrhythmia, ischemia, and hemodynamic instability; to provide the patient with a calm, supportive, and reassuring environment; to control the level of activity; to begin the education process for a lifetime of living with coronary heart disease; to control pain and inappropriate anxiety; and to treat adverse events promptly. It is assumed, as previously discussed, that oxygen therapy, beta-adrenergic blockers, aspirin, thrombolytics, unfactionated heparin, low-molecular-weight heparin, and nitroglycerin have been begun or given as appropriate in the emergency department. Also, it is assumed that a decision has been made about the appropriateness of adding glycoprotein IIb/IIIa inhibitors.

MONITORING

The patient must have continuous electrocardiographic monitoring and frequent hemodynamic evaluation by the assessment of blood pressure and heart rate. Electrocardiographic monitoring leads should be selected to maximize the ability of the CCU staff to detect and diagnose arrhythmias and recurrent ischemic ST-segment changes. Thus, the lead selected should ideally permit identification of the P wave as well as providing a QRS complex of adequate size. Furthermore, the lead should be selected to interrogate the area of known infarction or ischemia.[1] Blood pressure and pulse rate should be monitored with a frequency to be determined by the perceived level of acuity, but generally every one-half hour until stable and then every 4 h. Pulse oximetry is becoming standard. Precise orders should be given to notify the physician of, for example, systolic pressures >150 and <90 mmHg, heart rates >110 or <60 beats per minute, respiratory rate of >22 or <8 per minute, or significant decreases in blood oxygen saturation.[1]

ACTIVITY

Minimizing physical exertion is an important approach, in addition to minimizing sympathetic nervous system drive by administering beta-adrenergic blockers and by controlling pain and excessive anxiety, so as to decrease myocardial oxygen demand and thus decrease myocardial ischemia and necrosis. *Prolonged bed rest and a severe limitation of activities such as self-feeding are no longer recommended except in the case of continuing ischemic pain and/or hemodynamic instability because of evidence that cardiovascular deconditioning and unfavorable shifts in intravascular volume develop very rapidly in immmobilized patients in the supine position.*[381] Losses of plasma volume occur that decrease preload and stimulate compensatory reflexes, enhancing sympathetic activity. These fluid shifts may be the major cause of cardiovascular dysfunction with prolonged bed rest.[382] It is prudent to prescribe about 12 h of bed rest and a bedside commode for the patient with uncomplicated AMI.[1] Subsequently, low-level activities such as routine self-care, assisted bathing, and brief ambulation should be permitted to prevent deconditioning.

The major coronary precaution that should be strictly adhered to is the avoidance of the Valsalva maneuver, which increases cardiac wall stress because of increases in systolic blood pressure and heart rate.[1] These changes in wall stress may cause localized repolarization abnormalities in the infarct zone that may precipitate ventricular arrhythmias.[383,384] Constipation should be avoided and stool softeners routinely prescribed. A bedside commode is preferable to a bedpan in all but the most unstable patients.

ANALGESICS AND ANXIOLYTICS

The importance of controlling chest pain and excessive anxiety and the use of morphine and diazepam were discussed previously (see "Evaluation and Management of the Patient with Chest Pain in the Emergency Department"). Morphine is sometimes used in inadequate doses because of fear of side effects, and anxiolytics may be overused. Ischemic chest pain, heart rate, blood pressure, and perceived anxiety level have not been found to be different in patients treated with diazepam or with a placebo.[385] Conversely, strong psychological support in hospitals has prolonged effects to prevent anxiety and depression after AMI.[386] Anxiolytics may be useful in treating symptoms of nicotine withdrawal in smokers during hospitalization. Psychosis manifesting as delirium and agitation is not uncommon, particularly in the elderly, during prolonged stays in the ICU ("ICU psychosis"). Intravenous haloperidol can be useful and safe in this setting. Drug-induced psychosis or delirium caused by lidocaine, for example, should be considered.

EDUCATION

Education of the AMI patient by both the CCU staff and the physician are essential components of medical management and should be begun early during hospitalization. Presenting the patient with information about the management of symptoms and prevention of a recurrence gives a sense of empowerment associated with changes in behavior[387] and decreased anxiety.[388] Information should be presented in a direct fashion at a relatively simple level and should emphasize issues relevant to patient behavior, such as control of chest pain, diet, smoking, and exercise, rather than the pathophysiology of the disease. Family members, and, in particular, the spouse should participate in the education process. Because of the substantial risk of cardiac arrest in the 18 months after AMI, family members should be taught cardiopulmonary resuscitation.[389,390] Ideally, educational materials can be presented in a permanent printed form so that the self-education process can continue after discharge and can supplement that given by health care professionals during cardiac rehabilitation and physician visits.

Adjunctive Therapy during the Early In-Hospital Period

ANGIOTENSIN-CONVERTING ENZYME INHIBITORS

Recommendations[1]:

Class I

1. Patients within the first 24 h of a suspected AMI with ST-segment elevation in two or more anterior precordial leads or with clinical heart failure in the absence of significant hypotension or known contraindications to the use of ACE inhibitors
2. Patients with AMI and a left ventricular ejection fraction (LVEF) <40 percent or patients with clinical heart failure on the basis of systolic pump dysfunction during and after convalescence from AMI

Class IIa

1. All other patients within the first 24 h of a suspected or established AMI provided that significant hypotension or other clear-cut contraindications are absent
2. Asymptomatic patients with mildly impaired left ventricular function (ejection fraction of 40 to 50 percent and a history of old myocardial infarction)

Class IIb

1. Patients who have recently recovered from myocardial infarction but have normal or mildly abnormal global left ventricular function.

A number of clinical trials have shown that ACE inhibitors reduce left ventricular dysfunction and dilatation and slow the progression to congestive heart failure in patients with left ventricular dysfunction after AMI.[391–393]

The ACE inhibitors have also been shown, with few exceptions, to reduce mortality after AMI. Meta-analysis of 4 major and 11 minor trials involving, collectively, more than 100,000 patients showed an odds reduction in the ACE-inhibitor group of 6.5 percent ($2p = 0.006$).[394] Originally, there was some doubt about the timing of initiation of the ACE inhibitor after AMI because of the results of the Cooperative New Scandinavian Enalapril Survival Study (CONSENSUS) II.[395] In this randomized study, patients were assigned to intravenous placebo or enalapril during the first day of AMI and were subsequently given an oral placebo or enalapril. The trial was stopped in its early stages by the Safety Monitoring Committee because it was unlikely to show a positive effect and because of hypotension in elderly patients. The issue of timing of the initiation of ACE inhibitor therapy has been clarified subsequently. In GISSI-3, patients with either ST-segment elevation or depression were given oral lisinopril or were assigned to an open control group starting on the first day of AMI.[260] There was a significant reduction in mortality at 6 weeks (odds ratio 0.88), and the majority (60 percent) of lives saved were in the first 5 days. In ISIS-4, patients were assigned to an oral placebo or to captopril within the first 24 h, and a 7 percent mortality reduction was seen at 5 weeks in the captopril group.[261] The majority of the decrease in deaths was seen in the first 2 days. There was no increase in adverse events in the elderly in ISIS-4 or in GISSI-3. Thus, the hypotension in CONSENSUS II may be attributed to the use of intravenous enalapril.

Initiation of ACE-inhibitor therapy within the first few days after AMI in patients with left ventricular dysfunction and continuation of therapy over the long term was associated with a decrease in mortality and in fatal and severe nonfatal cardiovascular events in three other trials: Survival and Ventricular Enlargement (SAVE), captopril[392]; Acute Infarction Ramipril Efficacy (AIRE2), ramipril[396]; and Trandolapril Cardiac Evaluation (TRACE), trandolapril.[397]

Thus, trials of ACE inhibitors have shown clear evidence of benefit in AMI from their use early in the course of AMI. Efficacy may be greatest in those at highest risk, that is, patients with prior MI, anterior MI, tachycardia, or CHF. Therapy should begin within the first 24 h after hemodynamic stabilization, whether or not thrombolytic therapy has been administered. Intravenous forms should be avoided, and therapy should be started with low doses. The ACE inhibitors should not be given if systolic blood pressure is below 100 mmHg or if there are contraindications—that is, bilateral renal artery stenosis, renal failure, history of severe cough, or angioedema with previous treatment.[1] In the presence of significant left ventricular dysfunction, therapy should probably be continued indefinitely. Evidence from the Heart Outcomes Prevention Evaluation (HOPE) trial using the ACE inhibitor ramipril has shown significant decreases in cardiovascular events in high-risk individuals including, but not limited to, those with prior AMI.[398] These data, which will be discussed in more detail subsequently, provide support for the strategy of using ACE inhibitors in most patients indefinitely after acute MI.

MAGNESIUM

Recommendations[1]:

Class I

1. None.

Class IIa

1. Correction of documented magnesium (and/or potassium) deficits, especially in patients receiving diuretics before the onset of infarction.
2. Episodes of VT—torsades de pointes type—associated with a prolonged QT interval should be treated with 1 to 2 g of magnesium administered as a bolus over 5 min.

Class IIb

1. Magnesium bolus and infusion in high-risk patients such as the elderly and/or those for whom reperfusion therapy is not suitable.

The available data are conflicting but suggest that early (<6 h) administration of magnesium in high-risk patients may be associated with mortality reduction.

Magnesium has a number of potential cardioprotective effects, including vasodilatation,[399] inhibition of platelet function,[400] stabilization of cell membranes,[401] and protection against the cardiotoxic effects of catecholamines.[402]

Meta-analysis of 7 early randomized trials of the effects of magnesium in AMI was consistent with a significant benefit in mortality (odds ratio 0.44).[403,404] The Second Leicester Intravenous Magnesium Intervention Trial (LIMIT-2) was consistent with this interpretation in that the magnesium-treated patients in comparison with those not receiving magnesium had a 24 percent reduction in overall mortality ($p < 0.04$), a 25 percent decrease in the incidence of congestive heart failure in the CCU, and a 21 percent lower rate of coronary artery disease mortality at 4 years.[405,406] The large ISIS-4 trial, however, was negative and even raised the possibility of some harm.[261] Incorporation of the ISIS-4 data with that of the previous randomized trials and performance of meta-analysis resulted in the loss of the benefit that was previously apparent. It has been speculated that the lack of benefit in ISIS-4 was due to the relatively late administration of magnesium,[407] since the time to randomization in ISIS-4 was 8 h, as contrasted with 3 h in LIMIT-2. It may also have been a consequence of the low control-group mortality in ISIS-4 (7.2 percent) and the statistical inability to detect a treatment effect at this level.[408] That only 36 percent of patients in LIMIT-2 received thrombolytic therapy as opposed to 70 percent in ISIS-4 complicates interpretation further. Analysis of subgroups in ISIS-4 in which magnesium was administered within 6 h of the onset of symptoms or within 2 h of thrombolytic therapy also failed to demonstrate a therapeutic effect. Another randomized trial of intravenous magnesium in AMI patients who were not candidates for thrombolysis demonstrated a significant reduction of mortality in the treated group (4.2 versus 17.3 percent, $p < 0.01$), due primarily to a decrease in cardiogenic shock and congestive heart failure.[409]

The conflicting data that are available do not permit a recommendation that magnesium be used as standard general therapy in AMI. Magnesium should be used in situations where it would otherwise be recommended, as in the presence of magnesium deficiency or VT of the torsades de pointes type with a prolonged QT interval. Intravenous magnesium can be considered in high-risk patients, such as the elderly and in those for whom reperfusion is not suitable. Ongoing clinical trials are investigating the question further.

Management of the Low-Risk Patient

As discussed previously, there are increasing pressures to minimize resource utilization while not compromising safety in the patient with ischemic-type chest discomfort. As a practical matter, this means matching patient acuity and risk appropriately with the hospital facilities required to deal with their situation and to appropriately control time spent in these units. For example, the patient who is at low risk for AMI may be evaluated in the emergency department or in a chest pain evaluation unit, and if AMI or unstable angina are excluded, may be discharged within a matter of hours without having been formally admitted to the hospital. The patient with AMI who has an uncomplicated initial course and is at low risk for development of complications is a candidate for transfer out of the CCU within 24 to 36 h.[410–413] *Such a low-risk patient does not have a history of prior AMI and has not had recurrent ischemic pain, hypotension, congestive heart failure, persistent sinus tachycardia, heart block, or sustained VT. This patient may be a candidate for early discharge at 3 to 4 days.*

Patients who have been treated with thrombolytics are frequently candidates for early discharge from the CCU.[414–417] In this setting, the *absence* of early sustained VT or VF, as well as the absence of early sustained hypotension or shock, and the *presence* of a LVEF > 40 percent and of only one- or two-vessel coronary artery disease are independent predictors of freedom from late complications.[416]

Approaches to risk stratification and noninvasive testing, to guide management decisions in the post-AMI patient, are discussed subsequently (see "Noninvasive Risk Stratification in Patients Surviving Acute Myocardial Infarction"). Excessive diagnostic testing in all post-AMI patients, especially those at low risk, should be discouraged. The variability in practice in this regard, without demonstrable correlative changes in outcomes, suggests the need for more rigorous adherence to guidelines and protocols.[1]

As discussed previously, AMI can be diagnosed rapidly using serum cardiac markers. If AMI is effectively ruled out and the patient is at low risk (i.e., normal ECG and absence of the characteristics noted earlier, especially the absence of prolonged initial pain or the recurrence of pain), then noninvasive testing can establish the safety of early discharge (3 to 12 h) from the emergency department, chest pain evaluation unit, or CCU, for further evaluation as an outpatient.[217] In general, such patients do not necessarily need to be admitted to the CCU unless noninvasive testing is positive for ischemic heart disease. Patients with ischemic-type chest discomfort and intermediate probabilities of AMI—that is, duration of chest pain >20 to 30 min and nondiagnostic ECG changes (without significant ST-segment elevation or depression, T-wave inversion, or bundle branch block), without known coronary artery disease—should be admitted to an observation unit or to the CCU if an intermediate unit is unavailable. They should be placed on a fast track to rule in AMI or unstable angina, as previously outlined. If the clinical course is unrevealing and if early imaging is negative, then stress testing and further evaluation can be planned. Clinical decisions can usually be made within 12 h in this setting.[217]

Management of the High-Risk Patient with Acute Myocardial Infarction

The AMI patient at low risk is defined in the previous section by the absence of certain characteristics. By contrast, the *high-risk AMI patient is defined by the presence of one or more of these clinical features, which include recurrent chest pain; congestive heart failure and low cardiac output; arrhythmias and, in particular, recurrent or sustained VT or VF; mechanical cardiac complications of AMI such as ruptured papillary muscle or intraventricular septum; and/or inducible ischemia and extensive coronary artery disease.*

RECURRENT CHEST PAIN

The most common causes of recurrent chest pain after AMI are coronary ischemia and pericarditis.

Recommendations for diagnosis and treatment of recurrent chest discomfort[1]:

Class I

1. Aspirin for pericarditis
2. Beta-adrenergic blocking drugs (continue or initiate) intravenously, then orally for ischemic-type chest discomfort
3. (Re)administration of thrombolytic therapy (r-PA or rt-PA) for patients with recurrent ST-segment elevation
4. Coronary arteriography for ischemic-type chest discomfort recurring after hours to days after initial therapy and associated with objective evidence of ischemia in patients who are candidates for revascularization

Class IIa

1. Nitroglycerin intravenously for 24 h, then topically or orally for ischemic-type chest discomfort

Class IIb

1. Corticosteroids for pericarditis
2. Indomethacin for pericarditis

Recurrent Ischemia Recurrence of chest pain in the patient who has had an AMI is a serious development and requires immediate attention to establish the correct diagnosis and initiate treatment, especially if the pain represents recurrent ischemia, which is a more serious development than if the pain is a manifestation of pericarditis. Early postinfarction angina is an important predictor of the severity of coronary artery disease and has an overall incidence of about 18 percent.[418] Postinfarction angina is defined as chest pain that is frequently similar to the original discomfort, occurring at rest or with limited activity during hospitalization 24 h or more after onset of the AMI. The pain may or may not be associated with ST-segment elevation or depression or with pseudonormalization of inverted T waves on the postmyocardial ischemia ECG.[419] The pain is usually a result of ischemia in the territory of the myocardium supplied by the vessel that precipitated the initial myocardial ischemia. At least three categories of patients are at high risk for postinfarction angina: (1) patients with NQWMI; (2) patients who have received thrombolysis; and (3) patients with multiple risk factors.[420–422] The incidence of postinfarction angina is almost twice as high after NQWMI (25 to 35 percent) than after Q-wave myocardial infarction. Thrombolytic therapy for AMI created a new high-risk group for postinfarction angina (35 to 45 percent incidence), with a 12 to 15 percent incidence of reinfarction during the early experience with lytic therapy for reperfusion.[423] Regardless of whether postinfarction angina occurs after Q-wave myocardial infarction, NQWMI, or thrombolytic therapy, it is more likely to occur in patients with two- or three-vessel disease than in patients with single-vessel disease.[418] Postinfarction angina is important because it is associated with a twofold increase in the incidence of reinfarction. The 1-year mortality rate and acute risk of reinfarction is two- to fourfold greater in patients with postinfarction angina associated with ECG changes than in patients without chest pain or in patients with chest pain but without associated ST-T changes.[424,425]

The incidence of reinfarction following NQWMI has previously been reported to be as high as 40 percent within the first month following the event,[426] but with current treatments with glycoprotein IIb/IIIa inhibitors and fractionated heparins and possibly diltiazem, the incidence is less than 10 percent, as discussed previously. The incidence of reinfarction following thrombolytic therapy has been reduced from 12 to 15 percent to 5 to 7 percent with the use of adjunctive therapy, including heparin, aspirin, nitroglycerin, and beta blockers, as discussed previously. Nevertheless, reinfarction, despite the use of heparin and aspirin, still accounts for one-quarter of all deaths that occur following thrombolytic therapy and thus remains a major concern.[427] Patients with Q-wave myocardial infarction who do not receive thrombolytic therapy were previously likely to have an incidence of postinfarction angina of only about 12 to 15 percent and a reinfarction rate of about 5 to 7 percent, although these absolute rates have probably decreased with the more widespread use of adjunctive therapy with beta blockers, aspirin, and ACE inhibitors. Death, ventricular arrhythmias, and severe congestive heart failure are early sequelae of reinfarction, and there is an increased rate of sudden death and cardiogenic shock.[110,113]

Diagnosis of reinfarction within 18 h after thrombolytic therapy is based upon the recurrence of ischemic-type chest pain, as noted, lasting at least 30 min, which may be associated with ST-T-wave changes. There is a reelevation of MB-CK, and the diagnostic criteria were discussed previously. Adequate beta-adrenergic blockade should be achieved. Sublingual nitroglycerin should be administered, and restarting of intravenous infusion should be considered. Pain should be controlled. Coronary arteriography generally should be performed early after the redevelopment of ischemic chest pain, and it is common that a high-grade stenosis is found. If the lesion is suitable, PTCA should be performed, or additional thrombolysis should be administered if mechanical reperfusion is not feasible or available. With appropriate ECG changes—that is, ST-segment elevation—thrombolysis should be considered if cardiac catheterization and PTCA are not immediately available. If either APSAC or SK was used originally, it should not be readministered and rt-PA or r-PA should be utilized. These latter agents can be readministered. If multiple high-grade stenoses are found, coronary artery bypass grafting should be considered.

Pericarditis Pericardial involvement associated with AMI assumes one of two forms. By far the most common type is pericardial inflammation overlying the necrotic segment of a transmural myocardial infarction. This particular pericarditis is usually an incidental finding in the course of a more significant illness. The less frequent form of postinfarction pericarditis is generally a delayed complication, which may represent an immunologic or autoimmune reaction. This pericarditis, a component of Dressler's syndrome, generally represents a major complication that often outlasts the basic illness (see also Chap. 72).

EARLY POSTINFARCTION PERICARDITIS The prevalence of early postinfarction pericarditis, as reflected by the presence of typical symptoms and a friction rub, is 6 to 11 percent.[428,429] However, the general consensus among cardiologists is that this entity occurs far more frequently than is clinically recognized. This suspicion is supported by postmortem studies finding evidence of postinfarction pericarditis when it was not recognized clinically.[430] The pericarditis usually becomes evident between the second and fourth day following the AMI, but it may occur up to several weeks later. In comparison to post-AMI patients without pericarditis, those who develop the condition have larger infarcts, a lower ejection fraction, and a higher incidence of congestive heart failure.[431,432]

The most common manifestation of pericarditis other than the chest pain is a scratchy two- or three-component friction rub along the left sternal border. The friction rub may have only a single component and may be dismissed erroneously as a systolic murmur. The rub is evanescent, generally lasting 1 to 6 days. The pain of pericarditis is generally perceived by the patient to be different from that of the AMI. The location of the pain may be the same, but any radiation is usually to the neck, shoulder, or scapula rather than to the arms or jaw. Characteristically, the pain is aggravated by inspiration, swallowing, coughing, or recumbency. Fever, usually less than 39°C, frequently accompanies the pericardial inflammation and typically lasts longer than 3 days, unlike the fever in an uncomplicated myocardial infarction.[433] The ECG is frequently not helpful in these patients, partially because it is usually distorted by the infarction and perhaps because of the localized nature of the inflammation. The cardiac rhythm is generally sinus, but there is an increased prevalence of atrial fibrillation.[434] Since significant effusion is unusual with this form of pericarditis, the echocardiogram is of limited diagnostic value.

The treatment of choice is aspirin (160 to 325 mg daily), although higher doses (650 mg every 4 to 6 h) may be required.[1,435,436] Indomethacin is effective in relieving symptoms,[1] but experimentally causes thinning of scar formation.[437] Corticosteroids and ibuprofen provide pain relief but also have been associated with thinning of scar formation as well as with cardiac rupture.[438,439] The use of anticoagulants is relatively contraindicated in AMI complicated by pericarditis. Situations ordinarily calling for anticoagulation, such as mural thrombosis seen on echocardiography, require excellent clinical judgment in assessing the risk-benefit ratio if pericarditis is also present.

POSTMYOCARDIAL INFARCTION SYNDROME (DRESSLER'S SYNDROME) The clinical features of this syndrome are fever, chest pain, evidence of polyserositis, and a tendency to recur.[435] The reported frequency is 1 to 3 percent of AMIs.[434,435] The incidence, however, has appeared to diminish dramatically in the reperfusion era.[440] While there is usually a latency period of at least 1 week before its appearance, the pleuropericarditis may develop within the first week following the AMI.[441] The syndrome can occur in association with NQWMI, and it is usually associated with fever in the range of 38 to 39°C and occasionally up to 40°C. The chest pain is the most sensitive index of this syndrome and often precedes the fever. Aggravation of the pain by deep inspiration and turning is its most distinctive feature. The pericarditis is manifest by a friction rub, usually occurring between the second and eleventh week after the infarction and lasting from 3 days to 3 weeks. Pericardial effusion is common. While pericarditis is the dominant feature, as many as two-thirds of patients have pleural effusions. These effusions are usually small and are frequently bilateral but may be large and hemorrhagic. About one-quarter of patients have linear or patchy infiltrates in the lung bases.

The clinical features, pathologic findings, and prompt response to steroids all suggest an immunologic or autoimmune reaction. The presence of antimyocardial antibodies has been demonstrated in the majority of patients tested with the syndrome.

Treatment is similar to that of early postinfarction pericarditis but is more likely to require a course of oral corticosteroids. Recurrences are common for several months and require the reinstitution of corticosteroids with a more gradual tapering. Anticoagulants should generally be discontinued in the presence of postmyocardial infarction syndrome.[442]

HEART FAILURE IN ACUTE MYOCARDIAL INFARCTION

Pathophysiology and Hemodynamics The immediate hemodynamic consequences of myocardial infarction include both systolic and diastolic dysfunction. Systolic dysfunction is secondary to a loss of contractile function of the infarcted and ischemic myocardium.[443] Experimentally, over a period of 1 to 3 min, the regional disturbance of contraction progresses from dyssynchrony (disturbed temporal sequence of contraction) through hypokinesis (diminished motion) and akinesis (total lack of motion) to dyskinesia (paradoxical systolic expansion).[444] This loss of contractile function results in a decreased systolic ejection, increased end-systolic volume, increased end-diastolic volume, and a secondary increase in diastolic filling pressure caused by the increase in ventricular volume. The diastolic impairment often precedes the systolic dysfunction, which is characterized immediately by a transient increase in left ventricular diastolic distensibility,[445,446] followed by decreased distensibility due in part to adenosine triphosphate depletion and restraint by the pericardium and perhaps ultimately by the infiltration of inflammatory fluid and cells. The hemodynamic consequence of the reduced distensibility is increased diastolic pressure. The systolic stress on the ischemic segment, which contributes to "cell stretch" and "cell slippage," results in expansion of the infarcted segment[447] and provides the stimulus for volume overload hypertrophy, characterized by sarcomere replication, fiber elongation, and chamber enlargement. The chamber enlargement accommodates the increased volume and allows the diastolic pressure to return toward normal.[444]

Cardiac failure develops when left ventricular function is reduced to 30 percent or more of normal and usually occurs within minutes or hours of the onset of a large infarction. Since even with sustained coronary occlusion only 60 to 70 percent of the ischemic region undergoes necrosis, compromise of cardiac function associated with AMI is transient (24 to 72 h) in perhaps more than two-thirds of the cases. *Unlike the situation with chronic heart failure, the circulatory volume is normal or decreased in acute ventricular dysfunction associated with myocar-*

dial infarction. The usual clinical scenario is one of left ventricular dysfunction with pulmonary congestion and without hypoperfusion. There is sometimes biventricular failure, and in about 5 to 10 percent of cases there is predominantly right ventricular failure, as discussed later. The severity of the failure, its duration, and whether or not it is reversible are predominantly dependent on infarct size.[448,449] If more than 40 percent of the myocardium is destroyed, decompensation occurs, resulting in shock.[450–452] In a few patients, failure develops later as a consequence of expansion of the infarcted segment, reinfarction, or ischemia.[445] Less commonly, failure is precipitated by papillary muscle dysfunction or ventricular septal rupture. The compromised heart will also be negatively affected by supraventricular or ventricular arrhythmias, conduction disturbances, drugs with negative inotropic effects, fever, and hypovolemia.

Left ventricular dysfunction with the clinical signs of failure is said to occur in 30 to 40 percent of patients and usually develops when the abnormally contracting segment exceeds 30 percent of the left ventricular circumference.[453] Another factor contributing to cardiac failure is residual scarring from previous episodes of infarction, which limits the extent of compensation. After myocardial infarction, adjacent normal myocardium increases its contractility because of increased stimulation by catecholamines and also utilizes the Starling mechanism in an attempt to maintain cardiac output. The pathophysiology of heart failure is discussed in Chap. 20. That intravascular volume may be normal or decreased in acute heart failure in AMI is important in considering the therapeutic approach to low cardiac output and pulmonary congestion in acute infarction.

Right Ventricular Infarction Until about 15 to 20 years ago, right ventricular infarction was recognized infrequently and was usually thought not to be of great consequence. Subsequently, it was shown that the majority of patients with acute inferior infarction had abnormal regional function of the right ventricle,[454–456] although typical hemodynamic abnormalities are seen in only 10 to 15 percent of patients.[457,458] Right ventricular function returns to normal in most of these patients, suggesting that substantial stunning, rather than massive infarction, has occurred[1] (see also Chap. 37).

Inferior myocardial infarction associated with right ventricular infarction defines a high-risk subset with a mortality rate of 25 to 30 percent, as opposed to an overall mortality of about 6 percent in inferior myocardial infarction.[457] This group should be approached aggressively with consideration for reperfusion therapy. *Right ventricular involvement should always be considered and should be specifically sought out in inferior myocardial infarction with clinical evidence of low cardiac output because the therapeutic approaches are quite different in the presence of right ventricular involvement from those for predominantly left ventricular failure.*

Pathophysiology of Right Ventricular Infarction Right ventricular infarction is unusual in the absence of inferior infarction because occlusion of the right coronary artery proximal to the right ventricular branches usually also causes infarction in the inferior left ventricle, which is supplied by the distal distribution of the vessel.[459] The infarction usually involves the posterior septum and posterior wall rather than the right ventricular free wall. The relative sparing of the free wall results from the high degree of collateralization of the right ventricular arterial blood supply, from the blood flow derived from thebesian vessels, and from diffusion of oxygen from the ventricular cavity as well as from the fact that it is thin and has comparatively low oxygen demands because of its mass and low workload.[460–463]

The hemodynamic consequences of right ventricular ischemia or infarction share features previously described for the left ventricle. Thus, there is impairment of contractility and diastolic dysfunction related to dilatation and pericardial restraint. In a low-pressure volume pump, such as the right ventricle, this combination has even more deleterious effects than in the left ventricle and causes substantial increases in diastolic pressure and decreases in systolic pressure. If the right ventricular afterload is also increased because of left ventricular dysfunction, then right-sided output can decrease dramatically and the driving force becomes essentially the right atrial pressure. Under these circumstances, right atrial transport essentially becomes critical, and anything decreasing it, such as diminished volume and filling pressure or loss of AV synchrony, may cause severe decreases of right and, secondarily, left ventricular output.[422,464,465]

Diagnosis of Right Ventricular Infarction As noted, right ventricular infarction should be considered in all cases of acute inferior myocardial infarction, especially in the setting of low cardiac output. A typical presentation would include inferior myocardial infarction, clear lung fields, and jugular venous distention. Jugular venous distention that is enhanced by inspiration (Kussmaul's sign) in the setting of inferior myocardial infarction is highly suggestive of right ventricular involvement but may not be manifest with volume depletion and might only become apparent with repletion.[466] A right atrial pressure >10 mmHg that is >80 percent of the pulmonary wedge pressure is a sensitive and specific sign of right ventricular infarction.[467]

The differential diagnosis of heart failure or low cardiac output in inferior infarction includes (1) arrhythmia, such as atrial fibrillation, sustained ventricular arrhythmia, or high-degree AV block; (2) ongoing ischemia, such as ischemia at a distance if the occluded artery to the inferior wall was also supplying, through collaterals, the anterior wall; (3) previous infarction at another location; (4) a mechanical complication such as papillary muscle dysfunction or, less commonly, a ventricular septal defect; or (5) right ventricular infarction.[468] This differential diagnosis of causes of congestive heart failure in inferior AMI is summarized in Table 42-13.

TABLE 42-13 Differential Diagnosis of Congestive Heart Failure in Inferior AMI

Arrhythmia: high-degree AV block, atrial fibrillation, or sustained ventricular tachycardia
Ischemia at a distance, with the occluded artery to the inferior wall supplying the anterior wall via collaterals
Previous infarction at another location
Mechanical complication, such as papillary muscle dysfunction
Right ventricular infarction

ST-segment elevation in lead V_{4R} is the single most powerful predictor of right ventricular involvement in inferior infarction and identifies a patient subset with a markedly increased in-hospital mortality.[457] All patients with inferior infarction should be screened by recording ECG lead V_{4R}. Echocardiography can also be useful as an adjunctive diagnostic approach[179] and can be particularly valuable in detecting right-to-left shunting of blood through the foramen ovale, which can occur because of the high right atrial pressures in right ventricular ischemia. Such shunting can be a cause of hypoxemia unresponsive to oxygen administration in this setting.[469]

TREATMENT OF RIGHT VENTRICULAR ISCHEMIA AND INFARCTION The major objectives in treating right ventricular infarction are to maintain right ventricular preload, provide inotropic support, reduce afterload of the right ventricle, and achieve early reperfusion.[262] The recommendations are summarized in Table 42-14.[1] Venodilators such as nitrates should be avoided, and diuretics should be used with caution. Volume loading with 1 to 2 L of saline will frequently restore cardiac output and correct hypotension; this should be the initial step. Excessive volume loading, however, may dilate the ventricle and decrease output. Inotropic support should be initiated if saline administration does not restore output and correct hypotension.[1] Dobutamine is an ideal initial choice.

The critical role of atrial transport in maintaining output in right ventricular infarction and the need to maintain AV synchrony have been discussed. High-degree AV block occurs in about 50 percent of patients in this setting, and AV sequential pacing can restore cardiac output.[470,471] Atrial fibrillation occurs in up to one-third of these patients, in whom prompt cardioversion should be considered if there is any evidence of hemodynamic compromise.[472] If there is significant left ventricular dysfunction, which may further compromise right ventricular function, as noted, afterload reduction by nitroprusside infusion or intraaortic balloon pumping is indicated.[1]

Reperfusion with thrombolytic therapy or primary PTCA improves right ventricular ejection fraction and hemodynamic status[473] and decreases the incidence of complete heart block.[473-475] Coronary artery bypass grafting should be considered if multivessel disease is found.

TABLE 42-14 Treatment Strategy for Right Ventricular Ischemia/Infarction

Maintain right ventricular preload
Volume loading (IV normal saline)
Avoid use of nitrates and diuretics
Maintain AV synchrony
AV sequential pacing for symptomatic high-degree heart block unresponsive to atropine
Prompt cardioversion for hemodynamically significant SVT
Inotropic support
Dobutamine (if cardiac output fails to increase after volume loading)
Reduce right ventricular afterload with left ventricular dysfunction
Intra-aortic balloon pump
Arterial vasodilators (sodium nitroprusside, hydralazine)
ACE inhibitors
Reperfusion
Thrombolytic agents
Primary PTCA
CABG (in selected patients with multivessel disease)

ABBREVIATIONS: IV = intravenous; AV = atrioventricular; SVT = supraventricular tachycardia; ACE = angiotensin converting enzyme; PTCA = percutaneous transluminal coronary angioplasty; CABG = coronary artery bypass graft.
SOURCE: Ryan et al.,[1] with permission.

MANAGEMENT OF CONGESTIVE HEART FAILURE IN ACUTE MYOCARDIAL INFARCTION: GENERAL ISSUES

Hemodynamic Monitoring Recommendations for balloon flotation right side of the heart catheter monitoring[1]:

Class I

1. Severe or progressive congestive heart failure or pulmonary edema
2. Cardiogenic shock or progressive hypotension
3. Suspected mechanical complications of acute infarction, i.e., ventricular septal defect, papillary muscle rupture, or pericardial tamponade

Class IIa

1. Hypotension that does not respond promptly to fluid administration in a patient without pulmonary congestion

Class III

1. Patients with acute infarction without evidence of cardiac or pulmonary complications

The balloon flotation (Swan-Ganz) catheter fundamentally permits one, in the setting of low cardiac output, to distinguish between inadequate ventricular filling pressures and inadequate systolic function. The former is treated with volume expansion and the latter with inotropic support and frequently afterload reduction. The catheter, even when used correctly, is not totally benign and during manipulation may precipitate VT and pulmonary hemorrhage or infarction. To minimize the risk of infection, the catheter should not be left in place longer than 5 days.[1]

INTRAARTERIAL PRESSURE MONITORING Recommendations[1]:

Class I

1. Patients with severe hypotension (systolic arterial pressure less than 80 mmHg) and/or cardiogenic shock
2. Patients receiving vasopressor agents

Class IIa

1. Patients receiving intravenous sodium nitroprusside or other potent vasodilators

Class IIb

1. Hemodynamically stable patients receiving intravenous nitroglycerin for myocardial ischemia

2. Patients receiving intravenous inotropic agents

Class III

1. Patients with acute infarction who are hemodynamically stable. Arterial monitoring in AMI is useful in all hypotensive patients but especially in those who are in shock. The radial artery is the preferred site, although the brachial and femoral arteries can be used. Intraarterial catheters should not be left in place longer than 72 h because of the risk of thrombosis and infection.[1]

Intraortic Balloon Counterpulsation Recommendations[1]:

Class I

1. Cardiogenic shock not quickly reversed with pharmacologic therapy as a stabilizing measure for angiography and prompt revascularization
2. Acute mitral regurgitation or ventricular septal defect complicating myocardial infarction as a stabilizing therapy for angiography and repair and revascularization
3. Recurrent intractable ventricular arrhythmias with hemodynamic instability
4. Refractory postmyocardial infarction angina as a bridge to angiography and revascularization

Class IIa

1. Signs of hemodynamic instability, poor left ventricular function, or persistent ischemia in patients with large areas of the myocardium at risk

Class IIb

1. In patients with successful PTCA after failed thrombolysis or those with three-vessel coronary disease, to prevent reocclusion
2. In patients known to have large areas of myocardium at risk, with or without active ischemia

By inflating in the aorta during diastole and by deflating during systole, the intraaortic balloon pump reduces afterload during ventricular systole and increases coronary perfusion during diastole. The decrease in afterload and increased coronary perfusion account for its efficacy in cardiogenic shock and ischemia. It is particularly useful as a stabilizing bridge to facilitate diagnostic angiography and revascularization and repair of mechanical complications of AMI. The use of the intraaortic baloon pump after AMI postthrombolysis or post-PTCA has not been uniformly successful in improving clinical outcome, including reocclusion rate or global or regional left ventricular function.[476] Thus, the routine use of the intraaortic baloon pump after either drug or mechanical reperfusion cannot be recommended.[1]

Diuretics and Positive Inotropic Agents Diuretics and Cardiac Failure in Acute Myocardial Infarction As previously mentioned, patients with failure due to AMI have normal total body water, and the transudation of fluid into the lungs may induce hypovolemia. As ventricular compliance is decreased, an increased left ventricular end-diastolic pressure is necessary to maintain cardiac output, since the heart operates on the steep portion of the ascending limb of Starling's curve.[477,478] The administration of a diuretic in this setting may be associated with a decrease in cardiac output.[479–481] Thus, diuretics should not be the drugs used initially in the treatment of pulmonary congestion in AMI. Their use early in the course should usually be guided by hemodynamic measurements from a Swan-Ganz catheter. Diuretic therapy may become appropriate later if salt and water retention occur and left ventricular filling pressures become excessively high—>18 to 20 mmHg, for example.

Inotropic Agents in Congestive Heart Failure Associated with Acute Myocardial Infarction Digoxin is a relatively weak inotropic agent and is not the drug of choice in acute heart failure in myocardial infarction. In a direct comparison, dobutamine was shown to increase cardiac output by 40 percent and to decrease left ventricular filling pressure, whereas digoxin increased cardiac output by only 10 percent and did not decrease filling pressure.[482] Since endogenous catecholamine levels can be quite elevated, digoxin may contribute little. The primary use of digoxin in AMI is to control heart rate in atrial fibrillation.

Dobutamine has favorable pharmacologic properties for use in heart failure in myocardial infarction (see Chap. 21). It has a rapid onset of action and increases cardiac output because of its positive inotropic properties. It is a vasodilator and increases coronary flow. It decreases filling pressure, as noted. Dopamine has a tendency to increase heart rate more than dobutamine. With higher doses, dopamine may increase peripheral resistance and filling pressures, offsetting some of the positive inotropic effects. The phosphodiesterase inhibitor amrinone increases contractility and is a vasodilator that has been used in patients with heart failure due to AMI. There is concern that positive inotropic agents may increase infarct size. Evaluation of dobutamine in AMI showed that, as long as heart rate was not increased more than 10 percent above baseline, there was no increase in infarct size or in the incidence of reinfarction or arrhythmia.[483]

Management of Uncomplicated Cardiac Failure after Acute Myocardial Infarction The major determinant of left ventricular dysfunction is the extent of myocardial injury.[448,449,484] The loss of contractile function in the initial minutes or hours (1 to 4) is potentially reversible and accounts in part for the transient nature of cardiac failure in the setting of uncomplicated AMI, as noted above. The presence of cardiac failure and its severity depend not only on the extent of damage but also upon the extent of injury from previous episodes.

Since the introduction of the Swan-Ganz catheter, considerable data have accumulated correlating hemodynamics with clinical features. In 1967, prior to invasive monitoring, Killip and Kimball[485] devised a clinical classification based on physical findings present on admission that provided a prognostic guide. That guide was followed by the classification of Forrester and colleagues,[486,487] based on extensive data obtained from invasive monitoring of patients with acute MI (Table 42-15). The latter classification combined the presence or absence of pulmonary congestion with the presence or absence of systemic hypoperfusion. They added the underlying hemodynamics to this classification based on the pulmonary arterial occlusive (wedge) pressure and the cardiac index. These classifications also provide important diagnostic and therapeutic guidelines, despite the observation that patients frequently cross over from one class to the other and are seldom restricted to one particular hemodynamic subset. Each classification illustrated that with increasing severity of ventricular dysfunction, there is an increased risk

TABLE 42-15 Clinical and Hemodynamic Subsets in AMI

Subset	Clinical Features	Approximate % of Patients with AMI	Hospital Mortality, %
	Killip Class		
1	No signs of congestive heart failure	40–50	6
2	S_3 gallop and bibasilar rales	30–40	17
3	Acute pulmonary edema	10–15	38
4	Cardiogenic shock	5–10	81
	Cedars-Sinai Clinical Subsets		
1	No pulmonary congestion or tissue hypoperfusion	25	1
2	Pulmonary congestion only	25	11
3	Tissue hypoperfusion only	15	18
4	Pulmonary congestion and tissue hypoperfusion	35	60
	Cedars-Sinai Hemodynamic Subsets		
	Hemodynamic features		
1	PCW ≤ 18; CI > 2.2	25	3
2	PCW > 18; CI > 2.2	25	9
3	PCW ≤ 18; CI ≤ 2.2	15	23
4	PCW > 18; CI ≤ 2.2	35	51

Abbreviations: CI = cardiac index (L/min/m^2); PCW = pulmonary capillary wedge pressure (mmHg).

of mortality. Nevertheless, there is imprecision in predicting mortality rates from hemodynamics. Rackley and coworkers[488] observed that patients with a ventricular filling pressure >29 mmHg had a 100 percent mortality rate; those with a filling pressure >15 mmHg and a cardiac index <2 L/min per square meter of body surface had a mortality rate of 93 percent; while those with a ventricular filling pressure <15 and a cardiac index <2 L/min per square meter of body surface had a mortality rate of 63 percent.

In patients with uncomplicated AMI, there is no need to perform invasive monitoring if careful clinical observations are made. There should be repeated assessment of the heart and lungs; examination of the skin and mucous membranes; monitoring of the systemic arterial pressure, cardiac rhythm, and heart rate; and routine laboratory examinations, including chest x-ray and determinations of urine output and arterial blood-gas values. If there are clinical indications of pulmonary congestion and/or decreased peripheral perfusion, invasive monitoring includes the insertion of a Swan-Ganz catheter in order to monitor right ventricular hemodynamics and pulmonary artery occlusive pressure (which will reflect ventricular end-diastolic pressure) and to obtain serial determinations of the cardiac output. Occasionally, it may be necessary to insert an arterial catheter to measure the arterial pressure; however, one can usually follow the pressure adequately with the use of a sphygmomanometer or an automatic blood pressure monitoring device. Frequently, it is also essential to insert a Foley catheter to follow the urine output, particularly in patients with sustained hypotension or cardiogenic shock.

In most patients in whom cardiac failure is not complicated by mechanical factors—such as mitral valve rupture, ventricular septal rupture, pulmonary embolus, or tamponade—the failure is transient and of mild-to-moderate severity. If the cardiac output is normal, aggressive treatment is often not recommended.[149] In patients with rales at the base of the lungs with only minimal increase in heart rate and no other signs of hypoxemia (Killip class III), conventional therapy with morphine; nasal oxygen; intravenous, oral, or transdermal nitrates; and bed rest is adequate without any specific therapy for failure. In patients with extensive pulmonary edema who are normotensive and exhibit hypoxia and dyspnea (Forrester class II), the treatment of choice is nitroglycerin given intravenously at 0.1 μg/kg per minute and increased in increments of 5 to 10 μg/min, stopping at a dose that does not decrease the systolic blood pressure below 100 mmHg. On the average, nitroglycerin in a dose of 0.5 μg/kg per minute is required in patients with evolving acute infarction and failure. Another vasodilator that has been used extensively in the past in AMI is sodium nitroprusside, which is initiated at 0.5 μg/kg per minute and increased by 10- to 20-μg/min increments every 10 to 15 min until the desired therapeutic point or a maximum of 10 μg/kg per minute is reached. Nevertheless, nitroglycerin is the preferred agent, since it has been shown to offer some cardioprotection when given in the early phase of myocardial infarction and to be both reliable and safe. In contrast, in experimental infarction in the dog, it has been shown that nitroprusside is more likely to redirect coronary flow away from the ischemic area to normal areas and to induce coronary steal.[253] The effect of nitroprusside on cardioprotection has been inconsistent and in one large study was shown to be detrimental.[489] In view of the data showing ACE inhibitors to be effective in cardiac failure, these agents are being used more generally in this setting. It is preferable that hemodynamics be monitored invasively (by Swan-Ganz catheter) when one gives a vasodilator to reduce the ventricular filling pressure to 15 to 17 mmHg while maintaining adequate cardiac output and coronary perfusion. Whether or not one monitors hemodynamics invasively will depend in part on the confidence that clinical features reflect the volume status. Mitral valve regurgitation due to papillary muscle dysfunction is commonly an aggravating factor even in mild-to-moderate cardiac failure and responds well to a vasodilator, as does systemic hypertension. Usually a vasodilator is not adequate, in which case an intravenous inotropic agent should be added. The inotropic agents are generally those of sympathomimetic drugs, including dobutamine, dopamine, and norepinephrine (see Chaps. 21 and 49). Dobutamine, a synthetic direct-acting agent, is preferred, as noted, and has actions that include vasodilatation, increased cardiac output, decreased ventricular filling pressure, and increased coronary flow.[490] The infusion should be initiated at 2 to 5 mg/kg per minute and should be increased such that adequate systemic pressure is maintained and the heart rate does not increase by more than 10 to 15 percent. Dobutamine is preferably titrated to cardiac output and ventricular filling pressure. The ventricular filling pressure should be decreased to a range of 14 to 18 mmHg while maintaining adequate cardiac output and blood pressure. In general, the objective is to maintain adequate cardiac output and blood pressure without inducing tachycardia while maintaining a filling pressure that is normal or minimally increased.

In patients with inferior infarction and low cardiac output, right ventricular infarction should be suspected, as discussed. If it is present, a Swan-Ganz catheter should be inserted to determine the filling pressure. Therapy with a positive inotropic agent, such as dobutamine, should be used after assuring that there is appropriate intravascular volume to facilitate right ventricular filling.[491,492]

In patients with borderline blood pressure and evidence of peripheral hypoperfusion, therapy should be initiated with an inotropic agent and not a vasodilator. Similarly, in patients with left ventricular failure and frank hypotension (<95 mmHg), a vasodilator must be avoided and initial therapy should be with a positive inotropic agent. Dopamine would frequently be the choice under these circumstances, since it exerts cardiovascular effects similar to those of dobutamine, but it also possesses an alpha$_1$-adrenergic activity and releases endogenous norepinephrine from sympathetic nerve endings. Low doses of dopamine (2 to 7 mg/kg per minute) are associated with increased stroke volume, cardiac output, and renal blood flow and moderate effects to increase peripheral resistance. High doses of dopamine induce significant vasoconstriction and may increase the left ventricular filling pressure due to increased afterload, which further exacerbates pulmonary congestion. Dopamine also has a more positive chronotropic effect than does dobutamine, which can be a disadvantage in AMI. Norepinephrine, which produces potent arteriolar and venous constriction, is used for hypotension in other settings but is otherwise relatively contraindicated in AMI. It is seldom used unless patients are hypotensive and do not respond to dopamine, amrinone or milrinone, or dobutamine. It is used in cardiogenic shock after dopamine has failed, since it is the major alternative that can be used for maintaining adequate perfusion pressure.

As indicated earlier, diuretics should be used with more caution in acute heart failure associated with AMI than in chronic heart failure, since volume expansion is usually not the primary problem. If high filling pressure (>18 to 20 mmHg) persists after adequate output is achieved with positive inotropic agents and/or vasodilators, diuretics may be added. However, this effect can be achieved by vasodilator therapy, which avoids the hypovolemia and hypotension that may occur secondary to the subsequent diuresis (1 to 2 h). The preferred diuretics are intravenous furosemide or ethacrynic acid.[493] These drugs also provide some acute venodilation.

Complicated Heart Failure after Myocardial Infarction Some AMI patients present with acute, fulminating pulmonary edema (with severe respiratory distress; generalized inspiratory crackles and wheezing; expectoration of pink, frothy sputum; cool, clammy, diaphoretic skin; and cyanosis) and require much more aggressive therapy than do patients with uncomplicated AMI. The condition is usually associated with pulmonary artery wedge pressure exceeding 25 mmHg and an in-hospital mortality rate of at least 15 to 20 percent.[494] The systolic blood pressure is usually either low normal or borderline normal (95 to 105 mmHg). The maintenance of adequate oxygenation must be the primary concern. Administration of high concentrations (60 to 100 percent) of oxygen via a face mask is essential. If the patient appears moribund, endotracheal intubation should be performed. While an assessment of arterial blood gases is appropriate, the speed with which clinical events change in these emergent situations may demand that decisions be made without benefit of these values. After the institution of mechanical ventilation, positive end-expiratory pressure may be needed to maintain adequate oxygenation while keeping the inspired oxygen concentration within safe levels (FI_{O_2} < 60 percent). Positive end-expiratory pressure should be applied only with an awareness of its risks of pneumothorax and reduction in cardiac output secondary to decreased left ventricular preload.[494] Invasive hemodynamic monitoring is particularly useful in these patients. Therapeutic interventions, however, should not be delayed until the monitoring is established. The therapy for severe pulmonary edema should include intravenous morphine unless the patient is known to have chronic CO_2 retention. From 5 to 10 mg of morphine sulfate should be given slowly with careful observation for evidence of respiratory depression. If the systolic blood pressure is adequate (≥100 mmHg), nitroglycerin is administered intravenously. In the patient with severe pulmonary edema, the improvement in left ventricular pump performance afforded by the prompt reduction in systemic vascular resistance by nitroprusside[495] may be essential for the rapid reversal of this life-threatening situation (particularly if systemic hypertension had been present). Either nitroglycerin or nitroprusside will provide a reduction in preload. If the systolic blood pressure is 100 mmHg or less, treatment with a positive inotropic agent should probably be initiated, with the subsequent addition of a vasodilator or an agent to improve cardiac output. The adjunctive use of intravenous diuretics is the same as outlined for mild degrees of heart failure.

Peripheral Hypoperfusion without Pulmonary Congestion Patients with clinical hypoperfusion without pulmonary congestion (with cool, cyanotic extremities, somnolence or confusion, and decreased urine flow) usually have a cardiac index <2.2 L/min. The mortality rate in these patients is four times greater than that in patients without hypoperfusion.[494] Invasive hemodynamic monitoring of the pulmonary capillary wedge pressure is essential. Volume augmentation is the initial therapeutic step in patients with a pulmonary capillary wedge pressure <15 mmHg. If possible, this pressure should be maintained below the level of pulmonary congestion (>20 mmHg). Vasodilators are usually not indicated at least until adequate filling pressures have been achieved and cardiac output is augmented with positive inotropic agents. This situation is commonly seen with severe biventricular infarction and thus should be suspected with inferior and right ventricular infarction. In this case, bradycardia should be treated with atropine if it is thought to be contributing to the systemic hypoperfusion. Excessive treatment with nitroglycerin and volume contraction from previous diuretic therapy can also contribute to systemic hypotension.

HYPOTENSION AND CARDIOGENIC SHOCK Cardiogenic shock may occur when 40 percent or more of the left ventricle is destroyed.[450,451,496] It is the most common cause of in-hospital death with myocardial infarction. The incidence of cardiogenic shock was about 15 percent in the early 1970s, but it has now decreased to approximately 5 to 7 percent.[494] The mortality rate is frequently over 80 percent.[497] The most effective therapy in the treatment of cardiogenic shock is prevention, since its major determinant is infarct size.[448,498] Cardiogenic shock usually occurs within hours of the onset of infarction due to massive ischemia and necrosis.[498] In other cases, a relatively small infarction that is superimposed on extensive previous damage may precipitate cardiogenic shock. Less commonly, cardiogenic shock may develop days after the initial event. This occurrence is almost always due to development of new necrosis (extension or early reinfarction) in the area of the preceding infarction. The decrease in the incidence of cardiogenic shock is believed to be in part due to better treatment of angina and ischemia, together with the widespread use of thrombolytic therapy and other cardioprotective agents. Cardiogenic shock by definition represents a more severe form of cardiac failure, resulting in decreased organ perfusion in addition to the conventional features of pulmonary congestion and left ventricular dysfunction. Cardiac failure with hypoperfusion and that regarded as cardiogenic shock may differ only in the severity of decreased perfusion. Clearly, every effort must be made to treat hypoperfusion whether or not it satisfies the strict criteria of cardiogenic shock. Characteristics of cardiogenic shock are (Table 42-16) (1) evidence of organ hypoperfusion with cold, clammy skin, especially on the feet and hands, that may be associated with peripheral cyanosis of the nail beds; (2) oliguria, disordered mentation, and systolic blood pressure <80 to 90 mmHg; (3) left ventricular end-diastolic pressure or, more commonly, pulmonary capillary wedge pressure >18 mmHg; (4) evidence of a primary cardiac abnormality; and (5) a cardiac index *not* >1.8 L/min per square meter of body surface. Hypotension or shock due to a primary abnormality of cardiac rhythm or conduction is not considered cardiogenic shock.

The advantage of early revascularization in reducing mortality in the acute setting (SHOCK trial)[299] was discussed earlier. Since the prognosis is extremely poor for patients with cardiogenic shock due primarily to loss of muscle mass, reversible causes associated with a better prognosis must be excluded. Potentially reversible causes include mitral valve rupture, ventricular septal rupture, right ventricular infarction, pulmonary embolus, and cardiac tamponade. While the mortality associated with surgical correction of infarct-associated mitral rupture or ventricular septal defect is still high, it is far less than that associated with cardiogenic shock due solely to myocardial injury. The details of management of these mechanical causes of shock are discussed later. Hypotension may be due to inadequate fluid administration, to vasodilatation induced by such drugs as morphine and vasodilators, and occasionally to depressed contractility due to antiarrhythmic therapy. Inadequate filling pressure is a very important cause of hypotension and should be corrected immediately. It is particularly common in patients with inferior infarction, as noted. A Swan-Ganz catheter should be inserted to determine the circulatory status and assess the response to therapy.

Therapeutic objectives are to establish and maintain a systemic arterial pressure adequate for perfusing the vital organs and for reducing pulmonary congestion. The approaches to pulmonary congestion include the judicious use of morphine, and the maintenance of adequate oxygenation, together with endotracheal intubation and mechanical ventilation if necessary. In addition to instituting hemodynamic monitoring, one should assess urinary output using an indwelling catheter. If the pulmonary artery wedge pressure is <15 mmHg, prompt volume expansion to raise the capillary pressure to 18 to 20 mmHg should be initiated. The cornerstones of therapy are inotropic and vasopressor agents. If the systemic arterial pressure is below 80 to 90 mmHg, a pressor agent such as dopamine should be infused.[499] At relatively low doses of 2 to 5 mg/kg per minute, increases in stroke volume and cardiac output are mediated by beta-adrenergic stimulation and increases in renal blood flow are mediated by the dopaminergic-specific receptors. The alpha-adrenergic vasoconstrictor effects are manifest progressively at doses above 5 mg/kg per minute. The use of intravenous dopamine requires careful titration, beginning with a low dose and gradually increasing until an adequate (90 to 100 mmHg) systemic pressure is achieved. If high doses of dopamine are necessary to maintain adequate perfusion, a change to norepinephrine infusion should be considered. This drug is a potent arteriolar and venous constrictor that is mediated through alpha-adrenergic stimulation. It demonstrates relatively modest beta-adrenergic stimulation. It is, therefore, a very potent pressor agent with less chronotropic or arrhythmogenic effects than dopamine.[267] The drug should be started at low doses of 1 to 4 mg/min. Extravasation should be avoided, since it will produce tissue sloughing.

When the systemic blood pressure is 90 mmHg or more, dobutamine is frequently the preferred agent. By increasing cardiac output, dobutamine may produce a rise in systemic blood pressure, but this increase would not be expected to be >10 to 15 mmHg.[500,501] Dobutamine will not support arterial pressure except by its effect on cardiac output. As the cardiac output rises, the left ventricular filling pressure should decline. Dobutamine therapy should begin with a dose of 2 to 5 mg/kg per minute with increases every 5 to 10 min. Inappropriate increases in heart rate are unlikely to occur with doses <15 to 20 mg/kg per minute.[483]

On occasion, the severity of cardiac pump dysfunction will require the use of two divergent therapeutic modalities in order to facilitate left ventricular emptying.[502] The most commonly utilized of these combined therapies is nitroprusside and dopamine. The principal advantage offered by nitroprusside in this combination is a reduction in left ventricular preload. The cardiac output is not appreciably increased by the addition of

TABLE 42-16 Characteristics of Cardiogenic Shock

Evidence of hypoperfusion: cold clammy skin, especially of feet and hands; impaired mentation; and oliguria
Systolic blood pressure <80–90 mmHg
LVED pressure (or PCW pressure) ≥18mmHg
Evidence of primary cardiac abnormality
Cardiac index ≤1.8 L/m/m^2

ABBREVIATIONS: LVED = left ventricular end-diastolic; PCW = pulmonary capillary wedge.

nitroprusside to dopamine therapy. The advantage offered by dopamine in this combination is an augmentation of cardiac output and the maintenance of systemic arterial pressure.[503] A less frequently used combination, dobutamine and nitroprusside, has been shown to result in higher cardiac output and lower pulmonary capillary wedge pressures than has resulted with either drug alone.[502] Stabilization of the patient with cardiogenic shock may be achieved by mechanical circulatory assist devices, such as the intraaortic balloon as demonstrated in the completed SHOCK Trial.[299] Aortic balloon counterpulsation reduces afterload while simultaneously improving coronary perfusion by increasing diastolic aortic pressure, as discussed. It is the only intervention that will increase diastolic aortic pressure without increasing myocardial oxygen demand. Aortic counterpulsation is often helpful for patients in cardiogenic shock due to a potentially reversible condition or in whom cardiac transplantation is being considered. Such conditions include an acute but still evolving MI or AMI with a severe mechanical complication (e.g., mitral regurgitation or ventricular septal defect). In such cases, aortic counterpulsation should be used to stabilize the patient's condition in preparation for salvage of the jeopardized but still viable myocardium or correction of the mechanical defect.[267] Intraaortic counterpulsation in patients without a reversible defect is now being used with greater frequency, especially in patients <75 years of age based on the compelling data emerging from the long-term follow-up of the SHOCK Trial patients.[299]

Restoration of coronary blood flow is the most effective therapy in salvaging patients with cardiogenic shock who are unresponsive to fluid and pharmacologic management in the early hours after a myocardial infarction. If angioplasty and/or coronary artery bypass grafting are not readily available, thrombolytic therapy should be tried if it has not already been utilized—although it has not been shown to improve survival in this setting.[504,505] These patients should be transferred quickly to a tertiary care center. Blood pressure should be stabilized with an intraaortic balloon pump, and cardiac catheterization should be performed as soon as possible. Assessment of correctable mechanical lesions, such as ruptured papillary muscles, can be made together with evaluation of coronary anatomy. Depending upon this anatomy, a judgment can be made as to whether to attempt PTCA or to proceed to coronary artery bypass surgery. Mechanical revascularization appears to improve survival in cardiogenic shock complicating AMI.[299,506]

Mechanical Dysfunction Contributing to Cardiac Failure PAPILLARY MUSCLE RUPTURE Rupture of the left ventricular papillary muscle occurs in approximately 1 percent of myocardial infarctions and accounts for 0.4 to 5.0 percent of infarct-related deaths.[507] It occurs slightly less frequently than ventricular septal rupture. The posteromedial papillary muscle is involved 6 to 12 times more frequently than is the anterolateral muscle.[508] Thus, papillary muscle rupture with an acute anterior myocardial infarction is uncommon. The rupture may occur distally and may involve one or several of the smaller heads of the muscle or, less commonly, may occur proximally and produce complete dehiscence of the papillary muscle.

Papillary muscle rupture is manifest by the sudden appearance of pulmonary edema, usually 2 to 7 days after the infarction. The abruptness of onset and severity of pulmonary edema are usually greater than seen with ventricular septal rupture. A mid- or holosystolic murmur with wide radiation is usually audible. Although the murmur is generally loud, a thrill is rarely present, and the murmur may seem inconsequential. The diagnosis can be established by Doppler echocardiographic studies (see Chap. 13). The two-dimensional echocardiogram will generally show a flail mitral leaflet and may reveal a portion of the papillary muscle visualized as a mass attached to the chordae. Even when the flail leaflet is not observed, documentation of relatively intact ventricular systolic function in the postinfarction patient with pulmonary edema should suggest the diagnosis. The Doppler study will establish the presence and severity of the mitral regurgitation. Bedside right side of the heart catheterization can be used to exclude an oxygen step-up from the right atrium to the right ventricle, indicative of ventricular septal rupture, and to confirm elevated pulmonary capillary wedge pressures with tall V (regurgitant) waves characteristic of acute mitral regurgitation.

Studies in the presurgical era demonstrated a poor prognosis for these patients, with a 50 percent mortality rate in the first 24 h and a 6 percent survival rate for longer than 2 months.[442] Thus, immediate recognition and treatment are essential. Intraaortic counterpulsation alone or with vasodilator and inotropic therapy may frequently be required for temporary stabilization. During this period, the patient should undergo cardiac catheterization to define coronary anatomy and should be transferred to surgery for mitral valve replacement or repair.

PAPILLARY MUSCLE DYSFUNCTION The sudden development of an apical systolic murmur after a myocardial infarction is much more often secondary to papillary muscle dysfunction than it is to rupture. Twenty percent of patients who die from infarction have histologic evidence of papillary muscle necrosis, usually without rupture.[509] Papillary muscle dysfunction is frequently compatible with long-term survival.

The posteromedial papillary muscle is involved with ischemia or infarction more commonly than the anterolateral muscle because the latter receives blood from two arteries (left anterior descending and circumflex), whereas the posteromedial muscle is supplied predominantly from the circumflex.[510] Dysfunction may be transient during ischemia. Papillary muscle ischemia is usually accompanied by ischemia of the contiguous ventricular wall.[511] Involvement of the contiguous ventricular wall is a key factor in the development of significant mitral regurgitation, since isolated papillary muscle ischemia or even infarction is usually not sufficient to cause important mitral regurgitation.[512]

Papillary muscle dysfunction typically presents with an apical systolic murmur. The murmur may be holosystolic, late systolic, or even early systolic. Echocardiography coupled with Doppler flow studies will confirm the presence of mitral regurgitation, grade its severity, and permit assessment of left ventricular function. There is generally no hemodynamic deterioration associated with the appearance of the murmur. It is the unusual patient who develops pulmonary edema, and these patients usually have concomitant significant left ventricular dysfunction. The ordinary patient with papillary muscle dysfunction will require no specific therapy for the regurgitation, while the unusual patient with severe regurgitation should be treated as in the case of papillary muscle rupture. In intermediate cases with moderate to moderately severe regurgitation where cardiac surgery is not contemplated, afterload reduction with ACE inhibitors should be considered.

VENTRICULAR SEPTAL RUPTURE Rupture of the interventricular septum is estimated to occur in 1 to 3 percent of AMIs and accounts for approximately 5 percent of all infarct-related deaths.[513] Ventricular septal rupture occurs with an approximately equal frequency between anterior and inferior infarctions. There is a higher prevalence in first infarctions and the majority occur within the first week. Some 20 to 30 percent may develop as early as the first 24 h after the infarction.[514,515] Septal rupture rarely occurs after 2 weeks. Ventricular septal rupture is usually manifest by the appearance of a new harsh, holosystolic murmur along the left sternal border (often associated with a thrill) and sudden clinical deterioration with hypotension and pulmonary congestion. Right ventricular volume overload secondary to the shunt may produce signs of systemic venous congestion out of proportion to those of pulmonary venous congestion. Often the event is heralded by a recurrence of chest pain.

The diagnosis can be established by two-dimensional and Doppler echocardiographic studies that will demonstrate the site and approximate size of the rupture as well as the left-to-right shunt. Right-sided heart catheterization is useful in confirming the diagnosis (an increase in O_2 saturation of >5 percent from right atrium to right ventricle) and is an aid in managing the patient. The primary diagnostic concern is to exclude rupture of the papillary muscle. The presence of a thrill or an anterior infarction would be unusual with papillary muscle rupture, and results of the Doppler echocardiographic studies and/or the oxygen step-up on right side of the heart catheterization would confirm the presence of septal rupture.

When medical therapy alone is used, most patients with ventricular septal rupture deteriorate rapidly and virtually all patients die, many within 24 h after rupture. Except for the rare case in which there is no clinical or hemodynamic deterioration, medical therapy can be expected to be ineffective. *It is now axiomatic, that upon discovery of rupture of the ventricular septum, prompt surgical repair should take place, even for those patients who are clinically stable.* Inotropic and vasopressor agents may be required to sustain arterial blood pressure but can increase the left-to-right shunt. Prompt but temporary stabilization can be achieved with intraaortic balloon counterpulsation alone or in conjunction with vasodilator and inotropic drug therapy. Cardiac catheterization should be performed in an expeditious manner to define cardiac anatomy, left ventricular function, and mitral valve competence. An aggressive approach of immediate operative repair of these patients results in a short-term survival rate of 42 to 75 percent.[516–518] The 5-year actuarial survival rate for the operative survivors has been reported to be as high as 88 percent.[519] Surgical results are worse when ventricular septal rupture complicates inferior infarction and when there is combined right ventricular and septal dysfunction.[518]

CARDIAC RUPTURE Cardiorrhexis, or rupture of the heart, occurs in up to 24 percent of fatal AMIs. After cardiogenic shock and arrhythmias, it is the most common cause of death. The free wall of the ventricle is the most common site of rupture.[520]

Rupture of the free wall generally occurs within the first 2 weeks of the infarction and may occur within the first 24 h.[514,515] Rupture occurring after this interval usually represents extension of the infarction or rupture through a false aneurysm.[521]

The rupture occurs primarily in the left ventricle, with a fairly even distribution between the anterior, inferior, and lateral walls. Given the relatively smaller number of lateral infarctions, the incidence of rupture with lateral wall infarctions would presumably be relatively smaller than at other sites.[522] Free wall rupture is more likely to occur with the initial myocardial infarction, in women, in the sixth decade of life or later, and in patients with systemic arterial hypertension, particularly if there is no associated ventricular hypertrophy.[514] The prolonged use of corticosteroids might predispose a patient to cardiac rupture.

Cardiac rupture generally presents as sudden, unanticipated death. Symptoms such as pain, agitation, sinus tachycardia, or vagally mediated bradycardia seldom precede death by more than minutes. Occasionally, intermittent chest pain and/or transient hypotension may precede and portend the final catastrophic event. Cardiac rupture is diagnosed terminally by the development of electromechanical disassociation in the setting of recurrent chest pain. Few cases, and only those with immediate recognition, can be salvaged. Even these few cases require heroic measures, such as immediate pericardiocentesis, emergency thoracotomy, and surgical repair.

OTHER COMPLICATIONS OF ACUTE MYOCARDIAL INFARCTION

Pulmonary Embolism The prevalence of deep venous thrombosis in AMI is reported to be between 12 and 38 percent. Patients with large infarctions in any location, anterior infarctions, evidence of congestive heart failure, and complicated infarctions have a greater frequency of deep venous thrombosis.[523,524] Reduced cardiac output and immobilization are additional predisposing factors for deep venous thrombosis (see Chap. 90).

Venous thrombosis is usually a minor and frequently unrecognized complication of infarction but is potentially life-threatening. A prevalence of pulmonary embolism of 10 to 15 percent and a prevalence of fatal embolism in 3 to 6 percent of cases has been reported in the past.[525] More recently, pulmonary embolism has been reported to account for less than 1 percent of deaths in myocardial infarction, probably because of earlier ambulation and better therapy of low output.[521]

Early mobilization combined with therapy directed toward improving cardiac output, when appropriate, is probably the most effective means of preventing pulmonary emboli. Prophylactic anticoagulant therapy is not routinely recommended for all patients after a myocardial infarction but is advisable for patients with increased risk factors for deep venous thrombosis and pulmonary embolism.

Systemic Emboli Emboli to the cerebrovascular, renal, mesenteric, iliofemoral, or other arterial systems may complicate the AMI. The reported prevalence of clinically apparent systemic emboli in patients with myocardial infarction varies from 0.6 to 6.4 percent.[526,527] These emboli result from dislodgement of left ventricular thrombi, which are found in 20 to 40 percent of anterior myocardial infarctions. A ventricular thrombus is unusual in patients with an inferior infarction.[527,528] The predilection of the apical wall for thrombus development appears to be related to a combination of stagnant blood flow and poor wall contractility. Severe depression of left ventricular function is not a prerequisite for thrombus formation. The development of a mural thrombus in a small infarction (CK < 1000 U), however, is unusual.[529,530] Thrombus morphology and mobility would seem to correlate with systemic embolization.[526,531,532] Pedunculated and freely mobile thrombi have been thought to have a greater chance of embolization. At least two studies, however, could not correlate risk of embolization to any particular thrombus morphology.[527,530]

Left ventricular thrombosis usually occurs within the first 3 days after a myocardial infarction,[530,533] but may occur at any time during the hospital course. Early mural thrombosis occurs in large infarctions that have an unfavorable prognosis.[530] Systemic embolization occurs an average of 14 days after AMI and is unlikely to occur after more than 4 to 6 weeks.[534] Anticoagulation appears to reduce the incidence of mural thrombus formation[535] and the prevalence of systemic embolization.[526,528,529] All patients with an anterior myocardial infarction should have two-dimensional echocardiography performed within 24 to 72 h following the infarction, with particular emphasis on the two- and four-chamber apical views. Those with a severe apical wall contraction abnormality (akinesis or dyskinesis) should receive heparin for several days, followed by warfarin (INR 2 to 3) for 1 to 3 months. In patients with a left ventricular thrombus demonstrated by echocardiographic studies, chronic warfarin therapy (Chap. 44) is continued for approximately 3 months. Warfarin administration should be maintained indefinitely for atrial fibrillation.

Two-dimensional echocardiography has a sensitivity of 83 to 95 percent and a specificity of 86 to 90 percent in diagnosing a mural thrombus.[527,529,531,536] Angiography has a sensitivity of 20 to 63 percent and a specificity of 67 to 75 percent.[526,537] Occasionally, a technically unsatisfactory echocardiogram may require the use of alternative noninvasive imaging modalities. Both computed tomography and magnetic resonance imaging offer a similar sensitivity and perhaps superior specificity to echocardiography in this setting.[537]

Ventricular Aneurysm The true prevalence of ventricular aneurysm after myocardial infarction is not well defined. Probably the best approximation comes from postmortem studies estimating a 3 to 15 percent prevalence.[533,538] The CASS registry documented angiographically defined left ventricular aneurysms in 7.6 percent of patients with coronary artery disease. The location of the aneurysm is usually anterior, anteroapical, or apical. True posterior ventricular aneurysms located in the diaphragmatic wall between the septum and insertion of the posterior papillary muscle have been observed but are quite uncommon.[539]

Pathologically, the aneurysmal area is characterized by a thinned-out transmural scar that has completely lost its trabecular pattern. The scar, which may eventually calcify, is clearly delineated from surrounding ventricular muscle. Aneurysms characteristically have a wide base (the diameter of the mouth is equal to or larger than its greatest internal diameter), and one-half are lined by a laminated thrombus.[540]

As many as 80 percent of chronic ventricular aneurysms can be diagnosed clinically by the presence of an abnormal precordial impulse, most often located in the third left intercostal space at the midclavicular line; a typical bulge on the left ventricular border on chest x-ray, frequently with calcification around the apex; and ECG evidence of a large anterior infarction with ST-segment elevation persisting beyond 2 weeks following the infarction. Two-dimensional echocardiographic studies can confirm the diagnosis.[527] Left ventricular aneurysms are associated with a reduced survival rate. The prognosis for these patients, however, is primarily related to the left ventricular dysfunction and not to the presence of the aneurysm. True ventricular aneurysms rarely rupture. In fact, the survival rate for patients with an aneurysm is no different than that for patients without an aneurysm but with a similar degree of left ventricular dysfunction. Moreover, the incidence of sudden death is no different. Whether or not clinical recognition of the presence of a ventricular aneurysm is important in the management of the patient after an AMI remains to be answered.[536]

Most patients with ventricular aneurysms should be treated the same as any other postinfarction patient with a similar degree of left ventricular dysfunction. Vasodilators, digoxin, anticoagulants, and antiarrhythmics should be used, based not on the presence of the aneurysm but as dictated by presence of heart failure, mural thrombi, and life-threatening arrhythmias. Occasionally, surgical resection of the aneurysm is justified in order to correct refractory heart failure, recurrent life-threatening arrhythmias, or multiple systemic emboli. The aneurysm resection should usually be combined with coronary bypass grafting and, in cases of ventricular arrhythmias, should be guided by electrophysiologic mapping.

Pseudoaneurysm A pseudoaneurysm is a rare complication of myocardial infarction, the prevalence of which is not known. The probable sequence of events in the development of a pseudoaneurysm is as follows: occurrence of a transmural infarction with localized pericarditis arising at the site of infarction; development of adhesions between the visceral and parietal pericardium; rupture of the infarcted myocardium, with the extravasated blood confined by the adherent pericardium; progressive enlargement of the aneurysmal sac; and development of thrombus within the sac.[521]

Unlike a true ventricular aneurysm, a pseudoaneurysm has a narrow base (site of rupture). The wall is composed only of a thrombus and pericardium, and the risk of rupture is high.[541] While the neck is small (its diameter is <50 percent of the diameter of the fundus), the pseudoaneurysm may progressively enlarge to become larger than the left ventricle. The pseudoaneurysm may be clinically silent or may present as progressively worsening heart failure, an abnormal bulge on the cardiac border, persistent ST-segment elevation in the area overlying the infarction, or systolic murmurs.[542]

The diagnosis can be established by two-dimensional echocardiographic studies, ventriculographic radionuclide studies, MRI, or left ventriculographic contrast studies.[541] Surgical resection is always indicated.

ARRHYTHMIAS AND CONDUCTION DISTURBANCES COMPLICATING ACUTE MYOCARDIAL INFARCTION

Arrhythmias and conduction disturbances that are likely to be significant problems during the early phases of AMI and their management have been discussed earlier, under "Evaluation and Management of the Patients with Chest Pain in the Emergency Department." The arrhythmias and conduction abnormalities discussed include sinus bradycardia, AV block, idioventricular rhythm, VT, and VF. In general, the acute management of these rhythm disturbances is the same in the early and in the late phases of AMI. Sustained VT and VF are exceptions, however, in that their occurrence after the first 24 h has more ominous implications for long-term electrical instability and sudden cardiac death. Other rhythm and conduction abnormalities that may be manifest throughout the course of AMI and are not characteristically associated with the early phases, are discussed here.

Ventricular Ectopy, Ventricular Tachycardia, and Ventricular Fibrillation The management of VT and VF after the first 24 h of hospitalization for AMI is similar to that discussed for the early phase. The occurrence of symptomatic, sustained VT or VF in the later phases of the hospital course, however, suggests that a chronic arrhythmogenic focus may be developing in the damaged ventricle. These ventricular arrhythmias are classified as secondary and indicate increased risk for subsequent sudden cardiac death.

Sinus Tachycardia or Atrial Premature Beats Sinus tachycardia following AMI is common and is frequently an unfavorable prognostic sign. The increased heart rate enhances myocardial oxygen demand, while the decreased diastolic time decreases diastolic coronary flow. Patients with a large area of infarcted myocardium may have sinus tachycardia on the basis of left ventricular dysfunction, which causes reflex sympathetic nervous system activation. Other obvious causes of sinus tachycardia—such as fever, anxiety, pain, pulmonary embolism, anemia, hypovolemia, or hypoxemia—must be evaluated and treated. Sinus tachycardia may occur as a result of the effects of drugs, such as dobutamine, dopamine, theophylline, and atropine.[543] In the absence of precipitating causes, a persistent sinus tachycardia most likely reflects progressive left ventricular dysfunction, which should be evaluated and managed accordingly.

Frequent atrial premature complexes are relatively common in AMI and are caused by atrial ischemia or infarction and pericarditis.[543–547] No specific therapy is indicated; rather, attention should be given to the underlying disease process.

Paroxysmal Supraventricular Tachycardia Episodes of paroxysmal supraventricular tachycardia occur rather commonly in AMI and are usually transient.[544] Underlying causes are similar to those of atrial premature complexes. For reasons discussed, the tachycardia may worsen ischemia. Rate control is essential, and the therapeutic approaches—which may include carotid sinus massage, adenosine, digoxin, verapamil, or diltiazem—are discussed in Chaps. 23 and 24.

Atrial Flutter and Atrial Fibrillation Atrial flutter is relatively uncommon in AMI, whereas atrial fibrillation has an incidence of 10 to 15 percent.[544,545] Atrial fibrillation is associated with an increased in-hospital mortality rate, probably because it is associated with large infarcts and is seen relatively more commonly in older patients and those with cardiac failure, complex ventricular arrhythmias, advanced AV block, atrial infarction, and pericarditis.[548] The pathophysiologic implications are similar to those for paroxysmal supraventricular tachycardia in that a rapid ventricular response can worsen ischemia and infarction by increasing oxygen consumption. Furthermore, the loss of atrial transport can worsen cardiac output and lead to hemodynamic instability.

Atrial fibrillation increases in incidence with age; it occurs in less than 5 percent of patients with AMI under the age of 60 and in about 16 percent of those over age 70.[1] The incidence of atrial fibrillation has been reported to be lower in patients receiving thrombolytic therapy than in control patients.[549]

Systemic embolization occurs more commonly in AMI in the presence of atrial fibrillation (1.7 percent) than in its absence (0.6 percent). Fifty percent of these emboli occur during the first hospital day and 90 percent have occurred by the fourth day.[550] Thus, heparin therapy is indicated in patients not already receiving it, despite that the rhythm is usually transient.

If the patient experiences new or worsening pain, ischemic ST changes, or hemodynamic instability during atrial fibrillation with a rapid ventricular response rate, immediate electrical cardioversion is indicated. In the conscious patient, brief anesthesia is indicated (see Chaps. 24 and 29).

If the clinical situation is less urgent, the ventricular rate can be reduced with drugs. Rapid digitalization with intravenous digoxin is effective but will not result in an immediate response, which may take 1 to 2 h. In the absence of contraindications such as congestive heart failure or bronchospastic pulmonary disease, intravenously administered beta-blocking drugs are highly effective in slowing the ventricular rate. Intravenous administration of the calcium channel blockers, verapamil or diltiazem, can also be effective in slowing the ventricular response, but these are not considered to be first-line drugs (except possibly in the setting of NQWMI).

Firm recommendations have not been made about the use of class I and III antiarrhythmics to prevent the recurrence of atrial fibrillation in AMI.[1] Since recurrence is associated with a worse prognosis, however, it seems prudent to consider amiodarone or sotalol or, alternatively, quinidine or procainamide. Neither anticoagulation nor antiarrhythmic therapy should be continued for the long term. With stable sinus rhythm, either or both, as the case may be, should be stopped after 6 weeks.

Junctional Rhythm An escape AV junctional rhythm at a rate of 40 to 60 beats per minute in patients with inferior myocardial infarction and high-degree heart block is not uncommon.[544] Therapy usually is not required. Accelerated junctional rhythms are occasionally seen in AMI, more likely at rates of 70 to 130 beats per minute,[551] but are rarely seen at considerably higher rates. Treatment generally focuses on the underlying conditions, such as ischemia or digitalis toxicity.

Heart Block First-, second-, and third-degree AV blocks have been discussed briefly. First-degree block is frequently seen in AMI, and especially in inferior myocardial infarction. This is attributable to ischemia or enhanced vagal activity. It can be worsened by drugs such as beta blockers. Treatment is seldom required.

Second-degree AV block is also relatively common, especially Mobitz type I or Wenckebach block. This block, characterized by progressive lengthening of the PR interval before the atrial beat, is not conducted and may occur in as many as 10 percent of AMI patients.[552] It is associated with a narrow QRS and frequently is the result of AV node ischemia in inferior myocardial infarction. It is usually transient, and its presence does not affect the prognosis. Mobitz type II block is uncommon but is associated with more serious complications and a worse prognosis. It usually occurs with anterior myocardial infarction and reflects trifascicular block. It is characterized by a wide QRS and a nonvarying PR interval before a nonconducted atrial beat. Heart block may develop suddenly and is an ominous sign, with a mortality of about 80 percent. It is usually permanent.

Third-degree AV block, or complete heart block, occurs in about 5 percent of patients with AMI and is most commonly seen with inferior infarction, usually with block at the AV node. As indicated, complete heart block in inferior myocardial infarction is usually transient and may occur early or late in the hospital course with the same implications for prognosis. There is some increase in in-hospital mortality rates in this setting, but complete heart block in inferior myocardial infarction is not an independent predictor of poor long-term prognosis.[328] In contrast, patients with anterior infarction who develop third-degree AV block have a mortality rate of 80 percent.[553] Implications for temporary and permanent pacing are discussed subsequently.

Intraventricular Conduction Disturbances The development of bundle branch block during AMI usually signifies an extensive infarct. In one multicenter trial, the presence of bundle branch block was associated with a twofold increase in the in-hospital mortality rate (28 versus 14 percent), compared with the absence of bundle branch block.[331,554] Data indicate that the presence of bundle branch block identifies patients who (1) are more likely to develop congestive heart failure, (2) are more likely to develop high-degree heart block, (3) are more likely to have an episode of ventricular fibrillation, and (4) have a higher mortality rate.[554]

Indications for Temporary Transvenous Pacing Recommendations[1]:

Class I

1. Asystole
2. Symptomatic bradycardia (including sinus bradycardia with hypotension and type I second-degree AV block with hypotension not responsive to atropine)
3. Bilateral bundle branch block (alternating or right bundle branch block with alternating left anterior fascicular/posterior fascicular block; any age)
4. New or indeterminate-age bifascicular block (right bundle branch block with left anterior or posterior fascicular block) with first-degree AV block
5. Mobitz type II second-degree AV block

Class IIa

1. Right bundle branch block and left anterior or left posterior fascicular block (new or indeterminate)
2. Right bundle branch block with first-degree AV block
3. Left bundle branch block, new or indeterminate
4. Incessant VT, for atrial or ventricular overdrive pacing
5. Recurrent sinus pauses (greater than 3 s) not responsive to atropine

Class IIb

1. Bifascicular block of indeterminate age
2. New or age-indeterminant isolated right bundle branch block

Class III

1. First-degree heart block
2. Type I second-degree AV block with normal hemodynamics
3. Accelerated idioventricular rhythm
4. Bundle branch block or fascicular block known to exist before acute myocardial infarction

Cardiac pacing is discussed in Chap. 31. The indications generally agreed on for temporary pacemaker insertion in AMI include asystole, complete heart block in the setting of anterior myocardial infarction, new onset of right or left bundle branch block with persistent Mobitz II second-degree AV block in the setting of anterior myocardial infarction, or other symptomatic bradycardias unresponsive to atropine.[200]

Bundle branch block in the setting of AMI, as noted, identifies a population at risk for both electrical and mechanical complications. Such patients must be monitored for evidence of transient high-degree heart block. Prolonged intermediate care with telemetry monitoring and repeat assessments of heart failure status are important.

Permanent Pacing Recommendations[1]:

Class I

1. Persistent second-degree AV block in the His-Purkinje system with bilateral bundle branch block or complete heart block after AMI
2. Transient advanced (second- or third-degree) AV block and associated bundle branch block
3. Symptomatic AV block at any level

Class IIb

1. Persistent advanced (second- or third-degree) block at the level of the AV node

Class III

1. Transient AV conduction disturbances in the absence of intraventricular conduction defects
2. Transient AV block in the presence of isolated left anterior fascicular block
3. Acquired left anterior fascicular block in the absence of AV block
4. Persistent first-degree AV block in the presence of bundle branch block that is old or age-indeterminate

The use of permanent pacemakers is discussed in detail in Chap. 31. The subject is reviewed extensively in the ACC/AHA guidelines for pacemaker implantation.[555] That temporary pacing may have been required in the course of AMI does not necessarily indicate a need for permanent pacing. Patients who have had permanent pacemakers inserted after AMI usually have a relatively unfavorable prognosis primarily related to the extensiveness of the underlying disease and myocardial damage.[1] Thus, these patients are at increased risk for death from progressive congestive heart failure and VTs. The generally accepted indications for insertion of a permanent pacemaker after AMI are summarized in the previous recommendations.

DISCHARGE FROM THE CORONARY CARE UNIT

The length of stay in the CCU should be based on the risk of developing VT and VF. The risk of developing primary VF after AMI decreases exponentially, with the majority of arrhythmic deaths occurring within the first 24 h. After the third day, the episodes of life-threatening arrhythmias are fairly evenly distributed over the remainder of the hospitalization.[556] Thus, a patient with an uncomplicated infarction can be transferred from the CCU on the third day. Since 31 to 34 percent of in-hospital deaths from AMI occur after discharge from the CCU and half of them are sudden and unexpected, certain patients need more prolonged cardiac monitoring.[557,558] Those patients who are prime candidates for late-hospital sudden deaths manifest, while in the CCU, one or more of the following: (1) the arrhythmias of pump failure (sinus tachycardia, atrial flutter, or atrial fibrillation); (2) the arrhythmias of electrical instability (VT or VF); (3) acute interventricular conduction disturbances; (4) evidence of circulatory failure (congestive heart failure, pulmonary edema, or significant hypotension); or (5) large anterior infarction. The effectiveness of prolonged monitoring of this select group of patients in an intermediate care unit following CCU discharge is evident in a doubling of the rate of successful resuscitations.[559,560] Patients who do not fit into these high-risk subgroups can be discharged from the CCU to a medical unit without continuous monitoring. The wide availability of continuous monitoring in many hospitals in nonacute care units, however, permits easy further monitoring even on lower-risk patients and is preferable if available.

The activity permitted the patient with uncomplicated infarction has changed immensely during the last two decades. In an uncomplicated myocardial infarction, the patient does not need to be confined to the bed for longer than 24 h. In fact, the patient may use a bedside commode from the time of admission. The safety and benefits of chair rest were initially promoted by Samuel Levine and Bernard Lown in 1951.[561] Upon transfer from a CCU, the patient should be started on a program of progressive ambulation. The speed with which the patient progresses from one stage to the next depends on the severity of the infarction, the presence or absence of complications, the patient's age, and the presence of comorbid conditions. The length of hospitalization following an AMI should likewise depend on these same factors. If the patient has not manifested the arrhythmias of pump failure or electrical instability, evidence of circulatory failure, or advanced AV block during the first 4 days of hospitalization, he or she is very unlikely to do so at any later time.[562] This patient could probably be discharged after 7 or fewer days in the hospital.[563] The last 2 to 3 days of the hospitalization are generally necessary to resolve the questions pertaining to residual ventricular function, the presence or absence of ventricular ectopy, and the adequacy of the remainder of the coronary circulation. In addition, time is needed for instruction in risk-factor modification (see Chap. 50). As discussed previously, time in the hospital is being shortened, especially after successful thrombolysis.

Noninvasive Risk Stratification in Patients Surviving Acute Myocardial Infarction

The purpose of risk stratification of patients surviving AMI assumes that the information provided will enhance decision making, resulting in improved long-term outcome. While numerous tests provide prognostic information, only some have resulted in a treatment strategy that improves outcome. No single noninvasive cardiac test better exemplifies this potential "benefit gap" than ventricular premature beats after AMI which are associated with an increased risk of death; however, no antiarrhythmic intervention has been demonstrated to reduce mortality; some have even paradoxically increased the mortality rate.

Survivors of AMI have a substantial risk of incurring subsequent cardiovascular events. Noninvasive risk assessment provides useful information to individualize the extent of further workup and therapy by: (1) targeting specific long-term therapies that are established to alter mortality and morbidity; (2) identifying high-risk patients requiring aggressive diagnostic tests and therapies; (3) identifying low-risk groups as targets for a conservative approach emphasizing established long-term prophylactic therapies; (4) providing information that facilitates counseling the patient on prognosis; (5) provide data to recommend an exercise program; and (6) provide information used in planning and prioritizing modifications of lifestyle.

Three interrelated prognostic factors are the focus of predischarge assessment: (1) assessment of left ventricular function, (2) detection of residual myocardial ischemia (jeopardized myocardium), and (3) assessment of the risk of arrhythmic (sudden cardiac) death. Most proposed algorithms of noninvasive test selection focus on these three important clinical areas.[564,565] High-risk patients can be clinically identified, as previously discussed, without such noninvasive assessments because of evidence of one or more of the following: decompensated congestive heart failure, angina associated with electrocardiographic changes, in-hospital cardiac arrest, spontaneous sustained VT, or the development of a high-degree heart block.[566–569] In contrast to these high-risk groups, the majority of postinfarct patients have a relatively benign hospital course. In these patients, noninvasive testing can accurately identify a group at very low risk whose annual mortality is 1 to 3 percent.[416,417,570,571] The practical consequences of identifying a low-risk group is that emphasis is focused on early discharge, lifestyle modification and targeted prophylactic medical therapy rather than expensive, invasive diagnostic testing.

As discussed previously, there is general agreement that early coronary angiography and aggressive interventional therapy are indicated for patients with recurrent episodes of spontaneous angina or ischemia, in patients with evidence of persistent decompensated congestive heart failure or cardiogenic shock. In the following sections, the emphasis is on the noninvasive evaluation of asymptomatic patients.

ASSESSMENT OF LEFT VENTRICULAR FUNCTION AND LEFT VENTRICULAR EJECTION FRACTION

Many clinical features are associated with an increased risk for the development of congestive heart failure, including anterior and anterolateral infarction, papillary muscle dysfunction, and recurrent AMI as well as the development of transient episodes of high-degree heart block. Congestive heart failure in the setting of inferior AMI associated with right ventricular infarction is also a prognostically important category, necessitating an aggressive management strategy, as discussed. Measurement of LVEF is mandatory in such patients but also useful in patients without such obvious left ventricular dysfunction. Left ventricular ejection fraction can be assessed by either echocardiographic, radionuclide, or angiographic techniques.[572,573] Left ventricular ejection fraction is an important determinant of survival after AMI regardless of reperfusion status. In-hospital mortality is directly related to the severity of left ventricular dysfunction. In the absence of significant ischemia or ventricular arrhythmias, patients with a LVEF ≥40 percent have mortality rates in the range of 5 percent over 1 to 2 years, whereas a LVEF of 30 to 39 percent or <30 percent have mortality rates that increase to 10 to 15 percent compared to 20 to 25 percent, respectively.[564,572,573] Although measured much less frequently, the end-systolic volume index is also an accurate predictor of survival following AMI.[573,574]

Clinical reflections of the degree of left ventricular systolic dysfunction include the patient's exercise capacity as judged by exercise testing and/or the New York Heart Association clinical classification, which is an independent predictor of outcome. Patients with good exercise capacity, even in the presence of a reduced ejection fraction, have a superior long-term outcome in comparison with those who cannot perform mild-to-moderate exercise.[575]

ASSESSMENT OF MYOCARDIAL ISCHEMIA

Exercise Testing: Timing and Protocol Selection During hospitalization, in patients recovering from AMI, a practical and safe approach to exercise testing has been to utilize a submaximal treadmill exercise protocol (modified Naughton or modified Bruce protocol) rather than the standard Bruce protocol.[576] The target for completing the test is often symptom-limited exercise to a specific heart rate goal (e.g., 70 to 75 percent age-predicted) or to a peak work level (e.g., 5 metabolic equivalents, or METs) unless other factors (≥2 mm ST depression, chest pain, ventricular arrhythmia, or hypotension) arise first (see Chap. 14). The exercise ECG most accurately reflects the risk of subsequent ischemic events when baseline ECG is normal.

Exercise testing is also useful in planning the exercise prescription for a cardiac rehabilitation program (see Chap. 50). For safety, patients should be angina-free and free of cardiac failure before exercise testing. Patients selected in this fashion under the supervision of a physician are at minimal risk for complications.[570,571,577,578] One caveat is that in most of these studies, patients exercised 1 to 2 weeks after AMI, a time frame incompatible with managed care early discharge strategies.[577,578]

CLINICAL SIGNIFICANCE OF PREDISCHARGE SUBMAXIMAL EXERCISE TESTING Numerous studies have analyzed the predictive value of predischarge exercise testing during a 6- to 12-month follow-up after AMI.[570,571] Exercise variables of prognostic significance are exercise-induced ST-segment depression, ST-segment elevation, development of angina during exercise, inadequate blood pressure response to exercise, or exercise of short duration. From the practical standpoint, it is important to consider all of these exercise variables rather than to focus solely on the presence or absence of ST-segment depression. Done appropriately, submaximal exercise testing consistently identifies a high-risk group for recurrent cardiac events (AMI, unstable angina) or mortality in the first year after the AMI. However, the relative risk for mortality or cardiac events associated with a "positive exercise test" varies greatly between studies (twofold to more than 15-fold versus a "negative test"). A normal submaximal exercise test identifies a very low risk group (1 to 3 percent mortality rate for the first year).[570,571,578] Thus, a negative test result is adequately reassuring to encourage early discharge as well as discourage an aggressive diagnostic approach. The ACC/AHA guidelines support the widespread use of submaximal exercise testing in uncomplicated patients before discharge.[1]

For patients with a normal exercise test before discharge, symptom-limited maximal exercise testing can be repeated 2 to 6 weeks after AMI. The maximal exercise test can be used to identify additional high-risk patients.[579,580] The magnitude of this additional ischemia detection, however, as compared to a submaximal exercise test prior to hospital discharge, appears to be modest. Since many cardiovascular events can occur in the first 4 to 6 weeks, predischarge assessment of ischemia is preferred. Evidence of exercise-induced ischemia generally mandates cardiac catheterization to define the coronary anatomy and the consideration of revascularization (see algorithm in Fig. 42-11).[1] The consensus opinion of the ACC/AHA guidelines management group is that exercise testing is still useful in the risk stratification of patients who have received thrombolytic therapy, and it retains a class I indication in uncomplicated patients postinfarction.[1,581,582]

The clinical inference is that the detection of ischemia should lead to coronary arteriography. A randomized trial supports the performance of coronary arteriography in post-myocardial infarction patients with evidence of inducible ischemia before hospital discharge. In the DANAMI trials of 503 patients that survived AMI who were randomized to receive thrombolytic therapy, those patients with evidence of inducible ischemia prior to discharge had a nearly twofold higher cardiac event rate than did a group receiving early invasive intervention.[583] These study results are supportive of the usefulness of coronary arteriography in asymptomatic AMI patients with inducible ischemia.

Ambulatory Electrocardiographic Detection of Myocardial Ischemia A number of studies have assessed the presence of silent myocardial ischemia (usually defined as ≥1-mm ST-segment depression for ≥30 s) using 24-h ambulatory electrocardiographic monitoring in patients who have survived AMI. Some of the episodes of transient ST-segment depression on ambulatory ECGs are associated with chest pain and typical angina symptoms, but the majority of these ischemic episodes are silent. Many of these episodes of "silent ischemia" occur during levels of low activity and/or mental stress.[584–587] As with other modalities to measure ischemia, the detection of ambulatory electrocardiographic ischemia has been predictive of a poor outcome in long-term follow-up trials in patients surviving AMI. The correlations among exercise testing, ambulatory ECGs, and ischemia detected by thallium appear to overlap but are not identical.[588] No studies show that the reduction in episodes of silent ischemia result in an improved outcome. Thus, routine ambulatory electrocardiographic assessment of ischemia is not recommended.[1]

Alternatives for Evaluating Myocardial Ischemia THALLIUM-201 SCINTIGRAPHY There are several alternatives to standard

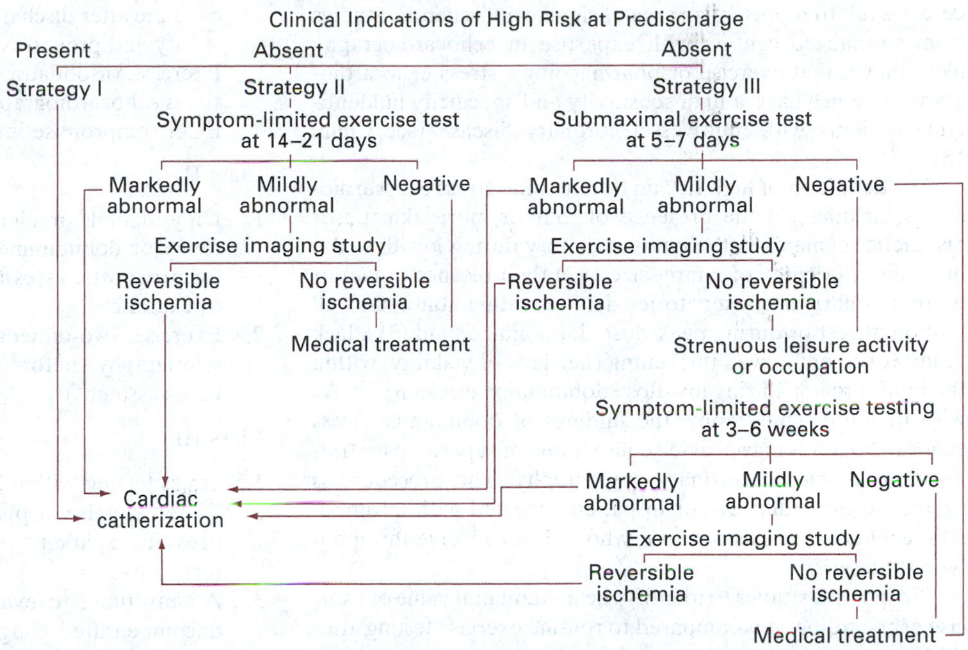

FIGURE 42-11 Strategies for exercise test evaluations soon after myocardial infarction. If patients are at high risk for ischemic events based on clinical criteria, they should undergo invasive evaluation to determine if they are candidates for coronary revascularization procedures (strategy I). For patients initially deemed to be at low risk at time of discharge after myocardial infarction, two strategies for performing exercise testing can be used. One is a symptom-limited test at 14 to 21 days (strategy II). If the patient is on digoxin or if the baseline ECG precludes accurate interpretation of ST-segment changes (e.g., baseline left bundle branch block or left ventricular hypertrophy), then an initial exercise imaging study can be performed. Results of exercise testing should be stratified to determine need for additional invasive or exercise perfusion studies. A third strategy is to perform a submaximal exercise test at 5 to 7 days after myocardial infarction or just before hospital discharge. The exercise test results could be stratified using the guidelines in strategy I. If exercise test studies are negative, a second symptom-limited exercise test could be repeated at 3 to 6 weeks for patients undergoing vigorous activity during leisure or at work. (From Ryan et al.,[1] with permission.)

exercise testing. One well-studied technique is exercise thallium-201 scintigraphy, as discussed previously (see Chap. 16). Exercise thallium-201 scintigraphy has a number of potential advantages over routine exercise testing: (1) it can be used when the 12-lead ECG is uninterpretable for ischemic ST-segment shifts because of baseline changes such as a left bundle branch block where it has a class I indication; (2) it allows assessment of reversible and irreversible perfusion defects, both within and outside the vascular region involved in the AMI; (3) the technique of single-photon emission computed tomography (SPECT) thallium scintigraphy provides a semiquantitative evaluation of ischemia; (4) exercise thallium-201 scintigraphy offers superior sensitivity and specificity for the detection of multivessel disease when compared with standard exercise testing; and (5) if pharmacologic adenosine stress is used, it can be safely performed on day 3 or 4 after myocardial infarction.[589,590]

High-risk patients are identified if (1) perfusion defects exist in more than one discrete vascular zone; (2) there is distinct evidence of redistribution; or (3) there was evidence of increased lung uptake. Low-risk patients are defined by thallium scintigraphy showing involvement of a single vascular region without redistribution, with no evidence of increased lung uptake. A high-risk thallium-201 scintigram is correlated with multivessel coronary disease. Thallium scintigraphy has been shown to be excellent at identifying high-grade stenoses of 90 percent or greater, especially high-grade lesions of the left anterior descending coronary artery.[590]

As in routine exercise testing, a limited number of studies have evaluated the value of pharmacologic stress thallium tomography in patients with thrombolytic therapy, with some conflicting results. Provocative pharmacologic studies using thallium-201 tomography also predicted risk of subsequent ischemic events after AMI.[589] Adenosine tomography also offers the advantage of allowing the safe assessment of ischemia as early as 3 to 4 days following AMI. In the era of cost containment and pressure for early hospital discharge, this approach, although not proven, may be beneficial in identifying patients who can safely be discharged early.[589]

Since adenosine single photon emission computed tomography (SPECT) can safely be performed early in asymptomatic post-myocardial infarction patients,[591] it may gain more general acceptance as the preferred test for post-myocardial infarction ischemia. At present ACC/AHA guidelines only give a class I indication to performing this test when the 12-lead ECG is abnormal (uninterpretable). Adenosine SPECT imaging can identify high-risk patients and also can track the relation between therapeutic changes and subsequent changes in risk of cardiac events by tracking changes in perfusion defect size. In a preliminary trial, cardiac event-free survival was 96 percent at 1 year for patients in whom the ischemic burden could be reduced to ≤9 percent by pharmacologic and/or invasive therapy.[591]

Other radionuclide techniques are useful in the evaluation of patients after AMI, but the focus here has been on thallium scintigraphy, which provides prognostic information by the detection of myocardial ischemia. Other techniques include the use of radionuclide angiography for the assessment of ventricular function, including the evaluation of right ventricular infarction, and the use of technetium pyrophosphate to estimate myocardial infarct size and hibernating myocardium. These are summarized in Table 42-6.[185] Only exercise and pharmacologic thallium studies have a class I indication for the evaluation of ischemia.[1] The choice between stress thallium and standard exercise testing depends on ECG interpretability, availability, cost, and clinical experience.[591]

EXERCISE ECHOCARDIOGRAPHY Exercise two-dimensional echocardiography is an alternative technique for identifying postinfarction ischemia. A reversible segmental wall motion defect is felt to represent an area of significant ischemia. Studies from specialized centers with expertise in echocardiography have shown that exercise or pharmacologic stress echocardiographic studies have a high sensitivity and specificity in identifying patients with multivessel coronary disease (see Chap. 13).[592–594]

The definition of high risk on dobutamine stress echocardiograms includes (1) the presence of four or more akinetic or diskinetic segments in the infarct territory during low-dose dobutamine (an index of infarct size); (2) the presence of two or more coronary artery territories demonstrating abnormal wall motion at rest or during peak-dose dobutamine; and (3) a lack of improvement in wall thickening (i.e., lack of viability) within the infarct region during low-dose dobutamine infusion.[592,593] As with thallium scintigraphy, the findings of dobutamine stress echocardiograms may provide comparable or superior risk stratification to that of coronary angiography. The procedure is predictive of cardiac events in patients treated with thrombolytic agents as well as in those who did not receive thrombolytic therapy.[594]

Prospective studies to identify the incremental value of exercise echocardiograms compared to routine exercise testing after AMI have not been performed. In general, negative tests with exercise, dipyridamole, or dobutamine echocardiography are associated with a low rate of cardiac events.[592–595] Variation among institutions in expertise in the quality of echocardiographic study and interpretation are limitations to a widespread recommendation for the preferred use of echocardiography.

A multinational study provides long-term verification for the use of pharmacologic stress echocardiography in post-myocardial infarction patients with single-vessel coronary artery disease.[596] Either persantine or dobutamine stress resulted in useful long-term prognostic information, with stress echocardiographic "ischemia" detection associated with high 4-year rates of myocardial infarction. The investigators emphasized that stress echocardiography provided effective risk stratification at a relatively low cost.[596]

META-ANALYSIS OF VARIOUS METHODOLOGIES OF EXERCISE TESTING POST-MYOCARDIAL INFARCTION In their comprehensive meta-analysis of alternative methodologies of post-myocardial infarction exercise testing by Peterson and colleagues, a few general patterns are apparent (Table 42-17). All exercise testing modalities share a high negative predictive value. However, all testing modalities have a rather dismal positive predictive value. None of the more sophisticated technologies appear to have a positive predictive value for subsequent cardiac events that substantially exceed simple stress echocardiography. The prognostic value of the testing modalities appear equally valid in patients with thrombolytic therapy.[597]

Exercise Testing in Uncomplicated Patients Recommendations[1]:

Class I

1. Stress electrocardiography
   a. Before discharge, for prognostic assessment or functional capacity (submaximal at 4 to 6 days or symptom-limited at 10 to 14 days)
   b. Early after discharge for prognostic assessment and functional capacity (14 to 21 days)
   c. Late after discharge (3 to 6 weeks) for functional capacity and prognosis if early stress was submaximal
2. Exercise, vasodilator stress nuclear scintigraphy, or exercise stress echocardiography when baseline abnormalities of the ECG compromise interpretation

Class IIa

1. Dipyridamole or adenosine stress perfusion nuclear scintigraphy or dobutamine echocardiography before discharge, for prognostic assessment in patients judged to be unable to exercise
2. Exercise two-dimensional echocardiography or nuclear scintigraphy (before or early after discharge for prognostic assessment)

Class III

1. Stress testing within 2 to 3 days of AMI.
2. Either exercise or pharmacologic stress testing at any time to evaluate patients with unstable postinfarction angina pectoris.
3. At any time, to evaluate patients with AMI, who have uncompensated congestive heart failure, cardiac arrhythmia, or noncardiac conditions that severely limit their ability to exercise.
4. Before discharge, to evaluate patients who have been selected for cardiac catheterization. In this situation, the exercise test may be useful after catheterization to evaluate function or identify ischemia in a distribution to correlate with coronary stenoses judged to be of borderline severity.

Suggested Algorithm for the Evaluation of Myocardial Ischemia after Myocardial Infarction Based on all of the evaluable data, the task force on practice guidelines for the management of AMI created a strategy for the evaluation of myocardial ischemia after AMI in low-risk patients, presented in Fig. 42-11.[1] If there are clinical indications of a high-risk patient, as detailed earlier, such patients are considered for early cardiac catheterization and coronary angiography (strategy I).[1] The evaluation of myocardial ischemia in low-risk patients is alternatively presented for strategies II and III. Strategy III favors using a submaximal exercise test or alternative imaging study prior to hospital discharge. Strategy II alternatively suggests that a symptom-limited exercise test be performed soon after hospital discharge. Regardless of whether exercise testing or a more sophisticated exercise imaging study is ordered in the hospital, a negative test does not preclude the repeat evaluation for myocardial ischemia once the patient is fully ambulatory, after 3 to 6 weeks.

ASSESSMENT OF THE RISK OF ARRHYTHMIC (SUDDEN CARDIAC) DEATH: OVERVIEW

Although the technology to assess the risk of arrhythmic death in patients after AMI has improved in sophistication, antiarrhythmic therapies to reduce risk have thus far proved disappointing. For comparison, there is consensus that the identification of postinfarction patients with a LVEF of ≤40 percent mandates the use of ACE inhibitors.[392,393,598] Likewise, the identification of asymptomatic postinfarction patients with ischemia indicates the need for early performance of coronary angiography to assess the potential for PTCA or coronary artery bypass surgery.[1] Unfortunately, the identification of asymptomatic but

TABLE 42-17 Predischarge Risk Stratification Done Using Noninvasive Testing*

	Sensitivity		Specificity		Positive Predictive Value		Negative Predictive Value	
Test Result	Cardiac Death	Cardiac Death or MI	Cardiac Death	Cardiac Death or MI	Cardiac Death	Cardiac Death or MI	Cardiac Death	Cardiac Death or MI
Exercise electrocardiography†								
ST-segment depression	0.42	0.44	0.75	0.70	0.04	0.16	0.98	0.91
Impaired systolic blood pressure	0.44	0.23	0.79	0.87	0.11	0.21	0.96	0.88
Limited exercise duration	0.56	0.53	0.62	0.65	0.10	0.18	0.95	0.91
Chest pain on exercise	0.23	0.29	0.83	0.82	0.08	0.19	0.94	0.89
Exercise myocardial perfusion imaging‡								
Reversible perfusion defect	0.89	0.80	0.38	0.48	0.07	0.16	0.98	0.95
Multiple perfusion defects	0.64	0.75	0.71	0.76	0.07	0.17	0.98	0.97
Exercise ventricular function imaging								
Exercise radionuclide angiography§								
Peak EF <40%	0.63	0.60	0.77	0.75	0.27	0.31	0.94	0.91
Change in EF <5%	0.80	0.55	0.67	0.74	0.15	0.18	0.98	0.94
New dyssynergy	—	0.78	—	0.50	—	0.17	—	0.94
Exercise echocardiography¶								
Change in EF <5%	—	0.56	—	0.60	—	0.14	—	0.92
New dyssynergy	1.00	0.62	0.62	0.79	0.18	0.48	1.00	0.86
Pharmacologic stress imaging								
Myocardial perfusion imaging‖								
Reversible perfusion defect	0.56	0.71	0.46	0.49	0.10	0.19	0.90	0.91
Multiple perfusion defects	—	0.50	—	0.64	—	0.17	—	0.90
Echocardiography**								
New dyssynergy	0.67	0.55	0.56	0.54	0.05	0.08	0.98	0.94

*All event rates are for 1 year after infarction. EF = ejection fraction; MI = myocardial infarction.
†Rate of cardiac death, 3.3%; rate of cardiac death or MI, 7.8%.
‡Rate of cardiac death, 4.6%; rate of cardiac death or MI, 13.1%.
§Rate of cardiac death, 9.3%; rate of cardiac death or MI, 13.2%.
¶Rate of cardiac death, 5.6%; rate of cardiac death or MI, 15.9%.
‖Rate of cardiac death, 6.6%; rate of cardiac death or MI, 15.0%.
**Rate of cardiac death, 2.5%; rate of cardiac death or MI, 5.0%.
SOURCE: Peterson et al.,[597] with permission.

high-risk patients for arrhythmic death after AMI is not similarly associated with a successful treatment strategy. This section addresses AMI patients who are asymptomatic and have not had sustained VT or VF—identifiers that all agree require aggressive management, most commonly the placement of an implantable cardioverter defibrillator (ICD).

The preponderance of evidence is that the majority of asymptomatic AMI patients who experienced arrhythmic (sudden cardiac) death have had sustained VT and/or VF.[599] A review of selected clinical trials of antiarrhythmic therapy focusing on patients after AMI is presented in Table 42-18[392,393,598,600–605] for the purpose of demonstrating the total deaths attributable to arrhythmic or sudden cardiac death, which vary widely in the placebo groups of these trials. The Cardiac Arrhythmia Suppression (CAST) trials[600,601] and the Canadian Amiodarone Myocardial Infarction Arrhythmia Trial (CAMIAT)[604] identified high-risk patients after AMI using the criteria of ventricular arrhythmia on ambulatory ECGs. In the placebo groups, the range of death attributable to arrhythmia varied from 48 to 66 percent. The Survival and Ventricular Enlargement (SAVE) trial,[392] the European Myocardial Infarction Amiodarone Trial (EMIAT),[603] and the Survival With Oral d-sotalol (SWORD)[602] trial identified patients after AMI using an ejection fraction cutoff. The range of deaths attributable to arrhythmia in the placebo group was 45 to 67 percent. Patients in trials with a mixture of etiologies of left ventricular dysfunction including old AMI, such as the Studies of Left Ventricular Dysfunction (SOLVD) prevention and SOLVD treatment trials, have a lower percentage of deaths attributable to arrhythmia.[393,598] The wide discrepancy in arrhythmic death rates and the variety of screening tests used to identify "high-risk" patients highlight a significant deficit in current arrhythmic death classification.[605]

The changing proportion of deaths attributable to arrhythmia and other causes after AMI is conceptually depicted in Fig. 42-12. Sustained VT and VF occur most frequently in the first year following AMI.[564] As ischemic cardiomyopathy develops over many years, deaths attributable to VT/VF decrease and proportionately more "sudden deaths" are attributable to asystole, electromechanical dissociation, or a high-degree heart block.[606] Also, noncardiac conditions emulate the circumstances of VT or VF (for instance, massive pulmonary embolism, ruptured abdominal or thoracic aortic aneurysm, or massive

TABLE 42-18 Review of Representative Clinical Trials: Placebo Cause-Specific Mortality

Trial (No. of Placebo Patients), Entrance Criteria	Mean Follow-up (months)	Annualized Mortality, %	Arrhythmia/SCD, %
CAST I[600] (743), VPC ≥6/VT/AMI	10	4.2	62
CAST II[601] (574), VPC ≥6/VT/AMI/EF ≤40%	18	6.4	66
SAVE[392] (1116), EF ≤40%/AMI 3–16 d	42	7.1	45
SOLVD PREV[598] (2117), No CHF/EF ≤35%	37	5.3	31
SOLVD Rx[393] (1294), CHF (II/III) + EF ≤35%	41	11.7	22
SWORD[602] (1572), MI, EF ≤40%	5	1.5	67
EMIAT[603] (743), MI + <40%	21	7.8	49
CAMIAT[604] (596), MI + VPC ≥10 or VT	20	4.7	48

ABBREVIATIONS: SCD = sudden cardiac death; CAST = Cardiac Arrhythmia Suppression Trial; VPC = ventricular premature complexes; VT = ventricular tachycardia; AMI = acute myocardial infarction; EF = ejection fraction; SAVE = Survival and Ventricular Enlargement; SOLVD = Studies of Left Ventricular Dysfunction; PREV = prevention; CHF = congestive heart failure; Rx = treatment; SWORD = Survival With Oral d-Sotalol; EMIAT = European Myocardial Infarction Amiodarone Trial; CAMIAT = Canadian Amiodarone Myocardial Infarction Arrhythmia Trial.

SOURCE: Adapted from Pratt et al.,[605] with permission.

stroke).[605] Thus, the temporal influence on cause-specific mortality after AMI is an important consideration. Risk stratification for arrhythmic death is clearly more relevant immediately following myocardial infarction (Fig. 42-12).

This discussion is limited to tests available for evaluating asymptomatic patients. The preponderance of evidence does not support a class I or even a class IIa indication for any of the modalities to be discussed: ambulatory ECG, heart rate variability, signal averaged ECG, or electrophysiologic testing. What is lacking in each is the absence of compelling data that the identification of "arrhythmic death risk" is coupled with a strategy to improve outcome.[1]

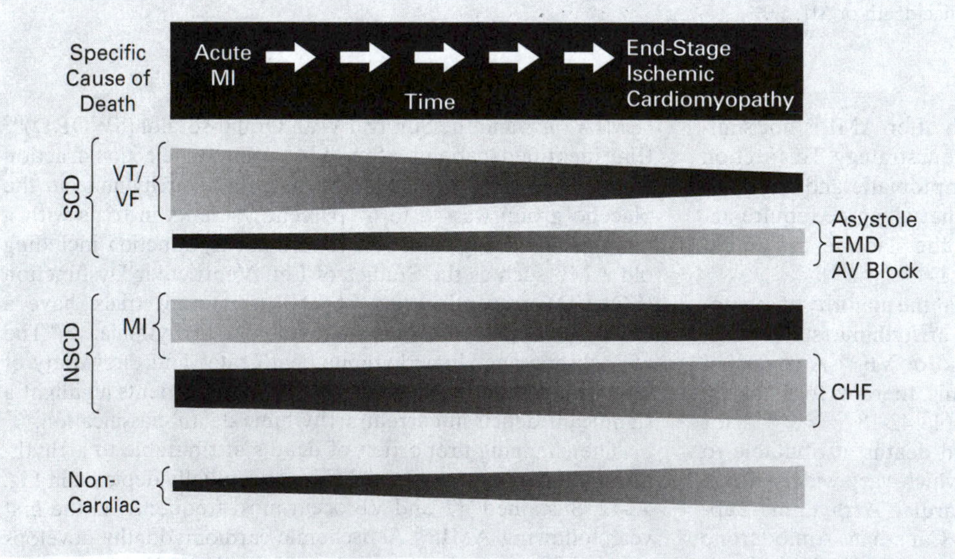

FIGURE 42-12 A theoretical view of approaches to identify a postmyocardial infarction population dying of ventricular tachycardia/fibrillation. This concept is presented in a qualitative fashion and represents estimates based on the literature (see text). SCD, sudden cardiac death; NSCD, non-sudden cardiac death; VT, ventricular tachycardia; VF, ventricular fibrillation; MI, myocardial infarction; EMD, electromechanical dissociation; CHF, congestive heart failure.

Ambulatory Electrocardiographic Recordings: Ventricular Arrhythmias Asymptomatic spontaneous ventricular arrhythmias detected on ambulatory ECGs are predictive of an increased risk of arrhythmic (sudden) death in the first 1 to 2 years following AMI.[564,607] The mechanism responsible for the majority of arrhythmic deaths in post–myocardial infarction patients is, as noted, sustained VT or VF.[599] Vulnerability for arrhythmic death appears to be highest in the first year after AMI, probably accounting for one-half of the first-year mortality.[564,607] Thus, it appears that arrhythmic death risk should be assessed prior to hospital discharge. The use of ambulatory electrocardiographic recording to identify a "high-risk" group, however, has a poor positive predictive value.[600,608] As seen in Table 42-19, postinfarction patients with no baseline ventricular arrhythmia on ambulatory electrocardiographic recording uniformly have a low risk for arrhythmic death.[564,608] Frequent premature ventricular complexes and nonsustained VT are generally associated with a two- and threefold increased risk, respectively.[13,564,607,608] As can be deduced from the data in Table 42-19, for every 100 patients identified with "warning arrhythmias," only 4 to 7 will have arrhythmic death in the following 1 to 2 years. Thus, a treatment strategy that would include routine prophylactic administration of an antiarrhythmic drug would necessitate a superb safety profile, since approximately 95 percent of the patients cannot benefit but all would be exposed to potentially lethal proarrhythmic risk. Such hazards have been documented in prophylactic antiarrhythmic drug trials.[600–602] Thus, ambulatory ECG has an adequate negative predictive value, but a poor positive predictive value, consistent with its class IIb rating.

TABLE 42-19 Risk of Sudden Death Based on VPCs Detected on AECG in Patients Surviving Acute Myocardial Infarction

Trial	Sample Size	Arrhythmic Death Mortality Rate, %[a]	Total Mortality Rate, %[a]	Actual Follow-up Months
CAST[600] (≥6 VPCs/h)				10
Encainide or flecainide	730	5.4[b]	9.2[b]	
Placebo	725	1.5	3.6	
CAPS[608] (≥10 VPCs/h)				12
All patients	502	4.6	9.0	
Placebo	100	—	7.0	
Bigger et al.[564]				24
All patients	819	3.8	5.9	
0 VPC	112	1.5	3.0	
>3 VPCs/h	2456	6.1	9.8	
>10 VPCs/h	162	6.3	9.4	
>30 VPCs/h	89	7.0	10.5	
BHAT[13] (placebo group)				25
0 VPCs	260	1.2	2.5	
Any VPCs	1380	2.6	5.5	
≤10 VPCs/h	211	4.5	10.0	
≥10 VPCs/h	1429	2.0	4.3	
Moss et al.[607]	759	6.8	11.6	6
Ruberman et al.[607a]				24
≤10 VPCs/h	1285	2.3	6.4	
≥10 VPCs/h	454	7.6	13.6	

[a]All corrected to an estimated 1-year mortality rate.
[b]End point of death or cardiac arrest.
ABBREVIATIONS: VPCs = ventricular premature complexes; AECG = ambulatory ECG.

Ambulatory Electrocardiogram Recordings: Heart Rate Variability Heart rate variability, measured by the standard deviation of the RR interval on monitored electrocardiographic leads, is an indirect assessment of proportional autonomic tone. Extensive variability in the heart rate connotes a preponderance of parasympathetic activity, whereas less variability in the heart rate is consistent with proportionately more sympathetic activity.[609–611] In animal models, enhanced sympathetic activity increases the vulnerability of the ischemic myocardium to the development of VF.[612]

Clinical trials have assessed the relation of heart rate variability to mortality rate in patients surviving AMI. Depressed heart rate variability is associated with an increased risk of death. Multivariate analysis has identified reduced heart rate variability as an independent predictor of arrhythmic death.[609–611,613] In one study, patients selected for depressed heart rate variability and ventricular arrhythmias, excluding patients with the lowest ejection fractions, identified a patient population in whom 75 percent of the deaths were presumed arrhythmic.[614] Heart rate variability measured after thrombolytic therapy still has clinical relevance, and an improvement in heart rate variability correlated with TIMI grade 3 flow.[615]

Practical approaches to minimizing cost, while focusing noninvasive testing on a targeted group, are under evaluation. In a study of 729 survivors of AMI prior to hospital discharge from St. George's Hospital in London, a 24-h heart rate variability index was compared to a 5-min analysis of an ectopic-free segment of the Holter recording, measuring the standard deviation of normal-to-normal RR intervals (SDNN).[616] The 5-min analysis of SDNN measurement was a useful and inexpensive tool to select patients for more extensive 24-h heart rate variability index evaluation.[4]

At present, while heart rate variability is a very promising method of evaluating parasympathetic and sympathetic effects in the heart, it cannot be recommended as a standard clinical test in AMI patients, unless and until trials demonstrate clinical benefits of a treatment strategy based upon the knowledge of this marker of sudden cardiac death.[1,617]

Baroreflex Sensitivity Baroreflex sensitivity is another autonomic marker that is a measure of the change in heart rate (anticipated reduction) to an increase in blood pressure. In this respect, it provides an index of the ability to reflexly increase cardiac vagal activity. Heart rate variability, in contrast, is a marker of vagal tone.[618]

The importance of these two autonomic markers is demonstrated by the results of the Autonomic Tone and Reflexes After Myocardial Infarction (ATRAMI) trial, a study of 1284 patients with a recent (≤28 days) myocardial infarction.[619] One-year mortality was increased in patients with a reduced baroreflex sensitivity as well as a low heart rate variability (see Table 42-20).[618] There was an additive value to the measurement of the two markers: If both are low there is a 15-fold increased risk of death than if both markers are normal (15 versus 1 percent; $p < 0.0001$). The interaction of LVEF and these autonomic markers is also apparent from Table 42-20, each being associated with a twofold greater risk of death in patients with LVEF <35 percent than it is in those with better preserved left ventricular systolic function. It is reasonable to conclude that both baroreflex sensitivity and heart rate variability have independent prognostic value for stratifying the risk of death after myocardial infarction.[74]

Signal-Average Electrocardiogram Time-domain analysis of the signal-averaged ECG can be used to detect low-amplitude, high-frequency potentials at the end of the QRS complex, termed *ventricular late potentials*. The presence of late potentials identifies patients likely to have inducible sustained monomor-

TABLE 42-20 Multivariate Analysis of Influence of Baroreceptor Sensitivity and Heart Rate Variability on Relative One-Year Mortality Risk after AMI

Variable Examined	Variable in Analysis	Groups	RR	95% CI	P
Baroreflex sensitivity	LVEF	35–50%	2.1	0.90–4.69	0.08
		<35%	4.7	2.04–10.9	0.0003
	BRS (ms/mmHg)	3.0–6.1	1.7	0.81–3.69	0.15
		<3.0	2.8	1.24–6.16	0.01
	VPCs per h	≥10	1.8	0.94–3.46	0.07
Heart rate variability	LVEF (%)	35–50%	1.9	0.87–4.49	0.10
		<35%	3.9	1.69–9.25	0.001
	SDNN	70–105	1.9	0.86–4.04	0.11
		<70	3.2	1.42–7.36	0.005
	VPCs per h	≥10	1.8	0.97–3.50	0.06

ABBREVIATIONS: RR = relative rate; CI = confidence interval; LVEF = left ventricular ejection fraction; BRS = baroreflex sensitivity; VPC = ventricular premature complex; SDNN = standard deviation of all normal beats.

SOURCE: Schwartz,[618] with permission.

phic VT during programmed electrical stimulation and is associated with an increased risk of subsequent arrhythmic events.[609,620,621] The predictive value of late potentials is best established in patients with AMI and is of less established value in other patient populations.

In some studies, the presence of an abnormal signal-averaged ECG, of frequent ventricular premature complexes on the ambulatory electrocardiographic recording, and left ventricular aneurysm were independent predictors of VT, regardless of whether or not a patient had received thrombolytic therapy.[621] If results of the signal-averaged ECG are negative—that is, there are no afterdepolarizations—the negative predictive value in this population is good and the likelihood of subsequent arrhythmic death is low. As with the evaluation of heart rate variability, the interpretation of the signal-averaged ECG can be improved by combining it with other variables, especially the LVEF. Even when multiple tests are combined for assessing the risk of sudden cardiac death, the strength is in their negative predictive value rather than their positive predictive value, which usually falls below 50 percent.[620,621] There is an adverse prognostic consequence of a positive signal-averaged ECG and an occluded infarct-related artery.[622] The routine use of signal-averaged ECGs in AMI is not at present recommended.[1]

Invasive Electrophysiologic Testing (Programmed Electrical Stimulation) Invasive electrophysiologic assessment has been evaluated in two distinct populations who survived AMI. The first and relatively small group had a cardiac arrest or an episode of sustained VT following an AMI. In such patients, the risk of recurrent cardiac arrest or arrhythmic events is high, and electrophysiologic studies are an alternative for assisting in therapy selection.[623]

The much larger patient population are those with an increased risk of arrhythmic death based upon the results of one or more noninvasive tests, as discussed previously. Performing electrophysiologic studies on all asymptomatic "high-risk" patients is not justified.[1] Reports on the utility of electrophysiologic studies have been inconsistent in predicting total mortality and are only slightly more consistent in identifying patients likely to have subsequent arrhythmic events.[624,625]

Results from the Multicenter Automatic Defibrillation Implantation Trial (MADIT) are somewhat relevant to this issue.[626] Patients in MADIT had had a prior Q-wave infarction with a LVEF of <35 percent and were selected if programmed electrical stimulation induced sustained VT that was nonsuppressible with intravenous procainamide. Patients were randomized to an implantable cardioverter-defibrillator group and/or conventional arrhythmic therapy. Although total mortality was less in the cardioverter-defibrillator group, the relevant point is that this invasive screening appeared to identify a high-risk group for subsequent arrhythmic death.[626] This study alone is not sufficient, however, to support the wider use of electrophysiologic testing in asymptomatic postinfarction patients for at least two reasons: (1) imbalances in the use of beta blockers between the two treatment strategies cloud the results, and (2) these patients were many years from their index infarction. Therefore, the relevance to predischarge risk assessment of AMI is tenuous.

Assessing Arrhythmic Death: Conclusions In the ACC/AHA guidelines, none of the noninvasive techniques is generally agreed upon to be beneficial, useful, and effective, either unequivocally (class I) or based upon the weight of evidence or opinion (class IIa) for predicting arrhythmic death. These techniques have class IIb indications, meaning that their usefulness and efficacy are not well established by either scientific evidence and/or general opinion.[1] In addition to their poor positive predictive value, no clinical trial has demonstrated that the use of any one or a combination of these modalities of testing identifies a high-risk population in whom an intervention strategy results in clinical benefit. Unless and until such studies are carried out to show that targeting a high-risk population and using the data to direct subsequent prophylactic therapy result in patient benefit, these modalities of risk assessment remain interesting tools for investigational studies and for use on selected individual patients. Other assessments of risk for sudden death, such as QT dispersion, are in an even earlier investigational stage, and at present, there is little supporting evidence that they are useful and effective in improving the management and outcome of AMI patients.[1,627]

Coronary Angiography and Percutaneous Transluminal Coronary Angioplasty

Recommendations[1]:

Class I

1. Patients with spontaneous episodes of myocardial ischemia or episodes of myocardial ischemia provoked by minimal exertion during recovery from infarction

2. Before definitive therapy of a mechanical complication of infarction such as acute mitral regurgitation, VSD, pseudoaneurysm, or left ventricular aneurysm
3. Patients with persistent hemodynamic instability

Class IIa

1. When myocardial infarction is suspected to have occurred by a mechanism other than thrombotic occlusion at an atherosclerotic plaque. This would include coronary embolism, certain metabolic or hematologic diseases, or coronary artery spasm.
2. Survivors of AMI with depressed left ventricular systolic function (left ventricular ejection fraction less than or equal to 40 percent), congestive heart failure, prior revascularization, or malignant ventricular arrhythmias.
3. Survivors of AMI who had clinical heart failure during the acute episode but subsequently demonstrated well-preserved left ventricular function.

Class IIb

1. Coronary angiography performed in all patients after infarction to find persistently occluded infarct-related arteries in an attempt to revascularize the artery or identify patients with three-vessel disease
2. All patients after a non-Q-wave myocardial infarction
3. Recurrent VT or VF or both, despite antiarrhythmic therapy, in patients without evidence of ongoing myocardial ischemia

Class III

1. Routine use of coronary angiography and subsequent PTCA of the infarct-related artery within days after thrombolytic therapy
2. Survivors of myocardial infarction who are thought not to be candidates for coronary revascularization

The selection of patients for cardiac catheterization and coronary angiographic studies prior to hospital discharge should be based on identifying patients at risk for ischemic events and on whether the information provided by cardiac catheterization and coronary angiography will change patient management.

Studies analyzing the prognostic utility of cardiac catheterization prior to hospital discharge are from the prethrombolytic era and demonstrate that the angiographic extent of coronary artery disease was related to survival.[628,629] Other trials have addressed the utility of routine coronary angiographic studies in patients who have received thrombolytic therapy.[630–633] The timing of cardiac catheterization during hospitalization has been addressed in several studies. In general, studies that have compared acute or early cardiac catheterization to a more conservative approach of performing cardiac catheterization and coronary angiographic studies only for patients with spontaneous recurrent angina or exercise-induced ischemia have demonstrated no benefit to the strategy of routine catheterization.[1,271]

Figure 42-11 presents a strategy for identifying symptomatic and asymptomatic high-risk patients who should have cardiac catheterization and coronary angiographic studies before discharge. Patients who have a complicated clinical course characterized by refractory cardiac failure, unstable angina, an episode of sustained VT, or cardiac arrest should be studied, as discussed previously. An aggressive approach to these patients is justified because of the observed 1-year mortality rate, ranging from 10 to 25 percent.[634] In the case of patients with symptomatic cardiac failure, right heart catheterization should be included.

The recommended algorithm for selecting asymptomatic, uncomplicated post-AMI patients for cardiac catheterization is also presented in Fig. 42-11. Decision making focuses on the presence or absence of myocardial ischemia. Because of the high incidence of residual ischemia in patients with a non-Q-wave infarction, the task force for guidelines for coronary angiographic studies after myocardial infarction recommended such studies in all non-Q-wave infarctions.[635] The more conservative recommendation here emphasizes evidence of objective ischemia. Where patients have received thrombolytic therapy, it seems reasonable that those who have evidence of residual ischemia are still at increased risk of future ischemic events and should undergo coronary angiography prior to discharge. Consideration of PTCA following coronary angiographic studies should be based on established clinical and anatomic guidelines[1,636] (see Chap. 45). Coronary artery bypass surgery should be considered in those groups in whom it has been shown to be of proven benefit: patients with triple-vessel disease, patients with ischemia, and those with significant left ventricular dysfunction (see also Chap. 48).[637]

SECONDARY PREVENTION AND CARDIAC REHABILITATION

Risk Factor Reduction

The relation between the level of activity of the inflammatory response in the arterial wall (which is the characteristic feature of atherosclerosis) and the tendency of the structural integrity of the artery to break down, with the resultant exposure of thrombogenic material and clot formation, is discussed in Chap. 35. The inflammatory response is caused and/or exacerbated by the presence of the classic risk factors. It follows that favorably modifying the risk factors would, intuitively, reduce coronary events. There is now abundant evidence that this is the case. Thus, since those who have had AMI are among those at highest risk for recurrence, management strategies to mitigate this risk are very important in patient management.[638]

SMOKING

Smoking has multiple cardiovascular effects that can promote AMI, including enhanced platelet aggregation, coronary vasospasm, and vascular inflammation. Smoking cessation is an essential goal after AMI, since the recurrence rate and death rate after AMI are doubled by the continuation of smoking (see also Chap. 38).[639] After AMI, however, risk associated with smoking declines rapidly to that of the nonsmoking cohort survivors within 3 years.[640] The psychological and physiologic aspects of smoking should be addressed, and a number of programs have been developed to deal with these needs. Most smokers who have quit, however, have done so without an organized program.[641] The role of the physician in motivating the patient to quit smoking is extremely important and the likelihood of success appears to be directly related to the extent of his or her involvement. Transdermal nicotine patches and oral preparations can be used to aid withdrawal but are not risk-free and should be used temporarily and adjunctively with physician counseling and/or a formal program in behavior modification.[642] The transdermal patches or oral nicotine preparations should not be used during the period just after AMI and should not be used concurrently with smoking. Difficult cases are probably handled best by referral to a formal smoking cessation program. Clonidine hydrochloride has also been used to ameliorate symptoms of smoking withdrawal as well as in conjunction with behavioral intervention.[638]

DYSLIPIDEMIA

Recommendations[1]:

Class I

1. Institute of the American Heart Association (AHA) step II diet, which consists of <7 percent of total calories as saturated fat and <200 mg/day of cholesterol in all patients after recovery from AMI.
2. Patients with low-density lipoprotein (LDL) cholesterol levels >125 mg/dL, despite consuming the AHA step II diet, should be placed on drug therapy with the goal of achieving a target LDL cholesterol <100 mg/dL.
3. Patients with normal plasma cholesterol levels who have a high-density lipoprotein (HDL) of less than 35 mg/dL should be placed on an exercise regimen to atttempt to increase it.

Class IIa

1. Drug therapy may be added to diet therapy in patients with LDL cholesterol levels <130 mg/dL but >100 mg/dL after an appropriate trial of the AHA step II diet alone.
2. Patients with normal total cholesterol levels, but with HDL cholesterol <35 mg/dL despite dietary and other nonpharmacologic therapy, may be started on drugs such as niacin in an attempt to raise HDL levels to more protective levels.

Class IIb

1. Drug therapy using either niacin or gemfibrozil may be added to diet regardless of LDL and HDL levels when triglyceride levels are >200 mg/dL.

The β-hydroxy- β-methylglutaryl-CoA (HMG-CoA) reductase inhibitors are the most effective drugs in lowering LDL cholesterol. Niacin is effective in raising HDL and, in combination with resins, is also effective in lowering LDL. Triple therapy with a reductase inhibitor, niacin, and resin can be useful in resistant cases. Drug therapy of dyslipidemias is discussed in Chap. 38.

As mentioned earlier, patients who have had an AMI are generally at high risk for recurrence. Furthermore, an abnormally elevated serum cholesterol level is a powerful risk factor for death in this group.[643,644] Early primary prevention studies and relatively small angiographic trials showed decreases in cardiovascular event rates with cholesterol-lowering therapy (see Chap. 38). Large secondary prevention trials have provided compelling evidence that in patients who have had an AMI, therapy with HMG-CoA reductase inhibitors to lower serum cholesterol levels that were either initially elevated—as in the Scandinavian Simvastatin Survival Study (4S)[645] or within "average" range as in the Cholesterol and Recurrent Events (CARE) trial[646]—was effective in reducing both cardiovascular and total mortality as well as cardiovascular events. In CARE, a treatment effect was not observed in the group with baseline LDL values <125 mg/dL. The guidelines of the expert panel of the National Cholesterol Education Program provide target goals for patients with manifest coronary artery disease. These goals are as follows: LDL cholesterol, 100 mg/dL (2.59 mmol/L); HDL cholesterol, >35 mg/dL (0.91 mmol/L).[647]

Serum lipid levels are decreased within several hours after AMI, presumably by the inflammatory response to tissue necrosis.[648] Evaluation of serum lipid levels should be made within the first 6 to 8 h from onset of symptoms or after recovery at 6 to 8 weeks. All AMI patients should have serum lipids evaluated and treated intensively in order to achieve target goals. Treatment should start in the hospital with initiation of the AHA step II diet. With established very high lipid levels (for example, LDL cholesterol >200 mg/dL), many clinicians would have a low threshold for initiating drug therapy early on, anticipating that diet therapy alone might not be sufficient for achieving target LDL goals. Although low HDL is a powerful risk factor for AMI, the benefit of treating it is unproven. It seems prudent to attempt to raise HDL levels by prescribing an exercise regimen. Niacin is also efficacious in raising HDL levels; it may be used, especially if indicated as adjunctive therapy with HMG-CoA reductase inhibitors or with resins, to lower LDL. There is less certainty about indications for treating elevated triglycerides, but it seems prudent to treat levels >400 mg/dL with diet and perhaps with fibrates or niacin (see Chap. 38).

INACTIVITY

There have been numerous studies of post-AMI patients documenting the beneficial effects of aerobic exercise on functional capacity and myocardial oxygen demand at a given submaximal workload.[649] Such exercise can decrease angina pectoris and ischemia. Conversely, a sedentary lifestyle is a risk factor for coronary artery disease. Meta-analysis of cardiac rehabilitation studies has shown a reduction in mortality in the exercise group as opposed to a control group.[649] These analyses have not permitted separating the effects of exercise per se from the other beneficial aspects of the programs. The greatest benefits of exercise are those observed with moderate, regular exercise as contrasted with the nonexercise group. The benefit can be obtained by exercising about 4200 kJ a week, which can be achieved by walking about 1.5 miles (2.4 km) per day. Long-term, regular exercise training can best be sustained by participating in a supervised exercise program beginning several weeks after discharge from the hospital.[638,649] A standard exercise program might involve three 20- to 30-min sessions three to four times per week at 60 to 75 percent of maximal aerobic capacity. This target activity level should be achieved progressively over several weeks, and progress should be monitored by the physician at regular intervals. The exercise regimen should be initiated and guided by monitored exercise testing.

Regular aerobic exercise should be prescribed for post-AMI patients in stable condition at an intensity, duration, and frequency as determined by formal testing and clinical judgment. Optimum benefit is achieved in a supervised program, although asymptomatic, stable patients can exercise without direct supervision but should receive regular monitoring by a physician (see also Chap. 50).

LOW-ESTROGEN STATES (FEMALES)

Recommendations[1]:

Class IIa

1. Hormone replacement therapy (HRT) with estrogen plus progestin for secondary prevention of coronary events should not be given de novo to postmenopausal women after myocardial infarction.
2. Postmenopausal women who are already taking HRT with estrogen plus progestin at the time of an AMI can continue this therapy.

Estrogen replacement therapy and the primary or secondary prevention of cardiovascular disease continues to be a somewhat contentious and emotional issue that involves weighing the potential efficacy of ERT in reducing cardiovascular risk against the possible increases in breast cancer rates.[650,651] Clinical trials have demonstrated that estrogen with or without progestins lowers both LDL cholesterol and fibrinogen,[652] an effect that would be expected to reduce cardiovascular risk. Contrary to conventional wisdom and expectations, the first large double-blind, placebo-controlled trial to assess the effects of estrogen and progestin treatment on the secondary prevention of coronary heart disease in postmenopausal women showed no reduction in any cardiovascular outcome after 4.1 years of follow-up.[653] Furthermore, the Heart and Estrogen-Progestin Replacement Study (HERS) Research Group reported a significant trend for more primary cardiac events in the treatment group than it did in the placebo group in year 1, although there were fewer events in years 4 and 5 in the treatment group than there were in the placebo group.[653] These observations led to the recommendation that, post-AMI, women on hormone replacement therapy at the time of the event should continue but that initiation of therapy could not be recommended[1].

Drug Therapy

BETA-ADRENERGIC BLOCKERS

Recommendations for long-term therapy in post-AMI patients[1]:

Class I

1. All post-AMI patients except those at low risk without clear contraindications should receive long-term therapy. Treatment should begin early in the course, preferably acutely, and should be continued indefinitely.

Class IIa

1. Low-risk patients without definite contraindications should be considered for beta-adrenergic blocker therapy
2. Survivors of non-ST elevation myocardial infarction

Class IIb

1. Patients with moderate or severe left ventricular failure or other relative contraindications of beta-adrenoceptor blocker therapy, provided they can be monitored closely

Class III

1. None

The benefits of beta-blocker therapy given early in the course of AMI were previously discussed. Multiple clinical trials have also demonstrated the benefits of long-term treatment of post-AMI patients with beta blockers.[654] Long-term efficacy has been demonstrated for propranolol,[13] timolol,[655] and metoprolol.[656] Mortality has been shown to be reduced by about 25 to 35 percent. The beneficial effect is highest in high-risk patients with large (usually anterior) myocardial infarction, and compensated left ventricular dysfunction. The beneficial effects in low-risk patients are less clear, but the consensus is that these patients should probably be treated because of the relatively favorable side-effect profile.[1] This recommendation extends to the patient with NQWMI although, as discussed, the data are less compelling. Beta blockers with intrinsic sympathomimetic activity should not be used in this context.

ASPIRIN

The role of aspirin during the early phases of AMI was discussed earlier. Aspirin use over the long term after AMI is also associated with a reduction in mortality. Meta-analysis of 6 major trials of aspirin treatment showed an overall reduction in vascular mortality in the treated group of 13 percent, with 31 and 42 percent reductions in nonfatal infarction and nonfatal stroke, respectively.[657] These trials used relatively large aspirin doses (300 to 1500 mg/day), but one trial showed efficacy at only 75 mg/day,[658] suggesting that long-term use of more modest doses would be effective. Thus, aspirin at relatively low doses is recommended for all patients with AMI in the absence of contraindications (see also Chap. 44).

ANTICOAGULATION

Anticoagulation can reduce mortality, recurrent myocardial infarction, and stroke after AMI, as indicated by an analysis of multiple trials.[654] Because of relatively high rates of bleeding with warfarin, the need for monitoring, and, in particular, the efficacy and low risk of aspirin, the role of warfarin is rather limited to those at increased risk for developing mural thrombi.[638] In addition, those post-AMI patients with demonstrable left ventricular thrombus and atrial fibrillation should be anticoagulated. The duration of anticoagulation should be limited to 3 months in the case of left ventricular thrombus.

ANGIOTENSIN-CONVERTING ENZYME INHIBITORS

The ACE inhibitors and recommendations for their use early in the course of AMI were previously discussed. Studies have documented their efficacy in secondary prevention. The reduction in late morbidity and mortality was most obvious in those with large infarctions with reduced ejection fraction and in those with anterior myocardial infarction. In these patients, left ventricular remodeling and progression to heart failure were reduced.[392,396,659] The beneficial effects of ACE inhibitors have been less obvious when low-risk patients were included.[660] The decrease in ischemic events in the SAVE trial[392] and in other ACE-inhibitor trials suggests that the threshold for use of ACE inhibitors for long-term therapy may be lowered by many clinicians to include those with only modest left ventricular dysfunction. Thus, ACE inhibitors have been recommended for chronic use after AMI in those patients with significant left ventricular dysfunction, and their use should be considered in those with only mild-to-moderate left ventricular dysfunction (ejection fraction <45 percent).

The publication of the Heart Outcomes Prevention Evaluation (HOPE) trial in patients with significant risk factors for cardiovascular events showed significant reduction in new events and new-onset diabetes mellitus in those treated with the ACE-inhibitor ramipril.[398] It is likely that the recommendations for use of ACE inhibitors will be extended to all patients at high risk for cardiovascular events regardless of blood pressure or left ventricular function.

Modification of Lifestyle and Cardiac Rehabilitation after Acute Myocardial Infarction

Because of the relatively high risk of recurrence and the need for lifelong modification of lifestyles and risk factors, most post-AMI patients should be enrolled in a cardiac rehabilitation program that emphasizes dietary modification, risk factor reduction, and exercise. The low-risk patient does not require prolonged supervised exercise, as previously discussed. All patients, however, can benefit from a structured environment to launch a lifetime of healthy living. Cardiac rehabilitation is discussed in Chap. 50 and risk factors and the prevention of coronary artery disease are discussed in Chap. 38.

There has been considerable reinvigoration of interest in the potential of dietary interventions in secondary prevention after AMI since the publication of the results of the Lyon Diet Study[661] and of the GISSI-Prevention Study.[662] Both of these studies showed dramatic (>30 percent) reduction in recurrence of cardiovascular events in patients in whom a diet and supplements rich in omega-3 fatty acids was added to adequate conventional therapy. Thus, in view of the minimal or absent risk it seems prudent to recommend that patients incorporate into their dietary regimes sources of omega-3 fatty acids (fish: especially tuna, salmon, and sardines; nuts such as walnuts; and probably fish oil supplements).

References

1. Ryan TJ, Antman EM, Brooks NH, et al. 1999 Update: ACC/AHA guidelines for the management of patients with acute myocardial infarction: A report of the American College of Cardiology/American Heart Association Task Force on Practice Guidelines (Committee on Management of Acute Myocardial Infarction). *J Am Coll Cardiol* 1999; 34:904.
2. Ryan TJ, Anderson JL, Antman EM, et al. ACC/AHA guidelines for the management of patients with acute myocardial infarction: A report of the American College of Cardiology/American Heart Association Task Force on Practice Guidelines (Committee on Management of Acute Myocardial Infarction). *J Am Coll Cardiol* 1996; 28:1328.
3. Osler W. *The Principles and Practice of Medicine*. New York: Appleton and Company; 1892.
4. Herrick JB. Clinical features of sudden obstruction of the coronary arteries. *JAMA* 1912; 59:2015.
5. Roberts WC, Buja LM. The frequency and significance of coronary arterial thrombi and other observations in fatal acute myocardial infarction. *Am J Med* 1972; 52:425.
6. Rentrop KP, Blanke H, Karsch KR, et al. Coronary angiographic findings and left ventricular pump function in acute infarction and changes in chronic stage infarction. *Z Kardiol* 1979; 68:335.
7. DeWood MA, Spores J, Notske R, et al. Prevalence of total coronary occlusion during the early hours of transmural myocardial infarction. *N Engl J Med* 1980; 303:897.
8. Bristow JD, Burchell HB, Campbell RW, et al. Report of the ad hoc committee on the indications for coronary arteriography. *Circulation* 1977; 55:969A.
9. Rentrop KP, Blanke H, Karsch KR, et al. Acute myocardial infarction: Intracoronary application of nitroglycerine and streptokinase. *Clin Cardiol* 1979; 2:354.
10. European Cooperative Study Group for Streptokinase Treatment in Acute Myocardial Infarction: Streptokinase in acute myocardial infarction. *N Engl J Med* 1979; 301:797.
11. Mathey DG, Kuck K-H, Tilsner V, et al. Nonsurgical coronary artery recanalization in acute transmural myocardial infarction. *Circulation* 1981; 63:489.
12. Stampfer MJ, Goldhaber SZ, Yusuf S, et al. Effect of intravenous streptokinase on acute myocardial infarction: Pooled results from randomized trials. *N Engl J Med* 1982; 307:1180.
13. Beta-Blocker Heart Attack Study Group. The beta-blocker heart attack trial. *JAMA* 1981; 246:2073.
14. GISSI: Gruppo Italiano per lo Studio della Streptochinasi nell'Infarto Miocardio. Effectiveness of intravenous thrombolytic treatment in acute myocardial infarction. *Lancet* 1986; 1:397.
15. GUSTO Investigators. An international randomized trial comparing four thrombolytic strategies for acute myocardial infarction. *N Engl J Med* 1993; 329:673.
16. Gunnar (ACC/AHA) RM, Passamani ER, Bourdillon PD, et al. Guidelines for the early management of patients with acute myocardial infarction. *J Am Coll Cardiol* 1990; 16:249.
17. Herlitz J, Blohm M, Hartford M, et al. Delay time in suspected acute myocardial infarction and the importance of its modification. *Clin Cardiol* 1989; 12:370.
18. National Heart, Lung, and Blood Institute *Morbidity and Mortality: Chartbook on Cardiovascular, Lung, and Blood Diseases.* Bethesda, MD: U.S. Department of Health and Human Services. Public Health Service, National Institutes of Health; May 1992.
19. Galis ZS, Sukhova GK, Lark MW, et al. Increased expression of matrix metalloproteinases and matrix degrading activity in vulnerable regions of human atherosclerotic plaques. *J Clin Invest* 1994; 94:2493.
20. Friesinger GC. The natural history of atherosclerotic coronary heart disease. In: Schlant RC, Alexander RW, eds. *The Heart,* 8th ed. New York: McGraw-Hill; 1994:1185.
21. van der Wal AC, Becker AE, van der Loos CM, et al. Site of intimal rupture or erosion of thrombosed coronary atherosclerotic plaques is characterized by an inflammatory process irrespective of the dominant plaque morphology. *Circulation* 1994; 89:36.
22. Mounsey P. Prodromal symptoms in myocardial infarction. *Br Heart J* 1951; 13:215.
23. Berk BC, Weintraub WS, Alexander RW. Elevaton of C-reactive protein in "active" coronary artery disease. *Am J Cardiol* 1990; 65:168.
24. Liuzzo G, Biasucci LM, Gallimore JR, et al. The prognostic value of C-reactive protein and serum amyloid a protein in severe unstable angina. *N Engl J Med* 1994; 331:417.
25. Ridker PM, Cushman M, Stampfer MJ, et al. Inflammation, aspirin, and the risk of cardiovascular disease in apparently healthy men. *N Engl J Med* 1997; 336:973.
26. Spodick DH, Flessas AP, Johnson MM. Association of acute respiratory symptoms with onset of acute myocardial infarction: Prospective investigation of 150 consecutive patients and matched controls. *Am J Cardiol* 1984; 53:481.
27. Saikku P. *Chlamydia pneumoniae* infection as a risk factor in acute myocardial infarction. *Eur Heart J* 1993; 14:62.
28. Miettinen H, Lehto S, Saikku P, et al. Association of *Chlamydia pneumoniae* and acute coronary heart disease events in non-insulin dependent diabetic and non-diabetic subjects in Finland. *Eur Heart J* 1996; 17:682.
29. Patel P, Mendall MA, Carrington D, et al. Association of *Helicobacter pylori* and *Chlamydia pneumoniae* infections with coro-

nary heart disease and cardiovascular risk factors. *Br Med J* 1995; 311:711.

30. Jackson LA, Campbell LA, Schmidt RA, et al. Specificity of detection of *Chlamydia pneumoniae* in cardiovascular atheroma: Evaluation of the innocent bystander hypothesis. *Am J Pathol* 1997; 150:1785.
31. Willich SN, Lewis M, Lowel H, et al. Physical exertion as a trigger of acute myocardial infarction. Triggers and mechanisms of myocardial infarction study group. *N Engl J Med* 1993; 329:1684.
32. Mittleman MA, Maclure M, Tofler GH, et al. Triggering of acute myocardial infarction by heavy physical exertion. Protection against triggering by regular exertion. Determinants of Myocardial Infarction Onset Study Investigators. *N Engl J Med* 1993; 329:1677.
33. Mittleman MA, Maclure M, Sherwood JB, et al. Triggering of acute myocardial infarction onset by episodes of anger. Determinants of Myocardial Infarction Onset Study Investigators. *Circulation* 1995; 92:1720.
34. Rahe RH, Romo M, Siltanen P. Recent life changes, myocardial infarction, and abrupt coronary death. *Arch Intern Med* 1974; 133:221.
35. Lundberg U, Theorell T, Lind E. Life changes and myocardial infarction: individual differences in life changes scaling. *J Psychosom Res* 1975; 37:27.
36. Jenkins CD. Recent evidence supporting psychologic and social risk factors for coronary disease. *N Engl J Med* 1976; 294:1033.
37. Mangano DT. Perioperative cardiac morbidity. *Anesthesiology* 1990; 72:153.
38. Leiberman RW, Orkin KF, Jobes DR, et al. Hemodynamic predictors of myocardial ischemia during halothane anesthesia for coronary artery revascularization. *Anesthesiology* 1983; 59:36.
39. Nelson AH, Fleisher LA, Rosenbaum SH. Relationship between postoperative anemia and cardiac morbidity in high risk vascular patients in the intensive care unit. *Crit Care Med* 1993; 21:860.
40. Frank SM, Beattie C, Christopherson R, et al. Unintentional hypothermia is associated with post-operative myocardial ischemia. *Anesthesiology* 1993; 78:468.
41. Frank SM, Fleisher LA, Breslow MD, et al. Perioperative maintenance of normothermia reduces the incidence of morbid cardiac events. *JAMA* 1997; 277:1127.
42. Zainea M, Duvernoy WF, Chauhan A, et al. Acute myocardial infarction in angiographically normal coronary arteries following induction of general anesthesia. *Arch Int Med* 1994; 154:2495.
43. Moliterno DJ, Willard JE, Lange RA, et al. Coronary-artery vasoconstriction induced by cocaine, cigarette smoking, or both. *N Engl J Med* 1994; 330:454.
44. Friedman M, Rosenman RH. Type A Behavior Pattern: Its association with coronary heart disease. *Ann Clin Res* 1971; 3:300.
45. Dimsdale JE. A perspective on type A behavior and coronary disease. *N Engl J Med* 1988; 318:110.
46. Muller JE, Stone PH, Turzi ZG, et al. Circadian variation in the frequency of onset of acute myocardial infarction. *N Engl J Med* 1985; 313:1315.
47. Mitler MM, Kripke DF. Circadian variation in myocardial infarction. *N Engl J Med* 1986; 314:1187.
48. Petralito A, Mangiafico RA, Giblino S, et al. Daily modifications of plasma fibrinogen, platelet aggregation, Howell's time, PTT, PT, and antithrombin III in normal subjects and in patients with vascular disease. *Chronobiologia* 1982; 9:195.
49. Rosing DR, Brakma P, Redwood DR, et al. Blood fibrinolytic activity in man: Diurnal variation and the response to varying intensities of exercise. *Circ Res* 1970; 27:171.
50. Marshall J. Diurnal variation in occurrence of strokes. *Stroke* 1977; 8:230.
51. Sayer JW, Wilkinson P, Ranjadayalan K, et al. Attenuation or absence of circadian and seasonal rhythms of acute myocardial infarction. *Heart* 1977; 77:325.
52. Quyyumi AA, Mockus L, Wright C, et al. Morphology of ambulatory ST segment changes in patients with varying severity of coronary artery disease: Investigation of the frequency of nocturnal ischemia and coronary spasm. *Br Heart J* 1985; 53:186.
53. el-Tamimi H, Mansour M, Pepine CJ, et al. Circadian variation in coronary tone in patients with stable angina. Protective role of the endothelium. *Circulation* 1995; 92:3201.
54. Millar-Craig MW, Bishop CN, Raftery EB. Circadian variation of blood pressure. *Lancet* 1978; 1:795.
55. Turton MB, Deegan T. Circadian variations of plasma catecholamine, cortisol, and immunoreactive insulin concentrations in supine subjects. *Clin Chim Acta* 1974; 55:389.
56. Willich SN, Lowel H, Lewis M, et al. Weekly variation of acute myocardial infarction. Increased Monday risk in the working population. *Circulation* 1994; 90:87.
57. Spielberg C, Falkenhahn D, Willich SN, et al. Circadian, day-of-week, and seasonal variability in myocardial infarction: Comparison between working and retired patients. *Am Heart J* 1996; 132:579.
58. Hofgren C, Karlson BW, Herlitz J. Prodromal symptoms in subsets of patients hospitalized for suspected acute myocardial infarction. *Heart Lung* 1995; 24:3.
59. Gill JB, Cairns JA, Roberts RS, et al. Prognostic importance of myocardial ischemia detected by ambulatory monitoring early after acute myocardial infarction. *N Engl J Med* 1996; 334:65.
60. Maseri A, Crea F, Kaski JC, et al. Mechanisms and significance of cardiac ischemic pain. *Prog Cardiovas Dis* 1992; 35:1.
61. Maseri A. The changing face of angina pectoris: Practical implications. *Lancet* 1983; 1:746.
62. Everts B, Karlson BW, Wahrborg P, et al. Localization of pain in suspected acute myocardial infarction in relation to final diagnosis, age and sex, and site and type of infarction in relation to final diagnosis, age and sex, and site and type of infarction. *Heart Lung* 1996; 25:430.
63. Herlitz J, Bang A, Isaksson L, et al. Ambulance dispatchers' estimation of intensity of pain and presence of associated symptoms in relation to outcome in patients who call for an ambulance because of acute chest pain. *Eur Heart J* 1995; 16:1789.
64. Margolis JR, Kannel WB, Feinleich M, et al. Clinical features of unrecognized myocardial infarction—silent and symptomatic. *Am J Cardiol* 1973; 32:1.
65. Bean WB. Masquerades of myocardial infarction. *Lancet* 1977; 1:1044.
66. Madias JE, Chintalapaly G, Choudry M, et al. Correlates and in-hospital outcome of painless presentation of acute myocardial infarction: A prospective study of a consecutive series of patients admitted to the coronary care unit. *J Invest Med* 1995; 43:567.
67. Jaffe AS, Roberts R. Precordial inspection and palpation in patients with acute myocardial infarction. *Prac Cardiol* 1981; 7:46.
68. Fowler NO. Physical signs in acute myocardial infarction and its complications. *Prog Cardiovasc Dis* 1968; 10:287.
69. Harvey WP. Some pertinent physical findings in the clinical evaluation of acute myocardial infarction. *Circulation* 1969; 40 (Suppl 4):175.
69a. Killip T III, Kimball JT. Treatment of myocardial infarction in a coronary care unit: A two year experience with 250 patients. *Am J Cardiol* 1967; 20:457.
70. Goldman L, Cook EF, Brand DA, et al. A computer protocol to predict myocardial infarction in emergency department patients with chest pain. *N Engl J Med* 1988; 318:797.
71. Lee TH, Rouan GW, Weisberg MC, et al. Sensitivity of routine clinical criteria for diagnosing myocardial infarction within 24 hours of hospitalization. *Ann Intern Med* 1987; 106:181.

72. Lee TH, Juarez G, Cook EF, et al. Ruling out acute myocardial infarction. *N Engl J Med* 1991; 324:1239.
73. Lee TH, Weisberg MC, Brand DA, et al. Candidates for thrombolysis among emergency room patients with acute chest pain. *Ann Intern Med* 1989; 110:957.
74. Roberts R. The two out of three criteria for the diagnosis of infarction—Is it passe? *Chest* 1984; 86:511.
75. Parker AB III, Waller BF, Gering LE. Usefulness of the 12-lead electrocardiogram in detection of myocardial infarction: Electrocardiographic, anatomic correlations, Part I. *Clin Cardiol* 1999; 19:55.
76. Cook RW, Edwards JE, Pruitt RD. Electrocardiographic changes in acute subendocardial infarction. I. Large subendocardial and large transmural infarcts. *Circulation* 1958; 18:603.
77. Gunnar RM, Pietras RJ, Blackaller J, et al. Correlation of vectocardiographic criteria for myocardial infarction with autopsy findings. *Circulation* 1967; 35:158.
78. Wagner NB, White RD, Wagner GS. The 12-lead ECG and the extent of myocardium at risk of acute infarction: Cardiac anatomy and lead locations, and the phases of serial changes during acute occlusion. In Califf RM, Mark DB, Wagner GS, eds. *Acute Coronary Care in the Thrombolytic Era.* Chicago: Year Book Medical Publishers; 1988:31.
79. Ambos HD, Moore P, Roberts R. A database for analysis of patient diagnostic data. In *Computers in Cardiology*. Long Beach, CA: IEEE Computer Society; 1978.
80. Gibson RS, Boden WE, Theroux P, et al. Diltiazem and reinfarction in patients with non-Q-wave myocardial infarction. Results of a double-blind, randomized, multicenter trial. *N Engl J Med* 1986; 315:423.
81. Bodenheimer MM, Banka VS, Trout RG, et al. Relationship between myocardial fibrosis and epicardial and surface electrocardiographic Q-waves in man. *J Electrocardiol* 1979; 12:205.
82. Pratt CM, Roberts R. Non-Q-wave myocardial infarction: Recognition, pathogenesis, prognosis and management. In McIntosh HD, eds. *Baylor Cardiology Series,* 8th ed. Houston: Baylor College of Medicine; 1985:5.
83. Wilson FN, Johnston FD, Hill IGW. The form of the electrocardiogram in experimental myocardial infarction. IV. Additional observations with later effects produced by ligation of the anterior descending branch on the left coronary artery. *Am Heart J* 1935; 10:1025.
84. Spodick DH. Q-wave infarction versus S-T infarction: Nonspecificity of electrocardiographic criteria for differentiating transmural and nontransmural lesions. *Am J Cardiol* 1983; 51: 913.
85. Roberts R. Nontransmural myocardial infarction. *Newsletter of the Council on Clinical Cardiology, American Heart Association* 1985; 11:1–17.
86. Eaton LW, Bulkley HG. Extension of acute myocardial infarction: Its relationship to infarct morphology in a canine model. *Circ Res* 1981; 49:80.
87. Gibson RS. Non-Q-wave myocardial infarction diagnosis, prognosis and management. *Curr Probl Cardiol* 1988; 13:9.
88. Marmor A, Sobel BE, Roberts R. Factors presaging early recurrent myocardial infarction ("extension"). *Am J Cardiol* 1981; 48:603.
89. Marmor A, Geltman EM, Schechtman K, et al. Recurrent myocardial infarction: Clinical predictors and prognostic implications. *Circulation* 1982; 66:415.
90. Schaer DH, Ross AM, Wasserman AG. Reinfarction, recurrent angina and reocclusion after thrombolytic therapy. *Circulation* 1987; 76(2 Pt 2):II.
91. Sgarbossa EB, Pinski SL, Barbagelata A, et al. Electrocardiographic diagnosis of evolving acute myocardial infarction in the presence of left bundle branch block. GUSTO-1 (Global Utilization of Streptokinase and Tissue Plasminogen Activator for Occluded Coronary Arteries) Investigators. *N Engl J Med* 1996; 334:481.
92. Helfant RH, Banka VS. *A Clinical and Angiographic Approach to Coronary Heart Disease.* Philadelphia: Davis; 1978.
93. Fenichel NM, Kugell VH. The large Q wave of the electrocardiogram. A correlation with pathologic observations. *Am Heart J* 1931; 7:235.
94. Rude RE, Poole WK, Muller JE, et al. Electrocardiographic and clinical criteria for recognition of acute myocardial infarction based on analysis of 3,697 patients. *Am J Cardiol* 1983; 52:936.
95. Bodenheimer MM, Banka VS, Helfant RH. Q-waves and ventricular asynergy: Predictive value and hemodynamic significance of anatomic localization. *Am J Cardiol* 1975; 35:615.
96. Schamroth L. Posterior Wall Myocardial Infarction. In *The 12-Lead Electrocardiogram, Book 1 (of 2).* Boston: Blackwell Scientific Publications; 1989:176.
97. Geft IL, Shah PK, Rodriguez L, et al. ST elevations in leads V_1 to V_5 may be caused by right coronary artery occlusion and acute right ventricular infarction. *Am J Cardiol* 1984; 53:991.
98. Lopez-Sendon J, Coma-Canella I, Alcasena S, et al. Electrocardiographic findings in acute right ventricular infarction: Sensitivity and specificity of electrocardiographic alterations in right precordial leads V4R, V3R, V1, V2, and V3. *J Am Coll Cardiol* 1985; 6:1273.
99. Erhardt L, Sjogren A, Wahlberg I. Single right-sided precordial lead in the diagnosis of right ventricular involvement in inferior myocardial infarction. *Am Heart J* 1976; 91:571.
100. Sivertssen E, Hoel B, Bay G, et al. Electrocardiographic atrial complex and acute atrial myocardial infarction. *Am J Cardiol* 1973; 31:450.
101. Mirvis DM. Physiologic bases for anterior ST segment depression in patients with acute inferior wall myocardial infarction. *Am Heart J* 1988; 116:1308.
102. Muller DW, Topol EJ, Califf RM, et al. Relationship between antecedent angina pectoris and short-term prognosis after thrombolytic therapy for acute myocardial infarction. Thrombolysis and Angioplasty in Myocardial Infarction (TAMI) Study Group. *Am Heart J* 1990; 119(2 Pt 1):224.
103. Roberts R, Gowda KS, Ludbrook PA, et al. Specificity of elevated serum MB CPK activity in the diagnosis of acute myocardial infarction. *Am J Cardiol* 1975; 36:433.
104. Klein MS, Shell WE, Sobel BE. Serum creatine phosphokinase (CPK) isoenzymes after intramuscular injections, surgery, and myocardial infarction. Experimental and clinical studies. *Cardiovasc Res* 1973; 7:412.
105. Perryman MB, Kerner SA, Bohlmeyer TJ, et al. Isolation and sequence analysis of a full-length cDNA for human M creatine kinase. *Biochem Biophys Res Commun* 1986; 140:981.
106. Villarreal-Levy G, Ma TS, Kerner SA, et al. Human creatine kinase: Isolation and sequence analysis of cDNA closes for the B subunit, development of subunit specific probes and determination of gene copy number. *Biochem Biophys Res Commun* 1987; 144:1116.
107. Tsung JS, Tsung SS. Creatine kinase isoenzymes in extracts of various human skeletal muscles. *Clin Chem* 1986; 32:1568.
108. Wilhelm AH, Albers KM, Todd JK. Creatine phosphokinase isoenzyme distribution in human skeletal and heart muscles. *IRCS Med Sci* 1976; 4:418.
109. Roberts R, Henry PD, Witteveen SAGJ, et al. Quantification of serum creatine phosphokinase (CPK) isoenzyme activity. *Am J Cardiol* 1974; 33:650.
110. Yasmineh WG, Ibrahim GA, Abbasnezhad MA, et al. Isoenzyme distribution of creatine kinase and lactate dehydrogenase in serum and skeletal muscle in Duchenne muscular dystrophy, collagen disease, and other muscular disorders. *Clin Chem* 1978; 24:1985.

111. Apple FS, Rogers MA, Sherman WM, et al. Profile of creatine kinase isoenzymes in skeletal muscles of marathon runners. *Clin Chem* 1984; 30:413.
112. Siegel AJ, Silverman LM, Evans WJ. Elevated skeletal muscle creatine kinase MB isoenzyme levels in marathon runners. *JAMA* 1983; 250:2835.
113. Keshgegian AA, Feiberg NW. Serum creatine kinase MB isoenzyme in chronic muscle disease. *Clin Chem* 1984; 30:575.
114. Shahangian S, Ash KO, Wahlstrom NO Jr, et al. Creatine kinase and lactate dehydrogenase isoenzymes in serum of patients suffering burns, blunt trauma, or myocardial infarction. *Clin Chem* 1984; 30:1332.
115. McBride JW, Labrosse KR, McCoy HG, et al. Is serum creatine kinase MB in electrically injured patients predictive of myocardial injury? *JAMA* 1986; 255:764.
116. Foxall CD, Emery AE. Changes in creatine kinase and its isoenzymes in human fetal muscle during development. *J Neurol Sci* 1975; 24:483.
117. Tzvetanova E. Creatine kinase isoenzymes in muscle tissue of patients with neuromuscular diseases and human fetuses. *Enzyme* 1971; 12:279.
118. Sadeh M, Stern LZ, Czyzewski K, et al. Alterations of creatine kinase, ornithine decarboxylase, and transglutaminase during muscle regeneration. *Life Sci* 1984; 34:483.
119. Plebani M, Zaninotto M. Diagnostic strategies in myocardial infarction using myoglobin measurement. *Eur Heart J* 1998; 19:N12.
120. Hartmann F, Kampmann MF, Frey N, et al. Biochemical markers in the diagnosis of coronary artery disease. *Eur Heart J* 1998; 19:N2.
121. Apple FS, Ricchiuti V, Voss EM, et al. Expression of cardiac troponin T isoforms in skeletal muscle of renal disease patients will not cause false-positive serum results by the second generation cardiac troponin T assay. *Eur Heart J* 1998; 19:N31.
122. Adams JE, Bodor GS, Davila-Roman VG, et al. Cardiac Troponin I: A marker with high specificity for cardiac injury. *Circulation* 1993; 88:101.
123. Bodor GS, Porterfield D, Voss EM, et al. Cardiac troponin I is not expressed in fetal and healthy or diseased adult human skeletal muscle tissue. *Clin Chem* 1995; 41:1710.
124. Zimmerman J, Fromm R, Meyer D, et al. Diagnostic marker cooperative study (DMCS) for the diagnosis of myocardial infarction. *Circulation* 1999; 99:1671.
125. HCIA. *Diagnostic Regional Groupings Handbook.* Washington DC; 1993.
126. Guadagnoli E, Hauptman PJ, Ayanian JZ, et al. Variation in the use of cardiac procedures after acute myocardial infarction. *N Engl J Med* 1995; 333:573.
127. Wevers RA, Delsing M, Klein-Gebbink JA, et al. Post-synthetic changes in creatine kinase isoenzymes. *Clin Chim Acta* 1978; 86:323.
128. George S, Ishikawa Y, Perryman MB, et al. Purification and characterization of naturally occurring and in vitro induced multiple forms of MM creatine kinase. *J Biol Chem* 1984; 259:2667.
129. Perryman MB, Knell JD, Roberts R. Carboxypeptidase-catalyzed hydrolysis of Cxterminal lysine: Mechanism for in vivo production of multiple forms of creatine kinase in plasma. *Clin Chem* 1984; 30:662.
130. Puleo PR, Guadagno PA, Roberts R, et al. Sensitive, rapid assay of subforms of creatine kinase MB in plasma. *Clin Chem* 1989; 35:1452.
131. Puleo PR, Meyer D, Wathen C, et al. Use of rapid assay of subforms of creatine kinase MB to diagnose or rule out acute myocardial infarction. *N Engl J Med* 1994; 331:561.
132. Somer H, Dubowitz V, Donner M. Creatine kinase isoenzymes in neuromuscular diseases. *J Neurol Sci* 1976; 29:129.
133. Goldman J, Matz R, Mortimer R, et al. High elevations of creatine phosphokinase in hypothyroidism: An isoenzyme analysis. *JAMA* 1977; 238:325.
134. Muller JE, Morrison J, Stone PH, et al. Nifedipine therapy for patients with threatened and acute myocardial infarction: A randomized, double-blind, placebo-controlled comparison. *Circulation* 1984; 69:740.
135. Urdal P, Landaas S. Macro creatine kinase BB in serum, and some data on its prevalence. *Clin Chem* 1979; 25:461.
136. Jaffe AS, Ritter C, Meltzer V, et al. Unmasking artifactual increases in creatine kinase isoenzymes in patients with renal failure. *J Lab Clin Med* 1984; 104:193.
137. Cummins B, Auckland M, Cummins P. Cardiac-specific troponin I radioimmunoassay in the diagnosis of acute myocardial infarction. *Am Heart J* 1987; 113:1333.
138. Cummings P, Young A, Auckland ML, et al. Comparison of serum cardiac specific troponin I with creatine kinase, creatine kinase-MB isoenzyme, tropomyosin, myoglobin and C-reactive protein release in marathon runners: Cardiac or skeletal muscle trauma? *Eur J Clin Invest* 1987; 17:317.
139. Adams JE, Sicard GA, Allen BT, et al. Diagnosis of perioperative myocardial infarction with measurement of cardiac troponin I. *N Engl J Med* 1994; 330:670.
140. Kobayashi S, Tanaka M, Tamura N, et al. Serum cardiac troponin T in polymyositis/dermatomyositis. *Lancet* 1992; 340:726.
141. Wu AHB, Valdes R, Apple FS, et al. Cardiac troponin-T immunoassay for diagnosis of acute myocardial infarction. *Clin Chem* 1994; 40:900.
142. Katus HA, Looser S, Hallermayer K, et al. Development and in vitro characterization of a new immunoassay of cardiac troponin T. *Clin Chem* 1992; 38:386.
143. Abdelmeguid AE, Topol EJ, Whitlow PL, et al. Significance of mild transient release of creatine kinase MB fraction after percutaneous interventions. *Circulation* 1996; 94:1528.
144. Abdelmeguid AE, Ellis SG, Sapp SK, et al. Defining the appropriate threshold of creatine kinase elevation after percutaneous interventions. *Am Heart J* 1996; 131:1097.
145. Kini A, Marmur JD, Kini S, et al. Creatine kinase-MB elevation after coronary intervention correlates with diffuse atherosclerosis, and low-to-medium level elevation has a benign clinical course: Implications for early discharge after coronary intervention. *J Am Coll Cardiol* 1999; 34:663.
146. Abdelmeguid AE, Topol EJ. The myth of the myocardial 'infarctlet' during percutaneous coronary revascularization procedures. *Circulation* 1996; 94:3369.
147. Roberts R. Recognition, diagnosis, and prognosis of early reinfarction: The role of calcium channel blockers. *Circulation* 1987; 75:V139.
148. Turi ZG, Rutherford JD, Roberts R, et al. Electrocardiographic, enzymatic and scintigraphic criteria of acute myocardial infarction as determined from study of 726 patients (a MILIS Study). *Am J Cardiol* 1985; 55:1463.
149. Roberts R. Enzymatic diagnosis of acute myocardial infarction. *Chest* 1988; 93:3S.
150. MILIS Study Group, eds. *Nationl Heart, Lung, and Blood Institute Multicenter Investigation of the Limitation of Infarct Size (MILIS): Design and Methods of the Clinical Trial. An Investigation of Beta-Blockade and Hyaluronidase for Treatment of Acute Myocardial Infarction.* Monograph 100. Dallas: American Heart Association; 1984.
151. Ohman EM, Armstrong PW, Christenson RH, et al. Cardiac troponin T levels for risk stratification in acute myocardial ischemia. GUSTO IIA Investigators. *N Engl J Med* 1996; 335:1333.
152. Antman EM, Tanasijevic MJ, Thompson B, et al. Cardiac-specific troponin I levels to predict the risk of mortality in patients with acute coronary syndromes. *N Engl J Med* 1996; 335:1342.
153. Lindahl B, Venge P, Wallentin L, et al. Relation between tropo-

nin T and the risk of subsequent cardiac events in unstable coronary artery disease. *Circulation* 1996; 93:1651.
154. Roberts R, From R, Beaudreaux A, et al. Multi-center blinded trial utilizing multiple diagnostic markers to exclude myocardial infarction in patients presenting consecutively to the ER with chest pain (abs). *Circulation* 1996; 94:I.
155. Ishikawa Y, Saffitz JE, Mealman JE, et al. Reversible myocardial ischemic injury is not associated with increased creatine kinase activities in plasma. *Clin Chem* 1997; 43:467.
156. Hamburg RJ, Verani MS, Mahmarian JJ, et al. Absence of trace MB creatine kinase release following stress-induced myocardial ischemia (Abs). *J Am Coll Cardiol* 1993; 21:161A.
157. TIMI IIIB Investigators. Effects of tissue plasminogen activator and a comparison of early invasive and conservative strategies in unstable angina and non-Q-wave myocardial infarction: Results of the TIMI IIIB Trial. Thrombolysis in Myocardial Ischemia. *Circulation* 1994; 89:1545.
158. Roberts R, Sobel BE. Elevated plasma MB creatine phosphokinase activity. A specific marker for myocardial infarction in perioperative patients. *Arch Intern Med* 1976; 136:421.
159. Klein MS, Coleman RE, Weldon CS, et al. Concordance of electrocardiographic and scintigraphic criteria of myocardial injury after cardiac surgery. *J Thorac Cardiovasc Surg* 1976; 71:934.
160. Righetti A, O'Rourke RA, Schelbert H, et al. Usefulness of preoperative and postoperative Tc-99m (Sn)-pyrophosphate scans in patients with ischemic and valvular heart disease. *Am J Cardiol* 1977; 39:43.
161. Goldberger AL. *Myocardial Infarction: Electrocardiographic Differential Diagnosis.* New York: CV Mosby; 1979:18–20.
162. Sullivan W, Vlodaver Z, Tuna N, et al. Correlation of electrocardiographic and pathologic findings in healed myocardial infarction. *Am J Cardiol* 1978; 42:724.
163. Tiefenbrunn AJ, Biello DR, Geltman EM, et al. Gated cardiac blood pool imaging and thallium-201 myocardial for detection of remote myocardial infarction. *Am J Cardiol* 1981; 47:1.
164. Gore JM, Goldberg RJ, Matsumoto AS, et al. Validity of serum total cholesterol level obtained within 24 hours of acute myocardial infarction. *Am J Cardiol* 1984; 54:722.
165. Ryder RE, Hayes TM, Mulligan IP, et al. How soon after myocardial infarction should plasma lipid values be assessed? *Br Med J* 1984; 289:1651.
166. Ceremuzynski L. Hormonal and metabolic reactions evoked by acute myocardial infarction. *Circ Res* 1981; 48:767.
167. Goldberger E, Alesio J, Woll F. The significance of hyperglycemia in myocardial infarction. *NY State Med J* 1945; 45:391.
168. Katz AS, Harrigan P, Parisi AF. The value and promise of echocardiography in acute myocardial infarction and coronary artery disease. *Clin Cardiol* 1992; 15:401.
169. Nisimura RA. Acute myocardial infarction: The role of echocardiography. In: Fuster V, Ross R, Topol EJ, eds. *Atherosclerosis and Coronary Artery Disease.* Philadelphia: Lippincott-Raven; 1996:855.
170. Harrison JK, Bashore TM. Assessment and management of the critically ill patient with valvular heart disease. In: Califf RM, Mark DB, Wagner GS, eds. *Acute Coronary Care.* St Louis: Mosby-Year Book; 1995:719.
171. Horowitz RS, Morganroth J, Parrotto C, et al. Immediate diagnosis of acute myocardial infarction by two-dimensional echocardiograpy. *Am Heart J* 1982; 103:814.
172. Berning J, Steensgaard-Hansen F. Early estimation of risk by echocardiographic determination of wall motion index in an unselected population with acute myocardial infarction. *Am J Cardiol* 1990; 65:567.
173. Sabia P, Abbott RD, Afrookteh A, et al. Importance of two-dimensional echocardiographic assessment of left ventricular function in patients presenting to the emergency room with cardiac-related symptoms. *Circulation* 1991; 84:1615.
174. Hepner AM, Armstrong WF. Echocardiography in acute myocardial infarction. In: Francis GS, Alpert JS, eds. *Coronary Care.* Boston: Little, Brown & Co.; 1995:473.
175. Sabia P, Afrookteh A, Touchstone DA, et al. Value of regional wall motion abnormality in the emergency room diagnosis of acute myocardial infarction: A prospective study using two-dimensional echocardiography. *Circulation* 1991; 84(Suppl I):I.
176. Kuhn MB, Egeblad H, Hojberg S, et al. Prognostic value of echocardiography compared to other clinical findings: Multivariate analysis based on long-term survival in 456 patients. *Cardiology* 1995; 86:157.
177. D'Arcy B, Nanda NC. Two-dimensional echocardiographic features of right ventricular ejection fraction in patients with coronary artery disease. *J Am Coll Cardiol* 1983; 2:911.
178. Tice FD, Kisslo J. Echocardiographic assessment and monitoring of the patient with acute myocardial infarction. Prospects for the Thrombolytic Era. In: Califf RM, Mark DB, Wagner GS, eds. *Acute Coronary Care,* St Louis: Mosby-Yearbook; 1994:49.
179. Cheitlin MD, Alpert JS, Armstrong WF, et al. ACC/AHA Guidelines for the Clinical Application of Echocardiography. A report of the American College of Cardiology/American Heart Association Task Force on Practice Guidelines (Committee on Clinical Application of Echocardiography). Developed in collaboration with the American Society of Echocardiography. *Circulation* 1997; 95:1686.
180. Johnston DL, Gupta VK, Wendt RE, et al. Detection of viable myocardium in segments with fixed defects on thallium-201 scintigraphy: Usefulness of magnetic resonance imaging early after acute myocardial infarction. *Magn Reson Imag* 1993; 11:949.
181. Holman ER, van Jonbergen HP, van Dijkman PR, et al. Comparison of magnetic resonance imaging studies with enzymatic indexes of myocardial necrosis for quantification of myocardial infarct size. *Am J Cardiol* 1993; 71:1036.
182. Kantor HL, Toussaint JF. Acute myocardial infarction: The role of magnetic resonance. In: Fuster V, Ross R, Topol EJ, eds. *Atherosclerosis and Coronary Artery Disease.* Philadelphia: Lippincott-Raven; 1996:905.
183. Hirose K, Reed JE, Rumberger JA. Serial changes in regional right ventricular free wall and left ventricular septal wall lengths during the first 4 to 5 years after index anterior wall myocardial infarction. *J Am Coll Cardiol* 1995; 26:394.
184. Foster CJ, Sekiya T, Love HG, et al. Identification of intracardiac thrombus: Comparison of computed tomography and cross-sectional echocardiography. *Br J Radiol* 1987; 60:327.
185. Ritchie JL, Bateman TM, Bonow RO, et al. Guidelines for clinical use of cardiac radionuclide imaging: Report of the American College of Cardiology/American Heart Association Task Force on Assessment of Diagnostic and Therapeutic Cardiovascular Procedures (Committee on Radionuclide Imaging), developed in collaboration with The American Society of Nuclear Cardiology. *J Am Coll Cardiol* 1995; 25:521.
186. Reduto LA, Berger HJ, Cohen LS, et al. Sequential radionuclide assessment of left and right ventricular performance after acute transmural myocardial infarction. *Ann Intern Med* 1978; 89:441.
187. Gibson WS, Christian TF, Pellikka PA, et al. Serial tomographic imaging with technetium-99m-sestamibi for the assessment of infarct-related arterial patency following reperfusion therapy. *J Nucl Med* 1992; 33:2080.
188. Christian TF, Schwartz RS, Gibbons RJ. Determinants of infarct size in reperfusion therapy for acute myocardial infarction. *Circulation* 1992; 86:81.
189. McCallister BD Jr, Christian TF, Gersh BJ, et al. Prognosis of myocardial infarctions involving more than 40% of the left ventricle after acute reperfusion therapy. *Circulation* 1993; 88:1470.
190. Miller TD, Christian TF, Hopfenspirger MR, et al. Infarct size after acute myocardial infarction measured by quantitative to-

mographic 99mTc sestamibi imaging predicts subsequent mortality. *Circulation* 1995; 92:334.
191. Fulton M, Julian DG, Oliver MF. Sudden death and myocardial infarction. *Circulation* 1969; 40:182.
192. Kuller L. Sudden death in arteriosclerotic heart disease: The case for preventive medicine. *Am J Cardiol* 1969; 24:617.
193. Adgey AAJ, Allen JD, Geddes JS, et al. Acute phase of myocardial infarction. *Lancet* 1971; 2:501.
194. Simon AB, Feinleib M, Thompson HK Jr. Components of delay in the prehospital phase of acute myocardial infarction. *Am J Cardiol* 1972; 30:476.
195. National Heart, Lung and Blood Institute. 9-1-1: *Rapid Identification and Treatment of Acute Myocardial Infarction.* NIH Publication 94-3302. Bethesda, MD: U.S. Department of Health and Human Services, Public Health Service, National Institutes of Health; 1994.
196. National Heart, Lung and Blood Institute. Patient/bystander recognition and action: Rapid identification and treatment of acute myocardial infarction. In: *National Heart Attack Alert Program* (*NHAAP*). NIH Publication NO. 93-3303. Bethesda, MD: National Institutes of Health; 1993.
197. Pressley JC, Severance HW Jr, Raney MP, et al. A comparison of paramedic versus basic emergency medical care of patients at high and low risk during acute myocardial infarction. *J Am Coll Cardiol* 1988; 12:1555.
198. Kareiakes DJ, Weaver WD, Anderson JL, et al. Time delays in the diagnosis and treatment of acute myocardial infarction: A tale of eight cities. Report from the Prehospital Study Group and the Cincinnati Heart Project. *Am Heart J* 1990; 120:773.
199. Goldstein S, Moss AJ, Greene W. Sudden death in acute myocardial infarction: Relationship to factors affecting delay in hospitalization. *Arch Intern Med* 1972; 129:720.
200. ACC/AHA Task Force, Gunnar RM, et al. ACC/AHA Guidelines for the early management of patients with acute myocardial infarction. *Circulation* 1990; 82:664.
201. Lewis RP, Lanese RR, Stang JM, et al. Reduction of mortality from prehospital myocardial infarction by prudent patient activation of mobile coronary care system. *Am Heart J* 1982; 103:123.
202. Eisenberg MS, Horwood BT, Cummins RO, et al. Cardiac arrest and resuscitation: A tale of 29 cities. *Ann Emerg Med* 1990; 19:179.
203. Cummins RO, Eisenberg MS, Litwin PE, et al. Automatic external defibrillators used by emergency medical technicians: A controlled clinical trial. *JAMA* 1987; 257:1605.
204. Kerber RE. *Statement on Early Defibrillation: AHA Medical/Scientific Statement.* Emergency Cardiac Care Committee. Chicago: American Heart Association; 1991.
205. Weaver WD, Hill D, Fahrenbruch CE, et al. Use of the automatic external defibrillator in the management of out-of-hospital cardiac arrest. *N Engl J Med* 1988; 319:661.
206. Stults KR, Brown DD, Schug VL, et al. Prehospital defibrillation performed by emergency medical technicians in rural communities. *N Engl J Med* 1984; 310:219.
207. Weaver WD, Cerqueira M, Hallstrom AP, et al. Prehospital-initiated vs. hospital-initiated thrombolytic therapy: The Myocardial Infarction Triage and Intervention Trial. *JAMA* 1993; 270:1211.
208. Weaver WD, Litwin PE, Martin JS, et al. Effect of age on use of thrombolytic therapy and mortality in acute myocardial infarction: The MITI Project Group. *J Am Coll Cardiol* 1991; 18:657.
209. Karagounis L, Ipsen SK, Jessop MR, et al. Impact of field-transmitted electrocardiography on time to in-hospital thrombolytic therapy in acute myocardial infarction. *Am J Cardiol* 1990; 66:786.
210. Fibrinolytic Therapy Trialists' (FTT) Collaborative Group. Indications for fibrinolytic therapy in suspected acute myocardial infarction: Collaborative overview of early mortality and major morbidity results from all randomized trials of more than one-thousand patients. *Lancet* 1994; 343:311.
211. ISIS-2 (Second International Study of Infarct Survival) Collaborative Group. Randomised trial of intravenous streptokinase, oral aspirin, both, or neither among 17,187 cases of suspected acute myocardial infarction: ISIS-2. *Lancet* 1988; 2:349.
212. GREAT Group. Feasibility, safety, and efficacy of domiciliary thrombolysis by general practitioners: Grampian Region Early Anistreplase Trial. *BMJ* 1992; 305:548.
213. Castaigne AD, Herve C, Duval-Moulin AM, et al. Prehospital use of APSAC: Results of a placebo-controlled study. *Am J Cardiol* 1989; 64(Suppl 2):30A.
214. Schofer J, Buttner J, Geng G, et al. Prehospital thrombolysis in acute myocardial infarction. *Am J Cardiol* 1990; 66:1429.
215. European Myocardial Infarction Project Group. Prehospital thrombolytic therapy in patients with suspected acute myocardial infarction. *N Engl J Med* 1993; 329:383.
216. Gibler WB, Kereiakes DJ, Dean EN, et al. Prehospital diagnosis and treatment of acute myocardial infarction: A North-South perspective. The Cincinnati Heart Project and the Nashville Prehospital TPA Trial. *Am Heart J* 1991; 121:1.
217. Jesse RL, Kontos MC. Evaluation of chest pain in the emergency department. *Current Problems in Cardiology* 1997; 22:149.
218. Stark ME, Vacek JL. The initial electrocardiogram during admission for myocardial infarction. *Arch Intern Med* 1987; 147:843.
219. Karlson BW, Herlitz J, Wiklund O, et al. Early prediction of acute myocardial infarction from clinical history, examination and electrocardiogram in the emergency room. *Am J Cardiol* 1991; 68:171.
220. Lee TH, Rouan GW, Weisberg MC, et al. Clinical characteristics natural history of patients with acute myocardial infarction sent home from the emergency room. *Am J Cardiol* 1987; 60:219.
221. Rouan GW, Hedges JR, Tolzis R, et al. A chest pain clinic to improve the follow-up of patients released from an urban university teaching hospital emergency department. *Ann Emerg Med* 1987; 16:1145.
222. Tierney WM, Roth BJ, Psaty B, et al. Predictors of myocardial infarction in emergency room patients. *Critical Care Med* 1985; 13:526.
223. McCarthy BD, Beshansky JR, D'Agostino RB, et al. Missed diagnoses of acute myocardial infarction in the emergency department: Results from a multicenter study. *Ann Emerg Med* 1993; 22:579.
224. Rusnak RA, Stair TO, Hansen K, et al. Litigation against the emergency physician: Common features in cases of missed myocardial infarction. *Ann Emerg Med* 1989; 18:1029.
225. Goldman L, Weinberg M, Weisberg M, et al. A computer-derived protocol to aid in the diagnosis of emergency room patients with acute chest pain. *N Engl J Med* 1982; 307:588.
226. Schroeder JS, Lamb IH, Hu M. Do patients in whom myocardial infarction has been ruled out have a better prognosis after hospitalization than those surviving infarction? *N Engl J Med* 1980; 303:1.
227. Kahn JK. Inadvertent thrombolytic therapy for cardiovascular diseases masquerading as acute coronary thrombosis. *Clin Cardiol* 1993; 16:67.
228. Butler J, Davies AH, Westaby S. Streptokinase in acute aortic dissection. *BMJ* 1990; 300:517.
229. Eriksen UH, Molgaard H, Ingerslev J, et al. Fatal haemostatic complications due to thrombolytic therapy in patients falsely diagnosed as acute myocardial infarction. *Eur Heart J* 1992; 13:840.
230. Katz PO, Dalton CB, Richter JE, et al. Esophageal testing of patients with noncardiac chest pain or dysphagia. *Ann Intern Med* 1987; 106:593.

231. Goyal RK. Changing focus on unexplained esophageal chest pain. *Ann Intern Med* 1996; 124:1008.
232. Nevens F, Janssens J, Piessens J, et al. Prospective study on prevalence of esophageal chest pain in patients referred on an elective basis to a cardiac unit for suspected myocardial ischemia. *Dig Dis Sci* 1991; 36:229.
233. Hewson EG, Sinclair JW, Dalton CB, et al. Twenty-four-hour esophageal pH monitoring: The most useful test for evaluating noncardiac chest pain. *Am J Med* 1991; 90:576.
234. Fruergaard P, Launbjerg J, Hesse B, et al. The diagnoses of patients admitted with acute myocardial infarction: A comparison between patients with and without confirmed myocardial infarction. *Eur Heart J* 1996; 17:1028.
235. Levene DL. Chest pain: Prophet of doom or nagging neurosis? *Acta Med Scand Supplementum* 1981; 644:11.
236. Ornato JP, Jesse RL, Tatum JL, et al. Lack of correlation between relief of chest pain after sublingual nitroglycerin and reversible radionuclide perfusion defects or presence of significant coronary atherosclerosis on coronary angiography (abs). *J Am Coll Cardiol* 1995; 25:12A.
237. Gibler W, Lewis L, Erb R, et al. Early detection of acute myocardial infarction in patients presenting with chest pain and nondiagnostic ECGs: Serial CK-MB sampling in the emergency department [published erratum appears in *Ann Emerg Med* 1991; 20(4):420]. *Ann Emerg Med* 1990; 19:1359.
238. Goldberg R, Gore J, Alpert J, et al. Incidence and case fatality rates of acute myocardial infarction (1975–1984): The Worcester Heart Attack Study. *Am Heart J* 1988; 115:761.
239. Marin MM, Teichman SL. Use of rapid serial sampling of creatine kinase MB for very early detection of myocardial infarction in patients with acute chest pain. *Am Heart J* 1992; 123:354.
240. Mauri F, Gasparini M, Barbonaglia L, et al. Prognostic significance of the extent of myocardial injury in acute myocardial infarction treated by streptokinase (the GISSI Trial). *Am J Cardiol* 1989; 63:1291.
241. Cohen M, Hawkins L, Greenberg S, et al. Usefulness of ST-segment changes in greater than or equal to 2 leads on the emergency room electrocardiogram in either unstable angina pectoris or non-Q-wave myocardial infarction in predicting outcome. *Am J Cardiol* 1991; 67:1368.
242. Slater DK, Hlatky MA, Mark DB, et al. Outcome in suspected acute myocardial infarction with normal or minimally abnormal admission electrocardiographic findings. *Am J Cardiol* 1987; 60:766.
243. Brush JE Jr, Brand DA, Acampora D, et al. Use of the initial electrocardiogram to predict in-hospital complications of acute myocardial infarction. *N Engl J Med* 1985; 312:1137.
244. Goldman L, Cook EF, Johnson PA, et al. Prediction of the need for intensive care in patients who come to emergency departments with acute chest pain. *N Engl J Med* 1996; 334:1498.
245. Pozen MW, D'Agostino RB, Selker HP, et al. A predictive instrument to improve coronary-care-unit admission practices in acute ischemic heart disease. *N Engl J Med* 1984; 310:1273.
246. Selker HP, Griffith JL, D'Agostino RB. A tool for judging coronary care unit admission appropriateness, valid for both real-time and retrospective use. *Med Care* 1991; 29:610.
247. Grijseels EWM, Deckers JW, Hoes AW, et al. Pre-hospital triage of patients with suspected myocardial infarction. *Eur Heart J* 1995; 16:325.
248. Fillmore SJ, Shapiro M, Killip T. Arterial oxygen tension in acute myocardial infarction: Serial analysis of clinical state and blood gas changes. *Am Heart J* 1970; 79:620.
249. Madias JE, Hood WB Jr. Reduction of precordial ST-segment elevation in patients with anterior myocardial infarction by oxygen breathing. *Circulation* 1976; 53(Suppl I):I.
250. Lowenstein E. Morphine "anesthesia"—a perspective. *Anesthesiology* 1971; 35:563.
251. Herlitz J. Analgesia in myocardial infarction. *Drugs* 1989; 37:939.
252. Antman EM. General hospital management. In: Julian DG, Braunwald E, eds. *Management of Acute Myocardial Infarction*. London, England: WB Saunders; 1994:42.
253. Chiariello M, Gold HK, Leinbach RC, et al. Comparison between the effects of nitroprusside and nitroglycerin on ischemic injury during acute myocardial infarction. *Circulation* 1976; 54:766.
254. Mann T, Cohn PF, Holman L, et al. Effect of nitroprusside on regional myocardial blood flow in coronary artery disease: Results in 25 patients in comparison with nitroglycerin. *Circulation* 1978; 57:732.
255. Bussmann WD, Passek D, Seidel W, et al. Reduction of CK and CK-MB indexes of infarct size by intravenous nitroglycerin. *Circulation* 1981; 63:615.
256. Flaherty JT, Becker LC, Bulkley BH, et al. A randomized prospective trial of intravenous nitroglycerin in patients with acute myocardial infarction. *Circulation* 1983; 68:576.
257. Jugdutt BI, Becker LC, Hutchins GM, et al. Effect of intravenous nitroglycerin on collateral blood flow and infarct size in the conscious dog. *Circulation* 1981; 63:17.
258. Jugdutt BI, Khan MI, Jugdutt SJ, et al. Impact of left ventricular unloading after late reperfusion of canine anterior myocardial infarction on remodeling and function using isosorbide-5-mononitrate. *Circulation* 1995; 92:926.
259. Yusuf S, Collins R, MacMahon S, et al. Effect of intravenous nitrates on mortality in acute myocardial infarction: An overview of the randomized trials. *Lancet* 1989; 1:1088.
260. GISSI-3, Gruppo Italiano per lo Studio della Streptochinasi nell'Infarto Miocardico. Effects of lisinopril and transdermal glycerol trinitrate singly and together on 6-week mortality and ventricular function after acute myocardial infarction. *Lancet* 1994; 343:1115.
261. ISIS-4 Collaborative Group. ISIS-4: A randomized factorial trial assessing early oral captopril, oral mononitrate, and intravenous magnesium sulphate in 58,050 patients with suspected acute myocardial infarction. *Lancet* 1995; 345:669.
262. Kinch JW, Ryan TJ. Right ventricular infarction. *N Engl J Med* 1994; 330:1211.
263. Come PC, Pitt B. Nitroglycerin-induced severe hypotension and bradycardia in patients with acute myocardial infarction. *Circulation* 1976; 54:624.
264. Fourth American College of Chest Physicians Consensus Conference on Antithrombotic Therapy. Consensus Conference on Antithrombotic Therapy. *Chest* 1995; 108(Suppl):225S.
265. Monocada S, Vane JR. The role of prostacyclin in vascular tissue. *Fed Proc* 1979; 38:66.
266. CAPRIE Steering Committee. A randomised, blinded, trial of clopidogrel versus aspirin in patients at risk of ischaemic events (CAPRIE). *Lancet* 1996; 348:1329.
267. Reimer KA, Lowe JE, Rasmussen MM, et al. The wavefront phenomenon of ischemic cell death. I. Myocardial infarct size vs duration of coronary occlusion in dog. *Circulation* 1977; 56:786.
268. Reimer KA, Jennings RB. The "wave front phenomenon" of myocardial ischemia cell death. II. Transmural progression of necrosis within the framework of ischemic bed size (myocardium at risk) and collateral flow. *Lab Invest* 1979; 40:633.
269. Lau J, Antman EN, Jimenez-Silva J, et al. Cumulative meta-analysis of therapeutic trials for myocardial infarction. *N Engl J Med* 1992; 327:248.
270. MIAMI Trial Research Group. Metoprolol in acute myocardial infarction: Patient population. *Am J Cardiol* 1985; 56:1G.
271. TIMI Study Group. Comparison of invasive and conservative strategies after treatment with intravenous tissue plasminogen activator in acute myocardial infarction. Results of thrombolysis in myocardial infarction (TIMI) phase II trial. *N Engl J Med* 1989; 320:618.

272. Langer A, Goodman SG, Topol EJ, et al. Late Assessment of Thrombolytic Efficacy (LATE) Study: Prognosis in patients with non-Q wave myocardial infarction. *J Am Coll Cardiol* 1996; 27:1333.
273. Collins R, Peto R, Baigent C, et al. Aspirin, heparin, and fibrinolytic therapy in suspected acute myocardial infarction. *Drug Therapy* 1997; 36:847.
274. ISIS-2 (Second International Study of Infarct Survival) Collaborative Group. Randomized trial of intravenous streptokinase, oral aspirin, both, or neither among 17,187 cases of suspected acute myocardial infarction: ISIS-2. *J Am Coll Cardiol* 1988; 12:3A.
275. ISIS-3 Collaborative Group. A randomized comparison of streptokinase vs tissue plasminogen activator vs anistreplase and of aspirin plus heparin vs aspirin alone among 41,299 cases of suspected acute myocardial infarction. *Lancet* 1992; 339:753.
276. GISSI-2 Gruppo Italiano per lo Studio della Streptochinasi nell'Infarto Miocardico. A factorial randomised trial of alteplace versus streptokinase and heparin versus no heparin among 12,490 patients with acute myocardial infarction. *Lancet* 1990; 336:65.
277. GUSTO III Investigators. A comparison of reteplase with alteplase for acute myocardial infarction. *N Engl J Med* 1997; 337:1118.
278. Gurfinkel EP, Manos EJ, Mejail RI, et al. Low molecular weight heparin versus regular heparin or aspirin in the treatment of unstable angina and silent ischemia. *J Am Coll Cardiol* 1995; 26:313.
279. Piegas LS, Canon SJF, Avezum AJ. Arterial patency and ejection fraction after late thrombolysis with streptokinase. Results from EMERAS (abs). *Eur Heart J* 1991; 12:97.
280. Wilcox R. LATE assessment of thrombolytic efficacy: Randomized trial of altepase or placebo 6–24 hours after symptoms of acute myocardial infarction. *Eur Heart J* 1992; 13:423(Abs).
281. GUSTO IIb Angioplasty Substudy Investigators. A clinical trial comparing primary coronary angioplasty with tissue plasminogen activator for acute myocardial infarction. *N Engl J Med* 1997; 336:1621.
282. Grines CL, De Maria AN. Optimal utilization of thrombolytic therapy for acute myocardial infarction: Concepts and controversies. *J Am Coll Cardiol* 1990; 16:223.
283. Califf RM, Topol EJ, Kereiakes DJ, et al. Cardiac resuscitation should not be a contraindication to thrombolytic therapy for myocardial infarction. *Circulation* 1988; 78:II.
284. Hsia J, Hamilton WP, et al. For HART Investigators. A comparison between heparin and low-dose aspirin as adjunctive therapy with tissue plasminogen activator for acute myocardial infarction. Heparin-Aspirin Reperfusion Trial (HART) Investigators. *N Engl J Med* 1990; 323:1433.
285. Roberts R, Kleiman NS. *The Open Artery: Perspectives on Coronary Reperfusion in Acute Myocardial Infarction.* Hamilton, Ontario, Canada: Decker Periodicals; 1992.
286. Granger CG, Califf RM, Hirsch J, et al. APTTs after thrombolysis and standard intravenous heparin are often low and correlate with body weight, age and sex: Experience from the GUSTO Trial. *Circulation* 1992; 86:I.
287. Roberts R. La difference: Long-term benefit of one thrombolytic over another. *Circulation* 1996; 94:1203.
288. Bode C, Smalling RW, Berg G, et al. Randomized comparison of coronary thrombolysis achieved with double-bolus reteplase (recombinant plasminogen activator) and front-loaded, accelerated alteplase (recombinant tissue plasminogen activator) in patients with acute myocardial infarction. *Circulation* 1996; 94:891.
289. Smalling RW, Bode C, Kalbfleisch J, et al. More rapid, complete, and stable coronary thrombolysis with bolus administration of reteplase compared with alteplase infusion in acute myocardial infarction. *Circulation* 1995; 91:2725.
290. Hampton JR, Schroder R, Wilcox RG, et al. Randomised, double-blind comparison of reteplase double-bolus administration with streptokinase in acute myocardial infarction (INJECT): trial to investigate equivalence. *Lancet* 1995; 346:329.
291. Cody RJ. Results from late breaking clinical trials sessions at ACC '97. *J Am Coll Cardiol* 1997; 30:1.
292. Cannon CP, Gibson CM, McCabe C, et al. TNK-tissue plasminogen activator compared with front-loaded alteplase in acute myocardial infarction. Results of the TIMI 10B Trial. *Circulation* 1998; 98:2805.
293. Van de Werf F. Assessment of the safety and efficacy of a new thrombolytic: TNK-tPA (ASSENT-2). unpublished work. 1999.
294. Van de Werf F, Cannon CP, Luyten A, et al. Safety assessment of single-bolus administration of TNK tissue-plasminogen activator in acute myocardial infarction: The ASSENT-1 trial. The ASSENT-1 Investigators. *Am Heart J* 1999; 137:786.
295. Neuhaus KL. A phase III trial of novel bolus thrombolytic lanoteplase. Intravenous plasminogen activator for early treatment of infarcting myocardium. Handout at 48th Scientific Session, American College of Cardiology, New Orleans; 1999.
296. Ryan TJ, Bauman WB, Kennedy JW, et al. ACC/AHA guidelines for percutaneous transluminal coronary angioplasty: A report of the American College of Cardiology/American Heart Association Task Force on Assessment of Diagnostic and Therapeutic Cardiovascular Procedures (Committee on Percutaneous Transluminal Coronary Angioplasty). *J Am Coll Cardiol* 1993; 22:2033.
297. Weaver WD, Simes RJ, Betriu A, et al. Comparison of primary coronary angioplasty and intravenous thrombolytic therapy for acute myocardial infarction: A quantitative review [published erratum appears in *JAMA* 1998; 279:1876]. *JAMA* 1997; 278:2093.
298. Tiefenbrunn AJ, Chandra NC, French WJ, et al. Clinical experience with primary percutaneous transluminal coronary angioplasty compared with alteplase (recombinant tissue-type plasminogen activator) in patients with acute myocardial infarction: A report from the Second National Registry of Myocardial Infarction (NRMI-2). *J Am Coll Cardiol* 1998; 31:1240.
299. Hochman JS, Sleeper LA, Webb JG, et al. Early revascularization in acute myocardial infarction complicated by cardiogenic shock. *N Engl J Med* 1999; 341:625.
300. Brodie BR, Stuckey TD, Wall TC, et al. Importance of time to reperfusion for 30-day and late survival and recovery of left ventricular function after primary angioplasty for acute myocardial infarction. *J Am Coll Cardiol* 1998; 32:1312.
301. Grines CL, Browne KF, Marco J, et al. A comparison of immediate angioplasty with thrombolytic therapy for acute myocardial infarction: The Primary Angioplasty in Myocardial Infarction Study Group. *N Engl J Med* 1993; 328:673.
302. Zijlstra F, deBoer MJ, Hoorntje JC, et al. A comparison of immediate coronary angioplasty with intravenous streptokinase in acute myocardial infarction. *N Engl J Med* 1993; 328:680.
303. Roberts R. Heparin and aspirin in thrombolysis: Biological and clinical issues. *Clin Challenges* 1992; 1:1.
304. Francis CW, Markham RE Jr, Barlow GH, et al. Thrombin activity of fibrin thrombi and soluble plasmic derivatives. *J Lab Clin Med* 1983; 102:220.
305. Funk CD, Funk LB, Kennedy ME, et al. Human platelet/erythroleukemia cell prostaglandin G/H synthase: cDNA cloning, expression, and gene chromosomal assignment. *FASEB J* 1991; 5:2304.
306. Hsia J, Kleiman N, et al. for HART Investigators. Heparin-induced prolongation of partial thromboplastin time after thrombolysis: Relation to coronary artery patency. *J Am Coll Cardiol* 1992; 20:31.

307. Bleich SD, Nochols TC, Schumacher RR, et al. Effect of heparin on coronary arterial patency after thrombolysis with tissue plasminogen activator in acute myocardial infarction. *Am J Cardiol* 1990; 66:1412.
308. National Heart Foundation of Australia Coronary Thrombolysis Group. Coronary thrombolysis and myocardial salvage by tissue plasminogen activator given up to four hours after onset of myocardial infarction. *Lancet* 1988; 1:203.
309. Kander NH, Holland KJ, Pitt B, et al. A randomized pilot trial of brief versus prolonged heparin after successful reperfusion in acute myocardial infarction. *Am J Cardiol* 1990; 65:139.
310. Topol EJ, George BS, Kereiakes DJ, et al. A randomized controlled trial of intravenous tissue plasminogen activator and early intravenous heparin in acute myocardial infarction. *Circulation* 1989; 79:281.
311. Hull RD, Raskob GE, Hirsch J, et al. Continuous intravenous heparin compared with intermittent subcutaneous heparin in the initial treatment of proximal vein thrombosis. *N Engl J Med* 1986; 315:1109.
312. Prins MH, Hirsch J. Heparin as an adjunctive treatment after thrombolytic therapy for acute myocardial infarction. *Am J Cardiol* 1991; 67:3A.
313. SCATI Group. Randomised controlled trial of subcutaneous calcium-heparin in acute myocardial infarction. *Lancet* 1989; 2:182.
314. Komrad MS, Coffey CE, Coffey KS, et al. Myocardial infarction and stroke. *Neurology* 1984; 34:1403.
315. Simoons MS, Arnold AER, Betriu A, et al. Thrombolysis with tissue plasminogen activator in acute myocardial infarction. No additional benefit from immediate percutaneous coronary angioplasty. *Lancet* 1988; 1:197.
316. Verstraete M, Bory M, Collen D, et al. Randomized trial of intravenous recombinant tissue-type plasminogen activity versus intravenous streptokinase in active myocardial infarction. Report from the European Cooperative Study Group for Recombinant Tissue-Type Plasminogen Activator. *Lancet* 1985; 1:842.
317. SWIFT Trial Study Group. SWIFT Trial of delayed elective intervention versus conservative treatment after thrombolysis with anistreplase in acute myocardial infarction. *BMJ* 1991; 302:555.
318. Williams DO, Braunwald E, Knatterud G, et al. One-year results of the Thrombolysis in Myocardial Infarction (TIMI) Phase II Trial. *Circulation* 1992; 85:533.
319. Juliard JM, Himbert D, Golmard JL, et al. Can we provide reperfusion therapy to all unselected patients admitted with acute myocardial infarction? *J Am Coll Cardiol* 1997; 30:157.
320. Gibson CM, Cannon CP, Greene RM, et al. Rescue angioplasty in the thrombolysis in myocardial infarction (TIMI) 4 Trial. *Am J Cardiol* 1997; 80:21.
321. Lemmer JH, Ferguson DW, Rakel BA, et al. Clinical outcome of emergency repeat coronary artery bypass surgery. *J Cardiovas Surg (Torino)* 1990; 31:492.
322. O'Connor GT, Plume SK, Olmstead EM, et al. Multivariate prediction of in-hospital mortality associated with coronary artery bypass graft surgery: Northern New England Cardiovascular Disease Study Group. *Circulation* 1992; 85:2110.
323. Hochman JS, Boland J, Sleeper LA, et al. Current spectrum of cardiogenic shock and effect of early revascularization on mortality: Results of an International Registry. SHOCK Registry Investigators. *Circulation* 1995; 91:873.
324. Das G, Talmers FN, Weissler AM. New observations on the effects of atropine on the sinoatrial and atrioventricular nodes in man. *Am J Cardiol* 1975; 36:281.
325. Kent KM, Smith ER, Redwood DR, et al. Electrical stability of acutely ischemic myocardium: Influences of heart rate and vagal stimulation. *Circulation* 1973; 47:291.
326. Kottmeier CA, Gravenstein JS. The parasympathomimetic activity of atropine and atropine methylbromide. *Anesthesiology* 1968; 29:1125.
327. Berger PB, Ruocco NA Jr, Ryan TJ, et al. Incidence and prognostic implications of heart block complicating inferior myocardial infarction treated with thrombolytic therapy: Results from TIMI-II. *J Am Coll Cardiol* 1992; 20:533.
328. Nicod P, Gilpin E, Dittrich H, et al. Long-term outcome in patients with inferior myocardial infarction and complete atrioventricular block. *J Am Coll Cardiol* 1988; 12:589.
329. McDonald K, O'Sullivan JJ, Conroy M, et al. Heart block as predictor of in-hospital death in both acute inferior and acute anterior myocardial infarction. *Am J Med* 1990; 74:277.
330. Fisch GR, Zipes DP, Fisch C. Bundle branch block in sudden death. *Prog Cardiovasc Dis* 1980; 23:187.
331. Hindman MC, Wagner GS, JaRo M, et al. The clinical significance of bundle branch block complicating acute myocardial infarction: Part I: Clinical characteristics, hospital mortality, and one-year follow-up. *Circulation* 1978; 58:679.
332. Zoll PM, Zoll RH, Falk RH, et al. External noninvasive temporary cardiac pacing: Clinical trials. *Circulation* 1985; 71:937.
333. Emergency Cardiac Care Committee and Subcommittees, American Heart Association. Guidelines for cardiopulmonary resuscitation and emergency cardiac care, Part III: Adult advanced cardiac life support. *JAMA* 1992; 268:2199.
334. Wood MA. Temporary transvenous pacing. In: Ellenbogen KA, Kay GN, Wilkoff BL, eds. *Clinical Cardiac Pacing.* Philadelphia: WB Saunders; 1995:687.
335. Campbell RW, Murray A, Julian DG. Ventricular arrhythmias in first 12 hours of acute myocardial infarction: Natural history study. *Br Heart J* 1981; 46:351.
336. Campbell RWF. Arrhythmias. In: Julian DG, Braunwald E, eds. *Management of Acute Myocardial Infarction.* London: WB Saunders; 1994:223.
337. Nordrehaug JE, von der Lippe G. Hypokalaemia and ventricular fibrillation in acute myocardial infarction. *Br Heart J* 1983; 50:525.
338. Higham PD, Adams PC, Murray A, et al. Plasma potassium, serum magnesium and ventricular fibrillation: A prospective study. *Q J Med* 1993; 86:609.
339. Antman EM, Berlin JA. Declining incidence of ventricular fibrillation in myocardial infarction: Implications for the prophylactic use of lidocaine. *Circulation* 1992; 86:764.
340. Behar S, Goldbourt U, Reicher-Reiss H, et al. Prognosis of acute myocardial infarction complicated by primary ventricular fibrillation: Principal investigators of the SPRINT Study. *Am J Cardiol* 1990; 66:1208.
341. Reeder GS, Gersh BJ. Modern management of acute myocardial infarction. *Current Problems in Cardiology* 1996; 21:591.
342. Dhurandhar RW, MacMillan RL, Brown KW. Primary ventricular fibrillation complicating acute myocardial infarction. *Am J Cardiol* 1990; 66:1208.
343. Lie KI, Wellens HJ, Durrer D. Characteristics and predictability of primary ventricular fibrillation. *Eur J Cardiol* 1974; 1:379.
344. Solomon SD, Ridker PM, Antman EM. Ventricular arrhythmias in trials of thrombolytic therapy for acute myocardial infarction: A meta-analysis. *Circulation* 1993; 88:2575.
345. MacMahon S, Collins R, Peto R, et al. Effects of prophylactic lidocaine in suspected acute myocardial infarction: An overview of results from the randomized controlled trials. *JAMA* 1992; 260:1910.
346. Scheinman MM, Levine JH, Cannom DS, et al. Dose-ranging study of intravenous amiodarone in patients with life-threatening ventricular tachyarrhythmias. The Intravenous Amiodarone Multicenter Investigators Group. *Circulation* 1995; 92:3264.
347. Huey BL, Gheorghiade M, Crampton RS, et al. Acute non-Q wave myocardial infarction associated with early ST segment

elevation: Evidence for spontaneous coronary reperfusion and implications for thrombolytic trials. *J Am Coll Cardiol* 1987; 9:18.

348. Chouhan L, Hajar HA, George T, et al. Non-Q and Q-wave infarction after thrombolytic therapy with intravenous streptokinase for chest pain and anterior ST-segment elevation. *Am J Cardiol* 1991; 68:446.
349. DeWood MA, Stifter WF, Simpson CS, et al. Coronary arteriographic findings soon after non-Q-wave myocardial infarction. *N Engl J Med* 1986; 315:417.
350. Fuster V, Badimon L, Badimon JJ, et al. The pathogenesis of coronary artery disease and the acute coronary syndromes (2). *N Engl J Med* 1992; 326:310.
351. Decanay S, Kennedy HL, Uretz E, et al. Morphological and quantitative angiographic analyses of progression of coronary stenoses: A comparison of Q-wave and non-Q-wave myocardial infarction. *Circulation* 1994; 90:1739.
352. Kennedy JW. Non-Q-wave myocardial infarction. *N Engl J Med* 1986; 315:451.
353. Klein LW, Helfant RH. The Q-wave and non-Q wave myocardial infarction: Differences and similarities. *Prog Cardiovas Dis* 1986; 29:205.
354. Savonitto S, Ardissino D, Granger CB, et al. Prognostic value of the admission electrocardiogram in acute coronary syndromes. *JAMA* 1999; 281:707.
355. Coller BS, Folts JD, Smith SR, et al. Abolition of in vivo platelet thrombus formation in primates with monoclonal antibodies to the platelet GPIIb/IIIa receptor: Correlation with bleeding time, platelet aggregation, and blockade of GPIIb/IIIa receptors. *Circulation* 1989; 80:1766.
356. Lefkovits J, Plow EF, Topol EJ. Platelet glycoprotein IIb/IIIa receptors in cardiovascular medicine. *New Engl J Med* 1995; 332:1553.
357. CAPTURE Study. Randomised placebo-controlled trial of abciximab before and during coronary intervention in refractory unstable angina: The CAPTURE Study [published erratum appears in *Lancet* 1997; 350:744]. *Lancet* 1997; 349:1429.
358. EPIC Investigation. Use of a monoclonal antibody directed against the platelet glycoprotein IIb/IIIa receptor in high-risk coronary angioplasty: The EPIC investigation. *N Engl J Med* 1994; 330:956.
359. EPILOG Investigators. Platelet glycoprotein IIb/IIIa receptor blockade and low-dose heparin during percutaneous coronary revascularization: The EPILOG investigators. *N Engl J Med* 1997; 336:1689.
360. Brener SJ, Barr LA, Burchenal JE, et al. Randomized, placebo-controlled trial of platelet glycoprotein IIb/IIIa blockade with primary angioplasty for acute myocardial infarction: ReoPro and Primary PTCA Organization and Randomized Trial (RAPPORT) Investigators. *Circulation* 1998; 98:734.
361. PURSUIT Trial Investigators. Inhibition of platelet glycoprotein IIb/IIIa with eptifibatide in patients with acute coronary syndromes. *N Engl J Med* 1998; 339:436.
362. PRISM Study Investigators. A comparison of aspirin plus tirofiban with aspirin plus heparin for unstable angina. Platelet Receptor Inhibition in Ischemic Syndrome Management (PRISM). *N Engl J Med* 1998; 338:1498.
363. PRISM-PLUS Study Investigators. Inhibition of the platelet glycoprotein IIb/IIIa receptor with tirofiban in unstable angina and non-Q-wave myocardial infarction. Platelet Receptor Inhibition in Ischemic Syndrome Management in Patients Limited by Unstable Signs and Symptoms (PRISM-PLUS) Study Investigators. *N Engl J Med* 1998; 338:1488.
364. Kong DF, Califf RM, Miller DP, et al. Clinical outcomes of therapeutic agents that block the platelet glycoprotein IIb/IIIa integrin in ischemic heart disease. *Circulation* 1998; 98:2829.

364a. FRISC Study Group. Low-molecular-weight heparin during instability in coronary artery disease, Fragmin during Instability in Coronary Artery Disease (FRISC) Study Group. *Lancet* 1996; 347(9001)561.

365. Klein W, Buchwald A, Hillis SE, et al. Comparison of low-molecular weight heparin with unfractionated heparin acutely and with placebo for 6 weeks in the management of unstable coronary artery disease. Fragmin in unstable coronary artery disease study. *Circulation* 1997; 96:61.

365a. Cohen M, Demers C, Gurfinkel EP, et al. A comparison of low-molecular-weight heparin with unfractionated heparin for unstable coronary artery disease. *N Eng J Med* 1977; 337:447.

366. TIMI IIA Trial Investigators. Dose-ranging trial of enoxaparin for unstable angina: Results of TIMI IIA. *J Am Coll Cardiol* 1997; 29:1474.
367. Antman EM, McCabe CH, Gurfinkel EP, et al. Enoxaparin prevents death and cardiac ischemic events in unstable angina/non-Q-wave myocardial infarction: Results of the thrombolysis in myocardial infarctions (TIMI) 11B trial. *Circulation* 1999; 100:1593.
368. Klimt CR, Knatterud GL, Stamler J, et al. Persantine-aspirin reinfarction study. Part II. Secondary coronary prevention with persantine and aspirin. *J Am Coll Cardiol* 1986; 7:251.
369. Campbell RWF, Murray A, Julian DG. Ventricular arrhythmias and ventricular fibrillation in acute myocardial infarction (abs). *Am J Cardiol* 1979; 45:462.
370. Gheorghiade M, Schultz L, Tilley B, et al. Natural history of the first non-Q-wave myocardial infarction in the placebo arm of the Beta-Blocker Heart Attack Trial. *Am Heart J* 1991; 122:1548.
371. Boden WE, Krone RJ, Oakes D, et al. Electrocardiographic subset analysis of diltiazem administration on long-term outcome after acute myocardial infarction. *Am J Cardiol* 1991; 67:335.
372. Multicenter Diltiazem Postinfarction Trial Research Group. The effect of diltiazem on mortality and reinfarction after myocardial infarction. *N Engl J Med* 1988; 319:385.
373. Boden WE, Messerli FH, Hansen JF, et al. Heart rate-lowering calcium channel blockers (diltiazem, verapamil) do not adversely affect long-term cardiac death or non-fatal infarction in post-infarction patients: Data pooled from 3 randomized, placebo-controlled clinical trials of 5,677 patients (abs). *J Am Coll Cardiol* 1996; 27:319A.
374. Danish Verapamil Infarction Trial II-DAVIT II. Effect of verapamil on mortality and major events after acute myocardial infarction. *Am J Cardiol* 1990; 66:779.
375. Danish Study Group on Verapamil in Myocardial Infarction. Verapamil in acute myocardial infarction. *Eur Heart J* 1984; 5:516.
376. Gheorghiade M. Calcium channel blockers in the management of myocardial infarction patients. *Henry Ford Hosp Med J* 1991; 39:210.
377. Boden WE, Scheldewaert R, Walters EG, et al. Design of a placebo-controlled clinical trial of long-acting diltiazem and aspirin versus aspirin alone in patients receiving thrombolysis with a first acute myocardial infarction. Incomplete Infarction Trial of Europena Research Collaborators Evaluating Prognosis Post-Thrombolysis (diltiazem) (INTERCEPT) Research Group. *Am J Cardiol* 1995; 75:1120.
378. FRISC II Investigators. Invasive compared with non-invasive treatment in unstable coronary-artery disease: FRISC II prospective randomised multicentre study. FRagmin and Fast Revascularisation during InStability in Coronary artery disease (FRISC II). *Lancet* 1999; 354:708.
379. Tosteson ANA, Goldman L, Udvarhelyi IS, et al. Cost-effectiveness of a Coronary Care Unit versus an Intermediate Care Unit for emergency department patients with chest pain. *Circulation* 1996; 94:143.
380. Tatum JL, Jesse RL, Kontos MC, et al. Comprehensive strategy

for the evaluation and triage of the chest pain patient. *Ann Emerg Med* 1997; 29:116.

381. Chobanian AV, Lille RD, Tercyak A, et al. The metabolic and hemodynamic effects of prolonged bed rest in normal subjects. *Circulation* 1974; 49:551.

382. Winslow EH. Cardiovascular consequences of bed rest. *Heart Lung* 1985; 14:236.

383. Metzger BL, Therrien B. Effect of position on cardiovascular response during the Valsalva maneuver. *Nurs Res* 1990; 39:198.

384. Taggart P, Sutton P, John R, et al. Monophasic action potential recordings during acute changes in ventricular loading induced by the Valsalva manoeuvre. *Br Heart J* 1992; 67:221.

385. Dixon RA, Edwards IR, Pilcher J. Diazepam in immediate post-myocardial infarct period: A double blind trial. *Br Heart J* 1980; 43:535.

386. Thompson DR, Meddis R. A prospective evaluation of in-hospital counselling for first time myocardial infarction in men. *J Psychosom Res* 1990; 34:237.

387. Duryee R. The efficacy of inpatient education after myocardial infarction. *Heart Lung* 1992; 21:217.

388. Fletcher V. An individualized teaching programme following primary uncomplicated myocardial infarction. *J Adv Nurs* 1987; 12:195.

389. Dracup K, Moser DK, Guzy PM, et al. Is cardiopulmonary resuscitation training deleterious for family members of cardiac patients? *Am J Public Health* 1994; 84:116.

390. Myerburg RJ, Kessler KM, Castellanos A. Sudden cardiac death: Epidemiology, transient risk, and intervention assessment. *Ann Intern Med* 1993; 119:1187.

391. Pfeffer MA, Lamas GA, Vaughan DE, et al. Effect of captopril on progressive ventricular dilatation after anterior myocardial infarction. *N Engl J Med* 1988; 319:80.

392. Pfeffer MA, Braunwald E, Moye LA, et al. Effect of captopril on morbidity and mortality in patients with left ventricular dysfunction after myocardial infarction: Results of the Survival and Ventricular Enlargement Trial. The SAVE Investigators. *N Engl J Med* 1992; 327:669.

393. SOLVD Investigators. Effect of enalapril on survival in patients with reduced left ventricular ejection fractions and congestive heart failure. *N Engl J Med* 1991; 325:293.

394. Latini R, Maggioni AP, Flather M, et al. Ace-inhibitor use in patients with myocardial infarction; summary of evidence from clinical trials. *Circulation* 1995; 92:3132.

395. Sigurdsson A, Swedberg K. Left ventricular remodelling, neurohormonal activation and early treatment with enalapril (CONSENSUS II) following myocardial infarction. *Eur Heart J* 1994; 15(Suppl B):14.

396. Acute Infarction Ramipril Efficacy (AIRE) Study Investigators. Effect of ramipril on mortality and morbidity of survivors of acute myocardial infarction with clinical evidence of heart failure. *Lancet* 1993; 342:821.

397. Kober L, Torp-Pedersen C, Carlsen JE, et al. A clinical trial of the angiotensin-converting-enzyme inhibitor trandolapril in patients with left ventricular dysfunction after myocardial infarction. Trandolapril Cardiac Evaluation (TRACE) Study Group. *N Engl J Med* 1995; 333:1670.

398. HOPE Investigators. Effects of an angiotensin-converting-enzyme inhibitor, ramipril, on cardiovascular events in high-risk patients. The Heart Outcomes Prevention Evaluation Study Investigators. *N Engl J Med* 2000; 342:145.

399. Turlapaty P, Altura BM. Magnesium deficiency produces spasms of coronary arteries: Relationship to etiology of sudden death ischemic heart disease. *Science* 1980; 208:198.

400. Adams JH, Mitchell JRA. The effect of agents which modify platelet behaviour and of magnesium ions on thrombus formation in vivo. *Thromb Haemost* 1979; 42:603.

401. Watanabe Y, Dreifus LS. Electrophysiological effects of magnesium and its interactions with potassium. *Cardiovasc Res* 1972; 6:79.

402. Vormann J, Fischer G, Classen HG, et al. Influence of decreased and increased magnesium supply on the cardiotoxic effects of epinephrine in rats. *Arzneimittelforschung* 1983; 33:205.

403. Teo KK, Yusuf S, Collins R, et al. Effects of intravenous magnesium in suspected acute myocardial infarction: Overview of randomised trials. *Brit Med J* 1991; 303:1499.

404. Antman EM, Lau J, Kupelnick B, et al. A comparison of results of meta-analyses of randomized control trials and recommendations of clinical experts: Treatments for myocardial infarction. *JAMA* 1992; 268:240.

405. Woods KL, Fletcher S, Roffe C, et al. Intravenous magnesium sulphate in suspected acute myocardial infarction: Results of the second Leicester Intravenous Magnesium Intervention Trial (LIMIT-2). *Lancet* 1992; 339:1553.

406. Woods KL, Flecher S. Long-term outcome after intravenous magnesium sulphate in suspected acute myocardial infarction: The second Leicester Intravenous Magnesium Intervention Trial (LIMIT-2). *Lancet* 1994; 343:816.

407. Antman EM. Magnesium in acute MI: Timing is critical. *Circulation* 1995; 92:2367.

408. Antman EM. Randomized trials of magnesium in acute myocardial infarction: Big numbers do not tell the whole story. *Am J Cardiol* 1995; 75:391.

409. Shechter M, Hod H, Chouraqui P, et al. Magnesium therapy in acute myocardial infarction when patients are not candidates for thrombolytic therapy. *Am J Cardiol* 1995; 75:321.

410. Gheorghiade M, Anderson J, Rosman H, et al. Risk identification at the time of admission to coronary care unit in patients with suspected myocardial infarction. *Am Heart J* 1988; 116:1212.

411. Pozen MW, Stechmiller JK, Voigt GC. Prognosis efficacy of early clinical categorization of myocardial infarction patients. *Circulation* 1977; 56:816.

412. Krone RJ. The role of risk stratification in the early management of a myocardial infarction. *Ann Intern Med* 1992; 116:223.

413. Kloner RA, Parisi AF. Acute myocardial infarction: Diagnostic and prognostic applications of two-dimensional echocardiography. *Circulation* 1987; 75:521.

414. Hopkins LE, Crabbe SJ, Chase SL. Use of a proprietary database to examine lengths of hospital stay of patients who received drug therapy for acute myocardial infarction. *Am J Hosp Pharm* 1989; 46:957.

415. Topol EJ, Burek K, O'Neill WW, et al. A randomized controlled trial of hospital discharge three days after myocardial infarction in the era of reperfusion. *N Engl J Med* 1988; 318:1083.

416. Mark DB, Sigmon K, Topol EJ, et al. Identification of acute myocardial infarction patients suitable for early hospital discharge after aggressive interventional therapy: Results from the Thrombolysis and Angioplasty in Acute Myocardial Infarction Registry. *Circulation* 1991; 83:1186.

417. Newby LK, Califf RM, Guerci A, et al. Early discharge in the thrombolytic era: An analysis of criteria for uncomplicated infarction from the Global Utilization of Streptokinase and t-PA for Occluded Coronary Arteries (GUSTO) Trial. *J Am Coll Cardiol* 1996; 27:625.

418. Bosch X, Theroux P, Waters DD, et al. Early postinfarction ischemia: Clinical, angiographic, and prognostic significance. *Circulation* 1987; 5:988.

419. Oliva PB, Hammill SC. The clinical distinction between regional postinfarction pericarditis and other causes of postinfarction chest pain: Ancillary observations regarding the effect of lytic therapy upon the frequency of postinfarction pericarditis, postinfarction angina, and reinfarction. *Clin Cardiol* 1994; 17:471.

420. Kudenchuk PJ, Ho MT, Weaver WD, et al. Accuracy of computer-interpreted electrocardiography in selecting patients for

thrombolytic therapy: MITI Project Investigators. *J Am Coll Cardiol* 1991; 17:1486.
421. Rothbaum DA, Linnemeier TJ, Landin RJ, et al. Emergency percutaneous transluminal coronary angioplasty in acute myocardial infarction: A 3-year experience. *J Am Coll Cardiol* 1987; 10:264.
422. Ferguson JJ, Diver DJ, Boldt M, et al. Significance of nitroglycerin-induced hypotension with inferior wall acute myocardial infarction. *Am J Cardiol* 1989; 64:311.
423. Cragg DR, Friedman HZ, Bonema JD, et al. Outcome of patients with acute myocardial infarction who are ineligible for thrombolytic therapy. *Ann Intern Med* 1991; 115:173.
424. Gibson RS, Young PM, Boden WE, et al. Prognostic significance and beneficial effect of diltiazem on the incidence of early recurrent ischemia after non-Q-wave myocardial infarction: Results of the Diltiazem Reinfarction Study. *Am J Cardiol* 1987; 60:203.
425. Schechtman KB, Capone RJ, Kleiger RE, et al. Differential risk patterns associated with 3 month as compared with 3 to 12 month mortality and reinfarction after non-Q-wave myocardial infarction. The Diltiazem Reinfarction Study Group. *J Am Coll Cardiol* 1990; 15:940.
426. Thanavaro S, Krone RJ, Kleiger RE, et al. In-hospital prognosis of patients with first nontransmural and transmural infarctions. *Circulation* 1980; 61:29.
427. Loop FD, Lytle BW, Cosgrove DM, et al. Reoperation for coronary atherosclerosis: Changing practice in 2509 consecutive patients. *Ann Surg* 1990; 212:378.
428. Krainin FM, Flessas AP, Spodick DH. Infarction-associated pericarditis: Rarity of diagnostic electrocardiogram. *N Engl J Med* 1984; 311:1211.
429. Thadani U, Chopra MP, Aber CP. Pericarditis after acute myocardial infarction. *Br Med J* 1971; 2:135.
430. Erhardt LR. Clinical and pathological observations in different types of acute myocardial infarction: A study of 84 patients deceased after treatment in a coronary care unit. *Acta Med Scand* 1974; 560:1.
431. Tofler GH, Muller JE, Stone PH, et al. Pericarditis in acute myocardial infarction: Characterization and clinical significance. *Am Heart J* 1989; 117:86.
432. Wall TC, Califf RM, Harrelson-Woodlief L, et al. Usefulness of a pericardial friction rub after thrombolytic therapy during acute myocardial infarction in predicting amount of myocardial damage: The TAMI Study Group. *Am J Cardiol* 1990; 66:1418.
433. Barman PC, Krishnaswami V, Geraci AR. Pericarditis in acute myocardial infarction. *NYS J Med* 1973; 73:645.
434. Guillevin L, Valere PE. Pericarditis in acute myocardial infarction (ltr). *Lancet* 1976; 1:429.
435. Berman J, Haffajee CI, Alpert JS. Therapy of symptomatic pericarditis after myocardial infarction: Retrospective and prospective studies of aspirin, indomethacin, prednisone, and spontaneous resolution. *Am Heart J* 1981; 101:750.
436. Lilavie CJ, Gersh PJ. Mechanical and electrical complication of acute myocardial infarction. *Mayo Clin Proc* 1990; 65:709.
437. Hammerman H, Schoen FJ, Braunwald E, et al. Drug-induced expansion of infarct: Morphological and functional correlations. *Circulation* 1984; 69:611.
438. Bulkley BH, Roberts WC. Steroid therapy during acute myocardial infarction: A cause of delayed healing of ventricular aneurysm. *Am J Med* 1974; 56:244.
439. Kloner RA, Fishbein MC, Lew H, et al. Mummification of the infarcted myocardium by high dose corticosteroids. *Circulation* 1978; 57:56.
440. Shahar A, Hod H, Barabash GM, et al. Disappearance of a syndrome: Dressler's syndrome in the era of thrombolysis. *Cardiology* 1994; 85:255.
441. Dressler W. The post-myocardial-infarction syndrome. *Arch Intern Med* 1959; 103:28.
442. Kossowsky WA, Epstein PJ, Levine RS. Post myocardial infarction syndrome: An early complication of acute myocardial infarction. *Chest* 1973; 63:35.
443. McKay RG, Pfeffer MA, Pasternak RC, et al. Left ventricular remodeling after myocardial infarction: A corollary to infarct expansion. *Circulation* 1986; 74:693.
444. Forrester JS, Wyatt HL, da Luz PL, et al. Functional significance of regional ischemic contraction abnormalities. *Circulation* 1976; 54:64.
445. Aroesty JM, McKay RG, Heller GV, et al. Simultaneous assessment of left ventricular systolic and diastolic dysfunction during pacing-induced ischemia. *Circulation* 1985; 71:889.
446. Tyberg JV, Forrester JS, Wyatt HL, et al. An analysis of segmental ischemic dysfunction utilizing the pressure-length loop. *Circulation* 1974; 49:748.
447. Weisman HF, Healey B. Myocardial infarct expansion, infarct extension, and reinfarction: Pathophysiologic concepts. *Prog Cardiovasc Dis* 1987; 30:73.
448. Sobel BE, Bresnahan GF, Shell WE, et al. Estimation of infarct size in man and its relation to prognosis. *Circulation* 1972; 46:640.
449. Roberts R, Henry PD, Sobel BE. An improved basis for enzymatic estimation of infarct size. *Circulation* 1975; 52:743.
450. Page DL, Caulfield JB, Kastor JA, et al. Myocardial changes associated with cardiogenic shock. *N Engl J Med* 1971; 285:133.
451. Alonso DR, Scheidt S, Post M, et al. Pathophysiology of cardiogenic shock: Quantification of myocardial necrosis, clinical, pathologic and electrocardiographic correlations. *Circulation* 1973; 48:588.
452. Harnarayan C, Bennett MA, Pentecost BL, et al. Quantitative study of infarcted myocardium in cardiogenic shock. *Br Heart J* 1970; 32:728.
453. Rigaud M, Rocha P, Boschat J, et al. Regional left ventricular function assessed by contrast angiography in acute myocardial infarction. *Circulation* 1979; 60:130.
454. Marmor A, Geltman EM, Biello DR, et al. Functional response of the right ventricle to myocardial infarction: Dependence on the site of left ventricular infarction. *Circulation* 1981; 64:1005.
455. Wackers FJT, Lie KI, Sokole EB, et al. Prevalence of right ventricular involvement in inferior wall infarction assessed with thallium 201 and technetium-99m pyrophosphate. *Am J Cardiol* 1978; 42:358.
456. Rigo P, Murray M, Taylor DR, et al. Right ventricular dysfunction detected by gated scintiphotography in patients with acute inferior myocardial infarction. *Circulation* 1975; 52:268.
457. Zehender M, Kasper W, Kauder E, et al. Right ventricular infarction as an independent predictor of prognosis after acute inferior myocardial infarction. *N Engl J Med* 1993; 328:981.
458. Berger PB, Ryan TJ. Inferior myocardial infarction: High-risk subgroups. *Circulation* 1990; 81:401.
459. Andersen HR, Falk E, Nielsen D. Right ventricular infarction: Frequency, size and topography in coronary heart disease: A prospective study comprising 107 consecutive autopsies from a coronary care unit. *J Am Coll Cardiol* 1987; 10:1223.
460. Lee FA. Hemodynamics of the right ventricle in normal and diseased states. *Cardiol Clin* 1992; 10:59.
461. Cross CE. Right ventricular pressure and coronary flow. *Am J Physiol* 1962; 202:12.
462. Haupt HM, Hutchins GM, Moore GW. Right ventricular infarction: Role of the moderator band artery in determining infarct size. *Circulation* 1983; 67:1268.
463. Setaro JF, Cabin HS. Right ventricular infarction. *Cardiol Clin* 1992; 10:69.
464. Goldstein JA, Barzilai B, Rosamond TL, et al. Determinants of hemodynamic compromise with severe right ventricular infarction. *Circulation* 1990; 82:359.
465. Goldstein JA, Tweddell JS, Barzilai B, et al. Importance of left ventricular function and systolic ventricular interaction to right

ventricular perfomance during acute right heart ischemia. *J Am Coll Cardiol* 1992; 19:704.

466. Dell'Italia LJ, Starling MR, Crawford MH, et al. Right ventricular infarction: Identification by hemodynamic measurements before and after volume loading and correlation with noninvasive techniques. *J Am Coll Cardiol* 1984; 4:931.
467. Cohn JN, Guiha NH, Broder MI, et al. Right ventricular infarction: Clinical and hemodynamic features. *Am J Cardiol* 1974; 33:209.
468. Wellens H. Right ventricular infarction (editorial). *N Engl J Med* 1993; 328:1036.
469. Manno BV, Bemis CE, Carver J, et al. Right ventricular infarction complicated by right to left shunt. *J Am Coll Cardiol* 1983; 1:554.
470. Braat SH, DeZwaan C, Brugada P, et al. Right ventricular involvement with acute inferior wall myocardial infarction identifies high risk of developing atrioventricular nodal conduction disturbances. *Am Heart J* 1984; 107:1183.
471. Love JC, Haffajee CI, Gore JM, et al. Reversibility of hypotension and shock by atrial or atrioventricular sequential pacing in patients with right ventricular infarction. *Am Heart J* 1984; 108:5.
472. Sugiura T, Iwasaka T, Takahashi N, et al. Atrial fibrillation in inferior wall Q-wave acute myocardial infarction. *Am J Cardiol* 1991; 67:1135.
473. Braat SH, Ramentol M, Halders S, et al. Reperfusion with streptokinase of an occluded right coronary artery: Effects on early and late right and left ventricular ejection fraction. *Am Heart J* 1987; 113:257.
474. Schuler G, Hofmann M, Schwarz F, et al. Effect of successful thrombolytic therapy on right ventricular function in acute inferior wall myocardial infarction. *Am J Cardiol* 1984; 54:951.
475. Moreyra AE, Suh C, Porway MN, et al. Rapid hemodynamic improvement in right ventricular infarction after coronary angioplasty. *Chest* 1988; 94:197.
476. Griffin J, Grines CL, Marsalese D, et al. A prospective, randomized trial evaluating the prophylactic use of balloon pumping in high risk myocardial infarction patients: PAMI-2 (Abs #715-2). *J Am Coll Cardiol* 1995; 25:86A.
477. Parmley WW, Chuck L, Chatterjee K, et al. Acute changes in the diastolic pressure-volume relationship of the left ventricle. *Eur J Cardiol* 1976; 4:105.
478. Smiseth OA, Rufsum H, Junemann J, et al. Ventricular diastolic pressure-volume shifts during acute ischemic left ventricular failure in dogs. *J Am Coll Cardiol* 1984; 3:966.
479. Dikshit K, Vyden JK, Forrester JS, et al. Renal and extrarenal hemodynamic effects of furosemide in congestive heart failure after acute myocardial infarction. *N Engl J Med* 1973; 288:1087.
480. Biddle TL, Yu PN. Effect of furosemide on hemodynamics and lung water in acute pulmonary edema secondary to myocardial infarction. *Am J Cardiol* 1979; 43:86.
481. Kiely J, Kelly DT, Taylor DR, et al. The role of furosemide in the treatment of left ventricular dysfunction associated with acute myocardial infarction. *Circulation* 1973; 48:581.
482. Goldstein RA, Passamani ER, Roberts R. A comparison of digoxin and dobutamine in patients with acute infarction and failure. *N Engl J Med* 1980; 303:846.
483. Gillespie TA, Ambos HD, Sobel BE, et al. Effects of dobutamine in patients with acute myocardial infarction. *Am J Cardiol* 1977; 39:588.
484. Kahn JC, Gueret P, Menier R, et al. Prognostic value of enzymatic (CPK) estimation of infarct size. *J Mol Med* 1977; 2:223.
485. Killip T III, Kimball JT. Treatment of myocardial infarction in a coronary care unit: A two year experience with 250 patients. *Am J Cardiol* 1967; 20:457.
486. Forrester JS, Diamond GA, Chatterjee K, et al. Medical therapy of acute myocardial infarction by application of hemodynamic subsets (first of two parts). *N Engl J Med* 1976; 295:1356.
487. Forrester JS, Diamond GA, Chatterjee K, et al. Medical therapy of adult myocardial infarction by application of hemodynamic subsets (second of two parts). *N Engl J Med* 1976; 295:1404.
488. Rackley CE, Satler LF, Pearle DL, et al. Use of hemodynamics measurements for management of acute myocardial infarction. *Cardiovasc Clin* 1976; 16:3.
489. Cohn JN, Franciosa JA, Francis GS, et al. Effect of short-term infusion of sodium nitroprusside on mortality rate in acute myocardial infarction complicated by left ventricular failure. *N Engl J Med* 1982; 306:1129.
490. Gillespie TA, Ambos HD, Sobel BE, Roberts R. Effects of dobutamine in patients with acute myocardial infarction. *Am J Cardiol* 1977; 39:588–594.
491. Clark G, Strauss HD, Roberts R. Dobutamine versus furosemide in the treatment of cardiac failure due to right ventricular function. *Chest* 1980; 77:220.
492. Roberts R. Inotropic therapy for cardiac failure associated with acute myocardial infarction. *Chest* 1988; 93:22S.
493. Young JB, Roberts R. Heart failure. In: Dirks JH, Sutton RAI, eds. *Diuretics: Physiology, Pharmacology and Clincial Use.* Philadelphia: Saunders; 1986:151.
494. Schreiber TL, Miller DH, Zola B. Management of myocardial infarction shock: Current status. *Am Heart J* 1989; 117:435.
495. Hill NS, Antman EM, Green LH, et al. Intravenous nitroglycerin: A review of pharmacology, indications, therapeutic effects and complications. *Chest* 1981; 79:69.
496. Wackers FJ, Lie KI, Becker AE, et al. Coronary artery disease in patients dying from cardiogenic shock or congestive heart failure in the setting of acute myocardial infarction. *Br Heart J* 1976; 38:906.
497. Cercek B, Shah PK. Complicated acute myocardial infarction: Heart failure, shock, mechanical complications. *Cardiol Clinics* 1991; 9:569.
498. Gutovitz AL, Sobel BE, Roberts R. The progressive nature of myocardial injury in selected patients with cardiogenic shock. *Am J Cardiol* 1978; 41:469.
499. Goldberg LI. Cardiovascular and renal actions of dopamine: Potential clinical application. *Pharmacol Rev* 1972; 21:1.
500. Gunnar R, Loeb HS. Shock in acute myocardial infarction: Evolution of physiologic therapy. *J Am Coll Cardiol* 1983; 1:154.
501. Mikulic E, Cohn JN, Franciosa JA. Comparative hemodynamic effects of inotropic and vasodilator drugs in severe heart failure. *Circulation* 1977; 56:528.
502. Miller RR, Awan NA, Joyce JA, et al. Combined dopamine and nitroprusside therapy in congestive heart failure. *Circulation* 1977; 5:881.
503. Richard C, Ricome JL, Rimailho A, et al. Combined hemodynamic effects of dopamine and dobutamine in cardiogenic shock. *Circulation* 1983; 67:620.
504. Lee L, Erbel R, Brown TM, et al. Multicenter registry of angioplasty therapy of cardiogenic shock: Initial and longterm survival. *J Am Coll Cardiol* 1991; 17:599.
505. Waller BF, Rothbaum DA, Pinkerton CA, et al. States of the myocardium and infarct-related coronary artery in 19 necropsy patients with acute recanalization using pharmacologic (Streptokinase, recombinant tissue plasminogen activator), mechanical (percutaneous transluminal coronary angioplasty) or combined types of reperfusion therapy. *J Am Coll Cardiol* 1987; 9:785.
506. Brodie BR, Weintraub RA, Stuckey TD, et al. Outcomes of direct coronary angioplasty for acute myocardial infarction in candidates and noncandidates for thrombolytic therapy. *Am J Cardiol* 1991; 67:7.
507. Wei JY, Hutchins GM, Buckley BH. Papillary muscle rupture

in fatal acute myocardial infarction: A potentially treatable form of cardiogenic shock. *Ann Intern Med* 1979; 90:149.
508. Nishimura RA, Schoff HV, Shub C, et al. Papillary muscle rupture complicating acute myocardial infarction: Analysis of 17 patients. *Am J Cardiol* 1983; 51:373.
509. Lie JT, Wright KE Jr, Titus JL. Sudden appearance of a systolic murmur after acute myocardial infarction. *Am Heart J* 1975; 90:507.
510. Shelburne JC, Rubinstein D, Gorlin R. A reappraisal of papillary muscle dysfunction: Correlative clinical and angiographic study. *Am J Med* 1969; 46:862.
511. DeBusk RF, Harrison DC. The clinical spectrum of papillary-muscle disease. *N Engl J Med* 1969; 281:1458.
512. Burch GE, DePasquale NP, Phillips JH. The syndrome of papillary muscle dysfunction. *Am Heart J* 1968; 75:399.
513. Radford MJ, Johnson RA, Daggett WM, et al. Ventricular septal rupture: A review of clinical and physiologic features and an analysis of survival. *Circulation* 1981; 64:545.
514. Rasmussen S, Leth A, Kjoller E, et al. Cardiac rupture in acute myocardial infarction: A review of 72 consecutive cases. *Acta Med Scand* 1979; 205:11.
515. Maker JF, Mallory GK, Laurenz GA. Rupture of the heart after myocardial infarction. *N Engl J Med* 1956; 255:1.
516. Held AC, Cole PL, Lipton B, et al. Rupture of the interventricular septum complicating acute myocardial infarction: A multicenter analysis of clinical findings and outcome. *Am Heart J* 1988; 116:1330.
517. Gaudiani VA, Miller DG, Stinson EB, et al. Postinfarction ventricular septal defect: An argument for early operation. *Surgery* 1981; 89:48.
518. Gray RJ, Sethna D, Matloff JM. The role of cardiac surgery in acute myocardial infarction. I. With mechanical complications. *Am Heart J* 1983; 106:723.
519. Moore CA, Nygard TW, Kaiser DS, et al. Postinfarction ventricular septal rupture: The importance of location of infarction and right ventricular function in determining survival. *Circulation* 1986; 74:45.
520. Bates RJ, Beutler S, Resnekor L, et al. Cardiac rupture—challenge in diagnosis and management. *Am J Cardiol* 1970; 40:429.
521. Roberts WG, Morrow AG. Pseudoaneurysm of the left ventricle: An unusual sequel of myocardial infarction and rupture of the heart. *Am J Med* 1967; 43:639.
522. Cabin HS, Roberts WC. Left ventricular aneurysm, intraaneurysmal thrombus and systemic embolus in coronary heart disease. *Chest* 1980; 77:586.
523. Hayes MJ, Morris GK, Hampton JR. Lack of effect of bed rest and cigarette smoking on development of deep venous thrombus after myocardial infarction. *Br Heart J* 1976; 38:981.
524. Miller RR, Lies JE, Carretta RF, et al. Prevention of lower extremity venous thrombus by early mobilization. *Ann Intern Med* 1976; 84:700.
525. Emerson PA, Marks P. Preventing thromboembolism after myocardial infarction: Effect of low-dose heparin or smoking. *Br Med J* 1977; 1:18.
526. Weinreich DJ, Burke JF, Pauletto FJ. Left ventricular mural thrombi complicating acute myocardial infarction. *Ann Intern Med* 1984; 100:789.
527. Visser CA, Kan G, Meltzer RS, et al. Embolic potential of left ventricular thrombus after myocardial infarction: A two-dimensional echocardiographic study of 119 patients. *J Am Coll Cardiol* 1985; 5:1276.
528. Kouvaras G, Chronopoulas G, Soufras G, et al. The effects of long term antithrombotic treatment of left ventricular thrombi in patients after an acute myocardial infarction. *Am Heart J* 1990; 119:73.
529. Keating EC, Gross SA, Schlamowitz RA, et al. Mural thrombi in myocardial infarctions: Prospective evaluation by two dimensional echocardiography. *Am J Med* 1983; 74:989.
530. Spirito P, Bellotti P, Chiarella F. Prognostic significance and natural history of left ventricular thrombi in patients with acute anterior myocardial infarction: A two-dimensional echocardiographic study. *Circulation* 1985; 72:774.
531. Jugdutt BI, Sivaram CA. Prospective two-dimensional echocardiographic evaluation of left ventricular thrombus and embolism after acute myocardial infarction. *J Am Coll Cardiol* 1989; 13:554.
532. Johannssen KA, Nordrehoug JE, Vonder Lippe G, et al. Risk factors for embolization in patients with left ventricular thrombi and acute myocardial infarction. *Br Heart J* 1988; 60:104.
533. Davis MJE, Ireland MA. Effect of early anticoagulation on the frequency of left ventricular thrombi after anterior wall acute myocardial infarction. *Am J Cardiol* 1986; 57:1244.
534. Lapeyre AC III, Steele PM, Kazmier FJ, et al. Systemic embolism in chronic left ventricular aneurysm: Incidence and the role of anticoagulation. *J Am Coll Cardiol* 1985; 6:534.
535. Turpie ACG, Robinson JG, Doyle DJ, et al. Comparison of high-dose with low-dose subcutaneous heparin to prevent left ventricular mural thrombosis in patients with acute transmural anterior myocardial infarction. *N Engl J Med* 1989; 320:352.
536. Takamoto T, Kim D, Urie PM, et al. Comparative recognition of left ventricular thrombi by echocardiography and cineangiography. *Br Heart J* 1985; 53:36.
537. Sechtem U, Theissen P, Heindel W, et al. Diagnosis of left ventricular thrombi by magnetic resonance imaging and comparison with angiocardiography, computed tomography and echocardiography. *Am J Cardiol* 1989; 64:1195.
538. Faxon DP, Ryan TJ, Davis KB, et al. Prognostic significance of angiographically documented left ventricular aneurysm from the coronary artery surgery study (CASS). *Am J Cardiol* 1982; 50:157.
539. Loop FD, Effler DB, Webster JS, et al. Posterior ventricular aneurysms. Etiologic factors and surgical treatment. *N Engl J Med* 1973; 288:237.
540. Loop FD, Effler DB, Navia JA, et al. Aneurysms of the left ventricle: Survival and results of a ten-year surgical experience. *Ann Surg* 1973; 178:399.
541. Catherwood E, Mintz GS, Kotler MN, et al. Two-dimensional echocardiographic recognition of left ventricular pseudo-aneurysm. *Circulation* 1980; 62:294.
542. Martin RH, Almond CH, Saab S, et al. True and false aneurysms of the left ventricle following myocardial infarction. *Am J Med* 1977; 62:418.
543. Liberthson RR, Salisbury KW, Hutter AM, et al. Atrial tachyarrhythmias in acute myocardial infarction. *Am J Med* 1976; 60:956.
544. Zoni-Berisso M, Carratino L, Ferroni A, et al. Frequency, characteristics and significance of supraventricular tachyarrhythmias detected by 24-hour electrocardiographic recording in the late hospital phase of acute myocardial infarction. *Am J Cardiol* 1990; 65:1064.
545. Gordon S, Finck DR, Perera RD, et al. Atrial infarction complicating an acute inferior myocardial infarction. *Arch Intern Med* 1984; 144:193(1).
546. Nielsen FE, Andersen HH, Gram-Hansen P, et al. The relationship between ECG signs of atrial infarction and the development of supraventricular arrhythmias in patients with acute myocardial infarction. *Am Heart J* 1992; 123:69.
547. James TN. Myocardial infarction and atrial arrhythmias. *Circulation* 1961; 24:761.
548. Goldberg RJ, Seeley D, Becker RC, et al. Impact of atrial fibrillation on the in-hospital and long-term survival of patients with acute myocardial infarction: A community-wide perspective. *Am Heart J* 1990; 119:996.

549. Nielsen FE, Sorensen HT, Christensen JH, et al. Reduced occurrence of atrial fibrillation in acute myocardial infarction treated with streptokinase. *Eur Heart J* 1991; 12:1081.
550. Behar S, Zahavi Z, Goldbourt U, et al. Long-term prognosis of patients with paroxysmal atrial fibrillation complicating acute myocardial infarction: SPRINT Study Group. *Eur Heart J* 1992; 13:45.
551. Konecke LL, Knoebel SB. Nonparoxysmal junctional tachycardia complicating acute myocardial infarction. *Circulation* 1972; 45:367.
552. Meltzer LE, Cohen HE. The incidence of arrhythmias associated with acute myocardial infarction. In: Meltzer LE, Dunning AJ, eds. *Textbook of Coronary Care.* Philadelphia: Charles Press; 1972,
553. Kostuk WJ, Beanlands DS. Complete heart block associated with acute myocardial infarction. *Am J Cardiol* 1970; 26:380.
554. Hindman MC, Wagner GS, JaRo M, et al. The clinical significance of bundle branch block complicating acute myocardial infarction: Part II Indications for temporary and permanent pacemaker insertion. *Circulation* 1978; 58:689.
555. Dreifus LS, Fisch C, Griffin JC, et al. Guidelines for implantation of cardiac pacemakers and antiarrhythmia devices: A report of the American College of Cardiology/American Heart Association Task Force on Assessment of Diagnostic and Therapeutic Cardiovascular Procedures (Committee on Pacemaker Implantation). *J Am Coll Cardiol* 1991; 18:1.
556. Goble AJ, Sloman G, Robinson JS. Mortality reduction in a coronary care unit. *Br Med J* 1966; 1:1005.
557. Graboys TB. In-hospital sudden death after coronary care unit discharge: A high risk profile. *Arch Intern Med* 1975; 135:512.
558. Grace WJ, Yarvote PM. Acute myocardial infarction: The course of the illness following discharge from the coronary care unit. A description of the intermediate coronary care unit. *Chest* 1971; 59:15.
559. Christensen D, Ford M, Reading J, et al. Sudden death in the late hospital phase of acute myocardial infarction. *Arch Intern Med* 1977; 137:1675.
560. Frieden J, Cooper JA. The role of the intermediate cardiac care unit. *JAMA* 1976; 235:816.
561. Levine A, Lown B. The "chair" treatment of coronary thrombosis. *Trans Assoc Am Phys* 1951; 64:316.
562. McNeer JF, Wagner GS, Ginsburg PB, et al. Hospital discharge one week after acute myocardial infarction. *N Engl J Med* 1978; 298:229.
563. Madsen EB, Hougaard P, Gilpin E, et al. The length of hospitalization after acute myocardial infarction determined by risk calculation. *Circulation* 1983; 68:9.
564. Bigger JT, Fleiss JL, Kleiger R, et al. The relationships among ventricular arrhythmias, left ventricular dysfunction, and mortality in the 2 years after myocardial infarction. The Multicenter Post-Infarction Research Group. *Circulation* 1984; 69:250.
565. Epstein SE, Palmeri ST, Patterson RE. Evaluation of patients after acute myocardial infarction: Indications for cardiac catheterization and surgical intervention. *N Engl J Med* 1982; 307:1487.
566. Hillis LD, Forman S, Braunwald E. Risk stratification before thrombolytic therapy in patients with acute myocardial infarction: The Thrombolysis in Myocardial Infarction (TIMI) Phase II co-investigators. *J Am Coll Cardiol* 1990; 16:313.
567. Schuster EH, Bulkley BH. Early post-infarction angina: Ischemia at a distance and ischemia in the infarct zone. *N Engl J Med* 1981; 305:1101.
568. Normand SL, Glickman ME, Sharma RG, et al. Using admission characteristics to predict short-term mortality from myocardial infarction in elderly patients: Results from the Cooperative Cardiovascular Project. *JAMA* 1996; 275:1322.
569. Lee KL, Woodleif LH, Topol EJ, et al. Predictors of 30-day mortality in the era of reperfusion for acute myocardial infarction: Results from an international trial of 41,021 patients. *Circulation* 1995; 91:1659.
570. Krone RJ, Miller JP, Gillespie JA, et al. Usefulness of low-level exercise testing early after acute myocardial infarction in patients taking beta-blocking agents. *Am J Cardiol* 1987; 60:23.
571. Krone RJ, Gillespie JA, Weld FM, et al. Low-level exercise testing after myocardial infarction: Usefulness in enhancing clinical risk stratification. *Circulation* 1984; 71:80.
572. Van Reet RE, Quinones MA, Poliner LR, et al. Comparison of two-dimensional echocardiography with gated radionuclide ventriculography in the evaluation of global and regional left ventricular function in acute myocardial infarction. *J Am Coll Cardiol* 1984; 3:243.
573. White HD, Norris RM, Brown MA, et al. Left ventricular end-systolic volume as the major determinant of survival after recovery from myocardial infarction. *Circulation* 1987; 76:44.
574. Mahmarian JJ, Moye L, Verani MS, et al. Criteria for the accurate interpretation of changes in left ventricular ejection fraction and cardiac volumes as assessed by rest and exercise gated radionuclide angiography. *J Am Coll Cardiol* 1991; 18:112.
575. Pilote L, Silberberg J, Lisbona R, et al. Prognosis in patients with low left ventricular ejection fraction after myocardial infarction. Importance of exercise capacity. *Circulation* 1989; 80:1636.
576. Fletcher GF, Balady G, Froelicher VF, et al. Exercise standards: A statement for healthcare professionals from the American Heart Association. *Circulation* 1995; 91:580.
577. Starling MR, Crawford MH, Kennedy GT, et al. Exercise testing early after myocardial infarction: Predictive value for subsequent unstable angina and death. *Am J Cardiol* 1980; 46:909.
578. Weld FM, Chu KL, Bigger JT, et al. Risk stratification with low-level exercise testing 2 weeks after acute myocardial infarction. *Circulation* 1981; 64:306.
579. Senaratne MPJ, Hsu L, Rossall RE, et al. Exercise testing after myocardial infarction: Relative values of the low level predischarge and the postdischarge exercise test. *J Am Coll Cardiol* 1988; 12:1416.
580. Starling MR, Crawford MH, Kennedy GT, et al. Treadmill exercise tests predischarge and six weeks post-myocardial infarction to detect abnormalities of known prognostic value. *Ann Intern Med* 1981; 94:721.
581. Villella A, Maggioni AP, Villella M, et al. Prognostic significance of maximal exercise testing àfter myocardial infarction treated with thrombolytic agents: The GISSI-2 data base. Gruppo Italiano per lo Studio della Sopravvivenza Nell'Infarto. *Lancet* 1995; 346:523.
582. Chaitman BR, McMahon RP, Terrin M, et al. Impact of treatment strategy on predischarge exercise test in the Thrombolysis in Myocardial Infarction (TIMI) II Trial. *Am J Cardiol* 1993; 71:131.
583. Madsen JK, Grande P, Saunamaki K, et al. Danish multicenter randomized study of invasive versus conservative treatment in patients with inducible ischemia after thrombolysis in acute myocardial infarction (DANAMI). *Circulation* 1997; 96:748.
584. Gottlieb SO, Gottlieb SH, Achuff SC, et al. Silent ischemia on Holter monitoring predicts mortality in high-risk postinfarction patients. *JAMA* 1988; 259:1030.
585. Jerczek M, Andresen D, Schroder J, et al. Prognostic value of ischemia during Holter monitoring and exercise testing after acute myocardial infarction. *Am J Cardiol* 1993; 72:8.
586. Currie P, Ashby D, Saltissi S. Prognostic significance of transient myocardial ischemia on ambulatory monitoring after acute myocardial infarction. *Am J Cardiol* 1996; 71:773.
587. Langer A, Minkowitz J, Dorian P, et al. Pathophysiology and prognostic significance of Holter-detected ST segment depression after myocardial infarction: The Tissue Plasminogen Acti-

vator Toronto (TPAT) Study Group. *J Am Coll Cardiol* 1992; 20:1313.
588. Mahmarian JJ, Steingart RM, Forman S, et al. Relationship between ambulatory electrocardiographic monitoring and myocardial perfusion imaging to detect coronary artery disease and myocardial ischemia. An ACIP ancillary study. *J Am Coll Cardiol* 1997; 29:764.
589. Mahmarian JJ, Mahmarian AC, Marks GF, et al. The role of adenosine thallium-201 tomography for precisely defining long-term risk in patients following acute myocardial infarction. *J Am Coll Cardiol* 1995; 25:1333.
590. Mahmarian JJ. Prediction of myocardium at risk. Clinical significance during acute infarction and in evaluating subsequent prognosis. *Cardiol Clin* 1995; 13:355.
591. Dakik HA, Kleiman NS, Farmer JA, et al. Intensive medical therapy versus coronary angioplasty for suppression of myocardial ischemia in survivors of acute myocardial infarction. *Circulation* 1998; 98:2017.
592. Carlos ME, Smart SC, Wynsen JC, et al. Dobutamine stress echocardiography for risk stratification after myocardial infarction. *Circulation* 1997; 95:1402.
593. Geleijnse ML, Elhendy A, VanDomburg RT, et al. Cardiac imaging for risk stratification with dobutamine-atropine stress testing in patients with chest pain: Echocardiography, perfusion scintigraphy, or both? *Circulation* 1997; 96:137.
594. Quinones MA. Risk stratification after myocardial infarction: Clinical science versus practice behavior. *Circulation* 1997; 95:1352.
595. Minardi G, Disegni M, Manzara C, et al. Diagnostic and prognostic value of dipyridamole and dobutamine stress echocardiography in patients with acute myocardial infarction. *Am J Cardiol* 1997; 80:847.
596. Cortigiani L, Picano E, Landi P, et al. Value of pharmacologic stress echocardiography in risk stratification of patients with single-vessel disease: A report from the echo-persantine and echo-dobutamine international cooperative studies. *J Am Coll Cardiol* 1998; 32:69.
597. Peterson ED, Shaw LJ, Califf RM. Risk stratification after myocardial infarction. *Ann Intern Med* 1997; 126:561.
598. SOLVD Investigators. Effect of enalapril on mortality and the development of heart failure in asymptomatic patients with reduced left ventricular ejection fraction. *N Engl J Med* 1992; 327:685.
599. Pratt CM, Francis MJ, Luck JC, et al. Analysis of ambulatory electrocardiograms in 15 patients during spontaneous ventricular fibrillation with special reference to preceding arrhythmic events. *J Am Coll Cardiol* 1983; 2:789.
600. Cardiac Arrhythmia Suppression Trial (CAST) Investigators. Preliminary report: Effect of encainide and flecainide on mortality in a randomized trial of arrhythmia suppression after myocardial infarction. *N Engl J Med* 1989; 321:406.
601. Cardiac Arrhythmia Suppression Trial II (CAST) Investigators. Effect of the antiarrhythmic agent moricizine on survival after myocardial infarction. *N Engl J Med* 1992; 327:227.
602. Waldo AL, Camm AJ, deRuyter H, et al. Effect of d-sotalol on mortality in patients with left ventricular dysfunction after recent and remote myocardial infarction. The SWORD Investigators. Survival With Oral d-Sotalol. *Lancet* 1996; 348:7.
603. Julian DG, Camm AJ, Fragin G, et al. Randomised trial of effect of amiodarone on mortality in patients with left-ventricular dysfunction after recent myocardial infarction: EMIAT. *Lancet* 1997; 349:667.
604. Cairns JA, Connolly SJ, Robert R, et al. Randomized trial of outcome after myocardial infarction in patients with frequent or repetitive ventricular premature depolarisations: CAMIAT. *Lancet* 1997; 349:675.
605. Pratt CM, Greenway PS, Schoenfeld MH, et al. An exploration of the precision of classifying sudden cardiac death: Implications for the interpretation of clinical trials. *Circulation* 1996; 93:519.
606. Luu M, Stevenson WG, Stevenson LW, et al. Diverse mechanisms of unexpected cardiac arrest in advanced heart failure. *Circulation* 1989; 80:1675.
607. Moss AJ, DeCamilla J, Davis H. Cardiac death in the first 6 months after myocardial infarction: Potential for mortality reduction in the early posthospital period. *Am J Cardiol* 1977; 39:816.
607a. Ruberman W, Weinblatt E, Goldberg JD, et al. Ventricular premature beats and mortality after myocardial infarction. *N Engl J Med* 1977; 297:750–757.
608. Cardiac Arrhythmia Pilot Study (CAPS) Investigators. Effects of encainide, flecainide, imipramine, and moricizine on ventricular arrhythmias during the year after acute myocardial infarction: The CAPS. *Am J Cardiol* 1988; 61:501.
609. Farrell TG, Bashir Y, Cripps T, et al. Risk stratification for arrhythmic events in postinfarction patients based on heart rate variability, ambulatory electrocardiographic variables and the signal-averaged electrocardiogram. *J Am Coll Cardiol* 1991; 18:687.
610. Bigger JT Jr, LaRovere MT, Steinman RC, et al. Comparison of baroreflex sensitivity and heart period variability after myocardial infarction. *J Am Coll Cardiol* 1989; 14:1511.
611. Odemuyiwa O, Malik M, Farrell T, et al. Comparison of the predictive characteristics of heart rate variability index and left ventricular ejection fraction for all-cause mortality, arrhythmic events and sudden death after acute myocardial infarction. *Am J Cardiol* 1991; 68:434.
612. Schwartz PJ, Vanol E, Stramba-Badiale M, et al. Autonomic mechanisms and sudden death: New insights from analysis of baroreceptor reflexes in conscious dogs with and without a myocardial infarction. *Circulation* 1988; 78:669.
613. Makikallio TH, Hoiber S, Kober L, et al. Fractal analysis of heart rate dynamics as a predictor of mortality in patients with depressed left ventricular function after acute myocardial infarction. *Am J Cardiol* 1999; 83:836.
614. Copie X, Hnatkova K, Staunton A, et al. Predictive power of increased heart rate versus depressed left ventricular ejection fraction and heart rate variability for risk stratification after myocardial infarction. Results of a two-year follow-up study. *J Am Coll Cardiol* 1996; 27:270.
615. Singh N, Mironov D, Armstrong PW, et al. Heart rate variability assessment early after acute myocardial infarction. Pathophysiological and prognostic correlates. GUSTO ECG substudy investigators. Global Utilization of Streptokinase and TPA for Occluded Arteries. *Circulation* 1996; 93:1388.
616. Faber TS, Staunton A, Hnatkova K, et al. Stepwise strategy of using short- and long-term heart rate variability for risk stratification after myocardial infarction. *Pacing Clin Electrophysiol* 1996; 19:1845.
617. American College of Cardiology Cardiovascular Technology Assessment Committee. Heart rate variability for risk stratification of life-threatening arrhythmias. *J Am Coll Cardiol* 1993; 22:948.
618. Schwartz PJ. The neural control of heart rate and risk stratification after myocardial infarction. *Eur Heart J* 1999; 1(Suppl H):H33.
619. LaRovere MT, Bigger JT Jr, Marcus FI, et al. Baro-reflex sensitivity and heart-rate variability in prediction of total cardiac mortality after myocardial infarction. *Lancet* 1998; 351:478.
620. Gomes JA, Winters SL, Martinson M, et al. The prognostic significance of quantitative signal-averaged variables relative to clinical variables, site of myocardial infarction, ejection fraction and ventricular premature beats: A prospective study. *J Am Coll Cardiol* 1989; 13:377.
621. Hohnloser SH, Franck P, Klingenheben T, et al. Open infarct

artery, late potentials, and other prognostic factors in patients after acute myocardial infarction in the thrombolytic era: A prospective trial. *Circulation* 1994; 90:1747.

622. Vatterott PJ, Hammill SC, Bailey KR, et al. Late potentials on signal-averaged electrocardiograms and patency of the infarct-related in survivors of acute myocardial infarction. *J Am Coll Cardiol* 1991; 17:330.
623. Zipes DP, Akhtar M, Denes P, et al. Guidelines for clinical intracardiac electrophysiologic studies: A report of the American College of Cardiology/American Heart Association Task Force on assessment of diagnostic and therapeutic cardiovascular procedures. *J Am Coll Cardiol* 1989; 14:1827.
624. Bourke JP, Richards DAB, Ross DL, et al. Routine programmed electrical stimulation in survivors of actue myocardial infarction for prediction of spontaneous ventricular tachyarrhythmias during follow-up: Results, optimal stimulation protocol and cost-effective screening. *J Am Coll Cardiol* 1991; 18:780.
625. Richards DA, Byth K, Ross DL, et al. What is the best predictor of spontaneous ventricular tachycardia and sudden death after myocardial infarction? *Circulation* 1991; 83:756.
626. Moss AJ, Hall J, Cannom DS, et al. Improved survival with an implanted defibrillator in patients with coronary disease at high risk for ventricular arrhythmia. *N Engl J Med* 1996; 335:1933.
627. Glancy JM, Garratt CJ, Woods KL, et al. QT dispersion and mortality after myocardial infarction. *Lancet* 1995; 345:945.
628. Gibson RS, Watson DD, Craddock GB, et al. Prediction of cardiac events after uncomplicated myocardial infarction: A prospective study comparing predischarge exercise thallium-201 scintigraphy and coronary angiography. *Circulation* 1983; 68:321.
629. De Feyter PJ, van Eenige MJ, Dighton DH, et al. Prognostic value of exercise testing, coronary angiography and left ventriculography 6–8 weeks after myocardial infarction. *Circulation* 1982; 66:527.
630. Grines CL, Topol EJ, Bates ER, et al. Infarct vessel status after intravenous tissue plasminogen activator and acute coronary angioplasty: Prediction of clinical outcome. *Am Heart J* 1988; 115:1.
631. Topol EJ, Califf RM, George BS, et al. A randomized trial of immediate versus delayed elective angioplasty after intravenous tissue plasminogen activator in acute myocardial infarction. *N Engl J Med* 1987; 317:581.
632. Muller DW, Topol EJ, Ellis EG, et al. Multivessel coronary artery disease: A key predictor of short-term prognosis after reperfusion therapy for acute myocardial infarction. *Am Heart J* 1991; 121:1042.
633. Aguirre FV, Kern MJ, Hsia J, et al. Importance of myocardial infarction artery patency on the prevalence of ventricular arrhythmia and late potentials after thrombolysis in acute myocardial infarction. *Am J Cardiol* 1991; 68:1410.
634. Multicenter Postinfarction Research Group. Risk stratification and survival after myocardial infarction. *N Engl J Med* 1983; 309:331.
635. Ross J Jr, Brandenburg RO, Dinsmore RE, et al. Guidelines for coronary angiography: A report of the American College of Cardiology/American Heart Association Task Force on assessment of diagnostic and therapeutic cardiovascular procedures. *J Am Coll Cardiol* 1987; 10:935.
636. Ryan TJ, Faxon DP, Gunnar RM, et al. Guidelines for percutaneous transluminal coronary angioplasty: A report of the American College of Cardiology/American Heart Association Task Force on the assessment of diagnostic and therapeutic cardiovascular procedures. *J Am Coll Cardiol* 1988; 1:889.
637. European Coronary Surgery Study Group. Prospective randomized study of coronary artery bypass surgery in stable angina pectoris: A progress report on survival. *Circulation* 1982; 65:II.
638. Deedwania PC, Amsterdam EA, Vagelos RH. Evidence-based, cost-effective risk stratification and management after myocardial infarction. *Arch Int Med* 1997; 157:273.
639. Ronnevik PK, Gundersen T, Abrahamsen AM. Effect of smoking habits and timolol treatment on mortality and reinfarction in patients surviving acute myocardial infarction. *Br Heart J* 1985; 54:134.
640. Rosenberg L, Kaufman DW, Helmrich SP, et al. The risk of myocardial infarction after quitting smoking in men under 55 years of age. *N Engl J Med* 1985; 313:1511.
641. Ockene JK. Smoking intervention: A behavioral, educational, and pharmacologic perspective. In: Okene IS, Ockene JK, eds. *Prevention of Coronary Heart Disease.* Boston, Mass: Little Brown & Co Inc; 1992:201.
642. Henningfield JE. Nicotine medications for smoking cessation. *N Engl J Med* 1995; 333:1196.
643. Pekkanen J, Linn S, Heiss G, et al. Ten-year mortality from cardiovascular disease in relation to cholesterol level among men with and without preexisting cardiovascular disease. *N Engl J Med* 1990; 322:1700.
644. Stampfer MJ, Sacks FM, Salvini S, et al. A prospective study of cholesterol, apolipoproteins, and the risk of myocardial infarction. *N Engl J Med* 1991; 325:373.
645. Scandinavian Simvastatin Survival Study Group. Randomised trial of cholesterol lowering in 4444 patients with coronary heart disease: The Scandinavian Simvastatin Survival Study (4S). *Lancet* 1994; 344:1383.
646. Sacks FM, Pfeffer MA, Moye LA, et al. The effect of pravastatin on coronary events after myocardial infarction in patients with average cholesterol levels. Cholesterol and Recurrent Events (CARE) Trial. *N Engl J Med* 1996; 335:1001.
647. Expert Panel on Detection E, and Treatment of High Blood Cholesterol in Adults. Summary of the second report of the National Cholesterol Education Program (NCEP) Expert Panel on Detection, Evaluation, and Treatment of High Blood Cholesterol in Adults (Adult Treatment Panel II). *JAMA* 1993; 22:933.
648. Rosenson RS. Myocardial injury: The acute phase response and lipoprotein metabolism. *J Am Coll Cardiol* 1993; 22:933.
649. Haskell WL. Sedentary lifestyle is a risk factor for coronary artery disease. In: Pearson TA, Criqui MH, Leupker RV, et al. eds. *Primer in Preventive Cardiology.* Dallas, TX: American Heart Association; 1994:173.
650. Stanford JL, Weiss NS, Voight LF, et al. Combined estrogen and progestin hormone replacement therapy in relation to risk of breast cancer in middle-aged women. *JAMA* 1995; 274:137.
651. Colditz GA, Hankinson SE, Hunter DJ, et al. The use of estrogens and progestins and the risk of breast cancer in postmenopausal women. *N Engl J Med* 1995; 332:1589.
652. Healy B. Effects of estrogen or estrogen/progestin regimes on heart disease risk factors in postmenopausal women: The Postmenopausal Estrogen/Progestin Interventions (PEPI) Trial. *JAMA* 1995; 273:199.
653. Hulley S, Grady D, Bush T, et al. Randomized trial of estrogen plus progestin for secondary prevention of coronary heart disease in postmenopausal women. Heart and Estrogen/Progestin Replacement Study (HERS) Research Group. *JAMA* 1998; 280:605.
654. Yusuf S, Lessem J, Jha P, et al. Primary and secondary prevention of myocardial infarction and strokes: An update of randomly allocated, controlled trials. *J Hypertens* 1993; 11(Suppl 4):S61.
655. Norwegian Multicenter Study Group. Timolol-induced reduction in mortality and reinfarction in patients surviving acute myocardial infarction. *N Engl J Med* 1981; 304:801.
656. Hjalmarson A, Elmfeldt D, Herlitz J, et al. Effect on mortality

of metoprolol in acute myocardial infarction: A double-blind randomised trial. *Lancet* 1981; 2:823.

657. Becker RC. Antiplatelet therapy in coronary heart disease: Emerging strategies for the treatment and prevention of acute myocardial infarction. *Arch Pathol Lab Med* 1993; 117:89.
658. Juul-Moller S, Edvardsson N, Jahnmatz B, et al. Double-blind trial of aspirin in primary prevention of myocardial infarction in patients with stable chronic angina pectoris: The Swedish Angina Pectoris Aspirin Trial (SAPAT) Group. *Lancet* 1992: 340:1421.
659. Ambrosioni E, Borghi C, Magnani B. The effect of the angiotensin-converting enzyme inhibitor zofenopril on mortality and morbidity after anterior myocardial infarction. *N Engl J Med* 1995; 332:80.
660. Ball SG, Hall AS. What to expect from ACE inhibitors after myocardial infarction. *Br Heart J* 1994; 72 (Suppl 3):S70.
661. deLorgeril M, Salen P, Martin J, et al. Mediterranean diet, traditional risk factors, and the rate of cardiovascular complications after myocardial infarction. Final report of the Lyon Diet Heart Study. *Circulation* 1999; 99:779.
662. GISSI Prevention Trial. Dietary supplementation with n-3 polyunsaturated fatty acids and vitamin E after myocardial infarction: Results of the GISSI-Prevention Trial. *Lancet* 1999; 354:447.

CHAPTER 43

THE ELECTROCARDIOGRAM IN ACUTE MYOCARDIAL INFARCTION

Anton P. Gorgels / Domien J. Engelen / Hein J. J. Wellens

The possibility of treating an acute coronary occlusion by thrombolytic therapy or intracoronary interventions such as percutaneous transluminal coronary angioplasty (PTCA) and stenting makes it necessary to determine, rapidly and precisely, which coronary artery is involved, the size of the area at risk, and the results of the intervention. The larger the area at risk, the more important the attempt to restore or improve perfusion of that area.

In recent years, much effort has been put into correlating electrocardiographic (ECG) changes during the acute ischemic episode with findings from coronary angiography performed at the same time. If specific ECG patterns can be recognized, it will be possible to determine, noninvasively, the culprit coronary artery and the size of the ventricular area that is jeopardized.

This chapter discusses the outcome of such studies. It shows that this information is helpful in decision making during acute myocardial infarction and the chapter is therefore placed in the section on coronary heart disease. Chapter 11 provides a general discussion on the value and limitations of the ECG in the diagnosis of cardiac disease (see also Chaps. 40–42).

CLINICAL PRESENTATION OF ACUTE MYOCARDIAL INFARCTION IN RELATION TO THE INFARCT VESSEL

The presentation of acute myocardial infarction is different depending on the coronary artery involved. The left anterior descending branch (LAD) is the most important coronary artery and supplies the anterior, lateral, septal, and frequently the inferoapical segments of the left ventricle. It also perfuses the proximal part of the bundle branches. The extent of ischemia and the prognosis is dependent on the site of occlusion in the LAD.[1] Involvement of the distal conduction system may result in impaired conduction, varying from right bundle-branch block (RBBB) with or without fascicular block to complete atrioventricular (AV) block.[2–4] The clinical picture may include heart failure and, in the subacute phase, ventricular tachycardia and fibrillation and an increased 1-year mortality.[5] The right coronary artery (RCA) perfuses the sinus node (in 55 percent of patients), the right ventricle, the AV node, the posteromedial papillary muscle, and the inferior part of the left ventricle and variably also the posterior and lateral segments.

Ischemia due to occlusion of the RCA leads to ST elevation in the inferior leads. Usually there is less extensive left ventricular (LV) involvement than in LAD occlusion, but the clinical picture may be impressive due to (1) activation of the vagal nervous system and/or (2) ischemia of the sinus and atrioventricular (AV) node, leading to sinus bradycardia and delay or block in the AV node, (3) right ventricular involvement with cardiogenic shock, and (4) ischemia of the papillary muscle, leading to mitral regurgitation.

The circumflex (CX) branch perfuses the posterior wall and variably the inferior and lateral segments. In case of predominant posterior wall involvement following occlusion of the CX, abnormalities in ventricular activation occur in the second half of the QRS complex and are therefore difficult to pick up on the 12-lead ECG, frequently causing underestimation of the area at risk and undertreatment of the patient.[6]

THE ELECTROCARDIOGRAM IN ANTERIOR WALL INFARCTION

The ECG signs of an anterior wall infarction are ST elevation in precordial leads V_2, V_3, and V_4. The behavior of the ST

TABLE 43-1 ECG Identifying the Site of Coronary Vessel Occlusion in Acute Infarction

Anterior wall infarction
Proximal to first septal and/or first diagonal branch of the LAD
Distal to first septal and/or first diagonal branch of the LAD
Inferoposterior wall infarction
1. Distinction between RCA and CX coronary artery
2. Proximal or distal in RCA RV infarction

ABBREVIATIONS: CX = circumflex; LAD = left anterior descending coronary artery; RCA = right coronary artery; RV = right ventricle.

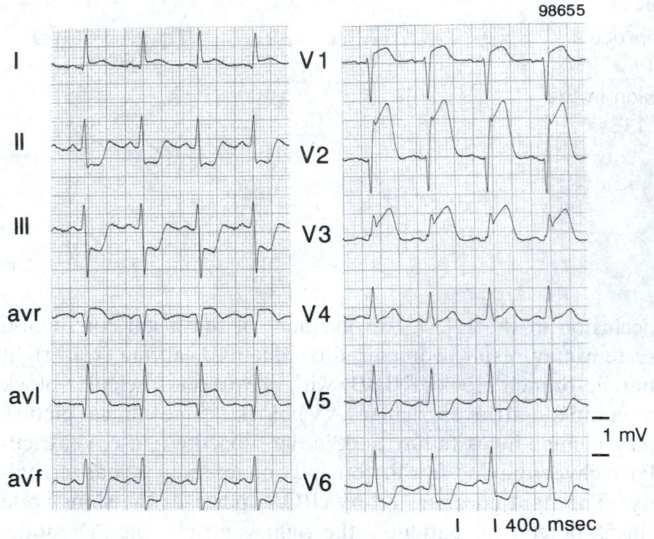

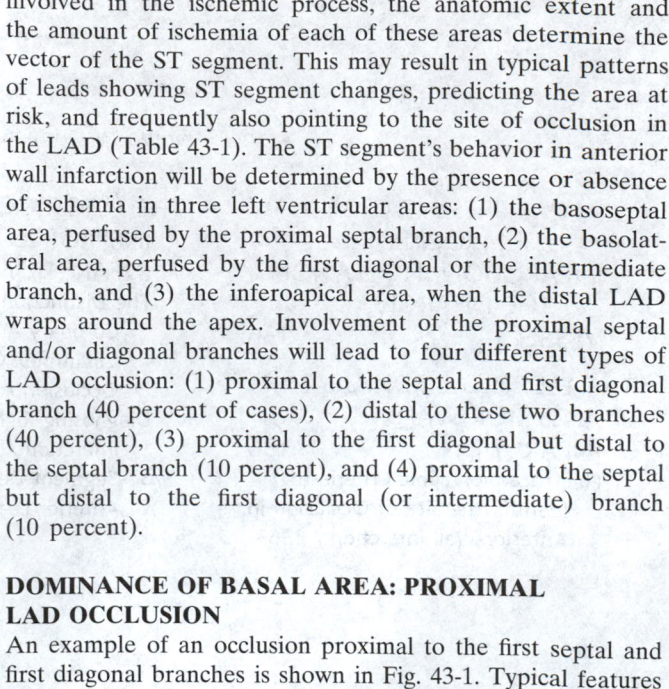

FIGURE 43-1 Acute anterior wall infarction in proximal LAD occlusion. Anterior wall infarction is present, as indicated by ST-segment elevation in leads V_2 and V_3. In addition, the precordial leads show marked ST-segment elevation in lead V_1 and ST-segment depression in leads V_5 and V_6. The extremity leads show ST-segment elevation in lead aV_R and ST-segment depression in inferior leads II, III, and aV_F.

segments in the other precordial and frontal leads is dependent not only on the anterior area but also on the contribution of the septal, lateral, and inferoapical areas. When they are involved in the ischemic process, the anatomic extent and the amount of ischemia of each of these areas determine the vector of the ST segment. This may result in typical patterns of leads showing ST segment changes, predicting the area at risk, and frequently also pointing to the site of occlusion in the LAD (Table 43-1). The ST segment's behavior in anterior wall infarction will be determined by the presence or absence of ischemia in three left ventricular areas: (1) the basoseptal area, perfused by the proximal septal branch, (2) the basolateral area, perfused by the first diagonal or the intermediate branch, and (3) the inferoapical area, when the distal LAD wraps around the apex. Involvement of the proximal septal and/or diagonal branches will lead to four different types of LAD occlusion: (1) proximal to the septal and first diagonal branch (40 percent of cases), (2) distal to these two branches (40 percent), (3) proximal to the first diagonal but distal to the septal branch (10 percent), and (4) proximal to the septal but distal to the first diagonal (or intermediate) branch (10 percent).

DOMINANCE OF BASAL AREA: PROXIMAL LAD OCCLUSION

An example of an occlusion proximal to the first septal and first diagonal branches is shown in Fig. 43-1. Typical features include ST elevation in aV_R and ST elevation of ≥2.5 mm in V_1, ST depression in the inferior leads and in V_5,[7–9] and an abnormal Q in aV_L. Figure 43-2, Plate 82, depicts the likely mechanism of these findings. There is global involvement of the left ventricle with a contribution to the ECG from all ischemic areas. Because of the larger mass of the basal part of the vector, the ST segment will point in a superior direction (Fig. 43-2, left panel). In the frontal plane, this results in ST elevation in leads aV_R and aV_L (Fig. 43-2, right panel). The cranially positioned lead V_1 will also record ST elevation. This upward orientation of the ST vector causes reciprocal ST depression in the inferior leads[10,11] and also sometimes in the lateral leads (V_5 and V_6). Local conduction delay in the lateral area will lead to widening of the Q wave in lead aV_L.

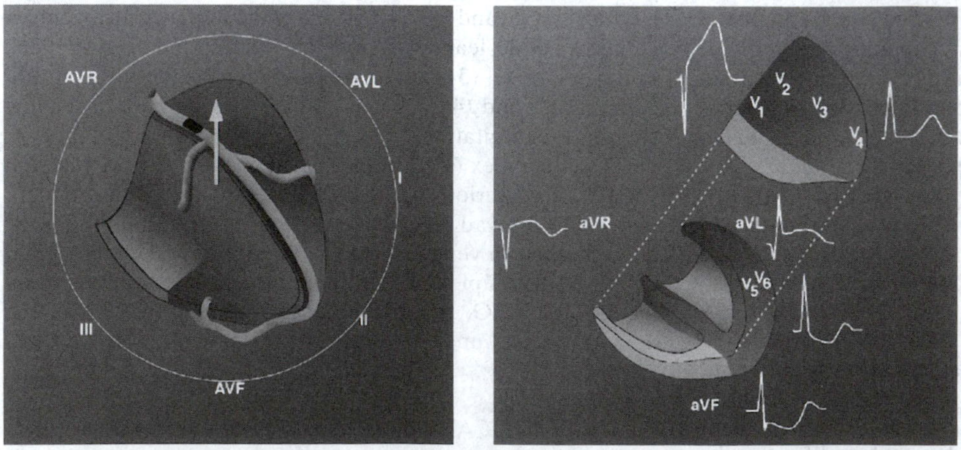

FIGURE 43-2 (Plate 82) Areas of left ventricular ischemia in LAD occlusion proximal to the first septal and first diagonal branch. *Left panel:* There is ischemia of the left ventricle. The ST-segment vector points in a superior direction because ischemia predominates in the basal areas. *Right panel:* The superiorly oriented ST vector leads to ST-segment elevation in lead aV_R and lead V_1 and ST-segment depression in the inferior leads and in V_5 and V_6.

DOMINANCE OF INFEROAPICAL AREA: DISTAL LAD OCCLUSION

Figure 43-3 shows an example of an acute anterior wall infarction due to a distal LAD occlusion (after the proximal septal and diagonal branches). Typical is the absence of ST-segment depression in the inferior leads.[12,13] Sometimes also, wide Q waves are recorded in V_4 through V_6.

In this situation, the inferoapical part is the dominant ischemic area, therefore the ST vector will point inferiorly (Fig. 43-4, left panel, Plate 83). The inferior leads will become isoelectric or even positive (Fig. 43-4, right panel, Plate 83, and Table 43-2). The Q

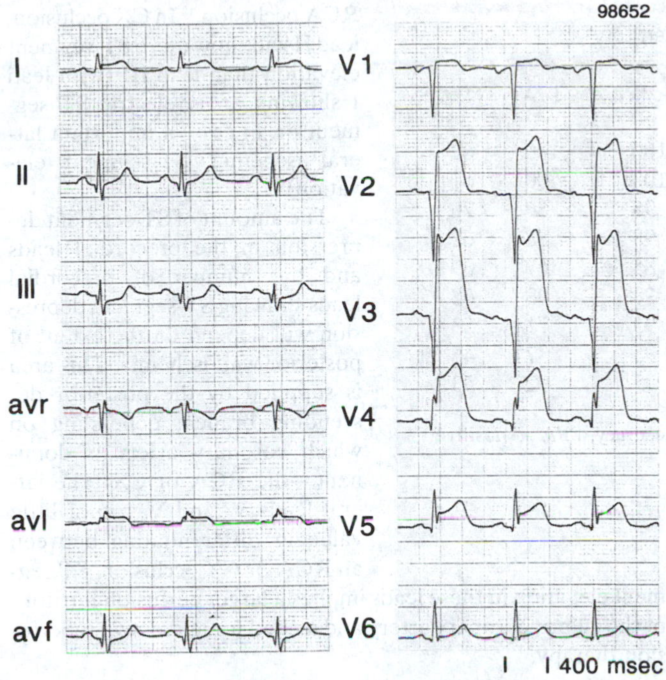

FIGURE 43-3 Acute anterior wall infarction in distal LAD occlusion. Signs of acute anterior wall infarction are seen, but ST-segment elevation is present in the inferior leads. Note also ST-segment depression in lead aV_R.

waves in the left precordial leads are likely caused by the combination of local conduction delay in that area combined with persistence of the regular septal Q wave in these leads.

DOMINANCE OF SEPTAL AREA: FIRST DIAGONAL (OR INTERMEDIATE) BRANCH NOT INCLUDED

Figure. 43-5 presents an example of a case in which a large anterobasal-lateral area is not involved because the occlusion is proximal to the first septal but distal to the first diagonal or intermediate branch. Signs of a proximal first septal branch occlusion are present, such as ST-segment elevation in aV_R, ST-segment elevation ≥2.5 mm in V_1, and ST-segment depression in V_5. As reported elsewhere, the right precordial lead V_{3R} may also show ST-segment elevation.[14] Lead aV_L now shows ST-segment depression and the inferior leads positive ST segments. Figure 43-6, Plate 84, is a diagrammatic presentation of this situation. The left panel shows the rightward orientation of the ST-segment vector, leading (right panel) to the greatest negativity of the ST segment in aV_L and most positivity in lead III, whereas leads aV_R and II are less positive—almost isoelectric. Negativity in lead aV_L is highly specific for an occlusion site behind the first diagonal branch (Table 43-2).

DOMINANCE OF THE LATERAL AREA, FIRST SEPTAL BRANCH NOT INCLUDED

Figure 43-7 shows the ECG of an acute anterior wall infarction with an occlusion site distal to the first septal but proximal to the first diagonal branch. Typical features are Q waves in the left lateral leads, ST-segment depression in lead III, and the absence of this finding in lead II. Figure 43-8, Plate 85, shows the distribution of ischemia in that situation, leading to the ST-segment vector, pointing in a left lateral direction (left panel), and leading to the described changes in the ST segment. Local conduction delay in the lateral area with persistence of the septal Q wave results in widening of the Q wave in leads aV_L and V_5 (right panel).

Electrocardiographic Criteria to Identify the Site of Occlusion in Anterior Wall Infarction

The ECG criteria to identify the site of occlusion in anterior wall infarction, summarized in Table 43-2, are particularly useful in patients presenting with a first acute anterior infarction.[15] In contrast to sensitivity, the specificity of these criteria is high, indicating that their presence accurately predicts the occlusion site, but their absence does not exclude it.

Right bundle-branch block remains, as previously described,[2] a very specific marker of an occlusion site before the first septal branch. ST-segment elevation in V_1 must be considerable to be sufficiently specific (≥ 2.5 mm) for that situation. In contrast, any ST-segment elevation in aV_R, apart from being specific, is the most sensitive marker. ST-segment depression in V_5 is not a very frequent marker, but it is specific. Lead aV_L is the most useful lead to identify an occlusion site, proximal (Q wave) or distal (negative ST segment) to the first diagonal branch.

THE ELECTROCARDIOGRAM IN INFEROPOSTERIOR WALL INFARCTION

The myocardium of the inferoposterior area of the left ventricle is perfused by the right coronary artery (RCA), and the circumflex (CX) coronary artery. The right ventricle and the AV node are usually supplied by the RCA. As indicated in Table 43-1, the objective of the ECG in inferoposterior infarction is to recognize not only the culprit coronary artery but also whether the right ventricle is involved secondary to an occlusion of the RCA proximal to the right ventricular branch.

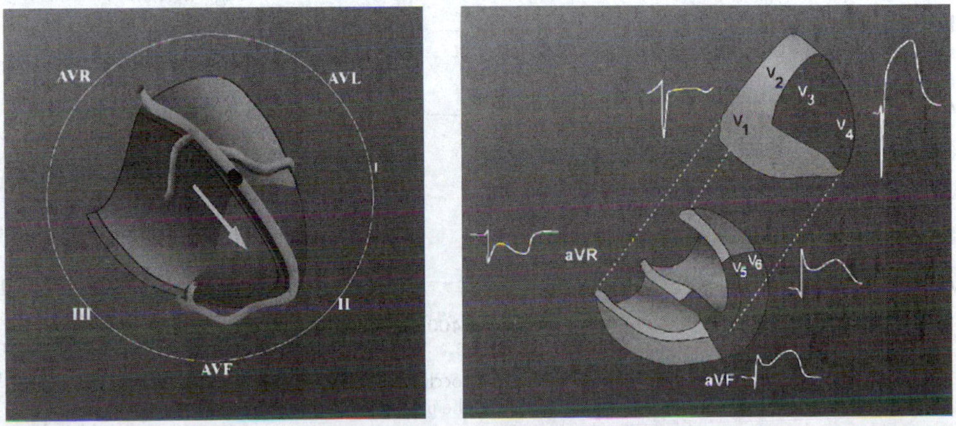

FIGURE 43-4 (Plate 83) Ischemic areas in distal LAD occlusion. *Left panel:* The ST vector points inferiorly due to ischemia of the inferoapical area. *Right panel:* The inferiorly directed ST vector leads to ST-segment depression in lead aV_R and ST-segment elevation in the inferior leads.

TABLE 43-2 ECG Criteria Identifying the Site of Occlusion in the LAD Territory

Criterion	Occlusion site	Sensitivity	Specificity	PPA	NPA
CRBBB	Proximal to S1	14	100	100	62
ST ↑ V_1 ≥2.5 mm	Proximal to S1	12	100	100	61
ST ↑ aV_R	Proximal to S1	43	95	86	70
ST ↓ V_5	Proximal to S1	17	98	88	62
Q aV_L	Proximal to D1	44	85	67	69
ST ↓ II ≥1.0 mm	Proximal to S1/D1	34	98	93	68
Q V_5	Distal to S1	24	93	71	53
ST ↓ aV_L	Distal to D1	22	95	87	46
No ST ↓ III	Distal to S1/D1	41	95	92	53

ABBREVIATIONS: D1 = first diagonal branch; NPA = negative predictive accuracy; PPA = positive predictive accuracy; S1 = first septal branch.
SOURCE: From Engelen et al.,[15] with permission.

The Distinction between a Right Coronary Artery and a Circumflex Coronary Artery Occlusion

As shown in Figs. 43-9 and 43-10, the distinction between an RCA or CX occlusion can be made by determining the ST-segment vector during the acute phase of myocardial infarction. Because RCA occlusion predominantly results in inferoseptal ischemia, the ST-segment vector is directed toward lead III; in CX occlusion, the ischemia is located in the inferoposterolateral region leading to an ST-segment vector pointing toward lead II. Therefore, in RCA occlusion, ST-segment elevation is greater in lead III than lead II (resulting in ST-segment depression in lead I and aV_L). A greater amount of ST-segment depression in aV_L than in lead I further improves the sensitivity in diagnosing an RCA occlusion.[16] In CX occlusion, lead II will show more ST-segment elevation than lead III (with lead I showing an isoelectric ST segment or, in case of important lateral ischemia, ST-segment elevation).

The amount of ST-segment depression in the precordial leads and the number of precordial leads showing ST-segment depression will depend on the extent of posterior wall ischemia. This area is supplied by the posterior descending branch, depending on which coronary artery is dominant—the RCA or CX. The lateral leads V_5 and V_6 are of little value in differentiating between an RCA or CX occlusion. ST-segment elevation in these leads implies a larger perfusion territory of the culprit coronary artery and a need for aggressive reperfusion therapy.[17]

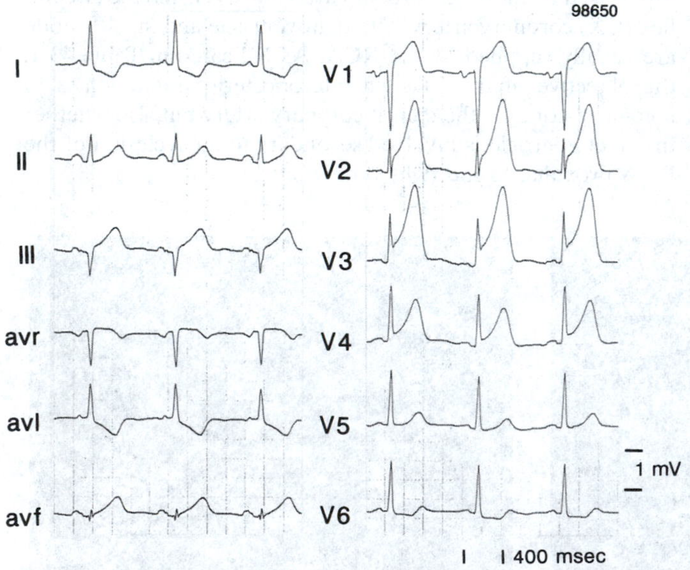

FIGURE 43-5 Acute anterior wall infarction due to LAD occlusion distal to the first diagonal but proximal to the first septal branch. The precordial leads show evidence of acute anterior wall infarction, but lead aV_L shows ST-segment depression.

Diagnosing Right Ventricular Infarction

Is the right ventricle (RV) involved in inferoposterior infarction? The RV is supplied by one or more branches of the RCA. Occlusions in the RCA have therefore been classified as occurring before (proximal) or after (distal) the RV branch(es) (Fig. 43-11). RV involvement is of importance because it may lead to cardiogenic shock due to underfilling of the left ventricle, an increased incidence of high degree AV nodal conduction delay during the actue phase, and a higher incidence of sustained ventricular tachycardia in the chronic (scar) phase of MI. As shown in Figs. 43-12 and 43-13, the best way to diagnose RV involvement is to record lead V_{4R}.[18] ST-segment elevation in lead V_{4R} with a positive T wave predicts an RCA occlusion proximal to the right ventricular branch, an isoelectric ST segment with a positive T wave points to a distal RCA occlusion, and a negative T wave indicates an occlusion of the CX.[19,20] Sufficient ST-segment elevation in the inferior leads of the standard ECG is needed to use the findings from V_{4R} reliably (Fig. 43-14).

ST-Segment Depression in the Anterior Leads

ST-segment depression in the anterior leads in inferior wall infarction reflects posterior wall involvement. ST-segment depression may extend from V_1 through V_6 (Fig. 43-10). Recent data indicate that larger infarctions with more postinfarction complications and a higher mortality rate are present in patients with precordial ST-segment depression.[21–23] The extent and amount of ST-segment depression should therefore play a role in decision making about the aggressiveness of reperfusion therapy. Maximal ST-segment depression in leads V_4 through V_6 is more frequently seen in patients with three-vessel disease, and they have a lower LV ejection fraction.[24] ST-segment depression in the precordial leads may occur both with RCA or CX involvement (Fig. 43-10). Absence of ST-segment depression points to

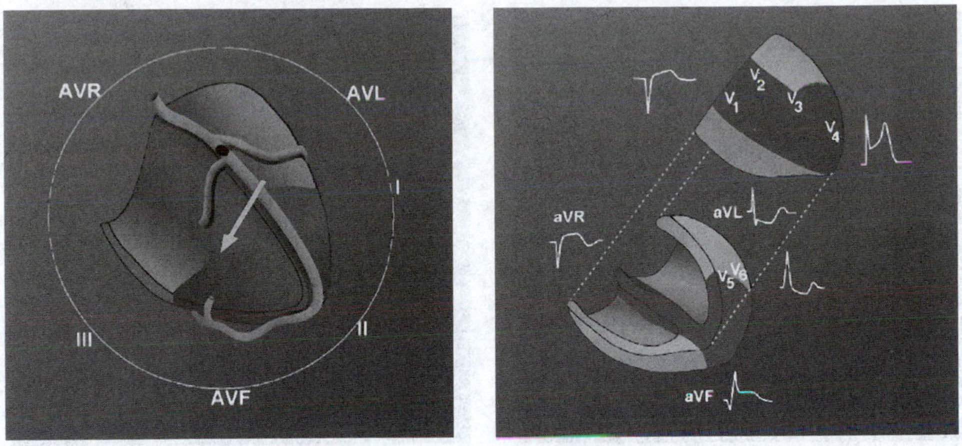

FIGURE 43-6 (Plate 84) Ischemic areas in LAD occlusion between the first diagonal (or intermediate) and first septal branch. *Left panel:* Predominance of ischemia in the septal-apical area leads to an ST-segment vector pointing in a rightward direction. *Right panel:* Apart from ST-segment elevation in the precordial leads, ST-segment elevation is also seen in leads III and aV_R. Negativity of the ST segment is seen in lead aV_L.

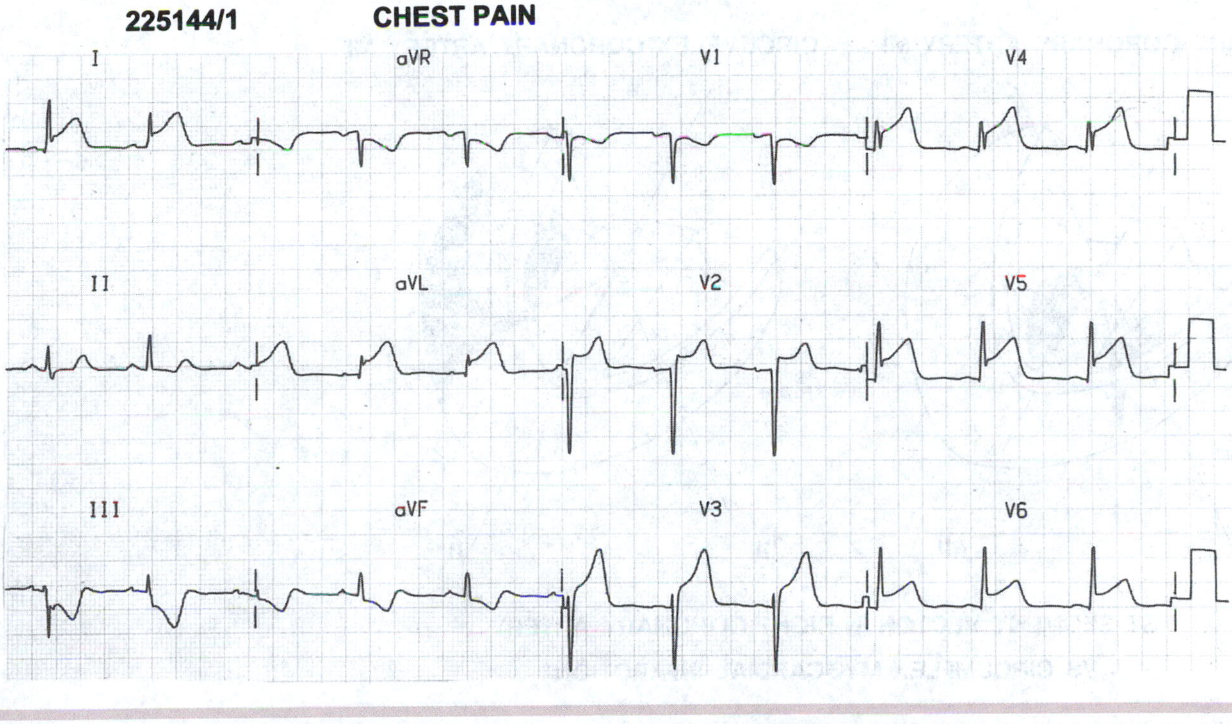

FIGURE 43-7 12-lead ECG with acute anterior wall infarction due to an occlusion site distal to the first septal branch. ST-segment elevation is present in the precordial leads and lead aV_L, whereas leads III and aV_R clearly show ST-segment depression.

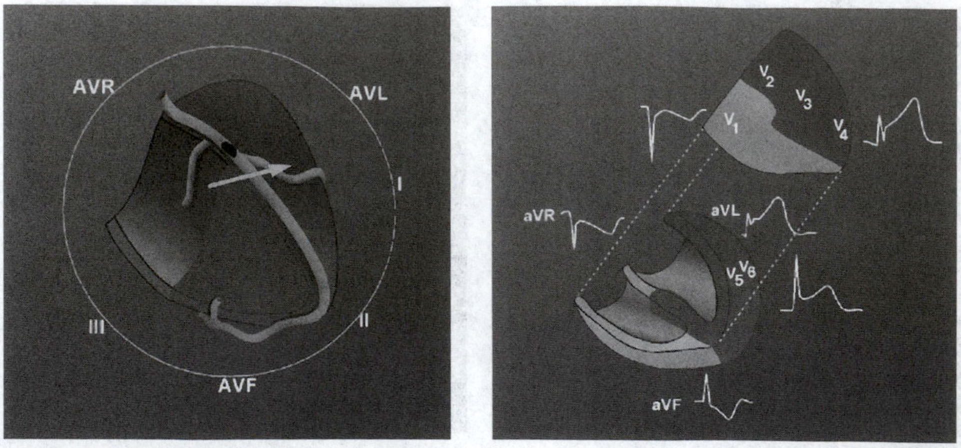

FIGURE 43-8 (Plate 85) Ischemic areas in LAD occlusion distal to the septal and proximal to the first diagonal branch. *Left panel:* Predominance of ischemia in the lateral area leading to an ST vector pointing in that direction. *Right panel:* The lateral orientation of the ST vector leads to ST-segment negativity of leads III and aV_R. Lead II is isoelectric due to the perpendicular orientation of the ST vector in that lead. The lateral leads I and aV_L show ST-segment elevation.

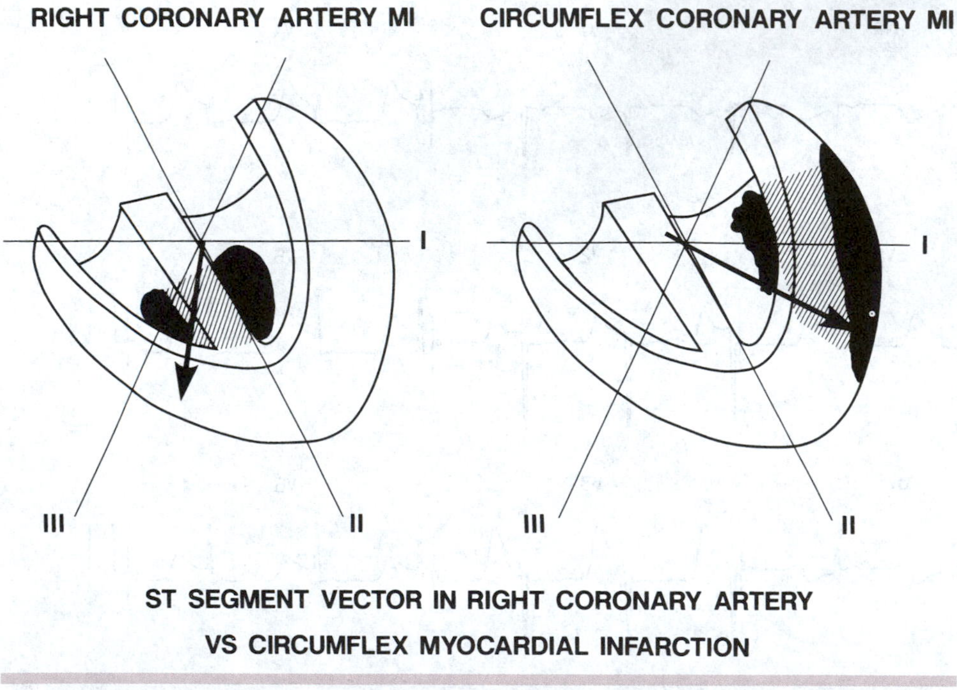

FIGURE 43-9 Schematic presentation of the ST-segment vector with inferoposterior infarction caused by a right coronary artery (RCA) or circumflex coronary artery (CX). As shown, RCA occlusion leads to predominant ischemia in the inferoseptal area with an ST-segment vector pointing toward lead III. In CX occlusion, the ischemic area is located posterolaterally, resulting in an ST-segment vector directed toward lead II.

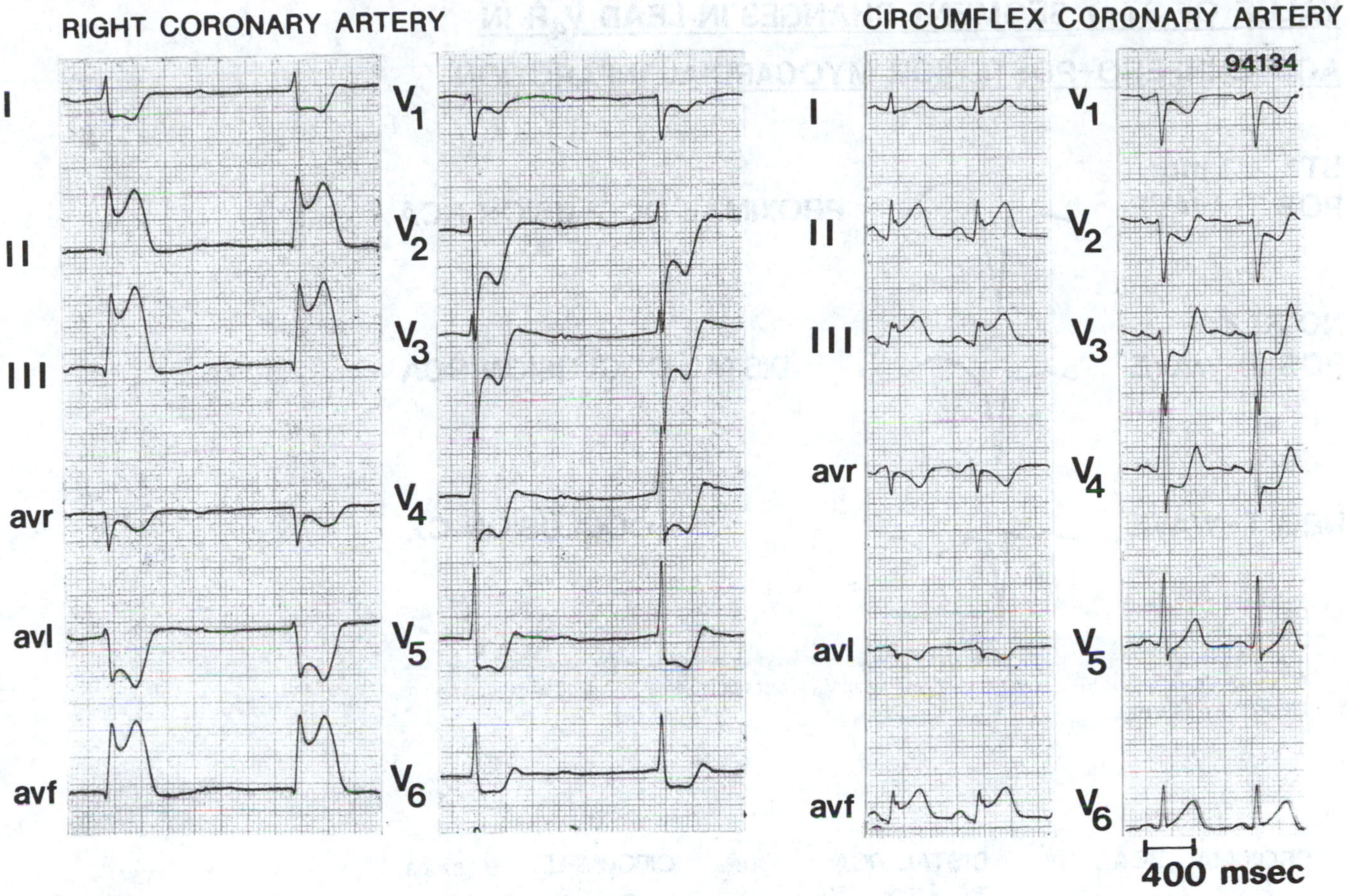

FIGURE 43-10 *Left panel:* The typical picture of a RCA occlusion. ST-segment elevation in lead III is higher than in lead II, resulting in ST-segment depression in lead I. In this patient with a dominant RCA complete AV block, right atrial and posterior wall infarction is also present. *Right panel:* An example of a CX occlusion. ST-segment elevation is more marked in lead II than in lead III, leading to a positive T wave in lead I.

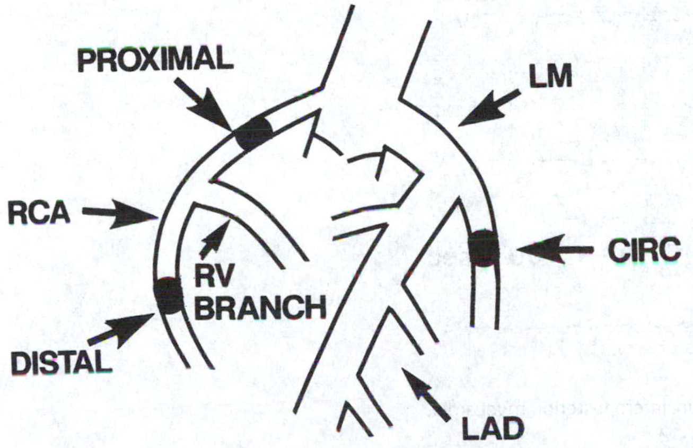

FIGURE 43-11 Diagram showing the coronary arteries and the possible sites of coronary artery occlusion leading to inferoposterior myocardial infarction. In the right coronary artery (RCA), the occlusion may be before (proximal) the right ventricular (RV) branch or after it (distal). As shown in proximal RCA occlusion, the RV is involved in the infarction.

the RCA as the infarct vessel.[25] Isolated ST-segment depression may present the difficulty of differentiating acute CX occlusion, resulting in true posterior wall infarction, from nonocclusive myocardial ischemia. In this regard, it has been suggested that localization of maximal ST-segment depression in V_2 or V_3 is predictive of acute CX occlusion.[26] Also, the use of additional leads V_7 through V_9 has been recommended.[27,28]

Isolated Right Ventricular Infarction

Rarely, the ECG shows only minor changes in the inferior leads and the predominant ST-segment elevation is seen in leads V_1, V_2, and the right precordial leads.[29] This picture reflects a predominant RV infarction and is found in case of a small RCA, a collaterally filled RCA, or an isolated occlusion of an RV branch.

Atrioventricular Conduction Disturbances in Acute Myocardial Infarction

ATRIOVENTRICULAR NODAL BLOCK

Different degrees of AV nodal conduction delay and block may occur in inferior wall infarction, especially when the proximal

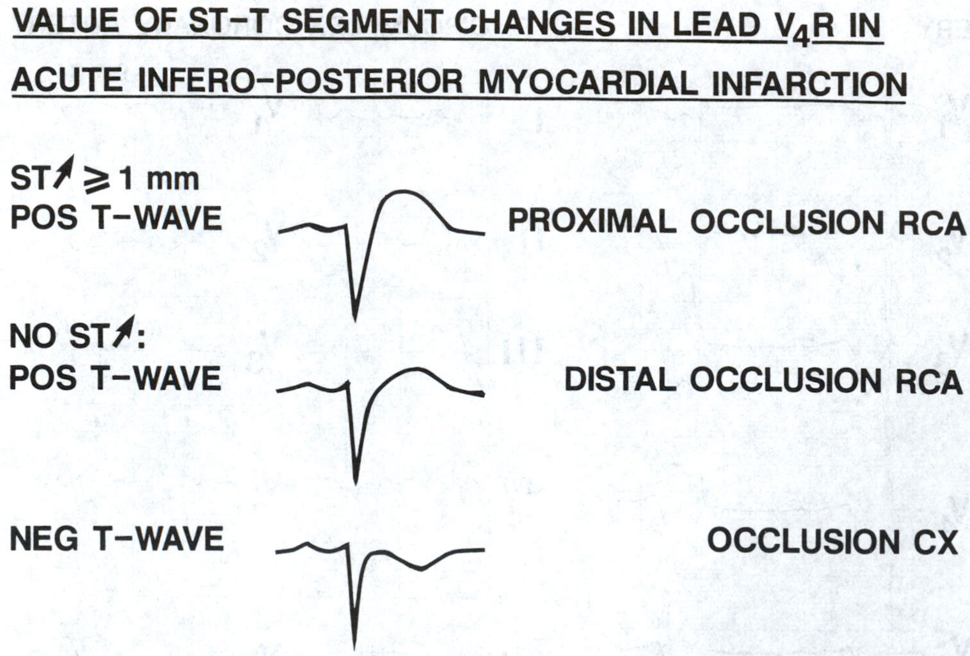

FIGURE 43-12 Characteristic ST-T-segment changes in lead V_{4R} in cases of proximal RCA, a distal RCA occlusion, or a CX occlusion (see text).

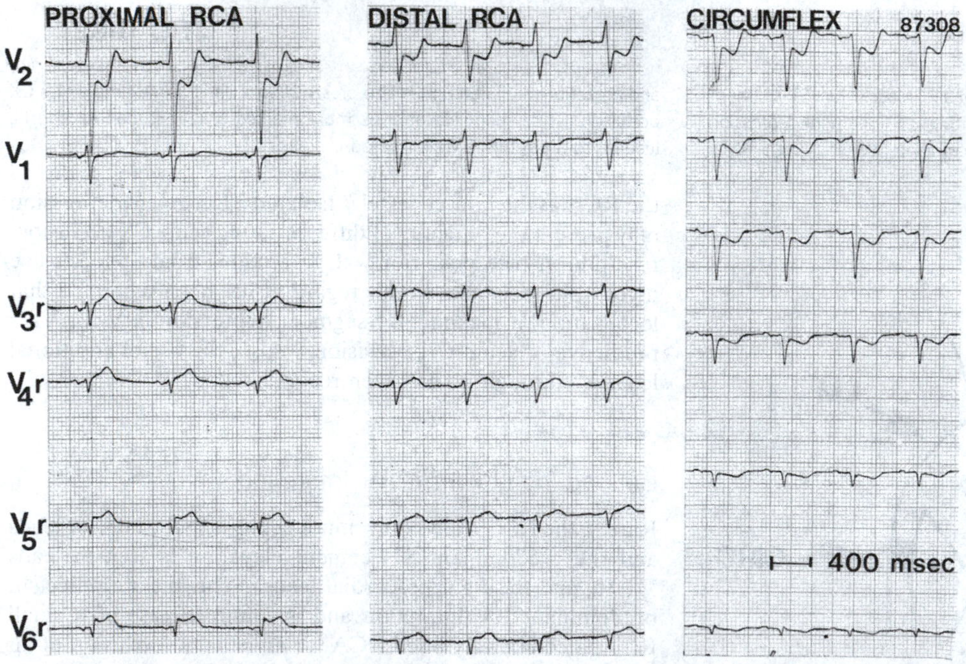

FIGURE 43-13 Three panels showing the behavior of the right precordial leads in inferoposterior myocardial infarction caused by a proximal RCA, distal RCA, or CX occlusion. See also Fig. 43-12.

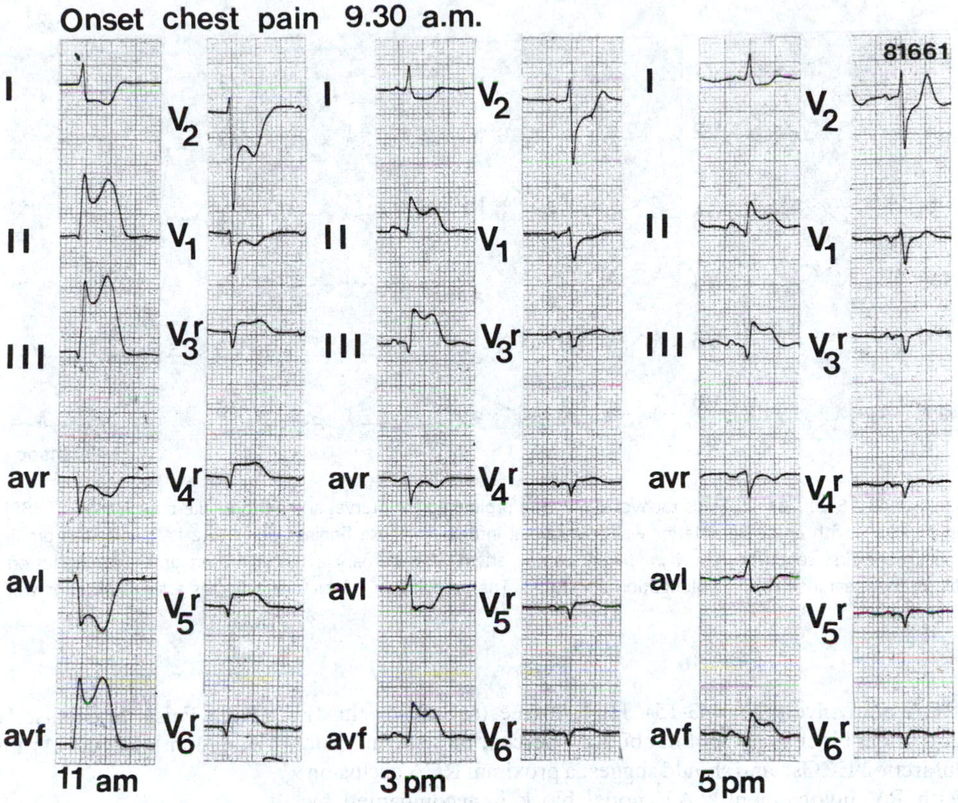

FIGURE 43-14 The relation between ST-segment elevation in leads II, III, and aV_F and in the right precordial leads in proximal RCA. Note that changes diagnostic for RV involvement in lead V_{4R} have disappeared $7\frac{1}{2}$ h after the onset of chest pain. As shown there is a relation between the amount of ST-segment elevation in the inferior leads and lead V_{4R}.

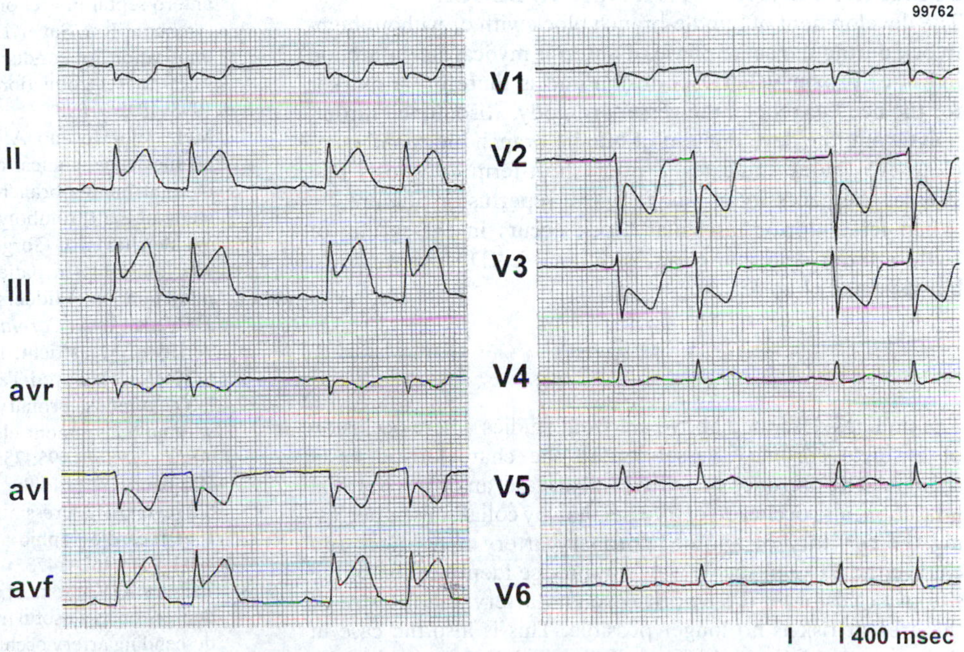

FIGURE 43-15 Three-to-two AV nodal Wenckebach phenomenon in a patient with an acute inferoposterior myocardial infarction. ST-segment elevation in lead III is higher than in lead II, indicating a right coronary artery (RCA) occlusion. Lead V4R (not shown) indicated an ST-segment elevation of 3 mm with a positive T wave, pointing to a proximal RCA with RV involvement.

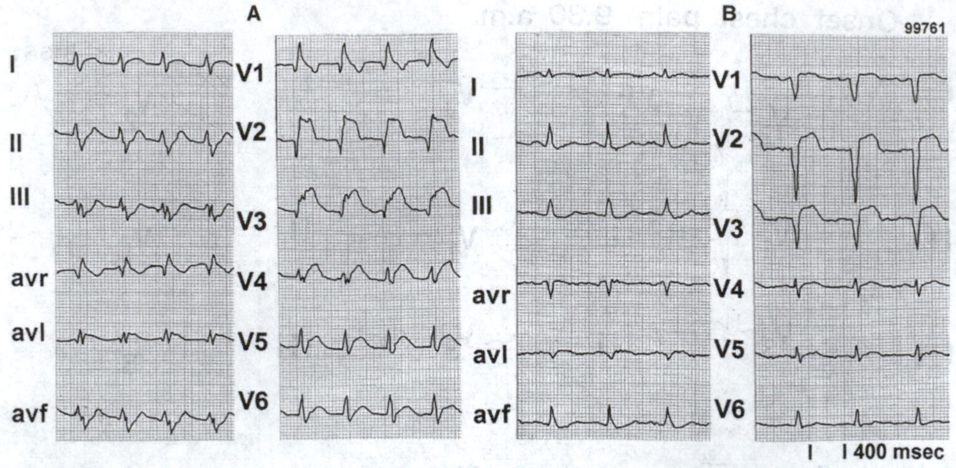

FIGURE 43-16 *Left panel:* Sinus tachycardia with a prolonged PR interval and right bundle-branch block (RBBB) in a patient with an acute anterior wall myocardial infarction. These findings point to a LAD occlusion proximal to the first septal branch. *Right panel:* Same patient after primary PTCA of the proximal LAD occlusion. Note disappearance of PR prolongation and RBBB. The precordial QRS picture indicates a small anterior wall infarction.

RCA is involved (Fig. 43-15). High-degree (second or third) AV nodal block is present in about 20 percent of acute inferior infarction ECGs[30] and should suggest a proximal RCA occlusion with RV involvement.[31] AV nodal block is accompanied by a higher in-hospital morbidity and mortality, not only in the prethrombolytic[32] but also in the thrombolytic era.[33] Early reperfusion is indicated to reduce infarct size and restore normal AV conduction.

SUBATRIOVENTRICULAR NODAL BLOCK

The development of bundle-branch block with or without hemiblock during the acute phase of anterior myocardial infarction indicates proximal LAD occlusion and is therefore a marker for the need to reopen the vessel promptly. Also, in the thrombolytic era, the development of bundle-branch block and complete AV block indicates a poor short-term prognosis and stresses the necessity of an aggressive reperfusion attempt.[34-36] When left anterior fascicular block occurs in the setting of acute inferior wall infarction, additional LAD disease should be suspected (Fig. 43-16).[37]

LIMITATIONS

The findings described above are from studies where occlusion of a single coronary vessel led to the characteristic ECG changes. The presence of multivessel disease, an old myocardial infarction, and occlusion of a vessel that, by collaterals, is perfusing the territory of another coronary artery may affect and change the ECG in such a way that precise identification of the site of occlusion in the culprit coronary artery and the size of the area at risk is no longer possible. This is also the case in the presence of a conal branch from the RCA protecting the superior portion of the interventricular septum in acute anterior wall myocardial infarction.[38] The ECG is also of limited value when ventricular activation is altered, as in preexistent left bundle-branch block, ventricular preexcitation, and a paced ventricular rhythm.

CONCLUSION

In acute cardiac ischemia the aggressiveness of (reperfusion) therapy should be determined by the size of the area at risk. As shown in this chapter, the inexpensive electrocardiogram can be of great help in providing that information.

ACKNOWLEDGMENT

The artwork of Ms. Adri van den Dool, Department of Cardiology, Academic Hospital Maastricht, the Netherlands, and of Ms. Mary-Ann Williams, Photographics Department (Head Mr. Peter Sell), King Faisal Specialist Hospital & Research Center, Riyadh, Kingdom of Saudi Arabia, is gratefully acknowledged.

References

1. Gaudron P, Eilles C, Kugler I, Ertl G. Progressive left ventricular dysfunction and remodeling after myocardial infarction: Potential mechanisms and early predictors. *Circulation* 1993; 87:755–763.
2. Lie KJ, Wellens HJJ, Schuilenburg RM, Durrer D. Factors influencing prognosis of bundle branch block complicating acute antero-septal infarction. *Circulation* 1974; 50:935–941.
3. Archbold RA, Sayer JW, Ray S, et al. Frequency and prognostic implications of conduction defects in acute myocardial infarction since the introduction of thrombolytic therapy. *Eur Heart J* 1998; 19:893–898.
4. Melgarejo-Moreno A, Galcera-Tomas J, Garcia-Alberola A, et al. Incidence, clinical characteristics, and prognostic significance of right bundle-branch block in acute myocardial infarction: A study in the thrombolytic era. *Circulation* 1997; 96:1139–1144.
5. Widdershoven J, Gorgels A, Vermeer F, et al. No change in one year mortality in patients discharged after an acute myocardial infarction. In: Widdershoven JMWG, De Vreede-Swagemakers JJM, eds. *Acute Coronary Syndromes in the Maastricht Area.* University of Maastricht; 1997; 4:67–75.
6. O'Keefe JH, Sayed-Taha K, Gibson W, et al. Do patients with left circumflex coronary artery-related acute myocardial infarction without ST-segment elevation benefit from reperfusion therapy? *Am J Cardiol* 1995; 75:718–720.
7. Birnbaum Y, Solodky A, Herz I, et al. Implications of inferior ST-segment depression in acute anterior myocardial infarction: Electrocardiographic and angiographic correlation. *Am Heart J* 1994; 127:1467–1473.
8. Tamura A, Kataoka H, Mikuriya Y, Nasu M. Inferior ST-segment depression as a useful marker for identifying proximal left anterior descending artery occlusion during acute anterior wall myocardial infarction. *Eur Heart J* 1995; 16:1795–1799.
9. Porter A, Sclarovsky S, Ben-Gal T, et al. Value of T wave direction with lead III ST-segment depression in acute anterior myocardial infarction: Electrocardiographic prediction of a wrapped left ante-

rior descending coronary artery. *Clin Cardiol* 1998; 21:562–566.
10. Tamura A, Kataoka H, Mikuriya Y, Nasu M. Inferior ST segment depression as a useful marker for identifying proximal left anterior descending artery occlusion during acute anterior myocardial infarction. *Eur Heart J* 1995; 16:1795–1799.
11. Birnbaum Y, Solodky A, Herz I, et al. Implications of inferior ST-segment depression in anterior acute myocardial infarction: Electrocardiographic and angiographic correlation. *Am Heart J* 1994; 127:1467–1473.
12. Sapin PM, Musselman DR, Dehmer GJ, Cascio WE. Implications of inferior ST-segment elevation accompanying anterior wall acute myocardial infarction for the angiographic morphology of the left anterior descending coronary artery morphology and site of occlusion. *Am J Cardiol* 1992; 69:860–865.
13. Tamura A, Kataoka H, Nagase K, et al. Clinical significance of inferior ST elevation during acute myocardial infarction. *Br Heart J* 1995; 74:611–614.
14. Kataoka H, Tamura A, Yano S, et al. ST elevation in the right chest leads in anterior wall ventricular acute myocardial infarction. *J Am Coll Cardiol* 1990; 66:1146–1147.
15. Engelen DJ, Gorgels AP, Cheriex EC, et al. Value of the electrocardiogram in localizing the occlusion site in the left coronary artery in acute anterior myocardial infarction. *J Am Coll Cardiol* 1999; 34:389–395.
16. Herz I, Assali AR, Adler Y, et al. New electrocardiographic criteria for predicting either the right or left circumflex artery as the culprit coronary artery in inferior wall acute myocardial infarction. *Am J Cardiol* 1997; 80:1343–1345.
17. Assali A, Sclarovsky S, Herz I, et al. Comparison of patients with inferior wall acute myocardial infarction with versus without ST-segment elevation in leads V_5 and V_6. *Am J Cardiol* 1998; 81:81–83.
18. Braat SH, Brugada P, de Zwaan C, Wellens HJJ. Value of electrocardiogram in diagnosing right ventricular involvement in patients with an acute inferior wall myocardial infarction. *Br Heart J* 1983; 49:368–372.
19. Klein HO, Tordjman T, Ninio R, et al. The early recognition of right ventricular infarction: Diagnostic accuracy of the electrocardiographic V4R lead. *Circulation* 1983; 67:558–565.
20. Braat SH, Gorgels APM, Bär FWHM. Value of the ST-T segment in lead V4R in inferior wall acute myocardial infarction to predict the site of coronary artery occlusion. *Am J Cardiol* 1988; 62:140–142.
21. Peterson ED, Hathaway WR, Zabel M, et al. Prognostic significance of precordial ST segment depression during inferior myocardial infarction in the thrombolytic era: Results in 16521 patients. *J Am Coll Cardiol* 1996; 28:305–312.
22. Birnbaum Y, Herz I, Sclarovsky S, et al. Prognostic significance of precordial ST segment depression on admission electrocardiogram in patients with inferior wall infarction. *J Am Coll Cardiol* 1996; 28:313–318.
23. Borgia MC, Gori F, Pellicelli A, et al. Influence of thrombolytic therapy on inferior acute myocardial infarction with concomitant anterior ST segment depression. *Angiology* 1999; 50:619–628.
24. Birnbaum Y, Wagner GS, Barbash GI, et al. Correlation of angiographic findings and right (V1-V3) versus left (V4-V6) precordial ST-segment depression in inferior wall acute myocardial infarction. *Am J Cardiol* 1999; 83:143–148.
25. Kontos M, Desai PV, Jesse RL, Ornato JP. Usefulness of the admission electrocardiogram for identifying the infarct related artery in inferior wall acute myocardial infarction. *Am J Cardiol* 1997; 79:182–184.
26. Shah A, Wagner GS, Green CL, et al. Electrocardiographic differentiation of the ST-segment depression of acute myocardial injury due to the left circumflex artery occlusion from that of myocardial ischemia of nonocclusive etiologies. *Am J Cardiol* 1997; 79: 512–513.
27. Casas R, Marriott HJL, Glancy L. Value of leads V7-V9 in diagnosing posterior wall acute myocardial infarction and other causes of tall R waves in V1-V2. *Am J Cardiol* 1997; 79:508–509.
28. Matetzky S, Freimark D, Chouraqui P, et al. Significance of ST segment elevations in posterior chest leads (V7 to V9) in patients with acute inferior myocardial infarction: Application for thrombolytic therapy. *J Am Coll Cardiol* 1998; 31:506–511.
29. Mittal SR. Isolated right ventricular infarction. *Int J Cardiol* 1994; 46:53–60.
30. Kimura K, Kosuge M, Ishikawa T, et al. Comparison of the results of early reperfusion in patients with inferior wall acute myocardial infarction with and without complete atrioventricular block. *Am J Cardiol* 1999; 84:731–733.
31. Braat S, de Zwaan C, Brugada P, et al. Right ventricular involvement with acute myocardial infarction identifies high risk of developing atrioventricular nodal conduction disturbances. *Am Heart J* 1984; 107:1183–1187.
32. Tans A, Lie K, Durrer D. Clinical setting and prognostic significance of high degree atrioventricular block in acute inferior myocardial infarction: A study of 144 patients. *Am Heart J* 1980; 99:4–8.
33. Berger P, Ruocco N, Ryan T, et al. Incidence and prognostic implications of heart block complicating acute inferior myocardial infarction treated with thrombolytic therapy: Results from TIMI II. *J Am Coll Cardiol* 1992; 20:533–540.
34. Newby KH, Pisano E, Krucoff MW, et al. Incidence and clinical relevance of the occurrence of bundle branch block in patients treated with thrombolytic therapy. *Circulation* 1996; 94:2424–2428.
35. Barron HV, Bowlby LJ, Breen T, et al. Use of reperfusion therapy for acute myocardial infarction in the United States: Data from the national registry of myocardial infarction. *Circulation* 1998; 97:1150–1156.
36. Harpaz D, Behar S, Gotlieb S, et al. Complete atrioventricular block complicating acute myocardial infarction in the thrombolytic era. *J Am Coll Cardiol* 1999; 34:1721–1728.
37. Assali A, Sclarovsky S, Herz I, et al. Importance of left anterior hemiblock development in inferior wall acute infarction. *Am J Cardiol* 1997; 79:672–674.
38. Ben-Gal T, Sclarovsky S, Herz I, et al. Importance of the conal branch of the right coronary artery in patients with acute anterior myocardial infarction: Electrocardiographic and angiographic correlation. *J Am Coll Cardiol* 1997; 29:506–511.

CHAPTER 44

THROMBOGENESIS, ANTITHROMBOTIC, AND THROMBOLYTIC THERAPY

Christopher P. Cannon / Valentin Fuster

IMPORTANCE OF THROMBOSIS IN ACUTE CORONARY SYNDROMES

Because nearly 2 million patients annually experience an acute coronary syndrome in the United States, with more than double that figure worldwide, cardiologists and other health care professionals have focused on improving the management of acute coronary syndromes, with one of the most prominent advances being thrombolytic therapy for patients with ST-segment elevation myocardial infarction (MI).[1] More recently, however, there have been numerous advances in antithrombotic therapy, for both patients with ST-elevation MI as well as the much larger group of patients with unstable angina and non-ST-elevation MI.

Rupture or erosion of an atherosclerotic plaque with superimposed nonocclusive thrombus is by far the most common cause of acute coronary syndromes (see also Chaps. 35 and 36). However, angiographic studies have shown a major difference in the severity of the thrombus, based on the presence or absence of ST-segment elevation: In ST-elevation MI the infarct-related artery usually has a 100 percent occlusion,[2,3] whereas in unstable angina/non-ST-elevation MI the culprit artery usually has a severe obstruction (80 to 95 percent) but is patent with coronary perfusion (Fig. 44-1).[4,5] Thus, because of the advent of acute reperfusion therapy, a classification of ST-elevation MI versus unstable angina/non-ST-elevation MI provides the critical information regarding the pathophysiology and acute management of acute coronary syndromes (Fig. 44-1).

Evolution of Athero(thrombo)sclerosis

Atherosclerosis is a silent process that usually commences 20 to 30 years prior to a patient's presentation with a clinical syndrome (see Chaps. 35 and 36).[6,7] Hypercholesterolemia, smoking, hypertension, and other coronary risk factors damage the endothelium and initiate the atherosclerotic process.[6–8] When the endothelium is dysfunctional, macrophages bind to endothelial adhesion molecules and can infiltrate the endothelial cell. Low-density lipoprotein (LDL) molecules are able to penetrate into the vessel wall, and the macrophages digest the LDL, becoming foam cells, which thereby create a lipid-filled atherosclerotic plaque.[7,9] Oxidized LDL may also have a direct toxic effect on the endothelium and smooth muscle cells, which contribute to instability of the atherosclerotic plaque. Such plaques, which usually are lesions with less than 50 percent stenosis, are more prone to rupture.[10–14]

Then, multiple factors contribute to plaque rupture, including endothelial dysfunction, plaque lipid content,[15] local inflammation causing breakdown of the thin shoulder of the plaque,[16] coronary vasoconstriction, local shear-stress forces, platelet activation,[17,18] and the status of the coagulation system (i.e., a potentially

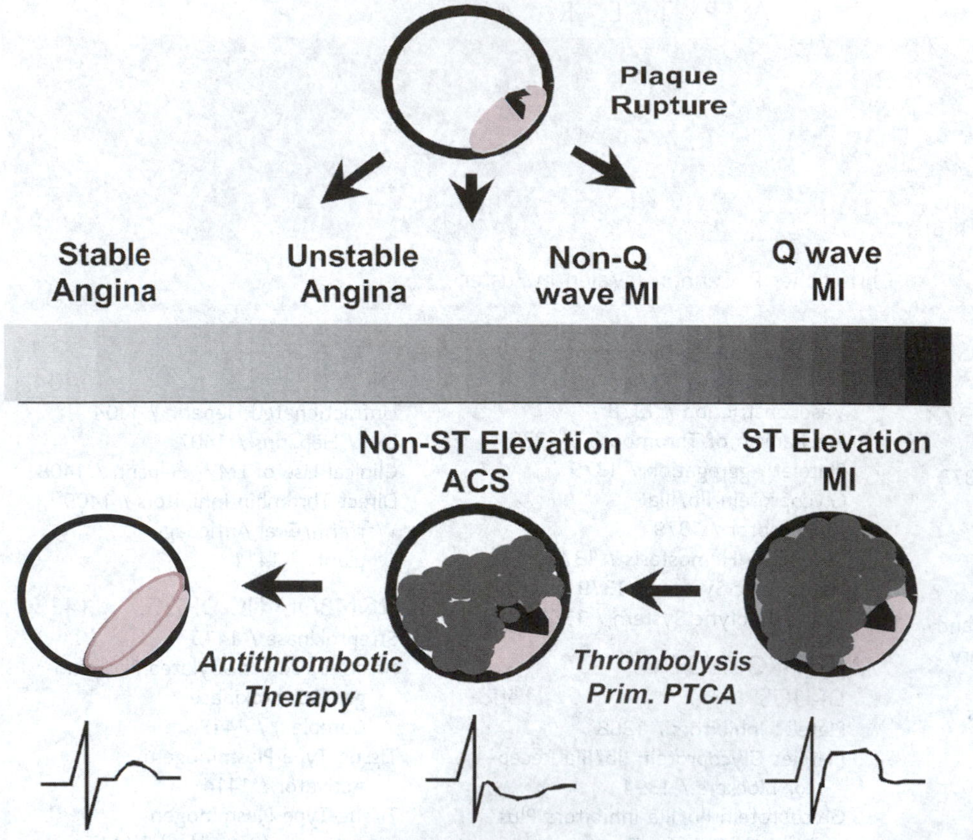

FIGURE 44-1 The new paradigm of acute coronary syndromes (ACS). The various clinical syndromes of coronary artery disease can be viewed as a spectrum, ranging from patients with stable angina to those with acute Q-wave myocardial infarction (MI). Across the spectrum of the acute coronary syndromes, atherosclerotic plaque rupture leads to coronary artery thrombosis: In acute Q-wave MI, which usually presents with ST-segment elevation on the electrocardiogram, complete coronary occlusion is present. In those with unstable angina or non-Q-wave MI, a flow-limiting thrombus is usually present. In patients with stable angina, thrombus is rarely seen. The overall treatment objective is to move the patients back to a stable lesion. In acute ST-elevation MI, the objective over the first minutes to hours is to open the artery and achieve reperfusion. In patients with unstable angina and non-ST-elevation MI, the goal is to stabilize or "passivate" the active thrombotic lesion over a period of hours to days. Then, over a period of months to years, the goal is to try to heal the lesion with risk factor reduction with treatment of hypercholesterolemia, hypertension, and diabetes, and with smoking cessation, in an attempt to reduce the likelihood of subsequent rupture of the coronary plaques. (Adapted from Cannon.[489] Reproduced with permission from the publisher and author.)

prothrombotic state),[19,20] all of which culminate in the formation of a platelet-rich thrombus on the disrupted plaque.[21–23]

It should be noted however, that more than 95 percent of all plaque ruptures are clinically silent.[24,25] Angiographic studies have shown that many high-grade lesions often appear in segments of the coronary artery that were previously normal.[26] The erratic and unpredictable growth of plaques is caused by plaque disruption or fissuring and intracoronary mural thrombosis.[27,28] The mural thrombus then undergoes fibrous organization and contributes, often asymptomatically, to the progression of the disease.[27,28] Thus, this process of plaque disruption and local thrombosis is ongoing in patients with clinically "stable" coronary artery disease, a point that reemphasizes the importance of long-term antithrombotic therapy in patients with coronary artery disease.

Percutaneous Coronary Intervention

Percutaneous coronary intervention (PCI) with angioplasty, stenting, or other modalities is associated with denudation of the endothelium and deep vessel injury. This results in exposure of thrombogenic elements in the atherosclerotic plaque and the vessel wall, which predisposes this area to platelet deposition and fibrin formation, leading to intravascular thrombosis.[29,195] Therefore, therapy to prevent acute occlusion following coronary intervention should be directed against both platelets and the coagulation cascade.

Saphenous Vein Bypass Grafting

Disease of the saphenous vein graft is a special case in coronary atherosclerosis. Occlusion rates are 8 to 18 percent per distal anastomosis 1 month postoperatively and 16 to 26 percent at 12 months.[30] Vein graft disease can be divided into three phases: an early postoperative phase (within 1 month after surgery) related to thrombotic occlusion, in which platelet activation and fibrin formation are implicated; an intermediate phase (within the first postoperative year) characterized by intimal hyperplasia, resulting in a form of accelerated atherosclerosis that may have a superimposed thrombotic tendency; and a late phase (after the first postoperative year) characterized by graft atherosclerosis similar to that of the native coronary arteries.[30,196] Therefore, the predominant pathogenetic mechanism in saphenous vein bypass grafting is related to both platelet activation and fibrin generation, particularly in the early postoperative phase.

Role of Endothelial Dysfunction and Inflammation in Early Coronary Atherosclerosis

At areas of plaque injury, there is early adherence of leukocytes and platelets.[31] These early cellular responses lead to the further migration and proliferation of smooth muscle cells, monocytes, and lymphocytes at areas of injury. Vascular endothelial cell injury leads to a cell-mediated response that is very similar to the inflammatory response, which leads to a complex cascade of events that culminate in atherosclerosis and eventually clinical vascular syndromes.[31,32] Activated T cells release cytokines, and monocyte chemotactic factor enhances the adhesion and migration of circulating monocytes and influences lipoprotein uptake by the macrophage and promotes foam cell formation.[31]

In postmortem studies of the atheromatous plaque, disrupted atheromatous plaque were found beneath thrombi in 84 percent of patients,[33] and these culprit lesions contained significantly more macrophages than quiescent lesions.[34] Furthermore, the macrophages and T lymphocytes at the site of plaque disruption were found to be in an activated state.[32] Other studies have localized matrix metalloproteinases to human atherosclerotic plaque, which may contribute to their disruption.[35] Studies of lymphocyte function and expression in patients with unstable angina revealed that this state is associated with the activation of a specific T-cell subset (CD-4$^+$/CD-28 null) that produces interferon-γ, an activator of monocytes, and the production of matrix metalloproteinases.[36] Other complement peptides, including C3-binding protein, localized in areas of endothelial injury and inflammation are chemotactic for monocytes. Clinical studies of patients with acute coronary syndromes have reflected a heightened systemic inflammatory response as measured by elevated circulating levels of markers such as C-reactive protein and other acute-phase reactants.[37–42]

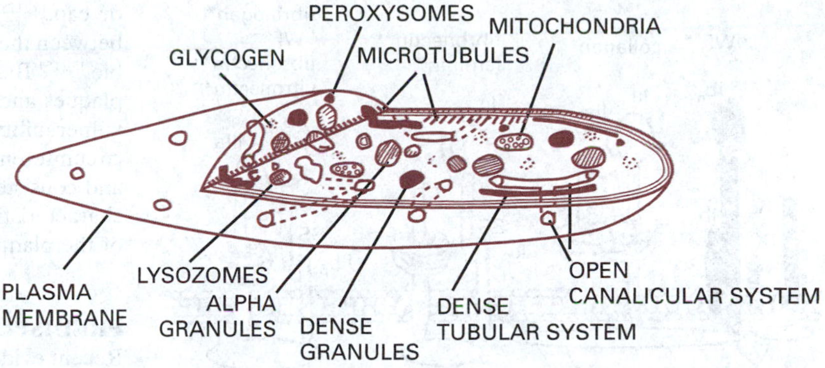

FIGURE 44-2 Platelet structure and main constituents: the dense granules [adenosine diphosphate (ADP), adenosine triphosphate (ATP), calcium, and serotonin]; alpha granules [β-thromboglobulin, platelet factor 4, platelet-derived growth factor (PDGF), von Willebrand factor, factor V, fibrinogen, plasminogen activator inhibitor (PAI-1), protease nexin II, thrombospondin, fibronectin, and P-selectin]; lysozomes (acid hydrolases and cathepsins D and E); and peroxysomes (catalase).

Role of Platelets and Thrombosis in the Progression to Acute Coronary Syndromes (Figs. 44-1 to 44-6)

The central role of coronary artery thrombosis in the pathogenesis of acute coronary syndromes is supported by six sets of observations: (1) at autopsy, thrombi can usually be identified at the site of a ruptured plaque;[21,22,24,43] (2) coronary atherectomy specimens obtained from patients with acute myocardial infarction (AMI) or unstable angina demonstrate a high incidence of acute thrombotic lesions;[44–47] (3) coronary angioscopic observations indicate that thrombus is frequently present;[48–54] (4) coronary angiography has demonstrated ulceration or irregularities suggesting a ruptured plaque[10,55] and/or thrombus in many patients;[5,56] and (5) evidence of ongoing thrombosis has been noted with elevation of several markers of platelet activity and fibrin formation;[6,57–64] and (6) the clinical outcome of patients with acute coronary syndromes is improved by antithrombotic therapy with aspirin,[65–68] heparin,[67–71] low molecular weight (LMW) heparin,[72–75] and platelet glycoprotein (GP) IIb/IIIa inhibitors.[76–78]

The thrombotic response to plaque disruption/fissuring is primarily determined by five local factors: (1) extent of plaque disruption (e.g., ulcer), (2) character of exposed contents (e.g., lipid pool), (3) degree of stenosis and surface irregularities that activate platelets (i.e., change in geometry after plaque disruption), (4) the surface of residual thrombus (recurrence), and (5) vasoconstriction. In addition, systemic factors appear to enhance thrombogenicity, which may occur in a very stenotic plaque denuded of endothelium without plaque fissuring.[24,79] This balance of local and systemic factors has important effects on outcome, as described below.

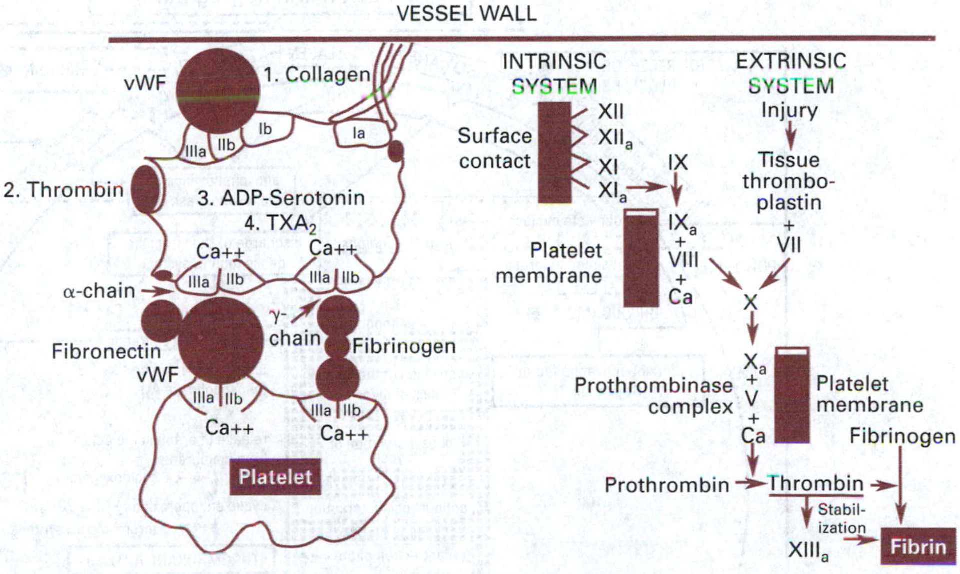

FIGURE 44-3 Interactions among platelet membrane receptors (glycoproteins Ia, Ib, and IIb/IIIa), adhesive macromolecules, and the disrupted vessel wall (*left panel*) and a flowchart of the intrinsic and extrinsic systems of the coagulation cascade (*right panel*). In the left panel, Arabic numerals indicate the pathways of platelet activation that are dependent on (1) collagen, (2) thrombin, (3) ADP and serotonin, and (4) thromboxane A_2 (TXA_2); there are also some reports suggesting the binding of von Willebrand factor (vWF) (polymeric protein) to collagen or heparin. Note the interaction of the right panel between clotting factors (XII, XIIa, XI, XIa, IX, IXa, VII, VIII, X, Xa, V, and XIIIa) and the platelet membrane. (From Fuster et al.[27,28] Copyright Massachusetts Medical Society. Reproduced with permission from the publisher and authors.)

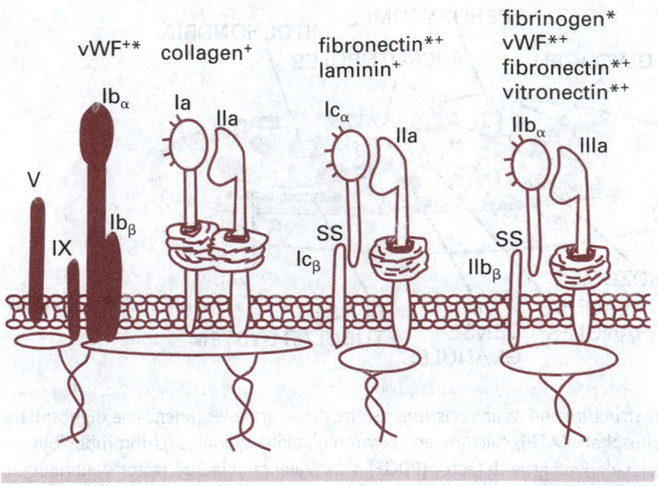

FIGURE 44-4 Interaction among platelet membrane receptors (glycoproteins) and adhesive macromolecules of plasma and/or disrupted vessel wall. *, present in plasma; +, present in vessel wall.

Plaque Disruption

NON-PLAQUE-RELATED FACTORS PREDISPOSING PLAQUE TO RUPTURE

Passive plaque disruption is related to physical forces, especially where the fibrous cap is thinnest, i.e., where it is most heavily infiltrated with foam cells and, as a result, the weakest. Pathologic studies have shown that vulnerable plaques are commonly composed of cellular elements and an atheromatous lipid-filled core separated from the arterial lumen by a fibrous membrane or cap.[15,24,25] For eccentric plaques, the shoulder region, that between the plaque and the adjacent vessel wall is most vulnerable.[15,24,54] Based on studies examining both intact and disrupted plaques and in vitro mechanical testing of isolated fibrous cap, vulnerability to rupture depends on three primary factors: (1) circumferential wall stress or cap "fatigue;" (2) location, size, and consistency of the atheromatous core; and (3) blood flow characteristics, such as the impact of flow on the proximal aspect of the plaque.[54]

PREDISPOSING FACTORS IN ACTIVE PLAQUE

Recent evidence points to a large number of inflammatory cells, notably monocyte-derived macrophages, as being present in disrupted plaque.[15,24,25] Macrophage-derived products, such as matrix metalloproteinases (MMPs), collagenases, and other proteolytic enzymes, degrade the matrix of the plaque, weaken the fibrous cap, and thus predispose plaque to rupture.[35] In culture, monocyte-derived macrophages have been found to degrade the collagen of the fibrous cap while simultaneously expressing MMP-1 (interstitial collagenase) and inducing MMP-2 (gelatinolytic).[80] Recent evidence has suggested that circulating oxidized LDL may influence matrix turnover in atherosclerotic plaque by causing macrophages to produce and release more matrix-degrading metalloproteinases (MMP-9), which increase matrix degradation, alter arterial remodeling, and thus predispose plaque to rupture.[81] It was also found that high-density lipoprotein (HDL) inhibited this process, thus possibly explaining HDL's favorable mechanism of action. When oxidized LDL overloading occurs, macrophages appear to enter into apoptotic death, periods during which induction of MMPs

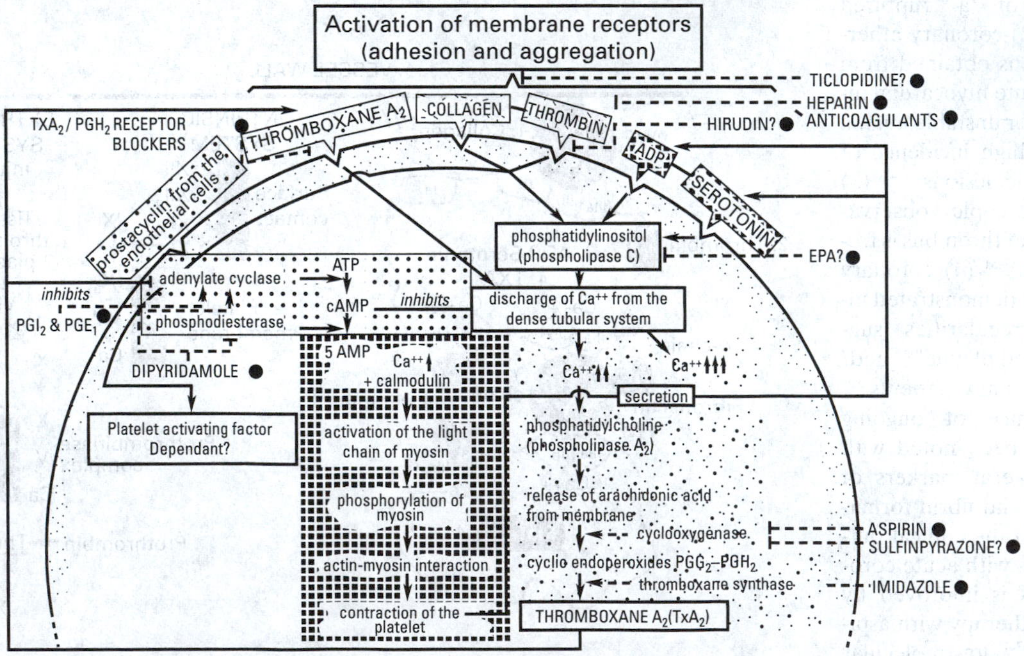

FIGURE 44-5 Mechanism of platelet activation and presumed sites of action of various platelet inhibitor agents. Platelet agonists lead to the mobilization of calcium (Ca^{2+}), which functions as a mediator of platelet activation through metabolic pathways dependent on adenosine diphosphate (ADP), thromboxane A_2 (TXA_2), thrombin, and collagen. Cyclic adenosine monophosphate (cAMP) inhibits calcium mobilization from the dense tubular system. Note that thrombin and collagen may independently activate platelets by means of platelet-activating factor. (●) = a platelet inhibitor; dashed line = a presumed site of drug action; ATP = adenosine triphosphate; EPA = eicosapentaenoic acid; PGE_1 = prostaglandin E_1; PGH_2 = prostaglandin H_2; = PGI_2 = prostaglandin I_2. (From Stein et al.[492] Reproduced with permission from the publisher and authors.)

and tissue factor appears to occur. The end result of plaque disruption is acute overlying thrombosis.

Inflammation/Infection

Recent evidence has also pointed to a role for inflammation, which appears to be key in the development of atherosclerosis[82,83] and in the development and recurrence of unstable angina.[37,39,84,85] Infectious agents, notably *Chlamydia pneumoniae*, appear to be one of the underlying causes of diffuse inflammation in the pathogenesis of coronary artery disease.[86–88] Others for which there is some, albeit less strong, evidence include *Heliobacter pylori* and *Cytomegalovirus*.[86] It is important to note that an etiologic relationship between these infectious agents to the development of acute coronary syndromes has not been definitively established.[88–90] On the other hand, evidence from several animal models,[91–94] and pilot treatment trials in patients,[95–97] suggests *Chlamydia pneumoniae* may be an important and *potentially treatable* cause of unstable angina or MI, and larger trials are ongoing.

Acute Thrombosis

Plaque disruption and thrombus formation/remodeling lead to a variable degree of luminal obstruction to blood flow and can present clinically as stable or unstable angina or acute MI or lead to sudden death (Fig. 44-1).[98] At the time of plaque disruption, a number of local and systemic thrombogenic factors may influence the degree and the duration of thrombus deposition. Such a thrombus may then either be partially lysed or become replaced in the process of organization by the vascular repair response.

Substrate and Tissue Factor–Dependent Thrombosis (Figs. 44-2 and 44-3)

The disruption of an atherosclerotic plaque exposes various vessel wall components to the circulating blood, and each have varying degrees of thrombogenicity. Among the various types of plaques, which included normal intima, fatty streaks, sclerotic plaques, fibrolipid lesions, and plaques with lipid-rich cores, it was the lipid-rich plaque (abundant in cholesterol ester) that displayed the highest thrombogenicity and the most intense tissue factor staining compared with the other plaque types.[99]

Tissue factor is a LMW glycoprotein that, after being exposed to circulating blood factors, initiates the extrinsic clotting cascade and is believed to be a major regulator of thrombosis and hemostasis (see Fig. 44-7). Tissue factor forms a high-affinity complex with coagulation factors VII/VII; the tissue factor–factor VIIa complex activates factors IX and X, which in turn lead to thrombin generation.[100] Atherectomy specimens from the culprit lesion in patients with unstable angina demonstrated a strong relationship between tissue factor and macrophages.[16] Experimental studies using a specific inhibitor of tissue factor (tissue factor pathway inhibitor) found that acute thrombus formation was reduced in lipid-rich plaques exposed to this specific inhibitor.[101] Such information supports the important role of tissue factor activity in acute thrombosis after coronary plaque rupture and opens new avenues of possible therapeutic intervention in the treatment and/or prevention of acute coronary syndromes.

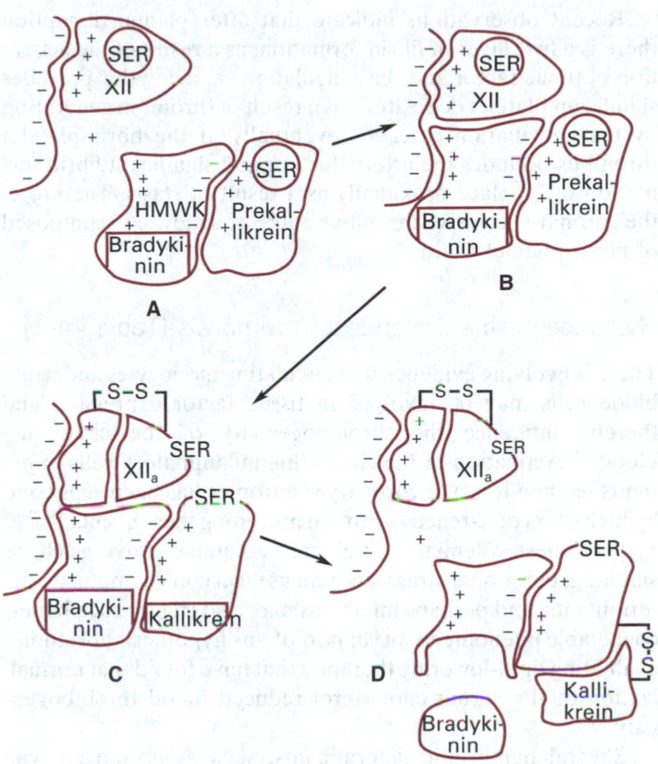

FIGURE 44-6 In the intrinsic pathway of coagulation, *contact activation* refers to a series of reactions following adsorption of factors XII and XI as well as prekallikrein and high molecular weight kininogen to highly negatively charged surfaces. The contact activation does not require calcium and results in surface-induced conformational changes of the molecules. *A–D*. Sequence of events. SER = serine protease.

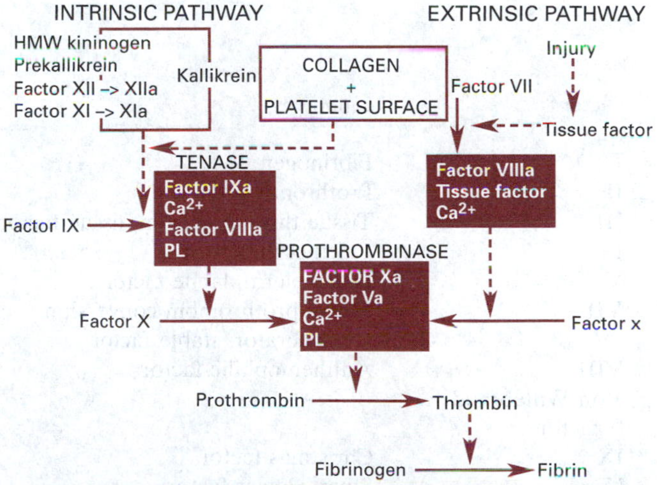

FIGURE 44-7 Clotting factor interactions. Coagulation is initiated by either an intrinsic or extrinsic pathway. In the intrinsic pathway, negatively charged surfaces initiate the contact activation and the phospholipid (PL) is furnished by platelets. In the extrinsic system, the phospholipid portion of tissue thromboplastin functions in conjunction with factor VIIa on the activation of factor X. From factor Xa on, both pathways converge upon a common path. Omitted from the diagram are inhibitors of the various steps, the augmentation of action of each pathway by activated factors, and the interaction between the intrinsic and extrinsic systems.

Recent observations indicate that after plaque disruption there is a first layer of fibrin formation, as a result of the activation of tissue factor and the coagulation cascade[1]; this precedes significant platelet deposition, as a result of thrombin generation by the coagulation cascade[1]; eventually, if the fibrin-platelet thrombus occludes the artery, further and significant fibrin formation takes place proximally as a result of stasis. Therefore, the coronary occlusive thrombus is like a "sandwich" composed of fibrin-platelet-fibrin.

Hypercoagulable-Dependent Thrombosis (Table 44-1)

There is evolving evidence that circulating monocytes and white blood cells may be involved in tissue factor expression and thereby influence the thrombogenicity of the circulating blood.[102] Activation of the circulating inflammatory cells in patients leading to acute coronary syndromes has been suggested by high titers of C-reactive protein preceding these events.[85,103–105] Hypercholesterolemia, a high-catecholamine drive such as smoking, emotional stress, cocaine use, certain chemotactic determinants, and perhaps infections may also trigger such hypercoagulable phenomena. In support of this hypothesis are studies evaluating lipid-lowering therapies that have found that normalization of the serum cholesterol reduced blood thrombogenicity.[106]

Several hemostatic determinants, such as fibrinogen, von Willebrand factor, and factor VIIa have been associated with an increased risk of cardiovascular disease. The association with fibrinogen is the most powerful and consistent. Abnormal levels of plasminogen activator inhibitor 1 (PAI-1) and tissue-type plasminogen activator (t-PA) antigen (a marker of endothelial dysfunction) are associated with an increased risk of cardiovascular events.[107] For instance, increased levels of PAI-1 have been found on young survivors of MI.[108] In a healthy cohort of patients, high baseline levels of endogenous t-PA have been found to be significant predictors of the risk of future MI.[108]

Vasoconstriction

Although the vast majority of acute coronary syndromes are caused by the disruption or erosion of a plaque with superimposed thrombus, other mechanisms that alter myocardial oxygen supply and demand must be considered. Studies by Maseri and colleagues have indicated that vasoconstriction has an important role.[109] In acute coronary syndromes, vasoconstriction may occur in response to a mildly dysfunctional endothelium near the culprit lesion or, more likely, may be a response to deep arterial damage or plaque disruption of the culprit lesion itself. Thus, with regard to this second type of vasoconstriction, it seems that a predisposition exists for platelet-dependent and thrombin-dependent vasoconstriction at the site of plaque disruption and thrombosis that may be significant but transient.[109] Thus, platelet-dependent vasoconstriction, mediated by serotonin and thromboxane A_2 (TXA_2),[110] and thrombin-mediated vasoconstriction occur if the vascular wall has been damaged substantially by deendothelialization, which suggests a direct interaction of these substances with the vascular smooth muscle cells.

Mechanism of Thrombosis

Thrombosis is comprised of two interrelated stages: primary hemostasis and secondary hemostasis.[111,112] The first stage of hemostasis is initiated by platelets as they adhere to damaged

TABLE 44-1 Glossary of the Coagulation Factors and Some of Their Properties

Factor	Synonyms	Molecular Weight	Plasma Concentration, mg/dL	In Vivo Half-Life, h	Inheritance
I	Fibrinogen	340,000	200–400	100–150	AD
II	Prothrombin	70,000	10	50–80	AD
III	Tissue thromboplastin, tissue factor	44,000	0		
IV	Calcium ion	40	9–10		
V	Proaccelerin, labile factor	330,000	1	24	AR
VII	Serum prothrombin conversion accelerator, stable factor	48,000	0.05	6	AR
VIII	Antihemophilic factor	330,000	0.01	12	SLR
Von Willebrand factor		(250,000)n[a]	1	24	AD
IX	Christmas factor	55,000	0.3	24	SLR
X	Stuart-Power factor	59,000	1	25–60	AR
XI	Plasma thromboplastin antecedent	160,000	0.5	40–80	AR
XII	Hageman factor	80,000	3	50–70	AR
XIII	Fibrin-stabilizing factor	320,000	1–2	150	AD
Prekallikrein	Fletcher factor	85,000	5	35	AR
High molecular weight kininogen	Fitzgerald, Flaujeac, Williams factor, contact activation cofactor	120,000	6	150	AR

[a]Multimers of the dimer subunit.
ABBREVIATIONS: AD = autosomal dominant; AR = autosomal recessive; SLR = sex-linked recessive.

vessels and form a platelet plug. The second phase involves activation of the coagulation system, which is comprised of a series of inactive proteins (zymogens) that are activated by proteolytic cleavage into active enzymes that ultimately cleave fibrinogen to fibrin to form a hemostatic clot (Fig. 44-7).[113] These two phases are dynamically interactive, however, since activated platelets can provide a surface for coagulation enzymes, and the ultimate enzyme of coagulation, thrombin, is a potent platelet activator.

Platelet Aggregation

Platelets play a key role in the transformation of a stable atherosclerotic plaque to an unstable lesion. With rupture or ulceration of an atherosclerotic plaque, the subendothelial matrix (e.g., collagen and tissue factor) is exposed to the circulating blood. Platelets mediate the "primary hemostasis" at the site of a ruptured plaque: the first step is *platelet adhesion* via the GP Ib receptor, as well as von Willebrand factor (Fig. 44-3). This is followed by *platelet activation*, which leads to (1) a shape change in the platelet (from a smooth discoid shape to a spiculated form, which increases the surface area upon which thrombin generation can occur); (2) degranulation of the alpha and dense granules, thereby releasing TXA_2, serotonin, and other platelet aggregatory and chemoattractant agents; and (3) expression of GP IIb/IIIa receptors on the platelet surface with activation of the receptor, such that it can bind fibrinogen. The final step is *platelet aggregation,* i.e., the formation of the platelet plug. Fibrinogen (or von Willebrand factor) binds to the activated GP IIb/IIIa receptors of two platelets, thereby creating a growing platelet aggregate.

Glycoprotein IIb/IIIa Receptor

The platelet GP IIb/IIIa receptor is a member of the integrin receptor superfamily of complexes that mediate cell-protein and cell-cell interactions.[114] The GP IIb/IIIa receptor is a calcium-dependent heterodimer, composed of two different subunits (α_{IIb} and β_3), both of which span the platelet membrane. The GP IIIa subunit contains a four-amino-acid sequence that is crucial for binding of fibrinogen and other ligands.[114] The first three amino acids are arginine-glycine-aspartic acid (abbreviated RGD). LMW peptide and nonpeptide GP IIb/IIIa inhibitors have been developed to bind to the RGD sequence of the receptor, thereby interfering with the binding of fibrinogen to the GP IIb/IIIa receptor (see page 1394).

Antiplatelet therapy has been directed at decreasing the formation of TXA_2 (e.g., aspirin), inhibiting the adenosine diphosphate (ADP) pathway of platelet activation (e.g., ticlopidine and clopidogrel), and directly inhibiting platelet aggregation (e.g., GP IIb/IIIa inhibitors).

Secondary Hemostasis

Simultaneously with formation of the platelet plug, the plasma coagulation system is activated. Traditionally, the coagulation cascade has been divided into two pathways: the *extrinsic* or contact system and the *intrinsic* system (Fig. 44-7). Recent evidence, however, has revised the understanding of coagulation into a single interrelated system.[115–117] The extrinsic pathway, initiated by release of tissue factor, is now felt to be the predominant mechanism of initiating hemostasis.[115,117] Ultimately, factor X is activated and leads to formation of thrombin, which in turn cleaves fibrinogen to fibrin (Fig. 44-3).

Thrombin plays a central role in arterial thrombosis: (1) it converts fibrinogen to fibrin in the final common pathway for clot formation, (2) it is a powerful stimulus for platelet aggregation, and (3) it activates factor XIII, which leads to cross-linking and stabilization of the fibrin clot.[111] Thrombin molecules are incorporated into coronary thrombi and can form the nidus of rethrombosis (i.e., reocclusion or reinfarction) as the thrombus undergoes fibrinolysis. Accordingly, effective thrombin inhibition is an important part of the therapy for acute coronary syndromes (see page 1394).

Hemostatic System

This is a complex, overlapping system that consists of blood vessels, platelets, procoagulants and anticoagulants, profibrinolytic components, and inhibitors. For clarity, the following sections deal with each component of the hemostatic mechanism individually. However, all of these processes are intimately related and inseparable.

ROLE OF VESSEL WALL CONTRACTION AND ENDOTHELIUM

The immediate control of bleeding from a small severed vessel is vasoconstriction, which is soon followed by local perivascular and intravascular activation of platelets and coagulation components. TXA_2 produced and released by activated platelets may play a role in persistent vasoconstriction, as do products released by stimulated endothelium (e.g., endothelin) or generated during coagulation (bradykinin generated by activated factor XII and fibrinopeptide B).

In normal vessels, circulating platelets do not adhere to normal (unstimulated) endothelial cells in vivo. This may relate to the fact that both platelets and endothelium have a negative charge and thus would be mutually repulsive. The negative electrical charge of endothelial cells is due to a pronounced glycocalyx, consisting of proteoglycans, of which heparan sulfate (a heparin-like substance that binds antithrombin III) is the most important. Stimulated or injured endothelial cells lose their negative surface charge. The nonthrombogenic nature of endothelium is also partly due to the lack of surface molecules as tissue factor.

The thromboresistance of normal endothelium also depends on several substances produced by endothelial cells. They include potent vasodilators and inhibitors of platelet function, such as prostacyclin [prostaglandin I_2 (PGI_2)] and nitric oxide (NO), which serve to prevent platelet adhesion to endothelium.[118,119] Anticoagulant properties include heparin-like glycosaminoglycans and a thrombin-binding protein called thrombomodulin.

The production of prostacyclin by endothelium is stimulated by contact with activated platelets or leukocytes by stretching of the arterial wall (pulsatile pressure) and by some drugs. PGI_1 has strong antiplatelet and vasodilator properties and thus acts as the biological antagonist of TXA_2. A direct link between impaired biosynthesis of PGI_2 in the vessel wall and thrombosis or atherosclerosis is suggested by the decreased capacity of endothelium to generate prostacyclin with age, atherosclerosis, and risk factors such as high cholesterol, heavy smoking, and diabetes. NO is formed from L-arginine by an oxidation pathway that requires several cofactors. NO relaxes smooth muscle cells through stimulation of guanylate cyclase, which, in turn, generates cyclic guanosine monophosphate (cyclic GMP).[120] By the same mechanism, it is also a potent inhibitor of adhesion and aggregation of platelets.

There is a clear synergism between prostacyclin and NO in preventing platelet activation. NO is effective only in the immediate vicinity of its site of release because hemoglobin almost immediately inactivates any NO that enters the bloodstream. It has been suggested that a deficiency in NO production contributes to the pathogenesis of atherosclerosis and to the development of complications of diabetes. Thrombomodulin is a transmembranous protein that serves as an endothelial receptor for free thrombin.[121] In the complex that is formed and which does not require calcium, thrombin loses its procoagulant activity and expresses its anticoagulant role by activating protein C.

ROLE OF PLATELETS

The exterior coat of platelets, the glycocalyx, contains many distinct glycoproteins that are important for platelet function. They include integrins and leucine-rich glycoproteins. These surface glycoproteins mediate platelet adhesion and aggregation as receptors for adhesive proteins and agonists. The platelets contain dense bodies, alpha granules, actin filaments, microtubules, and an open canalicular system, which all have their respective functions in the formation of a hemostatic plug (Fig. 44-2).

In normal conditions, platelets are quiescent and circulate freely in the blood because they do not attach to a normally functioning endothelium. Vessel injury, however, exposes subendothelial connective tissue to various elements to which platelets can adhere.[122,123] This phenomenon—platelet adhesion—is the initial event and one of the most crucial steps in platelet plug formation. The adhesive proteins collagen and fibronectin (and, to a lesser extent, laminin, microfibrils, and thrombospondin) are present in subendothelium and interact readily with von Willebrand factor, whereby this large protein changes its conformation. This allows platelets to bind to von Willebrand factor via their surface GP Ia/IIa and Ic/IIa receptors (Figs. 44-3 and 44-4). Particularly collagen, a ubiquitous structural component of the vessel wall, is important and may provide scaffolding on which other adhesive proteins assemble. Von Willebrand factor, which has two collagen-binding sites, is an absolute requirement for platelet adhesion but only at high shear rates, whereas fibronectin plays a significant role in platelet adhesion at lower shear rates.

After adhesion, platelets lose their discoid shape, form extended pseudopods, and spread out over the injured surface. Through the action of activators such as collagen and eventually thrombin and norepinephrine, the adhered platelets soon become activated, whereby other platelet receptors are expressed and several mediators stored in platelet granules are released.[124] This release reaction seems to be initiated by contraction of a circumferential band of microtubules. Stored granules are discharged through the open canalicular system after fusion of the granular membrane with the membranes of the open canalicular system. Among the granular agents released are ADP, serotonin, β-thromboglobulin, platelet factor 4, platelet growth factor, and TXA_2.[125,126]

These released substances, particularly ADP and TXA_2, induce binding of platelets to one another, a phenomenon called *platelet aggregation*. This process increases the size of the hemostatic plug at the site of injury and, by recruiting additional circulating platelets, transforms the initial monolayer of platelets into an aggregate. The platelet surface GP IIb/IIIa undergo a conformational change in the aggregation process, so that they can interact with plasma fibrinogen and other adhesive proteins as fibronectin and endothelial thrombospondin, which serve to link platelets together into a tighter aggregate (Fig. 44-7).[124,127]

The prostaglandins also play an important role in mediating the platelet release reaction and aggregation (Fig. 44-4). Collagen and epinephrine appear to trigger the activation of one or more phospholipases in the platelet membrane. Phospholipase A_2 acts on phosphatidylcholine to release arachidonic acid from the platelet membrane. Arachidonic acid is metabolized by cyclooxygenase to unstable proaggregating prostaglandin endoperoxide intermediates (prostaglandins G2 and H2). TXA_2 is formed by the action of thromboxane synthase on PGH_2; it further promotes platelet activation, thrombus growth, and local vasoconstriction.

On the other hand, the vascular endothelial cells synthesize prostacyclin (PGI_2), starting from arachidonic acid or from platelet-derived PGG_2. Prostacyclin stimulates adenylate cyclase and leads to an increased level of cyclic adenosine monophosphate (cyclic AMP) in the platelet (Fig. 44-5). Cyclic AMP, in turn, inhibits the discharge of calcium from the dense tubular system and thus prevents platelet aggregation and secretion. Phosphodiesterase enhances the breakdown of cyclic AMP.

Arachidonic acid also serves as a substrate for the formation of leukotrienes, a pathway mediated by lipoxygenase in the leukocytes. Thus, eicosanoids derived from arachidonic acid in platelets, endothelial cells, and leukocytes provide short-acting biological mediators that further promote not only platelet activation and local vasoconstriction but also platelet inhibition and vasodilatation. In addition, they intervene in local immune-mediated reactions.

ROLE OF BLOOD FLOW

Blood flow influences platelet function by shear stress. Exposure of platelets to very high shear stress leads to spontaneous aggregation even in the absence of exogenous agonists. Furthermore, some coagulation reactions are accelerated in the presence of high shear, and the ability of the endothelium to secrete tissue plasminogen activator over the basal level is increased two- to threefold.

ROLE OF BLOOD COAGULATION

Activated platelets provide a microenvironment that enhances the acceleration of fibrin formation at the site of injury. They rearrange their surface lipoproteins so that phospholipids, on which coagulation factors can concentrate, are now exposed to the bloodstream. This is accompanied by the exposure of high-affinity binding sites for the activated factors V, VIII, IX, and X. Thus, activated platelets provide a suitable surface on which the activation of prothrombin to thrombin is accelerated dramatically. Thrombin occupies a central position in the coagulation process. It is formed as the end product of a complex chain of reactions that transform, in sequence, a number of coagulation factors present as precursors (zymogens) in plasma into activated factors. Table 44-1 lists the well-recognized coagulation factors with their Roman numeral designations and synonyms and some of their properties. The coagulation factors are numbered roughly in the order of their discovery and do not reflect the sequence of reactions. Coagulation factors interact mainly on the membrane of activated platelets and other stimulated cells and tissue factor (a membrane protein exposed to the blood, e.g., after trauma) on which coagulation factors bind. Because of the low concentration of these factors in plasma and the abundant presence of circulating inhibitors, the interaction of procoagulants and their subsequent activation can proceed only slowly in the fluid phase of blood.

Coagulation factors are activated one by one, mainly through limited proteolysis. When the letter "a" accompanies a Roman numeral (e.g., factor VIIa), this indicates that the factor is in its activated form rather than in its naturally occurring precursor form (e.g., factor X). All activated factors are serine proteases: they split arginyl bonds in their specific substrate, and the latter then becomes another activated coagulation factor (waterfall or cascade sequence of events). In contrast, factors V and VIII, tissue factor and high molecular weight (HMW) kininogen are not proenzymes but function rather as cofactors. They can thus be considered as regulatory proteins (cofactors) that influence the reaction rate. These cofactors (except tissue factor) still require activation by minor proteolysis, while tissue factor X, present in extravascular spaces, must make contact with blood to function. The traditional coagulation scheme distinguishes an intrinsic from an extrinsic activation pathway.

The Intrinsic Pathway of the Coagulation System: Activation of Factors XII, XI, X, and IX All factors participating in the intrinsic pathway are present in circulating blood, and the reaction sequence is initiated by contact of platelets and/or coagulation components with a subendothelial tissue. Antigen-antibody complexes and activated platelets may also serve this purpose, as can fissured atherosclerotic plaques and foreign surfaces, such as those in an extracorporeal circulation or renal dialysis. In vitro, this initial contact phase involves the interaction of factor XII (Hageman factor), factor XI, prekallikrein, and HMW kininogen with a foreign surface (a surface other than normal endothelium or blood cells).

When circulating factor XII meets negatively charged surfaces such as glass and kaolin, it binds via its heavy chain to the surface. Upon adsorption, bound factor XII exerts traces of biological activity. For the mechanisms of this phenomenon, conformation changes of the molecule with exposure of the enzyme site in the light chain have been postulated (Fig. 44-6). Factor XI and prekallikrein exist in plasma as equimolar complexes with HMW kininogen, and these complexes are bound to initiating surfaces via the HMW kininogen moiety. HMW kininogen transports both factor XI and prekallikrein to an appropriate surface. Surface binding is assumed to serve to bring factor XII, prekallikrein, and factor XI to a close spatial orientation. Binding of factor XII to a negatively charged surface also makes the molecule more susceptible to proteolytic cleavage. Initially, traces of factor XIIa presumably generate traces of kallikrein from prekallikrein by splitting of a single peptide bond. Kallikrein will now activate more rapidly factor XII in a feedback loop, which, in turn, will generate more kallikrein, and the reciprocal activation of these two surface-bound molecules continues until the substrates are locally exhausted. Of note, a potent vasoactive substance, bradykinin, is released from HMW kininogen upon the activation of factor XII and generation of kallikrein. The latter also activates pro-urokinase, enhancing fibrinolytic activity.

Factor XIIa converts in vitro the next factor of the coagulation cascade, factor XI, from its zymogen form to its enzymatic constellation. Factor XI also circulates in plasma complexed with HMW kininogen; the latter protein thus serves as helper protein carrying factors XII and XI in the blood (Fig. 44-7). The in vivo activation of factor XI is less clear. It is possible that factor XII–independent activation of factor XI is mediated by thrombin. Both factor XIIa and thrombin cleave the same internal peptide bond (Arg369-Ile) in each of the two chains of the factor XI molecule, leading to the formation of two heavy and two light chains.

Factor XIa bound to the surfaces by HMW kininogen interacts upon activation with factor IX in a calcium-dependent two-step reaction. Each light chain of factor XIa contains a catalytic site, while its heavy chain has the binding site for factor IX and HMW kininogen. Binding of calcium ions to factor IX (a vitamin K–dependent protein) induces a conformational change in the molecule, which facilitates its binding to the heavy chain of factor XIa, which is essential for the optimal rate of factor IX activation. Platelets can also be reckoned to be important in the intrinsic system as they contain HMW kininogen, which can be expressed when the platelets are activated, as they indeed are on fissured and sclerotic plaques and foreign surfaces.

Activated factor IX, thrombin-modified factor VIII, negatively charged phospholipid (e.g., activated platelets), and calcium ions form a multimolecular complex coined *tenase* because it activates directly factor X; the glutamic acid (Gla) residues of factors IXa and Xa mediate their binding to phospholipid (Fig. 44-7).

Congenital deficiency of the three contact factors (factor XII, prekallikrein, and HMW kininogen) is not associated with bleeding, and only half of factor XI–deficient patients have bleeding problems with an intensity not related to the factor XI level. The significance of the contact phase is, therefore, speculative; however, it may become relevant in particular therapeutic settings. Indeed, extracorporeal circuits may be regarded as a giant test-tube condition, and the contact activation becomes important under these circumstances. Beyond the contact phase, the intrinsic activation system is important, already in physiologic conditions, as individuals with a severe deficiency of factor VIII or IX (two forms of hemophilia) have a serious bleeding condition.

The Extrinsic (Tissue Factor) Pathway of the Coagulation System: Activation of Factors VII and X In the extrinsic system, membrane-bound tissue factor starts off the chain of events by forming a complex with factor VII in the presence of calcium ions (Fig. 44-7). Tissue factor is as a dimer composed of two identical subunits with interacting enzyme-binding sites.[128,129] It is present on nonvascular cell surfaces and on microvesicles shed from cell surfaces. It was hypothesized that the normal distribution of tissue factor represents a hemostatic envelope ready to activate coagulation when vascular integrity is disrupted. Vascular endothelial cells and monocytes also can produce and express tissue factor activity upon stimulation with interleukin 1 or endotoxin, which suggests that cytokines may modulate tissue factor expression and fibrin deposition at the site of inflammation. Tissue factor is an integral membrane protein composed of protein and phospholipid components, both of which are required for its procoagulant activity. Factor VII is a single-chain protein that, in this form, already has some enzymatic activity and can complex with tissue factor. By cleavage of an Arg-Ile bond, however, the molecule of factor VII splits in a light chain and a heavy chain (containing the active site) linked by two disulfide bonds. This activation increases the coagulant activity of factor VII about 100-fold. However, the activation of factor VII occurs only after it has bound to tissue factor. The tissue factor–factor VIIa complex then combines with the substrate (factor X), producing a further conformational change in factor VIIa, so that it binds still more tightly to tissue factor, precluding dissociation of factor VIIa from tissue factor. The tissue factor–factor VIIa complex activates primarily factor X but also factors IX and XI, which interconnect the intrinsic and extrinsic activation pathways and play a prima ballerina role in the activation of coagulation.[13] Tissue factor accelerates these reactions as a cofactor, apparently by inducing a conformational change in factor VIIa.

It should be noted that phospholipids of the platelet membrane, in conjunction with factor Xa, can also activate factor VII—another bridge between the intrinsic and extrinsic pathways. Thus, the earlier concepts of a clearly separate intrinsic and extrinsic activation system are becoming obsolete. That factor VII is essential to ensure normal hemostasis is underlined by the bleeding condition of patients with severe congenital factor VII deficiency.

The Pathway in Common: The Formation of Prothrombinase, the Enzyme Converting Prothrombin to Thrombin Factor X stands at the crossroad of the extrinsic and intrinsic activation pathways.[130] This means that factor X can be activated either by the tenase complex (IXa, phospholipid, VIIIa, and Ca ions) or by the tissue factor–factor VIIa complex (Fig. 44-7). In both instances, activation of factor X results from the cleavage of a single peptide bond between Arg and Ile, releasing an activation peptide and unmasking an active site on the heavy chain.[131] This is brought about by the enzymatic activity residing in factor IXa, which is part of the tenase complex. The presence of proteolytically modified factor VIII—whether by thrombin, factor Xa, or factor IXa—by separation of factor VIII from von Willebrand factor enhances 10,000-fold the rate of activation of factor X by factor IXa. Factor VIIIa has no enzymatic activity and is thus a helper protein (a cofactor) which, to exert its function, binds to phospholipid vesicles, provided phosphatidylserine is available on the platelet membrane.[16,132] In fact, specific binding sites are available on activated platelets for factor VIII that are distinct from the binding sites for factor V expressed during stimulation of platelets. As shown below, activated protein C degrades factor VIIIa. Thus, factor VIII must be activated for hemostasis and inactivated for the maintenance of the fluidity of blood.

To be fully active, factor Xa has to form a stoichiometric 1:1 complex with factor Va; the latter molecule enhances the activation of prothrombin by factor Xa 300,000-fold. Normal plasma contains factor V in trace amounts (25 n*M*, while factor X is about 200 n*M*) and in an inactive state; its activation requires three specific enzymatic cleavages, which can be brought about by thrombin or less efficiently by factor Xa. The association of factor Va with factor Xa on an anionic phospholipid is termed *prothrombinase*. Factor Va increases the turnover (k_{cat}) 1000-fold, which means that the number of thrombin molecules generated by the enzyme upon saturation by the substrate is multiplied by a factor of approximately 1000. In contrast to the vitamin K–dependent procoagulation factors (prothrombin and factors VII, IX, and X), which bind to phospholipids via calcium bridges with their Gla domain, factor Va does not bind to phospholipids via calcium bridges but penetrates into the lipid bilayer.

The Action of Prothrombinase on Prothrombin The multimolecular complex prothrombinase initially cleaves one Arg-Ile bond in the prothrombin molecule, producing meizo-thrombin. This intermediate molecule remains membrane bound through the retained Gla domain linkage and activates the inhibitor protein C but lacks procoagulant properties either on platelets or on fibrinogen. To obtain the latter property, another arginine bond (Arg-Thr) has to be cleaved, yielding alpha-thrombin, which, lacking a Gla-containing region, is released from the cell surface.

For the different reactions pertaining to the coagulation cascade system, it is being assumed that all coagulation factors immobilize on phospholipids (stimulated platelets or perturbed endothelial or white cells) and that reaction products are shuttled between assembled complexes. An alternative but less efficient possibility is that reaction products dissociate from the phospholipid membranes to become free in solution. Single-membrane channeling protects critical enzymes from inactivation by plasma inhibitors (e.g., antithrombin III) as well as from dilution by blood flow.

The Pivotal Role of Thrombin Thrombin represents the culmination of the coagulation cascade; its action on fibrinogen is most dramatic, because thrombus formation is a visible process. Thrombin itself is responsible for its own nonlinear generation caused by positive feedback activation, whereby thrombin enhances neoformation of thrombin (Fig. 44-8). In addition, thrombin is a pivotal molecule for numerous other functions. The action of thrombin on platelets results in the release of platelet factor V exteriorization and in the transbilayer movement of its inner membrane surface (flip-flop reaction). Thrombin activates three of the four cofactor or helper proteins (factors V and VIII and thrombomodulin but not tissue factor). Thrombin furthermore activates factor XIII, which increases the strength and renders the fibrin more resistant to thrombolysis. Thrombin can increase the production and release of prostacyclin, NO, ADP, and PAI-1 from the normal endothelium, protecting the microcirculation against thrombosis. Thrombin inhibits its own production by a negative feedback mechanism via the thrombomodulin–protein C and S system. Thrombin is also involved in other biological effects, such as chemotaxis and mitogenesis. It also elicits a potent mitogenic response in fibroblasts and macrophages, thereby modulating inflammatory reactions at the site of vascular injury.

The Conversion of Fibrinogen to Fibrin Fibrinogen is a large paired molecule held together by disulfide bridges. Each symmetric half-molecule consists of one set of three different polypeptide chains termed $A\alpha$, $B\beta$, and γ. The two half-molecules are joined in the central amino-terminal domain in an antiparallel manner by three interchain disulfide bridges, two of which are between γ chains and the other between α chains.

Thrombin splits an arginine-glycine bond, first at the amino end of the two $A\alpha$ chains and later at the amino end of each of the two $B\beta$ chains so that each molecule releases in sequence two small aminopeptides A (FPA) and two small fibrinopeptides B (FPB) from fibrinogen and thus converts this molecule to fibrin monomers that are still soluble (Fig. 44-9). The FPA release exposes a polymerization site in the central region of the fibrinogen molecule (E domain) that subsequently aligns with a complementary site in the outer region (D domain) of another fibrin monomer to form staggered overlapping two-stranded fibrils. The slower FPB release exposes an independent site for noncovalent intermolecular interaction, resulting in complementary alignment of fibrin monomers. Subsequently, lateral association of fibrin monomers occurs, and the network becomes thicker and branched, still through a nonenzymatic process. These coupled monomers of fibrin, called *polymers*, are still soluble unless they become too large and precipitate; the resulting gel of fibrin forms the skeleton of a thrombus and traps red and white cells.

The structural stability of the fibrin network is achieved through covalent cross-linking.[133] Thrombin activates factor XIII (*fibrin-stabilizing factor*), a transglutaminase that, in the presence of calcium, forms peptide bonds between side chains of suitable lysine (donor) and Gla (acceptor) residues. The result of such a lysine cross-link is that the thrombus becomes firmer and more resistant to thrombolysis. It should be noted that fibrin-bound thrombin (approximately 40 percent of the thrombin generated) retains its coagulant and platelet-activating properties and is protected from inactivation by circulating heparin-antithrombin III.[134] During thrombolysis, fibrin-bound thrombin is released and can cause rethrombosis. Hirudin, hirulog, and similar antithrombin III-independent synthetic thrombin inhibitors, which are smaller than heparin, can inhibit fibrin-bound thrombin. Of note, two other plasma proteins (fibronectin and α2-plasmin inhibitor) are also covalently cross-linked to fibrin by factor XIIIa and are incorporated in the fibrin mesh.

Connections Between the Intrinsic and Extrinsic Pathways of Coagulation The concept of separating the two pathways of the coagulation system that merge in a common pathway from the activation of factor X on is a didactic schematization that is increasingly blurred as feedback mechanisms and interactions between the two pathways are found.[129] For example, the factor VIIa–tissue factor complex can activate factors IX and XI directly; factors IXa and Xa can activate factor VII. The extrinsic pathway seems to play a major role in the initiation of in vivo coagulation, while the intrinsic pathway is now thought to be required for continuous growth and maintenance of fibrin formation.

Activation of coagulation factors in successive stages is based on the classical cascade. It will be appreciated that the speed with which these reactions develop increases gradually, as in a system of electronic amplification. Also, here one should realize that nature acts in concert rather than in a sequence of solitary actions. Of course, this is a common feature in biological systems. In the case of the coagulation system, it is the more remarkable because it operates largely outside the cell without the controls imposed by intracellular compartmentation.

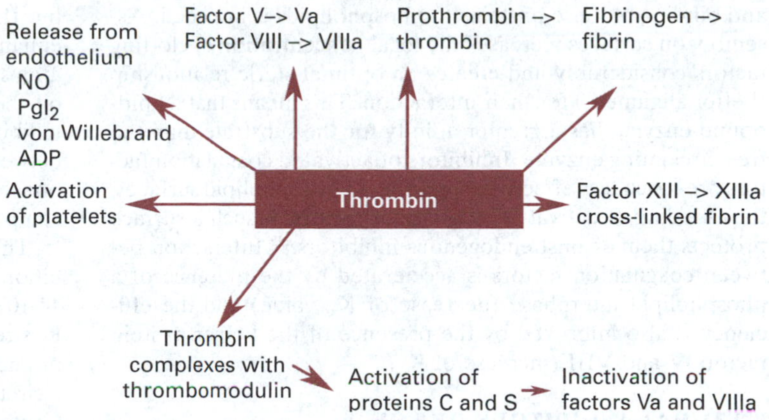

FIGURE 44-8 Thrombin is the pivotal enzyme in coagulation, being responsible for positive feedback activation, rapid activation of platelets and endothelial cells, and indirectly via thrombomodulin for its activation. ADP = adenosine diphosphate; PGI_2 = prostaglandin I_2.

Coagulation: A Series of Surface-Catalyzed Events With the exception of fibrinogen, prothrombin, and plasminogen, the coagulation factors are present in the fluid phase of blood at very low concentrations. Their encounter in solution is possible and their interaction slow, though this can be remarkably accelerated, up to 100,000-fold, after adsorption and concentration on surfaces. Modified endothelium, stimulated platelets, denuded subendothelial structures (e.g., collagen), fissured atherosclerotic plaques, and foreign surfaces (extracorporeal circulation conduits) allow the attachment of passing platelets (adhesion) and the absorption of coagulation proteins. One way for this to occur is by binding mediated through calcium bridges between negatively charged phospholipids (tissue factor, activated platelets, and microvesicles) and the γ-carboxyglutamic acid (Gla) residues of the four vitamin K–dependent procoagulants (prothrombin and factors VII, IX, and X), and two endogenous anticoagulants (proteins C and S). Coumarin drugs interfere in the vitamin K cycle, so that less glutamic acid is formed

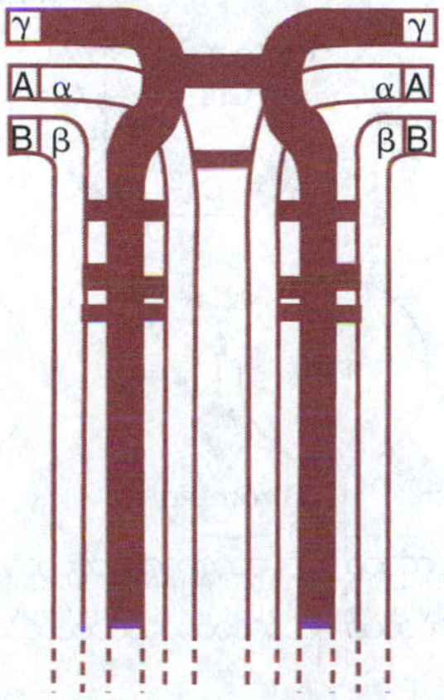

FIGURE 44-9 Structure of fibrinogen. This glycoprotein is a paired molecule, each half consisting of three homologous chains; $A\alpha$, $B\beta$, and γ. The horizontal connecting lines are disulfide bonds. Thrombin cleaves first the A peptide and then the B peptide. The disulfide knot of the dimer fibrinogen is clearly depicted. The entire sequence of 2946 amino acids has been elucidated.

and binding of these proteins to phospholipids is impeded. Assembly on surfaces increases the local concentration of clotting factors considerably and creates an optimal steric relationship (better alignment) for their interaction. This means that a lipid-bound enzyme has a greater affinity for the substrate than the free circulating enzyme. Inhibitors of activated coagulation factors are much less effective in binding to phospholipid surfaces; thus binding of activated coagulation factors to such a surface protects them against endogenous inhibitors.[135] Interaction between coagulation factors is accelerated by the presence of a phospholipid interphase (decrease of K_m value) and the efficiency is also improved by the presence of the helper protein factors V and VIII (increase of K_{cat}).

NATURAL INHIBITORS OF THE COAGULATION SYSTEM

Several mechanisms help to prevent uncontrolled formation of fibrin in the circulation. First, coagulation remains a strictly localized process because it requires negatively charged surfaces, which are in the first place provided by activated platelets. Platelet activation, in turn, is limited to sites of vessel injury and fissured atherosclerotic plaques. In addition, the flowing blood will rapidly dilute any inadvertently activated clotting factor before it perpetuates the reaction sequence to form fibrin. Finally, a number of proteins circulate in the blood to inhibit the coagulation process at various stages of the cascade. Four of them appear particularly important in preventing thrombosis: antithrombin III, protein C, tissue factor pathway inhibitor, and thrombomodulin.

Antithrombin III inhibits thrombin and the activated forms of several coagulation factors, but inhibition of thrombin and of factor Xa is particularly important and clinically relevant.[136] Thrombin forms a tightly bound, stable complex with antithrombin III; this occurs at a relatively slow rate that is enormously enhanced by heparin (see below) and also appreciably by heparan sulfate, a substance very similar to heparin, which is found on the intraluminal surface of vascular endothelial cells. The inhibition of thrombin is due to ternary complex formation between thrombin, antithrombin III, and heparin. The inhibition of factor Xa is the result of the formation of a binary complex between antithrombin III and factor Xa.

The protein C–thrombomodulin pathway of thrombin inhibition represents the major natural anticoagulant system (Fig. 44-10). Protein C is a proenzyme formed in the liver; vitamin K is required in its synthesis. On the surface of either platelets or endothelium, protein C is activated by thrombin to become a circulating serine protease that inhibits factors Va and VIIIa. Complex formation between thrombin and thrombomodulin, a potent cofactor present on the endothelial surface, catalyzes the activation of protein C. Protein S is another vitamin K–dependent protein that does not possess serine protease properties but appears to function as a cofactor for activated protein C by facilitating its binding to membrane phospholipids.[137] In plasma, protein S circulates free or bound to C4b-binding protein, a component of the complement system. Only free protein S serves as a cofactor of activated protein C. In addition to being a powerful anticoagulant, activated protein C initiates fibrinolysis by releasing t-PA from the endothelium and neutralizing PAI.

Tissue factor–factor VIIa complex is inactivated by the tissue factor pathway inhibitor (TFPI), previously called lipid protein–associated coagulation inhibitor.[129,130,135] TFPI appears to be the only plasma component inhibiting the catalytic activity of factor VIIa–tissue factor complex. Factor VIIa cannot be neutralized effectively unless it is bound to tissue factor.[129] This is in contrast to other coagulation components, which are neutralized more effectively as free reactants than after they interact in complexes.[138] TFPI first interacts with factor Xa to form Xa-TFPI complexes, which then form a quarternary Xa–TFPI–VIIa–tissue factor complex with resulting loss of the activity of VIIa–tissue factor complex. The plasma concentration of TFPI is low, but a larger pool of TFPI bound to vascular endothelium is present from which TFPI can be released into the blood by heparin.

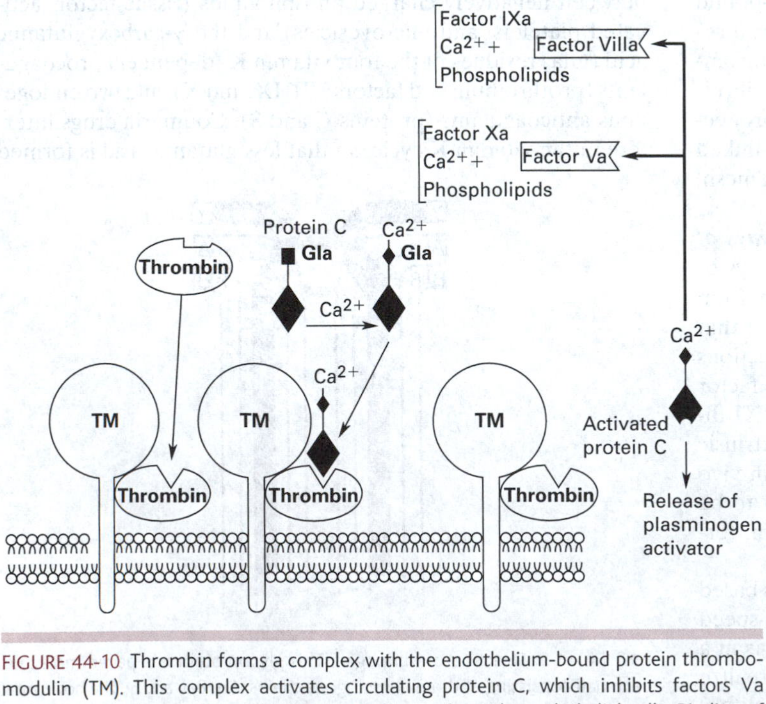

FIGURE 44-10 Thrombin forms a complex with the endothelium-bound protein thrombomodulin (TM). This complex activates circulating protein C, which inhibits factors Va and VIIIa and releases tissue-plasminogen activator from the endothelial cells. Binding of activated protein C to phospholipids is facilitated by protein S. Gla = γ-carboxyglutamic acid.

Thrombomodulin is located on the surface of all endothelial cells except those in the microcirculation of the human brain. When thrombin is generated within a vascular space, excess thrombin is bound to thrombomodulin. Thrombomodulin exerts three types of activities: (1) it inhibits thrombin-induced activation of platelets, factor V, and fibrinogen; (2) it promotes the activation of protein C after formation of the thrombomodulin-thrombin complex; and (3) it enhances the inhibition of thrombin by antithrombin III. Thus, thrombomodulin modifies the substrate specificity of thrombin; the procoagulant activity is switched off, and at the same time its anticoagulant activity is tremendously increased.

The Fibrinolytic System

This system is essential for removing excess fibrin deposits to preserve vascular patency. The role of fibrinolysis in the maintenance of blood fluidity is well illustrated by an increased incidence of venous thromboembolism in patients with abnormal, nonfunctional plasminogen. Similarly, the overproduction of PAI-1 in transgenic mice leads to an increased risk of venous embolism.

COMPONENTS OF THE FIBRINOLYTIC SYSTEM

Plasminogen This is present in human plasma at a concentration of about 2 μM, which is about twice the concentration of α_2-antiplasmin. The native molecule, denoted Glu-plasminogen, after its NH_2-terminal glutamic acid, is a single-chain glycoprotein, consisting of 791 amino acids.[23] Plasminogen is organized in seven structural domains (Fig. 44-11). From the NH2-terminal end, there is a *preactivation peptide,* five sequential, homologous, looped kringle structures, and the T-proteinase domain with the catalytic site composed of His^{603}, Asp^{646}, and Ser^{741}. The kringle domains contain lysine-binding sites that play a crucial role in the specific recognition of fibrin, cell surfaces, and α_2-antiplasmin.[139–141]

Plasminogen is converted to a two-chain serine protease called *plasmin* by cleavage of a single Arg^{561}-Val^{562} peptide bond between kringle 5 and the proteinase domain. The serine-containing active site is situated in the B or light chain. Plasmin may catalyze the release of the preactivation peptide from Glu-plasminogen, forming degraded plasminogen with amino-terminal lysine, valine, or methionine commonly called *Lys-plasminogen*. Lys-plasminogen is more easily activated to plasmin than Glu-plasminogen.[141] Plasmin digests a number of proteins, including fibrin, fibrinogen, and factors V and VIII, as well as a number of esters and amides.

Natural Plasminogen Activators Plasminogen may be converted to plasmin by a number of agents called *plasminogen activators*. The principal circulating plasminogen activator in humans is *tissue-type plasminogen activator* (t-PA). This a 70-kDa serine proteinase, which in its native form consists of a single polypeptide chain. t-PA is converted by plasmin to a two-chain form by hydrolysis of the Arg^{275}-Ile^{276} peptide bond. In contrast to most single-chain forms of serine proteinases, single-chain t-PA possesses significant catalytic activity. The amino-terminal region is composed of several domains with homologies to other proteins: a finger domain, a growth factor domain, and two looped kringle structures (Fig. 44-12). The region constituted by residues 276 to 527 represents the serine proteinase part with the catalytic site, composed of His^{322}, Asp^{371}, and Ser^{478}.[142] These distinct domains in t-PA are involved in several functions of the enzyme, including its binding to fibrin, fibrin-specific plasminogen activation, rapid clearance in vivo, and binding to endothelial cell receptors. Binding of t-PA to fibrin is mediated via the finger and the second kringle domains. The presence of fibrin markedly enhances the plasminogen-activating property of t-PA, as it not only binds t-PA and plasminogen but also greatly increases the affinity of t-PA for plasminogen. Thus, fibrin appears to concentrate both t-PA and plasminogen on its surface and to enhance their interaction (see Ambrose et al.[26] and Fuster et al.[28]). Plasmin so formed on fibrin surfaces has its lysine-binding and active sites occupied and is relatively protected from the inhibitory action of α_2-antiplasmin.

Single-chain urokinase-type plasminogen activator (scu-PA) is a 54-kDa glycoprotein containing 411 amino acids (Fig. 44-12). The plasma concentration of scu-PA is about 2 ng/mL.

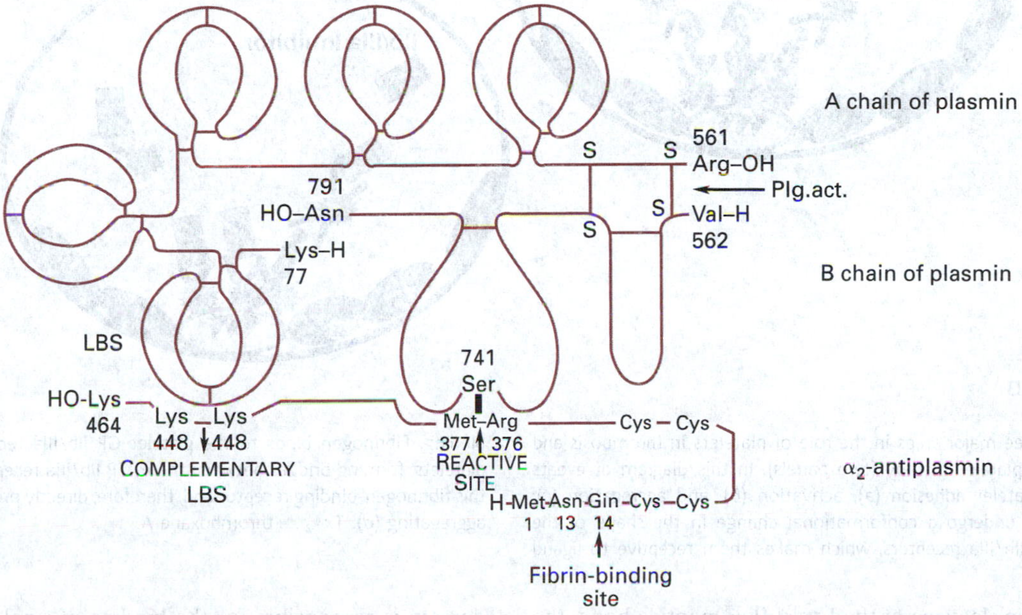

FIGURE 44-11 Schematic visualization of the molecular interactions regulating fibrinolysis. On the fibrin surface, plasminogen is efficiently converted to the proteolytic enzyme plasmin by bound plasminogen activator (Plg. act.). The plasmin generated is partially protected from inactivation by α_2-antiplasmin, while free plasmin in the blood is very rapidly inactivated. The lysine-binding sites (LBS) of plasminogen are important for the interaction between plasmin(ogen) and fibrin and between plasmin and α_2-antiplasmin. The heavy or A chain of plasminogen originates from the amino-terminal part of the molecule; the light or B chain constitutes the COOH-terminal part; the latter contains the active serine.

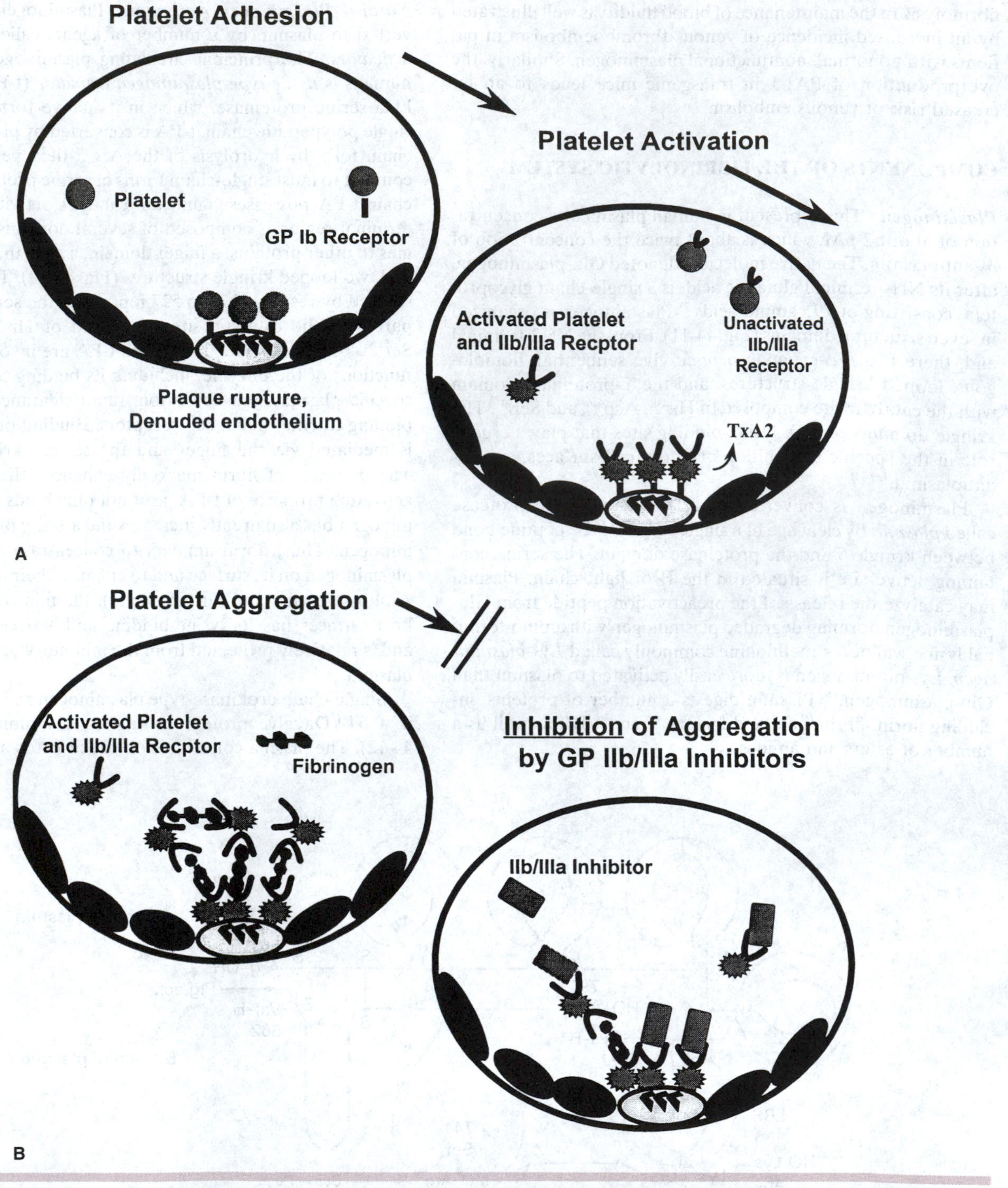

FIGURE 44-12 Three major steps in the role of platelets in thrombosis and the targets of antiplatelet therapy (two panels). In this diagram of events associated with platelet adhesion (*a*), activation (*b*), and aggregation (*c*), activated platelets undergo a conformational change in the shape of the glycoprotein (GP) IIb/IIIa receptors, which makes them receptive to ligand binding. Fibrinogen binds to the platelet GP IIb/IIIa receptors on adjacent platelets, forming bridges between them. GP IIb/IIIa receptor inhibitors block this fibrinogen-binding receptor and, therefore, directly prevent platelets from aggregating (*d*). TxA_2 = thromboxane A_2.

Upon proteolytic cleavage of the Lys^{158}-Ile^{159} peptide bond, the molecule is converted to a two-chain derivative (tcu-PA, urokinase). The catalytic triad is located in the carboxy-terminal polypeptide chain and is composed of Asp^{255}, His^{204}, and Ser^{356}. The amino-terminal chain contains an epidermal growth factor domain and one kringle domain. The epidermal growth factor domain is responsible for the binding of single-chain u-PA to its receptor, which is present on the surface of a variety of cells. The u-PA receptor is essential for localization of u-PA-mediated plasmin formation to the pericellular environment.[143,144] A LMW tcu-PA (33 kDa) can be generated from tcu-PA by hydrolysis of the Lys^{135}-Lys^{136} peptide with plasmin.

A LMW scu-PA (32 kDa) can be generated by proteolytic cleavage of the Glu^{143}-Leu^{144} peptide bond.[145]

ENDOGENOUS INHIBITORS OF THE FIBRINOLYTIC SYSTEM

α_2-Antiplasmin (α_2-plasmin inhibitor) belongs to the serine proteinase inhibitor superfamily (serpins). Like other inhibitors of this class, serpins react with their target proteinases by formation of a 1:1 molar reversible complex, followed by covalent binding between the hydroxyl group of the active-site serine residue of the proteinase and the carboxyl group of the P1 residue at the reactive site ("bait region") of the serpin (Fig. 44-11).

α_2-Antiplasmin is present in plasma at a concentration of about 1 μM. It is a 67-kDa glycoprotein containing 464 amino acids and about 13 percent carbohydrate.[146] The reactive site of the inhibitor is the Arg^{364}-Met^{365} peptide bond. α_2-Antiplasmin is unique among serpins by having a carboxy-terminal extension of 51 amino acid residues; this contains a secondary binding site that reacts with the lysine-binding sites of the kringles 1 to 3 of both plasminogen and plasmin. α_2-Antiplasmin (plasminogen-binding form) becomes partly converted in the circulating blood to a non-plasminogen-binding, less reactive form (about 30 percent of the total) that lacks the 26 carboxy-terminal residues. Two forms of α_2-antiplasmin are present in about equal amounts in purified preparations of the inhibitor. The amino-terminal Gln^{14} residue of α_2-antiplasmin can cross-link to Aa chains of fibrin, in a process that requires Ca^{2+} and is catalyzed by activated coagulation factor XIII. This renders the thrombus less sensitive to thrombolysis. Other serpins are α_2-macroglobulin and α_1-antitrypsin.

Two principal inhibitors specific for plasminogen activators have been identified in humans, and a number of additional subsidiary inhibitors of this type have been described. They are also members of the serine protease inhibitors (serpin) family.

PAI-1 is a 52-kDa single-chain glycoprotein consisting of 379 amino acids.[147,148] The reactive site of the inhibitor is the Arg^{346}-Met^{347} peptide bond. PAI-1 is stabilized by a tight binding to the cell-adhesive protein vitronectin. PAI-2 exists in two different forms with comparable kinetic properties and is detected only in pregnant women.[149]

REGULATION OF THE FIBRINOLYTIC SYSTEM

Formed fibrin, whether in normal wound seals or in tissue damaged by any stimulus, is lysed in the body as a result of its unique property of adsorbing small quantities of plasminogen and t-PA and local generation of plasmin, which is protected from inactivation by inhibitors.

Activation of plasminogen by t-PA is enhanced in the presence of fibrin or at the endothelial cell surface. Fibrinolysis may be inhibited at the level of plasminogen activation or at the level of plasmin. Fibrinolysis is also regulated as a result of increased or decreased synthesis and/or secretion of t-PA and of PAI-1 from the vessel wall[150] or by changes in their rates of elimination by the liver.[151]

Synthesis and Secretion of Tissue-Type Plasminogen Activator Vascular endothelial cells synthesize and secrete t-PA to the circulating blood.[150] The plasma concentration of free t-PA is less than 1 ng/mL. The half-life of t-PA in the circulation is only about 5 min because of rapid hepatic clearance; some t-PA is inactivated by PAI-1. Various stimuli—such as venous occlusion, physical exercise, catecholamines, bradykinin, or desmopressin—produce a rapid increase (within minutes) in the level of t-PA in the blood. This response is too rapid to represent increased synthesis but may reflect release of t-PA from cellular storage pools, as well as decrease in hepatic clearance due to a reduced hepatic blood flow.[152] A storage pool of t-PA in endothelial cells has not been conclusively identified.[153]

A variety of agents have been shown to increase the synthesis of t-PA by cultured endothelial cells, including thrombin, histamine, butyrate, phorbol myristate acetate, basic fibroblast growth factor, activated protein C, butanol and alcohol derivatives, and retinoids. The increase of t-PA induced by histamine, thrombin, and phorbol myristate acetate in endothelial cells is paralleled by increased levels of t-PA mRNA as a result of enhanced transcription of the t-PA gene.[153] Overexpression of t-PA in endothelial cells using a retroviral expression vector did not alter the morphology, attachment, proliferation, migration, or invasion in the in vitro systems. Potentially such t-PA-transduced cells could increase local fibrinolysis and may thus be useful for in vivo therapeutic interventions.[154]

Synthesis and Secretion of Plasminogen Activator Inhibitor 1 PAI-1 mRNA has been demonstrated in a large variety of tissues, suggesting that common cells in these tissues, such as endothelial or smooth muscle cells, may be the site of production.[155] PAI-1 is found in plasma, platelets, placenta, and extracellular matrix. The concentration in plasma is in the picomolar range but may increase to about 2 nM during pregnancy, most likely as a result of release of the inhibitor from placenta. Both active and latent PAI-1 are cleared rapidly, with half-lives in rabbits of approximately 15 and 5 min.[156,157] For unknown reasons, PAI-1 exhibits a circadian variation; the plasma concentration peaks in the morning and reaches a trough in the late afternoon and evening;[158] t-PA exhibits a diurnal variation, which is opposite to that observed for PAI-1.

PAI-1 mRNA is increased and PAI-1 protein detected in endothelial cells juxtaposed to thrombi, in smooth muscle cells adjacent to the neointima, and in macrophages. The augmented arterial wall expression of PAI-1 induced by thrombosis may shift the local balance between fibrinolysis and thrombosis toward the latter.[159]

Only a few studies have reported a downregulation of PAI-1 synthesis in endothelial cells, either by forskolin or by endothelial cell growth factor combined with heparin.[160] PAI-1 is not stored within cells but is rapidly and constitutively secreted after synthesis. An exception is formed by platelets that store PAI-1 in their alpha granules; activation of platelets thus results in release of PAI-1.

α_2-Antiplasmin This forms an inactive 1:1 stoichiometric complex with plasmin. The half-life of plasmin molecules on the fibrin surface, which have both their lysine-binding sites and active site occupied, is estimated to be 2 to 3 orders of magnitude longer than that of free plasmin (Fig. 44-11).

Plasminogen Activator Inhibitors PAI-1 reacts very rapidly with single-chain and two-chain t-PA and with two-chain u-PA (tcu-PA).[161,162] PAI-2 primarily inhibits tcu-PA. The inhibition rate of scu-PA, single-chain t-PA, and two-chain t-PA by

PAI-2 is about 10, 1200, and 150 times slower, respectively, than that by PAI-1. PAI-1 and PAI-2 do not react with scu-PA.[161]

Like other serpins, PAI-1 inhibits its target proteinases by formation of a 1:1 stoichiometric reversible complex, followed by covalent binding between the hydroxyl group of the active-site serine residue of the proteinase and the carboxyl group of the PI residue at the reactive center ("bait region") of the serpin. The rapid inhibition of both t-PA and u-PA by PAI-1 involves a reversible high-affinity second-site interaction that does not depend on a functional active site. In the presence of fibrin, single-chain t-PA is protected from rapid inhibition by PAI-1. It has, however, also been reported that PAI-1 binds to fibrin and that fibrin-bound PAI-1 may inhibit t-PA-mediated fibrin clot lysis.[163]

The active form of PAI-1 converts to a latent form that can be partially reactivated by denaturing agents. In addition, inhibitory PAI-1 may convert not only to latent PAI-1, which can be reactivated, but also to substrate PAI-1, which may be irreversibly degraded by target proteinases, including t-PA, u-PA, and thrombin.[164]

Plasminogen Activation by Tissue-Type Plasminogen Activator at the Fibrin Surface The main role of t-PA most likely is in the dissolution of fibrin.[139,165] t-PA is a poor enzyme in the absence of fibrin, but the presence of fibrin strikingly enhances the activation rate of plasminogen.[166] Plasmin formed on the fibrin surface has both its lysine-binding sites and active site occupied and is thus only slowly inactivated by α_2-antiplasmin (half-life of about 10 to 100 s); in contrast, free plasmin, when formed, is rapidly inhibited by α_2-antiplasmin (half-life of about 0.1 s).

During fibrin clot lysis, single-chain t-PA is converted to two-chain t-PA at the fibrin surface. This conversion is probably of little physiologic relevance, since the activity of single-chain t-PA and two-chain t-PA is enhanced to the same extent in the presence of fibrin or fragment-X polymer.[167] Fibrin-bound single-chain t-PA may adopt a conformation similar to that of two-chain t-PA. Whether conversion of Glu-plasminogen to the more easily activatable Lys-plasminogen contributes significantly to the increased plasminogen activation rate during fibrinolysis is still somewhat controversial.

Binding studies[168,169] as well as kinetic studies have revealed that lipoprotein(a) [Lp(a)] competes with plasminogen for binding to fibrin as a result of binding of Lp(a) to fibrin via its lysine-binding domains. As for plasminogen, binding of Lp(a) to fibrin is enhanced by partial proteolytic degradation of the fibrin surface.[168] As a functional consequence of the competition between Lp(a) and plasminogen for binding to fibrin, the fibrin-dependent enhancement of plasminogen activation by t-PA is inhibited.[169,170]

PATHOPHYSIOLOGY OF FIBRINOLYSIS

Increased levels of PAI-1 activity resulting in a decreased fibrinolytic capacity have been reported in several thrombotic disease states, including venous thromboembolism, obesity, sepsis, coronary artery disease, and acute MI.[158,171] Increased levels of PAI-1 have also been found in association with the insulin resistance syndrome in which a significant correlation was found between plasma PAI-1 levels and body mass index, triglyceride levels, insulin levels, and systolic blood pressure. Obese people—particularly those with android obesity—also have high PAI-1 levels.

Increased plasma levels of PAI-1 are one of the major disturbances of the hemostatic system in patients with coronary heart disease, and multiple interrelations with established metabolic risk factors have been observed. Increased PAI-1 levels have also been demonstrated in atherosclerotic lesions within the vessel wall. Therefore, both systemically and locally increased PAI-1 concentrations could have a pathogenic role in the development of atherosclerotic disease.

Many case-control or cross-sectional studies have demonstrated high plasma PAI-1 levels in patients who have had a MI or unstable angina. A relationship between deficient fibrinolysis due to high PAI activity levels and recurrent MI (within 3 years) was demonstrated in young men who had survived their first MI. On the other hand, PAI-1 activity was not predictive for recurrent infarction (nor was t-PA antigen) in a group of older patients followed over 5 years. In a cohort of patients with angina pectoris, high basal t-PA antigen levels were found to be associated with an increased risk of MI, while no correlation was observed with PAI activity.[172,173]

Attempts to demonstrate a relationship between plasma PAI-1 levels and the severity of vessel wall damage have led to conflicting results in cross-sectional studies. Analysis of the data of the European Concerted Action on Thrombosis (ECAT) angina pectoris study demonstrated that there was a weak distinction between patients with and patients without significant coronary stenosis; the former had significantly higher plasma levels of PAI-1. NO association could be observed with the extent of coronary atherosclerosis. There are multiple interrelations between plasma PAI-1 levels and other risk factors of atherothrombosis, such as those involved in the metabolic syndrome of insulin resistance. In the ECAT angina pectoris study, in which insulin determination was available for almost 1500 patients, two- to threefold differences in PAI-1 levels were observed in comparing the lowest and the highest quintile of insulin, body mass index, or triglyceride.[174]

ANTITHROMBOTIC DRUGS

Given the importance of thrombosis in acute coronary syndromes, thrombolytic and antithrombotic therapy has become the primary therapy for most conditions. This chapter reviews the numerous agents in clinical use or expected for clinical use in the coming years. The mechanism of action of the agent and the major evidence supporting its use in clinical medicine are reviewed; readers will also be referred to the specific chapter of that clinical syndrome for additional perspective on its use in context with the full treatment strategies.

Platelet Inhibitors

Platelet inhibition can be achieved in numerous ways (Fig. 44-12). These include inhibition of platelet cyclooxygenase (aspirin or sulfinpyrazone), inhibition of ADP receptors (ticlopidine or clopidogrel), or inhibition of the platelet GP IIb/IIIa receptor. Platelet inhibition can also be achieved by inhibition of thromboxane synthase with or without blockade of endoperoxide-thromboxane receptors, modulation of platelet adenylate or guanylate cyclase (prostacyclin analogs), interference with the function of the platelet GP Ib-IX receptor (monoclonal antibodies to GP Ib-IX), synthetic peptides to the A1 von Willebrand factor domain, recombinant von Willebrand fragments covering the A1 domain, and peptides that bind to but do not activate the platelet-receptor domain that interacts with thrombin. In this chapter, only platelet inhibitors that have been investigated in clinical trials are reviewed.

Aspirin This permanently acetylates cyclooxygenase, thereby blocking the synthesis of TXA_2 by the platelet (Fig. 44-5). By decreasing the amount of TXA_2 released, which would act to stimulate other platelets, this decreases overall platelet aggregation at the site of the thrombus. This inhibition of cyclooxygenase is permanent—and thus the antiplatelet effects last for the lifetime of the platelets—on order of 7 to 10 days. Aspirin selectively inhibits TXA_2 formation (Fig. 44-5) but only partially impedes platelet aggregation induced by ADP, collagen, and low concentrations of thrombin.[175]

Aspirin does not inhibit adherence of the initial layer of platelets to the subendothelium or atherosclerotic plaques, and the release of granule contents is not opposed. Thus, the effects of platelet-derived growth factors and other mitogens on smooth muscle cells are not inhibited.[176] Aspirin also impairs thrombosis by a mechanism that seems to be unrelated to platelet cyclooxygenase, as, for instance, the acetylation of guanosine triphosphate–binding proteins, thrombin receptors, and prothrombin.[177] The salicylate moiety of aspirin also antagonizes the lipoxygenase pathway of arachidonate metabolism in platelets, and the demonstration of two cyclooxygenase enzymes (COX-1 and COX-2)[178] may further elucidate the antithrombotic mechanism of aspirin.[179] Aspirin is known to have an anti-inflammatory effect at high doses, but whether an anti-inflammatory effect is present at doses used in acute coronary syndromes is not clear.

DOSE The ideal dose of aspirin for the primary or secondary prevention of cardiovascular disease is not determined. A dose of 40 mg was found to achieve maximal inhibition of TXA_2. Doses between 75 and 1300 mg/day have produced similar reductions in cardiovascular event.[65–68] Thus, there does not appear to be a dose response in efficacy of aspirin. In the Second International Study of Infarct Survival (ISIS-2), a dose of 160 mg/day was shown to have a mortality benefit, so this dose is the minimum initial dose recommended for acute therapy.[180] For safety (e.g., gastrointestinal bleeding), the rate of bleeding appears to be slightly higher with higher doses, and thus a dose of 75 to 81 mg daily could be an appropriate dose for long-term therapy, although major bleeding is relatively rare (<1 percent) even at a dose of 325 mg daily.[181]

ADVERSE EFFECTS Absolute contraindications for aspirin therapy are few but include documented aspirin allergy (e.g., asthma), active bleeding, severe thrombocytopenia (<20,000 cells/mL), or a known platelet disorder. In patients with gastrointestinal complaints (e.g., dyspepsia) with long-term aspirin therapy (i.e., aspirin intolerance), this would not be expected to be an acute problem of in-hospital treatment, and aspirin therapy is recommended for acute therapy, with evaluation of the cause of the disorder or consideration of alternate antithrombotic therapy in the subacute phase of the patient's acute coronary syndrome.

CLINICAL USE Aspirin is a critical antithrombotic agent in coronary artery disease. In the setting of acute ST-elevation MI, aspirin decreased reocclusion by over 50 percent in a meta-analysis of 32 angiographic trials[182] (Fig. 44-13). Aspirin also was found to decrease reinfarction significantly in the large ISIS-2 trial and most importantly reduced mortality by 23 percent.[180]

Several major studies have demonstrated clear beneficial effects of aspirin in patients with unstable angina and non-ST-elevation MI, with an approximately 50 percent reduction in the risk of death or MI in patients presenting with unstable angina or non-Q-wave MI (Fig. 44-13).[65–68] The first study from the Veterans Administration (VA) Cooperative Study Group documented a 51 percent reduction in the risk of death or MI in patients presenting with unstable angina, and the overall benefits of aspirin were maintained during the 1-year follow-up period.[65] The Canadian multicenter trial confirmed the large risk reduction by aspirin for the development of death or MI among patients with unstable angina/non-ST-elevation MI.[66] The Montreal Heart Institute study demonstrated the effectiveness of both aspirin, as well as heparin, in reducing the incidence of death or MI.[67] A more recent study by the Research on Instability in Coronary Artery Disease Group (RISC) extended these observations to all patients with acute coronary syndromes, showing an approximately 70 percent reduction by aspirin in subsequent risk of death or MI in patients with either unstable angina or non-ST-elevation MI.[68]

Following MI, aspirin reduces subsequent cardiac events, providing secondary prevention (Table 44-2).[183,184] These benefits have now been observed to persist for up to 4 years of follow-up with chronic antiplatelet therapy.[184] Thus, aspirin has had a dramatic effect in reducing adverse clinical events and is primary therapy for all acute coronary syndromes.

In PCI, aspirin has been used as background therapy in most trials, and one small trial did find a reduced rate of thrombotic cardiac events in patients randomized to aspirin compared with placebo.[185] In coronary artery bypass grafting (CABG), aspirin is also an important component of therapy. Without aspirin therapy, graft occlusion occurred in 16 to 26 percent of patients by 1 year.[30] The VA Cooperative Study randomized patients to five treatment arms: (1) aspirin 325 mg/day, (2) aspirin 325 mg three times daily, (3) 325 mg daily of aspirin and dipyridamole 75 mg daily, (4) sulfinpyrazone 267 mg daily, or (5) placebo. Early graft patency was significantly higher in patients randomized to aspirin at any dose, with benefit persisting at 1 year. The dose of 325 mg daily of aspirin was as effective as the 325 mg three times daily. Sulfinpyrazone and dipyridamole added no benefit to aspirin.[186]

PRIMARY PREVENTION OF ACUTE MYOCARDIAL INFARCTION Two studies examining the use of aspirin in primary prevention of MI (Table 44-3) were conducted. In the United States, in the Physicians' Health Study, more than 22,000 male physicians of ages 40 to 84 were randomized to receive 325 mg of aspirin every other day or placebo for 5 years. There was a 44 percent relative reduction in MI in the aspirin-treated group, although the absolute incidence of such event was less than 1 percent in the low-risk population (Fig. 44-13). This effect was limited to those older than 50 years. The incidence of cardiovascular death was not different.[187] In a British primary prevention trial of more than 5000 male physicians, two-thirds were randomized to receive 500 mg/day of aspirin and one-third were

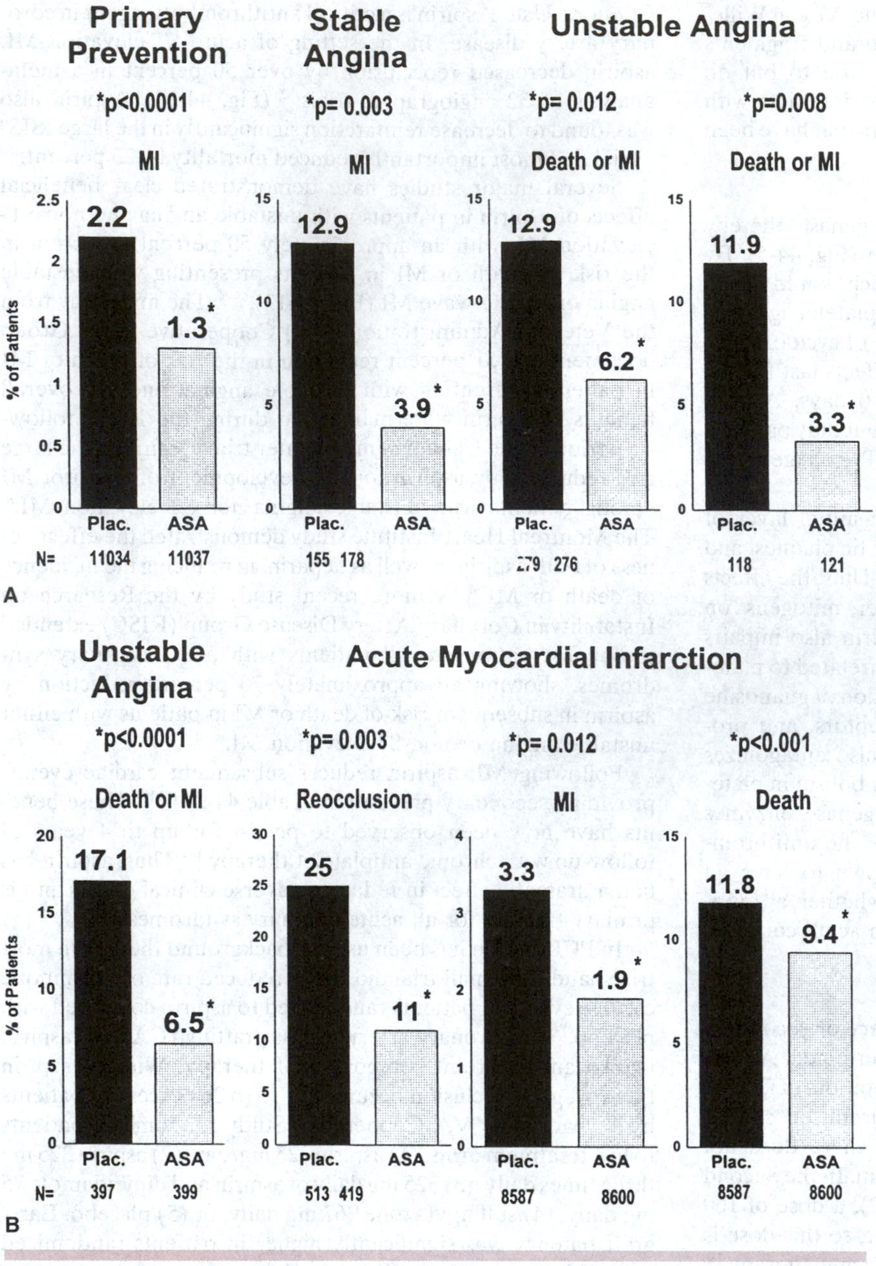

FIGURE 44-13 Benefit of aspirin across the spectrum of acute coronary syndromes. The risk of subsequent myocardial infarction (MI) was reduced by aspirin compared with placebo in healthy subjects and thus was effective in primary prevention.[187] Similarly, patients with stable angina had a reduced incidence of MI.[490] In unstable angina, the incidence of death or MI was reduced by over 50 percent in each of three trials shown.[66–68] In acute MI (AMI), aspirin reduced reocclusion of the infarct-related artery,[182] reinfarction, and mortality rates.[180] [Data are from the following trials, respectively: Steering Committee of the Physicians' Health Study Research Group,[187] Ridker et al.,[490] Cairns et al.,[66] Theroux et al.,[67] the RISC Group,[68] Roux et al.,[182] and ISIS-2 (Second International Study of Infarct Survival) Collaborative Group[180].]

advised to use no aspirin. After 6 years, there was no difference in the rate of MI.[188] However, a large number of protocol cross-overs (both physicians stopping aspirin in the aspirin group, and physicians taking aspirin in the placebo group) diluted the power of the study to show a significant difference.

In summary, aspirin has been shown to be beneficial in essentially every condition in which it has been tested. Its use is strongly recommended in all guidelines of management of coronary artery disease.[189,190]

Thienopyridines: Ticlopidine and Clopidogrel The thienopyridines are inactive in vitro but potent antiaggregating agents in vivo, indicating the importance of at least one active transient metabolite. The metabolic activation takes place in the liver as a portojugular shunt abolishes the antiaggregating effect. Ticlopidine and its chemical analog clopidogrel are noncompetitive but selective antagonists of ADP-induced platelet aggregation and act by specifically blocking GP IIb/IIIa activation (Fig. 44-5) specific for the ADP pathway. Since the two compounds are chemically related, their mechanisms of action are considered similar. Ex vivo studies indicate that the antiaggregating effect is concentration dependent; the rate of recovery is linked to platelet survival, suggesting a permanent effect on platelets.[191]

The two agents are believed to inhibit the binding of adenosine 5′-diphosphate (ADP) to its platelet receptor.[191–195] Initial studies reported that this ADP receptor blockade led to direct inhibition of fibrinogen binding to the GP IIb/IIIa complex.[196,197] There is also evidence that ticlopidine may interfere with von Willebrand factor, resulting in less binding of von Willebrand factor to platelet receptors.[197–199] Recent studies suggest there are at least two types of ADP receptors.[191,193,200] The first type is a low-affinity type 2 purinergic receptor that is G-protein coupled and results in mobilization of calcium from internal stores.[201] This leads to a conformational change in and activation of the GP IIb/IIIa receptor complex, fibrinogen binding, and platelet aggregation. The second type of ADP receptor (P2Y1) is of high affinity and is responsible for platelet shape change and rapid calcium influx.[201,202] Because ticlopidine and clopidogrel do not affect shape change or calcium influx, they appear to achieve their effect by interacting with the low-affinity type 2 purinergic receptor.[191,193,201] This interference with a specific ADP-dependent step of GP IIb/IIIa complex activation results in less platelet aggregation and, thus, ultimately impairs thrombus formation.[193,203,204] Despite these numerous in vitro studies, the mechanism(s) of action of ticlopidine and clopidogrel are still not fully characterized. Further insights would be greatly facilitated by the cloning of the type 2 purinergic ADP receptor.

Ticlopidine and clopidogrel have been tested in several animal models of platelet-dependent arterial or venous thrombosis

TABLE 44-2 Aspirin in Cardiovascular Disease

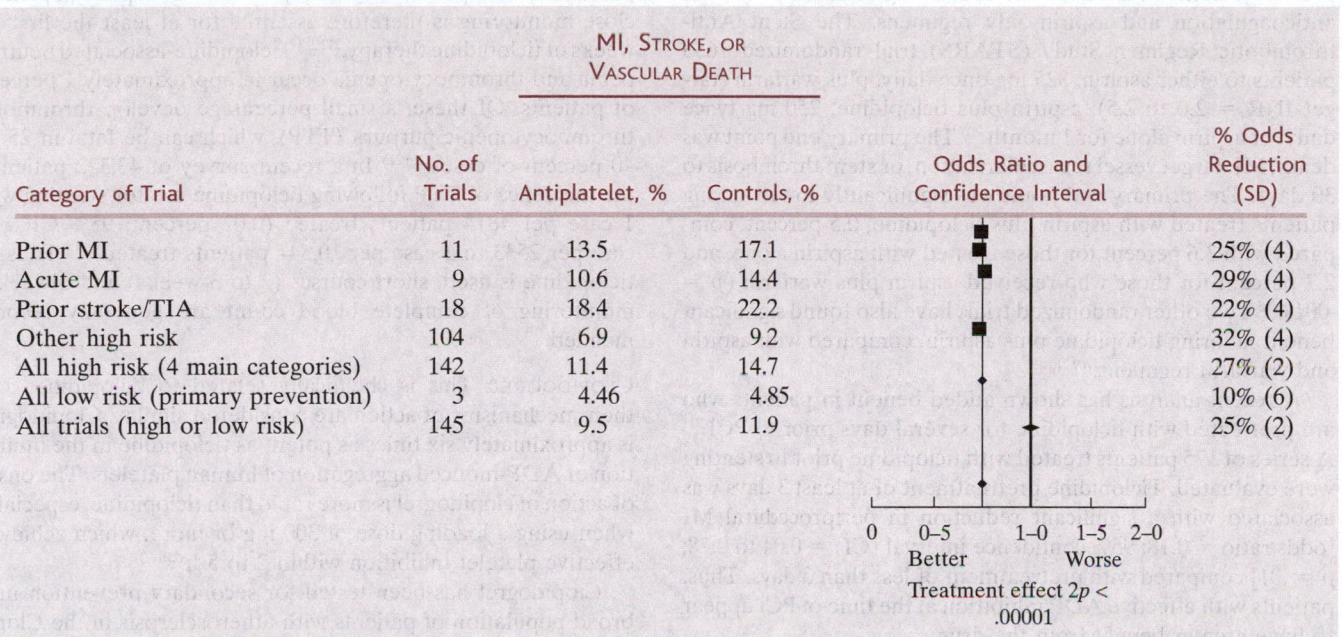

Category of Trial	No. of Trials	MI, Stroke, or Vascular Death: Antiplatelet, %	MI, Stroke, or Vascular Death: Controls, %	Odds Ratio and Confidence Interval	% Odds Reduction (SD)
Prior MI	11	13.5	17.1		25% (4)
Acute MI	9	10.6	14.4		29% (4)
Prior stroke/TIA	18	18.4	22.2		22% (4)
Other high risk	104	6.9	9.2		32% (4)
All high risk (4 main categories)	142	11.4	14.7		27% (2)
All low risk (primary prevention)	3	4.46	4.85		10% (6)
All trials (high or low risk)	145	9.5	11.9		25% (2)

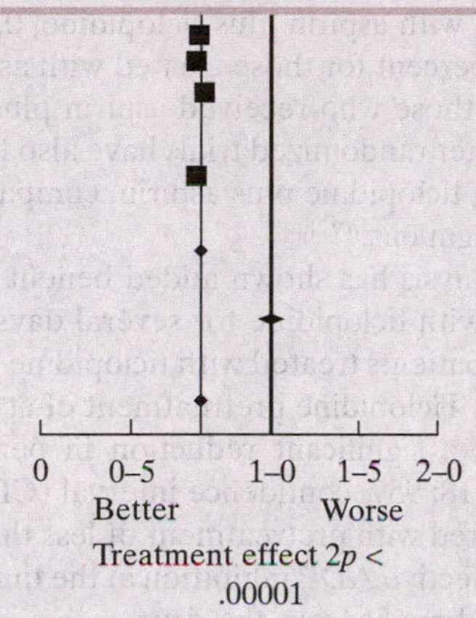

SOURCE: Antiplatelet Trialists' Collaboration,[184] with permission.
ABBREVIATIONS: MI = myocardial infarction; TIA = transient ischemic attack.

and found to be more effective than sulfinpyrazone, dipyridamole, and aspirin. Other effects are a reduction in fibrinogen levels and blood viscosity and improvement in decreased erythrocyte deformability.

TICLOPIDINE This was studied in a randomized trial of patients with unstable angina involving 652 patients. The control group did not receive aspirin because at the time of protocol design it was not routinely used to treat unstable angina. At 6-month follow-up, ticlopidine led to a significant 46 percent reduction in vascular death or nonfatal MI.[205] Of note, there was no difference in the number of events over the first 10 days, consistent with the delayed onset of the antiplatelet effect of ticlopidine. Thus, ticlopidine appears to be comparable to aspirin for secondary prevention of events after unstable angina/non-ST-elevation MI.

The effectiveness of ticlopidine has been shown in patients with transient ischemic cerebral attacks and stroke, and peripheral arterial or ischemic heart disease.[195] The first large trial of its effectiveness in 3069 patients with recent transient or mild persistent focal cerebral or retinal ischemia has shown that ticlopidine has a more pronounced effect on death from all causes or nonfatal stroke than aspirin.[206]

Ticlopidine has also been demonstrated to be effective in combination with aspirin for prevention of thrombosis and recurrent ischemic events in patients undergoing coronary stent implantation. The first randomized trial [Intracoronary Stenting and Antithrombotic Regimen (ISAR)] confirmed the advantage of an antiplatelet regimen over an anticoagulant regimen.[207] A total of 517 patients were randomized to intravenous heparin for only 12 h and ticlopidine, 250 mg twice daily, and aspirin, 100 mg twice daily, for 4 weeks; or to intravenous heparin for 5 to 10 days, aspirin, 100 mg twice daily, and phenprocoumon [target international normalized ratio (INR) = 3.5 to 4.5] for 4 weeks. At 30-day follow-up, the ticlopidine group had 75 percent fewer cardiac end points than the phenprocoumon group (1.6 versus 6.2 percent, $p = .01$) and no episodes of stent thrombosis (versus 5.0 percent, $p < 0.001$).

TABLE 44-3 Aspirin in Primary Prevention (U.S. Physicians' Health Study and British Doctors' Trial Results)

End Point	Reduction (% ± SD): United States — Physicians' Health Study	Reduction (% ± SD): British — Doctors' Trials	Reduction (% ± SD): Overview — Both Trials	p
Nonfatal myocardial infarction	44 ± 9	3 ± 19	32 ± 8	<.0001
Nonfatal stroke	↑19 ± 15	↑13 ± 24	↑18 ± 13	NS
Total cardiovascular deaths	2 ± 15	7 ± 14	5 ± 10	NS
Any vascular event	18 ± 7	4 ± 12	13 ± 6	NS

SOURCE: Fuster et al.,[493] with permission.

A larger, adequately powered study has now shown an impressive benefit of a ticlopidine-containing regimen over both anticoagulation and aspirin-only regimens. The Stent Antithrombotic Regimen Study (STARS) trial randomized 1653 patients to either aspirin, 325 mg once daily, plus warfarin (target INR = 2.0 to 2.5); aspirin plus ticlopidine, 250 mg twice daily; or aspirin alone for 1 month.[208] The primary end point was death, MI, target vessel revascularization, or stent thrombosis to 30 days. The primary end point was significantly lower among patients treated with aspirin plus ticlopidine, 0.5 percent, compared with 3.6 percent for those treated with aspirin alone, and 2.7 percent for those who received aspirin plus warfarin (p = .001).[208] Two other randomized trials have also found significant benefit favoring ticlopidine plus aspirin, compared with aspirin and warfarin regimens.[209,210]

A recent analysis has shown added benefit in patients who are pretreated with ticlopidine for several days prior to PCI.[211] A series of 175 patients treated with ticlopidine prior to stenting were evaluated. Ticlopidine pretreatment of at least 3 days was associated with a significant reduction in periprocedural MI [odds ratio = 0.18; 95% confidence interval (CI) = 0.04 to 0.78; p = .01] compared with pretreatment of less than 3 days. Thus, patients with effective ADP inhibition at the time of PCI appear to have greater benefit from the drug.

Side Effects The most common adverse effects associated with ticlopidine are gastrointestinal: diarrhea affects about 20 percent of treated patients. Other effects are skin reactions (urticaria, pruritus, and erythema) and hemorrhagic disorders (epistaxis, ecchymoses, and menorrhagia). These effects are generally not severe and resolve after discontinuation of ticlopidine. Ticlopidine has also been reported to increase total cholesterol by 9 percent.[206]

The most potentially serious problem is bone marrow depression (leukopenia, thrombocytopenia, and pancytopenia); close monitoring is therefore essential for at least the first 12 weeks of ticlopidine therapy.[212,213] Ticlopidine-associated neutropenia and thrombocytopenia occur in approximately 1 percent of patients. Of these, a small percentage develop thrombotic thrombocytopenic purpura (TTP), which can be fatal in 25 to 40 percent of cases.[214,215] In a recent survey of 43,322 patients, the incidence of TTP following ticlopidine use for stenting was 1 case per 4814 patients treated (0.02 percent; 95% CI = 1 case per 2533 to 1 case per 10,541 patients treated).[215] Thus, if ticlopidine is used, short courses (2 to 3 weeks) and biweekly monitoring of complete blood count are generally recommended.

Clopidogrel This is chemically related to ticlopidine, and their mechanisms of action are considered similar. Clopidogrel is approximately six times as potent as ticlopidine in the inhibition of ADP-induced aggregation of human platelets. The onset of action of clopidogrel is more rapid than ticlopidine, especially when using a loading dose of 300 mg or more, which achieves effective platelet inhibition within 2 to 5 h.[216]

Clopidogrel has been tested for secondary prevention in a broad population of patients with atherosclerosis in the Clopidogrel Versus Aspirin in Patients at Risk for Ischemic Events (CAPRIE) trial, which enrolled 19,185 patients, of which one-third had experienced an MI within 35 days and had documented peripheral arterial disease or an ischemic stroke from 1 week to 6 months prior to randomization.[181] Patients were randomized to either clopidogrel, 75 mg once daily, or aspirin, 325 mg once daily; mean follow-up was 1.9 years. Overall, clopidogrel was associated with an 8.7 percent reduction relative to aspirin in the combined end point of ischemic stroke, MI, or vascular death (5.32 versus 5.83 percent per year; p = .042) (Fig. 44-14).[181]

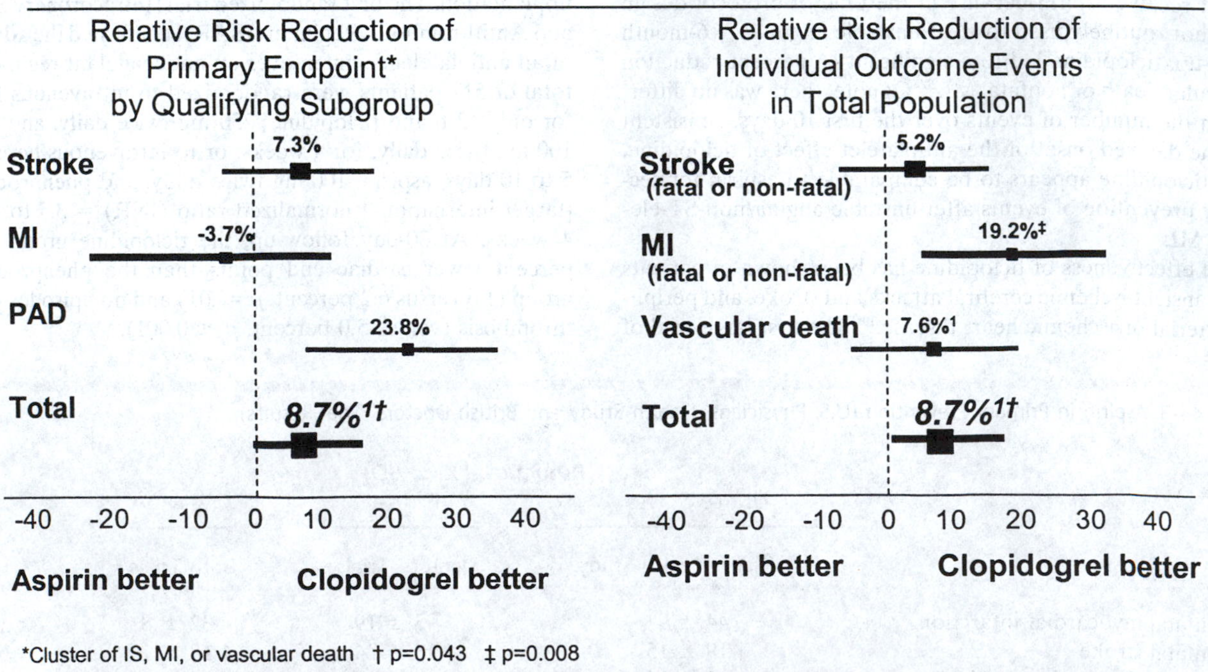

FIGURE 44-14 Benefit of clopidogrel compared with aspirin in patients with symptomatic atherosclerosis. Subgroups of patients are shown in the *left panel*, and outcome events in the total group are shown in the *right panel*. IS = ischemic stroke; MI = myocardial infarction; PAD = peripheral arterial disease. (Data are from the CAPRIE Steering Committee[181] and Gent.[217])

Curiously, among the 6302 patients who had an MI within 35 days of randomization (mean, 17.6 days), there was a statistically insignificant 3.7 percent increase in the combined end point of MI, stroke, and vascular death (p = .66).[181] Of the patients in the peripheral vascular disease and stroke strata, however, 2144 had a history of MI. In a post hoc secondary analysis of all 8446 patients with a history of MI, clopidogrel was associated with a 7.4 percent decrease in the combined end point, which is similar to the benefit of clopidogrel observed in the overall trial (combined end point reduction of 8.7 percent).[181] In addition, the relative benefit of clopidogrel on the components of the primary end point was greatest in preventing MI: clopidogrel produced a significant 19.2 percent reduction in MI (p = .008), while there were nonsignificant 5.2 and 7.6 percent reductions in stroke and vascular death, respectively (Fig. 44-14).[217] Based on these data, the Food and Drug Administration (FDA) approved clopidogrel for secondary prevention of vascular events among patients with symptomatic atherosclerosis. Very recent data have shown that selected high-risk subgroups of patients in the CAPRIE trial, such as those with prior CABG or diabetes, had a much greater benefit. For patients with prior CABG, clopidogrel reduced the annual rate of vascular death, MI, or stroke from 22.3 to 15.9 percent (p = .001).[218] Thus, clopidogrel is a suitable alternative to aspirin and appears to afford some benefit over aspirin. Clopidogrel is also the drug of choice in patients who have a true aspirin allergy.

Interest now has turned to the combination of clopidogrel plus aspirin. Experimental data have shown synergy between the two agents in their antithrombotic effects.[219] Trials are currently ongoing for patients with unstable angina/non-ST-elevation MI testing the combination of clopidogrel plus aspirin compared with aspirin alone.

Clopidogrel also appears to be as effective as ticlopidine in preventing stent thrombosis.[195,220-225] As previously noted, current regimens usually begin with a loading dose of 300 mg, which achieves effective platelet inhibition within 2 to 5 h,[216] followed by 75 mg daily. The current duration of treatment following stenting is 30 days, but a trial is currently examining whether there is added benefit from longer treatment.

Side Effects Clopidogrel is not associated with neutropenia and an extremely low (3 to 4 per million) rate of thrombotic thrombocytopenic purpura, and it was associated with a lower rate of gastrointestinal bleeding compared with aspirin.[181] In the CAPRIE study, adverse events with clopidogrel were proportionally less frequent than those previously reported for ticlopidine.[181] In CAPRIE, of 19,185 patients followed up for a mean of 1.91 years, only 0.10 percent in the clopidogrel group developed a significant reduction in neutrophil count ($<1.2 \times$ 10 g/L) compared with 0.17 percent in the aspirin group.

Thromboxane Synthase Inhibitors These have been developed with the expectation not only of suppressing TXA_2 biosynthesis (Fig. 44-5) but also of sparing or even enhancing the formation of prostacyclin by the vascular endothelium. Thromboxane synthase inhibition offers the potential advantage over aspirin-type cyclooxygenase inhibitors of reorienting the arachidonic cascade toward an overproduction of inhibitory prostanoids (PGI_2 and PGD_2) and a reduction in TXA_2 formation. However, specific inhibition of TXA_2 synthase produces an accumulation of cyclic prostaglandin endoperoxides, which occupy and activate TXA_2 and endoperoxide receptors on platelets and endothelium and thus attenuate the inhibitory effect of PGI_2 and PGD_2.

Most thromboxane synthase inhibitors have moderate potency and brief duration of action and do not result in a sufficiently sustained inhibition of TXA_2 production to be clinically effective. Moreover, some individuals are poor responders to drugs of this type. The increased generation of endoperoxides that share the same receptors as TXA_2 is another problem that will not be solved by more potent and long-acting drugs of this class.[226] Although thromboxane synthase inhibitors have shown some benefit in experimental models, their effects in clinical trials in patients with coronary artery disease have been disappointing.

Thromboxane Receptor Blockers The more recently developed thromboxane receptor blockers specifically impede the action of both TXA_2 and endoperoxides on their presumed common receptors on platelets (Fig. 44-5) and prevent vasoconstriction induced by TXA_2. These agents leave the normal pattern of thromboxane and prostacyclin formation unaltered. Thromboxane receptor antagonists prolong bleeding time more than thromboxane synthase inhibitors. As expected, TXA_2 synthesis is not inhibited and PGI_2 generation not augmented by specific thromboxane/endoperoxide receptor antagonists. Unfortunately, the results of the initial clinical studies with such agents have been disappointing.[227]

Combined Thromboxane Synthase Inhibitors and Receptor Blockers Some compounds have a dual activity. Ridogrel is a potent TXA_2 synthase inhibitor with modest additional TXA_2/prostaglandin endoperoxide receptor antagonist properties (at least 100-fold less).[228] Although the animal pharmacology was very promising, the preclinical evaluation was deceptive. Ridogrel was testing as adjunctive antiplatelet therapy with thrombolysis in the Ridogrel Aspirin Patency Trial (RAPT).[229] A total of 907 patients with acute MI treated with streptokinase were randomized to aspirin or ridogrel. The primary end point was coronary patency [Thrombolysis in Myocardial Infarction (TIMI) flow grades 2 and 3] at predischarge angiography to be performed between 7 and 14 days after admission. No difference was observed between the two groups: 72.2 percent in the ridogrel and 75.5 percent in the aspirin group. The incidence of major in-hospital clinical events during hospital stay was similar in both groups. However, in a post hoc analysis, a lower incidence of new ischemic events (reinfarction, recurrent angina, or ischemic stroke) was observed with ridogrel: 13 versus 19 percent in the aspirin group (p = .025). There was no excess in major bleeding complications, including hemorrhagic stroke. With only modest results, this agent has not been developed for widespread clinical use.

Dipyridamole This is a pyrimidopyrimidine compound whose antithrombotic action is not well understood. It is felt to decrease platelet aggregability but also decrease platelet adhesion to prosthetic valves, increase platelet survival, and decrease red blood cell deformability.[230] It has been shown in one study to reduce embolism from prosthetic cardiac valves when combined with warfarin.[230] In CABG, neither dipyridamole (nor sulfinpyrazone) added to the benefit of aspirin in maintaining graft patency.[186] Thus, its role in coronary artery disease is limited.

Sulfinpyrazone This is a weak antiplatelet agent that, after metabolism to a sulfide form, acts as an incomplete and reversible inhibitor of platelet cyclooxygenase, although other actions may exist. In one trial of unstable angina, patients were randomized to receive 1300 mg/day of aspirin, 800 mg/day of sulfinpyrazone, the combination of both, or placebo. After 18 months, the incidence of death and MI was reduced in the aspirin group, but sulfinpyrazone demonstrated no benefit.[231]

Platelet Glycoprotein IIb/IIIa Receptor Blockers

This is a potent class of platelet inhibitors. GP IIb/IIIa receptor antagonists block the binding of fibrinogen to specific membrane GP IIb/IIIa integrin receptors, thus preventing platelet aggregation induced by various platelet agonists. Whereas platelet activation is produced by a wide variety of stimuli, the final common step to platelet aggregation is fibrinogen binding. Thus, no matter what stimuli there are for platelet activation, the platelet is inhibited by the GP IIb/IIIa inhibitor—making it an order of magnitude more effective than aspirin (or ticlopidine) at inhibiting platelet aggregation. When testing platelet aggregation in the laboratory, aspirin inhibits ADP-induced platelet aggregation by approximately 5 to 10 percent, ticlopidine and clopidogrel inhibit platelet aggregation by approximately 30 percent, and the doses of the GP IIb/IIIa inhibitors being tested clinically inhibit platelet aggregation by approximately 80 to 90 percent.

Types of Glycoprotein IIb/IIIa Inhibitors There are three broad categories of GP IIb/IIIa inhibitors: (1) the monoclonal antibody fragment to the IIb/IIIa receptor, abciximab; (2) the intravenous peptide and nonpeptide small molecule inhibitors, such as eptifibatide and tirofiban; and (3) the oral GP IIb/IIIa inhibitors, such as xemilofiban, orbofiban, sibrafiban, and roxifiban (see page 1396).

The first platelet GP IIb/IIIa antagonists to be developed were murine monoclonal antibodies.[232] In vitro, these antibodies completely inhibit platelet aggregation and, in animal models of angioplasty injury and thrombolysis, prevent thrombosis and augment the activity of thrombolytic agents. Because of concerns about their immunogenicity, the derivative product chimeric monoclonal 7E3 Fab (c7E3 Fab, abciximab) was created via genetic recombination. This new molecule consists of the mouse-derived variable regions from the original molecule linked to the constant region derived from human immunoglobulin G. Abciximab binds to the GP IIb/IIIa receptor and to a broader group of integrins, such as the vitronectin receptor, which appears to be important in neointimal proliferation. In addition, abciximab has been shown to inhibit thrombin generation by tissue factor most likely due to its dual blockade of GP IIb/IIIa and $\alpha_v\beta_3$.[233]

Abciximab binds very tightly to the GP IIb/IIIa receptor.[234] Thus, the antiplatelet effect lasts much longer than the infusion period—a potential benefit on improving efficacy. On the other hand, if bleeding occurred, stopping the drug will not reverse the antiplatelet effect immediately; transfusion of platelets, however, will allow the antibodies to redistribute among all the platelets, thereby reducing the level of platelet inhibition. Abciximab also binds to other integrins on the platelet receptor, such as the vitronectin receptor,[114] but the clinical significance of this cross-reactivity is not yet established.

The peptide and peptidomimetic inhibitors (e.g., tirofiban and eptifibatide) are competitive inhibitors of the GP IIb/IIIa receptor.[235,236] Tirofiban and eptifibatide are RGD- and KGD-containing agents that bind to the fibrinogen binding site of the GP IIb/IIIa receptor. The level of platelet inhibition is directly related to the drug level in the blood. With these short-acting agents the ratio of drug molecules to GP IIb/IIIa receptors is greater than 250, whereas for the "tight-binding" agents (e.g., abciximab) the ratio is approximately 2.

Since both inhibitors have short half-lives, when the drug infusion is stopped,[235,236] the antiplatelet activity reverses after a few hours, which is a potential benefit for avoiding bleeding complications. On the other hand, for prolonged antiplatelet effect, the drug needs to be given intravenously for a longer period. The inhibitors developed to date have been specifically targeted to the GP IIb/IIIa receptor and not to cross-react other integrins.

The third group of GP IIb/IIIa inhibitors are the oral agents. These are also competitive inhibitors and are usually pro-drugs, which are absorbed and then converted to active compounds in the blood.[237–241] The oral agents all have longer half-lives, such that they can be given once, twice, or three times daily to achieve relatively steady levels of GP IIb/IIIa inhibition. With oral dosing, long-term therapy (i.e., longer than 1 year) is possible. As with the intravenous compounds, two major groups of drugs exist in the oral class: those with competitive inhibition and short "off time" from the receptor—where a high drug level is critical to achieving high levels of platelet inhibition—and those that have "tight" binding to the platelet (similar to abciximab) with the majority of the drug circulating bound to platelets.

Potential Mechanisms of Benefit of Glycoprotein IIb/IIIa Inhibitors Several potential mechanisms exist for how GP IIb/IIIa inhibition may improve clot resolution and clinical outcome in patients' acute coronary syndromes. First, by blocking platelet aggregation in the platelet-rich arterial thrombus, it prevents propagation of the thrombus. GP IIb/IIIa inhibitors may also be able to *disaggregate* a recently formed platelet plug. Second, by preventing accumulation of a large number of platelets at the lesion, it decreases the amount of platelet phospholipid membrane, a cofactor needed for thrombin generation in the clotting cascade. Third, a thrombus rich in platelets may resist thrombolysis (either thrombolytic therapy or endogenous thrombolysis), owing in part to the increased presence of PAI-1, a potent natural inhibitor of fibrinolysis that exists in high concentrations in platelets.

Glycoprotein IIb/IIIa Inhibition During Coronary Angioplasty The FDA had approved three agents for use during PCI, including abciximab (ReoPro) and eptifibatide (Integrilin) for elective and urgent PCI. In addition, tirofiban (Aggrastat) is approved for the treatment of patients with unstable angina and non-ST-elevation MI undergoing PCI. Abciximab is administered as a 0.25-mg/kg bolus and an infusion of 0.125 μg/kg per minute for 12 h following PCI. Although lower doses are approved, the most widely used dose is that from the unstable angina trial,[76] a dose of eptifibatide is 180-μg/kg bolus and infusion of 2.0 μg/kg per minute. A recent trial also showed benefit of this regimen with an added second bolus of 180 μg/kg 10 min after the first. The dose of tirofiban used in the angioplasty trial Randomized Efficacy Study of Tirofiban for Outcomes and Restenosis (RESTORE), and an ongoing trial, is a bolus of 10 μg/kg over 3 min followed by 0.15 μg/kg per minute.

Abciximab Initial testing of GP IIb/IIIa inhibitors began in patients undergoing PCI. In the Evaluation of c7E3 for the Prevention of Ischemic Complications (EPIC) trial of patients undergoing high-risk PCI, abciximab bolus and infusion had a 35 percent lower rate of death, MI, or urgent revascularization at 30 days compared with the placebo group (8.3 versus 12.8 percent, p = .008).[241a] In long-term follow-up, significant benefit has been observed at 6 months and 3 years.[242,243] Similar reductions in major cardiac events were observed in the Evaluation in PTCA to Improve Long-Term Outcomes with Abciximab Glycoprotein IIb/IIIa Blockade (EPILOG) trial of elective PCI. Death, MI, or urgent revascularization at 30 days for abciximab plus low-dose heparin group was 5.2 versus 11.7 percent for heparin alone, a 58 percent risk reduction ($p < 0.001$).[243a] The abciximab plus standard-dose heparin also had a significant reduction in ischemic complications to 5.4 percent ($p < 0.001$).[243a] Death or MI was similarly reduced by more than 50 percent when adding abciximab (Fig. 44-15). When using a lower dose of heparin with abciximab, there was no difference in the incidence of major bleeding or the need for transfusion between abciximab-treated patients and placebo. Thus, a low-dose heparin regimen can be recommended with abciximab (70-U/kg initial bolus with an additional 20 U/kg if the activated clotting time is less than 200 s).

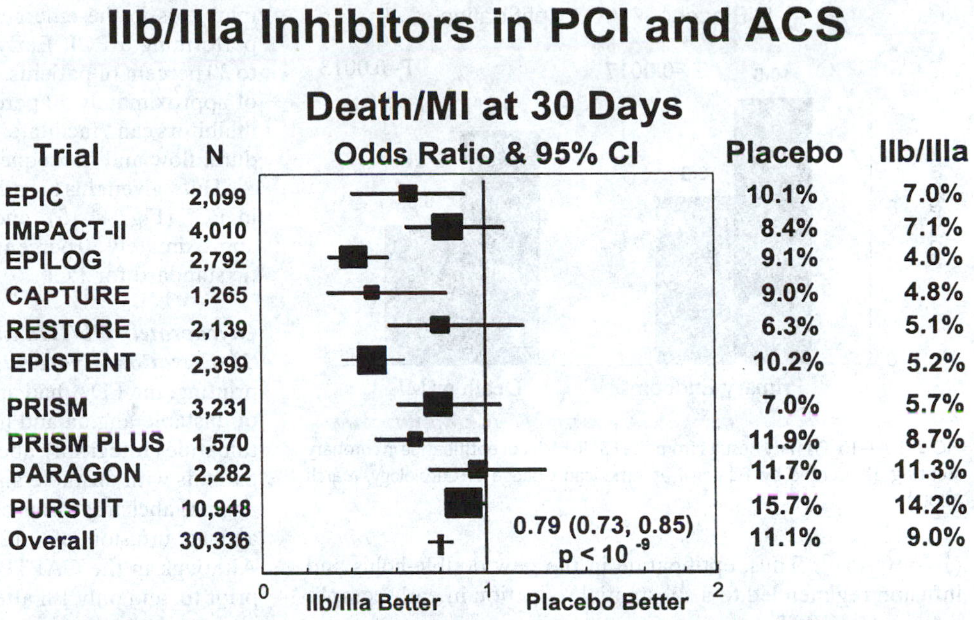
IIb/IIIa Inhibitors in PCI and ACS
Death/MI at 30 Days
Trial
N
Odds Ratio & 95% CI
Placebo
IIb/IIIa
EPIC 2,099 10.1% 7.0%
IMPACT-II 4,010 8.4% 7.1%
EPILOG 2,792 9.1% 4.0%
CAPTURE 1,265 9.0% 4.8%
RESTORE 2,139 6.3% 5.1%
EPISTENT 2,399 10.2% 5.2%
PRISM 3,231 7.0% 5.7%
PRISM PLUS 1,570 11.9% 8.7%
PARAGON 2,282 11.7% 11.3%
PURSUIT 10,948 15.7% 14.2%
Overall 30,336 11.1% 9.0%
0.79 (0.73, 0.85)
p < 10^-9
0
1
2
IIb/IIIa Better
Placebo Better

FIGURE 44-15 Meta-analysis of large Glycoprotein IIb/IIIa trials. (From Topol et al.[492] Reproduced with permission from the publisher and authors.)

Abciximab was also found to be beneficial when started 24 h *prior* to a PCI in the Chimeric 7E3 Fab Antiplatelet Therapy in Unstable Refractory Angina (CAPTURE) trial, which studied 1265 patients with refractory angina undergoing PCI.[253] All patients had undergone cardiac catheterization and had a planned PCI the following day. Death, MI, or urgent revascularization was reduced by abciximab from 15.9 to 11.3 percent (p = .012).[253] As in all the trials, the major benefit is in reductions of periprocedural MI as well as the need for urgent revascularization. A meta-analysis, however, has shown that there is a significant reduction in *mortality* when GP IIb/IIIa inhibition is used.[243b] These data highlight the clinical importance of thrombosis and of effective antithrombotic therapy in PCI.

The benefit of GP IIb/IIIa inhibition with coronary stenting was shown in the Evaluation of Platelet IIb/IIIa Inhibitor for Stenting (EPISTENT) trial.[243c] Compared with stenting alone, the rate of death, MI, or urgent revascularization at 30 days was significantly reduced in both abciximab groups—from 10.8 to 5.3 percent for stent plus abciximab ($p < 0.001$) and 6.9 percent for balloon angioplasty with abciximab (p = .007).[243c] Benefits were maintained at 6 months[244] and 1 year, with a significant reduction in 1-year mortality among patients treated with stent plus abciximab compared with stent alone.[245]

Eptifibatide This has been studied in two PCI trials and one large unstable angina trial. In the Integrilin to Minimize Platelet Aggregation and Coronary Thrombosis (IMPACT-II) trial of patients undergoing elective or urgent PCI, patients were randomized to eptifibatide at one of two doses or placebo, continued for 20 to 24 h after the procedure. These doses (infusion rates of 0.5 and 0.75 mg/kg per hour) however were found after the trial was completed to achieve only 50 to 60 percent platelet inhibition. The primary end point of the trial was a composite of death, MI, urgent need for revascularization, or stent placement for abrupt vessel closure at 30 days. There was a trend toward a lower composite event rate in the low-dose and high-dose eptifibatide-treated groups compared with placebo (9.2 and 9.9 percent versus 11.4 percent, respectively; p = .063 for low-dose eptifibatide).[8]

More recently, the Enhanced Suppression of the Platelet Receptor IIb/IIIa with Eptifibatide Therapy (ESPRIT) trial tested a higher dose, 180-μg/kg bolus followed by an infusion of 2.0 mg/kg per hour, with a second bolus of 180 μg/kg given 10 min after the first bolus. This dose was similar to that used in the Platelet IIb/IIIa Underpinning the Receptor for Suppression of Unstable Angina Trial (PURSUIT)[76] (see also page 1397) and was targeted to achieve 85 to 95 percent platelet inhibition. The second bolus was added to ensure no fall in the level of inhibition of platelet aggregation at the early periprocedural time point. In this trial, patients enrolled had either stable angina or unstable angina or a recent, but not acute, MI. The primary end point was death, MI urgent revascularization, or thrombotic bailout at 48 h. There was a 37 percent reduction in death or MI (10.5 versus 6.6 percent, p = .0017) (Fig. 44-16).[246] Death or MI at 48 h was reduced from 9.2 to 5.5 percent (p = .0013), a relative 40 percent reduction. Death, MI, or target vessel revascularization was reduced from 9.3 to 6.0 percent

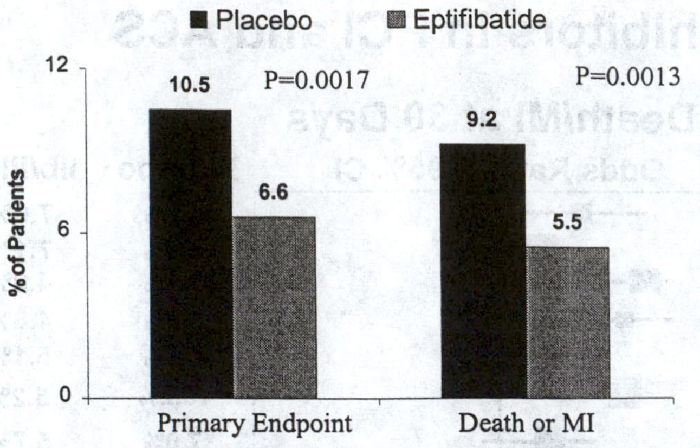

FIGURE 44-16 Primary Results from the ESPRIT trial of eptifibatide in coronary stenting. (Presented by Tcheng J at American College of Cardiology, March 2000.)

($p = .0045$).[246] Thus, eptifibatide in the new double-bolus and infusion regimen led to a substantial reduction in early complications from PCI.

TIROFIBAN This is a nonpeptide GP IIb/IIIa receptor antagonist. The compound has a short half-life (approximately 3 h).[247] Intravenous infusion of tirofiban for 1 or 4 h in healthy male volunteers dose-dependently inhibited ADP-, collagen-, arachidonic acid-, and thrombin-induced platelet aggregation.[247,248] Bleeding time was also significantly increased.

The RESTORE trial enrolled 2139 patients undergoing high-risk PCI and randomized patients to tirofiban (10-mg/kg bolus followed by infusion of 0.15-mg/kg per hour for 36 h). Tirofiban led to a lower, but not statistically significant, rate of the primary composite end point (death, MI, revascularization for target vessel ischemia, or stent placement for abrupt vessel closure at 30 days), (10.3 versus 12.2 percent, a 16 percent risk reduction, $p = .16$).[249] Death, MI, or urgent revascularization to 30 days was reduced by tirofiban by 24 percent (8.0 versus 10.5 percent, $p = .052$). In this trial, however, systematic collection of cardiac enzymes periprocedurally was not carried out, and thus a major end point was not ascertained as in the other trials. A trial is currently under way that will directly compare abciximab and tirofiban in PCI.

PRIMARY PERCUTANEOUS CORONARY INTERVENTION The final area of coronary intervention that has been tested is for *primary* PCI, i.e., for acute ST-elevation MI. After favorable results in a subgroup of the EPIC trial were observed,[250] the ReoPro and Primary PTCA Organization and Randomized Trial (RAPPORT) trial was conducted, comparing abciximab with placebo.[251] Although the prespecified 6-month end point of death, MI, or any target vessel revascularization was not significantly reduced, abciximab was able to reduce the 30-day incidence of death, MI, or urgent revascularization by 48 percent, from 11.2 to 5.8 percent ($p = .03$). This beneficial effect was sustained at 6 months (17.8 versus 11.6 percent, $p = .05$).[251] Two other randomized trials have also shown benefit of abciximab in primary PCI, each with a similar 50 percent reduction in death, MI, or urgent revascularization at 30 days.[251a,251b]

Another important observation has been made regarding treatment of patients with ST-elevation MI with GP IIb/IIIa inhibitors in the emergency department 30 to 90 min *prior* to performing a PCI. Early TIMI grade 3 flow is achieved in 20 to 30 percent of patients, with a TIMI grade 2 or 3 flow achieved of approximately 50 percent.[251a–c,281,283] Thus, use of GP IIb/IIIa inhibitors can "facilitate" the PCI by providing better preprocedural flow and consequently better procedural outcomes.

Thus, given this broad experience with GP IIb/IIIa inhibitors in PCI (Fig. 44-15), and with reductions in death or MI of approximately 50 percent, their use has become a new therapeutic standard for PCI.

Glycoprotein IIb/IIIa Inhibitors in Unstable Angina and Non-ST-Elevation Myocardial Infarction As of the time of this printing, the FDA had approved three agents for the treatment of unstable angina and non-ST-elevation MI: tirofiban and eptifibatide (Integrilin); abciximab (ReoPro) is approved for use in patients with unstable angina with a planned PCI. For unstable angina, abciximab can be administered as a 0.25-mg/kg bolus and an infusion of 0.125 μg/kg per minute for 12 to 24 h. Although in the CAPTURE trial it was administered for 24 h prior to, and only 1 h after, the procedure, in all the other trials abciximab was continued for 12 h after PCI. The approved dose of tirofiban is that used in the Platelet Receptor Inhibition for Ischemic Syndrome Management in Patients Limited by Unstable Signs and Symptoms (PRISM-PLUS) trial: a loading dose of 0.4 μg/kg per minute over 30 min, followed by 0.1 μg/kg per minute. Patients with renal insufficiency (creatinine clearance < 30 mL/min) should receive half the usual rate of infusion. The dose of eptifibatide is 180-μg/kg bolus and infusion of 2.0 μg/kg per minute.

TIROFIBAN PRISM-PLUS studied 1915 patients with documented unstable angina and non-ST-elevation MI with either electrocardiographic changes or positive enzymes.[78] The combination of tirofiban, heparin, and aspirin significantly lowered the rate of death, MI, or recurrent refractory ischemia at 7 days (primary end point) compared with heparin plus aspirin (12.9 versus 17.9 percent, respectively, a 32 percent risk reduction, $p = .004$).[78] This benefit was predominantly due to a 47 percent reduction in MI ($p = .006$) and a 30 percent reduction in refractory ischemia ($p = .02$). These benefits were achieved early and include a significant 66 percent reduction in death or MI at 48 h (0.9 versus 2.6 percent, $p = .01$).[78] Importantly, these benefits were preserved during follow-up: the 30-day rate of death or MI was also reduced by 30 percent (from 11.9 to 8.7 percent, $p = .03$).[78] Long-term follow-up to 6 months also showed a significant reduction in events (32.1 versus 27.7 percent, $p = .02$).[78]

The benefit of tirofiban plus heparin and aspirin was found across all subgroups evaluated, including men and women, elderly and young, unstable angina and non-ST-elevation MI patients, and those with ST-segment depression or elevation, *and* in those with no ST-segment or T-wave changes.[78] As expected, the absolute benefit in number of events prevented was greater in higher-risk patient subgroups, such as the elderly, diabetics, those who were already taking aspirin, and those with ST-segment changes or positive cardiac markers. The benefit of tirofiban plus heparin was also found in all types of management strategies: patients managed medically derived a 25 percent reduction in death or MI rate at 30 days, those who also had angioplasty had a 34 percent reduction, and those who were sent on to bypass surgery also derived a 30 percent benefit. Thus, benefit of adding tirofiban to aspirin plus heparin is derived in all patient groups treated.

A beneficial effect of tirofiban was also observed in the PRISM study, which randomized 3232 patients with unstable angina and non-ST-elevation MI to either heparin or tirofiban, with all patients receiving aspirin.[77] The primary goal of this study was to examine the effects of GP IIb/IIIa inhibition during medical therapy only; thus, the end point was a composite of death, MI, and refractory ischemic conditions at 48 h, and coronary procedures were not permitted by the protocol during the first 48 h. Tirofiban-treated patients had a significantly lower composite event rate than the placebo group (3.8 versus 5.6 percent, representing a 32 percent reduction, $p = .01$).[77] At 30 days, the improvement on the composite end point of death or MI was no longer statistically significant (death or MI, relative risk = 0.80, $p = .11$). Thus, the effects of GP IIb/IIIa inhibition with tirofiban appear to have greater long-term effects when used in conjunction with heparin (as was done in the PRISM-PLUS trial) (see below).

Eptifibatide This was studied in the PURSUIT trial involving 10,948 patients with unstable angina and non-Q-wave MI. Patients received aspirin and heparin and were randomized to in one of three arms: high-dose eptifibatide, low-dose eptifibatide, or placebo. By study design, the low dose was dropped after an interim analysis because of a reasonable safety profile of the high dose. Eptifibatide (180-μg/kg bolus and infusion of 2.0 μg/kg per minute) reduced the rate of death or MI at 30 days from 15.7 to 14.2 percent ($p = .042$).[76] This benefit of reducing 15 events per 1000 patients treated was achieved after only 72 h (while the patients were on study drug): 7.6 percent for placebo compared with 5.9 percent for eptifibatide ($p = .001$). Among patients undergoing early angioplasty or stenting while on study drug, benefits were more dramatic: 16.7 percent for placebo compared with 11.6 percent for eptifibatide ($p = .01$).[76] In this group, there were reductions in death or MI observed both prior to PCI and during the first 24 h after PCI.[252] Severe or moderate hemorrhage was more common in the eptifibatide group, 12.8 versus 9.9 percent ($p < 0.001$).

Abciximab The Global Use of Strategies to Open Occluded Coronary Arteries (GUSTO) IV–Acute Coronary Syndromes (ACS) trial recently reported (Topol, European Congress of Cardiology, Amsterdam 2000) no benefit of Abciximab in patients with unstable angina and non-Q-wave MI, who did not undergo PCI. On the other hand, among patients with unstable angina who undergo PCI (i.e., those managed with an early invasive strategy), abciximab has been shown to be beneficial. In the CAPTURE trial, 1265 patients with refractory angina had undergone cardiac catheterization and had a planned PCI the following day. They were then randomized to abciximab or placebo (in addition to aspirin and heparin) that was administered for 24 h *prior* to a PCI. Death, MI, or urgent revascularization was reduced by abciximab from 15.9 to 11.3 percent ($p = .012$).[253]

Lamifiban This nonpeptide synthetic compound that binds reversibly to the integrin IIb/IIIa with a K_D of 5 nM has been effective in several animal models of thrombosis.[254] The inhibition of the ADP-induced aggregation curve parallels the receptor occupancy obtained during in vitro radioligand-binding studies (approximately 50 percent inhibition with 50 percent receptor occupancy of GP IIb/IIIa). The half-life of the free drug is 40 min and that of the bound drug is 9 h. A dose-finding study was conducted in patients with unstable angina.[255]

The Canadian Lamifiban Study of 365 patients with unstable angina showed a lower rate of death or MI at 30 days (2.5 versus 8.19 percent for placebo, $p = .03$).[256] These results were not observed in the larger Platelet IIb/IIIa Antagonism for the Reduction of Acute Coronary Syndromes in a Global Organization Network (PARAGON) A study, which involved 2282 patients. In that study, death or MI at 30 days was 11.7 percent for placebo (aspirin plus heparin) compared with 10.6 percent for low-dose (1 μg/min) lamifiban and 12.0 percent for high-dose (5 μg/min) lamifiban (p = NS).[257] The findings on 6-month follow-up, however, suggest a possible benefit of low-dose lamifiban plus heparin: death or MI to 6 months was 12.6 percent for low-dose lamifiban plus heparin compared with 17.9 percent for placebo ($p = .025$).[257]

The PARAGON-B trial evaluated a dose of lamifiban based on renal function, so as to ensure optimal dose level. In this trial, 5225 patients with unstable angina or non-ST-elevation MI were enrolled and treated with lamifiban versus placebo. The primary end point, death, MI, or severe recurrent ischemia, was not significantly reduced in the overall group (11.8 versus 12.8 percent for heparin, $p = .329$).[258] In those with positive troponin T at baseline, however, there was a significant reduction in events (from 19 to 11 percent for lamifiban, $p = .018$). This agent is not being developed for commercial use.

Meta-analysis Figure 44-15 shows a meta-analysis of all the large GP IIb/IIIa inhibitor trials through 1999 in PCI or unstable angina.[259] The results show a consistent benefit on death or MI rate at 30 days (highly statistically significant, $p < 0.0000001$).[259] Although some differences exist in the relative benefits, it is currently believed that these may relate more to trial design and end-point assessment than differences between the drugs. Thus, it is felt that the benefit in reducing death or MI is a class effect of all the GP IIb/IIIa inhibitors. Direct comparisons between the agents are ongoing to determine the relative benefits of one agent compared with another. Thus, GP IIb/IIIa inhibition in patients with unstable angina/non-ST-elevation MI or PCI reduced death or MI rate at 30 days, representing a significant advance in the treatment of these acute coronary syndromes. These data highlight the importance of acute thrombosis and of platelet inhibition in acute coronary syndromes and establish GP IIb/IIIa inhibition as a new standard of care in the treatment of these conditions.

Need for Heparin with Glycoprotein IIb/IIIa Inhibitors The data from several of the trials suggest that GP IIb/IIIa inhibitors should be administered with concomitant heparin. This notion was first suggested by the dropping of the tirofiban-alone arm from the PRISM-PLUS trial, as compared with the superiority of the heparin plus tirofiban arm in that trial. Subsequently, the two other trials in unstable angina have found very similar results: In the PARAGON-A trial, there was a greater benefit when using triple antithrombotic therapy (aspirin, heparin, and the GP IIb/IIIa inhibitor), and this has also recently been reported in a dose-ranging study with lamifiban.[257] The third trial that recently demonstrated the need for heparin was the

PURSUIT. A recent abstract found that, among the 90 percent of patients in whom physicians decided to use heparin, a greater benefit on reduction in death or MI rate was observed (14 percent reduction, from 16.9 to 14.6 percent, $p = .013$) compared with a 41 percent *increase* in death or MI rate among the patients not treated with heparin.[260] Although these data may be confounded by other issues, they are consistent with the other trials. Thus, it appears important to use heparin with GP IIb/IIIa inhibitors when treating patients with unstable angina and non-ST-elevation MI. This fits our understanding of the pathophysiology of thrombus formation in acute coronary syndromes, which involves both platelets and the clotting cascade. Since one agent is a potent antiplatelet and the other is an anticoagulant, it follows that both together will have greater benefit. The next question in the field is the safety and efficacy of LMW heparin in combination with GP IIb/IIIa inhibitors.

Angiographic Observations: Establishing the Paradigm of Benefit Data on thrombus resolution are available from two trials: PRISM-PLUS and CAPTURE. An angiographic substudy was performed as part of the PRISM-PLUS trial to investigate the mechanism of benefit of tirofiban.[261] It was observed that the coronary thrombus was smaller in patients treated with tirofiban plus heparin and aspirin compared with heparin and aspirin. The percentage of patients who had definitive thrombus was reduced from 24 to 17 percent, and there was a 23 percent improvement in overall thrombus grade ($p = .022$).[261] Similarly, coronary flow, using the TIMI flow grading system,[3] was significantly improved, with TIMI grade 3 flow improving from 74.5 to 81.9 percent, with a 35 percent overall improvement in flow ($p = .002$).[261] Similar data are also available from the CAPTURE trial.[262] Together these data establish the pathophysiologic link between the potent platelet inhibition achieved by tirofiban, a reduction in thrombus, and improvement in coronary blood flow, and consequent improvement in clinical outcome for patients.

Reducing Infarct Size with Glycoprotein IIb/IIIa Inhibition A new concept in the field of GP IIb/IIIa inhibition is that these agents appear to be able to reduce the size of an evolving non-ST-elevation MI or even prevent the development of myocardial necrosis, based on evidence from two trials.[263,264] In the PRISM-PLUS troponin substudy, patients randomized to tirofiban plus heparin had a significantly lower peak troponin than did patients who received heparin and aspirin alone.[264] This was also true among patients who had a negative CK-MB on admission. In the PURSUIT trial, it was observed that the size of the MI (either index or recurrent MI) measured by peak CK-MB, was significantly smaller in patients treated with eptifibatide. Thus, these potent antiplatelet therapies appear to have an immediate effect in reducing the severity of the presenting illness, something that has been observed for patients who develop acute coronary syndromes while already taking aspirin.[265–267]

Another new concept in GP IIb/IIIa inhibition is that there appears to be a greater benefit of treatment when administered earlier relative to the onset of pain. In an analysis from PURSUIT, the absolute reduction in death or MI rate with eptifibatide was 2.8 percent for patients treated within 6 h from the onset of pain and was less for those treated between 6 to 12 and 12 to 24 h after onset of pain. No benefit was observed in patients treated 24 h after the onset of pain. Similar data have been observed in PRISM-PLUS (unpublished data).

Glycoprotein IIb/IIIa Inhibitors Plus Thrombolysis for Treatment of Acute Myocardial Infarction

Although thrombolytic therapy has proved to be a major advance in the treatment of patients with acute MI,[180,268] current thrombolytic regimens have several limitations: (1) failure of initial reperfusion,[269,270] (2) inadequate perfusion with delayed flow (TIMI grade 2 flow),[269,270] (3) imperfect myocardial perfusion,[271] and (4) infarct-related artery reocclusion/reinfarction in a significant percentage of patients.[270,272] Because platelets play a central role in coronary thrombosis—especially failed reperfusion, reocclusion, and reinfarction—attention has turned to the GP IIb/IIIa inhibitors as a means of improving current reperfusion regimens.[259,273]

MECHANISMS OF THROMBOLYTIC RESISTANCE

Lack of initial reperfusion, which could be termed *thrombolytic resistance,* appears to be due to several mechanisms (Table 44-4): (1) Fibrinolytic agents act only on the fibrin portion of the thrombus, leaving activated platelets as a source of rethrombosis. (2) Platelets elaborate PAI-1, which inhibits the action of the thrombolytic agent; platelets also release other agents, such as TXA_2, which causes local vasoconstriction.[274] (3) Lysis of clot-bound fibrin exposes clot-bound thrombin, which remains catalytically active and can cleave fibrinogen to fibrin, facilitating rethrombosis.[275] In addition, thrombosis can stimulate further thrombin production and activation of platelets.[276] (4) thrombolytic therapy also has a direct platelet-activating effect, leading to increased levels of TXA_2 and platelet-activating factor.[274,277] The presence of aspirin does not abolish the platelet-activating effect of fibrinolytic therapy.[274] Thus, thrombolysis promotes platelet activation and therefore actually creates an environment that may lead to subsequent rethrombosis and/or reocclusion.

INITIAL STUDIES

Preclinical studies were performed that first tested GP IIb/IIIa receptor inhibitors with thrombolytics to accelerate reperfusion time and reduce the risk of reocclusion.[278,279] The Thrombolysis and Angioplasty in Myocardial Infarction 8 (TAMI-8) trial[280] established the clinical feasibility of combining GP IIb/IIIa inhibitors with thrombolytic therapy. After receiving t-PA plus heparin and aspirin, patients received incremental doses of m7E3, a murine monoclonal antibody to the GP IIb/IIIa receptor. A consistent dose-dependent increase in platelet aggregation was observed, and a clear relationship between GP IIb/IIIa receptor occupancy and extent of platelet inhibition was established.[280]

TABLE 44-4 Potential Mechanisms of Thrombolytic Resistance

1) Only fibrin is lysed by thrombolytic agent
2) Plasminogen activator inhibitor 1
3) Thromboxane A_2
4) Clot-bound thrombin
5) Activation of platelets

Concomitant Full-Dose Thrombolytic Therapy Plus Glycoprotein IIb/IIIa Inhibition The combination of eptifibatide and t-PA, as tested in the Integrilin to Manage Platelet Aggregation and Combat Acute Myocardial Infarction (IMPACT-AMI) trial, significantly increased the rate of TIMI grade 3 infarct related artery (IRA) flow upon angiography at 90 min (66 percent, as compared with 39 percent in the placebo group, p = .006).[281] A subsequent trial combining full-dose streptokinase with ascending dosages of eptifibatide found modest improvements in TIMI grade 3 flow in the infarct-related artery, but there was an increased rate of major bleeding.

The Platelet Aggregation Receptor Antagonist Dose Investigation and Reperfusion Gain in Myocardial Infarction (PARADIGM) trial compared different lamifiban dosage levels to placebo in 353 patients presenting within 12 h of acute MI symptom onset. Patients received aspirin and heparin and either t-PA or streptokinase at standard doses.[282] Lamifiban was associated with improved myocardial reperfusion as measured by early resolution of ST-segment elevation, but no difference in the composite clinical end point was noted. Lamifiban also was associated with increased rates of gastrointestinal, coronary bypass related, and catheterization access-site bleeding complications.

In summary, with the strategy of concomitant full-dose thrombolytic therapy and full-dose GP IIb/IIIa inhibition, it has been difficult to balance efficacy and safety, so attention has turned to combining full-dose GP IIb/III inhibitors with reduced doses of thrombolytic agents.

Reduced-Dose Thrombolysis Plus Glycoprotein IIb/IIIa Inhibition The combination of a *reduced*-dose thrombolytic agent and a GP IIb/IIIa inhibitor was tested in the TIMI-14 trial using t-PA, streptokinase, and reteplase, and in Strategies for Patency Enhancement in the Emergency Department (SPEED) using reteplase.

The international TIMI-14 trial dose-ranging phase enrolled 681 patients with ST-elevation MI who met standard eligibility criteria.[283] The patients were randomized within 12 h of acute ST-elevation MI symptom onset to one of four reperfusion regimens (each encompassing several dosage levels): standard-dose t-PA alone (the control arm), reduced-dose t-PA plus abciximab, reduced-dose streptokinase plus abciximab, or abciximab alone. All patients received aspirin and heparin. The initial heparin dosage was a 70-U/kg bolus and an infusion of 15 U/kg per hour in the t-PA control arm, and a 60-U/kg bolus with an infusion of 7 U/kg per hour in the arms that included abciximab.

Abciximab alone was associated with 90-min TIMI grade 3 flow rates in 32 percent of patients and 90-min patency in 48 percent of patients.[283] The combination of streptokinase and abciximab produced only modest improvement in early TIMI grade 3 flow. TIMI grade 3 flow at 90 min was achieved in 42 percent of patients in the 0.5-MU (million units) group, 39 percent of patients in the 0.75-MU group, and 47 percent of patients in the 1.25-MU group. The 1.5-MU regimen, plus abciximab, was discontinued after four of six patients developed a major hemorrhage, one of whom developed an intracranial hemorrhage (ICH).

Dose ranging with t-PA found that the best angiographic results were obtained using a 50-mg dose given as a 15-mg bolus and a 35-mg infusion over 60 min. At 90 min, TIMI grade 3 flow was achieved in 77 percent of patients compared with 62 percent for t-PA alone (p = .02). Overall patency of the IRA was achieved in 93 percent of patients with the combination of abciximab and t-PA compared with 78 percent for t-PA (p = .09). An even greater difference was observed at 60 min when adding GP IIb/IIIa inhibition: the standard t-PA dose achieved only 43 percent TIMI grade 3 flow at 60 min compared with 72 percent for 50 mg t-PA plus abciximab (p = .0009). Major hemorrhage was similar among the t-PA plus abciximab and control groups, approximately 6 percent in each. In-hospital mortality was similar in all groups, ranging from 3 to 5 percent.

Thus, the addition of the GP IIb/IIIa receptor inhibitor abciximab to 50 mg of t-PA increased the rate of TIMI grade 3 flow at 60 min by an absolute 29 percent, representing a relative 67 percent improvement over standard therapy. At 90 min, the addition of the GP IIb/IIIa receptor inhibitor improved TIMI grade 3 flow by an absolute 15 percent (a relative 25 percent improvement). These results indicate that the combination of GP IIb/IIIa receptor inhibition with reduced-dose thrombolytic therapy appears to be a promising new regimen for enhancing both the speed and extent of reperfusion in acute ST-elevation MI.

Results from the SPEED trial[283a] similarly demonstrated improvements in early TIMI grade 3 flow with reteplase, indicating that the combination of low-dose thrombolytic therapy with t-PA or reteplase appears to be a potentially promising new regimen for improving both the speed and extent of thrombolysis in acute MI. There are numerous other ongoing angiographic and larger mortality trials that are exploring further the potential role of GP IIb/IIIa inhibitors with reduced-dose thrombolytic therapy.

SAFETY

One of the concerns with any antithrombotic agent is bleeding. Although the initial EPIC study showed increased bleeding when using abciximab plus heparin during angioplasty compared with heparin alone,[284] a strong interaction with the dose of heparin was observed. In the subsequent EPILOG trial, the rate of major bleeding was identical between heparin control patients and those receiving abciximab and low-dose heparin.[285] Similarly, the rate of major bleeding has generally not been significantly increased in other trials with intravenous administration.[77,78,249,286] Thus, use of lower doses of heparin and careful monitoring of the level of anticoagulation help avoid bleeding complications in patients receiving GP IIb/IIIa inhibitors. With regard to monitoring the degree of platelet inhibition, trials to date have used weight adjusted dosing of the GP IIb/IIIa inhibitors, but investigation is currently ongoing to determine when and where monitoring of platelet function might be useful clinically.[287,288]

Another concern, especially when adding GP IIb/IIIa inhibition to thrombolytic therapy, is the risk of ICH. Fortunately, GP IIb/IIIa inhibitors generally have a low risk of ICH when used alone, and no apparent increase compared with aspirin and heparin in the major trials.[76–78,249,257,284–286,289] The risk of ICH when combined with thrombolytic therapy may be largely due to the risk from the latter agent, but larger trials will be needed to define the exact rate.

THROMBOCYTOPENIA

This is an uncommon but important complication of GP IIb/IIIa inhibitors: For tirofiban in PRISM-PLUS, the rate of severe thrombocytopenia (<50,000 cells/mm^3) was 0.5 percent compared with 0.3 percent for heparin (p = NS)[78]; in the PURSUIT trial, thrombocytopenia (<20,000 cells/mm^3) occurred in 0.2 percent compared with <0.1 percent for heparin.[76] Thrombocytopenia is associated with increased bleeding and, in a smaller proportion of patients, recurrent thrombotic events.[290,291] This syndrome bears resemblance to heparin-induced thrombocytopenia (HIT) and indicates a need to monitor platelet count daily during the GP IIb/IIIa infusion.

Oral Glycoprotein IIb/IIIa Inhibition

Oral GP IIb/IIIa inhibitors are peptidomimetic agents that are competitive inhibitors of the GP IIb/IIIa receptor. They are usually pro-drugs, which are absorbed and then converted to active compounds in the blood.[237–241] The oral agents all have longer half-lives, such that they can be given once, twice, or three times daily to achieve relatively steady levels of GP IIb/IIIa inhibition. With oral dosing, long-term therapy (i.e., longer than 1 year) is possible. As with the intravenous compounds, two major groups of drugs exist in the oral class: those with competitive inhibition and short "off time" from the receptor (where a high drug level is critical to achieving high levels of platelet inhibition) and those which have "tight" binding to the platelet (similar to abciximab) with the majority of the drug circulating bound to platelets.

INITIAL CLINICAL EXPERIENCE

Pharmacokinetics and Pharmacodynamics A number of orally active platelet GP IIb/IIIa inhibitors have been studied in clinical trials (Table 44-5). Currently available data suggest that most of these agents inhibit ex vivo platelet aggregation in response to various agonists [ADP, collagen, or Thrombin Receptor Activator Peptide (TRAP)] that correlates closely with plasma level of active metabolite. In addition, the dose/concentration response is maintained without evidence for tolerance or tachyphylaxis over time. Differences in drug half-life may result in drug accumulation and more pronounced platelet inhibition during chronic therapy, depending on the dose interval employed. The pharmacokinetic and pharmacodynamic response to most oral GP IIb/IIIa inhibitors can be illustrated by comparing and contrasting the responses of short-acting (xemilofiban, half-life 4.1 h), moderate-acting (sibrafiban and orbofiban, half-lives approximately 10 to 11 h), and longer-acting agents (roxifiban and cromofiban, half-lives approximately 24 h).

Xemilofiban The first experience with oral GP IIb/IIIa inhibition was with xemilofiban.[237,292,293] High degrees of platelet inhibition were achieved with this oral GP IIb/IIIa inhibitor. It has a relatively short half-life and thus is given three times daily. The Oral Glycoprotein IIb/IIIa Receptor Blockade to Inhibit Thrombosis (ORBIT) trial was a randomized dose-ranging trial of xemilofiban in patients undergoing percutaneous intervention.[294] Peak inhibition of platelet aggregation was similar following the same dose of xemilofiban administered on days 14 and 28 of the trial. The time to peak blood level following the same dose of xemilofiban was reduced from 4 h following the first dose of drug to 2 h with steady-state dosing during chronic therapy.[294] Most bleeding events were observed during the first 2 weeks of therapy on a three-times daily dosing regimen.[294] Further bleeding events were uncommon during the final 2 weeks of treatment on a twice-daily dosing regimen, and the requirement for blood transfusion was infrequent.

TIMI-12 Trial This was a phase II, double-blind, dose-ranging trial designed to evaluate the pharmacokinetics, pharmacodynamics, safety, and tolerability of sibrafiban in 329 patients after acute coronary syndromes.[238] In the pharmacokinetics/pharmacodynamics cohort of TIMI-12, a total of 106 patients were randomized to receive one of seven dosing regimens of sibrafiban, ranging from 5 mg daily to 10 mg twice daily for 28 days. In the safety cohort, 223 patients were randomized to one of four dose regimens of sibrafiban (ranging from 5 mg twice daily to 15 mg once daily) or aspirin for 28 days.

High levels of platelet inhibition were achieved: mean peak values ranged from 47 to 97 percent inhibition of 20 μM ADP-

TABLE 44-5 Oral IIb/III Inhibitors That Have or Are Undergoing Clinical Testing

Oral Agent	Company	Trials	Phase	Study Population	Drug Half-Life, h
Xemilofiban	G.D. Searle	ORBIT EXCITE	II III	Coronary intervention	4.1
Sibrafiban	Roche and Genentech	TIMI-12 SYMPHONY	II III	Post-acute coronary syndromes	11
Orbofiban	G.D. Searle	SOAR OPUS–TIMI-16	II III	Acute coronary syndromes	10
Lotrafiban	Smith Kline Beecham	APLAUD BRAVO	II III	Acute coronary syndromes, TIA, postischemic stroke	4–8
Klerval	RPR	TIMI-15	II	Acute coronary syndromes CAD	4–5
Lefradifiban	Boehringer Ingelheim	FROST	II	Acute coronary syndromes	8–12
Cromofiban	Cor	NA	II	Acute coronary syndromes	12–24
Roxifiban	DuPont	ROCKET	II	Acute coronary syndromes	24

ABBREVIATIONS: CAD = coronary artery disease; TIA = transient ischemic attack; NA = not available.
SOURCE: Cannon CP. *Curr Opin Card Pulm Renal Invest Drugs* 2000; 2:114–123, with permission.

induced platelet aggregation on day 28 across the seven doses. Twice-daily dosing provided more sustained platelet inhibition (mean inhibition, 36 to 86 percent on day 28), while platelet inhibition returned to baseline levels by 24 h with once-daily dosing.[238] Major hemorrhage was rare in patients treated with sibrafiban (1.5 percent) or aspirin (1.9 percent). However, protocol-defined "minor" bleeding, usually mucocutaneous, occurred in 0 to 32 percent of patients in the various sibrafiban groups, compared with none of the aspirin-treated patients. In a multivariate model, minor bleeding was related to total daily dose ($p = .002$), once-daily compared with twice-daily dosing ($p < .0001$), renal function ($p < .0001$), and presentation with unstable angina ($p < .01$).[238]

Thus, the oral GP IIb/IIIa antagonist sibrafiban achieved effective, chronic platelet inhibition with a clear dose response but at the expense of a relatively high incidence of minor bleeding. The mucocutaneous bleeds appeared to be related to plasma drug concentrations, the degree of platelet inhibition, and other patient factors (weight and renal function). One lesson learned is that dosing of sibrafiban (or other oral agents) based on such clinical factors might help improve the safety profile of the drug with regard to minor bleeding.

Peak-to-Trough Ratios In TIMI-12, approximately double the rate of minor bleeding occurred with once-daily dosing, as compared with similar total daily dose of twice-daily dosing (e.g., 15 mg once daily versus 7 mg twice daily). This may indicate that the higher peak drug concentrations and degree of platelet inhibition (sometimes 100 percent) may be related to the bleeding episodes. The bleeding appeared to occur approximately 6 h after study drug ingestion, which correlates with the peak blood level. Thus, these data suggest that using dosing regimens that avoid high peaks may decrease the risk of bleeding.

Variability In addition, interpatient variability has been observed in drug level and degree of platelet inhibition. In contrast, the 24- to 72-h infusions of intravenous GP IIb/IIIa inhibitors have doses selected to achieve 80 to 95 percent inhibition—and a very steady level of inhibition is achieved. This is one of the major differences in the pharmacokinetics between the intravenous and oral GP IIb/IIIa inhibitors, and it may be an explanation for differences in clinical outcomes observed to date. This variability might lead to too low a level of inhibition at the trough level or too high a level of inhibition in some patients at peak times.

One potential strategy for dosing oral GP IIb/IIIa antagonists is to monitor the degree of platelet inhibition or drug level achieved in individual patients and adjust the dose to a target level, as is currently done with anticoagulant therapy. By avoiding higher levels of platelet inhibition, this strategy may reduce bleeding complications. This could potentially be accomplished with a bedside assay for platelet inhibition.[287] An alternate strategy for adjusting the dose of an oral GP IIb/IIIa inhibitor is to begin using fixed dose initially but lower the dose if the patient experiences minor bleeding. Such strategies may improve the overall safety profile of these potent platelet antagonists.

Thrombocytopenia This is another key area of tolerability. Data from the Orbofiban in Patients with Unstable Coronary Syndromes (OPUS)–TIMI-16 trial suggest that, with oral therapy, thrombocytopenia generally occurs early, within the first 2 weeks, with very low rates during long-term follow-up.[295] Among patients who developed thrombocytopenia, however, higher rates of both bleeding and cardiac events were seen. Thus, a very small percentage of patients treated with oral GP IIb/IIIa inhibitors developed thrombocytopenia, and a proportion of those developed thrombosis or bleeding. This pattern bears some resemblance to that for heparin and for intravenous GP IIb/IIIa inhibitors, suggesting the pathophysiology may relate to a more general drug-induced thrombocytopenia ± thrombosis (DITT) syndrome.

Degree of Platelet Inhibition and Efficacy Previous animal and clinical studies have suggested that the maximum benefit of GP IIb/IIIa inhibition occurs when the degree of platelet inhibition is greater than 80 percent.[284,285] Currently, it is not clear whether lower levels of platelet inhibition would also be beneficial. The IMPACT-II study showed a strong trend toward the reduction of recurrent ischemic events after coronary angioplasty at a dose of eptifibatide that achieved only 50 to 60 percent inhibition.[286] In contrast, a greater benefit was observed with a higher dose of eptifibatide (that targeted 85 to 90 percent platelet inhibition) in the ESPRIT trial (Tcheng J, presented at the American College of Cardiology, March 2000). Thus, it appears that greater benefit, at least in the acute setting, is achieved with doses that achieve more than 80 percent inhibition of 20 μM ADP-induced platelet aggregation, but this is not truly a "threshold" below which no benefit is achieved. For long-term therapy, a high level of blockade will need to be balanced with the potential of increased bleeding, and thus a slightly lower level of inhibition may be optimal.

Degree of Platelet Inhibition and Bleeding As observed in TIMI-12, increasing the degree of platelet inhibition may produce a higher incidence of minor bleeding events.[238] This suggests that a lower degree of platelet inhibition may be better tolerated during chronic, oral therapy. Nevertheless, major hemorrhage appears to be within an acceptable range in the initial trials with oral GP IIb/IIIa inhibitors, even at high levels of platelet inhibition. Therefore, one possible dosing strategy for GP IIb/IIIa inhibitors may be to tailor the dose to the risk of recurrent ischemic events, thus optimizing the degree of platelet inhibition and minimizing the risk of minor bleeding. For example, patients might be given a higher dose during the early phase of their acute coronary syndrome, when they are at highest risk of recurrent ischemic events. The dose could then be lowered during the chronic phase, when the risk of recurrent ischemic events is lower, thereby decreasing the risk of bleeding.

Need for Aspirin An important aspect of oral GP IIb/IIIa inhibition is concomitant therapy with aspirin. Several factors suggest the benefit of the combination of aspirin and an oral GP IIb/IIIa inhibitor. First, synergism has been demonstrated for inhibition of platelet aggregation in response to collagen, with a greater degree of platelet inhibition with the combination of aspirin plus the GP IIb/IIIa inhibitor.[296] Second, the action of aspirin is to decrease the synthesis of TXA_2 by the platelet, which decreases platelet *activation*, a step proximal to platelet aggregation. Thus, aspirin and GP IIb/IIIa inhibitors inhibit different steps in the formation of a platelet thrombus. In addition, reduction in TXA_2 reduces local coronary vasospasm, which helps reduce ischemia. Additional factors favoring the combination are aspirin's efficacy for primary and secondary prevention of ischemic events,[184] its relatively good safety profile, and its low cost. Finally, aspirin would provide antiplatelet effects during the troughs in GP IIb/IIIa blockade that may occur between doses. The potential adverse effect of concomitant aspirin is increased risk of bleeding, particularly gastrointestinal bleeding. In addition, it has been argued that the effects of a GP IIb/IIIa inhibitor are an order of magnitude stronger than those of aspirin—and thus adding aspirin is redundant to the antiplatelet effects of the GP IIb/IIIa inhibitor.

Four Large Phase III Trials The first phase III trial of an oral GP IIb/IIIa inhibitor in patients with acute coronary syndromes was the OPUS–TIMI-16. This trial involved 10,288 patients randomized at 888 hospitals in 28 countries worldwide. The inclusion criteria were onset within the last 72 h of an acute coronary syndrome defined as rest ischemic pain lasting at least 5 min associated with either ECG changes, positive cardiac markers, or a prior history of vascular disease. Major exclusion criteria included renal insufficiency (creatinine >1.6 mg/dL or an estimated creatinine clearance <40 mL/min, increased bleeding risk, or need for warfarin).

Eligible patients were treated with 150 to 162 mg of acetylsalicylic acid (aspirin) and were randomized, in double-blind fashion, to one of two dosing strategies of orbofiban given twice daily or to placebo. In one dose, orbofiban was given 50 mg twice daily throughout the trial (50/50 group); in the other, the 50 mg twice daily dose was given for the first 30 days (the highest risk period), and then the dose was reduced to 30 mg twice daily (50/30 group). Other medical and interventional therapy was at the discretion of the treating physician. Patients were seen at 14 and 30 days and every 3 months. The primary end point was a composite of death, MI, recurrent ischemia leading to rehospitalization or urgent revascularization, or stroke. The planned sample size was to be 12,000 patients, but the trial was stopped prematurely after an unexpected increased mortality rate at 30 days was observed in one of the orbofiban groups.[297]

The composite end-point rates at 30 days were 10.8 percent in the placebo group compared with 9.9 percent in the two orbofiban groups (p = 0.12).[297,298] The mortality rate at 30 days was 1.4 percent in the placebo group compared with 2.3 percent in the 50/30 group and 1.6 percent in the 50/50 group. Through follow-up, 10-month event rates were 22.9, 23.1 and 22.8 percent, respectively (p = NS).[297,298] The safety profile was acceptable, with the rate of major hemorrhage and thrombocytopenia (0.6 percent) greater than with aspirin but within the expected range for this class of drugs. Subsequent exploratory analyses found greater benefit for patients who underwent PCI while on study drug and those who were stable on admission (Killip class I).

Substudies from OPUS–TIMI-16 demonstrated that this agent led to increases in measures of platelet activation, such as P-selectin.[299,300] These data are consistent with the observations in vitro of an apparent prothrombotic effect, with increases in platelet activation and aggregation at low levels of platelet inhibition.[301] In contrast, in TIMI-12, no increase in P-selectin was observed with sibrafiban therapy.[18] Further research in this field is ongoing, but it appears that there may be differences among the oral GP IIb/IIIa inhibitors with regard to the potential prothrombotic effects.

Many lessons were learned from OPUS–TIMI-16, the first large trial of oral GP IIb/IIIa inhibition in acute coronary syndromes, which will be helpful in planning future trials of other GP IIb/IIIa inhibitors. First, it appears that it will be beneficial to optimize the dosing strategy used with the oral agents, potentially to mimic the stable antiplatelet effect achieved by the intravenous drugs. This would mean trying to reduce the interpatient and intrapatient variability, potentially adjusting the dose by weight and/or renal function. One might also use the plasma drug level and/or the bedside platelet function test to adjust the dose. Second, our data suggest that one could target stabilized patients. In addition, several new and planned trials will be testing different drugs (e.g., with tight IIb/IIIa receptor binding).

EXCITE Trial The Evaluation of Oral Xemilofiban in Controlling Thrombotic Events (EXCITE) trial studied the agent xemilofiban in patients undergoing PCI. This trial followed the promising results demonstrated by two pilot studies in PCI.[292,294] In the EXCITE trial, 7232 patients undergoing elective PCI (angioplasty or stent) without adjunctive intravenous GP IIb/IIIa inhibition were randomized in a double-blind fashion to receive one of two xemilofiban regimens or placebo: 20 mg of oral xemilofiban 30 to 90 min prior to percutaneous coronary revascularization, followed by 10 mg or 20 mg xemilofiban or placebo for both were subsequently administered three times daily for 6 months.[302]

Death, MI, or urgent revascularization at 6 months, the primary end point, occurred in 13.6 percent of patients in the placebo group, 14.1 percent of patients in the 10-mg xemilofiban group, and 12.6 percent of patients in the 20-mg xemilofiban group (p = NS).[302] A trend toward fewer periprocedural MIs in the first 48 h following PCI was not sustained.[302] On the other hand, mortality tended to be higher in 10-mg xemilofiban dose group: The mortality rate at 6 months was 1.0 percent for placebo, 1.6 percent for the 10-mg xemilofiban dose group, and 1.1 percent in the 20-mg dose group.[302] Major hemorrhagic events were significantly more common among the xemilofiban-treated patients.[302] Thus, administration of the oral GP IIb/IIIa receptor inhibitor xemilofiban immediately prior to percutaneous revascularization in patients with acute and stable coronary artery disease, and chronically for up to 6 months thereafter, did not significantly reduce the primary composite end point of death, MI, or need for urgent revascularization. Xemilofiban did reduce the incidence of periprocedural MIs during the first 48 h of dosing.

SYMPHONY-I Trial Following the phase II trial, TIMI-12,[238] the first Sibrafiban Versus Aspirin to Yield Maximum Protection from Ischemic Heart Events Post-acute Coronary Syndromes (SYMPHONY) trial was a randomized, double-blind, aspirin-controlled trial of two regimens of sibrafiban for the treatment of patients following an acute coronary syndrome. A total of 9233 patients with either AMI or high-risk unstable angina (with ST deviation of 0.5 mm or more) who were stabilized for at least 12 h were randomized to receive either aspirin (80 mg every 12 h) or high-dose or low-dose sibrafiban (without aspirin) every 12 h for a total of 3 months. The dose of sibrafiban was either 3, 4.5, or 6 mg, based on body weight and renal function. The primary efficacy end point was a composite of death, MI, and severe recurrent ischemia.

There was no difference in the primary end point between aspirin (9.8 percent), low-dose sibrafiban (10.1 percent), and high-dose sibrafiban (10.1 percent). Similarly there were no differences in mortality alone, MI, or recurrent ischemia. Major bleeding was more common with the two sibrafiban groups, high dose (5.7 percent) and low dose (5.2 percent) compared with aspirin (3.9 percent). In conclusion, sibrafiban without aspirin was not superior to aspirin alone for secondary prevention of cardiac events following acute coronary syndromes.

SYMPHONY-II Trial The second SYMPHONY trial, which was terminated early at the time the SYMPHONY-I results were available, studied the combination of low-dose sibrafiban plus aspirin, high-dose sibrafiban, and aspirin alone. A total of 6671 patients with stabilized acute coronary syndromes were randomized. Follow-up was on average for 90 days. The primary efficacy end point of death, MI, or severe recurrent ischemia showed no difference in the high-dose sibrafiban group (10.5 percent) compared with 9.3 percent for aspirin alone and 9.2 percent for low-dose sibrafiban plus aspirin. The mortality rate was significantly higher with the high-dose sibrafiban group: 2.4 compared with 1.3 percent for placebo and 1.7 percent for the low-dose sibrafiban plus aspirin group. A similar pattern was seen for recurrent MI: 6.9 percent for high-dose sibrafiban compared with 5.3 percent for aspirin and 5.3 percent for the low-dose plus aspirin group. Major bleeding was more common with the two sibrafiban groups, 4.6 percent with high-dose sibrafiban compared with 4.0 percent for aspirin and 5.7 percent for low-dose sibrafiban plus aspirin.

NEW AGENTS ON THE HORIZON

Another agent, lotrafiban, has been studied in phase II and is currently being studied in a large phase III trial—Blockade for the GP IIb/IIIa Receptor to Avoid Vascular Occlusion (BRAVO)—in which all patients will receive aspirin and be randomized to lotrafiban or placebo. Another agent, cromafiban, has a very long half-life and thus may have more predictable and stable levels of platelet inhibition. Lefradafiban has been tested in a phase II study, with intriguing trends toward benefit among patients with a positive troponin T at baseline,[303] which is similar to the findings seen with intravenous GP IIb/IIIa inhibitors in the CAPTURE[304] and PRISM trials.[305] These data suggest that identification of the ideal patients with risk-stratification methods may assist in targeting therapy to patients who will benefit most.

Two agents to date have been evaluated as both intravenous *and* oral compounds: Klerval[306,307] and (le)fradafiban.[308] In the TIMI-15B trial, a transition from initial intravenous treatment to prolonged oral treatment with Klerval achieved a smooth transition in the level of platelet inhibition in patients with acute coronary syndromes. Because of low bioavailability, however, the development of this drug was discontinued. Lefradafiban (oral) and fradafiban (intravenous) await further testing.

Roxifiban is an oral agent that binds tightly to platelet receptor and is slow to dissociate.[240,241,309,310] The half-life of dissociation is 7 min, more than 40 times longer than the short-acting molecules like tirofiban (approximately 10 to 20 s) (Table 44-6).[310] Roxifiban's tight binding is similar to that of abciximab, which also has a long half-life of dissociation.[310] This prolonged antiplatelet effect would avoid the possibility of "on-off" proaggregatory effects of the drug binding to the GP IIb/IIIa inhibitor,[301] which may have explained some of the findings from previous trials with oral GP IIb/IIIa inhibitors. Indeed, experimental models have shown that roxifiban has superior antithrombotic effects as compared with other short-acting GP IIb/IIIa inhibitors.[240] With its long half-life, roxifiban is administered once daily. It also has a very high potency and affinity for the GP IIb/IIIa receptor. As such, the oral doses needed are only 0.5 to 1.5 mg once daily. It has a very stable antiplatelet effect over time (i.e., a low peak to trough level of platelet inhibition), and blood levels do not appear to be affected significantly by renal function.

CONCLUSION

Thus, initial disappointment has been seen for the testing to date with oral GP IIb/IIIa inhibitors. Numerous questions re-

TABLE 44-6 Scorecard Comparing Oral Glycoprotein IIb/IIIa Inhibitors

	Second Generation	First Generation		
	Roxifiban	Orbofiban	Sibrafiban	Xemilofiban
Trial	ROCKET	OPUS–TIMI-16	SYMPHONY	EXCITE
IIb/IIIa selective	+++	+++	+++	+++
Binding	Tightly bound	Competitive	Competitive	Competitive
"Off rate"	7 min	Seconds	Seconds	Seconds
Peak of onset	3–6 h	4–6 h	4–6 h	2–3 h
Half-life	24 h	8–10 h	11 h	4–5 h
Excretion	Platelet dissociation	Renal	Renal	Renal
Dosing	q.d.	b.i.d.	b.i.d.	t.i.d.
Low peak/trough	+++	++	++	+
Intrapatient variability	+	++	++	++
Interpatient variability	++	++	++	++
Platelets <50,000	<0.5%	0.6%	<0.5%	0.5%

Source: Cannon CP. *Curr Opin Card Pulm Renal Invest Drugs* 2000; 2:114–123, with permission.

main, such as what level of platelet inhibition is optimal, how efficacy and safety can best be balanced, whether other adjunctive agents are needed, and whether monitoring of platelet function will assist in the use of these agents. In addition, identification of the optimal patients by using tools of risk stratification may assist in targeting therapy to patients who will benefit most. As with other classes of drug, such as beta blockers in congestive heart failure or cholesterol-lowering drugs (beginning with resin drugs 20 years ago), the road toward identifying appropriate patients, doses, and drugs is frequently a long one. With ongoing trials and "second generation" agents (Table 44-6) it is hoped that this class of drugs will be found to be clinically useful.

ANTICOAGULANT DRUGS

Unfractionated Heparin

Heparin refers not to a single molecule but rather to a family of mucopolysaccharide chains of varying length and composition. Heparin by itself has no anticoagulant property but rather is a cofactor to antithrombin (formerly referred to as antithrombin III). Heparin accelerates the action of two naturally occurring plasma inhibitors, forming a 1:1 stoichiometric complex with antithrombin III (an inhibitor of thrombin and activated factors X, IX, XI, and XII) and, at very high doses, with heparin cofactor II, which acts only on thrombin decay. Heparin contains a unique pentasaccharide that has a high-affinity binding sequence for antithrombin III. This sequence is present in only one-third of heparin molecules and is not required for binding to heparin cofactor II.

Factor Xa bound to platelets and thrombin bound to the endothelium or to fibrin (thrombus) are protected from inactivation by heparin-antithrombin III complex.[311,312] In plasma, approximately 20 times more heparin is needed to inactivate fibrin-bound thrombin than to inactivate free thrombin [311] This explains why more heparin is needed to prevent the extension of venous thrombosis than to prevent formation of the initial thrombus.

When in the bloodstream after parenteral administration, heparin binds to endothelial cells, mononuclear macrophages, and numerous plasma proteins. Some of these neutralize anticoagulant activity (e.g., platelet factor 4 and vitronectin), whereas others such as von Willebrand factor lose their function. Elevated levels of these heparin-binding proteins explain the different individual heparin dose requirements to obtain the same antithrombotic effect and the so-called "heparin resistance" in patients with inflammatory and malignant diseases.[312] Binding of heparin to the endothelium and various plasma proteins reduces bioavailability at low concentrations and causes variability of response to fixed doses of anticoagulant[312] (Table 44-7).

The pharmacokinetics of heparin are complicated. In brief, the anticoagulant response increases disproportionately in intensity and duration as the dose increases. This explains why the anticoagulant effect of heparin has to be closely monitored. At present, no completely satisfactory test measuring the generation of thrombin and the levels of antithrombin is available. The most commonly used test is the activated partial thromboplastin time (APTT), which is sensitive to the inhibitory effect of heparin on thrombin, factor X, and factor IX. Unfortunately, the different commercial APTT reagents vary in their response to heparin, and there are technical variables. The therapeutic level of the APTT should therefore be established in each clinical laboratory to correspond to 0.2 to 0.4 U of heparin per milliliter plasma by protamine titration or to 0.2 to 0.7 IU factor Xa per milliliter of plasma by the chromogenic substrate assay for the determination of anti-factor-Xa activity.

SIDE EFFECTS

The most common and major side effect of heparin is bleeding. The risk is higher when unfractionated heparin is given by

TABLE 44-7 Advantages and Disadvantages of Unfractionated Heparin, Low-Molecular-Weight Heparin, and Recombinant Hirudin

Unfractionated Heparin	LMW Heparin	Hirudin
Inhibits to the same extent thrombin and factor VII, much less IXa and XIa	Inhibits mainly factor Xa, thrombin to some extent	Specific and potent inhibitor of thrombin
Antithrombin III–dependent	Antithrombin III–dependent	Antithrombin III–independent
Neutralized by heparinase, several plasma proteins, platelet factor 4, and endothelium	Neutralized by heparinase, weak endothelium binding	Not neutralized by heparinase, endothelium, macrophages, fibrin monomer, and plasma proteins
Does not inactivate clot-bound thrombin and factor VII	Does not inactivate clot-bound thrombin and factor VII	Inactivates clot-bound thrombin
Inhibits platelet function	Inhibits platelet function	Prevents thrombin induced aggregation but not other platelet agonists
Induced thrombocytopenia is not rare	Can induce thrombocytopenia	Does not induce thrombocytopenia
Bioavailability after subcutaneous injection, 30%	Bioavailability after subcutaneous injection, >90%	Good bioavailability after subcutaneous injection, circa 85%
Poor dose-effect response	Fair dose-effect response	Fair dose-effect response
Not immunogenic	Not immunogenic	Not or barely immunogenic
Transient increase of liver enzymes is common	Transient increase of liver enzymes possible	No liver toxicity
Increases vascular permeability	No increase of vascular permeability	No increase of vascular permeability

intermittent infusion (14.2 percent) rather than continuous infusion (6.8 percent) or subcutaneously (4.1 percent). Also, the dose of heparin, the patient's anticoagulant response, serious concurrent illness, and chronic consumption of alcohol may predispose the patient to bleeding. HIT occurs in 2.4 percent of patients receiving therapeutic heparin and 0.3 percent for prophylactic heparin. In addition, vascular occlusion occurs in 0.4 percent. Rare complications are osteoporosis (usually with prolonged treatment), alopecia, skin necrosis, urticaria, and transient elevation of hepatic transaminases.

TABLE 44-8 Data from Direct Comparison of Antithrombotic Regimens: GISSI-2, ISIS-3, and GUSTO-I

	GISSI-2 and ISIS-3, Aspirin Plus Any Thrombolytic Agent		GUSTO-I, Aspirin Plus SK	
Outcome	No Heparin (*n* = 31,050), %	SC Heparin (*n* = 31,017), %	SC Heparin (*n* = 9971), %	IV Heparin (*n* = 10,377), %
Death	10.2	10.0	7.2	7.4
Reinfarction	3.3	3.0	3.4	4.0
Total stroke	1.2	1.2	1.3	1.4
Hemorrhagic stroke	0.4	0.5	0.5	0.5
Major bleeding	0.7	1.0	0.3	0.5

Abbreviations: SK = streptokinase; SC = subcutaneous; IV = intravenous.
Source: Hennekens et al.,[314] with permission.

CLINICAL USE

Adjunct to Thrombolytic Therapy: Subcutaneous Heparin Heparin has been studied in numerous trials in conjunction with thrombolytic therapy, and its role and dosing are still being debated. One of the first trials, which pre-dated the use of aspirin, was the Studio sulla Calciparina nell'Angina e nella Trombosi ventricolare nell'Infarto (SCATI)[224,313] group, which randomized 711 patients to either heparin or no heparin; 433 of these patients also received streptokinase. These patients did not receive aspirin. This study found a 44 percent reduction in mortality rate when 12,500 U subcutaneous heparin was given to patients with acute MI. This reduction in mortality was significant both in the group receiving streptokinase and in those who did not receive the thrombolytic agent.

The use of heparin in those receiving aspirin as adjunctive therapy with thrombolytic agents (Table 44-8) was examined in many studies, including Gruppo Italiano per lo Studio della Streptochinasi nell'Infarto Miocardico (GISSI) 2, ISIS-3, and GUSTO. In the GISSI-2/International Study, patients who received streptokinase and heparin beginning 12 h after the infusion of the thrombolytic agent had a non-statistically significant trend toward a decrease in mortality rate as compared with those who received streptokinase alone.[314] The mortality rate for those receiving t-PA was the same whether or not heparin was added to the regimen.[315,316]

ISIS-3 found that heparin given subcutaneously (12,500 U every 12 h starting 4 h after the start of thrombolytic therapy) and aspirin given with t-PA or streptokinase resulted in a nearly significant decrease in mortality.[317] There was also a trend toward a decrease in hospital reinfarction rate in the heparin group. However, this early benefit was lost when the primary end point of 35 days was reached. Heparin was associated with a very small excess of major bleeding (0.2 percent of patients: 1.0 percent compared with 0.8 percent for no heparin, $p < .01$). Intracerebral hemorrhage also seemed very slightly increased (0.056 versus 0.40 percent, $p < .05$).[317]

Intravenous Heparin This is an important adjunctive agent in decreasing reocclusion following t-PA for acute ST-elevation MI. Infarct-related artery patency has been studied in four angiographic trials evaluating whether heparin improves patency. No difference in patency was seen at 90 min.[318] Between 18 h and 5 days, however, there was higher patency among patients randomized to receive intravenous heparin.[319–321] Since early patency was similar, the benefit of heparin is felt to be due largely to decreased reocclusion. All trials with novel variants of t-PA [i.e., r-PA (reteplase) and TNK–t-PA, (tenecteplase)] have used adjunctive heparin in the clinical trials.

Following streptokinase or anistreplase (anisoylated plasminogen-streptokinase activator complex or APSAC), the role of heparin is less clear. One study with APSAC found no difference in coronary artery patency in those receiving heparin plus aspirin compared with aspirin alone.[322] In the GUSTO-I trial, patients treated with streptokinase with intravenous or subcutaneous heparin had similar infarct-related artery patency at 90 min and 24 h, but those receiving intravenous heparin had significantly higher patency at 5 to 7 days (84 versus 72 percent, $p = .04$).[270] Nonetheless, the overall 30-day mortality and the rate of clinical reinfarction were the same between these two groups.[323] It should be noted, however, that patients randomized to the subcutaneous arm did receive intravenous heparin when recurrent ischemia developed. Therefore, intravenous heparin may be considered optional in streptokinase-treated patients. Of note, however, the American College of Cardiology/American Heart Association guidelines do recommend intravenous heparin for patients receiving streptokinase or APSAC if they are at high risk of developing systemic emboli (e.g., large anterior MI or atrial fibrillation).

Very recent preliminary data on the 5-year follow-up of United States' patients only from GUSTO-I showed that the streptokinase group with intravenous heparin had a survival similar to that of t-PA. Thus, the late (days 5 to 7) patency advantage observed in the GUSTO angiographic substudy for intravenous heparin as compared with subcutaneous heparin might have translated into only a late mortality benefit. Further analysis of these preliminary data is needed, however.

Unstable Angina/Non-ST-Elevation Myocardial Infarction In unstable angina and non-ST-elevation MI, heparin is an important component of primary therapy. Two initial small studies suggested a reduction in cardiac events by heparin.[324,325] Three studies of heparin in unstable angina and non-ST-elevation MI also suggest benefit: The Montreal Heart Institute trial showed that heparin reduced refractory angina and MI compared with placebo.[67] A follow-up report extending enrollment in that trial found a reduction in the risk of subsequent MI by heparin compared with aspirin alone.[69] The RISC study failed to demonstrate a beneficial effect of heparin compared with aspirin but noted that, during heparin therapy, patients receiving both aspirin and heparin had the lowest rate of death or MI.[68]

The Antithrombotic Therapy for Acute Coronary Syndromes (ATACS) Study Group evaluated the role of combination antithrombotic therapy compared with aspirin alone in patients with acute ischemic syndromes who were not prior aspirin users.[70] They observed a trend toward fewer ischemic events (death, MI, or recurrent ischemia with ECG changes) in patients receiving aspirin and heparin and warfarin at 12 weeks (19 percent) compared with aspirin alone (28 percent) ($p = .09$).[70] They went on to perform a meta-analysis of the Theroux, RISC, and their own trial, and found that during the 5 days of active treatment with aspirin and heparin the risk of death or MI was lower than for aspirin alone (odds ratio = 0.44; 95% CI = 0.21 to 0.93).[70] A more recent and comprehensive meta-analysis showed a 33 percent reduction in death or MI at 2 to 12 weeks (7.9 versus 10.4 percent; relative risk = 0.67; 95% CI = 0.44 to 1.02) (Fig. 44-17).[71] These data support the use of aspirin plus heparin in unstable angina/non-ST elevation MI.

HEPARIN RESISTANCE

Variability in the anticoagulant effects of heparin, so-called heparin resistance,[326,327] is thought to be due to the heterogeneity of heparin molecules and to the neutralization of heparin by circulating plasma factors and by proteins released by activated platelets.[328-332] Clinically, frequent monitoring of the anticoagulant response by using APTT is recommended, with titrations made according to a standardized nomogram.[190] The use of a standardized nomogram minimizes the variability in the dosing adjustments given by various physicians and has been shown to improve the achievement of a target APTT.[328,333,334]

THERAPEUTIC RANGE

The exact level of anticoagulation that constitutes the therapeutic range is not yet established. Pilot studies in unstable angina[335] and acute MI[336-339] have suggested that lower APTT values are maybe related to recurrent ischemic events or lower infarct-related artery patency,[340,341] suggesting that the lower limit of the target range of APTT is at least 1.5 to 2 times control. On the upper boundary of the target range, higher APTT values are associated with an increased risk of hemorrhage.[342] In the large GUSTO-I trial of thrombolytic therapy, the lowest rate of bleeding (and mortality) was observed in patients who had a 12-h APTT between 50 and 70 s.[339] Furthermore, in unstable angina, in the TIMI-3B trial, there was no apparent benefit of higher levels of anticoagulation.[343]

HEPARIN DOSING

Standard heparin dosing involves a 5000-U bolus followed by a 1000-U/h infusion, which is then titrated according to the APTT.[328,344] The use of weight-adjusted heparin has been suggested as a means of improving APTT control and safety.[345] In one randomized trial, a high percentage of patients "overshot" in the initial APTT at 6 h (median, 150 s).[346] Another trial that examined a 60-U/kg bolus and an infusion of 12 U/kg per hour compared with fixed dosing found a higher percentage of patients within range without a large number of APTTs above range at 6 h.[347] A third trial that tested standard dosing versus weight-adjusted dosing (70-U/kg bolus and initial infusion of 15 U/kg per hour) found no significant difference in control of APTT with weight-adjusted dosing.[348] Another approach uses on-line feedback of APTT data to a computer algorithm using a pharmacodynamic model of heparin response in the individual patient, with promising results in an initial pilot trial.[349]

An important lesson learned from recent trials is that lower initial doses of heparin in the setting of thrombolytic therapy are associated with a lower rate of intracranial hemorrhage. In the TIMI-10B and Assessment of the Safety of a New Thrombolytic (ASSENT-I) trials,[350] and in TIMI-9 and GUSTO-II trials,[351-354] when the doses of heparin were reduced in the first part of the trial to the second part of the trial, the rates of ICH and major hemorrhage were reduced. A recent overview of all major thrombolytic trials, and of detailed information from the TIMI trials and the Intravenous n-PA for Treatment of Infarcting Myocardium

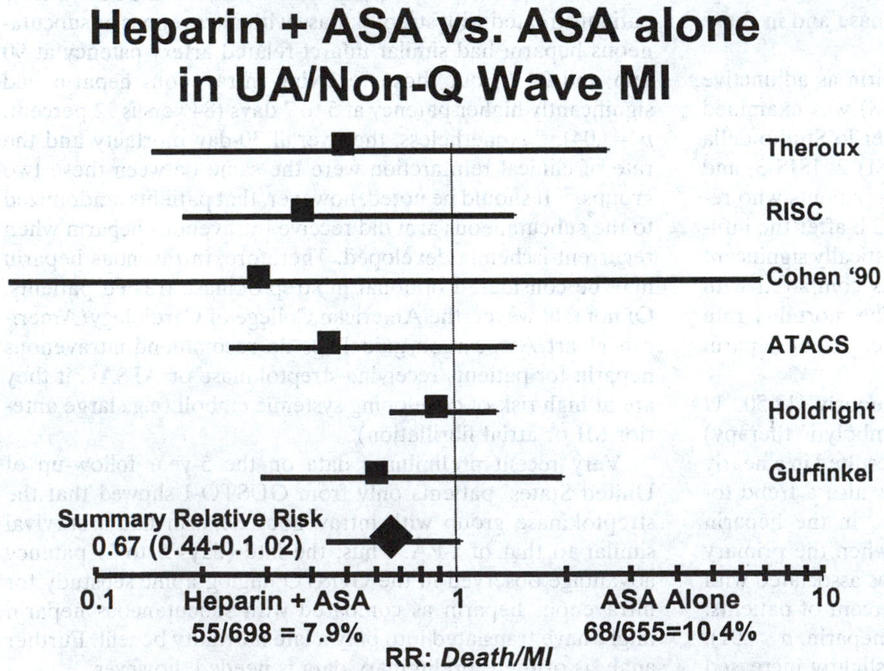

FIGURE 44-17 Meta-analysis of six randomized trials comparing unfractionated heparin plus aspirin compared with aspirin alone, showing benefit of the combination therapy. The rate of death or myocardial infarction (MI) during follow-up (2 to 12 weeks in the various studies) tended to be reduced in patients randomized to aspirin plus heparin. (Adapted from Oler et al.[71] Reproduced with permission from the publisher and authors.)

Early II (InTIME-II) trial, confirmed that lower doses of heparin are associated with reduced ICH.[355]

Further very compelling evidence of the benefit of lower doses of heparin comes from the InTIME-II trial, which compared the single-bolus thrombolytic agent, lanoteplase, and accelerated t-PA in 15,078 patients worldwide. The heparin dose was 70-U/kg bolus with a maximum of 4000 U (i.e., 4000 U/kg/h for all patients weighing more than 57 kg) and 15-U/h (max 1000 U/h) infusion. The rate of ICH for t-PA was the lowest ever reported in a large trial for accelerated t-PA: 0.62 percent.[355]

CURRENT RECOMMENDATION

Based on the emerging data, the 1999 update to the American College of Cardiology/American Heart Association guidelines for the management of acute MI will recommend a new lower dose of heparin: a bolus of 60 U/kg (maximum, 4000 U) and an initial infusion of 12 U/kg per hour (maximum, 1000 U/h).[356] No maximum is needed in nonthrombolytic treated patients. The guidelines also call for frequent monitoring of APTT (every 6 h until in the target range and every 12 to 24 h thereafter) and for titration of heparin by using a standardized nomogram, with a target range of APTT between 1.5 to 2 times control or approximately 50 and 70 s.[356]

CORONARY REVASCULARIZATION PROCEDURES

Use of adequate heparinization with aspirin throughout the procedure is strongly recommended.[357] The exact level of anticoagulation with unfractionated heparin has been debated, but current recommendations are to achieve an activated clotting time between 300 and 350 s in patients *not* receiving a GP IIb/IIIa inhibitor.[358] This can generally be achieved using a weight-adjusted dose of a 100-U/kg bolus, with 20-U/kg additional boluses if needed.[359] For patients who do receive a GP IIb/IIIa inhibitor, the target should be approximately 200 to 250 s, based on data from the EPILOG trial.[285]

LMW Heparins

Some of the limitations of unfractionated heparin can be overcome with LMW heparin (mean molecular weight, 4000 to 5000; range, 1000 to 10,000). LMW heparins produce their major anticoagulant effect by binding to antithrombin through the same high-affinity pentasaccharide sequence of unfractionated heparin, which, however, is present in only one-third of the LMW heparins. A minimum additional chain length of 15 saccharides (MW > 5400) is required for the inactivation of thrombin, but the inactivation of factor X requires only the pentasaccharide (Fig. 44-18). Unfractionated heparin has an anti–factor Xa to anti–factor II ratio of 1:1, which is between 4:1 and 2:1 for the various LMW heparins. Drugs with a high anti–factor Xa activity were indeed designed based on the hypothesis that inhibition of earlier steps in the blood coagulation system would be associated with a more potent antithrombotic effect than inhibition of subsequent steps. This is because of the amplification process inherent in the coagulation cascade; that is, a single factor Xa molecule can lead to the generation of hundreds of thrombin molecules.

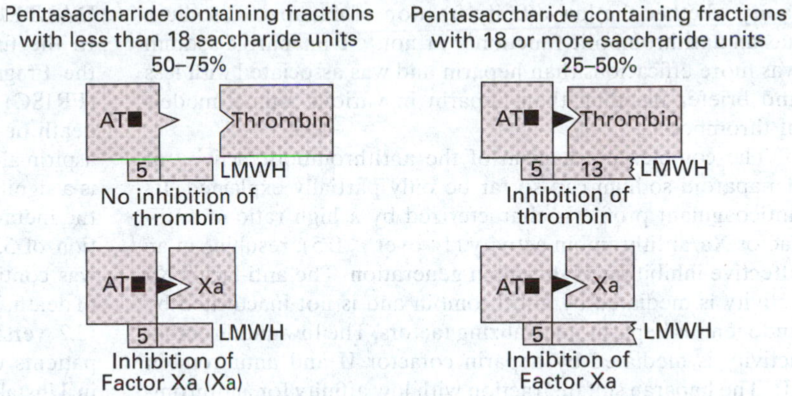

FIGURE 44-18 Mechanism of action of heparin and low molecular weight heparin (LMWH): Heparin acts as a cofactor to antithrombin to (1) change the conformation of its active site and (2) serve as a "bridge" to bring together an antithrombin (AT) and thrombin. Heparin is a catalyst: after it facilitates the binding of one pair of thrombin and antithrombin molecules, it is released and facilitates another thrombin-antithrombin interaction. LMWH also binds to antithrombin and changes the conformation of its active site, but does not act as a bridge to thrombin. Approximately 25 to 50 percent of the LMWH molecules of different commercial preparations contain at least 18 saccharide units, which allows binding to the heparin-binding site of thrombin, and thus both these molecules inhibit thrombin and factor Xa. The remaining 50 to 75 percent of LMWH molecules contain fewer than 18 saccharide units and inhibit only factor Xa.

The advantages of LMW heparins over unfractionated heparin are numerous (Table 44-7). Factor Xa bound to the platelet membrane in the prothrombinase complex is resistant to inactivation by unfractionated heparin but is not resistant to inactivation by LMW heparins. Also, LMW heparins have lesser binding characteristics to platelet factor 4, other plasma proteins, and endothelial cells, resulting in a higher bioavailability (after subcutaneous injection, greater than 90 versus 30 percent for unfractionated heparin); reduced plasma clearance, which is independent of dose and plasma concentration; a longer half-life (anti–factor Xa activity between 3 and 4 h for LMW heparins compared with 30 to 150 min for unfractionated heparin); and less interindividual variability of the anticoagulant response.[360] LMW heparins have a lower affinity for von Willebrand factor,[361] increase vascular permeability less than unfractionated heparin, and have a weak effect on platelet function. These differences could explain why LMW heparins produce less bleeding than unfractionated heparin with equivalent or higher antithrombotic effect in experimental animals[360] and in some clinical studies.

The long half-life of LMW heparins and their predictable anticoagulant response to weight-adjusted doses allow a twice daily subcutaneous administration without laboratory monitoring.[360]

HEPARINOIDS: MIXTURE OF LMW SULFATE GLYCOSAMINOGLYCANS

Danaparoid sodium (Org 10172) is a LMW heparinoid (6 kDa) and consists of a polydispersed mixture comprising sulfated glycosaminoglycuronides derived from animal mucosa; heparan sulfate (83% wt/wt), of which 4 to 5 percent has high affinity for antithrombin III; dermatan sulfate (12% wt/wt); and a minor amount of chondroitin sulfate (5% wt/wt).[362] There is uncertainty whether the low-affinity fraction of danaparoid sodium has an antithrombotic function[363] or not.[364] Danaparoid sodium was more efficacious than heparin and was associated with less and briefer bleeding than heparin in various animal models of thrombosis.

The complex mechanism of the antithrombotic activity of danaparoid sodium can so far be only partially explained. Its anticoagulant profile is characterized by a high ratio of anti–factor Xa/antithrombin activity (14 over < 0.5), resulting in an effective inhibition of thrombin generation. The anti-factor Xa activity is mediated by antithrombin and is not inactivated by endogenous heparin-neutralizing factors. The low antithrombin activity is mediated by heparin cofactor II and antithrombin III. The heparan sulfate fraction with low affinity for antithrombin III, despite lacking significant effects on coagulation factors Xa and IIa (thrombin) in vitro, has been shown in animal studies to contribute substantially to the antithrombotic activity. In contrast to heparin, danaparoid sodium shows hardly any or no effect on platelet function in vitro or in vivo. Danaparoid sodium is essentially free of contaminating heparin, has minimal cross-reactivity in in vitro assays for HIT, and has been used successfully in patients with this complication.

Pharmacokinetic studies have been primarily based on the kinetics of relevant anticoagulant activities because no specific chemical assay methods are available. In comparison with heparin, danaparoid sodium has a prolonged elimination half-life of anti–factor Xa activity. After intravenous and subcutaneous administration of danaparoid sodium, the antithrombin activity half-life is shorter (1.8 h) than its anti–factor Xa half-life (17.6 h). Danaparoid sodium has an absolute bioavailability of 100 percent after subcutaneous administration. The kidneys play an important role in the elimination of the anti–factor Xa activity of danaparoid sodium, but a cellular metabolism seems unlikely, since the liver does not affect the anti–factor Xa activity and there is only slight and reversible binding to the endothelium.[71,364]

Danaparoid sodium is effective in the prevention of deep venous thrombosis in patients with thrombotic stroke and after elective hip surgery or hip fracture.[365] The long half-life of danaparoid sodium, which is not effectively neutralized by protamine, has been rather difficult to manage clinically.

Clinical Use of LMW Heparin

LMW heparin has been studied extensively in the prevention and more recently for the treatment of venous thrombosis. In the United States, it is approved for prophylaxis against deep venous thrombosis based on results from several trials.[344,366–368] Other trials for the *treatment* of deep venous thrombosis have also been promising.[344,369–372] Several of these trials have demonstrated a lower rate of major hemorrhage with LMW heparin than with standard heparin.[344]

LMW HEPARIN IN UNSTABLE ANGINA

In recent years, LMW heparin has been studied extensively in unstable angina. Two pilot trials were encouraging.[373,374] A second, open-label pilot trial in unstable angina and non-Q-wave MI has also suggested that LMW heparin may be superior to aspirin and heparin.[375] This study used nadroparin (Fraxaparin), which has a 3:1 ratio of factor Xa–thrombin inhibition.

DALTEPARIN

In the first large trial of LMW heparin in unstable angina, the Fragmin During Instability in Coronary Artery Disease (FRISC) study, dalteparin plus aspirin was found to reduce death or MI dramatically over the first 6 days compared with aspirin alone (1.8 versus 4.8 percent, $p = .001$).[72] (Note that this is a significant reduction compared with aspirin alone, whereas the meta-analysis for unfractionated heparin had a risk reduction of 33 percent and $p = .06$.)[71] Beyond 6 days, dalteparin was continued versus placebo and, at 40 days, the composite of death, MI, or need revascularization was significantly reduced (2.2 versus 5.7 percent, $p < 0.001$).[72] A subsequent trial of patients with unstable angina for less than 72 h, the Fragmin in Unstable Coronary Artery Disease (FRIC) trial, found no difference in clinical outcomes between intravenous heparin and dalteparin, indicating it was a suitable alternative to unfractionated heparin, although it was not shown to be superior in this trial.[376]

ENOXAPARIN

The Evaluation of the Safety and Efficacy of Subcutaneous Enoxaparin in Non-Q Wave Coronary Events (ESSENCE) trial compared enoxaparin (a LMW heparin with 3.8:1 factor Xa–thrombin inhibition ratio) with intravenous heparin in 3000 patients with unstable angina and non-Q-wave MI. A 2 to 3 day course of enoxaparin was superior to unfractionated heparin with regard to the primary end point, the occurrence of death, MI, or recurrent ischemia at 14 days (16.6 versus 19.8 percent, $p = .019$).[73] The rates of this end point at 30 days were 19.8 versus 23.3 percent ($p = .016$).[73] Death or MI to 30 days also favored enoxaparin (6.2 versus 7.7 percent, $p = .08$).

Interestingly, in this double-blind trial, the rates of catheterization (43 versus 46 percent, $p = .08$ for enoxaparin compared with heparin) and PCI (13 versus 17 percent, respectively, $p = .001$) were lower in patients treated with enoxaparin. A subsequent cost-effectiveness analysis found that there was a minimal increase in the cost for the drug (enoxaparin compared with unfractionated heparin with APTT measurements) ($75)—but with lower rates of catheterization and revascularization, treatment with enoxaparin led to a *savings* of $1172 per patient treated. Thus, both improved outcomes, and lower costs were observed with enoxaparin compared with unfractionated heparin.

TIMI-11 Trials These also studied enoxaparin in unstable angina and non-Q-wave MI. In TIMI-11A, the first goal was to determine the appropriate dose of enoxaparin—whether to use a dose that previously had been shown to be effective in venous thrombosis (1.0 mg/kg subcutaneously twice daily) or whether higher doses would be beneficial in arterial thrombosis. In TIMI-11A, a higher dose (1.25 mg/kg) was found to have an unacceptably high rate of major hemorrhage, 6.5 percent to 14 days, as compared with a rate of 1.9 percent for patients treated with 1.0 mg/kg.[377] There was no difference in the rate of recurrent ischemic events between the two doses. Thus, the dose of 1.0 mg/kg appeared to be appropriate and was used in the TIMI-11B trial.

The TIMI-11B trial studied high-risk patients with unstable angina and non-ST-elevation MI. They were required to have ST deviation or positive cardiac serum markers (CK-MB or troponin) to be enrolled. TIMI-11B compared intravenous unfractionated heparin with enoxaparin (1.0 mg/kg subcutaneously twice daily in hospital and a fixed dose b.i.d. as an outpatient) for a total of 43 days. Death, MI, or severe recurrent ischemia requiring urgent revascularization through day 14 occurred in 16.6 percent of patients treated with heparin and in 14.2 percent of patients treated with enoxaparin (p = .03), a 15 percent relative risk reduction.[75] The rate of the primary end point to 43 days was 19.6 percent for unfractionated heparin and 17.3 percent for enoxaparin (p = .049).[75] Parallel reductions in death and MI were also observed.

A meta-analysis of the TIMI-11B and ESSENCE trials showed that, at 43 days, enoxaparin reduced the rate of death, MI, or urgent revascularization from 18.7 to 15.6 percent (p = .0006). Death or MI at 43 days was reduced from 8.6 to 7.1 percent (p = .02) (Fig. 44-19).[74] Thus, enoxaparin has been shown in two large randomized trials to be superior to unfractionated heparin for the treatment of unstable angina and non-ST-elevation MI. The FDA has approved enoxaparin for the treatment of patients with unstable angina and non-ST-elevation MI.

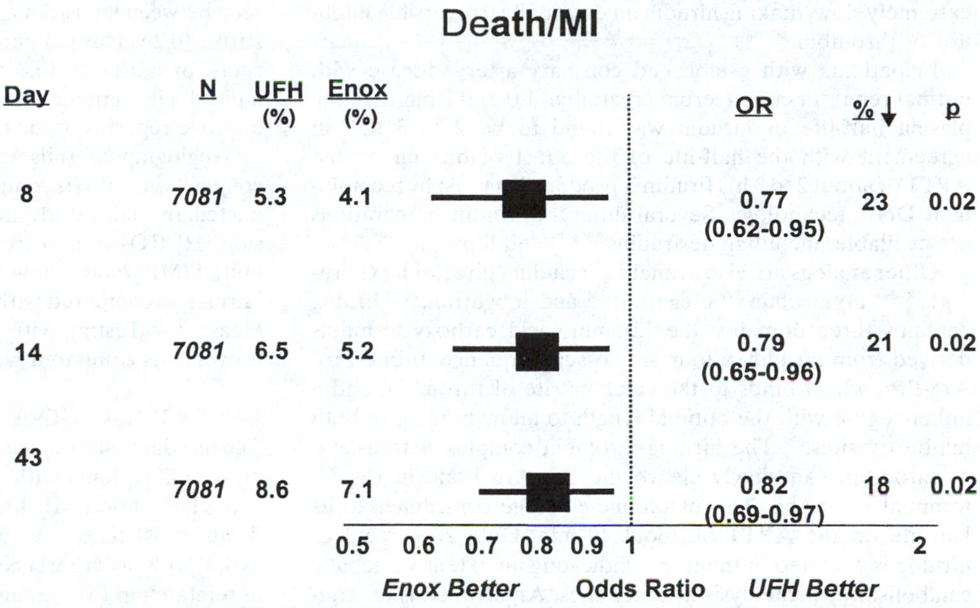

Death/MI
Day
N
UFH (%)
Enox (%)
OR
%↓
p
8
7081
5.3
4.1
0.77 (0.62-0.95)
23
0.02
14
7081
6.5
5.2
0.79 (0.65-0.96)
21
0.02
43
7081
8.6
7.1
0.82 (0.69-0.97)
18
0.02
0.5 0.6 0.7 0.8 0.9 1 2
Enox Better
Odds Ratio
UFH Better

FIGURE 44-19 TIMI-11B/ESSENCE meta-analysis (TESSMA): Data from over 7000 patients randomized in these two trials show a consistent and significant 20 percent reduction in the rate of death or myocardial infarction (MI) at each of the four time points in patients treated with enoxaparin compared with unfractionated heparin. (Adapted from Antman et al.[74] Reproduced with permission from the publisher and authors.)

LMW HEPARIN IN ANGIOPLASTY, STENTS, AND ACUTE MYOCARDIAL INFARCTION

There is emerging experience with LMW heparin in angioplasty. One study found that LMW heparin did not reduce restenosis.[378] However, LMW heparin may play a role in preventing thrombotic complications after complicated angioplasty. A recent nonrandomized experience of patients with suboptimal angioplasty or stent results treated some patients with LMW heparin for 4 weeks and others with standard care (aspirin). They found a reduced rate (1.5 versus 8.2 percent, $p < 0.05$) of death or recurrent MI during follow-up.[379] Thus, LMW heparin appears to have great promise and further randomized trials are under way.

Similarly, trials of LMW heparin in acute MI treated with thrombolytic therapy are under way.[380,381] In the setting of ST-elevation MI treated with thrombolytic therapy, one recent study found a significant reduction in the rate of death, MI, or readmission for an acute coronary syndrome.[380] A total of 300 patients treated with thrombolysis (predominantly streptokinase, but also anistreplase and t-PA) were randomized to intravenous unfractionated heparin (5000-U bolus and 1250 U/h titrated to an APTT of 2 to 2.5 times control) or enoxaparin (40-mg intravenous bolus, followed by 40 mg subcutaneously every 8 h) for 4 days. The rate of the composite end point at 3 months was 36.4 percent for heparin and 25.5 percent for enoxaparin (p = .04).[380] It appeared that rebound was reduced by enoxaparin, with the rate of reinfarction from days 4 to 6 of 6.6 percent for heparin and 2.2 percent for enoxaparin (p = .05).[380]

In a second recent study, dalteparin was compared with placebo in streptokinase-treated patients. TIMI grade 3 flow 20 to 28 h later tended to be higher in patients treated with dalteparin (68 versus 51 percent, p = .10), and the number of ischemic episodes on continuous ECG monitoring was lower (16 versus 38 percent, p = .04).[381]

Most recently, Heparin Aspirin Reinfarction (HART-II) trial compared enoxaparin with unfractionated heparin as adjuncts to t-PA and aspirin for patients with acute MI.[382] There was a strong trend toward improved early TIMI grade 3 flow with enoxaparin (53 versus 48 percent for unfractionated heparin, p = .06). There was an even greater effect on reocclusion (5.9 versus 9.8 percent).[382] Thus, LWM heparins appear to be beneficial in these pilot trials with thrombolysis, and larger studies are underway to try to confirm these results.

Direct Thrombin Inhibitors

These have also undergone extensive evaluation in conjunction with thrombolytic therapy. The prototypic agent is hirudin, a 65-amino-acid polypeptide that is derived from the leech *Hirudo medicinalis*, which acts as a potent and selective inhibitor of thrombin.[383] Hirudin selectively binds thrombin in a 1:1 fashion at two sites: (1) the carboxy terminus of hirudin binds to the substrate recognition site, the domain of thrombin that recognizes fibrinogen[384] or the platelet;[385] and (2) the amino terminus of hirudin binds to the catalytic site of thrombin.[384] Hirudin does not inhibit other enzymes in the coagulation or fibrinolytic pathways such as factor Xa, IX, kallikrein, activated protein C, plasmin, or tissue plasminogen activator.[383] Hirudin does not bind covalently to thrombin; however, the dissociation rate is extremely slow, making hirudin an essentially irreversible inhibitor of thrombin.[383,386]

In patients with established coronary artery disease with normal renal function (serum creatinine, 1.0 ± 0.2 mg/dL), the plasma half-life of hirudin was found to be 2 to 3 h,[387] in agreement with the half-life of the effect of hirudin on the APTT of about 2 to 3 h. Hirudin is produced in yeast by recombinant DNA technology. Several different hirudin preparations are available, including desirudin[352,354,388] and lepirudin.[389]

Other analogs are also available, including bivaluridin (Hirulog),[390–392] argatroban,[393] efegatran,[394] and inogatran.[395] Hirulog contains three domains: the 12-amino-acid carboxy terminus derived from hirudin; a four-amino-acid sequence, D-Phe-Pro-Arg-Pro, which binds to the catalytic site of thrombin; and a linker region with the optimal length to allow binding of both inhibitory sites.[390] The hirulog-thrombin complex is transient, as thrombin can slowly cleave the Pro-Arg bond in the N-terminal extension. This metabolic cleavage contributes to its half-life on the APTT of about 40 min. Only 20 percent of hirulog is excreted in the urine, indicating an extensive hepatic catabolism or proteolysis at other sites. Argatroban is an arginine derivative that binds to thrombin with intermediate affinity.

Direct thrombin inhibitors have been shown to inhibit all of the major actions of thrombin, including thrombin-induced generation of fibrin and thrombin-induced platelet activation, as well as thrombin's autocatalytic reaction.[383,396] Potential advantages of hirudin over heparin are that hirudin can inhibit clot-bound thrombin,[275] it is not inhibited by activated platelets,[397] and it does not require a cofactor and thus may provide a more stable anticoagulant response.[396]

ADJUNCT TO THROMBOLYTIC THERAPY

The effects of desirudin in the setting of thrombolysis were tested in TIMI-5, 6, and 9 and GUSTO-II.[352,354,388,398] Hirudin provided a more stable APTT, within the target range almost twice as frequently. No episodes of thrombocytopenia were reported for hirudin.

In TIMI-5, a lower rate of recurrent MI was observed (4.3 versus 11.9 percent, for hirudin and heparin, respectively, p = .03), as well as a trend toward lower reocclusion (1.6 versus 6.7 percent, p = .07).[388] In the phase III TIMI-9B trial, a similar trend in lower reinfarction was observed in hospital (2.3 versus 3.4 percent, p = .07), but no difference was observed in the primary end point (death, MI, or severe congestive heart failure/shock) at 30 days (12.9 percent for hirudin and 11.9 percent for heparin, p = NS).[352] Similarly, death or MI was not different between the two anticoagulants (9.7 versus 9.5 percent, p = NS).[352] Hirudin was tested in over 12,000 patients across the full spectrum of acute coronary syndromes in the GUSTO-IIb trial. There was a reduction in reinfarction (5.4 versus 6.3 percent for heparin, p = .04) but only a trend toward reduction in death or MI at 30 days (8.9 versus 9.8 percent, p = .06).[354] In patients with ST-elevation MI, death or MI was slightly lower (9.9 versus 11.3 percent, p = .13). An intriguing trend to benefit was seen in streptokinase-treated patients in GUSTO-II,[399] but this was not observed in TIMI-9B.[352]

In the HIT-III trial, excess ICH was observed with lepirudin (3.4 versus 0 percent). In the subsequent HIT-4 trial, involving 1208 patients and using a lower dose of lepirudin, TIMI flow grade 3 was observed in 40.7 percent in the lepirudin and in 33.5 percent in the heparin group (p = .16), No differences were seen between lepirudin and heparin in the rates of hemorrhagic stroke (0.2 versus 0.3 percent), reinfarction (4.6 versus 5.1 percent), or mortality (6.8 versus 6.4 percent) at 30 days. Thus, lepirudin in conjunction with streptokinase did not significantly improve reperfusion or clinical outcomes in this study.

Angiographic trials with other direct thrombin inhibitors in conjunction with thrombolytic therapy have also been conducted. In a pilot study and the Hirulog Early Rerfusion/Occlusion (HERO) trial, a trend toward improved early (90 to 120 min) TIMI grade 3 flow was observed with the higher dose of Hirulog as compared with heparin in patients receiving streptokinase.[391,392] Testing with other agents found modest or no improvements compared with heparin.[393,394,400]

UNSTABLE ANGINA

The hirudin desirudin was tested in the GUSTO-IIb trial involving 12,142 patients with unstable angina/non-ST-elevation MI and ST-elevation MI. In the entire cohort, the 30-day rate of death or MI tended to be lower (8.9 versus 9.8 percent, p = .06),[354] with no difference in mortality and a modest reduction in reinfarction (5.4 versus 6.3 percent for heparin, p = .04). In the 8011 patients with unstable angina or non-ST-elevation MI, the rate of death or MI was not significantly reduced at 30 days (8.3 versus 9.1 percent, p = .22).[354]

Lepirudin was compared with heparin in the Organisation to Assess Strategies for Ischemic Syndromes 2 (OASIS-2) trial,[389] and there was a strong trend toward reduction in cardiovascular death or MI at 7 days (3.6 versus 4.2 percent, respectively, p = .08). Major bleeding requiring transfusion was infrequent but more frequent with lepirudin (1.2 versus 0.7 percent for heparin, p = .01). The authors performed a meta-analysis of all the hirudin trials and observed a modest 10 percent benefit favoring hirudin, although this was not statistically significant for patients with unstable angina.

Other synthetic direct thrombin inhibitors have also been tested [e.g., argatroban and bivaluridin (Hirulog)], and again only modest or no improvements were observed compared with heparin,[400,401] although lower rates of bleeding have been observed with bivalirudin.[401] The direct thrombin inhibitors have been observed to provide a very stable level of anticoagulation, as measured by APTT,[354,402,403] and no episodes of thrombocytopenia were reported for the hirudin class. Of note, lepirudin is approved by the FDA for use as an anticoagulant in patients with HIT and associated thromboembolic disease.

USE DURING CORONARY ANGIOPLASTY

Following a pilot trial of hirudin in low-risk patients undergoing angioplasty, which showed a reduction in early abrupt closure,[404] a larger randomized, double-blind study compared hirudin (40-mg bolus followed by 0.2 mg/kg per hour) with heparin in the prevention of restenosis after coronary angioplasty.[405] The primary end point was event-free survival (freedom from cardiac death, MI, coronary bypass surgery, bailout procedure, repeat percutaneous transluminal coronary angioplasty, or elective stent placement). At 7 months, event-free survival was 67.3 percent in the group receiving heparin, 63.5 percent in the group receiving intravenous hirudin, and 68.0 percent in the group receiving both intravenous and subcutaneous hirudin (p = .61). However, the administration of hirudin was associated with a significant reduction in early cardiac events, which occurred in 11.0, 7.9, and 5.6 percent of patients in the respective groups.

Although significantly fewer early cardiac events occurred with hirudin than with heparin, hirudin had no apparent benefit with longer-term follow-up. Two retrospective analyses have recently shown that patients with unstable angina, treated with hirudin, and who undergo PCI on the study drug, have a dramatic reduction in death or MI. In the OASIS-2 trial, there was a 60 percent reduction in death or MI in those undergoing PCI compared with 5 percent in those who did not.[406] Thus, these data are consistent with those with GP IIb/IIIa inhibitors, which show a benefit both before and after the procedure.[407]

The direct thrombin inhibitor bivalirudin (Hirulog) was studied in a double-blind, randomized trial of over 4000 patients with unstable angina or recent MI undergoing angioplasty. Patients were assigned to receive either heparin or bivalirudin immediately before angioplasty. Overall, bivalirudin did not significantly reduce the incidence of the primary end point (death, MI, abrupt vessel closure, or rapid clinical deterioration of cardiac origin: 11.4 versus 12.2 percent for heparin). In the prospectively stratified subgroup of 704 patients with postinfarction angina, however, bivalirudin therapy did lead to a significant reduction in the primary end point (9.1 versus 14.2 percent, $p = .04$). In addition, bivalirudin was associated with a lower incidence of bleeding (3.8 versus 9.8 percent, p 0.001). No differences in recurrent ischemic events were seen at 6 months. Thus, bivalirudin appeared to be as effective as heparin but with a better safety profile during angioplasty. This study pre-dated coronary stenting and GP IIb/IIIa inhibitors, so more information is needed to assess its potential role. The FDA recently approved bivalirudin for use during angioplasty.

Thus, to date, the direct thrombin inhibitors have not produced a dramatic improvement in clinical outcome as adjuncts to thrombolytic therapy. The benefits in unstable angina have been modest and almost reached statistical significance on the primary end point in one trial and in angioplasty one agent is approved for use. There are several large ongoing trials evaluating the direct thrombin inhibitor bivalirudin HERO-2 is comparing bivalirudin with heparin as an adjunctive agent to streptokinase, and another is comparing bivalirudin plus bailout abciximab with heparin plus abciximab.

Warfarin/Oral Anticoagulants

Warfarin sodium and related coumarin congeners are effective antithrombotic compounds that differ in speed in the inhibition of vitamin K–2,3-epoxide within hepatic chromosomes. These compounds depress the synthesis of four vitamin K–dependent procoagulants (factors II, VII, IX, and X) and of two natural inhibitor proteins C and S (Fig. 44-20). The plasma concentration of these proteins will decrease in accord with their half-lives. The coagulation components with the shortest half-lives are the procoagulant factor VII and the endogenous anticoagulant protein C. This may cause a frank imbalance between procoagulants and anticoagulants at the start of treatment and lead to thrombosis of skin capillaries and venules with cutaneous necrosis.[408]

MONITORING OF WARFARIN TREATMENT

The intensity of the effect of warfarin on the synthesis of coagulation factors differs among patients; moreover, in the same individual, it may, over time, vary considerably. This explains the need for close monitoring by having daily blood tests in the first week of treatment with warfarin. The test used is the *prothrombin time*, a term that leads to confusion because the assay depends in fact on the global activity of five coagulation factors (prothrombin and factors V, VII, IX, and X). Among the six factors whose synthesis is inhibited by coumarin derivatives, three (prothrombin and factors VII and X) are effectively measured by this test, but not factor IX and the anticoagulant proteins C and S. On the other hand, the prothrombin time is also sensitive to factor V, a coagulation protein independent of vitamin K.

To perform the prothrombin time, a tissue extract (thromboplastin) and calcium are added to citrated plasma and the time to fibrin formation is measured. Commercial thromboplastin

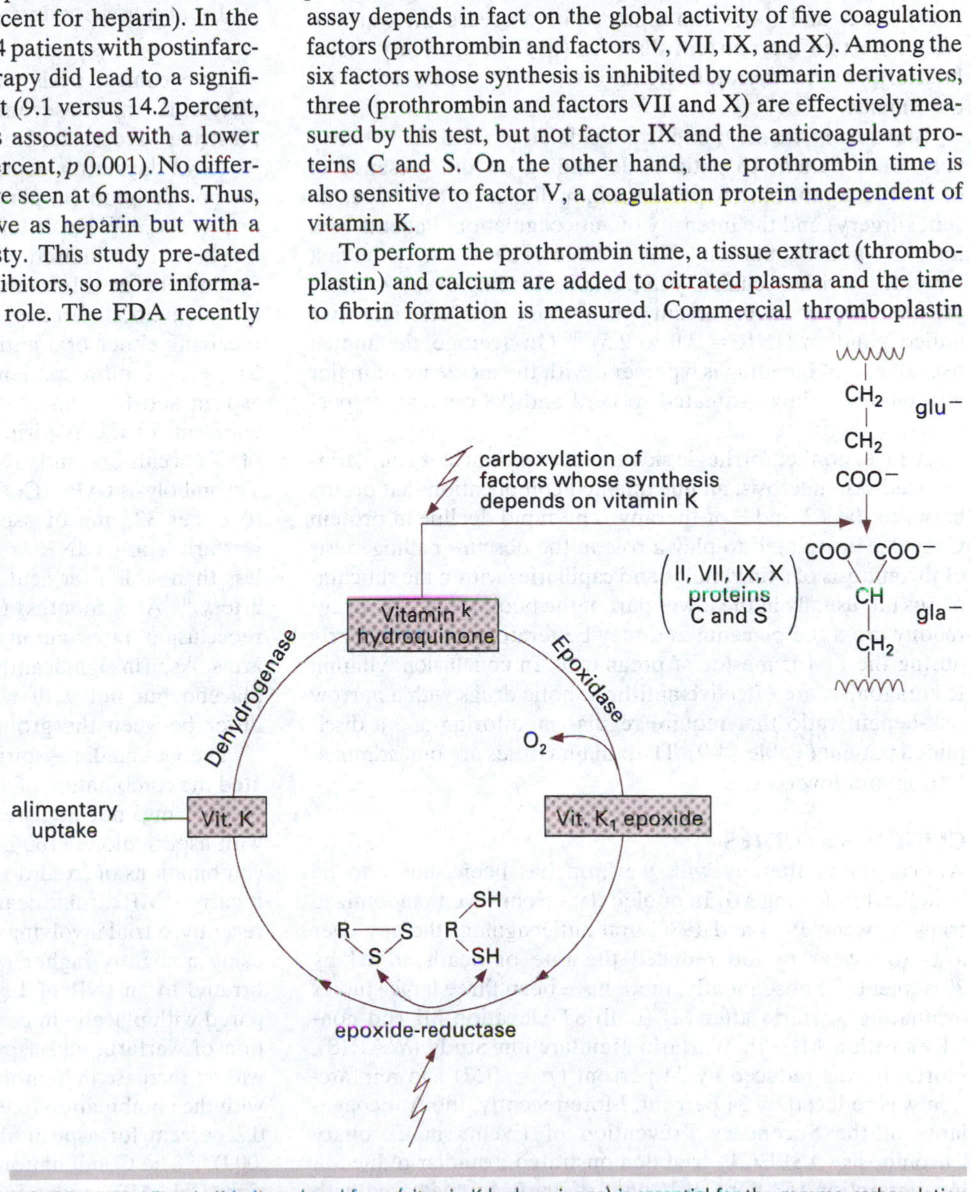

FIGURE 44-20 Vitamin K in its reduced form (vitamin K hydroquinone) is essential for the gamma-carboxylation reaction of glutamic acid (Glu)-to gamma-carboxyglutamic acid (Gla-). In this carboxylation, vitamin K hydroquinone is converted to vitamin K_1 epoxide and an epoxide-reductase regenerates active vitamin K hydroquinone. It is this regeneration step that is blocked by all coumarin-type anticoagulant drugs (e.g., warfarin).

reagents extracted by different methods from various organs and species vary extensively in their sensitivity to reductions in levels of vitamin K–dependent factors. To standardize determinations of prothrombin time and thus allow direct comparison of results obtained with different thromboplastins, the INR is recommended.[409]

At the start of warfarin treatment, the prothrombin time is first prolonged by factor VII depletion because factor VII has a half-life much shorter than that of the other vitamin K–dependent coagulation factors (prothrombin and factors IX and X). Thus, in the beginning of warfarin treatment, the prothrombin time is prolonged, while the intrinsic and common coagulation pathways are still uninfluenced. This explains why, in switching from heparin to warfarin, heparin should be continued unabated for at least 1 day after the prothrombin time (INR) has reached therapeutic values. Also, during long-term warfarin therapy, prothrombin times should be checked regularly, as many drugs and foods can enhance or decrease the warfarin effect. Certain intercurrent diseases (liver insufficiency, heart failure, and hyperthyroidism) may also modify warfarin dose requirements.

Bleeding is the most important side effect, and the risk may vary from patient to patient, depending on the presence of comorbid conditions (hypertension, malignancy, older age, recent surgery) and the intensity of anticoagulation. Patients with intensive anticoagulation (INR = 2.5 to 4) have, during the first 3 months, a risk of clinically important bleeding over two times greater (14 versus 6 percent) than those with less intensive anticoagulation (INR = 2.0 to 2.5).[410] On average, the annual overall risk of bleeding is 6 percent, with the incidence of major and fatal bleeding estimated to be 2 and 0.8 percent, respectively.

A rare, nonhemorrhagic side effect of warfarin is coumarin-induced skin necrosis, an unexplained complication that occurs between days 3 and 8 of therapy. The rapid decline in protein C level is postulated to play a role in the obscure pathogenesis of thrombosis of skin venules and capillaries within the subcutaneous fat, usually in the lower part of the body. Coumarin drugs readily cross the placenta and may be teratogenic, particularly during the first trimester of pregnancy. In conclusion, vitamin K antagonists are effective antithrombotic drugs with a narrow risk-benefit ratio that require regular monitoring and a disciplined patient (Table 44-9). Their main virtues are oral administration and low cost.

CLINICAL STUDIES

Anticoagulant therapy with warfarin has been shown to be beneficial following MI. In pooled data from seven randomized trials between 1964 and 1980, oral anticoagulant therapy over a 1- to 6-year period reduced the rate of death or MI by 20 percent.[411] Subsequently, there have been three large studies evaluating warfarin after MI (both ST-elevation MI and non-ST-elevation MI). In Warfarin Reinfarction Study (WARIS), mortality was reduced by 24 percent (p = .027) and reinfarction was reduced by 34 percent. More recently, the Anticoagulants in the Secondary Prevention of Events in Coronary Thrombosis (ASPECT) trial demonstrated a similar reduction in reinfarction (53 percent benefit of warfarin compared with placebo) in patients following acute MI.[412] Thus, warfarin monotherapy appears to be at least as effective as aspirin after MI.

TABLE 44-9 Drawbacks of Coumarin Drugs and Profile of an Ideal Antithrombotic Drug

Delayed action	
Need for blood monitoring prothrombin time (PT)	
PT test does not fully reflect the drug effect	
Interaction with many commonly used drugs leading to:	
Potentiation of anticoagulation	
Decreasing anticoagulation level	
Sometimes modifying the activity of the other interacting drug	
Anticoagulation level influenced by diet	
Annual risk of bleeding:	Total 6%
	Major 2%
	Fatal 0.8%
Narrow benefit-to-risk ratio	
Embryotoxicity during first trimester of pregnancy	

Two clinical trials compared warfarin therapy with antiplatelet therapy in secondary prevention of MI. In the German Austrian Myocardial Infarction Study (GAMIS), 946 patients 38 to 42 days after acute MI were randomized to open-label phenprocoumon (target INR = 2.5 to 5.0), aspirin 1.5 g/day, or placebo.[241,413] No difference was observed between groups in mortality or reinfarction. The French Enquete de Prevention Secondaire de l'Infarctus de Myocarde (EPSIM) study[243,414] revealed no difference in death or reinfarction in patients receiving either oral anticoagulants or aspirin, but there were 54 percent more patients with gastrointestinal events with aspirin and four times more severe hemorrhagic events with warfarin. In the Aspirin Versus Coumadin in the Prevention of Reocclusion and Recurrent Ischemia After Successful Thrombolysis (APRICOT) trial, 300 patients were randomized to either 325 mg of aspirin per day or heparin followed by warfarin (target INR = 2.8 to 4.0) after an initial angiogram less than 48 h after acute MI revealed a patent infarct-related artery.[414] At 3 months, there was no significant difference in reocclusion rates among the warfarin, aspirin, and placebo arms. Aspirin significantly reduced reinfarction compared with placebo but not with warfarin. The mortality rates did not differ between the groups.

The Coumadin Aspirin Reinfarction Study (CARS) evaluated the combination of aspirin (80 mg) and fixed-dose warfarin (1 or 3 mg, not adjusted to a prothrombin time) compared with aspirin alone (160 mg). No benefit was observed with the combinations of fixed-dose warfarin plus aspirin with regard to recurrent MI, cardiac death, or nonfatal ischemic stroke.[415] More recently, a trial involving men at risk for ischemic heart disease, using a slightly higher dose of warfarin (4.1 mg on average titrated to an INR of 1.5), found a significant reduction compared with placebo in coronary death or MI with the combination of warfarin and aspirin 75 mg daily.[416] In this trial, there was an increase in hemorrhagic strokes among patients treated with the combination (0.9 versus 0.1 percent for warfarin alone, 0.2 percent for aspirin alone, and 0 percent for placebo; p = .009).[416] The Combination Hemotherapy and Mortality Prevention (CHAMP) study randomized patients to receive either 160 mg/day of aspirin or 80 mg of aspirin plus coumadin to achieve an INR of 1.5 to 2.5. Results of this study found no difference in mortality or recurrent events with the addition of warfarin to aspirin.[417] Major bleeding was more common in the combination group: 1.25/100 patient years compared with 0.69/100 patient years for aspirin alone. Preliminary results of two studies (APRICOT II and ASPECT II) have shown benefit with the combination of coumadin (higher INR than in previous studies) plus aspirin as compared to aspirin alone (Verhevgt et al., European Congress of Cardiology, Amsterdam, 2000).[418]

There are several other areas for benefit or potential benefit with warfarin therapy. First, warfarin is superior to aspirin in prevention of systemic emboli in patients with atrial fibrillation.[411,419] In addition, beneficial effects in reducing systemic emboli have also been observed in patients after MI with documented left ventricular dysfunction.[420] Thus, in selected patients at risk for systemic emboli, warfarin affords a second beneficial effect. Thus, at present, warfarin is a suitable alternative to aspirin following MI, and is indicated if there is a risk for systemic embolization.

THROMBOLYTIC DRUGS

All thrombolytic drugs are plasminogen activators, and, as indicated in Fig. 44-21, some are natural activators endogenous to the human fibrinolytic system and others are not.

Streptokinase

Thus is a nonenzyme protein produced by several strains of hemolytic streptococci: it consists of a single polypeptide chain of 414 amino acids with a molecular weight of about 50,000.[421] Streptokinase cannot directly cleave peptide bonds, but it activates plasminogen to plasmin indirectly, following a three-step mechanism.[421] In the first step, streptokinase forms an equimolar complex with plasminogen. This complex undergoes a conformational change, resulting in the exposure of an active site in the plasminogen moiety. In the second step, this active site catalyzes the activation of plasminogen to plasmin. In a third step, plasminogen-streptokinase molecules are converted to plasmin-streptokinase complexes.[422] The active-site residues in the plasmin-streptokinase complex are the same as those in the plasmin molecule, but plasmin is unable to activate plasminogen, whereas the plasmin(ogen)-streptokinase complex is not inhibited by α_2-antiplasmin.

Most individuals have measurable circulating streptokinase-neutralizing antibodies, which may result from previous infections with B-hemolytic streptococci. Therefore, during thrombolytic therapy, sufficient streptokinase must be infused to neutralize these antibodies. A few days after streptokinase administration, the antistreptokinase titer rises rapidly to 50 to 100 times the preinfusion value and remains high for 4 to 6 months, during which renewed treatment with streptokinase is impracticable.[423]

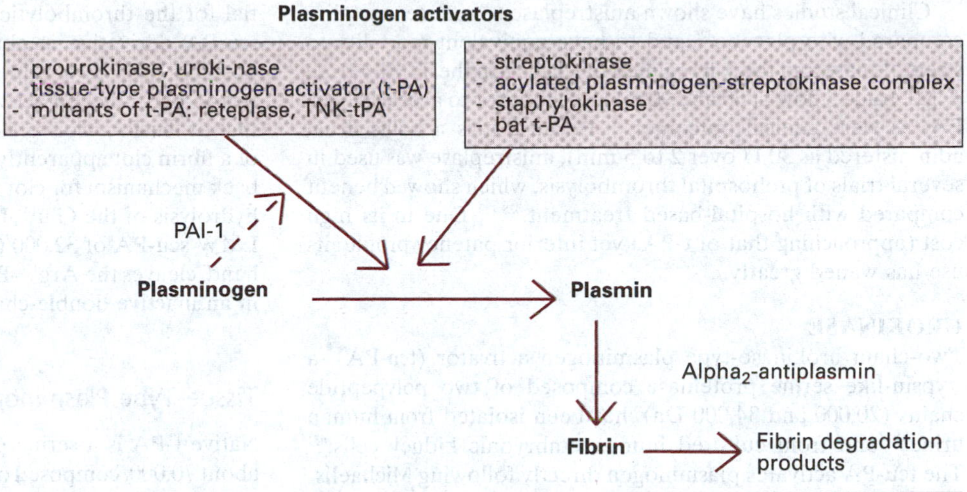

FIGURE 44-21 Components of the fibrinolytic system. In the *left top box*, natural plasminogen activators (endogenous to the human fibrinolytic system) and their mutants in clinical use are grouped separately from other plasminogen activators in clinical use (*right top box*).

Clinical trials have shown intravenous streptokinase, administered as an infusion of 1.5 million units over 1 h, leads to a significant reduction in mortality rate. In the GISSI-I trial, for patients with acute MI within 12 h, there was a 19 percent reduction in mortality rate.[268] In ISIS-2, there was a 25 percent reduction in mortality rate.[180] In the ISIS-3 trial, streptokinase was found to have an identical mortality rate as the 3-h regimen of t-PA with either subcutaneous or no heparin.[317] In the GUSTO-I trial, however, streptokinase was inferior to t-PA when the latter was administered as an accelerated 90-min bolus and infusion with concomitant intravenous heparin[323] (see also Chap. 42).

Anistreplase (Anisoylated Plasminogen-Streptokinase Complex)

APSAC (anistreplase) was constructed with the aim of controlling the enzymatic activity of the plasmin(ogen)-streptokinase complex by a specific reversible chemical protection of its catalytic center (i.e., by titration with a *p*-anisoyl group).[148,424] Anistreplase, which is an equimolar noncovalent complex between human Lys-plasminogen and streptokinase, has a catalytic center located in the carboxy-terminal region of the molecule, whereas the lysine-binding sites are found within the amino-terminal region of plasminogen. Reversible acylation of the catalytic center would thus not affect the weak fibrin-binding capacity of Lys-plasminogen in the complex. The plasmin(ogen)-streptokinase complex is an efficient activator of plasminogen. Deacylation of anistreplase uncovers the catalytic center, which converts plasminogen to plasmin. Deacylation of anistreplase does, however, occur both in the circulation and at the fibrin surface, and the fibrin specificity of thrombolysis with anistreplase is only marginal at best. A plasma half-life of 70 min was found for anistreplase, compared with 25 min for the plasminogen-streptokinase complex formed in vivo after administration of streptokinase.[425] Patients with high streptokinase antibodies do not respond to anistreplase, and anistreplase causes a marked increase in the streptokinase antibody titer within 2 to 3 weeks, which persists for months.

Clinical studies have shown anistreplase to reduce mortality compared with placebo[426] and to have equivalent mortality to streptokinase and the 3-h regimen of t-PA.[317] In the TIMI-4 trial, TIMI grade 3 flow at 60 and 90 min was inferior to accelerated t-PA, as were clinical outcomes.[427] Because it is a bolus drug, administered as 30 U over 2 to 5 min), anistreplase was used in several trials of prehospital thrombolysis, which showed benefit compared with hospital-based treatment.[428,429] Due to its high cost (approaching that of t-PA) yet inferior patency profile, its use has waned greatly.

UROKINASE

Two-chain urokinase-type plasminogen activator (tcu-PA), a trypsin-like serine proteinase composed of two polypeptide chains (20,000 and 34,000 Da), has been isolated from human urine[430] and from cultured human embryonic kidney cells.[431] The tcu-PA activates plasminogen directly following Michaelis-Menten kinetics but has no specific affinity for fibrin and activates fibrin-bound and circulating plasminogen relatively indiscriminantly. Extensive plasminogen activation and depletion of α_2-antiplasmin may occur following treatment of thromboembolic diseases with tcu-PA, leading to degradation of several plasma proteins, including fibrinogen, factor V, and factor VIII.

PRO-UROKINASE

Single-chain urokinase-type plasminogen activator (scu-PA, pro-urokinase) is a naturally occurring human protein first isolated from natural sources and then produced through recombinant DNA technology.[432] The human gene responsible for its synthesis is located on chromosome 10 and is about 6.4 kb long, organized in 11 exons; it gives rise to a 2.5-kb-long messenger RNA, which transcribes a single-chain glycosylated polypeptide. Evidence for the signal transduction pathways involved in regulation of the urokinase gene has to date demonstrated three mechanisms, which are dependent respectively on activation of c-AMP protein kinase, protein kinase C, and an as yet uncharacterized protein kinase.[433]

The single-chain protein is synthesized principally by renal and vascular endothelial cells but also by a variety of cultured normal, transformed, and malignant cell types. The protein scu-PA has also been expressed by gene-cloning techniques in *E. coli* bacteria[154,434] and mouse hybridoma cells.

The glycosylated natural scu-PA is a single-chain glycoprotein with a molecular weight of 54,000 Da and containing 411 amino acid residues. The N-terminal domain has a homology with the growth factor domain of other proteins, followed by a kringle domain, homologous to plasminogen, t-PA, and other proteins involved in coagulation.[435] However, the single-disulfide-bonded kringle domain of scu-PA does not contain a lysine-binding site, and it does not confer fibrin-binding properties to the enzyme. The single glycosylation site of the glycoprotein is located at asparagine 302. The molecule expressed by *E. coli* lacks the glycosyl group, which reduces the molecular weight to 47,000 Da.[434] The scu-PA is the native zymogenic precursor of urokinase. Limited hydrolysis by plasmin or kallikrein of the Lys^{158}-Ile^{159} peptide bond converts the molecule to tcu-PA (urokinase), which is held together by one disulfide bond essential for the thrombolytic activity[436] (Fig. 44-22). A fully active tcu-PA derivative is obtained after additional proteolysis at position Lys^{135}-Lys^{136}. In purified systems, scu-PA has some intrinsic plasminogen-activating potential, but it is 1 percent of that of tcu-PA. Conversion of scu-PA to tcu-PA in the vicinity of a fibrin clot apparently constitutes a significant positive feedback mechanism for clot lysis in human plasma in vitro. Specific hydrolysis of the Glu^{143}-Leu^{144} peptide bond in scu-PA yields a LMW scu-PA of 32,000 (scu-PA-32k). Thrombin, on the other hand, cleaves the Arg^{156}-Phe^{157} peptide bond in scu-PA, resulting in an inactive double-chain molecule.

Tissue-Type Plasminogen Activator

Native t-PA is a serine proteinase with a molecular weight of about 70,000, composed of one polypeptide chain containing 527 amino acids with serine as the amino-terminal amino acid.[142,157] t-PA is converted by plasmin to a two-chain form by hydrolysis of the Arg^{275}-Ile^{276} peptide bond. The two-chain form is held together by one interchain disulfide bond. t-PA for clinical use is presently produced by recombinant DNA technology [Activase (Genentech) or Actilyse (Boehringer Ingelheim)] and consists mainly of the single-chain form.

The NH_2-terminal region of t-PA is composed of four domains with homologies to other proteins: residues 4 to 50 (F domain) are homologous to the *finger domains* in fibronectin, residues 50 to 87 (E domain) are homologous to human epidermal growth factor, and two regions comprising residues 87 to 176 and 176 to 262 (K1 and K2 domains) are both homologous to the five "kringle" loop structures of plasminogen (Fig. 44-22). The region comprising residues 276 to 527 is homologous to that of other serine proteinases and contains the catalytic site, which is composed of His^{322}, Asp^{371}, and Ser^{478}. t-PA has a specific affinity for fibrin. The structures involved in the fibrin binding of t-PA are fully contained within the A (heavy) chain. Evidence obtained with deletion mutants suggests that binding of t-PA to fibrin is mediated both via the finger domain and via the second kringle region. A lysine-binding site is involved in the interaction of K2 domain with fibrin but not in the interaction of the finger domain with fibrin. The structures required for the enzymatic activity of t-PA are fully contained within the B chain.

The activation of plasminogen by t-PA, both in the presence and in the absence of fibrin, follows Michaelis-Menten kinetics.[166] There is a consensus that the presence of fibrin enhances the efficiency of plasminogen activation by t-PA by 2 to 3 orders of magnitude.[166] Fibrin provides a surface to which t-PA and plasminogen adsorb in a sequential and ordered way, yielding a cyclic ternary complex. Fibrin essentially increases the local plasminogen concentration by creating an additional interaction between t-PA and its substrate. The high affinity of t-PA for plasminogen in the presence of fibrin thus allows efficient activation on the fibrin clot, while no efficient plasminogen activation by t-PA occurs in plasma. Plasmin formed on the fibrin surface has both its lysine-binding sites and active site occupied and is thus only slowly inactivated by α_2-antiplasmin (a half-life of

FIGURE 44-22 Primary structure of tissue-type plasminogen (t-PA) activator (*A*) and pro-urokinase (*B*). The amino acids are represented by their single-letter symbols, and the black bars indicate disulfide bonds. ★ = active site residues His^{322}, Asp^{371}, and Ser^{478}; arrow in A = plasmin cleavage site for conversion of single-chain t-PA to the two-chain molecule; arrows in B = tcu-PA (Lys^{158}-Ile^{159}), and 54-kDa tcu-PA (Lys^{135}-Lys^{136}), the thrombin cleavage site (Arg^{156}-Phe^{157}) yielding inactive 54-kDa tcu-PA, and the conversion site to 32-kDa scu-PA (Glu^{143}-Leu^{144}).

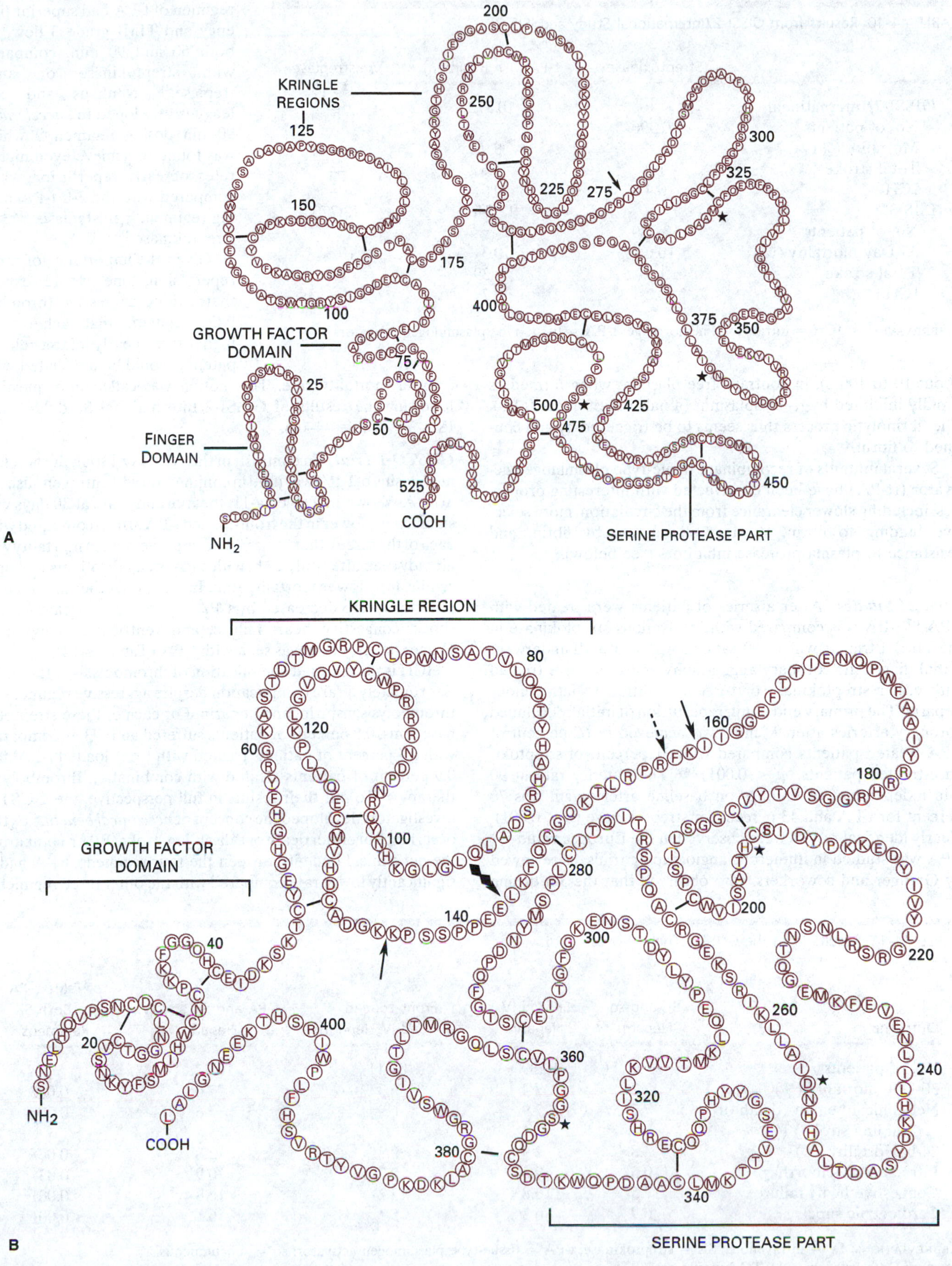
KRINGLE REGIONS
GROWTH FACTOR DOMAIN
FINGER DOMAIN
SERINE PROTEASE PART
NH$_2$
COOH
A
KRINGLE REGION
GROWTH FACTOR DOMAIN
SERINE PROTEASE PART
NH$_2$
COOH
B

TABLE 44-10 Results from GISSI-2/International Study and ISIS-3

	Streptokinase	t-PA (3-h Regimen)	Anistreplase
GISSI-2/International		10,372	—
No. of patients	10,396		
Mortality (%)	8.4	8.9	—
Total stroke	1.0	1.6	—
ICH	0.4	0.6	—
ISIS-3		13,746	13,773
No. of patients	13,780		
35-Day mortality (%)	10.6	10.3	10.5
Total stroke	1.04	1.39	1.26
ICH	0.2	0.7	0.6

ABBREVIATIONS: ICH = intracranial hemorrhage; t-PA = tissue-type plasminogen activator.

about 10 to 100 s); in contrast, free plasmin, when formed, is rapidly inhibited by α_2-antiplasmin (a half-life of about 0.1 s). The fibrinolytic process thus seems to be triggered by and confined to fibrin.

Several mutants of recombinant tissue-type plasminogen activator (rt-PA) have been constructed with interesting properties, including slower clearance from the circulation, more selective binding to fibrin, stronger stimulation by fibrin, and resistance to plasma protease inhibitors (see below).

Clinical Studies After a series of patients were treated with t-PA,[437] t-PA was compared with intravenous streptokinase in the TIMI-1 trial, in which 290 patients with acute MI underwent initial diagnostic coronary angiography and then were treated with either streptokinase or t-PA in addition to intravenous heparin. The primary end point, reperfusion of initially occluded coronary arteries after 90 min, was achieved in 62 percent of t-PA-treated patients compared with 31 percent of streptokinase-treated patients ($p < 0.001$).[3,438] The patency rate at 90 min independent of findings on baseline arteriogram was 70 percent for t-PA and 43 percent for streptokinase ($p < 0.001$). Nearly identical results were observed in the European study.[439] t-PA was studied in numerous angiographic trials, as reviewed by Granger and coworkers, who observed that the 3-h dosing regimen of t-PA had superior patency and TIMI grade 3 flow,[3] at both 60 and 90 min, compared with streptokinase or anistreplase.[440] Neuhaus and colleagues developed the *accelerated* 90-min dosing regimen,[441] which was found to achieve even higher rates of early reperfusion when compared with the 3-h t-PA dosing regimen,[442] anisteplase,[427,443] or streptokinase.[270]

Given the importance of rapid reperfusion, one would expect that a more aggressive thrombolytic regimen that achieves a higher rate of early infarct-related patency would be associated with a lower mortality rate. This notion was called into question following the results of GISSI-2/International Study[315,316] and ISIS-3[317] (Table 44-10).

GUSTO-I Trial In contrast, in the GUSTO-I trial, the accelerated dosing of t-PA was used in conjunction with intravenous heparin. As shown in Table 44-11, the mortality rate at 30 days was significantly lower in the front-loaded t-PA arm as compared with each of the three other arms.[323] The improvement in mortality was already seen after only 24 h, with t-PA-treated patients having a significantly lower mortality rate. In addition, other major complications were decreased by t-PA. There was less cardiogenic shock, congestive heart failure, and ventricular arrhythmia. Higher patency rate was seen with t-PA (Table 44-12).

ICH is the dreaded complication of thrombolysis, although it is fortunately a rare complication despite aggressive regimens of thrombolysis, aspirin, and heparin. For each of these streptokinase arms, 0.5 percent of patients suffered an ICH as compared with 0.7 percent of patients treated with front-loaded t-PA and 0.9 percent of patients treated with combination thrombolytic therapy.[323] To put their results in full perspective, the GUSTO investigators developed the concept of *net clinical benefit*, i.e., the occurrence of either death or a disabling stroke. When comparing the net clinical benefit between the four regimens, t-PA had a significantly lower rate compared with the other three regimens.

TABLE 44-11 Results from the GUSTO Trial

Outcome	SK and sq Heparin	SK and IV Heparin	Front-Loaded t-PA and IV Heparin	t-PA and SK and IV Heparin	*p* Value t-PA vs. Both SK Regimens
No. of patients	9796	10,377	10,344	10,328	
30-Day mortality (%)	7.2	7.4	6.3	7.0	0.005
Net clinical benefit (death or disabling stroke) (%)	7.7	7.9	6.9	7.6	0.006
24-h Mortality (%)	2.8	2.9	2.3	2.8	0.005
Intracranial hemorrhage	0.5	0.5	0.7	0.9	0.03
Congestive heart failure	17.5	16.8	15.2	16.8	<0.001
Cardiogenic shock	6.9	6.3	5.1	6.1	<0.001

ABBREVIATIONS: IV = intravenous; SK = streptokinase; t-PA = tissue-type plasminogen activator; sq = subcutaneous.
SOURCE: Data from the GUSTO Investigators.[270,323]

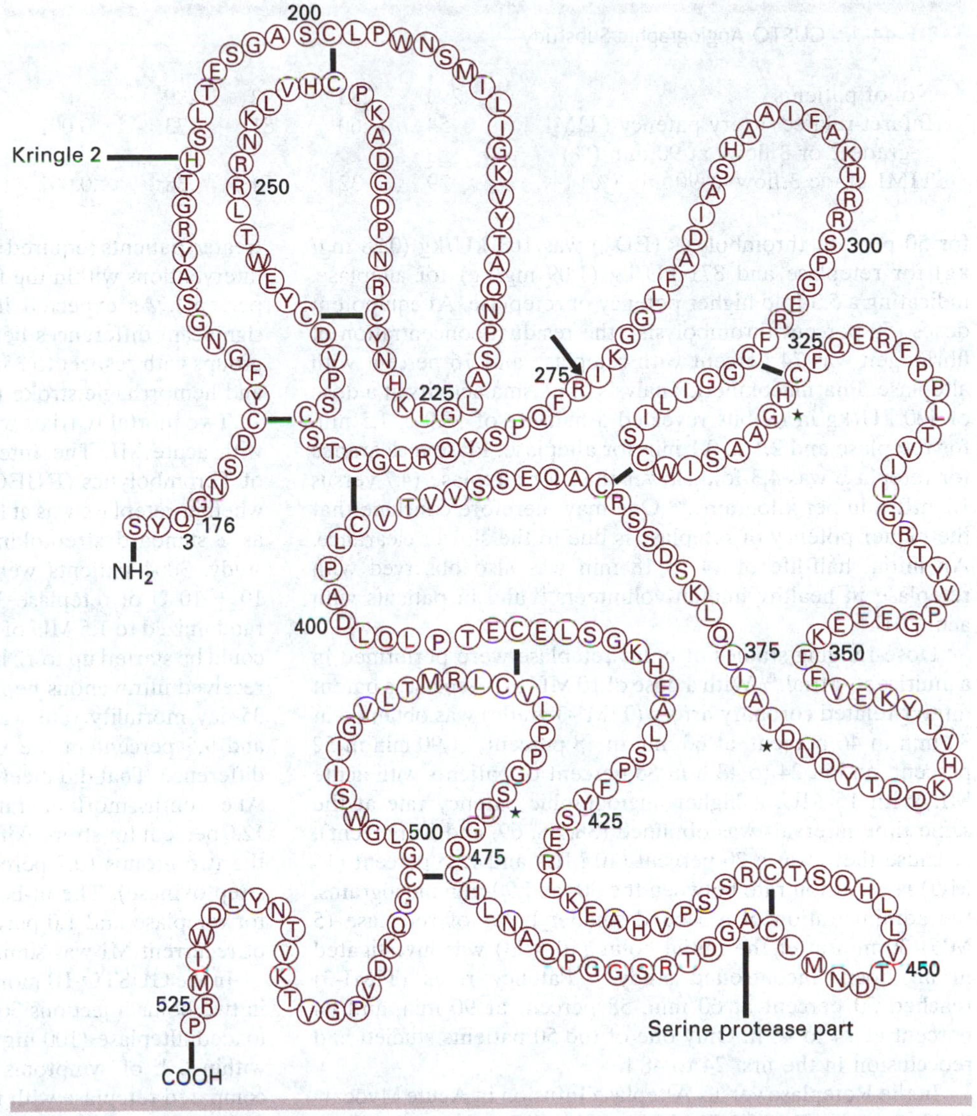

FIGURE 44-23 Schematic representation of the primary structure of reteplase (Retavase) (amino acids Ser^{1}-Gln^{3} and Gly^{176}-Pro^{527} of tissue-type plasminogen activator). The amino acids are represented by their single-letter symbols; black bars indicate disulfide bonds and the asterisks indicate the active-site residues in the protease part. The arrow indicates the plasmin cleavage site.

The explanation of the benefit of t-PA in the GUSTO and TIMI-4 trials and the lack of benefit in GISSI-2 and ISIS-3 is based on two factors: the t-PA regimen and the heparin dosing. The use of the front-loaded t-PA regimen achieves a higher rate of early patency compared with the older 3-h regimen.[440] The use of early intravenous heparin has been shown to improve late infarct-related artery patency (Table 44-12). In contrast, the GISSI-2 and ISIS-3 trials used the slower infusion regimen of t-PA and either no heparin or delayed, subcutaneous heparin, which does not elevate APTT until approximately 24 h after the start of treatment. Because the initial 24 h hold the highest risk of reocclusion of an open infarct-related artery (which is associated with a threefold increase in mortality), the subcutaneous heparin regimen is inadequate at preventing this important complication.

Double-Bolus Tissue-Type Plasminogen Activator Initial interest in a double-bolus regimen of t-PA came from a series of patients, in which two 50-mg boluses of t-PA were administered 30 min apart, and TIMI grade 3 flow was observed in 88 percent of patients.[444] In a subsequent randomized trial, however, double-bolus t-PA achieved only 58 percent TIMI grade 3 flow, compared with 66 percent for the accelerated 90-min infusion of t-PA.[445] The Continuous Infusion Versus Double-Bolus Administration of Alteplase (COBALT) trial compared double-bolus t-PA with the accelerated infusion of t-PA but was terminated prematurely because of concern about the safety of the double-bolus regimen. The 30-day mortality rate was higher in the double-bolus group than in the accelerated-infusion group: 7.98 percent as compared with 7.53 percent.[446] Rates of hemorrhagic stroke were 1.12 percent after double-bolus alteplase as compared with 0.81 percent after an accelerated infusion of alteplase (p = .23).[446] Statistically, double-bolus t-PA was *not* equivalent to t-PA.[446] Thus, based on this trial, double-bolus t-PA is not recommended for general clinical use,[446] and the accelerated, 90-min infusion of t-PA remains the current standard dosing for acute MI.

Tissue-Type Plasminogen Activator (Reteplase)

This is a single-chain nonglycosylated deletion variant of rt-PA consisting of only the K2 and the protease domains of human t-PA (Fig. 44-23). The active site of the protease domain of reteplase and that of t-PA, and their plasminogenolytic activity in the absence of a stimulator, do not differ, but the plasminogenolytic activity of reteplase in the presence of fragments of fibrinogen as a stimulator was fourfold lower compared with t-PA, whereas the binding of reteplase to fibrin was five times lower. These differences in plasminogenolytic activity and fibrin binding between the two molecules might be due to the missing finger domain in reteplase. It is known that fibrin binding is mediated through both the finger domain and the lysine-binding site in the K2 domain of t-PA. Reteplase and t-PA are inhibited by PAI-1 to a similar degree, but the affinity of reteplase for binding to endothelial cells and monocytes is reduced, probably as a consequence of deletion of the finger and epidermal growth factor domains in reteplase, which seem to be involved in the interaction with endothelial cell receptors. The thrombolytic properties of reteplase and alteplase (rt-PA) were compared in the rabbit jugular vein thrombosis model.[447] The effective dose

TABLE 44-12 GUSTO Angiographic Substudy

No. of patients	293	283	292	299	
Infarct-related artery patency (TIMI grade 2 or 3 flow) at 90 min (%)	54	60	81	73	<0.001
TIMI grade 3 flow at 90 min (%)	29	32	54	38	<0.001

for 50 percent thrombolysis (ED_{50}) was 163 kU/kg (0.28 mg/kg) for reteplase and 871 kU/kg (1.09 mg/kg) for alteplase, indicating a 5.3-fold higher potency of reteplase. At equipotent doses (50 percent thrombolysis), the residual concentration of fibrinogen was 74 percent with reteplase and 76 percent with alteplase. Pharmacokinetic analysis of plasma activity at a dose of 400 kU/kg in rabbits revealed a half-life of 18.9 ± 1.5 min for reteplase and 2.1 ± 0.1 min for alteplase. Plasma clearance for reteplase was 4.3-fold slower than for alteplase (4.7 versus 1.2 mL/min per kilogram).[448] One may therefore conclude that the higher potency of reteplase is due to the slower clearance. An initial half-life of 14 to 18 min was also observed with reteplase in healthy human volunteers[449] and in patients with acute MI.[450]

Dose-ranging studies of bolus reteplase were performed in a multicenter trial.[451] With a dose of 10 MU of reteplase, a patent infarct-related coronary artery (TIMI-3 grade) was obtained at 30 min in 46 percent, at 60 min in 48 percent, at 90 min in 52 percent, and at 24 to 48 h in 88 percent of patients with acute MI. With 15 MU, a higher angiographic patency rate at the same time intervals was obtained (38, 58, 69, and 85 percent). Because there was a 20 percent (10 MU) and 12.5 percent (15 MU) reocclusion rate between the 30- and 90-min angiograms, the administration of a second smaller bolus of reteplase (5 MU) 30 min after the initial bolus (10 MU) was investigated in an open uncontrolled study.[452] Patency rates (TIMI-3) reached 50 percent at 60 min, 58 percent at 90 min, and 84 percent at 24 to 48 h. Only one of the 50 patients studied had reocclusion in the first 24 to 48 h.

In the Reteplase versus Alteplase Infusion in Acute Myocardial Infarction (RAPID-I) trial involving 605 patients with acute MI, different bolus doses of reteplase (a single dose of 15 MU, 10 MU, and 5 MU 30 min later; and 10 MU and 10 MU 30 min later) were compared with the conventional dose regimen of alteplase (100 mg over 3 h). TIMI-3 patency rates at 90 min were obtained with the given reteplase regimen in 42.7, 45.4, and 62.9 percent, respectively, and in 47.6 percent of patients treated with alteplase.[453] The difference between the 10 MU + 10 MU reteplase and alteplase arms is significant (p = .01).

The RAPID-II trial was a randomized open-label angiographic study of 324 patients with acute MI that was designed to compare the effect of 10 + 10 U reteplase with that of an accelerated, front-loaded dose of alteplase (100 mg over 90 min) on the TIMI grade of the infarct-related coronary artery 90 min after the initiation of thrombolytic therapy.[454] There was no age limit, and patients were recruited up to 12 h after onset of symptoms; all received aspirin. The heparin regimen consisted of a 5000-IU intravenous bolus that was administered before thrombolytic therapy, followed by an infusion of 1000 IU/h for at least 24 h. In this study, reteplase achieved earlier and more complete reperfusion than did accelerated-dose alteplase.[454] TIMI grade 2 or 3 patency and TIMI grade 3 flow rates of the infarct-related artery at 90 min were significantly higher for reteplase relative to the alteplase control (83.4 versus 73.3 percent and 59.9 versus 45.2 percent, respectively).[454] At 60 min, both the TIMI grade 2 or 3 patency and the TIMI grade 3 flow rates were significantly higher for reteplase than for alteplase.[454] Reteplase-treated patients required significantly fewer additional coronary interventions within the first 6 h of treatment (13.3 versus 26.5 percent). As expected in a trial of this size, there were no significant differences between the reteplase and the alteplase groups with respect to 35-day mortality (4.1 versus 8.4 percent) and hemorrhagic stroke (1.2 versus 1.8 percent).[454]

Two mortality trials with reteplase were planned in patients with acute MI. The International Joint Efficacy Comparison of Thrombolytics (INJECT) study was designed to determine whether reteplase was at least as effective in mortality reduction as a standard streptokinase regimen.[455] In this double-blind study, 3004 patients were randomized to a double bolus of 10 + 10 U of reteplase 30 min apart, and 3006 patients were randomized to 1.5 MU of streptokinase over 60 min. Treatment could be started up to 12 h from onset of symptoms. All patients received intravenous heparin for at least 24 h and aspirin. The 35-day mortality rate was 9.0 percent in the reteplase group and 9.5 percent in the streptokinase group, a nonsignificant difference. That did meet predefined criteria for equivalence.[455] At 6 months, mortality rates were 11.0 percent for reteplase and 12.0 percent for streptokinase.[455] Bleeding events were similar in the two groups (0.7 percent for reteplase and 1.0 percent for streptokinase). The in-hospital stroke rates were 1.23 percent for reteplase and 1.0 percent for streptokinase. The incidence of recurrent MI was similar in the two groups.

In the GUSTO-III mortality trial, reteplase was administered in two bolus injections 30 min apart and compared with front-loaded alteplase (100 mg in 90 min) in 15,059 patients treated within 6 h of symptoms of acute MI. The GUSTO-III trial compared reteplase with front-loaded alteplase (t-PA).[456] Mortality (7.47 versus 7.24 percent, r-PA versus t-PA), ICH (0.91 versus 0.87 percent), and net clinical benefit (death or disabling stroke) were very similar clinically (7.9 percent in each group) between double-bolus reteplase and alteplase infusion, respectively.[456] When applying post hoc criteria for equivalence (evaluating the upper boundary of the 95% CI), reteplase is statistically equivalent for death or disabling stroke when a 1 percent absolute boundary is used [derived from the difference observed between streptokinase (SK) and t-PA]. Thus, clinically, the simpler double-bolus regimen of r-PA appears clinically equivalent to accelerated t-PA.

TNK–Tissue-Type Plasminogen Activator (Tenecteplase)

TNK–t-PA (tenecteplase) is a new thrombolytic agent that is a genetically engineered variant of t-PA (Fig. 44-24). TNK–t-PA is similar to wild-type t-PA, but has amino acid substitutions at three sites, which give it its name: a threonine (T) is replaced by asparagine, which adds a glycosylation site to position 103; an asparagine (N) is replaced by a glutamine, thereby removing a glycosylation site from site 117; and four amino acids—lysine (K), histidine, arginine, and arginine—are re-

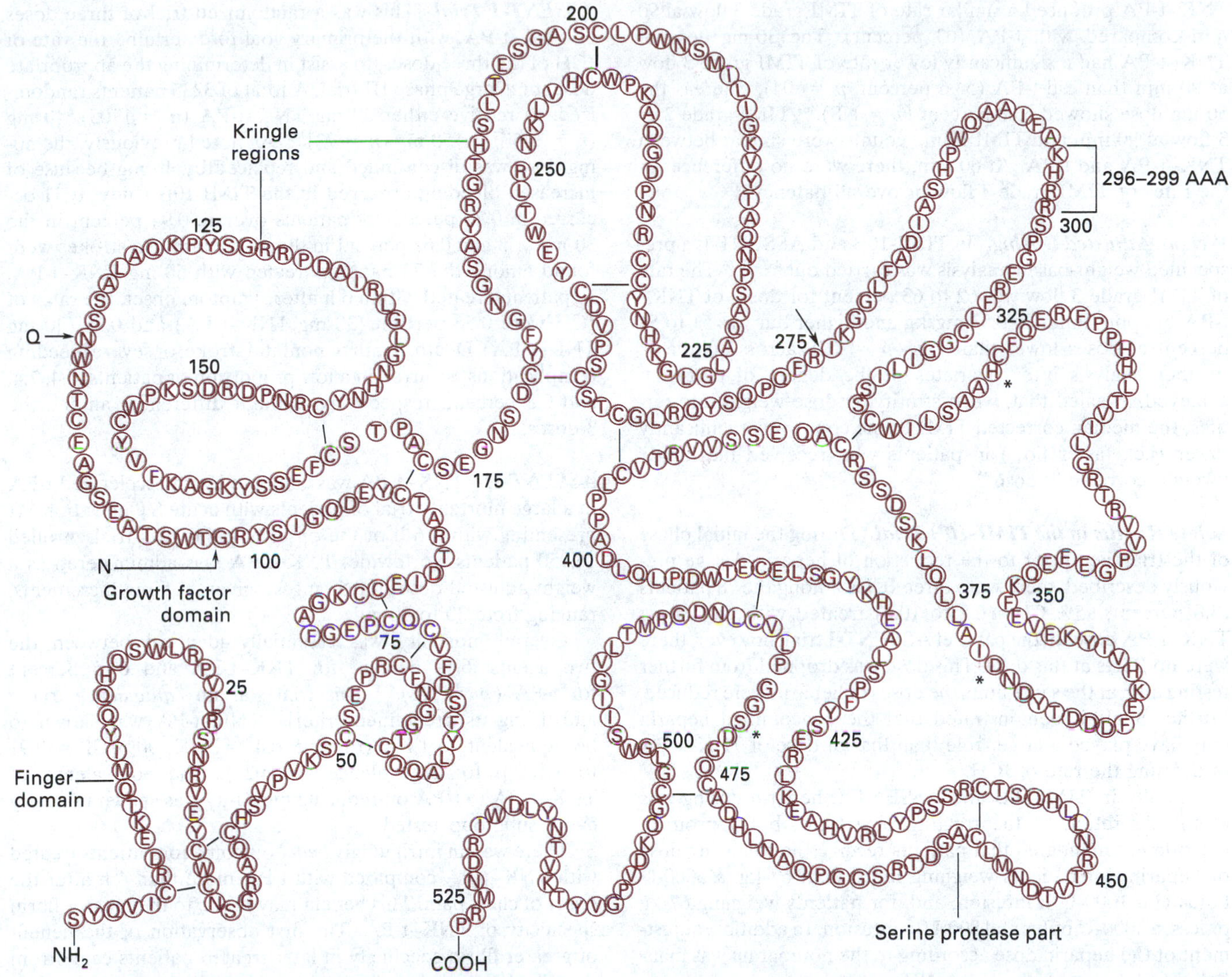

FIGURE 44-24 Schematic representation of the primary structure of recombinant tissue-type plasminogen activator–TNK (TNK–t-PA, tenecteplase) (substitution on rt-PA of Thr[103] by Asn, Asn[111] by Gln, and Lys[296]-His-Arg-Arg by Ala-Ala-Ala-Ala). The amino acids are represented by their single-letter symbols, black bars indicate disulfide bonds, and the asterisks indicate the active site residues in the protease part. The arrow indicates the plasmin cleavage site.

placed by four alanines at the third site. Together, these substitutions lead to, in animal models, a prolonged half-life of the molecule,[457,458] increased fibrin specificity,[457] and increased resistance to inhibition by PAI-1.[459–461]

Pharmacokinetics Clinical testing of TNK–t-PA began in the TIMI-10A trial, with doses ranging from 5 to 50 mg.[457] TNK–t-PA was demonstrated to have a slowed plasma clearance relative to values for t-PA. The corresponding plasma half-life of elimination of TNK–t-PA ranged from 11 to 20 min, as compared with 3.5 min as previously reported for t-PA.[462] These results were duplicated in the TIMI-10B trial.[458,463]

Fibrin Specificity TNK–t-PA is much more fibrin specific than t-PA, which is itself more fibrin specific than streptokinase or reteplase. Systemic fibrinogen and plasminogen levels fell by only 5 to 15 percent over the first 6 h at the 30- to 50-mg doses of TNK–t-PA compared with 40 to 50 percent drops following t-PA. Similarly, the consumption of α2-antiplasmin, the fluid-phase inhibitor of plasmin, and a resultant increase in plasmin–α2-antiplasmin complexes was four to five times greater with t-PA as compared with TNK–t-PA. This high level of fibrin specificity of TNK–t-PA compared with t-PA helps explain its efficacy when administered as a 5- to 10-s bolus, and the fact that it does not induce the *plasminogen steal* phenomenon.[464] Furthermore, these benefits in preserving the systemic coagulation factors appear to translate into lower rates of major bleeding in the large phase III trial (see below).

TIMI Grade 3 Flow In the dose-ranging trial TIMI-10A, the rate of TIMI grade 3 flow at 90 min was achieved in 57 to 64 percent of patients at the 30- to 50-mg TNK–t-PA doses, which was higher than in patients treated with the lower doses (p = .032).[457] In TIMI-10B, a total of 886 patients were randomized to receive either front-loaded (90-min infusion) t-PA or a single 5- to 10-s bolus of TNK–t-PA at 30- or 50-mg bolus.[463] The 50-mg dose was discontinued due to increased bleeding and replaced with a 40-mg dose of TNK–t-PA. The 40-mg dose of

TNK–t-PA produced a similar rate of TIMI grade 3 flow at 90 min compared with t-PA (63 percent). The 30-mg dose of TNK–t-PA had a significantly lower rate of TIMI grade 3 flow at 90 min than did t-PA (54.6 percent, $p = .04$), whereas the 50-mg dose showed 65.8 percent ($p =$ NS).[463] TIMI grade 2 or 3 flow at 90 min and TIMI frame counts were similar between TNK–t-PA and t-PA. At 60 min, there were no differences in the rates of TIMI grade 3 flow or overall patency.[463]

Weight-Adjusted Dosing In TIMI-10B and ASSENT-I, a prespecified weight-based analysis was carried out.[463,465,466] The rate of TIMI grade 3 flow was 62 to 63 percent for doses of TNK–t-PA of approximately 0.53 mg/kg and higher but was 51 to 54 percent at doses lower than this ($p = .028$ across quintiles). Further analysis into covariates of the degree of perfusion achieved revealed that, when stratifying dose/weight into tertiles, the median corrected TIMI frame count was significantly lower (i.e., faster flow) in patients who received the higher "weight corrected" dose.[465]

Safety Results in the TIMI-10B Trial During the initial phase of the trial, i.e., prior to the reduction of heparin dosage previously described, there were three ICHs among the 78 patients (3.8 percent, 95% CI = 0.8 to 10.8) treated with the 50 mg TNK–t-PA dose. In the parallel ASSENT-I trial, however, there were no ICHs at this dose. This dose was dropped from further testing and, at the same time, the doses of heparin were reduced. Further analysis demonstrated that the concomitant heparin may have played a larger role than that of dose of TNK–t-PA in defining the rate of ICH.

Initially in TIMI-10B and ASSENT-I, heparin dosing was at the discretion of the treating physicians, but a protocol amendment mandated that patients receive the following dose of heparin: for patients weighing more than 67 kg, a 5000-U bolus and 1000-U/h infusion, and, for patients weighing 67 kg or less, a 4000-U bolus and 800-U/h infusion. In addition, adjustment of the heparin dose according to the nomogram was mandated to begin with the 6-h APTT.

The rates of both ICH and serious bleeding were lower after the protocol amendment: for TNK–t-PA 30 mg, the ICH rate fell from 2.2 to 0 percent ($p = .047$), and, for t-PA, the rate fell from 2.8 to 1.2 percent ($p = .29$) (overall combined $p = .04$).[463] Similar observations and statistically significant reductions in ICH rate were observed in overall TNK–t-PA experience combining the TIMI-10B and ASSENT-I trials.[350] The rate of severe bleeding also decreased with the reduced heparin dosing: from 3 to 0 percent ($p = .02$) for 30 mg TNK–t-PA, and from 8 to 2 percent ($p = .01$) for t-PA (combined $p = .001$).[463] Thus, for the subsequent phase III trial (ASSENT-II), the lower heparin regimen was used.

Another observation on safety involved the rates of serious (noncerebral) bleeding in TIMI-10B, where lower rates of serious bleeding requiring transfusion were noted. For t-PA, 7.0 percent of patients required transfusion compared with 1.0 percent of TNK–t-PA patients treated with the 30-mg dose ($p < 0.001$) and 1.3 percent treated with the 40-mg dose ($p < 0.01$).[467] Similar low rates of serious bleeding requiring transfusion were observed in the ASSENT-I trial.[467] Thus, there appeared to be early evidence that the very fibrin specific agent TNK–t-PA might have lower rates of bleeding than t-PA.

ASSENT-I Trial This was a randomized trial of three doses of TNK–t-PA, with the primary goal to determine the rate of ICH of the three doses, to assist in determining the appropriate dose for a large phase III trial. A total of 3235 patients randomized: to receive either 30 mg TNK–t-PA ($n = 1705$), 40 mg ($n = 1457$), or 50 mg ($n = 73$).[468] As noted previously, the 50-mg dose was discontinued and replaced by 40 mg because of increased bleeding observed in the TIMI-10B study. ICH occurred in 0.77 percent of patients overall: 0.94 percent in the 30-mg arm and 0.62 percent in the 40-mg arm. No strokes were found among the 73 patients treated with 50 mg TNK–t-PA. In patients treated within 6 h after symptom onset, the rates of ICH were 0.56 percent (30 mg TNK–t-PA) and 0.58 (40 mg TNK–t-PA). Death, death or nonfatal stroke, or severe bleeding complications occurred in a low proportion of patients: 6.4, 7.4, and 2.8 percent, respectively, without differences among the 3 doses.

ASSENT-II TNK–t-PA was compared with accelerated t-PA in a large mortality trial of patients with acute ST-elevation MI presenting within 6 h of the onset of pain. This trial enrolled 16,950 patients worldwide. TNK–t-PA was administered as a weight-adjusted dose of 0.53 mg/kg given in 5-mg increments, ranging from 30 to 50 mg.

Overall mortality was essentially identical between the two agents: 6.17 percent for TNK–t-PA and 6.15 percent for t-PA ($p =$ NS).[469] This trial was an *equivalence* trial[470] and, using its predefined criteria, TNK–t-PA was shown to be equivalent to t-PA (relative risk = 1.00; 90% CI = 0.91 to 1.10; p for equivalence = 0.028). The equivalence of TNK–t-PA to t-PA on reducing mortality was shown in nearly every subgroup tested.

There was an intriguingly *better* outcome for patients treated with TNK–t-PA compared with t-PA more than 4 h after the onset of chest pain. This benefit may relate to the greater fibrin specificity of TNK–t-PA. The first observation of the benefit of greater fibrin specificity in later-treated patients came from the TIMI-1 trial, in which 90-min patency was preserved in patients treated with t-PA with time to treatment of less than or more than 4 h, whereas, for those treated with streptokinase, patency was significantly worse if time to treatment was more than 4 h.[3,438] Similar findings were seen in an analysis of the German angiographic thrombolytic trials.[471,472] The same pattern favoring the more fibrin-specific agent was seen in the GUSTO-III trial, where t-PA had significantly lower mortality than reteplase, a less fibrin-specific agent, in patients treated more than 4 h after the onset of pain.[456] It is hypothesized that the clot may be more resistant the longer it has been able to mature, and the greater fibrin specificity of the thrombolytic agent may enhance the ability to lyse the clot.

Safety Observations In ASSENT-II, the rate of ICH was also identical for TNK–t-PA and t-PA (0.93 versus 0.94 percent, $p =$ NS). Total stroke was also similar (1.78 percent for TNK–t-PA versus 1.66 percent for t-PA, $p =$ NS). However, there was an intriguingly lower rate (albeit not statistically significant) of ICH in patients older than 75 years of age treated with TNK–t-PA (1.7 percent versus 2.6 percent for those treated with t-PA). Further detailed analysis found that the highest-risk group for ICH was elderly female patients weighing 67 kg or less.[473] This group has been found in two previous multivariate analyses to be at high risk for ICH.[474,475] Most encouragingly, the rates for ICH in this high-risk group were only 1.1 percent following treatment with TNK–t-PA compared with 3.0 percent for those treated with t-PA. The multivariate adjusted odds ratio was 0.30 (95% CI = 0.09 to 0.98, $p < 0.05$).[473] In all other patients, the rates of ICH were similar between the two thrombolytic groups.

Importantly, these benefits on ICH were paralleled by significantly lower rates of major bleeding. In the trial as a whole, the rates of major bleeding were 4.7 percent for TNK–t-PA and 5.9 percent for t-PA ($p = .0002$).[469] Total bleeding also occurred in fewer patients ($p = .0003$).[469,476] Similarly, the rate of bleeding requiring transfusion was significantly lower with TNK–t-PA.

Desmodus Salivary Plasminogen Activator The subsistence of vampire bats on a diet of fresh blood is apparently contingent on their ability to interfere with the hemostatic system of the blood donor. The saliva of vampire bats contains a variety of factors that presumably satisfy two essential requirements: to maintain prolonged bleeding from the wound and to preserve blood fluidity following ingestion of a meal.[477] Different molecular forms of the *Desmodus* salivary plasminogen activator (DSPA) have been purified, characterized, cloned, and expressed. Two HMW forms exhibit about 85 percent homology to human t-PA: DSPAα1 (M_r 43) and DSPAα2 (M_r 39), which contain neither a kringle 2 domain nor a plasmin-sensitive processing site. DSPAβ lacks the finger-like structure and DSPAγ lacks the finger and epidermal growth factor structures.[405,478] The two HMW forms exhibit a specific activity in vitro equal to or higher than that of t-PA, a relative PAI-1 resistance, and a greatly enhanced fibrin specificity with a strict requirement for polymeric fibrin as a cofactor.[479–481] In animal models (rats, rabbits, and dogs) of thrombolysis, DSPAα1 is superior to t-PA in terms of potency (2.5 times higher), terminal half-life (three times longer), and clearance (four- to eightfold slower).[481] Interestingly, the fibrin cofactor requirement of DSPAα1 and DPSAα2, which both bind to fibrin, may not solely depend on fibrin binding, as the two smaller forms, DPSAβ and DSPAγ, are also fibrin dependent but lack fibrin affinity.[481]

ZK152387 is recombinant DSPAα1 produced in mammalian cell culture; its amino acid sequence is identical to that of its natural counterpart.[478] DSPAα1 may be suitable for bolus administration; its long half-life and high specific activity may allow a marked reduction of the absolute dose of drug required for effective thrombolysis as compared with t-PA.

Staphylokinase Mature staphylokinase consists of 136 amino acids in a single polypeptide chain without disulfide bridges. Staphylokinase, like streptokinase, is not an enzyme but forms a 1:1 stoichiometric complex with plasmin(ogen) that activates other plasminogen molecules. Streptokinase and plasminogen produce a complex that exposes the active site in the plasminogen molecule without proteolytic cleavage, whereas generation of plasmin is required for exposure of the active site in the complex with staphylokinase.[482,483]

Staphylokinase does not bind to fibrin, and fibrin stimulates the initial rate of plasminogen activation by staphylokinase only fourfold as compared with twofold by streptokinase. In purified systems α_2-antiplasmin rapidly inhibits the plasmin-staphylokinase complex (second-order inhibition rate constant of approximately $2 \times 10^6\ M^{-1}s^{-1}$), although it does not inhibit the plasmin(ogen)-streptokinase complex. Addition of 6-aminohexanoic acid or of fibrin-like substances (e.g., CNBr-digested fibrinogen) induces a more than 100-fold reduction of the inhibition rates of the plasmin-staphylokinase complex by α_2-antiplasmin. Rapid inhibition by α_2-antiplasmin indeed requires the availability of the lysine-binding sites in the plasminogen moiety of the complex. More detailed studies on the interaction between staphylokinase, plasmin(ogen), and α_2-antiplasmin have shown that neutralization of the plasmin-staphylokinase complex by α_2-antiplasmin results in dissociation of functionally active staphylokinase from the complex, followed by its recycling to other plasminogen molecules.[482]

In plasma, the conversion of plasminogen-staphylokinase to plasmin-staphylokinase complex does not occur at a significant rate because it is prevented by α_2-antiplasmin; without plasmin-staphylokinase complex, no significant plasminogen activation occurs. In the presence of fibrin, generation of the plasmin(ogen)-staphylokinase complex is facilitated, and inhibition of plasmin-staphylokinase by α_2-antiplasmin at the clot surface is delayed. Recycling of staphylokinase to fibrin-bound plasminogen, after neutralization of the complex, will result in more efficient generation of the active complex. This mechanism is mediated via the lysine-binding sites of plasminogen and results in significantly enhanced plasminogen activation at the fibrin surface. These regulatory properties of fibrin and α_2-antiplasmin suggest that the fibrin specificity of staphylokinase is due to rapid inhibition of generated plasmin-staphylokinase complex by α_2-antiplasmin and by a more than 100-fold reduced inhibition rate at the fibrin surface.[482,484]

Recombinant staphylokinase (STAR)[485] was found to have a potency for venous clot lysis in hamsters and rabbits comparable to that of streptokinase. Repeated administration of STAR, in contrast to streptokinase, did not induce resistance to clot lysis in this model. In addition, STAR was found to be significantly more efficient than streptokinase for the dissolution of platelet-rich arterial eversion graft thrombi.[485]

These encouraging results have formed the basis for the evaluation, on a pilot scale, of the pharmacokinetic, thrombolytic, and immunogenic properties of STAR in patients with acute MI.[486] In four of five patients with acute MI, 10 mg of STAR given intravenously over 30 min was found to induce angiographically documented coronary artery recanalization within 40 min. Plasma fibrinogen and α_2-antiplasmin levels were unaffected, and allergic reactions were not observed. In a second series of five patients with acute coronary occlusion, intravenous administration of 10 mg of STAR over 30 min induced recanalization in all patients within 20 min without associated fibrinogen degradation.[190,487] In these patients, however, neutralizing antibodies were consistently demonstrable in plasma at 14 to 35 days. Thus, with respect to immunogenicity, the initial observations in humans are not as encouraging as the experience in baboons. A subsequent trial was conducted in 100 patients with MI of less than 6-h duration who were allocated to accelerated and weight-adjusted t-PA over 90 min (52 patients) or to recombinant staphylokinase (STAR) (the first 25 patients to 10 mg and the next 23 patients to 20 mg given intravenously over 30 min).[488] All patients received aspirin and intravenous heparin. TIMI-3 flow grade at 90 min was achieved in 62 percent of STAR patients compared with 58 percent of t-PA patients (risk ratio = 1.1; 95% CI = 0.76 to 1.5). With 10 mg STAR, TIMI-3 patency was 50 percent (risk ratio = 0.86; 95% CI = 0.54 to 1.4 versus rt-PA); with 20 mg STAR, it was 74 percent (risk ratio = 1.3; 95% CI = 0.90 to 1.2 versus rt-PA). Residual fibrinogen levels at 0 min were 118 ± 47 percent (mean ± SD) of baseline with STAR and 68 ± 42 percent with rt-PA ($p < .0005$). STAR therapy was not associated with an excess mortality rate or electrical, hemorrhagic, mechanical, or allergic complications, but patients developed antibody-mediated STAR-neutralizing activity from week 2 after STAR treatment.

CONCLUSION

Thus, with an understanding of the pathogenesis of and risk of thrombus formation,[489] we can formulate a rational approach to the use of antiplatelet, anticoagulant, and thrombolytic agents.[489–491] Many advances have occurred in the treatment of acute coronary syndromes over the past 75 years.[492,493] In ST-elevation MI, new aggressive thrombolytic regimens improve early reperfusion and improve survival. The current focus is on bolus thrombolysis, the combination of reduced-dose thrombolytic therapy with GP IIb/IIIa inhibitors, and the use of LMW heparin in place of unfractionated heparin. In unstable angina and non-ST-elevation MI, two major advances are GP IIb/IIIa inhibition and LMW heparin. The direct thrombin inhibitors have also shown promise. Following acute coronary syndromes, use of the more potent antiplatelet agent than aspirin, clopidogrel, appears to decrease recurrent ischemic events, whereas disappointing results have come thus far from the oral GP IIb/IIIa inhibitors. With a great number of new thrombolytic and antithrombotic therapies for patients with acute coronary syndromes, it is hoped that their use will continue to improve clinical outcomes in the years ahead.

References

1. Fibrinolytic Therapy Trialists' (FTT) Collaborative Group. Indications for fibrinolytic therapy in suspected acute myocardial infarction: Collaborative overview of early mortality and major morbidity results from all randomised trials of more than 1000 patients. *Lancet* 1994; 343:311–322.
2. DeWood MA, Spores J, Notske R, et al. Prevalence of total coronary occlusion during the early hours of transmural myocardial infarction. *N Engl J Med* 1980; 303:897–902.
3. TIMI Study Group. The Thrombolysis in Myocardial Infarction (TIMI) trial: Phase I findings. *N Engl J Med* 1985; 312:932–936.
4. DeWood MA, Stifter WF, Simpson CS, et al. Coronary arteriographic findings soon after non-Q wave myocardial infarction. *N Engl J Med* 1986; 315:417–423.
5. TIMI IIIA Investigators. Early effects of tissue-type plasminogen activator added to conventional therapy on the culprit lesion in patients presenting with ischemic cardiac pain at rest: Results of the Thrombolysis in Myocardial Ischemia (TIMI IIIA) trial. *Circulation* 1993; 87:38–52.
6. Fuster V, Badimon L, Cohen M, et al. Insights into the pathogenesis of acute ischemic syndromes. *Circulation* 1988; 77:1213–1220.
7. Fuster V, Badimon L, Badimon JJ, Chesebro JH. The pathophysiology of coronary artery disease and the acute coronary syndromes. *N Engl J Med* 1992; 326:242–250 and 310–318.
8. Vita JA, Treasure CB, Nabel EG, et al. Coronary vasomotor response to acetylcholine relates to risk factors for coronary artery disease. *Circulation* 1990; 81:491–497.
9. Libby P. Molecular bases of the acute coronary syndromes. *Circulation* 1995; 91:2844–2850.
10. Ambrose JA, Winters SL, Arora RR, et al. Angiographic evolution of coronary artery morphology in unstable angina. *J Am Coll Cardiol* 1986; 7:472–478.
11. Little WC, Constantinescu M, Applegate RJ, et al. Can coronary angiography predict the site of a subsequent myocardial infarction in patients with mild-to-moderate coronary artery disease? *Circulation* 1988; 78:1157–1166.
12. Chester MR, Chen L, Kaski JC. Angiographic evidence for frequent "silent" plaque disruption in patients with stable angina (abstr). *J Am Coll Cardiol* 1995; 428A (special issue).
13. Webster MWI, Chesebro JH, Smith HC, et al. Myocardial infarction and coronary artery occlusion: A prospective 5-year angiographic study (abstr). *J Am Coll Cardiol* 1990; 15:218A.
14. Mann JM, Davies MJ. Vulnerable plaque: Relation of characteristics to degree of stenosis in human coronary arteries. *Circulation* 1996; 94:928–931.
15. Lee RT, Libby P. The unstable atheroma. *Arterioscler Thromb Vasc Biol* 1997;17:1859–1867.
16. Moreno PR, Bernardi VH, Lopez-Cuellar J, et al. Macrophages, smooth muscle cells, and tissue factor in unstable angina: Implications for cell-mediated thrombogenicity in acute coronary syndromes. *Circulation* 1996; 94:3090–3097.
17. Weiss EJ, Bray PF, Tayback M, et al. A polymorphism of a platelet glycoprotein receptor as an inherited risk factor for coronary thrombosis. *N Engl J Med* 1996; 334:1090–1094.
18. Ault K, Cannon CP, Mitchell J, et al. Platelet activation in patients after an acute coronary: Results from the TIMI 12 trial. *J Am Coll Cardiol* 1999; 33:634–639.
19. Merlini PA, Bauer KA, Oltrona L, et al. Presistent activation of coagulation mechanism in unstable angina and myocardial infarction. *Circulation* 1994; 90:61–68.
20. Rosenberg RD, Aird WC. Vascular-bed: Specific hemostasis and hypercoagulable states. *N Engl J Med* 1990; 340:1555–1564.
21. Falk E. Unstable angina with fatal outcome: Dynamic coronary thrombosis leading to infarction and/or sudden death. *Circulation* 1985; 71:699–708.
22. Davies MJ, Thomas A. Plaque fissuring: The cause of acute myocardial infarction, sudden ischemic death, and crescendo angina. *Br Heart J* 1985; 53:363–373.
23. Shah PK, Falk E, Badimon JJ, et al. Human monocyte-derived macrophages induce collagen breakdown in fibrous caps of atherosclerotic plaques: Potential role of matrix-degrading metalloproteinases and implications for plaque rupture. *Circulation* 1998; 92:1565–1569.
24. Falk E, Shah PK, Fuster V. Coronary plaque disruption. *Circulation* 1995; 92:657–671.
25. Davies MJ. Acute coronary thrombosis: The role of plaque disruption and its initiation and prevention. *Eur Heart J* 1995; 16(suppl L):3–7.
26. Ambrose JA, Tannenbaum MA, Alexopoulos D, et al. Angiographic progression of coronary artery disease and the development of myocardial infarction. *J Am Coll Cardiol* 1988; 12:56–62.
27. Fuster V, Badimon L, Badimon JJ, Chesebro JH. The pathogenesis of coronary artery disease and the acute coronary syndromes (1). *N Engl J Med* 1992; 326:242–250.
28. Fuster V, Badimon L, Badimon JJ, Chesebro JH. The pathogenesis of coronary artery disease and the acute coronary syndromes (2). *N Engl J Med* 1992; 326:310–318.
29. Califf R, Willerson J. Percutaneous transluminal angioplasty: Prevention of occlusion and restenosis. In: Fuster V, Verstraete M, eds. *Thrombosis in Cardiovascular Disorders*. Philadelphia: WB Saunders; 1992:389–408.
30. Fuster V, Chesebro JH. Role of platelets and platelet inhibitors

in aortocoronary artery vein-graft disease. *Circulation* 1986; 73:227–232.
31. Ross R. Atherosclerosis: An inflammatory disease. *N Engl J Med* 1999; 340:115–126.
32. Kovanen PT, Kaartinen M, Paavonen T. Infiltrates of activated mast cells at the site of coronary atheromatous erosion or rupture in myocardial infarction. *Circulation* 1995; 92:1084–1088.
33. Richardson PD, Davies MJ, Born GV. Influence of plaque configuration and stress distribution on fissuring of coronary atherosclerotic plaques. *Lancet* 1989; 2:941–944.
34. Moreno PR, Falk E, Palacios IF, et al. Macrophage infiltration in acute coronary syndromes: Implications for plaque rupture. *Circulation* 1994; 90:775–778.
35. Sukhova GK, Schonbeck U, Rabkin E, et al. Evidence for increased collagenolysis by interstitial collagenases-1 and -3 in vulnerable human atheromatous plaques. *Circulation* 1999; 99:2503–2509.
36. Liuzzo G, Kopecky SL, Frye RL, et al. Perturbation of the T-cell repertoire in patients with unstable angina. *Circulation* 1999; 100:2135–2139.
37. Liuzzo G, Biasucci LM, Gallimore JR, et al. The prognostic value of C-reactive protein and serum amyloid A protein in severe unstable angina. *N Engl J Med* 1994; 331:417–424.
38. Toss H, Lindahl B, Siegbahn A, Wallentin L, for the FRISC Study Group. Prognostic influence of increased fibrinogen and C-reactive protein levels in unstable coronary artery disease. *Circulation* 1997; 96:4204–4210.
39. Morrow DA, Rifai N, Antman EM, et al. C-reactive protein is a potent predictor of mortality independently and in combination with troponin T in acute coronary syndromes: A TIMI 11A substudy. *J Am Coll Cardiol* 1998; 31:1460–1465.
40. Benamer H, Steg PG, Benessiano J, et al. Comparison of the prognostic value of C-reactive protein and troponin I in patients with unstable angina pectoris. *Am J Cardiol* 1998; 82:845–850.
41. Ferreiros ER, Boissonnet CP, Pizarro R, et al. Independent prognostic value of elevated C-reactive protein in unstable angina. *Circulation* 1999; 100:1958–1963.
42. Morrow DA, Rifai N, Antman EM, et al. Serum amyloid A predicts early mortality in acute coronary syndromes: A TIMI 11A study. *J Am Coll Cardiol* 2000; 35:358–362.
43. Farb A, Burke AP, Tang AL, et al. Coronary plaque erosion without rupture into a lipid core: A frequent cause of coronary thrombosis in sudden coronary death. *Circulation* 1996; 93:1354–1363.
44. Escaned J, Van Suylen RJ, MacLeod DC, et al. Histologic characteristics of tissue excised during directional coronary atherectomy in stable and unstable angina pectoris. *Am J Cardiol* 1993; 71:1442–1447.
45. Sullivan E, Kearney M, Isner JM, et al. Pathology of unstable angina: Analysis of biopsies obtained by directional coronary atherectomy. *J Thromb Thrombolysis* 1994; 1:63–71.
46. Arbustini E, De Servi S, Bramucci E, et al. Comparison of coronary lesions obtained by directional coronary atherectomy in unstable angina, stable angina, and restenosis after either atherectomy or angioplasty. *Am J Cardiol* 1995; 75:675–682.
47. Harrington RA, Califf RM, Holmes DR Jr, et al. Is all unstable angina the same? Insights from the Coronary Angioplasty Versus Excisional Atherectomy Trial (CAVEAT-I). *Am Heart J* 1999; 137:227–233.
48. Sherman CT, Litvack F, Grundfest W, et al. Coronary angioscopy in patients with unstable angina pectoris. *N Engl J Med* 1986; 315:913–919.
49. Uchida Y, Fujimori Y, Hirose J, Oshima T. Percutaneous coronary angioscopy. *Jpn Heart J* 1992; 33:271–294.
50. Mizuno K, Satumo K, Miyamoto A, et al. Angioscopic evaluation of coronary artery thrombi in acute coronary syndromes. *N Engl J Med* 1992; 326:287–291.
51. De Feyter PJ, Ozaki Y, Baptista J, et al. Ischemia-related lesion characteristics in patients with stable or unstable angina: A study with intracoronary angioscopy and ultrasound. *Circulation* 1995; 92:1408–1413.
52. Silva JA, White CJ, Collins TJ, Ramee SR. Morphologic comparison of atherosclerotic lesions in native coronary arteries and saphenous vein graphs with intracoronary angioscopy in patients with unstable angina. *Am Heart J* 1998; 136:156–163.
53. Nesto RW, Waxman S, Mittleman MA, et al. Angioscopy of culprit coronary lesions in unstable angina pectoris and correlation of clinical presentation with plaque morphology. *Am J Cardiol* 1998; 81:225–228.
54. Van Belle E, Lablanche J-M, Bauters C, et al. Coronary angioscopic findings in the infarct-related vessel within 1 month of acute myocardial infarction: Natural history and the effect of thrombolysis. *Circulation* 1998; 97:26–33.
55. Ambrose JA, Hjemdahl-Monsen CE, Borrico S, et al. Angiographic demonstration of a common link between unstable angina and non-Q-wave myocardial infarction. *Am J Cardiol* 1988; 61:244–247.
56. Brunelli C, Spallarossa P, Ghigliotta G, et al. Thrombosis in refractory unstable angina. *Am J Cardiol* 1991; 68:110B–118B.
57. Fitzgerald DJ, Roy L, Catella F, Fitzgerald GA. Platelet activation in unstable coronary disease. *N Engl J Med* 1986; 315:983–989.
58. Theroux P, Latour JG, Leger-Gautier C, Delaria J. Fibrinopeptide A and platelet factor four levels in unstable angina. *Circulation* 1987; 75:156–162.
59. Robertson RM, Robertson D, Roberts LJ, et al. Thromboxane A_2 in vasotonic angina pectoris. *N Engl J Med* 1981; 304:998–1003.
60. Alexopoloulos D, Ambrose JA, Stump D, et al. Thrombosis-related markers in unstable angina. *J Am Coll Cardiol* 1991; 17:866–871.
61. Hirsch PD, Hillis LD, Campbell WB, et al. Release of prostaglandins and thromboxane into the coronary circulation in patients with ischemic heart disease. *N Engl J Med* 1981; 304:685–691.
62. Van der Berg EK, Schmitz JM, Benedict CR, et al. Transcardiac serotonin concentration is increased in selected patients with limiting angina complex coronary lesion morphology. *Circulation* 1989; 79:116–124.
63. Willerson JT, Golino P, Eidt J, et al. Specific platelet mediators and unstable coronary artery lesions: Experimental evidence and potential clinical implications. *Circulation* 1989; 80:198–205.
64. Becker RC, Tracy RP, Bovill EG, et al. for the TIMI-III Thrombosis and Anticoagulation Study Group. The clinical use of flow cytometry for assessing platelet activation in acute coronary syndromes. *Coron Artery Dis* 1994; 5:339–345.
65. Lewis HD, Davis JW, Archibald DG, et al. Protective effects of aspirin against acute myocardial infarction and death in men with unstable angina. *N Engl J Med* 1983; 309:396–403.
66. Cairns JA, Gent M, Singer J, et al. Aspirin, sulfinpyrazone, or both in unstable angina. *N Engl J Med* 1985; 313:1369–1375.
67. Theroux P, Ouimet H, McCans J, et al. Aspirin, heparin or both to treat unstable angina. *N Engl J Med* 1988; 319:1105–1111.
68. RISC Group. Risk of myocardial infarction and death during treatment with low dose aspirin and intravenous heparin in men with unstable coronary artery disease. *Lancet* 1990; 336:827–830.
69. Theroux P, Waters D, Qiu S, et al. Aspirin versus heparin to prevent myocardial infarction during the acute phase of unstable angina. *Circulation* 1993; 88:2045–2048.
70. Cohen M, Adams PC, Parry G, et al. Combination antithrombotic therapy in unstable rest angina and non-Q-wave infarction in nonprior aspirin users: Primary end points analysis from the ATACS trial. *Circulation* 1994; 89:81–88.
71. Oler A, Whooley MA, Oler J, Grady D. Adding heparin to

aspirin reduces the incidence of myocardial infarction and death in patients with unstable angina: A meta-analysis. *JAMA* 1996; 276:811–815.

72. Fragmin During Instability in Coronary Artery Disease (FRISC) Study Group. Low-molecular-weight heparin during instability in coronary artery disease. *Lancet* 1996; 347:561–568.
73. Cohen M, Demers C, Gurfinkel EP, et al. A comparison of low-molecular-weight heparin with unfractionated heparin for unstable coronary artery disease. *N Engl J Med* 1997; 337:447–452.
74. Antman EM, Cohen M, Radley D, et al. Assessment of the treatment effect of enoxaparin for unstable angina/non-Q-wave myocardial infarction: TIMI 11B-ESSENCE meta-analysis. *Circulation* 1999; 100:1602–1608.
75. Antman EM, McCabe CH, Gurfinkel EP, et al. Enoxaparin prevents death and cardiac ischemic events in unstable angina/non-Q-wave myocardial infarction: Results of the Thrombolysis in Myocardial Infarction (TIMI) 11B trial. *Circulation* 1999; 100: 1593–1601.
76. PURSUIT Trial Investigators. Inhibition of platelet glycoprotein IIb/IIIa with eptifibatide in patients with acute coronary syndromes. *N Engl J Med* 1998; 339:436–443.
77. Platelet Receptor Inhibition for Ischemic Syndrome Management (PRISM) Study Investigators. A comparison of aspirin plus tirofiban with aspirin plus heparin for unstable angina. *N Engl J Med* 1998; 338:1498–1505.
78. Platelet Receptor Inhibition for Ischemic Syndrome Management in Patients Limited by Unstable Signs and Symptoms (PRISM-PLUS) Trial Investigators. Inhibition of the platelet glycoprotein IIb/IIIa receptor with tirofiban in unstable angina and non-Q-wave myocardial infarction. *N Engl J Med* 1998; 338:1488–1497.
79. Van der Wal AC, Becker AE, Van der Loos CM, Das PK. Site of intimal rupture or erosion of thrombosed coronary atherosclerotic plaques is characterized by an inflammatory process irrespective of the dominant plaque morphology. *Circulation* 1994; 89:36–44.
80. Shah PK, Falk E, Badimon JJ, et al. Human monocyte-derived macrophages induce collagen breakdown in fibrous caps of atherosclerotic plaques: Potential role of matrix-degrading metalloproteinases and implications for plaque rupture. *Circulation* 1995; 92:1565–1569.
81. Xu XP, Meisel SR, Ong JM, et al. Oxidized low-density lipoprotein regulates matrix metalloproteinase-9 and its tissue inhibitor in human monocyte-derived macrophages. *Circulation* 1999; 99: 993–998.
82. Ridker PM, Cushman M, Stampfer MJ, et al. Inflammation, aspirin, and the risk of cardiovascular disease in apparently healthy men. *N Engl J Med* 1997; 336:973–979.
83. Anderson JL, Carlquist JF, Muhlestein JB, et al. Evaluation of C-reactive protein, an inflammatory marker, and infectious serology as risk factors for coronary artery disease and myocardial infarction. *J Am Coll Cardiol* 1998; 32:35–41.
84. Berk BC, Weintraub WS, Alexander RW. Elevation of C-reactive protein in "active" coronary artery disease. *Am J Cardiol* 1990; 65:168–172.
85. Haverkate F, Thompson SG, Pyke SDM, et al. for the European Concerted Action on Thrombosis and Disabilities Angina Pectoris Study Group. Production of C-reactive protein and risk of coronary events in stable and unstable angina. *Lancet* 1997; 349:462–466.
86. Danesh J, Collins R, Peto R. Chronic infection and coronary heart disease: Is there a link? *Lancet* 1997; 350:430–436.
87. Libby P, Egan D, Skarlatos S. Roles of infectious agents in atherosclerosis and restenosis: An assessment of the evidence and need for future research. *Circulation* 1997; 96:4095–4103.
88. Toss H, Gnarpe J, Gnarpe H, et al. Increased fibrinogen levels are associated with persistent *Chlamydia pneumoniae* infection in unstable coronary artery disease. *Eur Heart J* 1998; 19: 570–577.
89. Nobel M, De Torrente A, Peter O, Genne D. No serological evidence of association between chlamydia pneumonia infection and acute coronary heart disease. *Scand J Infect Dis* 1999; 31:261–264.
90. Ridker PM, Kundsin RB, Stampfer MJ, et al. Prospective study of *Chlamydia pneumoniae* IgG seropositivity and risks of future myocardial infarction. *Circulation* 1999; 99:1161–1164.
91. Fong IW, Chiu B, Viira E, et al. Rabbit model for *Chlamydia pneumoniae* infection. *J Clin Microbiol* 1997; 35:48–52.
92. Moazed TC, Kuo C, Grayston JT, Campbell LA. Murine models of *Chlamydia pneumoniae* infection and atherosclerosis. *J Infect Dis* 1997; 175:883–890.
93. Muhlestein JB, Anderson JL, Hammond EH, et al. Infection with *Chlamydia pneumoniae* accelerates the development of atherosclerosis and treatment with azithromycin prevents it in a rabbit model. *Circulation* 1998; 97:633–636.
94. Moazed TC, Campbell LA, Rosenfeld ME, et al. *Chlamydia pneumoniae* infection accelerates the progression of atherosclerosis in apolipoprotein E-deficient mice. *J Infect Dis* 1999; 180: 238–241.
95. Gurfinkel E, Bozovich G, Daroca A, et al., for the ROXIS Study Group. Randomised trial of roxithromycin in non-Q wave coronary syndromes: ROXIS pilot study. *Lancet* 1997; 350: 404–407.
96. Gupta S, Leathan EW, Carrington D, et al. Elevated *Chlamydia pneumoniae* antibodies, cardiovascular events, and azithromycin in male survivors of myocardial infarction. *Circulation* 1997; 96:404–407.
97. Anderson JL, Muhlestein JB, Carlquist J, et al. Randomized secondary prevention trial of azithromycin in patients with coronary artery disease and serological evidence for *Chlamydia pneumoniae* infection: The Azithromycin in Coronary Artery Disease—Elimination of Myocardial Infection with Chlamydia (ACADEMIC) study. *Circulation* 1999; 99:1540–1547.
98. Fuster V. Mechanisms leading to myocardial infarction: Insights from studies of vascular biology. *Circulation* 1994; 90:2126–2146 [published erratum appears in *Circulation* 1995; 91:256].
99. Fernandez-Ortiz A, Badimon JJ, Falk E, et al. Characterization of the relative thrombogenicity of atherosclerotic plaque components: Implications for consequences of plaque rupture. *J Am Coll Cardiol* 1994; 23:1562–1569.
100. Banner DW, D'Arcy A, Chene C, et al. The crystal structure of the complex of blood coagulation factor VIIa with soluble tissue factor. *Nature* 1996; 380:41–46.
101. Badimon JJ, Lettino M, Toschi V, et al. Local inhibition of tissue factor reduces the thrombogenicity of disrupted human atherosclerotic plaques: Effects of tissue factor pathway inhibitor on plaque thrombogenicity under flow conditions. *Circulation* 1999; 99:1780–1787.
102. Giesen PL, Rauch U, Bohrmann B, et al. Blood-borne tissue factor: Another view of thrombosis. *Proc Natl Acad Sci USA* 1999; 96:2311–2315.
103. Ridker PM. Evaluating novel cardiovascular risk factors: Can we better predict heart attacks? *Ann Intern Med* 1999; 130:933–937.
104. Koenig W, Sund M, Frohlich M, et al. C-reactive protein, a sensitive marker of inflammation, predicts future risk of coronary heart disease in initially healthy middle-aged men: Results from the MONICA (Monitoring Trends and Determinants in Cardiovascular Disease) Augsburg Cohort study, 1984 to 1992. *Circulation* 1999; 99:237–242.
105. Biasucci LM, Liuzzo G, Grillo RL, et al. Elevated levels of C-reactive protein at discharge in patients with unstable angina predict recurrent instability. *Circulation* 1999; 99:855–860.

106. Dangas G, Badimon JJ, Smith DA, et al. Pravastatin therapy in hyperlipidemia: Effects on thrombus formation and the systemic hemostatic profile. *J Am Coll Cardiol* 1999; 33:1294–1304.
107. Ridker PM, Vaughan DE, Stampfer MJ, et al. Endogenous tissue-type plasminogen activator and risk of myocardial infarction. *Lancet* 1993; 341:1165–1168.
108. Hamsten A, Wiman B, De Faire U, Blomback M. Increased plasma levels of a rapid inhibitor of tissue plasminogen activator in young survivors of myocardial infarction. *N Engl J Med* 1985; 313:1557–1563.
109. Maseri A, l'Abbate A, Baroldi G, et al. Coronary vasospasm as a possible cause of myocardial infarction: A conclusion derived from the study of "preinfarction" angina. *N Engl J Med* 1978; 299:1271–1277.
110. Bogaty P, Hackett D, Davies G, Maseri A. Vasoreactivity of the culprit lesion in unstable angina. *Circulation* 1994; 90:5–11.
111. Colman RW, Marder VJ, Salzman EW, Hirsh J. Overview of hemostasis. In: Colman RW, Hirsh J, Marder VJ, Salzman EW, eds. *Hemostasis and Thrombosis: Basic Principles and Clinical Practice*, 3rd ed. Philadelphia: JB Lippincott; 1994:3.
112. Handin RI, Loscalzo J. Hemostasis, thrombosis, fibrinolysis, and cardiovascular disease. In: Braunwald E, ed. *Heart Disease*, 4th ed. Philadelphia: WB Saunders; 1992:1767.
113. Verstraete M. Biology and chemistry of thrombosis. In: Haber E, Braunwald E, eds. *Thrombolysis: Basic Contributions and Clinical Progress*, vol 1. St Louis: CV Mosby Year Book; 1991:3.
114. Lefkovits J, Plow EF, Topol EJ. Platelet glycoprotein IIb/IIIa receptors in cardiovascular medicine. *N Engl J Med* 1995; 332:1553–1559.
115. Broze GJ Jr. The role of tissue factor pathway inhibitor in a revised coagulation cascade. *Semin Hematol* 1992; 29:159–169.
116. Osterud B, Rapaport S. Activation of factor IX of the reaction product of tissue factor and factor VII: Additional pathway for initiating blood coagulation. *Proc Natl Acad Sci USA* 1977; 74:5260–5264.
117. Furie B, Furie BC. Molecular and cellular biology of blood coagulation. *N Engl J Med* 1992; 326:800–806.
118. Vane JR, Anggard EE, Botting RM. Regulatory functions of the vascular endothelium. *N Engl J Med* 1990; 323:27–36.
119. Jaffe EA. Endothelial cell structure and function. In: Hoffmann R, Benz EJ, Shattil SJ, et al, eds. *Hematology: Basic Principles and Practice*. New York: Churchill Livingstone; 1991:1198.
120. Furchgott RF, Vanhoutte PM. Endothelium-derived relaxing and contracting factors. *FASEB J* 1989; 3:2007–2018.
121. Esmon CT. The roles of protein C and thrombomodulin in the regulation of blood coagulation. *J Biol Chem* 1989; 264:4743–4746.
122. Harker LA. Pathogenesis of thrombosis. In: Williams J, ed. *Hematology*, 4th ed. New York: McGraw-Hill; 1990:1559.
123. Ruoslahti E. Integrins. *J Clin Invest* 1991; 87:1–5.
124. Kieffer N, Phillips DR. Platelet membrane glycoproteins: Functions in cellular interactions. *Annu Rev Cell Biol* 1990; 6:329–357.
125. Lapetina EG. The signal transduction induced by thrombin in human platelets. *FEBS Lett* 1990; 268:400–404.
126. Rhee SG. Inositol phospholipid-specific phospholipase C: Interaction of the gamma 1 isoform with tyrosine kinase. *Trends Biochem Sci* 1991; 16:297–301.
127. Turitto VT, Baumgartner HR. Initial deposition of platelets and fibrin on vascular surfaces in flowing blood. In: Colman RW, Hirsh J, Marder VJ, Salzman EW, eds. *Hemostasis and Thrombosis: Basic Principles and Clinical Practice*, 3rd ed. Philadelphia: JB Lippincott; 1994:805.
128. Edgington TS, Mackman N, Brand K, Ruf W. The structural biology of expression and function of tissue factor. *Thromb Haemost* 1991; 66:67–79.
129. Rapaport SI, Rao LV. The tissue factor pathway: How it has become a "prima ballerina." *Thromb Haemost* 1995; 74:7–17.
130. Davie EW. Biochemical and molecular aspects of the coagulation cascade. *Thromb Haemost* 1995; 74:1–6.
131. Mann KG, Jenny RJ, Krishnaswamy S. Cofactor proteins in the assembly and expression of blood clotting enzyme complexes. *Annu Rev Biochem* 1988; 57:915–956.
132. Gilbert GE, Furie BC, Furie B. Binding of human factor VIII to phospholipid vesicles. *J Biol Chem* 1990; 265:815–822.
133. Mosesson MW. Fibrin polymerization and its regulatory role in hemostasis. *J Lab Clin Med* 1990; 116:8–117.
134. Hogg PJ, Jackson CM. Fibrin monomer protects thrombin from inactivation by heparin-antithrombin III: Implications for heparin efficacy. *Proc Natl Acad Sci USA* 1989; 86:3619–3623.
135. Harker LA, Mann KG. Thrombosis and fibrinolysis. In: Fuster V, Verstraete M, eds. *Thrombosis in Cardiovascular Disorders*. Philadelphia: WB Saunders; 1994:837.
136. Rosenberg RD, Bauer KA. The heparin-antithrombin system: A natural anticoagulant mechanism. In: Colman RW, Hirsh J, Marder VJ, Salzman EW, eds. *Hemostasis and Thrombosis: Basic Principles and Clinical Practice*. Philadelphia: JB Lippincott; 1994:837.
137. Dahlback B. Protein S and C4b-binding protein: Components involved in the regulation of the protein C anticoagulant system. *Thromb Haemost* 1991; 66:49–61.
138. Rapaport SI. The extrinsic pathway inhibitor: A regulator of tissue factor–dependent blood coagulation. *Thromb Haemost* 1991; 66:6–15.
139. Collen D. On the regulation and control of fibrinolysis: Edward Kowalski Memorial Lecture. *Thromb Haemost* 1980; 43:77–89.
140. Plow EF, Felez J, Miles LA. Cellular regulation of fibrinolysis. *Thromb Haemost* 1991; 66:32–36.
141. Thorsen S. The mechanism of plasminogen activation and the variability of the fibrin effector during tissue-type plasminogen activator–mediated fibrinolysis. *Ann NY Acad Sci* 1992; 667: 52–63.
142. Pennica D, Holmes WE, Kohr WJ, et al. Cloning and expression of human tissue-type plasminogen activator cDNA in *E. coli*. *Nature* 1983; 301:214–221.
143. Blasi F. Urokinase and urokinase receptor: A paracrine/autocrine system regulating cell migration and invasiveness. *Bioessays* 1993; 15:105–111.
144. Bachmann F. The plasminogen-plasmin enzyme system. In: Colman RW, Hirsh J, Marder VJ, Salzman EW, eds. *Hemostasis and Thrombosis: Basic Principles and Clinical Practice*, 3rd ed. Philadelphia: JB Lippincott; 1994:1592.
145. Huber R, Carrel RW. Implications of the three-dimensional structure of alpha 1-antitrypsin for structure and function of serpins. *Biochemistry* 1989; 28:8951–8966.
146. Sumi Y, Ichikawa Y, Nakamura Y, et al. Expression and characterization of pro alpha 2-plasmin inhibitor. *J Biochem (Tokyo)* 1989; 106:703–707.
147. Pannekoek H, Veerman H, Lambers H, et al. Endothelial plasminogen activator inhibitor (PAI): A new member of the Serpin gene family. *EMBO J* 1986; 5:2539–2544.
148. Kruithof EK, Vassalli JD, Schleuning WD, et al. Purification and characterization of a plasminogen activator inhibitor from the histiocytic lymphoma cell line U-937. *J Biol Chem* 1986; 261:11,207–11,213.
149. Bachmann F. The enigma PAI-2: Gene expression, evolutionary and functional aspects. *Thromb Haemost* 1995; 74:172–179.
150. Van Hinsbergh VW, Kooistra T, Emeis JJ, Koolwijk P. Regulation of plasminogen activator production by endothelial cells: Role in fibrinolysis and local proteolysis. *Int J Radiat Biol* 1991; 60:261–272.
151. Chandler WL, Levy WC, Veith RC, Stratton JR. A kinetic model of the circulatory regulation of tissue plasminogen activa-

tor during exercise, epinephrine infusion, and endurance training. *Blood* 1993; 81:3293–3302.
152. Collen D, Lijnen HR. Molecular basis of fibrinolysis, as relevant for thrombolytic therapy. *Thromb Haemost* 1995; 74:167–171.
153. Lijnen HR, Collen D. Regulation of the fibrinolytic system. In: Agnelli G, ed. *Year Book on Thrombolytic Therapy*. Amsterdam: Excerpta Medica; 1995:1.
154. Jaklitsch MT, Biro S, Casscells W, Dichek DA. Transduced endothelial cells expressing high levels of tissue plasminogen activator have an unaltered phenotype in vitro. *J Cell Physiol* 1993; 154:207–216.
155. Loskutoff DJ. Regulation of PAI-1 gene expression. *Fibrinolysis* 1991; 5:197–206.
156. Mayer EJ, Fujita T, Gardell SJ, et al. The pharmacokinetics of plasminogen activator inhibitor-1 in the rabbit. *Blood* 1990; 76:1514–1520.
157. Racanelli AL, Diemer MJ, Dobies AC, et al. Distribution and pharmacokinetics of active recombinant plasminogen activator inhibitor-1 in the rat and rabbit. *Fibrinolysis* 1992; 6:187–191.
158. Wiman B. Plasminogen activator inhibitor 1 (PAI-1) in plasma: Its role in thrombotic disease. *Thromb Haemost* 1995; 74:71–76.
159. Sawa H, Fujii S, Sobel BE. Augmented arterial wall expression of type-1 plasminogen activator inhibitor induced by thrombosis. *Arterioscler Thromb* 1992; 12:1507–1515.
160. Hajjar KA. Cellular receptors in the regulation of plasmin generation. *Thromb Haemost* 1995; 74:294–301.
161. Kruithof EK. Plasminogen activator inhibitors: A review. *Enzyme* 1988; 40:113–121.
162. Thorsen S, Philips M, Selmer J, et al. Kinetics of inhibition of tissue-type and urokinase-type plasminogen activator by plasminogen-activator inhibitor type 1 and type 2. *Eur J Biochem* 1988; 175:33–39.
163. Reilly CF, Hutzelmann JE. Plasminogen activator inhibitor-1 binds to fibrin and inhibits tissue-type plasminogen activator–mediated fibrin dissolution. *J Biol Chem* 1992; 267:17,128–17,135.
164. Declerck PJ, De Mol M, Vaughan DE, Collen D. Identification of a conformationally distinct form of plasminogen activator inhibitor-1, acting as a noninhibitory substrate for tissue-type plasminogen activator. *J Biol Chem* 1992; 267:11,693–11,696.
165. Suenson E, Bjerrum P, Holm A, et al. The role of fragment X polymers in the fibrin enhancement of tissue plasminogen activator–catalyzed plasmin formation. *J Biol Chem* 1990; 265: 22,228–22,237.
166. Hoylaerts M, Rijken DC, Lijnen HR, Collen D. Kinetics of the activation of plasminogen by human tissue plasminogen activator: Role of fibrin. *J Biol Chem* 1982; 257:2912–2919.
167. Andreasen PA, Petersen LC, Dan K. Diversity in catalytic properties of single chain and two chain tissue-type plasminogen activator. *Fibrinolysis* 1991; 5:207–215.
168. Harpel PC, Gordon BR, Parker TS. Plasmin catalyzes binding of lipoprotein (a) to immobilized fibrinogen and fibrin. *Proc Natl Acad Sci USA* 1989; 86:3847–3851.
169. Loscalzo J, Weinfeld M, Fless GM, Scanu AM. Lipoprotein(a), fibrin binding, and plasminogen activation. *Arteriosclerosis* 1990; 10:240–245.
170. Edelberg JM, Gonzalez-Gronow M, Pizzo SV. Lipoprotein(a) inhibition of plasminogen activation by tissue-type plasminogen activator. *Thromb Res* 1990; 57:155–162.
171. Juhan-Vague I, Alessi MC. Plasminogen activator inhibitor 1 and atherothrombosis. *Thromb Haemost* 1993; 70:138–143.
172. Prins MH, Hirsh J. A critical review of the relationship between impaired fibrinolysis and myocardial infarction. *Am Heart J* 1991; 122:545–551.
173. Jansson JH, Nilsson TK, Johnson O. Von Willebrand factor in plasma: A novel risk factor for recurrent myocardial infarction and death [see Comments]. *Br Heart J* 1991; 66:351–355.
174. Juhan-Vague I, Thompson SG, Jespersen J. Involvement of the hemostatic system in the insulin resistance syndrome: A study of 1500 patients with angina pectoris. The ECAT Angina Pectoris Study Group. *Arterioscler Thromb* 1993; 13:1865–1873.
175. Patrono C. Aspirin as an antiplatelet drug. *N Engl J Med* 1994; 330:1287–1294.
176. Clowes AW. Prevention and management of recurrent disease after arterial reconstruction: New prospects for pharmacological control. *Thromb Haemost* 1991; 66:62–66.
177. Szczeklik A. Thrombin generation in myocardial infarction and hypercholesterolemia: Effects of aspirin. *Thromb Haemost* 1995; 74:77–80.
178. Meade EA, Smith WL, DeWitt DL. Differential inhibition of prostaglandin endoperoxide synthase (cyclooxygenase) isozymes by aspirin and other non-steroidal anti-inflammatory drugs. *J Biol Chem* 1993; 268:6610–6614.
179. Marcus AJ, Safier LB, Broekman MJ, et al. Thrombosis and inflammation as multicellular processes: Significance of cell-cell interactions. *Thromb Haemost* 1995; 74:213–217.
180. ISIS-2 (Second International Study of Infarct Survival) Collaborative Group. Randomised trial of intravenous streptokinase, oral aspirin, both, or neither among 17,187 cases of suspected acute myocardial infarction: ISIS-2. *Lancet* 1988; 2:349–360.
181. CAPRIE Steering Committee. A randomised, blinded, trial of clopidogrel versus aspirin in patients at risk of ischaemic events (CAPRIE). *Lancet* 1996; 348:1329–1339.
182. Roux S, Christeller S, Ludin E. Effects of aspirin on coronary reocclusion and recurrent ischemia after thrombolysis: A meta-analysis. *J Am Coll Cardiol* 1992; 19:671–677.
183. Klimt CR, Knatterud GL, Stamler J, Meier P, for the PARIS II Investigator Group. Persantine-Aspirin Reinfarction Study: Part II. Secondary coronary prevention with persantine and aspirin. *J Am Coll Cardiol* 1986; 7:251–269.
184. Antiplatelet Trialist' Collaboration. Collaborative overview of randomised trials of antiplatelet therapy: I. Prevention of death, myocardial infarction and stroke by prolonged antiplatelet therapy in various categories of patients. *BMJ* 1994; 308:81–106.
185. Schwartz L, Bourassa MG, Lesperance J, et al. Aspirin and dipyridamole in the prevention of restenosis after percutaneous transluminal coronary angioplasty. *N Engl J Med* 1988; 318:1714–1719.
186. Goldman S, Copeland J, Moritz T, et al. Improvement in early saphenous vein graft patency after coronary artery bypass surgery with antiplatelet therapy: Results of a Veterans Administration cooperative study. *Circulation* 1988; 77:1324–1332.
187. Steering Committee of the Physicians' Health Study Research Group. Final report on the aspirin component of the ongoing Physicians' Health Study. *N Engl J Med* 1989; 321:129–135.
188. Peto R, Gray R, Collins R, et al. Randomised trial of prophylactic daily aspirin in British male doctors. *BMJ* 1988; 296:313–316.
189. Ryan TJ, Anderson JL, Antman EM, et al. ACC/AHA guidelines for the management of patients with acute myocardial infarction: A report of the American College of Cardiology/American Heart Association Task Force on Practice Guidelines (Committee on Management of Acute Myocardial Infarction). *J Am Coll Cardiol* 1996; 28:1328–1428.
190. Braunwald E, Mark DB, Jones RH, et al. *Unstable Angina: Diagnosis and Management. Clinical Practice Guideline Number 10*. Rockville, MD: Agency for Health Care Policy and Research and the National Heart, Lung, and Blood Institute, Public Health Service, US Department of Health and Human Services; 1994.
191. Mills DC, Puri R, Hu CJ, et al. Clopidogrel inhibits the binding of ADP analogues to the receptor mediating inhibition of platelet adenylate cyclase. *Arterioscler Thromb* 1992; 12:430–436.
192. Hardisty RM, Powling MJ, Nokes TJ. The action of ticlopidine on human platelets: Studies on aggregation, secretion, calcium

mobilization and membrane glycoproteins. *Thromb Haemost* 1990; 64:150–155.
193. Humbert M, Nurden P, Bihour C, et al. Ultrastructural studies of platelet aggregates from human subjects receiving clopidogrel and from a patient with an inherited defect of an ADP-dependent pathway of platelet activation. *Arterioscler Thromb Vasc Biol* 1996; 16:1532–1543.
194. Schafer AI. Antiplatelet therapy. *Am J Med* 1996; 101:199–209.
195. Sharis PJ, Cannon CP, Loscalzo J. The antiplatelet effects of ticlopidine and clopidogrel. *Ann Intern Med* 1998; 129:394–405.
196. Gachet C, Stierle A, Cazenave JP, et al. The thienopyridine PCR 4099 selectively inhibits ADP-induced platelet aggregation and fibrinogen binding without modifying the membrane glycoprotein IIb-IIIa complex in rat and in man. *Biochem Pharmacol* 1990; 40:229–238.
197. DiMinno G, Cerbone AM, Mattioli PL, et al. Functionally thrombasthenic state in normal platelets following administration of ticlopidine. *J Clin Inv* 1985; 75:328–338.
198. Desager JP. Clinical pharmacokinetics of ticlopidine. *Clin Pharmacokinet* 1994; 26:347–355.
199. Meyer D, Pietu G, Fressinaud E, Girma JP. Von Willebrand factor: Structure and function. *Mayo Clin Proc* 1991; 66:516–523.
200. Gachet C, Cattaneo M, Ohlmann P, et al. Purinoceptors on blood platelets: Further pharmacological and clinical evidence to suggest the presence of two ADP receptors. *Br J Haematol* 1995; 91:434–444.
201. Hourani SM, Hall DA. Receptors for ADP on human blood platelets. *Trends Pharmacol Sci* 1994; 15:103–108.
202. Savi P, Beauverger P, Labouret C, et al. Role of P2Y1 purinoceptor in ADP-induced platelet activation. *FEBS Lett* 1998; 422: 291–295.
203. Defreyn G, Gachet C, Savi P, et al. Ticlopidine and clopidogrel (SR 25990C) selectively neutralize ADP inhibition of PGE_1-activated platelet adenylate cyclase in rats and rabbits. *Thromb Haemost* 1991; 65:186–190.
204. Gachet C, Cazenave JP, Ohlmann P, et al. The thienopyridine ticlopidine selectively prevents the inhibitory effects of ADP but not of adrenaline on cAMP levels raised by stimulation of the adenylate cyclase of human platelets by PGE_1. *Biochem Pharmacol* 1990; 40:2683–2687.
205. Balsano F, Rizzon P, Violi F, et al. Antiplatelet treatment with ticlopidine in unstable angina: A controlled multicenter clinical trial. *Circulation* 1990; 82:17–26.
206. Hass WK, Easton JD, Adams HP Jr, et al. A randomized trial comparing ticlopidine hydrochloride with aspirin for the prevention of stroke in high-risk patients. Ticlopidine Aspirin Stroke Study Group [see Comments]. *N Engl J Med* 1989; 321:501–507.
207. Schömig A, Neumann F-J, Kastrati A, et al. A randomized comparison of antiplatelet and anticoagulant therapy after the placement of coronary-artery stents. *N Engl J Med* 1996; 334:1084–1089.
208. Leon MB, Baim DS, Popma JJ, et al. A clinical trial comparing three antithrombotic-drug regimens after coronary-artery stenting. Stent Anticoagulation Restenosis Study Investigators. *N Engl J Med* 1998; 339:1665–1671.
209. Hall P, Nakamura S, Maiello L, et al. A randomized comparison of combined ticlopidine and aspirin therapy versus aspirin therapy alone after successful intravascular ultrasound-guided stent implantation. *Circulation* 1996; 93:215–222.
210. Bertrand ME, Legrand V, Boland J, et al. Randomized multicenter comparison of conventional anticoagulation versus antiplatelet therapy in unplanned and elective coronary stenting. The full anticoagulation versus aspirin and ticlopidine (FANTASTIC) study. *Circulation* 1998; 98:1597–1603.
211. Steinhubl SR, Lauer MS, Mukherjee DP, et al. The duration of pretreatment with ticlopidine prior to stenting is associated with the risk of procedure-related non-Q-wave myocardial infarctions. *J Am Coll Cardiol* 1998; 32:1366–1370.
212. Noble S, Goa KL. Ticlopidine: A review of its pharmacology, clinical efficacy and tolerability in the prevention of cerebral ischaemia and stroke. *Drugs Aging* 1996; 8:214–232 [published erratum appears in *Drugs Aging* 1996; 8:444].
213. Verhaeghe R. Prophylactic antiplatelet therapy in peripheral arterial disease. *Drugs* 1991; 42(suppl 5):51–57.
214. Bennett CL, Weinberg PD, Rozenberg-Ben-Dror K, et al. Thrombotic thrombocytopenic purpura associated with ticlopidine: A review of 60 cases. *Ann Intern Med* 1998; 128:541–544.
215. Steinhubl SR, Tan WA, Foody JM, Topol EJ. Incidence and clinical course of thrombotic thrombocytopenic purpura due to ticlopidine following coronary stenting. EPISTENT Investigators: Evaluation of Platelet IIb/IIIa Inhibitor for Stenting. *JAMA* 1999; 281:806–810.
216. Savcic M, Hauert J, Bachmann F, et al. Clopidogrel loading dose regimens: Kinetic profile of pharmacodynamic response in healthy subjects. *Semin Thromb Hemost* 1999; 25(suppl 2):15–19.
217. Gent M. Benefit of clopidogrel in patients with coronary disease (abstr). *Circulation* 1997; 96(suppl I):I-467.
218. Bhatt DK, Hirsch AT, Chew DP, et al. Marked superiority of clopidogrel versus aspirin in patients with a history of previous cardiac surgery (abstr). *J Am Coll Cardiol* 2000; 35(suppl A):383A.
219. Herbert JM, Dol F, Bernat A, et al. The antiaggregating and antithrombotic activity of clopidogrel is potentiated by aspirin in several experimental models in the rabbit. *Thromb Haemost* 1998; 80:512–518.
220. Bertrand M. The CLASSICS trial. Presented at the American College of Cardiology Scientific Sessions. Orlando: FL; 1999.
221. Moussa I, Oetgen M, Roubin G, et al. Effectiveness of clopidogrel and aspirin versus ticlopidine and aspirin in preventing stent thrombosis after coronary stent implantation. *Circulation* 1999; 99:2364–2366.
222. Steinhubl SR, Topol EJ. Clopidogrel with aspirin is the optimal antiplatelet regimen for intracoronary stenting. *J Thromb Thrombolysis* 1999; 7:227–231.
223. Mishkel GJ, Aguirre FV, Ligon RW, et al. Clopidogrel as adjunctive antiplatelet therapy during coronary stenting. *J Am Coll Cardiol* 1999; 34:1884–1890.
224. Berger PB, Bell MR, Rihal CS, et al. Clopidogrel versus ticlopidine after intracoronary stent placement. *J Am Coll Cardiol* 1999; 34:1891–1894.
225. Muller C, Buttner HJ, Petersen J, Roskamm H. A randomized comparison of clopidogrel and aspirin versus ticlopidine and aspirin after the placement of coronary-artery stents. *Circulation* 2000; 101:590–593.
226. Verstraete M. Thromboxane synthase inhibition, thromboxane/endoperoxide receptor blockade and molecules with the dual property. *Drugs Today* 1993; 29:221–232.
227. Ritter JM, Doktor HS, Benjamin N, et al. On the mechanism of the prolonged action in man of GR32191, a thromboxane receptor antagonist. *Adv Prostaglandin Thromboxane Leukot Res* 1991; 351–354.
228. De Clerck F, Beetens J, De Chaffoy de Courcelles D, et al. R 68 070: Thromboxane A_2 synthetase inhibition and thromboxane A_2/prostaglandin endoperoxide receptor blockade combined in one molecule: I. Biochemical profile in vitro. *Thromb Haemost* 1989; 61:35–42.
229. RAPT Investigators. Randomized trial of ridogrel, a combined thromboxane A_2 synthase inhibitor and thromboxane A_2/prostaglandin endoperoxide receptor antagonist, versus aspirin as adjunction to thrombolysis in patients with acute myocardial infarction: The Ridogrel Aspirin Patency Trial (RAPT). *Circulation* 1994; 89:588–595.

230. DiSalveo TG, Webster MWI, Chesebro JH, Fuster V. Dipyridamole. In: Messerli FH, ed. *Cardiovascular Drug Therapy,* 2nd ed. Philadelphia: WB Saunders; 1996:1498.
231. Cairns JA, Gent M, Singer J, et al. Aspirin, sulfinpyrazone, or both in unstable angina: Results of a Canadian multicenter trial. *N Engl J Med* 1985; 313:1369–1375.
232. Coller BS. A new murine monoclonal antibody report an activation-dependent change in the conformation and/or microenvironment of the platelet glycoprotein IIb/IIIa complex. *J Clin Invest* 1985; 76:101–108.
233. Reverter JC, Béguin S, Kesseis H, et al. Inhibition of platelet-mediated, tissue factor–induced thrombin generation by the mouse/human chimeric 7E3 antibody. *J Clin Invest* 1996; 98: 863–874.
234. Coller BS, Folts JD, Scutter LE, Smith SR. Antithrombotic effect of a monoclonal antibody to the platelet glycoprotein IIb/IIIa receptor in an experimental model. *Blood* 1986; 68:783–786.
235. Kereiakes DJ, Kleiman NS, Ambrose J, et al. Randomized, double-blind, placebo-controlled dose-ranging study of tirofiban (MK-383) platelet IIb/III blockade in high risk patients undergoing coronary angioplasty. *J Am Coll Cardiol* 1996; 27:536–642.
236. Tcheng JE, Harrington RA, Kottke-Marchant K, et al. Multicenter, randomized, double-blind, placebo-controlled trial of the platelet integrin glycoprotein IIb/IIIa blocker integrelin in elective coronary intervention. *Circulation* 1995; 91:2151–2157.
237. Kereiakes DJ, Runyon JP, Kleiman NS, et al. Differential dose-response to oral xemilofiban after antecedent intravenous abciximab: Administration for complex coronary intervention. *Circulation* 1996; 94:906–910.
238. Cannon CP, McCabe CH, Borzak S, et al. A randomized trial of an oral platelet glycoprotein IIb/IIIa antagonist, sibrafiban, in patients after an acute coronary syndrome: Results of the TIMI 12 trial. *Circulation* 1998; 97:340–349.
239. Ferguson JJ, Deedwania PD, Kereiakes DJ, et al. Sustained platelet GP IIb/IIIa blockade with oral orbofiban: Interim pharmacodynamic results of the SOAR study (abstr). *J Am Coll Cardiol* 1998; 31(suppl A):185A.
240. Mousa SA, Kapil R, Mu DX. Intravenous and oral antithrombotic efficacy of the novel platelet GPIIb/IIIa antagonist roxifiban (DMP754) and its free acid form, XV459. *Arterioscler Thromb Vasc Biol* 1999; 19:2535–2541.
241. Mousa SA, Bozarth J, Youssef A, Levine B. Oral antiplatelet efficacy of the platelet GPIIb/IIIa antagonist, DMP754 in non-human primates. *Thromb Res* 1998; 89:217–225.
241a. The EPIC Investigators. Use of a monoclonal antibody directed against the platelet glycoprotein IIb/IIIa receptor in high risk angioplasty. *N Engl J Med* 1994; 330:956–961.
242. Topol EJ, Califf RM, Weisman HF, et al. Randomised trial of coronary intervention with antibody against platelet IIb/IIIa integrin for reduction of clinical restenosis: Results at six months. *Lancet* 1994; 343:881–886.
243. Topol EJ, Ferguson JJ, Weisman HF, et al. Long term protection from myocardial ischemic events after brief integrin B_3 blockade with percutaneous coronary intervention. *JAMA* 1997; 278: 479–484.
243a. The EPILOG Investigators. Platelet glycoprotein IIb/IIIa receptor blockade and low-dose heparin during percutaneous coronary revascularization. *N Engl J Med* 1997; 336:1689–1696.
243b. Anderson KM, Ferguson JJ, Stoner GL, et al. Long term mortality benefit with abciximab in patients undergoing percutaneous coronary intervention (PCI) (abstr). *Circulation* 1997; 96(suppl. I):I-162.
243c. The EPISTENT Investigators. Randomised placebo-controlled and balloon-angioplasty-controlled trial to assess the safety of coronary stenting with use of platelet glycoprotein-IIb/IIIa blockade. *Lancet* 1998; 352:87–92.
244. Lincoff AM, Califf RM, Moliterno DJ, et al. Complementary clinical benefits of coronary-artery stenting and blockade of platelet glycoprotein IIb/IIIa receptors: Evaluation of Platelet IIb/IIIa Inhibition in Stenting Investigators. *N Engl J Med* 1999; 341:319–327.
245. Topol EJ, Mark DB, Lincoff AM, et al. Outcomes at 1 year and economic implications of platelet glycoprotein IIb/IIIa blockade in patients undergoing coronary stenting: Results from a multicentre randomised trial. *Lancet* 1999; 354:2019–2024.
246. Tcheng JE. ESPRIT. Presented at the American College of Cardiology Scientific Sessions. Anaheim: CA; 2000.
247. Peerlinck K, De Lepeleire I, Goldberg M, et al. MK-383 (L-700,462), a selective nonpeptide platelet glycoprotein IIb/IIIa antagonist, is active in man. *Circulation* 1993; 88(4 pt 1):1512–1517.
248. Kereiakes DJ, Broderick TM, Roth EM, et al. Time course, magnitude, and consistency of platelet inhibition by abciximab, tirofiban, or eptifibatide in patients with unstable angina pectoris undergoing percutaneous coronary intervention. *Am J Cardiol* 1999; 84:391–395.
249. RESTORE Investigators. The effects of platelet glycoprotein IIb/IIIa blockade with tirofiban on adverse cardiac events in patients with unstable angina or acute myocardial infarction undergoing coronary angioplasty. *Circulation* 1997; 96:1445–1453.
250. Lefkovits J, Ivanhoe RJ, Califf RM, et al. Effects of platelet glycoprotein IIb/IIIa receptor blockade by a chimeric monoclonal antibody (abciximab) on acute and six-month outcomes after percutaneous transluminal coronary agioplasty for acute myocardial infarction. *Am J Cardiol* 1996; 77:1045–1051.
251. Brenner SJ, Barr LA, Burchenal JEB, et al. Randomized, placebo-controlled trial of platelet IIb/IIIa blockade with primary angioplasty for acute myocardial infarction. *Circulation* 1998; 98:734–741.
251a. Neumann F-J, Blasini R, Schmitt C, et al. Effect of glycoprotein IIb/IIIa receptor blockade on recovery of coronary flow and left ventricular function after placement of coronary-artery stents in acute myocardial infarction. *Circulation* 1998; 98:2695–2701.
251b. Montalescot G, Barragan P, Wittenberg O, et al. Abciximab associated with primary angioplasty and stenting in acute myocardial infarction: The ADMIRAL study, 30-day final results. *Circulation* 1999; 100(suppl. I):I-87.
251c. van den Merkhof LF, Zijlstra F, Olsson H, et al. Abciximab in the treatment of acute myocardial infarction eligible for primary percutaneous transluminal coronary angioplasty. Results of the Glycoprotein Receptor Antagonist Patency Evaluation (GRAPE) pilot study. *J Am Coll Cardiol* 1999; 33:1528–1532.
252. Kleiman NS, Tracy RP, Talley JD, et al. Inhibition of platelet aggregation with a glycoprotein IIb-IIIa antagonist does not prevent thrombin generation in patients undergoing thrombolysis for acute myocardial infarction. *J Thromb Thrombolysis* 2000; 9:5–12.
253. CAPTURE Investigators. Randomised placebo-controlled trial of abciximab before and during coronary intervention in refractory unstable angina: The CAPTURE study. *Lancet* 1997; 349:1429–1435.
254. Takiguchi Y, Asai F, Wada K, Nakashima M. Comparison of antithrombotic effects of GPIIb-IIIa receptor antagonist and TXA_2 receptor antagonist in the guinea-pig thrombosis model: Possible role of TXA_2 in reocclusion after thrombolysis. *Thromb Haemost* 1995; 73:683–688.
255. Theroux P, Kouz S, Knudtson ML, et al. A randomized double-blind controlled trial with the nor peptidic platelet GPI IIb/IIIa antagonist RO 44-9833 in unstable angina (abstr). *Circulation* 1994; 232.
256. Theroux P, Kouz S, Roy L, et al. Platelet membrane receptor glycoprotein IIb/IIIa antagonism in unstable angina: The Canadian Lamifiban study. *Circulation* 1996; 94:899–905.

257. PARAGON Investigators. International, randomized, controlled trial of lamifiban (a platelet glycoprotein IIb/IIIa inhibitor), heparin or both in unstable angina. *Circulation* 1998; 97:2386–2395.
258. Harrington RA, PARAGON B. Presented at the American College of Cardiology Scientific Sessions. Anaheim: CA; March 2000.
259. Topol EJ. Toward a new frontier in myocardial reperfusion therapy: Emerging platelet preeminence. *Circulation* 1998; 97: 211–218.
260. Peterson JG, Lauer MA, Sapp SK, Topol EJ. Heparin use is required for clinical benefit of GP IIb/IIIa inhibitor eptifibatide in acute coronary syndromes: Insights from the PURSUIT trial (abstr). *Circulation* 1998; 98(suppl I):I-360.
261. Zhao X-Q, Theroux P, Snapinn SM, Sax FL. for the PRISM-PLUS Investigators. Intracoronary thrombus and platelet glycoprotein IIb/IIIa receptor blockade with tirofiban in unstable angina or non-Q-wave myocardial infarction: Angiographic results from the PRISM-PLUS trial (Platelet Receptor Inhibition for Ischemic Syndrome Management in Patients Limited by Unstable Signs and Symptoms). *Circulation* 1999; 100:1609–1615.
262. Van den Brand M, Laarman GJ, Steg PG, et al. Assessment of coronary angiograms prior to and after treatment with abciximab, and the outcome of angioplasty in refractory unstable angina patients: Angiographic results from the CAPTURE trial. *Eur Heart J* 1999; 20:1572–1578.
263. Alexander JH, Sparapani RA, Mahaffey KW, et al. Eptifibatide reduces the size and incidence of myocardial infarction in patients with non-ST-elevation acute coronary syndromes (abstr). *J Am Coll Cardiol* 1999; 33(suppl A):331A.
264. Hahn SS, Chae C, Giugliano R, et al. Troponin I levels in unstable angina/non-Q wave myocardial infarction patients treated with tirofiban, a glycoprotein IIb/IIIa inhibitor (abstr). *J Am Coll Cardiol* 1998; 31(suppl A):229A.
265. Cannon CP, Thompson B, McCabe CH, et al. Predictors of non-Q-wave acute myocardial infarction in patients with acute ischemic syndromes: An analysis from the Thrombolysis in Myocardial Ischemia (TIMI) III trials. *Am J Cardiol* 1995; 75:977–981.
266. Borzak S, Cannon CP, Kraft PL, et al. Effects of prior aspirin and anti-ischemic therapy on outcome of patients with unstable angina. *Am J Cardiol* 1998; 81:678–681.
267. Garcia-Dorado D, Theroux P, Tornos P, et al. Previous aspirin use may attenuate the severity of the manifestation of acute ischemic syndromes. *Circulation* 1995; 92:1743–1748.
268. Gruppo Italiano per lo Studio della Streptochinasi nell'Infarto Miocardico (GISSI). Effectiveness of intravenous thrombolytic treatment in acute myocardial infarction. *Lancet* 1986; 1:397–401.
269. Cannon CP, Braunwald E. GUSTO, TIMI and the case for rapid reperfusion. *Acta Cardiol* 1994; 49:1–8.
270. GUSTO Angiographic Investigators. The comparative effects of tissue plasminogen activator, streptokinase, or both on coronary artery patency, ventricular function and survival after acute myocardial infarction. *N Engl J Med* 1993; 329:1615–1622.
271. Ito H, Tomooka T, Sakai N, et al. Lack of myocardial perfusion immediately after successful thrombolysis: A predictor of poor recovery of left ventricular function in anterior myocardial infarction. *Circulation* 1992; 85:1699–1705.
272. Ohman EM, Califf RM, Topol EJ, et al. Consequences of reocclusion after successful reperfusion therapy in acute myocardial infarction. *Circulation* 1990; 82:781–791.
273. Cannon CP. Overcoming thrombolytic resistance: Rationale and initial clinical experience combining thrombolytic therapy and glycoprotein IIb/IIIa receptor inhibition for acute myocardial infarction. *J Am Coll Cardiol* 1999; 34:1395–1402.
274. Coller BS. Platelets and thrombolytic therapy. *N Engl J Med* 1990; 322:33–42.
275. Weitz JI, Hudoba M, Massel D, et al. Clot-bound thrombin is protected from inhibition by heparin-antithrombin III but is susceptible to inactivation by antithrombin III–independent inhibitors. *J Clin Invest* 1990; 86:385–391.
276. Owen J, Friedman KD, Grossmann BA, et al. Thrombolytic therapy with tissue-plasminogen activator or streptokinase induces transient thrombin activity. *Blood* 1988; 72:616–620.
277. Gurbel P, Serebruany V, Shustov A, et al. Effects of reteplase and alteplase on platelet aggregation and major receptor expression during the first 24 hours of acute myocardial infarction treatment. *J Am Coll Cardiol* 1998; 21:1466–1473.
278. Gold HK, Coller BS, Yasuda T, et al. Rapid and sustained coronary artery recanalization with combined bolus injection of recombinant tissue-type plasminogen activator and monoclonal anti-platelet GPIIb/IIIa antibody in a dog model. *Circulation* 1988; 77:670–677.
279. Yasuda T, Gold HK, Leinbach RC, et al. Lysis of plasminogen activator–resistant platelet-rich coronary artery thrombus with combined bolus injection of recombinant tissue-type plasminogen activator and antiplatelet GPIIb/IIIa antibody. *J Am Coll Cardiol* 1990; 16:1728–1735.
280. Kleiman N, Ohman EM, Califf RM, et al. Profound inhibition of platelet aggregation with monoclonal antibody 7E3 Fab after thrombolytic therapy. Results of the Thrombolysis and Angioplasty in Myocardial Infarction (TAMI) 8 pilot study. *J Am Coll Cardiol* 1993; 22:381–389.
281. Ohman EM, Kleiman NS, Gacioch G, et al. Combined accelerated tissue-plasminogen activator and platelet glycoprotein IIb/IIIa integrin receptor blockade with integrilin in acute myocardial infarction. *Circulation* 1997; 95:846–854.
282. PARADIGM Investigators. Combining thrombolysis with the platelet glycoprotein IIb/IIIa inhibitor lamifiban: Results of the Platelet Aggregation Receptor Antagonist Dose Investigation and Reperfusion Gain in Myocardial Infarction (PARADIGM) trial. *J Am Coll Cardiol* 1998; 32:2003–2010.
283. Antman EM, Giugliano RP, Gibson CM, et al. Abciximab facilitates the rate and extent of thrombolysis: Results of TIMI 14 trial. *Circulation* 1999; 90:2720–2732.
283a. Strategies for Patency Enhancement in the Emergency Department (SPEED) Group. Trial of abciximab with and without low-dose reteplase for acute myocardial infarction. *Circulation* 2000; 101:2788–2794.
284. EPIC Investigators. Use of a monoclonal antibody directed against the platelet glycoprotein IIb/IIIa receptor in high risk angioplasty. *N Engl J Med* 1994; 330:956–961.
285. EPILOG Investigators. Platelet glycoprotein IIb/IIIa receptor blockade and low-dose heparin during percutaneous coronary revascularization. *N Engl J Med* 1997; 336:1689–1696.
286. IMPACT-II Investigators. Randomised placebo-controlled trial of effect of eptifibatide on complications of percutaneous coronary intervention: IMPACT-II. *Lancet* 1997; 349:1422–1428.
287. Coller BS, Land D, Scudder LE. Rapid and simple platelet function assay to assess glycoprotein IIb/IIIa receptor blockade. *Circulation* 1997; 95:860–867.
288. Steinhubl SR, Kottke-Marchant K, Moliterno DJ, et al. Attainment and maintenance of platelet inhibition by standard dosing of abciximab in diabetic and nondiabetic patients undergoing percutaneous coronary intervention. *Circulation* 1999; 100: 1977–1982.
289. EPISTENT Investigators. Randomised placebo-controlled and balloon-angioplasty-controlled trial to assess the safety of coronary stenting with use of platelet glycoprotein-IIb/IIIa blockade. *Lancet* 1998; 352:87–92.
290. Berkowitz SD, Sane DC, Sigmon KN, et al. Occurrence and clinical significance of thrombocytopenia in a population under-

going high-risk percutaneous coronary revascularization: Evaluation of c7E3 for the Prevention of Ischemic Complications (EPIC) Study Group. *J Am Coll Cardiol* 1998; 32:311–319.
291. Mahaffey KW, Harrington RA, Simoons ML, et al. Stroke in patients with acute coronary syndromes: Incidence and outcomes in the platelet glycoprotein IIb/IIIa in unstable angina—Receptor suppression using integrilin therapy (PURSUIT) trial. The PURSUIT Investigators. *Circulation* 1999; 99:2371–2377.
292. Kereiakes DJ, Kleiman NS, Ferguson JJ, et al. Sustained platelet glycoprotein IIb/IIIa blockade with oral xemilofiban in 170 patients following coronary stent deployment. *Circulation* 1997; 96:1117–1121.
293. Simpfendorfer C, Kottke-Marchant K, Topol EJ. First experience with chronic platelet GPIIb/IIIa receptor blockade: A pilot study of xemlofiban, an orally active antagonist in unstable angina patients eligible for PTCA (abstr). *J Am Coll Cardiol* 1996; 27(suppl A):242A.
294. Kereiakes DJ, Kleiman NS, Ferguson JJ, et al. Pharmacodynamic efficacy, clinical safety, and outcomes after prolonged platelet glycoprotein IIb/IIIa receptor blockade with oral xemilofiban: Results of a multicenter, placebo-controlled, randomized trial. *Circulation* 1998; 98:1268–1278.
295. Coulter SA, Cannon CP, Cooper RA, et al. Thrombocytopenia, bleeding, and thrombotic events with oral glycoprotein IIb/IIIa inhibition: Results from OPUS-TIMI 16 (abstr). *J Am Coll Cardiol* 2000; 35(suppl A):393A.
296. Willerson JT, McNatt JM, Clubb FJ Jr, et al. Xemilofiban, an oral GP IIb/IIIa receptor antagonist is enhanced by aspirin in inhibiting neointimal proliferation following percutaneous coronary angioplasty (abstr). *Circulation* 1997; 96(suppl I):I-168.
297. Cannon CP, McCabe CH, Wilcox RG, et al. Oral glycoprotein IIb/IIIa inhibition with orbofiban in patients with unstable coronary syndromes (OPUS-TIMI 16) trial. *Circulation* 2000; 102:149–156.
298. Ferguson JJ. Meeting highlights: Highlights of the 48th Scientific Session of the American College of Cardiology. *Circulation* 1999; 100:570–575.
299. Holmes MB, Sobel BE, Cannon CP, Schneider DJ. Increased platelet reactivity in patients given orbofiban after an acute coronary syndrome: An OPUS-TIMI 16 substudy. *Am J Cardiol* 2000; 85:491–493.
300. Casey M, Fornari C, Bozovich G, et al. Increased expression of platelet P-selectin in patients treated with oral orbofiban in the OPUS TIMI 16 study (abstr). *Circulation* 1999; 100(suppl I):I-681.
301. Peter K, Schwarz M, Ylanne J, et al. Induction of fibrinogen binding and platelet aggregation as a potential intrinsic property of various glycoprotein IIb/IIIa ($\alpha_{IIb}\beta_3$) inhibitors. *Blood* 1998; 92:3240–3249.
302. O'Neill WW, Serruys P, Knudtson M, et al.. Long-term treatment with a platelet glycoprotein-receptor antagonist after percutaneous coronary revascularization. *N Engl J Med* 2000; 342:1316–1324.
303. Akkerhuis M, Van den Zwaan C, Wilcox RG, et al. Troponin-I identifies patients with unstable coronary artery disease who benefit from long-term oral glycoprotein IIb/IIIa inhibition: The FROST study (abstr). *Circulation* 1999; 100(suppl I):I-292.
304. Hamm CW, Heeschen C, Goldmann B, et al. Benefit of abciximab in patients with refractory unstable angina in relation to serum troponin T levels. The c7E3 Fab Antiplatelet Therapy in Unstable Refractory Angina (CAPTURE) Study Investigators. *N Engl J Med* 1999; 340:1623–1629.
305. Heeschen C, Hamm CW, Goldmann B, et al. Troponin concentrations for stratification of patients with acute coronary syndromes in relation to therapeutic efficacy of tirofiban. *Lancet* 1999; 354:1757–1762.
306. Giugliano RP, McCabe CH, Sequeira RF, et al. Dose ranging study of intravenous RPR 109891 in patients with acute coronary syndromes: Results of TIMI 15A (abstr). *J Am Coll Cardiol* 1998; 31(suppl A):93A.
307. Giugliano RP, McCabe CH, Sequeira RF, et al. First report of an intravenous and oral GP IIb/IIIa inhibitor (RPR 109891) in patients with recent acute coronary syndromes: Results of the TIMI 15A and 15B trials. *Am Heart J* 2000; 140:81–93.
308. Muller TH, Weisenberger H, Brickl R, et al. Profound and sustained inhibition of platelet aggregation by Fradafiban, a nonpeptide platelet glycoprotein IIb/IIIa antagonist, and its orally active prodrug, Lefradafiban, in men. *Circulation* 1997; 96:1130–1138.
309. Mousa SA, Forsythe M, Bozarth J, et al. XV454, a novel nonpeptide small-molecule platelet GIIb/IIIa antagonist with comparable platelet alpha(IIb)beta3-binding kinetics to c7E3. *J Cardiovasc Pharmacol* 1998; 32:736–744.
310. Mousa SA, Bozarth JM, Lorelli W, et al. Antiplatelet efficacy of XV459, a novel nonpeptide platelet GPIIb/IIIa antagonist: Comparative platelet binding profiles with c7E3. *J Pharmacol Exp Ther* 1998; 286:1277–1284.
311. Weitz JI, Hudoba M, Massel D, et al. Clot-bound thrombin is protected from inhibition by heparin-antithrombin III but is susceptible to inactivation by antithrombin III–independent inhibitors. *J Clin Invest* 1990; 86:385–391.
312. Hirsh J, Fuster V. Guide to anticoagulant therapy: Part 1. Heparin. American Heart Association. *Circulation* 1994; 89:1449–1468.
313. The SCATI (Studio sulla Calciparina nell'Angina e nella Trombosi Ventricolare nell'Infarto) Group. Randomised controlled trial of subcutaneous calcium-heparin in acute myocardial infarction. *Lancet* 1989; 2:182–186.
314. Hennekens CH, Albert CM, Godfried SL, et al. Adjunctive drug therapy of acute myocardial infarction: Evidence from clinical trials. *N Engl J Med* 1996; 335:1660–1667.
315. Gruppo Italiano per lo Studio della Sopravvivenza nell'Infarto Miocardico: GISSI-2. A factorial randomised trial of alteplase versus streptokinase and heparin versus no heparin among 12,490 patients with acute myocardial infarction. *Lancet* 1990; 336:65–71.
316. International Study Group. In-hospital mortality and clinical course of 20,891 patients with suspected acute myocardial infarction randomised between alteplase and streptokinase with or without heparin. *Lancet* 1990; 336:71–75.
317. ISIS-3 (Third International Study of Infarct Survival) Collaborative Group. ISIS-3: A randomised comparison of streptokinase vs tissue plasminogen activator vs anistreplase and of aspirin plus heparin vs aspirin alone among 41,299 cases of suspected acute myocardial infarction. *Lancet* 1992; 339:753–770.
318. Topol EJ, George BS, Kereiakes DJ, et al. A randomized controlled trial of intravenous tissue plasminogen activator and early intravenous heparin in acute myocardial infarction. *Circulation* 1989; 79:281–286.
319. Hsia J, Hamilton WP, Kleiman N, et al. A comparison between heparin and low-dose aspirin as adjunctive therapy with tissue plasminogen activator for acute myocardial infarction. *N Engl J Med* 1990; 323:1433–1437.
320. Bleich SD, Nichols T, Schumacher RR, et al. Effect of heparin on coronary patency after thrombolysis with tissue plasminogen activator in acute myocardial infarction. *Am J Cardiol* 1990; 66:1412–1417.
321. De Bono DP, Simoons MI, Tijssen J, et al. Effect of early intravenous heparin on coronary patency, infarct size, and bleeding complications after alteplase thrombolysis: Results of a randomized double blind European Cooperative Study Group trial. *Br Heart J* 1992; 67:122–128.
322. O'Connor CM, Meese R, Carney R, et al. A randomized trial of intravenous heparin in conjunction with anistreplase (anisoy-

lated plasminogen streptokinase activator complex) in acute myocardial infarction: The Duke University Clinical Cardiology Study (DUCCS) 1. *J Am Coll Cardiol* 1994; 23:11–18.
323. GUSTO Investigators. An international randomized trial comparing four thrombolytic strategies for acute myocardial infarction. *N Engl J Med* 1993; 329:673–682.
324. Williams DO, Kirby MG, McPhearson K, Phear DN. Anticoagulant treatment in unstable angina. *Br J Clin Pract* 1986; 40: 114–116.
325. Telford AM, Wilson C. Trial of heparin versus atenolol in prevention of myocardial infarction in intermediate coronary syndrome. *Lancet* 1981; 1:1225–1228.
326. Maraganore JM, Bourdon P, Adelman B, et al. Heparin variability and resistance: Comparisons with a direct thrombin inhibitor (abstr). *Circulation* 1992; 86(suppl I):I-386.
327. Young E, Prins M, Levine MN, Hirsh J. Heparin binding to plasma proteins, an important mechanism for heparin resistance. *Thromb Haemost* 1992; 67:639–643.
328. Hirsh J. Heparin. *N Engl J Med* 1991; 324:1565–1574.
329. Ogilby JD, Untereker WJ, Corin WJ, et al. Variability of effective anticoagulation for PTCA is dependent upon heparin potency (abstr). *Circulation* 1991; 84(suppl II):II-592.
330. Bock PE, Juscombe M, Marshall SE, et al. The multiple complexes formed by the interaction of platelet factor 4 with heparin. *Biochem J* 1980; 191:769–776.
331. Lijnen HR, Hoylaerts M, Collens D. Heparin binding properties of human histidinerich glycoprotein: Mechanism and role in the neutralization of heparin in plasma. *J Biol Chem* 1983; 258:3803–3808.
332. Preissner KT, Muller-Berghaus G. Neutralization and binding of heparin by S-protein/vitronectin in the inhibition of factor Xa by antithrombin III. *J Biol Chem* 1987; 262:12,247–12,253.
333. Cruikshank MK, Levine MN, Hirsh J, et al. A standard nomogram for the management of heparin therapy. *Arch Intern Med* 1991; 151:333–337.
334. Flaker GC, Bartolozzi J, Davis V, et al. Use of a standardized nomogram to achieve therapeutic anticoagulation after thrombolytic therapy in myocardial infarction. *Arch Intern Med* 1994; 154:1492–1496.
335. Melandri G, Branzi A, Traini AM, et al. On the value of the activated clotting time for monitoring heparin therapy in acute coronary syndromes. *Am J Cardiol* 1993; 71:469–471.
336. Kaplan K, Davison R, Parker M, et al. Role of heparin after intravenous thrombolytic therapy for acute myocardial infarction. *Am J Cardiol* 1987; 59:241–244.
337. Camilleri JF, Bonnet JL, Bouvier JL, et al. Thrombolyse intraveineuse dans l'infarctus du myocarde: Influence de la qualite de l'anticoagulation dur le taux de recidives precoces dangor ou d'infarctus. *Arch Mal Coeur* 1988; 81:1037–1041.
338. Tracy RP, Kleiman NS, Thompson B, et al. Relation of coagulation parameters to patency and recurrent ischemia in the Thrombolysis in Myocardial Infarction (TIMI) phase II trial. *Am Heart J* 1998; 135:29–37.
339. Granger CB, Hirsh J, Califf RM, et al. Activated partial thromboplastin time and outcome after thrombolytic therapy for acute myocardial infarction: Results from the GUSTO-I trial. *Circulation* 1996; 93:870–878.
340. Hsia J, Kleiman N, Aguirre F, et al. Heparin-induced prolongation of partial thromboplastin time after thrombolysis: Relationship to coronary artery patency. *J Am Coll Cardiol* 1992; 20: 31–35.
341. Arnout J, Simoons M, De Bono D, et al. Correlation between level of heparinization and patency of the infarct-related coronary artery after treatment of acute myocardial infarction with alteplase (rt-PA). *J Am Coll Cardiol* 1992; 20:513–519.
342. Landefeld CS, Cook EF, Flateley M, et al. Identification and preliminary validation of predictors of major bleeding in hospitalized patients starting anticoagulant therapy. *Am J Med* 1987; 82:703–713.
343. Becker RC, Cannon CP, Tracy RP, et al. Relationship between systemic anticoagulation as determined by activated partial thromboplastin time and heparin measurements and in-hospital clinical events in unstable angina and non-Q wave myocardial infarction. *Am Heart J* 1996; 131:421–433.
344. Hirsh J, Fuster V. Guide to anticoagulation therapy: Part 1. Heparin. *Circulation* 1994; 89:1449–1468.
345. Raschke RA, Reilly BM, Guidry JR, et al. The weight-based heparin dosing nomogram compared with a "standard care" nomogram. *Ann Intern Med* 1993; 119:874–881.
346. Hassan WM, Flaker GC, Feutz C, et al. Improved anticoagulation with a weight adjusted heparin nomogram in patients with acute coronary syndromes: A randomized trial. *J Thromb Thrombolysis* 1996; 2:245–249.
347. Hochman JS, Wali AU, Gavrila D, et al. A new regimen for heparin use in acute coronary syndromes. *Am Heart J* 1999; 138:313–318.
348. Becker RC, Ball SP, Eisenberg P, et al. A randomized, multicenter trial of weight-adjusted intravenous heparin dose titration and point-of-care coagulation monitoring in hospitalized patients with active thromboembolic disease. *Am Heart J* 1999; 137:59–71.
349. Cannon CP, Dingemanse J, Kleinbloesem CH, et al. An automated heparin titration device to control activated partial thromboplastin time: Evaluation in normal volunteers. *Circulation* 1999; 99:751–756.
350. Giugliano RP, Cannon CP, McCabe CH, et al. Lower dose heparin with thrombolysis is associated with lower rates of intracranial hemorrhage: Results from TIMI 10B and ASSENT I (abstr). *Circulation* 1997; 96(suppl I):I-535.
351. Antman EM, for the TIMI 9A Investigators. Hirudin in acute myocardial infarction: Safety report from the Thrombolysis and Thrombin Inhibition in Myocardial Infarction (TIMI) 9A trial. *Circulation* 1994; 90:1624–1630.
352. Antman EM, for the TIMI 9B Investigators. Hirudin in acute myocardial infarction: Thrombolysis and Thrombin Inhibition in Myocardial Infarction (TIMI) 9B trial. *Circulation* 1996; 94: 911–921.
353. Global Use of Strategies to Open Occluded Coronary Arteries (GUSTO) IIa Investigators. A randomized trial of intravenous heparin versus recombinant hirudin for acute coronary syndromes. *Circulation* 1994; 90:1631–1637.
354. Global Use of Strategies to Open Occluded Coronary Arteries (GUSTO) IIb Investigators. A comparison of recombinant hirudin with heparin for the treatment of acute coronary syndromes. *N Engl J Med* 1996; 335:775–782.
355. Giugliano RP, Cutler SS, Llevadot J. Risk of intracranial hemorrhage with accelerated tPA: Importance of heparin dose (abstr). *Circulation* 1999; 100(suppl I):I-650.
356. Ryan TJ, Anderson JL, Antman EM, et al. 1999 Update: ACC/AHA guidelines for the management of patients with acute myocardial infarction—Executive summary and recommendations. *Circulation* 1999; 100:1016–1030.
357. Popma JJ, Coller BS, Ohman EM, et al. Antithrombotic therapy in patients undergoing coronary angioplasty. *Chest* 1995; 108(suppl 4):486S–501S [published erratum appears in *Chest* 1996; 109:295–296].
358. Nairns CR, Hillegass WB, Nelson CL, et al. Relation between activated clotting time during angioplasty and abrupt closure. *Circulation* 1996; 93:667–671.
359. Bittl JA, Strony J, Brinker JA, et al. Treatment with bivalirudin (Hirulog) as compared with heparin during coronary angioplasty for unstable or post-infarction angina. *N Engl J Med* 1995; 333:764–769.

360. Hirsh J, Levine MN. Low molecular weight heparin. *Blood* 1992; 79:1–17.
361. Sobel M, McNeill PM, Carlson PL, et al. Heparin inhibition of von Willebrand factor–dependent platelet function in vitro and in vivo. *J Clin Invest* 1991; 87:1787–1793.
362. Meuleman DG. Orgaran (Org 10172): Its pharmacological profile in experimental models. *Haemostasis* 1992; 22:58–65.
363. Zammit A, Dawes J. Low-affinity material does not contribute to the antithrombotic activity of Orgaran (Org 10172) in human plasma. *Thromb Haemost* 1994; 71:759–767.
364. Stiekema JC, Wijnand HP, Van Dinther TG, et al. Safety and pharmacokinetics of the low molecular weight heparinoid Org 10172 administered to healthy elderly volunteers. *Br J Clin Pharmacol* 1989; 27:39–48.
365. Patrono C. Aspirin as an antiplatelet drug. *N Engl J Med* 1994; 330:1287–1294.
366. Turpie AG, Levine MN, Hirsh J, et al. A randomized controlled trial of a low-molecular weight heparin (enoxaparin) to prevent deep-vein thrombosis in patients undergoing elective hip surgery. *N Engl J Med* 1986; 315:925–929.
367. Levine MN, Hirsh J, Gent G, et al. Prevention of deep vein thrombosis after elective hip surgery: A randomized trial comparing low molecular weight heparin with standard unfractionated heparin. *Ann Intern Med* 1991; 114:545–551.
368. Pezzuoli G, Serneri GG, Settembrini P, et al. Prophylaxis of fatal pulmonary embolism in general surgery using low-molecular weight heparin Cy 216: A multicentre, double-blind, randomized, controlled, clinical trial versus placebo (STEP). *Int Surg* 1989; 74:205–210.
369. Hull RD, Raskob GE, Pineo GF, et al. Subcutaneous low-molecular-weight heparin compared with continuous intravenous heparin in the treatment of proximal-vein thrombosis. *N Engl J Med* 1992; 326:975–982.
370. Prandoni P, Lensing AW, Muller HR, et al. Comparison of subcutaneous low-molecular-weight heparin with intravenous standard heparin in the treatment of proximal-vein thrombosis. *Lancet* 1992; 339:441–445.
371. Levine M, Gent M, Hirsh J, et al. A comparison of low-molecular-weight heparin administered primarily at home with unfractionated heparin administered in the hospital for proximal deep-vein thrombosis. *N Engl J Med* 1996; 334:677–681.
372. Koopman MMW, Prandoni P, Piovella F, et al. Treatment of venous thrombosis with intravenous unfractionated heparin administered in the hospital as compared with subcutaneous low-molecular-weight heparin administered at home. *N Engl J Med* 1996; 334:682–687.
373. Nesvold A, Kontny F, Abildgaard U, Dale J. Safety of high doses of low molecular weight heparin (Fragmin) in acute myocardial infarction: A dose-finding study. *Thromb Res* 1991; 64:579–587.
374. Gurfinkel R, Mejail R, Dutonto E, et al. Heparina de bajo peso molecular en la angina inestable: Estudio piloto. *Cardiol Intercontinental* 1994; 3:83–86.
375. Gurfinkel EP, Manos EJ, Mejail RI, et al. Low molecular weight heparin versus regular heparin or aspirin in the treatment of unstable angina and silent ischemia. *J Am Coll Cardiol* 1995; 26:313–318.
376. Klein W, Buchwald A, Hillis SE, et al. Comparison of low-molecular-weight heparin with unfractionated heparin acutely and with placebo for 6 weeks in the management of unstable coronary artery disease: Fragmin in Unstable Coronary Artery Disease (FRIC) study. *Circulation* 1997; 96:61–68.
377. Thrombolysis in Myocardial Infarction (TIMI) 11A Trial Investigators. Doseranging trial of enoxaparin for unstable angina: Results of TIMI 11A. *J Am Coll Cardiol* 1997; 29:1474–1482.
378. Faxon DP, Spiro TE, Minor S, et al. Low molecular weight heparin in prevention of restenosis after angioplasty: Results of Enoxaparin Restenosis (ERA) trial. *Circulation* 1994; 90: 908–914.
379. Goods CM, Liu MW, Jain SP, et al. Low molecular weight heparin versus standard heparin in patients at high risk for stent thrombosis: Clinical outcomes (abstr). *Circulation* 1996; 94(suppl I):I-684.
380. Baird SH, McBride SJ, Trouton TG, Wilson C. Low-molecular-weight heparin versus unfractionated heparin following thrombolysis in myocardial infarction (abstr). *J Am Coll Cardiol* 1998; 31 (suppl A):191A.
381. Frostfeldt G, Ahlberg G, Gustafsson G, et al. Low molecular weight heparin (dalteparin) as adjuvant treatment of thrombolysis in acute myocardial infarction: A pilot study—Biochemical markers in acute coronary syndromes (BIOMACS II). *J Am Coll Cardiol* 1999; 33:627–633.
382. Ross AM. HART II. Presented at the American College of Cardiology Scientific Sessions. Anaheim: CA; March 2000.
383. Markwardt F. Past, present and future of hirudin. *Haemostasis* 1991; 21:11–26.
384. Rydel TJ, Ravichandran KG, Tulinsky A, et al. The structure of a complex of recombinant hirudin and human alpha-thrombin. *Science* 1990; 249:277–280.
385. Vu TH, Wheaton VI, Hung DT, et al. Domains specifying thrombin-receptor interaction. *Nature* 1991; 353:674–677.
386. Stone SR, Hofsteenge J. Kinetics of the inhibition of thrombin by hirudin. *Biochemistry* 1986; 825:4622–4628.
387. Zoldhelyi P, Webster MW, Fuster V, et al. Recombinant hirudin in patients with chronic, stable coronary artery disease: Safety, half-life, and effect on coagulation parameters *Circulation* 1993; 88(5 pt 1):2015–2022.
388. Cannon CP, McCabe CH, Henry TD, et al. A pilot trial of recombinant desulfatohirudin compared with heparin in conjunction with tissue-type plasminogen activator and aspirin for acute myocardial infarction: Results of the Thrombolysis in Myocardial Infarction (TIMI) 5 trial. *J Am Coll Cardiol* 1994; 23:993–1003.
389. Organisation to Assess Strategies for Ischemic Syndromes (OASIS-2) Investigators. Effects of recombinant hirudin (lepirudin) compared with heparin on death, myocardial infarction, refractory angina, and revascularisation procedures in patients with acute myocardial ischaemia without ST elevation: A randomised trial. *Lancet* 1999; 353:429–438.
390. Maraganore JM, Bourdon P, Jablonski J, et al. Design and characterization of hirulogs: A novel class of bivalent peptide inhibitors of thrombin. *Biochemistry* 1990; 29:7095–7101.
391. Theroux P, Perez-Villa F, Waters D, et al. Randomized double-blind comparison of two doses of hirulog with heparin as adjunctive therapy to streptokinase to promote early patency of the infarct-related artery in acute myocardial infarction. *Circulation* 1995; 91:2132–2139.
392. White HD, Aylward PE, Frey MJ, et al. Randomized, double-blind comparison of hirulog versus heparin in patients receiving streptokinase and aspirin for acute myocardial infarction (HERO). *Circulation* 1997; 96:2155–2161.
393. Jang IK, Brown DF, Giugliano RP, et al. A multicenter, randomized study of argatroban versus heparin as adjunct to tissue plasminogen activator (TPA) in acute myocardial infarction: Myocardial Infarction with Novastan and TPA (MINT) study. *J Am Coll Cardiol* 1999; 33:1879–1885.
394. Fung AY, Lorch G, Cambier PA, et al. Efegatran sulfate as an adjunct to streptokinase versus heparin as an adjunct to tissue plasminogen activator in patients with acute myocardial infarction. ESCALAT Investigators. *Am Heart J* 1999; 138(4 pt 1): 696–704.
395. Thrombin Inhibition in Myocardial Ischaemia (TRIM) Study Group. A low molecular weight, selective thrombin inhibitor, inogatran, vs heparin, in unstable coronary artery disease in

1209 patients: A double-blind, randomized, dose-finding study. *Eur Heart J* 1997; 18:1416–1425.

396. Talbot M. Biology of recombinant hirudin (CGP 39393): A new prospect in the treatment of thrombosis. *Semin Thromb Hemost* 1989; 15:293–301.
397. Fareed J, Walenga JM, Pifarre R, et al. Some objective considerations for the neutralization of the anticoagulant effects of recombinant hirudin. *Haemostasis* 1991;21(suppl 1):64–72.
398. Lee LV, for the TIMI 6 Investigators. Initial experience with hirudin and streptokinase in acute myocardial infarction: Results of the Thrombolysis in Myocardial Infarction (TIMI) 6 trial. *Am J Cardiol* 1995; 75:7–13.
399. Metz BK, White HD, Granger CB, et al. Randomized comparison of direct thrombin inhibition versus heparin in conjunction with fibrinolytic therapy for acute myocardial infarction: Results from the GUSTO-IIb trial. Global Use of Strategies to Open Occluded Coronary Arteries in Acute Coronary Syndromes (GUSTO-IIb) Investigators. *J Am Coll Cardiol* 1998; 31:1493–1498.
400. Gold HK, Torres FW, Garabedian HD, et al. Evidence of a rebound coagulation phenomenon after cessation of a 4-hour infusion of a specific thrombin inhibitor in patients with unstable angina pectoris. *J Am Coll Cardiol* 1993; 21:1039–1047.
401. Kong DF, Topol EJ, Bittl JA, et al. Clinical outcomes of bivalirudin for ischemic heart disease. *Circulation* 1999; 100:2049–2053.
402. Cannon CP, Braunwald E. Hirudin: Initial results in acute myocardial infarction, unstable angina, and angioplasty. *J Am Coll Cardiol* 1995; 25:30S–37S.
403. Fuchs J, Cannon CP, and the TIMI 7 Investigators. Hirulog in the treatment of unstable angina: Results of the Thrombin Inhibition in Myocardial Ischemia (TIMI) 7 trial. *Circulation* 1995; 92:727–733.
404. Van den Bos AA, Deckers JW, Heyndrickx GR, et al. Safety and efficacy of recombinant hirudin (CGP 39 393) versus heparin in patients with stable angina undergoing coronary angioplasty. *Circulation* 1993; 88(5 pt 1):2058–2066.
405. Serruys PW, Herrman JP, Simon R, et al. A comparison of hirudin with heparin in the prevention of restenosis after coronary angioplasty. Helvetica Investigators. *N Engl J Med* 1995; 333:757–763.
406. Mehta S, Yusuf S, Rupprecht J, et al. Substantial benefit of hirudin compared to heparin among unstable angina patients undergoing early percutaneous coronary intervention (abstr). *J Am Coll Cardiol* 2000; 35(suppl A):357.
407. Boersma E, Akkerhuis KM, Theroux P, et al. Platelet glycoprotein IIb/IIIa receptor inhibition in non-ST-elevation acute coronary syndromes: Early benefit during medical treatment only, with additional protection during percutaneous coronary intervention. *Circulation* 1999; 100:2045–2048.
408. Hirsh J, Fuster V. Guide to anticoagulant therapy: Part 2. Oral anticoagulants. American Heart Association. *Circulation* 1994; 89:1469–1480 [published erratum appears in *Circulation* 1995; 91:A55–A56].
409. Turpie AG, Gunstensen J, Hirsh J, et al. Randomised comparison of two intensities of oral anticoagulant therapy after tissue heart valve replacement. *Lancet* 1988; 1:1242–1245.
410. Samama MM, Acar J. *Traitements Antithrombolytiques*. Paris: Masson; 1993.
411. Hirsh J, Fuster V. Guide to anticoagulation therapy: Part 2. Oral anticoagulants. *Circulation* 1994; 89:1469–1480.
412. Anticoagulants in the Secondary Prevention of Events in Coronary Thrombosis (ASPECT) Research Group. Effect of long-term oral anticoagulant treatment on mortality and cardiovascular morbidity after myocardial infarction. *Lancet* 1994; 343: 499–503.
413. Breddin K, Loew D, Lechner K, et al. The German-Austrian aspirin trial: A comparison of acetylsalicylic acid, placebo and phenprocoumon in secondary prevention of myocardial infarction. On behalf of the German-Austrian Study Group. *Circulation* 1980; 62(6 pt 2):V63–V72.
414. Meijer A, Verheugt FW, Werter CJ, et al. Aspirin versus coumadin in the prevention of reocclusion and recurrent ischemia after successful thrombolysis: A prospective placebo-controlled angiographic study—Results of the APRICOT study. *Circulation* 1993; 87:1524–1530.
415. Coumadin Aspirin Reinfarction Study (CARS) Investigators. Randomised double-blind trial of fixed low-dose warfarin with aspirin after myocardial infarction. *Lancet* 1997; 350: 389–396.
416. Medical Research Council's General Practice Research Framework. Thrombosis prevention trial: Randomised trial of low-intensity oral anticoagulation with warfarin and low-dose aspirin in the primary prevention of ischaemic heart disease in men at increased risk. *Lancet* 1998; 351:233–241.
417. Fiore L. CHAMPS trial. Presented at the American Heart Association Scientific Sessions. Atlanta, November 1999.
418. Fiore L, Ezekowitz MD, Brophy MT, et al. The Veterans Administration cooperative study program trial: "Combination, Hemotherapy and Mortality Prevention" (CHAMP)—Rates of major hemorrhage (abstr). *J Am Coll Cardiol* 2000; 35(suppl A):373A.
419. Stroke Prevention in Atrial Fibrillation Investigators. Preliminary report of the Stroke Prevention in Atrial Fibrillation study. *N Engl J Med* 1990; 322:863–868.
420. Loh E, Sutton MS, Wun CC, et al. Ventricular dysfunction and the risk of stroke after myocardial infarction. *N Engl J Med* 1997; 336:251–257.
421. Jackson KW, Tang J. Complete amino acid sequence of streptokinase and its homology with serine proteases. *Biochemistry* 1982; 21:6620–6625.
422. Reddy KN. Streptokinase: Biochemistry and clinical application. *Enzyme* 1988; 40:79–89.
423. Battershill PE, Benfield P, Goa KL. Streptokinase: A review of its pharmacology and therapeutic efficacy in acute myocardial infarction in older patients. *Drugs Aging* 1994; 4:63–86.
424. Smith RA, Dupe RJ, English PD, Green J. Fibrinolysis with acyl-enzymes: A new approach to thrombolytic therapy. *Nature* 1981; 290:505–508.
425. Monk JP, Heel RC. Anisoylated plasminogen streptokinase activator complex (APSAC): A review of its mechanism of action, clinical pharmacology and therapeutic use in acute myocardial infarction. *Drugs* 1987; 34:25–49.
426. AIMS Trial Study Group. Effect of intravenous APSAC on mortality after acute myocardial infarction: Preliminary report of a placebo-controlled clinical trial. *Lancet* 1988; 545–549.
427. Cannon CP, McCabe CH, Diver DJ, et al. Comparison of front-loaded recombinant tissue-type plasminogen activator, anistreplase and combination thrombolytic therapy for acute myocardial infarction: Results of the Thrombolysis in Myocardial Infarction (TIMI) 4 trial. *J Am Coll Cardiol* 1994; 24:1602–1610.
428. European Myocardial Infarction Project Group. Prehospital thrombolytic therapy in patients with suspected acute myocardial infarction. *N Engl J Med* 1993; 329:383–389.
429. Rawles J, on behalf of the GREAT Group. Halving of mortality at 1 year by domiciliary thrombolysis in the Grampian Region Early Anistreplase Trial (GREAT). *J Am Coll Cardiol* 1994; 23:1–5.
430. White WF, Barlow GH, Mozen MM. The isolation and characterization of plasminogen activators (urokinase) from human urine. *Biochemistry* 1966; 5:2160–2169.
431. Barlow GH. Urinary and kidney cell plasminogen activator (urokinase). *Methods Enzymol* 1976; 45:239–244.
432. Nolli ML, Sarubbi E, Corti A, et al. Production and characteriza-

tion of human recombinant single chain urokinase-type plasminogen activator from mouse cells. *Fibrinolysis* 1989; 3:101–106.
433. Scully MF. Plasminogen activator–dependent pericellular proteolysis. *Br J Haematol* 1991; 79:537–543.
434. Holmes WE, Pennica D, Blaber M, et al. Cloning and expression of the gene for pro-urokinase in *Escherichia coli. Biotechnology* 1985; 3:923–929.
435. Declerck PJ, Lijnen HR, Verstreken M, et al. A monoclonal antibody specific for two-chain urokinase-type plasminogen activator: Application to the study of the mechanism of clot lysis with single-chain urokinase-type plasminogen activator in plasma. *Blood* 1990; 75:1794–1800.
436. Scully MF, Ellis V, Watahiki Y, Kakkar VV. Activation of pro-urokinase by plasmin: Non-Michaelian kinetics indicates a mechanism of negative cooperativity. *Arch Biochem Biophys* 1989; 268:438–446.
437. Van de Werf F, Bergmann SR, Fox KA, et al. Coronary thrombolysis with intravenously administered human tissue-type plasminogen activator produced by recombinant DNA technology. *Circulation* 1984; 69:605–610.
438. Chesebro JH, Knatterud G, Roberts R, et al. Thrombolysis in Myocardial Infarction (TIMI) trial, phase 1: A comparison between intravenous tissue plasminogen activator and intravenous streptokinase. *Circulation* 1987; 76:142–154.
439. Verstraete M, Bernard R, Bory M, et al. Randomised trial of intravenous recombinant tissue-type plasminogen activator versus intravenous streptokinase in acute myocardial infarction: Report from the European Cooperative Study Group for Recombinant Tissue-type Plasminogen Activator. *Lancet* 1985; 1:842–847.
440. Granger CB, Califf RM, Topol EJ. Thrombolytic therapy for acute myocardial infarction. *Drugs* 1992; 44:293–325.
441. Neuhaus K-L, Feuerer W, Jeep-Teebe S, et al. Improved thrombolysis with a modified dose regimen of recombinant tissue-type plasminogen activator. *J Am Coll Cardiol* 1989; 14:1566–1569.
442. Carney RJ, Murphy GA, Brandt TR, et al. Randomized angiographic trial of recombinant tissue-type plasminogen activator (alteplase) in myocardial infarction. *J Am Coll Cardiol* 1992; 20:17–23.
443. Neuhaus K-L, Von Essen R, Tebbe U, et al. Improved thrombolysis in acute myocardial infarction with front-loaded administration of alteplase: Results of the rt-PA-APSAC Patency Study (TAPS). *J Am Coll Cardiol* 1992; 19:885–891.
444. Purvis JA, McNeill AJ, Siddiqui RA, et al. Efficacy of 100 mg of double-bolus alteplase in achieving complete perfusion in the treatment of acute myocardial infarction. *J Am Coll Cardiol* 1994; 23:6–10.
445. Bleich SD, Adgey AAJ, McMechan SR, Love TW, for the DouBLE Study Investigators. An angiographic assessment of alteplase: Double-bolus and frontloaded infusion regimens in myocardial infarction. *Am Heart J* 1998; 136:741–748.
446. Continuous Infusion Versus Double-Bolus Administration of Alteplase (COBALT) Investigators. A comparison of continuous infusion of alteplase with double-bolus administration for acute myocardial infarction. *N Engl J Med* 1997; 337:1124–1130.
447. Martin U, Fischer S, Kohnert U, et al. Thrombolysis with an *Escherichia coli*-produced recombinant plasminogen activator (BM 06.022) in the rabbit model of jugular vein thrombosis. *Thromb Haemost* 1991; 65:560–564.
448. Martin U, Kohler J, Sponer G, Strein K. Pharmacokinetics of the novel recombinant plasminogen activator BM 06.022 in rats, dogs, and non-human primates. *Fibrinolysis* 1992; 6:39–43.
449. Martin U, Von Mollendorff E, Akpan W, et al. Dose-ranging study of the novel recombinant plasminogen activator BM 06.022 in healthy volunteers. *Clin Pharmacol Ther* 1991; 50: 429–436.
450. Muller M, Haerer W, Ellbruck D, et al. Pharmacokinetics and effects on the hemostatic system of bolus application of a novel recombinant plasminogen activator in AMI patients (abstr). *Fibrinolysis* 1992; 6(suppl 2):26.
451. Neuhaus KL, Von Essen R, Vogt A, et al. Dose finding with a novel recombinant plasminogen activator (BM 06.022) in patients with acute myocardial infarction: Results of the German Recombinant Plasminogen Activator Study—A study of the Arbeitsgemeinschaft leitender kardiologischer Krankenhausarzte (ALKK). *J Am Coll Cardiol* 1994; 24:55–60.
452. Tebbe U, Von Essen R, Smolarz A, et al. Open, noncontrolled dose-finding study with a novel recombinant plasminogen activator (BM 06.022) given as a double bolus in patients with acute myocardial infarction. *Am J Cardiol* 1993; 72:518–524.
453. Smalling RW, Bode C, Kalbfleisch J, et al. More rapid, complete and stable coronary thrombolysis with bolus administration of reteplase compared with alteplase infusion in acute myocardial infarction. *Circulation* 1995; 91:2725–2732.
454. Bode C, Smalling RW, Berg G, et al. Randomized comparison of coronary thrombolysis achieved with double-bolus reteplase (recombinant plasminogen activator) and front-loaded, accelerated alteplase (recombinant tissue plasminogen activator) in patients with acute myocardial infarction. *Circulation* 1996; 94: 891–898.
455. International Joint Efficacy Comparison of Thrombolytics. Randomised, doubleblind comparison of reteplase double-bolus administration with streptokinase in acute myocardial infarction (INJECT): Trial to investigate equivalence. *Lancet* 1995; 346: 329–336.
456. Global Use of Strategies to Open Occluded Coronary Arteries (GUSTO III) Investigators. A comparison of reteplase with alteplase for acute myocardial infarction. *N Engl J Med* 1997; 337:1118–1123.
457. Cannon CP, McCabe CH, Gibson CM, et al. TNK-tissue plasminogen activator in acute myocardial infarction: Results of the Thrombolysis in Myocardial Infarction (TIMI) 10A dose-ranging trial. *Circulation* 1997; 95:351–356.
458. Modi NB, Eppler S, Breed J, et al. Pharmacokinetics of a slower clearing tissue plasminogen activator variant, TNK-tPA, in patients with acute myocardial infarction. *Thromb Haemost* 1998; 79:134–139.
459. Keyt BA, Paoni NF, Refino CJ, et al. A faster-acting and more potent form of tissue plasminogen activator. *Proc Natl Acad Sci USA* 1994; 91:3670–3674.
460. Benedict CR, Refino CJ, Keyt BA, et al. New variant of human tissue plasminogen activator (TPA) with enhanced efficacy and lower incidence of bleeding compared with recombinant human TPA. *Circulation* 1995; 92:3032–3040.
461. Collen D, Stassen J-M, Yasuda T, et al. Comparative thrombolytic properties of tissue-type plasminogen activator and of a plasminogen activator inhibitor-1-resistant glycosylation variant, in a combined arterial and venous thrombosis model in the dog. *Thromb Haemost* 1994; 72:98–104.
462. Tanswell P, Tebbe U, Neuhaus K-L, et al. Pharmacokinetics and fibrin specificity of alteplase during accelerated infusions in acute myocardial infarction. *J Am Coll Cardiol* 1992; 19:1071–1075.
463. Cannon CP, Gibson CM, McCabe CH, et al. TNK-tissue plasminogen activator compared with front-loaded alteplase in acute myocardial infarction: Results of the TIMI 10B trial. *Circulation* 1998; 98:2805–2814.
464. Torr SR, Machowiak DA, Fujii S, Sobel BE. "Plasminogen steal" and clot lysis. *J Am Coll Cardiol* 1992; 19:1085–1090.
465. Gibson CM, Cannon CP, Murphy SA, et al. Weight-adjusted dosing of TNK–tissue plasminogen activator and its relation to angiographic outcomes in the Thrombolysis in Myocardial Infarction 10B trial. *Am J Cardiol* 1999; 84:976–980.
466. Wang-Clow F, Fox NL, Berioli S, et al. A simple, incremental

weight-adjusted dosing scheme for TNK-tPA, a bioengineered variant of the natural t-PA molecule (abstr). *Circulation* 1998; 98(suppl I):I-280.

467. Fox NL, Cannon CP, Berioli S, et al. Rates of serious bleeding requiring transfusion in AMI patients treated with TNK-tPA (abstr). *J Am Coll Cardiol* 1999; 33(suppl A):353A.
468. Van de Werf F, Cannon CP, Luyten A, et al. Safety assessment of single-bolus administration of TNK tissue-plasminogen activator in acute myocardial infarction: The ASSENT-I trial. *Am Heart J* 1999; 137:786–791.
469. Assessment of the Safety and Efficacy of a New Thrombolytic Investigators. Single-bolus tenecteplase compared with front-loaded alteplase in acute myocardial infarction: The ASSENT-2 double-blind randomised trial. *Lancet* 1999; 354: 716–722.
470. Ware JH, Antman EM. Equivalence trials (editorial). *N Engl J Med* 1997; 337:1159–1161.
471. Zeymer U, Tebbe U, Von Essen R, et al., for the ALKK Study Group. Influence of time-to-treatment on early infarct-related artery patency after different thrombolytic regimens. *Am Heart J* 1999; 137:34–38.
472. Cannon CP. Timely thrombolysis: Synergism to open arteries and reduce mortality rates (editorial). *Am Heart J* 1999; 137:1–3.
473. Barron HV, Fox NL, Berioli S, et al. Comparison of intracranial hemorrhage rates in patients treated with rt-PA and TNK-tPA: Impact of gender, age and low body weight. *Circulation* 1999; 100(suppl I):I-1.
474. Simoons ML, Maggioni AP, Knatterud G, et al. Individual risk assessment for intracranial hemorrhage during thrombolytic therapy. *Lancet* 1993; 342:1523–1528.
475. Gurwitz JH, Gore JM, Goldberg RJ, et al. Risk for intracranial hemorrhage after tissue plasminogen activator treatment for acute myocardial infarction. Participants in the National Registry of Myocardial Infarction 2. *Ann Intern Med* 1998; 129: 597–604.
476. Fox NL, Barron HV, Berioli S, et al. Risk of serious bleeding in AMI patients treated with TNK-tPA or rtPA (abstr). *Circulation* 1999; 100(suppl I):I-793.
477. Gardell SJ, Duong LT, Diehl RE, et al. Isolation, characterization, and cDNA cloning of a vampire bat salivary plasminogen activator. *J Biol Chem* 1989; 264:17,947–17,952.
478. Witt W, Maass B, Baldus B, et al. Coronary thrombolysis with *Desmodus* salivary plasminogen activator in dogs: Fast and persistent recanalization by intravenous bolus administration. *Circulation* 1994; 90:421–426.
479. Bergum PW, Gardell SJ. Vampire bat salivary plasminogen activator exhibits a strict and fastidious requirement for polymeric fibrin as its cofactor, unlike human tissue-type plasminogen activator: A kinetic analysis. *J Biol Chem* 1992; 267:17,726–17,731.
480. Gardell SJ, Hare TR, Bergum PW, et al. Vampire bat salivary plasminogen activator is quiescent in human plasma in the absence of fibrin unlike human tissue plasminogen activator. *Blood* 1990; 76:2560–2564.
481. Schleuning WD, Alagon A, Boidol W, et al. Plasminogen activators from the saliva of *Desmodus rotundus* (common vampire bat): Unique fibrin dependence. *Ann NY Acad Sci* 1993; 667: 395–403.
482. Collen D, Lijnen HR. Staphylokinase, a fibrin-specific plasminogen activator with therapeutic potential? *Blood* 1994; 84: 680–686.
483. Schlott B, Hartmann M, Guhrs KH, et al. Functional properties of recombinant staphylokinase variants obtained by site-specific mutagenesis of methionine-26. *Biochim Biophys Acta* 1994; 1204:235–242.
484. Lijnen HR, Van Hoef B, Vandenbossche L, Collen D. Biochemical properties of natural and recombinant staphylokinase. *Fibrinolysis* 1992; 6:214–225.
485. Schlott B, Hartmann M, Guhrs KH, et al. High yield production and purification of recombinant staphylokinase for thrombolytic therapy. *Biotechnology* 1994; 12:185–189.
486. Collen D, Van de Werf F. Coronary thrombolysis with recombinant staphylokinase in patients with evolving myocardial infarction. *Circulation* 1993; 87:1850–1853.
487. Vanderschueren SM, Stassen JM, Collen D. On the immunogenicity of recombinant staphylokinase in patients and in animal models. *Thromb Haemost* 1994; 72:297–301.
488. Vanderschueren S, Barrios L, Kerdsinchai P, et al. A randomized trial of recombinant staphylokinase versus alteplase for coronary artery patency in acute myocardial infarction. The STAR Trial Group. *Circulation* 1995; 92:2044–2049.
489. Stein B, Fuster V, Israel DH, et al. Platelet inhibitor agents in cardiovascular disease: An update. *J Am Coll Cardiol* 1989; 14:813–836.
490. Ridker PM, Manson JE, Gaziano JM, et al. Low-dose aspirin therapy for chronic stable angina: A randomized, placebo-controlled clinical trial. *Ann Intern Med* 1991; 114:835–839.
491. Fuster V, Dyken ML, Vokonas PS, Hennekens C. Aspirin as a therapeutic agent in cardiovascular disease. *Circulation* 1993; 87:659–675.
492. Cannon CP. Optimizing the treatment of unstable angina. *J Thromb Thrombolysis* 1995; 2:205–218.
493. Topol EJ, Byzora TV, Plow ER. Platelet GPIIb-IIIa blockers. *Lancet* 1999; 353:227–231.

CHAPTER 45

PERCUTANEOUS CORONARY INTERVENTION

John S. Douglas, Jr. / Spencer B. King III

The treatment of patients with coronary heart disease changed dramatically with the advent and refinement of coronary artery surgical techniques in the 1970s and percutaneous coronary intervention in the next decade. This chapter addresses the development and contemporary use of catheter-based coronary artery intervention, including selection of patients and devices, procedural issues, results, complications, and long-term outcome.

DEVELOPMENT OF BALLOON ANGIOPLASTY

Percutaneous transluminal coronary angioplasty (PTCA) was conceived and shepherded into worldwide acceptance and application by Andreas R. Gruentzig, but the stage was set by the pioneering effort of others. Gruentzig's ideas were a direct extension of the work of Dotter and Judkins,[1] who in 1964 mechanically dilated femoral arteries with a coaxial double-catheter system, and of Zeitler,[2] who applied this technique successfully in West Germany and introduced it to Gruentzig. After Gruentzig's development of a polyvinyl chloride balloon catheter with fixed maximal inflated diameters in 1974, modern balloon angioplasty evolved rapidly. With further balloon catheter miniaturization and building on the coronary arteriography techniques of Sones and Judkins, Gruentzig succeeded in dilating experimental stenoses in canine coronary arteries[3–5] and then in dilating human arteries during bypass surgery. In September 1977, the first PTCA was performed in Zurich in a 37-year-old insurance salesman with severe angina pectoris and high-grade stenosis of the proximal left anterior descending (LAD) coronary artery.[6–8] Balloon angioplasty was successful in relieving the stenosis, and on the tenth anniversary of this landmark procedure, coronary arteriography revealed angiographically normal coronary arteries (Fig. 45-1). Over 20 years later, the patient remained asymptomatic.

Following the report of Gruentzig's first five patients in 1978[9] and 50 patients in 1979,[10] worldwide interest in the technique was assured. Under the auspices of the National Heart, Lung, and Blood Institute (NHLBI), multicenter registries were formed to report experiences with the evolving technique of balloon coronary angioplasty.[11–13] Development of an over-the-wire balloon catheter by Simpson et al.,[14] combined with advances in guidewire and balloon catheter technology, resulted in a steerable balloon catheter system capable of crossing and dilating heretofore unreachable coronary stenoses (Fig. 45-2). The use of percutaneous revascularization increased dramatically, exceeding 130,000 procedures in the United States in 1986, 400,000 in 1995, and 600,000 in 1999. By 1986 at Emory University Hospital, catheter-based revascularization techniques were performed more frequently than coronary artery bypass grafting (CABG) for relief from symptoms of ischemic heart disease (Fig. 45-3).

Initially, coronary balloon angioplasty was performed for discrete, proximal, noncalcified, subtotal lesions located in one coronary artery. Gruentzig was able to dilate successfully 64 percent of the initial 50 patients and 78 percent of the first 169.[10,15] Most of the patients dilated successfully were improved symptomatically. A 10-year follow-up of Gruentzig's early Zurich series revealed an overall survival rate of 90 and 95 percent for those with single-vessel disease.[15,16] Five-year survival in the NHLBI Registry was 93 percent for single-vessel disease and 87 percent for patients with multivessel disease,[17] and 70 percent of patients were free of target vessel revascularization at 10 years.[18] Large observational studies comparing medical, surgical, and PTCA therapy suggested that revascularization surpassed medical therapy for most anatomic subsets and that surgery provided a survival benefit over PTCA in severe multivessel disease.[19,20] Recently published observational data

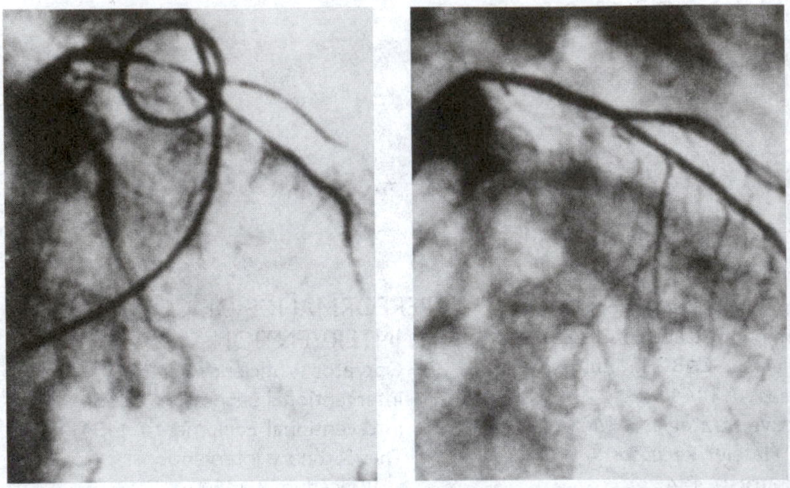

FIGURE 45-1 Right anterior oblique coronary arteriogram of the first patient who underwent transluminal coronary angioplasty on September 16, 1977 (*left*) and on September 16, 1987 (*right*). During this 10-year period, the patient remained completely asymptomatic, and the arteriogram at 10 years showed no narrowing in the coronary arteries. Over 20 years later, the patient is free of symptoms.

from the 1993–1995 New York State Cardiac Procedure Registry of 60,000 CABG and PTCA procedures reported better 3-year survival with CABG in patients with three-vessel disease and those patients with two-vessel disease/proximal LAD stenosis treated with CABG, whereas those with one-vessel disease/no LAD stenosis had better survival with PTCA. All other patients had similar survival with PTCA and CABG.[21] Only now are outcomes for similar anatomic subsets being reported from randomized trials,[22] and these results do not indicate a superiority of CABG over PTCA except in diabetics with three-vessel disease (see "Randomized Trials of Balloon Angioplasty," below).

RANDOMIZED TRIALS OF BALLOON ANGIOPLASTY

PTCA versus Medical Therapy

The favorable results of these observational studies and others reporting single-vessel and multivessel

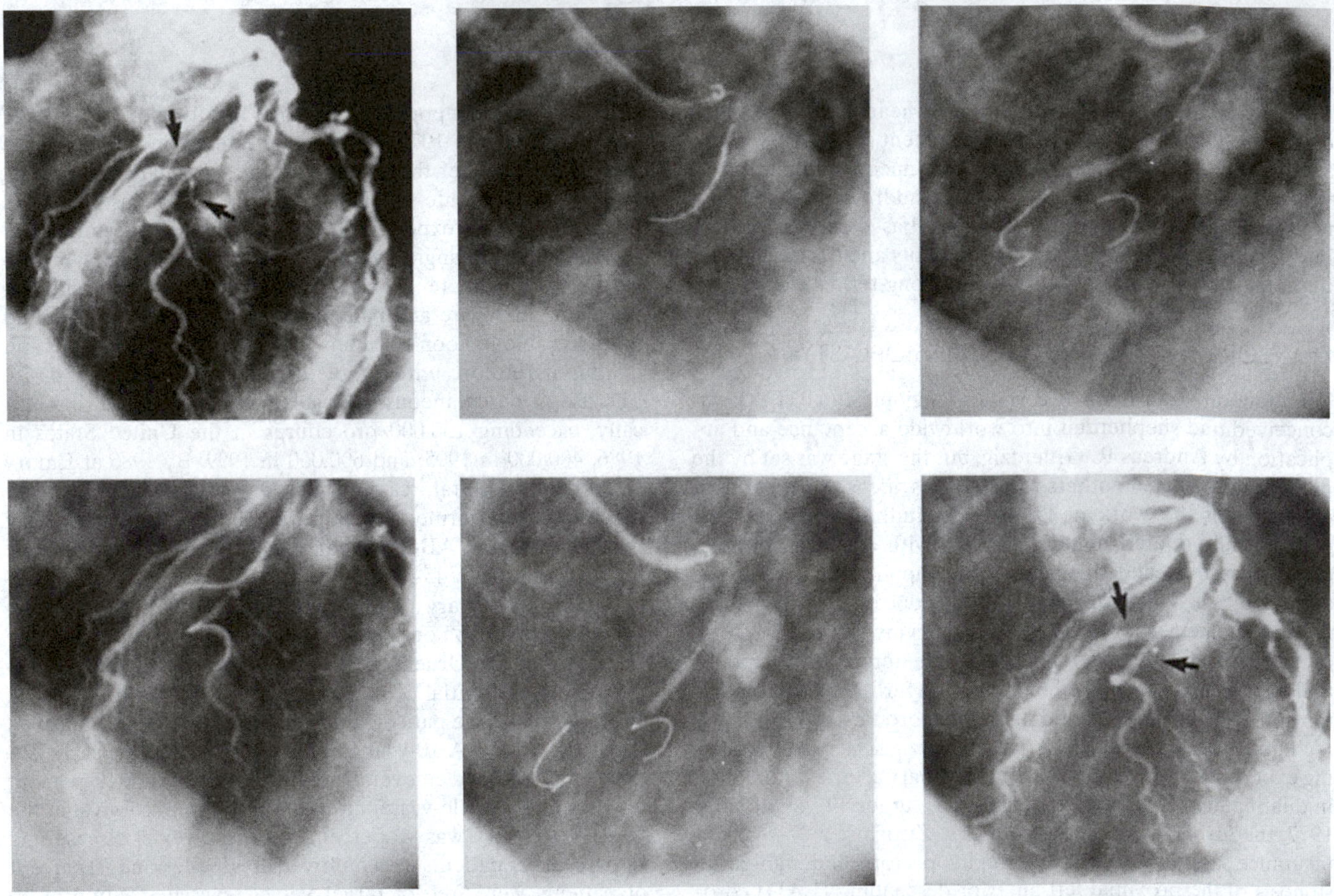

FIGURE 45-2 Angioplasty of high-grade stenoses of the LAD and diagonal bifurcation (*arrows*) using a single guiding catheter through which two dilatation devices were passed. The LAD artery was dilated with a 2.5-mm balloon (note "waist" of the balloon produced by the lesion), and the diagonal was dilated with a 2-mm balloon. Note the small intimal tear in the LAD artery following the procedure (*left anterior oblique views*). Treatment of bifurcation lesions continues to present a challenge due to relatively high subsequent cardiac events and restenosis even with the latest stent and/or atherectomy approaches.[57,58,63,64]

disease patients[23,24] led to a series of randomized trials comparing balloon angioplasty with medical therapy[25–31] and with CABG.[32–38] The Angioplasty Compared to Medical Therapy Evaluation (ACME), involving 212 patients with single-vessel disease and abnormal stress tests, revealed greater freedom from angina in the angioplasty group at 6 months (64 versus 46 percent) as well as better treadmill performance (2.1- versus 0.5-min increase). There was no difference in death or myocardial infarction (MI).[25] The Second Randomized Intervention Treatment of Angina (RITA-2) trial randomized 1018 patients with stable angina to PTCA or medical therapy.[28] The majority (60 percent) had single-vessel disease, and 33 percent had two-vessel disease. Angina relief and treadmill performance were significantly better in the PTCA patients, but complications also were more frequent; death or myocardial infarction occurred in 6.3 percent of PTCA patients compared with 3.3 percent of medically treated patients. Symptomatic benefit was greater in the patients with severe angina at baseline. In the Veterans Affairs Non-Q-Wave Infarction Strategies in Hospital (VANQWISH) trial, 920 patients were randomly assigned to either an invasive strategy (routine coronary angiography and myocardial revascularization) or conservative management (medical therapy and noninvasive testing).[26] Although there was no difference in mortality during 12 to 44 months of follow-up, there was a higher incidence of a composite end point (death or nonfatal infarction) in the invasive group at 1 month and at 1 year (111 versus 85 events; $p = 0.05$). Although stents, ticlopidine, and IIb/IIIa inhibitors were not used, there were no deaths at 30 days in the invasive group treated with PTCA but an 11.6 percent 30-day mortality in this group treated with CABG. Whereas the VANQWISH investigators recommended the conservative approach, the recently reported, larger Fast Revascularization During Instability in Coronary Disease (FRISC II) study strongly supported an invasive approach.[30,31] Among men at 6 months, the invasive strategy in FRISC II resulted in a 34 percent reduction in death or MI ($p = 0.002$) and a 52 percent reduction in mortality (1.5 versus 3.2 percent; $p = 0.03$). Although there was no reduction in death or MI in women, there was an approximately 50 percent reduction in symptoms of angina and need for readmissions during 6 months of follow-up.

In 341 mildly symptomatic patients (59 percent asymptomatic or class I, 40 percent class II) in the Atorvastatin versus Revascularization Treatment (AVERT) trial, PTCA was com-

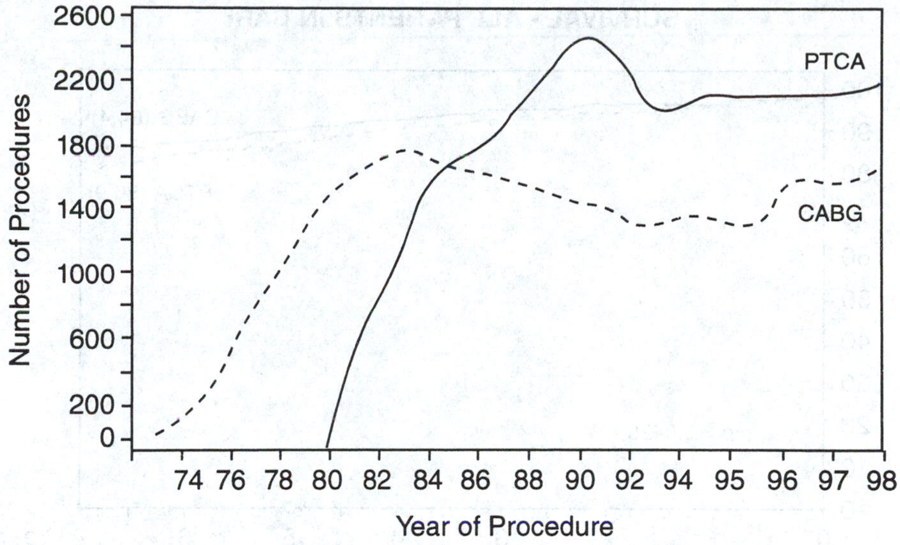

FIGURE 45-3 Coronary revascularization procedures at Emory University Hospitals from 1973 to 1998.

TABLE 45-1 Randomized Comparisons of PTCA and CABG

	EAST		BARI	
	PTCA	CABG	PTCA	CABG
Patient characteristics				
Age (years)	62	61	62	61
Ejection fraction, %	61	62	57	58
Heart failure, %	3	4	9	9
Prior MI, %	41	41	54	55
Diseased vessels, %				
Two	60	60	57	58
Three	40	40	41	41
In-hospital outcome, %				
Myocardial infarction	3	10	2.1	4.6
Death	1	1	1.1	1.3
Repeat revascularization				
PTCA	0	0	3.4	0
CABG	10	0	10.2	0.1
Five-year outcome, %				
Death	12.1	8.8	13.7	10.7
Additional PTCA	48.6	15.5	34.0	7.3
Additional CABG	25.1	0.5	31.3	1.1
Any additional revascularization	61.2	16.1	54.5	8.0

ABBREVIATIONS: EAST = Emory Angioplasty Surgery Trial;[32,37] BARI = Bypass Angioplasty Revascularization Investigation;[33] PTCA = percutaneous transluminal coronary angioplasty; CABG = coronary artery bypass graft surgery.

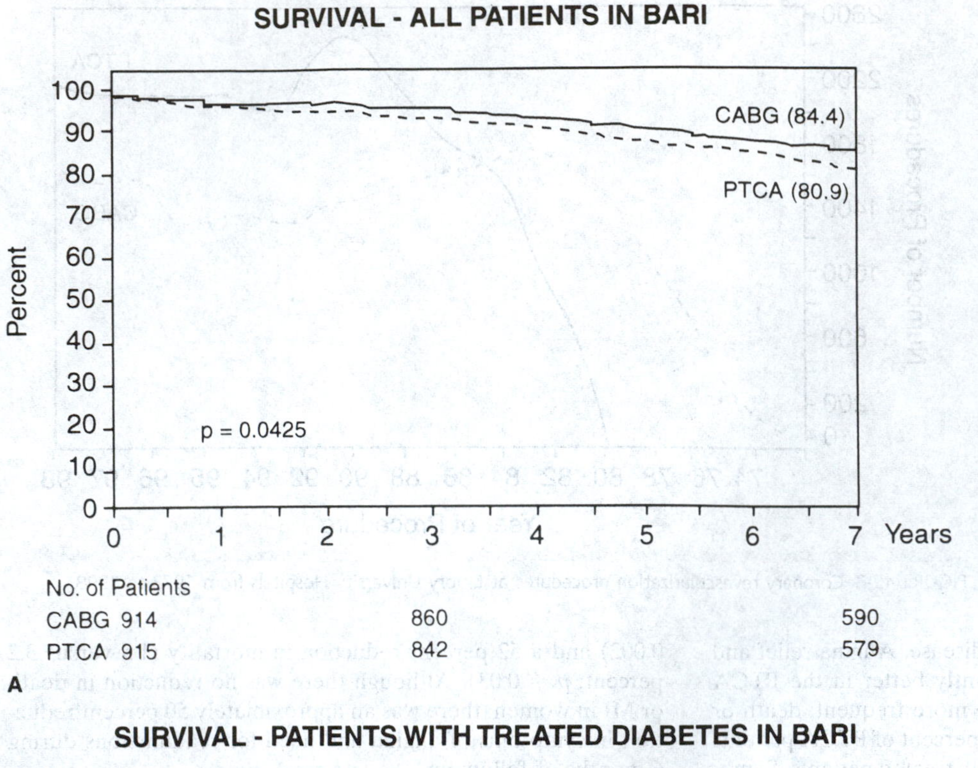

FIGURE 45-4 Survival curves for patients treated with CABG and coronary angioplasty (PTCA) in the Bypass Angioplasty Revascularization Investigation (BARI)[40] (*A-C*) and in the Emory Angioplasty versus Surgery Trial (EAST)[41] (*D-F*).

pared with aggressive lipid-lowering therapy (atorvastatin 80 mg).[29] At 18-month follow-up, angina relief was significantly better ($p < 0.009$) in the PTCA group, with 54 percent having improvement, versus 41 percent in the aggressive lipid-lowering group, but quality-of-life scores were similar, and there was a trend toward more events (primarily hospitalization for ischemia) in the PTCA group. In AVERT, stents were used in 30 percent of patients. This study suggests that in low-risk patients with no or mild symptoms, aggressive lipid lowering is as effective as PTCA in reducing subsequent ischemic events and emphasizes the importance of extending aggressive lipid lowering in all patients with obstructive coronary artery disease. The Medicine, Angioplasty or Surgery Study (MASS) randomized 214 patients with stable angina, normal left ventricular function, and severe proximal LAD stenosis to bypass surgery [with left internal mammary artery (LIMA) graft], PTCA, or medical therapy.[27] At 3 years, there was no difference in death or MI. Both revascularization strategies yielded better symptom relief, but subsequent procedures were more common in the PTCA group.

PTCA versus CABG

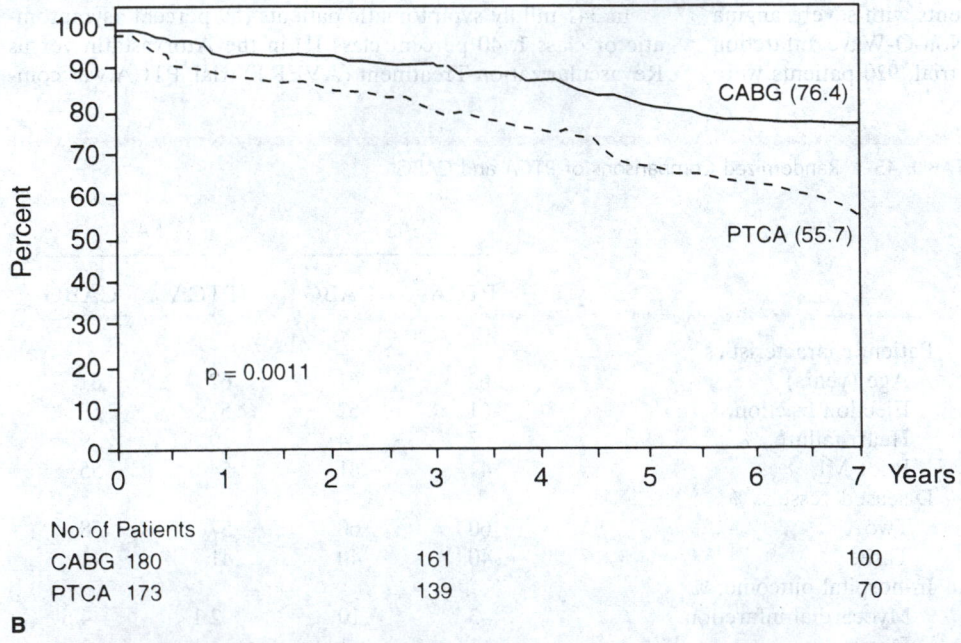

Over 5000 patients have been randomized in nine trials comparing angioplasty with CABG surgery. Two of these trials were sponsored by the NHLBI and performed in the United States. The first, the Emory Angioplasty versus Surgery Trial (EAST), was a single-center study,[32] whereas the larger Bypass Angioplasty Revascularization Investigation (BARI)[33,34] involved 18 centers. In-hospital mortality was similar for angioplasty and bypass surgery (approximately 1 percent) in these two studies of patients with multivessel disease, and 5-year survival also was similar (Table 45-1). Repeat revascularization procedures, however, were more common in the angioplasty group. Freedom from angina was better in the CABG group in both EAST and BARI. Meta-analyses of eight randomized published trials comparing PTCA and CABG (BARI not included) reported no difference in mortality or MI at 1 year after angioplasty or CABG, but 18 percent of the angioplasty patients had required bypass surgery and 20 percent had an additional angioplasty, a significantly higher rate of repeat revascularization than in the surgery group.[35,36] This increased need for additional revascularization procedures in angioplasty patients, largely due to restenosis, eroded the initial cost advantage of angioplasty; by 3 years in the EAST study, angioplasty had been 95 percent as costly as bypass surgery.[37,38]

Considerable interest was generated by a subset analysis of treated diabetics in BARI. Among the 353 diabetics treated with insulin or oral hypoglycemic agents, 5-year survival was significantly better in patients who underwent surgery compared with that of patients who underwent PTCA (80.6 versus 65.5 percent; $p = 0.003$).[39] Analysis of 7-year survival for all patients in BARI revealed for the first time a significantly better survival with CABG compared with PTCA-treated patients (84.4, 80.9 percent; $p = 0.0425$) (Fig. 45-4*A*). This difference was accounted for entirely by the poorer survival of treated diabetics revascularized with PTCA (55.7 versus 76.4 percent for CABG; $p = 0.0011$)[40] (see Fig. 45-4*B*). There was no difference in the survival of nondiabetics (see Fig. 45-4*C*). Further analysis of treated diabetics in BARI revealed that the survival benefit with CABG was conferred only to those patients who received an internal mammary artery (IMA) graft. The 7-year survival of patients treated with an IMA graft was 83.2 percent compared with 54.5 percent for saphenous vein graft only patients, a figure comparable with that attained with PTCA. EAST, which initially showed no difference between PTCA and CABG in diabetics, now at 8 years shows the same trend as BARI [41] (see Fig. 45-4*D*–*F*). Considering the rather late manifestation of these outcome differences, it is likely that factors other than early restenosis must be operative. Development of new lesions, perhaps unrecognized, probably accounts for those events occurring many years after revascularization. Poorer outcomes also were reported for diabetics in the BARI registry[42] and in the Emory University Hospital database.[43] In these randomized trials and observational reports, balloon angioplasty was the predominant interventional strategy. Use of stents has been shown to reduce restenosis, and their use in trials of stents versus CABG (see "Stents: After a Decade of Use the Dominant Strategy," below) and in diabetic patients is discussed below. Pending clarification by these trials, caution should exercised in the use of PTCA in diabetic patients with multivessel disease[44] and use of arterial grafts emphasized in diabetic patients.[45,46]

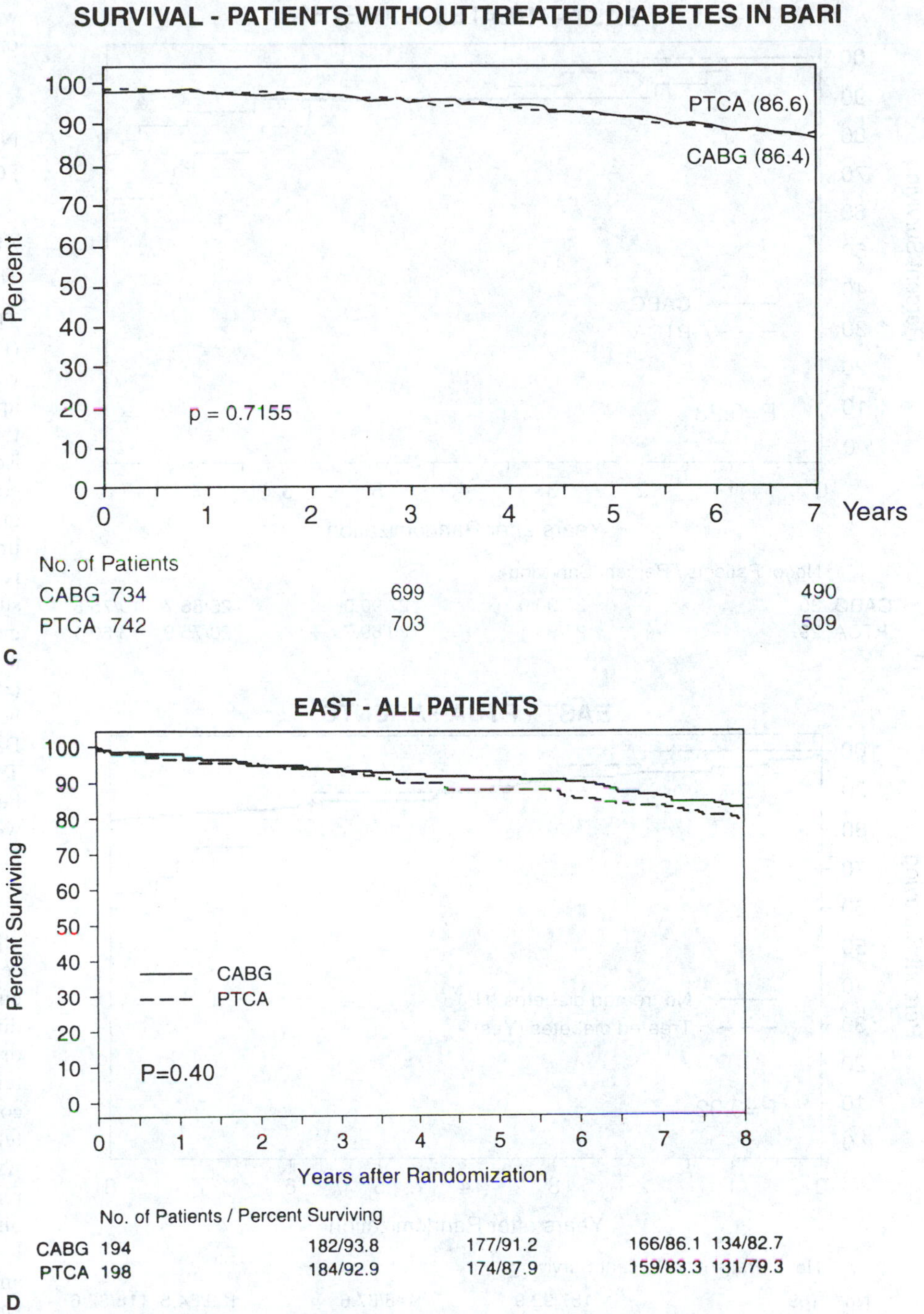

FIGURE 45-4 (*Continued*)

Only recently have data become available from BARI analyzing long-term outcomes based on more specific anatomic subsets.[22] At 7 years, there was no difference in survival of PTCA-treated versus CABG-treated patients with three-vessel disease without diabetes (85 versus 87 percent; $p = 0.4$, $n =$

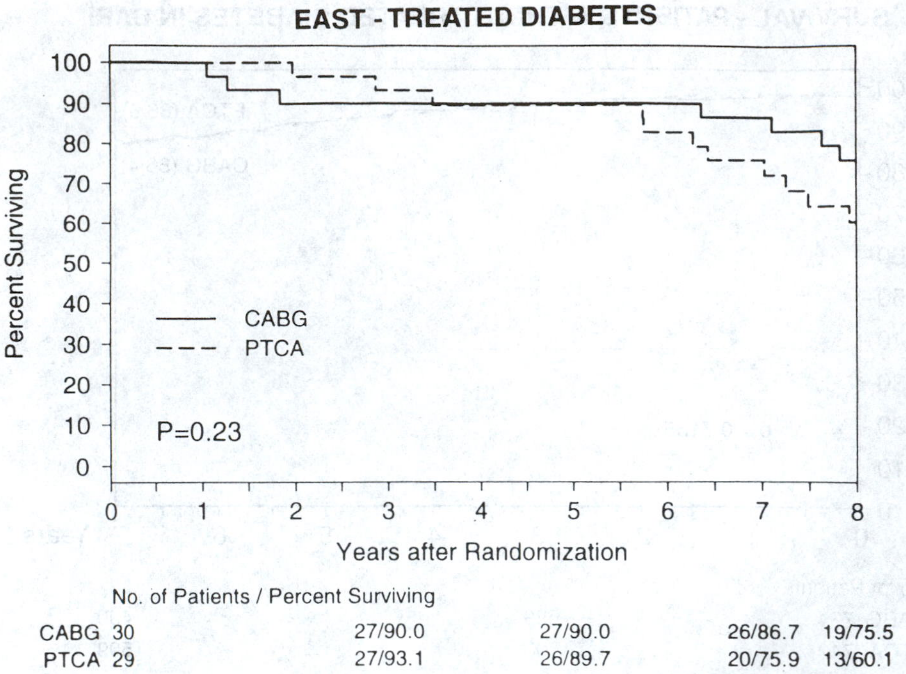

E

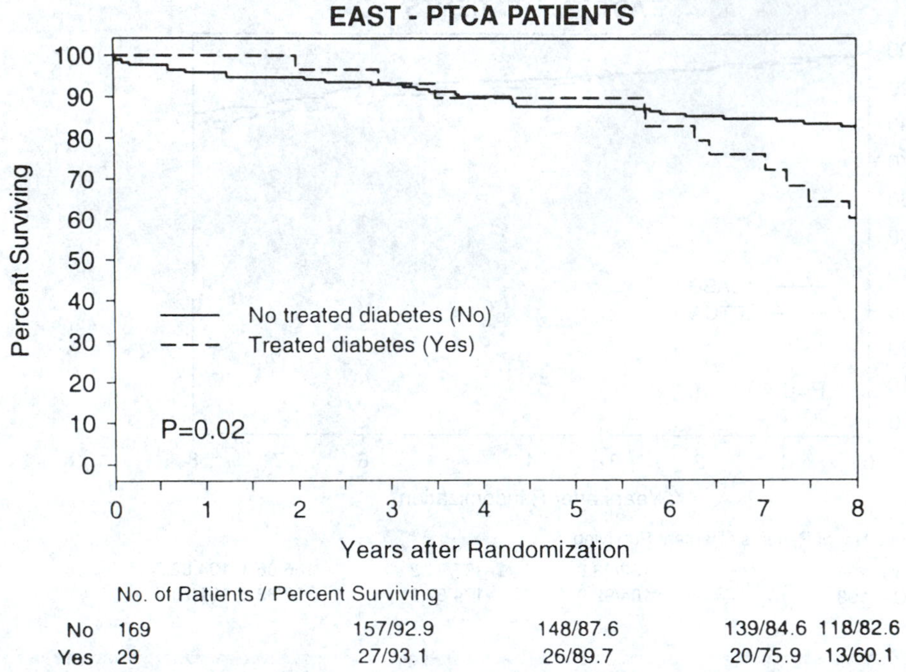

F

FIGURE 45-4 *(Continued)*

592), three-vessel disease with decreased left ventricular ejection fraction (LVEF) (70 versus 74 percent; $p = 0.6$, $n = 176$), two-vessel disease with proximal LAD stenosis (87 versus 84 percent; $p = 0.9$, $n = 352$), and two-vessel disease with proximal LAD stenosis and decreased LVEF (78 versus 71 percent; $p = 0.7$, $n = 72$). Contrary to the New York State Cardiac Procedure Registry data, these findings of a prospective, randomized trial tend to support the appropriateness of PTCA in nondiabetics with multivessel disease when the anatomy is permissive and the patient prefers a percutaneous approach.

NEW DEVICES AND STRATEGIES FOR CORONARY INTERVENTION

Atherectomy, Laser, and Thrombectomy Devices

The directional atherectomy catheter (Fig. 45-5*A*) developed by Simpson[47] was, in 1990, the first nonballoon device approved for coronary intervention and the first to undergo randomized comparison with balloon angioplasty. In native coronary artery[48,49] and saphenous vein graft lesions[50] judged suitable for either procedure, however, the more costly directional atherectomy did not show a substantive advantage over balloon angioplasty. Additional trials using techniques to achieve optimal atherectomy (<20 percent residual stenosis) have been completed.[51,52] The randomized Balloon versus Optimal Atherectomy Trial (BOAT) showed no increase in in-hospital death, Q-wave MI, or CABG with directional atherectomy, but a higher rate of non-Q-wave infarction occurred (16 versus 6 percent; $p < 0.0001$).[51] Restenosis was lower in the atherectomy arm (31 versus 39.8 percent; $p = 0.016$), but there was no difference in late clinical events. The use of directional atherectomy has declined dramatically in most but not all centers[53,54] because of its complexity, added cost, and marginal benefit. In some centers, this technique is used to debulk lesions prior to stenting with the hope of reducing restenosis[55,56] and for lesions at bifurcations and ostial lesions of the LAD coronary artery.[57,58] Excimer laser angioplasty was approved by the Food and Drug Administration (FDA) in 1992 for lesions not favorable for balloon angioplasty, but this technology has not been shown superior to balloon angioplasty[59] and is used infrequently in most centers and then primarily for treating in-stent restenosis, where it is safe and initially effective but has no proven superiority.[60] In 1994, two additional atherectomy devices, the Rotablator (Heart Technologies, Bellevue, WA; see Fig. 45-5*B*) and the Transluminal Extraction Catheter (TEC) (Interventional Technologies, San Diego, CA; see Fig. 45-5*C*) were approved for marketing by the FDA. The Rotablator's principal advantage is in the treatment of calcified and undilatable stenoses, but it is also used to treat bifurcation lesions and in-stent restenosis and to debulk

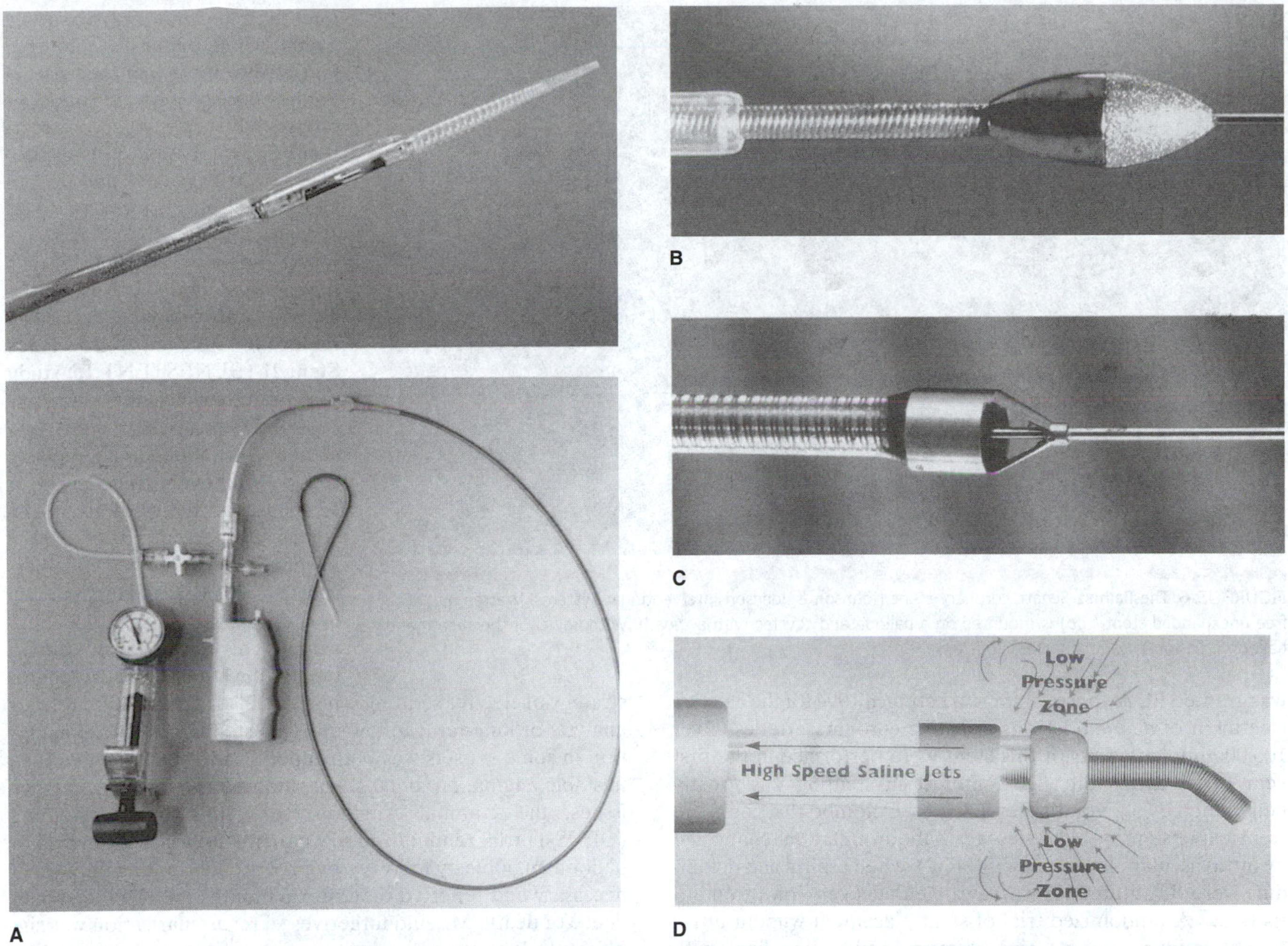

FIGURE 45-5 *A.* Directional atherectomy device (Simpson Atherocath, Devices for Vascular Intervention, Inc., Redwood City, CA). A battery-powered motor unit drives a cable that spins the cutter at approximately 2500 rev/min. *B.* Rotational atherectomy burr (Rotablator, Heart Technologies, Bellevue, WA) and the special 0.009-in. stainless steel guidewire over which the diamond-embedded burr spins at 150,000 to 200,000 rev/min. *C.* Transluminal Extraction Catheter (TEC, Interventional Technologies, Inc., San Diego, CA). The catheter rotates at 750 rev/min over a special 0.014-in. guidewire. Vacuum bottles aspirate plaque and thrombus cut by the blades of the conical head. *D.* Angiojet rheolytic thrombectomy catheter (POSSIS Medical, Inc., Minneapolis, MN); high-velocity jets, by virtue of the Bernoulli effect, pull thrombus into the catheter lumen, where it is evacuated.

prior to stenting.[61–64] The TEC device is used principally in saphenous vein grafts, where aspiration of thrombus is its unique attribute. In 1999, a rheolytic thrombectomy device known as the Angiojet (POSSIS Medical, Inc., Minneapolis, MN; see Fig. 45-5*D*) also became available for treatment of intracoronary thrombus, and it has proved useful in the setting of acute coronary syndromes associated with large thrombi and in treatment of stent thrombosis.[65–69]

Stents: After a Decade of Use, the Dominant Strategy

None of the devices described earlier had the impact on interventional cardiology that was produced by the development of the stainless steel intracoronary stent. The first coronary stents were implanted in patients in 1986 by Puel in Toulouse and Sigwart in Lausanne for restenosis prevention,[70,71] an unproven hypothesis at the time, whereas the initial implantation in a patient in the United States was performed by the authors at Emory University in 1987 in the setting of abrupt closure,[72,73] following encouraging results in a canine model by Roubin et al.[74] The initial European experience was with a self-expanding mesh stent, whereas the experience at Emory was with a balloon-mounted coil stent that subsequently was marketed as the Gianturco-Roubin flex stent (Cook, Inc., Bloomington, IN) following FDA approval for abrupt or threatened closure in 1993. This stent made balloon angioplasty considerably safer by providing effective therapy for coronary dissections and reducing the need for emergency coronary bypass surgery, but the use of this stent, despite intensive anticoagulation with heparin and warfarin, was complicated by stent thrombosis in 5 to 10 percent of patients, and bleeding was a common complication. The device that ultimately revolutionized interventional cardiology was the Palmaz-Schatz stent (Johnson & Johnson Interventional Systems, Warren, NJ) (Fig. 45-6). On the basis of two carefully conducted randomized trials that showed reduced restenosis compared with balloon angioplasty,[75,76] this device

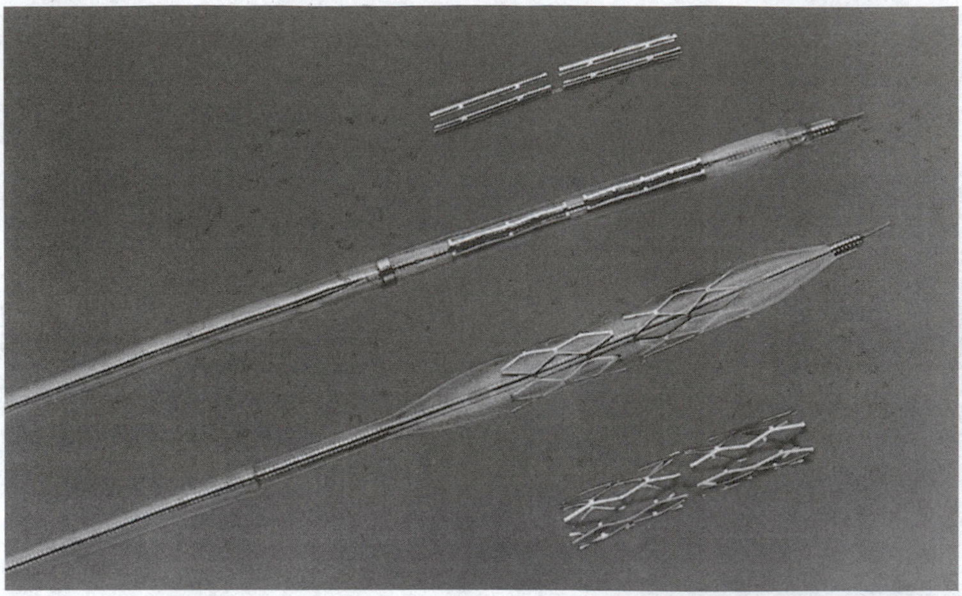

FIGURE 45-6 The Palmaz-Schatz coronary stent (Johnson & Johnson Interventional Systems, Warren, NJ). The free unexpanded stent (*top*) is mounted on a balloon and covered with a sheath. Withdrawal of the sheath and balloon inflation expand the stent (*bottom*).

was granted FDA approval for marketing in 1994 for the elective treatment of *de novo* lesions in native coronary arteries. Over 100,000 implantations of this stent were performed in the first year of its availability. The interest in stenting was greatly heightened by a pivotal observation by Colombo that complete stent expansion by high-pressure balloon inflation, confirmed by intravascular ultrasound (Fig. 45-7), when aspirin and ticlopidine were substituted for warfarin, yielded a very low thrombosis rate.[77] A randomized trial of stent placement without ultrasound guidance comparing aspirin and ticlopidine with phenprocoumon (a warfarin derivative) (ISAR) revealed a low 30-day incidence of cardiac events and bleeding rates in the aspirin-ticlopidine patients, supporting this simplified antithrombotic strategy[78,79] (Fig. 45-8). This finding was confirmed and extended by the Stent Anticoagulation Restenosis Study (STARS) investigation, which showed that aspirin and ticlopidine resulted in a lower rate of stent thrombosis than aspirin alone or a combination of aspirin and warfarin[80] (see Fig. 45-8), by a multicenter comparison of aspirin and ticlopidine with aspirin and oral anticoagulation in medium-risk (FANTASTIC, Fig. 45-8) and high-risk patients showing better outcome with the simpler approach,[81,82] and by a report of Mayo Clinic experience suggesting that 14 days of ticlopidine and aspirin was adequate for prophylaxis against stent thrombosis in most patients.[83] However, rare reports of thrombotic thrombocytopenia purpura related to ticlopidine use accounting for at least 20 deaths[84,85] led most centers to abandon ticlopidine in favor of clopidogrel, also an antagonist of platelet ADP receptors with similar pharmacologic activity but with far fewer side effects.[86] Clopidogrel proved equal to ticlopidine in observational reports,[87,88] and in a randomized investigation, the Clopidogrel Aspirin Stent Interventional Cooperative Study (CLASSICS), it was observed that neutropenia, thrombocytopenia, or early discontinuation of the drug was more common in the ticlopidine group (9.1 versus 2.9 percent) than in the clopidogrel group, which received 300 mg as a loading dose and 75 mg subsequently,[89] and that major cardiac events were similar at 1 month.[90] Currently, most centers use a loading dose of 300 to 525 mg clopidogrel when prolonged pretreatment is not possible plus aspirin 160 to 325 mg daily and 75 mg clopidogrel plus aspirin for 15 to 30 days after stent implantation.

A number of randomized trials have been conducted using the simpler antiplatelet therapy. The important Belgium Netherlands Stent II (BENESTENT II) study that randomized the heparin-coated Palmaz-Schatz stent and standard balloon angioplasty found better event-free survival at 12 months in the stent group (89 versus 79 percent; $p = 0.004$), lower restenosis (16 versus 31 percent; $p = 0.0008$), and higher costs in stent patients by $1020 at 1 year.[91] This study raised fundamental questions as to whether a strategy of elective stenting is justified in all patients, and further analysis of long-term follow-up suggested that stent implantation in some subsets was both superior and cost-effective (i.e., unstable angina, proximal LAD stenosis). To investigate these issues, the Optimal Angioplasty versus Primary Stenting (OPUS-1) trial randomized 479 patients to primary stenting or balloon angioplasty followed by provisional stenting only when necessary and reported that after 6 months the combined incidence of death, MI, and target-vessel revascularization was significantly lower in the primary stenting arm (6.1 versus 14.9 percent; $p = 0.003$), and at 6 months primary stenting was slightly less expensive ($10,206 versus $10,490).[92] This provocative study in which 99 percent of patients in the primary stent arm received a stent compared with 37 percent in the provisional stenting arm supported routine stenting when the anatomy is appropriate as opposed to primary balloon angioplasty with stent backup, a strategy that has been advocated by some investigators[93–95] and, of course, was the dominant strategy in the early days of stenting. The use of coronary stents was reviewed extensively in a recent American College of Cardiology Expert Consensus Document[96] and in other reports.[96a,96b] This document and these newer studies provide perspectives on which to base everyday decisions regarding contemporary coronary intervention.

Stents versus CABG in Multivessel Disease

The issue of whether to recommend CABG or PTCA in patients with multivessel disease will be significantly influenced by the long-term outcome of randomized trials comparing stents with bypass surgery. Intermediate-term data are available from the Arterial Revascularization Therapy Study (ARTS), which randomized 1205 multivessel disease patients in 68 clinical centers to stent or standard CABG. At 1 year, there was no difference in death or MI; however, repeat interventions were higher in the stent group.[97] One-year survival free of death, MI, and

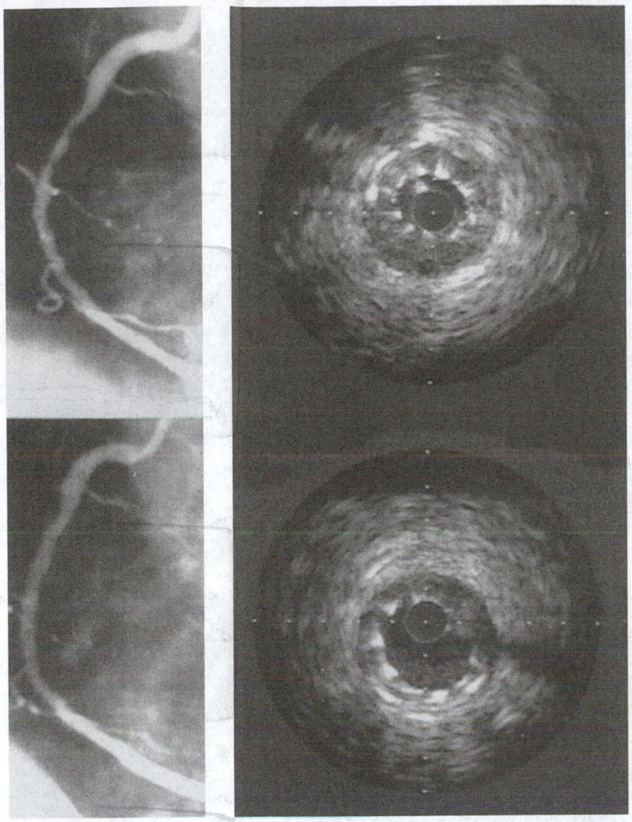

FIGURE 45-7 A 74-year-old woman developed early recurrence of angina after balloon angioplasty of the right coronary artery. Coronary arteriography revealed a severe, long stenosis of the right coronary artery (*top left*). Stenting was advised, and a Wallstent was deployed and dilated with a 3.5-mm balloon to 15 atm with an excellent angiographic result (*bottom left*). IVUS, however, showed that the distal end of the stent had been missed with the balloon and was poorly expanded (*top right*). This area was "redilated" to 16 atm with no change in the angiogram but much better stent expansion and wall apposition by ultrasound (*bottom right*). Following repeat dilation, the lumen cross-sectional area increased from 4.2 to 6.4 mm^2.

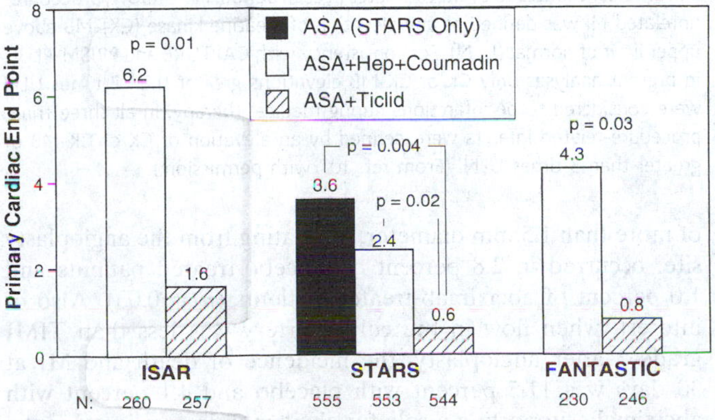

FIGURE 45-8 Results of three trials evaluating antiplatelet versus anticoagulant or aspirin alone therapy for stent prophylaxis. Aspirin and ticlopidine led to significant reduction of death, MI, or need for urgent revascularization. (Data from refs. 78, 80, and 82. Figure from ref. 79 with permission.)

reintervention was seen in 87.6 percent of the surgical group and 73.7 percent of the stent group ($p < 0.04$), but at a higher total 1-year cost (13,645 versus 10,860 euros). The occurrence of late events in 26 percent of ARTS stented patients was approximately one-half the incidence seen following balloon angioplasty in multivessel disease in BARI and EAST due to a reduced need for repeat revascularization in stented patients. As in BARI, the mortality rate in ARTS of diabetics treated percutaneously was significantly higher than that of nondiabetics (6.3 versus 3.1 percent; $p < 0.01$).[98] In the smaller Argentine Randomized Study of Stents versus CABG in Multivessel Disease (ERACI II), 450 patients were randomized, and at 14.7 months, survival was better in the stent group (97.4 versus 92.5 percent; $p < 0.015$) and freedom from MI was higher (97.7 versus 93.4 percent; $p < 0.017$), but repeat revascularization was needed more often in the stent group and costs were similar.[99] The Stent or Surgery Trial (SOS) will soon be completed and should offer additional insights.

Adjunctive Strategies

Intravascular ultrasound (IVUS) also has been used extensively in some centers to evaluate coronary lesions for device therapy and to assess the results of device and balloon treatment,[77,100] but the increased cost of this approach is a limiting factor. Although IVUS has had significant impact on the evolution of interventional cardiology, on the understanding of restenosis, and in evaluation of difficult lesions, its routine use in most centers is limited. See Chap. 47 for a detailed discussion.

IIb/IIIa Platelet Receptor Inhibitors

The latest arrows in the quiver of the interventionalist are the new, potent antiplatelet agents.[101–113] The first approved by the FDA was a monoclonal antibody directed against the platelet glycoprotein IIb/IIIa receptor. This agent, abciximab (ReoPro, Centocor, Malvern, PA), was shown to reduce ischemic complications and late clinical events in high-risk angioplasty.[105] The other IIb/IIIa receptor inhibitors approved by the FDA, unlike the antibody abciximab, are competitive inhibitors; eptifibatide (Integrilin, COR Therapeutics, San Francisco, CA) is a peptide, and tirofiban (Aggrastat, Merck, White House Station, NJ) is a small nonpeptide molecule. Each of these IIb/IIIa agents has been shown to consistently reduce a composite end point of death or nonfatal MI in the setting of coronary intervention and in acute coronary syndromes[79,101–105] (Fig. 45-9). Further, at 3-year follow-up in the EPIC trial, the first major study of abciximab during coronary intervention, a subgroup of 555 patients with acute coronary syndromes treated with bolus abciximab and infusion had a significant reduction in mortality at 3 years.[106] For a detailed discussion of IIb/IIIa platelet receptor inhibitors, see Chap. 44. In a recent review of the use of the three FDA-approved IIb/IIIa receptor inhibitor agents in acute coronary syndromes, it was noted that they were each effective in reducing a composite end point of death or MI when administered prior to or at the time of percutaneous coronary intervention[107] (Fig. 45-10). In most centers, the use of these agents, slowed initially by bleeding complications and high costs, has been increasing especially in high-risk patients. Also contributing to this trend is the favorable outcome of IIb/IIIa receptor inhibitor–treated patients in the Evaluation of Platelet IIb/IIIa

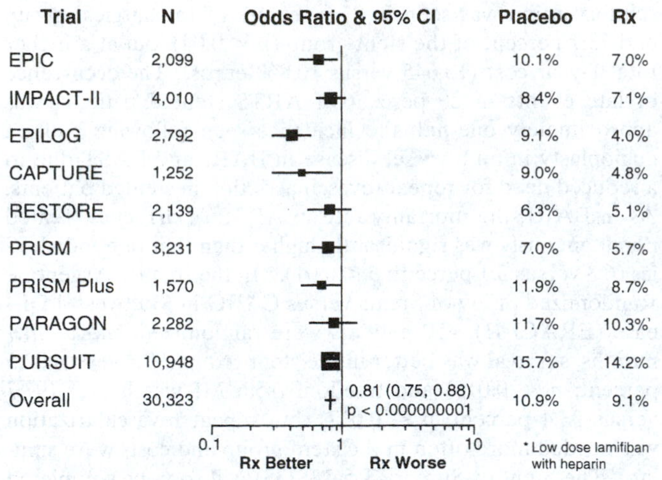
Trial
N
Odds Ratio & 95% CI
Placebo
Rx
EPIC 2,099 10.1% 7.0%
IMPACT-II 4,010 8.4% 7.1%
EPILOG 2,792 9.1% 4.0%
CAPTURE 1,252 9.0% 4.8%
RESTORE 2,139 6.3% 5.1%
PRISM 3,231 7.0% 5.7%
PRISM Plus 1,570 11.9% 8.7%
PARAGON 2,282 11.7% 10.3%*
PURSUIT 10,948 15.7% 14.2%
Overall 30,323 10.9% 9.1%
0.81 (0.75, 0.88)
p < 0.000000001
0.1
1
10
Rx Better
Rx Worse
* Low dose lamifiban with heparin

FIGURE 45-9 Odds ratios and 95 percent confidence intervals for nine large-scale randomized trials of IIb/IIIa platelet receptor inhibitors for percutaneous coronary interventions or unstable angina/non-Q-wave MI. Overall, in 30,323 patients, a 19 percent reduction in death or MI at 30 days was demonstrated. (From ref. 79 with permission.)

Inhibitors of Stenting (EPISTENT) trial, in which abciximab therapy in patients undergoing stent implantation or balloon angioplasty was evaluated.[108,109] At 6 months, the incidence of a composite end point of death or MI was 5.6 percent in patients receiving a stent and abciximab compared with 11.4 percent in those receiving a stent and placebo ($p < 0.001$) and 7.8 percent in patients treated with balloon angioplasty and abciximab (Fig. 45-11). There was a further advantage in diabetics, in whom the combination of abciximab and stenting was associated with a lower rate of repeat target vessel revascularization (8.1 percent) than was observed with stenting and placebo (16.6 percent; $p = 0.02$) or angioplasty and abciximab (18.4 percent; $p = 0.008$), and this benefit persisted through 1-year follow-up.[110] The mechanism by which target-vessel revascularization was reduced in the abciximab-treated patients is unclear.[111] Previous reports indicate that abciximab did not prevent neointimal proliferation or reduce in-stent restenosis.[112] EPISTENT does, however, raise the question regarding whether all diabetic patients and further all patients receiving stents should receive IIb/IIIa platelet inhibitors. Ongoing trials of these agents in stented patients may shed light on this important question. Clearly, however, these potent new strategies enhance the ability to provide safe and effective percutaneous revacularization.[113] Recently published data from CAPTURE indicated the presence of a gradient in the benefit obtained from IIb/IIIa receptor inhibition with abciximab in unstable angina. Death or MI was significantly less frequent in patients with elevated baseline troponin treated with abciximab compared with placebo (9.5 versus 23.9 percent; $p = 0.002$), but this end point was not different in troponin-negative patients (7.5 versus 9.4 percent; $p = 0.47$).[114] Stated differently, without an elevated troponin level, there was no benefit of treatment with respect to risk of death or MI. While there was no difference in death, MI, or urgent intervention in simple lesions, there was for complex lesions (ACC/AHA classes B2 and C) an incidence of this end point of 19.1 percent for placebo versus 11.5 percent for abciximab ($p = 0.055$).[115] The benefit gradient was steepest for bifurcation lesions in young patients. Occlusion of a side branch

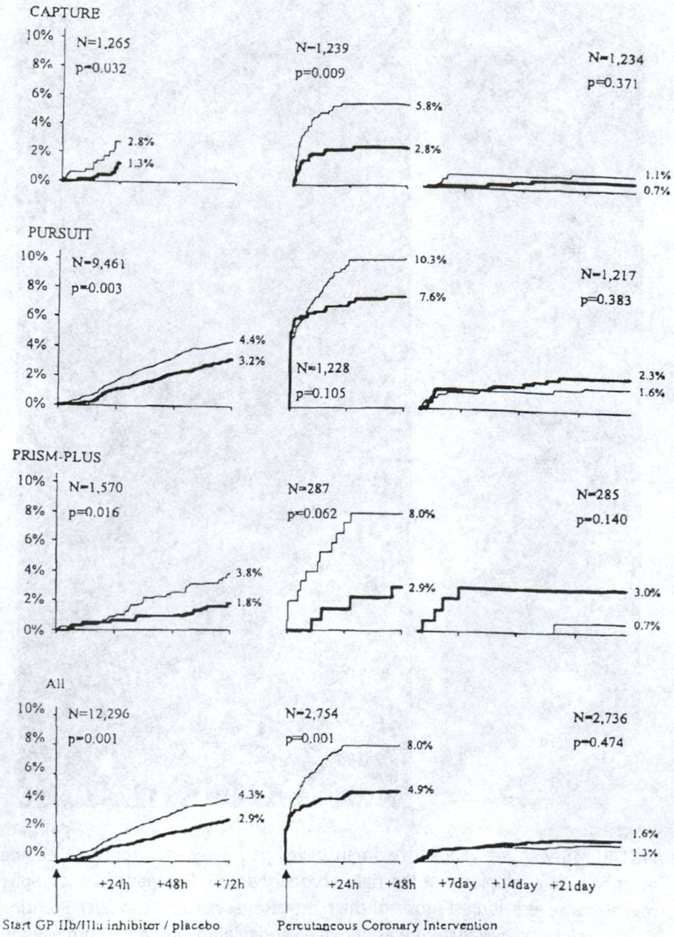

FIGURE 45-10 Kaplan-Meier curves showing cumulative incidence of death or nonfatal myocardial (re)infarction in patients randomly assigned to glycoprotein IIb/IIIa inhibition (*bold lines*) or placebo. Data were derived from CAPTURE, PURSUIT, and PRISM-PLUS.[101,102,103] (*Left*) Event rates during initial period of pharmacologic treatment until moment of a percutaneous coronary intervention (PCI) or coronary bypass grafting, if any. (*Center*) Event rates among PCI patients during 48-hour period after procedure. During and shortly after PCI, all patients were on study medication. (*Right*) Event rates in period starting 48 h after PCI, during which all patients were off study medication. At beginning of each period, event rates were (re)set at 0 percent. Any patient still alive contributes to event estimates in each period. In PURSUIT, procedure-unrelated MI was defined as any elevation of creatine kinase (CK)-MB above upper limit of normal (ULN). For consistency with CAPTURE and PRISM-PLUS, in present analyses only CK or CK-MB elevations greater than 2 times ULN were considered to be infarctions during medical therapy. In all three trials, procedure-related infarcts were defined by an elevation of CK or CK-MB of greater than 3 times ULN. (From ref. 107 with permission.)

of more than 1.5 mm diameter, orginating from the angioplasty site, occurred in 2.8 percent of placebo-treated patients and 1.0 percent of abciximab-treated patients ($p = 0.03$). Also of interest, when flow in the culprit artery was less than TIMI grade 3 after angioplasty, the incidence of death and MI at 30 days was 11.5 percent with placebo and 4.1 percent with abciximab, supporting a role for abciximab in ameliorating the consequences of postprocedure slow flow. These observations that IIb/IIIa receptor inhibitors appear to be more effective in patients with refractory unstable angina, complex anatomy, and slow flow, results not observed previously,[104,105,116] may help in the design of trials to better determine the place of these agents.

INDICATIONS FOR CORONARY INTERVENTION

In general, when one is selecting percutaneous coronary intervention, there should be assurance that the operator can treat, with a high probability of success, the coronary lesion(s) accounting for the symptoms or signs of myocardial ischemia. Further, the associated risk and durability of the revascularization should be acceptable as compared with bypass surgery or medical therapy during both early and long-term follow-up. The latter estimate requires consideration of the likelihood and consequences of abrupt vessel closure, restenosis, and incomplete revascularization. In addition, one cannot disregard the comparative costs of the initial intervention, its complications, and the need for subsequent revascularization procedures. The American College of Cardiology/American Heart Association Guidelines for Percutaneous Transluminal Coronary Angioplasty and Coronary Bypass Surgery provide a detailed analysis of many of these issues.[45,117,118]

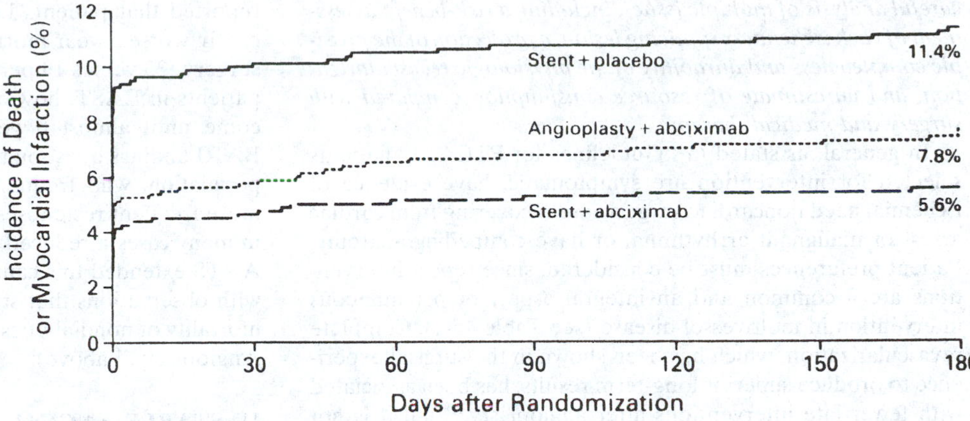

FIGURE 45-11 Kaplan-Meier estimates from EPISTENT of the incidence of the composite end point of death or MI within 6 months of randomization according to treatment assignment. For the composite end point of death or MI, $p < 0.001$ for the comparison between stent plus abciximab group and the stent plus placebo group, $p = 0.01$ for the comparison between angioplasty plus abciximab and stent plus placebo, and $p = 0.07$ for the comparison between stent plus abciximab and angioplasty plus abciximab. (From ref. 109 with permission.)

Selection of Patients

SINGLE-VESSEL DISEASE

Percutaneous revascularization is an attractive option for many symptomatic patients who are anatomically suitable, having single-vessel coronary disease. It is important, however, to remember that there are no large studies comparing angioplasty with surgery in this group of patients and none that show a statistically significant survival benefit of angioplasty compared with surgery or medical therapy. Data from Emory University indicate that of 692 single-vessel disease patients newly diagnosed in 1988, a total of 46 percent underwent angioplasty, 50 percent were treated medically, and 4 percent underwent coronary bypass surgery. Of 7604 patients with single-vessel disease treated at Emory with angioplasty between 1980 and 1991, angiographic success was 90 percent and complications were infrequent (Q-wave MI, 0.8 percent; emergency CABG, 1.7 percent; and death, 0.2 percent).[119] In these patients with single-vessel disease, 1-, 5-, and 10-year survival was 99, 93, and 86 percent, respectively, whereas 80, 69, and 58 percent were PTCA-free and 92, 87, and 77 percent were CABG-free at 1, 5, and 10 years. In the Duke Data Bank experience, 5-year survival with angioplasty in single-vessel disease compared favorably with bypass surgery (95 versus 93 percent with CABG).[120]

The ACME study showed that angioplasty in single-vessel disease can lead to improved quality of life compared with medical therapy at 6 months, with reduced angina and improved exercise performance out to 3 years.[25,121,122] Clearly, it is improvement in symptoms rather than prolongation of life that is achieved by angioplasty in this patient subset. The ACME data suggest, however, that using the angioplasty techniques available at that time resulted in a slightly increased risk of acute complications (2 percent emergency CABG, 1 percent Q-wave MI) and repeat revascularization (23 versus 9 percent) at 6 months but no difference in late revascularization at 3 years.[122]

In an observational report from Kansas City of 704 patients with single-vessel LAD artery revascularization, 2-year mortality was 3.9, 2.6, and 1 percent in PTCA, stent, and LIMA-LAD revascularization groups, respectively ($p = 0.33$), and repeat procedures occurred in 30, 24, and 5 percent, respectively ($p = 0.001$).[123] In the randomized Medicine, Angioplasty, or Surgery Study (MASS) of isolated LAD disease, there was no difference in MI or mortality at 5 years but fewer late events in the surgery group.[124] In a relatively small, randomized trial of angioplasty and IMA surgery for isolated disease of the LAD artery, there was no difference in mortality or MI, but angioplasty patients had more repeat revascularizations (25 versus 3 percent; $p < 0.01$).[125] Clear superiority of stenting over balloon angioplasty for isolated LAD disease was demonstrated in a randomized comparison of these strategies in 120 patients.[126] One-year rates of event-free survival were 87 percent after stenting and 70 percent after angioplasty ($p = 0.04$), and restenosis rates were 19 and 40 percent, respectively ($p = 0.02$).

Studies from the Cleveland Clinic analyzing the importance of repeat procedures in determining 2-year cardiac cost suggest that coronary intervention is more cost-effective than medical and surgical therapy when the probability of repeat procedures is low.[127] One would infer from this analysis that the presence of multiple or complex lesions, which are likely to recur, may tilt the scale sufficiently to modify adversely the favorable comparative cost-effectiveness of percutaneous intervention in single-vessel disease.

MULTIVESSEL DISEASE

A dramatic increase in the use of percutaneous intervention in multivessel disease, fueled by improved angioplasty technology and new devices, accounts for the growth in these procedures worldwide. *Rational selection of patients, however, requires a careful analysis of multiple issues, including a risk-benefit assessment of each ischemia-producing lesion, a projection of the possible completeness and durability of the physiologic revascularization, and an estimate of resource consumption compared with surgery and medical therapy.*

In general, as stated in "Guidelines for PTCA,"[118] patients selected for intervention are symptomatic, have evidence of ischemia, need noncardiac surgery, are recovering from cardiac arrest or malignant arrhythmia, or have compelling anatomy. Patient preferences must be considered, since repeat interventions are a common and an integral aspect of percutaneous intervention in multivessel disease (see Table 45-1). Complete revascularization, which has been shown in the surgical experience to produce superior long-term results, has been associated with fewer late interventions after angioplasty,[128] but it is not frequently attained due to the presence of total occlusions, noncritical stenoses, and diffuse disease. In the 1985–1986 NHLBI PTCA Registry, complete revascularization was achieved in 19 percent of multivessel patients.[129]

At Emory University among 10,783 patients who underwent coronary intervention, complete revascularization was achieved in 84 percent of patients with single-vessel disease and 25 percent with two-vessel disease but in only 5 percent with triple-vessel disease.[119] In the experience of EAST, 71 percent of index segments were revascularized in PTCA patients.[130] Culprit-lesion angioplasty is clearly an accepted strategy, but care must be taken to avoid significant residual ischemia after intervention. This approach was reflected in EAST, where revascularization was attempted in 96 percent of high-priority lesions in PTCA patients and in 99 percent of surgical patients. (*High-priority lesions* were defined as 70 to 100 percent stenoses located proximally or in large vessels $\geq$ 2.5 mm). This strategy yielded similar 3-year EAST primary end points for CABG and PTCA and an identical frequency of patients with all index segments free of stenosis of 70 to 100 percent (82 versus 82 percent).[130] Recently published data from BARI indicated that planned incomplete revascularization was unrelated to 5-year risk of cardiac death or death/MI but was related to risk of CABG.[131]

The risks of percutaneous coronary intervention are increased in the presence of unstable angina, advanced age, poor left ventricular function, extensive coronary artery disease, comorbid conditions, and female gender.[132] At Emory, in-hospital mortality for one-, two-, and three-vessel disease was 0.2, 0.4, and 1.2 percent, respectively ($p < 0.0001$), and emergency bypass surgery was needed in 1.7, 3.0, and 3.2 percent, respectively.[119] In general, the risk of intervention is directly related to the probability and consequences of abrupt closure. In multivessel disease, both are frequently higher, and impaired left ventricular function is commonly present. Recent application of stenting in multivessel percutaneous intervention has improved outcomes significantly.[133–136] In a report from the Washington Hospital Center, in-hospital and long-term outcomes of 398 consecutive patients undergoing multivessel stenting were quite similar to those of patients undergoing single-vessel stenting with respect to mortality (1.4 versus 0.7 percent; $p = 0.26$), repeat revascularization (20 versus 21 percent; $p = 0.73$), and Q-wave MI (0 versus 1.2 percent; $p = 0.02$). Overall event-free survival was similar.[135] Although the major randomized trials of angioplasty versus bypass surgery also showed no overall difference in mortality on long-term follow-up, BARI reported that patients being treated for diabetes had significantly worse 5-year mortality with angioplasty compared with surgery (35 versus 19 percent).[39] In a smaller cohort of diabetic patients in EAST, however, there were no differences in outcome until almost 8 years following revascularization. The BARI findings question the safety of angioplasty in the diabetic population, who frequently have diffuse multivessel disease, more frequent restenoses, more rapid disease progression, and in many cases a reduced recognition of recurrent ischemia.[44,137] ARTS extended this cautionary theme in multivessel diabetics with observations that stented diabetics had roughly twice the mortality of nondiabetics[98] (see "Randomized Trials of Balloon Angioplasty," above).

UNSTABLE ANGINA

Patients with unstable angina, who account for a majority of coronary interventions, are at increased risk for ischemic complications, particularly abrupt closure.[117,118,132] These complications, which are presumed to be related to the presence of thrombus and ruptured complex plaque[138] (see Chaps. 40 and 44), as demonstrated elegantly by angioscopy,[139,140] have led many operators to defer intervention for a few days while stabilizing the patient on aggressive antianginal therapy, including aspirin and heparin[141–143] (particularly in the presence of angiographic thrombus).[144] Alternatively, the favorable results achieved with angioplasty within 18 to 48 h after hospitalization in randomized trials of interventional strategies in unstable angina (96 percent angiographic success, 0.4 percent mortality, 2.9 percent MI, 0.7 percent emergency CABG, 2.2 percent abrupt closure)[145] and the recently reported FRISC II study of invasive management of non-Q-wave MI[30,31] have encouraged some to pursue a more aggressive approach, particularly in patients at highest risk of a coronary event—i.e., those with postinfarction angina[146] and angina refractory to medical therapy.[147] The use of direct antithrombins[148] and platelet glycoprotein IIb/IIIa inhibitors[105] has been shown to be effective in reducing complications of intervention in unstable angina, whereas the routine administration of thrombolytic agents has reduced the thrombus burden but with an unfavorable impact on complications (i.e., in hospital ischemic events; 12.9 versus 6.3 percent without thrombolytics; $p = 0.02$).[149] At present, the optimal adjunctive therapy in unstable angina is unclear, but recent trials of the currently available IIb/IIIa platelet receptor inhibitors and of low-molecular-weight heparin have shown important reductions in complications in patients with non-ST-segment elevation acute coronary syndromes during medical therapy[101–103,114–116,150–153] and additional protection with IIb/IIIa receptor inhibitors during coronary intervention[107,154] (see Fig. 45-10 and Chap. 41). Data from CAPTURE in patients with unstable angina indicated that the benefit of IIb/IIIa receptor inhibition was greatest in troponin-positive patients and those with complex coronary anatomy.[114,115,155]

Selection of Lesions

LESION CHARACTERISTICS

The importance of coronary stenosis angiographic morphology in predicting the outcome of coronary angioplasty is reflected in the American College of Cardiology/American Heart Association "PTCA Guidelines."[117,118] Lesions were classified as type

A for anticipated high success, low risk; type B for anticipated moderate success, moderate risk; and type C for anticipated low success, high risk (Table 45-2). The general validity of this classification in predicting outcome of balloon angioplasty was confirmed in low-risk patients,[156] in patients with multivessel disease,[157] and in patients undergoing directional atherectomy, in whom success and complication rates were 93 and 3 percent for type A lesions, 88 and 6 percent for type B_1, and 75 and 13 percent when more than one B characteristic was present (type B_2).[158] More recent analysis of this lesion scoring system using balloon angioplasty technology of the 1990s suggests rates of 96, 93, and 80 percent can be achieved with type A, B, and C lesions, respectively, and that certain morphologic characteristics (i.e., long lesions, calcified lesions, stenosis severity 80 to 90 percent, angulated lesions, and presence of thrombus)[159] may have higher predictive value in determining success and complications. The ABC classification also was reported to be useful in predicting outcome after contemporary angioplasty in a population of unstable angina patients in whom early adverse events occurred in 4 percent of type A, 7.7 percent of type B_1, 15.3 percent of type B_2, and 17.9 percent of type C lesions in patients treated with heparin.[160] It does appear, however, in many centers that the complexity of lesions being attempted has increased and that new devices (especially stents) and antithrombotic strategies have, to a certain extent, weakened the prognostic value of this scoring system. In one recent report of 1085 lesions treated in the era of new devices (type A, 8 percent; type B_1, 42 percent; type B_2, 35 percent; type C, 15 percent), procedural success was 100 percent for type A, 97.3 percent for type B_1, 97 percent for type B_2, and 87.4 percent for type C lesions. Predictors of procedural failure were lesion length greater than 20 mm, TIMI-I flow, calcification, angle greater than 90 percent, and chronic total occlusion.[161] In an effort to update this classification based on results of contemporary coronary intervention using stents and IIb/IIIa platelet receptor inhibitors, Ellis and colleagues analyzed results from 10,907 lesions and proposed a new classification scheme for risk stratification.[162] Over 4000 patients treated in 1995 through 1996 constituted a training set (40.7 percent received stents, 26 percent abciximab, 18.9 percent Rotablator, 0.9 percent directional atherectomy, 0.2 percent excimer laser, and 0.2 percent TEC). Nine preintervention variables were independently correlated with adverse outcome (nonchronic total occlusion, degenerated vein graft, vein graft age greater than 10 years, lesion length greater than 10 mm, severe calcium, lesion irregularity, large filling defect, angulated greater than 45 degrees plus calcium, and eccentricity). A proposed classification (Table 45-3) validated against 2146 patients treated in 1997 had greater predictive value than the ACC/AHA classification, but not by as much as expected. Importantly, lesion characteristics previously thought to be associated

TABLE 45-2 American College of Cardiology/American Heart Association Classification of Lesions

Type A Lesions (High Success, >85%, Low Risk)	
Discrete (<10 mm length)	Little or no calcification
Concentric	Less than totally occlusive
Readily accessible	Not ostial in location
Nonangulated segment, <45°	No major branch involvement
Smooth contour	Absence of thrombus
Type B Lesions (Moderate Success, 60 to 85%; Moderate Risk)	
Tubular (10–20 mm length)	Moderate to heavy calcification
Eccentric	Total occlusions <3 months old
Moderate tortuosity of proximal segment	Ostial in location
Moderately angulated segment, >45°, <90°	Bifurcation lesions requiring double guidewires
Irregular contour	Some thrombus present
Type C Lesions (Low Success, <60%; High Risk)	
Diffuse (>2 cm length)	Total occlusion >3 months old
Eccessive tortuosity of proximal segment	Inability to protect major side branches
Extremely angulated segments >90°	Degenerated vein grafts with friable lesions

Source: Ryan et al.[118] Reprinted with permission of the authors and the American College of Cardiology.

TABLE 45-3 New Risk-Assessment Schema Based on Analysis of 10,907 Lesions Treated in the Stent and IIb/IIIa Era

Strongest correlates:	Nonchronic total occlusion Degenerated saphenous vein graft (SVG)
Moderately strong correlates:	Length ≥10 mm Lumen irregularity Large filling defect Calcium + angle ≥45° Eccentric Severe calcification SVG age ≥10 years
Highest risk:	Either of strongest correlates
High risk:	≥3 moderate correlates and the absence of strong correlates
Moderate risk:	1–2 moderate correlates and the absence of strong correlates
Low risk:	No risk factors

Source: Ellis et al.[162]

with a heightened risk but absent in the new classification include lesion angulation per se, bifurcation location, ostial site, proximal tortuosity, and small thrombus. When the new model was tested against the 1997 validation set, adverse outcomes [death, MI > 3 × creatine kinase (CK) or emergency CABG] occurred in 2.1 percent of low-risk patients, 3.4 percent at moderate risk, 8.2 percent at high risk, and 12.7 at highest risk (compared with 2.5, 3.0, 5.2 and 6.6 percent for ACC/AHA types A, B_1, B_2, and C, respectively). Whether bifurcation location should be included as a predictor of complications is debatable. In our own experience, bifurcation has represented increased risk, and this was confirmed in CAPTURE, where placebo-treated patients with bifurcations had a higher rate of death, MI, or early revascularization than placebo-treated patients without bifurcations (23 versus 11.7 percent; $p < 0.05$).[115] Importantly, this increased risk of complications with bifurcations was neutralized by treatment with abciximab. It should be recognized, however, that other factors are important in determining risk in the stent and IIb/IIIa inhibitor era, including patient age, LVEF, acute MI presentation, and operator experience, and these also must be considered.[163–165]

LEFT MAIN CORONARY ARTERY LESIONS

Whereas percutaneous intervention in protected left main coronary artery disease has been an accepted strategy for many years,[166] significant narrowing of an unprotected left main coronary artery has been considered a contraindication to this approach since Gruentzig's early recognition of increased mortality.[9,10] With the advent of improved technology in the form of atherectomy devices and stents, percutaneous revascularization has been applied increasingly in patients with unprotected left main coronary artery lesions.[167–170] Although reports of unprotected left main angioplasty/stenting indicated reasonably good results in carefully selected patients,[168,170] CABG remains the treatment of choice according to ACC/AHA guidelines.[45] Patients considered for percutaneous intervention in an unprotected left main coronary artery lesion in our hospital include those with significant comorbidity, making CABG impractical, and patients experiencing abrupt left main coronary artery closure as a complication of coronary angiography or presenting in cardiogenic shock without immediately available surgery.[170,171]

PREDICTORS OF RESTENOSIS

Lesion characteristics that were associated with increased restenosis rates following balloon angioplasty alone or after stent implantation include length, total occlusion (Fig. 45-12), vessel size less than 3 mm, ostial location, previous angioplasty to the same site, and saphenous vein grafts.[172–174] The assessment of lesion characteristics by IVUS and angioscopy also has been shown to have prognostic value for determining angioplasty success and long-term outcome,[175–179] and in some centers these strategies are used frequently to guide therapy (see Chap. 47). Selection of lesions for intervention is strongly based on the operator's assessment of his or her ability to treat the ischemia-producing lesion safely and in a cost-conscious manner and to achieve long-term patency and symptomatic benefit.

IN-STENT RESTENOSIS

One of the most vexing lesions confronting the interventionalist is in-stent restenosis, a new "disease" created by the explosion of stent use worldwide. This lesion, solely the result of neointimal proliferation as opposed to a combination of negative remodeling and intimal proliferation seen in nonstented lesions,[179] was reported by Yokoi et al.[180] to have an overall recurrence rate of 37 percent, but this rate is up to 85 percent for diffuse in-stent restenosis. Among 288 lesions, recurrent restenosis was highly correlated with the pattern of restenosis (target lesion revascularization in 19 percent of focal lesions less than 10 mm, 35 percent for lesions larger than 10 mm but confined to the stent, 50 percent for lesion larger than 10 mm and extending beyond the stent, and 83 percent for total occlusions; $p < 0.0001$). Additional correlates were the presence of diabetes (odds ratio, 2.8) and previous in-stent restenosis (odds ratio, 2.7).[181] In-stent lesions have been shown by IVUS to have significant reintrusion of tissue shortly after catheter-based intervention not apparent by quantitative angiography.[182] Debulking with atherectomy and laser techniques has been advocated and, although safe and associated with a larger postprocedure minimal lumen diameter (MLD), has not been shown to be superior to balloon angioplasty.[183–186] Although preliminary results from a U.S.-based multicenter randomized comparison of rotational atherectomy and balloon angioplasty were encouraging,[187] results of ARTS indicated that rotablation was inferior to balloon angioplasty (restenosis in 70 percent compared with 50 percent with balloon; $p = 0.008$).[188] Yokoi[189] reported results of repeated balloon angioplasty of in-stent restenosis in 310 patients, observing a first recurrence in 51 percent and subsequent recurrences following repetitive procedures in 68, 78, 74, and 92 percent of patients. Although 98 percent of patients were free of death and 90 percent were free of death/MI/CABG at 3 years, the increasingly high restenosis rate makes this approach impractical. The investigational use of radiation to inhibit neointimal proliferation has produced the most promising strategy for potential use in the treatment of this difficult problem. In randomized trials, beta and gamma radiation has reduced restenosis rates of 50 to 60 percent to approximately 20 percent[190,191] with reduction in 2-year death, MI, or target vessel revascularization (TVR) from 52 to 23 percent ($p = 0.03$).[192]

Selection of Devices

Conventional balloon angioplasty is a simple, relatively low in cost, and effective method of reducing coronary stenosis, but new devices (especially stents) are being used with increasing frequency, particularly in conditions where balloon angioplasty has been proved not to be highly effective (Table 45-4). At Emory University Hospital in 1990, balloon angioplasty was the sole technique used in 88 percent of 1863 patients who underwent coronary intervention (directional atherectomy, 3 percent; excimer laser, 3 percent; stents, 2 percent; laser balloon, 1 percent), whereas in 1998, a majority of lesions that were discrete and not involving bifurcations were treated with stent implantation (66 percent of all patients), and the atherectomy procedures performed were principally with the Rotablator for calcified, rigid, or bifurcation lesions (accounting for 8 percent of patients). At the Cleveland Clinic in 1997, device use frequency was as follows: stents, 64 percent (62.6 percent planned and 1.6 percent bailout); rotational atherectomy, 18 percent; directional atherectomy, 0.6 percent; excimer laser, 0.5 percent; and TEC 0.1 percent.[162]

PROVISIONAL STENTING

The practice of performing balloon angioplasty as an initial strategy in a majority of patients and using stents for suboptimal

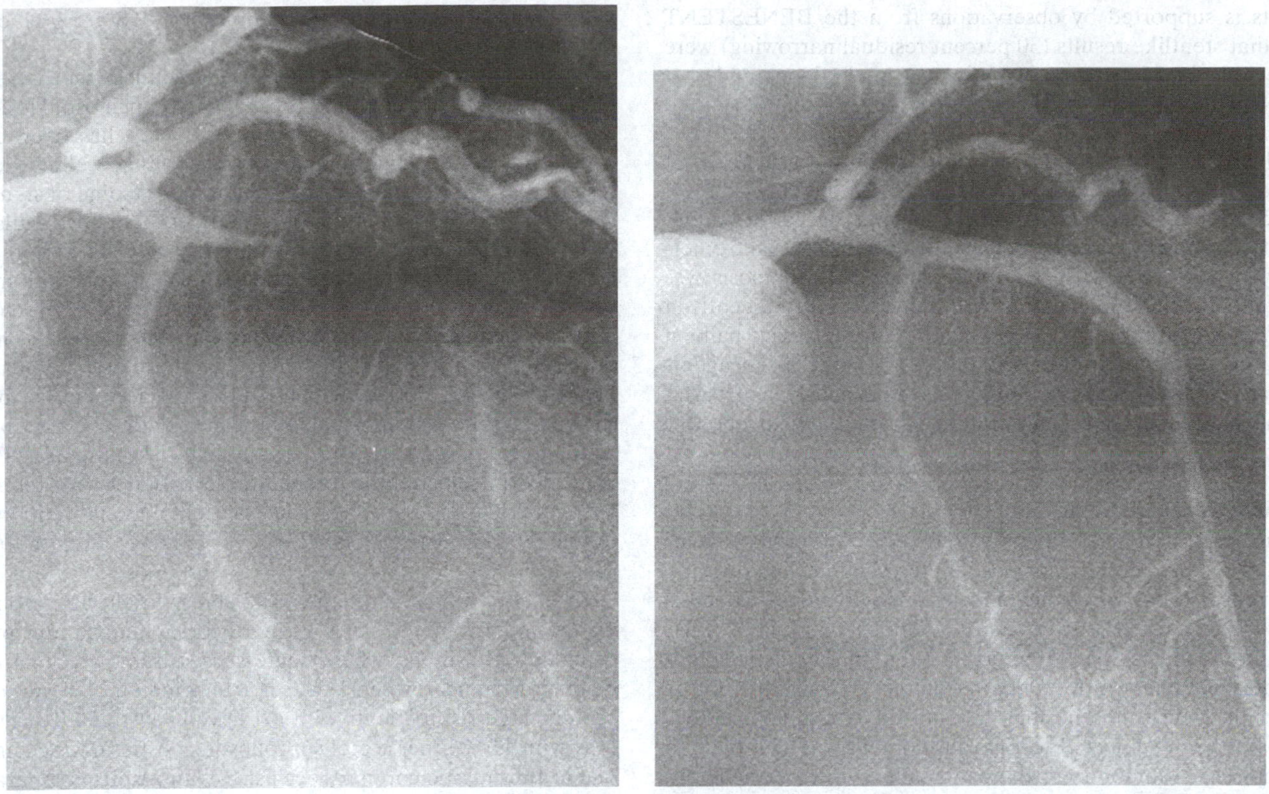

A B

FIGURE 45-12 An 82-year-old man with disabling angina and an occluded LAD artery of uncertain duration (*A*, right anterior oblique view). It was possible to recanalize the long LAD occlusion (*B*) using a hydrophilic-coated wire and conventional balloon angioplasty followed by placement of two Palmaz-Schatz stents. Stents have been shown to be superior to conventional balloon angioplasty in a randomized trial.[199]

TABLE 45-4 New Coronary Interventional Strategies Compared with Balloon Angioplasty

Technique	Indications	Contraindications	Advantages and Limitations
Balloon angioplasty	Focal stenosis	Insignificant narrowing, no ischemia, unimportant artery	Broad applicability, lower cost; poor outcome in thrombotic, ostial, and calcified lesions; significant restenosis
Stents	Focal stenosis	Heavy calcification or thrombus, vessel diameter <2.5 mm	Reduced emergency CABG and restenosis; more expensive, rare stent thrombosis
Directional atherectomy	Focal noncalcified	Diffuse disease, severe tortuosity or bend	Debulks, reduced restenosis; more frequent non-Q-wave MI, more expensive, technically difficult
Rotational atherectomy	Focal calcified stenosis, ostial site	Thrombus, large plaque burden, severe tortuosity or bend	Effective in calcified lesions, reduced elastic recoil; more expensive, similar restenosis, transient left ventricular dysfunction
Laser	Ostial lesion, SVG, in-stent restenosis	Severe calcification, tortuosity or bend	Debulks effectively; increased cost, similar restenosis
Transluminal extraction atherectomy	Thrombotic lesion, bulky SVG lesion	Severe tortuosity or bend, calcification	Thrombus and plaque removed; high complication rate in native vessels, distal embolization
Rheolytic thrombectomy	Thrombus	No thrombus	Effective thrombus removal; no plaque removal

results is supported by observations from the BENESTENT trial that stentlike results (30 percent residual narrowing) were achievable in 35 percent of patients with balloons and that they had a long-term outcome comparable with that of stented patients.[193] This strategy has been reported to be cost-effective,[194] but the recent OPUS-1 study of primary stenting suggested that primary stenting was cost-effective after 6 months because of reduced reinterventions.[92] Adjunctive stents placed for bailout have been shown clearly to reduce Q-wave infarction and emergency bypass surgery.[72,73] Although subacute thrombosis was substantially higher in patients with stents placed emergently in the early experience, the employment of high-pressure balloon inflations in recent studies and the use of antiplatelet agents such as ticlopidine and clopidogrel plus aspirin instead of warfarin have reduced this complication substantially to about 1 percent.[195]

PRIMARY STENTING

In our hospital, stents frequently are selected for primary treatment of complex lesions, aortoostial sites, shelflike lesions, early recurrence, total occlusions, and lesions with high restenosis rates (proximal LAD artery and saphenous vein grafts) (Figs. 45-7, 45-12, and 45-13). It is important to point out that restenosis rates obtained with stents in complex lesions are not as favorable as in simple lesions[196,197] and that these applications have not been subjected to rigorous comparison with balloon angioplasty. Randomized comparison has been carried out, however, in saphenous vein grafts, where 6-month MLD was significantly larger with stents (1.75 versus 1.47 mm; $p = 0.05$), and a composite end point of death, MI, CABG, or target lesion revascularization was less frequent (26 versus 38 percent; $p = 0.05$).[198] Stents also were shown in randomized trials to be superior to balloon angioplasty in total occlusions (TVR in 8.4 versus 15.4 percent; $p = 0.03$)[199] and in restenotic lesions (TVR in 10 versus 27 percent; $p = 0.001$).[200]

Given the superb results reported in the BENESTENT II study[91] with heparin-coated stents (overall clinical success 99 percent, stent thrombosis 0.2 percent, restenosis 16 percent, and 1-year mortality 1 percent) and the large number of new stent designs currently available, one would anticipate broadened use of improved and cheaper stents due to competitive market forces. Decreased cost may permit stenting to rival or prove more cost-effective than simple balloon angioplasty for most lesions.[201–203]

ATHERECTOMY

Currently, directional coronary atherectomy (DCA) is used infrequently in most centers as primary therapy but may be applied effectively in STRESS and BENESTENT-equivalent lesions[54] or used adjunctively prior to stent implantation based on registry data indicating that this strategy can yield restenosis rates as low as 11 percent.[56] Suitable lesions are generally proximal in vessels larger than 3 mm in diameter and have features that predict poor outcome with primary stenting such as high-bulk stenoses, ostial site, proximal LAD artery lesion, and protected left main coronary lesions[170,204] and include carefully selected bifurcation lesions[205–209] and complex postinfarction lesions (where histology frequently shows partially organized thrombus; see Fig. 45-10). Pretreatment of calcified lesions with rotational atherectomy may permit successful DCA in selected patients,[209] but in general moderate angiographic calcification and significant superficial calcification on IVUS are predictors of failure.[175]

Rotational atherectomy has proved useful in the presence of calcium, in treatment of aortoostial and branch ostial lesions, and in nondilatable lesions. In some series, it has been used in long, ulcerated, and complex lesions with excellent acute results,[210,211] and in some reports, long-term outcome of stenting was improved by rotablation pretreatment.[63] Highly angulated or thrombotic lesions or those with impaired distal runoff (recent infarction, fixed thallium defect) and segments with myocardial bridging should be avoided.[210–213] Rotational atherectomy also has been used in total occlusions, but restenosis rates have not been demonstrated to be better than those of balloon angioplasty. Elective intraaortic balloon pump placement has been shown to improve systemic blood pressure and to be associated with a lower non-Q-wave MI rate in high-risk patients.[214] Care is needed in selection of rotablation in patients with reduced left ventricular function due to the transient regional ventricular dysfunction shown to persist for over 2 hours after the procedure.[215]

The TEC, which is unique in its ability to cut and aspirate plaque and thrombus, is used primarily in saphenous vein grafts containing thrombus, where acute success rates are high, but embolic MI and restenosis are not uncommon.[216–218] In some centers, high-risk patients with MI have been treated successfully with TEC either acutely or following postinfarction angina due to thrombotic coronary occlusion with results comparable with those of balloon angioplasty.[219] When used in the treatment of complex native coronary artery lesions not associated with acute MI, the outcome also appears similar to that of balloon angioplasty,[220] but use of TEC doubles the cost. In carefully selected patients with large intracoronary thrombi and ongoing ischemia, TEC has proved useful, as has the Dispatch catheter (Scimed Life Systems, Maple Grove, MN), a device for localized intracoronary infusion.[221] The Angiojet (Possis Medical, Inc., Minneapolis, MN) is the most effective thrombectomy device currently available and is used principally to treat large intracoronary thrombi.[65–69,222]

LASER ANGIOPLASTY

Although ablative laser angioplasty (XeCl excimer and holmium Nd:YAG) has been shown to be effective in the treatment of aortoostial sites, undilatable lesions, total occlusions, calcification, long lesions, and saphenous vein grafts,[223–226] its superiority to simpler and less costly balloon strategies has not been demonstrated.[227–229] Lesions that should not be selected for ablative laser angioplasty include those on bend points or in tortuous segments, those associated with severe calcification or thrombus, or lesions with a suspected subintimal wire passage. In general, bifurcation lesions should not be selected for ablative laser therapy unless an eccentrically directed device can be used to avoid perforating at the flow divider of the vessel. The use of a laser guidewire to cross total occlusions has been advocated.[230]

PERFORMANCE OF CORONARY INTERVENTION

Operator Proficiency

Current guidelines recommend that cardiologists who wish to become competent in coronary intervention receive special

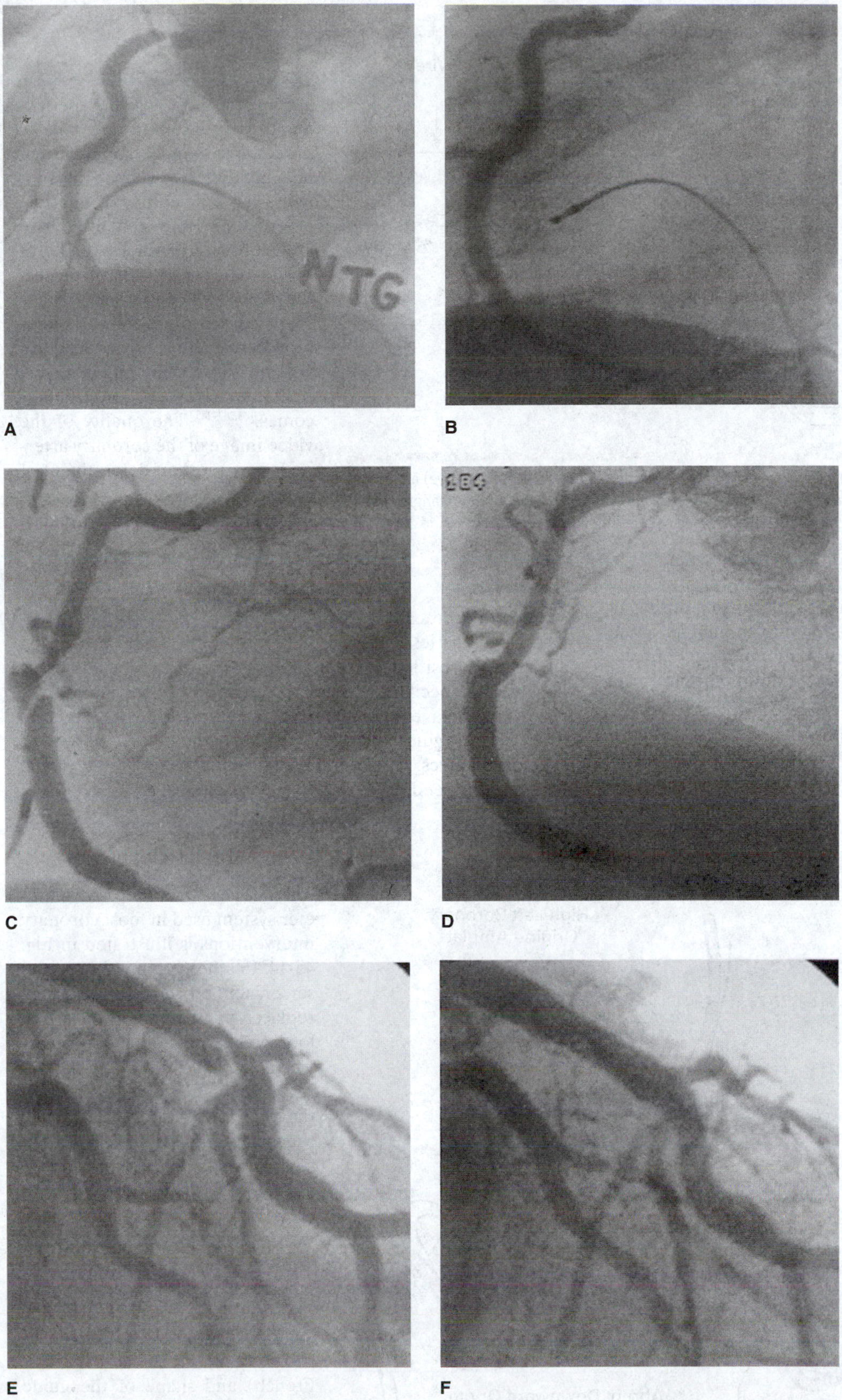

FIGURE 45-13 High-grade *de novo* stenosis of the ostium of the right coronary in a middle-aged man (*A*) was free of calcification. Percutaneous intervention was successful (*B*). This type of lesion is currently treated with stent implanation in most centers, preceded by rotational atherectomy if calcified. A very complex shelflike *de novo* stenosis of the right coronary artery (*C*) and the site 2 years after successful percutaneous intervention with directional atherectomy (*D*). Histology showed atheroma and organized thrombus. Flaplike *de novo* stenosis of the LAD (*E*). This type of lesion responds well to directional coronary atherectomy or stenting (*F*). Sites *A*, *C*, and *E* are poor lesions for conventional percutaneous balloon angioplasty.

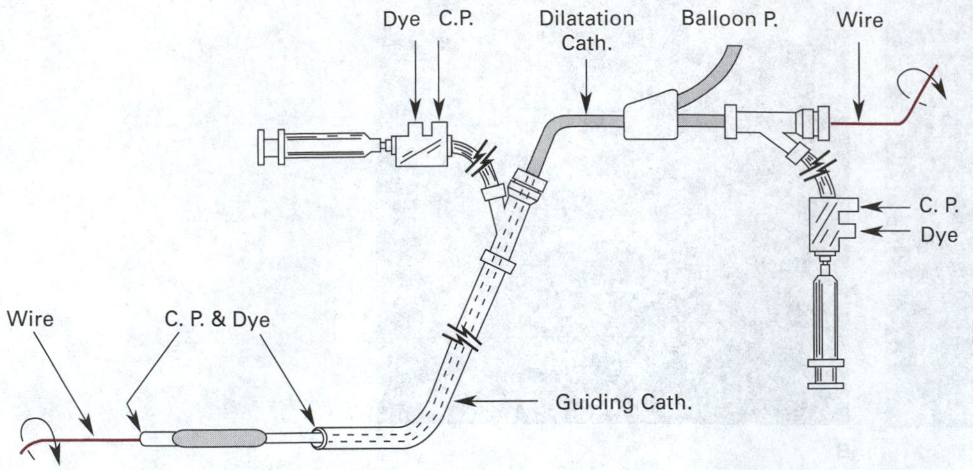

FIGURE 45-14 Diagram of the over-the-wire dilatation catheter with capacity for contract medium (dye) injection. The floppy guidewire is steerable. (From Aueron FM, Gruentzig AR. Percutaneous transluminal coronary angioplasty: Indications and current status. *Prim Cardiol* 1984; 10:91. Reproduced with permission of the publisher and authors.)

training in diagnostic and therapeutic catheterization during an additional year after the standard fellowship training program and maintain skills by performance of a minimum of 75 procedures per year.[231–237] Adequate case mix is an important aspect of a physician's training in interventional cardiology that has not yet been addressed by practice guidelines.[238,239] Assurance of quality by surveillance of procedural outcomes is made difficult by such complex issues as a need to adjust for high-risk patients, low incidence and subjectivity of major adverse events, and low volume of many operators.[163–165,240–242]

Interventional Laboratory

Optimal conditions for performance of coronary angioplasty procedures require sophisticated imaging systems; trained personnel; a large inventory of dilation, atherectomy, and stent hardware and software; and a variety of therapeutic safety nets to protect the patient when intervention fails or is complicated. Most studies suggest that laboratory procedural volume is important and inversely related to adverse procedural outcomes.[163,243–245] The quality of the video image of the coronary arteries is an important determinant of angioplasty success. A freeze-frame storage and display capability is required for use during the procedure, as is a high-quality video replay with slow-motion and stop-frame capability. The ability to solve specific problems—such as lesion eccentricity or rigidity, vessel tortuosity, and unusual position or orientation of the coronary ostia—often depends on specific device characteristics. Consequently, it is necessary to have available dilating catheters, stents, atherectomy devices, guidewires, and guiding catheters in a variety of shapes and sizes. Cardiac surgery should be available in the institution if needed for emergency situations.

Interventional Equipment

The over-the-wire steerable catheter system used in most coronary interventions is illustrated in Fig. 45-14. In atherectomy, ablative laser, or stent procedures, the device replaces or is mounted on a balloon catheter. The balloon or device is introduced through a guiding catheter that extends through the arterial puncture site (femoral, brachial, or radial) to the coronary artery or graft ostia, where coaxial alignment of the catheter and vessel is highly desirable. In the past, the Judkins right and left coronary shapes were used most frequently, but many other shapes are currently available to address specific anatomic problems (Figs. 45-15 and 45-16). The size (5–11 French) and shape of the guide catheter may be determined by the arterial size at the entry site, the guide catheter lumen requirement of the device used, and other factors such as a need for optimal vessel opacification. Balloon cath-

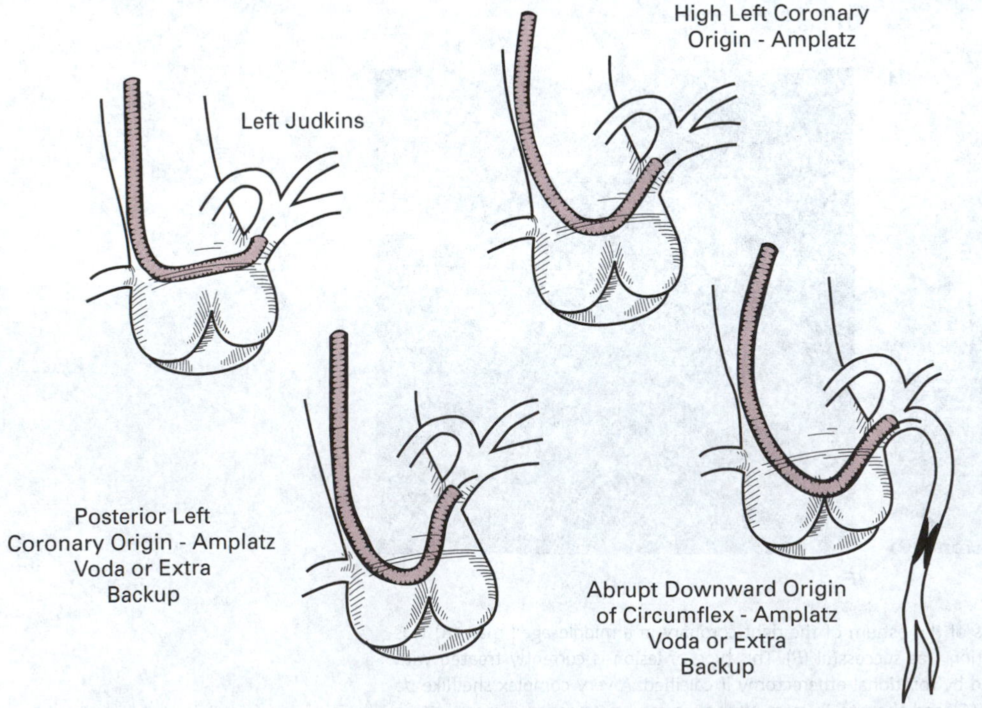

FIGURE 45-15 Guide catheter shapes commonly used for left coronary angioplasty.

eters for coronary use are available in an array of balloon lengths (8–40 mm), diameters (1.5–5 mm), shaft sizes, and special features, including active and passive perfusion, high-pressure capability, and local intracoronary infusion.

In the United States, the most frequently used stent in early experiences, the Palmaz-Schatz stent (see Fig. 45-6), was provided with a sheath delivery system that necessitated an 8 French guide catheter, whereas most currently used stents are accommodated by 6 French catheters, and use of these smaller catheters for radial artery or femoral approaches has increased dramatically.[246] A large number of new stent designs have cleared FDA approval and are available for use (Fig. 45-17). Although these new stent designs offer considerable advantage over first-generation devices in terms of their deliverability, profile, variety of sizes, and strength of balloon, stent versus stent comparisons have not been performed in a manner that helps the interventionalist in choosing the best device for a given problem.[247]

The high-speed rotational atherectomy device (see Fig. 45-5*B*), an olive-shaped burr with embedded diamond chips, requires a special 0.009-in. stainless steel guidewire, whereas the directional atherectomy cutter and laser catheters pass over conventional 0.014-in. steerable guidewires. The transluminal extraction catheter requires a unique 0.014-in. stainless steel guidewire that has a 0.21-in. ball at its tip.

The use of IVUS to guide therapy varies widely; it is almost routine practice in some centers and is rarely used in others. Ultrasound assessment of the adequacy of stent deployment (see Fig. 45-7), pioneered by Colombo and colleagues,[77] and evaluation of calcified lesions are probably the most frequent applications (see Chap. 47).

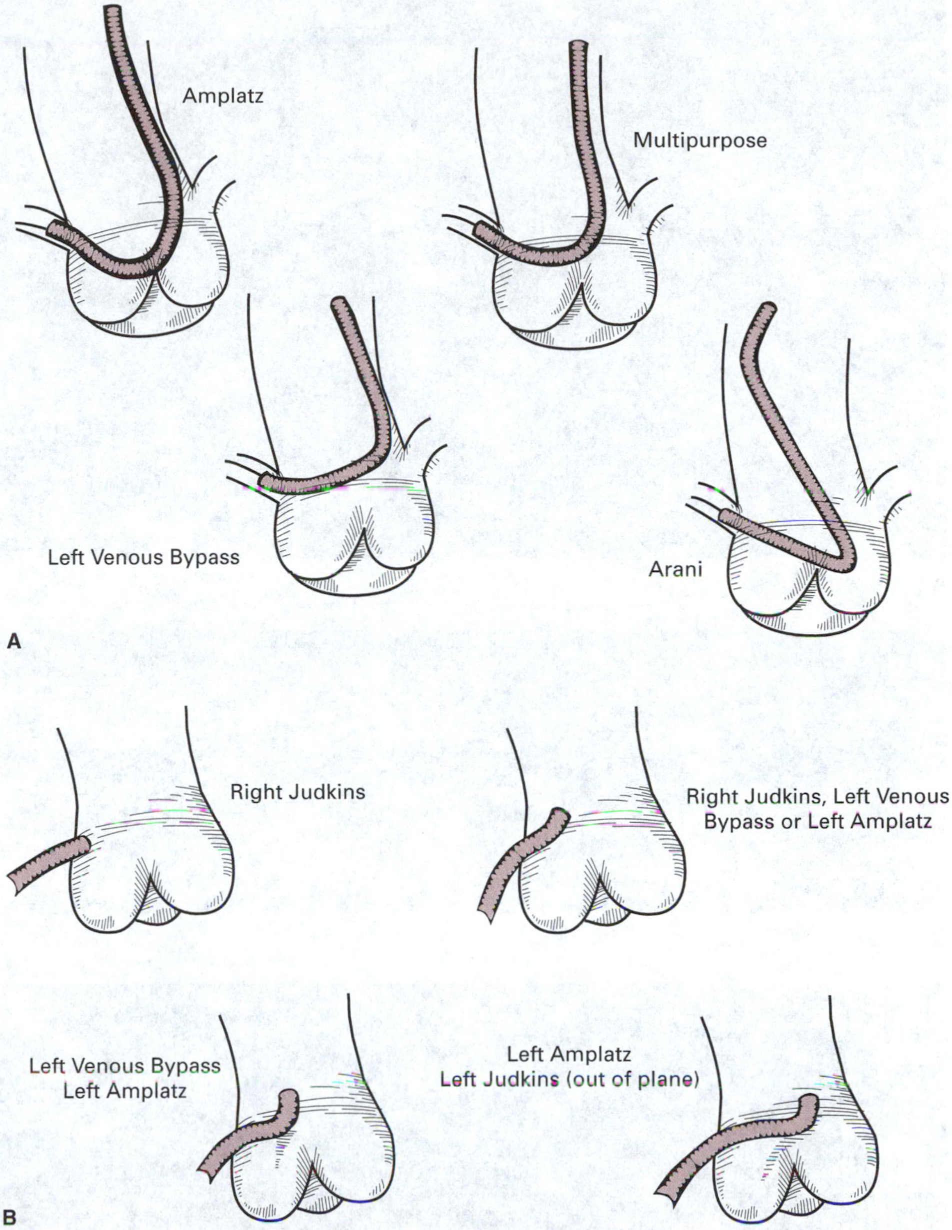

FIGURE 45-16 Guide catheter selection. *A*. Guide catheter shapes that are effective when the right coronary artery has a steep upward initial course. *B*. Guide catheter shapes that are effective when the right coronary artery has an anterior and leftward origin.

The Coronary Interventional Procedure

Prior to coronary intervention, patients receive an explanation of the procedure, including the operator's estimate of success, possible complications, risks, and benefits. A booklet and videotape describing the procedure and an explanation by the nursing staff help to reduce anxiety and ensure that both patient and family are well informed.

Antiplatelet therapy is used routinely. The therapy most widely used is aspirin 160 to 325 mg daily. Patients in whom stenting is planned also receive clopidogrel, usually in 300- to 525-mg loading dose unless pretreatment for several days has been performed. In a significant percentage of patients in our hospital, a platelet glycoprotein IIb/IIIa receptor antagonist is used when there is perceived to be an increased risk of abrupt closure or distal embolization (e.g., suspected or definite thrombus, acute coronary syndrome, complex lesion, diabetes, atherectomy procedure, or multisite intervention).[105] Restenosis trials have failed to show a clear advantage of one antiplatelet regi-

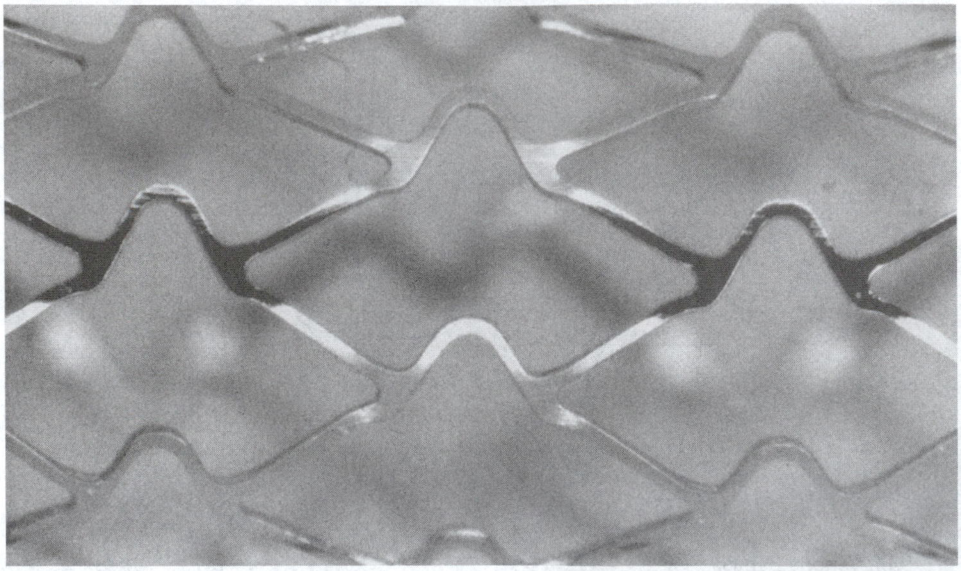

A

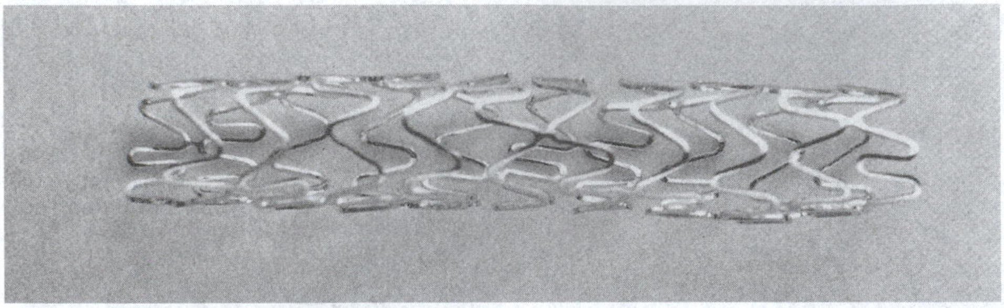

B

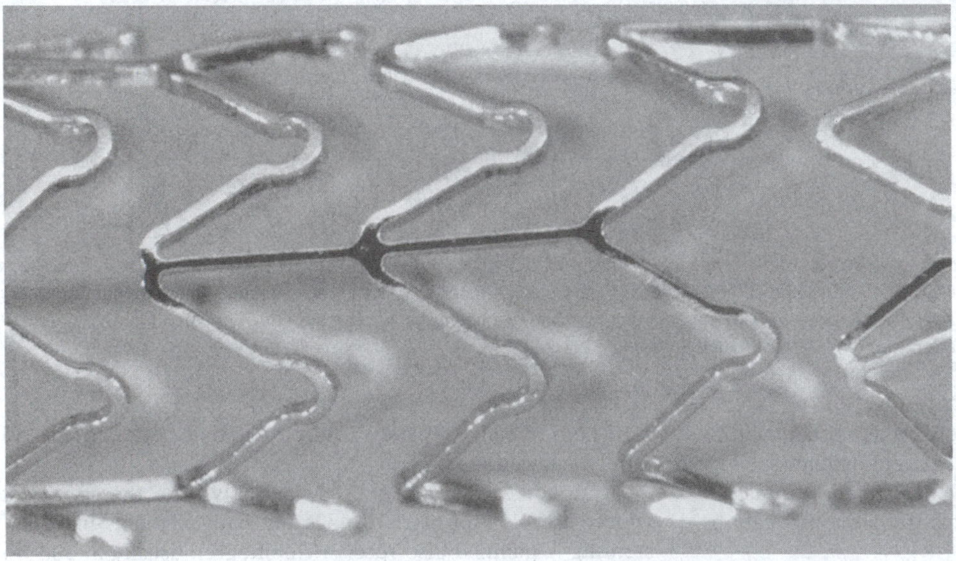

C

FIGURE 45-17 Currently available newer-generation stents. *A.* Nir stent (Medinol-Scimed, Maple Grove, MN). *B.* Cross-Flex LC stent (Cordis-Johnson & Johnson, Warren, NJ). *C.* Multi-Link Duet stent (Guidant, Santa Clara, CA). *D.* AVE-GFX stent (Medtronic-Applied Vascular Engineering, Santa Rosa, CA). *E.* Magic Wall stent (Schneider-Scimed, Maple Grove, MN). *F.* Radius stent (Scimed, Maple Grove, MN).

men over another and have not shown inhibition of restenosis by calcium channel-blocking agents, warfarin anticoagulation, angiotension-converting enzyme (ACE) inhibitors, steroids, or other agents.

Some operators administer a calcium channel-blocking agent prior to coronary intervention for prophylaxis against coronary artery spasm and to reduce ischemia during the procedure. Once the patient is in the catheterization laboratory, electrocardiographic monitoring leads are applied, a peripheral intravenous line is started, and midazolam 1 mg or an equivalent drug is given intravenously. In most laboratories, a femoral approach is employed; use of a radial artery approach, however, is increasing. Heparin is administered intravenously (100 units/kg, or 70 units/kg if IIb/IIIa receptor-inhibiting agents are used concomitantly). Maintenance of an activated clotting time (ACT) of greater than 300 s is recommended unless IIb/IIIa inhibitors are used, where 200 to 250 s is accepted. IIb/IIIa platelet receptor inhibitors are used selectively in our hospital for higher-risk patients (see "IIb/IIIa Platelet Receptor Inhibitors," above). Use of low-molecular-weight heparin during intervention is under investigation. Patients with a history of allergy to contrast material are premedicated with prednisone 40 to 60 mg orally the night before and the day of the procedure and with diphenhydramine (Benadryl) 50 mg intravenously at the time of the procedure. Ionic hyperosmolar contrast material is used commonly in our hospital for elective coronary angioplasty because of the extraordinary cost of low-osmolar agents and the lack of proved benefit to warrant their routine use.[248–250] Due to the reported increased thrombotic complications with nonionic agents (attributed to comparatively less thrombin inhibition and enhanced platelet activation), ionic agents have been preferred in patients with unstable ischemic syndromes or frank intracoronary thrombus.[249] Recently published studies comparing ionic (Ioxglate) and nonionic (Iomeprol) agents in a randomized format,[251] ionic versus nonionic contrast material in EPIC, EPILOG, and CAPTURE in a metaanalysis,[252] and ionic versus nonionic in stenting,[253] however, revealed no increase in thrombotic complications, whereas nonionic agents were associated with more bailout stenting in a randomized study.[254] These studies reported outcomes with contrast agents with osmolalities in the 600 to 700 mosmol/kg range. Recent preliminary reports of the use of the isosmolar nonionic dimer iodixanol in high-risk PTCA were promising,[255] and further evaluation of this agent is warranted. Contrast-induced bradycardia, more common with ionic agents, is treated with atropine. Patients selected for use of a low-osmolar contrast agent include those with renal insufficiency or severe left ventricular dysfunction. Nonionic agents generally are reserved for patients with known allergy to the available ionic agents or with a history of severe bradycardia with ionic agents.

Coronary arteriograms are performed in two approximately orthogonal views selected to demonstrate the lesion(s) to be treated and the course of the parent artery without overlap by other vessels. The angles chosen are recorded, and freeze frames demonstrating the anatomy are stored and displayed during the procedure. A balloon catheter or device is selected based on the diameter of the target coronary artery to be treated and the length of the stenotic segment as determined by comparison with the guiding catheter of known diameter. The balloon diameter is chosen to approximate closely the diameter of the normal adjacent vessel, since oversizing the angioplasty balloon has been associated with increased complications and no reduction in the rate of restenosis.[256] In general, an over-the-wire catheter system is preferred because of the ability to exchange easily for alternative

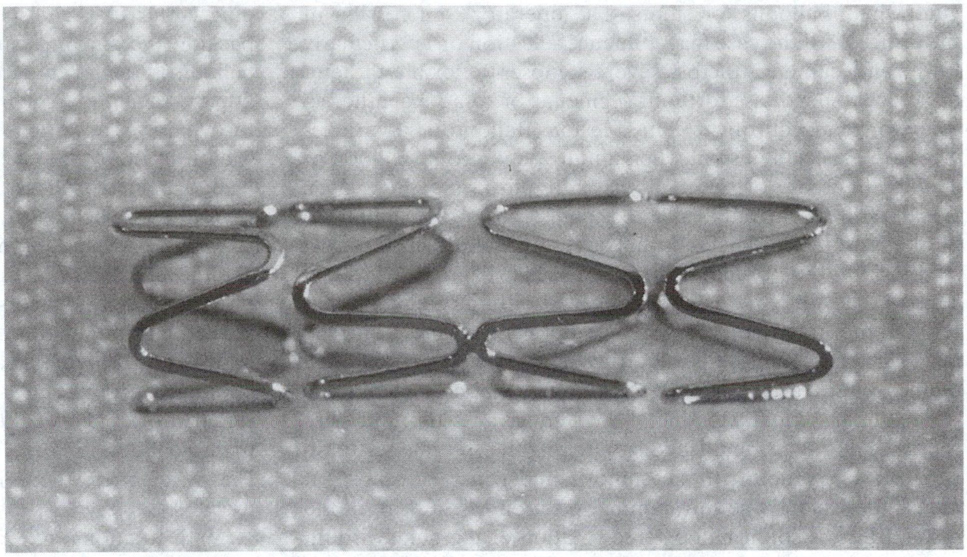

D

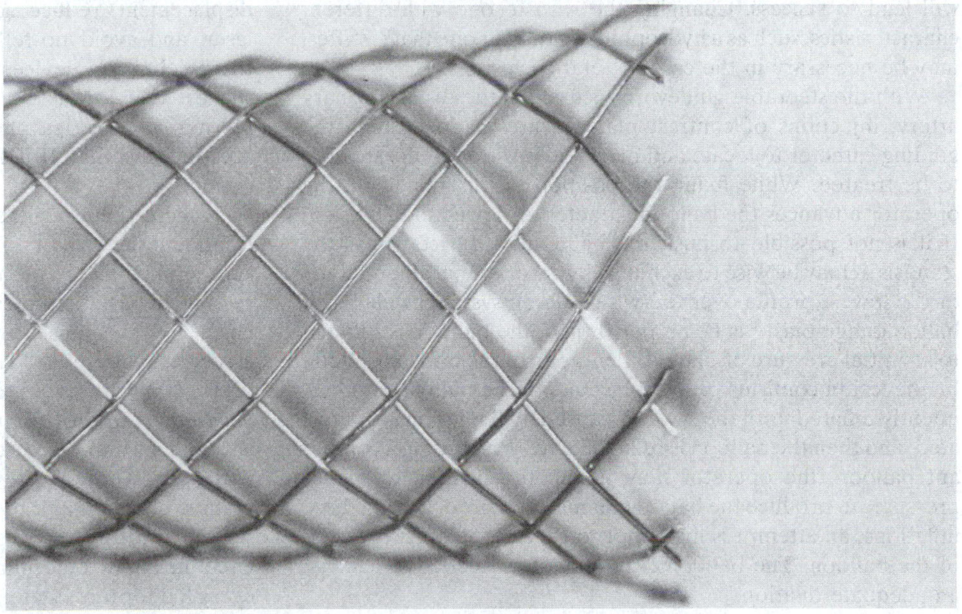

E

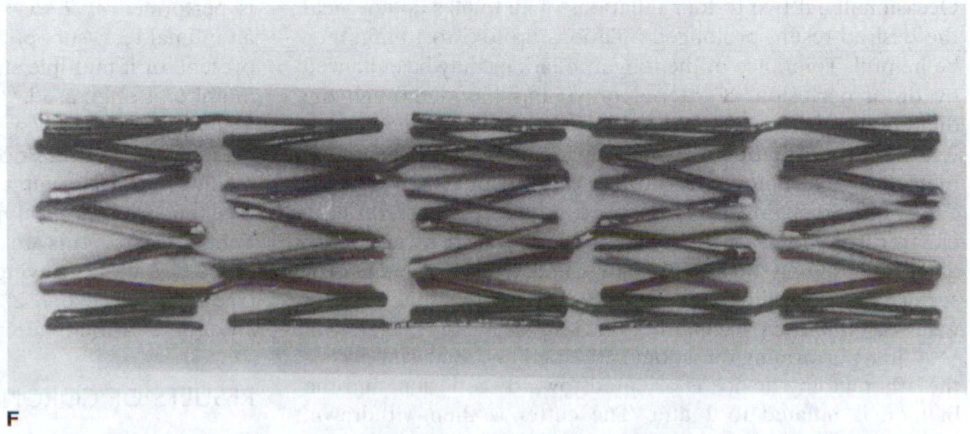

F

FIGURE 45-17 *(Continued)*

guidewires, balloons, or stents. The operator's impression of the difficulty of the case may influence selection of a particularly low profile catheter to cross severe stenoses, a flexible catheter or device to negotiate tortuous segments, or rotational atherectomy to treat a fibrotic, calcified lesion. Balloon-on-a-wire devices are especially useful when an ultra-low-profile balloon or simultaneous use of two balloons is required (see Fig. 45-2). Because of the current availability of very low profile and flexible balloon-mounted stents that are securely attached, direct stenting without predilating has increased dramatically in some centers. The coronary ostium is engaged with the guiding catheter, and the steerable guidewire is cautiously advanced into the target artery. In patients requiring angioplasty of more than one coronary artery, the most difficult lesion is commonly treated first. A clean crossing of the stenosis with the guidewire is critical and is accomplished by aligning the steerable wire tip with the entry point of the stenosis and gently advancing it across the lesion. The intraluminal position of the wire in the distal artery is confirmed by free rotation of the guidewire tip and by contrast angiography. If there is difficulty in crossing the stenosis with the guidewire, reshaping the tip commonly will lead to success. Changing the wire to one with different characteristics, such as a hydrophilic coating or one that is stiffer, may be necessary in the case of total occlusions.

With the steerable guidewire securely in the distal coronary artery, injections of contrast material are made through the guiding catheter to locate and mark the position of the stenosis to be treated. While fixing the position of the guidewire, the operator advances the balloon catheter or device to the lesion. If it is not possible to push the balloon or device across the stenosis, it may be wise to exchange it for rotational atherectomy or the lowest-profile over-the-wire balloon system available. If balloon angioplasty is being performed, the balloon is inflated to an initial pressure of 2 atm. Indentation of the inflated balloon by the lesion confirms proper placement. The balloon is subsequently inflated until the "waist" caused by the lesion is obliterated, and then the balloon is fully inflated. When using a compliant balloon, the operator may inflate the balloon to higher pressures to produce the balloon diameter desired. During these inflations, an attempt is made not to exceed the burst pressure of the balloon. The balloon is reinflated as needed to achieve an adequate dilation.

There is no clear evidence regarding the optimal number or duration of balloon inflations or the maximal balloon pressure. Occasionally, if two to four inflations of 30 to 60 s do not yield the desired result, prolonged inflations up to 5 to 10 min may be helpful. Tolerance of the longer inflations may be enhanced by distal perfusion of arterial or venous blood through the dilatation catheter or by use of an autoperfusion balloon catheter.[257] Balloon inflations are limited by evidence of ischemia, as indicated by symptoms of chest discomfort or by ST-segment elevation. Some investigators have monitored intracoronary electrocardiograms from the steerable intracoronary guidewire and found these to be more sensitive in detecting ischemia than surface electrocardiograms. One also can use the intracoronary wire for temporary pacing.[258]

When performing directional atherectomy, the "window" of the atherectomy device is oriented toward the lesion, and the balloon is inflated to 1 atm. The cutter is then withdrawn, allowing the lesion to enter the open window. The motor is activated, and a cut is performed by slowly advancing the spinning cutter to the distal end of the device housing, thereby packing the shavings into the nose cone of the device. The balloon is then deflated, the window reoriented, and the sequence repeated. To minimize the possibility of perforation, the window is not oriented toward normal portions of the vessel wall. It is important to note that overzealous atherectomy may lead to an increased risk of perforation or aneurysm formation.

Intracoronary stenting may be conducted either as a primary strategy or for suboptimal outcomes after balloon angioplasty or other interventions. Deployment strategies vary depending on stent designs, since some are balloon-mounted and others are self-expanding. Stent deployment with a properly sized balloon is performed (usually to >12 atm) to expand the stent optimally throughout its length. A recently reported randomized trial of stent implantation showed no advantage to inflation to more than 15 atm.[259] Although some operators advocate IVUS guidance, there is no consensus regarding its routine use.[260,261]

With rotational atherectomy and ablative laser procedures, many operators use special infusion or flushing strategies (using saline and/or vasodilators) to optimize laser debulking by blood displacement, reduce acoustic shock and dissection with the laser, and avoid no-reflow phenomena.[210,262] Proper sizing of these debulking devices is under investigation. Recent studies suggest that lower rotational atherectomy speeds (<160,000 rev/min) produce less platelet activation and comparable atheroablation and that IIb/IIIa receptor inhibitors block this activation.[263,264]

If there is concern about the adequacy of the lumen at the treatment site, use of a Doppler flow wire, angioscopy, or pressure gradients may be helpful in addition to ultrasound in assessing the result. Studies suggest that a normal coronary hyperemic flow response and a low transluminal gradient are associated with reduced risk of restenosis. *It is clear that optimizing the lumen size is the goal, since final lumen size is an important determinant of the probability of restenosis.* When the operator is confident that the best possible result has been obtained, the patient is returned to his or her room, where an electrocardiogram is obtained and the patient is placed on telemetry. Puncture-site closure devices are used with increasing frequency. Creatine kinase determinations are performed immediately and every 8 h for three determinations. Because of the dehydrating effect of the osmotic load, most patients receive at least 1 L of intravenous fluids after the procedure. Delayed sheath removal is performed at 2 to 4 h when the ACT is below 150 s. If an intimal tear, suboptimal result, or intraluminal thrombus is present, or if multiple stents are implanted, a IIb/IIIa receptor inhibitor is often used.[265] There is evidence that routine heparin administration following uncomplicated angioplasty is not helpful in reducing acute occlusion or restenosis.[266] Postprocedure medications in-hospital include aspirin, a calcium channel-blocking agent, topical nitrates, and clopidogrel in stented patients. Most patients are discharged on the first day following the procedure after receiving instructions on lipid-lowering therapy (see Chap. 38), exercise, and cessation of smoking and are given an outline of follow-up procedures.

RESULTS OF CORONARY INTERVENTION

The results obtained with coronary intervention procedures have been influenced significantly by technological advances, operator experience, and the difficulty of patients selected. With pioneering equipment, Gruentzig was able to dilate 64 percent of the first 50 patients and 78 percent of the first 169 patients.[10,15] Defining primary success as less than 50 percent residual stenosis and freedom from complications, a success rate of 91 percent in over 26,000 patients treated at Emory University Hospital was seen between 1980 and 1998 (Table 45-5). Note that complication rates generally declined despite increasingly difficult cases. Experienced operators should achieve primary success rates in excess of 95 percent in ideal proximal lesions compared with a reduced success rate of approximately 75 percent in recent (<3 months) total occlusions or when attempting to treat fibrotic, calcified, eccentric stenoses located distally in tortuous coronary arteries. In all techniques, including stenting,[196] lesion characteristics are a major determinant of the outcome of the procedure.[117,118,157–162] Long-term outcome has been reported out to 10 years in patients treated in Zurich, Atlanta, and Rotterdam,[15–17,119,267] and detailed 5- to 8-year follow-up data are available from randomized trials,[25–41,130,131] (see above and Table 45-1 and Fig. 45-4).

Complications

Patients undergoing coronary intervention are subject to the same complications encountered with the performance of coronary arteriography. In addition, because instrumentation of the atherosclerotic lesion takes place, coronary artery dissection, thrombus formation, and coronary artery spasm may occur, leading to acute occlusion of the coronary artery or of side branches arising from it. Atheroembolism may occur and lead to MI in an otherwise successful procedure. Occlusion of the treated artery is the most common serious complication of coronary angioplasty and accounts for most of the morbidity and mortality related to the procedure.

Of Gruentzig's first 50 patients, 5 experienced an acute deterioration necessitating emergency bypass surgery and 3 showed electrocardiographic evidence of MI.[10] The results of 3500 patients undergoing elective balloon angioplasty at Emory were analyzed and reported in detail.[268] Angioplasty was attempted in 3933 lesions, with a success rate of 91 percent. No complications occurred in 89 percent of patients, minor complications occurred in 6.9 percent, and major complications (emergency surgery, MI, death) occurred in 4.1 percent. Emergency CABG was performed in 2.7 percent of patients, who had an MI rate of 49 percent and a Q-wave MI rate of 23 percent. In patients sent for emergency surgery, the mortality rate was 2 percent. The overall MI rate was 2.6 percent. There were two nonsurgical deaths, giving a total mortality rate of 0.1 percent (4 of 3500). *Five preprocedural predictors of a major complication were identified: multivessel coronary artery disease, lesion eccentricity, presence of calcium in the lesion, female gender, and lesion length. The strongest predictor of a major complication was the appearance of an intimal dissection during the procedure.* Intimal dissection was evident in 29 percent of patients, and its presence resulted in a sixfold increase in the risk of a major complication. Minor complications tabulated in this study included the following: side branch occlusion (1.7 percent), ventricular arrhythmia requiring dc shock (1.5 percent), emergency recatheterization (0.8 percent), femoral artery repair (0.6 percent), transfusion requirement (0.3 percent), coronary embolus (0.1 percent), cardiac tamponade (0.1 percent), and stroke (0.03 percent). This early series of patients was treated with balloon angioplasty alone. In 1995 at Emory University Hospital, over 1600 patients were treated (76 percent with balloon alone), with angiographic success in 94 percent, Q-wave MI in 1.1 percent, non-Q-wave MI in 2.9 percent, and death in 0.6 percent. Stents have played an increasing role, being used in 66 percent of patients in 1998 with an improvement in acute outcome (see Table 45-5).

Although angiographic variables are important predictors of abrupt closure, of equal or greater importance is an estimate of the consequences of abrupt closure. This estimate is determined in large part by the amount of myocardium that is supplied by the artery in jeopardy. Occlusion of a small diagonal branch is of little consequence compared, for example, with the occlusion of a large LAD coronary artery that is also supplying collateral vessels to an occluded right coronary artery. In the first case, a small non-Q-wave MI is likely, whereas in the latter, occlusion would likely result in abrupt anterior and inferior ischemia and

TABLE 45-5 Results of Percutaneous Coronary Intervention, Emory University Hospital

	1980–1987	1988–1991	1992–1995	1996–1998	Total
Patients	7254	6591	6367	6417	26,629
Arterial segments treated	8885	9068	8321	8342	34,616
Initial success, %[a]	91	93	94	95	94
Complication-free success, %[b]	88	90	90	94	91
Single-vessel disease, %	67	49	35	43	48
Multivessel disease, %[c]	33	57	65	57	52
Multivessel PTCA, %[d]	7.8	11	9	9.5	9
Emergency CABG, %	3.4	2.1	1.3	1.5	2.1
Q-wave MI, %	1.6	1.0	0.8	0.3	1.0
In-hospital death, %	0.2	0.5	0.6	0.7	0.5

[a]Less than 50% residual stenosis.
[b]Less than 50% residual stenosis and freedom from complications.
[c]At least 50% stenosis of LAD + RCA, LAD + CIRC, CIRC + RCA, or LAD + RCA + CIRC.
[d]Dilatation of LAD + RCA, LAD + CIRC, CIRC + RCA, or LAD + CIRC + RCA.
ABBREVIATIONS: LAD = left anterior descending; RCA = right coronary artery; CIRC = circumflex artery; PTCA = percutaneous transluminal coronary angioplasty; CABG = coronary artery bypass graft; MI = myocardial infarction.

be associated with hypotension and possibly cardiogenic shock. Immediate stenting or bypass surgery may be lifesaving, but MI will occur in up to one-half of patients, and there is a significant risk of mortality in this subgroup of patients.

An analysis of 294 acute occlusions occurring during 8207 consecutive coronary angioplasty procedures performed in two centers revealed 13 cardiac deaths (4.4 percent of acute occlusions) and an overall cardiac mortality of 0.16 percent.[269] Of 13 patients who died, 12 were women. Multivariate analysis identified three independent predictors of death: collaterals originating from the dilated vessel, female gender, and multivessel disease. In an analysis of 32 deaths associated with 8052 PTCA procedures in three centers, left ventricular failure due to vessel occlusion, the most common cause of death, was independently correlated with female sex, "jeopardy score," and PTCA of a proximal right coronary artery (RCA) site but not ejection fraction or presence of multivessel disease.[270] Right ventricular failure due to occlusion of the proximal RCA and left main coronary dissections accounted for most of the remaining deaths.

The use of stents in the course of a failing angioplasty (Fig. 45-18) and prospectively in patients with unfavorable anatomy has significantly reduced the risk of urgent bypass surgery and Q-wave MI.[72,73,113] The increasing use of stents and adjunctive measures including new, powerful antithrombotic agents may herald a "new era" of coronary intervention.[113] New complications specifically related to the use of nonballoon devices include coronary perforation, distal atheroembolization, arterial access complications, and "domino stenting" (additional stents to treat end-of-stent dissections). The risk of coronary perforation is a limiting factor in achieving optimal atherectomy and significantly restricts use of the TEC device in native vessels. Among 8932 patients treated at William Beaumont Hospital, perforation was reported in 0.4 percent (balloon, 0.14 percent; TEC, 1.3 percent; DCA, 0.25 percent; excimer laser 2 percent).[271] This risk of perforation is highest in tortuous and smaller vessels and in laser angioplasty of right coronary lesions. In patients experiencing free perforations, Ellis reported that 75 percent required surgery, 29 percent had a Q-wave MI, and 14 percent died.[272] Perforation was reported in 10 of 432 stent patients (2.3 percent), resulting in cardiac tamponade (50 percent), MI (40 percent), emergency surgery (50 percent), and death (30 percent).[273] The manifestations of perforation were delayed (5–24 h) in 20 percent of patients. Angiographic features associated with stent-related perforation were complex lesion morphology, small vessel diameter (2.6 ± 0.2 mm), oversized stents (stent/artery ratio 1.4 ± 0.1), tapering vessel (40 percent), and recrossing dissections (20 percent).[273] These results should engender a cautious approach to stenting in small vessels and when there is uncertainty regarding wire position. One of the newest causes of perforation is the hydrophilic coronary guidewire, which easily penetrates the wall of small distal arteries causing bleeding and cardiac tamponade, especially when IIb/IIIa receptor inhibitors have been used. Prompt application of strategies for the management of vessel perforation can be lifesaving, and device angioplasty operators must be facile with them.

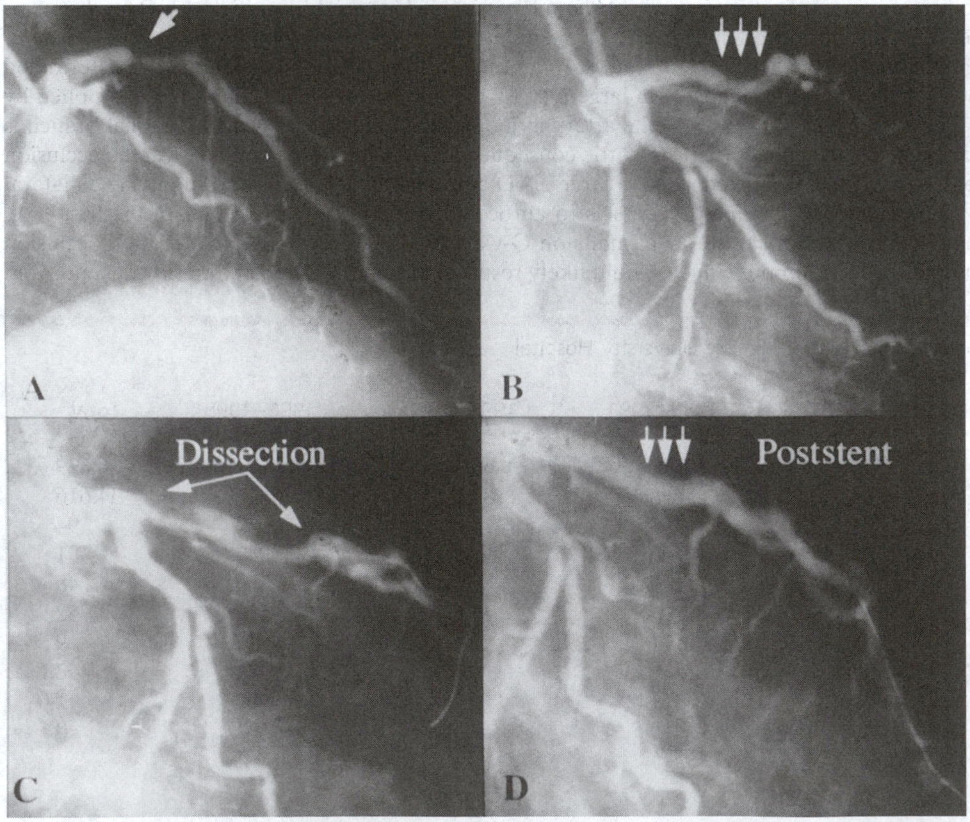

FIGURE 45-18 Complex stenosis of tortuous proximal LAD. *A.* Right anterior oblique, cranial angulation. *B.* Caudal angulation. Following an initial attempt at treatment of the lesion, a long dissection occurred. *C.* Prompt stent implantation stabilized the patient, preventing the need for emergency CABG (*D*).

Fortunately, the risk of vascular access-site complications, a frequent accompaniment of stenting when heparin and warfarin anticoagulation is used adjunctively, has been reduced with less aggressive antithrombotic strategies. In our experience, complications at the femoral artery puncture site were more often related to advanced age, female sex, hypertension, and postprocedure heparin use than to the size of the catheter.[274–276] Prolonged compression of pseudoaneurysms using ultrasound guidance and in some cases local thrombin injection obviates surgery in many patients with this complication.[277–279] Closure devices are used actively in some centers but add significantly to the cost of the procedure and have their own complications, including infection.

Distal coronary atheroembolization is only occasionally recognized clinically with balloon angioplasty but probably occurs moderately frequently[280] and is a clinically important limitation of debulking strategies such as atherectomy and laser ablation, where its manifestations are slow coronary flow, ischemia, and infarction.[281,282] Reports from CAVEAT indicate that creatine kinase elevations postprocedure were associated with worse long-term outcomes (death, MI, repeat intervention).[282] Although procedural modifications with rotational atherectomy appear to have reduced the immediate impact of microparticulate embolization,[210] the issue remains a source of concern and needs further study. Patients at increased risk include those with bulky or long native vessel lesions and nonfocal or thrombotic saphenous vein graft lesions, where embolization with TEC was noted in about 20 percent, and about one-third of patients with this complication died.[283,284] Atheroembolization also complicates stenting, accounting for an increased rate of non-Q-wave MI compared with balloon angioplasty. Particulate embolism to the coronary microcirculation may lead to otherwise silent infarction reflected by creatine kinase elevation, a topic of intense interest due to the finding of adverse late outcome, even with small elevations,[285] and the recognition that IIb/IIIa platelet receptor inhibitors, filters, and "occlusion-aspiration" systems can protect against this complication.[105,106,286,287] Not all studies, however, have found a correlation between enzyme elevations and adverse late outcome,[288] and this issue of when to use IIb/IIIa platelet receptors inhibitors is actively debated.[289]

Acute contrast nephropathy requiring dialysis is a costly complication of coronary intervention, which occurred in 15 of 1828 (0.8 percent) patients and was associated with a high (33.8 percent) in-hospital mortality.[290] Independent predictors of contrast nephropathy included decreased baseline creatinine clearance, diabetes, and contrast dose (no dialysis was required in patients receiving less than 100 mL of contrast material). Adequate periprocedural hydration and limitation of contrast volume are the most important measures in high-risk patients.[291]

FUTURE DIRECTIONS

The future of coronary intervention is bright indeed. The problem of subacute stent thrombosis, greatly diminished by current deployment strategies, should be solved by nonthrombogenic stents and/or more effective antithrombotic agents, thus opening the arena of small-vessel stenting (2- to 2.5-mm vessels) and further expanding intervention for multiple lesions in multiple vessels. The major impediments are cost and restenosis. The former should be ameliorated somewhat by market competition. Restenosis, which has been reduced by stenting of *de novo*[75,76,201] and restenotic lesions,[292] remains a challenge that is currently being addressed on multiple fronts with good prospects for meaningful solutions,[192,293–296] but new and sometimes unsuspected problems continue to arise, as in the recognition of the threat of late-late occlusion following brachytherapy.[297,298] Improved strategies to protect the microcirculation from atheroembolization are on the immediate horizon.[286]

References

1. Dotter CT, Judkins MP. Transluminal treatment of arteriosclerotic obstruction: Description of a new technique and a preliminary report of its application. *Circulation* 1964; 30:654–670.
2. Zeitler EJ, Schmidtke J, Schoop W. Die Perkutane Behandlung von Arteriellen Durchbluteungasstorungen der Estremiaten mit Katheter. *Vasa* 1973; 2:401–404.
3. Gruentzig AR, Turina MI, Schneider JA. Experimental percutaneous dilatation of coronary artery stenosis (abstract). *Circulation* 1976; 54(suppl II):II–81.
4. Gruentzig AR, Kumpe DA. Technique of percutaneous transluminal angioplasty with the Gruentzig balloon catheter. *AJR* 1979; 132:547–552.
5. Sheldon WC, Sones FM Jr. Stormy petrel of cardiology. *Clin Cardiol* 1994; 17:405–407.
6. Hurst JW. History of cardiac catheterization. In: King SB III, Douglas JS Jr, eds. *Coronary Arteriography and Angioplasty.* New York: McGraw-Hill; 1985:1–9.
7. King SB III. Angioplasty from bench to bedside to bench. *Circulation* 1996; 93:1621–1629.
8. King SB III. The development of interventional cardiology. *J Am Coll Cardiol* 1998; 31(suppl B):64B–88B.
9. Gruentzig A. Transluminal dilatation of coronary artery stenosis. *Lancet* 1978; 1:263.
10. Gruentzig AR, Senning A, Siegenthaler WE. Nonoperative dilatation of coronary artery stenosis: Percutaneous transluminal coronary angioplasty. *N Engl J Med* 1979; 301:61–68.
11. Kent KM, Bentivoglio LG, Block PC. Percutaneous transluminal coronary angioplasty: Report from the Registry of the National Heart, Lung, and Blood Institute. *Am J Cardiol* 1982; 49:2011–2020.
12. Detre K, Holubkov R, Kelsey S, et al. Percutaneous transluminal coronary angioplasty in 1985–1986 and 1977–1981: The National Heart, Lung, and Blood Institute Registry. *N Engl J Med* 1988; 318:265–270.
13. King SB III. Percutaneous transluminal coronary angioplasty. *J Am Coll Cardiol* 1999; 34:615–617.
14. Simpson JB, Baim DS, Robert EW, et al. A new catheter system for coronary angioplasty. *Am J Cardiol* 1982; 49:1216–1222.
15. Gruentzig AR, King SB III, Schlumpf M, et al. Long-term follow-up after percutaneous transluminal coronary angioplasty: The early Zurich experience. *N Engl J Med* 1987; 316:1127–1132.
16. King SB, Schlumpf M. Ten year completed follow-up after percutaneous transluminal coronary angioplasty: The early Zurich experience. *J Am Coll Cardiol* 1993; 22:353–360.
17. Detre K, Yeh W, Kelsey S, et al. Has improvement in PTCA intervention affected long-term prognosis? The NHLBI PTCA Registry experience. *Circulation* 1995; 91:2868–2875.
18. Cannan CR, Yeh W, Kelsey S, et al. Incidence and predictors of target vessel revascularization following percutaneous transluminal coronary angioplasty: A report from the National Heart, Lung, and Blood Institute Percutaneous Transluminal Coronary Angioplasty Registry. *Am J Cardiol* 1999; 84:170–175.
19. Jones RH, Kesler K, Phillips K, et al. Long-term survival benefits of coronary artery bypass grafting and percutaneous transluminal angioplasty in patients with coronary artery disease. *J Thorac Cardiovasc Surg* 1996; 111:1013.
20. Mark DB, Nelson CL, Califf RM, et al. Continuing evolution of therapy for coronary artery disease: Initial results from the era of coronary angioplasty. *Circulation* 1994; 89:2015–2025.
21. Hannan EL, Racz MJ, McCallister BD, et al. A comparison of three-year survival after coronary artery bypass graft surgery and percutaneous transluminal coronary angioplasty. *J Am Coll Cardiol* 1999; 33:63–72.
22. Velianou JL, Jacobs AK, Feit F, et al. Does angioplasty prolong survival in patients with multivessel disease? Results from the Bypass Angioplasty Revascularization Investigation (BARI). *Circulation* 1999; 100(suppl I):I-84.
23. Cowley MJ, Vetrovec GW, DiSciasio G, et al. Coronary angioplasty of multiple vessels: Short-term outcome and long-term results. *Circulation* 1985; 72:1314–1320.
24. O'Keefe JH Jr, Rutherford BD, McConahay DR, et al. Multivessel coronary angioplasty from 1980–1989: Procedural results and long-term outcome. *J Am Coll Cardiol* 1990; 16:1097–1102.
25. Parisi AF, Folland ED, Hartigan P. A comparison of angioplasty

with medical therapy in the treatment of single-vessel coronary artery disease. *N Engl J Med* 1992; 326:10–16.
26. Boden WE, O'Rourke RA, Crawford MH, et al. Outcomes in patients with acute non-Q-wave myocardial infarction randomly assigned to an invasive as compared with a conservative management strategy. *N Engl J Med* 1998; 338:1785–1792.
27. Hueb WA, Bellotti G, deOliveira SA, et al. The Medicine, Angioplasty or Surgery Study (MASS): A prospective, randomized trial of medical therapy, balloon angioplasty or bypass surgery for single proximal left anterior descending artery stenoses. *J Am Coll Cardiol* 1995; 26:1600–1605.
28. Coronary angioplasty versus medical therapy for angina: The Second Randomized Intervention Treatment of Angina (RITA-2) trial. *Lancet* 1997; 350:461–468.
29. Pitt B, Waters D, Brown WV, et al. Aggressive lipid-lowering therapy compared with angioplasty in stable coronary artery disease. *N Engl J Med* 1999; 341:70–76.
30. Wallentin L. Fast revascularization during instability in coronary artery disease (FRISC II): An early invasive versus early noninvasive strategy in unstable coronary artery disease. *J Am Coll Cardiol* 1999; 34:1.
31. Fragmin and Fast Revascularization during Instability in Coronary Artery Disease Investigators. Invasive compared with noninvasive treatment in unstable coronary-artery disease: FRISC II prospective randomised multicentre study. *Lancet* 1999; 354: 708–715.
32. King SB III, Lembo NJ, Weintraub WS, et al. A randomized trial comparing coronary angioplasty with coronary bypass surgery. *N Engl J Med* 1994; 331:1044–1050.
33. The Bypass Angioplasty Revascularization Investigation (BARI) Investigators. Comparison of coronary bypass surgery with angioplasty in patients with multivessel disease. *N Engl J Med* 1996; 335:217–225.
34. Chaitman BR, Schwartz L, Roubin GS, et al. Comparative 5 year incidence of ischemic events for PTCA and CABG in the Bypass Angioplasty Revascularization Investigation (BARI). *J Am Coll Cardiol* 1996; 27:55A.
35. Pocock SJ, Henderson RA, Rickards AF, et al. Metaanalysis of randomized trials comparing coronary angioplasty with bypass surgery. *Lancet* 1995; 346:1184–1189.
36. Sim I, Gupta M, McDonald K, et al. A meta-analysis of randomized trials comparing coronary artery bypass grafting with percutaneous transluminal coronary angioplasty in multivessel coronary artery disease. *Am J Cardiol* 1995; 76:1025–1029.
37. Kosinski AS, Barnharat HX, Weintraub WS, et al. Five year outcome after coronary surgery or coronary angioplasty: Results from the Emory Angioplasty versus Surgery Trial (EAST) (abstract). *Circulation* 1995; 92:I-543.
38. Weintraub WS, Mauldin PD, Becker E, et al. A comparison of the costs and quality of life after coronary angioplasty or coronary surgery for multivessel coronary artery disease: Results from the Emory Angioplasty versus Surgery Trial (EAST). *Circulation* 1995; 92:2831–2840.
39. The BARI Investigators. Influence of diabetes on 5-year mortality and morbidity in a randomized trial comparing CABG and PTCA in patients with multivessel disease: The Bypass Angioplasty Revascularization Investigation (BARI). *Circulation* 1997; 96:1761–1769.
40. The BARI Investigators. Seven year mortality in the Bypass Angioplasty Revascularization Investigation (BARI) by treatment and diabetic status. *J Am Coll Cardiol* 2000; 35:1122–1129.
41. King SB III, Kosinski AS, Guyton RA, et al. Eight-year mortality in the Emory Angioplasty versus Surgery Trial (EAST). *J Am Coll Cardiol* 2000; 35:1116–1121.
42. Detre KM, Guo P, Holubkov R, et al. Coronary revascularization in diabetic patients: A comparison of the randomized and observational components of the Bypass Angioplasty Revascularization Investigation (BARI). *Circulation* 1999; 99:633–640.
43. Weintraub WS, Stein B, Kosinski A, et al. Outcome of coronary bypass surgery versus coronary angioplasty in diabetic patients with multivessel coronary artery disease. *J Am Coll Cardiol* 1998; 31:10–19.
44. Kuntz RE. Importance of considering atherosclerosis progression when choosing a coronary revascularization strategy: The diabetics-percutaneous transluminal coronary angioplasty dilemma. *Circulation* 1999; 99:847–851.
45. Eagle KA, Guyton RA, Davidoff R, et al. ACC/AHA guidelines for coronary artery bypass graft surgery: Executive summary and recommendations. A report of the American College of Cardiology/American Heart Association Task Force on Practice Guidelines (Committee to Revise the 1991 Guidelines for Coronary Artery Bypass Graft Surgery). *Circulation* 1999; 100:1464–1480.
46. Hirotani T, Kameda T, Kumamoto T, et al. Effects of coronary artery bypass grafting using internal mammary arteries for diabetic patients. *J Am Coll Cardiol* 1999; 34:532–538.
47. Robertson GC, Simpson JB, Selmon MR, et al. Experience of directional coronary atherectomy over four years. *J Am Coll Cardiol* 1991; 17:384A.
48. Topol EJ, Leya F, Pinkerton CA, et al. A comparison of directional coronary atherectomy with coronary angioplasty in patients with coronary artery disease. *N Engl J Med* 1993; 329:221–227.
49. Adelman AG, Cohen EA, Kimball BP, et al. A comparison of directional atherectomy with balloon angioplasty for lesions of the left anterior descending coronary artery. *N Engl J Med* 1993; 329:228–233.
50. Holmes DR Jr, Topol EJ, Califf RM, et al. A multicenter, randomized trial of coronary angioplasty versus directional atherectomy for patients with saphenous vein bypass graft lesions. *Circulation* 1995; 91:1966–1974.
51. Baim DS, Cutlip DE, Sharma SK, et al. Final results of the balloon versus optimal atherectomy trial (BOAT). *Circulation* 1998; 97:322–331.
52. Simonton CA, Leon MB, Baim DS, et al. "Optimal" directional coronary atherectomy: Final results of the Optimal Atherectomy Restenosis Study (OARS). *Circulation* 1998; 97:332–339.
53. Williams DO, Fahrenbach MC. Directional coronary atherectomy: But wait, there's more. *Circulation* 1998; 97:309–311.
54. Tsuchikane E, Kobayashi T, Kirino M, et al. Which is better for STRESS and BENESTENT equivalent lesions, stenting or atherectomy?: Results of Stent versus Directional Atherectomy Randomized Trial (START). *Circulation* 1999; 100(suppl I): I-727.
55. Goldberg S, Aji J. Plaque excision combined with stent placement: Can a poor "finisher" become a good "starter"? *Circulation* 1998; 98:1591–1593.
56. Moussa I, Moses J, Di Mario C, et al. Stenting after optimal lesion debulking (SOLD) registry: Angiographic and clinical outcomes. *Circulation* 1998; 98:1604–1609.
57. Oesterle SN. Coronary interventions at a crossroads: The bifurcation stenosis. *J Am Coll Cardiol* 1998; 32:1853–1854.
58. Dauerman HL, Higgins PJ, Sparano AM, et al. Mechanical debulking versus balloon angioplasty for the treatment of true bifurcation lesions. *J Am Coll Cardiol* 1998; 32:1845–1852.
59. Reifart N, Vandormael M, Krajcar M, et al. Randomized comparison of angioplasty of complex coronary lesions at a single center: Excimer Laser, Rotational Atherectomy, and Balloon Angioplasty Comparison (ERBAC) study. *Circulation* 1997; 96:91–98.
60. Koster R, Hamm CW, Seabra-Comes R, et al. Laser angioplasty of restenosed coronary stents: Results of a multicenter surveillance trial. *Am Coll Cardiol* 1999; 34:25–32.
61. Bersin RM, Cedarholm JC, Kowalchuk GJ, et al. Long-term clinical follow-up of patients treated with the coronary Rotabla-

tor: A single-center experience. *Cathet Cardiovasc Intervent* 1999; 46:399–405.

62. Kini A, Marmur JD, Duvvuri S, et al. Rotational atherectomy: Improved procedural outcome with evolution of technique and equipment: Single-center results of first 1000 patients. *Cathet Cardiovasc Intervent* 1999; 46:305–311.
63. Kobayashi Y, De Gregorio J, Kobayashi N, et al. Lower restenosis rate with stenting following aggressive versus less aggressive rotational atherectomy. *Cathet Cardiovasc Intervent* 1999; 46:406–414.
64. Sharma SK, Bhalla N, Dangas G, et al. Rotational atherectomy prior to coronary stenting prevents side branch occlusion. *J Am Coll Cardiol* 1997; 29(suppl A):498A.
65. Whisenant BK, Baim DS, Kuntz RE, et al. Rheolytic thrombectomy with the Possis AngioJet: Technical considerations and initial clinical experience. *J Invas Cardiol* 1999; 11:421–426.
66. Scott LRP, Silva JA, White C, et al. Rheolytic thrombectomy: A new treatment for stent thrombosis. *Cathet Cardiovas Intervent* 1999; 47:97–101.
67. Nakagawa Y, Matsuo S, Yokoi H, et al. Stenting after thrombectomy with the AngioJet catheter for acute myocardial infarction. *Cathet Cardiovasc Diagn* 1998; 43:327–330.
68. Rodes J, Bilodeau L, Bonan R, et al. Angioscopic evaluation of thrombus removal by the Possis AngioJet thrombectomy catheter. *Cathet Cardiovasc Diagn* 1998; 43:338–343.
69. Nakaawa Y, Matsuo S, Kimura T, et al. Thrombectomy with Angiojet catheter in native coronary arteries for patients with acute or recent myocardial infarction. *Am J Cardiol* 1999; 83:994–999.
70. Sigwart U, Puel J, Mirkovitch V, et al. Intravascular stents to prevent occlusion and restenosis after transluminal angioplasty. *N Engl J Med* 1987; 316:701–706.
71. Puel J, Joffre F, Rousseau H, et al. Endo-protheses coronanennes and auto-expansive dans la preventions des restenoses apres angioplastie transluminale. *Arch Mal Coeur* 1987; 8:131–132.
72. Roubin GS, King SB III, Douglas JS Jr, et al. Intracoronary stenting during percutaneous transluminal coronary angioplasty. *Circulation* 1990; 81(suppl IV):IV-92–IV-100.
73. Hearn JA, King SB III, Douglas JS Jr, et al. Clinical and angiographic outcomes after coronary artery stenting for acute or threatened closure after percutaneous transluminal coronary angioplasty: Initial results with a balloon-expandable, stainless steel design. *Circulation* 1993; 88:2086–2096.
74. Roubin GS, Robinson KA, King SB, et al. Early and late results of intracoronary arterial stenting after coronary angioplasty in dogs. *Circulation* 1987; 76:891–897.
75. Fischman DL, Leon MB, Baim DS, et al. A randomized comparison of coronary-stent placement and balloon angioplasty in treatment of coronary artery disease. *N Engl J Med* 1994; 331:496–501.
76. Serruys PW, de Jaegere P, Kiemeneij F, et al. A comparison of balloon-expandable-stent implantation with balloon angioplasty in patients with coronary artery disease. *N Engl J Med* 1994; 331:489–495.
77. Colombo A, Hall P, Nakamura S, et al. Intracoronary stenting without anticoagulation accomplished with intravascular ultrasound guidance. *Circulation* 1995; 91:1676–1688.
78. Schoemig A, Newmann FJ, Kastrati A, et al. A randomized comparison of antiplatelet and anticoagulant therapy after the placement of coronary artery stents. *N Engl J Med* 1996; 334:1084–1089.
79. Topol EJ. Toward a new frontier in myocardial reperfusion therapy: Emerging platelet preeminence. *Circulation* 1998; 97:211–218.
80. Leon MB, Baim DS, Popma JJ, et at. A clinical trial comparing three antithrombotic-drug regimens after coronary-artery stenting. *N Engl J Med* 1998; 339:1665–1671.
81. Urban P, Macaya C, Rupprecht HJ, et al. Randomized evaluation of anticoagulation versus antiplatelet therapy after coronary stent implantation in high-risk patients: The Multicenter Aspirin and Ticlopidine Trial after Intracoronary Stenting (MATTIS). *Circulation* 1998; 98:2126–2132.
82. Bertrand M, Legrand V, Boland J, et al. Randomized multicenter comparison of conventional anticoagulation versus antiplatelet therapy in unplanned and elective coronary stenting: The Full Anticoagulation versus Aspirin and Ticlopidine (FANTASTIC) study. *Circulation* 1998; 98:1597–1603.
83. Berger PB, Bell MR, Hasdai D, et al. Safety and efficacy of ticlopidine for only 2 weeks after successful intracoronary stent placement. *Circulation* 1999; 99:248–253.
84. Steinhubl SR, Tan WA, Foody JM, et al. Incidence and clinical course of thrombotic thrombocytopenic purpura due to ticlopidine following coronary stenting. *JAMA* 1999; 281:806–810.
85. Bennett CL, Davidson CJ, Raisch DW, et al. Thrombotic thrombocytopenic purpura associated with ticlopidine in the setting of coronary artery stents and stroke prevention. *Arch Intern Med* 1999; 159:2524–2528.
86. Quinn MJ, Fitzgerald DJ. Ticlopidine and clopidogrel. *Circulation* 1999; 100:1667–1672.
87. Berger PB, Bellot V, Melby S, et al. Clopidogrel versus ticlopidine for coronary stents. *J Am Coll Cardiol* 1999; 33:34A.
88. Moussa I, Oetgen M, Roubin G, et al. Effectiveness of clopidogrel and aspirin versus ticlopidine and aspirin in preventing stent thrombosis after coronary stent implantation. *Circulation* 1999; 99:2364–2366.
89. Bertrand ME. Clopidogrel aspirin stent international study (CLASSICS) trial. *J Am Coll Cardiol* 1999; 34:7.
90. Urban P, Gershlick AH, Rupprecht HJ, et al. Efficacy of ticlopidine and clopidogrel on the rate of cardiac events after stent implantation: Evidence from CLASSICS. *Circulation* 1999; 100(suppl I):I-379.
91. Serruys PW, van Hout B, Bonnier H, et al. Randomised comparison of implantation of heparin-coated stents with balloon angioplasty in selected patients with coronary artery disease (Benestent II). *Lancet* 1998; 352:673–681.
92. Weaver WD. Late-breaking trials in interventional cardiology: Optimal angioplasty versus primary stenting (OPUS). *J Am Coll Cardiol* 1999; 34:1.
93. Narins CR, Holmes DR, Topol EJ. A call for provisional stenting: The balloon is back! *Circulation* 1998; 97:1298–1305.
94. Ten Berg JM, Kelder JC, Suttorp M, et al. A plea for plain old balloon angioplasty with a low rate of provisional stenting: An unselected consecutive group of 1058 patients. *Circulation* 1999; 100(suppl I):I-455.
95. Rodriquez A. Optimal coronary balloon angioplasty versus stent. *J Am Coll Cardiol* 1998; 32:1351–1357.
96. Holmes DR, Hirshfeld J, Faxon D, et al. ACC expert consensus document on coronary artery stents: Document of the American College of Cardiology. *J Am Coll Cardiol* 1998; 32:1471–1482.
96a. Rankin JM, Spinelli JJ, Carere RG, et al. Improved clinical outcome after widespread use of coronary-artery stenting in Canada. *N Engl J Med* 1999; 341:1957–1965.
96b. Jacobs AK. Coronary stents: Have they fulfilled their promise? *N Engl J Med* 1999; 341:2005–2006.
97. Verheugt FWA. Hotline sessions of the 21st European Congress of Cardiology. *Eur Heart J* 1999; 20:1603.
98. Serruys PW, Costa MA, Betriu A, et al. The influence of diabetes mellitus on clinical outcome following multivessel stenting or CABG in the ARTS Trial. *Circulation* 1999; 100(suppl I): I–364.
99. Rodriquez A, Palacios IF, Navia J, et al. Argentine randomized study: Coronary angioplasty with stenting versus coronary artery bypass surgery in patients with multiple vessel disease (ERACI II): 30-day and long-term follow-up results. *Circulation* 1999; 100(suppl I):I-234.
100. Oesterle SN, Limpljankit T, Yeung AC, et al. Ultrasound logic:

The value of intracoronary imaging for the interventionalist. *Cathet Cardiovasc Intervent* 1999; 47:475–490.
101. The PURSUIT Investigators. Inhibition of platelet glycoprotein IIb/IIIa with eptifibatide in patients with acute coronary syndromes. *N Engl J Med* 1998; 339:436–443.
102. PRISM-PLUS Investigators. Inhibition of the platelet glycoprotein IIb/IIIa receptor with tirofiban in unstable anigna and non-Q wave myocardial infarction. *N Engl J Med* 1998; 338:1488–1497.
103. The CAPTURE Investigators. Randomized placebo-controlled trial of abciximab before and during coronary intervention in refractory unstable angina: The CAPTURE study. *Lancet* 1997; 349:1429–1435.
104. The EPILOG Investigators. Platelet glycoprotein IIb/IIIa receptor blockade and low-dose heparin during percutaneous coronary revascularization. *N Engl J Med* 1997; 336:1689–1696.
105. The EPIC Investigators. Use of a monoclonal antibody directed against the platelet glycoprotein IIb/IIIa receptor in high-risk coronary angioplasty. *N Engl J Med* 1994; 330:956–961.
106. Topol EJ, Ferguson JJ, Weisman HF, et al. Long term protection from myocardial ischemic events after brief integrin β_3 blockade with percutaneous coronary intervention. *JAMA* 1997; 278: 479–484.
107. Boersma E, Akkerhuis M, Theroux P, et al. Platelet glycoprotein IIb/IIIa receptor inhibition in non-ST-elevation acute coronary syndromes: Early benefit during medical treatment only, with additional protection during percutaneous coronary intervention. *Circulation* 1999; 100:2045–2048.
108. The EPISTENT Investigators. Randomized placebo-controlled and balloon angioplasty-controlled trial to access safety of coronary stenting with use of platelet glycoprotein-IIb/IIIa blockade. *Lancet* 1998; 352:87–92.
109. Lincoff AM, Califf RM, Moliterno DJ, et al. Complementary clinical benefits of coronary artery stenting and blockade of platelet glycoprotein IIb/IIIa receptors. *N Engl J Med* 1999; 341:319–327.
110. Marso SP, Bhatt DL, Tanguay JF, et al. Synergy of stenting plus abciximab in diabetic patients: Persistence through 1-year follow-up from EPISTENT. *Circulation* 1999; 100(suppl I):365.
111. King SB III, Mahmud E. Will blocking the platelet save the diabetic? *Circulation* 1999; 100:2466–2468.
112. The ERASER Investigators. Acute platelet inhibition with abciximab does not reduce in-stent restenosis (ERASER study). *Circulation* 1999; 100:799–806.
113. Ellis SG, Whitlow PL, Guetta V, et al. A highly significant 40 percent reduction in ischemic complications of percutaneous coronary intervention in 1995: Beginning of a new era. *J Am Coll Cardiol* 1996; 27(suppl A):253A.
114. Hamm CW, Heeschen C, Goldman B, et al. Benefit of abciximab in patients with refractory unstable angina in relation to serum troponin T levels. *N Engl J Med* 1999; 340:1623–1629.
115. Van den Brand M, Laarman GJ, Steg PG, et al. Assessment of coronary angiograms prior to and after treatment with abciximab, and the outcome of angioplasty in refractory unstable angina patients: Angiographic results from the CAPTURE trial. *Eur Heart J* 1999; 20:1572–1578.
116. Ellis SG, Lincoff AM, Miller D, et al. Reduction in complications of angioplasty with abciximab occurs largely independent of baseline lesion morphology. *J Am Coll Cardiol* 1998; 32:1619–1623.
117. Ryan TJ, Faxon DP, Gunnar RM, et al. Guidelines for percutaneous transluminal coronary angioplasty: A report of the American College of Cardiology/American Heart Association Task Force on Assessment of Diagnostic and Therapeutic Cardiovascular Procedures (Subcommittee of Percutaneous Transluminal Coronary Angioplasty). *J Am Coll Cardiol* 1988; 12:519–540.
118. Ryan TJ, Bauman WB, Kennedy JW, et al. Guidelines for percutaneous transluminal coronary angioplasty: A report of the American Heart Association/American College of Cardiology Task Force on Assessment of Diagnostic and Therapeutic Cardiovascular Procedures (Committee on Percutaneous Transluminal Coronary Angioplasty). *Circulation* 1993; 88:2987–3007.
119. Weintraub WS, King SB III, Douglas JS Jr, et al. Percutaneous transluminal coronary angioplasty as a first revascularization procedure in single, double, and triple-vessel coronary artery disease. *J Am Coll Cardiol* 1995; 26:142–151.
120. Mark DB, Nelson CL, Califf RM, et al. Continuing evaluation and therapy for coronary artery disease: Initial results from the era of coronary angioplasty. *Circulation* 1994; 89:2015–2025.
121. Strauss WE, Fortin T, Hartigan P, et al. A comparison of quality of life scores in patients with angina pectoris after angioplasty compared with after medical therapy: Outcomes of a randomized clinical trial. *Circulation* 1995; 92:1710–1719.
122. Giacomini JC, Parisi AF, Folland ED, et al. Three year follow-up of patients in the VA ACME trial (abstract). *Circulation* 1993; 88(suppl I):I-218.
123. O'Keefe JH, Kreamer TR, Jones PG, et al. Isolated left anterior descending coronary artery disease: Percutaneous transluminal coronary angioplasty versus stenting versus left internal mammary artery bypass grafting. *Circulation* 1999; (suppl II):II-114–II-118.
124. Hueb WA, Soares PR, de Oliveiras A, et al. Five-year follow-up of the Medicine, Angioplasty, or Surgery Study (MASS): A prospective, randomized trial of medical therapy, balloon angioplasty, or bypass surgery for single proximal left anterior descending coronary artery stenosis. *Circulation* 1999; 100(suppl II):II-107–II-113.
125. Goy JJ, Eickhout E, Burnand B. Coronary angioplasty versus left internal mammary artery grafting for isolated proximal left anterior descending artery stenosis. *Lancet* 1994; 343:1449–1454.
126. Versaci F, Gaspardone A, Fabrizio P, et al. A comparison of coronary artery stenting with angioplasty for isolated stenosis of the proximal left anterior descending coronary artery. *N Engl J Med* 1997; 336:817–822.
127. Ellis SG, Brown K, Howell G, et al. Two-year cardiac cost after cardiac catheterization: Profound impact of revascularization after first PTCA compared with initial medical or surgical therapy. *J Am Coll Cardiol* 1996; 27(suppl A):72A.
128. Cowley MJ, Vandermael M, Topol EJ. Is traditionally defined complete revascularization needed for patients with multivessel disease treated with elective coronary angioplasty? *J Am Coll Cardiol* 1993; 22:1289–1297.
129. Bourassa MG, Holubkov R, Yeh W, et al. Strategy of complete revascularization in patients with multivessel coronary artery disease: A report from the 1985–1986 NHLBI PTCA Registry. *Am J Cardiol* 1992; 70:174–178.
130. Zhao XQ, Brown BG, Stewart DK, et al. Effectiveness of revascularization in the Emory Angioplasty versus Surgery Trial: A randomized comparison of coronary angioplasty with bypass surgery. *Circulation* 1996; 93:1954–1962.
131. Kip KE, Bourassa MG, Jacobs AK, et al. Influence of pre-PTCA strategy and initial PTCA result in patients with multivessel disease: The Bypass Angioplasty Revascularization Investigation (BARI). *Circulation* 1999; 100:910–917.
132. Ellis SG, Roubin GS, King SB III, et al. Angiographic and clinical predictors of acute closure after native vessel coronary angioplasty. *Circulation* 1988; 77:372–379.
133. Laham RJ, Ho KL, Baim DS, et al. Palmaz-Schatz stenting: Early results and one-year outcome. *J Am Coll Cardiol* 1997; 30: 180–185.
134. Moussa I, Reiners B, Moses J, et al. A long-term angiographic and clinical outcome of patients undergoing multivessel coronary stenting. *Circulation* 1997; 96:3873–3979.
135. Kornowski R, Mehran R, Satler LF, et al. Procedural results and late clinical outcomes following multivessel coronary stenting. *J Am Coll Cardiol* 1999; 33:420–426.

136. Hernandez-Antolin RA, Alfonso F, Goicolea J, et al. Results (>6 months) of stenting of >1 major coronary artery in multivessel coronary artery disease. *Am J Cardiol* 1999; 84:147–151.
137. O'Neill W. Multivessel balloon angioplasty should be abandoned in diabetic patients! *J Am Coll Cardiol* 1998; 31:20–22.
138. Fuster V, Badimon L, Badimon JJ, et al. The pathogenesis of coronary artery disease and acute coronary syndromes. *N Engl J Med* 1991; 326:242–250, 320–328.
139. Mizuno K, Satomura K, Miyamoto A, et al. Angioscopic evaluation of coronary artery thrombi in acute coronary syndromes. *N Engl J Med* 1992; 326:287–291.
140. Waxman S, Mittleman MA, Manzok , et al. Culprit lesion morphology in subtypes of unstable angina as assessed by angioscopy. *Circulation* 1995; 92(suppl I):I-79.
141. Laskey MA, Deutsch E, Hirshfield JWJ, et al. Influence of herapin therapy on percutaneous transluminal coronary angioplasty outcome in patients with coronary arterial thrombus. *Am J Cardiol* 1990; 65:179–182.
142. Laskey MA, Deutsch E, Barnathan E, et al. Influence of herapin therapy on percutaneous transluminal coronary angioplasty outcome in unstable angina pectoris. *Am J Cardiol* 1990; 65:1425–1429.
143. Rosenman Y, Gilon D, Zelingher J, et al. Importance of delaying balloon angioplasty in patients with unstable angina pectoris. *Clin Cardiol* 1996; 19:111–114.
144. Douglas JS Jr, Lutz JF, Clements SD, et al. Therapy of large intracoronary thrombi in candidates for percutaneous transluminal coronary angioplasty. *J Am Coll Cardiol* 1988; 11:238.
145. The TIMI-IIIB Investigators. Effects of tissue plasminogen activator and a comparison of early invasive and conservative strategies in unstable angina and non-Q wave myocardial infarction. *Circulation* 1994; 89:1545–1556.
146. Cannon CP, McCabe CH, Stone PH, et al. Prospective validation of the Braunwald classification of unstable angina: Results from the Thrombolysis in Myocardial Ischemia (TIMI) III Registry. *Circulation* 1995; 92(suppl I):I-19.
147. Ghigliotti G, Brunelli C, Corsiglia L, et al. Identification of high-risk patients with unstable angina. *J Am Coll Cardiol* 1996; 27(suppl A):332A.
148. Serruys PW, Herrman J-PR, Simon R, et al. A comparison of hirudin with herapin in the prevention of restenosis after coronary angioplasty. *N Engl J Med* 1995; 333:757–763.
149. Ambrose JA, Almeida OD, Sharma SK, et al. Adjunctive thrombolytic therapy during angioplasty for ischemic rest angina: Results of the TAUSA trial. *Circulation* 1994; 90:69–77.
150. Antman EM, McCabe CH, Gurfinkel EP, et al. Enoxaparin prevents death and cardiac ischemic events in unstable angina/non-Q-wave myocardial infarction: Results of the Thrombolysis in Myocardial Infarction (TIMI) IIB Trial. *Circulation* 1999; 100:1593–1601.
151. Antman EM, Cohen M, Radley D,et al. Assessment of the treatment effect of enoxaparin for unstable angina/non-Q-wave myocardial infarction: TIMI IIb-ESSENCE meta-analysis. *Circulation* 1999; 100:1602–1608.
152. Armstrong PW. Pursuing progress in acute coronary syndromes. *Circulation* 1999; 100:1586–1589.
153. Purcell H, Fox KM. Improving outcome in acute coronary syndromes: As good as it gets? *Eur Heart J* 1999; 20:1533–1537.
154. Ferguson JJ. EPILOG and CAPTURE trials halted because of positive interim results. *Circulation* 1996; 93:637.
155. Hamm CW. Unstable angina: The breakthrough. *Eur Heart J* 1999; 20:1517–1519.
156. Cragg DR, Friedman HZ, Almany SL, et al. Early hospital discharge after percutaneous transluminal coronary angioplasty. *Am J Cardiol* 1989; 64:1270–1274.
157. Ellis SG, Vandormael MG, Cowley MJ, et al. Coronary morphologic and clinical determinants of procedural outcome with angioplasty for multivessel coronary disease. *Circulation* 1990; 82:1193–1203.
158. Ellis SG, de Cesare NB, Pinkerton CA, et al. Relation of stenosis morphology and clinical presentation to the procedural results of directional coronary atherectomy. *Circulation* 1991; 84:644–653.
159. Tan K, Sulke N, Taub N, et al. Clinical and lesion morphologic determinants of coronary angioplasty success and complications: Current experience. *J Am Coll Cardiol* 1995; 25:855–865.
160. Herrman JR, Melkert R, Simon R, et al. ABC-lesion type as a risk factor for the occurrence of early and late clinical events in unstable patients following transluminal coronary angioplasty (PTCA). *J Am Coll Cardiol* 1996; 27(suppl A):390A.
161. Fry ET, Hermiller JB, Peters TF, et al. Is ACC/AHA classification predictive of successful coronary intervention in the era of new devices? *J Am Coll Cardiol* 1996; 27(suppl A):152A.
162. Ellis SG, Guetta V, Miller D, et al. Relation between lesion characteristics and risk with percutaneous intervention in the stent and glycoprotein IIb/IIIa era: An analysis of results from 10,907 lesions and proposal for new classification scheme. *Circulation* 1999; 100:1971–1976.
163. Hannan EL, Racz M, Rytan TJ, et al. Coronary angioplasty volume-outcome relationships for hospitals and cardiologists. *JAMA* 1997; 279:892–898.
164. Ellis SG, Weintraub W, Holmes D, et al. Relation of operator volume and experience to procedural outcome with percutaneous coronary revascularization at hospitals with high intervention volumes. *Circulation* 1997; 95:2479–2484.
165. Kastrati A, Neumann FJ, Schomig A. Operator volume and outcome of patients undergoing coronary stent placement. *J Am Coll Cardiol* 1998; 32:970–976.
166. O'Keefe JH, Hartzler GO, Rutherford BD, et al. Left main coronary angioplasty: Early and late results of 127 acute and elective procedures. *Am J Cardiol* 1989; 64:144–147.
167. Ellis SG, Tamai H, Nobuyoshi M, et al. Contemporary percutaneous treatment of unprotected left main coronary stenoses: Initial results from a multicenter registry analysis 1994–1996. *Circulation* 1997; 96:3867–3872.
168. Park SJ, Park SW, Hong MK, et al. Stenting of unprotected left main coronary artery stenoses: Immediate and late outcomes. *J Am Coll Cardiol* 1998; 31:37–42.
169. Macaya C, Alfonso F, Iniques GJ, et al. Stenting for elastic recoil during coronary angioplasty of the left main coronary artery. *Am J Cardiol* 1992; 70:105–107.
170. Keeley EC, Aliabadi D, O'Neill WW, et al. Immediate and long-term results of elective and emergent percutaneous interventions on protected and unprotected severely narrowed left main coronary arteries. *Am J Cardiol* 1999; 83:242–246.
171. Marso SP, Gabriel S, Plokker T, et al. Catheter-based reperfusion of unprotected left main stenosis during an acute myocardial infarction (the ULTIMA experience). *Am J Cardiol* 1999; 83:1513–1517.
172. Kobayashi N, Finci L, Ferraro M, et al. Restenosis after coronary stenting: Clinical and angiographic predictors in 1906 lesions. *J Am Coll Cardiol* 1999; 33(suppl A):32A.
173. Kastrati A, Elezi S, Dirschinger J, et al. Influence of lesion length on restenosis after coronary stent placement. *Am J Cardiol* 1999; 83:1617–1622.
174. Topol EJ, Nissen SE. Our preoccupation with coronary luminology: The dissociation between clinical and angiographic findings in ischemic heart disease. *Circulation* 1995; 92:2333–2342.
175. Tuzcu EM, Berkalp B, De Franco AC, et al. The dilemma of diagnosing coronary calcification: Angiography versus intravascular ultrasound. *J Am Coll Cardiol* 1996; 27:832–838.
176. Mintz GS, Popma JJ, Pichard AD, et al. Intravascular ultrasound predictors of restenosis after percutaneous transcatheter coronary revascularization. *J Am Coll Cardiol* 1996; 27:1678–1687.
177. Stone GW, Linnemeier T, St Goar FG, et al. Improved outcome

of balloon angioplasty with intracoronary ultrasound guidance: Core lab angiographic and ultrasound results from the Clout study. *J Am Coll Cardiol* 1996; 27(suppl A):155A.

178. Bauters C, LaBlanche JM, McFadden E, et al. Angioscopic thrombus is associated with a high risk of angiographic restenosis. *Circulation* 1995; 92(suppl I):I-401.
179. Hoffman R, Mintz GS, Dussaillant GR, et al. Patterns and mechanisms of in-stent restenosis: A serial intravascular ultrasound study. *Circulation* 1996; 94:1247–1254.
180. Yokoi H, Kimura T, Nakagawa Y, et al. Long-term clinical and quantitative angiographic follow-up after the Palmaz-Schatz stent restenosis. *J Am Coll Cardiol* 1996; 27:224.
181. Mehran R, Dangas G, Abizaid AS, et al. Angiographic patterns of in-stent restenosis: Classification and implications for long-term outcome. *Circulation* 1999; 100:1872–1878.
182. Shiran A, Mintz GS, Waksman R, et al. Early lumen loss after treatment of in-stent restenosis: An intravascular ultrasound study. *Circulation* 1998; 98:200–203.
183. Sharma SK, Duvvuri S, Dangas G, et al. Rotational atherectomy for in-stent restenosis: Acute and long-term results of the first 100 cases. *J Am Coll Cardiol* 1998; 32:1358–1365.
184. Radke PW, Klues HG, Haager PK, et al. Mechanisms of acute lumen gain and recurrent restenosis after rotational atherectomy of diffuse in-stent restenosis: A quantitative angiographic and intravascular ultrasound study. *J Am Coll Cardiol* 1999; 34:33–39.
185. Mehran R, Mintz GS, Satler LF, et al. Treatment of in-stent restenosis with excimer laser coronary angioplasty: Mechanisms and results compared with PTCA alone. *Circulation* 1997; 96:2183–2189.
186. Sakamoto T, Kawarabayashi T, Taguchi H, et al. Intravascular ultrasound-guided balloon angioplasty for treatment of in-stent restenosis. *Cathet Cardiovasc Intervent* 1999; 47:298–303.
187. Sharma SK, Kini A, Duvvuri S, et al. Randomized trial of rotational atherectomy versus balloon angioplasty for in-stent restenosis (ROSTER): Interim analysis of 100 cases. *Circulation* 1998; 98(suppl I):I-717.
188. Verheugt FWA. Hotline sessions of the 21st European Congress of Cardiology. *Eur Heart J* 1999; 20:1603–1606.
189. Yokoi H, Tamurat, Nakagawa Y, et al. Refractory stent restenosis following balloon angioplasty. *Circulation* 1999; 100(suppl I): I-301.
190. Waksman R, White LR, Chan RC, et al. Intracoronary beta radiation therapy for patients with in-stent restenosis: The 6 months clinical and angiographic results. *Circulation* 1999; 100(suppl I):I-75.
191. Leon MB, Moses JW, Lansky AJ, et al. Intracoronary gamma radiation for prevention of recurrent in-stent restenosis: Final results from the Gamma-1 Trial. *Circulation* 1999; 100(suppl I):I-75.
192. Teirstein PS, Massullo V, Jani S, et al. Two-year follow-up after catheter-based radiotherapy to inhibit coronary restenosis. *Circulation* 1999; 99:243–247.
193. Serruys PW, Azar AJ, Sigwart U, et al. Long term follow-up of "stent-like" (30 percent diameter stent post) angioplasty: A case for provisional stenting. *J Am Coll Cardiol* 1996; 27(suppl A):15A.
194. Eccleston DS, Eisenberg MJ. Primary, "French" or restenosis stenting or balloon angioplasty? Relative outcome and costs using a decision analytic model. *Circulation* 1995; 92(suppl I):I-662.
195. Mak K, Belli G, Ellis SG, et al. Subacute stent thrombosis: Evolving issues and current concepts. *J Am Coll Cardiol* 1996; 27:494–503.
196. Sawada Y, Nosaka H, Kimura T, et al. Initial and six month outcome of Palmaz-Schatz stent implantation: Stress/Benestent equivalent versus non-equivalent lesions (abstract). *J Am Coll Cardiol* 1996; 27(suppl A):252A.
197. Pan M, de Lezo JS, Medina A, et al. Simple and complex stent strategies for bifurcated coronary arterial stenosis involving the side branch origin. *Am J Cardiol* 1999; 83:1320–1325.
198. Savage MP, Douglas JS Jr, Fischman DL, et al. Stent placement compared with balloon angioplasty for obstructed coronary bypass grafts. *N Engl J Med* 1997; 337:740–747.
199. Buller CE, Dzavik V, Carere RG, et al. Primary stenting versus balloon angioplasty in occluded coronary arteries: The Total Occlusion Study of Canada (TOSCA). *Circulation* 1999; 100: 236–242.
200. Erbel R, Haude M, Hopp HW, et al. Coronary-artery stenting compared with balloon angioplasty for restenosis after initial balloon angioplasty. *N Engl J Med* 1998; 339:1672–1678.
201. Serruys PW, Emanuelsson H, van der Giessen W, et al. Heparin-coated Palmaz-Schatz stents in human coronary arteries: Early outcome of the Benestent-II Pilot Study. *Circulation* 1996; 93:412–422.
202. Cohen DJ, Krumholz HM, Sukin CA, et al. In-hospital and one-year economic outcomes after coronary stenting or balloon angioplasty: Results from a randomized clinical trial. *Circulation* 1995; 92:2480–2487.
203. Eeckout E, Kapenberger L, Goy J. Stents for intracoronary placement: Current status and future directions. *J Am Coll Cardiol* 1996; 27:757–765.
204. Laster SB, Rutherford BD, McConahay DR, et al. Directional atherectomy of the left main coronary artery: Acute and long term results (abstract). *J Am Coll Cardiol* 1994; 23:386A.
205. Lewis BE, Leya FS, Johnson SA, et al. Outcomes of angioplasty (PTCA) and atherectomy (DCA) for bifurcation and non-bifurcation lesions in CAVEAT (abstract). *Circulation* 1993; 88(suppl I):I-601.
206. Leya FS, Lewis BE, Sumida CW, et al. Modified "kissing" atherectomy procedure with dependable protection of side branches by two-wire technique. *Cathet Cardiovasc Diagn* 1992; 27:155–161.
207. Kimball BP, Cohen EA, Adelman AG, et al. Influence of stenotic lesion morphology on immediate and long-term (6 months) angiographic outcome: Comparative analysis of directional coronary atherectomy versus standard balloon angioplasty. *J Am Coll Cardiol* 1996; 27:543–551.
208. Boehrer JD, Ellis SG, Keeler GP, et al. Differential benefit of directional atherectomy over angioplasty for left anterior descending in proximal, non-ostial lesions: Result from CAVEAT. *J Am Coll Cardiol* 1994; 23:386A.
209. Mintz GS, Pichard AD, Popma JJ, et al. Preliminary experience with adjunct directional coronary atherectomy after high-speed rotational atherectomy in the treatment of calcific coronary artery disease. *Am J Cardiol* 1993; 71:799–804.
210. Stertzer SH, Pomerantsev EV, Fitzgerald PJ, et al. Effects of technique modification on immediate results of high speed rotational atherectomy in 710 procedures on 656 patients. *Cathet Cardiovasc Diagn* 1995; 36:304–310.
211. MacIsaac AI, Bass TA, Buchbinder M, et al. High speed rotational atherectomy: Outcome in calcified and non-calcified coronary artery lesions. *J Am Coll Cardiol* 1995; 26:731–736.
212. Ellis SG, Popma JJ, Buchbinder M, et al. Relation of clinical presentation, stenosis morphology, and operator technique to the procedural results of rotational atherectomy and rotational atherectomy-facilitated angioplasty. *Circulation* 1994; 89:882–892.
213. Broderick TM, Kereiakes DJ, Whang DD, et al. Myocardial bridging may predispose to coronary perforation during rotational atherectomy. *J Invas Cardiol* 1996; 8:161–163
214. O'Murchu B, Foreman RD, Shaw RE, et al. Role of intraaortic balloon pump counterpulsation in high risk coronary rotational atherectomy. *J Am Coll Cardiol* 1995; 26:1270–1275.
215. Williams MJA, Dow CJ, Newell JB, et al. Prevalence and timing of regional myocardial dysfunction after rotational coronary atherectomy. *J Am Coll Cardiol* 1996; 28:861–869.

216. Moses JW, Tierstein PS, Sketch MH Jr, et al. Angiographic determinants of risk and outcome of coronary embolus and myocardial infarction (MI) with the transluminal extraction catheter (TEC): A report from the New Approaches to Coronary Intervention (NACI) Registry (abstract). *J Am Coll Cardiol* 1994; 23:220A.
217. Safian RD, Grines CL, May MA, et al. Clinical and angiographic results of transluminal extraction coronary atherectomy in saphenous vein bypass grafts. *Circulation* 1994; 89:302–312.
218. Baim DS, Kent KM, King SB III, et al. Evaluating new devices: Acute (in-hospital) results from the New Approaches to Coronary Intervention Registry. *Circulation* 1994; 89:471–481.
219. Kaplan BM, O'Neill WW, Safian RD, et al. Clinical and angiographic follow-up to a prospective study of transluminal extraction atherectomy in high risk patients with myocardial infarction (abstract). *J Am Coll Cardiol* 1995; 25(suppl A):331A.
220. Safian RD, May MA, Lichtenberg A, et al. Detailed clinical and angiographic analysis of transluminal extraction coronary atherectomy for complex lesions in native coronary arteries. *J Am Coll Cardiol* 1995; 25:848–854.
221. Groh WC, Kurnik PB, Matthai WH, et al. Initial experience with an intracoronary flow support device providing localized drug infusion: The Scimed dispatch catheter. *Cathet Cardiovasc Diagn* 1995; 36:67–73.
222. Fajadet J, Bar O, Jordan C. Human percutaneous thrombectomy using the new hydrolyzer catheter: Preliminary results in saphenous vein grafts (abstract). *J Am Coll Cardiol* 1994; 23:220A.
223. Douglas JS Jr, Ghazzal ZMG, Ba'albaki HA, et al. Excimer laser coronary angioplasty of ostial lesions: Acute success and complications. *Cathet Cardiovasc Diagn* 1991; 23:75.
224. Eigler NL, Douglas JS Jr, Margolis JR, et al. Excimer laser coronary angioplasty of aorto-ostial stenosis: Results of the ELCA Registry. *Circulation* 1993; 88:2049–2057.
225. de Marchena EJ, Mallon SM, Knopf WD, et al. Effectiveness of holmium laser-assisted coronary angioplasty. *Am J Cardiol* 1994; 73:117–121.
226. Litvack F, Eigler N, Margolis J, et al. Percutaneous excimer laser coronary angioplasty: Results in the first consecutive 3000 patients. *J Am Coll Cardiol* 1994; 23:323–329.
227. Appelman YE, Piek JJ, deFeyter PJ, et al. Excimer laser coronary angioplasty versus balloon angioplasty used in long-term lesions: The long-term results of the AMRO Trial. *J Am Coll Cardiol* 1995; 25(suppl A):329A.
228. Appelman JY, Koolen JJ, deFeyter PJ, et al. Long-term outcome of excimer laser angioplasty versus balloon angioplasty in functional and total coronary occlusions. *J Am Coll Cardiol* 1995; 25(suppl A):330A.
229. Vandormael M, Riefart N, Preusler W. Six month follow-up results following excimer laser angioplasty, rotational atherectomy and balloon angioplasty for complex lesions: ERBAC study. *Circulation* 1994; 90(suppl I):I-213.
230. Serruys PW, Hamburger J, Fleck E, et al. Laser guide wire: A powerful tool in recanalization of chronic total coronary occlusion. *Circulation* 1995; 92(suppl I):I-76.
231. Pepine CJ, Babb JD, Brinker JA, et al. Task Force 3: Training in cardiac catheterization and interventional cardiology. *J Am Coll Cardiol* 1995; 25:14–16.
232. Cowley MJ, Faxon DP, Holmes DR Jr. Guidelines for training, credentialing, and maintenance of competence for the performance of coronary angioplasty: A report from the Interventional Cardiology Committee and the Training Program Standards Committee of the Society for Cardiac Angiography and Interventions. *Cathet Cardiovasc Diagn* 1993; 30:1–4.
233. Douglas JS Jr, Pepine CJ, Block PC, et al. Recommendations for development and maintenance of competence in coronary interventional procedures. *J Am Coll Cardiol* 1993; 22:629–631.
234. Ryan TJ, Klocke FJ, Reynolds WA, et al. Clinical competence in percutaneous transluminal coronary angioplasty: A statement for physicians from the ACP/ACC/AHA Task Force on Clinical Privileges in Cardiology. *J Am Coll Cardiol* 1990; 15:1469–1474.
235. Conti CR. Credentialing cardiologists who perform therapeutic cardiac interventions. *Clin Cardiol* 1995; 18:689–691.
236. Hirshfield JW, Ellis SG, Faxon DP, et al. Recommendations for the assessment and maintenance of proficiency in coronary interventional procedures: Statement of the American College of Cardiology. *J Am Coll Cardiol* 1998; 31:722–743.
237. Teirstein PS. Credentialing for coronary interventions: Practice makes perfect. *Circulation* 1997; 95:2467–2470.
238. Eisenberg MJ, Rice S, Schiller NB. Guidelines for physician training in advanced cardiac procedures: The importance of case mix. *J Am Coll Cardiol* 1994; 23:1723–1725.
239. Eisenberg MJ, St Claire DA, Mak K, et al. Importance of case mix during training in interventional cardiology. *Am J Cardiol* 1996; 77:1010–1013.
240. Ellis SG, Nowamagbe O, Bittl JA, et al. Analysis and comparison of operator-specific outcomes in interventional cardiology. *Circulation* 1996; 93:431–439.
241. Califf RM, Jollis JG, Peterson ED. Operator-specific outcomes: A call to professional responsibility. *Circulation* 1996; 93:403–406.
242. McGrath PD, Wennberg WE, Malenka DJ, et al. Operator volume and outcomes in 12,988 percutaneous coronary interventions. *J Am Coll Cardiol* 1998; 31:570–576.
243. Ritchie JL, Phillips KA, Luft HS. Coronary angioplasty: Statewide experience in California. *Circulation* 1993; 88:2735–2743.
244. Jollis JG, Peterson ED, DeLong ER, et al. The relation between the volume of coronary angioplasty procedures at hospitals treating Medicare beneficiaries and short-term mortality. *N Engl J Med* 1995; 331:1625–1629.
245. Ryan TJ. The critical question of procedure volume minimums for coronary angioplasty. *JAMA* 1995; 274:1169–1170.
246. Fajadet J, Brunel P, Jordan C, et al. Transradial approach for interventional coronary procedures: Analysis of complications (abstract). *J Am Coll Cardiol* 1996; 27(suppl A):392A.
247. Edelman ER, Rogers C. Stent-versus-stent equivalency trials: Are some stents more equal than others? *Circulation* 1999; 100:896–898.
248. Ritchie JL, Nissen SE, Douglas JS Jr, et al. Use of nonionic or low osmolar contrast agents in cardiovascular procedures. *J Am Coll Cardiol* 1993; 21:269–273.
249. Grines CL, Schreiber TL, Savas V, et al. A randomized trial of low osmolar ionic versus nonionic contrast media in patients with myocardial infarction or unstable angina undergoing percutaneous transluminal coronary angioplasty. *J Am Coll Cardiol* 1996; 27:1381–1386.
250. Lembo NJ, King SB III, Roubin GS, et al. Effects of nonionic contrast media on complications of percutaneous transluminal coronary angioplasty. *Am J Cardiol* 1991; 67:1046–1050.
251. Shrader R, Esch I, Ensslen R, et al. A randomized trial comparing the impact of a nonionic (Iomeprol) versus an ionic (Ioxaglate) low osmolar contrast medium on abrupt vessel closure and ischemic complications after coronary angioplasty. *J Am Coll Cardiol* 1999; 33:395–402.
252. Aguirre FV, Simoons ML, Ferguson JJ, et al. Impact of contrast media on clinical outcomes following percutaneous coronary interventions with platelet glycoprotein IIb/IIIa inhibition: Meta-analysis of clinical trials with abciximab. *Circulation* 1997; 96(suppl I):I–161.
253. Chevalier B, Royer T, Glatt B, et al. Does nonionic contrast medium still modify angioplasty results in the stent era? *J Am Coll Cardiol* 1999; 33(suppl A):85A.
254. Fleisch M, Mulhauser B, Garachemani A, et al. Impact of ionic (Ioxaglate) and nonionic (Loversol) contrast media on PTCA related complications. *J Am Coll Cardiol* 1999; 33(suppl A): 85A.

255. Davidson CJ, Laskey WK, Harrison JK, et al. A randomized trial of contrast media utilization in high risk PTCA (the COURT trial). *J Am Coll Cardiol* 1999; 33(suppl A):11A.
256. Roubin GS, Douglas JS Jr, King SB III, et al. Influence of balloon size in initial success, acute complications and restenosis after percutaneous transluminal coronary angioplasty: A prospective, randomized study. *Circulation* 1988; 78:557–565.
257. Waksman R, Ghazzal ZMB, Scott NA, et al. Efficacy and safety of using perfusion dilatation catheter as initial balloon in coronary angioplasty. *Cathet Cardiovasc Diagn* 1994; 32:319–322.
258. Meier B, Rutishauser W. Coronary pacing during percutaneous transluminal coronary angioplasty. *Circulation* 1985; 72:557–561.
259. Dirschinger J, Kastrati A, Neumann F, et al. Influence of balloon pressure during stent placement in native coronary arteries on early and late angiographic and clinical outcome: A randomized evaluation of high-pressure inflation. *Circulation* 1999; 100: 918–923.
260. Tobis JM, Colombo A. Do you need IVUS guidance for coronary stent deployment? *Cathet Cardiovasc Diagn* 1996; 37:360–361.
261. Russo RJ, Teirstein PS, for the AVID Investigators. Angiography versus intravascular ultrasound-directed stent placement (abstract). *J Am Coll Cardiol* 1996; 27(suppl A):306A.
262. Deckelbaum LI, Natarajan K, Bittl JA, et al. Effect of intracoronary saline infusion on dissection during excimer laser coronary angioplasty: A randomized trial. *J Am Coll Cardiol* 1995; 26:1264–1269.
263. Williams MS, Coller BS, Vaananen HJ, et al. Activation of platelets in platelet-rich plasma by rotablation is speed-dependent and can be inhibited by abciximab (c7E3 Fab; ReoPro). *Circulation* 1998; 98:742–748.
264. Reisman M, Katopodis J, Whitlow P, et al. Analysis of low speed rotational atherectomy in a multicenter registry: Implications for device utilization. *Circulation* 1998; 98(suppl I):I-351.
265. Kereiakes DJ, Lincoff M, Miller DP, et al. Abciximab therapy and unplanned coronary stent deployment: Favorable effects on stent use, clinical outcomes, and bleeding complications. *Circulation* 1998; 97:857–864.
266. Ellis SG, Roubin GS, Wilentz J, et al. Results of a randomized trial of heparin and aspirin vs aspirin alone for prevention of acute closure and restenosis after angioplasty (abstract). *Circulation* 1987; 76(suppl IV):IV-213.
267. Ruygrok PN, De Jaegere PT, Van Domburg RT, et al. Clinical outcome 10 years after attempted percutaneous transluminal coronary angioplasty in 856 patients. *J Am Coll Cardiol* 1996; 27:1669–1677.
268. Bredlau CE, Roubin GS, Leimbruger PP, et al. In-hospital morbidity and mortality in patients undergoing elective coronary angioplasty. *Circulation* 1985; 72:1044–1052.
269. Ellis SG, Roubin GS, King SB III, et al. In-hospital cardiac mortality following acute closure after percutaneous transluminal coronary angioplasty: Analysis of risk factors from 8207 procedures. *J Am Coll Cardiol* 1988; 11:211–216.
270. Ellis SG, Myler RK, King SB III, et al. Causes and correlates of death after unsupported coronary angioplasty: Implications for use of angioplasty and advanced support techniques in high-risk settings. *Am J Cardiol* 1991; 68:1447–1451.
271. Ajluni SC, Glazier S, Blankenship L, et al. Perforations after percutaneous coronary interventions: Clinical, angiographic, and therapeutic observations. *Cathet Cardiovasc Diagn* 1994; 32: 206–212.
272. Ellis SG, Arnold AZ, Raymond RE, et al. Increased coronary perforation in the new device era: Incidence, classification, management and outcome. *Circulation* 86(suppl I):I-787.
273. Bensuly KH, Glazier S, Grines CL, et al. Coronary perforation: An unreported complication after intracoronary stent implantation (abstract). *J Am Coll Cardiol* 1996; 27(suppl A):252A.
274. Waksman R, King SB III, Douglas JS Jr, et al. Predictors of groin complications after balloon and new-device coronary intervention. *Am J Cardiol* 1995; 75:886–889.
275. Moscucci M, Mansour KA, Kent C, et al. Peripheral vascular complications of directional coronary atherectomy and stenting: Predictors, management, and outcome. *Am J Cardiol* 1994; 74:448–453.
276. Popma JJ, Satler LF, Pichard AD, et al. Vascular complications after balloon and new device angioplasty. *Circulation* 1993; 88:1569–1578.
277. Rocha-Singh KJ, Schwend RB, Otis SM, et al. Frequency and nonsurgical therapy of femoral artery pseudoaneurysm complicating interventional cardiology procedures. *Am J Cardiol* 1994; 73:1012–1014.
278. Kang SS, Labropoulos N, Mansour MA, et al. Percutaneous ultrasound guided thrombin injection: A new method for treating postcatheterization femoral pseudoaneurysms. *J Vasc Surg* 1998; 27:1032–1038.
279. Liau C, Ho F, Chen M, et al. Treatment of iatrogenic femoral artery pseudoaneurysm with percutaneous thrombin injection. *J Vasc Surg* 1997; 26:18–23.
280. Saber RS, Edwards WD, Bailey KR, et al. Coronary embolization after balloon angioplasty or thrombolytic therapy: An autopsy study of 32 cases. *J Am Coll Cardiol* 1993; 22:1283–1288.
281. Waksman R, Scott NA, Douglas JS Jr, et al. Distal embolization is common after directional atherectomy in coronary arteries and vein grafts. *Circulation* 1993; 88(suppl I):I-299.
282. Harrington RA, Lincoff AM, Califf RM, et al. Characteristics and consequences of myocardial infarction after percutaneous coronary intervention: Insights from the Coronary Angioplasty versus Excisional Atherectomy Trial (CAVEAT). *J Am Coll Cardiol* 1995; 25:1693–1699.
283. Moses JW, Teirstein PS, Sketch MR Jr, et al. Angiographic determinants of risk and outcome of coronary embolus and myocardial infarction (MI) with the transluminal extraction catheter (TEC): A report from the New Approaches to Coronary Intervention (NACI) Registry (abstract). *J Am Coll Cardiol* 1994; 23:220A.
284. Safian RD, Grines CL, May MA, et al. Clinical and angiographic results of transluminal extraction coronary atherectomy in saphenous vein bypass grafts. *Circulation* 1994; 89:302–312.
285. Abdelmeguid AE, Topol EJ, Whitlow PL, et al. Significance of mild transient release of creatine kinase-MB fraction after percutaneous coronary interventions. *Circulation* 1996; 4:1528–1536.
286. Carlino M, De Gregoria J, Di Mario C, et al. Prevention of distal embolization during saphenous vein graft lesion angioplasty: Experience with a new temporary occlusion and aspiration system. *Circulation* 1999; 99:3221–3223.
287. Kong TQ, Davidson CJ, Meyers SN, et al. Prognostic implication of creatine kinase elevation following elective coronary artery interventions. *JAMA* 1997; 277:461–466.
288. Kini A, Marmur JD, Dangas G, et al. Creatine kinase-MB elevation after coronary intervention correlates with diffuse atherosclerosis, and low-to-medium level elevation has a benign clinical course: Implications for early discharge after coronary intervention. *J Am Coll Cardiol* 1999; 34:663–671.
289. Colombo A. Different benefits, different risks, equal cost. *Eur Heart J* 1999; 20:1531–1532.
290. McCullough PA, Wolyn R, Rocher LL, et al. Acute contrast nephropathy after coronary intervention: Incidence, risk factors and relationship to mortality. *J Am Coll Cardiol* 1996; 17(suppl A):304A.
291. Stevens MA, McCullough PA, Tobin KJ, et al. A prospective randomized trial of prevention measures in patients at high risk for contrast nephropathy. *J Am Coll Cardiol* 1999; 33:403–411.
292. Savage M, Fischman D, Teirstein P, et al. Utility of coronary

stents in the management of incessant restenosis. *Circulation* 1993; 88(suppl I):I-640.

293. Pratt RE, Dzau VJ. Pharmacological strategies to prevent restenosis. *Circulation* 1996; 93:848–852.

294. Waksman R, Robinson KA, Croker IR, et al. Intracoronary low-dose B-irradiation inhibits neointima formation after coronary artery balloon injury in the swine restenosis model. *Circulation* 1995; 92:3025–3031.

295. Waksman R, Robinson KA, Croker IR, et al. Intracoronary radiation before stent implantation inhibits neointima formation in stented porcine coronary arteries. *Circulation* 1995; 92:1383–1386.

296. Hehrlein C, Stintz M, Kinscherf R, et al. Pure B-particle-emitting stents inhibit neointima formation in rabbits. *Circulation* 1996; 93:641–645.

297. Waksman R. Late thrombosis after radiation: Sitting on a time bomb. *Circulation* 1999; 100:780–782.

298. Costa MA, Sabate M, van der Giessen WJ, et al. Late coronary occlusion after intracoronary brachytherapy. *Circulation* 1999; 100:789–792.

CHAPTER 46

MECHANICAL INTERVENTIONS IN ACUTE MYOCARDIAL INFARCTION

William O'Neill / Bruce R. Brodie

The history of mechanical reperfusion therapy is fascinating and has important lessons concerning the application of radical new treatments in modern medicine. Confluences of pathologic, clinical, and technical advances were required for this treatment to be initiated and validated. Lack of understanding of the pathophysiologic basis for acute myocardial infarction (AMI), lack of adequate understanding of clinical subsets, and lack of adequate medical devices led to multiple early pioneering attempts that were akin to the early rocket programs of the late 1950s. Ultimately, however, this treatment modality has been refined, tested, and validated and has the promise to dramatically decrease mortality for increasingly large segments of the population. This chapter will review the historical development of mechanical reperfusion, summarize the results of randomized clinical trials, define subsets most likely to be benefited or harmed by this approach, and offer a glimpse into future research directions.

HISTORICAL DEVELOPMENT

Mechanical reperfusion had its inception with the initial treatise of Fletcher et al.[1] that described the use of intravenous thrombolytic therapy in thromboembolic disorders, including myocardial infarction. The authors presented results on their experience with treatment of 22 patients with AMI. Unfortunately, no methodology for testing efficacy existed. A suggestion that the SGOT enzyme curves peaked earlier was entertained. Crude descriptors including chest pain relief, blood pressure response, and electrocardiographic changes were highly variable and did not provide consistent patterns to demonstrate harm or benefit. Importantly, autopsies were performed in three of the four patients who died. The autopsy results were confusing. One patient who died suddenly 3 weeks after treatment had evidence of a large healing infarction but no evidence of residual thrombus in the infarct artery. A fresh thrombus in a separate artery was perceived to be the cause of death. A second patient died shortly after cessation of streptokinase infusion, and at autopsy, a very fresh microscopic thrombus was found in an ulcerated plaque in the left main artery. A third patient with a history of atrial fibrillation was found to have a massive posterolateral infarction but only mild atherosclerotic plaque and no residual thrombus. These autopsy findings failed to demonstrate that failure of therapy to recanalize vessels lead to death or that thrombus was in fact related to any of these cases. The results of this initial study helped fuel a controversy that raged for 20 years in the scientific community on the role of thrombus formation in myocardial infarction.

Bouchek et al.[2] published the second pioneering observation concerning reperfusion therapy and the initial attempt at developing a platform for local treatment in 1960. This intrepid group performed emergency brachial cut-downs and used subselective catheters to apply fibrinolytic therapy to the aortic root of patients presenting with AMI. Unfortunately, they were unaware of Sones[3] work in selective coronary angiography. Bouchek et al. were astute enough to use the electrocardiogram (ECG) as a localizing tool so that right or left coronary subselective infusions could occur. Although this group presented similar enzymatic results, like Fletcher, they could not clearly establish that their treatment was beneficial. If only their catheters could have been advanced another 3 or 4 mm and angiographic documentation of clot lysis established, the history of reperfusion therapy would have been accelerated by 20 years!

Thus the lack of consensus concerning the inciting role of thrombotic occlusion in AMI, lack of equipment to visualize thrombus in vivo, and lack of clearly defined subgroups for treatment lead investigators to abandon invasive approaches in the 1960s. Later that decade, Favaloro[4] et al. made major contributions to the development of saphenous vein aortocoronary bypass and early on applied it to patients presenting with AMI.[4,5] This group quickly realized that due to enormous logistic and time constraints, this treatment was not practical in referral centers. Fortunately, two groups, one in Spokane[6] and one in Goettingen,[7] attempted to apply emergency surgical revascularization as management for myocardial infarction in a community setting. Preoperative emergency catheterization was required, and thus, for the first time, knowledge of the coronary anatomy during AMI became available. Both groups made seminal observations that served as cornerstones for reperfusion therapy. DeWood et al.[8] described the high prevalence of total coronary occlusion in the early hours after acute transmural myocardial infarction and the decreased incidence of total occlusion in the later hours of presentation. These authors concluded that total coronary occlusion occurred early and that spontaneous lysis explained the lower prevalence during later presentation. They concluded that total thrombotic occlusion was the cause and not the consequence of AMI. Perhaps equally important, this initial report and a subsequent report[9] clearly defined the role of electrocardiographic transmural injury current in identifying a population of patients most likely to have acute total occlusion and thus most likely to benefit from emergency revascularization.

At the same time that the Spokane group was testing surgical revascularization, Rentrop and associates were developing techniques to safely catheterize and study patients with AMI and cardiogenic shock. In June 1978, based on lessons learned from balloon angioplasty, they performed emergency guidewire recanalization of a catheter-related acute thrombotic coronary occlusion.[10] The instantaneous gratifying clinical and electrocardiographic results led this group to initiate mechanical reperfusion in AMI. They reported on the first 13 patients treated with mechanical reperfusion in 1979.[11] In June 1979, this group initiated a second phase of their investigation, selective catheter infusion of intracoronary streptokinase. They presented their work at the American Heart Association Meetings in November of 1979, and the modern era of reperfusion therapy was born. American investigators were largely uninterested in thrombolytic therapy of AMI in the 1960s and 1970s. The pathologic findings of Roberts and Buja[12] and the National Heart Lung and Blood Institute (NHLBI) consensus conference[13] swayed scientific conventional wisdom. The importance of thrombotic occlusion was unclear, and attention was focused on methods to limit infarct size by decreasing oxygen demand.[14] Once the works of DeWood et al. and Rentrop et al. were disseminated, enormous research interest was generated in both Europe and the United States. Randomized trials were quickly organized. Khaja et al.[15] first demonstrated the efficacy of intracoronary streptokinase administration. The western Washington group demonstrated the mortality advantage of intracoronary streptokinase therapy.[16] Because of the necessity of selective coronary angiography for this treatment, it became apparent that a severe residual stenosis persisted in most patients after successful recanalization. The Ann Arbor group first demonstrated that balloon angioplasty could more effectively relieve the residual stenosis than could thrombolytic therapy alone.[17] This resulted in less recurrent ischemia, less exercise-induced ischemia,[18] and more effective preservation of ventricular function.[19] Lack of trained operators, lack of catheterization facilities, and logistic constraints, however, led most investigators to abandon primary angioplasty in the mid-1980s.

Both intracoronary streptokinase and primary percutaneous transluminal coronary angioplasty (PTCA) lost momentum once intravenous thrombolytic therapy was validated in the mid-1980s.[20] Research interest focused on new thrombolytic drugs that could be administered intravenously. Many investigators were still concerned about the severe underlying residual stenosis remaining after thrombolytic therapy. Therefore, three major randomized trials the TAMI, TIMI-2a, and European Cooperative trials were performed.[21–23] Each trial attempted to determine the value of routine PTCA after thrombolytic therapy. In aggregate,[24,25] these studies gave surprising and disappointing results. Routine PTCA not only failed to improve results but actually appeared to be harmful. Angioplasty thus was abandoned as an adjunct to thrombolytic therapy in 1990.

Although routine, postthrombolytic PTCA was proven to be detrimental, interest still persisted in the use of PTCA without antecedent thrombolytic therapy and in cases of persistent chest pain after thrombolytic therapy. A great deal of the credit must be given to the pioneering work of Hartzler et al.[26] This group demonstrated that angioplasty alone may have outcomes superior to thrombolytic therapy.[27] At the same time, Brodie et al.[28] and O'Neill et al.[29] concluded that lone angioplasty had been inadequately tested as a reperfusion modality. These three groups joined forces and organized the original Primary Angioplasty in Myocardial Infarction (PAMI) study group. This group first formally compared intravenous thrombolytic therapy with primary PTCA. The results of this trial and the Zwolle and Mayo Clinic studies have largely defined the value of mechanical reperfusion in the 1990s.

RESCUE ANGIOPLASTY

In the early 1990s, intravenous thrombolytic therapy became the overwhelmingly preferred reperfusion strategy.[30–32] Unfortunately, with current fibrinolytic regimens, successful reperfusion after thrombolytic therapy is achieved in only 54 to 81 percent of patients, and TIMI 3 flow is achieved in only 29 to 54 percent of patients.[33] The achievement of successful reperfusion (especially TIMI 3 flow) in the infarct artery after thrombolytic therapy is the most important determinant of 30-day mortality and recovery of left ventricular function.[33] Rescue angioplasty, the mechanical reopening of an occluded infarct artery after failed thrombolysis, has been used as adjunctive therapy in an attempt to improve outcomes in patients with failed thrombolysis. Despite the intuitive benefit of this approach, the value of rescue angioplasty remains controversial, especially given the disappointing results of the TAMI, TIMI-2a, and European Cooperative studies.

Numerous observational studies have documented that rescue angioplasty can achieve successful reperfusion in 82 to 92 percent of patients with occluded infarct arteries after failed thrombolysis,[34–38] but reocclusion of the infarct artery has been common (18 percent in Ellis's meta-analysis),[39] and recovery of left ventricular function has been variable.[34,36,37] Mortality associated with unsuccessful rescue angioplasty has been very high, and mortality associated with all rescue angioplasties (successful and unsuccessful) has been no better than in patients with failed thrombolysis who do not undergo rescue angioplasty and has been higher than in patients with successful thrombolysis[34–37] (Table 46-1). The lack of benefit in these observational studies with rescue angioplasty may be related to selection bias, since rescue angioplasty often is selected for higher-risk patients.[39] The relatively high mortality after rescue angioplasty compared with successful thrombolysis is not surprising because patients with failed thrombolysis are a high-risk subgroup who have demonstrated resistance to pharmacologic reperfusion, possibly due to hypotension, large thrombus burden, or extensive intimal disruption, all of which are unfavorable to the success of coronary angioplasty. Also, reperfusion after rescue

TABLE 46-1 Observational Data Comparing Mortality* in Patients Undergoing Rescue Angioplasty (PTCA) for Failed Thrombolysis versus No Rescue Angioplasty versus Successful Thrombolysis

Trial	Successful Rescue PTCA	Failed Rescue PTCA	All Rescue PTCA	No Rescue PTCA	Successful Thrombolysis
TAMI 1–5 Trials (n = 192)[35]	10/169 (5.9%)	9/23 (39%)	19/192 (9.9%)	3/43 (7.0%)	28/607 (4.6%)
TIMI I and II Trials (n = 33)[36]	2/27 (7.4%)	2/6 (33%)	4/33 (12%)	7/100 (7%)	
TIMI IV Trial (n = 58)[37]	5/52 (9.6%)	2/6 (33%)	7/58 (12%)	4/37 (11%)	9/307 (2.9%)
GUSTO-I Trial (n = 198)[34]	15/175 (8.6%)	7/23 (30%)	22/198 (11.1%)	21/266 (7.9%)	55/1058 (5.2%)
TOTAL	32/423 (7.6%)	20/58 (34%)	52/481 (10.8%)	35/446 (7.8%)	92/1972 (4.7%)

* Mortality is in-hospital mortality for TIMI-IV and TAMI 1–5, 21 days for TIMI-I and II, and 30 days for GUSTO-I.

angioplasty, by definition, occurs later than reperfusion by successful thrombolysis, and this inherent delay decreases the extent of myocardial salvage. It is not clear if the particularly high mortality in patients with failed rescue angioplasty is due to additional associated high-risk features or if there may be harmful effects from the rescue angioplasty procedure itself.

Two moderately sized randomized trials have evaluated the efficacy of rescue angioplasty. The TAMI-5 trial[40] randomized 575 patients with AMI treated with tissue-type plasminogen activator (tPA) or urokinase or both to emergency angiography with rescue angioplasty for failed thrombolysis versus conservative care. Rescue angioplasty was performed in 18 percent of the emergency catheterization group with a success rate of 83 percent. At hospital discharge, the emergency catheterization group had a slightly higher infarct artery patency rate (94 versus 90 percent; p = 0.07), better regional wall motion, and less recurrent ischemia, but there were no differences in mortality, reinfarction, or global left ventricular ejection fraction.

The Randomized Evaluation of Salvage Angioplasty with Combined Utilization of Endpoints (RESCUE) trial[41] randomized 151 patients who had their first anterior wall myocardial infarction treated with thrombolytic therapy and had an occluded infarct artery demonstrated within 8 h of the onset of chest pain to rescue angioplasty versus conservative care. There was no difference in left ventricular ejection fraction at 30 days (40 versus 39 percent; p = NS), but the rescue angioplasty group tended toward a lower mortality (5.1 versus 9.6 percent; p = 0.18), less congestive heart failure (1.3 versus 7.0 percent; p = 0.11), had a lower composite of death and congestive heart failure (6.4 versus 16.6 percent; p = 0.05), and better exercise left ventricular ejection fraction (43 versus 38 percent; p = 0.04). These benefits occurred despite what the authors felt was a strong investigator bias not to randomize patients presenting very early in the course of their infarction.

Rescue angioplasty, especially after tPA, is associated with lower angiographic success rates and higher reocclusion rates than primary angioplasty and this limits its effectiveness. This may occur because infarct artery occlusion refractory to thrombolysis may have more extensive intimal disruption. In addition, platelet and thrombin activation that occurs with thrombolytic therapy may adversely affect the efficacy of PTCA.[42–44] Recent studies using coronary stenting with rescue angioplasty have reported high procedural success rates and low reocclusion rates.[45–47] The largest of these studies reported a success rate of 98 percent in 167 patients, a reocclusion rate of only 1.2 percent, and a combined end point of death or reinfarction of 1.4 percent at 30 days in nonshock patients.[47] Glycoprotein IIb/IIIa platelet inhibitors also may enhance outcomes with rescue angioplasty, but this has not been well studied, and the risk of bleeding when aspirin, heparin, ticlopidine, or clopidogrel and glycoprotein IIb/IIIa platelet inhibitors are used in conjunction with thrombolytic therapy is not established.[46]

A major limitation of the rescue angioplasty approach is the lack of a reliable noninvasive method to detect reperfusion after thrombolytic therapy. The ECG is very specific in predicting patency of the infarct artery when there is complete (>70 percent) resolution of ST-segment elevation at 90 min after thrombolytic therapy.[48] This occurs in only a minority of patients, however; in most patients there is only partial or no resolution of ST-segment elevation, and the patency status of the infarct artery is uncertain.[49] Similarly, enzyme rise or enzyme curves lack sufficient, rapid diagnostic accuracy.[50] Consequently, acute angiography is usually required to determine infarct artery patency.

Based on the available data, acute angiography with rescue angioplasty should be considered in patients with anterior or large myocardial infarction who are thought to have failed thrombolysis, as evidenced by persistent chest pain, lack of resolution of ST-segment elevation, or hemodynamic compromise 90 min or more after treatment.

The recently reported PACT trial[50a] of bolus tPA and transfer to the catheterization laboratory for rescue angioplasty for those without TIMI 3 flow showed that angioplasty could be performed safely following administration of a short-acting thrombolytic agent. Since transfer to the catheterization laboratory was very fast in this trial, no improvement in left ventricular function could be shown in the thrombolyzed cohort. An important question is whether in real-life situations, where transfer to the catheterization laboratory takes longer, will upstream thrombolysis be helpful.

PRIMARY ANGIOPLASTY

In the early 1990s, great controversy still existed about the routine use of angioplasty for treatment of AMI. Angioplasty after thrombolytic therapy was abandoned except for its use as a rescue after failed thrombolytic therapy. In centers where interventional programs existed, controversy existed about the use of immediate PTCA without antecedent thrombolytic therapy as an alternative to routine thrombolytic therapy. This controversy has now been largely settled based on a number of randomized trials of these reperfusion modalities.

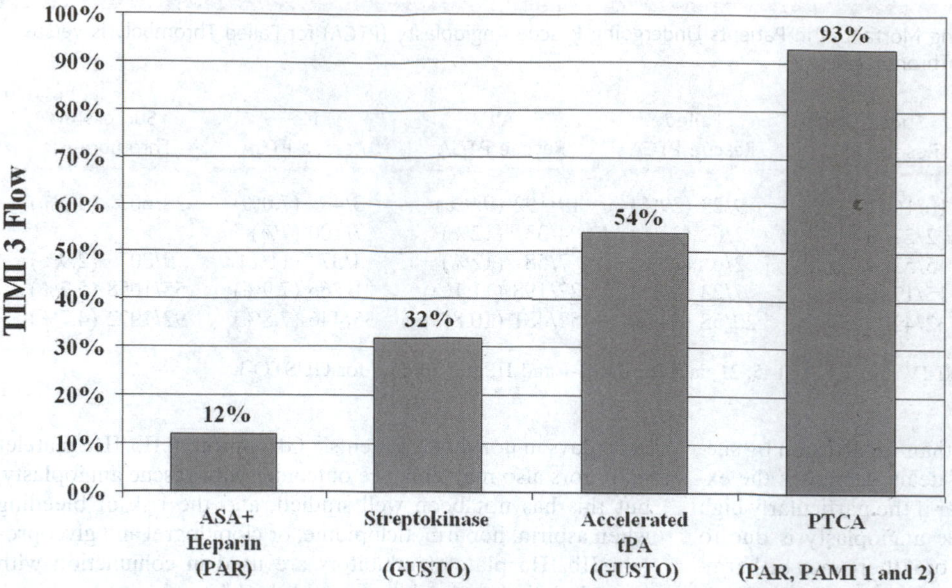

FIGURE 46-1 Frequency of achieving TIMI 3 flow in the infarct artery with aspirin and heparin,[84] thrombolytic therapy (measured 90 min after treatment),[72] and primary angioplasty (PTCA, measured immediately after intervention).[73]

Comparison of Outcomes with Thrombolytic Therapy

RANDOMIZED TRIALS

In 1997, Weaver et al. published a meta-analysis of 10 randomized trials[51–60] in a total of 2606 patients comparing thrombolytic therapy with primary angioplasty[61] (Fig. 46-1). The largest of these trials were the PAMI-1 trial,[52] the Zwolle trial,[53] and the GUSTO-IIb trial.[58] In this meta-analysis, primary angioplasty was associated with a lower in-hospital mortality (4.4 versus 6.5 percent; $p = 0.02$), a lower incidence of nonfatal reinfarction (2.9 versus 5.3 percent; $p = 0.002$), and a lower incidence of death or nonfatal reinfarction (7.2 versus 11.9 percent; $p = 0.001$). Primary angioplasty also was associated with a significantly lower incidence of stroke (0.7 versus 2.0 percent; $p = 0.007$) and hemorrhagic stroke (0.01 versus 1.1 percent; $p = 0.0005$). The survival benefit of primary angioplasty compared with thrombolytic therapy reported in this meta-analysis was substantial (21 lives saved per 1000 patients treated) and compared favorably with the survival benefit of thrombolytic therapy compared with placebo reported by the Fibrinolytic Therapy Trialists' (FTT) Collaborative Group (19 lives saved per 1000 patients treated).[62]

OUTCOMES IN HIGH-RISK PATIENTS

Patients with AMI at highest risk for mortality include patients with cardiogenic shock, elderly patients, patients with anterior wall myocardial infarction, and women. Data from randomized trials indicate that the greatest mortality benefit with primary angioplasty is seen in these high-risk patients (Table 46-2). The PAMI-1 investigators found a significant mortality benefit with primary angioplasty compared with tPA in non-low-risk patients (patients older than 70 years, anterior infarction, or heart rate >100 beats per minute) but no difference in mortality in low-risk patients.[52] Likewise, elderly patients showed a substantial mortality benefit with primary angioplasty compared with tPA in both the PAMI-1 trial[63] and the GUSTO-IIb trial,[64] whereas younger patients showed no mortality difference. The PAMI-1 investigators also found a substantial mortality benefit with primary angioplasty versus thrombolytic therapy in patients with anterior wall myocardial infarction but no mortality benefit in nonanterior wall myocardial infarction.[65] Garcia et al.[60] also found mortality benefit with primary angioplasty in patients with anterior wall myocardial infarction, but the GUSTO-IIb trial did not.[66] The lack of benefit in the GUSTO-IIb trial may be related to the lower rates of achieving TIMI 3 flow in the GUSTO-IIb trial.[67] Women are also at high risk for mortality with AMI partly related to more baseline risk factors. In the PAMI-1 trial, mortality in women was lower with primary angioplasty compared with tPA[68] (see Table 46-2). Patients with cardiogenic shock are the highest-risk subgroup of patients with AMI

TABLE 46-2 Mortality in High- and Low-Risk Patients with AMI Treated with Primary PTCA versus Lytic Therapy in Randomized Trials

Study	PTCA (%)	Lytic (%)	*p* Value
PAMI-1			
Not low risk (n = 206)[52]	2.0	10.4	0.01
Low risk (n = 189)	3.1	2.2	NS
Age >65 yrs (n = 150)[63]	5.7	15.0	0.07
Age <65 yrs (n = 245)	0.8	0.8	NS
Anterior MI (n = 138)[65]	1.4	11.9	0.01
Nonanterior MI (n = 257)	3.2	3.8	NS
Women (n = 107)[68]	4.0	14.0	0.07
Men (n = 288)	2.1	3.5	NS
GUSTO-IIb			
Age >70 yrs (n = 314)[64]	11.0	20.7	0.02
Age <70 yrs (n = 824)	3.6	3.5	NS
Anterior MI (n = 473)[66]	6.8	6.8	NS
Garcia et al.			
Anterior MI (n = 220)[60]	2.8	10.8	0.02

ABBREVATIONS: PAMI = Primary Angioplasty in Myocardial Infarction; GUSTO = Global Use of Strategies to Open Occluded Arteries; MI = myocardial infarction.

and appear to benefit most from primary angioplasty. Unfortunately, thrombolytic therapy is not very effective in patients with cardiogenic shock. In the GISSI-1 trial,[20] there was no difference in mortality in patients with cardiogenic shock treated with intravenous streptokinase versus placebo (70 percent in each), and the International Study Group found that mortality was high with both streptokinase and tPA (65 and 78 percent, respectively).[69] In contrast, pooled data from 19 observational studies with primary angioplasty for cardiogenic shock showed an overall mortality of 44 percent.[70] Recently, the SHOCK trial,[71] which randomized patients with cardiogenic shock to emergency revascularization versus medical stabilization, found a decreased mortality rate in favor of emergency revascularization at 6 months (50 versus 63 percent; $p = 0.03$). Survival benefit was especially pronounced in patients treated within 6 h of symptom onset and in patients under age 75 years. These data and previous observational data strongly support the use of primary angioplasty to provide survival benefit in patients with AMI complicated by cardiogenic shock, especially in young patients who present early after symptom onset.

OUTCOMES IN LOW-RISK PATIENTS

While the survival benefit with primary angioplasty versus thrombolytic therapy is limited to high-risk patients, low-risk patients benefit from a reduction in the incidence of reinfarction and recurrent ischemia. In a randomized comparison, the PAMI-1 trial[65] found a lower incidence of recurrent ischemia (9.7 versus 27.8 percent; $p = 0.0002$) and the Zwolle group[57] found a lower incidence of reinfarction (0 versus 16 percent; $p < 0.01$) in patients with non-anterior wall myocardial infarction treated with primary angioplasty. Similarly, Ribichini et al.,[59] in a randomized comparison of primary angioplasty versus thrombolytic therapy in patients with inferior infarction, found a lower incidence of reinfarction (1.8 versus 9.1 percent; $p = 0.10$) and recurrent ischemia (1.8 versus 20.0 percent; $p = 0.002$), higher infarct artery patency (100 versus 71 percent; $p = 0.0001$), and better left ventricular ejection fraction (55.2 versus 48.2 percent; $p = 0.001$) at hospital discharge in patients treated with primary angioplasty.

Thus, while low-risk patients have no survival benefit with primary angioplasty, they do benefit from less reinfarction, less recurrent ischemia, higher infarct artery patency rates, and better left ventricular function without the risk of intracranial hemorrhage.

IMPORTANCE OF TIMI FLOW

The importance of achieving timely restoration of normal blood flow in the infarct artery in patients with AMI was convincingly demonstrated in the GUSTO trial.[72] Patients with normal (TIMI 3) antegrade flow in the infarct artery at 90 min after treatment had the highest left ventricular ejection fraction at follow-up catheterization and the lowest 30-day mortality (Table 46-3). Patients with slow (TIMI 2) flow had a left ventricular ejection fraction and 30-day mortality that was significantly worse than patients with TIMI 3 flow and similar to patients with no flow (TIMI 0–1). A similar relationship between TIMI flow and mortality has been found with primary angioplasty[73] (see Table 46-3). These data indicate that only restoration of TIMI 3 flow is associated with optimal outcomes and that only TIMI 3 flow should be regarded as "true patency." A comparison of the rates of TIMI 3 flow with various reperfusion strategies in the GUSTO trial and with primary angioplasty from the PAMI-1 and PAMI-2 trials are shown in Fig. 46-1.[72,73] The ability of primary angioplasty to achieve significantly higher TIMI 3 flow rates than thrombolytic therapy probably explains most of the mortality advantage seen with primary angioplasty. Indeed, there appears to be a tight inverse relationship between short-term mortality and the ability to achieve TIMI 3 flow with various thrombolytic regimens and with primary angioplasty (Fig. 46-2). Newer thrombolytic strategies combining low-dose thrombolytics with platelet glycoprotein IIb/IIIa receptor inhib-

TABLE 46-3 Relationship Between TIMI Flow and 30-Day Mortality after Reperfusion Therapy for AMI

	30-Day Mortality	
TIMI Flow	GUSTO-I[72] (Lytic Therapy)	PAMI-1 and PAMI-2[73] (Primary PTCA)
TIMI 0–1	8.9%	17.2%
TIMI 2	7.4%	7.6%
TIMI 3	4.4%	2.1%

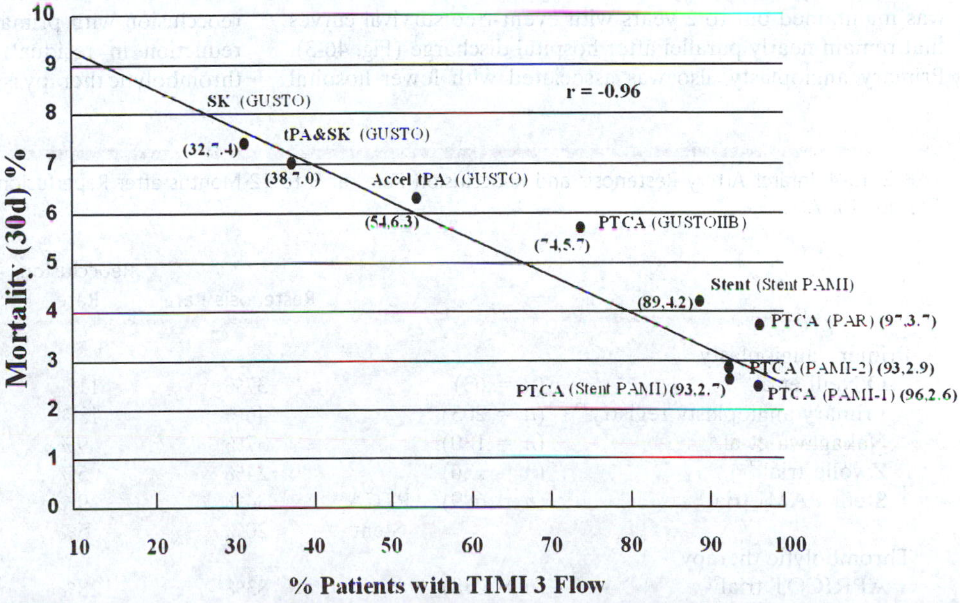

FIGURE 46-2 Relationship between in-hospital or 30-day mortality and the frequency of achieving TIMI 3 flow measured acutely in the infarct artery with several thrombolytic strategies from the GUSTO trial[72] and several primary angioplasty (PTCA) trials.[73,84,87]

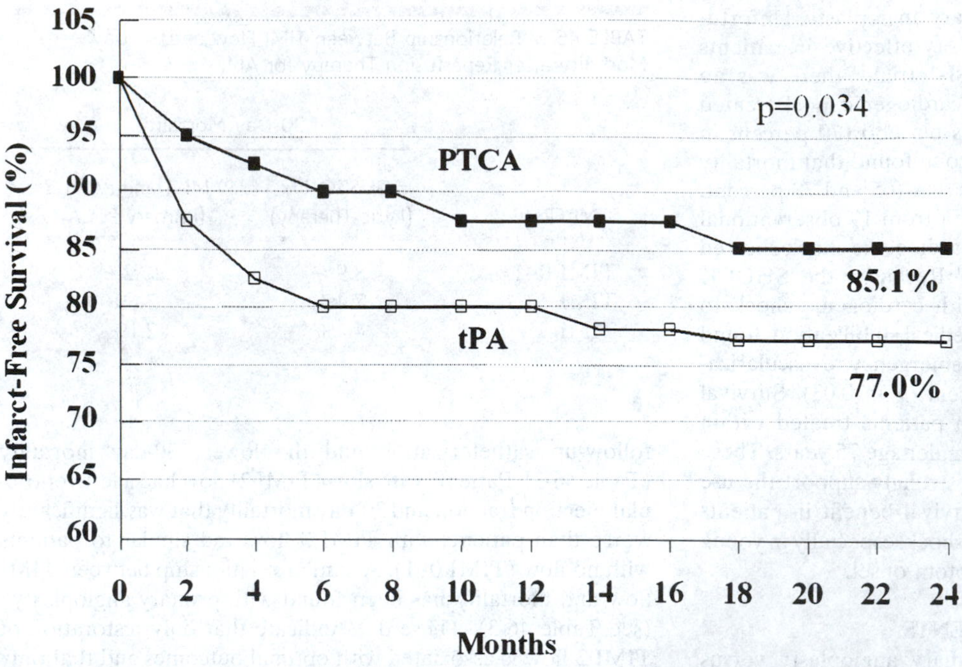

FIGURE 46-3 Actuarial infarction-free survival curves for patients with AMI treated with primary angioplasty [PTCA (*solid boxes*) versus tPA (*open boxes*)]. (Reproduced with permission from Nunn et al.[75])

itors have shown improved TIMI 3 flow rates[74] (see Chap. 42), but these rates are still well below the TIMI 3 flow rates achieved with primary angioplasty, and these strategies remain to be tested in large clinical trials.

LATE CLINICAL AND ANGIOGRAPHIC OUTCOMES

A comparison of late clinical outcomes of patients with AMI treated with primary angioplasty versus thrombolytic therapy has been provided by the PAMI investigators.[75] The initial benefit of primary angioplasty in reducing death and reinfarction was maintained out to 2 years with event-free survival curves that remain nearly parallel after hospital discharge (Fig. 46-3). Primary angioplasty also was associated with lower hospital readmission rates (59 versus 69 percent; $p = 0.035$) and lower rates of target-vessel revascularization with either angioplasty or bypass surgery (33 versus 54 percent; $p = 0.001$) compared with tPA. More recently, the Zwolle group has demonstrated that the early mortality and reinfarction benefit is maintained over 5-year follow-up.[76]

Reocclusion of the infarct artery at follow-up angiography occurs frequently after thrombolytic therapy when adjunctive percutaneous coronary intervention is not employed. The Antithrombotics in the Prevention of Reocclusion in Coronary Thrombolysis (APRICOT) study performed follow-up angiography at 3 months in patients with AMI treated with intravenous streptokinase who had a patent infarct artery at catheterization at 24 to 48 h and found a late reocclusion rate of 28 percent.[77] Similarly, White et al. found that 25 percent of patients with an initially patent infarct artery after thrombolytic therapy at 4 weeks had an occluded artery at 1 year.[78] In contrast, reocclusion rates at 6-month follow-up angiography after primary angioplasty have ranged from 5 to 13 percent[29,77,79–81] (Table 46-4). In a randomized comparison of primary angioplasty with streptokinase from the Zwolle group, reocclusion rates were significantly lower with primary angioplasty (9 versus 32 percent; $p = 0.001$).[53] With the use of coronary stenting, reocclusion rates at 6-month angiography have been reduced to about 5 percent.[81] The lower rates of reocclusion with primary angioplasty are likely related to the reduction in residual stenosis, since residual stenosis after thrombolytic therapy is highly correlated with late reocclusion.[77]

TABLE 46-4 Infarct Artery Restenosis and Reocclusion Rates at 3 to 12 Months after Reperfusion Therapy for AMI

			Restenosis Rate	Reocclusion Rate
Primary angioplasty				
O'Neill et al.[29]	(n = 63)		37%	11%
Primary angioplasty registry[79]	(n = 203)		46%	13%
Nakagawa et al.[80]	(n = 130)		37%	9%
Zwolle trial[77]	(n = 136)		24%	5%
Stent PAMI trial[81]	(n = 689)	PTCA	34%	9%
		Stent	20%	5%
Thrombolytic therapy				
APRICOT trial[77]	(n = 248)		83%*	28%
White et al.[78]	(n = 215)		—	25%

*Residual stenosis at 3-month angiography after thrombolytic therapy, like primary angioplasty, was defined as >50 percent luminal diameter narrowing.

Infarct artery patency is important for recovery of left ventricular function[79] and may be important for late survival. Several observational studies with thrombolytic therapy and primary angioplasty have found that both left ventricular function and infarct artery patency are strong independent predictors of late cardiac survival.[82,83] This suggests that the late angiographic outcomes after primary angioplasty may translate into better long-term clinical outcomes.

The restenosis rate at 6-month follow-up angiography after primary angioplasty is similar to that after elective angioplasty and occurs in 24 to 46 percent of patients.[29,77,79–81] While this remains a significant clinical and economic problem with primary angioplasty, only about one-half of patients with restenosis require repeat target-vessel revascularization, and restenosis does not interfere with recovery of left ventricular function as long as the infarct artery remains patent.[79] The use of stents with primary angioplasty, like elective angioplasty, has significantly reduced restenosis rates. The Stent PAMI trial showed a reduction in restenosis rates from 34 percent with angioplasty to 20 percent with stenting.[81] In comparison with primary angioplasty, the frequency of significant residual stenosis (>50 percent diameter narrowing) at 3-month follow-up angiography after thrombolytic therapy remains quite high[77] (Table 46-4).

Role of Cardiac Surgery in the Primary Angioplasty Approach

Not all patients with AMI brought to the cardiac catheterization laboratory undergo percutaneous coronary intervention.[52,84] Approximately 10 percent of patients are triaged to either medical treatment or are treated with coronary bypass surgery as the primary reperfusion strategy, i.e., primary coronary artery bypass grafting (CABG). Patients may be selected for primary CABG when there is severe left main coronary artery disease or severe three-vessel coronary artery disease with preserved (TIMI 3) flow in the infarct artery that allows time for transfer to the operating room. These patients frequently undergo operation emergently and comprise a little less than half the patients not undergoing percutaneous coronary intervention. The remaining patients not treated with percutaneous coronary intervention are treated medically. These include patients with no myocardial infarction (mistaken diagnosis), patients with no significant stenosis in the infarct artery (resolution of spasm or thrombus), patients in whom the infarct artery cannot be identified, and occasionally patients with unsuitable anatomy or a very small infarct-related artery.

Bypass surgery is also performed emergently after failed angioplasty, urgently for reinfarction or recurrent ischemia, and electively for definitive treatment of left main or severe multivessel disease. With recent experience and with the availability of stents, emergency bypass surgery is rare (~0.4 percent), and the need for urgent bypass surgery for reinfarction or recurrent ischemia that cannot be managed with repeat percutaneous coronary intervention is very infrequent (<1 percent).[81] Elective bypass surgery for treatment of residual coronary artery disease after initial successful primary angioplasty has been used in about 4 to 5 percent of patients. Altogether, bypass surgery is performed in about 7 to 10 percent of patients with the primary angioplasty approach.[84,85] Considering the severity of illness of these patients, surgical mortality has been relatively low (6.4 percent with emergency or urgent bypass surgery and 2.0 percent with elective bypass surgery in the PAMI-2 trial).[85]

Cardiac surgery is also used in patients with mechanical complications of AMI. Patients with ventricular septal rupture and acute mitral regurgitation from papillary muscle rupture usually develop cardiogenic shock and have a very poor outcome without surgical intervention and are candidates for emergency surgery. Patients with cardiogenic shock with severe left main disease (without mechanical complications) also may be candidates for emergency bypass surgery.[71]

Although cardiac surgery is an integral part of the primary angioplasty approach, it has been demonstrated that primary angioplasty can be performed safely and effectively at some community hospitals without on-site cardiac surgery when rigorous program criteria are established.[86,87] These criteria include the availability of experienced interventionists, a well-stocked and well-equipped catheterization laboratory, an experienced catheterization laboratory team, rigorous case-selection criteria, the establishment of good lines of communication between the interventional cardiologist and the cardiovascular surgeon at the referring institute, and an efficient emergency transport system. In many hospitals, transfer to an angioplasty/surgical center for those requiring an intervention may be a preferable approach.

Primary Angioplasty in Thrombolytic-Ineligible Patients

In most U.S. thrombolytic trials, 70 to 85 percent of patients with AMI screened have been considered ineligible for thrombolytic therapy because of advanced age, late presentation, prior bypass surgery, cardiogenic shock, or bleeding predisposition.[88] These patients constitute a high-risk subset with a significantly increased in-hospital mortality. Despite recommendations to broaden thrombolytic therapy to patients of any age and to patients presenting up to 12 h after the onset of symptoms, data from the National Registry of Myocardial Infarction (NRMI-2) have found that only 31 percent of patients with AMI are considered eligible for thrombolytic therapy, and only 75 percent of these patients are currently receiving thrombolytic therapy[89] (Fig. 46-4).

One of the major advantages of primary angioplasty compared with thrombolytic therapy is that primary angioplasty can be applied to a majority of patients with AMI.[90] The only contraindications to primary angioplasty are lack of vascular access, renal insufficiency, and active hemorrhage. Among patients who are usually not considered candidates for thrombolytic therapy but who may benefit greatly from reperfusion therapy with primary angioplasty are patients with cardiogenic shock, elderly patients, and patients with a predisposition to bleeding. Elderly patients are frequently excluded from thrombolytic trials, but those who have been enrolled in trials comparing thrombolytic therapy with primary angioplasty have had a substantial mortality benefit with primary angioplasty.[63,64] Patients with AMI and contraindications to thrombolytic therapy due to bleeding risk have a high mortality, and observational data suggest that mortality may be reduced by reperfusion with primary angioplasty.[91]

There are very little data supporting benefit of reperfusion therapy in patients who present more than 12 h after the onset of symptoms. One exception to this is patients who present late but have persistent ischemic chest pain. These patients frequently have collateral flow to the infarct zone and show substantial recovery of left ventricular function following reperfusion with primary angioplasty.[92] It is also possible that late restoration of patency of the infarct artery could enhance late survival independent of myocardial salvage by preventing left ventricular dilatation, promoting electrical stability, and serving as a source for collateral flow,[93,94] but this remains to be tested in prospective studies. Patients with AMI who do not have electrocardiographic ST-segment elevation or left bundle-

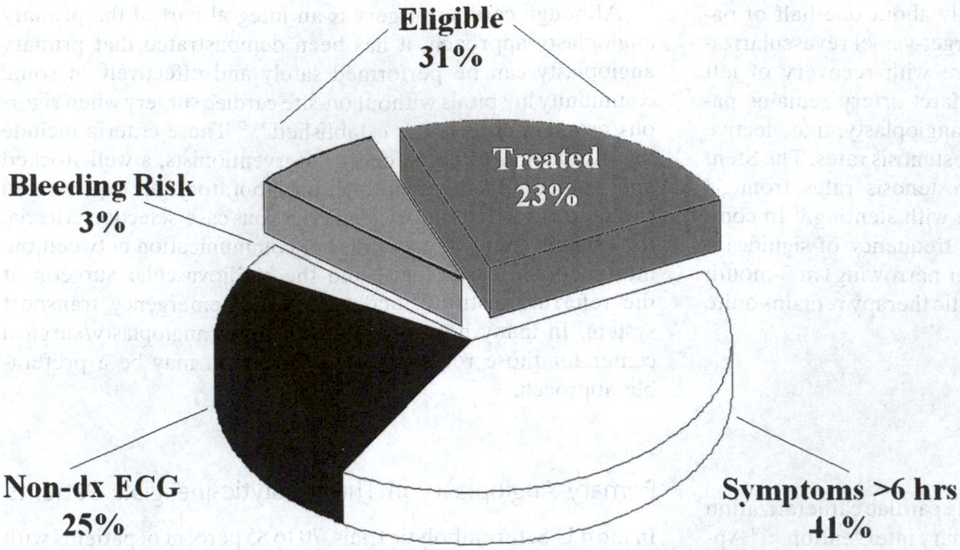

FIGURE 46-4 Distribution of patients with AMI (n = 272,651) who are considered eligible for thrombolytic therapy and those who are excluded. Patients were excluded in a sequential manner, with patients presenting more than 6 h from symptom onset excluded first, then patients with nondiagnostic ECGs, and then patients with bleeding risks. (Adapted from Barron et al.,[89] with permission.)

branch block have shown no benefit with thrombolytic therapy in randomized trials[62] and appropriately are not considered candidates for thrombolytic therapy. There are little data regarding benefit from primary angioplasty in this group of patients. McCullough et al.[95] demonstrated that patients with acute ischemic syndromes, including non-ST-segment elevation infarction, randomized to triage angiography with angioplasty when appropriate versus conservative care have less recurrent ischemia but have no mortality or reinfarction benefit.

Although prior bypass surgery is not a contraindication to thrombolytic therapy, these patients frequently have been excluded from thrombolytic trials. Reperfusion rates with thrombolytic therapy in patients with AMI due to saphenous vein graft occlusion are significantly less than with native vessel occlusion (TIMI 2–3 flow in the GUSTO trial: 48 versus 69 percent, respectively; $p < 0.01$).[96] Reperfusion rates with primary angioplasty in patients with saphenous vein graft occlusion are better than with thrombolytic therapy but are not as good as with primary angioplasty in native vessel occlusion. The PAMI-2 trial achieved TIMI 3 flow in 70 percent of patients with saphenous vein graft occlusion compared with 94 percent of patients with native coronary artery occlusion.[97] Patients with prior bypass surgery also had higher in-hospital mortality compared with patients without prior bypass surgery (6.9 versus 2.6 percent; $p = 0.05$).[97] While primary angioplasty appears to have an advantage over thrombolytic therapy in treating patients with AMI due to saphenous vein graft occlusion, new approaches are still needed to improve outcomes.

Cost Issues

RANDOMIZED COMPARISONS WITH THROMBOLYTIC THERAPY

There has been the perception that a strategy of primary angioplasty is more expensive than thrombolytic therapy in the treatment of AMI because of the initial cost of cardiac catheterization and coronary intervention. There are now data from several randomized trials that provide direct cost and length-of-stay comparisons between primary angioplasty and thrombolytic therapy.[98–100] The Mayo Clinic trial,[98] the PAMI-1 trial,[99] and the GUSTO-IIb trial[100] all showed a shorter length of hospital stay with primary angioplasty, which is likely due to a less complicated hospital course with less reinfarction and less recurrent ischemia (Table 46-5). The same randomized trials have shown comparable or lower hospital costs (charges) with primary angioplasty compared with thrombolytic therapy (see Table 46-5). A breakdown of the hospital charges from the PAMI-1 trial comparing primary angioplasty with tPA is shown in Fig. 46-5).[99] As expected, catheterization laboratory charges are higher with primary angioplasty, but the differences are not as great as expected because of the high use of catheterization and angioplasty in tPA-treated patients (63 and 36 percent, respectively). Initial catheterization laboratory charges with primary angioplasty are offset by higher drug charges in tPA patients due primarily to the charge for tPA. Other charges are slightly less with primary angioplasty, reflecting a shorter, less complicated hospital course. The cost advantages are not confined to hospital stay or American centers. The Zwolle group has shown similar decreases in cost during a 5-year follow-up.[76]

EARLY-DISCHARGE STRATEGIES

A strategy of early discharge with primary angioplasty may reduce costs further. Primary angioplasty appears to have two advantages over thrombolytic therapy in allowing a strategy for early discharge. First, the incidence of recurrent ischemic events and reinfarction is substantially less with primary angioplasty,

TABLE 46-5 Hospital Length of Stay and Hospital Charges/Costs Comparing Primary Angioplasty versus Lytic Therapy with tPA

	PTCA	tPA	*p* Value
Mayo Clinic trial[98]			
Length of stay (days)	8.1	10.5	0.08
Hospital charges ($)	21,000	26,700	0.09
PAMI-1 trial[99]			
Length of stay (days)	7.6	8.4	0.04
Hospital charges* ($)	23,468	26,904	0.04
GUSTO-IIb trial[100]			
Length of stay (days)	7.0	7.7	0.0009
Hospital costs* ($)	13,337	14,236	0.004

*PAMI-1 and GUSTO-IIb do not include professional charges.

and unlike thrombolytic therapy, ischemic events are usually confined to the first 2 days.[101] Second, angiographic data obtained at cardiac catheterization with primary angioplasty provide powerful information for risk stratification. These data include left ventricular ejection fraction, number of diseased vessels, and the reperfusion status or TIMI flow in the infarct artery after intervention. The PAMI-2 trial has documented the safety and cost savings of early discharge in low-risk patients treated with primary angioplasty.[102] Patients were classified as low risk if they met all the following clinical and angiographic criteria: age less than 70 years, ejection fraction greater than 45 percent, one- or two-vessel coronary artery disease, successful angioplasty, no saphenous vein graft occlusion, no persistent arrhythmias, and no congestive heart failure. Using these criteria, an extremely low risk group of patients was identified comprising about one-half the study population with an in-hospital mortality of 0.4 percent. The study documented that a strategy of targeting early discharge on day 3 in these low-risk patients was safe and reduced length of stay from 7.0 to 4.2 days and hospital costs from $11,604 to $9658.

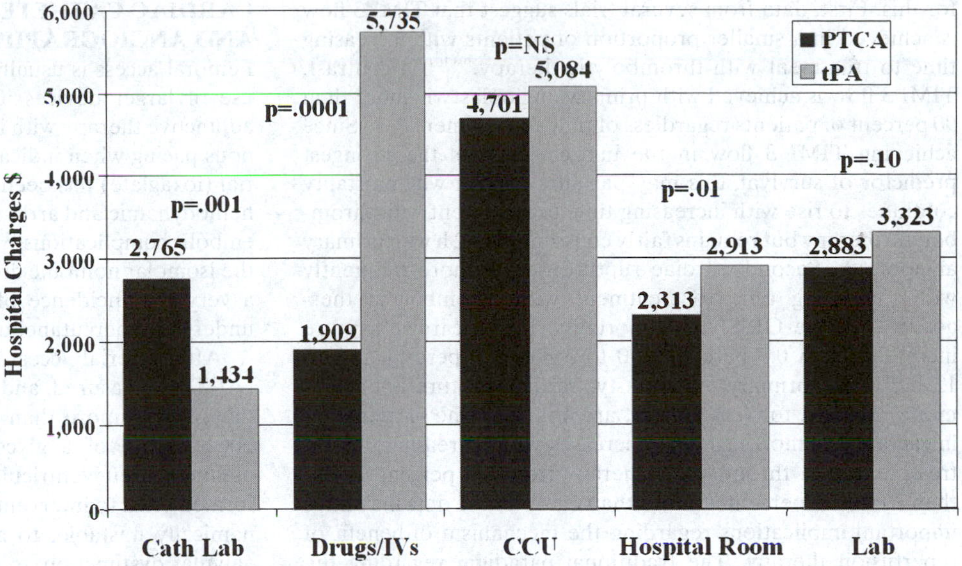

FIGURE 46-5 A breakdown of hospital charges from the PAMI-1 trial comparing thrombolytic therapy (tPA) with primary angioplasty. (Adapted with permission from Stone et al.[99])

COST-EFFECTIVENESS OF ADJUNCTIVE THERAPY

The impact of adjunctive treatment with coronary stents and platelet inhibitors on costs with primary angioplasty is evolving. Initial data from the Stent PAMI trial[103] suggest that the initial increased costs of stenting versus angioplasty alone ($2185) are partially recovered by decreased post-hospital costs due to less target-vessel revascularization (−$974). This makes the total 1-year costs $1211 higher with stenting compared with angioplasty alone. The costs and effectiveness of stenting patients with AMI appear comparable with those of elective stenting. The incremental costs and effectiveness of glycoprotein IIb/IIIa platelet receptor inhibitors in the setting of primary angioplasty is currently being evaluated.

Importance of Time to Reperfusion

Data from a number of randomized trials have shown that the mortality benefit of thrombolytic therapy is strongly dependent on the time from symptom onset until treatment up to 12 h.[62,72,104] Recent observations suggest that time to treatment may be less important with primary angioplasty.[105–107] The PAMI-2 trial found that mortality was lowest when patients were treated very early (<2 h) but that mortality was relatively independent of time to treatment after 2 h[105] (Fig. 46-6). Brodie et al.[107] also found that mortality was significantly lower when patients were reperfused at less than 2 h with primary angioplasty but that mortality was relatively constant after 2 h regardless of further increases in time to treatment[107] (see Fig. 46-6). (One exception to this is in patients with cardiogenic shock, who continue to have increasing mortality with increasing time to reperfusion.[71]) There are several possible explanations

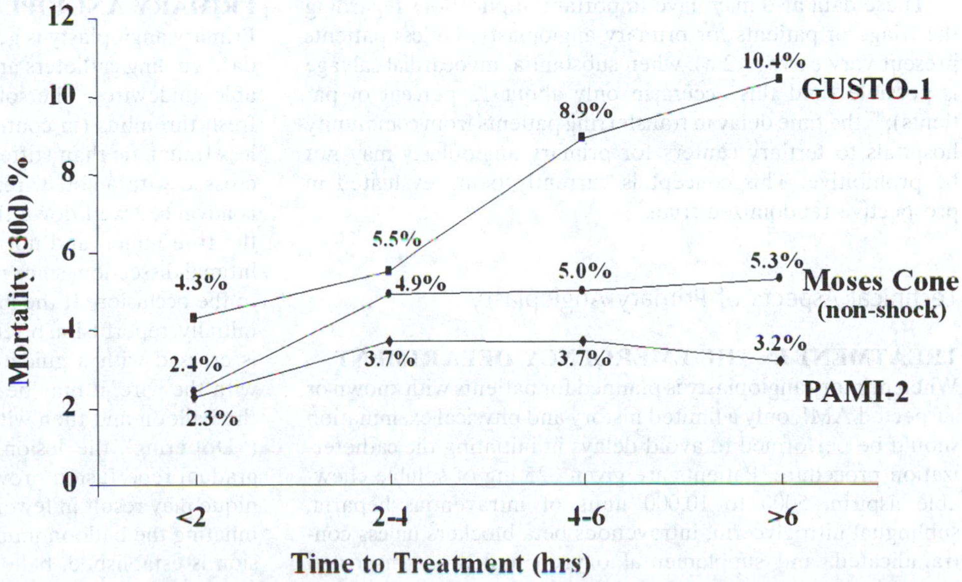

FIGURE 46-6 Thirty-day mortality in patients with AMI based on time to treatment comparing primary angioplasty (Moses Cone,[107] PAMI-2[105]) with tPA (GUSTO-1[72]). Mortality increases with increasing time to treatment with thrombolytic therapy but is relatively independent of time to treatment after 2 h with primary angioplasty.

for this. First, data from several trials suggest that TIMI 3 flow is achieved in a smaller proportion of patients with increasing time to treatment with thrombolytic therapy.[108,109] In contrast, TIMI 3 flow is achieved with primary angioplasty in more than 90 percent of patients regardless of time to treatment.[105–107] Since achieving TIMI 3 flow in the infarct artery is the strongest predictor of survival, this may partially explain why mortality continues to rise with increasing time to treatment with thrombolytic therapy but remains fairly constant after 2 h with primary angioplasty. Second, cardiac rupture occurs more frequently with increasing time to treatment with thrombolytic therapy.[110,111] In the GISSI trial, mortality due to cardiac rupture increased from 0.7 percent at 0 to 3 h to 2.0 percent at 8 to 12 h.[111] With primary angioplasty, cardiac rupture is uncommon.[112] Finally, for reasons that are not clear, the incidence of intracranial hemorrhage also increases with increasing time to treatment with thrombolytic therapy from 0.5 percent at less than 2 h to 1.0 percent at more than 6 h.[113] These data may have important implications regarding the mechanism of benefit of reperfusion therapy. The traditional paradigm regarding the mechanism of benefit of reperfusion therapy is that early reperfusion results in myocardial salvage, which results in improved left ventricular function and better survival. This paradigm has been expanded to include benefit of late reperfusion when myocardial salvage is no longer expected. An open infarct artery, even if opened too late for myocardial salvage, may result in survival benefit by preventing ventricular dilatation, promoting electrical stability, and providing a source of collateral flow.[93,94] The survival benefit due to myocardial salvage is felt to be strongly time-dependent, whereas the survival benefit due to late reperfusion not related to myocardial salvage is felt to be relatively independent of time to reperfusion. The data with primary angioplasty are consistent with this expanded paradigm, but studies with primary angioplasty suggest that the time period for significant myocardial salvage and recovery of left ventricular function is relatively short (<2 h).[107,114,115]

These data also may have important implications regarding the triage of patients for primary angioplasty. Unless patients present very early (<2 h), when substantial myocardial salvage is possible (and this occurs in only about 12 percent of patients),[107] the time delay in transferring patients from community hospitals to tertiary centers for primary angioplasty may not be prohibitive. This concept is currently being evaluated in prospective randomized trials.

Technical Aspects of Primary Angioplasty

TREATMENT IN THE EMERGENCY DEPARTMENT

When primary angioplasty is planned for patients with known or suspected AMI, only a limited history and physical examination should be performed to avoid delays in initiating the catheterization procedure. Patients are given 325 mg of soluble chewable aspirin, 5000 to 10,000 units of intravenous heparin, sublingual nitroglycerin, intravenous beta blockers unless contraindicated, and supplemental oxygen and are transported promptly from the emergency department to the catheterization laboratory. A lower weight-adjusted dose of heparin should be given if the use of a glycoprotein IIb/IIIa receptor blocker is considered.

CARDIAC CATHETERIZATION AND ANGIOGRAPHY

Femoral access is usually preferred because this allows for the use of larger devices if necessary and facilitates the use of adjunctive therapy with intraaortic balloon pumping or transvenous pacing when indicated. Low-osmolar ionic contrast material (ioxaglate) has been recommended to minimize the risk of hemodynamic and arrhythmic disturbances, as well as thromboembolic complications.[116,117] Recent studies also have shown that the isomolar nonionic dimer iodixanol has been associated with a very low incidence of adverse events in high-risk patients undergoing percutaneous coronary intervention.[118]

After arterial access is obtained, an activated clotting time (ACT) is measured, and additional heparin is given to prolong the ACT to more than 350 s prior to balloon inflation (200–300 s if use of a glycoprotein IIb/IIIa receptor blocker is planned). Left ventriculography is clinically useful when performed prior to intervention, even in patients who are hemodynamically unstable, to assess the severity of ventricular and valvular dysfunction, to help in identification of the infarct artery (if this is uncertain), and to aid in making decisions regarding the need for adjunctive therapy, such as intraaortic balloon pumping and pulmonary artery catheter insertion. Occasionally, papillary muscle rupture, ventricular septal defect, or rarely even frank free wall rupture will be demonstrated, prompting urgent surgery. Alternatively, demonstration of normal left ventricular function may raise early concerns of nonischemic diagnoses such as aortic dissection or pericarditis. A femoral venous sheath may be helpful in patients with occlusion of the right coronary artery to allow access for temporary transvenous pacing if necessary. In patients with hypotension or hemodynamic instability, placement of a pulmonary artery catheter is important to define and monitor hemodynamics. The use of a pulse oximeter to monitor oxygen saturation is also useful. Following diagnostic coronary and left ventricular angiography, patients are triaged to the most appropriate therapy.

PRIMARY ANGIOPLASTY PROCEDURE

Primary angioplasty is generally performed with 7 French standard guiding catheters and soft or floppy-tipped 0.014-in. steerable guidewires. The soft tip almost always can cross the soft fresh thrombus (in contrast to chronic total occlusions) and is less traumatic than stiffer wires. If the infarct lesion cannot be crossed with a soft wire, a stiffer wire is used. The guidewire is advanced well down the infarct artery to ensure that it is in the true lumen and not in the small side branch or under an intimal dissection, since navigation is usually done blindly distal to the occlusion. If the infarct-related artery is totally occluded initially, reperfusion often will be established after the occlusion is crossed with a guidewire. If reperfusion is not established with the wire, it may be preferable to cross the occlusion with the balloon and then withdraw the balloon without inflating it ("Dottering" the lesion) to establish reperfusion. The more gradual reperfusion provided with the wire or Dottering technique may result in fewer reperfusion arrhythmias than rapidly inflating the balloon immediately after crossing. Once reperfusion is established, balloon angioplasty of the infarct lesion is performed with similar technique to conventional angioplasty. Infarct lesions usually are soft and do not require high balloon pressures. The operator should strive for an optimal result with less than 30 percent residual luminal narrowing and TIMI 3 flow. If a significant residual stenosis remains, or if there is a dissection, coronary stenting is indicated because these features are predictive of recurrent ischemia or reocclusion.[119] As soon as the decision to perform coronary stenting is made, 500 mg ticlopidine or 150 to 300 mg clopidogrel should be given as a loading dose. As an alternative to stenting for suboptimal results, or if there is large residual thrombus, a glycoprotein IIb/IIIa platelet receptor inhibitor may be used (although if glycoprotein IIb/IIIa receptor blocker use is likely, it is preferable to use this agent prior to balloon inflation). The use of intracoronary thrombolytic therapy is not recommended because this results in increased rates of infarct artery occlusion when used as an adjunct to angioplasty in acute ischemic syndromes.[120] No flow (TIMI 0–1 flow) or slow flow (TIMI 2 flow) may occur after successful opening of the epicardial infarct artery obstruction. This is generally due to microvascular dysfunction from spasm, distal emboli, or endothelial injury and should be treated with intracoronary nitroglycerin, verapamil, and/or adenosine, which often helps to improve flow. Glycoprotein IIb/IIIa receptor blocking agents also may help with no reflow. With rare exceptions (such as refractory cardiogenic shock), a cardinal rule with primary angioplasty is to dilate only the infarct artery. Tandem lesions in the infarct vessel can be dilated, but dilating a noninfarct artery places too much myocardium acutely in jeopardy.

TABLE 46-6 Acute Catheterization Laboratory Complications with Primary Angioplasty (PTCA) and Primary Stenting in Nonshock Patients

Complication	Stent (n = 451) (%)	PTCA (n = 448) (%)	Combined (n = 899) (%)
Laboratory death	0.2	0	0.1
Emergency bypass surgery	0.2	0.2	0.2
Cardiac arrest			
Ventricular tachycardia/fibrillation*	3.1	4.7	3.9
Cardiopulmonary resusitation†	0.9	0.4	0.7
Intubation	0.2	0.7	0.4
Asystole/bradycardia‡	9.3	8.5	8.9
Sustained hypotension§	7.8	8.3	8.0

*Requiring electric cardioversion.
†Requiring chest compression.
‡Requiring atropine or temporary pacing.
§Requiring vasopressors or intraaortic balloon counterpulsation.
SOURCE: From the Stent PAMI trial.[76]

ACUTE CATHETERIZATION LABORATORY COMPLICATIONS

With increasing operator experience, improved equipment and patient selection, and the availability of stents, major catheterization laboratory complications with primary angioplasty have become infrequent. Acute catheterization laboratory complications from the Stent PAMI trial[121] in nonshock patients are shown in Table 46-6. Laboratory death and emergency bypass surgery for failed angioplasty are rare. Ventricular tachycardia or fibrillation requiring cardioversion, asystole and bradycardia including second- and third-degree atrioventricular (AV) block, and hypotension are the most common complications and usually occur immediately after reperfusion. These complications, which occur more often with right coronary artery infarction, historically were a problem with primary angioplasty, but with increased experience, they occur less frequently and are manageable.[84]

POSTANGIOPLASTY CARE

Following the interventional procedure, heparin should be held for 2 to 4 h until the ACT is less than 170 s, at which time the sheath should be removed. Heparin is resumed 2 h after sheath removal with a bolus at 15 units/kg per hour and titrated to maintain the activated partial thromboplastin time (aPTT) at 60 to 80 s. Full-dose heparin is continued until 48 h after the intervention, then is decreased to one-half dose for 12 h to prevent a rebound hypercoagulable state, and then is discontinued. In patients who receive abciximab, no postprocedural heparin is given. When tirofiban or eptifibatide is used, low-dose heparin is recommended. Low-risk patients (as defined earlier) can be transferred from the catheterization laboratory directly to the subacute unit (rather than the coronary care unit) and can be targeted for discharge on day 3 (day 0 = day of admission).[102] Aspirin should be given routinely. Ticlopidine 250 mg orally twice daily or clopidogrel 75 mg orally daily should be given in stented patients and continued for 2 to 4 weeks. If no contraindications are present, angiotensin-converting enzyme (ACE) inhibitors should be used in patients with congestive heart failure, hypertension, or low ejection fraction (<40 percent). Oral beta blockade also should be administered routinely in the absence of contraindications. Patients who develop symptoms or electrocardiographic changes suggestive of recurrent ischemia or reinfarction should undergo emergency repeat catheterization and intervention as indicated.

Adjunctive Therapy

STENTS

The use of stenting with percutaneous coronary intervention in AMI initially was thought to be contraindicated due to the presence of thrombus in the infarct artery and concern regarding the risks of subacute thrombosis. The use of platelet inhibition with aspirin plus ticlopidine or clopidogrel and high-pressure balloon deployment have greatly reduced the incidence of subacute thrombosis, and numerous studies have now documented the safety of stent deployment in the setting of AMI.[81,122,123] Several studies with first-generation stents have documented superior outcomes with stenting compared with angioplasty alone, with lower composite end points due primarily to less target-vessel revascularization or less recurrent ischemia[123–125] (Table 46-7). The largest randomized trial, the Stent PAMI trial[121] with 900 patients, has documented lower restenosis rates (20 versus 34 percent; $p = 0.001$), including less reocclusion (5

TABLE 46-7 Randomized Trials Comparing Primary Stenting with Primary Angioplasty for AMI

	PTCA %	Stent %	*p* Value
Zwolle trial (*n* = 227)[123]			
Death	2.7	1.7	NS
Reinfarction	7.0	0.9	0.04
TVR	17.4	3.6	0.002
Composite	20.0	5.4	0.001
GRAMI trial (*n* = 104)[124]			
Death	7.6	3.8	NS
Reinfarction	7.6	0	NS
TVR	7.6	0	NS
Composite	19.2	3.8	0.03
FRESCO trial (*n* = 150)[125]			
Death	0	1.3	NS
Reinfarction	2.7	1.3	NS
TVR	25.3	6.7	0.002
Composite	28.0	9.3	0.003
Stent PAMI trial (*n* = 900)[81]			
Death	2.7	4.2	NS
Reinfarction	2.2	2.4	NS
Ischemic TVR	17.0	7.7	0.0001
Composite	20.1	12.6	0.01

NOTE: Outcomes are at 6 months in all trials except the GRAMI trial, which lists in-hospital outcoms. The Gianturco-Rubin stent was used in the GRAMI and FRESCO trials, the Palmaz-Shatz stent in the Zwolle trial, and the heparin coated Palmaz-Shatz stent in the Stent PAMI trial. TVR = target vessel revascularization.

TABLE 46-8 Randomized Trials Comparing Abciximab versus Placebo with Primary Angioplasty or Primary Stenting for AMI

	Abciximab (%)	Placebo (%)	*p* Value
RAPPORT trial (30 days) (*n* = 483)[129]			
Death	2.5	2.1	NS
Reinfarction	3.3	4.1	NS
Urgent TVR	1.7	6.6	0.006
Composite	5.8	11.2	0.03
RAPPORT trial (6 months) (*n* = 483)[129]			
Death	4.1	4.5	NS
Reinfarction	6.6	7.4	NS
Any TVR	20.7	21.9	NS
Composite	28.2	28.1	NS
ADMIRAL trial (30 days) (*n* = 300)[130]			
Death	3.3	4.4	
Reinfarction	2.0	4.7	
Urgent TVR	4.7	10.0	
Composite	10.0	19.3	0.03
Munich trial (30 days) (*n* = 401)[131]			
Death	2.0	4.5	NS
Reinfarction	0.5	1.5	NS
TLR	3.0	5.0	NS
Composite	5.0	10.5	0.04

NOTE: Patients in the ADMIRAL and Munich trials were treated with primary stenting; TVR = target vessel revascularization; TLR = target lesion revascularization.

versus 9 percent; $p = 0.04$) and less ischemia-driven target-vessel revascularization (8 versus 17 percent; $p = 0.0001$) with stenting versus angioplasty alone but no difference in mortality or reinfarction (see Table 46-7). Currently, stenting cannot be recommended for routine use with primary angioplasty but should be used in selected patients, especially when there are suboptimal results or dissection following angioplasty. The results of large ongoing trials with newer stents may provide data that will extend these indications.

PLATELET INHIBITORS

Several trials have documented the efficacy of glycoprotein IIb/IIIa platelet receptor inhibition during elective coronary intervention.[126–128] The RAPPORT trial evaluated platelet inhibition with abciximab in patients with AMI undergoing primary angioplasty and found a significant reduction in the 30-day composite end point[129] (Table 46-8). However, by 6 months, there was no difference in outcomes (see Table 46-8). Also, the use of high-dose heparin in concert with prolonged sheath dwell times resulted in an excess of major bleeding episodes. Two European trials, the ADMIRAL trial[130] and the Munich trial,[131] have evaluated abciximab in patients with AMI undergoing primary stenting, and both have found a significant reduction in composite end points with abciximab compared with placebo (see Table 46-8). The CADILLAC trial has evaluated the efficacy of abciximab in 2000 patients with AMI undergoing either primary angioplasty or primary stenting. This study should provide efficacy as well as cost data that will help to define the role of platelet inhibition with primary angioplasty for AMI.[132]

INTRAAORTIC BALLOON COUNTERPULSATION

Clinical studies have shown that the use of intraaortic balloon counterpulsation results in augmentation of systemic pressure, reduction in preload and afterload, and an increase in coronary blood flow velocity.[133,134] This has given hope that intraaortic balloon counterpulsation may improve outcomes in patients with AMI. Unfortunately, randomized trials in high-risk patients with AMI have shown little or no benefit when intraaortic balloon counterpulsation is used alone without concomitant reperfusion or revascularization.[135,136] Several studies have evaluated the prophylactic use of intraaortic balloon counterpulsation after reperfusion with primary or rescue angioplasty in high-risk patients[137,138] (Table 46-9). Initial studies[137] suggested benefit in terms of less infarct artery reocclusion and less recurrent ischemia, but larger, more recent studies including the large PAMI-2 trial have shown little or no benefit.[138,139] The results of these trials and the advent of coronary stenting, which has reduced the incidence of reocclusion and recurrent ischemia, have diminished the role of intraaortic balloon counterpulsation after primary angioplasty in hemodynamically stable patients. Intraaortic balloon counterpulsation still has a role in hemodynamically unstable patients with congestive heart failure or shock prior to primary angioplasty and in patients with mechanical complications of AMI or anatomy that is unsuitable for percutaneous coronary intervention as a bridge to surgery. There also may be a role for prophylactic intraaortic balloon pumping before primary angioplasty in selected high-risk patients to prevent hemodynamic deterioration.[140]

TABLE 46-9 Randomized Trials Evaluating Prophylactic Intraaortic Balloon Pumping (IABP) after Primary or Rescue Angioplasty for AMI

	IABP (%)	No IABP (%)	*p* Value
Ohman et al. (*n* = 182)[137]			
Death	2.1	2.3	NS
Reinfarction	3.1	8.1	NS
Recurrent ischemia	4.2	20.9	0.001
Infarct artery reocclusion	8.2	20.8	<0.03
Composite*	12.5	24.4	<0.04
PAMI-2 trial (*n* = 437)[138]			
Death	4.3	3.1	NS
Reinfarction	6.2	8.0	NS
Recurrent ischemia	13.3	19.6	0.08
Infarct artery reocclusion	6.7	5.5	NS
Composite†	28.9	29.2	NS
Zwolle trial (*n* = 238)[139]			
Death	10.2	7.5	NS
Reinfarction	5.9	2.5	NS
6-Month ejection fraction	42 + 13	40 + 14	NS
Composite‡	26.3	25.8	NS

*In-hospital death, reinfarction, recurrent ischemia, emergency revascularization, or stroke.
†In-hospital death, reinfarction, infarct artery reocclusion, stroke, new congestive heart failure, or sustained hypotension.
‡Six-month death, reinfarction, stroke, ejection fraction <30%.

FUTURE RESEARCH DIRECTIONS: BEYOND TIMI 3 FLOW

The superior TIMI 3 flow rates achieved by mechanical reperfusion largely explain the mortality advantage of this strategy. Today, TIMI 3 flow rates of 90 percent or more are expected for optimal clinical benefit. It must be emphasized, however, that TIMI flow is a subjective, qualitative assessment of relative contrast velocity in major epicardial coronary vessels. Observations using myocardial contrast echocardiography suggest that effective myocardial perfusion may occur in only 70 percent of patients with TIMI 3 flow.[141] Similarly, the Zwolle group has shown that myocardial contrast blush grade is impaired in a large number of patients with normal TIMI flow.[142] Finally, Tsunoda et al.[143] have shown that up to one-third of patients with TIMI 2 flow have abnormal Doppler wave flows with a systolic flow reversal and diminished diastolic flow pattern. The reason for concern is that each of these techniques measures myocardial perfusion, and each has shown that ventricular function is only improved in those patients with normal myocardial perfusion.

The cause for abnormal perfusion after PTCA is unknown. Most myocardium is stunned after prolonged ischemia, but lack of demand alone does not explain the abnormal flow. Distal embolization of macroscopic thrombotic and plaque debris and reperfusion injury after reperfusion may be contributory. Extensive myocardial edema with capillary constriction and leukoaggregation or platelet macroemboli may prevent capillary perfusion.

Exciting new research modalities will test each of these potential mechanisms. The goal is to normalize myocardial perfusion and thus optimize salvage after reperfusion. Agents such as adenosine will be tested to decrease reperfusion injury.[144] Filtered leukocytes and complement-depleted blood have been used to reperfuse patients.[145] Supersaturated oxygen is being employed to limit myocardial injury during reperfusion.[146] Mechanical traps[147] will be employed to prevent macroembolization of debris during angioplasty and stent placement. Even glucose-insulin-potassium solutions may be of value.[148] Finally, glycoprotein receptor blockade may prevent platelet-rich thrombi from impairing microcirculatory function. Two trials have demonstrated significant improvement in ejection fraction when abciximab is added to stent therapy of AMI.[130,131] Mechanical reperfusion not only has demonstrated improvement in clinical outcome but also will contribute to an understanding of mechanisms involved in myocardial injury.

CONCLUSION

Mechanical reperfusion therapy of AMI has developed as an alternative to thrombolytic therapy. Reperfusion rates are significantly higher, rates of death and reinfarction are significantly lower, rates of intracranial hemorrhage are dramatically lower, and long-term survival is significantly greater compared with thrombolytic therapy. This treatment thus may be the preferred therapy for patients presenting to institutions equipped to perform it. Ongoing clinical trials will further elucidate the role of mechanical reperfusion after failed thrombolytic therapy and the role of transport of high-risk patients to referral institutions. The potential for mechanical reperfusion therapy is great. The major challenge for clinicians will be to find methods to apply this treatment to larger segments of the population.

References

1. Fletcher AP, Sherry S, Alkjaersig N, et al. The maintenance of a sustained thrombolytic state in man: II. Clinical observations on patients with myocardial infarction and other thromboembolic disorders. *J Clin Invest* 1959; 38:1111–1119.
2. Boucek RJ, Murphy WP Jr. Segmental perfusion of the coronary arteries with fibrinolysin in man following a myocardial infarction. *Am J Cardiol* 1960; 6:525–533.
3. Proudfit WJ, Bruschke AV, MacMillan JP, et al. Fifteen year survival study of patients with obstructive coronary artery disease. *Circulation* 1983; 68:986–997.
4. Favaloro RG. Surgical treatment of acute myocardial infarction. *J Am Coll Cardiol* 1999; 33:1435–1441.
5. Favaloro RG, Effler DB, Cheanvechai C, et al. Acute coronary insufficiency (impending myocardial infarction and myocardial infarction): Surgical treatment by saphenous vein graft technique. *Am J Cardiol* 1971; 28:598–607.
6. Berg R, Everhart FJ, Duvoisin G, et al. Operation for acute coronary occlusion. *Am Surg* 1976; 42:517–521.
7. Rentrop KP. Development and pathophysiological basis of thrombolytic therapy in acute myocardial infarction: Part II, 1977–1980. The pathogenetic role of thrombus is established by the Goettingen pilot studies of mechanical interventions and intracoronary thrombolysis in acute myocardial infarction. *J Intervent Cardiol* 1998; 11:265–285.
8. DeWood MA, Spores J, Notske R, et al. Prevalence of total coronary occlusion during the early hours of transmural myocardial infarction. *N Engl J Med* 1980; 303:897–902.
9. DeWood MA, Stifter WF, Simpson CS, et al. Coronary arteriographic findings soon after non-Q-wave myocardial infarction. *N Engl J Med* 1986; 315:417–423.
10. Rentrop P, DeVivie ER, Karsch KR, et al. Acute coronary occlusion with impending infarction as an angiographic complication relieved by a guide-wire recanalization. *Clin Cardiol* 1978; 1:101–106.
11. Rentrop KP, Blanke H, Karsch KR. Initial experience with transluminal recanalization of the recently occluded infarct-related coronary artery in acute myocardial infarction: Comparison with conventionally treated patients. *Clin Cardiol* 1979; 2:92–105.
12. Roberts WC, Buja LM. The frequency and significance of coronary arterial thrombi and other observations in fatal acute myocardial infarction. *Am J Med* 1972; 52:425–443.
13. Roberts WC. Coronary arteries in fatal acute myocardial infarction. *Circulation* 1972; 45:215–230.
14. Rude RE, Muller JE, Braunwald E. Efforts to limit the size of infarctions. *Ann Intern Med* 1981; 95:736–761.
15. Khaja F, Walton JA Jr, Brymer JF, et al. Intracoronary fibrinolytic therapy in acute myocardial infarction: Report of a prospective randomized trial. *N Engl J Med* 1983; 308:1305–1311.
16. Kennedy JW, Ritchie JL, Davis KB, et al. Western Washington randomized trial of intracoronary streptokinase in acute myocardial infarction. *N Engl J Med* 1983; 390:1477–1482.
17. O'Neill W, Timmis G, Bourdillon P, et al. A prospective randomized clinical trial of intracoronary streptokinase versus coronary angioplasty for acute myocardial infarction. *N Engl J Med* 1986; 314:812–818.
18. Fung AY, Lai P, Juni JE, et al. Prevention of subsequent exercise-induced peri-infarct ischemia by emergency coronary angioplasty in acute myocardial infarction: Comparison with intracoronary streptokinase. *J Am Coll Cardiol* 1986; 8:496–503.
19. O'Neill WW, Topol EJ, Fung A, et al. Coronary angioplasty as therapy for acute myocardial infarction: University of Michigan experience (abstract). *Circulation* 1987; 76(suppl II):II-79–II-87.
20. Gruppo Italiano per lo Studio della Streptochinasi nell'Infarto Miocardico (GISSI). Effectiveness of intravenous thrombolytic treatment in acute myocardial infarction. *Lancet* 1986; 1:397–402.
21. TIMI Research Group. Immediate vs delayed catheterization and angioplasty following thrombolytic therapy for acute myocardial infarction. *JAMA* 1988; 260:2849–2858.
22. Topol EJ, Califf RM, George BS, et al. A randomized trial of immediate versus delayed elective angioplasty after intravenous tissue plasminogen activator in acute myocardial infarction. *N Engl J Med* 1987; 317:581–588.
23. Simoons ML, Arnold AER, Betriu A, et al. Thrombolysis with tissue plasminogen activator in acute myocardial infarction: No additional benefit from immediate percutaneous coronary angioplasty. *Lancet* 1988; 1:197–203.
24. Holmes DR Jr, Topol EJ. Reperfusion momentum: Lessons from the randomized trials of immediate coronary angioplasty for myocardial infarction. *J Am Col Cardiol* 1989; 14:1572–1578.
25. Veen G, Verheugt FWA. PTCA after thrombolytic therapy for acute myocardial infarction: A meta-analysis (abstract). *Circulation* 1991; 84(suppl II):II-537.
26. Hartzler GO, Rutherford BD, McConahay DR, et al. Percutaneous transluminal coronary angioplasty with and without thrombolytic therapy for treatment of acute myocardial infarction. *Am Heart J* 1983; 106:965–973.
27. O'Keefe JH Jr, Rutherford BD, McConahay DR, et al. Early and late results of coronary angioplasty without antecedent thrombolytic therapy for acute myocardial infarction. *Am J Cardiol* 1989; 64:1221–1230.
28. Brodie B, Weintraub R, Stuckey T, et al. Outcomes of direct coronary angioplasty for acute myocardial infarction in candidates and noncandidates for thrombolytic therapy. *Am J Cardiol* 1991; 67:7–12.
29. O'Neill WW, Weintraub R, Grines CL, et al. A prospective, placebo-controlled, randomized trial of intravenous streptokinase and angioplasty versus lone angioplasty therapy of acute myocardial infarction. *Circulation* 1992; 86:1710–1717.
30. Conti CR. Clinical trials and decisions for thrombolytic therapy in patients with acute myocardial infarction (editor's note). *Clin Cardiol* 1990; 13:307–308.
31. SWIFT Trial Study Group. SWIFT trial of delayed elective intervention versus conservative treatment after thrombolysis with Anistreplase in acute myocardial infarction. *Br Heart J* 1991; 302:555–560.
32. Lieu TA, Gurley RJ, Lundstrom RJ, et al. Primary angioplasty and thrombolysis for acute myocardial infarction: An evidence summary. *J Am Coll Cardiol* 1996; 27:737–750.
33. GUSTO Angiographic Investigators. The effects of tissue plasminogen activator, streptokinase, or both, on coronary artery patency, ventricular function, and survival after acute myocardial infarction. *N Engl J Med* 1993; 329:1615–1622.
34. Ross AM, Lundergan CF, Rohrbeck SC, et al. for the GUSTO-1 Angiographic Investigators. Rescue angioplasty after failed thrombolysis: Technical and clinical outcomes in a large thrombolysis trial. *J Am Coll Cardiol* 1998; 31:1511–1517.
35. Abbottsmith CW, Topol EJ, George BS, et al. Fate of patients with acute myocardial infarction with patency of the infarct related vessel achieved with successful thrombolysis versus rescue angioplasty. *J Am Coll Cardiol* 1990; 16:770–778.

36. McKendall GR, Forman S, Sopko G, et al. Value of rescue percutaneous transluminal coronary angioplasty following unsuccessful thrombolytic therapy in patients with acute myocardial infarction. *Am J Cardiol* 1995; 76:1108–1111.
37. Gibson CM, Cannon CP, Grenne RM, et al. Rescue angioplasty in the Thrombolysis in Myocardial Infarction (TIMI-4) trial. *Am J Cardiol* 1997; 80:21–26.
38. Flachskampf FA, Ellis SG. Rescue percutaneous transluminal coronary angioplasty. *Curr Opin Cardiol* 1998; 13:289–293.
39. Ellis SG, Van de Werf, Ribeiro-daSilva E, et al. Present status of rescue coronary angioplasty: Current polarization of opinion in randomized trials. *J Am Coll Cardiol* 1992; 19:681–686.
40. Califf RM, Topol EJ, Stack RS, et al. Evaluation of combination thrombolytic therapy and timing of cardiac catheterization in acute myocardial infarction: Results of Thrombolysis and Angioplasty in Myocardial Infarction—Phase 5 randomized trial. *Circulation* 1991; 83:1543–1556.
41. Ellis SG, Ribeiro-da Silva E, Heyndrickx G, et al. Randomized comparison of rescue angioplasty with conservative management of patients with early failure of thrombolysis for acute anterior myocardial infarction. *Circulation* 1994; 90:2280–2284.
42. Rapold JH. Promotion of thrombin activity by thrombolytic therapy without simultaneous anticoagulation. *Lancet* 1990; 1:481–482.
43. Eisenberg PR, Sobel BE, Jasse AS. Activation of prothrombin accompanying thrombolysis with recombinant tissue-type plasminogen activator. *J Am Coll Cardiol* 1992; 19:1065–1069.
44. Coller BS. Platelet activation and thrombolytic therapy. *N Engl J Med* 1990; 322:33–42.
45. Cafri C, Denktas AE, Crystal E, et al. Contribution of stenting to the results of rescue PTCA. *Cathet Cardiovasc Intervent* 1999; 47:411–414.
46. Moreno R, Garcia E, Abeytua M, et al. Coronary stenting during rescue angioplasty after failed thrombolysis. *Cathet Cardiovasc Intervent* 1999; 47:1–5.
47. Dirschinger J, Pocat J, Kastrati A, et al. Clinical outcome after rescue stenting in patients with acute myocardial infarction (abstract). *J Am Coll Cardiol* 1999; 33(2, suppl A):30A.
48. Zeymer U, Schroder R, Molhoek P, et al. Noninvasive assessment of infarct-related artery patency after thrombolysis for acute myocardial infarction by ST resolution: Results of the HIT-4 angiographic substudy (abstract). *J Am Coll Cardiol* 1999; 33(2, suppl A):324A.
49. Kircher BJ, Topol EJ, O'Neill W, et al. Prediction of infarct coronary artery recanalization after intravenous thrombolytic therapy. *Am J Cardiol* 1987; 59:513–515.
50. Stewart JT, French JK, Theroux P, et al. Early noninvasive identification of failed reperfusion after intravenous thrombolytic therapy in acute myocardial infarction. *J Am Coll Cardiol* 1998; 31:1499–1505.
50a. Ross AM, Karin SC, Reiner JS, et al. A randomized trial comparing primary angioplasty with a strategy of short-acting thrombolysis and immediate planned rescue angioplasty in acute myocardial infarction: The PACT trial. *J Am Coll Cardiol* 1999; 34:1954–1962.
51. DeWood MA. Direct PTCA versus intravenous t-PA in acute myocardial infarction: Results from a prospective randomized trial. In: *Proceeding from the Thrombolysis and Interventional Therapy in Acute Infarction Symposium VI*. Washington: George Washington University Press; 1990:28.
52. Grines CL, Brown KF, Marco J, et al. A comparison of immediate angioplasty with thrombolytic therapy for acute myocardial infarction. *N Engl J Med* 1993; 328:673–679.
53. Zijlstra F, Jan de Boer M, Hoorntje JCA, et al. A comparison of immediate coronary angioplasty with intravenous streptokinase in acute myocardial infarction. *N Engl J Med* 1993; 328:680–684.
54. Gibbons RJ, Holmes ZR, Reeder GS, et al. Immediate angioplasty compared with the administration of a thrombolytic agent followed by conservative treatment for myocardial infarction. *N Engl J Med* 1993; 328:685–691.
55. Ribeiro EE, Silva LA, Carneiro R, et al. Randomized trial of direct coronary angioplasty versus intravenous streptokinase in acute myocardial infarction. *J Am Coll Cardiol* 1993; 22:376–380.
56. Grinfeld L, Berrocal B, Belardi J, et al. Fibrinolytics versus primary angioplasty in acute myocardial infarction (FAP) (abstract). *J Am Coll Cardiol* 1996; 27(suppl):A-222.
57. Zijlstra F, Beukema WP, van't Hof AWJ, et al. Randomized comparison of primary coronary angioplasty with thrombolytic therapy in low risk patients with acute myocardial infarction. *J Am Coll Cardiol* 1997; 29:908–912.
58. The Global Use of Strategies to Open Occluded Coronary Arteries in Acute Coronary Syndromes (GUSTO IIb) Angioplasty Substudy Investigators. A clinical trial comparing primary coronary angioplasty with tissue plasminogen activator for acute myocardial infarction. *N Engl J Med* 1997; 336:1621–1628.
59. Ribichini F, Steffenino G, Dellavalle A, et al. Comparison of thrombolytic therapy and primary coronary angioplasty with liberal stenting for inferior myocardial infarction with precordial ST-segment depression. *J Am Coll Cardiol* 1998; 32:1687–1694.
60. Garcia E, Elizaga J, Perez-Castellano N, et al. Primary angioplasty versus systemic thrombolysis in anterior myocardial infarction. *J Am Coll Cardiol* 1999; 33:605–611.
61. Weaver WD, Simes RJ, Betriu A, et al. Comparison of primary coronary angioplasty and intravenous thrombolytic therapy for acute myocardial infarction: A quantitative review. *JAMA* 1997; 278:2093–2098.
62. Fibrinolytic Therapy Trialists' (FTT) Collaborative Group. Indications for fibrinolytic therapy in suspected acute myocardial infarction: Collaborative overview of early mortality and major morbidity results from all randomized trials of more than 1000 patients. *Lancet* 1994; 343:311–322.
63. Stone GW, Grines CL, Browne KF, et al. Predictors of in-hospital and six-month outcome after acute myocardial infarction in the reperfusion era: The Primary Angioplasty and Myocardial Infarction (PAMI) trial. *J Am Coll Cardiol* 1995; 25:370–377.
64. Holmes DR Jr, White HD, Pieper KS, et al. Effect of age on outcome with primary angioplasty versus thrombolysis. *J Am Coll Cardiol* 1999; 33:412–419.
65. Stone GW, Grines CL, Browne KF, et al. Influence of acute myocardial infarction location on in-hospital and late outcome after primary percutaneous transluminal coronary angioplasty versus tissue plasminogen activator therapy. *Am J Cardiol* 1996; 78:19–25.
66. Vassanelli C, Ellis SG, Phillips HR, et al. No greater benefit with PTCA in patients with anterior infarction: Updated 30-day results of the GUSTO IIb Substudy (abstract). *Circulation* 1996; 94(8, suppl I):I-329.
67. Stone GW, Grines CL, O'Neill WW, et al. Primary coronary angioplasty versus thrombolysis (letter). *N Engl J Med* 1997; 337:1168.
68. Stone GW, Grines CL, Browne KF, et al. Comparison of in-hospital outcome in men versus women treated by either thrombolytic therapy or primary coronary angioplasty for acute myocardial infarction. *Am J Cardiol* 1995; 75:987–992.
69. The International Study Group. In-hospital mortality and clinical course in 2891 patients with suspected acute myocardial infarction randomized between alteplase and streptokinase with or without heparin. *Lancet* 1990; 336:71–75.
70. Moscucci M, Bates ER. Treatment of acute myocardial infarction: Cardiogenic shock. *Cardiol Clin* 1995; 13(3):391–406.
71. Hochman JS, Sleeper LA, Webb JG, et al. Early revascularization in acute myocardial infarction complicated by cardiogenic shock. *N Engl J Med* 1999; 341:625–634.

72. GUSTO Angiographic Investigators. The effects of tissue plasminogen activator, streptokinase, or both, on coronary artery patency, ventricular function, and survival after acute myocardial infarction. *N Engl J Med* 1993; 329:1615–1622.
73. Stone GW, O'Neill WW, Jones B, et al. The central unifying concept of TIMI-3 flow after primary PTCA and thrombolytic therapy in acute myocardial infarction (abstract). *Circulation* 1996; 94(8, suppl I):I-515.
74. Antman EM, Giugliano RP, Gibson CM, et al. Abciximab facilitates the rate and extent of thrombolysis: Results of the Thrombolysis in Myocardial Infarctions (TIMI) 14 trial. *Circulation* 1999; 99:2720–2732.
75. Nunn CM, O'Neill WW, Rothbaum D, et al. Long-term outcome after primary angioplasty: Report from the Primary Angioplasty in Myocardial Infarction (PAMI-I) trial. *J Am Coll Cardiol* 1999; 33:640–646.
76. Zijlstra F, Hoorntje JCA, de Boer M-J, et al. Long-term benefit of primary angioplasty as compared with thrombolytic therapy for acute myocardial infarction. *N Engl J Med* 1999; 341:1413–1419.
77. Veen G, de Boer MJ, Zijlstra F, et al. Improvement in three-month angiographic outcome suggested after primary angioplasty for acute myocardial infarction (Zwolle trial) compared with successful thrombolysis (APRICOT trial). *Am J Cardiol* 1999; 84:763–767.
78. White HD, French JK, Hamer AW, et al. Frequent re-occlusion of patent infarct-related arteries between four weeks and one year: Effects of anti-platelet therapy. *J Am Coll Cardiol* 1995; 25:218–223.
79. Brodie BR, Grines CL, Ivanhoe R, et al. Six month clinical and angiographic follow-up after direct angioplasty for acute myocardial infarction: Final results from the Primary Angioplasty Registry. *Circulation* 1994; 25:155–162.
80. Nakagawa Y, Iwasaki Y, Kimura T, et al. Serial angiographic follow-up after successful direct angioplasty for acute myocardial infarction. *Am J Cardiol* 1996; 78:980–984.
81. Grines C, Cox D, Stone G, et al. Coronary angioplasty with or without stent implantation for acute myocardial infarction. *N Engl J Med* 1999; 341:1949–1956.
82. White HD, Cross DB, Elliott JM, et al. Long-term prognostic importance of patency of the infarct-related coronary artery after thrombolytic therapy for acute myocardial infarction. *Circulation* 1994; 89:61–67.
83. Brodie BR, Stuckey TD, Kissling G, et al. Importance of infarct-related artery patency for recovery of left ventricular function and late survival after primary angioplasty for acute myocardial infarction. *J Am Coll Cardiol* 1996; 28:319–325.
84. O'Neill WW, Brodie BR, Ivanhoe R, et al. Primary coronary angioplasty for acute myocardial infarction (The Primary Angioplasty Registry). *Am J Cardiol* 1994; 73:627–634.
85. Stone GW, Brodie BR, Griffin JJ, et al. The role of cardiac surgery in the hospital phase management of patients treated with primary angioplasty for acute myocardial infarction. *J Am Coll Cardiol* 2000; 85:1292–1296.
86. Weaver WB, Litwin PE, Martin JS. Use of direct angioplasty for the treatment of patients for acute myocardial infarction in hospitals with and without on-site cardiac surgery. *Circulation* 1993; 88:2067–2075.
87. Wharton TP Jr, McNamara NS, Febele FA, et al. Primary angioplasty for the treatment of acute myocardial infarction: Experience at two community hospitals without cardiac surgery. *J Am Coll Cardiol* 1999; 33:1257–1265.
88. Cragg BR, Friedman HC, Bonema JD, et al. Outcome of patients with acute myocardial infarction who are ineligible for thrombolytic therapy. *Ann Intern Med* 1991; 115:173–177.
89. Barron HD, Bowlby LJ, Breen T, et al. Use of reperfusion therapy for acute myocardial infarction in the United States: Data from the National Registry of Myocardial Infarction 2. *Circulation* 1998; 97:1150–1156.
90. Brodie BR. Primary angioplasty in a community hospital in the USA: Insights into the advantages and limitations. *Br Heart J* 1995; 73:411–412.
91. Zahn R, Schuster S, Gottwik M, et al. Comparison of primary angioplasty with conservative therapy in patients with acute myocardial infarction and contraindications for thrombolytic therapy (abstract). *Circulation* 1998; 98(17, suppl I):I-558.
92. Brodie BR, Stuckey TD, Hansen C, et al. Benefit of late coronary reperfusion in patients with acute myocardial infarction and persistent ischemic chest pain. *Am J Cardiol* 1994; 74:538–543.
93. Braunwald E. Myocardial reperfusion, limitation of infarct size, reduction of left ventricular dysfunction, and improved survival: Should the paradigm be expanded? *Circulation* 1989; 79(2): 441–444.
94. Califf RM, Topol EJ, Gersh BJ. From myocardial salvage to patient salvage in acute myocardial infarction: The role of reperfusion therapy. *J Am Coll Cardiol* 1989; 14(5):1382–1388.
95. McCullough PA, O'Neill WW, Graham M, et al. A prospective randomized trial of triage angiography in acute coronary syndromes ineligible for thrombolytic therapy: Results of the Medicine versus Angiography in Thrombolytic Exclusion (MATE) trial. *J Am Coll Cardiol* 1998; 32:596–605.
96. Reiner JS, Lundergan CF, Kopecky SL, et al. Ineffectiveness of thrombolysis for acute myocardial infarction following vein graft occlusion (abstract). *Circulation* 1996; 94(8, suppl I):I-570.
97. Stone GW, Brodie BR, Griffin JJ, et al. Clinical and angiographic outcomes in patients with prior coronary artery bypass grafting treated with primary angioplasty for acute myocardial infarction. *J Am Coll Cardiol* 2000; 35:605–611.
98. Reeder GS, Bailey KR, Gersh BJ, et al. Cost comparison of immediate angioplasty versus thrombolysis followed by conservative therapy for acute myocardial infarction: A randomized, prospective trial. *Mayo Clin Proc* 1994; 69:5–12.
99. Stone G, Grines C, Rothbaum D, et al. Analysis of the relative cost and effectiveness of primary angioplasty versus tissue type plasminogen activator: The Primary Angioplasty in Myocardial Infarction (PAMI) trial. *J Am Coll Cardiol* 1997; 29: 901–907.
100. Mark B, Granger C, Ellis S, et al. Cost of direct angioplasty versus thrombolysis for acute myocardial infarction: Results from the GUSTO II randomized trial (abstract). *Circulation* 1996; 94(8, suppl I): I-168.
101. Stone GW, Grines CL, Browne KS, et al. Implications of recurrent ischemia after reperfusion therapy in acute myocardial infarction: A comparison of thrombolytic therapy and primary angioplasty. *J Am Coll Cardiol* 1995; 26:66–72.
102. Grines CL, Marsalese DL, Brodie BR, et al. Safety and cost-effectiveness of early discharge after primary angioplasty in low risk patients with acute myocardial infarction. *J Am Coll Cardiol* 1998; 31:967–972.
103. Cohen DJ, Grines CL, Cox D, et al. The cost-effectiveness of coronary stenting in acute myocardial infarction: Results from the PAMI stent trial (abstract). *Circulation* 1999; 100(18, suppl I):I-87.
104. Goldberg RJ, Morradd M, Gerwitz JH, et al. Impact of time to treatment with tissue plasminogen activator on morbidity and mortality following acute myocardial infarction (The Second National Registry of Myocardial Infarction). *Am J Cardiol* 1998; 82:259–264.
105. Stone GW, Brodie BR, Griffin J, et al. Should the risk of delaying reperfusion prohibit interhospital transfer to perform primary PTCA in acute myocardial infarction? (abstract). *Circulation* 1996; 94(8, suppl I):I-330.
106. Brodie BR, Stone GW, Claude-Marice M, et al. Importance of time to reperfusion on outcomes after primary PTCA for acute

myocardial infarction: Results from stent PAMI (abstract). *J Am Coll Cardiol* 1999; 33(2, suppl A):353-A.

107. Brodie BR, Stuckey TD, Wall TC, et al. Importance of time to reperfusion for 30-day and late survival and recovery of left ventricular function after primary angioplasty for acute myocardial infarction. *J Am Coll Cardiol* 1998; 32:1312–1319.
108. Cheseboro JH, Knatterud G, Roberts R, et al. Thrombolysis in Myocardial Infarction (TIMI) trial, phase 1: A comparison between intravenous tissue plasminogen activator and intravenous streptokinase. *Circulation* 1987; 76(1):142–154.
109. Bode C, Smalling RW, Berg G, et al. Randomized comparisons of coronary thrombolysis achieved with double bolus reteplase (recombinant plasminogen activator) and front loaded, accelerated alteplase (recombinant tissue plasminogen activator) in patients with acute myocardial infarction. *Circulation* 1996; 94: 891–898.
110. Honan MB, Harrell FE, Reimer KA, et al. Cardiac rupture, mortality and the timing of thrombolytic therapy: A meta-analysis. *J Am Coll Cardiol* 1990; 16:359–367.
111. Mauri F, DeBiase AM, Franziosi MG, et al. Analisi delle cause di morte intraospedaleria. *G Ital Cardio* 1987; 17:37–44.
112. Brodie BR, Stuckey TD, Hansen CJ, et al. Timing and mechanism of death determined clinically after primary angioplasty for acute myocardial infarction. *Am J Cardiol* 1997; 79:1586–1591.
113. Newby LK, Rutsh WR, Califf RM, et al. Time from symptom onset to treatment and outcomes after thrombolytic therapy. *J Am Coll Cardiol* 1996; 27:1646–1655.
114. O'Keefe JH Jr, Grines CL, DeWood MA, et al. Factors influencing myocardial salvage with primary angioplasty. *J Nucl Cardiol* 1995; 2:35–41.
115. Milavetz JJ, Giebel BW, Christian TF, et al. Time to therapy and salvage in myocardial infarction. *J Am Coll Cardiol* 1998; 31: 1246–1251.
116. Grines CL, Schreiber TL, Savas V, et al. A randomized trial of low osmolar ionic versus nonionic contrast media in patients with myocardial infarction or unstable angina undergoing percutaneous transluminal coronary angioplasty. *J Am Coll Cardiol* 1996; 27:1381–1386.
117. Batchelor WB, Granger CB, Phillips HR, et al. Ionic low osmolar contrast is associated with better outcome following direct PTCA: Results from GUSTO IIb (abstract). *Circulation* 1997; 96(suppl I):I-531.
118. Davidson CJ, Hermiller JB, Harrison JK, et al. A randomized trial of contrast media utilization in high risk PTCA (The COURT Trial) (abstract). *Circulation* 1998; 98(17, suppl I):I-88.
119. Grines CL, Brodie BR, Griffin J, et al. Which primary PTCA patients may benefit from new technologies? (abstract). *Circulation* 1995; 92(8, suppl I):I-146.
120. Mehran R, Ambrose JA, Bongu RM, et al. for the TAUSA Study Group. Angioplasty of complex lesions in ischemic rest angina: Results of the Thrombolysis and Angioplasty in Unstable Angina (TAUSA) trial. *J Am Coll Cardiol* 1995; 26:961–966.
121. Grines CL, Cox DA, Stone GW, et al. for the Stent PAMI Study Group. Coronary angioplasty with or without stent implantation for acute myocardial infarction. *N Engl J Med* 1999; 341:1949–1956.
122. Stone GW, Brodie BR, Griffin JJ, et al. Prospective, multicenter study of the safety and feasibility of primary stenting in acute myocardial infarction: In-hospital and thirty-day results of the PAMI stent pilot trial. *J Am Coll Cardiol* 1998; 31: 23–30.
123. Suryapranata H, van't Hof AWJ, Hoorntje JCA, et al. Randomized comparison of coronary stenting with balloon angioplasty in selected patients with acute myocardial infarction. *Circulation* 1998; 97:2502–2505.
124. Rodriguez A, Bernardi V, Fernandez M, et al. In-hospital and late results of coronary stents versus conventional balloon angioplasty in acute myocardial infarction (GRAMI trial). *Am J Cardiol* 1998; 81:1283–1291.
125. Antoniucci D, Santoro GM, Bolognese L, et al. A clinical trial comparing primary stenting of the infarct-related artery with optimal primary angioplasty for acute myocardial infarction: Results from the Florence Randomized Elective Stenting in Acute Coronary Occlusions (FRESCO) trial. *J Am Coll Cardiol* 1998; 31:1234–1239.
126. The EPIC Investigators. The use of a monoclonal antibody directed against the platelet glycoprotein IIb/IIIa receptor in high-risk coronary angioplasty. *N Engl J Med* 1994; 330:956–961.
127. The EPILOG Investigators. Platelet glycoprotein IIb/IIIa receptor blockade and low-dose heparin during percutaneous coronary revascularization. *N Engl J Med* 1997; 336:1689–1696.
128. The EPISTENT Investigators. Randomized placebo-controlled and balloon-angioplasty-controlled trial to assess safety of coronary stenting with use of platelet glycoprotein IIb/IIIa blockade. *Lancet* 1998; 352:87–92.
129. Brener SJ, Barr LA, Burchenal JEB, et al. Randomized, placebo-controlled trial of platelet glycoprotein IIb/IIIa blockade with primary angioplasty for acute myocardial infarction. *Circulation* 1998; 98:734–741.
130. The ADMIRAL Trial. Presented at the Annual Scientific Session of the American College of Cardiology, New Orleans, LA, 1999.
131. Neumann SJ, Kastrati A, Dirschinger J, et al. Use of platelet glycoprotein IIb/IIIa blockade in acute myocardial infarction treated with intracoronary stenting: 30-day clinical results of a randomized study (abstract). *J Am Coll Cardiol* 1999; 33(2, suppl A):338-A.
132. The CADILLAC Trial. Presented at the Annual Scientific Session of the American Heart Association, Atlanta, GA, 1999.
133. Kern MJ, Aguirre F, Bach R. Augmentation of coronary blood flow by intraaortic balloon pumping in patients after coronary angioplasty. *Circulation* 1993; 87:500–511.
134. Kern MJ, Aguirre FV, Tatineni S, et al. Enhanced coronary blood flow velocity during intraaortic balloon counterpulsation in critically ill patients. *J Am Coll Cardiol* 1993; 21:359–368.
135. O'Rourke M, Norris RM, Campbell TJ, et al. Randomized controlled trial of intraaortic balloon counterpulsation in early myocardial infarction with acute heart failure. *Am J Cardiol* 1981; 47:815–820.
136. Flaherty JT, Becker LC, Weiss JL, et al. Results of a randomized prospective trial of intraaortic balloon counterpulsation and intravenous nitroglycerin in patients with acute myocardial infarction. *J Am Coll Cardiol* 1985; 6:434–446.
137. Ohman EM, George BS, White CJ, et al. The use of aortic counterpulsation to improve sustained coronary artery patency during acute myocardial infarction: Results of a randomized trial. *Circulation* 1994; 90:792–799.
138. Stone GW, Marsalese D, Brodie BR. A prospective, randomized evaluation of prophylactic intraaortic balloon counterpulsation in high risk patients with acute myocardial infarction treated with primary angioplasty. *J Am Coll Cardiol* 1997; 29:1459–1467.
139. van't Hof AWJ, Liem AM, de Boer MJ, et al. A randomized comparison of intraaortic balloon pumping after primary coronary angioplasty in high risk patients with acute myocardial infarction. *Eur Heart J* 1999; 20:659–665.
140. Brodie BR, Stuckey TD, Hansen C, et al. Intraaortic balloon counterpulsation before primary percutaneous transluminal coronary angioplasty reduces catheterization laboratory events in high-risk patients with acute myocardial infarction. *Am J Cardiol* 1999; 84:18–23.
141. Ito H, Maruyama A, Iwakura K, et al. Clinical implications of the "no reflow" phenomenon: A predictor of complications and left ventricular remodeling in reperfused anterior wall myocardial infarction. *Circulation* 1996; 93:223–228.
142. Van't Hof AWJ, Liem A, Suryapranata H, et al. Angiographic

assessment of myocardial reperfusion in patients treated with primary angioplasty for acute myocardial infarction. *Circulation* 1998; 97:2302–2306.

143. Tsunoda T, Nakamura M, Wakatsuki T, et al. The pattern of alteration in flow velocity in the recanalized artery is related to left ventricular recovery in patients with acute infarction and successful direct balloon angioplasty. *J Am Coll Cardiol* 1998; 32:338–344.

144. Mentzer RM Jr, Birjiniuk V, Khuri S. Adenosine myocardial protection: Preliminary results of a phase II clinical trial. *Ann Surg* 1999; 229:643–649; discussion, 649–650.

145. Sawa Y, Matsuda H, Shimazaki Y, et al. Evaluation of leukocyte-depleted terminal blood cardioplegic solution in patients undergoing elective and emergency coronary artery bypass grafting. *J Thorac Cardiovasc Surg* 1994; 108:1125–1131.

146. Spears JR, Wang B, Wu X, et al. Aqueous oxygen: A highly O_2-supersaturated infusate for regional correction of hypoxemia and production of hyperoxemia. *Circulation* 1997; 96:4385–4391.

147. Webb JG, Carere RG, Virmani R, et al. Retrieval and analysis of particulate debris after saphenous vein graft intervention. *J Am Coll Cardiol* 1999; 34:468–475.

148. Diaz R, Paolasso EA, Piegas LS, et al. Metabolic modulation of acute myocardial infarction: The ECLA (Estudios Cardiologicos Latinoamerica) Collaborative Group. *Circulation* 1998; 98:2227–2234.

CHAPTER 47

CORONARY INTRAVASCULAR ULTRASOUND IMAGING

Steven E. Nissen

Although angiography continues to serve as the primary imaging modality used to assess the anatomy of coronary artery disease, intravascular ultrasound has matured into an important alternative method for examination of the coronaries during diagnostic or interventional catheterization.[1-8] Studies comparing angiography and intravascular ultrasound have demonstrated important differences in quantitative and qualitative findings.[7-11] Unlike angiography, which portrays the vessel as a silhouette of the lumen, intravascular ultrasound provides tomographic images that portray not only the lumen but also the deeper intramural structures within the vessel wall. The ability of ultrasound to penetrate and image soft tissue enables direct visualization of the atheroma, providing insights into the pathophysiology of coronary disease not obtainable by any other technique. Accordingly, intraluminal ultrasound imaging is now commonly utilized to confirm, refute, or supplement angiographic data in patients with coronary disease.[8]

RATIONALE FOR INTRAVASCULAR ULTRASOUND

Limitations of Angiography

Visual interpretation of angiograms exhibits significant observer variability, and necropsy examination is often discordant with the apparent angiographic severity of lesions.[12-18] In comparison to postmortem evaluation, angiography often significantly underestimates the extent of atherosclerosis.[13,18] Angiographic assessment of lesion severity is strikingly discordant with measurements of the physiologic effects of stenoses.[19] Angiography depicts coronary anatomy from a planar two-dimensional silhouette of the contrast-filled lumen. However, coronary lesions are often complex, with markedly distorted or eccentric luminal shapes, and mechanical interventions (other than stenting) exaggerate luminal eccentricity by fracturing or dissecting the atheroma.[9,20,21] The angiographic appearance of the postintervention vessel often reveals an enlarged but "hazy" lumen. This indistinct, broadened angiographic silhouette may overestimate actual vessel diameter and misrepresent the gain in lumen size.[21]

The traditional method for characterizing angiographic lesion severity depends upon visual or computer measurements of the percentage stenosis. This process requires comparison of luminal dimensions within both the lesion and an adjacent, uninvolved "normal" reference segment. However, necropsy studies demonstrate that coronary disease is frequently diffuse and contains no truly normal reference segment.[18] In the presence of diffuse disease, calculation of percent stenosis will predictably underestimate disease severity. Diffuse, concentric, and symmetrical disease affecting the entire vessel may result in the angiographic appearance of a small but normal artery.[21] Angiography is also confounded by the phenomenon of coronary "remodeling," observed histologically as the outward displacement of the external vessel wall in segments with atherosclerosis.[22] This adventitial enlargement attenuates lumen encroachment, thereby concealing the presence of the atheroma on angiography. Although such lesions do not restrict blood flow, clinical studies have demonstrated that these minimal, nonobstructive lesions represent an important cause of acute coronary syndromes.[23] Angiographically unrecognized disease virtually always underlies an ergonovine-positive response in symptomatic patients with a "normal" coronary angiogram.[24]

Theoretical Advantages of Ultrasound

Intravascular ultrasound has several unique properties of theoretical value in the detection and quantitation of coronary disease.[25,26] The cross-sectional perspective of ultrasound permits visualization of the full 360-degree circumference of the vessel wall. Accordingly, measurement of lumen area can be determined by planimetry independent of the radiographic projection or magnification.[7,21,25,26] The tomographic perspective of ultrasound enables evaluation of vessels difficult to assess by angiographic techniques, including diffusely diseased segments and bifurcation or ostial lesions. The ability to directly image the atheroma represents a truly unique capability not possible using any other commonly available imaging modality.

IMAGING TECHNOLOGY

Catheter Design

Intracoronary ultrasound equipment consists of two major components: a catheter incorporating a miniaturized transducer and a console containing the electronics necessary to reconstruct the image. High frequencies (20 to 50 MHz) are employed, resulting in excellent theoretical resolution (axially $<100\ \mu m$ and laterally $<250\ \mu m$). Two dissimilar technical approaches to transducer design exist: mechanically rotated devices and multielement electronic arrays[1–5] (Fig. 47-1). Each design has yielded small intravascular devices suitable for coronary imaging, typically ranging in size from 2.6 to 3.5 Fr (diameter of 0.86 to 1.17 mm). To facilitate subselective coronary cannulation and catheter exchanges, ultrasound catheters provide a lumen for a movable guidewire. Most systems generate images at a temporal frequency of 30 frames per second for recording on videotape.

Limitations and Artifacts

Intravascular ultrasound devices generate artifacts that may adversely affect image quality, alter interpretation, or reduce quantitative accuracy.[27] Ring-down artifact arises from acoustic oscillations in the piezoelectric transducer, resulting in high-amplitude signals that preclude imaging close to the transducer surface. Accordingly, the "acoustic" size of catheters is slightly larger than their physical size. Since the minimum size of current devices is approximately 0.9 mm, some severe stenoses cannot be imaged prior to intervention. Geometric distortion can result from imaging in an oblique plane (not perpendicular to the long axis of the vessel), resulting in an elliptical rather than circular imaging plane.[28]

Mechanical, but not electronic, transducers may exhibit cyclical oscillations in rotational speed, resulting in an artifact known as nonuniform rotational distortion (NURD).[27] This artifact arises from mechanical friction within the catheter drive shaft during the portions of its rotational cycle. This speed variation produces readily visible distortion often observed as circumferential stretching of a portion of the image with compression of the contralateral vessel wall. NURD is most evident when the drive shaft is bent into a small radius of curvature by a tortuous vessel. Improvements in the mechanical precision of ultrasound devices have reduced the impact of the artifact, but it still remains troublesome during some examinations.

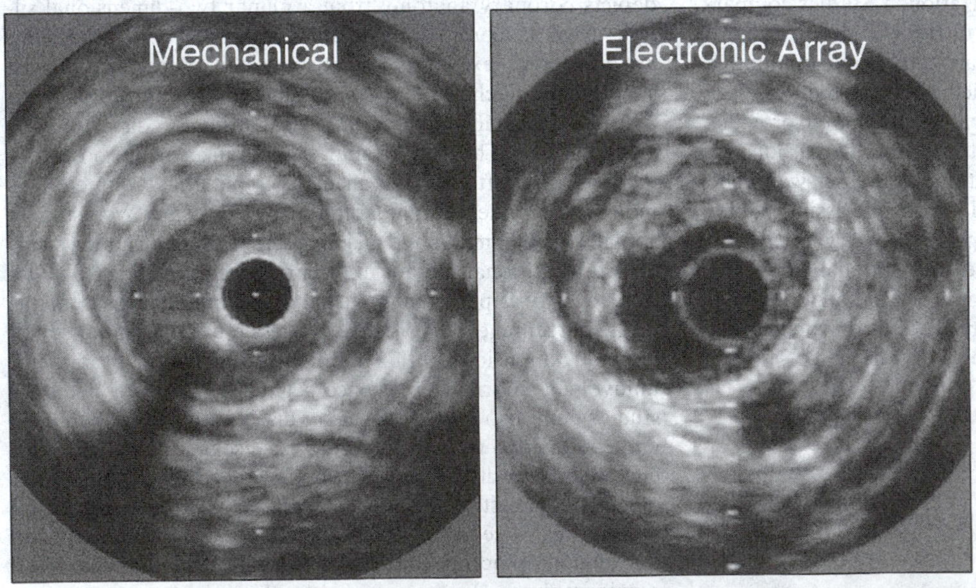

FIGURE 47-1 Mechanical and electronic array of intravascular ultrasound images. In the left panel, an intravascular ultrasound image produced using a mechanical type of catheter is illustrated. In the right panel, a similar plaque in a different patient illustrates an image acquired using a multiple-element electronic array.

CORONARY IMAGING

Examination Technique

Standard interventional techniques for intracoronary catheter delivery are used for intraluminal ultrasound examination. Intravenous heparin [to maintain activated clotting time (ACT) >200 to 250 s] and intracoronary nitroglycerin (100 to 300 μg) are routinely administered, although there are no controlled studies documenting the necessity for anticoagulation. Using a 7- or 8-Fr guiding catheter, the operator advances a steerable guidewire to subselectively cannulate the vessel. A stable guiding catheter position with good support is desirable, since current ultrasound catheters have less trackability and a larger profile than modern balloon angioplasty catheters. The operator carefully advances or retracts the imaging catheter over the wire to examine the vessel in real time, recording images on videotape for subsequent quantitative or qualitative analysis.

Some centers use a motorized pullback device to withdraw the catheter at a constant speed (between 0.25 and 1 mm/s, most frequently 0.5 mm/s). However, a single pullback, even when controlled by a precise motor, may be insufficient for a complete diagnostic ultrasound examination. Accordingly, motorized pullback is most often used to "survey" the coronary prior to more prolonged and thorough examination of sites of interest. Side branches, visualized with both angiography and ultrasound, are often used as landmarks to facilitate interpretation. Some practitioners advocate use of a uniform format, electronically rotating the ultrasound image so that branches appear in a standardized orientation. For example, imaging of the left anterior descending is often performed with the septal branches at 6 o'clock and the left circumflex appearing at about 9 o'clock.

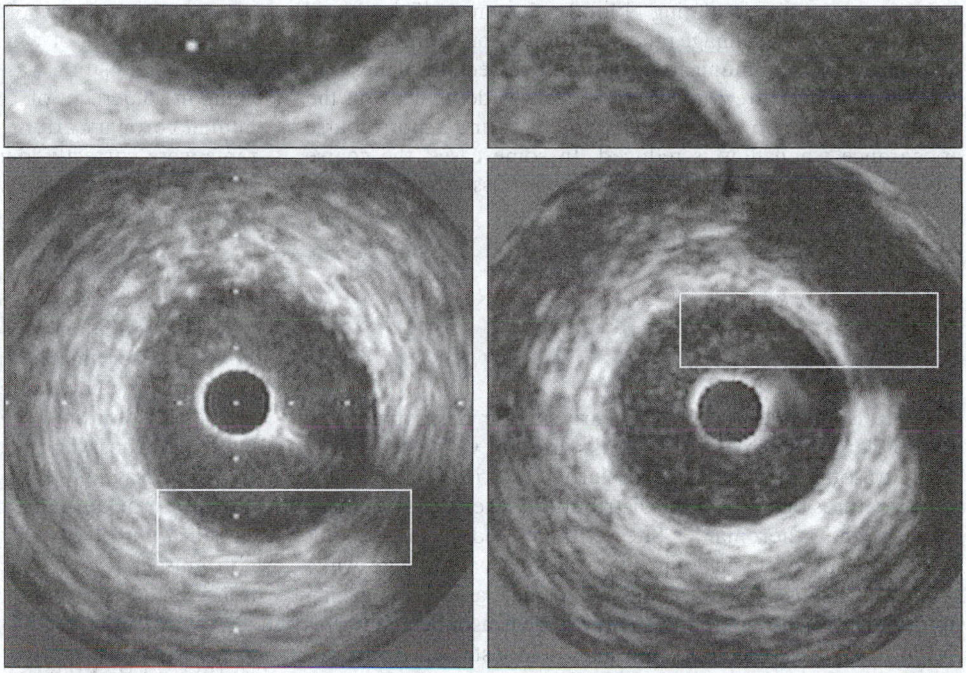

FIGURE 47-2 Two variants of normal coronary anatomy by intravascular ultrasound. In both images, a magnified view of the area contained within the rectangle is shown at the top. In the left panel, there is a monolayered artery; in the right panel, the artery has a trilaminar structure.

Safety of Coronary Ultrasound

Although intravascular ultrasound requires intracoronary instrumentation, studies have demonstrated few serious untoward effects.[29-31] The most frequently encountered complication is focal coronary spasm, which usually responds rapidly to intracoronary nitroglycerin. Data from European centers reported a 1.1 percent complication rate in 718 ultrasound examinations.[30] Another report from 28 centers (2207 studies) documented spasm in 2.9 percent and major complications such as occlusion or dissection judged to have a "certain relation" to instrumentation in 0.4 percent.[29] In both studies, complications (spasm, vessel dissection, or guidewire entrapment) occurred in patients undergoing angioplasty rather than diagnostic imaging.[44] In 170 cardiac transplant recipients (240 studies), there was no morbidity, but spasm occurred in 20 patients (8.3 percent) despite pretreatment with nitroglycerin.[31] Any intracoronary instrumentation carries the potential risk of intimal injury or vessel dissection. Accordingly, most laboratories limit credentialing for this procedure to personnel with interventional training.

Normal Coronary Anatomy

Studies performed either in vivo or using excised, pressure-distended vessels have characterized the appearance of normal coronaries by intravascular ultrasound.[32-36] Important determinants of vessel wall appearance include both the normal arterial structure and the inherent properties of ultrasound. An ultrasound reflection occurs at a tissue boundary whenever there is an abrupt change in acoustic impedance. Normally, two strong acoustic interfaces are visualized by ultrasound—the leading edge of the intima (at the interface between the blood-filled lumen and the endothelium) and the outer border of the media (at the junction of media and external elastic membrane). Underlying the trailing edge of the intima, a middle sonolucent layer is usually evident, which is composed principally of the tunica media. The echodense intima and adventitia with a sonolucent medial layer often give the wall a trilaminar appearance. However, this pattern is not a universal finding; in 30 to 50 percent of normal segments, a thin intimal layer reflects ultrasound poorly, which results in a monolayer appearance[35] (Fig. 47-2).

In a necropsy study, the ultrasound-derived intimal thickness in segments with three layers was significantly greater than for monolayered sites (0.24 ± 0.1 versus 0.11 ± 0.06 mm, $p < 0.001$). The mean age in the three-layered group was greater, 42.8 ± 9.8 versus 27.1 ± 8.5 years ($p < 0.001$).[37] Other studies demonstrate that a trilaminar appearance is dependent not only on the age but also on the histologic characteristics of the vessel. A three-layered appearance is consistently observed if an internal elastic membrane state is present.[38] However, if an internal elastic membrane is absent, a trilaminar appearance is observed only when the collagen content of the media is low. In older "normal" subjects, intimal thickening usually results in a pattern of two distinct echogenic layers sandwiching a sonolucent intermediate layer. In nearly all cases, the deepest arterial layers exhibit a characteristic "onionskin" pattern, representing the adventitia and periadventitial tissues with an indistinct outer vessel border.

In both normal and abnormal arteries, the lumen exhibits faint, finely textured, swirling echoes that arise from acoustic reflections from circulating blood elements. This blood "speckle" may assist image interpretation by providing a means to confirm the communication between dissection planes and the lumen. The pattern of blood speckle is dependent on the velocity of flow, showing increased intensity and a more coarse appearance when flow is reduced. In some cases, the coarse blood speckle can mimic the appearance of tissue, complicating image interpretation.

CHARACTERIZATION OF ATHEROSCLEROSIS

Atheroma Composition

The subtle changes that occur early in the development of atherosclerosis, such as fatty streaks, are not visible using current ultrasound devices. Atherosclerotic arteries exhibit a variety of features that reflect the distribution, severity, and composition of the atheroma.[32–34] Sites with limited disease exhibit generalized or focal thickening of the intimal leading edge, while advanced lesions appear as large echogenic masses encroaching upon the lumen. A comparative study of ultrasound and histology in 1100 fresh necropsy sections demonstrated that lipid-laden lesions are usually hypoechoic.[32] Soft, low-intensity echoes most often represent fibromuscular lesions and very bright echoes are observed within dense fibrous or calcified tissues (Fig. 47-3). In highly echogenic plaques, foci of calcification are recognized by attenuation of ultrasound penetration, which obscures deeper layers, a phenomenon known as "acoustic shadowing." In lipid-laden or fibromuscular lesions, a prominent echogenic overlying fibrous "cap" may be observed.

The echogenicity of the plaque components is dependent not only on the acoustic properties of tissue but also on the acquisition settings (gain, compression, etc.). Accordingly, most classification schemes compare the echogenicity of the plaque to the surrounding adventitia to correct for differences in ultrasound technique. However, in plaques containing a zone of reduced echogenicity, it is not possible to determine whether these represent areas of lipid deposition, thrombus, or necrotic degeneration, all of which can appear as zones of low density. Plaque composition was accurately predicted by ultrasound imaging in 96 percent of 112 quadrants from 21 freshly explanted human coronary arteries.[29] Fibrous and calcified plaque quadrants were correctly identified in almost all incidences (100 of 103, or 97 percent), but only 7 of 9 quadrants (78 percent) with predominantly lipid deposits were correctly identified.

Accordingly, some caution is warranted in the intravascular ultrasound classification of atheroma composition. Although currently available devices produce detailed views of the vessel wall, interpretation employs visual inspection of acoustic reflections to determine morphology. Different histologic features may exhibit comparable acoustic properties, and methods do not yet exist for objective or automated classification of atheromatous lesions. Thus, intravascular ultrasound can delineate the thickness and echogenicity of vessel wall structures but does not provide actual histology. Despite these limitations, the classification of coronary plaques into the categories of soft, fibromuscular, and calcified has important clinical implications.

Detection of Calcification

Ultrasound imaging has shown superiority over fluoroscopy or angiography in the detection of coronary calcification. In a series of 110 patients undergoing intervention, target lesion calcification was detected by ultrasound and fluoroscopy in 84 and 50 patients, respectively (76 versus 14 percent, $p < 0.001$).[39] Another retrospective study analyzed calcification by angiography and ultrasound in 183 interventional patients.[40] Assessment by the two techniques was concordant in 92 and discordant in 91 cases. Calcification was detected in 138 patients by ultrasound and 63 by fluoroscopy, showing a sensitivity and specificity for angiography of 46 and 82 percent, respectively. When calcium was detected angiographically, calcification by ultrasound often subtended >90 degrees and was superficial to the lumen in location. If no calcification could be visualized on the angiogram, the chance of detecting a large superficial arc of calcium by ultrasound was low (12 percent).

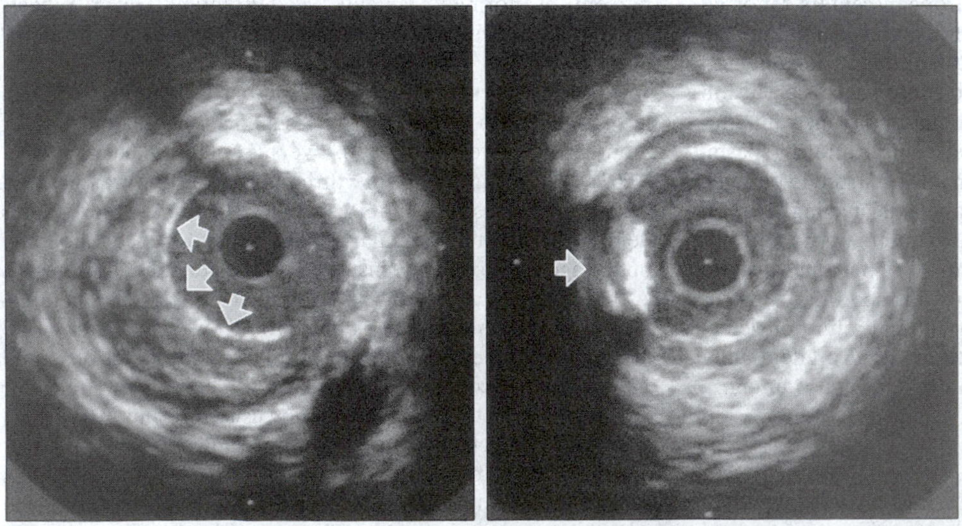

FIGURE 47-3 Atheroma morphology by intravascular ultrasound. In the left panel, a large, "soft," lipid-laden atheroma with a thin fibrous cap is shown (*arrows*). It is eccentric, involving only about 50 percent of the vessel wall. In the right panel, a circumferential atheroma with an area of focal calcification is evident (*arrow*).

Ultrasound calcification is a major determinant of the arterial response to intervention, portending a greater risk of dissection following balloon angioplasty, less tissue retrieval with directional atherectomy, and greater benefit with the use of rotational atherectomy.[41,42] Because of the importance of calcium in the selection of interventional devices, most classification schemes quantify calcification, usually by measuring the circumferential angle subtended by calcified plaque.[39] Commonly, the axial length of the calcified portion of the lesion is also reported and the depth of calcification assessed, described as superficial when the calcium remains in contact with the luminal surface and deep if no portion of the calcium deposit is superficial.

Arterial Remodeling

This term refers to a change in arterial dimensions associated with the development of atherosclerosis. In a necropsy study of 136 human left main coronary arteries, Glagov et al. originally described focal arterial enlargement at atherosclerotic sites, reporting a positive correlation between external elastic membrane (EEM) area and the area occupied by atheroma ($r = 0.44$, $p < 0.001$).[22] At sites with area stenosis less than 40 percent, the increase in arterial size "overcompensated" for the plaque deposition, leading to an increase in absolute lumen area. With more advanced lesions (area stenosis >40 percent), the degree of arterial enlargement or remodeling was blunted, resulting in a smaller lumen area. The authors hypothesized that this phenomenon represented a compensatory mechanism to preserve lumen size.

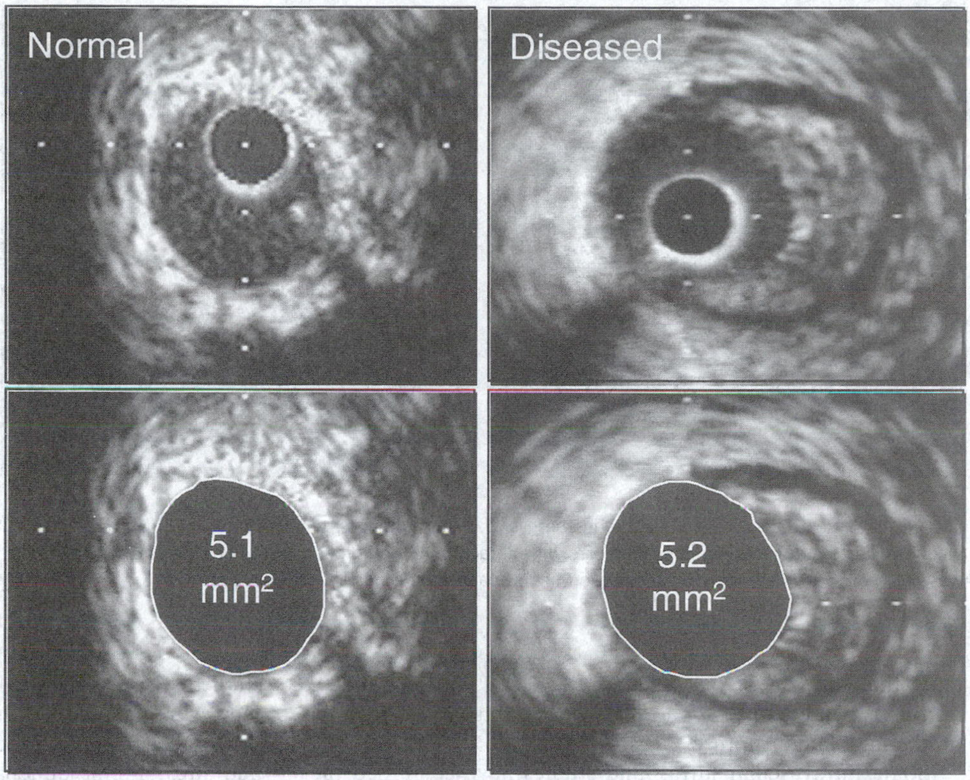

FIGURE 47-4 Example of coronary remodeling. In the left upper panel, a normal segment of the circumflex coronary is illustrated. In the right upper panel, an atherosclerotic segment of the coronary a few millimeters proximal to the normal segment is shown. In the bottom two panels, measurements taken at each of the sites show very similar cross-sectional areas. The preservation of lumen area results in a coronary angiogram that is normal despite the presence of a large atherosclerotic plaque in the involved segment.

The findings of Glagov et al. were later confirmed in vivo by intravascular ultrasound imaging[43,44] (Fig. 47-4). In 80 ultrasound cross sections obtained from 44 patients undergoing coronary interventions, EEM area correlated closely with plaque area ($r = 0.79$, $p = 0.0001$). In this study, lumen area increased with early atherosclerosis, confirming the phenomenon of overcompensation in early stages of the disease. With more advanced atherosclerosis, there was a correlation between increasing area stenosis and decreasing lumen area ($r = 0.58$, $p = 0.0001$).[43] Compensatory enlargement has also been demonstrated by ultrasound in superficial femoral arteries; however, there was no difference between lesions less than and greater than 40 percent stenosis.[45]

In recent years, ultrasound studies have demonstrated a new dimension to arterial remodeling: negative remodeling.[46,47] At diseased sites, the EEM area may actually be reduced in size, contributing to luminal narrowing rather than compensating for it. In 51 femoral arteries, EEM area was smaller at lesions than adjacent reference sites, with a negative correlation between stenosis severity and EEM area reduction ($r = 0.62$ by histology and 0.66 by ultrasound, $p < 0.001$ for both).[46] "Inadequate" remodeling, defined as an EEM area within the lesion less than 78 percent of a proximal reference site, has also been described in the coronaries of patients with stable angina.[47] Although 91 of 603 lesions (15 percent) fit this definition, there was a highly variable response among lesions within the same patient. However, when remodeling is defined in this fashion, there is an assumption that the reference EEM area represents the original vessel size, which may not be correct, since angiographic reference sites are invariably diseased according to ultrasound.

Although the exact mechanisms of compensatory or negative remodeling remain unclear, these phenomena have important clinical implications. Compensatory remodeling represents an important factor in the underestimation of the severity of atherosclerosis by angiography. Remodeling may influence the estimation of the vessel size during coronary interventions. Recently, negative remodeling has been implicated in restenosis following debulking and balloon angioplasty.[48]

Unstable Plaque and Thrombi

An emerging application of intracoronary ultrasound is the characterization of the atheroma associated with acute coronary syndromes (Fig. 47-5). The typical angiographic appearance of a ruptured plaque is a stenosis with an eccentric or ulcerated lumen, often with overhanging edges (Ambrose type II lesion).[49-54] However, retrospective reviews of angiograms of patients performed before an episode of unstable angina usually reveal minimal disease within the culprit lesion segment.[51] These studies highlight the inability of angiography to identify "rupture-prone" lesions. Histologic examination of unstable plaques after rupture usually reveals a lipid-laden plaque with a thin fibrous cap.[49] Based on these observations, it has been postu-

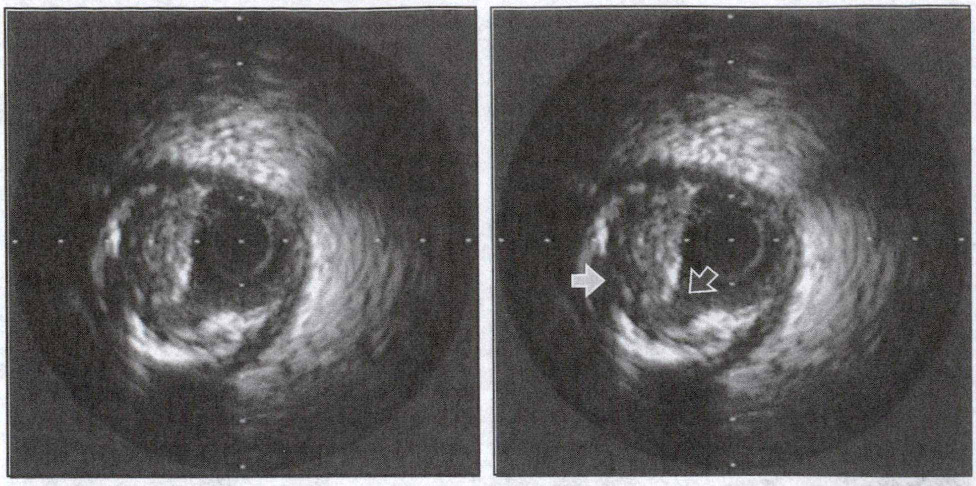

FIGURE 47-5 Ruptured coronary plaque. In these two identical images, the anatomy of a ruptured coronary plaque is illustrated. There is a large lipid core with a fracture of the fibrous cap (*right panel, arrow*). This image was obtained a few days after hospitalization of this patient for a unstable coronary syndrome.

lated that the size of the lipid pool and the thickness of the fibrous cap are more important than severity of stenosis in predicting plaque rupture.[52]

Some intravascular ultrasound studies have confirmed the presence of an echolucent atheroma within culprit lesions in patients with acute coronary syndromes. In a small study of 22 stable and 43 unstable angina patients, type II eccentric lesions were detected on the angiograms in 18 percent of stable and 40 percent of unstable angina patients. Echolucent plaques were more frequently observed in patients with unstable than in those with stable angina syndromes (74 versus 41 percent, $p < 0.01$).[11] Recent and intriguing intravascular ultrasound studies have examined the relationship between remodeling and the type of clinical presentation. The culprit lesions in 76 patients with acute coronary syndromes were compared with lesions in 40 patients with stable angina. In the unstable patients, both EEM and plaque areas were significantly larger than the corresponding measurements in the stable patients ($p = 0.02$ for both). Positive remodeling was more prevalent in the unstable group (51 versus 18 percent, $p = 0.002$) and negative remodeling more prevalent in the stable group (58 versus 33 percent, $p = 0.002$).[55]

The formation of intraluminal thrombi at a ruptured or fissured plaque is considered to be the hallmark of acute coronary syndromes.[56] Angiographic criteria for diagnosis of a coronary thrombus, the presence of haziness, an intraluminal filling defect, and/or irregular lumen contour are not sensitive.[54] Small observational studies have attempted to differentiate the ultrasound appearance of thrombus, defined as hypoechoic material projecting into the lumen with a slight synchronous pulsation and a distinct acoustic interface, from more echogenic plaque[57,58] (Fig. 47-6). However, in vitro studies have revealed limitations in the reliability of intravascular ultrasound diagnosis of thrombi (sensitivity of 57 percent and specificity of 91 percent), considerably inferior to angioscopy (sensitivity and specificity of 100 percent).[56] Radiofrequency analysis of ultrasound signals has shown some promise in differentiating between thrombus and plaque, although the clinical application is not yet feasible.[59,60]

DIAGNOSTIC CLINICAL APPLICATIONS

Quantitative Luminal Measurements

A broad spectrum of therapeutic decisions hinge upon assessment of coronary luminal dimensions. Accordingly, in diagnostic and interventional practice, quantitation of vascular dimensions represents an important clinical application of intravascular ultrasound. Several studies have compared luminal measurements by intravascular ultrasound and quantitative angiography.[6,7] For vessels without atherosclerosis, most studies document a close correlation between angiographic and ultrasonic coronary dimensions, although a few studies suggest slightly larger measurements by ultrasound.[7] However, in patients with atherosclerotic arteries, most investigators report only a moderate correlation between ultrasonic and angiographic dimensions, with the greatest disparities in vessel segments with a noncircular lumen shape.[5,7,10] This reduced correlation is probably explained by the irregular, noncircular cross-sectional profile of diseased vessels, which cannot be adequately measured using angiography.[10]

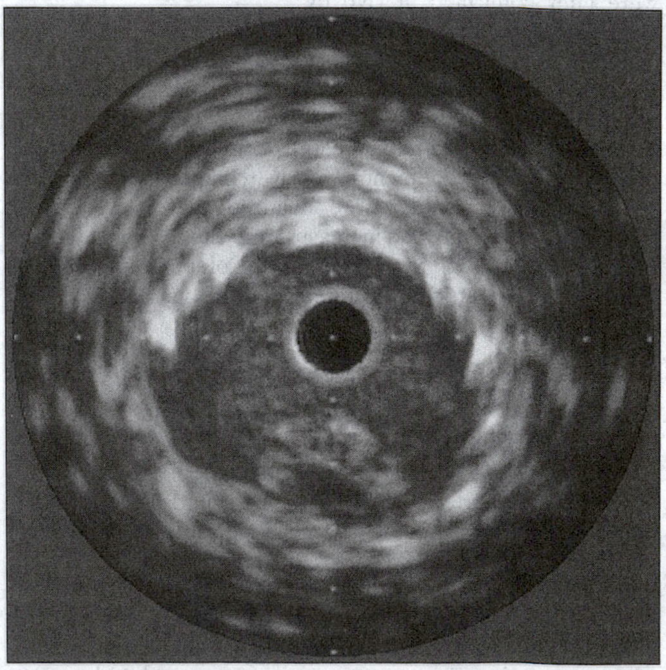

FIGURE 47-6 Thrombus within a coronary stent. In this intravascular ultrasound image, a stent is well visualized. There is a globular mass projecting into the lumen at 6 o'clock; it probably represents a large thrombus.

Quantitation of Atherosclerosis

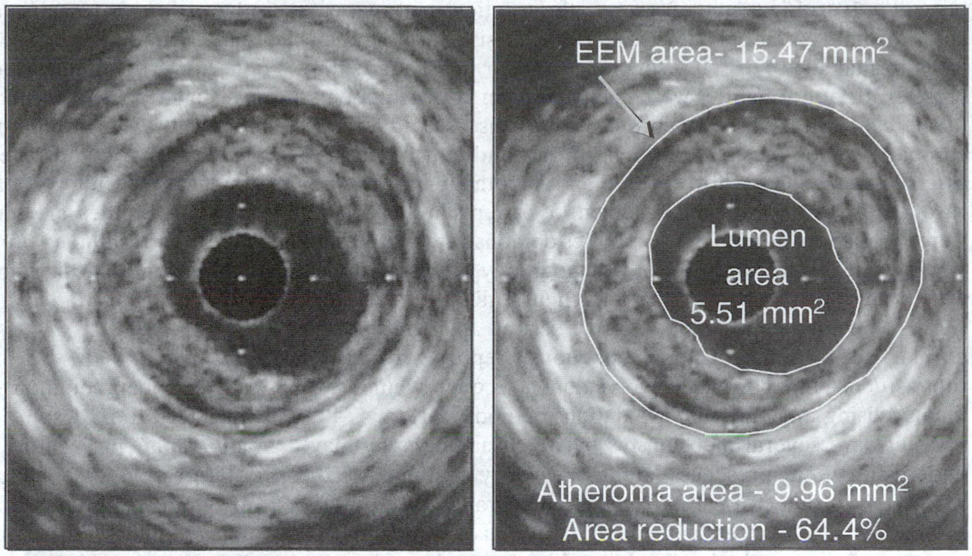

FIGURE 47-7 Boundaries for intravascular ultrasound measurements. In these two identical images, an athersclerotic plaque is well visualized. The right panel illustrates the planimetry typically employed to measure the extent of the atherosclerotic disease. Both the lumen and external elastic membrane (EEM) are measured. The atheroma area represents the difference between the EEM and the lumen areas. The area reduction is calculated as the atheroma area divided by the EEM area multiplied by 100.

Analysis of intravascular ultrasound images permits quantitative measurements of the extent and severity of coronary atherosclerosis[26] (Fig. 47-7). However, the inherent properties of ultrasound require utilization of different anatomic landmarks than those serving classic histology. In all ultrasound imaging, reflections at the leading edge of any interface are located precisely at the boundary where acoustic impedance abruptly changes. However, the position of the trailing edge of any anatomic structure is determined by multiple nonanatomic factors, including ultrasound beam properties, particularly the wavelength (frequency). Thus, leading-edge measurements accurately describe the location of a boundary, whereas trailing-edge measurements are unreliable. As previously noted, strong reflections are generally produced at two locations, the leading edge of the intima and the border between the media and the external elastic membrane. The position of the trailing edge of the intima is not accurately localized in intravascular ultrasound images. Accordingly, quantitative measurements must calculate the atheroma's cross-sectional area by subtracting the area bounded by the intimal leading edge from the area enclosed by the external elastic membrane. This approach results in a slight overestimation of atheroma volume (in comparison to histology) by including the area of the media within the calculation.

NORMAL INTIMAL THICKNESS

The threshold for abnormal intimal thickness by intravascular ultrasound is controversial, particularly since the categorical classification of a continuous variable, intimal thickness, as normal and abnormal is inherently arbitrary. In various histologic and ultrasound studies, normal intimal thickness ranges between 0.10 and 0.35 mm and the normal medial thickness ranges from 0.15 to 0.25 mm. In a necropsy study, normal intimal thickness not including media was age-dependent, averaging 0.21 mm in 21- to 25-year-olds, 0.22 mm in 26- to 30-year-olds, and 0.25 mm in 36- to 40-year-olds.[37] In a comparative study, intravascular ultrasound measurements of the intima plus media averaged 20 percent greater than histological measurements.[61,62] Considering the histologic and ultrasound data, most clinical studies have defined the ultrasound measurement threshold for coronary disease as an intimal thickness ≥0.5 mm.[63-67] Currently, there is no well-defined threshold for normal values for other measures, like intimal cross-sectional area.

The tomographic orientation of intravascular ultrasound represents an additional problem in quantifying atherosclerosis. Since each image contains information from only a thin "slice" of the vessel, global measures of atheroma burden require the integration of multiple cross sections. One successful approach to this conundrum employs a motorized device to steadily and progressively withdraw the ultrasound catheter through the interrogated vessel, typically at 0.5 to 1.0 mm/s. Since motor speed is kept constant, the operator can obtain a series of cross sections separated by a constant, recurring time interval; these are individually measured and then summated to approximate total atheroma burden using Simpson's rule. A second approach to atheroma quantitation employs three-dimensional (3D) reconstruction of the vessel from the two-dimensional ultrasound tomograms.[68] Unfortunately 3D methods are exceedingly complex, have many unresolved confounding variables, and remain largely unvalidated.

Atheroma Distribution

The circumferential distribution of the atheroma varies from nearly symmetrical plaques to very eccentric lesions in which the entire atheroma is located on one side of the artery. Assessed by ultrasound, the majority of plaques are eccentric, with a maximum atheroma thickness more than twice the minimum plaque thickness.[69] Studies have demonstrated a poor correlation between the apparent circumferential pattern by angiography and the actual plaque distribution revealed by ultrasound examination.[69] Such studies demonstrate the inaccuracy inherent in determining plaque distribution from the projected two-dimensional silhouette of the lumen (angiography). This observation has important implications for guidance of coronary interventions, particularly techniques for selective plaque removal, such as directional atherectomy.

Angiographically Unrecognized Disease

In patients undergoing angiography for clinically suspected coronary artery disease, no angiographic evidence of narrowing is present in 10 to 15 percent of cases. In these patients, intravascular ultrasound commonly detects atherosclerosis at angiographically normal sites.[21,25,26,70,71] Using intravascular ultrasound, atherosclerotic abnormalities were documented in 21 of 44 patients (48 percent) with suspected coronary artery disease and normal coronary angiograms.[70] Combining ultrasound and functional assessment (coronary flow reserve and endothelium-mediated vasodilator response), only 36 percent of patients in this cohort were completely normal. Other studies demonstrate that, if any luminal irregularity is present by angiography, ultrasound will usually demonstrate atherosclerosis at nearly all other examined sites.[21] The prevalence of atherosclerosis at angiographically normal sites confirms the finding, previously reported from necropsy studies, that coronary involvement is frequently underestimated using angiographic evaluation methods[12,13] (Fig. 47-8).

There are several mechanisms by which angiography may underestimate the presence, extent, or severity of atherosclerosis.[21] First, to detect focal narrowing, angiography relies upon comparison of the interrogated site to an adjacent uninvolved segment. However, the involved vessel is often reduced in caliber along its entire length, containing no truly normal segment for comparison. The angiographer may erroneously conclude that the vessel is simply "small in caliber." Overlapping structures and mechanical limits in x-ray positioning may prevent the angiographer from obtaining optimal radiographic projections (orthogonal to the lesion). Accordingly, eccentric plaques that occupy only a portion of the vessel circumference represent an important source of false-negative angiography. At atherosclerotic sites, compensatory enlargement of the vessel wall overlying the plaque often preserves lumen diameter, resulting in false-negative angiography because the lumen size in the involved segment is identical to that of adjacent, uninvolved segments. Finally, radiographic foreshortening can conceal short "napkin-ring" lesions.

For each of these mechanisms of false-negative angiography, intravascular ultrasound has been employed to confirm the presence and estimate the extent of atherosclerosis.[21] However, the long-term clinical implications of angiographically unrecognized atherosclerosis remain uncertain since no outcomes-based research has demonstrated a worse prognosis for patients with atherosclerosis detected only by ultrasound. However, several investigators have demonstrated that plaques with minimal to moderate angiographic narrowing are the most likely lead to acute coronary syndromes. Accordingly, the presence of angiographically occult coronary disease may have prognostic significance. Studies are currently under way to determine the value of ultrasound in predicting the clinical outcome in patients with angiographically unrecognized coronary disease.

Lesions of Uncertain Severity

Angiographers commonly encounter lesions that elude accurate characterization despite thorough examination using multiple radiographic projections. Difficult-to-assess sites include ostial or bifurcation lesions and moderate stenoses (angiographic severity ranging from 40 to 75 percent) in patients whose symptomatic status is difficult to evaluate. For ambiguous lesions, ultrasound provides a tomographic perspective, independent of the radiographic projection, that may permit quantification of the lesion. In two prospective series, intracoronary ultrasound changed the management strategy in approximately 20 percent of the examinations performed immediately prior to coronary intervention.[72,73] In both studies, however, operator selection of patients for ultrasound examination may have resulted in an overestimation of the true impact of ultrasound imaging on clinical decision making.

Angiographic assessment of left main coronary artery (LMCA) obstruction represents a particularly vexing clinical problem.[14] Radiographic contrast in the aortic cusp can obscure the ostium, and "streaming" of contrast from the injection vortex can result in a false impression of luminal narrowing. The LMCA is often short in length, leaving no normal "reference" segment. The bifurcation or trifurcation of the LMCA into daughter branches may produce vessel overlap, thereby concealing a stenosis. Intravascular ultrasound is commonly used to quantify LMCA lesions when angiographic interpretation is uncertain.[74] The technique for examination consists of subselective placement of the ultrasound transducer in the circumflex or anterior descending, followed by slow pullback to the aorta with the guiding catheter disengaged. There is no consensus regarding the threshold for critical LMCA obstruction. However, an area stenosis >50 percent or an absolute area <9 mm^2 has been proposed as a threshold.[74]

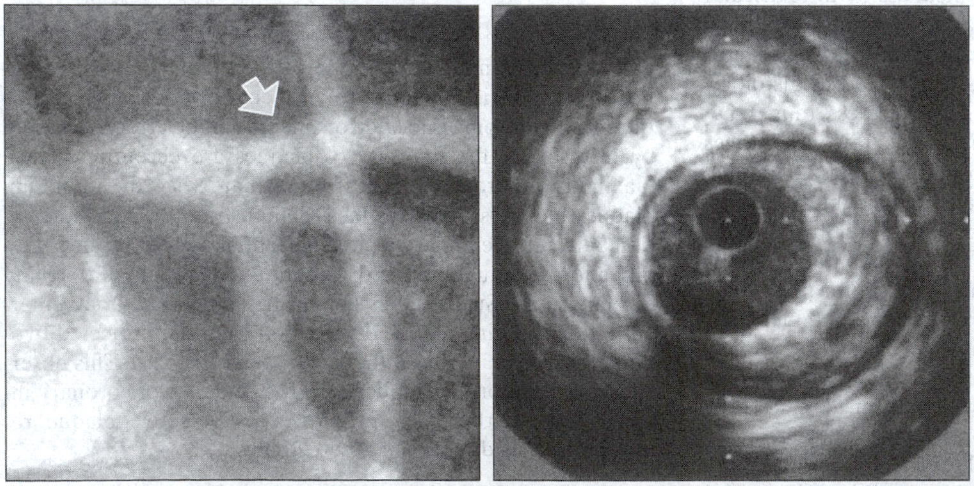

FIGURE 47-8 Underestimation of coronary atherosclerosis by angiography. In the angiogram in the left panel, a relatively minor lesion of the left anterior descending coronary is illustrated (*arrow*). In the right panel, this lesion is depicted by intravascular ultrasound and consists of a large eccentric atherosclerotic plaque that appears much more extensive than would be suspected from the angiogram.

Cardiac Allograft Disease

Transplant coronary artery disease is the leading cause of death beyond the first year after cardiac transplantation, with a reported incidence of 15 to 20 percent per year.[75] Although most transplant centers perform arteriograms annually for screening, these surveillance studies often fail to detect atherosclerosis prior to a clinical event.[76,77] Necropsy studies have demonstrated that angiography systematically underestimates coronary atherosclerosis in transplant recipients.[77] Patients may have diffuse vessel involvement that, for reasons already enumerated, conceals the atherosclerosis from the angiographer. Many active transplant centers now routinely perform intravascular ultrasound at the time of annual catheterization in all recipients. Investigations using ultrasound to detect transplant vasculopathy report a very high incidence of abnormal intimal thickening in 80 percent of patients at 1 year and in more than 92 percent studied 4 or more years after transplantation.[65–67,79–83]

Recent studies have revealed two pathways to transplant-associated atherosclerosis. Some patients receive atherosclerotic plaques transmitted via the donor heart, while others develop an immune-mediated vasculopathy.[67,81] Despite a young donor age, lesions of conventional atherosclerosis are frequently present in donor hearts. At a mean donor age of only 32 years, atherosclerosis, defined as a maximal intimal thickness ≥0.5 mm, was evident in 56 percent of patients.[67] Multivariate analysis demonstrated donor age ($p = 0.0001$) and male donor gender ($p = 0.0006$) to be important predictors of atherosclerosis. Ultrasound imaging was a necessity for accurate detection of donor lesions, since the sensitivity of angiography was only 43 percent. The natural history of donor lesions after transplantation is largely unknown. Since angiography is relatively insensitive, ultrasound remains the most important method used to study the early atherosclerotic lesion. In the first year after transplantation, progression occurred in 42 percent of patients.[82]

INTERVENTIONAL CLINICAL APPLICATIONS

Preinterventional Imaging

Several studies have demonstrated that ultrasound imaging of interventional target lesions may influence the approach to therapy. In one study (313 lesions), the intended revascularization strategy before ultrasound imaging was compared with the treatment actually performed.[42] In 40 percent of cases, the intended strategy was altered based on the ultrasound findings, most often ultrasound assessment of lesion composition or eccentricity (26 percent). Although there was a relatively close correlation between angiographic and ultrasonic lumen diameter ($r = 0.83$), a disagreement between the two methods was cited as the reason for altering the procedure in 13 percent of lesions. In another small, nonrandomized study ($n = 56$) of ultrasound guidance of balloon angioplasty or directional atherectomy, operators reclassified lesion characteristics after ultrasound in 68 percent of patients and the therapeutic approach was modified in 48 percent. Ultrasound measurements revealed a smaller lumen diameter than expected from angiography, leading to balloon upsizing in 34 percent of angioplasty cases.[84]

Several studies have purported to show benefits of ultrasound imaging prior to implantation of coronary stents.[85,86] The preliminary results of one prospective study identified vessel calcification as one of the predictors of "inadequate" stent expansion.[85] For ostial lesions, ultrasound imaging is sometimes used to determine whether the lesion involves the "true" ostium or spares the most proximal few millimeters, which may assist optimal stent positioning. When stents are used to treat dissections, ultrasound may reveal involvement of a longer segment than can be appreciated by angiography. This may be particularly relevant in "bailout" stenting for threatened abrupt closure, where it may be preferred to cover the full length of the dissection.[86] Despite promising data, reports on preinterventional imaging must be interpreted with caution. There are no prospective, controlled trials demonstrating a superior outcome using an ultrasound-guided approach. Study patients were not randomized, allowing for bias in selection of more complex cases for ultrasound guidance, which would likely emphasize the contributions of imaging. Furthermore, cases in which the operators were unable to advance the ultrasound catheter through the lesion were systematically excluded.

Imaging during Specific Interventions

BALLOON ANGIOPLASTY

Ultrasound guidance of balloon sizing has been proposed as a means to improve procedural result and late clinical outcome for percutaneous transluminal coronary angioplasty (PTCA).[87] In a study of 104 lesions, ultrasound was performed after obtaining a "satisfactory" angiographic result and revealed remodeling at the lesion or extensive plaque within the reference segment in 73 percent of the cases. In this subset, the balloon-to-artery ratio was increased from 1.12 ± 0.15 to 1.30 ± 0.17 ($p < 0.0001$) and the resulting angiographic minimal lumen diameter increased from 1.95 ± 0.5 to 2.21 ± 0.5 mm. Ultrasound lumen area improved from 3.16 ± 1.0 to 4.52 ± 1.1 mm^2 ($p > 0.0001$). Following ultrasound-guided balloon upsizing, the incidence of angiographic dissection was not increased (37 versus 40 percent, $p = 0.67$). However, the study was too small to demonstrate any effect upon intermediate or long-term clinical restenosis rates.

Intravascular ultrasound studies have evaluated the mechanisms of luminal enlargement following balloon angioplasty. Prior necropsy studies in patients who expired shortly after balloon angioplasty have described plaque fracture or disruption as the most common mechanism of dilatation.[20] Most ultrasound studies have confirmed that dissection is the most important mechanism of luminal enlargement, occurring in 40 to 80 percent of patients.[9,41,88–92] Identification of dissection or fracture is based on the visualization of blood flow in the newly created lumen, sometimes aided by injection of saline or iodinated contrast to opacify the lumen via microbubbles. Wall disruptions can be further defined by measuring the circumferential extent, length, and/or maximal depth of the dissection. One small study reported that calcified lesions had a higher incidence of dissection (67 versus 25 percent, $p = 0.03$) with a trend toward restenosis in lesions with no dissection.[41] Following iliac artery angioplasty, ultrasound evidence of dissection was noted in all 40 cases, accounting for 72 percent of the total lumen gain.[89]

Several alternative mechanisms for luminal enlargement not discernible by angiography have been identified using ultrasound, including arterial wall stretching and plaque compression, or "axial redistribution."[93–95] The contribution of vessel stretch to lumen gain following balloon angioplasty has been validated in experimental and clinical investigations. A peripheral angioplasty study reported that plaque area was reduced by 33 percent, accounting for only 20 percent of lumen gain.[89]

However, studies using automatic pullback devices have shown that "compression" actually represents redistribution of plaque along the long axis of the vessel.[95] The prognostic significance of different mechanisms of luminal enlargement remains under investigation.

DIRECTIONAL ATHERECTOMY

Directional coronary atherectomy (DCA) is currently performed relatively uncommonly. DCA devices incorporate a rotating circular blade to remove atherosclerotic plaque from the luminal surface. This process requires the inflation of a balloon within the housing of the cutter, leading to invagination of the plaque into the open window on the cutting surface.[96] Because angiographic and/or ultrasound calcification is a well-documented predictor of failure of directional atherectomy, ultrasound imaging has been advocated for guidance of atherectomy, particularly for preintervention lesion selection.[97,98] Ultrasound imaging can differentiate between superficial calcium, which predicts poor tissue retrieval, and deep calcium, which does not appear detrimental to favorable results. In 70 atherectomy patients, lesion calcification was detected by ultrasound in 63 percent, compared with 22 percent by angiography. Ultrasound-detected calcification resulted in reduced lumen gain and a smaller final lumen area.[97]

The additional spatial perspective provided by ultrasound may assist in the orientation of atherectomy cuts. However, successful application is complex because precise orientation of the ultrasound image remains difficult, relying primarily upon anatomic features such as side branches to orient the image. Repeated ultrasound examinations are sometimes performed between passes of the DCA device to determine the extent of plaque removal and the need for additional cuts. Ultrasound studies before and after directional atherectomy confirm that plaque removal is the primary mechanism of luminal enlargement[91,97] (Fig. 47-9). In 25 treated lesions, plaque reduction accounted for 78 percent of total lumen gain. Plaque area was reduced from 14.3 ± 0.8 to 10.5 ± 0.7 mm^2, whereas EEM area increased only slightly, from 16.7 ± 0.8 to 17.5 ± 0.8 mm^2, $p < 0.02$. Ultrasound studies show that despite a successful angiographic result, 40 to 60 percent of the target site is still occupied by atheroma.

Some investigators have proposed that achieving a larger lumen after atherectomy using ultrasound guidance would result in a lower restenosis rate. This hypothesis was tested in a multicenter registry (the Optimal Atherectomy Restenosis Study, or OARS) in which residual stenosis was reduced from 64 to 7 percent with ultrasound guidance.[98] The angiographic restenosis rate at 6 months was 28.9 percent and the 1-year target lesion revascularization rate was 17.8 percent. In the CAVEAT trial, DCA failed to reduce late events as compared with PTCA with or without ultrasound guidance.[99] Moreover, most atherectomy trials were performed without adjuvant therapy with GPIIb/IIIa inhibitors. It remains untested whether a larger postprocedure lumen and lower restenosis rate can be achieved using ultrasound guidance without a concomitant increase in complications.

ROTATIONAL ABLATION

Rotational ablation employs a high-speed (up to 200,000 rpm) diamond-coated burr to debulk atheroma. Theoretically, this device minimizes injury to the normal arterial wall by "differential cutting," in which normal elastic tissue is deflected away from the burr while relatively inelastic atheroma is not displaced and is therefore abraded by rotation of the burr. Clinical indications for rotational ablation include calcified segments or lesions that resist balloon dilatation. Rotational ablation is also sometimes used in long lesions, ostial lesions, and in-stent restenosis.[100-104] Demonstration of a heavily calcified vessel by angiography or ultrasound is often cited by operators as an indication for rotational ablation. However, there is a poor correlation between ultrasound and fluoroscopy in assessing the presence or extent of calcification. Accordingly, ultrasound is sometimes employed prior to rotational ablation to confirm or refute the presence of calcification. Vessels revascularized using rotational ablation are often diffusely diseased, and the "normal" dimension can be difficult to determine by angiography. Therefore, ultrasound is sometimes used to size the vessel and determine the largest burr that can be safely employed.

Intravascular ultrasound studies have confirmed the principle of selective plaque removal or differential cutting. In 48 lesions treated with rotational ablation, atheroma area decreased from 15.7 ± 4 to 13.0 ± 5 mm^2 and the arc of calcium decreased slightly from 227 ± 107 to 209 ± 107 degrees, $p < 0.05$.[104] Vessel expansion or dissection was noted in a minority of cases and did not contribute significantly to lumen gain. The residual narrowing of the cross-sectional area measured by ultrasound averaged 74 percent. Following rotational ablation, the residual lumen is usually round or ellipsoid and may have a 15 to 20

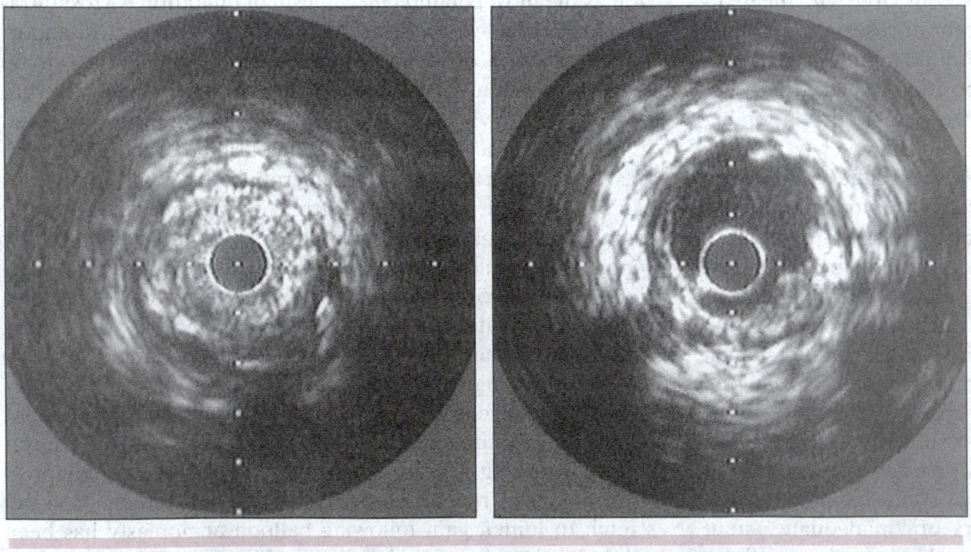

FIGURE 47-9 Directional coronary atherectomy. In the left panel, an intravascular ultrasound prior to atherectomy is shown. In the right panel, following directional atherectomy, extensive plaque removal is evident with a slightly irregular surface produced by the cutting action of the atherectomy device.

percent greater area than the largest burr used, presumably due to lateral movement of the burr during the procedure.

Luminal Measurements Postintervention

A poor correlation has been reported for comparisons of ultrasound and angiography in assessment of residual stenosis following balloon angioplasty, with measurements that are usually smaller by ultrasound than by angiography.[9,41,88–92] Two factors probably influence the overly optimistic tendency of angiographic imaging.[21] At the reference site, angiography tends to underestimate the diameter of the normal "reference" vessel because of the frequent presence of unrecognized atherosclerosis. At the target site, angiography tends to overestimate the actual gain in luminal diameter because contrast material penetrates into complex cracks and fissures produced by the intervention, giving the appearance of an enlarged lumen. To calculate a postprocedure percent diameter stenosis, the diameter at the target site (an overestimate) is divided by the reference diameter (an underestimate), resulting in a more favorable impression of the actual gain in luminal dimensions. Quantitative angiography showing a residual stenosis of 10 to 15 percent is commonly associated with a 60 to 80 percent atheroma burden.

Coronary Stent Deployment

INITIAL STUDIES OF ULTRASOUND GUIDANCE

The use of stents in percutaneous revascularization has increased exponentially over the last few years. Intravascular ultrasound imaging has played a pivotal role in understanding and optimizing the benefits of stent therapy.[105–107] In initial trials leading to FDA approval, articulated slotted-tube stents were deployed using moderate balloon pressures (6 to 10 atm).[108,109] To reduce subacute thrombosis, patients received aggressive anticoagulation with both antiplatelet and antithrombotic agents, including warfarin, for 3 to 6 months. Initial studies demonstrated a reduction in the restenosis rate compared with balloon angioplasty but reported a high incidence of hemorrhagic complications and longer hospital stays. A pioneering report detailing the intravascular ultrasound experience of Colombo et al. in Milan, Italy, significantly altered the understanding of optimal stent deployment and prevention of subacute thrombosis.[107] Ultrasound examination revealed a mean residual stenosis of 51 percent following angiographically guided stent deployment, with frequent incomplete stent apposition (Fig. 47-10).

Because stents are porous structures, angiographic contrast can flow outside of a partially deployed stent, resulting in the angiographic appearance of full deployment, despite the presence of incomplete apposition. In the Milan study, the operators performed additional balloon inflations at higher pressures (typically 18 to 20 atm) or used a larger balloon (or both), reducing final ultrasound residual stenosis to 34 percent and reporting a subacute thrombosis rate of only 0.3 percent with the use of no systemic antithrombotic agents (antiplatelet therapy only). It is now widely accepted that high-pressure deployment of the stents dramatically reduces the incidence of subacute thrombosis and obviates the need for acute and chronic administration of antithrombotic agents.[110,111] Subsequently, routine high-pressure deployment without ultrasound imaging became the standard of therapy.

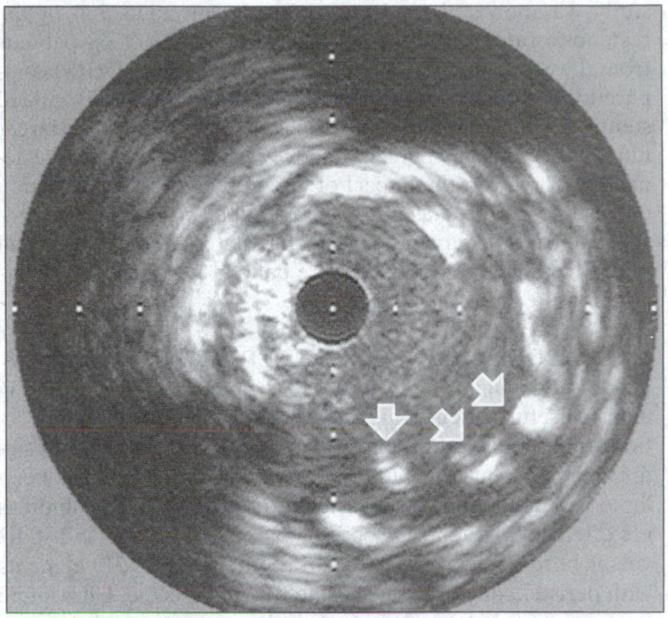

FIGURE 47-10 Underdeployed coronary stent. In this example, intravascular ultrasound images show several stent struts (*arrows*) that are not in full contact with the underlying vessel wall. This process is referred to as incomplete stent apposition.

ROUTINE VERSUS NONROUTINE ULTRASOUND

Following the widespread acceptance of high-pressure postdilatation with antiplatelet rather than anticoagulation regimens, the further benefit of ultrasound imaging has been debated.[86,110–114] Some investigators have suggested that despite routine use of high-pressure postdilatation, ultrasound-guided therapy can improve procedural results.[86,114] In a retrospective analysis of 315 lesions treated by high-pressure stenting, ultrasound was defined as "beneficial" if imaging resulted in further interventions that increased stent area by >25 percent or identified other lesions that required treatment.[115] Prior to ultrasound, the mean inflation pressure was 14.7 ± 3.2 atm, but only 47 percent of stents were considered "optimally" deployed. Additional ultrasound-triggered inflations improved in-stent lumen area by more than 25 percent in 83 lesions (26 percent of patients), and additional procedures were performed in lesions identified by ultrasound in 51 (16 percent). Final in-stent area improved from 6.9 ± 2.2 to 8.0 ± 1.93 mm² ($p < 0.001$). Procedural results were "improved" in 39 percent of the cases following ultrasound imaging.[115] It is now generally accepted that after high-pressure coronary stenting, ultrasound imaging results in additional procedures in approximately 20 to 40 percent of cases.

Since in-stent restenosis is predominantly determined by the degree of intimal hyperplasia, a larger lumen can theoretically accommodate more tissue growth without flow-limiting obstruction.[116] However, it remains uncertain whether ultrasound-guided "optimal" expansion translates into better clinical outcome. A randomized trial in 164 patients of ultrasound-guided stenting demonstrated a 6.3 percent absolute reduction in restenosis rate, which was not statistically significant because the study was powered to detect a 50 percent reduction of the restenosis rate.[117] A nonrandomized substudy of 538 patients from the Stent Anticoagulation Regimen Study (STARS) compared the outcome of ultrasound and angiographically guided stenting. The ultrasound arm achieved a significantly larger lumen area and a 39 percent relative reduction in clinical restenosis.[118] However, the impact of the more aggressive dilatation on restenosis rates has not been adequately examined by prospective trials. It remains conceivable that increased vessel wall injury from a larger high-pressure balloon will yield less favorable long-term results.

ULTRASOUND IMAGING OF PERISTENT SEGMENTS

Ultrasound imaging of "reference" segments following stenting may be useful in identifying reference segment disease or dissections that require additional interventions. The presence of significant peristent flow-limiting lesions or dissections has been linked to higher likelihood of stent thrombosis.[119] These findings are often angiographically occult or appear as areas of indistinct vessel border "haziness." In 201 stent patients, 31 segments with peristent angiographic haziness were detected. Ultrasound imaging revealed an angiographically inapparent obstructive lesion in 15, a peristent wall injury in 14, and mild intimal thickening in the remaining 2 segments.[120] The extent of neointimal hyperplasia at the stent margins has been linked to preexisting reference-segment disease.[121] In stenting as a "bailout" for dissection, intravascular ultrasound is more sensitive in detecting the extent of dissection, often revealing a greater true length than is evident from angiography, which may be helpful in guiding vessel salvage.

OPTIMAL PROCEDURAL GOALS OF ULTRASOUND GUIDED STENTING

Although ultrasound guidance of stenting has been practiced for several years, there is no consensus regarding optimal procedural end points. Colombo initially recommended achieving ≥60 percent of the average proximal and distal reference areas but later altered the definition to ≥100 percent of the distal reference lumen area.[105–107] Other definitions of optimal expansion include ≥90 percent of the distal reference area, ≥80 percent or ≥90 percent of the average reference area, a "lumen symmetry index" >0.7, and/or full coverage of reference-segment disease or dissections.[122,123] In most clinical trials, procedural end points are not achieved in the majority of cases. In the Optimal Stent Implantation Trial, the target of >90 percent of the average reference or >100 percent of the smaller reference area were not achieved in half the patients at an inflation pressure of 15 atm and only 60 percent of patients at 18 atm.[122] In the Angiography Versus Intravascular Ultrasound Directed Stent Placement (AVID) trial, the target end point of ≥90 percent of the distal reference area was not achieved in >70 percent of 225 patients.[124]

Recent reports have questioned the clinical relevance of using the stent-to-reference ratios as target for ultrasound-guided stenting. In 165 patients, target vessel revascularization was predicted by final in-stent lumen area (OR 1.4, 95 percent CI 1.1–1.9) and not the ratio of stent-to-reference area (OR 1.1, 95 percent CI 0.85–1.6).[112] Repeat revascularization was required in 30 percent of patients with a minimum in-stent lumen area <5 mm^2 but only 3 percent of cases with an area exceeding 9 mm^2. In another large cohort undergoing ultrasound-guided stenting, restenosis was inversely related to the minimum in-stent area.[125] An area of 9 mm^2 was achieved in 23 percent, but the incidence of restenosis in this subgroup was only 8 percent, compared with 29 percent in the remaining patients, $p < 0.0001$. Thus, commonly employed ultrasound end points based upon a predefined stent-to-reference ratio are both difficult to achieve and correlate weakly with clinical outcome.[125–127] Ultrasound studies have demonstrated that the degree of in-stent neointimal hyperplasia is independent of final lumen size, which may explain the higher restenosis rates in smaller vessels and poorly expanded stents.[116] If acute lumen gain is not adequate to accommodate subsequent tissue proliferation, there is significant late loss and restenosis.

Intravascular Ultrasound and Restenosis

A more complete understanding of restenosis has evolved from serial ultrasound measurements of plaque and lumen areas following balloon angioplasty and directional atherectomy.[128,129] In some studies, serial ultrasound examinations have shown that a late reduction in total vessel area (chronic negative remodeling) is an important mechanism of restenosis after interventional procedures.[129] These observations suggest that mechanical interventions to prevent chronic recoil (such as stenting) may be more important in preventing restenosis than interventions designed to prevent intimal hyperplasia. If further validated, this concept may explain the lower restenosis rate observed in randomized multicenter studies comparing balloon angioplasty and stent implantation.[108,109]

In 212 native coronary lesions in 209 patients following intervention, the ultrasound cross-sectional area with the smallest lumen area at late follow-up was compared with the matching site obtained immediately following the intervention.[129] At follow-up examination, there was a significant decrease in EEM area and an increase in plaque area ($p < 0.0001$ for both) that combined to reduce lumen area. More than 70 percent of lumen loss was attributable to the decrease in EEM area, whereas the neointimal area accounted for only 23 percent of the decrease in lumen area. The change in lumen area correlated more strongly with the change in EEM area ($r = 0.75$, $p < 0.0001$) than with the change in plaque area ($r = 0.28$, $p < 0.0001$). At lesions that demonstrated an increase in EEM area at follow-up (47 percent), there was no change or an actual gain in lumen area and a reduction in angiographic restenosis (26 versus 62 percent for lesions with a decrease in EEM area at follow-up, $p < 0.0001$).

Other investigators have suggested a bidirectional remodeling response following percutaneous coronary interventions: early adaptive enlargement and late shrinkage of the vessel. In a unique study, 61 lesions in 57 patients who underwent balloon angioplasty or atherectomy were examined by intravascular ultrasound in a serial manner—before and immediately after the intervention and after 24 h, 1 month, and 6 months.[48] The lumen area significantly improved during the first month following the intervention but significantly decreased at 6 months. Simultaneously, the EEM area increased in the first month but later decreased at 6 months. However, plaque area steadily increased from immediately postintervention to the 6-month follow-up. Thus the changes in lumen size closely tracked the changes in EEM area ($r = 0.72$, $p = 0.0001$). Although the increase in plaque area correlated with lumen loss, the correlation was not as strong ($r = 0.34$, $p = 0.0008$). The lumen gain observed during the first month was solely due to the compensatory vessel enlargement, whereas the late lumen loss was mostly caused by vessel shrinkage but also by progressive neointimal hyperplasia.

Investigations employing quantitative angiography have demonstrated that late lumen loss is significantly greater with stents than with balloon angioplasty. This, however, is offset by the much larger acute lumen gain, such that the net gain at follow-up is significantly greater with stenting.[108,109] Intravascular ultrasound has been employed to examine the mechanism of stent restenosis. Unlike the restenotic response to other percutaneous devices, which is a mixture of arterial remodeling and neointimal growth, stent restenosis is almost exclusively due to the neointimal proliferation.[129] In a serial study using intravascular ultrasound of stented coronary segments, there was no significant change in the area bound by stent struts, indicating that stents can withstand and resist the arterial remodeling process.[130] In some cases, restenosis develops at the margins of the stent. Predictors of stent restenosis have been identified by multivariate analysis, including the smaller reference vessel and lumen size, the larger plaque burden at the reference segments, and the smaller achieved in-stent lumen area at the stent margins.[121]

FUTURE DIRECTIONS

The technology and clinical role for intravascular ultrasound examination of the coronaries continues to evolve. Technological advances in intravascular imaging are anticipated, including further reductions in the size of imaging catheters and higher-frequency ultrasound catheters, yielding significantly better spatial resolution.[131,132] Although high-frequency probes enable better axial and lateral resolution, there are significant trade-offs in moving beyond the current 30-MHz frequency. For example, penetration is likely to be impaired in comparison with more conventional devices, and greater backscatter from blood cells at high frequencies may interfere with discrimination of the interface between lumen and vessel wall. However, if catheter miniaturization continues, a shorter wavelength will be important in preserving near-field image quality. It remains apparent that the physical limits of intravascular imaging technology have not been reached. Accordingly, further improvements in the performance of these devices are anticipated.

Analysis of backscattered ultrasound signals has been used by several investigators to perform "tissue characterization" of coronary plaques. Intrinsic characteristics of the backscattered ultrasound signals—including the amplitude distribution, frequency response, and power spectrum of the signal—convey specific information about tissue types.[133] Soft plaque consists of an amorphous collection of lipid substances, fibrosis, cholesterol clefts, and a variable amount of collagen and elastin. Thrombus, on the other hand, consists of a fairly organized layering of fibrous strands packed with a dense collection of red blood cells. The ability of computer-based analysis of the unprocessed radiofrequency backscatter to differentiate the histologic layers of the normal vessel wall remains investigational.

Three-dimensional reconstruction of intravascular ultrasound has been proposed as a means to facilitate understanding of the spatial relationship between the structures within different tomographic cross sections.[134] Despite the promise of these methods, many unresolved problems remain. The algorithms applied for 3D reconstruction do not consider the presence of curvatures of the vessel and assume that the catheter passes in a straight line through the center of consecutive cross sections. The systolic expansion of the coronary vessel and the movements of the catheter within the vessel during the cardiac cycle also generate artifacts. Accordingly, the reconstructed images should not be considered faithful representations of the vessel and should not be used for volumetric plaque determination. Simultaneous digitization of biplane fluoroscopic tracking of the radiopaque transducer and catheter tip has the potential to overcome some of these limitations, but is practical only for small-scale research purposes.[135]

SUMMARY

The equipment, technique, and applications for intravascular ultrasound imaging continue to evolve, finding increasingly common usage in clinical practice and research. The insights provided by the unique ability of intravascular ultrasound to directly image coronary plaques have contributed greatly to our understanding of the nature of atherosclerosis and the effects of interventional devices.

References

1. Bom N, Lancee CT, Van Egmond FC. An ultrasonic intracardiac scanner. *Ultrasonics* 1972; 10:72–76.
2. Yock PG, Johnson EL, Linker DT. Intravascular ultrasound: Development and clinical potential. *Am J Cardiac Imaging* 1988; 2:185–193.
3. Roelandt JR, Bom NY, Serruys PW. Intravascular high-resolution real-time, two-dimensional echocardiography. *Int J Cardiac Imaging* 1989; 4:63–67.
4. Hodgson JM, Graham SP, Savakus AD, et al. Clinical percutaneous imaging of coronary anatomy using an over-the-wire ultrasound catheter system. *Int J Cardiac Imaging* 1989; 4:187–193.
5. Nissen SE, Grines CL, Gurley JC, et al. Application of a new phased-array ultrasound imaging catheter in the assessment of vascular dimensions: In vivo comparison to cineangiography. *Circulation* 1990; 81:660–666.
6. Tobis JM, Mallery J, Mahon D, et al. Intravascular ultrasound imaging of human coronary arteries in vivo. *Circulation* 1991; 83:913–926.
7. Nissen SE, Gurley JC, Grines CL, et al. Intravascular ultrasound assessment of lumen size and wall morphology in normal subjects and patients with coronary artery disease. *Circulation* 1991; 84:1087–1099.
8. Nissen SE, Di Mario C, Tuzcu EM. Intravascular ultrasound, angioscopy, doppler, and pressure measurement. In: *Topol Cardiovascular Medicine*. Philadelphia: Lippincott-Raven Publishers; 1997.
9. Tobis JM, Mallery JA, Gessert J, et al. Intravascular ultrasound cross-sectional arterial imaging before and after balloon angioplasty in vitro. *Circulation* 1989; 80:873–882.
10. Topol EJ, Nissen SE. Our preoccupation with coronary luminology: The dissociation between clinical and angiographic findings in ischemic heart disease. *Circulation* 1995; 92:2333–2342.
11. Hodgson JM, Reddy KG, Suneja R, et al. Intracoronary ultrasound imaging: Correlation of plaque morphology with angiography, clinical syndrome and procedural results in patients undergoing coronary angioplasty. *J Am Coll Cardiol* 1993; 21:35–44.
12. Arnett EN, Isner JM, Redwood CR, et al. Coronary artery narrowing in coronary heart disease: Comparison of cineangiographic and necropsy findings. *Ann Intern Med* 1979; 91:350–356.

13. Grodin CM, Dydra I, Pastgernac A, et al. Discrepancies between cineangiographic and post-mortem findings in patients with coronary artery disease and recent myocardial revascularization. *Circulation* 1974; 49:703–709.
14. Isner JM, Kishel J, Kent KM. Accuracy of angiographic determination of left main coronary arterial narrowing. *Circulation* 1981; 63:1056–1061.
15. Vlodaver Z, Frech R, van Tassel RA, Edwards JE. Correlation of the antemortem coronary angiogram and the postmortem specimen. *Circulation* 1973; 47:162–168.
16. Zir LM, Miller SW, Dinsmore RE, et al. Interobserver variability in coronary angiography. *Circulation* 1976; 53:627–632.
17. Galbraith JE, Murphy ML, Desoyza N. Coronary angiogram interpretation: Interobserver variability. *JAMA* 1981; 240:2053–2059.
18. Roberts WC, Jones AA. Quantitation of coronary arterial narrowing at necropsy in sudden coronary death. *Am J Cardiol* 1979; 44:39–44.
19. White CW, Wright CB, Doty DB, et al. Does visual interpretation of the coronary arteriogram predict the physiologic importance of a coronary stenosis? *N Engl J Med* 1984; 310:819–824.
20. Waller BF. "Crackers, breakers, stretchers, drillers, scrapers, shavers, burners, welders, and melters": The future treatment of atherosclerotic coronary artery disease? A clinical-morphologic assessment. *J Am Coll Cardiol* 1989; 13:969–987.
21. Topol EJ, Nissen SE. Our preoccupation with coronary luminology: The dissociation between clinical and angiographic findings in ischemic heart disease. *Circulation* 1995; 92:2333–2342.
22. Glagov S, Weisenberg E, Zarins CK, et al. Compensatory enlargement of human coronary arteries. *N Engl J Med* 1987; 316:1371–1375.
23. Little WC, Constantinescu M, Applegate RJ, et al. Can arteriography predict the site of a subsequent myocardial infarction in patients with mild-to-moderate coronary artery disease? *Circulation* 1988; 78:1157–1166.
24. Yamagishi M, Miyatake K, Tamai J, et al. Detection of atherosclerosis at the site of focal vasospasm in angiographically normal or minimally narrowed coronary segments by intravascular ultrasound. *J Am Coll Cardiol* 1994; 23:352–357.
25. Nissen SE, Gurley JC. Application of intravascular ultrasound to detection and quantitation of coronary atherosclerosis. *Int J Cardiac Imaging* 1991; 6:165–177.
26. Nissen SE, DeFranco A, Tuzcu EM. Detection and quantification of atherosclerosis: The emerging role for intravascular ultrasound. In: Fuster V, ed., *Syndromes of Atherosclerosis: Correlations of Clinical Imaging and Pathology*. Armonk, NY; Futura; 1996:291.
27. TenHoff H, Korbijn A, Smit ThH, et al. Image artifacts in mechanically driven ultrasound catheters. *Int J Cardiac Imaging* 1989; 4:195–199.
28. Di Mario C, Madretsma S, Linker D, et al. The angle of incidence of the ultrasonic beam: A critical factor for the image quality in intravascular ultrasonography. *Am Heart J* 1993; 125: 442–448.
29. Hausmann D, Erbel R, Alibelli-Chemarin MJ, et al. The safety of intracoronary ultrasound: A multicenter survey of 2207 examinations. *Circulation* 1995; 91:623–630.
30. Batkoff BW, Linker DT. Safety of intracoronary ultrasound: Data from a multicenter European registry. *Cathet Cardiovasc Diagn* 1996; 38:238–241.
31. Pinto FJ, St Goar FG, Gao SZ, et al. Immediate and one-year safety of intracoronary ultrasonic imaging: Evaluation with serial quantitative angiography. *Circulation* 1993; 88:1709–1714.
32. Gussenhoven EJ, Essed CE, Lancee CT, et al. Arterial wall characteristics determined by intravascular ultrasound imaging: An in vitro study. *J Am Coll Cardiol* 1989; 4:947–952.
33. Potkin BN, Bartorelli AL, Gessert JM, et al. Coronary artery imaging with intravascular high-frequency ultrasound. *Circulation* 1990; 81:1575–1585.
34. Nishimura RA, Edwards WD, Warnes CA, et al. Intravascular ultrasound imaging: In vitro validation and pathologic correlation. *J Am Coll Cardiol* 1990; 16:145–154.
35. Fitzgerald PJ, St Goar FG, Connolly AJ, et al. Intravascular ultrasound imaging of coronary arteries: Are three layers the norm? *Circulation* 1992; 86:154–158.
36. St Goar FG, Pinto FJ, Alderman EL, et al. Intravascular ultrasound imaging of angiographically normal coronary arteries: An in vivo comparison with quantitative angiography. *J Am Coll Cardiol* 1991; 18:952–958.
37. Velican D, Velican C. Comparative study on age-related changes and atherosclerotic involvement of the coronary arteries of male and female subjects up to 40 years of age. *Atherosclerosis* 1981; 38:39–50.
38. Maheswaran B, Leung CY, Gutfinger DE, et al. Intravascular ultrasound appearance of normal and mildly diseased coronary arteries: Correlation with histologic specimens. *Am Heart J* 1995; 130:976–986.
39. Mintz GS, Popma JJ, Pichard AD, et al. Patterns of calcification in coronary artery disease: A statistical analysis of intravascular ultrasound and coronary angiography in 1,155 lesions. *Circulation* 1995; 91:1959–1965.
40. Tuzcu EM, Berkalp B, DeFranco AC, et al. The dilemma of diagnosing coronary calcification: Angiography versus intravascular ultrasound. *J Am Coll Cardiol* 1996; 27:832–838.
41. Honye J, Mahon DJ, Jain A, et al. Morphological effects of coronary balloon angioplasty in vivo assessed by intravascular ultrasound imaging. *Circulation* 1992; 85:1012–1025.
42. Mintz GS, Pichard AD, Kovach JA, et al. Impact of preintervention intravascular ultrasound imaging on transcatheter treatment strategies in coronary artery disease. *Am J Cardiol* 1994; 73:423–430.
43. Hermiller JB, Tenaglia AN, Kisslo KB, et al. In vivo validation of compensatory enlargement of atherosclerotic coronary arteries. *Am J Cardiol* 1993; 71:665–668.
44. Ge J, Erbel R., Zamorano J, et al. Coronary artery remodeling in atherosclerotic disease: An intravascular ultrasonic study in vivo. *Coron Artery Dis* 1993; 4:981–986.
45. Losordo DW, Rosenfield K, Kaufman J, et al. Focal compensatory enlargement of human arteries in response to progressive atherosclerosis: In vivo documentation using intravascular ultrasound. *Circulation* 1994; 89:2570–2577.
46. Pasterkamp G, Wensing PJ, Post MJ, et al. Paradoxical arterial wall shrinkage may contribute to luminal narrowing of human atherosclerotic femoral arteries. *Circulation* 1995; 91:1444–1449.
47. Mintz GS, Kent KM, Pichard AD, et al. Contribution of inadequate arterial remodeling to the development of focal coronary artery stenoses: An intravascular ultrasound study. *Circulation* 1997; 95:1791–1798.
48. Kimura T, Kaburagi S, Tamura T, et al. Remodeling of human coronary arteries undergoing coronary angioplasty or atherectomy. *Circulation* 1997; 96:475–483.
49. Richardson PD, Davies MJ, Born GV. Influence of plaque configuration and stress distribution on fissuring of coronary atherosclerotic plaques. *Lancet* 1989; 2:941–944.
50. Kalbfleisch SJ, McGillem MJ, Simon SB, et al. Automated quantitation of indexes of coronary lesion complexity: Comparison between patients with stable and unstable angina. *Circulation* 1990; 82:439–447.
51. Ambrose JA, Winters SL, Arora RR, et al. Angiographic evolution of coronary artery morphology in unstable angina. *J Am Coll Cardiol* 1986; 7:472–478.
52. Loree HM, Kamm RD, Stringfellow RG, Lee RT. Effects of fibrous cap thickness on peak circumferential stress in model atherosclerotic vessels. *Circ Res* 1992; 71:850–858.

53. Levin DC, Fallon JT. Significance of the angiographic morphology of localized coronary stenoses: Histopathologic correlations. *Circulation* 1982; 66:316–320.
54. Ambrose JA, Winters SL, Stern A, et al. Angiographic morphology and the pathogenesis of unstable angina pectoris. *J Am Coll Cardiol* 1985; 5:609–616.
55. Shoenhagen P, Ziada KM, Kapadia SR, et al. Extent and direction of arterial remodeling in stable versus unstable coronary syndromes: An intravascular ultrasound study. *Circulation* 2000; 101:598–603.
56. Siegel RJ, Ariani M, Fishbein MC, et al. Histopathologic validation of angioscopy and intravascular ultrasound. *Circulation* 1991; 84:109–117.
57. Kearney P, Erbel R, Rupprecht HJ, et al. Differences in the morphology of unstable and stable coronary lesions and their impact on the mechanisms of angioplasty: An in vivo study with intravascular ultrasound. *Eur Heart J* 1996; 17:721–730.
58. Bocksch W, Schartl M, Beckmann S, et al. Intravascular ultrasound imaging in patients with acute myocardial infarction. *Eur Heart J* 1995; 16(suppl J):46–52.
59. Bridal SL, Fornes P, Bruneval P, Berger G. Parametric (integrated backscatter and attenuation) images constructed using backscattered radio frequency signals (25–56 MHz) from human aortae in vitro. *Ultrasound Med Biol* 1997; 23:215–229.
60. Hiro T, Leung CY, Karimi H, et al. Angle dependence of intravascular ultrasound imaging and its feasibility in tissue characterization of human atherosclerotic tissue. *Am Heart J* 1999; 137:476–481.
61. Wong M, Edelstein J, Wollman J, Bond MG. Ultrasonic-pathological comparison of the human arterial wall: Verification of intima-media thickness. *Arterioscler Thromb* 1993; 13:482–486.
62. Potkin BN, Bartorelli AL, Gessert JM, et al. Coronary artery imaging with intravascular high-frequency ultrasound. *Circulation* 1990; 81:1575–1585.
63. Tuzcu EM, Hobbs H, Rincon G, et al. Occult and frequent transmission of atherosclerosis coronary disease with cardiac transplantation. *Circulation* 1995; 91:1706–1713.
64. Mehra MR, Ventura HO, Stapleton DD, Smart FW. The prognostic significance of intimal proliferation in cardiac allograft vasculopathy: A paradigm shift (review). *J Heart Lung Transplant* 1995; 14:6 Pt. 2, S207–S211.
65. Escobar A, Ventura HO, Stapleton DD, et al. Cardiac allograft vasculopathy assessed by intravascular ultrasonography and nonimmunologic risk factors. *Am J Cardiol* 1994; 74: 1042–1046.
66. Rickenbacher PR, Pinto FJ, Chenzbraun A, et al. Incidence and severity of transplant coronary artery disease early and up to 15 years after transplantation as detected by intravascular ultrasound. *J Am Coll Cardiol* 1995; 25:171–177.
67. Tuzcu EM. DeFranco AC, Goormastic M, et al. Dichotomous pattern of coronary atherosclerosis 1 to 9 years after transplantation: Insights from systematic intravascular ultrasound imaging. *J Am Coll Cardiol* 1996; 27:839–846.
68. Gil R, von Birgelen C, Prati F, et al. Usefulness of three-dimensional reconstruction for interpretation and quantitative analysis of intracoronary ultrasound during stent deployment. *Am J Cardiol* 1996; 77:761–764.
69. Mintz GS, Popma JJ, Pichard AD, et al. Limitations of angiography in the assessment of plaque distribution in coronary artery disease: A systematic study of target lesion eccentricity in 1446 lesions. *Circulation* 1996; 93:924–931.
70. Erbel R, Ge J, Bockisch A, et al. Value of intracoronary ultrasound and Doppler in the differentiation of angiographically normal coronary arteries: A prospective study in patients with angina pectoris. *Eur Heart J* 1996; 17:880–889.
71. Mintz GS, Painter JA, Pichard AD, et al. Atherosclerosis in angiographically "normal" coronary artery reference segments: An intravascular ultrasound study with clinical correlations. *J Am Coll Cardiol* 1995; 25:1479–1485.
72. Lee DY, Eigler N, Luo H, et al. Effect of intracoronary ultrasound imaging on clinical decision making. *Am Heart J* 1995; 129:1084–1093.
73. Mintz GS, Pichard AD, Kovach JA, et al. Impact of preintervention intravascular ultrasound imaging on transcatheter treatment strategies in coronary artery disease. *Am J Cardiol* 1994; 73:423–430.
74. Hermiller JB, Buller CE, Tenaglia AN, et al. Unrecognized left main coronary artery disease in patients undergoing interventional procedures. *Am J Cardiol* 1993; 71:173–176.
75. Uretsky BF, Kormos RL, Zerbe TR, et al. Cardiac events after heart transplantation: Incidence and predictive value of coronary arteriography. *J Heart Transplant* 1992; 11:S45–S50.
76. O'Neill BJ, Pflugfelder PW, Single NR, et al. Frequency of angiographic detection and quantitative assessment of coronary arterial disease one and three years after cardiac transplantation. *Am J Cardiol* 1989; 63:1221–1226.
77. Dressler FA, Miller LW. Necropsy versus angiography: How accurate is angiography? *J Heart Lung Transplant* 1992; 11(part2):S56–S59.
78. Johnson DE, Alderman EL, Schroeder JS, et al. Transplant coronary artery disease: Histopathological correlations with angiographic morphology. *J Am Coll Cardiol* 1991; 17:449–457.
79. Yeung AC, Davis SF, Hauptman PJ, et al. Incidence and progression of transplant coronary artery disease over 1 year: Results of a multicenter trial with use of intravascular ultrasound. Multicenter Intravascular Ultrasound Transplant Study Group. *J Heart Lung Transplant* 1995; 14:6, S215–S220.
80. Kerber S, Rahmel A, Heinemann-Vechtel O, et al. Angiographic, intravascular ultrasound and functional findings early after orthotopic heart transplantation. *Int J Cardiol* 1995; 49:119–129.
81. St Goar FG, Pinto FJ, Alderman EL, et al. Detection of coronary atherosclerosis in young adult hearts using intravascular ultrasound. *Circulation* 1992; 86:756–763.
82. Kapadia SR, Nissen SE, Ziada KM, et al. Development of transplant vasculopathy and progression of donor-transmitted atherosclerosis: A comparison by serial intravascular ultrasound imaging. *Circulation* 1998; 98:2672–2678.
83. Kapadia SR, Crowe TD, Ziada KM, et al. Natural history of donor transmitted atherosclerosis in transplant patients: Serial intravascular ultrasound study. *J Am Coll Cardiol* 1998; 31:856–862.
84. Impact of intravascular ultrasound on device selection and endpoint assessment of interventions: Phase I of the GUIDE trial (abstr). *J Am Coll Cardiol* 1993; 21:134A.
85. Hoffmann R, Mintz GS, Popma JJ, et al. Treatment of calcified coronary lesions with Palmaz-Schatz stents: An intravascular ultrasound study. *Eur Heart J* 1998; 19:1224–1231.
86. Russo RJ. Ultrasound-guided stent placement. *Cardiol Clin* 1997; 15:49–61.
87. Stone GW, Hodgson JM, St Goar FG, et al. Improved procedural results of coronary angioplasty with intravascular ultrasound-guided balloon sizing: The CLOUT pilot trial: Clinical Outcomes with Ultrasound Trial (CLOUT) investigators. *Circulation* 1997; 95:2044–2052.
88. Gil R, Di Mario C, Prati F, et al. Influence of plaque composition on mechanisms of percutaneous transluminal coronary balloon angioplasty assessed by ultrasound imaging. *Am Heart J* 1996; 131:591–597.
89. Losordo DW, Rosenfield K, Pieczek A, et al. How does angioplasty work? Serial analysis of human iliac arteries using intravascular ultrasound. *Circulation* 1992; 86:1845–1858.
90. Potkin BN, Keren G, Mintz GS, et al. Arterial responses to balloon coronary angioplasty: An intravascular ultrasound study. *J Am Coll Cardiol* 1992; 20:942–951.

91. Braden GA, Herrington DM, Downes TR, et al. Qualitative and quantitative contrasts in the mechanisms of lumen enlargement by coronary balloon angioplasty and directional coronary atherectomy. *J Am Coll Cardiol* 1994; 23:40–48.
92. van der Lugt A, Gussenhoven EJ, Stijnen T, et al. Comparison of intravascular ultrasonic findings after coronary balloon angioplasty evaluated in vitro with histology. *Am J Cardiol* 1995; 76:661–666.
93. Mintz GS, Pichard AD, Kent KM, et al. Axial plaque redistribution as a mechanism of percutaneous transluminal coronary angioplasty. *Am J Cardiol* 1996; 77:427–430.
94. Botas J, Clark DA, Pinto F, et al. Balloon angioplasty results in increased segmental coronary distensibility: A likely mechanism of percutaneous transluminal coronary angioplasty. *J Am Coll Cardiol* 1994; 23:1043–1052.
95. Mintz GS, Pichard AD, Kent KM, et al. Axial plaque redistribution as a mechanism of percutaneous transluminal coronary angioplasty. *Am J Cardiol* 1996; 77:427–430.
96. Simpson JB, Selmon MR, Robertson GC, et al.Transluminal atherectomy for occlusive peripheral vascular disease. *Am J Cardiol* 1988; 61:96G–101G.
97. Matar FA, Mintz GS, Pinnow E, et al. Multivariate predictors of intravascular ultrasound end points after directional coronary atherectomy. *J Am Coll Cardiol* 1995; 25:318–324.
98. Simonton CA, Leon MB. Baim DS, et al. "Optimal" directional coronary atherectomy: Final results of the Optimal Atherectomy Restenosis Study (OARS). *Circulation* 1998; 97:332–339.
99. Topol EJ, Leya F, Pinkerton CA, et al., on behalf of the CAVEAT Study Group. A comparison of coronary angioplasty with directional atherectomy in patients with coronary artery disease. *N Engl J Med* 1993; 329:221–227.
100. MacIsaac AI, Bass TA, Buchbinder M, et al. High speed rotational atherectomy: Outcome in calcified and noncalcified coronary artery lesions. *J Am Coll Cardiol* 1995; 26:731–736.
101. De Franco AC, Nissen SE, Tuzcu EM, Whitlow PL. Incremental value of intravascular ultrasound during rotational coronary atherectomy. *Cathet Cardiovasc Diagn* 1996; (suppl. 3): 23–33.
102. Sharma SK, Duvvuri S, Dangas G, et al. Rotational atherectomy for in-stent restenosis: Acute and long-term results of the first 100 cases. *J Am Coll Cardiol* 1998; 32:1358–1365.
103. Schiele F, Meneveau N, Vuillemenot A, et al. Treatment of in-stent restenosis with high speed rotational atherectomy and IVUS guidance in small 3.0 mm vessels. *Cathet Cardiovasc Diagn* 1998; 44:77–82.
104. Kovach JA, Mintz GS, Pichard AD, et al. Sequential intravascular ultrasound characterization of the mechanisms of rotational atherectomy and adjunct balloon angioplasty. *J Am Coll Cardiol* 1993; 22:1024–1032.
105. Nakamura S, Colombo A, Galglione S, et al. Intracoronary ultrasound observations during stent implantation. *Circulation* 1994; 89:2026–2034.
106. Goldberg SL, Colombo A, Nakamura S, et al. Benefit of intracoronary ultrasound in the deployment of Palmaz-Schatz stents. *J Am Coll Cardiol* 1994; 24:996–1003.
107. Colombo A, Hall P, Nakamura S, et al. Intracoronary stenting without anticoagulation accomplished with intravascular ultrasound guidance. *Circulation* 1995; 91:1676–1688.
108. Serruys PW, de Jaegere P, Kiemeneij F, et al., on behalf of the Benestent Study Group. A comparison of balloon-expandable-stent implantation with balloon angioplasty in patients with coronary artery disease. *N Engl J Med* 1994; 331:489–495.
109. Fischman DL, Leon MB, Baim DS, et al. A randomized comparison of coronary-stent placement and balloon angioplasty in the treatment of coronary artery disease. *N Engl J Med* 1994; 331:496–501.
110. Morice MC, Breton C, Bunouf P, et al. Coronary stenting without anticoagulation, without intravascular ultrasound: Results of the French registry. *Circulation* 1995; 92(suppl I):I-796.
111. Sandardas MA, McEniery PT, Aroney CN, Bett JHN. Elective implantation of intracoronary stents without intravascular ultrasound guidance or subsequent warfarin. *Cathet Cardiovasc Diagn* 1996; 37:355–359.
112. Goods CM, Al-Shaibi KF, Yadav SS, et al. Utilization of the coronary balloon-expandable coil stent without anticoagulation or intravascular ultrasound. *Circulation* 1996; 93:1803–1808.
113. Karrillon GJ, Morice MC, Benveniste E, et al. Intracoronary stent implantation without ultrasound guidance and with replacement of conventional anticoagulation by antiplatelet therapy. 30-day clinical outcome of the French Multicenter Registry. *Circulation* 1996; 94:1519–1527.
114. Prati F, Gil R, Di Mario C, et al. Is quantitative angiography sufficient to guide stent implantation? A comparison with three-dimensional reconstruction of intracoronary ultrasound images. *G Ital Cardiol* 1997; 27:328–336.
115. Allen KM, Undemir C, Shaknovich A, et al. Is there need for intravascular ultrasound after high pressure dilatation of Palmaz-Schatz stents (abstr). *J Am Coll Cardiol* 1996; 27:138A.
116. Hoffmann R, Mintz GS, Pichard AD, et al. Intimal hyperplasia thickness at follow-up is independent of stent size: A serial intravascular ultrasound study. *Am J Cardiol* 1998; 82:1168–1172.
117. Schiele F, Meneveau N, Vuillemenot A, et al. Impact of intravascular ultrasound guidance in stent deployment on 6-month restenosis rate: A multicenter, randomized study comparing two strategies—with and without intravascular ultrasound guidance. RESIST Study Group (REStenosis after Ivus guided STenting). *J Am Coll Cardiol* 1998; 32:320–328.
118. Fitzgerald PJ, Hayase M, Mintz GS, et al. CRUISE: Can routine intravascular ultrasound influence stent expansion? Analysis of outcomes. *J Am Coll Cardiol* 1998; 31:396A.
119. Schuhlen H, Hadamitzky M, Walter H, et al. Major benefit from antiplatelet therapy for patients at high risk for adverse cardiac events after coronary Palmaz-Schatz stent placement: Analysis of a prospective risk stratification protocol in the Intracoronary Stenting and Antithrombotic Regimen (ISAR) trial. *Circulation* 1997; 95:2015–2021.
120. Ziada KM, Tuzcu EM, De Franco AC, et al. Intravascular ultrasound assessment of the prevalence and causes of angiographic "haziness" following high-pressure coronary stenting. *Am J Cardiol* 1997; 80:116–121.
121. Hoffmann R, Mintz GS, Kent KM, et al. Serial intravascular ultrasound predictors of restenosis at the margins of Palmaz-Schatz stents. *Am J Cardiol* 1997; 79:951–953.
122. de Jaegere P, Mudra H, Figulla H, et al. Intravascular ultrasound-guided optimized stent deployment: Immediate and 6 months clinical and angiographic results from the Multicenter Ultrasound Stenting in Coronaries Study (MUSIC Study). *Eur Heart J* 1998; 19:1214–1223.
123. Stone GW, St Goar F, Fitzgerald P, et al. The Optimal Stent Implantation Trial: Final core lab angiographic and ultrasound analysis (abstr). *J Am Coll Cardiol* 1997; 29:369A.
124. Russo RJ, Nicosia A, Teirstein PS, Investigators AVID. Angiography versus intravascular ultrasound-directed stent placement. *J Am Coll Cardiol* 1997; 29:369A.
125. Kasaoka S, Tobis JM, Akiyama T, et al. Angiographic and intravascular ultrasound predictors of in-stent restenosis. *J Am Coll Cardiol* 1998; 32:1630–1635.
126. Ziada KM, Tuzcu EM, De Franco AC, et al. Absolute, not relative, post-stent lumen area is a better predictor of clinical events (abstr). *Circulation* 1996; 94:I-453.
127. Moussa I, Di Mario C, Moses J, et al. The predictive value of different intravascular ultrasound criteria for restenosis after coronary stenting (abstr). *J Am Coll Cardiol* 1997; 29:60A.
128. Mintz GS, Popma JJ, Pichard AD, et al. Intravascular ultrasound

predictors of restenosis after percutaneous transcatheter coronary revascularization. *J Am Coll Cardiol* 1996; 27:1678–1687.

129. Mintz GS, Popma JJ, Pichard AD, et al. Arterial remodeling after coronary angioplasty: A serial intravascular ultrasound study. *Circulation* 1996; 94:35–43.
130. Painter JA, Mintz GS, Wong SC, et al. Serial intravascular ultrasound studies fail to show evidence of chronic Palmaz-Schatz stent recoil. *Am J Cardiol* 1995; 75:398–400.
131. Lockwood GR, Ryan LK, Foster FS. A 45 to 55 MHz needle-based ultrasound system for invasive imaging. *Ultrason Imaging* 1993; 15:1–13.
132. Foster FS, Knapik DA, Machado JC, et al. High-frequency intracoronary ultrasound imaging. *Semin Intervent Cardiol* 1997; 2:33–41.
133. Linker DT, Kleven A, Gronningsaether A, et al. Tissue characterization with intra-arterial ultrasound: Special promise and problems. *Int J Cardiol Imaging* 1991; 6:255–263.
134. von Birgelen C, de Vrey EA, Mintz GS, et al. ECG-gated three-dimensional intravascular ultrasound: Feasibility and reproducibility of the automated analysis of coronary lumen and atherosclerotic plaque dimensions in humans. *Circulation* 1997; 96:2944–2952.
135. Evans JL, Ng KH, Wiet SG, et al. Accurate three-dimensional reconstruction of intravascular ultrasound data: Spatially correct three-dimensional reconstructions. *Circulation* 1996; 93:567–576.

CHAPTER 48

CORONARY BYPASS SURGERY

Bruce W. Lytle

Coronary bypass surgery as a planned consistent approach for the treatment of patients with angiographically documented coronary atherosclerosis was begun by Sones, Favaloro, and colleagues in 1967. Many previous schemes for surgical myocardial revascularization, direct and indirect, had been attempted, including pericardial pouderage, mammary artery implantation (Vineberg operation), coronary endarterectomy, and "blind" bypass grafting without the angiographic definition of coronary lesions.[1,2] The concept behind the concerted effort undertaken by cardiologists and cardiac surgeons at The Cleveland Clinic Foundation in 1967 was that the symptoms and clinical events associated with coronary artery disease (CAD) were related to stenotic coronary artery lesions that could be specifically identified by coronary angiography, and if those lesions could be treated with bypass grafting, unfavorable symptoms and events would be less common. Experience has shown that concept to be correct but also has shown that atherosclerosis is a progressive disease.

In the early years of coronary bypass grafting, the vast majority of grafts were reversed segments of saphenous vein anastomosed to the aorta and to the coronary arteries distal to coronary stenoses (Fig. 48-1*A*). It was rapidly obvious that effective bypass surgery relieved symptoms of angina, and during the decade 1970–1980, the practice of coronary artery surgery exploded. Improvements in instrumentation, technology, and surgical training were rapid, and by 1980, bypass surgery had evolved into a microsurgical procedure usually performed with optical assistance at many hundreds of medical centers around the world.

EARLY RANDOMIZED TRIALS OF BYPASS SURGERY VERSUS MEDICAL TREATMENT

During the 1970s, multiple investigations were initiated to examine the long-term outcomes of patients receiving initial bypass grafting compared with those treated initially with medical management. The most influential were multicenter, randomized trials of patients with chronic stable angina: the Veteran's Administration study of patients with chronic stable angina (VA study),[3] the European Coronary Surgery Study (ECSS),[4] and the Coronary Artery Surgery Study (CASS).[5,6] These trials randomized patients with angiographically documented coronary stenoses to either initial medical management or initial treatment with bypass surgery, and their primary emphasis was survival. In the two largest trials (ECSS and CASS), severely symptomatic patients were excluded from randomization, and in all these trials, patients who experienced the onset or persistence of severe symptoms were allowed to change from medical to surgical treatment, a phenomenon called *crossover*. Analyses of outcomes were performed on an "intention to treat" basis. That is, patients who were randomized to the medical treatment group but who later decided to have surgery were still considered part of the medically treated group, and patients randomized to surgery who did not actually receive surgery were still considered part of the surgically treated group.

All these trials showed there were some patient subsets that experienced a higher survival rate if they received initial surgical management rather than initial medical treatment, although those subsets varied among the trials. Not surprisingly, the patients who benefited the most from surgery in terms of survival were patients at the highest risk of death without operation. Individual trials noted improved survival rates for patients with significant left main stenosis, three-vessel disease with abnormal left ventricular (LV) function, and two- or three-vessel disease with a more than 75 percent stenosis in the proximal left anterior descending (LAD) coronary artery. The clinical descriptors of an abnormal baseline electrocardiogram (ECG) or a strongly positive exercise test helped to define patient subsets with improved survival rates with surgery. Recently, a metaanalysis that included the three major trials and some smaller ones

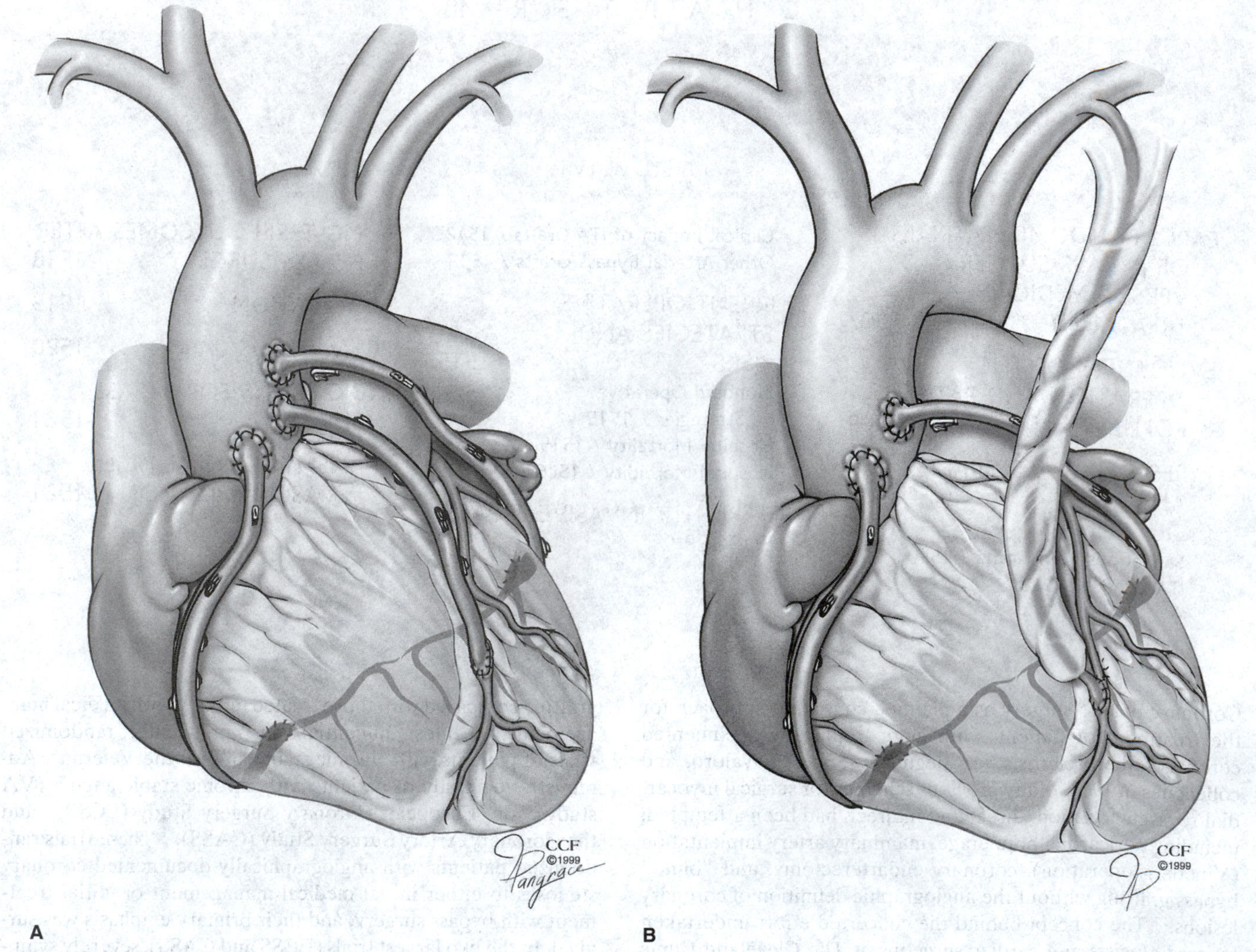

FIGURE 48-1 *A.* Most early coronary bypass operations involved only aorta to coronary saphenous vein grafts. *B.* The use of a left ITA to LAD artery graft improves clinical outcomes, and combining this strategy with vein grafts to other coronary arteries has become the standard bypass operation.

confirmed the observations of the individual trials but also seemed to show a significant survival benefit for patients with triple-, double-, or even single-vessel disease that included a proximal LAD stenosis regardless of whether they had normal or abnormal LV function. For patients without a proximal LAD stenosis, surgery improved the survival rate for only patients with left main stenosis or triple-vessel disease. In addition, the surgically treated patients had fewer symptoms at 5 postoperative years and took fewer antianginal medications.

The degree of benefit achieved with initial bypass surgery diminished with time both in terms of survival and with regard to symptom status.[8] There were multiple reasons for this. First, the status of the surgically treated patients deteriorated based on late graft failure and the progression of native vessel atherosclerosis. Very few patients in these early trials received internal thoracic artery (ITA) grafts or were treated with platelet inhibitors or lipid-lowering agents, strategies we now know significantly improved long-term outcomes after surgery. Second, the status of the "medically treated" patients actually improved slightly because a large proportion of those patients "crossed over" and underwent bypass surgery, although they were still analyzed as part of the medically treated group. In the three major studies, 40 to 44 percent of the total medically treated patient population had undergone bypass surgery by 10 postoperative years, including 65 percent of patients with left main disease and 48 percent of patients with three-vessel disease.[7] Finally, when all-cause mortality is the end point, any two survival curves eventually will meet at zero.

Randomized clinical trials as described earlier have the advantage that they lessen the influence of bias in the selection of treatment once patients are entered into the study, but they have the disadvantage that bias may be exerted at the point of inclusion into the trial. In all these trials, a minority of patients presenting for evaluation met the criteria for entry into the trial, and of those who met the criteria for entry, a minority actually were randomized. In the case of CASS, however, patients who were not randomized were followed prospectively in a registry, and that registry has produced observational studies that continue to provide useful information.

Among the important conclusions from the CASS Registry are that asymptomatic patients with 50 percent or more of left main stenosis and patients with left main equivalent (70 percent or more stenosis of the proximal LAD and circumflex vessels) have improved survival with surgery.[9,10] For severely symptomatic patients, bypass surgery improved the survival rates of those with three-vessel disease regardless of whether they had normal or abnormal LV function, even if those patients did not have severe proximal coronary artery stenoses.[11] Also, surgically treated patients who were completely revascularized fared better than incompletely revascularized patients, particularly if they had abnormal LV function.[12]

Outcomes for patients with unstable angina based on either progressive symptoms or rest angina with electrocardiographic changes were tested in the Veterans Administration Cooperative Study. Patients with rest angina and abnormal LV function had greatly improved survival with initial surgery. Patients with progressive angina did not appear to have a worse survival rate if they were treated initially with medical therapy, but 19 percent of this group crossed over to surgery within 30 days of randomization, and by 96 months, 45 percent had crossed over to surgery.[13]

Although these trials were undertaken relatively early in the history of coronary bypass surgery and today we can expect lower operative mortality rates and improved long-term outcomes after operation based on the use of arterial grafts, platelet inhibitors, and lipid-lowering agents, the observations from these studies provide the fundamental basis for the development of indications for bypass surgery even today.[2,14]

EVOLUTION OF THE OPERATION AND PATIENT POPULATION

In the early years of bypass surgery, surgical candidates usually were relatively young, had limited coronary artery disease, good LV function, and few comorbid conditions. The operation was almost always performed through a median sternotomy with the use of cardiopulmonary bypass. To achieve a surgical field and allow operations to be done on a still heart, either cold fibrillation or intermittent ischemic arrest was a common strategy. The operation involved bypass grafts of reversed segments of greater saphenous vein from the aorta to the distal coronary arteries (see Fig. 48-1*A*). In a small number of centers, the left ITA was used as a bypass graft, usually as a graft to the LAD artery (see Fig. 48-1*B*), but this strategy was not common.

Throughout the 1970s and 1980s, operations for bypass surgery became progressively safer for multiple reasons. Surgeons became better trained, and surgical experience increased. Optical assistance became routine, and microsurgical instrumentation improved. Cardiac anesthesia developed as a subspecialty, and postoperative care protocols became more routinized. Intraoperative myocardial protection improved with the use of cardioplegia, a strategy whereby a combination of cardiac standstill and effective myocardial protection was achieved by injecting cardioplegic solution (usually containing high potassium concentrations) into the coronary circulation. The use of this strategy allowed extensive coronary reconstructions to be achieved consistent with effective myocardial protection and made surgical treatment of extensive and severe coronary atherosclerosis possible with safety.

In addition, the population of patients undergoing bypass surgery changed to an older population with more extensive coronary stenoses, a higher incidence of left main stenoses, abnormal LV function, and more frequent comorbid conditions. Table 48-1 shows the changes in preoperative descriptors for patients undergoing primary coronary surgery at The Cleveland Clinic Foundation for selected years from 1967 to 1996, and Table 48-2 shows similar changes between 1980 and 1990 in a countrywide population as recorded by the Society of Thoracic Surgeons National Database.[15] The bypass surgery population changed for multiple reasons. Improved technology and experience made it possible to operate on more complex and sicker patients with reasonable risk. Also, the randomized trials demonstrated that the patients who have the most to gain from surgery were patients with left main or multivessel disease and abnormal LV function. Furthermore, the U.S. population has been aging, and older patients have high expectations for their activity level. Finally, in the early 1980s, the advent of percutaneous anatomic treatments for coronary stenoses (i.e., PCTA) provided an alternative treatment for patients with limited coro-

TABLE 48-1 Preoperative Clinical Characteristics for the First 1000 Patients per Year Undergoing Elective Primary Isolated Coronary Bypass Grafting (The Cleveland Clinic Foundation)

Clinical Variable	1967–1970	1973	1976	1979	1982	1985	1988	1990	1994	1996
Age (yr, median)	50	53	55	56	59	62	64	65	64	65
Men (%)	85	89	89	88	84	80	78	76	75	71
Severe angina (T)	19	21	24	20	17	23	26	34	30	34
Diabetes (%)	7	7	6	7	9	13	19	24	24	27
Age ≥70 yr (%)	0.2	0.5	3	4	10	17	26	32	28	34
Single-vessel disease* (%)	56	17	15	10	8	5	3	5	9	9
Double-vessel disease* (%)	31	33	28	28	25	25	19	25	29	26
Triple-vessel disease* (%)	13	50	57	62	67	71	78	70	60	63
Left main coronary stenosis (≥50%) (%)	9	8	12	12	13	13	16	17	19	19
Left ventricular asynergy (%)	41	41	45	54	55	56	57	51	48	39

The terms *single, double-*, and *triple-vessel disease* refer to the number of the three main coronary vessels (left anterior descending, circumflex, and right coronary arteries) that have stenoses ≥50%.

TABLE 48-2 Comparison of Patient Characteristics 1980 to 1990, The Society of Thoracic Surgery Database*

Characteristic	1980	1990	*P* Value
Age (y)	58.5 ± 9.11	64.1 ± 10.2	<0.001
EF	0.62 ± 0.15	0.51 ± 0.14	<0.001
Female	17.04	26.98	<0.005
Diabetes mellitus	11.73	22.8	<0.005
MI <21 days before CABG	0.34	12.47	<0.005
Cardiogenic shock	0.51	1.61	<0.010
Unstable angina	28.51	47.84	<0.005
Left main disease	6.93	11.7	<0.005
Reoperation	1.88	7.01	<0.005
Nonelective operation	4.11	18.22	<0.005

*Values are shown as percentages except for age and EF, which are shown as mean ± standard deviation.

ABBREVIATIONS: CABG = coronary artery bypass grafting; EF = ejection fraction; IABP = intraaortic balloon pump; MI = myocardial infarction.

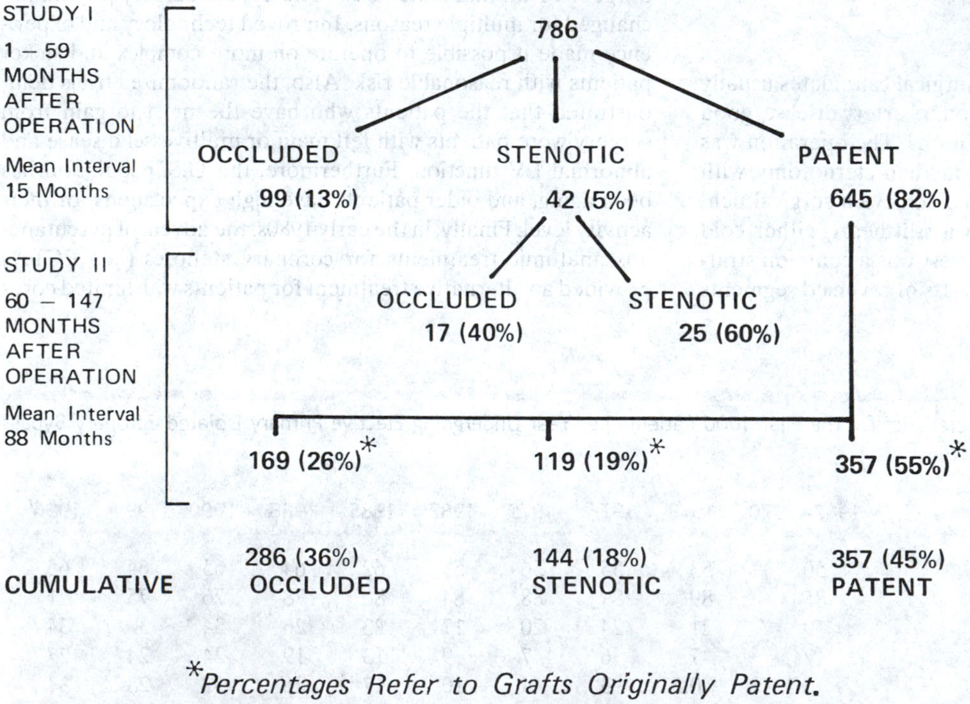

FIGURE 48-2 Data from serial postoperative angiography of saphenous vein to coronary artery grafts. Any graft narrowing was considered a stenosis. Percentages not marked with an asterisk refer to the total number of grafts (786). Percentages marked with an asterisk refer to grafts originally patent. Treatment with postoperative platelet inhibitors and lipid-lowering agents was not used for these patients. (Used with permission from Lytle BW, Loop FD, Cosgrove DM, et al. Long-term (5 to 12 years) serial studies of internal mammary artery and saphenous vein coronary bypass grafts. *J Thorac Cardiovasc Surg* 1985; 89:250.)

nary lesions, removing many of those patients from the surgical population.

TYPES OF BYPASS GRAFTS AND THEIR OUTCOMES

Saphenous Vein Grafts

The most important technical change in coronary surgery has been in the types of grafts that are used. By 1980, angiographic studies at multiple centers had shown that early vein graft patency rates were favorable (80–90 percent within the first postoperative year). Early patency rates were influenced by surgical technique, gender (men experienced better patency rates), the coronary artery grafted (LAD artery patency rates were better than circumflex and right coronary artery rates), the size of the vessel grafted, and the indications for repeat study (routine studies demonstrating better patency rates than studies performed because of symptoms). Coronary risk factors did not appear to influence early patency rates.[1,16–20] However, sequential studies of patent vein grafts demonstrated substantial late attrition. Fitzgibbon et al.[17] studied 590 vein grafts that were patent at 1 postoperative year and found that when studied late (>5 years after operation) 30 percent of patent grafts had become occluded, and 76 percent had angiographic evidence of pathologic changes. Fitzgibbon et al.[17] and Bourassa et al.[16] found a 2.1 percent yearly rate of occlusion of vein grafts up to 5 years after operation, but Bourassa et al.[20] noted a 5.3 percent yearly occlusion rate between 6 and 11 years after operation. Data from sequential The Cleveland Clinic Foundation studies (Fig. 48-2) showed that of vein grafts patent without stenosis 1 to 5 years after operation, only 55 percent remained angiographically perfect 6 to 12 years after surgery.[19] In addition, the attrition rate of patent grafts was not related to the coronary vessel grafted but was related to coronary risk factors such as diabetes and hyperlipidemia.[18,19]

The pathologic changes found in stenotic or occluded vein grafts are different at different postoperative intervals.[21–25] Grafts occluded within 1 or 2 months of surgery exhibit thrombosis, often associated with endothelial disruption. Grafts examined more than a few months after surgery consistently exhibit a hypercellular, proliferative hyperplasia involving the intima—intimal fibroplasia. Intimal fibroplasia is a concentric lesion that evolves into a more fibrotic lesion. It may cause fixed stenoses and may be associated with occlusion but usually is not. However, it appears to be the substrate for the development of vein graft atherosclerosis (VGA), the process that leads to many late graft stenoses or occlusions.

VGA is different from native coronary atherosclerosis. Native coronary artery atherosclerosis is a proximal, eccentric, and intermittent lesion that usually is covered by a fibrous cap. VGA is distributed throughout the length of vein grafts, it is circumferential, it is not encapsulated, and it is extremely friable. With time, the early circumferential lesion often progresses to eccentric lesions causing severe stenoses (Fig. 48-3). Because of its friability and nonencapsulated nature, VGA is a dangerous lesion. Embolization of atherosclerotic debris is a major risk during percutaneous interventions on vein grafts and during reoperations, and it is probable that spontaneous embolization may occur.[20,26] VGA usually is not recognized before 2 to 3 years after operation and does not appear to cause much graft attrition before 5 postoperative years. However, grafts that become occluded more than 5 years after operation usually exhibit thrombosis superimposed on VGA, and the increased rate of graft attrition seen more than 5 years after operation appears to be due in large part to VGA.

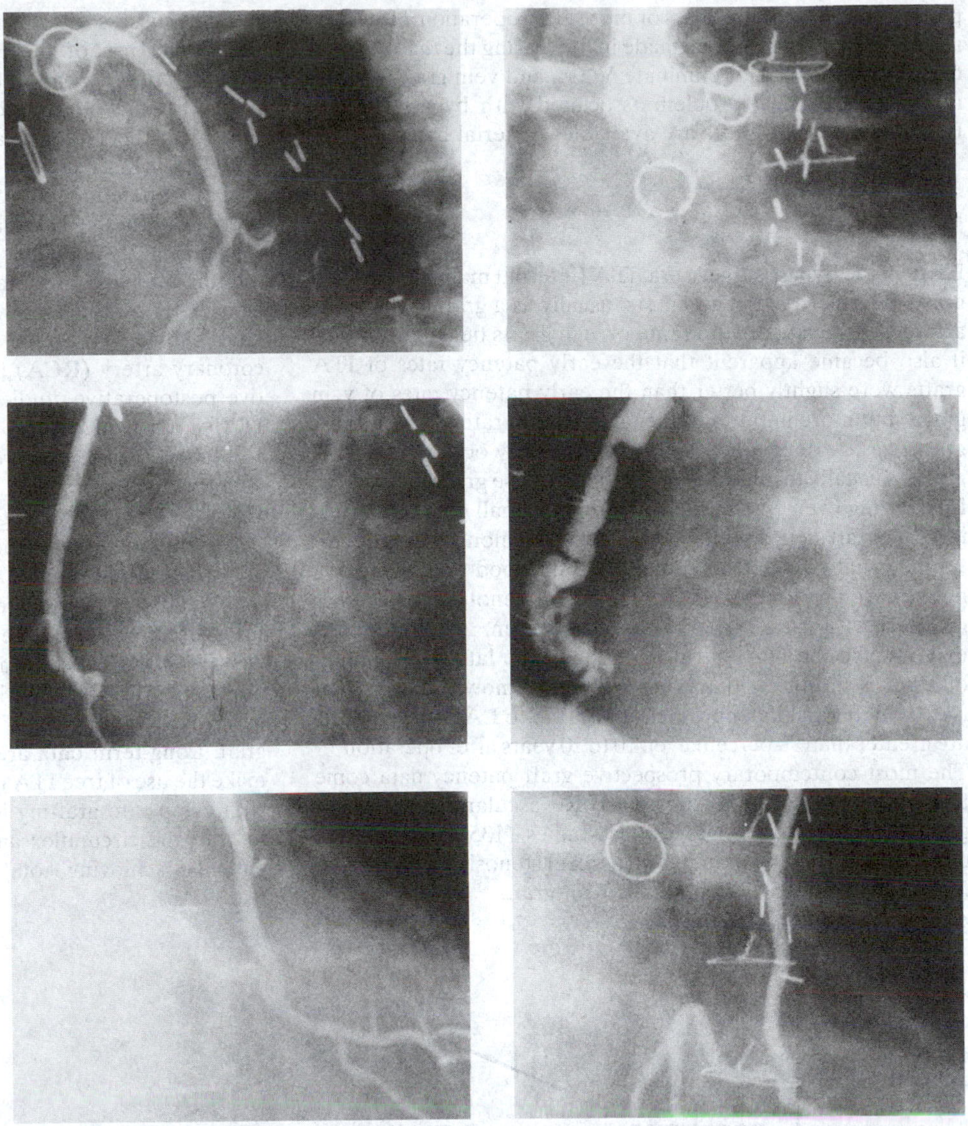

FIGURE 48-3 Angiographic anatomy 1 year after operation (*left*) showing patent vein grafts to the LAD artery and RCA and an ITA graft to the circumflex artery. Seven years later, the LAD artery vein graft is occluded, the RCA graft exhibits diffuse irregular stenoses characteristic of VGA, and the ITA graft is unchanged. (Used with permission from Lytle BW, Loop FD, Cosgrove DM, et al. Long-term (5 to 12 years) serial studies of internal mammary artery and saphenous vein coronary bypass grafts. *Thoracic Cardiovasc Surg* 1985; 89:250.)

Since the early studies of vein grafts cited earlier, substantial progress has been made in the prevention of vein graft attrition. First, multiple randomized, prospective trials have shown that the perioperative and long-term treatment of patients who received vein grafts with platelet inhibitors have significantly decreased the occlusion rate of saphenous vein grafts at 1 year after operation to 6 to 11 percent.[27,28] Second, lipid-lowering trials using a cholesterol-niacin combination or using an aggressive regimen of Pravastatin to lower low-density lipoprotein cholesterol levels have been shown to decrease the progression of angiographic lesions in vein grafts, including a decrease in the rate of occlusion 5 to 15 years after operation.[29,30] Importantly, a clinical trial (CARE trial) of 1091 patients who survived a myocardial infarction (MI), had average cholesterol levels, and underwent bypass surgery showed that treatment with Pravastatin decreased the risk of death and nonfatal MI over a 5-year follow-up.[31] Thus multiple studies appear to show that outcomes for patients receiving vein grafts today can be expected to be better than those noted in studies from the 1970s. Furthermore, some vein grafts provide very long-term benefit. For patients studied 16 to 20 years after operation Lawrie et al.[32] noted 46 percent vein graft patency and Fitzgibbon et al.[20] noted a 50 percent patency rate 15 years or more after operation. However, although progress has been made in decreasing the *rate* of VGA, these strategies do not eliminate VGA, and vein graft attrition remains the biggest problem associated with bypass surgery. Fortunately, other grafts are available—arterial bypass grafts.

ITA Grafts

Early in the bypass surgery era, ITA (internal mammary artery) grafts were used in a few centers, usually as a graft to the LAD artery. As the late attrition rate of vein grafts began to surface, it also became apparent that the early patency rates of ITA grafts were slightly better than the early patency rates of vein grafts, but more important, the late attrition rate of patent ITA grafts was extremely low[1,19] (Fig. 48-4). Early occlusion of ITA grafts is usually technically related, since these grafts can remain functioning even when used to graft very small coronary arteries. ITA graft stenosis or occlusion beyond 6 months after operation is usually related to competition in blood flow through a native coronary artery that is not severely stenotic and becomes manifest as a "string sign" or diffuse spasm. Atherosclerosis may involve the ITA, but it is rare, and the late development of atherosclerotic lesions in an ITA graft known to be patent is extremely rare. Patency rates of left ITA to LAD artery grafts are greater than 90 percent even 10 to 20 years after operation.[1,19] The most contemporary prospective graft patency data come from the Bypass Surgery Angioplasty Revascularization Investigation (BARI) trial angiographic studies (135 patients) that documented 1-year patency (<50 percent stenosis) of 98 percent for ITA grafts and 87 percent for vein grafts.[33]

The success of the left ITA to LAD artery graft has led to the use of the right ITA as a bypass graft, usually simultaneously with the left ITA (bilateral ITA grafting). The right ITA has been used as an in situ graft and as a "free" graft with the proximal anastomosis constructed either to the left ITA (Fig. 48-5*A*) or to the aorta (see Fig. 48-5*B*). Although patency rates of ITA grafts have been highest when used to graft the LAD artery–diagonal system, Dion et al.[34] restudied 135 pedicled ITA to circumflex artery grafts 13 months after operation and noted a 95 percent patency rate. Longer-term studies of ITA to circumflex artery grafts also have showed favorable outcomes.[1] ITA grafts to the right coronary artery (RCA) have been less frequent and prospective postoperative studies are rare, but long-term patency of ITA grafts to the RCA is possible.

Studies of aorta to coronary ITA grafts have tended to show patency rates not quite as good as those of pedicled grafts. However, these types of grafts can exhibit 20-year patency, and once they are patent, they appear to remain free from graft atherosclerosis.[1,34]

A relatively new strategy is composite arterial grafting with the right ITA used as a free graft anastomosed to the left ITA[35,36] (see Fig. 48-4*B*). This strategy allows more flexibility in the use of the right ITA, and early data show patency rates of 91 to 95 percent within a year of operation for this type of free ITA graft. Long-term data are not available, but this strategy may make the use of free ITA grafts more effective. Once experience with composite grafting is gained, the right ITA may be used to graft the circumflex and right coronary systems in selected patients, achieving total arterial revascularization with the two ITAs.

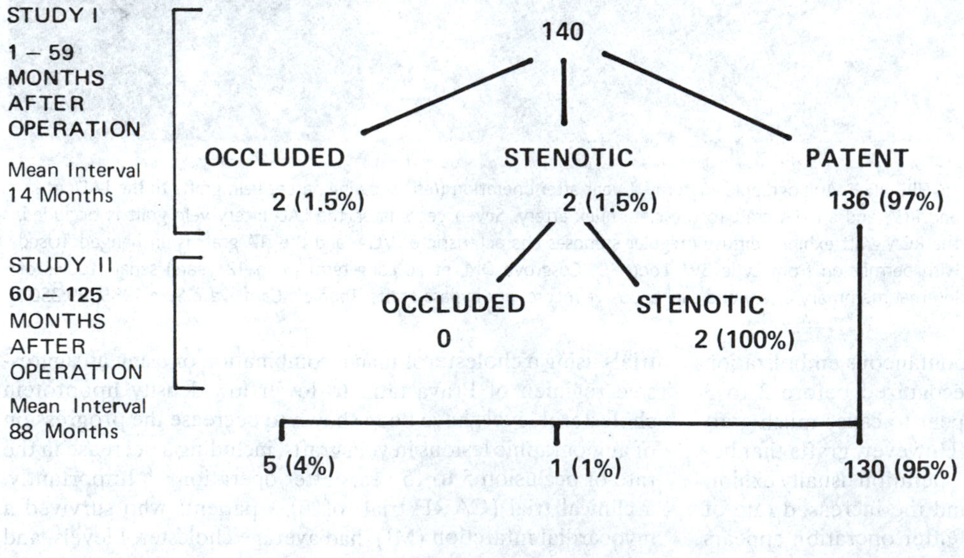

FIGURE 48-4 Data from serial postoperative angiography of ITA to coronary artery grafts. Percentages not marked with an asterisk refer to the total number of grafts (140). Percentages marked with an asterisk refer to grafts originally patent. (Used with permission from Lytle BW, Loop FD, Cosgrove DM, et al. Long-term (5 to 12 years) serial studies of internal mammary artery and saphenous vein coronary bypass grafts. *J Thorac Cardiovasc Surg* 1985; 89:252.)

Clinical Impact of ITA Grafts

The high and stable patency rate of the left ITA to LAD artery graft also produces improved clinical outcomes. No large randomized studies have compared ITA and vein grafts, but in a large observational study published in 1986, Loop et al.[37] showed that patients who received a left ITA to LAD artery graft (with or without vein grafts to the circumflex and RCA branches) had better 10-year survival rates when compared with patients who received only vein grafts (Fig. 48-6). This observation was true for patients with single-, double-, or triple-vessel disease. In addition, the ITA graft patients underwent fewer reoperations (4 versus 8 percent) and had fewer cardiac-related hospitalizations. Data from CASS have extended the observed benefits of ITA grafting to 15 to 18 years after operation.[38]

Logic seems to dictate that if one ITA graft is good, two ITA

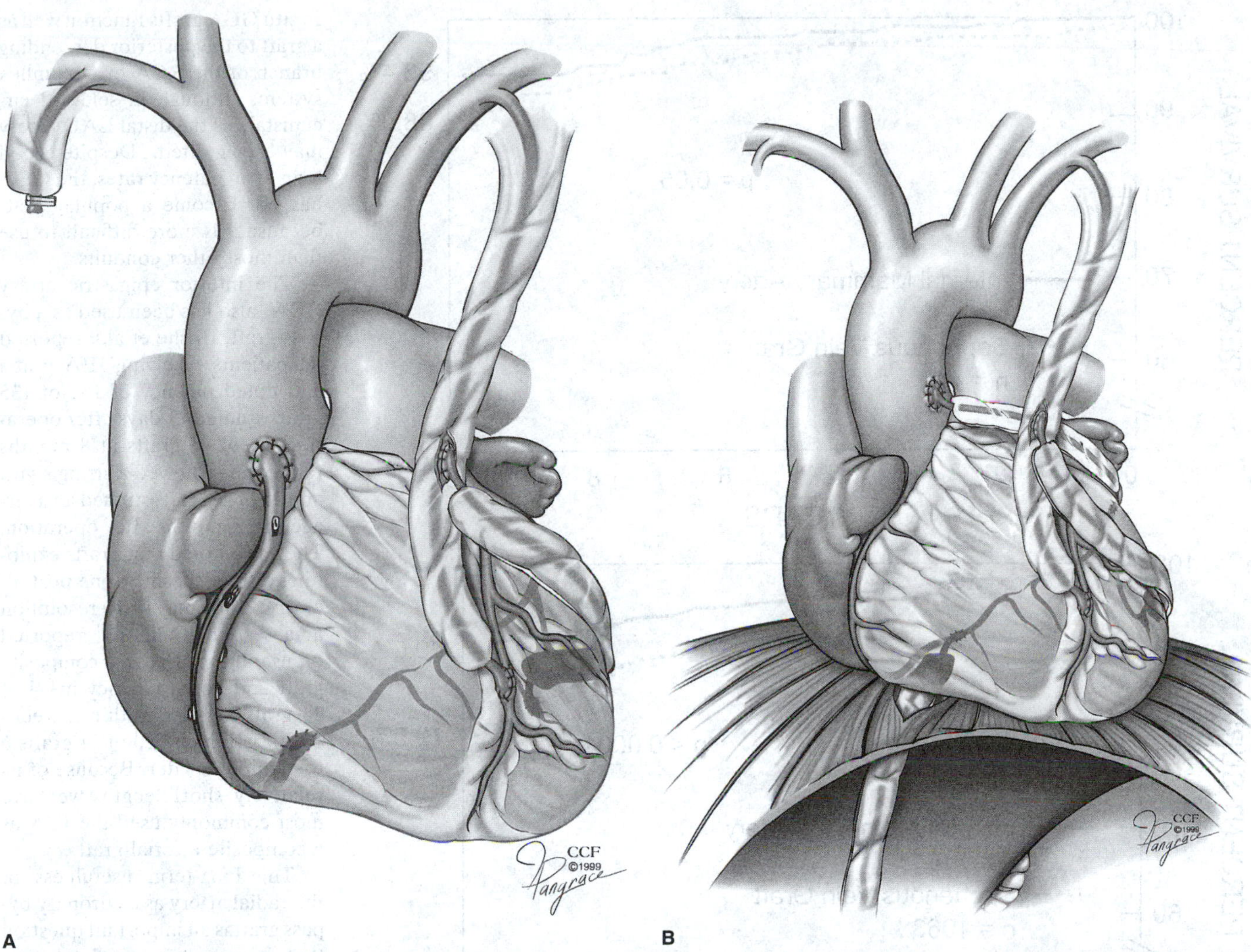

FIGURE 48-5 *A.* Bilateral ITA grafting with the right ITA used as a composite (from left ITA) graft to the circumflex coronary artery and a vein graft to the RCA. *B.* Total arterial revascularization with an aorta to coronary right ITA to circumflex graft, the radial artery used as a composite graft from the left ITA to diagonal coronary artery, the left ITA used as a graft to the anterior descending coronary artery, and an in situ GEA graft to the RCA.

grafts may improve outcomes further. However, the strategy of bilateral ITA grafting has not become widespread. Bilateral ITA grafting makes the bypass operation more difficult, some studies have shown an increase in the risk of wound complications, and the outcomes for patients receiving a single ITA to LAD artery graft are very good, particularly over the first postoperative decade. Furthermore, because of the importance of the LAD coronary artery in many patients, improved results may be difficult to show if LAD artery revascularization is secure. And indeed, a number of retrospective studies have shown either no benefit or relatively little incremental benefit of bilateral ITA grafting over single ITA grafting. These studies involved either small patient numbers or relatively short follow-up intervals. Recently, we retrospectively reviewed a large series of patients receiving single or bilateral ITA grafts and found an improved 12-year survival rate for the patients receiving bilateral ITA grafts, as well as a decreased risk of reoperation or percutaneous intervention over that same time frame[39] (Fig. 48-7). Another recent study that confirmed these observations also involves relatively large patient numbers.[40] It is probable that the incremental benefit of bilateral ITA grafting over single ITA grafting may be less than the benefit of a left ITA to LAD artery graft over only vein grafts. Nonetheless, it does appear that bilateral ITA grafting does offer incremental benefit.

Other Arterial Bypass Grafts

The gastroepiploic artery (GEA) was used for Vineberg-type myocardial implantation prior to the bypass grafting era, and its use as a coronary bypass graft was begun by Suma and Pym in 1986. Suma reported a 94 percent (253 of 268) patency rate within 2 months of operation and 47 of 50 GEA grafts (94 percent) patent at 2 to 5 postoperative years.[41] In situ GEA grafts have had better patency rates than free grafts. When late attrition has occurred, it has appeared to be related to native coronary artery competitive flow. Anecdotal angiographic studies have documented the patency of GEA grafts 9 to 10 years after operation and have not shown evidence of the occurrence of graft atherosclerosis. The GEA is prone to spasm, and intraluminal vasodilators have been used by many of its proponents.

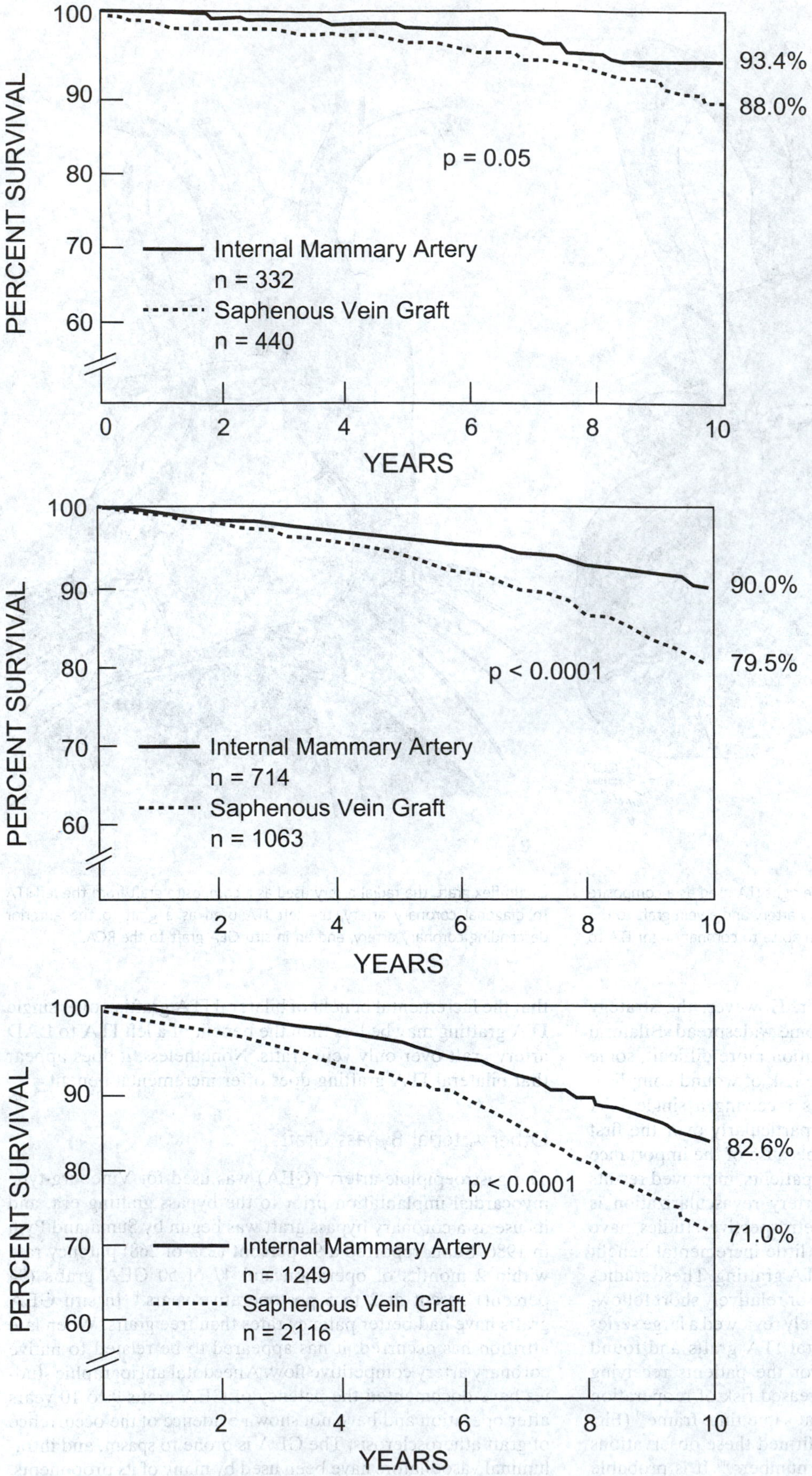

In situ GEA grafts function well as a graft to the posterior descending branch of the RCA or circumflex system, although in selected circumstances the distal LAD artery may be grafted. Despite good long-term patency rates, the GEA has not become a popular graft because it is more difficult to use than most other conduits.

The inferior epigastric artery (IEA) also has been used as a bypass graft. Buche et al.[42] reported on patients receiving IEA grafts and noted patency of 132 of 135 grafts studied 11 days after operation, 44 of 48 grafts at 8 months (although 8 showed a string sign), and 25 of 29 grafts studied an average of 25 months after operation. They also noted that grafts exhibiting diffuse spasm at one postoperative study may show resolution at a second. Califiore[36] reported on use of the IEA as a composite graft and noted patency in 34 of 34 grafts studied within 2 weeks of operation and 20 of 21 grafts 6 to 14 months later. Because of its relatively short length, we have most commonly used the IEA as a composite arterial graft.

The long-term usefulness of the radial artery as a coronary bypass graft is an important question that is as yet incompletely answered. The radial artery is a long graft that is easily procured and has very favorable size and handling characteristics. However, it is a thicker, more muscular artery than the ITA, and when it was used by Carpentier[44] and others[43] in the early 1970s, patency rates were not favorable. Recently, its use has been revisited along with the use of calcium-channel

FIGURE 48-6 Survival for patients with an ITA to LAD artery graft with and without vein grafts to other coronary vessels compared with survival for patients with only vein grafts. An ITA to LAD artery graft was associated with significantly better survival for patients with single- (*top*), double- (*middle*), or triple-vessel (*bottom*) disease. (Used with permission from Loop FD, Lytle BW, Cosgrove DM, et al. Influence of the internal-mammary-artery graft on 10-year survival and other cardiac events. *N Engl J Med* 1986; 314:106.)

blocking agents to prevent postoperative spasm, and Broadman et al.[45] and Acar et al.[46] have reported early (<6 months) patency rates of greater than 90 percent. Acar et al.[46] reported 75 radial grafts studied within 2 weeks of operation with 1 occluded graft and 4 with spasm. At 1 year, 61 grafts were restudied, with 4 occluded and 2 stenotic. At 4 to 7 years after operation, 50 patients underwent repeat study, and of 64 radial artery grafts, 10 were occluded, 1 had a string sign, and 53 (83 percent) looked perfect. In the same patients, 91 percent of left ITA grafts were patent. Possati et al.[47] performed serial studies after radial artery grafting and documented an 87 percent perfect patency at 5 postoperative years, compared with 98 percent left ITA patency and 69 percent vein graft patency in the same patients. Early diffuse radial artery graft abnormalities in 7 patients disappeared by the 5-year angiogram.[47] At this point the jury is still out on radial artery grafts. They are not as reliable in terms of patency as left ITA grafts are but may be superior to vein grafts over the long term if they are resistant to late graft atherosclerosis.

Total arterial revascularization is an appealing concept, but its clinical importance is not yet certain. For some patients, total arterial revascularization can be achieved solely with the use of ITA grafts, but for many others, other arterial grafts are needed. Bergsma et al.[48] reported on a group of 256 selected patients with triple-vessel disease revascularized with two ITA grafts and a GEA graft. These relatively good-risk patients experienced an expected good survival rate, but it was also noted that over a mean follow-up period of 51 months, 85.7 percent experienced no angina, an impressive figure. Much longer-term follow-up is needed. Realistically, it is unlikely that most coronary surgeons will use GEA grafts routinely, but if the long-term patency rates of radial artery grafts are superior to vein grafts, total arterial revascularization will become common.

CURRENT OPERATIVE STRATEGIES AND RISKS

Standard Operative Strategies

Currently, most operations for primary isolated coronary revascularization are still performed through a median sternotomy with the aid of cardiopulmonary bypass. Aortic occlusion and cold potassium-based cardioplegia (delivered antegrade through the aortic root or retrograde through a catheter in the coronary sinus) are used to achieve an immobile surgical field consistent with intraoperative myocardial protection. Standard revascularization techniques involve the use of an in situ left ITA to graft the coronary artery, and in most centers, vein grafts are then employed to graft the other vessels.

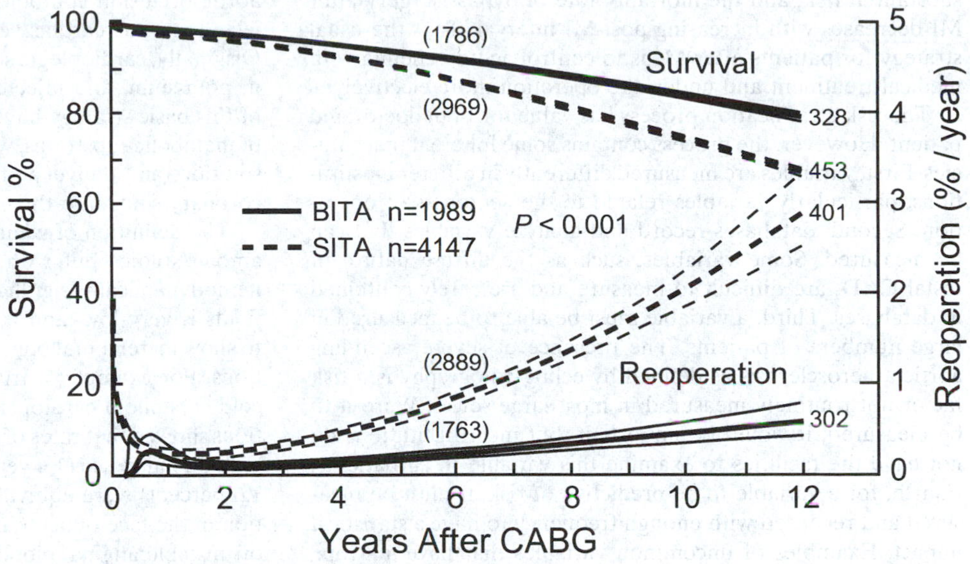

FIGURE 48-7 Comparison of survival and reoperation hazard function curves in propensity-matched patients receiving bilateral ITA grafts (BITA) and single ITA grafts (SITA) with or without additional vein grafts. CABG, coronary artery bypass grafting. (Used with permission from Lytle BW, Blackstone EH, Loop FD, et al. Two internal thoracic artery grafts are better than one. *J Thorac Cardiovasc Surg* 1999; 117:855–872.)

Hospital Mortality

Overall hospital mortality rates for primary bypass surgery vary between 1 and 4 percent. Mortality rates in the voluntary countrywide Society of Thoracic Surgeons Database ranged from 3.46 to 3.78 percent (including reoperations) from 1990 to 1994.[49] The unadjusted mortality rate for patients undergoing primary operations in New York State (a compulsory registry with subsequent public disclosure) from 1993 to 1995 was 1.9 percent,[50] and single-institution reviews have noted overall mortality rates of 1 percent or less for elective patients.[1] Multiple database analyses have been devoted to the identification of variables that can be used to predict in-hospital outcomes and adjust for patient selection. A recent review of the seven largest data sets available in the literature found that 7 variables were predictive of in-hospital death in all data sets: acuteness of operation, age, prior cardiac surgery, gender, LV ejection fraction, left main coronary artery percent stenosis, and number of coronary systems with more than 70 percent stenosis.[51] Acuteness of operation, age, and previous surgery had the greatest predictive value. Also identified were 13 variables that added some predictive value to the core variables: percutaneous transluminal angioplasty (PCTA) during the same admission, MI less than 1 week prior to operation, angina, ventricular arrhythmia, congestive heart failure, mitral regurgitation, diabetes, cerebral vascular disease, peripheral vascular disease, chronic obstructive pulmonary disease (COPD), and serum creatinine.

In the spectrum of clinical settings ranging from stable angina, to unstable angina with electrocardiographic changes, to recent subendocardial infarction, to recent Q-wave MI, and to cardiogenic shock, there has been an increased operative risk associated with increasing degrees of ischemia and decreasing degrees of LV function. Modern methods of myocardial protection have diminished the impact of unstable angina. However, operations for postinfarction ischemia and shock still generate substantial risk, and the mortality rate of bypass surgery after MI decreases with increasing post-MI interval. Thus the usual strategy for patients after MI is to control acute ischemia with medical treatment and undertake operation more electively.

The risk-stratification process has value for both doctor and patient. However, the process contains some inherent inaccuracies. First, variables are measured differently in different institutions, particularly variables related to the acuteness of operation. Second, databases record and analyze variables that can be measured. Some variables, such as the diffuse nature of distal CAD, are difficult to measure and are rarely contained in databases. Third, a variable must be able to be measured in large numbers of patients. The presence of severe ascending aortic atherosclerosis as defined by echocardiography is a risk factor not routinely measured in most large series. Were it to be measured, it would be important, but most institutions do not have the facilities to examine this variable in all patients. Fourth, for a variable to be predictive of risk, it must be measured and recorded with enough frequency to have a statistical impact. Examples of uncommon variables that have a strong impact on operative mortality include hepatic cirrhosis, congenital clotting disorders, severe protamine allergies, and previous mediastinal radiation therapy.

Coronary bypass surgery is a very scrutinized treatment. Overall mortality rates tend to be maintained in a narrow range in part because that scrutiny engenders careful patient selection if overall mortality rates begin to rise. Burack et al.[52] studied the New York State Department of Health Cardiac Surgery Reporting System (CSRS) and found evidence that high-risk patients were being denied bypass surgery. Certainly, not all institutions should perform all operations, and it probably is of benefit for high-risk patients to undergo surgery in selected institutions. However, in a milieu of medical economics where patient mobility may be limited, care must be exerted such that high-risk patients are not denied potentially lifesaving operations.

One operation-related variable that has been associated with decreased in-hospital risk is the use of ITA grafts. At one time there was concern that ITA use would increase risk. However, multiple retrospective studies from different data sets and during different surgical periods have shown that use of the ITA graft is associated with a decrease in hospital mortality rather than an increase.[53,54]

One advantage of identifying characteristics that predict high risk is that patients who are at extremely low risk also may be identified. For example, during the years 1995–1998, the STS Database recorded 25,776 patients who underwent a primary elective bypass operation, had a LV ejection fraction of greater than 50 percent, and did not have peripheral vascular disease, carotid disease, renal failure, a prior MI, or an intraaortic balloon pump. For these good-risk patients, 98 deaths occurred for a 0.38 percent mortality rate.[55]

Hospital Morbidity

PERIOPERATIVE MI

Since the early years of bypass surgery, improved strategies for myocardial protection have evolved, and significant perioperative MI has become less frequent. Today most surgeons employ aortic occlusion combined with some type of cardioplegia injected into the cardiac vascular system to produce a still heart. Originally, cardioplegic solutions were asanguineous, cold, high in potassium, and injected into the aortic root. Modifications of this basic strategy have included addition of blood, addition of metabolic substrates, warming some or all of the cardioplegic solution, and delivery of cardioplegia retrograde through the coronary sinus into the cardiac venous system.

The definition of what constitutes a perioperative MI varies among studies but with the use of cardioplegia, the risk of hemodynamically significant perioperative MI in elective patients is very low, and it has become difficult in such patients to show incremental benefit of any of the cardioplegia modifications. For example, a trial of warm blood cardioplegia versus cold crystalloid cardioplegia in primary elective bypass operations showed that rates of MI (1.4 versus 0.8 percent), intraaortic balloon pump use (1.4 versus 2.0 percent), and death (1.0 versus 1.6 percent) were equivalent.[56] For patients undergoing operation in the face of acute ischemia based either on failed PCTA or unstable angina, blood cardioplegia does appear to provide incremental benefit.[57,58] Retrograde delivery through the coronary sinus and coronary venous system provides more effective delivery during reoperations, in the setting of acute coronary ischemia, or if the aortic valve is insufficient.[59]

For the period of time needed to complete even extensive coronary revascularization operations using standard techniques, the metabolic environment created by these cardioplegic strategies appears to be sufficient for protection. Significant perioperative MI, when it occurs, appears to be based on anatomic causes, acute coronary occlusion, graft failure, or incomplete revascularization.

NEUROLOGIC COMPLICATIONS

Adverse neurologic events after coronary bypass surgery may negatively affect overall outcomes, and at a period in time where myocardial protection has diminished the impact of perioperative MI, the perioperative risk of cerebral complications is still under intense investigation. A recent multicenter study authored by Roach et al.[60] separated postoperative neurologic abnormalities into focal strokes (type I) and diffuse encephalopathies (type II). In this study, the total number of adverse outcomes was 6.1 percent, divided between type I (3.1 percent) and type II (3.0 percent). Advanced age and hypertension predicted an increased risk for both types of deficits.

Focal strokes (type I) appear to have multiple causes, including carotid or intracranial vascular disease, embolic phenomena based on interventricular or atrial thrombi or postoperative atrial fibrillation, and atheroembolization from the aorta, probably the most common cause. In fact, in the study by Roach et al.,[60] the greatest predictor of a type I deficit was proximal aortic atherosclerosis as noted by the surgeon. Hartman et al.[61] have associated the risk of stroke with the severity of aortic atherosclerosis as defined by transesophageal echocardiography, and Blauth et al.[62] associated the presence of ascending aortic atherosclerosis with evidence of atherosclerotic emboli to multiple organ systems. There are multiple techniques available to diminish the impact of aortic atherosclerosis, including alternative arterial cannulation sites, single aortic cross-clamping, circulatory arrest and aortic replacement, and surgery without cardiopulmonary bypass. Which strategy will produce the best outcomes will vary according to the particular pathology involved, but the most important point is recognition by the surgeon of the existence of the problem. Other predictors of type I deficit have included a history of stroke, diabetes, unstable angina, peripheral vascular disease, and a total carotid occlusion.

Variables that were predictive of type II deficits in the Roach et al. study included a history of alcohol abuse, atrial fibrillation, prior coronary artery bypass grafting (CABG), peripheral vascular disease, and congestive heart failure. The anatomic basis of type II deficits is not known, but many authors have noted some evidence of gaseous or particulate embolization associated with cardiopulmonary bypass. Strategies designed to minimize microembolization associated with cardiopulmonary bypass includes the use of membrane oxygenators, arterial filters, alpha-stat extracorporeal circulation acid-base management, and avoidance of cerebral hyperthermia. Another appealing concept is the performance of bypass surgery without the use of cardiopulmonary bypass, and logic would seem to dictate that this strategy would decrease the incidence of both types of neurologic complications. This issue is currently being intensively investigated.

The presence of carotid stenoses, symptomatic or asymptomatic, in a patient undergoing bypass surgery creates both a short- and a long-term risk of stroke. Studies of patients over age 65 with carotid Duplex scans have defined the predictors of 80 percent or more carotid stenoses as female gender, peripheral vascular disease, previous transient ischemic attack (TIA) or stroke, smoking history, and left main stenoses.[63] The majority of patients aged 65 or older had one of these characteristics, and it may be logical to screen all patients in that age group undergoing bypass surgery. Regardless of age, patients with a previous stroke, TIA, or carotid bruit should undergo Duplex screening, and any patients evidencing symptoms characteristic of vertebrobasilar insufficiency should have further studies.

The patient with simultaneous carotid and coronary disease is at higher risk than the patient with only CAD regardless of which therapeutic approach is used. Staged operations with carotid endarterectomy performed first has been shown to be safe but has been applied in very selected patients with less severe CAD. Patients undergoing bypass surgery in the face of a severe uncorrected carotid stenosis are at increased risk of stroke, and patients with bilateral stenoses are at a greatly increased risk of stroke.[64,65] Many experienced centers recommend combined carotid endarterectomy and coronary surgery for patients with carotid stenoses who are undergoing primary bypass operations, although even with this approach stroke and mortality rates are slightly worse than those for patients with isolated CAD.[66]

WOUND COMPLICATIONS

Deep sternal wound complications represent a serious adverse outcome and occur in 0.5 to 4 percent of cases depending on patient selection. Obesity and diabetes have been implicated in multiple studies as factors increasing the risk of sternal complications. There is some evidence that aggressive treatment of blood glucose levels with intravenous insulin may decrease the risk of infection in diabetic patients. No studies have shown that the use of a single ITA graft increases the risk of sternal wound complications, but some authors have implicated bilateral ITA grafting, particularly for diabetic patients.[67] Dissection of the ITA as a skeletonized artery rather than as a pedicle may leave collateral circulation to the sternum intact and diminish the impact of ITA use.

DIFFERENTLY INVASIVE BYPASS SURGERY

New concepts in how bypass surgery is being performed are now under exploration: operations done through small incisions (minimally invasive bypass surgery) and operations performed without the use of cardiopulmonary bypass (beating-heart or off-pump surgery). Stimuli for these changes include the maturation of small incision or endoscopic technology for the performance of thoracic and general surgery and the desire to decrease incision-related and cardiopulmonary bypass–related morbidity (and perhaps mortality) related to coronary surgery.

Small-incision and beating-heart concepts have been combined in an operation during which a small left anterior thoracotomy is used to prepare a left ITA graft that is then anastomosed to the LAD coronary artery under direct vision (MIDCAB or LAST operation) (Fig. 48-8). Endoscopic technologies sometimes have been used for the ITA preparation but usually not for creation of the anastomosis. Early studies showed that this approach was possible but also noted an increased risk of ITA graft failure associated with this strategy. However, with increased surgical experience, results clearly have improved.[68,69] Because the left ITA-LAD operation using standard techniques (median sternotomy and cardiopulmonary bypass) is extremely safe and produces excellent 20-year outcomes, the only major risks of bypass surgery that are likely to be diminished with the MIDCAB approach are wound complications. However, it is the hope that this less invasive approach may have cosmetic,

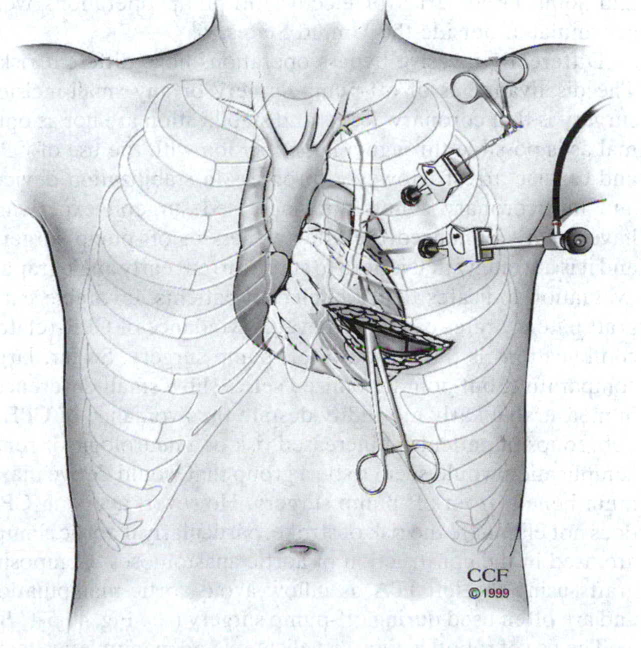

FIGURE 48-8 A small left anterior thoracotomy may be used to construct a limited anastomosis without the use of CPB, or with the use of percutaneous CPB, more vessels are accessible through this small incision. Endoscopic preparation of the left ITA graft may be employed.

hospital stay, time loss from work, and cost advantages. The disadvantage of a limited-access, off-pump operation is that a limited number of coronary vessels can be grafted through any one incision. To approach this issue, three directions are being pursued: small-incision surgery with cardiopulmonary bypass (CPB), large-incision surgery without CPB, and robotics surgery.

A percutaneous CPB system has been developed that involves femoral arterial and venous cannulation and percutaneous cannulas that allow balloon occlusion of the ascending aorta and the delivery of antegrade and retrograde cardioplegia. This approach allows aortic occlusion, cardiac arrest, and decompression, making the coronary vessels more accessible through a small left thoracotomy. The disadvantages of this approach are that coronary exposure may not be ideal, the right ITA and GEA arteries are difficult to use as grafts, the patient undergoes the risks of CPB, and the patient is exposed to vascular-related risks of catheter placement such as aortic dissection and atherosclerotic embolization. Industry sources appear to show that an early increased risk of aortic dissection has lessened with experience and that the risks of death and stroke are not obviously out of line.[70] The possible benefits of this approach are a decrease in wound complications and a faster return to full activity. In carefully selected patients, these goals seem achievable.

A more common differently invasive strategy is to use a median sternotomy incision to improve coronary artery access but avoid the use of CPB, bypass surgery being performed on the beating heart. Beating-heart surgery was employed in the early years of bypass surgery, and although poor angiographic outcomes led to its decline, it never disappeared completely. Many surgeons continued to perform small numbers of off-pump operations for patients at particularly high risk for CPB, and some large series of elective off-pump operations were accumulated outside the United States.[71,72]

Differently invasive bypass operations have different risks. The disadvantages of off-pump surgery or any small-incision surgery is that coronary access and stabilization are not as optimal as is possible through a large incision with the use of CPB and cardiac arrest. However, progress in stabilization devices and intracoronary shunts and increased surgeon experience have greatly enhanced the effectiveness of off-pump surgery, and it is a strategy that is here to stay. Current early angiographic evaluation indicates that for selected patients, favorable early graft patency rates can be achieved. Avoidance of CPB-related complications is the upside of off-pump surgery. So far, large comparative, but nonrandomized series show small differences in measurable early morbidity despite the avoidance of CPB.[73] Subgroups of patients at increased risk of a neurologic or renal complication would seem to be a group that would derive maximum benefit from off-pump surgery. However, avoiding CPB does not eliminate the risk of stroke, particularly if aortic clamps are used in the construction of aortic anastomoses. Composite grafts using the left ITA as inflow avoid aortic manipulation and are often used during off-pump surgery (see Fig. 48-5*A*, *B*).

The use of robotics-type visualization and manipulative technology is in its infancy but offers the possibility of expanding the extent of operations that can be performed through small incisions with or without CPB. The development of effective anastomotic stapling devices will greatly expand the possibilities for robotics bypass surgery.

LONG-TERM OUTCOMES AFTER BYPASS SURGERY

Late survival after bypass surgery is related to the patient's cardiac status at the time of operation, the bypass operation, progression of atherosclerosis, noncardiac comorbidity, and fate. Recent follow-up of 8221 surgical patients from the CASS Registry documented overall survival of 96, 90, 74, 56, and 45 percent at 1, 5, 10, 15, and 18 postoperative years, respectively.[74] These figures are inferior to those for the age-sex-matched U.S. population. Noted in other follow-up studies is that 55 percent of deaths over the first postoperative decade were cardiac in nature.[75]

Age is a major determinant of survival. In the CASS review, very young and very elderly patients had a decreased survival rate. The lack of ITA grafting in the CASS population almost certainly had a detrimental effect on the survival of young patients, but no studies of patients 40 years of age or under have ever shown survival rates equivalent to age-matched controls. However, elderly patients, while having a diminished survival when compared with younger patients, actually have survival rates better than those for age-matched controls, an effect that begins to be observed around age 60.[74]

LV function is the cardiac-related variable most closely related to long-term survival. In addition, left main stenosis, a proximal LAD artery stenosis, and the number of significantly stenotic coronary arteries all have influenced survival in most studies. The late survival of patients treated medically is dramatically influenced by these cardiac variables, but bypass surgery at least partially ameliorates their impact.[74] In our study analyzing the impact of arterial revascularization, a proximal LAD artery stenosis had no effect on late survival, and left main disease and the number of systems diseased had minor influence.[39] In no long-term study has bypass surgery completely obliterated the impact of abnormal LV function on late survival.

Risk factors for atherosclerosis also decrease late survival, most particularly cigarette smoking, hypercholesterolemia, hypertension, and diabetes. Smoking decreases the survival rate, and stopping smoking returns the patient to a nonsmoker's prognosis.[76] High elevations in total cholesterol are related to a decreased survival in some studies,[77] and there is suggestive evidence that pharmacologic treatment may improve the survival rate for these patients. Diabetes severe enough to require treatment is associated with a decreased late survival rate, but it is not yet clear whether or not glycemic control will improve the late survival rate of surgically treated patients. However, it has been shown that close control of diabetes does improve long-term outcomes for medically treated patients, and logic would dictate the importance of this approach despite bypass surgery.

As discussed previously, the surgical strategies of the left ITA-LAD artery graft and bilateral ITA grafting incrementally improve the late survival.

The impact of incomplete revascularization on long-term outcome is of increasing importance with the emergence of PCTA and minimally invasive bypass operations, strategies that may involve less complete revascularization than can be achieved with standard bypass surgical techniques. Definitions of what *incomplete revascularization* is have varied, and it is difficult to separate incomplete revascularization as a surgical strategy from incomplete revascularization as a marker of bad coronary and noncoronary atherosclerosis. Retrospective multivariate analyses of The Cleveland Clinic Foundation data identified incomplete revascularization as a risk factor for late death, but not a strong one.[77] A CASS Registry study by Bell et al.[12] noted a strong negative effect of incomplete revascularization on the late survival of patients with abnormal LV function who underwent bypass surgery, and Jones and Weintraub[78] observed a negative effect on patients with normal LV function.

Incomplete revascularization as a surgical strategy was examined in a study by Tasdemir et al.[72] that reviewed patients having off-pump bypass surgery. In this study, incomplete revascularization (usually of the circumflex system) was sometimes accepted in order to be able to perform bypass surgery without CPB. Failure to revascularize the circumflex system was a risk factor for early death and cardiac events, but late follow-up was not available.

REOPERATION

Atherosclerosis is a progressive disease, and some patients eventually will undergo repeat bypass surgery. A study reviewing patients undergoing primary bypass surgery in the 1970s noted a cumulative incidence of reoperation of 2.7, 11.4, and 17.3 percent at 5, 10, and 12 years after bypass, respectively.[79] Young age, normal LV function, single- or double-vessel disease, severe symptoms, incomplete revascularization, and not having an ITA graft were all factors increasing the likelihood of a reoperation. Today, the availability of PCTA, use of arterial grafts, and possibly risk factor control will diminish the rate of reoperation. However, recurrent ischemic syndromes will develop in some patients with previous surgery, and reoperation will sometimes be required.

Patients who are candidates for reoperation are different from those having primary surgery. Today, the typical candidate for reoperation underwent primary surgery more than 10 years ago, had triple-vessel disease at that time, and needs reoperation at least in part because of graft failure. The atherosclerotic process is advanced, and such patients have a high incidence of noncardiac atherosclerosis. Their cardiac atherosclerosis is severe, and they have a higher prevalence of aortic atherosclerosis, left main stenosis, severe distal CAD, and abnormal LV function than patients undergoing primary surgery. They usually have the unique characteristics of having their myocardial blood supply dependent on ITA grafts, being at risk for injury, or having atherosclerotic vein grafts that create the possibility of coronary atheroembolism. In addition, few data are available that help to define the indications for reoperation, particularly for patients who are not severely symptomatic. None of the randomized trials included patients with previous bypass surgery, and since their myocardium is usually jeopardized at least in part by vascular pathology different from native coronary artery atherosclerosis, generalization from the randomized studies is unwise.

To examine outcomes for patients with prior surgery who developed recurrent ischemic syndromes, we performed two retrospective, nonrandomized studies of patients who underwent repeat angiography after primary bypass surgery. The first involved patients who did not undergo prompt reoperation and compared outcomes with patients with vein graft stenoses with patients without vein graft stenoses.[80] This study showed that late (≥5 years) stenoses in vein grafts are more dangerous lesions than are native coronary lesions. For example, patients 5 years or more after operation with a 50 percent or greater stenosis in the LAD artery vein graft had survival of 70 and 50 percent 2 and 5 years after angiography compared with survival rates of 97 and 70 percent for patients whose LAD coronary artery was jeopardized by a 50 percent or greater native vessel stenosis.

The second study involved patients with stenotic vein grafts and compared outcomes for those who underwent repeat surgery with those who were treated without initial reoperation.[81] Treatment was not randomized, and the patients who underwent repeat surgery were more symptomatic. Patients with late (≥5 years) stenoses in vein grafts had better survival rates with surgery, and the patients who particularly benefited were those with an atherosclerotic vein graft to the LAD coronary artery. The patients with a 50 percent or greater LAD artery graft stenosis had immediate and obvious benefit, but even those with a 20 to 50 percent stenosis had an improved survival rate with surgery when followed for 5 years (Fig. 48-9). Patients with late stenoses in non-LAD artery grafts also appeared to have improved late survival unless they had a patent ITA to LAD artery graft. Patients with early vein graft stenoses did not have an improved late survival rate with surgery, although patients who underwent reoperation had fewer symptoms at late follow-up.

All studies that have examined large numbers of patients undergoing reoperation have noted an increased in-hospital risk when compared with patients undergoing primary surgery. The STS National Database noted an overall risk of 7.14 percent for reoperations from 1980 to 1990,[15] and The Cleveland Clinic Foundation studies have documented a risk of 3 to 4 percent for a first reoperation from 1967 through the present.[82–84]

The increased risk of reoperation is related in large part to an increased risk of perioperative MI. Graft injury, atherosclerotic embolization from vein grafts or the aorta, incomplete revascularization due to diffuse disease or lack of bypass conduit, and technical difficulty with severely atherosclerotic coronary vessels are anatomic causes of perioperative MI that are either unique to reoperation or more common in that setting. The use of retrograde cardioplegia has been of major benefit in the management of atherosclerotic vein grafts and patent ITA grafts, but avoiding perioperative MI during reoperation still represents a challenge.

In the reoperative setting, emergency operation produces a large increase in risk. Definitions of *emergency* vary among studies, but the lesson is the same. For example, in the STS National Database, primary operation had a risk of 2.24 percent for elective operation versus 5.7 percent for emergencies, whereas elective reoperations had a 5.33 percent risk compared with 12.69 percent for emergencies.[15] Left main stenosis, advanced age, congestive heart failure, female gender, and numbers of stenotic vein grafts have been other factors associated with increased risk.

In general, the long-term outcomes after reoperation are slightly inferior to those after primary surgery. Loop et al.[83] noted a 69 percent 10-year survival for 2429 hospital survivors of a first reoperation. LV function was the variable having the strongest impact on survival. Reoperations tend to achieve less perfect revascularization than primary procedures, and by 5 to 6 postoperative years, about 50 percent of reoperative patients have some angina, although in few patients is it severe.[82]

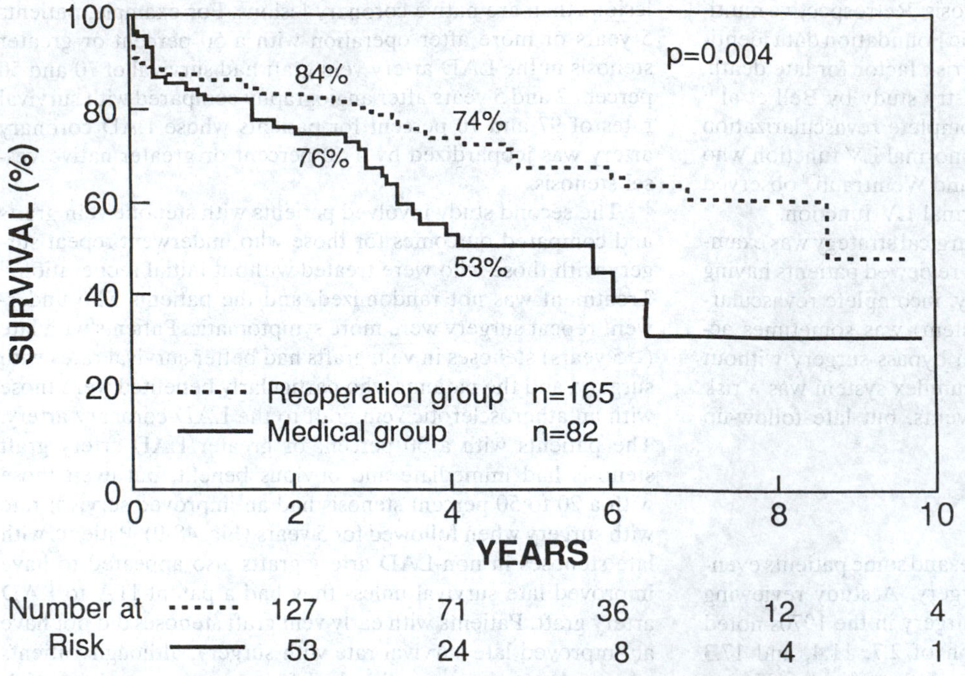

FIGURE 48-9 Patients with late (>5 years after operation) stenoses in venous grafts to the LAD coronary artery have better survival with reoperation than with medical treatment. (Used with permission from Lytle BW, Loop FD, Taylor PC, et al. The effect of coronary reoperation on the survival of patients with stenoses in saphenous vein bypass grafts to coronary arteries. *J Thorac Cardiovasc Surg* 1993; 605-14.)

PCTA VERSUS CABG

The advent of PCTA brought another invasive treatment for coronary atherosclerosis into the arena. Observational studies have identified many of the benefits (low procedure-related morbidity, early return to full activity, feasibility of multiple procedures) and disadvantages (not feasible for many patients, incomplete revascularization, restenosis, acute coronary occlusion) of PCTA. To compare PCTA and surgery for selected patient subgroups, multiple randomized trials have been undertaken.

A three-armed trial [The Medicine, Angioplasty or Surgery Study (MASS)] randomized 214 patients with severe (>80 percent) proximal LAD artery stenoses to medical treatment, PCTA, or bypass surgery (CABG).[85] During a 5-year follow-up, the primary end points of MI, death, and refractory angina occurred for 6 CABG patients, 29 PCTA patients, and 17 medically treated patients ($p = 0.001$). Considering repeat revascularization, death, and MI as events, event-free survival at 5 years was 98.6 percent after CABG, 93.9 percent after PCTA, and 88.9 percent for medically treated patients. The percentage of patients free of angina were CABG, 72.7 percent; PCTA, 64.7 percent; and medically treated, 25.8 percent. There was no difference, however, among the groups in the likelihood of death.

Multiple randomized, prospective trials have compared PCTA versus CABG for the treatment of multivessel CAD. The design of these trials has been to test the question of whether or not an initial strategy of PCTA compromises patient survival. The multicenter Bypass Angioplasty Revascularization Investigation (BARI) trial is the largest such trial (1792 patients randomized in 18 centers), and the single-center Emory Angioplasty Surgery Trial (EAST) is the other U.S. study.[86,87] Included in these trials were patients with stable or unstable angina who were good angiographic candidates for PCTA.

Of the spectrum of patients with coronary atherosclerosis who are considered for revascularization, a minority were included in these trials. Patients with left main stenosis of 50 percent or more were purposely excluded. In the BARI trial, more than half the patients who were potentially randomizable were excluded because of anatomy unfavorable for PCTA, and of the patients judged suitable, only half were randomized. A majority of BARI patients had two-vessel disease (59 percent) and normal LV function, and a minority (37 percent) had a proximal LAD artery lesion. Thus the BARI trial (and EAST patients had similar baseline characteristics) included very few patients who had been shown to have improved survival with CABG in the medicine versus surgery trials of the 1970s. In particular, the PCTA versus CABG trials are underpowered to detect a difference in survival for patients with multivessel disease and abnormal LV function because very few of such patients were randomized.

At approximately a 5-year follow-up interval, overall survival rates have been equivalent for the PCTA and CABG groups in both BARI and EAST. In the BARI trial, the subgroup of patients with treated diabetes had much worse survival with PCTA (Fig. 48-10). The survival advantage of the CABG group was present only if an ITA graft was used. Nondiabetic patients had equivalent survival.[88]

There were large differences between the PCTA and CABG groups in the need for repeat revascularization. Repeat revascularization was required in 54 percent of PCTA patients in both BARI and EAST versus 8 percent in the BARI CABG group and 13 percent in the EAST CABG group. There were smaller differences in symptom status and the need to take antianginal medications in favor of CABG. Detailed discussion of the limitation of these trials and the limitations in the conclusions that can be drawn from these trials have been described in detail by American College of Cardiology/American Heart Association task forces.[2,14] However, among the limitations of these trials in terms of current recommendations for the treatment of a broad spectrum of patients with multivessel CAD are the following: (1) The benefit of PCTA for high-risk patients (those subsets for whom surgery prolongs survival) has not been established because of the small number of such patients included in these randomized trials. (2) Only good angiographic candidates for PCTA were included, and the results of these trials cannot be extended to patients with more marginal suitability for PCTA. (3) Few PCTA patients received intracoronary stents. (4) Few surgical patients had extensive arterial revascularization. (5) None of the protocols included lipid-lowering therapy.

Observational studies have the disadvantage of bias in treatment selection but may have an advantage of being more inclusive. A recent large study from the New York State Cardiac Procedure Registries detailed a 3-year outcome of 29,646 CABG patients and 29,930 PCTA patients.[50] This study found a survival advantage for CABG for all patients with a proximal LAD artery lesion regardless of whether they had single-, double-, or triple-vessel disease.

Comparative trials of PCTA and CABG have involved patients with stable or unstable angina but not "beat the clock" treatment of acute MI. Currently, thrombolysis, PCTA, or both are the strategies employed for the vast majority of patients with acute MI.

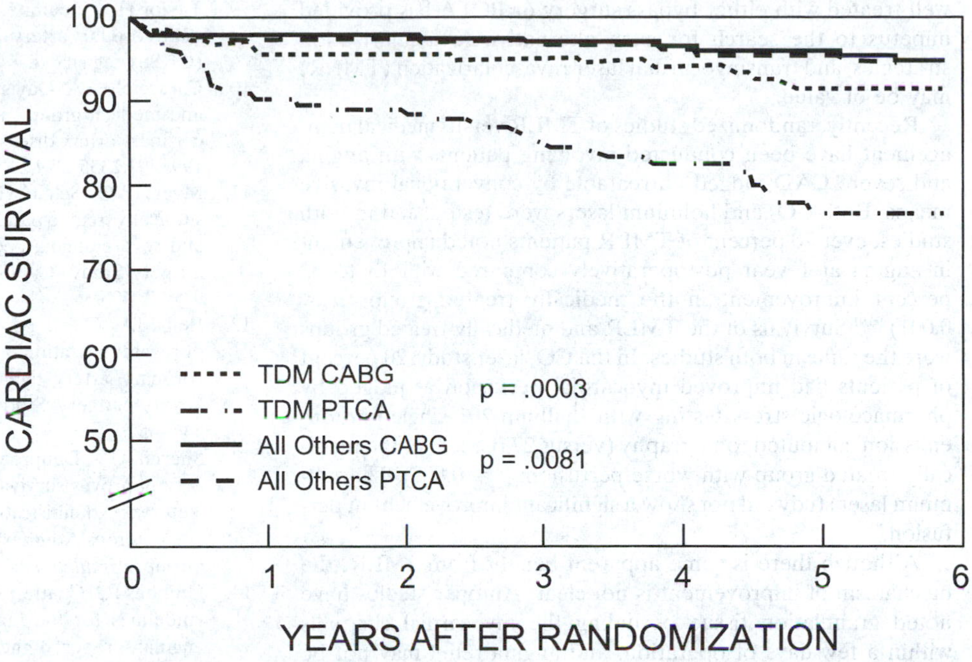

FIGURE 48-10 BARI trial patients with treated diabetes had worse survival following PCTA than following CABG ($p = 0.003$). Patients without diabetes had equivalent survival. (Used with permission from BARI Investigators. Influence of diabetes on 5-year mortality and morbidity in a randomized trial comparing CABG and PTCA in patients with multivessel disease. *Circulation* 1997; 96:1761–1769.)

There are no randomized studies of PCTA versus CABG for patients with previous bypass surgery. The percutaneous treatment of VGA usually has not been effective. Despite the use of stents, there is a high rate of restenosis and cardiac events.[89] Furthermore, it appears that these cardiac events are often serious ones, MI and/or death. Pathologies that are not based on VGA may be treated effectively with PCTA, including graft anastomotic stenoses, early vein graft stenoses, and native vessel stenoses. Patients with large amounts of myocardium jeopardized by atherosclerotic vein grafts usually should be treated with reoperation. However, generalizations are difficult for these complex patients, and therapeutic decisions are best made by interventional cardiologists, cardiac surgeons, and clinical cardiologists working in concert.

INDICATIONS FOR BYPASS SURGERY

In the individual case, recommendations concerning bypass surgery may be influenced by comorbid conditions that greatly increase operative risk or that limit the patient's ultimate life span. However, some generalizations can be made.[2,14] Patients with 50 percent or greater left main stenosis or multivessel disease with a proximal LAD artery stenosis and abnormal LV function should have a recommendation of surgery regardless of their symptom status. Individual randomized trials and meta-analyses have shown clearly a survival benefit for these patients, and there is no evidence that PCTA is safe in these subgroups.

Diabetic patients with multilesion, multivessel disease including a proximal LAD artery lesion should have surgery regardless of LV function and symptom status. Survival is better with CABG than with medical treatment, and PCTA is clearly not an equivalent intervention in terms of survival.

Patients with multivessel disease that include a proximal LAD artery lesion and demonstrable ischemia should have a recommendation for revascularization. If these patients are nondiabetic with normal LV function and are good angiographic candidates for PCTA, it appears that PCTA does not compromise 5-year survival, and the options of PCTA and CABG should be discussed with the patient.

For patients with single-vessel disease based on a proximal LAD artery lesion, survival appears equivalent with medical therapy, PCTA, and CABG, and all options are reasonable, although CABG patients have had fewer events and symptoms over 5 years.

For other subsets of patients with multivessel disease, surgery may be a reasonable choice for the treatment of symptoms in the face of demonstrable ischemia. The choice between PCTA and CABG for these patients should be based on coronary vascular anatomy and patient preference.

For patients with previous bypass surgery and a significant (≥50 percent) late stenosis in a vein graft to the LAD coronary artery, surgery should be recommended regardless of symptoms. For patients in other anatomic subgroups, the risk-benefit situation is complex. Usually reoperation is undertaken to treat severe symptoms and/or large areas of ischemic jeopardy.

TRANSMYOCARDIAL LASER REVASCULARIZATION

The concept of achieving myocardial revascularization by the creation of channels in the myocardium to allow perfusion of blood directly from the LV cavity to coronary sinusoids has been investigated since the 1950s. Early experiments involved mechanically created channels, but more recently, lasers of various wavelengths have been used. The increasing population of patients with severe distal native vessel atherosclerosis (usually occurring years after previous bypass surgery) who may not be well treated with either bypass surgery or PCTA has provided impetus to the search for such alternative revascularization strategies, and transmyocardial laser revascularization (TMLR) may be of value.

Recently, randomized studies of TMLR versus medical management have been conducted involving patients with angina and severe CAD judged untreatable by conventional invasive means. Both CO_2 and holmium lasers were tested, and in both studies, over 70 percent of TMLR patients noted improvement in angina at 1 year postoperatively compared with 13 to 32 percent improvement in the medically treated group ($p < 0.001$).[90,91] Survivals of the TMLR and medically treated groups were the same in both studies. In the CO_2 laser study, 20 percent of patients had improved myocardial perfusion as judged by pharmacologic stress testing with thallium-201 single-photon-emission computed tomography (versus 27 percent of the medically treated group with worse perfusion; $p = 0.002$). The holmium laser study did not show a significant improvement in perfusion.

Although there is some apparent benefit from TMLR, the mechanism of improvement is not clear. Autopsy studies have noted granulation tissue occluding the myocardial channels within a few days of operation, and angina relief may not be immediate. Denervation and microcollateral stimulation have been suggested as possible mechanisms of angina relief. TMLR appears to have a role in revascularization but currently does not appear to produce the degree or the consistency of improved myocardial perfusion that can be achieved when bypass surgery or PCTA is possible. The indications for TMLR are still in evolution.

References

1. Lytle BW, Cosgrove DM. Coronary artery bypass surgery. In: Wells SA, ed. *Current Problems in Surgery*. St. Louis: Mosby–Year Book; 1992; 29:733–807.
2. Eagle KA, Guyton RA, Davidoff R, et al. ACC/AHA guidelines for coronary artery bypass graft surgery: Executive summary and recommendations: A report of the American College of Cardiology/American Heart Association Task Force on Practice Guidelines (Committee to Revise the 1991 Guidelines for Coronary Artery Bypass Graft Surgery). *J Am Coll Cardiol* 1999; 34:1262–1346.
3. Peduzzi P. Eighteen-year follow-up in the Veterans Affairs Cooperative Study of coronary artery bypass surgery for stable angina: The VA Coronary Artery Bypass Surgery Cooperative Study Group. *Circulation* 1992; 86:121–130.
4. Varnauskas E and The European Coronary Surgery Study Group. Twelve-year follow-up of survival in the randomized European Coronary Surgery Study. *N Engl J Med* 1988; 319:332–337.
5. Passamani E, Davis KB, Gillespie MJ, et al. A randomized trial of coronary artery bypass surgery: Survival of patients with a low ejection fraction. *N Engl J Med* 1985; 312:1665–1671.
6. Alderman EL, Bourassi MG, Cohen LS, et al. Ten-year follow-up of survival and myocardial infarction in the randomized Coronary Artery Surgery Study. *Circulation* 1990; 82:1629–1646.
7. Yusuf S, Zucker D, Peduzzi P, et al. Effect of coronary artery bypass graft surgery on survival: Overview of 10-year results from randomised trials by the Coronary Artery Bypass Graft Surgery Trialists Collaboration. *Lancet* 1994; 344:563–570.
8. Rogers WJ, Coggin CJ, Gersh BJ, et al. Ten-year follow-up of quality of life in patients randomized to receive medical therapy or coronary artery bypass graft surgery: The Coronary Artery Surgery Study (CASS). *Circulation* 1990; 82:1647–1658.
9. Taylor HA, Deumite NJ, Chaitman BR, et al. Asymptomatic left main coronary artery disease in the Coronary Artery Surgery Study (CASS) registry. *Circulation* 1989; 79:1171–1179.
10. Caracciolo EA, Davis KB, Sopko G, et al. Comparison of surgical and medical group survival in patients with left main equivalent coronary artery disease: Long-term CASS experience. *Circulation* 1995; 91:2335–2344.
11. Myers WO, Schaff HV, Gersh BJ, et al. Improved survival of surgically treated patients with triple vessel coronary artery disease and severe angina pectoris: A report from the Coronary Artery Surgery Study (CASS) registry. *J Thorac Cardiovasc Surg* 1989; 97:487–495.
12. Bell MA, Gersh BJ, Schaff HV, et al. Effect of completeness of revascularization on long-term outcome of patients undergoing coronary artery bypass surgery: A report from the Coronary Artery Surgery Study (CASS) Registry. *Circulation* 1992; 86: 446–457.
13. Sharma GV, Deupree RH, Khuri SF, et al. Coronary bypass surgery improves survival in high-risk unstable angina: Results of a Veterans Administration Cooperative study with an 8-year follow-up. Veterans Administration Unstable Angina Cooperative Study Group. *Circulation* 1991; 84(suppl III):III-260–III-267.
14. Gibbons RJ, Chatterjee K, Daley J, et al. ACC/AHA/ACP-ASIM guidelines for the management of patients with chronic stable angina: A report of the American College of Cardiology/American Heart Association Task Force on Practice Guidelines (Committee on Management of Patients with Chronic Stable Angina). *J Am Coll Cardiol* 1999; 33:2092–2197.
15. Edwards FH, Clark RE, Schwartz M. Coronary artery bypass grafting: The Society of Thoracic Surgeons National Database experience. *Ann Thorac Surg* 1994; 57:12–19.
16. Bourassa MG, Campeau L, Lesperance J. Changes in grafts and coronary arteries after coronary bypass surgery. *Cardiovasc Clin* 1991; 21:83–100.
17. Fitzgibbon GM, Leach AJ, Kafka HP, et al. Coronary bypass graft fate: Long-term angiographic study. *J Am Coll Cardiol* 1991; 17:1075.
18. Campeau L, Enjalbert M, Lesperance M, et al. The relation of risk factors to the development of atherosclerosis in saphenous vein bypass grafts and the progression of disease in the native circulation. *N Engl J Med* 1984; 311:1329–1332.
19. Lytle BW, Loop FD, Cosgrove DM, et al. Long-term (5 to 12 years) serial studies of internal mammary artery and saphenous vein coronary bypass grafts. *J Thorac Cardiovasc Surg* 1985; 89:248–258.
20. Fitzgibbon GM, Kafka HP, Leach AJ, et al. Coronary bypass graft fate and patient outcome: angiographic follow-up of 5065 grafts related to survival and reoperation in 1388 patients during 25 years. *J Am Coll Cardiol* 1996; 28:616–626.
21. Vlodaver Z, Edward JE. Pathologic changes in aortic-coronary arterial saphenous vein grafts. *Circulation* 1971; 44:719–728.
22. Ratliff NB, Myles JL. Rapidly progressive atherosclerosis in aortocoronary saphenous vein grafts: Possible immuno-mediated disease. *Arch Pathol Lab Med* 1989; 113:772–776.
23. Fitzmaurice M, Ratliff NB. Immunoglobulin deposition in atherosclerotic aortocoronary saphenous vein grafts. *Arch Pathol Lab Med* 1990; 114:388–393.
24. Barboriak JJ, Pintar K, Korns ME. Atherosclerosis in aortocoronary vein grafts. *Lancet* 1974; 2:611–614.
25. Neitzel GF, Barboriak JJ, Pintar K, et al. Atherosclerosis in aortocoronary bypass grafts: Morphologic study and risk factor analysis 6 to 12 years after surgery. *Arteriosclerosis* 1986; 6:594–600.
26. Keon WJ, Heggtveit HA, Leduc J. Perioperative myocardial infarctions caused by atheroembolization. *J Thorac Cardiovasc Surg* 1982; 84:849–855.
27. Gavaghan TP, Gebski V, Baron DW. Immediate postoperative aspirin improves vein graft patency early and late after coronary

artery bypass graft surgery: A placebo-controlled, randomized study. *Circulation* 1991; 83:1526–1533.
28. Goldman S, Copeland J, Moritz T, et al. Starting aspirin therapy after operation: Effects on early graft patency. *Circulation* 1991; 84:520–526.
29. The Post Coronary Artery Bypass Graft Trial Investigators. The effect of aggressive lowering of low-density lipoprotein cholesterol levels and low-dose anticoagulation on obstructive changes in saphenous-vein coronary-artery bypass grafts. *N Engl J Med* 1997; 336:153–162.
30. Blankenhorn DH, Nessim SA, Johnson RL, et al. Beneficial effects of combined colestipol-niacin therapy on coronary atherosclerosis and coronary venous bypass grafts. *JAMA* 1987; 257: 3233–3240.
31. Flaker GC, Warnica JW, Sacks FM. et al. Pravastatin prevents clinical events in revascularized patients with average cholesterol concentrations: Cholesterol and Recurrent Events (CARE) investigators. *J Am Coll Cardiol* 1999; 34:106–112.
32. Lawrie GM, Morris GC Jr., Earle N. Long-term results of coronary bypass surgery: Analysis of 1698 patients followed 15 to 20 years. *Ann Surg* 1991; 213:377–385.
33. Whitlow PL, Dimas AP, Bashore TM, et al. Relationship of extent of revascularization with angina at one year in the Bypass Angioplasty Revascularization Investigation (BARI). *J Am Coll Cardiol* 1999; 34:1750–1759.
34. Dion R, Etienne PY, Verhelst R, et al. Bilateral mammary grafting: Clinical, functional, and angiographic assessment in 400 consecutive cases. *Eur J Cardiothorac Surg* 1993; 7:287–294.
35. Tector AJ, Amundsen S, Schmahl TM, et al. Total revascularization with T grafts. *Ann Thorac Surg* 1994; 57:33–39.
36. Califiore AM, DiGiammarco G, Lucimi N, et al. Composite arterial conduits for a wide arterial myocardial revascularization. *Ann Thorac Surg* 1994; 58:185–190.
37. Loop FD, Lytle BW, Cosgrove DM, et al. Influence of the internal-mammary artery graft on 10-year survival and other cardiac events. *N Engl J Med* 1986; 314:1–6.
38. Cameron A, Davis KB, Green G, et al. Coronary bypass surgery with internal-thoracic-artery grafts: Effects on survival over a 15-year period. *N Engl J Med* 1996; 334:216–219.
39. Lytle BW, Blackstone EH, Loop FD, et al. Two internal thoracic artery grafts are better than one. *J Thorac Cardiovasc Surg* 1999; 117:855–872.
40. Buxton BF, Komeda M, Fuller JA, Gordon I. Bilateral internal thoracic artery grafting may improve outcome of coronary artery surgery: Risk-adjusted survival. *Circulation* 1998; 98:III-1–III-6.
41. Suma H, Amano A, Horii T, et al. Gastroepiploic artery graft in 400 patients. *Eur J Cardiothorac Surg* 1996; 10:6–11.
42. Buche M, Schroeder E, Gurne O, et al. Coronary artery bypass grafting with the inferior epigastric artery: Midterm clinical and angiographic results. *J Thorac Cardiovasc Surg* 1995; 109:553–560.
43. Fisk RL, Brooks CH, Callaghan JC, et al. Experience with the radial artery for coronary artery bypass. *Ann Thorac Surg* 1976; 21:513–518.
44. Carpentier A. Selection of coronary bypass: Anatomic, physiological and angiographic consideration of vein and mannary artery bypass. *J Thorac Cardiovasc Surg* 1975; 70:414–431.
45. Brodman RF, Frame R, Camacho M, et al. Routine use of unilateral and bilateral radial arteries for coronary bypass graft surgery. *J Am Coll Cardiol* 1996; 28:959–963.
46. Acar C, Ramsheyi A, Pagny J. et al. The radial artery for coronary artery bypass grafting: Clinical and angiographic results at five years. *J Thorac Cardiovasc Surg* 1998; 116:981–989.
47. Possati G, Gardino M, Alessandrini F, et al. Mid-term clinical and angiographic results of radial artery grafts used for myocardial revascularization. *J Thorac Cardiovasc Surg* 1998; 116:1015–1021.
48. Bergsma TM, Grandjean JG, Voors AA, et al. Low recurrence of angina pectoris after coronary artery bypass graft surgery with bilateral internal thoracic and right gastroepiploic arteries. *Circulation* 1998; 97:2402–2405.
49. Edwards FH, Grover FL, Shroyer AL, et al. The Society of Thoracic Surgeons National Cardiac Surgery Database: Current risk assessment. *Ann Thorac Surg* 1977; 63:903–908.
50. Hannan EL, Racz MJ, McCallister BD, et al. A comparison of three-year survival after coronary artery bypass graft surgery and percutaneous transluminal coronary angioplasty. *J Am Coll Cardiol* 1999; 33:63–72.
51. Jones RH, Hannan EL, Hammermeister KE, et al. Identification of preoperative variables needed for risk adjustment of short-term mortality after coronary bypass graft surgery: The Working Group Panel on the Cooperative CABG Database Project. *J Am Coll Cardiol* 1996; 28:1478–1487.
52. Burack JH, Impellizzai P, Homel P, et al. Public reporting of surgical mortality: A survey of New York State cardiothoracic surgeons. *Ann Thorac Surg* 1999; 68:1195–1202.
53. Cosgrove DM, Loop FD, Lytle BW, et al. Does internal mammary artery grafting increase surgical risk? *Circulation* 1985; 72(suppl 2):170–174.
54. Grover FL, Johnson RR, Marshall G, et al. Impact of mammary grafts on coronary bypass operation mortality and morbidity. *Ann Thorac Surg* 1994; 57:559–569.
55. Edwards FH for STS Database. Personal communication, 1999.
56. Martin TD, Craver JM, Gott JP, et al. Prospective, randomized trial of retrograde warm blood cardioplegia: Myocardial benefit and neurologic threat. *Ann Thorac Surg* 1994; 57:298–302.
57. Bottner RK, Wallace RB, Visner MS, et al. Reduction of myocardial infarction after emergency coronary artery bypass grafting for failed coronary angioplasty with use of a normothermic perfusion cardioplegia protocol. *J Thorac Cardiovasc Surg* 1971; 101:1069–1075.
58. Christakis GT, Fremes SE, Weisel RD, et al. Reducing the risk of urgent revascularization for unstable angina: A randomized clinical trial. *J Vasc Surg* 1986; 3:764–772.
59. Buckberg GD. Strategies and logic of cardioplegic delivery to prevent, avoid and reverse ischemic and reperfusion damage. *J Thorac Cardiovasc Surg* 1987; 93:127–139.
60. Roach GW, Kanchuger M, Mangano CM, et al. Adverse cerebral outcomes after coronary bypass surgery: Multicenter study of Perioperative Ischemia Research Group and the Ischemia Research and Education Foundation investigators. *N Engl J Med* 1996; 335:1857–1863.
61. Hartman GS, Yao FS, Bruefach M III. Severity of aortic atheromatous disease diagnosed by transesophageal echocardiography predicts stroke and other outcomes associated with coronary artery surgery: A prospective study. *Anesth Analg* 1996; 83:701–708.
62. Blauth CI, Cosgrove DM, Webb BW, et al. Atheroembolism from the ascending aorta: An emerging problem in cardiac surgery. *J Thorac Cardiovasc Surg* 1992; 103:1104–1112.
63. Berens ES, Kouchoukos NT, Murphy SF, Wareing TH. Preoperative carotid artery screening in elderly patients undergoing cardiac surgery. *J Vasc Surg* 1992; 15:313–321.
64. Salasidis GC, Latter DA, Steinmetz OK, et al. Carotid artery duplex scanning in preoperative assessment for coronary artery revascularization: The association between peripheral vascular disease, carotid artery stenosis and stroke. *J Vasc Surg* 1995; 21:154–160.
65. Hertzer NR, Loop FD, Beven EG, et al. Surgical strategy for simultaneous coronary and carotid disease: A study including prospective randomization. *J Vasc Surg* 1989; 9:455–463.
66. Akins CW, Moncure AC, Daggett WM, et al. Safety and efficacy of concomitant carotid and coronary artery operations. *Ann Thorac Surg* 1995; 60:311–317.
67. Loop FD, Lytle BW, Cosgrove DM, et al. Sternal wound complications after isolated coronary bypass grafting: Early and late mortal-

ity, morbidity and cost of care. *Ann Thorac Surg* 1990; 49:179–187.

68. Possati G, Gandino M, Alessandrini F, et al. Systematic clinical and angiographic follow-up of patients undergoing minimally invasive coronary artery bypass. *J Thorac Cardiovasc Surg* 1998; 115: 785–790.
69. Calafiore AM, Teodori G, DiGiammao G, et al. Minimally invasive coronary artery surgery: The LAST operation. *Semin Thorac Cardiovasc Surg* 1997; 9:305–311.
70. Galloway AC, Shemin R, Glower DD et al. First report of the Port-Access International Registry. *Ann Thorac Surg* 1999; 67:51–58.
71. Buffolo E, deAndrade CS, Branco JN, et al. Coronary artery bypass grafting without cardiopulmonary bypass. *Ann Thorac Surg* 1996; 61:63–66.
72. Tasdemir O, Vural KM, Karagoz H, et al. Coronary artery bypass grafting on the beating heart without the use of extracorporeal circulation: Review of 2052 cases. *J Thorac Cardiovasc Surg* 1998; 116:68–73.
73. Iaco AL, Contini M, Teodori G, et al. Off or on bypass: What is the safety threshold? *Ann Thorac Surg* 1999; 68:1486–1489.
74. Myers WO, Blackstone EH, Davis K, et al. CASS Registry. Long term surgical survival. *J Am Coll Cardiol* 1999; 33:488–498.
75. Kirklin JW, et al. ACC/AHA Task Force Report: Guidelines and indications for coronary artery bypass surgery. *J Am Coll Cardiol* 1991; 17:543.
76. Cavender JB, Rogers WJ, Fisher LD, et al. Effects of smoking on survival and morbidity in patients randomized to medical or surgical therapy in the Coronary Artery Surgery Study (CASS): 10-year follow-up. *J Am Coll Cardiol* 1992; 20:287–294.
77. Cosgrove DM, Loop FD, Lytle BW, et al. Determinants of 10-year survival after primary myocardial revascularization. *Ann Surg* 1985; 202:480–490.
78. Jones EL, Weintraub WS. The importance of completeness of revascularization during long-term follow-up after coronary artery operation. *J Thorac Cardiovasc Surg* 1996; 112:227–237.
79. Cosgrove DM, Loop FD, Lytle BW, et al. Predictors of reoperation after myocardial revascularization. *J Thorac Cardiovasc Surg* 1986; 92:811–821.
80. Lytle BW, Loop FD, Taylor PC, et al. Vein graft disease: The clinical impact of stenoses in saphenous vein grafts to coronary arteries. *J Thorac Cardiovasc Surg* 1992; 103:831–840.
81. Lytle BW, Loop FD, Taylor PC, et al. The effect of coronary reoperation on the survival of patients with stenoses in saphenous vein to coronary bypass grafts. *J Thorac Cardiovasc Surg* 1993; 105:605–614.
82. Lytle BW, Loop FD, Cosgrove DM, et al. Fifteen hundred coronary reoperations: Results and determinants of early and late survival. *J Thorac Cardiovasc Surg* 1987; 93:847–859.
83. Loop FD, Lytle BW, Cosgrove DM, et al. Reoperation for coronary atherosclerosis: Changing practice in 2509 consecutive patients. *Ann Surg* 1990; 212:378–386.
84. Lytle BW, McElroy D, McCarthy PM, et al. Influence of arterial coronary bypass grafts on the mortality in coronary reoperations. *J Thorac Cardiovasc Surg* 1994; 107:675–683.
85. Hueb WA, Sowes PR, deOliveira SA, et al. Five-year follow-up of the Medicine, Angioplasty, or Surgery Study (MASS): A prospective, randomized trial of medical therapy. Balloon angioplasty or bypass surgery for single proximal left anterior descending coronary artery stenosis. *Circulation* 1999; 100(supp II):II-107–II-113.
86. Bypass Angioplasty Revascularization Investigation (BARI). Comparison of coronary bypass surgery with angioplasty in patients with multivessel disease. *N Engl J Med* 1996; 335: 217–225.
87. King SB, Lembo NJ, Weintraub WS, et al. A randomized trial comparing coronary angioplasty with coronary bypass surgery: Emory Angioplasty versus Surgery Trial (EAST). *N Engl J Med* 1994; 331:1044–1050.
88. BARI Investigators. Influence of diabetes on 5-year mortality and morbidity in a randomized trial comparing CABG and PTCA in patients with multivessel disease. *Circulation* 1997; 96:1761–1769.
89. Savage MP, Douglas JS Jr., Fischman DL, et al. Stent placement compared with balloon angioplasty for obstructed coronary bypass grafts. Saphenous Vein De Novo Trial Investigators. *N Engl J Med* 1997; 337:740–747.
90. Frazier OH, March RJ, Horvath KA, et al. Transmyocardial revascularization with a carbon dioxide laser in patients with end-stage coronary artery disease. *N Engl J Med* 1999; 341:1021–1028.
91. Allen KB, Dowling RD, Fudge TL, et al. Comparison of transmyocardial revascularization with medical therapy in patients with refractory angina. *N Engl J Med* 1999; 341:1029–1036.

CHAPTER 49

MANAGEMENT OF THE PATIENT AFTER CARDIAC SURGERY

Douglas C. Morris / Stephen D. Clements, Jr. / Carl C. Hug, Jr.

The initial management of the patient following cardiac surgery is primarily focused in specialized intensive care units. The unique pathophysiologic alterations associated with hypothermia and cardiopulmonary bypass (CPB)[1] mandated that a specialized environment, including intensive monitoring and offering sophisticated electrophysiologic, hemodynamic, and mechanical intervention supervised by specially trained critical care nurses, be available. While CPB is no longer universally applied in cardiac surgery, the multiple management problems posed by cardiac patients as a consequence of their preoperative status, effects of residual anesthetic drugs, success of the operative procedure, and intraoperative complications continue to demand specialized treatment. When direct coronary artery bypass grafting is done without CPB, the primary concerns are bleeding (residual heparin, surgical hemostasis), hypothermia, myocardial ischemia, and injury. The use of CPB accentuates these concerns and adds those of a generalized inflammatory response.

ROLE OF VASCULAR CANNULAE, LIFE SUPPORT, AND MONITORING IN THE IMMEDIATE POSTOPERATIVE PERIOD

On arrival in the ICU, the patient is still under the effects of anesthesia and hypothermia, often receiving one or more drugs affecting the systemic circulation, and, in most cases, mechanically ventilated. The patient typically arrives from the operating room with the necessary apparatus for monitoring the following parameters: heart rate and rhythm; arterial, central venous, pulmonary artery, and pulmonary artery occlusion pressures (PAOP); cardiac output; urinary output; mediastinal drainage; body temperature; and arterial oxygen saturation (SpO_2) and end-tidal carbon dioxide tension ($ETCO_2$). Immediately upon arrival in the ICU, reliable monitoring of the previously mentioned variables should be instituted. Once the patient is satisfactorily connected to the bedside monitors and ventilator, all the hemodynamic measurements should be recorded, the patient's level of consciousness and comfort should be assessed, a portable supine chest x-ray should be acquired, and a 12-lead electrocardiogram obtained.

Most of the apparatus attached to the patient upon arrival in the ICU serves a dual purpose. A pulmonary artery catheter not only allows monitoring of pulmonary artery pressures but can also be used to estimate the filling pressure of the left ventricle, cardiac output, and body core temperature. The peripheral arterial cannula provides a continuous pulse-wave tracing of systemic blood pressure and ready access to arterial blood sampling for laboratory analysis. *Regular periodic assessments of arterial blood gases, especially after a major change in ventilator settings, are essential unless continuous $ETCO_2$ and SpO_2 by pulse oximetry are being monitored.* $ETCO_2$ and SpO_2 are reliable in guiding the weaning of mechanical ventilation and tracheal extubation. Monitoring of these parameters has been used very effectively in "fast-track" protocols. Assessment of volume loss is based on chest and mediastinal tube drainage plus urine output. The endotracheal tube secured in the correct position with an appropriately inflated cuff is essential for positive-pressure ventilation of the lungs. Confirmation of bilateral breath sounds and absence of tracheal air leak versus cuff inflation should be made upon arrival in the ICU and after suctioning secretions from the oropharynx. The endotracheal tube's position should be ascertained on the initial chest x-ray. The endotracheal tube also allows for suctioning of bronchial secretions and reduces (but does not eliminate) the risk of oropharyngeal and gastric reflux secretions entering the trachea and bronchi. The endotracheal tube can often be removed the evening of surgery if the patient is conscious, is able to protect the airway, has good ventilatory mechanics and muscle strength, and is able to take on the work of breathing. Most patients can have the pulmonary artery catheter removed within 12 to 24 h if cardiovascular drug therapy is at minimum levels. The peripheral arterial cannula can be removed once cardiovascular function is satisfactory and the need for blood sampling is at a routine daily level. The urinary catheter is usually removed when the patient is ambulatory unless there is a vigorous diuresis or an increased risk of urinary retention. Chest tubes are generally removed when the total drainage is less than 100 mL per tube over 8 h.

The primary factor that differentiates cardiac surgery from other forms of surgery is CPB. With such improvements in extracorporeal technology as membrane oxygenation, arterial blood filtration, and blood sparing techniques, the noncardiac complications have been significantly reduced. Major improvements in myocardial protection technology coupled with changes in anesthetic and CPB techniques now frequently allow extubation within several hours of surgery.[2] Intraoperative management has now evolved to the point of minimizing the need for cardiopulmonary support after surgery, thereby allowing the patient to recover satisfactory vital function more rapidly than before. As a consequence, mechanical ventilation and other measures can be discontinued much earlier, and the patient can be safely and comfortably transferred from the ICU within the first 6 to 24 h, a process that has been termed *fast-tracking*.[3]

Individuals undergoing "off pump" procedures also have the potential for rapid recovery and early extubation and removal of catheters and chest tubes, and can be sitting up in the chair the next morning ready for transfer.

Fast-tracking describes efforts to minimize the duration of the patient's stay in the ICU or postanesthesia care unit and to allow the early, safe transfer of the cardiac surgical patient to a so-called step-down level of monitored care. Early extubation and transfer should require that the patient's status is characterized as follows: awake or easily aroused, neurologically intact, cooperative, and comfortable; stable, satisfactory hemodynamics; normothermia; satisfactory spontaneous ventilation; normal coagulation with minimal chest tube drainage; satisfactory urine output, electrolyte, and acid-base balance.[4]

EARLY POSTOPERATIVE MANAGEMENT

Pathophysiologic Consequences of Cardiopulmonary Bypass

The basic pathophysiology during the early postoperative period revolves around the following variables: transient left ventricular dysfunction, capillary leak, warming from hypothermia, mediastinal bleeding, and emergence from anesthesia.

The likely presence of left ventricular dysfunction during the first 24 h postoperatively with a gradual recovery to preoperative levels is suggested by studies based upon hemodynamic data, nuclear scanning, and metabolic techniques. While improvements in surgical techniques, cardioplegia delivery, and other myocardial protection measures achieved in the past decade would have been expected to lessen this complication, the reported prevalence of early ventricular dysfunction (90 percent) did not change between 1979 and 1990.[5] This transient myocardial depression has been attributed by some authors to inadequate myocardial protection or the effects of cold cardioplegia,[6,7] but the bulk of the evidence incriminates the inflammatory state induced by CPB as the primary causative factor.[1]

The inflammatory state induced by CPB involves platelet-endothelial cell interactions and vasospastic responses that result in low-flow states in the coronary circulation.[8] The inflammatory reaction causes vascular endothelial adhesion molecules to attract inflammatory cells that subsequently adhere to the vascular endothelium. These inflammatory cells mediate much of the subsequent injury by the release of oxygen radicals or proteolytic enzymes.[9] This release of oxygen-free radicals in response to reperfusion injury is now generally accepted as the explanation for the transient postoperative ventricular dysfunction.[10–12] Depressed myocardial function seems to be unrelated to CPB time, number of coronary artery grafts, preoperative medications, or postoperative core temperature. Ventricular function is generally depressed by 2 h and is at its worse at 4 to 5 h after CPB. Significant recovery of function usually occurs by 8 to 10 h, and full recovery is reached by 24 to 48 h.[13] Systemic vascular resistance, while not rising immediately after surgery, increases as ventricular function worsens. This rise in systemic vascular resistance is likely secondary to reduced ventricular function and the need to maintain systemic blood pressure and, per se, is not a major causative factor of depressed cardiac contractility. The confounding effect of vasopressor drugs used in an attempt to increase systemic blood pressure must be recognized.

The inflammation-mediated production of oxygen-free radicals and release of proteolytic enzymes by neutrophils also damages the endothelial cells. The "gatekeeper" function of the endothelium is disturbed and capillary permeability increases, resulting in edema.[9] The capillary leak syndrome may last from a few hours up to 1 to 2 days, depending to a large degree on the duration of CPB. When the capillary leak ceases and interstitial edema fluid is mobilized, intravascular volume overload is a threat. At this time, diuretics are beneficial to eliminate excessive fluid.

Hypothermia predisposes the patient to cardiac dysrhythmias, increases systemic vascular resistance, precipitates shivering (which increases O_2 consumption and CO_2 production), and impairs coagulation.[13] Hypothermia with the patient's core temperature below 35°C frequently recurs after rewarming to 37°C (98.6°F) at the end of CPB. This fall in core temperature reflects the loss of heat from the surgical field after CPB, exposure of the patient to ambient temperature, and incomplete rewarming of peripheral tissues, especially fat and muscle. If the patient is hypothermic upon arrival in the ICU, monitoring the temperature of noncore body sites such as a finger or toe can assure complete assessment of rewarming. Hypothermia causes peripheral vasoconstriction and contributes to the hypertension frequently seen after cardiac surgery. Furthermore, hypothermia causes a decrease in cardiac output by producing bradycardia along with the increase in vascular resistance. As the patient is rewarmed, large increases in O_2 consumption, and CO_2 production can occur, with a consequent increase in demand on cardiovascular and pulmonary functions.[14]

Hypercarbia will cause catecholamine release, tachycardia, and pulmonary hypertension. If the patient cannot increase the cardiac output and O_2 delivery, venous hemoglobin desaturation and metabolic acidosis will result. Most believe that the patient should be passively rewarmed by warm air (e.g., Bear Hugger) and that shivering should be eliminated by the administration of meperidine (25 to 50 mg) and muscle relaxants.[15] As body temperature increases, the vasoconstriction and hypertension associated with hypothermia are replaced by vasodilatation, tachycardia, and hypotension. Volume loading during the rewarming process helps reduce the rapid swings in blood pressure. Vasopressors (e.g., norepinephrine) may be required to maintain an adequate systemic blood pressure.

The commonly reported prevalence of severe postoperative bleeding (more than 10 U of blood transfused) following cardiac surgery is between 3 and 5 percent. In some hospitals, 25 percent of all blood products are dedicated to cardiac surgery.[16] While approximately one-half of the patients who undergo reoperation for excessive bleeding exhibit incomplete surgical hemostasis, the remainder bleed because of various acquired hemostatic defects, most often related to acquired platelet dysfunction.[17] The factors that predispose to bleeding following CPB are residual heparin effect, platelet dysfunction (which may be intensified by preoperative drug therapy, e.g., aspirin and $GPII_bIII_a$ inhibitors), clotting-factor depletion, inadequate surgical hemostasis, hypothermia, and postoperative hypertension. CPB decreases both platelet count and function. Hemodilution causes platelet counts to fall rapidly to about 50 percent of preoperative values. Within minutes after instituting CPB, the bleeding time is prolonged and platelet aggregation is impaired. The bleeding time usually normalizes by 2 to 4 h after CPB. The platelet count usually requires several days to return to normal levels. While the exact mechanism responsible for the transient platelet dysfunction remains undefined, it appears to be related to contact of platelets with the synthetic surfaces of the extracorporeal oxygenator and to hypothermia. Reductions in the plasma concentrations of coagulation factors II, V, VII, IX, X, and XIII due to hemodilution occur during CPB, but these coagulation factors remain well above levels considered adequate for hemostasis and generally normalize within the first 12 h after surgery. Moreover, while bleeding after CPB is often attributed to excessive fibrinolysis, the decrease in both plasminogen and fibrinogen levels during CPB is due to hemodilution and not consumption.[17] Upon returning from the operating room after exploration for bleeding, a common report is that no localized site of bleeding occurred and only diffuse oozing was found. Less frequently, a specific site such as an internal mammary pedicle will be identified.

MANAGEMENT OF COMMON POSTOPERATIVE SYNDROMES

Vasoconstriction with Hypertension and Borderline Cardiac Output

Increased arteriolar resistance as a consequence of hypothermia and increased levels of circulating catecholamines, plasma renin, or angiotensin II is present in most postoperative cardiac patients. The usual criterion for pharmacologic lowering of blood pressure in postoperative patients is a mean arterial blood pressure 10 percent above the upper level of normal (>90 mmHg). Patients with a friable aorta or friable suture lines might be subjected to a lower mean arterial pressure to prevent dehiscence. The mean arterial blood pressure is monitored because it is most reflective of systemic vascular resistance. As the hypothermic patient is rewarmed, a short-acting vasodilator (nitroprusside, nitroglycerin, or nicardipine) can be infused intravenously to maintain mean arterial pressure at 80 to 90 mmHg. Intravascular volume should be maintained at a relatively high level (PAOP of 14 to 16 mmHg) in anticipation of vasodilation upon rewarming and to enhance cardiac output and peripheral perfusion. If the cardiac index is marginal (2.0 to 2.2 L/min/m^2), an inotropic drug should be administered in addition to the vasodilator.

Vasodilatation and Hypotension

This condition, which generally appears during rewarming, is most effectively prevented and best treated by fluid administration. The specific volume expander selected should be based upon a determination of the predominant factor leading to the hypovolemia. If the predominant factor is a capillary leak syndrome with generalized edema, the use of colloids could aggravate the situation as the oncotic elements pass into the interstitium and exacerbate tissue edema. If vasodilatation with increased venous capacitance is the major problem, colloids will provide longer-lasting augmentation of intravascular volume. Hetastarch (administered in 250- to 500-mL increments) provides sustained volume expansion equal to 5 percent albumin, at a significant reduction in cost. It does, however, have a tendency to increase bleeding. If fluid administration has increased PAOP appropriately (e.g., 14 to 16 mmHg for a normal ventricle or 18 to 22 mmHg for a noncompliant ventricle) and systemic blood pressure remains marginal, vasopressor or inotropic drugs should be administered. Generally, a PAOP above 15 mmHg in the postoperative period is of little benefit due to a "flattening" of the diastolic function curve, which accompanies the decline in systolic function.[18] An inotropic vasopressor should be infused if more than 1 or 2 L of fluid have been administered and the PAOP is not rising. In some patients after cardiac surgery, fluid administration produces a substantial increase in left ventricular end-diastolic volume without changing PAOP. Whether this is due to an open pericardium with overdistension of the left ventricle or some other factor is unclear.[19] If the blood pressure is marginal and the cardiac index is over 2.0 L/min/m^2, norepinephrine or dopamine is the preferable agent. If the cardiac index is less than 2.0 L/min/m^2, an inotropic agent should be administered initially.

Normal Ventricular Systolic Function and Low Cardiac Output

This set of circumstances is often noted in small women with systemic hypertension and in patients undergoing aortic valve replacement for aortic stenosis. The likely explanation is diastolic dysfunction. The problem should be managed by volume expansion with the intent to elevate PAOP to levels as high as 20 to 25 mmHg if necessary. Sinus rhythm and atrioventricular synchrony are essential and, if not present, should be restored.

In the absence of other reasons for diastolic dysfunction, the possibility of cardiac compression from clots in the mediastinum and pericardial space should be considered. If volume expansion does not lead to hemodynamic improvement, transesophageal echocardiography (TEE) should be used to establish or exclude the presence of clots or other causes of low output. If the information derived from TEE does not permit explanation and/or resolution of the problem, the patient should return to the operating room for exploration.

A rather characteristic presentation of cardiac compression is the patient who initially has significant mediastinal bleeding that ceases rather abruptly. The patient then becomes hypotensive, with high PAOP and central venous pressure and progressively increasing inotropic drug requirements. Cardiac compression from clots in the pericardial space should be suspected and, if time allows, confirmed by TEE. Rapid clinical deterioration demands immediate exploration of the pericardial space.

APPROACH TO POSTOPERATIVE CARDIOVASCULAR PROBLEMS

Low Cardiac Output Syndrome

Satisfactory cardiac performance following cardiac surgery is usually indicated by a cardiac index greater than 2.2, L/min/m^2 with a heart rate below 100 beats per minute. Marginal cardiac function is present with a cardiac index between 2.0 and 2.2 L/min/m^2. A cardiac index below 2.0 L/min/m^2 is unacceptably low, and therapeutic intervention is indicated. Clinical signs of the adequacy or inadequacy of organ perfusion must be incorporated into any assessment of cardiac performance.

ASSESSMENT

The most common causes of low cardiac output postoperatively are related to a decreased left ventricular preload. The decreased preload, in turn, can likely be attributed to hypovolemia (due to bleeding or to vasodilatation as a consequence of warming or of drugs), cardiac tamponade, or right ventricular dysfunction. Alternative explanations for low cardiac output include decreased contractility due to a preexisting low ejection fraction or to intra- or postoperative ischemia or infarction. Perioperative myocardial ischemia or infarction is usually due to poor intraoperative myocardial protection, incomplete myocardial revascularization, coronary artery spasm, coronary embolism of atherosclerotic debris or air, prolonged systemic hypotension, or severe acute anemia. Tachy- or bradyarrhythmias decrease cardiac output by reducing ventricular preload (e.g., decreased diastolic filling time, loss of atrial contraction or atrioventricular synchrony) or by reducing the number of effective ventricular contractions per minute. Substantial increases in systemic vascular resistance (i.e., vasoconstriction) impede ventricular ejection and lower cardiac output. Vasodilatation from sepsis or anaphylaxis resulting in systemic hypotension could lead to reduced coronary blood flow and myocardial ischemia. Sepsis (an unlikely occurrence in the immediate postoperative period) is also associated with the production of myocardial depressant factors. Anemia may result in reduced blood viscosity (a major determinant of total peripheral resistance) leading to hypotension and decreased oxygen delivery to the heart. The hypotension in anemia, however, is most often due to changes in effective blood volume rather than to the changes in viscosity.

ETIOLOGY AND MANAGEMENT

The multiple variables constantly monitored usually provide sufficient clues as to the cause of low cardiac output. If there is no obvious noncardiac cause such as anaphylaxis or anaphylactoid reaction, acidosis, severe anemia, or marked alterations in body temperature, then the first step is to optimize the preload (PAOP of 15 to 18 mmHg). The next step is to optimize the heart rate by either cardiac pacing or antiarrhythmic drugs. Postoperative myocardial performance is usually best at a rate of 90 to 100 beats per minute. If these measures prove unsuccessful, pharmacologic intervention with inotropic agents, vasodilators, vasopressors, or a combination of these drugs must be considered. The selection of drugs should be based upon the balance of their effects on heart rate, contractility, ventricular preload, and systemic vasculature resistance (Table 49-1). The presence of elevated left- and right-sided filling pressures, a recent cessation of mediastinal drainage, and progressively increasing inotropic drug-dosage requirements suggests tamponade, which should be relieved emergently. TEE has been very helpful in clarifying these situations. The final therapeutic step, if the preceding measures have proved inadequate, is the use of aortic counterpulsation (i.e., intraaortic balloon pump) or another type of cardiac assist device.

TABLE 49-1 Medications Used in Low Cardiac Output Syndrome

Medication	Hemodynamic Properties	Dosage Range
Dopamine	Low dose—dopaminergic effect Moderate dose—inotropic effect High dose—vasopressor effect	2–20 μg/kg/min
Dobutamine	Positive inotropic agent	2–20 μg/kg/min
Epinephrine	Positive inotropic agent	1–4 μg/min
Amrinone	Positive inotropic agent	10–15 μg/kg/min
Isoproterenol	Potent inotropic agent Pronounced chronotropic effect	0.5–10 μg/min
Norepinephrine	Potent vasopressor effect; inotropic effect	1–100 μg/min
Phenylephrine	Potent vasopressor agent	10–500 μg/min

Hypertension

MANAGEMENT

A variety of medications are available for control of hypertension, and the drug selected should depend on the hemodynamic status of the patient, the cardiovascular effects of the drug, and the patient's other medical problems. Systemic hypertension in the presence of a high left ventricular filling pressure and marginal cardiac output is most appropriately treated by an arterial vasodilator. Nitroprusside relaxes vascular smooth muscle in arterial resistance vessels (both systemic and pulmonary) and in venous capacitance vessels. The potential exists with nitroprusside for dilation of the coronary resistance vessels and production of a coronary steal syndrome by shunting blood away from any ischemic areas. The advantages of the drug are its very rapid onset and the rapid dissipation of its effects. The risks with this agent are rapid and excessive hypotension and the potential for either acute cyanide toxicity or thiocyanate toxicity with prolonged use.[19]

Nitroglycerin is primarily a venous dilator, although it produces varying degrees of arterial vasodilatation, especially at high doses. Its major role in treating systemic hypertension is in the patient with high filling pressures and active myocardial ischemia.[20] Nicardipine is a potent systemic and coronary vasodilator without the risk of coronary steal, and it has no significant effect on the venous system. It can, therefore, effectively control postoperative hypertension without reducing the filling pressures or causing a coronary steal. While its onset of action is rapid (1 to 2 min), its elimination half-life is about 40 min. Unlike some calcium channel blockers, this agent lacks a negative inotropic effect and has no effect on atrioventricular conduction.[21] Hydralazine is a direct arterial vasodilator, which is usually administered in intermittent intravenous or intramuscular doses. Hydralazine-induced arterial vasodilation may produce a compensatory tachycardia. This drug is frequently resorted to in patients who are hemodynamically stable but remain hypertensive several days after surgery and cannot yet take or absorb oral medications.

When the hypertension is associated with a normal cardiac output and a relatively rapid sinus heart rate or a propensity toward dysrhythmias, a drug with negative inotropic and chronotropic properties is desirable. Esmolol is a cardioselective, ultrashort-acting beta blocker, which also produces a rapid and titratable control of the blood pressure accompanied by a decrease in heart rate. The drug is usually tolerated satisfactorily by patients with a history of bronchospasm because of its relatively high selectivity for $beta_1$-type adrenergic receptors. It is not ideal for patients with impaired cardiac contractility, particularly in the presence of elevated filling pressures.[22] Diltiazem is an arterial vasodilator that has a mild negative inotropic effect and a more potent negative chronotropic effect. Verapamil is a less potent vasodilator but with more potent negative inotropic, chronotropic, and dromotropic effects. It can be administered intravenously by either boluses or continuous infusion. Labetalol has both alpha- and beta-blocking properties as well as a direct vasodilatory effect. Its predominant effect is as a beta blocker, especially in the intravenous form. The angiotensin-converting enzyme inhibitor enalaprilat, which is the active form of enalapril, can be administered intermittently by the intravenous route. This agent is usually reserved for the patient who is hemodynamically stable with either a normal or reduced cardiac output but with hypertension expected to persist (Table 49-2).

Arrhythmias

GENERAL CONSIDERATIONS AND SINUS TACHYCARDIA

The most common rhythm disturbance immediately after cardiac surgery is sinus tachycardia. This condition is appropriately treated by searching for and correcting the underlying cause (pain, anxiety, low cardiac output, anemia, fever, or beta-blocker withdrawal). The second most common arrhythmia is ventricular ectopy. Again, an underlying cause such as myocardial ischemia, hypokalemia, hypomagnesemia, hypoxia, or administration of sympathomimetic drugs must be sought and corrected if possible. It is also important to review the patient's preoperative record to determine if the patient had preexisting ectopy. Patients with chronic ventricular ectopy frequently have their ectopy exaggerated postoperatively.[23] In the presence of active myocardial ischemia, pharmacologic suppression is advisable for complex ventricular ectopy. In the first 12 h after coronary bypass surgery, myocardial ischemia must be suspected and is difficult to exclude; accordingly, the preceding policy for ectopy suppression should be adhered to with the possible exception of those with known chronic ectopy. Lidocaine is the drug of choice in most instances. The loading dose of lidocaine is approximately 3 mg per kilogram of ideal body weight given over 20 min. One approach is to give an initial bolus of 75 mg, following by 50 mg every 5 min to a total dose of 225 mg. An alternative is to give a priming dose of 75 mg, followed by a loading infusion of 150 mg over 20 min. The usual initial maintenance infusion is 1.5 to 2.5 mg/min. If the arrhythmia is uncontrolled, one can give another bolus of 25 to 50 mg and increase the infusion rate. The chances of toxicity rise signifi-

TABLE 49-2 Intravenous Antihypertensive Agents

Drug	Peak Effect	Duration	Dosage
Nitroprusside	Immediate	2–5 min	0.3–1.0 μg/kg/min
Nitroglycerine	Immediate	2–5 min	5–100 μg/min infusion
Nicardipine	5–60 min	20–40 min	2.5 mg over 5 min; may repeat times 4 at 10-min intervals; infusion 2–15 mg/h
Esmolol	2–5 min	8–10 min	1-min loading infusion of 0.25–0.5 mg/kg; sustained infusion of 50–200 μg/kg/min
Enalaprilat	15–30 min	6 h or more	0.625–1.25 mg slowly over 5 min every 6 h
Hydralazine	15–20 min	3–4 h	5- to 10-mg bolus may be repeated every 15 min; up to total of 40 mg
Diltiazem	3–30 min	3 h	20- to 25-mg bolus may repeat; infusion of 10–20 mg/h
Verapamil	2–3 min	20–40 min	5- to 10-mg bolus; may repeat in 10 min; infusion of 3–25 mg/h
Labetalol	5–15 min	2–6 h	20-mg bolus over 2 min; then 40- to 80-mg boluses every 15 min until effect achieved (to total dose of 300 mg)

cantly at infusion rates above 4 mg/min, especially in individuals greater than 65 years of age. If the ectopy does not respond to lidocaine, the option is to not use an antiarrhythmic agent unless ventricular tachycardia occurs *or* to use intravenous amiodarone. Pacing the heart at a faster rate may prove successful in suppressing the ectopy.

VENTRICULAR TACHYCARDIA AND FIBRILLATION

After cardiac surgery, a few patients develop sustained ventricular tachycardia (either monomorphic or polymorphic) or ventricular fibrillation. These profound rhythm disturbances may develop in the absence of evidence of acute myocardial ischemia or infarction or electrolyte imbalance. In most cases the patients have had previous myocardial infarction and have undergone "complete" revascularization, including regions likely to be nonviable. Reperfusion of these areas that probably include viable as well as nonviable myofibrils embedded in the healed infarct may lead to altered dispersion of repolarization. These changes support development of reentry arrhythmias.[23] The ventricular tachycardia in these patients uncommonly responds to lidocaine and usually requires amiodarone. In some instances, a combination of amiodarone and a beta blocker is required. In a rare circumstance, aortic counterpulsation has seemed to be of benefit.

Every encounter with a wide complex tachycardia requires careful consideration as to the possibility of supraventricular tachycardia with aberrant conduction. In the presence of atrial fibrillation with a rapid ventricular response, right bundle branch aberrant conduction often mimics ventricular tachycardia. Care must be given to avoid lidocaine in these situations, because it may result in an even more rapid ventricular rate.

Wide complex tachyarrhythmias in the range of 250 to 300 beats per minute should suggest the presence of an anomalous conduction pathway. The mechanism of this arrhythmia usually involves atrial flutter, with one-to-one conduction or atrial fibrillation with a very fast ventricular response involving an anomalous pathway. Once this is recognized, procainamide becomes the drug of choice, since it does have favorable therapeutic effects on the bypass track tissue. Lidocaine and verapamil should be avoided if the presence of an anomalous pathway is suspected (see also Chap. 24).

SUPRAVENTRICULAR ARRHYTHMIAS

The most common supraventricular dysrhythmias, with the exception of sinus tachycardia, are atrial fibrillation and atrial flutter. These rhythm disturbances occur in 10 to 30 percent of patients following cardiac surgery. The predominant predisposing factor in the development of atrial fibrillation is the patient's age. The prevalence of atrial fibrillation in postoperative cardiac patients <40 years of age is as low as 3.7 percent, while the prevalence is at least 28 percent in patients >70 years. Atrial fibrillation is most likely to appear on the second postoperative day. Within 1 to 3 days, 80 percent of these patients will return to sinus rhythm with only digoxin or beta-blocker therapy.[24–26] The prophylactic use of beta blockers has a protective effect against the development of atrial fibrillation or flutter. This beneficial effect has been demonstrated with any one of several beta blockers, administered in low or high doses and started preoperatively or postoperatively. Neither digoxin nor verapamil has demonstrated effective prophylaxis against atrial fibrillation or flutter.[27]

Preoperative oral administration of amiodarone also reduces the prevalence of postoperative atrial fibrillation.[28] The major limitation to the widespread application of this prophylactic approach is the apparent need for a 7-day preoperative treatment period. An accelerated loading regimen over 1 to 2 days may be effective, but is unproved.[29]

Intravenous infusions of either esmolol or diltiazem can be used to control the ventricular rate with atrial fibrillation or flutter. Esmolol is given as a 1-min loading infusion of 0.25 to 0.5 mg/kg, followed by a sustained infusion of 50 to 200 μg/kg/min. Diltiazem is administered as a bolus of 20 to 25 mg (which may be repeated), followed by an infusion of 10 to 15 mg/h.

Atrial epicardial pacing wires provide the means of atrial pacing to convert some cases of atrial flutter to sinus rhythm.[25] Short bursts (15 to 30 s) of atrial pacing at rates of 300 to 600 per minute may be effective in converting atrial flutter. Approximately 10 percent of patients with atrial fibrillation require electrical cardioversion to restore sinus rhythm. If hemodynamic compromise is present and aggravated by a supraventricular tachyarrhythmia, cardioversion should be used immediately rather than later.

Intravenous ibutilide (1 mg infused over 10 min to be repeated once if necessary) is the most effective pharmacologic means of converting recent-onset atrial flutter. The drug is much less effective (in the range of 30 to 50 percent) for conversion of recent-onset atrial fibrillation. The disadvantage of ibutilide is the propensity for causing torsades de pointes in 2 to 4 percent of patients.[29]

CONDUCTION DEFECTS

The prevalence of intraventricular conduction abnormalities after coronary bypass surgery is reported to be from 1 to 45 percent, with approximately 10 percent being the most commonly reported frequency. The most common conduction defect is right bundle branch block, which may be due to selective sensitivity of the right bundle to the effects of hypothermia and the extracorporeal circulation process. Only about 5 percent of the patients are left with a permanent conduction abnormality, and the prognosis for these patients is no worse than it is for comparable patients with no conduction defect.[30,31] The development of high-degree (second- or third-degree) atrioventricular block is an indication for temporary pacing via epicardial pacing wires. Atrioventricular block is not as common as either bundle branch block or fascicular block, but it does occur, especially after aortic valve surgery.

Respiratory Management

EXPECTED RESPIRATORY CHANGES AFTER CARDIAC SURGERY

Pulmonary problems are the most significant cause of morbidity following cardiac surgery. The pain associated with sternotomy and, especially, with thoracotomy has a deleterious effect on the patient's willingness to breathe deeply and cough. Pain caused by the presence of chest tubes may also interfere with normal respiratory function. Phrenic nerve damage can result in diaphragmatic dysfunction. More commonly, the diaphragm is passively displaced cephalad by abdominal contents (gastrointestinal intraluminal air and fluid and edematous bowel) in the anesthetized, paralyzed patient supported by mechanical ventilation. Elevated left side of the heart filling pressures may cause alveolar edema and, in some patients, increased capillary permeability may exist. Insertion of an oro- or nasogastric tube by the anesthesiologist while the patient is under general anesthesia is recommended.

Atelectasis is the most common pulmonary complication, occurring in about 70 percent of patients following cardiac surgery with CPB.[32] During CPB, the lungs are not perfused and are usually allowed to collapse. Once the lungs are reexpanded, a variable amount of atelectasis remains. While the atelectasis might be microscopic, intermediate degrees (subsegmental and segmental) are common. The preponderance of atelectasis occurs in the left lower lobe because of its compression during cardiac surgery, the tendency to suction more thoroughly the right mainstem bronchus during blind naso-orotracheal suctioning, and the frequent surgical practice of opening the left pleural space to facilitate dissection of the left internal mammary artery. Evidence for a depletion of surfactant after cardiopulmonary bypass is lacking.[33]

After thoracotomy, both lung and chest wall compliance decrease significantly. The maximum decrease occurs at approximately 3 days, but the decrease persists to a lesser degree 6 or more days after sternotomy. Alterations in chest wall mechanics lead to a decrease in the forced expiratory volume (FEV_1) and the functional residual capacity (FRC). The changes in the FEV_1 may persist for 6 weeks. In addition to these changes in flows and volumes, reduced inspiratory strength and uncoordinated rib cage expansion occur. These changes result in an increase in respiratory rate and a decrease in tidal volume, a decrease in respiratory efficiency, and an increase in oxygen cost of breathing. The atelectasis and decrease in lung volume result in ventilation:perfusion mismatch and shunting. The clinical manifestation is a decrease in arterial PO_2 and hemoglobin saturation.[33]

There is little evidence of a significant increase in lung water after routine CPB. When increased capillary permeability exists, it is usually related to elevated cardiac filling pressures.[33]

BASIC CONCEPTS OF OXYGENATION AND ALVEOLAR VENTILATION

The goals of mechanical ventilation are the maintenance of satisfactory arterial oxygenation and CO_2 removal. Direct measurement of PaO_2 is generally used to assess the overall adequacy of blood oxygenation, while pulse oximetry (SpO_2) is used to monitor peripheral arterial hemoglobin saturation on a continuous basis. An $SpO_2 > 90$ percent is considered to be acceptable, but it may be associated with a marginal PaO_2. The oxygen-hemoglobin dissociation curve portrays this relationship (Fig. 49-1). The shoulder of this sigmoid curve lies at a PaO_2 of approximately 65 mmHg. A PaO_2 below this level will result in a precipitous fall in the oxygen saturation of hemoglobin. With hypothermia or with profound respiratory alkalosis, the curve will shift to the left, resulting in more avid binding of oxygen to hemoglobin and less release of oxygen to the tissues. The patient will likely be receiving 100 percent oxygen during transfer from the operating room to the ICU or postanesthesia care unit. The FIO_2 should be gradually decreased to 0.4 as tolerated to minimize adsorption atelectasis and pulmonary O_2 toxicity. Mechanical ventilation is also used to maintain alveolar ventilation, which regulates the arterial blood CO_2 tension

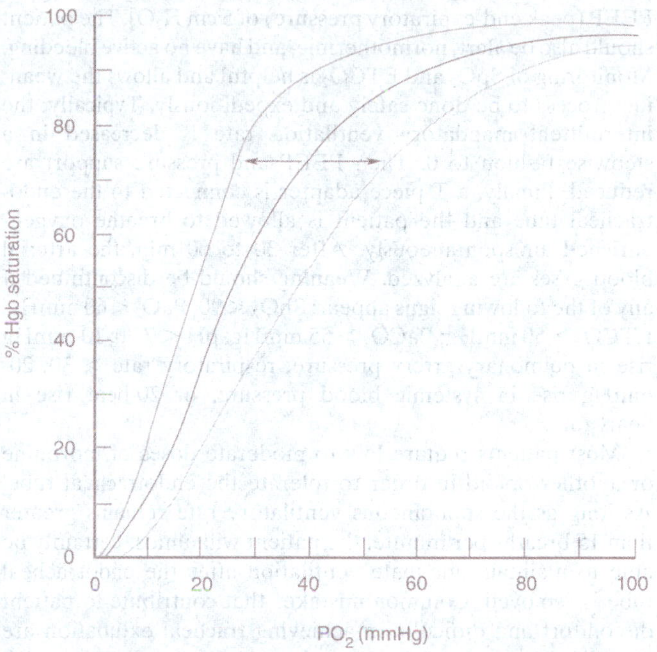

FIGURE 49-1 Oxygen-hemoglobin dissociation curve. The curve depicts the saturation of hemoglobin at increasing levels of PaO_2. A shift of the curve to the left increases the affinity of hemoglobin for oxygen and a shift to the right decreases the affinity.

($PaCO_2$). Alveolar ventilation is regulated by controlling the tidal volume and the respiratory rate. Generally, the ventilator should maintain an exhaled minute ventilation of 6 to 8 L/min. Decreasing the tidal volume below 8 to 10 mL/kg may result in alveolar hypoventilation and atelectasis. Mild hypocarbia ($PaCO_2$ of 30 to 35 mmHg) is satisfactory immediately after surgery, but more profound respiratory alkalosis should be avoided because it leads to hypokalemia and a leftward shift of the oxygen-hemoglobin dissociation curve (decreased oxygen release to the tissues). Hypocarbia is best corrected by reducing the ventilator rate.

Hypercarbia in the immediate postoperative period usually indicates that minute ventilation is inadequate. The problem can be rectified primarily by increasing the ventilator rate; in some cases it is appropriate to increase the tidal volume as well. Later, as the patient is weaned from the ventilator, hypercarbia may reflect opioid analgesia (a necessary side effect of satisfactory analgesia) or compensatory hypoventilation in response to a metabolic alkalosis, most likely due to excessive diuresis. Acetazolamide (Diamox), 250 to 500 mg intravenously every 6 h, is beneficial in correcting a primary metabolic alkalosis. Severe hypercarbia should raise a concern about mechanical problems such as ventilator malfunction, endotracheal tube malposition, or a pneumothorax.[5] Occasionally, hypoxemia and even hypotension may develop in the mechanically ventilated patient due to a tension pneumothorax or hemothorax. If the latter are suspected, assessment of breath sounds and a chest x-ray are indicated for confirmation.

VENTILATORY WEANING AND EXTUBATION

Ventilatory support should be reduced as tolerated when the cardiovascular system has become stable and the arterial oxygen tension is satisfactory [$PaO_2 > 70$ mmHg, with FIO_2 of 0.5 and

PEEP (peak end-expiratory pressure) of 5 cm H_2O]. The patient should also be alert, normothermic, and have no active bleeding. Monitoring of SpO_2 and $ETCO_2$ is helpful and allows the weaning process to be done safely and expeditiously. Typically, the intermittent mandatory ventilation rate is decreased in a stepwise fashion to 0. Then PEEP and pressure support are reduced. Finally, a T-piece adapter is connected to the endotracheal tube and the patient is allowed to breathe oxygen-enriched air spontaneously. After 30 to 60 min, the arterial blood gases are analyzed. Weaning should be discontinued if any of the following signs appear: $SpO_2 < 90$; $PaO_2 < 60$ mmHg; $ETCO_2 > 50$ mmHg; $PaCO_2 > 55$ mmHg; pH < 7.30; 10-mmHg rise in pulmonary artery pressure; respiratory rate > 30; 20-mmHg rise in systemic blood pressure; or 20-beat rise in heart rate.[5]

Most patients require low to moderate doses of morphine or another opioid in order to tolerate the endotracheal tube. As long as the spontaneous ventilatory rate remains greater than 15 breaths per minute, the patient will almost certainly be able to maintain adequate ventilation after the endotracheal tube is removed. Common mistakes that contribute to patient discomfort and difficulty in achieving tracheal extubation are (1) trying to sedate the patient with benzodiazepines only, which have no antitussive effect and (2) avoiding opioids for fear of respiratory depression.

BRONCHOSPASM

Severe bronchospasm during CPB is an unusual event, but it can occur. A few patients cannot have their chest cavity closed at the end of surgery because of hyperinflated lungs. The most likely cause of this fulminant bronchospasm is activation of human C5a anaphylatoxin by the extracorporeal circulation. Other likely causes of bronchospasm in the postoperative period are cardiogenic pulmonary edema; simple exacerbation of preexisting bronchospastic disease triggered by instrumentation, secretions, or cold anesthetic gas; beta-adrenergic blockers in susceptible individuals; and allergic reaction to protamine.[32]

The initial therapy of bronchospasm in the postoperative patient, once a diagnosis of heart failure is excluded, should be inhaled $beta_2$-agonists (terbutaline, metaproterenol, albuterol) and/or inhaled cholinergic agents (ipratropium bromide or glycopyrrolate). In the inhaled form these rather potent bronchodilators have minimal cardiovascular effects. In addition to their bronchodilator effect, these agents may augment mucociliary transport and aid in clearing secretions. A combination of $beta_2$-agonists and cholinergic agents should be tried in the patient refractory to a single agent. Even more refractory bronchospasm requires either a short course of systemic steroids or intravenous aminophylline. In addition to being a bronchodilator, aminophylline is a mild diuretic, increases the central nervous system respiratory drive, improves respiratory muscle function, and may decrease pulmonary artery pressure. It is, however, arrhythmogenic and chronotropic.

Postoperative Oliguria and Renal Insufficiency

ETIOLOGY

The use of radiocontrast agents in the days immediately preceding cardiac surgery may embarrass renal function, as manifested by a rise in blood urea nitrogen and serum creatinine values. Following CPB, there is a substantial incidence of postoperative renal dysfunction (up to 30 percent) but a relatively low incidence of severe renal impairment requiring dialysis (1 to 5 percent). Renal blood flow and glomerular filtration rate are reduced by 25 to 75 percent during bypass, with partial but not complete recovery in the first day after CPB. This reduction in renal function is attributed to renal artery vasoconstriction, hypothermia, and loss of pulsatile perfusion during CPB. Angiotensin II levels are higher with nonpulsatile flow as compared to pulsatile flow. While renal dysfunction cannot be consistently related to the systemic blood pressure and pump flow rate during nonpulsatile bypass, there is a definite relation between the incidence of postbypass renal dysfunction and the duration of CPB. In addition to the duration of CPB, the risk of developing postbypass renal failure seems to be a function of the patient's underlying renal function (also affected by age) and the perioperative circulatory status. The histologic changes that accompany renal impairment after cardiopulmonary bypass are characteristic of tubular necrosis. The tubular cells seem to be the most susceptible to acute reductions in renal perfusion.[33]

MANAGEMENT

There are three agents (so-called renoprotective drugs) that might be used during CPB to prevent an ischemic insult to the kidneys. Mannitol used in the CPB priming fluid may moderate ischemic insult, probably by volume expansion and hemodilution. It also initiates an osmotic diuresis, which prevents tubular obstruction and may serve as a free radical scavenger. Furosemide appears to improve renal blood flow when given during bypass. So-called renal dose dopamine (1 to 2.5 μg/kg/min based on ideal body weight) may maintain renal blood flow and urine output. Once renal failure has developed, none of these drugs is likely to offer any beneficial effect. A megadose of furosemide (200 to 300 mg) may be tried, but if there is no diuretic response, it should not be repeated. Similarly, a single dose of mannitol (12.5 to 25 mg) either with or without furosemide could be tried but not repeated if there is no effect. Whenever possible, it is advisable to avoid potentially nephrotoxic agents in the early postoperative period. Examples of such include radiologic contrast agents, aminoglycoside antibiotics, and angiotensin-converting enzyme inhibitors.

Postoperative Gastrointestinal Dysfunction

GASTROINTESTINAL CONSEQUENCES OF CARDIOPULMONARY BYPASS

The gastrointestinal consequences of CPB appear to be minimal. Reviews of the subject report a 1 percent prevalence.[32,33] Most patients eat within 24 to 48 h after an uncomplicated elective procedure. The limited investigations of the gastrointestinal tract after cardiac surgery have found a slight decrease in hepatic and pancreatic blood flow during cooling and rewarming on bypass and a decrease in gastric pH.[32,34] Transient elevations in liver function tests and hyperamylasemia may occur after cardiac surgery, and the risk factors include long CPB time, multiple transfusions, and multiple valve replacements. Appearance of jaundice portends a poor prognosis.[35] Severe gastrointestinal complications are usually ischemic in nature and are often associated with a low-output syndrome.[32] The use of opioids as part of general anesthesia and postoperative pain management contributes to gastrointestinal dysfunction (cramping, ileus, and constipation) and to postoperative nausea and vomiting. The nausea and vomiting can be minimized by use of a naso- or orogastric tube to maintain gastric decompression intraoperatively and early in the postoperative period, with the additional benefit of improving thoracoabdominal compliance to positive-pressure ventilation.

Postoperative Metabolic Disorders

POTASSIUM IMBALANCE

There are multiple factors that can produce large and rapid shifts in the serum potassium levels during and after CPB. These factors include the following: (1) high-potassium cardioplegia solution used during surgery; (2) renal dysfunction with associated oliguria and decreased clearance of potassium; (3) low cardiac output states accompanied by oliguria and acidosis; (4) hemolyzed red blood cells' release of potassium; (5) potassium lost by diuresis; and (6) diabetes mellitus interference with cellular uptake of potassium, unless insulin is infused intra- and postoperatively. The principal detrimental effects of these potassium shifts is on the electrical activity of the heart. The electrocardiographic signs of hyperkalemia and hypokalemia are described in Chap. 11. The electrocardiographic changes of hyperkalemia do not necessarily appear in the classic progressive manner; they are more related to the rate of rise in serum potassium rather than to the absolute serum concentration. The therapy of severe hyperkalemia should include counteracting the toxic cardiac effects of the elevated potassium with intravenous calcium gluconate or calcium chloride and lowering the serum level of potassium with sodium bicarbonate and/or administration of regular insulin and glucose. Hypokalemia does not usually become clinically evident until the serum potassium concentration is <2.5 meq/L, and at these levels it can be associated with severe ventricular tachyarrhythmias. Another consequence of potassium depletion is metabolic alkalosis as the hydrogen ions replace potassium ions within the cells. Hypokalemia is treated with the intravenous administration of KCl at a rate of no more than 10 to 15 meq/h. The serum potassium rises approximately 0.1 meq/L for each 2 meq of KCl administered. Large doses of KCl should be administered by a central venous catheter because of the caustic effect of potassium on peripheral veins.

HYPOMAGNESEMIA

Hypomagnesemia is common following cardiac surgery using CPB. Magnesium mimics potassium in its effects on the electrical activity of the heart. The cause of the hypomagnesemia is unknown, but it is probably multifactorial. Many patients will be hypomagnesemic preoperatively due to the use of loop diuretics, thiazides, digoxin, or alcohol and to the effects of type I diabetes mellitus. Magnesium is usually lost in the urine during CPB. Patients with postoperative hypomagnesemia develop atrial and ventricular dysrhythmias more frequently and require more prolonged mechanical ventilatory support than do patients with normal magnesium levels.[36] Magnesium administration also seems to improve stroke volume and cardiac index in the early postoperative period.[37] Magnesium can be administered as magnesium sulfate (2 g in 100-mL solution) to raise serum levels to 2 meq/L.

HYPERGLYCEMIA

During CPB there is a rise in blood glucose levels. The elevation is modest during hypothermia and becomes more marked during rewarming. This rise in glucose is due in part to increased glucose mobilization related to dramatic increases in cortisol, catecholamine, and growth hormone levels during CPB. Also, there is an apparent failure of insulin secretion, particularly during hypothermia, probably related to inhibition of the insulin secretory response by the elevated catecholamines. This blunting of the insulin response persists for the first 24 h after surgery. These changes are exaggerated in the diabetic patient.[38] Insulin requirements are likely to be 7 times greater than the preoperative requirements during the first 4 h postoperatively. Furthermore, such insulin resistance is exacerbated by catecholamines, diuretics, and blood transfusions.[39] These multiple factors make the diabetic patient susceptible to hyperosmolar, hyperglycemia, nonketotic diabetic coma.[40]

Postoperative Fever

Fever is a common occurrence in the postoperative patient. It is generally a consequence of pleuropericarditis, atelectasis, or phlebitis. Since 70 percent of patients have atelectasis after cardiac surgery, it is the most likely etiology of postoperative fever.[32] A reasonable assumption in a patient with a core temperature <38°C (100.4°F) and no evidence of phlebitis or presence of a pericardial or pleural rub is that the source of the fever is atelectasis. The appropriate therapeutic approach is to encourage intensified efforts at incentive spirometry and coughing. Any fever >38.5°C (101.3°F) warrants blood, sputum, and urine cultures. A white blood cell count (total and differential) and a chest x-ray should also be obtained.

Sternal wound infections occur in 0.4 to 5 percent of patients after sternotomy.[41–43] Multiple factors have been identified as increasing the risk of developing sternal wound infection. These include pneumonia, prolonged mechanical ventilation (especially with tracheostomy), emergency operations, postoperative hemorrhage with mediastinal hematoma, early reexploration, obesity, diabetes mellitus, and use of bilateral internal mammary grafts. While some studies have not found a higher prevalence of sternal wound infections with bilateral mammary grafts, the bulk of the evidence argues to the contrary. Perhaps some of the conflicting results can be explained by the fact that different degrees of devascularization of the sternum occur, depending on the particular technique used to harvest the internal mammary artery. The greatest risk for sternal infection seems to be in diabetic patients who receive bilateral internal mammary grafts.[43] Debate continues as to whether the most appropriate initial treatment is debridement and closure or open packing and subsequent plastic surgical closure with a muscle flap.

Approximately 1 percent of patients who have had coronary artery bypass surgery experience leg wound infections that necessitate extra care. Leg infections seem to occur more frequently in obese women, especially if the thigh veins are harvested.[44]

Neurologic and Neurophysiologic Dysfunction

MECHANISM

The mechanisms thought to account for most cerebral injury during cardiac surgery are macroembolization of air, debris from aortic atheroma, or left ventricular thrombus; microembolization of aggregates of granulocytes, platelets, and fibrin; and cerebral hypoperfusion. Death or disabling stroke occurs in about 2 percent of patients, with another 3 percent experiencing transient or minor functional disability secondary to cerebral infarction.[45] Focal neurologic deficits resulting from intraoperative events are usually noted within the first 24 to 48 h after surgery.

ENCEPHALOPATHY AND DELIRIUM

Alteration of mental status (encephalopathy and delirium) will be seen in approximately 30 percent of patients after cardiopulmonary bypass.[45] While the appearance of these encephalopathic symptoms likely reflects cerebral injury, other causes must be excluded, including drugs, sepsis, fever, hypoxemia, ethanol withdrawal, renal failure, and hyperosmolar state. Postoperative encephalopathic changes, varying from mild confusion and disorientation to protracted somnolence or agitation and hallucinations, may appear at any time during the hospital stay.[46] In fact, some physicians will not accept a diagnosis of postcardiotomy delirium unless the delirium develops following a lucid interval of 2 to 5 days after surgery. Studies of this condition have not identified any consistent risk factors, but advancing age, duration of CPB, and sleep deprivation have been frequently associated. The prevalence of this condition has remained rather constant since the early days of cardiac surgery involving CPB, but there has been a shift in the clinical presentation. Currently, the condition seems to present with disorientation rather than with hallucinations, paranoid ideation, and agitation noted earlier.[46] Recognition of this entity is important because the family can be assured that the patient's mental status is likely to recover. Agitation and acute psychosis in these patients usually respond to intravenous haloperidol, 2 to 10 mg, repeated as needed to produce adequate sedation.

BRACHIAL PLEXOPATHY AND ULNAR NERVE DYSFUNCTION

Another serious neurologic complication of cardiac surgery is brachial plexopathy. This neurologic dysfunction, involving C8 and T1, usually results from mechanical trauma secondary to sternal retraction but may be due to penetration by a posterior fractured segment of the first rib or injury during internal jugular cannulation. There is no specific therapy for this condition, and recovery can take as long as 6 months, with a few cases being permanent.[47] Ulnar nerve dysfunction may result from malpositioning of the upper extremities during surgery, which results in pressure being exerted on the ulnar nerve at the elbow.

References

1. Cameron D. Initiation of white cell activation during cardiopulmonary bypass: Cytokines and receptors. *J Cardiovasc Pharmacol* 1996; 27(suppl 1):S1–S5.
2. Chong JL, Pillai R, Fisher A, et al. Cardiac surgery, moving away from intensive care. *Br Heart J* 1992; 68:430–433.
3. Aps C. Fast-tracking in cardiac surgery. *Br J Hosp Med* 1995; 54:139–142.
4. Jindosi A, Aps C, Neville E, et al. Postoperative cardiac surgical care: An alternative approach. *Br Heart J* 1993; 69:59–64.
5. Bojar RM. *Manual of Perioperative Care in Cardiac and Thoracic Surgery*, 2d ed. Boston: Blackwell Scientific; 1994.
6. Levy JH, Salemenpera MT, Bailey JM, Ramsey JG. Postoperative circulatory control. In: Kaplan JA, ed. *Cardiac Anesthesia*, 3d ed. Philadelphia: Saunders; 1993:1168–1193.
7. Swanson DK, Myerowitz PD. Effect of reperfusion temperature and pressure on the functional and metabolic recovery of preserved hearts. *J Thorac Cardiovasc Surg* 1983; 86:242–251.
8. Gold JP, Roberts AJ, Hoover EL, et al. Effects of prolonged aortic cross clamping with potassium cardioplegia on myocardial contractility in man. *Surg Forum* 1979; 30:252–254.
9. Spiess BD. Ischemia—a coagulation problem? *J Cardiovasc Pharmacol* 1996; 27(suppl 1):S38–S41.
10. Verrier E. The microvascular cell and ischemia-reperfusion injury. *J Cardiovasc Pharmacol* 1996; 27(suppl 1):S26–S30.
11. Bolli R. Oxygen derived free radicals and postischemic myocardial dysfunction. *J Am Coll Cardiol* 1988; 12:239–249.
12. Przyklenk K, Kloner RA. "Reperfusion injury" by oxygen derived free radicals? *Circ Res* 1989; 64:86–96.
13. Breisblatt WM, Stein KI, Wolfe CJ, et al. Acute myocardial dysfunction and recovery: A common occurrence after coronary bypass surgery. *J Am Coll Cardiol* 1990; 15:1261–1269.
14. Donati F, Maille JG, Blain R, et al. End-tidal carbon dioxide tension and temperature changes after coronary artery bypass surgery. *Can Anaesth Soc J* 1985; 32:272–277.
15. Ralley FE, Wynando JE, Rams JG, et al. The effects of shivering on oxygen consumption and carbon dioxide production in patients rewarming from hypothermic cardiopulmonary bypass. *Can J Anaesth* 1988; 35:332–337.
16. Woodman RC, Harker LA. Bleeding complications associated with cardiopulmonary bypass. *Blood* 1990; 76:1680–1697.
17. Harker L, Malpass TW, Branson HE, et al. Mechanism of abnormal bleeding in patients undergoing cardiopulmonary bypass: Acquired transient platelet dysfunction associated with selective alpha-granule release. *Blood* 1980; 56:824–834.
18. Ellis RJ, Mangano DT, Van Dyke DC. Relationship of wedge pressure to end diastolic volume in patients undergoing myocardial revascularization. *J Thorac Cardiovasc Surg* 1979; 78:605–613.
19. Palmer RF, Lasseter KC. Drug therapy: Sodium nitroprusside. *N Engl J Med* 1975; 292:294–297.
20. Flaherty JT, Magee PA, Gardner TL, et al. Comparison of intravenous nitroglycerin and sodium nitroprusside for treatment of acute hypertension developing after coronary bypass surgery. *Circulation* 1982; 65:1072–1077.
21. Lambert CR, Hill JA, Feldman RL, et al. Effects of nicardipine on exercise- and pacing-induced myocardial ischemia in angina pectoris. *Am J Cardiol* 1987; 60:471–476.
22. Gray RJ, Bateman TM, Czer LS, et al. Comparison of esmolol and nitroprusside for acute postcardiac surgical hypertension. *Am J Cardiol* 1987; 59:887–891.
23. Topol EJ, Lerman BB, Baughman KL, et al. De novo refractory ventricular tachyarrhythmias after coronary revascularization. *Am J Cardiol* 1986; 57:57–59.
24. Leith JW, Thomson D, Baird DK, Harris PJ. The importance of age as a predictor of atrial fibrillation and flutter after coronary artery bypass grafting. *J Thorac Cardiovasc Surg* 1990; 100: 338–342.
25. Hashimoto K, Ilstrup DM, Schaff HV. Influence of clinical and hemodynamic variables on risk of supraventricular tachycardia after coronary artery bypass. *J Thorac Cardiovasc Surg* 1991; 101:56–65.
26. Fuller JA, Adams GG, Buxton B. Atrial fibrillation after coronary artery bypass grafting. Is it a disorder of the elderly? *J Thorac Cardiovasc Surg* 1989; 97:821–825.
27. Andrews TC, Reimold SC, Berlin JA, Antman EM. Prevention of supraventricular arrhythmias after coronary artery bypass surgery. A meta-analysis of randomized controlled trials. *Circulation* 1991; 84(suppl III):III-236–III-244.
28. Baerman JM, Kirsch MM, de Buitleir M, et al. Natural history

and determinates of conduction defects following coronary artery bypass surgery. *Ann Thorac Surg* 1987; 44:150–153.

29. Tuzcu EM, Emre A, Goormastic M, Loop FD. Incidence and prognostic significance of intraventricular conduction abnormalities after coronary bypass surgery. *J Am Coll Cardiol* 1990; 16:607–610.
30. Sladden RN, Berkowitz DE. Cardiopulmonary bypass and the lung. In: Gravlee GP, Davis RF, Utley IR, eds. *Cardiopulmonary Bypass*. Baltimore: Williams & Wilkins; 1993:468–487.
31. Ramsey J. The respiratory, renal and hepatic systems: Effects of cardiac surgery and cardiopulmonary bypass. In: Mora CT, ed. *Cardiopulmonary Bypass*. New York: Springer; 1995:147–168.
32. Hanks JB, Curtis SE, Hanks BB, et al. Gastrointestinal complications after cardiopulmonary bypass. *Surgery* 1982; 92:394–400.
33. Welling RE, Rath R, Albers JE, Glaser RS. Gastrointestinal complications after cardiac surgery. *Arch Surg* 1986; 121:1178–1180.
34. Mori A, Watanabe K, Onoe M, et al. Regional blood flow in the liver, pancreas, and kidney during pulsatile and nonpulsatile perfusion under profound hypothermia. *Jpn Circ J* 1988; 52: 219–227.
35. Collins JD, Bassendine MF, Ferner R, et al. Incidence and prognostic importance of jaundice after cardiopulmonary bypass surgery. *Lancet* 1983; 1:1119–1123.
36. Aglio LS, Stanford GG, Maddi R, et al. Hypomagnesemia is common following cardiac surgery. *J Cardiothorac Anesth* 1991; 5:201–208.
37. England MR, Gordon G, Salem M, Chernow B. Magnesium administration and dysrhythmias after cardiac surgery: A placebo-controlled, double-blind, randomized trial. *JAMA* 1993; 269:2369–2370.
38. Frater RW, Oka Y, Kadish A, et al. Diabetes and coronary artery surgery. *Mt Sinai J Med* 1982; 49:237–240.
39. Elliott MJ, Gill GV, Home PD, et al. A comparison of two regimens for the management of diabetes during open-heart surgery. *Anesthesiology* 1984; 60:364–368.
40. Seki S. Clinical features of hyperglycemia, nonketotic diabetic coma associated with cardiac operations. *J Thorac Cardiovasc Surg* 1986; 91:8678–8687.
41. Ulicny KS, Hiradzka SF. The risk factors of median sternotomy infection: A current review. *J Cardiac Surg* 1991; 6:338–351.
42. Hazelrigg SR, Wellons HA, Schneider JA, Kolm P. Wound complications after median sternotomy: Relationship to internal mammary grafting. *J Thorac Cardiovasc Surg* 1989; 98:1096–1099.
43. Grossi EA, Esposito R, Harris LJ, et al. Sternal wound infections and use of internal mammary artery grafts. *J Thorac Cardiovasc Surg* 1991; 102:342–347.
44. De Laria GA, Hunter JA, Goldin MD, et al. Leg wound complications associated with coronary revascularization. *J Thorac Cardiovasc Surg* 1981; 81:403–407.
45. Breuer AC, Furlan AJ, Hanson MR, et al. Central nervous system complications of coronary artery bypass graft surgery: Prospective analysis of 421 patients. *Stroke* 1983; 14:82–87.
46. Smith LW, Dimsdale JE. Postcardiotomy delirium: Conclusions after 25 years? *Am J Psychiatry* 1989; 146:452–458.
47. Shaw PJ, Bates D, Cartlidge NE, et al. Early neurological complications of coronary artery bypass surgery. *Br Med J* 1985; 91:1384–1387.

CHAPTER 50

REHABILITATION OF THE PATIENT WITH CORONARY HEART DISEASE

Nanette K. Wenger

Cardiac rehabilitation, an essential component of the long-term comprehensive management strategy for coronary patients, includes an individualized regimen of physical activity and health education and counseling appropriate for the individual patient's needs and specific cardiac problem.[1] *Cardiac rehabilitation* is described by the American College of Cardiology as "those exercise and counseling services which reduce symptoms or improve cardiac function"[2] and by the U.S. Public Health Service as "comprehensive, long-term programs involving medical evaluation, prescribed exercise, cardiac risk factor modification, education, and counseling." Initially, these services were recommended for patients following myocardial infarction (MI); subsequently, they were applied after coronary artery bypass graft (CABG) surgery or for patients with chronic stable angina pectoris. More recently, the U.S. Health Care Financing Administration concluded[3] that heart transplant patients and patients who had undergone percutaneous transluminal coronary angioplasty (PTCA) could benefit from prescribed cardiac rehabilitation. The Clinical Practice Guideline *Cardiac Rehabilitation*[4] documented the benefits of rehabilitative services for patients with heart failure and left ventricular (LV) systolic dysfunction and recommended their application.

The current short hospital stay for uncomplicated MI necessitates early ambulation and an accelerated educational regimen, with deferral of most teaching and counseling to the outpatient setting. Early discharge from the hospital is characteristic for patients after successful myocardial reperfusion by coronary thrombolysis or acute primary angioplasty. Patients recovering from CABG surgery typically undergo rapid ambulation, have a short hospital stay, and constitute an increasing percentage of patients referred for cardiac rehabilitation.[5] Such patients without prior MI characteristically have good ventricular function and favorable survival and are at low risk for proximate coronary events. Many require protracted guidance for coronary risk reduction; early counseling appears to aid in averting physiologic and psychological disability. Most patients following successful PTCA have brief hospital stays, good functional status, and early resumption of employment and other activities.[6,7] Patients with stable angina without recent MI constitute almost one-fourth of the total coronary population but are undeserved in terms of rehabilitative care. They are frequently not referred for formal rehabilitative services, often due to lack of insurance reimbursement. This population often has substantial loss of productivity and reduction in the quality of life and requires comprehensive medical management, with needs that may exceed those of patients after uncomplicated MI. With the aging of the U.S. population, coronary rehabilitative care is now provided to many elderly patients,[8,9] as well as to many patients with severe and complicated coronary illness. There is increasing contemporary emphasis on education and counseling as additional cornerstones of rehabilitative care, using the behavioral approach to assist patients in coronary risk reduction and other cardiovascular health-related goals[10–12]; on psychosocial assessment and interventions; and on occupational assessment and vocational counseling.

Each year almost 1 million survivors of MI are candidates for cardiac rehabilitation services in the United States, in addition to more than 7 million patients with stable angina pectoris and patients following revascularization with CABG surgery (367,000 patients in 1996, 44 percent under age 65) or PTCA and other transcatheter interventional procedures (482,000 in 1996, 51 percent younger than age 65). Of these several million patients with coronary heart disease for whom benefits can be anticipated from cardiac rehabilitation, only 11 to 20 percent participated in formal rehabilitation programs.[4,13] Among patients with acute MI enrolled in the Global Utilization of Streptokinase and tPA for Occluded Coronary Arteries (GUSTO) trial, 38 percent of U.S. patients and 32 percent of Canadian patients attended cardiac rehabilitation programs.[14] A U.S. national survey of 500 cardiac rehabilitation programs highlighted the underrepresentation of women, nonwhites, and those older than age 65.[15] Heart failure is the most common discharge diagnosis for hospitalized Medicare patients in the United States and the fourth most common discharge diagnosis for all hospitalized patients. Although coronary heart disease (CHD) is not etiologic in all these patients, it is a substantial contributor to heart failure. Application of cardiac rehabilitation services to patients with heart failure (as well as after cardiac transplantation) has gained increasing acceptance as its benefits and safety have been documented. An estimated 4.7 million patients with heart failure are potential candidates for cardiac rehabilitation.[4]

Nonetheless, this component of cardiac care is underutilized despite its efficacy and cost-effectiveness.[16,17]

EXERCISE TRAINING

Although no single randomized trial of exercise training demonstrated a reduction in mortality and morbidity in patients following MI, in part owing to inadequate sample size and/or duration of follow-up, to high dropout rates, etc., favorable trends occurred in several. Metaanalysis[16,18] of pooled data from large prospective, randomized exercise trials suggest as much as a 25 percent survival advantage for exercising subjects at 3-year follow-up following MI. This benefit cannot be attributed solely to exercise training, since many studies included coronary risk reduction as well as exercise. The reduction in mortality approaches that resulting from pharmacologic management of patients following MI with beta-blocking drugs and of patients with LV systolic dysfunction with angiotensin-converting enzyme (ACE) inhibitor therapy. The reduction in cardiovascular mortality was 26 percent in multifactorial randomized trials of cardiac rehabilitation as compared with 15 percent in trials that involved solely exercise training. There is no evidence that cardiac rehabilitation exercise training changes the rates of nonfatal reinfarction.[4,11]

The evidence-based Clinical Practice Guideline *Cardiac Rehabilitation* of the U.S. Department of Health and Human Services[4] highlights the beneficial effect of cardiac rehabilitation exercise training on exercise tolerance as one of the most clearly established favorable outcomes for coronary patients with angina pectoris, MI, CABG surgery, and PTCA and for patients with compensated heart failure or a decreased LV ejection fraction. This approach particularly benefits patients with decreased exercise tolerance.[19] Improved exercise tolerance was evident for both women and men and also occurred in elderly patients. The most consistent benefit resulted from exercise training at least three times weekly for 12 or more weeks' duration. The duration of aerobic exercise sessions varied from 20 to 40 min, at an intensity approximating 70 to 85 percent of the baseline exercise test heart rate. Improvement in exercise tolerance occurred with lower-intensity exercise as well.[20-22] Maintenance of exercise training is required to sustain improvement in exercise tolerance.

No significant increase in cardiovascular complications or other serious adverse outcomes was reported in any randomized, controlled trial of exercise training in coronary patients. These randomized, controlled trials involved 3932 patients following MI, 745 patients with catheterization-documented coronary disease, 215 patients following CABG surgery, and 139 following PTCA. No deterioration in measures of exercise tolerance was reported in any patients undergoing exercise training, nor did any controlled study document significantly greater improvement in exercise tolerance in control patient groups compared with exercising patients.

The improvement in functional capacity with exercise training, averaging 20 percent after recovery from MI, is associated with a reduction in activity-related symptoms: angina, dyspnea, fatigue, and at times claudication. Exercise training results in (1) an improvement in oxygen transport, evident as an increase in maximal cardiac output and oxygen consumption, (2) a reduction in heart rate, systolic blood pressure, and thereby myocardial oxygen requirement at rest and at submaximal work levels, and (3) and more rapid return to normal of the exercise heart rate.

The improvement in functional capacity and decrease in activity-related symptoms following usual moderate-intensity exercise training appear to be related primarily to peripheral adaptations. These include an increase in oxygen extraction and use by trained skeletal muscle, with a decrease in myocardial oxygen demand and requirement for coronary blood flow at submaximal exercise. The redistribution of cardiac output, decrease in systemic vascular resistance, and autonomic nervous system adaptations (particularly lowering of the heart rate) result in a decreased rate-pressure product at submaximal levels of exertion. High-intensity, long-term endurance exercise may effect cardiac (central) adaptations, possibly including improved ventricular contractility and increased maximal stroke volume in selected coronary patients[23]; such intensive exercise training is feasible for only a small subset of coronary patients. There is no evidence that exercise training as a sole intervention alters the angiographic characteristics of coronary lesions, increases coronary blood flow or myocardial oxygen supply, or stimulates the formation of a coronary collateral circulation in humans. No consistent improvement in cardiac hemodynamic measurements or ventricular systolic function has resulted from exercise training.[24,25] Exercise training, however, may improve skeletal muscle functioning in patients with heart failure.[26] Exercise training can decrease evidence of myocardial ischemia, as measured by exercise electrocardiogram (ECG) testing, ambulatory ECG recording, and radionuclide perfusion imaging.[27,28] In several randomized clinical trials, apparently spontaneous improvement in resting ejection fraction after MI occurred in both exercising and control populations, rendering suspect the improvements in ejection fraction described in observational studies of exercise training. There were no consistent changes in ventricular arrhythmia related to exercise rehabilitation.

Clinical benefits of exercise training include a decrease in the symptoms of angina pectoris in patients with coronary disease[27] and the symptoms of heart failure in patients with LV systolic dysfunction.[29,30] The improvement in electrocardiographic and nuclear cardiology measures of myocardial ischemia provides objective support for the symptomatic improvement.

Exercise training of patients with LV systolic dysfunction provided added symptomatic improvement to that achieved by appropriate medication.[30]

The decrease in symptoms and improvement in functional status that result from exercise training can enable a return to remunerative employment as well as to leisure and recreational activities.[31] For more impaired coronary patients, including many elderly ones, even a modest increase in functional capacity can help maintain independence.[8,9,32–35]

Guidelines for Prescriptive Exercise Training[36]

Individualized medically prescribed physical activity is the hallmark of rehabilitative exercise training. Standards and guidelines have been promulgated by a number of professional organizations.[2,37–43] The prescriptive components of exercise training include its "dosage," determined by the intensity, frequency, and duration of exercise; the types of exercise; and the rate of progression of exercise intensity. Coronary patients should not exercise at a level higher than that documented to produce an appropriate cardiovascular response during testing. The predischarge (or early posthospitalization) exercise test, typically performed for risk stratification, can serve as the basis for initial exercise recommendations. It is inappropriate to use age-predicted target heart rates for coronary patients; disease, therapies, and prior levels of training or fitness may influence the heart rate response to exercise.

Prescription of target heart rate range is based on the results of exercise testing. Although in prior years patients were advised to exercise to a target heart rate range between 70 and 85 percent of the highest level safely achieved at exercise testing,[44] exercise intensities in the 50 to 70 percent heart rate range have produced comparable improvement in functional capacity and endurance and may provide greater safety because of the lower risk of cardiovascular complications with unsupervised exercise.[21,22,45] These lower rates are less likely to produce discomfort that may deter long-term exercise adherence. The documented efficacy of lower-intensity exercise training to improve aerobic capacity has increased both its applicability and acceptance.[1,21,22] Particularly for unfit patients or those with lower exercise capacities, the increased comfort of lower-intensity exercise may encourage adherence, although increased duration of training may be required. Comparable favorable effects on quality of life occurred with low- and high-intensity exercise.[46] An alternative method for calculating target heart rate involves 70 to 85 percent of the difference between peak exercise test heart rate and resting heart rate, added to resting rate. This method may be advantageous in patients whose heart rate is attenuated by beta-blocking or other drugs.

The basic design of an exercise session involves an initial 5 to 10 min of warm-up exercise, i.e., stretching and range-of-motion activities that enable musculoskeletal and circulatory readiness for exercise. This is followed by a 20- to 40-min endurance component that initially involves walk-run sequences or exercise on a stationary bicycle or treadmill; for these activities, skill is a minimal component of the intensity of work demand.

When space for exercise is limited, "station" training may be preferable, with participants serially using bicycle ergometry, arm ergometry, rowing machines, and treadmills. When more space is available, gymnasium-type programs can accommodate larger numbers of patients for walk-jog activities and floor exercises; some facilities have indoor or outdoor tracks. A final 5- to 10-min cool-down period entails a gradual decrease in intensity that allows the heart rate to slow and averts postexercise hypotension. Three exercise sessions weekly appear adequate, and a greater frequency does not significantly improve aerobic capacity. Aerobic games, as a recreational component, add variety to an exercise program and improve adherence; they also provide upper body exercise. Because the oxygen cost of these activities varies with each patient's skills and competitiveness, they should be limited early in exercise training.

As the level of training increases, recreational activities in which skill often influences the intensity of work may add variety to the exercise regimen. Enjoyable, effective endurance activities include rope skipping, bicycling, skating, swimming, rowing, and aerobic dancing; both rope-skipping and swimming (for unskilled swimmers) impose higher workloads and should be undertaken carefully.

Characteristics of Aerobic (Dynamic) and Strength (Isometric) Exercise Training

Aerobic (dynamic) exercise, rhythmic repetitive movements of large muscle groups, traditionally is prescribed for coronary patients. The physiologic response, an increase in heart rate, parallels the intensity of activity, and an increase in stroke volume occurs in young and middle-aged patients. In most elderly patients, the increase in heart rate predominates, with little increase in stroke volume. Systolic blood pressure increases progressively with exercise intensity, with maintenance of or slight decrease in diastolic blood pressure and widening of the pulse pressure.

By contrast, with strength (isometric) training, the increase in heart rate is modest, and the increase in cardiac output is slight. There is a substantial increase in systolic blood pressure with high-intensity isometric activity, particularly in unfit individuals; this may provoke angina, ventricular dysfunction, and/or arrhythmias and is the basis for limiting isometric activity in coronary patients with a low exercise capacity. Once a reasonable aerobic capacity is achieved, combined aerobic and strength training exercises in coronary patients may produce substantial training effects and improve muscle strength,[47] with resulting improvement in endurance and the ability to return to active occupational and recreational lifestyles.[48] Studies document the effectiveness of mild to moderate resistive exercise training in selected patients with coronary heart disease.[49–52] The absence of signs or symptoms of myocardial ischemia, abnormal hemodynamic changes, and cardiovascular complications suggests that resistance exercise training is safe for coronary patients who have previously participated in aerobic exercise training. A major change in contemporary exercise programs is the inclusion of strength training for appropriately selected coronary patients. Most reported studies have involved small numbers of low-risk male patients, 70 years or younger, with minimal functional aerobic impairment and with normal or near-normal LV function. The extent to which the safety and effectiveness of resistance training demonstrated by these studies can be extrapolated to other populations of coronary patients (e.g., women, older patients of both genders with low aerobic fitness, or patients at moderate to high cardiovascular risk) is not known.[4]

Arm versus Leg Exercise Training

Because exercise training is predominantly muscle-specific, both arm and leg exercises should be included in exercise rehabilitation.[53] The heart rate and blood pressure responses to leg work decrease following leg training, with only modest improvement in the response to arm work. Following arm training, the most prominent decreases in heart rate and blood pressure response occur with arm work. In one study, improvement in exercise response of the untrained limb was only 50 to 75 percent of the trained limb, suggesting that about half the increase in trained-limb performance is due to a generalized training effect; the remainder reflects predominantly improved oxygen extraction by trained skeletal muscle.

Since walk-run sequences or exercise on a stationary bicycle or treadmill train primarily leg muscles, supplementary arm exercise training is accomplished by selected repetitive calisthenics, shoulder wheels, rowing machines, and arm ergometers. When data from leg exercise testing are used to prescribe arm exercise, a reduction of about 10 beats per minute in target heart rate range is appropriate. The workload for arm training is about half that for leg training.[53] Since most occupational and recreational activities entail both arm and leg work (and often predominantly arm work), arm exercise training should be included in rehabilitative exercise.

The Effect of Cardiovascular Drugs on Exercise Training

Exercise training can occur in patients receiving antianginal drugs, which may lessen symptoms and improve the ability to exercise.[54] Although beta-blocking drugs decrease the heart rate and blood pressure response to exercise, they do not attenuate the improvement in physical work capacity that results from exercise training. Exercise testing undertaken to prescribe exercise should be performed with patients receiving medications that are planned for their training.

The Role of Exercise Testing in Coronary Rehabilitation

Graded exercise testing, using either a treadmill or a bicycle protocol, is safely performed within the initial weeks following MI.[55] Most centers currently test patients to a sign- or symptom-limited end point because heart rate limits are often inaccurate as a result of antianginal therapy effects on heart rate. Treadmill testing typically entails serial 3-min stages of walking, beginning at slow speed, initially on the level, and then at increasing speed and elevations; comparable test protocols are available for a bicycle ergometer (see Chap. 14). Arm testing may be undertaken in patients with claudication or musculoskeletal problems that make leg testing not feasible.[56]

The results of predischarge exercise tests, performed with or without radionuclide studies, contribute independent prognostic information for risk stratification.[55] High-risk patients are characterized by having a low exercise capacity [peak workload below 4 to 6 metabolic equivalents (METs)]; the occurrence of angina, ischemic ST-segment abnormalities, and/or exercise-induced hypotension at low levels of exercise; and the development of ventricular arrhythmias at low levels of exercise. Radionuclide evidence of myocardial ischemia or LV dysfunction with exercise also indicates an adverse prognosis. Predischarge exercise testing also identifies low-risk patients with a favorable prognosis who do not require additional diagnostic testing, are well-suited for accelerated rehabilitation, and for whom early discharge home and prompt resumption of preinfarction activities, including return to work, can be recommended.[55,57] The exercise test can help define safe levels of activity and guide the surveillance necessary during exercise rehabilitation. This permits simple, effective, accelerated, and less costly rehabilitation for low-risk coronary patients, reserving financial and personnel resources for high-risk patients who may derive substantial benefit from supervised exercise training. Satisfactory performance of an exercise test, coupled with explanation of its relationship to activities to be undertaken at home, may lessen the common fear of postinfarction patients that physical activity may result in reinfarction or death.[58] Such counseling also has been associated with an early return to work.[31]

Safety of Rehabilitative Exercise Training

The Clinical Practice Guideline *Cardiac Rehabilitation*[4] highlights the safety of cardiac rehabilitation exercise training in that randomized, controlled trials involving over 4500 coronary patients showed no increase in morbidity or mortality. A questionnaire survey of 142 U.S. cardiac rehabilitation programs, involving patients participating in exercise rehabilitation between 1980 and 1984, reported a low rate of nonfatal MI of 1 per 294,000 patient-hours and a cardiac mortality rate of 1 per 784,000 patient-hours.[59] Twenty-one episodes of cardiac arrest occurred, with successful resuscitation of 17 patients. A 1978 report[44] also described a low rate of fatal cardiac events during or immediately following exercise training: 1 per 116,400 patient-hours of participation. Definitive information is not available regarding the effect of levels of supervision and of ECG monitoring of exercise training on safety.

IMPLEMENTATION OF CARDIAC REHABILITATIVE CARE

Inpatient, or Hospital, Phase

The major components of rehabilitative care for patients hospitalized for a coronary event include progressive resumption of physical activity (early ambulation) and education and counseling of both patient and family (see also Chap. 42).

EARLY AMBULATION

Early ambulation is designed to limit the detrimental effects of deconditioning: reduced physical work capacity and maximal oxygen uptake; orthostatic intolerance, characterized by orthostatic hypotension and tachycardia (due both to hypovolemia and to a lessened cardiovascular reflex response); increase in blood viscosity owing to a decrease in plasma volume disproportionate to the decrease in red blood cell mass; and decrease in pulmonary ventilation. The decrease in muscle mass and muscular contractile strength renders muscular contraction inefficient, with more oxygen required for comparable work.

Guidelines[60] for physical activity in the coronary or surgical intensive care unit are for initial low-intensity exercise (1–2 METs), with gradual progression in work demand; supervision of progressive ambulation permits detection of inappropriate responses. Patients are encouraged to feed themselves, perform personal care, use a bedside commode, and sit in a bedside chair. Cardiac work is less in the seated than in the supine position. Sitting in a chair two or three times daily limits the hypovolemia of immobilization and resulting orthostatic hypotension. Exposure to gravitational stress, rather than physical activity intensity, appears to be the determinant in limiting hypovolemia, cardiac underfilling, and deterioration of oxygen transport capacity with effort intolerance.[61] Patients perform selected arm and leg exercises designed to maintain muscle tone and increase flexibility and joint mobility. Incentive spirometry is important for postoperative patients.

Disproportionate responses[60] to low-level activity include chest discomfort, dyspnea, or palpitations; a heart rate in excess of 100 beats per minute or lower than 50 beats per minute; ST-segment displacement on the electrocardiographic monitor; appearance of arrhythmias; or a decrease of more than 10 to 15 mmHg in systolic blood pressure. Although the latter usually indicates ischemic ventricular dysfunction, the vasodilator effect of nitrate, calcium channel blocking drugs, or ACE inhibitor therapy also must be considered. A systolic blood pressure response during low-level activity of more than 180 mmHg or a diastolic pressure response of more than 110 mmHg is an indication for antihypertensive therapy. Appropriate responses to ambulation indicate that the patient can progress to higher-intensity activity; disproportionate responses require activity restriction and clinical reassessment for unrecognized cardiac ischemia or ventricular dysfunction.

The major prescriptive hospital activity is walking, with stepwise increases in pace and distance. Patients who must climb steps at home should practice this in the hospital. Most household tasks require a work intensity of 2 to 3 METs. Electrocardiographic telemetry monitoring during ambulation is indicated for selected patients, e.g., those with serious ventricular arrhythmias or asymptomatic myocardial ischemia. A protocol for early ambulation and concomitant educational activities for patients with MI is applicable, with minor modifications, to postoperative coronary patients (Table 50-1).

Neither early ambulation nor early hospital discharge adversely affects the short- or long-term morbidity or mortality of appropriately selected coronary patients.[60,62] Benefits include prevention of deconditioning, decrease in pulmonary atelectasis and thromboembolic complications, lessened anxiety and depression, and an enhanced sense of well-being, related to improved functional status. Improved functional status of patients at hospital discharge has been associated with an earlier and more complete return to work.

EDUCATION AND COUNSELING OF HOSPITALIZED PATIENTS AND THEIR FAMILIES[63]

The current abbreviated hospital stay limits the ability of health professionals to address the informational and learning needs of the patient, spouse, and family; to assist them through recovery; and to prepare them adequately for convalescence. Answering the questions or concerns of patients in a coronary or surgical intensive care unit (or during the preprocedure phase for elective coronary angioplasty or bypass surgery) can provide reassurance. Education includes a brief explanation of the medical or surgical problem(s), tests anticipated in subsequent days, and familiarization with procedures and equipment; this information helps patients adjust to a situation perceived as life-threatening. The temporary nature of most restrictions should be emphasized, citing that improved coronary status with recovery lessens the intensity of surveillance and care.

During the remainder of the hospitalization, providing more information and planning for discharge are appropriate. Increased knowledge can lessen anxiety and improve adherence to recommendations. Patients should be instructed about medications—the purpose, dosage, desired effects, and potential adverse responses of each. Many patients have not taken medications prior to a coronary event and may be unfamiliar with the problems of taking medications. Patients and family members should be taught the appropriate response to new or recurrent symptoms and how to gain access to emergency medical care.

Outpatient, or Ambulatory, Phase

About 70 percent of contemporary survivors of MI are younger than 70 years of age[10] and many patients following successful myocardial revascularization procedures are at low risk for proximate coronary events. Exercise rehabilitation for most low-risk coronary patients, particularly following myocardial revascularization, begins shortly after discharge from the hospital; these patients usually progress rapidly in increasing their intensity and duration of exercise, often without supervision. Coronary patients who are elderly; those with significant comorbidity, myocardial ischemia, heart failure, or serious arrhythmias; those with complications of MI or CABG surgery; or those with severe angina may require exercise surveillance of variable duration.[2,37,39,55] Outpatient exercise rehabilitation is best described by the characteristics of the exercise training and the requirements, duration, and complexity of surveillance, based on the patient's clinical and risk factor status, rather than by traditional phases of earlier years that typically had fixed durations and composition. This is concordant with responding to an individual patient's needs for exercise training rather than requiring a patient to conform to program phases or requirements.

THERAPEUTIC EXERCISE TRAINING

Therapeutic exercise training typically lasts for 8 to 12 weeks. Initial home exercise may involve progressive walking and walk-jog sequences or serial increases in the intensity and duration of use of a stationary bicycle. Videotapes may help guide and pace home exercise and are available for varying intensities of exercise training. Home-based exercise rehabilitation optimally includes planned communication and management by rehabilitation nurses and other specially trained personnel.[10,11]

In the early years of outpatient exercise rehabilitation, few patients had continuous ECG monitoring because ECG telemetry was not widely available. In subsequent years, complication rates were described as being lower in exercise programs with continuous ECG monitoring.[44] It remains unknown, however, whether ECG monitoring, closer medical supervision, and/or differences in exercise intensity were the safety determinants. More recently, continuous ECG monitoring has not been shown to provide added safety for low-risk patients during supervised exercise[59]; as a result, ECG monitoring is currently recommended only for high-risk patients and other selected patients with problems in exercising,[1,2,4,39] although some recommend more extensive ECG monitoring. Often, ECG monitoring is

TABLE 50-1 Inpatient Rehabilitation: Five-Step Myocardial Infarction Program (Revised 1996: Grady Memorial Hospital/Emory University School of Medicine)

Step	Date	M.D. Initials	Nurse/ Exer Specialist Notes	Supervised Exercise	CCU/Step Down Unit Activity	Educational Activity
				CCU		
1	____			Active and passive ROM all extremities in bed Teach patient ankle plantar and dorsiflexion—repeat hourly when awake	Partial self-care Feed self Dangle legs on side of bed Use bedside commode Sit in chair 15 min, 1–2 times/day	Orientation to CCU Personal emergencies, social service aid as needed Bedside teaching (CCU staff)
2	____			Active ROM all extremities, sitting on side of bed or bedside chair	Sit in chair 15–30 min, 2–3 times/day Complete self-care	Orientation to rehabilitation team, program Smoking cessation Educational literature if requested Planning transfer from CCU
				Step Down Unit		
3	____			Warm-up exercises, 2–2.5 METs: Stretching ROM Calisthenics Walk in hall 50–75 ft and back at slow pace	Sit in chair ad lib Walk in room Walk to class with supervision Out of bed as tolerated	Normal cardiac anatomy and function Development of atherosclerosis What happens when myocardial infarction occurs Coronary risk factors and their control Diet
4	____			Teach pulse counting, Borg Scale ROM and calisthenics, 3 METs Practice walking few stair-steps Walk 300–500 ft bid Instruct on home exercise	Tepid shower or tub bath, with supervision Walk in corridor prn	Heart attack management: Medications Exercise Surgery Response to symptoms Family, community adjustments on return home Work simplification techniques (as needed)
5	____			Continue above activities Check pulse counting Walk up flight of steps Walk 500 ft bid Continue home exercise instruction; present information regarding outpatient exercise program	Continue all previous activities Predischarge exercise test (as appropriate)	Discharge planning Medications, diet, activity Return appointments Schedules tests Return to work Community resources Educational literature Medication cards

NOTE: 1 foot = 0.30 meter.

SOURCE: Reprinted with permission of Grady Memorial Hospital/Emory University School of Medicine.

undertaken solely owing to its requirement for insurance reimbursement rather than based on medical need. Many patients in supervised exercise programs without continuous ECG monitoring or patients exercising independently can be taught either to check their heart rate response intermittently to ensure that it remains in the prescribed target heart rate range or to estimate exercise intensity by the rating of perceived exertion, as described by Borg.[64] In supervised settings, heart rate response can be documented by intermittent use of defibrillator paddles as ECG leads. A technique of value in maintaining appropriate exercise intensity in unsupervised settings is the "talk test," wherein patients exercise only to the level that permits continued conversation with an exercising companion, a level generally below the anaerobic threshold at which respiratory rate accelerates.

High-risk coronary patients may require supervised and often ECG-monitored exercise. These patients are characterized by having a markedly reduced exercise capacity, severely depressed ventricular function, complex ventricular arrhythmias, exercise-induced angina, ischemia, or hypotension at low exercise intensities, and/or the inability to self-monitor exercise heart rate. Because of their increased risk for adverse events, exercise training should occur, at least initially, in a medically supervised and probably ECG-monitored setting.[65] Because exercise-related cardiac complications may be increased not only in proximity to an acute coronary event, the need and duration of ECG surveillance of exercise for these high-risk patients remain uncertain. The uniform success of resuscitation with supervised exercise, despite the rarity of its application, suggests that exercise supervision may be beneficial for selected patients.[59]

Although recent studies document the efficacy of home-based exercise training and risk reduction guided by a specialized cardiac nurse manager, data are not available as to the efficacy of long-term risk reduction or long-term compliance with unsupervised exercise in the absence of management and supervision strategies. Several studies showed that all training regimens appeared to increase functional capacity more rapidly than occurred spontaneously.[11,29,30,47] Supervision of exercise may not entail an "all or nothing" approach; intermittent supervision may be feasible in a community facility, there may be periodic telephone transmission of the exercise ECG of patients who exercise at home, patients may use inexpensive heart rate monitors during home exercise, or a combination of these techniques may be used. It is not known whether any of these approaches improves adherence to exercise or exercise safety; several studies of independent exercise showed a lack of coronary risk reduction.

The Clinical Practice Guideline *Cardiac Rehabilitation*[4] highlights alternative approaches to the delivery of cardiac rehabilitation services, other than traditional supervised group interventions, as effective and safe for carefully selected clinically stable patients. Transtelephonic and other means of monitoring and surveillance of patients can extend cardiac rehabilitation beyond the setting of supervised, structured, group-based rehabilitation. The feasibility, safety, and efficacy of these alternative strategies for exercise rehabilitation must be assessed in more diverse populations of patients with stable coronary heart disease, particularly elderly patients, those with ventricular dysfunction, and other patients of higher risk status.

MAINTENANCE EXERCISE TRAINING

Once patients attain their initial exercise goals, maintenance training can be undertaken or continued in community recreational facilities or at home. Because lifetime regular physical activity is necessary to maintain physical fitness, patients must achieve reasonable independence in exercising and remain involved in an exercise regimen that is social, enjoyable, convenient, and appropriate. Most coronary patients with prior exercise restrictions who can safely attain a 7- to 8-MET level of performance can safely progress to unsupervised exercise. Patients leaving supervised exercise programs may require counseling regarding the selection and initiation of long-term exercise in the community or at home.

EDUCATION AND COUNSELING OF AMBULATORY CORONARY PATIENTS[36]

The behavioral approach to coronary risk reduction encourages and enables coronary patients to manage their illness, adopt and maintain healthy lifestyles, and improve adherence to medications and other recommended regimens.[66,67] Metaanalysis of 28 controlled trials of patient education showed that "education programs have demonstrated a measurable impact on blood pressure, mortality, exercise, [and] diet" and that other parameters are positively affected, although less consistently.[68] A combination of education, counseling, and behavioral intervention strategies seems most effective in promoting health, reducing risk, and favorably altering lifestyle.[4,10,66] Whether the same interventions are equally effective for men and women and across the life span remains unanswered because few studies have enrolled patients over 70 years of age or included women.

Patients with diagnosed coronary disease are at the highest risk for disability and death and thus constitute patients for whom untreated risk factors are most damaging.[69] Cardiac rehabilitation services provide an integrating structure for the multiple risk-reduction components of secondary prevention.

There is no evidence that the performance of CABG surgery per se encourages favorable modification of coronary risk status postoperatively.[70,71] Postoperative recurrence of coronary symptoms or deterioration of function following saphenous vein CABG surgery relates predominantly to progression of the underlying atherosclerosis both in the graft vessels and in the native circulation. Control of hypertension, diabetes, hyperlipidemia, and obesity and cessation of cigarette smoking,[72,73] with adoption of a physically active lifestyle, even at advanced age, may slow progression or induce regression of atherosclerosis and decrease the occurrence of subsequent coronary events.

Community resources that may be helpful in rehabilitation should be identified: counseling and guidance services, home-care agencies, vocational rehabilitation facilities and services for job training and placement, services for financial aid, outpatient coronary rehabilitation programs, and postcoronary groups or clubs. Participation in community heart clubs or educational groups may further facilitate rehabilitation; coronary risk reduction and other skills learned and practiced in these settings may encourage health-related behaviors and aid in reinforcing maintenance of these changes. Acquisition of knowledge appears to affect favorably both behaviors involving implementing recommendations for care and coping behaviors.[63]

CORONARY POPULATIONS WITH SPECIAL REHABILITATION NEEDS

Elderly Coronary Patients

Elderly patients constitute a high percentage of those with MI, CABG surgery, and PTCA and other transcatheter revascularization procedures. Complications of MI and myocardial revascularization are more frequent in the elderly, with prolongation of both immobilization and hospitalization predisposing to deconditioning; early ambulation can limit functional deterioration and decrease depression. In both medical and surgical coronary intensive care settings, the major educational strategy involves concise and repeated explanations, reassurance, and time and place orientation to help avert confusion and delirium. Teaching energy-conserving techniques for self-care and performance of household tasks helps maintain independent living, an outcome valued by elderly patients. Modification of conventional coronary risk factors is feasible and warranted, given the greater prevalence and severity of coronary disease at elderly age.

Elderly patients are also at high risk of disability following a coronary event. Recent trials of exercise rehabilitation have begun to include patients over 65 years of age and to evaluate outcomes in the elderly coronary population specifically. Although few studies and no randomized, controlled trials have addressed the efficacy and safety of exercise training and multifactorial rehabilitation in the elderly, the available studies provide important new information for clinical practice.

Elderly coronary patients in posthospital exercise regimens have exercise trainability comparable with that of younger patients participating in similar exercise rehabilitation,[35,74] with elderly women and men showing comparable improvement. One report found that exercise testing before hospital discharge was feasible in about half of patients aged 70 years or older with MI, enabling accurate risk stratification and exercise prescription.[75] No complications or adverse outcomes of exercise training in elderly patients were described in any cardiac rehabilitation study. Nonetheless, rates of entry referral to and participation in exercise rehabilitation were substantially lower among elderly than among younger patients,[9,33] and older women were even less likely to be referred than were older men.[34] Elderly patients are less fit after a coronary event, in part because of decreased fitness prior to the event. Adherence to exercise training was high (90 percent) in the reported studies,[35] and significant reduction in coronary risk factors occurred in elderly patients who participated in multifactorial cardiac rehabilitation.[9]

For elderly patients who exercise independently, emphasis should be placed on the importance of warm-up and cool-down activities because of the delayed return of the exercise heart rate to normal at elderly age. Walking provides an adequate training stimulus for many elderly patients because it constitutes a significant percentage of the decreased aerobic capacity of aging.[76] Running, jumping, and other high-impact activities should be limited to avoid musculoskeletal complications. Walking, bicycle ergometry, and/or walking in a pool in shallow water can favorably modify the decreased joint mobility of aging; enhance neuromuscular coordination, balance, and stability and thereby lessen propensity for falls; and improve endurance. Elderly individuals who exercise independently should be cautioned to decrease their exercise intensity in hot and humid environments.

Coronary Patients with Heart Failure

Impairment of exercise capacity with heart failure appears in part due to inadequate nutritive blood flow to skeletal muscle; factors other than lack of increase in cardiac output with exercise seem important, including the ability to decrease peripheral vascular resistance and possibly the adequacy of right ventricular function (see also Chap. 20). Patients with heart failure and normal cardiac output responses to exercise frequently improve their functional capacity with exercise training, whereas those with severe hemodynamic dysfunction with exercise often do not.[77] A combination of LV systolic dysfunction and residual myocardial ischemia may limit trainability. The ventricular ejection fraction predicts poorly both exercise capacity and the potential for improvement of exercise performance with training; some patients with substantial ventricular dysfunction have a normal exercise capacity and no symptoms or impairment of lifestyle.[78]

Most studies of exercise training of patients with heart failure and moderate to severe LV systolic dysfunction do not demonstrate deterioration in LV volume, wall thickness, or function.[79,80] Randomized, controlled clinical trial data of exercise training in postinfarction patients with an ejection fraction less than 40 percent showed that long-term home-based exercise may attenuate the unfavorable remodeling response and even improve ventricular function over time.[79] Peripheral (skeletal muscle) adaptations appear to mediate the improvement in exercise tolerance; exercise training can substantially correct the impaired oxidative capacity of skeletal muscle in chronic heart failure.[81] Exercise training also may improve peripheral artery endothelial function in patients with chronic heart failure.[82] Exercise training can augment both the symptomatic and functional benefits of ACE inhibitor therapy.[30] Even small improvements in symptomatic status and functional capacity can exert a substantial favorable impact on quality of life. Improved clinical outcomes are also described.[83] In both the supervised and at-home settings, low- to moderate-intensity exercise regimens provide benefit, although adverse events may occur in this high-risk patient group.[4]

Although the initial exercise training programs of patients with ventricular systolic dysfunction were predominantly supervised, typically with continuous ECG monitoring, other studies have described moderate-intensity, unsupervised exercise as safe and effective.[84,85] The optimal duration of exercise supervision and the duration and need for ECG monitoring of these patients remain uncertain but should be guided by clinical evidence of exercise-related ischemia and/or arrhythmia.[29] In a study of 105 ambulatory cardiac transplant candidates, nonsupervised prescribed walking at a target heart rate range close to baseline exercise test-determined anaerobic threshold produced significant improvement in peak maximal oxygen consumption and peak exercise tolerance in 38 of 68 clinically stable patients without adverse effects. After an average of 6 months of such exercise, 31 of these 38 patients improved sufficiently to be removed from the transplant list, with improvement persisting to 2 years.[86]

Additional important components of rehabilitative care for patients with significant activity limitations include teaching work simplification, particularly the pacing of daily living activities; working in a seated rather than a standing position; and taking frequent rest periods between activities.

Patients with Implanted Pacemakers and Cardioverter-Defibrillators

Exercise prescription is determined by the characteristics of the implanted pacemaker. Because most patients likely to exercise currently receive rate-responsive pacemakers, exercise testing can ascertain the appropriateness of the sensor response to the exercise intensity,[87] and reprogramming can be undertaken as needed.

The exercise target heart rate range for patients with implanted cardioverter-defibrillators should be set at 20 to 30 beats per minute below the threshold rate of the device to fire. This also enables appropriate work-related activities.[88] Coparticipants in the exercise setting must be reassured that they cannot be harmed by physical contact with a patient whose cardioverter-defibrillator discharges.

PSYCHOLOGICAL ASPECTS OF CORONARY REHABILITATION[36]

The importance of psychosocial variables in the prognosis of patients with established coronary disease has received increasing attention during the past decade. Although the type A behavior pattern previously received emphasis, currently the hostility component of type A behavior is regarded as its most adverse feature. High levels of anger and hostility appear associated with increased cardiac morbidity and mortality.[89,90]

Other major psychological problems in coronary patients involve anxiety, depression, denial, and dependence.[91] Denial of presenting symptoms may limit or delay access to care, often with adverse outcomes. "Appropriate" denial, characterized by confidence in a favorable outcome, often an effective coping strategy of patients with a coronary event, is associated with a favorable prognosis. Anxiety, which is often the initial psychological manifestation at hospitalization, is related to a fear of dying and may progress to depression as patients contemplate their potential inability to resume former family, occupational, and community roles. Anxiety and depression, the most common psychological complications of infarction, contribute to the failure to make satisfactory life adjustments, to return to work, to return to sexual function, and to engage in social activities subsequent to hospital discharge. Depression is reported to precede MI in 30 to 50 percent of patients. Depression is associated with increased morbidity and mortality following MI and CABG surgery[92,93]; patients with depression were five times more likely to die during the initial 6 months following MI than nondepressed patients.[94] Depression may be associated with social isolation, which may serve as an independent risk factor. The 6-month mortality of patients living alone was double that of patients living with others (16 versus 8 percent), and follow-up study of patients with angiographically documented coronary disease showed a 50 percent 5-year mortality rate among those most socially isolated, compared with 17 percent among those without these characteristics. The impact of social isolation on prognosis appeared independent of ventricular ejection fraction and other physiologic prognostic factors. Interventions against depression and social isolation following MI are currently being evaluated.

Many patients with successful physical recovery following MI or myocardial revascularization often have residual psychological impairment.[91] Two major strategies that appear to limit this complication are education and counseling and the initiation of a physical activity regimen. Many patients remain psychologically disabled because, inappropriately, they perceive an excessive severity of infarction and vulnerability to sudden death; safe resumption of physical activity provides reassurance and restores self-confidence.[58] In randomized exercise trials, exercising patients returned to sexual activity, to work, and to a near-normal lifestyle more rapidly and had greater improvements in work capacity, income, and job responsibility.[95] Both physical and psychosocial benefits occurred even with low-intensity exercise, particularly among older and sicker coronary patients. Despite the paucity of controlled studies, consistent moderate psychosocial benefit appears to result from combinations of structured exercise, education, and counseling.[63,96] Although the contribution of peer support in a group program has not been ascertained, it may be helpful given the predictive power of social isolation for coronary mortality.[97]

VOCATIONAL ASPECTS OF CORONARY REHABILITATION[36]

A major goal of rehabilitative care for nonelderly patients recovered from MI or myocardial revascularization is resumption of gainful employment, a change in occupation if needed, and the resulting economic and psychological benefits. In the 1980s, about 80 percent of patients who recovered from uncomplicated MI and who were younger than 65 years of age and employed at the time of infarction returned to work within 2 to 3 months, typically resuming former jobs.[98] Despite this favorable early return to work, subsequent cessation of employment was high, with as much as a 20 percent decrement in continued employment between 6 months and 1 year. Comparable data are not available for patients with complications of MI or residual functional impairment, although their return to work is estimated at 25 to 33 percent.

These data contrast markedly with work resumption following CABG surgery. Despite a substantial decrease in symptoms, improvement in functional capacity, and reported enhancement of life quality and participation in leisure activities, return to work following coronary bypass surgery has been much less favorable than anticipated.[99,100] No difference in 10-year employment status was described between patients randomized to medical and surgical treatment in the Coronary Artery Surgery Study (CASS).[101] Return to work following PTCA is comparable with that following CABG surgery, although PTCA patients are reported to return to work more promptly.[100] Other reports described lack of confidence in the ability to return to work following PTCA, even when patients were physically able to do so.[102]

Most studies of the return to work have involved predominantly or exclusively men; recent examination of working women with coronary disease showed them to have a longer convalescence and even lesser return to work; whether this is a gender issue or reflects older age or greater occurrence of depression among women warrants study.[103]

For patients younger than 65 years of age following MI or myocardial revascularization, the indirect health care costs of disability, including lessened productivity, loss of income, welfare payments, and unemployment insurance costs, must be considered when the cost-effectiveness of rehabilitation is determined.[57,104–106] Coronary heart disease is the leading problem in the United States for which adults receive premature disability benefits under the Social Security system; almost one-fourth of men and women receiving Social Security disability allowances have permanent disability due to coronary disease. Following both MI and myocardial revascularization, symptomatic and functional improvement correlates poorly with the return to work and resumption of preillness lifestyle, with psychosocial status appearing as a more important determinant.[99] Since only about 15 percent of the U.S. labor force currently performs manual labor and this percentage decreases with older age, the severity of angina or heart failure in coronary patients only rarely precludes or delays return to work. Many nonmedical factors negatively influence resumption of employment: older age, adequate nonwork income, anxiety or depression, activity-induced symptoms, lower social class and less education, jobs involving high-level physical activity (more common among blue-collar workers), and perception of the coronary illness as job-related. Patients who fail to resume employment within 6 months after a coronary event are unlikely ever to do so.[107]

Among the medical reasons for failure to return to work are unwarranted medical restrictions or, even more commonly, lack of professional assurance of the safety of so doing.[107] Exercise testing performed for risk stratification also can be used for work evaluation; it permits a relatively precise assessment of function that may help allay the apprehensions of the patient,[58] family,[108] physician, and employer about the capability and safety of return to work.[109] One randomized, controlled trial of occupational work assessment in a health maintenance organization population early following MI, identifying low-risk patients and counseling them about the appropriateness of prompt return to work, effected a 32 percent reduction in the duration of convalescence.[31] Extrapolation of exercise test data to job requirements should include an analysis of the job to be performed and differences in temperature, environment, intellectual demands, relation to meals, travel requirements, and emotional stress, among others. Nonetheless, patients without evidence of ischemia or arrhythmia during a symptom-limited standard exercise test typically are free of these problems when occupational static and dynamic work are combined.[110] Arm ergometry may be preferable for occupational assessment of patients who perform predominantly arm work.[53]

Furthermore, since most occupational work is intermittent, with brief periods of strenuous activity and longer intervals of low-level activity or rest, occupational myocardial work demand is lower than for the same level of steady-state exercise; cardiac output, blood pressure, and oxygen uptake do not approach steady state until about 2 min after the onset of work, explaining the tolerance of patients with modest cardiac impairment and limitation of cardiac output for significant workloads of short duration, when adequate rest periods are interspersed. Recommendations for full-time work should be for work levels approximating 30 percent of measured physical work capacity. Guidelines are available to assist physicians in assessing and establishing the employment of patients with coronary heart disease.[111]

Other nonmedical considerations also influence postinfarction or postrevascularization employment, particularly the financial, social, disability, and compensation benefits of not returning to work. Although appropriate physician and employer attitudes may facilitate reemployment, the viewpoint of the patient appears the major determinant. In a number of studies, the patient's preoperative perception about ability to return to work appeared to be the most important determinant.

Benefits to employers of cardiac rehabilitative care for their employees include earlier return to work, less disability, less absenteeism, reduced financial expenditures for sickness and disability payments, reduced training costs for replacement of personnel, and greater productivity.[1] Employers thus should encourage coronary rehabilitative care as a component of their managed care plans.

References

1. Report of the WHO Expert Committee, Wenger NK, Expert Committee Chairman. *Rehabilitation after Cardiovascular Diseases, with Special Emphasis on Developing Countries.* WHO Tech. Rep. Series No. 831, Geneva: World Health Organization; 1993.
2. American College of Cardiology. Position report on cardiac rehabilitation: Recommendations of the American College of Cardiology on cardiovascular rehabilitation. *J Am Coll Cardiol* 1986; 7:451.
3. Agency for Health Care Policy and Research. *Cardiac Rehabilitation Programs.* Health Technology Assessment Report No. 3, DHHS Publication No. AHCPR 92-0015. Rockville, MD: U.S. Department of Health and Human Services, Public Health Service, Agency for Health Care Policy and Research; December 1991.
4. Wenger NK, Froelicher ES, Smith LK, et al. *Cardiac Rehabilitation.* Clinical Practice Guideline No. 17, AHCPR Publication No. 96-0672. Rockville, MD: U.S. Department of Health and Human Services, Public Health Service, Agency for Health Care Policy and Research and the National Heart, Lung, and Blood Institute; October 1995.
5. Ben-Ari E, Kellermann JJ, Fishman EZ, et al. Benefits of long-term physical training in patients after coronary artery bypass grafting: A 58-month follow-up and comparison with a nontrained group. *J Cardiopulm Rehabil* 1986; 6:165.
6. Raft D, McKee DC, Popio KA, et al. Life adaptation after percutaneous transluminal coronary angioplasty and coronary artery bypass grafting. *Am J Cardiol* 1985; 56:395.
7. Ben-Ari E, Rothbaum DA, Linnemeir TJ, et al. Benefits of a monitored rehabilitation program versus physician care after emergency percutaneous transluminal coronary angioplasty: Follow-up of risk factors and rate of stenosis. *J Cardiopulm Rehabil* 1989; 7:281.
8. Ades PA, Waldmann ML, Gillespie C. A controlled trial of exercise training in older patients. *J Gerontol* 1995; 50A:M7.
9. Lavie CJ, Milani RV, Littman AB. Benefits of cardiac rehabilitation and exercise training in secondary coronary prevention in the elderly. *J Am Coll Cardiol* 1993; 22:678.
10. DeBusk RF, Houston Miller N, Superko HR, et al. A case-management system for coronary risk factor modification after acute myocardial infarction. *Ann Intern Med* 1994; 120:721.
11. Haskell WL, Alderman EL, Fair JM, et al. Effects of intensive multiple risk factor reduction on coronary atherosclerosis and

clinical cardiac events in men and women with coronary artery disease. The Stanford Coronary Risk Intervention Project (SCRIP). *Circulation* 1994; 89:975.

12. Schuler G, Hambrecht R, Schlierf G, et al. Regular physical exercise and low-fat diet: Effects on progression of coronary artery disease. *Circulation* 1992; 86:1.
13. Leon AS, Certo C, Comoss P, et al. Scientific evidence of the value of cardiac rehabilitation services with emphasis on patients following myocardial infarction: I. Exercise conditioning component (position paper). *J Cardiopulm Rehabil* 1990; 10:79.
14. Mark DB, Naylor CD, Hlatky MA, et al. Use of medical resources and quality of life after acute myocardial infarction in Canada and the United States. *N Engl J Med* 1994; 331:1130.
15. Thomas RJ, Houston Miller N, Lamendola C, et al. National survey on gender differences in cardiac rehabilitation programs: Patient characteristics and enrollment patterns. *J Cardiopulm Rehabil* 1996; 16:402.
16. O'Connor GT, Buring JE, Yusuf S, et al. An overview of randomized trials of rehabilitation with exercise after myocardial infarction. *Circulation* 1989; 80:234.
17. Oldridge N, Furlong W, Feeny D, et al. Economic evaluation of cardiac rehabilitation soon after acute myocardial infarction. *Am J Cardiol* 1993; 72:154.
18. Oldridge NB, Guyatt GH, Fischer ME, et al. Cardiac rehabilitation after myocardial infarction: Combined experience of randomized clinical trials. *JAMA* 1988; 260:945.
19. Balady GJ, Jette D, Scheer J, et al, and the Massachusetts Association of Cardiovascular and Pulmonary Rehabilitation Database Co-Investigators. Changes in exercise capacity following cardiac rehabilitation in patients stratified according to age and gender: Results of the Massachusetts Association of Cardiovascular and Pulmonary Rehabilitation Multicenter Database. *J Cardiopulm Rehabil* 1996; 16:38.
20. Rechnitzer PA, Cunningham DA, Andrew GM, et al. Relation of exercise to the recurrence rate of myocardial infarction in men: Ontario Exercise-Heart Collaborative Study. *Am J Cardiol* 1983; 51:65.
21. Blumenthal JA, Rejeski WJ, Walsh-Riddle M, et al. Comparison of high and low-intensity exercise training early after acute myocardial infarction. *Am J Cardiol* 1988; 61:26.
22. Goble AJ, Hare DL, Macdonald PS, et al. Effect of early programmes of high and low intensity exercise on physical performance after transmural acute myocardial infarction. *Br Heart J* 1991; 65:126.
23. Ehsani AA, Biello DR, Schultz J, et al. Improvement of left ventricular contractile function by exercise training in patients with coronary artery disease. *Circulation* 1986; 74:350.
24. Kennedy CC, Spiekerman RE, Lindsay MI Jr, et al. One-year graduated exercise program for men with angina pectoris: Evaluation by physiologic studies and coronary arteriography. *Mayo Clin Proc* 1976; 51:231.
25. Hung J, Gordon EP, Houston N, et al. Changes in rest and exercise myocardial perfusion and left ventricular function 3 to 26 weeks after clinically uncomplicated acute myocardial infarction: Effects of exercise training. *Am J Cardiol* 1984; 54:943.
26. Sullivan MJ, Higginbotham MB, Cobb FR. Exercise training in patients with severe left ventricular dysfunction: Hemodynamic and metabolic effects. *Circulation* 1988; 78:506.
27. Todd IC, Ballantyne D. Effect of exercise training on the total ischaemic burden: An assessment by 24-hour ambulatory electrocardiographic monitoring. *Br Heart J* 1992; 68:560.
28. Sebrechts CP, Klein JL, Ahnve S, et al. Myocardial perfusion changes following 1 year of exercise training assessed by thallium-201 circumferential count profiles. *Am Heart J* 1986; 112:1217.
29. Coats AJS, Adamopoulos S, Meyer TE, et al. Effects of physical training in chronic heart failure. *Lancet* 1990; 335:63.
30. Meyer TE, Casadei B, Coats AJS, et al. Angiotensin-converting enzyme inhibition and physical training in heart failure. *J Intern Med* 1991; 230:407.
31. Dennis C, Houston-Miller N, Schwartz RG, et al. Early return to work after uncomplicated myocardial infarction: Results of a randomized trial. *JAMA* 1988; 260:214.
32. Ades PA, Grunvald MH. Cardiopulmonary exercise testing before and after conditioning in older coronary patients. *Am Heart J* 1990; 120:585.
33. Ades PA, Hanson JS, Gunther PGS, et al. Exercise conditioning in the elderly coronary patient. *J Am Geriatr Soc* 1987; 35:121.
34. Ades PA, Waldman ML, Polk DM, et al. Referral patterns and exercise response in the rehabilitation of female coronary patients aged ≥62 years. *Am J Cardiol* 1992; 69:1422.
35. Williams MA, Maresh CM, Esterbrooks DJ, et al. Early exercise training in patients older than age 65 years compared with that in younger patients after acute myocardial infarction or coronary artery bypass grafting. *Am J Cardiol* 1985; 55:263.
36. Wenger NK, Smith LK, Froelicher ES, et al, eds. *Cardiac Rehabilitation: A Guide to Practice in the 21st Century*. New York: Marcel Dekker; 1999.
37. Balady GJ, Fletcher BJ, Froelicher ES, et al. Cardiac rehabilitation programs: A statement for healthcare professionals from the American Heart Association. *Circulation* 1994; 90:1602.
38. American College of Sports Medicine Position Stand. Exercise for patients with coronary artery disease. *Med Sci Sports Exerc* 1994; 26:i.
39. Health and Public Policy Committee, American College of Physicians. Cardiac rehabilitation services. *Ann Intern Med* 1988; 109:671.
40. American Association of Cardiovascular and Pulmonary Rehabilitation. *Guidelines for Cardiac Rehabilitation Programs*. Champaign, IL: Human Kinetics; 1991.
41. Wenger NK, Balady GJ, Cohn LH, et al. Ad Hoc Task Force on Cardiac Rehabilitation: Cardiac rehabilitation services following PTCA and valvular surgery. Guidelines for use. *Cardiology* 1990; 19:4.
42. Wenger NK, Haskell WL, Kanter K, et al. Ad Hoc Task Force on Cardiac Rehabilitation: Cardiac rehabilitation services after cardiac transplantation. Guidelines for use. *Cardiology* 1991; 20:4.
43. NIH Consensus Development Panel on Physical Activity and Cardiovascular Health. Physical activity and cardiovascular health. *JAMA* 1996; 276:241.
44. Haskell WL. Cardiovascular complications during exercise training of cardiac patients. *Circulation* 1978; 57:920.
45. DeBusk RF, Haskell WL, Miller NH, et al. Medically directed at-home rehabilitation soon after uncomplicated acute myocardial infarction: A new model for patient care. *Am J Cardiol* 1985; 55:251.
46. Worcester MC, Hare DL, Oliver RG, et al. Early programmes of high and low intensity exercise and quality of life after acute myocardial infarction. *B Med J* 1993; 307:1244.
47. Kelemen MH, Stewart KJ, Gillian RE, et al. Circuit weight training in cardiac patients. *J Am Coll Cardiol* 1986; 7:38.
48. Franklin BA, Bonzheim K, Gordon S, et al. Resistance training in cardiac rehabilitation. *J Cardiopulm Rehabil* 1991; 11:99.
49. Kelemen MH. Resistive training safety and assessment guidelines for cardiac and coronary prone patients. *Med Sci Sports Exerc* 1989; 21:675.
50. Sparling PB, Cantwell JD, Dolan CM, et al. Strength training in a cardiac rehabilitation program: A six-month follow-up. *Arch Phys Med Rehabil* 1990; 71:148.
51. Stewart KJ, Mason M, Keleman MH. Three-year participation in circuit weight training improves muscular strength and self-efficacy in cardiac patients. *J Cardiopulm Rehabil* 1988; 8:292.
52. Wilke NA, Sheldahl LM, Levandoski SG, et al. Transfer effect of upper extremity training to weight carrying in men with ischemic heart disease. *J Cardiopulm Rehabil* 1991; 11:365.

53. Franklin BA. Exercise testing, training and arm ergometry. *Sports Med* 1985; 2:100.
54. Wenger NK. Ischemic heart disease: Exercise training, selected aspects of pharmacologic therapy, and drug-exercise interactions. *Emory J Med* 1989; 3:253.
55. Ryan TJ, Antman EM, Brooks NH, et al. 1999 Update: ACC/AHA guidelines for the management of patients with acute myocardial infarction. A report of the American College of Cardiology/American Heart Association Task Force on Practice Guidelines (Committee on Management of Acute Myocardial Infarction). *J Am Coll Cardiol* 1999; 34:890; Executive Summary and Recommendations. *Circulation* 1999; 100: 1016.
56. Balady GJ, Weiner DA, Rose L, et al. Physiologic responses to arm ergometry exercise relative to age and gender. *J Am Coll Cardiol* 1990; 16:130.
57. Picard MH, Dennis C, Schwartz RG, et al. Cost-benefit analysis of early return to work after uncomplicated acute myocardial infarction. *Am J Cardiol* 1989; 63:1308.
58. Ewart CK, Taylor CB, Reese LB, et al. Effects of early postmyocardial infarction exercise testing on self-perception and subsequent physical activity. *Am J Cardiol* 1983; 51:1076.
59. Van Camp SP, Peterson RA. Cardiovascular complications of outpatient cardiac rehabilitation programs. *JAMA* 1986; 256:1160.
60. Wenger NK. In-hospital exercise rehabilitation after myocardial infarction and myocardial revascularization: Physiologic basis, methodology, and results. In: Wenger NK, Hellerstein H, eds. *Rehabilitation of the Coronary Patient,* 3d ed. New York: Churchill-Livingstone; 1992:351.
61. Hung J, Goldwater D, Convertino VA, et al. Mechanisms for decreased exercise capacity after bed rest in normal middle-aged men. *Am J Cardiol* 1983; 51:344.
62. Rowe MH, Jelinek MV, Liddell N, et al. Effect of rapid mobilization on ejection fractions and ventricular volumes after acute myocardial infarction. *Am J Cardiol* 1989; 63:1037.
63. Maeland JG, Havik OE. The effects of an in-hospital educational programme for myocardial infarction patients. *Scand J Rehabil Med* 1987; 19:57.
64. Borg GA. Psychophysical bases of perceived exertion. *Med Sci Sports Exerc* 1982; 14:377.
65. Williams RS, Miller H, Koisch FP Jr, et al. Guidelines for unsupervised exercise in patients with ischemic heart disease. *J Cardiac Rehabil* 1981; 1:213.
66. Blumenthal JA, Levenson RM. Behavioral approaches to secondary prevention of coronary heart disease. *Circulation* 1987; 76(suppl I):I-130.
67. Ornish D, Brown SE, Scherwitz LW, et al. Can lifestyle changes reverse coronary heart disease? The Lifestyle Heart Trial. *Lancet* 1990; 336:129.
68. Mullen PD, Mains DA, Velez R. A meta-analysis of controlled trials of cardiac patient education. *Patient Educ Couns* 1992; 19:143.
69. Fuster V, Pearson TA. 27th Bethesda Conference: Matching the intensity of risk factor management with the hazard for coronary disease events. *J Am Coll Cardiol* 1996; 27:957.
70. CASS Principal Investigators and Their Associates. Coronary Artery Surgery Study (CASS): A randomized trial of coronary artery bypass surgery. Quality of life in patients randomly assigned to treatment groups. *Circulation* 1993; 68:951.
71. Leaman DM, Brower RW, Meester GT. Coronary artery bypass surgery: A stimulus to modify existing risk factors? *Chest* 1982; 81:16.
72. Kottke TE, Battista RN, DeFriese GH, et al. Attributes of successful smoking cessation interventions in medical practice: A meta-analysis of 39 controlled trials. *JAMA* 1988; 259:2883.
73. Fiore MC, Smith SS, Jorenby DE, et al. The effectiveness of the nicotine patch for smoking cessation: A meta-analysis. *JAMA* 1994; 271:1940.
74. Shephard RJ. The scientific basis of exercise prescribing for the very old. *J Am Geriatr Soc* 1990; 38:62.
75. Saunamaki KI. Early post-myocardial infarction exercise testing in subjects 70 years or more of age: Functional and prognostic evaluation. *Eur Heart J* 1984; 5(suppl E):93.
76. Bruce RA, Larson EB, Stratton J. Physical fitness, functional aerobic capacity, aging, and responses to physical training or bypass surgery in coronary patients. *J Cardiopulm Rehabil* 1989; 9:24.
77. Wilson JR, Groves J, Rayos G. Circulatory status and response to cardiac rehabilitation in patients with heart failure. *Circulation* 1996; 94:1567.
78. Litchfield RL, Kerber RE, Benge JW, et al. Normal exercise capacity in patients with severe left ventricular dysfunction: Compensatory mechanisms. *Circulation* 1982; 66:129.
79. Giannuzzi P, Temporelli PL, Corrà U, et al., for the ELVD Study Group. Attenuation of unfavorable remodeling by exercise training in postinfarction patients with left ventricular dysfunction: Results of the Exercise in Left Ventricular Dysfunction (ELVD) Trial. *Circulation* 1997; 96:1790.
80. Dubach P, Myers J, Dziekan G, et al. Effect of exercise training on myocardial remodeling in patients with reduced left ventricular function after myocardial infarction: Application of magnetic resonance imaging. *Circulation* 1997; 95:2060.
81. Adamopoulos S, Coats AJS, Brunotte F, et al. Physical training improves skeletal muscle metabolism in patients with chronic heart failure. *J Am Coll Cardiol* 1993; 21:1101.
82. Hornig B, Maier V, Drexler H. Physical training improves endothelial function in patients with chronic heart failure. *Circulation* 1996; 93:210.
83. Belardinelli R, Georgiou D, Cianci G, et al. Randomized, controlled trail of long-term moderate exercise training in chronic heart failure: Effects on functional capacity, quality of life, and clinical outcome. *Circulation* 1999; 99:1173.
84. Squires RW, Lavie CJ, Brandt TR, et al. Cardiac rehabilitation in patients with severe ischemic left ventricular dysfunction. *Mayo Clin Proc* 1987; 62:997.
85. Williams RS. Exercise training of patients with ventricular dysfunction and heart failure. In: Wenger NK, ed. *Exercise and the Heart,* 2d ed. Philadelphia: Davis; 1985:219.
86. Stevenson LW, Steimle E, Fonarow G, et al. Improvement in exercise capacity of candidates awaiting heart transplantation. *J Am Coll Cardiol* 1995; 25:163.
87. Tamarisk NK. Enhancing activity levels of patients with permanent cardiac pacemakers. *Heart Lung* 1988; 17:698.
88. Kalbfleisch KR, Lehmann MH, Steinman RT, et al. Reemployment following implantation of the automatic cardioverter defibrillator. *Am J Cardiol* 1989; 64:199.
89. Williams RB Jr, Barefoot JC, Haney TL, et al. Type A behavior and angiographically documented coronary atherosclerosis in a sample of 2289 patients. *Psychosom Med* 1988; 50:139.
90. Helmers KF, Krantz DS, Howell RH, et al. Hostility and myocardial ischemia in coronary artery disease patients: Evaluation by gender and ischemic index. *Psychosom Med* 1993; 55:29.
91. Razin AM. Psychosocial intervention in coronary artery disease: A review. *Psychosom Med* 1982; 44:363.
92. Schleifer SL, Macari-Hinson MM, Coyle DA, et al. The nature and course of depression following myocardial infarction. *Arch Intern Med* 1989; 149:1785.
93. Frasure-Smith N, Lesperance F, Talajic M. Depression and 18-month prognosis after myocardial infarction. *Circulation* 1995; 91:999.
94. Frasure-Smith N, Lesperance F, Talajic M. Depression following myocardial infarction: Impact on 6-month survival. *JAMA* 1993; 270:1819.

95. Stern MJ, Cleary P. National Exercise and Heart Disease Project: Psychosocial changes observed during a low-level exercise program. *Arch Intern Med* 1981; 141:1463.
96. Maeland JG, Havlik OE. Psychological predictors for return to work after a myocardial infarction. *J Psychosom Res* 1987; 31:471.
97. Orth-Gomer K, Unden A-L, Edwards M-E. Social isolation and mortality in ischemic heart disease: A 10-year follow-up study of 150 middle-aged men. *Acta Med Scand* 1988; 224:205.
98. Wenger NK, Hellerstein HK, Blackburn H, et al. Physician practice in the management of patients with uncomplicated myocardial infarction: Changes in the past decade. *Circulation* 1982; 65:421.
99. Walter PJ, ed. *Return to Work after Coronary Artery Bypass Surgery: Psychosocial and Economic Aspects.* Berlin: Springer-Verlag; 1985.
100. Russell RO Jr, Abi-Mansour P, Wenger NK. Return to work after coronary bypass surgery and percutaneous transluminal angioplasty: Issues and potential solutions. *Cardiology* 1986; 73:306.
101. Rogers WJ, Coggin CJ, Gersh BJ, et al, for the CASS Investigators. Ten-year follow-up of quality of life in patients randomized to receive medical therapy or coronary artery bypass graft surgery. The Coronary Artery Surgery Study (CASS). *Circulation* 1990; 82:1647.
102. Fitzgerald ST, Becker DM, Celentano DD, et al. Return to work after percutaneous transluminal coronary angioplasty. *Am J Cardiol* 1989; 64:1108.
103. Walling A, Tremblay GJ, Jobin J, et al. Evaluating the rehabilitation potential of a large population of post-myocardial infarction patients: Adverse prognosis for women. *J Cardiopulm Rehabil* 1988; 8:99.
104. Ades PA, Huang D, Weaver SO. Cardiac rehabilitation participation predicts lower rehospitalization costs. *Am Heart J* 1992; 123:916.
105. Levin LA, Perk J, Hedback B. Cardiac rehabilitation: A cost analysis. *J Intern Med* 1991; 230:427.
106. Oldridge N, Furlong W, Feeny D, et al. Economic evaluation of cardiac rehabilitation soon after acute myocardial infarction. *Am J Cardiol* 1993; 72:154.
107. Almeida D, Bradford JM, Wenger NK, et al. Return to work after coronary bypass surgery. *Circulation* 1983; 68(suppl II):II-205.
108. Taylor CB, Bandura A, Ewart CK, et al. Exercise testing to enhance wives' confidence in their husbands' cardiac capability soon after clinically uncomplicated acute myocardial infarction. *Am J Cardiol* 1995; 55:635.
109. Hellerstein HK. Vocational aspects of rehabilitation: Work evaluation.In: Wenger NK, Hellerstein HK, eds. *Rehabilitation of the Coronary Patient,* 3d ed. New York: Churchill-Livingstone; 1992:523.
110. Hung J, McKillip J, Savin W, et al. Comparison of cardiovascular response to combined static-dynamic effort, postprandial dynamic effort and dynamic effort alone in patients with chronic ischemic heart disease. *Circulation* 1982; 65:1411.
111. 20th Bethesda Conference. Insurability and employability of the patient with ischemic heart disease, October 3–4, 1988. *J Am Coll Cardiol* 1989; 14:1003.

PART SEVEN

SYSTEMIC ARTERIAL HYPERTENSION

CHAPTER 51

HYPERTENSION: EPIDEMIOLOGY, PATHOPHYSIOLOGY, DIAGNOSIS, AND TREATMENT

Henry R. Black / George L. Bakris / William J. Elliott

INTRODUCTION

Hypertension is the most common disease-specific reason for which Americans visit a physician. It is currently among the leading causes of morbidity and mortality in the world and is expected to have an even greater impact on the health of the public as more of the world becomes developed.[1] In addition to the morbidity and mortality directly attributable to hypertension, high blood pressure (BP) is a powerful risk factor (a condition or characteristic of an individual or a population) that in this case increases the likelihood that an individual or population will develop a wide variety of cardiovascular (CV) diseases (Table 51-1).[2–5] Hypertension even has been associated with an increased risk of certain cancers.[6–8] Some authors have failed to appreciate this relationship when attributing certain cancers to particular antihypertensive treatments.[9]

All health care providers routinely encounter patients whose BP is elevated. In patients with definite hypertension (see below), the paramount consideration is the choice of treatment, but in an increasing number of individuals, lowering BP may be beneficial even if definite hypertension cannot be diagnosed. In the next decade, it is expected that more and more patients will become candidates for antihypertensive therapy, especially as trials demonstrate the benefits of treatment and pharmacologic approaches become safer and more effective. Furthermore, many citizens, perhaps of the majority of those over 40 years of age, who do not yet meet the criteria for pharmacologic treatment for hypertension will benefit from lifestyle modification, a presumably safe and cost-effective public health approach to reducing BP. Many of the lifestyle habits that lower BP or slow the rate of rise of BP probably should be incorporated into everyone's lifestyle very early.

This chapter reviews the risks imparted by elevated BP, discusses the pathophysiology of hypertension, and analyzes currently available and recommended tools to measure BP and evaluate patients with hypertension. Treatment both with and without drugs is discussed in light of the explosion of information furnished by clinical trials and the newer approaches to lowering BP created by an enhanced understanding of the mechanisms responsible for raising it. The techniques of molecular biology and the contribution of genetics to hypertension have dramatically increased physicians' appreciation of the complexity of the problem.

Hypertension is a disorder of circulatory regulation. The now-classic mosaic theory of the etiology of hypertension, which first was proposed in 1949 by Page, can be endorsed even more

TABLE 51-1 Risks Associated with Hypertension

Cerebrovascular disease	Renal insufficiency
Coronary artery disease	Peripheral vascular disease
Heart failure	Premature mortality

enthusiastically in light of current knowledge.[10] No longer can one expect a simple explanation of why BP is elevated in an individual patient or expect that a single approach to therapy will be successful in the majority of those who are treated.

However, with all the progress that has been made in identifying the risks associated with elevated BP and all the efforts to develop ways to lower BP and prove that they work, the situation in the United States leaves much to be accomplished.[11,12] Only 27.4 percent of hypertensive Americans ages 18 to 74 in the period 1991 to 1994 had a BP of <140/90 mmHg, the current goal.[11] The data are still worse for those ≥75 years of age, and the goal may well be too high in some subpopulations of hypertensives, particularly those with diabetes mellitus (DM) and/or renal disease with proteinuria. The record in the rest of the world is much worse.[13–17] Although the United States does better than other countries, much still needs to be done here and elsewhere. One must understand hypertension better to give optimal care to the 1.2 billion hypertensives estimated to be living by the year 2010. Physicians must strive to prevent as much of the enormous morbidity and premature mortality that one can predict will result.

DEFINITION

Blood pressure is a continuous variable, and whatever number is used to define hypertension will be arbitrary. In the past several decades, the levels at which definite hypertension is defined as beginning have changed from >160/95 mmHg to >140/90 mmHg. Although there is still some disagreement, most authorities now agree on several important principles:

- Hypertension should be defined by both systolic and diastolic BP levels.
- Simply defining and consequently categorizing individuals as hypertensive or not only on the basis of their BP levels neglects the value of using the presence or absence of other risk factors, comorbidity, and target organ damage (TOD) to assess prognosis and ultimately to guide therapy. Thus, the Sixth Joint National Committee on Prevention, Detection, Evaluation and Treatment of High Blood Pressure (JNC VI), the World Health Organization/International Society of Hypertension (WHO/ISH), and the British Hypertension Society (BHS) use a more comprehensive system to define hypertension[11,18,19] (Table 51-2). These definitions are based on properly measured office readings (see below). The definitions of hypertension for home and ambulatory measurements are different. Blood pressure >135/85 mmHg for 24-h ambulatory monitoring or home monitoring is the usual level considered to be where hypertension starts.[20,21] Although home or ambulatory measurements are useful, it is not appropriate routinely to use those values to diagnose most individuals. Office readings remain the standard. In certain situations, especially when an individual claims to have multiple "normal" readings outside the physician's office (see below), it may be reasonable to rely more on out-of-office measurements.
- The treatment approach to individuals with elevated BP should not focus simply on the BP level, which assesses the relative risk that is imparted by that BP, but also on the remainder of the CV risk profile, which estimates the absolute risk of events that an individual with that particular BP and risk profile will face. In the JNC VI classification and stratification of hypertension, for example, the stages (optimal to normal to high normal through stages 1 to 3) represent increasing relative risk as BP rises, while risk group A-C denotes increasing absolute risk as other risk factors and TOD are superimposed on the level of BP[11] (Table 51-3).

TABLE 51-2 Threshold Values for "Normal" versus "Abnormal" BP (in mmHg)

Source	Office Readings	Home Readings	ABPM Readings
JNC VI	140/90		
Ohasama	140/90	137/84	
French	140/90	127/83	
ASH	140/90	135/85	135/85
Staessen	140/90		133/82

SOURCE: Adapted from JNC VI: The sixth report on the Joint National Committee on Prevention, Detection, Evaluation, and Treatment of High Blood Pressure (JNC VI). *Arch Intern Med* 1997; 157:2413–2443. Ohasama: Tsuji I, Imai Y, Nagai K, et al. Proposal of reference values for home blood pressure measurement: Prognostic criteria based on a prospective observation of the general population in Ohasama, Japan. *Am J Hypertens* 1997; 10:409–418. French Society of Hypertension: De Gaudemaris R, Chau NP, Maillion JM. Home blood pressure variability, comparison with office readings and proposal for reference values: Groupe de la Mesure, French Society of Hypertension. *J Hypertens* 1994; 12:831–838. ASH: Pickering T. Recommendations for use of home (self) and ambulatory blood pressure monitoring: American Society of Hypertension Ad Hoc Panel. *Am J Hypertens* 1996; 9:1–11. Staessen: Staessen JA, O'Brien ET, Atkins N, Amery AK. Short report: Ambulatory blood pressure in normotensive compared with hypertensive subjects: The Ad-Hoc Working Group. *J Hypertens* 1993; 11:1289–1297.

It is not of major significance whether hypertensives are classified as being in a stage as recommended by JNC VI or a class per WHO/ISH.[11,18] What is important is that one base the evaluation and care of hypertensive patients on more than the BP number. Black and Yi have suggested that reimbursement for care of a hypertensive patient be based on the stage and risk group into which that patient falls, but to date such a system has not been implemented.[22]

EPIDEMIOLOGY AND RISK

Physicians generally do not concern themselves with reducing BP when it is elevated because of the specific clinical problems they can attribute to that elevation. Instead, hypertension is treated because of the increased risk of mortality and CV disease that results from having an elevated BP (Table 51-1).

These risks have been well documented in numerous epidemiologic studies, beginning with the Framingham Heart Study and many others in the 1950s and 1960s and extending to the present.[23–29] More recently, meta-analyses of pooled data have confirmed the robust, continuous relationship between BP level

TABLE 51-3 JNC VI Stratification of Cardiovascular Risk and Links to Initial Treatment Strategy

		Risk Group		
		A	B	C
	No. of Risk Factors	0	1 (not DM[a])	≥2 (or DM)
	Target organ damage	Absent	Absent	Present
BP stage	Cardiovascular disease	Absent	Absent	Present
High normal (130–139/85–89)		LM[b] only	LM only	LM plus drug therapy
Stage 1 (140–159/90–99)		LM for 12 months	LM for 6 months	LM plus drug therapy
Stage 2 (160–179/100–109)		LM plus drug therapy	LM plus drug therapy	LM plus drug therapy
Stage 3 (≥180/≥110)		LM plus drug therapy	LM plus drug therapy	LM plus drug therapy

[a]DM = diabetes mellitus.
[b]LM = lifestyle modifications.

and cerebrovascular disease and coronary artery disease (CAD) in both western and eastern populations.[30,31] In addition, BP is directly related to left ventricular hypertrophy (LVH) and heart failure (HF), peripheral vascular disease (PVD), carotid atherosclerosis, renal disease, and "subclinical disease."[4,5,32,33] Kannel and colleagues in the Framingham Heart Study have documented the fact that CV risk factors tend to cluster in hypertensives.[34] Hypertensives are more likely to have dyslipidemias, especially elevated serum triglycerides and low levels of high-density lipoprotein cholesterol (HDL-C), and type 2 DM. The common denominator may be insulin resistance, perhaps as a result of the frequent association of hypertension and obesity.[35]

In the last several years, it has become increasingly clear that the risks attributed to hypertension are much more strongly related to the level of systolic BP than to diastolic BP, especially in those over age 50 or 60 years.[36,37] The observation that systolic BP predicts events and TOD better than diastolic BP was persuasively argued in the early 1970s, but it took until 1993, in the Fifth Report of the Joint National Committee on the Detection, Evaluation and Treatment of Hypertension, before systolic BP was given even equal weight to diastolic BP in classification systems.[36,38]

Some have argued that one should not measure diastolic BP other than perhaps to calculate pulse pressure (PP).[39,40] Pulse pressure, the difference between systolic and diastolic BP, is an even better predictor of risk than is systolic BP in most of the epidemiologic studies done to date.[41–46] A wide PP, unless it is a result of aortic insufficiency or an arteriovenous malformation, is a simple clinical indicator of stiffer and less compliant large central arteries and significant arterial damage. Franklin and colleagues, again using data from the Framingham Heart Study cohort, showed that at all levels of systolic BP (even as low as 110 to 130 mmHg), risk is less with higher diastolic BPs.[46] More recent analyses by this group have suggested that these findings may be relevant only in those over age 60, and so it is not appropriate to ignore those with elevated diastolic BP level if their systolic readings are not above normal. The classification systems cited above have been careful not to include PP either in defining the risks of hypertension or in recommending treatment. A recently published position paper from the National High Blood Pressure Education Program has cautioned physicians not to rely on PP measurements until more support is gathered for this position.[47]

With the exception of hypertensive encephalopathy, it has long been felt that few, if any, clinical symptoms can be attributed to increased BP levels. This may have to be reevaluated, however, as newer and very well tolerated drugs are developed and as improved methods of assessing subtle symptoms are perfected. Clinical trials with angiotensin receptor blockers (ARBs), for example, consistently show that the members of the actively treated group have fewer adverse reactions than do those given placebo.[48,49] Furthermore, in the Treatment of Mild Hypertension Study (TOMHS) and the Hypertension Optimum Treatment (HOT) trial, the group with the lowest BP had the fewest complaints.[50,51] These trials utilized a wide variety of drugs to reduce BP and clearly showed not only that lowering BP is safe but that hypertensives treated to lower levels feel better. Hypertension may not be the asymptomatic condition it has long been thought to be.

ECONOMICS

Cost considerations are playing an increasingly important role in the pharmacologic management of hypertension in the United States, and they have always been a major consideration in the rest of the world. No regimen, no matter how carefully and appropriately selected, will be effective if the patient cannot afford it. Moreover, if antihypertensive agents do not appear on the national formulary or the formulary of the insurance company from which a patient gets medication, the cost will not be covered and the patient may not be willing or able to purchase them. Generic preparations are available for every class of antihypertensive agent except ARBs, and these generic preparations tend to be the least expensive options for initial therapy. In general, branded calcium antagonists (CAs) are the most expensive, with ARBs and angiotensin-converting enzyme inhibitors (ACE-Is) the next most expensive drugs. For many of the fixed-dose combinations now available, the cost is less than what would be paid for the individual components if they were purchased separately. It is also customary for fixed-dose combinations that include a thiazide diuretic to cost no more than does the nondiuretic component alone.

A careful analysis of the economics of hypertension treatment has to include more than what is spent on drugs, patient visits, or laboratory tests.[52,53] For many affected (and especially high-risk) patients, the extremely expensive complications of under- and/or untreated hypertension far outweigh the inconvenience and costs associated with effective treatment.[53] Current estimates are that in the United States in the year 2000, hypertension will cost approximately $37.2 billion.[54] Nearly half this total is spent on indirect costs (death benefits for the families of those who die from untreated hypertension, disability payments for stroke survivors, time away from work, and transportation costs, to name a few) and payments to hospitals and nursing homes.[54] Both of these expenses could be reduced if hypertension treatment were more effective in controlling BP and reducing the risk of the clinical sequelae of hypertension, including myocardial infarction (MI), HF, stroke, and end-stage renal disease (ESRD).[55]

PATHOPHYSIOLOGY

Hypertension is a disorder of BP regulation and results from a multitude of causes. Control of BP involves a complex interaction among the kidneys, the central nervous system (CNS) and peripheral nervous system (PNS), and the vascular endothelium thoughout the body as well as a variety of the other organs, such as the adrenal and pituitary glands. The heart is the organ that responds to many of the changes mediated by these systems. It also secretes hormones locally and systemically that interact with substances produced elsewhere and help regulate BP levels. In those genetically predisposed to develop hypertension, an imbalance occurs among the various systems that modulate the level of BP. The sympathetic nervous system (SNS), the renin-angiotensin-aldosterone (RAA) system, vasopressin (VP), nitric oxide (NO), and a host of vasoactive peptides, including endothelin, adrenomedullin, and others produced by the heart and a host of different cells (endothelial and vascular smooth cells, for example), modulate the responses of these systems and help maintain BP over a range commensurate with optimum physical and mental activity. Additionally, these systems affect the ability of the kidney to handle sodium (Na^+) and volume, which Guyton and colleagues feel is the primary controller of BP.[56]

Sympathetic Nervous System and Renal Sodium Handling

Guyton and colleagues noted that while the SNS and the RAA system are important for short-term changes in BP, ultimately it is the kidney that is responsible for long-term blood volume and BP control.[56] High-pressure baroreceptors in the carotid sinus and aortic arch respond to acute elevations in systemic BP by causing a reflex vagal bradycardia that is mediated though the parasympathetic system and inhibition of sympathetic output from the CNS. Low-pressure cardiopulmonary receptors in the atria and ventricles likewise respond to increases in atrial filling by increasing heart rate (HR) through inhibition of the cardiac SNS, increasing atrial natriuretic peptide (ANP) release, and inhibiting VP release.[57–59] These reflexes are largely controlled centrally, particularly in the nucleus tractus solitarii of the dorsal medulla. This vasomotor center also receives input from the limbic system and hypothalamus in response to emotional or psychological stress.

The consequences of SNS stimulation are peripheral vasoconstriction, an increase in HR, release of norepinephrine from the adrenals, and a resultant rise in systemic BP. The increase in SNS activity also plays a role in mediating local vascular hypertrophy and stiffness. Renal efferent sympathetics also are activated and cause internal vasoconstriction with a fall in renal blood flow and an increase in renal vascular resistance.[60] The renal SNS also directly stimulates Na^+ reabsorption and renin release from the juxtaglomerular apparatus.[60–62] Thus, the SNS and CNS have effects on renal handling of Na^+.

Hyperactivity of the SNS has been described in patients with essential hypertension, particularly in the young and those with "high-normal" BP (130 to 139/80 to 89 mmHg).[63,64] Elevated plasma norepinephrine levels with increased HR and cardiac indexes have been described in people with newly diagnosed hypertension.[64] These individuals frequently show exaggerated BP responses to emotional (mental arthimetic) and physical stressors such as ice-water immersion. Additionally, a subset of these patients exhibit elevated plasma renin levels that may reflect beta-adrenergic stimulation of renin secretion.

A defect in baroreceptor sensitivity has been postulated to be responsible for abnormal responsiveness of the SNS and thus may contribute to the increase in BP and HR variability noted in some hypertensive patients.[65] SNS activity also is increased in certain high-risk groups with hypertension, including African-Americans, those with obesity, those with insulin resistance, and those who ingest or inhale certain agents, such as nicotine, alcohol, cyclosporine, and cocaine.[66–68] A very small subset of patients may have hypertension caused by compression of the lateral medulla by cranial nerves and/or vessels.[60] This results in increased SNS activity. Selective decompression of these nerves may ameliorate the hypertension in rare instances. Activation of the CNS/SNS also may result from renal afferent sympathetics from the kidney in hypertensive patients. In experimental models of hypertension, renal sympathectomy resulted in a reduction in BP.[60,64]

The influence of the SNS on Na^+ handling in the kidney also has been examined in detail.[69] Several studies have linked SNS hyperactivity with greater than normal increases in BP in response to a given Na^+ load.[70–73] Indeed, Dahl and Heine were the first to show that hypertension can be transferred from a hypertensive Dahl salt-sensitive rat to a nonhypertensive Dahl salt-resistant rat by transplantation of the kidney.[70] Patients with essential hypertension and associated renal failure have been cured of the underlying hypertension by renal transplantation from a normotensive donor.[74]

Most authorities believe that the mechanism by which the kidney causes hypertension is impairment in the excretion of Na^+.[60,61,71,75–78] This impairment may be related to genetic changes in various Na^+ exchangers in the proximal and distal tubules that result in altered responses to stimulation by the SNS and the RAA system. Epidemiologic studies have linked the relative Na^+ content in the diet with the prevalence of hypertension in various populations, although the value of dietary Na^+ restriction in reducing BP remains controversial (see below).[79,80] Interventional studies with Na^+ restriction and/or loading have revealed that the BP responses in many hypertensive patients are "salt-sensitive": Their BP rises with a salt load.[81,82] In addition, several studies have shown that salt loading of patients with essential hypertension results in a net total body Na^+ accumulation. Three genetic diseases associated with hypertension in childhood (Liddle's syndrome, the syndrome of apparent mineralocorticoid excess, and glucocorticoid-remediable aldosteronism) all are associated with increased reabsorption of Na^+ by the kidney.[83]

A genetically mediated defect in the ability of the kidney to excrete Na^+ does not readily explain certain observations:

- Young hypertensive subjects appear to excrete Na^+ normally or supernormally.
- Individuals with high-normal BP may have a low blood volume.
- As many as 40 percent of people with hypertension do not show a change in BP with Na^+ loading ("salt resistance").
- With aging, salt sensitivity increases both in frequency and in degree such that by age 70, the majority of hypertensive patients are salt-sensitive.

In fact, it has been argued from meta-analyses that salt restriction is not important either in normotensives or in patients with hypertension under age 40.[84,85] All these findings are consistent with the possibility that the defect in Na^+ excretion in hypertensive patients is acquired rather than genetically determined. It should be kept in mind, however, that abnormal Na^+ handling is a mechanism that contributes to elevating BP in many but probably not all patients with hypertension.

The Renin-Angiotensin-Aldosterone System

The RAA system is one of the most important physiologic mediators that regulate blood volume and BP. Plasma angiotensinogen, which is released primarily from the liver, is acted on by renin from the kidney to generate angiotensin I, which is further degraded in the presence of angiotensin-converting enzyme to angiotensin II (AII). In addition to the systemic RAA system, there is now evidence that a local RAA system is present in blood vessels, the heart, the kidney, and elsewhere, where it may mediate local effects (such as tissue remodeling) independent of circulating renin or angiotensinogen levels.

Most of the actions of AII are mediated by the AT_1 receptor and include stimulating vascular smooth muscle contraction and hypertrophy, increasing cardiac contractility, stimulating the SNS in the CNS and PNS, increasing NO production, causing aldosterone and VP release, and increasing thirst (Table 51-4).[86] Within the kidney, stimulation of the AT_1 receptor by AII also causes renal vasoconstriction (especially of the efferent arteriole and vasa rectae), a fall in renal blood flow, and an increase in renal vascular resistance.[87] Angiotensin II also increases Na^+ reabsorption both by increasing aldosterone release and through direct effects on the proximal tubule. Additionally, AII increases the sensitivity of the tubuloglomerular (TG) feedback response.

Angiotensin subtype 2 (AT_2) receptors also are stimulated by angiotensin II. These receptors produce virtually opposite actions in some experimental systems and are clearly active during fetal development (Table 51-4). Their role in healthy adults and even in those with cardiac or vascular damage is still uncertain.

The role of the RAA system in essential hypertension is complex. Whereas plasma renin activity (PRA) is elevated in 20 percent of hypertensive patients, PRA is either normal (50 percent) or low (30 percent) in the majority. However, in many patients with normal plasma renin levels, PRA may be inappropriately high in relation to total body Na^+. This has been suggested by the observation that Na^+ depletion accentuates and Na^+ infusion blunts changes in PRA levels in patients with hypertension. Additional evidence to support this concept comes from the observation that BP in these patients frequently is reduced after the use of ACE-Is or ARBs.[88]

TABLE 51-4 Characteristics and Functions of AT_1 and AT_2 Receptors

AT_1 Receptors
Always expressed
Mediate vasoconstriction
Mediate growth
Smooth muscle proliferation
Stimulate connective tissue deposit in media
Facilitate low-density lipoprotein cholesterol transport to media
Inhibit endothelial function
Mediate renal tubular sodium reabsorption
AT_2 Receptors
Increased expression during stress or injury
Mediate vasodilatation
Inhibit growth (antiproliferation)
Decreased renal absorption of sodium

Sealey and colleagues have suggested that the reason for widely varying PRA levels may be nephron heterogeneity within individual kidneys, in which there are some ischemic nephrons that make excess renin and other hyperfiltering nephrons in which renin secretion is suppressed.[89] They postulated that the increased renin release from the ischemic nephrons enters the circulation and then leads to AII generation, which causes inappropriate vasoconstriction and Na^+ reabsorption in the other hyperfiltering nephrons. This results in Na^+ retention and the development of hypertension.

Unfortunately, this is only part of the explanation, since PRA is relatively low in African-Americans and the elderly, two populations with a high prevalence of hypertension and a high rate of complications from hypertension. Low PRA, however, does not necessarily mean that the RAA is not active, since tissue effects and local actions are not necessarily evident from PRA alone.

Vasopressin

While VP has been clearly shown *not* to play a role in the genesis of essential hypertension, it does play an important role in the maintenance of established hypertension, especially in African-Americans.[90] In African-Americans, studies have shown that selective inhibition of V_1A receptors reduces systolic BP by an additional 8 to 12 mmHg in the presence of a high-salt diet (suppression of the RAA system) and clonidine (suppression of SNS).[91,92] Interestingly, this is not observed in whites. In light of the interaction between arginine vasopressin (AVP), AII, and endothelin on cellular growth and vascular responsiveness, it appears that AVP may have a potentiating effect on one of these other hormones.[93]

Endothelin

Endothelin is known to be the most potent vasoconstrictor in humans.[94] Comparative studies with AII have demonstrated not only that the endothelin family of hormones has cellular actions similar to those of AII but that the two hormones work in concert to potentiate each other's vascular and cellular effects.[95] Given this, however, the specific role of endothelin in the etiology of essential hypertension is minimal.[96] It plays a far more important role in cyclosporine-induced hypertension and decreased renal function as well as in maintaining BP in people with HF.[97]

Endothelin is the major mechanism by which cyclosporine constricts the afferent arteriole of the kidney and reduces renal function. Calcium antagonists and endothelin receptor blockade prevent this reduction. Additionally, endothelin A receptors have been shown to play a major role in contributing to the maintenance of elevated renal perfusion pressure in patients with HF.[98]

Nitric Oxide

Nitric oxide is the vasodilator produced by the endothelium in response to vasoconstrictor hormones, and so the contribution of NO to the maintenance of normal BP is vitally important.[99,100] Defects in NO release or synthesis that are induced by atherosclerosis or that are genetically programmed are a major determinant in predisposing individuals to the development of atherosclerosis and hypertension.[101] NO serves as a major counterbalancing factor that maintains BP within the range necessary to maintain organ perfusion but avoid injury. It counterbalances vasoconstrictive hormones, cytokines such as AII, platelet-derived growth factor (PDGF), tumor necrosis factor-alpha, and other hormones that stimulate its release. Transgenic animal models that do not have the ability to synthesize NO have very high BP and die of CV causes earlier than do animals that can produce NO.

Additionally, NO plays a major role in the genesis of hypertension in people who are insulin-resistant. The underlying mechanisms and the factors that may govern the interaction between insulin and NO have been studied extensively in healthy people and insulin-resistant subjects. It appears that a genetic and/or acquired defect of NO synthesis could represent a central defect that triggers many of the metabolic, vascular, and sympathetic abnormalities characteristic of insulin-resistant states, all of which may predispose to CV.[102]

Ion Transport Abnormalities

A number of dietary factors affect the SNS, the CNS, and the RAA system in those genetically predisposed to develop hypertension. These dietary factors, such as high Na^+ intake and low potassium (K^+), Ca^{2+}, and/or magnesium (Mg^{2+}) intake, may produce, worsen, or attenuate changes in BP. Substantial evidence from animal models of hypertension as well as diabetic and nondiabetic hypertensive individuals supports an association between the hypertension and changes in intracellular pH as well as electrolyte composition.[103–121] These observations have led to various hypotheses regarding the importance of one ion relative to others.

Numerous investigators have documented increases in cytosolic free Na^+ concentrations in cells of hypertensive or diabetic patients compared with age- and sex-matched normotensive or nondiabetic controls.[103–105] These increases result from altered activity of the Na^+/H^+ antiporter and the Na^+/Li^+ countertransporter. These increases in intracellular Na^+ are highly correlated with the presence of an elevated diastolic BP.

The relationship between intracellular Mg^{2+} and BP is less clearly defined. Data from experimental models of hypertension as well as from patients with hypertension demonstrate an inverse relation between intracellular Mg^{2+} concentration and BP elevation.[106,107] The primary mechanism responsible for this relative reduction in intracellular Mg^{2+} relates to Na^+-dependent Mg^{2+} efflux through the plasmalemma membrane.[112]

Increases in the intracellular Ca^{2+} concentration are seen commonly in obese and essential hypertensive subjects.[105,110] Like Na^+, these changes reflect altered membrane ion transport activity. Early clinical studies demonstrated that oral Ca^{2+} ingestion reduces BP, but the results from clinical trials do not consistently show a reduction in BP after Ca^{2+} supplementation.[120,121]

Increased K^+ intake is well known to have effects on BP control through multiple mechanisms, including opening K^+ channels in the vasculature, altering sympathetic neuronal output, and increasing vasodilatory prostaglandins.[122–125] This is exemplified by the fact that hypokalemia in patients will blunt reductions in blood pressure by antihypertensive medication, perhaps because it results in the closure of K^+ channels.

Potassium also plays a role in modulating vascular responsiveness in salt-sensitive individuals. In a recent clinical study, increasing dietary K^+ for 3 weeks in 16 predefined salt-sensitive subjects and 42 salt-resistant subjects resulted in the conversion of all salt-sensitive subjects from nocturnal nondipping to dipping status[126] (see below). These results suggest that a positive relationship between dietary K^+ intake and BP modulation can exist even when daytime BP is unchanged by a high-K^+ diet.[126]

Taken together, these data suggest that both univalent and divalent cations affect vascular responses to stimuli such as those mediated by the RAA and the SNS. Changes in vascular responses are linked to altered function of membrane ion transporters (Na^+/H^+ antiporter, Na^+/K^+/ATPase, Mg^{2+}/Na^+ exchanger, Ca^{2+}/H^+ exchanger, Ca^{2+} ATPase, and others). Both the Na^+/K^+/ATPase and the Ca^{2+}/ATPase pumps are important in maintaining the Ca^{2+} homeostasis of the cell.

Extracellular Volume Homeostasis

Whereas an acute infusion of saline administered to animals with experimentally induced hypertension will initially raise blood volume and cardiac output, the increase in cardiac output is transient and is replaced by a rise in systemic vascular resistance (SVR).[71,72]

There are several potential mechanisms for this observation. First, the normal response to a salt load is inhibition of the SNS. However, it is known that in salt-sensitive patients, the SNS is not inhibited and even may be activated with a salt load.[127,128] A possible explanation is that in the setting of renal dysfunction or intrarenal ischemia, salt loading triggers an intense tuboglomerular feedback signal that activates the renal afferent SNS. This renal response subsequently triggers a CNS response. Indeed, there is evidence that renal afferent nerves activate CNS sympathetic activity in both experimental hypertension and chronic renal disease.

Second, parabiotic experiments have suggested there may be circulating factors in salt-loaded animals with hypertension that are responsible for some of the increase in SVR. One class of factors is circulating Na^+/K^+/ATPase inhibitors, which have been documented in some patients with essential hypertension.[129–131] These substances, one of which is ouabain, are digitalis-like and adrenally derived. Blaustein has suggested that these substances, which presumably are secreted in an attempt to facilitate Na^+ excretion, may have the adverse consequence of increasing intracellular Na^+ and thus facilitating Na^+-Ca^{2+} exchange in vascular smooth muscle cells. This would lead to a rise in intracellular Ca^{2+} and stimulate vascular smooth muscle contraction, vasoconstriction, and a rise in SVR.[110]

A third mechanism is the loss of a vasodepressor substance. There is good evidence that a lipid-like vasodepressor factor termed adrenomedullin is expressed in some of the interstitial cells in the renal medulla and the juxtamedullary region. Release of this factor into the circulation appears to depend on medullary blood flow and can be inhibited if activation of renal SNS or inhibition of NO reduces blood flow.[60] Thus, one might expect to see lower circulating levels of this substance in the setting of tubulointerstitial (TI) injury and intrarenal ischemia.

Fourth, the increase in pressure associated with a saline load could cause increased tension in the peripheral vasculature, leading to microvascular rarefaction (which has been observed in the forearms and nail beds of patients with essential hypertension) that could raise the SVR. An increased pressure load on the vessels also could result in compensatory vascular hypertrophy mediated by local growth factors and the local RAA system. Indeed, there is evidence that AII, PDGF, and basic fibroblast growth factor are involved in these processes.

Mechanisms of Na^+ Retention in Essential Hypertension

A rise in systemic BP normally is associated with brisk natriuresis. This is thought to be due to a transient rise in pressure in the peritubular capillaries in the juxtamedullary region, with a subsequent increase in interstitial pressure and a backflow of Na^+ through the paracellular space of the proximal tubule. Numerous studies have confirmed that most patients with essential hypertension have a defect in the pressure natriuresis curve, in which higher systemic pressures are required to excrete a Na^+ load.[132,133]

A second mechanism for decreased Na^+ excretion is an enhancement of TG feedback. Tubuloglomerular feedback is a reflex vasoconstriction that occurs with chloride delivery to the macula densa, and the vasoconstrictive response will reduce glomerular filtration and Na^+ excretion. TG feedback can be enhanced in the setting of increased local vasoconstrictors such as AII and adenosine or by a reduction in local vasodilators such as NO. TG feedback appears to be enhanced in models of experimental hypertension.[132,134]

Finally, alterations in intrarenal vasoactive mediators may be involved in the impairment of Na^+ excretion in patients with hypertension. In both experimental and human hypertension, there may be low levels of renal vasodilators, such as prostaglandins, dopamine, and NO as well as elevated levels of renal vasoconstrictors such as AII and adenosine and increased activity of the renal SNS. In addition to their effects of enhancing TG feedback, alterations in the levels of these agents could contribute to net Na^+ reabsorption because of their direct effects on tubular Na^+ transport.

Some studies have shown that TI injury can be induced in rats with either catecholamine (phenylephrine) or AII infusion and that subsequently these animals will develop hypertension when placed on a high-salt diet.[134] Evaluation of these biopsies demonstrated focal areas of peritubular capillary rarefaction. This also has been observed in kidney biopsies of patients with essential hypertension. The loss of peritubular capillaries could help explain the impairment of pressure natriuresis. The ischemia related to the vasoconstriction and capillary loss could lead to alterations in the various vasoactive mediators. Indeed, there is some evidence that NO levels fall and adenosine levels rise with TI injury and ischemia, and this could contribute to the enhanced TG feedback that has been observed.[135,136]

While this pathway links a hyperactive SNS or RAA system with TI injury and salt-dependent hypertension, it is likely that TI injury induced in other ways could result in salt-sensitive hypertension. Indeed, it is of interest that TI disease is associated with reflux nephropathy, chronic pyelonephritis, DM, cyclosporine, radiation, lead and analgesic nephropathy, hypercalcemia/nephrocalcinosis, and gout, all of which are strongly associated with hypertension. In addition, it is noteworthy that many high-risk groups associated with salt-dependent essential hypertension, such as aged persons, obese persons, and African-Americans, have a high prevalence of TI disease.

Insulin Resistance

Insulin resistance is a metabolic disorder that is manifested by a reduction in peripheral skeletal muscle utilization of glucose.[35] To fully understand the contribution of insulin resistance to the genesis of hypertension, one has to evaluate the effects of insulin resistance and hyperinsulinemia on factors that contribute to BP elevation. High levels of insulin cause sodium retention and other vascular effects, such as cellular proliferation and matrix expansion.[137] In the presence of hyperinsulinemia, neurohumoral factors such as AII, endothelin, and VP also potentiate proliferation of endothelial and vascular smooth muscle cells.[138] Lastly, the effect of insulin on various growth factors contributes to the development of vascular injury through its potentiation of the atherosclerotic process.[139] These factors in a person genetically predisposed to develop nephropathy can potentiate injury to the vasculature and end organs.

It should be noted, however, that not all subjects with insulin resistance have all the associated components of insulin resistance syndrome or syndrome X, i.e., lipid abnormalities, hyperuricemia, type 2 DM, glucose intolerance, hypertension, microalbuminuria, left ventricular hypertrophy, salt sensitivity, and obesity, among others. Studies in the normotensive offspring of hypertensive nondiabetic parents demonstrate the presence of insulin resistance.[140,141] This is also true for nondiabetic first-degree relatives of patients with type 2 DM.[142] Thus, a genetic predisposition seems to be needed to develop this syndrome.

TABLE 51-5 Candidate Genes Associated with Hypertension and Cardiovascular Risk

Monogenic forms
Glucocorticoid-remediable aldosteronism
Liddle's syndrome
Polygenic forms that affect
Angiotensinogen gene
Na^+-Li^+ countertransport
Epithelial amiloride-sensitive sodium channel
Nitric oxide generation
Alpha-adducin
G_3 beta subunit (intracellular signal transduction)
Insertion/deletion of ACE gene

Genetic Factors

Commonly accepted candidate genes associated with the genesis of hypertension are summarized in Table 51-5. Insulin resistance is clearly associated with hypertension. A possible genetic link between the presence of insulin resistance and the development of hypertension has been proposed.[143–146] Recent studies also have identified insulin resistance in the normotensive offspring of parents with essential hypertension. Saad and coworkers evaluated the association between insulin resistance and the propensity to develop hypertension in different racial groups.[147] Those investigators examined Pima Indians, whites, and blacks who were normotensive and nondiabetic. They noted that Pima Indians had higher fasting plasma insulin concentrations than did whites or blacks and lower whole body glucose disposal. They also noted a strong correlation between fasting plasma insulin concentrations and the rate of glucose disposal in whites but not in Pima Indians or blacks. Thus, the development of hypertension does not necessarily correlate with the presence of either hyperinsulinemia or insulin resistance in certain racial groups.

Work by various investigators to isolate a "hypertensive gene" or group of genes has been ongoing for many years. Abnormalities in the angiotensinogen gene identified by Caufield and coworkers provide evidence to link mutations in the angiotensinogen gene to the pathogenesis of essential hypertension.[148] A study of 179 hypertensive sibpairs from 69 type 2 diabetic kindreds showed that specific changes in the linkage of the angiotensinogen gene were highly correlated with the presence of hypertension.[149]

The delineation of a gene profile that will predict who will develop hypertension is near. A number of federally funded studies to gather sib pairs and families to identify candidate genes that predispose individuals to the development of hypertension are under way. Data from these studies may lead to the identification of such genes within the next 5 to 10 years. Thus, until these genetic profiles are delineated, it will be necessary to rely on the data garnered from epidemiologic studies to identify subjects at risk for the development of hypertension and CV events.

These are several clear examples of genetic influences in hypertension.

GLUCOCORTICOID-REMEDIABLE ALDOSTERONISM

This is an inherited autosomal dominant disorder that mimics an aldosterone-producing adenoma.[150] An important clinical clue to diagnosing this disease is the age at onset of hypertension. Patients with glucocorticoid-remediable aldosteronism (GRA) typically are diagnosed with high BP as children, whereas patients with other mineralocorticoid excess states, such as aldosterone-producing adenomas (APA) and idiopathic adrenal hyperplasia, usually are diagnosed in the third through sixth decades of life. A strong family history of hypertension is the rule, often associated with early death of affected family members from cerebrovascular accidents, as is seen characteristically in some GRA families.

In GRA, the RAA system is suppressed and aldosterone secretion is regulated solely by ACTH. As a result, plasma aldosterone levels usually decline during the course of an upright posture study, similar to what is seen in patients with APA.[151–153] The administration of exogenous ACTH to patients with GRA is associated with aldosterone hyperresponsiveness compared with normal subjects.[153] Moreover, in contrast to normal subjects in whom continuous ACTH administration is associated with a rise and a subsequent fall in aldosterone to basal levels over days, patients with GRA exhibit an exuberant aldosterone response that is sustained as long as ACTH is infused.

GRA is caused by a genetic mutation that results in a hybrid or chimeric gene product fusing nucleotide sequences of the 11-hydroxylase and aldosterone synthase genes.[154,155] Characterization of this chimeric gene indicates that it arose from unequal crossing between 11-hydroxylase and aldosterone synthase genes.[155] These two genes are located in close proximity on human chromosome 8, are 95 percent homologous in nucleotide sequence, and have an identical intron-exon structure. The structure of the duplicated gene contains the 5′ regulatory sequences that confer the ACTH responsiveness of 11-hydroxylase fused to more distal coding sequences of the aldosterone synthase gene.[153,154] Therefore, this hybrid gene is expected to be regulated by ACTH and have aldosterone synthase activity. This hybrid gene allows ectopic expression of aldosterone synthase activity in the ACTH-regulated zona fasciculata, which normally produces cortisol.[156,157] This abnormal gene duplication can be detected readily by southern blotting, allowing for direct genetic screening for this disorder with a small blood sample.

GLUCOCORTICOID RESISTANCE

The structure, growth, and secretory activity of the adrenal cortical zona fasciculata are regulated largely by ACTH. Only cortisol can inhibit ACTH release. An increase in ACTH release raises the levels of cortisol, which then inhibits the release of ACTH. This continuous inhibitory feedback effect of cortisol on ACTH release is interrupted in patients with glucocorticoid resistance. In this disorder, although cortisol levels are exceedingly high, ACTH release is not inhibited, leading to uninhibited ACTH secretion, which in turn stimulates the adrenal cortex to produce 11-deoxycorticosterone (DOC).[157] If sufficient DOC is secreted, salt and water retention ensue, precipitating hypertension and hypokalemia. Animal studies indicate that the mechanism for this may in part be related to changes in hippocampal steroid receptor building.[158]

Animal studies also indicate that an expressional downregulation of endothelial cell nitric oxide synthase (NOS III) may contribute to the hypertension caused by glucocorticoids. Ingestion of dexamethasone by telemetrically instrumented rats increased BP progressively over 7 days. Plasma oxidation products of NO decreased to 40 percent, and the expression of endothelial NOS III was found to be downregulated in the aorta and several other tissues in glucocorticoid-treated rats. Dexamethasone treatment significantly attenuated the relaxation to the endothelium-dependent vasodilator acetylcholine but not to the endothelium-independent vasodilator S-nitroso-*N*-acetyl-D,L-penicillamine. Additionally, incubation of human umbilical vein endothelial cells or bovine aortic endothelial cells with several glucocorticoids reduced NOS III mRNA and protein expression to 60 to 70 percent of control, an effect that was prevented by the glucocorticoid receptor antagonist mifepristone.[159]

LIDDLE'S SYNDROME

Liddle's syndrome is an autosomal dominant disorder that mimics the signs and symptoms of mineralocorticoid excess.[160] The fault appears to lie with continuously avid Na^+ channels in the distal nephron, resulting in excessive salt absorption and K^+ wasting (despite negligible aldosterone production) and severe hypertension.[161,162] A prominent feature is premature death from stroke or HF. The clinical manifestations can be corrected by triamterene and amiloride but not by spironolactone. Triamterene and amiloride directly block the Na^+ channel, whereas spironolactone inhibits Na^+ absorption by binding the aldosterone receptor.

The cellular defect associated with this syndrome is located on the apical portion of the tubule where the epithelial Na^+ channel (EnaC) located on the apical membrane plays a critical role in Na^+ absorption. Mutations in this channel cause diseases of Na^+ homeostasis, including a genetic form of hypertension (Liddle's syndrome inhibits cAMP-mediated stimulation of EnaC). Thus, the apical Na^+ channels and transepithelial Na^+ current are inhibited. Experimental data indicate that cAMP-mediated translocation of EnaC to the cell surface is defective in patients with Liddle's syndrome.[163]

DIAGNOSIS OF HYPERTENSION

Estimation of the pressure generated by the heart during its normal contractile cycle has been measured for more than 100 years. The value of such readings in predicting prognosis was recognized in the early 1930s by insurance companies, which probably have the best data correlating causal BP measurements and the risk of future disability and death.[164] Since the second half of the 1800s, palpation of the pulse and appreciation of the contour and pressure within a peripheral artery were skills learned only through extensive experience. Such subjective observations were supplanted by objective (albeit indirect) measurements after the introduction of the Riva-Rocci sphygmomanometer in the late nineteenth century.[165,166] This instrument was refined by Janeway and Korotkoff, who characterized the sounds heard when using a stethoscope placed over the compressed artery in 1906.[167–169] Even today, the terminology introduced by Korotkoff is still used: Systolic BP is recognized when clear and repetitive tapping sounds are heard; diastolic BP is recorded when the sounds disappear. Exceptions to these general rules are still recognized among patients who have audible sounds even down to zero mmHg and in obstetric patients: In both situations, the "muffling" of the sounds (Korotkoff phase IV) is recorded either in addition to the phase V measurement or as the diastolic BP, respectively.[170]

Techniques of Measuring Blood Pressure

The proper technique for accurate BP measurement typically is taught very early during medical training but then seldom is followed.[171–173] Many expert panels have made recommendations regarding the methodology of BP measurement, that frequently do not agree in all details, but several general principles can be extracted[174–177]:

TABLE 51-6 Blood Pressure Cuff Names and Sizes

Cuff	Width, cm	Length, cm
Newborn	2.5–4.0	5.0–9.0
Infant	4.0–6.0	11.5–18.0
Child	7.5–9.0	17.0–19.0
Normal adult	11.5–13.0	22.0–26.0
Large adult	14.0–15.0	30.5–33.0
Thigh	18.0–19.0	36.0–38.0

- There are six sizes of commonly available BP cuffs (Table 51-6). Using a smaller than recommended cuff on a larger arm typically results in an overestimation of casual BP. In obese or muscular persons, the large adult-size cuff is required for all those with an arm circumference at the mid-humerus over 38 cm. In very large individuals, a "thigh" cuff is often necessary.[178]
- In accurately measuring BP, the deflation rate of the column of mercury should be 2 to 3 mmHg/s. The lower rate of deflation should be used for persons with HRs less than 72 beats per minute (bpm); the more rapid deflation is appropriate only for those with resting tachycardia. If the precision of measurement is to be at least 2 mmHg, the observer should have the opportunity to hear at least one Korotkoff sound at each 2-mmHg gradation of the mercury column. Thus, the proper deflation rate depends on the HR of the subject and is unlikely to be more than 3 mmHg/s if a precise BP measurement is desired.
- It is unusual for a single BP measurement to be an accurate indicator of future CV risk; multiple measurements made on different occasions are more likely to be helpful in deciding whether a particular person ought to have his or her BP lowered. Although it is traditional to average the second and third of a series of BP measurements in a single position (e.g., supine, seated, or standing) and record this as the "average BP" at a given visit, recent "quality care guidelines" mandate instead the recording of individual BP measurements, with the lowest on a given date being the one of greatest interest to auditors. For these reasons, it is quickly becoming "standard practice" to record individual readings and is especially important to measure BP in several positions (including standing), since the auditors record only the lowest BP reading (in any position) as the "BP taken at that visit."[179] The BP readings of many physicians participating in managed care audits are being judged as a "quality of care" indicator, and recording the largest number of BP measurements in several positions offers the greatest opportunity to have at least one which is deemed "acceptable."[179]
- Most of the long-term data on hypertension and its treatment were derived from "casual" measurements made with a mercury sphygmomanometer and stethoscope in a health care provider's office. Physicians and patients often are more interested and impressed by BP readings taken in other settings (e.g., home monitors or ambulatory BP monitoring devices, both of which are discussed further below), but the great

majority of data linking BP measurements to adverse clinical sequelae (including MI, stroke, and death) were made in the traditional fashion in the physician's office, and for now, office readings taken by a trained professional should be the BP used for diagnosing and treating hypertensives in all but a few special situations.

Blood pressure is subject to a large degree of intrinsic variability. Several steps can be taken to minimize this variability, including the following:

- Taking multiple measurements, especially when the pulse is irregular (e.g., atrial fibrillation). This is necessary because ventricular filling pressures vary considerably as a result of variability of diastolic filling time.[180] Blood pressure variability is especially pronounced in older persons with primarily or exclusively systolic BP evaluations.
- Centering the bladder of the cuff over the brachial artery with its lower edge within 2.5 cm of the antecubital fossa. This leaves enough space so that the stethoscope head can be applied inferiorly without touching the cuff (and generating background noise).
- Having the subject rest silently and comfortably (with back support if seated) for at least 5 min before the measurement.
- Abstaining from drinking caffeine or alcohol-containing beverages or tobacco use within 30 min before a BP measurement.
- Questioning the subject regarding the most recent meal or evacuation of bowels or bladder. Distended abdominal viscera not only are painful but routinely cause elevations in BP, presumably related to anxiety and pain. Older persons typically have a lower BP postprandially; thus, it is often necessary to inquire about and record when the last meal was eaten.
- Assuring that the arm is supported at the level of the heart. Both muscular work (of tensed muscles around the elbow) and hydrostatic pressure caused by a "dangling arm" increase the pressure necessary to obliterate the pulse and lead to overestimates of systolic BP.
- Listening over the brachial artery by using the bell of the stethoscope with minimal pressure exerted on the skin. At the conclusion of the BP measurement, there should be no lasting indentations in the area where the head of the stethoscope was placed. Otherwise the systolic BP is likely to be overestimated and the diastolic BP to be underestimated because too great a pressure was exerted directly over the artery.
- The "peak inflation level" of the mercury column should be determined by using palpation of the radial artery before the stethoscope is applied. For all subsequent BP measurements, the cuff typically should be inflated 20 mmHg higher than the pressure at which the palpable pulse at the radial artery disappears. Important prognostic information may be missed if the "auscultatory gap" is not detected; this risk is minimized by determining the peak inflation level by palpation before the stethoscope is applied.[181]
- Although mercury columns traditionally have been used in the measurement of BP, environmental concerns associated with elemental mercury are increasing. In Sweden and many other countries, elemental mercury is forbidden in the workplace. Nonetheless, sphygmomanometers used in the measurement of BP should be calibrated frequently and routinely against such standards (typically every 6 months) to assure accuracy.
- Attempting to avoid "terminal digit preference." Traditionally, BP measurements have been made to the nearest 2 mmHg (the typical markings on a mercury sphygmomanometer). Theoretically, in a large collection of systolic and diastolic BP measurements, there should be an equal number of readings ending in 0, 2, 4, 6, or 8 mmHg. It is often instructive to compare the actual distribution of terminal digits with the 20 percent expected for each one. This typically reveals a preference for 0 (in inpatient medical services, where BP readings are typically precise to ±10 mmHg) or 8 (for outpatients in a managed care organization being graded on how many people are <140/90 mmHg).
- Measurements of BP in both arms typically are obtained at the initial visit, and the arm with the higher BP is used thereafter if the difference is greater than 10/5 mmHg. In such situations, there is often concern about coarctation of the aorta or Takayasu's arteritis or moyamoya disease, but seldom is this seen on ultrasonography or other confirmatory testing. Blood pressure measurement in a leg should be commonplace in all young hypertensives at the first visit and may be useful in older people as a peripheral indicator of aortic insufficiency ("Hill's sign").
- Assuring that the equipment used to measure BP is in good working order. Many sphygmomanometers (even in hospitals) are in poor repair and should be cleaned, calibrated, and fitted with nonleaking tubing and properly sized cuffs. The interest in BP measurements recently demonstrated by agencies that certify health systems for quality has improved the chance that any given patient will be hospitalized in a bed with properly maintained BP-measuring equipment.

Home Blood Pressure Measurements

The technology for obtaining accurate and reproducible BP measurements outside the traditional medical environment has improved greatly in the last 20 years. Many types of machines now exist (Table 51-7) that are convenient, inexpensive, and relatively accurate. Even persons with hearing difficulties, problems with hand-eye coordination, and other disabilities can operate semiautomatic devices with digital readouts and printers to estimate BP. Some authorities feel that such devices should be provided to every person with elevated BP, but others are concerned about overinterpretation of the data, which generally have not been used commonly in clinical decision making in clinical trials and should not be used routinely in practice to make diagnostic or therapeutic decisions.

Home BP readings are typically lower (by an average of 12/7 mmHg) than measurements taken in the traditional medical environment, even in normotensive subjects.[21] Home readings tend to be better correlated with both the extent of TOD and the risk of future mortality than are readings taken in the physician's office.[182] Home readings can be helpful in evaluating symptoms suggestive of hypotension, especially if the symptoms are intermittent or infrequent. During treatment, reliable home readings can lower costs by substituting for multiple visits to health care providers.[183] Persons who routinely measure BP at home probably have a better prognosis than do those who do not because of both selection bias (they tend to be more interested in their BP than are those who refuse to purchase and use a home BP machine) and social support (when a friend or

TABLE 51-7 Advantages and Disadvantages of Methods of BP Measurement Available to Patients in the Outpatient Setting

Attribute	Anaeroid with Stethoscope	Oscillometric with Stethoscope	Oscillometric with Digital Readout
Coordination necessary	Yes	Yes	Less so
Affected by presbyacusis	Yes	Yes	No
Affected by presbyopia	Yes	Less so	Less so
Widely available	Yes	Less so	Increasingly
Inexpensive	Yes	Less so	Increasingly
Good-quality results	Yes, with effort	Yes, with effort	Yes
Increases patients' interest in managing BP	Yes	Yes	Yes
Battery-powered	No	Yes	Yes
Affected by impaired grip strength	Yes	No	No
Independently validated by prospective studies	No	No	No

spouse becomes involved in measurement and overseeing pill-taking and appointment-keeping behaviors).

Home BP readings should be interpreted cautiously, carefully, and conservatively.[184] There are no data from long-term clinical studies that based all treatment decisions solely on home readings, but several preliminary reports show benefit from supplementing office BP measurements with home readings.[185,186] Several studies have shown that prognosis is better predicted by home readings than by one or two "casual" BP measurements.[187–189] Many of the factors that contribute to BP variability are more difficult to control in the home environment, including intrinsic circadian variation, food and alcohol ingestion, exercise, and stress. The possibility that home BP measurements will become an obsession is also a disadvantage. If home readings are to be taken, most authorities recommend that the instrument be calibrated against a mercury sphygmomanometer by using a Y-tube and that the technique of the measurer be checked. Home readings can be a useful adjunct to information obtained in the physician's office, especially when the two are widely disparate. One long-term study showed that people with much lower home BP readings (compared with those in the physician's office) suffer fewer major CV events than do people who have elevated readings both in the office and at home.[187,190] The authors recommend that patients who are interested in and capable of measuring their BP at home do it at a fixed time of the day and record all the readings obtained. The physician then can review them during the office visit and strive to educate the patients about the difficulties of interpretation of the readings.

Ambulatory Blood Pressure Monitoring

Extensive research has led to a better definition of the role of automatic recorders that measure BP frequently over a 24-h period during a person's usual daily activities (including sleep). Despite the acquisition and dissemination of excellent data, however, the use of these devices by practitioners in the United States has been extremely limited, mostly because of a lack of reimbursement by third-party payers. As a research tool, however, the advantages and disadvantages of ambulatory blood pressure monitoring (ABPM) have been well documented (Table 51-8), normal values have been defined (Table 51-2), and multiple publications correlating abnormal patterns of ABPM with adverse outcomes have appeared.[191,192] Several expert panels have defined the special situations in which ABPM is particularly useful (Table 51-9).

Several varieties of ABPM devices are currently available. In the United States, those which measure BP indirectly (i.e., without arterial cannulation) use either an auscultatory or an oscillometric technique. The former type uses a microphone placed over the artery to detect Korotkoff sounds in the traditional fashion. The latter measures biophysical oscillations of the brachial artery, which are compared (using a standardized algorithm) with those observed with a mercury sphygmomanometer: Systolic BP is determined directly from the threshold oscillation, mean arterial pressure is estimated, and diastolic

TABLE 51-8 Advantages and Disadvantages of Ambulatory Blood Pressure Monitoring

Advantages

- Many BP and pulse measurements during 24-h period
- Measures diurnal variation (including during sleep)
- Measures BP and pulse during daily activities
- Can identify "white coat" hypertension
- No "alerting response"
- No placebo effect
- Better correlation with target organ damage than other methods

Disadvantages

- Cost
- Limited availability of equipment
- Disruption of daily activities from noise/discomfort (e.g., sleep quality, flaccid arm during measurement)
- Limited "normative" data
- Limited guidelines (or consensus) for interpretation of data in individuals
- Few long-term prospective studies demonstrating utility compared with traditional (and much less expensive) BP measurements

Source: Adapted from Elliott WJ, Black HR. Special situations and special considerations. In: Hollenberg NK, ed. *Hypertension: Mechanism and Treatment.* Volume 1 of Braunwald EB, ed. *Atlas of Heart Disease.* Philadelphia: Current Medicine; 1995:12-1.

TABLE 51-9 Situations in Which ABPM is Useful

"High-normal" blood pressure without target organ damage
Office or "white coat" hypertension
Refractory hypertension
Episodic hypertension
Symptoms consistent with hypotension associated with antihypertensive medication
Hypertension with autonomic dysfunction
Nocturnal hypertension
Evaluation of efficacy of antihypertensive drugs in clinical research

SOURCE: Adapted from the National High Blood Pressure Education Program's Working Group Report on Ambulatory Blood Pressure Monitoring. *Arch Intern Med* 1990; 150:2270–2280.

BP is calculated. Both types of monitors are small (<450 g), simple to apply and use, accurate, relatively quiet and tolerable, and powered by two to four small batteries. Data from 80 to 120 measurements of BP and pulse typically are stored in a small microprocessor and then downloaded into a desktop computer, which then edits the readings and prints the report.

None of the currently available ABPM devices is completely without problems. Devices that rely on direct measurements require 24 h of arterial cannulation, which is potentially dangerous, and rarely are used even for research. Indirect measurements of BP using auscultatory techniques can be confused by ambient noise levels even if R-wave gating is used (this requires the electrocardiographic leads to be attached to the chest). Oscillometric techniques require that the subject keep the arm straight and flaccid during the measurement and can be completely confused if the subject has a tremor. The interpretation of ABPM readings may be enhanced by a diary of the subject's activities, but such diaries are not always completed.

ABPM makes it possible to measure BP routinely during sleep and has reawakened interest in the circadian variation of HR and BP. Most normotensives and perhaps 80 percent of hypertensives have at least a 10 percent drop in BP during sleep compared with the daytime average. Although there may be some important demographic confounders (blacks and the elderly have less prominent "dips"[193,194]), several prospective studies have shown an increased risk of CV events among those with a "nondipping" BP or pulse pattern.[195–197] However, there is concern, based on several Japanese studies, that elderly persons with more than a 20 percent difference between nighttime and daytime average BPs ("excessive dippers") may suffer unrecognized ischemia in "watershed areas" (of the brain and other organs) during sleep if their BP declines below the autoregulatory threshold.[198]

During the last 15 years, research has demonstrated an important correlation between ABPM readings and the prevalence and extent of TOD in hypertensives. Compared with "casual" BP measurements (obtained in the health care provider's office), ABPM measurements clearly are a better predictor of LVH, cardiac function, and overall scores summing optic, carotid, cardiac, renal, and peripheral vascular damage resulting from elevated BP.[199–201] Ambulatory BP monitoring also may be useful in identifying the small minority of typically unrecognized patients [61 of 234 (26 percent) in New York City] with "white coat normotension" who have normal BP readings in the physician's office but elevated ABPM readings with LVH and carotid wall thickening similar to that usually seen in sustained hypertensives.[202]

Perhaps the most important data demonstrating the value of ABPM have come from recent end-point studies of CV events (death, MI, stroke). In the first published study of outcomes in central Italy, ABPM was the best predictor of future CV events; "nondipper hypertensives" had approximately three times the risk of hypertensives whose BP was ≥10 percent lower at night compared to daytime ("dippers").[195] A population-based study involving 1572 men and women of ABPM versus casual and home BPs has been ongoing since 1987 in Ohasama, Japan.[188] After an average of approximately 5 years of follow-up, there was no significant relationship between one casual BP measurement and future CV mortality. However, there was a highly significantly increased risk of CV death in the quintile with the highest ABPM, and the lowest risk was found in those in the lowest quintile of ABPM.[189] The value of ABPM in refractory hypertension was demonstrated in a study of 86 hypertensive people taking on average three antihypertensive medications daily.[203] Follow-up data were collected approximately 4 years after an ABPM was performed; the patients having ABPM results in the lowest tertile had significantly lower rates of CV complications: 2.2 versus 9.5 versus 13.5 events per 100 patient-years. These data suggest that ABPM may be helpful in sorting out which patients with elevated office BP measurements who already are taking multiple antihypertensive medications ought to have intensified treatment and which ones can be spared the additional expense and risk. A subsidy of the Systolic Hypertension in Europe (Syst-EUR) trial involved 808 patients who had ABPM in addition to the usual clinic BP measurements before randomization to placebo or active treatment.[197] In the group randomized to placebo, ABPM was clearly a better predictor of future CV events than was the office BP measurement. Active treatment reduced the difference in prognosis among ambulatory and office measurements. Furthermore, the risk of a CV event was much higher in patients who did not display a nocturnal decline in BP. These data suggest (but do not prove) that the poor prognosis seen with nondipping hypertension can be mitigated by active antihypertensive treatment.

White Coat Hypertension

Since the advent of technology that allows accurate BP measurement outside the health care provider's office, it has been estimated by many but not all reports that 10 to 20 percent of American hypertensives have substantially lower BP measurements in other settings.[204] The name *white coat hypertension* has been given to the situation in which BP measurements outside the health care setting are considerably lower than those in it even though the "white coat" itself is unlikely to be the only factor that increases BP. Careful studies originally done in Italy and later corroborated in other countries show that BP rises in response to an approaching physician who is not previously known to the subject. This apparently does not happen if the subject is approached by a nurse even if she or he is wearing a white coat.

The clinical consequences and prognostic significance of white coat hypertension have been hotly debated in the medical literature for some years. One school of thought suggests that if a person has an acute rise in BP caused by stress related to an approaching physician, similar elevations in BP are likely whenever a stressful stimulus is encountered. Thus, some of the literature supports the concept that the white coat response is merely a precursor to "more substantial and more sustained hypertension."[205] This point of view is buttressed by the realization that in several clinical and population-based studies, white coat hypertension also is found in people with a greater prevalence of subclinical risk factors for CV, including LVH, a family history of hypertension and heart disease, hypertriglyceridemia, elevated fasting insulin levels, and lower HDL-C levels.[205–208]

A second school of thought, based on more careful and conservative definitions of the white coat effect, proposes that some individuals consistently show a similar and marked elevation in BP in response to the health care environment. Using somewhat more stringent criteria than the studies cited above, several long-term studies have shown a greatly reduced risk of either TOD or major CV sequelae among people with lower BPs measured either at home or by 24-h BP monitoring compared with measurements taken in the same person in the physician's office.[187,190,195] Whether the future risk of such individuals for CV events is similar (or even identical) to that of completely normotensive people is open to question. A third group has claimed that white coat hypertension simply represents regression to the mean in those with considerable BP variability.[204]

The best approach to the treatment of white coat hypertension is unresolved. Clearly, such individuals would benefit from lifestyle modification, which presumably would reduce the probability of progression to sustained hypertension. Completely abstaining from antihypertensive medication in "white coat hypertensives" appears unwise. Verdecchia and colleagues have published data indicating that in the long term, the risk of future CV events did not differ between white coat and sustained hypertensives when both were treated with antihypertensive medications.[209] Whether intensive treatment with continuous antihypertensive medication is warranted for only temporary increases in BP is debatable. Clearly, the treatment and repeated ABPM sessions required to monitor therapy would not be very cost-effective. The cost-effectiveness of ABPM to diagnose and monitor people with white coat hypertension has been estimated by several groups, primarily because 10 to 20 percent of hypertensives might be spared the cost of treatment and close follow-up.[210–212] One ABPM session annually has been set as the upper limit of what most American health plans could afford.[213] Several authoritative groups have recommended that ABPM be used sparingly in the general antihypertensive population but may be more widely used in managed care, veterans' hospitals, and other situations where minimal incremental direct costs are involved.[213,214]

EVALUATION OF THE HYPERTENSIVE PATIENT

Six key issues must be addressed during the initial office evaluation of a person with elevated BP readings:

- Documenting an accurate diagnosis of hypertension (see above)
- Defining the presence or absence of TOD related to hypertension
- Screening for other CV risk factors that often accompany hypertension
- Stratifying risk for CVD (according to risk Group A, B, or C in JNC VI)[11]
- Assessing whether the person is likely to have an identifiable cause of hypertension (secondary hypertension) and should have further diagnostic testing to confirm or exclude the diagnosis
- Obtaining data that may be helpful in the initial choice and subsequent choice of therapy

There are many diagnostic possibilities for explaining a single set of elevated BP readings (Tables 51-10 and 51-11). Aside from those who take one of several types of drugs known to elevate BP, many persons with only one elevated BP reading will have their BP decline and return to the normal range. This is the reason for recommending multiple encounters (at least two or three) before a diagnosis of hypertension is firmly established.

Routine Evaluation in All Hypertensive Patients

The recommendations of JNC VI and other national and international expert panels limit the number of and the expense related to initial tests for the routine evaluation of a hypertensive patient[11,18,19] (Table 51-12). Those which are used in assessing the presence or absence of TOD include physical examination, blood urea nitrogen (BUN)/creatinine, electrolytes, urinalysis, and an electrocardiogram (ECG). Assessing the number of CV risk factors can be accomplished with the medical history, chemistry panel [glucose, total cholesterol (TC), triglycerides], and urinalysis. The JNC VI suggests stratifying patients' risk for CV into three risk groups (Table 51-3). Other national expert panels have even more elaborate systems for linking the assessment of CV risk and the intensity of antihypertensive treatment.[19,215]

Several elements of the evaluation of a hypertensive patient warrant further comment. The physical examination needs to be "directed" toward looking for clues that might indicate an identifiable secondary cause of hypertension such as an abdominal or flank bruit, which would be a sign of visceral atherosclerosis or perhaps renal artery fibromuscular disease, or an abdominal or flank mass that might be a pheochromocytoma or a polycystic kidney.

Proper examination of the optic fundus often is neglected even though it is a valuable tool for evaluating hypertensive patients. In the years before effective antihypertensive drug therapy became available, the most important predictor of future CV mortality and morbidity was not the level of BP but in the appearance of TOD in the optic fundi.[216] Although the prognosis of hypertensive patients has improved greatly since that time, the appreciation of hypertension-related changes in the optic fundus is still important in the assessment of both the severity and the duration of elevated BP. The optic fundus is the only site in the entire body where blood vessels can be examined directly. Very few patients with a recent onset of hypertension have Keith-Wagener-Barker (KWB) grade III or IV fundi (Table 51-13).

Arteriosclerosis can be directly recognized, and the severity and duration of previous hypertension can be estimated through the appreciation of abnormalities of the retinal arteries.[217] The

TABLE 51-10 Causes of Hypertension

- I. Systolic and diastolic hypertension
  - A. Primary, essential or idiopathic
  - B. Secondary
    - 1. Renal
      - a. Renal parenchymal disease
        - (1) Acute glomerulonephritis
        - (2) Chronic nephritis
        - (3) Polycystic disease
        - (4) Diabetic nephropathy
        - (5) Hydronephrosis
      - b. Renovascular
        - (1) Renal artery stenosis
        - (2) Intrarenal vaculitis
      - c. Renin-producing tumors
      - d. Renoprival
      - e. Primary sodium retention (Liddle's syndrome, Gordon's syndrome)
    - 2. Endocrine
      - a. Acromegaly
      - b. Hypothyroidism
      - c. Hyperthyroidism
      - d. Hypercalcemia (hyperparathyroidism)
      - e. Adrenal
        - (1) Cortical
          - (a) Cushing's syndrome
          - (b) Primary aldosteronism
          - (c) Congenital adrenal hyperplasia
          - (d) Apparent mineralocorticoid excess (licorice)
        - (2) Medullary: pheochromocytoma
      - f. Extraadrenal chromaffin tumors
      - g. Carcinoid
      - h. Exogenous hormones
        - (1) Estrogen
        - (2) Glucocorticoids
        - (3) Mineralocorticoids
        - (4) Sympathomimetics
        - (5) Tyramine-containing foods and monoamine oxidase inhibitors
    - 3. Coarctation of the aorta
    - 4. Pregnancy-induced hypertension
    - 5. Neurologic disorders
      - a. Increased intracranial pressure
        - (1) Brain tumor
        - (2) Encephalitis
        - (3) Respiratory acidosis
      - b. Sleep apnea
      - c. Quadriplegia
      - d. Acute porphyria
      - e. Familial dysautonomia
      - f. Lead poisoning
      - g. Guillain-Barré syndrome
    - 6. Acute stress, including surgery
      - a. Psychogenic hyperventilation
      - b. Hypoglycemia
      - c. Burns
      - d. Pancreatitis
      - e. Alcohol withdrawal
      - f. Sickle cell crisis
      - g. After resuscitation
      - h. Postoperative
    - 7. Increased intravascular volume
    - 8. Alcohol and drug use
- II. Systolic hypertension
  - A. Increased cardiac output
    - 1. Aortic valvular insufficiency
    - 2. Arteriovenous fistula, patent ductus arteriosus
    - 3. Thyrotoxicosis
    - 4. Paget's disease of bone
    - 5. Beriberi
    - 6. Hyperkinetic circulation
  - B. Rigidity of aorta
- III. Iatrogenic hypertension (see Table 51-11)

SOURCE: Kaplan NM. Systemic hypertension: Mechanisms and diagnosis. In: Braunwald E, ed. *Heart Disease,* 5th ed. Philadelphia: Saunders; 1997:807.

TABLE 51-11 Drugs Known to Elevate Blood Pressure

- Nonsteroidal anti-inflammatory drugs
- Sympathomimetic amines (e.g., phenylpropanolamines)
- Estrogen and estrogen analogs (e.g., oral contraceptive pills and hormone replacement therapy)
- Methylxanthines (e.g., theophylline, caffeine, theobromine)
- Cyclosporine
- Erythropoietin
- Cocaine
- Nicotine
- Phencyclidine ("angel dust")
- "Herbal ecstasy" (and other ephedra-containing substances)
- Withdrawal from certain drugs (e.g., beta blockers, alpha agonists, opioids, ethanol, calcium antagonists)

TABLE 51-12 Routine Tests Recommended by JNC VI for the Initial Evaluation of a Hypertensive Patient

- Serum chemistry (glucose, potassium, creatinine)
- Urinalysis
- Electrocardiogram

TABLE 51-13 Keith-Wagener-Barker Classification of Optic Fundi

Grade	Characteristic Finding
I	Arterial tortuosity, localized arterial spasm or narrowing (relative to neighboring vein), "silver wiring"
II	Extensive or generalized arteriolar narrowing, resulting in arteriovenous crossing changes ("arterial nicking")
III	Hemorrhages or exudates
IV	Papilledema

normal yellowish-white color of the retinal arteries gradually changes to a reddish-brown tone ("copper wire"), and the ratio of artery/vein diameters is reduced from the normal 2:3 to less than 1:3. Over time, the column of blood within the artery gradually diminishes and the artery is reduced to a whitish thread ("silver wire") despite a persistent (albeit reduced) flow of blood. "AV nicking" is perhaps the most easily recognized ocular abnormality in hypertension. When the thickened artery containing blood at elevated pressure compresses a low-pressure, thin-walled vein within the shared adventitial sheath, the vein disappears from view. Hypertension is therefore both epidemiologically and pathophysiologically a risk factor for retinal vein occlusion, although this is not a common occurrence.[218,219] When arterial blood flow is reduced sufficiently to cause infarction of underlying retinal tissue, round to oval white patches with fluffy borders are formed ("cytoid bodies" or "cotton-wool spots"). When there is breakdown in the blood-retinal barrier (caused by a ruptured aneurysm, neovascularization—typically in diabetics—or "blowout" hemorrhages resulting from hypertension), intraretinal "flame-shaped" hemorrhages can be recognized on direct ophthalmoscopy. The leakage of plasma into the macular space often causes an acute reduction in vision and leaves behind the "macular star figure" for years thereafter. Grade IV retinopathy (papilledema), which is the hallmark of either retinal vein occlusion or a hypertensive emergency, usually is caused by ischemia in the optic nerve circulation resulting from increased intraocular or intracranial pressure and diminished axoplasmic flow in the optic nerve fibers. In some cases, particularly when BP is not exceedingly high and there is no other evidence of acute TOD from a hypertensive emergency, another cause should be sought. Papilledema without other evidence of hypertensive retinopathy generally is due to another etiology.

The impact of controlling hypertension on ophthalmic end points (e.g., vision loss, retinal hemorrhages, and laser photocoagulation procedures) has not received much attention in the general medical literature. There are nonetheless several reports of reduced risk of these end points in several clinical trials that assessed their incidence prospectively, particularly among diabetic hypertensives.[220–222]

Cardiac Evaluation

One of the most important elements of the physical examination of hypertensive patients is the cardiac examination. An atrial (S_4) gallop is an extremely common finding and may be a vital clue to the presence of hypertensive heart disease.

A key part of the laboratory evaluation is directed at determining whether LVH is present. The ECG is currently recommended by nearly all authorities as part of the initial evaluation of persons with hypertension. Not only is the ECG useful in documenting previously undetected MI, myocardial ischemia, and/or cardiac rhythm disturbances, it is the least expensive and possibly the most cost-effective way to diagnose and/or exclude LVH. Although several studies have suggested that compared with echocardiography, computed axial tomography (CAT), or magnetic resonance imaging (MRI) of the heart, the ECG is perhaps only 10 to 50 percent sensitive (depending on which criteria are used) and at best 80 percent specific, the expense of these more accurate methods of screening for LVH limits their use.[223–225] A "limited echocardiogram" that accurately calculates left ventricular (LV) size at a very affordable price and also provides information about ventricular geometry has been recommended by several authorities but has not been commonly endorsed by third-party or other payers.[226]

The prognostic significance of LVH among hypertensive patients is well established. Left ventricular hypertrophy often is thought of as the "hemoglobin A_{1c} of BP," since it is an objective measure of both the severity and the duration of elevations in BP. In the Framingham Heart Study, ECG evidence of LVH was associated with an approximately threefold increase in the incidence of CV events.[227] Echocardiographically detected LVH appears to predict an even greater incremental increase in the risk of future CV events, although the geometry of the ventricle also may play a role.[228,229] Hypertension typically is associated with concentric hypertrophy of the ventricle, perhaps as a result of concentric remodeling, which in one series carried a fourfold increased risk of cardiac morbidity and mortality (compared with nonhypertrophied hearts).[230] Eccentric hypertrophy, which is seen in response to exercise in athletes, imparted only a twofold increased risk of events in the same series.[229] In several reports from various locales, in both univariate and multivariate models, LVH was the most powerful of any of the traditional CV risk factors in predicting not only death or MI but also stroke, HF, and other CV end points.[228,229,231,232] Although research studies including thousands of people have demonstrated the importance of echocardiographically determined measurements of LV mass, there is concern that the intrinsic variability of a single echocardiogram is sufficiently high (perhaps 10 to 15 percent) that serial determinations in a usual hypertensive individual are unlikely to be cost-effective. The exception may be a person with stage 1 hypertension, in whom the presence of this form of LVH would lead to a reclassification of the patient and indicate the need for antihypertensive drug therapy earlier than it might have been given if the clinician had thought the patient was free of TOD.

LVH is associated both epidemiologically and pathophysiologically with intimal hyperplasia of the epicardial coronary arteries, increased coronary vascular resistance, increased severity and frequency of ventricular dysrhythmias, decreased flow reserve, and reduced diastolic relaxation. At the extreme, diastolic dysfunction and restrictive cardiomyopathy result clinically in "flash pulmonary edema" despite a normal ejection fraction. Although this phenomenon is not well understood, some feel that hypertension plays the major role in the pathogenesis of this syndrome, which has been identified in up to 40 percent of patients presenting to the hospital with HF.[233] The important prognostic role of LVH was demonstrated and separated from possible subclinical coronary disease in a consecutive series of 785 patients who had cardiac catheterization.[234] After

4 years of follow-up in patients with echocardiographically documented LVH, the risk of dying was increased twofold if there was coronary artery disease (CAD) but more than fourfold if CAD was not present.[234] Echocardiographically defined LVH was the most powerful risk factor for death.

The most contentious aspect of LVH is the importance of its reversal and how to achieve it. While early data from several centers indicate a better prognosis among patients with echocardiographically determined LVH whose LV mass index is reduced (typically by pharmacologic treatment of hypertension) compared with those whose index increases over time, the large therapeutic trials directed primarily at this question are still ongoing. There are major controversies, supported by separate meta-analyses with differing conclusions, about whether certain classes of antihypertensive drug therapy are more effective at quickly reducing LV mass, but these changes have not been correlated with a reduced risk of CV events in large numbers of patients.[235–237] Most studies agree that LVH is unlikely to regress without reducing BP; most authorities therefore recommend spending resources on achieving BP control rather than on serial echocardiograms to see if the LV mass index is returning toward normal.

Renal Evaluation

Current recommendations for the evaluation of renal function include just a measure of BUN and serum creatinine and a dipstick to detect heavy proteinuria. A more extensive search for microalbuminuria (MA), as defined by the presence of albumin in the urine above the normal range of less than 30 mg/day but below the detectable range with the conventional dipstick methodology, i.e., 300 mg/day, is also warranted.[238] Data from several pioneering studies done over the last two decades have demonstrated that MA is not only a predictor of diabetic complications but also a powerful independent risk factor for CV disease.[238–240] Moreover, MA predicts the development of ischemic CV events related to the development of atherosclerosis. Numerous clinical studies in persons with either type 1 or type 2 DM as well as those with renal disease have demonstrated higher CV mortality in those with MA.[239–244]

The prevalence of MA in patients with type 2 DM is about 20 percent (range, 12 to 36 percent) and affects about 30 percent of people with type 2 DM older than 55 years of age.[242–244] The prevalence of MA ranges from 5 to 40 percent among nondiabetic persons with essential hypertension.[244] The reason for this high variability in MA prevalence among those with essential hypertension relates to both the duration of BP control and associated lipid abnormalities, especially low-density lipoprotein cholesterol (LDL-C) levels.[245] A second related predictor is the duration of hypertension.[246] In this way, MA may be a marker of BP control, since BP control with all agents, except dihydropyridine CA and central or peripheral sympathetic blockers, reduces albuminuria.[247] Subsequent chronic renal failure occurs at a rate of 1 percent per annum in those with type 2 DM; the risk for those with type 1 DM approaches 75 percent after 10 years, while for those with essential hypertension, it is less than 1 percent over 5 years.[247,248]

Some studies have shown that the amount of MA present in a person is proportional to the severity of systolic, diastolic, and mean BP elevation as measured by either clinic or 24-h ambulatory BP monitoring.[249,250] This observation has been corroborated by the results of a clinical study of 211 untreated men with MA and essential hypertension.[251] This study agreed with the findings of previous investigators and showed that patients with MA had higher BP levels.[249] Another Italian population study with 1567 participants revealed an 18-mmHg higher systolic BP in the group of nondiabetic people with MA.[252] Lastly, circadian abnormalities of BP seen in nondippers (see above), who are known to be at higher risk for CV, also have a higher prevalence of MA.[253,254]

The exact pathophysiology of how MA contributes to or accelerates the atherosclerotic process is uncertain. The current understanding, however, suggests that MA is an indicator of increased vascular permeability and, hence, altered barrier function of the endothelium.[249,250,252–255] People with MA have an elevated transcapillary escape rate of albumin regardless of whether they have preexisting DM. Moreover, it has been argued that when albumin leaks into the interstitial space, cellular injury occurs secondary to free radicals and cytokine production enhanced by the presence of albumin. More recently, some authors have suggested that MA is another element of the metabolic components of syndrome X[256–258] (see above).

Simply using a conventional dipstick that can detect only higher levels of urinary protein (>300 mg/24 h) means that the clinician will miss the opportunity to characterize a patients' prognosis more precisely at the initial visit. Dipsticks that detect MA are available and inexpensive. Perhaps all hypertensives with "trace" proteinuria (generally 300 to 500 mg/day) when measured by conventional dipsticks should have a spot urine measurement of the albumin/creatinine ratio.[238] Routine assessment of MA in diabetic patients is well advised, but in hypertensives without DM, its value is still debatable. In part, this is due to the relatively low prevalence of MA in the nondiabetic population and the uncertainty of the significance of its modification in these groups.

Studies found that subjects with MA and type 2 DM have approximated total mortality of 8 percent and CV mortality of 4 percent annually. These values are up to four times higher than those of patients without MA.[258] Similar increases in CV mortality also are present in people with MA and without diabetes. In several series, the CV event rate in nondiabetic people with MA and hypertensives was twofold to fourfold higher than it was in those without MA.[259]

In several studies, people with MA had larger LV mass and higher degrees of LVH.[260–262] This has been documented by both ECG and echocardiographic criteria. However, this finding was not consistent in other populations that were relatively young (age between 18 and 45) and had stage 1 hypertension. This association of MA with LVH may be related to a higher BP load.

Evaluation of the Vasculature

One of the hallmarks of the hypertensive circulation is decreased vascular compliance. Acutely, elevated BP affects the elastic behavior of both large and small arteries such that the muscular layers of the arterial wall are unable to relax as quickly and transmit pressure waves as easily and reproducibly as they can when BP is lower. This is a passive and reversible phenomenon that typically lasts minutes to hours. Over a prolonged period, however, there is a gradual infiltration of the internal elastic lamina of blood vessels with thinned, split, and frayed elastic fibers and a laying down of new intercellular matrix; in extreme cases, medial necrosis is found within the arterial wall. This process, which is attributed to aging, hypertension, or a combination of the two, often is described as "arteriosclerosis," since it leads to chronic and generally irreversible stiffening of the arterial tree.[263]

There are several methods of assessing arterial compliance (Table 51-14), but most are invasive, expensive, or not widely used in clinical medicine.[264] Several new methods for calculating total arterial compliance are based on pulse contour analysis but have not been tested in large population-based studies to prove their value in estimating CV risk.[265,266] Blacher and associates showed in 710 subjects from the Framingham Heart Study that pulse wave velocity is higher in subjects with known atherosclerotic CV.[267] Whether this measure will be used routinely to evaluate hypertensives remains to be seen.

Pseudohypertension is the name given to the rare circumstance in which BP measurements by the usual indirect sphygmomanometry are much higher than direct intraarterial measurements; these differences usually are attributed to very "stiff" and calcified arteries that are nearly impossible to compress with the bladder in the usual BP cuff. The "Osler maneuver" (palpating the walls of the brachial artery when blood flow has been interrupted by inflating the cuff higher than systolic pressure) has been recommended as a simple measure to diagnose this condition, but several reports have found it less sensitive and specific than was reported initially, and the authors do not recommend using it.[268] Because making the diagnosis of pseudohypertension requires a potentially dangerous and expensive intraarterial measurement (and perhaps an infusion of an intravenous antihypertensive agent to "calibrate" the difference between indirect and direct BP measurements), few clinicians routinely check for and diagnose pseudohypertension.

The benefits of lowering BP in older patients with "stiff" arteries, however, are well established. Three clinical trials specifically in isolated systolic hypertension [systolic blood pressure (SBP) ≥160 mmHg with diastolic blood pressure (DBP) <90 or <95 mmHg] proved that older individuals with BP elevations only in systolic BP (a typical finding in patients with reduced vascular compliance) have a reduced risk of CV events with pharmacologic treatment.[269–271] Whether arterial compliance should be measured as a predictor of CV risk and measured serially over time is controversial; perhaps it would not be as cost-effective as serial BP determinations during treatment.

Other Evaluation

Other blood tests such as PRA and serum insulin or newly appreciated markers of CV risk such as C-reactive protein have been abandoned for routine or even specialized evaluation or have not been proved to be sensitive or specific enough to warrant inclusion in the evaluation of all hypertensive patients.[272]

Evaluation for Identifiable Causes of Hypertension

There are many identifiable causes of hypertension (secondary hypertension). In patients with some of these causes, the elevation of BP can be eliminated with specific treatment such as angioplasty or surgery therapy or by removing the agent that caused the hypertension. By far the most common identifiable cause is chronic renal failure. Although chronic renal disease almost never can be cured, the hypertension associated with it often can be controlled with adequate dialysis without the use of drugs. Renal artery stenosis, pheochromocytoma, and primary aldosteronism, however, are potentially curable. These conditions are encountered commonly enough that the clinician seeing a hypertensive patient must have a high index of suspicion in the appropriate clinical setting and should order the specialized tests necessary to screen for and confirm the diagnosis. Other etiologies, such as specific enzyme deficiencies, coarctation of the aorta, and Ask-Upmark kidney, are distinctly rare. This section will cover only the most common etiologies listed in Table 51-10. If a secondary cause of hypertension is suspected, a referral to a hypertension specialist may be appropriate.[11,19]

RENOVASCULAR HYPERTENSION

Patients with this form of secondary hypertension often have stage 3 hypertension and considerable TOD and are at risk of losing renal function. At least 90 percent of cases of renovascular hypertension now are due to renal artery atherosclerosis, with only 10 percent being due to fibromuscular dysplasia or unusual causes.[273,274] Atherosclerotic renal artery stenosis is a disease

TABLE 51-14 Methods for Determining Arterial Compliance

	Measured in	Invasive?	Drawbacks
Direct methods			
Angiography	Aorta	Yes	Expensive
Echocardiography	Aorta	No	Expensive
Echo tracking	Peripheral arteries	No	Not widely available
Intravascular ultrasound	Peripheral arteries	Yes	Expensive
Venous occlusion plethysmography	Peripheral arteries	No	Time- and operator-intensive
Indirect methods			
Stroke volume/pulse pressure ratio	Total arterial compliance	No	Reproducibility questionable
Pulse wave velocity	Segmental arteries	No	Limited to large arteries
Fourier pulse analysis	Peripheral arteries	No	Reproducibility questionable
Total compliance	Total arterial compliance	No	Expensive
Pulse contour analysis	Total arterial compliance	No	Time- and operator-intensive

TABLE 51-15 Testing for Renovascular Hypertension: Clinical Index of Suspicion as a Guide to Selecting Patients for Workup

- Low (should not be tested)
  - Stage 1 or 2 hypertension in the absence of clinical clues
- Moderate (noninvasive test recommended)
  - Stage 3 hypertension
  - Hypertension refractory to standard therapy
  - Abrupt onset of sustained stages 2–3 hypertension at age <20 years
  - Hypertension with a suggestive abdominal bruit (long, high-pitched, and localized to the region of the renal artery)
  - Stages 2–3 hypertension (diastolic BP exceeding 105 mmHg) in a smoker, a patient with evidence of occlusive vascular disease (cerebrovascular, coronary, peripheral, vascular), or a patient with unexplained but stable elevation of serum creatinine
- High (may consider proceeding directly to arteriography)
  - Stage 3 hypertension with either progressive renal insufficiency or refractoriness to aggressive treatment, particularly in a patient who has been a smoker or has other evidence of occlusive arterial disease
  - Accelerated or malignant hypertension (grade III or IV retinopathy)
  - Hypertension with recent elevation of serum creatinine, either unexplained or reversibly induced by an angiotensin-converting enzyme inhibitor
  - Moderate to severe hypertension with incidentally detected ansymmetry of renal size

SOURCE: Modified from Mann SL, Pickering TG. Detection of renovascular hypertension: State of the art: 1992. *Ann Intern Med* 1992; 117:845.

of older individuals. Characteristically, these patients develop hypertension after age 50 or have a history of hypertension that had been relatively easy to control and became refractory. A large proportion of these patients have evidence of vascular disease elsewhere (carotids, coronaries, and peripheral circulation, in particular), and the majority are cigarette smokers, often heavy smokers.[275] Although it is more common in whites, blacks also can develop atherosclerotic renovascular hypertension.[276,277] Fibromuscular dysplasia tends to affect young white women in whom BP tends to rise abruptly to stage 3 during the third decade of life. Abdominal or frank bruits are heard commonly, and renal function is usually normal when the diagnosis is entertained.

Laboratory Testing The objective of laboratory testing in patients suspected of having renovascular hypertension is not only to verify that arterial lesions are present but also to determine that the lesion that is discovered is in fact the cause of the patient's hypertension.[273] The clinical situations in which renovascular disease should be suspected are listed in Table 51-15.

The tests used to confirm the clinical suspicion that a patient has renovascular hypertension are biochemical or depend on a variety of imaging techniques (Table 51-16).

Biochemical Measurement of serum K^+ (which, if low, may indicate hyperaldosteronism) or PRA (which, if high, may confirm activation of the RAA system) plays no role in the further case finding for renovascular hypertension because the sensitivity and specificity are too low.[278] Even measuring the PRA after captopril (the so-called captopril test) has a sensitivity of only 60 to 70 percent, although better results have been obtained in some series.[278] Measuring the concentration and activity of renin simultaneously from each renal vein and computing the renal vein renin ratio was a very popular approach at one time, but the sensitivity and specificity for detection of renovascular hypertension with this test are both approximately 75 percent, unacceptably low for an invasive procedure that requires special expertise and sophisticated measurements.[278] This ratio may still be useful to help prove that an anatomic lesion is also the cause of a patient's hypertension but should not be used as a screening tool.

Imaging Rapid-sequence intravenous pyelography and standard renal scanning were the earliest noninvasive imaging studies used for diagnosing renovascular hypertension.[278] Even though in expert hands each has reasonable sensitivity (65 to 70 percent for scanning and 75 percent for pyelography), neither has a place in the diagnostic approach any longer. Renal duplex ultrasound has the advantage of being noninvasive and widely available. In some laboratories, the sensitivity of this test approaches 90 to 95 percent.[279] However, the presence of abdominal gas or fat may make it difficult to visualize the renal arteries, and the test is very operator-dependent. In specialized centers with special expertise and in selected patients, it may be a useful test. In most settings, however, little is gained by using this technique. Magnetic resonance angiography with gadolinium is a new approach to visualization of the renal arteries that is becoming widely available and is noninvasive.[280] However, until the quality of the images improves and the cost becomes lower, this technique is not likely to replace angiography when visualization of the renal arteries is felt to be necessary.

The two imaging modalities currently favored are isotopic renography with labeled dethylenetriamine pentaacetic acid (DTPA) (a measure of glomerular filtration) of MAG-3 (a

TABLE 51-16 Detection of Renovascular Hypertension

- Biochemical
  - Serum K^+
  - PRA
  - Renal vein renin activity
  - Split renal function tests
- Imaging
  - Rapid-sequence intravenous pyelography
  - Renography
  - Captopril or enalaprilat renography
  - Intraarterial digital substraction angiography
  - Standard angiography
  - Duplex renal ultrasound
  - Magnetic resonance angiography

measure of renal blood flow) with captopril and intraarterial digital subtraction angiography.[273] Isotopic renography with captopril is a minimally invasive test that detects a discrepancy between perfusion and function of the kidneys. The overall sensitivity and specificity are 90 percent when done carefully, especially in patients whose prior probability of having renovascular hypertension is judged to be high.[273,278] Only ACE-Is and ARBs need to be stopped before the test is performed, and adverse reactions from the single dose of captopril are rare. Isotopic renography with captopril also provides functional information. If the time to peak activity is initially normal and becomes abnormal after captopril ("captopril-induced changes"), the likelihood of cure or improvement after revascularization is high.[273]

Intraarterial digital subtraction angiography has become the invasive procedure of choice to demonstrate definitively the renal artery anatomy and determine whether an arterial lesion is present. Although an arterial puncture is required, the needle used is small and the dye load is modest. In addition, the type of lesion (ostial, nonostial, or branch) can be determined. In some centers, percutaneous renal angioplasty is done at the same time if it is felt to be indicated. The authors are not in favor of doing revascularization unless evidence has been obtained (a positive captopril renogram with captopril-induced changes or a renal vein renin ratio >1.5) that the lesion is functionally significant. The presence of anatomic renal artery stenosis does not mean that the lesion is responsible for the elevation in BP (functional renal artery stenosis).[273]

When considering whether to proceed with these studies, the clinician must consider how the data will be used. In a number of hypertensive patients with renovascular hypertension, BP is controlled adequately with medical therapy. If the risk of surgery or angioplasty is viewed as unacceptably high or if the patient will not consent to having a revascularization procedure if a remediable lesion is discovered, any specific further evaluation may not be appropriate.

PHEOCHROMOCYTOMA

Patients with pheochromocytoma are almost always symptomatic on presentation.[281] These patients usually have a characteristic cluster of complaints that occur in paroxysms or "spells." The description of the spell tends to be typical and is usually the same in each patient. The spells may occur many times a day or may be separated by weeks or months.[282] Often there is a characteristic trigger (change in position, certain foods, trauma, pain, or drugs) that if present should greatly increase the clinician's index of suspicion of pheochromocytoma. Hypertension is not usually paroxysmal, as has often been stated, with some BP readings elevated and some normal. Most measurements are in fact in the hypertensive range, although wide variability is the rule. The three most common symptoms of pheochromocytoma are headache, diaphoresis, and palpitations[282] (Table 51-17). Many other symptoms, particularly anxiety, weakness, and tremulousness, are also quite common. The pattern of symptoms can provide guidance about the predominant hormone secreted by the tumor. When norepinephrine is the primary hormone produced, pallor is usually the symptom. Flushing is more likely if substantial amounts of epinephrine are produced.

TABLE 51-17 Symptoms and Signs of Pheochromocytoma

Symptoms[a]	Frequency, %
Headaches	40–96
Diaphoresis	40–74
Palpitations	45–70
Pallor	40–45
Nervousness and/or anxiety	22–43
Tremulousness	29–31
Signs[b]	**Frequency, %**
Hypertension	>90
Sustained	50–60
Intermittent	2–50
Paroxysms	50
Weight loss (hypermetabolic state)	80
Funduscopic changes	50–70
Orthostatic hypotension	40–70

[a]Infrequent symptoms: flushing, Raynaud's phenomenon, nausea, seizures, dizziness, dyspnea, and abdominal, chest, or arm pain.
[b]Infrequent signs: acrocyanosis, bradycardia, fever, and glucose intolerance.

Laboratory Testing for Pheochromocytoma Whereas it is possible and sometimes desirable to manage hypertensive patients with renovascular hypertension or mineralocorticoid-excess states with medical therapy, it is almost always imperative to remove a pheochromocytoma. As with renovascular hypertension, once the clinical presentation suggests that a pheochromocytoma may be the cause of a patient's hypertension, a variety of tests are available to confirm the diagnosis (Table 51-18). If a pheochromocytoma is suspected, the next step is to obtain biochemical confirmation of an increase in catecholamine production. The authors prefer to measure 24-h urinary excretion of total catecholamines (norepinephrine, epinephrine, or dopamine) or their metabolites (vanillylmandelic acid or metanephrine).[282] In some laboratories, 24-h urinary metanephrines are the most sensitive and specific in the diagnosis (both approximately 85 percent and 90 percent), but when done precisely, there is little to choose in regard to which should be measured. When the two or three of these compounds are quantitated and several samples are analyzed, both the sensitivity and the

TABLE 51-18 Diagnostic Tests for Pheochromocytoma

Biochemical
Urinary free catecholamines
Urinary vanilylmandelic acid
Urinary metanephrines
Plasma catecholamines (or metanephrines)
Clonidine suppression test
Imaging studies
Computed axial tomography
Magnetic resonance imaging
^{131}I-meta-iodobenzylguanidine
Abdominal ultrasound
Adrenal vein or vena caval drainage
Angiography

specificity of the tests improve. Attention must be paid to the conditions under which the sample is collected, and urinary creatinine also should be measured to verify that the collection represents the 24-h excretion. To reduce the number of false-positive results, the patient should be in a nonstressful situation when the sample is obtained.

In the authors' view, only when the urinary assays are borderline can the measurement of plasma catecholamines be useful. If plasma catecholamines (norepinephrine plus epinephrine) levels exceed 2000 pg/mL in the basal state, the presence of a pheochromocytoma is highly likely. If the levels are less than 1000 pg/mL, the diagnosis is very unlikely, whereas in patients with plasma catecholamine levels between 1000 and 2000 pg/mL, the clonidine suppression test may be useful.[283] If plasma catecholamine levels do not suppress after the administration of 0.3 mg of oral clonidine in an appropriately prepared and monitored patient, a further aggressive search for a pheochromocytoma is warranted.

The choice of which initial imaging procedure to obtain is also somewhat controversial. CT scanning is a highly sensitive imaging modality that will locate nearly all pheochromocytomas, especially those in the adrenal gland or the abdomen. MRI has the advantage of not requiring contrast material (which is sometimes necessary with CT scanning) and is also helpful in localizing nonadrenal or nonabdominal pheochromocytomas. Enhancement of the T2-weighted images happens virtually only with pheochromocytomas and adrenal carcinomas, helping distinguish adrenal masses that are not biochemically active (so-called incidentalomas) from metabolically active or malignant tumors.

The use of I-meta-iodobenzylguanidine scanning has been particularly helpful when a pheochromocytoma is suspected but is not clearly located with CT or MRI. This radiopharmaceutical is a guanethidine analog that is concentrated in pheochromocytomas and other neural crest tumors.[284] Using total-body scanning helps localize the tumor if the initial CT or MRI scans are negative or equivocal. The sensitivity of this test exceeds 90 percent, but it is not uniformly available.

PRIMARY ALDOSTERONISM

In a hypertensive patient receiving no treatment who demonstrates significant hypokalemia (serum K^+ ≤3.2 meq/L) with renal K^+ wasting (24-h urinary K^+ >30 meq), PRA below 1 ng/mL, and elevated plasma or urinary aldosterone values, the diagnosis is unequivocal. Often, however, the diagnosis is not obvious because the values are not as definitive; in such cases, multiple measurements are needed during salt loading.

The single best test in people with normal renal function for identifying patients with primary aldosteronism is the measurement of 24-h urinary aldosterone excretion during salt loading[285,286] (Table 51-19). An excretion rate of >14 μg of aldosterone in 24 h after 3 days of salt loading (greater than 200 meq/day) distinguishes most patients with primary aldosteronism from those with essential hypertension. Only 7 percent of patients with primary aldosteronism have values that fall within the range for essential hypertension. In contrast, a substantial number (about 39 percent) of patients with primary aldosteronism have plasma aldosterone values that fall within the range for essential hypertension.[287] The findings of hypokalemia and suppressed PRA provide corroborative evidence, but the absence of either or both does not preclude the diagnosis.

TABLE 51-19 Diagnostic Studies for Mineralocorticoid Excess States

Biochemical
Serum potassium
Plasma renin activity
Plasma aldosterone
Plasma aldosterone/renin ratio
24-h urinary aldosterone excretion
Plasma 18-hydroxycorticosterone
Plasma 18-oxocortisol
Plasma 18-hydroxycortisol
Adrenal vein sampling for aldosterone
Imaging studies
Abdominal ultrasound
Computed axial tomography
Iodocholesterol scanning
Adrenal venography

A substantial number of patients with primary aldosteronism, however, do not present with hypokalemia; serum K^+ concentration is normal in 7 to 38 percent of reported cases.[288,289] In addition, 10 to 12 percent of patients with proven tumors may not have hypokalemia during short-term salt loading. Plasma renin activity <1 ng/mL per hour or one that fails to rise above 2 ng/mL per hour after salt and water depletion and upright posture has been used as an additional test to exclude primary aldosteronism.[288] However, a significant number (about 35 percent) of patients with the disease have values that rise >2 ng/mL per hour when appropriately stimulated.[286] In addition, about 40 percent of subjects with essential hypertension have suppressed PRA, and 15 to 20 percent of these patients have values <2 ng/mL per hour under conditions of stimulation.

The plasma aldosterone/renin ratio has been used to define the appropriateness of PRA for the circulating concentrations of aldosterone.[286] It is assumed that the volume expansion associated with excessive aldosterone production inhibits the synthesis of renin without affecting the autonomous production of aldosterone. Both tests are subject to the same limitations: First, there is inherent variability of plasma levels of aldosterone even in the presence of a tumor, and this translates into variability in the absolute value of the ratio; second, the use of drugs that result in marked and prolonged stimulation of renin long after their discontinuation may alter the ratio.

The most common cause of primary aldosteronism is an aldosterone-producing adenoma (70 to 80 percent of all proven cases). Approximately 20 to 30 percent of cases are caused by hyperplasia of the zona glomerulosa layer of the adrenal cortex (bilateral adrenal hyperplasia). Some reports suggest the occurrence of a syndrome intermediate between adenoma and hyperplasia.[288] The distinction between these two processes is important because surgical intervention is likely to be curative in the majority of adenomas and fails to reduce BP in patients with bilateral adrenal hyperplasia.

An adenoma is likely in the presence of spontaneous hypokalemia <3.0 meq/L, plasma 18-hydroxycorticosterone values >100 ng/dL, and an anomalous postural decrease in plasma aldosterone concentration.[289,290] In addition, adenomas are largely unresponsive to changes in sodium balance and appear to be exquisitely sensitive to ACTH, unlike hyperplasias, which are more sensitive to angiotensin II infusions.[290] Plasma 18-hydroxycorticosterone values <100 ng/dL, a postural increase in aldosterone, or both, are findings usually associated with hyperplasia, but they do not completely rule out the presence of an adenoma.[291]

An adrenal CT scan should be considered the initial step in tumor localization. It is noninvasive, and all adenomas ≥1.5 cm in diameter can be located accurately. Only 60 percent of nodules measuring between 1 and 1.4 cm in diameter are detected by CT scanning. Nodules <1 cm in diameter are very difficult, if not impossible, to demonstrate. The overall sensitivity of localizing adenomas by high-resolution CT scanning exceeds 90 percent.[292] Adrenal venous aldosterone levels should be measured when the biochemical findings are highly suggestive of an adenoma, but the adrenal CT scan is ambiguous.[293]

Medical therapy is indicated in patients with adrenal hyperplasia, patients with adenoma who are poor surgical risks, and patients with bilateral adrenal adenomas that may require bilateral adrenalectomy. Total bilateral adrenalectomy has no place in the management of primary aldosteronism.

The long-standing experience has been that the hypertension associated with primary aldosteronism is salt- and water-dependent and is best treated with sustained salt and water depletion.[294] The usual doses of diuretic agents are hydrochlorothiazide 25 to 50 mg/day or furosemide 80 to 160 mg/day in combination with either spironolactone 100 to 200 mg/day or amiloride 10 to 20 mg/day. These combinations usually result in prompt correction of hypokalemia and normalization of BP within 2 to 4 weeks.

In the majority of these patients, surgical excision of an aldosterone-producing adenoma leads to normotension as well as reversal of the biochemical defects. One year postoperatively, about 70 percent of patients are normotensive, but 5 years postoperatively, only 53 percent remain normotensive. The restoration of normal K^+ homeostasis is permanent. Patients undergoing surgery should receive drug treatment for a least 8 to 10 weeks both to decrease BP and to correct metabolic abnormalities. These patients have a significant K^+ deficiency that must be corrected preoperatively because hypokalemia increases the risk of cardiac arrhythmias during anesthesia.

After the removal of an aldosterone-producing adenoma, selective hypoaldosteronism usually occurs even in patients whose PRA had been stimulated with chronic diuretic therapy. Potassium supplementation therefore should be given cautiously, and serum K^+ values should be monitored closely. Sufficient residual mineralocorticoid activity often is left to prevent excessive renal retention of K^+ provided that Na^+ intake is adequate. Abnormalities in aldosterone production can persist for as long as 3 months after tumor removal.

OTHER FORMS OF IDENTIFIABLE SECONDARY HYPERTENSION

In addition to these three most common and potentially curable forms of identifiable secondary hypertension, there are a vast number of rare conditions in which the cause of the hypertension cannot be found (Table 51-10). These include enzyme deficiencies such as 17-β-hydroxylase deficiency and 17-α-hydroxylase deficiency, other congenital disorders such as the Ask-Upmark kidney, trauma such as the Page kidney, urologic causes such as hydronephrosis, endocrine abnormalities such as Cushing's syndrome and Cushing's disease, and even infectious etiologies such as renal tuberculosis.[274] Although the practicing clinician may never encounter a patient with any of these disorders, it is incumbent on him or her to know that these unusual conditions may present with hypertension and that the elevated BP may be the first clue to the diagnosis. Two causes of identifiable hypertension are not rare, and all clinicians will see patients with iatrogenic hypertension and those with sleep apnea (Table 51-11). Any of the drugs or other substances listed in the table should be stopped before one concludes that a patient has hypertension. The relation of sleep apnea to hypertension and obesity has long been recognized.[295,296] The typical clinical presentation of sleep apnea (daytime drowsiness, snoring) in an obese hypertensive should alert the clinician to this disorder.

TREATMENT OF HYPERTENSION

Patients with JNC VI stage 2 or 3 hypertension (SBP ≥160 mmHg or DBP ≥100 mmHg) and those in risk group C (those with DM and those with clinical CV) should receive drug therapy once their hypertension has been diagnosed and confirmed.[11] Furthermore, the length of time the clinician should rely on lifestyle modifications before starting drug therapy has been clarified in JNC VI and is based on risk estimates, not just on the level of BP (Table 51-3). Those with stage 1 hypertension (SBP 140 to 159 mmHg and/or DBP 90 to 99 mmHg) who have no other risk factors or end-organ damage (so-called risk group A) can be treated only with lifestyle modification for up to 1 year even if goal BP is not reached before drug therapy should be considered necessary. Since male sex and age over 60 years are considered risk factors, only women under 60 years of age are in group A.

Patients with stage 1 hypertension who are in risk group B (other CV risk factors but no TOD or DM) should receive pharmacologic therapy after only a 6-month trial of lifestyle modification unless goal BP is achieved without drugs. Those in risk group C [TOD, clinical cardiovascular disease (CVD), and/or DM) should be treated with pharmacologic agents and lifestyle modification even if they have high-normal BP (SBP 130 to 139 mmHg and/or DBP 85 to 89 mmHg).

Lifestyle Modification

The JNC VI recommended weight loss for obese hypertensive patients, modification of dietary Na^+ intake to ≤100 mmol/day, and modification of alcohol intake to no more than two drinks per day.[11] It also recommended an increase in physical activity for all patients with hypertension who have no specific condition that would make such a recommendation not applicable or safe. However, for many of the authors' patients these suggestions are not practicable or already are being implemented. For such patients, drug therapy may be indicated even sooner in group A and group B hypertensive patients.

There is little doubt that lifestyle factors such as diet, exercise, and stress can affect BP. There is a strong positive correlation between the level of body weight and body mass index (weight/height) and the level of BP.[297] The relationship of dietary Na^+ and BP is equally clear, especially at low and modest intakes of Na^+ and in those deemed to be salt-sensitive. Other nutrients, such as K^+, the omega-3 fatty acids present in fish oil, and possibly Ca^{2+} and Mg^{2+}, are inversely related to BP level. Sedentary individuals who do little, if any, aerobic exercise usually have higher BPs than do appropriately matched controls even when one controls for other confounding variables.[298] The relationship of stress to BP is somewhat less clear. Physical or mental stress will raise BP temporarily, but the relationship of chronic anxiety and stress has been more difficult to demonstrate.

The appreciation of these relationships has naturally led to numerous attempts to lower BP by modifying lifestyle (Table 51-20). The most important trial that evaluated the benefits of lifestyle modification, including weight loss, was the Trial of Hypertension Prevention (TOHP-1).[299] This study was large ($n = 2182$) and randomized and compared the benefits of weight loss, Na^+ reduction, or stress reduction to usual care and also compared K^+ supplements at 60 meq/day or Ca^{2+} at 1.0 g/day or Mg^{2+} at 15 mmol/day or fish oil at 3.0 g of omega-3 fatty acid to placebos. The weight loss, Na^+ reduction, and stress management were given to 308, 327, and 240 participants, respectively, for 18 months. The group assigned to supplementation (Mg^{2+}, Ca^{2+}, or placebo) then was rerandomized to fish oil, K^+, or placebo. In addition, 589 participants received usual care, giving this trial the ability to judge the efficacy of these treatments more objectively than any prior studies could. The nutritional treatments were delivered by trained nutritionists using group and individual sessions to maximize the adherence to the regimen and presumably its efficacy. The long period of treatment and observation in TOHP-1 also provided important information about the "natural history" of the efficacy of these therapies. TOHP-1 showed that weight loss was the most effective lifestyle modification, reducing BP by 2.9/2.3 mmHg in association with an average weight loss of 3.9 kg. Sodium reduction was the only other therapeutic modality that reduced BP a significant amount (1.7/0.9 mmHg) with a reduction of 44 meq/day of Na^+. All the other arms of the study (K^+, Ca^{2+}, Mg^{2+}, fish oil supplements, and stress management) failed to demonstrate any reduction in BP compared with placebo or usual care. Whereas there were physiologic markers that indicated that the nutritional approaches and weight loss did at least partially achieve their objectives, the stress management techniques used were not effective. Perhaps successful stress management might lower BP.

TOMHS also evaluated the long-term benefit of lifestyle modification.[300] This study compared five classes of antihypertensives (diuretics, CAs, ACE-Is, alpha blockers, and beta blockers) to placebo in middle-aged subjects with minimal elevations of BP (average BP of 140/91 mmHg when the study started) and superimposed these pharmacologic treatments on a comprehensive lifestyle regimen that included weight loss, Na^+ restriction, alcohol reduction, and exercise. A subgroup of the cohort got lifestyle modification with placebo. In TOMHS, the nutritional advice and the exercise program were presented to the participants and monitored by certified nutritionists and trained exercise physiologists. The subjects were seen frequently in group and individual sessions. The group given placebo reduced BP from 140/91 to 132/82 mmHg (a reduction of 9.1/8.6 mmHg) and sustained that level for the 4.4 years of study follow-up, even though the reduction of the Na^+ intake, amount of weight loss, and the increase in exercise did not reach study goals. Perhaps the most important finding in TOMHS was the statistically significantly fewer number of CV events ($p < .03$), in the group given

TABLE 51-20 Lifestyle Modifications That Lower Blood Pressure

PRIMARY LIFESTYLE MODIFICATIONS

1. Reduction of body weight (5-kg threshold; 10 kg reduces BP ~10/8 mmHg)
2. Reduction in dietary salt consumption (target 100 mmol/day; can lower BP ~12/10 mmHg, but individual responses vary)
3. Increase physical activity to 30–45 min, four times a week (can lower BP 8/4 mmHg and often helps control weight)
4. Increased consumption of fruits and vegetables (at least 4 servings/day; can lower BP ~6/3 mmHg and often helps reduce salt consumption)
5. Moderation of alcohol consumption (target 10–20 g ethanol for women, 20–30 g for men; can lower BP up to 8/4 mmHg in those who have more than 5 drinks/day)
6. Stress management (randomized clinical trials outside the workplace have been unconvincing, but many psychologists still recommend the approach despite a lack of detailed protocols that uniformly lower BP)

OTHER LIFESTYLE MODIFICATIONS THAT ARE ROUTINELY RECOMMENDED

1. Tobacco avoidance (lowers cardiovascular risk independently of any effect on BP)
2. Fish consumption (improves lipid profiles and cardiovascular risk more than expected if BP effect alone is operative)
3. Increasing dietary fiber (improves lipid profiles and cancer risk independently of effect on BP)

LIFESTYLE MODIFICATIONS THAT ARE NOT ROUTINELY RECOMMENDED

1. Biofeedback
2. Dietary calcium supplementation
3. Dietary magnesium supplementation
4. Micronutrient supplements

SOURCE: Whelton PK, Appel LJ, Espeland MA, et al., for the TONE Collaborative Research Group. Sodium restriction and weight loss in the treatment of hypertension in older persons: A randomized controlled trial of nonpharmacologic interventions in the Elderly (TONE). *JAMA* 1998; 279:839–846. Appel LJ, Moore TJ, Obarzanek E, et al. A clinical trial of the effects of dietary patterns on blood pressure. *N Engl J Med* 1997; 336:1117–1124. Bao DG, Mori TA, Burke V, et al. Effects of dietary fish and weight reduction on ambulatory blood pressure in overweight hypertensives. *Hypertension* 1998; 32:710–717. Arakawa K. Antihypertensive mechanism of exercise. *J Hypertens* 1993; 11:223–229. Beilin LJ. Stress, coping, lifestyle and hypertension: A paradigm for research, prevention and non-pharmacological management of hypertension. *Clin Exp Hypertens* 1997; 19:739–752.

pharmacologic treatment plus lifestyle modification. These patients achieved an average BP of 125/79 mmHg, a reduction of 16/12 mmHg. Even though the lifestyle modification was successful and sustained, the group given drugs had statistically significantly fewer CV events ($p < .03$), probably because their BP was lower.

The inevitable conclusion from this trial is that even successful lifestyle modification that brings BP to the current goals does not reduce morbidity and probably mortality as well as does the combination of drugs and lifestyle adjustments that brings BP down even further. The fact that the value of BP reduction in preventing CV complications with pharmacologic agents could be demonstrated in a group at such low risk calls into question the current emphasis on delaying treatment with drugs even in low-risk individuals while the patient and provider try to get BP to goal without them. In a subsequent paper, Grimm and colleagues also showed that quality of life, as assessed by a very extensive questionnaire delivered on multiple occasions during TOMHS, showed that subjects felt best in all the ways studied when their BP was lowest.[50] This result was seen whether they were on active pharmacologic treatment with lifestyle modification or on lifestyle modification alone. These data lead the authors to believe that physicians should strive to get the maximum BP reduction that can be achieved safely and do so by combining treatments and not restrict their approach to one modality or the other.

More recent studies have combined the two most successful lifestyle modifications (weight loss and Na^+ restriction) in prospective, randomized, and well-controlled long-term trials. The Trials of Hypertension Prevention-2 (TOHP-2) studied the value of weight loss and Na^+ restriction in a 2×2 factorial design against usual care.[301] The group assigned to both Na^+ reduction and weight loss did the best at 6 months [BP fell 4.0/2.8 mmHg (usual care subtracted)], while those receiving a single modality did not experience as much of a BP reduction (3.7/2.7 mmHg for the weight loss only group, 2.9/1.6 mmHg for the Na^+ reduction only group, also usual care subtracted). The disturbing finding here was that most of this reduction was gone by the 3-year follow-up, with the combined treatment having reduced BP by only 1.1/0.6 mmHg at that time. This finding highlights another difficulty with lifestyle modification: the high recidivism rate seen in virtually all long-term studies. While adherence to a drug regimen is notoriously poor, adherence to lifestyle modification is, if anything, even worse. As in TOHP-1, the regimen was delivered by highly trained nutritionists in group and individual sessions and is consequently not an inexpensive way to reduce BP.

The second long-term, randomized, and well-controlled study directly assessing the value of lifestyle modification was the Trial of Nonpharmacologic Interventions in the Elderly (TONE).[302] This study also evaluated the efficacy of weight loss and Na^+ reduction, but in a different population and with a somewhat different objective. Only hypertensives 60 to 80 years of age were enrolled, and all already were on single-drug pharmacologic treatment. The objective of TONE was to see whether the imposition of a formal lifestyle approach, again taught by highly trained professionals, would allow hypertensives to go off their medications. The results were equally disappointing. After 30 months, when the study ended, 44 percent of the actively treated subjects were able to stay off antihypertensives (they did not have a CV event or have BP rise to levels that were considered too high not to be given drugs: >150/90 mmHg) compared with 38 percent of those not getting active lifestyle modification. While this was statistically significant ($p < .001$), it means that 56 percent of successfully treated hypertensives needed to resume drug therapy even when given the best possible lifestyle regimen available administered by experts.

The value of alcohol reduction also has been addressed by a recently published clinical trial (PATHSI).[303] This study took 641 patients at seven Department of Veterans Affairs clinics who were actively employed and completely functional but had at least six alcoholic drinks per day. The subjects reduced their alcohol intake nearly 20 percent once they entered into the study and before their randomization to intensive counseling or usual care was done. Those in the intensive counseling group were seen frequently and were able to reduce their average alcohol consumption to 2.0 drinks per day, which was significantly better than the usual care group (3.3 drinks per day). In spite of this, BP and events were not different at the end of this 2-year trial.

Appel and associates showed in the Dietary Approaches to Stop Hypertension (DASH) trial that a diet rich in fruit and vegetables lowered BP by 2.8/1.1 mmHg more than did the control diet.[304] The fruit and vegetable diet was designed to contain K^+ and Mg^{2+} at the 75th percentile of the usual American diet, while the control diet was at the 25th percentile. A "combination" diet that also contained foods rich in Ca^{2+} and was lower in total and saturated fat content lowered BP by 5.5/3.0 mmHg more than did the control diet. In the hypertensive subjects in DASH ($n = 133$ of 459), the BP reduction was impressive (11.4/5.5 mmHg). Although this study was short (only 8 weeks) and may not be generalizable to the population since it was carried out in four centers with special expertise, this approach offers great promise for using nutritional management to prevent hypertension in individuals with high-normal BP. The DASH diet provides high amounts of K^+, Mg^{2+}, and Ca^{2+} in the food eaten, not as supplements, and also limits the dietary fat and saturated fat intake in a diet only modestly low in Na^+ (3000 mg/24 h). Further studies done over longer periods in a less highly selected cohort will be needed to verify these results and determine whether the DASH diet will be a valuable therapeutic tool for the general population.

While treatment modalities such as K^+, Ca^{2+}, and/or Mg^{2+} supplements, fish oil, and garlic have advocates, careful and objective assessment of the data leads one to the conclusion that lifestyle modification should be primarily adjunctive to drug therapy in hypertensives, especially now that so many well-tolerated agents have been developed and it has been proved that lowering BP with drugs reduces morbidity and mortality.[305-309] No study of lifestyle modification in hypertensives has demonstrated that life is prolonged or CV events prevented.

The recommendations for lifestyle modification from JNC VI and other guideline committees also include smoking cessation.[11] The reason for the inclusion of this recommendation was to improve CV health rather than because of a proven direct relationship between smoking and hypertension. A direct relationship between smoking and BP, in fact, had not been demonstrated in epidemiologic studies, and often the opposite (BP lower in smokers) was observed.[310] It is now clear, however, that cigarette smoking increases BP and HR transiently (for about 15 min) and that the rise in both is gone by 30 min. The mechanism is the increase in catecholamine secretion induced by smoking. Since the authors recommend that office readings be taken no sooner than 30 min after smoking and caffeine ingestion (another substance that transiently raises BP), one may well miss the elevation of BP caused by smoking if it is measured when the patient has not smoked. Indeed, ABPM studies have shown that smokers have significantly higher BP on days when they smoke compared with days when they do not.[311] The recommendation not to smoke is clearly appropriate, and it is worthwhile not only because of enhanced CV health but also because smoking induces a rise in BP.

The lack of proof of efficacy or effectiveness when using lifestyle modification to treat or even prevent hypertension does not mean that physicians should abandon their efforts to encourage patients to lose weight; restrict their Na^+ intake; eat generous amounts of K^+, Mg^{2+}, Ca^{2+}, and fish; exercise regularly; drink only moderately if they wish to; stop smoking; and reduce stress. What one needs to realize is that the most important thing is to lower BP, perhaps to the lowest tolerable level, and to do so safely and without excessive personal or societal cost. The tension between advocates of lifestyle modification and those who consider it at best no more than an adjunct is not useful. The recommendations for modifying lifestyle are still very appropriate for the general population. If adopted, they will prevent or delay the virtually inevitable rise in BP that occurs with age and many hypertensives will be able to reduce BP further than might be achieved with drugs alone. Lifestyle modification is the primary public heath approach to trying to reduce the prevalence of hypertension and the average BP in the society. If successful, such modification is likely to save more lives and prevent more MIs, strokes, and episodes of HF than can be prevented by using drugs in those who are already hypertensive.

PHARMACOLOGIC THERAPY

The primary goal of BP reduction is to achieve the recommended goal BP by using the least intrusive means possible.[11] *Intrusive* has several interpretations: economic, office visits, adverse effects, and convenience. The choice of the drug with which to begin therapy is probably the most important decision the clinician must make when treating hypertensive patients. Approximately half the patients physicians treat will respond to the first choice and can tolerate most rational options. If physicians choose wisely, the first choice will be successful in getting BP to goal, and that will be the drug on which the patient remains for what is usually an indefinite period of therapy. Since the remainder will need additional treatment, the choice of the first drug must be done with an eye toward what can be added to achieve that goal.

Classification of Antihypertensive Agents

Antihypertensive agents can be classified in a number of ways. Some are effective parentally and are indicated only for a hypertensive crisis, and others (the overwhelming majority) are used orally for chronic therapy. Antihypertensive agents are further classified by pharmacologic class and alleged primary mechanism of action (Table 51-21). There are more than 80 effective antihypertensive drugs and 40 fixed-dose combinations from which to choose. This provides physicians with many options but can make the choice seem more perplexing than it should be. All the drugs that are available lower BP safely and, in appropriate doses, essentially to the same degree. Some classes are more likely than others to reduce BP to goal with monotherapy and with acceptable tolerability. Those agents are appropriate choices for initial treatment.

Surrogate versus Clinical End Points

Physicians are no longer willing simply to look at the degree of BP reduction when making a choice of antihypertensive therapy. Clinical end points are the events that physicians are trying to prevent in treating hypertension. So-called surrogate (or intermediate) end points are factors that may contribute to clinical end points and can be affected favorably or unfavorably by treatment. Blood pressure reduction is a surrogate or intermediate end point, since the reason for treating hypertension is to reduce the morbidity and mortality associated with elevated BP, not simply to lower BP. Physicians now expect and demand proof that the selection made will prevent hypertension-related clinical end points. Data from large and prospective clinical trials that are designed to evaluate the ability of a drug to reduce hypertension-related CV events as well as or better than an otherwise reasonably alternative drug are the reliable means to use in choosing from among the otherwise bewildering number of options.

Before 1997, only diuretics and beta blockers had been shown to reduce the morbidity and mortality in clinical trials in hypertension. Dihydropyridine (DHP), CAs, and ACE-Is were added to the list after the Syst-EUR trial was completed.[270] This trial used the DHP CA nitrendipine, followed by enalapril and hydrochlorothiazide, if needed, to get BP to goal. It was only in 1999, when the Captopril Prevention Project (CAPPP) was published, that the ability of an ACE-I to reduce morbidity and mortality in a trial that enrolled subjects because they were hypertensive was demonstrated.[312] That project showed that a regimen starting with the ACE-I captopril achieved the same overall benefit in reducing morbidity and mortality as did one that began with diuretics or beta blockers (so-called conventional therapy).[312] Certain interesting findings need further study. For example, the group randomized to conventional therapy had statistically significantly fewer strokes, and the group given the ACE-I had a lower incidence of new DM and better outcomes in those with known type 2 DM. A more recent active comparison study, the second Swedish Trial of Hypertension in Older Persons (STOP-2), again confirmed that both ACE-Is and DHP CA reduce morbidity and mortality as well as but clearly not better than do diuretics and beta blockers.[313] In STOP-2, conventional treatment was not better than newer agents at preventing strokes, and the ACE-I group did not have less incident DM. This trial failed to confirm the intriguing findings from CAPPP.

Numerous studies have shown the value of ACE-Is in saving the lives of patients with HF, in those with an MI, and in those with type 1 DM with nephropathy and proteinuria.[314–317] Many of the subjects in these trials had hypertension but were enrolled in the studies because they had these other conditions, and so one needs to be cautious about whether these data can be extrapolated to hypertensives who do not have these complications. A major new trial, the Heart Outcome Prevention Evaluation (HOPE) trial, was published in 2000.[318] This trial demonstrated that treatment with the ACE-I ramapril significantly reduced CV events compared with placebo in participants with multiple CV risk factors who had an average BP of 138/78 mmHg.[318] However, HOPE did not have an active comparator, and the group on ramapril did have a modestly lower BP (3/2 mmHg). Although the investigators claimed that this small difference in BP could not explain most of the benefit of ramapril, it is still possible that it was the reduction in BP rather than the ACE-I that was responsible for the dramatic reduction in events.

In the next few years, approximately 30 more events trials will be completed.[319] Table 51-22 lists some of the more important trials in progress. When some or all of these trials are published, it should be known with some degree of certainty whether lowering BP is all that matters or whether a particular drug or class of drugs should be selected because it or they prevent hypertension-related events more effectively. The largest of these trials (42,448 subjects), the Antihypertensive and Lipid Lowering Trial to Prevent Heart Attack (ALLHAT), is due to be completed in 2003.[320] ALLHAT compares diuretics to DHP CAs, ACE-Is, and alpha blockers. Acute MI in the primary end point. In February 2000, the alpha-blocker arm of the ALLHAT trial was stopped because of a 25 percent higher CV mortality and twofold increase in HF when doxazosin was compared to chlorthalidone.[321] The primary end point was not different between the two groups. Here too, there was a difference in BP control. The chlorthalidone group had a 3/0 mmHg lower BP almost from the start compared with those getting doxazosin. Thus, the question of the degree BP reduction versus how one chooses to achieve it remains open.

It is of great interest that the participants receiving the alpha blocker had lower TC, triglycerides, and serum glucose and higher serum K^+ than did those on the diuretic.[321] If metabolic surrogate end points are important, all these changes would predict that alpha-blocker-treated subjects should have fewer events than do those on chlorthalidone. The opposite was the case. Another trial, the Controlled ONset Verapamil INvestigation of Cardiovascular Endpoints (CONVINCE), will be completed in 2002.[322] This study compares a nondihydropyridine CA (verapamil) to diuretics/beta blockers in 16,600 older hypertensives. This trial will indicate whether this class of CA will prevent mortality and morbidity as well as or better than conventional therapy does. It also will evaluate the importance of circadian variation in BP since the verapamil preparation used is designed to be given at night and released in concert with the morning rise in BP (see below). Event trials of ARBs in older high-risk hypertensives [Valsartan Amlodipine Long Term Use Evaluation (VALUE)] in hypertensives with ECG LVH (the Losartan Intervention for End Point Reduction–LIFE), and in those with diuretic nephropathy are in progress and will be finished in the next few years.[319,323]

Individualizing Therapy

In view of the many effective options available, the physician must pay very close attention to each patient's needs and plan his or her regimen accordingly. Each patient must be treated as an individual, not as a member of a population, and so the drug chosen must be compatible with that individual patient's preferences, lifestyle, and job requirements. Whatever is selected, it must be affordable. No amount of therapeutic wisdom will be effective if the patient does not have the funds to purchase the physician's choice.

Goal of Therapy

One must strive to reduce SBP to below 140 mmHg and to reduce DBP to below 90 mmHg, the goal currently articulated by several guidelines committees.[11,18,19] In diabetic patients, the recommended goal is lower (SBP <130 mmHg and DBP <85 mmHg). JNC VI recommended these more stringent goals for those with DM without proof from a clinical trial to support this aggressive approach. The subsequent publication of the HOT study and the United Kingdom Diabetes Prevention Study (UKDPS) provided the solid evidence that was needed to support this recommendation.[324,325] In patients with renal disease and at least 1 g of proteinuria per day, JNC VI recommended an even lower goal (SBP <125 mmHg and DBP <75 mmHg). This too was not an "evidence-based" recommendation but was based on the expectation that a still lower BP would be helpful in preventing morbidity and mortality in this population of hypertensives.[326] The African-American Study of Kidney Disease (AASK) will provide definitive evidence for or against this very stringent goal.[327] Whether this more aggressive goal should be extended to other subpopulations, such as those with prevalent CVD, remains to be proved.

One of the perceived limitations to achieving this lower level of BP control was the fear that lowering BP too far might be harmful, the concept of the "J" curve. Several investigators had pointed out that subjects treated to diastolic BP level below 85 mmHg had higher rates of MI than did those whose on-treatment diastolic BP was between 85 and 90 mmHg.[328,329] However, an increased risk for those with low diastolic BP is also evident in populations and in the placebo groups of several trials.[330,331] Furthermore, the Systolic Hypertension in the Elderly Program (SHEP) treated individuals down to an average diastolic BP of 67 mmHg and prevented MIs compared with those with an average of 71 mmHg.[269] Definite proof that aggressive treatment is not harmful has come from the HOT and UKPDS trials.[324,325] These studies showed no increase in the incidence of CV events in the groups randomized to the lowest levels of BP control, but HOT could not show that those treated to the lowest goal necessarily did the best. Both demonstrated reduced risk in hypertensives with DM and did not support the contention that hypertensives with known CAD would be at risk if treated aggressively. Both support the more aggressive BP treatment goals now recommended by guidelines committees (Table 51-23).

While the benefits of this level of aggressive therapy have not been proved conclusively, clinical trial results suggest that more events would be prevented with these treatment goals than with higher levels, with little if any harm to the patient. Another aspect, that of cost, was addressed in an analysis by Elliott and colleagues.[332] They compared the putative cost/effectiveness ratio of treating to a goal of [140/90 mmHg (JNC V) compared with 130/85 mmHg (JNC VI)] in hypertensives with type 2 DM.[11,38] Their theoretical analysis suggested that the

TABLE 51-21 Pharmacologic Properties of Commonly Used Antihypertensive Agents

Drug	Dose, mg/day	Doses per Day	Mechanisms of Action	Special Considerations
Diuretics				
Thiazides and related drugs	12.5–25	1	Decreased body sodium and extracellular fluid volume	More effective antihypertensive agents than loop diuretics unless serum creatinine is ≥2.0 mL/min or creatinine clearance is ≤50 mL/min
Hydrochlorothiazide				
Loop diuretics				
Furosemide	20–320	2	Inhibit $2Cl^-Na^+$ pump	Effective even in patients with advanced renal or congestive heart failure
Bumetanide	0.5–5	2	Ascending loop of Henle	
Ethacrynic acid	25–100	2		
Torsemide	5–20	1		
Fixed-dose diuretics (potassium-sparing)			Increase K^+ reabsorption	Weak diuretics
Hydrochlorothiazide/amiloride				
HCTZ/triamterene				
Spironolactone	25–100	2–3	Aldosterone antagonist	May cause hyperkalemia in patients with serum creatinine >2.5 mg/dL, particularly when combined with ACE inhibitors, K^+ supplements, or NSAIDs
Triamterene	50–100	2		
Adrenergic inhibitors				
Beta blockers				
Cardioselective			Inhibit $beta_1$ receptors, decrease CO	In higher doses, also inhibit $beta_2$ receptors
Atenolol	25–100	1	Increase SVR, decrease plasma renin activity (PRA)	
Metoprolol	50–200	1–2		
Noncardioselective			Inhibit $beta_1$ and $beta_2$ receptors	More likely to cause metabolic side effects
Nadolol	20–240	1		
Propranolol	40–240	1–2		
Timolol	20–40	2		
With intrinsic sympathomimetic activity (ISA)				
Acebutolol	200–1200	2	Partial agonist activity on beta-adrenergic receptors	No clear advantage except for less bradycardia and metabolic side effects than other beta blockers
Pindolol	10–60	2		
Antiadrenergic agents				
Centrally acting				
α-Methyldopa	250–1500	2	Stimulate $alpha_2$-adrenergic receptors in the brainstem, resulting in inhibition of efferent sympathetic activity; decrease SVR	Sudden withdrawal may result in hypertensive crisis
Clonidine	0.1–0.6	2		
Clonidine TTS	0.1–0.3	Once a week		
Guanfacine	1–3	1		
Peripherally acting				
Guanethidine	10–100	1	Inhibit norepinephrine release from sympathetic nerve terminals Decrease SVR	Frequently cause orthostatic hypotension and sexual dysfunction

Reserpine	0.05–0.25	1	Depletion of norepinephrine	Causes frequent neurologic symptoms; $alpha_1$-receptor blockers
Doxazosin	2–16	1	Inhibit $alpha_1$-adrenergic receptors.	First-dose effect; postural hypotension; useful for prostatic hypertrophy
Prazosin	2–20	1–2	Decrease SVR; CO same or increases	
Terazosin	1–20	1		
Alpha/beta blockers				
Labetalol	200–800	2–3	Blocks alpha- and beta-adrenergic receptors (7:1 beta:alpha blockade)	Same as beta blockers
Carvedilol	3.75–25	2	Blocks alpha- and beta-adrenergic receptors (3:1 beta:alpha blockade)	Same as beta blockers
ACE inhibitors				
Benazepril	10–40	1–2	Block conversion of angiotensin I to angiotensin II; decrease aldosterone; may increase bradykinin and vasodilatory prostaglandins; decrease SVR; no change in CO	When added to diuretics, may cause hypotension; may cause hyperkalemia in patients with renal failure, those with hypoaldosteronism, those receiving K-sparing diuretics or NSAIDs
Captopril	12.5–100	2–3		
Cilazapril	2.5–5	1–2		
Enalapril	2.5–40	1–2		
Fosinopril	10–40	1		
Lisinopril	5–40	1		
Perindopril	1–16	1–2		Can cause acute renal failure in patients with bilateral renal artery stenosis, renal artery stenosis of a solitary kidney, creatinine >3 mg/dL, or severe heart failure
Quinapril	5–80	1–2		
Ramipril	1.25–20	1		
Spirapril	12.5–50	1–2		
Trandolapril	1–4	1		
Calcium antagonists			Blocks entry of calcium into smooth muscle cells, resulting in vasodilation; decreases SVR; blunts increases in exercise heart rate	
Diltiazem	90–360	3–4		
Diltiazem CD	180–360	1		
Verapamil	80–480	2–3		May cause heart block, particularly when combined with beta blocker
Verapamil SR	120–480	1–2		
Verapamil-Covera HS	180–240	1 (at bedtime)		
Dihydropyridines				
Amlodipine	2.5–10	1	Same as diltiazem and verapamil	More potent vasodilators than diltiazem and verapamil; may cause dizziness, headache, tachycardia, flushing, edema
Felodipine	5–20	1	Do not blunt increase in exerise heart rate	
Isradipine	2.5–10	2		
Nicardipine	60–120	3		
Nifedipine	30–120	3		
Nifedipine (GITS)	30–120	1		
Nisoldipine	10–10	1–2		
Direct vasodilators				
Hydralazine	50–200	2–4	Direct relaxation of smooth muscle cells, causing arteriolar vasodilation secondary to opening [K^+] channels	Limited efficacy if given alone due to fluid retention and reflex vasodilation; should be combined with a diuretic and a beta blocker to prevent edema and tachycardia
Minoxidil	2.5–80	1		

TABLE 51-21 Pharmacologic Properties of Commonly Used Antihypertensive Agents (*Continued*)

Combination Drugs for Hypertension	
Drug	Trade Name
Beta-adrenergic blockers and diuretics	
Atenolol 50 or 100 mg and chlorthalidone 25 mg	Tenoretic
Bisoprolol fumarate 2.5, 5, or 10 mg, and hydrochlorothiazide 6.25 mg	Ziac[a]
Metoprolol tartrate 50 or 100 mg and hydrochlorothiazide 25 or 50 mg	Lopressor HCT
Nadolol 40 or 80 mg and bendroflumethiazide 5 mg	Corzide
Propranolol hydrochloride 40 or 80 mg and hydrochlorothiazide 25 mg	Inderide
Propranolol hydrochloride (extended release) 80, 120, or 160 mg and hydrochlorothiazide 50 mg	Inderide LA
Timolol maleate 10 mg and hydrochlorothiazide 25 mg	Timolide
ACE inhibitors and diuretics	
Benazepril hydrochloride 5, 10, or 20 mg, and hydrochlorothiazide 6.25, 12.5, or 25 mg	Lotensin HCT
Captopril 25 or 50 mg and hydrochlorothiazide 15 or 25 mg	Capozide[a]
Enalapril maleate 5 or 10 mg and hydrochlorothiazide 12.5 or 25 mg	Vaseretic
Lisinopril 10 or 20 mg and hydrochlorothiazide 12.5 or 25 mg	Prinzide, Zestoretic
Angiotensin II receptor antagonists and diuretics	
Losartan potassium 50 mg and hydrochlorothiazide 12.5 mg	Hyzaar
Calcium antagonists and ACE inhibitors	
Amlodipine besylate 2.5 or 5 mg and benazepril hydrochloride 10 or 20 mg	Lotrel
Diltiazem hydrochloride 180 mg and enalapril maleate 5 mg	Teczem
Verapamil hydrochloride (extended release) 180 or 240 mg and trandolapril 1, 2, or 4 mg	Tarka
Felodipine 5 mg and enalapril maleate 5 mg	Lexxel
Other combinations	
Triamterene 37.5, 50, or 75 mg, and hydrochlorothiazide 25 or 50 mg	Dyazide, Maxide
Spironolactone 25 or 50 mg and hydrochlorothiazide 25 or 50 mg	Aldactazide
Amiloride hydrochloride 5 mg and hydrochlorothiazide 50 mg	Moduretic
Guanethidine monosulfate 10 mg and hydrochlorothiazide 25 mg	Esimil
Hydralazine hydrochloride 25, 50, or 100 mg, and hydrochlorothiazide 25 or 50 mg	Apresazide
Methyldopa 250 or 500 mg and hydrochlorothiazide 15, 25, 30, or 50 mg	Aldoril
Reserpine 0.125 mg and hydrochlorothiazide 25 or 50 mg	Hydropres
Reserpine 0.10 mg, hydralazine hydrochloride 25 mg, and hydrochlorothiazide 15 mg	Ser-Ap-Es
Clonidine hydrochloride 0.1, 0.2, or 0.3 mg, and chlorthalidone 15 mg	Combipres
Methyldopa 250 mg and chlorothiazide 150 or 250 mg	Aldochlor
Reserpine 0.125 or 0.25 mg and chlorthalidone 25 or 50 mg	Demi-Regroton
Reserpine 0.125 or 0.25 mg and chlorothiazide 250 or 500 mg	Diupres
Prazosin hydrochloride 1, 2, or 5 mg, and polythiazide 0.5 mg	Minizide

[a]Approved first-line medications.

TABLE 51-22 Long-Term Outcome–Based Clinical Trials of Antihypertensive Agents in Progress

Acronym (Name)	First-Line Agent	Comparator	Patients	Comments
ALLHAT (Antihypertensive and Lipid Lowering Prevention of Heart Attack Trial)	Amlodipine, Doxazosin, Lisinopril	Chlorthalidone	42,448 in 625 centers in United States and Canada	Doxazosin arm stopped prematurely; 6-year follow-up planned
ANBP-2 (Australian National Blood Pressure Trial No. 2)	ACE inhibitor	Diuretic	6000 65–84-year-old Australians	5-year follow-up planned
ASCOT (Anglo-Scandinavian Cardiac Outcomes Trial)	Calcium antagonist or ACE inhibitor	Diuretic or beta blocker	18,000 residents of Scandinavia or United Kingdom	5-year follow-up planned
CONVINCE (Controlled-Onset Verapamil Investigation of Cardiovascular Endpoints)	COER-verapamil	HCTZ or atenolol	16,602 in 661 centers worldwide	5-year follow-up planned
ELSA (European Lacidipine Study of Atherosclerosis)	Lacidipine	Beta blocker	2251 European patients with known atherosclerosis	4-year follow-up planned
HYVET (Hypertension in the Very Elderly Trial)	ACE inhibitor (± diuretic)	Placebo	2100 patients >80 years old	5-year follow-up planned
INSIGHT (International Nifedipine GITS Study Intervention as a Goal in Hypertension Treatment)	Nifedipine GITS	HCTZ plus amiloride	6592 patients in nine European countries	3-year minimum follow-up planned
LIFE (Losartan Intervention for Endpoint Reduction)	Losartan	Atenolol	9194 patients in >300 centers worldwide	ECG LVH only; 4-year follow-up planned
NICS-EH (National Intervention Cooperative Study in Elderly Hypertensives)	Calcium antagonist	Diuretic	1000 Japanese >60 years old	5 year follow-up planned
NORDIL (Nordic Diltiazem Study)	Diltiazem	Diuretic or beta blocker	11,000 patients in 480 centers in Sweden and Norway	5-year follow-up planned
SHELL (Systolic Hypertension in the Elderly Long-Term Lacidipine Trial)	Lacidipine	Diuretic	4800 Europeans with isolated systolic hypertension	Compares 3.5-year incidence of cardiovascular morbidity/mortality
VALUE (Valsartan Amlodipine Long-Term Utilization Evaluation)	Valsartan (±HCTZ)	Amlodipine (±HCTZ)	14,400 patients in 1000 centers in 31 countries	6 years follow-up, 1450 primary end points expected

aggressive approach would save money. Even though more drugs would be needed, the reduction in both direct costs (hospitalization for the greater number of events that would occur in those with higher BP) and indirect costs (lost work) would more than balance the money spent for additional antihypertensives, any costs related to adverse reactions, and the extra visits to providers necessary to get BP to the lower goal.

TABLE 51-23 Goal Blood Pressure

General population without diabetes or renal disease	<140/90 mmHg
Diabetes	<130/85 mmHg
Renal disease with >1 g proteinuria	<125/75 mmHg
Isolated systolic hypertension	<140 mmHg

Factors to Consider in Choosing an Initial Antihypertensive Agent

There are 10 factors that should always be considered when initial therapy is chosen and other drugs are added (if additional agents are needed to reduce BP to goal) (Table 51-24).

EFFICACY

JNC VI made the distinction between surrogate and clinical end points when it provided guidelines for selecting treatment that were based on efficacy, defined as the reduction of morbid-

TABLE 51-24 Factors in the Choice of Agents for Antihypertensive Therapy

1. Efficacy
2. Comorbidity and other risk factors
3. Safety (adverse reactions and side effects)
4. Demographic considerations
5. Special situations
6. Dose schedule (dosage and chronotherapy)
7. Drug interactions
8. Adherence
9. Mechanism of action of drug and pathophysiology of patient's hypertension
10. Cost

TABLE 51-25 Considerations in Individualizing Antihypertensive Drug Therapy

Indication[a]	Drug Therapy
DM (type 1) with proteinuria	ACE-I
HF (systolic)	ACE-I, diuretics, beta blockers, aldosterone receptor blockers
Isolated systolic hypertension (older patients)	Diuretics (preferred), DHP CAs
MI	Beta blockers (non-ISA), ACE-Is (systolic dysfunction)

[a]Compelling indications unless contraindicated.
SOURCE: Modified from JNC VI.

ity and mortality. Now four classes of drugs (thiazide diuretics, beta blockers, long-acting DHP CAs, and ACE-Is) have been shown to reduce CV end points when used as the initial therapy for hypertension in appropriately designed and implemented clinical trials. Other agents, such as peripheral sympatholytics (reserpine and guanethidine), centrally acting alpha agonists (alpha-methyldopa), and vasodilators (hydralazine), also have been used in clinical trials as the second, third, or even fourth agent to be added to get BP under control. None is an option for initial therapy because they are relatively poorly tolerated compared with the agents that are recommended as initial therapy or need to be taken together with diuretics to lower BP effectively in the long term. Other drugs, such as alpha/beta blockers and ARBs, that are effective as monotherapy and are well tolerated, have not yet been shown to reduce clinical end points. Alpha blockers are valuable as adjunctive therapy, but the early data from ALLHAT have shown that this class should not be used as the initial treatment for hypertension unless symptomatic relief of benign prostatic hypertrophy (BPH) is needed.[321] Many would now recommend that a man with hypertension and BPH get another drug along with the alpha blocker as part of an antihypertensive regimen.

COMORBIDITY AND OTHER RISK FACTORS

JNC VI has recognized two other factors that may alter the correct choice of initial treatment in an individual hypertensive patient:

- Data from events trials that were conducted in subjects with other conditions (e.g., type 1 DM, acute MI, HF, and after HOPE, those considered to be at high risk for CV events) but in which many subjects with hypertension were enrolled. These trials were the basis for the JNC VI designation of a "compelling" indication (Table 51-25)
- Individual patients may have certain comorbid conditions for which a specific agent may be appropriate even though no trial has been completed in which that agent has been compared to drugs for which clinical trial data are currently available. This was the basis of the JNC VI recommendation for a drug to be indicated or contraindicated as a "specific" indication even though randomized clinical trials might not be available to support that decision (Table 51-26). A "specific" indication tries to codify clinical judgment, or that which any reasonable clinician would do to care for all the health needs of his or her patients. For the most part, these recommendations do not add classes of drugs to the list of those which are favored because of a reduction in clinical end points but instead alter the choice of which class should be selected for initial therapy. Good examples are osteoporosis and thiazide diuretics and angina pectoris and beta blockers.

The factors that influence the specific indications are generally the presence of other risk factors and active clinical problems. These conditions may and often should alter the initial and subsequent choice of antihypertensive therapy in an individual patient. An appreciation of the fact that the drugs prescribed to reduce BP can improve or adversely affect other clinical conditions is the basis for the JNC VI recommendation that although diuretics and beta blockers should be used when a patient has "uncomplicated" hypertension, the presence of these comorbid conditions clearly affects that decision.

This approach was also used by the BHS.[19] In those guidelines, similar language to that in JNC VI was used, but the BHS considered the presence of some of these comorbid conditions to be a compelling reason rather than a specific one to choose a particular class of drugs even though a trial had not been completed proving the value of those agents in patients with these conditions. The lessons from the Evaluation of Losartan in the Elderly II trial (ELITE II), which failed to show any advantage of an ARB over an ACE-I (see below), and ALLHAT are that it is best to demand and wait for evidence that an agent prevents events before recommending to clinicians that they should feel "compelled" to prescribe that class.

Dyslipidemias Hypertensive patients who have lipid abnormalities (which may be present in as many as 50 percent of those treated for hypertension) probably should not be treated with drugs that worsen their particular dyslipidemia. Although it has not been proved that the changes in serum lipids caused by certain classes of antihypertensive agents are harmful, it is certainly reasonable to choose an equally effective drug that is lipid-neutral or one that may improve the lipid profile.[333] In large doses (>25 mg/day), thiazide diuretics and related compounds such as chlorthalidone raise TC and LDL-C 5 to 10 percent at least transiently and may lower HDL-C 2 to 4 percent. Serum triglycerides are increased 15 to 30 percent.[334] With the

TABLE 51-26 Drugs That May Have Favorable or Unfavorable Effects on Comorbid Conditions

Favorable	
Angina	Beta blockers, Ca^{2+} antagonists
Atrial tachycardia and fibrillation	Beta blockers, CA nondihydropyridines
Cyclosporine-induced hypertension	Ca^{2+} antagonists (caution with the dose of cyclosporine)
DM (types 1 and 2) with proteinuria	ACE-Is (preferred), CAs (nondihydropyridines), low-dose diuretics
HF	ACE-Is, losartan, K^+-sparing agents, beta-blockers
Liver disease	Beta blockers
Peripheral vascular disease	Alpha-blockers, CAs
Pregnancy	Labetalol hydrochloride, methyldopa
DM (type 2)	ACE-Is
Dyslipidemia	Alpha blockers
Essential tremor	Beta blockers
Hyperthyroidism	Beta blockers
Migraine	Beta blockers (noncardioselective), Ca^{2+} antagonists (nondihydropyridine)
MI	Beta blockers (cardioselective)
Osteoporosis	Thiazide diuretics
Preoperative hypertension	Beta blockade
Prostatism (benign prostatic hyperplasia)	Alpha blockers
Renal insufficiency (caution in renovascular disease)	ACE-Is, ARBs, K^+-sparing agents for hypertension and creatinine >3 mg/dL
Unfavorable	
Bronchospastic disease	Beta blockers
Depression	Beta blockers, central alpha agonists, reserpine
DM (types 1 and 2)	Beta blockers, high-dose diuretics
Dyslipidemia	Beta blockers (non-ISA), diuretics (high-dose)
Gout	Diuretics
Second- or third-degree heart block	Beta blockers, Ca^{2+} antagonists (nondihydropyridine)
Renal insufficiency, renovascular disease	ACE-Is, ARBs

doses that are currently recommended (using up to but no more than 25 mg of hydrochlorothiazide), there is little if any alterations in these parameters. The beta blockers that do not have intrinsic sympathomimetic activity lower HDL-C even more (10 percent) and also raise triglycerides (approximately 20 percent) without affecting TC or LDL.[335] Beta blockers that do have intrinsic sympathomimetic activity and alpha/beta blockers are lipid-neutral.

Conversely, one could choose to add to therapy using a peripheral alpha blocker in patients with dyslipidemias who are already being treated with agents known to reduce CV events, such as beta blockers, ACE-Is, and diuretics.[333,336] These drugs reduce TC and LDL cholesterol approximately 8 to 10 percent, triglycerides 15 percent, and HDL-C 10 to 15 percent. The ALLHAT results mentioned above call into question the wisdom of this approach.[321] ACE-Is do not affect serum lipids, and in some studies benefits similar to those seen with alpha blockers have been observed. ARBs and CAs are lipid-neutral.[334,335]

Other sympatholytics do not affect the lipid profile, and direct vasodilators (e.g., hydralazine) raise HDL-C and lower triglycerides and TG even when used in combination with thiazide diuretics.

Glucose and Insulin and Diabetes Mellitus Antihypertensive drugs may affect glucose metabolism and worsen or improve insulin sensitivity.[333] The magnitude and direction of the drug-induced changes seen in glucose and insulin are very similar to what occurs with lipids. Peripheral alpha blockers and some ACE-Is (captopril, enalapril, trandolapril, and perindopril) may improve insulin sensitivity.[337] Not only do some ACE-Is improve insulin sensitivity, all have been shown to reduce urinary protein excretion, which may contribute to the renal benefit seen in patients with DM. Both moderate- to high-dose thiazides and beta blockers worsen insulin sensitivity and occasionally precipitate glucose intolerance. Beta blockers increase the risk of developing clinical DM by up to 25 percent.[338] In spite of these metabolic changes, in SHEP, treatment with low-dose chlorthalidone (plus atenolol or reserpine in some volunteers) reduced clinical events in the diabetic subgroup even more than it did in nondiabetics.[339] In the HOPE trial and in CAPPP, incident diabetes was prevented.[312,318] These findings, if confirmed by ALLHAT (STOP-2 did not demonstrate that ACE-Is prevented new DM), indicate that patients at high risk of becoming diabetic (the obese and those with glucose intolerance or other components of syndrome X) also might benefit from treatment with ramapril or an ACE-I.

Hypertensives with Diabetes Mellitus The combination of hypertension and DM confers much more risk for CV events and renal failure than does either one alone. Angiotensin-converting enzyme inhibitors, diuretics, and beta blockers have been shown consistently to reduce CV and renal risk. There are very few data on other classes of antihypertensive agents, although there are some preliminary studies with ARBs and CAs. JNC VI recommended that clinicians should feel "compelled" to give hypertensive patients with type 1 DM an ACE-I only because the only randomized clinical trial that has clearly demonstrated the utility of ACE-Is in reducing clinical events was done in a group of type 1 diabetic patients with hypertension.[316] Although no large, long-term events trials have been completed that have proved the special value of ACE-Is in patients with type 2 DM, many feel that the benefit shown for type I diabetic patients also can be assumed to occur for type 2 diabetic patients, and so ACE-Is were recommended by JNC VI as a specific indication.[11] Others argue that if BP control is achieved, it does not matter what drug or drugs are used. In UKPDS, the group that received the ACE inhibitor captopril did no better than did the group that received atenolol. This lends some support to the argument that BP control, not how it is accomplished, is the key factor in reducing events in type 2 diabetic patients.[325]

Although some experts have raised concern about the safety of DHP CAs in type 2 diabetic patients, the Syst-EUR study, in which these drugs were the initial therapy, demonstrated that the benefit accrued was greater in diabetic patients than it was in other patients.[340] Just as with SHEP, the results of a properly done clinical trial disproved surrogate end-point-based hypotheses from other sources of data such as observational studies, case-control studies, and meta-analyses of smaller trials.

Trials of CV mortality involving nondihydropyridine CAs in high-risk hypertensive patients have not been completed. However, nondihydropyridine CAs have been shown to reduce CV mortality after an MI and slow the progression of diabetic nephropathy.[341,342] Moreover, their use in combination with ACE-Is lowers urinary protein excretion, and unlike DHP CAs, they have additive effects to reduce proteinuria independent of BP reduction.[343,344] This combination appears to be particularly useful in diabetic patients with nephropathy and proteinuria.

From the available data, it would appear that in people with DM, the most important factor in reducing mortality and preserving renal function is reducing BP to goal (Table 51-23).

Left Ventricular Hypertrophy and Heart Failure Left ventricular hypertrophy results from chronic elevations in arterial pressure that cause cardiac myocyte hypertrophy and remodeling of the coronary resistance vessels. This leads to perivascular fibrosis of the intramyocardial arteries and arterioles. Over time, these changes in the myocardium contribute to the development of ventricular wall stiffness and diastolic dysfunction.[345]

Left ventricular hypertrophy is a robust independent risk factor for CV and premature mortality.[227] It is especially common in the elderly, particularly in elderly women, and often is associated with diastolic dysfunction. It appears that all antihypertensive agents that are recommended for initial therapy reduce LV mass. Data from meta-analyses have suggested that agents that block the RAA system reduce LV mass better than do other antihypertensive agents.[235] However, TOMHS and the Veterans Administration (VA) study of monotherapy found that there was no difference among antihypertensive agents in their ability to regress LVH.[236,237] Moreover, in TOMHS, nutritional hygienic measures such as weight loss, reduced Na^+ and alcohol intake, and exercise were effective by themselves in regressing LV mass. Perhaps the most important factor responsible for LV mass regression is the prolonged reduction of systolic BP.

Heart Failure Hypertension has been identified as a major risk factor for the subsequent development of HF, the onset of which typically occurs many years later.[346] For many un- or undertreated hypertensives, LVH is an important intermediate step, resulting in "hypertensive heart disease" with impaired LV filling and increased ventricular stiffness. This type of HF (which has been seen in up to 40 percent of hospitalized patients with an antecedent history of hypertension) is commonly called diastolic dysfunction.[233] The more common type of "systolic dysfunction" associated with a reduced LV ejection fraction most often is due to previous MI (for which hypertension is also an important risk factor). In a meta-analysis of clinical trials in hypertension, there was a 42 percent reduction in HF incidence among hypertensives randomized to either a low-dose diuretic or a beta blocker.[342]

Distinguishing between the two subtypes of HF is most easily done by quantitation of the LV ejection fraction.[347] The results dictate the therapy. Patients with low ejection fractions ("systolic HF") improve both BP and long-term prognosis with ACE-Is and diuretics, to which are sometimes added beta blockers, spironolactone, and/or other drugs.[314,347–349] The role of ARBs is controversial unless cough or other adverse effects preclude an ACE-I. In the first (but small) direct comparison of captopril and losartan [Evaluation of Losartan In The Elderly (ELITE)], there was a survival benefit (a tertiary hypothesis) attributed to the ARBs, which the larger study (ELITE II), with exactly the same protocol, did not confirm.[350] If cough or other adverse effects of an ACE-I preclude its use, an ARB becomes the rational choice. Ongoing research may define the benefit of using both an ACE-I and an ARB simultaneously in patients with systolic HF. The role of DHP CAs and other direct-acting vasodilators (e.g., hydralazine in combination with isosorbide dinitrate) remains controversial.[351] Most authorities recommend these drugs as second- or third-line therapy (after maximum doses of ACE-Is and/or ARBs) if BP is still elevated. Recently, in the Randomized Aldactone Evaluation Study (RALES) trial, spironolactone, an aldosterone antagonist, in doses that do not lower BP reduced morbidity and mortality in patients with HF, most of whom were already taking ACE-Is, aspirin, and diuretics.[349] Many of these patients were also on beta blockers.

Treatment of hypertension with diastolic dysfunction and HF has not been as well studied, but most authorities recommend using drugs that reduce HR, increase diastolic filling time, and allow the heart muscle to relax more fully: beta blockers or nondihydropyridine CAs.[352,353] Although these options make physiologic sense, no randomized clinical trials have had outcomes that demonstrate their long-term efficacy.[352]

Valvular Disease The coexistence of hypertension and valvular heart disease is, for most affected patients, simply an occurrence of two common conditions in the same person. There are few syndromes or scenarios in which the two are pathophysiologically connected, but there are some circumstances in which their coexistence has clinical importance, especially in regard to choosing antihypertensive drug therapy.

A murmur of aortic sclerosis is found in approximately 21 to 26 percent of adults over 65 years of age. Recent data from the CV Health Study showed that 29 percent of the 5621 subjects age 65 and over had this valvular abnormality detected on echocardiography; it was found much more commonly among hypertensives and those with LVH.[354] Perhaps most important, its presence was associated with a 50 percent increased risk of CV events over an average of 5 years of follow-up. After adjustment for risk factor differences at baseline (e.g., hypertension), only one of four studied end points retained statistical significance. Calcific aortic stenosis is about 10 times less common but often must be evaluated more extensively, usually with an echocardiogram. Aortic insufficiency in hypertensives is found almost exclusively in patients with isolated systolic hypertension and is most easily recognized by the murmur and several peripheral signs.[355] Unloading the LV with arteriolar vasodilators has long been recommended on a pathophysiologic basis and has been shown in a long-term trial against digoxin to prolong the time until valvular replacement surgery was required.[356] Although nifedipine was used in the study, it is likely that any vasodilator would be more effective than a weakly positive inotropic agent.

Mitral valvular disease is less common than it was in past decades, primarily because of efforts to treat streptococcal pharyngitis. Mitral stenosis is still seen occasionally in citizens of developing countries but is not commonly associated with systemic hypertension. Since digoxin typically is used to control the ventricular rate in atrial fibrillation, antihypertensive drugs that interfere with the excretion of digoxin should be used cautiously. Mitral insufficiency is also less common than it was in the past, but there are few problems specific to this disease that affect hypertension and its therapy.

The right-sided cardiac valves seldom need be considered in the treatment of patients with systemic hypertension. In patients with primary (or secondary) pulmonary hypertension (which can be treated with the usual antihypertensive drugs, although with less success), the status of the right-sided heart valves takes on increased significance.[357] Occasionally, insufficiency of the tricuspid valve is the major diagnostic clue to carcinoid heart disease (associated with weight loss drugs but rarely associated with hypertension).[358]

Microalbuminuria MA is a predictor of CV and renal death in patients with DM.[359–361] The class of antihypertensive medications known to have the most potent effects on reducing MA is the ACE-Is.[317,359–363] These agents reduce albuminuria by reducing intraglomerular pressure as well as decreasing glomerular size selectivity and partially restoring membrane charge.[362,363] The effects of different classes of antihypertensive agents on MA as well as related metabolic parameters are summarized in Table 51-27.

TABLE 51-27 Effects of Drugs on Microalbuminuria and Proteinuria

Decrease levels
ACE inhibitors
Angiotensin receptor blockers
Alpha/beta blockers
Nondihydropyridine CAs
Beta blockers
Diuretics
Increase levels
Short-acting dihydropyridine CAs
Minoxidil
No effect
Dihydropyridine CAs (long acting)
Alpha blockers
Central alpha agonists (clonidine, methyldopa)

Both ACE-Is and nondihydropyridine CAs reduce albuminuria and together have additive antialbuminuric effects, in part independently of further reductions in BP.[359,364,365]

The ACE-Is and ARBs are the antihypertensive agents that most consistently reduce proteinuria in response to their BP-lowering effect. Moreover, in the absence of hypertension, these agents prevent the increase of MA to proteinuria and in many cases normalize protein excretion in patients with MA.[366] Nondihydropyridine CAs (diltiazem and verapamil) also have some utility in reducing urinary protein excretion in hypertensive patients with kidney disease.[364] In two studies, these drugs had antiproteinuric effects similar to those of ACE-Is in hypertensive diabetic patients with chronic renal disease and heavy proteinuria.[367,368] Some studies have shown that a high Na^+ intake blunts the antiproteinuric and antihypertensive effects of an ACE-I.[369,370] Increasing dietary salt despite not affecting BP appears to abolish the antiproteinuric effect of the nondihydropyridine CA diltiazem, and so attention should be paid to Na^+ intake in patients with MA/or proteinuria.[368,369] Since there are so many more data, including events data, about ACE-I than about any other agents, including ARBs, ACE-Is should be the first-line treatment of hypertension in DM and should be included in all antihypertensive regimens in such patients if tolerated.

Renal Dysfunction Any agent or group of agents that adequately lowers BP to levels <130/85 mmHg will slow the progression of nephropathy. Aggressive BP reduction (<125/75 mmHg) is needed to maximally slow the progression of renal disease, especially among patients with elevated serum creatinine. Aggressive BP reduction (<125/75 mmHg) is needed to maximally slow the progression of renal disease, especially among patients with an elevated serum creatinine ≥1.4 mg/dL.[11] ACE-Is will slow the progression of diabetic and nondiabetic nephropathy, assuming BP reduction to levels below 140/90 mmHg.

In spite of the evidence from many long-term clinical trials, there is a general hesitancy among clinicians to use ACE-Is in such patients. This stems from a rise in serum creatinine that predictably occurs when the drug is given. It is common to see increases in serum creatinine of up to 25 percent above baseline within 2 to 3 months of ACE-inhibitor initiation. An analysis of long-term clinical trials has confirmed that this reduction in renal function plateaus within a month.[371] In a study from Scandinavia, ACE-Is were discontinued after an average follow-up of 6 years of therapy. The glomerular filtration rate (GFR) returned to levels not significantly different from baseline even though within the first 4 months after ACE-I initiation there was a clear initial reduction in GFR by an average of 8 to 10 percent below baseline.[372] This return to baseline GFR has not been reported with any other class of antihypertensive agent studied and suggests that ACE-Is prevented the expected deterioration of renal function over time. If the serum creatinine continues to rise, especially after 1 month of therapy, evaluation for renal artery stenosis may be indicated.

There are also concerns about hyperkalemia. This should be worrisome only if the serum K^+ rises ≥0.5 meq/L.

The role of ARBs in the treatment of nephropathy and reducing CV events has not been settled. All animal studies and one completed clinical trial in patients with HF suggest that these agents are as good as ACE-Is in slowing the progression of renal disease and reducing proteinuria and CV events.[360,365] Whether ARBs are better than ACE-Is or even equivalent remains to be proved. Two ongoing clinical trials in subjects with diabetic nephropathy are scheduled to be completed by 2002 and will answer the question definitively.[319]

Thus, while any class of antihypertensive agent may be used to achieve this new recommended lower level of BP to preserve renal function, certain principles should be kept in mind.

- BP will never be controlled adequately in patients with significant renal insufficiency (serum creatinine >1.8 mg/dL) without the use of a diuretic (usually a loop diuretic).
- Long-acting loop diuretics are preferred, or if furosemide is used, it needs to be given twice a day.
- Various combinations of medications will be needed to achieve BP reduction. One of these drugs should contain an ACE-I. If side effects are noted with the ACE-I, an ARB may be substituted to ensure renal protection and BP reduction.

Since CV is the most common cause of death in people with renal disease, beta blockers clearly also have a role in therapy. These agents do not have synergistic or additive effects on BP in the presence of agents such as clonidine.[373]

Coronary Artery Disease Since hypertension is a major risk factor for CAD, it is not surprising that a large number of patients have both conditions. It is unlikely on ethical grounds that a placebo-controlled trial will be done with any single antihypertensive drug in such patients. The presence of CAD in a patient with hypertension is likely to influence both the choice of drugs used to treat the patient and the BP goal to be achieved. Because both beta blockers and CAs are effective antihypertensive agents with major antianginal efficacy, they are often the preferred agents for initial treatment, especially in the common setting of unstable angina pectoris.[374] A recent meta-analysis suggested that the former are more effective, although the latter are more commonly used.[375] The recent HOPE trial showed a large survival benefit for high-risk hypertensives (most of whom had known CAD) treated with ramapril.[318] None of the volunteers in HOPE had known HF at enrollment in which this degree of benefit would have been expected. This has been interpreted by some as evidence in favor of this class of medication or even for this specific agent for all hypertensive patients with CAD.

The issue of how low to reduce BP in the setting of CAD is controversial. The concept of the J-shaped curve has been supported by data in patients with coronary disease, mostly using beta blockers.[328] Diastolic pressures less than 82 mmHg were associated with a higher risk of coronary events, and the rationale proposed was that since coronary artery filling occurs during diastole, reducing perfusion pressure during this time might increase coronary ischemia. These and other data led to the HOT study, in which 18,790 hypertensive patients without known coronary disease were randomized to one of three diastolic BP goals: ≤90, ≤85, and ≤80 mmHg.[324] After 3.8 years, there were no significant differences in major CV events across the groups, suggesting that there is no increase in risk from lowering diastolic BPs below 80 mmHg. It is unlikely that a similar study in patients with CAD will be done, but some still recommend caution in lowering BP below 85 mmHg in patients with angina and/or known CAD. JNC VI indicates that "BP should be lowered to the usual target range (<140/90 mmHg), and even lower BP is desirable if angina persists."[11] The World Health Organization/International Society of Hypertension's Collaborative Trialists' Group is collecting patient-specific outcome data and eventually may have sufficient power from the clinical trials in this registry for a post hoc analysis comparing levels of achieved BP control among 270,000 hypertensives with or without CAD.[319] Even after such data become available, it probably will be advisable to use beta blockers, CAs, and perhaps nitrates for hypertensive patients with CAD to achieve a slightly lower than usual BP target and to recommend aspirin and intensive treatment of dyslipidemias. Appropriate precautions must be taken for hypertensives also using sildenafil citrate (Viagra). To date, no antihypertensives seem to confer any increased risks when used with this agent, but all nitrate-containing preparations are contraindicated.

After Stroke Although hypertension is perhaps the most powerful risk factor for acute stroke and "clinically evident cerebrovascular disease is an indication for antihypertensive treatment," optimal BP management depends on the nature, cause, and chronology of the neurologic symptoms.[376] In the immediate setting of acute ischemic stroke, there is controversy about the optimal level of acceptable BP. Appropriate concern has been expressed about possible reduction in blood flow to "watershed" areas of the brain that are already poorly perfused if BP is reduced pharmacologically.[377] Many neurologists have observed acute worsening of cerebrovascular function and evolving neurologic deficits when BP has been reduced "too much" or "too quickly." Most physicians therefore are uncomfortable reducing BP to <180/100 mmHg. Many do not institute treatment until mean arterial pressure is >130 mmHg (e.g., BP >200/100 mmHg), except in the setting of concomitant hemorrhagic transformation or another hypertensive emergency (e.g., aortic dissection, MI, renal failure with bleeding).[378] This level of BP is at least supported by the exclusion criterion from the National Institutes of Health (NIH)-sponsored rt-PA for acute stroke trial; patients with BP >185/110 mmHg were prohibited from getting the thrombolytic agent and were instead suggested to receive antihypertensive therapy.[379] The optimal drug therapy for acute stroke-related hypertension is also ill defined, but most authorities prefer intravenously administered, short-acting agents because they can be discontinued quickly if a patient's neurologic condition deteriorates acutely.[378]

SAFETY (ADVERSE REACTIONS AND SIDE EFFECTS)

The two primary types of adverse reactions and side effects that occur with antihypertensive therapy are clinical and biochemical (Table 51-21). Clinical side effects are directly evident to the patient and are perceived by the patient or the clinician to be related to the drug. The appearance of these adverse reactions requires that the drug be stopped, the dose be reduced, or the patient be willing to remain on therapy until he or she becomes able to tolerate the side effect or until it disappears. The drugs recommended for initial therapy generally cause fewer clinical side effects than do other drugs at doses that lower BP.[11,18,19]

Biochemical side effects may lead to clinically evident adverse reactions (e.g., hypokalemia from thiazide diuretics causing muscle weakness, palpitations, nocturia, or polyuria), but usually the biochemical problems that occur with antihypertensive agents are more troublesome to the clinician than they are to the patient.

The importance of biochemical side effects is usually not that they result in clinically evident problems but the danger that these drug-related permutations of lipids, glucose, or insulin may aggravate other risk factors and accelerate the clinical impact of dyslipidemias, glucose intolerance, or insulin resistance. Whether the minor and often short-term effects on triglycerides, HDL-C, or TG that result from therapy with thiazides or beta blockers are responsible for an increase in ischemic heart disease remains to be proved. It is of great interest that in ALLHAT the biochemical profile of the group receiving the alpha blocker seemed favorable (lower triglycerides, TG, and glucose and higher K^+) compared with the group on chlorthalidone, yet the diuretic prevented CV events more successfully.[321] The remaining treatment arms of ALLHAT (DHP CA and ACE-I versus diuretic) should definitely delineate the role of these metabolic changes.

At the doses that are now recommended, these changes and the electrolyte disturbances noted with thiazides are modest, although it is still possible that at high doses, thiazides could reduce serum K^+ sufficiently to increase the rate of sudden cardiac death. Whether the increases in insulin resistance that are seen with thiazide diuretics and beta blockers and the hypokalemia that is seen with thiazide diuretics have precipitated DM sooner or in patients who would not otherwise have become diabetic also remains to be proved. Although it is not certain that these metabolic adverse reactions are clinically relevant, it may be prudent to select another option for patients with DM or a dyslipidemia so long as BP is reduced to goal. Certain types of dual therapy also may ameliorate biochemical adverse reactions. Angiotensin-converting enzyme inhibitors and ARBs and thiazides, when given together, produce few, if any, of the metabolic abnormalities associated with thiazides alone.[380] Several fixed-dose combinations or these classes of drugs are available and may be appropriate as initial therapy[11] (Table 51-21).

The incidence of clinical side effects tends to rise with increasing doses with all classes of drugs, with the exception of ACE-Is and ARBs. Patients who develop an adverse reaction on a high dose of a drug or on a dose they previously tolerated do not necessarily need to have that drug discontinued. Instead, the dose can be lowered and another antihypertensive can be added to reduce BP to goal. The primary problems with ACE-Is are cough and angioedema, both of which tend to be idiosyncratic and occur with all representatives of that class of agents. Reducing the dose or changing to a different ACE-I is rarely helpful. Angiotensin-converting enzyme inhibitors should be increased to the maximum recommended dose before therapy is abandoned or another agent is added unless a low-dose fixed-dose combination is felt to be more appropriate. Angiotensin II receptor blockers as a class appear to be the best tolerated of all currently available antihypertensive agents.[381] Although some experts feel that they should be reserved for initial therapy only in patients who have developed a cough with ACE-Is, they are also an excellent option for patients who have no complaints when treatment is started and patients in whom a drug that primarily blocks the RAA system appears to be a good option. When VALUE and LIFE are completed, it will be known whether ARBs are as good a choice as the other four classes of antihypertensives available.

DEMOGRAPHIC CONSIDERATIONS

Blacks and Other Ethnic Minorities Some classes of antihypertensive agents reduce BP more or less effectively in certain ethnic groups. Thiazide diuretics, for example, are more effective in blacks than in whites, whereas ACE-Is, ARBs, and beta blockers are more effective at lower doses in whites. Many blacks respond to agents that block the RAA system, but they often need higher doses than do whites or Asians.[382] Studies in African-Americans have demonstrated that starting with higher doses of an ACE-I makes this class quite efficacious in lowering BP in this population.[383] Therefore, if a black hypertensive patient would benefit from the special properties that these drugs may have in type 1 diabetic patients or in HF, for example, they definitely should be used even if additional agents will be needed to get BP to goal. Peripheral alpha blockers, alpha/beta blockers, and CAs are equally effective in all types of hypertensive patients in all ethnic groups. In general, the response rates to antihypertensive agents in Hispanics is intermediate between that seen in whites and that seen in blacks, while east Asians, though not necessarily south Asians (patients from the Indian subcontinent), often need lower doses than do whites.

The Elderly All classes of antihypertensive agents lower BP effectively in older persons, although the doses needed to reach goal are often lower than the doses necessary in young and middle-aged hypertensive patients.[384,385] Certain drugs and certain classes of drugs, however, should be avoided or used with caution in older hypertensives. These include agents, such as peripheral alpha blockers, that can exacerbate the postural fall in BP seen more frequently in older individuals with baroreceptor dysfunction; nondihydropyridine CAs and beta blockers that may aggravate subtle or subclinical conduction defects or precipitate systolic dysfunction and HF; and verapamil, which may not be well tolerated in some older persons already bothered by constipation. Cough from an ACE-I may be more common in older women. Diuretics and dihydropyridine DHP CAs have both been shown to reduce morbidity and mortality in older persons with stage 2 or 3 isolated systolic hypertension, making them excellent choices in such patients.[269–271] What is often forgotten in regard to many classes is that the benefits of effective treatment are more evident in older hypertensives who are at higher risk than are younger hypertensives.[385] Therapy should not be withheld for fear of toxicity or lack of efficacy in the elderly.

Children The diagnosis and treatment of hypertension in children are different from those in adults, primarily because of the limited experience with antihypertensive drug therapy in children and the low risk of CV events in younger individuals.[386,387] Most pediatricians are very comfortable measuring and monitoring BP in their patients, but few nonnephrologists commit the expected 1 percent of their patients to drug therapy. Because of a higher incidence of secondary hypertension than there is in adults, most hypertensive children have at least an evaluation of the kidneys and urinary tract before beginning treatment.[387]

The diagnosis of hypertension in pediatric patients is truly population-based, since the 5 percent of children with the highest BP are diagnosed with "significant hypertension" and the highest 1 percent are deemed eligible for pharmacologic treat-

TABLE 51-28 Antihypertensive Drugs Frequently Used in Children

Drug	Initial Dose	Usual Maximum Dose
Intravenously administered		
Sodium nitroprusside	0.5 μg/kg/min	8 μg/kg/min
Labetalol	1 mg/kg/h	3 mg/kg/h
Orally administered		
Hydrochlorothiazide	1 mg/kg/day	2–3 mg/kg/day
Furosemide	1 mg/kg/day	12 mg/kg/day
Bumetanide	0.02–0.05 mg/kg/day	0.3 mg/kg/day
Propranolol	1 mg/kg/day	8 mg/kg/day
Atenolol	1 mg/kg/day	8 mg/kg/day
Captopril (for neonates)	0.03 mg/kg/day	2 mg/kg/day
Captopril (for children)	1.5 mg/kg/day	6 mg/kg/day
Enalapril	0.15 mg/kg/day	40 mg/day
Nifedipine (extended release)	0.25 mg/kg/day	3 mg/kg/day
Prazosin	0.05–0.1 mg/kg/day	0.5 mg/kg/day
Minoxidil	0.1–0.2 mg/kg/day	1 mg/kg/day

SOURCE: Adapted from Sinaiko AR. Current concepts: Hypertension in children. *N Engl J Med* 1996; 335:1968–1973.

ment.[387] The diagnostic cutoffs for hypertension in youth are age- and weight-dependent, and "growth charts" for plotting the progress of a child's BP against age often are completed by pediatricians for height, weight, and, more recently, BP. More frequent measurements and attention to BP are warranted when a child's BP exceeds the 90th percentile. Treatment of hypertension in children begins with lifestyle modifications, since they are likely to be beneficial as a child grows into adolescence and adulthood.[386,387] Because few registration studies of antihypertensive drugs include children (owing to informed consent complexities and risk management issues), there are limited data on the benefits of specific drugs in hypertensive children. Although the recommended treatment algorithm is based on time-tested drug use in adults, there is a growing awareness of the possibility of long-term adverse effects with diuretics and especially beta blockers (which make exercise more difficult and may lead to weight gain) and a growing use of both ACE-Is and CAs. Antihypertensive drugs that are used frequently in children are shown in Table 51-28; the doses typically are based on the body weight of the child.

SPECIAL SITUATIONS

Pregnancy Hypertension is found in about 10 percent of pregnancies and is the major cause of perinatal morbidity and mortality in most developed countries. Because of the unique patient population, hypertension in pregnancy has a special definition, four specific types, and a treatment algorithm that recognizes the need to assess outcomes in both mother and baby. Since most pregnancies are managed by obstetricians, most of the authoritative pronouncements about this condition have been advanced by expert panels drawn from that discipline.[388,389] In the United States, hypertension in pregnancy is defined as either BP >140/90 mmHg on two measurements at least 4 h apart or a diastolic BP >110 mmHg at any time during pregnancy or up to 6 weeks postpartum.[389]

The classification of hypertension in pregnancy typically requires some knowledge of BP status before conception. If there was preexisting hypertension, the patient is said to have "chronic hypertension," which can be diagnosed before 20 weeks' gestation and persists at least 42 days postpartum. Preeclampsia is hypertension appearing after 20 weeks' gestation, associated with proteinuria (at least 300 mg per 24-h collection or 2+ on a random dipstick), which typically resolves within 42 days after delivery. Hypertension with superimposed preeclampsia is a combination of the two. The term *Hypertension unclassified* typically is used only when none of the above criteria are met and the BP status before conception or during the first trimester is unknown.

There has been a great effort to elaborate both the cause and the effective treatment for preeclampsia, but neither has been identified. A large number of demographic, genetic, laboratory parameters, and other factors have been associated with a higher risk of preeclampsia, but none has been accepted as the underlying "cause" (Table 51-29). Even more interesting are recent clinical trials that attempted to prevent preeclampsia with low-dose aspirin or Ca^{2+} supplementation.[390,391] Despite a great deal of evidence in smaller studies, typically in high-risk women, the large NIH-sponsored megatrials have been unsuccessful in showing benefit from these inexpensive preventive measures. In addition, since aspirin tends to delay parturition and increase the likelihood of bleeding, few obstetricians routinely recommend it.

Treatment of elevated BP during pregnancy traditionally has begun with bed rest, followed by methyldopa as the primary drug, based on its long history of efficacy and lack of adverse

TABLE 51-29 Factors Associated with Altered Risk of Preeclampsia

Genetic markers
Angiotensinogen gene polymorphism
Tumor necrosis factor–alpha gene polymorphism
Mitochondrial transfer RNA gene mutation
Congenital thrombophelias
Resistance to activated protein C (factor V Leiden, perhaps the most common form of hereditary prothrombotic disorder)
Mutation in gene for prothrombin factor II
Hyperhomocysteinemia (mutation C677T)
Protein S deficiency
Antiphospholipid antibody syndrome
Protein C and antithrombin deficiencies

SOURCE: Adapted from Shear R, Leduc L, Rey E, Moutquin J-M. Hypertension in pregnancy: New recommendations for management. *Curr Hypertens Reports* 1999; 1:529–539.

effects on babies. For severe hypertension (BP >160 or 169/109 mmHg) in outpatients that is not controlled with these measures to a diastolic BP between 90 and 100 mmHg, hydralazine, labetalol, and nifedipine routinely are added in succession.[392,393] Angiotensin-converting enzyme inhibitors and ARBs are contraindicated because of renal abnormalities in the fetus, and diuretics typically are avoided because of the risk for oligohydramnios. For intrapartum management, until delivery can be achieved, intravenous Mg^{2+} sulfate has been a mainstay for the prevention of progression of preeclampsia to seizures and other more serious complications.

Hypertension during pregnancy also carries prognostic significance for future health problems as the woman ages. Sixty percent of women with early-onset preeclampsia have abnormalities on renal biopsy and a higher risk of persistent hypertension after delivery. Women who develop hypertension during pregnancy not only are at higher risk for hypertension later in life but also have a roughly twofold increase in the risk of death from CAD.

Hypertensive Emergencies and Urgencies Although great strides have been made in the treatment of hypertension since the First Report of the Joint National Committee on Detection, Evaluation, and Treatment of High Blood Pressure in 1977, some patients still present to physicians' offices and emergency departments with hypertensive crises.[393] Fortunately, there now are excellent medications available for both acute, in-hospital treatment and outpatient management; these improvements have led to a decrease in the 1-year mortality rate after a hypertensive emergency from 80 percent (1928) to 50 percent (1955) to only 10 percent (Fig. 51-1).

The primary pathophysiologic abnormality in patients who experience hypertensive crises is the alteration of autoregulation in certain vascular beds (especially cerebral and renal), which often is followed by frank arteritis and ischemia in vital organs.[394] Autoregulation is the ability of blood vessels to dilate or constrict to maintain normal organ perfusion. Normal arteries from normotensive individuals can maintain flow over a wide range of mean arterial pressures, usually 60 to 150 mmHg. Chronic elevations of BP cause compensatory functional and structural changes in the arterial circulation and shift the autoregulatory curve to the right; this allows hypertensive patients to maintain normal perfusion and avoid excessive blood flow at higher BP levels.[395] When BP increases above the autoregulatory range, tissue damage occurs. An understanding of autoregulation is also important for therapy, since the sudden lowering of BP into a range that would otherwise be considered normal may reduce BP below the autoregulatory capacity of the hypertensive circulation and lead to inadequate tissue perfusion (Fig. 51-2). In the later stages of a hypertensive crisis, pathologists can demonstrate cerebral edema and both acute and chronic inflammation of the medium and small arteries and arterioles, often associated with necrosis.

Hypertensive crises occur in a variety of clinical settings. The most common is a chronic and often untreated patient with stage 3 essential hypertension (i.e., usual BP ≥ 180/110) whose BP rises above the autoregulatory range, triggering the pathophysiologic sequence outlined above. Identical crises can occur, however, any time there is an acute or rapid rise in BP in a normotensive or minimally hypertensive individual, such as a child or a woman during pregnancy. Hypertensive crises can most easily be recognized by the association of an extremely

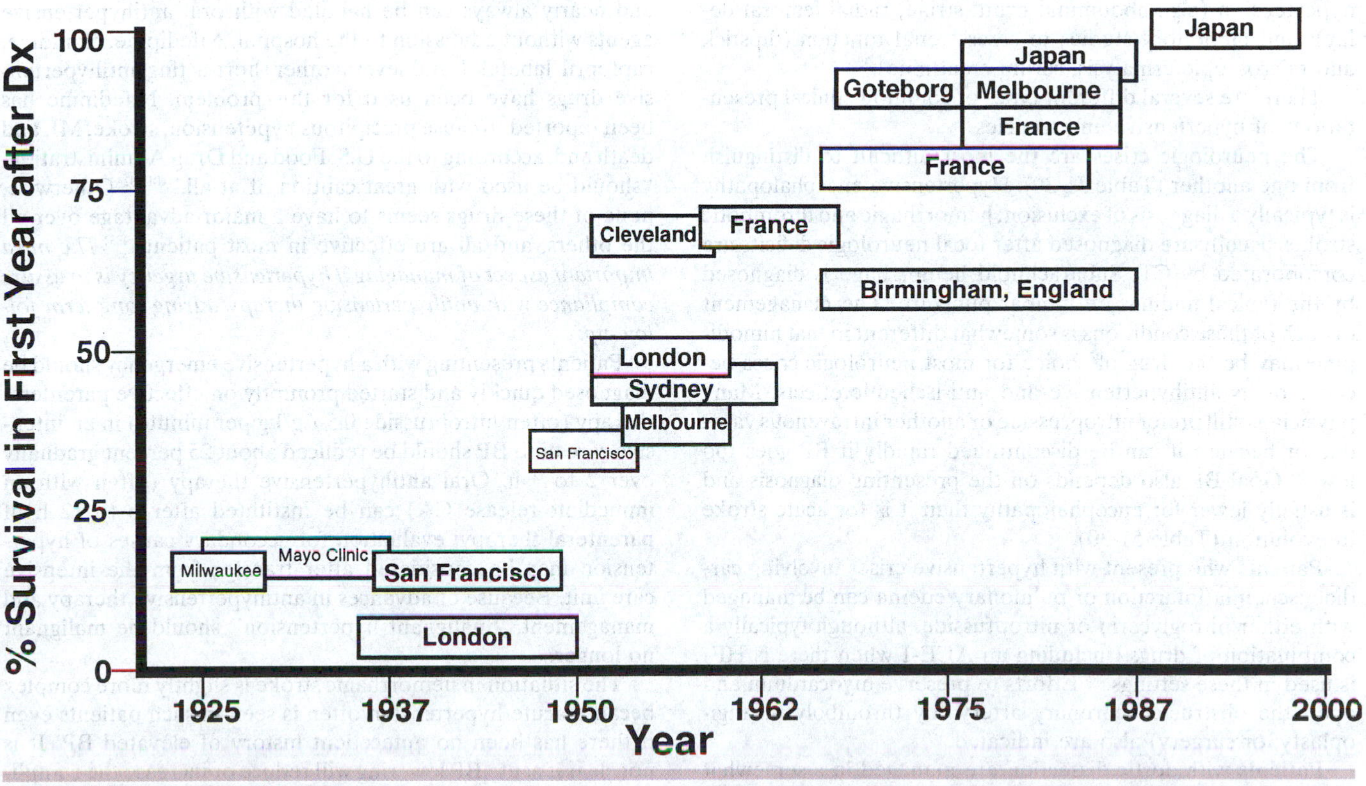

FIGURE 51-1 Improvement in 1-year survival from 1925 to 1999 among patients presenting with a hypertensive emergency. (From Elliott WJ. Hypertensive emergencies. In: Hollenberg SM, Kelly RF, eds. *Critical Care Clinics on Acute Cardiac Care*. New York: Saunders; in press.)

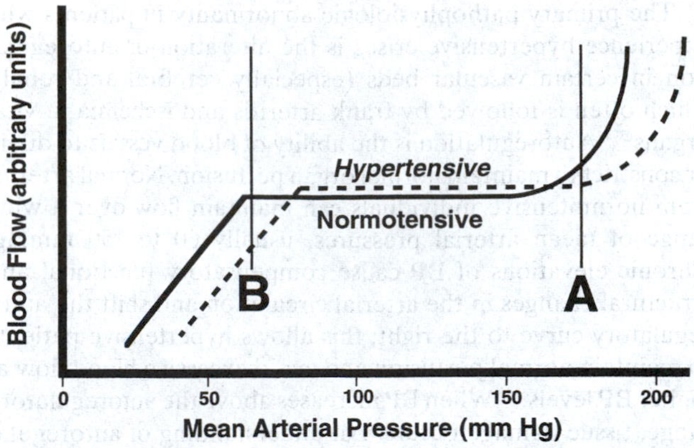

FIGURE 51-2 Blood pressure versus flow relationships in normotensive (*dark curve*) and hypertensive (*dotted curve*) persons, based on cerebral blood flow data of Strandgaard et al.[395] Chronically hypertensive persons can autoregulate their blood flow within the normal range despite higher blood pressures (e.g., vertical line "B"). Lowering BP in the setting of a hypertensive emergency to what might be considered "normal" (in a normotensive person, e.g., vertical line A) probably will put BP below the autoregulatory threshold and may compromise local circulation.

elevated BP with physical examination or laboratory findings that indicate acute TOD. The actual levels of BP are of little import.

The initial evaluation of a severely hypertensive patient includes a thorough inspection of the optic fundi (looking for acute hemorrhages, exudates, or papilledema); a mental status assessment; a careful cardiac, pulmonary, and neurologic examination; a quick search for clues that might indicate secondary hypertension (e.g., abdominal bruit, striae, radial-femoral delay); and laboratory studies to assess renal function (dipstick and microscopic urinalysis, serum creatinine).[394]

There are several different types of common clinical presentations of hypertensive emergencies.

The neurologic crises are the most difficult to distinguish from one another (Table 51-30). Hypertensive encephalopathy is typically a diagnosis of exclusion; hemorrhagic and thrombotic strokes usually are diagnosed after focal neurologic deficits are corroborated by CT. Subarachnoid hemorrhage is diagnosed by the typical findings on lumbar puncture. The management of each of these conditions is somewhat different in that nimodipine may be the drug of choice for most neurologic crises because of its antihypertensive and anti-ischemic effects. Many physicians still prefer nitroprusside or another intravenous vasodilator because it can be discontinued rapidly if BP goes too low.[396] Goal BP also depends on the presenting diagnosis and is usually lower for encephalopathy than it is for acute stroke in evolution (Table 51-30).

Patients who present with hypertensive crises involving cardiac ischemia/infarction or pulmonary edema can be managed with either nitroglycerin or nitroprusside, although typically a combination of drugs (including an ACE-I when there is HF) is used in these settings.[396] Efforts to preserve myocardium and open the obstructed coronary artery (by thrombolysis, angioplasty, or surgery) also are indicated.

Patients with aortic dissection are managed in a somewhat different fashion.[397] A beta blocker is added to the intravenous vasodilator, and the goal BP is much lower: Typically 120 mmHg systolic is recommended, but 100 mmHg systolic may be even better. Pharmacologic therapy is only a temporary adjunct to definitive surgical therapy, which should be planned with dispatch, although long-term medical therapy may be more appropriate in some patients.[398]

Hypertensive crises involving the kidney commonly are followed by a further deterioration in renal function even when BP is lowered properly. Some physicians prefer fenoldopam to nicardipine or nitroprusside in this setting because of its lack of toxic metabolites and specific renal vasodilating effects.[396,399,400] Blood pressure should be reduced about 10 percent during the first hour and a further 10 to 15 percent during the next 1 to 3 h. The need for acute dialysis often is precipitated by BP reduction, but many patients are able to avoid dialysis in the long term if BP is carefully and well controlled during follow-up.

Hypertensive crises resulting from catecholamine excess states [pheochromocytoma, monoamine oxidase (MAO) inhibitor crisis, cocaine intoxication, etc.] are best managed with an intravenous alpha blocker (phentolamine), with the beta blocker added later, if necessary. Many patients with severe hypertension caused by sudden withdrawal of antihypertensive agents (e.g., clonidine) are easily managed by reinstituting such therapy.

Hypertensive crises during pregnancy must be managed in a more careful and conservative manner because of the presence of the fetus. Magnesium sulfate, methyldopa, and hydralazine are the drugs of choice, with oral labetalol and nifedipine being drugs of second choice in the United States. Delivery of the infant often assists in the management of hypertension in pregnancy and often is hastened by the obstetrician under these conditions.

Hypertensive urgencies are situations in which acute TOD is not present; they require somewhat less aggressive management and nearly always can be handled with oral antihypertensive agents without admission to the hospital. Nifedipine, clonidine, captopril, labetalol, and several other short-acting antihypertensive drugs have been used for this problem. Nifedipine has been reported to cause precipitous hypotension, stroke, MI, and death and, according to the U.S. Food and Drug Administration, "should be used with great caution, if at all."[401,402] Otherwise, none of these drugs seems to have a major advantage over all the others, and all are effective in most patients.[403] *The most important aspect of managing a hypertensive urgency is to assure compliance with antihypertensive therapy during long-term follow-up.*

Patients presenting with a hypertensive emergency should be diagnosed quickly and started promptly on effective parenteral therapy (often nitroprusside 0.5 μg/kg per minute) in an intensive care unit. BP should be reduced about 25 percent gradually over 2 to 3 h. Oral antihypertensive therapy (often with an immediate-release CA) can be instituted after 6 to 12 h of parenteral therapy; evaluation for secondary causes of hypertension may be considered after transfer from the intensive care unit. Because of advances in antihypertensive therapy and management, "malignant hypertension" should be malignant no longer.

The situation in hemorrhagic stroke is slightly more complex because acute hypertension often is seen in such patients even if there has been no antecedent history of elevated BP. It is not clear if acute BP lowering will reduce or increase the complication rates (from worsened cerebral ischemia in other areas or making a zone surrounding the hemorrhage ischemic). As a result, it is recommended not to treat hypertension beyond a

TABLE 51-30 Types of Hypertension Crises with Suggested Drug Therapy and BP Targets

Type of Crisis	Drug of Choice	BP Target
Neurologic		
Hypertensive encephalopathy	Nitroprusside[a]	25% reduction in mean arterial pressure over 2–3 h
Intracranial hemorrhage or acute stroke in evolution	Nitroprusside[a] (controversial)	0–25% reduction in mean arterial pressure over 6–12 h (controversial)
Acute head injury/trauma	Nitroprusside[a]	0–25% reduction in mean arterial pressure over 2–3 h (controversial)
Subarachnoid hemorrhage	Nimodipine	Up to 25% reduction in mean arterial pressure in previously hypertensive patients, 130–160 systolic in normotensive patients
Cardiac		
Ischemia/infarction	Nitroglycerin or nicardipine	Reduction in ischemia
Heart failure	Nitroprusside[a] or nitroglycerin	Improvement in failure (typically 10–15% decrease in BP)
Aortic dissection	Beta blocker plus nitroprusside[a]	120 mmHg systolic in 30 min (if possible)
Renal		
Hematuria or acute renal impairment	Fenoldopam	0–25% reduction in mean arterial pressure over 1–12 h
Catecholamine excess states		
Pheochromocytoma	Phentolamine	To control paroxysms
Drug withdrawal	Drug withdrawn	Typically only one dose necessary
Pregnancy-related		
eclampsia	$MgSO_4$, methyldopa, hydralazine	Typically <90 mmHg diastolic but often lower

[a]Some physicians prefer an intravenous infusion or either fenoldopam or nicardipine, neither of which has potentially toxic metabolites, to nitroprusside. Recent studies have shown improvements in renal function during therapy with the former compared to nitroprusside.
SOURCE: Updated from Elliott WJ, Black HR. Hypertension crises. In: Parillo JE, Bone RC, eds. *Clinical Care Medicine: Principles of Diagnosis and Management.* Philadelphia: Mosby Year Book; 1990:565.

mean arterial pressure of >130 mmHg, and even then it is controlled rather more slowly into an intermediate range (e.g., 160/100 mmHg). Some have claimed that previously hypertensive patients with acute intracerebral hemorrhage should be managed even less aggressively.

Appropriate BP reduction in the setting of acute subarachnoid hemorrhage is even more controversial.[379] Even associating higher BP levels with higher rates of rebleeding has been difficult. If BP lowering is desired (e.g., if mean arterial pressure is >130 mmHg), a short-acting intravenous drug (e.g., nitroprusside) typically is recommended, since it can be discontinued quickly and the patient can be given fluids to restore the previous BP level if the neurologic status worsens.

DOSE SCHEDULE (DOSAGE AND CHRONOTHERAPY)

It is clear that BP needs to be controlled for 24 h. Preparations that are active once a day are easier for patients to remember to take, but adherence to treatment may not be substantially worse if twice-a-day preparations are used. In fact, patients may be better protected if they fail to remember to take one dose of a twice-a-day medication and be uncovered for 12 hours than if they skip a once-a-day pill and are unprotected for a considerably longer period.

In addition to "controlling BP" over 24 h, regimens should pay some attention to the circadian rhythm of BP and HR. Many of the sequelae of hypertension have a strong circadian variation, with a peak incidence in the early morning. Recent meta-analyses have quantitated the excess risk of heart attack during the period from 6 A.M. to noon at 40 percent, sudden cardiac death at 29 percent, and stroke at 49 percent compared with what would be expected if these events happened evenly or randomly throughout the day.[404,405] Since most patients administer antihypertensive agents in the morning, most authorities recommend long-acting drugs that should cover the early-morning period, when blood pressure, pulse, and cardiovascular risk are highest. Although many of the currently used medications have short intrinsic elimination half-lives, pharmaceutical technology has made available several methods of making sustained-release compounds from short-acting drugs.[406,407]

Recently, a chronobiological approach to antihypertensive therapy has become available.[407] This is currently available only for two preparations of verapamil.[408] These drug-delivery systems release active drug for 18 to 20 h, beginning between 2 A.M. and 4 A.M., leaving the patient with no active drug in the circulation from about 10 P.M. to 2 A.M. The rationale for this approach is that BP falls normally at night coincident with the usual circadian rhythm and active drug might cause excessive lowering of BP during the middle of the night.[409] These sustained-release preparations provide adequate active drug as the BP rises before awakening and during the peak time of CV events (the period between 6 A.M. and noon). The same matching of drug delivery to BP is not achieved by giving "homeostatically" designed drugs (i.e., all the others) at night. Such agents were designed for morning use, and giving them at night causes the risk of lowering BP too far during sleep.[198]

The putative advantage of such a system is that it would not excessively lower BP during sleep (when BP is typically at its nadir anyway) and would deliver an agent that is both hypotensive and HR-lowering at the time of day when BP, HR, and CV risk are nearly maximal.[198] The long-term consequences of this strategy are being tested in the CONVINCE trial with 16,602 subjects; conclusions may be available in 2002.[322]

DRUG INTERACTIONS

The selection of the initial agent to treat hypertension must be done with the understanding that many hypertensive patients may not reach goal BP on that agent alone and will therefore need additional antihypertensive therapy. Furthermore, many hypertensive patients need to take medications for other conditions, and so the problem of drug–drug interactions is particularly pertinent.

Certain combinations of antihypertensive agents are particularly effective, such as thiazide diuretics with beta blockers, ACE-Is, or ARBs.[380] Combinations of ACE-Is with CAs (both DHP and non-DHP) are also effective. Moreover, combinations of the two subtypes of CAs are synergistic with regard to BP reduction.[409] Dihydropyridine CAs and beta blockers are also very effective combinations. Nondihydropyridine CAs and beta blockers should not be used because of the risk of excessive bradycardia and conduction defects. Thiazide diuretics are also effective with all other antihypertensive drugs, including CAs, and always should be included in a triple-drug regimen. Little is known about the efficacy of combining alpha blockers with central and peripheral sympatholytics or with ACE-Is or ARBs.

Recently, a series of low-dose fixed-dose combinations have been introduced that have fewer clinical side effects than occur when the components are used as monotherapy (Table 51-21). The best example is the combination of a DHP CA with an ACE-I. These fixed-dose combinations have a significantly lower incidence of edema than that seen when a DHP CA is given alone.[380] The incidence of cough, however, is not lessened when these drugs are combined. The appeal of a low-dose fixed-dose combination is that BP can be reduced further with fewer adverse reactions with two drugs at lower doses than might occur when one or the other component is pushed to the full dose. The added advantage is that the patient needs to take fewer pills to get BP to goal and so adherence to the regimen tends to improve (see below).

Most commonly used antihypertensives do not have any serious drug–drug interactions with anticoagulants, platelet inhibitors, or antibiotics. Nondihydropyridine CAs, beta blockers, and possibly telmisartan (an ARB) must be used with care in patients who are taking digitalis preparations.[381] Nonsteroidal anti-inflammatory agents may raise BP and interfere with the activity of all antihypertensive agents because of their Na^+-retaining properties.[410]

ADHERENCE

Fewer than 50 percent of patients continue taking the initially prescribed antihypertensive drug therapy for a year.[411,412] The proportion who properly adhere to therapy improves only modestly when the drugs and medical care are provided free of charge. Recent estimates indicate that about 10 percent of the overall expenditures on hypertension in the United States are wasted because of nonadherence to medical advice and antihypertensive drug therapy.[413] Patients who do not follow the advice of their physicians and do not take their medications correctly have an *infinite* cost/benefit ratio because they incur all the cost associated with the therapy but derive *none* of the benefits of treatment.

TABLE 51-31 Strategies to Improve Medication Adherence

Educate patient regarding proper use of medications
Improve patient's social support network (e.g., spouse or caretaker)
Increase patient's autonomy and involvement in decision making (when appropriate)
Remove barriers to compliance with pill taking
Integrate into activities of daily living (e.g., brushing teeth)
Avoid large ("horse") pills
Avoid bad-tasting formulations (e.g., lactulose, quinine)
Simplify the therapeutic regimen
Minimize number of pills
Minimize frequency of pill taking
Minimize inconvenience of pill taking
Provide positive attitude and positive reinforcement about achieving therapeutic goals
Maintain continuity of care with same practitioner
Use well-tolerated antihypertensive drug therapy individualized for each patient

Assessing adherence with antihypertensive medications is generally difficult, but several simple measures often are recommended.[11,38,414] Some medications induce physical signs that are absent in those who have not recently taken them, e.g., bradycardia with beta blockers, orthostatic BP change with alpha blockers, and an increase in serum urate with diuretics. A telephone call to the patient's pharmacy generally will reveal how many times the prescribed medications have been refilled during the last year.[415] Several interventions have been advocated to improve adherence with medications (Table 51-31).

There is concern, however, that administering long-acting drugs will lower blood pressure to a relatively constant degree during the day and night. This may lead to hypoperfusion of vital organs during the night that will not be symptomatic.[408]

MECHANISM OF ACTION OF THE DRUG AND PATHOPHYSIOLOGY OF THE PATIENT'S HYPERTENSION

Some have felt that physicians could be much more successful in treating hypertensive patients if they could base therapy on the reason why the patient is hypertensive (the pathophysiologic abnormality responsible for the patient's hypertension) and match that information to the mechanism of action of antihypertensive drugs. If physcians truly could know precisely why an individual was hypertensive and easily and safely obtain such information, treating hypertension would be not be complicated. If it really were known exactly how drugs work, those decisions would be much simpler. This approach, while intellectually appealing, has problems.

The first difficulty is that attempts to profile patients either biochemically using PRA, for example, or hemodynamically by measuring cardiac output and peripheral vascular resistance are too expensive and potentially invasive to do in everyone. In addition, these methods are not precise enough to provide the kind of necessarily definitive information needed to predict the response to therapy in a particular patient. Furthermore, trying to base therapy on the presumed pathophysiology in an individual or group of individuals would be expected to have is also imprecise. This approach runs the risk of denying certain patients the potential benefits of certain classes of drugs. Although it is true that blacks and older persons tend on the average to have low or suppressed PRA, many do not. Also, many patients with a low PRA will respond to drugs, such as ACE-Is or ARBs, that are less effective on the average in hypertensives with this renin profile. In the VA trial of monotherapy, selecting initial treatment on the basis of PRA was less effective than simply using age and ethnicity (thiazide diuretics and CAs for older patients and blacks and ACE-Is and beta blockers for whites and in those less than 60 years of age).[382] However, neither method correctly predicted a good response in more than 63 percent of the patients.

The second issue that complicates this approach is that many, if not all, drugs have more complex mechanisms of action than they were originally thought to have and work well in patient subgroups in whom they were supposed to be ineffective. For example, thiazide diuretics not only reduce plasma volume but also are vasodilators after 4 weeks of therapy. It should not have been surprising that these agents are effective and very well tolerated in older persons even though many of those patients tend to have a modestly decreased plasma volume compared with younger hypertensives. Although it is true that ACE-Is usually suppress the endocrine RAA system, the antihypertensive effect is still evident even when plasma AII concentration returns to pretreatment levels. This is good evidence that there is a tissue site of action for these drugs or that other mechanisms, perhaps the stimulation of bradykinin or NO, participate in how ACE-Is lower BP and that the initial formulation of their mechanism of action was incomplete. This also explains why some patients with low PRA (a measure of the activity of the *endocrine* RAA system) respond well to these agents or to ARBs, which suppress the RAA system at the angiotensin AT_1 receptor in tissues throughout the body. Calcium antagonists were presumed to work best in older hypertensives and in those with suppressed PRA, but these agents are equally effective in all subgroups of hypertensives.[237]

Perhaps the major flaw in the reasoning that drugs can be used to "probe" the pathophysiologic abnormality causing a patient's hypertension is the concept that there is one overriding abnormality responsible for that patient's elevated BP. In all likelihood, more than one, if not many, of the systems that control BP, many of which are discussed in this chapter, are dysfunctional simultaneously and single or combinations of pharmacologic agents that reduce BP do so by correcting more than one abnormality.[10]

The choice of initial therapy therefore should be based primarily on evidence from clinical trials that document a reduction in CV events and/or renal disease progression. However, despite the fact that one cannot precisely determine the mechanism or mechanisms of action of drugs and that it is impossible to elucidate precisely why a particular patient is hypertensive, the empirical approach to treating hypertension dramatically reduced the rate of stroke and CAD after physicians began to treat hypertension aggressively. This approach, though far from perfect, has paid dividends.

COST

The economics of hypertension and its therapy are complex, but the simple fact is that if a person cannot afford to pay for the drug chosen by the health care provider, the completed prescription will do little good in the long term.[52,53] Many pharmacists and businesspeople associated with health care believe that the agent with the lowest purchase price is the best, but this oversimplification omits the costs of extra visits to health care providers, laboratory testing, and adverse drug experiences that result in emergency room visits or hospitalization.[415] Such global evaluations of the economics of hypertension and its therapy are rare. It is possible for a more expensive but better-tolerated drug (e.g., an ARB) to actually be less expensive in the long term than another agent that produces many side effects, some of which must be evaluated by laboratory testing, physician visits, and even hospitalization. There is also the possibility that some of the newer (and currently more expensive) agents are more effective in lowering BP and reducing cardiovascular events (which currently account for 82 percent of expenditures related to hypertension in the United States) than are some of the older agents; this alone may be sufficient to make them more cost-effective than the time-tested agents.

Generically available drugs are usually less expensive to purchase than their branded counterparts and are strongly favored in most managed care pharmacy plans by both mandates to physicians and lower copayments by patients.[416] Some organized health care plans insist that the first month of antihypertensive therapy always involve a low-dose thiazide diuretic because of its proven efficacy and low cost. Although JNC VI "favored" low-dose diuretics and beta blockers for uncomplicated hypertension, it did, for the first time, suggest that hypertensives with another "compelling condition" would benefit even more from other classes of antihypertensive agents. There are now more data to suggest that in the long term it matters more what BP level is achieved during treatment than which agent is chosen initially to begin the lowering.

Many authorities are concerned that achieving the new, lower target BPs for diabetic and renally impaired hypertensives will cost more, as it will require more visits to health care providers and more antihypertensive medications. These increases in short-term expenditures are likely, however, to be offset by a lower future incidence of expensive outcomes, including heart attack, stroke, ESRD, and HF, at least for diabetic patients over age 60 in the United States.[332]

Many proposals for reducing the high cost of antihypertensive therapy have been advanced. JNC VI has suggested withholding drug therapy for 6 to 12 months from those at low risk (risk groups A and B) with stage 1 hypertension and giving it instead to patients in risk group C with BP ≥130/85 mmHg.[11] In stage 2 to 3 hypertension, wider use of combination drug tablets has been advocated, as these tablets typically cost much less than two separate prescriptions for the same doses of individual agents. Some formularies and pharmacy benefits managers prefer agents that have all doses priced identically, with the theory that a pill splitter can then be used to divide one tablet into two or more days' treatment. Aggressive health care plans have implemented strategies that prohibit the use of more expensive medications (e.g., ARBs) unless two physicians independently ascribe an adverse effect to a less expensive drug (e.g., an ACE-I), and others require three separate ACE-Is to be administered sequentially before an ARB can be dispensed.

Until a universal pharmacy benefits program is instituted, there are likely to be wide variations in the pricing and cost of antihypertensive agents. Although it is difficult for physicians to stay abreast of fluctuations in these costs, it is important that all health care providers attempt to provide tolerable antihypertensive medications at the lowest possible cost for the benefit of the patient, the health plan, and the national budget.

SUMMARY AND RECOMMENDATIONS

Although there are numerous options and many sources of error, the successful pharmacologic treatment of a hypertensive patient need not be too complicated, although it also should not be oversimplified. Once the diagnosis has been established and the routine evaluation and any more complex tests believed to be necessary have been completed, lifestyle modification should begin. Lifestyle modification should be given time to work unless the patient is in a group for which drug therapy is indicated (together with lifestyle modifications at the initiation of treatment). Drug therapy is indicated in all hypertensive patients if goal BP is not reached with lifestyle modification alone.

The following steps are recommended for choosing a regimen and then altering it until the goal is reached:

- Deal first with cost. If the patient is unable to afford any but the least expensive drugs or cannot pay for the one that is selected, price becomes the primary issue.
- Ascertain whether other risk factors or comorbidity is present. Avoid drugs that may worsen these factors or conditions and choose the ones that may tend to improve them.
- Find out what clinical adverse reactions the patient would find the most troublesome and avoid agents that are more likely to cause or exacerbate these problems. Some patients are not concerned by certain side effects that are very troublesome for others.
- Consider demographic issues and select the class of drug with a higher probability of success if options are available.
- Start with the lowest effective dose and plan to see the patient within 2 to 4 weeks unless the severity of the patient's hypertension or another problem warrants an earlier visit. Carry out appropriate biochemical monitoring when necessary. In some patients, start with a fixed-dose combination when it appears appropriate.
- Increase the dose if goal BP has not been reached or if there has been only a minimal response. Do not increase the first dose or any dose prematurely. Give each dose adequate time to be fully effective. If intolerable side effects occur and are likely to be drug-related or if there has been no response, only then switch to another appropriate agent for monotherapy.
- Continue the process of dose titration and monitoring until the maximum recommended dose has been reached. Stopping before the full dose has been reached leads to a situation in which the patient is treated with multiple agents at subtherapeutic doses when only one or two drugs are necessary.
- If the drug of first choice fails to reduce BP to goal, add a second agent that has a different mechanism of action and is known to have additive antihypertensive effects to the first-choice agent. A fixed-dose combination that combines two drugs in the desired doses also could be used at this time.
- Titrate the second drug to the full dose, as was done for the first drug, and continue appropriate monitoring. If the two-drug combination fails, consider a specific cause for the patient's refractory hypertension, and if none is evident, add a third drug, being sure that a diuretic is part of the regimen. Consider a referral to a hypertension specialist.
- Plan to see a patient who is at goal at least once every 3 months to be sure that BP control is sustained.
- Reinforce the need for adherence to the regimen and always question each patient carefully about adverse reactions. Although some patients will not reach goal with this approach even with the many effective treatment options that are available, most will come under control or close to it. Patients who do this can anticipate substantial long-term benefit with an extended life expectancy and a much reduced risk of stroke, ischemic heart disease, HF, and probably renal failure and dementia.

CONCLUSION

Although treating high BP can be costly and at times seem unrewarding, the benefits to individual patients and to society make the effort worthwhile. Physicians must be careful not to become apathetic about hypertension. The problem has not been solved and will not be solved until all hypertensive patients are able to avail themselves of what has been among the most successful examples of preventive medicine.

References

1. Murray CJ, Lope AD. Evidence-based health policy—lessons from the Global Burden of Disease Study. *Science* 1996; 274(5288):740–743.
2. Kannel WB. Blood pressure as a cardiovascular risk factor: Prevention and treatment. *JAMA* 1996; 275:1571–1576.
3. MacMahon S, Rodgers A. The epidemiological association between blood pressure and stroke: Implications for primary and secondary prevention. *Hypertens Res* 1994; 17(suppl I):S23–S32.
4. Klag MJ, Whelton PK, Randall BL, et al. Blood pressure and end-stage renal disease in men. *N Engl J Med* 1996; 334:13–18.
5. Criqui MH, Langer RD, Fronek A, et al. Large vessel and isolated small vessel peripheral arterial disease. In: Fowkes FCR, ed. *Epidemiology of Peripheral Vascular Disease.* Ireland: Springer-Verlag; 1991:85.
6. Xie L, Wu K, Xu N, et al. Hypertension is associated with a high risk of cancer. *J Hum Hypertens* 1999; 13(5):295–301.
7. Rosengren A, Himmelmann A, Wihelmsen L, et al. Hypertension and long-term cancer incidence and mortality among Swedish men. *J Hypertens* 1998; 16(7):933–940.
8. Hamet P. Cancer and hypertension: A potential for crosswalk? *J Hypertens* 1997; 15(12 part 2):1573–1577.
9. Grossman E, Messerli FH, Goldbourt U. Does diuretic therapy increase the risk of renal cell carcinoma? *Am J Cardiol* 1999; 83(7):1090–1093.
10. Page IH. The mosaic theory. In: Page IH, ed. *Hypertension Mechanisms.* Orlando, FL: Grune & Stratton; 1987:910.
11. The Sixth Report of the Joint National Committee on Prevention, Detection, Evaluation, and Treatment of High Blood Pressure (JNC VI). *Arch Intern Med* 1997; 157:2413–2446.
12. Berlowitz DR, Ash AS, Hickey EC, et al. Inadequate management of blood pressure in a hypertensive population. *N Engl J Med* 1998; 339(27):1957–1963.

13. Colhoun HM, Dong W, Poulter NR. Blood pressure screening, management, and control in England: Results from the health survey for England 1994. *J Hypertens* 1998; 16:747–752.
14. De Backer G, Myny K, De Henauw S, et al. Prevalence, awareness, treatment and control of arterial hypertension in an elderly population in Belgium. *J Hum Hypertens* 1998; 12:701–706.
15. Stergiou GS, Thomopoulou GC, Skeva I, Moutokalakis TD. Prevalence, awareness, treatment, and control of hypertension in Greece: The Didima study. *Am J Hypertens* 1999; 12:959–965.
16. Joffres MR, Ghardirian P, Fondor JG, et al. Awareness, treatment, and control of hypertension in Canada. *Am J Hypertens* 1997; 10:1097–1102.
17. Zanchetti A. Antihypertensive therapy: Pride and prejudice. *J Hypertens* 1995; 13:1522–1528.
18. 1999 World Health Organization–International Society of Hypertension Guidelines for the Management of Hypertension: Guidelines Subcommittee. *J Hypertens* 1999; 17(2):151–183.
19. Ramsay LE, Williams B, Johnston GD, et al. British Hypertension Society guidelines for hypertension management 1999: Summary. *BMJ* 1999; 319:630–635.
20. Pickering T. Recommendations for use of home (self) and ambulatory blood pressure monitoring: American Society of Hypertension Ad Hoc Panel. *Am J Hypertens* 1996; 9:1–11.
21. Tsuji I, Imai Y, Nagai K, et al. Proposal of reference values for home blood pressure measurement: Prognostic criteria based on a prospective observation of the general population in Ohasama, Japan. *Am J Hypertens* 1997; 10:409–418.
22. Black HR, Yi JY. A new classification for hypertension based on relative and absolute risk with implications for treatment and reimbursement. *Hypertension* 1996; 28:719–724.
23. Kannel WB. Blood pressure as a cardiovascular risk factor: Prevention and treatment. *JAMA* 1996; 275(20):1571–1576.
24. Van den Hoogen PCW, Feskens EJM, Nagelkerke NJD, et al., for the Seven Countries Study Research Group. The relation between blood pressure and mortality due to coronary heart disease among men in different parts of the world. *N Engl J Med* 2000; 342:1–8.
25. Cholesterol, diastolic blood pressure, and stroke: 13,000 strokes in 450,000 people in 45 prospective cohorts: Prospective studies collaboration. *Lancet* 1995; 346(8991–8992):1647–1653.
26. MacMahon S, Peto R, Cutler J, et al. Blood pressure, stroke, and coronary heart disease: I. Prolonged differences in blood pressure: Prospective observational studies corrected for the regression dilution bias. *Lancet* 1990; 335(8692):756–774.
27. Stamler J, Stamler R, Neaton JD. Blood pressure, systolic and diastolic, and cardiovascular risks: US population data. *Arch Intern Med* 1993; 153:598–615.
28. Psaty BM, Furberg CD, Kuller LH, et al. Isolated systolic hypertension and subclinical CVD in the elderly: Initial findings from the Cardiovascular Health Study. *JAMA* 1992; 268:1287–1291.
29. Lee ML, Rosner BA, Weiss ST. Relationship of blood pressure to cardiovascular death: The effects of pulse pressure in the elderly. *Ann Epidemiol* 1999; 9:101–107.
30. Collins R, Peto R, MacMahon S, et al. Blood pressure, stroke, and coronary heart disease: II. Short-term reductions in blood pressure: Overview of randomized drug trials in their epidemiologic context. *Lancet* 1990; 335:827–838.
31. Blood pressure, cholesterol, and stroke in eastern Asia: Eastern Stroke and Coronary Heart Disease Collaborative Research Group. *Lancet* 1998; 352(9143):1801–1807.
32. Kannel WB, Gordon T, Castelli WP, Margolis JR. Electrocardiographic left ventricular hypertrophy and risk of coronary heart disease: The Framingham Study. *Ann Intern Med* 1970; 72:813–822.
33. Kuller LH, Shemanski L, Psaty BM, et al. Subclinical disease as an independent risk factor for cardiovascular disease. *Circulation* 1995; 92:720–726.
34. Kannel WB. Risk stratification in hypertension: New insights from the Framingham Study. *Am J Hypertens* 2000; 13:3S–10S.
35. Ferrannini E, Natali A, Capaldo B, et al. Insulin resistance, hyperinsulinemia, and blood pressure. *Hypertension* 1997; 30:1144–1149.
36. Kannel WB, Gordon T, Schwartz MJ. Systolic versus diastolic blood pressure and risk of coronary heart disease: The Framingham Study. *Am J Cardiol* 1971; 27:335–346.
37. Black HR, Kuller LH, O'Rourke MF, et al. The first report of the Systolic and Pulse Pressure (SYPP) Working Group on systolic and pulse pressure. *J Hypertens* 1999; 17(suppl 5):S3–S14.
38. Joint National Committee on Detection, Evaluation, and Treatment of High Blood Pressure. The Fifth Report of the Joint National Committee on Detection, Evaluation, and Treatment of High Blood Pressure (JNC V). *Arch Intern Med* 1993; 153:154–183.
39. Fisher CM. The ascendancy of diastolic blood pressure over systolic. *Lancet* 1985; 2:1349–1350.
40. Black HR. The paradigm has shifted, to systolic blood pressure. *Hypertension* 1999; 34:386–387.
41. Madhavan S, Ooi WL, Cohen J, Alderman MH. Relation of pulse pressure and blood pressure reduction to the incidence of myocardial infarction. *Hypertension* 1994; 23:395–401.
42. Pannier B, Brunel P, el Aroussy WE, et al. Pulse pressure and echocardiographic findings in essential hypertension. *J Hypertens* 1989; 7:127–132.
43. Verdecchia P, Schillaci G, Borgioni C, et al. Ambulatory pulse pressure: A potent predictor of total cardiovascular risk in hypertension. *Hypertension* 1998; 32:983–988.
44. Benetos A, Safar M, Rudnichi A, et al. Pulse pressure: A predictor of long-term cardiovascular mortality in a French male population. *Hypertension* 1997; 30:1410–1415.
45. Benetos A, Rudnichi A, Safar M, Guise L. Pulse pressure and cardiovascular mortality in normotensive and hypertensive subjects. *Hypertension* 1998; 32:560–564.
46. Franklin SS, Khan SA, Wong ND, et al. Is pulse pressure useful in predicting risk for coronary heart disease? The Framingham Heart Study. *Circulation* 1999; 100:354–360.
47. Izzo JL, Levy D, Black HR. Clinical advisory statement: Importance of systolic blood pressure in older Americans. *Hypertension* 2000; 35:1021–1024.
48. Messerli FH, Weber MA, Brunner HR. Angiotensin II receptor inhibition: A new therapeutic principle. *Arch Intern Med* 1996; 156:1957–1965.
49. Bauer JH, Reams GP. The angiotensin II type 1 receptor antagonist: A new class of antihypertensive drugs. *Arch Intern Med* 1995; 155:1361–1368.
50. Grimm RH, Grandits GA, Cutler JA, et al., for the TOMHS Research Group. Relationships of quality of life measures to long-term lifestyle and drug treatment in the Treatment of Mild Hypertension Study. (TOMHS) *Arch Intern Med* 1997; 157: 638–648.
51. Wiklund I, Halling K, Ryden-Bergsten T, Fletcher A. Does lowering the blood pressure improve the mood? Quality-of-life results from the Hypertension Optimal Treatment (HOT) study. *Blood Pressure* 1997; 6(6):357–364.
52. Stason WB. Economic impact of blood pressure. In: Black HR, Izzo JL Jr, eds. *Hypertension Primer*, 2d ed. Dallas, TX: American Heart Association; 1999:286.
53. Elliott WJ. Economic considerations in the management of hypertension. In: Black HR, Izzo JL Jr, eds. *Hypertension Primer,* 2d ed. Dallas, TX: American Heart Association; 1999:289.
54. *American Heart Association's Heart & Stroke Facts. Statistical Supplement.* Dallas, TX: American Heart Association; 2000:24.
55. Elliott WJ. The current inadequate control of hypertension: How

can we do better? In: Kaplan NM, ed. *Hypertension Therapy Annual.* London: Martin Dunitz; 2000:1.

56. Guyton AC, Coleman TG, Cowley AW, et al. Arterial pressure regulation: Overriding dominance of the kidneys. *Am J Med* 1972; 52:584–594.
57. Morimoto S, Sasaki S, Itoh H, et al. Sympathetic activation and contribution of genetic factors in hypertension with neurovascular compression of the rostral ventrolateral medulla. *J Hypertens* 1999; 17(11):1577–1582.
58. Laitinen T, Hartikainen J, Niskanen L, et al. Sympathovagal balance is major determinant of short-term blood pressure variability in healthy subjects. *Am J Physiol* 1999; 276(4 part 2): H1245–H1252.
59. Adamopoulos S, Rosano GM, Ponikowski P, et al. Impaired baroreflex sensitivity and sympathovagal balance in syndrome X. *Am J Cardiol* 1998; 82(7):862–868.
60. DiBona GF, Kopp UC. Neural control of renal function. *Physiol Rev* 1997; 77:76–97.
61. Kurokawa K. Kidney, salt and hypertension: How and why. *Kidney Int* 1996; 49(suppl 55):S46–S51.
62. Muirhead EE. Renal vasodepressor mechanisms: The medullipin system. *J Hypertens* 1993; 5:S53–S58.
63. Julius S, Schork MA. Predictors of hypertension. *Ann NY Acad Sci* 1978; 304:38–58.
64. Julius S, Valentini M. Continuing on J. P. Henry's path: Studies of physiology and pathophysiology of cardiopulmonary receptors in humans. *Acta Physiol Scand Suppl* 1997; 640:122–124.
65. Narkiewicz K, Pesek CA, Kato M, et al. Baroreflex control of sympathetic nerve activity and heart rate in obstructive sleep apnea. *Hypertension* 1998; 32(6):1039–1043.
66. Ryuzaki M, Stahl LK, Lyson T, et al. Sympathoexcitatory response to cyclosporin A and baroreflex resetting. *Hypertension* 1997; 29(2):576–582.
67. Ligtenberg G, Blankestijn PJ, Oey PL, et al. Reduction of sympathetic hyperactivity by enalapril in patients with chronic renal failure. *N Engl J Med* 1999; 340(17):1321–1328.
68. Watanabe K, Sekiya M, Tsuruoka T, et al. Relationship between insulin resistance and cardiac sympathetic nervous function in essential hypertension. *J Hypertens* 1999; 17(8):1161–1168.
69. Yuasa S, Li X, Hitomi H, et al. Sodium sensitivity and sympathetic nervous system in hypertension induced by long-term nitric oxide blockade in rats. *Clin Exp Pharmacol Physiol* 2000; 27(1–2): 18–24.
70. Dahl LK, Heine M, Primary role of renal homografts in setting chronic blood pressure levels in rats. *Circ Res* 1975; 36:692–696.
71. Muntzel M, Drueke T. A comprehensive review of the salt and blood pressure relationship. *Am J Hypertens* 1992; 5:1s–42s.
72. Luft FC, Rankin LI, Bloch R, et al. Cardiovascular and humoral responses to extremes of sodium intake in normal black and white men. *Circulation* 1979; 60:697–706.
73. Folkow B, Ely DL. Cardiovascular and sympathetic effects of 240-fold salt intake variations—studies in rats with implications to man. *Acta Physiol Scand* 1989; 136:89–96.
74. Rettig R, Schmitt B, Pelzl B, Speck T. The kidney and primary hypertension: Contributions from renal transplantation studies in animals and humans. *J Hypertens* 1993; 11(9):883–891.
75. Weir MR. Impact of salt intake on blood pressure and proteinuria in diabetes: Importance of the renin-angiotensin system. *Miner Electrolyte Metab* 1998; 24(6):438–445.
76. Sever PS, Poulter NR. A hypothesis for the pathogenesis of essential hypertension: The initiating factors. *J Hypertens* 1989; 7(suppl 1):9s–12s.
77. Joseph JG, Prior IAM, Salmond CE, Stanley D. Elevation of systolic and diastolic blood pressure associated with migration: The Tokelau Island Migrant Study. *J Chronic Dis* 1983; 36: 507–516.
78. Weinberger M, Fineberg N. Sodium and volume sensitivity of blood pressure: Age and pressure change over time. *Hypertension* 1991; 18:67–71.
79. Sanchez RA, Gimenez MI, Migliorini M, et al. Erythrocyte sodium-lithium countertransport in non-modulating offspring and essential hypertensive individuals: Response to enalapril. *Hypertension* 1997; 30(1 part 1):99–105.
80. Aviv A. Recent advances in cellular Ca^{++} homeostasis: Implications to altered regulations of cellular Ca^{++} and Na^+-H^+ exchange in essential hypertension. *Curr Opin Cardiol* 1996; 11(5):477–482.
81. Cappuccio FP, Markandu ND, Carney C, et al. Double-blind randomized trial of modest salt restriction in older people. *Lancet* 1997; 350(9081):850–854.
82. Wedler G, Brier M, Wiersbitsky M, et al. Sodium kinetics in salt-sensitive and salt-resistant normotensive and hypertensive subjects. *J Hypertens* 1992; 10:663–669.
83. Lifton R. Molecular genetics of human blood pressure variation. *Science* 1996; 272:676–680.
84. Alam S, Johnson AG. A meta-analysis of randomized controlled trials (RCT) among healthy normotensive and essential hypertensive elderly patients to determine the effect of high salt (NaCl) diet of blood pressure. *J Hum Hypertens* 1999; 13(6):367–374.
85. He J, Whelton PK, Appel LJ, et al. Long-term effects of weight loss and dietary sodium reduction on incidence of hypertension. *Hypertension* 2000; 35(2):544–549.
86. Timmermans PB. Angiotensin II receptor antagonists: An emerging new class of cardiovascular therapeutics. *Hypertens Res* 1999; 22(2):147–153.
87. Myers BD, Deen WM, Brenner BM. Effects of norepinephrine and angiotensin II on the determinants of glomerular ultrafiltration and proximal tubule fluid reabsorption in the rat. *Circ Res* 1975; 25:663–673.
88. Weber MA. Angiotensin II receptor antagonist in the treatment of hypertension. *Cardiol Rev* 1997; 5:72–80.
89. Sealey JE, Blumenfeld JD, Bell GM, et al. On the renal basis for essential hypertension: Nephron heterogeneity with discordant renin secretion and sodium excretion causing a hypertensive vasoconstriction-volume relationship. *J Hypertens* 1988; 6(10): 763–777.
90. Thibonnier M, Kilani A, Rahman M, et al. Effects of the nonpeptide V(1) vasopressin receptor antagonist SR49059 in hypertensive patients. *Hypertension* 1999; 34(6):1293–1300.
91. Bakris GL, Kusmirek SL, Smith AC, et al. Calcium antagonism abolishes the antipressor action of vasopressin (V1) receptor antagonism. *Am J Hypertens* 1997; 10(10 part 1):1153–1158.
92. Bakris G, Bursztyn M, Gavras I, et al. Role of vasopressin in essential hypertension: Racial differences. *J Hypertens* 1997; 15(5):545–550.
93. Bakris GL, Re RN. Endothelin modulates angiotensin II-induced mitogenesis of human mesangial cells. *Am J Physiol* 1993; 264(6 part 2):F937–F942.
94. Yanagisawa M, Kurihara H, Kimura S, et al. A novel potent vasoconstrictor peptide produced by vascular endothelial cells. *Nature* 1988; 332(6163):411–415.
95. Gardener SM, March JE, Kemp PA, Bennett T. Cardiovascular responses to angiotensins I and II in normotensive and hypertensive rats: Effects of NO synthase inhibition or ET receptor antagonism. *Br J Pharmacol* 1999; 128(8):1795–1803.
96. Krum H, Viskoper RJ, Lacourciere Y, et al. The effect of an endothelin-receptor antagonist, bosentan, on blood pressure in patients with essential hypertension: Bosentan Hypertension Investigators. *N Engl J Med* 1998; 338(12):784–790.
97. Taler SJ, Textor SC, Canzanello VJ, Schwartz L. Cyclosporin-induced hypertension: Incidence, pathogenesis and management. *Drug Saf* 1999; 20(5):437–449.
98. Moe GW, Albermaz A, Naik GO, et al. Beneficial effects of long-

term selective endothelin type A receptor blockade in canine experimental heart failure. *Cardiovasc Res* 1998; 39(3):571–579.

99. Higashi Y, Oshima T, Ozono R, et al. Effect of L-arginine infusion on systemic and renal hemodynamics in hypertensive patients. *Am J Hypertens* 1999; 12(1 part 1):8–15.
100. Cardillo C, Panza JA. Impaired endothelial regulation of vascular tone in patients with systemic arterial hypertension. *Vasc Med* 1998; 3(2):138–144.
101. Vogel RA. Cholesterol lowering and endothelial function. *Am J Med* 1999; 107(5):479–487.
102. Sartori C, Scherrer U. Insulin, nitric oxide and the sympathetic nervous system: At the crossroads of metabolic and cardiovascular regulation. *J Hypertens* 1999; 17(11):1517–1525.
103. Canessa M, Spalvins A, Adragna N, Falkner B. Red cell sodium cotransport and countransport in normotensive and hypertensive blacks. *Hypertension* 1984; 6:344–351.
104. Garay RP, Dagher G, Permollet MG, et al. Inherited defect in Na^+-K^+ cotransport system in erythrocytes from essential hypertensive patients. *Nature* 1980; 284:281–283.
105. Hilton PJ. Cellular sodium transport in essential hypertension. *N Engl J Med* 1986; 314:22–29.
106. Resnick LM. Ionic basis of hypertension, insulin resistance, vascular disease and related disorders. *Am J Hypertens* 1993; 6:123S–134S.
107. Resnick L, Gupta R, Sosa R, et al. Intracellular pH in human and experimental hypertension. *Proc Natl Acad Sci USA* 1987; 84:7663–7667.
108. Batlle DC, Sharma AM, Alsheikha MW, et al. Renal acid excretion and intracellular pH in salt sensitive genetic hypertension. *J Clin Invest* 1993; 91:2178–2184.
109. Tepel M, Bauer S, Husseini S, et al. Increased cytosolic free sodium in platlets from type 2 diabetic patients is associated with hypertension. *J Endocrinol* 1993; 138:565–572.
110. Draznin B. Cytosolic calcium and insulin resistance. *Am J Kidney Dis* 1993; 21(suppl 3):32–38.
111. Andronico G, Mangano MT, Piazza G, et al. Cellular cation exchange in arterial hypertension: Effects of insulin resistance. *J Hypertens* 1993; 11(suppl 5):S274–S275.
112. Picado MJ, de la Sierra A, Aguilera MT, et al. Increased activity of the Mg^{++}/Na^+ exchanger in red blood cells from essential hypertensive patients. *Hypertension* 1994; 23(6 part 2):987–991.
113. Ng LL, Dudley C, Bomford J, Hawley D. Leukocyte intracellular pH and Na^+/H^+ antiport activity in human hypertension. *J Hypertens* 1989; 7:471–475.
114. Resnick LM, Barbagallo M, Gupta RK, Laragh JH. Ionic basis of hypertension in diabetes mellitus: Role of hyperglycemia. *Am J Hypertens* 1993; 6(5 part 1):413–417.
115. Papageorgiou P, Morgan KP. Intracellular free Ca^{2+} is elevated in hypertrophic aortic muscle from hypertensive rats. *Am J Physiol* 1991; 29:H507–H515.
116. Ruiz-Palomo F, Toledo T. Primary Na^+/H^+ exchanger dysfunction: A possible explanation for insulin resistance syndrome. *Med Hypotheses* 1993; 41:186–189.
117. Williams B, Howard RL. Glucose-induced changes in Na^+/H^+ antiport activity and gene expression in cultured vascular smooth muscle cells: Role of protein kinase C. *J Clin Invest* 1994; 93:2623–2631.
118. Ng LL, Davies JE. Abnormalities in Na^+/H^+ antiporter activity in diabetic nephropathy. *J Am Soc Nephrol* 1992; 3(suppl 4):S50–S55.
119. Aviv A. Cytosolic Ca^{2+}, Na^+/H^+ antiport, protein kinase C trio in essential hypertension. *Am J Hypertens* 1994; 7:205–212.
120. McCarron DA, Reusser ME. Finding consensus in the dietary calcium-blood pressure debate. *J Am Coll Nutr* 1999; 18(suppl 5):398S–405S.
121. Kotchen TA, McCarron DA. Dietary electrolytes and blood pressure: A statement for healthcare professionals from the American Heart Association Nutrition Committee. *Circulation* 1998; 98(6):613–617.
122. Ishimitsu T, Tobian L. High potassium diets reduce endothelial permeability in stroke-prone spontaneously hypertensive rats. *Clin Exp Pharmacol Physiol* 1996; 23(3):241–245.
123. Tobian L. Dietary sodium chloride and potassium have effects on the pathophysiology of hypertension in humans and animals. *Am J Clin Nutr* 1997; 65(suppl 2):606S–611S.
124. Ishimitsu T, Tobian L, Uehara Y, et al. Effect of high potassium diets on the vascular and renal prostaglandin system in stroke-prone spontaneously hypertensive rats. *Prostaglandins Leukot Essent Fatty Acids* 1995; 53(4):255–260.
125. Fujimoto S, Ikegami Y, Isaka M, et al. K(+) channel blockers and cytochrome P450 inhibitors on acetylcholine-induced, endothelium-dependent relaxation in rabbit mesenteric artery. *Eur J Pharmacol* 1999; 384(1):7–15.
126. Wilson DK, Sica DA, Miller SB. Effects of potassium on blood pressure in salt-sensitive and salt-resistant black adolescents. *Hypertension* 1999; 34(2):181–186.
127. Campese VM. Salt-sensitive hypertension: Renal and cardiovascular implications. *Nutr Metab Cardiovasc Dis* 1999; 9(3):143–156.
128. Luft FC, Grim CE, Higgins JT, Weinberger MH. Differences in response to sodium administration in normotensive white and black subjects. *J Lab Clin Med* 1977; 90:555–562.
129. Blaustein MP, Hamlyn JM. Role of a natriuretic factor in essential hypertension: A hypothesis. *Ann Intern Med* 1983; 98:785–792.
130. McCarron DA, Morris CD, Henry HJ, Stanton JL. Blood pressure and nutrient intake in the United States. *Science* 1984; 224:1392–1398.
131. De Wardener HE, MacGregor GA. The relation of a circulating sodium transport inhibitor (the natriuretic hormone?) to hypertension. *Medicine (Baltimore)* 1983; 62:310–326.
132. Guyton AC, Langston JB, Navar G. Theory for renal autoregulation by feedback at the juxtaglomerular apparatus. *Circ Res* 1964; 14/15(suppl I):1187–1197.
133. Campese VM, Parise M, Karubian F, Bigazzi R. Abnormal renal hemodynamics in black salt sensitive patients with hypertension. *Hypertension* 1991; 18:805–821.
134. Johnson RJ, Schreiner GF. Hypothesis: The role of acquired tubulointerstitial disease in the pathogenesis of salt-dependent hypertension. *Kidney Int* 1997; 52:1169–1179.
135. Zou AP, Nithipatikom K, Li PL, Cowley AW Jr. Role of renal medullary adenosine in the control of blood flow and sodium excretion. *Am J Physiol* 1999; 276(3 part 2):R790–R798.
136. Szentivanyi M Jr, Zou AP, Maeda CY, et al. Increase in renal medullary nitric oxide synthase activity protects from norepinephrine-induced hypertension. *Hypertension* 2000; 35(1 part 2):418–423.
137. Stehouwer CDA, Lambert J, Donker AJM, Van Hinsbergh VWM. Endothelial dysfunction and pathogenesis of diabetic angiopathy. *Cardiovasc Res* 1997; 34:55–68.
138. Bakris GL, Walsh MF, Sowers JR. Endothelium/mesangium interactions: Role of insulin-like growth factors. In: Sowers JR, ed. *Endocrinology of the Vasculature.* Totowa, NJ: Humana Press; 1996:341.
139. Sowers JR, Sowers PS, Peuler JD. Role of insulin resistance and hyperinsulinemia in the development of hypertension and atherosclerosis. *J Lab Clin Med* 1994; 123:647–652.
140. Forsblom CM, Eriksson JG, Ekstrand AV, et al. Insulin resistance and abnormal albumin excretion in non-diabetic first-degree relatives of patients with NIDDM. *Diabetologia* 1995; 38:363–369.
141. Andersen UB, Dige-Petersen H, Frandsen EK, et al. Basal insulin-level oscillations in normotensive individuals with genetic predisposition to essential hypertension exhibit an irregular pattern. *J Hypertens* 1997; 15(10):1167–1173.
142. Forsblom CM, Eriksson JG, Ekstrand AV, et al. Insulin resistance

and abnormal albumin excretion in non-diabetic first-degree relatives of patients with NIDDM. *Diabetologia* 1995; 38:363–369.

143. Kurtz TW, Spence MA. Genetics of essential hypertension. *Am J Med* 1993; 94:77–84.
144. Dowse GK, Collins VR, Alberti KG, et al. Insulin and blood pressure levels are not independently related in Maritians of Asian Indian, Creole or Chinese origin: The Maritius noncommunicable disease study group. *J Hypertens* 1993; 11:297–307.
145. Charles MA, Pettitt DJ, Hanson RL, et al. Familial and metabolic factors related to blood pressure in Pima Indian children. *Am J Epidemiol* 1994; 140:123–131.
146. Ferrannini E, Guzzigoli G, Bonadonna R, et al. Insulin resistance in essential hypertension. *N Engl J Med* 1987; 317:350–357.
147. Saad MF, Lillioja S, Nyomba BL, et al. Racial differences in the relation between blood pressure and insulin resistance. *N Engl J Med* 1991; 324(11):733–739.
148. Caufield M, Lavender P, Farrall M, et al. Linkage of the angiotensinogen gene to essential hypertension. *N Engl J Med* 1994; 330:1629–1633.
149. Lesage S, Velho G, Vionnet N, et al. Genetic studies of the renin-angiotensin system in arterial hypertension associated with non-insulin-dependent diabetes mellitus. *J Hypertens* 1997; 15(6): 601–606.
150. Bravo EL, Tarazi RC, Dustan HP, et al. The changing clinical spectrum of primary aldosteronism. *Am J Med* 1983; 74:641–652.
151. Bravo EL, Dustan HP, Tarazi RC, et al. Clinical implications of primary aldosteronism with resistant hypertension. *Hypertension* 1988; 11(suppl I):1–207.
152. Ganguly A, Grim CE, Weinberger MH. Anomalous postural response in glucocorticoid-suppressible hyperaldosteronism. *N Engl J Med* 1981; 305:991–993.
153. Ganguly A, Weinberger MH, Guthrie GP, et al. Adrenal steroid response to ACTH in glucocorticoid-suppressible hyperaldosteronism. *Hypertension* 1984; 6:563–567.
154. Lifton RP, Dluhy RG, Powers M, et al. A chimeric 11-hydroxylase/aldosterone synthase gene causes glucocorticoid-remediable aldosteronism and human hypertension. *Nature* 1992; 355:262–265.
155. Lifton RP, Dluhy RG, Powers M, et al. Hereditary hypertension caused by chimeric gene duplications and ectopic expression of aldosterone synthase. *Nat Genet* 1992; 2:66–74.
156. Pascoe L, Curnow KM, Slutsker L, et al. Glucocorticoid-suppressible hyperaldosteronism results from hybrid genes created by unequal crossovers between CYP11B1 and CYP11B2. *Proc Natl Acad Sci USA* 1992; 89:8327–8331.
157. Woodland E, Tunny TJ, Hamlet SM, et al. Hypertension corrected and aldosterone responsiveness to renin-angiotensin restored by long-term dexamethasone in glucocorticoid-suppressible hyperaldosteronism. *Clin Exp Pharmacol Physiol* 1985; 12:245–248.
158. Hastings NB, Orchinik M, Aubourg MV, McEven BS. Pharmacological characterization of central and peripheral type I and type II adrenal steroid receptors in the prairie vole, a glucocorticoid-resistant rodent. *Endocrinology* 1999; 140(10):4459–4469.
159. Wallerath T, Witte K, Schafer SC, et al. Down-regulation of the expression of endothelial NO synthase is likely to continue to glucocorticol-mediated hypertension. *Proc Natl Acad Sci USA* 1999; 96(23):13,357–13,362.
160. Kondo K, Saruta T, Saito I, et al. Benign deoxycorticosterone producing adrenal tumor. *JAMA* 1976; 236:1042.
161. Liddle GW, Bledsoe T, Coppage WS. A familial renal disorder simulating primary aldosteronism but with negligible aldosterone secretion. *Trans Assoc Am Phys* 1963; 76:199.
162. Botero-Velez M, Curtiss JJ, Warnock DG. Liddle's syndrome revisited: A disorder of sodium reabsorption in the distal tubule. *N Eng J Med* 1994; 300:178.
163. Kellenberger S, Gautschi I, Rossier BC, Schild L. Mutations causing Liddle syndrome reduce sodium-dependent downregulation of the epithelial sodium channel in the Xenopus oocyte expression system. *J Clin Invest* 1998; 101:2741–2750.
164. Gubner RS. Systolic hypertension: A pathogenetic entity: Significance and therapeutic considerations. *Am J Cardiol* 1962; 9:773–776.
165. Brown WC, O'Brien ET, Semple PF. The sphygmomanometer of Riva Rocci 1896–1996. *J Hum Hypertens* 1996; 10:723–724.
166. Mancia G. Scipione Riva-Rocci. *Clin Cardiol* 1997; 20:503–504.
167. Janeway TC. A clinical study of hypertensive cardiovascular disease. *Arch Intern Med* 1913; 12:752–786.
168. Laher M, O'Brien E. In search of Korotkoff. *BMJ* 1982; 285:1796–1798.
169. Segall HN. How Korotkoff, the surgeon, discovered the auscultatory method of measuring arterial pressure. *Ann Intern Med* 1975; 83:561–562.
170. Franx A, Evers IM, van der Pant KA, et al. The fourth sound of Korotkoff in pregnancy: A myth. *Eur J Obstet Gynecol Reprod Biol* 1998; 76:53–59.
171. Bailey RH, Bauer JH. A review of common errors in the indirect measurement of blood pressure. *Arch Intern Med* 1993; 153:2741–2748.
172. Villegas I, Arias IC, Botero A, Escobar A. Evaluation of the technique used by health-care workers for taking blood pressure. *Hypertension* 1995; 26:1204–1206.
173. Practice imperfect [editorial]. *Lancet* 1991; 337:1195–1196.
174. Abbott D, Campbell N, Carruthers-Czyzewski P, et al. Guidelines for measurement of blood pressure, follow-up and lifestyle counseling: Canadian Coalition for High Blood Pressure Prevention and Control. *Can J Public Health* 1994; 85(suppl 2):S29–S43.
175. Cooper KM. Measuring blood pressure: The right way. *Nursing* 1992; 22:75.
176. Frohlich ED, Grim C, Labarthe DR, et al. Recommendations for Human Blood Pressure Determination by Sphygmomanometers: Report of a Special Task Force Appointed by the Steering Committee, American Heart Association. *Hypertension* 1988; 11:210A–222A.
177. Baker RH, Ende J. Confounders of auscultatory blood pressure measurement. *J Gen Intern Med* 1995; 10:223–231.
178. Stolt M, Sjonell G, Astrom H, et al. Improved accuracy of indirect blood pressure measurement in patients with obese arms. *Am J Hypertens* 1993; 6:66–71.
179. National Committee for Quality Assurance (NCQA). *HEDIS 3.0, Vol. 1* Washington, DC: NCQA; 1997.
180. Stewart MJ, Gough K, Padfield PL. The accuracy of automated blood pressure measuring devices in patients with controlled atrial fibrillation. *J Hypertens* 1995; 13:297–300.
181. Cavallini MC, Roman MJ, Blank SG, et al. Association of the auscultatory gap with vascular disease in hypertensive patients. *Ann Intern Med* 1996; 124:877–883.
182. Ohkubo T, Imai Y, Tsuji I, et al. Home blood pressure measurement has a stronger predictive power for mortality than does screening blood pressure measurement: A population-based observation in Ohasama, Japan. *J Hypertens* 1998; 16:971–975.
183. Soghikian K, Casper SM, Fireman BH, et al. Home blood pressure monitoring: Effect on use of medical services and medical costs. *Med Care* 1992; 30:855–865.
184. Appel LJ, Stason WB. Ambulatory blood pressure monitoring and blood pressure self-measurement in the diagnosis and management of hypertension. *Ann Intern Med* 1993; 118:867–882.
185. Gerin W, Pickering TG, Holland JK, Alter R. Telephone-linked home blood pressure monitoring may improve management [abstract]. *Am J Hypertens* 1999; 12:163.
186. Mengden T, Beltran B, Weisser B, et al. Long-term control of blood pressure guided by daily self-measurement is superior to usual office-based care [abstract]. *J Hypertens* 1999; 17 (suppl 3):30.

187. Perloff D, Sokolow M, Cowan R. The prognostic value of ambulatory blood pressures. *JAMA* 1983; 249:2792–2798.
188. Imai Y, Ohkubo T, Tsuji I, et al. Prognostic value of ambulatory and home blood pressure measurements in comparison to screening blood pressure measurements: A pilot study in Ohasama. *Blood Press Monit* 1996; 1(suppl 2):51–58.
189. Ohkubo T, Imai Y, Tsuji I, et al. Prediction of mortality by ambulatory blood pressure monitoring versus screening blood pressure measurements: A pilot study in Ohasama. *J Hypertens* 1997; 15:357–364.
190. Perloff D, Sokolow M, Cowan RM, Juster RP. Prognostic value of ambulatory blood pressure measurements: Further analyses. *J Hypertens* 1989; 7(suppl 3):S3–S10.
191. Staessen JA, O'Brien ET, Atkins N, Amery AK. Short report: Ambulatory blood pressure in normotensive compared with hypertensive subjects: The Ad-Hoc Working Group. *J Hypertens* 1993; 11:1289–1297.
192. Rasmussen SL, Torp-Pedersen C, Borch-Johnsen K, Ibsen H. Normal values for ambulatory blood pressure and differences between casual blood pressure and ambulatory blood pressure: Results from a Danish population survey. *J Hypertens* 1998; 16:1415–1424.
193. Gretler DD, Fumo MT, Nelson KS, Murphy MB. Ethnic differences in circadian hemodynamic profile. *Am J Hypertens* 1994; 7:7–14.
194. Staessen JA, Bieniaszewski L, O'Brien E, et al. Nocturnal blood pressure fall on ambulatory monitoring in a large international database. *Hypertension* 1997; 29:30–39.
195. Verdecchia P, Porcellati C, Schillaci G, et al. Ambulatory blood pressure: An independent predictor of prognosis in essential hypertension. *Hypertension* 1994; 24:793–801.
196. Verdecchia P, Schillaci G, Borgioni C, et al. Adverse prognostic value of a blunted circadian rhythm of heart rate in essential hypertension. *J Hypertens* 1998; 16:1335–1343.
197. Staessen JA, Thijs L, Fagard R, et al. Predicting cardiovascular risk using conventional vs. ambulatory blood pressure in older patients with systolic hypertension. *JAMA* 1999; 282:589–596.
198. Elliott WJ. Circadian variation in blood pressure: Implications for elderly patients. *Am J Hypertens* 1999; 12:43S–49S.
199. Kleinert HD, Harshfield GA, Pickering TG, et al. What is the value of home blood pressure measurement in patients with mild hypertension? *Hypertension* 1984; 6:574–578.
200. White WB, Schulman P, McCabe EM, Day HM. Average daily blood pressure, not office pressure, determines cardiac function in patients with hypertension. *JAMA* 1989; 261:873–877.
201. Palatini P, Penzo M, Ricioppa A, et al. Clinical relevance of nighttime blood pressure and of daytime blood pressure variability. *Arch Intern Med* 1992; 152:1855–1860.
202. Liu JE, Roman MJ, Pini R, et al. Cardiac and arterial target organ damage in adults with elevated ambulatory and normal office blood pressure. *Ann Intern Med* 1999; 131:564–572.
203. Redon J, Campos C, Narciso ML, et al. Prognostic value of ambulatory blood pressure monitoring in refractory hypertension: A prospective study. *Hypertension* 1998; 31:712–718.
204. Pearce KA, Grimm RH Jr, Rao S, et al. Population-derived comparisons of ambulatory and office blood pressures: Implications for the determination of usual blood pressure and the concept of white coat hypertension. *Arch Intern Med* 1992; 152: 750–756.
205. Weber MA, Neutel JM, Smith DHG, Graettinger WF. Diagnosis of mild hypertension by ambulatory blood pressure monitoring. *Circulation* 1994; 90:2291–2298.
206. Muscholl MW, Hense HW, Brockel U, et al. Changes in left ventricular structure and function in patients with white coat hypertension: Cross sectional survey. *BMJ* 1998; 317:565–570.
207. Owens PE, Lyons SP, Rodriguez SA, O'Brien ET. Is elevation of clinic blood pressure in patients with white coat hypertension who have normal ambulatory blood pressure associated with target organ changes? *J Hum Hypertens* 1998; 12:743–748.
208. Julius S, Jamerson K, Mejia A, et al. The association of borderline hypertension with target organ changes and higher coronary risk: The Tecumseh Blood Pressure Study. *JAMA* 1990; 264:354–358.
209. Verdecchia P, Schillaci G, Borgioni C, et al. Prognostic significance of the white coat effect. *Hypertension* 1997; 29:1218–1224.
210. Krakoff LR, Schechter C, Fahs M, Andre M. Ambulatory blood pressure monitoring: Is it cost-effective? *J Hypertens* 1991; 9(suppl):S28–S30.
211. Krakoff LR. Ambulatory blood pressure monitoring can improve cost-effective management of hypertension. *Am J Hypertens* 1993; 6(suppl):220S–224S.
212. Yarows SA, Khoury S, Sowers JR. Cost effectiveness of 24-hour ambulatory blood pressure monitoring in evaluation and treatment of essential hypertension. *Am J Hypertens* 1994; 7:464–468.
213. Appel LJ, Stason WB. Ambulatory blood pressure monitoring and blood pressure self-measurement in the diagnosis and management of hypertension. *Ann Intern Med* 1993; 118:867–882.
214. Sheps SG, Clement DL, Pickering TG, et al. Ambulatory blood pressure monitoring: Hypertensive Diseases Committee, American College of Cardiology position statement. *J Am Coll Cardiol* 1994; 23:1511–1513.
215. Jackson R, Barham P, Bills J, et al. Management of raised blood pressure in New Zealand: A discussion document. *BMJ* 1993; 307:107–110.
216. Keith NM, Wagener HP, Barker NW. Some different types of essential hypertension: Their course and prognosis. *Am J Med Sci* 1939; 197:332–343.
217. Tso MOM, Jampol LM. Pathophysiology of hypertensive retinopathy. *Ophthalmology* 1982; 89:1132–1145.
218. The Eye Disease Case-Control Study Group. Risk factors for branch retinal vein occlusion. *Am J Ophthalmol* 1993; 116: 286–296.
219. The Eye Disease Case-Control Study Group. Risk factors for central retinal vein occlusion. *Arch Ophthalmol* 1996; 114: 545–554.
220. Macular Photocoagulation Study Group. Laser photocoagulation for justrafoveal choroidal neovascularization: Five-year results from randomized clinical trials. *Arch Ophthalmol* 1994; 112: 500–509.
221. Knowler WC, Bennett PH, Ballintine EJ. Increased incidence of retinopathy in diabetics with elevated blood pressure: A six-year follow-up study in Pima Indians. *N Engl J Med* 1980; 302:645–650.
222. Turner R, Holman R, Stratton I, et al., for the United Kingdom Prospective Diabetes Study Group. Tight blood pressure control and risk of macrovascular and microvascular complications in type 2 diabetes: UKPDS 38. *BMJ* 1998; 317:707–713.
223. Levy D, Labib SB, Anderson KM, et al. Determinants of sensitivity and specificity of electrocardiographic criteria for left ventricular hypertrophy. *Circulation* 1990; 81:815–820.
224. Molloy TJ, Okin PM, Devereux RB, Kligfield P. Electrocardiographic detection of left ventricular hypertrophy by the simple QRS-voltage duration product. *J Am Coll Cardiol* 1992; 20:1180–1186.
225. Okin PM, Roman MJ, Devereux RB, Kligfield P. Electrocardiographic identification of increased left ventricular mass by simple voltage duration products. *J Am Coll Cardiol* 1995; 25:417–423.
226. Black HR, Weltin G, Jaffe CC. The limited echocardiogram: A modification of standard echocardiography for use in the routine evaluation of patients with systemic hypertension. *Am J Cardiol* 1991; 67:1027–1030.
227. Levy D, Salomon MS, D'Agostino RB, et al. Prognostic implications of baseline electrocardiographic features and their serial changes in subjects with left ventricular hypertrophy. *Circulation* 1994; 90:1786–1793.

228. Levy D, Garrison RJ, Savage DD, et al. Prognostic implications of echocardiographically determined left ventricular mass in the Framingham Heart Study. *N Engl J Med* 1990; 322:1561–1566.
229. Koren MJ, Devereux RB, Casale PN, et al. Relation of left ventricular mass and geometry to morbidity and mortality in uncomplicated essential hypertension. *Ann Intern Med* 1991; 114: 345–352.
230. Devereux RB, de Simone G, Ganau A, et al. Left ventricular hypertrophy and hypertension. *Clin Exp Hypertens* 1993; 15: 1025–1032.
231. Bikkina M, Levy D, Evans JC, et al. Left ventricular mass and risk of stroke in an elderly cohort: The Framingham Heart Study. *JAMA* 1994; 272:33–36.
232. Verdecchia P, Schillaci G, Borgioni C, et al. Prognostic significance of serial changes in left ventricular mass in essential hypertension. *Circulation* 1998; 97:48–54.
233. Soufer R, Wohlgelernter D, Vita NA, et al. Intact systolic ventricular function in clinical congestive heart failure. *Am J Cardiol* 1985; 55:1032–1036.
234. Liao Y, Cooper RS, McGee DL, et al. The relative effects of left ventricular hypertrophy, coronary artery disease, and ventricular dysfunction on survival among black adults. *JAMA* 1995; 273:1592–1597.
235. Dahlöf B, Pennert K, Hansson L. Reversal of left ventricular hypertrophy in hypertensive patients: A metaanalysis of 109 treatment studies. *Am J Hypertens* 1992; 5:95–110.
236. Liebson PR, Grandits GA, Dianzumba S, et al, for the Treatment of Hypertension Study Research Group. Comparison of five antihypertensive monotherapies and placebo for change in left ventricular mass in patients receiving nutritional hygienic therapy in the Treatment of Mild Hypertension Study (TOMHS). *Circulation* 1995; 91:698–706.
237. Gottdiener JS, Reda DJ, Massie BM, et al, for the VA Cooperative Study Group on Antihypertensive Agents. Effect of single-drug therapy on reduction of left ventricular mass in mild to moderate hypertension: Comparison of six antihypertensive agents; The Department of Veterans Affairs Cooperative Study Group on Antihypertensive Agents. *Circulation* 1997; 95:2007–2014.
238. Keane WF, Eknoyan G. Proteinuria, albuminuria, risk, assessment, detection, elimination (PARADE): A position paper of the National Kidney Foundation. *Am J Kidney Dis* 1999; 33(5):1004–1010.
239. Yudkin JS, Forest RD, Jackson CA. Microalbuminuria as predictor of vascular disease in non-diabetic subjects: Islington Diabetes Survey. *Lancet* 1988; 2:530–533.
240. Borch-Johnsen K, Feldt-Rasmussen B, Strandgaard S, et al. Urinary albumin excretion: An independent predictor of ischemic heart disease. *Arterioscler Thromb Vasc Biol* 1999; 19(8):1992–1997.
241. Mogensen CE. Microalbuminuria predicts clinical proteinuria and early mortality in maturity-onset diabetes. *N Engl J Med* 1984; 310:356–360.
242. Stephespon JM, Kenny S, Stevens LK, et al, and the WHO Multinational Study Group. Proteinuria and mortality in diabetes: The WHO multinational study of vascular disease in diabetes. *Diabetes Med* 1995; 12:149–155.
243. Gosling P. Microalbuminuria and cardiovascular risk: A word of caution. *J Hum Hypertens* 1998; 12:211–213.
244. Dinneen SF, Gerstein HC. The association of microalbuminuria and mortality in non-insulin-dependent diabetes mellitus: A systemic overview of the literature. *Arch Intern Med* 1997; 157: 1413–1418.
245. Bakris GL, Randall O, Rahman M, et al, for the AASK Study Group. Associations between cardiovascular risk factors and glomerular filtration rate at baseline in the African American Study of Kidney Disease (AASK) trial (abstract). *J Am Soc Nephrol* 1998; 9:139.
246. Mimran A, Ribstein J, Du Cailar G, Halimi JM. Albuminuria in normals and essential hypertension. *J Diabet Complications* 1994; 8:150–156.
247. Tarif N, Bakris GL. Preservation of renal function: The spectrum of effects by calcium channel blockers. *Nephrol Dial Transplant* 1997; 12:2244–2250.
248. Pontremoli R. Microalbuminuria in essential hypertension—its relation to cardiovascular risk factors. *Nephrol Dial Transplant* 1996; 11:2113–2134.
249. Bigazzi R, Bianchi S. Microalbuminuria as a marker of cardiovascular and renal disease in essential hypertension. *Nephrol Dial Transplant* 1995; 10(suppl 6):10–14.
250. Pontremoli R, Sofia A, Ravera M, et al. Prevalence and clinical correlates of microalbuminuria in essential hypertension: The MAGIC study. *Hypertension* 1997; 30:1135–1143.
251. Pedrinelli R, Dell'Omo G, Penno G, et al. Microalbuminuria and pulse pressure in hypertensive and atherosclerotic men. *Hypertension* 2000; 35(1 part 1):48–54.
252. Cirillo M, Senigalliese L, Laurenzi M, et al. Microalbuminuria in nondiabetic adults: Relation of blood pressure, body mass index, plasma cholesterol levels, and smoking: The Gubbio Population Study. *Arch Intern Med* 1998; 158:1933–1939.
253. Bianchi S, Bigazzi R, Baldari G, et al. Diurnal variations of blood pressure and microalbuminuria in essential hypertension. *Am J Hypertens* 1994; 7:23–29.
254. Redon J, Liao Y, Lozano JV, et al. Ambulatory blood pressure and microalbuminuria in essential hypertension: Role of circadian variability. *J Hypertens* 1994; 12:947–953.
255. Jensen JS. Renal and systemic transvascular albumin leakage in severe atherosclerosis. *Arterioscler Thromb Vasc Biol* 1995; 15:1324–1329.
256. Alzaid AA. Microalbuminuria in patients with type 2 diabetes: An overview. *Diabetes Care* 1996; 19:79–89.
257. Stehouwer CDA, Lambet J, Donker AJM, van Hinsberg VWM. Endothelial dysfunction and pathogenesis of diabetic angiopathy. *Cardiovasc Res* 1997; 34:55–68.
258. Gosling P. Microalbuminuria: A marker of systemic disease. *Br J Hosp Med* 1995; 54:285–290.
259. Agewall S, Wikstrand J, Ljungman S, Fagerberg B. Usefulness of microalbuminuria in predicting cardiovascular mortality in treated hypertensive men with and without diabetes mellitus. *Am J Cardiol* 1997; 80:164–169.
260. Cerasola G, Cottone S, D'lgnoto G, et al. Microalbuminuria as a predictor of cardiovascular damage in essential hypertension. *J Hypertens* 1989; 7:S332–S333.
261. Pedrinelli R, Di Bello V, Catapano G, et al. Microalbuminuria is a marker of left ventricular hypertrophy but not hyperinsulinemia in non-diabetic atherosclerotic patients. *Arterioscler Thromb* 1993; 12:947–953.
262. Palatini P, Graniero GR, Mormino P, et al. Prevalence and clinical correlates of microalbuminuria in stage I hypertension: Results from the Hypertension and Ambulatory Recording Venetian Study (HARVES). *Am J Hypertens* 1996; 9:334–341.
263. Virmani R, Avolio AP, Mergner WJ, et al. Effect of aging on aortic morphology in populations with high and low prevalence of hypertension and atherosclerosis: Comparison between Occidental and Chinese communities. *Am J Pathol* 1991; 139:1119–1129.
264. Glasser SP, Arnett DK, McVeigh GE, et al. Vascular compliance and cardiovascular disease: A risk factor or marker? *Am J Hypertens* 1997; 10:1175–1189.
265. Simon A, Megnien JL, Levenson J. Detection of preclinical atherosclerosis may optimize the management of hypertension. *Am J Hypertens* 1997; 10:813–824.
266. Kelly R, Hayward C, Avolio A, O'Rourke M. Noninvasive deter-

mination of age-related changes in the human arterial pulse. *Circulation* 1989; 80:1652–1659.

267. Blacher J, Asmar R, Djane S, London GM. Aortic pulse wave velocity as a marker of cardiovascular risk in hypertensive patients. *Hypertension* 1999; 33(5):1111–1117.
268. Messerli FH, Ventura HO, Amodeo C. Osler's maneuver and pseudohypertension. *N Engl J Med* 1985; 312:1548–1551.
269. The SHEP Cooperative Study Group. Prevention of stroke by antihypertensive drug treatment in older persons with isolated systolic hypertension. *JAMA* 1991; 265:3255–3264.
270. Staessen JA, Fagard R, Thijs L, et al, for the Systolic Hypertension in Europe (Syst-EUR) Trial Investigators. Morbidity and mortality in the placebo-controlled European Trial on Isolated Systolic Hypertension in the Elderly. *Lancet* 1997; 360:757–764.
271. Liu L, Wang J, Gong L, et al, for the Systolic Hypertension in China (Syst-China) Collaborative Group. Comparison of active treatment and placebo in older Chinese patients with isolated systolic hypertension. *J Hypertens* 1998; 16:1823–1829.
272. Ridker PM, Glynn RJ, Hennekens CH. C-reative protein adds to the predictive value of total and HDL-cholesterol in determining risk of first myocardial infarction. *Circulation* 1998; 97:2007–2011.
273. Setaro JF, Saddler MC, Chen CC, et al. Simplified captopril renography in diagnosis and treatment of renal artery stenosis. *Hypertension* 1991; 18:289–298.
274. Stair DC, Rios WA, Black HR. Atypical causes of curable renovascular hypertension: A review. *Prog Cardiovasc Dis* 1990; 33(3)185–210.
275. Black HR, Cooper KA. Cigarette smoking and atherosclerotic renal artery stenosis. *J Clin Hypertens* 1986; 2(4):322–330.
276. Emovon OE, Klotman PE, Dunnick NR, et al. Renovascular hypertension in blacks. *Am J Hypertens* 1996; 9(1):18–23.
277. Setaro JF, Chen CC, Hoffer PB, Black HR. Captopril renography in the diagnosis of renal artery stenosis and the prediction of improvement with revascularization. *Am J Hypertens* 1991; 4(12 part 2):698S–705S.
278. Mann SL, Pickering TG. Detection of renovascular hypertension: State of the art: 1992. *Ann Intern Med* 1992; 117:845.
279. Helenon O, Melki P, Correas JM, et al. Renovascular disease: Doppler ultrasound. *Semin Ultrasound CT MR* 1997; 18(2): 136–146.
280. Leung DA, Hoffman U, Pfammatter T, et al. Magnetic resonance angiography versus duplex sonography for diagnosing renovascular disease. *Hypertension* 1999; 33(2):726–731.
281. Yi J, Bakris GL. Pheochromocytoma. In: Conn RB, Borer WZ, Snyder JW, eds. *Current Diagnosis 9*. New York: Saunders; 1997:794.
282. Stein PP, Black HR. A simplified diagnostic approach to pheochromocytoma: A review of the literature and report of one institution's experience. *Medicine (Baltimore)* 1991; 70:46–66.
283. Bravo EL. Evolving concepts in the pathophysiology, diagnosis, and treatment of pheochromocytoma. *Endocr Rev* 1994; 15: 356–368.
284. Jalil N, Pattou FN, Combemale F, et al. Effectiveness and limits of preoperative imaging studies for the localization of pheochromocytomas and paragangliomas: A review of 282 cases: French Association of Surgery (AFC), The French Association of Endocrine Surgeons (AFCE). *Eur J Surg* 1998; 164(1):23–28.
285. Ferriss JB, Beevers DG, Brown JJ, et al. Clinical, biochemical, and pathological features of low renin ("primary") hyperaldosteronism. *Am Heart J* 1978; 95:375–381.
286. Lins PW, Adamson U. Plasma aldosterone-plasma renin activity ratio: A simple test to identify patients with primary aldosteronism. *Acta Endocrinol (Copenh)* 1986; 113:564.
287. Ganguly A. Primary aldosteronism. *N Engl J Med* 1998; 339(25):1828–1834.
288. Biglieri EG, Irony I, Kater Cl. Identification and implications of new types of mineralocorticoid hypertension. *J Steroid Biochem* 1989; 32:199.
289. Biglieri EG, Schambelan M. The significance of elevated levels of plasma 18-hydroxycorticosterone in patients with primary aldosteronism. *J Clin Endocrinol Metab* 1979; 49:87.
290. Ganguly A, Melada GA, Luetscher JA, et al. Control of plasma aldosterone in primary aldosteronism: Distinction between adenoma and hyperplasia. *J Clin Endocrinol Metab* 1973; 37:765.
291. Fraser R, Beretta-Piccoli C, Brown JJ, et al. Response of aldosterone and 18-hydroxycorticosterone to angiotensin II in normal subjects and patients with essential hypertension: Conn's syndrome and non-tumorous hyperaldosteronism. *Hypertension* 1991; 3(suppl I):87.
292. Geisinger MA, Zelch MA, Bravo EL, et al. Primary hyperaldosteronism: Comparison of CT, adrenal venography, and venous sampling. *AJR* 1983; 141:299.
293. Melby JC, Spark RF, Dale S, et al. Diagnosis and localization of aldosterone-producing adenomas by adrenal vein catheterization. *N Engl J Med* 1967; 277:1050.
294. Bravo EL, Dustan HP, Tarazi RC. Spironolactone as a nonspecific treatment for primary aldosteronism. *Circulation* 1973; 48:491.
295. Stradling JR, Crosby JH. Relation between systemic hypertension and sleep hypoxaemia or snoring: Analysis in 748 men drawn from general practice. *BMJ* 1990; 300:75–78.
296. Nieto FJ, Young TB, Lind BK, et al. Association of sleep-disordered breathing, sleep apnea, and hypertension in a large community-based study. *JAMA* 2000; 283:1829–1836.
297. Ledoux M, Lambert J, Reeder BA, Depres JP. Correlation between cardiovascular disease risk factors and simple anthropometic measures: Canadian Heart Health Surveys Research Group. *Can Med Assoc J* 1997; 157(suppl 1):S46–S53.
298. Fagard RH. Physical fitness, and blood pressure. *J Hypertens* 1993; 11(suppl 5):S47–S52.
299. The Trials of Hypertension Prevention Collaborative Research Group. The effects of nonpharmacologic interventions on blood pressure of persons with high normal levels: Results of the Trials of Hypertension Prevention, phase I [published erratum appears in *JAMA* 1992; 267:2330]. *JAMA* 1992; 267:1213–1220.
300. Neaton JD, Grimm RH, Prineas RJ, et al. Treatment of mild hypertension study: Final results. *JAMA* 1993; 270:713–724.
301. The Trials of Hypertension Prevention Collaborative Research Group. Effects of weight loss and sodium reduction intervention on blood pressure and hypertension incidence in overweight people with high-normal blood pressure: The Trials of Hypertension Prevention, phase II. *Arch Intern Med* 1997; 157:657–667.
302. Whelton PK, Appel LJ, Espeland MA, et al., for the TONE Collaborative Research Group. Sodium restriction and weight loss in the treatment of hypertension in older persons: A randomized controlled trial of nonpharmacologic interventions in the Elderly (TONE). *JAMA* 1998; 279:839–846.
303. Cushman WC, Cutler JA, Hanna E, et al., for the PATHS Group. The Prevention and Treatment of Hypertension Study (PATHS): Effects of an alcohol treatment program on blood pressure. *Arch Intern Med* 1998; 152:1197–1207.
304. Appel LJ, Moore TJ, Obarzanek E, et al. A clinical trial of the effects of dietary patterns on blood pressure. *N Engl J Med* 1997; 336:1117–1124.
305. Whelton PK, He J, Cutler JA, et al. Effects of oral potassium on blood pressure: Meta-analysis of randomized controlled clinical trials. *JAMA* 1997; 277:1624–1632.
306. Sacks FM, Brown LE, Appel L, et al. Combinations of potassium, calcium, and magnesium supplements in hypertension. *Hypertension* 1995; 26:950–956.
307. Sacks FM, Willett WC, Smith A, et al. Effect of blood pressure of potassium, calcium, and magnesium in women with low habitual intake. *Hypertension* 1998; 31:131–138.

308. Morris MC, Sacks FM, Rosner B. Does fish oil lower blood pressure: A meta-analysis of controlled trials. *Circulation* 1993; 88:523–533.
309. Issacsohn JL, Moser M, Stein EA, et al. Garlic powder and plasma lipids and lipoproteins: A multicenter, randomized, placebo-controlled trial. *Arch Intern Med* 1998; 158(11):1189–1194.
310. Minami J, Ishimitus T, Matsouka H. Effects of smoking cessation on blood pressure and heart and heart rate variability in habitual smokers. *Hypertension* 1999; 33(1 part 2):586–590.
311. Bolinder G, de Faire U. Ambulatory 24 hour blood pressure monitoring in healthy, middle-aged smokeless tobacco users, smokers, and nontobacco users. *Am J Hypertens* 1998; 11(10):1153–1163.
312. Hansson L, Lindholm LH, Niskanen L, et al. Effect of angiotensin-converting-enzyme inhibition compared with conventional therapy on cardiovascular morbidity and mortality in hypertension: The Captopril Prevention Project (CAPPP) randomised trial. *Lancet* 1999; 353(9153):611–616.
313. Hansson L, Lindholm LH, Ekborn T, et al. Randomised trial of old and new antihypertensive drugs in elderly patients: Cardiovascular mortality and morbidity. The Swedish Trial in Old Patients with Hypertension-2 study. *Lancet* 1999; 354(9192):1751–1756.
314. Garg R, Yusuf S, for the Collaborative Group on ACE Inhibitor Trials. Overview of randomized trials of angiotensin-converting enzyme inhibitors on mortality and morbidity in patients with heart failure. *JAMA* 1995; 273:1450–1456.
315. Pfeffer MA, Braunwald E, Moyé LA, et al, for the SAVE investigators. Effect of captopril on mortality and morbidity in patients with left ventricular dysfunction after myocardial infarction: Results of the Survival and Ventricular Enlargement Trials. *N Engl J Med* 1992; 327:669–677.
316. Lewis EJ, Hunsicker LG, Bain RP, Rohde RD, for the Collaborative Study Group. The effect of angiotensin-converting-enzyme inhibition on diabetic nephropathy. *N Engl J Med* 1993; 329:1456–1462.
317. Maschio G, Alberti D, Janin G, et al, for the Angiotensin-Converting-Enzyme Inhibition in Progressive Renal Insufficiency Study Group. Effect of the angiotensin-converting-enzyme inhibitor benazepril on the progression of chronic renal insufficiency. *N Engl J Med* 1996; 334:939–945.
318. Yusuf S, Sleight P, Pogue J, et al. Effects of an angiotensin-converting-enzyme inhibitor, ramipril, on death from cardiovascular causes, myocardial infarction, and stroke in high-risk patients: The Heart Outcomes Prevention Evaluation (HOPE) study investigators. *N Engl J Med* 2000; 342:145–153.
319. 1999 World Health Organization–International Society of Hypertension Guidelines for the management of hypertension: Guidelines Subcommittee. *J Hypertens* 1999; 17(2):151–183.
320. Davis BR, Cutler JA, Gordon DJ, et al. Rationale and design for the antihypertensive and lipid lowering treatment to prevent heart attack trial (ALLHAT). *Am J Hypertens* 1996; 9:342–360.
321. The ALLHAT Officers and Coordinators for the ALLHAT Collaborative Research Group. Major cardiovascular events in hypertensive patients randomized to doxazosin vs. chlorthalidone: The Antihypertensive and Lipid-Lowering Treatment to Prevent Heart Attack Trial (ALLHAT). *JAMA* 2000; 283:1967–1975.
322. Black HR, Elliott WJ, Neaton JD, et al. Rationale and design for the Controlled ONset Verapamil INvestigation of Cardiovascular Endpoints (CONVINCE) trial. *Controlled Clin Trials* 1998; 19(4):370–390.
323. Dahlof B, Devereux RB, Julius S, et al. Characteristics of 9194 patients with left ventricular hypertrophy: The LIFE study: Losartan Intervention For Endpoint Reduction in Hypertension. *Hypertension* 1998; 32(6):989–997.
324. Hansson L, Zandretti A, Carruthers SG, et al. Effects of intensive blood pressure lowering and low-dose aspirin in patients with hypertension: Principal results of the Hypertension Optimal Treatment (HOT) randomised trial: The HOT Study Group. *Lancet* 1998; 351:1755–1762.
325. Tight blood pressure control and risk of macrovascular and microvascular complications in type 2 diabetes: UKPDS 38: UK Prospective Diabetes Study Group. *BMJ* 1998; 317:703–713.
326. Lazarus JM, Bourgoignie JJ, Buckalew VM, et al. Achievement and safety of a low blood pressure goal in chronic renal disease: The Modification of Diet in Renal Disease Study Group. *Hypertension* 1997; 29:641–650.
327. Wright JS Jr, Kusek JW, Toto RD, et al. Design and baseline characteristics of participants in the African-American Study of Kidney Disease and Hypertension Pilot Study for the AASK pilot study investigators. *Controlled Clin Trials* 1996; 17:3S–16S.
328. Cruickshank JM, Thorpe JM, Zacharias FJ. Benefits and potential harm of lowering high blood pressure. *Lancet* 1987; 1:581–584.
329. Farnett L, Murlow CD, Linn WD, et al. The J curve phenomenon and the treatment of hypertension: Is there a point beyond which pressure reduction is dangerous? *JAMA* 1991; 265:489–495.
330. D'Agostino RB, Belanger AJ, Kannel WB, Cruickshank JM. Relation of low diastolic blood pressure to coronary heart disease death in presence of myocardial infarction: The Framingham Study. *BMJ* 1991; 303(6799):385–389.
331. Fletcher AE, Bulpitt CJ. How far should blood pressure be lowered? *N Engl J Med* 1992; 326:251–254.
332. Elliott WJ, Weir DR, Black HR. Cost-effectiveness of lowering treatment goal of JNC VI for diabetic hypertensives. *Arch Intern Med* 2000; 160:1277–1283.
333. Black HR. Metabolic considerations in the choice of therapy for the hypertensive patient. *Am Heart J* 1991; 121:707–715.
334. Kasiske BL, Ma JZ, Kalil R, Louis TA. Effects of antihypertensive therapy on serum lipids. *Ann Intern Med* 1995; 122:133–141.
335. Grimm RH, Flack JM, Grandits GA, et al, for the TOMHS Research Group. Long term effects on plasma lipids of diet and drugs to treat hypertension. *JAMA* 1996; 275:1549–1556.
336. Jones DW, Sands CD. Effects of doxazosin and hydrochlorothiazide on lipid levels in Korean patients with essential hypertension. *J Cardiovasc Pharmacol* 1993; 22(3):431–437.
337. Elisaf MS, Theodorou J, Pappas H, et al. Effectiveness and metabolic effects of perindopril and diuretics combination in primary hypertension. *J Hum Hypertens* 1999; 13(11):787–791.
338. Gress TW, Nieto FJ, Shahar E, et al, for the Atherosclerosis Risk in Communities Study. Hypertension and antihypertensive therapy and the risk factors for the type 2 diabetes mellitus. *N Engl J Med* 2000; 342:905–912.
339. Curb JD, Pressel SL, Cutler J, et al. Effect of diuretic-based antihypertensive treatment on cardiovascular disease risk in older diabetics with isolated systolic hypertension *JAMA* 1996; 276(23):1886–1892.
340. Tuomilehto J, Rastenyte D, Birkenhager WH, et al. Effects of calcium-channel blockade in older patients with diabetes and systolic hypertension: Systolic Hypertension in Europe Trial Investigators (Syst-Eur). *N Engl J Med* 1999; 340(9):677–684.
341. Yusuf S, Held P, Furberg C. Update of effects of calcium channel antagonists in myocardial infarction or angina in light of the second Danish Verapamil infarction trial (DAVIT-II) and other recent studies. *J Am Col Cardiol* 1991; 67:1295–1297.
342. Psaty BM, Smith NL, Siscovick DS, et al. Health outcomes associated with antihypertensive therapies used as first-line agents: A systematic review and meta-analysis. *JAMA* 1997; 277:739–745.
343. Bakris GL, Weir MR, DeQuattro V, McMahon FG. Effects of an ACE inhibitor/calcium antagonist combination on proteinuria in diabetic nephropathy. *Kidney Int* 1998; 54:1283–1289.
344. Bakris GL, Griffin KA, Picken MM, Bidani AK. Combined effects of an angiotensin converting enzyme inhibitor and a calcium antagonist on renal injury. *J Hypertens* 1997; 15:1181–1185.
345. Weber KT, Sun Y, Guarda E. Structural remodeling in hyperten-

sive heart disease and the role of hormones. *Hypertension* 1994; 23(part 2):869–877.

346. Douglas PS. Diastolic dysfunction: Old dog, new tricks [editorial]. *Am Heart J* 1999; 37:777–778.

347. Konstam MA, Dracup K, Baker DW, et al. Heart Failure: Evaluation and Care of Patients with Left Ventricular Systolic Dysfunction: Clinical Practice Guideline. No. 11. (AHCPR Publication #94-0612). Rockville, MD: Agency for Healthcare Policy and Research; 1994.

348. Hjalmarson A, Goldstein S, Faberberg B, et al. Effects of controlled-release metoprolol on total mortality, hospitalizations, and well-being in patients with heart failure: The Metoprolol CR/XL Randomized Intervention Trial in Congestive Heart Failure (MERIT-HF). *JAMA* 2000; 283:1295–1302.

349. Pitt B, Zannad F, Remme WJ, et al, for the Randomized Aldactone Evaluation Study (RALES) investigators. The effect of spironolactone on morbidity and mortality in patients with severe heart failure. *N Engl J Med* 1999; 341:709–717.

350. Pitt B, for the ELITE investigators. Results of the Evaluation of Losartan In The Elderly (ELITE) Trial. *Lancet* 1997; 349:757–762.

351. Packer MA, for the PRAISE Study Group. Final results of the Prospective Randomized Amlodipine Ischemia and Survival Evaluation Study. *N Engl J Med* 1996; 335:1107–1111.

352. Williams JF, Bristow MR, Fowler MB, et al. Guidelines for the evaluation and management of heart failure: Report of the American College of Cardiology/American Heart Association Task Force on Practice Guidelines (Committee on Evaluation and Management of Heart Failure). *J Am Coll Cardiol* 1995; 26:1376–1398.

353. Setaro JF, Zaret BL, Schulman DS, et al. Usefulness of verapamil for congestive heart failure associated with abnormal left ventricular diastolic filling and normal left ventricular systolic performance. *Am J Cardiol* 1990; 66:981–986.

354. Otto CM, Lind BK, Kitzman DW, et al. Association of aortic-valve sclerosis with cardiovascular mortality and morbidity in the elderly. *N Engl J Med* 1999; 341:142–147.

355. Sapira JD. Quincke, de Musset, Duroziez and Hill: Some aortic regurgitations. *South Med J* 1981; 74:459–467.

356. Scognamiglio R, Rahimtoola SH, Fasoli G, et al. Nifedipine in asymptomatic patients with severe aortic regurgitation and normal left ventricular function. *N Engl J Med* 1994; 331:689–694.

357. Rich S, Kaufmann E, Levy PS. The effect of high doses of calcium-channel blockers on survival in primary pulmonary hypertension. *N Engl J Med* 1992; 327:76–81.

358. Khan MA, Herzog CA, St. Peter JV, et al. The prevalence of cardiac valvular insufficiency assessed by transthoracic echocardiography in obese patients treated with appetite-suppressant drugs. *N Engl J Med* 1999; 339:713–718.

359. Remuzzi G, Ruggenenti P, Benigni A. Understanding the nature of renal disease progression. *Kidney Int* 1997; 51:2–15.

360. Tarif N, Bakris GL. Renal components of the hypertensive syndrome. *J Cardiovas Risk* 1997; 4(4):271–278.

361. The GISEN group. Randomized placebo-controlled trial of effect of ramipril on decline in glomerular filtration rate and risk of terminal renal failure in proteinuric, non-diabetic nephropathy. *Lancet* 1997; 349:1857–1863.

362. Benigni A, Remuzzi G. Glomerular protein trafficking and progression of renal disease to terminal uremia. *Semin Nephrol* 1996; 16(3):151–159.

363. Brown S, Walton C, Crawford P, Bakris GL. Comparative renal hemodynamic effects of an ACE inhibitor or calcium antagonist on progression of diabetic nephropathy in the dog. *Kidney Int* 1993; 43:1210–1218.

364. Kloke HJ, Branten AJ, Huysmans FT, Wetzels JF. Antihypertensive treatment of patients with proteinuric renal diseases: Risks or benefits of calcium channel blockers? *Kidney Int* 1998; 53(6):1559–1573.

365. Tarif N, Bakris GL. Angiotensin II receptor blockade and progression of renal disease in nondiabetic patients. *Kidney Int* 1997; 52(suppl 63):S-67–S-70.

366. Ravid M, Brosh D, Levi Z, et al. Use of enalapril to attenuate decline in renal function in normotensive, normoalbuminuric patients with type 2 diabetes mellitus: A randomized, controlled trial. *Ann Intern Med* 1998; 128(12 part 1):982–988.

367. Abbott K, Smith AC, Bakris GL. Effects of dihydropyridine calcium antagonists on albuminuria in diabetic subjects. *J Clin Pharmacol* 1996; 36:274–279.

368. Bakris GL, Smith AC. Effects of sodium intake on albumin excretion in patients with diabetic nephropathy treated with long-acting calcium antagonists. *Ann Intern Med* 1996; 125(3):201–203.

369. Bakris GL, Weir MR. Salt intake and reductions in arterial pressure and proteinuria: Is there a direct link? *Am J Hypertens* 1996; 9:200S–206S.

370. Heeg JE, de Jong PE, van der Hem GK, de Zeeuw D. Efficacy and variability of the antiproteinuric effect of ACE inhibition by lisinopril. *Kidney Int* 1989; 36(2):272–279.

371. Bakris GL, Weir MR. ACE inhibitor associated elevations in serum creatinine: Is this a cause for concern? *Arch Intern Med* 2000; 160:685–693.

372. Parving HH, Rossing P, Hommel E, Smidt UM. Angiotensin-converting enzyme inhibition in diabetic nephropathy: Ten years' experience. *Am J Kidney Dis* 1995; 26(1):99–107.

373. The National Kidney Foundation Hypertension and Diabetes Executive Committee Working Group. Treatment of hypertension in adults with diabetes to preserve renal function: A position paper. *Am J Kidney Dis*, in press.

374. Yeghiazarians Y, Braunstein JB, Askari A, Stone PH. Medical progress: Unstable angina pectoris. *N Engl J Med* 2000; 342:101–114.

375. Heidenreich PA, McDonald KM, Hastie T, et al. Meta-analysis of trials comparing beta-blockers, calcium antagonists, and nitrates for stable angina. *JAMA* 1999; 281:1927–1936.

376. Powers WJ. Acute hypertension after stroke: The scientific basis for treatment decisions. *Neurology* 1994; 43:461–467.

377. Adams HP, Brott TG, Crowell RM, et al. Guidelines for the management of patients with acute ischemic stroke: A statement for healthcare professionals from a special writing group of the Stroke Council, American Heart Association. *Stroke* 1994; 25:1901–1914.

378. The National Institute of Neurological Disorders and Stroke rt-PA Stroke Study Group. Tissue plasminogen activator for acute ischemic stroke. *N Engl J Med* 1995; 333:1581–1587.

379. Mayberg MR, Batjer HH, Dacey R, et al. Guidelines for the management of aneurysmal subarachnoid hemorrhage: A statement for healthcare professionals from a special writing group of the Stroke Council, American Heart Association. *Circulation* 1994; 90:2592–2605.

380. Epstein M, Bakris GL. Newer approaches to antihypertensive therapy: Use fixed dose combination therapy. *Arch Intern Med* 1996; 156:1969–1978.

381. Bakris GL, Weber MA, Black HR, Weir MR. Clinical efficacy and safety profiles of AT1 receptor antagonists. *Cardiovasc Rev Reports* 1999; 20:77–100.

382. Preston RA, Materson BJ, Reda DJ, et al, for the Department of Veterans Affairs Cooperative Study Group on Antihypertensive Agents. Age-race subgroup compared to renin profile as predictors of blood pressure response to antihypertensive therapy in 1031 patients: Results of the VA cooperative study. *JAMA* 1998; 280(13):1168–1172.

383. Weir MR, Gray JM, Paster R, Saunders E. Differing mechanisms of action of angiotensin-converting enzyme inhibition in black

and white hypertensive patients: The Trandolapril Multicenter Study Group. *Hypertension* 1995; 26(1):124–130.
384. National High Blood Pressure Education Program Working Group. National High Blood Pressure Education Program Working Group Report on Hypertension in the Elderly. *Hypertension* 1994; 23:275–285.
385. Lever AF, Ramsay LE. Treatment of hypertension in the elderly. *J Hypertens* 1995; 13:571–579.
386. Update on the Task Force Report (1987) on High Blood Pressure in Children and Adolescents: A Working Group Report from the National High Blood Pressure Education Program: National High Blood Pressure Education Program Working Group on Hypertension Control in Children and Adolescents. *Pediatrics* 1996; 98:649–658.
387. Sinaiko AR. Current concepts: Hypertension in children. *N Engl J Med* 1996; 335:1968–1973.
388. National High Blood Pressure Education Program Working Group on Hypertension in Pregnancy. Report of the National High Blood Pressure Education Program Working Group on Hypertension in Pregnancy. *Am J Obstet Gynecol* 1990; 163:1689–1712.
389. Helewa ME, Burrows RF, Smith J, et al. Report of the Canadian Hypertension Society Consensus Conference: Definition, evaluation, and classification of hypertensive disorders in pregnancy. *Can Med Assoc J* 1997; 157:715–725.
390. Caritis S, Sibai B, Hauth J, et al. Low-dose aspirin to prevent preeclampsia in women at high risk. *N Engl J Med* 1998; 338:701–705.
391. Levine RJ, Hauth JC, Curet LB, et al. Trial of calcium to prevent preeclampsia. *N Engl J Med* 1997; 337:69–76.
392. Kaplan NM. Management of hypertensive emergencies. *Lancet* 1994; 344:1335–1338.
393. Gifford RW Jr. Management of hypertensive crises. *JAMA* 1991; 266:829–835.
394. Elliott WJ, Black HR. Hypertensive emergencies and aortic dissection. *Curr Ther Crit Care Med* 1997; 185–191.
395. Strandgaard S, Paulson OR. Hypertensive disease and the cerebral circulation. In: Laragh JH, Brenner BM, eds. *Hypertension: Pharphysiology, Diagnosis, and Management*, Vol 1. New York: Raven Press; 1990:399.
396. Cohn JN, Burke LP. Nitroprusside. *Ann Intern Med* 1979; 91:752–757.
397. Dmowski AT, Carey MJ. Aortic dissection. *Am J Emerg Med* 1999; 17:372–375.
398. Chen K, Varon J, Wenker OC, et al. Acute thoracic aortic dissection: The basics. *J Emerg Med* 1997; 15:859–867.
399. Post JB IV, Frishman WH. Fenoldopam: A new dopamine agonist for the treatment of hypertensive urgencies and emergencies. *J Clin Pharmacol* 1998; 38:2–13.
400. Wallin JD, Fletcher E, Ram CV, et al. Intravenous nicardipine for the treatment of severe hypertension. *Arch Intern Med* 1989; 149:2662–2669.
401. Grossman E, Messerli FH, Grodzicki T, et al. Should a moratorium be placed on sublingual nifedipine capsules given for hypertensive emergencies and pseudoemergencies? *JAMA* 1996; 276:1328–1331.
402. Stason WB, Schmid CH, Niedzwiecki D, et al. Safety of nifedipine in patients with hypertension: A meta-analysis. *Hypertension* 1997; 30:7–14.
403. Grossman E, Ironi AN, Messerli FH. Comparative tolerability profile of hypertensive crises treatments. *Drug Saf* 1998; 19: 99–122.
404. Cohen MC, Rohtla KM, Lavery CE, et al. Meta-analysis of the morning excess of acute myocardial infarction and sudden cardiac death. *Circulation* 1997; 79:1512–1515.
405. Elliott WJ. Circadian variation in the timing of stroke onset: A meta-analysis. *Stroke* 1998; 29:992–996.
406. Elliott WJ, Prisant LM. Drug delivery systems for antihypertensive agents. *Blood Pressure Monit* 1997; 2:53–60.
407. Smolensky MH, Portaluppi F. Chronopharmacology and chronotherapy of cardiovascular medications: Relevance to prevention and treatment of coronary heart disease. *Am Heart J* 1999; 137(4 part 2):S14–S24.
408. White WB, Black HR, Elliott W, et al. Comparison of effects of controlled onset extended release verapamil at bedtime and nifedipine gastrointestinal therapeutic system on arising on early morning blood pressure, heart rate, and the heart rate–blood pressure product. *Am J Cardiol* 1998; 81:424–431.
409. Saseen JJ, Carter BL, Brown TE, et al. Comparison of nifedipine alone and with diltiazem or verapamil in hypertension. *Hypertension* 1996; 28(1):109–114.
410. Matersson HRB, Pope JE, Anderson JJ, Felson DT. A meta-analysis of the effects of nonsteroidal anti-inflammatory drugs on blood pressure. *Arch Intern Med* 1993; 153(4): 477–484.
411. Jones JK, Gorkin L, Lian JF, et al. Discontinuation of and changes in treatment after start of new courses of antihypertensive drugs: A study of a United Kingdom population. *BMJ* 1995; 311:293–296.
412. Bloom BS. Continuation of initial antihypertensive medication after one year of therapy. *Clin Ther* 1998; 20:671–681.
413. Levine M. Costs associated with noncompliance. In: Leenen, FHH, ed. *Patient Compliance and the Long-Term Management of Hypertension.* Montréal: STA Communications; 1996:21.
414. Elliott WJ. Compliance Strategies. In: Alderman MH, Mitch WE, eds. *Current Opinion in Nephrology and Hypertension*, Vol 3. Philadelphia: Current Science; 1994:271.
415. Hilleman DE, Mohiuddin SM, Lucas BD Jr, et al. Cost-minimization analysis of initial antihypertensive therapy in patients with mild-to-moderate essential diastolic hypertension. *Clin Ther* 1994; 16:88–102.
416. Drugs for Hypertension. *The Medical Letter on Drugs & Therapeutics.* 1999; 41:23–28.

PART EIGHT

PULMONARY HYPERTENSION AND PULMONARY DISEASE

CHAPTER 52

PULMONARY HYPERTENSION

Lewis J. Rubin

Pulmonary hypertension is a hemodynamic abnormality common to a variety of conditions that is characterized by increased right ventricular (RV) afterload and work. The clinical manifestations, natural history, and reversibility of pulmonary hypertension depend heavily on the nature of the pulmonary vascular lesions and the etiology and severity of the hemodynamic disorder. For example, subacute or chronic hypoxia predominantly causes increased muscularization of the small muscular pulmonary arteries and arterioles while leaving the intima relatively intact. Relief of the hypoxia improves or occasionally reverses the process with little or no pathologic residue.[1,2] In contrast, the lesions of systemic sclerosis (scleroderma), which tend to be confined to the intima of the small pulmonary arteries and arterioles, are usually progressive and irreversible. In contrast to scleroderma and chronic hypoxia, which spare the pulmonary capillary bed, the pulmonary capillaries are the primary site of involvement in pulmonary capillary hemangiomatosis.[3] Because of its large capacity, its great distensibility, its low resistance to blood flow, and the modest amounts of smooth muscle in the small arteries and arterioles, the pulmonary circulation is not predisposed to become hypertensive. When total cross-sectional area is decreased, such as by destruction or obliteration of lung tissue or occlusive lesions in the resistance vessels, pulmonary arterial pressures increase. The degree of pulmonary hypertension that develops is a function of the amount of the pulmonary vascular tree that has been eliminated. Pulmonary hypertension is usually secondary to cardiac or pulmonary disease. Although primary pulmonary hypertension (PPH) is uncommon, it has attracted considerable attention as a distinctive clinical entity in which intrinsic pulmonary vascular disease is free of the complicating features of secondary pulmonary hypertension contributed by diseases of the heart and/or lungs. Mild or even moderate pulmonary hypertension can exist for a lifetime without becoming evident clinically. For example, native residents at high altitude, in whom mild to moderate pulmonary hypertension is a natural result of sustained exposure to hypoxia, can function normally. When pulmonary hypertension does become manifest clinically, the symptoms tend to be nonspecific (Table 52-1).

DEFINITIONS

Pulmonary *arterial* hypertension can be either acute or chronic. The acute form is usually a result of either pulmonary embolism (see Chap. 53) or the adult respiratory distress syndrome. This chapter deals with *chronic* pulmonary arterial hypertension.

Pulmonary *venous* hypertension usually is encountered clinically as a consequence of left ventricular (LV) failure or mitral valvular disease. Occasionally, it may occur in the course of fibrosing mediastinitis. Only rarely is the entity known as pulmonary veno-occlusive disease (PVOD) encountered. Even though pulmonary hypertension may be confined, at the outset, to the pulmonary veins (e.g., in acute mitral insufficiency), sooner or later pulmonary arterial hypertension supervenes. The hallmarks of pulmonary venous hypertension are pulmonary congestion and edema. For practical purposes, pulmonary venous hypertension is said to exist when pulmonary venous (or left atrial) pressure rises above 15 mmHg.

Cor pulmonale signifies the presence of pulmonary hypertension in the setting of chronic respiratory disease.[4] The degree of pulmonary hypertension that develops in patients with chronic lung disease tends to be less severe than in connective tissue diseases, chronic thromboembolic disease, or primary pulmonary hypertension. Pulmonary hypertension may be severe, however, in some patients with interstitial lung disease.

TABLE 52-1 Symptoms of Primary Pulmonary Hypertension

Dyspnea	Palpitations
Fatigue	Orthopnea
Dizziness	Cough
Syncope	Hoarseness
Chest pain	

NORMAL PULMONARY CIRCULATION

Structure

Immediately before birth, pulmonary and systemic arterial blood pressures are about equal and on the order of 70/40 mmHg, with a mean of 50 mmHg. Immediately after birth, with closure of the ductus arteriosus and initiation of ventilation, pulmonary arterial pressure falls rapidly to about one-half of systemic levels. Thereafter, pulmonary arterial pressures gradually decrease over several weeks to reach adult levels[5] (see also Chap. 70).

In some neonates, the normal pulmonary hypertension of the fetus fails to recede normally, generally due to either a developmental anomaly or a relentless increase in pulmonary vascular tone. In such infants, the persistent pulmonary hypertension and RV failure may become life-threatening. Surgical intervention or temporizing measures, such as the use of inhaled nitric oxide (NO) or extracorporeal membrane oxygenation (ECMO), may be useful in reversing the pulmonary vascular abnormalities.[6]

In the normal adult at sea level, the small muscular arteries and arterioles in the lungs are thin-walled and contain very little smooth muscle. In contrast, in the fetus or the adult who has lived under hypoxic conditions (e.g., native residents at high altitude), the media of the arterioles are thickened, and the muscle extends distally into precapillary vessels that are ordinarily devoid of muscle; i.e., the precapillary vessels undergo "remodeling."[7]

Endothelium and Endothelium–Smooth Muscle Interactions

In addition to its role as a semipermeable barrier between blood and interstitium, the endothelium serves a wide array of biologically important functions, the net effect of which is the processing of blood flowing through the lungs. Among these functions are the synthesis, uptake, storage, release, and metabolism of vasoactive substances; transduction of blood-borne signals; modulation of coagulation and thrombolysis; regulation of cell proliferation; engagement in the local inflammatory and proliferative reactions to injury; involvement in immune reactions; and angiogenesis (see also Chap. 4). Some of the enzymes involved in these processes, such as the angiotensin-converting enzyme, are found on the surface of endothelial cells; others, such as 5′-nucleotidase, are found within the cell.[8] Hence it is appropriate to regard endothelium as an organ with diverse metabolic and endocrine functions, one that is unique because of its strategic location as a continuous, monolayered lining of blood vessels throughout the body. It is also important to bear in mind that the lungs contain the largest expanse of endothelium in the body.

The cells that comprise the monolayered endothelial lining communicate not only with each other by anatomic junctions and bridges but also with the underlying smooth muscle by way of biologically active substances.[9] This interaction participates in regulating normal vasomotor tone as well as in response to the administration of vasoactive substances. It is not difficult to imagine that damage to the lining cells, proliferation of the intima, or hypertrophy of the smooth muscle will upset the normal interplay.

Hemodynamics

For the adult pulmonary circulation, the definition of *normal* depends on the altitude. The normal pulmonary hemodynamics of adults residing at sea level and above sea level are compared in Table 52-2. At *sea level,* a cardiac output of 5 to 6 L/min is associated with a pulmonary arterial pressure of about 20/12 mmHg, with a mean of about 15 mmHg. At an altitude of 15,000 ft, the same level of blood flow is associated with somewhat higher pressures (see Table 52-2). Pulmonary arterial pressures also tend to increase somewhat with age.

A pressure drop of only 5 to 10 mmHg between the pulmonary artery and left atrium accompanies the cardiac output of 5 to 6 L/min (see Table 52-2). Determination of pulmonary vascular resistance, calculated as the ratio of the difference in mean pressure at the two ends of the pulmonary vascular bed (pulmonary arterial pressure minus left atrial pressure divided by the cardiac output; see Table 52-2), has proved to be a practical clinical tool for assessing the hemodynamic state of the pulmonary circulation and for distinguishing between active and passive changes in the pulmonary resistance vessels (e.g., the effect of administering a vasodilator agent to a patient with pulmonary hypertension). In practice, since the left atrium may not be readily accessible, pulmonary wedge pressure generally is substituted for left atrial pressure.

Another approach to defining certain characteristics and the behavior of the pulmonary arterial tree, i.e., elastic properties and geometry, is the calculation of pulmonary arterial input

TABLE 52-2 Values for Normal Pulmonary Circulation at Sea Level and Altitude

	Sea Level	Altitude (~15,000 ft)
Pulmonary arterial pressure (P_{PA}), mmHg	20/12, 15	38/14, 25
Cardiac output (Q), L/min	6.0	6.0
Left atrial pressure (P_{LA}), mmHg	5.0	5.0
Pulmonary vascular resistance (PVR),[a] (mmHg/L)/min (R units)	1.7	3.3

[a] $PVR = \frac{P_{PA} - P_{LA}}{Q} = \frac{15-5}{6} = 1.67$ R units. To convert T units to CGS units (dynes·s/cm^5), multiply R units by 80.

impedance. This approach has more physiologic than clinical value. It takes into account the pulsatile nature of pulmonary arterial pressures and flow. Like vascular resistance, it is defined as a ratio. But instead of a ratio involving *mean* pressures and blood flow, the ratio is of the amplitudes of pulsatile pressure to oscillatory flow near the beginning of the pulmonary artery at a particular frequency. Values for the ratio are obtained by resolving mathematically the pulsatile pressure and flow curves into their sinusoidal components.

Although calculated pulmonary vascular resistance has proved useful in assessing the state of the normal and abnormal pulmonary circulation, and even though a change in calculated resistance often can be helpful in deciding whether pulmonary vasoconstriction or vasodilatation has occurred, translation of a calculated ratio into vasomotor activity has to be made with caution.[4] For example, changes in calculated pulmonary vascular resistance are not readily interpretable when a vasodilator agent evokes multiple hemodynamic changes simultaneously (e.g., simultaneous changes in pulmonary vascular pressures and blood flow). Also, a clinical shortcut, such as the substitution in the numerator of the pulmonary arterial pressure for the pressure *drop* between the pulmonary artery and left atrium, may be useful empirically but deprives the calculation of any physiologic meaning. Finally, the clinical significance of a value calculated for pulmonary vascular resistance depends heavily on the implications of the hemodynamic changes on the work of the right ventricle. For example, the same decrease in calculated pulmonary vascular resistance brought about by two different pulmonary vasodilators may affect the work of the right ventricle differently: Should one agent elicit a *decrease* in pulmonary arterial pressure along with an *increase* in cardiac output (an ideal response), it is more apt to be of long-term benefit than another agent that, while increasing the cardiac output, fails to decrease the pulmonary arterial pressure.

In the normal lung, a considerable increase in cardiac output, i.e., two to three times that at rest, generally increases pulmonary arterial pressure by only a few millimeters of mercury. On the other hand, in pulmonary hypertensive states, in which the distensibility and extent of the pulmonary vascular bed have been restricted by disease, pulmonary arterial pressure increases along with even small increments in pulmonary blood flow. Changes in pulmonary blood volume are much more subtle than changes in blood pressure or flow in their hemodynamic effects; they are also much more difficult to quantify. Clinical clues can be helpful in recognizing that the pulmonary blood volume has increased. Often a fullness of the pulmonary vascular pattern on the chest radiograph along with evidences of interstitial edema suggests that pulmonary blood volume has increased acutely. In chronic mitral stenosis or LV failure, the pulmonary blood volume is not only increased but is also redistributed toward the apices of the lungs, i.e., "cephalization."

Autonomic innervation of the pulmonary vascular tree plays much less of a role in modulating vasomotor tone than do local stimuli, particularly hypoxia. Indeed, hypoxia can exert its pulmonary pressor effect in the isolated lung, i.e., one that is devoid of external innervation. The mechanism by which hypoxia exerts its local pressor effect is not fully characterized but appears to involve altered smooth muscle cell membrane ion channel activity.[2] Acidosis potentiates the hypoxic pressor effect. Hypercapnia also exerts a pulmonary pressor effect, presumably by way of the local acidosis that it generates, but it is less powerful than hypoxia as a pulmonary vasoconstrictor agent.

PULMONARY HYPERTENSION: GENERAL FEATURES

Clinical Manifestations

Pulmonary hypertension is a final common hemodynamic consequence of multiple etiologies and diverse mechanisms. As noted earlier, most cases of pulmonary hypertension are secondary (Table 52-3). Among the underlying causes of pulmonary hypertension are mechanical compression and distortion of the resistance vessels of the lungs (e.g., by diffuse pulmonary fibrosis), hypoxic vasoconstriction (e.g., in severe obstructive airways or diffuse parenchymal diseases), intravascular obstruction (e.g., thromboemboli or tumor emboli), and combinations of mechanical and vasoconstrictive influences. The significance of pulmonary hypertension, however, is that if it is uncontrolled, it leads to RV failure. Once pulmonary arterial pressures reach systemic levels, RV failure becomes inevitable.

Special Studies

The "gold standard" for the diagnosis of pulmonary hypertension is right-sided heart catheterization. This technique enables the direct determination of right atrial and ventricular pressures, pulmonary arterial pressure, pulmonary wedge pressure (as an approximation of pulmonary venous pressure), pulmonary blood flow (cardiac output), and the responses of these parameters to interventions (vasodilators, oxygen, exercise). From the measurements and samples obtained during cardiac catheterization, pulmonary vascular resistance can be calculated (see Table 52-2). As a rule, noninvasive methods are less reliable and less informative.

CHEST RADIOGRAPHY

The findings on the chest radiograph depend on the duration of the pulmonary hypertension and the etiology. The characteristic findings of pulmonary hypertension are enlargement of the pulmonary trunk and hilar vessels in association with attenuation (pruning) of the peripheral pulmonary arterial tree (Fig. 52-1). Right-sided heart enlargement can be best detected radiographically on the lateral view as fullness in the retrosternal airspace. In secondary pulmonary hypertension, changes in the lungs (e.g., hyperinflation, fibrosis) and in the position of the heart and diaphragm often mask the radiologic changes of pulmonary hypertension. Contrast angiography has a role in the workup for pulmonary hypertension when chronic thromboembolic disease, which may be treated surgically, is suspected.[8]

THE ELECTROCARDIOGRAM

The electrocardiogram (ECG) can disclose hypertrophy of the right ventricle and is more reliable in respiratory disorders that do not involve the parenchyma of the lungs (e.g., alveolar hypoventilation and sleep apnea) than in obstructive airways disease or parenchymal lung disease.

ECHOCARDIOGRAPHY

The amount of reliable information obtained by Doppler and two-dimensional echocardiography depends greatly on the com-

TABLE 52-3 Nomenclature and Classification of Pulmonary Hypertension

DIAGNOSTIC CLASSIFICATION

1. Pulmonary arterial hypertension
   1.1 Primary pulmonary hypertension
      (a) Sporadic
      (b) Familial
   1.2 Related to
      (a) Collagen-vascular disease
      (b) Congenital systemic to pulmonary shunts
      (c) Portal hypertension
      (d) HIV infection
      (e) Drugs/toxins
         (1) Anorexigens
         (2) Other
      (f) Persistent pulmonary hypertension of the newborn
      (g) Other
2. Pulmonary venous hypertension
   2.1 Left-side atrial or ventricular heart disease
   2.2 Left-side valvular heart disease
   2.3 Extrinsic compression of central pulmonary veins
      (a) Fibrosing mediastinitis
      (b) Adenopathy/tumors
   2.4 Pulmonary veno-occlusive disease
   2.5 Other
3. Pulmonary hypertension associated with disorders of the respiratory system and/or hypoxemia
   3.1 Chronic obstructive pulmonary disease
   3.2 Interstitial lung disease
   3.3 Sleep-disordered breathing
   3.4 Alveolar hypoventilatory disorders
   3.5 Chronic exposure to high altitude
   3.6 Neonatal lung disease
   3.7 Alveolar-capillary dysplasia
   3.8 Other
4. Pulmonary hypertension due to chronic thrombotic and/or embolic disease
   4.1 Thromboembolic obstruction of proximal pulmonary arteries
   4.2 Obstruction of distal pulmonary arteries
      (a) Pulmonary embolism (thrombus, tumor, ova and/or parasites, foreign material)
      (b) In-situ thrombosis
      (c) Sickle cell disease
5. Pulmonary hypertension due to disorders directly affecting the pulmonary vasculature
   5.1 Inflammatory
      (a) Schistosomiasis
      (b) Sarcoidosis
      (c) Other
   5.2 Pulmonary capillary hemangiomatosis

mitment of individual clinics to standardizing and perfecting these noninvasive techniques. In general, echocardiographic techniques have proved useful in providing a measure of RV thickness as an index of RV hypertension. In some clinics, reliable estimates of the level of pulmonary hypertension have been obtained by determining regurgitant flows across the tricuspid and pulmonic valves using continuous-wave Doppler echocardiography.[9] In patients in whom the pulmonic valve has been visualized, its behavior during the cardiac cycle also has been used to estimate the level of pulmonary arterial pressure. Probably one of the more rewarding applications of echocardiography has been as an alternative to repeated cardiac catheterization in tracing the course of the disease and in assessing the effects of therapeutic interventions (e.g., pulmonary vasodilators) in some patients (see also Chap. 13).

LUNG SCANS

Ventilation-perfusion scans are of most value in the diagnosis and exclusion of pulmonary thromboembolic disease (see below).

RADIONUCLIDE STUDIES

The response of the RV ejection fraction to exercise is assessed in some clinics using radionuclide angiography. Scintigraphy using thallium-201 also has been useful in detecting hypertrophy of the right ventricle due to pulmonary hypertension (see also Chap. 16).

LUNG BIOPSY

The sampling of lung tissue by open thoracotomy or thoracoscopy occasionally is helpful in identifying the etiology of the pulmonary hypertension, e.g., in the setting of suspected pulmonary vasculitis. However, the procedure carries substantial risk in these hemodynamically compromised individuals. Attempts to predict responsiveness to vasodilators on the basis of lung biopsy have met with limited success.[10]

SECONDARY PULMONARY HYPERTENSION

Cardiac and/or respiratory diseases are the most common causes of secondary pulmonary hypertension. Pulmonary thromboembolic disease ranks third. Cardiac disease leads to pulmonary hypertension by increasing pulmonary blood flow (e.g., large left-to-right shunts) or by increasing pulmonary venous pressure (e.g., LV failure). Almost invariably, secondary influences such as intimal proliferation in the pulmonary resistance vessels add a component of obstructive pulmonary vascular disease.[11] In respiratory disease, the predominant mechanism for the pulmonary hypertension is an increase in resistance to pulmonary blood flow arising from perivascular parenchymal changes coupled with pulmonary vasoconstriction due to hypoxia. In pulmonary thromboembolic disease, clots in various stages of organization and affecting pulmonary vessels of different size increase resistance to blood flow.[11]

Cardiac Disease

The mechanisms of pulmonary hypertension usually are quite different in acquired disorders of the left side of the heart than in those of congenital heart disease.

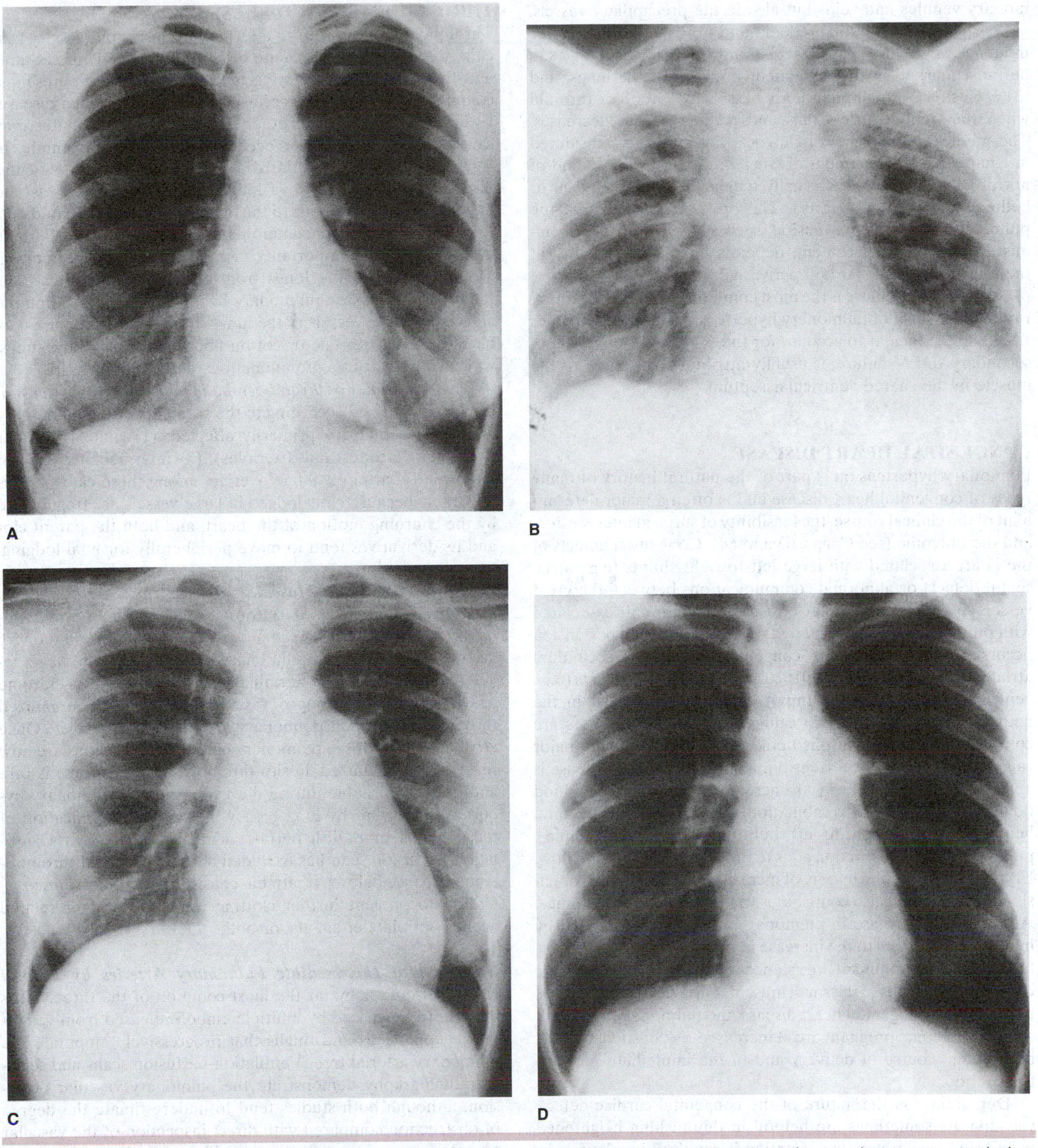

FIGURE 52-1 Cardiac silhouette in four patients with severe pulmonary hypertension on admission to the hospital: *A,B.* Primary pulmonary hypertension showing different stages in the evolution of right-sided heart failure. *C.* Widespread pulmonary fibrosis. *D.* Systemic lupus erythematosus proven by lung biopsy. This radiograph is indistinguishable from that of primary pulmonary hypertension.

ACQUIRED DISORDERS OF THE LEFT SIDE OF THE HEART

LV failure is the most common cause of pulmonary hypertension. Among the various etiologies, myocardial disorders and lesions of the mitral and aortic valves predominate. Both categories of lesions lead to an increase in pulmonary venous pressure that, in turn, evokes an increase in pulmonary arterial pressure. Presumably, the increase in pulmonary arterial pressure is reflex in origin. In time, three types of morphologic changes supervene: (1) occlusive intimal and medial changes not only in pulmonary venules and veins but also in the precapillary vessels, (2) perivascular interstitial edema and fibrosis that, under the influence of gravity, cause vascular and perivascular changes to be most marked in the dependent portions of the lungs, and (3) occlusion of small pulmonary vessels by emboli or thrombi when the right ventricle fails and cardiac output decreases. The medical management of myocardial failure is considered in Chap. 21. The treatment of congenital heart disease and of mitral valvular disease is usually mechanical (e.g., surgical or balloon mitral valvuloplasty). The prospect for relief of the pulmonary venous hypertension, such as by mitral valve commissurotomy or replacement, depends on the reversibility of the pulmonary vascular and perivascular lesions.

Although LV failure is the most common cause of RV failure, rarely is the level of pulmonary hypertension that accompanies LV failure sufficient to account for the RV failure. RV failure, secondary to LV failure, is usually attributed to failure of the muscle in the shared ventricular septum.

CONGENITAL HEART DISEASE

Pulmonary hypertension is part of the natural history of many types of congenital heart disease and is often a major determinant of the clinical course, the feasibility of surgical intervention, and the outcome (see Chaps. 63 and 64). Congenital defects of the heart associated with large left-to-right shunts (e.g., atrial septal defect) or abnormal communications between the great vessels (e.g., patent ductus arteriosus) are commonly associated with pulmonary arterial hypertension. Pulmonary hypertension occurs in both "pretricuspid" congenital defects (e.g., secundum atrial septal defect) and "posttricuspid" congenital defects (e.g., ventricular septal defect). Important differences exist in the natural history of these two categories. Their differences are considered elsewhere in this book (see Chap. 70). The major cause of pulmonary hypertension in congenital heart disease is an increase in blood flow, an increase in resistance to blood flow, or most often, a combination of the two. In congenital heart disease with right-to-left shunting (systemic hypoxemia), pulmonary vasoconstriction adds to the resistance to blood flow. Erythrocytosis, acting by way of increased viscosity and propensity to thrombosis, also contributes to the increase in resistance. Although the increase in pulmonary vascular tone elicited by hypoxia contributes to the increase in pulmonary vascular resistance, the predominant resistance is offered by anatomic changes in the walls of the small muscular arteries and arterioles. Patients with congenital heart disease and pulmonary hypertension who become pregnant are at increased risk of sudden death both in the course of delivery and in the immediate postpartum period.

Depending on the nature of the congenital cardiac defect, vasodilators sometimes are helpful in diminishing heightened pulmonary vasomotor tone. Caution is required in administering such agents to patients with congenital heart disease because of the potential to increase right-to-left shunting by reducing systemic vascular resistance to a greater degree than its pulmonary counterpart. Phlebotomy, with replacement of fluid (e.g., plasma or albumin), is helpful in congenital cyanotic heart disease in which severe hypoxemia has evoked a large increase in red cell mass. Once again, caution is required to avoid depletion of iron stores and to avoid reduction in the circulating blood volume.

THROMBOEMBOLIC DISEASE

Thromboembolic disease is a form of occlusive pulmonary vascular disease. It may be acute or chronic. In the United States and Europe, clots originating in peripheral veins represent a common cause of chronic occlusive pulmonary vascular disease. Elsewhere in the world, other intravascular particulates may cause pulmonary vascular occlusive disease. For example, in Egypt, where schistosomiasis is endemic, pulmonary vascular disease stemming from ova lodged in pulmonary vessels and hypersensitivity reactions to the organism (usually situated outside the lungs) is not uncommon. In some parts of Asia, filariasis is reputed to be an important cause of pulmonary hypertension. Tumor emboli to the lungs from extrapulmonary sites (e.g., the breast) can cause pulmonary hypertension by invading the adjacent minute vessels of the lungs. Intravenous drug use may be associated with talc or cotton fiber embolism to the lungs, which can result in a granulomatous pulmonary arteritis.

The *syndromes of thromboembolic pulmonary hypertension* can be categorized according to the segments of the pulmonary arterial tree that are primarily affected: (1) small (muscular pulmonary arteries and arterioles), (2) intermediate, and (3) large central arteries. Some overlap among these categories is inevitable because clots lodged in large vessels are fragmented by the churning motion of the heart, and both the parent clot and its derivatives tend to move peripherally for final lodging.

Occlusion of Small Muscular Arteries and Arterioles by Organized Thrombi At autopsy, small thrombi, predominantly recent in origin, are commonplace in the small pulmonary vessels of patients with pulmonary hypertension who have developed heart failure preterminally. In contrast is the syndrome of widespread pulmonary vascular occlusion by organized thrombi in the small pulmonary arteries and arterioles. Once attributed to multiple pulmonary emboli, these lesions are now regarded as organized, in situ thrombi.[12] The syndrome is rare and indistinguishable during life from primary pulmonary hypertension except by lung biopsy. Histologic identification of these lesions serves little purpose in management. After a ventilation-perfusion scan has excluded chronic proximal thromboembolism (see below), treatment consists of long-term anticoagulation to prevent further clotting using warfarin or related agents, antiplatelet agents, or both.

Occlusion of Intermediate Pulmonary Arteries by Emboli This syndrome is by far the most common of the three.[12] It is thought to be caused by multiple emboli released from vessels in the upper legs and thighs that progressively amputate the pulmonary arterial tree. Ventilation-perfusion scans and selective angiography demonstrate the pulmonary vascular occlusion, although both studies tend to underestimate the degree of obstruction compared with direct inspection of the vascular tree at surgery or postmortem (see Chap. 53). The major therapeutic concern in these patients is to exclude chronic proximal pulmonary thromboembolism (see below) and to prevent recurrent thromboemboli. Treatment involves the use of anticoagulants of the warfarin type and antiplatelet agents.

Chronic Proximal Pulmonary Thromboembolism In some patients who have survived large to massive pulmonary emboli, resolution fails to occur, and the clots become organized and incorporated into the walls of the major pulmonary arteries,

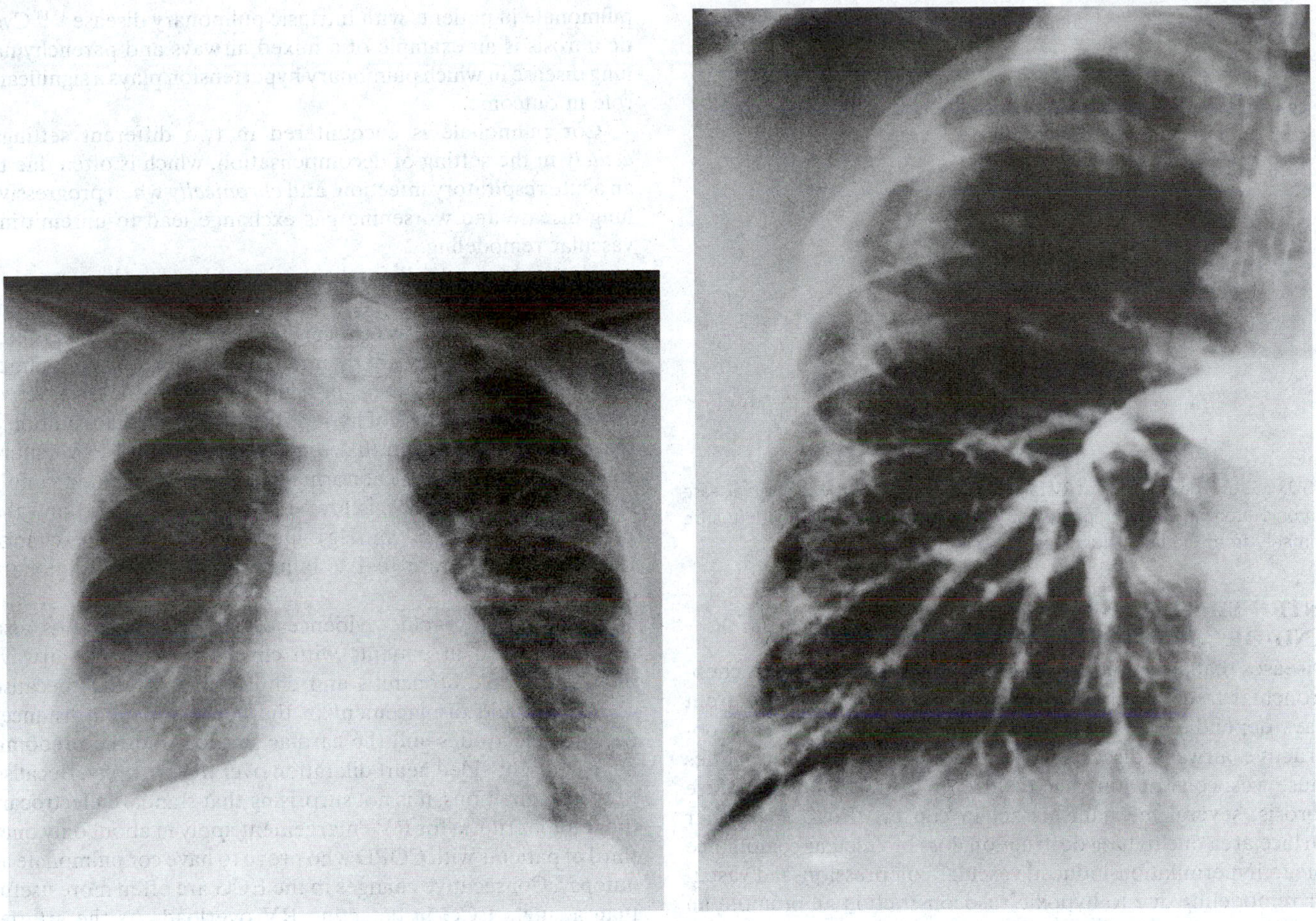

FIGURE 52-2 Pulmonary hypertension due to organized clot in central pulmonary arteries. Dramatic relief after pulmonary thromboendarterectomy. *A.* Chest radiograph. The right upper lobe is strikingly hypoperfused, and the vasculature on the left is quite prominent, reflecting redirection of the pulmonary blood flow to open vessels. *B.* Angiogram. The flow to the right upper lung is interrupted by the large central clot.

leading to pulmonary hypertension (Fig. 52-2). Overwhelming the capacity of the local fibrinolytic mechanisms also allows the clot to propagate, to obstruct large segments of the pulmonary vascular bed, and to decrease the compliance of the central pulmonary vessels. By the time the diagnosis is made, the obstructing lesions in the central pulmonary arteries have become an integral part of the vascular wall through the processes of endothelialization and recanalization.[12]

The importance of recognizing *proximal* pulmonary thromboembolism as a cause of pulmonary hypertension is the possibility of relieving the pulmonary hypertension by surgical intervention, i.e., by pulmonary thromboendarterectomy. Ventilation-perfusion lung scanning is the critical diagnostic test. As a rule, patients with proximal pulmonary thromboembolism show two or more segmental perfusion defects. If the perfusion defects are segmental or larger, selective pulmonary angiography is called for to define the location, extent, and number of pulmonary vascular occlusions.[13,14] Cardiac catheterization for selective pulmonary angiography also enables hemodynamic assessment. Fiberoptic angioscopy, helical computed tomographic scanning, and magnetic resonance imaging may be helpful in defining the lesions of proximal thromboembolic pulmonary hypertension[15] (see also Chap. 53).

Surgery is advocated for patients with pulmonary hypertension who have persistent clot in lobar or more proximal pulmonary arteries after at least 6 months of anticoagulation. Thromboendarterectomy is done via a median sternotomy using deep hypothermic cardiopulmonary bypass with intermittent periods of circulatory arrest. Postoperatively, hemodynamic improvement is usually quite dramatic.[8,14] Reperfusion pulmonary edema can be a severe complication immediately after the obstruction has been relieved. In experienced hands, mortality is on the order of 5 percent. After the operation, patients are placed on lifelong anticoagulants. A filter is usually placed in the inferior vena cava to further prevent recurrence.

Respiratory Diseases and Disorders

In addition to intrinsic pulmonary diseases, disturbances in respiratory muscle function or in the control of breathing also can lead to pulmonary hypertension. Among the intrinsic lung diseases are those affecting the airways (e.g., chronic bronchitis) as well as those affecting the parenchyma (i.e., emphysema, pulmonary fibrosis). Among the ventilatory disorders are the syndromes of alveolar hypoventilation due to respiratory muscle weakness and sleep-disordered breathing.

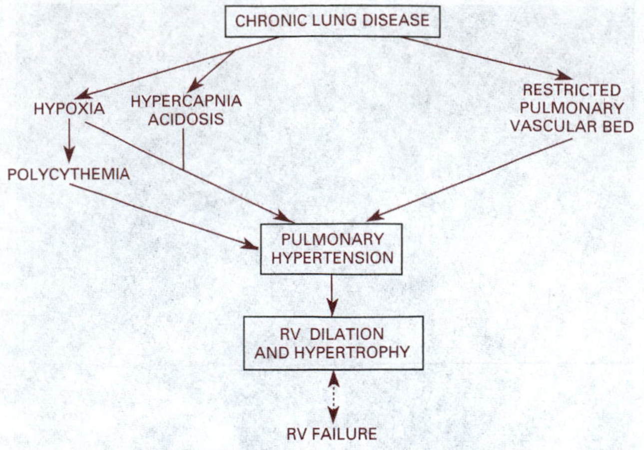

FIGURE 52-3 The evolution of RV failure in chronic obstructive airways disease (chronic bronchitis and emphysema; COPD). The factors on the left arise primarily from the bronchitis; those on the right from emphysema.

INTRINSIC DISEASES OF THE LUNGS AND/OR AIRWAYS

Diseases that affect the parenchyma of the lungs or the tracheobronchial tree can elicit pulmonary hypertension in different ways depending on the underlying disease (Fig. 52-3). In obstructive airways disease, ventilation-perfusion abnormalities cause vasoconstriction due to arterial hypoxemia. In diffuse fibrosis, several mechanisms act in concert: Loss of vascular surface area due to lung destruction, loss of vascular compliance due to hyperinflation-induced vascular compression, and vascular remodeling due to hypoxic vasoconstriction all promote an increased pulmonary vascular resistance.

INTERSTITIAL FIBROSIS

Pulmonary sarcoidosis, asbestosis, and idiopathic and radiation-induced fibrosis are common causes of widespread pulmonary fibrosis that culminates in cor pulmonale. Dyspnea and tachypnea generally dominate the clinical picture of interstitial fibrosis; cough is rarely prominent. As a rule, severe pulmonary hypertension occurs toward the end of the illness, when hypoxemia and hypercapnia are present at rest (see Fig. 52-1). RV failure is a common sequel.

Systemically administered vasodilators have no proven place in dealing with the pulmonary hypertension associated with interstitial fibrosis and may worsen intrapulmonary gas exchange. Recent experience with inhaled vasodilators, such as the prostacyclin analogue iloprost, is encouraging and suggests the possibility of producing selective pulmonary vasodilator and/or antiproliferative effects in this population.[16] Oxygen therapy, particularly during daily activity or sleep, can be important in attenuating the hypoxic pulmonary pressor response. Glucocorticoids and other potent immunosuppressive agents are the mainstay of therapy and often effect some symptomatic relief. The advent of lung transplantation has widened greatly the therapeutic horizons for dealing with widespread interstitial fibrosis.

CHRONIC OBSTRUCTIVE AIRWAYS DISEASE

Chronic bronchitis and emphysema [chronic obstructive pulmonary disease (COPD)] are the most common causes of cor pulmonale in patients with intrinsic pulmonary disease.[17,18] Cystic fibrosis is an example of a mixed airways and parenchymal lung disease in which pulmonary hypertension plays a significant role in outcome.

Cor pulmonale is encountered in two different settings: *acutely* in the setting of decompensation, which is often due to an acute respiratory infection, and *chronically* when progressive lung disease and worsening gas exchange lead to unremitting vascular remodeling.

The "gold standard" for diagnosing pulmonary hypertension in patients with COPD is right-sided heart catheterization. Noninvasive studies, such as echocardiography, have proved useful in some centers.[19,20] RV enlargement, the cardinal sign of pulmonary hypertension, can be difficult to discern in obstructive airways disease because of hyperinflation and cardiac rotation.[21] Once suspicion is raised that the clinical picture of RV failure stems from gas exchange abnormalities, an arterial blood sample will confirm that the P_{O_2} is low ($P_{O_2} < 40–50$ mmHg) and the P_{CO_2} is high ($P_{CO_2} > 50$ mmHg). Derangement in gas exchange to this degree is rare in LV failure unless overt pulmonary edema is present.

Electrocardiographic evidence of RV hypertrophy is also often equivocal in patients with chronic obstructive airways disease (chronic bronchitis and emphysema, COPD) because of rotation and displacement of the heart, widened distances between electrodes and the cardiac surface, and the predominance of right-sided heart dilatation over hypertrophy. Because of these limitations, it is not surprising that standard electrocardiographic criteria for RV enlargement apply in about only one-third of patients with COPD who prove to have cor pulmonale at autopsy. Consecutive changes in the ECG are often more useful than a single ECG in detecting RV overload. As the arterial P_{O_2} drops to abnormal levels (e.g., <60–70 mmHg while awake), T waves tend to become inverted, biphasic, or flat in the right, precordial leads (V_1 to V_3); the mean electrical axis of the QRS shifts 30° or more to the right of the patient's usual axis; ST segments become depressed in leads II, III, and aV_F; and right bundle-branch block (incomplete or complete) often appears. These changes tend to reverse as arterial oxygenation improves (see also Chap. 11).

In the patient with COPD with acute cor pulmonale precipitated by a bout of bronchitis or pneumonia, the goal of therapy is to maintain tolerable levels of arterial oxygenation while waiting for the upper respiratory infection to subside. Supplemental oxygen, such as 28% oxygen delivered by a Venturi mask, generally suffices to relieve arterial hypoxemia and to restore pulmonary arterial pressures to normal. Considerable improvement also may be accomplished even in the individual who has chronic pulmonary hypertension by sustained (>18 h/day) breathing of oxygen-enriched air.

Once the right ventricle has failed, inotropic agents should be used cautiously because of the threat of arrhythmias posed by arterial hypoxemia and respiratory acidosis. Moreover, after adequate oxygenation has been achieved, the need for digitalis and diuretics often decreases because the hemodynamic burden on the right ventricle decreases. Even though acute cor pulmonale is largely reversible, each bout appears to leave behind a slightly higher level of pulmonary hypertension after recovery.[17]

Arterial blood gas composition is the therapeutic compass to the control of pulmonary hypertension in COPD. The degree of hypoxia may be underestimated by blood sampling while the patient is awake and at rest, since hypoxemia is more marked during sleep and with physical activity. Determinations of the oxygen saturation during sleep or with ambulation using pulse oximetry are helpful in optimally prescribing supplemental oxygen.

Ensuring the return of arterial oxygenation toward normal is much more vital than is the administration of inotropic agents.[22] When respiratory infection has triggered the episode of pulmonary hypertension, a vital strategy for achieving a lasting improvement in arterial oxygenation is the administration of an appropriate antibiotic. While awaiting the salutary effects of antibiotic therapy, attention is paid to hydration, to postural drainage, and to adequate alveolar ventilation.

Phlebotomy, once popular because of the prospect that increased blood viscosity contributes importantly to the pulmonary hypertension, has fallen into disuse. Polycythemia is rarely severe enough to be a serious problem in cor pulmonale associated with bronchitis and emphysema, and when its is present, it is usually indicative of inadequate relief of hypoxemia with optimal use of supplemental oxygen.

Vasodilators recently have been tried in various types of secondary pulmonary hypertension, including that due to COPD.[23] The agents tried are the same as those outlined for *primary* pulmonary hypertension. They run the risk of aggravating arterial hypoxemia by exaggerating ventilation-perfusion abnormalities. Unfortunately, the efficacy of vasodilator agents in secondary pulmonary hypertension has proved to be far less impressive or predictable than in primary pulmonary hypertension. To date, the safest and most effective approach to pulmonary vasodilatation in obstructive lung disease with arterial hypoxemia is the use of supplemental oxygen.[23]

CONNECTIVE TISSUE DISEASES

Pulmonary vascular disease is an important component of certain connective tissue diseases. Among these, the more common are systemic lupus erythematosus (SLE), the scleroderma spectrum of diseases, and dermatomyositis.[24] The lesions may take the form of interstitial inflammation and fibrosis, obliterative disease, or vasculitis, either singly or in combination. Although pulmonary hypertension can complicate many connective tissue diseases, it has been documented most often in SLE and progressive systemic sclerosis (scleroderma) and its variant syndromes. The possibility has been raised that primary pulmonary hypertension is an inflammatory, or autoimmune, disease. This prospect has gained support from the occasional instances in which the lesions are confined to the pulmonary arterial tree without interstitial involvement and similarities in the histologic appearance of the vascular lesions. The high frequency of both collagen-vascular disease and primary pulmonary hypertension in women and the occurrence of Raynaud's phenomenon in up to 20 percent of patients with primary pulmonary hypertension has been used as additional evidence.[25] Finally, there is a high incidence of positive serologic tests for antibodies (ANA, anti-Ku), particularly in women with primary pulmonary hypertension. With respect to the pathogenesis of the two disorders, the idea has been raised that both the Raynaud's phenomenon and an increase in pulmonary vascular tone represent a widespread vasoconstrictive pulmonary-systemic disorder. However, this hypothesis has not gained universal support.

The lungs and pleura are frequently involved in SLE, with a reported frequency of up to 70 percent. Patients with pulmonary hypertension and SLE are predominantly women; most of these patients also exhibit Raynaud's phenomenon.

The histopathologic lesions in these patients resemble those of primary pulmonary hypertension. Pulmonary hypertension in these patients may originate in microthrombi secondary to the hypercoagulable state caused by lupus anticoagulant or anticardiolipin antibodies in the blood. Less likely is the hypothesis of generalized vasoconstriction noted earlier. Unfortunately, treatment of pulmonary hypertension associated with SLE using either anticoagulants or pulmonary vasodilators has had only modest success. This poor outcome contrasts with the results obtained in patients with active pulmonary vasculitis, who may either improve or stabilize their vascular disease with immunosuppressive agents.

In progressive systemic sclerosis (scleroderma) and its variants, such as the CREST syndrome (*c*alcinosis, *R*aynaud's syndrome, *e*sophageal involvement, *s*clerodactyly, and *t*elangiectasia) and in overlap syndromes (e.g., mixed connective tissue disease), the incidence of pulmonary vascular disease is high. In these patients, pulmonary hypertension is the cause of considerable morbidity and mortality. In a prospective study involving cardiac catheterization of patients with progressive systemic sclerosis or the CREST syndrome variant, pulmonary hypertension, either as an isolated finding or in association with pulmonary parenchymal or cardiac disease, was found in up to one-third of patients with progressive systemic sclerosis and in up to one-half of patients with the CREST syndrome.[26] The pulmonary vascular disease may be independent of pulmonary or other visceral disease. As in the case of SLE, the pathology of these lesions is often indistinguishable from that of primary pulmonary hypertension. Vasodilator therapy has not proved to be highly effective; however, continuous intravenous epoprostenol recently has been shown to improve hemodynamics and exercise tolerance.[27]

ALVEOLAR HYPOVENTILATION IN PATIENTS WITH NORMAL LUNGS

In patients who hypoventilate despite normal lungs (alveolar hypoventilation), the primary pathogenetic mechanism is alveolar hypoxia potentiated by respiratory acidosis.[28] These abnormal alveolar and arterial blood gases play the same role in eliciting pulmonary hypertension in patients with alveolar hypoventilation as in those in whom the abnormal alveolar and blood gases are the result of ventilation-perfusion abnormalities. In individuals with normal lungs, the alveolar hypoventilation generally originates from an inadequate ventilatory drive (e.g., after encephalitis), covert obstruction of the upper airways (e.g., in the sleep apnea syndromes), an ineffective chest bellows (e.g., after poliomyelitis or polymyositis), or lungs entrapped by neoplasm or fibrosis (e.g., in trapped lung caused by asbestosis).

Regardless of etiology, whether pulmonary hypertension will occur in patients with alveolar hypoventilation and normal lungs depends on the whether there is sufficient alveolar and arterial hypoxia to raise pulmonary arterial pressures considerably. In the sleep apnea syndromes, severe arterial hypoxemia and pulmonary hypertension that develop initially only during sleep may become self-perpetuating and carry over into wakefulness, although this only occurs in those with severe disturbances in respiration during sleep.[29]

For the patient with alveolar hypoventilation with combined respiratory and cardiac (right ventricular) failure, the highest therapeutic priority is to improve oxygenation. Assisted ventilation, particularly during sleep, may be particularly helpful in improving oxygenation and reducing hypercapnia (e.g., continuous positive airway pressure) breathing. Pharmacologic therapy is rarely needed for patients with alveolar hypoventilation because of the efficiency of assisted ventilation coupled with oxygen therapy in promoting pulmonary vasodilatation.

PRIMARY (UNEXPLAINED) PULMONARY HYPERTENSION

Definition

PPH is a disorder intrinsic to the pulmonary vascular bed that is characterized by sustained elevations in pulmonary artery pressure and vascular resistance that generally lead to RV failure and death.[25] The diagnosis of PPH requires the exclusion on clinical grounds of other conditions that can result in pulmonary artery hypertension[30] (see Table 52-3). PPH is a rare disease, with an incidence of 1 to 2 per million.[31] Its prevalence is about 0.1 to 0.2 percent of all patients who come to autopsy.

The clinical diagnosis of PPH rests on three different types of evidence: (1) clinical, radiographic, and electrocardiographic manifestations of pulmonary hypertension, (2) hemodynamic features consisting of abnormally high pulmonary arterial pressures and pulmonary vascular resistance in association with normal left-sided filling pressures and a normal or low cardiac output, and (3) exclusion of the causes of secondary pulmonary hypertension.

SPECIAL TYPES

Certain associations of PPH have attracted interest because of their prospects for shedding light on some etiologies. These include so-called anorexigen-induced pulmonary hypertension, familial pulmonary hypertension, human immunodeficiency virus (HIV) infection–associated pulmonary hypertension, and portal-pulmonary hypertension.[30-33] In each of these, the clinical findings and the histologic appearance of the lungs at autopsy are identical to those which characterize the sporadic form of PPH. This diversity in associations underscores the likelihood that so-called PPH is the final common expression of heterogeneous etiologies.

General Features

After puberty, females predominate, those between 10 and 40 years of age being most often affected. Before puberty, no sex difference is discernible. The textbook picture of a patient with PPH is that of a young woman in the prime of life who develops one or more of the symptoms in Table 52-1 without discernible cause. Sex and age are sometimes useful in distinguishing clinically between the likelihood of PPH and pulmonary thromboembolic disease. The latter generally favors men, particularly in their later years.[25]

As a rule, median survival of patients can be predicted on the basis of the New York Heart Association functional classification: 6 months for class IV, 2½ years for class III, and 6 years for classes I and II. Unless interrupted by sudden death, which occurs in approximately 15 percent of patients, the usual downhill course terminates in intractable RV failure.[34]

Etiology

The common denominator in the pathogenesis of PPH appears to be injury to the layers of the vascular wall of the small muscular pulmonary arteries and arterioles.[35] In response to injury, the intima of these vessels proliferates so that the endothelium changes from a single flat layer to a piled-up projection that narrows the caliber of the vascular lumen. Along with intimal proliferation, the media of the affected vessels hypertrophy.[36]

The primary site of injury in PPH remains uncertain. Recent studies have implicated an intrinsic defect in ion channel function and calcium homeostasis in vascular smooth muscle,[37] whereas others have shown that endothelial function is disturbed, leading to altered production or handling of a variety of endothelial-derived vasoactive substances.[35] These abnormalities, coupled with altered platelet-endothelial interactions that predispose to intravascular thrombosis, lead to an inexorable course of enhanced vascular reactivity, proliferation and remodeling, and progressive obliterative vasculopathy. Diverse etiologies seem to be capable of eliciting PPH[38] (Table 52-4). For example, ingestion of the anorexigens fenfluramine and its isomer dexfenfluramine has been demonstrated to markedly increase the risk of PPH,[31] ingestion of toxic oil elicited an outbreak of pulmonary hypertension in Spain,[39] and HIV infection, even in the absence of the acquired immune deficiency syndrome, also has been implicated.[32]

For a long while, virtually all reports of PPH dealt with sporadic cases. An epidemic in Europe between 1967 and 1970 that was linked to the use of Aminorex, an anorectic agent, raised the prospect of hereditary predisposition, since only 1 in 1000 who took the drug developed pulmonary hypertension. More recently, the fenfluramines have been associated with both severe pulmonary hypertension and valvular heart disease.[31,40] The recent toxic oil epidemic in Spain has reinforced

TABLE 52-4 Suggested Mechanisms for Primary Pulmonary Hypertension

Proposed Mechanism	Evidence
Early/sustained vasoconstriction kinetics	Altered smooth muscle cell calcium Endothelial dysfunction
Genetic predisposition identified	Familial disease with gene locus ?Susceptibility with exposures, e.g., anorexigens, HIV, portal hypertension
Pulmonary thrombosis/embolism arteries/arterioles	Widespread occlusion of ?Altered endothelial-platelet interaction
Autoimmune disease	Raynaud's phenomenon and antinuclear antibodies common, female gender predilection

the concept of individual susceptibility to pulmonary vasotoxic agents.[39]

In recent years, an increasing number of patients have been identified in whom PPH is genetically linked.[41] In these individuals, the hereditary pattern is that of autosomal dominance with incomplete penetrance. The locus of the familial gene recently has been localized to the long arm of chromosome 2.[42] One major insight provided by the families with PPH is the diversity of pulmonary vascular lesions in members of the same family.[41]

Pathology

The evolution of PPH depends on progressive attenuation of the pulmonary arterial tree, which gradually increases pulmonary vascular resistance to the point of eliciting RV strain and failure. The seat of the disease is in the small pulmonary arteries (between 40 and 100 mm in diameter) and arterioles. The obliterative lesions can affect one or more layers of these vessels. In some instances, medial hypertrophy predominates; in others, it is the intima that proliferates. In addition, evidence of inflammation also may be present[36] (Fig. 52-4).

Histologic examination of the lung identifies a constellation of pulmonary precapillary lesions that are consistent with the clinical diagnosis of PPH, i.e., plexiform lesions, angiomatoid lesions, concentric intimal fibrosis, and necrotizing arteritis. The pathologist is often hard-pressed to distinguish between organized clots in small vessels that initiate the pulmonary hypertension and those which result from the obliterative pulmonary vascular disease. Recent clots in small pulmonary arteries and arterioles are common at autopsy in patients with PPH, particularly when the right ventricle has failed and cardiac output falls. Although similar clots may not have initiated the pulmonary hypertension process in PPH, it seems reasonable that more often they are complicating features that aggravate and exaggerate pulmonary vascular obstruction.

Pathophysiology

The hemodynamic hallmarks of PPH in the resting patient were indicated earlier: a combination of a high pulmonary arterial pressure, a normal or low cardiac output, and a normal left atrial (pulmonary wedge) pressure. As a result of this hemodynamic pattern, calculated pulmonary vascular resistance is high, generally leading to the logical conclusion that the resistance vessels, i.e., the small muscular arteries and arterioles, are the predominant sites of vascular obstruction. During exercise, as cardiac output increases, pulmonary arterial pressures increase further; the increments in pressure in the pulmonary hypertensive circuit are much more striking than in the normotensive pulmonary circulation owing to the inability to dilate existing vasculature or recruit unused vessels to accommodate the rise in pulmonary blood flow.

Pulmonary vasodilators are currently administered acutely for testing the responsiveness of the pulmonary circulation.[30] Among these, inhaled NO and intravenous prostacyclin have become the "gold standards." Several clinical and hemodynamic changes are sought as desirable end points: (1) improvement in exercise tolerance and in the quality of life; the increase in physical capacity, attributable to an increase in cardiac output, in turn improves oxygen delivery to peripheral organs and tissues; (2) a decrease in the level of pulmonary arterial hypertension, with evidence of regression of RV hypertrophy or dilatation, or both; (3) a decrease in calculated pulmonary vascular resistance; optimally, this decrease should entail an increase in cardiac output (with minimal increase in heart rate) accompanied by a decrease in pulmonary arterial pressure; and (4) since pulmonary vasodilators are also systemic vasodilators, pulmonary vasodilatation has to be effected without evoking undue systemic hypotension and tachycardia.

The combination of right-sided heart catheterization and vasodilator testing is particularly useful not only for defining the hemodynamic state of the patient but also in providing a hemodynamic baseline for future invasive and noninvasive studies, such as serial echocardiograms.

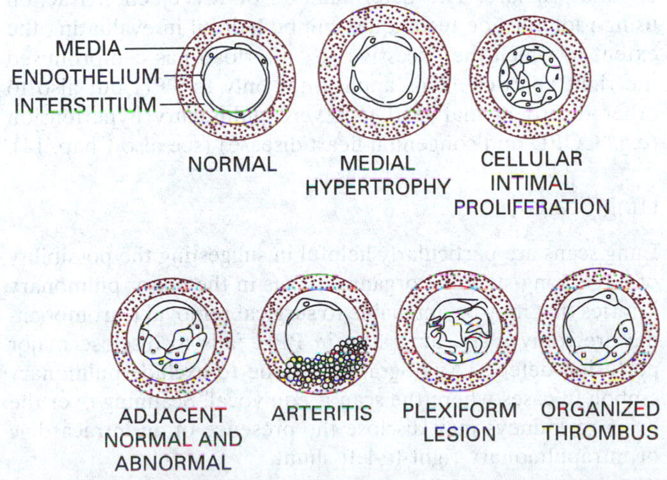

FIGURE 52-4 Vascular lesions in primary pulmonary hypertension. The plexiform lesion, once believed to be the histologic hallmark of primary pulmonary hypertension, has emerged as only one feature of a constellation of lesions.

Clinical Picture

In its early stages, the disease is difficult to recognize. In the sporadic case, the first clue is often an abnormal chest radiograph (see Fig. 52-1) or ECG indicative of RV hypertrophy (Fig. 52-5). Both are late manifestations. The existence of RV enlargement is generally confirmed by echocardiography. By the time these changes appear, however, pulmonary hypertension is moderate to severe. Initial complaints, particularly easy fatigability and dyspnea, tend to be discounted, i.e., attributed to being "out of shape," except when the index of suspicion is high, e.g., with a history of ingestion of anorectic agents or of familial pulmonary hypertension (see Table 52-1).

When the disease is advanced, the activities of daily life are progressively circumscribed by increasing nonspecific discomfort. Dyspnea, particularly during physical activity, becomes incapacitating. Some patients develop an angina type of chest pain along with breathlessness. Other common symptoms are weakness, fatigue, and exertional or postexertional syncope (see Table 52-1). Infrequently, an enlarged pulmonary artery causes hoarseness because of compression of the left recurrent laryngeal nerve. In time, right-sided heart failure develops.

Patients with severe pulmonary hypertension seem prone to sudden death. Death has occurred unexpectedly during normal activities, cardiac catheterization, and surgical procedures and after the administration of barbiturates or anesthetic agents.

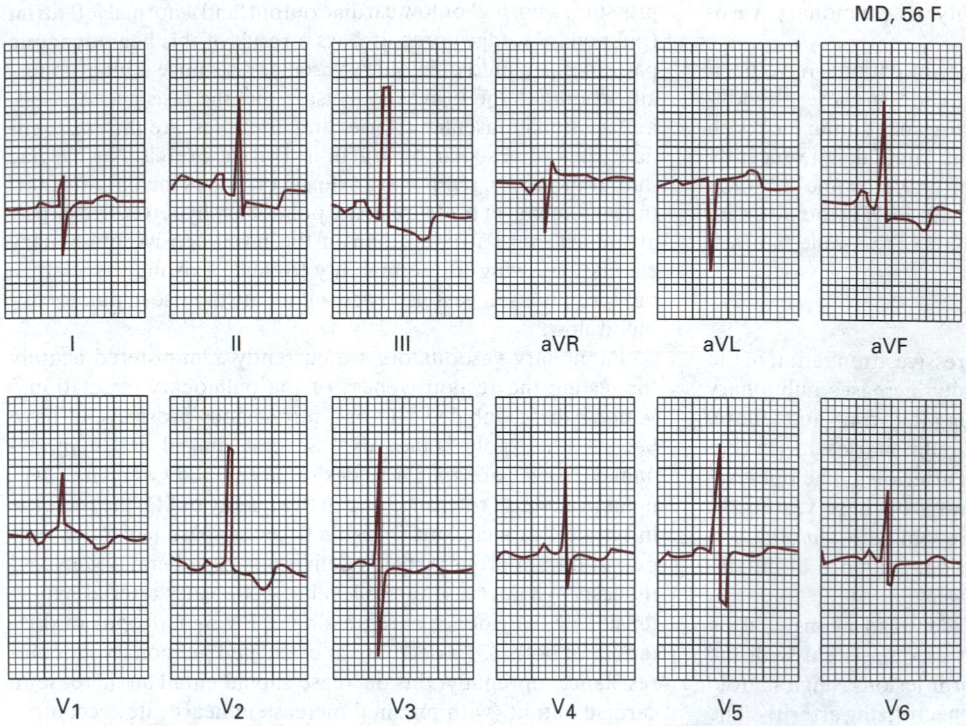

FIGURE 52-5 ECGs in patients with primary pulmonary hypertension and cor pulmonale.

The mechanisms for sudden death are not clear and may include arrhythmias or acute pulmonary thromboembolism. In a few instances, severe bradycardia and atrioventricular (AV) dissociation have preceded cardiac arrest.

It was noted earlier that as far as clinical manifestations and physical examination are concerned, PPH has an advantage over secondary pulmonary hypertension in that its manifestations are not obscured by those of underlying cardiac or respiratory disease. On physical examination, the jugular venous pulse usually shows a prominent *a* wave. RV hypertrophy causes a heave along the left sternal border, and a distinct systolic impulse is palpable over the region of the main pulmonary artery (see Chap. 10). The pulmonic component of the second sound is markedly accentuated, the second heart sound is narrowly split, and an ejection click is heard in the pulmonic area. Often a fourth heart sound emanating from the hypertrophied right ventricle is heard at the lower left sternal border. The murmur of tricuspid regurgitation is best heard along the sternal border with the patient in the supine position and can be accentuated with inspiration. In some patients, a midsystolic murmur is audible at the pulmonic area; as pulmonary arterial pressures approximate systemic arterial levels, the murmur of pulmonary valvular regurgitation often appears (see also Chap. 10).

The onset of RV failure is accompanied by jugular venous distention and a gallop (S_3); inspiration intensifies the gallop. The liver becomes enlarged and tender, and hepatojugular reflux can be elicited. Hydrothorax and ascites are seen as RV failure progresses.

Special Studies

Direct determination of pulmonary circulatory pressures by right-sided heart catheterization is the only way to definitively establish the diagnosis of pulmonary hypertension; however, other studies that are less direct can strongly suggest that it is present. Since the diagnosis of "primary" is one of exclusion, a number of tests are undertaken, usually in the hope of identifying a more treatable disease than PPH.[38]

CHEST RADIOGRAPHY AND ELECTROCARDIOGRAPHY

In the early stages, the chest radiograph is generally normal. Later it shows cardiac enlargement in association with enlargement of the pulmonary trunk, while the peripheral pulmonary arterial branches are attenuated; the lung fields appear oligemic (see Fig. 52-1). Although fullness of the central pulmonary arterial trunks and peripheral "pruning" are distinctive, appearances vary somewhat from patient to patient in accord with the level and pace of the pulmonary hypertension and the age of the patient. Radiographic evidence of RV enlargement usually becomes overt only late in the course of the pulmonary hypertension. The ECG almost always shows right axis deviation, RV hypertrophy, and, usually, right atrial enlargement (see Chap. 11).

THE ECHOCARDIOGRAM

Two-dimensional echocardiography confirms the enlargement and hypertrophy of the right atrium and ventricle, tricuspid regurgitation, and pulmonic valvular regurgitation. At the same time, LV structure and function are normal. The magnitude of the velocity of the tricuspid regurgitant jet using Doppler techniques can provide a noninvasive estimate of RV peak systolic pressure. The determination of RV ejection fraction using radionuclide techniques can be helpful in evaluating the extent to which the excessive RV afterload has compromised the right ventricle. This applies not only to PPH but also to other disorders that lead to severe pulmonary hypertension (e.g., COPD and congenital heart disease) (see also Chap. 14).

Lung Scans

Lung scans are particularly helpful in suggesting the possibility of large, long-standing organized clots in the major pulmonary arteries that may be amenable to surgical removal (thromboendarterectomy). The lung scan in PPH fails to disclose major perfusion defects. Angiography is done to exclude pulmonary emboli in cases where the scan is equivocal. Scanning over the brain or kidneys may disclose the presence of an intracardiac or intrapulmonary right-to-left shunt.

RIGHT-SIDED HEART CATHETERIZATION

Cardiac catheterization is invaluable in quantifying the hemodynamic abnormalities, in excluding cardiac causes of pulmonary arterial hypertension, and in assessing the hemodynamic responses of the heart and pulmonary circulation to vasodilator agents.[4]

Diagnosis

The diagnosis of PPH rests on two pillars: (1) the detection of pulmonary hypertension and (2) the exclusion of known causes of high pulmonary arterial pressure. The history is of utmost importance. Before categorizing pulmonary hypertension as "primary" or "unexplained," due regard must be paid to the exclusion of known etiologies (see Table 52-3), particularly thromboembolic disease and connective tissue disorders. Account also should be taken of the likelihood of familial disease. Pulmonary function tests are useful in excluding diffuse pulmonary disorders, particularly interstitial fibrosis and granuloma. Serologic testing can point the way to covert connective tissue disorders. Abnormal liver function tests can signal the coexistence of portal and pulmonary hypertension. The value of cardiac catheterization in eliminating acquired or congenital heart disease was indicated earlier. Unfortunately, by the time pulmonary hypertension complicating heart disease is recognized, the anatomic lesions often are too far advanced for the obliterative pulmonary vascular disease to be reversible. One notable exception is the dramatic improvement that often follows surgical removal of organized clots from the walls of major pulmonary arteries.

Treatment

For the past few decades, treatment of PPH has repeatedly turned to the use of vasodilators in the hope that an increase in pulmonary vascular tone contributed importantly to the high pulmonary arterial pressures. Although the bulk of the pulmonary vascular obstruction was clearly anatomic, vasodilators offered the prospect not only of decreasing pulmonary arterial pressures somewhat, and therefore the hemodynamic burden on the right ventricle, but also of prompting reversibility of the anatomic lesions, such as muscular hypertrophy, that resulted simply from the high pulmonary arterial pressures. Unfortunately, the use of vasodilators, which could affect the systemic as well as the pulmonary circulation and which often were accompanied by undesirable side effects, led to progressive disenchantment with one agent after another.

The situation has changed considerably during the past decade. The introduction of acute vasodilator testing for responsiveness helped to confirm the idea that in about one-third of patients, heightened pulmonary vasomotor tone helped to sustain the pulmonary hypertension. An optimal "responder" to acute testing manifested an increase in cardiac output along with a decrease in pulmonary arterial pressure and in pulmonary vascular resistance without affecting systemic arterial pressure unduly. Improvement in exercise tolerance accompanied the increase in cardiac output. Another landmark was the introduction of calcium channel blocking agents that could be taken orally, and in general, those who were highly responsive during acute testing could be maintained at lower pulmonary arterial pressures by these agents. A third insight was that even patients who failed to satisfy the criteria for a good hemodynamic response to acute vasodilator testing might respond to continuous infusion of epoprostenol. Indeed, a substantial number of such patients have been treated in this way for years, and even more have used continuous intravenous epoprostenol as a transition to transplantation of the lung or lungs or of heart and lungs. During this evolution, heart-lung and then lung transplantation became increasingly feasible and available, although the donor supply is still a limiting factor.

As a result of these advances, a patient with PPH has several therapeutic options, ranging from oral calcium channel blocking agents to continuous infusion of prostacyclin to lung transplantation. However, none of these modalities is free of complications. The oral calcium channel blocking agents generally have to be administered in large doses that are often accompanied by undesirable side effects.[43] The continuous infusion of a vasodilator, such as prostacyclin, runs the risks not only of a permanently placed intravenous catheter but also of drug-related side effects that can preclude dose increases.[44,45] Transplantation offers the substitution of immunosuppression and its attendant risk of infection as a better option than chronic cor pulmonale and RV failure.[46] Despite the limitations of each of these therapeutic modalities, together they provide a graduated therapeutic approach that has provided, at each stage, a better quality of life for many individuals with PPH. Moreover, they have prompted the search for agents that can be used in place of prostacyclin, which, until now, has required intravenous infusion; prostacyclin analogues that are delivered subcutaneously and by aerosol are currently under investigation. Other novel approaches include chronic ambulatory NO, which can be administered by inhalation.

VASODILATOR AGENTS

Various agents have been tried over the years as pulmonary vasodilators. These include α-adrenergic antagonists, β-adrenergic agonists, diazoxide, hydralazine, nitrates, and angiotensin-converting enzyme inhibitors. In general, these have not withstood the test of time. Experience has taught that untoward reactions can occur with any pulmonary vasodilator, even when low doses are used. Three categories of agents continue to hold promise, however: calcium channel blocking agents, arachidonic acid metabolites, and NO.

DRUGS THAT BLOCK CALCIUM TRANSPORT

The designation *calcium channel blocker* refers to a heterogeneous group of agents of different structural, pharmacologic, and electrophysiologic properties. The agents in this category currently receiving the most clinical attention as potential pulmonary vasodilators are nifedipine and diltiazem. Of the two, nifedipine is the more popular. Verapamil generally is not used because of its undesirable negative inotropic effect.

Nifedipine Note that this use is not listed in the manufacturer's directive. Nifedipine is a synthetic agent that is unrelated to other vasoactive or cardiotonic drugs. It is a potent systemic vasodilator that is used for the treatment of coronary vasospasm. Although it has significant direct negative inotropic effects, these are usually not prominent clinically because of the reflex sympathetic stimulation of the heart; it does not possess antiarrhythmic properties. It is now the preferred agent for therapy of patients who manifest acute vasoreactivity when tested with short-acting agents under hemodynamic monitoring.

Sustained-release preparations are used, with the dosage generally titrated to the maximal tolerable level based on avoiding untoward systemic effects, i.e., hypotension, headache, dizziness, and flushing. Considerable caution is necessary in administering the higher dosages, however, because side effects can occur precipitously and be life-threatening. In one study, 64 patients with PPH were treated acutely with high doses of calcium channel blockers. Seventeen patients responded to treatment with nifedipine (13 patients) or diltiazem (4 patients) and were alive after 5 years.[46]

In experienced centers, the trial of nifedipine or diltiazem orally is preceded by use of testing of acute vasoreactivity using one or more of three agents: (1) inhaled NO, in concentrations of 10 to 40 ppm for 5 to 10 min, (2) prostacyclin (PGI_2, Epoprostenol, Flolan), administered intravenously in increasing doses (starting dose of 1–2 ng/kg/min followed by successive increments every 15 min of 2 ng/kg/min until a maximal dose of 12 ng/kg/min is reached or until side effects preclude further increases), and (3) adenosine (50–200 ng/kg/min). Only patients who manifest significant reductions in pulmonary vascular resistance (usually >20–30 percent), resulting from a fall in pulmonary artery pressure without systemic hypotension and accompanied by an unchanged or increased cardiac output, are considered candidates for chronic therapy with oral calcium channel antagonists.

Arachidonic Acid Metabolites Epoprostenol (Flolan, prostacyclin, PGI_2), a metabolite of arachidonic acid, and its analogues continue to be a major focus of attention as treatments for a variety of forms of pulmonary hypertension. The pulmonary endothelium elaborates prostacyclin into the bloodstream, where it has a short biologic half-life, i.e., 2 to 3 min. In principle, it is attractive for the treatment of pulmonary hypertension on several accounts: (1) it is a pulmonary vasodilator, (2) it inhibits platelet aggregation, and (3) it inhibits proliferation of vascular smooth muscle. Unfortunately, it suffers the disadvantage of requiring continuous intravenous infusion, which is currently being done using portable pumps.[44,45] Analogues that can be given orally, subcutaneously, or by the inhaled route are under investigation. Success in long-term management recently has been reported using aerosolized iloprost, a stable prostacyclin analogue.[16,47] Currently, its most effective use is for long-term management in patients with severe (NYHA classes III or IV) primary pulmonary hypertension who are unresponsive to or are not candidates for therapy with calcium channel blockers.[44,45,48]

Nitric Oxide NO is synthesized in endothelial cells from one of the guanidine nitrogens of L-arginine by the enzyme NO synthase. It has proved to be the endothelial-derived relaxing factor that contributes to the low initial tone of the pulmonary circulation. It has the advantage of other vasodilators of selectively relaxing pulmonary vessels without affecting systemic arterial pressure. It is currently being used as a test of vasoreactivity in a wide variety of pulmonary hypertensive states including PPH and also has been used to control pulmonary hypertension in the syndrome of persistent pulmonary hypertension in the newborn.[49,50,51]

Anticoagulants Since 1984, when Fuster et al.[52] in a nonrandomized clinical trial showed that long-term survival was improved in patients with PPH by anticoagulant therapy (warfarin in low doses), the use of anticoagulants has been incorporated into the therapeutic regimen in patients with PPH. This practice is supported by the high incidence of antemortem clots found at autopsy in the small pulmonary arteries and arterioles of patients with PPH. Moreover, in a recent trial that separated "responders" from "nonresponders" to calcium channel blockers, survival was significantly better in those given warfarin than in those who were not anticoagulated.[43] The advent of RV failure increases the propensity for clotting in the pulmonary circulation. The usual goal of anticoagulation is to achieve and maintain an INR of 2 to 2.5.[53]

ATRIAL SEPTOSTOMY

Blade-balloon atrial septostomy has been performed in patients with severe RV pressure and volume overload refractory to maximal medical therapy.[54] The goal of this approach is to decompress the overloaded right heart and improve systemic output of the underfilled left ventricle. Improvements in exercise function and signs of severe right-sided heart dysfunction such as syncope and ascites have been observed. Since the creation of an interatrial communication will result in an increased venous admixture, worsening hypoxemia is an expected outcome. The size of the septostomy that is created should be monitored carefully to achieve the ideal balance of optimizing systemic oxygen transport and reducing right-sided heart filling pressures without overfilling a noncompliant left ventricle or producing extreme degrees of venous admixture.

LUNG TRANSPLANTATION

Only one-third of patients with PPH are responsive to long-term oral vasodilator therapy. Of the remainder, approximately 65 to 75 percent maintain sustained clinical improvement with long-term continuous intravenous therapy using prostacyclin. When pulmonary hypertensive disease has progressed, or threatens to progress, to the stage of RV failure, the physician and patient are left with few therapeutic options other than lung transplantation. Lung transplantation is currently being done at specialized centers and is almost invariably handicapped by a shortage of donor lungs, which can lead to long delays. Single- or double-lung transplantation has largely replaced heart-lung transplantation. Often, hemodynamic improvement is dramatic,[55] but transplantation for PPH poses not only a considerable surgical risk but also the prospect of opportunistic infections that accompanies lifelong immunosuppression.[56] Rejection phenomena, notably bronchiolitis obliterans, are the major limiting factor to prolonged survival. The median survival after lung transplantation is approximately 3 years.[46] Recurrence of PPH after transplantation has not been reported.

Prognosis

The diagnosis of PPH carries with it a poor prognosis unless medical or surgical therapy succeeds in decreasing pulmonary vascular resistance. Although death usually occurs within a few years after the onset of symptoms, instances of long-term survival do occur. Although sudden death accounts for 10 to 15 percent of all PPH-related deaths, the prognosis is largely determined by the severity of pulmonary hypertension and right-sided heart dysfunction.[34]

PULMONARY VENO-OCCLUSIVE DISEASE AND PULMONARY CAPILLARY HEMANGIOMATOSIS

These are the least common of all types of unexplained pulmonary hypertension. Not infrequently, the patient is thought to have primary pulmonary hypertension until manifestations inconsistent with pulmonary precapillary disease, such as pulmonary congestion and edema or severe hypoxemia, redirect attention to the vascular bed distal to the arterioles, i.e., the capillaries, pulmonary small veins, and venules. The pathogenetic mechanism of POVD is unknown but may begin as an inflammatory-thrombotic process in the small pulmonary veins and venules and ends in fibrous obliteration of the venous and venular lumens. Presumably as a secondary phenomenon, the distal pulmonary arterial tree also develops obstructive lesions that are generally proliferative ("reactive") rather than inflammatory in nature; the intervening capillary bed is generally normal. The pulmonary veno-occlusive lesions have been attributed to an inflammatory response to vascular injury, followed by thrombosis and scarring. Among the postulated etiologies (based on exceedingly sparse evidence) are viral illness, chemotherapy, toxins, autoimmune disease, and mediastinal fibrosis.[36]

Both POVD and capillary hemangiomatosis can be familial. When the pulmonary hypertension is suspected of originating distal to the pulmonary capillary bed, mitral valve disease, myocardial dysfunction, or even left atrial myxoma has a greater likelihood of being the cause than does POVD.

Clinical Picture

Predominantly children and young adults are affected, but the age has ranged from infancy to 48 years. Clinical suspicion of this disorder generally arises when a patient with congested and edematous lungs proves to have a normal mitral valve and left ventricle.

The cardinal signs are dyspnea and fatigue on exertion in conjunction with evidence of pulmonary hypertension; the pulmonary venous rather than pulmonary arterial etiology is suggested by radiologic evidence of postcapillary pulmonary hypertension without evidence of involvement of the left side of the heart (Fig. 52-6*A*). Pleural effusions are common. Cyanosis, syncope, hemoptysis, and finger clubbing have been inconsistent findings. Moderate to severe hypoxemia, due to intrapulmonary shunting through the abnormal capillary network, is a hallmark of capillary hemangiomatosis. Rarely, systemic embolization may occur.

Hemodynamics

Cardiac catheterization discloses a high pulmonary arterial pressure with a normal pulmonary wedge (and LV end-diastolic) pressure. The low wedge pressure has been attributed to discontinuities and channels of high resistance between the pulmonary capillaries and the pulmonary and bronchial venous channels so that wedging interrupts all sources of flow distal to the area blocked by the catheter.[30] When epoprostenol is administered to a patient with POVD, an acute pulmonary edema pattern

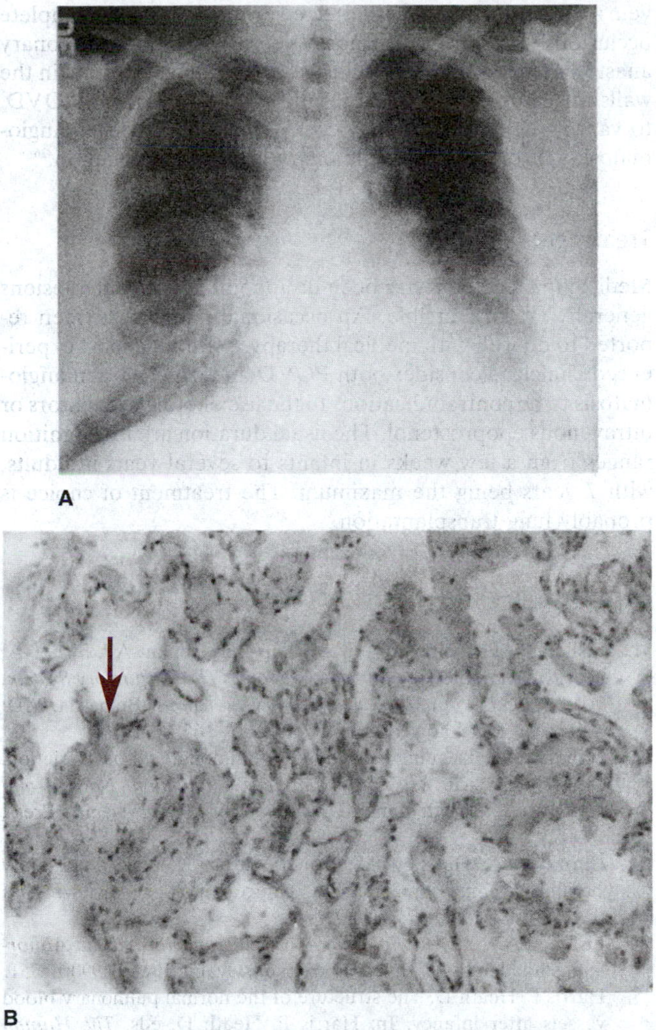

FIGURE 52-6 POVD proven by open lung biopsy. *A*. Chest radiography. Pulmonary interstitial edema is marked at both bases. *B*. Lung biopsy. In addition to obliterative pulmonary venular disease, the pulmonary arterioles (*arrow*) showed intimal proliferation and medical hypertrophy. (Courtesy of Dr. G. G. Pietra.)

may ensue, resulting from increasing pulmonary blood flow in the face of downstream vascular obstruction.[48,57] Although not universally present, this response is virtually diagnostic of POVD. Patients with capillary hemangiomatosis may experience worsening hypoxemia with epoprostenol, attributable to increased shunting through the low-resistance capillary meshwork.

Pathology

Few lung biopsies have been done during life. At autopsy, both lungs are involved. The lungs are the seat of congestion, edema, and focal fibrosis, which may become extensive. The venous lesions may be more marked in one region than in another. Although the small pulmonary arteries as well as the small pulmonary veins are affected, the lesions are different (see Fig. 52-6*B*). Most striking are the morphologic changes in the pulmonary veins and venules, which are narrowed or occluded by intimal proliferation and fibrosis; up to 95 percent of the veins and venules may be affected in this way, but complete occlusion is uncommon. Bronchial veins and bronchopulmonary anastomoses share in the occlusive process. Hypertrophy in the walls of the pulmonary arteries may be quite striking. POVD, to varying degrees, also may coexist with capillary hemangiomatosis. Thrombi in the pulmonary arteries are common.[36]

Treatment

Medical management has been disappointing, since the lesions generally are irreversible. An occasional patient has been reported to do well with medical therapy,[58] although most experienced clinicians consider both POVD and capillary hemangiomatosis to be contraindications to the use of oral vasodilators or intravenous epoprostenol. The usual duration after recognition ranges from a few weeks in infants to several years in adults, with 7 years being the maximum. The treatment of choice is probably lung transplantation.

References

1. Fishman AP. Pulmonary circulation. In: Fishman AP, Fisher A, eds. *The Handbook of Physiology*, Sec 3: *The Respiratory System*, vol I: *Circulation and Nonrespiratory Functions*. Bethesda, MD: American Physiological Society; 1985:93–165.
2. Fishman AP. The enigma of hypoxic pulmonary vasoconstriction. In: Fishman AP, ed. *The Pulmonary Circulation: Normal and Abnormal*. Philadelphia: University of Pennsylvania Press; 1990:109–130.
3. Eltorky MA, Headley AS, Winer-Muram H, et al. Pulmonary capillary hemangiomatosis: A clinicopathologic review. *Ann Thorac Surg* 1994; 57:772–776.
4. Fishman AP, ed. *The Pulmonary Circulation: Normal and Abnormal*. Philadelphia: University of Pennsylvania Press; 1990:1–551.
5. Harris P, Heath D. The structure of the normal pulmonary blood vessels after infancy. In: Harris P, Heath D, eds. *The Human Circulation: Its Form and Function in Health and Disease*. Edinburgh: Churchill-Livingstone; 1986:30–47.
6. Kinsella JP, Abman SH. Recent developments in the pathophysiology and treatment of persistent pulmonary hypertension of the newborn. *J Pediatr* 1995; 126:853–864.
7. Reid LM. Vascular remodeling. In: Fishman AP, ed. *The Pulmonary Circulation: Normal and Abnormal*. Philadelphia: University of Pennsylvania Press; 1990:259–282.
8. Moser KM, Auger WR, Fedullo PF. Chronic major vessel thromboembolic pulmonary hypertension. *Circulation* 1990; 81:1735–1743.
9. Beard JT II, Bryd BF III. Saline contrast enhancement of trivial Doppler tricuspid regurgitation signals for estimating pulmonary arterial pressure. *Am J Cardiol* 1988; 62:486–488.
10. Palevsky HI, Schloo BL, Pietra GG, et al. Primary pulmonary hypertension: Vascular structure, morphometry, and responsiveness to vasodilator agents. *Circulation* 1989; 80:1207–1221.
11. Edwards WD. The pathology of secondary pulmonary hypertension. In: Fishman AP, ed. *The Pulmonary Circulation: Normal and Abnormal*. Philadelphia: University of Pennsylvania Press; 1990:329–342.
12. Fedullo PF, Auger WR, Channick RN, et al. Chronic thromboembolic pulmonary hypertension. *Clin Chest Med* 1995; 16:353–374.
13. Ryan KL, Fedullo PF, Davis GB, et al. Perfusion scans underestimate the severity of angiographic and hemodynamic compromise in chronic thromboembolic pulmonary hypertension. *Chest* 1988; 93:1180–1185.
14. Jamieson SW, Auger WR, Fedullo PF, et al. Experience and results with 150 pulmonary thromboendarterectomy operations over a 29-month period. *J Thorac Cardiovasc Surg* 1993; 106:116–127.
15. Ricou F, Nicod PH, Moser KM, Peterson KL. Catheter-based intravascular ultrasound imaging of chronic thromboembolic pulmonary disease. *Am J Cardiol* 1991; 67:749–752.
16. Olschewski H, Ardeschir H, Walmrath D, et al. Inhaled prostacyclin and iloprost in severe pulmonary hypertension secondary to lung fibrosis. *Am J Respir Crit Care Med* 1999; 160:600–603.
17. Weitzenblum E, Oswald M, Mirhom R, et al. Evolution of pulmonary haemodynamics in COPD patients under long-term oxygen therapy. *Eur Respir J* 1989; 2(suppl 7):669S–673S.
18. Fishman AP. A century of primary pulmonary hypertension. In: Rubin LJ, Rich S, eds. *Primary Pulmonary Hypertension*. New York: Marcel Dekker; 1997:1–18.
19. Matthay RA, Shub C. Imaging techniques for assessing pulmonary artery hypertension and right ventricular performance with special reference to COPD. *J Thorac Imag* 1990; 5:47–67.
20. Tramarin R, Torbicki A, Marchandise B, et al. Doppler echocardiographic evaluation of pulmonary artery pressure in chronic obstructive pulmonary disease: A European multicentre study. *Eur Heart J* 1991; 12:103–111.
21. Maeda S, Katsura H, Chida K, et al. Lack of correlation between P pulmonale and right atrial overload in chronic obstructive airways disease. *Br Heart J* 1991; 65:132–136.
22. Weitzenblum E, Sautegeau A, Ehrhart M, et al. Long-term oxygen therapy can reverse the progression of pulmonary hypertension in patients with chronic obstructive pulmonary disease. *Am Rev Respir Dis* 1985; 131:493–498.
23. Brown G. Pharmacologic treatment of primary and secondary pulmonary hypertension. *Pharmacotherapy* 1991; 11:137–156.
24. Yousem SA. The pulmonary pathologic manifestations of the CREST syndrome. *Hum Pathol* 1990; 21:467–474.
25. Rich S, Dantzker DR, Ayres SM, et al. Primary pulmonary hypertension: A national prospective study. *Ann Intern Med* 1987; 107:216–223.
26. Shuck JW, Oetgen WJ, Tesar JT. Pulmonary vascular response during Raynaud's phenomenon in progressive systemic sclerosis. *Am J Med* 1985; 78:221–227.
27. Badesch D, Brundage B, Tapson V, et al. Continuous intravenous epoprostenol for pulmonary hypertension due to scleroderma: Spectrum of disease. *Ann Intern Med* 2000; 132:425–434.
28. Fishman AP. Pulmonary hypertension and cor pulmonale. In: Fishman AP, ed. *Pulmonary Diseases and Disorders*, 2d ed. New York: McGraw-Hill; 1988:999–1048.
29. Chaouat AE, Weitzenblum E, Krieger J, et al. Pulmonary hemodynamics in the obstructive sleep apnea syndrome: Results in 220 consecutive patients. *Chest* 1996; 109:380–386.
30. Rubin LJ. Primary pulmonary hypertension. *N Eng J Med* 1997; 336:111–117.
31. Abenhaim L, Moride Y, Brenot F, et al. Appetite-suppressant drugs and the risk of primary pulmonary hypertension. *N Engl J Med* 1996; 335:609–616.
32. Speich R, Jenni R, Opravil M, et al. Primary pulmonary hypertension in HIV infection. *Chest* 1991; 100:1268–1271.
33. Kuo PC, Plotkin JS, Rubin LJ. Distinctive clinical features of portopulmonary hypertension. *Chest* 1997; 112:980–986.
34. D'Alonzo GE, Barst RJ, Ayres SM, et al. Survival in patients with primary pulmonary hypertension. *Ann Intern Med* 1991; 115:343–349.
35. Voelkel NF, Tuder RM, Weir EK. Pathophysiology of primary pulmonary hypertension: In Rubin LJ, Rich S, eds. *Primary Pulmonary Hypertension*. New York: Marcel Dekker; 1997:83–133.
36. Pietra G. Pathology of primary pulmonary hypertension. In: Rubin LJ, Rich S, eds. *Primary Pulmonary Hypertension*. New York: Marcel Dekker, 1997:19–62.
37. Yuan JXJ, Aldinger AM, Juhaszova M, et al. Dysfunctional voltage-gated K^+ channels in pulmonary artery smooth muscle cells

of patients with primary pulmonary hypertension. *Circulation* 1998; 98:1400–1406.

38. Gaine SP, Rubin LJ. Primary pulmonary hypertension. *Lancet* 1998; 353:719–725.
39. Lopez-Sendon J, Sanchez MAG, De Juan MJM, Coma-Canella I. Pulmonary hypertension in the toxic oil syndrome. In: Fishman AP, ed. *The Pulmonary Circulation: Normal and Abnormal*. Philadelphia: University of Pennsylvania Press; 1990:385–396.
40. Connolly HD, Crary JL, McGoon MD, et al. Valvular heart disease associated with fenfluramine-phentermine. *N Engl J Med* 1997; 337:581–588.
41. Loyd J, Newman J. Familial primary pulmonary hypertension: Clinical patterns. *Am Rev Respir Dis* 1984; 129:194–197.
42. Nichols W, Koller D, Slovis B, et al. Localization of the gene for familial primary pulmonary hypertension to chromosome 2q31-32. *Nature Gen* 1997; 15:277–280.
43. Rich S, Kaufmann E, Levy PS. The effect of high doses of calcium-channel blockers on survival in primary pulmonary hypertension. *N Engl J Med* 1992; 327:76–81.
44. Barst RJ, Rubin LJ, McGoon MD, et al. Survival in primary pulmonary hypertension with long-term continuous intravenous prostacyclin. *Ann Intern Med* 1994; 121:409–415.
45. Rubin LJ, Mendoza J, Hood M, et al. Treatment of primary pulmonary hypertension with continuous intravenous prostacyclin (epoprostenol). *Ann Intern Med* 1991; 112:485–591.
46. Arcasoy SM, Kohoff RM. Lung transplantation. *N Engl J Med* 1999; 340:1081–1091.
47. Olschewski H, Walmrath D, Schermuly R, et al. Aerosolized prostacyclin and iloprost in severe pulmonary hypertension. *Ann Intern Med* 1996; 124:820–824.
48. Barst RJ, Rubin LJ, Long WA, et al. A comparison of continuous intravenous epoprostenol (prostacyclin) with conventional therapy for primary pulmnary hypertension. *N Engl J Med* 1996; 334:296–302.
49. Sitbon O, Brenot F, Denjean A, et al. Inhalednitric oxide as a screening vasodilator agent in primary pulmonary hypertension: A dose-response study and comparison with prostacyclin. *Am J Respir Crit Care Med* 1995; 151:384–389.
50. Lunn RJ. Inhaled nitric oxide therapy. *Mayo Clin Proc* 1995; 70:247–255.
51. Pepke-Zaba J, Higenbottam T, Dinh-Xuan AT, et al. Inhaled nitric oxide as a cause of selective pulmonary vasodilation in pulmonary hypertension. *Lancet* 1991; 338:1173–1174.
52. Fuster V, Steele PM, Edwards WD, et al. Primary pulmonary hypertension: Natural history and the importance of thrombosis. *Circulation* 1984; 70:580–585.
53. Medical management. In: Rubin LJ, Rich S, eds. *Primary Pulmonary Hypertension*. New York: Marcel Dekker; 1996:271–286.
54. Kerstein D, Levy PS, Hsu DT, et al. Blade balloon atrial septostomy in patients with severe primary pulmonary hypertension. *Circulation* 1995; 91:2028–2035.
55. Pasque MK, Kaiser LR, Dresler CM, et al. Single lung transplantation for pulmonary hypertension. *J Thorac Cardiovasc Surg* 1992; 103:475–481.
56. Katayama Y, Cremona G, Wallwork J, Higenbottam T. Transplantation for primary pulmonary hypertension. In: Rubin LJ, Rich S, eds. *Primary Pulmonary Hypertension*. New York: Marcel Dekker; 1996:287–304.
57. Davis LL, deBoisblanc BP, Glynn CE, et al. Effect of prostacyclin on microvascular pressures in a patient with pulmonary veno-occlusive disease. *Chest* 1995; 108:1754–1756.
58. Palevsky HI, Pietra GG, Fishman AP. Pulmonary veno-occlusive disease and its response to vasodilator agents. *Am Rev Respir Dis* 1990; 142:426–429.

CHAPTER 53

PULMONARY EMBOLISM

Victor F. Tapson

Approximately 100,000 patients in the United States die each year directly due to acute pulmonary embolism (PE), with another 100,000 deaths occurring in patients with concomitant disease in whom PE contributes significantly to the demise of the patient.[1,2] A substantial number of patients die from PE prior to being diagnosed. Many of these deaths appear to be preventable. Autopsy studies have repeatedly documented the high frequency with which PE has gone unsuspected and undetected.[3] Despite advances in diagnostic technology and therapeutic approaches, PE remains underdiagnosed and prophylaxis continues to be dramatically underutilized. Pulmonary embolism nearly always results from deep venous thrombosis (DVT) of the proximal deep veins of the legs, that is, including the popliteal veins, and their vicinity, although axillary and subclavian vein thrombi may also embolize. Venous thromboembolism (VTE) represents the clinical spectrum of DVT and PE and occurs extraordinarily commonly in hospitalized patients, particularly after major surgery.

Because DVT and PE are so commonly clinically unsuspected, considerable diagnostic and therapeutic delays result and substantial morbidity and mortality are the ultimate consequence. The risk factors for DVT are discussed below, followed by the pathophysiology of acute PE. Because of the potential overlap with regard to the diagnostic approach to suspected DVT and PE, these are discussed in the same section. The principles of management of DVT and PE are addressed. Finally, the less common entity of chronic thromboembolic pulmonary hypertension is reviewed.

ACUTE DEEP VENOUS THROMBOSIS: RISK FACTORS AND PATHOGENESIS

Virchow proposed that the pathogenesis of DVT was based upon several potential initiating events, including stasis, venous injury, and hypercoagulability. Risk factors for DVT are based upon these processes (Table 53-1). Thrombosis may develop within the lumen of any vein as well as in the right side of the heart. Extensive investigation has been undertaken of the veins of the lower extremities, since most significant PE originate from this location. Although thrombi may form at any point along the vein wall, most originate in valve pockets. The veins of the calf are the most common site of origin, with subsequent extension of the clot prior to embolization.[4] If the clot does propagate, it usually remains attached at its base and floats in the vein more proximally. Eventually, it may expand to fill the vessel entirely, with both retrograde and further proximal extension. If embolization does not occur, the thrombosis can partially or completely resolve via three mechanisms, which include recanalization, organization, and lysis. Fatal PE is the most feared complication of DVT. Chronic thrombophlebitis with recurrent pain and swelling can be incapacitating. Fre-

TABLE 53-1 Risk Factors for Venous Thromboembolism

Acquired factors
Age greater than 40
Prior history of venous thromboembolism
Prior major surgical procedure
Trauma
Hip fracture
Immobilization/paralysis
Venous stasis
Varicose veins
Congestive heart failure
Myocardial infarction
Obesity
Pregnancy/postpartum period
Oral contraceptive therapy
Cerebrovascular accident
Malignancy
Severe thrombocythemia
Paroxysmal nocturnal hemoglobinuria
Antiphospholipid antibody syndrome (including lupus anticoagulant)
Inherited factors
Antithrombin III deficiency
Factor V Leiden (activated protein C resistance)
Prothrombin gene (G20210A) defect
Protein C deficiency
Protein S deficiency
Dysfibrinogenemia
Disorders of plasminogen
Hyperhomocysteinemia

quently more than one risk factor for venous thrombosis is present and knowledge of these risk factors provides the rationale for both prophylaxis and clinical suspicion.

Acquired Risk Factors

Most venous thrombi arise in venous valves, where blood flow tends to stagnate. The increased frequency of thrombosis with advanced age and immobilization further emphasizes the importance of stasis in thrombogenesis. Immobility, regardless of the cause, discourages venous return and contributes to stasis. Acute paraplegia significantly increases the risk of DVT (particularly in the paralyzed limb), and the period of highest risk appears to be the first 2 weeks after the onset of the paralysis.[5] Prolonged bed rest or long automobile or airplane trips may be the only obvious risk factors in patients developing thromboemboli. Obesity also appears to increase the risk of VTE. Information extrapolated from the Prospective Investigation of Pulmonary Embolism Diagnosis (PIOPED) suggests that the relationship of obesity and VTE are not entirely understood and that further clarification would be useful.[6] Although obesity is commonly believed to be a significant risk, it is likely that immobility and stasis are contributing factors. Age appears to increase mortality due to PE,[7] and it appears that PE is suspected less commonly prior to death in the elderly patient.[8] The risk of VTE is particularly high in those of the elderly with concomitant cardiac disease or cancer.

Antecedent pulmonary thromboembolism forecasts an appreciable risk of recurrence in the hospitalized patient. Surgical patients with a previous history of VTE who do not receive prophylaxis develop postoperative DVT in more than 50 percent of cases.[9] Surgery itself significantly enhances the risk. Even surgery patients without significant additional risk factors develop venography-proven DVT in nearly 20 percent of cases if neither pharmacologic nor mechanical prophylaxis is applied.[10] Prophylactic anticoagulation is initiated either prior to surgery or shortly thereafter to prevent the development of intraoperative and early postoperative thrombosis. Total hip and total knee replacement patients not receiving prophylaxis develop DVT in more than 50 percent of cases.[11] These orthopedic settings have been comprehensively investigated, prompted by the increasing use of low-molecular-weight heparin (LMWH). Spinal or pelvic surgery place patients at particularly high risk for VTE.

Trauma, particularly of the lower extremities and pelvis, heightens the risk of DVT. Pulmonary embolism has been identified at autopsy in as many as 60 percent of patients with lower extremity fractures,[12] and mortality has been attributed to PE in as many as 50 percent of patients dying after hip fracture.[13] The incidence of VTE increases with time after the traumatic event. Autopsy-confirmed PE in patients surviving for less than 24 h after trauma has been demonstrated in 3.3 percent, increasing to 5.5 percent in those surviving up to 7 days. Pulmonary emboli occurred in 18.6 percent of those surviving for a longer period.[14] Venous catheters (particularly in the jugular, subclavian, or femoral veins) traumatize veins as well as serving as potential nidi for thrombosis. Associated cancer or immobility is often present in these individuals. Symptomatic PE can originate from catheter-induced (or non-catheter-induced) upper extremity thrombi, although this appears much less commonly than when the leg or pelvic veins are the source. Upper extremity (axillary-subclavian) thrombosis may also occur due to the effort-induced syndrome described by Paget-Schroetter.[15]

Recent epidemiologic analyses as well as autopsy data suggest that patients with cardiac and malignant disease are particularly predisposed to VTE.[7,16] Although myocardial infarction without anticoagulation has been associated with a significant incidence of DVT, more recent therapeutic strategies have had a beneficial impact.[17] Several of the large, multicenter, placebo-controlled acute myocardial infarction trials have indicated that the use of thrombolytic therapy has reduced the incidence of VTE.[18,19]

Malignancies clearly augment the risk of VTE, although the precise pathogenesis of thromboembolism in cancer is not well understood.[16] It is clear, however, that numerous mechanisms—including intrinsic tumor procoagulant activity and extrinsic factors such as chemotherapeutic agents and indwelling access catheters—contribute to this process. The thrombophilic tendency associated with cancer is often amplified by weakness and reduced ambulation with venous stasis. A recent analysis, based upon data from the PIOPED trial, revealed that of 399 patients with PE, 73 (18.3 percent) had cancer.[7] Pancreatic, lung, gastric, genitourinary tract, and breast malignancies are associated with a particularly high risk of DVT and PE. It appears that about half of all cancer patients and about 90 percent of those with metastases exhibit abnormalities of one or more coagulation parameter. The most common abnormalities include elevation of clotting factor levels (fibrinogen, factors

V, VIII, IX, and XI), fibrinogen and fibrin degradation products, and thrombocytosis.[16]

Most tumor cells produce both tissue factor and cancer procoagulant.[16,20] Tissue factor appears to be the primary coagulant factor implicated in promoting fibrin deposition and is expressed in situ as well as in isolated cells of numerous cancers.[21] Tumor cell expression of tissue factor also promotes metastatic dissemination.[21] Cancer procoagulant is a cysteine protease that activates factor X. Mucin, a glycoprotein produced by certain tumors, possesses a sialic acid moiety that may nonenzymatically cleave factor X to Xa. Plasminogen activator inhibitor type 1 (PAI-1) is secreted by numerous tumor cells and inhibits plasmin generation, augmenting the thrombophilic state as well as possibly also promoting tumor metastasis dissemination.[21] Other procoagulant properties of tumor cells include expression of cytokines such as IL-1β and tumor necrosis factor alpha (TNF-α), which, in turn, regulate expression of procoagulants and mediate interactions between tumor cells, platelets, leukocytes, and endothelial cells. Thrombin, certain cytokines, and growth factors such as vascular endothelial growth factor (VEGF) can stimulate endothelial cells to synthesize tissue factor, further potentiating a procoagulant surface and leading to fibrin deposition on vessel walls. Activated protein C inhibitor may contribute to a prothrombotic state, as it can inhibit both fibrinolysis and the protein C anticoagulant pathway.[21]

Chemotherapy, with resulting neutropenia and sepsis, often necessitates hospitalization and bed rest, which contributes further to the high risk of VTE. Following the administration of various chemotherapeutic agents, changes in the levels of coagulation factors, suppression of anticoagulant and fibrinolytic activity, and direct endothelial damage have been documented clinically and experimentally.[22] Hormonal therapy, particularly tamoxifen in breast cancer adjuvant therapy, is also associated with an increased risk of thromboembolism, particularly when combined with chemotherapy. The thrombophilic state induced by chemotherapeutic agents has recently been reviewed.[22] Further comprehensive research will more clearly elucidate the mechanisms underlying thrombophilia in cancer patients. In spite of the clear association, there is no convincing evidence that an aggressive search for cancer is warranted in patients presenting with apparently idiopathic DVT.[23]

Pregnancy and the postpartum period are the most common settings in which women under age 40 acquire thromboembolic disease. Venous thrombosis develops in these settings five times more often than in age-matched women not on oral contraceptives.[24] Although DVT appears to be more common in the third-trimester and postpartum than prior to delivery, the risk is clearly considerable throughout pregnancy.[24] Cesarean section further augments the risk. Oral contraceptives are associated with the development of VTE, although the precise risk has been controversial.[25] The risk increases with third-generation agents (agents containing desogestrel or gestodene as the progestogen component).[26,27] Results from a clinical trial evaluating hormonal replacement therapy indicated that such therapy increased the incidence of VTE in women 45 to 64 years of age. A yearly total of 16.5 cases of VTE per 100,000 women may be attributed to hormonal replacement therapy.[28] The risk of VTE also appears to be highest during the first year of exposure to hormonal replacement.[29] It has not been clearly established that previous use increases the risk.[30] Although such therapy is associated with obvious benefits, physicians must consider other potential risk factors for VTE before prescribing hormonal replacement therapy.

Other disease states and clinical settings enhance the risk of VTE. Most intensive care unit patients can be considered at risk for VTE because of their multiple risk factors, including significant underlying disease, immobility, and venous injury due to trauma or central venous catheters. These patients should receive some form of DVT prophylaxis and a high index of suspicion for VTE should be maintained in appropriate clinical circumstances.

Inherited Risk Factors

Inherited thrombophilias result in variable degrees of VTE risk. Individuals with, for example, antithrombin III or factor V Leiden deficiency without significant superimposed risk factors such as surgery or immobilization often do not suffer from VTE until an additional risk factor develops. The factor V Leiden mutation is a common genetic polymorphism associated with activated protein C resistance and appears to be present in approximately 4 to 6 percent of the general population.[31] The relative risk of a first idiopathic venous thrombosis among men heterozygous for the mutation has been shown to be three- to sevenfold higher than that of those not affected.[31] Another thrombophilic mutation has been identified in the 3′ untranslated region of the prothrombin gene (substitution of A for G at position 20210), and this mutant allele is present in 2 percent of the general population.[32] This prothrombin gene defect increases the risk of DVT by a factor of 2.7 to 3.8.[32–33] It appears that carriers of both factor V Leiden and the prothrombin G20210A defect have an increased risk of recurrent DVT after a first episode and are candidates for lifelong anticoagulation.[34] There has been increasing interest in the potential role of homocysteine in VTE. In vitro, homocysteine has potentially thrombogenic effects, including injury to vascular endothelium and antagonism of the synthesis and function of nitric oxide.[35] Coexisting hyperhomocysteinemia has been shown to increase the risk for thrombosis in patients with factor V Leiden.[36] However, the thermolabile methylenetetrahydrofolate reductase gene variant is not independently associated with thrombosis, emphasizing that the precise role of homocysteine in venous thrombosis is unclear. Thus, interactions between the genetic factors (defects in enzymes) that control homocysteine metabolism and nutritional factors (folate, vitamin B_6, and vitamin B_{12} deficiencies) that affect homocysteine metabolism appear to warrant additional investigation with regard to VTE. It would appear certain that additional inherited thrombophilic disorders will be identified that may explain some of the "idiopathic" cases.

ACUTE PULMONARY EMBOLISM: PATHOPHYSIOLOGY

Gas-Exchange Abnormalities

The effect of PE on oxygenation and hemodynamics depends upon the extent of obstruction of the pulmonary vascular bed and the severity of underlying cardiopulmonary disease. Hypoxemia develops in the preponderance of patients with PE and has been attributed to various mechanisms. When no previous cardiopulmonary disease is present, lung regions with low ventilation/perfusion ratios and shunting due to perfusion of atelectatic areas appear to be the predominant mechanisms of hypoxemia. Hypoxemia leads to an increase in sympathetic tone with systemic vasoconstriction and may actually increase venous return with augmentation of stroke volume, at least initially, if there is no significant underlying cardiac or pulmonary pathology already present.

Hemodynamic Alterations

Massive emboli can cause profound hemodynamic compromise. In the setting of massive emboli, cardiac output is diminished but may be initially sustained as the mean right atrial pressure increases. The increased pulmonary vascular resistance impedes right ventricular outflow with a reduction in left ventricular preload. When no underlying cardiopulmonary disease is present, occlusion of 25 to 30 percent of the vascular bed by emboli results in a rise in pulmonary artery pressure (PAP). As the extent of vascular obstruction increases, hypoxemia worsens, stimulating vasoconstriction and a further rise in PAP. Greater than 50 percent obstruction of the pulmonary arterial bed is generally present before there is substantial elevation of the mean pulmonary artery pressure. When the extent of embolic occlusion approaches 75 percent, the right ventricle must generate a systolic pressure in excess of 50 mmHg and a mean PAP of greater than 40 mmHg to preserve pulmonary perfusion.[37] Although a hypertrophied right ventricle (in an otherwise normal patient) may theoretically be capable of achieving pressures this high, a normal right ventricle is unable to and will fail.[37] In reality, individuals with significant underlying cardiopulmonary disease and superimposed PE are more inclined to develop a more profound deterioration in cardiac output than normal individuals with PE, whether or not right ventricular hypertrophy is present. Furthermore, a depressed cardiac output in the absence of an elevated right atrial pressure suggests that the PE is superimposed upon preexisting cardiac disease. Right ventricular failure develops more frequently in the setting of PE when the patient has underlying coronary artery disease.[38] Aggressive hemodynamic support may sustain some patients with massive embolism at least temporarily, even when the right ventricle is dilated and hypocontractile, but any further increment in embolic burden may be fatal.

DIAGNOSIS OF DEEP VENOUS THROMBOSIS AND PULMONARY EMBOLISM

Venous thromboembolism represents the spectrum of one disease. Most clinically significant PE arise from the prior development of DVT in the lower extremities, with subsequent embolization to the lungs. Patients may present with symptoms of either DVT, PE, or both. At the present time, the diagnostic strategy involves recognition of certain symptoms and signs of DVT and/or PE and usually involves an imaging study directed at either the legs or the lungs, depending upon the presentation. Ventilation/perfusion ($\dot{V}/\dot{Q}$) scanning has been the diagnostic cornerstone for patients with suspected PE for decades. However, the contrast-enhanced computed tomography (CT) scan is being used increasingly as experience and technology improve. The diagnostic approach to acute DVT and PE has recently been exhaustively reviewed and presented as clinical practice guidelines by the American Thoracic Society.[39]

Lower extremity ultrasound is the most common leg study utilized, and the $\dot{V}/\dot{Q}$ scan still appears to be the most frequently utilized lung imaging study. It is important to realize that an increasingly common diagnostic strategy in patients presenting with suspected PE but with a nondiagnostic lung imaging study is to perform a lower extremity study in hopes of proving that DVT is present.

History and Physical Examination

The clinical diagnosis of both DVT and PE, based upon the history and physical examination, are insensitive and nonspecific. Patients with lower extremity DVT may be asymptomatic or may have erythema, warmth, pain, swelling, and/or tenderness. These findings are not specific for DVT but suggest the need for further evaluation. The differential diagnosis of DVT includes cellulitis, edema from other causes, musculoskeletal pain, or trauma (some of these may be concomitant and may or may not be related). Pulmonary embolism must always be considered when unexplained dyspnea is present. Dyspnea as well as pleuritic chest pain and hemoptysis are common in PE but are nonspecific. Coughing may be present, and while sometimes caused by PE, it more commonly occurs with bronchitis or pneumonia. It is far less common than shortness of breath. Anxiety, light-headedness, and syncope are all symptoms that may be caused by PE but may also be due to a number of other entities that result in hypoxemia or hypotension. Tachypnea and tachycardia are the most common signs of PE but are also nonspecific. Syncope or sudden hypotension should suggest the possibility of massive PE. The cardiac and pulmonary physical examinations are both nonspecific. A pleural rub or accentuated pulmonic component of the second heart sound may suggest PE but can also be explained by other disorders. In spite of the limitations of the history and physical examination for DVT and PE, the index of clinical suspicion becomes a more useful parameter when considered in conjunction with additional studies and $\dot{V}/\dot{Q}$ scanning.[40] Dyspnea, tachypnea, clear lung fields, and hypoxemia may often be attributed to a flare of chronic obstructive disease or asthma when underlying PE is present. Thus, diagnostic efforts aimed at possible VTE should still be considered despite alternative explanations if risk factors and the clinical setting are suggestive.

Laboratory Testing

Routine laboratory testing is not useful in proving or refuting the presence of DVT or PE but may be helpful in confirming or excluding alternative or concomitant diagnoses. For example, leukocytosis and pulmonary infiltrates may suggest pneumonia, and worsening hypercapnia in a patient with known chronic obstructive lung disease may suggest a flare of the underlying lung disease. It is important to realize, however, that acute PE can develop in the setting of other cardiopulmonary disorders that do not exclude the possibility of concomitant PE.

D-DIMER TESTING

The D-dimer is a specific derivative of cross-linked fibrin. Measurement of circulating plasma D-dimer has been comprehensively evaluated as a diagnostic test for acute VTE, both independently and together with other diagnostic measures. A normal enzyme-linked immunosorbent assay (ELISA) appears to be sensitive in excluding PE. When the D-dimer level is 500 μg/L or greater, the sensitivity and specificity for PE have been shown to be 98 and 39 percent, respectively.[41] The sensitivity of the plasma D-dimer appears to remain high up to 1 week after presentation. In another prospective analysis, 96 percent of 79 patients with high-probability $\dot{V}/\dot{Q}$ scans had an elevated D-dimer concentration.[42] Thus, increased levels of cross-linked fibrin degradation products are an indirect but suggestive marker of intravascular thrombosis in addition to indicating fibrinolysis. Although the sensitivity of the D-dimer appears high, the specificity is not high enough to be diagnostic. Patients with both suspected and proven DVT and PE often have underlying disease states that also cause the D-dimer to be elevated.

When clinical studies comparing D-dimer with the results of other diagnostic tests for VTE are reviewed, there appear to be appreciable differences in assay performance, heterogeneity among the patient population, and inconsistent use of definitive diagnostic criteria for venous thromboembolism.[43,44] The number of available D-dimer assays, including rapid bedside assays, is increasing. It appears that results of clinical studies utilizing one manufacturer's D-dimer assay cannot be extrapolated to another study using another manufacturer's assay. No single assay has been established as superior to all the others. The ELISA assays are sensitive but cannot be performed rapidly. The latex tests, while rapid, have not been proven to be sufficiently sensitive. A rapid, quantitative, immunoturbidimetric technique has been evaluated that recognizes the D-dimer epitope by using antibody-coated latex particles.[45] In at least one study, the degree of abnormality of this D-dimer test appeared to correlate with the extent of the DVT, with proximal thrombosis producing higher D-dimer levels.[45] In addition, patients presenting immediately after the onset of symptoms were found to have higher D-dimer levels than patients examined after a few days. Thus, certain quantitative D-dimer tests may prove to offer additional information regarding the acuity and extent of thromboembolic disease. Future studies of D-dimer techniques should be rigorous with regard to the definitive presence or absence of DVT and/or PE as well as addressing issues such as duration of symptoms, presence of comorbid disease, and extent of thrombosis.

Recently, both DVT and PE management studies have been performed, with therapeutic decisions based, to some extent, upon D-dimer results. When a bedside whole-blood agglutination D-dimer assay and impedance plethysmography were both negative in patients with suspected DVT and anticoagulation was withheld, the negative predictive value was 98.5 percent (95 percent confidence interval, 96.3–99.6) based upon 3 months of follow-up.[46] For the D-dimer test alone, the negative predictive value was 97.2 percent. A diagnostic protocol including an assessment of clinical probability, $\dot{V}/\dot{Q}$ scan, ELISA plasma D-dimer, and lower extremity ultrasound (US) was utilized in 308 consecutive patients presenting to the emergency room with suspected PE.[47] Of these patients, 106 (34 percent) had diagnostic $\dot{V}/\dot{Q}$ scans (high probability in 63 and normal in 43). The noninvasive evaluation was diagnostic in 125 patients (62 percent). In 48 patients, PE was ruled out by a nondiagnostic lung scan together with low clinical probability. In 53 cases, it was ruled out by a quantitative D-dimer of less than 500 μg/L. Only 77 of the 202 patients with nondiagnostic $\dot{V}/\dot{Q}$ scans required pulmonary angiography. At 6 months follow-up, only 2 of the 199 patients in whom the diagnostic protocol had ruled out PE had a VTE event. Using the same cutoff value for the quantitative D-dimer, these investigators subsequently reported that of 198 patients with suspected PE and a D-dimer <500 μg/L, 196 were free of PE, one had PE, and one was lost to follow-up.[48] Thus, the negative predictive value of the D-dimer was approximately 196 of 198 (99 percent). Although these data represent the work of only one group of investigators, they are promising. Rapid bedside assays are becoming more available and additional outcome studies will help to clarify their role. At present, plasma D-dimer measurements should be interpreted with caution and in the context of other diagnostic tests.

ARTERIAL BLOOD GAS ANALYSIS

Hypoxemia, while not universal, is extremely common in acute PE. Some patients, particularly young individuals without underlying cardiopulmonary disease may have a normal Pa_{O_2}. In a retrospective study of hospitalized patients with PE, the Pa_{O_2} was greater than 80 mmHg in 29 percent of patients less than 40 years old, compared with 3 percent in the older group.[49] However, the alveolar-arterial (A-a) difference was elevated in all patients. Thus, as age increases, it becomes even less likely that a patient with PE will have a normal room air Pa_{O_2}. In the PIOPED, a subset of patients suspected of PE without a history or evidence of underlying cardiac or pulmonary disease was evaluated, and the Pa_{O_2} and A-a difference values were compared.[50] Patients with and without PE could not be distinguished based upon either of these values. However, the A-a difference was elevated by more than 20 mmHg in 76 of 88 (86 percent) patients with PE. The diagnosis of acute PE cannot be excluded based upon a normal Pa_{O_2}, and although the A-a difference is usually elevated, it may very rarely be normal in patients without preexisting cardiopulmonary disease. An important tenet should be that unexplained hypoxemia, particularly in the setting of risk factors for DVT, should suggest the possibility of PE.

Electrocardiography

Electrocardiography (ECG) cannot be relied upon to rule in or rule out PE, though ECG proof of a clear alternative diagnosis, such as myocardial infarction, is useful when PE is among the possible diagnoses. The potential coexistence of PE together with another process must, however, be a consideration. ECG findings in acute PE are generally nonspecific and include T-wave changes, ST-segment abnormalities, and left- or right-axis deviation. The changes that do occur are likely caused by right ventricular dilation. The "classic" S1Q3T3 pattern described by McGinn and White[51] in 1935 in seven patients with acute cor pulmonale secondary to PE was subsequently demonstrated to be present in about 10 percent of PE cases.[52] In patients without underlying cardiac or pulmonary disease from the Urokinase Pulmonary Embolism Trial (UPET), electrocardiographic abnormalities were documented in 87 percent of patients with proven PE.[53] These findings were not specific for PE, however. In this clinical trial, 26 percent of patients with massive or submassive PE and 32 percent of those with massive PE had manifestations of acute cor pulmonale, such as the S1 Q3 T3 pattern, right bundle-branch block, P-wave pulmonale, or right axis deviation. Such changes are thus seen in a minority of patients. The low frequency of specific ECG changes associated with PE was confirmed in the PIOPED study.[50] It has been recently suggested that the anterior subepicardial ischemic pattern is the most frequent ECG sign of massive PE.[54]

Chest Radiography

The chest radiograph is abnormal in the majority of patients with PE, but the findings are nonspecific. Atelectasis, pulmonary infiltrates, pleural effusion, and mild elevation of a hemidiaphragm may be present.[50] Classic radiographic evidence of pulmonary infarction (Hampton's hump) or decreased vascularity (Westermark's sign) are suggestive but uncommon. A normal chest radiograph in the presence of significant dyspnea and hypoxemia without evidence of bronchospasm or anatomic cardiac shunt is strongly suggestive of PE. In most situations, however, the chest radiograph cannot be used to definitively diagnose or exclude PE. Although exclusion of other processes such as pneumonia, congestive heart failure, pneumothorax, or rib fracture (which may cause symptoms similar to acute PE) is important, PE often coexists with other underlying lung diseases.

Imaging Studies for Pulmonary Embolism

VENTILATION/PERFUSION SCANNING

Ventilation/perfusion scanning has been the pivotal diagnostic test for approaching suspected PE for many years. However, even in patients in whom PE is ultimately proven, the $\dot{V}/\dot{Q}$ scan is most commonly nondiagnostic. Certain $\dot{V}/\dot{Q}$ scan readings are of substantial utility, however. Normal and high-probability scans are considered diagnostic. A normal perfusion scan excludes the diagnosis of PE with enough certainty that further diagnostic testing is unnecessary. Matching areas of decreased ventilation and perfusion in the presence of a normal chest radiograph suggests a process other than PE. However, low- or intermediate-probability (nondiagnostic) scans are commonly found with PE, and particularly when clinical suspicion is high, additional testing is necessary. In the PIOPED study, the utility of $\dot{V}/\dot{Q}$ scanning combined with clinical assessment of patients with suspected PE was prospectively evaluated.[40] Patients with PE had scans that were of high, intermediate, or low probability, but so did most individuals without PE. Although the specificity of high-probability scans was 97 percent, the sensitivity was only 41 percent. Of interest, 33 percent of patients with intermediate-probability scans and 12 percent of patients with low-probability scans were diagnosed definitively with PE by pulmonary arteriography. When the clinical suspicion of PE was considered very high, the positive predictive value of high-probability scans for PE was 96 percent. More interestingly, in those with high clinical suspicion and intermediate- and low-probability scans, it was 66 and 40 percent, respectively. Thus, further diagnostic testing for PE should be performed even when the lung scan is of low or intermediate probability if the clinical setting suggests PE. Although the $\dot{V}/\dot{Q}$ scan may sometimes be diagnostic of PE or exclude the possibility with sufficient certainty, it is often nondiagnostic. The latter fact emphasizes the need to further improve our diagnostic resources.

PULMONARY ARTERIOGRAPHY

Pulmonary arteriography is the established "gold standard" diagnostic technique for the diagnosis of PE. It is a very sensitive and specific test. However, for smaller (subsegmental) emboli, it appears less accurate. Two referee readers from the PIOPED agreed on the presence or absence of subsegmental emboli in only 66 percent of cases.[55] In another study, using selective pulmonary arteriography, there was excellent agreement on main, lobar, and segmental emboli but only 13 percent agreement on subsegmental emboli.[56] The significance of such emboli is unclear, however, and may depend upon the presence of underlying cardiopulmonary disease, the extent of concurrent DVT, and the continued presence or absence of risk factors for DVT. Arteriography is safe in most instances. Complications related to this technique among 1111 patients suspected of PE in the PIOPED study included death in 0.5 percent and major nonfatal complications in 1 percent.[55] An increasingly utilized alternative to pulmonary arteriography is to perform lower extremity studies when the $\dot{V}/\dot{Q}$ scan is nondiagnostic; if DVT is discovered, the therapeutic approach is generally the same as if an arteriogram were positive for PE. If serial lower extremity testing is negative, the chances of significant PE or morbidity from a subsequent event appears unlikely.[57] However, the ease with which serial testing can be performed is variable, and arteriography is often the best alternative when the leg test is negative, since the sensitivity of ultrasound for DVT is substantially lower in patients with asymptomatic DVT. Lower extremity testing is being increasingly utilized in patients with nondiagnostic lung scans and in stable patients; this appears to be appropriate.[39] Pulmonary arteriography has also been performed at the bedside utilizing a Swan-Ganz catheter.[58] However, accurate interpretation of arteriography, particularly in the case of submassive emboli, is crucial.

ECHOCARDIOGRAPHY

Echocardiography is not usually used for approaching the patient with suspected PE, although it may suggest its presence in some clinical settings, and it has been suggested as a potential means by which to determine the need for thrombolytic therapy.[59] Echocardiography can often be performed more rapidly than either $\dot{V}/\dot{Q}$ scanning or pulmonary arteriography and may suggest hemodynamically significant PE.[60] Studies of patients with documented PE have revealed that more than 80 percent of patients have imaging or Doppler abnormalities of right-ventricular size or function that may suggest acute PE.[60,61] However, patients who are acutely ill with suspected PE often have underlying cardiac or pulmonary disorders such as chronic obstructive lung disease, and neither right-ventricular dilation nor hypokinesis can be reliably used even as indirect evidence of PE in these settings. Intravascular ultrasound imaging has been utilized in both the experimental and clinical setting to image large emboli.[62–64] This technique can be performed at the bedside. Although the technique may be less sensitive and specific and more time-consuming in the setting of smaller emboli, further investigation may be warranted.

COMPUTED TOMOGRAPHY

Contrast-enhanced spiral (helical) CT scanning has been increasingly investigated and utilized in patients with clinically suspected acute and chronic PE. This technique involves continuous movement of the patient through the scanner with concurrent scanning by a constantly rotating gantry and detector system.[65] A helix of projecting data is obtained. Continuous volume acquisitions can be obtained during a single breath, and with newer scanners, breath-holding may be less important. Rapid scans can be obtained, facilitating imaging in critically ill patients. Limitations of helical CT scanning in early clinical studies included poor visualization of horizontally oriented vessels in the right middle lobe and lingula because of volume averaging.[66] The peripheral areas of the upper and lower lobes may be inadequately scanned and the presence of intersegmental lymph nodes may result in false-positive studies. Multiplanar reconstructions in coronal, sagittal, or oblique planes aid in distinguishing lymph nodes from emboli (see also Chap. 17).

Computed tomography scanning may reveal emboli in the main, lobar or segmental pulmonary arteries with >90 percent sensitivity and specificity.[66-69] Accurate results have been reported for large PE.[70,71] However, for subsegmental emboli, the sensitivity and specificity appear to be lower. The incidence of isolated subsegmental emboli appears to be approximately 6 to 30 percent, with the former figure likely being more representative.[55,72] Of note, even with the gold standard diagnostic test (arteriography), two referee readers from the PIOPED agreed on the presence or absence of subsegmental emboli in only 66 percent of cases.[55] Another study, using selective pulmonary arteriography, indicated excellent agreement on main, lobar, and segmental emboli but only 13 percent agreement on subsegmental emboli.[56] Thus, this apparent limitation with spiral CT scanning is also a concern with angiography. The incorporation of CT scanning into diagnostic algorithms for PE is being endorsed increasingly.[73] However, no prospective multicenter randomized clinical trials large enough to unequivocally prove the sensitivity and specificity of contrast-enhanced CT scanning in patients with suspected PE have been performed. Most have been single-center trials of moderate size. The value of CT for large emboli appears clear, however.

TABLE 53-2 Sensitivity and Specificity for Contrast-Enhanced CT Scanning for Acute Pulmonary Embolism

References	Number of Patients	Sensitivity (%)	Specificity (%)
Spiral CT			
Remy-Jardin[66]	72	90	86
Remy-Jardin[67]	42	100	96
Goodman[68]	20	86[a]	92[a]
		63[b]	89[b]
van Rossum[70]	124	97	98
van Rossum[71]	45	95	97
Sostman[77]	28	73	97
Electron-beam CT			
Teigen[69]	60	65	97
Teigen[74]	25	95	80

[a]Main, lobar and segmental emboli.
[b]All emboli including peripheral.

Sensitivity and specificity data from several large studies evaluating helical CT scanning for acute PE are shown in Table 53-2. Contrast-enhanced electron-beam CT also appears useful in diagnosing acute PE.[69,74] In one comparison with pulmonary angiography, only 8 of 720 vascular zones (1.1 percent) were considered inadequately visualized with electron-beam CT. As with spiral CT, three-dimensional reconstruction techniques can be applied to the pulmonary vessels to better define vessels located within the plane that has been sectioned. Another important advantage of these CT techniques over the V̇/Q̇ scan is the concomitant ability to define nonvascular structures such as airway, parenchymal, and pleural abnormalities, lymphadenopathy, and cardiac and pericardial disease. Prospective randomized clinical trials comparing these techniques with the standard diagnostic approach to PE will help to determine their precise role. It appears that CT scanning is being increasingly utilized.

MAGNETIC RESONANCE IMAGING

Magnetic resonance imaging (MRI) is also being utilized to evaluate clinically suspected PE at some centers.[75,76] One clinical trial compared MRI with spiral CT: the average sensitivity of CT for five observers was 75 percent and of MRI 46 percent.[77] The average specificity of CT was 89 percent, compared with 90 percent for MRI. Sensitivity and specificity values for expert readers were higher, however. Spiral CT may be somewhat more useful than MRI for detecting PE at the present time, but MRI has several attractive advantages, including excellent sensitivity and specificity for the diagnosis of DVT. As in the case of CT scanning, the diagnosis of entities other than PE using MRI is a major advantage over the V̇/Q̇ scan.

Diagnostic algorithms for patients presenting with suspected DVT and PE have been recommended in the American Thoracic Society Consensus Statement and allow for a certain degree of flexibility with regard to specific diagnostic modalities utilized.[39]

Imaging Studies for Deep Venous Thrombosis

A number of diagnostic techniques can be utilized to evaluate the patient with suspected DVT. Compression US is the most common technique used in the United States and in many other areas of the world. Impedance plethysmography is used at some centers, and a number of important clinical trials have been performed utilizing this technique. MRI appears to have some important advantages, but it has not generally been used as a first-line test. Venography remains the gold standard, but has been necessary less often at many centers in view of the accuracy of US. Each diagnostic technique has advantages and limitations. Although diagnostic algorithms may be suggested for suspected DVT, these are institution-specific, depending upon resources and available expertise with certain techniques. Newer diagnostic testing modalities, such as scanning with technetium 99m–labeled glycopeptide IIb/IIIa receptor antagonists, appear promising but will not be discussed.[78]

CONTRAST VENOGRAPHY

Although contrast venography remains the gold standard for the diagnosis of DVT, it has been less commonly used since the advent of US. Venography should be performed whenever noninvasive testing is nondiagnostic or impossible to perform. It is an invasive procedure that may result in superficial phlebitis or hypersensitivity reactions, but it is generally safe and accurate.

IMPEDANCE PLETHYSMOGRAPHY

Impedance plethysmography has been carefully studied in patients presenting with suspected acute DVT. It has proven reliable for the detection of proximal DVT (including that occurring in and above the popliteal vein). Preliminary studies suggested greater than 90 percent sensitivity and 97 percent specificity for DVT involving the proximal lower extremity, although less than 30 percent of isolated calf vein thromboses were detected.[79,80] Although this modality is sometimes portable, it does require access to the calf and thigh for electrode and cuff placement. The specificity of IPG is affected by disorders that obstruct venous outflow, such as tumor or hematoma. Plaster casts or external fixation of extremities limits the utility of this technique. Some investigators have emphasized the potential limitations of IPG.[81] Among the limitations of the technique are its inability to detect asymptomatic/nonobstructive proximal DVT, or calf DVT and its lack of utility for diagnoses other than DVT.[39] It is used much less commonly than compression US.

ULTRASONOGRAPHY

Compression US with venous imaging is a portable, accurate, and widely available diagnostic technique for proximal lower extremity DVT. Combined with a Doppler reading, this technique is referred to as *duplex ultrasonography*. Ultrasound technology has been further sophisticated by the development of color duplex instrumentation that display Doppler frequency shifts as color superimposed on the gray-scale image. The color duplex images display both mean blood flow *velocity*, expressed as a change in hue or saturation, and *direction* of blood flow, displayed as red or blue. US imaging techniques can also identify or suggest the presence of pathology other than DVT—for example, Baker's cysts, hematomas, lymphadenopathy, arterial aneurysms, superficial thrombophlebitis, and abscesses may be suggested or diagnosed.[82] The sensitivity and specificity of US for symptomatic proximal DVT has been well above 90 percent in most recent clinical trials.[83,84] There are limitations, including insensitivity for asymptomatic DVT (less than 50 percent), operator dependence, the inability to accurately distinguish acute from chronic DVT in symptomatic patients, and insensitivity for calf vein thrombosis.[85–87] Compared with other technology, it is relatively inexpensive and is the preferred diagnostic modality for the straightforward case of symptomatic suspected proximal DVT.

MAGNETIC RESONANCE IMAGING

Magnetic resonance imaging (MRI) has clear advantages as a diagnostic test for suspected DVT and appears to be an accurate noninvasive alternative to venography.[88] A major feature of this technique is excellent resolution of the inferior vena cava and pelvic veins.[89,90] Preliminary experience with MRI suggests that it is at least as accurate as contrast venography or US imaging and more sensitive than US for pelvic vein thrombosis.[88–90] Simultaneous bilateral lower extremity imaging can be accomplished, and MRI appears to accurately distinguish acute from chronic DVT. This technique appears to be useful in distinguishing other entities such as cellulitis or a Baker's cyst from acute DVT. As with many other diagnostic techniques, its utility depends to a certain degree on the experience on the part of the reader. There is the additional advantage of evaluating a patient for the entire spectrum of VTE in one imaging session by scanning the legs and pelvis as well as the lungs. MRI is used by some medical centers when the initial diagnostic test (usually US) is nondiagnostic (see also Chap. 18).

PREVENTION OF DEEP VENOUS THROMBOSIS

Background

Prophylaxis for DVT is effective.[91] A substantial reduction in the incidence of DVT can be accomplished when individuals at risk receive appropriate preventive care, as such measures appear to be grossly underutilized. A review of the use of prophylaxis for DVT in 16 Massachusetts hospitals revealed that such therapy was administered to only 44 precent of high-risk patients in teaching hospitals and only 19 percent in nonteaching hospitals.[92] The frequency of prophylaxis ranged from 9 to 56 percent among hospitals. Another retrospective analysis revealed that only 97 of 250 patients (39 percent) at *very high risk* for DVT received any form of prophylaxis and that of these 97, only 64 (66 percent) received appropriate care.[93] Prophylaxis can be pharmacologic (anticoagulation) or nonpharmacologic. Low-molecular-weight heparin (LMWH) products have been increasingly utilized in clinical practice for both prevention and treatment of established VTE. Extensive literature is now available supporting the use of these preparations for DVT prevention. The LMWH preparations are advantageous in that they produce a more predictable dose response and are administered subcutaneously only once or twice daily (without monitoring) depending on the preparation (see "Management of Established Venous Thromboembolism," below).[94] Early ambulation whenever possible is always recommended in postoperative patients.

General Medical Patients

Patients are stratified according to DVT risk, and certain prophylactic measures are more appropriate for some patients than for others. Generally, low-dose anticoagulation with standard, unfractionated heparin or LMWH is indicated in medical or surgical patients deemed at risk for DVT. When standard heparin is used for prophylaxis in general medical patients, 5000 U delivered subcutaneously every 8 to 12 h is generally adequate. LMWHs have also been studied in general medical patients. In a large double-blind, randomized clinical study comparing two different doses of subcutaneous LMWH (enoxaparin) delivered once daily to acutely ill medical patients, the higher dose (40 mg) proved more effective than the lower dose (20 mg).[95] The incidence of DVT was 5.5 percent in the former group and 14.9 percent in the latter.

When prophylactic anticoagulation is contraindicated, mechanical devices (intermittent pneumatic compression) are utilized. Anticoagulation together with pneumatic compression is appropriate in patients deemed at exceptionally high risk or with multiple risk factors for DVT.

General Surgical Patients

In general surgery patients, a number of prophylactic strategies have been employed. An overview of the results of randomized trials in surgical patients demonstrated the substantial benefit of DVT prophylaxis.[91] In this review of more than 70 randomized trials involving 16,000 patients, it was demonstrated that perioperative use of subcutaneous heparin could prevent about half of all PE and about two-thirds of all DVT. In a large meta-analysis, the value of prophylaxis to reduce the incidence of DVT was confirmed; it was also suggested that intermittent pneumatic compression plus the use of gradient compression stockings may result in the lowest incidence of postoperative DVT.[96] Other combined treatments were associated with lower rates than heparin alone and appear appropriate in patients at exceptionally high risk. For those patients undergoing minor operations who are less than 40 years old and have no additional risk factors for DVT, no prophylaxis other than early ambulation is recommended. Older patients undergoing major operations without additional risk factors should receive either standard, unfractionated heparin, LMWH, or intermittent pneumatic compression. When additional risk factors are present in the latter group, standard heparin every 8 h or LMWH should be administered. Enoxaparin has been FDA-approved for prophylaxis in patients undergoing elective abdominal surgery (40 mg subcutaneously once daily). A second preparation, dalteparin, has also been approved in the United States for once-daily use as prophylaxis for elective abdominal surgery.

Other High-Risk Patients

Certain orthopedic populations at particularly high risk for acute DVT have been carefully studied with well-designed randomized clinical trials, which led to the approval of enoxaparin by the FDA for prophylaxis against DVT in patients undergoing elective total hip or knee replacement. The approved dosing regimens are 30 mg subcutaneously twice daily initiated within 12 to 24 h after surgery, and 40 mg once daily initiated preoperatively. The duration of prophylaxis depends upon whether the patient is ambulatory and upon additional risk factors. At least one large randomized, placebo-controlled clinical trial suggested a lower incidence of DVT with more prolonged (1 month) outpatient prophylaxis in this patient population.[97] LMWHs have also been evaluated in trauma patients at risk for DVT and have proven efficacious in this patient population.[98] Intermittent pneumatic compression should be utilized if anticoagulation prophylaxis is contraindicated.

A number of LMWH preparations are currently being investigated. It is important to realize that these preparations are not identical and the results of clinical trials with one agent cannot be extrapolated to another. Detailed recommendations for DVT prophylaxis are published and updated every 2 to 3 years (American College of Chest Physicians Consensus).[99]

MANAGEMENT OF ESTABLISHED VENOUS THROMBOEMBOLISM

Assuring adequate oxygenation and hemodynamic support for PE is of paramount importance. Such supportive measures for massive PE are discussed further on in this chapter (see "Hemodynamic Management of Massive Pulmonary Embolism," below). Pain control and elevation of the leg are recommended for DVT, particularly severe, symptomatic acute iliofemoral DVT. Certain recommendations, such as bed rest in patients with established DVT, have not been well substantiated, but this measure should be instituted when significant symptoms are present. The major focus for effective therapy of VTE involves anticoagulation.

Anticoagulation

When DVT or PE is diagnosed or strongly suspected, anticoagulation therapy should be initiated immediately unless contraindications exist. The diagnosis must be confirmed if anticoagulation is to be continued.

STANDARD, UNFRACTIONATED HEPARIN

Standard heparin has been the time-honored parenteral anticoagulant based upon its prompt antithrombotic effect in preventing thrombus growth. The major anticoagulant effect of heparin is accounted for by a unique pentasaccharide with a high-affinity binding sequence to antithrombin III, which is present on only one-third of heparin molecules.[100] The interaction of heparin with antithrombin III markedly accelerates its ability to inactivate thrombin, factor Xa, and factor IXa. Heparin also catalyzes the inactivation of thrombin by a second plasma cofactor, heparin cofactor II. Heparin does not directly dissolve thrombus, but it allows the fibrinolytic system to act unopposed and more readily reduces the size of the thromboembolic burden.[100] Although thrombus growth can be prevented, early recurrence can develop even during therapeutic anticoagulation.

When intravenous standard, unfractionated heparin is instituted, the activated partial thromboplastin time (APTT) should be aggressively followed at 6-h intervals until it is consistently in the therapeutic range of 1.5 to 2.0 times control values.[101] This range corresponds to a heparin level of 0.2 to 0.4 U/mL as measured by protamine sulfate titration. Heparin can be administered by several protocols, but a weight-based approach has been shown to substantially enhance the chances of attaining the therapeutic range quickly. Heparin can be administered as an intravenous bolus of 5000 U followed by a maintenance dose of at least 30,000 to 40,000 U every 24 h by continuous infusion.[102] The lower dose is administered if the patient is considered at high risk for bleeding. This aggressive approach decreases the risk of subtherapeutic anticoagulation and, although supratherapeutic levels are sometimes achieved initially, bleeding complications do not appear to be increased.[102] More recent data continue to support aggressive heparin dosing. An alternative regimen consisting of a bolus of 80 U/kg followed by 18 U/kg/h has been recommended.[103,104] Subsequent adjusting of the heparin dose should also be weight-based (Table 53-3). This approach was recommended by the recent American College of Chest Physicians (ACCP) Consensus Conference on Antithrombotic Therapy.[104] Warfarin therapy may be initiated as soon as the APTT is therapeutic and heparin should be maintained until a therapeutic International Normalized Ratio (INR) of 2.0 to 3.0 has been overlapped with a therapeutic APTT for 2 consecutive days. This initial anticoagulation approach applies to both acute DVT and PE. Although proximal lower extremity thrombus is more likely to result in PE, calf thrombi should still be treated aggressively with anticoagulation or followed with noninvasive testing over 10 to 14 days for extension into the popliteal vein.[105,106] The spectrum of upper extremity venous thrombosis is variable and includes patients with peripherally and centrally placed intravenous catheters as

TABLE 53-3 Nomogram for Heparin Therapy in Acute Venous Thromboembolism

The initial heparin dose is 80 U/kg bolus, then 18 U/kg/h. Subsequent dose modifications, based on APTT as follows:

APTT		
(Sec)	(Times Control)	Heparin Dose Adjustment
<35	<1.2	80 U/kg bolus, then increase by 4 U/kg/h
35 to 45	1.2 to 1.5	40 U/kg bolus, then increase by 2 U/kg/h
46 to 70	1.5 to 2.3	No change
71 to 90	2.3 to 3	Decrease infusion rate by 2 U/kg/h
>90	>3	Hold infusion 1 h, then decrease rate by 3 U/kg/h

SOURCE: American College of Chest Physicians Guidelines[104] and Raschke et al.[103]

well as those with underlying malignancy. Symptomatic patients with documented upper extremity DVT should be anticoagulated.[107] Prophylacticanticoagulation in patients with long-term indwelling catheters should also be instituted.[104,108]

LOW-MOLECULAR-WEIGHT HEPARIN

Mechanisms of Action and Pharmacology Low-molecular-weight heparin is being utilized increasingly for acute venous thromboembolism. These agents differ in a number of respects from standard, unfractionated heparin. Standard heparin consists of lengthy glycosaminoglycan polymers that are heterogenous in size, with a mean molecular weight of approximately 15,000 Da. LMWHs, also glycosaminoglycans, are prepared by chemical or enzymatic depolymerization and are approximately one-third of the size of unfractionated heparin. These LMWH fractions are also diverse, with a mean molecular weight of 4000 to 5000 Da. The difference in size between unfractionated heparin and LMWH results in an altered anticoagulant profile.[109] Only one-third of the LMWH molecules contain the pentasaccharide required for antithrombin III binding. Maximal inhibition of thrombin requires the binding of heparin to both antithrombin III and the activated enzyme. In contrast, the accelerated inactivation of factor Xa by the heparin/antithrombin III combination requires only the binding of unfractionated heparin to antithrombin III and does not require the formation of the ternary complex. Heparin molecules smaller than 18 saccharide units are unable to bind thrombin and antithrombin III simultaneously, precluding maximal acceleration of the inactivation of thrombin by antithrombin III. These smaller LMWH molecules do, however, retain their ability to catalyze the inhibition of factor Xa by antithrombin III. For this reason, LMWH fractions appear to have relatively more anti-Xa than antithrombin activity and significantly less effect upon the APTT. While the ratio of anti-Xa to antithrombin of heparin is 1:1, the LMWH preparations have significantly higher ratios. In addition, other anticoagulant properties such as stimulation of tissue factor pathway–inhibitor release appear to be responsible for the effect of these agents, suggesting more reason for variability among them.[109] While the different preparation methods result in products with similar molecular profiles, structural variations remain, which impart significant differences in their biologic actions. Chemical modifications of various portions of the molecules, charge density, and the degree of desulfation all affect the characteristics of the final product. Because of these differences, antithrombin III activity, the effects on tissue-factor-pathway inhibitor, platelet factor 4, and heparin cofactor II would be expected to be different for the different preparations. Other potential dissimilarities between heparin and LMWH and between the individual LMWH preparations include differences in stimulation of the release of tissue plasminogen activator and prostacyclin. A major advantage of these preparations over unfractionated heparin is substantially enhanced bioavailability. This has been shown to differ for different LMWH preparations as well. Each of the LMWH compounds should be considered a distinct agent and they should not, at the present time, be considered interchangeable. Important characteristics and advantages of the LMWH preparations are shown in Tables 53-4 and 53-5.

Clinical Trials and Indications Numerous clinical trials have strongly suggested the efficacy and safety of LMWH for treatment of established acute proximal DVT, using recurrent symptomatic VTE as the primary outcome measure.[110–116] Treatment with LMWH is more convenient for the patient and for the nursing staff for several reasons. A continuous intravenous line is not required, as these agents can be administered once or twice per day subcutaneously at therapeutic doses. In most cases monitoring of the APTT is not required. Patients can be monitored by measuring levels of factor X, and certain patient populations, such as significantly obese individuals or those with renal insufficiency, are probably best managed with such monitoring. There has not been com-

TABLE 53-4 A Comparison of Low-Molecular-Weight Heparin with Unfractionated Heparin

Characteristic	UFH[a]	LMWH[b]
Mean molecular weight	12,000–15,000	4000–6000
Protein binding	Substantial	Minimal
Anti-Xa activity	Substantial	Substantial
Anti-IIa activity	Substantial	Minimal
Platelet inhibition	Substantial	Minimal
Vascular permeability	Moderate	None
Microvascular permeability	Substantial	Minimal
Elimination (predominant)	Hepatic/macrophages	Renal

[a]Unfractionated heparin.
[b]Low-molecular-weight heparin.

TABLE 53-5 Potential Advantages of Low-Molecular-Weight Heparins over Unfractionated Heparin

- Efficacy: Comparable or superior[a]
- Safety: Comparable or superior[b]
- Bioavailability: Superior
- Subcutaneous administration
- Once or twice daily dosing
- No laboratory monitoring[c]
- Less phlebotomy
- Earlier ambulation
- Home therapy in certain patient subsets

[a]Based upon objectively documented recurrence rates in clinical trials.
[b]Based upon rates of major and minor bleeding in clinical trials.
[c]In certain patient populations (significant obesity, renal insufficiency), monitoring has been suggested.

plete agreement on the approach to these individuals. Outpatient therapy for stable patients with DVT is increasing significantly. In two large, randomized (Canadian and European) trials, therapy with LMWH (enoxaparin and fraxiparine, respectively) was compared with that using standard weight-based unfractionated heparin.[110,111] The LMWH patients were treated entirely as outpatients or continued at home after a brief hospitalization. The outpatient LMWH regimens proved safe and effective. Three meta-analyses examined the use of LMWH compared with unfractionated heparin in the initial treatment of acute proximal DVT.[117–119] Although there was overlap among the clinical trials included in the analyses, they have helped to confirm the efficacy and safety of LMWH for the treatment of established DVT. At the present time, only one LMWH (enoxaparin) is FDA-approved for use in the United States for treatment of established DVT in the outpatient setting or for DVT (with or without PE) in the inpatient setting. Unlike the regimen for prophylaxis, in which a fixed dose of enoxaparin is utilized, a weight-based dosing regimen is employed for treatment of established VTE. For outpatient therapy, the recommended dose of enoxaparin is 30 mg subcutaneously every 12 h, while for inpatient treatment both 30 mg every 12 h and 40 mg once daily have been studied and FDA-approved. In addition to being more convenient, the LMWH preparations appear to be cost-effective, particularly when outpatient therapy is utilized.[120] Some of the different LMWH products and their prophylaxis and treatment regimens are listed in Table 53-6. The appropriate steps in instituting anticoagulation with enoxaparin for established VTE, including outpatient therapy, are shown in Table 53-7.

LONG-TERM THERAPY FOR DEEP VENOUS THROMBOSIS AND PULMONARY EMBOLISM

Documented proximal DVT or PE should be treated for 3 months with oral warfarin, keeping the INR at 2.0 to 3.0. Individuals unable to take warfarin can be treated with long-term subcutaneous heparin or LMWH. More prolonged therapy is indicated when significant risk factors persist. Furthermore, patients in whom no clear risk factors exist (idiopathic VTE) appear to benefit from more prolonged anticoagulation.[121] In a double-blind study, patients completing 3 months of anticoagulation for a first episode of idiopathic VTE were randomized to receive either warfarin (INR 2.0 to 3.0) or placebo for an additional 24 months, and there was a substantial reduction in recurrences in the warfarin group without a statistically significant increase in bleeding.[121] Both short- and long-term anticoagulation guidelines are outlined in the ACCP Consensus Conference guidelines.[104]

OTHER ANTICOAGULANTS

Newer anticoagulants are being explored. Heparin works indirectly, requiring antithrombin III as a cofactor, and its effects vary considerably between patients. Hirudin is a direct thrombin inhibitor that has several advantages over heparin, including efficacy against fibrin clot–bound thrombin. It does not require any cofactors and is not inactivated by platelet factor 4 or plasma proteins. This drug, derived from the saliva of the medicinal leach (*Hirudo medicinalis*), appears promising. Data from several clinical myocardial infarction trials suggested that hirudin is at least as safe as heparin.[122,123] Recombinant hirudin has been examined for prophylaxis of DVT in patients receiving total hip replacement and resulted in a low rate of proximal DVT.[124] As with heparin, these direct thrombin inhibitors have very narrow therapeutic indices. Other direct thrombin inhibitors and substances such as selective factor Xa inhibitors and tissue factor pathway inhibitor (TFPI) merit further investigation in the treatment of acute VTE.[125–130]

TABLE 53-6 Doses of Low-Molecular-Weight for Prevention and Treatment of Venous Thromboembolism

LMWH	Prevention	Treatment
Enoxaparin	30 mg q12h or 40 mg qd	1 mg/kg bid, 1.5 mg/kg qd[a]
Dalteparin	2500 to 5000 Xa U qd	200 Xa U/kg qd
Tinzaparin	75 Xa U/kg qd	175 Xa U/kg qd
Nadroparin	41 to 62 U/kg qd	<50 kg 4100 Xa U q12h 50 to 75 kg 6150 Xa U q12h >70 kg 9200 Xa U q12h
Reviparin	4200 Xa U qd	35 to 45 kg 3500 Xa U q12h 46 to 60 kg 4200 Xa U q12h >60 kg 6300 Xa U q12h
Ardeparin	50 Xa U/kg q 12h	Not evaluated

[a]Enoxaparin is the only LMWH approved for use in the United States for established DVT. It is indicated in patients who present with DVT (with or without concomitant PE). A dose of either 1.5 mg/kg or 1 mg/kg q12h has proven effective for inpatients with DVT +/− PE. Outpatient studies have been with 1 mg/kg q12h. It would appear highly likely that the once-daily dose would be adequate for outpatients, particularly since these patients tend to be stable and *may* have smaller thrombotic burdens.

TABLE 53-7 Initiating Low-Molecular-Weight Heparin for Established Deep Venous Thrombosis

Establish diagnosis of DVT[a] (with or without pulmonary embolism)
Be certain that no contraindications to anticoagulation exist
If diagnosis is strongly *suspected* but not yet proven and the patient is at low bleeding risk, initiate therapy (be certain that proof of thrombosis is established as quickly as possible)
If *outpatient therapy* is being considered, be certain patient is appropriate (medically stable, no massive DVT, pulmonary embolism absent, compliant, ability to self-administer LMWH[b] or have family or home health access for this)
Outpatient program established (patient must know who to contact, where/when to follow up)
Regimen
Enoxaparin initiated administered subcutaneously[c,d]
Warfarin initiated at 5 to 10 mg qd on day 1
The INR[e] checked and goal is 2.0 to 3.0
The APTT is not monitored (consider checking platelet count at day 3 to 5)
Enoxaparin continued for at least 5 days or until the INR is therapeutic for 2 consecutive days

[a]Deep venous thrombosis.
[b]Low-molecular-weight heparin.
[c]This is the only FDA-approved LMWH for treatment of established DVT with or without pulmonary embolism.
[d]1 mg/kg q12h is the FDA-approved dose for inpatient or outpatient therapy, while 1.5 mg/kg qd is approved for inpatient use.
[e]International Normalized Ratio.

COMPLICATIONS OF ANTICOAGULATION

Complications of heparin include bleeding and heparin-induced thrombocytopenia (HIT). The rates of major bleeding in recent trials using standard heparin by continuous infusion or high-dose subcutaneous injection have been less than 5 percent.[104] Heparin-induced thrombocytopenia typically develops 5 or more days after the initiation of heparin therapy, and occurs in 5 to 10 percent of patients.[131–133] If a patient is placed on heparin for VTE and the platelet count progressively decreases to 100,000/mm^3 or less, heparin therapy should be discontinued. Although the risk of HIT appears to be lower with LMWH, it is important for clinicians to realize that HIT can occur with the use of either form of heparin.[134] Over the past decade, there have been many important advances in the pathogenesis, diagnosis, and treatment of HIT, which represents one of the most common immune-mediated adverse drug reactions.[135] This entity is caused by heparin-dependent IgG antibodies that recognize complexes of heparin and platelet factor 4, leading to activation of platelets via platelet Fc gamma IIa receptors. Formation of procoagulant, platelet-derived microparticles, and, possibly, activation of endothelium generate thrombin in vivo. The generation of thrombin helps to account for the strong association between HIT and thrombosis, including the recently recognized syndrome of warfarin-induced venous limb gangrene. This syndrome develops during warfarin treatment of HIT and deep venous thrombosis when acquired protein-C deficiency leads to the inability to regulate thrombin generation in the microvasculature. The diagnosis of HIT can be made confidently when one or more typical clinical events (most frequently, thrombocytopenia with or without thrombosis) occur in a patient with detectable HIT antibodies. The pivotal role of thrombin generation in this syndrome provides a rationale for the use of anticoagulants that reduce thrombin generation (danaparoid) or inhibit thrombin (lepirudin).

Vena Cava Interruption

In patients with established VTE in whom heparin therapy cannot be continued, inferior vena cava (IVC) filter placement can be undertaken to prevent lower extremity thrombi from embolizing to the lungs. These devices have been widely used for nearly two decades. The essential indications for filter placement include contraindications to anticoagulation, recurrent embolism while on adequate therapy, and significant bleeding complications during anticoagulation.[136] Filters are sometimes placed in the setting of massive PE when it is believed that any further emboli might be lethal.[136] A number of filter devices exist, but the Greenfield filter design has been most widely used. These devices can be inserted via the jugular or femoral vein and are effective. Complications are unusual.[137] Possible mechanisms of IVC filter failure include filter migration; improper filter positioning, allowing thrombi to bypass the filter; and formation of thrombosis proximal to the filter or on the proximal tip of the filter with subsequent embolization. Rare complications include clinically significant perforation of the IVC, migration to the heart, and displacement of the filter during insertion. Rarely, these devices may erode into the wall of the IVC. Occasionally, IVC obstruction due to thrombosis at the filter site may occur. Deaths due to filter placement are extraordinarily uncommon. Anticoagulation is generally continued when a filter is placed unless it is contraindicated. Temporary filters have been placed in individuals deemed at extremely high risk for DVT yet unable to receive anticoagulant prophylaxis, such as certain trauma patients.[138]

Thrombolytic Therapy

Acceleration of clot lysis in PE using thrombolytic therapy was first documented several decades ago.[139–141] The prospective, multicenter, randomized UPET evaluated 160 patients with arteriographically proven PE.[53] Thrombolysis was accelerated in patients receiving urokinase compared with those on heparin when pulmonary arteriograms and lung perfusion scans were examined 24 h after treatment. Subsequently, the difference between the two groups diminished and by day 5 the improvement in each group was similar. There were no differences in the frequency of recurrent PE or mortality rate within 2 weeks of treatment. The lack of reduction in mortality may have been explained by the fact that only 7 percent of the patients in the clinical trial were classified as having massive PE with shock. The second phase of this clinical trial also documented the efficacy of streptokinase administered over 24 h.

Both urokinase and streptokinase were approved for use in pulmonary embolism. In 1980, the National Institutes of Health issued consensus guidelines for PE thrombolysis and recommended thrombolytic therapy for patients with obstruction of blood flow to a lobe or multiple pulmonary segments and for patients with hemodynamic compromise regardless of the size of the PE.[142] Recombinant tissue plasminogen activator (t-PA) was subsequently approved for use for the treatment of PE and is administered as a 100-mg intravenous infusion delivered over 2 h.[143] Even shorter infusion durations have been evaluated, and future clinical trials may lead to wider acceptance of these regimens. At present, the above t-PA regimen is the most rapidly administered protocol that is currently approved for use.

At the present time, the clearest indication for the use of thrombolytic therapy is in patients with hemodynamic instability (hypotension) when there are no concomitant contraindications.[144,145] Patients with severely compromised oxygenation should also be considered.[144] Stable patients with a significant embolic load are individualized, often receiving treatment in the absence of absolute or relative contraindications. For example, a strong case for thrombolytic therapy can be made when the embolic load visualized on the imaging study is extensive (defect involving the equivalent of half of the pulmonary vascular bed) or with echocardiographic evidence of right ventricular dysfunction without clear hemodynamic instability.[146,147] Another setting in which thrombolytic therapy may be considered is when extensive DVT accompanies a submassive PE. No clinical studies have been undertaken to support this indication. Perhaps future trials will clarify more controversial guidelines.

The recommendations for use of thrombolytic therapy in PE have been carefully reviewed.[146] Potential indications are presented in Table 53-8. Approved regimens for the treatment of PE are presented in Table 53-9. Coagulation assays are not necessary during thrombolysis, since the approved regimens are administered as fixed doses. Heparin should be withheld until the thrombolytic infusion is completed. The APTT is then determined and heparin is initiated without a loading dose if this value is less than twice the upper limit of normal. If the APTT exceeds this value, the test is repeated every 4 h until it is safe to proceed with heparin. The method of delivery of thrombolytic agents has also been investigated. Although a number of investigators have employed standard or low-dose intrapulmonary arterial thrombolytic infusions in order to deliver a high concentration of drug in close proximity to the clot,[148,149] intravenous therapy appears adequate in most settings.[150] More direct techniques, such as catheter-directed administration of intraembolic thrombolytic therapy are discussed below.

TABLE 53-8 Thrombolytic Therapy in Venous Thromboembolism: Potential Indications[a]

Hypotension related to PE[b]
Severe hypoxemia
Lobar or greater perfusion defect[c]
Right ventricular dysfunction associated with PE
Extensive deep vein thrombosis

[a]All indications require careful review of contraindications to thrombolytic therapy.
[b]This indication is widely accepted.
[c]This indication was supported by NIH guidelines in 1980.[142] However, administration of thrombolytic therapy based upon a lobar defect alone *in the absence of other indications* is not widely practiced.

TABLE 53-9 Thrombolytic Therapy for Acute Pulmonary Embolism: Approved Regimens

Streptokinase: 250,000 U IV (loading dose over 30 min); then 100,000 U/h for 24 h[a]
Urokinase: 2000 U/lb IV (loading dose over 10 min); then 2000 U/lb/h for 12 to 24 h
Tissue-type plasminogen activator: 100 mg IV over 2 h

[a]Streptokinase administered over 24 to 72 h at this loading dose and rate has also been approved for use in patients with extensive DVT.

The use of thrombolytic therapy for DVT without PE is more controversial. A comprehensive review of the literature suggests that use of streptokinase may be associated with a reduction in postphlebitic syndrome when used for acute DVT, although bleeding is increased with thrombolytic therapy.[151] Future studies may clarify the role of thrombolytic therapy for DVT. It is reasonable to consider systemic thrombolytic therapy in patients with proximal occlusive DVT associated with significant swelling and symptoms when there are no absolute or relative contraindications.

The major complication resulting from thrombolytic therapy is bleeding. These agents are not fibrin-specific and any clot, whether pathologic or protective, is subject to lysis. Although hemorrhagic complications in the UPET were relatively high, further experience with thrombolytic therapy has suggested that adverse effects are reduced when venous cut-downs and unnecessary arterial phlebotomy are avoided.[152] Thus, when thrombolytic therapy is administered, invasive procedures should be minimized. The most devastating complication associated with this treatment is the development of intracranial hemorrhage.[153] Clinical trials have suggested that this occurs in significantly less than 1 percent of patients. Contraindications to systemic thrombolytic therapy in VTE are listed in Table 53-10. Bleeding related to thrombolytic therapy requires immediate management. Bleeding from vascular puncture sites should be addressed with manual compression followed by a pressure dressing. Intracranial bleeding requires immediate discontinuation of thrombolytics or anticoagulants, and emergent neurologic and neurosurgical consultation should be obtained. A noncontrasted brain CT scan should be performed. Retroperitoneal hemorrhage may develop from a vascular puncture above the inguinal ligament and may be life-threatening. Severe or refractory bleeding should be addressed with transfusion of 10 U of cryoprecipitate and 2 U of fresh frozen plasma, and heparin

TABLE 53-10 Thrombolytic Therapy for Acute Pulmonary Embolism: Contraindications

Absolute
Intracranial tumor or hemorrhagic stroke
Previous head trauma or cranial surgery
Active or recent gastrointestinal/internal bleeding
Relative
Thrombocytopenia or coagulopathy
Uncontrolled severe hypertension
Cardiopulmonary resuscitation
Surgery or biopsy within the previous 10 days

can be reversed with protamine. A comprehensive review of thrombolytic therapy for acute VTE has been published.[154]

Catheter-Directed Techniques

The intravenous route has been the primary method of delivery, but local thrombolytic therapy has been utilized in massive PE. Intrapulmonary arterial delivery of thrombolytic agents by bolus or prolonged infusion with or without concomitant heparin has been utilized for massive PE (see "Thrombolytic Therapy," above).[148,149] These studies have generally been small and uncontrolled. Although intrapulmonary arterial delivery of thrombolytic agents appears to offer no advantage over the intravenous route,[150] *intraembolic* thrombolytic infusions may offer advantages over merely infusing the agents into the pulmonary artery. Such techniques have been applied in both animal models of PE and in patients, with enhanced thrombolysis.[155,156] Lower than conventional doses of t-PA or urokinase are delivered via a catheter imbedded directly within massive emboli over 10 to 20 min.[155,156] Combining thrombolytic therapy via direct delivery (at low doses) with the possible mechanical benefits of direct intraembolic infusion could prove advantageous over the intravenous route, particularly in the setting of contraindications to thrombolytic therapy. Larger randomized studies would be needed to demonstrate the efficacy, potential advantages, and safety of such techniques. The implementation of these techniques, as well as the catheter-directed administration of intraembolic thrombolytic therapy described above, depend upon the experience of the medical team involved. Transvenous embolectomy without thrombolysis, via a suction-catheter device, has been proven quite effective by some[157,158] but is not widely performed. In an experience spanning 7 years, one group successfully extracted emboli in 11 of 18 patients with massive PE utilizing this technique; 13 survived their hospital stay while 5 died.[158]

Catheter-directed techniques have been successfully employed in the setting of acute iliofemoral DVT utilizing urokinase doses ranging from 1.4 to 16 million U delivered over an average of 30 h.[159,160] Results from a national registry of patients with iliofemoral thrombosis treated with local, catheter-directed therapy indicates that this approach is frequently successful.[160] Randomized trials may be appropriate.

Surgical Embolectomy

Pulmonary embolectomy may be performed in the setting of acute massive PE. The advent of thrombolytic therapy has reduced the number of potential candidates, but contraindications to these agents are relatively common. Although many patients die from PE before surgical embolectomy can be performed, some deteriorate hours after the initial episode, suggesting that surgery may occasionally be appropriate. In one case series of 71 embolectomies performed for acute PE using cardiopulmonary bypass, hospital mortality was 29 percent.[161] However, the mortality in those patients who had not sustained a cardiac arrest preoperatively was only 11 percent.

Hemodynamic Management of Massive Pulmonary Embolism

Massive PE should always be a consideration in the setting of the sudden onset of hypotension or extreme hypoxemia. Electromechanical dissociation or sudden cardiac arrest should always make massive PE suspect. If the patient is stable enough, lung imaging (generally $\dot{V}/\dot{Q}$ scan or spiral CT scan) should be performed when possible. Echocardiography may support the diagnosis of massive PE and may also suggest that aggressive intervention including thrombolytic therapy be considered.[146,147] When massive PE associated with hypotension and/or severe hypoxemia is suspected, supportive treatment is immediately initiated. Intravenous saline can be rapidly infused, but caution is recommended because right ventricular function is often markedly compromised. Dopamine or norepinephrine appear to be the favored choices of vasoactive therapy in massive PE and should be administered if the blood pressure is not rapidly restored.[162] Death from massive PE results from right ventricular failure, and dobutamine has been recommended by some as a means by which to augment right ventricular output.[163,164] A vasopressor such as norepinephrine combined with dobutamine might offer optimal results, and further exploration of such combined therapy would prove enlightening. Oxygen therapy is administered and thrombolytic therapy should be administered if hypotension is present and there are no contraindications. Intubation and mechanical ventilation are instituted as needed to support respiratory failure. Surgical embolectomy may be indicated, particularly if thrombolytic therapy cannot be administered.

CHRONIC THROMBOEMBOLIC PULMONARY HYPERTENSION

In the majority of cases of acute PE, the patient either dies or completely recovers; however, a substantial residual thromboembolic burden occasionally remains and/or continues to form.[165,166] In these patients, the clot becomes organized and adherent and is not amenable to thrombolysis. If the obstruction becomes extensive, pulmonary hypertension develops. At least 50 percent of patients who develop chronic thromboembolic pulmonary hypertension have no documented history of DVT or PE, and this feature greatly impedes the diagnosis. Most patients have no identifiable coagulopathy. Dyspnea with exertion and fatigue are the most common complaints. The nonspecific nature of these findings may substantially delay the correct diagnosis. The physical examination generally reveals a right ventricular heave, a loud P_2, a right ventricular S_3, and tricuspid regurgitation consistent with pulmonary hypertension. In 20 percent of patients, one or more murmurs may be auscultated over the lung fields.

The chest radiograph usually reveals right ventricular enlargement and enlarged main pulmonary arteries. ECG changes are consistent with pulmonary hypertension. Arterial blood gases generally reveal hypoxemia with a widened A-a difference, although some patients may only demonstrate exercise-induced hypoxemia. Echocardiography documents pulmonary hypertension and enlargement of the right ventricle. Chest CT scanning is prudent and may reveal other rare causes of pulmonary hypertension, such as mediastinal fibrosis, and may, in fact, demonstrate evidence of chronic thrombi. With chronic thromboembolic pulmonary hypertension, the $\dot{V}/\dot{Q}$ scan nearly always indicates a high probability of PE, but occasionally it is less impressive. Right heart catheterization and pulmonary arteriography are performed, both to establish the diagnosis with certainty and to determine operability. Pulmonary angioscopy has frequently proven complementary to arteriography in assessing these patients.

Although anticoagulation should be instituted and IVC filters are recommended in patients with chronic thromboembolic pulmonary hypertension, the only means by which to alleviate symptoms and affect survival is with surgery. The University of California at San Diego has been a leading center for the evaluation and surgical therapy of these patients. Pulmonary thromboendarterectomy is performed via median sternotomy on cardiopulmonary bypass, and the overall mortality, which has continued to improve, is now less than 5 percent. Lung transplantation can sometimes be performed in patients in whom thrombi are too distal to extract.

SUMMARY

Venous thromboembolism represents a spectrum consisting of DVT and PE. It is a common cause of death, particularly in hospitalized patients with significant risk factors, and is frequently not diagnosed until autopsy. The history and physical examination for both DVT and PE consist of suggestive but generally very nonspecific findings. These findings, particularly in the setting of risk factors for VTE, are important in raising the level of suspicion for VTE, leading to diagnostic testing. Preventive measures in patients at risk are crucial. Anticoagulation represents appropriate therapy for most patients with VTE. Low-molecular-weight heparins are being used increasingly in established VTE as well as for prophylaxis. Thrombolytic therapy should be considered in massive PE in the absence of contraindications, and guidelines for the use of these agents is evolving. Placement of a filter in the inferior vena cava is indicated when anticoagulation is contraindicated. Newer agents such as direct thrombin inhibitors are being explored. Future clinical trials will help to clarify the roles of both the newer diagnostic modalities and therapeutic strategies.

References

1. Anderson FA, Wheeler HB. Venous thromboembolism: Risk factors and prophylaxis. *Clin Chest Med* 1995; 16:235–251.
2. Dalen JE, Alpert JS. Natural history of pulmonary embolism. *Prog Cardiovasc Dis* 1975; 17:257–270.
3. Lindblad B, Eriksson A, Bergquist D. Autopsy-verified pulmonary embolism in a surgical department: Analysis of the period from 1951 to 1988. *Br J Surg* 1991; 78:849–852.
4. Cotton LT, Clark C. Anatomical localization of venous thrombosis. *Ann R Coll Surg Engl* 1965; 36:214–224.
5. Lamb GC, Tomski MH, Kaufman J, et al. Is chronic spinal cord injury associated with increased risk of venous thromboembolism? *J Am Paraplegia Soc* 1993; 16:153–156.
6. Layish DT, DeLong DM, Tapson VF. Relationship between obesity and pulmonary embolism: A review of the PIOPED data. *Chest* 1996; 110:53S.
7. Carson JL, Kelley MA, Duffy A, et al. The clinical course of pulmonary embolism. *N Engl J Med* 1992; 326:1240–1245.
8. Goldhaber SZ, Hennekens CH, Evans DA, et al. Factors associated with correct antemortem diagnosis of major pulmonary embolism. *Am J Med* 1982; 73:822–826.
9. Kakkar VV, Howe CT, Nicolaides AN, et al. Deep vein thrombosis of the legs: Is there a "high risk" group? *Am J Surg* 1970; 120:527–530.
10. Clagett GP, Reisch JS. Prevention of venous thromboembolism in general surgical patients: Results of a meta-analysis. *Ann Surg* 1988; 208:227–240.
11. Clagett GP, Anderson FA Jr, Geerts W, et al. Prevention of venous thromboembolism. *Chest* 1998; 114:531S–560S.
12. Fisher M, Michele A, McCann W. Thrombophlebitis and pulmonary infarction associated with fractured hip. *Clin Res* 1963; 11:407.
13. Fitts, WT Jr, Lehr HB, Bitner RL, et al. An analysis of 950 fatal injuries. *Surgery* 1964; 56:663–668.
14. Coon WW. Risk factors in pulmonary embolism. *Surg Gynecol Obstet* 1976; 143:385–390.
15. Haire WD. Arm vein thrombosis. *Clin Chest Med* 1995; 16:341.
16. Falanga A, Rickles FR. Pathophysiology of the thrombophilic state in the cancer patient. *Semin Thromb Hemostas* 1999; 25:173–182.
17. Handley AJ, Emerson PA, Fleming PR. Heparin in the prevention of deep vein thrombosis after myocardial infarction. *BMJ* 1972; 2:436–438.
18. Gruppo Italiano per lo Studio della Streptochinasi nell'Infarto Miocardico (GISSI). Effectiveness of intravenous thrombolytic treatment in acute myocardial infarction. *Lancet* 1986; 1:397–402.
19. ISIS-2 Collaborative Group. Randomized trial of IV streptokinase, oral aspirin, both or neither among 17,187 cases of suspected acute myocardial infarction. *Lancet* 1988; 2:349–360.
20. Rickles FR, Levine MN, Edwards RL. Hemostatic alterations in cancer patients. *Cancer Met Rev* 1992; 11:291–311.
21. Carroll VA, Binder BR. The role of the plasminogen activation system in cancer. *Semin Thromb Hemostas* 1999; 25:183–198.
22. Lee AYY, Levine MN. The thrombophilic state induced by therapeutic agents in the cancer patient. *Semin Thromb Hemostas* 1999; 25:137–146.
23. Sorensen HT, Mellemkjaer L, Steffensen FH, et al. The risk of a diagnosis of cancer after primary deep venous thrombosis or pulmonary embolism. *N Engl J Med* 1993; 38:1169–1173.
24. Toglia MR, Weg JG. Current concepts: Venous thromboembolism during pregnancy. *N Engl J Med* 1996; 335:108–114.
25. Stadel BV. Oral contraceptives and cardiovascular disease. *N Engl J Med* 1981; 305:672–677.
26. Weiss N. Third-generation oral contraceptives: How risky? *Lancet* 1995; 346:1570.
27. World Health Organization Collaborative Study of Cardiovascular Disease and Steroid Hormone Contraception. Venous thromboembolic disease and combined oral contraceptives: Results of international multicentre case-control study. *Lancet* 1995; 346: 1575–1582.
28. Daly E, Vessey MP, Hawkins MM, et al. Risk of venous thromboembolism in users of hormone replacement therapy. *Lancet* 1996; 348:977–980.
29. Jick H, Derby LE, Wald MyersM, et al. Risk of hospital admission for idiopathic venous thromboembolism among users of postmenopausal estrogens. *Lancet* 1996; 348:981–983.
30. Grodstein F, Stampfer MJ, Goldhaber SZ, et al. Prospective study of exogenous hormones and risk of pulmonary embolism in women. *Lancet* 1996; 348:983–987.
31. Ridker PM, Hennekens CH, Lindpainter K, et al. Mutation in the gene coding for coagulation factor V and the risk of myocardial infarction, stroke, and venous thrombosis in apparently healthy men. *N Engl J Med* 1995; 332:912.
32. Poort SR, Rosendaal FR, Reitsma PH, et al. A common genetic variation in the 3′-untranslated region of the prothrombin gene is associated with elevated plasma prothrombin levels and an increase in venous thrombosis. *Blood* 1996; 88:3698–3703.
33. Hillarp A, Zoller B, Svensson PJ, Dahlback B. The 20210A of the prothrombin gene is a common risk factor among Swedish outpatients with verified deep venous thrombosis. *Thromb Haemostas* 1997; 78:990–992.
34. DeStefano V, Martinelli I, Mannucci PM, et al. The risk of recur-

rent deep venous thrombosis among heterozygous carriers of both factor V Leiden and the G20210A prothrombin mutation. *N Engl J Med* 1999; 341:801–806.

35. D'Angelo A, Selhub J. Homocysteine and thrombotic disease. *Blood* 1997; 90:1–11.
36. Ridker PM, Hennekens CH, Selhub J, et al. Interrelation of hyperhomocysteinemia, factor V Leiden, and risk of future venous thromboembolism. *Circulation* 1997; 95:1777–1782.
37. Benotti JR, Dalen JE. The natural history of pulmonary embolism. *Clin Chest Med* 1984; 5:403.
38. McIntyre KM, Sasahara AA. The ratio of pulmonary artery pressure to pulmonary vascular obstruction. *Chest* 1977; 71:692.
39. Tapson VF, Carroll BA, Davidson BL, et al. The Diagnostic Approach to Acute Venous Thromboembolism. American Thoracic Society Consensus Statement and Clinical Practice Guidelines. *Am J Resp Crit Care Med* 1999; 160:1043–1066.
40. The PIOPED Investigators. Value of the ventilation/perfusion scan in acute pulmonary embolism: Results of the prospective investigation of pulmonary embolism diagnosis. *JAMA* 1990; 263:2753–2759.
41. Bounameaux H, Cirafici P, DeMoerloose P, et al. Measurement of D-dimer in plasma as diagnostic aid in suspected pulmonary embolism. *Lancet* 1991; 337:196.
42. Rowbotham BJ, Egerton-Vernon J, Whitaker AN, et al. Plasma cross-linked fibrin degradation products in pulmonary embolism. *Thorax* 1990; 45:684–687.
43. Becker DM, Philbrick JT, Bachhuber TL, Humphries JE. D-dimer testing and acute venous thromboembolism: A shortcut to accurate diagnosis? *Arch Intern Med* 1996; 156:939–946.
44. Moser KM. Diagnosing pulmonary embolism: D-dimer needs rigorous evaluation. *BMJ* 1994; 309:1525–1526.
45. Knecht MF, Heinrich F. Clinical evaluation of an immunoturbidimetric D-dimer assay in the diagnostic procedure of deep vein thrombosis and pulmonary embolism. *Thromb Res* 1997; 88: 413–417.
46. Ginsberg JS, Kearon C, Douketis J, et al. The use of D-dimer testing and impedance plethysmographic examination in patients with clinical indications of deep venous thrombosis. *Arch Intern Med* 1997; 157:1077–1081.
47. Perrier A, Bounameaux H, Morabia A, et al. Diagnosis of pulmonary embolism by a decision analysis-based strategy including clinical probability, D-dimer levels, and ultrasonography: A management study. *Arch Intern Med* 1996; 156:531–536.
48. Perrier A, Desmarais S, Goehring C, et al. D-dimer testing for suspected pulmonary embolism in outpatients. *Am J Respir Crit Care Med* 1997; 156:492–496.
49. Green RM, Meyer TJ, Dunn M, Glassroth J. Pulmonary embolism in younger adults. *Chest* 1992; 101:1507–1511.
50. Stein PD, Terrin ML, Hales CA, et al. Clinical, laboratory, roentgenographic, and electrocardiographic findings in patients with acute pulmonary embolism and no pre-existing cardiac or pulmonary disease. *Chest* 1991; 100:598–603.
51. McGinn S, White PD. Acute cor pulmonale resulting from pulmonary embolism. *JAMA* 1935; 104:1473–1480.
52. Sokolow M, Katz LN, Muscovitz AN. The electrocardiogram in acute pulmonary embolism. *Am Heart J* 1940; 19:166–184.
53. The Urokinase Pulmonary Embolism Trial; A national cooperative study. *Circulation* 1973; 47(suppl. II):1–108.
54. Ferrari E, Imbert A, Chevalier T, et al. The ECG in pulmonary embolism. Predictive value of negative T waves in precordial leads: 80 case reports. *Chest* 1997; 111:537–543.
55. Stein PD, Athanasoulis C, Alavi A, et al. Complications and validity of pulmonary angiography in acute pulmonary embolism. *Circulation* 1992; 85:462–468.
56. Quinn MF, Lundell CJ, Klotz TA, et al. Reliability of selective pulmonary arteriography in the diagnosis of acute pulmonary embolism. *AJR* 1987; 149:469–471.
57. Hull RD, Raskob G, Ginsberg JS, et al. A noninvasive strategy for the treatment of patients with suspected pulmonary embolism. *Arch Intern Med* 1994; 154:289–297.
58. Rosengarten PL, Tuxen DV, Weeks AM. Whole lung pulmonary angiography in the intensive care unit with two portable chest x-rays. *Crit Care Med* 1990; 18:459–460.
59. Nass N, McConnell MV, Goldhaber SZ, et al. Recovery of regional right ventricular function after thrombolysis for pulmonary embolism. *Am J Cardiol* 1999; 83:804–806.
60. Come PC. Echocardiographic evaluation of pulmonary embolism and its response to therapeutic interventions. *Chest* 1992; 101: 151S–162S.
61. Kasper W, Meinertz T, Kersting F, et al. Echocardiography in assessing acute pulmonary hypertension due to pulmonary embolism. *Am J Cardiol* 1980; 45:567–572.
62. Tapson VF, Davidson CJ, Gurbel PA, et al. Rapid and accurate diagnosis of pulmonary emboli in a canine model using intravascular ultrasound imaging. *Chest* 1991; 100:1410–1413.
63. Tapson VF, Davidson CJ, Kisslo KB, et al. Rapid visualization of massive pulmonary emboli utilizing intravascular ultrasound. *Chest* 1994; 105:888–890.
64. Ricou F, Nicod PH, Moser KM, Peterson KL. Catheter-based intravascular ultrasound imaging of chronic thromboembolic pulmonary disease. *Am J Cardiol* 1991; 67:749–752.
65. Remy-Jardin M, Remy J. Spiral CT angiography of the pulmonary circulation. *Radiology* 1999; 212:615–636.
66. Remy-Jardin M, Remy J, Wattinne L, Giraud F. Central pulmonary thromboembolism: Diagnosis with spiral volumetric CT with the single-breath-hold technique: Comparison with pulmonary angiography. *Radiology* 1992; 185:381–387.
67. Remy-Jardin M, Remy J, Deschildre F, et al. Diagnosis of pulmonary embolism with spiral CT: Comparison with pulmonary angiography and scintigraphy. *Radiology* 1996; 200:699–706.
68. Goodman LR, Curtin JJ, Mewissen MW, et al. Detection of pulmonary embolism in patients with unresolved clinical and scintigraphic diagnosis: Helical CT versus angiography. *AJR* 1995; 164:1369–1374.
69. Teigen CL, Maus TP, Sheedy PF, et al. Pulmonary embolism: Diagnosis with contrast-enhanced electron-beam CT and comparison with pulmonary angiography. *Radiology* 1995; 194: 313–319.
70. van Rossum AB, Pattynama PM, Treurniat FE, et al. Spiral CT angiography for detection of pulmonary embolism: Validation in 124 patients. *Radiology* 1995; 197(P):303.
71. van Rossum AB, Treurniat FE, Kieft GJ, et al. Role of spiral volumetric computed tomographic scanning in the assessment of patients with clinical suspicion of pulmonary embolism and an abnormal ventilation perfusion scan. *Thorax* 1996; 51:23–28.
72. Oser RF, Zuckerman DA, Gutirrez FR, Brink JA. Anatomic distribution of pulmonary embolism at pulmonary arteriography: Implications for spiral and electron-beam CT. *Radiology* 1996; 199:31–35.
73. Goodman LR, Lipchik RJ. Diagnosis of acute pulmonary embolism: Time for a new approach. *Radiology* 1996; 199:25–27.
74. Teigen CL, Maus TP, Sheedy PF, et al. Pulmonary embolism: Diagnosis with electron-beam CT. *Radiology* 1993; 188:839–845.
75. Meaney JFM, Weg JG, Chenevert TL, et al. Diagnosis of pulmonary embolism with magnetic resonance angiography. *N Engl J Med* 1997; 336:1422–1427.
76. Tapson VF. Pulmonary embolism—New diagnostic approaches. *N Engl J Med* 1997; 336:1449–1451.
77. Sostman HD, Layish DT, Tapson VF, et al. Prospective comparison of helical CT and MR imaging in clinically suspected acute pulmonary embolism. *JMRI* 1996; 6:275.
78. Mousa SA, Bozarth JM, Edwards S, et al. Novel technetium-99m–labeled platelet GPIIb/IIIa receptor antagonists as poten-

tial imaging agents for venous and arterial thrombosis. *Coron Artery Dis* 1998; 9:131–141.
79. Hull R, Hirsh J, Powers P. Impedance plethysmography: The relationship between venous filling and sensitivity and specificity for proximal vein thrombosis. *Circulation* 1978; 58:898–902.
80. Hull R, van Aken WG, Hirsh J, et al. Impedance plethysmography using the occlusive cuff technique in the diagnosis of venous thrombosis. *Circulation* 1976; 53:696–700.
81. Anderson DR, Lensing AWA, Wells PS, et al. Limitations of impedance plethysmography in the diagnosis of clinically suspected deep-vein thrombosis. *Ann Intern Med* 1993; 118:25–30.
82. Borgstede JP, Clagett GE. Types, frequency, and significance of alternative diagnoses found during duplex Doppler venous examinations of the lower extremities. *J Ultrasound Med* 1992; 11:85–89.
83. Lensing AW, Levi MM, Buller HR, et al. Diagnosis of deep-vein thrombosis using an objective Doppler method. *Ann Intern Med* 1990; 113:9–13.
84. White R, McGahan JP, Daschbach MM, Hartling MM. Diagnosis of deep-vein thrombosis using duplex ultrasound. *Ann Intern Med* 1989; 111:297–304.
85. Cronan JJ, Leen V. Recurrent deep venous thrombosis: Limitations of ultrasound. *Radiology* 1989; 170:739–742.
86. Killewich LA, Bedford GR, Beach KW, Strandness DE. Diagnosis of deep venous thrombosis: A prospective study comparing duplex scanning to contrast venography. *Circulation* 1989; 79: 810–814.
87. Davidson BL, Elliott CG, Lensing AWA. Low accuracy of color Doppler ultrasound in the detection of proximal leg vein thrombosis in asymptomatic high-risk patients. *Ann Intern Med* 1992; 117:735–738.
88. Evans AJ, Tapson VF, Sostman HD, et al. The diagnosis of deep venous thrombosis: A prospective comparison of venography and magnetic resonance imaging. *Chest* 1992; 102:120S.
89. Witty LA, Tapson VF, Evans AJ, et al. MRI versus ultrasound: A radiologic and clinical evaluation of DVT. *Am Rev Respir Dis* 1993; 147:A998.
90. Burke B, Sostman HD, Carroll BA, Witty LA. The diagnostic approach to deep venous thrombosis: Which technique? *Clin Chest Med* 1995; 16:253–268.
91. Collins R, Scrimgeour A, Yusuf S, Peto R. Reduction in fatal pulmonary embolism and venous thrombosis by perioperative administration of subcutaneous heparin. *N Engl J Med* 1988; 318:1162–1173.
92. Anderson FA Jr, Brownell W, Goldberg RJ, et al. Physician practices in the prevention of venous thromboembolism. *Ann Intern Med* 1991; 115:591–595.
93. Bratzler DW, Raskob GE, Murray CK, et al. Underuse of venous thromboembolism prophylaxis for general surgery patients: Physician practices in the community hospital setting. *Arch Intern Med* 1998; 158:1909–1912.
94. Tapson VF, Hull R. Management of venous thromboembolic disease: The impact of low-molecular-weight heparin. *Clin Chest Med* 1995; 16:281–294.
95. Samama MM, Cohen AT, Darmon JY, et al. A comparison of enoxaparin with placebo for the prevention of venous thromboembolism in acutely ill medical patients. *N Engl J Med* 1999; 341:793–800.
96. Colditz GA, Tuden RL, Oster G. Rates of venous thrombosis after general surgery: Combined results of randomised clinical trials. *Lancet* 1986; 2:143.
97. Bergqvist D, Benoni G, Bjorgello XX, et al. Low-molecular-weight heparin (enoxaparin) as prophylaxis against venous thromboembolism after total hip replacement. *N Engl J Med* 1996; 335:696–700.
98. Geerts WH, Jay RM, Code KI, et al. A comparison of low-dose heparin with low-molecular-weight heparin as prophylaxis against venous thromboembolism after major trauma. *N Engl J Med* 1996; 335:701–707.
99. Clagett GP, Anderson FA Jr, Geerts WH, et al. Prevention of venous thromboembolism. *Chest* 1998; 114(suppl):531S–560S.
100. Hirsh J, Warkentin TE, Raschke R, et al. Heparin and low-molecular-weight heparin. Mechanisms of action, pharmacokinetics, dosing considerations, monitoring, efficacy, and safety. *Chest* 1998; 114:489S–510S.
101. Hull RD, Raskob GE, Hirsh J, et al. Continuous intravenous heparin compared with intermittent subcutaneous heparin in the initial treatment of proximal vein thrombosis. *N Engl J Med* 1986; 315:1109–1114.
102. Hull R, Raskob G, Rosenbloom D, et al. Optimal therapeutic level of heparin therapy in patients with venous thrombosis. *Arch Intern Med* 1992; 152:1589–1595.
103. Raschke RA, Reilly BM, Guidry JR, et al. The weight-based heparin dosing nomogram compared with a "standard care" nomogram. *Ann Intern Med* 1993; 119:874.
104. Hyers TM, Agnelli G, Hull RD, et al. Antithrombotic therapy for venous thromboembolic disease. *Chest* 1998; 114:561S–578S.
105. Lagerstedt CI, Olsson C-G, Fagher BO, Oqvist BW. Need for long-term anticoagulant treatment in symptomatic calf-vein thrombosis. *Lancet* 1985; 2:515–518.
106. Moser KM et al. Is embolic risk conditioned by location of deep venous thrombosis? *Ann Intern Med* 1981; 94:439–444.
107. Prandoni P, Polistena P, Bernardi E, et al. Upper extremity deep vein thrombosis. *Arch Intern Med* 1997; 157:57–62.
108. Randolph AG, Cook DJ, Gonzalez CA, et al. Benefit of heparin in central venous and pulmonary artery catheters: A meta-analysis of randomized controlled trials. *Chest* 1998; 113:165–171.
109. Nader HB, Walenga JM, Berkowitz SD, et al. Preclinical differentiation of low molecular weight heparins. *Semin Thromb Hemost* 1999; 25(suppl 3):63–72.
110. Levine M, Gent M, Hirsh J, et al. A comparison of low molecular-weight-heparin administered primarily at home with unfractionated heparin administered in the hospital for proximal deep vein thrombosis. *N Engl J Med* 1996; 334:677–681.
111. Koopman MM, Prandoni P, Piovella F, et al. Low molecular-weight-heparin versus heparin for proximal deep vein thrombosis. *N Engl J Med* 1996; 334:682–687.
112. A Collaborative European Multicentre Study. A randomized trial of subcutaneous low-molecular-weight heparin (CY216) compared with intravenous unfractionated heparin in the treatment of deep vein thrombosis. *Thromb Haemostas* 1991; 65:251–256.
113. Hull RD, Raskob GE, Pineo GF, et al. Subcutaneous low molecular-weight heparin compared with continuous intravenous heparin in the treatment of proximal-vein thrombosis. *N Engl J Med* 1992; 326:975–983.
114. Prandoni P, Lensing AWA, Buller HR, et al. Comparison of subcutaneous low-molecular-weight heparin with intravenous standard heparin in proximal deep vein thrombosis. *Lancet* 1992; 339:441–445.
115. Simonneau G, Charbonnier B, Decousus H, et al. Subcutaneous low-molecular-weight heparin compared with continuous intravenous unfractionated heparin in the treatment of proximal deep vein thrombosis. *Arch Intern Med* 1993; 153:1541–1546.
116. Lindmarker P, Holmstrom M, Granqvist S, et al. Fragmin once daily subcutaneously in a fixed dose compared with continuous intravenous unfractionated heparin in the treatment of deep venous thrombosis. *Thromb Haemostas* 1993; 69:648.
117. Siragusa S, Cosmi B, Piovella F, et al. Low-molecular-weight heparins and unfractionated heparin in the treatment of patients with acute venous thromboembolism: Results of a meta-analysis. *Am J Med* 1996; 100:269–270.
118. Lensing AWA, Prins MH, Davidson BL, Hirsh J. Treatment of deep venous thrombosis with low-molecular-weight heparins: A meta-analysis. *Arch Intern Med* 1995; 155:601–607.

119. Leizorovicz A, Simonneau G, Decousus H, Boissel JP. Comparison of efficacy and safety of low molecular weight heparins and unfractionated heparin in initial treatment of deep venous thrombosis. *BMJ* 1994; 309:299–304.
120. O'Brien B, Levine M, Willan A, et al. Economic evaluation of outpatient treatment with low-molecular-weight heparin for proximal vein thrombosis. *Arch Intern Med* 1999; 159:2298–2304.
121. Kearon C, Gent M, Hirsh J, et al. A comparison of three months of anticoagulation with extended anticoagulation for a first episode of idiopathic venous thromboembolism. *N Engl J Med* 1999; 340:901–907.
122. The Global Use of Strategies to Open Occluded Coronary Arteries (GUSTO) IIB Investigators. A comparison of recombinant hirudin with heparin for the treatment of acute coronary syndromes. *N Engl J Med* 1996; 335:775–782.
123. Antman EM for the TIMI 9B Investigators. Hirudin in acute myocardial infarction: Thrombolysis and thrombin inhibition in MI (TIMI) 9B trial. *Circulation* 1996; 94:911–921.
124. Eriksson BI, Wille-Jorgensen P, Kalebo P, et al. A comparison of recombinant hirudin with a low-molecular-weight heparin to prevent thromboembolic complications after total hip replacement. *N Engl J Med* 1997; 337:1329–1335.
125. Gustafsson D, Elg M, Lenfors S, et al. Effects of inogatran, a new low molecular weight thrombin inhibitor, in rat models of venous and arterial thrombosis, thrombolysis and bleeding time. *Blood Coagul Fibrinolysis* 1996; 7:69–79.
126. Roux S, Tschopp T, Baumgartner HR. Effects of napsagatran, a new synthetic thrombin inhibitor and of heparin in a canine model of coronary artery thrombosis: Comparison with a ex vivo annular perfusion chamber model. *J Pharmacol Exp Ther* 1996; 277:71–78.
127. Valjii K, Arun K, Bookstein JJ. Use of a direct thrombin inhibitor (argatroban) during pulse-spray thrombolysis in experimental thrombosis. *J Vasc Intervent Radiol* 1995; 6:91–95.
128. Nicolini FA, Lee P, Malycky JL, et al. Selective inhibition of factor Xa during thrombolytic therapy markedly improves coronary artery patency in a canine model of coronary thrombosis. *Blood Coagul Fibrinolysis* 1996; 7:39–48.
129. Abildgaard U. Relative roles of tissue factor pathway inhibitor and antithrombin in the control of thrombogenesis. *Blood Coagul Fibrinolysis* 1995; 6(suppl 1):S45–S49.
130. Pineo GF, Hull RD. Thrombin inhibitors as anticoagulant agents. *Curr Opin Hematol* 1999; 6:298–303.
131. Kelton JG, Sheridan D, Santos A, et al. Heparin-associated thrombocytopenia: Laboratory studies. *Blood* 1988; 79:925–930.
132. Amiral J, Bridey F, Dreyfus M, et al. Platelet factor 4 complexed to heparin is the target for antibodies generated in heparin-induced thrombocytopenia. *Thromb Haemost* 1992; 68:95–96.
133. Visentin GP, Ford SE, Scott JP, Aster RH. Antibodies from patients with heparin-induced thrombocytopenia/thrombosis are specific for platelet factor 4 complexed with heparin or bound to endothelial cells. *J Clin Invest* 1994; 93:81–88.
134. Warkentin TE, Levine MN, Hirsh J, et al. Heparin-induced thrombocytopenia in patients treated with low-molecular-weight heparin or unfractionated heparin. *N Engl J Med* 1995; 332:1330–1335.
135. Warkentin TE. Heparin-induced thrombocytopenia: A ten-year retrospective. *Annu Rev Med* 1999; 50:129–147.
136. Greenfield LJ. Vena caval interruption and pulmonary embolectomy. *Clin Chest Med* 1984; 5:495–505.
137. Becker DM, Philbrick JT, Selby JB. Inferior vena cava filters: Indications, safety, effectiveness. *Arch Intern Med* 1992; 152: 1985–1994.
138. Hughes GC, Smith TP, Eachempati SR, et al. The use of a temporary vena caval interruption device in high-risk trauma patients unable to receive standard venous thromboembolism prophylaxis. *J Trauma* 1999; 46:246–249.
139. Johnson AJ, McCarthy WR. The lysis of artificially induced intravascular clots in man by intravenous infusion of streptokinase. *J Clin Invest* 1959; 38:1627–1643.
140. Miller GAH, Gibson RV, Sutton GC. Treatment of pulmonary embolism with streptokinase. *BMJ* 1969; 1:812–815.
141. Sasahara AA, Cannilla JE, Belks JJ, et al. Urokinase therapy in clinical pulmonary embolism. *N Engl J Med* 1969; 277:1168–1173.
142. NIH: Symposium: Thrombolytic therapy in thrombosis: A National Institutes of Health Consensus Development Conference. *Ann Intern Med* 1980; 93:141–143.
143. Goldhaber SZ, Kessler CM, Heit J, et al. A randomized controlled trial of recombinant tissue plasminogen activator versus urokinase in the treatment of acute pulmonary embolism. *Lancet* 1988; 2:293–298.
144. Witty LA, Steinfeld AD, Tapson VF. Thrombolytic therapy in acute pulmonary embolism: Physician attitudes. *Arch Intern Med* 1994; 154:1601–1604.
145. Goldhaber SZ. Evolving concepts in thrombolytic therapy for pulmonary embolism. *Chest* 1992; 101(suppl):183S–185S.
146. Goldhaber SZ, Haire WD, Feldstein ML, et al. Alteplase versus heparin in acute pulmonary embolism: Randomized trial assessing right ventricular function and pulmonary perfusion. *Lancet* 1993; 341:507–510.
147. Nass N, McConnell MV, Goldhaber SZ, et al. Recovery of regional right ventricular function after thrombolysis for pulmonary embolism. *Am J Cardiol* 1999; 83:804–806.
148. Leeper KV Jr, Popovich J Jr, Lesser BA, et al. Treatment of massive acute pulmonary embolism. The use of low doses of intrapulmonary arterial streptokinase combined with full doses of systemic heparin. *Chest* 1988; 93:234–240.
149. The UKEP study. Multicentre clinical trial on two local regimens of urokinase in massive pulmonary embolism. *Eur Heart J* 1987; 8:2–10.
150. Verstraete M, Miller GAH, Bounameaux H, et al. Intravenous and intrapulmonary recombinant tissue-type plasminogen activator in the treatment of acute massive pulmonary embolism. *Circulation* 1988; 77:353–360.
151. Rogers LQ, Lutcher CL. Streptokinase therapy for deep vein thrombosis: A comprehensive review of the literature. *Am J Med* 1990; 88:389–395.
152. Sane DC, Califf RM, Topol EJ, et al. Bleeding during thrombolytic therapy for acute myocardial infarction: Mechanisms and management. *Ann Intern Med* 1989; 111:1010–1022.
153. Gore JM. Prevention of severe neurologic events in the thrombolytic era. *Chest* 1992; 101:124S–130S.
154. Dalen JE, Alpert JS, Hirsh J. Thrombolytic therapy for pulmonary embolism. Is it safe? Is it effective? *Arch Intern Med* 1997; 157:2550–2556.
155. Tapson VF, Gurbel PA, Royster R, et al. Pharmacomechanical thrombolysis of experimental pulmonary emboli: Rapid low-dose intraembolic therapy. *Chest* 1994; 106:1558–1562.
156. Tapson VF, Davidson CJ, Bauman R, et al. Rapid thrombolysis of massive pulmonary emboli without systemic fibrinogenolysis: Intra-embolic infusion of thrombolytic therapy. *Am Rev Respir Dis* 1992; 145:A719.
157. Greenfield LJ, Kimmell GO, McCurdy WC. Transvenous removal of pulmonary emboli by vacuum-cup catheter technique. *J Surg Res* 1969; 9:347–352.
158. Timsit JF, Reynaud P, Meyer G, Sors H. Pulmonary embolectomy by catheter device in massive PE. *Chest* 1991; 100:655–658.
159. Semba CP, Dake MD. Iliofemoral deep venous thrombosis: Aggressive therapy with catheter-directed thrombolysis. *Radiology* 1994; 191:487–494.
160. Mewissen MW, Seabrook GR, Meissner MH, et al. Catheter-directed thrombolysis for lower extremity deep venous thrombosis: Report of a national multicenter registry. *Radiology* 1999; 211:39–49.

161. Gray HH, Morgan JM, Paneth M, Miller GAH. Pulmonary embolectomy: Indications and results. *Br Heart J* 1987; 57:572.
162. Tapson VF, Witty LA. Massive pulmonary embolism: Diagnostic and therapeutic strategies. *Clin Chest Med* 1996; 16:329.
163. Jardin F, Genevray B, Brun-ney D, Margairaz A. Dobutamine: a hemodynamic evaluation in pulmonary embolism shock. *Crit Care Med* 1985; 13:1009–1012.
164. Manier G, Castaing Y. Influence of cardiac output on oxygen exchange in acute pulmonary embolism. *Am Rev Respir Dis* 1992; 145:130–136.
165. Shure D. Chronic thromboembolic pulmonary hypertension: Diagnosis and treatment. *Semin Respir Crit Care Med* 1996; 17:7.
166. Fedullo PF, Auger WR, Channick RN, et al. Chronic thromboembolic pulmonary hypertension. *Clin Chest Med* 1995; 16: 353–374.

CHAPTER 54

CHRONIC COR PULMONALE

John H. Newman

DEFINITION

Cor pulmonale is a term that describes the pathologic effects of lung dysfunction on the right side of the heart. Pulmonary hypertension is the link between lung dysfunction and the heart in cor pulmonale. Cor pulmonale occurs as a late manifestation of many diseases of the lung, but the common thread in each case is increased right ventricular afterload. Cor pulmonale can be an elusive clinical diagnosis because pulmonary hypertension can exist without clinical manifestations and because clinical signs, such as dyspnea, may be shared with the underlying disease. Acute pulmonary hypertension leads to acute dilatation of the right ventricle; chronic pulmonary hypertension leads to ventricular hypertrophy followed by dilatation. The presence of overt right-sided heart failure is not essential to make the diagnosis of cor pulmonale, but right-sided heart failure is a common consequence. The clinical manifestations of cor pulmonale relate to alterations in cardiac output, salt and water homeostasis, and in most cases, gas exchange in the lung. Right-sided heart dysfunction secondary to left-sided heart failure, valvular dysfunction, or congenital heart disease is excluded in the definition of cor pulmonale.[1] Pulmonary venous obstruction is a cause of cor pulmonale; pulmonary venoocclusive disease is usually considered in the spectrum of primary pulmonary hypertension.

As a concept, cor pulmonale was introduced over 200 years ago, but the exact origin of the term is uncertain.[2] Osler[3] commented in the first edition of his textbook that "hypertrophy of the right ventricle . . . results from increased resistance in the pulmonary circulation, as in cirrhosis of the lung and emphysema." McGinn and White[4] apparently were the first to use the term *acute cor pulmonale* in the discussion of a case of acute, massive thromboembolism in 1935. William Harvey's discussion of the relationship of the lung and right side of the heart in *De Motu Cordis*[5] showed remarkable insight into the limitations of the right ventricle.

INCIDENCE, ETIOLOGIES, AND PATHOLOGY

Emphysema and chronic bronchitis cause over 50 percent of cases of cor pulmonale in the United States. The prevalence of cor pulmonale is difficult to determine because cor pulmonale does not occur in all cases of chronic lung disease and because routine physical examination and laboratory tests are relatively insensitive to the presence of pulmonary hypertension. The prevalence of chronic obstructive lung disease in the United States is about 15 million, directly resulting in approximately 70,000 deaths per year and contributing to about 160,000 other deaths.[6] It has been estimated that cor pulmonale accounts for 5 to 10 percent of organic heart disease. Cor pulmonale was present in 20 to 30 percent of admissions for heart failure in one study.[7] It is likely that cor pulmonale is a complication in a high percentage of cases. Gazes[8] found that 9.2 percent of cases of heart disease that came to autopsy had right heart abnormalities.

Chronic cor pulmonale occurs most frequently in adult male smokers, although the incidence in women is increasing as heavy smoking in females becomes more prevalent. A list of all diseases that may lead to cor pulmonale would be extensive and is not included in this chapter, but the major types of disease processes are listed in Table 54-1. Two important causes of cor pulmonale, thromboembolism and primary pulmonary hypertension, are discussed in Chaps. 52 and 53.

Chronic Obstructive Pulmonary Disease

Chronic obstructive pulmonary disease (COPD) causes cor pulmonale through several interrelated mechanisms, including hypoventilation, hypoxemia from ventilation-perfusion ($\dot{V}/\dot{Q}$) mismatch, and reduction of perfused surface area.[9,10] Patients with more prominent hypoxemia and alveolar hypoventilation develop erythrocytosis, edema, and early onset of cor pulmonale ("blue bloaters").[10] Patients in whom dyspnea on exertion is

TABLE 54-1 Etiologies of Chronic Cor Pulmonale by Mechanism of Pulmonary Hypertension

I. Hypoxic vasoconstriction
   A. Chronic bronchitis and emphysema, cystic fibrosis
   B. Chronic hypoventilation
      1. Obesity
      2. Sleep apnea
      3. Neuromuscular disease
      4. Chest wall dysfunction
   C. High-altitude dwelling and chronic mountain sickness (Monge's disease)
II. Occlusion of the pulmonary vascular bed
   A. Pulmonary thromboembolism, parasitic ova, tumor emboli
   B. Primary pulmonary hypertension
   C. Pulmonary venocclusive disease/pulmonary capillary hemangioma
   D. Sickle cell disease/sickle crisis/marrow embolism
   E. Fibrosing mediastinitis, mediastinal tumor
   F. Pulmonary angiitis from systemic disease
      1. Collagen vascular diseases
      2. Drug-induced lung disease
      3. Necrotizing and granulomatous arteritis
III. Parenchymal disease with loss of vascular surface area
   A. Bullous emphysema, alpha$_1$ antiproteinase deficiency, hyperinflation
   B. Diffuse bronchiectasis, cystic fibrosis
   C. Diffuse interstitial disease
      1. Pneumoconiosis
      2. Sarcoid, idiopathic pulmonary fibrosis, histiocytosis X
      3. Tuberculosis, chronic fungal infection
      4. Adult respiratory distress syndrome
      5. Collagen vascular disease (autoimmune lung disease)
      6. Hypersensitivity pneumonitis

the most prominent symptom have less hypoventilation and less hypoxemia at rest and therefore develop cor pulmonale later ("pink puffers"). Some of the differences between blue bloaters and pink puffers may relate to ventilatory drives; patients with low drives may be more likely to fit the blue-bloater category, whereas pink puffers strive to maintain normal arterial pH and gas tensions.[12] Another hypothesis is that blue bloaters have more inflammatory bronchitis and that pink puffers suffer more from pure emphysema.[10] *Physical examination* in advanced COPD shows an increase in the thoracic diameter, flattened diaphragms, hyperresonance to percussion, decreased breath sounds with expiratory wheezes, distant heart sounds, distended neck veins during expiration, and a palpable liver. Liver enlargement and leg edema are manifestations of fluid retention, and right-sided heart failure and may or may not be present. The *chest roentgenogram* may show characteristic changes of emphysema such as hyperlucent lungs, bullae, increased anteroposterior (AP) diameter, and flattened diaphragms. In some cases, increased bronchovascular markings and air bronchograms suggest the presence of thickened or inflamed airways. On the other hand, the chest roentgenogram may not show characteristic findings or be indicative of the severity of the physiologic impairment. Pulmonary function tests show an increased residual volume and total lung capacity, decreased forced vital capacity (FVC), and markedly decreased expiratory flow rates (FEV_1, FEF_{25-75}). Arterial blood studies at rest can be normal when disease is mild but in severe disease show decreased P_{O_2}, increased P_{CO_2}, and decreased pH. With cor pulmonale, P_{O_2} is likely to be below 55 mmHg. Desaturation increases with exercise and frequently during sleep. The $\dot{V}/\dot{Q}$ inequality and alveolar hypoventilation both contribute to the hypoxemia. A P_{CO_2} above 45 mmHg at rest defines net alveolar hypoventilation. Asthma is a form of COPD that rarely, if ever, leads to chronic cor pulmonale, probably because asthma is usually a disease of intermittent airways obstruction.

Cor pulmonale in COPD is related to the severity of lung dysfunction, and pulmonary hypertension is a manifestation of advanced disease. Exercise limitation in COPD is usually due to limitation of ventilatory capacity, not cardiac reserve, although sedentary patients develop deconditioning, which reduces exercise performance. No single test of lung function—such as spirometry, lung volumes, carbon monoxide diffusing capacity (DL_{CO}), blood gas tension, or radiography—is highly predictive of cor pulmonale because abnormalities such as reduced surface area and hypoxic vasoconstriction add independently to pulmonary artery pressure.[10]

Diffuse Interstitial Lung Disease

These patients have dyspnea, tachypnea, exercise intolerance, and occasionally clubbing of the digits. Basilar crackles are heard frequently on auscultation of the chest and may persist throughout inspiration. The *chest roentgenogram* shows diffuse reticular, reticulonodular, or fibrotic lesions, but the appearance does not always correlate well with physiologic impairment. In some disease presentations, such as desquamative interstitial pneumonitis, there may be an alveolar filling pattern with air bronchograms. A lung biopsy frequently is required to identify the basic pathologic process, and even then the exact etiology may not always be determined. Transbronchial biopsy can be diagnostic in some interstitial diseases such as sarcoidosis, and bronchoalveolar lavage may point to a diagnosis in many cases.[13] *Pulmonary function tests* show a restrictive process with reduced lung volumes, decreased compliance, and decreased diffusing capacity without airway obstruction. The vital capacity is reduced, and the forced expiratory volume in 1 s (FEV_1) as a percentage of FVC is usually at least 80 percent. At first, P_{O_2} decreases during exercise but is kept at normal levels at rest by hyperventilation. As the disease becomes more severe, P_{O_2} is low at rest. The course and prognosis of interstitial lung disease depend on the specific etiology, and there is wide variation among and within diseases.[13]

The presence of cor pulmonale in interstitial lung disease implies extensive lung dysfunction, perhaps with vascular involvement (as in systemic lupus erythematosus), and cor pulmonale may not occur even in end-stage disease. Treatment of idiopathic pulmonary fibrosis frequently is unsatisfactory despite the use of high-dose corticosteroids and either cyclophosphamide or azathiopirine. Recent trials using interferon-alpha with corticosteroids show promise of improved efficacy.[14]

Hypoventilation Syndromes

Some disorders (i.e., kyphoscoliosis) may impair or restrict mechanisms of ventilation, causing general alveolar hypoventilation and alveolar hypoxia.[15] Extreme obesity may be associated with hypoventilation, cyanosis, polycythemia, and somnolence (without intrinsic lung disease), often called the *pickwickian syndrome*.[16] Patients with daytime somnolence, morning headaches, and personality disturbances have been found to have periodic apnea during sleep associated with sleep deprivation, loud snoring, hypoxemia, and hypercapnia caused by upper airway obstruction (i.e., by the tongue, enlarged tonsils, or collapse of pharyngeal walls). Brainstem abnormalities such as Arnold-Chiari malformation also may cause respiratory center depression and primary hypoventilation. Neuromuscular diseases such as postpolio syndrome and chronic Guillain-Barré syndrome may present with cor pulmonale and right-sided heart failure.[17] Diagnosis of hypoventilation is confirmed by blood gas analysis, a depressed ventilatory response to inhaled CO_2, tests of pulmonary hypoventilation, or sleep studies. It has become apparent that disordered ventilation during sleep is a major component of many hypoventilation syndromes.[18] In all cases of hypoventilation, the main stimulus for pulmonary hypertension is hypoxic vasoconstriction, a response of the pulmonary arterioles to alveolar hypoxia. The respiratory acidosis that may accompany hypoventilation augments the vasoconstrictor response to hypoxia. Noninvasive assisted nocturnal ventilation with continuous positive airway pressure (CPAP), with or without added O_2 is the most efficacious therapy in most patients with nocturnal hypoventilation.[17]

Pulmonary Vascular Disease

Chronic cor pulmonale is a consequence of several diseases that involve the pulmonary vessels. Primary pulmonary hypertension and recurrent (or unresolved) pulmonary emboli are described in detail in Chaps. 59 and 60. Sickle cell disease, from SS or SC hemoglobinopathy, can cause cor pulmonale after multiple episodes of pulmonary infarction from focal pulmonary sickling, fat embolism, or thromboembolism.[18,19] Pulmonary venoocclusive disease is a rare disease of the pulmonary veins that presents with pulmonary hypertension and variable pulmonary infiltrates. It occasionally occurs in human immune deficiency virus (HIV) infection and after bone marrow transplantation.[20]

Cirrhosis of the liver is usually associated with pulmonary vasodilatation, but occasionally a disorder clinically and pathologically identical to primary pulmonary hypertension emerges.[21] HIV infection is a new cause of pulmonary vascular disease resembling primary pulmonary hypertension.[22] Collagen-vascular disease can cause cor pulmonale by primary vasculitis as well as by diffuse interstitial fibrosis. Systemic sclerosis, systemic lupus erythematosus (SLE), and rheumatoid arthritis (RA) are the collagen-vascular diseases that most commonly cause pulmonary arteritis. Patients with SLE and RA frequently present with primary interstitial lung disease. Occasionally, the presentation is that of cor pulmonale without interstitial disease but with primary pulmonary arteritis.[23] Cor pulmonale is not reported as a feature of Goodpasture's syndrome or idiopathic pulmonary hemosiderosis. Historically, dietary pulmonary hypertension has occurred as a result of the use of Aminorex in Europe, contaminated canola oil in Spain, and in eosinophilia myalgia syndrome in the United States related to contaminated tryptophan.[24] The new anorectic drug dexfenfluramine has caused pulmonary hypertension in France and recently has been banned in the United States by the Food and Drug Administration (FDA) because of its association with primary pulmonary hypertension and perhaps valvular dysfunction.[25]

PATHOPHYSIOLOGY

Increased pulmonary vascular resistance (PVR) and pulmonary hypertension are central mechanisms in all cases of cor pulmonale.[10] Physiologic mechanisms of pulmonary arterial pressure are shown in Table 54-2. These variables can be described in part by Poiseuille's law. Fortunately, most pulmonary diseases and disorders do not produce enough pulmonary hypertension to cause cor pulmonale.

Normal Pulmonary Circulation

The primary function of this unique high-flow, low-pressure, low-resistance system is to provide blood for gas exchange, and it is ideally structured for this function. It receives and transmits the entire cardiac output at low hydrostatic pressures primarily because of three characteristics: (1) the pulmonary arteries are thin-walled with little resting muscular tone, (2) there is negligible vasomotor control by the autonomic nervous system at rest in the adult, and (3) many small arterioles and alveolar capillaries produce a high surface area that can be recruited when needed to expand the pulmonary vascular bed, resulting in a decreased PVR. Normal mean pulmonary artery pressure (PAP) is about 12 to 17 mmHg; PAP above 20 mmHg at rest

TABLE 54-2 Genesis of Pulmonary Vascular Pressure: Poiseuille's Law

$$\text{Ppa} = \text{CO}\left(\frac{8}{\pi} \times n \times \frac{1}{N} \times \frac{1}{r^4}\right) + \text{Pla}$$

Flow = cardiac output (usually ↑ elevated in COPD; if PRV is fixed. ↑ CO will ↑ PAP).

$\frac{8}{\pi}$ = numerical constant related to tubular structure of vessels.

n = blood viscosity (increased in polycythemia vera, secondary erythrocytosis, and cryoglobulinemia).

N = number of perfused vessels of a particular radius. N is decreased in any occlusive or destructive disease (see Table 61-1). N for pulmonary capillaries is >200 million.

$\frac{1}{r^4}$ = radius of a vessel is a critical determinant of flow (r is decreased by vasoconstriction, luminal obstruction, or hyperinflation. A change in r from 1 to 2 units changes resistance 16-fold).

Pla = left atrial pressure. Passive pulmonary hypertension can result from left atrial pressure elevation due to either LV or valvular disease.

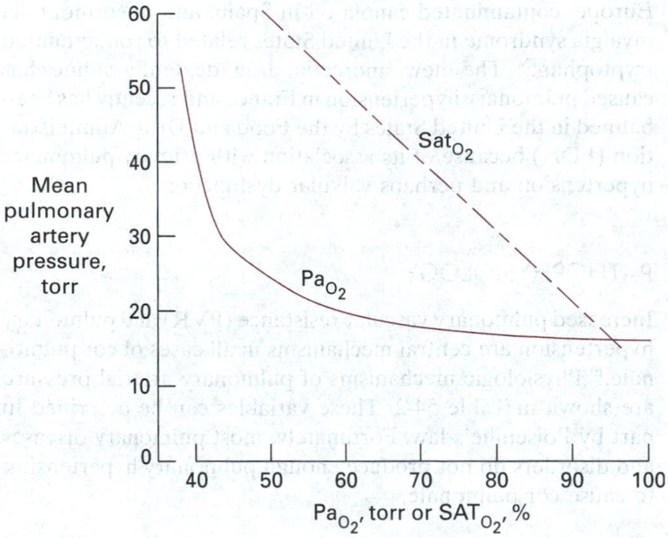

FIGURE 54-1 Pulmonary arterial pressure as a function of Pa_{O_2} or oxyhemoglobin saturation in humans. Pulmonary arterial pressure rises sharply as Pa_{O_2} decreases below 55 mmHg. (Redrawn from Reeves JT, Grover RF. High altitude pulmonary hypertension and pulmonary edema. *Prog Cardiol* 1975; 4:105, and from Burrows B. Anaerobic infections of the lung and pleural space. *Am Rev Respir Dis* 1974; 110:64, with permission.)

suggests pulmonary hypertension. Flow of blood from the main pulmonary artery (PA) through the pulmonary capillaries to the left atrium is accomplished by a pressure drop of only 5 to 9 mmHg, compared with an arterial-to-venous gradient of 90 mmHg in the systemic circuit. Thus normal PVR is 10- to 20-fold less than systemic vascular resistance.

Pulmonary Hypertension

The effective cross-sectional area of the pulmonary vascular bed must be reduced by 25 to 50 percent before any change in PAP can be detected at rest. Exercise causes increased PAP because of increased pulmonary blood flow in the normal bed, and exercise will dramatically raise PAP if the vascular bed is reduced. Obliterative vascular diseases increase PVR by vascular luminal occlusion, whereas diffuse interstitial diseases act primarily by compression and obliteration of small vessels. Hyperinflation in COPD increases PVR partly by compressing intraalveolar vessels, reducing the cross-sectional area of the bed. It is now well established, however, that arteriolar constriction resulting from alveolar hypoxia is the predominant cause of pulmonary hypertension in chronic airways diseases.[1,10,26,27]

PULMONARY ARTERIOLAR CONSTRICTION

The most important cause of pulmonary vasoconstriction is alveolar hypoxia. The mechanism of hypoxic pulmonary vasoconstriction is unknown. It is thought to be due either to mediator release from some unknown effector cell or a direct action of hypoxia on pulmonary vascular smooth muscle K channels.[28,29] The degree of hypoxic vasoconstriction depends primarily on the alveolar P_{O_2}, and when alveolar P_{O_2} is less than 55 mmHg, PAP rises sharply (Fig. 54-1). When PAP is greater than 40 mmHg due to hypoxia, arterial oxygen saturation is very likely less than 75 percent.[26] There is large individual variability in the hypoxic pressor response, and hypoxic vasoconstriction is enhanced by acidosis and blunted by alkalosis. Acidosis also has a mild direct pressor effect on the pulmonary circulation.[28] Extensive investigations into the mechanism of hypoxic vasoconstriction have shown that many local and circulating mediators of pulmonary vascular tone are capable of modulating the hypoxic pressor response but that no single mediator yet discovered is solely or predominantly responsible[28] (Table 54-3).

Hypoxic vasoconstriction in a region of lung where ventilation is diminished probably serves to maximize net arterial oxygenation by diverting blood from the hypoxic region to better-ventilated areas. Because the pulmonary vascular bed is capable of significant recruitment, localized hypoxic vasoconstriction does not cause pulmonary hypertension. Generalized hypoxia causes generalized hypoxic vasoconstriction and the development of pulmonary hypertension (Fig. 54-2). In COPD, the first episodes of alveolar hypoxia may occur during sleep, and it gradually becomes more prevalent thereafter.[30] Any cause of alveolar hypoventilation (see Table 54-1) can result in chronic cor pulmonale through the mechanism of hypoxic pulmonary vasoconstriction, including entities as different as diffuse emphysema and kyphoscoliosis[9,15] (see also Chap. 59).

OTHER CONTRIBUTIONS TO PULMONARY HYPERTENSION

Increases in cardiac output and blood volume or direct effects of acidosis and/or hypoxia on the myocardium may contribute to pulmonary hypertension. Increased blood flow such as occurs with exercise engenders an increased PAP, and in such a situation, the effects of hypoxia and acidosis also will be exaggerated.[26] Sustained or repetitive severe hypoxemia causes secondary erythrocytosis. Blood viscosity increases rapidly after the hematocrit exceeds about 55 percent, raising PVR and also decreasing cerebral function. If left ventricular failure (LVF) is superimposed on an already reduced pulmonary vascular bed, pulmonary hypertension will be augmented by elevated downstream left atrial pressure. Once established, pulmonary hypertension may be self-perpetuating. A sustained increase in PAP in patients with diffuse lung disease causes muscular hypertrophy in the walls of small arteries, with extension of muscle toward alveolar vessels, further increasing PVR and

TABLE 54-3 Endogenous Pulmonary Vasomotor Tone

Dilator	Constrictor
Beta-adrenergic	Alpha-adrenergic agonists
Histamine H_2	Histamine H_1
Prostacyclin (PGI_2), PGE_1	PGE_2, PGF_{1a}, Thromboxane A_2PGD_2
Acetylcholine*	Serotonin
Oxygen	Hypoxia
Bradykinin	Angiotensin II
Vasoactive intestinal polypeptide	Platelet activating factor
	Endothelin
Nitric oxide	Leukotriene C_4/D_4
Atrial natriuretic peptide	Vasopressin
Adenosine	

*The response of the pulmonary vascular bed is tone-dependent. When the pulmonary circulation is preconstricted, acetylcholine is a vasodilator through the release of endothelium-derived NO.

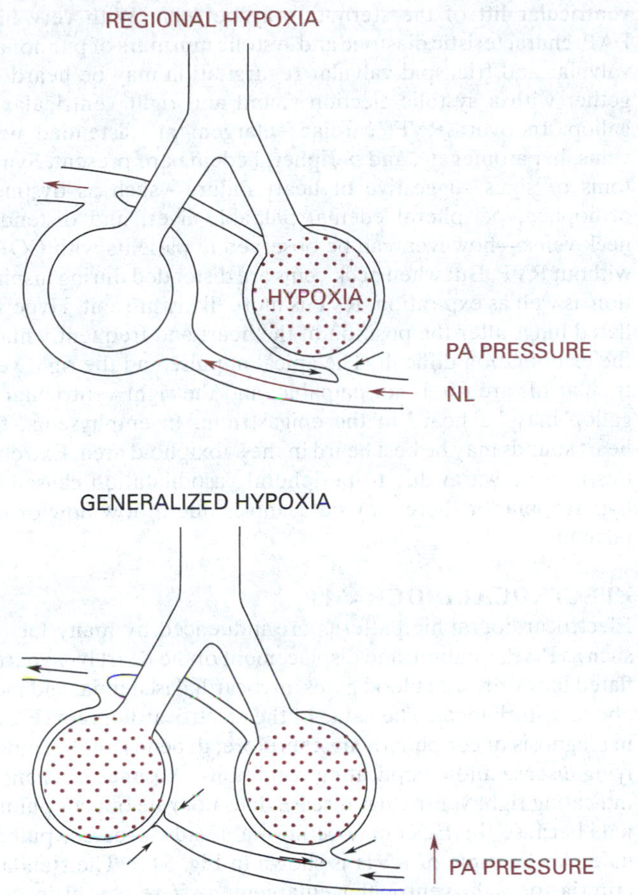

FIGURE 54-2 Hypoxic pulmonary vasoconstriction maximizes arterial oxygenation by diverting blood away from areas of regional hypoxia toward better-ventilated zones. Generalized hypoxia causes generalized hypoxic vasoconstriction and results in pulmonary hypertension. (From Newman JH. Pulmonary vascular reactivity in primary pulmonary edema. *Semin Respir Med* 1983; 4:299; reproduced with permission of the publisher. Courtesy of J. V. Weil.)

PAP. Chronic hypoxia alone results in muscularization of pulmonary arterioles and exaggerated increases in PAP with stimuli.[26,31]

Right Ventricular Response to Pulmonary Hypertension

The right ventricle is thin-walled and eccentric and better able to handle an increase in volume load than to meet an increased pressure load.[10] The primary cause of right ventricular strain and failure (RVF), therefore, is a chronic pressure load (afterload). Small increases in PAP may result in large increases in right ventricular work. Pulmonary hypertension at rest indicates a high baseline resistance, and small changes in blood flow will cause large increases in PAP.

Response of the right ventricle to pulmonary hypertension depends on the acuteness and severity of the pressure load. Acute cor pulmonale (see Chaps. 59 and 60) occurs after a sudden and severe stimulus (i.e., massive pulmonary emboli) with ventricular dilatation and failure but without hypertrophy. Acute cor pulmonale may develop within minutes to hours. Chronic cor pulmonale, however, is associated with a more slowly evolving and slowly progressive hypertension,[33] and the response involves increased protein synthesis and right ventricular hypertrophy (RVH).[34] The severity of the hypertension, the rapidity with which it becomes severe, and the possible eventual onset of RVF are influenced by factors that intercede intermittently, such as (1) *alterations in ventilatory function,* causing alveolar pressure changes with effects on chamber function, (2) *alterations in gas exchange,* with more or less severe hypoxemia, hypercapnia, and acidosis, and (3) *alterations in volume load,* as influenced by exercise, heart rate, polycythemia, or renal retention of salt and water associated with cor pulmonale. At some stage, the myocardium is unable to function at the high-pressure load, dilates, and fails. RVF may occur relatively early in some patients with chronic bronchitis and emphysema because of sustained hypoxemia and hypercarbia, but it occurs later in patients with diffuse interstitial lung disease because the degree of RVH helps to maintain blood flow even when PAP is high.[33] Extreme pulmonary hypertension and RVH can occur in normal persons living at high altitude (>10,000 ft, or 3033 m) with no evidence for heart failure.[34] Thus the right ventricle can develop into an efficient high-pressure pump over time and sustain normal function for months to years.

Left Ventricular Function in Cor Pulmonale

Dysfunction of the left ventricle occurs in some patients with cor pulmonale, but the evidence available indicates that cor pulmonale per se does not cause disease of the left side of the heart. The likelihood in most cases is that left-sided heart dysfunction coexisting with cor pulmonale results from other known causes, such as coronary ischemia or systemic hypertension. Left ventricular failure is a serious complication in cor pulmonale because the increase in left atrial pressure and in lung water further impairs lung function, increases the work of breathing, increases PAP, impairs gas exchange, and may induce respiratory failure. When underlying disease of the left ventricle is present, the direct effects of hypoxia, hypercapnia, and acidosis arising from primary lung disease may precipitate left ventricular failure.[10,35,36]

Several lines of evidence point to mechanical effects of lung dysfunction and right ventricular dilatation on performance of the left ventricle.[36,37] Wide swings in transpulmonary pressure in obstructive lung disease can reduce left ventricular filling and increase left ventricular afterload.[38] Hypertrophy and elevated end-diastolic pressure of the right ventricle in cor pulmonale can reduce left ventricular compliance and impair left ventricular filling through effects on the shared ventricular septum.[39] Despite these effects, most patients with chronic cor pulmonale demonstrate normal resting cardiac output, normal pulmonary artery wedge pressure, and normal resting left ventricular ejection fraction.[40] The majority of patients with abnormal left ventricular ejection fraction in either compensated or decompensated chronic lung disease probably have demonstrable coronary artery disease.

Edema Formation and Cor Pulmonale

Peripheral edema occurs in some cases of chronic cor pulmonale. The mechanism of edema formation is poorly understood but is probably related to increased systemic venous pressure, hypercarbia, and hypoxemia.[10,41] The presence of pulmonary hypertension per se does not appear to be sufficient to cause fluid retention until right atrial pressure becomes elevated. Decreased clearance of aldosterone from the passively congested liver contributes to salt retention but is likely not an initiating event. Plasma volume is increased, however, in chronic cor pulmonale.[10]

Hypercarbia stimulates plasma renin activity, and hypercarbic, edematous patients with COPD have increased plasma levels of aldosterone and antidiuretic hormone.[42,43] This pattern occurs despite oxygen therapy in these patients. Thus not only increased salt retention but also impaired water excretion contributes to edema in chronic hypercapnia. Atrial natriuretic peptide is elevated in cor pulmonale in response to elevated right atrial pressure and perhaps acidosis.[10] Severe hypoxemia is associated with reduced renal blood flow and glomerular filtration rate and a decrease in urine sodium excretion.[10] Other mechanisms of edema formation are increased systemic capillary hydrostatic pressure, related to increased venous pressure and blood volume; and perhaps inappropriate release of arginine vasopressin.[10] Many mechanisms appear to be operating to produce edema in chronic cor pulmonale, several of which are related to the primary pulmonary dysfunction, especially in COPD. The exact mechanisms and sequence of events leading to edema are difficult to determine in any specific case. Pulmonary edema and pleural effusion are not seen as a consequence of chronic cor pulmonale.

CLINICAL MANIFESTATIONS OF COR PULMONALE

Symptoms

Clinical manifestations of cor pulmonale are often obscured by the signs and symptoms of underlying disease and therefore are closely related to the pulmonary disease or disorder. It is necessary first to recognize the type and severity of lung disease and then to look for cor pulmonale.

There is no history that is specific for cor pulmonale. Episodes of leg edema, atypical chest pain, dyspnea on exertion, exercise-induced peripheral cyanosis, prior respiratory failure, and excessive daytime somnolence are all historical clues suggesting the presence of cor pulmonale. Chest pain may be due to strain or distortion of the chest wall (musculoskeletal) or may be related to right ventricular ischemia. Cough and complaints of easy fatigability are common. Some patients with nocturnal hypoventilation and sleep apnea may present with personality changes, mild systemic hypertension, and headache. Shortness of breath is nearly a universal symptom in cor pulmonale. The degree of activity that leads to dyspnea should be quantified because patients reduce activities to avoid dyspnea. Thus the naive question of whether a patient is short of breath may lead to a negative reply because the patient is less and less active. Abdominal pain may result from liver and bowel congestion if RVF is present.

Physical Examination

The earliest signs are those associated with long-standing pulmonary hypertension. The most sensitive sign for pulmonary hypertension is an accentuated pulmonary component of S_2, which also may be palpable in the pulmonic area, and right ventricular lift of the sternum may be seen. With very high PAP, characteristic diastolic and systolic murmurs of pulmonary valvular and tricuspid valvular regurgitation may be heard together with a systolic ejection sound and right ventricular S_3 gallop. In overt RVF, cardiac enlargement, distended neck veins, hepatomegaly, and peripheral edema are present. Symptoms or signs suggestive of heart failure—such as dyspnea, orthopnea, peripheral edema, palpable liver, and distended neck veins—however, can be observed in patients with COPD without RVF. But when neck veins are distended during inspiration as well as expiration, RVF is more likely present. Hyperinflated lungs alter the position of the heart and frequently make the examination difficult. The apical impulse and the right ventricular lift are often not palpable, and the right ventricular S_3 gallop may be heard in the epigastrium. In emphysema, the heart sounds may be best heard in the subxiphoid area. Extremities may be warm due to peripheral vasodilatation caused by hypercapnia, or there may be cyanosis due to low flow or hypoxemia.

ELECTROCARDIOGRAM

Electrocardiographic patterns are influenced by many factors such as PAP, rotation, and displacement of the heart by hyperinflated lungs, arterial blood gases, myocardial ischemia, and metabolic disturbances. The value of the electrocardiogram (ECG) in diagnosis of cor pulmonale, therefore, depends on the underlying disease and complicating conditions. Absence of changes indicating right ventricular disease does not rule out cor pulmonale because the ECG may be normal in advanced cor pulmonale. An example of RVH is shown in Fig. 54-3. The standard criteria for right ventricular enlargement were absent in two-thirds of patients with COPD who had RVH on postmortem examination.[1] It has been suggested that when classic RVH changes are absent, diagnosis should be based on the combination of rS in V_5 to V_6, RAD, qR in aV_R, and P pulmonale.[44] Tall peaked P waves in leads II and aV_F may reflect positional changes rather than right atrial enlargement. Right bundle-branch block occurs in about 15 percent of patients. A pattern of S_1, Q_3, and T_3 carries reasonable sensitivity and specificity for cor pulmonale in COPD.[45] Arrhythmias are infrequent in uncomplicated cor pulmonale, but when present, they are mostly supraventricular and may reflect blood gas abnormalities, hypokalemia, or excess of drugs such as digitalis, theophylline, and beta agonists. Multifocal atrial tachycardia is associated with decompensated COPD and is best treated by attention to the underlying disease rather than by antiarrhythmic drugs. Ventricular arrhythmias, when they occur, are associated with a high mortality.

CHEST ROENTGENOGRAM

The radiographic findings of pulmonary hypertension in patients with normal lung parenchyma (such as in primary pulmonary hypertension) are well described[46,47] (Fig. 54-4). Most diseases that cause cor pulmonale have grossly abnormal chest roentgenograms, and the radiologic diagnosis of pulmonary hypertension in these diseases is more difficult. Right ventricular enlargement may be difficult to detect in the vertical heart of emphysema, and comparison with previous films may be helpful. In the most obvious cases of cor pulmonale, there is right ventricular and PA enlargement, but pulmonary hypertension precedes right ventricular dilatation. One indicator of pulmonary hypertension is measurement of the dimensions of the right and left PAs. Enlargement is considered to exist if the diameter of the right descending PA is greater than 16 mm and the left descending PA is greater than 18 mm.[48] These findings occurred in 43 of 46 patients with known pulmonary hypertension, but the true sensitivity and specificity of these measurements are not known.

ECHOCARDIOGRAM

Advances in echocardiography make this a useful test where cor pulmonale is suspected.[49] The standard M mode reliably detects right ventricular dilatation and is best able to display the anteriormost right ventricular wall near the interventricular septum. Two-dimensional echocardiography allows improved visualization of right ventricular chamber size and wall thickness, as well as changes in the interventricular septum resulting from RVH.[49,50] Because the right ventricle is asymmetric, measurement of right ventricular volume is difficult even with two-dimensional views. Right ventricular pressure overload usually is detected by hypertrophy of the anterior right ventricular wall and by dilatation of the chamber. Hypertrophy of the septum can be found, and paradoxical septal encroachment into the left ventricular chamber can be seen in severe cor pulmonale.[53] Right ventricular volume overload, as in atrial septal defect, causes dilatation as the predominant finding, often in association with abnormal ventricular septal motion.[51]

Echo-Doppler techniques have become the noninvasive standard to detect pulmonary hypertension and to measure cardiac output. These techniques are relatively accurate when PAP is above 30 mmHg, but they may not detect milder but pathologic pulmonary hypertension.[52–53] Echo Doppler is useful for longitudinal follow-up of pharmacologic treatment of pulmonary hypertension and cor pulmonale.

RIGHT-SIDED HEART CATHETERIZATION

Right-sided catheterization is the only technique available for the direct measurement of PAP, PA wedge pressure, and cardiac output. It is occasionally important in differentiating cor pulmonale from left ventricular dysfunction when the clinical presentation is confusing. This is especially true in patients with primary pulmonary hypertension (PPH) or unresolved pulmonary emboli, where airway function may appear normal, or with restrictive cardiomyopathy (see Chap. 75). In cor pulmonale, PA diastolic pressure is usually significantly higher than wedge pressure, unlike LVF or mitral stenosis, where the diastolic–wedge pressure gradient is smaller in most patients. Mean PAP

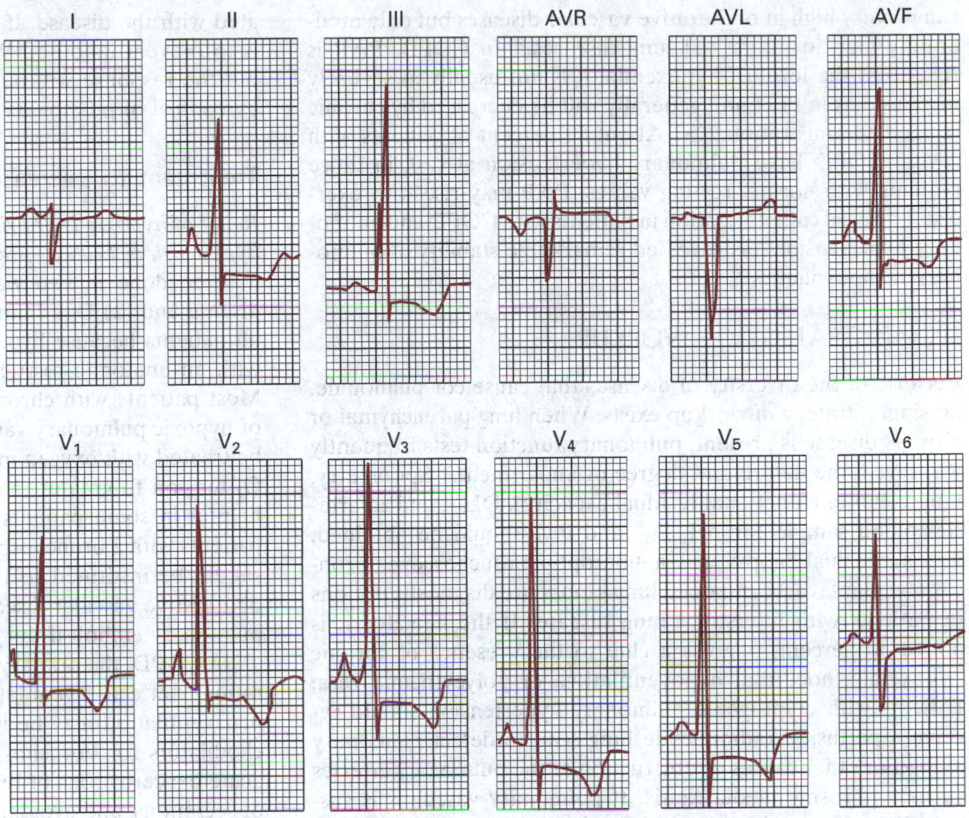

FIGURE 54-3 Electrocardiogram in a patient with cor pulmonale. The mean QRS axis is +120°. The tall, peaked P waves indicate right atrial enlargement. The tall R waves in leads V_1 to V_3 and deep S wave in V_6 and the associated T-wave changes indicate RVH. (From Voelkel NF, Reeves JT. Primary pulmonary hypertension. In: Moser KM, ed. *Pulmonary Vascular Diseases*. New York: Marcel Dekker; 1979; reproduced with permission of the publisher and the author. Courtesy of J. R. Pryor.)

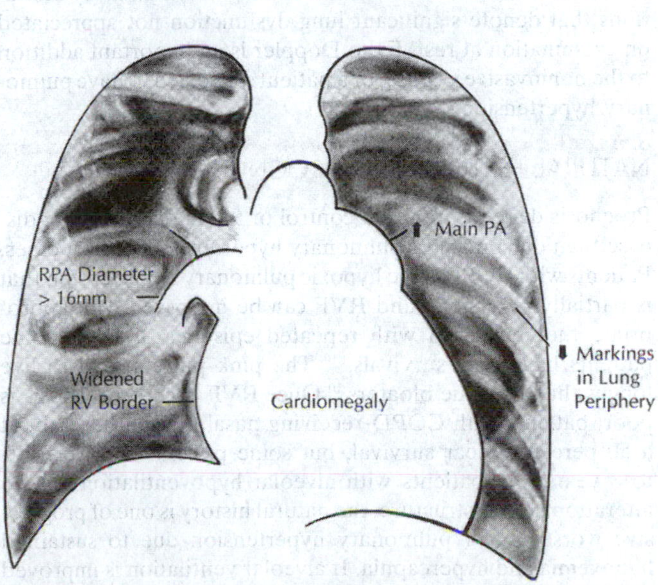

FIGURE 54-4 Classic features of the chest radiograph in severe pulmonary hypertension. The enlarged pulmonary arteries can be mistaken for hilar adenopathy, and the large main pulmonary artery obscures the aortic arch. Right descending PA diameter greater than 16 mm suggests severe pulmonary hypertension.

can be very high in obliterative vascular diseases but only moderately high in interstitial lung diseases.[36] In COPD, PAP is related to the level of hypoxemia; it is not usually as severely increased as in PPH and generally will be decreased by chronic oxygen administration.[26,54,55] About 50 percent of patients with severe COPD have pulmonary hypertension at rest; in those patients with normal resting values, PAP may rise with exercise.[10,54] Serial catheterization in patients with COPD and pulmonary hypertension has revealed remarkable stability of pulmonary hemodynamics.[56]

USUAL STRATEGY OF WORKUP

Because of the diversity of diseases that cause cor pulmonale, no single strategy of workup exists. When lung parenchymal or airways disease is present, pulmonary function tests frequently will reveal the nature and degree of impairment.[57] Spirometry, lung volumes (functional residual capacity), DL_{CO}, and an arterial blood sample for pH, P_{O_2}, and P_{CO_2} should be obtained. Transbronchial biopsy via a fiberoptic bronchoscope, bronchoalveolar lavage, and open lung biopsy are diagnostic options in patients with interstitial lung disease. If the hematocrit is above 50 percent, it gives a clue to the presence of chronic hypoxemia, nocturnal hypoventilation, or polycythemia vera. Patients with cryptogenic pulmonary hypertension should receive a perfusion radionuclide lung scan to detect pulmonary emboli or other causes of obstruction of the pulmonary arteries such as fibrosing mediastinitis. If pulmonary vasculitis is suspected, serum can be screened for the presence of antinuclear antibody, hepatitis B surface antigen, rheumatoid factor, and cryoglobulins. Factor V_{Leiden} is likely to be a frequent abnormality in thrombotic pulmonary hypertension,[58] and the antiphospholipid antibody syndrome may cause cor pulmonale.[59]

Polysomnography should be performed in patients with cor pulmonale and any sign or symptoms of sleep apnea. Exercise tests occasionally will reveal desaturation or ventilatory limitations that denote significant lung dysfunction not appreciated on examination at rest. Echo Doppler is an important addition to the noninvasive workup of a patient suspected to have pulmonary hypertension.

NATURAL HISTORY AND PROGNOSIS

Prognosis depends more on control of the underlying lung disease than on control of pulmonary hypertension in most cases. Patients with COPD have hypoxic pulmonary hypertension that is partially reversible, and RVF can be improved with appropriate therapy. Even with repeated episodes of RVF, some patients have long survivals.[1,10] The pink puffers tend to live longer than the blue bloaters.[10] Once RVF occurs, prognosis is poor; patients with COPD receiving nasal oxygen have about a 50 percent 2-year survival, but some patients survive for 5 to 8 years.[27] In patients with alveolar hypoventilation but no alteration in lung structure, the natural history is one of progressive worsening of pulmonary hypertension due to sustained hypoxemia and hypercapnia. If alveolar ventilation is improved prior to the development of nonreversible changes in vessel walls, the prognosis is good.

MEDICAL TREATMENT

The underlying lung disease is the focus of therapy and is the best way to reduce the right ventricular pressure work associated with the disease. If RVF has not appeared, a major goal is to prevent its onset. When it appears, it should be treated, but the response will be poor unless cardiac work is reduced by control of pulmonary hypertension.

Treatment to Decrease Pulmonary Hypertension

Relief of hypoxia is of prime importance in reducing pulmonary hypertension, both to prevent and to treat cor pulmonale. This may be done in two ways: (1) treatment of the underlying disease and (2) O_2 administration.[55] Neither will lower PAP in all patients because hypertension is often intractable in those with an anatomic restriction of the pulmonary vascular bed. Most patients with chronic cor pulmonale have a component of hypoxic pulmonary vasoconstriction, and all patients should be treated with oxygen in amounts adequate to restore arterial O_2 tension to greater than 60 mmHg. Corticosteroids may be helpful in some patients with interstitial lung disease and in patients with a bronchospastic component of COPD. Measures should be instituted to treat the systemic disease with which obliterative vascular disease is associated or to prevent further pulmonary emboli if this is the problem.

In COPD, the primary focus is relief of hypoxemia by restoration of effective ventilation or by O_2 administration. Net alveolar ventilation may be improved by therapy, including bronchodilators for bronchospasm, antibiotics to prevent or treat acute exacerbations of bronchitis, bronchial toilet for removal of secretions, and avoidance of airway irritants such as tobacco smoke. Nocturnal aspiration of gastric fluid is now known to be a common cause of exacerbation of chronic lung disease. Tranquilizers, sedatives, and narcotics should be avoided in unstable patients and patients with hypoventilation. Correction of hypoxia and acidosis may produce a striking reduction in PAP. In diseases that alter lung function but not structure, effective alveolar ventilation must be restored by treatment of the underlying disease or by use of mechanical ventilation. Short-term ventilatory stimulants may be useful in some cases of decreased ventilatory drives, although nasal CPAP has become the first choice in most cases of sleep apnea.[10]

Adequate oxygenation may prevent the onset of heart failure, both acutely and over a long period of time. Any patient with cor pulmonale and RVF should be given sufficient O_2 to restore P_{O_2} to levels above 60 mmHg, but it should be given cautiously when P_{CO_2} is high and the threat of respiratory acidosis is present. Oxygen therapy is usually well tolerated in patients with stable lung disease but not in patients with acute acidosis or respiratory muscle fatigue. When low-flow nasal O_2 causes significant increases in P_{CO_2}, mechanical ventilation may be required to relieve hypoxia. Studies have shown conclusively that home oxygen therapy, nocturnal or continuous, is beneficial in keeping patients with severe COPD functioning better for longer periods of time; it may be effective both in treating cor pulmonale and in postponing its onset.[27,55] Continuous 24 h/day oxygen therapy is the desired goal in most patients, because desaturation occurs during both sleep and physical activity.

Treatment of Heart Failure

Cor pulmonale is heart disease, and while treatment of the lung disease and relief of hypoxia are necessary to reduce cardiac work, general principles of management of heart failure apply. Diuretics and phlebotomy can be appropriate measures for treatment of RVF. Pulmonary vasodilators are efficacious in some patients with primary pulmonary hypertension but are of unproven value in cor pulmonale from COPD.[61]

Beneficial effects of digitalis are not as obvious as in LVF, and arrhythmias caused by digitalis may occur at relatively low serum levels in patients with hypoxia and acidosis. Susceptibility to digitalis intoxication is enhanced in pulmonary disease.[62] Its use in cor pulmonale therefore has been controversial. Nevertheless, studies have shown that *digitalis improves right ventricular function in cor pulmonale, and it is an appropriate drug for treatment of RVF when given cautiously and at carefully controlled dosage levels.*[63] It should not be used during the acute phases of respiratory insufficiency when there are large fluctuations in levels of hypoxemia and acidosis but is reserved for the time when the patient is stabilized. Heart rate in this setting cannot be used as a guide for the level of digitalization. It is also reasonable to question whether or not patients with cor pulmonale who continue to have overt RVF after relief of hypoxemia in intensive therapy for the underlying lung disease will benefit from the use of digitalis. Digitalis is appropriate if there is known or suspected concurrent left ventricular systolic dysfunction.

Vasodilator therapy to reduce right ventricular afterload has been recognized as a potential treatment strategy for several years. Vasodilator therapy has the disadvantage of being secondary therapy that is not aimed at the primary lung dysfunction. Vasodilator use has not become widespread because of small observed reductions in pulmonary hypertension and occasional worsening of gas exchange.[61]

Diuretics are effective in the treatment of RVF, and indications for their use are the same as in other forms of heart disease. Pulmonary function is improved by diuretics in patients with COPD who have hypervolemia.[64] The effects of diuretics should be monitored carefully by measurement of arterial P_{O_2}, P_{CO_2}, and pH because acid-base abnormalities are often present in cor pulmonale. Contraction alkalosis can be a problem in hypercarbic patients with a large buffer base who have had vigorous diuresis.

When the hematocrit is above 55 to 60 percent, phlebotomy may reduce PAP and PVR and possibly improve right ventricular function.[65] The phlebotomy should be in small volumes (200–300 mL) and done cautiously.

SURGICAL TREATMENT

There is no surgical treatment for most diseases that cause chronic cor pulmonale. Pulmonary embolectomy is extremely efficacious for unresolved pulmonary emboli causing chronic thrombotic pulmonary hypertension (see Chap. 60). Adenoidectomy in children with chronic airways obstruction and uvulopalatopharyngcoplasty in selected patients with sleep apnea can relieve cor pulmonale related to hypoventilation. Single-lung, double-lung, and heart-lung transplantations are all used for salvage in the terminal phase of several diseases complicated by cor pulmonale.[66] *The diseases most commonly treated by lung transplantation are primary pulmonary hypertension, emphysema, idiopathic pulmonary fibrosis, and cystic fibrosis.* Two-year survival for single- and double-lung transplant has risen to 60 percent, still lower than the approximately 80 percent for heart transplant alone. One interesting finding is that the right ventricle can recover function after lung transplant even after the chronic stress of severe pulmonary hypertension. Volume-reduction surgery for selected patients with emphysema improves ventilatory function and gas exchange, and the long-term benefit of this approach is under study.[67]

References

1. Palevsky HI, Fishman AP. Chronic cor pulmonale. *JAMA* 1990; 263:2347–2354.
2. Richards DW. The right heart and the lung with some observations on teleology: The J. Burns Amberson Lecture. *Am Rev Respir Dis* 1966; 94:691–702.
3. Osler W. *The Principles and Practice of Medicine.* New York: Appleton; 1892:628–640.
4. McGinn S, White PD. Acute cor pulmonale resulting from pulmonary embolism, its clinical recognition. *JAMA* 1935; 104:1473–1480.
5. Harvey W. *Exercitatio de Motu Cordis et Sanguinis in Animalibus.* Francofurti: Guilielem Fitzeri; 1628 (Leake CD, transl). Springfield, IL: Charles C Thomas; 1928.
6. Standards for the diagnosis and care of patients with chronic obstructive pulmonary disease: ATS statement. *Am J Respir Crit Care Med* 1995; 152(55):S77–S120.
7. A report of the Surgeon General. *Chronic Obstructive Lung Disease: The Health Consequences of Smoking.* Rockville, MD: U.S. Department of Health and Human Services; 1984:189.
8. Gazes PC. *Clinical Cardiology: A Bedside Approach.* Philadelphia: Lea & Febiger; 1990:301–320.
9. Thurlbeck WM. Pathophysiology of chronic obstructive pulmonary disease. *Clin Chest Med* 1990; 11:389–403.
10. MacNee W. Pathophysiology of cor pulmonale in chronic obstructive pulmonary disease. State of the art. *Am J Pulm Crit Care Med* 1994; 150(4):833–892, 1158–1163.
11. Jamal K, Fleetham JA, Thurlbeck WM. Cor pulmonale: Correlation with central airway lesions, peripheral airway lesions, emphysema and control of breathing. *Am Rev Respir Dis* 1990; 141:1172–1177.
12. Mountain R, Zwillich C, Weil J. Hypoventilation in obstructive lung disease. *N Engl J Med* 1978; 298:521–525.
13. Schwarz MI, King TE Jr, eds. *Interstitial Lung Diseases.* St Louis: Mosby–Year Book; 1998.
14. Ziesche R, Hofbauer E, Wittman K, et al. A preliminary study of long-term IF gamma 1-b and low dose prednisolone in pulmonary fibrosis. *N Engl J Med* 1999; 341:1264–1270.
15. Bergofsky EH. Respiratory failure in disorders of the thoracic cage. *Am Rev Respir Dis* 1979; 119:643–669.
16. Burwell CS, Robin ED, Whaley RD, Bickelmann AG. Extreme obesity associated with alveolar hypoventilation—A Pickwickian syndrome. *Am J Med* 1956; 21:811–818.
17. Strohl KP, Rogers RM. Obstructive sleep apnea. *N Engl J Med* 1996; 334:99–104.
18. Gerry JL, Buckley BH, Hutchins GM. Clinicopathologic analysis of cardiac dysfunction in 52 patients with sickle cell anemia. *Am J Cardiol* 1978; 42:211–216.
19. Weil JV, Castro O, Malik AB, et al. Pathogenesis of lung disease in sickle hemoglobinopathies. *Am Rev Respir Dis* 1993; 148:249–256.
20. Swenson SJ, Tashjian JH, Myers JL, et al. Pulmonary veno-occlusive disease: CT findings in eight patients. *AJR* 1996; 167:937–940.
21. Lange PA, Stoller JK. The hepatopulmonary syndrome. *Ann Intern Med* 1995; 122:521–529.
22. Coplan N, Shinony R, Ioachim H. Primary pulmonary hypertension associated with human immunodeficiency viral infection. *Am J Med* 1990; 89:96–99.
23. Winslow TM, Ossipov MA, Fazio GP, et al. Five year follow-up of the prevalence and progression of pulmonary hypertension in systemic lupus erythematosus. *Am Heart J* 1995; 129:510–515.
24. Brenot F, Simonneau G. Risk factors for primary pulmonary hypertension. In: Rubin LJ, Rich S, eds. *Primary Pulmonary Hyper-*

tension, Vol 99: *Lung Biology in Health and Disease*. New York: Marcel Dekker; 1997:131–147.
25. Mark EJ, Patalas ED, Chang HT, et al. Fatal pulmonary hypertension associated with short term use of fenfluramine and phentermine. *N Engl J Med* 1997; 337:602–606.
26. Burrows B. Arterial oxygenation and pulmonary hemodynamics in patients with chronic airways obstruction. *Am Rev Respir Dis* 1974; 110(suppl):64–70.
27. Nocturnal Oxygen Therapy Trial Group. Continuous or nocturnal oxygen therapy in hypoxemic chronic obstructive lung disease: A clinical trial. *Ann Intern Med* 1980; 93:391–398.
28. Voelkel N. Mechanisms of hypoxic pulmonary vasoconstriction. *Am Rev Respir Dis* 1986; 133:1186.
29. Michelakis ED, Archer SL, Weir EK. Acute hypoxic pulmonary vasoconstriction: A model of O_2 sensing. *Physiol Res* 1995; 44:361–367.
30. Douglas NJ, Flenley DC. Breathing during sleep in patients with obstructive lung disease. *Am Rev Respir Dis* 1990; 141:1065–1070.
31. Enson Y. Pulmonary heart disease: Relation of pulmonary hypertension to abnormal lung structure and function. *Bull NY Acad Med* 1977; 53:551–566.
32. Meerson FX. *The Failing Heart: Adaptation and Maladaptation*. New York: Raven Press; 1983:51.
33. Enson Y, Thomas HM, Bosken CH, et al. Pulmonary hypertension in interstitial lung disease: Relation of vascular resistance to abnormal lung structure. *Trans Assoc Am Phys* 1975; 88:248–255.
34. Grover RF. Pulmonary circulation in animals and man in high altitude. *Ann NY Acad Sci* 1965; 127:632–639.
35. Fishman AP. The left ventricle in chronic bronchitis and emphysema. *N Engl J Med* 1971; 285:402–404.
36. Murphy ML, Adamson J, Hutcheson F. Left ventricular hypertrophy in patients with chronic bronchitis and emphysema. *Ann Intern Med* 1974; 81:307–313.
37. Matthay RA, Berger HO. Cardiovascular function in cor pulmonale. *Clin Chest Med* 1983; 4:269–295.
38. Buda AJ, Pinsky MR, Ingels NB, et al. Effect of intrathoracic pressure on left ventricular performance. *N Engl J Med* 1979; 301:453–459.
39. Bermis CE, Sehur JR, Borkenhagen D, et al. Influence of right ventricular filling pressure on left ventricular pressure and dimension. *Circ Res* 1974; 34:498–504.
40. Santamore WB, Dell-Italia LJ. Ventricular interdependence: Significant left ventricular contributions to right ventricular systolic function. *Prog Cardiovasc Dis* 1998; 40:289–308.
41. Bichet D, Schrier RS. Cardiac failure, liver disease and nephrotic syndrome. In: Schrier JR, Gottschalk C, eds. *Diseases of the Kidney*. Boston: Little, Brown; 1993:2453–2491.
42. Farber MO, Roberts LR, Weinberger MH, et al. Abnormalities of sodium and H_2O handling in chronic obstructive lung disease. *Arch Intern Med* 1982; 142:1326–1330.
43. Stewart AG, Waterhouse JC, Billings CG, et al. Effects of ACE inhibition on sodium excretion in patients with hypoxemic COPD. *Thorax* 1994; 49:995–998.
44. Lehtonen J, Sutinen S, Ikaheimo P, Paako P. Electrocardiographic criteria for the diagnosis of right ventricular hypertrophy verified at autopsy. *Chest* 1988; 93:839–842.
45. Murphy ML, Hutcheson F. The electrocardiographic diagnosis of right ventricular hypertrophy in chronic obstructive pulmonary disease. *Chest* 1974; 65:622–627.
46. Moore CB, Kraus WL, Dork DS. The relationship between pulmonary arterial pressure and roentgenographic appearance in mitral stenosis. *Am Heart J* 1959; 58:576–581.
47. Chang CH. The normal roentgenographic measurement of the right descending pulmonary artery in 1,085 cases. *AJR* 1962; 87:929–935.
48. Matthay RA, Schwarz MI, Ellis JH. Pulmonary artery hypertension in chronic obstructive pulmonary disease: Chest radiographic assessment. *Invest Radiol* 1981; 16:95–100.
49. Cacho A, Prokash R, Sarne R, Kaushik VS. Usefulness of two-dimensional echocardiography in diagnosing right ventricular hypertrophy. *Chest* 1983; 84:154–157.
50. Hagan A, DeMaria A. Diseases of the right heart. In: *Clinical Applications of Two Dimensional Echocardiography*. Boston: Little, Brown; 1985:270.
51. Louie EK, Rich S, Levitshy S, Brundage BH. Doppler echocardiographic demonstration of the differential effects of RV pressure and volume overload on LV geometry and filling. *J Am Coll Cardiol* 1992; 19:84–91.
52. Kitabatake A, Michitoshi I, Asao M, et al. Noninvasive evaluation of pulmonary hypertension by a pulsed Doppler technique. *Circulation* 1983; 68:302–309.
53. Schiller N. Pulmonary artery pressure estimation by Doppler and two-dimensional echocardiography. *Cardiol Clin* 1990; 8:277–287.
54. Kawakami Y, Kishi F, Yamamoto H, et al. Relation of oxygen delivery, mixed venous oxygenation and pulmonary hemodynamics to prognosis in COPD. *N Engl J Med* 1983; 308:1045–1049.
55. Tarpy SP, Edlli BR. Long-term oxygen therapy. *N Engl J Med* 1995; 333:710–715.
56. Weitzenblum E, Loiseau A, Hirth C, et al. Course of pulmonary hemodynamics in patients with chronic obstructive pulmonary disease. *Chest* 1979; 75:656–662.
57. Crapo RO. Pulmonary function testing. *N Engl J Med* 1994; 331:25–31.
58. Ridker P, Hennekens CH, Lindpaintner K, et al. Mutation in the gene coding for coagulation factor V and the risk of infarction, stroke, and venous thrombosis in apparently healthy men. *N Engl J Med* 1995; 332:912–917.
59. Asherson RA, Khamashta MA, Ordi-Ros, et al. The primary antiphospholipid syndrome: Major clinical and serological features. *Medicine* 1989; 68:366–374.
60. Kryger MH. Management of obstructive sleep apnea. *Clin Chest Med* 1992; 13:481–492.
61. Wiedemann H, Matthay R. Cor pulmonale in chronic obstructive pulmonary disease circulatory pathophysiology and management. *Clin Chest Med* 1990; 11:523–545.
62. Green LH, Smith TW. The use of digitalis in patients with pulmonary disease. *Ann Intern Med* 1977; 87:459–465.
63. Smith DE, Bissett JK, Phillips JR, et al. Improved right ventricular systolic time intervals after digitalis in patients with cor pulmonale and chronic obstructive pulmonary disease. *Am J Cardiol* 1978; 41:1299–1304.
64. Gertz I, Hedenstierna G, Wester PO. Improvement in pulmonary function with diuretic therapy in the hypervolemic and polycythemic patient with chronic obstructive pulmonary disease. *Chest* 1979; 75:146–151.
65. Weisse AB, Moschos CB, Frank MJ, et al. Hemodynamic effects of staged hematocrit reduction in patients with stable cor pulmonale and severely elevated hematocrit levels. *Am J Med* 1975; 58:92–98.
66. Patterson GA, Cooper JD. Lung transplantation. *Chest Surg Clin North Am* 1995; 3:1.
67. Cooper JD, Trulock EP, Triantafillon AN, et al. Bilateral pneumectomy (volume reduction) for chronic obstructive pulmonary disease. *J Thorac Cardiovasc Surg* 1995; 109:106–116.

PART NINE

Valvular Heart Disease

CHAPTER 55

ACUTE RHEUMATIC FEVER

Simon Chakko / Alan L. Bisno

DEFINITION

Rheumatic fever is an inflammatory disease that occurs as a delayed nonsuppurative sequel to group A streptococcal infection of the pharynx. It involves the heart, joints, central nervous system, skin, and subcutaneous tissues with varying frequency. Its clinical manifestations include migratory polyarthritis, fever, carditis, and, less frequently, Sydenham's chorea, subcutaneous nodules, and erythema marginatum. Rheumatic fever is a clinical syndrome for which no specific diagnostic test exists. No symptom, sign, or laboratory test result is pathognomonic, although several combinations of them are diagnostic. Its importance relates to involvement of the heart, which, though rarely fatal during the acute stage, may lead to rheumatic valvular disease, a chronic and progressive condition that causes cardiac disability or death many years after the initial event.

ETIOLOGY

Antecedent infection of the upper respiratory tract with the group A streptococcus is necessary for the development of rheumatic fever. Cutaneous streptococcal infection may lead to acute glomerulonephritis but has never been demonstrated to cause rheumatic fever. The evidence establishing the group A streptococcus as the etiologic agent of rheumatic fever is only indirect, because the organism cannot be recovered from the lesions and there is no experimental animal model. Nevertheless, the evidence from clinical, immunologic and epidemiologic studies is overwhelming.

At least one-third of patients deny previous sore throat, and cultures of the pharynx are often negative for group A streptococci at the onset of rheumatic fever. However, an antibody response to streptococcal extracellular products can be demonstrated in almost all cases,[1] and the attack rate of acute rheumatic fever is strongly correlated with the magnitude of the antibody response.[2]

A clear sequential relationship between outbreaks of streptococcal pharyngitis or scarlet fever and rheumatic fever has been demonstrated in epidemiologic studies of military recruit camps, and such outbreaks can be eradicated when streptococcal infection is controlled by chemotherapy.[3] Prompt and effective penicillin therapy of streptococcal pharyngitis prevents the initial attack of rheumatic fever (so-called primary prevention),[4] and continuous chemoprophylaxis against streptococcal infection (secondary prophylaxis) prevents its recurrences.[5]

EPIDEMIOLOGY

Rheumatic fever is a major health problem in the developing countries of Asia, Africa, the Middle East, and Latin America. It is difficult for physicians trained in North America to comprehend the magnitude of the problem. A World Health Organization survey conducted between 1986 and 1990 estimated the prevalence of rheumatic fever and chronic rheumatic heart disease per 1000 schoolchildren to be 12.6 in Zambia, 10.2 in Sudan, and 7.9 in Bolivia.[6] Hospital statistics from many developing countries reveal that 10 to 35 percent of all cardiac admissions are for rheumatic fever and rheumatic heart disease.[6,7] It has been estimated that there are at least 50,000 cases of rheumatic fever annually in India and more than 1 million people with rheumatic heart disease.[7] Exceedingly high attack rates have been reported among aboriginal populations in New Zealand and Australia.[8]

Acute rheumatic fever is most common among children in the 5- to 15-year age group. There is no clear-cut sex predilection, although there is a female preponderance in rheumatic mitral stenosis and in Sydenham's chorea. The attack rate of acute rheumatic fever following untreated exudative tonsillitis varies, depending upon the epidemiologic circumstances and the rheumatogenic potential of prevalent streptococcal strains. This rate has been reported to approximate 3 percent during epidemics in military recruit camps[9] but only 0.4 percent after endemically occurring infections in untreated children in civilian populations.[10] Acute rheumatic fever is more likely to occur after those streptococcal infections judged to be more severe by clinical and immunologic criteria (i.e., exudative tonsillopharyngitis, vigorous rises in serum titers of antistreptolysin O, and prolonged convalescent streptococcal throat carriage). Nevertheless, approximately one-third of the cases occur after asymptomatic streptococcal infections. A striking feature of the epidemiology of acute rheumatic fever is the propensity of patients who have suffered an initial attack to experience recurrences of the disease following group A streptococcal infections.

Strains of group A streptococci vary in their propensity to elicit acute rheumatic fever. Although the precise factor or factors that confer this property are unknown, highly rheumatogenic strains share certain biological characteristics. Only a limited number of the more than 90 streptococcal M-protein types have been strongly and repetitively associated with rheumatic fever.[11] These strains are often heavily encapsulated, a feature manifest by the formation of mucoid colonies on blood-agar plates. Their M-protein molecules share a particular surface-exposed antigenic domain against which rheumatic fever patients mount a strong immunoglobulin G response.[12] These characteristics were established, however, by study of rheumatic fever cases and outbreaks in the United States and Great Britain; they remain to be validated for cases occurring in third-world countries or among aboriginal populations.

The twentieth century witnessed a dramatic decline in the incidence of rheumatic fever and rheumatic heart disease in the industrialized nations.[13] The incidence of rheumatic fever and the prevalence of rheumatic heart disease are now very low in North America and western Europe. Rates fewer than 2 per 100,000 schoolchildren have been reported from several areas in the United States. The disease is very rare in affluent suburban populations[14] but persists among disadvantaged families dwelling in the crowded inner cities.[14,15] The higher incidence rates reported among blacks than among whites appear to be due to socioeconomic rather than genetic factors.

The reasons for the recent decline in the incidence of rheumatic fever in developed countries are multifactorial. One of the factors was likely an improvement in living standards, including a decrease in household crowding. Crowding favors interpersonal spread of group A streptococci and probably enhances streptococcal virulence by human passage. Although the diminution was well under way prior to the introduction of penicillin, this highly effective antimicrobial may have contributed to the decline in initial attacks of rheumatic fever and clearly contributed to a decrease in mortality by preventing repetitive attacks in patients compliant with programs of secondary prophylaxis.

There is no evidence of a decline in the frequency of streptococcal pharyngitis concomitant with the dramatic decline in rheumatic fever incidence. This strongly suggests that there have been changes in the rheumatogenicity of streptococcal strains currently prevalent in civilian populations of North America and western Europe. This concept was further validated by the isolation of strains manifesting the above-mentioned rheumatogenic phenotypic characteristics during a resurgence of rheumatic fever that occurred in certain American communities toward the end of the century (see below).

In the mid-1980s, after decades of decline, outbreaks of rheumatic fever occurred in numerous cities and in two military recruit camps in the United States.[13,16] Strains of group A streptococci recovered from patients with acute rheumatic fever and their families and those found in community and training camp surveys were generally high-mucoid and often belonged to well-established rheumatogenic serotypes (serotypes 3 and 18). A survey of hospitals conducted by the American Heart Association indicated that the reported outbreaks were focal and not nationwide.[17] The largest epidemic occurred in Salt Lake City, Utah, and the surrounding intermountain area,[18] where over 500 cases were diagnosed between 1985 and 1999.

Surprisingly, the epidemiologic features of several of the civilian outbreaks—including the largest one in Salt Lake City—differed from the traditional patterns described above in that the victims were predominantly white middle-class children living in the suburbs. Only one-third of the children with rheumatic fever in Salt Lake City had a sore throat of sufficient severity that the parents considered taking them to a physician.[19] Most such outbreaks appear to have subsided during the 1990s, but that in Salt Lake City is continuing as of this writing.

PATHOGENESIS

The exact mechanism by which the group A streptococcus causes rheumatic fever remains unexplained. Possibilities include (1) toxic effects of streptococcal products, particularly streptolysins S or O, which are capable of inducing tissue injury; (2) a serum sickness–like reaction; and (3) autoimmune phenomena induced by the similarity or identity of certain streptococcal antigens to wide variety of human tissue antigens.[20] Although no mechanism has been unequivocally proven, autoimmunity or, more precisely, molecular mimicry appears to be most likely.[21] There are shared epitopes between cardiac myosin and streptococcal M protein that lead to cross-reactive humoral and T-cell immunity against group A streptococci and the heart.[22] Epitopes of streptococcal M protein also share antigenic determinants with heart valves, sarcolemmal membrane proteins, synovium, and articular cartilage.[23] Circulating antibodies that react with neurons of the caudate and subthalamic nuclei and with group A streptococcal cell membranes have been found in many children with Sydenham's chorea.[24] Injection of streptococcal mucopeptide-polysaccharide cell wall complex can induce chronic nodular lesions in the dermal connective tissue in experimental animals.[25] These cross-reactive and toxic phenomena could explain many of the clinical manifestations of rheumatic fever, but, in the absence of a credible animal model of the disease, there is no direct proof that they do so.

During active rheumatic carditis both the number of helper (CD4) lymphocytes and the ratio of CD4 to CD8 cells are increased in the heart valves, and the production of interleukin-1 and interleukin-2 is reportedly increased.[26,27] Scarring and collagen deposition in the valves and destruction of myocytes may result.

The fact that, even in severe epidemics of exudative pharyngitis, rheumatic fever affects only a small proportion of infected persons, coupled with the known familial aggregation of rheumatic fever cases, has long suggested the possibility of a genetic predisposition to rheumatic attacks. Studies of the distribution of class 1 HLA antigens in rheumatics versus controls have been inconclusive. A statistically significant association has been reported between certain of the class II HLA antigens (HLA-DR2 in blacks[28] and HLA-DR4 in whites[29]) and rheumatic fever. An intriguing potential link between the genetic constitution of the human host and susceptibility to rheumatic fever is the identification of certain alloantigens that are expressed in a higher proportion of circulating B lymphocytes of rheumatic subjects and their family members than in those of patients with poststreptococcal glomerulonephritis or normal controls.[30]

PATHOLOGY

Acute rheumatic fever is characterized by exudative and proliferative inflammatory lesions of the connective tissue, most notably of the heart, joints, and subcutaneous tissue. When carditis ensues, all layers of the heart are involved. Pericarditis is common and fibrinous pericarditis is occasionally present. The pericardial inflammation usually resolves over time with no clinically significant sequelae, and tamponade is rare. In fatal cases, myocardial involvement leads to globular enlargement involving all four chambers of the heart. In the myocardium, initially there is fragmentation of collagen fibers, lymphocytic infiltration, and fibrinoid degeneration. This is followed by the appearance of myocardial Aschoff nodules, which are considered pathognomonic of acute rheumatic fever. The Aschoff nodule consists of an area of central necrosis surrounded by lymphocytes, plasma cells, and large mononuclear and giant multinucleate cells. Many of these cells have an elongated nucleus with a clear area just within the nuclear membrane ("owl-eyed nucleus"). These cells are called *Anitschkow myocytes*, although histochemical studies suggest that they are of macrophage-histiocyte origin.[31] Aschoff nodules may also be found in endomyocardial biopsy specimens obtained from patients with acute rheumatic carditis.[32]

Endocardial involvement is responsible for chronic rheumatic valvulitis.[33] Small fibrinous, verrucous vegetations, 1 to 2 mm in diameter, are seen on the atrial surface at sites of valve coaptation and on the chordae tendineae. Even when no vegetations are present, there is edema and inflammation of the valve leaflets. A thickened and fibrotic patch (MacCallum's patch) may be found in the posterior left atrial wall. It is believed to be the effect of the mitral regurgitant jet impinging on the left atrial wall.[33] Healing of the valvulitis leads to granulation and fibrosis of the leaflets and fusion of the chordae. Valvular stenosis or incompetence may result. The mitral valve is involved most frequently, followed by the aortic valve. Tricuspid and pulmonic valves are usually spared.

CLINICAL MANIFESTATIONS

Rheumatic fever may involve different organ systems such as heart, joints, skin, and central nervous system. The clinical picture depends upon the systems involved, and the manifestations may appear singly or in various combinations (Table 55-1). Five clinical features (carditis, polyarthritis, chorea, subcutaneous nodules, and erythema marginatum) are so characteristic of the disease that they are classified as major manifestations according to the Jones criteria (Table 55-2).[34] Additional findings such as fever, arthralgia, heart block, and acute-phase reactants in the blood (i.e., elevation of erythrocyte sedimentation rate and serum concentration of C-reactive protein) are commonly present in acute rheumatic fever but are nonspecific in nature and are therefore classified as minor manifestations.

The latent period from the onset of streptococcal sore throat to the onset of initial and recurrent attacks of rheumatic fever varies between 1 and 5 weeks with a median of 19 days. The mode of onset is quite variable. An abrupt onset with fever and toxicity is common in patients in whom acute polyarthritis is the presenting complaint. The onset may be insidious or even subclinical when mild carditis is the initial manifestation. Most attacks begin with polyarthritis, and occasionally this may be preceded by abdominal pain and fleeting signs of peritoneal inflammation, which may be misdiagnosed as acute appendicitis.

TABLE 55-1 Clinical Manifestations of Acute Rheumatic Fever

General	
	High fever, lassitude, prostration, tachycardia
Cardiac	
	Cardiomegaly, congestive heart failure
	Acute pericarditis, pericardial effusion
	Apical pansystolic murmur (mitral regurgitation)
	Apical middiastolic murmur (Carey Coombs)
	Basal diastolic (aortic regurgitation)
Dermatologic	
	Subcutaneous nodules
	Erythema marginatum
Rheumatologic	
	Arthralgia
	Migratory polyarthritis
Neurologic	
	Sydenham's chorea

TABLE 55-2 Guidelines for the Diagnosis of the Initial Attack of Rheumatic Fever (Jones criteria, updated in 1992)[a]

Major Manifestations	Minor Manifestations	Supporting Evidence for Antecedent Group A Streptococcal Infection
Carditis	Clinical findings	Positive throat culture or rapid streptococcal antigen test
Polyarthritis	Arthralgia	
Chorea	Fever	
Erythema marginatum	Laboratory findings	Elevated or rising streptococcal antibody titer
Subcutaneous nodules	Elevated acute phase reactants	
	Erthrocyte sedimentation rate	
	C-reactive protein	
	Prolonged P-R interval	

[a]If supported by evidence of preceding group A streptococcal infection, the presence of two major manifestations or one major and two minor manifestations indicates a high probability of acute rheumatic fever.

SOURCE: From Dajani et al.[34] Reproduced by permission of *JAMA* 1992; 268:2069–2073, copyrighted 1992, American Medical Association.

Overall, arthritis occurs in approximately 75 percent of first attacks, carditis in 40 to 50 percent, chorea in 15 percent, and subcutaneous nodules and erythema marginatum in less than 10 percent.[35] These figures may vary widely, however.

Carditis

Carditis is the only manifestation of acute rheumatic fever that has the potential to cause long-term disability and death. Severe mitral regurgitation (or, possibly, severe myocarditis) may precipitate intractable heart failure and may be fatal during the acute phase of the disease. Fortunately, this complication is quite rare. Carditis, if present, usually appears within the first 3 weeks of the illness. The cardiac involvement is frequently mild or even asymptomatic, but occasionally the course can be fulminant. The diagnosis of carditis requires the presence of one of the following four manifestations: (1) organic cardiac murmurs not previously present, (2) cardiomegaly, (3) pericarditis, (4) congestive heart failure.

Valvulitis is associated with characteristic murmurs that are almost always present unless they are obscured by a loud pericardial friction rub, a large pericardial effusion, or low cardiac output. Mitral regurgitation leads to a blowing holosystolic murmur best heard at the apex and radiating to the axilla and occasionally to the base of the heart or the back. Hemodynamic and surgical pathologic studies conducted in South African patients suggest that mitral annular dilatation is usually the initial abnormality and predisposes to lengthening or rupture of the chordae tendineae and prolapse of the anterior leaflet.[36,37] Increased flow across the mitral valve in the presence of valvulitis may produce a middiastolic murmur (Carey Coombs murmur) that follows an S_3 gallop. This murmur is always accompanied by a systolic murmur of mitral regurgitation. It is not diagnostic of rheumatic fever because other conditions that lead to increased flow across the mitral valve can cause a similar murmur, and in children an S_3 gallop can be physiologic. The Carey Coombs murmur can be differentiated from the diastolic rumble of mitral stenosis by the absence of an opening snap, presystolic accentuation, and loud first sound. A high-pitched decrescendo basal diastolic murmur of aortic regurgitation may also be heard. It is best heard along the left sternal border, over the aortic area, in expiration with the patient leaning forward (see also Chap. 57).

Myocarditis in the absence of valvulitis is not likely to be rheumatic in origin. Tachycardia is common. S_3, S_4, or summation gallops may be audible. Cardiomegaly may be noted on the chest roentgenogram or echocardiogram. In acute congestive heart failure, rapid distention of the hepatic capsule may lead to right-upper-quadrant discomfort and tenderness. Congestive heart failure is usually caused by left ventricular volume overload associated with severe mitral or aortic regurgitation.

In the presence of pericarditis, a pericardial friction rub or muffled heart sounds due to a large effusion may be noted. The presence of effusion should be confirmed by echocardiography. Large effusions leading to tamponade are rare. Pericarditis in the absence of valvular involvement is rarely due to acute rheumatic fever, and other causes should be sought.[34]

Polyarthritis

Arthritis is the most frequent major manifestation of rheumatic fever.[38] Any joint may be affected, but involvement of larger joints such as knees, ankles, elbows, and wrists is more common. The spine is only rarely affected. Several joints are involved in quick succession, and each for a brief period of time, resulting in the typical picture of migratory polyarthritis accompanied by signs and symptoms of an acute febrile illness. A striking feature of rheumatic arthritis is its dramatic response to salicylate therapy. Thus, the typical migratory polyarthritis pattern may not be present if effective anti-inflammatory therapy is administered early in the course of the disease.

The synovial fluid contains numerous white blood cells with a marked preponderance of polymorphonuclear leukocytes. Bacterial cultures are sterile. Inflammation of any one joint subsides spontaneously within a week and the entire bout of polyathritis rarely lasts more than 4 weeks. Resolution is complete with no residual joint damage. A possible exception is the so-called Jaccoud deformity of the metacarpophalangeal joints. This is a periarticular fibrosis and not a true synovitis, and its relation to rheumatic fever is unclear.[39]

Subcutaneous Nodules

These nodules are seen in only 1 to 21 percent of patients with rheumatic fever.[38] They are most often associated with carditis and rarely appear as an isolated manifestation of rheumatic fever. They are round, firm, painless, freely movable subcutaneous lesions varying in size from 0.5 to 2.0 cm. They occur in crops and are usually found over bony surfaces and over tendons such as elbows, knees, and wrists, the occiput and vertebrae (Fig. 55-1). They last for a week or two and disappear spontaneously. Similar nodules also occur in rheumatoid arthritis and systemic lupus erythematosus.

Erythema Marginatum

This rash is usually found on the trunk and proximal parts of the extremities, with the face being spared. It begins as an

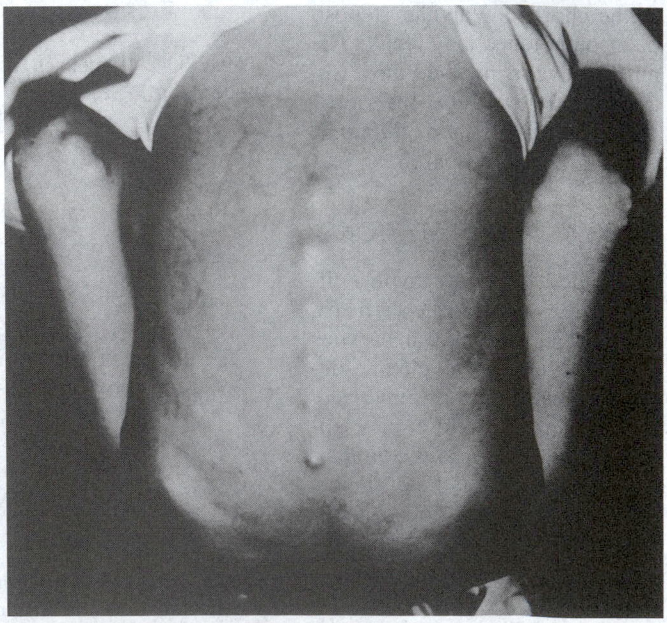

FIGURE 55-1 Subcutaneous nodules on the spine and elbows. (Courtesy of Dr. Benedict F. Massell.)

erythematous macule or papule that extends outward while skin in the center returns to normal. Lesions may merge and form serpiginous patterns. They are never pruritic or indurated, blanch on pressure, and are not influenced by anti-inflammatory therapy. The rash is evanescent, migrating from place to place and leaving no residual scarring. Individual lesions may appear and disappear in minutes to hours. Erythema marginatum has also been reported in sepsis, drug reactions, and glomerulonephritis.

Sydenham's Chorea (St. Vitus Dance)

This neurologic disorder often occurs in isolation, either unaccompanied by other major manifestations of rheumatic fever or after a latent period of several months, at a time when all other manifestations of rheumatic fever have subsided. It is characterized by rapid, purposeless, involuntary movements, most noticable in the extremities and face. The arms and legs flail about in erratic, jerky, uncoordinated movements. The speech is usually slurred and jerky. The involuntary movements disappear during sleep and may be suppressed by sedation. The patient is unable to sustain a tetanic muscular contraction. Emotional lability is characteristic of Sydenham's chorea and may often precede other neurologic manifestations. The duration of the chorea is variable, and its severity may wax and wane. Most patients recover in 6 months. Long-term sequelae such as convulsions, learning disabilities, and behavior problems are rare but have been reported in a small number of patients. Experience with brain imaging is limited but isolated case reports suggest that magnetic resonance imaging or computed tomographic scans may reveal abnormalities in the caudate nuclei, putamen, and substantia nigra.[40]

Rarely, chorea may be due to other conditions that affect the basal ganglia, including collagen vascular, endocrine, neoplastic, genetic, metabolic, and infectious disorders.[41] Perhaps the most frequent differential diagnostic consideration is systemic lupus erythematosus. The relationship of chorea occurring during pregnancy (chorea gravidarum) to acute rheumatic fever remains unclear.

Minor Manifestations

Minor manifestations of rheumatic fever include fever, arthralgia, and laboratory evidences of inflammation (Table 55-2). Fever usually ranges from 38.4 to 40°C and rarely lasts for more than 3 to 4 weeks. Arthralgia is pain in one or more joints without objective evidence of inflammation. In diagnosing rheumatic fever using the Jones criteria, arthralgia should not be considered a minor manifestation when arthritis is present.

Other Clinical Features

Abdominal pain in rheumatic fever is the result of peritoneal inflammation and may be confused with acute appendicitis or sickle cell crisis. Because it occurs at the onset of the illness, other manifestations of rheumatic fever may not yet be present. Epistaxis has been reported as a manifestation of rheumatic fever, but it is not clear to what extent it may be attributable to the large doses of aspirin administered for treatment of the disease. Tachycardia may be out of proportion to fever and persists during sleep.

LABORATORY FINDINGS

A mild to moderate normochromic normocytic anemia and leukocytosis with an increased proportion of polymorphonuclear leukocytes are common. Elevated serum levels of C-reactive protein and an increased erythrocyte sedimentation rate are almost always present, indicating acute inflammation. An exception is "pure" chorea, which may appear after these markers of inflammation have returned to normal.

Throat cultures are usually negative for group A streptococci by the time rheumatic fever appears. Streptococcal antibody tests provide evidence for antecedent streptococcal infection and include antistreptolysin O (ASO), anti-DNAse B, and antihyaluronidase. These antibodies reach peak titer at about the time of onset of acute rheumatic fever. The ASO is elevated in 80 percent or more of patients with rheumatic fever. A battery of these three tests will establish the presence of immunologically significant infection with group A streptococcus in 95 percent of patients.[42] The normal ranges for these titers vary depending upon the test used, patient's age, and geographic locale. ASO titers greater than 200 Todd units per milliliter in adults and 320 Todd units in children are generally considered elevated. In patients seen early during the course of rheumatic fever, rising antibody titers may be seen. An elevated streptococcal antibody titer is not diagnostic of rheumatic fever, but the diagnosis is very unlikely if all three tests (ASO, anti-DNAse B, and antihyaluronidase) are negative (see section on "Diagnosis" below (or exceptions).

Electrocardiogram

Persistent sinus tachycardia that does not resolve during sleep is common in the presence of carditis.[43] Sinus bradycardia and sinus arrhythmia may be present in some patients and can be abolished by the administration of atropine. Prolongation of the PR interval is a common abnormality. In various studies, the incidence varied from 10 to 84 percent.[43] A recent study of the resurgence of rheumatic fever[18] described the electrocardiographic findings in 232 patients. Alterations in atrioventricular conduction were noted in 74 patients (32 percent). Of these, 66 had a prolonged PR interval, 4 had transient episodes of AV block, and 4 had transient episodes of AV dissociation.

Some investigators have suggested that the AV conduction delay is a manifestation of carditis.[43] However, the response to atropine and the lack of correlation with clinical carditis suggests that this is a nonspecific finding.[34] Transient complete heart block that causes Stokes-Adams attacks has been described. Bundle-branch blocks are rare. Atrial flutter and fibrillation have been described in the presence of carditis. Low QRS voltage may be noted if a large pericardial effusion is present.

Echocardiogram

Few studies have used echocardiography to evaluate and follow up patients with rheumatic carditis.[44] During the resurgence of rheumatic fever in Salt Lake City, two-dimensional and Doppler echocardiograms were performed in children with rheumatic fever.[18] During the acute phase of rheumatic carditis, echocardiographic evidence of mitral regurgitation ws often found even when a murmur was not audible ("silent mitral regurgitation").

Valvular thickening and the presence of nodular lesions on the body and tips of the mitral leaflet have been described.[45] These are most likely echocardiographic equivalents of rheumatic verrucae. The key features of rheumatic mitral valvulitis were annular dilation and elongation of the chordae to the anterior leaflet, resulting in mitral regurgitation with a posterolaterally directed jet.[18] In an echocardiographic study of 73 patients with active rheumatic carditis and mitral regurgitation, it was noted that 90 percent of patients had elongated mitral valve chordae, 94 percent had prolapse of the anterior leaflet of the mitral valve, and 96 percent had annular dilation.[46] The resulting mitral regurgitant jet was directed toward the posterolateral wall of the left atrium. The site where this jet strikes the posterior left atrial wall corresponds with the site of endocardial thickening described at autopsy as MacCallum's patch. Rheumatic carditis can be differentiated from the common mitral valve prolapse syndrome because only the coapting portion of the anterior mitral leaflet prolapses and there is no billowing of the medial portion of the leaflet.

In the past congestive heart failure seen in acute rheumatic fever was attributed to myocarditis. Recent echocardiographic studies have shown that patients with rheumatic fever and congestive heart failure have preserved left ventricular systolic function and severe mitral regurgitation.[45,47] Thus the etiology of heart failure appears to be acute mitral regurgitation and not myocarditis.[19,44] Although these findings are interesting, experience is limited, and it is not yet clear the extent to which echocardiography has incremental diagnostic value when added to the clinical findings in the diagnosis of carditis or in ascertaining the likelihood of development of chronic rheumatic heart disease.

Endomyocardial Biopsy

Rheumatic fever is basically a clinical syndrome for which no specific diagnostic test exists. However, the presence of Aschoff nodules on histologic specimens obtained at surgery and autopsy can be considered diagnostic of rheumatic fever. Percutaneous transvenous myocardial biopsy is now feasible and may be useful in the diagnosis.[48] Aschoff nodules and interstitial mononuclear infiltrates with or without myocyte necrosis have been described in the myocardial biopsy specimens of four patients with acute rheumatic fever.[49–52] To determine the role of myocardial biopsy in the diagnosis of rheumatic carditis, a prospective study was performed in 54 patients.[32] Among 11 patients with definite clinical rheumatic carditis, 3 (27 percent) had Aschoff nodules in the biopsy specimen; the remainder had evidence of myocarditis, but the abnormalities were not diagnostic of rheumatic carditis. Among patients with suspected rheumatic carditis, myocardial specimens were diagnostic only in a minority of cases. The investigators concluded that the role of myocardial biopsy in the diagnosis of rheumatic fever was limited.

DIAGNOSIS

The diagnostic criteria for acute rheumatic fever were originally proposed by T. Duckett Jones 1944 and have been later modified and updated by the American Heart Association (Table 55-2).[34] Based on their diagnostic importance, clinical and laboratory findings are divided into major and minor manifestations. If supported by evidence of a preceding group A streptococcal infection, the presence of two major manifestations, or of one major and two minor manifestations indicates a high probability of acute rheumatic fever. Supporting evidence of a previous group A streptococcal infection is a prerequisite for fulfilling the criteria.

There are some circumstances in which the diagnosis of rheumatic fever can be made without strictly adhering to the Jones criteria. Chorea may not occur until several months after the antecedent streptococcal pharyngeal infection. Isolated carditis that does not provoke congestive failure may not be recognized during the acute phase of illness yet may persist for months. In these situations, markers of inflammation may no longer be present and antistreptococcal antibody titers may have returned to normal by the time the illness comes to light. Moreover, in patients with previous rheumatic fever or established rheumatic heart disease, recurrences are common and a presumptive diagnosis of a recurrence may be made in the presence of a single major or several minor manifestations.[34]

Overdiagnosis must be avoided. Following well-documented group A streptococcal pharyngitis, vague signs and symptoms and nonspecific laboratory abnormalities may appear. Discomfort in the extremities, borderline temperature elevation, increased intensity of functional murmurs, tachycardia, elevated erythrocyte sedimentation rate, and prolonged PR interval may occur in the absence of major manifestations. These patients do not develop rheumatic heart disease on follow-up.[34] Thus the diagnosis of rheumatic fever should not be made in the absence of major manifestations. There is no evidence that temporarily withholding salicylates or corticosteriods has any adverse effect on the long-term prognosis. Thus premature administration of these drugs before the symptoms become distinct should be avoided.

Because acute rheumatic fever can have such diverse manifestations (acute polyarthritis, congestive heart failure, chorea, or combinations of these) and because there is no specific diagnostic test for the disease, the differential diagnostic possibilities in an individual case may be quite broad. Among the diseases that need most frequently to be differentiated are rheumatoid arthritis, juvenile rheumatoid arthritis, systemic lupus erythematosus, serum sickness, sickle cell crisis or cardiopathy, rubella arthritis, septic arthritis (especially gonococcal arthritis in adolescent patients), Lyme disease, infective endocarditis, viral myocarditis, and early stages of Henoch-Schönlein purpura. Less frequent differential diagnostic considerations include gout, sarcoidosis, Hodgkin's disease, and leukemia. Choreiform movements have been described in patients with systemic lupus erythematosus, neoplasms involving the basal ganglia, Legionnaire's disease, hypoparathyroidism, antiphospholipid syndrome, Wilson's disease, and Huntington's disease. Chorea is also seen occasionally in women taking oral contraceptives, and during pregnancy ("chorea gravidarum").

In areas of low rheumatic fever incidence, the Jones criteria are perhaps most useful in excluding the diagnosis. The specificity of the criteria is most problematic when the diagnosis is based upon acute polyarthritis as a single major manifestation plus laboratory findings indicative of acute inflammation. In such cases, there must be clear-cut supporting laboratory evidence of recent streptococcal infection and alternative diagnoses must be carefully ruled out.

TREATMENT

Antibiotics neither modify the course of the disease nor prevent the development of rheumatic carditis. Nevertheless, a course of antibiotics to eradicate group A streptococci remaining in the pharynx and tonsils is usually given. Penicillin G benzathine (1.2 million units intramuscularly as a single injection) is the treatment of choice for patients who are not allergic to penicillin. Erythromycin is prescribed for the penicillin-allergic patient. An oral cephalosporin is an acceptable alternative if the penicillin allergy is not of the immediate type. Following this, continuous prophylactic therapy is given to prevent streptococcal pharyngitis (see below).

Anti-inflammatory drugs provide dramatic clinical improvement but are not curative and do not prevent development of rheumatic heart disease.[53] Aspirin is very effective in reducing fever, toxicity, and inflammation of the joints. It is given as tolerated in a dosage of 90 to 100 mg/kg/day in children and 6 to 8 g/day in adults in divided doses every 4 h. A serum salicylate level of 20 to 25 mg/dL is adequate. Adverse effects include salicylism and gastrointestinal bleeding. The precise dose of aspirin is determined by the severity of symptoms, clinical response, salicylate levels, and tolerance to the drug. After 2 weeks of therapy, a reduced dose of aspirin may be used for another 6 weeks.

Corticosteroids are used in patients with carditis manifest by heart failure and in patients who do not tolerate aspirin or whose symptoms do not respond well to this drug. Prednisone 40 to 60 mg a day in divided doses is given for 2 to 3 weeks and the dosage is gradually reduced over the following 3 weeks. In some patients symptoms of rheumatic fever may reappear when the anti-inflammatory therapy, especially steroids, is stopped. Continuing aspirin therapy for 1 month after steroids are discontinued can prevent this. Although the use of nonsteroidal anti-inflammatory drugs seems reasonable in patients who cannot tolerate salicylates and who do not require corticosteroids, there is a paucity of data on the use of these agents in acute rheumatic fever. Thus, their role in management remains to be defined.

Congestive heart failure is managed in the conventional manner. Digoxin should be used cautiously in the presence of myocarditis. After the acute attack subsides, the level of physical activity is determined by the cardiac status. Patients without residual cardiac disease do not require restriction of physical activity. In the rare instances in which patients with acute rheumatic fever develop intractable heart failure, mitral valve repair or replacement may be life-saving (see also Chap. 57).

TABLE 55-3 Secondary Prevention of Rheumatic Fever (Prevention of Recurrent Attacks)

Agent	Dose	Mode
Benzathine penicillin G	1 200 000 U every 4 weeks[a]	Intramuscular
	or	
Penicillin V	250 mg twice daily	Oral
	or	
Sulfadiazine	0.5 g once daily for patients ≤27 kg (60 lb)	Oral
	1.0 g once daily for patients >27 kg (60 lb)	
For individuals allergic to penicillin and sulfadiazine		
Erythromycin	250 mg twice daily	Oral

[a]In high-risk situations, administration every 3 weeks is justified and recommended.
SOURCE: From Dajani et al.[55] Reproduced by permission of *Pediatrics* 1995; 96:758–764.

PROGNOSIS

Manifestations of chronic rheumatic heart disease include mitral and aortic insufficiency or stenosis, congestive heart failure, and atrial fibrillation. The ultimate cardiac prognosis of an individual rheumatic fever attack is rather directly related to the severity of cardiac involvement during the acute phase provided that the patient is protected from recurrent attacks (see below). In the United Kingdom—United States Collaborative Study,[54] only 6 percent of the patients with no carditis or only questionable carditis during their attack of acute rheumatic fever were found to have heart murmurs when reexamined 10 years later. Heart disease was present at follow-up in 30 percent of the patients initially found to have only apical systolic murmurs, in 40 percent of those with basal diastolic murmurs during the acute phase, and in 68 percent of those who initially suffered from congestive heart failure, pericarditis, or both. Some patients with "pure" chorea may later develop rheumatic heart disease, even though carditis was not recognized during the

TABLE 55-4 Duration of Secondary Rheumatic Fever Prophylaxis

Category	Duration
Rheumatic fever with carditis and residual heart disease (persistent valvular disease[a])	At least 10 years since last episode and at least until age 40 years, sometimes lifelong prophylaxis
Rheumatic fever with carditis but no residual heart disease (no valvular disease[a])	10 years or well into adulthood, whichever is longer
Rheumatic fever without carditis	5 years or until age 21 years, whichever is longer

[a]Clinical or echocardiographic evidence.
SOURCE: From Dajani et al.[55] Reproduced by permission of *Pediatrics* 1995; 96:758–764.

initial attack. In such cases, however, it may be that the initial findings of carditis were no longer prominent by the time that chorea (which often occurs after a long latent period) manifested itself.

Prevention

The risk of developing rheumatic fever following a symptomatic or asymptomatic streptococcal infection is much higher in patients who have experienced a previous attack than in nonrheumatic individuals. In some studies the recurrence rate following immunologically confirmed streptococcal upper respiratory infection has been as high as 16 percent.[2] In patients with rheumatic heart disease, recurrent attacks lead to progressive damage. Although patients who did not suffer carditis initially are less prone to develop it in the event of a recurrence, exceptions do occur. It is therefore crucial that rheumatic fever patients be protected optimally from streptococcal infections. This is accomplished by continuous antimicrobial prophylaxis.[55]

The recommended prophylactic regimens are shown in Table 55-3. The optimal duration of antibiotic prophylaxis remains controversial. The risk of acute rheumatic fever declines with age and the number of years since previous attack. The recommendations of the American Heart Association for the duration of secondary prophylaxis are given in Table 55-4. The decision to discontinue rheumatic fever prophylaxis must be individualized on the basis of risk of recurrence and the probable consequence of a recurrence. It should be noted that health care workers, individuals who have contact with schoolchildren, military recruits, and residents of areas with a high incidence of rheumatic fever are at increased risk for streptococcal infection. This fact should be taken into account when considering discontinuation of prophylaxis.

References

1. Stollerman GH. The epidemiology of primary and secondary rheumatic fever. In: Uhr JW, ed. *The Streptococcus, Rheumatic Fever and Glomerulonephritis*. Baltimore: Williams & Wilkins; 1964: 311–337.
2. Taranta A, Wood HF, Feinstein AR, et al. Rheumatic fever in children and adolescents. A long-term epidemiologic study of subsequent prophylaxis, streptococcal infections, and clinical sequelae. IV. Relation of the rheumatic fever recurrence rate per streptococcal infection to the titers of streptococcal antibodies. *Ann Intern Med* 1964; 60(suppl 5):47–57.
3. Frank PF, Stollerman GH, Miller LF. Protection of a military population from rheumatic fever. *JAMA* 1965; 193:755–783.
4. Wannamaker LW, Rammelkamp CH Jr, Denny FW, et al. Prophylaxis of acute rheumatic fever by treatment of preceding streptococcal infection with various amounts of depot penicillin. *Am J Med* 1951; 10:673–695.
5. Wood HF, Feinstein AR, Taranta A, et al. Rheumatic fever in children and adolescents. A long-term epidemiologic study of subsequent prophylaxis, streptococcal infections, and clinical sequelae: III. Comparative effectiveness of three prophylaxis regimens in preventing streptococcal infections and rheumatic recurrences. *Ann Intern Med* 1964; 60(suppl 5):31–46.
6. World Health Organization. WHO programme for the prevention of rheumatic fever/rheumatic heart disease in 16 developing countries: Report from phase I (1986–90). *Bull WHO* 1992; 70:213–218.
7. Vijaykumar M, Narula J, Reddy KS, Kaplan EL. Incidence of rheumatic fever and prevalence of rheumatic fever disease in India. *Int J Cardiol* 1994; 43:221–228.
8. Carapetis JR, Wolff DR, Currie BJ. Acute rheumatic fever and rheumatic heart disease in the top end of Australia's Northern Territory. *Med J Aust* 1996; 164:146–149.
9. Rammelkamp CH, Denny FW, Wannamaker LW. Studies on the epidemiology of rheumatic fever in the armed services. In: Thomas L, ed. *Rheumatic Fever*. Minneapolis: University of Minnesota Press; 1952:72–89.
10. Siegel AC, Johnson EE, Stollerman GH. Controlled studies of streptococcal pharyngitis in a pediatric population: I. Factors related to the attack rate of rheumatic fever. *N Engl J Med* 1961; 265:559–566.
11. Bisno AL. The concept of rheumatogenic and non-rheumatogenic group A streptococci. In: Read SE, Zabriskie JB, eds. *Streptococcal Diseases and the Immune Response*. New York: Academic Press; 1980:789–803.
12. Bessen DE, Veasy LG, Hill HR, et al. Serologic evidence for a class I group A streptococcal infection among rheumatic fever patients. *J Infect Dis* 1995; 172:1608–1611.
13. Bisno AL. Group A streptococcal infections and acute rheumatic fever. *N Engl J Med* 1991; 325:783–793.
14. Land MA, Bisno AL. Acute rheumatic fever: A vanishing disease in suburbia. *JAMA* 1983; 249:895–898.
15. Ferguson GW, Shultz JM, Bisno AL. Epidemiology of acute rheumatic fever in a multi-ethnic, multi-racial U.S. urban community: The Miami-Dade experience. *J Infect Dis* 1991; 164:720–725.
16. Wallace MR, Garst PD, Papadimos TJ, Oldfield EC. The return of acute rheumatic fever in young adults. *JAMA* 1989; 262:2557–2561.
17. Taubert KA, Rowley AH, Shulman ST. Seven-year national survey of Kawasaki disease and acute rheumatic fever. *Pediatr Infect Dis J* 1994; 13:704–708.
18. Veasy LG, Tani LY, Hill HR. Persistence of acute rheumatic fever in the intermountain area of the United States. *J Pediatr* 1994; 124:9–16.
19. Veasy LG. Lessons learned from the resurgence of rheumatic fever in the United States. In: Narula J, Virmani R, Reddy KS, Tandon R, eds. *Rheumatic Fever*. Washington, DC: Armed Forces Institute of Pathology; 1999:69–78.
20. Stollerman GH. Rheumatogenic streptococci and autoimmunity. *Clin Immunol Immunopathol* 1991; 61:131–142.
21. Zabriskie JB. Rheumatic fever: A model for the pathological consequences of microbial-host mimicry. *Clin Exp Rheumatol* 1986; 4:65–73.
22. Cunningham M. Molecular mimicry between group A streptococci and myosin in the pathogenesis of acute rheumatic fever. In: Narula J, Virmani R, Reddy KS, Tandon R, eds. *Rheumatic Fever*. Washington, DC: Armed Forces Institute of Pathology; 1999:135–165.
23. Baird RW, Bronze MS, Kraus W, et al. Epitopes of group A streptococcal M protein shared with antigens of articular cartilage and synovium. *J Immunol* 1991; 146:3132–3137.
24. Husby G, van de Rijn I, Zabriskie JB, et al. Antibodies reacting with cytoplasm of subthalamic and caudate nuclei neurons in chorea and rheumatic fever. *J Exp Med* 1976; 144:1094–1110.
25. Schwab JH, Cromartie WJ. Immunological studies on a C polysaccharide complex of group A streptococci having a direct toxic effect on connective tissue. *J Exp Med* 1960; 111:295–307.
26. Morris K, Mohan C, Wahi PL, et al. Increase in activated T cells and reduction in suppressor/cytotoxic T cells in acute rheumatic fever and active heart disease: A longitudinal study. *J Infect Dis* 1993; 167:979–983.
27. Morris K, Mohan C, Wahi PL, et al. Enhancement of IL-1, IL-2 production and IL-2 receptor generation in patients with acute rheumatic fever and active rheumatic heart disease: A prospective study. *Clin Exp Immunol* 1993; 91:429–436.
28. Ayoub EM, Barrett DJ, Maclaren NK, Krischer JP. Association

of class II human histocompatibility leukocyte antigens with rheumatic fever. *J Clin Invest* 1986; 77:2019–2026.
29. Anastasiou-Nana MI, Anderson JL, Carlquist JF, Nanas JN. HLA-DR typing and lymphocyte subset evaluation in rheumatic heart disease: A search for immune response factors. *Am Heart J* 1986; 112:992–997.
30. Khanna AK, Buskirk DR, Williams RC Jr, et al. Presence of a non-HLA B cell antigen in rheumatic fever patients and their families as defined by a monoclonal antibody. *J Clin Invest* 1989; 83:1710–1716.
31. Chopra P, Wanniang J, Kumar AS. Immunochemical and histochemical profile of Aschoff bodies in rheumatic carditis in excised left atrial appendages: An immunoperoxidase study in fresh and paraffin-embedded tissue. *Int J Cardiol* 1992; 34:199–207.
32. Narula J, Chopra P, Talwar KK, et al. Does endomyocardial biopsy aid in the diagnosis of active rheumatic carditis? *Circulation* 1993; 88(part 1):2198–2205.
33. Virmani R, Farb A, Burke AP, Narula J. Pathology of acute rheumatic carditis. In: Narula J, Virmani R, Reddy KS, Tandon R, eds. *Rheumatic Fever*. Washington, DC: Armed Forces Institute of Pathology; 1999:217–234.
34. Dajani AS, Ayoub E, Bierman FZ, et al. Guidelines for the diagnosis of rheumatic fever: Jones criteria, updated 1992. *JAMA* 1992; 268:2069–2073.
35. Sanyal SK, Thapar MK, Ahmed SH, et al. The initial attack of acute rheumatic fever during childhood in North India: A prospective study of the clinical profile. *Circulation* 1974; 49:7–12.
36. Barlow JB. Aspects of active rheumatic carditis. *Aust N Z J Med* 1992; 22:592–600.
37. Marcus RH, Sareli P, Pocock WA, Barlow JB. The spectrum of severe rheumatic mitral valve disease in a developing country: Correlations among clinical presentation, surgical pathologic findings, and hemodynamic sequelae. *Ann Intern Med* 1994; 120:177–183.
38. Bisno AL. Noncardiac manifestations of rheumatic fever. In: Narula J, Virmani R, Reddy KS, Tandon R, eds. *Rheumatic Fever*. Washington, DC: Armed Forces Institute of Pathology; 1999:245–256.
39. Stollerman GH. *Rheumatic Fever and Streptococcal Infection*. New York: Grune & Stratton; 1975:147–180.
40. Heye N, Jergas M, Hotzinger H, et al. Sydenham chorea: Clinical, EEG, MRI and SPECT findings in the early stage of the disease. *J Neurol* 1993; 240:121–123.
41. Swedo SE. Sydenham's chorea: A model for childhood autoimmune neuropsychiatric disorders. *JAMA* 1994; 272:1788–1791.
42. Stollerman GH, Lewis AJ, Schultz I, Taranta A. Relationship of immune response to group A streptococci to the course of acute, chronic and recurrent rheumatic fever. *Am J Med* 1956; 20:163–169.
43. Krishnan SC, Kushwaha SS, Josephson ME. Electrocardiographic abnormalities and arrhythmias in patients with acute rheumatic fever. In: Narula J, Virmani R, Reddy KS, Tandon R, eds. *Rheumatic Fever*. Washington, DC: Armed Forces Institute of Pathology; 1999:287–298.
44. Minich LL, Tani LY, Veasy LG. Role of echocardiography in the diagnosis and follow-up evaluation of rheumatic fever. In: Narula N, Virmani R, Reddy KS, Tandon R, eds. *Rheumatic Fever*. Washington, DC: Armed Forces Institute of Pathology; 1999:307–318.
45. Vasan RS, Shrivastava S, Vijayakumar M, et al. Echocardiographic evaluation of patients with acute rheumatic fever and rheumatic carditis. *Circulation* 1996; 94:73–82.
46. Marcus RH, Sareli P, Pocock WA, et al. Functional anatomy of severe mitral regurgitation in active rheumatic carditis. *Am J Cardiol* 1989; 63:577–584.
47. Essop MR, Wisenbaugh T, Sareli P. Evidence against a myocardiac factor as the cause of left ventricular dilation in active rheumatic carditis. *J Am Coll Cardiol* 1993; 22:826–829.
48. Narula J, Narula N, Southern JF, Chopra P. Endomyocardial biopsy for the diagnosis of rheumatic carditis. In: Narula J, Virmani R, Reddy KS, Tandon R, eds. *Rheumatic Fever*. Washington, DC: Armed Forces Institute of Pathology; 1999:319–328.
49. Echigo S, Kamiya T, Baba K, et al. A case of congestive cardiomyopathy with histological findings suggesting rheumatic carditis by endomyocardial biopsy. *Jpn Circ J* 1980; 44:823–826.
50. Ursell PC, Alballa A, Fenoglio JJ Jr. Diagnosis of acute rheumatic carditis by endomyocardial biopsy. *Hum Pathol* 1982; 13:677–679.
51. Marboe CC, Knowles DMII, Weiss MB, Fenoglio JJ Jr. Monoclonal antibody identification of mononuclear cells in endomyocardial biopsy specimens from a patient with rheumatic carditis. *Hum Pathol* 1985; 16:332–338.
52. Byck PL, Listinsky CM, Cooper TB, Papapeitro SE. Acute congestive heart failure in a 55-year-old man. Rheumatic carditis diagnosed by endomyocardial biopsy. *Arch Pathol Lab Med* 1990; 114:526–527.
53. Thatai D, Turi ZG. Current guidelines for the treatment of patients with rheumatic fever. *Drugs* 1999; 57:545–555.
54. United Kingdom and United States Joint Report on Rheumatic Heart Disease. The natural history of rheumatic fever and rheumatic heart disease: Ten-year report of a cooperative clinical trial of ACTH, cortisone and aspirin. *Circulation* 1965; 32:457–476.
55. Dajani A, Taubert K, Ferrieri P, et al. Treatment of acute streptococcal pharyngitis and prevention of rheumatic fever: A statement for health professionals. Committee on Rheumatic Fever, Endocarditis, and Kawasaki Disease of the Council on Cardiovascular Disease in the Young, the American Heart Association. *Pediatrics* 1995; 96:758–764.

C H A P T E R 56

AORTIC VALVE DISEASE

Shahbudin H. Rahimtoola

The assessment and management of patients with valvular heart disease has undergone many changes in the past four decades. The incidence of acute rheumatic fever has declined, and as a result rheumatic heart disease is not the most important cause of valve disease in the developed countries. Prolapse of the mitral valve and congenital aortic valve disease are now the most common valvular lesions. Valve surgery has been the major therapeutic advance in treating patients with severe valve disease; in fact, most patients with severe valve disease are now considered candidates for surgery. Echocardiography/Doppler ultrasound has a very important role in the diagnosis and follow-up of these patients. Cardiac catheterization/angiography remains an extremely important diagnostic procedure that is needed in almost all patients being considered for interventional therapy. Catheter balloon valvuloplasty is a useful technique for the treatment of some stenotic cardiac valves.

AORTIC VALVE STENOSIS

Aortic stenosis (AS) is obstruction to outflow of blood flow from the left ventricle to the aorta. The obstruction may be at the valve, above the valve (supravalvular), or below the valve (subvalvular).[1] Supravalvular AS is a congenital lesion. Subvalvular AS results either from a discrete fibromuscular obstruction, which is a congenital lesion, or from a muscular obstruction (hypertrophic cardiomyopathy).

Etiology

The most common causes of AS are congenital,[2,3] rheumatic, and calcific (degenerative) (Table 56-1). Calcific AS is seen in patients 35 years of age or older and is the result of calcification of a congenital or rheumatic valve or of a normal valve that has undergone "degenerative" changes.[4] Recent data suggest that degenerative/calcific AS may represent an immune reaction to antigens present in the valve[5] and is related to atherosclerosis.[6]

Rare causes of AS include obstructive, infective vegetations that are usually large, e.g., those seen in fungal endocarditis. Atherosclerotic AS is seen most frequently in patients with severe hypercholesterolemia and is observed in children and young adults with homozygous type II hyperlipoproteinemia.[7,8] Paget's disease of the bone,[9] end-stage renal disease,[10,11] systemic lupus erythematosus, rheumatoid involvement, ochronosis,[12] and irradiation are other rare causes of AS.

At the present time, calcific AS in the older patient is the most common valve lesion requiring valve replacement.[4,13] Among patients under the age of 70, congenital bicuspid valve accounted for one-half of the surgical cases; degenerative changes were the cause in 18 percent.[4] In contrast, in those aged 70 or older, degenerative changes accounted for almost one-half of the surgical cases and a congenital bicuspid valve for approximately one-quarter of the cases (Fig. 56-1).

Pathology

In congenital AS, the valve may be unicuspid, bicuspid, or tricuspid, depending on the patient's age.[14] In patients under the age of 15 years, over 80 percent of stenotic valves are either unicuspid or bicuspid and 15 to 20 percent are tricuspid. In patients aged 15 to 65 years, 60 percent are bicuspid, 10 percent are unicuspid, and 25 to 30 percent are tricuspid. In patients 65 years of age or over, 90 percent of the valves are tricuspid and 10 percent are bicuspid. Unicuspid valves produce severe obstruction in infancy and are the most frequent malformation found in fatal valvular AS in children under the age of 1 year.[2] Congenital bicuspid valves can produce severe obstruction to left ventricular (LV) outflow after the first few years of life.[3] The valvular abnormality produces turbulent flow, which traumatizes the leaflets and eventually leads to fibrosis, rigidity, and calcification of the valve. In a congenitally abnormal tricuspid aortic valve, the cusps are of unequal size and have some degree of commissural fusion; the third cusp may be diminutive. Eventually, the abnormal structure leads to changes similar to those seen in a bicuspid valve, and significant LV outflow obstruction often results. In calcific AS (so called "degenerative") early

TABLE 56-1 Etiology of Aortic Valve Stenosis

I. Congenital
II. Acquired
  A. Rheumatic
  B. Calcific (degenerative/autoimmune)
  C. Rare causes
    1. Obstructive infective vegetations
    2. Homozygous type II hyperlipoproteinemia
    3. Paget's disease of bone
    4. Systemic lupus erythematosus
    5. Rheumatoid involvement
    6. Ochronosis (alkaptonuria)
    7. Irradiation

changes show chronic inflammatory cell infiltrate (macrophages and T lymphocytes), lipid in lesion and in adjacent fibrosa and thickening of fibrosa with collagen and elastin.[6] These patients also have a higher incidence of risk factors for coronary atherosclerosis.[15]

Rheumatic AS results from adhesions and fusion of the commissures and cusps. The leaflets and the valve ring become vascularized, which leads to retraction and stiffening of the cusps. Calcification occurs, and the aortic valve orifice is reduced to a small triangular or round opening, which is frequently regurgitant as well as stenotic. Importantly, the heart exhibits other evidence of rheumatic heart disease—namely, involvement of the mitral valve and presence of Aschoff's nodules in the myocardium.

Rheumatoid AS is extremely rare and results from nodular thickening of the valve leaflets and the involvement of the proximal part of the aorta. In severe forms of hypercholesterolemia, lipid deposits occur not only in the aortic wall but also in the aortic valve and occasionally produce AS.

The LV is concentrically hypertrophied.[16] The hypertrophied cardiac muscle cells are increased in size, with their transverse diameters ranging from 15 to 70 μm (normal, 10 to 15 μm). There is an increase of connective tissue,[17–19] and a variable amount of fibrous tissue (collagen fibrils) in the interstitial tissue. Usually, the cardiac muscle cells do not degenerate in patients with AS. Myocardial ultrastructural changes[20] may account for the LV systolic dysfunction that occurs late in the disease; such changes include unusually large nuclei, loss of myofibrils, accumulation of mitochondria, large cytoplasmic areas devoid of contractile material, and proliferation of fibroblasts and collagen fibers in the interstitial space.

Subclinical calcific emboli are commonly found in calcific AS if diligently sought at autopsy.

Pathophysiology

With reduction in the *aortic valve area* (AVA), energy is dissipated during the transport of blood from the LV to the aorta. The AVA has to be reduced by about 50 percent of normal before a measurable gradient can be demonstrated in humans.[21] When a pressure gradient develops between the left ventricle and the ascending aorta, LV pressure rises; aortic pressure remains within the normal range until end-stage heart failure occurs. The relationship of the AVA to cardiac output and pressure gradient is discussed in Chap. 57. As LV pressure rises, ventricular wall stress increases, which leads to impaired LV function. The heart normalizes wall stress by becoming hypertrophic. Since AS develops slowly, hypertrophy develops in proportion to increased intraventricular pressure, and myocardial stress remains normal.[22] *Thus, the major compensatory mechanism by which the heart copes with LV outflow obstruction is ventricular hypertrophy*. LV mass in patients with severe AS undergoing valve replacement averages 229 g/m^2 (normal, 105 g/m^2);[22] at autopsy, left ventricles weighing as much as 1000 g have been reported. LV volume, however, is within the normal range,[22] and so there is a considerable thickening of the LV wall.

The diastolic properties of the LV are affected in AS.[23–27] This diastolic abnormality results from a combination of impaired myocardial relaxation with altered chamber compliance because the hypertrophied LV per se offers increased resistance to filling, and from increased myocardial stiffness because of structural alterations.[27] As a result, LV end-diastolic pressure is elevated, but this is not necessarily a measure of LV failure. Powerful atrial contraction produces the required LV filling and results in an elevated LV end-diastolic pressure (atrial booster pump function).[28,29] The necessary LV filling and fiber length to achieve an adequate stroke volume are achieved by atrial systole, which occupies only a small part of the cardiac cycle. Therefore there is a transient increase in left atrial pressure due to the large *a* wave, but mean left atrial pressure remains in the normal range or is only minimally increased (Fig. 56-2).

Left atrial contraction is therefore of considerable benefit to these patients.

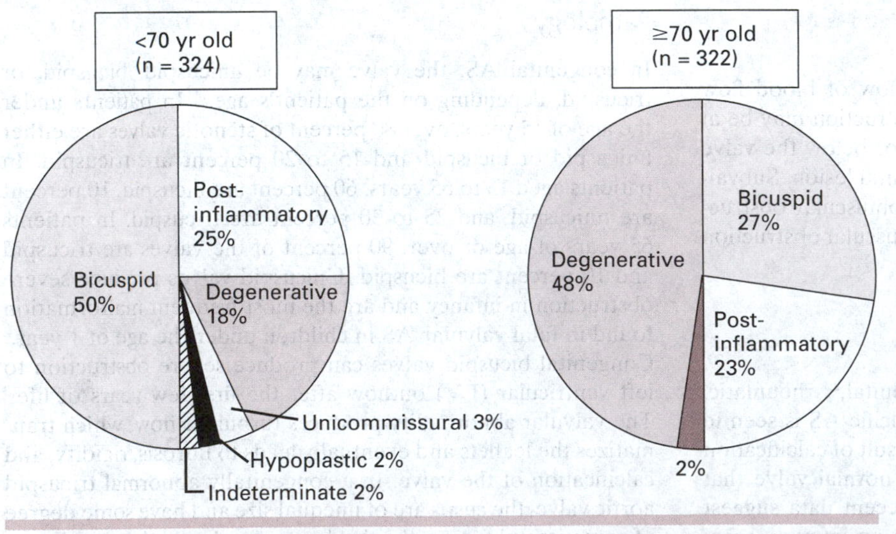

FIGURE 56-1 Etiology of aortic stenosis in patients under the age of 70 years (*left panel*); congenital bicuspid valve accounted for one-half of the surgical cases. In those aged 70 or older (*right panel*), "degenerative" changes accounted for almost one-half of the surgical cases. (From Passik et al.,[4] with permission.)

Loss of effective atrial contraction, either because of atrial fibrillation or because of an inappropriately timed atrial contraction [e.g., that associated with first-degree heart block or with atrioventricular (AV) dissociation], results in elevations of mean left atrial pressure, reduction of cardiac output, or both and may precipitate clinical heart failure with pulmonary congestion.

Patients with severe LV hypertrophy may exhibit LV diastolic dysfunction, which may produce the syndrome of clinical heart failure (paroxysmal nocturnal dyspnea, orthopnea, and even pulmonary edema) even if LV systolic pump function is normal. In patients 60 years of age or older, a higher percentage of women (41 percent) than men (14 percent) have "excessive" hypertrophy, that is, greater amounts of hypertrophy in spite of similar degrees of severity of AS.[30] They have "supernormal" LV systolic pump function (high LV ejection fraction) and a small, thick-walled chamber with lower end-systolic wall stress (Table 56-2).

LV systolic pump function is determined by myocardial (muscle) function and by a combination of LV afterload and preload. Thus, impaired LV systolic pump function (as measured by ejection fraction) may be the result of afterload-preload mismatch,[31] impaired myocardial function, or both. LV systolic pump function is normal in most patients with severe AS. When the LV hypertrophy alone is not adequate to overcome the outflow obstruction, the left ventricle uses the Frank-Starling mechanism (preload reserve) to maintain systolic pump function. When the preload reserve is no longer adequate, a reduction of LV systolic pump function occurs (Fig. 56-2). In AS, major use of the preload reserve is not a good compensatory mechanism. Even small increases in LV volume may result in major increases in LV end-diastolic pressure because the LV is on the very steep portion of its diastolic pressure-volume curve, and the corresponding increase in mean left atrial pressure produces pulmonary edema. Thus, clinical heart failure may be a result of either LV diastolic dysfunction in the presence of normal LV systolic function or impaired myocardial function producing LV systolic dysfunction, with or without associated LV diastolic dysfunction. Eventually, pulmonary artery, right ventricular, and right atrial pressures are elevated. Peripheral edema results from increases in systemic venous pressure and salt and water retention.

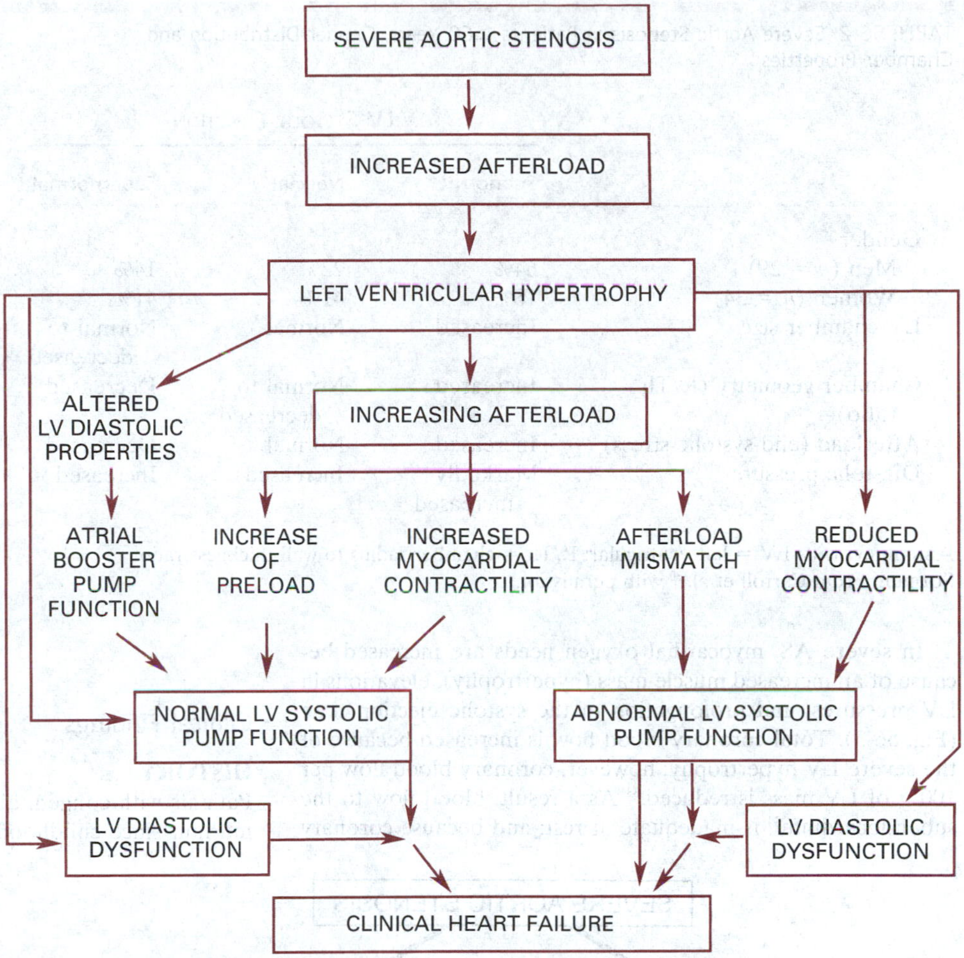

FIGURE 56-2 Illustration of some aspects of the pathophysiology in severe aortic stenosis (see text). The heart responds to AS by hypertrophy, and LV systolic pump function remains normal. LV hypertrophy may alter the LV diastolic properties. As a result, LV end-diastolic pressure is elevated; but powerful atrial contraction produces the required LV filling and fiber length (atrial booster pump function).

As LV afterload continues to increase, the LV uses two additional compensatory mechanisms, namely, increase of preload and increase of myocardial contractility. Both of these help maintain normal LV systolic pump function.

When the limit of the preload reserve has been reached (afterload mismatch) or myocardial contractility is reduced, LV systolic pump function becomes abnormal.

Clinical heart failure is usually a result of abnormal LV systolic pump function; diastolic dysfunction may also be present in some patients. Clinical heart failure in those with normal LV systolic pump function is a result of LV diastolic dysfunction. (Copyright © by S. H. Rahimtoola, M.B., F.R.C.P., M.A.C.P., M.A.C.C. See Ref. 93.)

In most patients with AS, cardiac output is in the normal range and initially increases normally with exercise. Later, as the severity of AS increases progressively, the cardiac output remains within the normal range at rest, but, on exercise, it no longer increases in proportion to the amount of exercise undertaken or does not increase at all (fixed cardiac output). With the development of heart failure, there is a reduction in the resting cardiac output and a tachycardia. As a result, stroke volume may be so lowered that it results in a small gradient across the LV outflow tract in spite of severe AS. As the patient's age increases, there is a progressive decrease of cardiac output with exercise and a progressive increase of LV end-diastolic pressure at equal levels of AVA. This may be related only to LV diastolic dysfunction and is most marked in the older patient.[32]

TABLE 56-2 Severe Aortic Stenosis in Patients ≥60 Years, Gender Distribution and Chamber Properties

	LV Systolic Function		
	Subnormal	Normal	Supernormal
Gender			
Men (n = 29)	64%	22%	14%
Women (n = 34)	18%	41%	41%
LV chamber size	Increased	Normal	Normal to decreased
Chamber geometry (R/Th ratio)	Increased	Normal to decreased	Decreased
Afterload (end-systolic stress)	Increased	Normal	Decreased
Diastolic pressure	Markedly increased	Increased	Increased

Abbreviations: LV = left ventricular; R/Th = chamber radius to wall thickness ratio.
Source: From Carroll et al.,[30] with permission.

In severe AS, myocardial oxygen needs are increased because of an increased muscle mass (hypertrophy), elevations in LV pressures, and prolongation of the systolic ejection time (Fig. 56-3). Total coronary blood flow is increased because of the severe LV hypertrophy; however, coronary blood flow per 100 g of LV mass is reduced.[33] As a result, blood flow to the subendocardium[34] is inadequate at rest; and because coronary vasodilator reserve is reduced,[35] myocardial blood flow is also reduced further, relative to need, on exercise. Coronary blood flow is reduced because of a reduced coronary perfusion pressure (the elevated LV end-diastolic pressure lowers the diastolic aortic-LV pressure gradient) and also because the hypertrophied myocardium compresses the coronary arteries as they traverse the myocardium to supply blood to the subendocardium (systolic "milking" of intramural arteries). As a result, patients may have classic angina pectoris even in the absence of *coronary artery disease* (CAD). Associated obstructive CAD from atherosclerosis further increases the imbalance between myocardial oxygen needs and supply (Fig. 56-2).

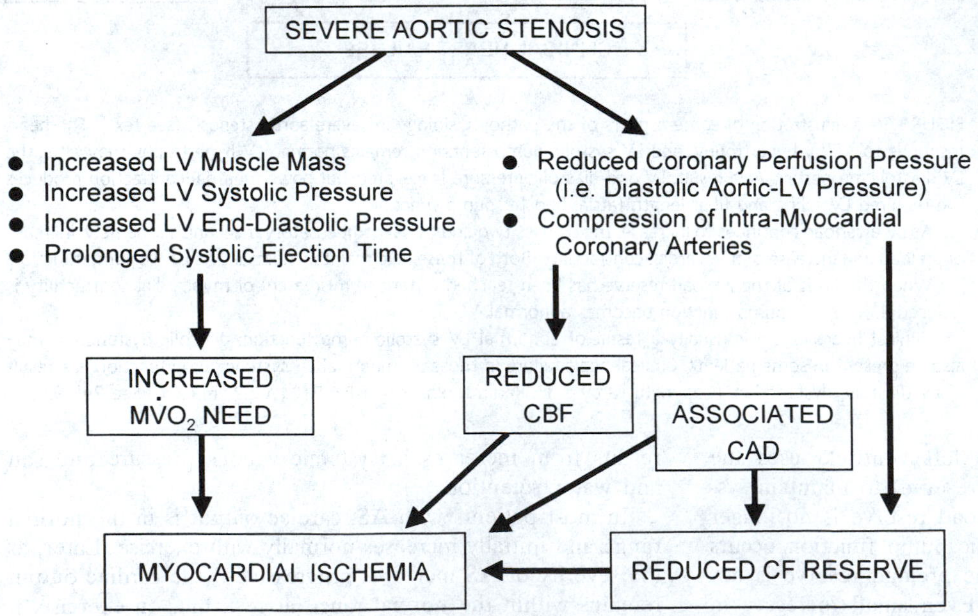

FIGURE 56-3 In severe aortic stenosis, myocardial oxygen needs are increased because of increased muscle mass (hypertrophy), increases in LV pressures, and prolongation of the systolic ejection time. Total coronary blood flow is increased; however, coronary blood flow per 100 g of LV mass is reduced because of a reduction in diastolic aortic-LV pressure gradient and "systolic milking" of the coronary arteries in the hypertrophied LV as they traverse the myocardium from the epicardium to endocardium to supply the subendocardial myocardial region. Thus, these patients may have myocardial ischemia, particularly in the subendocardial region. Coronary vasodilator reserve, i.e., the ability of the coronary blood flow to increase with vasodilatation, is also significantly reduced, and thus the myocardial ischemia can be markedly exacerbated on effort. Associated obstructive coronary artery disease can be expected to further exacerbate the myocardial ischemia. (Copyright © by S. H. Rahimtoola, M.B., F.R.C.P., M.A.C.P., M.A.C.C. See Ref. 93.)

Clinical Findings

HISTORY

Patients with congenital valve stenosis may give a history of a murmur since childhood or infancy; those with rheumatic stenosis may have a history of rheumatic fever. Most patients with valvular AS, including some with severe valve stenosis, are asymptomatic. The symptoms of AS are angina pectoris, syncope, exertional presyncope, dyspnea (on exertion, orthopnea, paroxysmal nocturnal dyspnea, pulmonary edema), and the symptoms of heart failure. Once symptoms occur in a patient with severe AS, the life span of the patient is very short without surgical treatment. Sudden cardiac death is stated to occur in 5 percent of patients with AS. It occurs only in those with severe valve stenosis, most of whom have had some cardiac symptoms before the fatal episode. Typical angina pectoris occurs with or without associated CAD and results from an imbalance between myocardial oxygen needs and supply (Fig. 56-3).

Syncope is the result of reduced cerebral perfusion. Syncope occurring on effort is caused by either systemic vasodilatation in the presence of a fixed or inadequate cardiac output, an arrhythmia, or both.[36-38] Syncope at rest is usually due to a transient ventricular tachyarrhythmia, from which the patient recovers spontaneously. Other possible causes of syncope include transient atrial fibrillation or transient AV block, during which the ventricle is deprived of the powerful atrial booster pump function and/or the ventricular rate is slow.

Dyspnea on exertion, orthopnea, paroxysmal nocturnal dyspnea, and pulmonary edema result from varying degrees of pulmonary venous hypertension. Systemic venous congestion with enlargement of the liver and peripheral edema result from increased systemic venous pressure and salt and water retention. There is an increased incidence of gastrointestinal arteriovenous malformations.[39,40] As a result, these patients are susceptible to gastrointestinal hemorrhage and anemia. Calcific systemic embolism may occur.[41,42]

PHYSICAL FINDINGS

There is a spectrum of physical findings in patients with AS, depending on the severity of the stenosis, stroke volume, LV function, and the rigidity and calcification of the valve (Table 56-3). The arterial pulse rises slowly, taking a longer time than normal to reach peak pressure, and the peak is reduced (*parvus et tardus*);[43] the pulse pressure may be narrowed. The anacrotic notch on the upstroke is best appreciated in the carotid arteries. The more severe the valve stenosis, the lower the anacrotic notch on the arterial pulse. A systolic thrill may be felt in the carotid arteries. The jugular venous pulse is normal unless the patient is in heart failure. In the absence of heart failure, the heart size is normal. The cardiac impulse is heaving and sustained in character, and there may be a palpable fourth heart sound (S_4). An aortic systolic thrill is often present at the base of the heart. In 80 to 90 percent of adult patients with severe AS, there is an S_4 gallop sound, a midsystolic ejection murmur that peaks late in systole, and a single second heart sound (S_2) because A_2 and P_2 are superimposed or A_2 is absent or soft. There is often a faint early diastolic murmur of minimal aortic regurgitation. In the young patient with valvular AS, a systolic ejection sound (systolic ejection click) initiates the systolic murmur but later tends to disappear as AS becomes severe. The S_2 may be paradoxically split due to late A_2, and there may be no early diastolic murmur. In many patients, particularly the elderly, the systolic ejection murmur is atypical, may be soft, is described as a seagull sound (or musical, or cooing), and may be heard only at the apex of the heart (Gallavardin phenomenon). In the presence of heart failure, the jugular venous pressure is often increased, the left ventricle is dilated, a third heart sound is present, and the systolic murmur may be very soft or absent. Thus, the clinical features on physical examination may resemble those of heart failure from a variety of causes, such as dilated cardiomyopathy, rather than AS (see also Chap. 10).

Severe valvular AS is common in patients 60 years of age or older.[13,44] The clinical features in many of these patients tend to be somewhat different from those typical of younger patients.[44] Systemic hypertension is common, being present in about 20 percent of the patients, half of whom have moderate or severe systolic and diastolic hypertension. A fifth of the patients first present in congestive heart failure. The male: female ratio is 2:1. Because of thickening of the arterial wall and its associated lack of dispensability, the arterial pulse rises normally or even rapidly, and the pulse pressure is wide. The S_2 is either absent or single. As noted above, the murmur may be high-pitched and musical and may radiate from the base to the apex or may be heard best at the apex, mimicking mitral regurgitation.

CHEST X-RAY

The characteristic finding is a normal-sized heart with a dilated proximal ascending aorta (poststenotic dilation). Calcium in the aortic valve can be seen on the lateral film but is better appreciated by fluoroscopy with image intensification. In the current era, calcification is most easily recognized on two-

TABLE 56-3 Physical Examination of Patients with Varying Severity of Aortic Valve Stenosis

	Mild	Moderate	Severe + Normal LV Function	Severe + LV Dysfunction	Severe + Heart Failure[a]
Arterial pulse	Normal	Slowly rising	*Parvus et tardus*	*Parvus et tardus*	Small volume
Jugular venous pulse	Normal	Normal	Normal	Normal	±
Carotid thrill	±	±	±	±	±
Cardiac impulse	Normal	Heaving	Heaving, sustained palpable *a* wave	Heaving	Heaving or reduced
Precordial thrill	±	±	Usually ++	±	−
Auscultation					
S_4	−	±	++	+	−
S_3	−	−	−	±	+
ESS	+	±	−	−	−
Peak of ESM	Early systole	Mid-systole	Late systole	Late to mid-systole, soft	Mid-systole, soft or absent
S_2	Normal	Normal or single	Single or paradoxical	Single	Single

[a]There may be signs of mitral and tricuspid regurgitation and of pulmonary hypertension.

ABBREVIATIONS: S_4 = fourth heart sounds (presystolic gallop); S_3 = third heart sound (diastolic gallop); ESS = ejection systolic sound; ESM = ejection systolic murmur; S_2 = second heart sound.

dimensional echocardiography. Calcium in the aortic valve is the hallmark of AS in adults 40 to 45 years of age.[45,46] In patients aged 45 years or above, the diagnosis of severe AS is doubtful if there is no calcium in the aortic valve. The presence of calcium, however, does not necessarily mean that the valve is stenotic or that the AS is severe. In patients with heart failure, the cardiac size is increased because of dilatation of the left ventricle and left atrium; the lung fields show pulmonary edema and pulmonary venous congestion with redistribution of blood flow. In the presence of heart failure, the right ventricle and the right atrium may be dilated.

ELECTROCARDIOGRAM

The *electrocardiogram* (ECG) in severe AS shows LV hypertrophy with or without secondary ST-T-wave changes. It is important to recognize, however, that in about 10 to 15 percent of patients with severe AS, LV hypertrophy cannot be appreciated on the ECG. In fact, the ECG may be entirely normal in some of these patients. The P-wave abnormality (P = 0.12 s) of left atrial enlargement and/or hypertrophy and/or conduction delay is present in over 80 percent.[47] The ECG may show left bundle branch block, right bundle branch block with left or right axis deviation, or, occasionally, isolated right bundle branch block.[48–50] In some patients, the conduction abnormality results from aortic valve calcification extending into the specialized conducting tissue, which may even produce heart block. The patients are usually in sinus rhythm. The presence of atrial fibrillation indicates the presence of either associated mitral valve disease, CAD, or heart failure secondary to aortic valve disease. Atrial fibrillation is relatively common in the elderly with calcific AS, probably because of the increased presence of associated diseases.

Laboratory Investigations

ECHOCARDIOGRAPHY/DOPPLER ULTRASOUND

Echocardiography/Doppler (echo/Doppler) ultrasound (Chap. 13) is an extremely important and useful noninvasive test. On the echocardiogram, the aortic valve leaflets normally are barely visible in systole, and the normal range of aortic valve opening is 1.6 to 2.6 cm. In the presence of a bicuspid aortic valve, eccentric valve leaflets may be seen. The aortic valve leaflets may appear to be thickened as a result of calcification and/or fibrosis; however, the older patient without valve stenosis may also have thickened cusps. The aortic valve may have a reduced opening, but this also occurs in other conditions in which the cardiac output is reduced. The LV hypertrophy often results in thickening of both the interventricular septum and the posterior LV wall. The LV cavity size is normal. All these abnormalities are better appreciated on two-dimensional echocardiography. When LV systolic function is impaired, the left ventricle and left atrium are dilated and the percentage of dimensional shortening is reduced.

In many patients, the severity of AS is incorrectly estimated by M-mode or two-dimensional echocardiography. Neither is a completely reliable technique for assessing the severity of AS. The presence of normal movement of thin aortic leaflets on the echocardiogram, however, is strong evidence against severe AS in adults.

Echo/Doppler, when properly applied, is extremely useful for estimating the valve gradient and AVA noninvasively.[50–56] When compared with results obtained at cardiac catheterization, the standard error of the estimate of mean gradient in the best laboratories is 10 mmHg.[57] Thus, the mean gradient by Doppler can be expected to be within ±20 mmHg (95 percent confidence level) of that obtained at catheterization.[57] Similarly, the AVA will be within ±0.3 cm^2 of that obtained at cardiac catheterization.[57] A recent study of 156 patients compared AVA obtained by cardiac catheterization with that obtained by Doppler ultrasound.[58] Of 125 patients with AVA 0.8 cm^2 at cardiac catheterization, in 36 (29 percent) Doppler-estimated AVA was ≥0.9 cm^2. In all 7 patients with AVA >1.0 cm^2 by cardiac catheterization, Doppler-estimated AVA was 1.0 cm^2; the findings in these 7 patients must be interpreted cautiously because they were likely to be a highly selected subgroup. Guidelines for assessing severity of AS based on Doppler-obtained gradients are shown in Table 56-4. In a study of 636 patients studied by cardiac catheterization, no single aortic valve gradient was found to be both sensitive and specific for severe AS. A mean gradient of ≥50 mmHg or a peak gradient ≥60 mmHg were "specific" with a 90 percent or more positive predictive value. It was not possible to find a lower limit with 90 percent negative predictive value.[59] Thus, a mean gradient of <50 mmHg is compatible with mild, moderate, or severe AS.

TABLE 56-4 Suggested Conservative Guidelines for Relating Severity of Aortic Stenosis to Doppler Gradients in Adults with Normal Cardiac Output and Normal Average Heart Rate

Peak Gradient, mmHg	Mean Gradient, mmHg	Severe AS
≥80	≥70	Highly likely
60–79	50–69	Probable
<60	<50	Uncertain

SOURCE: From Rahimtoola,[57] with permission.

Transesophageal echo/Doppler ultrasound is very useful in defining the aortic valve abnormality and in assessing its severity when an adequate examination cannot be obtained with the transthoracic technique.

CARDIAC CATHETERIZATION/ANGIOGRAPHY

Cardiac catheterization remains the standard technique to assess the severity of AS "accurately." This is done by measuring simultaneous LV and ascending aortic pressures and measuring

TABLE 56-5 A Suggested Grading of the Degree of Aortic Stenosis

Aortic Stenosis	AVA, cm^2	AVA Index, cm^2/m^2
Mild	>1.5	>0.9
Moderate	>1.0–1.5	>0.6–0.9
Severe[a]	≤0.8–1.0	≤0.4–0.6

[a]Patients with AVAs that are at borderline values between the moderate and severe grades (0.9–1.1 cm^2; 0.55–0.65 cm^2/m^2) should be considered individually.

ABBREVIATIONS: AVA = aortic valve area.

SOURCE: From Rahimtoola,[57] with permission.

TABLE 56-6 Aortic Valve Disease: Indications for Coronary Arteriography

Patients ≥35 years
Patients <35 years:
- Left ventricular dysfunction
- Symptoms or signs suggesting CAD
- Two or more risk factors for premature CAD (excluding gender)

ABBREVIATIONS: CAD = coronary artery disease.
SOURCE: From Rahimtoola,[57] with permission.

cardiac output by either the Fick principle or the indicator dilution technique. The AVA can be calculated (see Chap. 15). It is important to calculate AVA.[59] AS can be considered to be severe when the valve area is 1.0 cm^2 or less or the AVA index is 0.6 cm^2 per square meter or less (Table 56-5).[57] The state of LV systolic pump function can be quantitated by measuring LV end-diastolic and end-systolic volumes and ejection fraction. *It must be recognized that ejection fraction may underestimate myocardial function in the presence of the increased afterload of severe AS.*

The presence of CAD and its site and severity can be estimated only by selective coronary angiography, which should be performed in all patients 35 years of age or older being considered for valve surgery and in those <35 years if they have LV systolic dysfunction, symptoms or signs suggesting CAD, or two or more risk factors for premature CAD (excluding gender) (Table 56-6). The incidence of associated CAD will vary considerably depending on the prevalence of CAD in the population.[57,60] It was reported to be 50 percent in patients with AS and 20 percent in patients with aortic regurgitation.[57] In general, in persons 50 years of age or older, it is about 50 percent (Table 56-7).[44,61–63]

TABLE 56-7 Isolated Aortic Valve Replacement: Incidence of Associated Coronary Artery Disease

	VA Co-op Study[a]	Mayo Clinic[b]	MGH[c] (80–89 years)
Total number of patients	643	618	64
Patients with coronary artery disease	312	321	37
%	49%	52%	58%
1 VD	17%	22%	27%
2 VD	17%	14%	19%
3 VD	15%	17%	13%
Additional LMCAD	—	5%	3%

[a]Sethi GK et al.[61]
[b]Mullany CJ et al.[62]
[c]Levinson JR et al.[63]
ABBREVIATIONS: LMCAD = left main coronary artery disease; MGH = Massachusetts General Hospital; VA = Veterans Administration; VD = vessel disease.

GATED BLOOD POOL RADIONUCLIDE SCANS

Gated blood pool radionuclide scans provide information on ventricular function similar to that provided by two-dimensional echocardiography and LV cineangiography. These studies are of particular value in the occasional patient in whom LV cineangiography is unsuccessful and echocardiographic studies are suboptimal.

EXERCISE TESTS

It is usually recommended that exercise tests of any kind not be undertaken in patients with severe AS unless there is a specific reason for such studies. Exercise tests in these patients may precipitate ventricular tachyarrhythmias and ventricular fibrillation. If there is doubt about the severity of AS and concern that the patient's symptoms may not be caused by AS, it is usually wise to document the absence of severe AS before performing an exercise test. Occasionally, in a patient with severe AS who denies all symptoms, a closely monitored exercise test by experienced and skilled physician(s) may be needed to assess exercise capacity but should usually *only* be undertaken after exclusion of associated significantly obstructive CAD.

AMBULATORY ECG RECORDING

Ambulatory ECG recordings may be needed in an occasional patient suspected of having an arrhythmia[64,65] or painless ischemia. Occasionally, patients with mild or moderate AS who are symptomatic may be suspected of having an arrhythmia or painless ischemia as a cause of the symptoms. At times, in asymptomatic patients with severe AS, one may need to determine if the patient has painless ischemia (see also Chap. 25).

PROVOCATIVE DIAGNOSTIC TEST

In an occasional patient, the severity of the AS may be in doubt because of a small stroke volume and small mean aortic valve gradient. The AS may be severe or mild to moderate, and the calculated AVA may be very small because of severe stenosis or because the small stroke volume only opens the valve to a limited extent; thus, the AVA will be determined to be small even on echo/Doppler ultrasound. Infusion of an inotropic agent such as dobutamine, which results in increases of stroke volume and heart rate, usually helps one to make a correct diagnosis. In these circumstances, it is important to measure cardiac output and LV and aortic pressures simultaneously and meticulously, both before and during dobutamine infusion. Whether the AS is mild or severe the gradient increases with dobutamine infusion; however, in mild AS the AVA increases significantly; but in severe AS the AVA does not increase or increases minimally (approximately 10 percent).

Clinical Decision Making

There are a number of steps involved in clinical decision making in patients with valvular heart disease (Table 56-8).[57] The first is a complete clinical evaluation, which includes history, physical examination, ECG, and chest x-ray. Next, disease of all cardiac valves, ventricular function, and hemodynamic effects as well as CAD, other cardiovascular disease, and disease of other organs should be diagnosed and the severity assessed. Before proceeding to additional testing, it is important to list the question(s) to be answered and to be reasonably certain that these

TABLE 56-8 Steps in Clinical Decision Making in Patients with Valvular Heart Disease

1. Perform a complete clinical evaluation
   History
   Physical examination
   Electrocardiogram
   Chest x-ray film
2. Diagnose and assess severity of disease
   All valves
   Ventricular function
   Hemodynamic effects
   Coronary artery disease
   Other cardiovascular disease
   Effects on other body organs
   Other organ diseases
3. List questions that need answering
4. Be reasonably certain these questions need to be answered
5. Perform test(s) most likely to provide these answers in one's own institution with the following criteria:
   Reliability
   Accuracy
   Lowest risk to patients
   Reasonable (or lowest) cost
6. Review results of test(s)
7. Make an overall assessment of patient
8. Make recommendations regarding management

SOURCE: From Rahimtoola,[57] with permission.

questions need to be answered. The test(s) that are most likely to provide these answers *in the clinician's own institution* should then be performed, with the following criteria being kept in mind: reliability, accuracy, lowest risk to patient, and reasonable (lowest) cost. The results of the test(s) should be reviewed as they become available, and an overall evaluation/assessment of the patient and, finally, recommendations regarding management should be made.

In a prospective, blinded study of consecutive patients with valvular heart disease, the sensitivity and specificity of diagnosis of AS and the accuracy of assessment of severity of AS were determined (Table 56-9).[66] This study revealed the following important points: (1) Clinical evaluation was sensitive, highly specific, and reasonably accurate in diagnosing AS and was very accurate in assessing its severity when AS was moderate or severe. This emphasizes the importance of a thorough clinical evaluation of the patient. (2) Echo/Doppler ultrasound improved the accuracy of this assessment to a certain extent. (3) The reason clinical evaluation and echo/Doppler do not have a 100 percent specificity is the inability in an occasional patient to distinguish mild AS from turbulence across a normal or slightly diseased aortic valve. (4) Both clinical evaluation and echo/Doppler ultrasound are excellent in diagnosing the AS as being at least moderate or severe. (5) An important difficulty in diagnosis by clinical evaluation and by echo/Doppler is in not being able to separate accurately all patients with moderate AS from those with severe AS.

TABLE 56-9 Clinical Decision Making Utilizing Clinical Evaluation and Echo/Doppler in Patients with Aortic Stenosis

	After Clinical Evaluation, %	After Echo/Doppler, %
Diagnosis of AS		
Sensitivity	78	100
Specificity	92	92
Accuracy of diagnosis		
All levels of severity	48	65
Moderate or severe AS	100	100

SOURCE: From Kotlewski et al.,[66] with permission.

Natural History and Prognosis

Valvular AS is frequently a progressive disease, the severity increasing over time.[67–71] The factors that control this progression and the time it takes for severe outflow obstruction to develop are unknown; however, it appears that in the older patient, AS may progress at about twice the rate that it does in the younger patient.[72] In a study of 142 patients with "mild" stenosis (catheterization-proven AVA >1.5 cm^2),[73] the rate of progression to severe stenosis was 8 percent in 10 years, 22 percent in 20 years, and 38 percent in 25 years. At 25 years, 38 percent still had mild AS (Table 56-10). The duration of the asymptomatic period after the development of severe AS is also unknown; some recent data suggest that it may be less than 2 years. The outcome of the asymptomatic patient with severe AS is not known. In the study of 123 asymptomatic patients aged 63 ± 16 years, the actuarial probability of death or aortic valve surgery was 7 ± 5 percent at 1 year, 38 ± 8 percent at 3 years, and 74 ± 10 percent at 5 years.[74] The event rate at 2 years for peak aortic jet velocity by Doppler ultrasound of >4 m/s was 79 ± 18 percent, for 3 to 4 m/s was 66 ± 13 percent, and for <3 m/s was 16 ± 16 percent. However, the limitations of gradients and of aortic peak velocity obtained by Doppler ultrasound should be kept in mind.[75] The overwhelming majority of adults with severe AS who are seen by cardiologists have symptoms.

Severe disease in adults is lethal, particularly if the patient is symptomatic, with a prognosis that is worse than for many forms of neoplastic disease.[57] The 3-year mortality is approximately 36 to 52 percent, the 5-year mortality is about 52 to 80 percent, and the 10-year mortality is 80 to 90 percent.[57] A recent study of elderly patients (average age 77 years) showed 1-year and 3-year mortalities were 44 and 75 percent, respectively.[76] With the onset of severe symptoms (angina, syncope, or heart

TABLE 56-10 Natural History of Mild[a] Aortic Stenosis (n = 142)

	10 Years	20 Years	25 Years
Mild	88%	63%	38%
Moderate	4%	15%	25%
Severe	8%	22%	38%

[a]Mild stenosis is defined here as an aortic valve area >1.5 cm^2.
SOURCE: From Horstkotte and Loogen,[73] with permission.

TABLE 56-11 Average Survival of Symptomatic Patients with Severe AS

	Autopsy Data,[a] Years	Post Cardiac Catheterization,[b] Months
Overall	3	23
Angina	5	45
Syncope	3	27
Heart failure	<2	11

[a]From Ross and Braunwald.[77]
[b]From Horstkotte and Loogen.[73]

failure), the average life expectancy is 2 to 3 years (Table 56-11).[73,77] Almost all patients with heart failure are dead in 1 to 2 years.[73,77] A combination of symptoms is much more ominous, a sign of a greatly reduced survival. Sudden death, like syncope, occurs in the presence of severe AS. Its exact incidence is difficult to determine but may be about 5 percent.[77] Most but not all of these patients have had some cardiac symptoms before the fatal episode; at times, the only symptom has been exertional presyncope. Patients with aortic valve "sclerosis" have an approximately 50 percent increase in cardiovascular mortality and myocardial infarction.[78] This incidence is lower than in patients with AS, and aortic sclerosis appears to be a marker for vascular atherosclerosis.

Management

All patients with AS need antibiotic prophylaxis against infective endocarditis (see Chap. 73). Those in whom the valve lesion is of rheumatic origin need additional prophylaxis against recurrence of rheumatic fever. Patients with mild or moderate stenosis rarely have symptoms or complications and do not need any specific medical therapy (Table 56-12). In mild stenosis, the patient should be encouraged to lead a normal life. Those with moderate AS should avoid moderate to severe physical exertion and competitive sports. In patients with mild or moderate AS, if atrial fibrillation should occur, it should be reverted rapidly to sinus rhythm. In severe AS, reversion to sinus rhythm often becomes a matter of some urgency.

Operation should be advised for the symptomatic patient who has severe AS. In young patients, if the valve is pliable and mobile, simple commissurotomy or valve repair may be feasible; the operative mortality is <1 percent.[79] It will relieve outflow obstruction to a major degree. In such patients, catheter balloon valvuloplasty is the procedure of choice in experienced and skilled centers. Both of these are palliative procedures that postpone valve replacement for many years. Older patients and even young patients with calcified, rigid valves need valve replacement. The natural history of symptomatic patients with severe AS is dismal, i.e., a 10-year mortality of 80 to 90 percent, but there is good outcome after surgery, particularly in patients without any comorbid cardiac and noncardiac conditions. Given the unknown natural history of the asymptomatic patient with severe AS, which may not be benign,[57] it is reasonable to recommend surgery even to the asymptomatic patient. There is, however, no consensus about valve replacement in the truly asymptomatic patient. Clearly, if the patient has LV dysfunction, then valve replacement should be performed. Some recommend

TABLE 56-12 Medical Treatment of Patients with Aortic Valve Stenosis

I. Antibiotic prophylaxis
   A. Infective endocarditis (Chap. 82)
   B. Recurrent rheumatic carditis (Chap. 62)
II. Restriction of activities
   A. Severe exercise
   B. Competitive sports
III. Arrhythmias
   A. Prevent and/or control
   B. Restore sinus rhythm, if possible
IV. Cardiac medications (only if essential)
   A. Avoid negative inotropic and proarrhythmic agents if possible
   B. Diuretics—use cautiously
   C. Arteriolar and venodilators—use cautiously
V. Follow-up of asymptomatic patients
   A. Mild AS: Every 2–5 years
   B. Moderate AS: Every 6–12 months
   C. Develop symptoms: Immediate

TABLE 56-13 Severe Aortic Valve Stenosis: Indications for Surgery

I. All symptomatic patients
   A. LV function normal: as soon as possible
   B. LV dysfunction: urgent
   C. Heart failure: emergent
II. Asymptomatic patients
   A. Patients undergoing surgery for CAD, aorta, other valves
   B. Associated significantly obstructed CAD
   C. LV dysfunction
   D. Progressive decline of LVEF
   E. Marked or excessive LVH:
      1. ≥11–12 mm in smaller people, e.g., women
      2. ≥13–14 mm in larger people, e.g., men
   F. Patients aged ≥60–65 years
   G. "Very" severe AS ≤0.7 cm^2; 0.4 cm^2/m^2
   H. Others:
      1. Abnormal response to exercise
         a. Hypotension/no or minimal increase of BP
         b. Ischemia
         c. LV dysfunction
         d. Arrhythmias
      2. Arrhythmias
         a. Ventricular/Atrial tachyarrhythmias
         b. A-V block >1° AVB

ABBREVIATIONS: LV = left ventricular; AVA = aortic valve area; CAD = Coronary artery disease.

TABLE 56-14 Aortic Valve Replacement (AVR) Operative Mortality and Late Survival: Effect of Coronary Bypass Surgery (CBS)

	1982–1983	1967–1976					
	Operative Mortality, %	Operative Mortality, %	All Patients, %	1 VD, %	2 VD, %	3 VD, %	LMCAD, %
AVR + no CAD	1.4	4.5	63	—	—	—	—
AVR + CAD + CBS	4.0	6.3	49	38	28	34	11
AVR + CAD + no CBS	9.4	10.3	36	65	22	13	1

ABBREVIATIONS: CAD = coronary artery disease, VD = vessel disease, LMCAD = left main coronary artery disease.
SOURCE: From Mullany et al.,[62] with permission.

valve replacement in all asymptomatic patients with severe AS, while others would recommend it in those with AVA ≤0.7 cm² and in selected patients with AVA of 0.76 to 1.0 cm² (Table 56-13).

The operative mortality of valve replacement is about 5 percent or less (see Chap. 61).[57,61,62] In patients without associated CAD, heart failure, or other comorbid factors, it may be 1 to 2 percent in centers with experienced and skilled staff.[62] Patients with associated CAD should have coronary bypass surgery at the same time as valve surgery because it results in a lower operative and late mortality (Table 56-14). The operative mortality in octogenarians or older is much higher: up to 6 percent for isolated aortic valve replacement and up to 10 percent for those undergoing aortic valve replacement and associated coronary bypass surgery.

In severe AS, valve replacement results in an improvement of survival (Fig. 56-4),[73,80] even in those with normal preoperative LV function. LV function remains normal postoperatively if perioperative myocardial damage has not occurred.[22,57,81,82] LV hypertrophy regresses toward normal;[22,57,81,82] after 2 years, the regression continues at a slower rate for up to 8 to 10 years after valve replacement.[82] In those with excessive LV hypertrophy preoperatively,[30] the hypertrophy may regress slowly or not at all. These patients may have persistent severe LV diastolic dysfunction, which may be a difficult clinical problem both in the early postoperative period and after hospital discharge. Their clinical picture subsequently resembles that of patients with hypertrophic cardiomyopathy without outflow obstruction, and they may have to be treated as such. Surviving patients are functionally improved. After aortic valve replacement, the 10-year survival is 60 percent or better and the 15-year survival is 45 percent or better.[83] Approximately one-half of the late deaths are not related to the prosthesis but to associated cardiac abnormalities and other comorbid conditions.[83] Thus, the late survival will vary in different subgroups of patients. The older patients (≥65 years) have a relative 10-year survival (actual survival compared to an age- and gender-matched person in the population) after valve replacement that is significantly better than that of those who are younger (<65 years)—94 percent versus 81 percent (Fig. 56-5).[84]

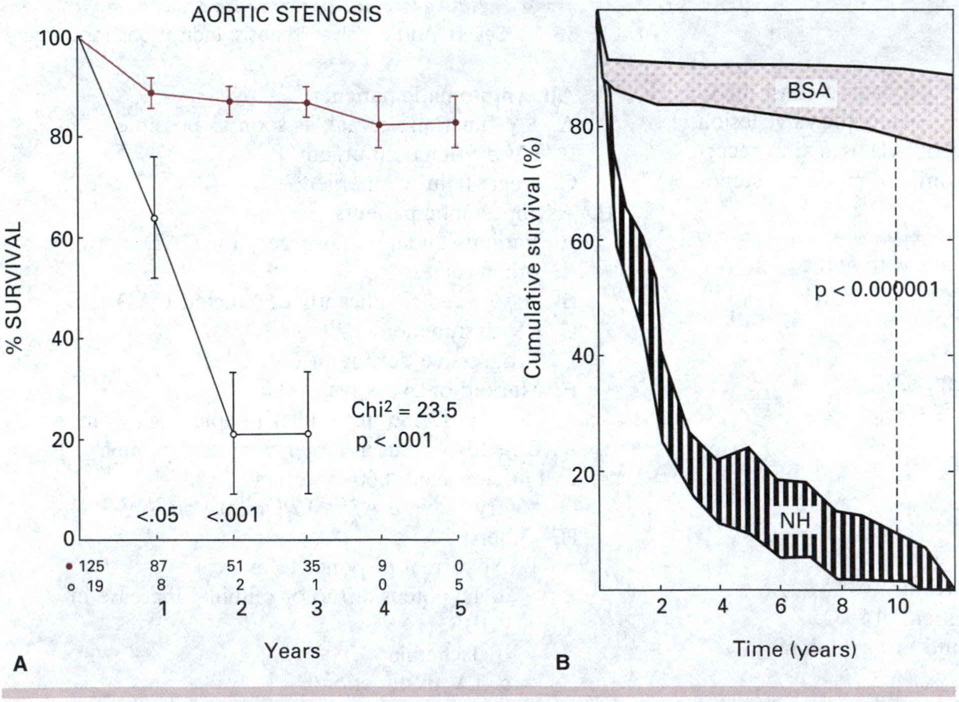

FIGURE 56-4 There are no prospective randomized trials of aortic valve replacement in severe aortic stenosis, and there are unlikely to be any in the near future. Two studies have compared the results of aortic valve replacement with medical treatment during the same time period in symptomatic patients with normal LV systolic pump function. *Panel A.* Patients who had valve replacement (*closed circles*) had a much better survival than those treated medically (*open circles*). (From Schwarz et al.,[80] with permission.)

Panel B. Patients who were treated with valve replacement (BSA) had a better survival than those treated medically (NH). (From Horstkotte and Loogen,[73] with permission.)

These differences in survival between those treated medically and surgically are so large that there is a great deal of confidence that aortic valve replacement significantly improves the survival of those with severe AS.

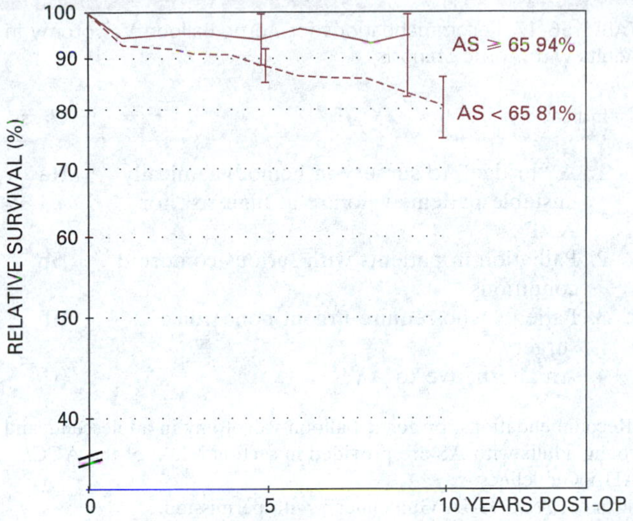

FIGURE 56-5 Data from the Karolinska Institute in Sweden provided an interesting perspective on the long-term survival after valve replacement in patients aged ≥65 years. They examined the relative survival, i.e., compared the survival of the patient who had undergone aortic valve replacement with another age- and sex-matched person in the same population. Patients under the age of 65 had a relative survival of 81 percent, significantly lower than 100 percent. On the other hand, patients aged ≥65 years who underwent valve replacement had a relative survival of 94 percent at the end of 10 years—not significantly different from 100 percent. These data indicate that (1) survival following valve replacement for AS in patients aged ≥65 years is identical to an age- and sex-matched individual in the population who does not have AS and (2) the late relative survival of patients aged 65 years or greater is much better than that of patients under the age of 65. (From Lindblom et al.,[84] with permission.)

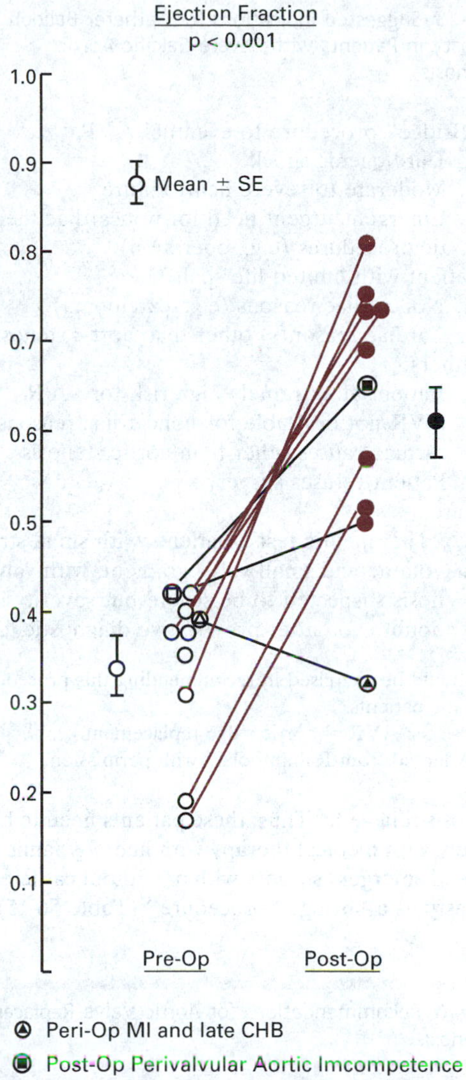

FIGURE 56-6 Examination of changes in LV ejection fraction in each individual patient. In those who had aortic stenosis with LV systolic dysfunction and clinical heart failure, the LV ejection fraction after aortic valve replacement increased from 0.34 to 0.63. All but one patient showed an improvement in LV ejection fraction; the only patient who showed a deterioration in ejection fraction suffered a perioperative myocardial infarction and had complete heart block, and the only patient who showed only a small increase in ejection fraction had had a myocardial infarct prior to valve replacement. Note that ejection fraction normalized in two-thirds of the patients, and in the two patients with the lowest ejection fraction (0.18 and 0.19), the ejection fraction normalized in both.

These data indicate that there is probably no lower limit of ejection fraction at which time these patients become inoperable. This also indicates that the lower the ejection fraction, the more urgent the need for valve replacement. (From Smith et al.,[88] with permission.)

Patients who present with heart failure should be hospitalized and treated with digitalis, diuretics, and *angiotensin-converting enzyme* (ACE) inhibitors and should undergo surgery as soon as possible. ACE inhibitors should be used extremely cautiously if at all. The patient must be monitored and hypotension avoided; a "significant" fall in blood pressure is an indication to discontinue or reduce the dose of ACE inhibitor. If heart failure does not respond satisfactorily and rapidly to medical therapy, surgery becomes a matter of considerable urgency.[85] Catheter balloon valvuloplasty can be an important bridge procedure in selected critically ill patients.[85] It usually improves the patients' hemodynamics and makes them better candidates for valve replacement. Valve replacement in patients with AS and heart failure can be performed at an operative mortality of 10 percent or less.[86] Although this is higher than in patients not in heart failure, the risk is justified because late survival in those who survive the operation is excellent and is far superior to that which can be expected with medical therapy; the 7-year survival of patients who survive operation is 84 percent.[87] The survival is lower in those with associated CAD.[86] The impaired LV function improves in all such patients provided that there has been no perioperative myocardial damage; it becomes normal in two-thirds of the patients (Fig. 56-6).[88] In some patients the improvement is less marked.[86] This is more likely in those with longer duration of preoperative LV dysfunction and in those with associated CAD. In addition, the operative survivors are functionally much improved. LV hypertrophy and dilatation (if present preoperatively) regress toward normal. Despite the excellent results of valve replacements in patients with severe AS who are in heart failure, it is important to recognize that surgery should *not* be delayed until heart failure develops.

In the data bases of older patients who underwent catheter balloon valvuloplasty, 6 percent of the patients were in cardiogenic shock.[89,90] The hospital mortality in such patients was very high, almost 50 percent. After hospital discharge, the subsequent mortality is also very high if the patients have not had

TABLE 56-15 Suggested Indications for Catheter Balloon Valvuloplasty in Patients with Severe Calcific Aortic Valve Stenosis[a]

I. "Bridge" procedure to eventual AVR
   A. Cardiogenic shock
   B. Moderate to severe heart failure
   C. Emergent/urgent need for noncardiac therapeutic procedures (e.g., operation)
II. Patient with limited life span
   A. Noncardiac reasons (e.g., carcinoma)
   B. Cardiac reason(s) other than aortic stenosis
III. Others
   A. Patient at extremely high risk for AVR
   B. AVR not desirable for noncardiac reasons or cardiac causes other than aortic stenosis
   C. Patient refuses surgery
IV. Rare
   A. "Therapeutic test": patients with small stroke volume and small valve gradient, with valve stenosis suspected to be severe but severity in doubt even after provocative diagnostic tests

[a]Caution should be exercised in recommending this procedure in asymptomatic patients.
ABBREVIATIONS: AVR = aortic valve replacement.
SOURCE: Adapted from Rahimtoola,[85] with permission.

their stenosis relieved.[90] Thus, these patients need to be treated aggressively with medical therapy with hemodynamic monitoring and need emergent surgery with or without catheter balloon valvuloplasty as a "bridge" procedure[85] (Table 56-15).

TABLE 56-16 Recommendations for Aortic Valve Replacement in Aortic Stenosis

Indication	Class
1. Symptomatic patients with severe AS	I
2. Patients with severe AS undergoing coronary artery bypass surgery	I
3. Patients with severe AS undergoing surgery on the aorta or other heart valves	I
4. Patients with moderate AS undergoing coronary artery bypass surgery or surgery on the aorta or other heart valves (see sections III.F.6., III.F.7., and VIII.D. of the ACC/AHA Guidelines)	IIa
5. Asymptomatic patients with severe AS and	
• LV systolic dysfunction	IIa
• Abnormal response to exercise (e.g., hypotension)	IIa
• Ventricular tachycardia	IIb
• Marked or excessive LV hypertrophy (≥15 mm)	IIb
• Valve area <0.6 cm^2	IIb
6. Prevention of sudden death in asymptomatic patients with none of the findings listed under indication 5	III

SOURCE: ACC/AHA Guidelines,[91] with permission.

TABLE 56-17 Recommendations for Aortic Balloon Valvotomy in Adults with Aortic Stenosis[a]

Indication	Class
1. A "bridge" to surgery in hemodynamically unstable patients who are at high risk for AVR	IIa
2. Palliation in patients with serious comorbid conditions	IIb
3. Patients who require urgent noncardiac surgery	IIb
4. An alternative to AVR	III

[a]Recommendations for aortic balloon valvotomy in adolescents and young adults with AS are provided in section VI.A. of the ACC/AHA Guidelines.
SOURCE: ACC/AHA Guidelines,[91] with permission.

The role of catheter balloon valvuloplasty in the older patient has now been clarified.[57,85] In calcific AS after catheter balloon valvuloplasty, the average increase in AVA is 0.3 cm^2 and the final AVA usually averages 0.8 cm^2; thus, many patients continue to have severe AS.[57,85,89] The 30-day, 1-year, and 3-year mortalities average 14, 35, and 71 percent, respectively, in the older patient (average age 78 ± 9 years) with calcific AS,[89] a mortality rate that may be similar to the natural history of this lesion. This technique is indicated[85] as a bridge procedure in those who need emergent noncardiac surgery and in those who are in heart failure (or in cardiogenic shock), who have an expected limited short life span when operative risks are considered to be prohibitively high, and who refuse surgery. When performed as a bridge procedure, valve surgery should not be unduly delayed. On rare occasions, it may be considered as a therapeutic test in patients in whom AS is suspected to be severe but the severity of the AS is in doubt after all standard tests have been performed (Table 56-15), including provocative diagnostic tests to assess mean aortic gradient, stroke volume, and AVA before and after infusion of dobutamine. Catheter balloon valvuloplasty is the procedure of choice in young patients who have pliable, noncalcified valves with commissural fusion (see Chap. 63).

The recommendations of the American College of Cardiology/American Heart Association (ACC/AHA) Practice Guidelines are shown in Tables 56-16 and 56-17.[91] Guidelines *are not* and *should not* be the law. Application of these guidelines to clinical practice should be based on the following principles: (1) classes I and III applies to all patients in these classes unless there is a specific clinical circumstance not to do so; (2) class II applies to patients in this class depending on the clinical conditions of the patients and the skill and experience at the individual medical center.

ACUTE AORTIC REGURGITATION

Etiology

The two most common causes of acute *aortic regurgitation* (AR) are infective endocarditis and prosthetic valve dysfunction.[92] Other causes include dissection of the aorta, systemic hypertension, and trauma.[93,94] AR associated with dissection of the aorta indicates that the dissection involves the ascending aorta down to the aortic valve annulus/root. AR associated with systemic hypertension is usually mild and transient; it is associated with severe elevation of aortic pressure, and, when the systemic hypertension is controlled, the AR usually disappears unless permanent changes have occurred in the aortic valve annulus/root or valve leaflets.

Pathophysiology

The LV diastolic pressure-volume relationship plays a very important role in the pathophysiology of acute valve regurgitation (Fig. 56-7).[95,96] Two features should be considered:[92] (1) The ability of the left ventricle to dilate acutely is limited; as a result, the volume overload of acute AR produces a rapid increase of LV diastolic pressure (curve B in Fig. 56-7). (2) The LV diastolic pressure-volume relationship before the onset of acute AR. If the left ventricle is already stiff or less compliant than normal from an associated lesion (e.g., AS or systemic hypertension), the LV diastolic pressure will rise more precipitously as a result of the volume overload of acute AR (curve A) than if the LV were normal (curve B). On the other hand, if the left ventricle is somewhat dilated from a previous lesion, for example, mild AR (curve C), initially the LV pressure will rise more gradually with acute AR but may subsequently rise to the same high levels as that seen with a normal or stiff LV.

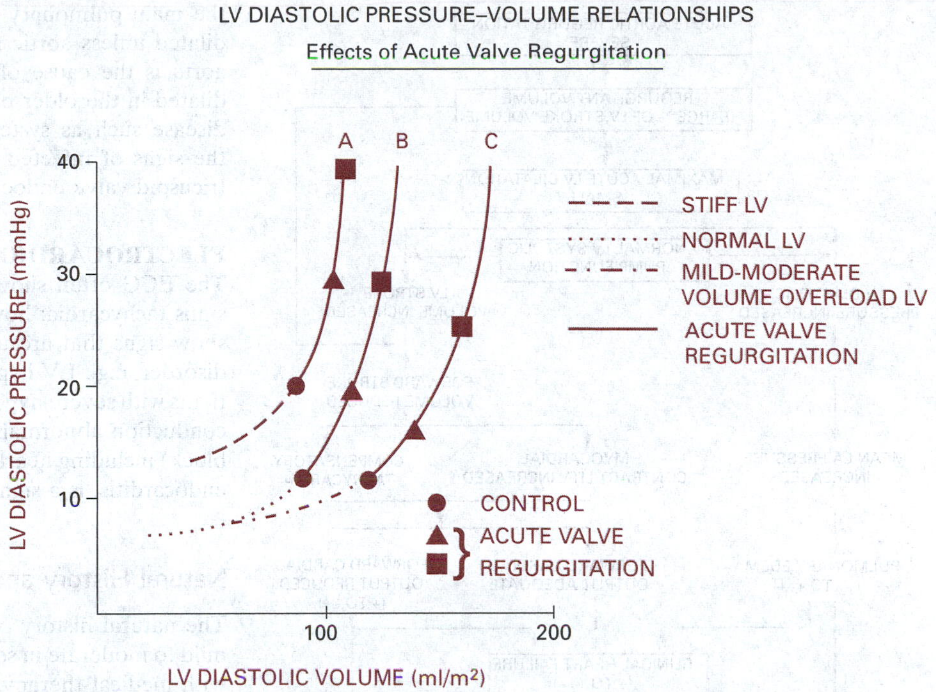

FIGURE 56-7 The left ventricular (LV) diastolic pressure-volume (P-V) relationship in acute valve regurgitation. The volume overload of acute AR produces a rapid increase of LV diastolic pressure in a patient with normal LV diastolic P-V prior to the acute AR (*curve B*). The LV diastolic pressure will rise more or less precipitously as a result of the volume overload of acute AR, depending on whether the LV is already stiff (*curve A*) or is somewhat dilated from a previous volume overload (*curve C*). (From Rahimtoola,[98] with permission.)

Acute AR that is mild produces little or no hemodynamic abnormality, for example, when associated with systemic hypertension. Increasing severity of regurgitation produces greater degrees of hemodynamic abnormalities, and severe AR often produces the clinical picture of "heart failure."

Acute AR that is severe results in a large volume of regurgitant blood; therefore, the volume of blood in the LV in diastole is increased. In an acute situation, the LV end-diastolic volume can only increase mildly (no more than 20 to 30 percent) and the LV diastolic pressure-volume relationships are particularly important. The LV systolic pump function is initially normal (Fig. 56-8). The increased LV diastolic pressure results in increases in mean left atrial and pulmonary venous pressures and produces varying degrees of pulmonary edema.[97] The normal LV systolic pump function in the presence of LV dilatation results in an increase of LV stroke volume. A large percentage of the LV stroke volume is returned to the LV in diastole, however; as a result, the forward stroke volume is reduced. The LV uses two mechanisms: an increase of myocardial contractility and, importantly, a compensatory tachycardia to maintain an adequate forward cardiac output. As a result, the forward cardiac output may be appropriate initially. If the compensatory mechanisms are inadequate, however, forward cardiac output is reduced. Pulmonary edema, with or without an adequate cardiac output, produces the picture of clinical heart failure.[97] Subsequently, LV systolic pump function may become abnormal; when that occurs, the pulmonary edema is further increased and the forward cardiac output is further reduced, leading to more severe manifestations of clinical heart failure.

Clinical Findings

HISTORY, PHYSICAL FINDINGS

The clinical presentations of patients with acute AR are those relating to preexisting disorders that have caused the acute AR. For example, patients may have peripheral signs of infective endocarditis, a history of trauma, or severe chest pain of aortic dissection. The other clinical presentations are those related to the AR itself. If the AR is mild, the patient is usually asymptomatic. In the symptomatic patient, the symptoms are those of heart failure.

On physical examination, the symptomatic patient with acute severe AR usually has a tachycardia. The arterial pulse shows an increased rate of rise of pressure. Systolic pressure is usually normal unless there is very severe heart failure; however, the diastolic pressure is in the normal range or may be decreased. The pulse pressure is usually normal. Thus, although the classic peripheral signs of chronic, severe AR are often absent, an important diagnostic clue is the rapid rate of rise of arterial pressure. The usual clinical signs of heart failure may be present. On examination of the precordium, the LV impulse is normal or slightly displaced to the left; it is usually hyperkinetic unless LV systolic dysfunction is present. The first heart sound is soft, and the second heart sound is often single and is soft. If pulmonary hypertension is present, P_2 is loud and there is a loud S_3

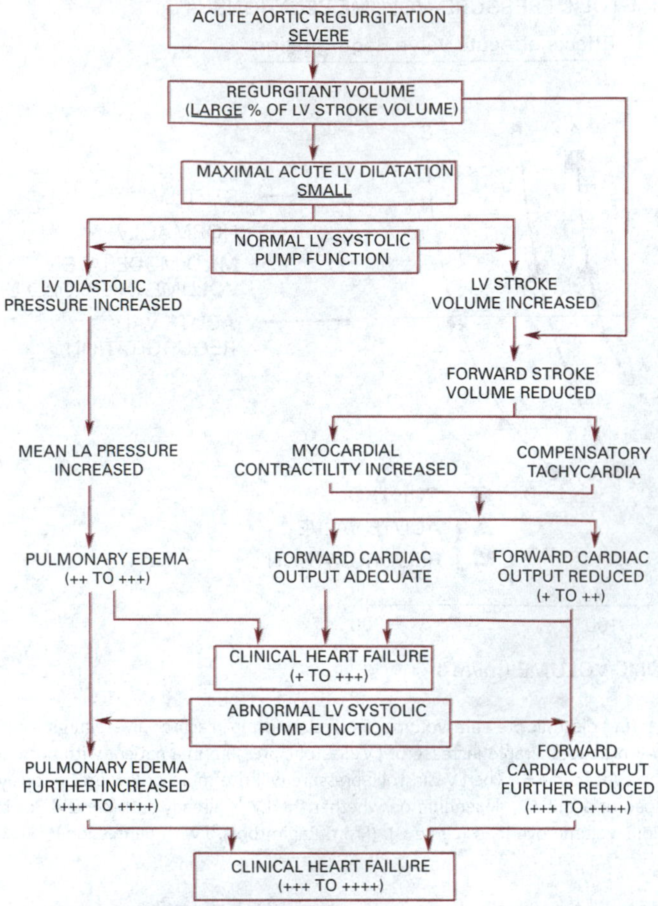

FIGURE 56-8 Pathophysiology of acute severe aortic regurgitation. Acute AR that is severe results in a large volume of regurgitant blood; therefore, the volume of blood in the left ventricle in diastole is increased. In an acute situation, the LV end-diastolic volume can only increase mildly (no more than 20 to 30 percent) and the LV diastolic pressure-volume relationships are particularly important (see Fig. 56-1). The subsequent findings are dependent on LV systolic pump function, LV diastolic pressure-volume relationship, myocardial contractile state, and compensatory tachycardia (see text for details). (Copyright © by S. H. Rahimtoola, M.B., F.R.C.P., M.A.C.P., M.A.C.C. See Ref. 93.)

gallop sound, but an S_4 gallop sound is absent. The clinical sine qua non of AR is the AR murmur, an early or immediate, blowing, decrescendo diastolic murmur beginning after A_2 that is best heard with the diaphragm of the stethoscope. Having the patient sit up and lean forward with the breath held in expiration facilitates the audibility of the murmur in difficult cases. The murmur may be short and soft if the ascending aortic pressure equalizes with LV pressure in early or middiastole. An Austin Flint murmur, if present, occurs in middiastole (see also Chap. 10).

An important clinical picture in intravenous drug abusers[92] includes: (1) a peripheral arterial pulse that has a rapid rate of rise and fall, even though the pulse pressure is small; (2) the telltale signs of intravenous drug abuse; (3) sinus tachycardia; and (4) "normal" heart size with pulmonary edema on chest x-ray.

CHEST X-RAY

The chest x-ray shows a "normal" heart size with pulmonary edema; however, some enlargement of all cardiac chambers and the main pulmonary artery may be present. The aorta is not dilated unless aortic annular/root disease or dissection of the aorta is the cause of the acute AR. The aorta may also be dilated in the older patient and/or in those with an associated disease such as systemic hypertension. The lungs may show the signs of infected pulmonary emboli if there is associated tricuspid valve endocarditis.

ELECTROCARDIOGRAM

The ECG often shows nonspecific ST-T-wave changes and a sinus tachycardia; however, it may be normal. The ECG may show signs that are usually found in the associated causative disorder, e.g., LV hypertrophy with ST-T-wave changes in patients with severe hypertension. The ECG may show a variety of conduction abnormalities (atrioventricular and bundle branch block) including heart block, which, in the presence of infective endocarditis, is a sign of paravalvular/myocardial abscess.

Natural History and Prognosis

The natural history of this condition is variable. If the AR is mild to moderate in severity, these patients are likely to do well with medical therapy. Eventually, the changes of chronic AR will be seen. In patients with severe AR, the natural history depends on whether or not they have heart failure.[98] If heart failure is present, which is common, the prognosis is very poor without valve surgery unless the heart failure can be very easily controlled with medical therapy.

Management

DIAGNOSIS OF AORTIC REGURGITATION

In most instances, the diagnosis can be made by clinical evaluation, which includes the history, physical examination, electrocardiography, and chest x-ray. The diagnosis by physical examination in an acutely ill patient who is in extremis may be difficult.

Transthoracic echo/Doppler ultrasound is an important and valuable noninvasive procedure that should be used in every instance. It will demonstrate the AR and its severity and will provide useful information about the size and function of the left ventricle and other valvular and cardiac abnormalities. If the transthoracic method is not adequate, for example, in the very ill patient, then the transesophageal method should be used (see Chap. 13).

Echocardiography shows the diastolic flutter of the anterior leaflet of the mitral valve. In addition, the echocardiogram may show vegetations on the aortic valve, prolapse of an aortic valve leaflet into the left ventricle in diastole, and premature mitral valve closure. The mitral valve may be seen to open for only a short time because the stroke volume is limited. Occasionally, the aortic valve leaflets have been totally destroyed, and none are seen on the echocardiogram. Doppler ultrasound can easily demonstrate the AR and provides an estimate of its severity.

Cardiac catheterization and angiography, including coronary arteriography, show the abnormal physiology described, and aortography shows gross AR. These modalities may be needed to make the diagnosis and are usually indicated before surgical intervention. Coronary arteriography is indicated in the appropriate patient (see above). In the extremely ill patient, there is often a need for clinical judgment with regard to the tests that are essential.

Other tests (cine-computed tomography, including fast cine-computed tomography, radionuclide gated blood scan, or ambulatory ECG) may be needed in very special conditions.

DIAGNOSIS OF THE ETIOLOGY OF ACUTE AORTIC REGURGITATION

The diagnosis of the etiology is usually made during the clinical evaluation by finding the usual clinical characteristics of the underlying lesion. Additional laboratory tests will be needed to confirm the diagnosis—for example, blood cultures in those with suspected infective endocarditis.

Echo/Doppler ultrasound (transthoracic and transesophageal) examination is also extremely valuable in diagnosing the underlying lesion. Its widespread availability and comparative ease of use, especially in the very acutely ill patient, make it the noninvasive procedure of choice. The availability of biplane and omniplane transesophageal probes further enhances its value as a diagnostic tool.

Magnetic resonance imaging (MRI) has a very high specificity for the diagnosis of dissection of the aorta[99,100] and, if available, should be used in all hemodynamically stable patients if the diagnosis has not already been made. The availability of biplane or omniplane transesophageal echocardiography markedly improves the specificity and diagnostic accuracy of transesophageal echocardiography. Angiography is also an effective and time-honored method of diagnosing dissection of the aorta.

In summary, clinical evaluation is available in all institutions; echo/Doppler ultrasound is available in almost all institutions. The use of the other tests depends on the availability of equipment and the skill and experience of personnel using the equipment for this purpose at each institution.

BEDSIDE HEMODYNAMIC MONITORING

In acute disorders affecting the left ventricle, there may be a phase lag between the rise in pulmonary venous pressure and the appearance of pulmonary edema on the chest x-ray film. As a result, the reliability of the chest x-ray in demonstrating the presence and severity of elevated left atrial pressure initially is less than satisfactory in the acutely ill patient.[101] If the assessment of left atrial pressure is made by physical examination and chest x-ray, a significant number of errors may be made in these patients with an acute cardiac problem. Therapeutic decisions based on incorrect assessments may result in significant problems; for example, inappropriate diuresis may result in a fall of cardiac output, or inappropriate volume loading may result in a further increase in left atrial pressure. Furthermore, the optimization of filling pressures and cardiac output may not be made accurately in acute heart failure without measuring their actual values. Thus, use of a balloon flotation catheter for bedside hemodynamic monitoring is required in most if not almost all acutely ill patients with acute AR.

TREATMENT

Treatment of the heart failure is directed toward reducing pulmonary venous pressure and increasing cardiac output. In all patients, treatment is also directed toward correcting or controlling the etiologic disease/disorder and/or the altered pathophysiologic state (Table 56-18).[92,98]

TABLE 56-18 Treatment of Heart Failure in Acute Valve Regurgitation

I. Correct or control altered pathophysiologic state
   - A. Reduce pulmonary venous pressure
     1. Diuresis
     2. Vasodilation
     3. Control heart rate and maintain sinus rhythm (digitalis, cardioversion, antiarrhythmics)
   - B. Increase cardiac output
     1. Reduction of valve regurgitation (vasodilators)
     2. Inotropic stimulation (digitalis, dobutamine)
   - C. Improve left ventricular systolic dysfunction
     1. Reduce pulmonary venous pressure
     2. Increase cardiac output
     3. ACE inhibitors

II. Correct or control underlying disease or disorder
   - A. Antibiotics for infective endocarditis
   - B. Pharmacologic therapy for systemic hypertension
   - C. Surgery for valve regurgitation in infective endocarditis, prosthetic valve dysfunction, dissection of the aorta, trauma

SOURCE: From Rahimtoola,[92] with permission.

Vasodilators (intravenous nitroprusside for an acute, severe condition) are useful and important in the management of these patients.[102] Vasodilators will produce a reduction of left atrial v wave and mean left atrial pressure. They produce a reduction in LV end-diastolic and end-systolic volumes and an increase in LV ejection fraction. The regurgitant fraction and regurgitant volume are reduced; as a result, the forward stroke volume and cardiac output are increased.[102] Digitalis therapy is of significant benefit in the management of heart failure. The combination of various agents (vasodilators, diuretics, and digitalis) tends to produce the maximum benefit in an individual patient; intravenous nitroprusside is often necessary in the acutely ill patient.

Surgical therapy (valve replacement/valve repair or appropriate surgery for dissection of the aorta) is the cornerstone of the most definitive therapy currently available for heart failure in these patients. The management of the patient with heart failure or suspected heart failure is outlined in Fig. 56-9.[98] If the valve regurgitation is due to *dissection of the aorta,* the need for cardiac surgery is an emergency, even if the regurgitation is mild or moderate, because AR indicates involvement of the ascending aorta down to the region of the aortic valve annulus/root (see also Chap. 88). The outcome of the patient with heart failure due to infective endocarditis is very poor with medical therapy but is improved with valve replacement.[103] The indications for surgery in *infective endocarditis* are listed in Table 56-19.[81] Infective endocarditis due to special organisms (e.g., fungi) can only rarely be controlled by pharmacologic therapy alone, and surgery is almost always needed. In these and some other conditions, valve surgery may be needed even if the AR is only mild or moderate. It must be recognized, however, that in 90 to 95 percent of patients needing surgery for endocarditis, the indication for valve surgery is heart failure. When the heart failure is a result of *prosthetic valve dysfunction* or *trauma,* the need for surgery can be an emergency, an urgent situation, or

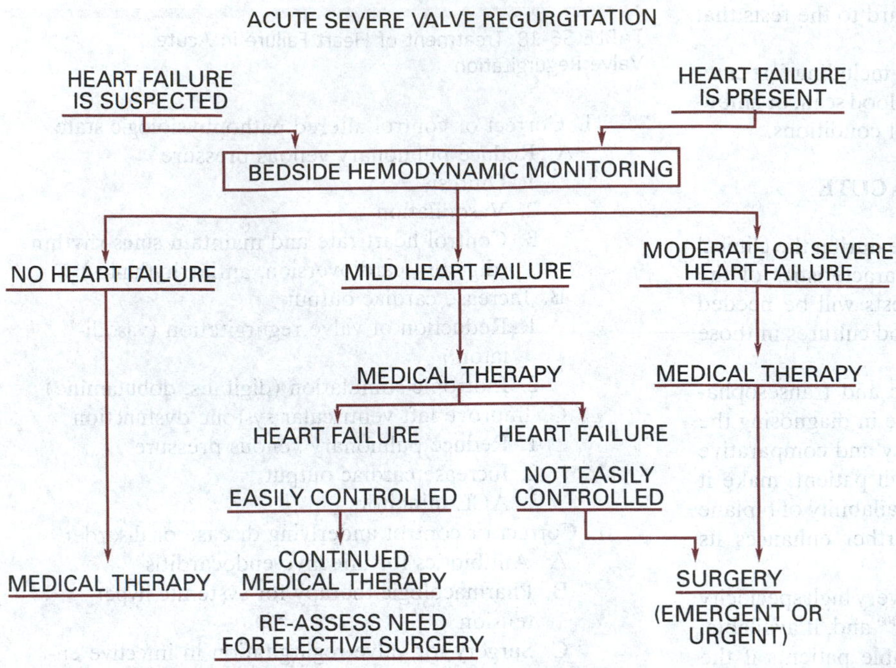

FIGURE 56-9 Role of bedside hemodynamic monitoring in acute aortic regurgitation. All patients with acute AR probably should have this procedure. If the AR is mild and there are no significant hemodynamic abnormalities, then the balloon flotation catheter can be withdrawn. On the other hand, if the AR is moderate to severe and there are significant hemodynamic abnormalities, then the balloon flotation catheter is left in place to guide therapy in the management of these acutely ill patients. If the hemodynamic abnormalities are mild, the patient is treated medically. If these abnormalities are easily controlled, medical therapy is continued and periodic reassessments are made to assess the need for elective surgery. If the hemodynamic abnormalities are not easily corrected or the hemodynamic abnormalities initially are moderate/severe, then surgery is undertaken either emergently or urgently. (From Rahimtoola,[98] with permission.)

an elective procedure. Prosthetic valves are inherently stenotic. When regurgitation is superimposed, it produces a pressure plus volume overload on the left ventricle that the ventricle may not handle very well acutely. Furthermore, valve regurgitation may be a sign of bioprosthetic valve degeneration or prosthetic endocarditis; in both conditions, prosthetic valve replacement is usually needed even if the valve regurgitation is mild to moderate. Trauma may result in AR from damage to valve leaflets or aortic annulus/root or from dissection of the aorta. If trauma produces dissection of the aorta and AR, the need for surgery may be an emergent one.

In some instances, the heart failure can be controlled completely with pharmacologic therapy, and the left ventricle and left atrium are able to dilate and adapt to the volume overload; in such instances, surgical therapy may be delayed, perhaps for a considerable period of time.

CHRONIC AORTIC REGURGITATION

Etiology

In North America, the most common cause of chronic, isolated severe AR is aortic root/annular dilatation that is presumably the result of medial disease. Other common causes include a congenital (bicuspid) valve, previous infective endocarditis, and rheumatic disease.[93,94] Chronic AR also occurs in association with a variety of other diseases (Table 56-20). Between 40 and 60 percent of the surgically removed valves from patients with isolated severe regurgitation are classified as idiopathic. Half of these (or 20 to 30 percent of all the valves removed) show histologic criteria of myxomatous degeneration.[104]

Pathology

During systole the aortic root/annulus expands by an increase of 14 to 16 percent of the diameter (twice the radius).[105] This

TABLE 56-19 Indications for Surgery in Infective Endocarditis

Congestive heart failure
Infection
Uncontrolled by antibiotic therapy
Fungal
Usually with staphylococcal infection of aortic or mitral valves
Serratia
Usually with gram-negative bacillary infection
Recurrent septic systemic emboli despite adequate antibiotic therapy
Perivalvular and myocardial abscesses
Structural damage to valve in association with other catastrophes (e.g., ruptured sinus of Valsalva)
Very large mobile vegetation

SOURCE: From Rahimtoola,[81] with permission.

TABLE 56-20 Etiology of Chronic Aortic Valve Regurgitation

Aortic root dilatation
Congenital bicuspid valve
Previous infective endocarditis
Rheumatic
In association with other diseases
Congenital lesions, e.g., supravalvular or discrete subvalvular AS, ventricular septal defect, and aneurysm of the sinus of Valsalva
Connective tissue disease, e.g., Marfan syndrome, osteogenesis imperfecta, and Ehlers-Danlos syndrome
Autoimmune diseases, e.g., ankylosing spondylitis, rheumatoid arthritis, and systemic lupus erythematosus
Various forms of aortitis and arteritis, e.g., giant-cell arteritis and Takayasu's disease
Syphilis

causes the commissural attachments to spread apart, initiating the opening of the valves. These movements are continued during LV systole, which produces the forward motion of the blood. The length of the free edge of the cusps equals the diameter of the aortic root/annulus, or roughly one-third of the perimeter. Therefore, dilatation of the aortic root/annulus, if it is not accompanied by an enlargement of the cusps, results in AR.[104]

Depending on the cause, the valve cusps may show thickening, shortening, commissural lesions, or calcification (Fig. 56-10).[106] Regardless of the cause, the LV is dilated and hypertrophied; some of the largest ventricles have been described in association with chronic severe AR. Little pockets may be seen in the LV outflow tract. These are pouches out of the endocardial lining formed by the regurgitant jet(s) striking the left ventricle.

The myocardium is hypertrophied, with replication of sarcomeres in series, elongation of fibers, and wall thickening. The wall is not as thickened as in patients with AS. Ultrastructural changes in the myocardial cells are similar to those seen in AS; an important difference, however, is the frequent presence of degenerated cardiac muscle cells in patients with severe AR. Cardiac muscle cells with mild degeneration show focal myofibrillar lysis, with preferential loss of thick myofilament and focal proliferation of tubules of the sarcoplasmic reticulum. Moderately degenerated muscle cells show a marked decrease

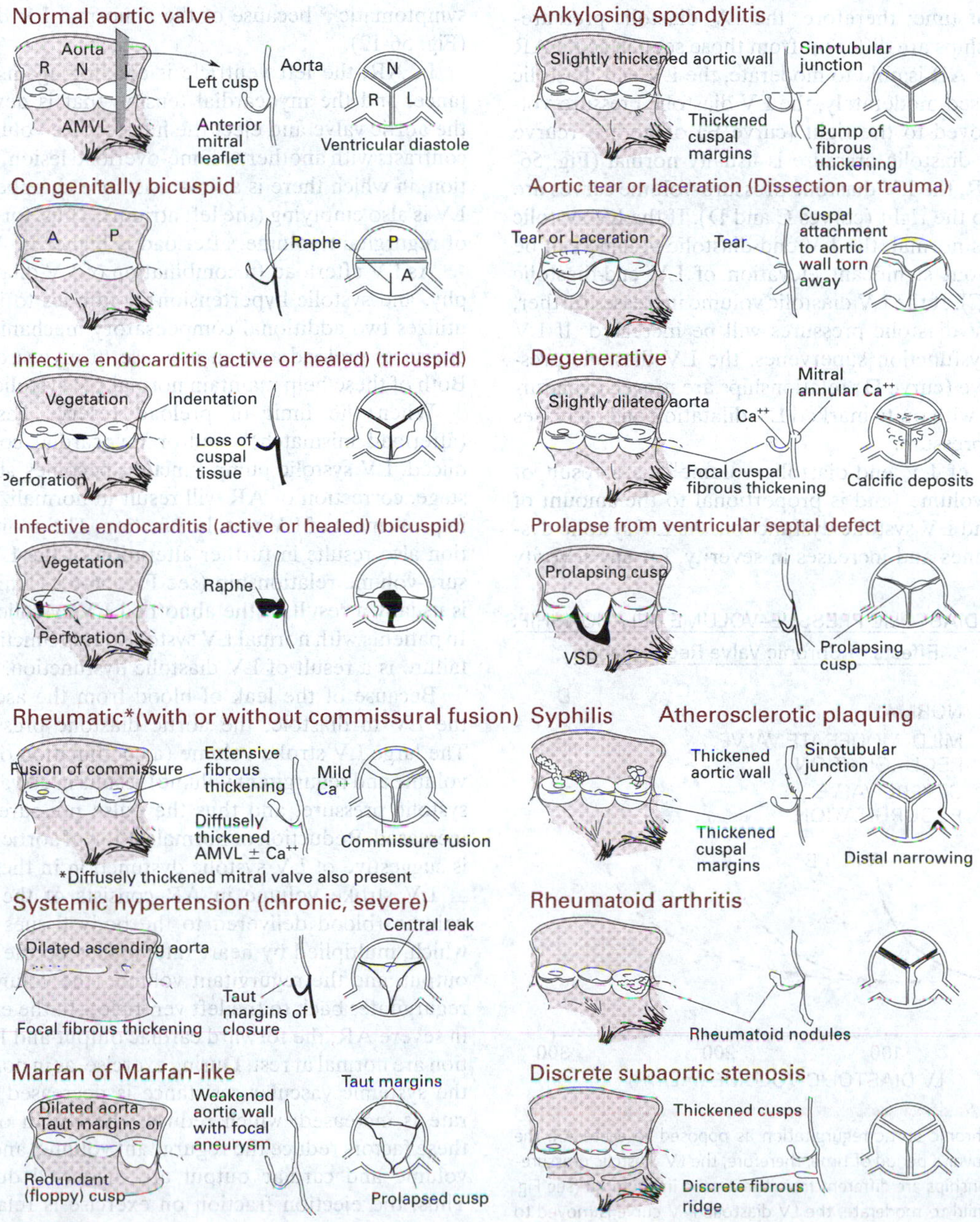

FIGURE 56-10 Pathologic findings in aortic regurgitation depending on the etiology of the AR. (From Waller,[106] with permission.)

in the number of myofibrils and T tubules and proliferation of sarcoplasmic reticulum, mitochondria, or both. Severely degenerated muscle cells usually are present in areas of marked fibrosis; they are often atrophic, have thickened basement membranes, and have lost their intercellular connections. These degenerated cardiac muscle cells may represent the ultrastructural basis for impaired LV function, which is seen more commonly in severe AR than in severe AS.

In patients with rheumatoid arthritis and ankylosing spondylitis, nodules on the outer surface of the anterior leaflet of the mitral valve have been described.

Pathophysiology

In chronic as opposed to acute AR, the AR becomes severe over a period of time; therefore, the LV diastolic pressure-volume relationships are different from those seen in acute AR (Fig. 56-7). If the AR is mild to moderate, the LV end-diastolic volume is increased moderately, the LV diastolic pressure-volume curve is moved to the right (curve B) of normal (curve A), and the LV diastolic pressure is usually normal (Fig. 56-11). In severe AR, the LV diastolic pressure-volume curves are moved further to the right (curves C and D). If the LV systolic pump function is normal, the LV end-diastolic volume can be quite large without significant elevation of LV end-diastolic pressure (curve C). If the LV diastolic volume increases further, however, the LV diastolic pressures will be increased. If LV systolic pump dysfunction supervenes, the LV diastolic pressure-volume curve (curve D) relationships are moved even further to the right, with quite marked LV dilatation and increases in LV diastolic pressure.

The increase of LV end-diastolic volume[107] is a result of the regurgitant volume (and is proportional to the amount of regurgitation) and LV systolic dysfunction. As LV systolic dysfunction supervenes and increases in severity, for any severity of regurgitant volume the LV end-diastolic volume increases further in an attempt to maintain LV stroke volume.

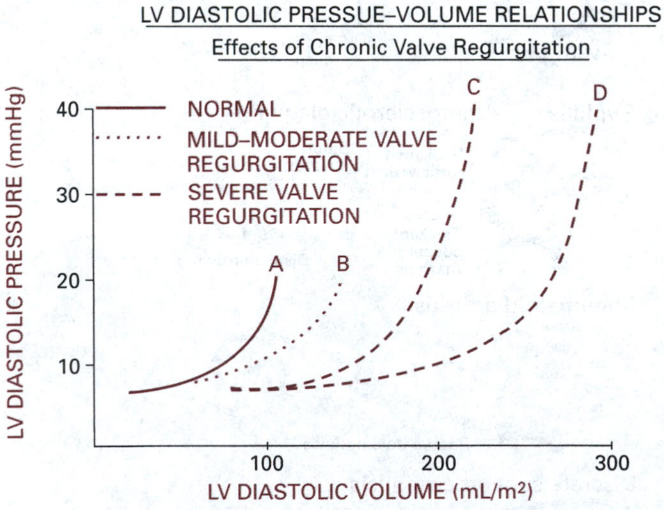

FIGURE 56-11 In chronic aortic regurgitation as opposed to acute AR, the AR becomes severe over a period of time; therefore, the LV diastolic pressure-volume (P-V) relationships are different from those seen in acute AR (see Fig. 56-7). If the AR is mild to moderate, the LV diastolic P-V curve is moved to the right (*curve B*). In severe AR, the LV diastolic P-V curves are moved further to the right, depending on whether the LV systolic pump function is normal (*curve C*) or abnormal (*curve D*). (From Rahimtoola,[98] with permission.)

Severe chronic AR results in a large regurgitant volume (a large percentage of LV stroke volume). The left ventricle responds by dilating (average LV end-diastolic volume in patients undergoing surgery was 205 mL/m^2);[22] the dilatation is proportional to the amount of the regurgitant volume. The subsequent large LV stroke volume produces LV systolic hypertension. Both of these increase LV wall stress (afterload), which can result in an impairment of LV function. The heart responds by becoming hypertrophied (average LV mass in patients undergoing valve surgery was 222 g/m^2),[22] and LV systolic pump function remains normal. There is also an alteration of the LV diastolic pressure-volume relationship (Fig. 63-11). As a result, some patients with normal LV systolic pump function become symptomatic[108] because of the abnormal LV diastolic function (Fig. 56-12).

In AR, the left ventricle is ejecting against systemic resistance, and the myocardial tension that is developed to open the aortic valve and eject the huge stroke volume is great. This contrasts with another volume-overload lesion, mitral regurgitation, in which there is a low-resistance chamber into which the LV is also emptying (the left atrium). Thus, for the same degree of regurgitant volume, afterload is higher in AR.

As LV afterload (a combination of LV dilatation, hypertrophy, and systolic hypertension) continues to increase, the LV utilizes two additional compensatory mechanisms, namely, increase of preload and an increase of myocardial contractility. Both of these help maintain normal LV systolic pump function.

When the limit of preload reserve has been reached (afterload mismatch)[31] and/or myocardial contractility is reduced, LV systolic pump function becomes abnormal. At this stage, correction of AR will result in normalization or marked improvement of LV systolic function. The additional LV dilatation also results in further alteration of the LV diastolic pressure-volume relationship (see Fig. 56-6). Clinical heart failure is usually a result of the abnormal LV systolic pump function. In patients with normal LV systolic pump function, clinical heart failure is a result of LV diastolic dysfunction.

Because of the leak of blood from the ascending aorta to the LV in diastole, the aortic diastolic pressure is reduced. The large LV stroke volume (a combination of forward stroke volume and regurgitant volume) results in elevation of the aortic systolic pressure, and thus the pulse pressure is considerably increased. Reduction or normalization of aortic systolic pressure is suggestive of LV systolic dysfunction in these patients.

LV stroke volume in AR consists of the forward stroke volume (blood delivered to the body tissues and the heart), which, multiplied by heart rate, makes up the forward cardiac output, and the regurgitant volume (the volume of blood that regurgitates back to the left ventricle). In the early stages, even in severe AR, the forward cardiac output and LV ejection fraction are normal at rest. During exercise, as in normal individuals, the systemic vascular resistance is decreased[109] and the heart rate is increased, which reduces the length of diastole. Both these factors reduce the regurgitant volume, and forward stroke volume and cardiac output are increased during exercise.[109] Thus, the ejection fraction on exercise is related to both the myocardial contractile state[110] and the fall in systemic vascular resistance.[109] Accordingly, a decline in ejection fraction on exercise cannot be used as a specific marker of LV function in these patients unless the change in systemic vascular resistance has also been measured. A fall of normal resting ejection fraction to less than 0.50 on exercise, however, has been shown to correlate with reduced total body oxygen consumption[103] and increased left atrial pressure during exercise.[109,111] Further impairment of LV function produces demonstrable abnormalities at rest; there is a further increase in LV end-diastolic volume, which helps to maintain forward stroke volume. The resting LV ejection fraction is reduced, and mean left atrial pressure begins to increase. Even at this stage, the forward cardiac output may be maintained in the normal range. The increases in left atrial pressure may produce various grades of pulmonary edema. Finally, in the state of severe heart failure, the ejection fraction may be low, LV end-diastolic volume is large, and LV end-diastolic pressure is greatly increased and is associated with increases in left atrial, pulmonary, right ventricular, and right atrial pressures. Forward cardiac output is no longer normal. An increase in systemic venous pressure in association with salt and water retention produces engorgement of systemic organs (e.g., the liver) as well as peripheral edema.

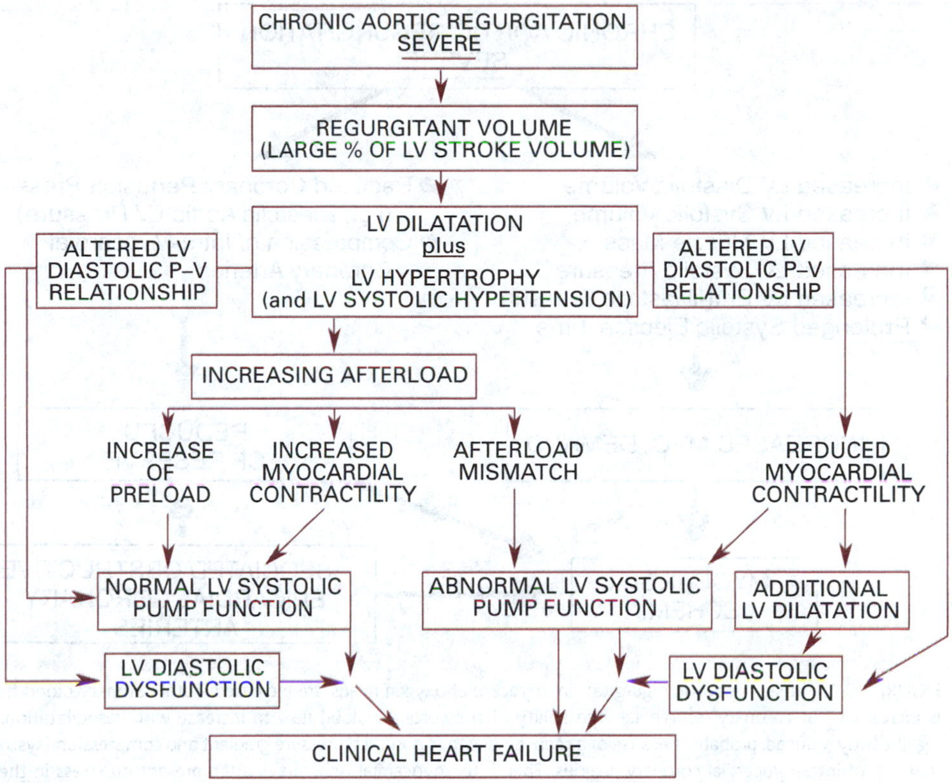

FIGURE 56-12 Severe chronic aortic regurgitation results in a large regurgitant volume (a large percentage of LV stroke volume). The left ventricle responds by dilating; the subsequent large LV stroke volume results in the production of LV systolic hypertension. There is an alteration of the LV diastolic pressure-volume (P-V) relationship. However, some patients with normal LV systolic pump function become symptomatic because of the abnormal LV diastolic function. As LV afterload (a result of LV dilatation, hypertrophy, and systolic hypertension) continues to increase, the LV utilizes two additional compensatory mechanisms, i.e., increase of preload and an increase of myocardial contractility. Both of these help maintain normal LV systolic pump function.

When the limit of preload reserve has been reached (afterload mismatch) and/or myocardial contractility is reduced, LV systolic pump function becomes abnormal. The additional LV dilatation also results in further alteration of the LV diastolic P-V relationship.

Clinical heart failure is usually a result of the abnormal LV systolic pump function; diastolic dysfunction may also be present in some patients. Clinical heart failure in those with normal LV systolic pump function is a result of LV diastolic dysfunction. (Copyright © by S. H. Rahimtoola, M.B., F.R.C.P., M.A.C.P., M.A.C.C. See Ref. 93.)

In severe AR, myocardial oxygen needs are increased because of increases in LV diastolic and systolic volumes, LV muscle mass (hypertrophy), and LV pressures as well as by prolongation of systolic ejection time. Total coronary blood flow is increased. Coronary reserve, the ability of the coronary blood flow to increase with vasodilatation, however, is significantly reduced,[112–114] probably because of a reduced diastolic aortic-LV pressure gradient and compression of intramyocardial coronary arteries (systolic "milking" of intramural arteries). Therefore, myocardial ischemia is often present on stress in these patients.[112–114] Some patients with severe AR may complain of angina pectoris on effort even in the absence of epicardial CAD. Associated obstructive CAD can be expected to exacerbate further the myocardial ischemia (see Fig. 56-13).

Clinical Features

HISTORY

Patients with mild to moderate AR usually do not have symptoms that can be attributed to the heart. Even patients with severe AR may be asymptomatic. They may complain of pounding of the head or palpitations, which result from their awareness of the beating of a dilated left ventricle that undergoes a large volume change in systole, during either sinus beats or postectopic beats. The main symptoms of severe AR result from elevated pulmonary venous pressures and include dyspnea on exertion, orthopnea, and paroxysmal nocturnal dyspnea. When congestive heart failure occurs, patients complain of fatigue and weakness. Angina pectoris occurs in 20 percent of such patients and may be present even if the coronary arteries are normal. Angina associated with syphilitic AR may be due to associated ostial stenosis of the coronary arteries. In such patients, angina often occurs at rest and is difficult to control.

PHYSICAL EXAMINATION

A variety of interesting but not very useful clinical signs may be present in patients with chronic severe AR. These include *de Musset's sign* (bobbing of the head with each heartbeat), *Traube's sign* (pistol-shot sound heard over the femoral artery), *Duroziez's sign* (systolic murmur over the femoral artery when

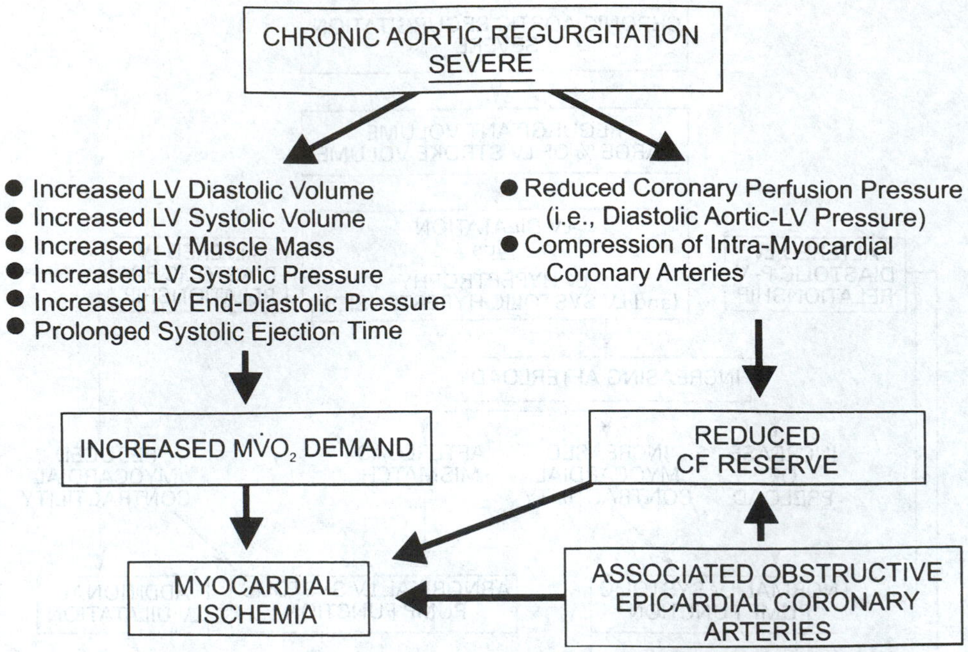

FIGURE 56-13 In severe aortic regurgitation, myocardial oxygen needs are increased. Total coronary blood flow is increased, but coronary reserve, i.e., the ability of the coronary blood flow to increase with vasodilatation, is significantly reduced, probably because of a reduced diastolic aortic-LV pressure gradient and compression (systolic milking) of intramyocardial coronary arteries. Therefore, myocardial ischemia is often present on stress in these patients. Associated obstructive coronary artery disease can be expected to further exacerbate the myocardial ischemia. (Copyright © by S. H. Rahimtoola, M.B., F.R.C.P., M.A.C.P., M.A.C.C. See Ref. 93.)

it is compressed proximally and diastolic murmur when it is compressed distally), and *Quincke's pulse* (capillary pulsations that can be detected by pressing a glass slide on the patient's lip or transmitting a light through the patient's fingertips).

The arterial pulse is very characteristic and consists of an abrupt distention with a rapid rise and a quick collapse *(Corrigan's pulse)*. The arterial pulse may be bisferiens, a double impulse during systole. The systolic arterial pressure is increased (in severe AR it averages 145 to 160 mmHg), the diastolic pressure is reduced (in severe AR it averages 45 to 60 mmHg), and the Korotkoff's sounds persist down to 0 mmHg. Even in such instances, however, the recorded intraarterial pressure rarely falls below 30 mmHg. The vasoconstriction that occurs in the presence of heart failure may result in some elevation of the arterial diastolic pressure and should not be interpreted as an improvement in severity of AR. Similarly, LV systolic dysfunction can produce a fall of systolic blood pressure that should not be considered to be an improvement of the AR. The fall of systolic pressure along with elevation of diastolic pressures tends to normalize the pulse pressure. The jugular venous pressure is normal except in heart failure and in those rare instances in which the greatly dilated ascending aorta obstructs the superior vena cava.

On inspection, the chest may rock and the cardiac impulse may be visible. The cardiac impulse is hyperdynamic (Table 56-21). There may be a systolic thrill at the base of the heart, over the carotids, and in the suprasternal notch. This results from a large LV stroke volume across a diseased aortic valve. A diastolic thrill signifies severe AR. The first heart sound is usually soft because the mitral valve leaflets are close to each other at the onset of systole, or there may be premature valve closure. This is exaggerated if the PR interval is prolonged. The S_2 is usually single because the aortic valve does not close properly[115] or because the LV ejection time is prolonged and the P_2 may not be heard. Often, a systolic ejection murmur, which is sometimes very loud, is present. The clinical sine qua non of AR is an early or immediate, blowing, decrescendo diastolic murmur beginning after A_2. It is best heard with the diaphragm of the stethoscope at the left sternal border or, in difficult instances, by having the patient sit up and lean forward and by auscultating in held respiration at the end of a deep expiration. In severe AR, the murmur may be holodiastolic. When it is soft, its intensity can be increased by having the patient perform isometric exercise, for example, a handgrip, which increases aortic diastolic pressure. At times, this murmur is better heard along the right sternal border, which should draw attention to the possibility that the cause of the AR is aortic root/annular disease (see also Chap. 10). Classically, rupture of the sinus of Valsalva into the right heart chambers produces a continuous murmur.

In many patients with severe AR, an Austin Flint murmur[116] (see Chap. 10) is present in presystole and/or mid-diastole. Two inferences can be drawn from the presence of an Austin Flint murmur: (1) it signifies that the AR is severe and (2) it requires that associated mitral stenosis be excluded. The most helpful sign at the bedside is the response of the murmur to the inhalation of amyl nitrite. The vasodilatation produced by amyl nitrite increases forward flow, reduces the regurgitant volume, and results in the Austin Flint murmur becoming much softer or disappearing. On the other hand, the increased cardiac output and the tachycardia accentuate or increase the murmur of mitral stenosis. Alternatively, echocardiography can easily demonstrate the presence of organic mitral stenosis.

With severe LV dilatation and/or LV systolic dysfunction, secondary mitral regurgitation may be present with the characteristic holosystolic murmur. Heart failure may be associated with pulmonary congestion/edema, pulmonary hypertension, right ventricular enlargement, tricuspid regurgitation, elevated jugular venous pressure, hepatomegaly, and peripheral edema (see Chap. 20).

CHEST X-RAY

The LV is increased in size, and this can be appreciated on the chest x-ray by an increase in the cardiothoracic ratio. Since the upper limit of normal of the cardiothoracic ratio is 0.49, many patients with increased LV size have an enlarged ventricular volume and may still have a cardiothoracic ratio within the normal range. A better noninvasive quantification of LV size

TABLE 56-21 Physical Examination of Patients with Varying Severity of Chronic Aortic Valve Regurgitation

	Mild	Moderate	Severe	Severe + LV Systolic Dysfunction	Severe + Heart Failure + LV Systolic Dysfunction
Arterial pulse	Normal	Corrigan's + to + +	Corrigan's + + +	Corrigan's + +	Corrigan's +
Arterial pressure					
Systolic	Normal	Increased + to + +	Increased + + +	Increased + +	Normal/+
Diastolic	Normal	Decreased + to + +	Decreased + + + to + + + + +	Decreased + + to + + +	Decreased + +
Pulse pressure	Often normal	Increased + to + +	Increased + + + to + + + +	Increased + + to + + +	Increased +
Cardiac impulse	Often normal	Hyperdynamic	Very hyperdynamic visible ± chest may rock	Hyperdynamic	May be hypodynamic
Precordial thrill:					
Systolic	−	±	±	±	−
Diastolic	−	−	±	±	−
Auscultation:					
S_4	−	−	−	−	−
S_1	Normal	Often soft	Soft	Soft	Soft
S_2	Normal	Normal or single	Often single	Often single	Often single
S_3	−	+	+ + to + + +	+ + +	+ + +
ESM	±	+	+ to + +	+ to + +	+
AoDM	+	+ +	+ + + to + + + +	+ + to + + +	+ to + +
Austin Flint murmur	−	−	±	−	−

ABBREVIATIONS: S_1 and S_2 = first and second heart sounds; S_3 = third heart sound (diastolic gallop); S_4 = fourth heart sound (presystolic gallop); ESM = ejection systolic murmur; AoDM = aortic diastolic murmur; − absent; + + + + most prominent; ± present or absent.

can be obtained by echocardiography. The ascending aorta is dilated throughout, and there may be calcium in the aortic valve. With increased filling pressures in the later stages, there might be evidence of an enlarged left atrium and an increased left atrial and pulmonary venous pressure, which are manifested in the pulmonary vascular shadows by a redistribution of blood flow, pulmonary congestion, and pulmonary edema. In the presence of heart failure, enlargement of the right atrium and superior vena cava may be appreciated. Calcification that is limited to the ascending aorta is strongly suggestive of luetic aortitis.

ELECTROCARDIOGRAM

The ECG shows LV hypertrophy with or without associated secondary ST-T-wave changes. In a small percentage of patients, ECG evidence of LV hypertrophy is absent in spite of severe AR. Conduction abnormalities, such as atrioventricular block or left or right bundle branch block with or without axis deviation, may be present. The PR interval may be prolonged,[117] particularly in patients with ankylosing spondylitis. The rhythm is usually sinus. The presence of atrial fibrillation should make one suspect the presence of associated mitral valve disease or heart failure.

ECHOCARDIOGRAPHY

The sign of AR on echocardiography is diastolic fluttering of the anterior leaflet of the mitral valve. Echocardiography is of particular value for excluding the presence of associated mitral stenosis in patients with an Austin Flint diastolic murmur. LV dimensions are increased, and if ventricular function is normal, the percentage of dimensional shortening is normal. Because of the increase in LV dimensions caused by volume overload, there is separation between the open anterior leaflet of the mitral valve and the endocardial surface of the interventricular septum (septal–E point separation), but this does not necessarily indicate impaired LV function when AR is present. In AR, as in other volume-overload lesions, the response in mild volume overload is an elongation of the heart. Since M-mode echocardiography takes a pencil look at the short axis of the heart, LV dimensions by M-mode echocardiography may appear to be normal. In such patients, two-dimensional echocardiography is much superior to the M-mode technique for assessing LV volumes and systolic function. A dilated ascending aorta can be detected on echocardiography, as can an enlarged left atrium. Aortic valve vegetations suggest infective endocarditis. Some other conditions can easily be detected by echocardiography, for example, prolapse of the aortic leaflet into the left ventricle in diastole. Doppler ultrasound is useful for diagnosing and assessing the severity of AR. There is a significant incidence of false-positive mild regurgitation. There is also an overlap between the various grades of severity of assessment of AR by Doppler when compared to angiography. Transesophageal echocardiography is a useful technique when transthoracic echocardiogram is unsatisfactory and in certain instances for identifying the anatomy of the valve leaflets and aortic root/

annulus; it is essential to evaluate if the valve is suitable for repair. Echo/Doppler ultrasound is also very useful for assessing disease of other valves.

CARDIAC CATHETERIZATION/ANGIOGRAPHY

Cardiac catheterization allows the measurement of intracardiac and intravascular pressures and cardiac output, both at rest and during exercise, and can demonstrate the changes described under "Pathophysiology," above. In addition, other valvular disease—for example, mitral stenosis, aortic stenosis, and mitral regurgitation—can be excluded. LV angiography demonstrates enlarged LV volumes and allows the calculation of LV volumes and LV ejection fraction. Angiography performed with injection of contrast medium in the ascending aorta demonstrates AR and allows a semiquantitative assessment of the degree of AR. In addition, the angiogram demonstrates the dimensions of the aortic root and the state of the ascending aorta. The indications for selective coronary angiography are the same as for aortic stenosis (see Table 56-6).

GATED BLOOD POOL RADIONUCLIDE SCANS

Gated blood pool radionuclide scans also allow the measurement of LV volumes and ejection fraction. In addition, with this technique, it is possible to quantify the amount of AR. These scans, however, assess regurgitation present at both the aortic and mitral valves. Thus, if both valves are incompetent, the total amount of regurgitation present at both valves will be measured. This technique also allows measurement of LV ejection fraction on exercise and on serial studies.

TREADMILL EXERCISE TEST

A treadmill exercise test provides an objective assessment of the degree of functional impairment and documentation of arrhythmias related to exertion. In some patients, however, the exercise test may remain normal despite deterioration of LV function.

AMBULATORY ECG RECORDING

Ambulatory ECG recording may be needed in an occasional patient suspected of having an arrhythmia.

MAGNETIC RESONANCE IMAGING

MRI can demonstrate AR but is rarely needed clinically.

Clinical Decision Making

Please see the equivalent section under "Aortic Valve Stenosis," above. The sensitivity, specificity, and accuracy of diagnosis of chronic AR are shown in (Table 56-22).[66] The following should be noted: (1) The sensitivity, specificity, and accuracy of diagnosing AR after clinical evaluation are good but not quite as good as in AS; (2) echo/Doppler ultrasound improves these criteria to a greater extent than in AS; (3) the difficulties lie in accurately distinguishing patients with mild AR from normal individuals and those with moderate AR and in distinguishing between moderate AR and severe AR; and (4) both clinical evaluation and echo/Doppler ultrasound are excellent in diagnosing the AR as being moderate or severe.

TABLE 56-22 Clinical Decision Making Utilizing Clinical Evaluation versus Echo/Doppler in Patients with Aortic Regurgitation

	After Clinical Evaluation, %	After Echo/Doppler, %
Diagnosis of AR		
Sensitivity	66	79
Specificity	76	74
Accuracy of diagnosis		
All levels of severity	43	57
Moderate or severe AR	91	100

SOURCE: From Kotlewski et al.,[66] with permission.

Natural History and Prognosis

Patients with mild AR that does not progress should have a normal life expectancy. Their major risk is the development of infective endocarditis and further valve destruction. Patients with moderate AR, if their disease does not progress, would be expected to have a life expectancy that is reasonably close to the normal range. The disease does progress, however, and mortality at the end of 10 years appears to be about 15 percent.

Patients with severe AR are known to have a long asymptomatic period before the condition is discovered. In asymptomatic patients with normal LV function at rest, symptoms and/or LV dysfunction (and/or sudden death) develop at the rate of about 3 to 6 percent per year. The predictor of development of symptoms is LV systolic dysfunction at rest.[118–122] In patients with normal LV systolic function at rest (Table 56-23), the predictors of development of LV systolic dysfunction and/or symptoms are an increased LV size (LV dimension at end-diastole of ≥70 mm and at end-systole of ≥50 mm,[119–121] and LV end-diastolic volume index of ≥150 mL/m^2),[123] and abnormal LV ejection fraction on exercise of <0.50.[111] In smaller people, for example, in women,[122] these values are too large and have to be corrected for body size. The corrected dimensions for end diastole and end systole are 35 mm/m^2 and 25 mm/m^2, respectively. Sudden death in asymptomatic patients appears to occur only in those with a massively dilated left ventricle (LV end-diastolic dimension of ≥80 mm).[119] It is likely that LV dysfunction first appears on exercise and later also at rest; eventually, heart failure ensues.

TABLE 56-23 Chronic Severe Aortic Regurgitation: Asymptomatic + Normal LV Function at Rest

		Likelihood of Symptoms or LV Dysfunction or Death, % per Year
LV end-diastolic dimension	≥70 mm	10
	<70 mm	2
LV end-systolic dimension	≥50 mm	19
	40–49 mm	6
	<40 mm	0

SOURCE: From Bonow et al.,[119] with permission.

Severe symptoms, however, may occur even when LV systolic pump function is normal at rest (see "Pathophysiology," above). The 5-year mortality of symptomatic patients with severe AR is about 25 percent, and the 10-year mortality averages 50 percent.[118] Once symptoms occur in patients with AR, it is likely that the rate of deterioration will be rapid. Most patients with angina are dead within 4 years.[124] The 2- to 3-year mortality of those with heart failure is 50 to 70 percent. In a recent study, the mortality was 4.7 percent per year, in the symptomatic patient it was 9.4 percent per year[125] and in the asymptomatic patient 2.8 percent, which was not significantly different from age- and gender-matched individuals in the population. In the symptomatic patient, those in the New York Heart Association (NYHA) classes III and IV had an annual mortality of 24.6 percent per year, while in the class II patient it was 6.3 percent per year. In asymptomatic patients, those with LV ejection fraction <0.55, the annual mortality was 5.8 percent per year, and in those with LV end-systolic dimension ≥25 mm/m², it was 7.8 percent per year.[125]

Management

All patients with AR need antibiotic prophylaxis to prevent infective endocarditis. Patients with AR of a rheumatic origin need antibiotic prophylaxis to prevent recurrences of rheumatic carditis. Patients with syphilitic AR need a course of antibiotics to treat syphilis.

Patients with mild AR need no specific therapy (Table 56-24). They do not need to restrict their activities and can lead a normal life. Patients with moderate AR also usually need no specific therapy. These patients, however, should avoid heavy physical exertion, competitive sports, and isometric exercise.

The value of long-term vasodilators to produce an improvement in LV size and function has been evaluated in two placebo-controlled randomized trials. In the hydralazine trial,[126] 36 percent of the patients were in NYHA functional class II, and patients had moderate to severe AR. Hydralazine produced modest reduction of LV end-diastolic volume and a small increase in ejection fraction at the end of 2 years; however, because of side effects, long-term compliance was poor,[126] which probably accounted for the extremely modest beneficial effects.[127] In asymptomatic patients with severe AR,[128] a calcium channel blocking agent, long-acting nifedipine, produced significant reductions in blood pressure and LV end-diastolic volume and mass and major increases in LV ejection fraction at the end of 1 year. Almost all patients completed the trial. Recently, a prospective randomized trial in *asymptomatic* patients with *normal LV systolic* function[120] showed that at the end of 6 years, 34 ± 6 percent of patients treated with digoxin developed LV systolic dysfunction and/or symptoms and thus needed valve replacement, compared to 15 ± 3 percent of patients treated with long-acting nifedipine ($p < .001$) (Fig. 56-14); 90 percent (23 of 26) of those who needed valve replacement had developed LV systolic dysfunction with or without symptoms; only 3 had become symptomatic without developing LV systolic dysfunction. Accordingly, all asymptomatic patients with severe AR and normal LV systolic function should be treated with a vasodilator (calcium antagonists long-acting nifedipine) unless there is a contraindication to its use.

The role of nifedipine in patients with moderate AR has not been studied. In view of its beneficial effects in severe AR, long-acting nifedipine could be used in selected patients with moderate AR if there are no contraindications to its use. An acute study showed that nifedipine was superior to an ACE inhibitor,[129] and a 6-month trial showed that the results with captopril were similar to placebo.[130] One study with quinapril involved 10 patients, many of whom had moderate AR.[131] In another study with enalapril, most patients had mild to moderate AR and many had severe systemic hypertension.[132] Moreover, there are no published data to show that ACE inhibitor therapy reduces the need for valve surgery. In brief, ACE inhibitors are not of proven benefit in asymptomatic patients with AR and with normal LV systolic function.

Symptomatic patients with severe AR need medical and surgical treatment. Medical treatment (Table 56-24) consists of the administration of digitalis, diuretics, and vasodilators. Digitalis acts by increasing myocardial contractility, often reducing LV end-diastolic volume while increasing the LV ejection fraction and also the cardiac output if it is reduced in the resting state. Digitalis is clearly indicated in patients with symptoms.

TABLE 56-24 Medical Treatment of Patients with Aortic Regurgitation

I. Antibiotic prophylaxis
  A. Infective endocarditis
  B. Recurrent rheumatic carditis
II. Restriction of activities (moderate/severe AR)
  A. Severe exercise
  B. Competitive sports
III. Arrhythmias
  A. Prevent and/or control
  B. Restore sinus rhythm, if possible
IV. Cardiac medications
  A. Asymptomatic, normal LV function
    1. Mild AR: None
    2. Moderate AR: ? Nifedipine long-acting
    3. Severe AR: Nifedipine long-acting
  B. Severe AR symptomatic (while waiting for surgery)
    1. Normal LV function: Nifedipine long-acting
    2. LV dysfunction: Digitalis; ACE inhibitors; Hydralazine ± nitrates, if needed; Diuretics, if needed; Dobutamine, if needed
  C. Severe AR + heart failure:
    Digitalis, diuretics, ACE inhibitors
    Hydralazine + nitrates
    IV nitroprusside, if IV therapy needed
    Dobutamine, if needed
V. Follow-up of asymptomatic patient
  A. Mild AR: Every 2–5 years
  B. Moderate AR: Every 1–2 years
  C. Severe AR: Every 6–12 months
  D. Develop symptoms: Early or immediate

SOURCE: Copyright © by S. H. Rahimtoola, M.B., F.R.C.P., M.A.C.P., M.A.C.C. See Ref. 93.

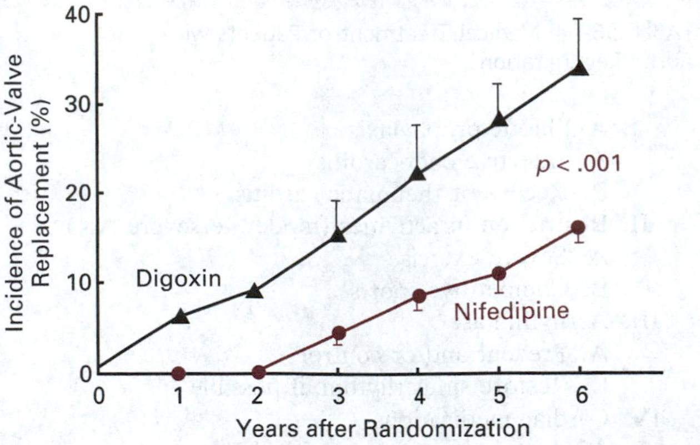

FIGURE 56-14 The role of long-term nifedipine therapy in asymptomatic patients with severe AR and normal LV systolic pump function was evaluated in 143 asymptomatic patients in a prospective randomized trial. By actuarial analysis, at 6 years, 34 ± 6 percent of patients in the digoxin group underwent valve replacement, versus 15 ± 3 percent of those in the nifedipine group, $p < .001$.

This randomized trial demonstrates that long-term vasodilator therapy with nifedipine reduces and/or delays the need for aortic valve replacement in asymptomatic patients with severe AR and normal LV systolic pump function. (From Scognamiglio et al.,[120] with permission.)

The need for and benefits of this therapy in asymptomatic patients have not been well documented. Diuretics are of value when the left atrial pressure is elevated and in the presence of heart failure.

Vasodilators are either arterial, venous, or both. Vasodilators act by reducing the peripheral arterial resistance, which favors forward cardiac output and reduces regurgitant volume; initially, the total LV stroke volume remains unchanged. If the left atrial pressure is elevated and LV ejection fraction reduced, vasodilators frequently result in an improvement in both.

Long-term hydralazine therapy in symptomatic patients results in significant benefit in only 20 to 35 percent of patients.[57] Those who are likely to benefit cannot be predicted. Vasodilators are indicated in patients who refuse surgery or are not operative candidates for any reason.

Vasodilators are also indicated for short-term therapy in patients awaiting valve replacement to optimize their hemodynamics (reduce filling pressures and increase cardiac output) and thus reduce their operative risks. If LV systolic function is normal, they can be given long-acting nifedipine. If they have abnormal LV systolic function, they should be treated with digitalis and ACE inhibitors; diuretics and hydralazine, with or without nitrates, can be used if needed. Small doses of hydralazine (50 mg) are without therapeutic effect in AR, and larger doses (≥100 mg) need to be given only twice daily;[133] the twice-daily regimen reduces the incidence of side effects. Hydralazine should be started in small doses and gradually increased, depending on patient tolerance of the drug.

Vasodilators are of considerable short-term benefit in patients in functional classes III and IV or heart failure. All such patients need digitalis, diuretics, and ACE inhibitors. In patients in functional class IV with heart failure, vasodilators should ideally be started after the institution of bedside hemodynamic monitoring—that is, measurement of pulmonary artery wedge pressure and cardiac output with the use of balloon flotation catheters. Hemodynamic monitoring accurately identifies patients who need the therapy, since clinical judgments can be wrong. It establishes whether arterial dilators alone will suffice or whether additional venodilators are needed. Finally, it provides information on the optimum dosage of vasodilator therapy. After the initial hemodynamic measurements are made, arterial dilators are given in progressively increasing dosage until an optimum effect on cardiac output has been obtained. If cardiac output does not show any further increase but left atrial pressure is still very high, additional venodilator therapy should be given. If the patient is very ill or the hemodynamic abnormalities are marked, intravenous therapy (e.g., sodium nitroprusside) is the vasodilator of first choice. In this situation, intravenous vasodilator therapy should be used only with bedside hemodynamic monitoring. Inotropic agents, such as dobutamine, may be needed to improve LV function and increase cardiac output. Low-dose dopamine may be of value to increase urinary output.

Patients with severe chronic AR need valve surgery. The correct timing of surgical therapy is now better defined but is not fully clarified. Valve replacement should be performed before irreversible LV dysfunction occurs. The major problem, however, is identifying the precise point at which LV dysfunction will occur. Here, two major difficulties are encountered: (1) patients may already have impaired LV systolic pump function at rest when they first present or at the time of the first symptom and (2) patients with severe symptoms may have normal LV systolic pump function. Patients may be in NYHA functional class III (symptoms with less than ordinary activity), with a normal LV ejection fraction,[108] or they may be in functional class I (asymptomatic), with a reduced LV ejection fraction.[108] A reduced LV ejection fraction demonstrated by two-dimensional echocardiography and/or radionuclide ventriculography is the best noninvasive indicator of depressed LV systolic function.

Decisions about surgery in AR should be based on the clinical functional class and on the LV ejection fraction at rest (Table 56-25).[134] Patients with chronic severe AR who are symptomatic (NYHA functional classes II to IV) need valve replacement. Although there may be some disagreement about recommending valve replacement to patients with normal ejection fraction who are in functional class II, we currently would do so. The benefit from valve replacement has been demonstrated even when the LV ejection fraction is 0.25 or less.[135] As opposed to AS, in which there is no lower level of ejection fraction that indicates inoperability, it is likely that some patients with AR and a very low ejection fraction become inoperable. This level has not been precisely defined but may be about 0.15 or less. There is a need to individualize the need for valve replacement in those with very severe LV systolic dysfunction at rest, in those with very severe LV dilatation (LV end-diastolic volume index ≥300 mL/m^2),[136] and in those with a small regurgitant volume, with a ratio of regurgitant volume to end-diastolic volume of 0.14[137] (Table 56-25). Recent data indicate that patients with severe AR, LV end-diastolic dimension on echocardiography of ≥80 mm, and mild to moderate reduction of LV ejection fraction (mean 0.43) can obtain benefit from valve replacement.[138] Postoperatively, they are symptomatically improved, LV ejection fraction increases, and LV size is reduced; the 5- and 10-year survivals are 87 and 71 percent, respectively.

Although the issue is controversial in some countries, we believe that patients who are in NYHA functional class I

TABLE 56-25 Chronic Severe Aortic Regurgitation: Indications for Surgery[a]

I. Symptomatic patients
  A. LV function normal: As soon as possible
  B. LV dysfunction: Urgent
  C. Heart failure: Emergent
  D. Individualize if:
    1. Very severe LV dysfunction (LVEF ≤0.20)
    2. Severe LV dilatation (LVEDD ≥80 mm with severe LV dysfunction; LVEDVI ≥300 ml/m²)
    3. Small RgV (RgV/EDV ≤0.14)
II. Asymptomatic patients
  A. LV systolic dysfunction (LVEF ≤0.50–0.54)
  B. Normal LV systolic function
    1. Associated cardiovascular diseases requiring surgery
      a. CAD
      b. Other valve disease
      c. Ascending aortic aneurysm
    2. Large LV
      LVEDD ≥70–75 mm; 35–38 mm/m²
      LVESD ≥50–55 mm; 25–27 mm/m²
      LVEDVI ≥150 ml/m²
      PLUS PA wedge on exercise ≥20–22 mmHg
    3. Progressive changes in LV size and function
      Increase of LVEDD and/or LVESD
      Decrease of LVEF

[a]Valve replacement/valve repair.
ABBREVIATIONS: CAD = coronary artery disease; EF = ejection fraction; EDD = end-diastolic dimension; EDVI = end-diastolic volume index; RgV = regurgitant volume; EDV = end-diastolic volume; PAW = pulmonary artery wedge.
SOURCE: Copyright © by S. H. Rahimtoola, M.B., F.R.C.P., M.A.C.P., M.A.C.C. See Ref. 93.

(asymptomatic) and have a reduced ejection fraction at rest should be offered aortic valve replacement. If the ejection fraction is normal at rest, one should consider valve replacement in NYHA functional class I patients if they have severe obstructive CAD and/or need surgery for other valve disease (Table 56-25). It is suggested that patients undergo an exercise test during right heart catheterization if the left ventricle is large (LV end-diastolic volume ≥150 mL/m², LV internal dimension on M-mode echocardiography of ≥70 mm at end diastole and ≥50 mm at end systole) and/or the LV ejection fraction shows a new, persistent reduction to 0.54 to 0.60; if the patients have reduced exercise capacity on treadmill testing; or if ambulatory ECG monitoring demonstrates ventricular tachyarrhythmias. Valve replacement is recommended if the pulmonary artery wedge pressure during exercise ≥20 to 24 mmHg. Patients with associated significant CAD should have coronary bypass surgery performed at the time of valvular surgery (see "Aortic Valve Stenosis," above, and Table 56-14).

Aortic valve replacement, with or without associated coronary bypass surgery for obstructive CAD, can be performed at many surgical centers with an operative mortality of 5 percent or less (see Chap. 66). In those without associated CAD or reduced LV systolic function, the operative mortality may be

TABLE 56-26 Recommendations for Aortic Valve Replacement in Chronic Severe Aortic Regurgitation

Indication	Class
1. Patients with NYHA functional Class III or IV symptoms and preserved LV systolic function, defined as normal ejection fraction at rest (ejection fraction ≥0.50)	I
2. Patients with NYHA functional class II symptoms and preserved LV systolic function (ejection fraction ≥0.50 at rest) but with progressive LV dilatation or declining ejection fraction at rest on serial studies or declining effort tolerance on exercise testing	I
3. Patients with Canadian Heart Association functional Class II or greater angina with or without CAD	I
4. Asymptomatic or symptomatic patients with mild to moderate LV dysfunction at rest (ejection fraction 0.25 to 0.49)	I
5. Patients undergoing coronary artery bypass surgery or surgery on the aorta or other heart valves	I
6. Patients with NYHA functional Class II symptoms and preserved LV systolic function (ejection fraction ≥0.50 at rest) with stable LV size and systolic function on serial studies and stable exercise tolerance	IIa
7. Asymptomatic patients with normal LV systolic function (ejection fraction >0.50) but with severe LV dilatation (end-diastolic dimension >75 mm or end-systolic dimension >55 mm)[a]	IIa
8. Patients with severe LV dysfunction (ejection fraction <0.25)	IIb
9. Asymptomatic patients with normal systolic function at rest (ejection fraction >0.50) and progressive LV dilatation when the degree of dilatation is moderately severe (end-diastolic dimension 70 to 75 mm, end-systolic dimension 50 to 55 mm)	IIb
10. Asymptomatic patients with normal systolic function at rest (ejection fraction >0.50) but with decline in ejection fraction during	
• Exercise radionuclide angiography	IIb
• Stress echocardiography	III
11. Asymptomatic patients with normal systolic function at rest (ejection fraction >0.50) and LV dilatation when degree of dilatation is not severe (end-diastolic dimension <70 mm, end-systolic dimension <50 mm)	III

[a]Consider lower threshold values for patients of small stature of either gender. Clinical judgment is required.
SOURCE: ACC/AHA Guidelines,[91] with permission.

in the range of 1 to 2 percent. If aortic valve replacement is successful and uncomplicated, LV volume and hypertrophy regress but do not return to normal; the beneficial effects on LV size, volume, and mass continue to be seen up to 5 years after surgery.[82,139,140] Impaired LV systolic pump function improves postoperatively in 50 percent or more of patients;[135] this improvement is more likely to occur if LV dysfunction has been present preoperatively for 12 months or less, and in this subgroup LV ejection fraction usually normalizes.[140] Even if LV systolic pump function does not improve, there is a reduction in end-diastolic volume and hypertrophy;[125] from a cardiac point of view, this is advantageous to the patient. The 5-year survival of patients undergoing aortic valve replacement in severe AR is 85 percent (this figure includes operative and late cardiac deaths).[134] The 5-year survival of patients with LV ejection fraction $\geq$0.45 is 87 percent, versus 54 percent in patients with an ejection fraction <0.45.[134] Late survival after valve replacement for chronic severe AR is best predicted by variables indicative of LV systolic pump function. Both the operative mortality and late survival are dependent on cardiac and LV function and associated noncardiac comorbid factors (see "Aortic Valve Stenosis," above, and Chap. 66).

Indeed, in general, the major factors influencing outcome in patients with valvular heart disease are: LV dysfunction and its magnitude, duration of LV dysfunction, degree of LV dilatation, greater NYHA functional class, older age, associated CAD, and comorbid conditions.

New techniques of aortic valve repair are being developed and evaluated, and early results are encouraging in selected subgroups.[105,141,142] It is possible that selected patients may eventually need to have valve repair rather than valve replacement for AR.

The recommendations of the ACC/AHA Practice Guidelines are shown in Table 56-26.[91] Guidelines are *not* and should *not* be the Law. Application of such guidelines to clinical practice should be based on the following principles: (1) classes I and III applies to all patients in these classes unless there is a specific clinical circumstance not to do so; (2) class II applies to patients in this class depending on the clinical conditions of the patients and the skill and experience at the individual medical center.

References

1. Roberts WC. Valvular, subvalvular and supravalvular aortic stenosis: Morphologic features. *Cardiovasc Clin* 1973; 5:97.
2. Moller JH, Nakib A, Elliott RS, Edwards JE. Symptomatic congenital aortic stenosis in the first year of life. *J Pediatr* 1966; 69:728–734.
3. Braunwald E, Goldblatt A, Aygen MM, et al. Congenital aortic stenosis: I. Clinical and hemodynamic findings in 100 patients. II. Surgical treatment and the results of operation. *Circulation* 1963; 27:426–462.
4. Passik CS, Ackerman DM, Pluth JR, Edwards WD. Temporal changes in the causes of aortic stenosis: A surgical pathological study of 646 cases. *Mayo Clin Proc* 1987; 62:119–123.
5. Olsson N, Dalsgaaro C-J, Haegerstrand A, et al. Accumulation of T lymphocytes and expression of interleukin-2 receptors in nonrheumatic stenotic aortic valves. *J Am Coll Cardiol* 1994; 23:1162–1170.
6. Otto CM, Knusisto J, Reichenbach D, et al. Characterization of the early lesion of "degenerative" valvular aortic stenosis: Historical and immunohistochemical studies. *Circulation* 1994; 90:844–853.
7. Narang NK, Andrew AMR, Chaudhury HR, Gaba BS. Aortic stenosis due to familial hypercholesterolemic xanthomatosis: A case report with brief review of literature. *Indian Heart J* 1978; 30:189–192.
8. Deutscher S, Rockette HE, Krishnaswami V. Diabetes and hypercholesterolemia among patients with calcific aortic stenosis. *J Chronic Dis* 1984; 37:407–415.
9. Strickberger SA, Schulman SP, Hutchins GM. Association of Paget's disease of bone with calcific aortic valve disease. *Am J Med* 1987; 82:953–956.
10. Maher ER, Pazianas M, Curtis JR. Calcific aortic stenosis: A complication of chronic uraemia. *Nephron* 1987; 47:119–122.
11. Maher ER, Young G, Smyth-Walsh B, et al. Aortic and mitral valve calcification in patients with end-stage renal disease. *Lancet* 1987; 2:875–877.
12. Dereymaeker L, Van Parijs G, Bayart M, et al. Ochronosis and alkaptonuria: Report of a new case with calcified aortic valve stenosis. *Acta Cardiol* 1990; 45:87–92.
13. Selzer A. Changing aspects of the natural history of valvular aortic stenosis. *N Engl J Med* 1987; 31:91–98.
14. Roberts WC. The structural basis of abnormal cardiac function: A look at coronary, hypertensive, valvular, idiopathic myocardial, and pericardial heart disease. In: Levine JJ, ed. *Clinical Cardiovascular Physiology*. New York: Grune & Stratton; 1976.
15. Stewart BF, Siscovick P, Lind B, et al. Clinical factors associated with calcific aortic valve disease. *J Am Coll Cardiol* 1997; 29: 630–634.
16. Kennedy JW, Twiss RD, Blackmon JR, Dodge HT. Quantitative angiography: III. Relationships of left ventricular pressure, volume, and mass in aortic valve disease. *Circulation* 1968; 38:838–845.
17. Bertrand ME, LaBlanche JM, Tilmant PY, et al. Coronary sinus blood flow at rest and during isometric exercise in patients with aortic valve disease: Mechanism of angina pectoris in presence of normal coronary arteries. *Am J Cardiol* 1981; 47:199–205.
18. Bonow RO. Left ventricular structure and function in aortic valve disease. *Circulation* 1989; 79:966–969.
19. Krayenbuehl HP, Hess OM, Monrad ES, et al. Left ventricular myocardial structure in aortic valve disease before, intermediate, and later after aortic valve replacement. *Circulation* 1989; 79:744–755.
20. Schwarz F, Flameng W, Schaper J, et al. Myocardial structure and function in patients with aortic valve disease and their relation to postoperative results. *Am J Cardiol* 1978; 41:661–669.
21. Tobin JR Jr, Rahimtoola SH, Blundell PE, Swan HJC. Percentage of left ventricular stroke work loss: A simple hemodynamic concept for estimation of severity in valvular aortic stenosis. *Circulation* 1967; 35:868–879.
22. Pantely G, Morton MJ, Rahimtoola SH. Effects of successful, uncomplicated valve replacement on ventricular hypertrophy, volume, and performance in aortic stenosis and aortic incompetence. *J Thorac Cardiovasc Surg* 1978; 75:383–391.
23. Hess OM, Ritter M, Schneider J, et al. Diastolic stiffness and myocardial structure in aortic valve disease before and after replacement. *Circulation* 1984; 69:855–865.
24. Murakami T, Hess O, Gage JE, et al. Diastolic filling dynamics in patients with aortic stenosis. *Circulation* 1986; 73:1162–1174.
25. Dineen E, Brent BN. Aortic valve stenosis: Comparison of patients to those without chronic congestive heart failure. *Am J Cardiol* 1986; 57:419–422.
26. Fifer MA, Borow KM, Colan SD, Lorell BH. Early diastolic left ventricular function in children and adults with aortic stenosis. *J Am Coll Cardiol* 1985; 5:1147–1154.
27. Hess OM, Villari B, Krayenbuehl HP. Diastolic dysfunction in aortic stenosis. *Circulation* 1993; 87(suppl IV):73–76.

28. Braunwald E, Frahm CJ. Studies on the Starling's law of the heart. IV: Observations on the hemodynamic functions of the left atrium in man. *Circulation* 1961; 24:633–642.
29. Stott DK, Marpole DGF, Bristow JD, et al. The role of left atrial transport in aortic and mitral stenosis. *Circulation* 1970; 41:1031–1041.
30. Carroll JD, Carroll EP, Feldman T, et al. Sex-associated differences in left ventricular function in aortic stenosis of the elderly. *Circulation* 1992; 86:1099–1107.
31. Ross J Jr. Afterload mismatch and preload reserve: A conceptual framework for the analysis of ventricular function. *Prog Cardiovasc Dis* 1976; 18:255–264.
32. Bache RJ, Wang Y, Jorgensen CR. Hemodynamic effects of exercise in isolated valvular aortic stenosis. *Circulation* 1971; 44:1003.
33. Johnson LL, Sciacca RR, Ellis K, et al. Reduced left ventricular myocardial blood flow per unit mass in aortic stenosis. *Circulation* 1978; 57:582–590.
34. Vinten-Johansen J, Weiss HR. Oxygen consumption in subepicardial and subendocardial regions of the canine left ventricle—The effect of experimental acute valvular aortic stenosis. *Circ Res* 1980; 46:139–145.
35. Marcus ML, Doty DB, Horatzka LF, et al. Decreased coronary reserve: A mechanism for angina pectoris in patients with aortic stenosis and normal coronary arteries. *N Engl J Med* 1982; 307:1362–1366.
36. Grech ED, Ramsdale DR. Exertional syncope in aortic stenosis: Evidence to support inappropriate left ventricular baroreceptor response. *Am Heart J* 1991; 121:603–606.
37. Schwartz LS, Goldfischer J, Sprague GJ, Schwartz SP. Syncope and sudden death in aortic stenosis. *Am J Cardiol* 1969; 23: 647–658.
38. Kulbertus HE. Ventricular arrhythmias, syncope and sudden death in aortic stenosis. *Eur Heart J* 1988; 9(suppl E):51–52.
39. Shoenfeld Y, Eldar M, Bedazovsky B, et al. Aortic stenosis associated with gastrointestinal bleeding: A survey of 612 patients. *AmHeart J* 1980; 100:179–182.
40. Love JW. The syndrome of calcific aortic stenosis and gastrointestinal bleeding: Resolution following aortic valve replacement. *J Thorac Cardiovasc Surg* 1982; 83:779–783.
41. Pleet AB, Massey EW, Vengrow ME. TIA, stroke, and the bicuspid aortic valve. *Neurology* 1981; 31:1540–1542.
42. Brockmeier LB, Adolph RJ, Gustin BW, et al. Calcium emboli to the retinal artery in calcific aortic stenosis. *Am Heart J* 1981; 101:32–37.
43. Wood P. Aortic stenosis. *Am J Cardiol* 1958; 1:553–571.
44. Murphy ES, Lawson RM, Starr A, Rahimtoola SH. Severe aortic stenosis in the elderly: State of left ventricular function and result of valve replacement on ten-year survival. *Circulation* 1981; 64(suppl II):184–188.
45. Szamosi A, Wassberg B. Radiologic detection of aortic stenosis. *Acta Radiol Diagn* 1983; 24:201.
46. Siegel RJ, Maurer G, Navatpumin T, Shah PK. Accurate noninvasive assessment of critical aortic valve stenosis in the elderly (abstr). *J Am Coll Cardiol* 1983; 1:639.
47. Gooch AS, Calatayud JB, Rogers PA, Garman PA. Analysis of the P wave in severe aortic stenosis. *Dis Chest* 1966; 49:459–463.
48. Thompson R, Mitchell A, Ahmed M, et al. Conduction defects in aortic valve disease. *Am Heart J* 1979; 98:3–10.
49. Nair CK, Aronow WS, Stokke K, et al. Cardiac conduction defects in patients older than 60 years with aortic stenosis and without mitral annular calcium. *Am J Cardiol* 1984; 53:169–172.
50. Rosenbaum M, Elizari M, Lazari J. *Los Hemibloques*. Buenos Aires: Paidos; 1968:363.
51. Galan A, Zoghbi WA, Quiñones MA. Determination of severity of valvular aortic stenosis by Doppler echocardiography and relation of findings to clinical outcome and agreement with hemodynamic measurements determined at cardiac catheterization. *Am J Cardiol* 1991; 67:1007–1012.
52. Agatston AS, Chengot M, Rao A, et al. Doppler diagnosis of valvular aortic stenosis in patients over 60 years of age. *Am J Cardiol* 1985; 56:106–109.
53. Skjaerpe T, Hegrenaes L, Hatle L. Noninvasive estimation of valve area in patients with aortic stenosis by Doppler ultrasound and two-dimensional echocardiography. *Circulation* 1985; 72: 810–815.
54. Yeager M, Yock PG, Popp RL. Comparison of Doppler-derived pressure gradient to that determined at cardiac catheterization in adults with aortic valve stenosis: Implications for management. *Am J Cardiol* 1986; 57:644–648.
55. Currie PJ, Seward JB, Reeder GS, et al. Continuous-wave Doppler echocardiographic assessment of severity of calcific aortic stenosis: A simultaneous Doppler-catheter correlative study in 100 adult patients. *Circulation* 1985; 71:1162–1169.
56. Oh JK, Taliercio CP, Holmes DR Jr, et al. Prediction of the severity of aortic stenosis by Doppler aortic valve area determination: Prospective Doppler-catheterization in 100 patients. *J Am Coll Cardiol* 1988; 11:1227–1234.
57. Rahimtoola SH. Perspective on valvular heart disease: Update II. In: Knoebel S, ed. *An Era in Cardiovascular Medicine*. New York: Elsevier; 1991:45–70.
58. Roger VL, Tajik AJ, Reeder GS, et al. Effect of Doppler echocardiography on utilization of hemodynamic cardiac catheterization in the preoperative evaluation of aortic stenosis. *Mayo Clin Proc* 1996; 71:141–149.
59. Griffith MJ, Carey C, Coltart DJ, et al. Inaccuracies of using aortic valve gradients alone to grade severity of aortic stenosis. *Br Heart J* 1989; 62:372–378.
60. Enriquez-Sarano M, Klodas E, Garratt KN, et al. Secular trends in coronary atherosclerosis—Analysis in patients with valve regurgitation. *N Engl J Med* 1996; 335:316–322.
61. Sethi GK, Miller DC, Sonchek J, et al. Clinical, hemodynamic and angiographic predictors of operative mortality in patients undergoing single valve replacement. *J Thorac Cardiovasc Surg* 1987; 93:884–887.
62. Mullany CJ, Elveback ER, Frye RL, et al. Coronary artery disease and its management: Influence on survival in patients undergoing aortic valve replacement. *J Am Coll Cardiol* 1987; 10:66–72.
63. Levinson JR, Akins CW, Buckley MJ, et al. Octogenarians with aortic stenosis: Outcome after aortic valve replacement. *Circulation* 1989; 80(suppl I):49–56.
64. Klein RC. Ventricular arrhythmias in aortic valve disease: Analysis of 102 patients. *Am J Cardiol* 1984; 53:1079–1083.
65. von Olshausen K, Schwarz F, Apfelbach J, et al. Determinants of the incidence and severity of ventricular arrhythmias in aortic valve disease. *Am J Cardiol* 1983; 51:1103–1109.
66. Kotlewski A, Kawanishi DT, McKay CR, et al. The relative value of clinical examination, echocardiography with Doppler and cardiac catheterization with angiography in the evaluation of aortic valve disease. In: Bodnar E, ed. *Surgery for Heart Valve Disease*. London: ICR; 1990:66–72.
67. Jonasson R, Jonsson B, Nordlander R, et al. Rate of progression of severity of valvular aortic stenosis. *Acta Med Scand* 1983; 213:51–54.
68. Nestico PF, DePace NL, Kimbiris D, et al. Progression of isolated aortic stenosis: Analysis of 29 patients having more than one cardiac catheterization. *Am J Cardiol* 1983; 52:1054–1058.
69. Hoagland PM, Cook EF, Wynne J, Goldman L. Value of noninvasive testing in adults with suspected aortic stenosis. *Am J Med* 1986; 80:1041–1050.
70. Cohen LS, Friedman WF, Braunwald E. Natural history of mild congenital aortic stenosis elucidated by serial hemodynamic studies. *Am J Cardiol* 1972; 30:1–5.
71. Cheitlin MD, Gertz EW, Brundage BH, et al. Rate of progression

of severity of valvular aortic stenosis in the adult. *Am Heart J* 1979; 98:689–700.
72. Wagner S, Selzer A. Patterns of progression of aortic stenosis: A longitudinal hemodynamic study. *Circulation* 1982; 65:709–712.
73. Horstkotte D, Loogen F. The natural history of aortic valve stenosis. *Eur Heart J* 1988; 9(suppl E):57–64.
74. Otto CM, Burwash JG, Legget ME, et al. Prospective study of asymptomatic valvular aortic stenosis: Clinical, echocardiographic, and exercise predictors of outcome. *Circulation* 1997; 95:2262–2270.
75. Rahimtoola SH. Prophylactic valve replacement for mild aortic valve disease at time of surgery for other cardiovascular disease? . . . NO. *J Am Coll Cardiol* 1999; 33:2009–2015.
76. Holmes DR Jr, Nishimura RA, Reeder GS. In-hospital mortality after balloon valvuloplasty: Frequency and associated factors. *J Am Coll Cardiol* 1991; 17:189–192.
77. Ross J Jr, Braunwald E. Aortic stenosis. *Circulation* 1968; 36(suppl IV):61–67.
78. Otto CM, Lind BK, Kitzman DW, et al. Association of aortic valve sclerosis with cardiovascular mortality and morbidity in the elderly. *N Engl J Med* 1999; 341:142–147.
79. Kirklin JW, Barratt-Boyes BG. Congenital valvular aortic stenosis. In: *Cardiac Surgery*. New York: Wiley; 1986:972–988.
80. Schwarz F, Banmann P, Manthey J, et al. The effect of aortic valve replacement on survival. *Circulation* 1982; 66:1105–1110.
81. Rahimtoola SH. Valvular heart disease: A perspective. *J Am Coll Cardiol* 1983; 1:199–215.
82. Monrad ES, Hess OM, Murakami T, et al. Time course of regression of left ventricular hypertrophy after aortic valve replacement. *Circulation* 1988; 77:1345–1355.
83. Hammermeister KL, Sethi GK, Henderson WG, et al. A comparison of outcomes in men 11 years after heart-valve replacement with a mechanical valve or bioprosthesis. *N Engl J Med* 1993; 328:1289–1296.
84. Lindblom D, Lindblom U, Qvist J, Lundström H. Long-term relative survival rates after heart valve replacement. *J Am Coll Cardiol* 1990; 15:566–573.
85. Rahimtoola SH. Catheter balloon valvuloplasty for severe calcific aortic stenosis: A limited role. *J Am Coll Cardiol* 1994; 23:1076–1078.
86. Connolly HM, Oh JK, Orszulak TA, et al. Aortic valve replacement for aortic stenosis with severe left ventricular dysfunction: Prognostic indicators. *Circulation* 1997; 95:2395–2400.
87. Rahimtoola SH, Starr A. Valvular surgery. In: Braunwald E, Mock M, Watson J, eds. *Congestive Heart Failure: Current Research and Clinical Applications*. Orlando, FL: Grune & Stratton; 1982:89–93.
88. Smith N, McAnulty JH, Rahimtoola SH. Severe aortic stenosis with impaired left ventricular function and clinical heart failure: Results of valve replacement. *Circulation* 1978; 58:255–264.
89. Otto CM, Mickel MC, Kennedy JW, et al. Three-year outcome after balloon aortic valvuloplasty: Insights into prognosis of valvular aortic stenosis. *Circulation* 1994; 89:642–650.
90. Moreno PR, Jang I-K, Newell JB, et al. The role of percutaneous aortic balloon valvuloplasty in patients with cardiogenic shock and critical aortic stenosis. *J Am Coll Cardiol* 1994; 23:1071–1075.
91. Bonow RO, Carabello B, de Leon AC Jr, et al. ACC/AHA guidelines for the management of patients with valvular heart disease: A report of the American College of Cardiology/American Heart Association Task Force on Practice Guidelines (Committee on Management of Patients with Valvular Heart Disease). *J Am Coll Cardiol* 1998; 32:1486–1588.
92. Rahimtoola SH. Recognition and management of acute aortic regurgitation. *Heart Dis Stroke* 1993; 2:217–221.
93. Braunwald E. Valvular heart disease. In: Braunwald E, ed. *Heart Disease*, 4th ed. Philadelphia: Saunders; 1992:1007–1077.
94. Rahimtoola SH. Valvular heart disease. In: Stein J, ed. (O'Rourke RA, Cardiology Section ed). *Internal Medicine*, 4th ed. St. Louis: Mosby–Year Book; 1994:202–234.
95. Belenkie I, Rademaker A. Acute and chronic changes after aortic valve damage in the intact dog. *Am J Physiol* 1981; 241:H95–H103.
96. Welch GH Jr, Braunwald E, Sarnoff SJ. Hemodynamic effects of quantitatively varied experimental aortic regurgitation. *Circ Res* 1957; 5:546–551.
97. Rahimtoola SH. Aortic regurgitation. In: Rahimtoola SH, ed. *Atlas of Heart Diseases: Valvular Heart Disease*. Vol XI. Philadelphia: Current Medicine; 1997:7.1–7.26.
98. Rahimtoola SH. Management of heart failure in valve regurgitation. *Clin Cardiol* 1992; 15(suppl I):22–27.
99. Nienaber CA, von Kodolitsch Y, Nicholas V, et al. The diagnosis of thoracic aortic dissection by noninvasive imaging procedures. *N Engl J Med* 1993; 328:1–9.
100. Cigarroa JE, Isselbacher EM, De Sanctis RW, Eagle KA. Diagnostic imaging in the evaluation of suspected aortic dissection: Old standards and new directions. *N Engl J Med* 1993; 328:35–43.
101. Kostuk W, Barr JW, Simon AL, Ross J Jr. Correlations between the chest film and hemodynamics in acute myocardial infarction. *Circulation* 1973; 48:624–632.
102. Chatterjee K, Parmley WW, Swan HJC, et al. Beneficial effects of vasodilator agents in severe mitral regurgitation due to dysfunction of subvalvular apparatus. *Circulation* 1973; 48:684–690.
103. Richardson JV, Karp RB, Kirklin JW, Dismukes WE. Treatment of infective endocarditis: A 10-year comparative analysis. *Circulation* 1978; 58:589–597.
104. Tonnemacher D, Reid CL, Kawanishi DT, et al. Frequency of myxomatous degeneration of the aortic valve as a cause of isolated aortic regurgitation severe enough to warrant aortic valve replacement. *Am J Cardiol* 1987; 60:1194–1196.
105. Antunes M. Repair for acquired valvular heart disease. In: Rahimtoola SH, ed. *Atlas of Heart Diseases: Valvular Heart Disease*. Vol XI. Philadelphia: Current Medicine; 1997:12.1–12.23.
106. Waller BF. Rheumatic and nonrheumatic conditions producing valvular heart disease. In: Frankl WS, Brest AN, eds. *Cardiovascular Clinics—Valvular Heart Disease: Comprehensive Evaluation and Management*. Philadelphia: Davis; 1986:30–31.
107. Miller GAH, Kirklin JW, Swan HJC. Myocardial function and left ventricular volumes in acquired valvular insufficiency. *Circulation* 1965; 31:374–384.
108. Karaian CH, Greenberg BH, Rahimtoola SH. The relationship between functional class and cardiac performance in patients with chronic aortic insufficiency. *Chest* 1985; 88:553–557.
109. Kawanishi DT, McKay CR, Chandraratna PAN, et al. Cardiovascular response to dynamic exercise in patients with chronic symptomatic mild-to-moderate and severe aortic regurgitation. *Circulation* 1986; 73:62–72.
110. Shen WF, Roubin GS, Choong CY-P, et al. Evaluation of relationship between myocardial contractile state and left ventricular function in patients with aortic regurgitation. *Circulation* 1985; 71:31–38.
111. Boucher CA, Wilson RA, Kanarek DJ, et al. Exercise testing in asymptomatic or minimally symptomatic aortic regurgitation: Relationship of left ventricular ejection fraction to left ventricular filling pressure during exercise. *Circulation* 1983; 67:1091–1100.
112. Falsetti HL, Carroll RJ, Cramer JA. Total and regional myocardial blood flow in aortic regurgitation. *Am Heart J* 1979; 97:485–493.
113. Uhl GS, Boucher CA, Oliveros RA, Murgo JP. Exercise-induced myocardial oxygen supply-demand imbalance in asymptomatic or mildly symptomatic aortic regurgitation. *Chest* 1981; 80:686–691.
114. Nittenburg A, Foult JM, Antony I, et al. Coronary flow and resistance reserve in patients with chronic aortic regurgitation, angina pectoris, and normal coronary arteries. *J Am Coll Cardiol* 1988; 11:478–486.

115. Sabbah HN, Khaja F, Anbe DT, Stein PD. The aortic closure sound in pure aortic insufficiency. *Circulation* 1977; 56:859–863.
116. Schaefer RA, McAnulty JH, Starr A, Rahimtoola SH. Diastolic murmurs in the presence of Starr-Edwards mitral prosthesis: With emphasis on the genesis of the Austin Flint murmur. *Circulation* 1975; 51:402–409.
117. Roberts WC, Day PJ. Electrocardiographic observations in clinically isolated, pure, and chronic, severe aortic regurgitation: Analysis of 30 necropsy patients aged 19 to 65 years. *Am J Cardiol* 1985; 55:431–438.
118. Rapaport E. Natural history of aortic and mitral valve disease. *Am J Cardiol* 1975; 35:221–227.
119. Bonow RO, Lakatos E, Maron BJ, Epstein SE. Serial long-term assessment of the natural history of asymptomatic patients with chronic aortic regurgitation and normal left ventricular systolic function. *Circulation* 1991; 84:1625–1635.
120. Scognamiglio R, Rahimtoola SH, Fasoli G, et al. Nifedipine in asymptomatic patients with severe aortic regurgitation and normal left ventricular function. *N Engl J Med* 1994; 331:689–695.
121. Tornos MP, Olona M, Permanyer-Miralda G, et al. Clinical outcome of severe asymptomatic chronic aortic regurgitation: A long-term prospective follow-up study. *Am Heart J* 1995; 130:333–339.
122. Klodas E, Enrique-Sarano M, Tajik AJ, Mullany CJ, et al. Surgery for aortic regurgitation in women: Contrasting indications and outcomes compared with men. *Circulation* 1996; 94:2472–2478.
123. Siemienczuk D, Greenberg B, Morris C, et al. Chronic aortic insufficiency: Factors associated with progression to aortic valve replacement. *Ann Intern Med* 1989; 110:587–592.
124. McKay CR, Rahimtoola SH. Natural history of aortic regurgitation. In: Gaasch WH, Levine HJ, eds. *Chronic Aortic Regurgitation*. Boston: Kluwer Academic; 1980:1–17.
125. Dujardin KS, Enriquez-Sarano M, Schaff HV, et al. Mortality and morbidilty of aortic regurgitation in clinical practice: A long-term follow-up study. *Circulation* 1999; 99:1851–1857.
126. Greenberg B, Massie B, Bristow JD, et al. Long-term vasodilator therapy of chronic aortic insufficiency: A randomized double-blinded, placebo-controlled clinical trial. *Circulation* 1988; 78:92–103.
127. Rahimtoola SH. Vasodilator therapy in chronic severe aortic regurgitation. *J Am Coll Cardiol* 1990; 16:430–432.
128. Scognamiglio R, Rasoli G, Ponchia A, Dalla-Volta S. Long-term nifedipine unloading therapy in asymptomatic patients with chronic severe aortic regurgitation. *J Am Coll Cardiol* 1990; 16:424–429.
129. Rothlisberger C, Sareli P, Wisenbaugh T. Comparison of single-dose nifedipine and captopril for chronic severe aortic regurgitation. *Am J Cardiol* 1993; 72:799–804.
130. Wisenbaugh T, Sinovich V, Dullabh A, Sareli P. Six month pilot study of captopril for mildly symptomatic, severe isolated mitral and isolated aortic regurgitation. *J Heart Valve Dis* 1994; 3:197–204.
131. Schon HR, Dorn R, Barthel P, Schömig A. Effects of 12 months quinapril therapy in asymptomatic patients with chronic aortic regurgitation. *J Heart Valve Dis* 1994; 3:500–509.
132. Lin M, Chian H-T, Lin S-L, et al. Vasodilator therapy in chronic asymptomatic aortic regurgitation: Enalapril versus hydralazine. *J Am Coll Cardiol* 1994; 24:1046–1053.
133. McKay CR, Nanna M, Kawanishi DT, et al. Importance of internal controls, statistical methods, and side effects in acute vasodilator trials: A study of hydralazine kinetics in patients with aortic regurgitation. *Circulation* 1985; 72:865–872.
134. Greves J, Rahimtoola SH, McAnulty JH, et al. Preoperative criteria predictive of late survival following valve replacement for severe aortic regurgitation. *Am Heart J* 1981; 101:300–308.
135. Clark DG, McAnulty JH, Rahimtoola SH. Valve replacement in aortic insufficiency with left ventricular dysfunction. *Circulation* 1980; 61:411–421.
136. Taniguchi K, Nakano S, Hirose H, et al. Preoperative left ventricular function: Minimal requirement for successful late results of valve replacement for aortic regurgitation. *J Am Coll Cardiol* 1987; 10:510–518.
137. Levine HJ, Gaasch WH. Ratio of regurgitant volume to end-diastolic volume: A major determinant of ventricular response to surgical correction of chronic volume overload. *Am J Cardiol* 1983; 52:406–410.
138. Klodas E, Enriquez-Sarano M, Tajik AJ, et al. Aortic regurgitation complicated by extreme left ventricular dilation: Long-term outcome after surgical correction. *J Am Coll Cardiol* 1996; 27:670–677.
139. Gaasch WH, Carroll JD, Levine HJ, Criscitiello MG. Chronic aortic regurgitation: Prognostic value of left ventricular end-systolic dimension and end-diastolic radius/thickness ratio. *J Am Coll Cardiol* 1983; 1:775–782.
140. Bonow RO, Dodd JT, Maron BJ, et al. Long-term serial changes in left ventricular function and reversal of ventricular dilatation after valve replacement for chronic aortic regurgitation. *Circulation* 1988; 78:1108–1120.
141. Cosgrove DM, Rosenkranz ER, Hendren WG, et al. Valvuloplasty for aortic insufficiency. *J Thorac Cardiovasc Surg* 1991; 102:571–577.
142. Duran C, Kumar N, Gometza B, Al Halees Z. Indications and limitations of aortic valve reconstruction. *Ann Thorac Surg* 1991; 52:447–454.

C H A P T E R 57

MITRAL VALVE DISEASE*

Shahbudin H. Rahimtoola / Maurice Enriquez-Sarano / Hartzell V. Schaff / Robert L. Frye

MITRAL STENOSIS

Etiology

Mitral stenosis (MS), an obstruction to blood flow between the left atrium (LA) and the left ventricle (LV), is caused by abnormal mitral valve function. In virtually all adult patients, the cause of MS is previous rheumatic carditis.[1] About 60 percent of patients with rheumatic mitral valve disease do not give a history of rheumatic fever or chorea, and about 50 percent of patients with acute rheumatic carditis do not eventually have clinical valvular heart disease.[2] Other causes of MS are all uncommon or rare and are listed in Table 57-1.[2-10] Congenital MS is uncommon. It is usually caused by a "parachute" deformity of the valve, in which shortened chordae tendineae insert in a large, single papillary muscle. MS, usually rheumatic, in association with atrial septal defect is called *Lutembacher's syndrome*. A rare cause of MS is massive mitral valve annular calcification. This process occurs most frequently in elderly patients and produces MS by limiting leaflet motion. When stenosis is present, it is usually mild in degree. Other causes of obstruction to LA outflow include a LA myxoma, massive LA ball thrombus, and cor triatriatum, in which a congenital membrane is present in the LA.

Pathology

Acute rheumatic carditis is a pancarditis involving the pericardium, myocardium, and endocardium. In temperate climates and developed countries, there is usually a long interval (averaging 10 to 20 years) between an episode of rheumatic carditis and the clinical presentation of symptomatic MS. In tropical and subtropical climates and in less developed countries, the latent period is often shorter, and MS may occur during childhood or adolescence (see Chap. 55).

The pathologic hallmark of rheumatic carditis is an Aschoff's nodule. The most common lesion of acute rheumatic endocarditis is mitral valvulitis. In this condition the mitral valve has vegetations along the line of closure and the chordae tendineae. Mitral regurgitation (MR) may be present during the acute episode of rheumatic carditis.

MS is usually the result of repeated episodes of carditis alternating with healing and is characterized by the deposition of fibrous tissue. MS may result from fusion of the commissures, cusps, or chordae, or a combination of these.[9,10] Ultimately, the deformed valve is subject to nonspecific fibrosis and calcification. Lesions along the line of closure result in fusion of the commissures and contracture and thickening of the valve leaflets. The chordal lesions are manifest as shortening and fusion of these structures. The combination of commissural fusion, valve leaflet contracture, and fusion of the chordae tendineae results in a narrow, funnel-shaped orifice, which restricts the flow of blood from the LA to the LV. The rapidity with which patients become symptomatic may depend on the number and severity of repeated bouts of rheumatic valvulitis. Frequently, the rheumatic episodes are not clinically apparent.

In pure MS, the LV is usually normal, but there may be evidence of previous carditis with deposition of fibrous tissue. The LA is enlarged and hypertrophied as a consequence of LA hypertension. Mural thrombi are often found in the LA, particularly if atrial fibrillation has been present. Calcification of the mitral valve frequently also involves the mitral annulus.

Pathophysiology

The pathophysiologic features of MS all result from obstruction of the flow of blood between the LA and the LV. With reduction in valve area, energy is lost to friction during the transport of blood from the LA to the LV. Accordingly, a pressure gradient is present across the stenotic valve. The relationship between valve area, cardiac output, flow period, and average diastolic gradient between the LA and the LV is defined by the formula of Gorlin and Gorlin (Chap. 15).

It is readily apparent that maintaining cardiac output when

* Mitral stenosis section written by Dr. Rahimtoola. Mitral regurgitation section written by Drs. Enriquez-Sarano, Schaff, and Frye.

TABLE 57-1 Causes of Mitral Stenosis

Cause	Involved Structure(s)			
	Leaflet	Chordae	Commissures	Other
Rheumatic fever	+	+	+	
Congenital	+	+		Single papillary muscle
Active infective endocarditis	+			Vegetation
Neoplasm				Mass, pulmonary vein obstruction
Massive annular calcification	+	0	0	Rigid annulus
Systemic lupus erythematosus	+	+	+	Verrucous vegetations may extend into papillary muscles
Carcinoid				Atrial septal defect or lung tumor in order to affect left heart
Methysergide therapy	+	+		Serotonin agonist/antagonist
Hunter-Hurler syndromes				Mucopolysaccharide deposits
Fabry's disease				Aramide trihexoxide deposits
Whipple's disease				PAS-positive macrophage deposits
Rheumatoid arthritis	+	+	+	PAS-positive plasma cell infiltrate

SOURCE: From Kawanishi DT, Rahimtoola SH. Mitral stenosis. In: Rahimtoola SH, ed. *Valvular Heart Disease. II.* St. Louis: Mosby; 1996:8.1–8.24.

the valve area is small requires a large gradient and thus an elevated LA pressure. Similarly, an increased demand for cardiac output (CO), such as occurs during exercise or pregnancy, results in an increase in gradient and high LA pressures. More subtle is the effect of the length of the diastolic flow period on the relationship between CO and gradient. The time available for diastole is that part of the cardiac cycle occupied by isovolumic contraction and relaxation or by ejection. As the heart rate increases, the total amount of time spent during systole increases despite a reduction in the systolic time per beat.[11,12] *Thus, time available for diastole decreases as the heart rate increases.* Because blood can flow through the mitral valve only during diastole, the flow rate is inversely proportional to the duration of the flow period at a constant stroke volume. Of course, a higher flow rate results in a greater loss of energy to friction and requires a larger gradient and higher LA pressures. It is important to remember that the gradient from LA to LV is a function per beat, not per minute. Thus, the gradient is dependent on the stroke volume and the diastolic filling time as well as the LV diastolic pressure.

The pressure gradient between the LA and the LV, which increases markedly with increased heart rate or CO, is responsible for LA hypertension. The LA gradually enlarges and hypertrophies. Pulmonary venous pressure rises with LA pressure increase and is passively associated with an increase in pulmonary arterial (PA) pressure (Fig. 57-1). In up to 20 percent of patients, the pulmonary vascular resistance is also elevated,[13] which further increases PA pressure. PA hypertension results in *right ventricular* (RV) hypertrophy and RV enlargement. The changes in RV function eventually result in *right atrial* (RA) hypertension and enlargement and systemic venous congestion; frequently, tricuspid regurgitation also occurs. In a small percentage of patients, there may be regional or global LV systolic dysfunction, the cause or causes of which are not fully understood.[14–18]

Pulmonary venous hypertension alters lung function in several ways. Distribution of blood flow in the lung is altered, with a relative increase in flow to the upper lobes and therefore in physiologic dead space. Pulmonary compliance generally decreases with increasing pulmonary capillary pressure, increasing the work of breathing, particularly during exercise. Chronic changes in the pulmonary capillaries and pulmonary arteries include fibrosis and thickening. These changes protect the lungs from the transudation of fluid into the alveoli (alveolar pulmonary edema). Indeed, it is not uncommon to find patients with severe MS whose resting PA wedge pressure (indirect LA pressure) exceeds 25 to 30 mmHg. Capillary and alveolar thickening, which help protect against pulmonary edema, further add to the abnormalities of ventilation and perfusion. Pulmonary vascular changes cause an elevated pulmonary vascular resistance.

In some patients with high pulmonary vascular resistance and RV dysfunction, CO may be low. The body maintains oxygen consumption by extracting more oxygen from the arterial blood, and the mixed venous oxygen content falls. The hemoglobin-O_2 dissociation curve is shifted to the right, facilitating the unloading of oxygen from hemoglobin to the tissues. The reduced CO may result in a *surprisingly small gradient* across the mitral valve despite severe stenosis. Although pulmonary congestion may be less striking in these patients, the CO does not increase normally with exercise, and, typically, the patients are severely limited by fatigue.

Long-standing MS with severe PA hypertension and resultant RV dysfunction may be accompanied by chronic systemic venous hypertension. Tricuspid regurgitation is frequently present, even in the absence of intrinsic disease of this valve. Functional pulmonic regurgitation may also be present. Dependent edema formation and visceral congestion directly reflect elevated systemic venous pressure and salt and water retention. Chronic passive congestion in the liver leads to central lobular necrosis and eventually to cardiac cirrhosis.

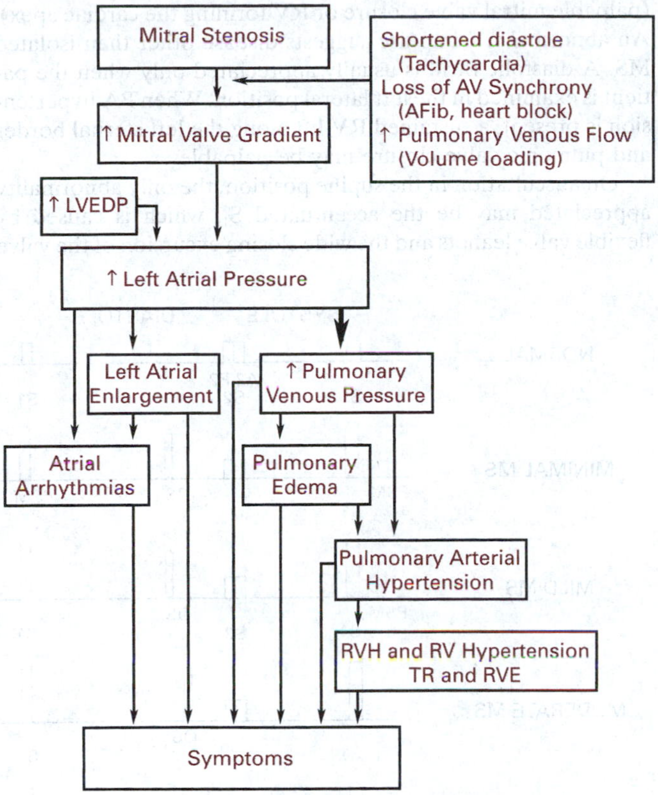

FIGURE 57-1 Pathophysiology of mitral stenosis. Mitral stenosis results in a diastolic pressure gradient from the LA to the LV. The actual gradient is dependent on the mitral valve area and the mitral valve *flow per diastolic second*. As a result, there is an elevation of LA pressure and therefore also of pulmonary venous pressure. Physiologic and pathologic changes—such as tachycardia and atrial fibrillation (which shorten diastole and may also result in loss of effective atrial contraction) or pregnancy, volume loading, and left-to-right shunts (at ventricular and aortopulmonary levels), which increase pulmonary venous flow—will increase the mitral valve gradient as well as LA and pulmonary venous pressures. An increased LV diastolic pressure will also result in further increase of LA pressure. An elevated LA pressure has several important effects; these include enlargement of the left atrium, atrial arrhythmias, and an increase of pulmonary venous pressure. Pulmonary venous hypertension may result in pulmonary edema and pulmonary arterial hypertension. PA hypertension and RV ventricular hypertension results in RV hypertrophy and may result in tricuspid regurgitation and RV enlargement. All of these changes contribute to producing symptoms. In addition, a fixed or even reduced cardiac output will also contribute to the symptomatic state of the patient. [Copyright by S. H. Rahimtoola. M.B., F.R.C.P., M.A.C.P., M.A.C.C. (Ref. 10).]

Clinical Findings

HISTORY

An asymptomatic interval is usually present between the initiating event of acute rheumatic fever and the presentation of symptomatic MS (averaging 10 to 20 years).[13,19] During this interval, the patient feels well (Table 57-2). Initially, there is little or no gradient at rest, but with increased cardiac output, LA pressure rises and exertional dyspnea develops. As mitral valve obstruction increases, dyspnea occurs at lower work levels. The progression of disability is so subtle and so protracted that patients may adapt by circumscribing their lifestyles. It becomes

TABLE 57-2 Symptoms Associated with Mitral Stenosis

On exertion
Dyspnea, wheezing, cough
Fatigue
Diminished activity/or pace of activity
Palpitations
Feeling faint, presyncope, syncope
At rest
Cough, wheezing
Paroxysmal nocturnal dyspnea
Orthopnea
Hemoptysis
Hoarseness (Ortner's syndrome)
From complications of MS

SOURCE: Copyright S. H. Rahimtoola, M.B., F.R.C.P, M.A.C.P., M.A.C.C. (Ref. 10).

imperative, then, to document what activities the patient can perform without symptoms and at what activity level symptoms begin; failure to do this often results in an underestimation of disability.

As obstruction progresses, the patients note orthopnea and paroxysmal nocturnal dyspnea that apparently results from redistribution of blood to the thorax on assuming the supine position. With severe MS and elevated pulmonary vascular resistance, fatigue rather than dyspnea may be the predominant symptom. Dependent edema, nausea, anorexia, and right-upper-quadrant pain reflect systemic venous congestion resulting from elevated systemic venous pressure and salt and water retention.

Palpitations are a frequent complaint in patients with MS and may represent frequent premature atrial contractions or paroxysmal atrial fibrillation/flutter. Of patients with severe symptomatic MS, 50 percent or more have chronic atrial fibrillation. Paroxysmal atrial fibrillation may produce pulmonary edema in some patients with MS. The acute increase in LA pressure that produces pulmonary edema results both from a decrease in the diastolic flow period caused by increased heart rate and from a loss of atrial transport function.

Systemic embolism, a frequent complication of MS, may result in stroke, occlusion of extremity arterial supply, occlusion of the aortic bifurcation, and visceral or myocardial infarction. Atrial fibrillation, increasing age of the patient, increasing LA size, and a previous history of embolism are associated with an increased incidence of systemic embolism[13] (Table 57-3).

Hemoptysis may result from a variety of causes. It is usually due to increased pulmonary venous pressure. Sputum may be blood-stained with paroxysmal nocturnal dyspnea, pink frothy sputum may result from rupture of alveolar capillaries associated with acute pulmonary edema or from pulmonary infarction due to pulmonary embolism, or hemoptysis may be severe and profuse (pulmonary apoplexy). The latter results from rupture of thin-walled, dilated bronchial veins, and although usually not fatal, it may be life-threatening because of aspiration pneumonia or massive hemorrhage. The edematous bronchial mucosa is more likely to be associated with chronic bronchitis, especially in cold and wet climates; it can also result in blood-stained sputum.

TABLE 57-3 Complications of Mitral Stenosis

Arrhythmias
Atrial flutter/fibrillation
Embolism
Systemic-cerebral, coronary, abnormal, peripheral, pulmonary
Acute pulmonary edema
Pulmonary arterial hypertension
Right ventricular hypertrophy/dilatation
Tricuspid regurgitation
Clinical heart failure
Left ventricular dysfunction
Chest pain/angina
Infective endocarditis

SOURCE: Copyright by S. H. Rahimtoola, M.B., F.R.C.P., M.A.C.P., M.A.C.C. (Ref. 10).

Exertional chest pain, typical of angina pectoris, may be present in some patients with severe MS but normal coronary arteries. Severe PA hypertension has been postulated as a cause. Infective endocarditis is an uncommon complication of pure MS.

Progression of symptoms in MS is generally slow but relentless. Thus, a sudden change in symptoms rarely reflects a change in valve obstruction. Rather, there is usually a noncardiac precipitating event or paroxysmal atrial fibrillation. Fever, pregnancy, hyperthyroidism, and noncardiac surgery, all of which increase CO, can precipitate decompensation in patients with moderate to severe MS.

PHYSICAL FINDINGS

During the latent, presymptomatic interval, incidental physical findings may be normal or may provide evidence of mild MS. Frequently, the only characteristic finding noted at rest will be a loud S_1 and a presystolic murmur. A short diastolic decrescendo rumble may be heard only with exercise. In patients with symptomatic stenosis, the findings are more obvious, and careful physical examination usually leads to the correct diagnosis (Chap. 10).

The general appearance of the patient in MS is usually normal. The MS facies, characterized by malar flush (pinkish-purple patches on the cheeks),[13] is uncommon and is caused by peripheral cyanosis, which is usually associated with a low CO, systemic vasoconstriction, and severe PA hypertension. Tachypnea may be present if LA pressure is high. The arterial pulse is normal except for irregularity in atrial fibrillation and is of low volume when CO is reduced. All peripheral pulses should be carefully examined because of the frequency of systemic embolism. The jugular venous pressure may be normal or may show evidence of elevated RA pressure. A prominent *a* wave is a result of RV hypertension/hypertrophy or of associated tricuspid stenosis. A prominent *v* wave is caused by tricuspid regurgitation. Atrial fibrillation produces an irregular venous pulse with absent *a* waves. The chest findings may be normal or may reveal signs of pulmonary congestion with rales or pleural fluid (dullness and absent breath sounds). Marked LA enlargement may produce egophony at the tip of the left scapula.

The precordium is usually unremarkable on inspection. On palpation, the apical impulse should feel normal or is tapping (palpable mitral valve closure or RV forming the cardiac apex). An abnormal LV impulse suggests disease other than isolated MS. A diastolic thrill is usually appreciated only when the patient is examined in the left lateral position. When PA hypertension is present, a sustained RV lift along the left sternal border and pulmonic valve closure may be palpable.

On auscultation in the supine position, the only abnormality appreciated may be the accentuated S_1, which is caused by flexible valve leaflets and the wide closing excursion of the valve

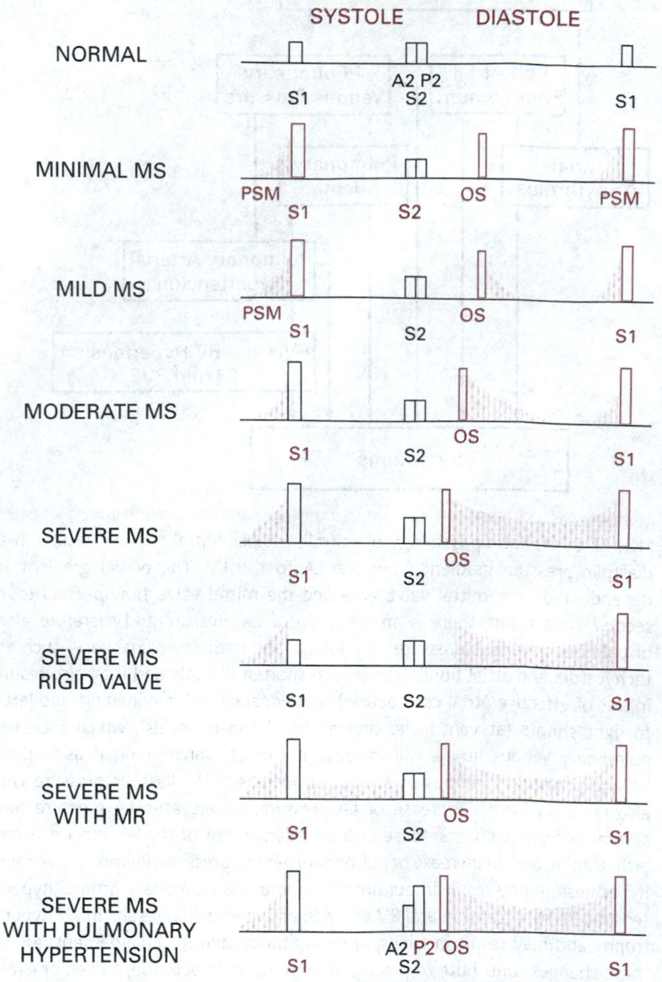

FIGURE 57-2 Auscultatory signs of MS in patients in sinus rhythm are illustrated. These include a presystolic murmur, loud first heart sound (S_1), an opening snap (OS), and a middiastolic murmur (low-pitched, decrescendo diastolic rumble, rumbling murmur). These signs may be accentuated or at times may be heard only by placing the patient in the left lateral decubitus position. Importantly, these signs are helpful in assessing the severity of the MS; as the MS becomes more severe, the S_2-OS interval is shortened and the length of the middiastolic rumble is increased. In mild OS, the S_2-OS interval is long and the diastolic murmur is short. In moderate MS, the S_2-OS interval is shorter, and although the diastolic murmur is longer at rest, there is usually a gap between the end of the murmur and the onset of the presystolic murmur. In severe MS, the S_2-OS interval is short (usually 0.04 to 0.06 s) and the diastolic murmur is a full-length murmur. With PA hypertension, P_2 is increased in intensity. In the presence of a rigid mitral valve (with or without calcification), S_2 is soft and the OS is usually not heard. A holosystolic murmur of mitral regurgitation may be present. (Adapted and modified from Kawanishi DT, Rahimtoola SH. Mitral stenosis. In: Rahimtoola SH, ed. *Valvular Heart Disease II*. St. Louis: Mosby; 1996:8.1–8.24. Copyright by S. H. Rahimtoola, M.B., F.R.C.P., M.A.C.P., M.A.C.C.)

leaflets[20] (see also Chap. 10). Failure to examine the patient in the left lateral position accounts for most of the missed diagnoses of symptomatic MS. The diastolic rumble is heard best with the bell of the stethoscope applied at the apical impulse. Nevertheless, the murmur may be localized, and the region around the apical impulse also should be auscultated. The *opening snap* (OS) occurs when the movement of the domed mitral valve into the LV is suddenly stopped.[20] It is heard best with the diaphragm and is often most easily appreciated midway between the apex and the left sternal border. In this intermediate region, the S_1, the pulmonary component of the second heart sound (P_2), and the OS can be identified. The auscultatory signs of MS in sinus rhythm and in atrial fibrillation are illustrated in Figs. 57-2 and 57-3.

The OS occurs after the LV pressure falls below LA pressure in early diastole. When LA pressure is high, as in severe MS, the snap occurs earlier in diastole (Fig. 57-2). The converse is true with mild MS. The interval between A_2 and the OS varies from 40 to 120 ms. Although the OS is present in most cases of MS, it is absent in patients with stiff, fibrotic, or calcified leaflets. Thus, absence of the OS in severe MS suggests that mitral valve replacement rather than commissurotomy may be necessary.

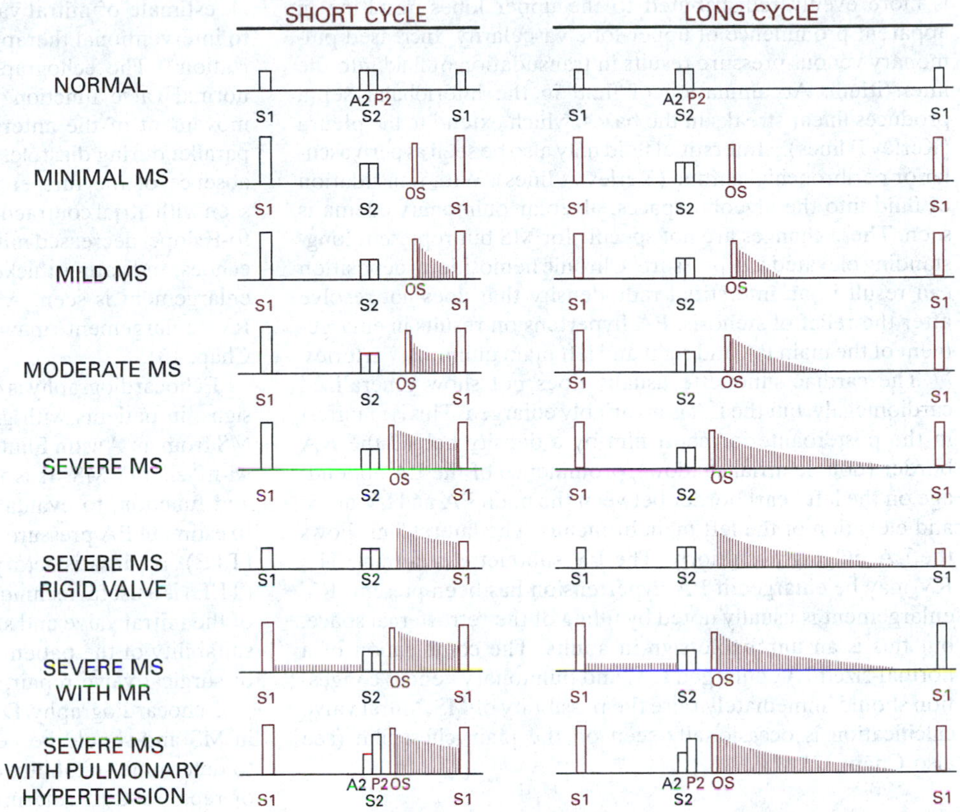

FIGURE 57-3 Auscultatory signs of MS in atrial fibrillation are illustrated. The presystolic murmur is absent. The loud S_1 and the OS are still heard. In the short cycles, the duration of diastole is short and the middiastolic rumble occupies the whole of diastole (*left panel*). In the long cycles (*right panel*), the length of middiastolic murmur is related to the severity of MS. As the MS becomes more severe, the length of this murmur is increased. In atrial fibrillation, with a slow ventricular response and very long R-R intervals, the middiastolic rumble may not occupy the whole diastolic period and the presystolic murmur is usually absent. Thus, one may get the impression that the MS is moderate rather than severe. Increasing the heart rate—for example, with brief physical exertion—may produce more characteristic auscultatory findings. Alternatively, when the ventricular rate in atrial fibrillation is rapid or in short cycles, the auscultatory findings may suggest a more severe degree of MS than is really the case (*left panel*). (Adapted and modified from Kawanishi DT, Rahimtoola SH. Mitral stenosis. In: Rahimtoola SH, ed. *Valvular Heart Disease. II*. St. Louis: Mosby; 1996:8.1–8.24. Copyright 1996 by S. H. Rahimtoola, M.B., F.R.C.P., M.A.C.P., M.A.C.C.)

The low-pitched diastolic rumble follows the OS and is best heard with the bell of the stethoscope. In some patients with low cardiac output or mild MS, brief exercise, such as situps or walking, is adequate to increase flow and bring out the murmur. The murmur is low-pitched, rumbling, and decrescendo. In general, the more severe the MS, the longer the murmur (Fig. 57-2). Presystolic accentuation of the murmur occurs in sinus rhythm and has been reported even in atrial fibrillation. In the latter situation, a brief "presystolic" accentuation is due to narrowing of the mitral orifice produced by ventricular systole before the final, completeclosure of the mitral valve and the mitral component of S_1. A diastolic rumble is not diagnostic of MS and may be heard with increased flow across a normal mitral valve—for example, in ventricular septal defect with a large left-to-right shunt.

The two most important auscultatory signs of severe MS are a short A_2-OS interval (usually 40 to 60 ms) and a full-length diastolic rumble. The A_2-OS interval may be longer if there is associated moderate/severe aortic regurgitation, and the OS may be absent when the mitral valve is rigid. The diastolic murmur may not be full-length in severe MS if the stroke volume is low and there is no tachycardia.

Systolic murmurs also may be heard in association with the murmur of MS. A blowing, holosystolic murmur at the apex suggests associated MR; whereas a systolic blowing murmur heard best at the lower left sternal border that increases with inspiration usually signifies tricuspid regurgitation. The Graham Steell murmur is a high-pitched diastolic decrescendo murmur of pulmonic regurgitation caused by severe PA hypertension. In most patients with MS, such a murmur usually indicates AR instead. In general, a left-sided S_3 is not compatible with severe MS with the possible exception of concomitant severe AR and/or significant LV systolic dysfunction. If an S_3 and a rumble are present, MR is usually the predominant lesion (see also Chap. 10).

ROENTGENOGRAM

The posteroanterior and lateral chest films are often so typical that experienced clinicians can make the tentative diagnosis from them. The thoracic cage is normal. The lung fields show evidence of elevated pulmonary venous pressure. Blood flow is more evenly redistributed to the upper lobes, resulting in apparent prominence of upper-lobe vascularity. Increased pulmonary venous pressure results in transudation of fluid into the interstitium. Accumulation of fluid in the interlobular septa produces linear streaks in the bases, which extend to the pleura (Kerley B lines).[21] Interstitial fluid may also be seen as perivascular or peribronchial cuffing (Kerley A lines). With transudation of fluid into the alveolar spaces, alveolar pulmonary edema is seen. These changes are not specific for MS but represent longstanding elevated LA pressure. Chronic hemosiderin deposition can result in an interstitial radiodensity that does not resolve after the relief of stenosis. PA hypertension results in enlargement of the main PA and right and left main pulmonary arteries.

The cardiac silhouette usually does not show generalized cardiomegaly, but the LA is invariably enlarged. This is manifest in the posteroanterior chest film by a density behind the RA border (double atrial shadow), prominence of the LA appendage on the left heart border between the main PA and LV apex, and elevation of the left main bronchus. The lateral film shows the LA bulging posteriorly. The LV silhouette is normal. The RV may be enlarged if PA hypertension has been present. RV enlargement is usually noted by filling of the retrosternal space, but this is an unreliable sign in adults. The combination of a normal-sized LV, enlarged LA, and pulmonary venous congestion should immediately raise the possibility of MS. Mitral valve calcification is occasionally seen on the plain chest film (see also Chap. 12).

ELECTROCARDIOGRAM

The *electrocardiogram* (ECG) is not usually as helpful as the chest x-ray. Patients in sinus rhythm may have a widened P wave caused by interatrial conduction delay and/or prolonged LA depolarization. Classically, the P wave is broad and notched in lead II and biphasic in lead V_1; it measures 0.12 s or more. Atrial fibrillation is common. LV hypertrophy is almost never present unless there are associated lesions. RV hypertrophy may be present if PA hypertension is marked (see also Chap. 11).

CLINICAL INDICATIONS OF SEVERE MITRAL STENOSIS

Some clinical features make it virtually certain that MS is severe. These include (1) moderate to severe PA hypertension as indicated by clinical and ECG evidence of RV hypertrophy or PA hypertension or both and/or (2) moderate to severe elevation of LA pressure as indicated by orthopnea, a short P_2-OS interval, a diastolic rumble that occupies the whole length of a long diastolic interval in patients with atrial fibrillation, and pulmonary edema on the chest x-ray. In both these clinical circumstances, one must be certain that there is no other cause for elevated LA pressure and that LA hypertension is not caused mainly by a correctable transient elevation of LV diastolic pressure.

Laboratory Tests

ECHOCARDIOGRAPHY/DOPPLER ULTRASOUND

Echocardiography/Doppler ultrasound has proved to be both sensitive and specific for MS when adequate studies are done (Chap. 13).[22-25] False-positive and false-negative results are uncommon. M-mode and two-dimensional echocardiography do not reliably predict the severity of MS. Doppler studies provide an estimate of mitral valve area that is within $\pm 0.4\ cm^2$ (prior to interventional therapy) of that obtained by cardiac catheterization.[26] The echographic findings of MS reflect the loss of normal valve function. The fusion of commissures results in movement of the anterior and posterior leaflets anteriorly in parallel during diastole. In patients in sinus rhythm, there is an absence of the further opening of the valve that is normally seen with atrial contraction. Other findings include decreased E-to-F slope, decreased mitral valve leaflet excursion, and multiple echoes, indicating thickening or calcification of the valve. LA enlargement is seen. Abnormal pulmonary valve motion and RV enlargement may signify PA hypertension (see also Chap. 13).

Echocardiography is of great value in patients with equivocal signs, in patients with gross PA hypertension, to differentiate MS from an Austin Flint murmur of AR, and in the rare patient with "silent" MS. It is used to assess LV, RV, and atrial size and function; to evaluate the aortic and tricuspid valves; and to estimate PA pressure. When transthoracic echocardiography (TTE) is unsatisfactory, transesophageal echocardiography (TEE) is a useful technique to assess LA thrombus, the anatomy of the mitral valve and subvalvular apparatus, and to assess the suitability of the patient for catheter balloon commissurotomy or surgical valve repair.

Echocardiography/Doppler ultrasound is a most useful test in MS and should be performed in all patients. It is essential to determine suitability of the valve for commissurotomy and/or repair and to determine the likely result.

CARDIAC CATHETERIZATION/ANGIOGRAPHY

In most patients with disabling symptoms from presumed MS, right and left heart catheterization should be performed as part of a preoperative assessment. Simultaneous measurement of cardiac output and the gradient between the LA and the LV and calculation of valve area remain the "gold standard" for assessing the severity of MS (Chap. 15). LV angiography assesses the competence of the mitral valve, an important determinant of operability for mitral commissurotomy. Quantification of LV function provides a useful prognostic indicator of operative and late survival and of the expected functional result. Aortic valve function should be evaluated in all patients. Selective supraventricular aortography should be performed in all patients unless there is a contraindication. Tricuspid valve function can be assessed when there is a question of coexisting lesions. In certain circumstances—for example, in a patient with suspected severe MS who has a small gradient and mildly elevated LA pressure—dynamic exercise in the catheterization laboratory with measurement of mitral valve gradient, CO and LA and PA pressures can be extremely useful. Another example is a patient with significant symptoms in whom the findings at rest suggest moderate (or even mild) MS. Selective coronary arteriography establishes the site, severity, and extent of coronary artery disease and should be performed in patients with angina, in those with LV dysfunction, in those with risk factors for coronary artery disease, and in those 35 years of age or older who are being considered for interventional therapy.

OTHER INVESTIGATIONS

In most clinical situations, other investigations are not needed. Occasionally, a treadmill exercise test to evaluate functional capacity may be very useful clinically—for example, when a patient denies symptoms in spite of severe hemodynamic abnormalities.

Clinical Decision Making

The reader is referred to the section on aortic stenosis in Chap. 57. In a prospective blinded study of consecutive patients with valvular heart disease, the sensitivity and specificity of diagnosis of MS by clinical evaluation was 86 and 87 percent, respectively. The accuracy of diagnosis of MS for moderate to severe stenosis was 92 percent by clinical evaluation and 97 percent by echocardiography/Doppler ultrasound.[27] This emphasizes the importance of a thorough clinical evaluation. The principal difficulty with both clinical evaluation and echocardiography/Doppler ultrasound is being able to accurately separate in all instances mild from moderate MS and moderate from severe MS.

Natural History and Prognosis

The population presenting with MS is changing because of the sharp decline in the incidence of acute rheumatic fever in the past 40 years (see also Chap. 55). Native-born American citizens with symptomatic MS are presenting at an older age. Young adults in the third and fourth decades with symptomatic MS are more likely to come from low socioeconomic backgrounds and from the inner city or to be immigrants, particularly from Latin America, the Middle East, Africa, or Asia. Therefore, the latent period between acute rheumatic fever and symptomatic MS is variable and appears to be related to the presence of repeated streptococcal infection. Women with MS outnumber men by almost two to one. The most important feature of the asymptomatic interval is the susceptibility to repeated bouts of both rheumatic valvulitis and streptococcal infection. The mechanism for the progression from no symptoms to mild to severe symptoms is progressive stenosis of the mitral valve.

With the onset of exertional dyspnea and fatigue, the valve area is usually reduced to one-half to one-third its normal size. Further small reductions in valve area markedly obstruct flow and result in symptoms with minimal exertion. The interval from initial mild symptoms to disabling symptoms may be 10 years. During this time, the patient is at some risk of death (see below). Permanent injury may result from atrial fibrillation with rapid ventricular rate, resulting in pulmonary edema, and from systemic embolus. Unfortunately, it is not possible to predict who is at risk of embolism. When late functional class II or functional class III symptoms are present, the valve area is usually 1.0 cm^2 or less (in an occasional patient the valve area is 1.2 or 1.3 cm^2), and both rest and exercise hemodynamics are deranged.[2] Further small reductions in valve area result in symptoms at rest.

The 10-year survival of patients with MS who are asymptomatic is approximately 84 percent and that of those who are mildly symptomatic is 34 to 42 percent (Fig. 57-4).[28–30] The 10-year survival of patients who are moderately or severely symptomatic and who do not have therapy is 40 percent or less, and the survival at 20 years is less than 10 percent.[28–30] Patients in the New York Heart Association functional class IV have a very poor survival without treatment[28]: 42 percent at 1 year and 10 percent or less at 5 years. All are dead by 10 years (Fig. 57-5).

Management

MS can be prevented through two approaches (Table 57-4). First, all streptococcal infections should be diagnosed rapidly and correctly treated (Chap. 55). This prevents most initial episodes of acute rheumatic fever. Second, all patients with known previous acute rheumatic fever/rheumatic carditis with or without obvious valve disease should receive appropriate antibiotic prophylaxis against recurrent streptococcal infection (Chap. 55).

Although the incidence of infective endocarditis is low in isolated MS, all patients exposed to bacteremia should receive appropriate prophylaxis against infective endocarditis (Chap. 73). Family and vocational planning should be considered. Women with this disease should consider bearing children before symptoms occur, since pregnancy is usually well tolerated with mild MS. Occupations that require strenuous exertion in middle age and later should probably be avoided if possible. In patients with moderate or severe MS, activities such as strenuous exercise and competitive sports should be restricted.[9]

When patients reach the symptomatic threshold, medical treatment may be of some benefit. Digitalis offers no improvement for the patient with normal sinus rhythm and normal LV function. When atrial fibrillation is present, however, digitalis plays a critical role in controlling ventricular rate. In selected patients, beta-adrenergic blocking agents, diltiazem, or amiodarone may be added if digoxin alone is not satisfactory in controlling ventricular rate at rest or on exercise. Beta-adrenergic blocking agents should be used with great caution or not at all in patients with impaired LV function, associated significant aortic stenosis, or other associated severe valvular disease. Digoxin and diltiazem or digoxin and low-dose amiodarone are probably the two best combined regimens. Diuretics reduce pulmonary congestion and peripheral edema and allow most patients freedom from severe salt restriction. For the patient with mild symptoms, maintenance of sinus rhythm is desirable. Cardioversion of atrial fibrillation and maintenance of sinus rhythm using antiarrhythmic therapy with either digitalis and quinidine or digitalis and amiodarone should be offered to these patients. In patients who need interventional therapy, cardioversion is usually performed after completion of the procedure. Anticoagulation with warfarin is usually begun about 3 weeks in advance of cardioversion and for 4 weeks after the procedure.[31] Patients with chronic atrial fibrillation and those with a previous history of embolism should receive anticoagulation with warfarin (International Normalized Ratio, or INR, of 2 to 3) unless there is a specific contraindication.

There are no randomized trials of surgery versus medical therapy. Roy and Gopinath's study[29] showed that in comparable patients, surgical commissurotomy was associated with a better survival than medical therapy in patients with class II symptoms as well as in those with class III and IV symptoms (Fig. 57-6).

Unless there is a contraindication, surgery should be recommended to an MS patient with functional class III or IV symptoms (Table 57-5). For younger patients with a pliable, noncalcified valve and without important mitral regurgitation, this means valve repair. The hemodynamic results of surgical commissurotomy are excellent.[9,32,33] Because of the low morbidity and mortality of mitral commissurotomy/valve repair,[9,32–34] surgery is also offered to those patients when functional class II symptoms are present. The results of successful commissurot-

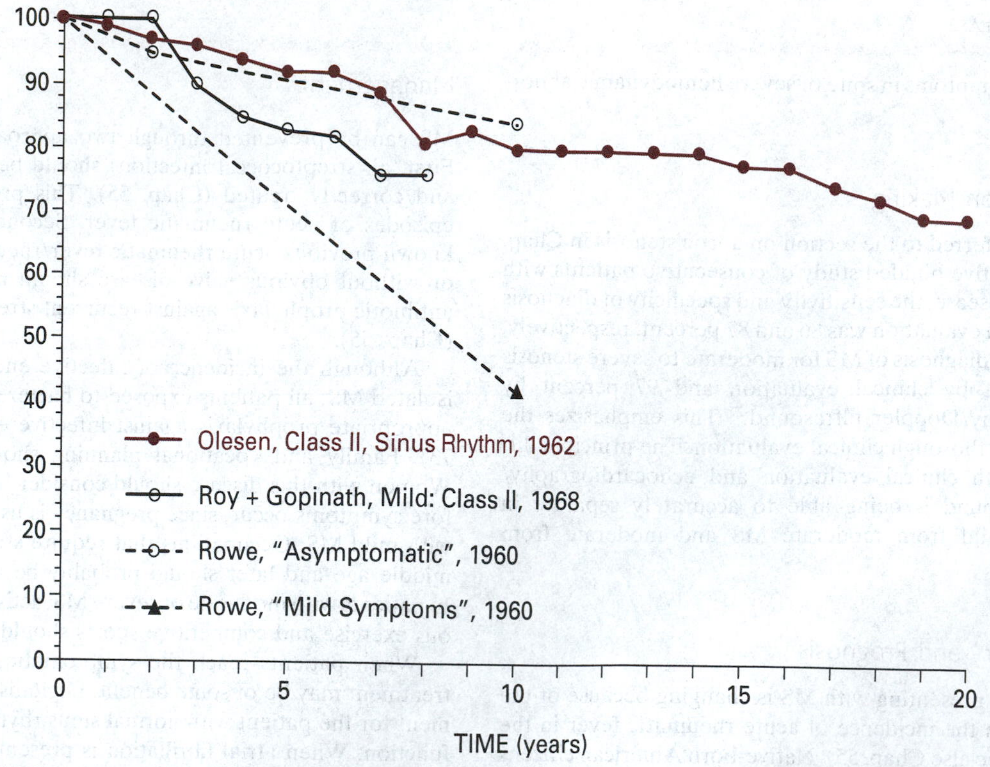

FIGURE 57-4 This figure depicts the survival of patients with MS who initially where asymptomatic or had mild symptoms and were treated medically. In the 1960 study of Rowe and coworkers[30] (*dashed lines*), 52 percent of 250 patients with "auscultatory MS" who presented between 1925 and 1947 were asymptomatic; their 10-year survival was 84 percent. The lower dashed line represents the survival in the 42 percent of patients who had mild symptoms on clinical presentation; their 10-year survival was 42 percent.[30] The data of Olesen, 1962[27] (*upper solid curve connecting solid symbols*), show the survival in the 21 percent of 271 symptomatic MS patients who had class II symptoms. Their 10- and 20-year survival was 34 and 14 percent, respectively. The data of Roy and Gopinath, 1968[29] (*lower solid curve connecting open symbols*), also show the survival in patients with class II symptoms. (From Kawanishi DT, Rahimtoola SH. Mitral stenosis. In: Rahimtoola SH, ed. *Valvular Heart Disease. II*. St. Louis: Mosby; 1996:8.1–8.24.)

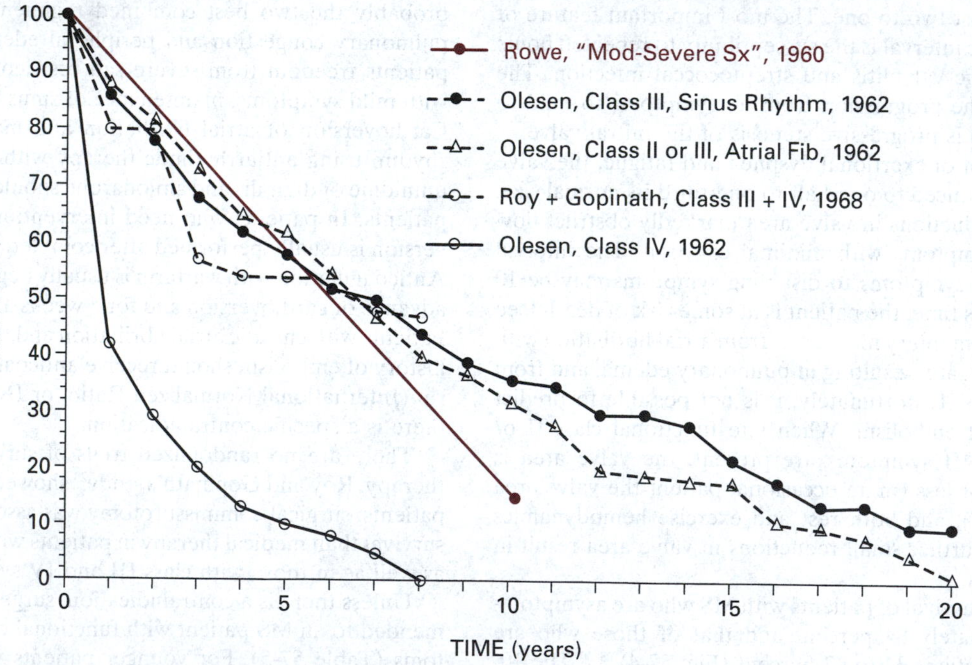

FIGURE 57-5 Survival of patients with MS and moderate or advanced (severe) symptoms is shown. Patients who were in NYHA functional class IV (Olesen, class IV, 1962)[28] had a 42 percent 1-year survival and all patients had died within 8 years. The other four survival curves are of patients who were in functional classes II to IV, and their survival curves are similar, with 5-, 10-, and 15-year approximate survivals of 60, 40, and 20 percent, respectively; at 20 years, less than 10 percent of the patients were still alive.[28–30] Thus, the survival in this group of patients with more advanced symptoms is much worse than that of patients who were initially asymptomatic or minimally symptomatic (see Fig. 57-4). (From Kawanishi DT, Rahimtoola SH. Mitral stenosis. In: Rahimtoola SH, ed. *Valvular Heart Disease. II*. St. Louis: Mosby; 1996:8.1–8.24.)

TABLE 57-4 Medical Treatment of Mitral Stenosis

- Prevention
  - Primary
    - Treatment of streptococcal group A infection
  - Secondary (antibiotic prophylaxis)
    - Recurrent rheumatic fever
    - Infective endocarditis
- Restrict activities (moderate/severe MS)
  - Severe exercise
  - Competitive sports
- Arrhythmias
  - Prevent and/or control
  - Restore sinus rhythm if possible
- Cardiac medications
  - Use only if essential
  - Diuretics—use cautiously
  - Anticoagulants for systemic/pulmonary emboli
  - Elevated pulmonary venous pressure—diuretics
  - Heart failure—digitalis, diuretics, ACE inhibitors
- Follow-up of asymptomatic patients

Mild MS	Every 2–5 years
Moderate MS	Every 1–2 years
Severe MS	Every 6–12 months if interventional therapy not performed
Development of symptoms	Early or "immediate"

SOURCE: Copyright by S. H. Rahimtoola, M.B., F.R.C.P., M.A.C.P., M.A.C.C. (Ref. 10).

TABLE 57-5 Indications for Interventional Therapy for Severe Mitral Stenosis

- All severely symptomatic patients (functional classes III and IV)
- All mildly symptomatic patients (functional class II)[a,b]
- Asymptomatic patients[a,b]
  - Pulmonary artery hypertension
  - Episodic pulmonary edema
  - Atrial fibrillation (persistent or repeated episodes)
  - Thromboembolism (systemic/pulmonary)
  - Severe mitral stenosis (valve suitable for CBC/surgical valve repair)

[a]Catheter balloon commissurotomy (CBC)/surgery.
[b]Individualize depending on patient characteristics; suitability of patient for CBC/surgical valve repair versus valve replacement, skill and experience of interventional team.
SOURCE: Copyright by S. H. Rahimtoola, M.B., F.R.C.P., M.A.C.P., M.A.C.C. (Ref. 10).

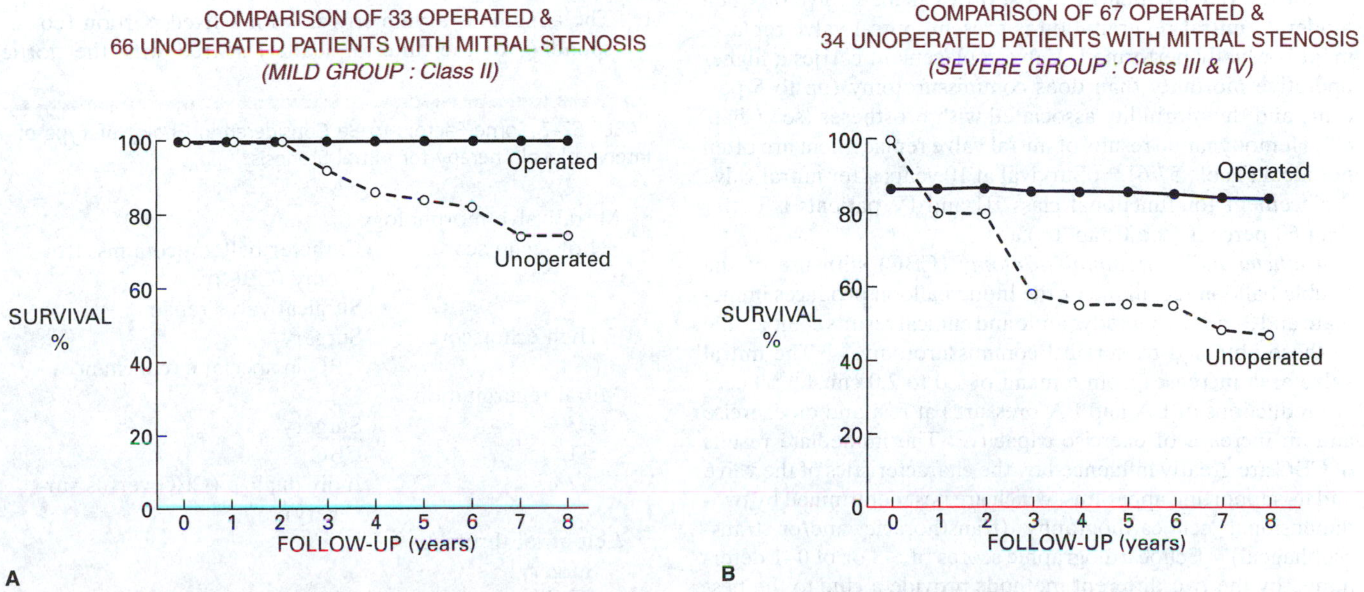

FIGURE 57-6 Comparison of survival of patients with class II symptoms (*left panel*) and class III and IV symptoms due to MS (*right panel*).[29] Survival of patients treated medically (unoperated) is indicated by the broken line and with surgical closed mitral commissurotomy (operated) by the solid line. In patients treated by surgical commissurotomy, there were no operative or late deaths in those with mild symptoms and no late deaths in those with class III and IV symptoms. There is a clear improvement in survival in operated patients. The 5-year mortality with medical treatment alone in those with class III and IV symptoms approaches 50 percent (also see Fig. 57-5); with surgery, there is no appreciable mortality following recovery from the procedure. [From Roy SB, Gopinath N. Mitral stenosis. *Circulation* 1968; 38(suppl v):68–76.]

TABLE 57-6 Mitral Stenosis: Results of Mitral Valve Replacement in 33 Patients

	Mitral Stenosis	
	Pre-MVR[a]	Post-MVR
LV end-diastolic pressure, mmHg	11 ± 5	12 ± 6
Mean PA wedge pressure, mmHg	36 ± 15	28 ± 14[b]
Mean systolic PA pressure, mmHg	54 ± 24	42 ± 22[c]
Cardiac index, L/min/m^2	2.1 ± 1.5	2.3 ± 0.6
LV EDVI, mL/m^2	79 ± 18	72 ± 24
LV ESVI, mL/m^2	41 ± 13	39 ± 21
LVEF	0.48 ± 0.10	0.47 ± 0.14
Mitral regurgitant volume, mL	—	—
Regurgitant volume/end-diastolic volume	—	—
Mitral valve gradient, mmHg	15 ± 7	8 ± 3[b]
Mitral valve area, cm^2	1.2 ± 0.4	1.8 ± 0.6[b]

[a]MVR = mitral valve replacement.
[b]$p < .001$.
[c]$p < .01$ comparing before and after mitral valve replacement artery.
SOURCE: Crawford MH et al.[36]

vival was 65 ± 6 percent.[47] The 7-year event-free survival ranged from 13 to 90 percent in various subgroups. The 7-year event-free survival was best predicted by the post-CBC mitral valve area (≥1.5 cm^2) and PA wedge pressure (18 mmHg); the 7-year event-free survival was 90 ± 6 percent.[47] In the appropriate patient and in centers with skilled and experienced staff, CBC is the procedure of first choice for relief of severe MS. Factors to be taken into account choosing between surgery and CBC in an individual patient are shown in Table 57-7.

The recommendations of the ACC/AHA Practice Guidelines are shown in Tables 57-8, 57-9, and 57-10.[48] Guidelines are *not* and should *not* be the law. Application of guidelines to clinical practice should be based on the following principles: (1) classes I and III apply to all patients in these classes unless there is a specific clinical circumstance contradicting this and (2) class II applies to patients in this class depending on the clinical condition of the patient and the skill and experience at the individual medical center.

omy are excellent; in experienced and skilled centers, surgical mortality is less that 1 percent. Late mortality at 10 years is less than 5 percent, the thromboembolism rate is 2 percent per year or less, and the reoperation rate ranges from 0.5 to 4.5 percent per year. The return of symptoms after commissurotomy/valve repair is usually the result of an incomplete operation, other valvular lesions, refusion of mitral commissures, or deterioration of myocardial function. In less developed countries, excellent results have been reported in a very high percentage of young patients for up to 25 years.[35]

For the older patient with a stiff or calcified valve or when moderate mitral regurgitation is present, mitral valve replacement is usually performed. Valve replacement carries a higher operative mortality than does commissurotomy (up to 5 percent) and the morbidity associated with prostheses (see Chap. 60). Hemodynamic results of mitral valve replacement are often not ideal (Table 57-6).[36,37] Survival at 10 years after mitral valve replacement for functional class III and IV patients is better than 60 percent (see Chap. 60).

Catheter balloon commissurotomy (CBC) with use of the double balloon technique or the Inoue balloon produces immediate and 3-month hemodynamic and clinical results comparable to those obtained by surgical commissurotomy.[38–41] The mitral valve area increases from a mean of 1.0 to 2.0 cm^2.[26,32,38] There are reductions of LA and PA pressures at rest and on exercise and an increase of exercise capacity.[39] The immediate results of CBC are greatly influenced by the characteristics of the valve and its supporting apparatus, which are best determined by two-dimensional echocardiography (transthoracic and/or transesophageal).[22] Echocardiographic scores of ≤8 or of 0–1 determined by the two different methods provide a clue to the best immediate results. Repeat CBC or mitral valve replacement is needed in 20 percent of patients within 5 to 7 years. Late survival is poorer in those in whom functional class IV, higher echocardiographic score, higher LV end-diastolic pressure, or higher PA systolic pressure is present prior to the CBC.[42–47] In one study, the 7-year survival was 95 ± 1 percent and the event-free sur-

NORMAL MITRAL STRUCTURE AND FUNCTION

The mitral valve is a complex structure formed by four elements[49,50]:

1. The annulus is asymmetrical, with a fixed portion (corresponding to the anterior leaflet) shared with the aortic

TABLE 57-7 Some Factors to Be Considered in Choice of Type of Interventional Therapy for Mitral Stenosis[a]

Mitral valve morphology	
Low echo score:	Catheter balloon commissurotomy (CBC)
	Surgical valve repair
High echo score:	Surgery
	CBC in special circumstances
Mitral regurgitation	
≥3+:	Surgery
≤1+:	CBC
2+:	Individualize (CBC versus surgery)
Left atrial thrombus	
Surgery	
CBC in special circumstances	
Need for other cardiac surgery	
Surgery	
CBC in special circumstances	

[a]In centers with skilled and experienced interventional teams.
SOURCE: Copyright by S. H. Rahimtoola. M.B., F.R.C.P., M.A.C.P., M.A.C.C. (Ref. 10).

TABLE 57-8 Recommendations for Percutaneous Mitral Balloon Valvotomy

Indication	Class
1. Symptomatic patients (NYHA functional class II, III, or IV), moderate or severe MS (mitral valve area ≤1.5 cm^2),[a] and valve morphology favorable for percutaneous balloon valvotomy in the absence of left atrial thrombus or moderate to severe MR	I
2. Asymptomatic patients with moderate or severe MS (mitral valve area ≤1.5 cm^2)[a] and valve morphology favorable for percutaneous balloon valvotomy who have pulmonary hypertension (pulmonary artery systolic pressure >50 mmHg at rest or 60 mmHg with exercise) in the absence of left atrial thrombus or moderate to severe MR	IIa
3. Patients with NYHA functional class III–IV symptoms, moderate or severe MS (mitral valve area ≤1.5 cm^2),[a] and a nonpliable calcified valve who are at high risk for surgery in the absence of left atrial thrombus or moderate to severe MR	IIa
4. Asymptomatic patients, moderate or severe MS (mitral valve area ≤1.5 cm^2)[a] and valve morphology favorable for percutaneous balloon valvotomy who have new onset of atrial fibrillation in the absence of left atrial thrombus or moderate to severe MR	IIb
5. Patients in NYHA functional class III–IV, moderate or severe MS (MVA ≤1.5 cm^2), and a nonpliable calcified valve who are low-risk candidates for surgery	IIb
6. Patients with mild MS	III

[a]The committee recognizes that there may be variability in the measurement of mitral valve area and that the mean transmitral gradient, pulmonary artery wedge pressure, and pulmonary artery pressure at rest or during exercise should also be taken into consideration.
SOURCE: ACC/AHA Guidelines,[48] with permission.

TABLE 57-9 Recommendations for Mitral Valve Repair for Mitral Stenosis

Indication	Class
1. Patients with NYHA functional class III–IV symptoms, moderate or severe MS (mitral valve area ≤1.5 cm^2),[a] and valve morphology favorable for repair if percutaneous mitral balloon valvotomy is not available	I
2. Patients with NYHA functional class III–IV symptoms, moderate or severe MS (mitral valve area ≤1.5 cm^2),[a] and valve morphology favorable for repair if a left atrial thrombus is present despite anticoagulation	I
3. Patients with NYHA functional class III–IV symptoms, moderate or severe MS (mitral valve area ≤1.5 cm^2),[a] and a nonpliable or calcified valve with the decision to proceed with either repair or replacement made at the time of the operation	I
4. Patients in NYHA functional class I, moderate or severe MS (mitral valve area ≤1.5 cm^2),[a] and valve morphology favorable for repair who have had recurrent episodes of embolic events on adequate anticoagulation	IIb
5. Patients with NYHA functional class I–IV symptoms and mild MS	III

[a]The committee recognizes that there may be a variability in the measurement of mitral valve area and that the mean transmitral gradient, pulmonary artery wedge pressure, and pulmonary artery pressure at rest or during exercise should also be considered.
SOURCE: ACC/AHA Guidelines,[48] with permission.

TABLE 57-10 Recommendations for Mitral Valve Replacement for Mitral Stenosis

Indication	Class
1. Patients with moderate or severe MS (mitral valve area ≤1.5 cm^2)[a] and NYHA functional class III–IV symptoms who are not considered candidates for percutaneous balloon valvotomy or mitral valve repair	I
2. Patients with severe MS (mitral valve area ≤1 cm^2)[a] and severe pulmonary hypertension (pulmonary artery systolic pressure >60 to 80 mmHg) with NYHA functional class I–II symptoms who are not considered candidates for percutaneous balloon valvotomy or mitral valve repair	IIa

[a]The committee recognizes that there may be a variability in the measurement of mitral valve area and that the mean transmitral gradient, pulmonary artery wedge pressure, and pulmonary artery pressure should also be considered.
SOURCE: ACC/AHA Guidelines,[48] with permission.

annulus and a dynamic portion (corresponding to the posterior leaflet) that represents most of the circumference of the annulus.

2. The two leaflets are asymmetrical; the anterior has the greater length of tissue but occupies a smaller portion of the circumference of the annulus than the posterior.
3. The chordae join each papillary muscle to the corresponding commissure and the adjoining halves of both leaflets and maintain the two leaflets in a position allowing coaptation.
4. The two papillary muscles and the adjacent wall attach the mitral apparatus to the LV.

Mitral competence during systole is normally ensured, first, by a large area of coaptation between leaflets allowing high friction resistance to abnormal valve movement and, second, by the systolic position to the anterior leaflet parallel to the direction of blood flow. The mechanism of MR frequently combines abnormal function of more than one anatomic element, which fact underlines the complexity of conservative surgery for restoration of normal mitral function.

MITRAL REGURGITATION

Mitral regurgitation (MR) is characterized by an abnormal reversed blood flow from the left ventricle (LV) to the left atrium (LA). The etiologic profile of MR is now dominated by degenerative and ischemic causes in developed countries. The development of noninvasive assessment with transesophageal echocardiography, color-flow imaging and Doppler methods of quantitation of regurgitation has transformed diagnostic approaches. With improved understanding of the impact of LV dysfunction on outcome, and most importantly with major advances in conservative surgery, the management of MR has become far more proactive.

Etiology and Mechanism (Table 57-11)

MR is often referred to as *organic* if there is an intrinsic valve disease or *functional* if the valve is structurally normal but leaks due to an extravalvular abnormality. Ischemic MR may be organic (ruptured papillary muscle) or functional (LV dysfunction). Nonischemic MR may be organic (e.g., rheumatic) or functional (e.g., cardiomyopathy).

RHEUMATIC DISEASE

Rheumatic MR is rarely pure, and in most cases is associated with stenosis and fusion of the commissures (Fig. 57-7, Plate 86). Severe rheumatic MR requiring surgical correction is still frequent in developing countries but is now rare in developed countries.[51] The underlying lesion is retractile fibrosis of leaflets and chordae, causing loss of coaptation. The secondary dilatation of the mitral annulus tends to further decrease the contract between leaflets. Elongated or ruptured chordae are infrequent.

DEGENERATIVE MITRAL REGURGITATION

These causes are often associated with valve prolapse, an abnormal movement of the leaflets into the LA during systole due to inadequate chordal support (elongation or rupture) and excessive valvular tissue. In western countries, mitral prolapse represents the most frequent causes leading to surgery for severe MR.[51] Degenerative MR can be separated in three categories:

- The mitral valve prolapse syndrome, characterized by diffuse myxomatous infiltration, discussed in detail in Chap. 58 (Fig. 57-8, Plate 87).
- The degenerative "primary" ruptured chordae, which involves the posterior more often than the anterior leaflet and occurs more often in men than in women. There is usually no excessive tissue, but enlargement of the annulus may occur as in any MR. The involved leaflet may present with a myxomatous infiltration,[52] but the other leaflet usually remains normal. Calcification of the mitral annulus or systemic hypertension may precede the occurrence of the ruptured chordae. Isolated ruptured cord may occasionally be due to blunt thoracic trauma and endocarditis (secondary forms).
- Degenerative MR without prolapse, which is usually mild and due to valve sclerosis or isolated annular calcification; here regurgitation is secondary to deformation of the valves of annulus (Fig. 57-9, Plate 88).

INFECTIVE ENDOCARDITIS

Infective endocarditis accounts for about 5 percent of cases of severe MR. Vegetations may produce mild MR by interposition between leaflets. Severe endocarditic MR is usually related to ruptured chordae and less frequently to destruction of mitral tissue involving either the leaflet's edges or a perforation (Fig. 57-10, Plate 89).

ISCHEMIC AND FUNCTIONAL MITRAL REGURGITATION

Ischemic and functional MR—i.e., due to LV wall dysfunction secondary to ischemia, scarring, aneurysm, cardiomyopathy, or myocarditis—have in common the same mechanism: the coaptation of intrinsically normal leaflets is incomplete. Rupture of

TABLE 57-11 Mitral Regurgitation: Mechanisms

Etiology	Mechanism	Echocardiographic Appearance
Rheumatic	Retraction	Thickened chordae/ leaflets
Lupus erythematosus	Thickening	Normal or restricted motion
Anticardiolipin syndrome		
Carcinoid		
Ergot lesions		
Postradiation		
Degenerative	Prolapsed leaflets	Prolapsing/flail leaflets
Marfan syndrome	Ruptured chords	Redundant tissue
Ehlers-Danlos syndrome		Ruptured chords
Traumatic MR		
Ischemic (infarction)	Ruptured papillary muscle	Flail leaflet
Myocardial disease	Dilatation of annulus	Normal leaflets
Ischemic (chronic)	Traction anterior leaflet	Reduced motion of leaflets
Cardiomyopathies		
Infiltrative disease	Thickened leaflet	Thickened leaflets
Hypereosinophilic syndrome	Loss of coaptation	Reduced motion
Endomyocardial fibrosis		
Hurler's disease		
Endocarditis	Destructive lesions	Perforations
		Flail leaflets
Congenital	Cleft leaflet	Cleft leaflet
	Transposed valve	Tricuspid valve

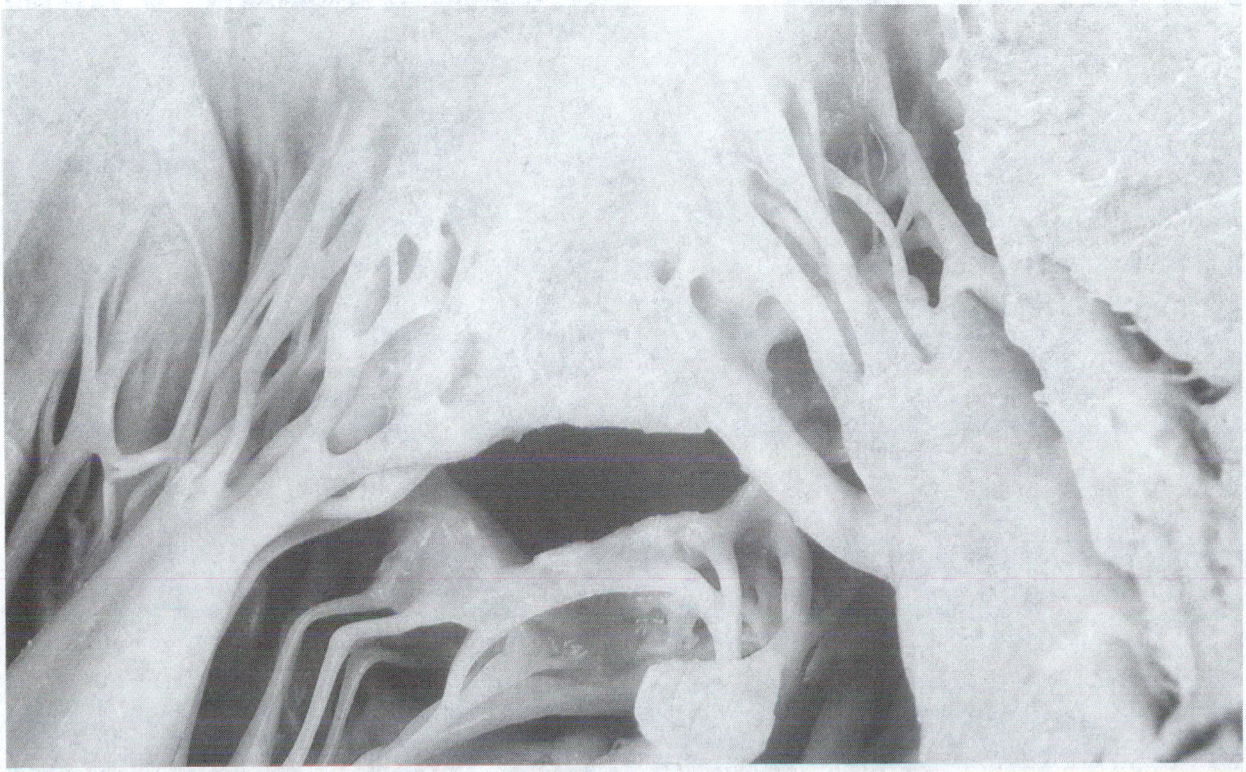

FIGURE 57-7 (Plate 86) Anatomic example of rheumatic MR. Note the thickening of the leaflet and chordae and the retraction of the mitral tissue. (Courtesy of Dr. W. D. Edwards.)

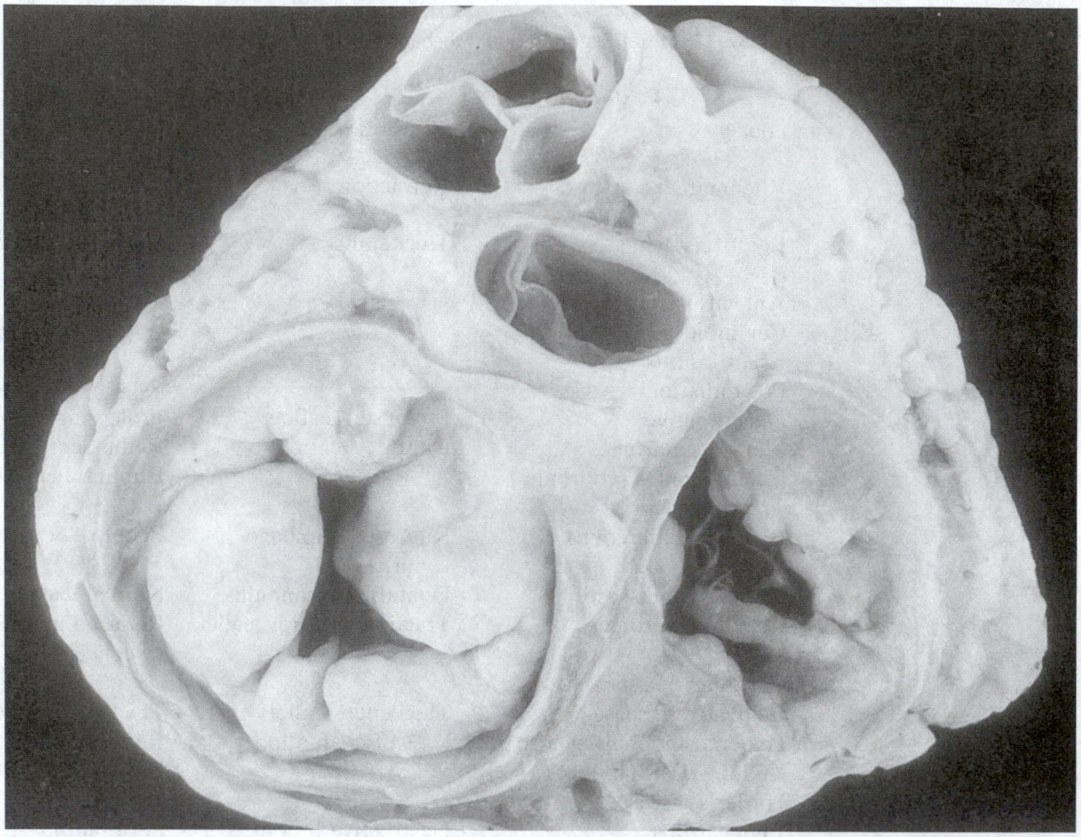

FIGURE 57-8 (Plate 87) Anatomic example of MR due to mitral valve prolapse seen from the atrial view (the mitral orifice is on the left of picture). Note the redundancy of the leaflets with excess tissue. (Courtesy of Dr. W. D. Edwards.)

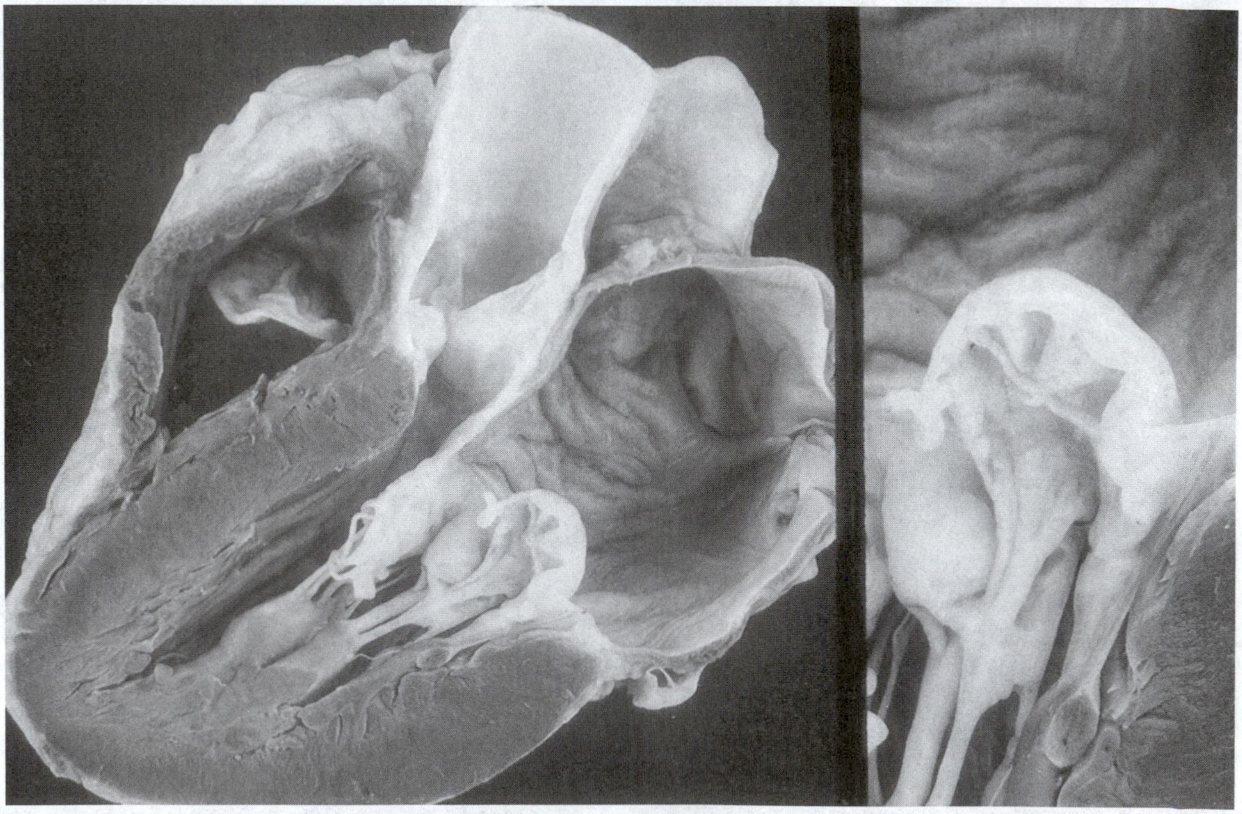

FIGURE 57-9 (Plate 88) Anatomic example of a flail posterior leaflet with ruptured chord. On the right of the picture, closeup view of the ruptured chord. Otherwise the left atrium is enlarged and the valvular tissue normal. (Courtesy of Dr. W. D. Edwards.)

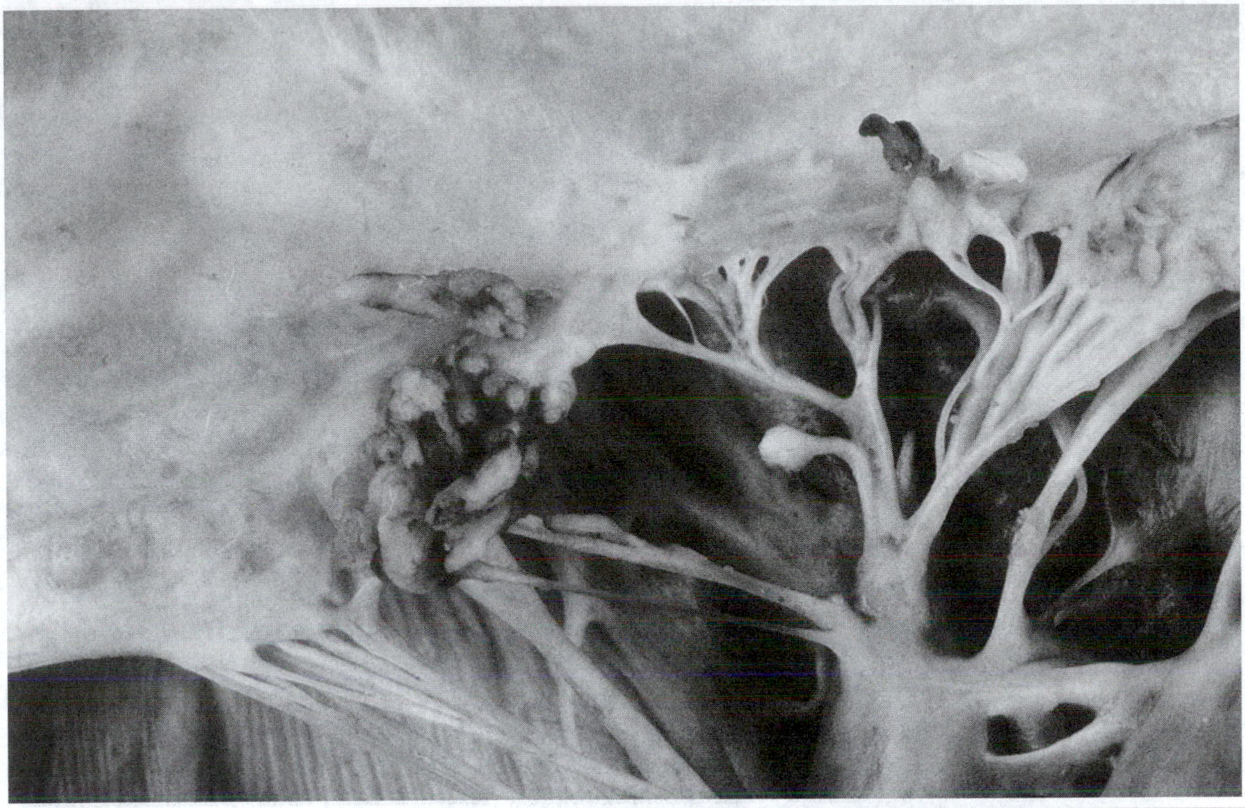

FIGURE 57-10 (Plate 89) Anatomic example of MR due to endocarditis. Note the vegetations of the anterior leaflet and the ruptured chords. (Courtesy of Dr. W. D. Edwards.)

papillary muscle produces MR because of the flail leaflet and involves in 80 percent of cases the posteromedial papillary muscle and is most often associated with infarction of the adjacent ventricular wall.[53] It is the rarest form of heart rupture and of ischemic MR. Complete rupture is rapidly fatal without surgery, and partial or single-head rupture of the papillary muscle more often allows emergency surgery[53] (Fig. 57-11, Plate 90).

OTHER CAUSES OF MITRAL REGURGITATION

MR is observed very frequently with color-flow imaging, even in patients without cardiac disease. However, clinically significant MR may be found in (1) *connective tissue disorder,* Marfan syndrome, Ehlers-Danlos syndrome, pseudoxanthum elasticum, osteogenesis imperfecta, Hurler's disease, systemic lupus erythematosus, and anticardiolipin syndrome; (2) penetrating or nonpenetrating *cardiac trauma;* (3) *myocardial disease*—hypertrophic cardiomyopathy or sarcoidosis; (4) *endocardial lesions* due to hypereosinophilic syndrome, endocardial fibroelastosis, carcinoid tumors, ergot toxicity, radiation toxicity, diet or drug toxicity[54]; (5) *congenital* lesions such as cleft mitral valve isolated or associated with persistent atrioventricular canal, corrected transposition with or without Ebstein's abnormality of the left atrioventricular valve, and (6) *cardiac tumors.*

Pathophysiology

The abnormal coaptation of the mitral leaflets creates a *regurgitant orifice* during systole. The systolic pressure gradient between the LV and LA is the driving force of the regurgitant flow, which results in a *regurgitant volume.* This regurgitant volume represents a percentage of the total ejection of the LV and may be expressed as the *regurgitant fraction.* The regurgitant volume creates a volume overload by entering the LA in systole and the LV in diastole, modifying LV loading and function.

CHRONOLOGY OF REGURGITATION

The pressure gradient between the LV and atrium begins with mitral closure (simultaneous to S_1) and persists after closure of the aortic valve (S_2) until the mitral valve opens.[55] Thus, timing of regurgitant flow is determined by that of the regurgitant orifice and is most often holosystolic. Various dynamic changes in the regurgitant orifice can be observed depending on its cause.[56] With small regurgitant orifices, the regurgitant orifice declines with the ventricular volume tending to limit regurgitation to early systole.[55] Conversely, in valve prolapse, the regurgitant orifice appears or increases late in systole and variations of regurgitant flow throughout systole are the complex results of combined effects of changes of regurgitant orifice and gradient.[56,57]

DEGREE AND CONSEQUENCES OF REGURGITATION

The degree of volume overload depends on three factors, the area of the regurgitant orifice,[58] the regurgitant gradient, and the regurgitant duration. The volume overload is usually less severe in mitral than in aortic regurgitation, despite a usually

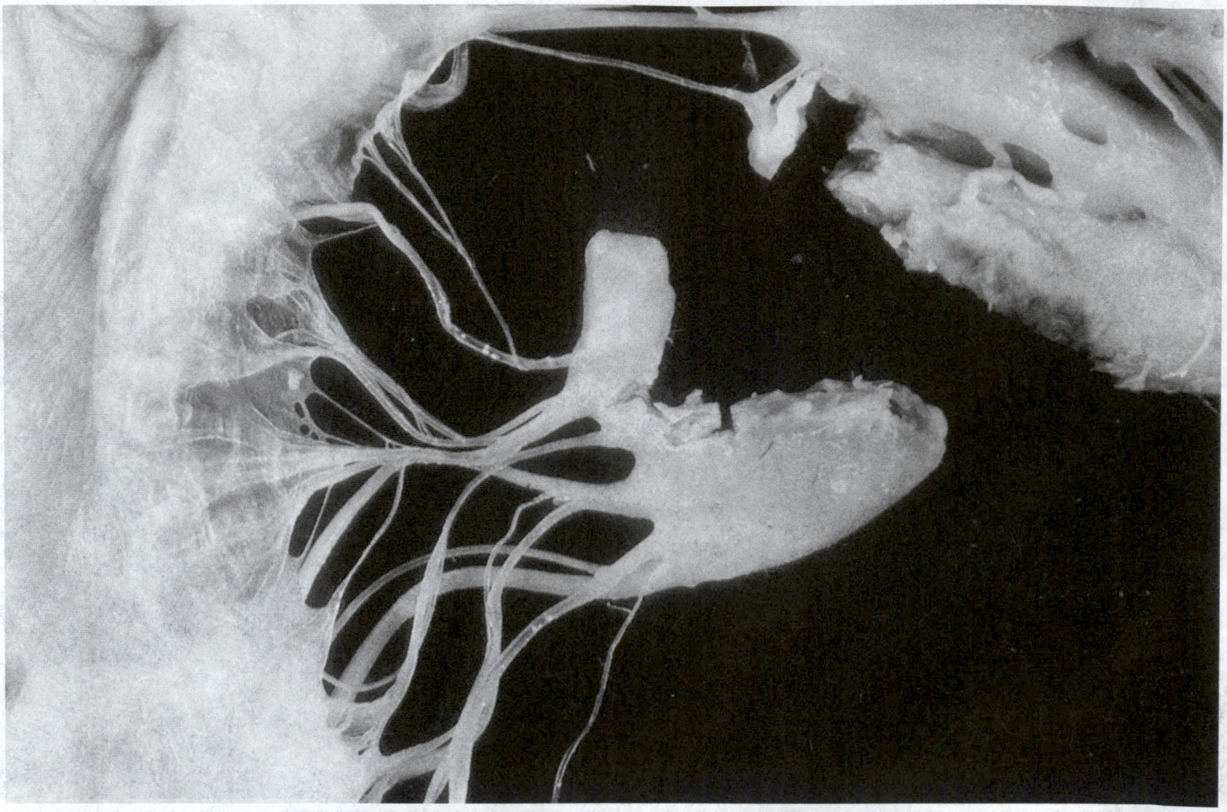

FIGURE 57-11 (Plate 90) Anatomic example of a ruptured posterior papillary muscle. Note the normal valvular tissue otherwise. (Courtesy of Dr. W. D. Edwards.)

larger regurgitant gradient and orifice.[58] Such differences are related to a shorter duration of MR during the cardiac cycle in mitral than in aortic regurgitation.[58]

The degree of MR is not fixed and may vary with interventions. Vasodilators may be beneficial,[59] but the change in regurgitant orifice area rather than that of ventriculoatrial gradient is the main mechanism of this effect. In functional[60] and organic MR,[61] the regurgitant orifice increases with increased afterload or ventricular volume and decreases with decreased afterload or improved contractility, but it is not influenced by changes in heart rate.[61]

The regurgitant energy produced by the LV translates into two components: the kinetic energy (regurgitant volume) and the potential energy (elevation of atrial pressure). The typical left atrial pressure change is the V wave,[62] which nevertheless, is not specific for MR. The height of the V wave and more generally left atrial pressure is mainly determined by left atrial compliance.[62] In acute MR, the LA is less compliant than in chronic MR and the MR produces a marked increase in LA pressure. The atrial V wave, in turn, decreases the ventriculoatrial gradient and, thus, for any effective regurgitant orifice,[58] tends to limit the regurgitant volume. When MR becomes chronic, the LA dilates, the V wave is less prominent, and it does not limit the regurgitant volume; the LA pressure may be normal even with severe MR.[63] At that stage, usually the cardiac output is decreased but the pulmonary pressures are often normal. Pulmonary hypertension in MR is poorly understood and mostly observed in elderly patients.

LEFT VENTRICULAR FUNCTION

With MR the LV is dilated, but less so than in aortic regurgitation of comparable degree.[64] LV end-diastolic volume and wall stress are increased,[64] and the ventricle's shape becomes spherical. End-systolic volume is increased in chronic MR but end-systolic wall stress is usually normal.[65] The myocardial mass is increased proportionately to LV dilatation.[66]

LV function is difficult to characterize because of the changes in preload and afterload. It has been suggested that normalization of ejection fraction (EF) to the preload would provide an appropriate assessment of LV function. Afterload is more difficult to assess because the MR may decrease the instantaneous impedance to ejection, but the measure of afterload provided by end-systolic wall stress is within the normal range.[65] However the usual inverse correlation between end-systolic wall stress and EF is also observed in MR.[67] Complex indices using the afterload—such as the end systolic wall stress,[68] or maximum elastance,[65] normalized to the LV volume—have been proposed and may be sensitive to subtle changes in function.

LV dysfunction is a frequent and dismal complication of MR.[69,70] The mechanism of LV hypertrophy is a reduction in protein degradation, but the mechanisms leading to interstitial fibrosis and LV dysfunction remain mysterious. Experimentally, LV dysfunction is not due to changes in coronary blood flow. The changes in myofiber contractility parallel those in LV function[71] and are associated with reduced myofiber content,[72] but the cause of the myofiber dysfunction and the explanation of its high incidence have not been clarified.

During diastole, LV relaxation is prolonged but chamber stiffness is reduced.[73] Age and decreased systolic function[73] are associated with increased chamber stiffness. The significance of the diastolic abnormalities is unclear.

ISCHEMIC AND FUNCTIONAL MITRAL REGURGITATION

The pathophysiology of ruptured papillary muscles is poorly known. In chronic ischemic or functional MR, the primary disease involves the LV, which is often contracting poorly. However, MR may be determined more by localized LV deformation than by the systolic function. The apical and inferior traction on papillary muscles leads to leaflet tethering and tenting and subsequently to MR.[74,75] In ischemic or functional as opposed to organic (due to primary valvular disease) MR, the regurgitant volume is usually small,[76] and the LV and atrial dilatation is in excess to the degree of MR.[58] Nevertheless, MR is associated with elevated left atrial pressure[58] and poor outcome[77]; it is also a marker of sensitivity to vasodilators.

HORMONAL ACTIVATION

In organic MR, natriuretic peptides are elevated in experimental[78] and clinical[79] studies. The main determinant of elevation of atrial natriuretic peptide is the elevation of atrial pressures.[79] In our experience, brain natriuretic peptide is more a marker of LV remodeling than of altered hemodynamics. The value of natriuretic peptide levels as markers of hemodynamics, LV function, and prognosis is not established yet.

The activation of the renin-angiotensin system is not fully understood. In dogs with organic MR, systemic activation of the renin-angiotensin system is rare,[80] but tissue levels of angiotensin II are markedly elevated.[81,82] The role of angiotensin in the development of hypertrophy and fibrosis are not fully clarified.

Clinical Presentation

The sex distribution has changed in parallel to the changes in etiology of MR. With the decrease in rheumatic heart disease, severe MR is now predominantly seen in males (65 to 75 percent). The prevalence of MR increases with age[83]; therefore, patients with severe MR most often present in the sixth decade of life.[84]

The clinical presentation—including symptoms, physical findings, electrocardiographic and radiographic change—is determined by the degree, rapidity of development, and cause of MR and by LA and LV function and compliance.

SYMPTOMS

Patients with mild MR usually have no symptoms. Severe MR is diagnosed most often because of the murmur when no or minimal symptoms are present.[84] Fatigue and mild dyspnea on exertion are the most usual symptoms and are rapidly improved by rest. The administration of diuretics and progressive self-limitation of physical activity may prevent the occurrence of more severe symptoms. Severe dyspnea on exertion or, more rarely, paroxysmal nocturnal dyspnea, frank pulmonary edema, or even hemoptysis may be observed later in the course of the disease. Such severe symptoms may be triggered by a new onset of atrial fibrillation, or increase in degree of MR, the occurrence of endocarditis or ruptured chordae, or a change in LV compliance or function.

With severe MR of *acute onset,* symptoms are usually more dramatic—pulmonary edema or congestive heart failure—but will progressively subside with administration of diuretic and increased LA compliance. A syndrome of sudden onset of atypical chest pain and dyspnea may occur with abrupt chordal rupture. Rupture of papillary muscle usually has a dramatic presentation, with cardiogenic shock or a severe pulmonary edema. Pulmonary edema may also be observed in transient severe papillary muscle dysfunction.

Sudden death as the initial presentation of MR is rare.[85]

PHYSICAL EXAMINATION

Blood pressure is usually normal. Carotid upstroke is brisk.

Cardiac palpation may show laterally displaced, diffuse, and brief apical impulse with enlarged LV. An apical thrill is characteristic of severe MR. The left sternal border lift is observed with right ventricular dilatation and may be difficult to distinguish from the left atrial lift due to the dilated, expansive LA, which is more substernal and lower.

S_1 is included in the murmur and is usually normal but may be increased in rheumatic disease. S_2 is usually normal but may be paradoxically split if the LV ejection time is markedly shortened. The presence of a third heart sound (S_3) is directly related to the volume of the regurgitation in patients with organic MR.[86] It is often associated with an early diastolic rumble due to the increased mitral flow in diastole even without mitral stenosis (Chap. 10). The S_3 and diastolic rumble are low-pitched sounds and may be difficult to detect without careful auscultation in the left lateral decubitus position. The S_3 increases with expiration. In ischemic-functional MR, S_3 corresponds more often to restrictive LV filling. An atrial gallop (S_4) is heard mainly in MR of recent onset and in ischemic/functional MR in sinus rhythm. Midsystolic clicks are markers of valve prolapse (Chaps. 10 and 11).

The hallmark of MR is the systolic murmur, most often holosystolic, including first and second heart sounds. If an opening snap or S_3 is mistakenly interpreted as S_2, the murmur may appear midsystolic. Only a careful examination beginning at the base of the heart to identify the second heart sound and progressing toward the apex will allow clear recognition of the nature of the murmur. The murmur is of the blowing type but may be harsh, especially in valve prolapse. The maximum intensity is usually at the apex, and it may radiate to the axilla in rheumatic or anterior leaflet prolapse, affecting primarily the anterior leaflet. In posterior leaflet prolapse, the jet is usually superiorly and medially directed and the murmur radiates towards the base of the heart.[87] The murmur may be heard in the back, in the neck, and sometimes on the skull. In the cases where the murmur radiates to the base, it may be difficult to distinguish from the murmur of aortic stenosis or obstructive cardiomyopathy, and pharmacologic maneuvers showing that the murmur decreases with amyl nitrite and increases with methoxamine strongly suggest MR. Murmur intensity does not increase with postextrasystolic beats and usually parallels the degree of MR,[88] but in myocardial infarction severe MR may be totally silent[89] (see Chap. 10).

Murmurs of shorter duration usually correspond to mild MR; they may be mid or late systolic in mitral valve prolapse or early systolic in functional MR.

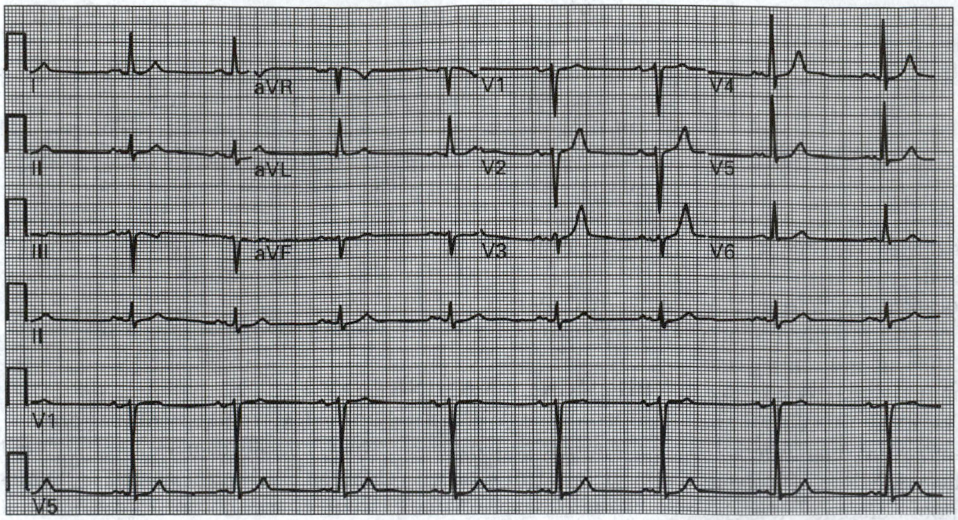

FIGURE 57-12 Electrocardiogram of a patient with severe MR. Note LA enlargement, as indicated by notched p waves (lead I and rhythm strip lead II).

ELECTROCARDIOGRAM

The most frequent feature of MR is atrial fibrillation which was found in approximately 50 to 60 percent of earlier series and is now present in approximately 50 percent of surgically corrected MR.[90] Patients in sinus rhythm may present with signs of left atrial enlargement (Fig. 57-12). LV hypertrophy is more rarely seen and may be associated with secondary ST-T abnormalities.[91] Right ventricular hypertrophy is uncommon. The electrocardiogram, especially in acute MR, may be entirely normal. In ischemic MR, Q waves in the inferior leads or left bundle-branch block is often noted.

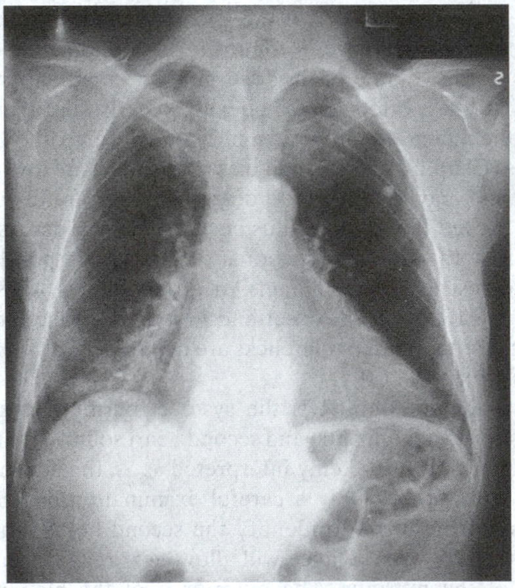

FIGURE 57-13 Chest roentgenogram of a patient with severe MR. Note the cardiomegaly and enlargement of the LA body and appendage.

CHEST ROENTGENOGRAM

Cardiomegaly may be present in chronic MR or in ischemic/functional MR (Fig. 57-13). LA body and appendage dilatation is frequent but giant LA is rare and is usually seen in severe mixed valve disease. Although valvular calcifications are rare, annular calcification seen as a C-shaped density below the posterior leaflet is frequent. Because LA pressure is frequently normal even with severe MR, signs of pulmonary hypertension or pulmonary edema are rarely observed.

CLINICAL SYNDROMES

The clinical presentation of patients with MR can be schematically separated in four syndromes, summarized in Table 57-12.

Laboratory Tests

DOPPLER ECHOCARDIOGRAPHY

Doppler echocardiography has an important role in the assessment of MR using two-dimensional echocardiography with directed M-mode measurements, color-flow imaging, pulsed and continuous-wave Doppler, and transesophageal echocardiography (TEE). Quantitative measurements of flow and detailed hemodynamic assessment should be routinely performed. The goals of Doppler echocardiography are (1) to assess the mor-

TABLE 57-12 Mitral Regurgitation: Clinical Presentations

	MVP Syndrome	Chronic MR	Acute MR	Ischemic/Functional MR
Symptoms	Chest pain	Fatigue	Pulmonary edema	CHF
Physical examination	Midsystolic click, murmur	Loud murmur S_3	Loud murmur S_4	Soft murmur S_3, S_4
Electrocardiogram	ST-T changes	Atrial fibrillation	Normal	Q waves, left bundle-branch block
Chest x-ray	Pectus excavatum	Cardiomegaly	Normal heart size, pulmonary edema	Cardiomegaly, pulmonary edema

phology of the mitral valve (etiology and mechanism), (2) to assess the degree of MR, and (3) to assess ventricular and atrial function (see also Chap. 13).

Morphology The features of the most common causes are indicated below.

Rheumatic MR is characterized by thickening of the leaflets and chordae. The posterior leaflet has reduced mobility whereas the anterior leaflet may be doming if commissural fusion is associated. A valvular prolapse is usually not present unless a ruptured chordae or active rheumatic carditis are present. Similar lesions are observed in lupus or anticardiolipin syndrome, in which transesophageal echocardiography may also show small vegetations.

In *degenerative MR,* prolapse is observed with the passage of valvular tissue beyond the annulus plane in the long-axis view (Fig. 57-14). Some features are important:

- Myxomatous changes with diffusely thickened leaflets and excessive valvular tissue
- Localization of the leaflet involved (most often the posterior) confirmed by the initial direction of the jet
- The presence of mitral annular calcification, which may represent a limitation for conservative surgery if extensive and severe
- Flail segments appearing as complete eversion of the segment with or without the small floating echo of ruptured chordae[92] (Fig. 57-15)

The usual mechanism in endocarditic MR, flail leaflets, is relatively easy to diagnose.[92] Perforations are more difficult to diagnose. Mitral annular abscesses are rare and are best detected by TEE. Vegetations can be seen on leaflets or on ruptured chords with superior sensitivity by TEE.[93]

In ischemic/functional MR, the finding of a dilated annulus[94,95] is nonspecific[76] and annular descent is reduced. The features of ischemic heart disease may be observed as regional wall motion abnormalities.[94] The leaflet tissue is normal. The mitral tenting due to the abnormal traction by the principal chordae on the anterior leaflet reduces the area of coaptation of the two leaflets and therefore allows for a central jet of MR.[94,95]

With papillary muscle rupture,[53] MR is due to the flail leaflet. The diagnosis is based on visualization of a small mass of muscle attached to chordae and floating freely during the cardiac cycle.

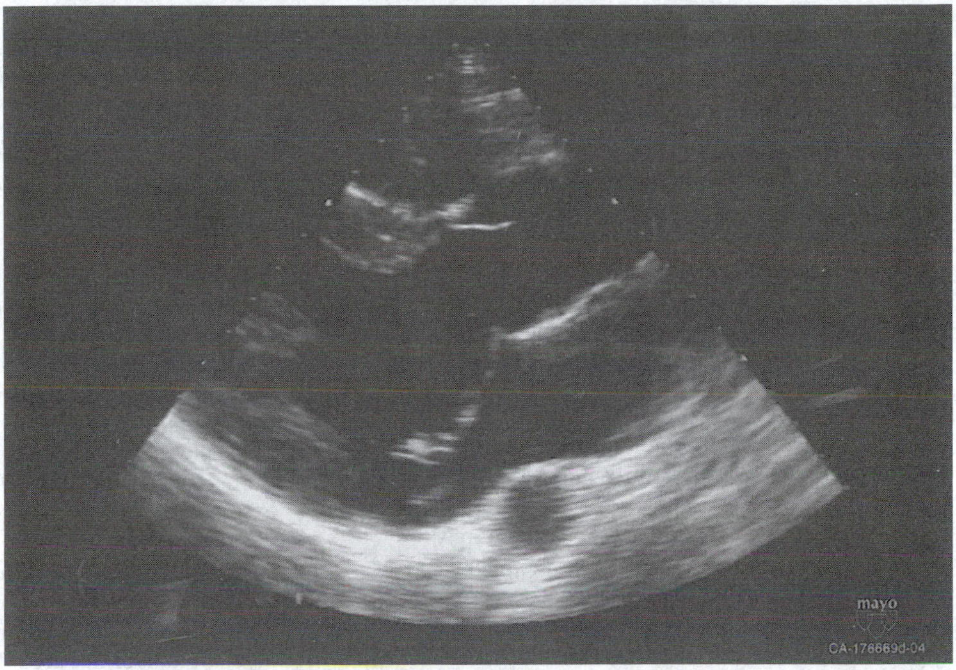

FIGURE 57-14 Echocardiogram of a bileaflet mitral valve prolapse seen from the parasternal long-axis view.

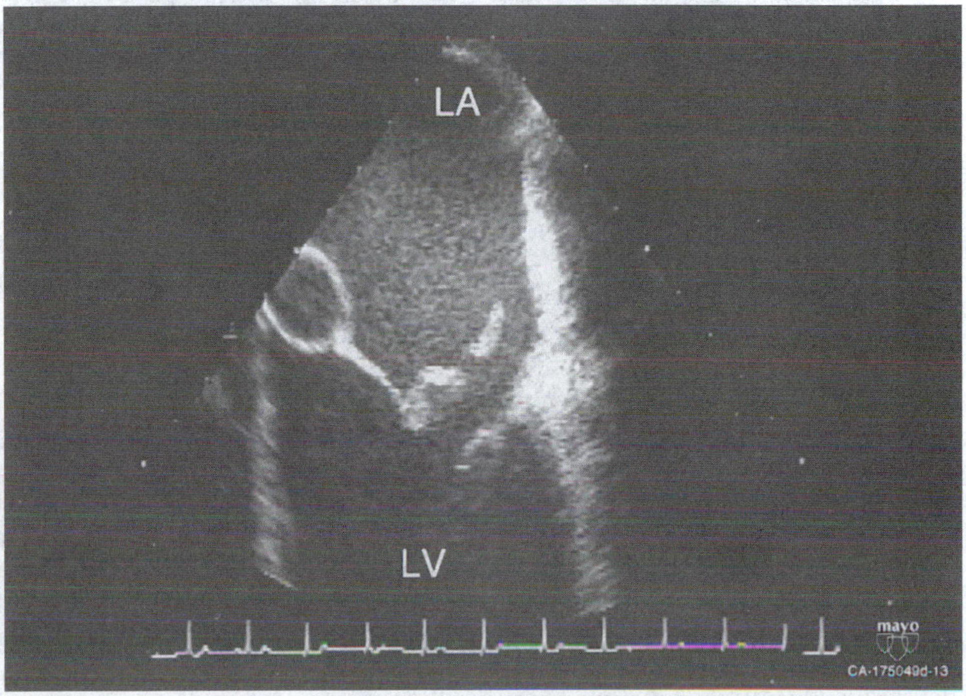

FIGURE 57-15 Transesophageal echocardiography (*horizontal plane*) of a flail anterior leaflet. The ruptured chord is seen at the tip of the anterior leaflet.

TABLE 57-13 Assessment of Severity of Mitral Regurgitation

Clinical		
Systolic thrill		
Murmur intensity		
S_3		
Diastolic rumble		
Laboratory		
Qualitative		
Large jet ≥8 cm² (echo-Doppler)		
Pulmonary vein reversal (Doppler, angiography)		
Dense contrast in LA (angiography)		
Quantitative		
Criteria:	Regurgitant volume ≥60 mL	
	Regurgitant fraction ≥50%	
	Effective regurgitant orifice ≥40 mm²	
Method:	Doppler echocardiography	
		Quantitative Doppler
		Quantitative 2D echo
		Amplitude weighted mean velocity
		Proximal isovelocity surface area (PISA)
		Radionuclide angiography
		Quantitative LV angiography

Assessment of Severity of Regurgitation (Table 57-13)
SEMIQUANTITATIVE METHODS COLOR-FLOW IMAGING JET ANALYSIS The origin and direction of the jet is related to etiology. Jet length and ratio of jet to left atrial area (or more simply jet area)[96] have been suggested as good indices of MR severity. Small jets consistently correspond to mild MR.[76] However, color-flow imaging has significant limitations, intrinsically related to the nature of regurgitant jets (Chap. 13). The extent of a jet is determined by its momentum and thus as much by regurgitant velocity as by regurgitant flow. Also, jets are constrained by the LA and expand more in large LAs.[76] The eccentric jets of valve prolapse[97] impinge on the LA wall and tend to underestimate MR[76] (Fig. 57-16, Plate 91). Central jets of functional MR expand markedly in the enlarged LA, and this tends to overestimate MR[76] (Fig. 57-17, Plate 92). TEE usually shows larger jets but does not suppress these limitations of color-flow imaging (Chap. 13).

VENA CONTRACTA MEASUREMENT The vena contracta is the region of the regurgitant flow immediately below the flow convergence through the regurgitant orifice.[98] Therefore, direct measurement of vena contracta width provides an index of the regurgitant orifice area. The vena contracta width appears superior to jet measurements and can be obtained either through transesophageal[98] or transthoracic echocardiography.[99]

The *pulmonary venous velocity profile* is useful to assess the degree of MR.[100] Systolic reversal in pulmonary veins is a strong argument for severe MR but is related not only to MR severity but also to jet direction and LA pressure.[101] Consequently, pul-

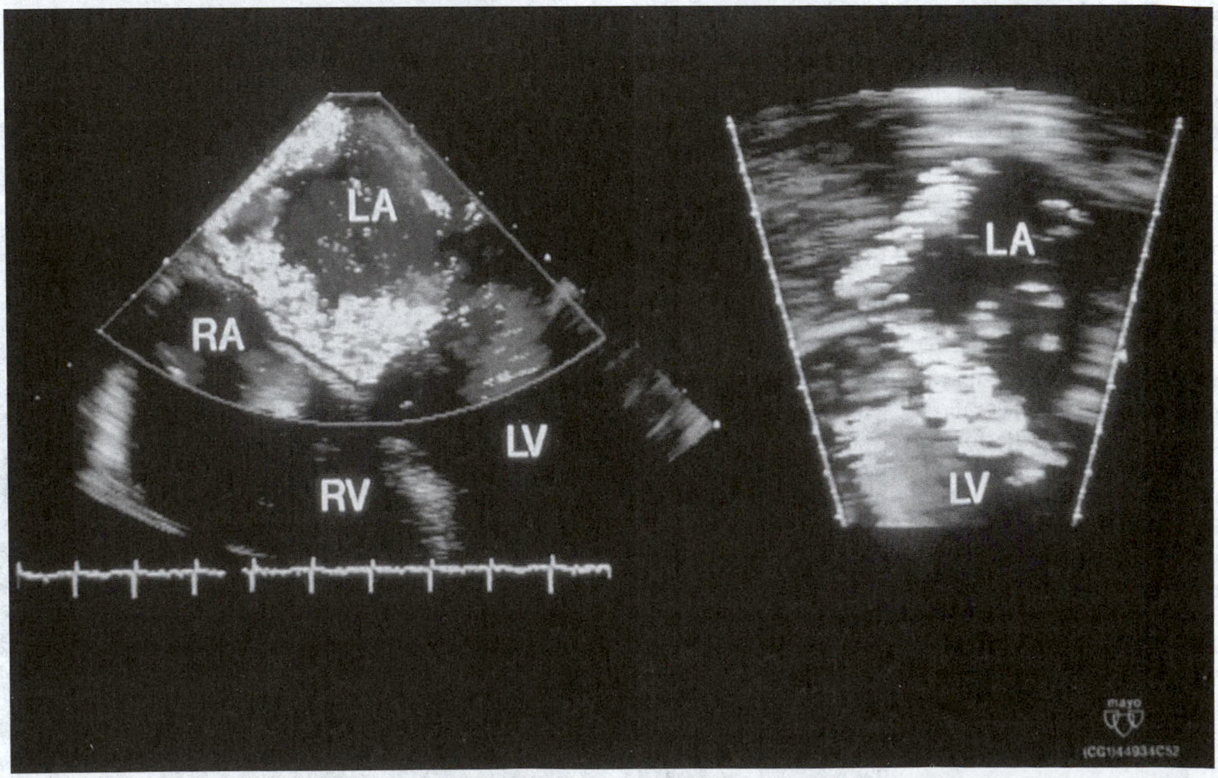

FIGURE 57-16 (Plate 91) Color-flow imaging of an eccentric jet (flail posterior leaflet). *Left:* Transesophageal (*horizontal plane*) echocardiography. *Right:* Transthoracic echocardiography. Note that with both modalities the jet is thinned, impinging on the atrial wall and tending to underestimate this severe regurgitation.

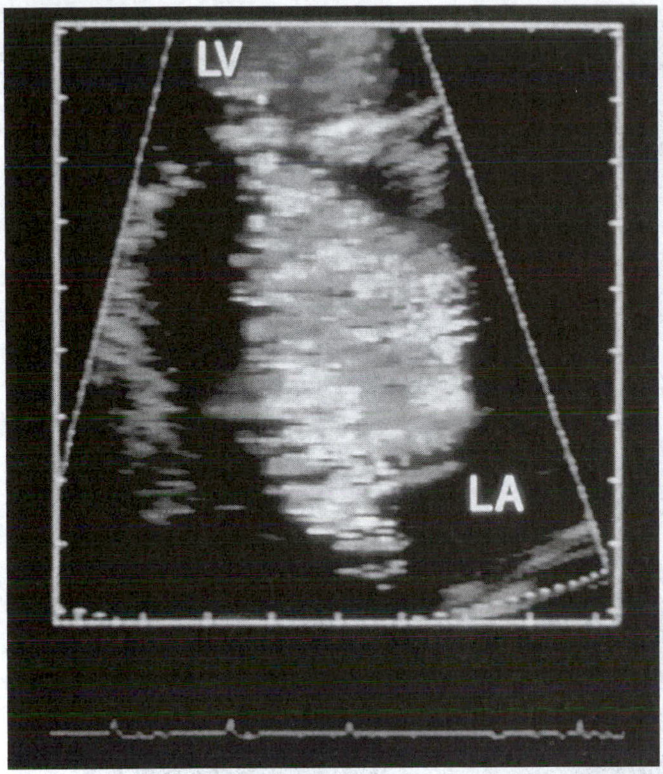

FIGURE 57-17 (Plate 92) Color flow imaging of a central jet of a functional mitral regurgitation by transthoracic echocardiography. Note that the jet is free, expands in the left atrium, and tends to overestimate this moderate regurgitation.

monary venous reversal may be absent or asymmetric in severe MR[101] (Fig. 57-18).

QUANTITATIVE METHODS *The goal* of quantitative methods is to measure the volume overload expressed as the regurgitant volume (difference between the total and forward stroke volume) or fraction (proportion of LV ejection volume regurgitated in the LA). The lesion's severity is expressed as the effective regurgitant orifice (ERO) area and calculated as follows[58,102]: ERO = regurgitant flow/regurgitant velocity or ERO = regurgitant volume/regurgitant TVI, where the TVI is the time velocity integral of the regurgitant jet.

The *practical* quantitation of MR can be performed using various methods:

- *Quantitative Doppler* is based on the calculation of the mitral and aortic stroke volumes using pulsed-wave Doppler.[103] The principle is simple and applicable in most cases, but the measurement of the mitral stroke volume is technically demanding, with a significant learning phase.[103]
- *Quantitative two-dimensional echocardiography* is of similar principle but is based on measurement of LV volumes for total stroke volume calculation.[104]
- The *proximal isovelocity surface area* (PISA) method, conversely, directly measures regurgitant flow by analyzing the flow convergence proximal to the regurgitant orifice (Fig. 57-19, Plate 93) and is based on the principle of conservation of mass. Because color-flow mapping allows precise determination of velocity in the flow-convergence region, the regurgitant flow can be calculated. Using regurgitant flow and velocity, regurgitant orifice and volume can be calculated.[102] This method is simple and accurate if the assumptions are respected. (See also Chap. 13.)

Assessment of Left Ventricular and Atrial Function The technique of guided M-mode diameters is used for assessment of LV size, mass, and wall stress.[90,105,106] LV volumes can be reliably measured by two-dimensional echocardiography. The EF can be calculated or estimated. M-mode diameter or volume can assess the LA size by two-dimensional echocardiography.

RADIONUCLIDE STUDIES

Radionuclide angiography can be used to estimate the LV end-diastolic and end-systolic volume as well as the right and LV EF. The detection of exercise-induced LV dysfunction is frequent. However the significance of such measurement on the long-term prognosis has not been analyzed in large series of patients. A comparison of the counts measured over the RV and LV allows the calculation of the regurgitant fraction.

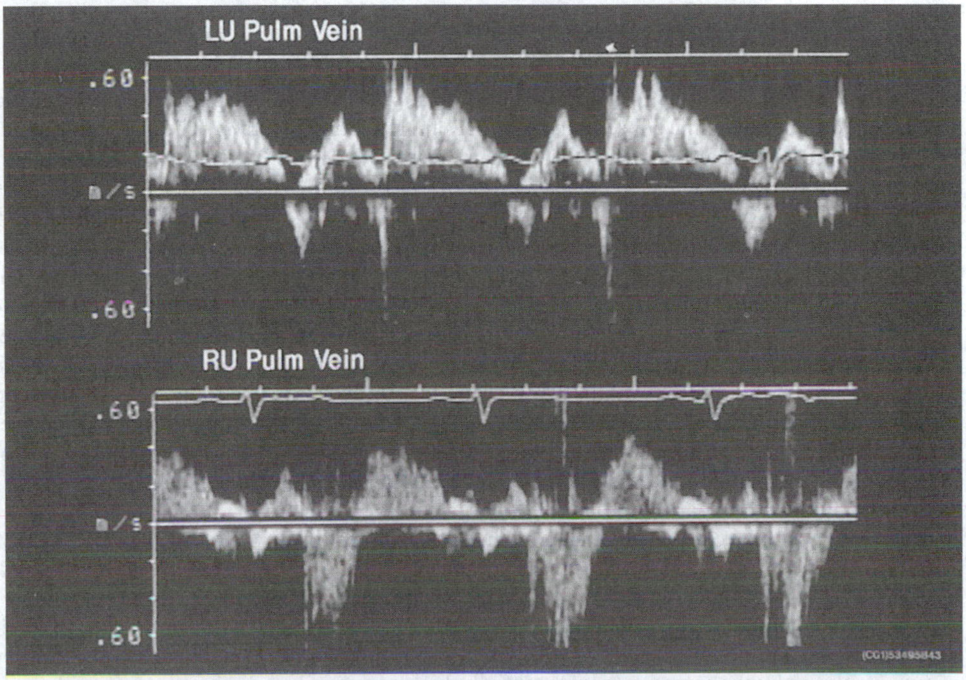

FIGURE 57-18 Pulmonary venous flow of a patient with MR due to a flail posterior leaflet (by transesophageal echocardiography). Note that the flow is asymmetrical, with preserved systolic flow in the left upper pulmonary vein and systolic reversal in the right upper pulmonary vein.

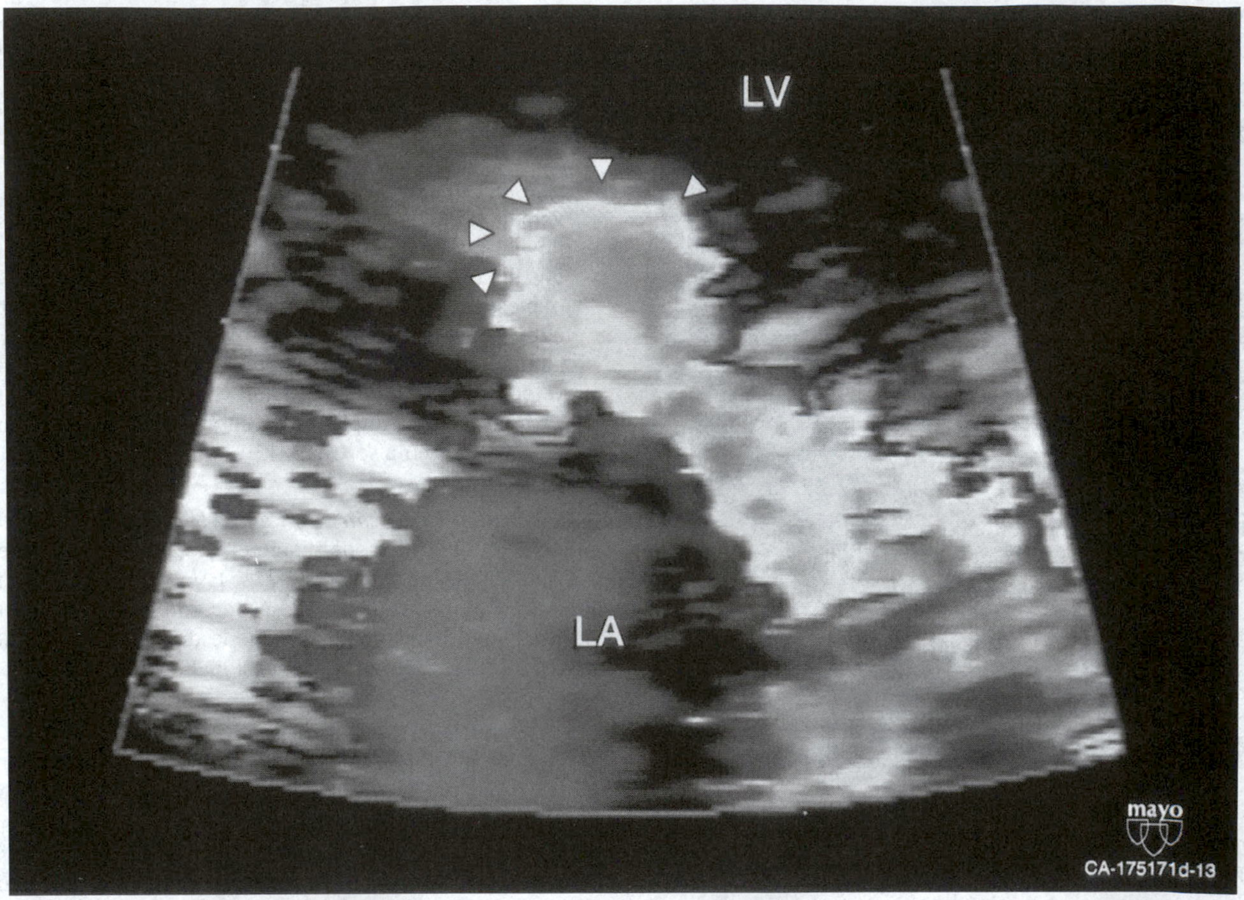

FIGURE 57-19 (Plate 93) Color flow imaging of the proximal flow convergence of a mitral regurgitation due to a flail posterior leaflet (by transthoracic echocardiography). The downward baseline shift of the color-flow scale enlarges the size of the flow convergence, which is easily measurable.

CARDIAC CATHETERIZATION

Cardiac catheterization is utilized to assess hemodynamic status, the severity of MR, LV function, and coronary anatomy.

The major hemodynamic consequences of MR are reduction of cardiac output and elevation of pulmonary artery wedge pressure. Marked pulmonary hypertension is rarely present. The large V wave of the pulmonary wedge pressure is more frequent in acute than in chronic MR but can be observed in other disease such as ventricular septal defect or heart failure with reduced left atrial compliance without MR (Fig. 57-20).

The assessment of MR degree can be obtained by LV selective angiography and can be qualitatively graded in three or four grades on the basis of the degree and persistence of opacification of the LA.[107] Although time-honored, this method has limitations, like all qualitative methods.[108] Quantitation of MR can be obtained by comparing the angiographic stroke volume to the forward stroke volume, calculated by the Fick or thermodilution methods,[109] to calculate the regurgitant volume and fraction. The angiographic stroke volume usually overestimates the true stroke volume and corrections have been used to minimize the overestimation of the regurgitant volume. Subtraction of two stroke volumes introduces a potentially high range of error, which cannot be verified by combined methods or by repeating the measurements; therefore this method is rarely utilized.

The assessment of LV function can be performed using quantitative angiography. LV volumes correlate strongly to the regurgitant volume, duration and etiology of MR, and LV function. The most frequently utilized indices of LV function are end-systolic volume and EF, which are useful prognostic indices.[70,110] High-fidelity pressure recording with LV angiography allows calculation of more complex indices of LV distensibility in diastole[73] and of wall stress, maximum LV elastance, and LV systolic stiffness. The additional value of these complex measurements has been investigated in small groups of patients and remains to be defined in larger populations.

Selective coronary angiography allows definition of coronary anatomy. Obstructive coronary atherosclerosis continues to be frequent even in the absence of angina,[111] and coronary angiography is ordinarily performed in patients more than 40 to 50 years of age.

STRATEGY OF UTILIZATION OF LABORATORY TESTING

Not all the tests should be performed in all patients[112] (Fig. 57-21). Because transthoracic Doppler echocardiography confirms the diagnosis and degree of MR and of associated valvular diseases and provides a unique assessment of mitral lesions, it is performed in most cases for the initial diagnostic assessment, for follow-up, and for presurgical assessment. TEE provides superior imaging quality, but its incremental value is notable

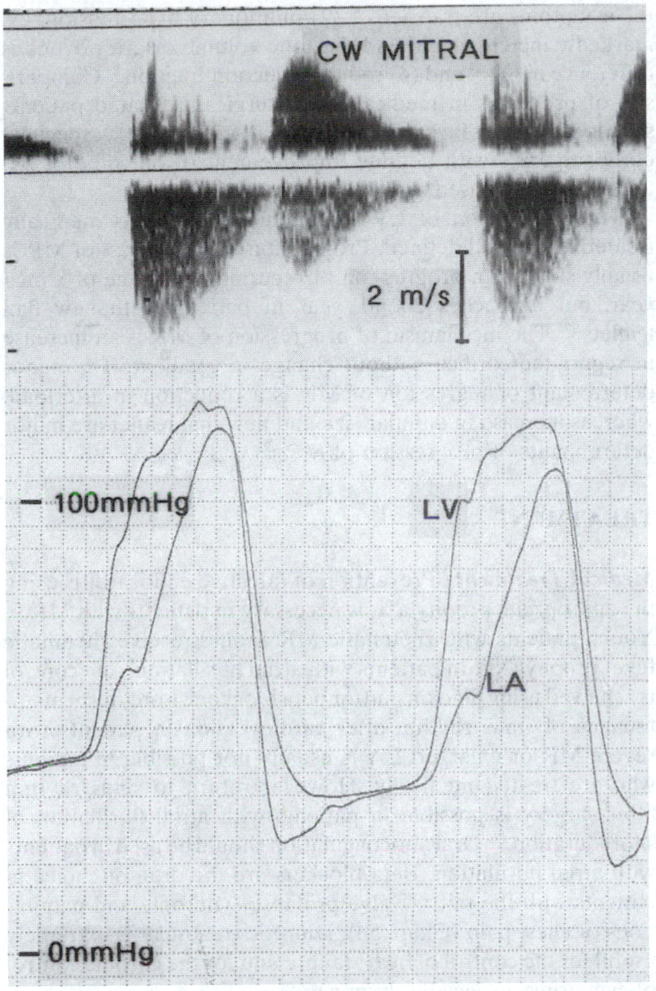

FIGURE 57-20 Simultaneous recording of LV and LA pressures and continuous-wave Doppler (CW) in a patient with severe MR. Note the large V wave on the left atrial pressure recording, with a triangular shape of the mitral regurgitant jet obtained by CW. (Courtesy of Dr. Rick Nishimura, Mayo Clinic.)

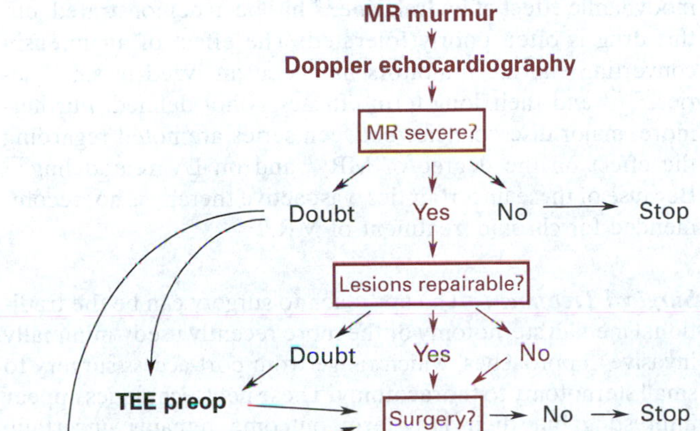

FIGURE 57-21 Strategy of utilization of tests in patients with mitral regurgitation.

only when the transthoracic information is incomplete.[92] In our practice it is reserved preoperatively to the patients in whom a doubt persists regarding the lesions (especially if endocarditis is suspected) or regarding the severity of regurgitation, but it is utilized on a large scale intraoperatively to monitor the results of valve repair.[113]

Coronary angiography is indicated as a presurgical procedure depending on age. LV angiography is not required unless there is concern regarding validity of echocardiographic studies.[114] Although color-flow Doppler showed a significant number of discrepancies as compared to angiography,[115] the understanding of its pitfalls[76] and more recently introduced quantitative methods have reduced the need for redundant tests. Also, the analysis of LV function provided by routine LV angiography does not appear to add significant information to the noninvasive data.[90] However, the utilization of tests should be individualized based on the patient's characteristics and the results of noninvasive studies.

Management

PRINCIPLES

Surgical treatment is reserved for patients with severe MR. Criteria most often used for severe MR are angiographic 4+ grade or color flow jet ≥8 cm^2,[96] with the intrinsic limitations of these definitions. Using quantitative techniques, thresholds for severe MR are 60 mL per beat for regurgitant volume, 50 percent for regurgitant fraction, and 40 mm^2 for effective regurgitant orifice.[116] Patients with severe MR will require surgery at some point during their follow-up. In these patients, the most relevant question is the timing of the surgical indication, which is influenced by the natural history of MR and by the outcome after surgical correction of MR. The determinants of outcome are listed in Table 57-14.

NATURAL HISTORY

Because of the qualitative and imprecise assessment of the degree of MR, the natural history of MR is ill defined. Patients with mild rheumatic MR appear to have a good prognosis,[117] whereas in those with more severe MR a higher mortality has been noted.[84,118] In patients with unoperated clinically significant MR, the late survival has been found as high 60 percent at 10 years[119] or as low as 46 percent[120] or even 27 percent[121] at 5 years. In our experience with flail mitral leaflets, at 10 years, survival was 57 percent, which represents an excess mortality as compared to the expected survival.[84]

The probability of sudden death is important to consider

TABLE 57-14 Determinants of Outcome

Unoperated Patients	Operated Patients
Symptoms	Age
Pulmonary hypertension	Preoperative symptoms
LV end-diastolic volume	Coronary disease
AV-O_2 difference	End-systolic dimensions
Ejection fraction	Ejection fraction
	LA size?
	Valve repair

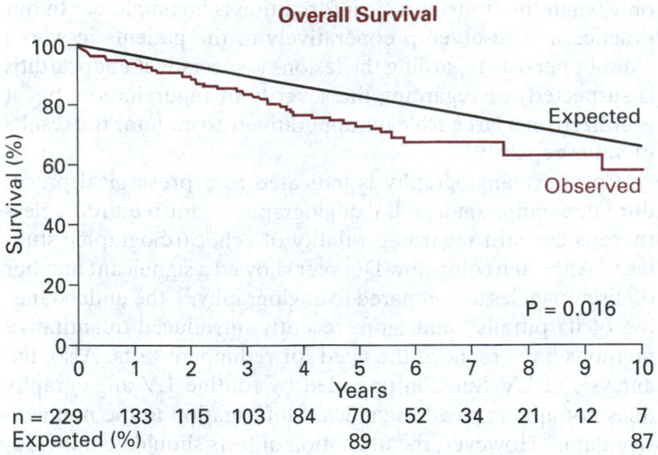

FIGURE 57-22 Survival with medical treatment of patients diagnosed with MR due to flail leaflets. Note the excess mortality in comparison to the expected survival. (Reprinted by permission of the *New England Journal of Medicine* from Ling LH, et al. 1996; 335:1417–1423. Copyright 1996, Massachusetts Medical Society.)

before delaying surgery. Such a devastating complication occurs more often if the ventricular function is decreased[84] but may also occur in patients with normal EF who are asymptomatic.[118] In our experience, sudden death in patients with MR due to flail leaflets occurs at a rate of 1.8 percent per year.[122] The rates are higher in patients with symptoms or reduced ejection fraction, but even in the absence of these risk factors the rate is 0.8 percent per year.[122]

Morbidity in patients with severe MR is also high. Of patients who are initially asymptomatic, approximately 10 percent per year develop symptoms,[123] which may be hastened by atrial fibrillation. In patients with flail leaflets 10 years after diagnosis, heart failure occurred in 63 percent, and permanent atrial fibrillation in 30 percent of those initially in sinus rhythm[84] (Fig. 57-22). Also at 10 years, 90 percent of the patients had either died or undergone surgery,[84] confirming that in these patients surgery is almost unavoidable (Fig. 57-23).

The predictors of poor outcome in patients medically treated are (1) severe symptoms (NYHA classes III to IV),[120] even if

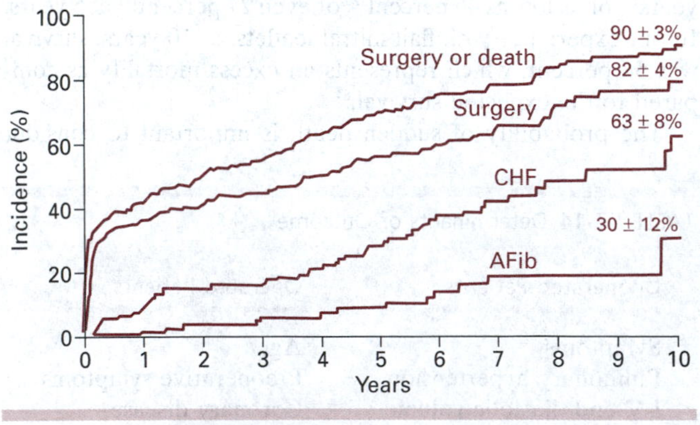

FIGURE 57-23 Cardiac morbidity with medical treatment in patients diagnosed with MR due to flail leaflets. CHF, congestive heart failure, Afib, atrial fibrillation. (Reprinted by permission of the *New England Journal of Medicine* from Ling LH, et al. 1996; 335:1417–1423. Copyright 1996, Massachusetts Medical Society.)

the symptoms are transient,[84] (2) pulmonary hypertension, (3) markedly increased LV end-diastolic volume or arteriovenous difference in O_2,[124] and (4) reduced ejection fraction.[84] Comparison of prognosis in medically and surgically treated patients shows a trend in favor of the surgical treatment,[118] especially early surgery,[84] with definite improvement of outcome of patients with decreased systolic LV function.[124]

The progression of LV dysfunction in patients medically treated is not well defined. Progression of the degree of MR is usually slow, with progression of regurgitant volume of 8 mL/year, but it reaches 20 mL/year in patients with new flail leaflets.[125] The mechanism of progression of MR is an increase in regurgitant orifice without change in gradient. The major determinant of regression of MR is a reduction in afterload, whereas increase in annular size and new flail leaflet are major determinants of progression of MR.[125]

TREATMENT

Medical Treatment Prevention of infective endocarditis using the appropriate prophylaxis is necessary in patients with MR.[126] Young patients with rheumatic MR should receive rheumatic fever prophylaxis. In patients with atrial fibrillation, rate control is achieved using digoxin and/or beta blockers. Long-term maintenance of sinus rhythm after cardioversion in patients with severe MR or enlarged LA is usually not possible in patients who are treated medically. However return to sinus rhythm after surgery is possible in patients with atrial fibrillation of short duration.[127] Oral anticoagulation should be used in patients with atrial fibrillation. Beta blockers are the drug of choice in patients with the mitral valve prolapse syndrome and palpitations or chest pain (Chap. 58). Diuretic treatment is extremely useful for the control of heart failure and for the chronic control of symptoms, especially dyspnea.

Acute afterload reduction may decrease the degree of MR.[59] This effect is achieved by reducing the LV systolic pressure but also by decreasing the effective regurgitant orifice area.[60] Acute utilization of sodium nitroprusside in unstable patients with severe MR, especially in the context of myocardial infarction, may be lifesaving in preparation for surgery.[60]

Chronic afterload reduction is more controversial. The hemodynamic effect of hydralazine,[128] has been demonstrated, but this drug is often poorly tolerated. The effect of angiotensin converting enzyme inhibitors has been analyzed in small series,[129–131] and their long-term efficacy is not defined. Furthermore, major discrepancies between series are noted regarding the effect on the degree of MR[132] and on LV remodeling.[133] Because of these uncertainties, vasoactive therapy is not recommended for chronic treatment of MR.[112]

Surgical Treatment The approach to surgery can be the traditional median sternotomy or the more recently used "minimally invasive" approaches, which range from port-access surgery to small sternotomy to thoracotomy. These new techniques appear interesting but their long-term outcome remains uncertain. There are two main valvular surgical options: mitral valve reconstruction and mitral valve replacement.

MITRAL VALVE RECONSTRUCTION Reconstruction of the incompetent mitral valve is almost always possible (approximately

90 percent of patients referred for primary correction of acquired MR at the Mayo Clinic). The frequency with which valve repair can be used varies with experience of the operating team and the spectrum of underlying valve disease; repair is more often feasible with degenerative valve disease than with rheumatic valvulitis or endocarditis.

The *valvular procedure* is as follows. With leaflet prolapse immobilization of this prolapsing section can be obtained by plicating or by excising it and then repairing the leaflet. This will overcome the problem of localized prolapse. However, the resulting reduction in area of the leaflet could reduce coaptation and induce residual MR; therefore, annuloplasty is a routine part of the repair. Resection or plication of prolapsing sections is most successful with posterior leaflet prolapse. With anterior leaflet prolapse the risk of residual MR is higher if the plication or resection is not combined with subvalvular procedures.[113] Other repairable leaflet abnormalities include congenital clefts and acquired perforation, which may be closed by using a patch of pericardium or synthetic material.

In the *subvalvular procedure,* chordal shortening may be necessary in patients with elongated chordae to ensure the appropriate coaptation of the leaflets, but the durability of this procedure has been criticized.[134] A major recent progress has been the introduction of transposition of chordae and of artificial chordae which have made the anterior leaflet prolapse as repairable as the posterior leaflet prolapse.[135,136]

Annular dilatation, almost constantly associated with MR, is treated by reduction of mitral circumference, i.e., *annuloplasty*. The annuloplasty should be placed in the region supporting the posterior leaflet to preserve the area of anterior leaflet. A cloth-covered rigid ring was originally developed by Carpentier. Recently, flexible annuloplasty rings have been developed to preserve the normal systolic contraction of the mitral annulus.[137] In general, results with the Carpentier ring annuloplasty have been favorable, but LV outflow obstruction associated with abnormal systolic anterior motion of the anterior mitral leaflet has been reported in 6 to 10 percent of patients.[138] This complication is mainly due to hypovolemia and excessive use of inotropes[113] but may be lower with flexible rings.[139]

It is important to assess the adequacy of mitral valve reconstruction before completion of the operation. When satisfactory repair cannot be achieved, it is preferable to replace the valve immediately. To assess adequacy of mitral repair (residual stenosis, regurgitation, or systolic anterior motion), TEE, which does not interfere with the surgical procedure, is performed routinely.[113]

Valve Replacement When mitral reconstruction is considered impossible or is unsuccessful, replacement must be performed. The dilemma is the choice between a mechanical valve of excellent durability but with the hazard of thromboembolism and a biological valve with undefined long-term durability[140] but less tendency to cause thromboembolism. With atrial fibrillation, chronic anticoagulant therapy is necessary even with a bioprosthesis, so that avoiding anticoagulation is not relevant in choosing a prosthesis.

Postoperative Outcome Valve repair, by preserving the normal valvular tissue, is preferable to valve replacement. Compared to prosthetic replacement, mitral valve reconstruction has a lower operative mortality.[141,142] Direct comparison of the results of valve repair and replacement is difficult[142] because the patients undergoing a valve repair are usually at a less advanced stage of the disease than patients undergoing valve replacement.[141] However, survival and LV function after valve repair are better than after insertion of a prosthetic valve.[141] Better ventricular function with valvuloplasty may be due to preservation of chordae and papillary muscles.[143] Durability of valve repair for degenerative disease is excellent if no more than mild residual MR is accepted.[134] Valve repair has the same low rate of reoperation than valve replacement.[141] MR post-repair is due in two-thirds of the cases to new lesions and in one-third to an inadequate primary correction.[144] *Therefore valve repair should be the preferred procedure for surgical correction of MR* (Fig. 57-24).

Operative mortality has been reported between 5 and 12 percent[140] in earlier series, but most patients had prosthetic valve replacement rather than reconstruction. The operative risk is lower in the current era, around 1 to 2 percent in patients younger than 75 years with organic MR operated on at the Mayo Clinic whether they had valve repair or replacement.[90] LV function is not a predictor of operative mortality and patients with organtic MR even with markedly depressed function have a reasonable chance of surviving surgery.[90] Age symptoms and coronary disease are the most important predictors of operative mortality.[90] Some important points should be noted: First,

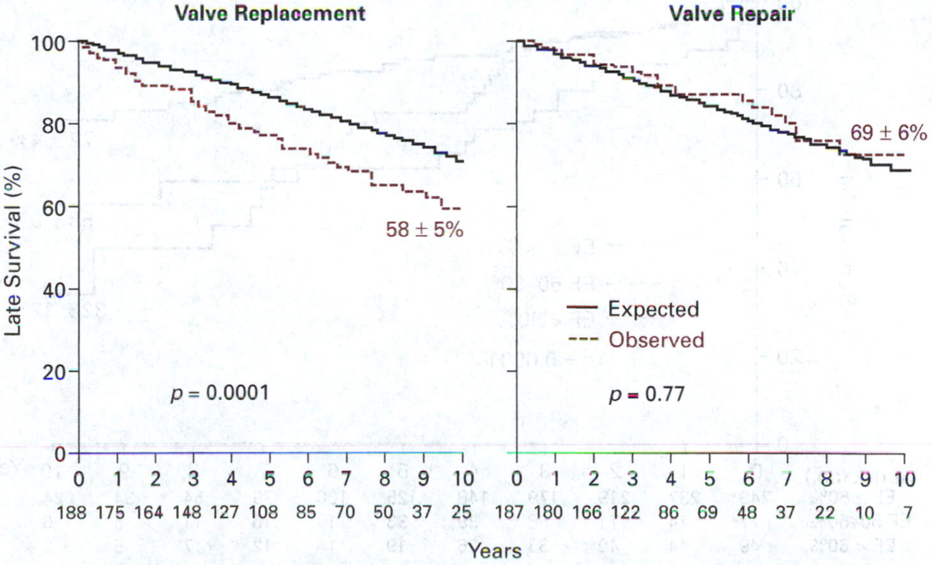

FIGURE 57-24 Late survival after surgical correction of organic MR. Note the excess mortality in comparison to the expected survival after valve replacement (*left*) in contrast to the survival identical to expected after valve repair (*right*). (From Enriquez-Sarano M, Schaff H, Orszulak T, et al. Valve repair improves the outcome of surgery for mitral regurgitation. *Circulation* 1995; 91:1264–1265, with the authorization of the American Heart Association.)

the risk of surgery has become progressively similar in patients 65 to 75 years old as compared to younger patients. Second, operative mortality has decreased recently in patients 75 and older but remains relatively high, around 5 percent. Third, in ischemic MR the operative mortality remains high, around 10 percent.

Postoperative survival has considerably improved and in our recent experience, with a population of mean age 62, the 5- and 10-year survivals were 83 and 68 percent after valve repair and 69 and 52 percent after valve replacement. Remarkably, the survival after valve repair is not different from the expected survival, whereas it represents 77 percent of the expected survival after valve replacement.[141]

A large majority of long-term survivors after mitral valve replacement for MR show a symptomatic improvement by at least one functional class and some become asymptomatic. However, with time postoperative heart failure and symptomatic deterioration tend to occur at a progressively increasing rate (38 percent at 10 years in operative survivors) and is most often (in two thirds of the cases) due to residual LV dysfunction.[145] Valvular or prosthetic dysfunction explain the heart failure in approximately one-third of the cases.[145] Postoperative congestive heart failure has a dismal prognosis and should be prevented as much as possible[145] by early correction of the MR.

The most frequent cause of mortality after surgical correction of MR is LV dysfunction[90] due to chronic irreversible myocardial damage.[66,69,70] LV dysfunction occurs, in our experience in 40 percent of patients overall and 32 percent of those with organic MR.[69] The majority of patients demonstrate a decrease in EF after successful valve replacement.[66,69] This decline may be the result of several factors: cumulative permanent myocardial damage, occasional myocardial insult sustained at the time of operation, diminished preload, and probably increase in impedance to ejection after elimination of the MR. However, the relationships between pre- and postoperative LV function[65,66,69,70,110] and between preoperative LV function and postoperative survival[68,90,105] underline the fact that LV dysfunction is most often already present preoperatively. Because of the modified loading conditions, multiple and complex indices of LV function have been proposed.[65,67,68] Despite these altered loading conditions preoperative EF is an acceptable independent predictor of postoperative EF[66,69,70] and survival.[90] In general, one can estimate that the postoperative EF likely will decrease by approximately 10 percent early after valve replacement.[66,69,70] However, there is a significant individual variation and more decline is observed with markedly increased end-systolic diameter,[69,105] volume,[70,110] or wall stress[69] or in patients with severe symptoms, prolonged duration of MR or coronary disease.[69] A markedly reduced preoperative EF (<50 percent) is associated with a high late mortality,[90] but nevertheless surgery provides a better outcome than medical treatment.[124] Even a "borderline" EF (50 to 60 percent) is associated with an excess late mortality.[90] Therefore, *currently the widely accepted signs of overt LV dysfunction in MR are LV diameter ≥45 mm or ejection fraction <60 percent.*[112] Nevertheless, the end-systolic diameter rarely and belatedly reaches 45 mm and the best outcome of surgery is obtained in patients with both end-systolic diameter <45 mm and ejection fraction ≥60 percent[69,90] (Fig. 57-25).

Another issue, which has been controversial, has been the impact on postoperative outcome of preoperative symptoms. Patients with severe preoperative symptoms, NYHA class III or IV, incur an excess postoperative mortality independently of all baseline characteristics, in particular age, EF, and the type of surgery performed.[146] Importantly, patients preoperatively in class I or II incur a very low operative risk,[146,147] and an excellent long term survival, identical to the expected survival.[146] These data suggest that *in centers and patients at low operative risk, timing of surgery when there are no or minimal symptoms offers distinctive advantages*.

Atrial fibrillation when present preoperatively usually persists postoperatively, unless of brief duration[127] but the excess risk due this arrhythmia appears modest,[90,127] although it requires anticoagulation. Conversely, the association of a Maze procedure to mitral valve repair can be accomplished with minimal risk.[148]

Late risk of thromboembolism after mitral replacement for MR is not different from it as in other mitral valve diseases. Differences in thromboembolic risk after valve repair and valve replacement have been variably estimated[141,142] but appear to favor valve repair. In addition, because following valve repair, anticoagulation is recommended permanently only if atrial

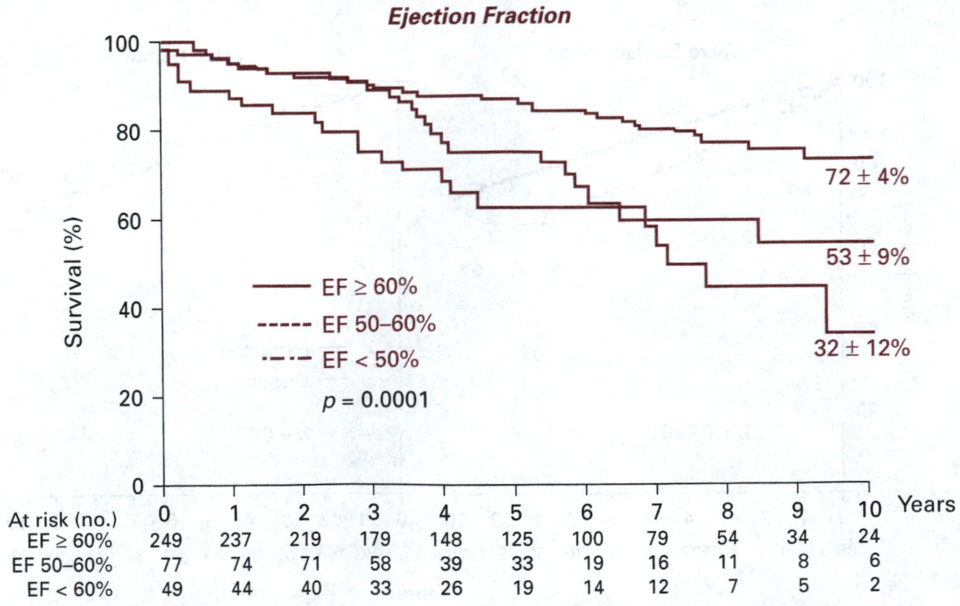

FIGURE 57-25 Survival after surgical correction of organic mitral regurgitation. Note the excess mortality in patients with preoperative ejection fraction above 50 percent but also in patients with preoperative ejection fractions of 50 to 60 percent. (From Enriquez-Sarano M, Tajik A, Schaff H, et al. Echocardiographic prediction of survival after surgical correction of organic mitral regurgitation. *Circulation* 1994; 90:830–837, with the authorization of the American Heart Association.)

fibrillation persists, the occurrence of bleeding is less common than following prosthetic replacement.[141]

Indications for Surgery Based on the most recent data regarding the natural history of MR treated with and without surgery, the indications for surgery have evolved[112] and can be outlined as follows:

Traditional Indications Patients with severe symptoms (functional NYHA class III or IV). Patients with transient severe symptoms even if they markedly improve with medical treatment should be considered at high risk and offered surgery within that category.

Advanced Indications These apply to patients with NYHA class II symptoms and to patients with no symptoms (class NYHA I) but with either signs of overt LV dysfunction (LV ejection fraction <60 percent, end-systolic diameter ≥45 mm) or with pulmonary hypertension or with atrial fibrillation.

Early Indications Patients with no symptoms (NYHA class I) and no sign of LV dysfunction (ejection fraction ≥60 percent). These patients can expect the best results of surgery and in particular, after the immediate postoperative phase, a survival identical to the expected survival.[90,146] Therefore, the authors consider surgery to be a reasonable option in this subgroup. However because surgery in these patients is justified neither by symptoms nor by LV dysfunction certain conditions should be fulfilled:

- *Low operative risk:* Both the operative mortality in the institution where such an indication is contemplated and the operative risk for the individual patient involved should be minimal (1 to 2 percent).
- *Reparability:* The valvular lesions as determined by echocardiography should be in all probability repairable and the surgeon performing the intervention should have a high degree of experience with all forms of valve repair.
- *Intraoperative TEE should be performed* by experienced physicians to monitor the repair procedure and help with decisions warranted by an imperfect result.
- *Quantitation of MR should be performed* systematically in these patients preoperatively using multiple noninvasive techniques to determine objectively the degree of MR and affirm that surgery is warranted.

Therefore, despite the considerable progress recently accomplished, currently *not all patients and not all institutions* are candidates for these early indications of surgical correction of MR, but surgery should be considered early in the course of MR when severe MR has been thoroughly documented.

References

1. Waller BE. Rheumatic and nonrheumatic conditions producing valvular heart disease. *Cardiovasc Clin* 1986; 16:3–104.
2. Rahimtoola SH. Valvular heart disease. In: Stein J, ed. *Internal Medicine*, 4th ed. St. Louis: Mosby-Year Book; 1994:202–234.
3. Braunwald E. Valvular heart disease. In: Braunwald E, ed. *Heart Disease*, 4th ed. Philadelphia: Saunders; 1992:1007–1018.
4. Davies JJ. *Pathology of Cardiac Valves*. London: Butterworth; 1980.
5. Fowler NO. Mitral stenosis and left atrial myxoma. In: *Diagnosis of Heart Disease*. New York: Springer-Verlag; 1991:146–159.
6. Osterberger LE, Goldstein S, Khaja F, Lakier JB. Functional mitral stenosis in patients with massive mitral annular calcification. *Circulation* 1981; 64:472–476.
7. Libman E, Sacks B. A hitherto undescribed form of valvular and mitral endocarditis. *Arch Intern Med* 1924; 33:701–737.
8. Galve E, Candell-Riera J, Pigrau C, et al. Prevalence, morphologic types, and evolution of cardiac valvular disease in systemic lupus erythematosus. *N Engl J Med* 1988; 319:817–823.
9. Schoen FJ, St. John Sutton M. Contemporary pathologic considerations in valvular disease. In: Virmani B, Atkinson JB, Feuoglio JJ, eds. *Cardiovascular Pathology*. Philadelphia: Saunders; 1991: 334–353.
10. Kawanishi DT, Rahimtoola SH. Mitral stenosis. In: Rahimtoola SH, ed. *Valvular Heart Disease II*. St. Louis: Mosby; 1996:8.1–8.24.
11. Leavitt JL, Coats MH, Falk RH. Effects of exercise on transmitral gradient and pulmonary artery pressure in patients with mitral stenosis or a prosthetic mitral valve: A Doppler echocardiographic study. *J Am Coll Cardiol* 1991; 17:1520–1526.
12. Selzer A. Effects of atrial fibrillation upon the circulation in patients with mitral stenosis. *Am Heart J* 1960; 59:518–526.
13. Wood P. An appreciation of mitral stenosis: Part 1. Clinical features. *BMJ* 1954; 1:1051–1063. An appreciation of mitral stenosis: Part 2. Investigations and results. *BMJ* 1954; 1:1113–1124.
14. Gash AK, Carabello BA, Cepin D, Spann JE. Left ventricular ejection performance and systolic muscle function in patients with mitral stenosis. *Circulation* 1983; 67:148–154.
15. Colle JP, Rahal S, Ohayon J, et al. Global left ventricular function and regional wall motion in pure mitral stenosis. *Clin Cardiol* 1984; 7:573–580.
16. Gaasch WH, Folland ED. Left ventricular function in rheumatic mitral stenosis. *Eur Heart J* 1991; 12(suppl B):66–69.
17. Harvey RM, Ferrer MI, Samet P, et al. Mechanical and myocardial factors in rheumatic heart disease in mitral stenosis. *Circulation* 1955; 11:531–551.
18. Mohan JC, Khalilullah M, Arora R. Left ventricular intrinsic contractility in pure rheumatic mitral stenosis. *Am J Cardiol* 1989; 64:240–242.
19. Bowe JC, Bland EF, Sprague HB, White PD. The course of mitral stenosis without surgery: 10 and 20 year perspective. *Ann Intern Med* 1960; 52:741–749.
20. Barrington WW, Bashore T, Wooley CE. Mitral stenosis: Mitral dome excursion at M_1 and the mitral opening snap—the concept of reciprocal heart sounds. *Am Heart J* 1988; 115:1280–1290.
21. Melhem RE, Dunbar JD, Booth RW. The "B" lines of Kerley and left atrial size in mitral valve disease: Their correlation with mean atrial pressure as measured by left atrial puncture. *Radiology* 1991; 76:65–69.
22. Reid CL, Chandraratna PAN, Kawanishi DT, et al. Influence of mitral valve morphology on double-balloon catheter balloon valvuloplasty in patients with mitral stenosis: An analysis of factors predicting immediate and 3-month results. *Circulation* 1989; 80:515–524.
23. Gordon PF, Douglas PS, Come PC, Manning WJ. Two-dimensional and Doppler echocardiographic determinants of the natural history of mitral valve narrowing in patients with rheumatic mitral stenosis: Implications for follow-up. *J Am Coll Cardiol* 1992; 19:968–973.
24. Shapiro ML. Echocardiography of the mitral valve. In: Wells PC, Shapiro LN, eds. *Mitral Valve Disease*, 2nd ed. London: Butterworth; 1996:47–50.
25. Khandheria BK, Tajik AJ, Reeder GS, et al. Doppler color flow imaging: A new technique for visualization and characterization of the blood flow jet in mitral stenosis. *Mayo Clin Proc* 1986; 61:623–630.

26. Rahimtoola SH. Perspective on valvular heart disease: An update. *J Am Coll Cardiol* 1989; 14:1–23.
27. Kawanishi DT, Kotlewski A, McKay CR, et al. The relative value of clinical examination, echocardiography with Doppler and cardiac catheterization with angiography in the evaluation of mitral valve disease. In: Bodnar E, ed. *Surgery for Heart Valve Disease.* London: ICR Publishers; 1990:73–78.
28. Olesen KH. The natural history of 271 patients with mitral stenosis under medical treatment. *Br Heart J* 1962; 24:349–357.
29. Roy SB, Gopinath N. Mitral stenosis. *Circulation* 1968; 38(suppl V):68–76.
30. Rowe JC, Bland EF, Sprague HB, White P. The course of mitral stenosis without surgery: Ten- and twenty-year perspectives. *Ann Intern Med* 1960; 52:741–749.
31. Prystowsky EN, Benson W Jr, Fuster V, et al. Management of patients with atrial fibrillation: A statement for healthcare professionals from the Subcommittee on Electrocardiography and Electrophysiology, American Heart Association. *Circulation* 1996; 93:1262–1277.
32. Kulick DL, Reid CL, Kawanishi DT, Rahimtoola SH. Catheter balloon commissurotomy in adults: Part II. Mitral and other stenoses. *Curr Probl Cardiol* 1990; 15:403–470.
33. Hickey MSJ, Blackstone EH, Kirklin JW, Dean LW. Outcome probabilities and life history after surgical mitral commissurotomy: Implications for balloon commissurotomy. *J Am Coll Cardiol* 1991; 17:29–42.
34. Scalia D, Rizzoli G, Campanile F, et al. Long-term results of mitral commissurotomy. *J Thorac Cardiovasc Surg* 1993; 105:633–642.
35. John S, Bashi VV, Jairaj PS, et al. Closed mitral valvotomy: Early results and long-term follow-up of 3724 consecutive patients. *Circulation* 1983; 68:891–896.
36. Crawford MH, Souchek J, Oprian CA, et al. Determinants of survival and left ventricular performance after mitral valve replacement. *Circulation* 1990; 81:1173–1181.
37. Rahimtoola SH. The problem of valve prosthesis—Patient mismatch. *Circulation* 1978; 58:20–24.
38. Turi ZG, Reyes VP, Raju S, et al. Percutaneous balloon versus surgical closed commissurotomy for mitral stenosis: A prospective, randomized trial. *Circulation* 1991; 83:1179–1185.
39. Patel JJ, Shama D, Mitha AS, et al. Balloon valvuloplasty versus closed commissurotomy for pliable mitral stenosis: A prospective hemodynamic study. *J Am Coll Cardiol* 1991; 18:1318–1322.
40. Arora R, Nair M, Kalra GS, et al. Immediate and long-term results of balloon and surgical closed mitral valvotomy: A randomized comparative study. *Am Heart J* 1993; 125:1091–1094.
41. Reyes VP, Raju BS, Wynne J, et al. Percutaneous balloon valvuloplasty compared with open surgical commissurotomy for mitral stenosis. *N Engl J Med* 1994; 331:961–967.
42. NHLBI Valvuloplasty Participants. Multicenter experience with balloon mitral commissurotomy—NHLBI Balloon Valvuloplasty Registry report on immediate and 30-day follow-up results. *Circulation* 1992; 85:448–461.
43. McKay CR, Kawanishi DT, Kotlewski A, et al. Improvement in exercise capacity and exercise hemodynamics 3 months after double-balloon catheter balloon valvuloplasty in the treatment of patients with symptomatic mitral stenosis. *Circulation* 1988; 77:1013–1021.
44. Cohen DJ, Kuntz RE, Gordon SPF, et al. Predictors of long-term outcome after percutaneous balloon mitral valvuloplasty. *N Engl J Med* 1992; 327:1329–1335.
45. Palacios I, Tuzcu ME, Weyman AE, et al. Clinical follow-up of patients undergoing percutaneous mitral balloon valvotomy. *Circulation* 1995; 91:671–676.
46. Dean LS, Mickel M, Bonan R, et al. Four year follow-up of patients undergoing percutaneous balloon mitral commissurotomy: A report from the National Heart, Lung and Blood Institute Balloon Valvuloplasty Registry. *J Am Coll Cardiol* 1996; 28:1452–1457.
47. Orrange SE, Kawanishi DT, Lopez BM, et al. Actuarial outcome after catheter balloon commissurotomy in patients with mitral stenosis. *Circulation* 1997; 95:382–389.
48. Bonow RO, Carabello B, de Leon AC Jr, et al. ACC/AHA Guidelines for the management of patients with valvular heart disease: A report of the American College of Cardiology/American Heart Association Task Force on Practice Guidelines (Committee on Management of Patients With Valvular Heart Disease). *J Am Coll Cardiol* 1998; 32:1486–1588.
49. Lam J, Ranganathan N, Wigle E, Silver M. Morphology of the human mitral valve: I. Chordae tendineae: A new classification. *Circulation* 1970; 41:449–458.
50. Ranganathan N, Lam J, Wigle E, Silver M. Morphology of the human mitral valve: II. The valve leaflets. *Circulation* 1970; 41:459–467.
51. Olson L, Subramanian R, Ackermann D, Orszulak T, Edwards W. Surgical pathology of the mitral valve: A study of 712 cases spanning 21 years. *Mayo Clin Proc* 1987; 62:22–34.
52. Hickey A, Wilcken D, Wright J, Warren B. Primary (spontaneous) chordal rupture: Relation to myxomatous valve disease and mitral valve prolapse. *J Am Coll Cardiol* 1985; 5:1341–1346.
53. Kishon Y, Oh J, Schaff H, Mullany C, Tajik A, Gersh B. Mitral valve operation in postinfarction rupture of a papillary muscle: Immediate results and long-term follow-up of 22 patients. *Mayo Clin Proc* 1992; 67:1023–1030.
54. Connolly H, Crary J, McGoon M, et al. Valvular heart disease associated with fenfluramine-phentermine. *N Engl J Med* 1997; 337:581–588.
55. Yellin E, Yoran C, Sonnenblick E, et al. Dynamic changes in the canine mitral regurgitant orifice area during ventricular ejection. *Circ Res* 1979; 45:677–683.
56. Schwammenthal E, Chen C, Benning F, et al. Dynamics of mitral regurgitant flow and orifice area. Physiologic application of the proximal flow convergence method: Clinical data and experimental testing. *Circulation* 1994; 90:307–322.
57. Enriquez-Sarano M, Sinak L, Tajik A, et al. Changes in effective regurgitant orifice throughout systole in patients with mitral valve prolapse: A clinical study using the proximal isovelocity surface area method. *Circulation* 1995; 92:2951–2958.
58. Enriquez-Sarano M, Seward J, Bailey K, Tajik A. Effective regurgitant orifice area: A noninvasive doppler development of an old hemodynamic concept. *J Am Coll Cardiol* 1994; 23:443–451.
59. Chatterjee K, Parmley W, Swan H, et al. Beneficial effects of vasodilator agents in severe mitral regurgitation due to dysfunction of subvalvular apparatus. *Circulation* 1973; 48:684–690.
60. Keren G, Bier A, Strom J, et al. Dynamics of mitral regurgitation during nitroglycerin therapy: A Doppler echocardiographic study. *Am Heart J* 1986; 112:517–525.
61. Yoran C, Yellin E, Becker R, et al. Dynamic aspects of acute mitral regurgitation: Effects of ventricular volume, pressure and contractility on the effective regurgitant orifice area. *Circulation* 1979; 60:170–176.
62. Grose R, Strain J, Cohen M. Pulmonary arterial V waves in mitral regurgitation: Clinical and experimental observations. *Circulation* 1984; 69:214–222.
63. Braunwald E, Awe W. The syndrome of severe mitral regurgitation with normal left atrial pressure. *Circulation* 1963; 27:29–35.
64. Wisenbaugh T, Spann J, Carabello B. Differences in myocardial performance and load between patients with similar amounts of chronic aortic versus chronic mitral regurgitation. *J Am Coll Cardiol* 1984; 3:916–923.
65. Starling M, Kirsch M, Montgomery D, Gross M. Impaired left ventricular contractile function in patients with long-term mitral regurgitation and normal ejection fraction. *J Am Coll Cardiol* 1993; 22:239–250.

66. Enriquez-Sarano M, Hannachi M, Jais J, Acar J. Résultats hémodynamiques et angiographiques après correction chirurgicale de l'insuffisance mitrale: A propos de 51 cathétérismes itératifs. *Arch Mal Coeur* 1983; 76:1194–1203.
67. Corin W, Monrad E, Murakami T, et al. The relationship of afterload to ejection performance in chronic mitral regurgitation. *Circulation* 1987; 76:59–67.
68. Carabello B, Nolan S, McGuire L. Assessment of preoperative left ventricular function in patients with mitral regurgitation: Value of the end-systolic wall stress-end-systolic volume ratio. *Circulation* 1981; 64:1212–1217.
69. Enriquez-Sarano M, Tajik A, Schaff H, et al. Echocardiographic prediction of left ventricular function after correction of mitral regurgitation: Results and clinical implications. *J Am Coll Cardiol* 1994; 24:1536–1543.
70. Crawford M, Souchek J, Oprian C, et al. Determinants of survival and left ventricular performance after mitral valve replacement. *Circulation* 1990; 81:1173–1181.
71. Urabe Y, Mann D, Kent R, et al. Cellular and ventricular contractile dysfunction in experimental canine mitral regurgitation. *Circ Res* 1992; 70:131–147.
72. Spinale F, Ishihra K, Zile M, et al. Structural basis for changes in left ventricular function and geometry because of chronic mitral regurgitation and after correction of volume overload. *J Thorac Cardiovasc Surg* 1993; 106:1147–1157.
73. Corin W, Murakami T, Monrad E, et al. Left ventricular passive diastolic properties in chronic mitral regurgitation. *Circulation* 1991; 83:797–807.
74. He S, Fontaine A, Schwammenthal E, et al. Integrated mechanism for functional mitral regurgitation. *Circulation* 1997; 96:1826–1834.
75. Otsuji Y, Handschumacher M, Schwammenthal E, et al. Insights from three dimensional echocardiography into the mechanism of functional mitral regurgitation. *Circulation* 1997; 96:1999–2008.
76. Enriquez-Sarano M, Tajik A, Bailey K, Seward J. Color flow imaging compared with quantitative doppler assessment of severity of mitral regurgitation: Influence of eccentricity of jet and mechanism of regurgitation. *J Am Coll Cardiol* 1993; 21:1211–1219.
77. Lamas G, Mitchell G, Flaker G, et al. Clinical significance of mitral regurgitation after acute myocardial infarction. *Circulation* 1997; 96:827–833.
78. Haggstrom J, Hansson K, Karlberg B, et al. Plasma concentration of atrial natriuretic peptide in relation to severity of mitral regurgitation in Cavalier King Charles spaniels. *Am J Vet Res* 1994; 55:698–703.
79. Brookes CI, Kemp MW, Hooper J, et al. Plasma brain natriuretic peptide concentrations in patients with chronic mitral regurgitation. *J Heart Valve Dis* 1997; 6:608–612.
80. Pedersen H, Koch J, Poulsen K. Activation of the renin-angiotensin system in dogs with asymptomatic and mildly symptomatic mitral valvular insufficiency. *J Vet Int Med* 1995; 9:328–331.
81. Dell'Italia L, Meng Q, Balcells E, et al. Increased ACE and chymase-like activity in cardiac tissue of dogs with chronic mitral regurgitation. *Am J Physiol* 1995; 269:H2065–H2073.
82. Dell'Italia L, Meng Q, Balcells E, et al. Compartmentalization of angiotensin II generation in the dog heart: Evidence for independent mechanisms in intravascular and interstitial spaces. *J Clin Invest* 1997; 100:253–258.
83. Singh J, Evans J, Levy D, et al. Prevalence and clinical determinants of mitral, tricuspid and aortic regurgitation *Am J Cardiol* 1999; 83:897–902.
84. Ling H, Enriquez-Sarano M, Seward J, et al. Clinical outcome of mitral regurgitation due to flail leaflets. *N Engl J Med* 1996; 335:1417–1423.
85. Kligfield P, Hochreiter C, Niles N, et al. Relation of sudden death in pure mitral regurgitation, with and without mitral valve prolapse, to repetitive ventricular arrythmias and right and left ventricular ejection fractions. *Am J Cardiol* 1987; 60:397–399.
86. Folland E, Kriegel B, Henderson W, et al. Implications of third heart sounds in patients with valvular heart disease: The Veterans Affairs Cooperative Study on Valvular Heart Disease. *N Engl J Med* 1992; 327:458–462.
87. Antman E, Angoff G, Sloss L. Demonstration of the mechanism by which mitral regurgitation mimics aortic stenosis. *Am J Cardiol* 1978; 42:1044–1048.
88. Desjardins V, Enriquez-Sarano M, Tajik A, et al. Intensity of murmurs correlates with severity of valvular regurgitation. *Am J Med* 1996; 100:149–156.
89. Forrester J, Diamond G, Freedman S, et al. Silent mitral insufficiency in acute myocardial infarction. *Circulation* 1971; 44: 877–883.
90. Enriquez-Sarano M, Tajik A, Schaff H, et al. Echocardiographic prediction of survival after surgical correction of organic mitral regurgitation. *Circulation* 1994; 90:830–837.
91. Glick B, Roberts W. Usefulness of total 12-lead QRS voltage in diagnosing left ventricular hypertrophy in clinically isolated, pure, chronic, severe mitral regurgitation. *Am J Cardiol* 1992; 70:1088–1092.
92. Enriquez-Sarano M, Freeman W, Tribouilloy C, et al. Functional anatomy of mitral regurgitation: Echocardiographic assessment and implications on outcome. *J Am Coll Cardiol* 1999; 34:1129–1136.
93. Shively B, Gurule F, Roldan C, et al. Diagnostic value of transesophageal compared with transthoracic endocardiography in infective endocarditis. *J Am Coll Cardiol* 1991; 18:391–397.
94. Izumi S, Miyatake K, Beppu S, et al. Mechanism of mitral regurgitation in patients with myocardial infarction: A study using realtime two-dimensional Doppler flow imaging and echocardiography. *Circulation* 1987; 76:777–785.
95. Boltwood C, Tei C, Wong M, Shah P. Quantitative echocardiography of the mitral complex in dilated cardiomyopathy: The mechanism of functional mitral regurgitation. *Circulation* 1983; 68: 498–508.
96. Spain M, Smith M, Grayburn P, et al. Quantitative assessment of mitral regurgitation by Doppler color flow imaging: Angiographic and hemodynamic correlations. *J Am Coll Cardiol* 1989; 13:585–590.
97. Pearson A, St. Vrain J, Mrosek D, Labovitz A. Color Doppler echocardiographic evaluation of patients with a flail mitral leaflet. *J Am Coll Cardiol* 1990; 16:232–239.
98. Tribouilloy C, Shen W, Quere J, et al. Assessment of severity of mitral regurgitation by measuring regurgitant jet width at its origin with transesophageal Doppler color flow imaging. *Circulation* 1992; 85:1248–1253.
99. Mele D, Vandervoort P, Palacios I, et al. Proximal jet size by Doppler color flow mapping predicts severity of mitral regurgitation. *Circulation* 1995; 91:746–754.
100. Klein A, Obarski T, Stewart W, et al. Transesophageal Doppler echocardiography of pulmonary venous flow: A new marker of mitral regurgitation severity. *J Am Coll Cardiol* 1991; 18:518–526.
101. Enriquez-Sarano M, Dujardin K, Tribouilloy C, et al. Determinants of pulmonary venous flow reversal in mitral regurgitation and its usefulness in determining the severity of the mitral regurgitation. *Am J Cardiol* 1999; 83:535–541.
102. Vandervoort P, Rivera J, Mele D, et al. Application of color Doppler flow mapping to calculate effective regurgitant orifice area. An in vitro study and initial clinical observations. *Circulation* 1993; 88:1150–1156.
103. Enriquez-Sarano M, Bailey K, Seward J, et al. Quantitative Doppler assessment of valvular regurgitation. *Circulation* 1993; 87:841–848.

104. Blumlein S, Bouchard A, Schiller N, et al. Quantitation of mitral regurgitation by Doppler echocardiography. *Circulation* 1986; 74:306–314.

105. Wisenbaugh T, Skudicky D, Sareli P. Prediction of outcome after valve replacement for rheumatic mitral regurgitation in the era of chordal preservation. *Circulation* 1994; 89:191–197.

106. Zile M, Gaasch W, Carroll J, Levine J. Chronic mitral regurgitation: Predictive value of preoperative echocardiographic indexes of left ventricular function and wall stress. *J Am Coll Cardiol* 1984; 3:235–242.

107. Sellers R. Left retrograde cardioangiography in acquired heart disease: Technic, indications and interpretations in 700 cases. *Am J Cardiol* 1964; 14:437–447.

108. Croft C, Lipscomb K, Mathis K, et al. Limitations of qualitative angiographic grading in aortic or mitral regurgitation. *Am J Cardiol* 1984; 53:1593–1598.

109. Sandler H, Dodge H, Hay R, Rackley C. Quantitation of valvular insufficiency in man by angiocardiography. *Am Heart J* 1963; 65:501–513.

110. Borow K, Green L, Mann T, et al. End systolic volume as a predictor of postoperative left ventricular performance in volume overload from valvular regurgitation. *Am J Med* 1980; 68:655–663.

111. Enriquez-Sarano M, Klodas E, Garratt KN, et al. Secular trends in coronary atherosclerosis—analysis in patients with valvular regurgitation. *N Engl J Med* 1996; 335:316–322.

112. Bonow R, Carabello B, DeLeon A, et al. ACC/AHA guidelines for the management of patients with valvular heart disease. *Circulation* 1998; 98:1949–1984.

113. Freeman W, Schaff H, Khanderia B, et al. Intraoperative evaluation of mitral valve regurgitation and repair by tranesophageal echocardiography: Incidence and significance of systolic anterior motion. *J Am Coll Cardiol* 1992; 20:599–609.

114. Leitch J, Mitchell A, Harris P, et al. The effect of cardiac catheterization upon management of advanced aortic and mitral regurgitation. *Eur Heart J* 1991; 12:602–607.

115. Slater J, Gindea A, Freedberg R, et al. Comparison of cardiac catheterization and Doppler echocardiography in the decision to operate in aortic and mitral valve disease. *J Am Coll Cardiol* 1991; 17:1026–1036.

116. Dujardin K, Enriquez-Sarano M, Bailey K, et al. Grading of mitral regurgitation by quantitative Doppler echocardiography—Calibration by left ventricular angiography in routine clinical practice. *Circulation* 1997; 96:3409–3415.

117. Wilson M, Lim W. The natural history of rheumatic heart disease in the third, fourth, and fifth decades of life. I. Prognosis with special reference to survivorship. *Circulation* 1957; 16:700–712.

118. Delahaye J, Gare J, Viguier E, et al. Natural history of severe mitral regurgitation. *Eur Heart J* 1991; 12(suppl B):5–9.

119. Rappaport E. Natural history of aortic and mitral valve disease. *Am J Cardiol* 1975; 35:221–227.

120. Munoz S, Gallardo J, Diaz-Gorrin J, Medina O. Influence of surgery on the natural history of rheumatic mitral and aortic valve disease. *Am J Cardiol* 1975; 35:234–242.

121. Horstkotte D, Loogen F, Kleikamp G, et al. Effect of prosthetic heart valve replacement on the natural course of isolated mitral and aortic as well as multivalvular diseases: Clinical results in 783 patients up to 8 years following implantation of the Björk-Shiley tilting disc prosthesis. *Z Kardiol* 1983; 72:494–503.

122. Grigioni F, Enriquez-Sarano M, Ling L, et al. Sudden death in mitral regurgitation due to flail leaflet. *J Am Coll Cardiol* 1999; 34:2078–2085.

123. Rosen S, Borer J, Hochreiter C, et al. Natural History of the asymptomatic/minimally symptomatic patient with severe mitral regurgitation secondary to mitral valve prolapse and normal right and left ventricular performance. *Am J Cardiol* 1994; 74:374–380.

124. Hammermeister K, Fisher L, Kennedy W, et al. Prediction of late survival in patients with mitral valve disease from clinical, hemodynamic, and quantitative angiographic variables. *Circulation* 1978; 57:341–349.

125. Enriquez-Sarano M, Basmadjian A, Rossi A, et al. Progression of mitral regurgitation: A prospective Doppler echocardiographic study. *J Am Coll Cardiol* 1999; 34:1137–1144.

126. Shulman S, Amren D, Bisno A, et al. Prevention of bacterial endocarditis: A statement for health professionals by the Committee on Rheumatic Fever and Bacterial Endocarditis of the Council on Cardiovascular Diseases in the Young of the American Heart Association. *Am J Dis Child* 1985; 139:232–235.

127. Chua Y, Schaff H, Orszulak T, Morriss J. Outcome of mitral valve repair in patients with preoperative atrial fibrillation: Should the maze procedure be combined with mitral valvuloplasty? *J Thorac Cardiovasc Surg* 1994; 107:408–415.

128. Greenberg B, Massie B, Brundage B, et al. Beneficial effects of hydralazine in severe mitral regurgitation. *Circulation* 1978; 58:273–279.

129. Tishler M, Rowan M, LeWinter M. Effect of Enalapril on left ventricular mass and volumes in asymptomatic chronic, severe mitral regurgitation secondary to mitral valve prolapse. *Am J Cardiol* 1998; 82:242–245.

130. Marcotte F, Honos G, Walling A, et al. Effect of angiotensin converting enzyme inhibitor therapy in mitral regurgitation with normal left ventricular function. *Can J Cardiol* 1997; 13:479–485.

131. Host U, Kelbaek H, Hildebrandt P, et al. Effect of Ramilpril on mitral regurgitation secondary to mitral valve prolapse. *Am J Cardiol* 1997; 80:655–658.

132. Rothlisberger C, Sareli P, Wisenbaugh T. Comparison of single dose nifedipine and captopril for chronic severe mitral regurgitation. *Am J Cardiol* 1994; 73:978–981.

133. Wisenbaugh T, Sinovich V, Dullbh A, Sareli P. Six month pilot study of captopril for mildly symptomatic, severe isolated mitral and isolated aortic regurgitation. *J Heart Valve Dis* 1994; 3:197–204.

134. Gillinov A, Cosgrove D, Blackstone E, et al. Durability of mitral valve repair for degenerative disease. *J Thorac Cardiovasc Surg* 1998; 116:734–743.

135. Frater R, Gabbay S, Shore D, et al. Reproducible replacement of elongated or ruptured mitral valve chordae. *Ann Thorac Surg* 1983; 35:14–28.

136. Lessana A, Escorsin M, Romano M, et al. Transposition of posterior leaflet for treatment of ruptured main chordae of the anterior mitral leaflet. *J Thorac Cardiovasc Surg* 1985; 89:804–806.

137. Duran C, Revuelta J, Gaite L, et al. Stability of mitral reconstructive surgery at 10–12 years for predominantly rheumatic valvular disease. *Circulation* 1988; 78:I91–I96.

138. Mihaileanu S, Marino J, Chauvaud S, et al. Left ventricular outflow obstruction after mitral valve repair (Carpentier's technique). Proposed mechanisms of disease. *Circulation* 1988; 78:I78–I84.

139. David T, Komeda M, Pollick C, Burns R. Mitral valve annuloplasty: The effects of the type on left ventricular function. *Ann Thorac Surg* 1989; 47:524–528.

140. Cohn IH, Allred E, Cohn IA, et al. Early and late risk of mitral valve replacement: A 12-year concomitant comparison of the porcine bioprosthetic and prosthetic disc mitral valves. *J Thorac Cardiovasc Surg* 1985; 90:872–880.

141. Enriquez-Sarano M, Schaff H, Orszulak T, et al. Valve repair improves the outcome of surgery for mitral regurgitation. *Circulation* 1995; 91:1264–1265.

142. Perier P, Deloche A, Chauvaud S, et al. Comparative evaluation of mitral valve repair and replacement with Starr, Bjork, and porcine valve prostheses. *Circulation* 1984; 70:I187–I192.

143. David T, Burns R, Bacchus C, Druck M. Mitral regurgitation with and without preservation of chordae tendinae. *J Thorac Cardiovasc Surg* 1984; 88:718–725.
144. Cerfolio R, Orszulak T, Pluth J, et al. Reoperation after valve repair for mitral regurgitation: Early and intermediate results. *J Thorac Cardiovasc Surg* 1996; 111:1177–1183.
145. Enriquez-Sarano M, Schaff H, Orszulak T, et al. Congestive heart failure after surgical correction of mitral regurgitation. A long-term study. *Circulation* 1995; 92:2496–2503.
146. Tribouilloy C, Enriquez-Sarano M, Schaff H, et al. Impact of preoperative symptoms on survival after surgical correction of organic mitral regurgitation: Rationale for optimizing surgical indications. *Circulation* 1999; 99:400–500.
147. Sousa Uva M, Dreyfus G, Rescigno G, et al. Surgical treatment of asymptomatic and mildly symptomatic mitral regurgitation. *J Thorac Cardiovasc Surg* 1996; 112:1240–1249.
148. Handa N, Schaff HV, Morris JJ, et al. Outcome of valve repair and the cox maze procedure for mitral regurgitation and associated atrial fibrillation. *J Thorac Cardiovasc Surg* 1999; 118:628–635.

C H A P T E R 58

MITRAL VALVE PROLAPSE SYNDROME

Robert A. O'Rourke

The syndrome of mitral valve prolapse (MVP) is the most common form of valvular heart disease, occurring in 2 to 6 percent of the population, thus being more common than a bicuspid aortic valve. The incidence varies depending on the criteria used for its diagnosis.[1,2] MVP is commonly detected by cardiac auscultation, with one or more systolic clicks and/or a mid- to late-systolic murmur detected on a careful physical examination. Often the auscultatory complex is the only clinical manifestation of cardiac disease, and many patients are asymptomatic.

Midsystolic clicks were first described in the late nineteenth century and originally were attributed to a pericardial or extracardiac etiology. Subsequently, late-systolic murmurs were recognized to be present in apparently healthy people and were associated with a benign natural history. Thus the murmur also was considered to be extracardiac in origin.

In 1961, Reid[3] suggested that the midsystolic click and the late-systolic murmur were due to mitral regurgitation. In 1963, Barlow et al.[4] confirmed this hypothesis by left ventricular (LV) cineangiography. Subsequently, intracardiac phonocardiogram studies documented the mitral valve origin of a systolic click and late-systolic murmur.

During the past four decades, considerable new data obtained from pathologic studies, echocardiography, and cineventriculography have demonstrated that this common syndrome is associated with prolapse of one or both mitral valve leaflets into the atrium during LV systole.

Recognition of MVP (also known as the *systolic click–late systolic murmur syndrome*) is often difficult because of the extreme variability of its clinical manifestations. It is, however, an important cause of incapacitating chest pain and refractory arrhythmias in certain patients. The abnormal components of the mitral valve apparatus are a potential site for endocarditis, and some patients, particularly males in their sixties and seventies, can develop severe mitral regurgitation (MR) due to ruptured chordae tendineae.

DEFINITION, ETIOLOGY, AND TIMING

MVP refers to the systolic billowing of one or both mitral leaflets into the left atrium, with or without MR. MVP often occurs as a clinical entity with no or only mild MR, and it is frequently associated with unique clinical characteristics when compared with the other causes of MR.[5-9] Nevertheless, MVP is the most common cause of significant MR and the most frequent substrate for mitral valve endocarditis in the United States. The mitral valve apparatus is a complex structure composed of the mitral annulus, valve leaflets, chordae tendineae, papillary muscles, and the supporting left ventricle, left atrium, and aortic walls[10] (Fig. 58-1). Disease processes involving any one or more of these components may result in dysfunction of the valvular apparatus and prolapse of the mitral leaflets toward the left atrium during systole when LV pressure exceeds left atrial (LA) pressure.

The complexity of the mitral valve apparatus provides an explanation for the presence of secondary prolapse in many conditions that affect one or more of the components of the apparatus (e.g., ruptured mitral chordae). There is, however, considerable evidence that a disorder of the mitral valve leaflets exists in which there are specific pathologic changes causing redundancy of the mitral leaflets and their prolapse into the left atrium during systole. This is the primary form of MVP (Table 58-1).

In *primary* MVP, there is interchordal hooding due to leaflet redundancy that involves both the rough and clear zones of the involved leaflets[6] (Fig. 58-2). The height of the interchordal hooding usually exceeds 4 mm and involves at least one-half of the anterior leaflet or at least two-thirds of the posterior leaflet. The basic microscopic feature of primary MVP is marked proliferation of the *spongiosa,* the delicate myxomatous connective tissue between the *atrialis* (a thick layer of collagen and elastic tissue forming the atrial aspect of the leaflet) and the *fibrosa,* or *ventricularis,* which is composed of dense layers of

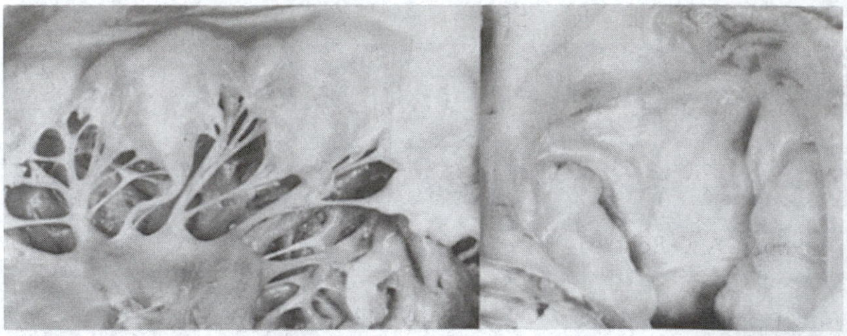

FIGURE 58-1 Myxomatous mitral valve. *A*. The opened mitral valve shows characteristic interchordal hooding and redundancy of the leaflets. *B*. The unopened mitral valve viewed from the left atrial side shows extensive scalloping that is characteristic of a myxomatous mitral valve. (From Guthrie and Edwards.[14] Reproduced with permission from the publisher and authors.)

TABLE 58-1 Classification of Mitral Valve Prolapse

Primary mitral valve prolapse
Familial
Nonfamilial
Marfan syndrome
Other connective tissue diseases
Secondary mitral valve prolapse
Coronary artery disease
Rheumatic heart disease
Cardiomyopathies
"Flail" mitral valve leaflet(s)
Normal variant
Inaccurate auscultation
"Echocardiographic heart disease"

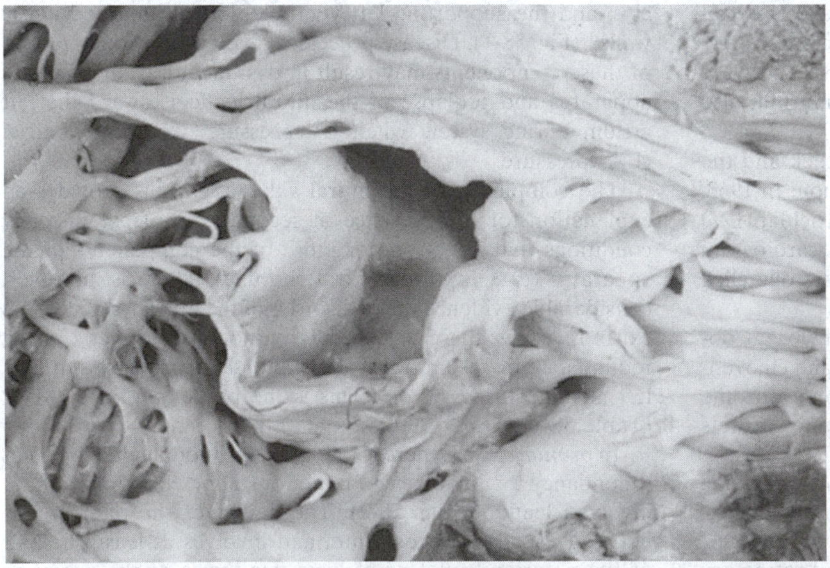

FIGURE 58-2 Myxomatous mitral valve with ruptured posterior leaflet chordae. The central part of the posterior leaflet (*lower center*) shows fragments of ruptured chordae. The intact chordae are elongated, and the leaflets show redundancy and fibrous thickening. (From Edwards F. Pathology of mitral incompetence. In: Silver MD, ed. *Cardiovascular Pathology*. New York: Churchill Livingstone; 1983. Reproduced with permission from the publisher and authors.)

collagen and forms the basic support of the leaflet.[6] In primary MVP, myxomatous proliferation of the acid mucopolysaccharide-containing spongiosa tissue causes focal interruption of the fibrosa. Secondary effects of the primary MVP syndrome include fibrosis of the surfaces of the mitral valve leaflets, thinning and/or elongation of chordae tendineae, and ventricular friction lesions. Fibrin deposits often form at the mitral valve–left atrial angle.

The primary form of MVP may occur in families, where it appears to be inherited as an autosomal dominant trait with varying penetrance.[11,12] No consistent chromosomal abnormalities have yet been identified in patients with MVP, which also often occurs in isolated cases.[13,14] Primary MVP has been found with increasing frequency in patients with Marfan syndrome, where it is almost always present, and in other heritable connective tissue diseases such as Ehlers-Danlos syndrome,[15] pseudoxanthoma elasticum,[16] and osteogenesis imperfecta.[17] Marfan syndrome also has an autosomal dominant mode of inheritance. It is possible that some genetic studies of MVP may have been tracking a more general connective tissue disorder such as Marfan syndrome (see also Chap. 76).

Many observers have speculated that primary MVP syndrome represents a generalized disorder of connective tissue. Thoracic skeletal abnormalities such as straight thoracic spine and pectus excavatum are commonly associated with this syndrome.[18] The mitral valve undergoes differentiation between the thirty-fifth and forty-second days of fetal life, when the vertebrae and thoracic cage are beginning chondrification and ossification.[19] Any adverse factors in this period may affect both the mitral valve and the bones of the thoracic cage. Of possible relevance, rats fed a diet containing large amounts of peas of the genus *Lathyrus* develop both bony abnormalities and myxomatous changes in their valve leaflets. Therefore, it has been postulated that the MVP syndrome is a connective tissue disorder resulting from fetal exposure to toxic substances during the early part of pregnancy.[20,21]

Others have suggested that MVP is a result of defective embryogenesis of cell lines of mesenchymal origin. The increased prevalence of primary MVP in patients with von Willebrand disease and other coagulopathies, primary hypomastia, and various connective tissue diseases has been used to support this concept.[21]

In *secondary* forms of MVP (see Table 58-1), myxomatous proliferation of the spongiosa portion of the mitral valve leaflet is absent. Tei et al.[22] were able to produce de novo echocardiographic evidence of MVP, often with MR, in closed-chest dogs undergoing transient coronary artery occlusion; MVP was attributed to relative displacement of ischemic papillary muscles. Also, serial studies in patients with known ischemic heart disease occasionally have documented unequivocal MVP following an acute coronary syndrome that was previously absent.[23] In most patients with coronary artery disease (CAD) and MVP, however, the two entities are coincident but unrelated.

More recent studies[24–26] indicate that MR caused by MVP may result from postinflammatory changes, including those following rheumatic fever. In histologic studies of surgically excised valves, fibrosis with vascularization and scattered infiltration of round cells, including lymphocytes and plasmacytes, was found *without myxomatous proliferation* of the spongiosa.[24] With rheumatic carditis, the anterior mitral leaflet is more likely to prolapse.[26]

MVP has been observed in patients with hypertrophic cardiomyopathy, in whom posterior MVP may result from a disproportionately small LV cavity, altered papillary muscle alignment, or a combination of factors.[21] The mitral valve leaflet is usually normal, but occasionally, the changes of primary MVP are present. Since LV segmental wall motion abnormalities and sometimes depressed global LV function occur in certain patients with echocardiographic and auscultatory evidence of MVP and MR, nonhypertrophic cardiomyopathy has been listed as a cause of mitral prolapse.[27] This is probably not the case; the ventricular wall motion abnormalities usually disappear when the mitral valve is repaired or replaced. In MVP patients, atrial septal defects, pulmonary hypertension, anorexia nervosa, dehydration, or straight-back syndrome may be secondary to the relatively small size of the left ventricle in this disorder, resulting in a mitral apparatus that is relatively large and redundant.[21,28] However, atrial septal defect may be associated with primary MVP.[16] Patients with primary and secondary MVP must be distinguished from those with normal variations on cardiac auscultation or echocardiography; these variations can result in an incorrect diagnosis of MVP, particularly in patients who are hyperkinetic or dehydrated during the physical examination or two-dimensional (2-D) echocardiography. Other auscultatory findings may be misinterpreted as midsystolic clicks or late-systolic murmurs.[8,21] Patients with mild to moderate billowing of one or more nonthickened leaflets toward the left atrium with the leaflet coaptation point on the ventricular side of the mitral annulus and no or minimal MR by Doppler echocardiography are probably normal. Unfortunately, many such patients with neither a nonejection click nor murmur of MR are frequently overdiagnosed as having the MVP syndrome.[1,2,29]

PATHOPHYSIOLOGY

In patients with MVP, there is frequently LA enlargement and LV enlargement, depending on the presence and severity of MR.[30] The supporting apparatus is often involved, and in patients with connective tissue syndromes such as Marfan syndrome, the mitral annulus is usually dilated, sometimes calcified, and does not decrease its circumference by the usual 30 percent during LV systole. The hemodynamic effects of mild to moderate MR are similar to those from other causes of MR.

Many studies suggest an increased prevalence of autonomic nervous system dysfunction in patients with primary MVP. In 1979, Gaffney et al.[31] reported a reduced heart rate slowing with intravenous phenylephrine and an abnormal diving reflex heart rate response in patients with MVP as compared with age-matched controls. Patients with MVP had a lesser lower extremity pooling of blood in response to lower body negative pressure. Increased vagal tone and prolonged QT intervals on the electrocardiogram (ECG) are more common in patients with MVP. Measurements of serum and 24-h urine epinephrine and norepinephrine levels are often increased in patients with symptomatic MVP as compared with controls.[32] Patients with MVP often have an increased heart rate and contractility response to intravenous isoproterenol.[33] An increased incidence of high-affinity beta receptors in the lymphocytes of patients with MVP has been reported, as well as greater than usual increases in cyclic adenosine monophosphate with isoproterenol stimulation as compared with normal individuals.[33] Patients with MVP often have postural phenomena such as orthostatic tachycardia and hypotension. Low intravascular volume and/or an abnormality in the renin-aldosterone axis may contribute to the orthostatic changes.[7,34]

ASSOCIATED CONDITIONS

Tricuspid valve prolapse, with similar interchordal hooding and histologic evidence of mucopolysaccharide proliferation and collagen dissolution, occurs in about 40 percent of patients with MVP.[6] Pulmonic valve prolapse and aortic valve prolapse occur in approximately 10 and 2 percent of patients with MVP, respectively.[6] The frequent findings of thoracic skeletal abnormalities in patients with MVP were noted earlier. There is an increased incidence of secundum atrial septal defect in patients with MVP and an increased incidence of MVP in patients with atrial septal defects that cannot be explained by a chance occurrence and does not represent only stretching of a patent fossa ovalis (see also Chaps. 63 and 64). An increased incidence of left-sided atrioventricular bypass tracts and supraventricular tachycardias also occurs in patients with MVP.[6,35]

CLINICAL MANIFESTATIONS

Symptoms

The diagnosis of MVP is most commonly made by cardiac auscultation in asymptomatic patients or by echocardiography being performed for some other purpose. The patient may be evaluated because of a family history of cardiac disease or occasionally may be referred because of an abnormal resting ECG. Some patients consult their physicians because of one or more of the common symptoms that occur in patients with this syndrome. The most common presenting complaint is *palpitation*. The source of palpitation is usually ventricular premature beats, but various supraventricular arrhythmias are also frequent, and the most common sustained tachycardia is paroxysmal reentry supraventricular tachycardia (see Chap. 24). Ventricular tachycardia occurs in some patients, and others have had symptomatic bradyarrhythmias. Palpitation is often reported by patients at a time when continuous ambulatory ECG recordings show no arrhythmias.

Chest pain is a frequent complaint in patients with MVP. It is atypical in most patients without coexisting ischemic heart disease and rarely resembles classic angina pectoris. Occasionally, it is recurrent and can be incapacitating. The etiology of the chest pain is unknown; sometimes it may represent true myocardial ischemia produced by abnormal tension on the papillary muscles and supporting ventricular wall by the prolapsing mitral leaflets.[36] Coronary artery spasm has been reported in patients with MVP, but it is unlikely to be the cause of most episodes of atypical chest pain.[37]

Dyspnea and *fatigue* are frequent symptoms in patients with MVP, including many without severe MR. Objective exercise testing often fails to show impaired exercise tolerance, and some patients exhibit distinct episodes of hyperventilation. Neuropsychiatric complaints occur in certain patients with MVP. Some have panic attacks (see Chap. 80), and others have frank manic-depressive syndromes. Transient cerebral ischemic episodes occur with increased incidence in patients with MVP, and some develop stroke syndromes.[38–42] One recent study showed no association between MVP and stroke.[43] Reports of amaurosis fugax, homonymous field loss, and retinal artery occlusion have been made; occasionally, the visual loss persists.[44] These signs likely are due to embolization of platelets and fibrin deposits that occur on the atrial side of the mitral valve leaflets.[45] *It is important to note that both MVP and panic attacks occur relatively frequently. Accordingly, the occurrence of the two syndromes in the same individual would be expected to occur frequently by chance, rather than panic attacks necessarily being part of the primary MVP syndrome.*

Physical Examination

The presence of thoracic skeletal abnormalities may suggest the diagnosis of MVP, the most common being scoliosis, pectus excavatum, straightened thoracic spine, and narrowed anteroposterior diameter of the chest.[16] Some patients with MVP may show signs, such as arachnodactyly, more typical of Marfan syndrome.

The principal cardiac auscultatory feature of this syndrome is the midsystolic click, a high-pitched sound of short duration (see Chap. 10). The click may vary considerably in intensity and location in systole according to LV loading conditions and contractility. It results from the sudden tensing of the mitral valve apparatus as the leaflets prolapse into the left atrium during systole. Multiple systolic clicks may be generated by different portions of the mitral leaflets prolapsing at varying times during systole.[46] The major differentiating feature of the midsystolic click of MVP from that due to other causes (e.g., aneurysm of the ventricular septum, atrial myxomas, or pericarditis) is that its timing during systole may be altered by maneuvers that change hemodynamic conditions (Table 58-2).

The midsystolic click is frequently followed by a late-systolic murmur, usually medium- to high-pitched and most audible at the apex. Occasionally, the murmur has a musical or honking quality. The character and intensity of the murmur also vary under certain conditions, from brief and almost inaudible to holosystolic and loud (Fig. 58-3).

Dynamic auscultation is often useful for establishing the clinical diagnosis of the MVP syndrome.[21] Changes in the LV end-diastolic volume lead to changes in the timing of the midsystolic click and murmur. When end-diastolic volume is decreased, the critical volume is achieved earlier in systole, and the click-murmur complex occurs shortly after the first heart sound (Fig. 58-4). In general, any maneuver that decreases the end-diastolic LV volume, increases the rate of ventricular contraction, or decreases the resistance to LV ejection of blood causes the MVP to occur early in systole, and the systolic click and murmur to move toward the first heart sound (see Table 58-2). By contrast, any maneuver that augments the volume of blood in the ventricle, reduces myocardial contractility, or increases LV afterload lengthens the time from the onset of systole to the initiation of MVP, and the systolic click and/or murmur move toward S_2. Maneuvers causing the click and/or murmur to occur earlier in systole include standing from the supine position, submaximal isometric handgrip exercise, the Valsalva maneuver, and amyl nitrite inhalation. Those which cause the click and murmur to move toward S_2 include squatting from the upright position and maneuvers that slow the heart rate.

TABLE 58-2 Response of the Murmur of Mitral Valve Prolapse to Interventions

Intervention	Timing	Intensity
Standing upright	←	↑
Recumbent	→	↓ or 0
Squatting	→	↓ or 0
Hand-grip	←	±
Valsalva	←	±
Amyl nitrite	±	↑

NOTE: ↑ = increase; ↓ = decrease; 0 = no change; ± = variable; ← = earlier; → = later.

Electrocardiogram

The ECG is usually normal in patients with MVP. The most common abnormality noted is the presence of ST-T-wave depression or T-wave inversion in the inferior leads (III, aV_F)[47] (Fig. 58-5). These changes may reflect ischemia of the inferior wall due to traction on the posteromedial papillary muscle by the prolapsing mitral leaflets. Sometimes ST-T-wave changes are present only during interventions that induce prolapse earlier in systole, as discussed earlier. More unusual electrocardiographic changes include prominent U waves, peaked T waves in the midprecordial leads, and prolongation of the QT interval.

MVP is associated with an increased incidence of false-positive exercise electrocardiographic results in patients with normal coronary arteries, especially females. Myocardial perfusion imaging with thallium or technetium sestamibi has been useful for differentiating false from true abnormal exercise electrocardiographic findings in patients with MVP (see Chap. 16).

Although arrhythmias may be observed on the resting ECG or during treadmill or bicycle exercise, they are detected more reliably by continuous ambulatory electrocardiographic recordings (see Chap. 13). The reported incidence of documented arrhythmias is higher in patients with MVP, ranging from 40 to 75 percent.[48] Most of the arrhythmias detected, however, are not life-threatening. Patients with ST-T-wave changes in the inferior electrocardiographic leads appear to have a higher incidence of serious ventricular arrhythmias on ambulatory recordings.[20]

Echocardiography

Echocardiography (see Chap. 13) is the most useful noninvasive test for defining MVP. The M-mode echocardiographic definition of MVP includes 2 mm or more of posterior displacement of one or both leaflets or holosystolic posterior "hammocking"

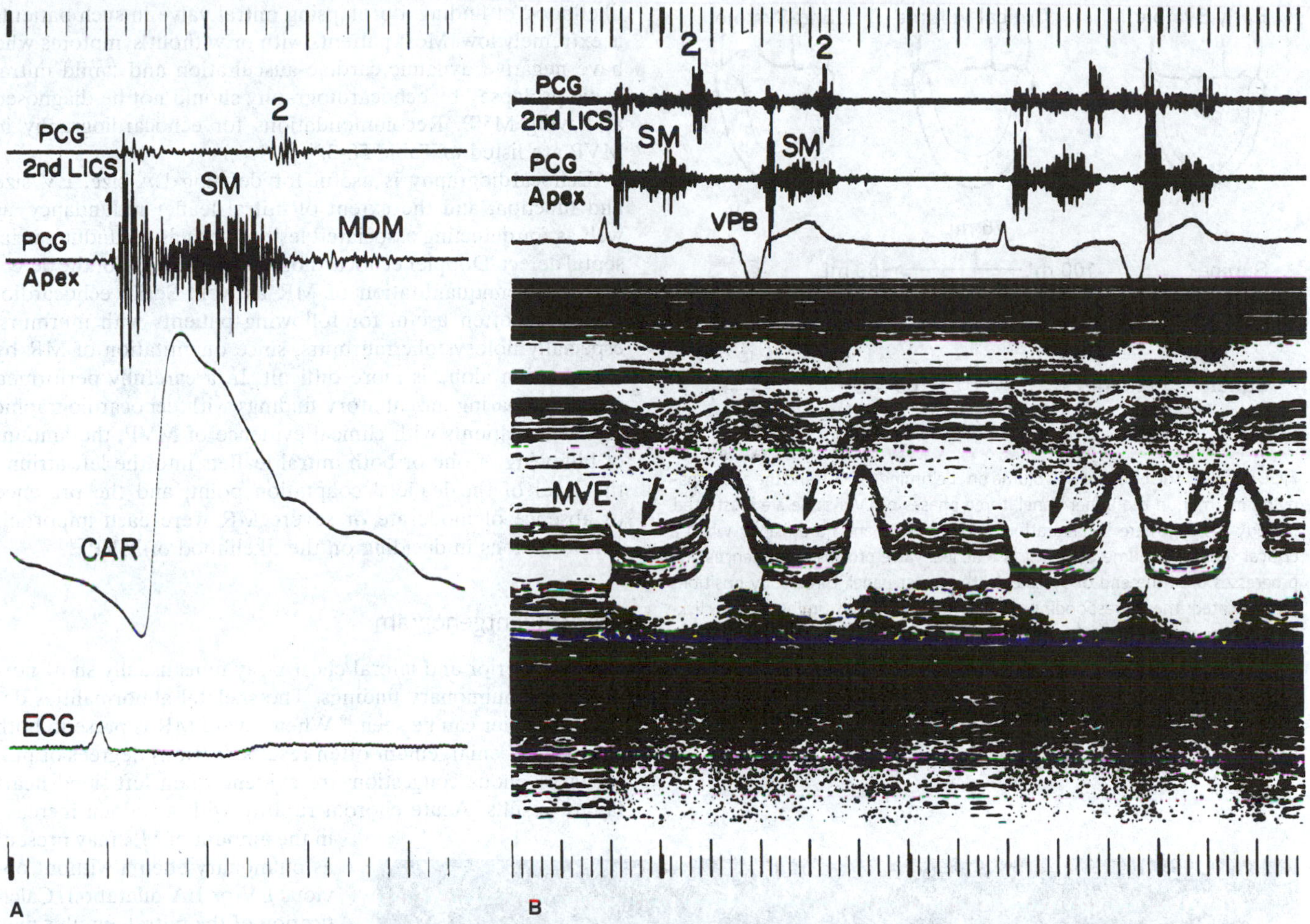

FIGURE 58-3 Phonocardiogram and echocardiogram in mitral valve prolapse. *A.* The phonocardiogram shows a high-frequency holosystolic murmur (HSM) with late-systolic accentuation. A low-frequency middiastolic murmur (MDM) is present at the apex. *B.* The echocardiogram demonstrates a hammock-shaped systolic motion of the valve leaflets. The rhythm is atrial fibrillation with bigeminy. 1, first heart sound; 2, second heart sound; MVE, mitral valve echogram. (Courtesy of Dr. Ernest Craige.)

of more than 3 mm (see Fig. 58-3). On 2-D echocardiography, systolic displacement of one or both mitral leaflets, particularly when they coapt on the LA side of the annular plane, in the parasternal long-axis view indicates a high likelihood of MVP[49] (see Fig. 58-5). There is disagreement concerning the reliability of an echocardiographic diagnosis of MVP when observed only in the apical four-chamber view. The diagnosis of MVP is even more certain when the leaflet thickness is greater than 5 mm during ventricular diastole. Leaflet redundancy is often associated with an elongated mitral annulus and elongated chordae tendineae. On Doppler velocity recordings, the presence or absence of MR is an important consideration, and MVP is more likely when the MR is detected as a high-velocity jet midway or more posterior in the left atrium.[29]

At present, there is no consensus on the 2-D echocardiographic criteria for MVP. Since echocardiography is a tomographic cross-sectional technique, no single view should be considered diagnostic. The parasternal long-axis view permits visualization of the medial aspect of the anterior mitral leaflet and middle scallop of the posterior leaflet. If the findings of prolapse are localized to the lateral scallop in the posterior leaflet, they would be best visualized by the apical four-chamber view.[49,50] All available echocardiographic views should be used, with the provision that anterior leaflet billowing alone in the four-chamber apical view is not evidence of prolapse; however, a displacement of the posterior leaflet or the coaptation point in any view including the apical views suggests the diagnosis of prolapse. The echocardiographic criteria for MVP should include structural changes such as leaflet thickening, redundancy, annular dilatation, and chordal elongation.

Patients with echocardiographic criteria for MVP but without evidence of thickened/redundant leaflets or definite MR are more difficult to classify. If such patients have auscultatory findings typical of MVP, the echocardiogram confirms the diagnosis. On the other hand, a patient with typical auscultatory findings but a negative echocardiogram likely also has MVP; in the past, as many as 10 percent of patients with MVP have had a nondiagnostic echocardiographic study. Currently, this percentage is lower because of more careful and complete echocardiographic studies. In clinical practice, a false diagnosis of MVP occurs too frequently. The use of echocardiography as a screening test for MVP in patients with and without symptoms who have no systolic click or murmur on serial, carefully performed auscultatory examinations *is not recommended.* The

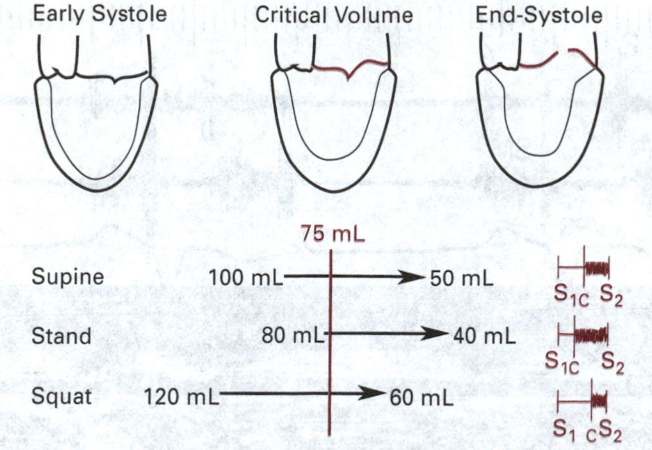

FIGURE 58-4 The effect of LV volume on the timing of MVP and the accompanying murmur. In the upper panel, three phases of LV systole are illustrated. In early systole, there is coaptation of the leaflets and no prolapse; when a critical ventricle volume of 75 mL is reached, valve prolapse commences and progresses until the end of systole. In the lower panel, three body positions are indicated; the corresponding change in volume and timing of the click-murmur are shown. The critical volume for prolapse remains constant. When the critical volume occurs earlier, the onset of the click-murmur is earlier. When the critical volume occurs later, the onset of the click-murmur is later. (From Crawford MH, O'Rourke RA. In: Isselbacher KJ et al., eds. *Harrison's Principles of Internal Medicine*, 9th ed. New York: McGraw-Hill; 1980:91–105. Reproduced with permission from the publisher, editors, and authors.)

likelihood of finding a prolapsing mitral valve in such patients is extremely low. Most patients with or without symptoms who have negative dynamic cardiac auscultation and "mild mitral valve prolapse" by echocardiography should not be diagnosed as having MVP. Recommendations for echocardiography in MVP are listed in Table 58-3.[51]

Echocardiography is useful for defining LA size, LV size and function, and the extent of mitral leaflet redundancy, as well as for detecting associated lesions such as secundum atrial septal defect. Doppler echocardiography is helpful for the detection and semiquantitation of MR as well. Serial echocardiograms are often useful for following patients with murmurs, especially holosystolic murmurs, since quantitation of MR by examination alone is more difficult. In a carefully performed study comparing auscultatory findings with echocardiographic results in patients with clinical evidence of MVP, the amount of billowing of one or both mitral leaflets into the left atrium, the level of the leaflets' coaptation point, and the presence or absence of moderate or severe MR were each important considerations in deciding on the likelihood of MVP.[29]

Chest Roentgenogram

Posteroanterior and lateral chest x-ray films usually show normal cardiopulmonary findings. The skeletal abnormalities described earlier can be seen.[19] When severe MR is present, both LA and LV enlargement often results. Various degrees of pulmonary venous congestion are evident when left-sided heart failure results. Acute chordal rupture with a sudden increase in the amount of MR may present as pulmonary edema without obvious LV or LA dilatation. Calcification of the mitral annulus may be seen, particularly in adults with Marfan syndrome (see Chap. 12).

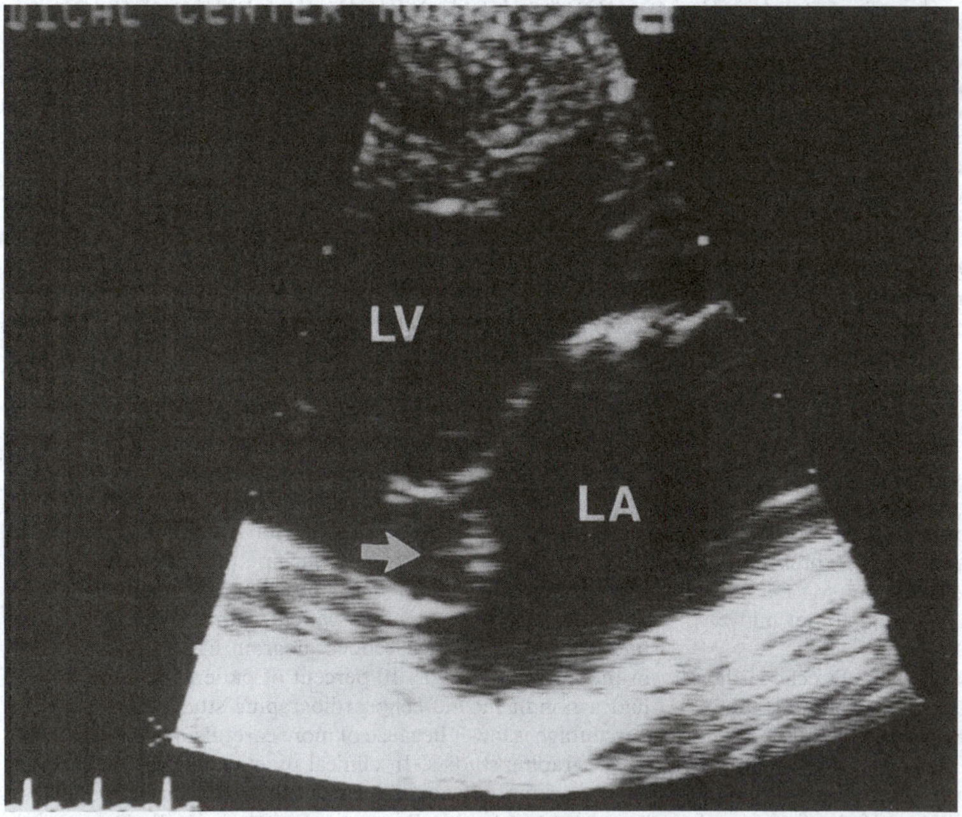

FIGURE 58-5 A parasternal 2-D echocardiographic view showing prolapse of a redundant posterior mitral leaflet toward the left atrium during systole. LV, left ventricle; LA, left atrium.

Myocardial Perfusion Scintigraphy

Exercise myocardial perfusion imaging with thallium or technetium sestamibi has been recommended as an adjunct to exercise ECG for determining the presence or absence of coexistent myocardial ischemia in patients with MVP.[52] Most MVP patients *with clinical evidence of CAD* have an abnormal exercise scintigram. On the other hand, a negative scintigram in these patients does not exclude ischemia as the basis for the chest pain, nor does it completely exclude CAD as the etiology (see Chap. 16).

Cardiac Catheterization

Cardiac catheterization is rarely used as a diagnostic technique for

MVP. Also, contrast ventriculography is unnecessary for determining LV function because it usually can be quantitated by 2-D echocardiography or radionuclide ventriculography. While contrast cineventriculography is often useful for assessing the severity of MR, cardiac catheterization and angiography are used most commonly in patients with MVP to exclude the possibility of CAD.

Intracardiac pressures and cardiac output are usually normal in uncomplicated MVP; however, these measurements become progressively more abnormal as MR becomes more severe.

LV cineangiography usually confirms the presence of prolapse of the mitral valve.[5,8] The right anterior oblique projection is best for observing prolapse of the three scallops of the posterior leaflet. The left anterior oblique view is necessary for the adequate evaluation of prolapse of the anterior leaflet.

LV wall motion is usually normal in patients with primary MVP, but some patients show abnormal contraction patterns in the absence of CAD.[5,27] These contraction abnormalities usually represent indentation of the left ventricle at the point of attachment of the papillary muscles; it is thought to be due to abnormal traction on the papillary muscles and buckling of the ventricular wall. Patients with the most severe prolapse more commonly exhibit misshapen ventricular cavities during systole, and wall motion abnormalities frequently disappear after successful mitral valve replacement or repair.[27]

Coronary arteriography is usually normal in patients with primary MVP, and no congenital anomalies of the coronary vessels have been associated with this syndrome.

TABLE 58-3 Recommendations for Echocardiography in Mitral Valve Prolapse

Indication	Class
1. Diagnosis, assessment of hemodynamic severity of MR, leaflet morphology, ventricular compensation in patients with physical signs of MVP.	I
2. To exclude MVP in patients who have been given the diagnosis where there is no clinical evidence to support the diagnosis.	I
3. To exclude MVP in patients with first-degree relatives with known myxomatous valve disease.	IIa
4. Risk stratification in patients with physical signs of MVP with no or mild regurgitation.	IIa
5. To exclude MVP in patients in the absence of physical findings suggestive of MVP a positive family history.	III
6. Routine repetition of echocardiography in patients with MVP with no MR and no changes in clinical signs or symptoms.	III

Class I: Conditions for which there is evidence and/or general agreement that a given procedure or treatment is useful and effective.

Class II: Conditions for which there is conflicting evidence and/or a divergence of opinion about the usefulness/efficacy of a procedure or treatment.

Class IIa: Weight of evidence/opinion is in favor of usefulness/efficacy.

Class IIb: Usefulness efficacy is less well established by evidence/opinion.

Class III: Conditions for which there is evidence and/or general agreement that the procedure/treatment is not useful/effective and in some cases may be harmful.

SOURCE: From ACC/AHA clinical practice guidelines for valvular heart disease. *J Am Coll Cardiol* 1998; 32:1486–1588.

Electrophysiologic Testing

The indications for electrophysiologic testing in a patient with MVP are similar to those in other patients (i.e., recurrent unexplained syncope, sudden death survivors, symptomatic complex ventricular ectopy, and the presence of the preexcitation syndromes) (see Chap. 26). Upright tilt studies with monitoring of blood pressure and rhythm may be valuable in patients with light-headedness or syncope and in diagnosing autonomic dysfunction (see Chap. 32).

NATURAL HISTORY, PROGNOSIS, AND COMPLICATIONS

In most patient studies, the MVP syndrome is associated with a benign prognosis[6,53–60] (Fig. 58-6). The age-adjusted survival rate for both males and females with MVP is similar to that

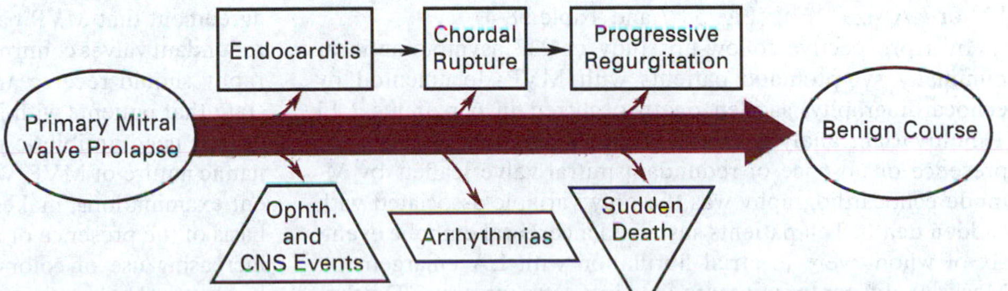

FIGURE 58-6 The course and possible complications of MVP. In most patients, the MVP syndrome is associated with a benign prognosis. CNS, central nervous system; Ophth, ophthalmologic. (From Crawford MH, O'Rourke RA. In: Isselbacher KJ et al., eds. *Harrison's Principles of Internal Medicine*, 9th ed. New York: McGraw-Hill; 1980:91–105. Reproduced with permission from the publisher, editors, and authors.)

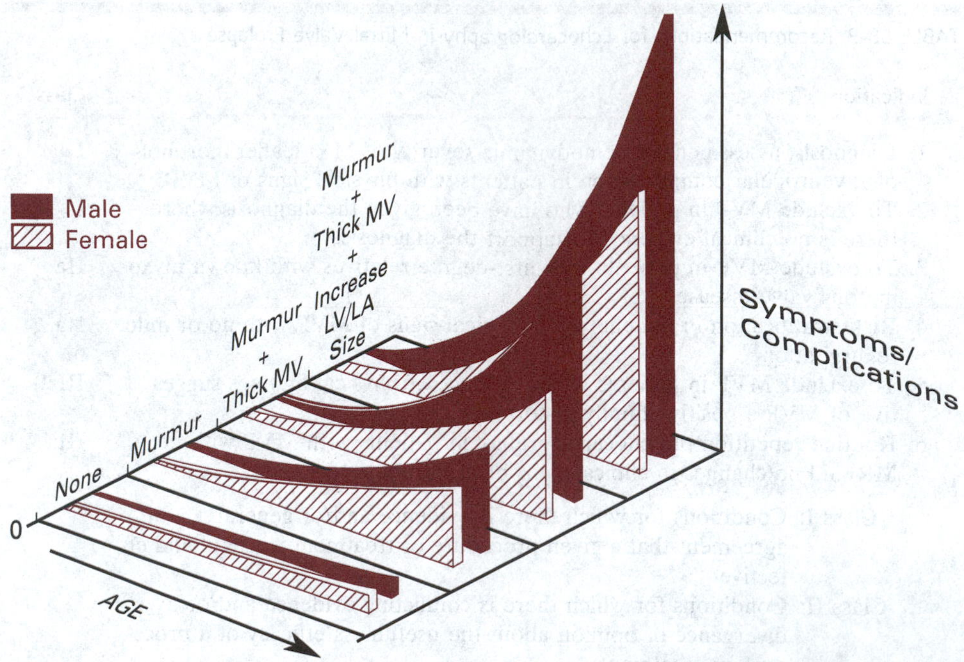

FIGURE 58-7 The relations between cardiac structure, age, and complications in the MVP syndrome. Patients with MVP, typical auscultatory findings, thickening of the valve leaflets, and LV or LA enlargement are at risk of developing complications. When two or more of these findings are present, the likelihood of complications is highest. By contrast, the absence of these features can be used to identify patients with MVP who have an exceedingly low risk. In general, complications increase with age and are more common in males than in females. (From Boudoulas et al.[57] Reproduced with permission from the publisher and authors.)

in patients without this common clinical entity. The gradual progression of MR in patients with mitral prolapse, however, may result in progressive dilatation of the left atrium and ventricle. LA dilatation often results in atrial fibrillation, and moderate to severe MR eventually results in LV dysfunction and the development of congestive heart failure. Pulmonary hypertension may occur with associated right ventricular dysfunction. In some patients with an initially prolonged asymptomatic interval, the entire process may enter an accelerated phase as a result of LA and LV dysfunction, atrial fibrillation, and in certain instances, ruptured mitral valve chordae. The latter occurs more commonly in males and with increasing age.[6,7]

Several long-term prognostic studies suggest that complications occur most commonly in patients with a mitral systolic murmur, thickened redundant mitral valve leaflets, or increased LV or LA size[30,57,58,62] (Fig. 58-7 and Table 58-4).

In a prospective follow-up study of 237 asymptomatic or minimally symptomatic patients with MVP documented by echocardiography, sudden death occurred in 6 patients.[55] In a multivariant analysis of the echocardiographic findings, the presence or absence of redundant mitral valve leaflets by M-mode echocardiography was the only variable associated with sudden death. Ten patients sustained a cerebral embolic event, six of whom were in atrial fibrillation with LA enlargement. Marks et al.[49] confirmed these data in a retrospective 2-D echocardiographic study from 456 patients with MVP. Two groups of patients were compared; those with thickening and redundancy of the mitral valve leaflet and those without leaflet thickening. Complications or a history of complications was more prevalent in those with leaflet thickening and redundancy compared with those without leaflet thickening. The incidence of stroke, however, was similar in the two groups. Long-term follow-up studies in patients with MVP associated with a floppy, myxomatous mitral valve permit several conclusions.[7] Serious complications occur in some patients with MVP, predominantly in those with diagnostic auscultatory findings. Also, redundant mitral valve leaflets and increased LV size are associated with a frequency of serious complications. Finally, men and those over 50 years of age are at increased risk of complications, including severe MR requiring surgery.

Sudden death is the least common but obviously the most severe complication of MVP (Table 58-5). While infrequent, the highest incidence of sudden death has been reported in the familial form of MVP. Some of these patients have been noted to have QT-interval prolongation. Also, patients with MVP with severe autonomic dysfunction and excessive vagotonia resulting in bradyarrhythmias and asystole have been reported.[63,64] Therefore, arrhythmias are likely to be the usual cause of sudden death in patients with MVP, so it seems prudent to limit ambulatory electrocardiographic recordings to those patients at highest risk. Many believe that patients with electrocardiographic ST-T-wave changes are more likely to have complex ventricular arrhythmias.[6,7] Certainly, any patients with symptoms suggestive of arrhythmia or who have arrhythmias noted during physical examination or on the resting ECG should be evaluated further (see Chap. 24).

Infective endocarditis is a serious complication of MVP, and MVP is the leading predisposing cardiovascular diagnosis in most series of patients reported with endocarditis.[6,7,65] Since the absolute incidence of endocarditis is extremely low for the entire MVP population, there has been much discussion concerning the risk of endocarditis in MVP.[66] While there is general agreement that MVP patients with murmurs and/or thickened redundant valves confirmed by echocardiography or cineangiography should receive antibiotic prophylaxis, some authorities state that patients with isolated systolic clicks and no murmurs do not need antibiotic prophylaxis for endocarditis.[67] The dynamic nature of MVP, with variable physical findings on different examinations, makes it difficult to make judgments on the basis of the presence or absence of a systolic murmur. With the increasing use of color-flow echo-Doppler studies, MR often has been observed in patients in whom no murmur is heard.[68] Recommendations for antibiotic endocarditis prophylaxis for patients with MVP undergoing procedures associated with bacteremia are listed in Table 58-6.

As indicated earlier, progressive MR occurs frequently in patients with long-standing MVP. Fibrin emboli are responsible

TABLE 58-4 Use of Echocardiography for Risk Stratification in Mitral Valve Prolapse

Study	No. of Patients	Features Examined	Outcome	P
Nishimura et al., 1985[55]	237	MV leaflet ≥5 mm	↑ sum of sudden death, endocarditis and cerebral embolus	P <0.02
		LVID ≥60 mm	↑ MVR (26 vs. 3.1%)	P <0.001
Zuppiroli et al., 1994[58]	119	MV leaflet >5 mm	↑ complex ventricular arrhythmia	P <0.001
Babuty et al., 1994[61]	58	Undefined MV thickening	No relation to complex ventricular arrhythmias	NS
Takamoto et al., 1991[59]	142	MV leaflet ≥3 mm redundant, low echo density	↑ ruptured chordae (48 vs. 5%)	NS
Marks et al., 1989[49]	456	MV leaflet ≥5 mm	↑ endocarditis (3.5 vs. 0%)	P <0.02
			↑ moderate-severe MR (11.9 vs. 0%)	P <0.001
			↑ MVR (6.6 vs. 0.7%)	P <0.02
			↑ stroke (7.5 vs. 5.8)	NS
Chandraratna et al., 1984[60]	86	MV leaflets >5.1 mm	↑ cardiovascular abnormalities (60 vs. 6%) (Marfan's syndrome, TVP, MR, dilated descending aorta)	P <0.001

NOTE: MV, mitral valve; LVID, left ventricular internal diameter; MVR, mitral valve replacement; MR, mitral regurgitation; TVP, tricuspid valve prolapse.
SOURCE: From ACC/AHA guidelines for the clinical application of echocardiography. *Circulation* 1997; 95:1686–1744.

in some patients for visual problems consistent with involvement of the ophthalmic or posterior cerebral circulation. Several studies have indicated an increased likelihood of cerebral vascular accidents of various types in patients under age 45 who have MVP than would have been expected in a similar population without MVP. Therefore, it has been recommended that antiplatelet drugs such as aspirin be administered to patients who have MVP and suspected cerebral nervous system emboli; however, neither antiplatelet drugs nor anticoagulants should be prescribed routinely for patients with MVP because the incidence of embolic phenomena is very low. Recommendations for aspirin and oral anticoagulants in MVP are listed in Table 58-7. *It is important to avoid the incorrect diagnosis of MVP syndrome. This mistake is especially likely to occur in patients with neuropsychiatric symptoms, in whom an incorrect diagnosis of MVP is made from the ECG. Such an improper diagnosis can form the foundation of a chronic, often disabling cardiac neurosis. Even if the diagnosis of MVP is properly made, it is not necessarily correct to attribute neuropsychiatric symptoms to the MVP* (see also Chap. 80).

TREATMENT

The majority of patients with MVP are asymptomatic and lack the high-risk profile described earlier. These patients with mild or no symptoms and findings of milder forms of prolapse should be assured of a benign prognosis. A normal lifestyle and regular exercise are encouraged.[5,7] For most patients in whom the *diag-*

TABLE 58-5 Mitral Valve Complications in 102 Hearts with Mitral Valve Prolapse

	No.	Percent
Sudden death	0	0
Primary rupture of chordae	7	7
Bacterial endocarditis	7	7
Mitral valve regurgitation	18	18
Primary rupture of chordae	(7)	—
Bacterial endocarditis	(4)	—
Severe prolapse	(4)	—
Entrapped chordae	(3)	—
Fibrin deposits	4	4

SOURCE; Modified from Lucas RV Jr, Edwards JE. The floppy mitral valve. *Curr Probl Cardiol* 1982; 7:1–48.

TABLE 58-6 Recommendations for Antibiotic Endocarditis Prophylaxis for Patients with Mitral Valve Prolapse Undergoing Procedures Associated with Bacteremia

Indication	Class
1. Patients with characteristic systolic click-murmur complex.	I
2. Patients with isolated systolic click and echo evidence of MVP and MR.	I
3. Patients with isolated systolic click, echo evidence of high-risk MVP.	IIa
4. Patients with isolated systolic click and no or equivocal evidence of MVP.	III

SOURCE: From ACC/AHA guidelines for the clinical application of echocardiography. *Circulation* 1997; 95:1686–1744.

TABLE 58-7 Recommendations for Aspirin and Oral Anticoagulants in Mitral Valve Prolapse

Indication	Class
1. Aspirin therapy for cerebral transient ischemic attacks (TIAs).	I
2. Warfarin therapy for patients in atrial fibrillation with age ≥65 yr, hypertension, MR murmur, or history of heart failure.	I
3. Aspirin therapy for patients in atrial fibrillation <65 years old with no history of MR, hypertension, or heart failure.	I
4. Warfarin therapy for poststroke patients.	I
5. Warfarin therapy patients for TIAs despite aspirin therapy.	IIa
6. Aspirin therapy in poststroke patients with contraindications to anticoagulants.	IIa
7. Aspirin therapy for patients in sinus rhythm with echocardiographic evidence of high-risk MVP	IIb

SOURCE: From ACC/AHA guidelines for the clinical application of echocardiography. *Circulation* 1997; 95:1686–1744.

nosis of MVP is definite, we recommend antibiotic prophylaxis for the prevention of infective endocarditis while undergoing procedures associated with bacteremia. Patients with MVP and palpitation associated with sinus tachycardia or mild tachyarrhythmias and those with chest pain, anxiety, or fatigue often respond to therapy with beta blockers.[5,7,69] In many cases, however, the cessation of catecholamine stimulants such as caffeine, alcohol, cigarettes, and certain drugs may be sufficient to control symptoms.

Orthostatic symptoms are best treated with volume expansion, preferably by liberalizing fluid and salt intake. Mineralocorticoid therapy may be needed in severe cases, and wearing support stockings may be beneficial.[7] In sudden death survivors and those patients with symptomatic complex arrhythmias, specific antiarrhythmic therapy should be guided by monitoring techniques, including electrophysiologic testing when indicated[7] (see Chap. 26).

Daily aspirin therapy (80–325 mg/day; see Table 58-7) is recommended for MVP patients with documented focal neurologic events. Such patients also should avoid cigarettes and oral contraceptives. Some clinicians use long-term anticoagulant therapy with warfarin in poststroke patients with prolapse, particularly when symptoms occur on aspirin therapy (see also Chap. 89).

Restriction from competitive sports is recommended when moderate LV enlargement, LV dysfunction, uncontrolled tachyarrhythmias, long QT interval, unexplained syncope, prior sudden death survival, or aortic root enlargement is present, individually or in combination.[7]

The familial occurrence of MVP should be explained to the patient and is particularly important in those with associated disease, who are at greater risk for complications. Screening relatives can uncover high-risk individuals and potentially prevent some complications. There is no contraindication to pregnancy based on the diagnosis of MVP alone.

Patients with severe MR with symptoms and/or impaired LV systolic function require cardiac catheterization studies and evaluation for mitral valve surgery.[70] The thickened, redundant mitral valve often can be repaired rather than replaced, with a low operative mortality and excellent long-term results.[71–79] Follow-up studies also suggest lower thromboembolic and endocarditis risk than with prosthetic valves.

Asymptomatic patients with MVP and no significant MR can be evaluated clinically every 2 to 3 years. Echocardiography has been suggested every 5 years in such patients to help determine the natural history and the likelihood of complications. Patients with MVP who have high-risk characteristics, including those with moderate to severe MR, should be followed more frequently, even if no symptoms are present.

Surgical Considerations

Management of the patient with MVP may require valve surgery, particularly in those patients who develop a flail mitral leaflet due to rupture of chordae tendineae or their marked elongation.[79] Most such valves can be repaired successfully by surgeons experienced with mitral valve repair, especially when the posterior leaflet valve is predominantly affected. Symptoms of heart failure, the severity of MR, the presence or absence of atrial fibrillation, LV systolic function, LV end-diastolic and end-systolic volumes, and pulmonary artery pressure (rest and exercise) all influence the decision to recommend mitral valve surgery. Recommendations for surgery in patients with MVP and MR are the same as for those with other forms of nonischemic severe MR and include class III–IV symptoms, LV ejection fraction less than 60 percent, and/or marked increases in LV end-diastolic and end-systolic volumes. If mitral repair is likely to be successful, severe MR with class II symptoms or atrial fibrillation may be an appropriate reason for surgical referral.[51]

References

1. Freed LA, Levy D, Levine RA, et al. Prevalence and clinical outcomes of mitral valve prolapse. *N Engl J Med* 1999; 341:1–7.
2. Nishimura R, McGoon MD. Perspectives on mitral-valve prolapse. *N Eng J Med* 1999; 341:48–58.
3. Reid JV. Mid-systolic clicks. *S Afr Med J* 1961; 35:353–357.
4. Barlow JB, Pocok WA, Marchand P, Denny M. The significance of late systolic murmurs. *Am Heart J* 1963; 66:443–452.
5. O'Rourke RA, Crawford MH. The systolic click-murmur syndrome: Clinical recognition and management. *Curr Probl Cardiol* 1976; 1(1):1.
6. Lucas RV Jr, Edwards JE. The floppy mitral valve. *Curr Probl Cardiol* 1982; 7:1–48.
7. Fontana ME, Sparks EA, Boudoulas H, Wooley CF. Mitral valve prolapse in the mitral valve prolapse syndrome. *Curr Probl Cardiol* 1991; 16:315–375.
8. O'Rourke RA. The mitral valve prolapse syndrome. In: Chizner MA, ed. *Classic Teachings in Clinical Cardiology*. Cedar Grove, NJ: Laennec; 1996:1049–1070.
9. Devereux RB. Recent developments in the diagnosis and management of mitral valve prolapse. *Curr Opin Cardiol* 1995; 10:107–116.
10. Perloff JK, Roberts WC. The mitral apparatus: Functional anatomy of mitral regurgitation. *Circulation* 1972; 46:227–239.
11. Devereux RB, Brown WT, Kramer-Fox R, Sachs I. Inheritance of mitral valve prolapse: Effect of age and sex on gene expression. *Ann Intern Med* 1982; 97:826–832.
12. Shell WE, Walton JA, Clifford ME, Willis PW III. The familial

occurrence of the syndrome of mid-late systolic click and late systolic murmur. *Circulation* 1969; 39:327–338.
13. Savage DD, Garrison RJ, Devereux RB, et al. Mitral valve prolapse in the general population: I. Epidemiologic features: The Framingham Study. *Am Heart J* 1983; 106:571–576.
14. Procacci PM, Savran SV, Schrieter SL, Bryson AL. Prevalence of clinical mitral valve prolapse in 1169 young women. *N Engl J Med* 1976; 294:1086–1088.
15. Leier CV, Call TD, Fulkerson PK, Wooley CF. The spectrum of cardiac defects in the Ehlers-Danlos syndrome, types I & III. *Ann Intern Med* 1980; 92:171–178.
16. Lebwohl MG, Distefano D, Prioleau PG, et al. Pseudoxanthoma elasticum and mitral valve prolapse. *N Engl J Med* 1982; 307:228–231.
17. Schwartz T, Gotsman MS. Mitral valve prolapse in osteogenesis imperfecta. *Isr J Med Sci* 1981; 17:1087–1088.
18. Udoshi MB, Shah A, Fisher VJ, Dolgin M. Incidence of mitral valve prolapse in subjects with thoracic skeletal abnormalities: A prospective study. *Am Heart J* 1979; 97:303–311.
19. Bon Tempo CP, Ronan JA Jr. Radiographic appearance of the thorax in systolic click: Late systolic murmur syndrome. *Am J Cardiol* 1975; 36:27–31.
20. Crawford MH, O'Rourke RA. Mitral valve prolapse syndrome. In: Isselbacher KJ, Adams RD, Braunwald E, et al, eds. *Update I: Harrison's Principles of Internal Medicine*. New York: McGraw-Hill; 1981:91–152.
21. O'Rourke RA. The syndrome of mitral valve prolapse. In: Albert JA, ed. *Valvular Heart Disease*. New York: Lippincott-Raven; 1999:157–182.
22. Tei C, Sakamaki T, Shah PM, et al. Mitral valve prolapse in short-term experimental coronary occlusion: A possible mechanism of ischemic mitral regurgitation. *Circulation* 1983; 68:183–189.
23. Crawford MH. Mitral valve prolapse due to coronary artery disease. *Am J Med* 1977; 62:447–451.
24. Tomaru T, Uchida Y, Mohri N. Post-inflammatory mitral and aortic valve prolapse: A clinical and pathological study. *Circulation* 1987; 76:68–76.
25. Lembo NJ, Dell'Italia LJ, Crawford MH, et al. Mitral valve prolapse in patients with prior rheumatic fever. *Circulation* 1988; 77:830–836.
26. Marcus RH, Sareli P, Pocock WA, et al. Functional anatomy of severe mitral regurgitation in active rheumatic carditis. *Am J Cardiol* 1986; 63:577–584.
27. Crawford MH, O'Rourke RA. Mitral valve prolapse: A cardiomyopathic state? *Prog Cardiovasc Dis* 1984; 27:133–139.
28. Lax D, Eicher M, Goldberg SJ. Mild dehydration induces echocardiographic signs of mitral valve prolapse in healthy females with prior normal cardiac findings. *Am Heart J* 1992; 124:1533–1540.
29. Krivokapich J, Child JS, Dadourian BJ, Perloff JK. Reassessment of echocardiographic criteria for the diagnosis of mitral valve prolapse. *Am J Cardiol* 1988; 61:131–135.
30. Fukuda N, Oki T, Iuchi A, et al. Predisposing factors for severe mitral regurgitation in idiopathic mitral valve prolapse. *Am J Cardiol* 1995; 76(7):503–507.
31. Gaffney FA, Karlsson ES, Campbell W, et al. Autonomic dysfunction in women with mitral valve prolapse. *Circulation* 1979; 59:894–899.
32. Boudoulas H, Reynolds JC, Mazzaferri E, Wooley CF. Metabolic studies in mitral valve prolapse syndrome. *Circulation* 1980; 61:1200–1205.
33. Anwar A, Kohn SR, Dunn JF, et al. Altered beta-adrenergic receptor function in subjects with symptomatic mitral valve prolapse. *Am J Med Sci* 1991; 302:89–97.
34. Santos AD, Puthenpurakal MK, Ahmad H, et al. Orthostatic hypotension: A commonly unrecognized cause of symptoms in mitral valve prolapse. *Am J Med* 1981; 71:746–750.
35. Betriu A, Wigle ED, Felderhof CH, McLoughlin MJ. Prolapse of the posterior leaflet of the mitral valve associated with secundum atrial septal defect. *Am J Cardiol* 1975; 35:363–369.
36. LeWinter MM, Hoffman JR, Shell WE, et al. Phuenylephrine-induced atypical chest pain in patients with prolapsing mitral valve leaflets. *Am J Cardiol* 1974; 34:12–18.
37. Sabom MB, Curry RC Jr, Pepine CJ, et al. Ergonovine testing for coronary artery spasm in patients with angiographic mitral valve prolapse. *Cathet Cardiovasc Diagn* 1978; 4:265–274.
38. Barnett HJM, Jones MW, Boughner DR, Kostuck WJ. Cerebral ischemic events associated with prolapsing mitral valve. *Arch Neurol* 1976; 33:777–782.
39. Barletta GA, Gagliardi R, Benvenuti L, Fantini F. Cerebral ischemic attacks as a complication of aortic and mitral valve prolapse. *Stroke* 1985; 16:219–223.
40. Barnett HJM, Boughner DR, Taylor DW, et al. Further evidence relating mitral valve prolapse to cerebral ischemic event. *N Engl J Med* 1980; 302:139–144.
41. Petty GW, Orencia AJ, Khandheria BK, Whisnant JP. A population-based study of stroke in the setting of mitral valve prolapse: Risk factors and infarct subtype classification. *Mayo Clin Proc* 1994; 69:632–634.
42. Orencia AJ, Petty GW, Khandheria BK, et al. Mitral valve prolapse and the risk of stroke after initial cerebral ischemia. *Neurology* 1995; 45:1083–1086.
43. Gilon D, Buonanno FS, Jaffee MM, et al. Lack of evidence of an association between mitral valve prolapse and stroke in young patients. *N Engl J Med* 1999; 341:8–13.
44. Wilson LA, Keeling PW, Malcolm AD, et al. Visual complications of mitral leaflet prolapse. *Br Med J* 1977; 2:86–88.
45. Chesler E, King RA, Edwards JE. The myxomatous mitral valve and sudden death. *Circulation* 1983; 67:632–639.
46. Weis AJ, Salcedo EE, Stewart WJ, et al. Anatomic explanation of mobile systolic clicks: Implications for the clinical and echocardiographic diagnosis of mitral valve prolapse. *Am Heart J* 1995; 129:314–320.
47. Bhutto ZR, Barron JT, Liebson PR, et al. Electrocardiographic abnormalities in mitral valve prolapse. *Am J Cardiol* 1992; 70:265–266.
48. Schaal SF. Ventricular arrhythmias in patients with mitral valve prolapse. *Cardiovasc Clin* 1992; 22(1):307–316.
49. Marks AR, Choong CY, Sanfilippo AJ, et al. Identification of high-risk and low-risk subgroups of patients with mitral valve prolapse. *N Engl J Med* 1989; 320:1031–1036.
50. Shah PM. Echocardiographic diagnosis of mitral valve prolapse. *J Am Soc Echocardiogr* 1994; 7(3 pt 1):286–293.
51. Bonow RO, Carabello B, De Leon AC Jr, et al. ACC/AHA guidelines for the management of patients with valvular heart disease. *J Am Coll Cardiol* 1998; 32:1486–1588.
52. Klein GJ, Kostuck WJ, Bougher DR, Chamberlain MJ. Stress myocardial imaging in mitral leaflet prolapse syndrome. *Am J Cardiol* 1978; 42:746–750.
53. Allen H, Harris A, Leatham A. Significance and prognosis of an isolated late systolic murmur: A 9- to 22-year follow-up. *Br Heart J* 1974; 36:525–532.
54. Mills P, Rose J, Hollingsworth J, et al. Long-term prognosis of mitral valve prolapse. *N Engl J Med* 1977; 297:13–18.
55. Nishimura RA, McGood MD, Shub C, et al. Echocardiographically documented mitral-valve prolapse: Long-term follow-up of 237 patients. *N Engl J Med* 1985; 313:1305–1309.
56. Düren DR, Becker AE, Dunning AJ. Long-term follow-up of idiopathic mitral valve prolapse in 300 patients: A prospective study. *J Am Coll Cardiol* 1988; 11:42–47.
57. Boudoulas H, Kolibash BH, Wooley CF. Mitral valve prolapse: A heterogenous disorder. *Prim Cardiol* 1991; 17:29–43.
58. Zuppiroli A, Rinaldi M, Kramer-Fox R, et al. Natural history of mitral valve prolapse. *Am J Cardiol* 1995; 75:1028–1032.
59. Takamoto T, Nitta M, Tsujibayashi T, et al. The prevalence and

clinical features of pathologically abnormal mitral valve leaflets (myxomatous mitral valve) in the mitral valve prolapse syndrome: An echocardiographic and pathologic comparative study. *J Cardiol Suppl* 1991; 25:75–86.
60. Chandraratna PAN, Nimalasuriya A, Kawanishi D, et al. Identification of the increased frequency of cardiovascular abnormalities associated with mitral valve prolapse by two-dimensional echocardiography. *Am J Cardiol* 1984; 54:1283–1285.
61. Babuty D, Cosnay P, Breuillac JC, et al. Ventricular arrhythmia factors in mitral valve prolapse. *PACE* 1994; 17:1090–1099.
62. Cheitlin MD, Alpert JS, Armstrong WF, et al. ACC/AHA guidelines for the clinical application of echocardiography. *Circulation* 1997; 95:1686–1744.
63. Cosgrove DM, Stewart WJ. Mitral valvuloplasty. *Curr Probl Cardiol* 1989; 14:359–415.
64. Kirklin JW. Mitral valve repair for mitral incompetence. *Mod Concepts Cardiovasc Dis* 1987; 56:7–11.
65. Marshall CE, Shappel SD. Sudden death and the ballooning posterior leaflet syndrome: Detailed anatomic and histochemical investigation. *Arch Pathol* 1974; 98:134–138.
66. Clemens JD, Horwitz RI, Jaffe CC, et al. A controlled evaluation of the risk of bacterial endocarditis in persons with mitral valve prolapse. *N Engl J Med* 1982; 307:776–781.
67. Devereux RB, Frary CJ, Kramer-Fox R, et al. Cost-effectiveness of infective endocarditis prophylaxis for mitral valve prolapse with or without a mitral regurgitant murmur. *Am J Cardiol* 1994; 74:1024–1029.
68. Dajani AS, Bisno AL, Chung KJ, et al. Prevention of bacterial endocarditis: Recommendations by the American Heart Association. *JAMA* 1990; 264:2919–2922.
69. Winkle RA, Lopes MG, Goodman DJ, et al. Propranolol for patients with mitral valve prolapse. *Am Heart J* 1977; 93:422–427.
70. Galloway AC, Colvin SB, Baumann FG, et al. Current concepts of mitral valve reconstruction for mitral insufficiency. *Circulation* 1988; 78:1087–1098.
71. Cheitlin MD. The timing of surgery in mitral and aortic valve disease. *Curr Probl Cardiol* 1987; 12:75–149.
72. Cosgrove DM, Stewart WJ. Mitral valvuloplasty. *Curr Probl Cardiol* 1989; 14:359–415.
73. Kirklin JW. Mitral valve repair for mitral incompetence. *Mod Concepts Cardiovasc Dis* 1987; 56:7–11.
74. Cohn LH, Couper GS, Aranki SF, et al. Long-term results of mitral valve reconstruction for regurgitation of the myxomatous mitral valve. *J Thorac Cardiovasc Surg* 1994; 107:143–150.
75. Eishi K, Kawazoe K, Sasako Y, et al. Comparison of repair techniques for mitral valve prolapse. *J Heart Valve Dis* 1994; 3:432–438.
76. Perier P, Clausnizer B, Mistarz K. Carpentier "sliding leaflet" technique for repair of the mitral valve: Early results. *Ann Thorac Surg* 1994; 57:383–386.
77. Eishi K, Kawazoe K, Sasako Y, et al. Comparison of repair techniques for mitral valve prolapse. *J Heart Valve Dis* 1994; 3:432–438.
78. Perier P, Clausnizer B, Mistarz K. Carpentier sliding leaflet technique for repair of the mitral valve: Early results. *Ann Thorac Surg* 1994; 57:383–386.
79. Ling LH, Enriquez-Sarano M, Seward JB, et al. Clinical outcome of mitral regurgitation due to flail leaflet. *N Engl J Med* 1996; 335;1417–1423.

CHAPTER 59

TRICUSPID VALVE, PULMONIC VALVE, AND MULTIVALVULAR DISEASE

Robert A. O'Rourke

DEFINITION, ETIOLOGY, AND PATHOLOGY

Tricuspid Valve Disease

Tricuspid valve dysfunction can occur with normal or abnormal valves.[1] When normal tricuspid values develop dysfunction, the resulting hemodynamic abnormality is almost always pure regurgitation. Tricuspid regurgitation (TR) occurs when the tricuspid valve allows blood to enter the right atrium (RA) during a right ventricular (RV) contraction. Tricuspid stenosis (TS) results from obstruction to diastolic flow across the valve during filling of the RV. A diagrammatic illustration of tricuspid valve disease and the prevalence of various pathologic etiologies are shown in Fig. 59-1*A* and *B*.

Diseases causing TR are more numerous than those causing TS. It is important to note that the normal tricuspid valve often does not completely coapt in systole, as is shown by the frequent occurrence of TR jets on Doppler ultrasound. Usually the volume of regurgitant blood is so small that the TR is silent; this finding occurs in 24 to 96 percent of normal individuals by Doppler ultrasound and thus must be considered a variant of normal.[2–4] Pathologic TR is most commonly due to diseases that cause RV dilatation and failure;[5] left ventricular (LV) failure and/or pulmonary hypertension can result in tricuspid regurgitation (Table 59-1). Primary diseases of the tricuspid valve apparatus, which includes the tricuspid annulus, the leaflets, the chordae, the papillary muscle, and the RV wall, also cause TR (Table 59-1).[6–8] The most common etiology of isolated TR is infective endocarditis in drug addicts[9] (see Chap. 73). Less common causes include myocardial infarction, trauma, carcinoid, leaflet prolapse, and such congenital abnormalities as atrial septal defect and Ebstein's anomaly[10–15] (see Chap. 63). TR also occurs in patients with rheumatoid arthritis, radiation therapy, and Marfan's syndrome.[6] Primary involvement of the tricuspid valve due to rheumatic fever results in TS, usually in association with TR (Fig. 59-2).

The most common cause of TS is rheumatic fever. This is usually associated with concomitant mitral stenosis (MS). Isolated TS can be seen with the carcinoid syndrome, infective endocarditis, endocardial fibroelastosis, endomyocardial fibrosis, and systemic lupus erythematosus, among other conditions[6–8] (Table 59-2). It has also been reported to occur in patients with Fabry's disease, or Whipple's disease and in patients receiving methysergide therapy.[6] Mechanical obstruction of the valve can be due to a RA myxoma, tumor metastases, and thrombi in the RA, each resulting in the hemodynamic abnormalities of TS.[16,17] In addition, RV inflow tract obstruction can result from thrombosis endocarditis, degeneration, or calcification affecting a prosthetic tricuspid valve.

In rheumatic tricuspid valve disease, alterations in the valve are characterized by fibrosis, with contracture of the leaflets and commissural fusion. The former leads to TR and the latter to TS.[18] The stenotic component of rheumatic tricuspid valve disease is often minor and would go unrecognized clinically if it were not for the high flow across the valve caused by the coexistent regurgitation. Whenever the tricuspid valve is affected by rheumatic disease, there is also involvement of left-sided valves.[19] Flammang and associates observed that 9.5 per-

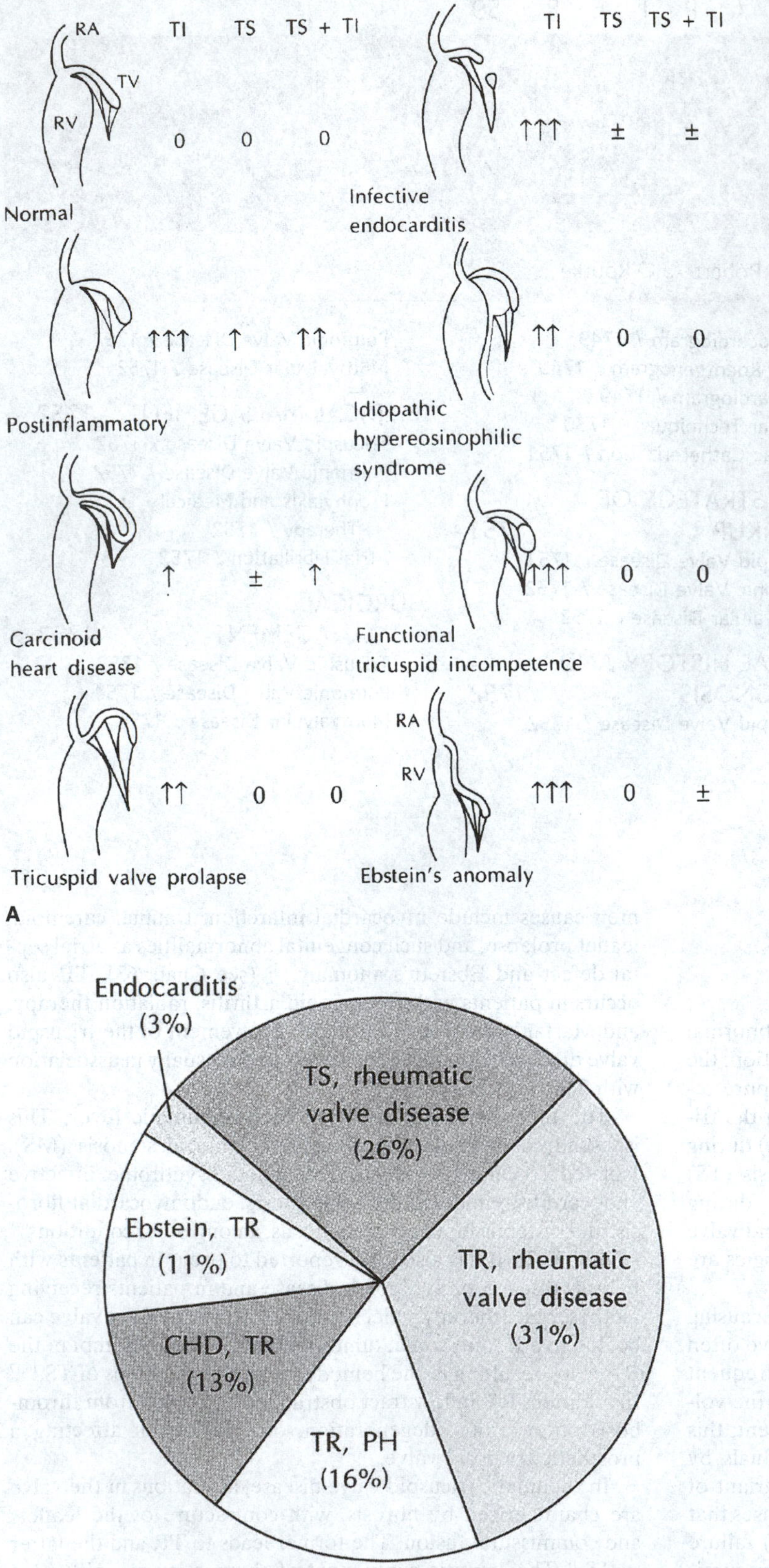

FIGURE 59-1 *A.* Tricuspid valve (TV) disease. Diagrammatic illustration of TV; TI, tricuspid insufficiency; TS, tricuspid stenosis; RA, right atrium; RV, right ventricle. *B.* Pathologic findings in TV. TR, tricuspid regurgitation; TS, tricuspid stenosis. [From Virmani R et al. Pathology of valvular heart diseases. In: Rahimtoola SH, ed. Philadelphia: Mosby (Current Medicine, Inc.), 1997:116, with permission.]

cent of cases requiring surgical replacement of *both* the mitral and aortic valves also had rheumatic involvement of the tricuspid valve.[20]

Carcinoid heart disease is present in up to 53 percent of patients with malignant carcinoid tumor (usually originating in the ileum) with extensive metastases[15] (see Chap. 77). Carcinoid usually causes TR and TS and, less often, pulmonic stenosis (PS) and pulmonic regurgitation (PR).[21,22] Changes include deposits of fibrous tissue on the surfaces of these valves. Fibrous plaques can also develop on the endocardial surfaces of the RA and RV as well as on the intima of the coronary sinus and the pulmonary artery.[23] The hemodynamic effects result from the rigidity and contracture of the fibrous tissues deposited on the valves. Although TS may result, the major functional abnormality is usually TR.

The most common type of TR is the secondary type that results from the enlargement of the orifice and annulus secondary to congestive heart failure with RV dilation due to LV disease (Table 59-1). TR may diminish when the heart failure is treated successfully but can be permanent with long-standing dilatation of the RV.[24–26] In infective endocarditis, the TR results from improper coaptation of the leaflets because of interposed vegetations (Table 59-1). Major degrees of regurgitation may be due to rupture of chordae tendineae of the RV or perforation of the valve leaflets.

Until recently, myocardial infarction was not considered a common cause of TR except when secondary to chronic congestive heart failure.[27] Rare cases have been described from rupture of an RV papillary muscle.[28,29] Currently, RV infarction is being recognized more often and is frequently associated with TR, as documented by echocardiography (see Chap. 42).

Various degrees of tricuspid valve prolapse are commonly present in the general population and may occur in 3 to 54 percent in patients with mitral valve prolapse[22] (see Chap. 58). The reported incidence of *severe* TR from prolapse is low.[30]

External blunt trauma, most often in motor vehicle accidents, is a classic cause of TR. Isolated instances of rupture of a tricuspid papillary muscle have been described from external cardiopulmonary resuscitation.[31] Traumatic TR usually results from rupture of one or more of the components of the tensor apparatus, with disruption of the papillary muscle occurring more often than rupture of the chordae.[13] Less frequently, there is a laceration of leaflet tissue.[32,33] Occasionally, traumatic TR and ruptured ventricular septum coexist[34] (Chap. 79). TR can also occur from iatrogenic trauma produced during an endomyocardial biopsy.[35,36] Mild TR often results when a pacemaker is placed across a normally functioning tricuspid valve or after extraction of permanent pacemaker leads.[37]

Tolerance to traumatic TR varies, with up to 39 years of survival reported.[38–40] Patients with rupture of a papillary muscle tend to tolerate the TR less well than do those in whom the trauma resulted in rupture of chordae.[39] Among reported cases of TR

TABLE 59-1 Diseases Causing Acquired Tricuspid Valve Regurgitation

Disease Causing Pulmonary Hypertension
All LV diseases with LV failure
Mitral stenosis or mitral regurgitation
Pulmonary venous obstruction
Diseases causing an increase in pulmonary vascular resistance
Primary pulmonary hypertension
Acquired pulmonary vascular disease (atrial septal defects), ventricular septal defects, and patent ductus arteriosus
Intrinsic pulmonary disease (chronic obstructive pulmonary disease, pulmonary fibrosis, and pulmonary resection)
Collagen vascular diseases
Pulmonary emboli, acute and chronic
Primary Diseases of the Tricuspid Valve
Rheumatic heart disease
Rheumatoid arthritis
Trauma, penetrating and nonpenetrating
Radiation therapy
Carcinoid heart disease
RA myxoma
Infective endocarditis
Eosinophilic myocarditis
Prosthetic and bioprosthetic valve malfunction, including thrombosis and calcification
RV myocardial infarction
Myxomatous tricuspid valve (tricuspid valve prolapse)

SOURCE: Modified from Cheitlin and MacGregor,[22] with permission.

resulting from the rupture of the chordae, a traumatic etiology is more common than is infective endocarditis.[41] Primary congenital lesions of the tricuspid valve that cause regurgitation are Ebstein's malformation and valvular dysplasia, as discussed in Chap. 64.

Pulmonic Valve Disease

Acquired lesions of the pulmonic valve generally cause PR (Table 59-3). On rare occasions, an inflammatory process can create stenosis and regurgitation of the valve. Pulmonary hypertension from any cause, such as MS, chronic lung disease, or pulmonary emboli, can produce PR. Inflammatory diseases, such as endocarditis, rheumatic fever, and, rarely, tuberculosis, can result in PR.[42–45]

PS is created by obstruction of systolic flow across the valve and is most commonly congenital (Fig. 59-3; see Chaps. 63 and 64). Sarcomas and myxomas can sometimes extend to the pulmonic valve, causing PS.[46] Previous cardiac surgery on a congenital pulmonic valve lesion can result in PR. The carcinoid syndrome with cardiac involvement can create mild PS and associated PR[44] (Fig. 59-4). Compression of the pulmonary artery can stimulate valvular stenosis and is rarely produced by tumor, aneurysm, or even constrictive pericarditis.

Multivalvular Disease

Multivalvular disease includes mixed single valve disease [e.g., aortic stenosis (AS) plus aortic regurgitation (AR)] or combined disease affecting two or more values (e.g., MS plus TR). Rheumatic fever remains an important cause of combined disease of the mitral and aortic valves. Primary involvement of the tricuspid valve in the rheumatic process is unusual, and more commonly TR results from RV failure secondary to LV decompensation in valvular heart disease. A high prevalence of anatomic lesions involving two or more valves is present when the characteristic Aschoff body is observed at necropsy.[47] Connective tissue diseases (see Chap. 76) can affect both the aortic and the mitral valves. For example, in Marfan's syndrome mitral valve prolapse, resulting in MR, often occurs together with the frequently observed changes in the aortic valve and ascending aorta. In the aging patient, calcification can develop in the aortic valve and the mitral valve apparatus as well as in the mitral annulus. Finally, infective endocarditis of the aortic or mitral valve can extend to the adjacent valve apparatus. In an autopsy series, combined aortic and mitral valve disease was observed in 33 percent of 996 patients with rheumatic fever.[48] In a 30-year follow-up of 1042 children with a history of rheumatic fever, multiple-valve involvement became apparent in 50 percent of

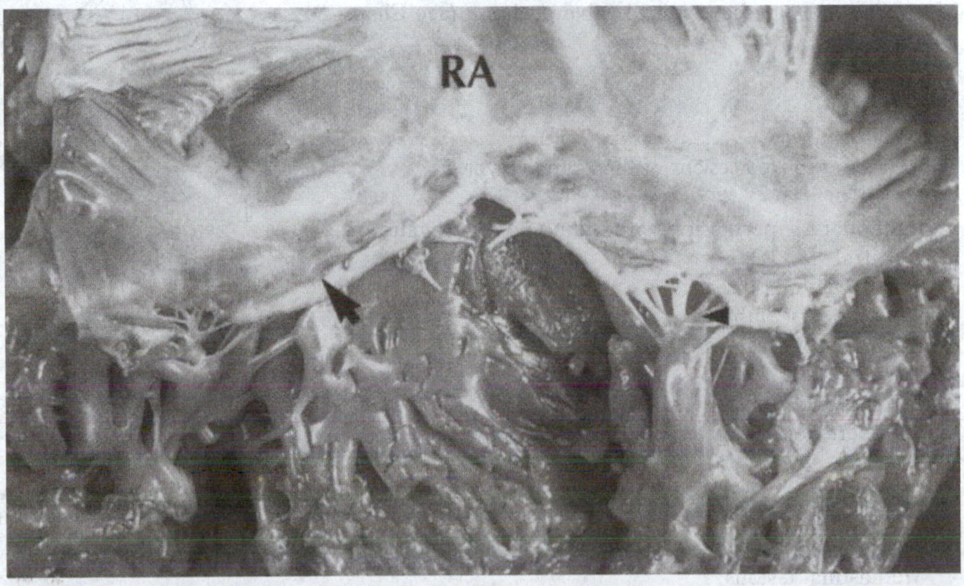

FIGURE 59-2 Heart displaying a tricuspid valve with fused, shortened chordae and rolled, thickened, fibrotic edge, consistent with chronic rheumatic heart disease. Isolated rheumatic TR or TS is very rare; it occurs almost always in the presence of concomitant MS. RA, right atrium. [From Farb A et al. Anatomy and pathology of the right ventricle (including acquired tricuspid and pulmonic valve disease). *Card Clin North Am* 1993; 10:1–2, with permission.]

TABLE 59-2 Diseases Causing Acquired Tricuspid Valve Stenosis

Rheumatic heart disease (usually with mitral stenosis)
Carcinoid heart disease
Fabry's disease
Whipple's disease
Endocardial fibroelastosis
Endomyocardial fibrosis
Methysergide therapy
Systemic lupus endocarditis
RA myxoma or thrombus
Prosthetic valve thrombosis
Prosthetic valve infective endocarditis
Paraprosthetic valve degeneration and calcification

SOURCE: Modified from Cheitlin and MacGregor,[22] with permission.

the individuals.[49] Bland and Jones followed 699 patients with cardiac involvement due to rheumatic fever for 20 years; 99 percent eventually exhibited aortic and mitral valve abnormalities.[50]

Rheumatic fever, myxomatous proliferation and prolapse, calcification in the aged, and infective endocarditis can impair both the aortic and mitral valves. The inflammatory process of rheumatic fever thickens and scars valve leaflets, which leads to fusion, fibrosis, and calcification (Fig. 59-5).

Myxomatous proliferation and valvular prolapse occur in the aortic, tricuspid, and pulmonic valves as well as in the mitral valve (Fig. 59-6). Fusiform aneurysms of the aortic sinus and ascending aorta can develop in Marfan's syndrome; a dilated annulus, prolapse, ruptured chordae, and annular calcification can affect the mitral valve (Fig. 59-7). Annular dilatation, with or without prolapse, is a major cause of mitral regurgitation (MR) in Marfan's syndrome,[51] and most of the patients with Marfan's syndrome have mitral valve prolapse (see Chaps. 60 and 76).

TABLE 59-3 Acquired Lesions of the Pulmonic Valve

Pulmonary hypertension with pulmonic regurgitation
Mitral stenosis
Chronic lung disease
Pulmonary emboli
Inflammatory lesions
Endocarditis
Rheumatic fever
Tuberculosis
Tumors
Sarcoma
Myxoma
Previous surgery or angioplasty for congenital lesions
Mediastinal lesions
Tumor
Aneurysm
Constrictive pericarditis
Miscellaneous
Carcinoid syndrome

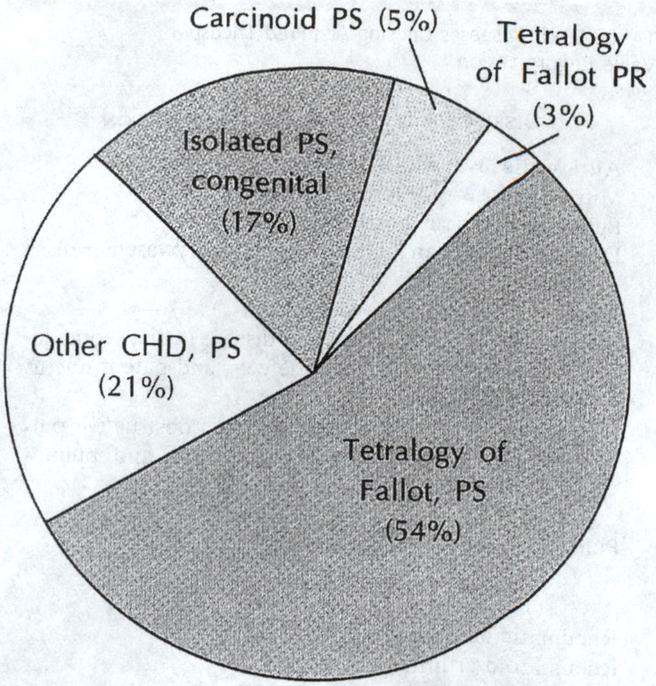

FIGURE 59-3 Pathologic findings in pulmonary valve (PV) replacement. CHD, congenital heart disease; PH, pulmonary hypertension; PR, pulmonary regurgitation; PS, pulmonary stenosis; TR, tricuspid regurgitation; TS, tricuspid stenosis. (Adapted from Altricher PM et al. Surgical pathology of the pulmonary valve; a study of 116 cases spanning 15 years. *Mayo Clin Proc* 1989; 64:1352–1360, with permission.)

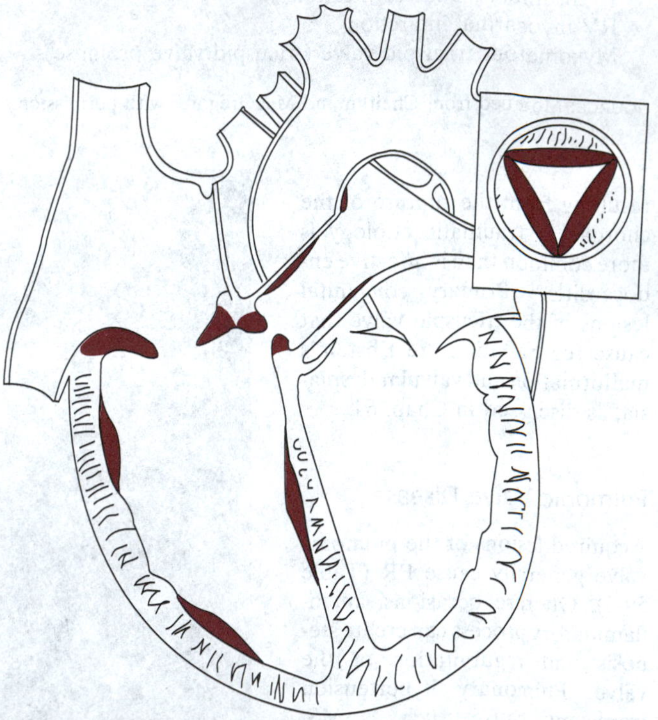

FIGURE 59-4 Carcinoid heart disease. The insert shows PS. The leaflets of the tricuspid valve are thickened. The valve is predominantly incompetent and causes PR. Fibrous plaques are deposited on the lining of the right ventricle and pulmonary trunk. (From Edwards JE. Effects of malignant noncardiac tumors upon the cardiovascular system. *Cardiovasc Clin* 1971; 4:282. Reproduced with permission from the publisher and author.)

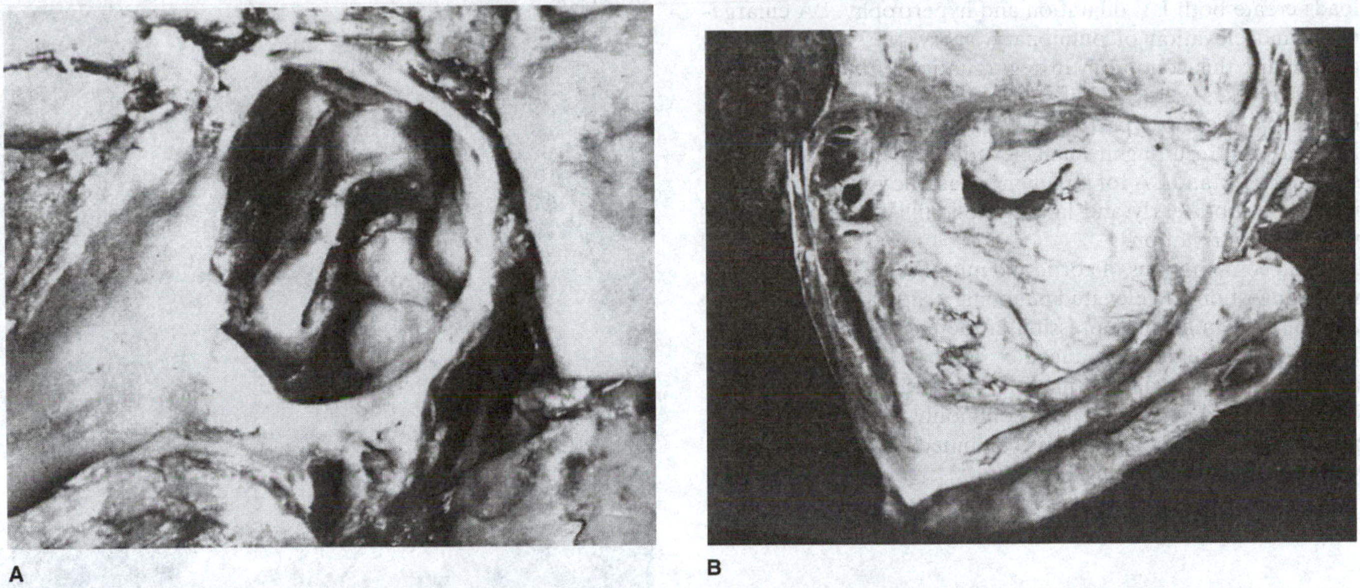

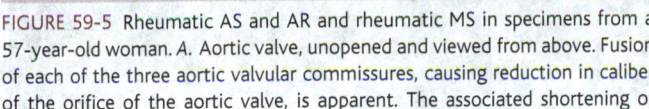

FIGURE 59-5 Rheumatic AS and AR and rheumatic MS in specimens from a 57-year-old woman. *A.* Aortic valve, unopened and viewed from above. Fusion of each of the three aortic valvular commissures, causing reduction in caliber of the orifice of the aortic valve, is apparent. The associated shortening of the cusps results in aortic regurgitation. *B.* Mitral valve, unopened and viewed from above, and opened LA. The mitral valve shows fusion at each of the commissures. The orifice is reduced in caliber. The LA is large, and calcification of the posterior part of the LA wall is present (lower part of figure).

In aging patients, calcification can involve the aortic and mitral valves. Aortic stenosis is common, whereas mitral annular calcification usually creates regurgitation (Fig. 59-8). Infective endocarditis can extend from either the aortic or the mitral valve to the adjacent valve through the inflammatory process (Fig. 59-9).

PATHOPHYSIOLOGY

Tricuspid Valve Disease

In TR, the systolic blood flow into the RA elevates the mean RA pressure.[52] Regurgitant flow produces a prominent *cv* wave reflected through the venous system. Diastolic volume overload of the RV causes further dilatation of the RV and movement of the intraventricular septum toward the LV during diastole. RV failure further raises the mean RA and vena caval pressures and results in systemic venous congestion and signs of RV failure.[22]

TR decreases diastolic flow across the valve, elevates the RA pressure, and reduces the cardiac output.[1,53,54] With TS, there is stiffening of the valve by fibrosis and commissural fusion, both of which narrow the effective valvular orifice.[1,22] Flow from systemic veins or RA into the RV is obstructed, and a pressure gradient develops in diastole between the RA and RV. The normal area of the tricuspid valve is 7 cm^2, and impairment of RV filling occurs when the valve area is reduced to less than 1.5 cm^2. Elevation of the mean RA pressure above 10 mmHg usually results in peripheral edema. Development of atrial fibrillation produces a higher RA pressure in TS than when sinus rhythm and normal RA contraction are present. The hemodynamic abnormalities in TS can be further influenced by coexisting MS. Reduced RV flow in tricuspid valve obstruction has been proposed as a mechanism for protection against severe pulmonary hypertension.

Pulmonic Valve Disease

Pulmonic regurgitation is the most frequently acquired lesion of the pulmonic valve (Table 59-3). Regurgitation may be secondary to pulmonary hypertension or may be caused by primary abnormalities in the leaflets. PR imposes a volume overload on the RV, and if pulmonic hypertension preexists, the overload is superimposed on hypertrophied myocardium. Volume overload of the RV may cause an increase in diastolic volume of the chamber, an increase in RV stroke volume, and subsequent RV failure, resulting in TR.[1,22] Fortunately, isolated PR can usually be tolerated for a long time without cardiac decompensation.[55]

Multivalvular Disease

Multiple valve diseases affecting the mitral and aortic valves can produce a pressure overload, volume overload, or combinations of the two.[1,22] In the presence of combined valvular lesions, the pressure overload will cause concentric LV hypertrophy, even if myocardial failure develops.[1,23] An LV volume overload will result from AR and MR, and further dilatation will follow, with development of heart failure.[1,22] The combination of MS and AR usually results in a volume overload on the LV associated with LV pressure-volume work and myocardial oxygen consumption.[56,57]

Important physiologic considerations in combined valvular disease are the predominance of a single valvular lesion in altering hemodynamics and the potential failure to identify the presence of a second abnormal valve. MS produces left atrial (LA) and pulmonary venous hypertension, with eventual pulmonary hypertension and RV failure, even though aortic stenosis may also be present. Despite the presence of MS, concomitant AS can create pressure overload and hypertrophy of the LV. When MR accompanies AS, the pressure and volume overloads create both LV dilatation and hypertrophy. LA enlargement and elevation of pulmonary artery pressure eventually accompany this condition. In regurgitation of both mitral and aortic valves, severe LV dilatation develops, accompanied by compensatory LV hypertrophy.[58] LV compliance increases in MR and AR, resulting in small elevations of end-diastolic pressure in the LV and LA for larger end-diastolic volumes.[59] Abnormalities in both early and late diastolic filling can accompany valvular regurgitation.[60]

In all combinations of aortic and mitral valve lesions, pulmonary congestion and elevated pulmonary capillary pressure usually follow significant depression of the contractile state of the LV. LA enlargement produced by either MS or MR is often associated with atrial fibrillation. Alterations in pulmonary blood flow and cardiac rhythm commonly accompany the LV pressure-volume overload in combined mitral and aortic valve disease.

TR usually accompanies RV dilatation secondary to pulmonary hypertension from any combination of mitral or aortic valve diseases. TS almost invariably is accompanied by disease of the mitral valve and can create significant elevations of the RA and central venous pressures.

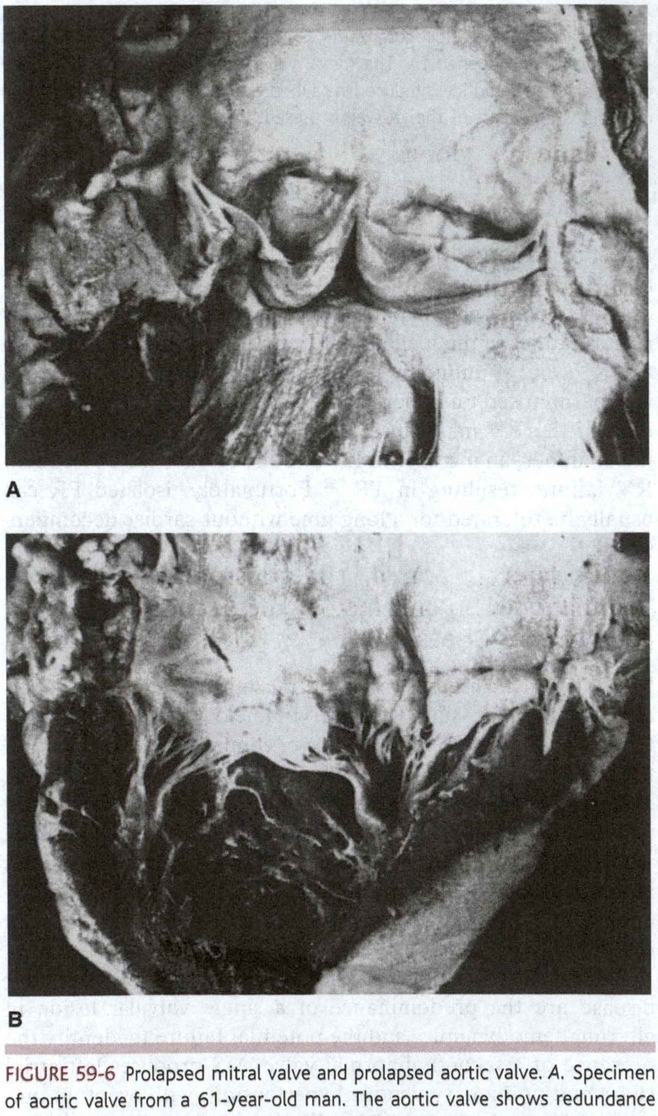

A B

FIGURE 59-6 Prolapsed mitral valve and prolapsed aortic valve. *A*. Specimen of aortic valve from a 61-year-old man. The aortic valve shows redundance or prolapse of its right cusp. *B*. Specimen of mitral valve from a 73-year-old woman. The mitral valve shows prominent evidence of prolapse involving the posterior leaflet (right) and the posterior half of the anterior leaflet.

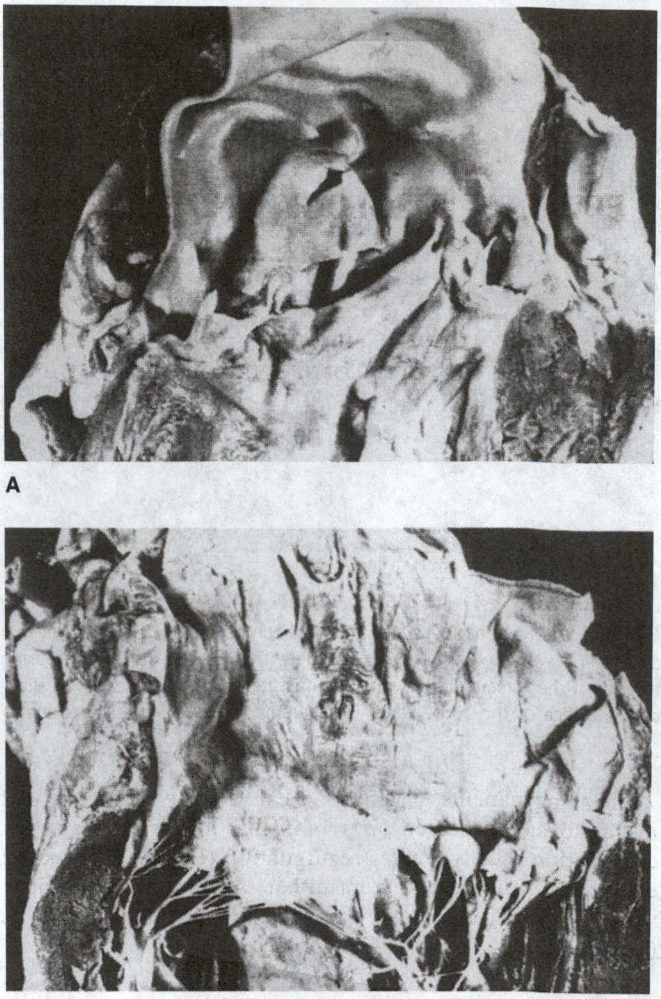

A B

FIGURE 59-7 Floppy mitral valve and limited dissecting aneurysm of the ascending aorta, leading to aortic regurgitation, in a specimen from a 60-year-old man. *A*. Ascending aorta and aortic valve. The ascending aorta exhibits a laceration leading to a false channel within the aortic wall in which a hematoma is present (seen on each side of the opened aorta). Secondary distortion of the aortic valvular mechanism caused aortic regurgitation. *B*. Mitral valve, LA, and a portion of the LV. The posterior leaflet of the mitral valve (right) shows several areas of prolapse.

CLINICAL MANIFESTATIONS

Symptoms

TRICUSPID VALVE DISEASE

Since TR generally accompanies LV failure or MS, presenting symptoms include dyspnea, orthopnea, and peripheral edema.[61] Even though LV failure is usually present, paroxysmal nocturnal

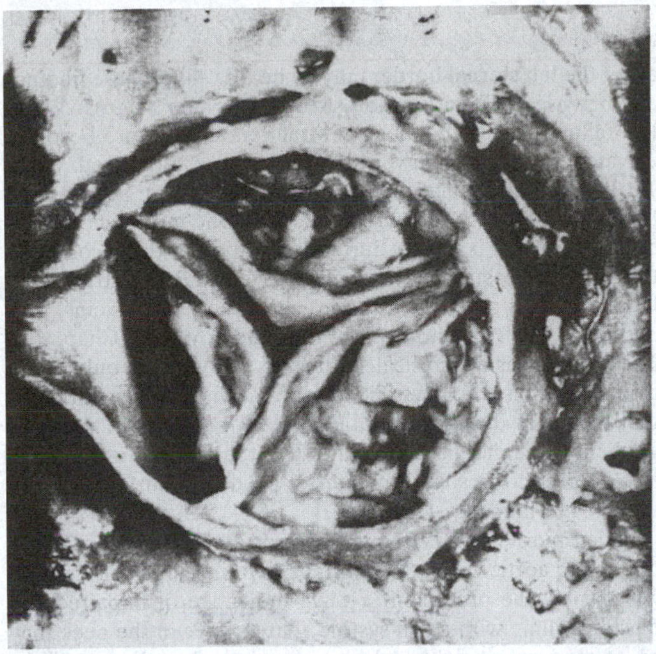

A

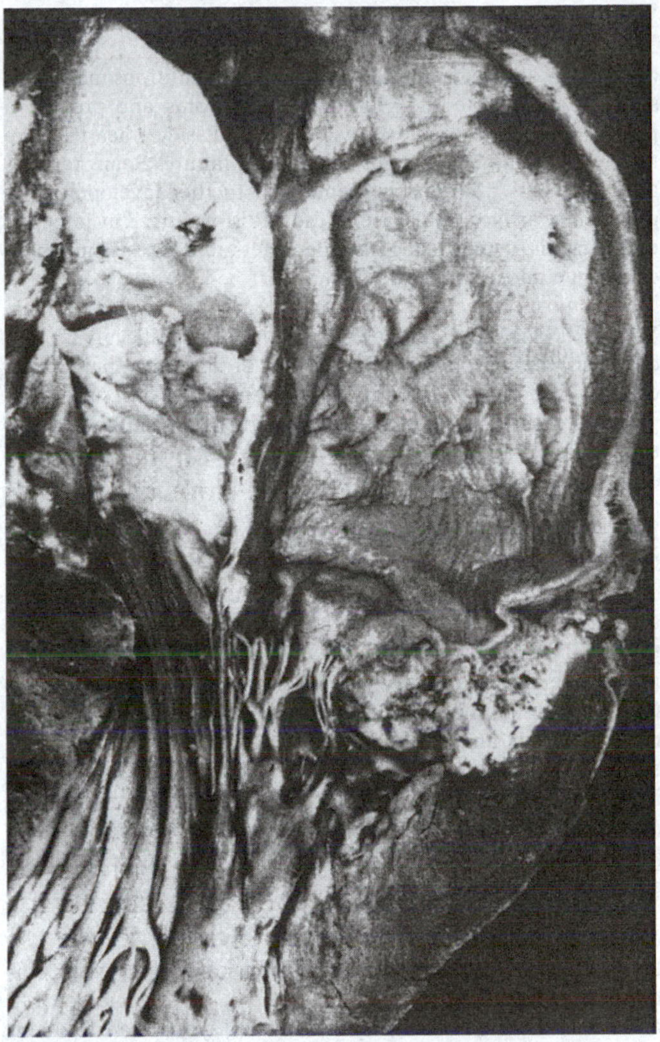

B

FIGURE 59-8 Senile calcific AS and calcification of the mitral ring in specimens from two individuals. *A.* Aortic valve. Classic example of senile calcific aortic stenosis in the unopened aortic valve viewed from above. *B.* LA, mitral valve, and lateral wall of LV. Sagittal section through LA and LV walls reveals a calcified mass at the junction of the LA, the LV, and the posterior mitral leaflet.

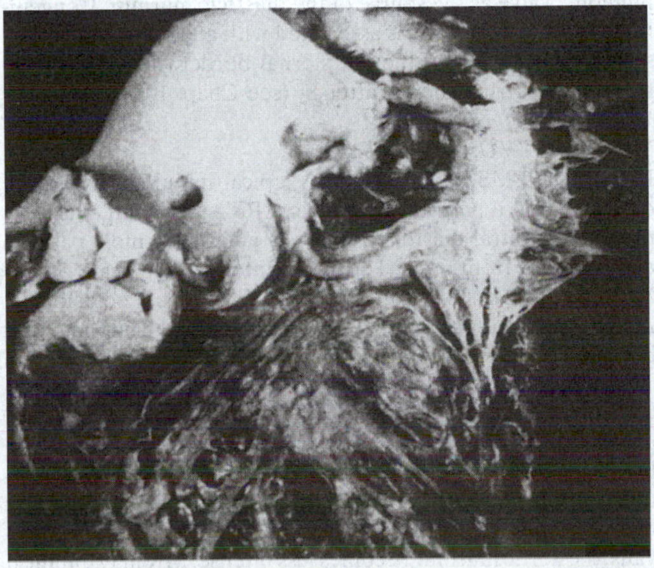

A

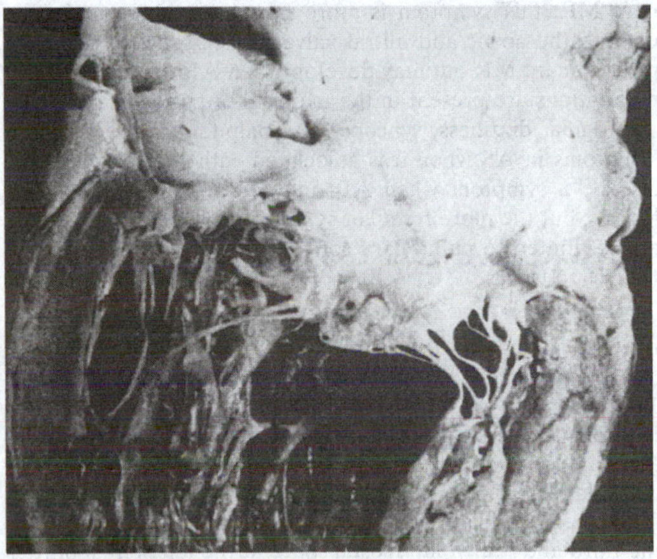

B

FIGURE 59-9 Bacterial endocarditis in specimens from a 36-year-old man. *A.* Aortic valve. The base of the aortic valve shows major destruction of a cusp with extension of inflammation onto the subjacent mitral valve. Near the free edge of the mitral valve, its ventricular aspect shows an ostium of a nonruptured mycotic aneurysm. *B.* Mitral valve, LA, and LV. The lobulated mycotic aneurysm of the mitral valve lies near its free edge.

dyspnea is often absent. TR under these conditions may occasionally ameliorate the pulmonary symptoms and provide a physiologic basis for the alleviation of left-sided heart failure by the development of right-sided heart failure. Some patients also have less pulmonary edema due to the development of pulmonary arteriolar disease. If the TR is produced by infective endocarditis, symptoms of febrile illness may be accompanied by fatigue and peripheral edema.

The most frequent symptoms in TS are dyspnea and fatigue. When MS coexists, the development of significant TS can diminish the paroxysmal symptoms of dyspnea, pulmonary congestion, and pulmonary hypertension.[16,17] Occasionally, patients with TS complain of prominent pulsations in the neck veins, which may precede the development of peripheral edema.

PULMONIC VALVE DISEASE

Clinical manifestations of acquired pulmonic valvular lesions depend on the severity of the hemodynamic impairment as well as on the extent of the underlying disease. Isolated PR can be tolerated without symptoms. Severe pulmonary hypertension may cause syncope in addition to shortness of breath and fatigue. With inflammatory lesions of the pulmonic valve, febrile manifestations and pulmonary infection may be present. The carcinoid syndrome is characterized by episodes of facial flushing, increased intestinal activity, diarrhea, and bronchospasm (see Chap. 77). Tumors involving the pulmonic valve may exert pressure from expansion and metastases that affect the heart and lungs.

MULTIVALVULAR DISEASE

Dyspnea is the most frequent complaint of patients with combined mitral and aortic valve disease.[1,22,62] With combined MS and AS, chest discomfort, palpitations, and syncope are frequent clinical manifestations. Symptoms of heart failure result from pulmonary congestion and usually include fluid retention. Although angina pectoris is uncommon in patients with predominant MR, this symptom is more frequent with regurgitation of both the aortic and mitral valves. Also, syncope is rare in predominant MR but may develop when AR and MR coexist; palpitations are present in the majority of patients.

Angina, dizziness, syncope, and palpitations are common symptoms in AS when it is associated with MR. Angina may also be a symptom when AR and MS are the predominant lesions; but the more frequent symptoms, dyspnea and fatigue, are attributed to pulmonary congestion and heart failure (see Chaps. 56 to 58).

Physical Examination

TRICUSPID VALVE DISEASE

In patients with primary TR not due to pulmonary hypertension, there are large *v* waves in the jugular venous pulse (JVP). There is a dilated RV with a precordial lift and right-sided third or fourth heart sounds. There is usually a long systolic murmur in the third and fourth intercostal space at the left sternal border that increases with inspiration. The murmur is often confined to early and mid-systole or may not be heard at all when there is small gradient between the RV and RA during systole and a large regurgitant orifice (see Chap. 10). When a large amount of blood returns to the RV in diastole, a short diastolic rumble along the left sternal border may be heard. All of these findings are increased with inspiration (Rivero Carvallo's sign).[63] When RV failure occurs, the mean central venous pressure becomes elevated, and the jugular veins are pulsatile and engorged. When TR is due to pulmonary hypertension, there is an accentuated P_2, and a high-pitched decrescendo diastolic murmur of PR is often heard that is louder during inspiration in the second and third left intercostal spaces. In patients with TR and atrial fibrillation, there is a prominent *cv* wave in the jugular veins, produced by the regurgitant flow into the RV (see Chap. 10). The characteristic physical finding of TR due to pulmonary hypertension is a holosystolic murmur at the left sternal border that increases during inspiration; there is a RV-RA pressure gradient throughout systole. Although the murmur of MR may also be present, respiration exerts a predominant influence on the TR murmur (see Chap. 10).

Tricuspid stenosis is frequently associated with lesions of the mitral and aortic valves. When sinus rhythm is present, the JVP will display the prominent *a* wave indicative of impaired RV diastolic filling with atrial systole. The *a* wave in the neck may be of moderate height and sometimes reaches the mandible. Auscultation of the heart is required to confirm that the rise of the venous *a* wave is simultaneous with the first heart sound. The *cv* wave is small, and the *y* descent is slow and insignificant (see Chap. 10).

PULMONIC VALVE DISEASE

If RV failure and TR have developed as a result of PR, a prominent *cv* wave will be present in the JVP. Increased RV activity may be visible and palpable along the left sternal border. If pulmonic hypertension is present, the pulmonic second sound will be accentuated over the left upper sternal border. The murmur of acquired PR is a high-pitched diastolic blow along the left sternal border. Thus, the murmur may be difficult to differentiate from the murmur of AR, but the absence of peripheral findings of AR is useful in identifying regurgitation of the pulmonic valve as the source of the diastolic murmur. Congenital PR characteristically is associated with a low-pitched, decrescendo murmur along the left sternal border, the peak of the murmur occurring shortly after P_2 (see Chap. 10).

MULTIVALVULAR DISEASE

In combined MS and AS, the LV apical impulse may not be displaced, but a palpable parasternal RV systolic lift is usually present. A mitral diastolic rumble is audible in most patients and can vary from grade I to III in intensity (on scale of I to VI). The aortic systolic murmur is usually loud, but occasionally may be faint with severe MS. A mitral opening snap may not be audible, and in some patients the diastolic rumble of MS cannot be heard.

When both AR and MR exist, the diastolic arterial blood pressure is usually less than 70 mmHg. In those with a diastolic blood pressure above 70 mmHg, there is usually a loud holosystolic mitral murmur. If AR is the dominant lesion, the early diastolic murmur is usually prominent, whereas when MR prevails, the aortic murmur becomes less intense. MR may diminish the AR due to the increased LV diastolic filling from the enlarged LA. Depending on the contractile state of the myocardium, loud regurgitant murmurs may be associated with mild regurgitation, whereas faint murmurs may accompany severe valvular regurgitation if myocardial failure has developed. A diastolic "flow murmur" across the mitral valve is heard in the majority of patients with combined MR and AR. If AR is important, a systolic murmur produced by the large forward flow across the aortic valve often is present (see Chap. 10).

When AR and MS are both present, the LV impulse is also displaced, sustained, and forceful. The early diastolic murmur at the apex may be prominent and may be accentuated by the AR flow striking the anterior leaflet of the stenotic mitral valve. Although the low-pitched diastolic murmur of MS and the diastolic flow murmur with AR are usually reliable diagnostic parameters, neither murmur correlates with the hemodynamic measurements when the two lesions coexist.

When AR is combined with MS, the systemic pulse pressure does not necessarily reflect the severity of AR. A prominent apical impulse in apparently pure MS indicates the likelihood of associated AR but may not indicate its severity. Finally, the intensity of the aortic diastolic murmur is of little value in predicting the severity of AR in the presence of MS (Chap. 10).

In the presence of AS and possible MR, an apical holosystolic murmur is reasonable evidence for associated MR, but the intensity of the murmur is not a reliable indicator in estimating severity.

While the murmur of TR often increases with inspiration, distinction from a concomitant MR murmur may be difficult. Identification of the rumble of TS requires careful auscultation during inspiration at the left lower sternal border. Detection by auscultation is more difficult because of the frequent association of MS and TS.

Electrocardiogram

TRICUSPID VALVE DISEASE

Atrial fibrillation is frequent in patients with TR. When TR results from myocardial infarction, acute or chronic electrocardiographic (ECG) changes will be seen in the inferior leads, and ST-segment elevation indicating RV infarction may be present in the right-sided precordial leads. The characteristic ECG finding in TS is a large P wave of RA enlargement in the absence of RV hypertrophy[1,22,64] (see Chap. 11).

PULMONIC VALVE DISEASE

Although there are no characteristic changes with pulmonic valvular lesions, preexisting pulmonary hypertension will produce RV hypertrophy, right-axis deviation, and changes in the *p* wave, suggesting RA enlargement. If pulmonary hypertension is secondary to mitral stenosis, P mitrale, with characteristic notches, will be present in lead II (see Chap. 11).

MULTIVALVULAR DISEASE

In combined MS and AS, ECG evidence of LV hypertrophy, LA enlargement, and atrial fibrillation is often present. Similar findings are observed in MR and AR, with a high likelihood of LA and LV enlargement along with atrial fibrillation. With AS and MR, LV hypertrophy is accompanied by a moderate incidence of atrial fibrillation. MS with severe AR also produces LV hypertrophy.

Chest Roentgenogram

TRICUSPID VALVE DISEASE

TR may produce some degree of RA enlargement, but there will usually be accompanying RV enlargement.[61] In TS, the most characteristic radiographic finding is prominence of the RA without significant pulmonary arterial enlargement or changes due to pulmonary hypertension[1,22] (see Chap. 12).

PULMONIC VALVE DISEASE

Patients with PR have pulmonary artery prominence along with an increase in RV dimensions. If PS is acquired, there may be poststenotic dilatation or prominence of the main pulmonary artery.

MULTIVALVULAR DISEASE

With combined MS and AS, the LA is always enlarged. LV chamber size may be significantly enlarged; however, prominent RV dimensions are usually present. Valvular calcification at either site is relatively uncommon. In AS accompanied by MR, heart size is increased, with both LV and LA enlargement. In MS with AR, marked LV enlargement is often present.

Echocardiogram

TRICUSPID VALVE DISEASE

With TR, there may be echocardiographic evidence of systolic prolapse, rupture of the chordae or papillary muscle, or vegetative lesions on the valve.[65] Increased RV dimensions indicate impaired RV function and the likelihood of secondary TR (see Chap. 13). Contrast echocardiography with peripheral venous injection can identify the back-and-forth flow across the valve.[66] The echo-Doppler technique can estimate the severity of the regurgitation and the systolic pressure in the RV[67] (Fig. 59-10). Color-flow Doppler imaging can delineate the patterns and sites of regurgitation across the valve apparatus[71] (see Chap. 13).

A characteristic pattern of TS can often be recorded with the echocardiogram. Fibrosis and calcification of the valve can be identified. Obstructive lesions, such as myxoma, thrombus, or other tumors, can be recognized echocardiographically. The two-dimensional echocardiogram of a patient with carcinoid syndrome with both TR and TS is shown in Fig. 59-11*A* and *B*. The echo-Doppler technique can be used to estimate the diastolic gradient across the valve with generally good accuracy (see Chap. 13).

PULMONIC VALVE DISEASE

Echocardiography can delineate the anatomy of the pulmonic valve as well as intrinsic or extrinsic lesions impinging on the valve apparatus. Sometimes a vegetative lesion or tumor can be detected in the pulmonic valve area. The echo-Doppler technique can estimate both the severity of both the regurgitation and the stenosis of the valve,[68] and analysis of echo-Doppler recordings can provide estimates of pulmonary artery pressure[69–71] (Fig. 59-12). Color-flow imaging can further confirm the patterns of regurgitation in the RV outflow tract (see Chap. 13).

MULTIVALVULAR DISEASE

Echocardiography provides information on valve anatomy, chamber dimensions, pressure gradients, valve size, patterns of regurgitation, and estimates of ventricular function. MS and AS produce characteristic echoes (see Chap. 13). Prolapse of mitral, aortic, and tricuspid valves can be characteristically recognized with echocardiography.[72] The number of aortic cusps can be identified, as can the presence of calcium in the aortic or mitral

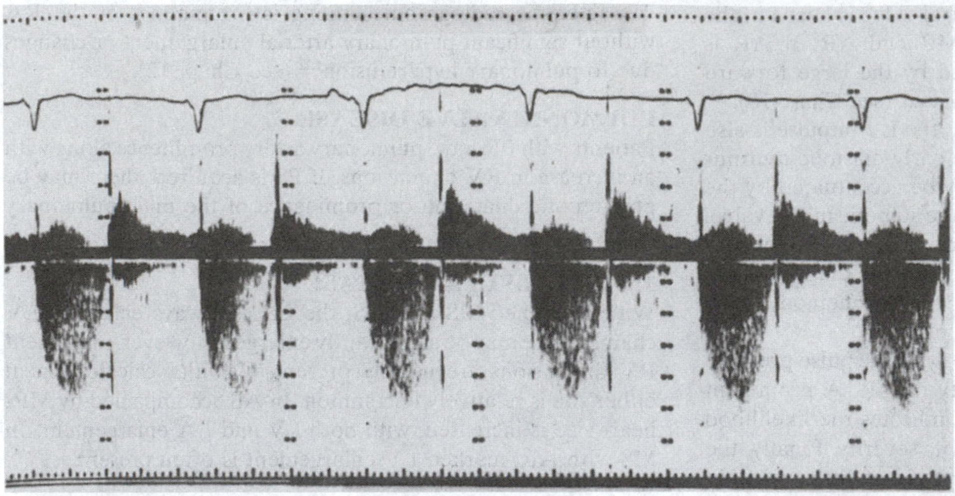

FIGURE 59-10 A continuous echo-Doppler recording in a patient with tricuspid valve disease illustrates TR in the lower portion and TS in the upper portion of the tracing. (Reproduced with permission from and courtesy of Dr. Pamela Sears-Rogan.)

valve apparatus. Dimensions of the LA, LV, and RV, together with LV wall thickness measurements and determinations of mass, are useful in estimating the extent of volume and pressure overload. Two-dimensional and Doppler echocardiographic techniques can assess the orifice size of the aortic and mitral valves and estimate the valve gradients accurately.[73,74] Even in the presence of AR, appropriate modifications in the mathematical analysis of the pressure gradient can yield reasonably accurate estimates of the aortic valve gradients (see Chap. 13). Color-flow Doppler readings can identify patterns and sites of valvular regurgitation across the aortic and mitral valves.[75,76] Also, thrombus formation in the LA and LV can be detected with various echocardiographic methods. Transesophageal echocardiography can accurately assess prosthetic valve function and valvular repair during the operative procedures.

Nuclear Techniques

A radionuclide ventriculogram (RNV) can delineate dimensions of the RA and RV, which may help differentiate between TS and TR (see Chap. 16). RV size and function can be evaluated in stenotic and regurgitant lesions of the pulmonic valve. Myocardial perfusion imaging techniques are useful in detecting RV infarction as a cause of TR as well as in providing estimates of RV function. RV size and function can be evaluated in stenotic and regurgitant lesions of the pulmonic valve.

Quantitative information on LV function at rest and during exercise can be provided by RNV (see Chap. 16). Segmental wall motion can be assessed at rest and during exercise and

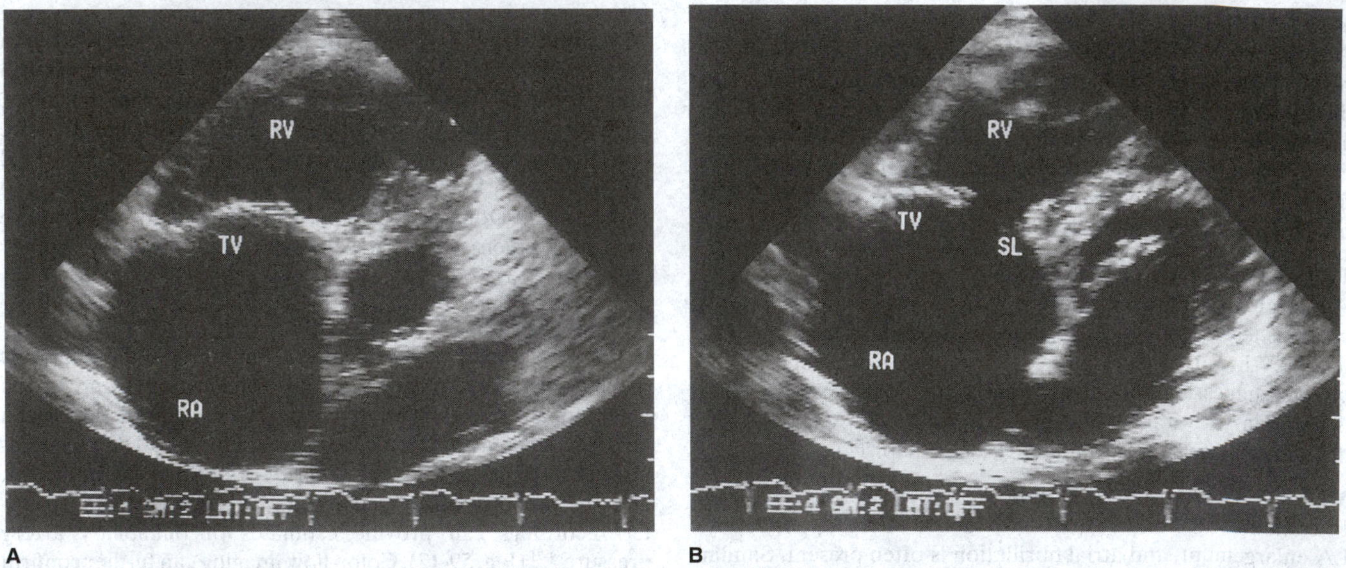

FIGURE 59-11 *A.* Two-dimensional echocardiogram of a 40-year-old patient, with carcinoid tumor of the testes without metastases. He presented with a testicular mass and was found to have a grade III/VI pansystolic murmur and grade III/VI diastolic murmur; both increased with inspiration. This four-chamber view shows a thickened stenotic tricuspid valve (TV) in diastole. The RA is enlarged, and the atrial septum bulges to the left, indicating a higher RA than LA pressure, which is consistent with tricuspid stenosis. The liver was normal because the humoral products of the carcinoid tumor bypassed the liver by the testicular venous drainage flowing directly to the inferior vena cava and renal veins. Carcinoid tumors arise from neuroendocrine cells known as enterochromaffin cells, which are found in organs derived from the embryonic gut. Because the liver detoxifies the humoral products of the carcinoid tumor, which most often arises in the ileum, it is extremely rare to see carcinoid heart disease in the absence of liver metastases, making this case extremely unusual.[4,5] Only about 20% of patients with carcinoid tumors develop cardiovascular symptoms. RV, right ventricle; SL, septal leaflet. *B.* Two-dimensional echocardiogram in diastole. This is from the same patient as in (*A*). Note the thickened tricuspid valve (TV) and the lack of excursion of the TV from diastole to systole. This washer-like, thickened TV is characteristic of carcinoid heart disease. It is common for a carcinoid TV to be both stenotic and insufficient. With carcinoid TV disease the valve becomes thickened, and its mobility and flexibility are reduced. RA, right atrium; RV, right ventricle. (From Cheitlin and MacGregor,[22] with permission.)

may assist in the recognition of underlying coronary artery disease. Since combined lesions of the aortic and mitral valves often create pulmonary hypertension and RV dysfunction, RNV is useful in estimating the RV ejection fraction[77] (see Chap. 16).

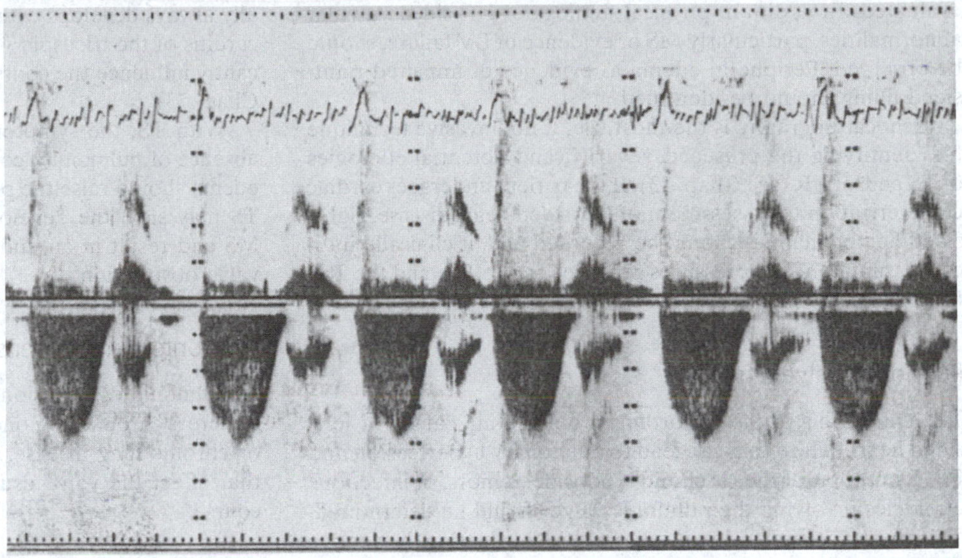

FIGURE 59-12 An echo-Doppler continuous tracing in a patient with TR. By employing the equation, the systolic gradient across the tricuspid valve can be calculated, and the addition of 10 mmHg yields an estimate of the pulmonary systolic pressure. Thus, in this patient, the level of pulmonary hypertension could be estimated from the echo-Doppler tracing of the TR. (Reproduced with permission from and courtesy of Dr. Pamela Sears-Rogan.)

Cardiac Catheterization

TRICUSPID VALVE DISEASE

Accurate angiographic documentation of TR is difficult to obtain because the catheter overrides the tricuspid valve, and ventricular irritability with an RV injection can induce TR. A prominent *cv* wave in the RA suggests TR, and an intracardiac phonocardiogram may record a regurgitation murmur in the absence of Rivero Carvallo's sign.[78]

If TS is clinically suspected, simultaneous pressures should be recorded in the RA and in the RV in order to measure the gradient across the valve accurately.[59] Since the normal gradient across the tricuspid valve is less than 1 mmHg, small gradients may not be detected if pullback pressure is recorded from the RV to the RA. The area of the tricuspid valve in TS is usually less than 1.5 cm^2; in severe TS, it is less than 1 cm^2.

PULMONIC VALVE DISEASE

PR is not readily demonstrated angiographically, but a right-sided injection can outline the pulmonary valve as well as show poststenotic dilatation. An aortic root injection can be helpful in the elimination of AR as the etiology of a diastolic murmur along the left sternal border. Nevertheless, this distinction is usually best made by echo-Doppler studies.

MULTIVALVULAR DISEASE

Cardiac catheterization is appropriate for most patients with combined valvular heart disease in order to calculate the stenotic and regurgitant status of each valve as well as to identify the predominant valvular lesion. Gradients across the valve can be measured with precision and the valve area calculated. Pulmonary hypertension is commonly present in these patients, and LV end-diastolic pressure is often elevated despite the presence of MS (see Chap. 15).

In MR plus AR, the LV end-diastolic pressure is elevated in most patients, and the central aortic pressure is generally greater than 40 mmHg. As noted, however, in approximately one-third of the patients the central aortic diastolic pressure may be above 70 mmHg. The *v* wave of MR can be recorded in the wedge position, and capillary and pulmonary arterial pressures are abnormally elevated in most of these patients.

In AS with MR, LV end-diastolic and pulmonary artery pressures are elevated; however, the extent of pressure elevation does not necessarily reflect the severity of the MR. When it is severe, forward cardiac output may be reduced; thus, a spuriously small pressure gradient may be recorded across a significantly stenotic aortic valve. In MS with AR, the LV end-diastolic pressure is abnormal and the central aortic diastolic pressure is usually less than 70 mmHg.

In combined valvular lesions, the measurement of total angiographic LV stroke volume is useful in calculating the regurgitant volume across each valve.[1,22] When both valves are regurgitant, it is more difficult to calculate the regurgitant volume across each valve.

Assessment of ventricular function is important in patients with combined valvular lesions; yet the ejection fraction may be spuriously normal or elevated in MR and, to a lesser extent, in AR. Measurements of LV end-systolic pressure, volume, and wall thickness permit calculation of end-systolic wall stress.[79] This parameter has been particularly helpful in pressure and volume overload conditions, since the end-systolic pressure-volume wall stress calculation is relatively independent of loading conditions.

Finally, coronary arteriography should be performed at the time of cardiac catheterization in patients above the age of 35, since coronary artery disease may be present without symptoms and may contribute to LV dysfunction. Coronary artery bypass grafting at the time of valve surgery is an important consideration.

USUAL STRATEGY OF WORKUP

Tricuspid Valve Disease

The history should identify underlying conditions, such as rheumatic fever, systemic disorders, and left-sided heart failure, as etiologies for tricuspid valve disease. The physical examination should carefully define the waveforms in the JVP. The auscultatory changes of systolic and diastolic murmurs at the left lower sternal border during the respiratory cycle should be carefully evaluated. In addition, physical findings of left-sided valvular abnormalities, particularly MS or evidence of LV failure, should be observed. Peripheral edema as evidence of impaired right-sided filling should be identified.

Echocardiography is the most useful noninvasive technique for identifying the presence, severity, and potential etiologies of TS and/or TR (see Chap. 13). If the patient undergoes cardiac catheterization for assessment of left-sided heart disease, right-sided hemodynamics should be recorded and, if clinically indicated, simultaneous pressures recorded in the RA and the RV (see Chap. 15).

Pulmonic Valve Disease

The clinical history is important in delineating causes of left-sided heart failure that can lead to pulmonary hypertension and PR. Symptoms of the carcinoid syndrome, tumors, or infectious etiologies involving the pulmonic valve should be determined. The physical examination is important in evaluating the venous pulsations in the neck veins as well as the pulmonic murmurs. RV prominence should be carefully evaluated, as should concomitant left-sided valve lesions and evidence of heart failure. Although an ECG and chest x-ray should be obtained to assess the pulmonic artery, RV outflow tract, and body of the RV, the most useful noninvasive technique is echocardiography. The anatomy, competence of the valve, extent of the regurgitation, and stenosis can be recognized and assessed by an echo-Doppler sudy. In addition, other valve lesions affecting the left side of the heart can be documented. Since PR can be relatively well tolerated, this specific lesion does not require such frequent follow-up, but underlying mechanisms for pulmonary hypertension or left-sided heart failure should be monitored closely.

Multivalvular Disease

Symptoms of dyspnea, exercise intolerance, chest discomfort, or syncope should be elicited during a carefully taken clinical history. On physical examination, special attention should be directed to the peripheral and central arterial pulses and the JVP. Heart size, precordial movement, and auscultatory findings should be carefully noted. A 12-lead ECG and posterior-anterior and lateral chest films should be obtained. Echocardiography is indicated to delineate valve anatomy, measure valve gradients, recognize regurgitant patterns, calculate orifice size, and estimate ventricular function and wall motion (see Chap. 13). A limited exercise test with or without radionuclide studies may help determine the exercise capacity as well as detect functional deterioration, chest pain, arrhythmias, deterioration of ventricular ejection fraction, or segmental wall motion abnormalities. If symptoms are atypical and the extent of valvular or LV function cannot be satisfactorily evaluated by noninvasive techniques, cardiac catheterization is indicated.

NATURAL HISTORY AND PROGNOSIS

Tricuspid Valve Disease

With TR due to RV hypertension, the symptoms and clinical course are primarily related to the left-sided heart conditions that produce a pressure-volume overload on the RV. TR virtually always develops with severe RV failure. In infective endocarditis of the tricuspid valve, the type of organism may significantly influence the course and the response to antibiotics (see Chap. 73).

With TS, the symptoms are usually those of MS, and the absence of pulmonary congestion in the presence of peripheral edema should raise the possibility of underlying TS. Significant TS may slow the development of characteristic symptoms of MS and result in an underestimation of the severity of mitral valve obstruction.

Pulmonic Valve Disease

In pulmonic valve lesions, the course will be more prolonged if there is chronic pulmonary hypertension due to mitral stenosis or chronic lung disease. Inflammatory conditions and tumors that affect the valve usually result in a much shorter clinical course.

Multivalvular Disease

When combined aortic and mitral valve disease are due to rheumatic fever, 10 years or more may elapse before the development of significant murmurs, and an additional decade (or more) may elapse before symptoms become manifest. If lesions of the aortic and mitral valves are due to degenerative collagen changes, symptoms may develop later in life. When combined lesions are due to calcific changes in the aortic valve and annulus as well as the mitral valve annulus, symptoms develop much later in life. There may, however, be rapid progression of degenerative aortic calcific stenosis over a 2- to 3-year period (see Chap. 56).

MEDICAL MANAGEMENT

Tricuspid Valve Disease

With TR, treatment of RV failure requires digitalis and diuretics, and vasodilating agents are also required for the management of LV failure (see Chap. 21). If failure of the right side of the heart is caused by MS, early intervention to enlarge or replace the mitral valve is appropriate (see Chap. 57).

In TS, the usual precautionary measures of antibiotic coverage and prevention of endocarditis apply. Peripheral edema may not respond well to administration of digitalis, diuretics, and vasodilator therapy, thus emphasizing the clinical importance of detecting underlying TS. Tricuspid balloon valvuloplasty has been used successfully in patients with predominant TS.[80]

Pulmonic Valve Disease

Patients with congenital pulmonic valve stenosis are usually best treated by catheter balloon valvotomy (see Chaps. 63 and 64).

Prophylaxis and Medical Therapy

Antibiotic prophylaxis against endocarditis (see Chap. 73) is appropriate for patients with either tricuspid or pulmonic valve lesions. If pulmonary emboli contribute to the pulmonary hypertension, anticoagulation is indicated (see Chap. 53). Further treatment of pulmonary hypertension may require managementof left heart failure, correction of MS, or the use of vasodilating agents that can lower pulmonary artery pressure. Vasodilating agents are often ineffective in treating primary pulmonary hypertension (see Chap. 52).

If rheumatic fever is the likely etiology of combined aortic and mitral valve disease, prophylactic penicillin should usually be continued until age 35 years (see Chap. 55). Dental prophylaxis with antibiotic coverage, using either amoxicillin or erythromycin, should be provided in all patient groups prior to dental procedures. For genitourinary or other abdominal procedures, gram-negative antibiotic coverage should be provided (see Chap. 82).

Atrial Fibrillation

If atrial fibrillation develops, chronic anticoagulation with low-dose warfarin [International Normalized Ratio (INR) 2.0 to 3.0] is warranted, since the accompanying incidence of systemic and cerebral emboli is estimated at 10 to 20 percent (see Chap. 61).

The early development of atrial fibrillation associated with hemodynamic deterioration warrants an initial attempt at electrical cardioversion. If this is successful, digitalis as well as antiarrhythmic preparations should be administered thereafter for prophylaxis against recurrence (see Chap. 24). Chronic atrial fibrillation should be controlled with digitalis, beta blockers, and calcium blockers as indicated. The development of symptoms, particularly dyspnea, limited exercise activity, chest pain, and syncope, warrants consideration for surgery. It is usually recommended for New York Heart Association (NYHA) class III symptoms despite adequate medical therapy.

SURGICAL MANAGEMENT

Tricuspid Valve Disease

The decision to proceed with valvular heart surgery is usually based on the severity of the aortic and mitral valve disease, rather than on the severity of the disease of the tricuspid valve. The usual decisions to be made regarding the tricuspid valve are (1) whether a procedure should be added to the mitral and/or aortic valve procedures and, (2) if so, which procedure—annuloplasty or valve replacement—should be performed. Patients may present with mild mitral valve disease but severe tricuspid valve dysfunction. Such patients may require an operation on the tricuspid valve only.

The severity of the symptoms and clinical signs of tricuspid valve disease are used to determine the indications for tricuspid valve surgery. If there are signs of TS and, particularly, if stenosis is demonstrated by cardiac catheterization and two-dimensional echocardiography, the tricuspid valve is directly visualized at operation with the anticipation of performing commissurotomy or valve replacement. Tricuspid valve balloon valvulotomy has been advocated for[80–84] TS of various etiologies.[82] However, severe TR is a common consequence of this procedure, and results are poor when severe TR develops.

When there are signs of severe TR secondary to MS, it is important to document the duration of the regurgitation and the severity and duration of pulmonary artery hypertension. If the TR is severe and long-standing and if there is chronic pulmonary artery hypertension, it is unlikely to resolve in the early postoperative period after mitral valve surgery alone. In this circumstance, tricuspid valve surgery is usually indicated. In contrast, if TR and pulmonary artery hypertension are of short duration, mitral valve replacement will usually reduce pulmonary artery pressure in the early postoperative period, and this will result in a decrease in the TR. Occasionally, severe TR will be present with only modest elevation of pulmonary artery pressure. In this circumstance, the tricuspid valve leaflets are usually deformed and valve replacement is necessary.[83]

The appearance of the heart at the time of surgery is helpful in assessing the severity of tricuspid valve disease. A thinned-out RA wall together with moderate to marked enlargement of the RA and venae cavae are indications of significant disease. The degree of stenosis and regurgitation can be estimated by palpation through the RA appendage. Intraoperative transesophageal echocardiography (see Chap. 13) provides more precise information as to the degree of residual valvular regurgitation after repair. The ACC/AHA guidelines recommendations for surgery for TR are listed in Table 59-4.

TS may be treated successfully by commissurotomy, which is usually performed under direct vision. The procedure may be combined with annuloplasty to correct valve regurgitation. Valve replacement is occasionally necessary if the changes in the leaflets and subvalvular structures are advanced or if severe TR cannot be relieved by annuloplasty. For TR, three basic reconstructive techniques have been described. The first procedure is used widely and consists of plication of the posterior leaflet,[84,85] thus converting the tricuspid valve into a functionally bicuspid valve.[84,85] De Vega described a second type of annuloplasty that narrows the annulus along the anterior and posterior leaflets with a pursestring suture.[86,87] The third major technique, described by Carpentier et al., consists of placing a carefully sized semiflexible ring along the anterior and posterior

TABLE 59-4 Recommendations for Surgery for Tricuspid Regurgitation

Indication	Class
Annuloplasty for severe TR and pulmonary hypertension in patients with mitral valve disease requiring mitral valve surgery	I
Valve replacement for severe TR secondary to diseased or abnormal tricuspid valve leaflets not amenable to annuloplasty or repair	IIa
Valve replacement of annuloplasty for severe TR with mean pulmonary artery pressure <60 mmHg when symptomatic	IIa
Annuloplasty for mild TR in patients with pulmonary hypertension secondary to mitral valve disease requiring mitral valve surgery	IIb
Valve replacement or annuloplasty for TR with pulmonary artery systolic pressure <60 mmHg in presence of a normal mitral valve in asymptomatic patients or in symptomatic patients who have not received a trial of diuretic therapy	III

aspects of the annulus.[88] It draws in and supports the tissue evenly. Follow-up studies have shown that annular dilatation occurs in these areas rather than along the leaflets.[89]

When the leaflets and subvalvular apparatus are severely deformed as a result of rheumatic fever, reconstruction may not be feasible. In such cases, replacement is performed with either a mechanical or tissue valve. Anticoagulation with warfarin (see Chap. 52) is generally advisable in patients with tricuspid valve replacement, and therefore the major advantage of a bioprosthetic valve is negated. If a mechanical valve is preferred and the cavity of the RV is not capacious, a low-profile, tilting disk-type prosthesis seems appropriate. Usually, however, if TR is severe, a ball-cage prosthesis functions better.

Mild TR does not seem to increase the risk of surgery involving the mitral valve or both aortic and mitral valves. When the TR is moderate to severe, however, the risk of operation is significantly increased. Although long-term improvement in TR after mitral valve replacement alone has been documented, a tricuspid procedure is generally employed in the setting of moderate to severe TR to enhance cardiac function in the critical early days after operation.[90] Mitral valve replacement alone does not invariably decrease TR, even several months after operation.[91]

In general, the early and late results of tricuspid annuloplasty have been superior to those of valve replacement, and valve replacement should be avoided when possible. There is a significant incidence of thrombosis with tricuspid prostheses, and the long-term functional results have been less favorable than those of aortic and mitral valve replacements.[92] Good early results have been obtained with all three methods of annuloplasty.[93–97] When tricuspid valve replacement is necessary, the 30-day perioperative mortality increases to 15 to 20 percent. Two preoperative factors—severity of edema and mean pulmonary artery pressure—as important predictors of long-term survival.[98] A variety of prostheses have been used for tricuspid valve replacement with variable results.[98–103]

Infective endocarditis of the tricuspid valve is relatively common because of the increased incidence of drug abuse. In general, the treatment of tricuspid valve endocarditis is medical. When septic pulmonary embolization occurs despite intensive antibiotic treatment, tricuspid valve surgery is indicated. Excision of the valve without replacement has been recommended, and reinfection of the new valve in intravenous drug users is an important risk.[104] Nevertheless, since valvulectomy alone carries an important risk of heart failure, tricuspid valve replacement has been recommended by others.[105]

The cardiac output is often marginal after tricuspid valve surgery, a reflection of persistent pulmonary arterial hypertension and long-standing RV dysfunction. Measurements of cardiac output and pulmonary artery pressure are used to guide postoperative care. If annuloplasty is performed, a pulmonary artery catheter can be used for such measurements (see Chap. 15). Nitroglycerin infused through a central venous catheter is a valuable adjunct in reducing pulmonary artery pressure. Prostaglandin E_1, in combination with pressor agents, may also be employed to treat severe postoperative pulmonary hypertension.[106] Intravenous dopamine and dobutamine may be used to enhance myocardial contractility. If cardiac output remains marginal, an intraaortic balloon pump may be used to reduce left-sided pressures. Pulmonary artery balloon counterpulsation has been employed for acute RV failure.[107] The use of a temporary circulatory assist device, such as a centrifugal pump, to bypass the RV may sustain adequate circulation when RV failure is unresponsive to other measures.

Digitalis and diuretics are usually employed for several months after tricuspid valve surgery. For patients with tricuspid valve replacement, warfarin and dipyridamole are used as anticoagulants.[108] The additional use of antiplatelet agents in this setting may improve the long-term results.[109] A serious late complication of tilting disk valves in the tricuspid position is thrombosis. Thrombolytic therapy with streptokinase has been used successfully to restore valve function.[110] Prophylaxis against infective endocarditis is also required (see Chap. 73).

Pulmonic Valve Disease

Pulmonic valve surgery for acquired disease is performed infrequently. PS on an acquired basis is rare. Although there are a variety of causes of PR, this hemodynamic condition is relatively well tolerated if pulmonary vascular resistance is normal. Pulmonic valve replacement may be performed for acquired conditions, such as carcinoid heart disease and infective endocarditis, but it usually is limited to cases where RV dysfunction has become severe after congenital heart disease surgery[111,112] (see Chaps. 63 and 64). In general, bioprosthetic valves have been preferred because of the tendency for mechanical valve thrombosis in this position. Pulmonic valve surgery is currently being performed earlier and more commonly, since studies indicate that RV dysfunction may be present in asymptomatic postoperative patients with PR.[113]

Infective endocarditis involves the pulmonic valve in about 1 percent of cases seen at autopsy. Isolated pulmonic valve infective endocarditis is even more uncommon but may be the cause of metastatic pulmonary infections. In a review of 28 cases of this entity, the overall mortality rate was 24 percent, with all those treated by operation surviving.[114] Valvulectomy in combination with antibiotic therapy is sometimes the most effective treatment (see Chap. 77).

Multivalvular Disease

Many patients with clinical evidence of combined disease of the mitral and aortic valves have severe and progressive symptoms. Experience indicates that both valves can be replaced, with a hospital mortality rate that is now between 5 and 10 percent.

Commonly, in the presence of aortic and mitral valve disease, repair, rather than replacement, of the stenotic or regurgitant mitral valve can be accomplished (see Chap. 57). Disease of the aortic valve in adults usually requires valve replacement. The combination of aortic valve replacement with mitral valve repair probably decreases early mortality rates and improves long-term survival. There have been marked subjective and objective improvements in surviving patients. When tricuspid valve replacement is added, the risk of the operation is higher (up to 20 percent), but even then the long-term results are considerably better than the life history of surgically untreated patients with triple-valve disease. The use, when possible, of tricuspid annuloplasty rather than replacement has greatly improved the early results of operation in this group of patients.

When hemodynamic derangement is significant at both mitral and aortic valves, the decision to repair or replace both is easily made, and the principles of surgical treatment are the same as when one valve alone requires operation.[115,116]

MULTIVALVULAR SURGERY

Combined MS and AR When mechanical correction is anticipated in predominant MS, balloon mitral valvotomy followed by aortic valve replacement (AVR) obviates the need for double-valve replacement, which has a higher risk of complications than does single-valve replacement.[117] In most cases, it is advisable to perform mitral valvotomy first and then follow the patient for symptomatic improvement. If symptoms disappear, correction of AR can be delayed.

Combined MS and TR If the mitral valve anatomy is favorable for percutaneous balloon valvotomy and there is concomitant pulmonary hypertension, valvotomy should be performed regardless of symptom status. After successful mitral valvotomy, pulmonary hypertension and TR almost always diminish.[118]

If mitral valve surgery is performed, concomitant tricuspid annuloplasty should be considered, especially if there are preoperative signs or symptoms of right-heart failure, rather than risking severe, persistent TR, which may necessitate a second operation. However, TR that seems severe on echocardiography but does not cause elevation of RA or RV diastolic pressure will generally improve greatly after mitral valve replacement (MVR). If intraoperative assessment suggests that TR is functional without significant dilatation of the tricuspid annulus, it may not be necessary to perform an annuloplasty.

Combined MS and AS If the degree of AS appears to be mild and the mitral valve is acceptable for balloon valvotomy, this should be attempted first. If mitral balloon valvotomy is successful, the aortic valve should then be reevaluated.

Combined AS and MR Noninvasive evaluation should be performed with two-dimensional and Doppler echocardiography to evaluate the severity of both AS and MR. Attention should be paid to LV size, wall thickness and function, LA size, right-heart function, and pulmonary artery pressure. Patients with severe AS and severe MR (with abnormal mitral valve morphology) with symptoms, LV dysfunction, or pulmonary hypertension should undergo combined AVR and MVR or mitral valve repair. However, in patients with severe AS and lesser degrees of MR, the severity of MR may improve greatly after isolated AVR, particularly when there is normal mitral valve morphology. Intraoperative transesophageal echocardiography and, if necessary, visual inspection of the mitral valve should be performed at the time of AVR to determine whether additional mitral valve surgery is warranted in such patients.

In patients with mild to moderate AS and severe MR in whom surgery on the mitral valve is indicated because of symptoms, LV dysfunction, or pulmonary hypertension, preoperative assessment of the severity of AS may be difficult because of reduced forward stroke volume. If the mean aortic valve gradient is greater than 30 mmHg, AVR should be performed. In patients with less severe aortic valve gradients, inspection of the aortic valve and its degree of opening on two-dimensional or transesophageal echocardiography as well as visual inspection by the surgeon may be important in determining the need for concomitant AVR.

References

1. Bonow RO, Carabello B, de Leon AC Jr, et al. ACC/AHA guidelines for the management of patients with valvular heart disease: A report of the American College of Cardiology/American Heart Association Task Force on Practice Guidelines (Committee on Management of Patients with Valvular Heart Disease). *J Am Coll Cardiol* 1998; 32:1486–1588.
2. Kostucki W, Vandenbossche JL, Friart A, Engbert H. Pulsed Doppler regurgitant flow patterns of normal valves. *Am J Cardiol* 1986; 58:309–313.
3. Sahn DJ, Maciel BC. Physiological valvular regurgitation: Doppler echocardiography and the potential for iatrogenic heart disease. *Circulation* 1988; 78:1075–1077.
4. Yoshida K, Yoshikawa J, Shakudo M. Color Doppler evaluation of valvular regurgitation in normals. *Circulation* 1988; 78: 840–847.
5. McMichael J, Shillingford JP. The role of valvular incompetence in heart failure. *Br Med J* 1957; 1:537–542.
6. Waller BF, Howard J, Fess S. Pathology of tricuspid valve stenosis and pure tricuspid regurgitation: III. *Clin Cardiol* 1995; 18: 225–230.
7. Waller BF, Howard J, Fess S. Pathology of tricuspid valve stenosis and pure tricuspid regurgitation: I. *Clin Cardiol* 1995; 18: 97–102.
8. Waller BF, Howard J, Fess S. Pathology of tricuspid valve stenosis and pure tricuspid regurgitation: II. *Clin Cardiol* 1995; 18: 167–174.
9. Glancy DL, Marcus FI, Cuadra M, et al. Isolated organic tricuspid valvular regurgitation. *Am J Med* 1969; 46:989–996.
10. Nishimura RA, Smith HC, Gersh BJ. Tricuspid regurgitation after myocardial infarction. *Am J Cardiol* 1994; 74:308.
11. Szyniszewski AM, Carson PE, Sakwa M, et al. Valve replacement for tricuspid regurgitation appearing late after healing of left ventricular posterior wall and right ventricular acute myocardial infarction. *Am J Cardiol* 1994; 73:616-617.
12. Chiu WC, Shindler DM, Scholz PM, Boyarsky AH. Traumatic tricuspid regurgitation with cyanosis: Diagnosis by transesophageal echocardiography. *Ann Thorac Surg* 1996; 63:992–993.
13. Chataline A, Agnew TM, Graham KJ, et al. Blunt chest trauma of the heart. *NZ Med J* 1999; 112:334–336.
14. Aziz TM, Burgess MI, Rahman AN, et al. Risk factors for tricuspid valve after orthotopic heart transplantation. *Ann Thorac Surg* 1999; 68:1247–1251.
15. Soga J, Yakyura Y, Osaka M. Carcinoid syndrome: A statistical evaluation of 748 reported cases. *J Exp Clin Cancer Res* 1999; 18:133–141.
16. Perloff JK, Harvey WP. Clinical recognition of tricuspid stenosis. *Circulation* 1960; 22:346–364.
17. Kitchin A, Turner R. Diagnosis and treatment of tricuspid stenosis. *Br Heart J* 1964; 26:354–379.
18. Edwards JE. The spectrum and clinical significance of tricuspid regurgitation. *Pract Cardiol* 1980; 6:86–90.
19. Roguin A, Reinkerich D, Milo S, et al. Long-term follow-up of patients with severe rheumatic tricuspid stenosis. *Am Heart J* 1998; 136:103–108.
20. Flammang D, Jaumin P, Kremer R. Organic tricuspid pathology in rheumatic valvulopathies. *Acta Cardiol* 1975; 30:155–170.
21. Pellikka PA, Tajik AJ, Khandheria BK, et al. Carcinoid heart disease: Clinical and echocardiographic spectrum in 74 patients. *Circulation* 1993; 87:1188–1196.
22. Cheitlin MD, MacGregor J. Acquired tricuspid and pulmonic

valve disease. In: Rahimtoola SH, ed. *Atlas of Heart Diseases: Valvular Heart Disease.* St. Louis: Mosby; 1997: 11.2–1.
23. Ludwig J. Cardiac vein involvement in carcinoid syndrome: Possible evidence of retrograde blood flow in cardiac veins in tricuspid insufficiency. *Am J Clin Pathol* 1971; 55:617–623.
24. McMichael J, Shillingford JP. The role of valvular incompetence in heart failure. *Br Med J* 1957; 1:537–541.
25. Boucek RJ Jr, Graham TP, Morgan JP, et al. Spontaneous resolution of massive congenital tricuspid insufficiency. *Circulation* 1976; 54:795–800.
26. Ajayi AA, Adigun AQ, Ojofeitim EO, et al. Arthrometric evaluation of cachexia in chronic congestive heart failure: The role of tricuspid regurgitation. *Int J Cardiol* 1999; 71:79–84.
27. Collins R, Daly JJ. Tricuspid incompetence complicating acute myocardial infarction. *Postgrad Med J* 1977; 53:51–52.
28. Zone DD, Botti RE. Right ventricular infarction with tricuspid insufficiency and chronic right heart failure. *Am J Cardiol* 1976; 37:445–448.
29. McAllister RG Jr, Friesinger GC, Sinclair-Smith BC. Tricuspid regurgitation following inferior myocardial infarction. *Arch Intern Med* 1976; 95:95–99.
30. Maranhao V, Gooch AS, Yang SS, et al. Prolapse of the tricuspid leaflets in the systolic murmur-click syndrome. *Cath Cardiovasc Diagn* 1975; 1:81–90.
31. Gerry JL Jr, Bulkley BH, Hutchins GM. Rupture of the papillary muscle of the tricuspid valve: A complication of cardiopulmonary resuscitation and a rare cause of tricuspid insufficiency. *Am J Cardiol* 1977; 40:825–828.
32. Jahnke EJ Jr, Nelson WP, Aaby GV, FitzGibbon GM. Tricuspid insufficiency: The result of nonpenetrating cardiac trauma. *Arch Surg* 1967; 95:880–886.
33. VanGilder JE, Jain AC, Weiss RB, et al. Traumatic right ventricular aneurysm presenting as tricuspid regurgitation. *WV Med J* 1979; 75:93–98.
34. Stephenson LW, MacVaugh H III, Kastor JA. Tricuspid valvular incompetence and rupture of the ventricular septum caused by nonpenetrating trauma. *J Thorac Cardiovasc Surg* 1979; 77:768–772.
35. Williams MJ, Lee MY, DiSalvo TG, et al. Biopsy-induced flail tricuspid leaflet and tricuspid regurgitation following orthotopic cardiac transplantation. *Am J Cardiol* 1996; 77:1339–1344.
36. Hausen B, Albes JM, Rohde R, et al. Tricuspid valve regurgitation attributable to endomyocardial biopsies and rejection in heart transplantation. *Ann Thorac Surg* 1995; 59:1134–1140.
37. Marvin RF, Schrank JP, Nolan SP. Traumatic tricuspid insufficiency. *Am J Cardiol* 1973; 32:723–727.
38. Brandenburg RO, McGoon DC, Campeau L, Giuliani ER. Traumatic rupture of the chordae tendineae of the tricuspid valve: Successful repair twenty-four years later. *Am J Cardiol* 1966; 18:911–915.
39. Morgan JR, Forker AD. Isolated tricuspid insufficiency. *Circulation* 1971; 43:559–564.
40. Croxson MS, O'Brien KP, Lowe JB. Traumatic tricuspid regurgitation: Long-term survival. *Br Heart J* 1971; 33:750–755.
41. Grubier M, Denis B, Martin-Noel O. Les ruptures de cordages tricuspidiens. *Coeur Med Int* 1976; 15:215–222.
42. Espino Vela J, Contreras R, Rustrian Rosa F. Rheumatic pulmonary valve disease. *Am J Cardiol* 1969; 23:12–18.
43. Roberts WC, Buchbinder NA. Right-sided valvular infective endocarditis. *Am J Med* 1972; 53:7–19.
44. Levitt MA, Snoey ER, Tamkin GW, Gee G. Prevalence of cardiac value anomalies in afebril injection drug users. *Acad Emerg Med* 1999; 9:911–915.
45. Seymour J, Emanuel R, Patterson N. Acquired pulmonary stenosis. *Br Heart J* 1968; 30:776–785.
46. Rossignol B, Machecourt J, Denis B, et al. Cardiopathie carcinoide secondaire a une tumeur du grêle: A propos d'un cas associat insuffisance tricuspidienne et insuffisance pulmonaire. *Arch Mal Coeur Vaiss* 1977; 70:1221–1226.
47. Roberts WC, Virmani R. Aschoff bodies at necroposy in valvular heart disease. *Circulation* 1978; 57:803–815.
48. Clausen BJ. Rheumatic heart disease: An analysis of 796 cases. *Am Heart J* 1940; 20:454–474.
49. Wilson MG, Lubschez R. Longevity in rheumatic fever. *JAMA* 1948; 138:794–798.
50. Bland EF, Jones TD. Rheumatic fever and rheumatic heart disease: A twenty-year report on 1000 patients followed since childhood. *Circulation* 1951; 4:836–843.
51. Roberts WC, Honig HS. The spectrum of cardiovascular disease in the Marfan's syndrome: A clinico-pathologic study of 18 necropsy patients and comparison to 151 previously reported patients. *Am Heart J* 1982; 104:115–135.
52. Hansing CE, Rowe GG. Tricuspid insufficiency: A study of hemodynamics and pathogenesis. *Circulation* 1972; 45:793–799.
53. Killip T, Lukas DS. Tricuspid stenosis: Physiologic criteria for diagnosis and hemodynamic abnormalities. *Circulation* 1957; 16:3–13.
54. El-Sherif N. Rheumatic tricuspid stenosis: A hemodynamic correlation. *Br Heart J* 1971; 33:16–31.
55. Holmes JC, Flowler NO, Kaplan S. Pulmonary valvular insufficiency. *Am J Med* 1968; 44:851–862.
56. Rackley CE, Bechar VS, Whalen RE, McIntosh HD. Biplane cineangiographic determinations of left ventricular function: Pressure-volume relationships. *Am Heart J* 1967; 74:766–779.
57. Baxley WA, Dodge HT, Rackley CE, et al. Left ventricular mechanical efficiency in man with heart disease. *Circulation* 1977; 55:564–568.
58. Jones JW, Rackley CE, Bruce RA, et al. Left ventricular volumes in valvular heart disease. *Circulation* 1964; 29:887–891.
59. Kern MJ, Aguirre F, Donohue T, Bach R. Interpretation of cardiac pathophysiology from pressure waveform analysis: Multivalvular regurgitant lesions. *Cath Cardiovasc Diagn* 1993; 28:167–172.
60. Rousseau MF, Pouleur H, Charlier AA, Bruseur LA. Assessment of left ventricular relaxation in patients with valvular regurgitation. *Am J Cardiol* 1982; 50:1028–1036.
61. Salazar E, Levine HD. Rheumatic tricuspid regurgitation: The clinical spectrum. *Am J Med* 1962; 33:111–129.
62. Terzaki AK, Cokkinos DV, Leachman RD, et al. Combined mitral and aortic valve disease. *Am J Cardiol* 1970; 25:588–601.
63. Rivero Carvallo JM. El diagnostica de la estenosis tricuspides. *Arch Inst Cardiol Mex* 1950; 20:1–11.
64. Killip T, Lukas DS. Tricuspid stenosis: Clinical features in twelve cases. *Am J Med* 1958; 24:836–852.
65. DePace NL, Ross J, Ashandrian AS, et al. Tricuspid regurgitation: Noninvasive techniques for determining causes and severity. *J Am Coll Cardiol* 1984; 3:1540–1550.
66. Meltzer RS, van Hoogenhuyze D, Serruys PW, et al. Diagnosis of tricuspid regurgitation by contrast echocardiography. *Circulation* 1981; 63:1093–1099.
67. Yock PG, Popp RL. Noninvasive estimation of right ventricular systolic pressure by Doppler ultrasound in patients with tricuspid regurgitation. *Circulation* 1984; 70:657–662.
68. Waggoner AD, Quinones MA, Young JB, et al. Pulsed Doppler echocardiographic detection of right-sided valve regurgitation: Experimental results and clinical significance. *Am J Cardiol* 1981; 47:279–286.
69. Masuyama T, Kodama K, Kitabatake A, et al. Continuous-wave Doppler echocardiographic detection of pulmonary regurgitation and its application to noninvasive estimation of pulmonary artery pressure. *Circulation* 1986;74:484–492.
70. Isobe M, Yazaki Y, Takaku F, et al. Prediction of pulmonary

arterial pressure in adults by pulsed Doppler echocardiography. *Am J Cardiol* 1986; 57:316–321.

71. Chan KL, Currie PJ, Seward JB, et al. Comparison of three Doppler ultrasound methods in the prediction of pulmonary artery pressure. *J Am Coll Cardiol* 1987; 9:549–554.
72. Ogawa S, Hayashi J, Sasaki H, et al. Evaluation of combined valvular prolapse syndrome by two-dimensional echocardiography. *Circulation* 1982; 65:174–180.
73. Otto CM, Pearlman AS, Comens KA, et al. Determination of the stenotic aortic valve area in adults using Doppler echocardiography. *J Am Coll Cardiol* 1986; 7:509–517.
74. Smith MD, Handshoe R, Handshoe S, et al. Comparative accuracy of two-dimensional echocardiography and Doppler pressure half-time methods in assessing severity of mitral stenosis in patients with and without prior commissurotomy. *Circulation* 1986; 78:100–107.
75. Perry GJ, Helmcke F, Nanda NC, et al. Evaluation of aortic insufficiency by Doppler color flow mapping. *J Am Coll Cardiol* 1987; 9:952–959.
76. Enriquez-Serano M, Bailey KP, Seward JB, et al. Quantitative Doppler assessment of valvular regurgitation. *Circulation* 1993; 87:841–848.
77. Winzelberg GG, Boucher CA, Pohost GM, et al. Right ventricular function in aortic and mitral valve disease: Relation of gated first-pass radionuclide angiography to clinical and hemodynamic findings. *Chest* 1981; 79:520–528.
78. Cha SD, Gooch AS, Maranhao V. Intracardiac phonocardiography in tricuspid regurgitation: Relation to clinical and angiographic findings. *Am J Cardiol* 1981; 48:573–583.
79. Rackley CE. Quantitative evaluation of left ventricular function by radiographic techniques. *Circulation* 1976; 54:862–879.
80. Patel TM, Sani SI, Shah SC, Patel TK. Tricuspid balloon valvuloplasty: A more simplified approach using Inoue balloon. *Cath Cardiovasc Diagn* 1996; 37:86–88.
81. Kratz J. Evaluation and management of tricuspid valve disease. *Cardiol Clin* 1991; 9:397–407.
82. Orbe LC, Sobrino N, Arcas R, et al. Initial outcome of percutaneous balloon valvuloplasty in rheumatic tricuspid valve stenosis. *Am J Cardiol* 1993; 71:353–354.
83. Onate A, Alcibar J, Inguanzo R, et al. Balloon dilatation of tricuspid and pulmonary valves in carcinoid heart disease. *Tex Heart Inst J* 1993; 20:115–119.
84. Kay JH, Maselli-Campagna G, Tsuji HK. Surgical treatment of tricuspid insufficiency. *Ann Surg* 1965; 162:53–58.
85. Boyd AD, Engelman RM, Isom OW, et al. Tricuspid annuloplasty: Five and one-half years' experience with 78 patients. *J Thorac Cardiovasc Surg* 1974; 68:344–351.
86. DeVega NF. La annulplastia selectiva: Reguable y permanente. *Rev Esp Cardiol* 1972; 25:55–60.
87. Abe T, Tsukamoto M, Morishita K, et al. 1989: De Vega's annuloplasty for acquired tricuspid disease: Early and late results in 110 patients, updated in 1996. *Ann Thorac Surg* 1996; 62:1876–1877.
88. Carpentier A, Deloche A, Hanania G, et al. Surgical management of acquired tricuspid valve disease. *J Thorac Cardiovasc Surg* 1974; 67:53–65.
89. Deloche A, Guerino J, Fabiani JN, et al. Étude anatomique des valvulopatheis rheumatismales tricuspidiennes. *Ann Chir Thorac Cardiovasc* 1973; 44:343–349.
90. Braunwald NS, Ross J, Morrow AG. Conservative management of tricuspid regurgitation in patients undergoing mitral valve replacement. *Circulation* 1967; 35(suppl 1):163–169.
91. Simon R, Oelert H, Borst HG, Lichtelen PR. Influence of mitral valve surgery on tricuspid incompetence concomitant with mitral valve disease. *Circulation* 1980; 62:1152–1157.
92. Thorburn CW, Morgan JJ, Shanahan MX, Chang VP. Long-term results of tricuspid valve replacement and the problem of prosthetic valve thrombosis. *Am J Cardiol* 1983; 51:1128–1132.
93. Grondin P, Meere C, Limet R, et al. Carpentier's annulus and De Vega's annuloplasty: The end of the tricuspid challenge. *J Thorac Cardiovasc Surg* 1975; 70:852–861.
94. Kay JH, Mendez AM, Zubiate P. A further look at tricuspid annuloplasty. *Ann Thorac Surg* 1976; 22:498–500.
95. Peterffy A, Jonasson R, Szamosi A, Henze A. Comparison of Kay's and De Vega's annuloplasty in surgical treatment of tricuspid incompetence. *Scand J Thorac Cardiovasc Surg* 1980; 14:249–255.
96. Rabago G, De Vega NG, Castillon L, et al. The new De Vega technique in tricuspid annuloplasty: Results in 150 patients. *J Cardiovasc Surg* 1980; 21:231–238.
97. Reed GE, Boyd AD, et al. Operative management of tricuspid regurgitation. *Circulation* 1976; 54(suppl 3):III96–III98.
98. Baughman K, Kallman C, Yurchak P, et al. Predictors of survival after tricuspid surgery. *Am J Cardiol* 1984; 54:137–141.
99. Breye RH, McClenathan JH, Michaelis LL, et al. Tricuspid regurgitation: A comparison of nonoperative management, tricuspid annuloplasty, and tricuspid valve replacement. *J Thorac Cardiovasc Surg* 1976; 72:867–874.
100. Jugdutt BI, Fraser RS, Lee SJK, et al. Long-term survival after tricuspid valve replacement: Results with seven different prostheses. *J Thorac Cardiovasc Surg* 1977; 74:20–27.
101. Kouchoukos NT, Stephenson LW. Indications for and results of tricuspid valve replacement. *Adv Cardiol* 1976; 17:199–206.
102. Sanfelippo PM, Giuliani ER, Danielson GK, et al. Tricuspid valve prosthetic replacement: Early and late results with the Starr-Edwards prosthesis. *J Thorac Cardiovasc Surg* 1976; 71: 441–445.
103. Singh AK, Christian FD, Williams DO, et al. Follow-up assessment of St. Jude medical prosthetic valve in the tricuspid position: Clinical and hemodynamic results. *Ann Thorac Surg* 1984; 37:324–327.
104. Arbulu A, Asfaw I. Tricuspid valvulectomy without prosthetic replacement: Ten years of clinical experience. *J Thorac Cardiovasc Surg* 1981; 82:684–691.
105. Stern H, Sisto D, Strom J, et al. Immediate tricuspid valve replacement for endocarditis. *J Thorac Cardiovasc Surg* 1986; 91: 163–167.
106. D'Ambra M, LaRaia P, Philbin D, et al. Prostaglandin E1: A new therapy for refractory right heart failure and pulmonary hypertension after mitral valve replacement. *J Thorac Cardiovasc Surg* 1985; 89:567–572.
107. Miller DD, Moreno-Cabral RJ, Stinson EB, et al. Pulmonary artery balloon counterpulsation for acute right ventricular failure. *J Thorac Cardiovasc Surg* 1980; 80:760–763.
108. Cannegieter SC, Rosendaal FR, Wintzen AR, et al. Optimal oral anticoagulant therapy in patients with mechanical heart valves. *N Engl J Med* 1995; 333:11–17.
109. Chesebro JH, Fuster V, Elveback LR, et al. Trial of combined warfarin plus dipyridamole of aspirin therapy in prosthetic heart valve replacement: Danger of aspirin compared with dipyridamole. *Am J Cardiol* 1983; 51:1537–1541.
110. Boskovic D, Elezovic I, Boskovic D, et al. Late thrombosis of the Björk-Shiley tilting disc valve in the tricuspid position. *J Thorac Cardiovasc Surg* 1986; 91:1–8.
111. DePace NL, Iskandrian AS, Morganroth J, et al. Infective endocarditis involving a presumably normal pulmonic valve. *Am J Cardiol* 1984; 53:385–387.
112. Misbach GA, Turley K, Ebert PA. Pulmonary valve replacement for regurgitation after repair of tetralogy of Fallot. *Ann Thorac Surg* 1983; 36:684–691.
113. Wessel HU, Cunningham WJ, Paul MH, et al. Exercise performance in tetralogy of Fallot after intracardiac repair. *J Thorac Cardiovasc Surg* 1980; 80:582–593.

114. Cassling R, Rogler W, McManus B. Isolated pulmonic valve infective endocarditis: A diagnostically elusive study. *Am Heart J* 1985; 109:558–567.
115. Stephenson LW, Edic RN, Harken AH, Edmunds H Jr. Combined aortic and mitral valve replacement: Changes in practice and prognosis. *Circulation* 1984; 69:640–644.
116. Kumar AS, Chander H, Trehan H. Surgical technique of multiple valve replacement with biological valves. *J Heart Valve Dis* 1995; 4:45–46.
117. Blackstone EH, Kirklin JW. Death and other time-related events after valve replacement. *Circulation* 1985; 72:753–767.
118. Skudicky D, Essop MR, Sareli P. Efficacy of mitral balloon valvotomy in reducing the severity of associate tricuspid valve regurgitation. *Am J Cardiol* 1994; 73:209–211.

C H A P T E R 60

CLINICAL PERFORMANCE OF PROSTHETIC HEART VALVES

Gary L. Grunkemeier / Albert Starr / Shahbudin H. Rahimtoola

A heart valve functions as a check valve: opening to permit forward blood flow and closing to prevent retrograde flow, about 40 million times per year. Heart valve prostheses consist of an orifice, through which blood flows, and an occluding mechanism that closes and opens the orifice. There are two classes of heart valves: *mechanical prostheses,* with rigid, manufactured occluders, and *biological* or *tissue valves,* with flexible leaflet occluders of animal or human origin. Among the mechanical valves there are three basic types, depending on whether the occluding mechanism is (1) a reciprocating ball, (2) a tilting disk, or (3) two semicircular hinged leaflets. The biological valves include those whose origin is from (1) the patient, (2) another human, or (3) another species. For each type there are several models available from different manufacturers. Selected frequently used valves are described.

PROSTHETIC HEART VALVES

Mechanical Valves

Ball valves appeared in the early 1960s, disk valves in the early 1970s, and bileaflet valves predominantly during the 1980s.

BALL VALVES

The first successful valve replacement devices, which led to long-term survivors and a design that has endured until today, used a ball-in-cage design.[1,2] Several modifications of this design have been used, but only the *Starr-Edwards* valve (Fig. 60-1, Plate 94) has endured; it has been used about 200,000 times.

DISK VALVES

Improvement on the clinical success of the ball valves was sought by developing designs with reduced height. The first successful low-profile design was the *Björk-Shiley* tilting-disk valve, introduced in 1969.[3] It evolved through several design refinements,[4] and about 360,000 valves were implanted. These refinements also introduced a structural failure mode caused by strut fracture in the Convexo-Concave model. Some results with the discontinued Björk-Shiley models are included because many patients are still alive with these valves. Tilting-disk valves employ a circular disk as an occluder. It is retained by wirelike arms or closed loops that project into the orifice. The disks are graphite with a coating of pyrolytic carbon, and the housings are stainless steel or titanium. With the disk open, the primary orifice is separated into two unequal (major and minor) orifices. The *Medtronic Hall* valve has been used clinically since 1977.

BILEAFLET VALVES

Current development in mechanical valves is based on the bileaflet design, introduced by St. Jude Medical in 1977. Unlike the free-floating occluders in ball and disk valves, the two semicircular leaflets of a bileaflet valve are connected to the orifice housing by a hinge mechanism. The leaflets swing apart during opening, creating three flow areas: one central and two peripheral. The *St. Jude* bileaflet valve (Fig. 60-2, Plate 95) has been used over 900,000 times and the *Carbomedics* valve has been used about 300,000 times since its clinical introduction in 1986.

Biological Valves

Biological valves include as wide a variety of models, as do mechanical valves:

1. An *autograft* valve is one that is translocated within the same individual—e.g., the pulmonary valve in the aortic valve position.
2. A *homograft* (or allograft) valve is one that has been transplanted from a donor of the same species—when, for example, a donor's aortic or pulmonary valve has been placed in a recipient's aortic or pulmonary position.

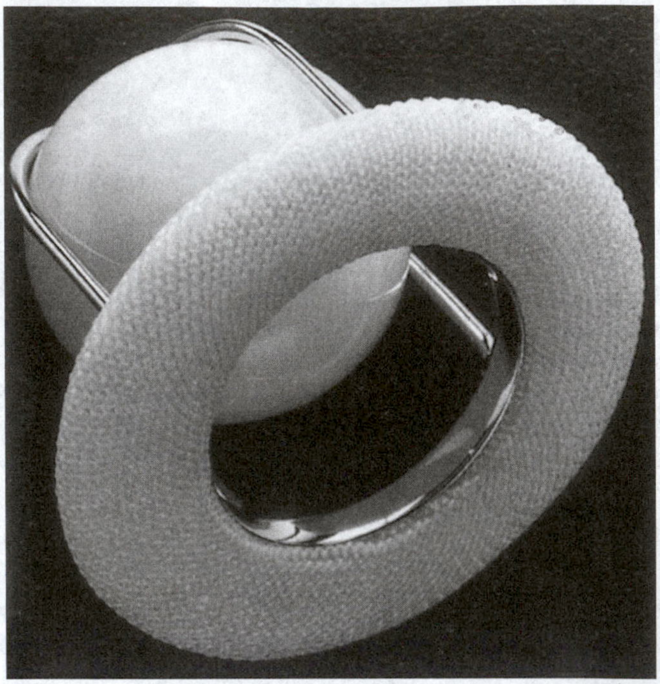

FIGURE 60-1 (Plate 94) Starr-Edwards caged ball valve. The ball is a silicone rubber polymer, impregnated with barium sulfate for radiopacity, which oscillates in a cage of cobalt-chromium alloy. When the valve opens, blood flows through the circular primary orifice and a secondary orifice between the ball and the housing. In the aortic position, there is a tertiary orifice between the ball and the aortic wall.

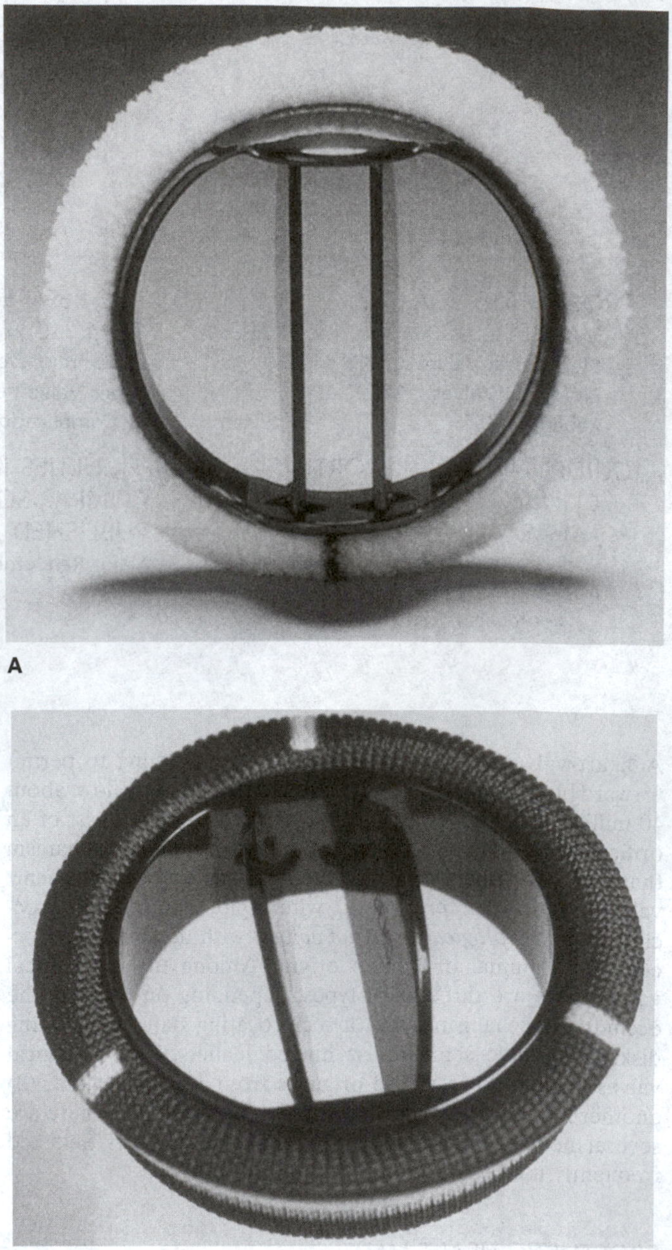

A

B

FIGURE 60-2 (Plate 95) Bileaflet valves. The St. Jude Medical valve (*A*) has leaflets that open to an angle of 85 degrees from the plane of the orifice and travel from 55 to 60 degrees to the fully closed position, depending on valve size. The original version, whose housing did not rotate within the sewing ring, has been supplemented by a model that does rotate for intraoperative adjustment. The Carbomedics valve (*B*) has flat leaflets that open to 78 to 80 degrees and close at an angle of 25 degrees with the horizontal and has a carbon-coated surface on the sewing ring to inhibit thrombus formation.

3. *Heterograft* (or xenograft) valve is a transplant from another species, either an intact valve (e.g., a porcine aortic valve) or a valve fashioned from heterologous tissue (e.g., bovine pericardium).

The point of using biological valves is to reduce the complications associated with thromboembolism and the need for anticoagulation. The first successful biological valves were homografts, pioneered by Ross[5] and Barratt-Boyes[6] in 1962.

AUTOGRAFT

The pulmonary autograft procedure consists of an autotransplant of the pulmonary valve to the aortic position; the pulmonary valve is then replaced by an aortic or pulmonary homograft. This operation was first described in 1967[7] and is called the Ross procedure; it is currently undergoing increased popularity,[8–12] but this operation involves a double valve replacement, with the attendant early and late risks. This procedure uses double valve replacement to solve a single valve problem; however, subsequent problems with pulmonary valve replacement may be easier to remedy and those related to autograft will be similar to those of aortic valve re-replacement.

HOMOGRAFT

The homograft valve is considered to be a preferred substitute for aortic valve replacement, especially in younger patients. It achieves excellent hemodynamics; there is no need for anticoagulation and it has low thrombogenicity. The drawbacks are a more technically demanding operation and a low availability; however, the latter drawback has been alleviated by its commercial availability from cryopreservation services. Several methods of procurement, sterilization, and preservation have been used.[13] Three surgical techniques are used for aortic valve replacement: (1) replacement of the valve only into the subcoronary position, (2) complete aortic root replacement with reimplantation of

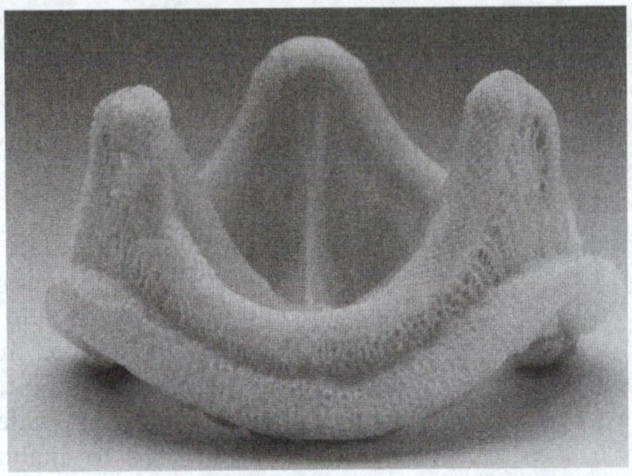

FIGURE 60-3 (Plate 96) Stented porcine valves. The Carpentier-Edwards SupraAnnular Valve is designed to be implanted above rather than within the aortic annulus. It has low-pressure fixation and a cone-shaped stent which flares out at the top to improve leaflet durability.

the coronary arteries, and (3) miniroot replacement with part of the donor aortic wall inserted within the host aorta.

PORCINE HETEROGRAFT

Glutaraldehyde sterilizes valve tissue, renders it bioacceptable by destroying antigenicity, and stabilizes the collagen cross-links for durability. The use of glutaraldehyde for tissue preservation was pioneered by Carpentier,[14] who introduced the term *bioprosthesis*[15] for nonviable valves of biological origin, such as the *Hancock II* and *Carpentier-Edwards SupraAnnular* (SAV) porcine valves (Fig. 60-3, Plate 96).

Most porcine valves are mounted on rigid or flexible stents, to which the leaflets and the sewing ring are attached. Unstented versions have also been devised by several manufacturers.[16–20] Their goal is to achieve some of the potential benefit of a homograft valve, especially hemodynamics and perhaps durability, with an easily available commercial product. The valve, however, is porcine and can be expected to have the same problems of primary valve failure as the stented porcine valve. As with homografts, there are potentially three ways of implanting a stentless porcine valve (valve only, aortic root replacement, and cylinder inclusion). The St. Jude Medical Toronto SPV (Fig. 60-4, Plate 97) and the Medtronic Freestyle (Fig. 60-5, Plate 98) stentless porcine valves were approved for marketing by the FDA in 1997.

BOVINE PERICARDIAL VALVE

Pericardial valves that are tailored and sewn into a valvular configuration using bovine pericardium as a fabric result in a valve that opens more completely than a porcine valve, providing better hemodynamics. They might also be expected to have better durability, because there is extra tissue to allow for shrinkage and a higher percentage of collagen to be cross-linked during fixation. Unfortunately, the Ionescu-Shiley, the first commercially available pericardial valve, did not bear out this promise and was taken off the market, as was the Hancock pericardial valve. These failures were due to aspects of the design, however, rather than to an intrinsic problem with pericardial tissue. The Carpentier-Edwards Perimount pericardial bioprosthesis (Fig. 60-6) has a method of construction that overcomes these design

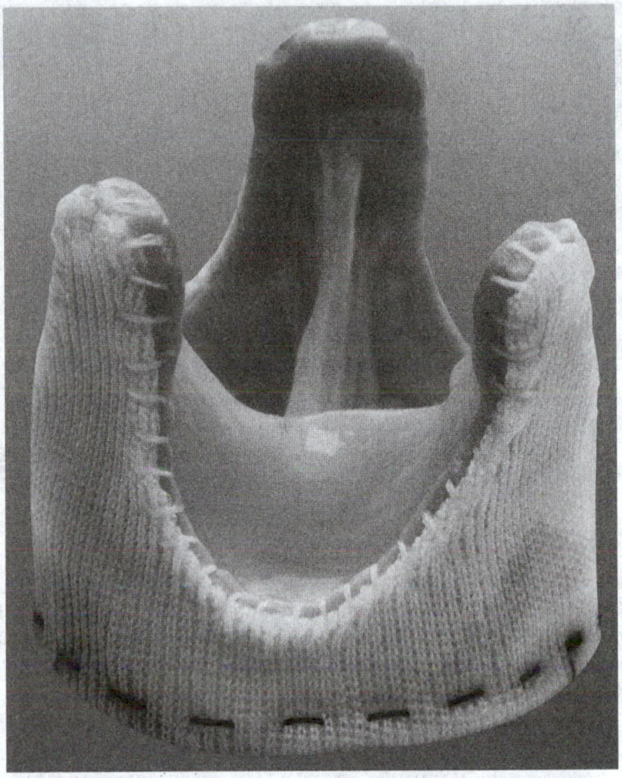

A

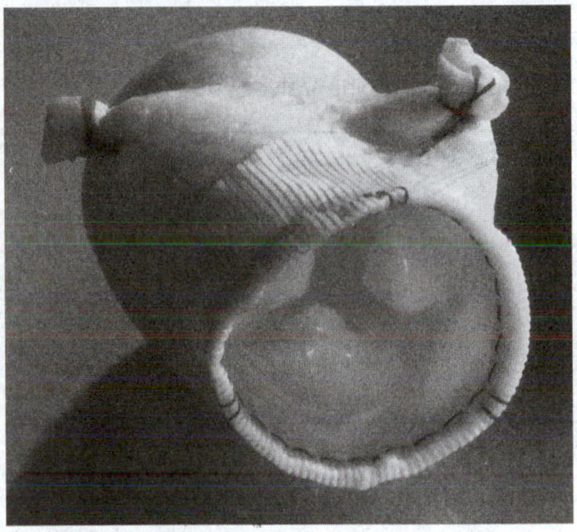

B

FIGURE 60-4 (Plate 97) St. Jude Toronto SPV (*A*) and Medtronic Freestyle (*B*) stentless porcine valves. The Toronto SPV is designed to be used as a subcoronary valve replacement. The Freestyle can be implanted using any of the methods of implantation used for homografts: subcoronary implantation of the valve alone, aortic root replacement, or cylinder (root) inclusion.

issues. It has been used clinically since 1982 and received FDA approval, for the aortic position only, in 1991.

Repair

When possible, valve repair[21–23] is generally preferable to replacement (see discussion below).

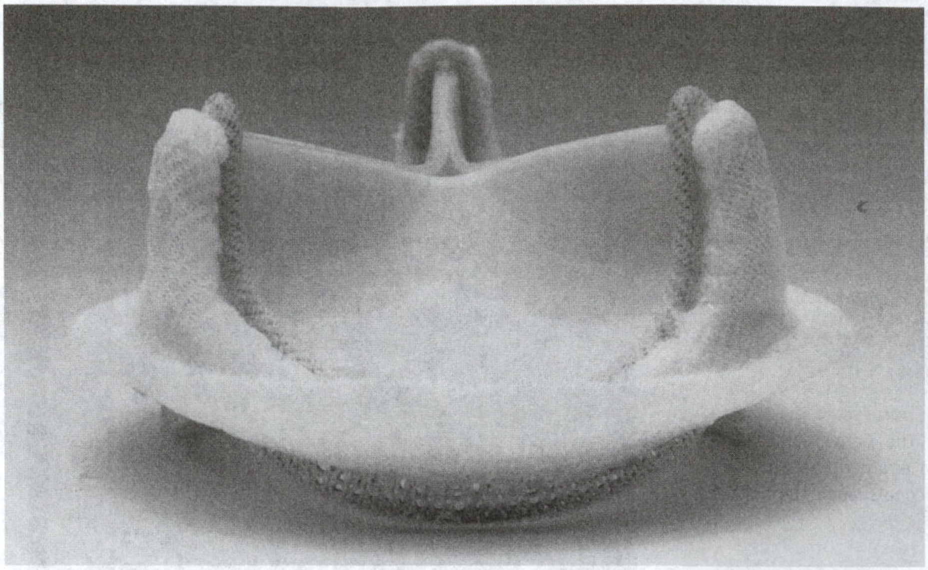

FIGURE 60-5 (Plate 98) The Carpentier-Edwards Perimount pericardial bioprosthesis uses a method of mounting the leaflets to the stent, which does not depend on retaining stitches passed through the pericardium—a design weakness of previous pericardial valves. Instead, the leaflets are anchored behind the stent pillars.

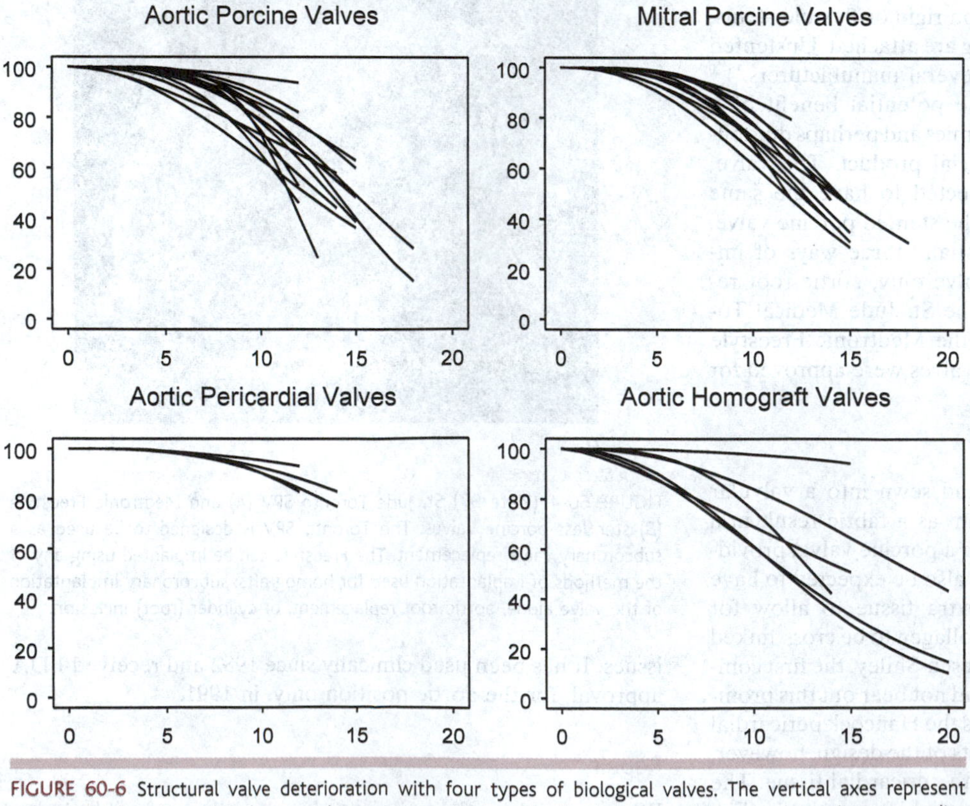

FIGURE 60-6 Structural valve deterioration with four types of biological valves. The vertical axes represent percent freedom from SVD; horizontal axes represent years after implant. These follow-up data relates to studies with minimum follow-up to 400 valve-years and conform to the FDA requirements for each location of valve. (From Grunkemeier et al.[61] Reproduced by permission of the publisher and authors.)

GUIDELINES FOR REPORTING CLINICAL RESULTS

The analytic aspects of the reporting of clinical results of heart valves have evolved consistently since the first successful implants in 1960. As late (posthospital) experience accumulated near the end of the first decade of implants, the need to analyze time-related events resulted in the introduction of actuarial analysis,[24] which had previously been used to analyze the results of cancer therapy.[25] Later, the use of linearized (constant hazard) rates,[26,27] Cox regression,[28] and multivariable parametric models[29] was advocated. The effectiveness of these refined statistical methods in comparing results from different series, however, was limited by the lack of standardization in definitions and follow-up methods.

AATS/STS Guidelines for Clinical Reporting

In 1988, standards that specified which complications should be collected and how they should be defined were proposed by the Ad Hoc Liaison Committee for Standardizing Definitions of Prosthetic Heart Valve Morbidity, a joint committee of the American Association for Thoracic Surgery (AATS) and the Society of Thoracic Surgeons (STS).[30] These guidelines were revised in 1996.[31,32] The complications that were determined to be of critical importance by these guidelines are as follows:

1. *Structural valvular deterioration,* or any change in function of an operated valve resulting from an intrinsic abnormality that causes stenosis or regurgitation.
2. *Nonstructural dysfunction,* a composite category that includes any abnormality that results in stenosis or regurgitation of the operated valve that is not intrinsic to the valve itself, exclusive of thrombosis and infection. This includes inappropriate sizing, also called *prosthesis-patient mismatch.*[33]

3. *Valve thrombosis* is any thrombus, in the absence of infection, attached to or near an operated valve that occludes part of the blood flow path or that interferes with the function of the valve.
4. *Embolism* is any embolic event that occurs in the absence of infection after the immediate perioperative period (when anesthesia-induced unconsciousness is completely reversed). These include any new, temporary or permanent, focal or global neurologic deficits and peripheral embolic events; emboli proven to consist of nonthrombotic material are excluded.
5. *Bleeding event* (*formerly anticoagulant hemorrhage*) is any episode of major internal or external bleeding that causes death, hospitalization, or permanent injury (e.g., vision loss) or requires transfusion. The complication "bleeding event" applies to all patients, whether or not they are taking anticoagulants or antiplatelet drugs.
6. *Operated valvular endocarditis* is any infection involving an operated valve. Morbidity associated with active infection—such as valve thrombosis, thrombotic embolus, bleeding event, or paravalvular leak—is included under this category but is not included in other categories of morbidity.

TABLE 60-1 Complications for Evaluating Clinical Performance of Replacement Heart Valves and Objective Performance Criteria (OPC)[a] Values for Complication Rates (Percent/Year)

Definitions of Morbidity	OPC, %/YEAR Mechanical	Biological
1. *Structural deterioration:* Valve deterioration, wear, stress fracture, poppet escape, clacification, leaflet tear, stent creep; *excludes* infected or thrombosed valves		
2. *Nonstructural dysfunction:* Entrapment by pannus or suture, leak, inappropriate sizing, hemolytic anemia; excludes thromboembolism and infection	(leak) 1.2 (major 0.6)	(leak) 1.2 (major 0.6)
3A. *Valve thrombosis:* Thrombosis proved by operation, autopsy, or clinical investigation; *excludes* infection	0.8	0.2
3B. *Thromboembolism:* Neurologic deficit, peripheral arterial emboli, acute myocardial infarction *after* operation in patients with known normal coronary arteries or those <40 years of age; *excludes* septic emboli, hemorrhage, immediate surgical events	3.0	2.5
4. *Anticoagulant-related hemorrhage:* Bleeding that causes death, stroke, operation, hospitalization, or transfusion in patients receiving anticoagulants and/or antiplatelet drugs	3.5 (major 1.5)	1.4 (major 0.9)
5. *Prosthetic valve endocarditis:* Based on blood cultures, clinical signs, and/or histologic evidence at reoperation or autopsy; *includes* valve thrombosis, embolus, or paravalvular leak associated with active infection	1.2	1.2

[a]Please see text for definition of OPC.
SOURCE: The complications and their definitions are adapted from Ref. 30, the OPC values are taken from Appendix K of Ref. 35.

The *consequences* of the above morbid events include reoperation, valve-related mortality, sudden unexpected unexplained death, cardiac death, total deaths, and permanent valve-related impairment.[31,32]

FDA Guidelines for New Valve Approvals

In 1976, medical devices including prosthetic heart valves came under the jurisdiction of the FDA,[34] which subsequently issued various guidelines for submission of premarket approval (PMA) applications for heart valves. The FDA issued a guidance document in December 1993[35] that used the analytical approach to clinical studies adapted from the work of Gersh et al.[36] These authors proposed a method for premarket clinical testing of heart valves that emphasizes confidence interval estimation and comparisons to objective performance criteria (OPC). *OPC are linearized rates for critical complications, representing averages achieved by the best currently used valves.* A *linearized rate* is calculated as the number of events divided by total patient-years and multiplied by 100 to convert it to units of "events per 100 years" or "percent per year."[27]

To determine OPC for contemporary use, the FDA screened the literature plus data submitted by clinical investigators of approved devices and identified OPC for the major morbidity categories.[35] They determined that these rates were similar for aortic and mitral positions but varied for some complications between mechanical and biological valves. The OPC for complications are given in Table 60-1 for mechanical and biological replacement heart valves. Several observations on these data are significant.

The category *Structural deterioration* was not included in the list of OPC because the clinical PMA investigation is not designed to detect intrinsic valve failure. Structural durability should be evaluated by in vitro testing, and the clinical realization of structural failure should be so small (mechanical valves) that the clinical study is of insufficient size or so long-term (tissue valves) that the clinical study is of insufficient duration to assess it adequately.

From the *Nonstructural dysfunction* category, the FDA included only leak, the most common and the most frequently reported subcategory, and derived OPC for major leaks ("as defined by AATS/STS, 1988")[30] and for all leaks.

The FDA separated *Thromboembolism* into the separate categories of valve thrombosis and thromboembolism, as had been strongly advocated,[37,38] and the FDA derived OPC both for major *Anticoagulant-related hemorrhage* events ("as defined by AATS/STS, 1988")[30] and for all bleeding events.

Based on the OPC values given in Table 60-1, the FDA has set the minimum amount of follow-up required for a PMA study at 800 valve-years.[39] The assumption of constant risk for heart valve complications, as embodied by the OPC formulation, is only an approximation; but if operative events are excluded (the intent of the FDA guidelines) and maximum follow-up is in the 2- to 3-year range, this assumption may be acceptable, at least for the purpose of sample size estimation.

VALVE-RELATED COMPLICATIONS

Actuarial valve failure–free curves[25] are used to describe tissue valve durability, and linearized rates[27] are used for all other complications.

Structural Deterioration

This category, the first one considered in the guidelines for reporting, virtually always results in death or valve explant. There is a dual standard with regard to this complication: for biological valves, structural deterioration is probably inevitable if the patient lives long enough; whereas for mechanical valves, the only acceptable rate is a very low one (near zero).

MECHANICAL VALVES

The durability of currently used mechanical valves is remarkable, given the harsh biological environment in which the valve must perform. For example, the current Starr-Edwards ball valve, now in use for 35 years and in over 200,000 patients, has had fewer than a dozen structural problems reported to the manufacturer, most of which did not cause clinical problems. Even the discontinued Björk-Shiley Convexo-Concave valve, whose strut fracture failures have been highly publicized, had fewer than 1 percent failures reported after 15 years of experience.[40] The Medtronic Hall valve had three leaflet fractures in a version that is not used in the United States. The problem was determined to be related to unequal coatings of pyrolytic carbon on the two faces of the leaflet and to be limited to a very small subset of valves. Since the manufacturing specifications were changed to ensure more equal coatings, the problem has not recurred. The St. Jude valve has had only 12 reported postoperative fractures of the disk or housing, which resulted in leaflet escape reported to the FDA—an excellent record considering that over 900,000 valves have been implanted.

BIOLOGICAL VALVES

Data on freedom from structural deterioration for several series of aortic porcine and pericardial bioprostheses and homografts are shown in Fig. 60-6. The mean age of patients in these older series is around 50 years. The current series of porcine valves, together with the tendency to select older patients,[41–44] should have improved durability. Design changes in some porcine valves,[45,46] such as stentless configurations,[16–20] may possibly improve durability.

Although the Carpentier-Edwards pericardial valve has been available for over 15 years, relatively few long-term results on the valve are available. Those that have been reported, however, show improved durability in the aortic position, as compared with the previously discontinued Ionescu-Shiley pericardial valve. The durability of the Carpentier-Edwards pericardial valve also compares favorably with that of porcine valves (Fig. 60-6; Table 60-2). The patients in the Carpentier-Edwards pericardial valve series were older than patients in previous series of pericardial and porcine valves, however, and it is unknown to what extent this has resulted in apparent improvement in the durability of the Carpentier-Edwards pericardial valve.

Structural durability is considered to be better with *homografts* than with other bioprostheses. From various published reports[13] for homografts used primarily in the aortic position, it is apparent that the variation among series is wide, the current methods of sterilization/preservation provide better results than those which have been discontinued, and the results do not appear better than those for porcine bioprostheses (Fig. 60-6).

The pulmonary autograft is considered an excellent aortic valve substitute, especially for young patients[10] and in the treatment of patients with endocarditis.[47] Freedom from reoperation has been reported as 100 percent in 33 patients from 8 to 47 years old followed to a maximum of 48 months[11] and 93 percent at 5.5 years in 51 patients from 2 to 21 years old.[10] Data from one center showed 48.5 percent freedom from reoperation at 19 years[47] and, after excluding patients from three hospitals, 85 percent freedom from reoperation at 20 years.[48] To evaluate complications of this procedure fully, problems with the valve used to replace the pulmonary valve must be combined with complications of the pulmonary autograft itself.

TABLE 60-2 14-Year Results with Carpentier-Edwards Pericardial Valve

		FDA-Mandated Patients[a] (*n* = 267) Actuarial (%)
Thromboembolism/thrombosis		19 ± 4
Anticoagulant-related bleeding		6 ± 2
Endocarditis/sepsis		7 ± 2
Valve dysfunction		70 ± 4
Explant due to structural valve deterioration:	Total	15 ± 3
	≤65 years of age	24 ± 5
	>65 years of age	4 ± 2
Mortality:	Total	60 ± 3.1
	Valve-related	21 ± 3.2

[a]FDA approval was based on 719 patients at 7 years. Data from FDA-mandated longer follow-up of selected patients are from Frater et al.[85]

VALVE REPAIR

Mitral valve repair is considered preferable to replacement, when practicable. It has been shown to improve ejection fraction[49] and to provide good results for treating bacterial endocarditis[50] and valve problems in elderly patients.[51,52] It has been strongly suggested that it improves survival; however, there are problems associated with the comparisons.[53]

The weakness of valve repair is durability. The 10-year actuarial reoperation rate has been reported to be 15 percent in nonrheumatic mitral disease.[54] The reoperation rate for patients with rheumatic mitral disease varies from 25 percent reoperation at 5 years[55] to 17 percent at 10 years in a large series in which calcium debridement[56] and anterior leaflet procedures were performed.[57] The reoperation rate at 10 years was 24 percent for patients less than 20 years of age and 9 percent at 10 years for patients over 20 years of age.[58]

Early results of aortic valve repair have been published,[23,59,60] but further follow-up is needed to assess the long-term results.

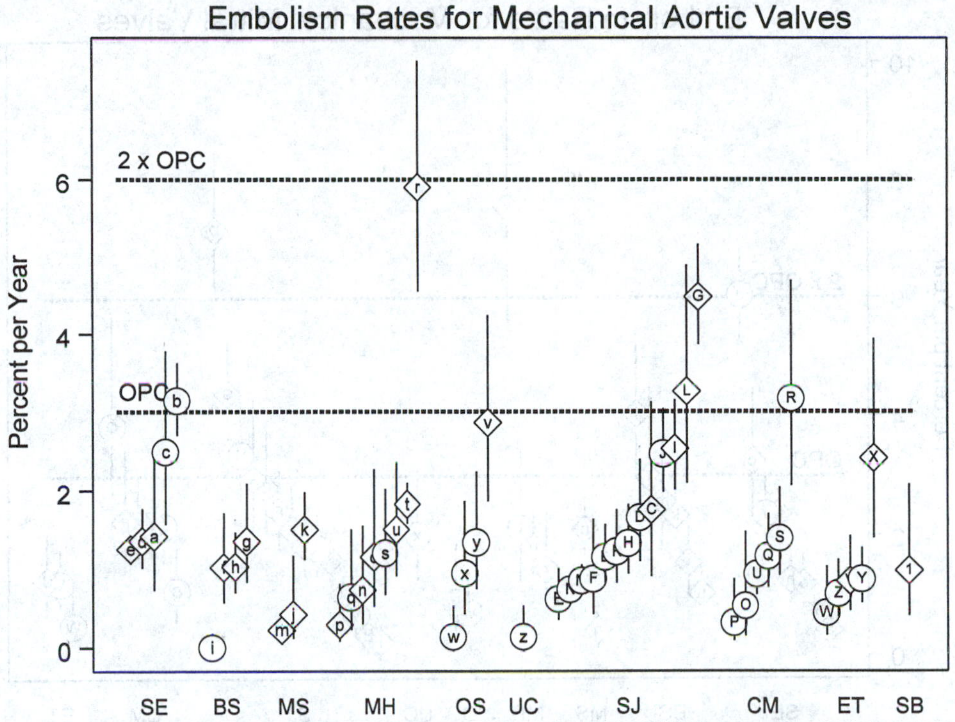

FIGURE 60-7 Embolism rates for mechanical aortic valves. Each open symbol represents a different series, and the height of the symbol is the linearized rate for the series. The vertical bar indicates the 95 percent confidence interval. There is a dashed line at the height of the FDA objective performance criteria (OPC); for approval of a new valve, the upper confidence limit should be less than twice the OPC (*upper dashed line*). Diamonds indicate that both early and late events were used to calculate the rates, circles indicate that only late events were used. Letters inside the symbols correspond to the cited references for the series in the original publication. The series are grouped by valve model, shown below the horizontal axis by two-letter abbreviations: SE = Star-Edwards caged-ball; BS = Björk-Shiley tilting disk; MS = Monostrut tilting disk; MH = Medtronic Hall tilting disk; OS = Omniscience and Omnicarbon tilting disk; UC = Ultracor tilting disk; SJ = St. Jude bileaflet; CM = Carbomedics bileaflet; ET = Edwards Tekna and Duromedics bileaflet; SB = Sorin Bicarbon bileaflet. (From Grunkemeier et al.[61] Reproduced by permission of the publisher and authors.)

Other Valve-Related Complications

Linearized rates are often used to describe the complications required by the AATS/STS guidelines for reporting.[30–32] The use of such rates assumes that the risks are constant, which is usually only approximately true. A review of a large number of published reports of the performance of prosthetic heart valves reveals a wide spread of results for every complication for every valve. In 172 series of heart valves covering 335,485 valve-years accumulated by 63,531 valves of 20 different models implanted in two positions (aortic, mitral), the linearized event rates ranged from 0 to 7.5 percent per year for thromboembolism, 0 to 0.6 percent per year for thrombosis, 0 to 9.3 percent per year for bleeding, 0 to 1.7 percent per year for infection, and 0 to 2.8 percent per year for paravalvular leak.[61] Caution must be exercised in directly comparing event rates among valves for many reasons, including the simplifications involved in the use of linearized rates, varying definitions of complications (many of these reports predate the standardized definitions), and differences in patient characteristics between series.[53,62]

DIFFICULTIES IN MAKING COMPARISONS BETWEEN PUBLISHED SERIES

As noted above, there is wide variation in the reported complication rates of series using the same valves. Figures 60-7 to 60-10 illustrate the wide range of embolism with use of the same heart valve in different series. This variation must be due to variations between series other than the *valve model*. These include factors associated with the following:

1. *Patients*—age, ventricular function, comorbidities, etc.
2. *Reporting center*—surgical variables, postoperative medical management, method, frequency and thoroughness of follow-up, definitions of complications, etc.
3. Problems with *data analysis*[63,64]—many patient-related factors are known to influence thromboembolism,[53,65] stroke rates in patients with atrial fibrillation and in the elderly are equal to those observed in prosthetic valve series,[66] and standardized definitions[30–32] were not in effect or were not employed when many of the available series were reported, etc.
4. *Published data*—these reports describe only a small fraction of the valves implanted and are probably not a representative subset.

Several types of bias can affect reported results. As examples, selection bias occurs in the collection and analysis of data and the decision to report them;[63] publication bias describes the fact that published series tend to be those with the best (or worst, but

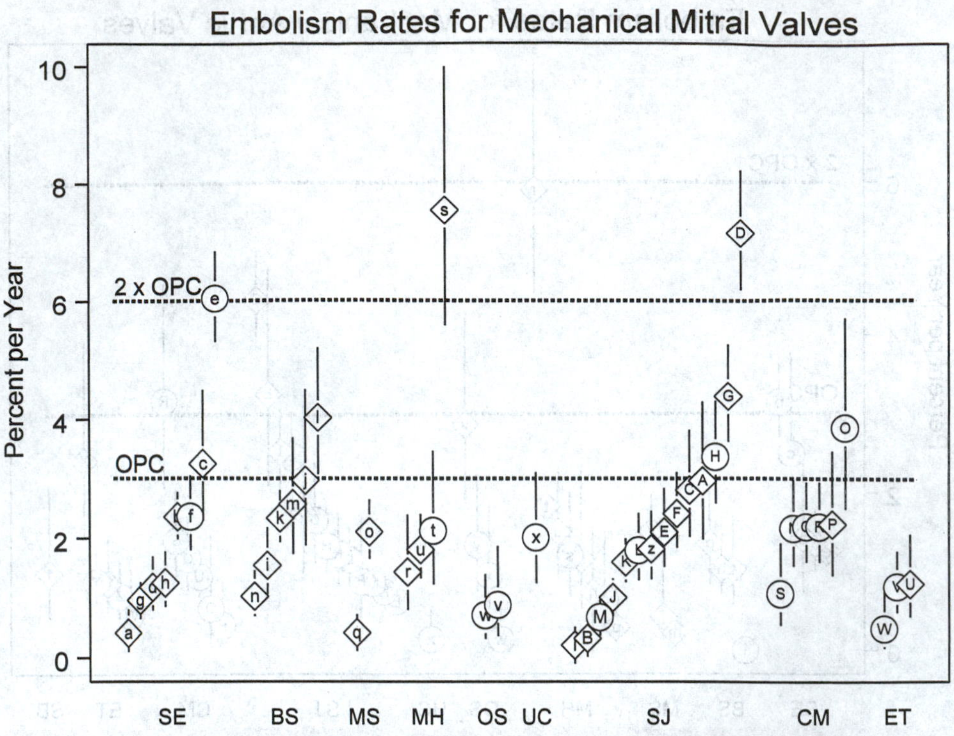

FIGURE 60-8 Embolism rates for mechanical mitral valves. For explanation of symbols and valve model abbreviations, see Fig. 60-7. (From Grunkemeier et al.[61] Reproduced by permission of the publisher and authors.)

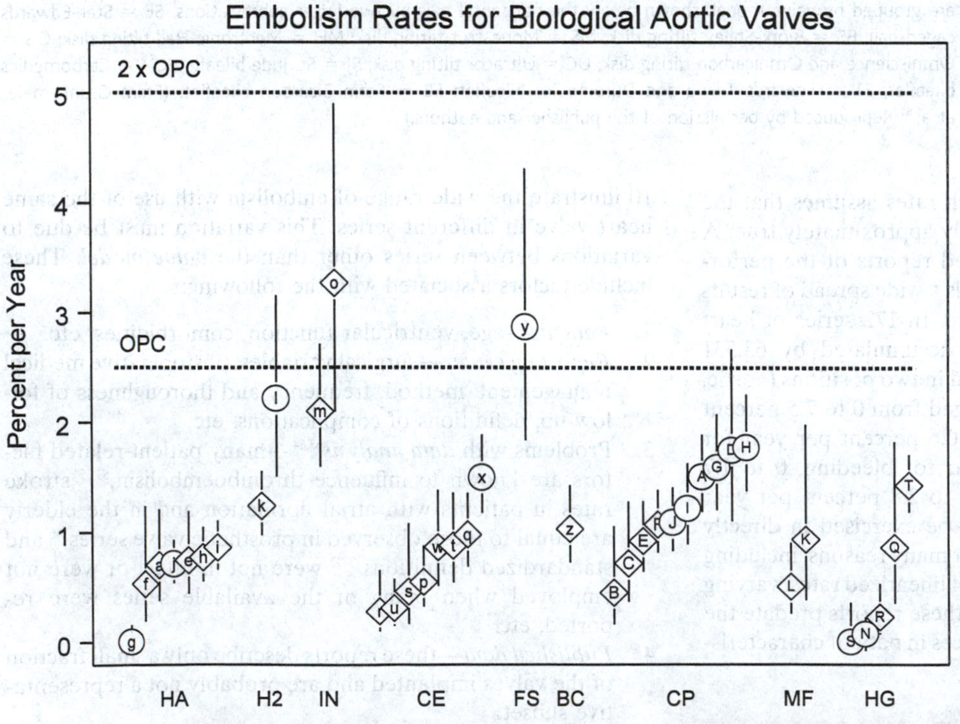

FIGURE 60-9 Embolism rates for biological aortic valves. For explanation of symbols, see Fig. 60-7. Valve model abbreviations: HA = Hancock I and Modified Orifice porcine; H2 = Hancock II porcine; IN = Intact porcine; CE = Carpentier-Edwards porcine; FS = Freestyle stentless porcine; BC = Biocor stentless porcine; CP = Carpentier-Edwards Perimount pericardial; MF = Mitroflow pericardial; HG = homograft. (From Grunkemeier et al.[61] Reproduced by permission of the publisher and authors.)

not typical) results.[67] If a random allocation of valves had been made among patients within a center, statistical methods could theoretically assess the effect on complication rates due to valve model. For logistic, financial, and ethical reasons, however, the number of randomized studies of valves is small, and the available studies are usually of insufficient size to show differences among valves. Although randomized studies provide the best internal validity or valve-specific comparison within centers, they may lack external validity or generalizability to patients outside of the study.[68]

A theoretically preferable way to answer this bias is to allocate patients randomly to different treatments (valves). Randomized trials, however, also have difficulties,[69] and as noted, there are logistic, financial, and ethical arguments against randomization of patients to different heart valves.[70] Consequently, the number of randomized studies of valves is small, and those that exist are usually of insufficient size to add to the knowledge already obtained from careful observational studies except for comparison of survival data with use of different types of prosthesis.

Major Randomized Trials

The two major randomized clinical trials that have been reported are the Edinburgh Heart Valve Trial[71] and the Veterans Administration (VA) Cooperative Study on Valvular Heart Disease.[72] Both studies compared mechanical valves to porcine bioprostheses.

The Edinburgh trial compared the Björk-Shiley Standard valve to porcine valves—initially the Hancock and later the Carpentier-Edwards.[71] It contains actuarial comparisons at 5 and 12 years for the 211 aortic and 261 mitral valve patients. The authors concluded that survival with a mechanical valve was better than with the bioprosthetic valve, but that this was somewhat offset by the increased risk of bleeding.

The VA trial compared the

standard Björk-Shiley valve to the Hancock Modified Orifice (size 21 to 23 mm aortic) or Hancock Standard (other sizes) porcine valves.[72] Table 60-3 contains actuarial comparisons of the endpoint variables at 15 years. The principal long-term findings of this randomized trial[73] are: (1) Use of a mechanical valve resulted in a lower mortality and a lower reoperation rate after aortic valve replacement (AVR); (2) The mortality after mitral valve replacement (MVR) was similar with use of the two prosthetic valve types; (3) There were virtually no primary valve failures with use of a mechanical valve; (4) Primary valve failure after AVR and MVR occurred more frequently in patients with a bioprosthetic valve especially in patients aged <65 years; (5) The primary valve failure rate between bioprosthesis and mechanical valve was not significantly different in those aged ≥65 years; (6) Use of a bioprosthetic valve resulted in a lower bleeding rate; and (7) There were no significant differences between the two valve types with regard to other valve related complications including thromboembolism, and all complications.

Comparison of the 12-year actuarial event rates between these two trials[72] showed that the bleeding and thromboembolism rates were higher in the VA study but that reoperation rates were higher in the Edinburgh study. These differences could be partially accounted for by the composition of the two patient populations: The Edinburgh patients (1) were younger and less heavily anticoagulated, (2) included women and those with double valve replacements, and (3) had a higher percentage of porcine valves in the mitral position. Late results show a better survival with mechanical valves than with bioprostheses in the mitral position with the original valve in the Edinburgh trial (42 versus 24 percent, $p < .05$), probably because of the high rate of bioprosthetic degeneration, and in the aortic position in the VA trial (23 versus 0 percent; $p = 0.0001$).

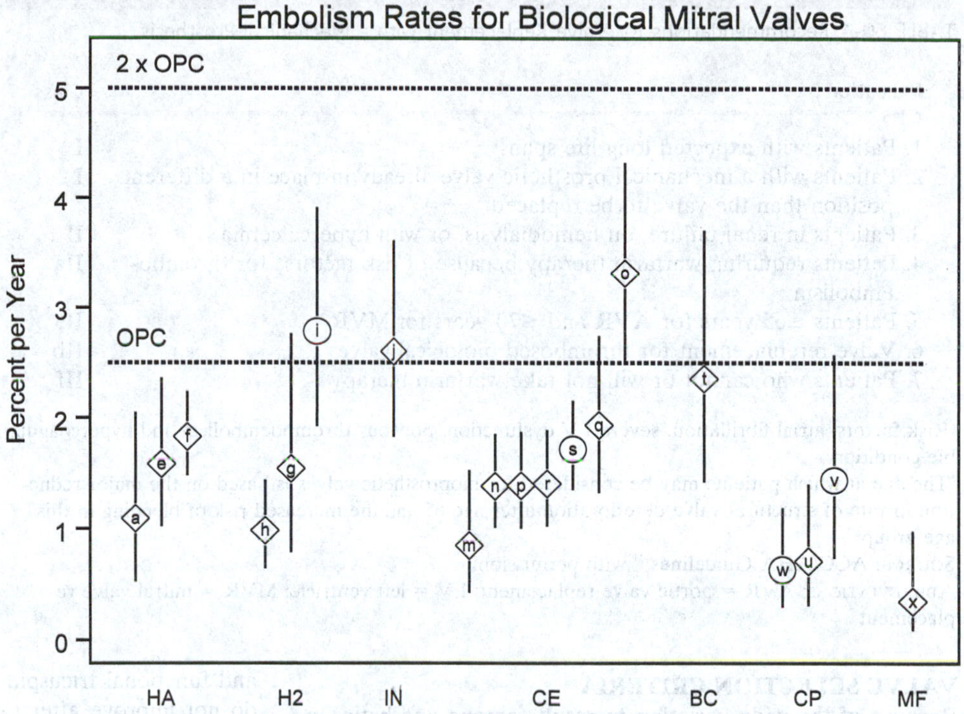

FIGURE 60-10 Embolism rates for biological mitral valves. For explanation of symbols, see Fig. 60-7. Valve model abbreviations: see Fig. 60-9. (From Grunkemeier et al.[61] Reproduced by permission of the publisher and authors.)

TABLE 60-3 Probability of Death due to Any Cause, Any Valve-Related Complication and Individual Valve-Related Complications 15 Years after Randomization[a]

	Aortic Valve Replacement			Mitral Valve Replacement		
Outcome Event	Mechanical $n = 198$	Bioprosthetic $n = 196$	p	Mechanical $n = 88$	Bioprosthesis $n = 93$	p
Death from any cause	66 ± 3%	79 ± 3%	0.02	81 ± 4%	79 ± 4%	0.30
Any valve-related complication	65 ± 4%	66 ± 5%	0.26	73 ± 6%	81 ± 5%	0.56
Systemic embolism	18 ± 4%	18 ± 4%	0.66	18 ± 5%	22 ± 5%	0.96
Bleeding	51 ± 4%	30 ± 4%	0.0001	53 ± 7%	31 ± 6%	0.01
Endocarditis	7 ± 2%	15 ± 5%	0.45	11 ± 4%	17 ± 5%	0.37
Valve thrombosis	2 ± 1%	1 ± 1%	0.33	1 ± 1%	1 ± 1%	0.95
Perivalvular regurgitation	8 ± 2%	2 ± 1%	0.09	17 ± 5%	7 ± 4%	0.05
Reoperation	10 ± 3%	29 ± 5%	0.0004	25 ± 6%	50 ± 8%	0.15
Primary valve failure	0 ± 0%	23 ± 5%	0.0001	5 ± 4%	44 ± 8%	0.0002

n = number of patients randomized.
*Values given are actuarial percentages ± standard error.
NOTE: p values are for differences between mechanical and porcine valves.
SOURCE: From Hammermeister et al.[73]

TABLE 60-4 Recommendations for Valve Replacement with a Mechanical Prosthesis

Indication	Class
1. Patients with expected long life spans	I
2. Patients with a mechanical prosthetic valve already in place in a different position than the valve to be replaced	I
3. Patients in renal failure, on hemodialysis, or with hypercalcemia	II
4. Patients requiring warfarin therapy because of risk factors[a] for thromboembolism	IIa
5. Patients ≤65 years for AVR and ≤70 years for MVR[b]	IIa
6. Valve rereplacement for thrombosed biological valve	IIb
7. Patients who cannot or will not take warfarin therapy	III

[a]Risk factors: atrial fibrillation, severe LV dysfunction, previous thromboembolism and hypercoagulable condition.
[b]The age at which patients may be considered for bioprosthetic valves is based on the major reduction in rate of structural valve deterioration after age 65 and the increased risk of bleeding in this age group.
SOURCE: ACC/AHA Guidelines,[74] with permission.
ABBREVIATIONS: AVR = aortic valve replacement; LV = left ventricle; MVR = mitral valve replacement.

VALVE SELECTION CRITERIA

Because of the wide variation in results among and between various valve models, it is impossible to rank valves within valve types on the basis of complication rates. Some general recommendations, however, can be made with regard to valve selection (Table 60-4).[74]

A biological valve should be used when the patient cannot or will not take anticoagulants or has a short life expectancy. Its use in relation to subsequent pregnancy is controversial (see Chap. 61). A mechanical valve should be used if the patient needs anticoagulant therapy (e.g., because of atrial fibrillation), has a mechanical valve in another position, previously had a stroke, requires double valve replacement, or has a long life expectancy. Mechanical valves should be considered for double valve replacement because the risk of structural deterioration for two porcine valves is additive,[75] whereas the thromboembolic risk of two mechanical valves is not additive.[76]

MANAGEMENT OF PATIENTS WITH PROSTHETIC HEART VALVES

Patients who have undergone valve replacement are *not* cured but still have serious heart disease. They have exchanged native valvular disease for prosthetic valvular disease and must be followed with the same care as patients with native valvular disease.[77] The clinical course of patients with prosthetic heart valves is influenced by several factors.[78]

Ventricular Dysfunction

Despite relief of valvular obstruction or regurgitation, some patients fail to improve after valve replacement or even deteriorate because of ventricular dysfunction. The cause of dysfunction may be carditis associated with rheumatic disease, myocardial degeneration and fibrosis from long-standing pressure or volume overload, ischemic damage at the time of valve replacement, coronary artery disease, or other associated diseases such as systemic hypertension or idiopathic dilated cardiomyopathy. Perioperative myocardial damage is an important cause of postoperative ventricular dysfunction. The importance of myocardial protection at the time of valve surgery is now recognized, and current operative techniques reduce myocardial oxygen consumption by hypothermic cardioplegia and use a variety of means for maintaining adequate myocardial perfusion and protection.

Other Cardiac Lesions

Cardiac diseases affecting primarily one valve often affect other valves, the conduction system, the coronary arteries, and the pulmonary vasculature. With the exception of pulmonary hypertension and functional tricuspid regurgitation, these disorders usually do not improve after isolated valve replacement. Rheumatic disease typically affects both mitral and aortic valves but not necessarily with the same severity at the same time. Therefore, patients who have mitral valve replacement may subsequently, years later, require aortic valve replacement, or vice versa. Calcification of the aortic and mitral valve annuli may extend to the conduction system. High-degree or complete atrioventricular block may occur at the time of surgery or during the late postoperative period, requiring pacemaker implantation. Coronary artery disease is very common in the age range of patients requiring valve replacement. Preoperative coronary arteriography should be performed in all patients with myocardial ischemic pain, in those with left ventricular dysfunction, in those with risk factors for coronary artery disease, and in those about 35 years of age or older.[78,79] Coronary bypass surgery of technically suitable vessels should be performed at the time of valve surgery if the patients have associated significant coronary artery disease.

Prosthesis-Related Problems

The incidence of problems with each prosthesis (see Tables 60-5 and 60-6) was discussed earlier. *Operative mortality* is related to older age of patient, New York Heart Association functional class III or IV, increased left ventricular size, left ventricular dysfunction, heart failure, pulmonary hypertension, low cardiac output, and presence of associated diseases such as systemic arterial hypertension, diabetes mellitus, peripheral and cerebral vascular disease, prior heart surgery, prior myocardial infarction, chronic obstructive pulmonary disease, and renal and hepatic failure. Coronary bypass surgery performed at the same time as valve replacement increases the operative mortality modestly (from 1.4 to 4.0 percent), but associated coronary artery disease, if not bypassed, significantly increases the operative mortality to 9.4 percent and the 10-year mortality to 64 percent.[80] Other very important factors include the occurrence of perioperative myocardial infarction, the duration of the operation, aortic cross-clamp time, and whether or not the patient needed reoperation within 1 to 2 weeks after the initial operation, and on an elective or emergency basis.

The risk of *prosthetic endocarditis* is about 3 percent in the first year and 0.5 percent in subsequent years. Infections in the early postoperative period (up to 2 to 12 months) are due to hospital-based organisms. Despite therapy, the infections are difficult to cure and have a high mortality (about 80 percent);[81,82] early reoperation is usually recommended. The mortality rate from late (2 to 12 months or later) postoperative infection is approximately 40 percent;[81,82] about half the patients can be treated successfully with medication alone. The infected valve should be replaced in patients who do not respond to medical treatment or who have evidence of heart failure, annular invasion, embolism, prosthetic dysfunction, unstable prosthesis, or gram-negative, staphylococcal, or fungal infection.[64] The importance of adequate antibiotic prophylaxis for the prevention of endocarditis cannot be overemphasized; the prevention and treatment of prosthetic valve endocarditis are discussed in Chap. 82.

TABLE 60-5 Recommendations for Valve Replacement with a Bioprosthesis

Indication	Class
1. Patients who cannot or will not take warfarin therapy	I
2. Patients ≥65 years[a] needing AVR who do not have risk factors for thromboembolism[b]	I
3. Patients considered to have possible compliance problems with warfarin therapy	IIa
4. Patients >70 years[a] needing MVR who do not have risk factors for thromboembolism[b]	IIa
5. Valve rereplacement for thrombosed mechanical valve	IIb
6. Patients <65 years[a]	IIb
7. Patients in renal failure, on hemodialysis, or with hypercalcemia	III
8. Adolescent patients who are still growing	III

[a]The age at which patients should be considered for bioprosthetic valves is based on the major reduction in rate of structural valve deterioration after age 65 and increased risk of bleeding in this age group.

[b]Risk factors: atrial fibrillation, severe LV dysfunction, previous thromboembolism, and hypercoagulable condition.

SOURCE: ACC/AHA Guidelines,[74] with permission.

ABBREVIATION: AVR = aortic valve replacement; LV = left ventricle; MVR = mitral valve replacement.

Long-term anticoagulant therapy is associated with *bleeding* episodes. The incidence of minor bleeding is about 2 to 4 percent per year or less. The incidence of major bleeding is about 1 to 2 percent per year or less, with a mortality rate of about 0.5 percent per year or less. The incidence of these complications is lower in patients who take their medications reliably, in those in whom smooth long-term anticoagulation can be achieved, and in those who receive low-dose warfarin therapy (INR 2 to 3 versus >3). With oral anticoagulants, low- or mid-dose warfarin therapy is combined with low-dose aspirin. Higher degrees of anticoagulation increase the incidence of bleeding without reducing the incidence of thromboembolism. The management of antithrombotic therapy is discussed in Chap. 68.

Prosthetic dehiscence is the result of sutures pulling out of the cardiac tissues. It may result from infection, inadequate surgical technique, or diseased cardiac tissue (e.g., edema, necrosis, calcification).

Because of the continued proliferation of new types and models of prostheses and their relatively brief history of clinical use, the natural history of *structured valve deterioration* is incompletely determined. Although some mechanical prostheses had initial problems with component failure, the most common cause for dysfunction of mechanical prosthetic valves is thrombotic obstruction. The incidence of thrombotic obstruction with the Björk-Shiley spherical occluder valve is higher than that seen with the Starr-Edwards or St. Jude valves, particularly in the mitral position. Failure of biological valves is more common than failure of mechanical prostheses because of leaflet deterioration or calcification; progressive prosthetic regurgitation and/or stenosis is the rule. Bioprosthesis failure is greater in younger patients, in older patients with chronic renal insufficiency, and in the mitral position. In younger patients (average age <60 years), failure of mitral prostheses usually starts at 5 to 8 years and of aortic prostheses at 8 to 10 years. It is unlikely that the tissue valves currently in use will be able to provide the long-term performance demonstrated by the ball-valve mechanical prosthesis.

Red cells are fractured by turbulence and contact with foreign surfaces. Some degree of *hemolysis* is present with all mechanical prostheses but not with bioprostheses. Important hemolysis, however, may occur with a perivalvular leak or severe prosthetic obstruction regardless of prosthesis type. Serum

TABLE 60-6 Major Complications of Valve Replacement

1. Operative mortality
2. Perioperative myocardial infarction
3. Prosthetic endocarditis
4. Prosthetic dehiscence
5. Prosthetic dysfunction
    a. Obstruction: Usually thrombotic, occasionally due to item 3, 4, or 8
    b. Regurgitation
    c. Hemolysis
    d. Structural failure
6. Thromboemboli
7. Hemorrhage with anticoagulant therapy
8. Valve prosthesis-patient mismatch
9. Prosthetic replacement often caused by item 3, 4, or 5, occasionally caused by item 6, 7, or 8
10. Late mortality, including sudden, unexplained death

SOURCE: Rahimtoola.[64] Reproduced with permission of the publisher and author.

lactic dehydrogenase (LDH) is usually the simplest and most reliable index of hemolysis to follow in patients with prosthetic valves. A sudden increase in LDH may indicate prosthesis dysfunction, perivalvular leak, or cloth tear. Iron and folate therapy usually correct the anemia. Valve rereplacement may be required for severe, refractory hemolytic anemia.

Important *systemic embolization* is an unfortunate complication of prosthetic valve replacement. Anticoagulation is recommended for all patients with mechanical prostheses. *Despite long-term anticoagulation, patients with prosthetic valves face an embolic rate from aortic prostheses of 1 to 2 percent or less per year and from mitral prostheses of 3 to 4 percent or less per year.*

No prosthesis currently employed has an effective orifice as large as that of the native valve, and valve prosthesis-patient mismatch[33] may occur. *All patients with prosthetic heart valves have mild to moderate stenosis.* Patients with aortic valve prostheses have obstruction to left ventricular outflow (aortic stenosis), and patients with mitral valve prostheses have obstruction to left atrial emptying (mitral stenosis). This is most important in a large patient in whom a prosthesis that is considered "small" in relation to body size must be placed for technical reasons. The resulting patient-prosthesis mismatch[33] contributes to incomplete relief of symptoms. The long-term effect of intrinsic prosthetic stenosis on survival and ventricular dysfunction is unknown but may lead to long-term effects similar to those of aortic or mitral stenosis.[83] The presence of intrinsic prosthetic stenosis must be considered when patients with prosthetic heart valves are being advised concerning activity.

Reoperation to replace a prosthetic heart valve is a serious complication. It is usually required for moderate to severe prosthetic dysfunction and dehiscence, prosthetic valve endocarditis, and occasionally recurrent thromboembolism, severe recurrent bleeding from anticoagulant therapy, or valve prosthesis–patient mismatch.

Late cardiac death may result from ventricular dysfunction, other cardiac lesions, or prosthesis-related causes. Late, sudden death is not uncommon. It may result from a bradyarrhythmia; a tachyarrhythmia that is often associated with ventricular dysfunction, prosthetic dysfunction, or mismatch; coronary artery disease; or a combination of these.

Management[78]

All patients with prosthetic valves need appropriate antibiotics for prophylaxis against infective endocarditis (Chap. 82). Patients with rheumatic heart disease continue to need antibiotics as prophylaxis against the recurrence of rheumatic carditis (Chap. 62). Adequate antithrombotic therapy is needed for appropriate patients (Chap. 68).

During the first 4 to 6 weeks after surgery, the physician and surgeon jointly manage the patient, directing their attention toward relieving postoperative discomfort, readjusting cardiac medications, and instituting anticoagulation if not contraindicated. A graduated plan of activity is started that, in most cases, enables the patient to return to full activity in 4 to 6 weeks.

Several syndromes are peculiar to the postoperative period. The *postperfusion syndrome* usually appears in the third or fourth postoperative week. It is characterized by fever, splenomegaly, and atypical lymphocytes; it is benign and self-limited. The *postpericardiotomy syndrome* is characterized by fever and pleuropericarditis. It usually develops in the second or third postoperative week but can appear as late as 1 year after surgery and sometimes recurs. Although this syndrome is usually self-limited, most patients benefit from taking anti-inflammatory drugs, such as aspirin or indomethacin; a short course of glucocorticoids is also occasionally required.

Even though the pericardium is left open at the end of surgery, *cardiac tamponade* has been known to occur during the first 6 weeks. The fact that a critically ill patient may improve promptly with pericardial drainage underscores the need to consider this uncommon postoperative complication. Usually, anticoagulants have been given and the fluid is hemorrhagic.

The *4- to 6-week postoperative visit* is critical, because by this time the patient's physical capabilities and expected improvement in functional capacity can usually be assessed. At this time, the physician should assemble essential records and data for the subsequent office follow-up, including the preoperative history, physical examination, chest roentgenogram, electrocardiogram (ECG) and indication for surgery, preoperative echocardiographic/Doppler ultrasound and cardiac catheterization/angiographic reports, surgeon's operative report, postoperative complications, and hospital discharge summary. The prosthesis model, serial number, and size should be recorded.

The workup on this visit should include an interval or complete initial history and physical examination, ECG, chest x-ray, echocardiography/Doppler ultrasound, complete blood count, and measurement of electrolytes, LDH, and international normalized ratio (INR) if indicated (Table 60-7). The examination's main focus is on physical signs that relate to functioning of the prosthesis or suggest the presence of a myocardial, conduction, or valvular disorder. The auscultatory findings to expect with some normally functioning prostheses have been described.[84]

TABLE 60-7 Recommendations for Follow-up Strategy of Patient with Prosthetic Heart Valves

Indication	Class
1. History, physical exam, ECG, chest x-ray, echocardiogram, complete blood count, serum chemistries, and INR (if indicated) at first postoperative outpatient evaluation[a]	I
2. Radionuclide angiography or magnetic resonance imaging to assess LV function if result of echocardiography is unsatisfactory	I
3. Routine follow-up visits at yearly intervals with earlier reevaluations for change in clinical status	I
4. Routine serial echocardiograms at time of annual follow-up visit in absence of change in clinical status	IIb
5. Routine serial fluoroscopy	III

[a]This evaluation should be performed 3 to 4 weeks after hospital discharge. In some settings, the outpatient echocardiogram may be difficult to obtain: if so, an inpatient echocardiogram may be obtained before hospital discharge.

SOURCE: ACC/AHA Guidelines,[73] with permission.

ABBREVIATIONS: INR = international normalized ratio; LV = left ventricle.

Severe perivalvular mitral regurgitation can be inaudible on physical examination, a fact to remember when considering possible causes of functional deterioration in a patient.

The interval between routine follow-up visits depends on the patient's needs. Anticoagulant regulation usually does not require office visits.

Multiple noninvasive tests have emerged for assessing valvular and ventricular function. Fluoroscopy can reveal abnormal rocking of a dehiscing prosthesis or limitation of the occluder if the latter is opaque as well as strut fracture of a Björk-Shiley valve. Radionuclide angiography, which is useful for determining whether or not functional deterioration is the result of reduced ventricular function, is performed if the same data cannot be obtained by echocardiography.

Echocardiography/Doppler ultrasound is the most useful noninvasive test. It provides information about prosthesis stenosis/regurgitation, valve area, assessment of other valve disease(s), pulmonary hypertension, atrial size, left ventricular hypertrophy, left ventricular size and function, and pericardial effusion/thickening. It is essential at the first postoperative visit because it allows an assessment of the effects and results of surgery and serves as a baseline for comparison should complications and/or deterioration occur later. Subsequently, it is performed as is needed in both symptomatic and asymptomatic patients at 1- to 2-year intervals. We recommend that in patients with a bioprosthesis in the mitral position, echocardiography/Doppler ultrasound should be performed annually after 5 years and in the aortic position annually after 8 years because of the increasing incidence of bioprosthetic structural valve deterioration.

"Heart failure" after valve replacement may be the result of (1) preoperative left ventricular dysfunction that improved partially or not at all, (2) perioperative myocardial damage, (3) progression of other valve disease, (4) complications of prosthetic heart valves, and (5) associated heart disease such as coronary artery disease and systemic arterial hypertension.

Any patient with a prosthetic heart valve who does not improve after the surgery or who later shows deterioration of functional capacity should undergo appropriate testing to determine the cause. Such studies are also usually necessary for patients who require reoperation for endocarditis or repeated embolism to determine the hemodynamics and anatomy.

The indications for reoperating on a patient with prosthetic valve endocarditis have already been discussed. A patient in stable condition, without prosthetic valve endocarditis, can usually undergo reoperation with only slightly greater risk than that of the initial surgery. For the patient with catastrophic dysfunction, surgery is clearly indicated and urgent. The patient without endocarditis or severe dysfunction requires careful hemodynamic evaluation; the decision about reoperation should then be based on the hemodynamic abnormalities, the symptoms, ventricular function, and current knowledge of the natural history of the particular prosthesis.

ACKNOWLEDGMENT

The authors wish to thank Hui-Hua Li, MD, and K. Jeanne Zerr, RN, MBA, for valuable assistance in the preparation of this chapter. We are also grateful to the heart valve manufacturers for supplying information about their products.

References

1. Harken D, Soroff HS, Taylor WJ. Partial and complete prosthesis in aortic insufficiency. *J Thorac Cardiovasc Surg* 1960; 40:744–762.
2. Starr A, Edwards M. Mitral replacement: Clinical experience with a ball valve prosthesis. *Ann Surg* 1961; 154:726–740.
3. Björk VO. A new tilting disc valve prosthesis. *Scand J Thorac Cardiovasc Surg* 1969; 3:1–10.
4. Björk VO. The improved Björk-Shiley tilting disc valve prosthesis. *Scand J Thorac Cardiovasc Surg* 1978; 12:81–84.
5. Ross DN. Homograft replacement of the aortic valve. *Lancet* 1962; 2:487.
6. Barratt-Boyes BG. Homograft aortic valve replacement in aortic incompetence and stenosis. *Thorax* 1964; 19:131–135.
7. Ross DN. Replacement of aortic and mitral valves with a pulmonary autograft. *Lancet* 1967; 2:956–958.
8. Elkins RC. Pulmonary autograft—The optimal substitute for the aortic valve? *N Engl J Med* 1994; 330:59–60.
9. Oury JH, Eddy AC, Cleveland JC. The Ross procedure: A progress report. *J Heart Valve Dis* 1994; 3:361–364.
10. Elkins RC, Santangelo K, Randolph JD, et al. Pulmonary autograft replacement in children. The ideal solution? *Ann Surg* 1992; 216:363–370; discussion, 370–371.
11. Kouchoukos NT, Davila-Román VG, Spray TL, et al. Replacement of the aortic root with a pulmonary autograft in children and young adults with aortic-valve disease. *N Engl J Med* 1994; 330:1–6.
12. Chambers JC, Somerville J, Stone S, Ross DN. Pulmonary autograft procedure for aortic valve disease: Long-term results of the pioneer series. *Circulation.* 1997; 96:2206–2214.
13. Grunkemeier GL, Bodnar E. Comparison of structural valve failure among different "models" of homograft valves. *J Heart Valve Dis* 1994; 3:556–560.
14. Carpentier A, Lemaigre G, Robert L. Biological factors affecting long-term results of valvular homografts. *J Thorac Cardiovasc Surg* 1969; 58:467–483.
15. Carpentier A, Dubost C. From xenograft to bioprosthesis. In: Ionescu MI, Ross DN, Wooler GH, eds. *Biological Tissue in Heart Valve Replacement*. London: Butterworth; 1971:515–541.
16. Hazekamp MG, Goffin YA, Huysmans HA. The value of the stentless biovalve prosthesis: An experimental study. *Eur J Thorac Cardiovasc Surg* 1993; 7:514–519.
17. Konertz W, Hamann P, Schwammenthal E, et al. Aortic valve replacement with stentless xenografts. *J Heart Valve Dis* 1992; 1:249–252.
18. David TE, Bos J, Rakowski H. Aortic valve replacement with the Toronto SPV bioprosthesis. *J Heart Valve Dis* 1992; 1:244–248.
19. Vrandecic MP, Gontijo BF, Fantini FA, et al. The new stentless aortic valve: Clinical results of the first 100 patients. *Cardiovasc Surg* 1994; 2:407–414.
20. Hvass U, Chatel D, Ouroudji M, et al. The O'Brien-Angell stentless valve: Early results of 100 implants. *Eur J Cardiothorac Surg* 1994; 8:384–387.
21. Carpentier A. Mitral reconstruction in predominant mitral incompetence. In: Duran C, Angell WW, Johnson AD, Oury JH, eds. *Recent Progress in Mitral Valve Disease*. London: Butterworth; 1984:265–276.
22. Duran C. Mitral reconstruction in predominant mitral stenosis. In: Duran C, Angell WW, Johnson AD, Oury JH, eds. *Recent Progress in Mitral Valve Disease*. London: Butterworth; 1984: 255–264.
23. Cosgrove DM, Rosenkranz ER, Hendren WG, et al. Valvuloplasty for aortic insufficiency. *J Thorac Cardiovasc Surg* 1991; 102:571–576; discussion, 576–577.
24. Duvoisin GE, Brandenburg RO, McGoon DC. Factors affecting

thromboembolism associated with prosthetic heart valves. *Circulation* 1967; 35,36(suppl I):70–76.
25. Kaplan EL, Meier P. Nonparametric estimation from incomplete observations. *J Am Stat Assn* 1958; 53:457–481.
26. Stinson EB, Griepp RB, Oyer PE, Shumway NE. Long-term experience with porcine xenografts. *J Thorac Cardiovasc Surg* 1977; 73:54–63.
27. Grunkemeier GL, Thomas DR, Starr A. Statistical considerations in the analysis and reporting of time-related events: Application to analysis of prosthetic valve-related thromboembolism and pacemaker failure. *Am J Cardiol* 1977; 39:257–258.
28. Grunkemeier GL, Macmanus Q, Thomas DR, Starr A. Regression analysis of late survival following mitral valve replacement. *J Thorac Cardiovasc Surg* 1978; 75:131–138.
29. Blackstone EH, Naftel DC, Turner ME Jr. The decomposition of time-varying hazard into separate phases, each incorporating a separate stream of concomitant information. *J Am Stat Assoc* 1986; 81:615–624.
30. Edmunds LH Jr, Clark RE, Cohn LH, et al. Guidelines for reporting morbidity and mortality after cardiac valvular operations. *Ann Thorac Surg* 1988; 46:257–259.
31. Edmunds LH Jr, Clark RE, Cohn LH, et al. Guidelines for reporting morbidity and mortality after cardiac valvular operations. *Ann Thorac Surg* 1996; 62:932–935.
32. Edmunds LH Jr, Clark RE, Cohn LH, et al. Guidelines for reporting morbidity and mortality after cardiac valvular operations. *J Thorac Cardiovasc Surg* 1996; 112:708–711.
33. Rahimtoola SH. The problem of prosthesis-patient mismatch. *Circulation* 1978; 58:20–24.
34. Rahimtoola SH, Rahmoeller GA. The law on cardiovascular devices: The role of the Food and Drug Administration and of physicians in its implementation. *Circulation* 1980; 62:919–924.
35. *Draft Replacement Heart Valve Guidance*. Rockville, MD: Prosthetic Devices Branch, Division of Cardiovascular, Respiratory and Neurological Devices, Office of Device Evaluation, Center of Devices and Radiological Health, Food and Drug Administration. December 7, 1993.
36. Gersh BJ, Fisher LD, Schaff HV, et al. Issues concerning the clinical evaluation of new prosthetic valves. *J Thorac Cardiovasc Surg* 1986; 91:460–466.
37. Nashef SAM. Reporting the results of heart valve operations (letter). *Ann Thorac Surg* 1989; 47:949–950.
38. Bodnar E, Butchart EG, Bamford J, et al. Proposal for reporting thrombosis, embolism and bleeding after heart valve replacement. *J Heart Valve Dis* 1994; 3:120–123.
39. Grunkemeier GL, Johnson D, Naftel DC. Sample size requirements for studying heart valves with constant risk events. *J Heart Valve Dis* 1994; 3:53–58.
40. Grunkemeier GL, Anderson WN. Passive surveillance of heart valve devices: Björk-Shiley outlet strut fracture rates. *J Long-Term Effects Med Implants* 1995; 5:155–168.
41. Jones LE, Weintraub WS, Craver JM, et al. Ten-year experience with the porcine bioprosthetic valve: Interrelationship of valve survival and patient survival in 1,050 valve replacements. *Ann Thorac Surg* 1990; 49:370–383; discussion, 383–384.
42. Jamieson WR, Tyers GF, Janusz MT, et al. Age as a determinant for selection of porcine bioprostheses for cardiac valve replacement: Experience with Carpentier-Edwards standard bioprosthesis. *Can J Cardiol* 1991; 7:181–188.
43. al-Khaja N, Belboul A, Rashid M, et al. The influence of age on the durability of Carpentier-Edwards biological valves: Thirteen years' follow-up. *Eur J Cardiothorac Surg* 1991; 5:635–640.
44. Pelletier LC, Carrier M, Leclerc Y, et al. Influence of age on late results of valve replacement with porcine bioprostheses. *J Cardiovasc Surg* 1992; 33:526–533.
45. Barratt-Boyes BG, Jaffe WM, Ko PH, Whitlock RM. The zero pressure, fixed Medtronic Intact porcine valve: An 8.5 year review. *J Heart Valve Dis* 1993; 2:604–611.
46. Munro AI, Jamieson WR, Tyers GF, Burr LH. The Medtronic Intact porcine bioprosthesis: Clinical performance to eight years. *J Heart Valve Dis* 1994; 3:634–640.
47. Matsuki O, Okita Y, Almeida RS, et al. Two decades' experience with aortic valve replacement with pulmonary autograft. *J Thorac Cardiovasc Surg* 1988; 95:705–711.
48. Ross D, Jackson M, Davies J. Pulmonary autograft aortic valve replacement: Long-term results. *J Cardiac Surg* 1991; 6(suppl 4):529–533.
49. Enriquez-Sarano M, Schaff HV, Orszulak TA, et al. Valve repair improves the outcome of surgery for mitral regurgitation: A multivariate analysis. *Circulation* 1995; 91:1022–1028; comments, 1264–1265.
50. Hendren WG, Morris AS, Rosenkranz ER, et al. Mitral valve repair for bacterial endocarditis. *J Thorac Cardiovasc Surg* 1992; 103:124–128; discussion, 128–129.
51. Azar H, Szentpetery S. Mitral valve repair in patients over the age of 70 years. *Eur J Cardiothorac Surg* 1994; 8:298–300.
52. Jebara VA, Dervanian P, Acar C, et al. Mitral valve repair using Carpentier techniques in patients more than 70 years old: Early and late results. *Circulation* 1992; 86(suppl II):53–59.
53. Rahimtoola SH. Lessons learned about the determinants of the results of valve surgery. *Circulation* 1988; 78:1503–1507.
54. Aoyagi S, Tanaka K, Kawara T, et al. Long-term results of mitral valve repair for non-rheumatic mitral regurgitation. *Cardiovasc Surg* 1995; 3:387–392.
55. Skoularigis J, Sinovich V, Joubert G, Sareli P. Evaluation of the long-term results of mitral valve repair in 254 young patients with rheumatic mitral regurgitation. *Circulation* 1994; 90(suppl II):167–174.
56. Grossi EA, Galloway AC, Steinberg BM, et al. Severe calcification does not affect long-term outcome of mitral valve repair. *Ann Thorac Surg* 1994; 58:685–687.
57. Grossi EA, Galloway AC, LeBoutillier M III, et al. Anterior leaflet procedures during mitral valve repair do not adversely influence long-term outcome. *J Am Coll Cardiol* 1995; 25:134–136.
58. Duran CM, Gometza B, Saad E. Valve repair in rheumatic mitral disease: An unsolved problem. *J Cardiac Surg* 1994; 9(suppl 2):282–285.
59. Cosgrove DM, Lytle BW, Taylor PC, et al. The Carpentier-Edwards pericardial aortic valve: Ten year results. *J Thorac Cardiovasc Surg* 1995; 110:651–662.
60. Waller DA, Essop AR, Scott PJ, Nair RU. Repair of asymptomatic aortic valve disease during other cardiac surgery. *Int J Cardiol* 1992; 36:309–314.
61. Grunkemeier GL, Li H-H, Starr A, Rahimtoola SH. Long-term performance of heart valve prostheses. *Curr Probl Cardiol* 2000; 25:75–154.
62. Grunkemeier GL, London MR. Reliability of comparative data from different sources. In: Butchart E, Bodnar E, eds. *Current Issues in Heart Valve Disease: Thrombosis, Embolism and Bleeding*. London: ICR; 1992:464–475.
63. Sackett DL. Bias in analytic research. *J Chronic Dis* 1979; 32:51–63.
64. Rahimtoola SH. Valvular heart disease: A perspective. *J Am Coll Cardiol* 1983; 3:199–215.
65. Edmunds LH Jr. Thrombotic and bleeding complications of prosthetic heart valves. *Ann Thorac Surg* 1987; 44:430–445.
66. Bamford J, Warlow C. Stroke and TIA in the general population. In: Butchart EG, Bodnar E, eds. *Thrombosis, Embolism and Bleeding*. London: ICR; 1992:3–15.
67. Berlin JA, Begg CB, Louis TA. An assessment of publication bias using a sample of published clinical trials. *J Am Stat Assoc* 1989; 84:381–392.

68. Kramer MS, Shapiro SH. Scientific challenges in the application of randomized trials. *JAMA* 1984; 252:2739–2745.
69. Rahimtoola SH. Some unexpected lessons from large multicenter randomized clinical trials. *Circulation* 1985; 72:449–455.
70. Grunkemeier GL, Starr A. Alternatives to randomization in surgical studies. *J Heart Valve Dis* 1992; 1:142–151.
71. Bloomfield P, Wheatley DJ, Prescott RJ, Miller HC. Twelve-year comparison of a Björk-Shiley mechanical heart valve with porcine bioprostheses. *N Engl J Med* 1991; 324:573–579.
72. Hammermeister KE, Sethi GK, Henderson WG, et al. A comparison of outcomes in men 11 years after heart-valve replacement with a mechanical valve or bioprosthesis. Veterans Affairs Cooperative Study on Valvular Heart Disease. *N Engl J Med* 1993; 328:1289–1296.
73. Hammermeister K, Sethi GK, Henderson WG, Grover FL, et al. Outcomes 15 years after valve replacement with a mechanical vs bioprosthetic valve: Final report of the VA randomized trial. *J Am Coll Cardiol.* In press, October 2000.
74. Bonow RO, Carabello B, de Leon AC Jr, et al. ACC/AHA guidelines for the management of patients with valvular heart disease: A report of the American College of Cardiology/American Heart Association Task Force on Practical Guidelines (Committee on Management of Patients with Valvular Heart Disease). *J Am Coll Cardiol* 1998; 32:1486–1588.
75. Grunkemeier GL, Jamieson WR, Miller DC, Starr A. Actuarial versus actual risk of porcine structural valve deterioration. *J Thorac Cardiovasc Surg* 1994; 108:709–718.
76. Starr A, Grunkemeier GL. Recurrent thromboembolism: Significance and management. In: Butchart EG, Bodnar E, eds. *Current Issues in Heart Valve Disease: Thrombosis, Thromboembolism and Bleeding*. London: ICR; 1992:402–415.
77. Rahimtoola SH. Valvular heart disease. In: Stein J, ed. *Internal Medicine*, 4th ed. *Cardiology*, O'Rourke RA, section ed. St. Louis: Mosby-Year Book; 1994:202–234.
78. Grunkemeier GL, Rahimtoola SH, Starr A. Prosthetic heart valves. In: Rahimtoola SH, ed. *Atlas of Heart Diseases, 11*. Philadelphia: Current Medicine; 1997:13.1–13.27.
79. Rahimtoola SH. Aortic valve stenosis. In: Rahimtoola SH, ed. *Valvular Heart Disease, II.* St. Louis: Mosby; 1997:7.02–7.26.
80. Mullany CJ, Elveback LR, Frye RL, et al. Coronary artery disease and its management: Influence on survival in patients undergoing aortic valve replacement. *J Am Coll Cardiol* 1987; 10:66–72.
81. Kloster FE. Infective prosthetic valve endocarditis. In: Rahimtoola SH, ed. *Infective Endocarditis*. New York: Grune & Stratton; 1978:291–305.
82. Douglas JL, Cobbs CG. Prosthetic valve endocarditis. In: Kaye D, ed. *Infective Endocarditis*, 2d ed. New York: Raven Press; 1992:375–396.
83. Rahimtoola SH, Murphy E. Valve prosthesis-patient mismatch: A long-term sequela. *Br Heart J* 1981; 45:331–335.
84. Vongpatawasin W, Hillis LD, Lange RA. Prosthetic heart valves. *N Engl J Med* 1996; 335:407–416.
85. Frater RWM, Furlong P, Cosgrove DM, et al. Long-term durability and patient functional status of the Carpentier-Edwards Perimount pericardial bioprosthesis in the aortic position. *J Heart Valve Dis* 1998; 7:48–53.

C H A P T E R 61

ANTITHROMBOTIC THERAPY FOR VALVULAR HEART DISEASE

John H. McAnulty / Shahbudin H. Rahimtoola

INTRODUCTION

The most important reason to address the issue of protection against thromboemboli in every patient with valve disease is the risk of a stroke. In addition, the consequences of valve thrombosis and of emboli to other organs make the risk of antithrombotic therapy reasonable to assume in many patients with valve disease. Treatment has to be individualized, but some issues and principles are widely applicable (Table 61-1).[1,2] Although some recommendations are appropriate for affluent American communities, the risk, benefit, and cost ratio may not be applicable in poorer areas, where the resources are simply not available. Thromboemboli are not ignored, but alternative therapy—for example, a greater use of antiplatelet agents, in particular aspirin—may, on balance, be more appropriate.

Intracardiac thrombosis most often presents as an embolic cerebrovascular event in over 80 percent of cases. Rarely, thrombosis becomes manifest by causing valve dysfunction. The physical examination should include careful attention to the peripheral pulses and to the skin, fundi, and soft tissues (mouth, conjunctiva), looking for clues of an embolus. A detailed neurologic assessment for focal deficits is essential. Although thrombosis most often occurs without any change in the cardiac examination, auscultation to assess for a change in a murmur or in the quality of heart sounds is important. Intracardiac thrombosis often is first diagnosed when cardiac catheterization or echocardiography is performed for other reasons.

Thrombus is the most common but not the exclusive cause of an embolus. Infective endocarditis must be considered and excluded as a cause, particularly in individuals with valve disease. Disruption of a vascular plaque in the ascending aorta, arch, or descending aorta and in the cerebral vessels may be a common cause of peripheral and cerebral emboli in patients with atherosclerotic disease. Intracardiac tumors or calcified emboli from the heart or aorta are other rare causes.

NATIVE VALVE DISEASE

The risk of thromboembolism in patients with native valve disease is most directly related to certain risk factors, including atrial fibrillation, a history of thromboembolism, left ventricular (LV) dysfunction, and known hypercoagulability. The risk is increased by the presence of certain types of native valve disease (e.g., mitral stenosis) and with prosthetic heart valves, particularly mechanical prostheses, which put a patient at risk even without other associated risk factors (Fig. 61-1).

Risk Factors for Thromboemboli with Native Valve Disease

ATRIAL FIBRILLATION

Most is known about the stroke risk with atrial fibrillation, which is common even without valve disease. Six recent large prospective randomized trials have assessed the value of antithrombotic therapy for primary prevention in patients with nonvalvular atrial fibrillation.[3-8] The term *nonvalvular* is not completely accurate, as at least some patients with aortic valve disease and with mitral regurgitation were included in the studies if the valve lesions were considered hemodynamically "insignificant."

In these trials, the embolic rate (essentially the rate of a stroke in untreated patients with nonvalvular atrial fibrillation) ranged from 3 to 8 percent per year. This was true whether the atrial fibrillation was constant or paroxysmal. Importantly, these trials indicated that warfarin therapy reduced the stroke rate to approximately 0.5 to 2 percent per year. One study, SPAF II,[7] demonstrated equal protection against an adverse neurologic event when aspirin (325 mg daily) was compared to warfarin. In SPAF III,[8] the aspirin was less protective if atrial fibrillation occurred in association with LV dysfunction or uncontrolled

TABLE 61-1 Valve Disease and Antithrombotic Therapy[a,b]

1. Prevention of thromboemboli should be addressed each time a patient with valve disease is seen.
2. Lifelong antithrombotic therapy is required in patients with atrial fibrillation (paroxysmal or persistent) (Table 61-2).
3. Warfarin therapy is required in all patients with a mechanical prothesis (Table 61-3).
4. Antithrombotic therapy should be started early after valve surgery.
5. Warfarin should be avoided in the first trimester of pregnancy.
6. Antithrombotic therapy should be individualized during noncardiac surgery and cardiovascular procedures (Table 61-5).

[a]See text for discussion.
[b]In general, whenever warfarin/aspirin therapy is recommended it is assumed that there is no specific contraindication to its use.

hypertension, if the patient was a woman over age 75, and most importantly, if the patient had had a previous thromboembolic event. Warfarin is indicated in these patients if they are reasonable candidates for the drug, with particular emphasis on its role in those who have had a previous embolic event, as secondary prevention;[6,8] the International Normalized Ratio (INR) should be in the 2.0 to 3.0 range (see also Chap. 44).

The exclusion of mitral stenosis in these prospective trials implies that the risks of emboli and the benefits of warfarin in these patients with associated atrial fibrillation are well understood; however, these are not thoroughly documented or proven. Retrospective assessment, however, suggests that such patients may have an embolic rate >5 percent per year. Until the role of warfarin is better defined, the authors recommend its use in patients with mitral stenosis and one or more risk factors.

LEFT VENTRICULAR DYSFUNCTION

Systemic or pulmonary thromboemboli occur at a rate of over 5 percent per year in patients with LV dysfunction. The type and degree of dysfunction indicating risk are not well defined, but LV systolic abnormalities have been related to emboli most often. However, antithrombotic therapy is of unproven value in preventing or reducing the embolic rate.[9,10] Still, the risk is sufficient that, with or without valve disease, consideration should be given to treatment. One approach (including the authors') is to use warfarin if the LV ejection fraction (EF) ≤0.30 and the patient is a reasonable candidate for this treatment.

PREVIOUS THROMBOEMBOLI

In other clinical situations (e.g., in patients with atrial fibrillation[6,8] or with a prosthetic valve[11–13]), a thromboembolic event defines patients at high risk for having an embolic event—i.e., a recurrent event. It is unclear whether this is true in patients with native valve disease, but we recommend lifelong warfarin therapy.

HYPERCOAGULABLE CONDITIONS

Reasons to consider anticoagulant therapy are the presence of protein C, protein S, or antithrombin III deficiencies; the anticardiolipin antibody syndrome; resistance to activated protein C; or an associated malignancy. This is also true in patients with native valve disease (see also Chap. 44).

Screening for Patients at High Risk for Thromboemboli

The risk factors described above define patients requiring antithrombotic therapy. Transthoracic (TTE) and transesophageal echocardiography (TEE) are often performed in patients with valvular heart disease and in those who have had a systemic embolic episode. The use of these procedures in determining which patients are at risk of thromboemboli is not yet well defined; left atrial (LA) thrombi, a patent foramen ovale, an atrial septal aneurysm, or spontaneous echo contrast are occasional findings of concern, but the value of treatment is unproven. Until more is known, it may not be appropriate to screen patients with native valve disease who do not have one of the obvious clinical risk factors listed above.

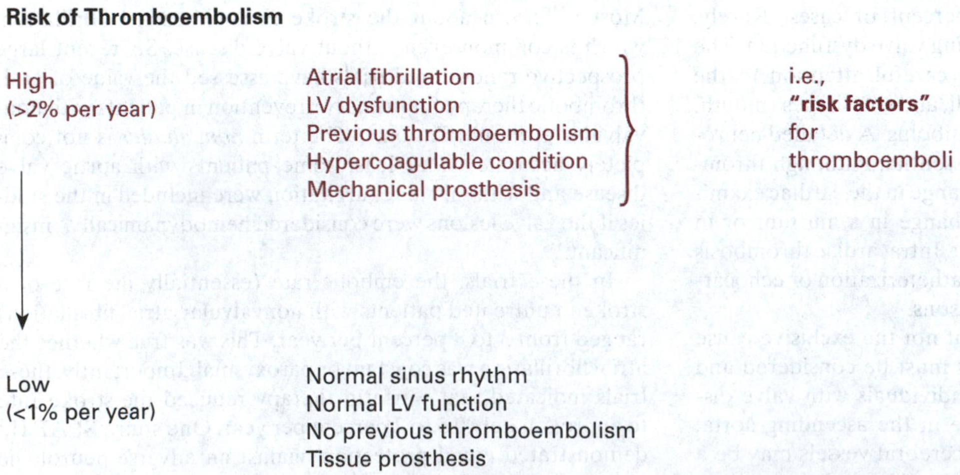

FIGURE 61-1 Risk of thromboembolism. Clinical variables define valve disease patients as being at high or low risk of thromboembolic events.

Antithrombotic Treatment for Native Valve Disease

Antithrombotic therapy is not required in patients with native valve disease (Table 61-2) unless there is an associated risk factor.[2,14] Theoretically, the risk of thrombosis is greater with mitral valve disease as compared to aortic valve disease: there is more blood stasis, the LA may be larger, and the frequency of atrial fibrillation is greater. Still, the presence of mitral valve stenosis or regurgitation by itself is not a reason to initiate antithrombotic therapy. If there is a risk factor, antithrombotic therapy should be considered as defined in Table 61-2. If the patient is a reasonable candidate for war-

TABLE 61-2 Antithrombotic Therapy—Native Valve Disease

I. *No therapy* if no thrombosis risk factor
II. *Therapy* if thrombosis risk factor present
   A. *Atrial fibrillation*
      1. Warfarin (INR 2–3) if congestive heart failure, hypertension, or previous thromboembolism
      2. Warfarin (INR 2–3) if valve lesion is mitral stenosis
      3. Aspirin (325 mg/day) or warfarin (INR 2–3) if valve lesion other than mitral stenosis
   B. *Previous thromboembolism*—warfarin (INR 2–3)
   C. *LV dysfunction* (ejection fraction ≤0.30—warfarin (INR 2–3)
   D. *Hypercoagulable state*—warfarin (INR 2–3)

Abbreviation: INR = International Normalized Ratio.

farin therapy, the use of warfarin (maintaining an INR of 2 to 3) is appropriate if a patient with valve disease has atrial fibrillation (constant or paroxysmal) in combination with reduced LV function (heart failure or LV EF ≤0.30) or with associated severe hypertension or if there is a history of thromboemboli. There is a suggestion that women over the age of 75 with atrial fibrillation might be better protected by warfarin than aspirin,[8] but the bleeding rate on warfarin is significant in this patient population; treatment should be individualized and the INR more closely monitored. If a patient with atrial fibrillation has reasonable LV function, has not had a previous thromboembolism, and does not have other risk factors, aspirin (325 mg/day) is just as likely as warfarin to be protective against thromboemboli, without the associated expense and risk of warfarin therapy.[7,15] Unrelated to atrial fibrillation, warfarin therapy is recommended if a patient has had a previous thromboembolism or has LV dysfunction (heart failure and an ejection fraction ≤0.30).

PROSTHETIC HEART VALVES

All patients with mechanical valves require warfarin therapy. Even with the use of warfarin, the risk of thromboemboli in these patients is 1 to 2 percent per year;[16–19] the risk is *considerably higher* without treatment with warfarin.[11] The risk of an embolus in patients with biological valves in sinus rhythm has been approximately 0.6 to 0.7 percent per year, and most of those patients were not on warfarin therapy.[16,17,19–21] Almost all studies have shown that the risk of embolism is greater with a valve in the mitral position (mechanical or biological) as compared to a valve in the aortic position;[11,16] however, this was not found in one study.[17] With either type of prosthesis or valve location, the risk of emboli is probably higher in the first few days and months after valve insertion,[20] before the valve is fully endothelialized.

Antithrombotic Treatment for Prosthetic Valves (Table 61-3)

MECHANICAL VALVES

All patients with mechanical valves require warfarin, and the INR should be maintained between 2.0 and 3.5.[16,17,22–24] In patients with an aortic prosthesis without risk factors for emboli the INR should be between 2.0 and 3.0; in those with risk factors and in those with a mitral prosthesis the INR should be between 2.5 and 3.5.[2] Some valves are thought to be more thrombogenic than others (particularly the tilting-disk valves), and a case could be made for increasing the INR to between 3 and 4.5, but this would be associated with an increased risk of bleeding.[22,25,26] The addition of low-dose aspirin (50 to 100 mg/day) to warfarin therapy may further decrease the risk of thromboembolism.[27,28] The authors recommend the addition of aspirin (50 to 100 mg/

TABLE 61-3 Antithrombotic Therapy[a]—Prosthetic Heart Valves

	Mechanical Prosthetic Valves			Biological Prosthetic Valves		
	Warfarin, INR 2–3	Warfarin, INR 2.5–3.5	Aspirin, 50–100 mg	Warfarin, INR 2–3	Warfarin, INR 2.5–3.5	Aspirin, 50-100 mg
First 3 months after valve replacement		+	+		+	+
After first 3 months						
Aortic valve	+		+			+
Aortic valve + risk factor[b]		+	+	+		
Mitral valve		+	+			+
Mitral valve + risk factor		+	+		+	+

[a]Depending on the clinical status of patient, antithrombotic therapy must be individualized (see special situations in text).
[b]Risk factors (see Fig. 61-1): atrial fibrillation, previous thromboembolus, LV dysfunction, hypercoagulable state.

day) to warfarin unless there is a contraindication to the use of aspirin (i.e., bleeding or aspirin intolerance). This combination is particularly appropriate in patients who have had an embolus while on warfarin therapy and/or who are known to be particularly hypercoagulable; for example, it is recommended by a committee addressing antithrombotic therapy in women during pregnancy.[29] It is important to note that the thromboembolic risk increases early after the insertion of the prosthetic valve; this is a reason to initiate heparin therapy within the first 24 to 48 h of surgery, with maintenance of the *activated partial thromboplastin time* (aPTT) at a "therapeutic effect" level (Table 61-4) until warfarin therapy has achieved the recommended INR level.

BIOLOGICAL (TISSUE) VALVES

Because of an increased risk of thromboemboli during the first 3 months after implantation of a biological prosthetic valve, anticoagulation with warfarin is indicated.[20] The risk is particularly high in the first few days after surgery, and heparin therapy should be started within 24 to 48 h, with maintenance of the aPTT at a "therapeutic effect" level (Table 61-4) until an INR of 2.0 to 3.0 is achieved with warfarin. After 3 months, the tissue valve can be treated like native valve disease (see Table 61-2), and warfarin can be discontinued in approximately two-thirds of patients with biological valves.[16,17,20,30] Associated atrial fibrillation or an LV EF ≤0.30 are reasons for lifelong warfarin therapy.

TABLE 61-4 "Therapeutic Effect" of Heparin

Unfractionated heparin	An aPTT at 8 h after a dose that has been calibrated[a] to reflect a heparin level of 0.35 to 0.70 anti-Xa units
Low-molecular-weight heparin	An aPTT at 8 h after a dose that has been calibrated[a] reflect a heparin level of 0.7 to 1.1 anti-Xa units
During pregnancy	A heparin level of 0.6 to 0.7 anti-Xa units with unfractionated heparin or 0.10 to 0.11 anti-Xa units with low-molecular-weight heparin[b] (aPTT measurements do not accurately reflect heparin levels during pregnancy)

[a]Calibration of aPTT to heparin levels is performed in each clinical laboratory; thus the time (number of seconds) of the aPTT reflecting the "therapeutic effect" levels will vary.

[b]*Important Note:* Although low-molecular-weight heparin is increasingly being utilized in many disorders, it is reemphasized here (see text) that its value in protecting against thromboemboli in patients with valve disease has *not* been proven. Therefore its use in patients with valve disease *cannot* be recommended at the present time.

SPECIAL CLINICAL SITUATIONS

Altered Native Valves

Valve disease is increasingly being treated by interventional catheter techniques or surgical valve repair. It is difficult to give firm recommendations about antithrombotic therapy in these patients, but the recommendations given for treatment of native valve disease would seem most applicable in patients who have had surgical valve repair or catheter valve procedures (see Table 61-2).

Pregnancy

Pregnancy makes decisions regarding antithrombotic therapy for valve disease more difficult. Warfarin should be avoided in the first trimester of pregnancy, particularly in weeks 6 through 12.[29,31,32] It crosses the placental barrier and is associated with, and is the clear cause of, an embryopathy manifest in the live born as mental impairment, ocular atrophy, and facial and digital abnormalities. Therefore, warfarin should be discontinued immediately when pregnancy is recognized and heparin therapy should be initiated. The value of switching from warfarin to heparin *before* conception is uncertain. We suggest this when pregnancies are planned, since little is known about the consequences of warfarin taken in the first 6 weeks of pregnancy; however, this is often not clinically practical or feasible. Currently, the estimated risk of an embryopathy in well-managed warfarin therapy is ≤5 percent. While a return to warfarin during the second and third trimesters is recommended, there is concern that this drug may continue to endanger the fetus.

Heparin does not cross the placenta. While not devoid of problems (maternal bleeding, heparin-initiated thrombocytopenia, an increased risk of osteoporosis when used for longer than 1 month), successful pregnancies have occurred when adequate doses of the drug are administered subcutaneously at home throughout gestation.[33] Thromboembolic complications have occurred with heparin use during pregnancy in women with a mechanical prosthesis.[34,35] To minimize this, it is important to give a dose that will result in high "therapeutic effect" heparin levels (Table 61-4) prior to the next dose (this usually requires 15,000 to 30,000 units every 12 h).[29,36] Activated PTT measurements do not accurately reflect heparin levels during pregnancy.

Low-molecular-weight heparin (LMWH) is currently approved *only* for treatment of venous thrombosis. Still, there is no reason to suspect that it will not result in effective anticoagulation in patients with valve disease. It has been used safely in pregnancy,[37,38] does not cross the placenta, can be given once or twice daily, does not require regular blood test monitoring, and is associated with less thrombocytopenia and osteoporosis. More studies are needed.[39] Since there are *no* data about use of LMWH in patients with native valve disease or with prosthetic heart valves, LMWH cannot be recommended in such patients at this time.

Aspirin crosses the placenta and has been implicated as a cause of abortion and fetal growth retardation,[40] but it has been used so frequently without problems and has even been considered for use in all pregnant women as prophylaxis against preclampsia[41] that, when required for valve disease (see Table 61-2), it should be continued.

The concern about the use of antithrombotic therapy during pregnancy makes the decision about management of valve disease more difficult in women of childbearing age. If valve surgery is required, commissurotomy or valve repair is preferable because subsequent antithrombotic therapy is not required unless the woman has one of the risk factors for thrombosis (see Fig. 61-1). If a prosthetic valve is required in a woman of childbearing age, the advantage of a mechanical prosthesis is its durability. On the other hand, it obligates the woman of childbearing age to anticoagulation with warfarin because aspirin therapy itself does not offer adequate protection against thromboembolism. The theoretical advantage of a biological prosthesis is that, except for the first 3 months after valve replacement, warfarin therapy is not required. However, as many as one-third of patients with biological valves have associated atrial fibrillation and require warfarin antithrombotic therapy. In addition, the rate of degeneration of biological valves accelerates dramatically in young patients and thus also in women of childbearing age.[42] Furthermore, some data suggest that the rate of structural valve degeneration is increased in pregnant women. The choice of a prosthesis should be individualized. A young woman capable of safely using warfarin when not pregnant and warfarin/heparin during pregnancy is best treated with a mechanical valve. If a woman's social situation or attention to her health is questionable in regard to the safe use of anticoagulation therapy, a biological valve may be considered. In young women needing aortic valve replacement, the Ross procedure should be considered (see also Chap. 60).

Surgery and Dental Care (Table 61-5)

The risk of increased bleeding during a procedure performed with a patient on antithrombotic therapy has to be weighed against the increased risk of a thromboembolism caused by stopping the therapy.

The risk of stopping warfarin can be estimated and is relatively low if the drug is withheld for only a few days. As an example, and using a *worst case* scenario (e.g., a patient with a mechanical prosthesis with previous thromboemboli), the risk of a thromboembolus off warfarin could be as high as 10 to 20 percent per year. Thus, if the therapy were stopped for 3 days, the risk of an embolus would be 3/365 times 0.10 to 0.20, which equals 0.08 to 0.16 percent. There are theoretical concerns that stopping the drug and then reinstituting it might result in hypercoagulability—with a thrombotic "rebound." An increase in markers for activation of thrombosis with abrupt discontinuation of warfarin therapy has been observed,[43] but it is not clear that these increase the clinical risk of thromboembolism.[44] In addition, when reinstituting warfarin therapy, there are theoretical concerns of a hypercoagulable state caused by suppression of proteins C and S before the drug affects the thrombotic factors. Although the risks are only hypothetical, this is a reason to treat individuals at very high risk with heparin therapy until the INR returns to the desired range.

Although antithrombotic therapy must be individualized, some generalizations apply (see Table 61-6). For procedures where bleeding is unlikely or would be inconsequential if it occurred, antithrombotic therapy should not be stopped. This can apply to surgery on the skin, dental prophylaxis, or simple treatment for dental caries. Eye surgery, in particular surgery for cataracts or glaucoma, is usually associated with very little bleeding; when bleeding is likely or its potential consequences are severe, antithrombotic treatment should be altered. If a patient is on aspirin, it should be discontinued 1 week before the procedure and restarted as soon as it is considered safe by the surgeon or dentist.

For most patients on warfarin, the drug should be stopped 48 to 72 h before the procedure to ensure the INR is ≤1.5 and restarted within 24 h after a procedure; admission to the hospital or a delay in discharge to give heparin is usually unnecessary.[2,27,44–47] Deciding who is at very high risk of thrombosis and thus should require heparin until warfarin can be reinstated may be difficult; clinical judgment is required. Heparin can usually be reserved for those who have had a recent thrombosis or embolus (arbitrarily within 1 year), those with demonstrated thrombotic problems when previously off therapy, and those with three or more risk factors. When used, unfractionated heparin should be started 24 h after warfarin is stopped (i.e., 48 h before surgery) and stopped 4 to 6 h before the procedure. The heparin should be restarted as early after surgery as bleeding stability allows and the aPPT maintained at a "therapeutic level" (Table 61-4) until warfarin is restarted and the desired INR can be achieved. Home administration and management of heparin (and warfarin) can be arranged to minimize time in the hospital. LMWH is even more easily utilized outside of the hospital (see also Chap. 48); however, there are no data with its use in patients with valve disease.

TABLE 61-5 Antithrombotic Therapy at the Time of Surgery

I. Usual approach
  A. If patient on warfarin
    Stop 72 h before procedure
    Restart on day of procedure or after control of active bleeding
  B. If patient on aspirin
    Stop 1 week before procedure
    Restart the day after procedure or after control of active bleeding
II. Unusual circumstances
  A. Very high risk of thrombosis if off warfarin[a]
    Stop warfarin 72 h before procedure
    Start heparin 48 h before procedure[b]
    Stop heparin 6 h before procedure
    Restart heparin within 24 h of procedure and continue until warfarin can be restarted and the INR is 2–3
  B. Surgery complicated by postoperative bleeding
    Start heparin as soon after surgery as deemed safe and maintain aPTT of 60–80 s until warfarin restarted and the INR is 2–3
  C. Very low risk from bleeding[c]
    Continue antithrombotic therapy

[a]Clinical judgment: consider this approach if recent thromboembolus or if three risk factors are present.
[b]Heparin can be given in outpatient setting before and after surgery.
[c]For example, local skin surgery, dental prophylaxis, and treatment for caries.
Abbreviation: aPTT = activated partial thromboplastin time.

TABLE 61-6 Antithrombotic Therapy at the Time of a Thromboembolic Event

I. Acute management
   A. *No* antithrombotic treatment for 72 h
   B. CT scan at 72 h
      1. *No (or little) hemorrhage* on CT:
         a. Heparin: aPTT in low "therapeutic effect" (Table 61-4)
         b. Warfarin: continue heparin until INR in desired range[a]
      2. *Hemorrhage* on CT:
         a. No treatment until bleed stabilized or treated (7–14 days), then heparin and warfarin as above
II. Chronic management
   A. If embolus occurred *off* antithrombotic therapy:
      1. Treat with warfarin[a]
   B. If embolus occurred *on* antithrombotic therapy:
      1. If patient was on aspirin, switch to warfarin[a]
      2. If patient was on warfarin but INR was low, increase dose until INR in high desired range[a]
      3. If patient was on warfarin and INR was in desired range, add aspirin 80–325 mg/day
      4. If recurrent embolus or bleed on warfarin plus aspirin, assess valve for possible surgery

[a]See Tables 61-2 and 61-3.
Abbreviation: CT = computed tomography.

Cardiac Catheterization and Angiography

Antiplatelet therapy or heparin need not be stopped for these procedures. Protamine can be given to the patient on heparin if bleeding occurs. In an emergent or semiemergent situation, cardiac catheterization can be performed with a patient on warfarin, but, preferably, the drug should be stopped 72 h before the procedure and restarted the day of the procedure. This is also true for most patients with prosthetic heart valves (mechanical as well as biological). If a patient is at very high risk of thromboembolism, heparin should be started 48 h before the procedure and continued until warfarin is restarted and the desired INR is achieved. If the catheterization procedure is to include a transseptal puncture (especially in a patient who has not had previous opening of the pericardium), patients should be off all antithrombotic therapy and the INR should be <1.2—the same is also true if an LV puncture is to be performed.[48]

Therapy at the Time of an Active Thromboembolic Event

VALVE THROMBOSIS

Thrombosis of a valve, usually a prosthetic valve, can result in severe hemodynamic compromise. If recognized (TEE can be diagnostic[49]), this complication may be treated with thrombolytic therapy, although the risk of bleeding and of emboli at the time of treatment is high.[50,51] Thrombolytic therapy is most effective for a "young thrombus." Many valves, however, have pannus formation and tissue ingrowth on the valve, which is not amenable to thrombolytic therapy. Therefore, we recommend emergency surgery rather than thrombolytic therapy in the patient with severe hemodynamic compromise. If a patient is not a surgical candidate, thrombolysis should be attempted.[2,52] Streptokinase or urokinase should be initiated but stopped at 24 h if there is no improvement by Doppler echocardiography and at 72 h even if hemodynamic recovery is incomplete.[2] This should be followed by heparin until high INR levels are achieved with concomitant warfarin therapy (INR 3 to 4 for aortic prostheses or 3.5 to 4.5 with mitral prostheses).

THROMBOEMBOLIC EVENT

An embolic event often indicates inadequate therapy for that patient's circumstances. Data and opinions about optimal timing for initiating or continuing anticoagulants in patients in whom an embolus is the presumed cause of a stroke are conflicting.[2,53–55] Ideally, treatment would be started early to prevent recurrent emboli, but the early use of heparin (within 72 h) is associated with a 15 to 25 percent chance of converting a nonhemorrhagic into a hemorrhagic stroke.[54] While a case can still be made for immediate use of heparin,[53,54] the early recurrence of an embolus in patients with valve disease while off anticoagulants has not been clearly documented. Data are insufficient to provide definitive treatment outlines, but the authors' practice is listed in Table 61-6.

ACUTE MANAGEMENT OF AN EMBOLIC EVENT

Antithrombotic therapy should be withheld or stopped for 72 h. If a computed tomography (CT) scan at that time reveals little or no hemorrhage, heparin should be administered to maintain an aPPT at the lower end of the therapeutic level (Table 61-4) until warfarin, started at the same time, results in the desired INR (see Tables 61-2 and 61-3). If the CT scan demonstrates significant hemorrhage, antithrombotic therapy should be withheld until the bleed is treated or has stabilized (7 to 14 days). Anticoagulation can then be started as just described.

LONG-TERM MANAGEMENT

If the embolic event occurs when a patient is *off* antithrombotic therapy, long-term warfarin therapy is required (see Tables 61-2 and 61-3). An exception may be those with mitral valve prolapse; aspirin (325 mg/day) is recommended for those who are judged to have had a minor event. If the embolic event occurs while the patient is *on* antithrombotic treatment, therapy should be individualized. Those who are on warfarin but in whom the INR was low at the time of the embolus should have the dose increased into the high end of the desired range (see Tables 61-2 and 61-3). If the embolus occurs in a patient despite an INR in the desirable range, aspirin (50 to 100 mg/day) should be added to the warfarin. Embolism recurring with this combination should lead to consideration of possible valve surgery if the valve is the likely source of the thrombus.

Therapy at the Time of a Bleed

With significant bleeding, antithrombotic therapy should be stopped and, if the patient is at risk, drug effects should be reversed. If possible, the site of bleeding should be corrected and antithrombotic therapy restarted as soon as possible. If this is not possible, treatment decisions are difficult. In patients with a mechanical prosthesis or multiple risk factors for thromboemboli, acceptance of intermittent bleeding with acute management for the bleeds may be necessary. In valve patients who are at lower risk of emboli or in whom the role of antithrombotic treatment is less clear (e.g., LV dysfunction), it may be optimal to withhold chronic therapy or, if a patient is on warfarin, to switch to aspirin. In some patients with mechanical valves, consideration should be given to replacing the mechanical valve with a biological valve, for example, in those who have had multiple, large life- or organ-threatening bleeds.

Antithrombotic Therapy in the Patient with Endocarditis

If a patient with valve disease develops endocarditis, antithrombotic therapy should be continued.[2,56] If the patient presents with or develops an embolic event involving the central nervous system, therapy should be as described above for acute embolic events. Additionally, the issue of whether or not the embolus is due to thrombus or infected vegetation should be addressed. If thrombus is likely, the chronic anticoagulation program will also require alteration.

References

1. Rahimtoola S. Lessons learned about the determinants of the results of valve surgery. *Circulation* 1988; 78:1503–1506.
2. Bonow RO, Carabello B, deLeon AC Jr, et al. ACCAHA guidelines for the management of patients with valvular heart disease: A report of the American College of Cardiology American Heart Association Task Force on Practice Guidelines (Committee on Management of Patients with Valvular Heart Disease). *J Am Coll Cardiol* 1998; 32:1486–1588.
3. Petersen P, Boysen G, Godtfredsen J, et al. Placebo controlled, randomized trial of warfarin and aspirin for prevention of thromboembolic complications in chronic atrial fibrillation. *Lancet* 1989; 1:175–179.
4. The Boston Area Anticoagulation Trial for Atrial Fibrillation Investigators. The effect of low-dose warfarin on the risk of stroke in patients with nonrheumatic atrial fibrillation. *N Engl J Med* 1990; 323:1505–1511.
5. Ezekowitz MD, Bridgers SL, James KE, et al. Warfarin in the prevention of stroke associated with nonrheumatic atrial fibrillation. *N Engl J Med* 1992; 327:1406–1412.
6. EAFT (European Atrial Fibrillation Trial) Study Group. Secondary prevention in nonrheumatic atrial fibrillation after transient ischemic attack or minor stroke. *Lancet* 1993; 342:1255–1262.
7. Stroke Prevention in Atrial Fibrillation Investigators. Warfarin versus aspirin for prevention of thromboembolism in atrial fibrillation: Stroke Prevention in Atrial Fibrillation II Study. *Lancet* 1994; 343:687–691.
8. Stroke Prevention in Atrial Fibrillation Investigators. Adjusted-dose warfarin versus low-intensity, fixed dose warfarin plus aspirin for high-risk patients with atrial fibrillation: Stroke Prevention in Atrial Fibrillation III randomized clinical trial. *Lancet* 1996; 348:633–638.
9. ACCAHA Task Force. Guidelines for the evaluation and management of heart failure. *Circulation* 1999; 92:2764–2784.
10. Al-Khadra AS, Salem DN, Rand WM, et al. Warfarin anticoagulation and survival: A cohort analysis from the Studies of Left Ventricular Dysfunction. *J Am Coll Cardiol* 1998; 31:749–753.
11. Cannegieter SC, Rosendaal FR, Briet E. Thromboembolic and bleeding complications in patients with mechanical heart valve prostheses. *Circulation* 1994; 89:635–641.
12. Starr A, Grunkemeier GL. Recurrent thromboembolism: Significance and management. In: Butchart EG, Bodnar E, eds. *Thrombosis, Embolism and Bleeding.* London: ICR; 1992: 402–415.
13. Blackstone EH. Analyses of thrombosis, embolism and bleeding as time-related outcome events. In: Butchart EG, Bodnar E, eds. *Thrombosis, Embolism and Bleeding.* London: ICR; 1992: 445–463.
14. Levin HJ, Pauler SG, Eckman MH. Antithrombotic therapy in valve disease: Fourth ACCP conference on antithrombolic therapy. *Chest* 1995; 108(suppl):360S–370S.
15. The SPAF III Writing Committee for the Stroke Prevention in Atrial Fibrillation Investigators. Patients with nonvalvular atrial fibrillation at low risk of stroke during treatment with aspirin: Stroke Prevention in Atrial Fibrillation III Study. *JAMA* 1998; 279:1273–1277.
16. Bloomfield P, Wheatley DJ, Prescott RJ, Miller HC. Twelve-year comparison of a Bjork-Shiley mechanical heart valve with porcine bioprostheses. *N Engl J Med* 1991; 324:573–579.
17. Hammermeister KE, Sethi GK, Henderson WG, et al. A comparison of outcomes in men 11 years after heart-valve replacement with a mechanical valve or bioprosthesis. *N Engl J Med* 1993; 328:1289–1296.
18. Cobanoglu A, Fessler CL, Guvendik L, et al. Aortic valve replacement with the Starr-Edwards prosthesis: A comparison of the first and second decades of follow-up. *Ann Thorac Surg* 1988; 45:248–252.
19. Vongpatanasin W, Hillis D, Lange RA. Prosthetic heart valves. *N Engl J Med* 1996; 335:407–416.
20. Geras M, Chesebro JH, Fuster V, et al. High risk of thromboemboli early after bioprosthetic cardiac valve replacement. *J Am Coll Cardiol* 1995; 25:1111–1119.
21. North RA, Sadler L, Stewart AW, et al. Long-term survival and valve-related complications in young women with cardiac valve replacements. *Circulation* 1999; 99:2669–2676.
22. Cannegieter SC, Rosendaal FR, Wintzen AR, et al. Optimal oral anticoagulant therapy in patients with mechanical heart valves. *N Engl J Med* 1995; 333:11–17.
23. Jegaden O, Eker A, Delahaye F, et al. Thromboembolic risk and late survival after mitral valve replacement with the St. Jude medical valve. *Ann Thorac Surg* 1994; 58:1721–1728.
24. Saour JN, Sieck JO, Mamo LAR, Gallus AS. Trial of different intensities of anticoagulation in patients with prosthetic heart valves. *N Engl J Med* 1990; 322:428–432.
25. Hylek EM, Skates SJ, Sheehan MA, Singer DE. An analysis of the lowest effective intensity of prophylactic anticoagulation for patients with nonrheumatic atrial fibrillation. *N Engl J Med* 1996; 335:540–546.
26. Acar J, Iung B, Boissel JP, et al. AREVA: Multicenter randomized comparison of low-dose versus standard-dose anticoagulation in patients with mechanical prosthetic heart valves. *Circulation* 1996; 94:2107–2112.
27. Hyashi J, Nakazawa S, Oguma F, et al. Combined warfarin and antiplatelet therapy after St. Jude medical valve replacement for mitral valve disease. *J Am Coll Cardiol* 1994; 23:672–677.
28. Turpie AG, Gent M, Laupacis A, et al. A comparison of aspirin with placebo in patients treated with warfarin after heart-valve replacement. *N Engl J Med* 1993; 329:524–529.
29. Ginsberg JS, Hirsh J. Use of antithrombotic agents during pregnancy. Fourth ACCP conference on antithrombolic therapy. *Chest* 1995; 108 (suppl):305S–311S.
30. Turpie AGG, Gunstensen J, Hirsh J, et al. Randomized comparison of two intensities of oral anticoagulant therapy after tissue heart valve replacement. *Lancet* 1988; 1:1242–1245.
31. Hall JR, Pauli RM, Wilson KM. Maternal and fetal sequelae of anticoagulation during pregnancy. *Am J Med* 1980; 68:122.
32. Iturbe-Alessio I, del Carmen Fonseca M, Mutchinick O, et al.

Risks of anticoagulant therapy in pregnant women with artificial heart valves. *N Engl J Med* 1986; 315:1390–1393.
33. Ginsberg JS, Kowalchuk G, Hirsh J, et al. Heparin therapy during pregnancy. *Arch Intern Med* 1989; 149:2233–2236.
34. Hanania G, Thomas D, Michel PL, et al. Pregnancy and prosthetic heart valves: A French cooperative retrospective study of 155 cases. *Eur Heart J* 1994; 15:1651–1658.
35. Salazar E, Iazguirre R, Verdejo J, Mutchinick O. Failure of adjusted doses of subcutaneous heparin to prevent thromboembolic phenomena in pregnant patients with mechanical cardiac valve prostheses. *J Am Coll Cardiol* 1996; 27:1698–1703.
36. Elkayam U. Anticoagulation in pregnant women with prosthetic heart valves: A double jeopardy (editorial). *J Am Coll Cardiol* 1996; 27:1704–1706.
37. Sturridge F, DeSwiet M, Letsky E. The use of low molecular weight heparin for thromboprophylaxis in pregnancy. *Br J Obstet Gynaecol* 1994; 101:69–71.
38. Nelson-Piercy C, Letsky EA, DeSweit M. Low-molecular weight heparin for obstetric thromboprophylaxis: Experience of sixty-nine pregnancies in sixty-one women at high risk. *Am J Obstet Gynecol* 1997; 176:1062–1068.
39. Sanson BJ, Lensing AW, Prins MH, et al. Safety of low-molecular-weight heparin in pregnancy: A systematic review. *Thromb Haemost* 1999; 81:668–672.
40. Corby DG. Aspirin in pregnancy and fetal effects. *Pediatrics* 1978; 62:930–937.
41. DuBard MB, Cutter GR. Low-dose aspirin therapy to prevent preeclampsia. *Am J Obstet Gynecol* 1993; 168:1083–1091.
42. Jamieson WR, Miller DC, Akins CW, et al. Pregnancy and bioprostheses: Influence on structural valve deterioration. *Ann Thorac Surg* 1995; 60:S282–S286.
43. Genewein U, Hasberli A, Werner S, Beer J. Rebound after cessation of oral anticoagulant therapy: The biochemical evidence. *Br J Haematol* 1996; 92:479–485.
44. Eckman MH, Beshansky JR, Durand-Zaleski I, et al. Anticoagulation for noncardiac procedures in patients with prosthetic heart valves: Does low risk mean high cost? *JAMA* 1990; 263:1513–1521.
45. Bryan AJ, Butchart EG. Prosthetic heart valves and anticoagulant management during non-cardiac surgery. *Br J Surg* 1995; 82: 577–578.
46. Busuttil WJ, Fabr BMI. The management of anticoagulation in patients with prosthetic heart valves undergoing non-cardiac operations. *Postgrad Med J* 1995; 71:390–392.
47. Tinker JH, Tarhan S. Discontinuing anticoagulant therapy in surgical patients with cardiac valve prostheses: Observations in 180 operations. *JAMA* 1978; 239:738–739.
48. Morton MJ, McAnulty JH, Rahimtoola SH, Ahuja N. Risks and benefits of postoperative cardiac catheterization in patients with ball-valve prostheses. *Am J Cardiol* 1977; 40:870–875.
49. Gueret P, Vignon P, Fournier P, et al. Transesophageal echocardiography for the diagnosis and management of nonobstructive thrombosis of mechanical mitral valve prosthesis. *Circulation* 1995; 91:103–110.
50. Silber H, Khan SS, Matloff JM, et al. The St. Jude valve: Thrombolysis as the first line of therapy of cardiac valve thrombosis. *Circulation* 1993; 887:30–37.
51. Reddy NK, Padmanabhan TNC, Singh S, et al. Thrombolysis in left-sided prosthetic valve occlusion: Immediate and follow-up results. *Ann Thorac Surg* 1994; 58:462–471.
52. Lengyel M, Fuster V, Keltai M, et al. Guidelines for management of lift-sided prosthetic valve thrombosis: A role for thrombolytic therapy: Consensus Conference on Prosthetic Valve Thrombosis. *J Am Coll Cardiol* 1997; 30:1521–1526.
53. Pessin MS, Estol CJ, Lafranchise F, Chaplan LR. Safety of anticoagulation after hemorrhagic infarction. *Neurology* 1994; 43:1289–1303.
54. Chamorro A, Vila N, Saiz A, et al. Early anticoagulation after large cerebral embolic infarction: A safety study. *Neurology* 1995; 45:861–865.
55. Sherman DJ, Dyken ML, Gent M, et al. Antithrombotic therapy for cerebrovascular disorders: Fourth ACCP consensus conference on antithrombotic therapy. *Chest* 1995; 108(suppl):444s–456s.
56. Wilson WR, Geraci JE, Danielson GK, et al. Anticoagulant therapy and central nervous system complication in patients with prosthetic valve endocarditis. *Circulation* 1978; 57:1004–1007.

PART TEN

CONGENITAL HEART DISEASE

C H A P T E R 62

CARDIOVASCULAR DISEASES DUE TO GENETIC ABNORMALITIES

Jeffrey A. Towbin / Robert Roberts

Genetic factors play a significant role in the pathogenesis of many if not all cardiovascular disorders. Malformations of the heart and blood vessels account for the largest number of human birth defects, occurring in about 1 percent of all live births; among stillbirths, the prevalence is estimated to be tenfold higher.[1,2] In conjunction with cytogenetics (the study of chromosomes and their abnormalities), molecular genetics provides an opportunity to decipher the genetic basis of cardiovascular diseases. Genetic diagnosis and screening for genetic disorders will soon be incorporated into standard practice.[3] The goal of the Human Genome Project[4] is to identify all of the genes by the year 2001 (see Chap. 7).[5] The challenge for the clinical and investigative cardiologist is to link these genes to their specific physiologic or pathologic function.[6] It is thus imperative that the cardiologist understand the basis for genetic disorders so as to have a better appreciation of the medical, ethical, and moral implications.[7]

BASIS FOR GENETIC TRANSMISSION

All hereditary information is transmitted through DNA, a linear polymer composed of purine (adenine, guanine) and pyrimidine (cytosine, thymine) bases (see Chap. 4). The basic hereditary unit is the gene, which consists of a distinct fragment of DNA that encodes for a specific polypeptide (protein). It is estimated there are only about 100,000 genes, although there is enough DNA to code for several hundred thousand genes. However, less than 5 percent of the DNA is used to code for genes. Each individual has two copies of each gene—called alleles. The genes are localized in linear sequence along 23 pairs of chromosomes, the rod-shaped bodies derived from the parents of each individual. Each parent contributes one member of each chromosome pair (the pair is referred to as *homologous chromosomes*) and thus one copy of each gene. The site at which a gene is located on a particular chromosome is called the *genetic locus*. A given gene always resides at the same specific locus on a particular chromosome, so the loci on homologous chromosomes are identical but the alleles residing at these loci may be the same or different. When the same loci on two homologous chromosomes have identical alleles, the individual is homozygous. When the two genes differ (i.e., two different alleles present at the locus), the individual is heterozygous at that locus. Each individual is homozygous at some loci and heterozygous at others, and, based on present knowledge, at least one-third of human genes have polymorphic forms. The gene, transmitted to each offspring during the union of sperm and ova, passes on the genetic information to the offspring (genotype), which, through the synthesis of their corresponding proteins, determines the observable characteristics of an individual (phenotype). The genetic information carried in the gene's DNA is coded by the sequence of the four bases. Translation of this information into protein is through a translational code passed on through messenger ribonucleic acid (mRNA), whereby each specific amino acid is encoded by three bases referred to as a *codon* (Chap. 4). The mRNA transcribed from the gene serves as the template that determines which amino acids are included and their sequence in the resulting polypeptide. Although it is true each gene encodes for a unique protein, it is preferable to use polypeptide, since many proteins are single polypeptides and other proteins consist of several polypeptides which may be from a single gene or multiple genes. The 23 pairs of chromosomes include 22 pairs of autosomes (chromosomes 1 to 22) and one pair of sex chromosomes, X and Y. Females have two X chromosomes, while males carry one X and one Y chromosome. Both autosomal alleles are potentially active in specifying RNA copies of their DNA sequences, but the expression of each gene depends on the cell type, developmental stage, and regulatory molecules that interact with promoter sequences, and enhancer sequences that control gene transcription. In cells that carry two X chromosomes, whether these are derived from normal females or XXY individuals with Klinefelter syndrome, only one X is active after early embryogenesis.

ORIGIN OF GENETIC DISEASE

The three broad categories of inherited diseases are chromosomal abnormalities, single gene disorders, and polygene disorders (Table 62-1). Thus, hereditary and congenital diseases may be due to chromosomal abnormalities or mutations within a single gene or multiple genes. A mutation is a stable, heritable alteration in DNA caused by a number of factors, including environmental agents such as radiation, chemicals, and viruses as well as baseline changes in the fidelity of transfer of sequences. Since offspring typically resemble their parents, it is assumed that the DNA nucleotide sequences remain stable. Base sequence changes do occur, however, albeit at a slow rate compared to the overall life span of humans, and these changes occur by a number of different mechanisms. Mutations can involve a visible alteration at the level of the chromosome, such as deletion or translocation of a portion of the chromosome, whereby often several genes are eliminated or altered. Chromosome alterations (discussed later), especially those involving too many or too few chromosomes (called an euploidy), are quite common in human development. The sequence of each codon determines the amino acid, and the linear sequence of the codons in the mRNA is collinear with the linear sequence of the amino acids in the protein. A change in even one amino acid, if critical to the function of the protein, will result in altered function or lack of function, with a concomitant change in the phenotype. Since proteins are the working molecules derived from genes, mutations in genes exert their deleterious effects via structural alteration of the proteins, whether they be enzymes, regulatory proteins, or structural proteins. On the average, a mutation occurs every 106 cell divisions, and, obviously, only mutations occurring in the gametes are transmitted. On the average, a gene undergoes one mutation per 200,000 years.

TABLE 62-1 Inherited Disorders

Chromosomal abnormalities	Polygene disorders
Single-gene disorders	

GENETICS OF SINGLE-GENE DISORDERS

Inherited disorders due to a single abnormal gene are transmitted to offspring in a predictable fashion termed *mendelian transmission*. These inheritance patterns produce phenotypes that are inherited according to Mendel's laws of inheritance. As previously noted, in each individual there exists two copies of each gene, referred to as alleles, one obtained from the mother and one from the father. Mendel's first law states that each of the two alleles located on separate chromosomes segregates independently and is passed unchanged into different gametes at the formation of the next generation. Thus, the odds of getting the mother's allele versus the father's are by chance alone, namely, 50 percent. Mendel's second law states that genes on the same chromosome also assert themselves independently through the process of crossover between chromosomes (discussed below). The greater the distance between two loci, the more likely they are to be separated during genetic transmission. As a result of gene mutations, abnormal genes located on any of the 22 autosomal pairs or the two sex chromosomes may produce phenotypes inherited by simple patterns classified as autosomal (dominant or recessive) or X-linked, respectively. When different genes induce the same phenotype, it is referred to as *genetic heterogeneity,* and most diseases in humans exhibit genetic heterogeneity. The same disease may be due to multiple mutations in the same gene (*allele heterogeneity*) or it may be due to a single or multiple mutations in two or more genes (*locus heterogeneity*). Within any one family, however, the gene and the mutation responsible for the disease are the same and only rarely would two genes be transmitted for the same disease. A good example is familial hypertrophic cardiac myopathy (HCM), in which eight different genes have been recognized with multiple mutations in each. Genetic heterogeneity is to be distinguished from polygenic disorders, such as atherosclerosis, which are due to the interaction of several genes. As noted above, mutations can involve a microscopically visible alter-

TABLE 62-2 Single-Gene Disorders

Alteration of a single nucleotide (point mutation)
Missense
Truncated
Elongated
Nonsense
Synonomous
Deletion of several nucleotides
Addition of several nucleotides

ation, such as deletion or translocation of a portion of the chromosome, or they can involve a minute change in one purine or pyrimidine base in the DNA sequence of a single codon. Mutations involving only a single nucleotide are known as point mutations and are responsible for 70 percent or more of all adult single gene disorders (Table 62-2). A point mutation may be a substitution of one nucleotide for another, resulting in a different amino acid being encoded (missense mutation); or it may change the codon from encoding for an amino acid to that of a stop codon, which will truncate the protein (truncated mutant); or it may eliminate a stop codon so the protein is elongated (elongated mutant). Finally, a nucleotide may be deleted or added, which results in a frame shift, and the gene is read entirely differently (nonsense mutation), resulting in a nonfunctioning protein. If a purine nucleotide is substituted for a pyrimidine, the mutation is referred to as a *transversion,* while if purine or pyrimidine substitutes for another purine or pyrimidine, respectively, it is called a *transition*. Other mutations may result from deletion or addition of several nucleotides. An example of the latter is the defect responsible for myotonic dystrophy, where a triplet repeat of several thousand nucleotides in length is inserted into the 3′ end of the gene. Another type of mutation is known as *gene conversion,* where two genes interact and part of the nucleotide sequence of one gene becomes incorporated into the other. Mutations in genes exert their deleterious effects via structural alteration of enzymes, regulatory proteins, or structural proteins. The terms *dominant inheritance* and *recessive inheritance* refer to characteristics of the phenotype and are not characteristics of the gene per se. Dominant inheritance implies that a person with one copy of a mutant allele and one copy of the normal allele develops a phenotype of the mutant allele. Recessive traits, on the other hand, require both alleles to be mutant to develop a phenotype. This situation usually occurs when the patients are consanguineous, with each carrying mutant alleles, or when the mutant allele is common in the population, as is seen in sickle cell anemia.

Genetic Penetrance and Expressivity

The percentage of individuals with a disease-related gene who have one or more features of the disease is referred to as *penetrance.* Penetrance is an all-or-none phenomenon, and any manifestation, however minute, indicates that the gene has full penetrance in that individual. Nonpenetrance refers to lack of any observable phenotype. This feature is to be distinguished from *expressivity,* which refers to the variable nature of the clinical features. Thus, by definition, to have expressivity, the trait must be penetrant. Numerous genetic and environmental factors can affect expression of a gene, making it nearly impossible to determine which factor is most important in a specific individual or specific disease. These factors include (1) genetic background, (2) age-dependency, (3) sex influence and sex limitation, (4) exogenous factors, (5) maternal factors, (6) modifying loci, and (7) gene alterations.

Patterns of Inheritance

AUTOSOMAL DOMINANT INHERITANCE

Dominant disorders are those that have phenotypic manifestations (disease) in heterozygous individuals—persons carrying only one abnormal allele, with the other allele on the homologous chromosome being normal. In autosomal dominant disorders, both males and females can be affected, and since alleles segregate independently at meiosis, there is a 50-50 chance that the offspring of an affected heterozygote will inherit the mutant allele. Not all affected individuals, however, must have an affected parent because, in all autosomal dominant diseases, a certain proportion of cases occur due to a new mutation (i.e., they are sporadic). The parent whose germ cells contain the new mutation will be clinically normal, since the mutation affects only a single germ cell, but will transmit the disease-causing allele to half of his or her offspring. Autosomal dominant inheritance can be misdiagnosed as sporadic if there is low expressivity in the phenotypically normal parent carrying the mutant allele or if extramarital paternity has occurred. The following features are characteristic of autosomal dominant inheritance (Fig. 62-1): (1) each affected individual has an affected parent unless the disease occurred due to a new mutation or the heterozygous parent has low expressivity; (2) equal proportions (i.e., 50-50) of normal and affected offspring are likely statistically to be born to an affected individual; (3) normal children of an affected individual bear only normal offspring; (4) equal proportions of males and females are affected; (5) both sexes are equally likely to transmit the abnormal allele to male and female offspring, and male-to-male transmission occurs; and (6) vertical transmission through successive generations occurs. Two other features are characteristically seen in autosomal dominant diseases that help to differentiate this type of inheritance from autosomal recessive disorders: delayed age of onset and variable clinical expression. The former is commonly seen in such disorders as familial HCM, while the latter may occur in Holt-Oram syndrome, in which the patient may present with an atrial septal defect (ASD) and skeletal abnormality of the upper extremity in combination or with either of these abnormalities individually. Examples of autosomal dominant primary heart disease include HCM and Romano-Ward long-QT syndrome.

AUTOSOMAL RECESSIVE INHERITANCE

Autosomal recessive phenotypes are clinically apparent when the patient carries two mutant alleles (i.e., is homozygous) at the locus responsible for the disease state. The disease-causing gene is found on one of the 22 autosomes, and thus both males and females will be equally affected. Clinical uniformity is typical, and disease onset generally occurs early in life. Recessive disorders are more commonly diagnosed in childhood than are dominant diseases. Only one in four children (25 percent) on average, will be affected. The following are characteristics of

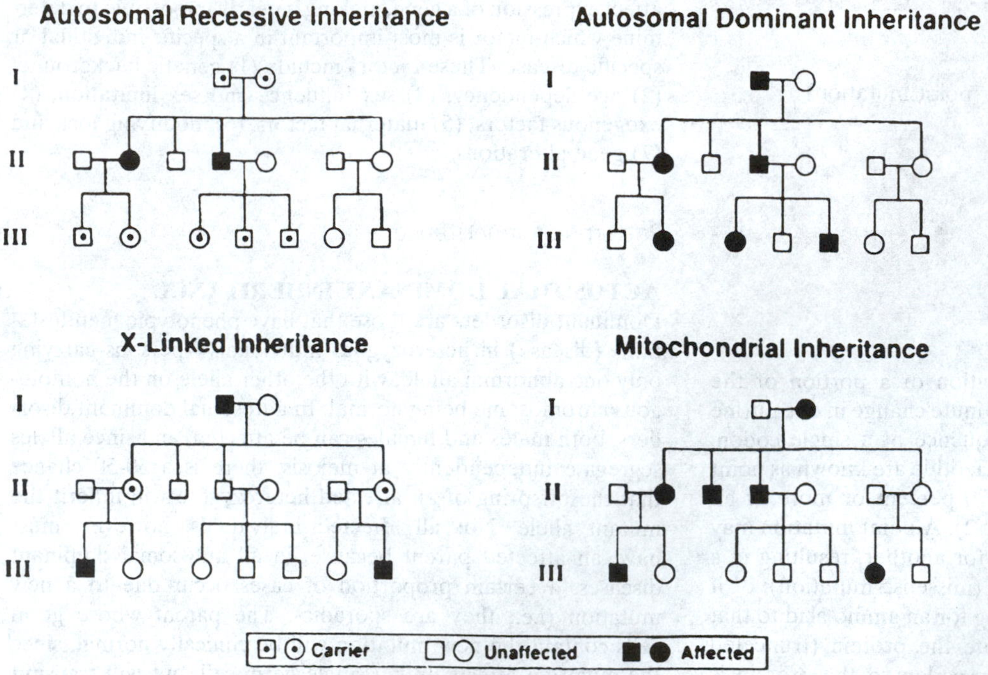

FIGURE 62-1 This typical set of pedigrees outlines the usual inheritance patterns for autosomal dominant and recessive traits, X-linked inheritance, and mitochondrial inheritance. Squares signify males and circles, females. Filled-in circles and squares are affected females and males, respectively. A slash line through a circle or square designates a deceased individual.

autosomal recessive disorders (Fig. 62-1): (1) parents are clinically normal heterozygotes; (2) alternate generations are affected, with no vertical transmission; (3) both sexes are affected with equal frequency; and (4) each offspring of heterozygous carriers has a 25 percent chance of being affected, a 50 percent chance of being an unaffected carrier, and a 25 percent chance of inheriting only normal alleles. Examples of autosomal recessive disorders affecting the heart include Jervell and Lange-Nielsen long-QT/deafness syndrome and Pompe's (type II glycogen storage) disease.

X-LINKED INHERITANCE

X-linked inherited disorders are caused by genes located on the X chromosome; therefore the clinical risk and severity of disease differ between the sexes. Since a female has two X chromosomes, she may carry either one mutant allele (heterozygote) or two mutant alleles (homozygote); the trait may therefore display dominant or recessive expression. Males have a single X chromosome (and one Y chromosome); therefore they are expected to display the full syndrome whenever they inherit the abnormal gene from their mother. This development of the trait occurs regardless of whether the mother carrying the mutant allele exhibits a recessive (i.e., clinically silent) or dominant (i.e., clinically apparent) trait. Hence, the terms *X-linked dominant* and *X-linked recessive* apply only to the expression of the gene in females. Since males must pass on their Y chromosome to all male offspring, they cannot pass on mutant X alleles to their sons; therefore no male-to-male transmission of X-linked disorders can occur. On the other hand, males must contribute their one X chromosome to all daughters. All females receiving a mutant X chromosome are known as *carriers,* and those who become affected clinically with the disease are known as *manifesting female carriers*. The characteristic features of X-linked inheritance (Fig. 62-1) include (1) no male-to-male transmission; (2) all daughters of affected males are carriers; (3) sons of carrier females have a 50 percent risk of being affected, and daughters have a 50 percent chance of being carriers; (4) affected homozygous females occur only when an affected male and carrier female have children; and (5) the pedigree pattern in X-linked recessive traits tends to be oblique because of the occurrence of the trait in the sons of normal carriers sisters of affected males (i.e., uncles and nephews affected). Examples of X-linked disorders of the heart include X-linked cardiomyopathy, X-linked cardioskeletal myopathy (Barth's syndrome) and those X-linked diseases in which the heart is affected, such as muscular dystrophy (MD) (e.g., Duchenne/Becker and Emery-Dreifuss MD).

MITOCHONDRIAL INHERITANCE

Another inheritance pattern described in patients with cardiovascular anomalies occurs because of abnormalities of the mitochondrial genome. Generation of energy is dependent on the oxidative phosphorylation process within the mitochondria. Within many mitochondria is a single chromosome that encodes for a number of the enzymes of oxidative phosphorylation (i.e., encodes for 13 of the 69 proteins required for oxidative metabolism) and the transfer RNAs (tRNAs) and ribosomal RNAs (rRNAs) required for their translation. The remaining enzymes of the oxidative-phosphorylation pathway are encoded by genes on the nuclear chromosomes, and the resultant proteins are transported into the mitochondrion. Genetic defects of oxidative phosphorylation, therefore, can be due either to gene mutations within the X chromosome or autosomes (i.e., nuclear chromosomes), resulting in diseases that behave as Mendelian recessive traits, or to mitochondrial genome defects that cause diseases with nonmendelian traits. These differences may be explained by events of conception, since the spermatocyte contributes few or no mitochondria to the zygote (Fig. 62-2). The entire mitochondrial complement present in a fetus must therefore be derived from the mitochondria already present in the cytoplasm of the oocyte. Thus, phenotypes due to mitochondrial DNA mutations demonstrate maternal inheritance only. The characteristic features of mitochondrial inheritance of disease (Fig. 62-1) include (1) equal frequency and severity of disease for each sex; (2) transmission through females only, with offspring of affected males being unaffected; (3) all offspring of affected females may be affected; (4) extreme variability of expression of disease within a family (may include apparent nonpenetrance); (5) phenotypes may be age-dependent; (6) or-

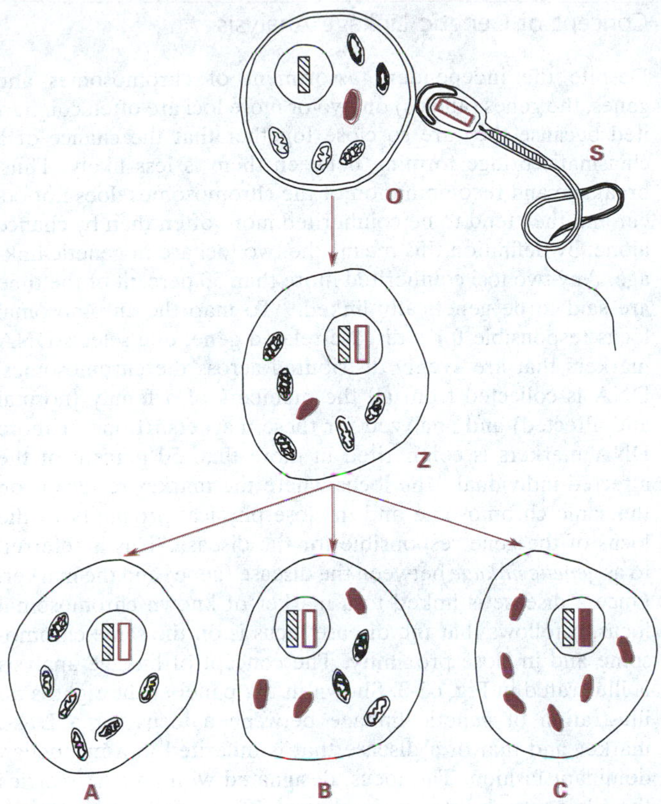

FIGURE 62-2 Cartoon (not to scale) illustrating maternal inheritance of mtDNA, compared with biparental inheritance of nuclear genes, and the random distribution of normal and mutant mitochondrial genomes in daughter cells of the zygote. It is assumed for simplicity that individual mitochondria contain either normal (open mitochondria) or mutant (filled mitochondria) mtDNA, not both. O = oocyte; S = sperm; Z = zygote; A, B, C = daughter cells of zygote, representing stem cells of different tissues. (Reprinted with permission from DiMauro S et al. Mitochondrial encephalomyopathies. *Neurol Clin* 1990; 8:494.)

gan mosaicism is common. An example of mitochondrial inherited cardiac disease is the cardiomyopathy of Kearns-Sayre syndrome.

POLYGENIC INHERITANCE OF CARDIAC DISEASE

Disorders such as hypertension or ischemic heart disease are believed to require concomitant mutations in several genes—i.e., they are polygenic hereditary disorders (discussed in Chap. 7). The genes responsible for polygenic hereditary disorders are difficult to map, since computational methods to describe their mode of inheritance are only now being explored.[8] Over the past two decades, this type of inheritance has been invoked for a large number of disorders, including coronary artery disease and congenital heart disease. In multifactorial, or polygenic, genetic diseases, multiple genes interact in a cumulative fashion to induce the disease or provide an increased risk of developing the disease. This multifaceted process is illustrated by coronary artery disease, in which one common phenotype is myocardial infarction due to thrombosis superimposed on atherosclerosis. There are many single-gene disorders that alter plasma lipoproteins and contribute to atherosclerosis (see Chaps. 7, 35, and 38). Several other genetic risk factors have been identified that predispose to atherosclerosis, such as the paraoxonase gene or homocysteine gene.[9] The phenotype of acute myocardial infarction is more likely if the individual, in addition to atherosclerosis, has a mutant form of fibrinogen[10] or mutant forms of other clotting factors, discussed in detail in Chap. 7.

OVERVIEW OF CHROMOSOMAL MAPPING AND IDENTIFICATION OF A DISEASE-RELATED GENE

Identification of a disease-causing gene, in the setting where the protein is unknown, was until the 1980s nearly impossible. Familial hypercholesterolemia and some of the thalassemias are disorders in which genes were isolated and cloned, knowing the protein. For the majority of diseases, however, neither the defect nor the protein is known. Technical advances[11] aiding chromosomal mapping include (1) computerized linkage analysis, (2) development of highly informative DNA markers, and (3) detection of markers by polymerase chain reaction (PCR).[11] The 46 chromosomes of the human genome contain 3 billion base pairs (bp). To locate a particular gene, one must first map the chromosomal location and its relative position. This process requires certain chromosomal landmarks. Identification of a particular locus is made possible by showing that the disease-related gene of interest is on the same chromosome and in close proximity to one of these landmarks, a method referred to as *genetic linkage analysis*. This technique requires a family with a disease that is transmitted over at least two generations (and preferably three) with at least 10 affected individuals, although even 6 or 7 affected individuals may be adequate, depending on the structure of the family. A landmark, referred to as a DNA or chromosomal *marker*, is a polymorphic sequence of DNA, the chromosomal position of which is known and can be detected by analyzing an individual's DNA (discussed in detail below). A major limitation until recently was the lack of markers evenly distributed across each of the chromosomes. Today there is a marker available at least every 1 million base pairs on all chromosomes.[12,13] Genetic distance is measured in terms of centimorgans (cM), named after the geneticist T. H. Morgan, and 1 cM approximates 1 million bp. Markers, like genes, have two alleles and are transmitted to offspring according to Mendel's law, with the individual being heterozygous or homozygous for that marker. If a marker is homozygous, it is not informative for genetic linkage. Hence, several markers in the same region may have to be analyzed to find one that is heterozygous in that individual. When all of the markers are placed together on each chromosome and the genetic distance between them is estimated, a *genetic map* is produced. A map of over 5000 highly informative markers has been developed, which has significantly accelerated the mapping of disease-related genes—an achievement that provides the foundation for genetic linkage analysis.[13] Each gene, allele, or marker is transmitted independently; thus, the odds of any two genes (or a marker and a gene) being coinherited are by chance alone (50 percent), even though they are on the same chromosome. The homologous pairs of chromosomes are assorted, and one from each parent is transmitted to the offspring by chance. Genetic diversity from homologous chromosomes segregating independently would produce 223 types of gametes; in other words, the probability of an offspring inheriting a set of chromosomes identical to those of a parent is one in 8,388,608.[14] If this were the only mechanism for diversity, all of the genes on a particular chromosome would be coinherited in the next progeny. This does not happen. Genes on the same chromosome are transmitted independently unless they are in close physical proximity to each other. Genes on the same chromosome are transmitted independently by the mechanism of crossover between homologous chromosomes (Fig. 62-3), which provides continual mixing of the genes during every meiosis and is the predominant reason why no two individuals have the same genotype unless they are identical twins. Prior to meiosis, the two homologous chromosomes come together and form bridges (*chiasmata*) such that segments of equal proportion are exchanged between them, giving rise to crossover of various genes. There is no net loss of chromosomal material or genes, but crossover leads to a constant intermixing of the chromosomes such that no two offspring will ever be identical. Crossovers occur only between homologous chromosomes. The loci occupy the same chromosomal position on the homologous chromosome on which they are combined as they had on their original homologous chromosome. On average there are 33 crossovers between homologous chromosome pairs per meiosis.[14] In genetic parlance, crossing over is referred to as recombination.

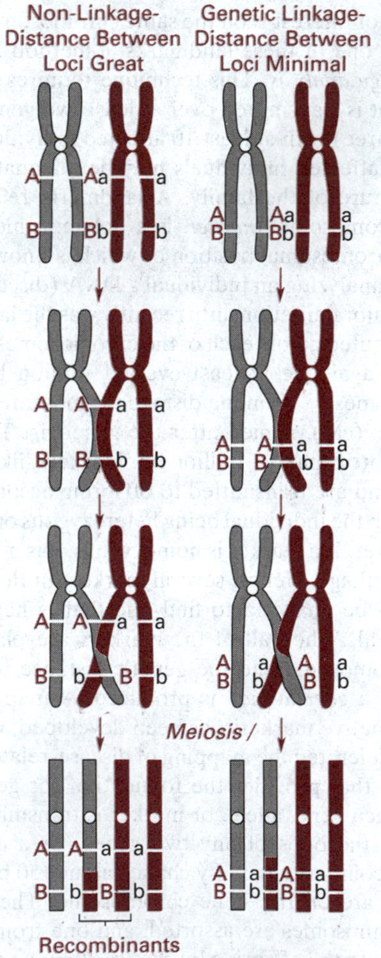

FIGURE 62-3 Comparison of nonlinked genes (*left*) and linked genes (*right*). In nonlinkage, the distance between loci is large, allowing crossing over to occur and resulting in recombinants after meiosis. The distance between linked genes is comparatively small, thereby minimizing the chance for recombinants.

Concept of Genetic Linkage Analysis

Despite the independent assortment of chromosomes and genes, the genes (alleles) on two or more loci are often coinherited because they are so close together that the chance of a chiasmatic bridge forming between them is less likely. Thus, breakage and recombination of the chromosomes does not occur and they tend to be coinherited more often than by chance alone; by definition this means the two loci are in genetic linkage. Any two loci coinherited more than 50 percent of the time are said to be genetically linked.[15] To map the chromosomal locus responsible for a disease-related gene, one selects DNA markers that are evenly distributed across the chromosomes. DNA is collected from all the members of a family (normal and affected) and analyzed for these markers. If one or more DNA markers is coinherited in more than 50 percent of the affected individuals, the locus where the marker resides is on the same chromosome and in close physical proximity to the locus of the gene responsible for the disease. This is referred to as *genetic linkage* between the disease (gene) and the marker. Once a disease is linked to a marker of known chromosomal locus, it follows that the disease locus is on the same chromosome and in close proximity. The concept of linkage analysis is illustrated in Fig. 62-3. Shown in the panel at the right is an illustration of genetic linkage between a locus for a DNA marker and that of a disease that is inherited in a mendelian dominant fashion. The locus, designated with an "A," carries the allele responsible for the disease. The corresponding locus, "a," on the homologous chromosome has the allele that codes for the same protein but has not undergone a mutation and is thus the normal allele. The loci designated "B" and "b" represent alleles of a DNA marker of known location that has nothing to do with the disease. In the panel on the right, the disease and the marker loci are so close that they tend to be coinherited within the family, whereas in the panel on the left, the DNA marker of known location is so far from the locus carrying the disease allele it is not coinherited but separate by chance. The calculation necessary to prove definitively that genetic linkage exists between a marker and a disease-related locus is sophisticated and requires advanced computer programs. The odds for and against linkage are calculated, and linkage exists if the odds in favor of linkage are at least 1000:1. To avoid the cumbersome ratio (1000:1), the logarithm to base 10 is derived, which is 3 (i.e., 10^3), and is referred to as the LOD score (log of the odds). If the LOD score is −2 (i.e., 10^{-2} or 100:1 odds against linkage), it excludes linkage. The likelihood of two genes being separated by recombination increases in proportion to the distance between them. The distance between a marker and a disease-causing gene when genetically linked is quite variable and may be anywhere from 1000 kilobase pairs (kbp) to 50,000 kbp but is usually within 1000 to 10,000 kbp.[16] The inherent resolution of genetic linkage analysis is never better than 1000 kbp. It is possible on the basis of linkage analysis alone to construct a chromosomal map of all the markers, with the distance between the various markers estimated in centimorgans. This is a complex calculation derived from the number of recombinations between the markers during meioses. The recombination frequency between two markers, two genes, or a gene and a marker is the ratio of the number of crossover events to the total number of meioses. The lower the recombination frequency between the locus of a marker and that of a disease-related gene, the closer those two must be in physical distance on the chromosome. Even though the locus of the marker and that of the disease-related gene are in close enough proximity to be genetically linked, recombination may occur, and the extent to which recombination does occur reflects roughly the physical distance between the two loci. The recombination fraction (or *theta*) is used to develop a means of estimating the genetic distance (in centimorgans) between genetically linked loci. A recombination frequency or crossover of 1 percent between two loci, whether occupied by two genes or one gene and a marker, reflects a physical distance between them of approximately 1 million bp (1 cM).[16] For a marker and a gene separated by 1 cM, this means the chance of a crossover between them during meiosis is only 1 percent; thus, the chance of being coinherited is 99 percent. This is a statistically derived genetic map, however, and the distances are only approximate. The correlation between the percent crossover and the physical distance in base pairs varies somewhat from chromosome to chromosome and from region to region even on the same chromosome. For example, recombination is more frequent in the telomeric than in the centromeric portion of the chromosome and is also more frequent in females. If the marker locus and the disease-related locus are close, such as 5 to 10 cM, then a single crossover may be uncommon and a double crossover rare. Two loci may be 20 to 40 cM apart, however, and a double crossover occurs, which recombines the locus with the original chromosome and leads to coinheritance of the two (linkage of the two loci). When this occurs, the genetic distance is misleading and represents a gross underestimation of the true physical distance between the two loci.

Chromosomal Markers and Their Identification

A chromosomal marker (as defined above) is any DNA sequence of known chromosomal location that is polymorphic for the population (two or more alleles). The greater the number of alleles, the more informative the marker. When compared between individuals in the population, the DNA of the human genome shows a difference in the nucleotide sequence (polymorphism) every 300 to 500 bp. Polymorphisms occur more frequently in the sequence of the unexpressed DNA (intron) than in DNA coding for proteins (exon). Until recently, the most common chromosomal marker was that of restriction fragment length polymorphism (RFLP)[17] identified by Southern blotting. These markers have been replaced by what are referred to as short tandem repeat polymorphisms (STRP),[18] which occur more frequently, are more informative, and are more conveniently and rapidly detected than are RFLPs[19] (Fig. 62-4). Distributed throughout the human genome are repeats of dinucleotides, trinucleotides, or tetranucleotides that are repeated in tandem (microsatellites) and may vary anywhere from 60 to 300 repeats. The number of tandem repeats of STRPs, which provide for marked polymorphism, occur about every 500 bp throughout the human genome. The dinucleotide repeats of cytosine-adenosine are more common than trinucleotide or tetranucleotide repeats. A major advantage of STRPs is rapid and convenient detection by PCR rather than requiring Southern blotting, as is necessary for RFLPs. PCR requires only a nanogram of DNA as opposed to a milligram for RFLPs, and results are available in only 1 to 24 h as opposed to 9 to 10 days for Southern blotting. The resolution of STRPs detected by PCR is much better than by Southern blotting and, since STRPs have multiple alleles (as opposed to RFLPs, which have only two alleles), they are much more informative for genetic linkage. A more recent marker is that of single nucleotide polymorphism, which may represent the markers of the future.[17–19]

Identification of the Gene

Once the chromosomal location of a gene has been mapped, the first technique in attempting to identify the gene is referred to as the *candidate gene approach.* Over 5000 loci have now been mapped for human genes and over 1000 genes recorded in a gene bank. In addition, there are over 50,000 expressed sequenced tags (ESTs) mapped. The ESTs are unique DNA sequences of 100 to 200 bp, each of which is believed to represent a unique gene.[20] These genes and ESTs are entered through a worldwide network of databases[21] in the United States, Europe, and Japan that is updated on a daily basis. Once a locus is identified on a chromosome, genes previously known to be localized to that region become candidate genes for the newly mapped locus. These genes are amplified, usually by PCR, to determine if there is a mutation that segregates with the disease. If none of the candidate genes in the region is shown to have a mutation that cosegregates with the disease, it may be necessary to clone the region. This approach is referred to as *posi-*

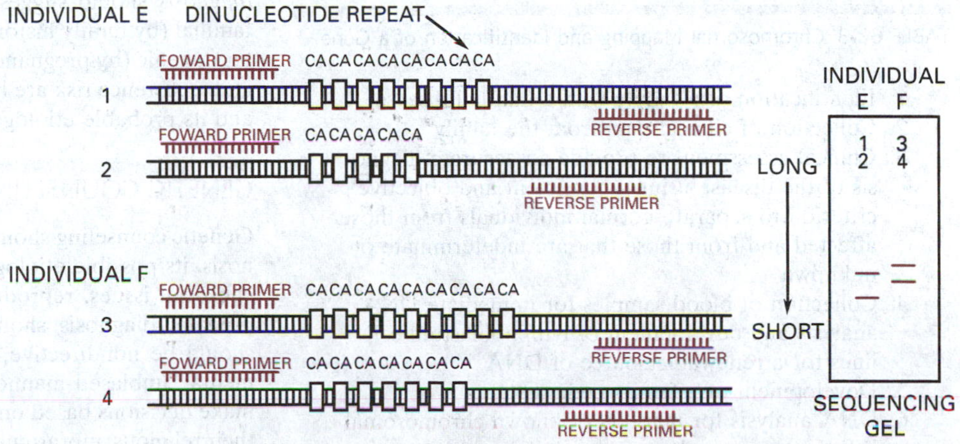

FIGURE 62-4 Sequence-based polymorphisms. This type of polymorphism is based on sequence variations caused by variable numbers of repeat sequence within a population. In this case, variable numbers of CA dinucleotide repeats are shown at one locus. These polymorphisms can be detected by use of specific oligonucleotide primers and the polymerase chain reaction (PCR). The resultant PCR products will vary in size and can be detected by polyacrylamide gel electrophoresis. These sequence-based PCR polymorphisms may be highly polymorphic, thus providing increased statistical strength to linkage analysis over two-allele polymorphisms seen in Southern blot restriction fragment length polymorphisms (RFLPs). (Reprinted with permission from Keating M. Linkage analysis and long QT syndrome. Using genetics to study cardiovascular disease. *Circulation* 1992; 85:1973–1986.)

tional cloning, so named because a region is cloned knowing only its position relative to the genetically linked marker. Positional cloning is usually not attempted unless the region (containing the gene) between the flanking markers is 1 cM or less. To reduce the region for cloning, it is necessary to expand the family with the hope of finding crossovers such that markers common to all affected would span only a short distance (<1 cM). This collection of markers in a region would represent the haplotype being inherited by the affected individual and contains the responsible gene. To prove that the gene causes the disease, the mutation must be identified and shown to cosegregate with the disease and not with the unaffected members in the family. The remaining task would be to determine the gene product (protein) and the pathophysiology of how the mutation induces the disease. In attempting to decipher the pathophysiology, one may transfect cells in culture with normal and mutant forms of the gene and compare the resulting phenotype. The other definitive approaches for determining causality are to overexpress the gene as a transgene in animals such as mice or to do homologous knockout, replacing the normal with the mutant gene to determine whether the disease phenotype is induced as have been done for familial hypertrophic cardiomyopathy (FHCM).[22-24] Chromosomal mapping of hereditary diseases by linkage analysis and subsequent isolation of the gene[25] are summarized in Table 62-3.

Family History and Evaluation

The most important part of an evaluation for genetic disease is the family history. First, the family history may give clues to the diagnosis of a particular disorder, information about possible inheritance patterns within an individual family, and information about conditions for which family members may be at an increased risk. An individual's ethnic background may, for instance, suggest the need for specific types of genetic screening such as for hemoglobinopathies in individuals of African or Mediterranean ancestry or for Tay-Sachs disease in individuals of eastern European (Ashkenazi) Jewish ancestry. The individual with the medical problem who brought the family to the attention of the physician is referred to as the *proband,* or *propositus* (proposita for females). Information generally should be collected on all individuals who are first-, second-, or third-degree relatives of the proband. First-degree relatives of the proband are the parents and children. Second-degree relatives are aunts and uncles, grandparents, and grandchildren of the proband. Third-degree relatives are first cousins, great aunts and uncles, great-grandparents, and great-grandchildren. A pedigree chart (as shown in Fig. 62-1) is useful in this task. This information should include medical problems and pregnancies. If relatives are deceased, the age at death and the cause of death should be recorded. With a pedigree chart and specific family information, more general questions are asked, including whether other family members have the same or similar problems. Information about various types of birth defects, mental retardation, early infant deaths, miscarriages, stillbirths, or other diseases or handicaps in the family is sought. With some disorders, there may be a variability of a particular condition (i.e., clinical heterogeneity), even within a family. For example, with a possible diagnosis of FHCM, one should ask about premature death or syncope. A pregnancy history may provide information to support a possible teratogenic exposure. The date of the last menstrual period, whether the pregnancy was planned, whether contraception was used immediately prior to pregnancy, the time when the pregnancy was recognized, and when the mother sought prenatal care should be noted. Problems during the pregnancy, such as bleeding, spotting, cramping, fevers, rashes, or illnesses; drug exposures (both prescribed and nonprescribed), alcohol intake, or "recreational" drug use; and exposures to potent chemicals in the workplace or while involved in various hobbies should be explored. Pregnancy and family histories can then be used in conjunction with the findings on physical examination to derive a potential etiologic diagnosis and to plan for further diagnostic studies. The term *etiologic diagnosis* should suggest whether a specific cardiac defect is familial (by family history), genetic but not familial (sporadic), teratogenic (by pregnancy history), or multifactorial. Prognosis and recurrence risk are linked strongly to an accurate diagnosis and its probable etiology.

TABLE 62-3 Chromosomal Mapping and Identification of a Gene

1. Identification of a family with a familial disease
2. Collection of clinical data from the family
3. Clinical assessment to provide an accurate diagnosis of the disease using a consistent and objective criterion to separate normal individuals from those affected and from those that are indeterminate or unknown
4. Collection of blood samples for immediate DNA analysis and development of lymphoblastoid cell lines for a renewable source of DNA
5. Development of a family pedigree
6. DNA analysis for markers of known chromosomal loci that span the human genome in an attempt to find a marker locus linked to the disease
7. Identification of the gene
8. Identification of mutation(s) causing the disease
9. Demonstration of a causal relationship between the mutant gene and the disease
10. Development of a convenient test to screen for the mutations

GENETIC COUNSELING PRINCIPLES

Genetic counseling should provide information about the diagnosis, its possible etiology, and its prognosis. In addition, psychosocial issues, reproductive options, and the availability of prenatal diagnosis should be discussed. Genetic counseling should be nondirective, providing information in a nonjudgmental, unbiased manner. The family should then be able to make decisions based on medical information in the context of their religious, moral, cultural, and social backgrounds and their financial situation. Although a genetic counselor may occasionally feel frustrated with a specific couple's decision, an effective counselor does not let personal biases interfere with the counseling role. Conflicts leading to major ethical issues and disputes may arise, however, and may be particularly apparent regarding issues of nonpaternity, sex selection, pregnancy termination, and selective nontreatment of malformed infants. Couples have many reproductive options, but not all may be acceptable religiously or culturally. Nevertheless, potential options should be mentioned in a sensitive manner. A common misunderstanding among families in genetic counseling is the issue of prenatal diagnosis and its relationship to abortion. Prenatal diagnosis does not imply that a parent should or would terminate the pregnancy. In many circumstances, the information from prenatal diagnosis may help to reassure a couple that their risk of having another handicapped child is in fact much lower than expected. Conversely, if defects are found, the subspecialist may use more diagnostic approaches to make rational decisions about medical management of the infant prior to or immediately after delivery.

Genetic Diagnosis and Health Insurance

The accelerated pace of gene discovery, molecular medicine, and molecular diagnostics has begun to allow for improved genetic counseling and portends the possibility of future genetic therapy. As knowledge about the genetic basis of disease grows, however, so does the potential for health insurance coverage discrimination to be used to exclude individuals at risk or to change prohibitively high rates on the basis of predetermined illness. For this reason, planners of the Human Genome Project recognized the need to protect individuals who volunteered for genetic study as well as those diagnosed by molecular methods in the future. Also for this reason, the National Institutes of Health–Department of Energy (NIH-DOE) Working Group on Ethical, Legal, and Social Implications (ELSI) of the Human Genome Project was developed. The Congress has passed a bill prohibiting companies from using DNA analysis to assess genetic risk as a basis for hiring. Only 11 states, however, prohibit the use of DNA analysis to determine who should get medical insurance or whether they qualify for high- or low-risk premiums.[7]

CARDIOVASCULAR DISEASE DUE TO SINGLE-GENE MUTATIONS

Compensatory Response of the Heart Is Limited to Hypertrophy, Dilatation, or a Combination

The heart responds to stimuli, physiologic or pathologic, which may be inherited or acquired, with hypertrophy, dilation, or a combination of the two.[26] The same mechanisms mediate the growth response to pressure overload, volume overload, or loss of contractile mass (myocardial infarction). In FHCM, hypertrophy occurs without altered workload. In familial dilated cardiomyopathy (DCM), the heart responds predominantly by dilatation, generally in association with diffuse loss of myocytes and fibrosis. Most inherited defects are associated with hypertrophy. Several mutations in the mitochondrial genome have been associated with cardiac hypertrophy or dilatation.[27,28] In mitochondrial DNA mutations, HCM or DCM is usually part of a general phenotypic expression of a systemic disease that is characterized by metabolic disorders and involving the central nervous and the skeletal muscle systems. Three clinical categories of primary cardiomyopathies exist: (1) hypertrophic, (2) dilated, and (3) restrictive forms. Most of the cardiomyopathies other than those caused by infection have a genetic basis, although many of the mutations may occur de novo and are not necessarily familial. Only when a genetic defect is present in the germline and transmitted to one or more generations is it familial. For a detailed discussion of the clinical features, diagnosis, and treatment of the cardiomyopathies refer to Chaps. 64 to 69.

Familial Hypertrophic Cardiomyopathy (FHCM)

GENETIC BASIS

Familial HCM is an autosomal dominant disorder characterized by myocardial hypertrophy with a wide spectrum of symptoms, including dyspnea, chest pain, and syncope. The annual mortality rate of 2 to 4 percent is primarily due to sudden death, which often occurs in asymptomatic individuals (see Chap. 67). This disorder is the leading cause of sudden death in the young and in athletes. The annual incidence of sudden death is higher in younger patients with FHCM (about 6 percent) than in the elderly (1 percent). The diagnosis is based on typical clinical features and the demonstration of unexplained left ventricular, right ventricular, or biventricular hypertrophy on two-dimensional echocardiography. The left ventricular hypertrophy is commonly asymmetrical, localized to the septum, but it may involve the entire ventricle in a concentric pattern. Isolated right ventricular hypertrophy occurs in fewer than 5 percent. Isolated apical hypertrophy is rare except in Japan, where it is claimed to account for 20 to 30 percent of the cases. Dynamic outflow tract obstruction occurs in about 30 percent.[29,30] Histologically, the myocardial hypertrophy consists of myocyte hypertrophy, cellular and myofibrillar disarray, and myocardial fibrosis. The literature suggests that the hallmark of FHCM is myocyte and myofibrillar disarray (see Chap. 66). The disorder exhibits marked variability of expressivity, even in the same family. FHCM was the first primary cardiomyopathy to yield to molecular genetics. Jarcho et al. in 1989 showed genetic linkage of the disease to the chromosomal locus of 14q1 in a large French/Canadian family.[31] The 14q1 locus subsequently was shown to be involved in FHCM in several families throughout North America.[32] The β-myosin heavy chain (βMHC) gene was identified as the responsible gene (Fig. 62-5), and over 50 mutations have been detected.[11,33,34] A total of eight genes have now been identified responsible for FHCM and a brief description of the loci and the proteins they encode, together with their function, is summarized in Table 62-4. Mutations in the βMHC gene may account for 30 to 50 percent of the families with FHCM.[33] While it remains to be determined for certain, these eight genes probably account for 80 to 90 percent of the disease of FHCM. Two other loci have been identified, one in a family with HCM and Wolff-Parkinson-White (WPW) syndrome mapped to 7q3[35] and the other to chromosome 11q in a Japanese family.[36] Since all of the genes identified to date involve the sarcomere, it has been proposed that FHCM is a disease of the sarcomere and perhaps should be referred to as *sarcomeropathy*.[34]

The βMHC is the most common gene for FHCM and over 50 mutations have been described. Almost all of the mutations are point mutations (a single base nucleotide) that result in substitution of one amino acid for another and are located in the globular head of the myosin molecule. These mutations appear to arise independently.[37] The frequency of each particular mutation is low. Two hot spots, codons 403 and 719, have been identified for mutations in the βMHC in patients with

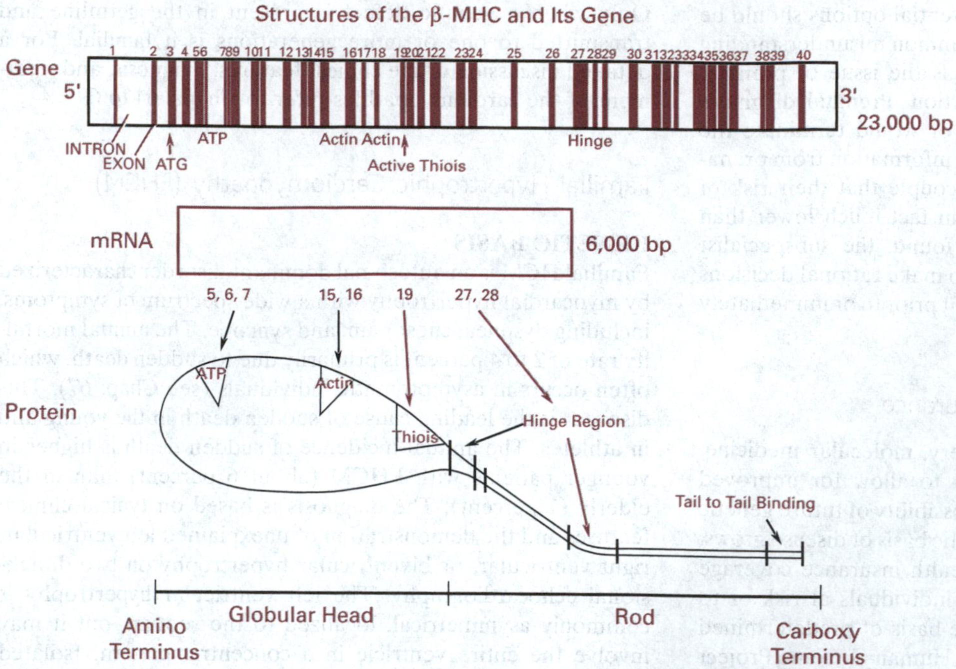

FIGURE 62-5 Structure of β-myosin heavy chain (β-MHC) and its gene.

with a high incidence of sudden death, yet there is often minimal hypertrophy.[44] The occurrence of palpitations, arrhythmias, or syncope are poor predictors of sudden death. A family history of sudden death usually indicates that the affected individuals in the family are at risk for sudden death. Several studies have now been performed correlating the genotype to the phenotype and several interesting observations have evolved pertinent to the diagnosis and treatment and future genetic screening. Results of these studies[45] have shown that the majority of families with the βMHC mutations Arg^{403}Gln, Arg^{453}Cys, and Arg^{719}Trp are associated with a poor prognosis and a high incidence of sudden cardiac death[34,42,43,46] (Fig. 62-6). In contrast, the βMHC mutations Leu^{908}-Val, Gly^{256}Glu, and Val^{606}Met are associated with near-normal life expectancy, and mutations Glu^{930}Lys and Arg^{249}Gln are associated with an intermediate risk of sudden cardiac death.[47] The incidence of premature death in affected individuals with Arg^{403}Gln is approximately 50 percent,[34] and the mean age of sudden cardiac death is 33 years. The life expectancy of affected individuals with the βMHC mutation Arg^{719}Gln appears to be about 38 years and in those with Arg^{453}Cys about 30 years. In contrast, the mutation Leu^{908}Val is associated with low penetrance, a benign course, and a low incidence of sudden cardiac death.[46] The cumulative survival rate at 60 years of age was 92 percent with this mutation. Similarly, the Gly^{256}Glu and Val^{606}-Met mutations are associated with a relatively benign course, with most individuals having a near-normal life span. In contrast, the two mutations Glu^{930}Lys and Arg^{249}Gln[46,47] show an intermediary prognosis, with an average age of onset of cardiac failure and severe symptoms around 49 years. These correla-

HCM.[38,39] Mutations in the rod region of the βMHC molecule have also been described but are uncommon and appear to induce a mild phenotype.[40]

PROGNOSIS FROM GENOTYPE-PHENOTYPE CORRELATIONS

The hypertrophy of FHCM is markedly variable in its degree, distribution, and age at onset as well as in the type and severity of its associated clinical manifestations.[41–43] The natural course of FHCM in certain families is riddled with sudden cardiac death, whereas in others, sudden cardiac death is almost absent and the life span is essentially normal.[34] None of the clinical features are reliable predictors of sudden death. Hypertrophy, while present in all individuals, since it is required for the clinical diagnosis, does not correlate with the incidence of sudden death. FHCM due to mutations in the troponin T gene is associated

TABLE 62-4 Hypertrophic Cardiomyopathy (HCM) Genes, mRNA, and Proteins

Gene	Chromosomal Locus	Frequency	Number of Mutations	Function and Location
β-MyHC	14q1	35–50%	>50	Contractile molecule that forms a thick filament of the sarcomere
MyBP-C	11q11	15–20%	>15	Binds to myosin and titin
Cardiac troponin T (cTnT)	1q3	15–20%	>20	Regulation of contraction via calcium binding
α-Tropomyosin	15q2	<5%	3	Binds the troponin complex to actin
Cardiac troponin 1	19q13	<1%	3	Inhibits contractility
MLC-1	3p	<1%	2	Unknown
MLC-2	12q	<1%	2	Unknown
α-Cardiac actin	15q11	?	2	Forms the actin thin filament of the sarcomere
Unknown	7q3	?	?	Unknown
Unknown	11q	?	?	Unknown

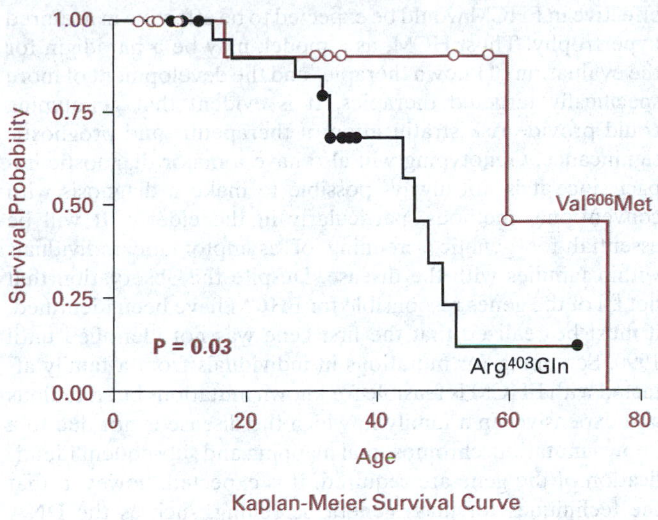

FIGURE 62-6 Kaplan-Meier survival curve in patients with hypertrophic cardiomyopathy depending on myosin heavy chain mutation.

tions must be interpreted with caution, however, as the number of families studied remains too small for definitive generalizations to be made. Although most individuals affected with FHCM due to the βMHC mutation manifest the disease in the second or third decade of life, those with FHCM due to myosin-binding protein C mutations frequently do not develop any evidence of the disease until the fourth or fifth decade.[48] This is a striking example of age-dependent penetrance based on 16 families involving over 500 individuals. However, once the disease develops, the particular mutation is highly predictive of risk for sudden death. Mutations in the essential light chain (3p) and the regulatory light chain of myosin (12q23-q24.3) of patients is associated with a peculiar form of HCM in which mid–left ventricular chamber thickening occurs due to massive hypertrophy of the papillary muscles and adjacent ventricular tissue, resulting in mid-cavitary obstruction.[49] In addition to the cardiac abnormalities described, the skeletal muscles of these patients were histologically abnormal and appeared as ragged-red fibers.

INFLUENCE OF OTHER GENES AND THE ENVIRONMENT

While a single-gene mutation appears to be the primary cause of the disease, there remain significant environmental and other genetic influences that determine whether or not the phenotype develops (penetrance) and its expressivity. A striking example of the influence of environment on FHCM is the observation that hypertrophy seldom develops in the right ventricle, yet the defective genes and their mutations are present to the same extent in the right as in the left ventricles.[34] Presumably, the increased workload and pressure in the left ventricle stimulate the development of the hypertrophy and phenotypic expression. There also appears to be more hypertrophy in males than females who have FHCM. βMHC is the major myosin and contractile unit of many skeletal muscles, yet the latter do not appear to be affected by this disease, again emphasizing the influence of either the environment or other genes.[50] Another example of presumably environmental or other genetic influences is the marked variability of the extent and degree of left ventricular hypertrophy that occurs even within the same family with the same mutation. In addition, there is a significant effect from other genes that predispose to features such as hypertrophy. An example of the influence of another gene on FHCM is afforded by the angiotensin converting enzyme (ACE) DD genotype. Patients with FHCM who also have the ACE DD genotype have a much higher incidence of sudden death[51] and more extensive hypertrophy,[52] which may be mediated through the mitogenic effect of angiotensin II. Individuals with FHCM who participate in combative reports seem to be more prone to develop hypertrophy and sudden death.[53] A similar effect is observed if they have a variance of the endothelin I gene.[54] It is not surprising that the phenotype of cardiac hypertrophy requires the coordination of probably hundreds of genes, and thus it is highly likely that other genes in addition to ACE will exert a minimal, yet significant influence on either the penetrance or expressivity of the primary genetic defect.

ELUCIDATION OF THE PATHOGENESIS FROM GENETIC MODELS

Based on in vitro and in vivo studies in genetic animal models of HCM, it now appears that the primary defect is impaired contractility. Analysis of a human heart from a patient with the Arg[403]Gln mutation showed the ratio of myosin to actin was normal,[55] indicating there is no deficiency of the βMHC protein. All of the responsible mutant genes encode for a sarcomeric protein and appear in some way to impair systolic contraction or diastolic relaxation. In feline adult cardiac myocytes, in which βMHC is the predominant myosin form, expression of human mutant βMHC gene, Arg[403]Gln, was associated with sarcomere disassembly.[56] Expression of the human mutant troponin T in this model also induced sarcomere disassembly and was associated with impaired rate of cell shortening as detected by laser.[24] Furthermore, it was shown the expressed mutant protein was incorporated into the sarcomere. In a transgenic mouse, expression of troponin T gene (cTnT-Gln[92])[57] exhibited sarcomere disarray, increased fibrous tissue, and sudden death, but only minimal hypertrophy. In this model it was also shown that increased expression of the mutant protein was associated with a more severe phenotype, confirming the mutant protein has a dominant-negative effect as expected. These results have been confirmed by several investigators.[56,58–60] Expression of the mutant myosin heavy chain gene or the troponin gene in the mouse has, in general, been associated with less hypertrophy than expected.[57] Recently, a transgenic rabbit model (rabbit has βMHC as its cardiac myosin) has been developed expressing the βMHC (Arg[403]Gln) mutation, which exhibits sarcomere disarray, hypertrophy, and increased fibrous tissue virtually identical to that observed in humans.[61] Thus, the overall postulated pathogenesis of FHCM may be summarized briefly as follows: The mutant protein is incorporated into the sarcomere and acts as a poison peptide which impairs contractility of that particular cell which, in turn, provides the stimulus for the mitogenic response (probably several growth factors) of compensatory hypertrophy. The growth stimulus, as in acquired disorders, appears highly localized and mediated by autocrine or intracrine factors, given that the hypertrophy is localized in many patients, primarily to the interventricular septum. The growth factors also stimulate fibroblast proliferation and increased matrix formation. The relationship between the hypertrophy and increased fibrous tissue response to sudden death and arrhythmias remains to be determined. It is postulated that the fibrous tissue leads to delayed electrical conduction and predisposes to arrhythmias and sudden death.[62,63] The future elucidation of the molecular basis for the pathogenesis of this disease, however, must provide a rationale for three puzzling, consistent features of the pathology of FHCM: (1) predominance of hypertrophy in the septum, (2) sarcomere and myocyte disarray, and (3) the supernormal systolic function. The diastolic stiffness or decreased compliance is expected with hypertrophy, whether it is primary or compensatory, but these other features are not seen in compensatory hypertrophy associated with myocardial infarction or pressure overload.

IMPLICATIONS FOR FUTURE THERAPIES

Based on clinical studies and experimental genetic models, certain important observations have evolved. FHCM is seldom manifested before puberty and when due to certain genes may not be manifested until the fourth or fifth decade. This provides a window for future therapeutic intervention as therapies become available. The observation that the DD genotype increases the extent of hypertrophy and the risk for sudden death in individuals with FHCM is of considerable therapeutic interest.[51] ACE inhibitors have been shown to either induce regression or prevent progression of hypertrophy due to pressure overload, in part due to a direct effect on the growth response. Therefore, it would be intriguing to know whether or not ACE inhibitors induce regression of hypertrophy in patients with FHCM and, perhaps more importantly, prevent hypertrophy in children genetically affected who are identified by genetic testing prior to the development of hypertrophy. There is no evidence to recommend such therapy for FHCM at this time. Elucidation that the hypertrophy is secondary and similar to the hypertrophy developed in response to pressure overload also has important implications; hence, therapies shown to be effective in FHCM would be expected to be effective in acquired hypertrophy. Thus, HCM, as a model, may be a paradigm for the evaluation of known therapies and the development of more specifically targeted therapies. It is evident that genotyping could provide risk stratification of therapeutic and prognostic significance. Genotyping will also have a major diagnostic impact since it is not always possible to make a diagnosis with conventional methods, particularly in the elderly. It will be essential for genetic screening of asymptomatic individuals within families with the disease. Despite the observation that not all of the genes responsible for FHCM have been identified, it must be realized that the first gene was not identified until 1990. Screening for mutations in individuals from a family affected with FHCM is feasible for known mutations but is tedious and expensive. In a family in which the disease is not due to a known mutation, chromosomal mapping and subsequent identification of the gene are required. It is expected, however, that the techniques for mass genetic screening, such as the DNA chip array, will make it possible to do routine genetic screening.[64] Ultimately, if gene therapy becomes available, genotyping will, of course, be essential. It is conceivable that regression of cardiac hypertrophy can be induced by inhibiting transcription of the mutant allele or translation of the mutant mRNA, thus abolishing synthesis of the mutant peptide. Thus, not only genetic diagnosis but also curative therapy may be possible. Since the heart, even in an adult, is renewed every 2 to 3 weeks, there is a tremendous potential for a cure with subsequent remodeling to normal.

Pompe's Disease (Type II Glycogen Storage Disease)

Genetic deficiency of acid α-1,4-glucosidase production results in a wide clinical spectrum ranging from the rapidly fatal infantile-onset of type II glycogen storage disease (GSD) to a slowly progressive adult-onset myopathy. The infantile-onset form (Pompe disease) typically manifests during the first months of life and patients usually die before their second year.[65] This rare inborn error of glycogen metabolism occurs in less than 1 per 100,000 persons. Massive glycogen accumulation occurs, leading to the clinical findings of enlarged tongue, striking hepatomegaly, hypotonia with decreased deep tendon reflexes, and hypertrophic cardiomyopathy[65] with cardiac failure (Table 62-5). The diagnosis may be predicted from the electrocardiogram (ECG), which demonstrates striking QRS complex voltage.[65] The diagnosis can also be made by analysis of α-glucosidase in blood lymphocytes or skin fibroblasts. Recently, urinary oligosaccharide identification using matrix-assisted laser desorption ionization time-of-flight mass spectrometry

TABLE 62-5 Cardiovascular Anomalies Associated with Selected Autosomal Recessive Syndromes

Syndrome	Cardiovascular Anomaly
Carpenter's syndrome	Patent ductus arteriosus
Cockayne's syndrome	Atherosclerosis
Cutis laxa	Pulmonary hypertension
Cystic fibrosis	Cor pulmonale
Ellis–van Creveld syndrome	Atrial septal defect
Friedreich's ataxia	Hypertrophic cardiomyopathy
Homocystinuria	Thromboses
MPS IH (Hurler's syndrome)	Coronary artery disease, aortic and mitral insufficiency, hypertrophic cardiomyopathy
MPS IS (Scheie's syndrome)	Aortic valve disease
MPS IV (Morquio's syndrome)	Aortic valve disease
MPS VI (Maroteaux-Lamy syndrome)	Aortic valve disease
Pompe's disease (GSD II)	Hypertrophic cardiomyopathy
Pseudoxanthoma elasticum	Coronary artery disease, mitral insufficiency
Refsum disease	Arrhythmias
Smith-Lemli-Opitz syndrome	Ventricular septal defect, patent ductus arteriosus
Thrombocytopenia–absent radii (TAR) syndrome	Atrial septal defect, tetralogy of Fallot

has been shown to allow facile and sensitive identification of the pathognomonic oligosacchariduria of this disorder.[66] The disease has autosomal recessive inheritance and is caused by mutations in this lysosomal gene found on chromosome 17q23-q25. Recently, the lysosomal-associated membrane protein (LAMP-1) was shown to be elevated in Pompe disease, which occurs due to altered trafficking and turnover of LAMP-1.[67]

In an attempt to better understand this metabolic disorder, animal models have been developed using targeted disruption of the murine acid α-glucosidase gene.[68,69] This model closely mimics the human disorder, particularly the cardiac phenotype. Also, using animal models such as quail and rat, gene therapy using recombinant α-glucosidase has been shown to correct the enzyme levels and clinical phenotype, suggesting that enzyme replacement by this method is promising therapy in humans.[70–72]

Beckwith-Wiedemann Syndrome (BWS)

The combination of macroglossia, exophthalmos, and visceromegaly has been designated the BWS.[73,74] Multiple other abnormalities have also been described, including fetal adrenocortical cytomegaly, hypoglycemia due to pancreatic islet hyperplasia, transverse linear creases of the ear lobules, hemihypertrophy, and accelerated osseous maturation. Infants with this syndrome are at particularly high risk, cumulatively estimated at between 5 and 20 percent, for development of Wilms' tumor, adrenocortical carcinomas, hepatoblastomas, and rhabdomyosarcomas.[75] The cardiovascular system is also commonly affected with the development of HCM. The BWS occurs with an incidence of 1 in 13,700 live births. Cases (about 85 percent) are generally sporadic, but familial disease (15 percent) has been described. Most of these familial cases have apparent autosomal dominant inheritance,[76] albeit with reduced, sex-dependent penetrance and variable expressivity. A variety of structural abnormalities of chromosome 11 have been shown, including partial duplication of 11p13, duplication of 11p15 only, deletion of 11p11-13, or deletion of 11p11. The extra chromosomal material is usually of paternal origin. The breakpoints found in BWS patients with balanced chromosomal translocation or inversion involving chromosome 11 lie in two regions: (1) close to the insulin/insulin-like growth factor II (INS/IGF2) genes in 11p15.5 or (2) proximal to β-hemoglobin (HBB). The recombinant chromosome was shown to be of maternal origin. Family studies showed that the gene responsible for familial BWS mapped to 11p15.5. For sporadic BWS, uniparental paternal disomy for 11p15.5 markers was found in approximately 20 percent of cases analyzed. Mutations in p57KIP2, a potent tight-binding of several G1 cyclin/cyclin-dependent kinase complexes, have been identified in cases of BWS,[77–80] and mice lacking this gene have been shown to have a phenotype similar to that seen in humans.[81] Clinical heterogeneity exists, however; potential mechanisms include a possible role for genomic imprinting (i.e., an epigenetic chromosomal modification in the gamete or zygote causing preferential expression of a specific parental allele in the somatic cells of the offspring) in 11p15, and this was later shown to occur with KVLQT1, a cardiac potassium channel gene known to cause long-QT syndrome when mutated.[82,83] This region of 11p15.5 has a cluster of imprinted genes, in fact, such as insulin-like growth factor II (IGF2),[84] H19,[85] LIT1,[86] and p57KIP2.[77–80] Animal models have been created using these as transgenes.[84]

Leopard Syndrome

This rare autosomal dominant disorder is characterized by the cardinal features leading to the pneumonic L (lentigenes), E (ECG conduction defects), O (ocular hypertelorism), P (pulmonic valve stenosis), A (abnormalities of genitals), R (retardation of growth), and D (deafness, sensorineural). Cardiac abnormalities are common and include both anatomic as well as conduction defects. Anatomically, PS is the most frequent, followed by HCM and endocardial fibroelastosis (Table 62-6). The most common ECG defects include first-degree AV block, left anterior hemiblock, and complete heart block. No cytogenetic or molecular genetic abnormalities have been identified.

Friedreich's Ataxia (FA)

FA is the most common of the hereditary spinal cerebellar degenerations, with an incidence of 1 in 50,000 and carrier frequency of 1 in 110.[87] This autosomal recessive form of spinocerebellar degeneration is characterized by progressive limb ataxia, loss of deep tendon reflexes, sensory abnormalities, and musculoskeletal deformities. The symptoms of FA usually appear insidiously during childhood or early adolescence. Progres-

TABLE 62-6 Cardiovascular Anomalies Associated with Selected Autosomal Dominant Syndromes

Syndrome	Cardiovascular Anomaly
Albright's hereditary osteodystrophy	Cardiomyopathy
Ehlers-Danlos syndrome	Rupture of large vessels
Holt-Oram syndrome	Atrial and ventricular septal defects
Leopard syndrome	Pulmonic stenosis, hypertrophic cardiomyopathy, prolonged PR interval
Marfan syndrome	Aortic aneurysm, aortic insufficiency, mitral valve prolapse
Myotonic dystrophy	Dilated cardiomyopathy, conduction abnormalities
Neurofibromatosis	Coarctation of the aorta, renal artery Stenosis
Treacher Collins syndrome	Atrial and ventricular septal defects, patent ductus arteriosus
Tuberous sclerosis	Myocardial rhabdomyoma, Wolff-Parkinson-White syndrome
Noonan's syndrome	Pulmonic stenosis, hypertrophic cardiomyopathy, atrial septal defect, aortic stenosis

sive weakness of the upper and lower extremities gradually becomes obvious. Gait difficulties are often the first symptom; they progress slowly, followed by unsteadiness in the arms and hands. Difficulty in writing and handling eating utensils subsequently becomes apparent.

Cardiac involvement[87] occurs in 50 to 90 percent of patients. The most common abnormality is hypertrophic cardiomyopathy (Table 62-5); dilated cardiomyopathy occurs rarely. Thus, the most common cardiac symptoms relate to cardiac failure and arrhythmias. Left ventricular outflow tract obstruction due to asymmetrical septal hypertrophy may be evident, and approximately 50 percent of patients die of cardiac disease. Patients are followed for development of arrhythmias and the signs and symptoms of cardiac failure. Treatment consists primarily of conventional drugs to relieve the symptoms and signs of heart failure.

Involvement of the heart is readily detected by electrocardiography and echocardiography. The electrocardiographic abnormalities are found in 90 percent of patients and include repolarization abnormalities manifesting as inverted or biphasic T waves in the inferior limb leads and left precordial leads, a short PR interval, left and right ventricular hypertrophy, as well as left and right axis deviation. Premature atrial contractions, atrial flutter/fibrillation, and premature ventricular contractions are common. Echocardiography detects cardiac involvement in 60 to 100 percent of patients with the most common finding of concentric hypertrophy, but asymmetrical septal hypertrophy accompanied by systolic anterior motion (SAM) of the mitral valve is also common. Left ventricular chamber diameter may be normal or decreased and fractional shortening or ejection fraction is usually normal, although dilated cardiomyopathy (left ventricular dilation and reduced contractility) is seen occasionally (see Chap. 10). There is no specific treatment for the cardiac manifestations except symptomatic treatment if cardiac failure ensues (see Chap. 23).

Friedreich's ataxia is inherited as an autosomal recessive disorder, and parental consanguinity has been noted in some cases. The gene was initially mapped to chromosome 9q13-31.1,[88] and in 1996 the gene was identified.[89] This gene is 40 kb, contains five exons, has a 1.3-kb transcript, and encodes a 210–amino acid protein called frataxin. The highest level of expression is within the heart, while intermediate levels are seen in liver, skeletal muscle, and pancreas; minimal levels are identified in other tissues, including the brain. Although a few affected patients were found to have a point mutation of frataxin, the majority (about 95 percent) are homozygous for an unstable GAA trinucleotide expansion in the first intron.[89] The remainder of patients are compound heterozygotes for the expansion. In patients homozygous for the expansion, there is a correlation between the number of GAA repeats on the smaller allele, age of onset, disease progression, and cardiomyopathy,[87,90-93] confirming that the expansion is the primary cause of disease. The expansion results in severely reduced levels of mature frataxin mRNA.[89]

Campuzano et al.[94] demonstrated that frataxin is localized to the mitochondria associated with the mitochondrial membranes and crests using immunocytofluorescence and immunocytoelectron microscopic evaluation. They suggested that reduction in frataxin results in oxidative damage. Subsequently, Rotig and colleagues[95] suggested that frataxin regulates mitochondrial iron transport and that deficiency of iron-sulfur cluster-containing subunits of mitochondrial respiratory complexes I and II and the iron-sulfur protein aconitase occurs. Hence, it appears that Friedreich's ataxia is a mitochondrial disorder.[96,97] As these patients have HCM, diabetes, ataxia, and apparent free radical toxicity, the mitochondrial basis of this disorder clarifies the clinical features.

Dilated Cardiomyopathy

IDIOPATHIC DILATED CARDIOMYOPATHY

Idiopathic DCM (DCM) is a disease of unknown etiology characterized by increased ventricular chamber size, decreased wall thickness, and impaired systolic ventricular function. The prevalence of idiopathic DCM has been estimated to be approximately 40 cases per 100,000.[98] The diagnosis of DCM is typically made by echocardiography (see Chap. 65), and symptoms usually are those of sudden death and heart failure. Familial DCM (FDCM) is estimated to account for 30 percent of patients with idiopathic DCM. In a large family with idiopathic DCM, an autosomal dominant pattern was determined and the disease was linked to chromosome 1q32.[99] Three other chromosomal loci have been identified: 9q13,[100] 2q31,[101] and 10q21-23.[102] Three additional chromosomal loci have been mapped—to 1p1-1q1,[103] 3p22-25,[104] and 6q23[105]—in families having DCM in association with conduction defects and 6q23 also has limb girdle dystrophy. In the family mapped to 1p1-1q1, transient arrhythmias, which presented in the second or third decade, become sustained and commonplace by the third or fourth decade. The abnormal rhythms included second- or third-degree AV block, atrial fibrillation, or marked bradycardia, commonly requiring a pacemaker. DCM usually developed in the fourth or fifth decade, generally out of proportion to the severity of the rhythm disturbance. Sudden death commonly occurred in the late stages of the disease. On autopsy, marked right and left ventricular dilatation, interstitial fibrosis, myocyte degeneration characterized by cytoplasmic vacuolization, and AV nodal cell replacement by fibrous tissue were noted. The gene and its characteristics have recently been described as lamin A/C, the same gene identified for autosomal dominant Emery-Dreifuss muscular dystrophy. None of the other genes residing at these loci responsible for FDCM have yet been identified. However, two genes have now been identified responsible for FDCM—actin[106] and desmin.[107] Three missense mutations have been identified in actin. Actin, in addition to forming the thin filaments of the sarcomere, essential to the generation of force, is also an important cytoskeletal protein involved in structural integrity and the transmission of force. Mutations in actin responsible for FDCM are located in the domain which is immobilized and attached to the Z-band or intercalated disk and involved with transmitting force. In contrast, it was recently shown that mutations in the actin domain affecting the myosin cross bridges and the generation of force (sarcomere) give rise to FHCM.[108] Desmin is the specific intermediate filament for muscle and an essential cytoskeletal protein for maintaining cardiac structure and for the transmission of force and other signals to the cytoplasm and the nucleus of the cell. Desmin stretches from its attachment to the sarcomere Z-band to the nuclear membrane and other organelles.[109] Mutations in desmin have been shown to be associated with cardiac and skeletal abnormalities.[110] A missense mutation ($Ile^{451}Met$) was recently found to be responsible for DCM in a family without any skeletal or smooth muscle abnormalities. Mutations leading to combined skeletal and cardiac abnormalities have all been in the rod region of desmin. In contrast, the Ile[451]Met mutation responsible for the restricted cardiac phenotype of DCM encodes for the tail domain of human desmin, located in codon 451 with cytosine substituting for guanine. This would suggest a possible unique cardiac function for the domain in this region. Elimination of the desmin gene in a knockout mouse was associated with a phenotype of DCM exhibiting impaired cardiac function and myocyte necrosis.[110] It is of note that DCM associated with musculoskeletal disorders such as Duchenne muscular dystrophy are due to dystrophin, α-dystroglycan, and α-sarcoglycan, all of which are cytoskeletal proteins[111] (Fig. 62-7). There is thus the strong suggestion that familial DCM may be a disease of the cytoskeletal proteins[107,112–114] analogous to HCM being a disease of the sarcomere. This has been termed by Towbin as the "final common pathway hypothesis"[113,114] (Fig. 62-8).

X-LINKED DILATED CARDIOMYOPATHY (XLCM)

Berko and Swift[2] reported a five-generation kindred with DCM and no clinical evidence of skeletal myopathy. Males presented in their teens or early twenties with clinical evidence of mitral regurgitation and an echocardiographic diagnosis of DCM. Episodes of ventricular tachycardia were noted in several patients. The males progressed rapidly (within 1 or 2 years) to death or cardiac transplantation. Manifesting female carriers developed mild cardiomyopathy in the fourth or fifth decade and progressed slowly. Right ventricular endomyocardial biopsy revealed minimal interstitial fibrosis, while postmortem evaluation showed marked dilatation, widespread patchy fibrosis (worst in the posterior wall), and normal mitochondria on electron microscopy. There were no pathognomonic findings differentiating this cardiomyopathy from other dilated forms except for the apparent X-linked inheritance and elevation of the muscle isoform of creatine kinase (CK-MM) in the serum of affected males and female carriers.

Towbin and colleagues[115] demonstrated linkage of XLCM to the dystrophin locus at Xp21 (i.e., the gene responsible for Duchenne and Becker muscular dystrophy) in the family described above as well as in a second family. Evaluation of the protein defect in XLCM showed absence (or low abundance) of the *N*-terminal and rod portion of the dystrophin protein, while skeletal muscle total protein was normal.[115] The 156-kDa dystrophin-associated glycoprotein (known as α-dystroglycan),[116,117] a membrane-bound constituent of the dystrophin-associated glycoprotein complex, was decreased in cardiac tissue as well.[116] This was later confirmed.[118] Diverse mutations leading to XLCM have been shown by Towbin and Ortiz-Lopez,[119,120] Yoshida et al.,[121] Muntoni et al.,[122] and Milasin et al.,[123] with most mutations residing in the 5′ portion of the gene. It appears that the DCM occurs due to mechanical destablization of the muscle membrane. Recently, novel mutations in the 5′ end of dystrophin, including a transposon[124] insertion and an *Alu*-rearrangement[125] were found to result in XLCM. Treatment of congestive heart failure and ventricular arrhythmias is necessary and transplantation is common (see Chap. 23).

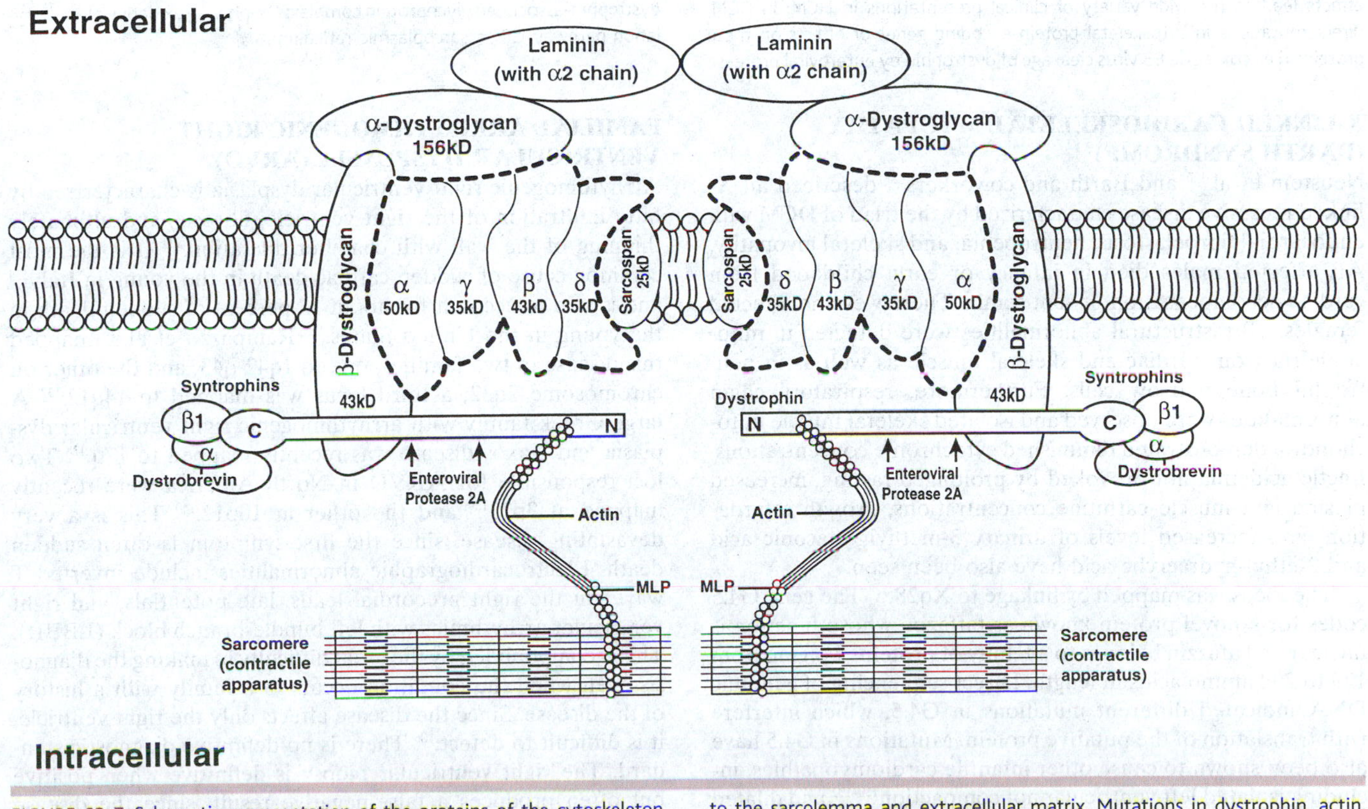

FIGURE 62-7 Schematic representation of the proteins of the cytoskeleton involved in development of dilated cardiomyopathy with or without skeletal myopathy and/or conduction defect. Note that dystrophin links the sarcomere to the sarcolemma and extracellular matrix. Mutations in dystrophin, actin, MLP, and the dystroglycan and sarcoglycan complexes have resulted in dilated cardiomyopathy in patients and animal models.

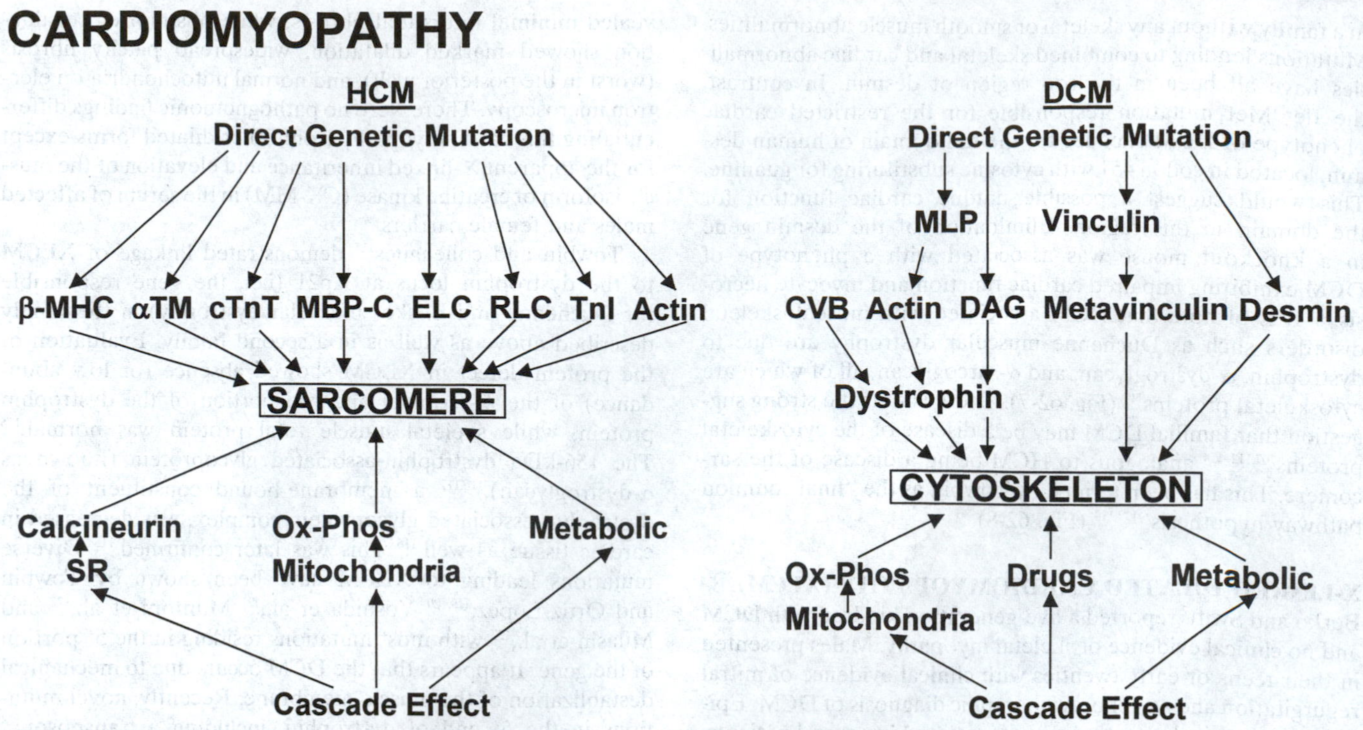

FIGURE 62-8 The "final common pathway hypothesis" described by Towbin, showing the pathways involved in development of hypertrophic (HCM) and dilated cardiomyopathy (DCM). In HCM, mutations in the sarcomeric protein-encoding genes result in the phenotype. In addition, the phenotype may be altered or modified by metabolic or mitochondrial derangements as well as by activation of a molecular pathway such as calcineurin. These cascade effects lead to the wide variety of clinical presentations in HCM. In DCM, direct mutations in cytoskeletal protein-encoding genes or effects on these proteins (i.e., coxsackie B3 virus cleavage of dystrophin by enteroviral protease 2A) also modify the clinical phenotype. Cascade effects via metabolism, mitochondrial abnormalities, or drug interactions are also influential in the severity of disease. HCM/DCM abbreviations: β-MHC = β-myosin heavy chain; αTM = α tropomyosin; cTnT = cardiac troponin T; MBP-c = myosin binding protein C; ELC = essential light chain; RLC = regulatory light chain; TNI = troponin I; CVB = coxsackie virus B; MLP = muscle LIM protein; DAG = dystrophin-associated glycoprotein complex; Ox-phos = oxidative phosphorylation pathway; SR = sarcoplasmic reticulum.

X-LINKED CARDIOSKELETAL MYOPATHY (BARTH SYNDROME)

Neustein et al.[126] and Barth and coworkers[127] described an X-linked recessive disease characterized by the triad of DCM with endocardial fibroelastosis, neutropenia, and skeletal myopathy. All affected males died in infancy or early childhood from cardiac decompensation or septicemia. There were no affected females. Ultrastructural abnormalities were detected in mitochondria from cardiac and skeletal muscle as well as in neutrophil bone marrow cells. Furthermore, respiratory chain abnormalities were observed and isolated skeletal muscle mitochondria demonstrated diminished cytochrome concentrations. Lactic acidemia not provoked by prolonged fasting, increased plasma and muscle carnitine concentrations, growth retardation, and increased levels of urinary 3-methylglutaconic acid and 2-ethyl-hydracrylic acid have also been seen.

The locus was mapped by linkage to Xq28.[128] The gene G4.5 codes for a novel protein known as taffazin, whose function is unclear.[129] Tafazzin belongs to a family of proteins ranging from 129 to 292 amino acids in length. Direct sequencing of genomic DNA indicated different mutations in G4.5, which interfere with translation of the putative protein. Mutations in G4.5 have also been shown to cause other infantile cardiomyopathies, including isolated left ventricular noncompaction[130–132] and dilated hypertrophic cardiomyopathy. Treatment is that for cardiac failure (see Chap. 23).

FAMILIAL ARRHYTHMOGENIC RIGHT VENTRICULAR DYSPLASIA (ARVD)

Arrhythmogenic right ventricular dysplasia is characterized by fatty infiltration of the right ventricle, fibrosis, and ultimately thinning of the wall with chamber dilatation.[133] It is the most common cause of sudden cardiac death in the young in Italy[134] and is said to account for about 17 percent of sudden death in the young in the United States.[135] Rampazzo et al.[136] mapped this disease in two families, one to 1q42-q43, and the other on chromosome 2q32; a third locus was mapped to 14q12.[137] A large Greek family with arrhythmogenic right ventricular dysplasia and Naxos disease was recently mapped to 17q.[138] Two loci responsible for ARVD in North America were recently mapped at 3p23[139] and the other at 10p12.[140] This is a very devastating disease, since the first symptom is often sudden death. Electrocardiographic abnormalities include inverted T waves in the right precordial leads, late potentials, and right ventricular arrhythmias with left bundle-branch block (LBBB). This is compounded by the great difficulty in making the diagnosis even when the condition occurs in a family with a history of the disease. Since the disease affects only the right ventricle, it is difficult to detect.[106] There is no definitive diagnostic standard. The right ventricular biopsy is definitive when positive but often produces a false-negative result, since the disease initiates in the epicardium and spreads to the endocardium of the right ventricular free wall, making it inaccessible to biopsy.

Consensus diagnostic criteria was developed that include right ventricular biopsy, magnetic resonance imaging (MRI), echocardiography, and electrocardiography.[141] Identification of the gene will have tremendous diagnostic impact and hopefully will provide an explanation as to why ARVD is restricted to the right ventricle. Is it a specific right ventricular chamber gene? Is there a stimulus that is unique or predominates in the right ventricle that precipitates the phenotype? What is the stimulus? There are data suggesting that apoptosis is the process leading to the development of fat and fibrosis in ARVD. Discovery of a gene should shed light on the apoptosis pathway.

RESTRICTIVE CARDIOMYOPATHY

In the western countries, restrictive cardiomyopathy (RCM) is the least common of the three major categories of cardiomyopathy (see Chap. 75). The most common cause of secondary restrictive cardiomyopathy in adults is myocardial amyloid. Patients manifest exercise intolerance due to their inability to increase cardiac output by tachycardia without further compromising ventricular filling. Weakness and dyspnea are often prominent, and chest pain may also occur. At end stage, the findings are those of cardiac failure with anasarca. Mutations in the transthyretin (TTR) gene[142,143] which codes for the TTR serum protein, has been found associated with RCM. This protein contains four subunits, each with 127 amino acids, encoded by four exons within a 7-kb gene. Many TTR point mutations cause TTR to form amyloid, which occurs primarily in the heart, leading to heart failure. The diagnosis is suspected by echo and confirmed by genetic analysis. Treatment is that of cardiac failure.

Familial forms of restrictive cardiomyopathy have also been seen. One such family was found to have mutations in the desmin gene[144] and mice have been created with desmin mutations that have a similar phenotype as the clinical condition.[110]

Mucopolysaccharidoses

The mucopolysaccharidoses (MPS) are a group of diseases caused by deficiency of lysosomal enzymes involved in the degradation of glycosaminoglycans.[145] Undegraded glycosaminoglycans accumulate in lysosomes and affect tissue function. MPS have been divided into seven major types. The classification (types I to VII) is based on the deficient enzyme responsible for the disorder. These disorders carry such eponyms as *Hurler, Scheie, Hurler-Scheie, Hunter, Sanfilippo, Morquio, Maroteaux-Lamy,* and *Sly*. They share many clinical features, including multiple system involvement, organomegaly, dysostosis multiplex, facial abnormalities, loss of hearing and vision, joint involvement, cardiac involvement, and central nervous system (CNS) involvement. Cardiac disease includes myocardial hypertrophy, pulmonary and systemic hypertension, valvular disease, coronary occlusion, and myocardial infarction. Congestive heart failure and sudden death are relatively frequent. The most common mucopolysaccharidosis with cardiac involvement is MPS I (Hurler syndrome). Valvular disease is prominent in the Scheie's syndrome (late-onset form). Less commonly, heart disease has been noted in Sanfilippo A syndrome with aortic regurgitation, as well as in severe Maroteaux-Lamy syndrome with valvular heart disease (Table 62-5). The diagnosis for either of these disorders is made by assaying the enzyme activity in cultured skin fibroblasts or leukocytes.

Hurler's Syndrome

Hurler's syndrome (MPS-I) is an autosomal recessive trait found on chromosome 22 (22q11), which occurs in approximately 1 of 40,000 people. It is caused by a deficiency of α-iduronidase (IDUA), which is required for the degradation of both heparan sulfate and dermatan sulfate.[146] The result is similar to that of Hunter's syndrome, with both dermatan and heparan sulfate in high concentrations in the urine. Myocardial infarction occurs in childhood (Table 62-5). *Severe* (Hurler, MPS-IH), *intermediate* (Hurler/Scleie, MPS-IH/S), and *mild* (Scheie) clinical subtypes of MPS-I occur.[145] MPS-IH patients usually present within the first year of life and progress with a combination of hepatosplenomegaly, skeletal deformities, corneal clouding, and severe mental retardation. Obstructive airway disease, respiratory infection, and cardiac complications usually result in death before age 10 years. Dangel[147] reported on 64 children with mucopolysasccharidoses, noting 72 percent with cardiac disease (valvular lesions, cardiomyopathy). Mitral valve thickening with regurgitation or stenosis, hypertrophic cardiomyopathy, aortic stenosis, and EFE were most common. MPS-IH/S is characterized by little neurologic involvement but most of the somatic involvement described for MPS-IH develops early in the teenage years, causing considerable loss of mobility. MPS-IS patients, those with the mildest symptoms, have little or no neurologic involvement, normal stature, and normal life span but do develop stiff joints, mild hepatosplenomegaly, aortic valve disease, and corneal clouding.[145] Diagnosis is confirmed in MPS-I by demonstration of mucopolysacchariduria and absence of IDUA activity in leukocytes and fibroblasts. Biochemical differentiation between subtypes is difficult. Gene identification[148] has allowed for mutation analysis; the broad range of clinical phenotypes is related to the types of mutations in the IDUA gene.[149] Allogenic bone marrow transplantation is the most effective treatment for Hurler's syndrome[150] and gene transfer is being evaluated.[151] Animal models are now available[152–154] for study.

Hunter's Syndrome

Hunter's syndrome, an X-linked disorder mapped to the Xq26-Xq28 region, is found in approximately 1 of 30,000 people.[145] It is caused by a deficiency of the enzyme iduronate sulfatase and results in excessive urinary excretion of dermatan and heparan sulfate and accumulation of mucopolysaccharides, which can result in coronary obstruction and subsequent myocardial infarction in childhood. Most patients die before the third decade. Mutations in this gene are heterogeneous, ranging from small microlesions to gross deletions and inversions[155–157] and, in some cases, involves neighboring genes. Therefore, wide clinical variation is common. Gene therapy has been reported.[158–160]

Morquio's Disease

Morquio's disease (MPS-IVA), an autosomal recessive disorder caused by a genetic deficiency in *N*-acetyl-galactosamine-6-sulfatase, is a prototypical chondroosteodystrophy.[145] The disorder is characterized by specific spondyloepiphyseal dysplasia, short-trunk dwarfism, coxa valga, odontoid hypoplasia, corneal opacities, normal intelligence, and excessive urinary excretion of keratan sulfate and chondroitin 6-sulfate. The deficient *N*-acetyl-galactosamine-6-sulfatase results in progressive accumulation of mucopolysaccharides in lysosomes of various tissues, leading to vertebral involvement and cardiac disease (Table 62-5) in the second decade of life. Tomatsu et al.[161] isolated and characterized the full-length cDNA of the gene and it was localized to chromosome 16q24.[162] This gene is approximately 50 kb in size and has 14 exons; mutations have been described.[163,164]

Maroteaux-Lamy Disease

The Maroteaux-Lamy syndrome is caused by the deficiency of the enzyme arylsulfatase B, which is required for degradation of the glycosaminoglycans, dermatan sulfate, and chondroitin 4-sulfate.[165] It is associated with aortic valve disease. This gene, located on 5q13-q14,[165] has been isolated and characterized.[166] Mutations have been identified, and different mutations cause different clinical phenotypes.[167] The clinical features are quite variable, occurring in infancy and consist of growth retardation, coarse facies, corneal clouding, and multiple skeletal changes, together with dilated cardiomyopathy and aortic or mitral value stenosis or insufficiency. Cardiac manifestations usually appear after the neurologic features but are usually present by adolescence. Molecular diagnosis is currently available. Bone marrow transplants are currently the treatment of choice.[150] All of these disorders can be diagnosed prenatally by enzyme assay in at-risk pregnancies.

MUSCULAR DYSTROPHIES WITH CARDIAC INVOLVEMENT

The muscular dystrophies are a heterogeneous group of diseases, the primary manifestations of which include progressive muscle wasting secondary to intrinsic defects of the muscle fiber. These defects have a wide spectrum of clinical expression and include Duchenne's muscular dystrophy, Becker's muscular dystrophy, Emery-Dreifuss muscular dystrophy, the limb-girdle muscular dystrophies, and myotonic dystrophy. Cardiac disease, especially DCM, is central to the morbidity and mortality associated with these disorders (Table 62-7).

Duchenne Muscular Dystrophy (DMD)

DMD is an X-linked disorder characterized by the early onset of progressive, generalized muscle weakness and "pseudohypertrophy" of certain muscle groups.[168] The incidence of DMD is estimated to be 1 in 3300 live male births with little ethnic variation, and the calculated mutation rate of 10^4 is an order of magnitude higher than for most other genetic diseases. About one-third of cases arise by spontaneous mutation, with the remaining two-thirds occurring by inheritance of the disease-causing gene from the carrier mother. Female carriers of DMD are usually asymptomatic but occasionally have a slowly progressive myopathy of moderate severity. This "manifesting female carrier" state occurs in approximately 8 percent of carriers and is thought to occur due to random X-inactivation. The disease may also be expressed in females with Turner syndrome having a single X chromosome and in females with X-autosome translocations that disrupt the DMD gene. In the latter case, the translocation not only disrupts the DMD gene but also causes the nonrandom inactivation of the normal allele on the other X chromosome, resulting in the expression of the disease phenotype.

Although evidence of skeletal muscle disease in boys with DMD is evident in the neonatal period, as seen by high serum muscle enzymes (particularly CK-MM), clinical disease is not. There may be mild developmental delay, walking later than expected, but weakness is usually not appreciated until at least 2 or 3 years of age. Early symptoms reported by parents include difficulty in running or climbing stairs, frequent falling, and enlargement of calf muscles. Pelvic-girdle weakness is more obvious than shoulder-girdle weakness in the early stages. The gait becomes lordotic and waddling, and the child usually walks with the heels raised slightly off the ground (i.e., toe walking). As pelvic girdle weakness increases, the child has increasing difficulty rising from a seated position. In order to rise from the floor to a standing position, the child must brace the arms against the front of the thigh and climb up the legs, the so-called Gowers sign. Muscle pseudohypertrophy usually appears by 5 to 6 years of age, with muscle enlargement most commonly occurring in the calf muscles; the quadriceps, infraspinatus, deltoid, and gluteal muscles may also be involved, however. The upper and lower extremities become progressively weaker with age, and joint contractures may appear due to uneven weakness of agonist and antagonist muscles. Contractures of the hip flexors, iliotibial bands, and heel cords develop in 70 percent of patients between 6 and 10 years of age. Most patients are wheelchair-bound by the end of the first decade of life. After ambulation is lost, fixed contractures occur and paraspinal muscle weakness leads to progressive kyphoscoliosis. Significant weakness of the respiratory muscles occurs early in the second decade and is a common cause of demise.

Although most cases of DMD can be recognized on the basis of the patient's history and clinical signs alone, laboratory evaluation is important to confirm the diagnosis.[168] As previously noted, extremely high levels of CK-MM are found in the early stages of disease, as early as birth, and precede evidence of clinical involvement. Other muscle enzymes—including aldolase, SGOT, lactic dehydrogenase (LDH), and pyruvate kinase—are also grossly elevated. In the end stages of the disease, enzyme levels fall but do not reach normal values. Electromyographic examination may also be useful, demonstrating the characteristic features of a myopathy. Insertional activity is normal or increased initially but decreases in the advanced stages of the disease, when fibrosis replaces muscle fibers. Fibrillation potentials and positive sharp waves occur in the early stages of the disease due to the splitting of muscle fibers. The motor unit potentials are small and polyphasic, and an early recruitment pattern with minimal effort is present. Mild intellectual impairment is common in patients with DMD. The retardation is present at an early age, is nonprogressive, and does not correlate well with the stage of the disease. Approximately one-third of patients have IQs below 75, characterized primarily by impaired verbal ability.

The heart is commonly involved in DMD, with electrocardiographic abnormalities and dilated cardiomyopathy being most typical.[168] Cardiac symptoms, however, are unusual before the terminal stages of the disease. Congestive heart failure tends to occur. A midsystolic click and late systolic murmur associated with mitral valve prolapse are also common. In addition, an S3 or S4 gallop, sinus tachycardia, and a mitral regurgitation murmur are usually heard; cardiomegaly and increased pulmonary vascular markings appear at this stage, and bilateral diaphragmatic elevations may be seen owing to diaphragmatic dystrophy. Unlike the late-onset findings of dilated cardiomyopathy, the electrocardiogram is abnormal early in the course of DMD, with a tall R-wave and an abnormally increased R/S ratio in the right precordial chest leads and a deep, narrow Q-wave in leads I, aV_L, V_5, and V_6. These abnormalities progress over time and are attributed to the finding of that the greatest dystrophic myocardial changes in the posterobasal and contiguous lateral left ventricular myocardium. In addition, P waves with negative terminal deflections in V_1 exceeding 20 ms and 0.1 mV appear in 20 to 45 percent of patients and, in the absence of left atrial enlargement on echocardiogram, are attributed to an intrinsic disorder of left atrial or intraatrial conduction. A short PR interval may be seen in up to 50 percent of patients but is not thought to be due to a bypass tract, as seen in Wolff-Parkinson-White syndrome. Infranodal conduction abnormalities, however, may be seen in patients with DMD, and these include complete or incomplete bundle-branch block, and left anterior or posterior fascicular block. Atrial and ventricular premature beats and atrial flutter are seen in some patients.

Echocardiography reveals left ventricular dilatation and dysfunction, with significantly reduced ejection fraction, and LV hypokinesis of the posterobasal ventricular wall is identified. Doppler and color Doppler commonly demonstrate mitral regurgitation, either secondary to the dilated cardiomyopathy or to the associated mitral valve prolapse, which occurs secondary to papillary muscle dysfunction. In some patients systolic function appears normal but diastolic dysfunction is present.

Histopathologic abnormalities of the heart and skeletal muscle are universal in patients with DMD, and those of skeletal muscle are widespread even in the early stages of disease.[168] Typical findings are rounding of the muscle fibers, increased variability in fiber size, increased central nucleation, and fiber splitting. Necrotic and regenerating fibers are present along with large, round hyaline fibers. In the late stages, muscle may be virtually replaced by fat and fibrous tissue. In the heart, degenerative changes in muscle fibers and areas of fibrosis in the ventricles, atria, and conduction system occur, with most pronounced changes in the posterobasal region and adjacent lateral wall of the left ventricle. The underlying cause of cardiac disease is not currently known, but it is speculated that the gene defect in DMD leads to instability of the translated cytoskeletal protein, leading to weakening of the myocyte membrane and subsequent myocyte death due to mechanical stress.

The dystrophin gene, on the short arm of the X chromosome,[168,169] is responsible for these disorders and when dystrophin abnormalities occur due to mutations, may cause either low level production of a nonfunctional protein or complete absence of dystrophin in the heart and skeletal muscle of affected patients. It is among the largest genes discovered thus far, comprising approximately 2.5 Mbp and transcribing a 14-kb mRNA molecule. This cytoskeletal protein-encoding gene is normally expressed in striated and smooth muscle as well as in brain. In muscle tissue, the dystrophin protein has been localized to the cytoplasmic surface of the sarcolemma and is associated with several integral membrane glycoproteins.[170] This glycoprotein/dystrophin complex—which involves the sarcoglycans, dystroglycans, syntrophins, and dystrobrevins—connects dystrophin to the sarcolemma and links to the extracellular matrix; it may be involved in the regulation of intracellular calcium, which is increased in dystrophin-deficient muscle, along with increased calcium channel transport.

The diagnostic approaches to DMD have changed dramatically over the past decade. Previously, serum CK-MM level and muscle biopsy were the standard approaches. Today DMD is diagnosed primarily by molecular analysis, which is rapid and accurate and may predict clinical course. Most commonly, dystrophin mutations that cause a frameshift[171] of the nucleotide sequence result in the severe form of muscular dystrophy, DMD.

Management of the congestive heart failure associated with the DCM seen in DMD is identical to that used for patients with other causes of heart failure and arrhythmias. Pacing is not usually necessary.

Becker's Muscular Dystrophy (BMD)

BMD is an X-linked disorder that differs in both severity and time of onset from DMD,[168] despite being due to allelic mutations in dystrophin, the gene responsible for DMD. BMD appears later and progresses more slowly than DMD, so that survival to middle age is seen. The pattern of muscle weakness, however, is identical to that in DMD, with early involvement of the pelvic girdle and proximal lower extremities.[168] The initial signs of weakness usually appear during the second decade but may be seen as late as the third decade. The weakness gradually progresses, with the upper extremities becoming involved after 5 to 10 years. Patients generally remain ambulatory until their mid-thirties. As in DMD, muscle hypertrophy is common; intellectual impairment, however, is less common and less severe. As in DMD, life expectancy is also reduced in BMD, with only 50 percent of patients surviving to 40 years of age.

Cardiac involvement may be seen in adolescence and ultimately affects 80 percent of patients.[172] As in DMD, dilated cardiomyopathy and cardiac failure are the usual abnormalities encountered (Table 62-7) and are often the ultimate cause of death. Conduction abnormalities manifesting as fascicular block or complete heart block are also seen. As in DMD, muscle enzyme activity is markedly elevated in BMD, and preclinical cases may be detected by elevated CK-MM. Electromyographic examination shows a "myopathic" pattern with small, polyphasic motor units and early recruitment of motor units. The histology of BMD is similar to that of other forms of muscular dystrophy. In contrast to DMD, hyaline fibers are rarely seen. Electrocardiographic changes are similar to those seen in DMD. Other electrocardiographic abnormalities encountered include left axis deviation, right bundle-branch block, left bundle-branch block, and complete heart block. The echocardiogram may demonstrate the features of dilated cardiomyopathy.

BMD is also due to mutations within the dystrophin gene; i.e., it is allelic with DMD. As is the case with DMD, more than 30 percent of patients with BMD have no family history of the disease, an indication that they represent spontaneous mutations. The phenotypic difference between DMD and BMD patients has been speculated to be due to frameshift mutations leading to more severe disease (DMD) while out-of-frame mutations cause less severe (BMD) disease.[171] The frameshift hypothesis explains more than 90 percent of the cases of DMD versus BMD. The cardiac abnormalities in BMD, like those

TABLE 62-7 Manifestations of Neurologic Cardiac Disorders

Neuromuscular Disorder	Mode of Inheritance	Incidence per 100,000	Age of Onset	Pathology: Cardiac	Pathology: Musculoskeletal	Clinical: Cardiac	Clinical: Musculoskeletal
Myotonic dystrophy	Autosomal dominant	10	Third to fourth decade	Atrophy, interstitial fibrosis and fatty infiltration of the conduction system	Atrophy, interstitial fibrosis and fatty infiltration	AV block, atrial arrhythmias, CHF (rare)	Myotonia, atrophy of strap muscles
Friedreich's ataxia	Autosomal recessive	2.0	Child/adolescent	Interstitial fibrosis, myocyte hypertrophy	Normal	Abnormal ECG axis and Q waves, atrial arrhythmias, hypertrophic cardiomyopathy (concentric, asymmetrical), dilated cardiomyopathy	Ataxia, kyphoscoliosis
Duchenne's muscular dystrophy	X-linked recessive	2.0	2–5 years	Myocardial fibrosis in posterobasal LV free wall, degeneration of conducting fibers, noninflammatory arteriopathy	Myofibril necrosis, interstitial accumulation of fat and fibrous tissue	Dysrhythmias, ECG abnormalities, dilated cardiomyopathy	Pseudohypertrophy, proximal limb and neck weakness, contractures, scoliosis and chest cage deformities
Becker's muscular dystrophy	X-linked recessive	0.4	Second to third decade	Focal areas of fatty infiltration and proliferating connective tissue	Same as Duchenne's	Dilated cardiomyopathy	Pseudohypertrophy, proximal limb-girdle weakness and atrophy

Kearns-Sayre syndrome	Maternal, nonmedelian (i.e., mitochondrial)	Rare	Childhood/adolescence	Ragged-red fibers	Ragged-red fibers, glycogen accumulation, proliferation of abnormal mitochondria	Progressive AV block, dilated cardiomyopathy, hypertrophic cardiomyopathy	Ptosis, ataxia
Emery-Dreifuss syndrome	X-linked recessive (? autosomal dominant)	Rare	Second to third decade	Focal myocardial fibrosis	Same as Duchenne's	Atrial standstill, progressive conduction block, malignant ventricular arrhythmias, dilated cardiomyopathy	Contractures of elbows, pericervical muscles, and Achilles tendon; humeroperoneal muscle weakness and atrophy
Fascioscapulohumeral muscular dystrophy	Autosomal dominant	0.6	Second to third decade	Unknown	Same as Duchenne's	Atrial abnormalities, conduction delays, atrial fibrillation/flutter	Proximal shoulder and facial weakness and atrophy; lower extremity weakness
Myotubular (centronuclear) myopathy	X-linked recessive	Rare	Variable	Myocardial fibrosis	Hypertrophic fibers with central nuclei	Dilated cardiomyopathy	Respiratory difficulty and hypotonia
Nemaline myopathy	Autosomal dominant with reduced penetrance	Rare	Birth/infancy	Nemaline bodies	Nemaline bodies	Dilated cardiomyopathy	Diffuse muscle weakness and hypotonia

SOURCE: From Berko and Swift,[2] Collins et al.,[3] and Brower,[4] with permission.

described for DMD, require further study.[173] The treatment of CHF and arrhythmias is similar to that of other patients with these signs and symptoms.

Animal models have been created during the past several years that help to characterize the roles of dystrophin and the associated complexes.[174–180] Loss-of-function mutations of dystrophin lead to a DMD or BMD phenotype, while utrophin-deficient mice have defects in the postsynaptic membrane folds at the neuromuscular junction. Mice lacking both dystrophin and utrophin display a severe muscular dystrophy with premature death.[177–180] Sarcoglycan-deficient mice also demonstrate severe muscular dystrophy but, in addition, severe hypertrophic and/or dilated cardiomyopathy has been seen.[174,175]

Various methods evaluating the possibility of gene therapy for dystrophinopathies have been reported over the past several years in mice, with varying degrees of success. Minigene and stem-cell transplantation have both been considered promising using dystrophin and utrophin.[181,182]

Emery-Dreifuss Muscular Dystrophy (EDMD)

EDMD is a relatively rare disorder[168] characterized by weakness in the humeroperoneal distribution, early joint contractures, and dilated cardiomyopathy, with X-linked (occasionally, autosomal dominant) inheritance. The onset of disease in these patients occurs between 2 and 10 years of age, with weakness initially noted in the shoulder girdles and upper extremities. Contractures of the elbows and posterior cervical muscles appear early. The disease is slowly progressive, with involvement of the distal leg musculature following that of the upper extremities; contractures of the knees and ankles follow contractures of the elbows. Unlike the case in DMD and BMD, muscle pseudohypertrophy does not occur. The disease evolves slowly and usually stabilizes in the third decade, with most patients remaining ambulatory. Dilated cardiomyopathy is a common occurrence, but the severity of disease varies from family to family. Varying degrees of atrioventricular block are common (Table 62-7) and atrial standstill may occur. These electrical abnormalities may lead to episodes of syncope, transient ischemic attacks, stroke, and sudden death. A pacemaker is commonly required. Atrial fibrillation has also been observed. As in DMD and BMD, muscle enzyme activity is elevated, albeit to a lesser extent. Skeletal muscle biopsy histopathologic findings are similar to those associated with other forms of muscular dystrophy. Type I fiber atrophy has been described in some cases (Fig. 62-9). The gene responsible for X-linked EDMD was localized to Xq28[184] before being cloned. The gene called emerin (or STA) was shown to have an open reading frame of 762 nucleotides that encodes a serine-rich 254–amino acid protein with probable mechanical/structural function.[185] Emerin mRNA shows ubiquitous tissue distribution, with the highest expression in skeletal and cardiac muscles. The cDNA sequence of emerin predicts a tail-anchor membrane protein with an amino acid sequence similar to that of the thymopoietins, a group of nuclear lamina-associated proteins.[186] Nagano et al.[187] and Manilal et al.[188] both showed that emerin is a 34-kDa nuclear membrane protein in skeletal and cardiac muscle, which is absent in EDMD.

The autosomal dominant form of EDMD was initially mapped to chromosome 1, and recently the gene was identified as lamin A/C.[189] The encoded protein is also thought to be a nuclear lamina-associated protein. The phenotypic spectrum of this gene appears to be broad when mutated. In some cases, only a DCM phenotype with conduction disease occurs in the absence of skeletal muscle disease clinically, similar to what is seen with dystrophin.

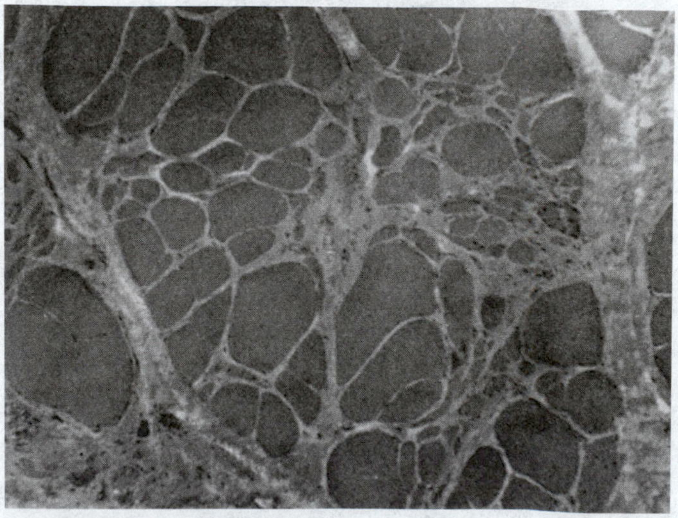

FIGURE 62-9 Skeletal muscle biopsy in Emery-Dreifuss muscular dystrophy. Increased endomysial and perimysial connective tissue, with marked variation in myofiber size, internal nuclei, and myofibers splitting (×153). (Reprinted with permission from Specht LA, McKee AC. MGH Case Records (case 34-1992): A 19-year-old man with progressive proximal muscle weakness, contractures, and cardiac abnormalities. *N Engl J Med* 1992; 327:558.)

Myotonic Dystrophy (Steinert's Disease)

Myotonic dystrophy (DM) is the most common form of inherited muscular dystrophy in adults, with an incidence of 1 in 8000 to 10,000 persons.[168] This autosomal dominant disorder affects multiple organ systems and its name is derived from the combined myopathy, dystrophy, and myotonia of skeletal muscle. Myotonia, an abnormality in relaxation after muscle contraction, is the primary feature of this disease. DM is variably expressed, and individuals may present with signs and symptoms involving many different organ systems. Penetrance varies with age and the disease may affect different tissues at different periods of life; a severe form of DM exists with symptoms at birth.

Classically, DM presents in a young adult with new-onset weakness of the hands or mild foot drop. Asymptomatic myotonia—namely, sustained contraction and depolarization of skeletal muscle in response to a percussive or electrical impulse—may be elicited. Myotonia is usually in the hands and tongue, while weakness involves the distal extremities predominantly. A typical facies usually accompanies these findings, including loss of temporal muscle and slight weakness of the lips and mouth with a "hatchet-like" shape, frontal balding, and ptosis (Fig. 62-10). Other systems including heart, eyes, CNS, endocrine system, gastrointestinal system and respiratory system may be involved (Table 62-5). Electromyographic abnormalities are frequent and subcapsular; punctuate iridescent cataracts are common in middle-aged patients.

Myotonia is best seen in the small muscles of the hand and in the tongue. There are repetitive discharges with gradual and

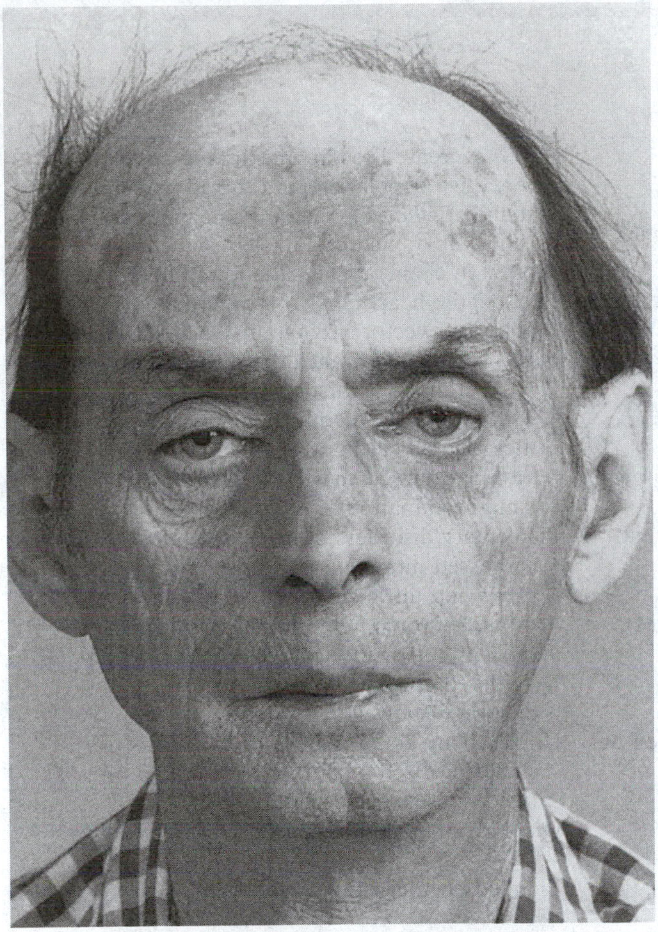

FIGURE 62-10 A 41-year-old man with myotonic dystrophy (DM). Muscle wasting of temporalis muscles with narrow small chin produces a "hatchet-like" facies. Baldness and ptosis (note droopy eyelids with pupils partially covered and sclerae visible) contribute to characteristic appearance. (Reprinted with permission from Roses AD, Pericak-Vance MA. In: *Molecular Basis of Neurology*. Cambridge, MA: Blackwell; 1993:147–159.)

uneven decay of amplitude on electromyography. Myotonic muscles undergo dystrophic changes, which may take years to several decades. In general, the younger the presentation, the more rapid the progression. Only a small percentage of affected individuals, probably less than 10 percent, progress to requiring a wheelchair for ambulation; many require a brace worn in the shoes to control foot drop.

Serious complications of DM involve the heart.[189] Cardiac conduction abnormalities are common (Tables 62-7 and 62-8) and may be progressive, particularly in younger patients. These are identified by periodic ECG monitoring and usually occur without obvious cardiac complaints. Sudden cardiac death in athletically inclined adolescents is relatively frequent. In studies of families with DM, cardiac findings may be the initial clinical manifestation of the disease, with bradycardia and first-degree heart block being common. Progression to complete heart block may occur over time and is not well tolerated, potentially ending in death and frequently requiring pacing. In some cases, ventricular tachycardia or dilated cardiomyopathy may also occur (Table 62-8). Typically, however, systolic function is preserved but diastolic dysfunction occurs.

DM patients may have a particular psychological profile that includes indifference, reticence, and hostility. Mild mental retardation may be seen, particularly in patients with congenital DM. Young and middle-aged patients may be hypersomnolent and indolent, sometimes sleeping up to 20 h daily. Testicular atrophy is common in males and amenorrhea and ovarian cysts may occur in females (Table 62-8). Increasing debilitation, handicap, and disability may occur in subsequent generations of a family; this increasing disease severity is known as *anticipation*.

The gene for myotonic dystrophy was localized to 19q13.3[190] and encodes for myotonin protein kinase (DMPK), a serine-threonine protein kinase.[191] The genetic basis for myotonic dystrophy consists of long stretches of three bases repeated in tandem. The triplet repeat present in the DMPK gene is CTG, which in the mRNA is CUG and is located in the 3′ end of the gene beyond the protein coding region. The severity of disease (neuromuscular, cardiac, and CNS) relates to the length of the repeats. Less than 50 triplet repeats is usually associated with no disease. Usually 100 to 250 repeats are required to cause disease and, if more than 250 repeats are present, the disease is usually seen at birth and reflects genetic anticipation (increasingly severe expression and earlier onset of disease through generations as a result of the increase in the number of CTG repeats with subsequent generations). Clinical cardiac symptoms (i.e., syncope) and ECG abnormalities (i.e., left bundle-branch block) correlate directly with CTG expansion size.[189] In addition, the incidence of malignant ventricular arrhythmias also correlate directly with the size of CTG expansion.

Myotonic dystrophy is one of the many familial neuromuscular diseases due to the genetic defect of multiple triplet repeats.[189] However, the mechanisms whereby the triplet repeats induce the disease remains an enigma. Myotonic dystrophy is somewhat unique since the triplet repeats are in the 3′ end of the gene beyond the protein coding region. DMPK levels are reduced in patients with myotonic dystrophy; when the gene for DMPK is eliminated in knockout mice, muscle weakness results, but none of the other organs are involved, such as the eyes or testes, as observed in myotonic dystrophy. This has led to an extensive search for other explanations, including adjacent genes. One by-product of this research was identification of a novel group of proteins that bind specifically to triplet repeats in DNA and RNA[192]; binding is determined by the sequence of the triplet repeat. A specific protein was identified that binds only to the CUG sequence in the mRNA of DMPK. The CUG-BP protein has a molecular weight of 52 kDa and three binding sites for CUG repeats.[192] The protein has several serine and threonine phosphorylation sites, which appear to be regulated by DMPK. Further studies indicated that this protein is identical to another protein (NB50) that is known to be responsible for mRNA transport from the nucleus to the cytoplasm.[193] This has given rise to the hypothesis that the CUG-BP is sequestered by the multiple CUG repeats and not available to other mRNAs for processing or transport from the nucleus. The involvement of several mRNAs would explain the multiple organs involved. This would also explain why, in the mouse with the DMPK gene knocked out, one observes only muscle weakness because in the absence of the multiple triplet repeats, the other mRNAs are properly transported by the CUG-BP protein and function

TABLE 62-8 Systemic Involvement in Myotonic Dystrophy

Organ or System	Clinical	Diagnostic Signs
Muscle	Myotonia, weakness, dystrophy	*EMG:* decreased resting membrane potential, repetitive depolarization ("dive bomber" sound) *Pathology:* sarcoplasmic masses, ringed fibers, internal nuclei frequent; nuclei often in chains; large variation in fiber size
Cardiac	Bradycardia common, complete heart block frequent, prolonged PR interval, dilated cardiomyopathy	First-degree heart block, bradycardia on ECG; abnormal vectorcardiogram; SA node, right and left bundle branch dysfunction; increased His-Purkinje conduction (His bundle studies) with progressive conduction system abnormalities; dilated cardiomyopathy
Lens	Posterior subcapsular, iridescent, or scintillating cataracts	Dust-like cataracts may be visible only on slit lamp examination
Eye	Decreased vision (independent of cataracts and diabetic retinopathy); diplopia	Pigmentary disorders of macula keratosis sicca; decreased intraocular pressure; frequent ptosis and ultraocular muscle weakness
CNS	Mental retardation (especially congenital DM); hypersomnia	Possible neuronal heterotopias; suspicious, reticent personality characteristics
Gastrointestinal	Dysphagia, abdominal pain	Disordered esophageal and gastric peristalsis; dilation of bowel
Skeletal	Cranial and facial abnormalities, malocclusion of dentition	Cranial bony abnormalities, hyperostosis of skull (localized or diffuse), small sella turcica, large sinuses, micrognathia
Respiratory	Hypoventilation, postanesthesia respiratory failure	Diaphragmatic and intercostal muscle weakness
Smooth muscle	Dilation of hollow-viscus organs and ureters, abnormal bowel motility	Thinned or interrupted smooth muscle

normally.[194,195] This hypothesis is now actively pursued by many investigators. Preliminary findings show an accumulation of the CUG-BP in the nuclei of cells from DM.[196,197] Another possible mechanism is variations in gene levels in the immediate vicinity, such as the homeobox gene DMPHP.

Relative to therapy, conduction disturbances typically require permanent pacemaker implantation and dilated cardiomyopathy requires treatment for heart failure.

Fascioscapulohumeral Dystrophy

Fascioscapulohumeral,[198] or Landouzy-Dejerine, muscular dystrophy exists as two clinical types. One type has autosomal dominant inheritance with onset at the end of the first or the beginning of the second decade. The weakness of the facial, shoulder, and upper arm muscles is slowly progressive, but wide variability is seen. The second clinical type of fascioscapulohumeral dystrophy is the infantile form. Onset is within the first 2 years of life, and many patients are wheelchair-bound by 1 year of age. Clinical manifestations of muscular dystrophy generally are absent in the parents.

The cardiac involvement involves progressive atrial dysfunction resulting in permanent paralysis of the atria, beginning with sinus bradycardia, junctional escape rhythm, and AV block (Table 62-7). Criteria for diagnosis of permanent paralysis of the atria include absence of P waves on surface ECG, esophageal electrogram, and intracardiac electrocardiogram, unresponsiveness of the atrium to electrical stimulation, and immobility of the atria on fluoroscopy and echocardiography. Focal abnormalities of the atria precede these events. Nonparalytic regions of the atrium may demonstrate enhanced activity, apparent clinically as atrial tachycardia or flutter. Therapy depends on the clinical features. The chromosomal locus has been identified on chromosome 4q35,[199] but the responsible gene(s) are unknown.

Nemaline Myopathy

Nemaline myopathy is named for the small rod-like particles found in striated muscle. Inheritance is probably autosomal dominant, although autosomal recessive inheritance may occur.[200] Clinical features include hypotonia with truncal and extremity weakness from an early age and a narrow arched palate. Conduction abnormalities and cardiac dilatation have been described[200,201] but are unusual (Table 62-7). Nemaline rods are demonstrable in the myocardium and conduction tissues. The genetic cause of this disease was recently discovered by Nowak et al.,[202] who identified mutations in the human skeletal muscle α-actin gene (ACTA1), all missense mutations. Interestingly, the clinical phenotype varied significantly, from mild disease to severe, infantile-onset disease. In addition, a different clinical disorder, actin myopathy (i.e., congenital myopathy with excessive thin filaments), was also found to carry mutations in ACTA1.[202,203]

Two other forms of nemaline myopathy have also been identified. Mutations in TPM3, encoding α-tropomyosin slow, has been found mutated in both dominant and recessive nemaline myopathy.[204] In addition, mutations in NEB, encoding nebulin, has been seen in slowly progressive congenital nemaline myopathy.[205] Therefore, the underlying cause for this phenotype are mutations in skeletal muscle sarcomeric genes, similar to that seen in HCM and cardiac sarcomeric genes. Therapy is required when the conduction abnormalities or cardiac dilatation causes clinical symptoms.

Endocardial Fibroelastosis (EFE)

This disorder is characterized by endocardial thickening, which leads to decreased compliance and impaired diastolic function. Primary forms are typically unassociated with other cardiac anomalies. Most commonly, this disease presents in infancy and early childhood with signs and symptoms of congestive heart failure.[206] The diagnosis is usually made by biopsy. The incidence of primary EFE in the United States in the past was relatively high—approximately one case in 5000 live births.[207] During the past decade, however, this incidence has decreased markedly, for unknown reasons. Treatment of children with primary EFE with anticongestive and inotropic measures has been ineffective, and the clinical course usually results in either death or transplantation. Postmortem examination typically demonstrates enlargement of the left ventricle. Histopathology commonly reveals extensive deposition of extracellular matrix, primarily collagen and elastic fibers, in the endocardium. Three inherited forms of EFE have been described: autosomal recessive, autosomal dominant, and an X-linked recessive disorder. The majority of cases, however, occur sporadically. The X-linked form shows mitochondrial abnormalities similar to Barth syndrome[127,128] with the exception that EFE patients have endocardial scarring. It is likely, however, that this form is caused by mutations in the G4.5 gene found in Barth syndrome and LV noncompaction.[129] It was hypothesized in the 1950s and 1960s that EFE is secondary to intrauterine myocarditis in sporadic cases, particularly as a result of mumps or Coxsackievirus. Ni et al.[208] recently identified mumps viral genome in the majority of autopsy specimens retrieved from infants dying between the 1950s and 1980s. This disease essentially disappeared after the program of vaccination (mumps-measles-rubella or MMR) began in the United States.

DEFECTS OF METABOLISM CAUSING CARDIOMYOPATHY

Carnitine Deficiency

L-Carnitine is a small, water-soluble molecule containing seven carbon atoms and is important in the shuttling of long-chain fatty acids and activated acetate across the inner mitochondrial membrane. A specific translocase facilitates the exchange of long-chain acylcarnitine and acetylcarnitine. Carnitine also serves as the shuttle for the end products of peroxisomal fatty acid oxidation and for α-ketoacids derived from branched chain amino acids. These metabolites are transferred into the mitochondrial matrix for terminal oxidation.

Primary carnitine deficiency syndrome is characterized by a profound decrease in carnitine in affected tissues. The mechanism underlying the primary disorder is defective transport of carnitine from the serum into the affected cells.[209] End-stage disease of many different organs, including the heart, may induce depletion of carnitine stores and must be differentiated from the chronic inherited type. Based on carnitine levels, carnitine defiency is usually divided into two forms: a myopathic form and a systemic form. In the myopathic form, carnitine levels are decreased only in muscle tissue; in the systemic form, multiple tissues are affected, including muscle, liver, and plasma.[209] The systemic form presents in infancy or early childhood with episodes of hypoglycemia, ammonemia, acidemia, hepatomegaly, and EFE. A gene for primary systemic "carnitine" deficiency was recently mapped to chromosome 5q31.1-5q32,[210] the SCD locus. A murine model with juvenile visceral steatosis (*jvs*) has been identified[211] in which homozygotes have low serum total and free carnitine levels but no reduction in urinary excretion of carnitines.[212] This gene was mapped to the *jvs* locus on chromosome 11 of the mouse, which is syntenic to human 5q.[213] The human gene was recently found to be a novel sodium ion-dependent carnitine transporter, OCTN2.[214]

Therapy includes oral carnitine, occasionally reversing the cardiomyopathy. Additional therapy includes bicarbonate to reverse the acidemia, intravenous glucose, and anticongestive measures. Intercurrent illness commonly causes acute decompensation and death.

Medium Chain Acyl-CoA Dehydrogenase (MCAD) Deficiency

This disorder appears to be the most common inborn error of fatty acid oxidation, estimated to occur in one per 6000 to 10,000 live Caucasian births. It is characterized by recurrent episodes of illness, provoked by fasting more than 12 h, with the first episode generally occurring between 6 and 24 months of life. The most common symptoms include vomiting and severe lethargy that can progress to coma, as well as the less striking symptoms of muscle weakness and exercise intolerance. Hypoglycemia is often present between episodes, when patients appear normal. Hepatomegaly and DCM (rarely) are also seen. Liver biopsy can show marked fatty infiltrate ranging from predominantly microvesicular to a macrovesicular pattern. This autosomal recessive disorder was localized to chromosome 1p31 and human and rat MCAD cDNAs were cloned and sequenced.[215] The coding region is 1263 bp and encodes a precursor protein containing 421 amino acids. A variety of mutations have been reported. An A-to-G nucleotide replacement at position 985 of MCAD cDNA appears to be the most prevalent mutation responsible for MCAD deficiency (greater than 90 percent).[216] This deletion is predicted to result in a truncated protein of 385 amino acids instead of the normal 421–amino acid product. The common A-to-G 985 mutation appears to be due to a founder effect. Poor genotype-phenotype correlation exists.[217]

The therapy for these patients includes treatment of the acidosis and, when present, treatment of heart failure. Glucose therapy is indicated for hypoglycemia while intravenous fluids are needed during episodes of vomiting.

Long-Chain Acyl-CoA Dehydrogenase (LCAD) Deficiency/Very Long Chain Acyl-CoA Dehydrogenase (VLCAD) Deficiency

First described in 1985, LCAD manifests itself as recurrent episodes of coma, vomiting, and hypoglycemia triggered by fasting. Some patients have much more severe illness with notable involvement of cardiac and skeletal muscle.[28] Both DCM and HCM have been seen. Like MCAD, LCAD patients have secondary carnitine deficiency, and their fasting urine organic acid profile is abnormal, with low ketones and increased levels of dicarboxylic acids. The LCAD gene was identified[218] in 1991. In addition to the well-known β-oxidation enzymes in the mitochondrial matrix, there are two additional membrane-bound enzymes of β-oxidation.[219,220] One of these has been called "very long chain acyl-CoA dehydrogenase" (VLCAD), while the other is known as the "trifunctional protein." VLCAD is a membrane-bound homodimer with monomers of larger size than the other enzymes of the complex. It catalyzes the initial rate limiting step in mitochondrial fatty acid β-oxidation. The human VLCAD cDNA[221,222] and genomic sequence[210] were identified over the past several years, with multiple mutations subsequently identified.[224] Andresen et al.[225] recently showed that clear correlation of genotype with disease phenotype exists. Patients with severe childhood phenotype, which has a high incidence of cardiomyopathy and mortality, have mutations that result in no residual enzyme activity. Those with milder childhood and adult phenotypes have mutations that may result in residual enzyme activity. This clear genotype-phenotype correlation sharply contrasts that seen in MCAD deficiency, in which no correlation has been established. This new understanding of the mitochondrial β-oxidation pathway has led to new insights of the disorder once thought to be due to LCAD deficiency but now thought to be VLCAD deficiency.

Therapy for these patients includes aggressive treatment with glucose and hemodynamic support. When cardiac disease persists, chronic therapy for the dilated or hypertrophic heart disease should be instituted.

Fabry's Disease

An X-linked recessive disorder with complete penetrance and variable clinical expressivity, this entity is due to a deficiency of the enzyme α-galactosidase A, a lysosomal enzyme that participates in the catabolism of neutral glycosphingolipids, and is found in one in 40,000 live births. The disease frequently has its onset in adolescence and typically manifests with sensations of burning pain in the hands and feet. These sensations tend to be associated with fever, heat, cold, and exercise. Multiple angiokeratomas are noticeable with increasing age, with the umbilical area and genitalia the sites most commonly affected. Progressive renal failure develops with age, and CNS manifestations commonly include seizures, headaches, hemiplegia, and stroke. Corneal opacities are also frequently seen.

The cardiac manifestations of Fabry's disease generally appear in young adulthood. Aortic root dilation, dilated or hypertrophic cardiomyopathy,[226] valve dysfunction (especially mitral valve),[227] and myocardial infarction occur in these patients. Recently, association with tetralogy of Fallot was reported,[228] as was restrictive cardiomyopathy.[229] Electrocardiographic abnormalities commonly include atrial fibrillation, intraventricular conduction delay, right bundle-branch block, ST-T wave changes, short PR interval, and left ventricular hypertrophy. The short PR interval can progressively shorten over time probably secondary to lipid deposition in the atrioventricular node. Chamber thickness and mitral valve prolapse are evident on echocardiographic examination. Light microscopy shows lipid accumulation in nearly all cardiac tissue. Concentric lamellae are seen within cells and contain the neutral glycophospholipid. Therapy for these cardiac abnormalities does not differ from that typically used for HCM, myocardial ischemia or infarction, or mitral insufficiency found in patients without Fabry's disease. Recently, cardiac transplantation has been reported.[230]

The disease-causing gene, lysosomal-galactosidase A (GLA), is localized to Xq12.1-Xq12.2. The full-length cDNA has 1393 bp with a 60-nucleotide 5′ untranslated region, encoding for a precursor peptide of 429 amino acids.[231] The gene was found to contain seven exons. Mutations have been described[232,233] and genotype-phenotypic correlation performed. Mouse models have been developed which closely mimic the human disorder.[234] Antenatal and postnatal diagnosis is available. Therapy is symptomatic at present, but enzyme replacement therapy is likely in the future. Recently, gene transfer studies have been reported that correct the enzymatic and lysosomal storage defects in Fabry-like mice.[235]

Homocystinuria

Homocystinuria, inherited as an autosomal recessive defect, occurs with a frequency of 1 in 75,000. There is a deficiency of cystathionine β-synthase (CBS), which leads to elevated methionine in the blood and homocystine and methionine in the urine[236] (see Chaps. 39 and 41). In the homozygous individuals, major clinical features include a marfanoid habitus with a thin, tall body build and arachnodactyly, pectus excavatum, kyphoscoliosis, and osteoporosis. Subluxation of the lens, usually in a downward position, is frequently seen by 10 years of age, and myopia is common. Approximately 60 percent of affected individuals are mentally retarded to some degree. Schizophrenic behavior has also been noted in some patients. Cardiovascular abnormalities consist primarily of arterial and venous thrombosis (Table 62-5), with medial degeneration of the aorta and large arteries and intimal hyperplasia and fibrosis. It is estimated that about one-third of patients with familial homocystinuria will experience arterial or venous thrombosis. It is interesting that even within the same family with the same mutation there is marked variability among affected siblings.[237] The thrombotic episodes usually occur before the age of 30 years and include deep vein thrombosis, pulmonary embolism, and arterial thrombosis in the cerebral, peripheral, and coronary arteries.[237] However, when this disease occurs in individuals with other thrombogenic risk factors such as factor V Leiden,[238] the incidence of thrombosis, both arterial and venous, is significantly increased. An increased risk of cardiovascular disease has also been observed in carriers of the gene for homocystinuria. The gene was initially assigned to the subtelomeric region of band 21q22.3 by in situ hybridization studies.[239] Three types of cDNAs differing in both their translated and untranslated regions were isolated, with the resultant differences due to alternative splicing. The human gene was cloned and complete-sequence, alternatively spliced forms, and mutations described.[240] Numerous mutations have now been identified and correlated with the phenotype. The gene is 28 kb in size, contains 23 exons, and contains many *alu* repeat sequences which predisposes the gene to rearrangements.[241] The defect can be treated in some cases by pyridoxine supplementation. The percentage of pyridoxine responders ranges between 13 and 47 percent. Betaine, low-methionine diet, and aspirin treatments have also been tried with varying success. Prenatal diagnosis is available by an enzyme assay and gene analysis. Recently, tandem spectrometry has been used in the diagnosis.[241]

Homocystinuria, while a rare disease, has received increased attention recently because of several studies indicating that homocysteine is an important and independent risk factor for atherosclerosis and thrombosis.[242,243] In one such study performed recently, of 269 patients with the first episode of deep vein thrombosis, 10 percent had elevated plasma homocysteine levels, compared with 4 percent in 269 matched controls.[243] Homocystinuria results from impaired enzyme activity in the metabolism of cobalamin, but may also occur from a deficiency of vitamin B_6, folate, or vitamin B_{12}. The mechanism whereby homocysteine induces atherosclerosis is postulated to be through induction of the cyclin A gene which induces vascular smooth muscle proliferation, a major component of atherosclerosis.[244] The mechanism whereby homocysteine induces thrombosis is probably through its known effect on activation of factor V in endothelial cells, inhibition of protein C, and decreased antithrombin III activity. It remains somewhat controversial as to how common hyperhomocysteinemia is as a risk factor for atherosclerosis and/or thrombosis. It is, however, very important to exclude hyperhomocysteinemia in patients with vascular disease such as myocardial infarction, strokes, or systemic thrombosis, particularly if these are occurring prematurely or there are no other risk factors, since, in the acquired form, the condition is relatively easy to treat by the administration of vitamins.

Mitochondrial Cardiomyopathies

The human mitochondrial genome[245] is a small, circular DNA molecule (Fig. 62-11) that is maternally inherited. Mitochondrial DNA (mtDNA) encodes 13 of the 69 proteins required for oxidative metabolism, 22 transfer RNAs (tRNAs), and 2 ribosomal RNAs (rRNAs) required for their translation. Since mtDNA has much less redundancy than the nuclear genome (in which essentially identical information is received from both parents), and tRNAs and rRNAs are present in multiple copies, the mitochondrial genome is an excellent target for mutations giving rise to human disease.[246,247] Mitochondria are dependent on nucleocytoplasmic mechanisms for most structural components, but do contribute vital peptides that are central to cellular respiration. The electron transport chain, which generates cellular ATP, is organized into complexes I to IV and the ATP synthase (complex V) (Fig. 62-12). The 13 mtDNA genes that encode enzymes in the respiratory chain include 7 complex I[246,248] subunits (ND1, 2, 3, 4L, 4, 5, and 6); 1 complex III subunit (cytochrome b); 3 complex IV subunits (COI, II, III); and 2 complex V subunits (ATPase 6 and 8). Each cell contains numerous mitochondria and each mitochondrion contains multiple copies of mtDNA. In most mitochondrial

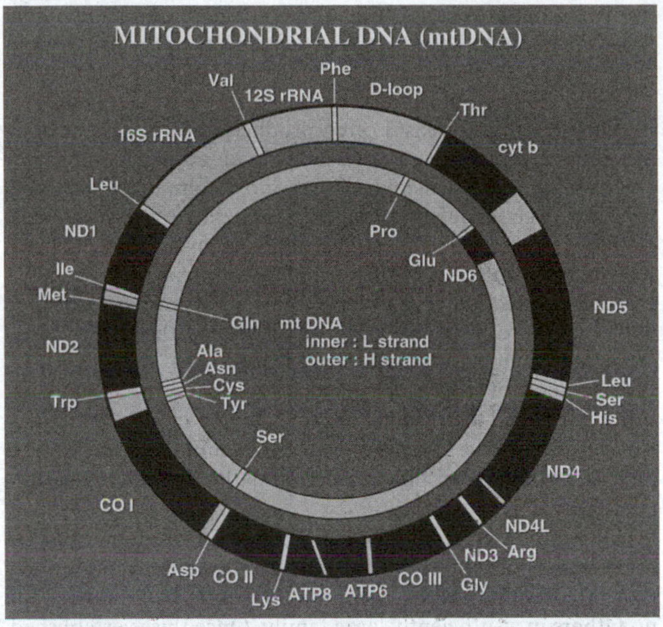

FIGURE 62-11 Mitochondrial genome. This small, circular DNA molecule encodes 13 enzymes of the respiratory chain, 22 tRNAs, and 2 rRNAs. When it is mutated, cardiac, neurologic, and myopathic disorders develop.

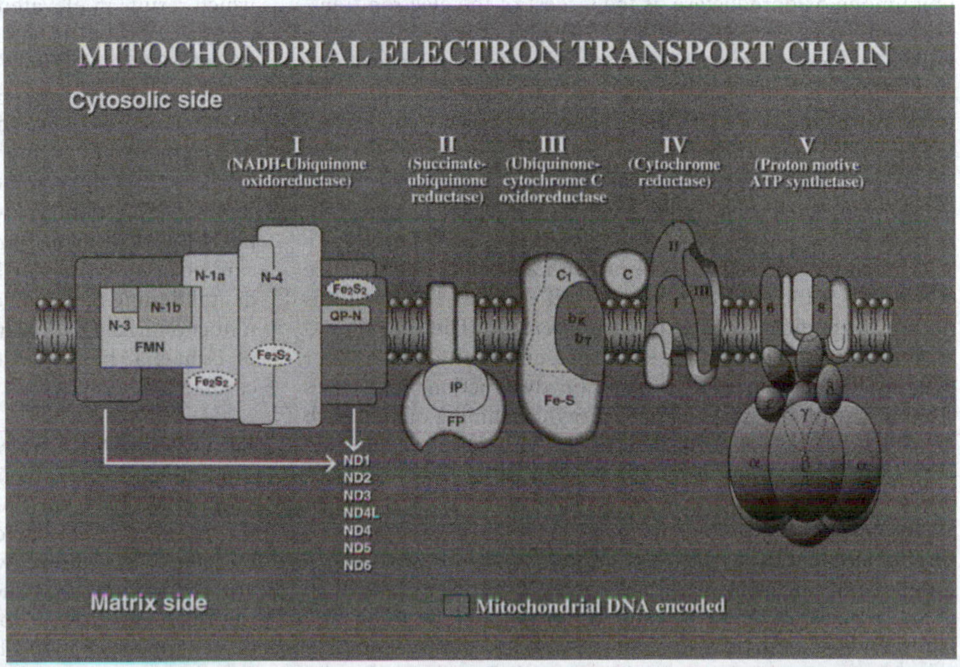

FIGURE 62-12 The electron transport chain enzyme complex (complexes I to V).

disorders, patients carry a mix of mutant and normal mitochondria—a condition known as *heteroplasmy,* with the proportions varying from tissue to tissue and individual to individual within a pedigree, in a manner correlating with severity of phenotype.

Mitochondrial diseases often produce disturbances of brain and muscle function and are usually evident during infancy or early childhood. Cardiac disease is most commonly seen with respiratory chain defects. Ragged-red fibers are present in muscle biopsy specimens almost invariably when the molecular defect involves mtDNA.[249] These defects represent the genetics of ATP production. The diverse clinical syndromes associated with various respiratory chain complexes are thought to result from involvement of tissue-specific isoforms in some cases, involvement of tissue-nonspecific (generalized) subunits in other cases, and the residual enzyme activity in affected tissues. The cardiac diseases seen associated with mitochondrial defects include both hypertrophic cardiomyopathy and dilated cardiomyopathy.[246]

Mitochondrial gene mapping, in contrast to the nuclear genome, does not require genetic linkage. One simply has to show that the disease exhibits transmission through all mothers and no fathers in a sufficiently large family. Once this is established, the mitochondrial genome can be sequenced to identify the mutation, which must be shown to segregate with the disease since there are many harmless polymorphisms.

Therapy for these disorders is generally symptom-based. Conduction disturbance generally requires placement of a permanent pacemaker, and heart failure is treated with the usual therapy. In some patients, beta-blockers may be useful. Hypertrophic heart disease is usually treated in a fashion similar to that of other forms of HCM. Mitochondrial-based therapy may include coenzyme Q10, carnitine, or vitamins, but these therapeutic approaches typically do not alter the clinical course.

COMPLEX I DEFICIENCY

Complex I, or nicotinamide adenine dinucleotide (NADH): ubiquinone oxidoreductase, is the largest of the electron transport chain complexes[250,251] (Fig. 62-12) with at least 35 complex I nuclear gene products and 7 mitochondrially encoded proteins. It is embedded in the inner mitochondrial membrane and serves to dehydrogenate NADH and shuttle electrons to coenzyme Q. This electron transport generates a protein gradient across the inner mitochondrial membrane, helping to synthesize ATP. When complex I abnormalities occur, significant health problems arise.

Mitochondriocytopathies occur with an estimated incidence of 1 per 10,000 live births, and isolated complex I deficiency is one of those most frequently encountered.[248] The first clinical symptoms of complex I deficiency, presenting either at birth or in early childhood, result from brain dysfunction, sometimes combined with defects in other energy-consuming organs, such as skeletal muscle and the heart. For this reason, complex I deficiencies are grouped among the mitochondrial encephalomyopathies.

Robinson[248] categorized complex I–deficient patients into three major clinical groups. The most common presentation is Leigh syndrome, with cardiomyopathy occuring in about 40 percent of cases.[252] A second category often seen is fatal neonatal lactic acidosis (MELAS—see below). A third but uncommon group present with hepatopathy and tubulopathy with mild symptoms, such as exercise intolerance, or with cataracts and cardiomyopathy. The most frequently observed pathologic mtDNA mutations are found in genes for mitochondrial tRNAs for leucine (T3271C, A3243G) and lysine (A8344G, T8356C) and in the protein-encoding subunits ND1 (T4160A, G3460A), ND4 (G11778A), and ND6 (T14484C, G14459A).

Treatment of these disorders is limited. Riboflavin, succinate supplements (since the metabolite enters the respiratory chain at complex II), ubiquonone, and idebanone have been recommended for therapy in patients with MELAS. Carnitine and coenzyme Q10 have also been used.

COMPLEX III DEFECTS

This results in a myopathic or multisystem disorder. Cardiomyopathy has been found both alone or in conjunction with skeletal myopathy. Encephalomyopathy also presents with retinopathy, ataxia, spasticity, dementia, weakness, sensorineural hearing loss, and exercise intolerance.

COMPLEX IV DEFECTS

This abnormality is similar clinically to complex I defects. The mitochondrial genome encodes for three subunits of cytochrome C oxidase, which represents the terminal portion of the respiratory chain (Fig. 62-12) and catalyzes conversion of molecular oxygen to water. A benign reversible infantile myopathy which normalizes by early childhood may occur, as may a fatal infantile myopathy manifested by profound weakness, hypotonia, respiratory insufficiency, and death. This myopathy may occur alone, or in association with severe renal tubular dysfunction or cardiomyopathy with red ragged fibers.

HYPOXEMIA, mtDNA DAMAGE, AND CARDIAC DISEASE

Since cardiac tissue relies on mitochondrial oxidative phosphorylation (ox-phos) for energy production, deficiency of portions of this system or its end-product may cause cardiac abnormalities.[248] Hypoxemia can increase oxygen radical production, which results in elevated mtDNA damage and altered ox-phos gene expression. In addition, these enzymes decline with age while mtDNA deletions increase with age, especially deletion at nucleotide 4977 bp. Ischemic hearts may be more likely to have increased chances of mtDNA deletion due to the effect of hypoxemia[253] and, using PCR amplification across the deletion breakpoint of the common mtDNA4977 deletion, it was found that mtDNA damage was increased in chronically ischemic hearts, as well as in some hearts with other forms of chronic cardiac disease (i.e., DCM, HCM), but this is probably an incidental finding and has no effect on cardiac function. Similarly, mitochondrial DNA damage increases with age independent of ischemia, but it is doubtful whether it in any way alters cardiac function.

KEARNS-SAYRE SYNDROME (KSS)

This mitochondrial myopathy is characterized by ptosis, chronic progressive external ophthalmoplegia, abnormal retinal pigmentation, and cardiac conduction defects as well as DCM.[255] Hearing loss and limb weakness are frequently associated, as are endocrinopathies such as diabetes mellitus, hypoparathyroidism, and growth hormone deficiency. Approximately 20 percent of KSS patients have cardiac involvement and of these, the majority usually have conduction defects causing progressive heart block (Table 62-7). These patients generally have large heterogeneous deletions in the mitochondrial genome, of which tRNA$^{leu(UUR)}$-3243 is most common.

Clinically, conduction abnormalities, bifascicular block, or progressive high-grade block may define the requirement for permanent pacemaker implantation. Symptomatic improvement using mitochondrial therapies may occasionally be seen with coenzyme Q10 therapy. The major function of coenzyme Q10 in mitochondria is to shuttle electrons from complexes I and II to complex III, while stabilizing the respiratory chain complexes. Vitamins such as phylloquinone (vitamin K_1), menadione (vitamin K_3), and ascorbic acid (vitamin C) have been used to donate electrons directly to cytochrome *c*. In addition, the endocrine abnormalities and heart failure should be treated in the usual way.

MERRF SYNDROME

This syndrome is characterized by *m*yoclonic *e*pilepsy with *r*agged-*r*ed muscle *f*ibers (MERRF) and is caused by a single nucleotide substitution in tRNA^{Lys}, which apparently interferes with mitochondrial translation.[256] The defining clinical features are myoclonus, generalized seizures, ataxia, and hypertrophic cardiomyopathy. Skeletal muscle biopsy demonstrates ragged-red fibers on microscopy. Symptoms usually begin in childhood, but adult onset has been described. Other common manifestations include impaired hearing, demential neuropathy, short stature, optic atrophy, lactic acidosis, and lipomas.

Shoffner et al.[256] showed an A-to-G transition mutation (position 8344) as the cause of the disease and associated with defects in complexes I and IV. This abnormality causes decline in ATP-generating capacity, with a resultant cardiomyopathy. Other reports have outlined various disease-causing mutations. Therapy is similar to other mitochondrial myopathies; anticonvulsant medications may also be indicated.

MELAS SYNDROME

*M*itochondrial *e*ncephalomypathy and *l*actic *a*cidosis with *s*troke-like episodes (MELAS) is clinically characterized by stroke before age 40 years; encephalopathy with seizures, dementia, or both; and lactic acidosis, ragged-red fibers, or both.[257] Recurrent headaches and recurrent vomiting are common. Other frequent manifestations include exercise intolerance, limb weakness, short stature, and elevated CSF protein. Hypertrophic cardiomyopathy or dilated cardiomyopathy may occur.

Variable respiratory chain defects have been described, but complex I abnormalities are most common. Between 80 and 90 percent of patients have an adenine-to-guanine point mutation in tRNA$^{Leu(UUR)}$ at position 3243. Therapy is similar to that described for MERRF.

THERAPY

Medical therapy for mitochondrial disorders has been disappointing and for that reason newer approaches have been sought. As most pathologic mtDNA mutations are heteroplasmic and there is a threshold whereby a certain level of mutated mtDNA is necessary before a disease becomes biochemically or clinically apparent, any approach that increases the proportion of wild-type to mutated mtDNA will reverse the phenotype and thus be a potentially useful treatment. When there is an extremely high level of the pathogenetic mutation in cells, as occurs with muscle necrosis, these necrotic cells form regenerated muscle. Clark et al.[258] took advantage of this phenomenon by inducing necrosis and regeneration in muscle by performing a muscle biopsy, which resulted in the absence of mutated mtDNA in the biopsied muscle. Due to the invasiveness of this approach, reduced utility of the therapy is anticipated unless other methods of inducing necrosis can be developed.

More recently, Taivassalo et al.[259] developed a novel therapy that they called *gene shifting,* which is similar to that described by Clark et al.[258] These authors enhanced the incorporation of new (satellite) cells through regeneration following injury or muscle hypertrophy induced by eccentric or concentric resistance exercise training. They were able to show a remarkable increase in the ratio of wild-type to mutant mtDNAs, and in the proportion of muscle fibers with normal respiratory chain activity. This work suggests that it might be possible to reverse the molecular events that led to the expression of metabolic myopathy and demonstrates that this form of "gene shifting" therapy could be effective.

Connective Tissue Disorders

The composition, structure, and function of normal and abnormal connective tissues are gradually being elucidated[260,261] (see Chap. 85). The annuli fibrosis that separate the atria and ventricles and support the two atrioventricular valves are largely type I collagen fiber bundles, while the blood vessel walls are elastin and collagen types I and III (50 percent), with lesser contributions from types IV, V, and VI collagen. Elastin in located at 7q11; collagen 1A1, at 17q21.13-17q22.05; collagen 1A2, at 7q21.3-7q22.1; collagen 2A1, at 12q13.1-12q13.3; collagen 3A1, at 2q31; and collagen 5A2, at 2q31.

MARFAN SYNDROME

Marfan syndrome is a heritable disorder of connective tissue caused by a defect in fibrillin protein encoded by the fibrillin-1 gene on chromosome 15 at 15q15-q20 (see Chap. 98). The Marfan syndrome occurs in approximately 1 in 10,000 individuals and is equally common in males and females. There is marked variation in clinical expression, and the diagnosis can be made at any age from the newborn period through adulthood.[263] Because of the variability in expression, overlap with nonpathologic features (such as tall stature) can be observed in the general population. Since fibrillin[264] is diffuse, Marfan syndrome affects skeletal, ocular, cardiovascular, skin, pulmonary, and central nervous system.[260,261] The skeletal manifestations of Marfan syndrome include tall stature, thin body build, long arms and legs (dolichostenomelia), long fingers and toes (arachnodactyly), hyperextensibility, pectus deformity, scoliosis, joint contractures, and narrow, high-arched palate. Cardiovascular abnormalities, particularly affecting the mitral apparatus and aorta, are also common. There may also be overlap with other disorders that share some of the same phenotypic features, such as the condition termed *congenital contractual arachnodactyly* (CCA).[265] Clinical manifestations of CCA include dolichostenomelia and arachnodactyly, contractures of large joints, and abnormal pinnae formation. In 1990, Marfan syndrome was mapped to the long arm of chromosome 15(15q15q-q20).[266] Subsequently, a defect in the gene for fibrillin-1 (FBN1)[267] was found to be the cause of Marfan syndrome. This large glycoprotein has a molecular weight of 350 kDa[264] and is a component of microfibrils that are ubiquitous in the connective frequently occurs or increases during adolescence. The mRNA transcript of this gene is approximately 10 kb. Not only do defects in this gene cause Marfan syndrome, but Milewicz and Duvic[268] also showed that severe neonatal Marfan syndrome is due to a specific 3-bp insertion in the fibrillin-1 cDNA. Furthermore, fibrillin defects have been found in patients with atypical phenotypes including autosomal dominant ectopia lentis with skeletal features[269] and milder forms such as the MASS phenotype (mitral valve, aorta, skeleton, and skin)[269] or isolated ascending aortic aneurysm with dissection.[270,271] Unfortunately, each family appears to have an individual mutation in the gene, making screening difficult and requiring that each new mutation case be studied individually.[272] This high impact disorder is estimated to be responsible for 1 to 2 percent of the deaths in industrialized societies, with death usually caused by rupture of an asymptomatic, undiagnosed aneurysm. Mutations in FBN1 also have been associated with the marfanoid craniosynostosis (Shprintzen-Goldberg) syndrome.[273] Recent data suggest that CCA is a separate disorder due to a fibrillin-2 gene (FBN2) defect on chromosome 5 (5q23-q31).[274]

Another locus for Marfan syndrome has also been mapped to 3p24.2-p25.[275] Marfan syndrome has been observed in all racial and ethnic groups, and approximately 55 percent are sporadic cases with no family history. There appears to be an increased effect of paternal age, with the mean age of fathers of sporadic cases being increased.

Some of the skeletal features can be analyzed anthropometrically. For example, the increased limb length can be measured by the length of the upper and lower segments and by the upper-lower segment ratio (US/UL). The lower segment is measured from the top of the pubic ramus to the floor, and the upper segment is measured from the pubic ramus to the top of the head. US/UL is reduced for classic Marfan syndrome at all ages. The ratio of arm span to height is usually increased in Marfan syndrome, although scoliosis may complicate the calculation of both ratios. Arachnodactyly can be assessed by the ratio of the middle finger length to total hand length or by analysis of the metacarpal index on hand radiographs.

Hyperextensibility can be assessed by several simple maneuvers. The Steinberg (thumb) sign is positive when the thumb projects through the clenched hand on the ulnar side. The Walker-Murdock (wrist) sign is positive when the first and fifth digit of one hand wrap completely around the wrist of the other hand. Pectus excavatum of variable severity is fairly common. Scoliosis can occur at any age. The ocular findings of Marfan syndrome classically include subluxation of the lenses (ectopia lentis), usually but not always in an upward direction. This occurs in 50 to 60 percent of patients. Myopia is very common, and retinal detachments have also occurred, especially after surgical removal of the lenses. Corneal flattening is also described. Loss of vision occurs in a significant number of patients. Other manifestations include an increase in the occurrence of inguinal hernias, which may recur, and the development of spontaneous pneumothorax and lung abnormalities in some patients. Sacral meningoceles and dilated cisterna magna have also been reported. A severe neonatal form of the Marfan syndrome has cardiovascular, skeletal, and ocular complications present at birth,[261] and patients typically succumb within the first year of life, often from congestive heart failure.

The majority of cardiac abnormalities associated with Marfan syndrome affect the ascending aorta, the aortic valve, and the mitral valve (Table 62-6). Physical examination alone is insufficient to detect subtle changes in the heart and in the aorta. The dilation of the ascending aorta may occur gradually before physical findings occur. Echocardiograms are recommended annually and beta-blocker therapy should be considered.[276] If the diameter of the aorta corrected for body surface area exceeds the upper limits of normal by 50 percent, the frequency of evaluations should be increased to at least every 6 months. Prophylactic repair with composite graft including aortic valve should be performed when ascending aortic dilation reaches a diameter of 6 cm[277] (see Chap. 98). Repair of a severe pectus excavatum may be indicated at an earlier stage, not only for cosmetic reasons, but to allow easier and safer aortic surgery, should it be indicated. After surgery, the use of beta blockers and anticoagulants should be maintained, and individuals should avoid contact sports and marked physical exertion. Surveillance of the aorta should continue after surgery. Some evidence suggests that beta blockers may reduce the rate of aortic dilation and the risk of serious complications.[276] Prophylactic antibiotics should be used on all patients to decrease the risk of bacterial endocarditis. In general, contact sports (e.g., football, basketball) should be avoided—along with isometric exercises, weight lifting, and extreme physical activity—and replaced with noncompetitive sports such as swimming and bicycling. Other abnormalities include mitral valve prolapse, mitral regurgitation, and aortic regurgitation. The cardiovascular abnormalities in neonatal Marfan syndrome differs somewhat from that seen in older patients, demonstrating significant mitral regurgitation as well as tricuspid and pulmonary valve regurgitation. In addition, these children have significant heart failure, as previously noted.

A special issue involves Marfan syndrome and pregnancy (see Chap. 92). In addition to the 50 percent recurrence risk in offspring, there is also a concern about the stress that pregnancy will put on the aorta. There are at least two dozen case reports of aortic dissection during pregnancy or shortly after delivery,[278] generally occurring with aortic regurgitation or other evidence of aortic dilatation. Pregnant women with Marfan syndrome should have echocardiograms every 6 to 8 weeks during pregnancy and should be followed as high-risk obstetrical patients.

The diagnosis of Marfan syndrome is currently made primarily on clinical grounds although molecular diagnosis is now feasible (although not useful).[279] Suspected patients with a positive family history should have positive clinical features in at least two organ systems. If the family history is negative for Marfan syndrome, positive findings should be present in the skeletal system and in at least two other organ systems. Suspected patients should also have a negative urine nitroprusside test to rule out homocystinuria, one of the disorders in the differential diagnosis. Management of patients with a negative family history and only suggestive skeletal features is unclear. In view of its implications, it may be unwise to inform such patients with minimal features that they have Marfan syndrome. Nonetheless, they should be followed clinically with perhaps periodic echocardiograms and ophthalmologic exams. In these individuals, strong consideration for molecular genetic evaluation is wise.

In terms of genetic counseling, families should be informed of the autosomal dominant inheritance pattern, with 50 percent recurrence in offspring. The rationale for patient follow-up and management should also be explained, along with psychosocial support and medical follow-up. Prenatal diagnosis may be possible.[263,268]

EHLERS-DANLOS SYNDROMES

There are at least 11 different forms of Ehlers-Danlos syndrome (EDS), which are generally given numerical designations.[279] The most common forms are types I through IV, as discussed here. Types II and III overlap with the features of type I, but both are progressively less severe; type III is sometimes known as *benign hypermobility syndrome*. The features of Ehlers-Danlos type I include hyperextensible and fragile skin with poor wound healing and "cigarette paper" scarring. Hyperextensibility of the joints increases susceptibility to dislocation of the hips, shoulders, elbows, knees, and clavicles. The ears tend to be hypermobile and are sometimes described as "lop ears." Scoliosis is a relatively common finding, as are clubfeet in infancy. There is an increased risk of premature birth resulting from premature rupture of membranes. Umbilical and diaphragmatic hemias tend to be relatively common.

The most common cardiac features include mitral valve prolapse, tricuspid valve prolapse, and dilation of the aortic root and/or sinus of Valsalva.[279] Atrial septal defects and other abnormalities of the aortic arch and mitral valve have also been seen. Probably the most significant cardiovascular defect is the increased susceptibility to dissecting aortic aneurysm (Table 62-6), which can lead to death. Poor wound healing and decreased vascular integrity have been noted. Surgical procedures are freqeuntly not tolerated well, and patients should probably avoid unnecessary surgery. In addition, patients should be cautioned to avoid tauma as much as possible. Type I Ehlers-Danlos is inherited as an autosomal dominant disorder with variability in expression. The presumed defect in this disorder involves synthesis of normal collagen with mutations identified in the $\alpha 2$ (V) chain of type V collagen.[279,280]

Ehlers-Danlos type IV is sometimes referred to as the "malignant" form of Ehlers-Danlos syndrome,[281] since there is marked susceptibility to spontaneous rupture of large blood vessels or bowel. The hyperelasticity and hyperextensibility tend to be less obvious than in type I. Easy bruisability and susceptibility to bleeding, however, are very prominent. Spontaneous rupture of any of the major vessels has been reported. Pregnancy-related complications are particularly striking, the overall risk of death with pregnancy being 25 percent. The basic defect in this autosomal dominant disorder is in the type III collagen gene located on chromosome 2 (2q31),[282] and defects have been reported.[283] Other Ehlers-Danlos genes thus far identified include types VI (1p36.3-1p36.2; lysyl hydroxylase),[284,285] VII A1 (17q21.31-q22), and VII A2 (7q22.1),[286] with mutations of the COLIA2 gene,[281] and the progeroid variant,[287] which is caused by galactosyl-transferase mutations.

Patients with types I and IV EDS require yearly cardiac examinations. Initial evaluation with chest radiography and echocardiography will enable the cardiologist to decide the frequency of follow-up and repeat echocardiograms depending on the level of aortic dilatation and mitral valve prolapse (MVP). Annual chest x-rays are cost-effective as a minimal approach, with echocardiograms necessary every 1 to 2 years. Antibiotic prophylaxis for subacute bacterial endocarditis (SBE) is also needed in patients with MVP or aortic abnormalities.

FAMILIAL ANEURYSMS

It has been recognized for some time that certain aneurysms in peripheral and central arteries (see Marfan's syndrome above) have a familial tendency.[288] As data accumulates on genetic defects in fibrillin[261,279] (Marfan's syndrome) and in the collagen disorders,[289,290] there appears to be overlap in the genetic defects of fibrilin and procollagen, particularly type III, as causes for aneurysms. Some have a defect in type II procollagen (COL3A1) similar to defects that have been reported in Ehlers-Danlos syndrome (EDS) type IV.[283] Familial incidence of aneurysms is said to account for 7 percent of aneurysms.[291] Since EDS is relatively rare, many of the more common familial procollagen abnormalities may represent phenotypic overlap. These findings have resulted in a reassessment of the traditional teaching that most aortic aneurysms result from atherosclerosis. Family history should be carefully assessed in all patients with aortic or cerebral aneurysms, and, if it is positive, other family members should be assessed. Many should be followed with noninvasive evaluation in a fashion similar to that described for Marfan's syndrome.

PSEUDOXANTHOMA ELASTICUM (PXE)

This is a genetic disease of the elastic tissue which involves the skin, eyes, and cardiovascular system.[292] The characteristic lesion is that of the skin consisting of a highly raised, yellowish papule known as a *pseudoxanthoma,* overlying areas of flexural stress such as the neck, cubital and popliteal fossae, and groin. The eye changes are slate-gray linear bands representing tears in Bruch's membrane and subsequent fibrosis leading to loss of central vision in 70 to 80 percent of cases. Calcification of peripheral arteries occurs frequently, most commonly in the femoral artery, but also in the coronary arteries. The heart is affected by myocardial ischemia and infarction, secondary to the coronary disease, which is the major cause of morbidity and mortality (Table 62-5). A restrictive cardiomyopathy is common due to endocardial fibrosis with mitral valve prolapse (MVP).[293,294] Two genetic variants having autosomal dominant inheritance and two others with autosomal recessive inheritance occur. The only difference between the recessive and dominant forms is the presence of affected parents and offspring. Bale recently mapped a gene to 16p13.1, but the gene remains unknown.[281] Because the basic defect is unknown, no specific treatment is available.

The cardiac features should be followed closely once abnormalities are noted. In stable patients, yearly examinations are required at a minimum. Myocardial dysfunction with or without heart failure requires anticongestive and inotropic support, while SBE prophylaxis is needed for those patients with MVP. Symptoms should be used to direct therapy.

CUTIS LAXA

This designation refers not only to a specific dermatologic sign but also to a variety of mendelian and nonmendelian congenital and acquired syndromes sharing the characteristic feature of lax, nonresilient skin. Two varieties of autosomal recessive cutis laxa exist. Death from pulmonary complications may occur in the first months of life and most patients die by the third year. Signs of right-sided heart failure are often seen in infancy and are generally due to pulmonary disease, although pulmonary artery stenosis also occurs[295] (Table 62-5). Histopathologically, the pulmonary artery lesions are due to medioelastic fiber paucity. MVP has also been notable. A gene that causes this spectrum of disease has been identified as elastin (ELN), the same gene previously shown to cause supravalvular aortic stenosis (SVAS).[296–298] As increased fibroblast activity in acquired cutis laxa has also been noted,[299] there is molecular and biochemical correlation. In addition, ultrastructural alterations of skin elastic fibers has been reported.[300]

Primary Disorders of Rhythm and Conduction

Virtually all rhythm and conduction abnormalities have been reported to be familial. However, many families have been small so that the mode of inheritance (or even whether the inheritance is mendelian) is uncertain. In many cases, these conduction defects have been associated with other cardiac and systemic disorders. For a detailed clinical discussion of arrhythmia and conduction disorders, see Chap. 27.

ROMANO-WARD LONG-QT SYNDROME (LQTS)

The association of stress-induced syncope, sudden death, and ventricular arrhythmias in families has long been noted, including a distinct syndrome[301] having prolongation of the QT interval and abnormal T waves on ECG. Multiple families with this syndrome have demonstrated autosomal dominant inheritance, with torsade de pointes polymorphic ventricular tachycardia, bradycardia and T-wave alternans (see Chap. 36). The diagnosis is made when the QT interval corrected for heart rate (QTc) is greater than 480 ms using Bazzett's formula; T-wave abnormalities are usually seen. In symptomatic patients (i.e., patients with syncope or "seizures"), the diagnosis may be made with shorter QTc (i.e., 470 ms). A diagnostic algorithm has been useful.[302] Two likely hypothetical pathogenetic mechanisms for Romano-Ward LQTS was proposed by Schwartz.[303] They include (1) sympathetic nervous system abnormalities and (2) potassium channel (or other ion channel) abnormalities.

In 1991, Keating and coworkers[304] provided evidence for tight molecular genetic linkage to chromosome 11p (11p15.5). Shortly thereafter, Towbin and colleagues demonstrated genetic heterogeneity in families with Romano-Ward LQTS.[305] Linkage evidence was found for loci on chromosome 7 (LQT2)[301] and chromosome 3 (LQT3) and another gene was linked to chromosome 4 (LQT4).[301] More recently, two other genes have been mapped for LQT5 and LQT6, both found on chromosome 21q22.[306]

The chromosome 11–linked (LQT1) gene was discovered to be KCNQ1, which encodes a potassium channel known as KVLQT1,[301] the slowly activated, delayed rectifier potassium channel I_{Ks}. Multiple mutations in KVLQT1 have been identified and this gene appears to be the most commonly mutated gene in LQTS. KVLQT1 was later shown to require a β-subunit to function normally. This β-subunit gene, KCNE1, encodes minK, which regulates the function of these combined channels, resulting in normal function of this slowly activated delayed rectifier potassium (I_{Ks}) channel. This gene, now also called LQT5, maps to chromosome 21q22. Mutations in either KVLQT1 or minK result in LQTS. The HERG gene, an I_{Kr} potassium channel, has been mapped to chromosome 7q35-q36 and mutations in a variety of domains of this channel were shown to be responsible for the disease in LQT2 families.[301] Another channel gene, the cardiac sodium channel called SCN5A, mapped to 3p21, was shown to be responsible for LQT3. Recently, LQT6 was discovered by Abbott and coworkers[306] to be the β-subunit, MiRP1 or KCNE2. This small channel protein regulates I_{Kr}, the rapidly activated delayed rectifier potassium channel, by interacting with HERG. Mutations in either MiRP1 or HERG result in the LQTS phenotype although the mutations in MiRP1 have been shown to also cause drug-induced (i.e., clarithromycin) VT or VF. The chromosome 4-linked (LQT4) gene remains undiscovered presently. The long-QT syndrome, therefore, appears to be an ion channelopathy, and multiple different ion-channel mutations could result in the long-QT syndrome (Fig. 62-13).

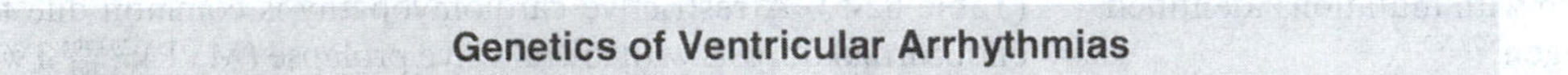

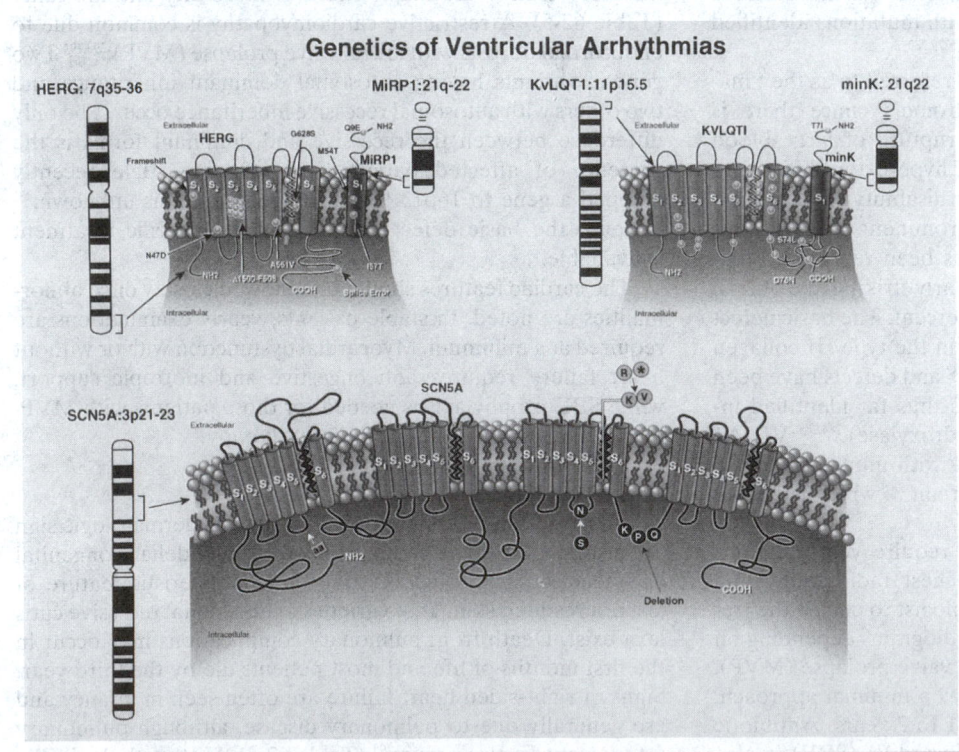

FIGURE 62-13 Genetic loci and ion channels encoded by the genes responsible for long-QT syndrome.

Phenotype-genotype studies have been reported in LQTS. Distinct ECG differences between patients have been demonstrated with mutations of different genes (LQT1-LQT3).[307] Important prognostic differences appear to occur with various mutations of the different genes.[301,308] Zareba et al.[308] recently provided genotype-phenotype correlation of mutations in LQT1, LQT2, and LQT3. In this study, mutations in LQT1 and LQT2 resulted in earlier onset of syncope than LQT3 (usually by age 15 years) and more frequent episodes of syncope. However,

LQT3 patients appeared to be at higher risk of death than either LQT1 or LQT2. The mode of symptoms and death also appears to be gene-specific to some extent. LQT1 mutations have been associated with episodes of syncope, seizures, or sudden death during diving/swimming or emotional upset. LQT2 also appears to be triggered by emotions but auditory triggers (i.e., phone or alarm clock ringing) are also important. LQT3, on the other hand, has a high incidence of events during sleep. LQT3 patients appear to shorten their QT intervals with exercise, while exercise seems to trigger events in LQT1 and LQT2 patients.

Recently, Schwartz et al.[309] have provided evidence that sudden infant death syndrome (SIDS) could be due to QT prolongation. Using ECGs on the third or fourth day of life in over 34,000 infants over a >20 year period, they found 34 infants died prior to their first birthday. In 24 of these cases, SIDS was diagnosed. Retrospective ECG analysis demonstrated that one-half of these infants had QTc prolongation on the initial screening ECG. Although no molecular analysis exists, it is speculated that ion channel mutations could be at play for a group of children with SIDS.[309,310]

Gene based therapy has been reported to improve the ECG features of LQTS, including QTc shortening and T-wave normalization. Schwartz et al.[311] treated patients with LQT2 and LQT3 with the sodium channel blocker mexiletine and showed significant QTc shortenting. Compton et al.[312] used exogenous potassium to increase the serum potassium in LQT2 patients with QTc shortening noted, while Shimizu et al.[313] used potassium channel openers to achieve similar results. However, no long-term results or outcomes have been reported with any of these therapies.

JERVELL AND LANGE-NIELSEN LONG-QT SYNDROME

This syndrome, described in 1957, is characterized by congenital deafness, syncope, prolonged QT interval, sudden death, and autosomal recessive inheritance[301] (see Chap. 36). Affected individuals are usually diagnosed in childhood with congenital, severe high-tone perceptive bilateral deafness; fainting spells precipitated by exertion, rage or fright; and ECG evidence of QT interval prolongation and T-wave abnormalities. As would be expected for rare autosomal recessive traits, the parents of affected individuals are more likely than usual to be consanguineous. Homozygous mutations or compound heterozygous mutations in either KVLQT1 or *minK* (i.e., I_{Ks}) have been shown to result in Jervell and Lange-Nielsen syndrome.[314–317] In this circumstance, the deafness requires a homozygous mutation, which results in abnormal production of endolymph, a potassium-rich fluid, in the inner ear. Thus, deafness is autosomal recessive while LQTS is autosomal dominant (i.e., heterozygous mutation results in LQTS; homozygous mutation results in longer QTc and worse outcome).

BRUGADA SYNDROME (IDIOPATHIC VENTRICULAR FIBRILLATION)

First described in detail in 1992, the Brugada syndrome is characterized by ST-segment elevation in leads V_1–V_3, with or without right bundle-branch block[318,319] (Fig. 62-14). Clinical symptoms occur due to ventricular fibrillation. In many patients, spontaneous resuscitation occurs. In others, sudden death occurs, particularly during sleep. This disorder appears to be relatively common in Europe and Southeast Asia and commonly is

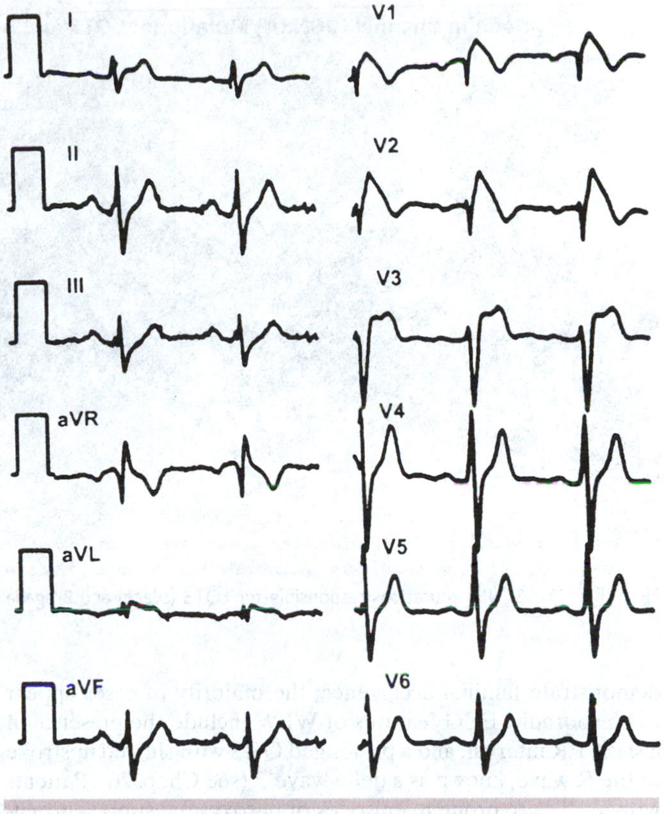

FIGURE 62-14 Electrocardiographic characteristics of Brugada syndrome. Note the ST-segment elevation in V_1 to V_3.

familial, usually with autosomal dominant inheritance.[320] Some patients do not have overt ECG manifestations and provocation studies in the catheterization laboratory using procainamide, flecainide, or ajmaline may be necessary for diagnosis.

The genetics of Brugada syndrome appear to involve mutations in ion channels as well. Mutations in SCN5A, the cardiac sodium channel gene previously shown to cause LQT3, have been identified[320,321] (Fig. 62-15). Although the surface ECG and biophysical characteristics of these patients differ from LQT3, it is interesting that symptoms occur during sleep in both disorders. There also appears to be a temperature-dependent effect on the electrophysiologic properties of some of these mutations.[322] Genetic heterogeneity appears to occur, but no other genes have been reported to date.

FAMILIAL ATRIAL FIBRILLATION

Familial atrial fibrillation appears to be rare, but a moderately sized family was identified and the gene responsible for the disease mapped to 10q22.[323] This family inherited the disease as an autosomal dominant trait, with the average age of onset of atrial fibrillation being 17 years. This family has a highly penetrant form of the disease, with most affected developing atrial fibrillation very early in childhood. The signs and symptoms are those related to atrial fibrillation which include palpitations, syncope, and dyspnea. Several other families with familial atrial fibrillation have since been identified due to the same locus.

WOLFF-PARKINSON-WHITE SYNDROME (WPW)

The preexcitation syndromes, including WPW, have been considered to be congenital, but only a small number of patients

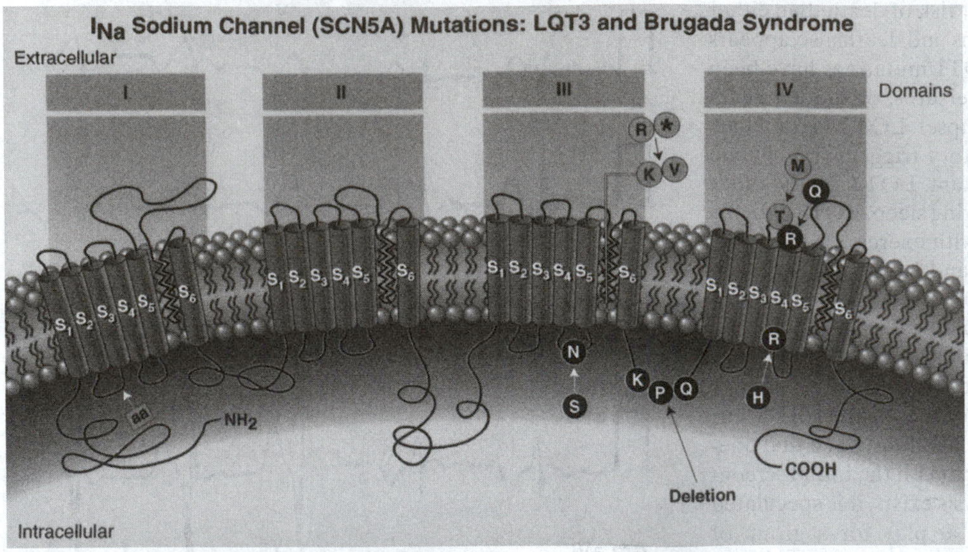

FIGURE 62-15 SCN5A mutations responsible for LQT3 (*black*) and Brugada syndrome (*gray*).

demonstrate familial occurrence; the majority of cases appear to be sporadic. ECG features of WPW include the presence of a short PR interval, and a prolonged QRS with slurred upstroke of the R wave, known as a delta wave[324] (see Chap. 26). Patients with WPW are prone to episodes of paroxysmal supraventricular tachycardia (see Chap. 27). An autosomal dominant pattern of inheritance of accessory pathways has been reported.[35] In a family with FHCM and WPW the locus was mapped to chromosome 7 (7q3) has been shown in patients with both FHCM and WPW.[35]

Autosomal Dominant Atrioventricular Block This disorder, when familial, presents with adult onset (age 20 to 50 years) and has an autosomal dominant inheritance pattern.[301,325] Approximately 50 families have been identified with this disorder which, in each transmission, is consistent with autosomal dominant inheritance with full penetrance and variable expression. Whether all of these conditions represent a single disorder is not known. The common presentation of this disease includes one of the following: (1) right bundle-branch block (RBBB) alone; (2) left axis deviation (LAD) alone; (3) RBBB plus LAD; or (4) complete heart block. In addition, atrioventricular block has been associated with DCM and skeletal myopathy, and several genetic loci have been identified.[105,326,327] Another gene has been mapped to chromosome 19q13 in a family with AV block but without DCM.[326]

Congenital Heart Disease with or without Genetic Syndromes

FAMILIAL ATRIAL SEPTAL DEFECT (ASD)

Two mendelian forms of ASD exist as autosomal dominant traits. One form has no other associated abnormalities and was initially speculated to be on chromosome 6p, linked to the HLA complex, as yet unconfirmed by genetic linkage analysis. Further analysis identified mutations in the transcription factor Nkx2.5 in families and sporadic cases of ASD.[327] This is likely to be genetically heterogeneous and search for other disease-causing genes is being pursued. The more common form of familial secundum ASD is associated with atrioventricular conduction delay, which rarely progresses to heart block. In these patients, attention should be directed to the upper limbs, particularly the thumbs, to rule out the Holt-Oram syndrome, which will be described below. Another form of familial ASD has also been described which is thought to be mitochondrially inherited.

HOLT-ORAM SYNDROME (HOS)

The cardinal manifestations of this autosomal dominant condition include upper limb dysplasia, ASD, and marked variability within families. The abnormalities of the arm demonstrate a wide spectrum in heterozygous individuals, ranging from undetectable, to distally placed thumbs and hypoplastic thenar eminences, triphylangeal thumbs, anomalies of the carpus, and radial aplasia, to phocomelia and hypoplasia of the clavicles and shoulders. The upper extremity deformity is typically bilateral, but the left side commonly is more severe than the right. In addition to the ASD, other cardiac malformations are occasionally found, the most frequent of which is a ventricular septal defect (VSD). Cardiac conduction disturbances, usually involving the AV node in patients with septal defects and hypoplastic peripheral arteries, are also found (Table 62-6). Other noncardiac manifestations include dermatoglyphic abnormalities and pectus excavatum. Since the noncardiac abnormalities have a very wide spectrum, all patients with ASD should be evaluated closely for upper limb deformities.

A male with features consistent with Holt-Oram syndrome in addition to mental retardation and other anomalies was found to have a deletion of chromosome 14 in the q23-q24.2 region. Linkage to chromosome 12 (12q213-q22) was later demonstrated in one family with Holt-Oram syndrome, while other families did not link to this region, indicative of heterogeneity.[328,329] The responsible gene for 12q21.3 was subsequently identified.[330,331] The chromosome 12–linked HOS was concomitantly reported by Basson et al.[330] and Li et al.[331] as TBX5, a member of the Brachyury (T) gene family, located at 12q24.1. This gene is a member of the T-box transcription factor family,[332,333] a group of genes that share a common DNA-binding motif (T box). Basson et al.[330] identified mutations in two families (nonsense, missense mutations) and suggested that haplo-insufficiency was the mechanism at play. Li et al.[331] identified mutations in three families and three sporadic cases, four of which encoded premature stop codons and two reading frame shift mutations. The authors pointed out that no obvious phenotype-genotype correlations existed. In fact, individuals with identical mutations had widely different skeletal and cardiac features. They also suggested that haplo-insufficiency was at play and occurred between days 26 and 52 of gestation.

SUPRAVALVULAR AORTIC STENOSIS (SVAS) AND WILLIAMS SYNDROME

SVAS occurs in three different situations, occurring with an estimated incidence of 1 in 20,000 births. The most common is associated with the Williams syndrome which is usually sporadic but may be a highly variable autosomal dominant condition. The full spectrum of Williams syndrome[334,335] includes dysmorphic facies, often called "elfin" facies, infantile hypercalcemia, mental retardation, short stature, SVAS, and multiple peripheral pulmonic stenoses.[279,334] Many of these individuals have robust (so-called cocktail party) personalities. Late-onset problems may include progressive joint contractures, gastrointestinal dysfunction, and genitourinary dysfunction.

Cardiovascular features of Williams syndrome are present in about 75 percent of patients,[279,335] the most characteristic of which is supravalvular aortic stenosis. Other findings include peripheral pulmonic arterial stenosis and pulmonic valvular stenosis. Occasionally, VSD or ASD may be present. Peripheral vascular anomalies, including renal arterial stenosis, diffuse narrowing of the aorta, and coarctation of the aorta, may be present and may be associated with systemic hypertension. Sudden death has occurred in children with Williams syndrome, especially after cardiac catheterization. Coronary arterial stenosis may occur and lead to myocardial infarction. Histopathology in these patients suggests the possibility of abnormal elastic fibers.[336]

A second setting for SVAS is the autosomal dominant entity which is distinct from that of Williams syndrome (WS). Mental retardation and abnormal facies are not found and these individuals present with SVAS and/or peripheral pulmonary artery stenoses.[279,334] In some cases, family members present with moderate pulmonic valve and branch pulmonary artery stenoses but without SVAS. Later, the valvular and branch pulmonary stenoses may disappear while SVAS becomes evident. The stenotic aortic lesion requires surgery in less than one-half of these patients. The diagnosis relies on echocardiography, but cardiac catheterization is sometimes required. Finally, SVAS may present as sporadic cases. Many investigators have long believed that the sporadic SVAS, WS, and autosomal dominant SVAS are all interrelated.

In 1993, WS was shown to result from a submicroscopic deletion involving chromosome 7q11.23 in the region of the elastin gene,[337] and subsequently confirmed.[338] Inherited or de novo deletion of one elastin allele was identified in each of the patients studied and suggested that hemizygosity at the elastin locus is responsible for the vascular pathology in WS. Concordance in monozygotic twins and occurrence in second cousins has been described and anecdotal reports of parent and child with WS have been reported. In addition, familial supravalvular aortic stenosis (SVAS) without WS, which appears to be inherited as an autosomal dominant trait, is well known. This autosomal dominant form of SVAS was found to be linked to the elastin gene at 7q11.23[334] as well, and deletions were identified. Baumer et al.[339] suggested that WS results from this deletion at 7q11.23 that arises from recombination between misaligned repeat sequences flanking the WS region. It is currently believed that this syndrome is a contiguous gene syndrome. The first deleted gene identified in the critical region, elastin (ELN), has been shown to cause the SVAS phenotype but not any of the other features of Williams syndrome (Fig. 62-16, Plate 99). Elastin gene (ELN) deletion is seen in 90 to 95 percent of WS patients and translocations also occur. ELN rearrangements, point mutations, splice mutations, and nonsense mutations have been found in families and sporadic cases of SVAS or Williams syndrome. However, a few patients with classic features of WS, usually without cardiac defects, do not have a deletion involving elastin. This fact suggests that, while deletion of elastin is necessary for the SVAS phenotype, it may not be necessary for Williams syndrome. Elastin is an extracellular matrix protein that comprises 90 percent of the elastic matrix that restores a vessel's shape after it has been stretched. Intense efforts to identify other deleted genes that contribute to the phenotype subsequently identified deletions of LIMK1 (a protein tyrosine kinase expressed in developing brain), syntaxin IA (a component of the synaptic apparatus), WBSCR1 (containing an RNA-binding motif), RFC2 (a subunit of the replication factor C complex involved in DNA replication), FKBP6 (a FK506-binding protein immunophilin which is thought to play a role in the calcium metabolism abnormalities and growth delay in these patients), WSTF (a putative transcription factor), WS-TRP (considered as playing a role in signal transduction), FZD3 (a gene homologous to *Drosophila* tissue polarity gene *frizzled*), and GTF21 (a multifunctional member of a widely expressed transcription factor complex that is phosphorylated by Bruton tyrosine kinase).[340–348] The roles of these genes in the Williams syndrome phenotype, however, is not known. In order to localize, isolate, and characterize the genes that contribute to the Williams syndrome phenotype, Hockenhull et al.[349] constructed a high-resolution integrated map of the critical region, established a panel of somatic cell hybrids from patients with classic clinical features, and defined deletion breakpoints and estimated the size of the deletions with classical Williams syndrome. They also identified two new genes, CPETR1 and CPETR2, which are deleted in these patients. A mouse knockout model has been created and is being studied.

NOONAN SYNDROME

In 1963, nine patients with valvular pulmonic stenosis, short stature, mild mental retardation, hypertelorism, and unusual facial features were described.[350] This disorder, sometimes confused with Turner syndrome, is distinct and females and males are equally affected. Noonan syndrome is relatively common, with an incidence of 1 in 1000 to 2500 live births. The diagnosis can sometimes be made prenatally. Postnatal growth, however, is generally delayed and tends to parallel the third percentile with normal growth velocity, although the adolescent growth spurt is usually blunted or absent. Facial features appear to change with age. The main features of the newborn period are hypertelorism with down-slanted palpebral fissures; low-set, posteriorly rotated ears with thickened helices; deeply grooved philtrum; micrognathia; and excess neck skin with low posterior hairline. As the infant ages, the head appears larger, with prominent eyes and thinning of the palpebral fissures and depression of the nasal root. The face appears more myopathic and becomes more triangular in shape. In some young adults, the eyes become less prominent. The neck length is relatively short, which exaggerates the webbing. Individuals tend to have prominent nasolabial folds, a high anterior hairline, and transparent, wrinkled skin. The hair is generally described as being curly

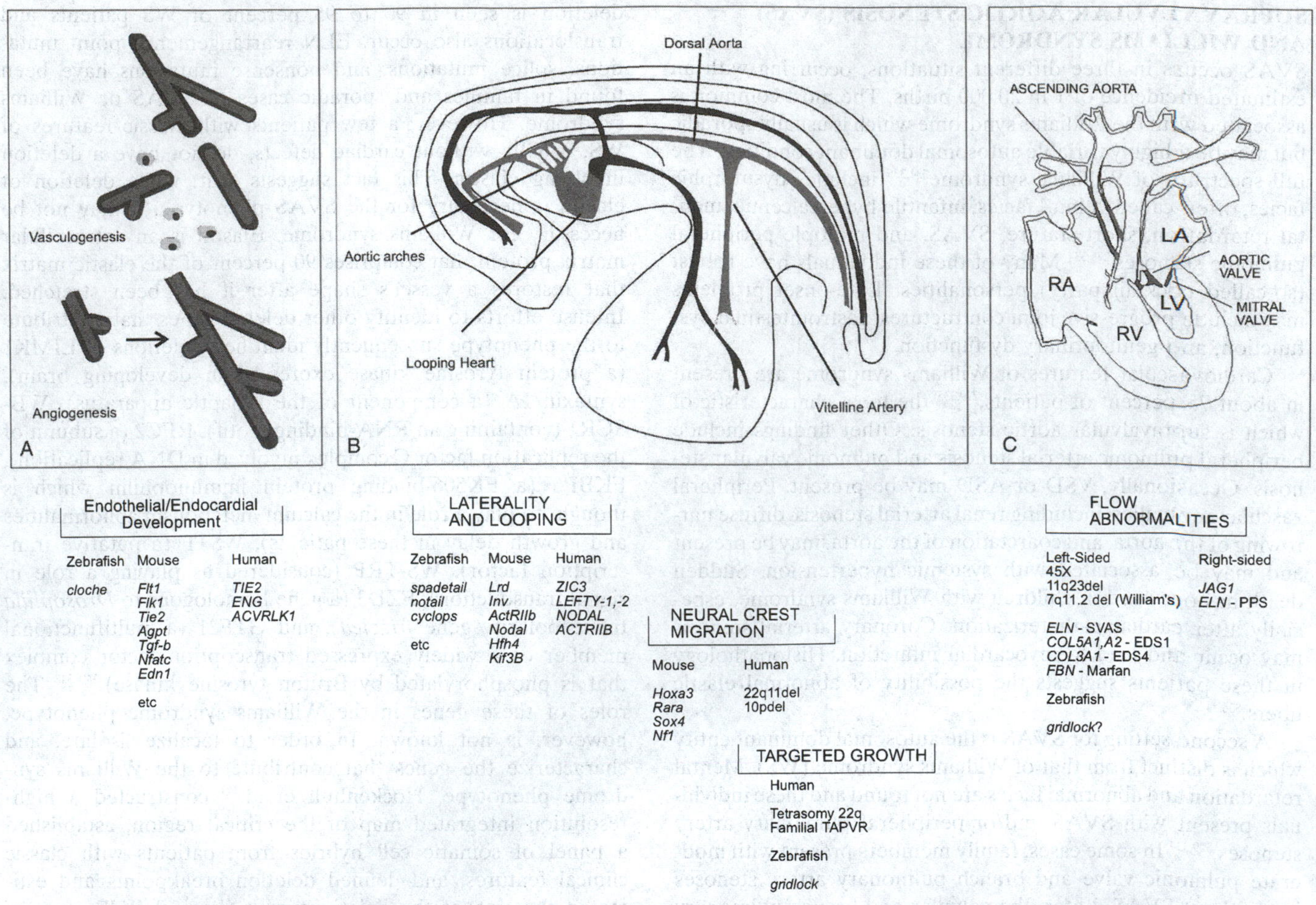

FIGURE 62-16 (Plate 99) Genetic defects causing congenital heart disease with or without genetic syndromes. Mutants from zebrafish, mouse, and human relating to primary developmental processes or maintenance of the vascular system are illustrated, including those of vasculogenesis and angiogenesis (*A*), embryonic development of the vascular system (*B*), and LV outflow tract obstruction (*C*).

or woolly in older children and adolescents. Approximately 60 percent of males have cryptorchidism. Sexual development is variable and may be delayed. Most females appear to be fertile. Pectus carinatum superiorly and pectus excavatum inferiorly appears to be present in about 70 percent of individuals. The chest appears to lengthen with age, giving the appearance of relatively low-set nipples. Other features include cubitus valgus, clinodactyly, vertebral anomalies, dental malocclusion, café-au-lait spots, pigmented nevi, bleeding disorders, lymphatic dysplasia, and pulmonary and intestinal lymphangiectasia. Mental retardation is present in 35 percent of cases.[351]

It appears that about two-thirds of patients with Noonan syndrome have some type of cardiac defect. Approximately half of these patients have valvular pulmonic stenosis. Other relatively common cardiac anomalies include hypertrophic cardiomyopathy, ASDs, VSDs, and persistent patent ductus arteriosus. Pulmonic arterial branch stenosis, mitral valve prolapse, Ebstein's anomaly, and single ventricle have also been reported (Table 62-6).

The clinical features of Noonan syndrome can overlap with a number of other conditions. Chromosome studies should be done in females to rule out Turner syndrome. Phenotypic overlap with WS, primidone teratogenicity syndrome, fetal alcohol syndrome, Aarskog syndrome, Leopard syndrome, neurofibromatosis, and malignant hyperthermia (King syndrome) have been reported.

Most cases of Noonan syndrome appear to be sporadic. Thus, the percentage of inherited cases may actually be much higher than the 30 percent previously reported. The majority of inherited cases are apparently inherited from the mother, thought to be the result of decreased fertility in males. Therefore, although the recurrence risk for offspring is expected to be 50 percent, it might actually be somewhat lower. A gene causing Noonan syndrome has been mapped to chromosome 12(12q22-qter),[352] but the gene has remained elusive. Genetic heterogeneity has also been demonstrated.

TUBEROUS SCLEROSIS (TS)

Classically, tuberous sclerosis consists of the triad of mental retardation, seizures, and adenoma sebaceum. These features, however, may not be present in all patients. The term *tuberous sclerosis* primarily refers to hamartomatous lesions in the brain as well as intracranial calcifications primarily in the area of the basal ganglia. These lesions appear to be present in about 90 percent of patients. Seizures are a frequent finding, being seen in about 90 percent, and have some correlation with mental retardation. About 60 percent of tuberous sclerosis patients are mentally retarded, close to 100 percent of whom have seizures; of those without mental retardation, only 75 percent have seizures. Seizures tend to occur earlier in patients with mental retardation than those without mental retardation. Ocular lesions, particularly benign astrocytoma, occur in about 50 percent of patients. Cutaneous lesions are common; 80 percent of patients develop angiofibromas of the face, usually referred to by the misnomer adenoma sebaceum. Depigmented skin patches that are especially apparent by Wood's light examination are seen in about 80 percent of patients, frequently from birth. Pulmonary disease may occur primarily in adult females and is likely to be severe and life-threatening. The primary cardiac finding is the presence of rhabdomyomata.[353,354] Wolff-Parkinson-White (WPW) syndrome and supraventricular tachycardia have also been reported.[354,355]

Tuberous sclerosis is an autosomal dominant condition in which about 80 percent of cases are suspected as resulting from new mutations with unaffected parents. A child diagnosed with tuberous sclerosis should be evaluated by computed tomography (CT) of the brain and electroencephalography for the presence of CNS lesions and also have renal ultrasound. Parents should be examined for the presence of depigmented patches (by Wood's light), dental abnormalities, retinal findings, and abdominal ultrasound for renal cysts. It is now apparent that there are at least two genes causing tuberous sclerosis: TSC1 on chromosome 9 at 9q34 (hamartin)[356] and TSC2 (tuberin) on chromosome 16 at 16p13. These two protein products co-localize to cytoplasmic vesicles[357] and interact with each other. TSC2 spans 43 kb of genomic DNA and encodes a number of alternatively spliced transcripts of 16 kb. Constitutional inactivating mutations of the TSC2 gene, including complete deletion, have been detected in patients with TS and the associated hamartomas show loss of heterozygosity for markers in the TSC2 region, indicating that TSC2 functions as a tumor suppressor gene and that loss of function of both alleles is normally required before cellular growth becomes dysregulated. Various cancers[358] have been found to occur due to mutations in the TS complex. In addition, large deletions in TSC2 and its neighboring gene PKD1 have been seen in children with polycystic kidney disease.[359] Genotype-phenotype correlations are not helpful.[360,361] Animal models have been developed with resultant tumors noted.[362–365]

FAMILIAL COARCTATION OF THE AORTA

Familial coarctation of the aorta (usually with autosomal dominant transmission) has been described but no locus or gene has been identified. This congenital lesion is the most common congenital anomaly of the aortic arch in humans, occurring in 5 to 8 percent of children with congenital heart defects. A recessive mutation, *gridlock,* in the zebrafish (*Danio rerio*) has been identified in which blood flow to the tail is impeded by a localized vascular defect.[366] There is some question as to whether this mutation is a model for human aortic coarctation,[367] but it may aid in learning about vascular obstruction. As coarctation of the aorta occurs in association with other left heart obstructive lesions in an individual or in members of a family with other left heart obstructive lesions, it is likely that the mechanism causing disease is complex. Other mutations, such as those of endothelin1, endothelin A receptor, Hand2, MFH-1, and retinoid receptor genes have been shown to lead to aortic arch malformations in mice (Fig. 62-16).

IVEMARK SYNDROME (ASPLENIA/POLYSPLENIA) OR HETEROTAXY SYNDROMES

Ivemark syndrome represents a group of defects that interferes with the normal establishment of laterality.[279,368] The more severe asplenia and polysplenia syndromes have an estimated incidence of 1 in 10,000 to 20,000 live births. The occurrence is usually sporadic, but familial cases have been described with autosomal recessive and X-linked transmission; chromosomal translocations (i.e., between chromosomes 12 and 13) and deletions (involving chromosomes 10 and 13) have been described, as has monozygotic twinning. Both forms tend to have similar cardiac defects, including ASDs, VSDs, endocardial cushion defects, and pulmonic stenosis as well as other defects.[369,370] Asplenia, however, tends to be more commonly associated with severe defects of the atrioventricular canal and VSDs, while polysplenia tends to be more associated with ASDs. In many cases, complex cardiac malformations occur, including single ventricle physiology. A total of 32 cases of asplenia were identified in 4059 autopsies, and all cases were sporadic with a male excess.

Rightward looping of the midline heart tube is the first overt manifestation of anatomic left-right differences, which eventually come to include the asymmetry of the lungs and most malformations associated with abnormal looping; therefore, they usually occur as one manifestation of a more global abnormality of left-right heart anomalies, abnormalities of spleen position and/or number, and some degree of malrotation of the gut. The overall left-right axis of the individual may be situs ambiguus (i.e., indeterminate sidedness) or situs inversus (complete left-right reversal), compared to normal sidedness (situs solitus).

Cardiac malformations attributable to abnormal laterality represent 3.4 percent of all heart defects.[371] Since there is familial clustering of situs, it appears that genetics contributes significantly to these abnormalities. This is supported by mutant mouse models with similar defects,[371] as well as gene defects in some humans.

The first gene locus for human situs defects was mapped to Xq26.2 in families with X-linked disease.[372] This gene was later shown to be a zinc-finger transcription factor Z1C3, and mutations were found in sporadic and familial cases.[371,372] Studies in other vertebrates yielded additional candidate genes as well. Several genes were found to be asymmetrically expressed along the left-right axis in chick prior to development of anatomic left-right asymmetry[274,368] and some of these same genes were also found to be asymmetrically expressed in the mouse (Fig. 62-16). These genes included nodal, pitx2, lefty-1 and lefty-2. Genetic studies in mice also implicated several additional genes that did not have asymmetric expression, such as HNF3, Actrllb, and Smad.[373–375] Mutation analysis in patients have identified a small number of mutations in all of these genes.[376,377]

Other Genetic Syndromes

A variety of other genetic syndromes with associated cardiovascular disease occur primarily in childhood. These include Ellis-Van Crevald syndrome, Treacher Collins syndrome, Alagille syndrome, Smith-Lemli-Opitz syndrome, thrombocytopenia-absent radii (TAR) syndrome, Goldenhar syndrome, Cornelia de Lange syndrome, Rubinstein-Taybi syndrome, VACTERL association, and CHARGE association. Since these are primarily pediatric diseases, they are not included in this discussion. For detailed descriptions of these and other pediatric genetic syndromes with cardiovascular abnormalities, see current reviews of this topic.[378]

CARDIOVASCULAR DISORDERS ASSOCIATED WITH CHROMOSOME ABNORMALITIES

Chromosomal Nomenclature

Cytogenetics is the study of chromosomes and chromosomal abnormalities. Chromosomes are classified according to their size and shape. Chromosomes have two arms, one long and one short. The short arm is usually referred to as the "p" arm, and the long arm is usually referred to as the "q" arm. For instance, the long arm of chromosome 22 is designated 22q and the short arm 22p. The arms of the chromosomes meet at the centromere or primary constriction, which is responsible for division of chromosome pairs during meiosis and mitosis. There are three shapes of human chromosomes based on the position of the centromere. Metacentric chromosomes have the centromere in a central position and the long and short arms are approximately equal. Submetacentric chromosomes have an eccentric centromere, producing arms of unequal lengths. Acrocentric chromosomes have a centromere close to one end of the chromosome. Acrocentric chromosomes have small pieces of chromatin known as satellites attached to their short arms.

Since 1971, banding of chromosomes has become routine and the banding patterns of each chromosome can be distinguished separately. For this reason, chromosome abnormalities are designated by the actual chromosome number rather than the chromosome group (e.g., trisomy 18 rather than trisomy E).

Classification of Chromosomal Alterations

Chromosome alterations, especially those involving too many or too few chromosomes (called aneuploidy), are quite common in human development. Chromosome aberrations most commonly cause structural defects of the cardiovascular system, and typically these are evident at birth. Approximately 50 percent of all fetuses conceived are spontaneously aborted (usually in the first trimester), with one-half of these being aneuploid. Among live-born infants, about 1 in 200 (0.5 percent) have a chromosome abnormality. The frequency of chromosome abnormalities among live-born children with congenital heart defects is in the range of 5 to 13 percent.[378] Hence, the vast majority of chromosomal aberrations are lost in early fetal life and, in most instances, occur as new mutations. For this reason, with both parents being normal, the risk of recurrence to relatives is usually low.

1. Aneuploidy, defined as the gain or loss of chromosomes resulting in too many or too few chromosomes, occurs most commonly by nondysjunction (failure of a homologous pair of chromosomes to separate). Nondisjunction occurs during meiosis in one parent (i.e., in spermatogenesis or oogenesis) or in the first mitotic cleavage of the zygote. In meiotic nondysjunction, when a pair of chromosomes does not normally separate, both members of the pair (or neither member of the pair) pass into one gamete. When an additional copy of the chromosome is added during fertilization, three copies of the same chromosome (or only one copy) are found in the new zygote instead of the chromosome pair. Two of the most common chromosomal disorders causing heart disease, Down syndrome (trisomy 21) and Turner syndrome (XO), are due to nondisjunction. Absence of one chromosome is called *monosomy;* all autosomal monosomies, as well as those containing only a Y sex chromosome, are lethal for the embryo. The presence of three chromosomes is called *trisomy,* as seen in Down syndrome, while the presence of an entire extra set of chromosomes is known as *triploidy*.

2. Chromosomal rearrangements occur when a chromosome breaks and rejoins within itself differently than normally occurs. This can potentially result in an inversion of genetic material. Typically there is no apparent phenotypic effect in persons carrying an inversion but their offspring may have severe abnormalities due to the disruption in chromosome pairing during meiosis that can take place.

3. Chromosome deletions, or loss of chromosomal material, may be seen by light microscopy and consists of deletion of 10^6 bp or greater. If there is a large amount of DNA lost, more than one gene may be affected (disrupted or lost), a series of abnormalities in a single individual may result due to interruptions in a series of genes within the loci of a single chromosome. These contiguous gene deletion syndromes[379] may be heritable and the occurrence of the disorder in a family behaves as a dominant disorder (X-linked or autosomal dominant). Most deletions occur de novo. Two breaks in the same chromosome that reunite with the intermediate segment being inverted is referred to as an inversion. Isochromes are formed when two short or long arms join with loss of the other arm. Chromosomal translations occur when breaks occur in two chromosomes and reunite after exchange of segments. These deletions are best appreciated at the DNA level by Southern analysis or polymerase chain reaction (PCR) analysis.

4. Chromosome duplications or gains of chromosomal material may also be associated with phenotypic abnormality but most commonly cause no obvious aberration.

Cytogenetics and Techniques

High-resolution cytogenetic techniques allow unambiguous identification of each human chromosome and detection of most structural abnormalities of the chromosomes. These structural abnormalities include translocations, deletions, and duplications. High-resolution chromosome analysis involves synchronization of lymphocyte cultures in order to accumulate all cells at one point in the cell cycle. Other cells that may be used include skin, fibroblasts, and amniotic cells. Enrichment of this cell population in prophase and prometaphase rather than the middle to late stages of metaphase, which is characteristic of conventional harvesting techniques, allows improved visualization of the subbanding patterns of chromosomes. Each band seen at metaphase actually represents multiple subbands in earlier stages that have fused together as the chromosome contracts. Whereas a typical metaphase cell contains 300 to 400 bands per haploid genome, synchronized chromosome preparations make it possible to visualize 500 to 1000 bands per haploid set. With the development of banding methods, the human karyotype could be divided into 300 to 400 descrete bands or approximately 7 to 10 × 10^6 bp per band, and a much greater number of deletions, duplications, and translocations could be detected. High-resolution techniques allow visualization of from 500 to 2000 bands per haploid genome, and have enabled the delineation of a number of microdeletion or microduplication syndromes (also known as contiguous gene syndromes), including the DiGeorge syndrome and Beckwith-Wiedemann syndrome.

FLUORESCENCE IN SITU HYBRIDIZATION (FISH)

Fluorescence in situ hybridization or FISH provides for the detection of submicroscopic chromosomal deletions or duplications. This technique uses DNA probes conjugated with a fluorescent dye visible under a fluorescence microscope derived from chromosomal regions that hybridize to the specific chromosomes. This method makes possible direct visualization of single sequences not only on chromosomes but also within decondensed interphase nuclei, providing a high-resolution (<1 mb) approach to gene mapping and analysis of nuclear organization.

INDICATIONS FOR CHROMOSOMAL ANALYSIS

Chromosomal studies can provide valuable information to the family and the physician and should be considered in any child who has a heart defect with (1) minor dysmorphic features, (2) growth retardation that cannot be explained by the heart defect, or (3) developmental delay. In addition, the practitioner might more strongly consider chromosome studies if there is a family history of multiple miscarriages or other infants with birth defects or mental retardation. A genetic consultant can help determine whether or not chromosome studies should be performed, and they can help to integrate the findings of the chromosome analysis with the clinical picture. The major disadvantage of doing chromosomal studies is the cost (generally between $300 to $500).

Chromosomal Disorders

Many chromosomal disorders have associated cardiovascular disease. The most common of these include Down's syndrome (trisomy 21), Patau syndrome (trisomy 13), Edwards syndrome (trisomy 18), and Turner syndrome. Since trisomy 13 and 18 usually result in death during infancy, these are not described. A significant number of other chromosomal abnormalities are also associated with cardiovascular disease and are seen primarily as pediatric disorders. These abnormalities include triploidy, aneuploidy (other than trisomy 21, trisomy 18, trisomy 13, and Turner syndrome), deletions, and duplications. The triploidy syndromes—which include 69,XXX, 69,XXY, or 69,XYY—have a greater than 50 percent incidence of congenital heart disease, the vast majority of which are atrial and ventricular septal defects (ASD, VSD). The aneuploidy syndromes, not discussed thus far, are varied and uncommon. These include mosaicism of chromosome 8 and chromosome 9, which clinically present with VSDs with or without other associated complex defects. Aortic root dilatation and MVP occur with partial monosomy of chromosome 22. Other cardiovascular abnormalities associated with partial trisomy of chromosome 7q includes VSD, pulmonic stenosis (PS), patent ductus arteriosus (PDA), coarctation of the aorta (CoA), and L-transposition of the great vessels. Partial trisomy of chromosome 7p also occurs and most commonly is associated with VSD, PS, or AV canal.

DOWN'S SYNDROME (TRISOMY 21)

Chromosome 21 is the smallest of all human chromosomes, containing less than 2 percent of the genomic DNA. Down's syndrome, however, is the most common phenotype caused by a human chromosome abnormality, occurring approximately once in every 500 to 600 births. This disorder is usually due to the presence of an extra chromosome 21 (i.e., trisomy 21), but in some cases it is caused by the presence of only the distal half of chromosome 21, band q22 (i.e., 21q22)—the "Down's syndrome critical region"—so-called due to the presence of a subset of major phenotypic features of Down's syndrome including mental retardation, congenital heart disease, characteristic facial appearance, hand and dermatoglyphic changes.[380-382] In order to produce this syndrome, the region of 21q22 must be triplicated. The gene or genes responsible for manifesting Down's syndrome are unknown, but the severity of the disease is believed to depend on the extent of the region q22 and beyond that is triplicated. Creation of a linkage map of chromosome 21 has allowed for consideration of potential candidate genes. Recently, several genes have been implicated in some of the phenotypic features, but the cardiac features currently have no known cause.

The typical trisomy 21 occurs in 95 percent of cases of Down's syndrome and results from chromosomal nondisjunction. Some 2 to 3 percent of Down's syndrome cases are mosaics, having one trisomy cell line and one normal cell line, and the remainder (1 to 4 percent) are due to an extra copy of all or part of the long arm of chromosome 21 being translocated to another chromosome. The risk of trisomy 21 is exponentially related to maternal age, with the lowest risk for young women, rising steeply after age 35 years, and reaching 4 percent for women older than 45 years.

The recurrence risk is generally quoted at 1 to 2 percent. When a child with a translocation type of Down's syndrome is discovered, parental chromosomal analysis should always be performed to determine whether the translocation was inherited. If the translocation was not inherited and both parents have normal chromosomes, the recurrence risk is probably low, although prenatal chromosome diagnosis may be considered for future pregnancies. If the mother carries translocation of chromosome 21, the recurrence risk is approximately 10 percent. If the father is determined to be the carrier of a D;21 translocation, the recurrence risk is about 2 percent.[378] If one of the parents is determined to specifically be a 21;21 translocation carrier, the parents have a 100 percent chance of recurrence of Down's syndrome and no possibility of having normal offspring.[378] Luckily, the latter occurs in only about 1 in every 2000 cases of Down's syndrome but clearly has a significant impact on family planning.

Some 40 to 50 percent of patients with Down's syndrome have congenital heart disease (40 to 60 percent of these are atrioventricular septal defects, AVSDs) and this, along with hematologic malignant disease and duodenal atresia, are among the most common causes of morbidity and mortality.[378] Patients who escape these problems generally survive into the fifth decade and beyond. The most characteristic cardiac defect in

TABLE 62-9 Chromosomal Abnormalities Associated with Specific Types of Congenital Heart Defects

Endocardial cushion defect	Trisomy 21
Coarctation of the aorta	Turner syndrome
Total anomalous pulmonary venous return	Partial trisomy 22q 49,XXXXX; 49,XXXXX
Patent ductus arteriosus	Partial trisomy 8q
Tetralogy of Fallot	Monosomy 22q11
Conotruncal abnormalities	Partial trisomy 5q
Conduction defect	Turner syndrome
Hypoplastic left heart	

Down's syndrome is the AVSD (also called *endocardial cushion defect* or *atrioventricular canal defect*) (Table 62-9).[378] In addition to problems of volume overload secondary to left-to-right shunting, these patients are predisposed to early pulmonary hypertension. Elevated pulmonary vascular resistance becomes a significant risk beyond 1 year of age. Once this occurs, these patients become unsuitable for surgical repair. Approximately one-third of patients with Down's syndrome and congenital heart defects have complex heart disease, increasing the morbidity and mortality further. Other clinical features of Down's syndrome include hypotonia and decreased Moro reflex with joint hyperextensibility in the newborn period, a flat facial profile with excessive, redundant skin in the posterior neck, antimongoloid slant (upward) of palpebral fissures, and small white Brushfield spots around the circumference of the irides in children with blue irides. The hands and feet may reveal a simian crease (50 percent), clinodyactyly, or incurving of the fifth finger, brachydactyly with short metacarpals and phalanges, and a wide gap between the first two toes. Individuals are mentally retarded to varying degrees, with IQs ranging from 25 to 70. Generally, males are infertile.

TURNER SYNDROME

This disorder, which is due to a single X chromosome in females (i.e., XO genotype), occurs in approximately 1 female in 2500.[378] The frequency of nonmosaic XO karotypes is significantly higher in spontaneous abortuses than in liveborns, with less than 2 percent of such conceptuses reaching term. Clinically, there is a variable and often mild phenotype, and the diagnosis may go unsuspected until a child's short stature is evaluated or a women complains of amenorrhea. The clinical findings[378] of patients with Turner syndrome includes lymphedema of hands and feet, inguinal hernias, short stature, primary amenorrhea, facial features including a slightly traingular face with down-slated palpebral fissures, epicanthal folds, and ptosis. Ears are frequently low-set and posteriorly rotated, and the mandible is commonly micrognathic. The neck is typically short with marked webbing and the posterior hairline may be low, extending to the upper shoulders. A broad thorax with widely spaced nipples is common, as is cubitus valgus and shortening of fourth and fifth metacarpals. Abnormalities of sexual development are usually associated, including hypogonadotropic hypogonadism with ovarian dysgenesis. Intelligence is normal. Many cases are mosaic for cell lines with the normal 46XX or 46XY makeup. The frequency of congenital cardiac disease varies from 20 to 50 percent, with at least one-half of these having CoA. A variety of other cardiac defects may also occur either singly or in combination with CoA. The majority of these include other left heart abnormalities including bicuspid aortic valve, aortic stenosis, dilated ascending aorta,[378] and hypoplastic left heart syndrome (HLHS). ASD and VSD as well as partial anomalous pulmonary venous return have also been reported (Table 62-9).

Coarctation of the aorta can usually be diagnosed clinically due to poor femoral pulses and differential blood pressure, with the arm blood pressure being consistently hypertensive, while the leg pressures are typically very low. Echocardiography or magnetic resonance imaging will confirm the diagnosis. Therapy may include surgical repair or, in some cases, balloon angioplasty. Infants may require prostaglandin E therapy to keep the ductus arteriosis patent; these young patients may present in heart failure or cardiac collapse if duct-dependent. Those patients with HLHS are duct-dependent and will die unless a Norwood operation or cardiac transplant is performed. Bicuspid aortic valves do not usually require therapy unless stenosis occurs. All cardiac defects require prophylaxis for subacute bacterial endocarditis (SBE). Chromosomal studies are recommended in all cases of Turner syndrome, since only about 60 percent of cases will have monosomy X. The remaining cases have mosaicism or various abnormalities of the X chromosome. Most cases of Turner syndrome are sporadic and the recurrence risk appears to be relatively low. However, parents may choose to have prenatal chromosomal diagnosis in subsequent pregnancies.

CATCH-22 Syndromes

DIGEORGE ANOMALY

First described in 1965,[383] the combination of thymic hypoplasia, parathyroid hypoplasia, and cardiac defects has been termed DiGeorge syndrome or DiGeorge anomaly. Because the disorder is of heterogeneous etiology, the term *DiGeorge anomaly* is currently preferred to *DiGeorge syndrome*. These thymic, parathyroid, and cardiac defects all result from developmental abnormalities of the third and fourth branchial arches.

Eighty percent of affected infants present with congenital heart defects within the first 48 h of life. According to the classification system of Clark,[384] the two types of defects associated with DiGeorge anomaly are conotruncal defects and branchial arch mesenchymal tissue defects. Among conotruncal defects, truncus arteriosus is the most common type. Among the branchial arch mesenchymal tissue defects, interrupted aortic arch type b and right aortic arch are the most common.[378]

The second key feature is persistent hypocalcemia, occurring either as the initial presenting feature or in combination with the cardiac defect. Parathyroid glands may be absent or reduced in size and number, and serum parathyroid hormone levels are decreased. Hypocalcemia may require continuous calcium infusions and/or frequent calcium supplementation. In cases of partial defect, the hypocalcemia may improve over time.

There are multiple etiologies for DiGeorge which include chromosome abnormalities, single-gene defects, teratogenic exposures, and association with other defects.[384] Approximately 5 to 10 percent of infants with features of DiGeorge anomaly will have an obvious abnormality of chromosome 22 with monosomy of the proximal portion of the long arm. However, approximately 70 percent of patients will have submicroscopic deletions of 22q11 detectable only by FISH.[384,385] In addition, many of these patients have features of the Sprintzen velocardiofacial (VCF) syndrome and the Takao conotruncal face syndrome.[386,387] These syndromes are currently referred to as a group by the mnemonic of CATCH-22 syndrome for the associated defects: *c*ardiac, *a*bnormal facies, *t*hymic hypoplasia, *c*left platate, *h*ypocalcemia, *22*q11 deletions). Approximately 15 percent of infants with DiGeorge anomaly can be found to have obvious chromosome abnormalities of which about two-thirds involve a monosomy 22q11.[388] This usually results from an unbalanced translocation involving chromosome 22 and another chromosome. More recent studies using fluorescence in situ hybridization (FISH) with probes from the critical region have shown that a total of about 85 percent of DiGeorge anomaly patients are deleted, with about 70 percent of patients having submicroscopic, molecular deletions, del22 (q11.21 q11.23). Although patients have different deletion endpoints, a 1.5-Mb region is deleted in most. Rarely, a syndrome of "partial" DiGeorge syndrome due to balanced translocation has been described. This translocation was cloned and a disrupted gene DNA-binding protein.[389] More recently, a variety of candidate genes have been identified, including the human homolog of the *Drosophila disheveled* segment-polarity gene,[390] the *clathrin heavy chain-like* gene (CLTCL),[391] *UFD1L* (a developmentally expressed ubiquitination gene),[392] *HIRA*,[393] *DGSI*,[394] and the *goosecoid-like* (GSCL) homeobox gene[395] (Fig. 62-16). The best of these candidate genes, fulfilling most of the criteria necessary to cause this complex, are *HIRA* and *UFD1L*. *HIRA* is a mammalian homolog of yeast proteins, which are corepressors of cell cycle–dependent histone gene transcription, expressed in neural crest and neural crest–derived tissues.[396] This gene has been shown to be required for outflow tract septation. However, mice with haploinsufficiency are normal. *UFD1L*, the homolog of a highly conserved yeast gene involved in degradation of ubiquinated proteins, results in the same craniofacial and cardiac defects seen in CATCH-22 when mutated.[397] Recently, Lindsay et al.[398] engineered a chromosomal deletion (Dfl) in mice that spanned the critical region. The heterozygous deleted animals developed heart disease identical to that seen in humans. They suggested that the cardiovascular lesions occurred due to inadequate formation, early regression, or growth failure of the fourth aortic arch arteries. It should be noted that Yamagishi et al.[397] reported a DGS and/or VCFS patient who is heterozygous for a de novo deletion spanning 20 kb of DNA, disrupting *CDC45L* and *UFD2L*, both candidate genes. The authors suggested these genes to be involved in the development of these syndromes and argued that these genes were regulated by dHAND, a basic helix-loop-helix transcription factor. They proposed a model whereby downregulation of UFD1L activity results in accumulation of certain proteins and excessive apoptosis or maldevelopment of neural crest cells. Based on their view, they suggested disruption of UFD1L function alone, or in combination with CDC45L and/or HIRA is the most likely etiology for most defects seen in DGS. This is currently being carefully studied.

Several therapies have been used to treat the profound T-cell immunodeficiency associated with the DiGeorge syndrome. These therapies have included bone-marrow transplantation. Recently, Market et al.[399] described use of cultured postnatal thymus tissue transplantation in five infants, with good results.

SHPRINTZEN VELOCARDIOFACIAL (VCF) SYNDROME

This condition was first recognized in 1978 with ascertainment primarily in children with palatal defects[386]; this is the most common syndrome associated with cleft palate and appears to be the same disorder as the Takao conotruncal anomaly face syndrome.[387] The clinical features include mild short stature, cleft palate especially of the secondary palate with submucous clefts, pharyngeal incompetence leading to speech disorders, and speech delay. Most cases are sporadic but some autosomal cases have been reported.

Cardiac defects are prominent in this disorder, the majority being conotruncal-type defects.[400–403] Ventricular septal defect occurs in 70 to 75 percent, while right-sided aortic arch occurs in about 50 percent and tetralogy of Fallot is found in 15 to 20 percent of children. Partial DiGeorge anomaly seems to be present in some cases. About 85 percent of VCF syndrome patients have deletions of chromosome 22q11, usually submicroscopic and visible only by FISH techniques.

Takao syndrome (conotruncal face anomaly syndrome) first described in 1976, has similarities to both DiGeorge and Shprintzen syndromes clinically,[387,402] hence its incorporation in the CATCH-22 association. These Japanese children were noted to have a specific dysmorphic facial appearance in association with conotruncal malformations. Deletions within the 22q11 region in these patients have been found,[402] confirming its similarity to the DiGeorge syndrome and VCF syndrome.

References

1. Hoffman JIE. Incidence of congenital heart disease: II. Prenatal incidence. *Pediatr Cardiol* 1995; 16:155–165.
2. Berko BA, Swift M. X-linked dilated cardiomyopathy. *N Engl J Med* 1987; 316:1186–1190.
3. Collins FS, Patrinos A, Jordan E, et al. New goals for the U.S. Human Genome Project: 1998–2003. *Science* 1998; 282:682–689.
4. Brower V. News in science. *Nature Biotech* 1998; 16:895.
5. Brower V. Genome II: The next frontier. *Nature Biotech* 1998; 16:104.
6. Roberts R. A glimpse of the future from present day molecular genetics. In Opie LH, Yellon DM, eds. *Cardiology at the Limits III*. Cape Town: Stanford Writers; 1999:105–120.
7. Roberts R, Ryan TJ. 29th Bethesda Conference-Task Force 3: Clinical research in a molecular era and the need to expand its ethical imperatives. *J Am Coll Cardiol* 1998; 31:917–949.
8. Haines JL, Perricak-Vance MA. Sibpair analysis. In Haines JL, Perricak-Vance MA, eds. *Approaches to Gene Mapping in Complex Human Diseases*. New York: Wiley-Liss; 1998:273–303.
9. Serrato M, Marian AJ. A variant of human paraoxonase/arylesterase (HUMPONA) gene is a risk factor for coronary artery disease. *J Clin Invest* 1995; 96:3005–3008.
10. Yu QT, Safavi F, Roberts R, et al. A variant of β-fibrinogen is a genetic risk factor for coronary artery disease and myocardial infarction. *J Invest Med* 1996; 44:154–159.
11. Roberts R, Marian AJ, Bachinski LL. Overview: Application of molecular biology to medical genetics. In Markwald RR, Clark EB, Takao A, eds. *Inborn Heart Disease—Developmental Mechanisms*. Mount Kisco, NY: Futura Press; 1994:87–111.
12. Weissenbach J. A second generation linkage map of the human genome based on highly informative microsatellite loci. *Gene* 1994; 135:275–278.
13. Cooperative Human Linkage Center (CHLC). A comprehensive human linkage map with centimorgan density. *Science* 1994; 265:2049–2054.

14. Cooper NG, ed. *The Human Genome Project: Deciphering the Blueprint of Heredity*. Mill Valley, CA: University Science Books; 1994.
15. Haines JL, Perricak-Vance MA. Lod score analysis. In: Haines JL, Perricak-Vance MA, eds. *Approaches to Gene Mapping in Complex Human Diseases*. New York: Wiley-Liss; 1998:253–272.
16. Roberts R, Towbin J. Principles and techniques of molecular biology. In: Roberts R, ed. *Molecular Basis of Cardiology*. Cambridge, MA: Blackwell; 1993:15–112.
17. Hagmann M. A good SNP may be hard to find. *Science* 1999; 285:21–22.
18. Halushka MK, Fan J-B, Bentley K, et al. Patterns of single-nucleotide polymorphisms in candidate genes for blood-pressure homeostasis. *Nature Genet* 1999; 22:239–247.
19. Cargill M, Altshuler D, Ireland J, et al. Characterization of single-nucleotide polymorphisms in coding regions of human genes. *Nature Genet* 1999; 22:231–238.
20. Adams MD, Kelley JM, Gocayne JD, et al. Complementary DNA sequencing: Expressed sequence tags and Human Genome Project. *Science* 1991; 252:1651–1656.
21. Collins FS. Shattuck lecture: Medical and societal consequences of the Human Genome Project. *N Engl J Med* 1999; 341:28–37.
22. Oberst L, Zhao G, Park JT, et al. Dominant-negative effect of a mutant cardiac troponin T on cardiac structure and function in transgenic mice. *J Clin Invest* 1998; 102:1498–1505.
23. Blanchard EM, Lizuka K, Christe M, et al. Targeted ablation of the murine α-tropomyosin gene. *Circ Res* 1997; 81:1005–1011.
24. Marian AJ, Zhao G, Seta Y, et al. Expression of a mutant (Arg92Gln) human cardiac troponin T, known to cause hypertrophic cardiomyopathy, impairs adult cardiac myocytes contractility. *Circ Res* 1997; 81:76–85.
25. Hejtmancik JF, Roberts R. Molecular genetics and the application of linkage analysis. In: Roberts R, ed. *Molecular Basis of Cardiology*. Cambridge, MA: Blackwell; 1993:355–381.
26. Roberts R, Bachinski LL, Yu QT, et al. Molecular analysis of genotype/phenotype correlations of hypertrophic cardiomyopathy. In: Dhalla NS, Singal PK, Beamish RE, eds. *Heart Hypertrophy and Failure*. Boston: Kluwer; 1995:3–19.
27. Ozawa T, Tanaka M, Sugiyama S, et al. Multiple mitochondrial DNA deletions exist in cardiomyocytes of patients with hypertrophic or dilated cardiomyopathy. *Biochem Biophys Res Comm* 1990; 170:830–836.
28. Kelly DP, Strauss AW. Inherited cardiomyopathies. *N Engl J Med* 1994; 330:913–919.
29. Lakkis NM, Nagueh SF, Kleiman NS, et al. Echocardiography guided ethanol septal reduction for hypertrophic obstructive cardiomyopathy. *Circulation* 1998; 98:1750–1755.
30. Nagueh SF, Lakkis NM, He Z-X, et al. Role of myocardial contrast echocardiography during nonsurgical septal reduction therapy for hypertrophic obstructive cardiomyopathy. *J Am Coll Cardiol* 1998; 32:225–229.
31. Jarcho JA, McKenna W, Pare JAP, et al. Mapping a gene for familial hypertrophic cardiomyopathy to chromosome 14q1. *N Engl J Med* 1989; 321:1372–1378.
32. Hejtmancik JF, Brink PA, Towbin J, et al. Localization of the gene for familial hypertrophic cardiomyopathy to chromosome 14q1 in a diverse U.S. population. *Circulation* 1991; 83:1592–1597.
33. Marian AJ, Roberts R. Familial hypertrophic cardiomyopathy: A paradigm of the cardiac response to injury. *Ann Med* 1998; 30:24–32.
34. Marian AJ, Roberts R. Recent advances in the molecular genetics of hypertrophic cardiomyopathy. *Circulation* 1995; 92:1336–1347.
35. MacRae C, Ghasia N, Kass S, et al. Familial hypertrophic cardiomyopathy with Wolfe-Parkinson-White syndrome maps to a locus on chromosome 7q3. *J Clin Invest* 1995; 96:1216–1220.
36. Ko Y-L, Chen J-J, Tang T-K, et al. Mapping the locus for familial hypertrophic cardiomyopathy to chromosome 11 in a family with a case of apical hypertrophic cardiomyopathy of the Japanese type. *Hum Genet* 1996; 97:457–461.
37. Watkins H, Thierfelder L, Anan R, et al. Independent origin of identical β-cardiac myosin heavy-chain mutations in hypertrophic cardiomyopathy. *Am J Hum Genet* 1993; 53:1180–1185.
38. Dausse E, Komajda M, Fetler L, et al. Familial hypertrophic cardiomyopathy: Microsatellite haplotyping and identification of a hot spot for mutations in the β-myosin heavy chain gene. *J Clin Invest* 1993; 92:2807–2813.
39. Consevage MW, Salada GC, Baylen BG, et al. A new missense mutation, Arg^{719}Gln, in the β-cardiac heavy chain myosin gene of patients with familial hypertrophic cardiomyopathy. *Hum Mol Genet* 1994; 3:1025–1026.
40. Marian AJ, Yu QT, Mares A Jr, et al. Detection of a new mutation in the β-myosin heavy chain gene in an individual with hypertrophic cardiomyopathy. *J Clin Invest* 1992; 90:2156–2165.
41. Abchee AB, Lechin M, Quinones MA, et al. The severity of left ventricular hypertrophy is greater in patients with hypertrophic cardiomyopathy due to malignant mutations (abstr). *J Am Coll Cardiol* 1995; 25:415A.
42. Marian AJ. Sudden cardiac death in patients with hypertrophic cardiomyopathy: From bench to bedside with an emphasis on genetic markers. *Clin Cardiol* 1995; 18:189–198.
43. Anan R, Greve G, Thierfelder L, et al. Prognostic implications of novel β-cardiac myosin heavy chain gene mutations that cause familial hypertrophic cardiomyopathy. *J Clin Invest* 1994; 93:280–285.
44. Moolman J, Corfield VA, Rosen B, et al. Sudden death due to troponin T mutations. *J Am Coll Cardiol* 1997; 29:549–555.
45. Roberts R. Molecular genetics: Therapy or terror? *Circulation* 1994; 89:499–502.
46. Epstein ND, Cohn GM, Cyran F, et al. Differences in clinical expression of hypertrophic cardiomyopathy associated with two distinct mutations in the β-myosin heavy chain gene: A 908 Leu-Val mutation and a 403 Arg-Gln mutation. *Circulation* 1992; 86:345–352.
47. Watkins H, Rosenzweig A, Hwang D, et al. Characteristics and prognostic implications of myosin missense mutations in familial hypertrophic cardiomyopathy. *N Engl J Med* 1992; 326:1108–1114.
48. Watkins H, McKenna W, Thierfelder L, et al. Mutations in the genes for cardiac troponin T and α-tropomyosin in hypertrophic cardiomyopathy. *N Engl J Med* 1995; 332:1058–1064.
49. Poetter K, Jiang H, Hassenzadeh S, et al. Mutations in either the essential or regulatory light chains of myosin are associated with a rare myopathy in human heart and skeletal muscle. *Nature Genet* 1996; 13:63–69.
50. Perryman MB, Yu QT, Marian AJ, et al. Expression of a missense mutation in the mRNA for β-myosin heavy chain in myocardial tissue in hypertrophic cardiomyopathy. *J Clin Invest* 1992; 90:271–277.
51. Marian AJ, Yu QT, Workman R, et al. Angiotensin converting enzyme polymorphism in hypertrophic cardiomyopathy and sudden cardiac death. *Lancet* 1993; 342:1085–1086.
52. Lechin M, Yu QT, Roberts R, et al. Angiotensin I converting enzyme geneotypes and left ventricular hypertrophy in patients with hypertrophic cardiomyopathy. *Circulation* 1995; 92:1808–1812.
53. Maron BJ. Cardiovascular preparticipation screening of competitive athletes. In: Williams RA, ed. *The Athlete and Heart Disease: Diagnosis, Evaluation & Management*. Philadelphia: Lippincott Williams & Wilkins; 1999:273–285.
54. Beohar N, Damaraju S, Prather A. Angiotensin-I converting enzyme genotype DD is a risk factor for coronary artery disease. *J Invest Med* 1995; 43:275–280.
55. Vybiral T, Roberts R, Deitiker PR, et al. Accumulation and

assembly of myosin in the Arg-Gln β-MHC hypertrophic cardiomyopathy mutant. *Circ Res* 1992; 71:1404–1409.
56. Marian AJ, Yu QT, Mann DL, et al. Expression of a mutation causing hypertrophic cardiomyopathy in adult feline cardiocytes disrupts sarcomere assembly in adult feline cardiac myocytes. *Circ Res* 1995; 77:98–106.
57. Oberst L, Zhao G, Park JT, et al. Dominant-negative effect of a mutant cardiac troponin T on cardiac structure and function in transgenic mice. *J Clin Invest* 1998; 102:1498–1505.
58. Vikstrom KL, Factor SM, Leinwand LA. Mice expressing mutant myosin heavy chains are a model for familial hypertrophic cardiomyopathy. *Mol Med Today* 1996; 2:556–567.
59. Geisterfer-Lowrance AA, Christe M, Conner DA, et al. A mouse model of familial hypertrophic cardiomyopathy. *Science* 1996; 272:731–734.
60. Becker KD, Gottshall KR, Hickey R, et al. Point mutations in human cardiac myosin heavy chain have differential effects on sarcomeric structure and assembly: An ATP binding site change disrupts both thick and think filaments, whereas hypertrophic cardiomyopathy mutations display normal assembly. *J Cell Biol* 1997; 137:137–140.
61. Marian J, Wu Y, McCluggage M. A transgenic rabbit model for human hypertrophic cardiomyopathy. *J Clin Invest* 1999; 104:1683–1692.
62. Berenfeld O, Jalife J. Purkinje-muscle reentry as a mechanism of polymorphic ventricular arrhythmias in a 3-dimensional model of the ventricles. *Circ Res* 1998; 82:1063–1077.
63. Pogwizd SM, McKenzie JP, Cain ME. Mechanisms underlying spontaneous and induced ventricular arrhythmias in patients with idiopathic dilated cardiomyopathy. *Circulation* 1998; 98:2404–2414.
64. Service R. DNA chips survey an entire genome. *Science* 1998; 281:1122.
65. Towbin JA. Molecular genetic aspects of cardiomyopathy. *Biochem Med Metab Biol* 1993; 49:285–320.
66. Klein A, Lebreton A, Lemoine J. Identification of urinary ligosaccharides by matrix-assisted laser desorption ionization time-of-flight mass spectrometry. *Clin Chem* 1998; 44:2422–2428.
67. Meikle PJ, Yan M, Ravenscroft EM, et al. Altered trafficking and turnover of LAMP-1 in Pompe disease-affected cells. *Mol Genet Metab* 1999; 66:179–188.
68. Bijvoet AJ, van de Kamp EH, Kroos MA, et al. Generalized glycogen storage and cardiomegaly in a knockout mouse model of Pompe disease. *Hum Mol Genet* 1998; 7:53–62.
69. Raben N, Nagaraju K, Lee E, et al. Targeted disruption of the acid α-glucosidase gene in mice causes an illness with critical features of both infantile and adult human glycogen storage disease type II. *J Biol Chem* 1998; 273:19086–19092.
70. Yang HW, Kikuchi T, Hagiwara Y, et al. Recombinant human acid α-glucosidase-deficient human fibroblasts, quail fibroblasts, and quail myoblasts. *Pediatr Res* 1998; 43:374–380.
71. Kikuchi T, Yang HW, Pennybacker M, et al. Clinical and metabolic correction of Pompe disease by enzyme therapy in acid maltase-deficient quail. *J Clin Invest* 1998; 101:827–833.
72. Pauly DF, Johns DC, Matelis LA, et al. Complete correction of acid α-glucosidase deficiency in Pompe disease fibroblats in vitro, and lysosomally targeted expression in neonatal rat cardiac and skeletal muscle. *Gene Ther* 1998; 5:473–480.
73. Wiedemann HR. Complexo malformatif familial avec hernie unbilicate et macroglossie: Un "syndrome nouveau"? *J Genet Hum* 1964; 13:223–232.
74. Beckwith JB. Macroglossia, omphalocele, adrenal cytomegaly, gigantism and hyperplastic visceromegaly. *Birth Defects* 1969; 2:188–196.
75. Sotelo-Avila C, Gonzalez-Crussi F, Fowler JW. Complete and incomplete forms of Beckwith-Wiedemann syndrome: Their oncogenic potential. *J Pediatr* 1980; 96:47–50.
76. Best LG, Hoekstra RE. Wiedemann-Beckwith syndrome: Autosomal dominant inheritance in a family. *Am J Med Genet* 1981; 9:291–299.
77. Bhuiyan ZA, Yatsuki H, Sasaguri T, et al. Functional analysis of the p57KIP2 gene mutation in Beckwith-Wiedemann syndrome. *Hum Genet* 1999; 104:205–210.
78. Hatada I, Nabetani A, Morisaki H, et al. New p57KIP2 mutations in Beckwith-Wiedemann syndrome. *Hum Genet* 1997; 100: 681–683.
79. Lam WW, Hatada I, Ohishi S, et al. Analysis of germlinie CDKNIC (p57KIP2) mutations in familial and sporadic Beckwith-Wiedemann syndrome (BWS) provides a novel genotype-phenotype correlation. *J Med Genet* 1999; 36:518–523.
80. Lee MP, De Baun M, Randhawa G, et al. Low frequency of p57KIP2 mutation in Beckwith-Wiedemann syndrome. *Am J Hum Genet* 1997; 61:304–309.
81. Zhang P, Liegeois NJ, Wong C, et al. Altered cell differentiation and proliferation in mice lacking p57KIP2 indicates a role in Beckwith-Wiedemann syndrome. *Nature* 1997; 387:151–158.
82. Lee MP, Hu RJ, Johnson LA, Feinberg AP. Human KVLQT1 gene shows tissue-specific imprinting and encompasses Beckwith-Wiedemann syndrome chromosomal rearrangements. *Nature Genet* 1997; 15:181–185.
83. Smilinich NJ, Day CD, Fitzpatrick GV, et al. A maternally methylated CpG island in KVLQT1 is associated with an antisense paternal transcript and loss of imprinting in Beckwith-Wiedemann syndrome. *Proc Natl Acad Sci USA* 1999; 96:8064–8069.
84. Sun FL, Dean WL, Kelsey G, et al. Transactivation of Igf2 in a mouse model of Beckwith-Wiedemann syndrome. *Nature* 1997; 389:809–815.
85. Catchpoole D, Lam WW, Valler D, et al. Epigenetic modification and uniparental inheritance of H19 in Beckwith-Wiedemann syndrome. *J Med Genet* 1997; 34:353–359.
86. Mitsuya K, Megura M, Lee MP, et al. LIT1, an imprinted antisense RNA in the human KVLQT1 locus identified by screening for differentially expressed transcripts using monochromosomal hybrids. *Human Mol Genet* 1999; 8:1209–1217.
87. Durr A, Cossee M, Agid Y, et al. Clinical and genetic abnormalities in patients with Friedreich's ataxia. *N Engl J Med* 1996; 335:1169–1175.
88. Chamberlain S, Shaw J, Rowland A, et al. Mapping of mutation causing Friedreich's ataxia to human chromosome 9. *Nature* 1988; 334:248–250.
89. Campuzano V, Montermini L, Mooto MD, et al. Friedreich's ataxia: 81. Autosomal recessive disease caused by an intronic GAA triplet repeat expansion. *Science* 1996; 271:1423–1427.
90. Filla A, De Michele G, Cavalcanti F, et al. The relationship between trinucleotide (GAA) repeat length and classical features in Friedreich ataxia. *Am J Hum Genet* 1996; 59:554–560.
91. Montermini L, Richter A, Morgan K, et al. Phenotypic variability in Friedreich ataxia: Role of the associated GAA triplet repeat expansion. *Ann Neurol* 1997; 41:675–682.
92. Lamont PJ, Davis MB, Wood NW. Identification and sizing of the GAA triplet repeat expansion of Friedreich ataxia in 56 patients: Clinical and genetic correlates. *Brain* 1997; 120:672–680.
93. Monros E, Molto MD, Martinez F, et al. Phenotype correlation and intergenerational dynamics of the Friedreich ataxia GAA trinucleotide repeat. *Am J Hum Genet* 1997; 61:101–110.
94. Campuzano V, Montermini L, Lutz Y, et al. Frataxin is reduced in Friedreich ataxia patients and is associated with mitochondrial membranes. *Hum Mol Genet* 1997; 11:1771–1780.
95. Rotig A, de Lonlay P, Chretien D, et al. Aconitase and mitochondrial iron-sulphur protein deficiency in Friedreich ataxia. *Nature Genet* 1997; 17:215–217.
96. Knight SAB, Kim R, Pain D, Dancis A. the yeast connection to Friedreich ataxia. *Am J Hum Genet* 1999; 64:365–371.
97. Koutnikova H, Campuzano V, Foury F, et al. Studies of human,

mouse and yeast homologues indicate a mitochondrial function for frataxin. *Nature Genet* 1997; 16:345–351.
98. Codd MB, Sugrue DD, Gersh BJ, et al. Epidemiology of idiopathic dilated and hypertrophic cardiomyopathy: A population-based study in Olmsted County, Minnesota, 1975–1984. *Circulation* 1989; 80:564–572.
99. Durand JB, Bachinski LL, Beiling L, et al. Localization of a gene responsible for familial idiopathic dilated cardiomyopathy to chromosome 1q32. *Circulation* 1995; 92:3387–3389.
100. Krajinovic M, Pinamonti B, Sinagra G, et al. Linkage of familial dilated cardiomyopathy to chromosome 9. *Am J Hum Genet* 1995; 57:846–852.
101. Siu BL, Nimura H, Osborne JA, et al. Familial dilated cardiiomyopathy locus maps to chromosome 2q31. *Circulation* 1999; 99:1022–1026.
102. Bowles KR, Gajarski R, Porter P, et al. Gene mapping of familial autosomal dominant dilated cardiomyopathy to chromosome 10q21-23. *J Clin Invest* 1996; 98:1355–1360.
103. Kass S, MacRae C, Graber HL, et al. A gene defect that causes conduction system disease and dilated cardiomyopathy maps to chromosome 1p1-1q1. *Nature Genet* 1994; 7:546–551.
104. Olson TM, Keating MT. Mapping a cardiomyopathy locus to chromosome 3p22-25. *J Clin Invest* 1996; 97:528–532.
105. Messina DN, Speer MC, Pericak-Vance MA, et al. Linkage of familial dilated cardiomyopathy with conduction defect and muscular dystrophy to chromosome 6q23. *Am J Hum Genet* 1997; 61:909–917.
106. Olson T, Michels VV, Thibodeau, SN, et al. Actin mutations in dilated cardiomypathy, a heritable form of heart failure. *Science* 1998; 280:750–752.
107. Li D, Tapscott T, Gonzalez O, et al. Desmin mutation responsible for idiopathic dilated cardiomyopathy. *Circulation* 1999; 100:461–464.
108. Morgensen J, Klausen C, Pedersen AK, et al. α-Cardiac actin is a novel disease gene in familial hypertrophic cardiomyopathy. *J Clin Invest* 1999; 103:R39–R43.
109. Fuchs E. Intermediate filaments and disease: Mutations that cripple cell strength. *J Cell Biol* 1994; 125:511–516.
110. Milner DJ, Weitzner G, Tran D, et al. Disruption of muscle architecture and myocardial degeneration in mice lacking desmin. *J Cell Biol* 1996; 1343:1255–1270.
111. Maeda M, Holder E, Lowes B, et al. Dilated cardiomyoapthy associated with deficiency of the cytoskeletal protein metavinculin. *Circulation* 1997; 95:17–20.
112. Marian AJ, Roberts R. Molecular pathophysiology of cardiomyopathies. In: Sperelakis N, ed. *Cardiac Physiology*. San Diego, CA: Academic Press; 1999.
113. Towbin JA. The role of cytoskeletal proteins in cardiomyopathies. *Curr Opin Cell Biol* 1998; 10:131–139.
114. Towbin JA, Bowles KR, Bowles NE. Etiologies of cardiomyopathy and heart failure: Evidence for a final common pathway for disorders of the myocardium. *Nature Med* 1999; 5:266–267.
115. Towbin JA, Hejtmancik JF, Brink P, et al. X-linked dilated cardiomyopathy (XLCM): Molecular genetic evidence of linkage to the Duchenne muscular dystrophy gene at the Xp21 locus. *Circulation* 1993; 87:1854–1865.
116. Towbin JA. Biochemical and molecular characterization of X-linked dilated cardiomyopathy. In: Clark EB, Markwald RR, Takao A, eds. *Developmental Mechanisms of Heart Disease*. New York: Futura; 1995:121–132.
117. Ohlendieck K, Matsumura K, lonasescu W, et al. Duchenne muscular dystrophy: Deficiency of dystrophin-associated proteins in the sarcolemma. *Neurology* 1993; 43:795–800.
118. Bies RD, Maeda M, Roberds SL, et al. A 5′ dystrophin duplication mutation causes membrane deficiency of alpha-dystroglycan in a family with X-linked cardiomyopathy. *J Mol Cell Cardiol* 1997; 29:3175–3188.
119. Towbin JA, Ortiz-Lopez R. X-linked dilated cardiomyopathy is not due to a muscle promoter deletion in dystrophin in 3 families. *N Engl J Med* 1994; 330:369–370.
120. Ortiz-Lopez R, Li H, Su J, et al. Evidence for a dystrophin missense mutation as a cause of X-linked dilated cardiomyopathy (XLCM). *Circulation* 1997; 95:2434–2440.
121. Yoshida K, Ikeda S, Nakamura A, et al. Molecular analysis of the Duchenne muscular dystrophy gene in patients with Becker muscular dystrophy presenting with dilated cardiomyopathy. *Muscle Nerve* 1993; 16:1161–1166.
122. Muntoni F, Cau M, Ganau A, Congi R, et al. Brief report: Deletion of the dystrophin muscle-promoter region associated with X-linked dilated cardiomyopathy. *N Engl J Med* 1993; 329:921–925.
123. Milasin J, Muntoni F, Severini GM, et al. A point mutation in the 5′ splice site of the dystrophin gene first intron responsible for X-linked dilated cardiomyopathy. *Hum Mol Genet* 1996; 5:73–79.
124. Yoshida K, Nakamura A, Yazaki M, et al. Insertional mutation by transposable element L1, in the DMD gene results in X-linked dilated cardiomyopathy. *Hum Mol Genet* 1998; 7:1120–1132.
125. Ferlini A, Galie N, Merlini L, et al. A novel Alu-like element rearranged in the dystrophin gene causes a splicing mutation in a family with X-linked dilated cardiomyopathy. *Am J Hum Genet* 1998; 63:436–446.
126. Neustein HB, Lurie PR, Dahms B, et al. An X-linked recessive cardiomyopathy with abnormal mitochondria. *Pediatrics* 1998; 64:24–29.
127. Barth PG, Schotte HR, Berden JA, et al. An X-linked mitochondrial disease affecting cardiac muscle skeletal muscle and neutrophil leukocytes. *J Neurol Sci* 1983; 62:327–355.
128. Bolhuis PA, Hensels GW, Hulsebos TJM, et al. Mapping of the locus for X-linked cardioskeletal myopathy with neutropenia and abnormal mitochondria (Barth syndrome) to Xq28. *Am J Hum Genet* 1991; 48:481–485.
129. Bione S, D'Adamo P, Maestrini E, et al. A novel X-linked gene, G4.5, is responsible for Barth syndrome. *Nature Genet* 1996; 12:385–389.
130. Bleyl SB, Mumford Thompson V, et al. Neonatal lethal noncompaction of the left ventricular myocardium is allelic with Barth syndrome. *Am J Hum Genet* 1997; 61:868–872.
131. Johnston J, Kelley, RI, Feigenbaum A, et al. Mutation characterization and genotype-phenotype correlation in Barth syndrome. *Am J Med Genet* 1997; 61:1053–1058.
132. D'Adamo P, Fassone L, Patton MA, et al. The X-linked gene G4.5 is responsible for different infantile dilated cardiomyopathies. *Am J Hum Genet* 1997; 61:862–867.
133. Thiene G, Basso C, Danieli G, et al. Arrhythmogenic right ventricular cardiomyopathy. *Trends Cardiovasc Med* 1997; 7:84–90.
134. Thiene G, Nava A, Corrado D, et al. Right ventricular cardiomyopathy and sudden death in young people. *N Engl J Med* 1988; 318:129–133.
135. Shen WK, Edwards WD, Hammill SC, et al. Right ventricular dysplasia: A need for precise pathological definition for interpretation of sudden death. *J Am Coll Cardiol* 1994; 23:34.
136. Rampazzo A, Nava A, Erne P, et al. A new locus for arrhythmogenic right ventricular cardiomyopathy (ARVD2) maps to chromosome 1q42-q43. *Hum Mol Genet* 1995; 4:2151–2154.
137. Severini GM, Krajinovic M, Pinamonti B, et al. A new locus for arrhythmogenic right ventricular dysplasia on the long arm of chromosome 14. *Genomics* 1996; 31:193–200.
138. Coonar AS, Protonotarios N, Tsatsopoulou A, et al. Gene for arrhythmogenic right ventricular cardiomyopathy with diffuse nonepidermolytic palmoplantar keratoderma and woolly hair wooly hair (Naxos disease) maps to 17q21. *Circulation* 1998; 97:2049–2058.
139. Ahmad F, Li D, Karibe A, et al. Localization of a gene responsible for arrhythmogenic right ventricular dysplasia to chromosome 3p23. *Circulation* 1998; 98:2791–2795.

140. Li D, Ahmad F, Gardner MJ, Weilbaecher D, et al. The locus of a novel gene responsible for arrhythmogenic right ventricular dysplasia characterized by early onset and high penetrance maps to chromosome 10p12-p14. *Am J Hum Genet* 2000; 66:148–156.
141. McKenna WJ, Thiere G, Nava AA, et al. Diagnosis of arrhythmogenic right ventricular dysplasis/cardiomyopathy. *Br Heart J* 1994; 71:215–218.
142. Jacobson DR, Pastore R, Yaghoubian R, et al. Variant-sequence transthyretin (isoleucine 122) in late-onset cardiac amyloidosis in black Americans. *N Engl J Med* 1997; 336:466–473.
143. Jacobson DR, Ittmann M, Buxbaum JN, et al. Transthyretin Ile 122 and cardiac arryloidosis in African-Americans; 2 case reports. *Tex Heart Inst J* 1997; 24:45–52.
144. Goldfarb LG, Park K-Y, Cervenakova L, et al. Missense mutations in desmin associated with familial cardiac and skeletal myopathy. *Nature Genet* 1998; 19:402–403.
145. Neufeld EF, Muenzer J. The mucopolysaccharidoses. In: Scriver CR, Beaudet AL, Sly NS, Valle D, ed. *The Metabolic and Molecular Basis of Inherited Disease*. New York: McGraw-Hill; 1995: 2465–2494.
146. Bach G, Freidman R, Weissmann B, et al. The defect in Hurler and Scheie syndromes: Deficiency of α-L-iduronidase. *Proc Natl Acad Sci USA* 1972; 69:2049–2051.
147. Dangel JH. Cardiovascular changes in children with mucopolysaccharide strorage diseases and related disorders—Clinical and echocardiographic findings in 64 patients. *Eur J Pediatr* 1998; 157:534–538.
148. Scott HS, Guo X, Hopwood JJ, et al. Structural and sequence of the human α-L-iduronidase gene. *Genomics* 1992; 13:1311–1313.
149. Scott HS, Litjens T, Nelson PV, et al. Identification of mutations in the α-L-iduronidase gene (IDUA) that cause Hurler and Scheie syndromes. *Am J Hum Genet* 1993; 53:973–986.
150. Krivit W, Peters C, Shapiro EG. Bone marrow transplantation as effective treatment of central nervous system disease in globoid cell leukodystrophy, metachromatic leukodystrophy, adenoleukodystrophy, mannosidosis, fucosidosis, aspartylglucosaminuria, Hurler, Maroteaux-Lamy, and Sly syndromes, and Gaucher disease type III. *Curr Opin Neurol* 1999; 12:167–176.
151. Huang MM, Wong A, Yu X, et al. Retrovirus-mediated transfer of the human α-L-iduronidase cDNA into human hematopoietic progenitor cells leads to correction in trans of Hurler fibroblasts. *Gene Ther* 1997; 4:1150–1159.
152. Russell C, Hendson G, Jevon G, et al. Murine MPS1: Insights into the pathogenesis of Hurler syndrome. *Clin Genet* 1998; 53:349–361.
153. Clarke LA, Russell CS, Pownall S, et al. Murine mucopolysaccharidoses type I: Targeted disruption of the murne α-L-iduronidase gene. *Hum Mol Genet* 1997; 6:503–511.
154. He X, Li CM, Simonaro CM, et al. Identification and characterization of the molecular lesion causing mucopolysaccharidoses type I in cats. *Mol Genet Metab* 1999; 67:106–112.
155. Hartog C, Fryer A, Upadhyaya M. Mutation analysis of iduronate-2-sulphatase gene in 24 patients with Hunter syndrome: characterization of 6 novel mutations. *Hum Mutat* 1999; 14:87.
156. Timms KM, Bondeson ML, Ansari-Lari MA, et al. Molecular and phenotypic variation in patients with severe Hunter syndrome. *Hum Mol Genet* 1997; 6:479–486.
157. Li P, Bellows AB, Thompson JN. Molecular basis of iduronate-2-sulphatase gene mutations in patients with mucopolysaccharidosis type II (Hunter syndrome). *J Med Genet* 1999; 36:21–27.
158. DiFrancesco C, Cracco C, Tomanin R, et al. In vitro correction of iduronate-2-sulphatase deficiency by adenovirus gene transfer. *Gene Ther* 1997; 4:442–448.
159. Marra BL, Medina CD, Hoang GKB, et al. Gene therapy for neurologic disease: Benchtop discoveries to bedside applications. 2. The bedside. *J Child Neurol* 1997; 12:77–84.
160. Stroncek DF, Hubel A, Shankar RA, et al. Retroviral transduction and expansion of peripheral blood lymphocytes for the treatment of mucopolysaccharidosis type II, Hunter's syndrome. *Transfusion* 1999; 39:343–350.
161. Tomatsu S, Fukuda S, Masue M, et al. Morquio disease: Isolation, characterization and expression of full-length cDNA for human N-acetyl-galactosamine-6-sulfate sulfatase. *Biochem Biophys Res Comm* 1991; 1871:677–683.
162. Masuno M, Tomatsu S, Nakashima Y, et al. Mucopolysaccharidosis IVA: Assignment of the human N-acetylgalactosamine-6-sulfatase (GALNS) gene to chromosome 16q24. *Genomics* 1993; 16:777–778.
163. Fukuda S, Tomatsu S, Masue M, et al. Mucopolysaccharidosis type IVA N-acetyl galactosamine-6-sulfate sulfatase exonic point mutations in classical Morquio and mild cases. *J Clin Invest* 1992; 90:1049–1053.
164. Yamada N, Fukuda S, Tomatsu S, et al. Molecular heterogeneity in mucopolysaccharidosis IVA in Australia and Northern Ireland: Nine novel mutations including T312S, a common allele that confers a mild phenotype. *Hum Mutat* 1998; 11:202–208.
165. Jackson CE, Yuhki N, Desnick RJ, et al. Feline arylsulfatase B (ARSB): Isolation and expression of the cDNA, comparison with human ARSB, and gene localization to feline chromosome A1. *Genomics* 1992; 14:403–411.
166. Mondaressi S, Rupp K, Von Figura K, et al. Structure of the human arylsulfatase B gene. *Biol Chem Hoppe Seyler* 1993; 374:327–335.
167. Voskoboeva E, Isbrandt D, Von Figura K, et al. Four novel mutant alleles of the arylsulfatase B gene in two patients with intermediate form of mucopolysaccharidosis VI (Maroteaux-Lamy syndrome). *Hum Genet* 1994; 93:259–264.
168. Cox GF, Kunkel LM. Dystrophies and heart disease. *Curr Opin Cardiol* 1997; 12:329–343.
169. Sadoulet-Puccio HM, Kunkel LM. Dystrophin and its isoforms. *Brain Pathol* 1996; 6:25–35.
170. Bonnemann CG, McNally EM, Kunkel LM. Beyond dystrophin: Current progress in the muscular dystrophies. *Curr Opin Pediatr* 1997; 8:569–582.
171. Malhotra SB, Hart KA, Klamut HJ, et al. Frame-shift deletions in patients with Duchenne and Becker muscular dystrophy. *Science* 1988; 242:755–759.
172. Melacini P, Fanin M, Danieli GA, et al. Myocardial involvement is very frequent among patients affected with subclinical Becker muscular dystrophy. *Circulation* 1996; 94:3168–3175.
173. Yoshida K, Ikeda S, Nakamura A, et al. Molecular analysis of the Duchenne muscular dystrophy gene in patients with Becker muscular dystrophy presenting with dilated cardiomyopathy. *Muscle Nerve* 1993; 16:1161–1166.
174. Nigro V, Okazaki Y, Belsito A, et al. Identification of the Syrian hamster cardiomyopathy gene. *Hum Mol Genet* 1997; 6:601–607.
175. Sakamoto A, Ono K, Abe M, et al. Both hypertrophic and dilated cardiomyopathies are caused by mutation of the same gene, α-sarcoglycan in hamsters: An animal model of disrupted dystrophin-associated glycoprotein complex. *Proc Natl Acad Sci USA* 1997; 94:13873–13878.
176. Deconinck KAE, Potter AC, Tinsley JM, et al. Postsynaptic abnormalities in the neuromuscular junctions of utrophin-deficient mice. *J Cell Biol* 1997; 136:883 894.
177. Grady RM, Merlie JP, Sanes SR. Subtle neuromuscular defects in utrophin-deficient mice. *J Cell Biol* 1997; 136:871–882.
178. Deconinck AE, Rafael JA, Skinner JA, et al. Utrophin-dystrophin-deficient mice as a model for Duchenne muscular dystrophy. *Cell* 1997; 90:717–727.
179. Grady RM, Teng HB, Nichol MC, et al. Skeletal and cardiac myopathies in mice lacking utrophin and dystrophin: A model for Duchenne muscular dystrophy. *Cell* 1997; 90:729–738.
180. Lumeng CN, Phelps SF, Rafael JA, et al. Characterization of

dystrophin and utrophin diversity in the mouse. *Hum Mol Genet* 1999; 8:593–599.
181. Tinsley JM, Potter AC, Phelps SR, et al. Amelioration of the dystrophic phenotype of *mdx* mice using a truncated utrophin transgene. *Nature* 1996; 384:349–353.
182. Rafael JA, Sunada Y, Cole NM, et al. Prevention of dystrophic pathology in *mdx* mice by a truncated dystrophin isoform. *Hum Mol Genet* 1994; 3:1725–1733.
183. Gussoni E, Soneoka Y, Strickland CD, et al. Dystrophin expression in the *mdx* mouse restored by stem cell transplantation. *Nature* 1999; 401:390–394.
184. Consalez GG, Thomas NST, Stayton CL, et al. Assignment of Emery-Dreifuss muscular dystrophy to the distal region of Xq28: The results of a collaborative study. *Am J Hum Genet* 1991; 48:468–480.
185. Bione S, Maestrini E, Rivella S, et al. Identification of a novel X-linked gene responsible for Emery-Dreifuss muscular dystrophy. *Nature Genet* 1994; 8:323–327.
186. Harris CA, Andryuk PJ, Cline SW, et al. Structure and mapping of the human thymopletin (TMPO) gene and relationship of the human TMPO-b to rat lamin-associated polypeptide-2. *Genomics* 1995; 28:198–205.
187. Nagano A, Koga R, Ogawa M, et al. Emerin deficiency at the nuclear membrane in patients with Emery-Dreifuss muscular dystrophy. *Nature Genet* 1996; 12:254–259.
188. Manilal S, thi Man N, Sewry CA, et al. The Emery-Dreifuss muscular dystrophy protein, emerin, is a nuclear membrane protein. *Hum Mol Genet* 1996; 5:801–808.
189. Bonne G, DiBarletta MR, Varnous S, et al. Mutations in the gene encoding lamin A/C cause autosomal dominant Emery-Dreifuss muscular dystrophy. *Nature Genet* 1999; 21:285–289.
190. Brunner H, Korneluk R, Coerwinkel-Driessen M, et al. Myotonic dystrophy is closely linked to the gene for muscle-type creatine kinase (CKMM). *Hum Genet* 1989; 81:308–310.
191. Timchenko LT. Myotonic dystrophy: The role of RNA CUG triplet repeats. *Am J Hum Genet* 1999; 64:360–364.
192. Timchenko LT, Timchenko NA, Caskey CT, et al. Novel proteins with binding specificity for DNA CTG repeats and RNA CUG repeats: Implications for myotonic dystrophy. *Hum Mol Genet* 1996; 5:115–121.
193. Timchenko LT, Miller JW, Timchenko NA, et al. Identification of a (CUG)n triplet repeat RNA-binding protein and its expression in myotonic dystrophy. *Nucleic Acids Res* 1996; 24:4407–4414.
194. Roberts R, Timchenko NA, Miller JW, et al. Altered phosphorylation and intracellular distribution of a (CUG) triplet repeat RNA-binding protein in patients with myotonic dystrophy and in myotonic protein kinase knock out mice. *Proc Natl Acad Sci USA* 1997; 94:13221–13226.
195. Jansen G, Groenen PJ, Bachner D, et al. Abnormal myotonic dystrophy protein kinase levels produce only mild myopathy in mice. *Nature Genet* 1996; 13:316–324.
196. Philips AV, Timchenko LT, Cooper T. Disruption of splicing regulated by a CUG-binding protein in myotonic dystrophy. *Science* 1998; 280:737–740.
197. Lu X, Timchenko NA, Timchenko LT. Cardiac elav-type RNA-binding protein (ETR-3) binds to RNA CUG repeats expanded in myotonic dystrophy. *Hum Mol Genet* 1999; 8:53–60.
198. Hanson PA, Rowland LP. Mobius syndrome and facioscapulohumeral muscular dystrophy. *Arch Neurol* 1971; 24:31–39.
199. Galluzzi G, Deidda G, Cacurri S, et al. Molecular analysis of 4q35 rearrangements in fascioscapulohumeral muscular dystrophy (FSHD): application to family studies for a correct genetic advice and a reliable prenatal diagnosis of the disease. *Neuromusc Disord* 1999; 9(3):190–198.
200. North KN, Laing NG, Wallgren-Pettersson C, et al. Nemaline myopathy: Current concepts. *J Med Genet* 1997; 34:705–713.
201. Wallgren-Patterson C. Congenital nemaline myopathy: A clinical follow-up study of twelve patients. *J Neurol Sci* 1989; 89:1–14.
202. Nowak KH, Wattansirichaigoon D, Goebel HH, et al. Mutations in the skeletal muscle α-actin gene in patients with actin myopathy and nemaline myopathy. *Nature Genet* 1999; 23:208–212.
203. Goebel HH, Anderson JR, Hubner C, et al. Congenital myopathy with excess of thin filaments. *Neuromusc Disord* 1997; 7:160–168.
204. Laing NG, Wilton SD, Akkari PA, et al. A mutation in the α-tropomyosin gene TPM3 associated with autosomal dominant nemaline myopathy. *Nature Genet* 1995; 9:75–79.
205. Pelin K, Hilpelä P, Donner K, et al. Mutations in the nebulin gene associated with autosomal recessive nemaline myopathy. *Proc Natl Acad Sci USA* 1999; 96:2305–2310.
206. Sellers FJ, Keith JD, Manning JA. The diagnosis of primary endocardial fibroelastosis. *Circulation* 1994; 29:49–59.
207. Opitiz JM. Genetic aspects of endocardial fibroelastosis. *Am J Med Genet* 1982; 11:92–96.
208. Ni J, Bowles NE, Kim Y, et al. Viral infection of the myocardium in endocardial fibroelastosis: Molecular evidence for the role of mumps virus as an etiological agent. *Circulation* 1997; 95:133–139.
209. Waber LJ, Valle D, Neill C, et al. Carnintine deficiency presenting as familial cardiomyopathy: A treatable defect in carnitine transport. *J Pediatr* 1982; 101:700–705.
210. Shoji Y, Koizumi A, Kayo T, et al. Evidence for linkage of human primary systemic carnitine deficiency with D5S436: A novel gene locus on chromosome 5q. *Am J Hum Genet* 1998; 63:101–108.
211. Koizumi T, Nikaido H, Hayakawa J, et al. Infantile disease with microvascular fatty infiltration of viscera spontaneously occuring in C3H-H2-2 strain of mouse with similarities to Reye's syndrome. *Lab Anim* 1988; 22:83–87.
212. Kuwajima M, Kono N, Horiuchi M, et al. Animal model of systemic carnitine deficiency: Analysis in C3H-H-2° strain of mouse associated with juvenile visceral steatosis. *Biochem Biophys Res Commun* 1991; 174:1090–1094.
213. Nikaido H, Horiuchi M, Hashimoto N, et al. Mapping the *jvs* (juvenlie steatosis) gene, which causes systemic carnitine deficiency in mice of chromosome 11. *Mamm Genome* 1995; 6:369–370.
214. Nezu J-i, Tamai I, Oku A, et al. Primary systemic carnitine deficiency is caused by mutations in a gene encoding sodium ion-dependent carnitine transporter. *Naure Genet* 1999; 21:91–94.
215. Kelly JP, Kim J, Billadello JJ, et al. Nucleotide sequence of medium-chain acyl-CoA dehydrogenase mRNA and its expression in enzyme-deficient human tissue. *Proc Natl Acad Sci USA* 1987; 84:4068–4072.
216. Romppanen EL, Mononen T, Monenen I. Molecular diagnosis of medium-chain acyl-CoA dehydrogenase deficiency by oligonucleotide ligation assay. *Clin Chem* 1998; 44:68–71.
217. Andresen BS, Bross P, Udvari S, et al. The molecular basis of medium-chain acyl-CoA dehydrogenase (MCAD) deficiency in compound heterozygous patients: Is there correlation between genotype and phenotype? *Hum Mol Genet* 1997; 6:695–707.
218. Indo Y, Yang-Feng T, Glassberg R, et al. Molecular cloning and nucleotide sequence of cDNAs encoding human long-chain acyl-CoA dehydrogenase and assignment of the location of its gene (ACADL) to chromosome 2. *Genomics* 1991; 11:609–620.
219. Izai K, Uchida Y, Orii T, et al. Novel fatty acid β-oxidation enzymes in rat liver mitochondria: I. Purification and properties of very long-chain acyl-coenzyme A dehydrogenase. *J Biol Chem* 1992; 267:1027–1033.
220. Uchida Y, Izai K, Orii T, et al. Novel fatty acid β-oxidation enzymes in rat liver mitochondria. II. Purification and properties of enoyl-coenzyme A (CoA) hydratase/3-hydroxyacyl-CoA dehydrogenase 3-ketoacyl-CoA thiolase trifunctional protein. *J Biol Chem* 1992; 267:1034–1041.
221. Andresen BS, Bross P, Vianey-Saban C, et al. Cloning and characterization of human very-long-chain acyl-CoA dehydrogenase

cDNA, chromosomal assignment of the gene and identification in four patients of nine different mutations within the VLCAD gene. *Hum Mol Genet* 1996; 5:461–472.
222. Aoyama T, Souri M, Ueno I, et al. Cloning of human very-long-chain acyl-coenzyme A dehydrogenase and molecular characterization of its deficiency in two patients. *Am J Hum Genet* 1995; 57:273–283.
223. Strauss AS, Powell CK, Hale DE, et al. Molecular basis of human mitochondrial very-long-chain acyl-CoA dehydrogenase deficiency causing cardiomyopathy and sudden death in childhood. *Proc Natl Acad Sci USA* 1995; 92:10196–10500.
224. Andresen BS, Vianey-Saban C, Bross P, et al. The mutational spectrum in very-long-chain acyl-CoA dehydrogenase (VLCAD) deficiency. *J Inherit Metab* 1996; 19:169–172.
225. Andresen BA, Olpin S, Poorthuis BJHM, et al. Clear correlation of genotype with disease phenotype in very-long chain acyl-CoA dehydrogenase deficiency. *Am J Hum Genet* 1999; 64:479–494.
226. Colucci WS, Lorell BH, Schoen FJ, et al. Hypertrophic obstructive cardiomyopathy due to Fabry's disease. *N Engl J Med* 1982; 307:926–928.
227. Becker AE, Schoorl R, Balk AG, van der Heide RM. Cardiac manifestations of Fabry's disease: Report of a case with mitral insufficiency and electrocardiographic evidence of myocardial infarction. *Am J Cardiol* 1975; 36:829–835.
228. Lewin MB, Belmont J, McNamara DG, et al. Further associations of congenital heart disease and genetic syndromes: Report of a case of tetralogy of Fallot and Fabry's disease. *Pediatr Cardiol* 1999; 20:236–237.
229. Cantor WJ, Butany J, Iwanochko M, et al. Restrictive cardiomyopathy secondary to Fabry's disease. *Circulation* 1998; 98:1457–1459.
230. Cantor WJ, Daly P, Iwanochko M, et al. Cardiac transplantation for Fabry's disease. *Can J Cardiol* 1998; 14:81–84.
231. Bishop DF, Calhoun DH, Bernstein HS, et al. Human alpha-galactosidase A: Nucleotide sequence of a cDNA clone encoding the mature enzyme. *Proc Natl Acad Sci USA* 1986; 83:4859–4863.
232. Eng CM, Desnick RJ. Molecular basis of Fabry disease: Mutations and polymorphisms in the human alpha-glactosidase A gene. *Proc Natl Acad Sci USA* 1994; 3:103–111.
233. Germain DP, Poenaru L. Fabry disease: Identification of novel α-galactosidase A mutations and molecular carrier detection by use of fluorescent chemical cleavage mismatches. *Biochem Biophys Res Commun* 1999; 257:708–713.
234. Suzuki K, Proia RL, Suzuki K. Mouse models of human lysosomal diseases. *Brain Pathol* 1998; 8:195–215.
235. Ziegler RJ, Yew NS, Li C, et al. Correction of enzymatic and lysosomal storage defects in Fabry mice by adenovirus-mediated gene transfer. *Hum Gene Ther* 1999; 10:1667–1682.
236. Skovby P. Homocystinuria: Clinical, biochemical and enetic aspects of cystathionine beta-synthase and its deficiency in man. *Acta Paediatr Scand* 1985; 321:14–21.
237. Mudd SH, Skovby F, Levy HL, et al. The natural history of homocystinuria due to cystathionine β-synthase deficiency. *Am J Hum Genet* 1985; 37:1–31.
238. Mandel H, Brenner B, Berant M, et al. Coexistence of hereditary homocystinuria and factor V Leiden: Effect on thrombosis. *N Engl J Med* 1996; 334:763–768.
239. Munke M, Kraus JP, Ohura T, Francke U. The gene for cystathionine beta-synthase (CBS) maps to the subtelomeric region on human chromosome 21q and to proximal mouse chromosome 17. *Am J Hum Genet* 1988; 42:550–559.
240. Kraus JP, Oliverusova J, Sokolova J, et al. The human cystathionine β-synthase (CBS) gene: Complete sequence, alternative splicing, and polymorphisms. *Genomics* 1998; 52:312–324.
241. Seashore MR. Tandem spectrometry in newborn screening. *Curr Opin Pediatr* 1998; 10:609–614.
242. Mayer EL, Jacobsen DW, Robinson K. Homocysteine and coronary atherosclerosis. *J Am Coll Cardiol* 1996; 27:517–527.
243. den Heijer M, Koster T, Blom HJ, et al. Hyperhomocysteinemia as a risk factor for deep-vein thrombosis. *N Engl J Med* 1996; 334:759–762.
244. Tsai J, Wang H, Perrella MA, et al. Induction of cyclin a gene expression by homocysteine in vascular smooth muscle cells. *J Clin Invest* 1996; 97:146–153.
245. Attardi G. The elucidation of human mitochondrial genome: A historical perspective. *Bioessays* 1994; 5:34–39.
246. Smeitink J, van den Heuvel L. Human mitochondrial complex I in health and disease. *Am J Hum Genet* 1999; 64:1505–1510.
247. Liang MH, Wong L. Yield on mtDNA mutation analysis in 2000 patients. *Am J Med Genet* 1998; 77:395–400.
248. Robinson BH. Human complex I deficiency: Clinical spectrum and involvement of oxygen free radicals in the pathogenicity of the defect. *Biochem Biophys Acta* 1998; 1364:271–286.
249. Chomyn A. The myoclonic epilepsy and ragged-red fiber mutation provides new insights into human mitochondria function and genetics. *Am J Hum Genet* 1998; 62:745–751.
250. Smeitink JAM, Loeffer JLCM, Triepels RH, et al. Nuclear genes of human complex I of the mitochondrial electron transport chain: State of the art. *Hum Mol Genet* 1998; 7:1573–1579.
251. Loeffen JL, Triepels RH, van den Heuvel LP, et al. cDNA of eight nuclear encoded subunits of NADH: Ubiquinone oxidoreductase: Human complex I cDNA characterization completed. *Biochem Biophys Res Commun* 1998; 253:415–422.
252. Morris AA, Leonard JV, Brown GK, et al. Deficiency of respiratory chain complex I is a common cause of Leigh disease. *Ann Neurol* 1996; 40:25–30.
253. Carral-Debrinski M, Stepien G. Shoffner JM, et al. Hypoxemia is associated with mitochondrial DNA damage and gene induction: Implications for cardiac disease. *JAMA* 1991; 266:1812–1816.
254. Rowland LP, Blake D, Kirano M, et al. Clinical syndromes associated with ragged-red fibers. *Rev Neurol* 1991; 147:467–473.
255. Tveskov C, Angelo-Nielsen K. Kearns-Sayre syndrome and dilated cardiomyopathy. *Neurology* 1990; 40:553–554.
256. Shoffner JM, Lott MI, Lezza AMS, et al. Myotonic epilepsy and ragged-red fiber disease (MERRF) is associated with a mitochondrial DNA $tRNA^{LYS}$ mutation. *Cell* 1990; 61:931–937.
257. Pavalakis SG, Phillips PC, DiMauro S, et al. Mitochondrial myopathy, encephalopathy, lactic acidosis, and strokelike episodes: A distinctive clinical syndrome. *Ann Neurol* 1984; 16:481–487.
258. Clark KM, Bindoff LA, Lightowlers RN, et al. Reversal of a mitochondrial DNA defect in human skeletal muscle. *Nature Genet* 1997; 16:222–224.
259. Taivassalu T, Fu K, Johns T, Arnold D, et al. Gene shifting: a novel therapy for mitochondrial myopathy. *Hum Mol Genet* 1999; 8:1047–1052.
260. Byers PH. Disorders of collagen biosynthesis and structure. In: Scriver CR, Beaudett AL, Sly NS, Valle D, eds. *The Metabolic and Molecular Basis of Inherited Disease*. New York: McGraw-Hill; 1995:4029–4077.
261. Milewicz DM, Molecular genetics of Marfan syndrome and Ehlers-Danlos type IV. *Curr Opin Cardiol* 1998; 13:198–204.
262. Tsipouras P, del Mastro R, Sarfarazi M, et al. Genetic linkage of the Marfan syndrome, ectopia lentis, and congential contractural arachnodatyly to the fabrillin genes on chromosomes 15 and 5. *N Engl J Med* 1992; 326:905–909.
263. Geva T, Sanders SP, Diogenes MS, et al. Two-dimensional and Doppler echocardiographic and pathologic characteristics of the infantile Marfan syndrome. *Am J Cardiol* 1990; 65:1230–1237.
264. Sakai LY, Keene DR, Engvall E. Fibrillin. a new 250-kD glycoprotein, is a component of extracellular microfibrils. *J Cell Biol* 1986; 103:2499–2509.
265. Huggon IC, Burke JP, Talbot JF. Contractural arachnodactyly

with mitral regurgitation and iridodonesis. *Arch Dis Child* 1990; 65:317–319.
266. Kainulainen K, Pulkkinen L, Savolainen A, et al. Location on chromosome 15 of the gene defect causing Marfan's syndrome. *N Engl J Med* 1990; 323:935–939.
267. Dietz HC, Cutting GR, Pyeritz RE, et al. Marfan syndrome caused by a recurrent de novo missense mutation in the fibrillin gene. *Nature* 1991; 352:337–339.
268. Milewicz DM, Duvic M. Severe neonatal Marfan syndrome resulting from a de novo three base pair insertion into the fibrillin gene on chromosome 15. *Am J Hum Genet* 1994; 54:447–453.
269. Lonnqvist L, Child A, Kainulainen K, et al. A novel mutation of the fibrillin gene causing ectopia lentis. *Genomics* 1994; 19:573–576.
270. Boileau C, Jondeau G, Babron M, et al. Autosomal dominant Marfan-like connective tissue disorder with aortic dilation and skeletal anomalies not linked to the fibrillin genes. *Am J Hum Genet* 1993; 53:46–54.
271. Francke U, Berg MA, Tynan K, et al. A Gly1127Ser mutation in an EGF-like domain of the fibrillin-1 gene is a risk factor for ascending aortic aneurysm and dissection. *Am J Hum Genet* 1994; 45:1287–1296.
272. Milewicz DM, Michael K, Fisher N, et al. Fibrillin-1 (FNB1) mutations in patients with thoracic aortic aneurysms. *Circulation* 1996; 94:2708–2711.
273. Sood SR, Eldadah ZA, Krause WL, et al. Mutation in fibrillin-1 and the marfanoid-craniosynostosis (Sprintzen-Goldberg) syndrome. *Nature Genet* 1996; 12:209–211.
274. Putnam EA, Zhang H, Ramirez F, Milewicz DM. Fibrillin-2 (RBN2) mutations result in the Marfan-like disorder, congenital contractural arachnodactyly. *Nature Genet* 1995; 11:456–458.
275. Collod G, Babron M, Jondeau G, et al. A second locus for Marfan syndrome maps to chromosome 3p24.2-p25. *Nature Genet* 1994; 8:264–268.
276. Shores J, Berger KR, Murphy EA, Pyeritz RE. Progression of aortic dilatation and the benefit of long-term beta-adrenergic blockade in Marfan's syndrome. *N Engl J Med* 1994; 330:1335–1341.
277. Gott VL, Gillinov AM, Pyeritz RE, et al. Aortic root replacement. Risk factor analysis of a seventeen-year experience with 270 patients. *J Thorac Cardiovasc Surg* 1995; 109:536–544.
278. Pyeritz RE. Maternal and fetal complications in pregnancy in the Marfan syndrome. *Am J Med* 1981; 71:784–790.
279. Towbin JA, Casey B, Belmont J. The molecular basis of vascular disorders. *Am J Hum Genet* 1999; 64:678–684.
280. Michalickova K, Susic M, Willing MC, et al. Mutations of the α-2(v) chain of type V collagen impair matrix assembly and produce Ehlers-Danlos syndrome type I. *Hum Mol Genet* 1998; 78: 249–255.
281. Giunta C, Superti Furga A, Spranger S, et al. Ehlers-Danlos type VII: clinical features and molecular defects. *J Bone Joint Surg Ann* 1999; 81:225–238.
282. Emanuel BS, Cannizzaro LA, Seyer JM, et al. Human A1 (III) and A2 (V) procollagen genes are located on the long arm of chromosome 2. *Proc Natl Acad Sci USA* 1985; 82:3385–3389.
283. Burrows NP. The molecular genetics of the Ehlers-Danlos syndrome. *Clin Exp Dermatol* 1999; 24:99–106.
284. Walker LC, Marini JC, Grange DK, et al. A patient with Ehlers-Danlos syndrome type VI is homozygous for a premature termination codon in exon 14 of the lysyl hydroxylase I gene. *Mol Genet Metab* 1999; 67:74–82.
285. Passoja K, Rautavuoma K, Ala-Kokko L, et al. Cloning and characterization of a third human lysyl hydroxylase isoform. *Proc Natl Acad Sci USA* 1998; 95:10482–10486.
286. Prockop DJ. Mutations in collagen genes as a cause of connective-tissue diseases. *N Engl J Med* 1992; 326:540–546.
287. Okajima T, Fukumoto S, Furukawa K, et al. Molecular basis for the progeroid variant of Ehlers-Danlos syndrome: Identification and characterization of two mutations in galactosyl transferase I gene. *J Biol Chem* 1999; 274:28841–28844.
288. Kontusaari S, Tromp G, Kuivaniemi H, et al. A mutation in the gene for type II procollagen (COL3AI) in a family with aortic aneurysms. *J Clin Invest* 1990; 86:1465–1473.
289. MacSweeney ST, Skidmore C, Turner RJ, et al. Unravelling the familial tendency to aneurysmal disease: Popliteal aneurysm, hypertension and fibrillin genotype. *Eur J Vasc Endosc Surg* 1996; 12:162–166.
290. McMillan WD, Patterson BK, Keen RR, et al. In situ localization and quantification of mRNA for 92-kD bype IV collagenase and its inhibitor in aneurysmal, occlusive, and normal aorta. *Athers Thromb Vasc Biol* 1995; 15:1139–1144.
291. Kuivaniemi H, Tromp G, Prockop DJ. Genetic causes of aortic aneurysms: Unlearning at least part of what the textbooks say. *J Clin Invest* 1991; 88:1441–1444.
292. Sherer DW, Sapadin AN, Lebwohl MG. Pseudoxanthoma elasticum: An update. *Dermatology* 1999; 199:3–7.
293. Challenor VF, Conway N, Munro JL. The surgical treatment of restrictive cardiomyopathy in pseudoxanthoma elasticum. *Br Heart J* 1988; 59:266–269.
294. Pyeritz RE, Weiss JL, Renie WE, et al. Pseudoxanthoma elasticum and mitral-valve prolapse. *N Engl J Med* 1982; 307:1451–1452.
295. Weir EK, Joffe HS, Blaufuss AH, Beighton P. Cardiovascular abnormalities in cutis laxa. *Eur J Cardiol* 1977; 5:255–261.
296. Bale SJ. Recent advances in gene mapping of skin diseases pseudoxanthorna elasticum: A satisfying sibling study. *J Cutan Med Surg* 1999; 3:154–156.
297. Zhang MC, He L, Giro M, et al. Cutis laxa arising from frameshift mutations in exon 30 of the elastin gene (ELN). *J Biol Chem* 1999; 274:981–986.
298. Tassabehji M, Metcalfe K, Hurst J, et al. An elastin gene mutation producing abnormal tropelastin and cutis laxa. *Hum Mol Genet* 1998; 7:1021–1028.
299. Bouloc A, Godeau G, Zeller J, et al. Increases fibroblast elastase activity in acquired cutis laxa. *Dermatology* 1999; 198:346–350.
300. Boente MC, Winik BC, Asial RA. Wrinkly skin syndrome: Ultrastructural alterations of the elastic fibers. *Pediatr Dermatol* 1999; 16:113–117.
301. Priori SG, Barhanin J, Hauer RNW, et al. Genetic and molecular basis of cardiac arrhythmias: Impact on clinical management (Parts I and II). *Circulation* 1999; 99:518–528.
302. Schwartz PJ, Moss AJ, Vincent GM, et al. Diagnostic criteria for the long QT syndrome: An update. *Circulation* 1993; 88:782–784.
303. Schwartz PJ, Locati EH, Napolitano C, et al. The long QT syndrome. In: Zipes DP, Halife J, eds. *Cardiac Electrophysiology: From Cell to Bedside.* Philadelphia: Saunders; 1996:788–811.
304. Keating M, Dunn C, Atkinson D, et al. Linkage of a cardiac arrhythmia, the long QT syndrome, and the Harvey ras-1 gene. *Science* 1991; 252:704–706.
305. Towbin JA, Li H, Taggart RT, et al. Evidence of genetic heterogeneity in Romano-Ward long QT syndrome: Analysis of 23 families. *Circulation* 1994; 90:2635–2644.
306. Abbott GW, Sesti F, Splawski I, et al. MiRP1 forms I_{Kr} potassium channels with HERG and is associated with cardiac arrhythmia. *Cell* 1999; 97:175–187.
307. Moss AJ, Zareba W, Benhorin J, et al. Electrocardiographic T-wave patterns in genetically distinct forms of the hereditary long-QT syndrome. *Circulation* 1995; 92:2929–2934.
308. Zareba W, Moss AJ, Schwartz PJ, et al. ECG T-wave patterns in genetically distinct forms of the hereditary long QT syndrome. *Circulation* 1995; 92:2929–2934.
309. Schwartz PJ, Stramba-Badiale M, Segantini A, et al. Prolongation of the QT interval and the sudden infant death syndrome. *N Engl J Med* 1998; 338:1709–1714.

310. Towbin JA, Friedman RA. Prolongation of the long QT syndrome and sudden infant death syndrome. *N Engl J Med* 1998; 338:1760–1761.
311. Schwartz PJ, Priori SG, Locati EH. Long QT syndrome patients with mutations of the SCN54 and HERG genes have differential response to Na+ channel blockade and to increases in heart rate: Implications for gene-specific therapy. *Circulation* 1995; 92:3373–3375.
312. Compton SJ, Lux RL, Ramsey MR, et al. Genetically defined therapy of inherited long-QT syndrome: Correction of abnormal repolarization by potassium. *Circulation* 1996; 94:1018–1022.
313. Shimzu W, Kurita T, Matsuo K, et al. Improvement of repolarization abnormalities by a K+ channel opener in LQT1 form of congenital long-QT syndrome. *Circulation* 1998; 97:1581–1588.
314. Neyroud N, Tesson F, Denjoy I, et al. A novel mutation on the potassium channel gene *KVLQT1* causes the Jervell and Lange-Nielsen cardioauditory syndrome. *Nature Genet* 1997; 15: 186–189.
315. Splawski I, Timothy KW, Vincent GM, et al. Brief report: Molecular basis of the long-QT syndrome associated with deafness. *N Engl J Med* 1997; 336:1562–1567.
316. Chen Q, Zhang D, Gingell RL, et al. Homozygous deletion in KVLQT1 associated with Jervell and Lange-Nielsen syndrome. *Circulation* 1999; 99:1344–1347.
317. Tyson J, Tranebjaerg L, Bellman S, et al. IsK and *KVLQT1:* mutation in either of the two subunits of the slow component of the delayed rectifier potassium channel can cause Jervell and Lange-Nielsen syndrome. *Hum Mol Genet* 1997; 12:2179–2185.
318. Brugada P, Brugada J. Right bundle-branch block, persistent ST segment elevation and sudden cardiac death: A distant clinical and electrocardiographic syndrome—A multicenter report. *J Am Coll Cardiol* 1992; 20:1391–1396.
319. Gussak I, Antzelevitch C, Bjerregaard P, et al. The Brugada syndrome: Clinical, electrophysiological, and genetic considerations. *J Am Coll Cardiol* 1999; 33:5–15.
320. Nademanee K, Veerakul G, Nimmannit S, et al. Arrhythmogenic marker for the sudden unexplained death syndrome in Thai men. *Circulation* 1997; 96:2595–2600.
321. Chen Q, Kirsch GE, Zhang D, et al. Genetic basis and molecular mechanism for idiopathic ventricular fibrillation. *Nature* 1998; 392:293–296.
322. Dumaine R, Towbin JA, Brugada P, et al. Ionic mechanisms responsible for the electrocardiographic phenotype of the Brugada syndrome are temperature dependent. *Circ Res* 1999; 85:803–809.
323. Brugada R, Tapscott T, Czernuszewicz GZ, et al. Identification of a genetic locus for familial atrial fibrillation. *N Engl J Med* 1997; 336:905–911.
324. Wolff L, Parkinson J, White PD. Bundle branch block with short PR interval in healthy young people prone to paroxysmal tachycardia. *Am Heart J* 1930; 5:686–704.
325. Waxman MB, Catching JD, Felderhof CH, et al. Familial atrioventricular heart block: An autosomal dominant trait. *Circulation* 1975; 51:226–233.
326. Brink PA, Ferreira A, Moolman JC, et al. Gene for progressive familial heart block type I maps to chromosome 19q13. *Circulation* 1995; 91:1633–1640.
327. Schott J-J, Benson DW, Basson CT, et al. Congenital heart disease caused by mutations in the transcription factor NKX2-5. *Science* 1998; 281:108–111.
328. Bonnet D, Pelet A, Legeai-Mallet L, et al. A gene for Holt-Oram syndrome maps to the distal long arm of chromosome 12. *Nature Genet* 1994; 6:405–408.
329. Basson CT, Cowley GS, Solomon SD, et al. The clinical and genetic spectrum of the Holt-Oram syndrome (heart-hand syndrome). *N Engl J Med* 1994; 330:885–891.
330. Basson CT, Bachinski DR, Lin RC, et al. Mutations in human cause limb and cardiac malformation in Holt-Oram syndrome. *Nature Genet* 1997; 15:30–35.
331. Li QY, Newbury-Ecog RA, Terrett JA, et al. Holt-Oram syndrome is caused by mutations in TBX5, a member of the *Brachyury* (*T*) gene family. *Nature Genet* 1997; 15:21–29.
332. Manouvrier-Hanu S, Holder-Espinasse M, Lyonnet S. Genetics of limb anomalies in humans. *Trends Genet* 1999; 15:409–417.
333. Smith J. T-box genes: What they do and how they do it? *Trends Genet* 1999; 15:154–158.
334. Morris CA. Genetic aspects of supravalvular aortic stenosis. *Curr Opin Cardiol* 1998; 13:214–219.
335. Hallidie-Smith KA, Karas S. Cardiac anomalies in Williams-Beuren syndrome. *Arch Dis Child* 1988; 63:809–813.
336. O'Connor WN, Davis JB, Geissler R, et al. Supravalvular aortic stenosis: Clinical and pathological observations in six patients. *Arch Pathol Lab Med* 1985; 109:179–185.
337. Ewart AK, Morris CA, Atkinson D, et al. Hemizygosity at the elastin locus in developmental disorders, Williams syndrome. *Nature Genet* 1993; 5:11–16.
338. Nickerson E, Greenberg F, Keating MT, et al. Deletions of the elastin gene at 7q11.23 occur in about 90% of patients with Williams syndrome. *Am J Hum Genet* 1995; 56:1156–1161.
339. Baumer, A, Dutly F. Balmer D, et al. High level of unequal meiotic crossovers at the origin of 22q11.2 and 7q11.23 deletions. *Hum Mol Genet* 1998; 7:887–894.
340. Frangiskakis JM, Ewart AK, Morris CA, et al. LIM-kinase I hemizygosity implicated in impaired visuospatial constructive cognition. *Cell* 1996; 86:59–69.
341. Tassabehji M, Metcalfe K, Ferguson WD, et al. LIM-kinase deleted in Williams syndrome. *Nature Genet* 1996; 13:272–273.
342. Osborne LR, Soder S, Shi X-M, et al. Hemizygous deletion of the syntaxin IA gene in individuals with Williams syndrome. *Am J Hum Genet* 1997; 61:449–452.
343. Meng X, Lu X, Li Z, Green ED, et al. Complete physical map of the common deletion region in Williams syndrome and identification and characterization of three novel genes. *Hum Genet* 1998; 103:590–599.
344. Osborne LR, Martindale D, Sherer SW, et al. Identification of genes from a 500-kb region at 7q11.23 that is commonly deleted in Williams syndrome patients. *Genomics* 1996; 36:328–336.
345. Peoples R, Perez-Jurado L, Wang Y-K, et al. The gene of replication factor C subunit 2 (RFC-2) is within the 7q11.23 Williams syndrome deletion. *Am J Hum Genet* 1996; 58:1370–1373.
346. Perez-Jurado LA, Wang Y-K, Peoples R, et al. A duplicated gene in the breakpoint regions of the 7q11.23 Williams-Beuren syndrome encodes the initiator binding protein TFII-I and BAP-135, a phosphorylation target of BTK. *Hum Mol Genet* 1998; 7:325–334.
347. Wang Y-K, Samos CH, Peoples R, et al. A novel human homologue of the *Drosophila frizzled wnt* receptor gene binds wingless protein and is in the Williams syndrome deletion at 7111.23. *Hum Mol Genet* 1997; 6:465–574.
348. Lu X, Meng X, Morris CA, et al. A novel human gene, WSTF, is deleted in Williams syndrome. *Genomics* 1998; 54:241–249.
349. Hockenhull EL, Carett MJ, Metcalfe K, et al. A complete physical contig and partial transcript map of the Williams syndrome critical region. *Genomics* 1999; 58:138–145.
350. Noonan JA, Ehmke DA. Associated noncardiac malformations in children with congenital heart disease. *J Pediatr* 1963; 63:468–470.
351. Sharland M, Burch M, McKenna WM, et al. A clinical study of Noonan syndrome. *Arch Dis Child* 1992; 67:178–183.
352. Jamieson CR, van der Burgt I, Brady AF, et al. Mapping a gene for Noonan syndrome to the long arm of chromosome 12. *Nature Genet* 1994; 8:357–360.
353. Quek SC, Yip W, Quek ST, et al. Cardiac manifestations in tuberous sclerosis: A 10-year review. *J Pediatr Child Health* 1998; 34:283–287.

354. Smith M, Sperling D. Novel 23-base-pair duplication in TSC1 exon 15 in an infant presenting with cardiac rhabdomyomas. *Am J Med Genet* 1999; 84:346–349.
355. O'Callaghan FJ, Clarke AC, Jaffe H, et al. Tuberous sclerosis complex and Wolff-Parkinson-White syndrome. *Arch Dis Child* 1998; 78:159–162.
356. Povey S, Burley MW, Attwood J, et al. Two loci for tuberous sclerosis: one on 9q34 and one on 16q13. *Ann Hum Genet* 1994; 58:107–127.
357. Plank TL, Yeung RS, Henske EP. Hamartin, the product of the tuberous sclerosis 1 (TSC1) gene, interacts with tuberin and appears to be localized to cytoplasmic vesicles. *Cancer Res* 1998; 58:4766–4770.
358. Hornigold N, Devlin J, Davies AM, et al. Mutation of the 9q34 gene TSC1 in sporadic bladder cancer. *Oncogene* 1999; 18:2657–2661.
359. Longa L, Scolari F, Brusco A, et al. A large TSC2 and PKD1 gene deletion is associated with renal and extrarenal signs of autosomal dominant polycystic kidney disease. *Nephrol Dial Transplant* 1997; 12:1900–1907.
360. Van Slegtenhorst M, et al. Mutational spectrum of the TSC1 gene in a cohort of 225 tuberous sclerosis complex patients: No evidence for genotype-phenotype correlation. *J Med Genet* 1999; 36:285–289.
361. Jones AC, Shyamsunder MM, Thomas MW, et al. Comprehensive mutation analysis of TSC1 and TSC2 and phenotypic correlatives in 150 families with tuberous sclerosis. *Am J Hum Genet* 1999; 64:1305–1315.
362. Onda H, Lueck A, Marks PW, et al. Tsc 2(+/−) mice develop tumors in multiple sites that express gelsolin and are influenced by genetic background. *J Clin Invest* 1999; 104:687–695.
363. Hino O, Fukuda T, Satake N, et al. TSC2 gene mutant (Eker) rat model of a dominantly inherited cancer. *Prog Exp Tumor Res* 1999; 35:95–108.
364. Yeung RS, Katsetos CD, Klein-Szanto A, et al. Subependymal astrocytic hamertome, in the Eker rat model of tuberous sclerosis. *Am J Pathol* 1997; 151:1477–1486.
365. Satake N, Kobayashi T, Kobayashi E, et al. Isolation and characterization of a rat homologue of the human tuberous sclerosis 1 gene (TSC1) and analyses of its mutations in rat renal carcinomas. *Cancer Res* 1999; 59:849–855.
366. Weinstein BM, Stemple DL, Driever W, et al. Gridlock, a localized heritable vascular patterning defect in the zebrafish. *Nature Med* 1995; 1:1143–1147.
367. Towbin JA, McQuinn TC. Gridlock: A model for coarctation of the aorta? *Nature Med* 1995; 1:1141–1142.
368. Yost HJ. The genetics of midline and cardiac laterality defects. *Curr Opin Cardiol* 1998; 13:185–189.
369. Rose V, Izukawa T, Moes CA. Syndromes of asplenia and polysplenia: A review of cardiac and noncardiac malformations in 60 cases with special references to diagnosis and prognosis. *Br Heart J* 1987; 37:840–852.
370. Seo J, Brown NA, Ho SY, et al. Abnormal laterality and congenital cardiac anomalies: Relations of visceral and cardiac morphologies in the *iv/iv* mouse. *Circulation* 1992; 86:642–650.
371. Casey B. Two rights make a wrong: human left-right malformations. *Hum Mol Genet* 1998; 7:1565–1571.
372. Gebbia M, Ferrero GB, Pilia G, et al. X-linked situs abnormalities result from mutations in *ZIC3*. *Nature Genet* 1997; 17:305–308.
373. Meno C, Saijoh Y, Fujii H, et al. Left-right asymmetric expression of the TGF β-family member lefty in mouse embryos. *Nature* 1996; 381:151–155.
374. Meno C, Shimono A, Saijoh Y, et al. Lefty-1 is required for left-right determination as a regulator of lefty-2 and nodal. *Cell* 1998; 94:287–297.
375. Nomura M, Li E, Smadz role in mesoderm formation, left-right patterning, and cranofacial development. *Nature* 1998; 393:786–790.
376. Kosaki K, Bassi MT, Kosaki R, et al. Characterization and mutation analysis of human LEFTY A and LEFTY B, homologues of murine genes implicated in left-right axis development. *Am J Hum Genet* 1999; 64:712–721.
377. Kosaki R, Gebbia M, Kosaki K, et al. Left-right axis malformations associated with nucleotide substitutions in ACVR2B, the gene for human activin receptor type IIB. *Am J Med Genet* 1999; 82:70–76.
378. Towbin JA, Greenberg F. Genetic syndromes and clinical molecular genetics. In: Bricker JT, Garson A Jr, Fisher DJ, Neish SR, eds. *The Science and Practice of Pediatric Cardiology*. Baltimore: Williams & Wilkins; 1998:2627–2700.
379. Emanuel BS. Molecular cytogenetics: Toward dissection of the contiguous gene syndromes. *Am J Hum Genet* 1988; 43:575–578.
380. Korenberg JR, Kawashima H, Pulst S-M, et al. Molecular definition of a region of chromosome 21 that causes features of the Down syndrome phenotype. *Am J Hum Genet* 1990; 47:236–246.
381. Korenberg JR, Bradley C, Disteche CM. Down syndrome: Molecular mapping of the congenital heart disease and duodenal stenosis. *Am J Hum Genet* 1992; 50:294–302.
382. Hubert R, Mitchell S, Chen XN, et al. BAC and PAC contig covering 3.5 Mb of the Down syndrome congenital heart disease region between DZIS5S and MX1 on chromosome 21. *Genomics* 1997; 41:218–226.
383. DiGeorge AM. Discussions on a new concept of the cellular base of immunology. *J Pediatr* 1965; 67:907–908.
384. Clark EB. Mechanisms in the pathogenesis of congenital heart defects. In: Pierpont ME, Moller JM, eds. *The Genetics of Cardiovascular Disease*. Boston: Martinus Nijhoff; 1985:3–36.
385. Emanuel BS, Budarf ML, Scambler PJ. The genetic basis of conotruncal cardiac defects: The chromosome 22q11.2 deletion. In: Harvey RP, Rosenthal N, eds. *Heart Development*. San Diego, CA: Academic Press; 1999:463–478.
386. Shprintzen RJ, Goldberg RB, Young D, et al. The velo-cardio-facial syndrome: A clinical and genetic analysis. *Pediatrics* 1981; 67:167–172.
387. Burn JA, Takao A, Wilson D, et al. Conotruncal anomaly face syndrome is associated with a deletion within chromosome 22q11. *J Med Genet* 1993; 30:822–824.
388. Greenberg F, Elder FFB, Haffner P, et al. Cytogenetic findings in a prospective series of patients with DiGeorge anomaly. *Am J Hum Genet* 1988; 43:605–611.
389. Budarf ML, Collins J, Gong W, et al. Cloning a balanced translocation associated with DiGeorge syndrome and identification of a disrupted candidate gene. *Nature Genet* 1994; 10:269–278.
390. Pizzuti A, Novelli G, Mari A, et al. Human homologue sequences to the *Drosophila disheveled segment-polarity* gene are deleted in the DiGeorge syndrome. *Am J Hum Genet* 1996; 58:722–729, 1996.
391. Holmes SE, Riazi MA, Gong W, et al. Disruption of the clathrin heavy chain-like gene (*CLTCL*) associated with features of DGS/VCFS: A balanced (21;22)(p12;q11) translocation. *Hum Mol Genet* 1997; 6:357–367.
392. Puzzuti A, Novelli G, Ratti A, et al. UFD1L, a developmentally expressed ubiquitination gene, is deleted in CATCH 22 syndrome. *Hum Mol Genet* 1997; 6:259–265.
393. Wilming LG, Snoeren CAS, Van Rijswijk A, et al. The murine homologue of HIRA, a DiGeorge syndrome candidate gene, is expressed in embryonic structures affected in human CATCH 22 patients. *Hum Mol Genet* 1997; 6:247–258.
394. Gong W, Emanuel BS, Galili N, et al. Structural and mutational analyses of a conserved gene (*DGSI*) from the minimal DiGeorge syndrome critical region. *Hum Mol Genet* 1997; 6:267–276.
395. Wakamiya M, Lindsay EA, Rivera-Perez JA, et al. Functional

analysis of *Gscl* in the pathogenesis of the DiGeorge and velocardiofacial syndromes. *Hum Mol Genet* 1998; 7:1835–1840.

396. Farrell MJ, Stadt H, Wallis KT, et al. HIRA, a DiGeorge syndrome candidate gene, is required for cardiac outflow tract septation. *Circ Res* 1999; 84:127–135.

397. Yamagishi H, Garg V, Matsuko R, et al. A molecular pathway revealing a genetic basis for human cardiac and craniofacial defects. *Science* 1999; 283:1158–1161.

398. Lindsay EA, Botta A, Jurecic V, et al. Congenital heart disease in mice deficient for the DiGeorge syndrome region. *Nature* 1999; 401:379–383.

399. Markert ML, Boeck A, Hale LP, et al. Transplantation of thymus tissue in complete DiGeorge syndrome. *N Engl J Med* 1999; 341:1180–1189.

400. Recto MR, Parness IA, Gelb BD, et al. Clinical implications and possible association of malposition of the branch pulmonary arteries with DiGeorge syndrome and microdeletion of chromosomal region 22q11. *Am J Cardiol* 1997; 80:1624–1627.

401. Lu J-H, Chung M-Y, Hwang B, et al. Prevalence and parental origin in tetralogy of Fallot associated with chromosome 22q11 microdeletion. *Pediatrics* 1999; 104:87–90.

402. Wulfsberg EA, Leara-Cox J, Neri G. What's in a name? Chromosome 22q11 abnormalities and the DiGeorge, velocardiofacial, and conotruncal anomalies face syndromes. *Am J Med Genet* 1997; 65:317–319.

403. Goldmuntz E, Clark BJ, Mitchell LE, et al. Frequency of 22q11 deletions in patients with conotruncal defects. *J Am Coll Cardiol* 1998; 32:492–498.

CHAPTER 63

THE PATHOLOGY, PATHOPHYSIOLOGY, RECOGNITION, AND TREATMENT OF CONGENITAL HEART DISEASE

Michael D. Freed

INCIDENCE AND ETIOLOGY

The incidence of congenital heart disease in the United States is approximately 8 per 1000 live births.[1,2] Many infants who are born alive with cardiac defects have anomalies that do not represent a threat to life, at least during infancy. Almost one-third of those infants, or 2.6 per 1000 live births, however, have critical disease, which is defined as a malformation severe enough to result in cardiac catheterization, cardiac surgery, or death within the first year of life.[3] Today, with early detection and proper management, the majority of infants with critical disease can be expected to survive the first year of life.[3] Most who now survive infancy will join the increasingly large cohort of adults with congenital heart disease.

Estimates of the incidence of specific lesions vary, depending on whether the data are drawn from infants or older children and whether the diagnosis is based on clinical, echocardiographic, catheterization, surgical, or postmortem studies.[1-4] The incidence in other countries is remarkably similar to that reported for the United States.[5,6]

Despite these differences in case material, except for bicuspid aortic valve and mitral valve prolapse, it is apparent that ventricular septal defect (VSD) is the most common malformation, occurring in 28 percent of all patients with congenital heart disease (Table 63-1).

Among 2251 infants with critical congenital heart disease in the New England Regional Infant Cardiac Program,[3] 53.7 percent were male. Certain defects, however, are considerably more common in one sex than in the other. Aortic stenosis occurs more commonly in boys (4:1), and atrial septal defects occur more frequently in girls (2.5:1).

Although earlier theories concerning the etiology of congenital heart diseases suggested that most defects were multifactorial—that is, the malformations are caused by a combination of a hereditary predisposition (presumably caused by abnormalities in the genetic code) and an environmental trigger[7]—more recent advances in molecular biology suggest that a much higher percentage are caused by point mutations.[8]

Some abnormalities are caused by chromosomal aberrations (see Chap. 62). Trisomy 21 (Down's syndrome) is highly associated with complete atrioventricular (AV) canal, VSDs, and tetralogy of Fallot, and children with Turner's syndrome (XO) frequently have coarctation of the aorta. Other anomalies are caused by teratogens: VSD in fetal alcohol syndrome, Ebstein's anomaly in a fetus with prenatal exposure to lithium, and patent ductus arteriosus (PDA) in mothers who contracted rubella during the first trimester are examples.

Some syndromes are inherited as single-gene defects and have congenital heart disease as one of their manifestations. Holt-Oram syndrome, an association of radial limb abnormalities and atrial septal defects (ASDs), is caused by an abnormality of a T-box transcription factor Tbx5, and the cardio-velo-facial syndrome, associated with abnormalities of the conotruncus, resulting in a high proportion of infants born with truncus arteriosus or interrupted aortic arch, is a result of a deletion on chromosome 22 (22 q 11)[9] (see Chap. 62).

It is clear now that a higher proportion of congenital heart disease than previously thought is due to single-gene defects and that the same malformation may be caused by mutant genes at different loci.[8] With increasing knowledge of molecular mechanisms, it seems inevitable that the etiology and pathogenesis of congenital heart disease will be clarified increasingly in the years ahead.

TABLE 63-1 Incidence of Specific Congenital Heart Defects

Defect	Percentage of Cases[a] Averaged
Ventricular septal defect	28.3
Pulmonary stenosis	9.5
Patent ductus arteriosus	8.7
Ventricular septal defect with pulmonary stenosis[b]	6.8
Atrial septal defect, secundum	6.7
Aortic stenosis	4.4
Coarctation of aorta	4.2
Atrioventricular canal[c]	3.5
Transposition of great arteries	3.4
Aortic atresia	2.4
Truncus arteriosus	1.6
Tricuspid atresia	1.2
Total anomalous pulmonary venous connection	1.1
Double-outlet right ventricle	0.8
Pulmonary atresia without ventricular septal defect	0.3

[a]Total number of cases = 103,590.
[b]Includes tetralogy of Fallot.
[c]Includes partial and complete.
SOURCE: References 1–3, 5, 6.

FETAL CIRCULATION AND THE TRANSITION TO NEONATAL AND ADULT CIRCULATION

The fetus obtains all metabolic necessities, including oxygen, from the placenta. The fetal circulation is an adaptation to allow most of the right ventricular output to bypass the lungs and go instead to the placenta to pick up oxygen. Most of the understanding of this adaptation comes from more than 40 years of research,[10–18] primarily on fetal lambs. The fetal circulation is arranged in parallel rather than in series, with mixing at the atrial (foramen ovale) and great vessel (ductus arteriosus) level (Fig. 63-1). Normally, blood returning from the body goes into the right atrium via the superior vena cava or inferior vena cava. Inferior vena cava blood is diverted by the crista dividens so that approximately 27 percent of combined ventricular output passes through the foramen ovale into the left atrium, with the remainder passing through the tricuspid valve to the right ventricle. Left atrial return is mixed with blood returning from the lungs into the left ventricle and then to the ascending aorta, where it goes to the coronary arteries, head, and upper body vessels, with a small proportion going across the arch into the descending aorta. Right ventricular blood passes out of the pulmonary artery, where approximately 90 percent (59 percent of combined ventricular output) is diverted through the ductus arteriosus into the descending aorta by the elevated pulmonary vascular resistance. Thus, approximately two-thirds of the blood passes through the right side of the heart and one-third passes through the left side of the heart.

The oxygen saturation of fetal blood is considerably lower than that in a newborn or infant because of the lower efficiency of the placenta compared with the lungs for oxygen exchange (Fig. 63-2). The blood with the highest saturation (approximately 70 percent) is that returning from the placenta. Some of this higher-saturation blood is diverted across the foramen ovale so that saturation on the left side of the heart (65 percent) is somewhat higher than it is on the right side (55 percent). This allows diversion of the lowest-saturation blood (~55 percent) through the ductus arteriosus to the placenta, increasing the efficiency of oxygen pickup. An additional fetal adaptation to oxygen transport at low oxygen saturation is the presence of high levels of fetal hemoglobin with a higher affinity for oxygen than normal hemoglobin. This leftward shift of the oxygen dissociation curve facilitates oxygen uptake at the relatively low P_{O_2} of the placenta vasculature.

The wide communication at the atrial level (foramen ovale) allows for near equalization of atrial and ventricular end-diastolic pressures. The wide communication at the great vessel level (ductus arteriosus) allows equalization of systolic pressures in the aorta and the pulmonary artery and, in the absence of aortic or pulmonic stenosis, at the ventricular level (Fig. 63-3).

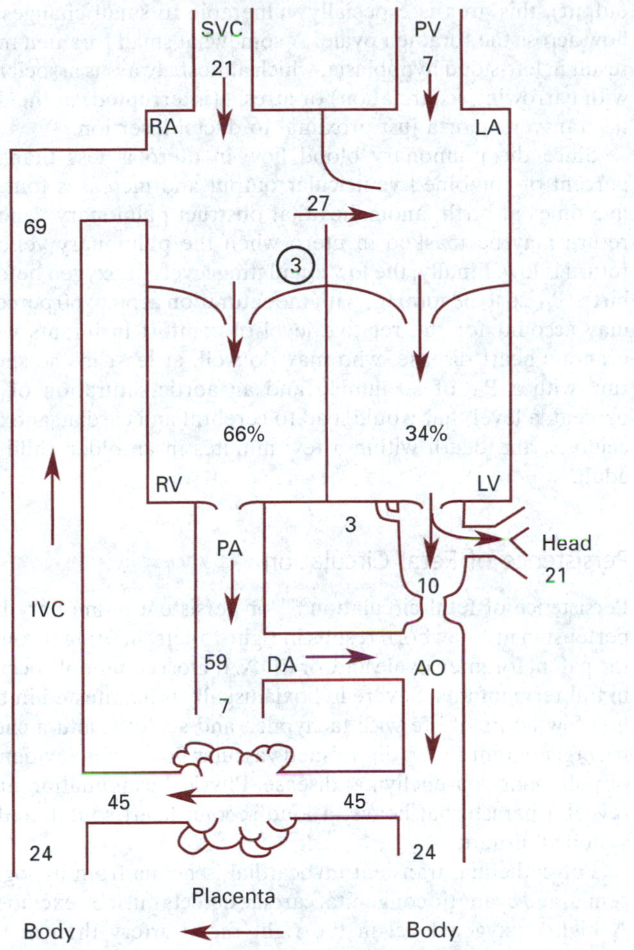

FIGURE 63-1 The course of the circulation in a late-gestation fetal lamb. *The numbers represent the percentage of combined ventricular output.* Some of the return from the inferior vena cava (IVC) is diverted by the crista dividens in the right atrium (RA) through the foramen ovale into the left atrium (LA), where it meets the pulmonary venous return (PV), passes into the left ventricle (LV), and is pumped into the ascending aorta. Most of the ascending aortic flow goes to the coronary, subclavian, and carotid arteries, with only 10 percent of combined ventricular output passing through the aortic arch (indicated by the narrowed point in the aorta) into the descending aorta (AO). The remainder of the inferior vena cava flow mixes with the return from the superior vena cava (SVC) and coronary veins, passes into the right atrium and right ventricle (RV), and is pumped into the pulmonary artery (PA). Because of the high pulmonary resistance, only 7 percent passes through the lungs (PV), with the rest going into the ductus arteriosus (DA) and then to the descending aorta (AO), the placenta, and the lower half of the body. (From Freed MD. Fetal and transitional circulation. In: Fyler DC, ed. *Nadas' Pediatric Cardiology*. Philadelphia: Hanley & Belfus; 1992. Reproduced with permission from the publisher and author.)

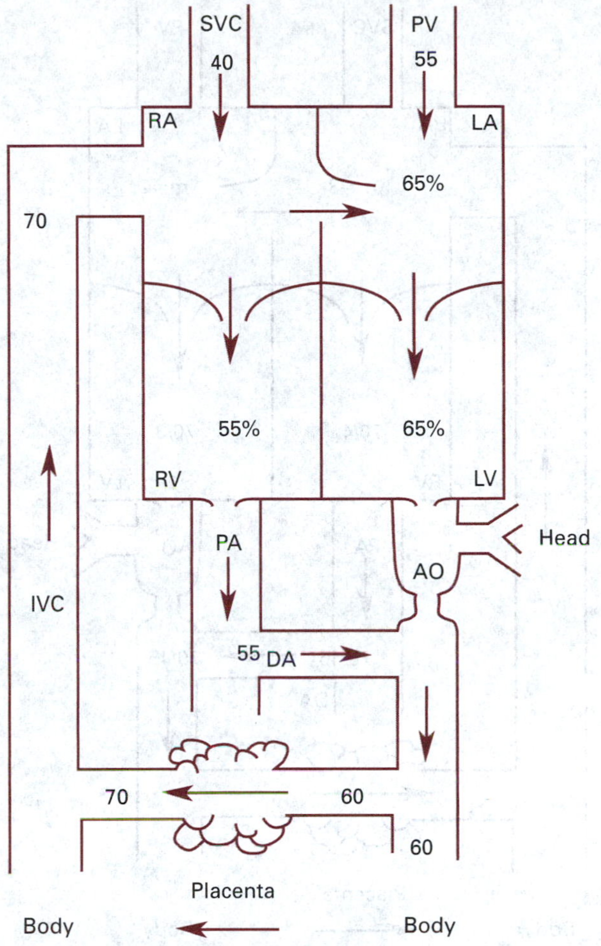

FIGURE 63-2 *The numbers indicate the percent of oxygen saturation in a late-gestation lamb.* The oxygen saturation is highest in the inferior vena cava, representing that primarily from the placenta. The saturation of blood in the heart is slightly higher on the left side than on the right side. The abbreviations in this diagram are the same as those in Fig. 63-1. (From Freed MD. Fetal and transitional circulation. In: Fyler DC, ed. *Nadas' Pediatric Cardiology*. Philadelphia: Hanley & Belfus; 1992. Reproduced with permission from the publisher and author.)

Within a few moments after birth, the circulatory physiology must switch rapidly from the placenta to the lung as the organ of oxygen exchange. Failure of any one of a number of a complex series of pulmonary and cardiac events may result in cerebral and then generalized hypoxemia, with lasting damage or death. With the onset of spontaneous respiration, the lungs are expanded and the pulmonary arterioles, which probably have been actively vasoconstricted, dilate. The reduction in pulmonary vascular resistance results from both simple physical expansion of the lung with the onset of respiration and the vasodilation of the pulmonary resistance vessels, probably partly as a result of the high level of oxygen in alveolar gas. Simultaneously, the placenta is removed from the circulation either by clamping the umbilical cord or by constriction of the umbilical arteries. This sudden increase in systemic vascular resistance and drop in pulmonary vascular resistance cause blood leaving the right ventricle to go out into the lung rather than through the ductus arteriosus. The sudden increase in left atrial return of blood now going through the lung increases left ventricular end-diastolic and left atrial pressure, shutting the flap valve of the foramen ovale against the edge of the cristae dividens, eliminating the atrial-level shunt.

With pulmonary vascular resistance lower than systemic vascular resistance, there may be some left-to-right (aorta to pulmonary artery) shunting through the ductus arteriosus. The mechanism for closure of the ductus arteriosus is not completely understood. The increased level of oxygen probably causes vasoconstriction of the ductus musculature, but there are strong

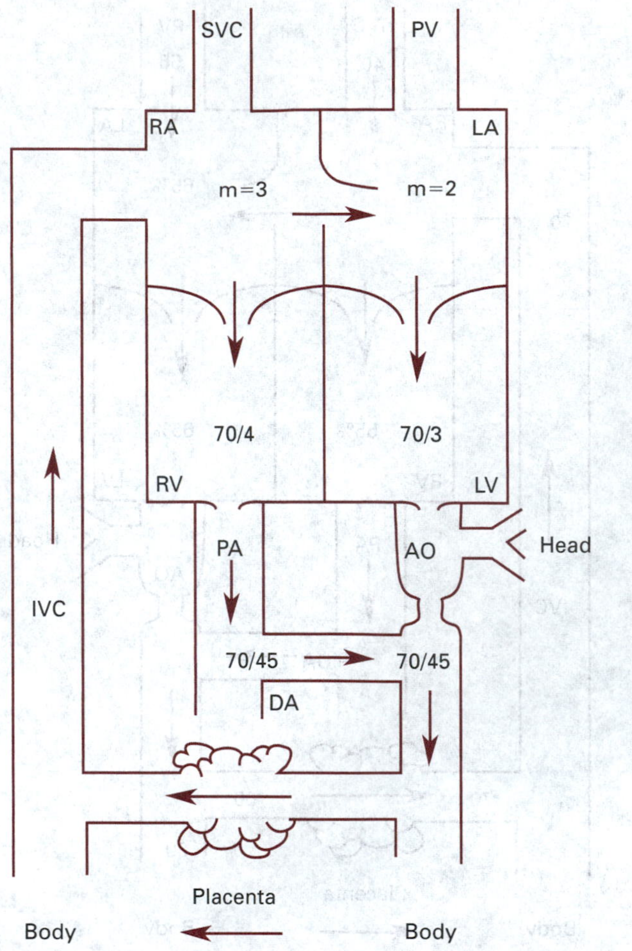

FIGURE 63-3 The numbers indicate the pressures observed in late-gestation lambs. Because large communications between the atrium and the great vessels are present, the pressures on both sides of the heart are virtually identical. The abbreviations are the same as those in Fig. 63-1. (From Freed MD. Fetal and transitional circulation. In: Fyler DC, ed. *Nadas' Pediatric Cardiology*. Philadelphia: Hanley & Belfus; 1992. Reproduced with permission from the publisher and author.)

suggestions that a reduction in circulating prostaglandins (PGs) of the E series plays a role. Within 3 or 4 days, the biochemical closure becomes irreversible when cellular necrosis of the endothelium leads to obliteration of the lumen. The pulmonary artery pressure drops to approximately half systemic levels within a day or so but takes another 2 to 6 weeks to drop down to adult levels.

The structure and hemodynamics of the field circulation have significant consequences in a neonate with congenital heart disease.[19] The parallel circulation with connections at the atrial and great vessel level allows a wide variety of congenital cardiac malformations to exist while still picking up oxygen at the placenta and delivering it to the tissues. For example, atresia of the tricuspid or mitral valve, while devastating after birth, does not have a significant effect in utero. Furthermore, since the right ventricle performs two-thirds of the cardiac work before birth, the left ventricle is underloaded; this may explain why congestive heart failure is seen not uncommonly with congenital defects. Because the normal flow across the aortic isthmus is relatively low (only about 10 percent of combined ventricular output), this area is especially vulnerable to small changes in flow across the foramen ovale. A somewhat small foramen may result in left-sided hypoplasia, which almost always is associated with narrowing (coarctation) or atresia (interrupted) at the distal transverse aorta just proximal to ductal insertion.

Since the pulmonary blood flow in utero is less than 10 percent of combined ventricular output and increases four to five times at birth, anomalies that obstruct pulmonary venous return may be masked in utero when the pulmonary venous return is low. Finally, the low circulating levels of oxygen before birth (P_{O_2} 26 to 38 mmHg) with the saturation at 50 to 60 percent may account for the relative level of comfort in infants with cyanotic heart disease, who may do well, at least in the short run, with a P_{O_2} of 30 mmHg and an aortic saturation of 50 percent, a level that would lead to cerebral and cardiac anoxia, acidosis, and death within a few minutes in an older child or adult.

Persistence of Fetal Circulation

Persistence of fetal circulation[20,21] or persistent pulmonary hypertension in a newborn results in right-to-left shunting through the patent foramen ovale and/or PDA. It most commonly occurs in full-term infants. Severe hypoxia usually is manifested in the first few hours of life with tachypnea and acidosis, and a chest roentgenogram shows diminished vascular flow but no evidence of pulmonary parenchymal disease. Physical examination may reveal a parasternal heave, a loud second heart sound, and a systolic murmur.

Polycythemia, transient myocardial ischemia from hypoglycemia, and cyanotic congenital cardiac defects must be excluded. A higher oxygen level in the right radial artery than in the umbilical artery confirms right-to-left shunting through the ductus arteriosus. Echocardiography and Doppler evaluation are of the utmost importance to rule out structural heart disease, especially total anomalous pulmonary venous connection.

The initial treatment[21] includes an increase in the inspired oxygen level and correction of acidosis with sodium bicarbonate. Frequently, artificial ventilation is required. Hyperventilation to diminish the partial pressure of carbon dioxide often is successful in lowering the pulmonary pressure and diminishing the right-to-left shunt. Recently, inhaled nitric oxide to reduce pulmonary vascular resistance has been found to be a useful adjunct to other therapies.[22] Treatment of severe disease with an extracorporeal membrane oxygenator is successful in a significant number of patients.[23] Similar hemodynamic alterations also may be seen in newborns with parenchymal lung disease.

COMPLICATIONS OF CONGENITAL HEART DISEASE

Complications associated with congenital heart disease are listed in Table 63-2.

TABLE 63-2 Complications of Congenital Heart Disease in Children

Congestive heart failure	Growth retardation
Hypoxemia	Pulmonary vascular disease

Congestive Heart Failure

Congestive heart failure is a potentially lethal complication of congenital heart disease and occurs in over 80 percent of infants who have malformations severe enough to require cardiac catheterization or surgery within the first year of life.[24] Its onset is usually a phenomenon of the first 6 months of life. Onset after 1 year of age is rare without a serious intercurrent problem such as infective endocarditis, pneumonia, or anemia.

Heart failure within the first 12 to 18 h of life usually is due to malformations that involve pressure or volume overload independent of pulmonary flow, as occurs with severe valvular regurgitation or a systemic arteriovenous fistula. Rarely, myocarditis may produce failure from the time of birth, as may congenital complete heart block or supraventricular tachycardia. Other causes in this age group include primary cardiomyopathy, severe polycythemia or anemia, and depressed myocardial contractility from neonatal asphyxia, hypocalcemia, hypoglycemia, or sepsis.

A majority of full-term infants presenting with severe heart failure during the remainder of the first week have critical obstruction to systemic arterial flow, which in virtually all cases has been unmasked by narrowing or closure of the ductus arteriosus. Examples are aortic atresia, coarctation of the aorta, interruption of the aortic arch, and critical aortic stenosis. *During the second week of life, aortic atresia and coarctation remain the most common causes of heart failure, but left ventricular volume overload from VSD, transposition of the great arteries with a VSD, and truncus arteriosus make their appearance.* These malformations present as the pulmonary vascular resistance falls, increasing the left-to-right shunt. *Statistically, VSD is the primary cause of congestive failure, followed by transposition, coarctation, complete AV canal, and PDA.*

The most common symptom of congestive heart failure is difficulty in breathing, with rapid, grunting, or gasping breathing or breathlessness with feeding. Observation of an undisturbed infant reveals dyspnea, the signs of which are nasal flaring and subcostal or intercostal retractions. A respiratory rate consistently above 60 is to be expected, and rates in the range of 90 to 100 are not uncommon. Poor weight gain is the rule. Cool moist skin, a subdued and rapid arterial pulse, and hepatic enlargement are common accompanying signs. A gallop rhythm, pulmonary rales, and expiratory wheezes may be present. It may be difficult to distinguish the pulmonary findings of heart failure from those of pneumonia or bronchiolitis; indeed, many infants develop heart failure during an intercurrent pulmonary infection. Edema, if present, usually is found in the periorbital area and on the dorsa of the feet and hands. Cardiac enlargement is confirmed by chest roentgenography. Infants with malformations such as coarctation of the aorta and total anomalous pulmonary venous connection, abnormalities that usually are not characterized by an impressive murmur, sometimes are referred only after weeks of tachypnea and failure to thrive, when a chest roentgenogram taken to explore the possibility of lung disease has revealed cardiac enlargement.

When a sizable systemic-to-pulmonary communication exists in a premature infant, usually as a result of a PDA, signs of heart failure usually are associated with signs of ventilatory failure.

Hospitalization is recommended for all infants with heart failure. Elevation of the head and chest to an angle of approximately 30° and administration of humidified oxygen by techniques that do not disturb the infant help relieve dyspnea and systemic arterial hypoxia as determined by pulse oximetry. Arterial oxygen saturation levels should be monitored in newborns, particularly the premature, to avoid the risk of retrolental fibroplasia. Rest, aided by sedation, is beneficial. With severe failure, oral feedings should be suspended temporarily to prevent aspiration and fluid intake should be restricted to 65 mL/kg per day intravenously for at least the first 24 h. Anemia, acidosis, hypoxia, hypercarbia, hypoglycemia, or hypocalcemia should be corrected; serum sodium, potassium, blood urea nitrogen, and creatinine concentrations should be monitored. A low threshold for the administration of antibiotics is appropriate.

Digoxin is recommended for the management of congestive failure in infants and children, especially those with decreased ventricular systolic function, because of its excellent absorption when given orally, rapid onset of action, relatively rapid excretion, and convenience of administration. The recommended oral maintenance doses of digoxin for the different age ranges of children, expressed in μg/kg per day, are as follows: for the premature, 5; for neonates, 10; for infants between 4 and 24 months of age, 15; for older children, 10; and for adolescents, 5. The daily maintenance dose usually is given in two divided doses approximately 12 h apart. The total digitalizing dose is three times the daily maintenance dose. Parenteral doses of digoxin are approximately 75 percent of oral doses for digitalization and maintenance. Half the digitalizing dose may be given initially, followed by the remaining two quarter doses at 4-, 8-, or 12-h intervals, depending on the desired speed of total digitalization. Maintenance therapy should be started 8 to 12 h after the last digitalizing dose. In a severely ill infant with decreased perfusion and unpredictable absorption, digitalization by the intravenous route is recommended. Impaired renal function leads to digoxin accumulation and toxicity, and so the initial and maintenance doses should be adjusted accordingly. Toxicity, if it is to occur, usually appears within the first week of therapy. If anorexia, nausea or vomiting, or electrocardiographic evidence of either atrial or ventricular ectopy or AV block appears, digoxin should be stopped and the serum digoxin level should be determined. Toxicity is probable if the level exceeds 3.0 ng/mL in an infant less than 6 months of age or 2.0 ng/mL in an older infant or child. If the need for digoxin continues, the dose is adjusted as the patient grows and gains weight.

The diuretic furosemide used intravenously in doses of 1.0 to 2.0 mg/kg or orally in doses of 1.5 to 2.0 mg/kg is very effective in the acute management of congestive heart failure. With severe failure, the dose may be increased by increments of 1.0 mg/kg intravenously if no urinary response has been achieved after 45 min. For long-term oral diuretic therapy, 1.5 to 2.0 mg/kg once daily or, if necessary, twice daily is recommended. Chlorothiazide, a slightly less potent diuretic but one with a longer duration of action, may be given orally in a dose of 20 to 50 mg/kg per day. Hypokalemia and hypochloremia can be induced with these potent diuretics, and a daily oral supplement of potassium chloride in the range of 1.0 to 1.5 meq/kg, with adjustment depending on the serum level, is recommended. Spironolactone, an aldosterone antagonist, has proved useful in supplementing the diuresis and preventing the hypokalemia induced by the diuretics described above. It may be given orally in a single daily dose of 2 to 3 mg/kg. A regimen of spironolactone 2 mg/kg given every day and furosemide

1 mg/kg is usually adequate for long-term diuretic therapy for mild to moderate heart failure and usually does not require potassium supplementation.

In emergency situations, it may be necessary to provide an immediate inotropic stimulus in the form of intravenous sympathomimetic amines administered by constant infusion pump. Isoproterenol in a dose of 0.1 μg/kg per minute exerts a powerful inotropic effect, but its usefulness may be limited by induced tachycardia and peripheral vasodilation, sometimes to the detriment of renal perfusion. Epinephrine in a dose of 0.1 to 1.0 μg/kg per minute or dobutamine or dopamine in a dose of 5 to 15 μg/kg per minute generally has been more helpful, with dopamine providing more adequate renal flow. The systemic arterial blood pressure, urinary output, and electrocardiogram (ECG) should be monitored continuously. Vasodilator therapy in the form of intravenous sodium nitroprusside may be of considerable help in patients with severe congestive failure that is not associated with large left-to-right shunts. The infusion rate at the start should be no higher than 0.5 μg/kg per minute, but it may be increased gradually to 4.0 μg/kg per minute to achieve the desired effect. Systemic arterial pressure should be monitored continuously to detect serious hypotension. The angiotensin-converting enzyme inhibitors captopril, enalapril, and lisinopril given orally have proved effective in selected patients: captopril starting at 0.1 to 0.4 mg/kg per dose in a neonate and 0.3 to 0.6 mg/kg per dose in an older child given one to four times per day, enalapril 0.16 to 0.25 mg/kg per day in two divided doses, or lisinopril 0.16 to 0.25 mg/kg per day in a single daily dose. Hypotension and/or hyperkalemia are the primary adverse effects of these agents.[25]

Infants with potentially exhausting respiratory effort or with hypoxia or hypercapnia secondary to pulmonary edema or respiratory failure benefit from endotracheal intubation and ventilation on a volume-controlled, positive-pressure respirator, usually with the addition of positive end-expiratory pressure. These measures may permit additional therapy, cardiac catheterization, and surgical intervention with a much greater margin of safety.

In newborns who have failure as a result of narrowing or closure of the ductus arteriosus in the presence of critical obstruction to flow from the left side of the heart, dramatic and lifesaving relief can be expected with reopening of the ductus by the infusion of PGE_1 at a dose of 0.1 μg/kg per minute.

Finally, infants or children in whom medical therapy is clearly inadequate or only temporarily successful may require prompt surgical intervention for control of heart failure. *As a rule, the earlier the onset of congestive failure, the more likely the need for surgery.*

Hypoxemia

The sequelae of hypoxemia are listed in Table 63-3. *Cyanosis,* a bluish tinge to the color of the skin caused by the presence of at least 3 to 5 g/dL of reduced hemoglobin, is frequently the initial sign of congenital heart disease in an infant. It also may be an early sign of pulmonary, central nervous system, or metabolic disease or methemoglobinemia. Nonsurgical palliation with PGE_1 and the rapid development of surgical techniques for infants make a prompt distinction between cardiac and noncardiac cyanosis, usually by echocardiography, extremely important.

TABLE 63-3 Sequelae of Hypoxemia

Cyanosis	Exercise intolerance
Clubbing	Hypoxic spells
Polycythemia	Brain abscess
Squatting	Cerebrovascular accidents

Hypoxia leading to cyanosis in congenital heart disease may be due to heart failure with pulmonary edema and pulmonary venous desaturation or to intracardiac right-to-left shunting. The hypoxia that is due either to heart failure or to lung disease with intrapulmonary shunting usually responds dramatically to oxygen administration, whereas hypoxia that is due to cyanotic defects does not. Since many infants are relatively anemic during the first few months of life (hemoglobin concentration, 10.4 to 12 g/dL), cyanosis may be subtle.

When cyanosis has been present in older children for several months, the distal tips of the fingers and toes become hyperemic. Eventually, the capillary end loop dilation causes *clubbing* of the fingers and toes with a loss of the normal angle of the base of the nail and fingers. Also, with long-standing hypoxemia, the hematocrit increases to maintain the oxygen-carrying capacity of the blood (*polycythemia*). The increased hemoglobin concentration at any given oxygen saturation will result in more reduced hemoglobin, exaggerating the cyanosis.

The central nervous system may be the target organ of cerebrovascular accidents or brain abcess. *Brain abcess* probably is due to bacteremia primarily with mouth organisms that cross from the venous system to the arterial system right-to-left from shunting. The incidence seems to be directly related to arterial saturation and occurs mostly in older children and adolescents.[26]

Cerebrovascular accidents are due directly to hypoxemia or indirectly in children who are polycythemic presumably secondary to sludging.[27] The former group usually consists of infants less than 2 years old who are anemic and thus may have markedly reduced oxygen levels. The latter group consists of children or young adults who are polycythemic and have sludging or in situ microthrombosis. Interestingly, iron deficiency leads to stiff red cells, and so sludging may occur with modest levels of polycythemia (hematocrit 55 to 60 percent) in the presence of iron deficiency. With hematocrits in the range of 65 percent or higher, increased viscocity may lead to a cerebrovascular accident. Maintaining a proper level of hemoglobin has a salutory effect on hemodynamics and oxygen delivery in the presence of significant hypoxemia.[28,29]

Other systems also may be affected by hypoxemia or polycythemia. In older adolescents, the increase in hemoglobin breakdown may result in hyperuricemia and can precipitate a secondary form of gout.[30]

Disturbances in hemostasis also occur with polycythemia. Coagulation factors are commonly abnormal in patients with hematocrits in excess of 60 percent.[31] Actual platelet counts may be normal but can be increased initially in some patients, with subsequent decreases related to persistent and worsening desaturation. There is evidence of shortened platelet survival time in patients with cyanotic heart disease.[32] Laboratory evaluation of coagulation status requires that correction be made for the diminished volume of plasma and for the volume of anticoagulant used in blood samples to avoid false results. Hematologic management of adults with cyanotic congenital heart disease requires special experience and knowledge.[33]

The major consequences of cyanosis can be avoided in many instances, although differences in intelligence have been demonstrated between cyanotic and acyanotic children.[34]

Retardation of Growth and Development

Children with severe cardiac malformations frequently exhibit retardation of growth and development, with height and weight near or below the third percentile or weight 20 percentile points below the mean percentile for height.[35]

Growth retardation is most severe among children with overt cyanosis and those with large left-to-right shunts that cause heart failure. Heart failure tends to cause a greater retardation of weight than of height. Skeletal retardation, reflected by bone age, usually occurs with height and weight retardation and, among children with cyanotic heart disease, correlates with the severity of hypoxemia.

Other factors contribute to growth retardation, including insufficient caloric intake, dyspnea, frequent infections, psychological disturbances, malabsorption, and hypermetabolism. Among infants with severe congenital heart disease recognized within the first year of life, there is a significantly increased incidence of subnormal birth weight, intrauterine growth retardation, and major extracardiac anomalies.[3] Finally, a relatively small number of children have associated syndromes known to be characterized by growth retardation, such as rubella and Noonan's, Turner's, and Down's syndromes.

Growth retardation related primarily to congenital heart disease usually responds to surgical correction or palliation, with an impressive acceleration of growth and a return to or toward normal.

Although cardiac surgery seldom is recommended on the basis of growth failure alone, decelerated growth should be recognized early and, until proved otherwise, considered an index of the severity of heart disease. In general, the more successful the surgery is, the less will be the retardation of growth and development, with its sequelae of physical, psychological, and intellectual problems.[36]

Pulmonary Arterial Hypertension and Pulmonary Vascular Obstructive Disease

Pulmonary arterial hypertension (PAH) and pulmonary vascular obstructive disease (PVOD) are serious complications of congenital heart disease. PAH usually results from direct transmission of systemic arterial pressure to the right ventricle or pulmonary arteries via a large communication. Less frequently, it is due to severe obstruction to blood flow through the left side of the heart at the pulmonary venous level or beyond. PVOD refers to a process involving structural and developmental changes in the smaller muscular arteries and arterioles of the lung that gradually diminishes and eventually destroys the ability of the pulmonary vascular bed to transport blood from the larger pulmonary arteries to the pulmonary veins without an abnormal elevation of proximal pulmonary arterial pressure.

Pulmonary resistance (R_p) may be as high as 8 to 10 Wood units immediately after birth but falls rapidly throughout the first week of life. Indexed Wood units, as a measure of resistance to flow across either the pulmonary or the systemic vascular bed, are obtained by dividing the mean pressure difference (in millimeters of mercury) across the pulmonary or systemic vascular beds by the blood flow index (expressed in liters per minute per square meter) across those respective beds. By 6 to 8 weeks, it usually has reached the normal adult level (1 to 3 Wood units). These changes are accompanied by a gradual dilatation of first the smaller and then the larger muscular pulmonary arteries and then, in the weeks and months that follow, a thinning of their muscular walls, the growth of existing arteries, and the development of new arteries and arterioles. The latter process contributes over 90 percent of the smaller or intraacinar pulmonary arterial vessels present in older children and adults.[37]

Increased pulmonary arterial pressure has an adverse effect on the normal maturation of the pulmonary vascular bed. Such pressure encourages a persistence of the thick muscular medial layer present in the smaller pulmonary arteries of term newborns, stimulates an extension of smooth muscle into smaller and more peripheral arteries than normal for age, and retards the growth of existing acinar arteries and the development of new ones.

In the presence of a large systemic-to-pulmonary communication, pulmonary arterial pressures remain at or near systemic levels, with the result that the diminution in pulmonary muscle mass and pulmonary resistance is less rapid and of a lesser magnitude than it is in a normal infant. Nevertheless, the diminution is usually sufficient to permit a large pulmonary blood flow and, as a result, congestive failure by the end of the first month. Exceptions are found among infants with a large systemic-to-pulmonary communication but with alveolar hypoxia, a stimulus for pulmonary vasoconstriction, in whom there is less than normal involution of the medial musculature and a diminution in pulmonary vascular resistance. Clinically, this is expressed by the lower incidence of congestive failure observed among infants with large VSDs born and living at high altitude and in some children with Down's syndrome and a large VSD or atrioventricular canal who may hypoventilate or have upper airway obstruction. Rarely, an infant will maintain a very high pulmonary vascular resistance in the face of an anatomically large systemic-to-pulmonary communication without evidence of significant hypoxemia or acidemia and remain free of the signs and symptoms of congestive failure. Conversely, in a premature infant in whom the medial muscle mass is less at birth than it is in a full-term infant, the fall in pulmonary vascular resistance is usually much more rapid than normal.

Chronic PAH, increased flow, or both produce a characteristic series of histologic changes in the smaller pulmonary arteries and arterioles originally described and graded by Heath and Edwards (grades I through VI below)[38] (Fig. 63-4, Plate 100) and, more recently, by Rabinovitch[37] (grades A through C below):

- Grade I—medial hypertrophy
- Grade II—concentric or eccentric cellular intimal proliferation
- Grade III—relatively acellular intimal fibrosis with occlusion of the smaller pulmonary arteries and arterioles
- Grade IV—progressive, generalized dilatation of the distal muscular arteries and the appearance of plexiform lesions, complex vascular structures composed of a network or plexus

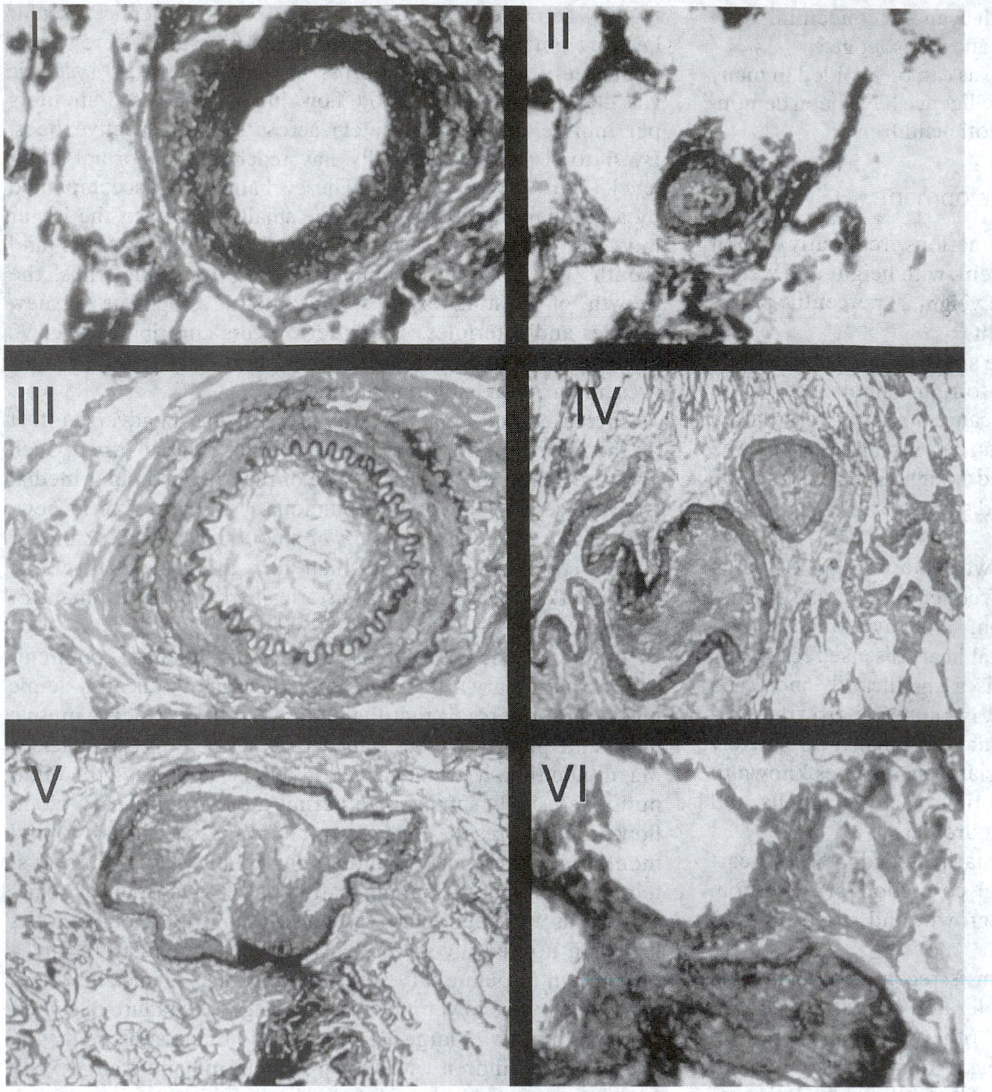

FIGURE 63-4 (Plate 100) Pulmonary vascular changes by the Heath and Edwards criteria (see text). Grades 1–6 are represented by panels I–VI, respectively.

of proliferating endothelial tissue, frequently accompanied by thrombus, within a dilated thin-walled sac

- Grade V—thinning and fibrosis of the media superimposed on the plexiform lesions
- Grade VI—necrotizing arteritis within the media
- Grade A—extension of muscle into normally nonmuscular peripheral arteries with or without a mild increase in medial wall thickness of normally muscular arteries (less than 1.5 times normal)
- Grade B—extension of muscle as described above with an even greater increase in medial wall thickness of normally muscular arteries (mild, 1.5–2 × normal; severe, >2 × normal)
- Grade C—changes seen in grade B (severe) but with a decreased arterial concentration relative to alveoli (mild, ≥1/2 normal; severe, <1/2 normal)

Grades A and B are partitions of Heath-Edwards grade I and may be seen with large left-to-right shunts with (B) or without increased pressure (A). Grade C criteria may be found with grades I and II, are invariable with grade III, and usually preclude a complete return to normal of pulmonary arterial pressures and resistance despite successful surgical correction of the systemic-to-pulmonary communication.

Estimation of pulmonary vascular resistance from data obtained at cardiac catheterization remains the most widely used means of assessing the state of the pulmonary vascular bed. Hypoxemia from oversedation, atelectasis, or pneumonitis at the time of study should be avoided scrupulously. If pulmonary vascular resistance is elevated, its responsiveness to vasodilation induced by the inhalation of 100% oxygen, the pulmonary arterial administration of prostacyclin, or the inhalation of nitric oxide should be tested.[39]

Values of $R_p \leq 3$ Wood units are considered normal. The status of the pulmonary vasculature also can be expressed as a ratio of pulmonary vascular resistance to systemic vascular resistance (R_p/R_s). *Pulmonary/systemic resistance ratios less than 0.2:1 are considered normal.*

As pulmonary vascular resistance increases, pulmonary blood flow generally decreases. Eventually, a point is reached where surgical closure of the defect will produce only a small diminution of blood flow, a proportionately small decrease in pulmonary arterial pressure, and no significant change in the factors contributing to the progression of vascular disease. At this point surgery usually is not recommended, since the benefits are minimal and closure of the defect may eliminate a useful "blow-off" for increasing resistance. *An R_p/R_s ratio of 0.7:1 or an R_p of 11 Wood units with a pulmonary/systemic blood flow ratio of 1.5:1 is the criterion generally used to define this situation.* Without surgery, these patients survive as examples of the Eisenmenger syndrome, in which $R_p \geq R_s$ and at least some right-to-left shunting occurs at rest or with exercise. Some of these patients can survive for several decades and lead productive lives, with relatively mild symptoms and few limitations.[40]

The decision regarding surgery for patients with less severe PVOD is a clinical one. The higher the calculated resistance is and the greater the structural changes in the pulmonary vasculature are, as judged by lung biopsy or quantitative pulmonary arterial wedge angiography, and the older the patient is with any given level of elevated resistance or grade of structural change, the less likely it is that the outcome will be satisfactory.[37]

The prevention of PVOD requires the identification of the patients at risk, i.e., all patients with a systemic-to-pulmonary communication and a pulmonary arterial systolic pressure higher than half the systemic arterial systolic pressure. Also included are all patients with transposition, regardless of pressure or flow, with the possible exception of those with severe pulmonary stenosis. Ideally, all patients at risk should undergo correction or pulmonary arterial banding unless there is proof that the pulmonary arterial systolic pressure has fallen to or is less than half the systemic systolic pressure before the end of the first year of life among those with normally related great arteries. Among patients with transposition with a large VSD or patent ductus arteriosis, action must be taken within the first 3 months of life.

Long-Term Problems with Surgically Corrected Defects

With the advances that have occurred in the surgical treatment of congenital heart defects, more of these patients are living to adulthood. This discussion of potential long-term problems is intended for those who follow these children after surgery and through adult life[41] (see Chap. 64).

There are residua, sequelae, and complications that result from most surgical procedures for congenital heart defects. A residual part of the original defect, such as mitral prolapse in repaired ASD, may purposefully not have been approached surgically. Some sequelae are unavoidable consequences of the surgery, such as pulmonary regurgitation after pulmonary valvotomy. There are also complications that occur as unexpected but related events after successful surgery, such as late complete heart block. When viewed with these possibilities in mind, only surgical correction of a PDA is likely to result in no long-term problems.

Most patients have residual murmurs after surgery for congenital heart defects. Determination of the origin of these murmurs and evaluation of the severity of the hemodynamic abnormalities they represent are important. Noninvasive diagnostic tools, especially Doppler and two-dimensional echocardiography, are often useful.

The risk of infective endocarditis to patients persists after surgery, with the exception of those who have undergone patent ductus ligation or division or repair of an ASD or VSD in whom there is no residual shunt. Patients in whom it has been necessary to place an artificial valve are at increased risk of endocarditis.[42,43]

There are specific problems related to some of the more common defects. For those with repaired ASDs, VSDs, and AV (canal) septal defects, a residual shunt may be present, but ordinarily it is small and not of hemodynamic significance. Those with repaired AV canal defects may have important AV valvular regurgitation. Repaired coarctation of the aorta can gradually become narrowed again, or patients may develop idiopathic hypertension. Surgery for valvular pulmonary stenosis usually results in mild residual stenosis and regurgitation, which are well tolerated and have little tendency to progress with time. The natural history of valvular aortic stenosis after surgery is not as benign.[44] Because significant regurgitation must be avoided, the initial results may not be as good in terms of the severity of residual stenosis. In addition, aortic stenosis tends to worsen with time; thus, proper follow-up is mandatory for these patients.

Few patients enter adulthood with the continued problem of cyanosis. Since those with residual defects amenable to surgical correction should have had surgery well before this time, only patients with complex and uncorrectable defects and those with pulmonary vascular disease should have problems of cyanosis during the adult years. Particularly important among these patients is management of any attendant psychosocial problems (employment, insurability,[45] and learning disabilities) and difficulties related to pregnancy.[46]

Those who have had surgery for cyanotic defects are more likely to have sequelae and complications. Some degree of exercise intolerance is not unusual in this group of patients, and exercise stress testing aids in their management.[47]

Dysrhythmias are particularly common among these patients. *In those who have had intraventricular repairs, most commonly for tetralogy of Fallot, late complete heart block and serious ventricular arrhythmias can occur and may result in sudden death.*[48] This risk appears to be highest in those who had transient complete heart block at the time of surgery and who develop right bundle branch block with left anterior hemiblock after surgery. Extensive interatrial surgical procedures for transposition of the great arteries also frequently lead to dysrhythmias, most commonly sick sinus syndrome with bradytachyarrhythmias and atrial flutter, with a high incidence of sudden death.[49] Ambulatory 24-h electrocardiographic monitoring (see Chap. 25) and stress testing (see Chap. 14) and intracardiac electrophysiologic studies are important in following patients who have had complex repairs. Atrial dilation after the Fontan operation has resulted in atrial flutter and/or fibrillation, which are frequently problematic therapeutically.[50]

Serious ventricular dysfunction[51] and venous obstructions also may occur, usually in those who had severe defects. Interatrial repairs for transposition of the great arteries leave the anatomic right ventricle to do the work of the systemic ventricle.[52] In addition, these repairs may lead to pulmonary and/or systemic venous obstruction. Atriopulmonary connections for the repair of tricuspid atresia and many types of univentricular hearts frequently leave an anatomically abnormal ventricle as the systemic ventricle. In this group of patients, the right atrium has become the "pulmonary ventricle," with an elevated right atrial pressure that may lead to problems of systemic venous hypertension such as protein-losing enteropathy.[53]

Finally, some children have had repairs in which synthetic prostheses were utilized. Artificial valves do not grow as the child does, and they must be much more durable in view of the child's life expectancy. There are also some surgical procedures that require the placement of conduits, with or without valves, that can degenerate and become obstructive with time. *Bioprosthetic valves undergo accelerated fibrosis and calcification in patients less than about 30 to 35 years of age.*

It should be kept in mind that in spite of these problems, the majority of patients who reach adulthood after surgical repair of congenital defects are relatively asymptomatic; they can and do lead productive lives.

INTRACARDIAC COMMUNICATIONS BETWEEN THE SYSTEMIC AND PULMONARY CIRCULATIONS, USUALLY WITHOUT CYANOSIS

Ventricular Septal Defect

PATHOLOGY AND INCIDENCE

A ventricular septal defect is the most common congenital cardiac anomaly (Table 63-4). It may be an isolated defect or part of a complex malformation. Approximately 80 percent of these defects are paramembranous but may extend into the inlet, trabecular, or outlet sections of the muscular septum. Less common are conal septal or subarterial doubly committed defects (5 to 7 percent), inlet defects lying beneath the septal leaflet of the tricuspid valve in the region of the atrioventricular canal (5 to 8 percent), and defects in the muscular septum that may be in the inlet, trabecular, or outlet area[54] (Fig. 63-5). Multiple muscular defects are not infrequently seen.

The incidence of VSDs is about 2 per 1000 live births, and its prevalence among school-age children has been estimated as 1 per 1000, constituting about one-quarter of the congenital cardiac malformations in combined series (Table 63-1). Males and females are affected equally.

VSDs may be isolated or associated with other congenital cardiac abnormalities. Malformations associated with VSD are, in order of decreasing frequency: (1) coarctation of the aorta, (2) additional shunts, most commonly ASD and PDA, (3) intracardiac obstructions such as subpulmonary or subaortic stenosis, mitral stenosis, and anomalous muscle bundle of the right ventricle, and (4) incompetent atrioventricular valves.

ABNORMAL PHYSIOLOGY

The consequences of a VSD depend on the size of the defect and the pulmonary vascular resistance. A small defect offers a large resistance to flow. There is no elevation of right ventricular or pulmonary arterial pressure, and the left-to-right shunt may be so small that it can be detected only by selective left ventricular angiography or two-dimensional imaging with Doppler color flow mapping. This type of defect imposes little physiologic burden on the heart, although there is always the danger of infective endocarditis.

A defect of moderate size still permits a difference between the right and left ventricular systolic pressures but may allow a large left-to-right shunt with resulting left atrial hypertension and dilatation and left ventricular volume overload. The development of pulmonary vascular disease among these patients is unusual but possible.

When the effective area of the defect is large, approximately equal to or greater than the aortic valve orifice, the defect offers virtually no resistance to flow and the systolic pressures in both ventricles, the aorta, and the pulmonary artery are essentially the same. The relative proportion of blood going to the two circulations is directly governed by the relative resistance of the two vascular beds.

TABLE 63-4 Communications with Predominant Left-to-Right Shunting

Ventricular septal defect	Atrioventricular canal
Atrial septal defect	Patent ductus arteriosus
Partial anomalous pulmonary venous connection	Sinus of Valsalva fistula

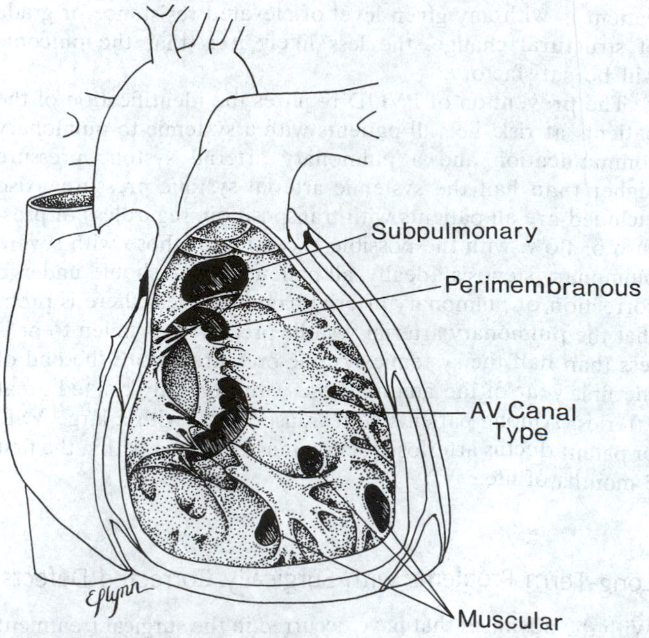

FIGURE 63-5 Different types of ventricular septal defects when viewed from the right ventricle. (From Fyler DC, ed. *Nadas' Pediatric Cardiology*. Philadelphia: Hanley & Belfus; 1992. Reproduced with permission from the publisher and author.)

At birth, pulmonary vascular resistance is high and there is little, if any, left-to-right shunt despite the presence of a large defect. This resistance to flow gradually falls over the first few weeks of life, permitting a progressively greater amount of blood to flow through the defect, through the lungs, and back to the left atrium and left ventricle. In most infants, the left ventricular volume overload eventually leads to left ventricular "failure" with elevated left ventricular end-diastolic and left atrial pressures and pulmonary congestion.

In term infants born at sea level with a large VSD, clinical deterioration may occur at any time from about 3 to 12 weeks after birth. In premature infants, in whom the less well developed pulmonary vascular hypertrophy regresses more rapidly, failure frequently is noted at 1 to 4 weeks.

History Infants or children with a small isolated defect are asymptomatic. The murmur of a small defect may be detected within the first 24 to 36 h of life, since the very restrictive opening permits the normal rapid fall in pulmonary arterial resistance and pressures. Infants with larger defects usually present between 3 and 12 weeks of age with congestive failure, frequently with associated lower respiratory tract infections. Parents describe tachypnea, grunting respirations, and fatigue, particularly with feedings. Weight gain is slow, and excessive sweating is common.

Physical Examination A child with a small defect is comfortable. With moderate holes, a systolic thrill at the lower left sternal border is common. If the defect is small, the pulmonary artery pressure is normal and so the second heart sound is not accentuated. The systolic murmur along the lower left sternal border is characteristically holosystolic but may be limited to early or midsystole. This latter feature suggests a defect in the muscular septum rather than the membranous septum.

Infants with large defects, large left-to-right shunt, and PAH tend to be restless, irritable, and underweight. Moderate respiratory distress may be present. Both the right and the left ventricular systolic impulses are impressively hyperdynamic to palpation. A thrill at the lower left sternal border is common. The second heart sound is narrowly split, with a loud, frequently palpable pulmonary component. Third heart sound gallops at the apex are common. Characteristically, the systolic murmur is holosystolic at the lower left sternal border and is accompanied by a middiastolic rumble of grade 2 to 3 intensity at the apex, with the latter indicating a pulmonary/systemic blood flow ratio (Q_p/Q_s) of 2:1 or greater. Hepatic enlargement can be identified below the right costal margin. Pulmonary rales may be seen with severe failure.

With the passage of time, one may observe signs of a diminishing left-to-right shunt with an improved rate of weight gain, less dyspnea, a diminution of the precordial hyperactivity, and disappearance of the apical diastolic flow rumble. This clinical improvement may be a result of the defect becoming smaller, the development of subvalvular pulmonary stenosis with little or no appreciable change in the size of the defect, or, most worrisome, the development of PVOD with continued severe PAH. With developing subpulmonary stenosis, the systolic murmur radiates more and more impressively to the upper left sternal border and the second heart sound becomes more widely split, with a progressive diminution in the intensity of the pulmonary component. Decreased flow resulting from pulmonary vascular disease is characterized by a gradual reduction in the intensity and duration of the systolic murmur, more narrow splitting of the second heart sound, and marked accentuation of the pulmonary component.

The clinical picture of advanced pulmonary vascular disease secondary to a congenital left-to-right shunt, or Eisenmenger's syndrome, is that of a relatively comfortable older child, adolescent, or young adult with mild cyanosis and clubbing in whom one finds a prominent a wave in the jugular venous pulse, a mild right ventricular lift, and a second heart sound that is narrowly split or virtually single with a very loud, usually palpable pulmonary component. An early pulmonary systolic ejection sound, reflecting dilatation of the main pulmonary artery, may be heard, and there may be no systolic murmur at all. In older adolescents and adults, an early diastolic murmur of pulmonary regurgitation or a holosystolic murmur of tricuspid regurgitation may appear.

Chest Roentgenogram In the presence of a small defect, the heart size and shape and the pulmonary blood flow are barely altered. With large defects, there is moderate to marked enlargement of the heart, with prominence of the main pulmonary arterial segment and impressive overcirculation in the peripheral lung fields. The left atrium is dilated unless an associated ASD is present, allowing decompression of the left atrium. With increasing pulmonary vascular disease, there is diminution in heart size toward normal while the central pulmonary arteries remain dilated. The peripheral pulmonary arterial markings become attenuated, and a "pruned" effect is produced in the outer third of the lung fields.

Electrocardiogram With a small defect, one can expect the normal progression of the mean QRS axis from right to left and the normal gradual diminution of the prominent right ventricular voltages characteristic of newborns. The left ventricular forces remain within normal limits or become slightly augmented as a reflection of the mild left ventricular volume overload. With large defects, the mean QRS axis tends to remain oriented to the right and there is little or no regression in right ventricular voltage. The left ventricular forces gradually increase, resulting in a pattern of biventricular hypertrophy within the first few weeks of life. Left atrial hypertrophy is usually present, and frequently right atrial hypertrophy as well. With the development of pulmonary vascular disease or significant pulmonary stenosis, the mean QRS axis tends to remain oriented to the right; there is no regression in right ventricular voltage, but the evidence of left ventricular and left atrial hypertrophy lessens or disappears.

Echocardiogram Two-dimensional imaging can distinguish an uncomplicated VSD from more complex malformations and is capable of imaging most defects directly when multiple transducer positions are used. The addition of pulsed-wave Doppler with color flow mapping permits the identification of small, multiple, muscular, and other less easily visualized defects. The position and size of the opening can be determined as well as its relationships to the aorta, pulmonary artery, and AV valves. Continuous-wave Doppler echocardiography can predict the systolic right ventricular pressure from the difference between the systolic pressure measured by a blood pressure cuff if there is no aortic stenosis and the Doppler gradient (Fig. 63-6). In the absence of associated pulmonic stenosis, the right ventricular

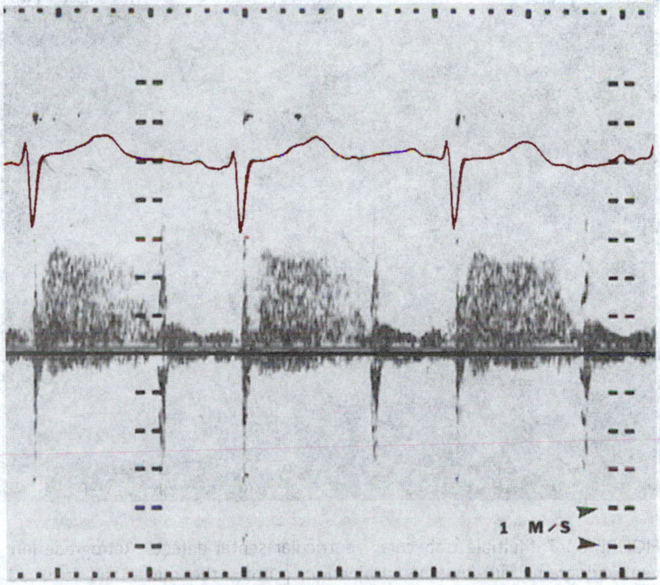

FIGURE 63-6 Continuous-wave Doppler with spectral display from the left lower sternal border of a child with a ventricular septal defect that demonstrates holosystolic turbulence with peak velocity = 2.8 m/s across the defect, compatible with an instantaneous systolic pressure difference of 31 mmHg between the right and left ventricles.

systolic pressure provides an estimate of the pulmonary artery pressure. An accurate approximation of right ventricular systolic pressure also can be made by estimating the right ventricular to right atrial systolic pressure gradient across the tricuspid valve if tricuspid regurgitation is present.

Cardiac Catheterization Cardiac catheterization is being done less commonly in VSDs not associated with other cardiac malformations. When it is performed, an increase in oxygen saturation at the right ventricular level reflects the left-to-right shunt via the VSD. With small defects, the right ventricular and pulmonary arterial systolic pressures are normal. With large defects, these pressures are at or near systemic levels, and the mean left atrial pressure may be elevated to the range of 10 to 15 mmHg.

Selective left ventricular angiography in the anteroposterior, lateral, and oblique views with craniocaudal angulation can be done to establish the spatial relations of the great arteries to each other and to the ventricles and also to determine the exact site, size, and number of septal defects (Fig. 63-7). Aortography is helpful in eliminating the possibility of an associated ductus arteriosus or unsuspected coarctation of the aorta if the arch cannot be well imaged by echocardiography.

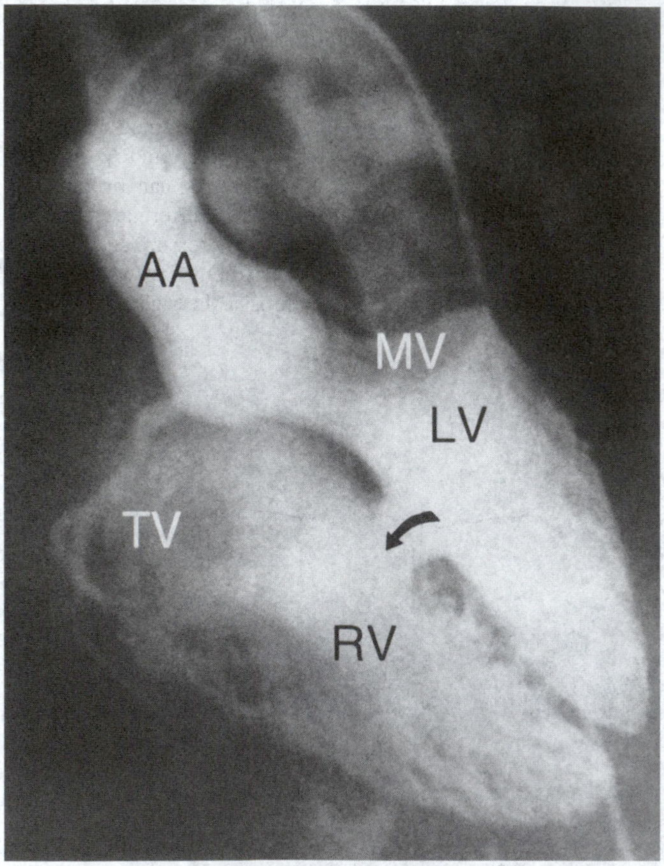

FIGURE 63-7 Multiple trabecular ventricular septal defects. Retrograde left ventriculogram, four-chamber projection, profiles the mitral and tricuspid valves and the midtrabecular VSD (*arrow*). Additional VSDs closer to the apex are more anterior in location and are not profiled in this projection. AA = ascending aorta; LV = left ventricle; MV = mitral valve; RV = right ventricle; TV = tricuspid valve. (From Lock JE, Keane JF, Perry SB. *Diagnostic and Interventional Catheterization in Congenital Heart Disease*, 2d. ed. Boston: Kluwer; 2000.)

NATURAL HISTORY AND PROGNOSIS

Fortunately, the majority of VSDs are small and do not present a serious clinical problem. Approximately 24 percent of these small defects close spontaneously by 18 months, 50 percent by 4 years, and 75 percent by 10 years.[55] A spontaneous closure rate approaching 45 percent within the first 12 to 14 months has been observed among infants with an uncomplicated paramembranous or muscular VSD in the neonatal period.[56] Even large defects tend to become smaller, but the likelihood of eventual spontaneous closure is much lower (probably in the range of 60 percent if judged large at 3 months of age and only 50 percent if it is still large at 6 months).[55]

Congestive failure is a threatening and almost inevitable complication of a large VSD. Almost 80 percent of infants with large defects require hospitalization by age 4 months.[3] The risk of death with congestive failure is in the range of 11 percent. Significant subvalvular pulmonary stenosis develops in approximately 3 percent of these individuals and may progress to the point of severe tetralogy of Fallot. PVOD is seldom severe and rarely is irreversible in the first 12 months of life, but thereafter it becomes progressively more common and less likely to regress. At risk of this complication are infants and children with a pulmonary systolic pressure in excess of 50 percent of the systemic arterial systolic pressure beyond the first year of life.[57] A very small number of infants with large VSDs maintain a high level of pulmonary vascular resistance throughout the first year of life and remain almost entirely free of symptoms and congestive heart failure. In these patients, irreversible pulmonary vascular disease may develop without the usual and expected clinical signs and symptoms described above.

A small number of children, 0.6 percent in a large group of carefully followed patients, will develop aortic regurgitation as a result of prolapse of the right, the posterior, or both aortic valve leaflets into the defect.[58] This complication is more prevalent among males, in a ratio of 2:1, and seems particularly likely to occur with defects of the subpulmonary type. Shunt size appears not to be related to the development of this complication. The characteristic aortic diastolic murmur may appear at any time between ages 6 months and 20 years. Regurgitation is usually progressive, sometimes rapidly so, and predisposes these individuals to infective endocarditis.

The risk of infective endocarditis in patients with an uncomplicated VSD that is managed medically lies somewhere between 4 and 10 percent for the first 30 years of life.[59] The development of aortic regurgitation more than doubles this risk. Attempts at surgical closure of the defect with or without aortic regurgitation reduce the risk to less than half that of unoperated patients.[60]

MEDICAL MANAGEMENT

The basis of the medical management of children with ventricular septal defects is an understanding that defects frequently get smaller and may close spontaneously. Approximately 70 percent of small ventricular septal defects probably close.[55] Even large muscular defects may get significantly smaller, and up to 25 percent of them will become hemodynamically insignificant if one can wait long enough. Nevertheless, significant complications can occur, and the decision whether to proceed with medical or surgical management must be reevaluated constantly.

For children with a large ventricular septal defect, the first decision point usually occurs before 8 to 12 weeks of age. Infants with large septal defects usually develop significant left-to-right shunts as the pulmonary resistance drops. Congestive heart failure ensues with tachypnea, tachycardia, and difficulty feeding. Digoxin and diuretics are occasionally useful, but if the left-to-right shunt is very large, feeding may be problematic. For children who cannot gain at least 15 g per day (30 g per day is normal) in whom no other cause is found for failure to thrive, surgical repair is indicated. Occasionally, in marginal cases, increasing the caloric density of the formula from 20 calories per ounce up to 30 to 32 calories per ounce may be useful. In children whom the increased work prevents from taking more than 10 to 12 ounces per day, however, caloric supplementation is unlikely to be sufficient and surgical repair is necessary.

The second decision point in children who do not fail to thrive occurs between 9 and 12 months of age. Children with unrestrictive or mildly restrictive ventricular septal defects have pulmonary artery hypertension that may lead to irreversible pulmonary vascular obstructive disease. If the pulmonary artery pressure is elevated at 9 to 12 months of age, surgery is indicated to prevent this serious life-shortening complication. In some children, the high-pitched nature of the murmur, the normal pulmonary component of the second heart sound, the absence of right ventricular hypertension on ECG, and the large intraventricular pressure gradient on echocardiography make the estimation of normal pulmonary artery pressure firm. Occasionally in children in whom the signs, symptoms, and laboratory findings are ambiguous or conflicting, cardiac catheterization may be necessary to assure that the pulmonary artery pressure is normal and that pulmonary vascular obstructive disease is not a risk.

The third decision point occurs somewhere in midchildhood (5 to 10 years of age). If the defect has not caused failure to thrive and is not associated with pulmonary hypertension, it still may be associated with a significant left-to-right shunt, causing a volume overload to the left ventricle. Eventually, congestive heart failure is possible, and some recommend surgical closure during childhood if there is a significant volume overload. There is no firm number that suggests a dangerous level of left ventricular volume overload. Some centers close the ventricular septal defect when the pulmonary-to-systemic flow ratio (measured by cardiac catheterization, radionuclide angiography, echocardiography or magnetic resonance imaging) is more than 2 to 1. Others use significant left atrial and left ventricular dilation by echo. A minority of centers do not recommend surgical closure as long as the pulmonary artery pressure is normal since there are few adults with a ventricular septal defect who develop problems with late congestive heart failure.

Unfortunately, not all patients with a large defect are encountered during the first or second year of life, when it is possible to prevent injury to the pulmonary vascular bed. If significant PAH is allowed to persist, one can expect progression to irreversible pulmonary obstructive disease. For this reason, *prompt surgical closure of defects is recommended in all individuals beyond the age of 2 years if the pulmonary arterial systolic pressure is greater than half the systemic arterial systolic pressure, the mean pulmonary pressure exceeds 25 mmHg, or the R_p/R_s ratio is higher than 0.3:1.* With severe pulmonary vascular disease, a point eventually is reached where the risk of death at operation or in the months or years immediately after the operation as a result of progressive vascular disease more than offsets the possible benefits from surgical closure. At present, surgery is recommended if the calculated R_p is less than 10 Wood units/m^2 or the R_p/R_s ratio is 0.7:1, provided that the Q_p/Q_s ratio is still 1.5:1. In adults, the upper limit of pulmonary vascular resistance for surgery is approximately 800 dynes, or 10 Wood units.

Patients in whom the defect is judged clinically to be small at 6 months of age may be reexamined at 1- or 2-year intervals to reassure the patient and family, reemphasize the importance of antibiotic protection against infective endocarditis, document further narrowing or closure of the defect, and (in a very small number of patients) detect the first signs of aortic valve prolapse.

In patients with Eisenmenger's complex,[40] stamina is limited by systemic arterial hypoxemia and, in some, right-sided heart failure. Complications to be anticipated include syncope, hemoptysis, brain abscess, hyperuricemia, and congestive failure. Pregnancy, with a maternal mortality of 30 to 60 percent, and oral contraceptives are contraindicated. Transient symptomatic relief from extreme polycythemia (usually >68 percent) may be achieved with careful erythropheresis. Travel to or living at high altitudes is poorly tolerated, and supplemental oxygen should be provided and used during air travel. The average age of death for individuals with Eisenmenger's complex is 33 years, with sudden death the mode of exit in the majority.

The risk of congenital heart disease for a subsequent sibling of a single affected child is on the order of 1 to 2 percent. The risk to a newborn who has one parent with VSD is approximately 3 percent.[61] Pregnancy in the presence of a small defect and normal pulmonary vascular resistance does not appear to carry an increased risk to the patient or infant, although precautions against infective endocarditis should be taken.

SURGICAL MANAGEMENT

Banding of the pulmonary artery to reduce pulmonary blood flow and pressures played an important role in the management of congestive heart failure and the prevention of PVOD before the era of predictably successful closure of VSDs in infants but now is used rarely. Complications of pulmonary arterial banding include deformity of the pulmonary arteries and/or pulmonary valve, progressive right ventricular hypertrophy with loss of ventricular compliance, and the development of subaortic left ventricular outflow tract obstruction.

VSDs are closed during a total cardiopulmonary bypass with cardioplegic arrest and moderate systemic hypothermia. Total circulatory arrest or minimal perfusion with profound hypothermia (18°C) is sometimes necessary in infants who weigh less than 5 kg.[62]

Paramembranous VSDs may be exposed through the right atrium and the tricuspid valve orifice. A transverse or longitudinal right ventriculotomy may be necessary for closure of high conal septal defects associated with aortic valve leaflet prolapse.

Care is required to prevent injury to the AV node near the ostium of the coronary sinus and to the bundle of His as it courses inferiorly, passing on the left side of the ventricular septum near the posterocaudal margin of the septal defect. Interoperative transesophageal echocardiography with Doppler color flow assessment can be used for the detection of significant residual or previously unsuspected problems that may be corrected in the operating room.

Results from primary surgical closure of VSDs are generally excellent, with surgical mortality less than 1 percent in centers with extensive experience, when surgery is performed during the early months of life before the evolution of PVOD. Operative risk should be even lower in older children if the pulmonary vascular resistance remains low. The pulmonary vascular bed responds favorably when the systemic-to-pulmonary shunt is eliminated before age 2 years. Normal life expectancy and functional capabilities should be anticipated postoperatively. Survival 25 years after the closure of a VSD is approximately 95 percent.[63] The mortality rate is unquestionably higher among patients who are operated on with $R_p > 7$ Wood units.

The surgical repair of a multiple muscular VSD has been problematic. The highly trabecular right ventricular septal surface can make the localization of all the defects difficult. Recently, techniques have become available to close these defects in the catheterization laboratory.[64] A device that can be anchored on the left ventricular and right ventricular septal surface was approved by the U.S. Food and Drug Administration in 1999 for this indication. Other devices are now in phase 2 testing.

Between February 1989 and July 1998, 148 transcatheter closures were preformed at Children's Hospital in Boston with no deaths or late morbidity resulting from catheter-related events. By echocardiography, 83 percent of the defects were closed or had trivial residual leaks.[64] The relative role of surgery versus interventional catheterization closure remains to be determined in this subset with multiple trabeculated septal defects.

Atrial Septal Defect

DEFINITION

An ASD is a through-and-through communication between the atria at the septal level. It is to be distinguished from a valvular-competent foramen ovale, which may persist into adulthood.

PATHOLOGY

ASDs are usually sufficiently large to allow free communication between the atria. They may be subdivided according to anatomic location[65] (Fig. 63-8).

ANATOMIC TYPES

Defect at the Fossa Ovalis (Ostium Secundum) This defect classically involves the region of the fossa ovalis and is the most common type (70 percent)[65,66] (Fig. 63-8*A* and *C*). Atrial septal tissue separates the inferior edge of the defect from the AV valves. Associated partial anomalous pulmonary venous connections are not uncommon, with one or more of the right pulmonary veins draining into the right atrium or one of its tributaries. Mitral valve prolapse is present in some cases.

Partial Atrioventricular Canal Defects Defects of the AV septum, which lies inferior to the fossa ovalis, constitute approximately 20 percent of ASDs and are part of a complex malformation known as *common atrioventricular canal defects*, which are considered below (Fig. 63-8*D*).

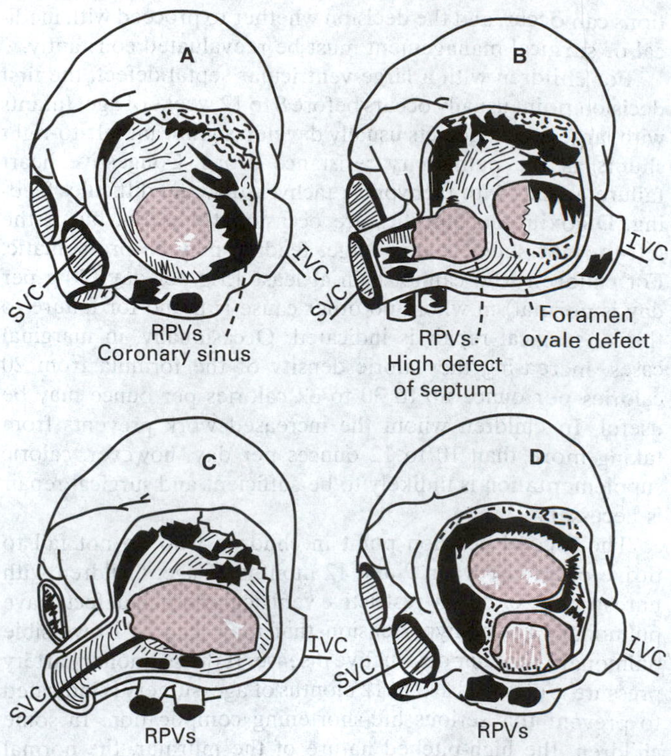

FIGURE 63-8 Types of interatrial communications. *A*. Large ostium secundum type of atrial septal defect. *B*. So-called sinus venosus type of defect—one high in the atrial septum associated with anomalous connection of the right superior pulmonary vein to the junctional area of the superior vena cava and right atrium. *C*. Very large ostium secundum type of atrial septal defect with absence of the posterior rim. *D*. Partial form of common atrioventricular canal with cleft mitral valve. SVC = superior vena cava; RPVs = right pulmonary veins; IVC = inferior vena cava. (From Lewis FJ et al.[65] Copyright 1957, American Medical Association. Reproduced with permission from the publisher and authors.)

Sinus Venosus Defects These defects, accounting for approximately 6 percent of the total, appear to represent a biatrial connection of the superior vena cava (or, in rare instances, the inferior vena cava), which straddles the otherwise normal intact atrial septum. Also involved is an anomalous termination of one or more of the right-sided pulmonary veins either into the vena cava or into the right atrium near its junction with the vena cava (Fig. 63-8*B*).

Coronary Sinus Defects A coronary sinus defect is an uncommon type of ASD located in the position normally occupied by the ostium of the coronary sinus. This defect is part of a developmental complex consisting of the absence of the coronary sinus and entry of the left superior vena cava directly into the left atrium.

Conditions Common to All Anatomic Types The right atrial and ventricular chambers as well as the central pulmonary arteries become enlarged. When pulmonary hypertension intervenes, it usually does not do so before the third decade. The earliest lesion is cellular fibrous intimal thickening in the proximal segments of arterioles. The pulmonary arterial pressure then rises, followed by the development of medial hypertrophy of muscular arteries and the appearance of plexiform lesions. The right ventricular wall hypertrophies, and atherosclerosis may occur in the major pulmonary arteries. Saccular aneurysm and thrombosis with dissecting aneurysm or rupture may occur (see above, "Pulmonary Arterial Hypertension and Pulmonary Vascular Obstructive Disease"). In the final state, the pulmonary vascular bed may be difficult to distinguish from that in VSD with PVOD.

ABNORMAL PHYSIOLOGY

Usually there is no resistance to blood flow across the defect and no significant pressure difference between the two atria. A left-to-right shunt of blood occurs (Fig. 63-9) because (1) the right atrial system is more distensible than the left, (2) the tricuspid valve is normally more capacious than the mitral valve, and (3) the thinner-walled right ventricular chamber more readily accommodates a larger volume of blood at the same filling pressure than does the left ventricle. A large left-to-right shunt may be found in a neonate or young infant before the right ventricular compliance has had time to change appreciably from that of the left ventricle. Presumably, this occurs because a rapid fall in pulmonary vascular resistance encourages a larger right ventricular stroke volume, a smaller end-systolic volume, and hence an increased ability of the right ventricle to accept a larger volume of blood during the diastolic filling phase of the cardiac cycle.[67]

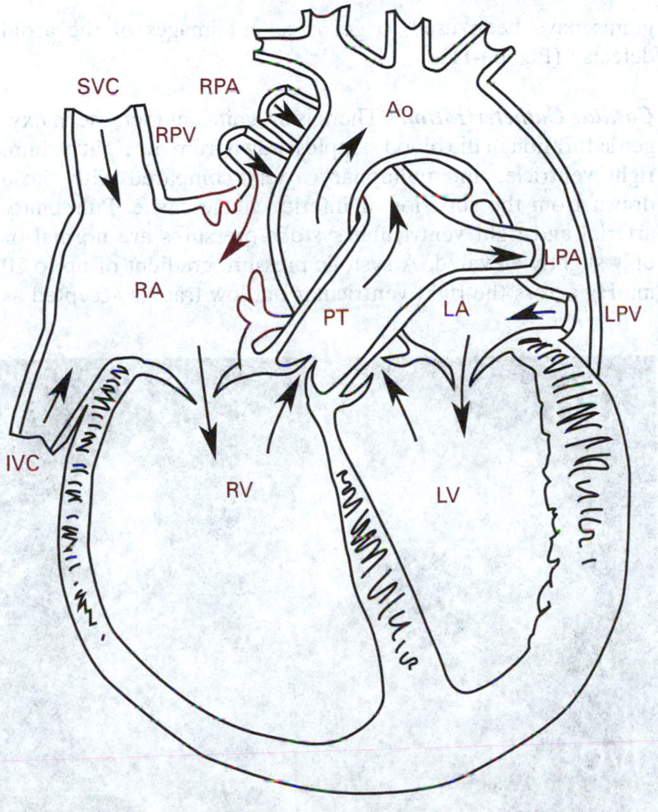

FIGURE 63-9 Atrial septal defect at fossa ovalis with left-to-right shunt. SVC = superior vena cava; IVC = inferior vena cava; RA = right atrium; RV = right ventricle; PT = main pulmonary arterial trunk; RPA = right pulmonary artery; LPA = left pulmonary artery; RPV = right pulmonary vein; LPV = left pulmonary vein; LA = left atrium; LV = left ventricle; AO = aorta. (From Edwards JE.[66] Reproduced with permission from the publisher and author.)

The pulmonary arterial system undergoes normal maturation after birth, with most patients tolerating the large volume load on the right ventricle and pulmonary circuit quite well for many years. With the development of pulmonary vascular disease and PAH, the left-to-right shunt decreases, largely because of the increased thickness and decreased compliance of the right ventricle. In some patients, this process continues until there is eventually shunt reversal, with arterial desaturation and cyanosis.

CLINICAL MANIFESTATIONS

ASD is found in approximately 6 percent of children who survive beyond the first year of life with congenital heart disease.[5] *If one excludes mitral valve prolapse and a congenitally bicuspid aortic valve, it is the most common form of congenital heart disease among adults.*

ASDs are more common among females, with a female/male ratio of approximately 2:1. The mode of transmission is best explained in most instances on a multifactorial basis, in which the risk would be approximately 2.5 percent for first-degree relatives of a single affected family member. However, examples of autosomal dominant transmission are recognized[68] either as an isolated entity associated with severe AV conduction disturbances or with upper extremity malformations as in the Holt-Oram syndrome. Examples of mendelian autosomal recessive transmission are found in the Ellis–van Creveld syndrome (see Chap. 62).

History The majority of these children are considered asymptomatic but probably most have some mild diminution of stamina, since it is not unusual for the patient or the parents to comment on the increased endurance that follows surgical correction. Symptoms of mild fatigue and dyspnea tend to be recognized in the late teens and early twenties, and at least three-quarters of these individuals will be definitely symptomatic as adults. Congestive heart failure is rare in childhood, but a few infants, perhaps 5 percent, have heart failure in the first year of life. Failure becomes more common again in the fourth and fifth decades, usually associated with the onset of arrhythmias.[69]

Physical Examination Many of these children have a slender habitus, but normal growth and development are the rule. Prominence of the left anterior chest is common, and a hyperdynamic right ventricular systolic lift usually can be felt. Looking at the jugular venous pulse demonstrates that the *v* wave is equal to the *a* wave instead of revealing the normal a wave predominance. The first heart sound may be slightly accentuated at the lower left sternal border. The two components of the second heart sound are characteristically widely split, with the interval of splitting fixed despite expiration or the Valsalva maneuver. The pulmonary component of the second heart sound may be accentuated even in the absence of PAH. With increasing pulmonary arterial pressure and resistance, the interval between the aortic and pulmonary components of the second heart sound narrows and the pulmonary component becomes louder, but the lack of respiratory influence on the interval between the two components persists. A midsystolic spindle-shaped murmur of grade 2 to 3 intensity at the left upper sternal border, reflecting increased right ventricular stroke volume and relative

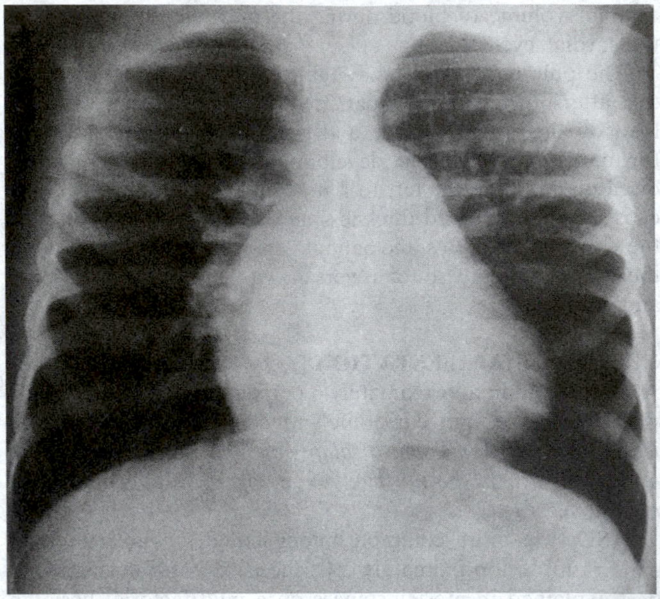

A

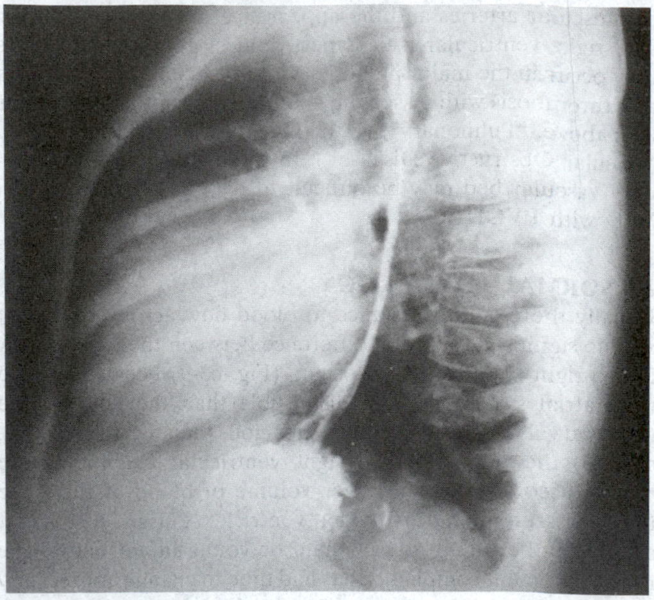

B

FIGURE 63-10 Chest roentgenogram of a 4-year-old child with a secundum atrial septal defect, a large left-to-right shunt, and normal pulmonary arterial pressures. *A.* Frontal. *B.* Lateral. Right ventricular enlargement (seen in the lateral view) accompanies prominence of the main pulmonary arterial segment and increased blood flow. No left atrial dilation is present.

pulmonary stenosis, is to be expected. A low- to medium-pitched early diastolic murmur over the lower left sternal border, denoting increased diastolic flow across the tricuspid valve, is present in most individuals with large shunts (see Chap. 10). Cyanosis and clubbing reflect right-to-left shunting. In this setting, the murmurs of tricuspid and pulmonary regurgitation are not uncommon.

Chest Roentgenogram Mild to moderate cardiac enlargement and prominence of the main and branch pulmonary arteries are characteristic. The absence of left atrial displacement of the barium-filled esophagus in the lateral view helps distinguish ASD from large left-to-right shunts at other levels (Fig. 63-10).

Electrocardiogram An rsR′ pattern over the right precordium indicating mild right ventricular conduction delay or mild right ventricular hypertrophy is characteristic in secundum-type ASD. The mean QRS axis in the frontal plane is 90° or greater in 60 percent of patients. Left-axis deviation is common in primum-type ASD. Abnormal leftward p axis is common in sinus venosus–type ASD. Serious arrhythmias are usually, though not invariably, limited to adults; atrial fibrillation and atrial flutter are the most common arrhythmias.

Echocardiogram M-mode studies reflect volume overload of the right side of the heart with increased right atrial and right ventricular dimensions and paradoxical ventricular septal motion. Two-dimensional and Doppler echocardiography with color flow mapping (see Chap. 13) permit identification and visualization of secundum, AV canal, and sinus venosus defects. Visualization of anomalous draining pulmonary veins is slightly more difficult. The transesophageal approach offers excellent images for those patients in whom the transthoracic approach is inadequate.[70] Recently three-dimensional (3-D) echocardiograms have been used to get excellent images of the atrial defects[71] (Fig. 63-11).

Cardiac Catheterization There is a significant increase in oxygen saturation in the blood samples drawn from the right atrium, right ventricle, and pulmonary artery compared with those drawn from the superior or inferior venae cavae. Pulmonary arterial and right ventricular systolic pressures are normal or only slightly elevated. A systolic pressure gradient of up to 20 mmHg across the right ventricular outflow tract is accepted as

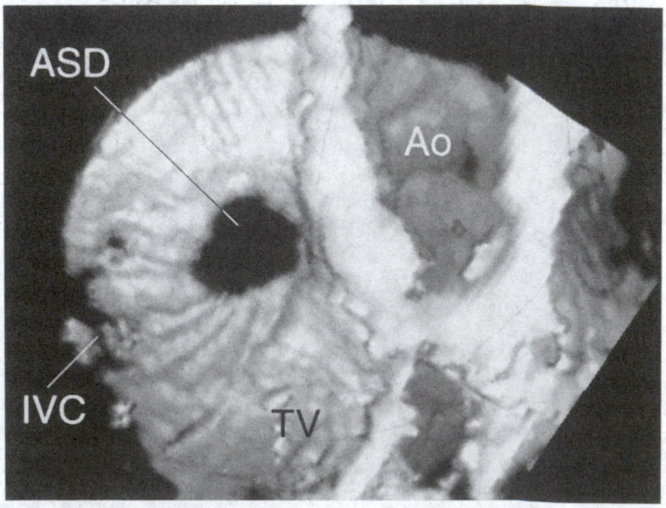

FIGURE 63-11 Three-dimensional echocardiogram of a secundum atrial septal defect (ASD). This is a right atrial en-face view that shows the size, shape, and position of the defect in relation to the right atrial septal surface. Ao = aortic valve; TV = tricuspid valve; IVC = inferior vena cava. Courtesy of Dr. Gerry Marx.

being secondary to flow rather than to organic obstruction. The right and left atrial mean and phasic pressures are virtually identical, with little, if any, elevation above normal (mean pressure gradient <3 mmHg) unless there are associated abnormalities.

NATURAL HISTORY AND PROGNOSIS

Defects of the secundum type usually go undetected in the first year or two of life because of the lack of symptoms and the unimpressive auscultatory findings. A soft systolic murmur is the usual reason for referral. Symptoms become more common in persons in their late teens and twenties, and by age 40 the majority of these individuals are symptomatic, some severely so.[72] Pulmonary vascular disease with serious pulmonary hypertension begins to make its appearance in the early twenties. *It affects approximately 15 percent of young adults, particularly women, and may be rapidly progressive, especially with pregnancy*. The incidence of atrial fibrillation or flutter also increases with each decade and is closely linked to the onset of congestive failure. Spontaneous closure of secundum defects is rare beyond the first 2 years of life.[69] Congestive heart failure is the most common cause of death among unoperated patients. Other causes of death include pulmonary embolism or thrombosis, paradoxical emboli, brain abscess, and infection.

MEDICAL MANAGEMENT

The few infants who present with symptoms of congestive failure are treated with digoxin and, if necessary, diuretics and are studied by cardiac catheterization. If the defect is uncomplicated and the symptoms persist despite a trial of therapy, surgical closure is advised without further delay. For asymptomatic infants and children, closure is recommended just before entry into school. Restrictions of activity or exercise are unnecessary. If the physical, laboratory, and echocardiographic findings are completely characteristic, preoperative catheterization is not necessary. Closure is recommended if the defect is large and if there is right ventricular volume overload on echocardiography. In those with pulmonary hypertension closure is recommended for patients with Q_p/Q_s ratios >1.5:1 by catheterization provided that the systemic arterial saturation is >92 percent and total R_p < 15 Wood units.[73] Closure would seem prudent before pregnancy or the use of contraceptives in view of the tendency to develop rapidly progressive PVOD in this setting. Transcatheter closure of centrally located secundum in selected older infants, children, and adults using a double-umbrella ("clamshell") or a buttoned device appears to be an acceptable alternative to surgical closure.[74–76] *Infective endocarditis is rare, and antibiotic coverage at times of possible bacteremia is recommended only if associated mitral valve disease is suspected.*

SURGICAL MANAGEMENT

Defects of the interatrial septum are exposed through the lateral wall of the right atrium.

Ostium secundum (fossa ovalis) defects frequently are closed by direct suturing; a very large defect or one with tenuous margins is closed with a patch, usually glutaraldehyde-treated autologous pericardium. Anomalous pulmonary veins are sought along the posterolateral aspect of the superior or inferior vena cava and from within the right atrium before closure of the defect. Sutures are placed with care along the posterior rim of the inferior vena caval orifice to prevent the creation of a tunnel from the inferior vena cava into the left atrium, which would cause postoperative hypoxemia.

High ASDs of the sinus venosus type, which often are associated with anomalous drainage of one or more right pulmonary veins into the superior vena cava, are corrected by means of the placement of a pericardial or tubular Dacron patch from above the abnormally draining vein or veins down to and around the ASD (Fig. 63-12). Pulmonary venous blood thus is diverted through the ASD into the left atrium. Pericardial gusset enlargement of the superior vena cava at the cavoatrial junction may be required. Anomalous right pulmonary veins draining to the right atrium are diverted into the left atrium by placement of a patch baffle well anterior and to the right of the pulmonary vein orifices. The risks of surgery are minimal (less than 0.5 percent), with virtually all these children home by the fourth postoperative day.

In adults, clinical benefit after closure of ASDs can be anticipated even in those with significant physiologic compromise,

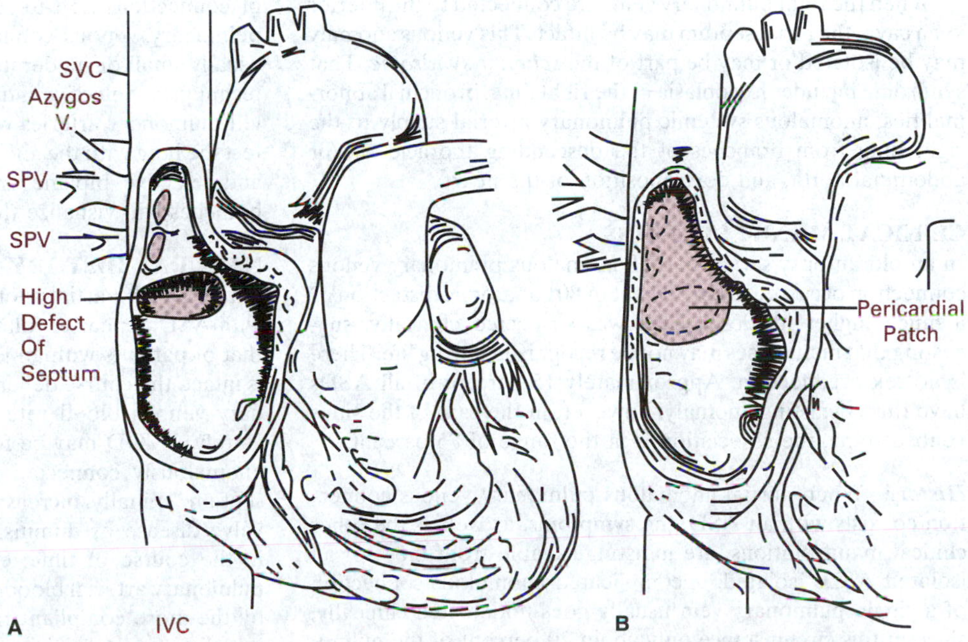

FIGURE 63-12 *A*. Sinus venosus type of atrial septal defect, with its constantly accompanying anomalous pulmonary venous connection of superior pulmonary vein (SPV) to superior vena cava (SVC). *B*. Repair is effected with a pericardial patch placed to divert pulmonary venous blood across the defect into the left atrium and to divert superior vena caval blood to the right atrium. (This illustration appeared originally in the first edition of *The Heart*, in 1966, and in all subsequent editions. It is reproduced here by courtesy of Dr. John W. Kirklin, Birmingham, Alabama.)

but mortality is higher than it is in the young and the magnitude of improvement is less certain. Nonetheless, surgical closure of ASDs is advised even when R_p approaches 15 Wood units because of the excessive morbidity and mortality associated with a persistent interatrial communication.[77] *Morbidity in adults and the low risk of surgical closure in young children mandate surgery in the preschool or preadolescent years.*

Although life-threatening complications after closure of ASDs in children are rare, transient postoperative atrial arrhythmias and postpericardiotomy syndrome with pericardial effusions occasionally are seen. The long-term prognosis for a normal life expectancy and functional capability is excellent for patients who have closure of an uncomplicated ASD during the first two decades of life.

Partial Anomalous Pulmonary Venous Connection

PATHOLOGY

In partial anomalous pulmonary venous connection, one or more, but not all, of the pulmonary veins enter the right atrium or its venous tributaries. The atrial septum may rarely be intact, but an ASD is usually present. There are many patterns of anomalous pulmonary venous connection, but the four most common, in order of decreasing frequency, are (1) pulmonary veins from the right upper and/or middle lobe to the superior vena cava, usually with a sinus venosus ASD, (2) all the right pulmonary veins to the right atrium, usually in the polysplenia syndrome, (3) all the right pulmonary veins to the inferior vena cava, entering this systemic vein just above or below the diaphragm, and (4) the left upper or both left pulmonary veins to an anomalous vertical vein draining to the left brachiocephalic vein.

When the right pulmonary veins are connected to the inferior vena cava, the atrial septum may be intact. This venous anomaly may be isolated or may be part of the *scimitar syndrome*. That syndrome includes hypoplasia of the right lung, bronchial abnormalities, anomalous systemic pulmonary arterial supply to the right lung from branches of the descending thoracic and/or abdominal aorta, and dextroposition of the heart.

CLINICAL MANIFESTATIONS

In an old autopsy series, partial anomalous pulmonary venous connection occurred in 0.6 percent of 801 anatomic dissections,[78] a much higher incidence than was suspected clinically, suggesting that many cases may not be recognized during life. There is no sex predilection. Approximately 15 percent of all ASDs have this coexisting anomaly; however, in the case of the sinus venosus type, the association is in the range of 85 percent.

History When partial anomalous pulmonary venous connection coexists with an ASD, the symptoms, as well as the other clinical manifestations, are indistinguishable from those of an isolated ASD. Isolated, uncomplicated anomalous connection of a single pulmonary vein usually goes undetected clinically, since in this circumstance only about 20 percent of the pulmonary venous flow returns to the right atrium or its tributaries. When the entire venous return from one lung or two pulmonary veins is connected anomalously, approximately 65 percent of the pulmonary venous flow returns to the right side of the heart and the symptoms are similar to those of an ASD with a comparable increase in pulmonary blood flow.

Physical Examination The findings are the same as those in patients with an ASD with the exception that *the two components of the second heart sound, though usually widely split, move normally with respiration if the atrial septum is intact.*

Chest Roentgenogram Right ventricular enlargement, pulmonary arterial dilatation, and increased pulmonary blood flow are characteristic when more than one pulmonary vein connects anomalously. With anomalous connection of the right pulmonary veins to the inferior vena cava, the pulmonary venous pattern may assume a crescent-shaped or scimitar curve in the right lower lung field along the right lower heart border (scimitar).

Electrocardiogram The ECG is normal (in the case of anomalous connection of a single pulmonary vein) or reflects volume overload of the right side of the heart, as was described above in "Atrial Septal Defect."

Echocardiogram If more than one pulmonary vein drains anomalously, the volume usually is sufficient to produce the characteristic pattern of right ventricular diastolic overload. Failure to visualize an atrial septal opening with two-dimensional imaging and color flow mapping from a subcostal coronal or high right-sided parasternal longitudinal view should arouse suspicion of an intact atrial septum. A variety of views supplemented by color flow mapping may be necessary to identify the anomalous connection.[79]

Cardiac Catheterization Anomalously connected pulmonary veins may be entered directly with the venous catheter. Selective biplane angiograms in these vessels will document their site of connection. Left-to-right shunting with partial anomalous pulmonary venous connection and an intact atrial septum is usually small or moderate and may go undetected by oximetry techniques. Selective indicator dilution curves in the right and left pulmonary arteries with systemic arterial sampling can detect the lung with the anomalous pulmonary venous connection, and selective biplane angiograms in the pulmonary arterial branches will visualize these connections.

NATURAL HISTORY AND PROGNOSIS

Patients with partial anomalous pulmonary venous connection with ASD appear to follow a course similar, if not identical, to that of patients with an isolated ASD. When the atrial septum is intact, the course depends primarily on the volume of pulmonary venous blood returning to the right side of the heart. Rarely, PVOD may be found even in the presence of a single anomalously connected pulmonary vein and an intact atrial septum.[80] Finally, increasing left atrial pressure caused by mitral valve disease or diminishing left ventricular compliance will, in the course of time, encourage a greater redistribution of pulmonary arterial blood flow to the portion of the lung drained by the more compliant right atrium. Thus, patients who were initially asymptomatic and had a very modest volume of anomalous pulmonary venous return in youth may become symptomatic and even develop congestive failure in adult life.

MEDICAL MANAGEMENT

Asymptomatic patients with small shunts require no treatment. Those with symptoms, larger pulmonary blood flows, congestive failure, or PAH require surgical correction. With an intact atrial septum, precise preoperative identification of the site of the anomalous venous connection is essential. Long-term follow-up in patients who have not had surgery is indicated to detect increasing flow or the appearance of PAH.

SURGICAL MANAGEMENT

Anomalous connection of a right pulmonary vein or veins to the superior vena cava usually is associated with a sinus venosus ASD (Fig. 63-12). (see "Atrial Septal Defect, Surgical Management," above.) Partial anomalous pulmonary veins draining to the superior vena cava, inferior vena cava, or right atrium are repaired by being diverted through the ASD into the left atrium, using an appropriately placed patch baffle. Isolated left-sided anomalous pulmonary veins draining to the left ascending vertical vein or the left superior vena cava are detached and anastomosed directly to the left atrial appendage. Long-term morbidity and mortality are minimal among patients with uncomplicated partial pulmonary venous connections, equivalent to those observed after closure of an ASD.

Common Atrioventricular Canal Defects

DEFINITION

Atrioventricular canal defects are characterized by an ASD in the lowermost part of the atrial septum (ostium primum), a cleft of the mitral valve (either alone or in combination with a cleft of the tricuspid valve), or deficiency of ventricular septal tissue or some combination. In the most severe form (complete AV canal defect), there is a large deficiency of the lower part of the atrial septum and the upper muscular portion of the ventricular septum and a common AV valve that straddles the ventricular septum. The condition appears to result from incomplete growth of the AV endocardial cushions and the AV septum.

PATHOLOGY

The ostium primum type of ASD is characterized by a crescent-shaped upper border and no septal tissue forming the lower border. The lower aspect of the defect is bounded by the atrial surfaces of the AV valves and, in the complete type (see below), in part by the upper edge of the ventricular septum. A small amount of septal tissue separates the defect from the posterior atrial wall.

ANATOMIC TYPES

Variations occur with respect to the nature of the AV valves. The terms *partial* and *complete* were first introduced to describe these types by Rogers and Edwards.[81]

Partial Type The ostium primum ASD is associated with a "cleft" in the anterior mitral leaflet or, probably more accurately, a septal commissure between the superior and inferior leaflets of the left AV valve (Figs. 63-8*D* and 63-13).[66] The tricuspid valve is not cleft or shows a minor central deficiency. The ventricular aspects of the anterior mitral valve elements are fused to the upper edge of the deficient ventricular septum, precluding an interventricular communication. If there is no atrial septal tissue or if the atrial septum is so rudimentary that it produces a common chamber involving both atria, the term *common atrium* or *single atrium* is applied.

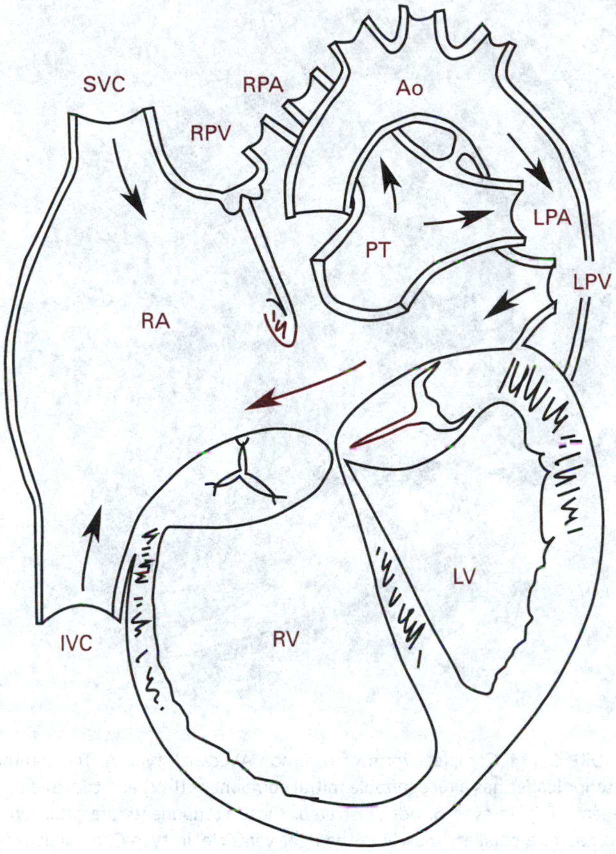

FIGURE 63-13 Common AV canal of the partial type. The mitral valve shows a cleft in its anterior leaflet, while the tricuspid valve is undisturbed. SVC = superior vena cava; IVC = inferior vena cava; RA = right pulmonary artery; LPA = left pulmonary artery; RPV = right pulmonary vein; LPV = left pulmonary vein; LV = left ventricle; Ao = aorta. (From Edwards JE.[66] Reproduced with permission from the publisher and author.)

Complete Type The complete type of common AV canal is characterized by failure of partitioning of the primitive canal into separate AV orifices. The orifice between the atria and the ventricles is guarded by a common valve, of which the anterior leaflet is derived from the ventral AV endocardial cushion and represents the anterior halves of the anterior mitral and septal tricuspid leaflets. The posterior leaflet is derived from the dorsal AV endocardial cushion and represents the posterior halves of the anterior mitral and septal tricuspid leaflets.

Usually, considerable space exists between the anterior and posterior leaflets above and the ventricular septum below; thus, in most cases of the complete type, there is free communication between the ventricles.

Rastelli and associates[82] subdivided the complete variety into three subgroups—types A, B, and C—on the basis of the structure of the common anterior leaflet and its chordal attachments to the ventricular septum and/or papillary muscles (Fig. 63-14). With regard to the posterior common leaflet, there is variation among the three types in regard to the presence or absence of subdivision and whether the posterior leaflet is attached to the ventricular septum by chordae or by an imperforate membrane.

Variations from the classic types of AV canal defects are recognized, the most common being the AV canal type of iso-

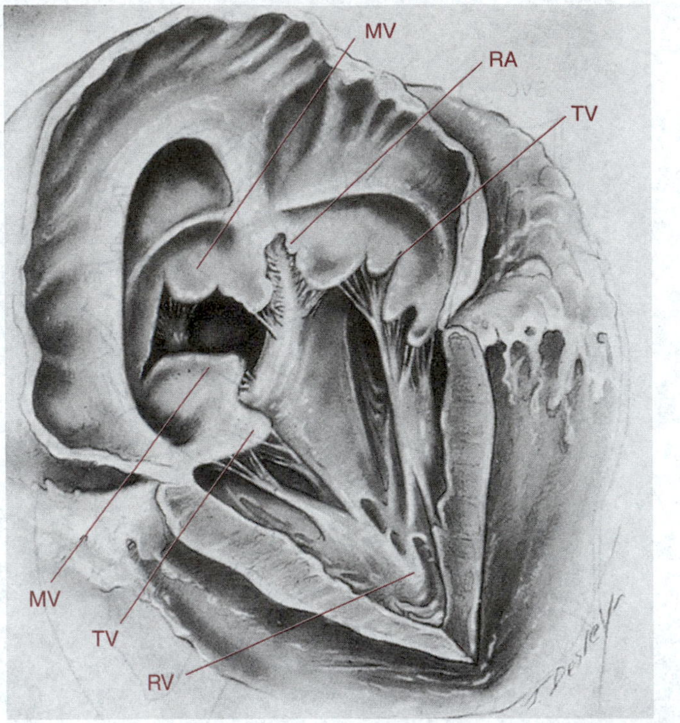

FIGURE 63-14 Complete form of common AV canal, type A. The common anterior leaflet has a recognizable mitral component (MV) and tricuspid component (TV). In type B, not illustrated, those components are attached by chordae to a papillary muscle in the right ventricle. In type C, not illustrated, the common anterior leaflet is a single unit without any attachment to the underlying ventricular septum. Type A is most amenable to repair. RV = right ventricle; RA = right atrium. (From Rastelli GC et al.[82] Reproduced with permission from the publisher and authors.)

lated VSD, isolated ostium primum ASD without malformed AV valves, and isolated cleft of the anterior mitral or septal tricuspid valve leaflets.

ASSOCIATED CONDITIONS

In the asplenia syndrome, the complete variety is almost universal; with polysplenia, it occurs in about one-quarter of cases.[83] An ASD of the secundum type is present in about half the cases. Double orifice of the mitral valve may be associated with the incomplete type, and tetralogy of Fallot may be associated with the complete type.

ABNORMAL PHYSIOLOGY

If the communication at the ventricular level is large, the right ventricular and pulmonary artery pressures will be elevated. These patients are similar to those with large VSDs. Patients with a communication at the atrial level usually have only normal or slightly elevated systolic pressures in the right side of the heart and a large pulmonary blood flow, as in the secundum type of ASD. Defects in the tricuspid valve, mitral valve, or both may result in severe regurgitation or direct shunting of blood from the left ventricle to the right atrium.

CLINICAL MANIFESTATIONS

Approximately 3 percent of infants and children with congenital heart disease have AV canal defects. The majority, some 60 to 70 percent, have the complete form. The female/male ratio is approximately 1.3:1. Well over half the patients with the complete form have associated Down's syndrome. Among children with Down's syndrome, 45 percent have some form of congenital heart disease. Malformations of the AV canal type, usually of the complete variety, account for approximately 50 percent of these abnormalities.[84]

History Only if the mitral valve is incompetent do the symptoms of patients with partial AV canal differ from those associated with a secundum type of ASD. The complete form of AV canal or the partial form connected with significant mitral regurgitation may be associated with poor weight gain, easy fatigue, dyspnea, repeated respiratory infections, and congestive heart failure. Patients with complete AV canal are almost invariably very sick.

Physical Examination The findings with a partial defect are those of an ASD. If the cleft anterior mitral leaflet is incompetent, the findings of mitral regurgitation also will be present.

The physical findings with the complete AV canal defect are those of a very large VSD, usually with full-blown congestive failure, but the second heart sound is split and fixed. The murmur of mitral regurgitation may not be heard or recognized as such.

Chest Roentgenogram Overall cardiac enlargement that is out of proportion to the degree of pulmonary plethora or a cardiac silhouette suggesting combined ventricular dilatation may serve to distinguish an uncomplicated secundum ASD from a primum defect with significant mitral regurgitation. Marked cardiac enlargement and severe pulmonary overcirculation are features of the complete AV canal defect.

Electrocardiogram One of the most helpful diagnostic features in distinguishing individuals with AV canal defects from those with isolated ASDs or VSDs is the characteristic superior orientation of the mean QRS axis in the frontal plane, with a right bundle branch delay in the precordial leads. Between 92 and 95 percent of both types of canal have a QRS axis lying between 0 and −150°. The patterns of atrial and ventricular hypertrophy reflect the underlying hemodynamic abnormalities.

Echocardiogram Two-dimensional echo is capable of visualizing the extent of septal defects and, with Doppler study and color flow mapping, left-to-right shunting at the atrial and/or ventricular level and associated mitral and/or tricuspid valvular regurgitation (Fig. 63-15). The anatomic features of the anterior AV leaflet and its connections may be visualized with sufficient clarity to permit subdivision of complete AV canal defects into types A, B, and C (Fig. 63-14). Straddling AV valves, a double-orifice mitral valve, single papillary muscles, and hypoplasia or outflow obstruction of the right or left ventricle also can be determined with this technique.[85]

Cardiac Catheterization Cardiac catheterization rarely is performed if the echocardiogram is characteristic and if the history, clinical examination, and echo suggest a large left-to-right shunt and low pulmonary resistance. When it is performed, a significant increase in oxygen saturation between the superior vena cava and the right atrium is present. A right ventricular or pulmonary arterial systolic pressure in excess of 60 percent of the systemic systolic pressure favors the presence of a complete canal. With a large communication between the two ventricles

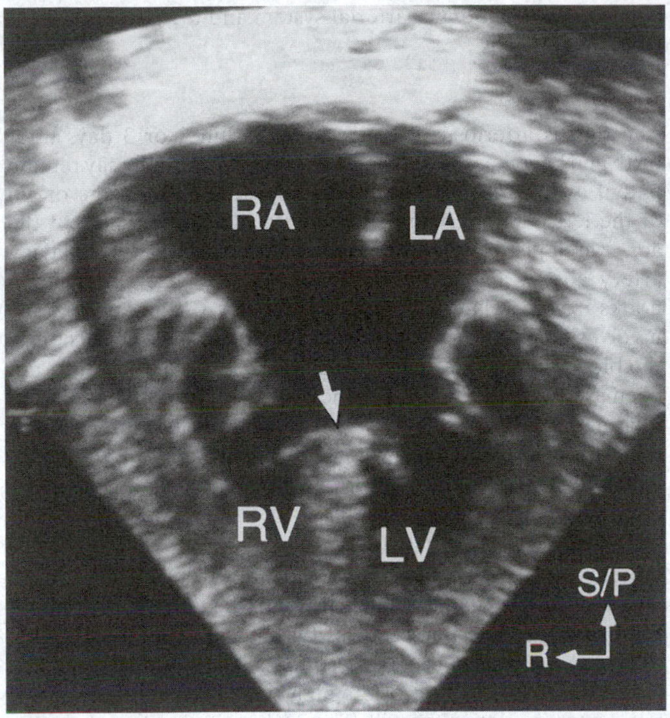

FIGURE 63-15 Apical four-chamber view of complete common AV canal. Note the large deficiency of both atrial and ventricular septa as well as apical displacement of the AV valves. The arrow points to the attachment of the inferior bridging leaflet to the ventricular septal crest. (From Levine J and Geva T.[85] Reproduced with permission.)

below the AV valves, the right ventricular, pulmonary arterial, and systemic arterial systolic pressures are virtually identical. Left ventricular angiography in the frontal view demonstrates the "gooseneck deformity" of the left ventricular outflow tract that is characteristic of AV canal malformations and allows a semiquantitative assessment of the degree of mitral regurgitation and shunting from the left ventricle to the right atrium. The left anterior oblique view with craniocaudal angulation is recommended for visualizing the interventricular defect and judging the extent of ventricular septal deficiency. Aortography is essential to eliminate the possibility of a PDA if the echocardiogram was not diagnostic.

NATURAL HISTORY AND PROGNOSIS

Partial defects without significant mitral regurgitation follow a course similar to that described for the secundum type of septal defects. An exception would be the greater likelihood of infective endocarditis because of the mitral valve deformity. Moderate or severe mitral regurgitation produces heart failure with resulting symptoms and growth retardation. Infants with a complete AV canal without protective pulmonary stenosis quickly develop and continue to have congestive failure until the course is altered by death, the development of PVOD, or surgical intervention.

MEDICAL MANAGEMENT

Children with an uncomplicated partial defect are managed in the same manner as children with an uncomplicated ASD. Those who are symptomatic should undergo early surgical closure of the primum ASD and, if possible, plication of the cleft in the septal commissure of the left AV ("mitral") valve. The few patients with significant residual mitral regurgitation after surgery are managed medically until mitral valve replacement is appropriate. Those without symptoms are repaired before they start school.

The approach to an infant with complete AV canal is the same as that for an infant with a large VSD but is tempered by the knowledge that spontaneous improvement is very unlikely except at the expense of the pulmonary vascular bed. Repair is recommended early if there is significant congestive heart failure or between 4 and 6 months of age if the pulmonary arterial systolic pressure is greater than half the systemic arterial systolic pressure. Elevation of pulmonary vascular resistance in the first year of life warrants surgical intervention without delay.

With regard to genetic counseling, the risk of a subsequent sibling having heart disease in the presence of a single affected family member is in the range of 2 percent; it is probably higher for the offspring of an affected parent, particularly if that parent is the mother.[86] Concordance for AV canal defects among affected siblings or offspring is much higher than it is with other forms of congenital heart disease and approaches 90 percent.

SURGICAL MANAGEMENT

The remarkable clinical improvement that follows anatomic repair of complete common AV septal defects in infancy encourages early correction within the first year of life. Banding of the pulmonary artery in a critically ill infant with a large interventricular defect was used in the past but has been replaced by a more reparative operation in most centers. The specifics of repair are dictated by anatomic detail: Individual variation is considerable (Fig. 63-16), but the creation of a competent, nonstenotic left-sided AV ("mitral") valve is essential for an acceptable early and long-term prognosis.

A patch usually is sutured to the right side of the ventricular septum to obliterate the interventricular communication. The anterior and posterior components of the common valve are divided, and the mitral valve is sutured to the patch at an appropriate level. The "cleft" between the left anterior and left posterior leaflets should be closed by suturing if approximation of these edges appears to increase competence without the creation of stenosis. Prosthetic valve implantation rarely is required during primary anatomic repair.[87] The right-sided AV ("tricuspid") apparatus, although less critical to survival, is repaired using the same principles. The interatrial communication usually is closed with a separate piece of pericardium to minimize hemolysis in the presence of residual mitral regurgitation.[87] Mitral valve competence is assessed by gentle distention of the left ventricle with cold saline.

A partial AV canal is repaired through a right atriotomy. The cleft may be closed with a few simple interrupted sutures to encourage inversion and coaptation of the leaflet margins. The ASD usually is closed with a pericardial patch.

Permanent complete heart block once contributed substantially to early mortality and morbidity but is now rare. Patients undergoing repair of a partial AV canal should be observed for the possible development of subaortic left ventricular outflow tract obstruction caused by redundant or residual endocardial cushion tissue.

In-hospital mortality after correction of a complete AV canal in infancy ranges from 3 to 10 percent;[88,89] the highest mortality is encountered during the first few months of life and in infants with severe AV valve regurgitation, elevated pulmonary vascular resistance, hypoplasia of the left or right ventricle, or other

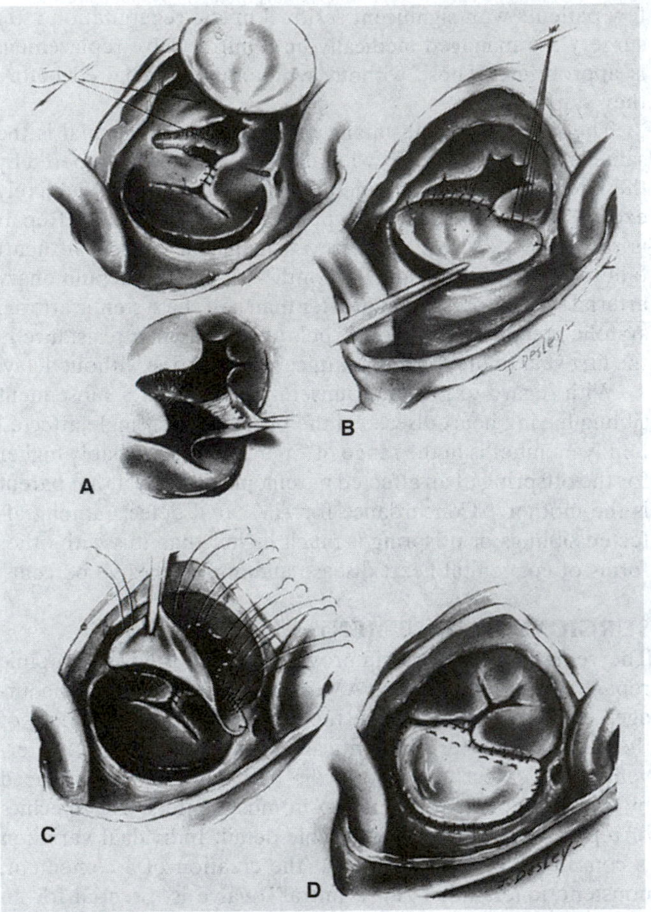

FIGURE 63-16 Steps in the repair of the complete form of common AV canal, type A. *A* and *B*. A pericardial patch is sutured to the ventricular septum. *C* and *D*. The anterior leaflet of the mitral valve is reconstructed and attached to the patch. A portion of the tricuspid leaflet is attached to the patch. (From Rastelli GC et al.[82] Reproduced with permission from the publisher and authors.)

cardiac malformations. At Children's Hospital in Boston, 191 children with a median age of 4.6 months were repaired between January 1990 and December 1998 with an operative mortality of 1.5 percent. Reoperation was necessary in 22 patients (11.7 percent), a mean of 20 months later: 18 for residual mitral regurgitation and 4 for left ventricular outflow tract obstruction.[90] Successful correction of a complete AV canal can be accomplished despite associated tetralogy of Fallot, double-outlet ventricle, and other complex anomalies.[87]

EXTRACARDIAC COMMUNICATIONS BETWEEN THE SYSTEMIC AND PULMONARY CIRCULATIONS, USUALLY WITHOUT CYANOSIS

Patent Ductus Arteriosus

DEFINITION

Patent ductus arteriosus, the most common type of extracardiac shunt, represents persistent patency of the vessel that normally connects the pulmonary arterial system and the aorta in a fetus (Fig. 63-17).

PATHOLOGY

The ductus arteriosus usually closes within 2 or 3 days after birth and becomes the *ligamentum arteriosum*, but it may remain patent as long as 8 weeks postnatally. It runs from the origin of the left pulmonary artery below to the lower aspect of the aortic arch just beyond the level of origin of the left subclavian artery above. The recurrent branch of the left vagus nerve hooks around its lateral and inferior aspects. Closure postnatally involves a complex interaction of increased oxygen tension in the blood and circulating prostaglandins. Exogenous PGE_1 has been used extensively to keep the ductus open postnatally,[91] and indomethacin, a prostaglandin inhibitor, can close the ductus in many premature infants in whom persistent patency is disadvantageous.[92]

ABNORMAL PHYSIOLOGY

Patients with PDA may be divided into groups according to whether the vascular resistance through the ductus is low, moderate, or high. The resistance of the ductus is related not only to its cross-sectional area but also to its length. In patients with a very small ductus that offers high resistance, the flow across the ductus is relatively small. The extra volume of work on the left ventricle is small, and the pulmonary pressure and resistance are not elevated. Patients with only moderate resistance in the

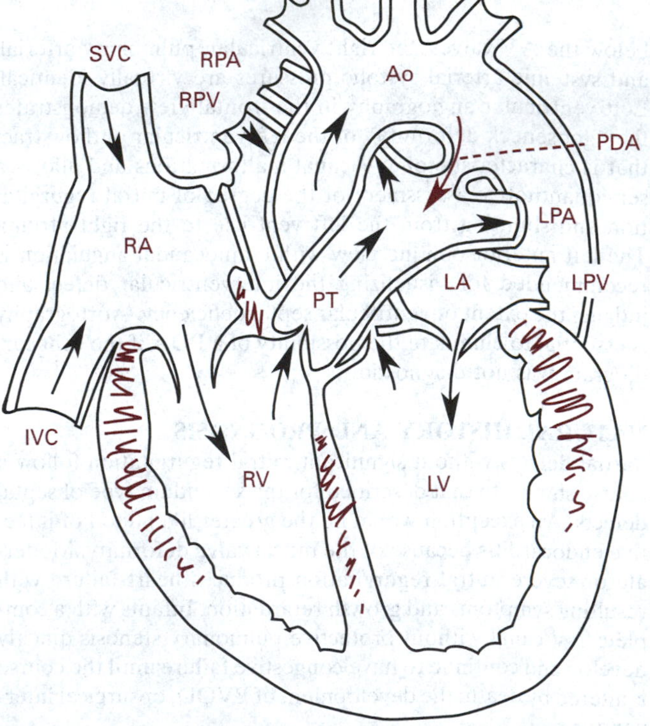

FIGURE 63-17 Patent ductus arteriosus (PDA). SVC = superior vena cava; IVC = inferior vena cava; RA = right atrium; RV = right ventricle; PT = main pulmonary arterial trunk; RPA = right pulmonary artery; LPA = left pulmonary artery; RPV = right pulmonary vein; LPV = left pulmonary vein; LA = left atrium; LV = left ventricle; Ao = aorta. (From Edwards JE.[66] Reproduced with permission from the publisher and author.)

ductus have some increase in pulmonary artery pressure, with a moderately greater volume of shunting across the ductus.

In patients with a large patent ductus, the aorta and pulmonary artery are essentially in free communication; the systolic pressure in the pulmonary artery is equal to that in the aorta. The volume load of blood recirculating through the lungs is on the left ventricle, with pulmonary congestion resulting from increased pulmonary flow and/or left ventricular failure. With time, the left ventricle compensates with dilation and hypertrophy to carry the volume load, and the pulmonary vasculature may respond to the high pressure (see the section on PAH, above). The right ventricle is burdened mainly by a pressure load.

If the pulmonary resistance equals or exceeds the resistance of the systemic circulation, there is shunting of unsaturated blood from the pulmonary artery to the aorta, resulting in hypoxemia, especially in the lower body and legs.

CLINICAL MANIFESTATIONS

History The history of the mother's pregnancy and of perinatal events may provide clues that are associated with a high incidence of PDA, such as exposure to rubella in the first trimester in a nonimmunized mother. PDA is also more common in premature infants, especially those with birth asphyxia or respiratory distress.[93]

Symptoms usually are restricted to patients with large shunts that produce heart failure or with other complicating problems, such as respiratory distress in a premature infant. The symptoms related to heart failure were discussed above. Heart failure is most likely to develop in the first few weeks or months of life. If it does not appear during infancy, it is unlikely to occur before the third decade. Growth may be affected in those with large shunts and failure. The clinical presentation in a premature infant is usually very different from that in a full-term infant, particularly in those with a birth weight under 1.5 kg, who are more likely to have moderate to severe respiratory distress. In these infants, the clinical features of respiratory distress often blend over the course of several days into those of heart failure. Increasing ventilatory or oxygen requirements with carbon dioxide retention or episodic apnea and bradycardia are often the first signs that a PDA may be complicating the picture.

Physical Examination In a full-term infant or child with PDA, there is frequently a systolic thrill over the pulmonary artery and in the suprasternal notch. The peripheral pulses are generally brisk and bounding, especially with the larger shunts secondary to runoff from the aorta to the pulmonary artery in diastole. A patient with elevated pulmonary vascular resistance and a right-to-left shunt will have "differential cyanosis," with cyanosis and clubbing of the toes but not the fingers, from shunting of hypoxemic blood from the pulmonary artery into the descending aorta. The apex impulse may be increased or displaced in those with large shunts. The right ventricular impulse is increased in a premature infant with respiratory distress and in infants and children with significant pulmonary hypertension. The typical murmur is a continuous, or "machinery," murmur that is best heard at the left upper sternal border and below the left clavicle. It is usually a rough murmur with eddy sounds, which are helpful in making the diagnosis, and it peaks at or near the second heart sound. In patients with at least a moderate shunt, there is a middiastolic rumble at the apex as a result of relative mitral stenosis from increased flow across the mitral valve. The second heart sound may be difficult to hear because of the continuous murmur, but it is usually normal. The pulmonary component is accentuated in those with pulmonary hypertension.

Chest Roentgenogram Findings on chest roentgenography also are dependent on the magnitude of the shunt. In patients with a small shunt, the chest roentgenogram is normal. With larger shunts, the left atrium and left ventricle are enlarged. Increases in pulmonary arterial flow on x-ray parallel the magnitude of the shunt. In the presence of heart failure, there are signs of pulmonary edema. In older patients who have developed Eisenmenger physiology, the only abnormality may be marked prominence of the central pulmonary arteries, with rapid tapering to the periphery of the lung fields.

Electrocardiogram With a small shunt, the ECG is normal. Left atrial hypertrophy is probably the most common abnormality found, but left ventricular hypertrophy of the volume overload type, with deep Q waves and increased R-wave voltage in the left precordial leads, is also common as the shunt size increases and left ventricular dilation occurs. Right ventricular hypertrophy is seen with pulmonary hypertension.

Echocardiogram There is left atrial enlargement, and the left ventricular end-diastolic dimension and mean velocity of circumferential fiber shortening are increased significantly. Small shunts can be detected with color Doppler imaging with a typical spectral flow pattern into the pulmonary artery, while a larger ductus can be visualized with two-dimensional echocardiography. Occasionally, a trivial amount of flow is seen through the ductus as an incidental finding in those with or without associated heart disease.

Cardiac Catheterization In those with typical, uncomplicated PDA, cardiac catheterization is not necessary. When catheterization is performed, the catheter usually passes preferentially from the left pulmonary artery into the descending aorta, except when the ductus is too small. The saturation is increased in the pulmonary artery compared with the right atrium and ventricle to a degree relative to the size of the shunt. The pulmonary arterial and right ventricular pressures are elevated in those with a large ductus. The pulmonary vascular resistance is elevated in older patients who have developed changes in the pulmonary vascular bed. These patients also have diminished saturation in the descending aorta once the pulmonary resistance reaches a level that will reverse the shunt. Aortography will opacify the ductus and pulmonary arteries.

NATURAL HISTORY AND PROGNOSIS

The complications related to PDA include infective endarteritis, heart failure, and pulmonary hypertension with vascular damage. Infection of the ductus is a risk regardless of its size. This risk increases with the length of survival. This can lead to the development of a mycotic aneurysm with the potential to compress the recurrent laryngeal nerve, embolize septic material to the lungs, or rupture. Calcification of the ductal wall is common in adults.

In patients with large shunts, heart failure can cause significant morbidity and mortality, particularly in a premature and young infant, and sudden death can occur. Progressive damage to the pulmonary vascular bed can occur in some, but it rarely occurs to an irreversible degree in the first year of life. Once irreversible damage occurs, premature death in late adolescence or early adulthood can be anticipated.

With improved technology, children without associated heart disease are noted to have a trivial amount of flow through a very small (<1 mm) patent ductus. Frequently, the shunt is too small to produce an audible murmur. The natural history of this echo-Doppler-discovered ductus arteriosus without clinical findings is unknown, but most think it is benign since cardiologists have not noted patients with endarteritis in a "silent" ductus.

MEDICAL MANAGEMENT

Interruption of flow through the PDA is the ultimate goal of management. For those in congestive heart failure, usually premature infants, medical management with digoxin and diuretics with fluid restriction may play a minor role, but the ultimate aim is closure to prevent heart failure and promote growth in infants and prevent infective endarteritis and pulmonary vascular disease in older children.

For premature infants, treatment with indomethacin is usually the first-line therapy.[94] Successful closure depends on both the dosage and the timing of treatment, although the major determinants seem to be gestational and postnatal age rather than the concentration of the drug. Because of ductal reopening, serial treatment regimens may be necessary, especially in those weighing less than 1000 g at birth. There is increasing evidence that the administration of "prophylactic" indomethacin in infants weighing less than 1000 g at birth may be associated with a higher closure rate and a better outcome.[92] Indomethacin therapy has been associated with an increased bleeding tendency resulting from platelet dysfunction, decreased urine output secondary to renal dysfunction, and necrotizing enterocolitis.[92] For the very premature with a PDA, however, a trial of indomethacin is preferable to the other options.

For premature infants who failed to close their PDA with a course of indomethacin or for term infants with a persistent PDA, closure has been recommended. If the PDA is large, there is usually a large left-to-right shunt with congestive heart failure. In these infants, the indication for closure is heart failure and usually failure to thrive. Even in the absence of these indications, when a large PDA is associated with PAH, closure is recommended to prevent PVOD. In children with a smaller PDA with an audible murmur but no evidence of significant hemodynamic embarrassment, closure usually is recommended because of the incidence of bacterial endarteritis, which over a lifetime is in the range of 30 percent. For children with a PDA without a heart murmur, which usually is discovered incidentally when an echocardiogram is performed for other reasons, the author does not currently recommend closure.

SURGICAL AND INTERVENTIONAL CATHETER CLOSURE

Surgery for a persistent PDA was first reported more than 60 years ago and is now done routinely in most centers. The safety and efficacy of this procedure even in very young children are well established, with risks that are very low (well under 1 percent), and success at interrupting flow is almost universal.

The PDA is exposed and mobilized through a small left thoracotomy in the fourth intercostal space.[95] Ductus obliteration is accomplished by division or ligation. A short, broad, or thin-walled ductus is divided between vascular clamps. The ends are closed with a continuous suture. A long, narrow, thick-walled ductus can be divided or ligated with two or three sutures spaced a few millimeters apart. The suture ligatures at each end are anchored superficially in the ductus wall to prevent migration and assure thrombosis and obliteration.

The fragile and thin-walled PDA of a premature infant is obliterated by gentle ligation with a thick suture to minimize disruption or, if small, by occlusion using metallic surgical clips. Extrapleural exposure is preferred by some surgeons. Ligation in the neonatal intensive care unit, avoiding transport to the operating room, is common. Transport from a remote intensive care unit to a cardiac surgical unit for ductus ligation on a "day-stay" basis is also efficacious.[96] Ductus obliteration offers clinical improvement in infants weighing as little as 500 g, with minimal operative risk, a reduced incidence of necrotizing enterocolitis, a reduced duration of intubation, and improvement in late survival.

Closure of a PDA in an adult requires particular caution; calcification and rigidity of the ductus wall complicate clamping. Placement of a Dacron patch over the aortic orifice of the ductus from within the aorta may be advisable.[97]

Recently, advances in less invasive surgery have been applied to the closure of a PDA using video-assisted thoracoscopic surgery. A miniaturized camera is inserted into the thorax, and through a separate tiny incision, a surgical stapler is inserted and a clip is placed across the PDA, interrupting flow. Among 230 patients, there was only 1 with minimal residual flow, 1 with persistent recurrent laryngeal nerve dysfunction, and no deaths, transfusions, or chylothoraces. The mean operating time was 20 min, and the hospital stay lasted only a couple of days.[98] At Children's Hospital in Boston, this procedure has been applied to premature infants as small as 575 g, with discharge from the hospital the day after the procedure in full-term infants and children.[99]

The PDA sometimes can be closed by interventional catheterization techniques. In 1971, Portsmann and Wierny introduced a rather complex methodology to plug a PDA by using a transarterial and transvenous approach employing very large catheters.[100] More recently, Rashkind and Cuaso introduced and others have since popularized the use of a double-umbrella device to plug a PDA,[101] but the large size of the delivery sheath of the Rashkind device makes it inapplicable to young and very small children. Gianturco coils—thin metallic wires glossed with Dacron that assume a coil configuration when released from a catheter—have become an attractive alternative (Fig. 63-18). They can be delivered through relatively small catheters and have been found to be quite effective, although their utility is limited in those <8 months of age with PDAs that are more than 3.5 or 4.0 mm at the narrowest point.[102] In the others using these coils, the results have been very promising, with a 90 percent success rate.

With several highly successful, low-risk, inexpensive, and minimally traumatic procedures available to close a persistent PDA in a neonate, child, adolescent, or adult without pulmonary vascular disease, local experience is likely to be the best guide to which option is preferable in an individual child.

Sinus of Valsalva Fistula

PATHOLOGY

Sinus of Valsalva fistula is uncommon; it also is referred to as *aortic sinus aneurysm* (see also Chap. 88). Because of an assumed intrinsic weakness at the union of the aorta with the heart, the aortic media may separate from the aortic annulus and retract upward. The structure that lies between becomes aneurysmal and may rupture to form a fistula. The usual sites of the defects are the posterior (noncoronary) sinus aneurysms that rupture through the atrial septal wall into the right atrium (Fig. 63-19*A*) and those of the right sinus that rupture into the right ventricular infundibulum (Fig. 63-19*B*).[103] The aneurysm is represented by a colored pouch with multiple perforations in the wall. The principal associated condition is a supracristal VSD in cases with aneurysms of the right sinus (about 50 percent).

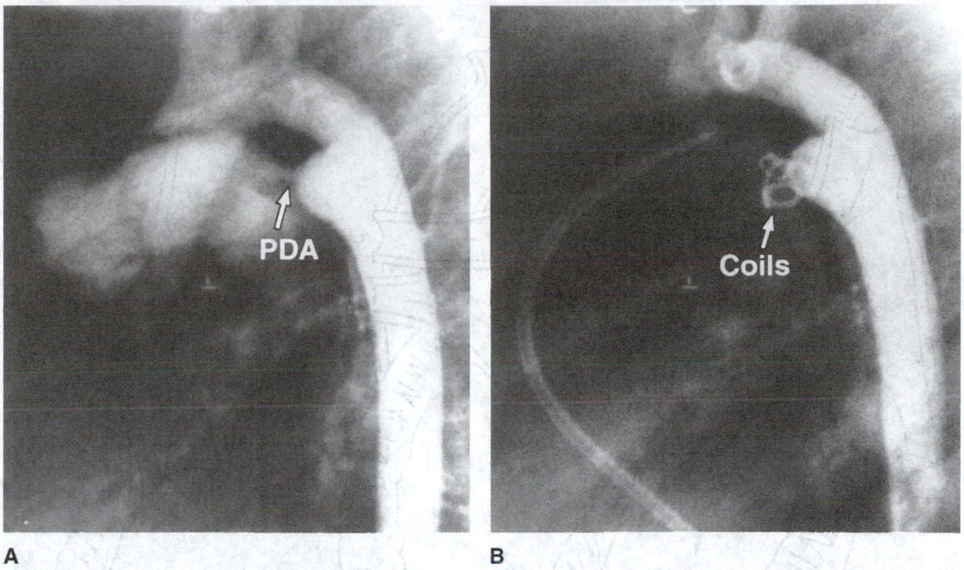

FIGURE 63-18 Lateral angiogram showing coil occlusion of a patent ductus arteriosus. *A*. Small PDA allows shunting from descending aorta to pulmonary artery. *B*. Shunting is eliminated by a coil placed in the ductus arteriosus. (Courtesy of John F. Keane, MD.)

CLINICAL MANIFESTATIONS

Sinus of Valsalva fistulas are most common in adults.[104] When the rupture is secondary to bacterial endocarditis, evidence of a preceding infection is found. If the rupture occurs slowly, a small fistulous tract into the right atrium or ventricle develops and presents recent-onset findings of a small left-to-right shunt. With sudden rupture, there is usually a tearing pain in the midchest associated with the dramatically rapid development of pulmonary congestion caused by the sudden onset of a large shunt. Characteristically, the murmur is loud and continuous but is heard lower on the chest than is the murmur of PDA. A to-and-fro murmur rather than a continuous one may be heard at times. The apex impulse is hyperdynamic, and the pulse pressure is widened. VSD may complicate the clinical picture. Cardiac catheterization will confirm the level of the shunt. A pressure difference across the right ventricular outflow tract may be present if the right sinus is involved. Aortography or Doppler echocardiography[105] will confirm the diagnosis.

NATURAL HISTORY AND PROGNOSIS

With slow rupture and a small shunt, the major risk is infective endocarditis or extension of the rupture with an increasing shunt. With a large shunt, the heart failure is usually rapidly progressive and may result in death very quickly. A few patients seem to stabilize in this situation.

MEDICAL MANAGEMENT

Appropriate cultures should be drawn and antibiotics should be begun if endocarditis is suspected. Treatment of heart failure should be instituted rapidly. *Because of the natural history, all patients should have this condition corrected surgically*.

SURGICAL MANAGEMENT

Aneurysms or fistulas from the noncoronary or right coronary sinuses are repaired through the aortic root while the patient is supported on total cardiopulmonary bypass with moderate hypothermia, using techniques similar to those employed for aortic valve replacement. The aortic valve leaflets, the margins of the aneurysm, and the coronary arterial orifices must be visualized precisely. Aneurysms of the noncoronary sinus can be repaired through the right atrium; those arising from the right coronary sinus are accessible through the right ventricle. In most cases, the orifice of the aneurysmal fistula is surgically obliterated, using a Dacron patch. In a recent series of 129 patients, reparative methods included plication (47 percent), patch repair (40 percent), and aortic root replacement (12 percent). Sixty percent of those patients needed aortic valve replacement at the same time.[104]

A conal, or supracristal (type I), VSD must be sought and closed through either the aortic valve or the right ventricular outflow tract when an aneurysm of the right coronary sinus extends into the right ventricle.

Surgical results are usually quite good. In the large series cited above, the operative survival was 96 percent with no late deaths in an average of 5.9 years of follow-up.[104]

VALVULAR AND VASCULAR MALFORMATIONS OF THE LEFT SIDE OF THE HEART WITH RIGHT-TO-LEFT, BIDIRECTIONAL, OR NO SHUNT

Coarctation of the Aorta

PATHOLOGY

Coarctation of the aorta is a discrete narrowing of the distal segment of the aortic arch. The characteristic lesion is a deformity of the media of the aorta that involves the anterior, supe-

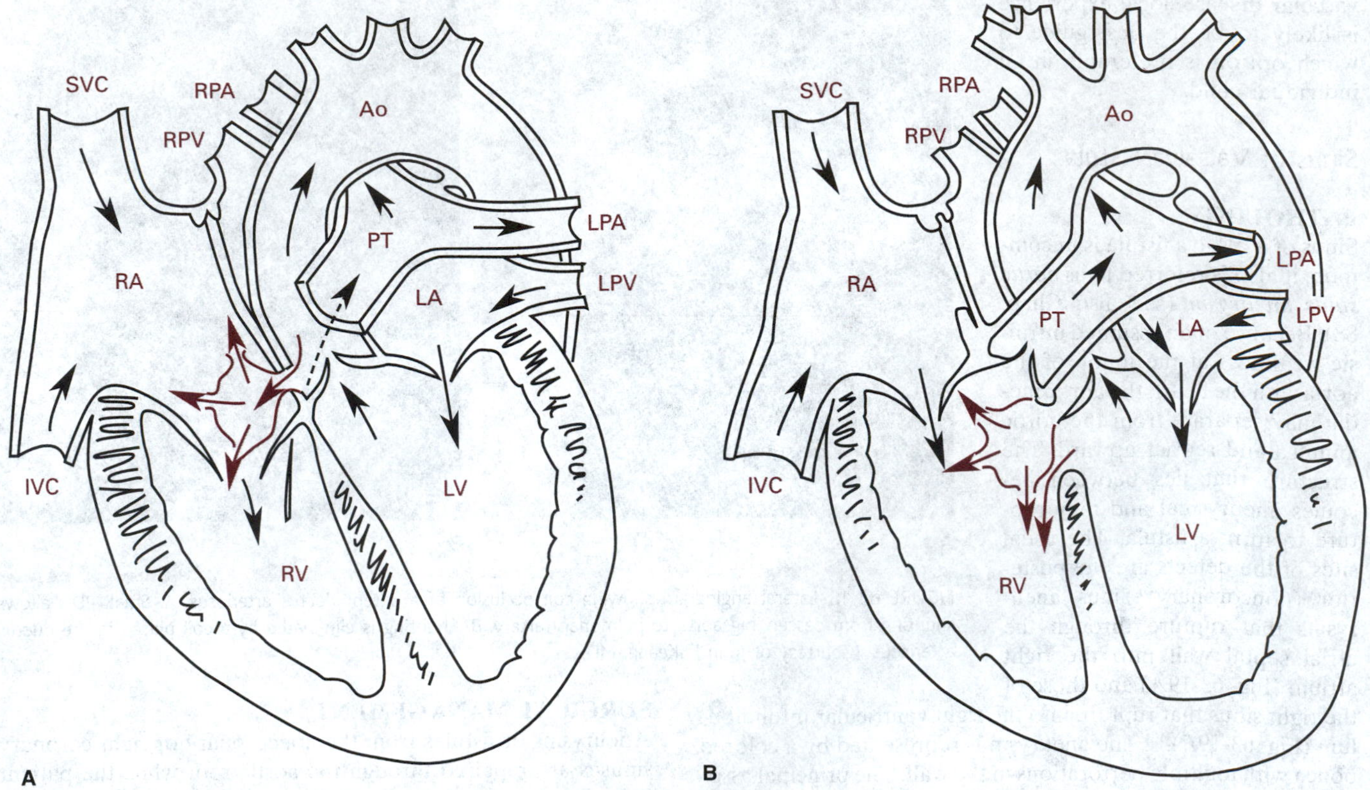

FIGURE 63-19 Sinus of Valsalva fistula. *A*. Aneurysm involves the posterior sinus and ruptures into the right atrium. *B*. Aneurysm involves the right aortic sinus and ruptures into the right ventricle. A ventricular septal defect is commonly associated, as illustrated. SVC = superior vena cava; IVC = inferior vena cava; RA = right atrium; RV = right ventricle; PT = main pulmonary arterial trunk; RPA = right pulmonary artery; LPA = left pulmonary artery; RPV = right pulmonary vein; LPV = left pulmonary vein; LA = left atrium; LV = left ventricle; Ao = aorta. (From Edwards JE.[66] Reproduced with permission from the publisher and author.)

rior, and posterior walls and is represented by a curtain-like infolding of the wall that causes the lumen to be narrowed and eccentric[106] (see Chap. 88).

In infants, the lesion lies either opposite the ductus or in a preductal location. In adolescents and adults, it is usually at the ligamentum arteriosum. An aberrant right subclavian artery may be associated. In rare cases, the narrowing lies proximal to the origin of the left common carotid artery or involves a segment of the abdominal aorta.

The principal cardiac abnormality is left ventricular hypertrophy. In some infants, left ventricular endocardial fibroelastosis may be associated. Tubular hypoplasia of the distal aortic arch and isthmus is very common, especially with associated cardiac abnormalities involving left heart obstruction.[107] The proximal aorta may show a moderate degree of cystic medial necrosis. Beyond the coarctation, the lining may show a localized jet lesion.

Prominent collaterals are characteristic in older infants, children, and adolescents. They may be divided into anterior and posterior systems, with the anterior system originating with the internal mammary arteries and making use of the epigastric arteries in the abdominal wall to supply the lower extremities. The posterior system involves parascapular arteries connected with the posterior intercostal arteries and carries blood to the distal aortic compartment principally for supply of the abdominal viscera. The anterior spinal artery, receiving branches from the proximal and distal compartments of the aorta, is also dilated and tortuous.

ASSOCIATED CONDITIONS

The most commonly associated defects are tubular hypoplasia of the aortic arch, PDA, VSD, and aortic stenosis (valvular and/or subvalvular). A bicuspid aortic valve is present in 46 percent of autopsy cases.[106]

ABNORMAL PHYSIOLOGY

In most instances, both the systolic and diastolic arterial pressures above the coarctation are elevated above normal levels. Below the coarctation, the systolic pressure is lower than that in the upper extremities, and the diastolic pressure is usually near or only slightly below the normal range. The mechanism of upper extremity hypertension appears to involve the increased resistance to aortic flow produced by the coarctation itself, the decreased capacity and distensibility of the vessels into which the left ventricle ejects, and humoral factors.[108]

CLINICAL MANIFESTATIONS

Coarctation of the aorta occurs in approximately 4 percent of all infants and children with congenital heart disease and is the predominant lesion in approximately 8 percent of infants presenting with critical heart disease in the first year of life. It ranks behind only VSD, dextrotransposition of the great arteries, and tetralogy of Fallot.[3] Among all individuals born with coarctation, approximately half present within the first month or two of life with heart failure. About 50 percent of infants so admitted have uncomplicated coarctation; the remaining half can be expected to have at least one complicating cardiac abnormality. VSD is the most common (64 percent), followed by left ventricular outflow tract obstruction (31 percent).[109] The timing of ductal tissue constriction in terms of both ductal closure and perhaps aortic constriction appears to play a decisive role in the onset or worsening of symptoms in most of these patients. The male/female ratio is approximately 3:1 for isolated coarctation but is only 1.1:1 for complicated coarctation. Approximately 45 percent of children with Turner's syndrome have coarctation.

History The clinical picture in a symptomatic infant is one of dyspnea, difficulty in feeding, and poor weight gain. Older children are for the most part asymptomatic, although a few complain of mild fatigue, dyspnea, or symptoms of claudication in the legs when running.

Physical Examination In a symptomatic infant, signs of congestive heart failure are characteristic. A gallop rhythm is common, and a murmur from associated defects or from the coarctation itself (posteriorly in the interscapular area) may be heard. Frequently, these murmurs are either inaudible or nondescript on admission and become characteristic only when congestive failure is brought under control. Prominent arterial pulsations may be visible in the suprasternal notch and carotid arteries, and the left ventricular impulse is forceful. An early systolic ejection click at the apex suggests the presence of a bicuspid aortic valve. The murmur from the coarctation is medium-pitched, systolic, and blowing in quality. It is best heard posteriorly in the interscapular area, usually with some degree of radiation to the left axilla, apex, and anterior precordium. Low-pitched, continuous murmurs of collateral circulation may be heard over the chest wall, particularly posteriorly, but seldom before adolescence. A short middiastolic rumble at the apex without clinical evidence of mitral disease is relatively common.

The characteristic systolic blood pressure difference between the upper and lower extremities may be difficult to appreciate or measure in infants with severe congestive failure or with a large VSD or PDA. With improved compensation, pulses in the upper extremities become readily palpable. The femoral pulses remain weak, delayed, or absent. In these very young infants, it is important that the pulses in both brachial and carotid arteries be assessed. Weak or absent pulses in all sites are more characteristic of critical aortic stenosis or aortic atresia.

In older children and adults, the radial arterial pulses typically are strong; those in the femoral arteries are diminished, delayed, or absent. A repeatedly measured systolic or mean pressure difference between the upper and lower extremities greater than 10 mmHg is diagnostic. The pulse pressure in the leg is reduced, and in some patients no pressure can be measured by auscultation or Doppler. Approximately one-third of older children have mild to severe hypertension, with severe hypertension defined as a systolic pressure above 150 mmHg, a diastolic pressure above 100 mmHg, or both. Some patients have only a mild pressure difference between the arms and the legs at rest but a much larger difference during treadmill exercise. A systolic pressure difference between the two arms suggests that the origin of one subclavian artery is at or below the obstruction, e.g., aberrent right subclavian from the descending aorta.

In light of the simplicity of measuring blood pressure in the upper and lower extremities of children and the importance of early detection, it is surprising and disappointing that approximately 95 percent of children and adolescents with coarctation are referred by pediatricians and other health care providers to a pediatric cardiologist for evaluation of a heart murmur and/or hypertension without this serious underlying malformation being recognized.[110]

Chest Roentgenogram For a symptomatic infant, the pattern is one of impressive cardiac enlargement and venous congestion. In an older and asymptomatic child, the heart size is generally at the upper limits of normal with a left ventricular prominence. A figure-three configuration of the left margin of the aorta at the level of the coarctation may be seen in overpenetrated films, with the upper curve formed by the slightly dilated aorta just above the coarctation, the central indentation by the coarctation itself, and the lower curve by the poststenotic dilatation below the coarctation. Notching of the inferior margin of the ribs by tortuous intercostal arteries acting as collaterals is seldom present before 7 or 8 years of age.

Electrocardiogram The ECG of a symptomatic infant reflects right or biventricular hypertrophy during the first 3 months of life. T-wave inversion in the left precordial leads is common. In older children, the ECG is usually normal or may indicate mild left ventricular and left atrial hypertrophy.

Echocardiogram Two-dimensional echocardiographic imaging of the aortic arch from the suprasternal notch permits visualization of the coarctation and detection of anatomic variations such as isthmic or transverse arch hypoplasia. The precordial and subxiphoid views are of great value in assessing the presence and severity of associated defects. Doppler flow studies are helpful for diagnostic confirmation. In infants with heart failure, left ventricular dilation and decreased contractility are common. The severity of the coarctation can be evaluated by Doppler gradients and the diminished pulsatile flow in the abdominal aorta.

Cardiac Catheterization Study of symptomatic infants characteristically reveals left atrial and left ventricular hypertension and a significant systolic pressure difference between the left ventricle and the femoral artery, particularly if the coarctation is isolated. In the presence of a large VSD and PDA, the left ventricular hypertension and the systolic pressure difference between the left ventricle and the femoral artery are less impressive and may not exist at all. Every attempt should be made to define the nature and severity of associated defects. Imaging is recommended in older children to demonstrate the exact site and length of the coarctation as well as to show unusual features of the collateral circulation that may be of importance to the surgeon. Magnetic resonance imaging is an excellent and in most instances preferable alternative to angiography today for demonstrating the site and length of the coarctation (Fig. 63-20).

NATURAL HISTORY AND PROGNOSIS

Approximately one-half of infants admitted with heart failure within the first weeks of life have coarctation without significant

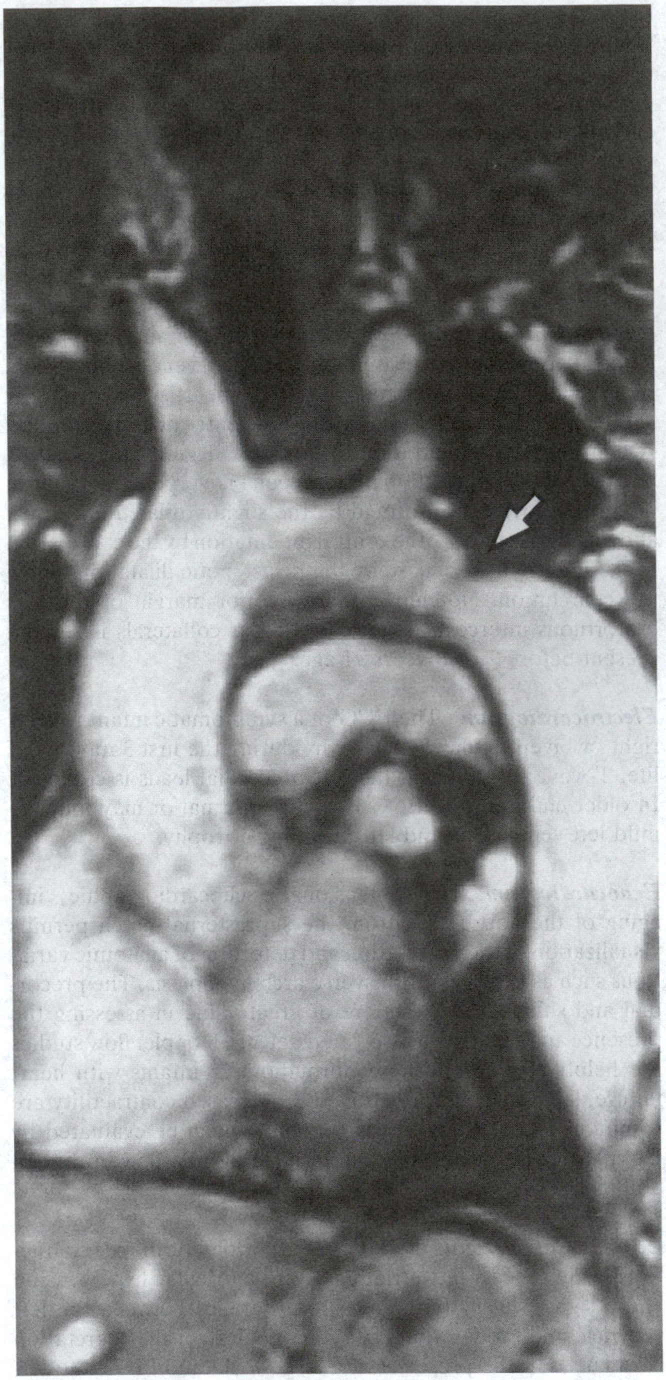

FIGURE 63-20 Selected frame from magnetic resonance angiogram in a child with discrete coarctation (*arrow*) distal to an enlarged left subclavian artery. (Courtesy of Andrew Powell, MD.)

associated defects.[109] The majority of these infants respond well to medical management and, if no repair is performed, reach a stage at 2 or 3 years of age where they are indistinguishable from asymptomatic children of the same age whose coarctation is first detected during a routine physical examination. Upper extremity hypertension usually increases during the first several months of life and then tends to diminish again as collateral circulation improves, while signs of failure diminish at the same time. For infants with severe failure and any serious associated defects, balloon dilation or surgery provides virtually the only chance of survival.

The consequences of persistent hypertension in an individual who has not undergone surgery appear in the second and third decades in the form of severe hypertension, aortic rupture, or intracranial hemorrhage from an aneurysm of the circle of Willis. Congestive heart failure that often is complicated by mitral or aortic valve disease, a dissecting aneurysm of the aorta, or atherosclerosis is seen in the fourth decade. The risk of endocarditis on the aortic or mitral valves or endarteritis at the site of coarctation appears to be spread relatively evenly over the years. The average age of death of patients who survive childhood with coarctation without surgery is 34 years.[111]

MEDICAL MANAGEMENT

Vigorous medical treatment is indicated for infants with severe heart failure. A newborn with severe failure may experience dramatic relief from the intravenous infusion of PGE_1 to reopen the closing ductus.[91] Prompt correction of the coarctation is recommended for all infants in whom there are one or more associated defects and for all infants with isolated coarctation unless the response to medical management has been dramatic and sustained.

The timing and type of correction of isolated discrete coarction of the aorta remain a topic of some dispute. There is general agreement that all children with congestive heart failure should be repaired after a brief period of stabilization and treatment of the failure. Since heart failure usually is limited to infants in the first few months of life and since balloon dilation of native coarctation in children under 6 months of age has had an unacceptable restenosis rate of up to 75 percent,[112] virtually all physicians would consider surgical repair the favored approach. For infants and children without congestive heart failure, the timing has been somewhat more problematic. Historically, the preferred approach was waiting until age 1 to 4 to avoid the problem of recoarctation that was found occasionally among patients corrected before 1 year of age[113] and residual or recurrent hypertension among patients without demonstrable recurrent coarctation, renal disease, or significant aortic regurgitation, which appears to be related to the duration of hypertension before surgery. More recently, the ability to reduce the restenosis rate has led some centers to reduce the age of elective surgical repair of coarctation to 3 to 6 months. For those in whom balloon dilation is contemplated, waiting until age 1 to 4 still seems appropriate.

Although there is general agreement that symptomatic children under 6 months of age with coarctation ought to be repaired surgically and that the first approach to those who develop restenosis at virtually any age should be balloon dilation or stent placement, the proper therapy for the treatment of native coarctation in children older than 1 year of age remains somewhat controversial. For balloon dilation, immediate success (defined as an increase in the coarctation diameter with a residual gradient of less than 20 mmHg) occurs in 80 to 95 percent of patients who are dilated, with the gradient reduction averaging 75 percent. However, long-term gradient relief after angioplasty has been somewhat less than that with surgery. Restenosis rates in the intermediate term seem to be directly related to the age at dilation, with 85 percent of neonates, 35 percent of infants, and 10 percent of children over 2 years of age developing restenosis.[112] Repeat dilation is almost invariably successful, and many advocate this approach even if it requires two dilations rather than a one-step surgical approach. Occasionally in older children a stent can be placed if the balloon dilation fails to persistently increase the luminal diameter (Fig. 63-21). In selected older children and adults, this has been very successful, with an average reduction in the gradient from 25 to 5 mm in 32 patients at Children's Hospital in Boston.[114] Complications usually have been related to associated diseases, although aneurysms, usually small, at the site of dilation have been reported in about 5 percent of cases. Large catheters are necessary, and trauma to the femoral artery is not uncommon.

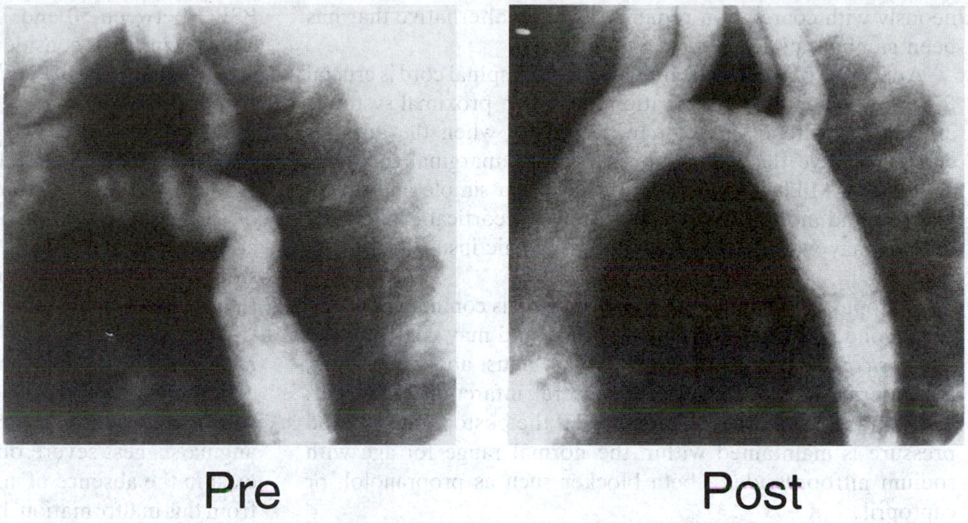

FIGURE 63-21 Repair of coarctation with a stent. *Left panel:* coarctation caused by kink with anterior indentation. *Right panel:* narrowing eliminated with stent. (Courtesy of Audrey Marshall, MD.)

Patients who have repaired coarctation need to be followed indefinitely. For those with significant recoarctation, expressed as a systolic pressure gradient between the upper and lower extremities of 20 mm or more at rest, balloon angioplasty and/or stent placement are recommended. Repeat surgery for recurrent coarctation is rarely necessary. Occasionally, patients are seen who have insignificant or small resting gradients but manifest abnormal upper extremity hypertension and significant gradients with exercise.[109] These patients probably should undergo balloon angioplasty and stent replacement with pharmacologic control of their hypertension if it is present at rest and beta blockade if the hypertension becomes significant with exercise.

SURGICAL MANAGEMENT

The coarctation is exposed and mobilized through a left posterolateral thoracotomy. It is usually possible to resect the narrow segment and restore continuity with a direct end-to-end anastomosis (Fig. 63-22). When the narrowed segment is longer, repair by subclavian flap aortoplasty or rarely a tubular vascular prosthesis to bridge the gap between the two ends of the aorta may be necessary. In adults with a relatively nonelastic or calcified aorta, a tubular vascular prosthesis can be used to bypass the unresected coarctation or the previous repair. Dacron patch repair of coarctation has an unacceptably high incidence of late aneurysm formation and is no longer advised.[115] Tension-free suture lines are essential. Postoperative bleeding, chylothorax, paraplegia, and injury to the phrenic and recurrent laryngeal nerves remain potential complications.[116]

If a significant VSD is also present, a pulmonary arterial band is placed at the time of coarctation repair during infancy. The VSD then may be repaired electively during the next several months, when the child's congestive heart failure is well controlled. Primary repair of the VSD shortly after or simulta-

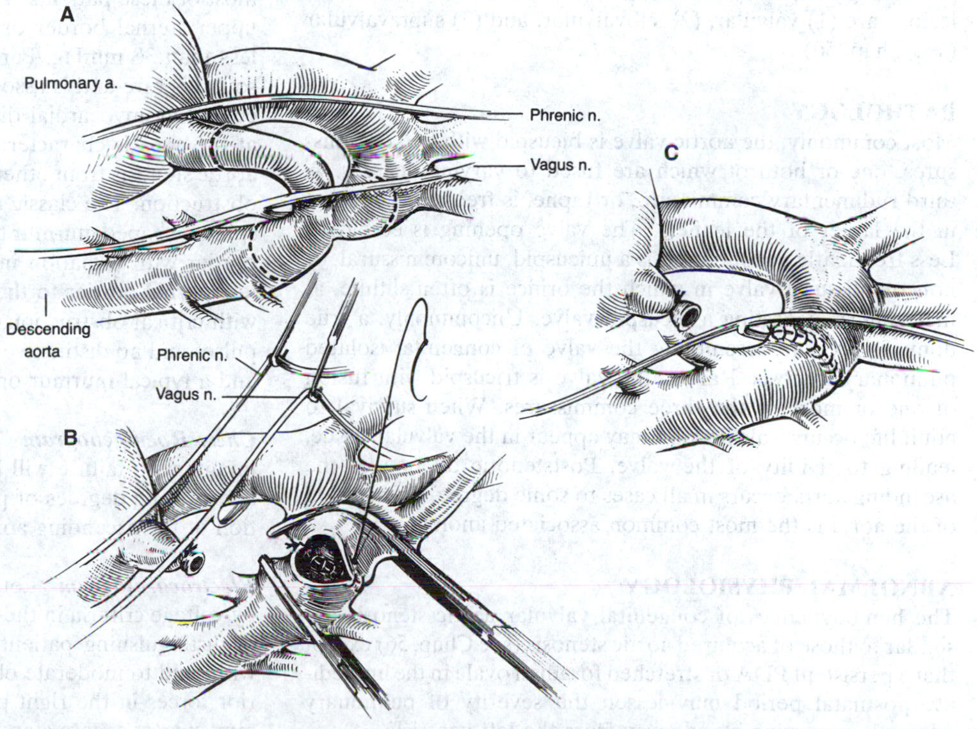

FIGURE 63-22 Repair of coarctation surgically. *A.* Discrete aortic coarctation in an infant with a small ductus arteriosus seen via left thoracotomy exposure. *B.* Repair technique using resection with end-to-end anastomosis. *C.* Complete repair. (From Castaneda AR, Jonas RA, Mayer JE Jr, Hanley FL. *Cardiac Surgery of the Neonate and Infant.* Philadelphia: Saunders; 1994: 333. Reproduced with permission from the publisher and author.)

neously with coarctation repair is a viable alternative that has been gaining favor recently.[117]

Adequacy of collateral circulation to the spinal cord is crucial for the safe repair of coarctation. A rise in proximal systemic arterial pressure of more than 20 mmHg when the aorta is clamped above the coarctation suggests a marginal collateral circulation. Mild systemic hypothermia is a simple and useful adjunct, and monitoring of somatosensory cortical evoked potentials may warn of an impending ischemic insult to the spinal cord.[118]

Postoperative paradoxical hypertension is common between the second and fifth postoperative days and may contribute to the *postcoarctation syndrome*, in which ileus, abdominal pain, mesenteric vasculitis, and even visceral infarction can occur. This syndrome rarely is encountered if the postoperative blood pressure is maintained within the normal range for age with sodium nitroprusside, a beta blocker such as propranolol, or captopril.

Operative mortality for infants with isolated coarctation is in the range of 0 to 3 percent [113,116,117] but is 10 percent or higher when other cardiovascular defects are present. Subsequent deaths are uncommon in surviving infants with isolated coarctation but are more likely in those with complicated associated defects.

Valvular Aortic Stenosis

DEFINITION

Aortic stenosis is defined as subtotal obstruction of varying severity in the channel of left ventricular outflow. In order of decreasing frequency, the sites of obstruction by congenital lesions are (1) valvular, (2) subvalvular, and (3) supravalvular (see Chap. 56).

PATHOLOGY

Most commonly, the aortic valve is bicuspid with two commissures, one or both of which are fused to varying degrees. A third rudimentary commissure, or raphe, is frequently present in the larger of the leaflets. The valve opening is eccentric. Less frequently encountered is a unicuspid, unicommissural, or noncommissural valve in which the orifice is often slitlike, at first glance suggesting a bicuspid valve. Uncommonly, a true dome is present, resembling the valve of congenital isolated pulmonary stenosis. Rarely, the valve is tricuspid with fusion of one or more of the three commissures. When survival to adult life occurs, calcification may appear in the valvular tissue, leading to rigidity of the valve. Poststenotic dilation of the ascending aorta occurs in all cases to some degree. Coarctation of the aorta is the most common associated anomaly.

ABNORMAL PHYSIOLOGY

The hemodynamics of congenital valvular aortic stenosis are similar to those of acquired aortic stenosis (see Chap. 56) except that a persistent PDA or stretched foramen ovale in the immediate postnatal period may lessen the severity of pulmonary edema by diverting blood away from the left ventricle.

Severity usually is judged by the peak systolic pressure gradient (PSPG) across the aortic valve, which is determined at cardiac catheterization, and the calculated aortic valve area. In the presence of a normal cardiac output, a PSPG $\geq$75 mmHg or an aortic valve area $<$0.5 cm^2/m^2 is considered severe, a PSPG between 50 and 75 mmHg or a valve area between 0.5 and 0.8 cm^2/m^2 is considered moderate, and a PSPG $<$50 mmHg or a valve area $>$0.9 cm^2/m^2 is considered mild (see Chaps. 15 and 56).

CLINICAL MANIFESTATIONS

About 7 percent of infants and children with congenital heart disease have aortic stenosis in one of its several forms, and approximately 80 percent of these patients have valvular aortic stenosis. Valvular stenosis is much more common among males than females, with a ratio of 4:1.

History The detection of a systolic murmur leads to the discovery of this malformation in most patients, the vast majority of whom are asymptomatic. Easy fatigue, dyspnea, syncope, and angina suggest severe obstruction, but severe obstruction may exist in the absence of any symptoms. Sudden death may occur from this malformation, but in most such cases death is preceded by either symptoms or ECG changes. Infants with critical stenosis from birth present with congestive failure within the first week or two of life and represent true emergencies. A similar small number of patients with less critical but still very severe obstruction are detected over the course of the next 4 to 6 months.

Physical Examination The arterial blood pressure and the quality of the peripheral arterial pulses of older infants and children are usually normal. A measured pulse pressure $<$20 mmHg suggests severe stenosis. The cardiac apex impulse may be forceful and sustained, and a systolic thrill along the right upper sternal border and over the carotid arteries is present in most of these patients. The absence of such a thrill at the right upper sternal border or suprasternal notch suggests a PSPG less than 30 mmHg. Paradoxical splitting of the second heart sound is rare and is associated with very severe obstruction or coexisting myocardial disease. An early systolic ejection click at the apex is characteristic and serves to distinguish valvular aortic stenosis from other forms of left ventricular outflow tract obstruction. The classic auscultatory finding is a harsh systolic spindle-shaped murmur that is loudest at the right upper sternal border with radiation into the carotid arteries and down the left sternal border to the apex (see Chap. 56). Among infants with critical obstruction, there may be no palpable peripheral pulses and no distinctive murmur, with a return of weak pulses and a typical murmur only after decongestive therapy.

Chest Roentgenogram The overall heart size is normal, but infants with failure will have generalized cardiac enlargement and varying degrees of pulmonary edema. Poststenotic dilatation of the ascending aorta is characteristic.

Electrocardiogram Left ventricular hypertrophy, as indicated by voltage criteria in the left precordial leads, is seldom helpful in distinguishing patients with severe obstruction from those with mild to moderate obstruction. However, diminished anterior forces in the right precordial leads and a deep $SV_1 \geq 30$ mm suggest severe stenosis, as does absence of the Q wave in V_6. Fifty percent of patients with severe obstruction have a flat, biphasic, or inverted T wave in V_6 (Fig. 63-23). Severe and even critical obstruction may be present with none of the ECG abnormalities mentioned above. Monitoring of the ST segment in leads V_5 through V_7 during cautious exercise testing appears to be a reliable method of detecting children in whom a significant PSPG (>50 mmHg) has developed and in whom that gradient may represent a threat of sudden death.[119] Symptomatic infants may show right, left, or biventricular hypertrophy, frequently with T-wave inversion over the left precordium.

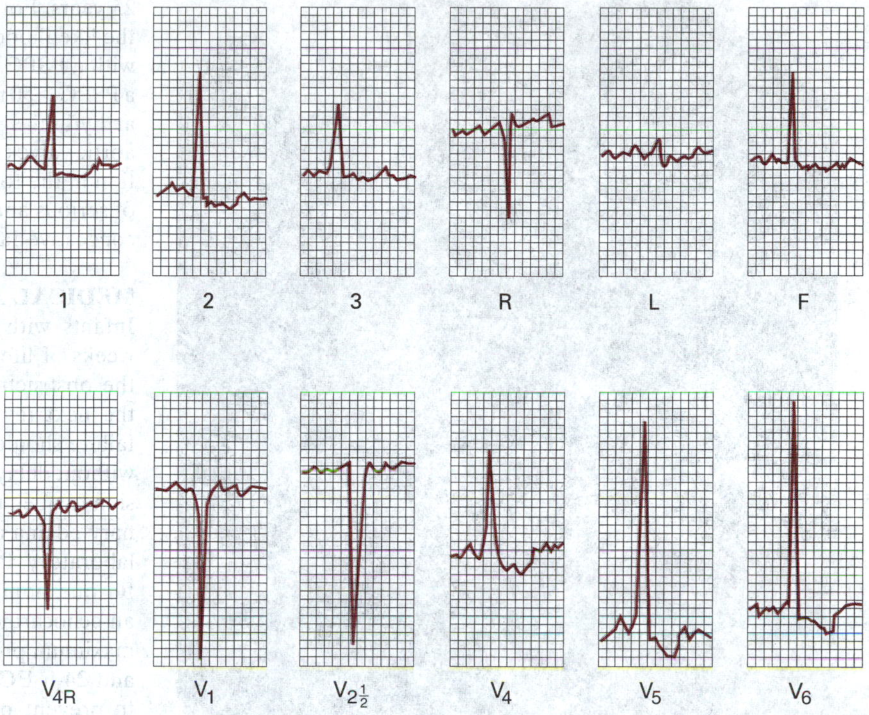

FIGURE 63-23 Electrocardiogram from an 8-year-old boy with valvular aortic stenosis and a 94-mmHg peak systolic pressure gradient. The small anterior QRS forces, abnormally large posterior forces, absent Q waves in leads V_5 and V_6, and abnormal T waves and ST segments reflect severe left ventricular systolic pressure overload with ischemia.

Echocardiogram Continuous-wave Doppler echocardiography guided by two-dimensional echocardiographic imaging predicts very accurately the peak and mean instantaneous systolic pressure gradient across discrete forms of left ventricular outflow tract obstruction (see Chap. 13) (Fig. 63-24). Two-dimensional echocardiography can distinguish valvular from supravalvular or subvalvular obstruction and identify critically ill infants in whom the size of the left ventricle, mitral valve annulus, or aortic root is hypoplastic to a degree that would preclude survival.[120,121]

Cardiac Catheterization Infants symptomatic with severe aortic obstruction often have a left-to-right shunt through a stretched foramen ovale, PAH, and a right-to-left shunt through a PDA. A marked increase in left ventricular end-diastolic pressure is usually present. The PSPG between the left ventricle and the central aorta should be documented whenever possible. If left ventricular output is markedly diminished, this gradient may be relatively small even in the presence of severe obstruction. Left ventricular angiography will confirm the site of obstruction and outline the size of the left ventricular cavity (Fig. 63-25*A*).

In older infants and children, pressures on the right side of the heart are usually normal. Simultaneous recording of central aortic and left ventricular pressures or a pressure tracing upon catheter withdrawal from the left ventricle to the aorta, coupled with an accurate estimate of cardiac output, is necessary for reliable assessment of severity. Left ventricular angiography will document the site of obstruction. The aortic leaflets typically are thickened and domed, with a central or eccentric jet of contrast material entering the ascending aorta. Poststenotic dilatation is characteristic. Supravalvular aortography is recommended to assess the presence and severity of aortic regurgitation.

NATURAL HISTORY AND PROGNOSIS

About half the infants born with severe valvular aortic stenosis are symptomatic enough to require hospitalization within the first week of life. Not uncommonly, the murmur is mistaken for that of a VSD. Congestive heart failure beyond infancy and before adolescence usually is not seen without the presence of complicating factors. Symptomatic infants require prompt relief of obstruction by balloon or surgical valvotomy, but the mortality rate remains significant. Endocardial fibroelastosis, papillary muscle necrosis, associated intra- and extracardiac deformities, and a small left ventricular cavity contribute to this mortality rate. Survivors may have significant aortic regurgitation, but the majority can be managed medically until valve replacement is feasible.

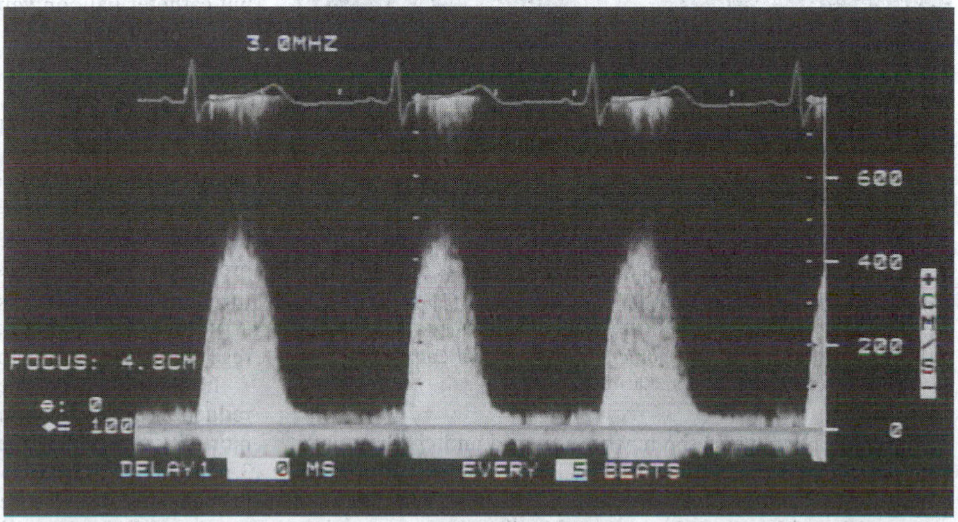

FIGURE 63-24 Doppler interrogation in the ascending aorta in a patient with valvar aortic stenosis. The peak velocity of 4.8 m/s correlates with a maximum instantaneous gradient of 92 mmHg across the aortic valve.

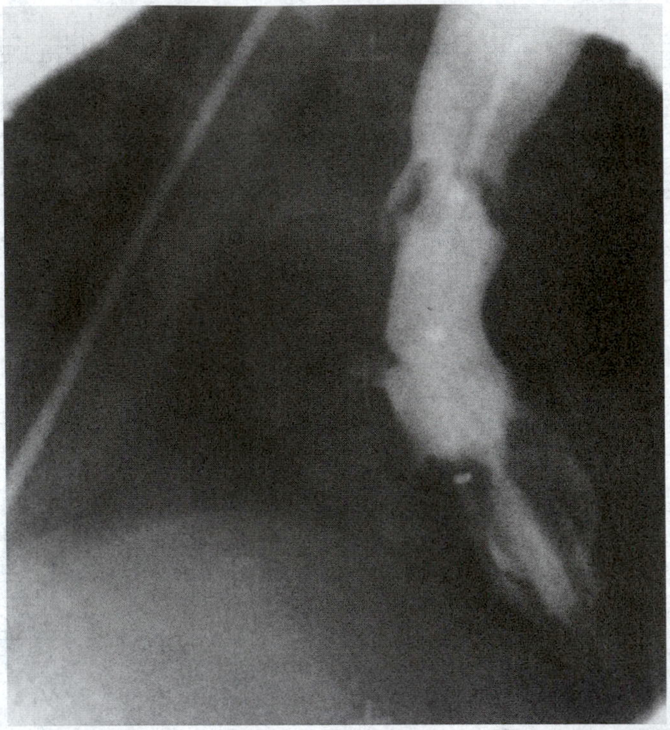

A

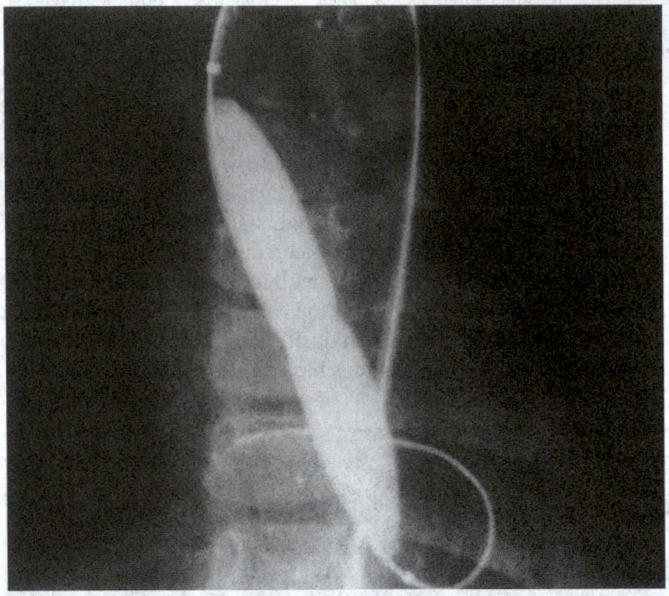

B

FIGURE 63-25 Balloon aortic valvuloplasty. *A.* Left ventricular angiogram showing a domed, thickened aortic valve with fusion of the right and left commissures. *B.* Balloon dilation using a retrograde technique. A waist is demonstrated in the midportion of the balloon before full inflation. (From Lock JE, Keane JF, Perry SB. *Diagnostic and Interventional Catheterization in Congenital Heart Disease*. Boston: Kluwer; 2000: 151.)

Most infants beyond the newborn period and children with mild aortic valvular stenosis (PSPG at catheterization <25 mmHg or a Doppler mean pressure gradient <25 mmHg) remain stable, with only a 21 percent likelihood of progression in severity and the need for intervention within the subsequent 25 years. For patients with a PSPG between 25 and 49 mmHg, the likelihood of significant progression rises to 41 percent, and with a PSPG >50 mmHg, it rises to 71 percent.[122] Patients with a PSPG >50 mmHg are judged to be at risk of serious ventricular arrhythmias and sudden death. Infective endocarditis on the aortic valve (see Chap. 73) poses an extremely serious complication in the form of systemic arterial emboli and the production of serious and sometimes catastrophic aortic regurgitation with congestive failure, shock, and death.[60]

MEDICAL AND SURGICAL MANAGEMENT

Infants with the characteristic murmur detected in the first weeks of life should be evaluated very carefully to be certain the obstruction is not severe and does not become severe in the next few weeks or months.[123] Those who develop heart failure should be operated on or undergo balloon valvuloplasty without delay. In a critically ill neonate, intravenous PGE_1 infusion to open the ductus may provide temporary relief of pulmonary edema en route to the operating room or catheterization laboratory. Beyond infancy, a plan of reexamination with careful questioning regarding symptoms and an ECG each year, an echocardiogram with Doppler assessment of the mean and maximum pressure gradient every year or two, exercise testing, and 24-h ECG monitoring about every 3 years should suffice to prevent progression from going unrecognized. Indications for cardiac catheterization for gradient assessment and possible balloon dilation include the appearance of symptoms or syncope, decreased anterior forces with an $SV_1 \geq 30$ mm or flattening or inversion of the T wave in V_6 in the resting ECG, abnormal ST-T segments on exercise testing, or an estimated maximum instantaneous gradient of 65 mmHg or a mean pressure gradient >60 mmHg by echocardiographic Doppler techniques.

Transluminal catheter balloon valvuloplasty has become the acceptable alternative to surgery. In skilled hands, it can provide effective reduction of the transvalvular gradient while producing only a mild increment in aortic regurgitation in most instances.[124,125] Elective balloon dilation is recommended if the PSPG is >50 mmHg at catheterization and aortic regurgitation is mild or nonexistent. For a neonate with critical valvular obstruction, some centers continue to rely on surgical intervention, but catheter balloon valvuloplasty has become a very competitive alternative and in the author's institution is the procedure of choice for these very sick infants.

Balloon dilation has been performed since the mid-1980s, and long-term follow-up studies are not yet available. Early studies and more recent experience suggest that the balloon diameter should not exceed that of the valve ring, and most centers now use balloons that are 85 to 90 percent of the diameter of the aortic annulus. The balloon usually is inflated to a pressure of 4 to 6 atmospheres until the "waist" produced by the stenotic valve has been abolished (Fig. 63-25*B*). Transient arrythmias are seen occasionally, but other than creating aortic regurgitation, other complications are uncommon.

In older children, the results are usually quite good, with a reduction of the peak gradient of approximately 60 percent, a mortality rate under 2 percent, and a complication rate of about 3 percent.[124,125] In neonates, the results are more problematic, probably because of severity of disease, unstable conditions, and the size of the patient, with 12 percent early and late mortality in one series. In this center, reintervention (usually repeat balloon dilation) was necessary in 40 percent with a mean follow-up of 4.3 years.[126]

When surgical intervention is required for critical aortic stenosis during infancy, the heart is exposed through a median sternotomy and the aortic valve is visualized through the ascending aorta during a brief period of low-flow perfusion with mild hypothermia. Standard cardiopulmonary bypass, mild hypothermia, and cardioplegia are used in older children.[127] The surgeon must discriminate between true commissures and abnormal raphes because incision of the latter produces intolerable aortic valvular regurgitation. Relief of valvular stenosis is accomplished with a carefully placed incision in the middle of each fused but well-supported true commissure.

A conservative attitude is essential during operation for aortic stenosis in an infant or small child. Mild valvular regurgitation almost always occurs consequent to commissurotomy but is usually well tolerated. Moderate residual stenosis is preferred to intolerable aortic valvular regurgitation, especially in infants in whom valve implantation is technically difficult. If valve replacement is necessary in an infant or small child, use of the autograft pulmonary valve in the aortic position offers the attractive possibility of continuing growth of this neoaortic valve that may parallel that of the patient.[128]

The risk of operation is high in critically ill infants, in the range of 10 to 15 percent, particularly in those with a low ejection fraction, high left ventricular end-diastolic pressure, endocardial fibroelastosis, marked congestive failure, or features of left ventricular hypoplasia.[129] Morbidity after aortic valvotomy in an older child is rare, and the likelihood of relief of left ventricular outflow tract obstruction and survival is good. The Natural History Study of Congenital Heart Defects, reporting on 133 children undergoing aortic commissurotomy after age 2 years, found that only 27 percent required a second operation in the subsequent 20 years, with 78 percent of those operations consisting of valve replacement. Aortic regurgitation was the indication for operation in 14 percent of those with valve replacements.[122]

Relief of aortic valve obstruction, whether by balloon valvuloplasty or surgical valvotomy, is palliative rather than curative. Gradual restenosis is the rule, with almost one-third of infants who undergo valvotomy requiring a second operation, usually valve replacement, within the next two decades. Aortic regurgitation, a well-recognized complication of valvuloplasty, valvulotomy, and/or infective endocarditis, may require surgical intervention as well. Endocarditis is a serious and lifelong hazard, with an incidence among patients followed for 20 years of approximately 5 percent, a mortality rate of just over 25 percent, and a predilection for patients in the second, rather than first, decade of life and with PSPGs >50 mmHg.[60,122]

Secondary valvulotomy by balloon or surgery for recurrent or residual stenosis can be attempted, but calcification and restenosis eventually force aortic valve replacement in almost all those requiring surgery on the aortic valve in infancy or childhood. A small aortic annulus severely limits the relief of left ventricular hypertension unless one resorts to Konno's operation, in which the annulus is divided, the upper ventricular septum resected creating a VSD, patching the VSD with prosthetic material, and replacing the valve (a homograft or pulmonary autograft) into the enlarged annulus. The ascending aorta and anterior right ventricular wall are reconstructed using a prosthetic graft, and in the case of an autograft, the main pulmonary artery and pulmonary valve are replaced with a cryopreserved pulmonary homograft.[130]

Children with more than mild aortic stenosis are restricted from strenuous organized athletics, isometric exercises, and activities that require a good deal of stamina and produce shortness of breath.[131]

Supravalvular Aortic Stenosis

PATHOLOGY

The obstruction in the ascending aorta includes the following three types: (1) hourglass (discrete), (2) hypoplastic (diffuse), and (3) membranous. Associated obstructions in the pulmonary trunk, peripheral pulmonary arteries, and branches of the aortic arch are common.[132] Hypertrophy of the coronary arterial walls and premature coronary atherosclerosis have been described.[133]

CLINICAL MANIFESTATIONS

Supravalvular stenosis may be familial, associated with characteristic facies and mental retardation, sporadic, or (rarely) the result of congenital rubella. All forms may be and usually are associated with varying degrees of peripheral or branch pulmonary arterial stenosis. The familial form is transmitted as an autosomal dominant trait with variable expression (see Chap. 62). Mental retardation is not present, and there are no characteristic facial features.[134] Supravalvular aortic stenosis associated with mental retardation, frequently called *Williams' syndrome*, is associated with a high and prominent forehead, epicanthal folds, underdevelopment of the bridge of the nose and mandible, and a broad, overhanging upper lip. It is due to a deletion of the elastin gene on chromosome 7 and can now be identified by florescent in situ hybridization studies. It has been linked with idiopathic hypercalcemia of infancy, but in the majority of patients recognized beyond infancy, hypercalcemia is not present.[135]

The symptoms of supravalvular aortic stenosis are similar to those of subvalvular aortic stenosis (see below). Patients with the familial form usually have a distinctive family history but one that seldom emerges in its entirety on initial questioning. The physical findings are also similar to those of subvalvular aortic stenosis, although a systolic blood pressure difference may be recorded between the two arms on occasion, with the right arm pressure being greater than the left (Coanda effect).[136] Chest roentgenography and ECG are not distinctive unless associated pulmonary arterial stenosis leads to right ventricular hypertrophy. Echocardiography can identify the narrowed aortic lumen just above the aortic valve and provide an estimate of the severity of the obstruction by the Doppler-derived instantaneous pressure gradient.

At cardiac catheterization, a systolic pressure gradient can be demonstrated just above the aortic valve by careful pullback. Supravalvular aortography or left ventricular angiography will visualize the supravalvular narrowing (Fig. 63-26). Pressure recordings in the branch pulmonary arteries should be obtained, and pulmonary arterial angiography should be performed in the presence of any significant stenoses. Narrowing at the branch points of major arteries (coronary, carotid, mesenteric, renal, etc.) is seen occasionally.

NATURAL HISTORY AND PROGNOSIS

The sequence of progressive obstruction, the appearance of symptoms and ECG changes, and the possibility of sudden

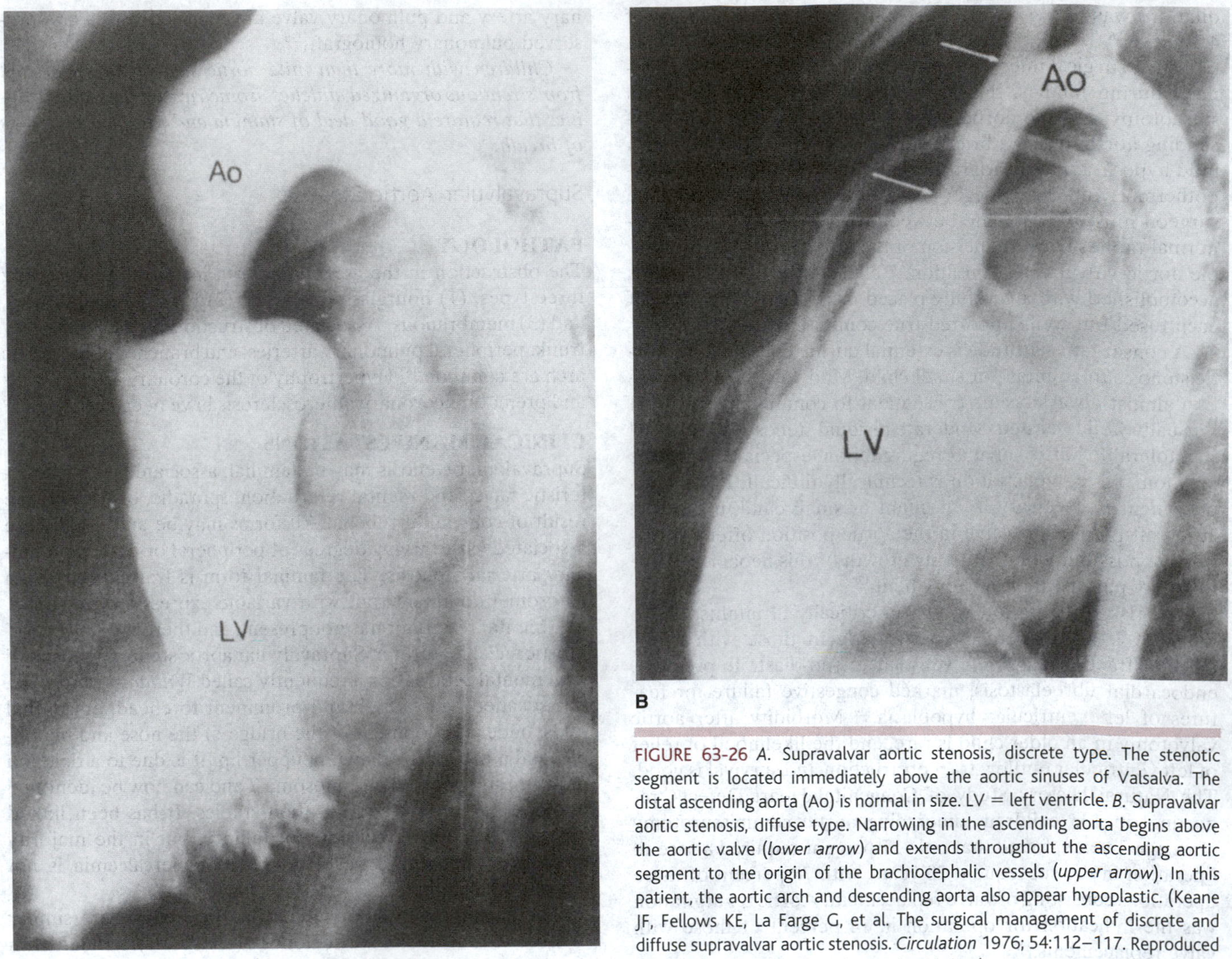

A

B

FIGURE 63-26 *A.* Supravalvar aortic stenosis, discrete type. The stenotic segment is located immediately above the aortic sinuses of Valsalva. The distal ascending aorta (Ao) is normal in size. LV = left ventricle. *B.* Supravalvar aortic stenosis, diffuse type. Narrowing in the ascending aorta begins above the aortic valve (*lower arrow*) and extends throughout the ascending aortic segment to the origin of the brachiocephalic vessels (*upper arrow*). In this patient, the aortic arch and descending aorta also appear hypoplastic. (Keane JF, Fellows KE, La Farge G, et al. The surgical management of discrete and diffuse supravalvar aortic stenosis. *Circulation* 1976; 54:112–117. Reproduced with permission of the author and publisher.)

death appear to apply for supravalvular aortic stenosis as well as for valvular aortic stenosis. Infective endocarditis represents a threat to these patients throughout life.

MANAGEMENT

The indications for cardiac catheterization and follow-up are the same as those with valvular aortic stenosis. Noninvasive imaging frequently suffices, but angiography may be necessary to evaluate the gradient and rule out arterial narrowing. Surgery usually is recommended if the gradient across the narrowing exceeds 40 mmHg.

Discrete supravalvular aortic stenosis is relieved by one or more incisions through the narrow segment of the ascending aorta, usually at the level of the sinotubular ridge at the top of the commissures. Incisions are extended well down into the aortic sinuses. Ridges of obstructing fibrous tissue are excised. The aorta is enlarged by the insertion of a gusset of prosthetic vascular graft material or pericardium to increase the circumference.[127] A favorable outcome can be anticipated postoperatively in most patients with supravalvular aortic stenosis if the arterial wall abnormality is localized.[137] Intimal obstruction of the coronary arterial ostia may require debridement, dilation, or even saphenous vein or internal mammary bypass grafting.

Diffuse tubular hypoplasia of the ascending aorta is a technically challenging problem that is associated with a higher mortality rate and usually poor postoperative hemodynamic results.

Subvalvular Aortic Stenosis

PATHOLOGY

Three classic varieties of subvalvular aortic stenosis involve the left ventricular outflow tract: the discrete, tunnel, and muscular types. The discrete type is characterized by a localized fibrous encirclement of the left ventricular outflow tract a short distance below the aortic valve (Fig. 63-27) or fibromuscular tissue that extends onto the mitral leaflet and also may attach to the aortic cusps. The tunnel type involves hypoplasia of the aortic annulus and a channel with a fibrous lining in the subjacent left ventricular outflow tract.[138,139] The muscular type also is known as *hypertrophic cardiomyopathy* (or idiopathic hypertrophic subaortic stenosis) and is discussed in Chap. 67.

More than half these patients have associated malformations, of which PDA, VSD, or coarctation are the most common.

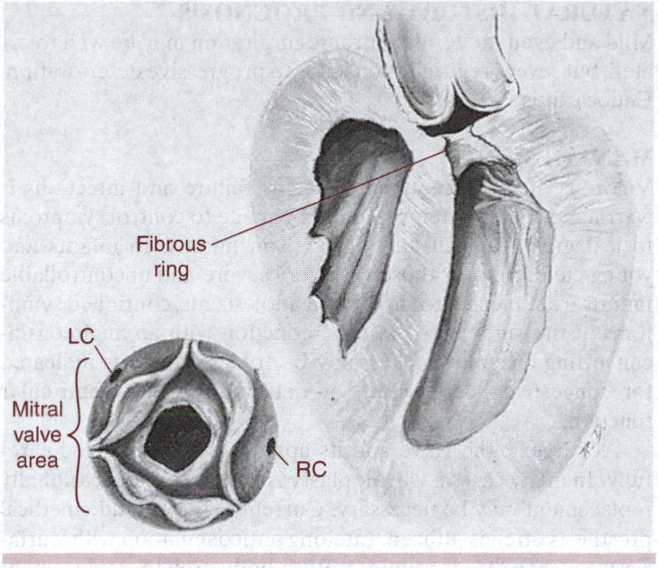

FIGURE 63-27 Localized subvalvular aortic stenosis. Obstruction is immediately upstream from the aortic valve. LC and RC = left and right coronary arteries. (From Kirklin JW and Ellis FH Jr.[144] Reproduced with permission from the publisher and authors.)

CLINICAL MANIFESTATIONS

Discrete stenosis is more common among males, with a male/female ratio of approximately 2.5:1. In the isolated forms, the majority of patients are referred because of the detection of a murmur that not uncommonly is mistaken initially for that of a VSD. The symptoms have the same implications as they do for valvular aortic stenosis.

The physical examination is similar to that of valvular aortic stenosis, with two exceptions: An early systolic ejection click is not heard, and an early diastolic murmur of aortic regurgitation is present in approximately one-half of these patients.

The roentgenographic features and ECG are also similar to those of valvular aortic stenosis except for the absence of poststenotic dilatation of the ascending aorta. Two-dimensional echocardiography permits excellent visualization of the anatomy of the obstruction. Estimation of the systolic pressure gradient can be obtained from Doppler echocardiographic studies.

When catheterization is performed, a careful pullback pressure tracing across the left ventricular outflow tract will document the severity of the gradient and establish the site of the obstruction. Left ventricular biplane angiography will outline the nature of the obstruction. Aortography is recommended to evaluate the degree of aortic regurgitation.

NATURAL HISTORY AND PROGNOSIS

Severe congestive failure in infancy is unusual and, if present, is almost invariably associated with complicating defects.[138] The obstruction is progressive in most instances, sometimes rapidly so. In one study, 75 percent of patients showed an increase of 25 mmHg or more in a 5-year period.[140] The cause of the progression is not known, but an intriguing theory suggests that distorted anatomy increases shear stress, leading to a stimulation of growth factors and cellular proliferation.[141] Associated aortic regurgitation also tends to be progressive and appears to result from damage from the jet of blood through the obstruction, with secondary thickening and deformity of the valve leaflets. The results of surgery depend on the extent of involvement of the left ventricular outflow tract, with the best results being obtained in patients with a thin, discrete subvalvular membrane. The least satisfactory results occur in patients with tunnel obstruction.

MANAGEMENT

Medical management is similar to that of patients with valvular aortic stenosis, but surgery for the discrete type usually is recommended for pressure gradients ≥30 mmHg because of the possibility of progression of obstruction, and the likelihood of progressive aortic valvular deformity and regurgitation.[142]

Continued follow-up for assessment of reobstruction and progression of aortic regurgitation and for reemphasis of the precautions against infective endocarditis is essential in all patients.[143]

Subvalvular fibromuscular (membranous) left ventricular outflow tract obstruction is exposed through the aortic root as was described for aortic valvular stenosis (Fig. 63-27). Small half-circle needles and sutures or hooks are placed into the abnormal fibromuscular tissue, pulling it into view for precise excision from the underlying ventricular septum and the anterior mitral valve leaflet. The area of the bundle of His, which usually is just beneath the anterior commissure between the right and noncoronary leaflets, is avoided. An additional septal myectomy or myotomy beneath and to the left of the commissure between the right and left leaflets may be required if secondary hypertrophy is significant. Immediate and early operative outcome is generally good, but *residual, recurrent, and progressive subaortic obstruction occurs in up to 25 percent of these patients, requiring long-term follow-up.*[144,145]

Diffuse tunnel obstruction in the left ventricular outflow tract poses a difficult technical problem that requires aortoseptoplasty, reconstruction of the left ventricular outflow (Konno's operation or a modification of it).[130,142]

Bicuspid Aortic Valve

PATHOLOGY

Classically, the two cusps are oriented anteriorly and posteriorly, with the anterior or conjoined cusp being the larger. A raphe, or ridge, is present along the aortic aspect of the larger cusp, running from the aortic wall to the free edge of the cusp. The most common associated condition of significance is coarctation of the aorta. The most common complication is calcification of the valve. *In about 85 percent of cases of calcific aortic stenosis in patients below age 70, the valve is congenitally bicuspid.* Aortic regurgitation from prolapse of the larger cusp is a less common complication and is usually not evident until adolescence or adult life.

CLINICAL MANIFESTATIONS

The incidence in the general population approaches 2 percent; therefore, it is the most common congenital abnormality of the heart or great vessels except possibly for mitral valve prolapse (see Chap. 58). Its importance lies in its frequent association with other forms of congenital heart disease: the predisposition of the valve to become stenotic as a result of fibrosis and deposition of calcium over the course of years, the tendency of the valve to become regurgitant, its association with aortic root dilatation and dissection,[146] and finally, the susceptibility of the valve to infective endocarditis. It is also common among patients with isolated or dominant aortic regurgitation, patients with infective endocarditis with or without a history of predisposing heart disease, and, probably most frequently, otherwise normal individuals who come to the physician's attention because of unrelated illnesses. Patients with uncomplicated bicuspid aortic valve are asymptomatic. The incidence among males is approximately 2.5 times that among females (see Chap. 56).

The characteristic feature is auscultatory and consists of an early systolic ejection click, which is best heard at the apex and does not vary with respiration. A soft, early, or midsystolic murmur is frequently present at the right upper sternal border. Less commonly, a soft murmur of aortic regurgitation may be heard. Two-dimensional echocardiography with adequate images can identify the bicuspid valve with a high degree of sensitivity and diagnostic accuracy.

NATURAL HISTORY AND PROGNOSIS

The majority of congenitally bicuspid aortic valves are nonobstructive at birth, but with the passage of time, a few of these valves become fibrotic, stiffer, and more obstructive and eventually become the site of calcium deposition, primarily among individuals between ages 15 and 65. Important calcium deposition is unusual before age 30, whereas grossly visible deposits of calcium are present in the valves of virtually all patients with severe stenosis beyond that age. A much smaller number of individuals born with a bicuspid aortic valve develop isolated aortic regurgitation. In approximately one-third, this is the result of fibrosis, prolapse, or retraction of one or both of the leaflets; in the remainder, regurgitation results from infective endocarditis on an apparently functionally normal bicuspid valve (see Chaps. 56 and 73).

Congenital Mitral Regurgitation

PATHOLOGY

Mitral regurgitation may be due to a primary valve abnormality or secondary to a more complex defect (see "Common Atrioventricular Canal Defects," above). There are a variety of rare primary malformations, including isolated cleft, fenestration, and double orifice. Mitral regurgitation also occurs frequently with conditions that cause left ventricular dilatation and failure.

CLINICAL MANIFESTATIONS

Poor growth, frequent respiratory infections, and failure occur with significant mitral regurgitation. The physical findings are generally similar to those with mitral regurgitation of other causes (see Chap. 10). There may be a prominent left precordial bulge if cardiomegaly has been present from infancy. The systolic murmur may radiate to the base of the heart. Left atrial and left ventricular enlargement correlate with the degree of volume overload. Echocardiography with Doppler color flow mapping will demonstrate these as well as left ventricular function and the severity of regurgitation. The specific defect may be outlined, such as an isolated cleft or a double-orifice valve. Findings at cardiac catheterization substantiate the hemodynamic alterations (see Chap. 15).

NATURAL HISTORY AND PROGNOSIS

Mild and even moderate mitral regurgitation may be well tolerated, but severe regurgitation leads to progressive deterioration. Endocarditis is a risk.

MANAGEMENT

Vigorous medical treatment of heart failure and infections is warranted. Every attempt should be made to control symptoms to a degree that will allow growth in infants. In infants and young children, only those with very severe and uncontrollable failure are subjected to surgery. In adolescents, continued symptoms justify surgery. Afterload reduction with an angiotensin-converting enzyme blocker may be tried. Surgery is indicated for congestive heart failure or deteriorating left ventricular function.

At surgery, the valve and its apparatus are inspected carefully. In many cases a valvuloplasty is possible, but occasionally replacement may be necessary. Currently, the St. Jude medical prosthesis often is utilized. Lifelong anticoagulation with warfarin (see Chap. 44) is required. With body growth, replacement with a larger prosthesis may be difficult, and no good annular enlarging operation exists.

VALVULAR AND VASCULAR MALFORMATIONS OF THE RIGHT SIDE OF THE HEART WITH RIGHT-TO-LEFT, BIDIRECTIONAL, OR NO SHUNT

Pulmonary Stenosis with Intact Ventricular Septum

PATHOLOGY

Valvular pulmonary stenosis with an intact ventricular septum usually is characterized by a dome-shaped stenosis of the pulmonary valve and less commonly by dysplasia of the valve. The valve may be unicuspid, bicuspid, or tricuspid. The annulus also may be narrow. The pulmonary trunk exhibits poststenotic dilatation. In adult patients, calcification of the valve may appear.

In pulmonary valvular dysplasia, the annulus of the valve may be abnormally narrow, but the most dramatic changes are related to the cusps, of which three are identifiable. The cusps are exceedingly thickened by mucoid and dense connective tissue.[147]

Concentric hypertrophy of the right ventricle is present, with its degree reflecting the degree of obstruction at the valve level. *The hypertrophy of the infundibular musculature may cause secondary infundibular stenosis.*

Less commonly, there may be isolated subvalvular pulmonary stenosis caused by infundibular narrowing or an anomalous muscle bundle across the middle of the right ventricle.[148] Both types may be associated with a VSD.

Isolated supravalvular pulmonary stenosis, or pulmonary arterial coarctations, also may occur. From angiographic studies, these are classified into four types: (1) *localized stenosis with poststenotic dilatation*, (2) *segmental stenosis*, (3) *diffuse hypoplasia*, and (4) *multiple peripheral stenoses*. The stenosis may be localized to any segment of the pulmonary arterial system. The process is unilateral in about one-third of cases and bilateral in two-thirds. Pulmonary arterial stenosis is commonly (about

75 percent), though not universally, associated with other cardiovascular abnormalities, such as tetralogy of Fallot. It also may be seen as a sequela of congenital rubella, Williams', Noonan's,[149] or Alagille's syndrome.

ABNORMAL PHYSIOLOGY

There is a pressure difference during systole between the main right ventricular cavity and the pulmonary artery. The area of the pulmonary valve orifice is normally 2 cm^2/m^2; it is about 0.5 cm^2 at birth and increases in size with body growth. In general, the effective valve area must be decreased about 60 percent before there is a hemodynamically significant obstruction to flow. PSPG may reach 150 to 240 mmHg in severe cases. The degree of obstruction is assessed by the peak and mean systolic pressure gradients and the amount of flow across the valve. In neonates, severe stenosis can be associated with a relatively small pressure difference if the flow is very low as a result of right ventricular failure. If pulmonary flow is normal, patients with PSPG at rest <40 mmHg have mild stenosis and patients with PSPG >75 mmHg have severe stenosis.

When the pulmonary stenosis is severe, the right ventricle may fail and the cardiac output may be decreased at rest; this is associated with elevation of both the right ventricular end-diastolic pressure and the right atrial mean pressure. This may cause the foramen ovale to open and allow shunting of blood from the right atrium to the left atrium, resulting in arterial oxygen desaturation and cyanosis. In most adolescent or adult patients with significant pulmonary stenosis, the resting cardiac output is within normal limits but usually does not increase normally during exercise. In contrast, younger children may be able to increase cardiac output during exercise, even with significant obstruction.[119,150]

CLINICAL MANIFESTATIONS

Pulmonary stenosis is one of the most common congenital heart defects and accounts for about 10 percent of patients in most large study populations (Table 63-1). The stenosis is at the level of the pulmonary valve in most instances, but it can occur within the right ventricle, in the pulmonary arteries, or in a combination of the two. Infants with severe stenosis with patency of the foramen ovale may have right-to-left shunting.

History Most infants and children are asymptomatic, but a small percentage with very severe obstruction manifest symptoms, usually mild fatigue or shortness of breath with exertion. Young infants with critical obstruction present with cyanosis if there is a patent foramen ovale or ASD. Squatting and syncope are rare in childhood.[151]

Physical Examination Patients with a dysplastic valve and occasional supravalvular stenosis have consistent noncardiac abnormalities in a familial syndrome described by Noonan,[149] with short stature, hypertelorism, ptosis, low-set ears, and mental retardation.

In older patients with valvular pulmonary stenosis, cyanosis is uncommon, except with severe obstruction and an atrial communication. Hepatomegaly and the murmur of tricuspid regurgitation may be present with severe obstruction. With at least moderate obstruction, a prominent a wave is seen on examination of the jugular venous pulse. A systolic thrill in the suprasternal notch and at the left upper sternal border is present with significant obstruction unless there is isolated subvalvular stenosis. The right ventricular parasternal impulse becomes increasingly forceful with more severe obstruction. *An early systolic click with expiration that disappears with inspiration heard at the left upper sternal border is the hallmark of valvular stenosis unless the obstruction is severe or the valve is dysplastic.* A click is not present with isolated stenosis at other levels. As the obstruction increases in severity, the pulmonary component of the second heart sound becomes progressively softer and more delayed, becoming inaudible when the right ventricular pressure reaches systemic levels or greater. The second heart sound is normal or accentuated with supravalvular stenosis. A fourth heart sound is heard if the obstruction is severe. The characteristic systolic murmur is harsh, crescendo-decrescendo in shape, and best heard at the left upper sternal border with radiation toward the left clavicle. The murmur radiates more to the axilla and back with supravalvular stenosis. The duration of the murmur and the timing of peak intensity correlate well with the severity of obstruction. With mild to moderate stenosis, the murmur peaks in midsystole and ends at or before the aortic component of the second heart sound. In patients with severe stenosis, the murmur peaks late in systole and extends beyond the aortic component of the second heart sound (see Chaps. 10 and 59).[151]

Chest Roentgenogram Most patients have a normal or only slightly increased heart size, primarily of the right ventricle. Significant enlargement is seen with critical obstruction and is an ominous sign. Characteristically, the main and proximal left pulmonary arteries are prominent as a result of poststenotic dilatation when the stenosis is valvular. This finding may be absent with very severe obstructions, with a dysplastic valve, in very young infants, or with stenosis above or below the valve. The pulmonary vascular pattern is normal in most of these patients, but the vascularity is diminished in those with a right-to-left shunt at the atrial level.

Electrocardiogram Right ventricular forces in the anterior precordial leads correlate reasonably well with the degree of obstruction.[151] They are normal or demonstrate mild hypertrophy with an rsR′ pattern if there is mild obstruction. With severe stenosis, there is right axis deviation, right atrial hypertrophy, and very tall pure R waves in the anterior precordial leads. The presence of a qR pattern in these leads is almost always a sign of very severe obstruction. Those with a dysplastic valve frequently have a superior QRS axis.

Echocardiogram Two-dimensional imaging allows identification of the level of obstruction, and Doppler studies provide an excellent measure of severity. Shunting at the atrial level also can be evaluated.[152]

Cardiac Catheterization Diagnostic catheterizations are rarely necessary, but data obtained before balloon dilation demonstrate an elevated right ventricular systolic pressure with a distinct systolic pressure difference across the narrowed segment, as demonstrated by slow withdrawal of the catheter from the distal pulmonary arterial branches to the proximal right ventricle. Simultaneous measurement of systemic arterial and right ventricular pressures with measurement of flow is necessary to assess severity accurately. The right ventricular end-

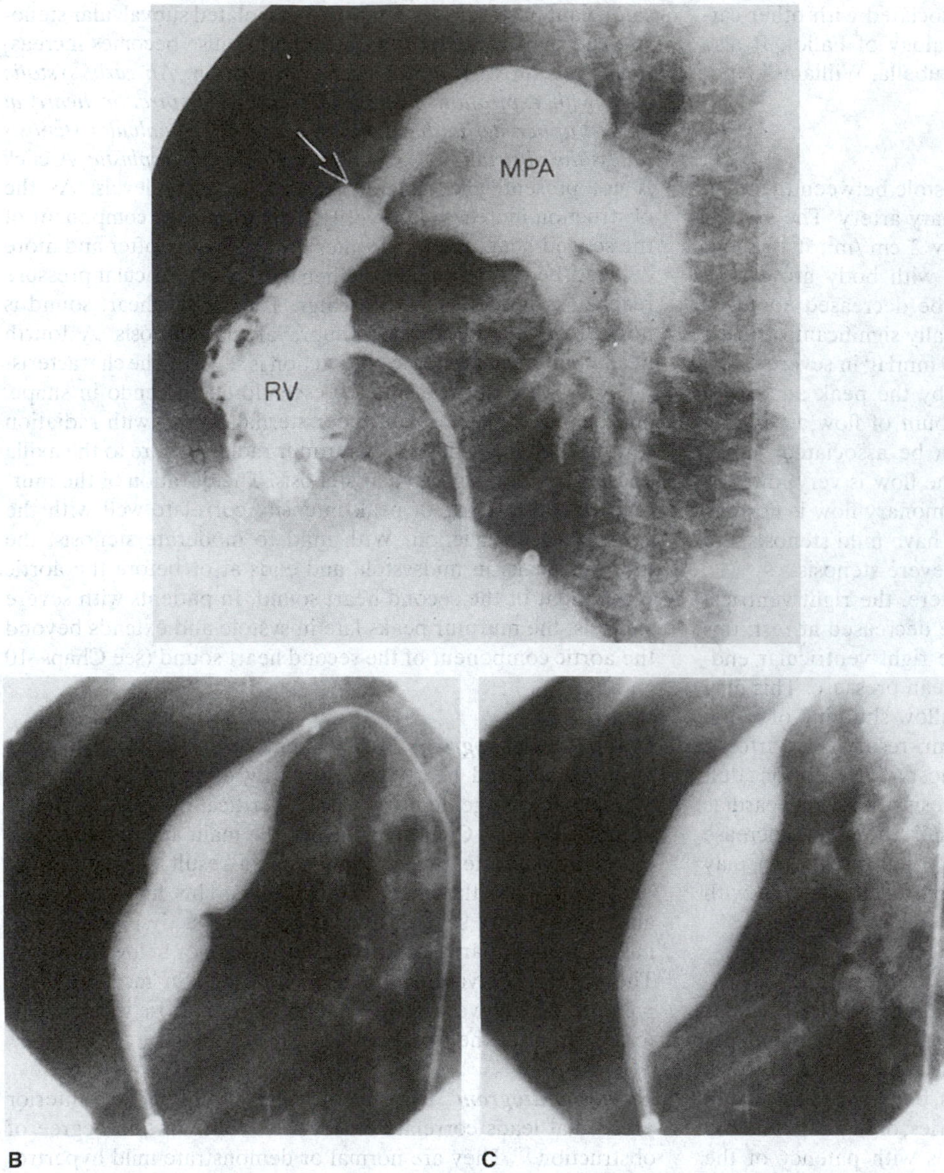

FIGURE 63-28 A. Lateral view of a right ventricular (RV) angiogram demonstrating the typical features of valvular pulmonary stenosis with doming of the pulmonary valve (*arrow*) and a narrow jet of contrast entering the dilated main pulmonary artery (MPA). *B.* An 18-mm balloon is inflated across the 14-mm annulus. A moderate waist is seen at 1 atmosphere of pressure. *C.* The waist is eliminated at 4 atmospheres of pressure. (From Lock JE, Keane JF, Perry SB. *Diagnostic and Interventional Catheterization in Congenital Heart Disease*. 2d ed. Boston: Kluwer; 2000.)

diastolic pressure and right atrial *a* wave may be elevated. Systemic oxygen saturation is diminished only in those with more severe obstruction and a patent foramen ovale or, less commonly, a true ASD. A left-to-right shunt at the atrial level is detected in some patients with mild to moderate obstruction. With valvular stenosis, right ventricular angiography demonstrates thickened and doming valve leaflets and a jet of contrast material entering the dilated pulmonary artery (Fig. 63-28*A*). Doming is not characteristic of the dysplastic valve. Infundibular subvalvular narrowing caused by muscular hypertrophy may occur secondary to the valvular stenosis or rarely as an isolated anomaly. Isolated anomalous muscle bundles in the right ventricle also may be seen. Pulmonary arterial angiography best demonstrates the sites of obstruction with supravalvular stenoses. Ventricular volume studies have demonstrated depressed ventricular function in patients with right-to-left shunts. Balloon dilation is discussed below under "Management."

NATURAL HISTORY AND PROGNOSIS

The clinical course of valvular stenosis is favorable in most patients with mild to moderate obstruction. In a national cooperative study,[153] 86 percent of patients had no significant increase in their pressure gradients over a 4- to 8-year interval. Those with a significant increase were less than 4 years of age and had at least moderate stenosis initially. Progression during the period of growth seems to be the likely explanation for most of the increases, but a few patients developed subvalvular muscular hypertrophy, which increased the obstruction. Even mild obstruction may progress significantly in some infants during the first year of life. The prognosis of those with severe obstruction without intervention is poor, especially in infants with critical obstruction. With severe obstruction, right ventricular damage and dysfunction can ensue over the years, and heart failure or arrhythmias can cause premature death in adults.[154] Tricuspid regurgitation also may result. Obstruction of the subvalvular type frequently increases with time, while supravalvular stenosis usually does not progress. Brain abscess can occur if a right-to-left shunt is present. Infective endocarditis with vegetations on the valve, pulmonary arterial wall, or infundibular region is also a risk. The children originally followed and treated as part of the national cooperative study cited above[151,153] were reevaluated 15 to 25 years later.[155] Among the 580 patients alive at the completion of the previous study, new data were available on 464 (78.4 percent). The probability of 25-year survival was 95.7 percent compared with an expected age- and sex-matched control group survival of 96.6 percent. Ninety-seven percent were asymptomatic. Although cardiac catheterization studies were not repeated, clinical examination and echocardiography at follow-up suggested no pulmonary stenosis in 2 percent, mild stenosis in 93 percent, moderate stenosis in 3 percent, and severe stenosis in only 1 percent. Pulmonary regurgitation was present in 40 percent, usually secondary to surgical valvotomy. Endocarditis was uncommon, as were ventricular arrhythmias.

MANAGEMENT

Management obviously depends on the severity of obstruction. For those with mild to moderate valvular pulmonary stenosis, periodic reexamination is indicated to detect any evidence of progression, with more frequent evaluation for those under 1 year of age. Measures to treat heart failure should be instituted in an infant with critical stenosis, but prompt intervention is mandatory. Cyanosis or a right ventricular systolic pressure well above systemic levels also is an indication for prompt intervention. Intervention is warranted in older children when the gradient exceeds 75 mmHg and is clearly not indicated when the gradient is less than 25 mmHg. *In the intermediate group, there is still some controversy, but general practice suggests valvuloplasty when the gradient exceeds 40 mmHg, although objective data to support therapy at this level are lacking.*

Balloon valvuloplasty has replaced surgical therapy as a first approach. Through the femoral vein, a balloon catheter is advanced across the valve and inflated to about 120 percent of the size of the pulmonary annulus, ripping the domed valve and thus relieving the obstruction (Fig. 63-28*B*).

The Valvuloplasty and Angioplasty of Congenital Anomalies Registry has published the combined results on 822 children.[156] Valvuloplasty resulted in improvement in most children with valvular obstruction, reducing the gradient from 71 ± 33 mmHg to 28 ± 24 mmHg. Valvuloplasty is, not surprisingly, less effective in children with a dysplastic pulmonary valve.[156,157] Complications were uncommon (5 in 822, or 0.6 percent), including two deaths. Valvuloplasty also has been performed in critical neonatal pulmonary stenosis with cyanosis caused by right-to-left shunting at the atrial level with a high success rate.[158,159] Subvalvular obstruction is less amenable to dilatation.

Peripheral pulmonary stenosis also has been occasionally amenable to dilatation, although the results are frequently less dramatic because of the multiple areas of stenosis and the fact that the complications, including pulmonary artery rupture, are more common.[160,161] Recently, stents have been used, with promising results,[161] in those with peripheral pulmonary artery stenosis in an attempt to keep open vessels that recoil back to normal size after the balloon is deflated. For those in whom there is isolated subvalvular stenosis or associated defects or in whom balloon dilatation has failed, surgical intervention is recommended.

The risk of death after pulmonary artery dilation is higher than that after dilation of the valve.[160] In the large collaborative study cited above, the death rate was 3 percent, although a more recent study from the author's institution found a mortality rate less than 1 percent among 400 cases.[162]

SURGICAL MANAGEMENT

Operation rarely is indicated for isolated pulmonary valvular stenosis; balloon valvuloplasty is virtually always successful in eliminating a clinically significant obstruction. A thickened, immobile, dysplastic pulmonary valve, however, is best treated by complete surgical excision (valvectomy). A small annulus is augmented with a pericardial or Dacron gusset.[163]

Subvalvular pulmonary stenosis is relieved through a right ventriculotomy, a main pulmonary arteriotomy, or a right atriotomy. Hypertrophic parietal and septal muscle bands constituting the fibrous orifice of the os infundibulum and obstructing moderator bands or muscle bundles within the body of the right ventricle are excised. Care is exercised to avoid injury to major coronary arterial branches. The right ventriculotomy usually can be closed by direct suturing, but a small oval patch of pericardium or Dacron can be used to prevent constriction of the outflow tract. Right ventricular function is compromised minimally by a small patch that does not extend across the annulus; larger patches to the pulmonary arterial bifurcation probably impair ventricular performance but may be necessary when there is associated annular or main pulmonary arterial hypoplasia. When possible, excision from the pulmonary artery or the right atrium is preferred to avoid ventricular injury. Excellent relief of right ventricular outflow tract obstruction can be expected after resection. Mortality and significant morbidity are rare.

Stenoses of main or extraparenchymal branch pulmonary arteries can be relieved by pericardial, synthetic, or homograft aortic or pulmonary arterial patches if the obstruction is proximal. Proximal coarctations in the larger portion of the arterial tree are more readily corrected than are those in small distal branches beyond the bifurcation of either the right or the left pulmonary artery, where results are poor.[164] In these instances, catheter balloon angioplasty, although certainly not without risk, offers nonsurgical relief of obstruction even in the small pulmonary arterial branches and should be considered the procedure of choice for distal pulmonary arterial stenoses.[160,161]

Prophylaxis against infective endocarditis is recommended for all patients whether or not surgery is performed, although the risks seem to be lower than they are with many other congenital anomalies.

Tetralogy of Fallot

PATHOLOGY

Tetralogy of Fallot is characterized by biventricular origin of the aorta above a large VSD (Fig. 63-29), obstruction to pulmonary blood flow, and right ventricular hypertrophy. Fibrous continuity of the aortic origin and the anterior mitral valve is maintained.[66]

The right ventricular infundibulum lies anterior to the position of the VSD and is bounded by the anterior and septal walls anteriorly and medially; the posterior wall is said to be a vertical crista supraventricularis or displaced conus septum.[165] The right ventricular infundibulum is a distinctive channel, but the caliber varies widely from only mild obstruction to atresia. Usually, it exhibits a significant degree of stenosis and is the dominant site of the obstruction to pulmonary flow that is characteristic of tetralogy.

The pulmonary valve is often malformed, usually being either bicuspid or unicuspid. That valve may contribute to pulmonary stenosis, but only uncommonly is it the only site of significant obstruction to pulmonary flow. Characteristically, the pulmonary trunk is thin-walled and its lumen is more narrow than normal, but usually it is wider than either the right ventricular infundibulum or the orifice of the pulmonary valve. The aorta is wider than normal, its change in caliber being roughly opposite to that of the pulmonary trunk. The foramen ovale is frequently patent in patients of all ages. In all cases of tetralogy with significant pulmonary obstruction, collateral branches to the lungs arise from the aorta.

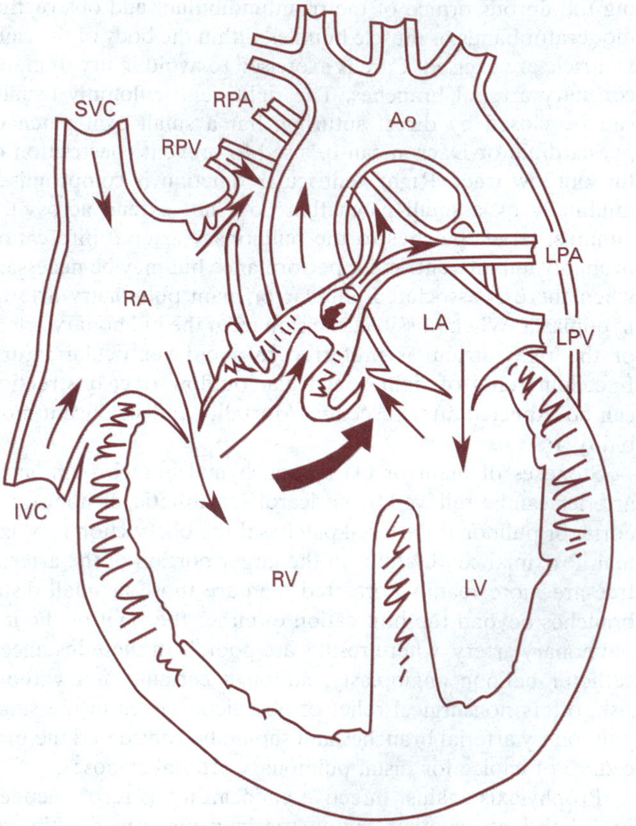

FIGURE 63-29 Classic tetralogy of Fallot. There are infundibular and pulmonary valvular stenoses. There is also right-to-left shunting at the atrial level. SVC = superior vena cava; IVC = inferior vena cava; RA = right atrium; RV = right ventricle; RPA = right pulmonary artery; LPA = left pulmonary artery; RPV = right pulmonary vein; LPV = left pulmonary vein; LA = left atrium; LV = left ventricle; Ao = aorta. (From Edwards.[66] Reproduced with permission from the publisher and author.)

There is invariably a large malalignment VSD. Anterior, middle, or apical muscular defects are also present in up to 5 percent of children seen as infants. Many close spontaneously, but if corrective surgery is to be performed successfully, they must be evaluated.

Coronary artery abnormalities are not uncommon. The anterior descending coronary artery in the interventricular septum may arise from the right instead of the left coronary artery. Although physiologically unimportant preoperatively, the course across the right ventricular outflow tract makes the usual site of right ventriculotomy and outflow patch unavailable during reparative surgery, frequently necessitating a conduit to "jump over" the vessel. The anatomy of the coronary circulation used to require angiography to establish, but more recently echocardiography with Doppler color flow has been sufficient to detail the distribution of the proximal coronary circulation in most cases.

ASSOCIATED CONDITIONS

The condition most commonly associated with tetralogy of Fallot is right aortic arch (about 30 percent).[166] A persistent left superior vena cava has been described in 10.6 percent of cases. When an associated ASD exists, this anomaly is referred to as *pentalogy of Fallot.* The ductus arteriosus may be absent, present unilaterally on either the right or the left side, or bilateral.

ABNORMAL PHYSIOLOGY

Since the VSD is usually large, with an area about as great as that of the aortic valve, both ventricles and the aorta have essentially the same systolic pressures. The most important hemodynamic factor is the ratio between the resistance to flow into the aorta and the resistance to flow across the stenotic right ventricular infundibulum. If the stenosis is not severe, the resistance to right ventricular outflow is not large, the pulmonary flow may be twice the systemic flow, and the arterial oxygen saturation may be normal (acyanotic tetralogy of Fallot). However, the resistance to the pulmonary flow may be increased markedly, causing right-to-left shunting, arterial desaturation, and subsequent polycythemia. When the pulmonary stenosis is very severe, the pulmonary blood flow may be by way of collateral vessels from the systemic arteries to the distal pulmonary arteries beyond the stenosis. The infundibular obstruction, which may be in part dynamic, is increased by drugs, heart rate maneuvers, and activities that increase myocardial contractility or decrease right ventricular volume. In addition, the infundibular hypertrophy may increase gradually over time. Since the systolic pressure in the right ventricle cannot exceed that in the left ventricle because of the large VSD, the right ventricle is "protected" from excessive pressure and work, and so congestive heart failure is uncommon.

Hypercyanotic episodes (spells) in patients with tetralogy are of uncertain origin. It is likely that some episodes are caused by unusual hyperactivity of muscular fibers in the right ventricular outflow tract that produce or exaggerate the infundibular stenosis, increasing pulmonary resistance and thus increasing the right-to-left shunting. Some spells may be caused by a decrease in peripheral resistance and systemic arterial pressure, which also may cause the right-to-left shunt to increase and pulmonary blood flow to decrease.

CLINICAL MANIFESTATIONS

Tetralogy of Fallot is the most common congenital cardiac defect that causes cyanosis. Tetralogy with an associated ASD, or pentalogy of Fallot, is not distinguishable clinically. For a discussion on the hypoxemia and the consequences in tetralogy, see the section on cyanosis and its complications earlier in this chapter.

History Most of these patients now are diagnosed prenatally by ultrasound or present in the first days or weeks of life with a heart murmur. If the right ventricular obstruction is severe, cyanosis is present at birth and is exacerbated when the ductus closes. If the obstruction is milder, the infant may be acyanotic with left-to-right flow through the VSD and occasionally may develop congestive heart failure. In this group, gradually increasing right ventricular obstruction may reduce the left-to-right shunt, and eventually, when infundibular resistance and pulmonary resistance exceed systemic resistance, right-to-left shunting develops, resulting in cyanosis.

Dyspnea with exertion occurs commonly in toddlers and older children with unrepaired defects. Attacks of suddenly increasing cyanosis associated with hyperpnea, or hypoxic spells,[167] are common between ages 2 months and 2 years. There are many precipitating events, including infection, exertion, and summer heat. They occur most often in the morning, with increasing irritability. The frequency and duration vary widely, but prolonged episodes can lead to syncope, seizures, and death. Squatting with exercise is common from 1.5 to 10 years of age in those not previously repaired. These problems are becoming uncommon as more and more children undergo early repair.

Physical Examination Growth is usually normal unless cyanosis is extreme. Clubbing of the fingers and toes occurs after 3 months of age and is proportional to the level of cyanosis. Signs of congestive heart failure do not appear in tetralogy of Fallot during childhood unless there is a superimposed illness such as anemia or infective endocarditis.

Increased right ventricular activity is observed. A systolic thrill may be palpable at the left midsternal border, with a harsh midsystolic murmur in that location. Softer murmurs signal more severe obstruction and are common when presentation is in the newborn period or during hypoxic spells. The murmur ends before the second heart sound, which is characteristically single. A continuous murmur is heard if a PDA or large collateral vessels are present. An early systolic ejection sound at the left sternal border and apex is uncommon; its presence suggests primarily valvular pulmonary stenosis.

Chest Roentgenogram The total heart size is usually normal on chest roentgenography, but right ventricular enlargement is present in the lateral view. The aorta arches to the right in many cases. Pulmonary flow is diminished. The pulmonary segment is concave and the apex is elevated, giving the *coeur en sabot* (boot-shaped) contour. A very young infant may have only diminished pulmonary flow.

Electrocardiogram In tetralogy of Fallot, the mean QRS axis of the ECG is usually to the right, between +90° and +210°. There is right ventricular hypertrophy, with a tall R wave in the right precordial leads and a deep S wave in the left leads. Some of these patients have right atrial hypertrophy.

Echocardiogram Two-dimensional echocardiography can delineate the anatomic components of tetralogy.[168] Anomalies of the coronary arteries can be demonstrated, and associated defects can be excluded.

Hematologic and Other Laboratory Studies Before surgical repair, the hemoglobin and hematocrit should be measured and pulse oximetry should be performed in all patients at initial evaluation and periodically thereafter for determination of the degree of polycythemia and the early detection of anemia relative to the degree of cyanosis. The latter is common, especially in those under 2 years of age, and may predispose a patient to cerebrovascular accidents. Platelet counts and clotting studies may be advisable in older unrepaired patients with marked polycythemia, particularly if a surgical procedure is planned. Serum uric acid levels should be measured if polycythemia is severe and long-standing.

Cardiac Catheterization In an increasing number of centers, the quality of echocardiography (especially when done in neonates or infants) is sufficiently diagnostic to outline the right ventricular and proximal pulmonary artery anatomy, rule out additional muscular VSDs, and establish the proximal coronary circulation. As a consequence, diagnostic cardiac catheterization and angiography are less commonly performed preoperatively than they were in the past in children with tetralogy of Fallot.

In those in whom the study is performed, the right ventricular systolic pressure is equal to the pressure in the left ventricle and aorta. If the pulmonary artery can be entered, the pressure will be normal or low. The level or levels of obstruction can be evaluated by careful pullback to the right ventricle. Caution should be observed if the pulmonary artery is entered, as the catheter may critically reduce the pulmonary flow and cause a hypoxic episode. Systemic arterial oxygen saturation is reduced because of right-to-left shunting from the right ventricle to the left ventricle. If a patent foramen ovale or ASD is present, there may be an additional right-to-left or bidirectional shunt at the atrial level. Selective biplane right ventricular angiography will demonstrate levels of obstruction, continuity and size of the pulmonary arteries, and size and position of the ventricular defect. If this is not demonstrated by echocardiography or aortography, selective coronary arteriography should be performed on all patients preoperatively to demonstrate the coronary arterial pattern.[169]

MEDICAL MANAGEMENT

Although the definitive treatment of tetralogy of Fallot is surgical, medical management plays a role before surgery and in the postoperative period. For a severely cyanotic newborn, prostaglandin administration is of benefit[91] to keep the ductus open until surgery can be done. Before surgery, the hematocrit and hemoglobin should be monitored and iron-deficiency anemia should be treated promptly to prevent strokes. Fever or other illness that would lead to dehydration and possible thrombotic complications should be treated promptly.

Hypoxic spells in an infant should be treated initially by placing the infant in the knee-chest position and administering a high concentration of oxygen and morphine sulfate. If acidosis is present and does not correct spontaneously and promptly, intravenous sodium bicarbonate and an alpha-adrenergic agonist should be given. Propranalol may be useful in preventing hypoxic spells.[170]

Bacterial endocarditis is a serious complication, especially in those who have had a systemic-to-pulmonary artery shunt. Meticulous care should be taken to maintain good dental hygiene, and prophylactic antibiotics at times of predictable risk are mandatory (see Chap. 73).

SURGICAL MANAGEMENT

Historically, the approach to tetralogy of Fallot has been either palliation or corrective surgery. The introduction of an aorta-to-pulmonary-artery shunt for the treatment of tetralogy of Fallot[171] truly can be called the beginning of effective treatment for pediatric cardiovascular disease. When open heart surgery was initiated in the 1950s, tetralogy of Fallot was among the first lesions to be corrected.[172] Over the years, the age at which corrective surgery can be performed has dropped so that in many centers primary repair is the procedure of choice at any age. Palliation, when it is now performed, almost inevitably involves a modified Blalock-Taussig shunt that interposes a graft between the subclavian artery and the ipsolateral pulmonary artery, usually on the side opposite the aortic arch.[173] Even in the perinatal period, the placement of a 4-mm tube will result in satisfactory palliation for a year in more than 90 percent of infants.

Surgical correction for those with pulmonary stenosis involves closing the VSD, usually through a right ventriculotomy, resecting infundibular muscle, and, if the infundibulum, pulmonary valve, and main pulmonary artery are hypoplastic, using a pericardial patch to open the narrowed area. Care must be taken to avoid heart block while closing the VSD and avoid cutting a major branch of the coronary artery. If a patent foramen ovale is present, it usually is left open to allow decompression in the perioperative period. If a true ASD is present (pentology of Fallot), it should be closed to avoid left-to-right shunting once the right ventricle has recovered from the perioperative insult.[174]

Children with tetralogy of Fallot and pulmonary atresia with good-sized pulmonary arteries usually are repaired by closing the VSD and interposing a conduit, frequently an aortic homograft, between the right ventricle and the pulmonary artery.[175] If this is done in children under 7 or 8 years of age, replacement of the conduit is to be expected secondary to somatic growth. Children with tetralogy of Fallot and hypoplastic and/or discontinuous pulmonary arteries require an individualized approach that frequently involves balloon dilation of hypoplastic vessels, unifocalization of discontinuous vessels, and, it is hoped, eventual repair with a conduit closing the VSD.[176] Operative and early mortality rates for repair of tetralogy of Fallot are now quite low in most centers. Kirklin and coworkers[173] in the early 1980s reported mortality rates of 1.6 percent with operations at 5 years of age to 4.1 percent at 1 year of age. At Children's Hospital in Boston, there was a 4.2 percent mortality rate among 330 children under 1 year of age operated on between 1973 and 1990, with a mortality rate of only 2.5 percent in the past 6 years of the study (1984–1990).[174] Late complications have included residual peripheral pulmonary stenosis, a small incidence of residual VSDs, and, rarely, aortic regurgitation. The long-term survivors have had atrial or, more commonly, ventricular arrhythmias and continue to be at risk for infective endocarditis.

Physicians at the Mayo Clinic, the first center to use the pump oxygenator to repair tetralogy of Fallot in the 1950s, have reported a minimum 30-year follow-up of the 162 30-day survivors of surgery.[177] The 32-year actuarial survival rate was 86 percent, with subgroup survival rates of those less then 5 years old, 5 to 7 years old, and 8 to 11 years old at the time of surgical repair being 90, 93, and 91 percent, respectively. Late sudden death from cardiac causes occurred in 10 patients during the 32-year period. The performance of some previous palliative operation (Waterston or Pott's shunts) but not a palliative Blalock-Taussig shunt was associated with higher mortality. With earlier surgery and less utilization of palliative procedures, it is hoped that the surgical results will be even better for children born in the 1980s and 1990s and beyond.

Ebstein's Anomaly

PATHOLOGY

In Ebstein's anomaly, the anterior leaflet of the tricuspid valve is attached normally to the annulus, but varying portions of the posterior and septal leaflets are displaced downward, being attached to the ventricular wall below the annulus. The proximal part of the right ventricle is thin-walled and continuous with the right atrium. The functional right ventricle is small and is made up of the apical and infundibular portions of the right ventricle. An additional common finding is that the papillary muscles and chordae are highly malformed, with great variation in the manner of attachment of the two involved leaflets to the right ventricular wall. Commonly, multiple direct attachments of valvular tissue to the right ventricular mural endocardium occur.[178,179]

An interatrial communication is present in most cases, usually taking the form of a patent foramen ovale. Continuity of right atrial and right ventricular myocardial tissues, in addition to the usual connections by way of the main conduction pathways, has been observed. *The presence of Ebstein's anomaly has been associated with maternal lithium use during pregnancy, although the risk ratio remains unclear.*[180]

ABNORMAL PHYSIOLOGY

Ebstein's anomaly results in obstruction to right ventricular filling because of a decrease in the size of the right ventricle, part of which is incorporated into the huge right atrium. The deformed tricuspid valve also frequently is associated with tricuspid regurgitation with a right-to-left shunt through the foramen ovale. In the perinatal period, when the pulmonary vascular resistance is high, the tricuspid regurgitation may be severe. This results in increased right atrial pressure and, when the patent foramen ovale is open, severe cyanosis. As the pulmonary vascular resistance falls, the right-to-left shunting is decreased and hypoxemia improves. In older children, right-sided congestive heart failure with edema and/or ascites may develop.

CLINICAL MANIFESTATIONS

History Approximately one-half of reported patients develop symptoms of cyanosis and right-sided heart failure in early infancy. The remainder present with a murmur or abnormal chest roentgenogram, but with no symptoms, in early childhood or because of gradual progression of symptoms through late childhood or adult life.[181] The most common symptom is dyspnea on exertion. The spectrum of exercise intolerance has been described.[182] Palpitations resulting from supraventricular tachyarrhythmias occur in 20 to 30 percent of these children. Occasionally, syncope occurs as a result of arrhythmia or low cardiac output if the atrial septum is intact.

Physical Examination A newborn with elevated pulmonary vascular resistance has severe cyanosis. In older infants and children, cyanosis and clubbing are mild. Only a small percentage do not have an ASD or patent foramen ovale and thus are not cyanotic. The precordium is generally quiet even in those with striking cardiomegaly. The liver is enlarged, and the jugular venous pulse may be elevated. The holosystolic murmur of tricuspid regurgitation is heard at the lower left sternal border and may be accompanied by a "scratchy" diastolic murmur of tricuspid stenosis. The first heart sound is split and loud, and the second heart sound is widely and persistently split. Loud third and fourth heart sounds are usual, especially in older patients.

Chest Roentgenogram Heart size, as shown by chest roentgenography, varies, but the heart is ordinarily very large because of the very dilated right atrium. In those with cyanosis, pulmonary blood flow is diminished correspondingly.

Electrocardiogram Giant, peaked P waves are common, along with a prolonged PQ interval and right ventricular conduction delay or complete right bundle branch block. In approximately 10 percent of these patients, the pattern of Wolff-Parkinson-White syndrome (with a short PQ interval and slurring of the initial QRS forces or a delta wave) is seen.[181]

Echocardiogram Two-dimensional echocardiography is very helpful in the diagnosis (Fig. 63-30), identifying the lesion, depicting the degree of displacement of the tricuspid valve into the right ventricle, and assessing the severity of the tricuspid regurgitation. In neonates, evaluation of the pulmonary valve usually allows a distinction between anatomic pulmonary atresia from absence of opening of the valve caused by severe tricuspid regurgitation and high pulmonary vascular resistance.[183]

Cardiac Catheterization There is a higher than usual risk associated with cardiac catheterization because of the frequency of rhythm disturbances. Proper precautions and prompt use of cardioversion when necessary minimize this risk. In most cases, echocardiography and color Doppler evaluation are sufficient, and catheterization is performed less commonly than it was previously.

There is usually right-to-left shunting at the atrial level. Right atrial hypertension is present. The characteristic right ventricular pressure recording is not obtained until the catheter is advanced to the apex or outflow tract. An intracardiac ECG demonstrates, on pullback from the right ventricle, an area where the ECG is ventricular but the pressure is atrial in contour.[184] This method is not infallible, but it provides good evidence of tricuspid displacement with an "atrialized" portion of the right ventricle.

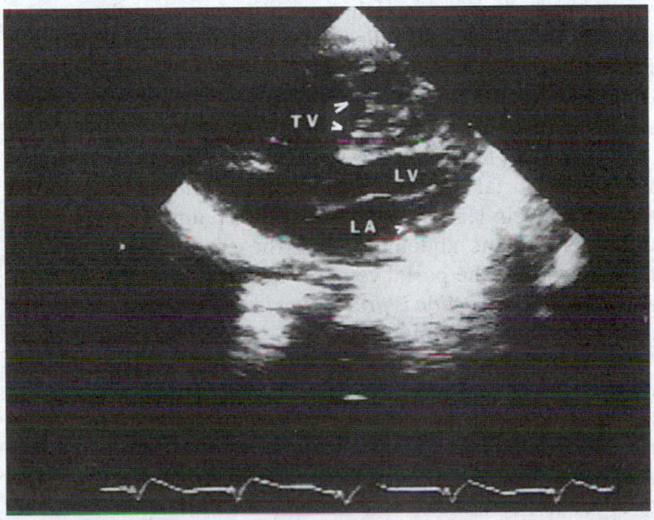

FIGURE 63-30 Two-dimensional echocardiogram in parasternal view in a patient with Ebstein's anomaly of the tricuspid valve (TV). Numerous attachments of the tricuspid valve (*arrowheads*) to the interventricular septum and right ventricular apex are seen. LV = left ventricle; LA = left atrium.

NATURAL HISTORY AND PROGNOSIS

The natural history varies greatly with the severity of the abnormality. In a study of 50 patients who presented in the neonatal period, 9 (18 percent) died in the perinatal period, with late deaths in another 15 (9 from hemodynamic deterioration, 5 sudden, and 1 noncardiac), for a 10-year actuarial survival of 61 percent.[185] In a study that included more children who presented after the perinatal period, the probability of survival was 50 percent at 47 years of age.[186] Predictors of poor outcome were New York Heart Association class III or IV, cardiothoracic ratio >65 percent, and atrial fibrillation.

For women who survive into adulthood without significant arrhythmias or cyanosis, successful pregnancy with good fetal outcome is possible.[187]

MEDICAL MANAGEMENT

Medical therapy varies depending on the severity of disease and the age at presentation. For those presenting with cyanosis in the perinatal period, procrastination until the pulmonary vascular resistance has decreased may be the best strategy. For those who are severely hypoxemic, maintaining the patency of the ductus with PGE_1 may be lifesaving. Reducing the pulmonary vascular resistance with nitric oxide may reduce right-to-left shunting and improve oxygenation.[188] Persistence of severe cyanosis beyond 1 week of age suggests pulmonary stenosis or pulmonary atresia in addition to Ebstein's deformity of the tricuspid valve.

For children with arrhythmias, an electrophysiologic study may be indicated. For those with disabling or life-threatening arrhythmias, radiofrequency ablation may be performed with initial success rates of about 80 percent but recurrences in 30 percent of patients.[189]

In older children who develop right-sided congestive heart failure, anticongestive measures with digoxin and diuretics may be tried, although this level of deterioration is usually an indication for surgical intervention.

SURGICAL MANAGEMENT

The surgical management of Ebstein's disease remains problematic. In the perinatal period, when the pulmonary vascular resistance is high, watchful waiting is probably the best approach. If the child remains severely hypoxemic (saturations <75 percent) after the pulmonary vascular resistance falls, palliation with a Blalock-Taussig shunt to improve pulmonary blood flow may be sufficient to relieve hypoxemia, and this should allow growth to an age at which other procedures can be considered.[190] For children in whom hypoxemia remains a significant problem, three approaches have been used. The first is a Glenn anastomosis connecting the superior vena cava to the right pulmonary artery, allowing inferior vena cava blood to go through the right atrium and ventricle to the pulmonary artery.[191] A more definitive procedure that eliminates hypoxemia that is used primarily for children with single ventricle but now is applied in this situation as well is the modified Fontan. In this approach, the tricuspid valve is oversewn and the patent foramen ovale is closed, diverting all systemic venous return to the pulmonary arteries by passing the right heart.[192] In a small group of patients, this has been done with success.

The more common approach has been tricuspid valve reconstruction or replacement, usually with a bioprosthesis. Among 189 patients operated on at the Mayo Clinic over a period of

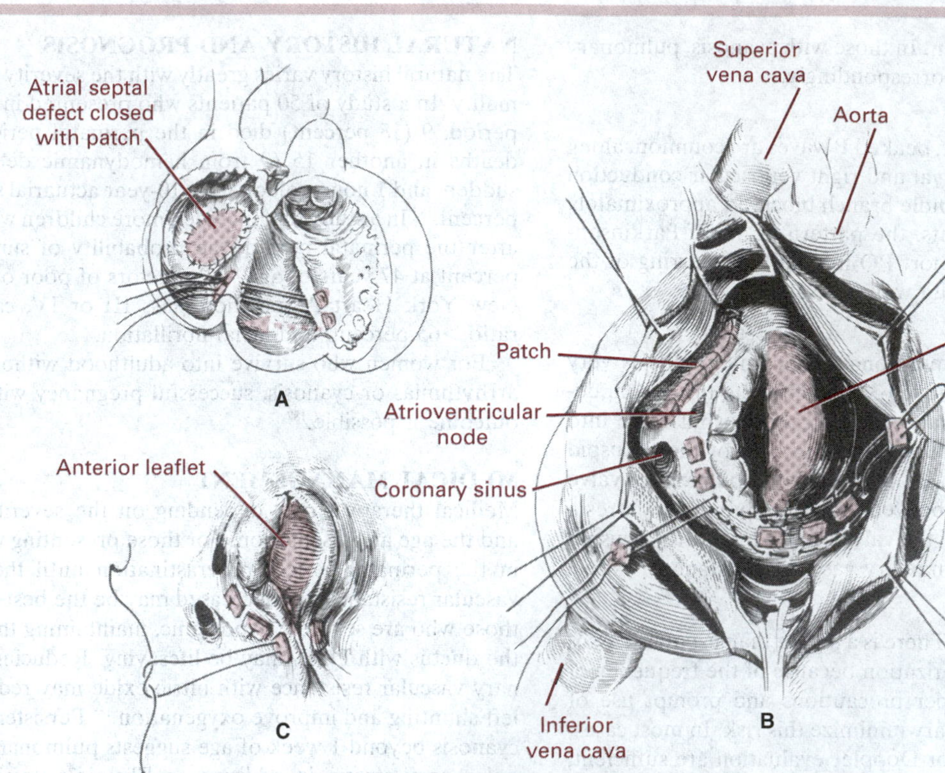

FIGURE 63-31 Danielson repair of Ebstein's malformation. *A.* Anterior cutaway drawing. The atrial septal defect is closed securely with a patch. Pledgeted sutures are placed to position the posterior leaflet at the annulus and imbricate the "atrialized" right ventricular chamber. *B* and *C.* Drawing of the right atrium showing the annuloplasty suture passed through two pledgets. Tying of this suture reduces dilation of the tricuspid valve so that the large anterior leaflet can meet the two smaller cusps and constitute a functional, essentially monocusp valve.

almost 20 years, there were 12 hospital deaths (6.3 percent) and an additional 10 late deaths. Among those followed more than 1 year after operation, more than 90 percent were in New York Heart Association class I or II.[193] More recently, other approaches have been suggested, including reconstruction of the normally shaped right ventricle with repositioning of the displaced leaflet of the tricuspid valve at the normal level[194] and reimplantation of the tricuspid valve leaflets with a vertical plication of the atrialized portion of the right ventricle to reduce its size (Fig. 63-31).[195] *Although the newer approaches seem promising in small numbers of patients in the short run, many patients with the milder form of the disease can live well into adulthood,*[196] *and so indications for the newer operations in patients who are asymptomatic or only mildly limited remain problematic.*

ABNORMALITIES OF THE PULMONARY VENOUS CONNECTIONS

Total Anomalous Pulmonary Venous Connection

PATHOLOGY

When all pulmonary veins terminate in a systemic vein or the right atrium, the term *total anomalous pulmonary venous connection* or *return* is applied (Fig. 63-32). Usually the pulmonary veins leave the lung and then join a chamber-like confluence posterior to the left atrium. From the confluence of veins, one primitive embryologic vessel persists and leads to the anomalous termination. Less commonly, two or more vessels lead to multiple sites of termination.

If the left cardinal vein persists, drainage flows superiorly into the innominate vein and then to the superior vena cava and right atrium or inferiorly into a persistent left superior vena cava and coronary sinus to the right atrium. If the right cardinal vein persists, drainage is to the superior vena cava, the azygous vein, or the right atrium directly. These types are sometimes referred to collectively as supracardiac or supradiaphragmatic drainage and almost never are associated with pulmonary venous obstruction.[197]

If the site of termination is infradiaphragmatic, with connection to the portal venous system or the inferior vena cava, the anomalous vein leaves the confluence of pulmonary veins and descends into the abdomen along the esophagus to join the ductus venosus, the portal vein, or the left gastric vein. *Pulmonary venous obstruction is present in virtually all cases of infradiaphragmatic connection.*[197]

In all cases of total anomalous pulmonary venous connection, there is a patent foramen ovale. The atrium and ventricle of the left side are small in comparison with the right-sided chambers but are within normal limits in regard to absolute size. In the absence of asplenia or polysplenia syndromes, associated anomalies are not common.

ABNORMAL PHYSIOLOGY

In this anomaly, all the blood from both the pulmonary and systemic circulations eventually returns to the right atrium. In neonates with the connection below the diaphragm, the increase

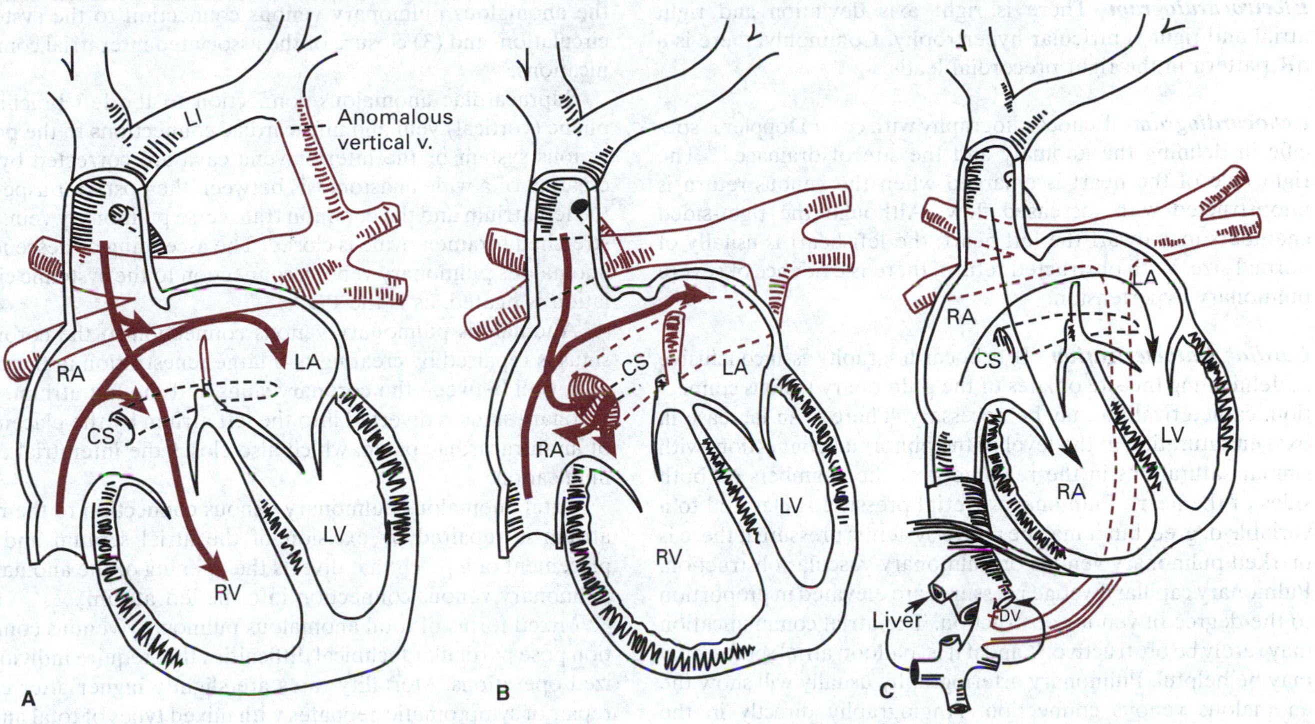

FIGURE 63-32 Three common types of total anomalous pulmonary venous connection. *A.* Total anomalous pulmonary venous connection to the left brachiocephalic (innominate) vein (LI). *B.* Total anomalous pulmonary venous connection to the coronary sinus (CS). *C.* Total anomalous pulmonary venous connection of the infradiaphragmatic type to the ductus venosus (DV). RA = right atrium; RV = right ventricle; LA = left atrium; LV = left ventricle.

in pulmonary flow as the pulmonary resistance decreases after birth cannot be accommodated and the obstruction to flow causes a marked increase in pulmonary venous pressure, resulting in a very high pulmonary vascular resistance. If the ductus arteriosus is still open, the pulmonary vascular resistance exceeds systemic vascular resistance with a right-to-left shunt at the ductal level. When the ductus closes, the increased pulmonary resistance results in increased right ventricular pressure. If the right ventricle fails, the right atrial pressure will increase, and right-to-left shunting at the atrial level may be present, often with profound hypoxemia.

In older children with unobstructed damage above the diaphragm (supracardiac), the pulmonary resistance is usually low. This low resistance facilitates a high pulmonary flow. With mixing of all pulmonary and systemic flow in the right atrium, the oxygen saturation is usually relatively high, resulting in physiology similar to that of an ASD and mild cyanosis.[198]

CLINICAL MANIFESTATIONS

Total Anomalous Pulmonary Venous Connection with Pulmonary Venous Obstruction Neonates with total anomalous pulmonary venous connection below the diaphragm who have pulmonary venous obstruction present with cyanosis, which may be severe, and dyspnea. Symptoms frequently develop beyond 12 h of age, allowing differentiation from respiratory distress syndrome. In addition to dyspnea, feeding difficulties and cardiac failure are seen.

The physical findings are usually unimpressive. The heart is not hyperactive, and thrills are absent. The second heart sound may be split, with an increased pulmonary component. Significant murmurs are uncommon.

Total Anomalous Pulmonary Venous Connection without Pulmonary Venous Obstruction These patients are usually asymptomatic at birth, although some may develop transient tachypnea. Presentation typically occurs during the first year of life. Some of these children have tachypnea and feeding difficulties, with frequent respiratory infections. Cyanosis often is mild and may not be clinically apparent. Other children may be asymptomatic and present with a heart murmur.

The cardiac examination is similar to that of an ASD with increased right-sided flow. The right ventricular impulse is usually hyperactive. The jugular venous pulse is elevated, and hepatomegaly appears early. There is a diffuse and hyperdynamic right ventricular impulse. The second heart sound is split and relatively fixed; the loudness of the pulmonary component may be increased. There is usually a grade 2 or 3 midsystolic flow murmur at the left sternal border. At the lower sternal border, there are a middiastolic rumble and prominent third and fourth heart sounds. Rales may be heard over the lung fields, and periorbital edema is common. A continuous murmur rarely may be heard over the common venous channel.

Chest Roentgenogram With the unobstructed types, the heart is enlarged with increased pulmonary flow. Pulmonary edema is uncommon. In patients with return to the left innominate vein, there may be a characteristic bulging of the superior mediastinum bilaterally, producing a "snowman," or figure-of-eight, contour. With obstructed types, the heart size is nearly normal; there is very marked pulmonary edema, which may give a granular appearance to the lungs, making differentiation from respiratory distress syndrome difficult in a newborn.

Electrocardiogram There is right axis deviation and right atrial and right ventricular hypertrophy. Commonly, there is a qR pattern in the right precordial leads.

Echocardiogram Echocardiography with color Doppler is specific in defining the anomaly and the site of drainage.[199] The right side of the heart is enlarged when the venous return is unobstructed with increased flow. Although the right-sided chambers may dwarf the left heart, the left heart is usually of normal size. With obstructed return, there is evidence of severe pulmonary hypertension.

Cardiac Catheterization If echocardiography is inconclusive in delineating the site or sites of the pulmonary venous connection, catheterization may be necessary. There is an increase in oxygen saturation at the level of the abnormal connection, with similar saturations in the remainder of the chambers on both sides of the heart. Pulmonary arterial pressure is elevated to a variable degree, but it may be above systemic pressure if there is marked pulmonary venous or pulmonary vascular obstruction. Pulmonary capillary wedge pressures are elevated in proportion to the degree of venous obstruction. The atrial communication may rarely be obstructive,[198] and if it is, balloon atrial septostomy may be helpful. Pulmonary arteriography usually will show the anomalous venous connection. Angiography directly in the common venous channel, if it is entered, will outline its course and any sites of obstruction optimally.

NATURAL HISTORY AND PROGNOSIS

The natural history varies depending on the degree of obstruction of egress of blood from the pulmonary veins.[198] Those who present in the perinatal period with severe cyanosis and respiratory distress, usually with pulmonary venous drainage below the diaphragm, represent a medical emergency and will die without early surgery.

Those with supracardiac drainage and some degree of obstruction and therefore pulmonary hypertension are frequently sufficiently tachypneic that feeding is problematic, and they fail to gain weight at a normal rate. They tolerate respiratory infections poorly and occasionally need emergency surgery for respiratory failure.

Those with no pulmonary venous obstruction have large left-to-right shunts and mild cyanosis but may have no or minimal symptoms at rest or exercise. If corrective surgery is not performed, they are at risk for pulmonary vascular disease.[200]

MEDICAL MANAGEMENT

For neonates with severe cyanosis and respiratory disease, oxygen, a respirator, and PGE_1 can be used to temporize but survival is dependent on early surgery. For those with mild pulmonary hypertension and failure to thrive, surgery usually is performed semielectively. For those with no pulmonary hypertension, who usually present with murmurs and findings similar to those of an atrial septal defect, surgery is more elective but little is gained by waiting, and more centers are advocating early repair in this group as well.[201]

SURGICAL MANAGEMENT

Correction of total anomalous pulmonary venous connection requires (1) creation of a large communication between the left atrium and the pulmonary venous system, (2) obliteration of the anomalous pulmonary venous connection to the systemic circulation, and (3) closure of the associated interatrial communications.[201]

Supracardiac anomalous connection to the left brachiocephalic (vertical) vein and infracardiac connections to the portal venous system or the inferior vena cava are corrected by the creation of a wide anastomosis between the posterior aspect of the left atrium and the common transverse pulmonary vein. The stretched foramen ovale is closed. The ascending or descending anomalous pulmonary venous connection to the systemic circulation is ligated, as is the PDA.

Anomalous pulmonary venous connection to the coronary sinus is repaired by creating of a large fenestration in the common wall between the coronary sinus and the left atrium. The coronary sinus is diverted into the left atrium by the placement of an intracardiac patch, which also closes the interatrial communication.

Total anomalous pulmonary venous connection to the right atrium is repaired by excision of the atrial septum and the placement of a patch that diverts the opening of the anomalous pulmonary venous connection into the left atrium.

Mixed forms of total anomalous pulmonary venous connection pose particular technical difficulties that require individualized operations. Mortality rates are slightly higher after early repair of symptomatic neonates with mixed types of total anomalous pulmonary venous connections.

Although the results of repair of total anomalous pulmonary venous connection without obstruction in an older child have always been quite good, until recently neonates with obstructed total venous return have been problematic. In the 1960s and early 1970s, the surgical mortality rate exceeded 50 percent.[202] Between 1970 and 1980, surgical techniques improved and the mortality rate was reduced to 10 to 20 percent.[203] More recently, surgical results have continued to improve, with no mortality among 27 infants who underwent reparative surgery at Children's Hospital in Boston in the late 1980s.[204] Late survival has been quite good, with 98 percent surviving a median of 87 months in one study.[205]

After a satisfactory operative course, the prognosis has been excellent in those in whom a large common pulmonary vein can be attached to the back wall of the left atrium with a relatively large anastomosis. For those initially with obstructed total anomalous pulmonary venous return, the left atrium may be small and the anastomosis may be more difficult. Late obstruction of one or more pulmonary veins has been seen. When present, the obstruction can be approached by balloon dilation, stent placement, or repeat surgery.[206]

MALPOSITION OF THE CARDIAC STRUCTURES

Definition and Terminology

The *segmental approach* to the diagnosis of complex congenital heart disease[207] provides an orderly, effective method for determining the anatomic and hemodynamic interrelationships of the cardiac chambers, valves, and great vessels. For this approach to be better understood, certain definitions are helpful. Positioning of viscera is described as situs solitus, inversus, or ambiguous. In *situs solitus* (S), the distribution of all the organs is recognized as normal, for example, a left-sided stomach and spleen, a predominantly right-sided liver, a trilobed right lung, and a bilobed left lung. In *situs inversus* (*totalis*) (I), the organs show a perfect mirror image in regard to left and right to that of situs solitus. Anteroposterior relations are not disturbed. When neither situs solitus nor situs inversus can be identified, *situs ambiguous* (A) is said to be present. This usually applies in cases of asplenia or polysplenia.

With the rarest of exceptions, the *atria follow the body situs* and are so designated (morphologic right atrium to the right of the left atrium in atrial situs solitus and to the left of the left atrium in atrial situs inversus). The AV canal consists of the tricuspid valve, the mitral valve, and the septum of the AV canal and connects the atrial portion with the ventricular portion of the heart. As a rule, *each AV valve is part of the specific ventricle into which it leads.* The valve situs may be solitus, inversus, or ambiguous.

The alignment or type of AV or ventriculoarterial (VA) connection addresses the issue of what flows into what. The connection may be described at the AV or VA level as concordant (e.g., right atrium to right ventricle, left ventricle to aorta) or discordant (e.g., right atrium to left ventricle, left ventricle to pulmonary artery) or may be considered an arrangement that requires a special description. In the case of AV alignment in which the atria are not lateralized, the alignment would be ambiguous. In the univentricular heart, the designation would be double-inlet, absent right, or absent left AV connection. Special descriptions in the case of VA alignment or type of VA connection include double-outlet and single-outlet VA connection. The mode of connections, either AV or VA, addresses the structural makeup of the connecting segments: the AV canal and the infundibulum or conus. The mode of AV connection may be normal, common, stenotic, imperforate, atretic, double-orifice, overriding, straddling, or unguarded. The mode of VA connection may be expressed in terms of the position and development of the conus or infundibulum, which, although normally incorporated into the right ventricle, is not an intrinsic part of the true right ventricle. It may be described as subpulmonary, subaortic, very deficient, or bilaterally present or absent.[208]

The position of the ventricles may be described by the terms *d loop* and *l loop*. When the morphologic right ventricle lies to the right of the morphologic left ventricle, the ventricular portion of the heart is said to exhibit a d loop (D). The ventricles are said to be noninverted or in the solitus position. When the ventricular relations are reversed, l loop (L) is said to be present. The ventricles are inverted or in the inversus position. *These relationships are independent of the visceral or atrial situs as well as the position of the heart or its chambers within the chest.*

The great arteries may deviate from the usual with respect to both their anteroposterior and lateral (left-to-right) relationships. In solitus (S) or *normally related great arteries* (NRGA), the aortic origin lies to the right of and posterior to the position of the pulmonary valve. In the inversus (I) relationship, the anteroposterior relationships are not disturbed but the aortic origin lies to the left of the pulmonary arterial origin. In *transposition of the great arteries* (TGA), the aorta arises from the anatomic right ventricle, the pulmonary artery arises from the anatomic left ventricle, and usually the aortic origin is more anterior than that of the pulmonary artery.

When the aortic origin lies to the right of the pulmonary origin, the transposition is called *dextro* or *d transposition* (D-TGA) (see the discussion of complete transposition of the great arteries, below). When the aortic origin lies to the left of the pulmonary origin, *levo transposition* (L-TGA) is said to be present (see the section on congenitally corrected transposition, below).

When the abnormal relationship of the great arteries is neither complete nor corrected transposition, the term *malposition of the great arteries* (MGA) may be used. Malpositions are designated as D-MGA or L-MGA, depending on the laterality in the relation between the origins of the two great arteries.[208] Within this group are found examples of the abnormal VA alignment, where one great artery arises from the appropriate ventricle and the other great artery also arises from the same (or inappropriate) ventricle. These are examples of *double-outlet right ventricle* (DORV) or *double-outlet left ventricle* (DOLV). Also included is the arterial malposition termed *anatomically corrected malposition* (ACM). This is characterized by the great arteries having a normal VA alignment (concordant), but with the aorta anterior to the pulmonary artery by virtue of an abnormal mode of VA connection: the presence of a well-developed conus lying beneath both the aorta and the pulmonary artery or only beneath the aorta. The route for the flow of blood in ACMs may be normal or abnormal, depending on the AV alignment.[208]

The Segmental Approach to Diagnosis

The segmental, or step-by-step, approach is a valuable tool for arriving at the correct diagnosis in patients with complex congenital heart disease and is independent of cardiac position. In order, one determines (1) the locations of the right and left atria and their venous connections, (2) the location of the right and left ventricles and their alignment with the atria, (3) the mode of connection of the AV valves to the ventricles, (4) the position of the great arteries and their alignment with the ventricles, and (5) the location and status of the infundibulum. In addition, one must search for associated malformations between and within each of these segments.

Determining atrial situs can be accomplished in most instances by taking advantage of the high degree of abdominal visceroatrial concordance. With abdominal situs solitus (S), the liver is on the right and the right atrium almost invariably is on the right as well; with abdominal situs inversus (I), the liver is on the left and the right atrium almost invariably is on the left. With abdominal situs ambiguous (A), the liver may be placed almost symmetrically across the midline and the atria may be located normally or inverted or both atria may have morphologic characteristics of either the right atrium or the left atrium (Fig. 12-4). A symmetric liver is found in approximately 60 percent of patients with situs ambiguous. Lateralization of the liver, which is evident in the remainder, may simulate either situs solitus or situs inversus.

When both atria have characteristics of a right atrium,[209] *dextroisomerism*, or "bilateral right-sidedness," is said to be present. This situation is usually, though not invariably, accompanied by asplenia. When both atria have characteristics of a left atrium, *levoisomerism*, or "bilateral left-sidedness," is said to exist. This usually, but again not invariably, is accompanied by polysplenia.

Bronchial situs, as determined by overpenetrated chest roentgenogram or bronchial tomography, is an excellent predictor of atrial situs, but the most accurate technique appears to be two-dimensional echocardiography with Doppler color flow mapping. The hepatic portion of the inferior vena cava, which almost always enters the morphologic right atrium, usually can be identified easily, as can the connections and structural details of the superior vena cava, coronary sinus, pulmonary veins, atrial septum, and atrial appendages.

Additional clinical clues to atrial situs may be obtained from the ECG, where a superior and leftward orientation of the P-wave vector suggests levoisomerism and polysplenia. Howell-Heinz and Howell-Jolly bodies in the peripheral blood smear are characteristic of dextroisomerism or asplenia.

For determination of the AV, ventricular, and VA relationships, high-quality selective biplane angiography, supplemented by equally high-quality two-dimensional echocardiography with Doppler color flow mapping, is essential.[209] Symbols used to designate the combination or sequence of segments are arranged in order as follows: (1) the visceroatrial or bronchoatrial situs, (2) the ventricular loop, and (3) the relations of the great arteries. These may be included within parentheses and preceded by abbreviations that indicate the VA alignment, for example, TGA, DORV, or single ventricle (SV). Associated malformations such as VSD, pulmonary stenosis, and straddling tricuspid valve may be listed after the parentheses. Thus, the typical or usual transposition of the great arteries with situs solitus, d-ventricular loop, and aorta arising from the right ventricle and to the right of the pulmonary artery, with an intact ventricular septum (IVS), would be designated TGA (SDD) IVS. The designation for typical corrected transposition (TGA) with situs solitus (S), l-ventricular loop (L), aorta arising from the morphologic right ventricle and lying to the left of the pulmonary artery (L), with VSD and pulmonary stenosis (PS), would be TGA (SLL), VSD, PS. This designation would apply to transposition with situs solitus, whether the heart lay in the right or left chest (dextrocardia or levocardia, respectively). It should be noted that the description of the position of the heart within the chest would offer no additional information referable to the intracardiac anatomy or great vessel alignment.[207]

Levocardia, Dextrocardia, and Mesocardia

The position of the cardiac apex indicates a condition of levocardia, dextrocardia, or mesocardia.

The trend today is to discard the terms *dextroposition, dextroversion, mirror-image dextrocardia*, and *isolated dextrocardia* because they do not provide any significant information beyond what is already known—that the cardiac apex is in the right chest—and to use the broad term *dextrocardia* for all right-sided hearts, followed by a description of the visceroatrial situs. In the case of patients in whom the heart appears to have been pulled or pushed into the right chest by massive atelectasis or hypoplasia of the right lung, diaphragmatic hernia, eventration of the diaphragm, pleural effusion, obstructive emphysema, or pneumothorax, an appropriate descriptive phrase should be added. The term *isolated levocardia* is applied to all left-sided hearts with situs inversus or situs ambiguous, and a description of the visceroatrial situs should follow.

Dextrocardia with complete situs inversus occurs in approximately 2 per 10,000 live births. *The incidence of congenital heart disease is relatively low among these individuals and is estimated to be about 3 percent.* Dextrocardia with situs solitus or situs ambiguous is considerably less common and occurs in perhaps 1 in 20,000 live births. The incidence of congenital heart disease is extremely high in this situation, however, probably in the range of 90 percent or greater. From these figures, one could project that approximately 12 percent of individuals found to have dextrocardia and congenital heart disease would have complete situs inversus. This estimate compares favorably with the figure of 18 percent observed in large autopsy series. About 50 percent of patients with dextrocardia and heart disease have situs solitus, and the remainder, perhaps 30 percent, have situs ambiguous.[207] An l-ventricular loop is found in the majority of patients with dextrocardia regardless of situs but is most common, as one might expect, among patients with situs inversus, in whom it approaches 80 percent. Cardiac malformations usually, although not invariably, are severe and complex. The most common lesions and their approximate frequency are as follows: transposition of the great arteries, 50 to 75 percent; double-outlet right ventricle, 10 to 18 percent; VSD, 60 to 80 percent; single ventricle, 15 to 40 percent; and pulmonary stenosis or atresia, 70 to 80 percent.[207] Approximately three-quarters of transposed great arteries have the segmental arrangement of corrected transposition. Tetralogy of Fallot is distinctly uncommon. Polysplenia or asplenia is found in about one-third of patients with dextrocardia and almost invariably with situs ambiguous. Kartagener's syndrome, the triad of situs inversus, sinusitis, and bronchiectasis, results from impaired ciliary movement. It is present in approximately 20 percent of patients with dextrocardia and situs inversus totalis.[210] The incidence of isolated levocardia has been estimated at approximately 0.6 per 10,000 live births. It is estimated that over 90 percent of affected individuals have associated heart disease. Situs inversus is present in approximately 15 percent, and the remainder have situs ambiguous, with the ratio of asplenia to polysplenia or accessory spleens being from 2.5:1 to 1.5:1. The associated defects are comparable in complexity and severity to those associated with dextrocardia. *Mesocardia* may exist as a variant position of the normal heart or a variant position of dextrocardia or isolated levocardia.

MEDICAL AND SURGICAL MANAGEMENT

Medical management of patients with cardiac malposition is similar to that of patients with normally located hearts, with the exceptions of continuous daily antibiotic coverage and pneumococcal vaccine for patients with asplenia and the particular attention to detail that is necessary to establish the correct diagnosis in individuals with unusual and complex malformations. Surgical management differs in the technical considerations imposed by the malposition of the heart itself, the frequency of occurrence of the l-ventricular loop, and the variability of the intracardiac conduction system.

Dextro Transposition of the Great Arteries

DEFINITION

In this condition, the aorta and the pulmonary artery are misplaced in relation to the ventricular septum, with the aorta arising from the right ventricle and the pulmonary artery arising from the left ventricle (discordant VA connection).

PATHOLOGY

In the majority of cases, there are situs solitus of the atria and viscera (S) and concordance of the AV connection and the right

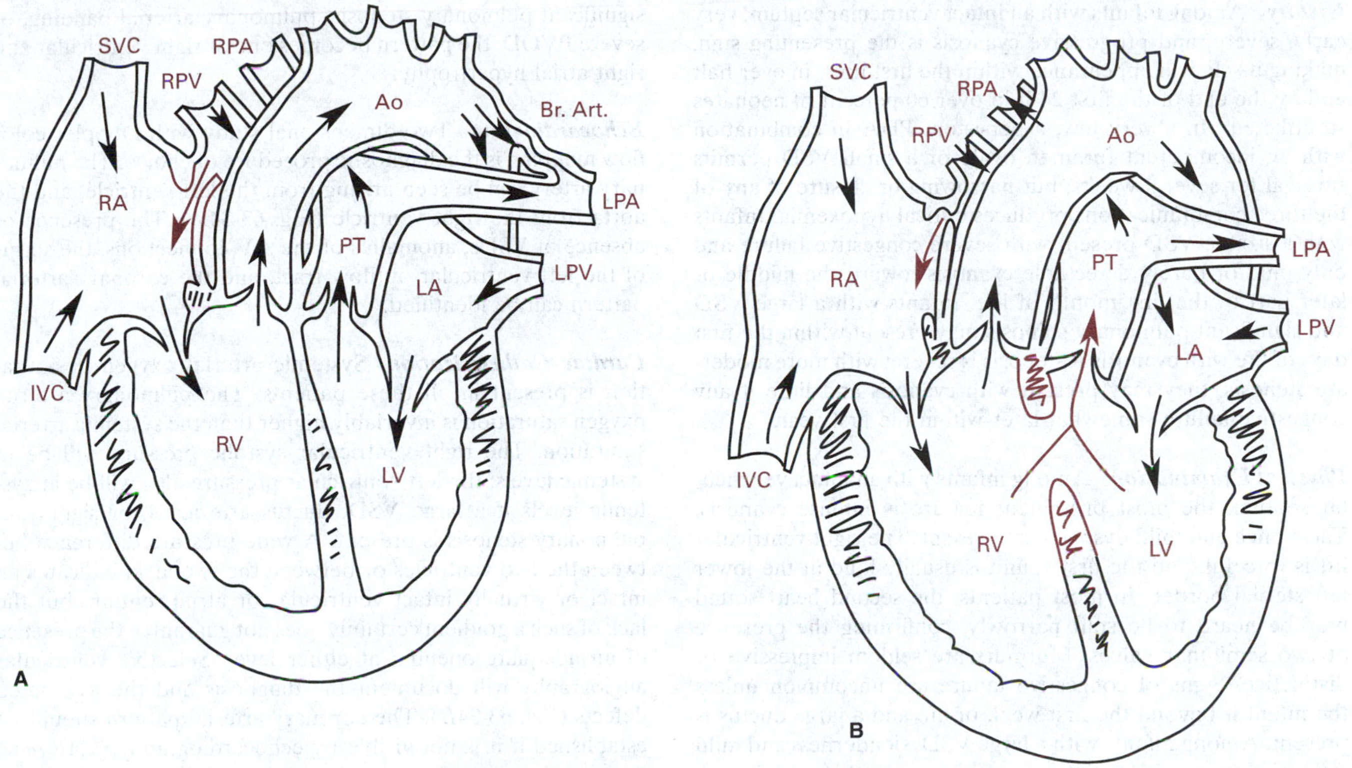

FIGURE 63-33 Complete D transposition of the great arteries. *A.* With intact ventricular septum. A patent foramen ovale and enlarged bronchial arteries (Br. Art.) are present. *B.* With ventricular septal defect and without pulmonary stenosis. SVC = superior vena cava; IVC = inferior vena cava; RA = right atrium; RV = right ventricle; Ao = aorta; LA = left atrium; LV = left ventricle.

ventricle lies to the right of the left ventricle (d loop, D) (Fig. 63-33). The aorta lies to the right of the pulmonary arterial origin (d transposition, D) and is anterior. Of the communications between the two sides of the circulation, a narrow patent foramen and PDA are common in very young infants. The ventricular septum is intact in approximately half these patients, and another 10 percent have only a very small VSD. The remainder have a large VSD or multiple VSDs.[211]

Pulmonary stenosis of significance is very uncommon among neonates with an intact ventricular septum but develops with the passage of time in approximately one-third of patients in whom the right ventricle continues to be the systemic ventricle. In most cases it is mild and usually, though not invariably, is the result of a bulging of the ventricular septum into the left ventricular outflow area. Approximately one-third of patients with a large VSD have significant left ventricular outflow tract obstruction (pulmonary stenosis). Causes of this obstruction include leftward malalignment of the infundibular septum, the presence of a membranous collar or ridge encircling the left ventricular outflow tract, anomalous adhesion of the anterior mitral leaflet to the ventricular septum, stenotic deformity of the pulmonary valve, and, rarely, an aneurysm of endocardial tissue related to the VSD.[212]

The coronary arteries usually arise from the two aortic sinuses adjacent to the pulmonary trunk—the "facing sinuses"—with the most common arrangement being the right coronary artery arising from the rightward sinus and the left coronary artery, with its anterior descending and circumflex branches, arising from the leftward sinus.

Hypertensive pulmonary vascular disease may occur at an inordinately early age and may occur even in patients with an intact ventricular septum and initially low left ventricular pressures. Three-quarters or more of patients with d transposition, situs solitus, and d loop [TGA (SDD)] either have no significant associated cardiac defects or have relatively simple malformations in the form of VSD, ASD, PDA, or pulmonary stenosis. The remainder have more complicated lesions and will not be discussed in this section.

ABNORMAL PHYSIOLOGY

The systemic and pulmonary circulations are arranged so that the systemic venous return is conducted back to the systemic arterial system and the pulmonary venous return is conducted back to the pulmonary arterial system, with no obligatory mixing or interchange. For survival, there must be communication between the two circulations in the form of a patent foramen ovale, a PDA, or a VSD. The hemodynamics are dependent on the combination of defects present and particularly on the amount of mixing between the systemic and pulmonary circulations. The right ventricle is the systemic ventricle, and its systolic pressure is the same as systemic arterial pressure.

CLINICAL MANIFESTATIONS

Approximately 3 to 4 percent of children with recognized congenital heart disease have transposition of the great arteries (Table 63-1). Males are more commonly afflicted than are females in a ratio between 2:1 and 3:1.

History Among infants with an intact ventricular septum, very early, severe, and progressive cyanosis is the presenting sign, making its clinical appearance within the first hour in over half and by the end of the first 24 h in over 60 percent of neonates so afflicted.[3] In a very few, a persistent PDA in combination with an incompetent foramen ovale or a small VSD permits survival for several weeks, but narrowing or closure of any of the three communications produces critical hypoxemia. Infants with a sizable VSD present with severe congestive failure and only mild or barely detectable cyanosis toward the middle or later part of the first month of life. Infants with a large VSD and significant pulmonary stenosis may present within the first days of life with cyanosis if stenosis is severe; with more moderate stenosis, they may present with cyanosis and little if any congestive failure somewhat later within the first year.

Physical Examination Among infants with an intact ventricular septum, the most prominent feature is intense cyanosis. Tachypnea and mild dyspnea are present. The right ventricular lift is forceful, and the first sound is usually loud at the lower left sternal border. In most patients, the second heart sound may be heard to be split narrowly, confirming the presence of two semilunar valves. Murmurs are seldom impressive or distinctive. Signs of congestive failure are uncommon unless the infant is beyond the first week of life and a large ductus is present. Among infants with a large VSD, slenderness and mild cyanosis or a grayish pallor are apparent. Breathing is labored, and both the right and left ventricular impulses are hyperactive. A thrill is uncommon. A systolic murmur at the lower left sternal border is usually present but is seldom loud or completely holosystolic. A gallop rhythm and a diastolic flow rumble at the apex are typical. Infants and children with VSD and significant pulmonary stenosis generally are severely cyanotic.

Chest Roentgenogram With an intact ventricular septum, the heart size and pulmonary vascularity appear normal or at the upper limits of normal during the first week. Later, a narrow base caused by the displaced pulmonary artery may give rise to the characteristic "egg-on-side" contour. Impressive cardiomegaly, pulmonary plethora, and this characteristic contour are more common during the second week and beyond. With a large VSD, marked cardiac enlargement involving all chambers, impressive pulmonary plethora, and the egg-on-side contour are present. With significant pulmonary stenosis, the heart resembles that of a patient with tetralogy of Fallot, but it is usually slightly larger and the pulmonary vascularity is less diminished than one would expect for a comparable degree of clinical cyanosis. A right aortic arch is present in 4 to 16 percent of those patients.

Electrocardiogram If the ventricular septum is intact, the ECG may reveal tall or peaked P waves by the second or third day of life; however, clearly abnormal right ventricular forces usually are not apparent until the latter part of the first week. The persistence of an upright T wave in leads V_1 and V_{3R} beyond 4 days of age provides an early clue that the right ventricular systolic pressure is at systemic levels. An older infant will have abnormal right axis deviation and marked right ventricular hypertrophy. A large VSD with a large pulmonary blood flow usually will produce biatrial and biventricular hypertrophy. If pulmonary blood flow is reduced toward normal, whether by significant pulmonary stenosis, pulmonary arterial banding, or severe PVOD, the pattern becomes one of right ventricular and right atrial hypertrophy.

Echocardiogram Two-dimensional study with Doppler color flow mapping is the diagnostic procedure of choice. The pulmonary artery can be seen arising from the left ventricle, and the aorta from the right ventricle (Fig. 63-34*A*). The presence or absence of VSDs, anomalies of the AV connections, the status of the left ventricular outflow tract, and the coronary arterial pattern can be identified.

Cardiac Catheterization Systemic arterial oxygen desaturation is present in all these patients. The pulmonary arterial oxygen saturation is invariably higher than the systemic arterial saturation. The right ventricular systolic pressure will be at systemic levels; the left ventricular pressure also will be at systemic levels if a large VSD, ductus arteriosus, or significant pulmonary stenosis is present. A wide pressure difference between the two ventricles or between the two atria indicates an intact or virtually intact ventricular or atrial septum, but the lack of such a gradient certainly does not guarantee the presence of an adequate opening at either level. Selective ventricular angiography will document the diagnosis and the associated defects (Fig. 63-34*B*). The coronary arterial pattern should be established if it is not visible by echocardiography.[213] *All newborns with transposition can benefit from balloon atrial septostomy at catheterization by virtue of the increased mixing of the pulmonary and systemic venous circulations and the decompression of the left atrium.*

NATURAL HISTORY AND PROGNOSIS

Without balloon septostomy or surgical intervention, 50 percent of infants with transposition die within the first month and 90 percent die within the first year of life.[214] Those with an intact ventricular septum die very early from hypoxemia. Those with a large VSD usually live somewhat longer, but the majority die in the first months of congestive failure; the few survivors have severe PVOD. Those with a large VSD and pulmonary stenosis have the best outlook, but the average life expectancy is barely 5 years even with this combination of defects. With an adequate interatrial opening, whether natural, balloon-induced, or surgically created, infants with an intact ventricular septum do relatively well during the first year. Increasing cyanosis during the first year in these patients may be due to a gradual diminution of the size of the atrial septal opening, narrowing or closure of a persistent PDA or small VSD, the gradual development of subvalvular pulmonary stenosis, or the development of PVOD. Before age 2 years, cerebrovascular accidents are a hazard to these hypoxemic infants and occur almost invariably in a setting of relative anemia rather than extreme polycythemia. The appearance of PVOD is unusual but can occur within the first 12 months of life. It becomes more common, approaching 40 percent, in the second year of life and thereafter. Infants with a large VSD and no significant pulmonary stenosis will develop PVOD and become prohibitive risks for corrective surgery by the end of the first year of life. Those with a VSD and severe pulmonary stenosis usually become progressively more cyanotic.

Palliative and subsequent corrective operations have enabled a relatively large group of patients to survive beyond infancy and early childhood. Among the survivors of the atrial switch operations, such as the Mustard and Senning procedures, are found residual abnormalities such as pulmonary stenosis and PVOD as well as complications that result from surgery. These complications include residual intraatrial baffle leaks, systemic and/or pulmonary venous obstruction, and arrhythmias. Late sudden death has been described in about 3 percent of survivors and very possibly results from arrhythmias. Finally, right ventricular dysfunction with or without progressive tricuspid regurgitation has been documented in many of the somewhat older survivors of atrial inversion operations and raises the question of whether the right ventricle can function adequately as the systemic arterial ventricle beyond adolescence and early adult life.

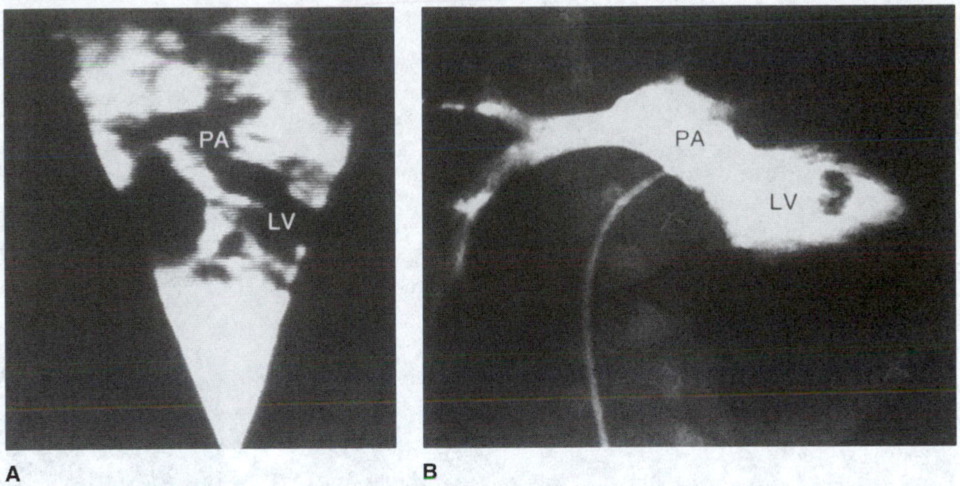

FIGURE 63-34 *A.* Two-dimensional echocardiogram. The left ventricle leads to a bifurcating great vessel (pulmonary artery, PA), confirming transposition. *B.* Anterolateral projection of an angiogram in the smooth-walled left ventricle (LV). The dye is ejected into the pulmonary artery.

While complications have been problematic for some, long-term follow-up of the group as a whole has been good. The Toronto experience is the oldest and largest. Among 534 children who underwent a "Mustard" procedure since 1962, there were 52 early deaths (9.7 percent). Survival at 5 years was 89 percent, and it was 76 percent at 20 years.[215] In a study from New Zealand of 113 hospital survivors of surgery performed between 1964 and 1982, survival at 10, 20, and 28 years was 90 80, and 80 percent, respectively, with 76 percent of survivors being New York Heart Association class I.[216] There has been less long-term follow-up of survivors of the "Senning" type of atrial repair. In a recent study of 100 patients, the actuarial survival at 13 years was 90 percent for those with simple transposition and 78 percent survival for those with complex disease.[217]

MEDICAL MANAGEMENT

The first step in the treatment of infants with an intact ventricular septum is to provide without delay an adequate systemic arterial oxygen saturation. This can be achieved in almost all instances by establishing an adequate interatrial opening with balloon atrial septostomy and providing adequate systemic arterial-to-pulmonary arterial shunting via the ductus with the use of intravenous PGE_1 infusion;[91] the latter procedure frequently is supplemented by endotracheal intubation to compensate for prostaglandin-related apnea. The adequacy of the atrial septostomy opening can be determined by a sustained increase in the systemic arterial oxygen saturation to above 60 percent and verified by direct visualization with two-dimensional echocardiography. If the relief of hypoxemia is unsatisfactory with PGE_1 alone and if the interatrial opening is judged by echocardiography to be small, the alternatives are to perform a balloon atrial septectomy without delay or to proceed directly with corrective surgery in the form of the arterial switch operation.

SURGICAL MANAGEMENT

Arterial switch repair is now the preferred surgical alternative to the atrial inversion procedures for a neonate with an intact ventricular septum and for a slightly older infant with a large VSD and without significant structural pulmonary stenosis (Fig. 63-35). Arterial switching should be performed within the first 2 to 3 weeks of life, before left ventricular systolic pressure falls significantly below that of the right ventricle. For infants beyond 3 weeks of age, if the ratio of left ventricular to right ventricular pressure has fallen below 0.60, a pulmonary arterial band may be applied with or without a systemic-to-pulmonary arterial shunt and the arterial switch operation may be performed approximately 1 week later. Most patterns of coronary arterial origin and course appear to be amenable to the operation, and infants as small as 2.0 kg may be repaired successfully.

In some centers, the surgical risks have been reduced to about 5 to 10 percent,[218] although in other centers, the surgical mortality continues to be higher.[219] Short- and medium-term prognosis is good,[220] but longer-term studies are awaited. The most common problem has been stenosis at the pulmonary artery anastomotic site.[221] When severe, this usually has been amenable to balloon dilation or stenting.[222]

For infants with transposition, a large VSD, and pulmonary hypertension, the arterial switch technique with VSD closure must be carried out within the first 2 months of life to prevent severe PVOD. Infants with a large VSD and severe pulmonary stenosis usually may be palliated with a systemic-to-pulmonary arterial shunt and repaired in later infancy or as young children,[175] although some centers are doing reparative surgery in infancy.[223] Finally, the severe hypoxemia present in children with a large VSD and severe PVOD may be reduced by an intraatrial repair performed as a palliative procedure, with no attempt at closure of the VSD.[224]

Double-Outlet Right Ventricle

PATHOLOGY

In this malformation, more than 50 percent of the semilunar valve orifices of both great arteries arise from the morphologic right ventricle. In most cases, the ventricles display a d loop, and the pulmonary arterial origin is normally positioned, arising from a conus above the right ventricle. The aorta also arises

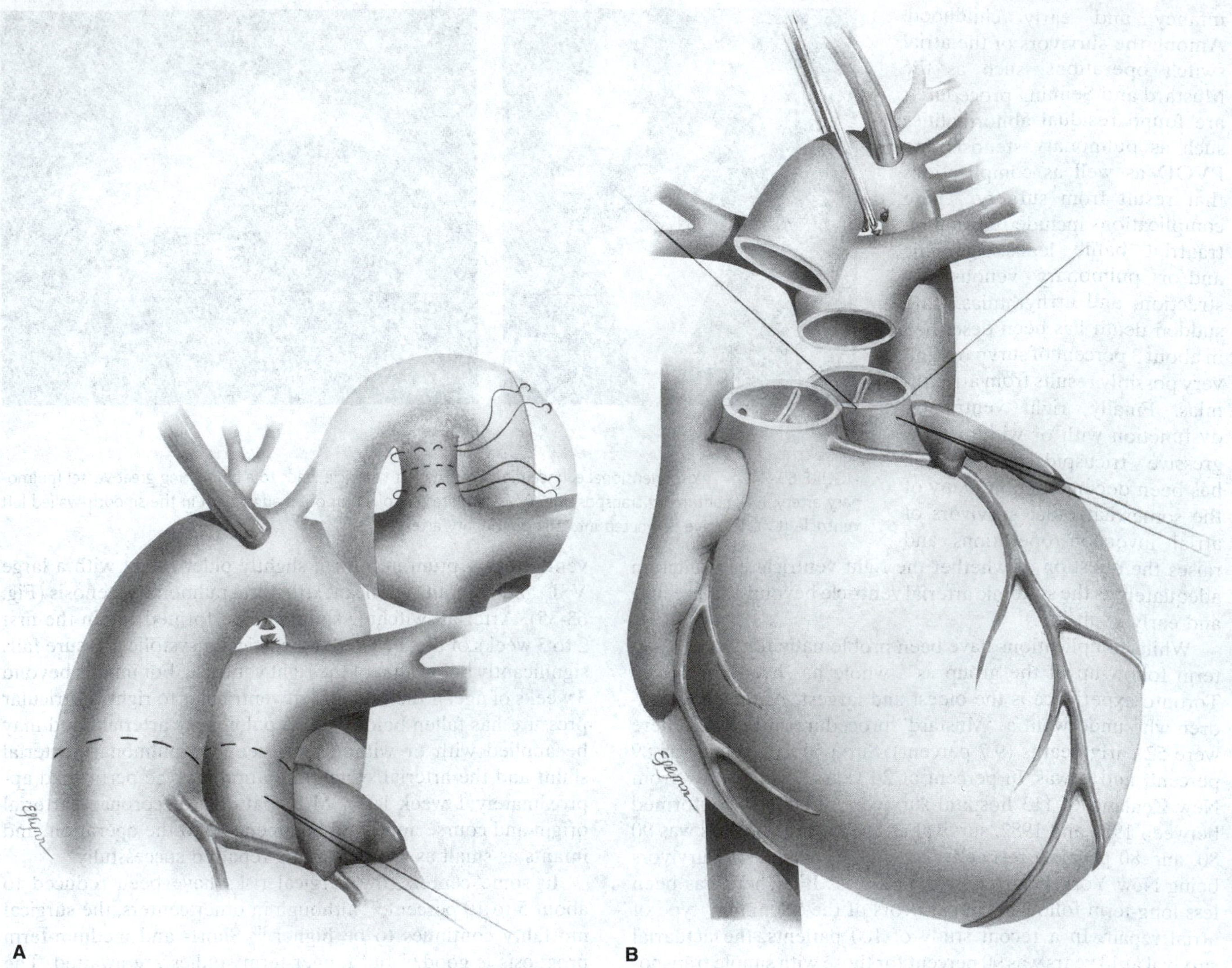

FIGURE 63-35 Surgical technique of the arterial switch operation. *A.* Aortic cannula is positioned distally in the ascending aorta, the ductus arteriosus is divided between suture ligatures, and the branch pulmonary arteries are dissected out to the hilum to provide adequate mobility for anterior translocation. The broken lines represent the levels of transection of the aorta and the main pulmonary artery. Marking sutures are placed in the anticipated sites of coronary transfer. *B.* Transection of the great arteries. The left ventricular outflow tract, neoaortic valve, and coronary arteries are inspected thoroughly. *C.* The coronary arterial buttons are excised from the free edge of the aorta to the base of the sinus of Valsalva. *D.* The coronary buttons are anastomosed to V-shaped excisions made in the neoaorta. *E.* The pulmonary artery is brought anterior to the aorta (Lecompte maneuver). Anastomosis of the proximal neoaorta is shown. *F* and *G.* The coronary donor sites are filled with autologous pericardial patches. A single U-shaped patch (*F*) or two separate patches (*G*) may be used. *H.* Completed anastomosis of the proximal neopulmonary artery and the distal pulmonary artery. (Modified from Castaneda AR. Anatomic correction of transposition of the great arteries at the arterial level. In: Sabiston DC Jr, Spencer FC, eds. *Surgery of the Chest.* 5th ed. Philadelphia: Saunders; 1990. Reproduced with permission from the authors and publisher.)

from the right ventricle above conal tissue. The two semilunar valves are at about the same level, and there is no fibrous continuity between the semilunar and mitral valves (Fig. 63-36).

In most cases, the aortic origin is to the right (d malposition) of the pulmonary arterial origin, with the two vessels usually displaying a side-by-side relationship. Uncommonly, the aortic origin is distinctly anterior to the pulmonary origin or the aorta arises to the left (l malposition) of the pulmonary artery.[225]

With rare exceptions, there is a VSD. The condition may be subdivided further on the basis of the relation of the VSD to the origin of the great arteries. The VSD is subaortic in approximately two-thirds of patients, subpulmonary (*Taussig-Bing heart*) in 18 percent, related to both great arteries (*doubly committed*) in 3 percent, and remote or unrelated to either great artery in about 7 percent.[225]

ASSOCIATED CONDITIONS

Pulmonary stenosis occurs in over half these cases, with the condition usually resulting from a narrow subpulmonary conus. ASD, subaortic stenosis, and coarctation of the aorta are also relatively common, with the latter particularly associated with the subpulmonary defect. Obstruction at the mitral valve may be observed in about one-fifth of cases of double-outlet right ventricle. Mitral valve straddling of the VSD and varying degrees of left ventricular hypoplasia also are encountered.

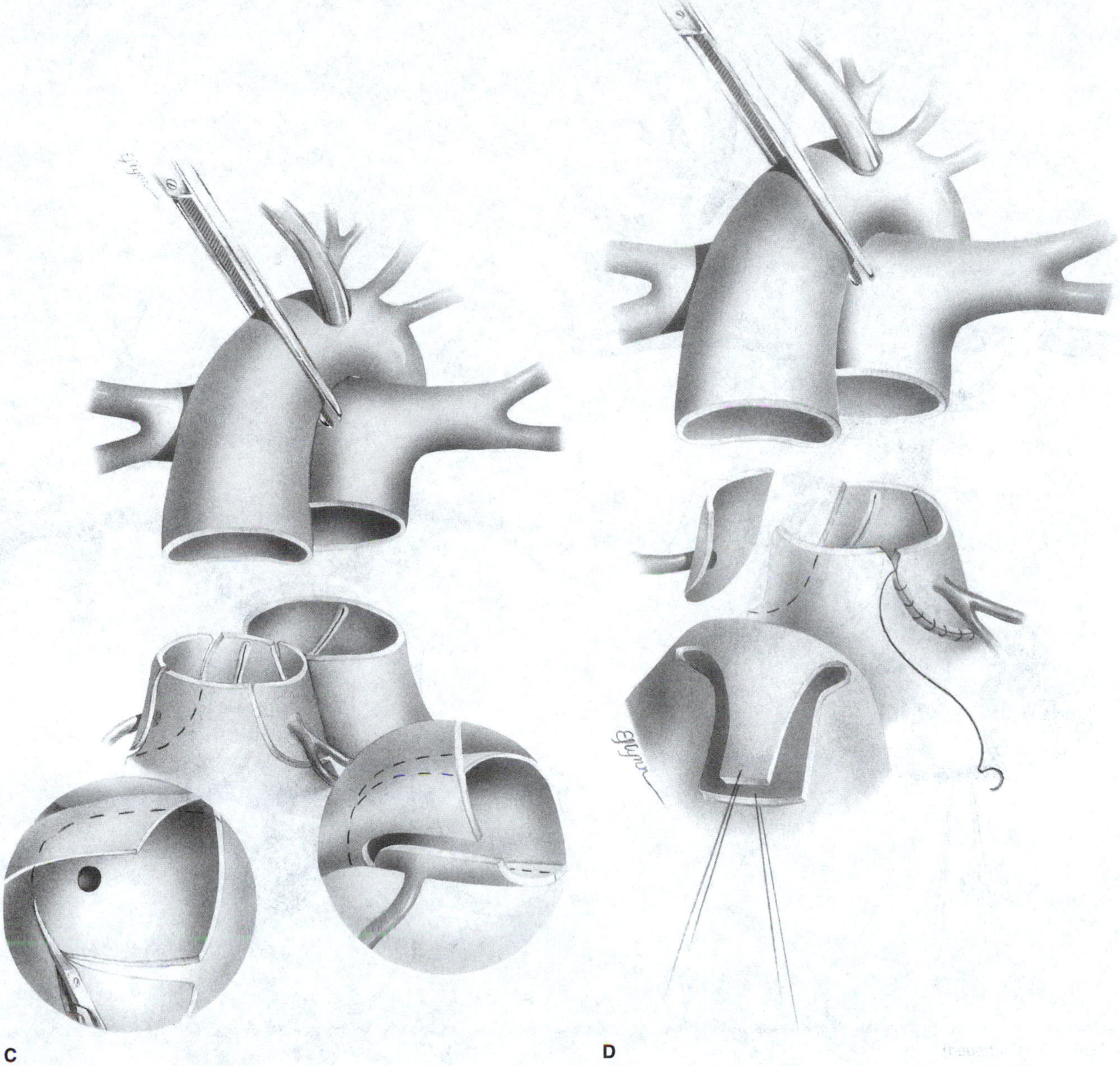

C D

FIGURE 63-35 *(Continued)*

CLINICAL MANIFESTATIONS

Double-outlet right ventricle, or origin of both great arteries from the right ventricle, is a relatively rare malformation that is found in only 0.8 percent of patients with congenital heart disease. It is of considerable importance, however, because its clinical and laboratory features frequently resemble those of more common and more easily correctable malformations. Double-outlet right ventricle reflects the relationship of the great vessels to the ventricular septum; the presentation and treatment of children with this condition depend on the associated anomalies.

History and Physical Examination Patients with a subaortic VSD without pulmonary stenosis (Fig. 63-36*A*) have the same findings on examination as do patients with a large isolated VSD. Congestive failure appears within a few weeks of birth, and cyanosis is seldom described. Those with a subaortic VSD and pulmonary stenosis (Fig. 63-36*B*) usually present after the newborn period and follow a course similar to that of patients with tetralogy of Fallot. Patients with a subpulmonary defect without pulmonary stenosis (Fig. 63-36*C*), the Taussig-Bing malformation, resemble patients with transposition of the great arteries and a large VSD without pulmonary stenosis. The findings are those of severe congestive failure and cyanosis.

Chest Roentgenogram Cardiomegaly with pulmonary overperfusion is characteristic of all types of this anomaly without pulmonary stenosis. Double-outlet right ventricle with subaortic VSD and pulmonary stenosis resembles tetralogy of Fallot. In the case of subpulmonary VSD without pulmonary stenosis,

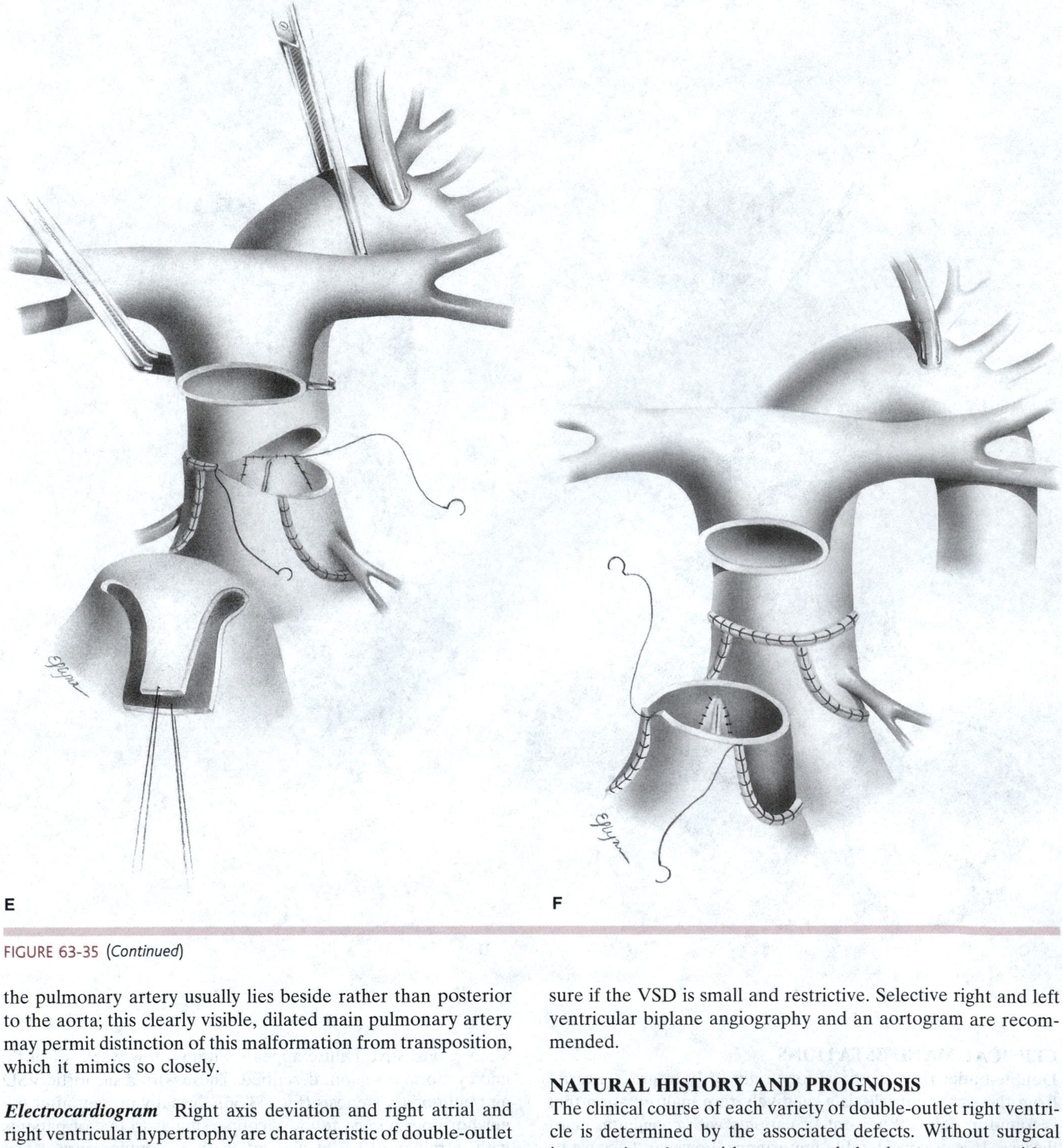

FIGURE 63-35 (*Continued*)

the pulmonary artery usually lies beside rather than posterior to the aorta; this clearly visible, dilated main pulmonary artery may permit distinction of this malformation from transposition, which it mimics so closely.

Electrocardiogram Right axis deviation and right atrial and right ventricular hypertrophy are characteristic of double-outlet right ventricle.

Echocardiogram Two-dimensional echocardiography is very useful in demonstrating the anatomic components and associated defects.[225,226]

Cardiac Catheterization There is an increase in oxygen saturation at the right ventricular level. The pulmonary arterial saturation is lower than that of the aorta in patients with a subaortic VSD and is invariably higher than that of the aorta in those with a subpulmonary septal defect and transposition physiology. Left ventricular systolic pressure may be higher than right pressure if the VSD is small and restrictive. Selective right and left ventricular biplane angiography and an aortogram are recommended.

NATURAL HISTORY AND PROGNOSIS

The clinical course of each variety of double-outlet right ventricle is determined by the associated defects. Without surgical intervention, those with an unguarded pulmonary artery either die in infancy with congestive failure or develop PVOD. Spontaneous narrowing or closure of the VSD may occur and is life-threatening. Increasing dyspnea, increasing intensity of the systolic murmur, and progressive left ventricular hypertrophy suggest this complication. Patients with pulmonary stenosis tend to have progressive obstruction and cyanosis.

MEDICAL MANAGEMENT

Vigorous treatment of heart failure is required for those without pulmonary stenosis. Almost all cases are best treated with surgical palliation or correction in infancy. If there is pulmonary

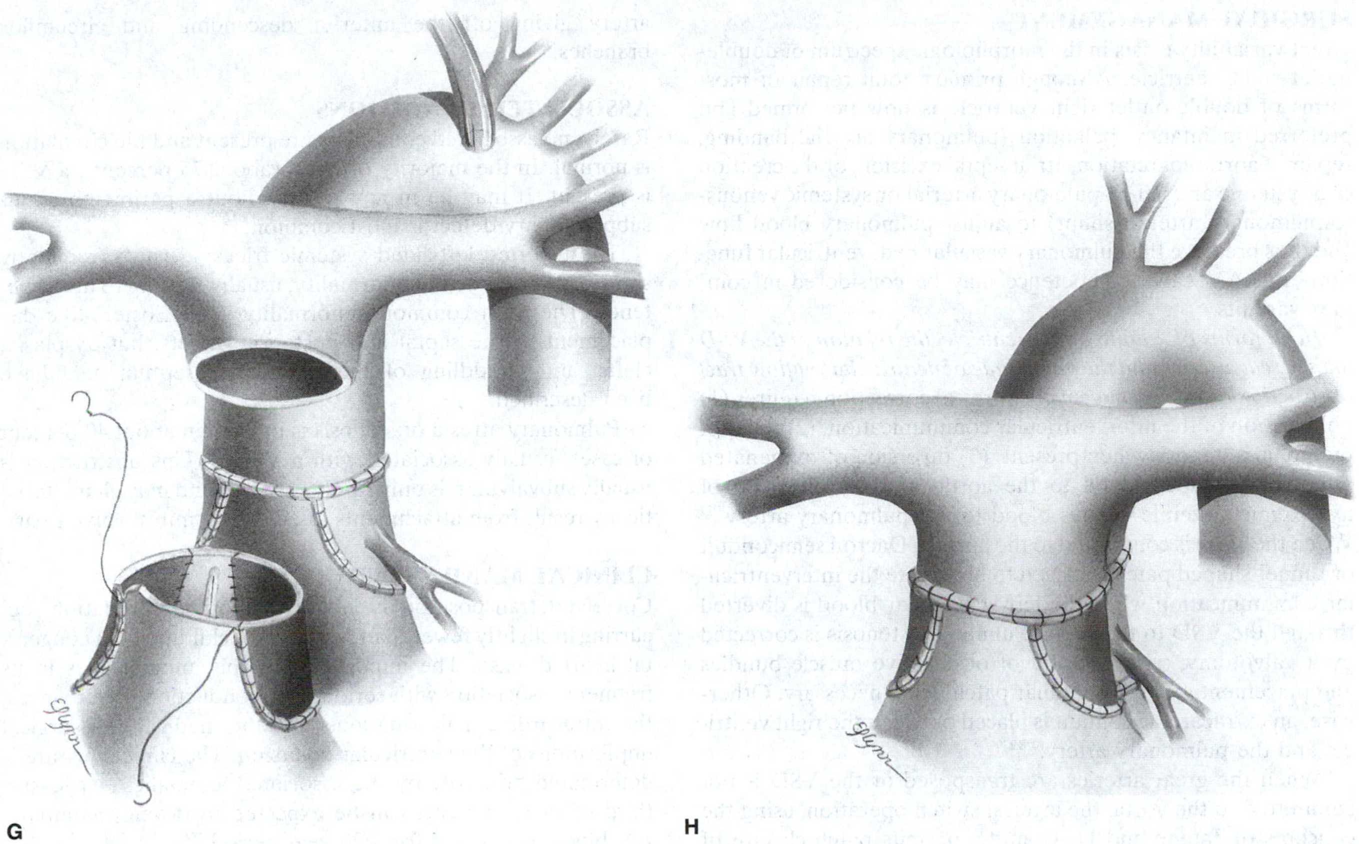

FIGURE 63-35 (*Continued*)

hypertension, banding or correction should be done by 2 to 3 months of age. Patients with ventricular hypoplasia, mitral stenoses, straddling AV valves, or a remote VSD are usually not candidates for biventricular repair, and initial palliation should prepare the child for a modification of the Fontan operation. Whether or not corrective surgery has been performed, all patients in whom the left ventricular output must pass through the VSD should be observed continuously for the possibility of spontaneous narrowing and obstruction at that site.

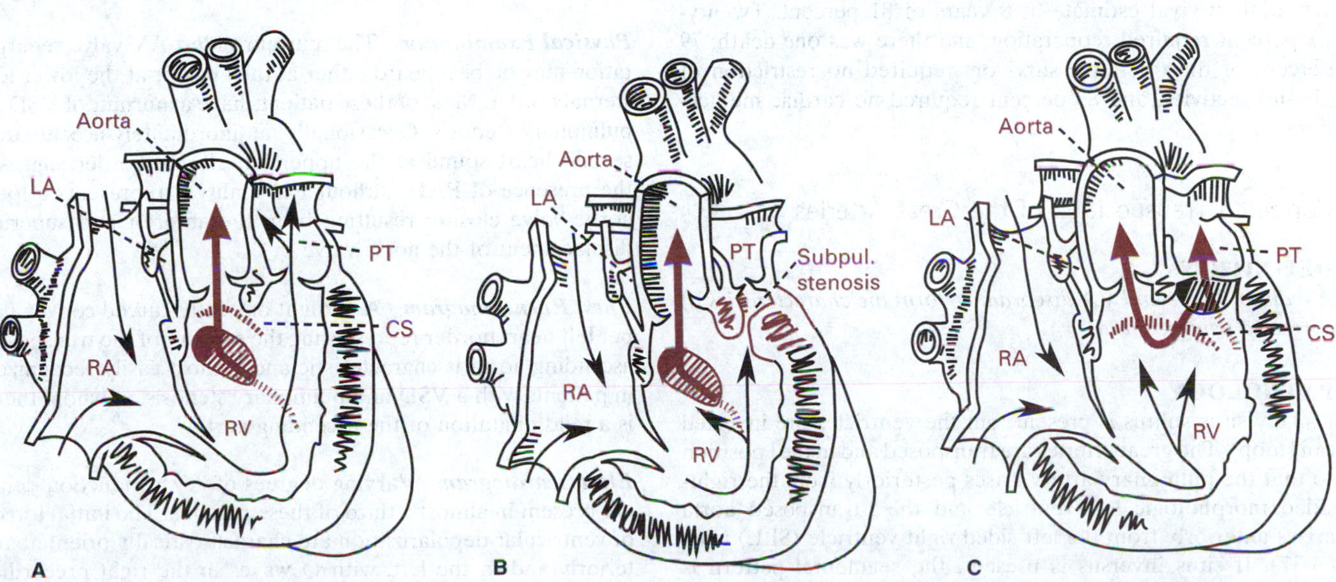

FIGURE 63-36 Double-outlet right ventricle. *A.* With subaortic ventricular septal defect without pulmonary stenosis. *B.* With subaortic ventricular septal defect and subpulmonary stenosis (Subpul. stenosis). *C.* With subpulmonary, supracristal ventricular septal defect. The so-called Taussig-Bing complex. RA = right atrium; RV = right ventricle; CS = crista supraventricularis; LA = left atrium; PT = main pulmonary arterial trunk.

SURGICAL MANAGEMENT

Great variability exists in the morphologic spectrum of double-outlet right ventricle. Although primary total repair of most forms of double-outlet right ventricle is now performed and preferred in infancy, palliation (pulmonary arterial banding, repair of aortic coarctation, atrial septal excision, or the creation of a systemic arterial-to-pulmonary arterial or systemic venous-to-pulmonary arterial shunt) to adjust pulmonary blood flow and thus preserve the pulmonary vascular bed, ventricular function, and AV valve competence may be considered in complex variants.

In all forms of double-outlet ventricle, the relation of the VSD to the great arteries and the magnitude of ventricular outflow tract obstruction dictate management. Surgical correction requires (1) obliteration of the interventricular communication, (2) relief of pulmonary stenosis when present, (3) diversion of oxygenated pulmonary venous blood to the aorta, and (4) diversion of hypoxemic systemic venous blood to the pulmonary artery.[227] When the VSD is committed to the aorta, a Dacron semiconduit or tunnel-shaped patch is placed to obliterate the interventricular communication while the left ventricular blood is diverted through the VSD to the aorta. Pulmonary stenosis is corrected by a valvotomy, with excision of obstructive muscle bundles and placement of a transannular patch when necessary. Otherwise, an extracardiac conduit is placed between the right ventricle and the pulmonary artery.[228,229]

When the great arteries are transposed or the VSD is not committed to the aorta, the arterial switch operation, using the concepts of Jatene and Le Compte, permits patch closure of the VSD, directing left ventricular blood into the neoaorta.[230] Further consideration of repair of double-outlet right ventricle associated with more complex defects is beyond the scope of this discussion. For a patient who is not a candidate for biventricular repair because of hypoplasia of a ventricle or a straddling AV valve, initial palliation should prepare the child for a modification of the Fontan operation.

In a 10-year review of repair of double-outlet right ventricle in 73 patients,[228] early mortality was 11 percent, with an overall actuarial survival estimate at 8 years of 81 percent. Twenty-six percent required reoperation, and there was one death; 79 percent of the operative survivors required no restriction of physical activity, and 83 percent required no cardiac medications.

Corrected Transposition of the Great Arteries

DEFINITION

AV discordance and VA discordance form the characteristics of corrected transposition.

PATHOLOGY

Usually situs solitus is present, but the ventricles are inverted (an l loop). The great arteries are transposed and in the l position so that the pulmonary artery arises posteriorly from the right-sided morphologic left ventricle and the l-transposed aorta arises anteriorly from the left-sided right ventricle (SLL) (Fig. 63-37). If situs inversus is present, the segmental pattern is IDD. Along with the ventricular inversion, there is AV valvular inversion. The two coronary arteries arise from the right and left (posteriorly facing) sinuses, with the right-sided coronary artery giving off the anterior descending and circumflex branches.[231]

ASSOCIATED CONDITIONS

Rarely, no associated conditions are present and the circulation is normal. In the majority of cases (about 75 percent), a VSD is present. It may be in any location, but a perimembranous subpulmonary defect is most common.

The inverted left-sided systemic tricuspid valve frequently shows some degree of abnormality, usually leading to incompetence. The most common abnormality is an Ebstein-like displacement of the septal and posterior leaflets, but dysplasia, clefts, and straddling of the ventricular septum also have been described.

Pulmonary atresia or stenosis is present in about 40 percent of cases, usually associated with a VSD.[231] This obstruction is usually subvalvular, is only rarely valvular, and may characteristically result from attachments of accessory mitral valve tissue.

CLINICAL MANIFESTATIONS

Corrected transposition is an uncommon malformation, occurring in slightly fewer than 1 percent of children with congenital heart disease. The importance of this anomaly lies in its frequent association with serious AV conduction disturbances, the intracardiac malformations, and the medical and surgical implications of the ventricular inversion. The clinical picture is determined primarily by the associated anomalies. At least a third of these patients can be expected to develop complete AV block if followed for a 20-year period.[232]

History A slow, irregular heart rate often is detected in utero, and 10 percent of patients with congenital complete block prove to have corrected transposition. Patients with a large VSD without pulmonary stenosis usually present within the first month or so of life with symptoms indistinguishable from those of infants with a large VSD alone. Patients with VSD and pulmonary stenosis may present with symptoms of cyanosis and resemble patients with tetralogy of Fallot.

Physical Examination The murmur of left AV valve regurgitation may be best heard either at the apex or at the lower left sternal border. Most of these patients have a murmur of VSD or pulmonary stenosis. Occasionally, an inordinately accentuated second heart sound at the upper left sternal border suggests the presence of PAH, although in reality it represents a loud aortic valve closure resulting from the anterior and superior displacement of the aorta valve.

Chest Roentgenogram A straight or gently curved convex upper left heart border representing the contour of the transposed ascending aorta is characteristic and is most easily recognized in patients with a VSD and pulmonary stenosis, in whom there is a mild dilatation of the ascending aorta.

Electrocardiogram Varying degrees of AV conduction delay are present in almost a third of these patients. The initial forces of ventricular depolarization are characteristically oriented anteriorly and to the left, with Q waves in the right precordial leads and not in leads I, V_5, and V_6 resulting from depolarization of the septum from the left side (right ventricle) to the right side (left ventricle). With normal or nearly normal pressure in

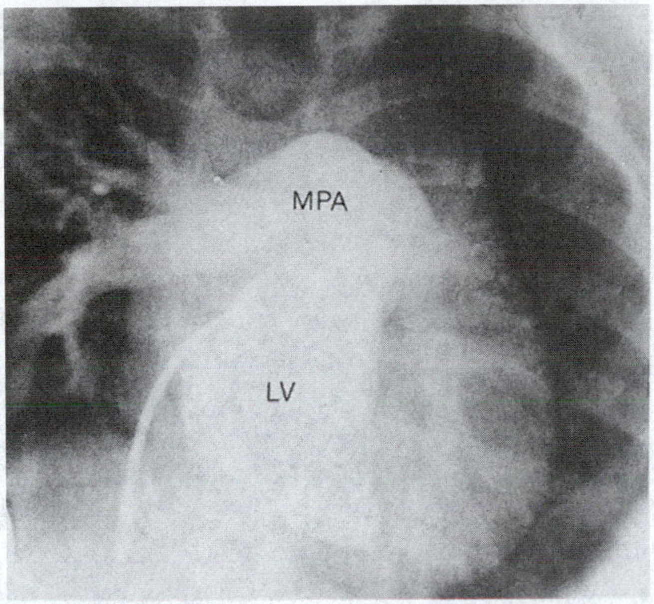

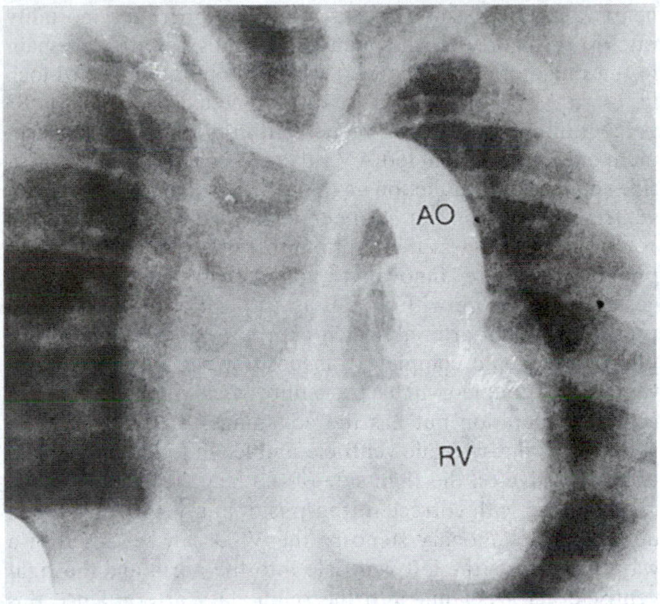

FIGURE 63-37 *A.* Posteroanterior view of the left ventricular (LV) angiogram in a child with corrected transposition of the great arteries. The main pulmonary artery (MPA) arises from the smooth-walled left ventricle, which receives the systemic venous blood. *B.* Posteroanterior view of the right ventricular angiogram (RV). The ascending aorta (AO) arises to the left of the pulmonary artery from the more heavily trabeculated right ventricle, which receives the pulmonary venous blood. The ventricular septum, seen here perpendicular to the frontal plane, is intact.

the systemic venous or morphologic left ventricle, a QS pattern in the right and an RS pattern in the left precordial leads are usual.

Echocardiogram Using a segmental approach, two-dimensional echocardiography permits identification of the anatomic components and associated defects.[233]

Cardiac Catheterization When diagnostic catheterization is performed, the morphologic left ventricle is entered from the right atrium, and in the presence of a VSD, the catheter may cross the defect, traverse the morphologic right ventricle, and enter the ascending aorta in the position normally occupied by the pulmonary artery. Entry into the medially placed pulmonary artery may be much more difficult, but the use of flow-guided catheters permits successful entry for the measurement of pressure. Selective angiography in both ventricles will outline the defects. The ventricular septum usually lies in the anteroposterior plane, and frequently a VSD may be imaged best angiographically in the frontal view (Fig. 63-37). Gentle manipulation of the catheter within the heart is indicated, since the production of varying degrees of transient AV block is not uncommon, and in rare instances, the block may prove permanent.

NATURAL HISTORY AND PROGNOSIS

The clinical course is determined primarily by the severity of the associated defects. It is estimated that only about 1 percent of individuals with corrected transposition have an otherwise normal heart. Even with complicating anomalies, survival to adulthood is possible.[234] Congestive heart failure associated with a large VSD has been the most common cause of death, with most fatalities occurring within the first year of life. AV conduction abnormalities tend to be progressive, and complete AV block may appear at any age. Similarly, left AV valve regurgitation may present at any age and significantly alters the long-term outcome.[235] Finally, the morphologic right ventricle may not be capable of sustaining adequate cardiac output over a normal life span.[236]

MEDICAL MANAGEMENT

Management of corrected transposition includes the treatment of congestive failure, cyanosis, and AV block and the prevention of infective endocarditis. Patients with severe pulmonary hypertension or congestive heart failure should undergo early banding of the pulmonary artery or repair of the defect. Similarly, patients with a VSD, severe pulmonary stenosis, and cyanosis benefit from systemic-to-pulmonary artery shunting procedures or total correction. Those with a congenital block require prompt pacemaker therapy. Patients with significant left AV valve regurgitation require valve replacement. Regularly scheduled follow-up examinations are recommended for all these patients to detect progressive AV conduction disorders and the progression or late appearance of left AV valve incompetence. Antibiotic coverage as protection against infective endocarditis is recommended, as is the introduction of an afterload reducer at the first appearance of AV valve regurgitation.[237]

SURGICAL MANAGEMENT

The conventional approach has been correction of the underlying lesion, closure of the ventricular septal defect in those with an isolated VSD, and closure of the VSD and a conduit from the left (pulmonary) ventricle to the pulmonary artery in those with L-TGA, VSD, and PS.[238] Unfortunately, this approach frequently has led to suboptimal results because of a very high incidence of complete heart block, increasing left AV valve regurgitation, and right systemic ventricular dysfunction and heart failure.[235] Despite recent advances, operative mortality rates for VSD or VSD and pulmonary stenosis or atresia remain in the range of 4 to 15 percent with postoperative heart block in 14 to 33 percent.[239,240] The 10-year actual survival was 83 percent in one study[239] and 55 percent in the other.[240] Replacement of the regurgitant left AV valve at the first sign of progressive ventricular dysfunction has been recommended to preserve ventricular function but has been of limited utility.[241]

In view of the less than optimum results with the standard procedures, more innovative approaches have been suggested.[242] For those with a VSD in association with corrected transposition, an arterial switch can be performed and, since this would create complete transposition, an atrial switch as well. This "double-switch" procedure is clearly a much more complex operation but has the advantage of leaving the left ventricle as the systemic ventricle and leaving the problematic tricuspid valve on the right side of the heart.

For those with corrected transposition, a ventricular septal defect, and pulmonary stenosis, the VSD can be closed in a way that diverts the left ventricle into the aorta and the right ventricle via a conduit into the pulmonary artery. Since this also would create transposition physiology, one needs to do an atrial switch by Mustard's or Senning's technique. Although the early mortality for this approach is about 10 percent,[243,244] it is hoped and expected that the long-term results will be superior to those of the more conventional approach.

Single Ventricle

DEFINITION

The univentricular heart, or single ventricle, is characterized by the entire flow from the two atria being carried directly through the left and/or right AV valves into the single ventricular chamber. The double-inlet type of AV connection may take the form of either one common or two separate AV valves; straddling of one AV valve sometimes is included. The VA connections may be concordant (pulmonary artery from right ventricle and aorta from left ventricle), discordant (pulmonary artery from left ventricle and aorta from right ventricle), double-outlet (both great arteries from either the left or the right ventricle), or single-outlet (atresia of one great artery). Alternatively, one of the AV valves may be atretic. This is associated with normally related great vessels or transposition of the great arteries.

PATHOLOGY

A common type of single ventricle is associated with triscupid atresia in which the ventricle has the morphology of a left ventricle. There may be normally related great vessels (type I), D transposition of the great arteries (type II), or L transposition (type III). Depending on the size of the ventricular communication with the hypoplastic right ventricle, there may be pulmonary atresia (A), pulmonary stenosis (B), or no pulmonary stenosis (C).

In a large series,[245] about two-thirds were type I, and of these about two-thirds had pulmonary stenosis (I B). Among the one-third with transposition, the most common variety is without pulmonary outflow obstruction (II C). L transposition accounts for less than 5 percent in almost all series of children with tricuspid valve atresia.

When the mitral valve is severly stenotic or atretic, the left ventricle and aorta are usually hypoplastic or atretic (hypoplastic left heart syndrome). In this situation, it is the right ventricle that is the predominant ventricle. Depending on the severity of the left-sided hypoplasia, the ascending aorta and aortic arch are usually hypoplastic as well.

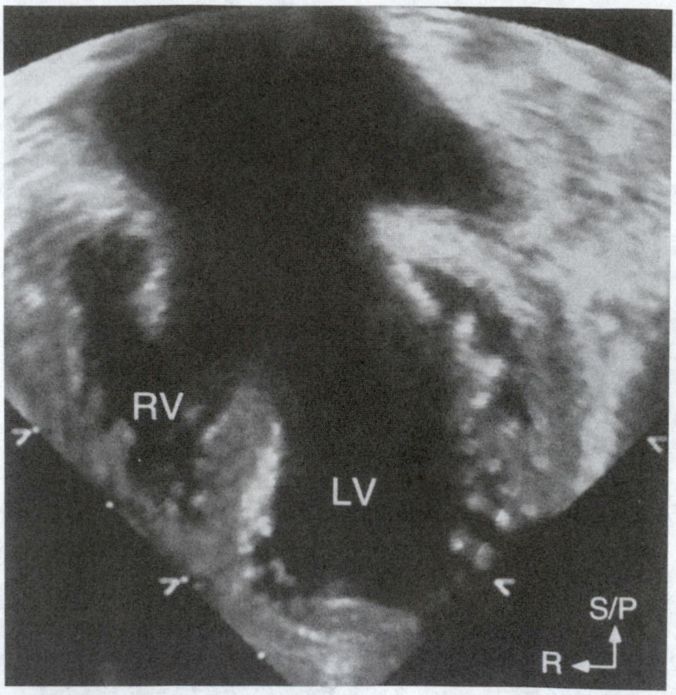

FIGURE 63-38 A malaligned atrioventricular canal with a large left ventricle (LV) and small right ventricle (RV). This would be repaired by a single ventricle approach (Fontan). (From Levine J and Geva T.[85] Reprinted with permission of the author and publisher.)

When there is one large atrioventricular valve or when both AV valves are present, the valve may straddle the ventricular septum, producing one large ventricle and one small ventricle (Fig. 63-38). The most common situation (65 to 70 percent of cases) is that in which the dominant ventricular chamber has the trabecular pattern of a left ventricle and communicates through an opening, the bulboventricular foramen, with a rudimentary right ventricle.[246] The VA connection is discordant (transposition of the great arteries) in about 90 percent of these patients. In about 20 percent of cases, the dominant ventricle shows the trabecular features of a right ventricle and the rudimentary chamber shows those of a left ventricle. The majority of these patients have a double-outlet VA connection from the main chamber, and a smaller number have a single-outlet connection with pulmonary atresia.[246] In 10 to 14 percent, neither ventricular sinus can be identified; this is the so-called primitive ventricle.

The term *Holmes' heart,* which is of historical interest, refers to a double-inlet left ventricle with situs solitus, normally related great arteries (SDS), an absent right ventricular sinus, and a subpulmonary infundibular outlet chamber communicating with the left ventricle via a restrictive bulboventricular foramen.[247]

ASSOCIATED CONDITIONS

Pulmonary stenosis or atresia is common. Subaortic stenosis and coarctation of the aorta occurs in association with L transposition and may result from a narrow bulboventricular foramen. In those with tricuspid or mitral atresia, an atrial communication is present.

CLINICAL MANIFESTATIONS

This complex and challenging malformation is relatively rare. The clinical picture is determined largely by the associated defects, among which pulmonary stenosis or atresia, which is present in a little over half of the patients, and obstruction to aortic flow are the most important.

All these patients have some degree of systemic hypoxemia because of mixing of the two sides of the circulation. If pulmonary stenosis or atresia is present, the presenting symptom is usually cyanosis. Without pulmonary stenosis, the presentation is usually congestive heart failure at 2 to 6 weeks of age as the pulmonary resistance falls. For those with subaortic stenosis and/or coarctation of the aorta, failure can occur within the first days of life as the ductus arteriosus closes. Physical examination depends on the combination of lesions present, but systolic ejection murmurs and a single second heart sound are very common.

Chest Roentgenogram Almost all these patients have at least some degree of cardiac enlargement. Those with little or no pulmonary stenosis generally have very large hearts with marked pulmonary plethora. Only patients with very severe pulmonary stenosis or atresia show a nearly normal heart size and diminished pulmonary arterial blood flow.

Electrocardiogram Evidence of right or left ventricular hypertrophy is common depending on which ventricle predominates.

Echocardiography Two-dimensional echocardiography with Doppler color flow studies can identify the morphologic and functional features of this malformation that are necessary to establish the diagnosis and formulate a plan for clinical management.[248]

Cardiac Catheterization A degree of systemic arterial oxygen desaturation is present in all these patients, although the severity appears to be related mainly to the volume of pulmonary blood flow. Careful recording of intracardiac and arterial pressures is essential to detect significant or potentially significant obstruction to blood flow across either AV valve, across the atrial septum, or between the ventricle and the aorta or pulmonary artery. The morphologic features of the ventricle, the relation of the aorta and the pulmonary artery, and other features can be established with high-quality selective ventricular angiography, using specially angled views to supplement conventional views.[249]

NATURAL HISTORY AND PROGNOSIS

Since by definition only one ventricle is "usable," treatment must be aimed at preserving the anatomy, physiology, and function to allow this single ventricle to support the circulation and establishing a method for systemic venous return to go to the lungs without a second pumping chamber.

These patients usually present as newborns with cyanosis, congestive failure, or a combination of both. Those in whom pulmonary arterial pressure and blood flow are increased require surgery to prevent death from congestive heart failure or progressive PVOD. Patients with severe pulmonary stenosis or atresia require systemic-to-pulmonary arterial shunting procedures. Among patients with univentricular heart, there is a propensity for the development of subaortic obstruction[250] and AV valve regurgitation.[251] Both threaten ventricular compliance and diminish the likelihood of successful long-term palliation.[252] Survivors are subject to the threats of infective endocarditis, brain abscess, and progressive PVOD.

MEDICAL MANAGEMENT

Early recognition and identification of patients with these complex defects are important so that successful palliative surgical procedures can be carried out for the relief of congestive failure or cyanosis. PGE_1 is useful in neonates with ductal-dependent defects.[91] An adequate interatrial communication is essential for those with mitral or tricuspid atresia. For those with pulmonary stenosis or atresia, a Blalock-Taussig shunt can be livesaving. Ventricular function and AV valvular competence are preserved by early creation of a bidirectional modified Glenn anastomosis (superior vena cava to undivided pulmonary artery).[253] Subaortic stenosis or obstruction at the bulboventricular foramen can be bypassed by anastomosis of the proximal pulmonary artery to the lateral aspect of the ascending aorta while pulmonary blood flow is delivered to the distal pulmonary arterial tree through a systemic arterial or systemic venous shunt.[254,255] Digitalis and diuretics may be necessary for patients with continuing heart failure. Care should be taken that anemia or severe polycythemia does not develop and that these patients are protected adequately against infective endocarditis. The pulmonary vascular bed must be protected and ventricular function and compliance must be preserved carefully if more definitive procedures are to be considered.

SURGICAL MANAGEMENT

Long-term palliation of children with a single ventricle is usually a three-stage approach: (1) initial palliation in the perinatal period, (2) a bidirectional Glenn at 6 to 18 months of age, and (3) a modified Fontan at 1 to 3 years of age. For complex problems, a heart transplant soon after birth has been suggested.[256]

Initial palliation for patients with univentricular AV connections requires adjustment of pulmonary blood flow with a pulmonary arterial band when it is excessive or the creation of a shunt when it is diminished. The modified Blalock-Taussig shunt is preferred in neonates. Relief of aortic stenosis and the creation of an adequate atrial communication frequently are necessary as well. The prognosis is affected adversely by a single ventricle of the right ventricular type[257] and the evolution of AV valvular regurgitation[258] or subaortic obstruction.[259]

Ventricular function and AV valvular competence are preserved by early creation of a bidirectional modified Glenn anastomosis, in which the superior vena cava is divided with the caudad portion patched closed; the cephalad portion is sutured to the top of the right pulmonary artery. If pulmonary atresia is not present, the main pulmonary artery is closed.[260] Subaortic stenosis or obstruction at the bulboventricular foramen can be palliated by anastomosis of the proximal pulmonary artery to the lateral aspect of the ascending aorta, while pulmonary blood flow is delivered to the distal pulmonary arterial tree through a systemic arterial or systemic venous shunt (the Damus-Kaye-Stansel operation). Other surgical options for the relief of subaortic obstruction are direct enlargement of the bulboventricular foramen (VSD), the modified Norwood operation,[255] and the arterial switch operation.[261]

Although initially some types of single ventricle were repaired by dividing the common chamber into the right and left ventricles, this has largely been abandoned because of unacceptably high initial mortality resulting from problems in connecting the ventricles to the appropriate great vessels without interfering with the atrioventricular valves and the high incidence of complete heart block.

The current approach is a modification of the principal suggested by Fontan and Baudet[262] to bypass the right side of the heart, directing systemic venous blood directly to the pulmonary arteries and allowing the single functioning ventricular chamber to pump blood to the systemic circulation. First, if it has not been done already, a bidirectional Glenn anastomosis is constructed (see above), and then an intraatrial tunnel is constructed to divert the inferior vena caval blood to the caudad portion of the superior vena cava, which then is connected to the underside of the right pulmonary artery (Fig. 63-39). A fenestration in the baffle sometimes is used to decompress the right side in the perioperative period. Recently, instead of tunnelling within the atrium, an external conduit has been used between the inferior vena cava (IVC) and the right pulmonary artery ligating the IVC–right atrial junction. The single ventricle is thus relieved of the burden of the volume overload and ventricular hypertrophy required to maintain the pulmonary circulation and is asked only to deliver systemic cardiac output.[262]

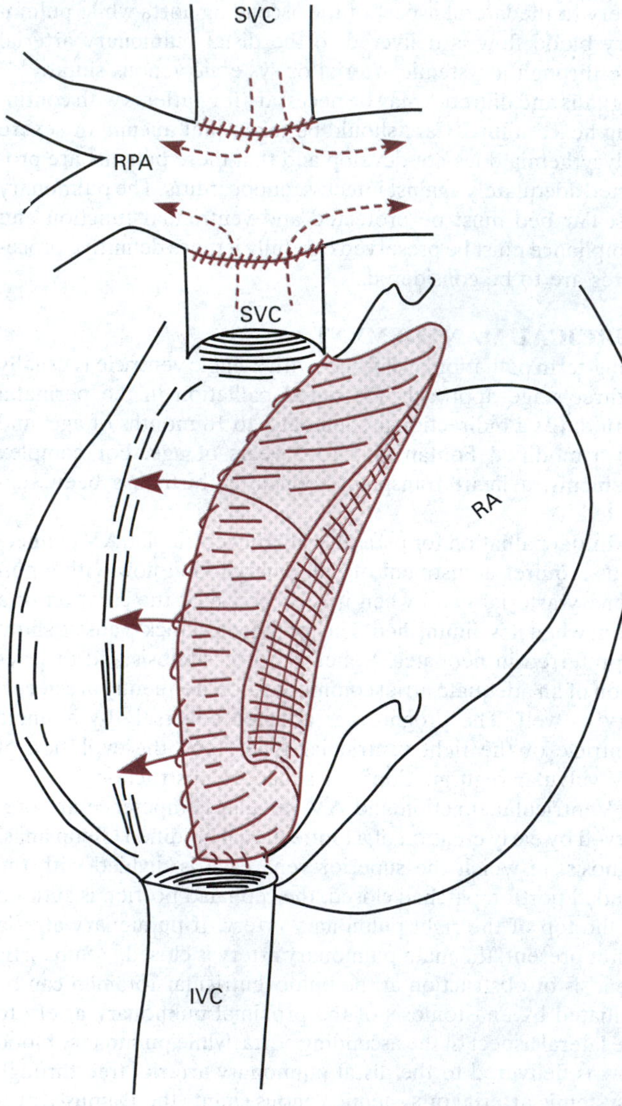

FIGURE 63-39 The modified Fontan operation. The superior vena cava (SVC) is divided. The cephalad portion is anastomosed to the superior aspect of the right pulmonary artery (RPA), and an intraatrial baffle is constructed from the inferior vena cava (IVC) to the superior vena cava along the lateral wall of the right atrium (RA). The caudad portion of the SVC then is connected to the inferior aspect of the right pulmonary artery.

The surgical risks depend on patient selection. For those with complex forms of single ventricle and those with elevated pulmonary pressure or resistance, ventricular dysfunction, or atrioventricular valve regurgitation, the risks are increased. For those without risk factors and with tricuspid atresia or double-inlet left ventricle, the risks are less than 5 percent.[263] Even for those with some risk factors or with more complex disease, at some centers the mortality is under 10 percent.[263,264]

For children with hypoplastic left heart syndrome, the survival from the three-stage procedure (initial Norwood, bidirectional Glenn, and Fontan) is approximately 50 percent,[265] although some centers are reporting a survival rate as high as 76 percent.[266] There does not seem to be any significant difference in survival in centers that use the three-stage anatomic "repair" from primary heart transplantation in the perinatal period at 36 months of age.[265]

Quality and length of life are clearly improved, but persistent problems (AV valvular regurgitation, systemic embolization, limitation of exercise tolerance, protein-losing enteropathy, atrial arrhythmias, and deterioration of ventricular function) occur with a frequency of about 1 percent per year.[263] For patients with progressive deterioration, cardiac transplantation is recommended.

CONGENITAL ABNORMALITIES OF THE CORONARY ARTERIAL CIRCULATION

Coronary Arteriovenous Fistula

PATHOLOGY

A coronary arteriovenous fistula is a fistulous communication between a coronary artery and a cardiac chamber, the coronary sinus, or the pulmonary trunk (Fig. 63-40).

The site of origin may involve any of the epicardial coronary arteries. *The right coronary artery is the site of origin in somewhat over half the cases, and the two most common sites into which the fistula feeds are a cardiac vein (usually the coronary sinus) and the right ventricle.* Although solitary communication is the rule, there may be multiple sites of termination. A fistula into the pulmonary trunk usually is characterized by one or more vessels opening into the pulmonary trunk and connecting with branches of each of the two main coronary arteries. The artery or arteries feeding the fistula are grossly enlarged and tortuous. Saccular aneurysms may develop in segments of dilated vessels; such aneurysms usually are observed in adults and frequently show calcification of the wall.

CLINICAL MANIFESTATIONS

Many patients with a coronary arteriovenous fistula are asymptomatic.[267,268] In some, the magnitude of the shunt into the right side of the heart is great enough to cause congestive heart

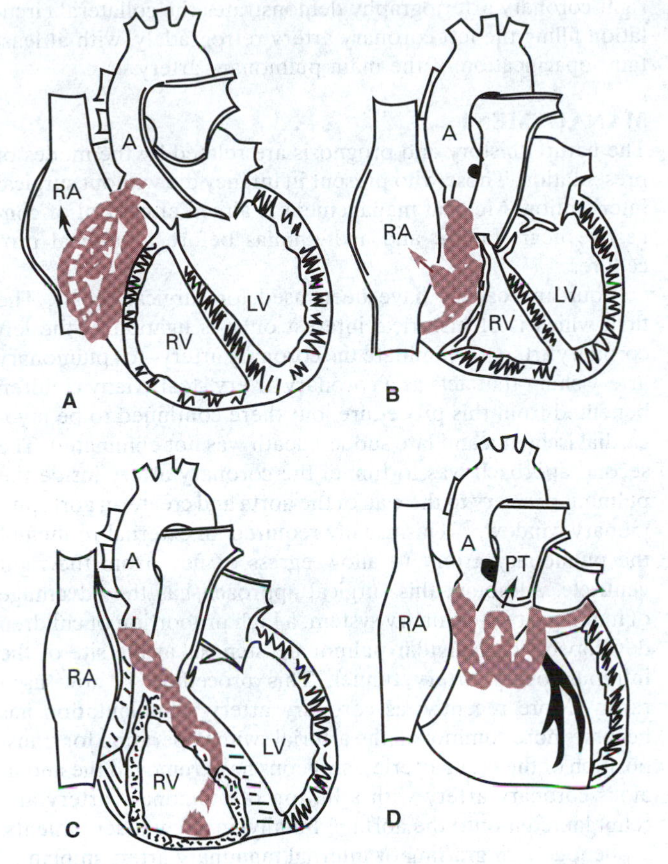

FIGURE 63-40 Anomalous communications of coronary arteries. *A.* Right coronary artery communicates with coronary sinus. *B.* Right coronary artery communicates with right atrium (RA). *C.* Anomalous communication of right coronary artery with right ventricle (RV). *D.* Two coronary arteries arise from the aorta (A) and make collateral communication with accessory coronary artery arising from pulmonary trunk (PT). LV = left ventricle.

failure, with a tendency for this to occur in early infancy or after 40 years of age. The classic finding is that of a continuous murmur with an unusual location, since it is loudest over the fistula. It may have a louder diastolic component, especially if communication is with the right ventricle. In those with large shunts, there may be cardiomegaly and increased pulmonary flow shown by chest roentgenography and right ventricular hypertrophy shown by ECG. Transthoracic echocardiography is usually diagnostic in children;[269] transesophageal studies may be necessary in adults. At cardiac catheterization, an increase in oxygen saturation may be encountered, usually in the right atrium or right ventricle, if the shunt is large enough. Selective coronary arteriography will demonstrate the involved coronary artery and the site of entry of the fistula. The most common complication is infective endocarditis, but thrombosis, myocardial ischemia, and rupture may occur.

SURGICAL MANAGEMENT

Except for very small fistulas, closure is recommended, since the flow tends to increase with age and these patients are at risk for infective endocarditis, congestive heart failure, and myocardial ischemia. Until relatively recently, closure was invariably surgical. Occasionally, closure was done without a coronary bypass by placing obliterating mattress sutures across the fistula beneath the coronary artery as it passes over the surface of the heart.[270] More commonly, cardiopulmonary bypass is preferred for safe exposure of large or multiple fistulas, such as those entering the right atrium near the junction of the superior vena cava and the right atrium, those arising from the artery to the sinoatrial node, and those between the left coronary artery and the left ventricle.[271] The orifice of the fistula is obliterated by direct suture or the placement of a Dacron or pericardial patch. Fistulas have been closed from within the open coronary artery; the artery then is repaired by direct suturing. Surgical mortality should be minimal;[271] the long-term results have been favorable.[272]

Fistulas have been closed by interventional catheterization techniques. Perry and associates[273] attempted to close fistulas in nine patients: four from the left circumflex artery, three from the left anterior descending artery, and two from the right coronary artery. Gianturco coils were used in six patients and a double-umbrella in two, with coils and an umbrella used in one. All were completely occluded. In three patients with multiple fistulas, no attempt was made in the catheterization laboratory and the patients were referred for surgery. This "noninvasive" technique seems to be applicable to some children and adults with coronary AV fistulas, although long-term follow-up is necessary to be certain that the fistulas do not recur.

Origin of the Left Coronary Artery from the Pulmonary Artery

PATHOLOGY AND PATHOPHYSIOLOGY

In this anomaly, the left coronary artery arises from the pulmonary artery rather than from the aorta (Fig. 63-41). In the perina-

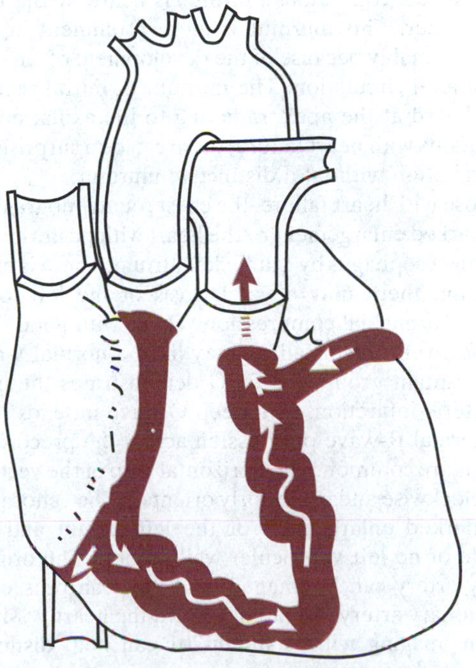

FIGURE 63-41 Anomalous origin of the left coronary artery from the pulmonary trunk. With time, wide collaterals develop between the two coronary systems so that right coronary arterial blood is shunted into the left coronary system and thence into the pulmonary trunk.

tal period, the pulmonary artery pressure is high and the left coronary is perfused with venous blood. Problems arise when the pulmonary resistance and pulmonary artery pressure fall and the diastolic pressure is insufficient to perfuse the left ventricular myocardium. In the absence of collateral vessels from the right coronary, left ventricular ischemia and eventually infarction of the left ventricular wall and papillary muscles occur. This in turn leads to congestive heart failure, usually by 3 to 8 weeks of age.

In a small group of children, extensive collaterals between the right coronary (arising normally from the aorta) and the left system develop. Perfusion via the right may be sufficient to oxygenate the left ventricular myocardium so that no ischemia develops. Over time, the higher perfusion pressure in the aorta may allow a left-to-right shunt into the pulmonary artery through the right and then the left coronary system. Eventually this may lead to a "steal" of blood from the myocardium into the lower-resistance pulmonary circuit.

CLINICAL MANIFESTATIONS

The clinical spectrum and mode of presentation in patients with this abnormality vary.[274,275] The majority of these patients present at 6 to 12 weeks of age. Acute episodes of irritability, profuse cold sweating, pallor (? angina), and respiratory distress occur, with evidence of heart failure. Less often, these patients present at an older age with mitral regurgitation and heart failure. A few reach adolescence or adulthood with no or relatively few symptoms other than occasional exertional angina or palpitations. Sudden death may be the first and only sign of this condition.

On physical examination, the heart is enlarged, with an abnormal left ventricular apex impulse. Other signs of failure are usually present. Pallor and clammy skin are common. In some patients, a soft continuous murmur is heard at the upper left sternal border. This murmur is more prominent in older patients, presumably because of the development of a more extensive collateral circulation. The murmur of mitral regurgitation may be heard at the apex, radiating to the axilla; however, in young infants with heart failure, there can be a surprising degree of regurgitation without a distinctive murmur.

In those with heart failure, the chest roentgenogram typically shows marked enlargement of the heart with posterior displacement of the esophagus by a large left atrium. There is pulmonary edema, and there may be atelectasis of the left lower lobe because of bronchial compression. Those with good collaterals and no left ventricular failure may have a normal x-ray.

In the infant group, the ECG demonstrates the pattern of anterolateral infarction, with deep Q wave in leads I and aVL and abnormal R-wave progression across the precordium. Arrhythmias are common. The horizontal loop of the vectorcardiogram is clockwise and posteriorly oriented. The echocardiogram shows marked enlargement of the left atrium and ventricle with little or no left ventricular wall motion. The origin of the coronary artery can be imaged, and flow can be seen toward the pulmonary artery instead of toward the heart.[276] Myocardial perfusion imaging with thallium-201 can help distinguish an anomalous coronary artery from congestive cardiomyopathy.[277]

At cardiac catheterization, there may be an increase in saturation in the pulmonary artery if there is enough retrograde flow. There is usually some pulmonary hypertension, with very elevated pulmonary wedge pressure. Aortography or selective right coronary arteriography demonstrates the collateral circulation filling the left coronary artery retrogradely, with at least faint opacification of the main pulmonary artery.

MANAGEMENT

The natural history and prognosis are related by the modes of presentation. Those who present in infancy die without surgical intervention. Medical management is aimed at control of congestive heart failure and arrhythmias before a surgical procedure.

Four approaches have been used for surgical repair. The first, which is of historical interest only, is ligation of the left coronary artery to eliminate the coronary artery–to–pulmonary artery shunt that acts as a coronary artery steal. Many children benefited from this procedure, but there continued to be myocardial ischemia and late sudden death was not eliminated. The second approach was to tunnel the coronary artery inside the pulmonary artery to the wall of the aorta and create an aortopulmonary window.[278] This usually required an external roofing of the pulmonary artery to allow egress of flow from the right ventricle. Although this surgical approach has the advantage of making a two-coronary system, a high proportion of children developed supravalvular pulmonary stenosis at the site of the intrapulmonary artery tunnel. This procedure is now used rarely. More recently, as coronary artery reimplantation has become more common in the arterial switch operation for transposition of the great arteries, surgeons have removed the anomalous coronary artery with a button of pulmonary artery and reimplanted it onto the aorta.[279] Finally, in a few older patients, saphenous vein grafting or internal mammary artery implantation has been used.[280]

The late results after surgery have been quite good.[279,281] The congestive heart failure frequently improves, the heart becomes smaller, the left ventricular shortening fraction improves, and mitral regurgitation tends to regress. Interestingly, the infarction pattern on ECG with deep anterolateral Q waves frequently disappears, suggesting that the poor function is due to extreme ischemia rather than infarction (hybernating myocardium).[282]

References

1. Mitchell SC, Korones SB, Berendes HW. Congenital heart disease in 56,109 births: Incidence and natural history. *Circulation* 1971; 43:323–332.
2. Hoffman JIE, Christianson R. Congenital heart disease in a cohort of 19,502 births with long-term follow-up. *Am J Cardiol* 1978; 42:641–647.
3. Fyler DC. Report of the New England Regional Infant Cardiac Program. *Pediatrics* 1980; 65:II375–II461.
4. Perry LW, Neill CA, Ferencz C, et al. Infants with congenital heart disease: The cases. In: Ferencz C, Rubin JD, Loffredo CA, Magee CA, eds. *Epidemiology of Congenital Heart Disease: The Baltimore-Washington Infant Heart Study 1981–1989.* Mount Kisco, NY: Futura; 1993:33–61.
5. Fyler DC, ed. *Nadas' Pediatric Cardiology.* Philadelphia: Hanley & Belfus; 1992:273.
6. Keith JD. Prevalence, incidence and epidemiology. In: Keith JD, Rowe RD, Vlad P, eds. *Heart Disease in Infancy and Childhood,* 3d ed. New York: Macmillan; 1978:3.
7. Nora JJ. Causes of CHD—old and new modes, mechanisms and models. *Am Heart J* 1993; 125:1409–1418.
8. Belmont JW. Recent progress in the molecular genetics of congenital heart defects. *Clin Genet* 1998; 54:11–9.

9. Hall JG. Catch 22. *J Med Genet* 1993; 30:801–802.
10. Dawes GS. *Foetal and Neonatal Physiology: A Comparative Study of the Changes at Birth.* Chicago: Year Book; 1968:90.
11. Lind J, Wegelius C. Human fetal circulation: Changes in the cardiovascular system at birth and disturbances in the postnatal closure of the foramen ovale and ductus arteriosus: Cold Spring Harbor Symposium. *Quant Biol* 1954; 19:109–125.
12. Rudolph AM, Heymann MA. The circulation of the fetus in utero. *Circ Res* 1967; 21:163–184.
13. Rudolph AM, Heymann MA. Circulatory changes with growth in the fetal lamb. *Circ Res* 1970; 26:289–299.
14. Rudolph AM, Heymann MA. Cardiac output in the fetal lamb: The effects of spontaneous and induced changes of heart rate on right and left ventricular output. *J Obstet Gynecol* 1976; 124:183–192.
15. Teitel DF, Iwamoto HS, Rudolph AM. Effects of birth-related events on central flow patterns. *Pediatr Res* 1987; 22:557–566.
16. Coceani F, Olley PM. Role of prostaglandins, prostacyclin, and thromboxanes in the control of prenatal patency and postnatal closure of the ductus arteriosus. In: Heymann MA, ed. *Prostaglandins in the Perinatal Period.* New York: Grune & Stratton; 1980:109.
17. Rudolph AM. Fetal and neonatal pulmonary circulation. *Annu Rev Physiol* 1979; 41:383–395.
18. Fineman JR, Soifer SJ, Heymann MA. Regulation of vascular tone in the perinatal period. *Annu Rev Physiol* 1995; 57:115–134.
19. Heymann MA, Rudolph AM. Effects of congenital heart disease on fetal and neonatal circulations. *Prog Cardiovasc Dis* 1972; 15:115–143.
20. Levin DL, Heymann MA, Kitterman JA, et al. Persistent pulmonary hypertension in the newborn infant. *J Pediatr* 1976; 89: 626–630.
21. Fox WW, Duara S. Persistent pulmonary hypertension in the neonate: Diagnosis and management. *J Pediatr* 1983; 103: 505–514.
22. Kinsella JP, Abman SH. Recent developments in inhaled nitric oxide therapy of the newborn. *Curr Opini Pediatr* 1999: 11:121–125.
23. UK Collaborative randomized trial of neonatal extracorporeal membrane oxygenation: UK Collaborative ECMO Trial Group. *Lancet* 1996: 348:75–82.
24. Talner NS. Heart failure. In: Emmanouilides GC, Riemenschneider TA, Gutgesell HP, eds. *Moss and Adams Heart Disease in Infants, Children, and Adolescents Including the Fetus and Young Adult,* 5th ed. Baltimore: Williams & Wilkins; 1995:1746.
25. Seguchi M, Nakazawa M, Momma K. Effect of enalapril on infants and children with congestive heart failure. *Cardiol Young* 1992; 2:14–19.
26. Fischbein CA, Rosenthal A, Fischer EG, et al. Risk factors of brain abscess in patients with congenital heart disease. *Am J Cardiol* 1974; 34:97–102.
27. Phornphutkul C, Rosenthal A, Nadas AS, Berenberg W. Cerebrovascular accidents in infants and children with cyanotic congenital heart disease. *Am J Cardiol* 1973; 32:329–334.
28. Beekman RH, Tuuri DT. Acute hemodynamic effects of increasing hemoglobin concentration in children with a right to left ventricular shunt and relative anemia. *J Am Coll Cardiol* 1985; 5:357–362.
29. Gidding SS, Stockman JA III. Effect of iron deficiency on tissue oxygen delivery in cyanotic congenital heart disease. *Am J Cardiol* 1988; 61:605–607.
30. Ross EA, Perloff JK, Danovitch GM, et al. Renal function and urate metabolism in late survivors with cyanotic congenital heart disease. *Circulation* 1986; 73:396–400.
31. Henriksson P, Varendh G, Lundstrom NR. Haemostatic defects in cyanotic congenital heart disease. *Br Heart J* 1979; 41:23–27.
32. Waldman JD, Czapek EE, Paul MH, et al. Shortened platelet survival in cyanotic heart disease. *J Pediatr* 1975; 87:77–79.
33. Territo MC, Rosove MH, Perloff JK. Cyanotic congenital heart disease: Hematologic management, renal function, and urate metabolism. In: Perloff JK, Child JS, eds. *Congenital Heart Disease in Adults.* Philadelphia: Saunders; 1991:93.
34. Aram DM, Ekelman BL, Ben Shachar G, Levinsohn MW. Intelligence and hypoxemia in children with congenital heart disease: Fact or artifact? *Am J Coll Cardiol* 1985; 6:889–893.
35. Cameron JW, Rosenthal A, Olson AD. Malnutrition in hospitalized children with congenital heart disease. *Arch Pediatr Adolesc Med* 1995; 149:1098–1102.
36. Schuurmans FM, Pulles-Heintzberger CF, Gerver WJ, et al. Longterm growth of children with congenital heart disease: A retrospect study. *Acta Paediatr* 1998; 87:1250–1255.
37. Rabinovitch M. Pathophysiology of pulmonary hypertension. In: Emmanouilides GC, Riemenschneider TA, Allen HD, Gutgesell HP, eds. *Moss and Adams Heart Disease in Infants, Children, and Adolescents,* 5th ed. Baltimore: Williams & Wilkins; 1995: 1659.
38. Heath D, Edwards JE. The pathology of hypertensive pulmonary vascular disease: A description of six grades of structural changes in the pulmonary arteries with special reference to congenital cardiac septal defects. *Circulation* 1958; 18:533.
39. Turanlahti MI, Laitinen PO, Sarna SJ, Pesonen E. Nitric oxide, oxygen and prostacyclin in children with pulmonary hypertension. *Heart* 1998; 79:169–174.
40. Nihill MR. Clinical management of patients with pulmonary hypertension. In: Emmanouilides GC, Riemenschneider TA, Allen HD, Gutgesell HP, eds. *Moss and Adams Heart Disease in Infants, Children, and Adolescents,* 5th ed. Baltimore: Williams & Wilkins; 1995:1695.
41. Gersony WM. Long-term follow-up of operated congenital heart disease. *Cardiol Clin* 1989; 7:915–923.
42. Freed MD. Infective endocarditis in the adult with congenital heart disease. *Cardiol Clin* 1993; 11:589–602.
43. Morris CD, Reller MD, Menashe VD. Thirty year incidence of infective endocarditis after surgery for congenital heart defect. *JAMA* 1998; 279:599–603.
44. Keane JF, Driscoll DJ, Gersony WM. Second Natural History Study of Congenital Heart Defects: Results of treatment of patients with aortic valvar stenosis. *Circulation* 1993; 87 (suppl):I16–I27.
45. Hart EM, Garson A Jr. Psychosocial concerns of adults with congenital heart disease: Employability and insurability. *Cardiac Clin* 1993; 11:711–715.
46. Schmaltz AA, Neudorf U, Winkler UH. Outcome of pregnancy in women with congenital heart disease. *Cardiol Young* 1999; 9:88–96.
47. Strong WB. Introduction: Pediatric cardiology exercise testing. *Pediatri Cardiol* 1999; 20:1–3.
48. Chandar JS, Wolff GS, Garson A Jr, et al. Ventricular arrhythmias in postoperative tetralogy of Fallot. *Am J Cardiol* 1990; 65:655–661.
49. Gelatt M, Hamilton RM, McCrindle BW, et al. Arrhythmia and mortality after the Mustard procedure: A 30-year single-center experience. *J Am Coll Cardiol* 1997; 29:194–201.
50. Fishberger SB, Wernovsky G, Gentiles TL, et al. Factors that influence the development of atrial flutter after the Fontan operation. *J Thorac Cardiovasc Surg* 1997; 113:80–86.
51. Moreau GA, Graham TP Jr. Clinical assessment of ventricular function after surgical treatment of congenital heart defects. *Cardiol Clin* 1989; 7:439–452.
52. Turina MI, Siebenmann R, von Segesser L, et al. Late functional deterioration after atrial correction for transposition of the great arteries. *Circulation* 1989; 80:I162–I167.
53. Mertens L, Hagler DJ, Sauer U, et al. Protein-losing enteropathy

after the Fontan operation: An international multicenter study: PLE study group. *J Thorac Cardiovasc Surg* 1998; 115:1063–1073.
54. Graham TP, Gutgesell HP. Ventricular septal defects. In: Emmanouilides GC, Riemenschneider TA, Allen HD, Gutgesell HP, eds. *Moss and Adams Heart Disease in Infants, Children, and Adolescents,* 5th ed. Baltimore: Williams & Wilkins; 1995:724.
55. Alpert BS, Cook DH, Varghese PJ, Rowe RD. Spontaneous closure of small ventricular septal defects: Ten-year follow-up. *Pediatrics* 1979; 63:204–206.
56. Trowitzsch E, Braun W, Stute M, Pielmeier W. Diagnosis, therapy, and outcome of ventricular septal defects in the 1st year of life: A two-dimensional colour-Doppler echocardiography study. *Eur J Pediatr* 1990; 149:758–761.
57. Weidman WH, Blount SG Jr, DuShane JW, et al. Clinical course in ventricular septal defect. *Circulation* 1977; 56:I156–I169.
58. Rhodes L, Keane JF, Keane JP, et al. Long follow-up (to 43 years) of ventricular septal defect with audible aortic regurgitation. *Am J Cardiol* 1990; 66:340–345.
59. Gersony WM, Hayes CJ. Bacterial endocarditis in patients with pulmonary stenosis, aortic stenosis or ventricular septal defect. *Circulation* 1977; 56:I84–I87.
60. Gersony WM, Hayes CJ, Driscoll DJ, et al. Bacterial endocarditis in patients with aortic stenosis, pulmonary stenosis or ventricular septal defect. *Circulation* 1993; 87(suppl I):I121–I126.
61. Driscoll DJ, Michels VV, Gersony WM, et al. Occurrence risk for congenital heart defects in relatives of patients with aortic stenosis, pulmonary stenosis, or ventricular septal defect. *Circulation* 1993; 87(suppl I):I114–I120.
62. Casteneda AR, Jonas RA, Mayer JE, Hanley FL. *Cardiac Surgery of the Neonate and Infant.* Philadelphia: Saunders; 1994:187–203.
63. Moller JH, Patton C, Varco RL, Lillchei CW. Late results (30–35 years) after operative closure of isolated ventricular septal defect from 1954–1960. *Am J Cardiol* 1991; 68:1491–1497.
64. Rocchini A, Lock JE. Defect closure: Umbrella devices. In: Lock JE, Keane JF, Perry SB, eds. *Diagnostic and Interventional Catheterization in Congenital Heart Disease.* Boston: Kluwer; 2000:179.
65. Lewis FJ, Winchell P, Bashour FA. Open repair of atrial septal defects: Results in sixty-three patients. *JAMA* 1957; 165:922.
66. Edwards JE. Classification of congenital heart disease in the adult. In: Roberts WC, ed. *Congenital Heart Disease in Adults.* Philadelphia: Davis; 1979:1.
67. Mahoney LT, Truesdell SC, Krzmarzick TR, Lauer RM. Atrial septal defects that present in infancy. *Am J Dis Child* 1986; 140:1115–1118.
68. Benson DW, Sharkey A, Fatkin D, et al. Reduced penetrance, variable expressivity, and genetic heterogeneity of familial atrial septal defects. *Circulation* 1998; 97:2043–2048.
69. Murphy JG, Gersh BJ, McGoon MD, et al. Long-term outcome after surgical repair of isolated atrial septal defect: Follow-up at 27–32 years. *N Engl J Med* 1990; 323:1645–1650.
70. Seward JB, Tajik AJ. Transesophageal echocardiography in congenital heart disease. *Am J Cardiol Imaging* 1990; 4:215–222.
71. Dall'Agata A, McGhie J, Taams MA, et al. Secundum atrial septal defect is a dynamic three dimensional entity. *Am Heart J* 1999; 137:1075–1086
72. Hamilton WT, Hattajee CE, Dalen JE, et al. Atrial septal defect secundum: Clinical profile with physiologic correlates. In: Roberts WC, ed. *Adult Congenital Heart Disease.* Philadelphia: Davis; 1987:395.
73. Steele PM, Fuster V, Cohen M, et al. Isolated atrial septal defect with pulmonary vascular obstructive disease, long-term follow-up and prediction of outcome after surgical correction. *Circulation* 1987; 76:1037–1042.
74. Prieto LR, Foreman CK, Cheatham JP, Latson LA. Intermediate-term outcome of transcatheter secundum atrial septal defect closure using the Bard Clamshell Septal Umbrella. *Am J Cardiol* 1996; 78:1310–1312.
75. Masura J, Lange PE, Wilkinson JL, et al. US/International multicenter trial of atrial septal catheter closure using the Amplatzer Septal Occluder: Initial results (abstract). *Am J Card* 1998; 31(supplement A):57A.
76. Zamora R, Rao PS, Lloyd TR, et al. Intermediate-term results of Phase I Food and Drug Administration Trials of buttoned device occlusion of secundum atrial septal defects. *J Am Coll Cardiol* 1998; 31:674–676.
77. St. John-Sutton MG, Tajik AJ, McGoon DC. Atrial septal defect in patients ages 60 years or older: Operative results and long-term postoperative follow-up. *Circulation* 1981; 64:402–409.
78. Healy JE Jr. An anatomic survey of anomalous pulmonary veins: Their clinical significance. *J Thorac Cardiovasc Surg* 1952; 23:433–444.
79. Silverman NH. Anomalous pulmonary venous connections. In: Silverman NH, ed. *Pediatric Echocardiography.* New York: Williams & Wilkins; 1993:179.
80. Saalouke MG, Shapiro SR, Perry LW, Scott LP III. Isolated partial anomalous pulmonary venous drainage associated with pulmonary vascular obstructive disease. *Am J Cardiol* 1977; 39:439–444.
81. Rogers HM, Edwards JE. Incomplete division of the atrioventricular canal with patent interatrial foramen primum (persistent common cardioventricular ostium): Report of five cases and review of the literature. *Am Heart J* 1948; 36:28.
82. Rastelli GC, Ongley PA, Kirklin JW, McGoon DC. Surgical repair of the complete form of persistent common atrioventricular canal. *J Thorac Cardiovasc Surg* 1968; 55:299–308.
83. Rose V, Izukawa T, Moes CA. Syndromes of asplenia and polysplenia: A review of cardiac and non-cardiac malformations in 60 cases with special reference to diagnosis and prognosis. *Br Heart J* 1975; 37:840–852.
84. Lacro RV. Dysmorphology. In: Fyler DC, ed. *Nadas' Pediatric Cardiology.* Philadelphia: Hanley & Belfus; 1992:37.
85. Levine J, Geva T. Echocardiographic assessment of common atrioventricular canal. *Prog Pediatr Cardiol* 1999; 10:137–151.
86. Nora JJ, Nora AH. Maternal transmission of congenital heart diseases: New recurrence risk figures and the questions of cytoplasmic inheritance and vulnerability to teratogens. *Am J Cardiol* 1987; 59:459–463.
87. Kirklin JW, Barratt-Boyes BG. Atrioventricular canal defect. In: Kirklin JW, Barratt-Boyes BG, eds. *Cardiac Surgery,* 2d ed. New York: Churchill Livingstone; 1993:693.
88. Hanley FL, Fenton KN, Jonas RA, et al. Surgical repair of complete atrioventricular canal defects in infancy: Twenty-year trends. *J Thorac Cardiovasc Surg* 1993; 106:387–397.
89. Alexi-Meskishvili V, Ishino K, Dahnert I, et al. Correction of complete atrioventricular septal defects with the double-patch technique and cleft closure. *Ann Thorac Surg* 1996; 62:519–525.
90. Daebritz S, del Nido PJ. Surgical management of common atrioventricular canal. *Prog Pediatri Cardiol* 1999; 10:161–171.
91. Freed MD, Heymann MA, Lewis AB, et al. Prostaglandin E-1 in infants with ductus arteriosus-dependent congenital heart disease. *Circulation* 1981; 64:899–905.
92. Gersony WM, Peckham GJ, Ellison RC, et al. Effects of indomethacin in premature infants with patent ductus arteriosus: Results of a national collaborative study. *J Pediatr* 1983; 102: 895–906.
93. Siassi B, Blanco C, Cabal LA, Coran AG. Incidence and clinical features of patent ductus arteriosus in low-birthweight infants: A prospective analysis of 150 consecutively born infants. *Pediatrics* 1976; 57:347–351.
94. Varvarigou A, Bardin CL, Beharry K, et al. Early ibuprofen administration to prevent patent ductus arteriosus in premature newborn infants. *JAMA* 1996; 275:539–544.
95. Castaneda AR, Jonas RA, Mayer JE, Hanley FL. *Cardiac Surgery of the Neonate and Infant.* Philadelphia: Saunders; 1994:203.

96. Satur CR, Walker DR, Dickinson DF. Day case ligation of patent ductus arteriosus in preterm infants: A 10-year review. *Arch Dis Child* 1991; 66:477–480.
97. Bell Thomson J, Jewell E, Ellis FH Jr, Schwaber JR. Surgical technique in the management of patent ductus arteriosus in the elderly patient. *Ann Thorac Surg* 1990; 30:80–83.
98. Laborde F, Folligvet T, Batisse A, et al. Video-assisted thoracoscopic surgical interruption: The technique of choice for patent ductus arteriosus. *J Thorac Cardiovasc Surg* 1995; 110:1681–1685.
99. Burke RP, Wernovsky G, van der Velde M, et al. Video-assisted thorascopic surgery for congenital heart disease. *J Thorac Cardiovasc Surg* 1995; 109:499–507.
100. Portsmann W, Wierny L. Percutaneous transfemoral closure of the patent ductus arteriosus: An alternative to surgery. *Semin Roentgenol* 1981; 16:95–102.
101. Rashkind WJ, Cuaso CC. Transcatheter closure of patent ductus arteriosus. *Pediatr Cardiol* 1979; 1:3–7.
102. Shim D, Fedderly RT, Beekman RH III, et al. Follow-up of coil occlusion of patent ductus arteriosis. *J Am Coll Cardio* 1996; 28:207–211.
103. Sakakibara S, Konno S. Congenital aneurysm of the sinus of Valsalva: Anatomy and classification. *Am Heart J* 1962; 63: 405–424.
104. Takach TJ, Reul GJ, Duncan JM, et al. Sinus of Valsalva aneurysm or fistula: Management and outcome. *Ann Thorac Surg* 1999; 68:1573–1577.
105. Shaffer EM, Snider AR, Beekman RH, et al. Sinus of Valsalva aneurysm complicating bacterial endocarditis in an infant: Diagnosis with two-dimensional and Doppler echocardiography. *J Am Coll Cardiol* 1987; 9:588–591.
106. Clagett OT, Kirklin JW, Edwards JE. Anatomic variations and pathologic changes in 124 cases of coarctation of the aorta. *Surg Gynecol Obstet* 1954; 98:103.
107. Bharati S, Lev M. The surgical anatomy of the heart in tubular hypoplasia of the transverse aorta (preductal coarctation). *J Thorac Cardiovasc Surg* 1986; 91:79–85.
108. Gardiner HM, Celermajer DS, Sorensen KE, et al. Arterial reactivity is significantly impaired in normotensive young adults after successful repair of aortic coarctation in childhood. *Circulation* 1994; 89:1745–1750.
109. Beekman RH. Coarctation of the aorta. In: Emmanouilides GC, Riemenschneider TA, Allen HD, Gutgesell HP, eds. *Moss and Adams Heart Disease in Infants, Children, and Adolescents,* 5th ed. Baltimore: Williams & Wilkins; 1995:1111.
110. Ing FF, Starc TJ, Griffiths SP, Gersony WM. Early diagnosis of coarctation of the aorta in children: A continuing dilemma. *Pediatrics* 1996; 98:378–382.
111. Campbell M. Natural history of coarctation of the aorta. *Br Heart J* 1970; 32:633–640.
112. Fletcher SE, Nihill MR, Grifka RG, et al. Balloon angioplasty of native coarctation of the aorta: Mid-term follow-up and prognostic factors. *J Am Coll Cardio* 1995; 25:730–734.
113. Zehr KJ, Gillinov AM, Redmond JM, et al. Repair of coarctation of the aorta in neonates and infants: A thirty-year experience. *Ann Thorac Surg* 1995; 59:33–41.
114. Kreutzer J, Perry SB. Stents. In Lock JE, Keane JF, Perry SB, eds. *Diagnostic and Interventional Catheterization in Congenital Heart Disease*, 2d ed. Boston, Kluwer; 2000:221.
115. Parks WJ, Ngo TD, Plauth WH, et al. Incidence of aneurysm formation after Dacron patch aortoplasty repair for coarctation of the aorta: Long-term results and assessment utilizing magnetic resonance angiography with three-dimensional surface rendering. *J Am Coll Cardiol* 1995; 26:266–271.
116. Kirklin JW, Barratt-Boyes BG. Coarctation of the aorta and interrupted aortic arch. In: Kirklin JW, Barratt Boyes BJ, eds. *Cardiac Surgery,* 2d ed. New York: Churchill Livingstone; 1993:1263.
117. Quaegebeur JM, Jonas RA, Weinberg AD, et al. Outcomes in seriously ill neonates with coarctation of the aorta: A multi-institutional study. *J Thorac Cardiovasc Surg* 1994; 108:841–854.
118. Pollock JC, Jamieson MP, McWilliam R. Somatosensory evoked potentials in the detection of spinal cord ischemia in aortic coarctation repair. *Ann Thorac Surg* 1986; 41:251–254.
119. Driscoll DJ, Wolfe RR, Gersony WM, et al. Cardiorespiratory responses to exercise of patients with aortic stenosis, pulmonary stenosis, and ventricular septal defect. *Circulation* 1993; 87(suppl I):I102–I113.
120. Silverman NH. *Pediatric Echocardiography.* New York: Williams & Wilkins; 1993:386.
121. Rhodes LA, Colan SD, Perry SB, et al. Predictors of survival in neonates with critical aortic stenosis. *Circulation* 1991; 84:2325–2335.
122. Keane JF, Driscoll DJ, Gersony WM, et al. Second Natural History Study of Congenital Heart Defects: Results of treatment of patients, with aortic valvular stenosis. *Circulation* 1993; 87(suppl I):I16–I27.
123. Yetman AT, Rosenberg HC, Joubert GI. Progression of asymptomatic aortic stenosis identified in the neonatal period. *Am J Cardiol* 1995; 75:636–637.
124. McCrindle BW, for the Valvuloplasty and Angioplasty of Congenital Anomalies (VACA) Registry investigators. Independent predictors of immediate results of percutaneous balloon aortic valvotomy in childhood. *Am J Cardiol* 1996; 77:286–293.
125. Moore P, Egito E, Mowrey H, et al. Midterm results of balloon dilatation of congenital aortic stenosis: Predictors of success. *J Am Coll Cardiol* 1996; 27:1257–1263.
126. Egito ES, Moore P, O'Sullivan J, et al. Transvascular balloon dilation for neonatal critical aortic stenosis: Early and midterm results. *J Am Coll Cardiol* 1997; 442–447.
127. Kirklin JW, Barratt-Boyes BG. Congenital aortic stenosis. In: Kirklin JW, Barratt-Boyes BH, eds. *Cardiac Surgery,* 2d ed. New York: Churchill Livingstone; 1993:1195.
128. Elkins RC, Knott-Craig CJ, Ward KE, Lane MM. The Ross operation in children: 10-year experience. *Ann Thorac Surg* 1998; 65:496–502.
129. Hawkins JA, Minich LL, Tani LY, et al. Late results and reintervention after aortic valvotomy for critical aortic stenosis in neonates and infants. *Ann Thorac Surg* 1998; 1758–1762.
130. Najm HK, Coles JG, Black MD, et al. Extended aortic root replacement with aortic allografts or pulmonary autografts in children. *J Thorac Cardiovasc Surg* 1999; 118:503–509.
131. Graham TP Jr, Bricker JT, James FW, Strong WB. 26th Bethesda conference: Recommendations for determining eligibility for competition in athletes with cardiovascular abnormalities: Task Force 1: Congenital heart disease. *J Am Coll Cardiol* 1994; 24:867–873.
132. Fyler DC. Aortic outflow abnormalities. In: Fyler DC, ed. *Nadas' Pediatric Cardiology.* Philadelphia: Hanley & Belfus; 1992:506.
133. Van Son JA, Edwards WD, Danielson GK. Pathology of coronary arteries, myocardium, and great arteries in supravalvular aortic stenosis. *J Thorac Cardiovasc Surg* 1994; 108:21–28.
134. Ensing GJ, Schmidt MA, Hagler DF, et al. Spectrum of findings in a family with nonsyndromic autosomal dominant supravalvular aortic stenosis: A Doppler echocardiographic study. *J Am Coll Cardiol* 1989; 13:413–419.
135. Zalzstein E, Moes CA, Musewe NN, Freedom RM. Spectrum of cardiovascular anomalies in Williams-Beuren syndrome. *Pediatr Cardiol* 1991; 12:219–223.
136. French JW, Guntheroth WG. An explanation of asymmetric upper extremity blood pressure in supravalvular aortic stenosis: The Coanda effect. *Circulation* 1970; 42:31–36.
137. Van Son JA, Danielson GK, Puga FJ, et al. Supravalvular aortic stenosis: Long term results of surgical treatment. *J Thorac Cardiovasc Surg* 1994; 107:103–114.
138. Wright GB, Keane JF, Nadas AS, et al. Fixed subaortic stenosis

in the young: Medical and surgical course in 83 patients. *Am J Cardiol* 1983; 52:830–835.
139. Choi JY, Sullivan ID. Fixed subaortic stenosis: Anatomic spectrum and nature of progression. *Br Heart J* 1991; 65:280–286.
140. Freedom RM, Pelech A, Brand A, et al. The progressive nature of subaortic stenosis in congenital heart disease. *Int J Cardiol* 1985; 8:137–148.
141. Cape EG, Vanauker MD, Sigfusson G, et al. Potential role of mechanical stress in the etiology of pediatric heart disease: Septal shear stress in subaortic stenosis. *J Am Coll Cardiol* 1997; 30:247–254.
142. Drinkwater DC, Laks H. Surgery for subvalvular aortic stenosis. *Prog Pediatr Cardiol* 1994; 3:189–201.
143. Maginot KR, Williams RG. Fixed subaortic stenosis. *Prog Pediatr Cardiol* 1994; 3:141–149.
144. Kirklin JW, Ellis FH Jr. Surgical relief of diffuse subvalvular aortic stenosis. *Circulation* 1961; 24:739.
145. DeVries AG, Hess J, Witsenburg M, et al. Management of fixed subaortic stenosis: A retrospective study of 57 cases. *J Am Coll Cardiol* 1992; 19:1013–1017.
146. Braverman AC. Bicuspid aortic valve and associated aortic wall abnormalities. *Curr Opin Cardiol* 1996; 11:501–503.
147. Koretzky ED, Moller JH, Korns ME, et al. Congenital pulmonary stenosis resulting from dysplasia of valve. *Circulation* 1969; 40:43–53.
148. Li MD, Coles JC, McDonald AC. Anomalous muscle bundle of the right ventricle: Its recognition and surgical treatment. *Br Heart J* 1978; 40:1040–1045.
149. Noonan JA. Hypertelorism with Turner phenotype, a new syndrome associated with congenital heart disease. *Am J Dis Child* 1968; 116:373–380.
150. Stone FM, Bessinger FB Jr, Lucas RV Jr, Moller JH. Pre- and postoperative rest and exercise hemodynamics in children with pulmonary stenosis. *Circulation* 1974; 49:1102–1106.
151. Ellison RC, Freedom RM, Keane JF, et al. Indirect assessment of severity in pulmonary stenosis. *Circulation* 1977; 56(suppl I):I14–I20.
152. Lima CO, Sahn DJ, Valdez-Cruz LM, et al. Noninvasive prediction of transvalvular pressure gradient in patients with pulmonary stenosis by quantitative two-dimensional echocardiographic Doppler studies. *Circulation* 1983; 67:866–871.
153. Nugent EW, Freedom RM, Nora JJ, et al. Clinical course in pulmonary stenosis. *Circulation* 1977; 56(suppl I):I38–I47.
154. Mody MR. The natural history of uncomplicated valvular pulmonic stenosis. *Am Heart J* 1975; 90:317–321.
155. Hayes CJ, Gersony WM, Driscoll DJ, et al. Second natural history of congenital heart defects: Results of treatment of patients with pulmonary valvular stenosis. *Circulation* 1993; 87(suppl I): I28–I37.
156. Stanger P, Cassidy SC, Girod DA, et al. Balloon pulmonary valvuloplasty: Results of the Valvuloplasty and Angioplasty of Congenital Anomalies Registry. *Am J Cardiol* 1990; 65:775–783.
157. Marantz PM, Huhta JC, Mullins CE, et al. Results of balloon valvuloplasty in typical and dysplastic pulmonary valve stenosis: Doppler echocardiographic follow-up. *J Am Coll Cardiol* 1988; 12:476–479.
158. Ali Khan MA, al-Yousef S, Huhta JC, et al. Critical pulmonary valve stenosis in patients less than 1 year of age: Treatment with percutaneous gradational balloon pulmonary valvuloplasty. *Am Heart J* 1989; 117:1008–1014.
159. Ladysans EJ, Qureshi SA, Parsons JM, et al. Balloon dilation of critical stenosis of the pulmonary valve in neonates. *Br Heart J* 1990; 63:362–367.
160. Kan JS, Marvin WJ Jr, Bass JL, et al. Balloon angioplasty—branch pulmonary artery stenosis: Results from the Valvuloplasty and Angioplasy of Congenital Anomalies Registry. *Am J Cardiol* 1990; 65:798–801.
161. O'Laughlin MP. Catheterization treatment of stenosis and hypoplasia of pulmonary arteries. *Pediatr Cardiol* 1998; 19:48–56.
162. Baker CM, McGowen FX, Lock JE, Keane JF. Management of pulmonary artery trauma due to balloon dilation. *J Am Coll Cardiol* 1998; 31(suppl A):57A.
163. Vancini M, Roberts KD, Silove ED, Singh SP. Surgical treatment of congenital pulmonary stenosis due to dysplastic leaflets and small valve annulus. *J Thorac Cardiovasc Surg* 1980; 79:464–468.
164. McGoon MD, Fulton RE, Davis GD, et al. Systemic collateral and pulmonary artery stenosis in patients with congenital pulmonary valve atresia and ventricular septal defect. *Circulation* 1977; 56:473–479.
165. Becker AE, Connor M, Anderson RH. Tetralogy of Fallot: A morphometric and geometric study. *Am J Cardiol* 1975; 35:402–412.
166. Rao BN, Anderson RC, Edwards JE. Anatomic variations in the tetralogy of Fallot. *Am Heart J* 1971; 81:361–371.
167. Morgan BC, Guntheroth WG, Bloom RS, Fyler DC. A clinical profile of paroxysmal hyperpnea in cyanotic congenital heart disease. *Circulation* 1965; 31:66–69.
168. Hagler DJ, Tajik AJ, Seward JB, et al. Wide-angle two-dimensional echocardiographic profiles of conotruncal abnormalities. *Mayo Clin Proc* 1980; 55:73–82.
169. Formanek A, Nath PH, Zollikofer C, Moller JH. Selective coronary arteriography in children. *Circulation* 1980; 61:84–95.
170. Ponce FE, Williams LC, Webb HM, et al. Propanolol palliation of tetralogy of Fallot: Experience with long-term drug treatment in pediatric patient. *Pediatrics* 1973; 52:100–108.
171. Blalock A, Taussig HB. The surgical treatment of malformations of the heart in which there is pulmonary stenosis or pulmonary atresia. *JAMA* 1945; 128:129.
172. Lillehei CW, Cohen M, Warden HE, et al. Direct vision intracardiac surgical correction of the tetralogy of Fallot, pentalogy of Fallot, and pulmonary atresia defects: Report of the first 10 cases. *Ann Surg* 1955; 142:418–442.
173. Kirklin JW, Blackstone EH, Kirklin JK, et al. Surgical results and protocols in the spectrum of tetralogy of Fallot. *Ann Surg* 1983; 198:251–265.
174. Castaneda AR, Jonas RA, Mayer JE, Hanley FL. Tetralogy of Fallot. In: *Cardiac Surgery of the Neonate and Infant.* Philadelphia: Saunders; 1994:215.
175. Rastelli GC, Wallace RB, Ongley PA. Complete repair of transposition of the great arteries with pulmonary stenosis: A review and report of a case corrected by using a new surgical technique. *Circulation* 1969; 39:83–95.
176. Kreutzer J, Perry SB, Jonas RA, et al. Tetralogy of Fallot with diminutive pulmonary arteries: Preoperative pulmonary valve dilation and transcatheter rehabilitation of pulmonary arteries. *J Am Coll Cardiol* 1996; 27:1741–1747.
177. Murphy JG, Gersh BJ, Mair DD, et al. Long-term outcome in patients undergoing surgical repair of tetralogy of Fallot. *N Engl J Med* 1993; 329:593–599.
178. Lev M, Liberthson RR, Joseph RH, et al. The pathologic anatomy of Ebstein's disease. *Arch Pathol* 1970; 90:334–343.
179. Schreiber C, Cook A., Ho SY, et al. Morphologic spectrum of Ebstein's malformation: Revisitation relative to surgical repair. *J Thorac Cardiovasc Surg* 1999; 117:148–155.
180. Cohen LS, Friedman JM, Jefferson JW, et al. A reevaluation of risk of in utero exposure to lithium. *JAMA* 1994; 271:146–150.
181. Watson H. Natural history of Ebstein's anomaly of tricuspid valve in childhood and adolescence: An international co-operative study of 505 cases. *Br Heart J* 1974; 36:417–427.
182. Driscoll DJ, Mottram CD, Danielson GK. Spectrum of exercise intolerance in 45 patients with Ebstein's anomaly and observations on exercise tolerance in 11 patients after surgical repair. *J Am Coll Cardiol* 1988; 11:831–836.

183. Roberson DA, Silverman NH. Ebstein's anomaly: Echocardiographic and clinical features in the fetus and neonate. *J Am Coll Cardiol* 1989; 14:1300–1307.
184. Hernandez FA, Richkind R, Cooper HR. The intracavitary electrocardiogram in the diagnosis of Ebstein's anomaly. *Am J Cardiol* 1958; 1:181–190.
185. Celermajer DS, Cullen S, Sullivan ID, et al. Outcome in neonates with Ebstein's anomaly. *J Am Coll Cardiol* 1992; 19:1041–1046.
186. Gentles TL, Calder AL, Clarkson PM, Neutze JM. Predictors of long-term survival with Ebstein's anomaly of the tricuspid valve. *Am J Cardiol* 1992; 69:377–381.
187. Donnelly JE, Brown JM, Radford DJ. Pregnancy outcome and Ebstein's anomaly. *Br Heart J* 1991; 66:368–371.
188. Kulik TJ. Inhaled nitric oxide in the management of congenital heart disease. *Curr Opin Cardiol* 1996; 11:75–80.
189. Reich JD, Auld D, Hulse E, et al. The Pediatric Radiofrequency Ablation Registry's experience with Ebstein's anomaly: Pediatric Electrophysiology Society. *J Cardiovasc Electrophysiol* 1998; 9:1370–1377.
190. Starnes VA, Pitlick PT, Bernstein D, et al. Ebstein's anomaly appearing in the neonate: A new surgical approach. *J Thorac Cardiovasc Surg* 1991; 101:1082–1087.
191. Marianeschi SM, McElhinney DB, Reddy VM, et al. Alternative approach to the repair of Ebstein's malformation: Intracardiac repair with ventricular unloading. *Ann Thorac Surg* 1998; 66:1546–1550.
192. Van Son JA, Falk V, Black MD, et al. Conversion of complex neonatal Ebstein's anomaly into functional tricuspid or pulmonary atresia. *Eur J Cardiothorac Surg* 1998; 13:280–284.
193. Danielson GK, Driscoll DJ, Mair DD, et al. Operative treatment of Ebstein's anomaly. *J Thorac Cardiovasc Surg* 1992; 104:1195–1202.
194. Carpentier A, Chauvaud S, Mace L, et al. A new reconstructive operation for Ebstein's anomaly of the tricuspid valve. *J Thorac Cardioasc Surg* 1988; 96:92–101.
195. Quaegebeur JM, Sreeram H, Fraser AG, et al. Surgery for Ebstein's anomaly: The clinical and echocardiographic evaluation of a new technique. *J Am Coll Cardiol* 1991; 17:722–728.
196. Radford DJ, Graff RF, Neilson GH. Diagnosis and natural history of Ebstein's anomaly. *Br Heart J* 1985; 54:517–522.
197. Lucas RV Jr, Lock JE, Tandon R, Edwards JE. Gross and histologic anatomy of total anomalous pulmonary venous connections. *Am J Cardiol* 1988; 62:292–300.
198. Gathman GE, Nadas AS. Total anomalous pulmonary venous connection: Clinical and physiologic observations of 75 pediatric patients. *Circulation* 1970; 42:143–154.
199. Chin AJ, Sanders S, Sherman F, et al. Accuracy of subcostal two-dimensional echocardiography in prospective diagnosis of total anomalous pulmonary venous connection. *Am Heart J* 1987; 113:1153–1159.
200. Newfeld EA, Wilson A, Paul MH, Reisch JS. Pulmonary vascular disease in total anomalous pulmonary venous drainage. *Circulation* 1980; 61:103–109.
201. Castaneda AR, Jonas RA, Mayer JE, Hanley FL. *Cardiac Surgery in the Neonate and Infant.* Philadelphia: Saunders; 1994:157.
202. Behrendt DM, Aberdeen E, Waterson DJ, Bonham-Carter RE. Total anomalous pulmonary venous drainage in infants: I. Clinical and hemodynamic findings, methods, and results of operation in 37 cases. *Circulation* 1972; 46:347–356.
203. Norwood WI, Hougen TJ, Castaneda AR. Total anomalous pulmonary venous connection: Surgical considerations. *Cardiovasc Clin* 1981; 11:353–364.
204. VanderVelde M, Parness IA, Colan SD, et al. Two-dimensional echocardiography in the pre- and postoperative management of total anomalous pulmonary venous connection. *J Am Coll Cardiol* 1991; 18:1746.
205. Bando K, Turrentine MW, Ensing GJ, et al. Surgical management of total anomalous pulmonary venous connection: Thirty-year trends. *Circulation* 1996; 94(suppl):II12–II26.
206. Lacour-Gayet F, Zoghbi J, Serraf AE, et al. Surgical management of progressive pulmonary venous obstruction after repair of total anomalous pulmonary venous connection. *J Thorac Cardiovasc Surg* 1999; 117:679–687.
207. Van Praagh R, Weinberg PM, Smith SD, et al. Malpositions of the heart. In: Adams FH, Emmanouilides GC, Riemenschneider TA, eds. *Moss' Heart Disease in Infants, Children, and Adolescents,* 4th ed. Baltimore: Williams & Wilkins; 1989:530.
208. Van Praagh R. Segmental approach to diagnosis. In: Fyler DC, ed. *Nadas' Pediatric Cardiology.* Philadelphia: Hanley & Belfus; 1992:27.
209. Van Praagh S, Santini F, Sanders SP. Cardiac malpositions with special emphasis on visceral heterotaxy (asplenia and polysplenia syndromes). In: Fyler DC, ed. *Nadas' Pediatric Cardiology.* Philadelphia: Hanley & Belfus; 1992:589.
210. Rooklin AR, McGeady SJ, Mikaelian DO, et al. The immotile cilia syndrome: A cause of recurrent pulmonary disease in children. *Pediatrics* 1980; 66:526–538.
211. Fyler DC. D-transposition of the great arteries. In: Fyler DC, ed. *Nadas' Pediatric Cardiology.* Philadelphia: Hanley & Belfus; 1992:557.
212. Paul MH, Wernovsky G. Transposition of the great arteries. In: Emmanouilides GC, Riemenschneider TA, Allen HD, Gutgesell HD, eds. *Moss and Adams Heart Disease in Infants, Children, and Adolescents,* 5th ed. Baltimore: Williams and Wilkins; 1995:1154.
213. Yoo S, Burrows PE, Moes CAF, et al. Evaluation of coronary arterial patterns in complete transposition by laidback aortography. *Cardiol Young* 1996; 6:149–155.
214. Liebman J, Cullum L, Belloc NB. Natural history of transposition of the great arteries: Anatomy and birth and death characteristics. *Circulation* 1969; 40:237–262.
215. Gelatt M, Hamilton RM, McCrindle BW, et al. Arrhythmia and mortality after the Mustard procedure: A 30-year single-center experience. *J Am Coll Cardiol* 1997; 29:194–201.
216. Wilson NJ, Clarkson PM, Barratt-Boyes BG, et al. Long-term outcome after the Mustard repair for simple transposition of the great arteries: 28-year follow-up. *J Am Coll Cardiol* 1998; 32:758–765.
217. Kirjavainen M, Happonen JM, Louhimo I. Late results of Senning operation. *J Thorac Cardiovasc Surg* 1999; 117:488–495.
218. Wernovsky G, Mayer JE Jr, Jonas RA, et al. Factors influencing early and late outcome of the arterial switch operation for transposition of the great arteries. *J Thorac Cardiovasc Surg* 1995; 109:289–301.
219. Gutgesell HP, Massaro TA, Kron IL. The arterial switch operation for transposition of the great arteries in a consortium of University Hospitals. *Am J Cardiol* 1994; 74:959–960.
220. Wernovsky G, Freed MD. Transposition of the great arteries: Results and outcome of the arterial switch operation. In: Freedom RM, ed. *Atlas of Heart Diseases,* vol XII, *Congenital Heart Disease.* Philadelphia: Current Medicine; 1997:16.1.
221. Williams WG, Quaegebeur JM, Kirklin JW, Blackstone EH. Outflow obstruction after the arterial switch operation: A multiinstitutional study: Congenital Heart Surgeons Society. *J Thorac Cardiovasc Surg* 1997; 114:975–987.
222. Nakanishi T, Matsumoto Y, Seguchi M, et al. Balloon angioplasty for postoperative pulmonary artery stenosis in transposition of the great arteries. *J Am Coll Cardiol* 1993; 22:859–866.
223. Castaneda AR, Jonas RA, Mayer JE, Hanley FL. *Cardiac Surgery of the Neonate and Infant.* Philadelphia: Saunders; 1994:444.
224. Sagin-Saylam G, Somerville J. Palliative Mustard operation for transposition of the great arteries: Late results after 15–20 years. *Heart* 1996; 75:72–77.
225. Hagler DJ. Double-outlet right ventricle. In: Emmanouilides TA, Riemenschneider TA, Allen HD, Gutgesell HP, eds. *Moss and*

Adams Heart Disease in Infants, Children, and Adolescents, 5th ed. Baltimore: Williams & Wilkins; 1995:1246–1270.
226. Snider AR, Serwer GA. *Echocardiography in Pediatric Heart Disease.* Chicago: Year Book; 1990:190–195.
227. Kirklin JW, Barratt-Boyes BG. Double outlet right ventricle. In: Kirklin JW, Barratt-Boyes BG, eds. *Cardiac Surgery,* 2d ed. New York: Churchill Livingstone; 1993:1469.
228. Aoki M, Forbess JM, Jonas RA, et al. Result of biventricular repair for double-outlet right ventricle. *J Thorac Cardiovasc Surg* 1994; 107:338–349.
229. Belli E, Serraf A, Lacour-Gayet F, et al. Surgical treatment of subaortic stenosis after biventricular repair of double-outlet right ventricle. *J Thorac Cardiovasc Surg* 1996; 112:1570–1580.
230. Mavroudis C, Backer CL, Muster AJ, et al. Taussig-Bing anomaly: Arterial switch versus Kawashima intraventricular repair. *Ann Thorac Surg* 1996; 61:1330–1338.
231. Freedom RM. Congenitally corrected transposition of the great arteries: Definitions and pathologic anatomy. *Pediatr Cardiol* 1999; 10:3–16.
232. Fischbach PS, Law IH, Serwer GS. Congenitally corrected l-transposition of the great arteries: Abnormalities of atrioventricular conduction. *Prog Pediatr Cardiol* 1999; 10:37–43.
233. Snider AR, Serwer GA, Ritter SB. Abnormalities in ventricular connection. In: Snider AR, Serwer GA, Ritter SB, eds. *Echocardiography in Pediatric Heart Disease.* St. Louis: Mosby; 1990: 317–323.
234. Connelly MS, Liu PP, Williams WG, et al. Congenitally corrected transposition of the great arteries in the adult: Functional status and complications. *J Am Coll Cardiol* 1996; 27:1238–1243.
235. Lundstrom U, Bull C, Wyse RK, Somerville J. The natural and "unnatural" history of congenitally corrected transposition. *Am J Cardiol* 1990; 65:1222–1229.
236. Cowley CG, Rosenthal A. Congenitally corrected transposition of the great arteries: The systemic right ventricle. *Prog Pediatr Cardiol* 1999; 10:31–35.
237. Warnes CA. Congenitally corrected transposition: The uncorrected misnomer (editorial comment). *J Am Coll Cardiol* 1996; 27:1244.
238. Kirklin JW, Barratt-Boyes BG. Congenitally corrected transposition of the great arteries. In: Kirklin JW, Barratt-Boyes BG, eds. *Cardiac Surgery,* 2d ed. New York: Churchill Livingstone; 1993:1511.
239. Sano T, Riesenfeld T, Karl TR, Wilkinson JL. Intermediate term outcome after intracardiac repair of associated cardiac defects in patients with atrioventricular and ventriculoarterial discordance. *Circulation* 1995; 92(suppl II):II272–II278.
240. Termignon JL, Leca F, Vouhe PR, et al. "Classic" repair of congenitally corrected transposition and ventricular septal defect. *Ann Thorac Surg* 1996; 62:199–206.
241. Van Son JA, Danielson GK, Huhta JC, et al. Late results of systemic atrioventricular valve replacement in corrected transposition. *J Thorac Cardiovasc Surg* 1995; 109:642–653.
242. Ilbawi MN, DeLeon SY, Backer CL, et al. An alternative approach to the surgical management of physiologically corrected transposition with ventricular septal defect and pulmonary stenosis or atresia. *J Thorac Cardiovasc Surg* 1990; 100:410–415.
243. Imai Y. Double-switch operation for congenitally corrected transposition. *Adv Cardiac Surg* 1997; 9:65–86.
244. Reddy VM, McElhinney DB, Silverman NH, Hanley FL. The double switch procedure for anatomical repair of congenitally corrected transposition of the great arteries in infants and children. *Euro Heart J* 1997; 18:1470–1477.
245. Rosenthal A, Dick M. Tricuspid atresia. In: Emmanouilides GC, Riemenschneider TA, Allen HD, Gutgesell HD, eds. *Moss and Adams Heart Disease in Infants, Children, and Adolescents,* 5th ed. Baltimore: Williams & Wilkins; 1995:902.
246. Hagler DJ, Edwards WD. Univentricular atrioventricular connection. In: Emmanouilides GC, Riemenschneider TA, Allen HD, Gutgesell HD, eds. *Moss and Adams Heart Disease in Infants, Children, and Adolescents,* 5th ed. Baltimore: Williams & Wilkins; 1995:1278.
247. Dobell ARC, Van Praagh R. The Holmes heart: Historic associations and pathologic anatomy. *Am Heart J* 1996; 132:437–445.
248. Silverman NH. *Pediatric Echocardiography.* New York: Williams & Wilkins: 1993:279.
249. Freedom RM, Culham JAG, Moes CAF. *Angiocardiography of Congenital Heart Disease.* New York: Macmillan; 1989.
250. George BL, Kaplan S. Single ventricle and subaortic obstruction. *Prog Pediatr Cardiol* 1994; 3:167–176.
251. Moak JP, Gersony WM. Progressive atrioventricular valvular regurgitation in single ventricle. *Am J Cardiol* 1987; 59:656–658.
252. Donofrio MT, Jacobs ML, Norwood WI, Rychik J. Early changes in ventricular septal defect size and ventricular geometry in the single left ventricle after volume-unloading surgery. *J Am Coll Cardiol* 1995; 26:1008–1015.
253. Mainwaring RD, Lamberti JJ, Moore JW. The bidirectional Glenn and Fontan procedures—integrated management of the patient with a functionally single ventricle. *Cardiol Young* 1996; 6:198–207.
254. Van Son JA, Reddy VM, Haas GS, Hanley FL. Modified surgical techniques for relief of aortic obstruction in (SLL) hearts with rudimentary right ventricle and restrictive bulboventricular foramen. *J Thorac Cardiovasc Surg* 1995; 110:909–915.
255. Norwood WI, Lang P, Hansen DD. Physiologic repair of aortic atresia-hypoplastic left heart syndrome. *N Engl J Med* 1983; 308:23–26.
256. Bailey LL, Nehlsen-Cannarella SL, Doroshow RW, et al. Cardiac allotransplantation in newborns as therapy for hypoplastic left heart syndrome. *N Engl J Med* 1986; 315:949–951.
257. Mayer JE, Bridges ND, Lock JE, et al. Factors associated with marked reduction in mortality for Fontan operation in patients with single ventricle. *J Thorac Cardiovasc Surg* 1992; 103:444–452.
258. Moak JP, Gersony WM. Progressive atrioventricular valvular regurgitation in single ventricle. *Am J Cardiol* 1987; 59:656–658.
259. Matitiau A, Geva T, Colan SD, et al. Bulboventricular foramen size in infants with double-inlet left ventricle or tricuspid atresia with transposed great arteries: Influence on initial palliative operation and rate of growth. *J Am Coll Cardiol* 1992; 19:142–148.
260. Jacobs ML, Rychik J, Rome JJ, et al. Early reduction of the volume work of the single ventricle: The hemi-Fontan operation. *Ann Thorac Surg* 1996; 62:456–462.
261. Van Son JA, Reddy VM, Haas GS, Hanley FL. Modified surgical techniques for relief of aortic obstruction in (SLL) hearts with rudimentary right ventricle and restrictive bulboventricular foramen. *J Thorac Cardiovasc Surg* 1995; 110:909–915.
262. Fontan F, Baudet E. Surgical repair of tricuspid atresia. *Thorax* 1971; 26:240–248.
263. Cetta F, Feldt RH, O'Leary PW, et al. Improved early morbidity and mortality after Fontan operation: The Mayo Clinic experience, 1987 to 1992. *J Am Coll Cardiol* 1996; 28:480–486.
264. Petrossian E, Reddy VM, McElhinney DB, et al. Early results of the extracardiac conduit Fontan operation. *J Thorac Cardiovasc Surg* 1999; 117:688–696.
265. Jacobs ML, Blackstone EH, Bailey LL. Intermediate survival in neonates with aortic atresia: A multi-institutional study: The Congenital Heart Surgeons Society. *J Thorac Cardiovasc Surg* 1998; 116; 417–434.
266. Bove EL. Surgical treatment for hypoplastic left heart syndrome. *Jpn J Thorac Cardiovasc Surg* 1999; 47:47–56.
267. Tkebuchava T, Von Segesser LK, Vogt PR, et al. Congenital coronary fistulas in children and adults: Diagnosis, surgical technique and results. *J Cardiovasc Surg* 1996; 37:29–34.
268. Vavuranakis M, Bush CA, Boudoulas H. Coronary artery fistulas

in adults: Incidence, angiographic characteristics, natural history. *Cathet Cardiovasc Diagn* 1995; 35:116–120.

269. Velvis H, Schmidt KG, Silverman NH, Turley K. Diagnosis of coronary artery fistula by two-dimensional echocardiography, pulsed Doppler ultrasound and color flow imaging. *J Am Coll Cardiol* 1989; 14:968–976.
270. Urruita SCO, Falashci G, Ott DA, Cooley DA. Surgical management of 56 patients with congenital coronary artery fistulas: Report of three cases. *Ann Thorac Surg* 1983; 35:300–307.
271. Mavroudis C, Backer CL, Rocchini AP, et al. Coronary artery fistulas in infants and children: A surgical review and discussion of coil embolization. *Ann Thorac Surg* 1997; 63:1235–1242.
272. Blanche C, Chaux A. Long-term results of surgery for coronary artery fistulas. *Int Surg* 1990; 75:238–239.
273. Perry SB, Rome J, Keane JF, et al. Transcatheter closure of coronary artery fistulas. *J Am Coll Cardiol* 1992; 20:205–209.
274. Hurwitz RA, Caldwell RL, Girod DA, et al. Clinical and hemodynamic course of infants and children with anomalous left coronary artery. *Am Heart J* 1989; 118:1176–1181.
275. Wesselhoeft H, Fawcett JS, Johnson AL. Anomalous origin of the left coronary artery from the pulmonary trunk: Its clinical spectrum, pathology, and pathophysiology, based on a review of 140 cases with seven further cases. *Circulation* 1968; 38:403–425.
276. Schmidt KG, Cooper MJ, Silverman NH, Stanger P. Pulmonary artery origin of the left coronary artery: Diagnosis by two-dimensional echocardiography, pulsed Doppler ultrasound and color flow mapping. *J Am Coll Cardiol* 1988; 11:396–402.
277. Gutgesell HP, Pinsky WW, DePuey EG. Thallium-201 myocardial perfusion imaging in infants and children: Value in distinguishing anomalous left coronary artery from congestive cardiomyopathy. *Circulation* 1980; 61:596–599.
278. Takeuchi S, Imamura H, Katsumoto K, et al. New surgical method for repair of anomalous left coronary artery from pulmonary artery. *J Thorac Cardiovasc Surg* 1979; 78:7–11.
279. Cochrane AD, Coleman DM, Davis AM, et al. Excellent long-term functional outcome after an operation for anomalous left coronary artery from the pulmonary artery. *J Thorac Cardiovasc Surg* 1999; 117:332–342.
280. El-Said GM, Ruzyllo W, Williams RL, et al. Early and late results of saphenous vein graft for anomalous origin of left coronary artery from pulmonary artery. *Circulation* 1973; 48(suppl III):2–6.
281. Rein AJ, Colan SD, Parness IA, Sanders SP. Regional and global left ventricular function in infants with anomalous origin of the left coronary artery from the pulmonary trunk: Preoperative and postoperative assessment. *Circulation* 1987; 75:115–123.
282. Rahimtoola SH. Concept and evaluation of hibernating myocardium. *Annu Rev Med* 1999; 50:75–86.

CHAPTER 64

CONGENITAL HEART DISEASE IN ADULTS

Carole A. Warnes / John E. Deanfield

Congenital heart disease occurs in 5 to 10 per 1000 live births.[1] Without early treatment, the majority of patients would die in infancy or childhood, with only 5 to 15 percent surviving until puberty.[2] The advent of surgical procedures, from ligation of a patent arterial duct[3] in 1939 to the innovations of the 1990s, as well as advances in medical treatment, has transformed the outlook for children with even complex defects. The majority now survive into adolescence and adult life (Chap. 63). This success story has radically altered both the size and complexity of the population of young adults with congenital heart disease. In the United States alone, well over a half-million patients with functionally important congenital cardiac malformations have reached adulthood in the past three decades.[4] Despite the fact that most patients now surviving to adult life will have undergone surgery during childhood, "total correction" is not the rule.[5] The term *total correction* is itself a misnomer, perhaps with the exception of the successfully ligated ductus arteriosus without residua. The misperception of "cure" leads adults not to seek understanding of their anomaly, to fail to follow endocarditis prophylaxis, and to fail in pursuing continued cardiac care. The majority, if not all, require long-term surveillance, and many need reoperation. Other adults may require their first operation for congenital heart lesions that were well tolerated during childhood.

Both the "natural" survivors and the postoperative patients require specialized medical care. Arrhythmia is common, as are residual or deteriorating hemodynamic problems and endocarditis. Although cardiologists specializing in the care of adults may be expert in one or more of these areas, the critical relationship between rhythm and hemodynamic status in hearts with complex circulations (as after a Fontan operation or after intra-atrial repair for transposition) may lead to treatment errors by those inexperienced in the treatment of congenital heart defects. Patients with cyanosis require special care because of erythrocytosis, bleeding, renal problems, and arthropathy; moreover, they require specific counseling and management regarding pregnancy. In addition to the medical problems, psychosocial problems such as the search for employment, life and health insurance, participation in sports, sexual activity, and contraception are of great importance to adolescents and young adults with congenital heart disease. Many of the "normal" ordeals of growing up are more difficult for this group, in whom chronic illness, embarrassing scars, and/or exercise limitation may inhibit normal social intercourse and maturation.

Over the last few years, the specialist needs of this growing population have begun to be appreciated. In addition to the challenge of continuing the expert care of their complex cardiac problems from the pediatric environment into the much wider adult medical community, knowledge of the long-term fate of patients with congenital heart disease is essential for pediatric cardiologists in order to refine initial management strategy. A rather short-term view of "success" or "failure" has been encouraged by rapid changes in medical and surgical policies over the last three decades. Nevertheless, there are clear examples, such as the management of transposition of the great arteries, where awareness of long-term problems has altered the primary surgical approach. The Mustard or Senning procedures (see below) provide a physiologic repair at acceptably low risk but may result in long-term systemic ventricular dysfunction, arrhythmias, and sudden death. This has enabled the introduction of anatomic repair by the arterial-switch procedure, despite high surgical mortality in the early series, with the expectation of a more satisfactory long-term outcome. Other debates, over such issues as the place of Fontan operations, cavopulmonary anastomosis, and systemic-to-pulmonary shunts, are not yet resolved and will be strongly influenced by the accumulation of rigorously collected outcome data, not merely for survival but also for morbidity and quality of life.

The optimal solutions for delivery of care to the adult with congenital heart disease will depend on the different medical systems in operation around the world. The common requirements include collaboration between pediatric and adult cardiologists; the establishment of a few specialist centers with appropriate medical, surgical, anesthetic, and nonmedical staff together with investigational facilities; the establishment of treatment guidelines, and centralization of accumulating knowledge.[6] The report of a consensus conference on adult congenital heart disease commissioned by the Canadian Cardiovascular Society represents an important step forward.[7] This includes recommendations for training and a hierarchy of care from the community to the specialist center. Similar training guidelines have been published in the United States.[8]

MEDICAL CONSIDERATIONS

Many young adults with congenital heart disease have mild lesions that have not required and may not ever require surgery. The commonest defects in this category are small ventricular septal defect, mild pulmonary valve stenosis, mild aortic valve stenosis, and mitral valve prolapse (Table 64-1). Such patients need infrequent follow-up (e.g., biannual) to assess any progression in severity of the lesion, to reinforce the need for antibiotic prophylaxis against infective endocarditis (Chap. 73), and to obtain psychosocial advice. Other patients reach adult life with more complex defects that are still unrepaired. Some may still be candidates for palliative or definitive surgery, whereas in others surgery may no longer be possible, often because of the presence of irreversible pulmonary vascular disease. More and more survivors of surgery in childhood are now reaching adult life; they now form the largest group of patients (Table 64-2). The majority need continuing medical surveillance, since late cardiovascular problems may result from hemodynamic disturbances, arrhythmia, and endocarditis. Such patients can also develop noncardiac problems as a consequence of their heart disease (e.g., secondary to cyanosis) and are, of course, susceptible to all the potential acquired "medical problems" of adulthood.

TABLE 64-1 Common Congenital Heart Defects Compatible with Survival to Adult Life without Surgery or Interventional Catheterization

Mild pulmonary valve stenosis
Peripheral pulmonary stenosis
Bicuspid aortic valve
Mild subaortic stenosis
Mild supravalvar aortic stenosis
Small atrial septal defect
Small ventricular septal defect
Small patent ductus arteriosus
Mitral valve prolapse
Ostium primum atrial septal defect (atrioventricular septal defect)
Marfan's syndrome
Ebstein's anomaly
Corrected transposition (atrioventricular-ventriculo-arterial discordance)
Balanced complex lesions (e.g, double-inlet ventricle with pulmonary stensosis)
Defects with pulmonary vascular obstructive disease (Eisenmenger's syndrome)

Hemodynamics

Study of the hemodynamic consequences of repaired and unrepaired congenital heart disease is a crucial aspect of long-term follow-up. Progressive congestive cardiac failure secondary to myocardial deterioration is the most common cause of disability and death in patients whose ventricles may have been subjected to many years of volume and pressure loading, often with chronic hypoxia. A significant number of the adult postoperative patients with congenital heart disease have been repaired at older ages than is the current practice. This may result in greater preoperative damage and pulmonary vascular disease, which may persist postoperatively. In the early era of open-heart surgery, myocardial protection was sometimes less than optimal, resulting in myocardial damage.

It should also be appreciated that postoperative circulations created by the repair of many congenital heart defects result in an adequate physiologic repair (e.g., deoxygenated blood to lungs and oxygenated blood to the body) but often have far from normal anatomy. For example, after the Mustard and Senning operation for transposition of the great arteries, the right ventricle remains on the systemic side of the circulation. Some of these patients have evidence of deteriorating right ventricular function, and there is increasing concern that this will become a major life-threatening problem with longer follow-up.[9] Similar concerns have been expressed for systemic ventricular function after the Fontan operation.[10] The different morphologic characteristics and loading conditions for these ventricles suggest that standard indices of ventricular function,

TABLE 64-2 Common Congenital Heart Defects Surviving to Adult Life after Surgery/Interventional Catheterization

Aortic valve disease, valvotomy or replacement
Pulmonary stenosis, valvotomy
Tetralogy of Fallot
Atrial septal defect
Ventricular septal defect
Atrioventricular septal defect
Transposition of the great arteries, atrial redirection
Complex transposition of the great arteries
Total anomalous pulmonary venous connection
Pulmonary atresia/ventricular septal defect
Fontan operation for complex congenital heart disease
Ebstein's anomaly
Coarctation of the aorta
Mitral valve disease

derived from studies of structurally normal hearts, may be inappropriate for such patients (see also Chap. 20).[11] Prospective serial studies are beginning to define "normal ranges" for congenital heart defects and to examine their "natural" and "unnatural" history.[12]

Residual hemodynamic defects are often present in repaired patients and may cause problems even many years after surgery. These may be amenable to further surgery (see below) or require long-term medical treatment. Medical management of cardiac failure in patients with congenital heart disease is adopting therapies shown to be of benefit in large-scale clinical trials of patients with heart failure from predominantly cardiomyopathy or ischemic heart disease.[13–15] Appreciation of ventricular "remodeling" and the effect of neurohumeral responses on symptoms and disease progression has led to increasing and earlier use of angiotensin-converting enzyme inhibitors and, in some cases, beta blockers and long-acting calcium antagonists in addition to standard therapy with digoxin and diuretics (see Chap. 21). These agents may also slow the rate of progressive deterioration in ventricular function reported in certain congenital heart diseases even when they have been adequately "corrected."

Cyanosis

Adults with congenital heart disease may have central cyanosis from right-to-left shunting secondary to their unrepaired cardiac defect or to pulmonary vascular disease (Eisenmenger's syndrome; see Chap. 63). The latter complication should be seen less frequently in years ahead as a result of the trend toward early recognition and repair of congenital heart disease in infancy. Currently, however, a significant number of patients reach adult life with pulmonary vascular disease as a result of lesions such as large ventricular septal defect, atrioventricular (AV) septal defect, truncus arteriosus, and double-outlet right ventricle. Their pulmonary vascular resistance may already have been too high for surgical repair at the time of diagnosis; in others, pulmonary vascular disease may have progressed despite repair of the congenital heart defect.

Chronic cyanosis may lead to erythrocytosis and hyperviscosity. Many patients with cyanotic congenital heart disease establish a stable high hematocrit but few symptoms of hyperviscosity.[16] They have a low risk of stroke and do not require venesection.[17] In others, the hemoglobin concentration may rise progressively. Once it exceeds 20 g/dL, they are at risk from thromboembolic complications and may suffer from headache, dizziness, and fatigue. Symptoms may be improved with judicious venesection by the removal of 500 mL of blood and volume replacement with normal saline or dextrose solution.[17,18] Overzealous venesection, however, may result in both acute and chronic problems, including cardiovascular collapse in patients with Eisenmenger's syndrome, iron depletion, microcytosis, and hyperviscosity in its own right.[19] The paradoxical anemia of erythrocytotic patients with iron deficiency due to repeated phlebotomy may be missed and indeed has been shown to increase the risk of stroke.[20] It has been demonstrated that phlebotomies and microcytosis were strongly associated with stroke, perhaps due to the fact that iron-deficient red blood cells are less deformable than are normal red blood cells and do not pass through the microcirculation as readily as do iron-replete cells.

Patients with chronic cyanosis also develop defective hemostasis from abnormalities in platelet function and in the coagulation and fibrinolytic systems,[19,20] especially patients with marked erythrocytosis. The risk of hemorrhage, especially at surgery, is well recognized and may be fatal. Hyperuricemia is common because of increased red cell turnover and renal dysfunction. Arthralgia is well recognized, but gouty arthritis is rare and may be misdiagnosed. Renal impairment can deteriorate to renal failure as a result of relatively minor interventions, such as injection of contrast medium at angiography or the injudicious use of nonsteroidal anti-inflammatory agents.[21,22] Patients with right-to-left shunts are at risk of paradoxic embolus, which may cause a cerebrovascular accident or renal infarction. Air filters must be utilized with all intravenous lines. A cerebral abscess is a well-known complication of a septic embolus and must always be considered in the cyanotic patient with any neurologic symptoms, however transient, or low-grade fever. Facial and truncal acne is common, and is not only a cosmetic problem but a potential source of sepsis. A specific concern has been the safety of air travel in adults with cyanotic congenital heart disease, since in-flight atmospheric conditions on commercial jets approach altitude equivalents of 6000 to 8000 ft (1829 to 2438 m). In a recent report, however, only modest (approximately 6 percent) decreases in systemic arterial oxygen saturation were found, with no adverse effects.[23]

Progressive kyphoscoliosis has been recognized for many years as a complication of congenital heart disease.[24] It is common in cyanotic patients and those with previous thoracotomy. The degree of deformity, if left untreated, may become profound and compromise pulmonary function. Treatment with bracing or insertion of a Harrington rod may be indicated, since the kyphoscoliosis may significantly reduce both the quality and quantity of life. Surgical repair is not possible, however, in those with Eisenmenger's syndrome, since the surgical risk is too high.

The prognosis for patients with Eisenmenger's syndrome depends on the site of the lesion and the medical and cardiac care they receive.[25–27] Death may result from right-sided heart failure, pulmonary hemorrhage, or arrhythmia. It can also occur prematurely due to potentially avoidable complication, such as inappropriate drug therapy or injudicious general anesthesia. Special care must be employed during noncardiac surgery, utilizing cardiac anesthesia, maintenance of preload, and cardiac monitoring.[28] Recent data suggest promise for chronic prostacyclin therapy in reducing pulmonary artery pressure, but this is preliminary.[29]

Infective Endocarditis

Patients with both unoperated and operated congenital heart disease are at risk from infective endocarditis. Lifelong antibiotic prophylaxis is recommended, but the specific indications and optimal regimens are still debated.[30,31] The American Heart Association Special Report on Prevention of Infective Endocarditis has stratified risk groups for the various lesions.[31] Prophylaxis is advocated for all lesions except isolated secundum atrial septal defect and repaired secundum atrial septal defect, ventricular septal defect, or patent ductus arteriosus without residua beyond 6 months (see Chap. 73). The wide variety of portals of entry includes dental work, skin sepsis, obstetric and gynecologic procedures, genitourinary and gastrointestinal interventions, and surgery.[32,33] There is also a risk of bacteremia and infective endocarditis in young adults who have their ears pierced or acquire a tattoo.[34] Patients must be educated and preferably should carry an information card with them. The symptoms of endocarditis may be subtle, and the diagnosis must be considered in any patient who experiences unexplained malaise or fever. Injudicious prescription of antibiotics without previous blood culture may mask the problem and make bacteriologic diagnosis and appropriate treatment difficult. Both general measures, such as oral hygiene as well as skin and nail care, and appropriate antibiotic treatment are important. Among 102 patients with congenital heart disease who filled in a questionnaire, there was a disturbing lack of knowledge about endocarditis prevention measures and indeed about their cardiac lesion in general.[35]

Electrophysiologic Problems

Arrhythmias and conduction defects have a major impact on the prognosis and management of both unoperated and operated patients and have been linked to sudden death in a number of conditions.[36,37] The principles of diagnosis and treatment are similar to those employed in patients with arrhythmia due to other causes (see Chap. 24), with some important exceptions. Rhythm disturbances that may be benign in a structurally normal heart may be life-threatening in congenital heart disease. Restoration of sinus rhythm is usually much more important, and rate control of atrial arrhythmias is usually not a good treatment option. Special consideration must be given before the use of therapies that may have negative inotropic properties. In unoperated patients, chamber dilatation, myocardial hypertrophy, and fibrosis may all contribute to the genesis of arrhythmia. In operated patients, additional sinus or AV node damage and atrial and/or ventricular scarring may cause electrophysiologic problems. The etiology is multifactorial, and the clinical significance of arrhythmia depends very much on the hemodynamic context in which it occurs.

Supraventricular arrhythmia and sinus node injury, not surprisingly, occur most often in conditions with "atrial defects" or those requiring atrial surgery.[38,39] Abnormalities of sinus node function are common in patients with atrial septal defect, particularly the sinus venosus type,[40] and are often seen after Mustard or Senning operation for transposition of the great arteries.[41] Sinus node dysfunction has also been reported after surgery for tetralogy of Fallot, the Fontan procedure, and many other operations for congenital heart lesions.[42] Clinical manifestations include sinus bradycardia, sinoatrial block, sinus arrest, and occasionally the tachybradycardia syndrome with paroxysmal atrial flutter and fibrillation. Although bradycardia has been postulated as the cause of sudden death in some conditions, current evidence indicates that tachyarrhythmia is usually a more likely explanation (see below).[41]

In sinus node disease, insertion of a pacemaker is indicated for patients with symptoms resulting from a slow heart rate, such as tiredness, dizziness, and syncope or for an extremely low heart rate (see Chap. 31). Indications in asymptomatic individuals are still controversial, since the arrhythmia is benign in many cases. It should be noted that pacing may be difficult because of the complex underlying anatomy and lack of a suitable site for endocardial lead fixation.[43] The choice of pacemaker will depend on the precise indication. The simplest VVI pacemaker may be adequate prophylaxis against bradycardia-related sudden death. In general, however, rate-responsive pacemakers are preferable, and dual-chamber pacing may provide the best hemodynamics (see also Chap. 31).[44,45]

Injury to the AV node and proximal conduction tissue may result from surgery for lesions such as ventricular septal defect, AV septal defect, or tetralogy of Fallot. Transient complete AV block in the postoperative period has been shown to have prognostic significance in some reports, particularly if the site of damage is below the bundle of His. In a 30-year follow-up of ventricular septal defect repair at the Mayo Clinic, the development of transient complete heart block for over 72 h followed by resumption of sinus rhythm was a strong independent predictor of late mortality.[46] Whether transient perioperative AV block warrants permanent pacing and whether an invasive electrophysiologic study can help stratify risk are unresolved.[38] Postoperative right bundle-branch block is frequent after ventriculotomy and may be due to injury related to closure of a ventricular septal defect or to interruption of distal Purkinje fibers by ventriculotomy or muscle resection.[37,38] Occasionally, the electrocardiographic (ECG) pattern of right bundle-branch block with left-axis deviation occurs (bifascicular block), and there may also be PR-interval prolongation (trifascicular block).[47,48] Early reports suggested that these findings were harbingers of sudden cardiac death due to complete heart block.[49] More recent studies, however, have not substantiated this adverse prognosis.[50]

Tachyarrhythmias can be life threatening. Late sudden death has been reported in several lesions, both before and after repair. In general, the worse the disease (i.e., more complex anatomy and/or more extensive surgery), the greater the incidence of sudden death, although aortic stenosis and coarctation are also represented in this group. Studies suggest that the risk increases incrementally 20 years after surgical repair.[51] The identification of patients at risk and their management are important but controversial issues. After the Mustard and Senning operation, atrial flutter with a rapid ventricular response is dangerous, especially when it occurs in association with right ventricular dysfunction or venous pathway obstruction.[52] Medical or electrical cardioversion should be promptly used to restore sinus rhythm, and drug therapy may need to be accompanied by pacemaker insertion. Recently, ablation (surgical or catheter) has been advocated for certain cases of atrial flutter (see Chap. 28). Atrial tachyarrhythmias are also common after the Fontan operation; sinus node injury, atrial suturing, and a dilated hypertensive right atrium probably contribute.[42,51] Modification of the operation to exclude the right atrium from the Fontan circuit, the total cavopulmonary connection, may reduce the incidence of potentially serious early and late rhythm disturbances.[53,54]

Ventricular arrhythmias are known to occur after open-heart surgery, particularly repair of tetralogy of Fallot.[48,55] Studies using ambulatory ECG monitoring in postoperative patients have documented asymptomatic complex ectopy and nonsustained ventricular tachycardia in up to 50 percent of patients,[55–57] and more than 20 percent have inducible ventricular tachycardia at electrophysiologic study.[58,59] Experimental and clinical studies have shown that the electrical substrate for reentry arrhythmia is present in the right ventricle.[60] In several reports, older age at surgery is a predisposing factor,[57,61] an observation that suggests factors present at the time of repair may be involved in the genesis of postoperative arrhythmia, in addition to the myocardial damage occurring at the time of surgery or during postoperative follow-up.[62] This is consistent with morphologic studies that have documented increasing fibrosis of the right ventricle as part of the natural history of defects such as tetralogy of Fallot.[63] The current practice of early surgical repair for tetralogy of Fallot may reduce the incidence of such postoperative ventricular arrhythmia, and encouraging preliminary data support this view.[62,64] Other postulated risk factors include elevated right ventricular systolic pressure, reduced right ventricular ejection fraction, pulmonary regurgitation, and a ventriculotomy scar.[65] The clinical significance of nonsustained ventricular tachycardia and especially the indications for prophylactic antiarrhythmic therapy remain unclear.[52] There is a disparity between the high frequency of ventricular arrhythmia and the much lower incidence of sudden death.[66,67] The predictive value of an abnormal ambulatory ECG or of electrophysiologic study has not been established. Furthermore, prophylactic antiarrhythmic therapy has not been shown to be of value in asymptomatic patients with congenital heart defects. Such therapy may have proarrhythmic potential, be negatively inotropic, or have serious extracardiac side effects. As a result, there is insufficient evidence to advocate prophylactic treatment for asymptomatic individuals with nonsustained arrhythmia. On the other hand, there are a few cases of sudden death, out-of-hospital ventricular fibrillation, and/or sustained ventricular tachycardia in almost all large series of patients after repair of tetralogy of Fallot. Identification of at-risk individuals and appropriate treatment remain a challenge. Recent reports have indicated a link between the electrical and mechanical properties of the right ventricle, which may have clinical relevance.[68] The QRS duration on the surface ECG correlates with cardiothoracic ratio and, in a retrospective review, a QRS greater than 180 ms was a sensitive and specific marker for sudden death or out-of-hospital cardiac arrest.[69] Others have not confirmed this.[70] Further refinements in risk stratification in adults with tetralogy of Fallot or other congenital heart lesions are necessary and probably will involve hemodynamic and electrophysiologic testing both at rest and after exercise, evaluation of ventricular late potentials (Chap. 26), and heart rate variability.[71] It should be remembered, however, that, despite the attention given to ventricular arrhythmia after repair of tetralogy of Fallot, a major source of morbidity in such patients is from atrial arrhythmia.[72]

Radiofrequency ablation, so successfully used to treat arrhythmia in patients with structurally normal hearts (Chap. 28), is being applied to patients with congenital heart disease. These applications represent some of the most challenging electrophysiologic procedures because of the complex cardiac anatomy, enlarged chamber size, and abnormal localization of the underlying conduction system. Nevertheless, ablation may have a role, not merely in subjects with accessory pathways or AV reentry tachycardia, but also in intraatrial reentry arrhythmias that may be present after operations such as Fontan and Mustard or Senning procedures.[73,74]

Pregnancy

An increasing number of women with complex and postoperative congenital heart defects are reaching childbearing age. Advice is sought on both maternal and fetal risk as well as on the incidence of congenital heart disease in the offspring. In the United States, most maternal cardiac disease is congenital in origin. Data are accumulating regarding outcomes of pregnancy in many complex anomalies.[75–80] Prepregnancy counseling is mandatory for all patients whether operated or unoperated. The evaluation should include a detailed history, physical examination, ECG, and chest x-ray along with a comprehensive echocardiogram to evaluate ventricular function, all valve lesions and defects, and pulmonary artery pressure. If pulmonary artery pressure and resistance is in doubt following noninvasive testing, a cardiac catheterization may be necessary. An exercise test may facilitate a detailed assessment of functional capacity.

There are profound changes in the maternal cardiovascular system during pregnancy, including a large (30 to 40 percent) increase in blood volume, a fall in peripheral vascular resistance, and an increase in cardiac output (approximately 40 percent; see also Chap. 82). In general, women with left-to-right shunts or valvular regurgitation tolerate pregnancy well, whereas those with right-to-left shunts or valvular stenosis do less well.[81,82] Asymptomatic young women with small or moderate left-to-right shunts and normal pulmonary artery pressures can expect an uncomplicated pregnancy and labor. In the presence of a large left-to-right shunt, however, heart failure may be provoked or aggravated by pregnancy. Patients with cyanosis have the most problems in carrying a fetus to term and have a high incidence of early spontaneous abortion. Early studies showed that, with higher degrees of cyanosis (as reflected by the maternal hemoglobin), the incidence of spontaneous abortion increased and the handicap to fetal growth became more pronounced. Infants are unlikely to survive if the maternal hemoglobin level is above 18 g/dL.[83] A study from Presbitero et al. demonstrated a clear relationship between the degree of hypoxia and fetal loss (Table 64-3).[84] When the maternal oxygen saturation was 85 percent, only 2 out of 17 pregnancies (12 percent) resulted in live-born infants. Only 41 of 96 pregnancies (43 percent) produced a live birth in 45 cyanosed mothers. There were 49 spontaneous abortions and 6 stillbirths in this series, again reflecting the high risk that maternal cyanotic congenital heart disease poses for the fetus. Meticulous care during pregnancy and delivery lessened the maternal complication rate,

TABLE 64-3 Fetal Outcome in Cynotic Congenital Heart Disease and Its Relation with Maternal Cyanosis

Hemoglobin, g/dL[a]	Pregnancy, no.	Live Births, no.	Live Born, %
≤16	28	20	71
17–19	40	18	45
≥20	26	2	8
Arterial Oxygen Saturation, %[b]	**Pregnancy, no.**	**Live Births, no.**	**Live Born, %**
≤85	17	2	12
85–89	22	10	45
≥90	13	12	92

[a]Hemoglobin level unknown in two pregnancies.
[b]Arterial oxygen saturation unknown in 44 pregnancies.
SOURCE: From Presbitero P, Somerville J, Stone S, et al. Pregnancy in cyanotic congenital heart disease: Outcome of mother and fetus. *Circulation* 1994; 89:2673–2676. Reproduced with permission from the publisher and authors.

but this was still considerable. Such patients require rest and a short labor as well as avoidance of dehydration and sepsis. In such situations, the decision as to whether to continue with the pregnancy depends on an assessment of the risk to the mother and fetus as compared with the patient's desire to have children.

An elevated pulmonary vascular resistance, from either Eisenmenger's syndrome or primary pulmonary hypertension, is a clear contraindication to pregnancy. Pregnancy for women with Eisenmenger's syndrome carries approximately a 50 percent mortality rate.[85] Termination of pregnancy is always preferable; ideally, this should be done with cardiac anesthesia. If such patients are seen late in pregnancy and termination is not feasible, management should concentrate on maintenance of adequate preload and avoidance of vasodilation. The ideal management around the time of delivery for these patients is controversial because individual experience is small. Vaginal delivery is usually associated with less blood loss than is cesarean section. The latter, however, can be done quickly with all medical personnel in attendance. One report has suggested an approach of elective delivery by cesarean section under general anesthesia.[86] The use of prophylactic heparin before and after delivery is also controversial, and there is no established consensus.[86,87] Even after successful delivery, however, death frequently occurs within the few days following from deteriorating hemodynamics or pulmonary infarction.[85] Patients with Marfan's syndrome and aortic root dilation (greater than 40 mm) are at greater risk of aortic dissection and rupture, and while those without preexisting cardiovascular disease whose aortic root is smaller often tolerate pregnancy well, the risk is unpredictable.[88,89] Patients with severe aortic stenosis are also at increased risk because of the fall in afterload that accompanies pregnancy and exaggerates the valve gradient.[90,91] While early reports suggested a high risk of aortic rupture and cerebral hemorrhage in patients with aortic coarctation,[92] recent data have been more encouraging.[93] Fetal risk is increased, however, presumably as a result of compromised placental blood supply.

The management of pregnant women with mechanical prosthetic cardiac valves is a special problem because of the risk to the mother of thromboembolism and the risk to the fetus of anticoagulants (warfarin crosses the placenta and is teratogenic).[94,95] Depending on the condition involved and the mother's motivation and compliance, the use of subcutaneous heparin in the first and third trimesters and warfarin in the midtrimester is one treatment option. Heparin, however, is a poor anticoagulant during pregnancy; even with meticulous control of anticoagulation, there is still an increased risk of valve thrombosis.[96] In addition, there is also an increased risk of fetal loss with this approach. Because of the poor results with heparin, some authors have advocated the use of warfarin throughout pregnancy despite the risk of fetal teratogenicity.[97] This risk may be less if the dose of warfarin is less than 5 mg/day.[98] Nonetheless, this approach is still very controversial, despite the fact that fetal teratogenicity with warfarin may have been overemphasized (see Chap. 44).[99] Before prescribing any cardiovascular drug during pregnancy, the effects on both mother and fetus must be considered.

Management of labor should be specifically directed toward avoidance of rapid changes in circulatory volume, blood pressure, or cardiac output. In most cases, vaginal delivery is recommended, with careful attention to maternal position and analgesic agents. The American Heart Association no longer recommends endocarditis prophylaxis for vaginal delivery.[31] This recommendation, however, is not based on controlled data, and most cardiologists recommend antibiotics under these circumstances for almost all congenital heart defects.

Genetic Counseling

The risk of recurrence is an increasingly important issue as more males and females with congenital heart disease reach reproductive age, and genetic counseling should be provided for all potential parents. Recent genetic advances are clarifying the etiology of a number of congenital heart diseases. It has been estimated that the cause of congenital heart disease is genetic in approximately 8 percent of cases (e.g., velocardiofacial syndrome and Holt-Oram syndrome with autosomal dominant transmission) and environmental in 2 percent (e.g., congenital rubella syndrome).[100] In the remainder, genetic and environmental factors are thought to interact.[101] The greater the number of affected first-degree relatives within the family, the greater the recurrence risk. Recurrence risks in siblings of patients with congenital heart disease are well documented and range between 1 and 8 percent.[102] For the affected potential parents, however, the risk of recurrence in offspring is the key information, and fewer data exist. Early reports suggested that recurrence risks were considerably higher in offspring compared to siblings. Studies, such as the Second Natural History of Congenital Heart Defects, have suggested a low risk (1.2 percent for aortic stenosis, 2.8 percent for pulmonary stenosis, and 2.9 percent for ventricular septal defects).[103] There is considerable variation in recurrence risks in reported series, and factors inherent in study design, ascertainment bias, and follow-up account for many of the differences. In addition, certain forms of congenital heart disease recur more frequently than others (e.g., left ventricular outflow tract obstruction), and the recurrence risk appears to be higher in pregnancies with affected mothers rather than fathers. Accumulation of further information will be invaluable for counseling of patients. Fetal cardiac ultrasound at approximately 18 weeks of pregnancy facilitates early diagnosis.

Investigation and Imaging

Transthoracic echocardiography and cardiac catheterization with angiocardiography are the principal investigations in pediatric cardiology. Transthoracic echocardiography is an invaluable tool in adults also, although image acquisition is more challenging because of body habitus and chest wall abnormalities as a result of previous surgeries.[104] Transesophageal echocardiography is becoming increasingly important for the definition of cardiac structure and function,[104–106] and multiplane probes with color-flow Doppler imaging allow simultaneous assessment of anatomy and physiology. Specific areas and lesions of the heart that are well imaged in this way include systemic and pulmonary venous drainage, atrial lesions (including baffle function), AV valve morphology and function, left ventricular outflow tract lesions (including the ascending aorta in Marfan's syndrome), and intracavity thrombus or vegetations (Fig. 64-1).[106,107]

Magnetic resonance imaging (MRI) can also provide valuable anatomic information, which in some cases is superior to that from ultrasound, even via a transesophageal approach. Rapid technologic advances—including three-dimensional image reconstruction; software to study hemodynamics, such as velocity mapping; and cine-MRI—may reduce the need for invasive investigation (Fig. 64-2).[108-110] The expertise required both to acquire and to interpret MRI information is likely to be confined to specialized regional centers, but access to the MRI facility should be available to all units managing adult patients with congenital heart disease.

In parallel with the decreasing need for diagnostic cardiac catheterization, there has been a dramatic rise in the indications for and scope of interventional procedures in adult patients with congenital heart disease.[111] Residual defects after repair that are amenable to treatment in the catheterization laboratory include coronary fistulas, paravalvular leaks, and pulmonary artery stenoses. Optimum management of patients with complex congenital heart disease can often be achieved by planned collaboration between surgeon and interventional cardiologist. In other patients with a range of relatively simple lesions—including patent ductus arteriosus, pulmonary valve stenosis, atrial septal defect/patent foramen ovale, and certain forms of ventricular septal defect—definitive treatment avoiding surgery may be achieved by interventional catheterization.

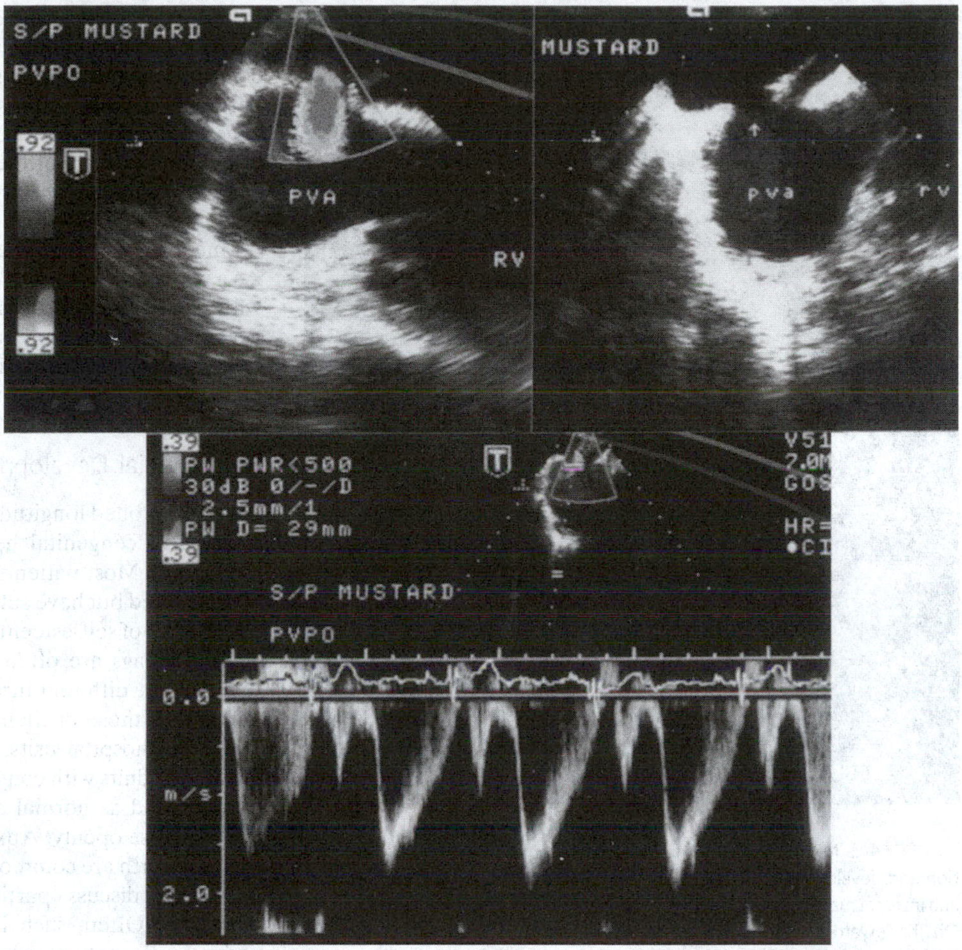

FIGURE 64-1 Transesophageal echocardiogram and Doppler evaluation after a Mustard operation for transposition of the great arteries. There is moderate pulmonary venous obstruction, indicated by the accelerated flow through the narrowing indicated by the arrow. PVA, pulmonary venous atrium; RV, right ventricle. (Courtesy of Dr. I. D. Sullivan, Great Ormond Street Hospital for Children, London.)

PSYCHOSOCIAL ASPECTS

During adolescence, a crucial transition occurs for the patient with congenital heart disease. By the end of the teenage years, the young adult must understand the nature and implications of his or her heart problem. Sensible advice and guidance must be available regarding employment, insurance, socialization, contraception, exercise, and sports.

Employment

Most patients can work and should have access to employment appropriate to their physical and intellectual capabilities. The report of the Natural History Study of Congenital Heart Defects suggested that, among patients with ventricular septal defect, pulmonary stenosis, and aortic stenosis, in comparison with national normal standards, a greater percentage achieved higher levels of education (college and beyond).[112] No similar data are yet available for large groups of patients with more complex defects, although their situation will undoubtedly prove worse.

Despite the excellent potential of many adults with congenital heart disease, job discrimination is frequently encountered, even when a patient has been cleared by a cardiologist. In the United States, the National Rehabilitation Act of 1973 seeks to prevent job discrimination by employers with 10 or more employees by obliging them to consider only the present capacity of applicants to perform a given job and not projections of future deterioration. In other countries, employers frequently take into account future prospects for absenteeism or premature career curtailment. In these circumstances, young adults with congenital heart defects are often at a disadvantage, particularly if they apply for jobs with long training periods.

Restrictions for employment exist for jobs in which the safety of others is the direct responsibility of an individual, such as driving a bus or truck. Most armed services exclude applicants with a cardiac history. The regulations for commercial airline pilots are clearer and subject to regular review. In Europe, a risk of sudden cardiac death or acute disability below 1 percent per annum is the maximum considered acceptable for multicrew flights and below 0.1 percent per annum for solo flights. The number of congenital heart defects in which low risk rates are clearly defined remains small.[113]

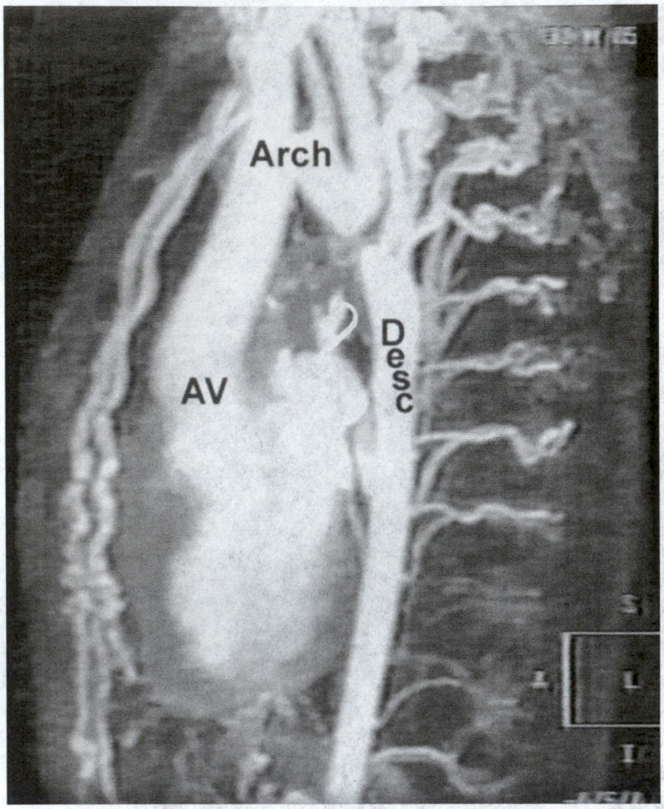

FIGURE 64-2 MRI angiogram of a 33-year-old man showing a severe coarctation and development of extensive collateralization involving the intercostal and internal mammary arteries. AV, aortic valve; Desc, descending aorta. (From Oh JK, Seward JB, Tajik AJ. Congenital heart disease. In: Oh JK, Seward JB, Tajik AJ, eds: *The Echo Manual*, 2d ed. Philadelphia: Lippincott-Raven, 1999: 233. Reproduced with permission from the publisher and authors.)

Insurance

Possession of adequate life insurance is often a prerequisite for a home mortgage. Insurance companies are of necessity fiscally conservative. As a result, life insurance is difficult to obtain for many young adults in the absence of adequate long-term survival data for their congenital heart lesions. Most of the data used to assess risk are either incorrect or out of date and do not apply to currently performed medical or surgical procedures. In 1986, a survey in the United States recorded that only patients with very simple lesions were insured at regular rates.[114] These included mild pulmonary valve stenosis, uncomplicated repaired atrial septal defect, ventricular septal defect, and patent ductus arteriosus. A similar survey in the United Kingdom in 1993 evaluated both employment status and insurability of young adults with congenital heart disease.[115] In general, policies were as restrictive as those in the earlier survey, with mitral valve prolapse (without regurgitation), postoperative patent ductus arteriosus, and coarctation insurable at standard rates and all other lesions being either insurable at higher rates or not insurable at all. Marked inconsistencies were found, making "shopping around" mandatory. This situation is likely to improve when health care professionals are able to provide high-quality follow-up data on morbidity and mortality rates relevant to current treatment protocols (see Chap. 104).

Despite surgical repair, long-term cardiac care into adult life is usually required for patients with congenital heart disease. In many countries, health care provision and financing are changing rapidly, with costs spiraling dramatically.[116] There are particular problems in systems that rely on private health insurance. Medical expenses incurred during childhood are usually reimbursed as part of the parents' policy. This coverage often ceases to be available once the patient reaches the age of majority. A new policy sought at this stage at best excludes benefits for medical or surgical treatment of the cardiac condition itself. As a result, the level of medical surveillance of the adult patient with congenital heart disease drops dramatically after age 21 years. This is a major problem, since, with adequate regular follow-up, costs for adults with congenital heart disease are considerably lower than those for other chronic diseases.

Psychosocial Development

Large controlled longitudinal studies of the psychosocial consequences of congenital heart disease are rare and difficult to interpret.[117] Most patients with congenital heart disease appear well adjusted but have subtle feelings of "difference" from their peers. Lack of self-esteem and fear of isolation are common.[118–120] These feelings are often compounded by frequent reminders that they are different through limitation of their activities compared with those of their peers, the presence of scars, cardiac symptoms, hospital visits, and family anxiety. As a result, adolescents and adults with congenital heart disease should be encouraged to lead as normal a life as possible and to discuss their heart disease openly. Anxieties about sexual activity, marriage, and childbirth are common, but patients often find these aspects difficult to discuss, particularly with the doctor in a regular clinic.[120–122] Often, such issues are best handled by the team caring for the patient, which may include a nurse, social worker, and psychologist. As the child with congenital heart disease matures, one of the most potent effects on his or her life is parental overprotection. In adolescents and young adults, this may result in enormous resentment and rebellion against all adult authority figures, including the doctor. Compliance with medical treatment and advice can be affected.

The impact of congenital heart disease on intellectual development is controversial. Interpretation of testing must take into account the very abnormal childhood experienced by many patients, with absences from school for medical reasons as well as decreased social interaction. In addition, patients have often had an overprotected childhood, and their attitude to testing procedures may be different from those of their peers. All studies of intellect exclude patients with genetic syndromes and other dysmorphic, somatic, or neurologic defects, but subtle abnormalities are easily missed.[123] Certain aspects of development appear to be more specifically affected by congenital heart disease. For example, walking is delayed in cyanotic children, but speech is not. This will affect the relevance of early IQ testing to later performance. Currently, data suggest that cyanosis is associated with mild intellectual impairment.[124–126] This association is reduced by early corrective surgery, even involving cardiopulmonary bypass.

Contraception

Sexually active adolescents and young adults should be given appropriate advice about contraception.[127,128] In general, the low-dose estrogen oral contraceptive pill is safe for young women with congenital heart disease.[129] Exceptions include women with hypertension (e.g., associated with coarctation of the aorta) and those with pulmonary vascular disease or cyanosis with associated erythrocytosis. Progesterone preparations are alternatives, although they have a lower contraceptive efficacy.[130] They are, however, inappropriate for patients with cardiac failure because of the tendency for fluid retention; moreover, progesterone-only pills can cause depression in adolescents. Barrier methods, either using condom or diaphragm, are safe and effective, but intrauterine devices should probably not be used because of the risk of endocarditis and of increased bleeding, particularly in cyanotic women.[131] In women with severe pulmonary vascular disease or with lesions in which pregnancy would result in high maternal risk, laparoscopic sterilization should be considered.

Exercise and Sports

Exercise is of both physical and psychological benefit. It leads to improved cardiovascular fitness and decreased likelihood of obesity, hypertension, and ischemic heart disease.[132,133] Furthermore, participation in exercise and sports is part of normal socialization in adolescent and adult life. In many adults with congenital heart disease, exercise capacity is diminished, even after surgery. Reduced performance may also reflect lack of regular exercise in protected individuals with congenital heart defects. This is often reinforced by doctors who, if in doubt, tend to limit exercise.

The Twenty-sixth Bethesda Conference provided recommendations for competition in athletics by patients with cardiovascular abnormalities.[134] Sports are broadly categorized into those involving dynamic exercise and those involving static exercise, although these two types of exercise are at two extremes of a continuum. Another important consideration is the danger of bodily injury from collision or the consequences of syncope. Significant disease or death precipitated by exercise in patients with congenital heart disease is rare, but the other consideration is whether prolonged long-term exercise might contribute to progressive hemodynamic deterioration (e.g., left ventricular hypertrophy and aortic stenosis). In some cases, exercise capacity is clearly normal and the risk is minimal, as after closure of a small patent ductus arteriosus. In others, exercise capacity is limited and the risk is high, as in severe pulmonary hypertension. Between these extremes is a gray area in which recommendations must take into account the individual, the underlying cardiac defect, hemodynamic status, and the type of sport and form of exercise contemplated (e.g., social or competitive, or contact or noncontact). Formal testing should be performed (preferably including measurement of oxygen uptake), both as a measure of the effects of submaximal and maximal exercise and also as a reassurance to the patient. A 12-min walking test provides a good guide to functional capacity, whereas a treadmill protocol with more strenuous effort is employed to assess risk by revealing occult arrhythmia, ischemia, or fall in blood pressure (Chap. 14). Subjective estimates of exercise capacity are often inaccurate.

In general, volume overload, valve regurgitation, and left-to-right shunts are associated with good exercise tolerance, while pressure overload, valve stenosis, and right-to-left shunt are not. The recommendations provided by the Bethesda Conference should be considered guidelines only. The physician with knowledge of the severity of the patient's lesion and physiologic and psychologic response to training and competition may choose to modify these recommendations.[134] Those patients with a history of symptomatic arrhythmia, syncope, pulmonary hypertension, or myocardial dysfunction deserve special attention, since they are probably at higher risk. Patients with fixed, elevated pulmonary vascular resistance have limited exercise capacity, and for them exercise has considerable risk. Walking should be encouraged but strenuous exercise avoided. The most controversial recommendations are those for aortic stenosis and Marfan's syndrome. It could be argued that exercise may increase the risk of sudden death or progression of left ventricular hypertrophy in the former (see Chap. 56) and of progressive aortic dilatation in the latter (see Chap. 76). Thus, patients with more than mild aortic stenosis should be counseled against moderate to strenuous activities. Patients with Marfan's syndrome, particularly those with aortic root dilatation, should be counseled against isometric exercise and activities with the potential for bodily collision. Supervised training programs for adults with congenital heart disease can improve aerobic fitness and increase the safe level at which they can participate in sports. Such programs also improve psychological adjustment and self-esteem.

SURGICAL CONSIDERATIONS

Reoperations

Reoperations in adults with congenital heart disease provide a particular challenge.[135,136] The risks are often higher than for primary procedures. Careful preoperative planning should include complete understanding of the cardiac anatomy and its relationships to neighboring structures, and study of previous operative reports. Sternal reentry is particularly risky when the ventricle immediately beneath the sternum is a high-pressure chamber or when an extracardiac conduit lies in this position. The use of Gore-Tex membranes under the sternum may reduce the difficulties of future repeat procedures. Postoperative hemodynamic and respiratory problems are particularly common after reoperation because of the increased duration of surgery, previously scarred myocardium and/or lung disease, and greater use of blood products. The need for reoperation may come as a shock to patients and relatives who may have believed that childhood surgery was curative. As a result, resentment is frequent, and tact is required. Indications for reoperation are shown in Table 64-4.

Inevitable Reoperation

Early repair of congenital heart defects that have involved insertion of a prosthetic valve or extracardiac conduit commonly results in a need for reoperation to replace prostheses that are either too small or have undergone degeneration. Extracardiac conduits are commonly used for repair of pulmonary atresia with ventricular septal defect, truncus arteriosus, transposition with left ventricular outflow tract obstruction and/or ventricular septal defect, congenitally corrected transposition with left ventricular outflow tract obstruction, and/or ventricular septal defect and were used in early Fontan operations. Development

TABLE 64-4 Indications for Reoperation in Adults with Congenital Heart Disease

1. Inevitable reoperation after definitive repair prosthetic valves, extracardiac conduits placed at an early age that become of inadequate size because of body growth
2. Residual defects after definitive repair: ventricular septal defect after tetralogy of Fallot and left AV valve regurgitation after AV septal defect repair
3. New/recurrent defects after definitive repair: subaortic stenosis, restenosis of aortic valve, pulmonary regurgitation in tetralogy of Fallot
4. Staged repair of complex defects: pulmonary atresia with ventricular septal defect
5. Unexpected complications: infective endocarditis
6. Heart/heart-lung transplantation for uncorrectable congenital heart disease
7. Patient operated on for congenital heart disease with new acquired heart disease: coronary disease

of obstruction is influenced by the type and size of conduit, technique of insertion, and timing of the original operation. In one series of 143 survivors of heterograft conduit insertion, all had to be replaced by 10 years.[137] A homograft aorta or pulmonary artery and valve have also been used for the repair of pulmonary atresia with ventricular septal defect.[138] Fresh or frozen homografts in childhood have not performed as well as initially hoped.[139] Calcification and obstruction remain significant complications. However, because of their favorable handling characteristics, homografts remain the conduits of choice for many reconstructions.[140,141] Besides the conduit itself, improved operative technique and the use of a large conduit have clear beneficial influence on the need for early replacement. This may be facilitated by utilizing a prosthetic roof of pericardium placed over the fibrous tissue bed of the explanted conduit, thus permitting a large tissue valve to be inserted.[142] Patients with right-sided conduits need careful follow-up, particularly toward the end of the expected life of the conduit. Although conduit obstruction may be suspected from clinical examination, the signs of severe obstruction may be subtle and may be missed. As a result, replacement may be performed too late. The consequent major deleterious effects on right ventricular function increase the risk of surgery and may not be fully reversible. Regular, noninvasive evaluation by transthoracic or transesophageal echocardiography or MRI is indicated in selected patients and may provide the information usually obtained by cardiac catheterization and angiography. Reoperation is usually indicated if the right ventricular pressure is 75 percent of the systemic or if there is evidence of deteriorating ventricular function.[143]

Residual and Recurrent Defects

Residual and recurrent defects may be difficult to distinguish unless careful assessment after the original repair has been performed. They may have a major impact on morbidity and mortality rates, as when major left AV valve regurgitation persists after repair of AV septal defect.[144] Much more long-term follow-up data are needed before guidelines for reoperation for relatively minor residual abnormalities, such as mild left AV valve regurgitation, in this situation can be established.

The reported need for reoperation after the commonly performed reparative operation for tetralogy of Fallot varies between 1.8 and 13 percent over a follow-up of up to 31 years.[145,146] Ventricular septal defect and right ventricular outflow tract obstruction are the commonest residual abnormalities. Pulmonary regurgitation is extremely common and inevitable after transannular patching as part of the original repair. The hemodynamic consequences of pulmonary regurgitation for the right ventricle are greater in the presence of other defects, such as residual obstruction and/or ventricular septal defect. Pulmonary valve replacement has not been frequently required in the first two decades after repair but may become increasingly performed because of the late deleterious effects of pulmonary regurgitation on the right ventricle.[147] Current indications include progressive right ventricular dilatation and a decrease in exercise tolerance.[148] This is often accompanied by progressive tricuspid regurgitation and atrial arrhythmias. When surgery is performed before the development of right ventricular failure, both clinical status and right ventricular function improve.[149] The optimal method for assessing pulmonary regurgitation in serial follow-up has not been determined; therefore, appropriate guidelines for intervention are still not established.

Several studies have emphasized the palliative nature of aortic valvotomy in childhood.[150–152] Isolated aortic stenosis most frequently results from a bicuspid aortic valve, although in neonates and infants the structural abnormality of the aortic valve is more severe and the results of surgery even worse (see Chap. 63). In a series of 59 patients who underwent open aortic valvotomy at over 1 year of age, the actuarial survival rate was 94 percent at 5 years but only 77 percent at 22 years. Reoperation was carried out in 36 percent, and the actuarial probability of reoperation was 44 percent at 22 years. When serious events, comprising death, reoperation, and endocarditis, were grouped together, 92 percent were free of events at 5 years but only 39 percent at 22 years. Others have reported a similar long-term outcome.[150] The causes of restenosis have not been studied in detail but appear to be related to the degree of residual obstruction.

Staged Repair

For complex congenital heart disease, definitive repair may not be possible until the anatomy and physiology of the circulation have been improved by one or more palliative procedures as part of a staged approach to "correction." This course is often necessary for patients with pulmonary atresia and ventricular septal defect, hypoplastic pulmonary arteries, and multifocal pulmonary blood supply. Palliative procedures to increase flow to the central pulmonary arteries and unifocalization of pulmonary flow by anastomosis (direct or indirect) of collateral vessels to the pulmonary arteries may eventually result in the ability to perform a repair (conduit insertion between the right ventricle and pulmonary artery and ventricular septal defect closure) with an acceptable postoperative right ventricular/left ventricular pressure ratio.[153,154] Good surgical results have been reported from such an approach, but the long-term outcome is not yet known.[155]

Other situations in which definitive repair may be indicated in the young adult include complex congenital heart defects with one functioning ventricle palliated by a systemic-pulmonary shunt or pulmonary artery banding in childhood. In selected patients who fulfill the stringent criteria for a Fontan operation, it is likely that long-term results will be better after a Fontan operation than when the ventricle is left with a chronically increased load resulting from a systemic pulmonary shunt.[12] The Fontan operation, however, should be considered palliative rather than curative: long-term problems are frequent.

Unexpected Reoperations

Indications for unexpected reoperation include thrombosis in a low-flow circulation such as the Fontan, prosthetic valve failure or thrombosis, and infective endocarditis. The latter may be particularly difficult to diagnose in complex congenital heart disease where the site of vegetations may not be easy to image (e.g., in a Blalock-Taussig shunt). Reoperation in the patient with uncontrolled endocarditis carries a particularly high risk.

Heart and Heart-Lung Transplantation

Despite the major successes of the last three decades, an increasing number of patients survive to adult life with deteriorating clinical status. Their only remaining prospect may be a heart or heart-and-lung transplant (see Chap. 22). These patients often present specific surgical problems of multiple previous chest incisions, complex venous anatomy, and borderline pulmonary vascular resistance. In addition, the young adult with end-stage heart disease may not have the ideal social milieu to cope with the demands of transplantation and may require considerable psychological support. Nonetheless, the results in this group of patients may be excellent.[156] The shortage of donors and the ability to monitor rejection in a single organ have stimulated great interest in single-lung transplantation for patients with primary pulmonary hypertension and Eisenmenger's syndrome (in conjunction with closure of the shunt).[157]

First Operations for Congenital Heart Disease in Adults

The first surgical repair of a congenital heart defect may be required in a teenager or an adult because the lesion was mild and of little hemodynamic significance in childhood but progressed in severity with time. Examples of such lesions include a bicuspid aortic valve with progressive stenosis (see Chap. 56), Marfan's syndrome with aortic root dilatation (see Chap. 76), and Ebstein's anomaly with worsening symptoms. Alternatively, lesions such as small to moderate atrial septal defects may have been missed or misdiagnosed until adult life. In certain complex congenital heart defects, the combination of lesions produces a balanced hemodynamic state compatible with prolonged survival without intervention. Patients with double-inlet ventricle and pulmonary stenosis, complex pulmonary atresia, and tetralogy of Fallot may remain well until the second and even third decades of life before deteriorating.[158] The contemplation of heart surgery in an adolescent or young adult is often terrifying, implying the acceptance of the presence of a serious heart problem by the patient and his or her immediate friends and family. The scar on the chest may cause embarrassment, and the patient may be discriminated against both socially and at work. All these issues need to be dealt with sympathetically by the physician.

Noncardiac Surgery

When performed without adequate preparation, noncardiac surgery in adults with congenital heart disease is a major cause of avoidable morbidity and death. All the anesthetic risks encountered for cardiac reoperation apply equally to noncardiac surgery, but in the latter the patient may be managed by medical staff who may be unfamiliar with the significance of the congenital heart disease. Many patients with congenital heart defects are at increased risk for arrhythmia and from agents that depress ventricular function. The surgeon must be aware of the presence of a pacemaker or pacing leads that may affect the safe use of diathermy. Prophylaxis against infective endocarditis is usually indicated, and the choice of antibiotic regimen is dictated by the surgical procedure or intervention being undertaken (see Chap. 73). In patients with pulmonary vascular disease, general anesthesia may have disastrous consequences, with a sudden fall in systemic vascular resistance.[28] Similar hemodynamic changes may induce a severe hypercyanotic spell in a patient with uncorrected tetralogy of Fallot, and meticulous pre-, intra-, and postoperative hemodynamic monitoring is mandatory, together with the avoidance of vasodilating anesthetic agents, hypoxia, hypoventilation, and blood or volume loss. Cyanotic patients also have impaired hemostasis, and some patients may be taking anticoagulants. Intravenous lines, drugs, and infusions must be managed carefully in patients with intracardiac shunts, since air or emboli may reach the systemic circulation. The safety of noncardiac surgery in adults with congenital heart disease is greatly increased when physicians, anesthesiologists, and surgeons familiarize themselves with these issues, seek specialized advice, and, if necessary, refer the patient to a team with more experience.

SPECIFIC LESIONS

General Considerations

Some lesions that are commonly seen in adult congenital heart disease, as a result of both natural and unnatural survival, are listed in Tables 64-1 and 64-2.

Interpretation of the literature on long-term outcome of congenital heart defects is hampered by a number of difficulties. First, follow-up is still short, and numbers of survivors are small for many defects. The era of open-heart surgery for congenital heart defects only began in the 1950s, and "correction" has only been attempted much more recently for many categories of patients now beginning to reach adult life (e.g., the Fontan operation). Second, surgical practice has undergone a process of evolution during this time, with new operations for some lesions (e.g., transposition of the great arteries) or major change in operative technique for others (e.g., the Fontan operation). Third, major advances in cardiopulmonary bypass and myocardial protection have accompanied improved preoperative diagnosis and recognition of intracardiac anatomy, particularly of the disposition of the conduction tissues. Finally, for almost all lesions, the management philosophy has changed, with a trend to early primary repair as opposed to initial palliation. For many defects, therefore, long-term outcome data relevant to current practice are not available.

Correct application of survival analysis is essential for interpretation of follow-up data. In particular, the use of hazard functions providing an estimate of *instantaneous risk* is particularly valuable. The following section deals with some specific defects seen in adults with congenital heart disease.

Atrial Septal Defect

Atrial septal defects are among the commonest congenital anomalies in adolescents and adults, accounting for up to 30 percent of congenital heart disease in this age group.[159,160] Approximately 75 percent of defects are ostium secundum defects, 20 percent ostium primum defects (discussed below), and 5 percent sinus venosus defects; defects at other sites are rare (see Chap. 63).[161,162] Associated lesions include pulmonary stenosis, mitral valve prolapse, and mitral regurgitation. Atrial septal defects may be associated with other syndromes, including the Holt-Oram syndrome (see Fig. 10-2)[163] and may be familial.[164] In the latter, conduction disease manifesting as prolongation of the PR interval and, rarely, heart block have been described.[164] Lutembacher syndrome (atrial septal defect coexisting with mitral stenosis) is now very uncommon.

NATURAL HISTORY

Survival into adulthood is the rule, and patients living into their eighties and nineties have been reported.[159] Life expectancy, however, is not normal. Death during the first 20 years of life is infrequent, but after the age of 40 years, the mortality rate increases to about 6 percent per year.[165,166] Defects may go unrecognized for many years because symptoms are rare until later life and physical signs may be subtle. Later, the natural history is characterized by progressive symptoms and cardiomegaly, the development of atrial arrhythmias, right ventricular hypertrophy, and pulmonary hypertension. The mechanisms for the development of symptoms are multifactorial[159] and include the following:

1. Change in left ventricular compliance from superimposed hypertension or coronary artery disease may increase the shunt with age. Long-standing right ventricular volume overload, although relatively well tolerated, ultimately leads to right ventricular dysfunction and progression of tricuspid regurgitation.
2. Supraventricular arrhythmias, particularly atrial fibrillation and flutter, increase with time and may cause symptoms and cardiac failure (Fig. 64-3).
3. Progressive pulmonary hypertension may become symptomatic after the third decade of life.
4. Rarer complications may occur, including systemic and pulmonary emboli, recurrent chest infections, and infective endocarditis (in patients with coexisting mitral valve disease).

MANAGEMENT

Surgical closure either by direct suture or use of a patch has been performed for more than 40 years (see Chap. 63). Surgery carries a low risk (less than 1 percent operative mortality rate),

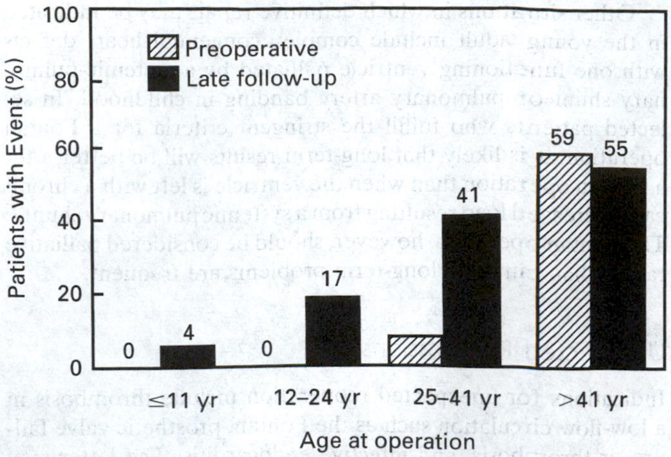

FIGURE 64-3 Incidence of atrial flutter or atrial fibrillation preoperatively and at late follow-up according to the age at operation after repair of atrial septal defect. (From Murphy JG, Gersh BJ, McGoon MD, et al. Long-term outcome after surgical repair of isolated atrial septal defects: Follow-up at 27–32 years. *N Engl J Med* 1990; 323:1645. Reproduced with permission from the publisher and authors.)

provided that the pulmonary vascular resistance is not significantly elevated.[162] In older patients, the indication for closure is a little more controversial. Shah et al. compared the outcome of patients treated medically and surgically when diagnosed after the age of 25 years.[167] This unrandomized study followed patients for more than 20 years and concluded that there was no difference in survival or symptoms between the two groups and no difference in the incidence of new arrhythmia, stroke, or other embolic phenomena in the follow-up period. Notably, however, more than 70 percent of patients in both the medical and surgical groups were asymptomatic at presentation, which may partly explain the favorable outcome of the medically treated group, who had a 91 percent survival. Konstantinides et al. evaluated 179 patients with secundum atrial septal defect 40 years of age or older and compared the outcome of medically and surgically treated groups.[168] They demonstrated a reduced mortality rate after surgical closure, with a 95 percent surgical survival versus an 84 percent medical survival at 10 years. Nonfatal cardiovascular complications, however, were similar, with atrial fibrillation and flutter occurring with a similar incidence in both groups. The functional status of the medically treated group deteriorated in 34 percent of patients and improved in many of the surgical patients, particularly those in class III or IV. It thus seems reasonable to conclude that symptomatic adult patients will improve after surgical repair, and the only real contraindication is severe pulmonary vascular disease. When surgery is delayed, symptoms are likely to be progressive, and surgical repair is less likely to prevent problems with atrial fibrillation and thromboembolic events. For those with preexisting atrial fibrillation, a concomitant right-sided maze procedure may facilitate restoration and maintenance of sinus rhythm.[169] The management of the asymptomatic adult patient is less clear, but certainly closure of the defect halts progression of right ventricular volume overload, tricuspid regurgitation, and progression of pulmonary vascular disease, and it can be accomplished with low surgical risk. The standard surgical approach remains a midline sternotomy, but patients should be made aware of the alternatives of thoracotomy or inframammary incision. Although morbidity rates may be higher, the resulting scar may be less offensive, especially to young women.

Closure of atrial septal defect has been achieved in selected patients by use of a variety of occlusion devices inserted at cardiac catheterization.[170–174] Several alternatives have been evaluated, but no large series with adequate follow-up are yet available for comparison with surgery. The attractions of closing defects without open-heart surgery are obvious. Eventually, the transcatheter technique may supplant surgery as the method of closure for atrial septal defects of appropriate size, morphologic characteristics, and location. In addition, the presence of a patent foramen ovale has been suggested as a risk factor for cerebral embolus. Determining the risk of clinical events in asymptomatic subjects with patent foramen ovale and indications for treatment are highly controversial areas. Catheter treatment may become the method of choice for patients who have a clear indication for intervention.

LATE RESULTS

In a recent study of patients undergoing surgical repair of an atrial septal defect between 1956 and 1960, late survival of patients undergoing operation at below 24 years of age was not significantly different from that of an age- and sex-matched control population. Late survival in patients aged 25 to 41 years was good but less than that of the control population, while repair after age 41 years was associated with significantly poorer late survival (see Fig. 64-3). The combination of older age at operation and pulmonary hypertension had an additive effect on late mortality rates.[175] In this and other series, the propensity for atrial fibrillation and flutter increased as a function of age both before and after operation (Fig. 64-4).[175,176] Twenty-two percent of late deaths were due to stroke, and all occurred in patients with postoperative atrial fibrillation or flutter. These data support the current policy of repair at a preschool age (Chap. 63). A separate study of 66 patients who underwent closure of atrial septal defect between 60 and 78 years of age implied a benefit in survival in patients discharged from the hospital compared with unoperated historical age- and sex-matched controls.[177] A study of patients over 70 years of age showed improved survival of patients in New York Heart Association (NYHA) class II and III when treated surgically compared to medical treatment. Patients in NYHA class IV did poorly with medical or surgical treatment.

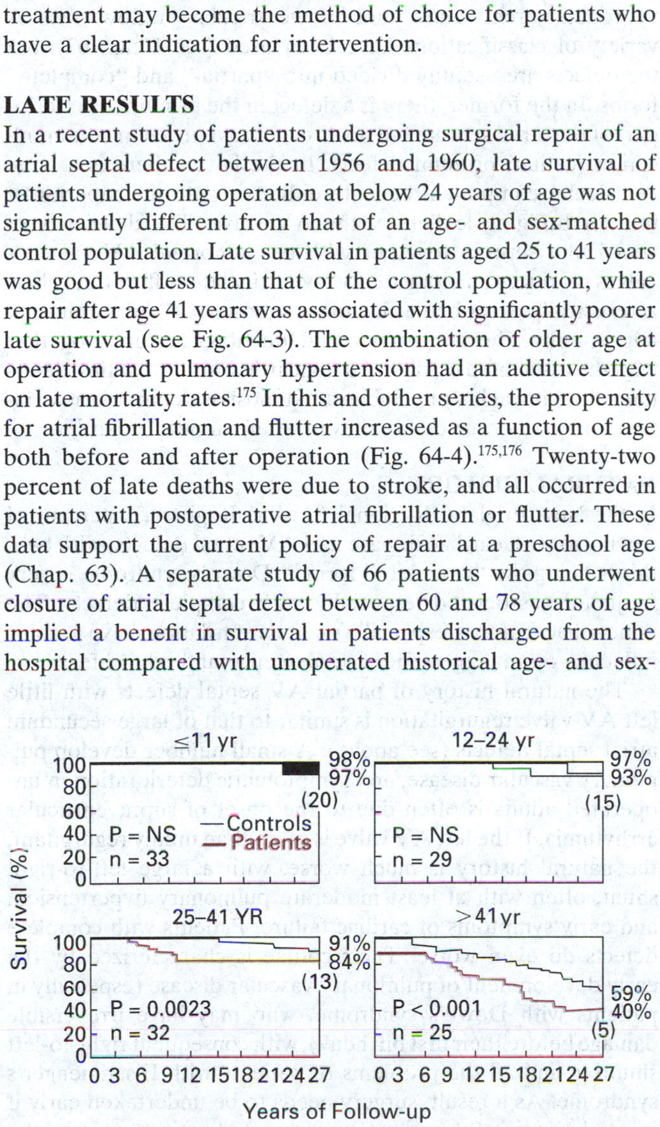

FIGURE 64-4 Long-term survival of perioperative survivors of atrial septal defect repair by age at time of operation. Controls are survival in an age- and sex-matched population. (From Murphy JG, Gersh BJ, McGoon MD, et al. Long-term outcome after surgical repair of isolated atrial septal defects: Follow-up at 27–32 years. *N Engl J Med* 1990; 323:1645. Reproduced with permission from the publisher and authors.)

The near-normal survival and low morbidity rates in patients undergoing repair within the first two decades of life have important implications for employment and insurance recommendations. Such patients should be encouraged to lead a normal life, and competitive sports should not be restricted in the absence of hemodynamic or electrophysiologic sequelae. Patients who have undergone repair in the third decade of life or later require careful regular surveillance. Although late survival is good, the development of supraventricular arrhythmia and risk of cerebrovascular accident are of concern. Anticoagulation is indicated in patients with atrial fibrillation and should be considered in those with supraventricular tachycardia or atrial flutter in the absence of other contraindications (see also Chaps. 24 and 44). Long-term follow-up is recommended for patients repaired in adult life who have increased pulmonary artery pressure at the end of operation, pre- and postoperative arrhythmia, ventricular dysfunction, or coexisting heart disease.

Ventricular Septal Defect

Isolated ventricular septal defect, although one of the commonest congenital abnormalities in infants and children, is far less frequent in the adolescent and adult for several reasons.[159] First, most patients with a hemodynamically significant defect will have undergone repair in childhood; second, spontaneous decrease in size and closure are common for small or moderate perimembranous or muscular defects (this decreases in frequency with increasing age); finally, patients with large, unoperated defects may die earlier in life.[178] The spectrum of isolated ventricular septal defects in the adult is thus limited to the following four groups of patients: (1) those with small, restrictive defects that were either small to begin with or have partially closed; (2) those with Eisenmenger's syndrome and a predominant right-to-left shunt with cyanosis,[179] who need to be distinguished from those who develop secondary infundibular pulmonary stenosis, which can also decrease the left-to-right shunt and may result in cyanosis with shunt reversal (see Chap. 63);[180] (3) the occasional patient with a moderately restrictive defect in whom the diagnosis has been overlooked or who has not had closure in childhood; and (4) those who have had their defects closed in childhood.

NATURAL HISTORY

The natural history of small, restrictive ventricular septal defects is very favorable. Nevertheless, the risk of infective endocarditis persists (developing in almost 4 percent of patients with ventricular septal defect), and lifelong prophylaxis is required. Spontaneous closure may occasionally still occur in adult life. A subset of patients with perimembranous defects or defects in the outlet septum may develop aortic cusp prolapse and aortic regurgitation. This may be progressive and is often severe by the end of the second decade of life. As incompetence increases, the ventricular septal defect may become "closed" by the prolapsing cusp; if it is left to develop, however, aortic valve replacement may be necessary.[181] Such defects are associated with a high risk of infective endocarditis. Severe and progressive pulmonary vascular disease is a feature of older patients with nonrestrictive large defects. Eisenmenger's syndrome is compatible with survival into young adult life, but the complications of right-sided heart failure, paradoxical emboli, and erythrocytosis usually result in death by the third decade (see Chap. 63). Occasionally, patients with moderate-sized ventricular septal defects and left-to-right shunts who did not develop pulmonary vascular disease present in adolescence and young adult life with symptoms of fatigue, effort intolerance, and respiratory infections.

MANAGEMENT

Patients with small ventricular septal defects are asymptomatic and should be managed conservatively. Continued medical follow-up is, however, helpful to remind patients about the need for prophylaxis against infective endocarditis and to minimize inappropriate discrimination during the search for employment and insurance. Ventricular septal defects associated with aortic cusp prolapse and aortic regurgitation should be repaired even when the shunt is small in an effort to prevent progressive deterioration of the aortic valve. Surgical repair is indicated in the rare adult with a significant left-to-right shunt (pulmonary/systemic flow ratio exceeding 2:1) and a low pulmonary vascular resistance. The management of patients with large defects and infundibular narrowing causing right-to-left shunting and cyanosis is similar to that for tetralogy of Fallot (see below).

Unfortunately, adults are still seen with a large ventricular septal defect and pulmonary vascular disease. In those with borderline pulmonary vascular resistance (7 to 10 U/m^2), surgery may be attempted, but the benefits are unpredictable, since the pulmonary vascular disease may progress despite closure of the defect (see Chap. 63).[182] Medical management and consideration for heart-lung or single-lung transplantation are the only realistic options for patients with established severe pulmonary vascular disease, although prostacyclin may hold some promise.[29]

LATE RESULTS

Late results of surgery are good, but the life expectancy for the whole group is not normal. In a study of 179 operative survivors between 1956 and 1959, 30-year survival was 82 percent, compared with 97 percent in age- and sex-matched controls.[180] Only 25 percent of patients in the series were over 10 years of age at surgery, and their 30-year survival of 70 percent was substantially lower than the 88 percent in patients under 2 years of age at operation. Thirty-year survival was 83 percent for patients aged 3 to 10 years at surgery. Older age at repair and preoperative pulmonary vascular disease are important predictors of late outcome. Postoperative conduction defects, especially right bundle-branch block, are common, but complete heart block, which was seen in the early surgical experience, is now rare. Late ventricular arrhythmia has been reported, as after repair of tetralogy of Fallot.[183] The incidence of late sudden death, however, is extremely low, and prophylactic antiarrhythmic therapy in asymptomatic patients is not indicated.

Certain selected ventricular septal defects may be closed with transcatheter devices. One report described closure of 21 muscular ventricular septal defects in 12 patients, half of whom had complex heart defects.[184] All the defects were closed successfully, and subsequent cardiac surgery for associated lesions was performed in 11 of 12 patients.

In postoperative patients, the risk of late infective endocarditis is very small, provided that the defect is isolated and is completely closed. Antibiotic prophylaxis, however, is often advised, particularly for 6 months postoperatively. Recommendations regarding physical activity and competitive sports require detailed evaluation, which may include exercise testing, cross-sectional echocardiography, and ambulatory ECG monitoring. The presence of abnormal left ventricular function, a more than trivial residual shunt, arrhythmia, or any degree of pulmonary hypertension mandates some restriction of physical activity.

Atrioventricular Septal Defect

The term *atrioventricular septal defect* describes the spectrum of lesions that involve a defect at the site of the normal AV septum, resulting in an abnormality involving the AV valves, ventricular architecture, and left ventricular outflow tract. A variety of classifications have been used (see Chap. 63), but the defects are usefully divided into "partial" and "complete" forms. In the former, there is a defect in the primum or inferior part of the atrial septum but no direct intraventricular communication (ostium primum defect). In the latter, there is a large ventricular component beneath either or both the superior or inferior bridging leaflets of the AV valve. The deficiency of ventricular septum together with the abnormal AV valve or valves produces an elongated left ventricular outflow tract characteristically described as having a "gooseneck" appearance at angiography. The morphologic and functional features, together with the associated cardiac and noncardiac abnormalities, determine the natural history. Subaortic stenosis is a common association and may occur de novo even after surgical repair.[185]

NATURAL HISTORY

In the New England Regional Cardiac Registry, 5 percent of newborns with cardiac disease had AV septal defects, with two-thirds being the "complete" form.[186] Down's syndrome is very frequently associated, especially with complete defects. The noncardiac features, especially mental retardation, have a major influence on management in adolescence and adult life.

The natural history of partial AV septal defects with little left AV valve regurgitation is similar to that of large secundum atrial septal defects (see above). A small number develop pulmonary vascular disease, and symptomatic deterioration in unoperated adults is often due to the onset of supraventricular arrhythmia. If the left AV valve is more than mildly regurgitant, the natural history is much worse, with a large left-to-right shunt, often with at least moderate pulmonary hypertension, and early symptoms of cardiac failure. Patients with complete defects do even worse. Their course is characterized by the early development of pulmonary vascular disease (especially in patients with Down's syndrome, who may have irreversible damage before their first birthday), with consequent right-to-left shunting and all the problems of patients with Eisenmenger's syndrome. As a result, surgery needs to be undertaken early if it is to be successful, and most uncorrected patients seen by the adolescent or adult cardiologist will have a pulmonary vascular resistance that is too high for repair (greater than 8 to 10 U/m^2; see Chaps. 15 and 63). Their outcome is poor, but survival into their thirties is possible. Uncorrected patients with partial AV septal defects may present to the adult cardiologist for consideration of surgery, which should be recommended for those with a significant left-to-right shunt in the absence of other contraindications.

MANAGEMENT

Surgical repair involves closure of the atrial and ventricular septal defects and restoration of a competent left AV valve as far as is possible (see Chap. 63).[187] The surgical mortality rate in experienced centers is approximately 10 percent for complete defects and less than 5 percent for partial defects.[162]

LATE RESULTS

Patients with repair of both partial and complete forms of AV septal defect have now been followed for more than 20 years. Late results are good in the absence of pulmonary vascular disease and significant residual left AV valve regurgitation. Some patients with complete defects who were corrected later in childhood, before the need for correction in early infancy was appreciated, have developed progressive pulmonary vascular disease. This late complication should be greatly reduced in patients undergoing repair in the first 6 months of life, as is now technically feasible (see Chap. 63). Even patients who are repaired late in adult life (at 40 years of age or more) can have excellent results, with an early mortality rate of only 6 percent and a good chance of left AV valve repair in experienced hands.[188]

During long-term follow-up, careful attention must be paid to the status of the left AV valve. If the regurgitation increases in severity, reoperation and mitral valve replacement may be necessary.[144] Monitoring for arrhythmia at intervals is also currently recommended; in general, little intervention is usually required, apart from lifelong infective endocarditis prophylaxis. Surgically repaired non-Down's patients without pulmonary vascular disease can often enjoy life without cardiovascular disability and should not be discouraged from competitive sports, pregnancy, or employment. Restrictions are clearly required for those with pulmonary vascular disease, left AV valve regurgitation, or mitral valve replacement on anticoagulants. Patients with Down's syndrome, both operated and unoperated, are demanding, and their families require considerable support from the physician as well as from educational and social services. The recurrence risk of congenital heart disease in offspring of mothers with AV septal defect is higher than average, and potential parents should be counseled.

Tetralogy of Fallot

Tetralogy of Fallot is the commonest form of cyanotic congenital heart disease seen in the adult. Nonetheless, in the developed world the unoperated patient with tetralogy of Fallot has, fortunately, become a rarity, since the overwhelming majority of patients will have undergone palliation or, more often, repair in childhood. From an anatomic and pathophysiologic standpoint, the manifestations of tetralogy of Fallot are similar in all age groups, although hypercyanotic spells, which are often seen in infants and young children, are rare in adults. The development of systemic hypertension with age is a problem, since it increases the afterload to both ventricles.[159,189] Although pulmonary blood flow may improve, this occurs at the expense of right ventricular failure. Acquired calcific aortic stenosis has similar effects. Aortic regurgitation may occur as a result of cusp prolapse into the subaortic ventricular septal defect, and the aorta itself may be dilated. The aortic regurgitation may also be exacerbated by infective endocarditis. Since the volume overload is transmitted to both ventricles, patients may present with right ventricular failure as a consequence of aortic regurgitation. The development of chronic obstructive lung disease is another manifestation of an acquired cardiopulmonary disease that may place the adult patient with tetralogy of Fallot at particular risk.

NATURAL HISTORY

Survival into the seventh decade is described,[190] but the natural history in the unoperated patient, which is determined by the severity of obstruction of the right ventricular outflow tract and pulmonary vasculature, is poor. Only 25 percent of patients reach the age of 10 years; 11 percent are alive at 20 years, 6 percent at age 30 years, and only 3 percent at age 40 years.[159,162,191] Complications of right-to-left shunting and erythrocytosis, which include stroke and cerebral abscess, are common and, in many instances, fatal. Patients are at continuing risk of infective endocarditis; the development of congestive heart failure in adolescence or early adult life is a major cause of death, as is arrhythmia. Myocardial fibrosis resulting from long-standing right ventricular pressure overload and hypoxemia are postulated mechanisms.[192] Prior palliative surgery with a Cooley or Waterston shunt (between the ascending aorta and right pulmonary artery) or a Potts shunt (between the descending aorta and the left pulmonary artery) can lead to the late development of pulmonary vascular disease.[193]

MANAGEMENT

The focus of medical treatment in unoperated patients is on the elevated hematocrit, bleeding disorders, and abnormal uric acid metabolism and the complications of pregnancy. Repair is indicated in all suitable patients, and the principles and techniques are not significantly different in adults than in children (see Chap. 63).[161] Most adults are suitable candidates for repair, but occasionally a patient with an underdeveloped pulmonary vascular bed may require a palliative shunt procedure. Intracardiac repair consists of closure of the ventricular septal defect and relief of right ventricular outflow tract obstruction. In some patients, this may require excision of the pulmonary valve and patch reconstruction of the anulus and outflow tract. In the occasional patient with an anomalous origin of the left coronary artery from the right coronary artery, a conduit between the right ventricle and pulmonary artery may be required.[162]

LATE RESULTS

Late survival is excellent, even in patients who underwent repair during the very early years of open heart surgery.[162] At the Mayo Clinic, the cumulative 30-year survival for patients undergoing successful surgery between 1956 and 1960 was 86 percent compared to 95 percent in age- and sex-matched controls (Fig. 64-4).[194] In a previous series of 396 hospital survivors of repair between 1955 and 1962 at the same institution, 91 percent were alive at 20 years. At 30 years, 77 percent of the initial cohort of 106 patients undergoing surgery between 1954 and 1960 by Lillehei and associates were alive, including 1 patient who was 45 years of age at the time of operation.[195] Surgery cannot be considered "curative," since survival, even in excellent series, is slightly but significantly worse than for a matched control population. The risk factors for an adverse late outcome include older age at surgery, preoperative congestive heart failure, a previous Potts shunt, persistent right ventricular systolic hypertension, and a residual ventricular septal defect.[175,193] Late death may be sudden, due to tachyarrhythmia or, very rarely in the current era, to conduction disease (see above).[50] Left and right ventricular failure due to right ventricular pressure overload or left ventricular volume overload is another important cause of late death in older patients.[159]

The late functional outcome is excellent for the majority of patients. Most lead normal lives, but the results appear to be better in those undergoing surgery at a younger age.[196] Persistent or recurrent symptoms are usually the result of incomplete relief of right ventricular systolic hypertension or recurrent or residual ventricular septal defects. These problems are often manifest within the first few years after surgery and may require reoperation. Progressive aortic dilatation and aortic regurgitation may also occur, requiring aortic valve replacement.[197] Pulmonary regurgitation may be well tolerated for decades but may be associated with late impairment of exercise capacity and, frequently, atrial arrhythmias. Right ventricular volume overload may also be well tolerated for years but ultimately results in right ventricular failure and progressive tricuspid regurgitation. Pulmonary valve replacement can be accomplished with a low risk.[149] In some patients, isolated right ventricular restrictive physiology may paradoxically improve exercise performance and reduce cardiac enlargement, due possibly to shortening of the duration of pulmonary regurgitation.[68]

Recent information links pulmonary regurgitation, cardiomegaly, QRS duration, and potentially life-threatening ventricular arrhythmia.[68,69] This may be important for identification of risk of late sudden death, which has been a rare event in most long-term follow-up series. Asymptomatic ventricular arrhythmia is very common during long-term follow-up. It is again related to older age at repair, but the link between nonsustained ventricular arrhythmia and adverse clinical outcome is uncertain (see above).[61,62] Objective testing has emphasized the effects of older age at operation on subsequent exercise performance. This is essentially normal for children repaired at below 5 years of age but is usually impaired when surgery is undertaken in adolescence or adulthood.[198]

Before unrestricted physical activity after repair of tetralogy of Fallot can be recommended, careful evaluation—including echocardiography, ECG monitoring, and exercise testing—should be undertaken. Normal activity, including competitive sports, seems reasonable if surgery has been performed at a young age, right and left ventricular function and size are normal, and there are no residual ventricular septal defect, significant right ventricular outflow tract obstruction, or worrisome arrhythmia. In those who do not fulfill these stringent criteria, the degree to which physical activity should be restricted must be individualized. Currently, long-term follow-up of all patients with tetralogy of Fallot is recommended.

Pulmonary Stenosis

Isolated pulmonary valve stenosis is a common form of adult congenital heart disease and is characterized typically by a trileaflet valve with fused commissures. A dysplastic valve without commissural fusion occurs infrequently in otherwise normal children but more commonly in patients with Noonan's syndrome (see Fig. 10-13).[159] Subvalvar stenosis due to infundibular hypertrophy is usually a secondary phenomenon in response to obstruction to right ventricular outflow but may occur as a rare isolated entity. Supravalvar or peripheral pulmonary artery stenosis is also extremely uncommon as an isolated entity but is associated with tetralogy of Fallot and supravalvar aortic stenosis in Williams' syndrome (see Fig. 10-25).

NATURAL HISTORY

Prolonged survival into adult life is common and depends upon the severity of obstruction. In patients with severe pulmonary stenosis, symptoms of right-sided failure increase with time because of progressive obstruction and alterations in right ventricular compliance.[199] In the Joint Study of the Natural History of Congenital Heart Disease, 19 percent of patients with severe stenosis aged 2 to 11 years and 37 percent aged 12 to 21 years were symptomatic. The natural history of moderate pulmonary stenosis in older patients is more favorable, with less tendency to progression.

MANAGEMENT

Patients with mild stenosis are asymptomatic and require no intervention other than antibiotic prophylaxis against infective endocarditis. In patients with more severe stenosis (>140-mm gradient between the right ventricle and pulmonary artery), intervention to reduce severity should be considered even if there are no symptoms.

Surgical valvotomy for isolated pulmonary stenosis has been successfully performed for more than 40 years. Perioperative morbidity and mortality rates are minimal beyond the neonatal period in patients without severe congestive cardiac failure or right ventricular dysplasia.[162] Late results are also excellent. In a study from the Mayo Clinic of patients undergoing surgery between 1956 and 1957, late survival for those undergoing valvotomy who are over 21 years of age was similar but not identical to that of an age- and sex-matched control population (Fig. 64-5). Among patients undergoing surgery at an older age, late survival, although still good, was less than that of the control population (Fig. 64-6).[200] This effect of age on late outcome, which was independent of the use of ventriculotomy and outflow patches and of pulmonary regurgitation, is likely the result of long-standing pressure overload on the right ventricle. Late functional results are excellent, and pulmonary regurgitation is well tolerated in the short and medium term. More severe pulmonary regurgitation may result when a pulmonary valvectomy or transanular patch is required, as may be the case for a small or dysplastic valve; the long-term consequences on the right ventricle and functional capacity are not yet well documented (see "Tetralogy of Fallot," above).

Surgical valvotomy is now rarely required after infancy because of the advent of catheter balloon pulmonary valvotomy. In most institutions, balloon valvotomy is the initial procedure of choice at all ages. In the series of 822 patients in the Valvuloplasty and Angioplasty of Congenital Heart Abnormalities registry, gradient reduction was substantially worse in patients with dysplastic valves.[201] Interventional catheter procedures should be confined to centers with experienced operators.

Long-term follow-up data are not yet available. It appears that the excellent early results are maintained for at least 5 years. The late effects of pulmonary regurgitation resulting from the use of large balloons need to be determined. The risk of infective endocarditis in patients with mild pulmonary stenosis

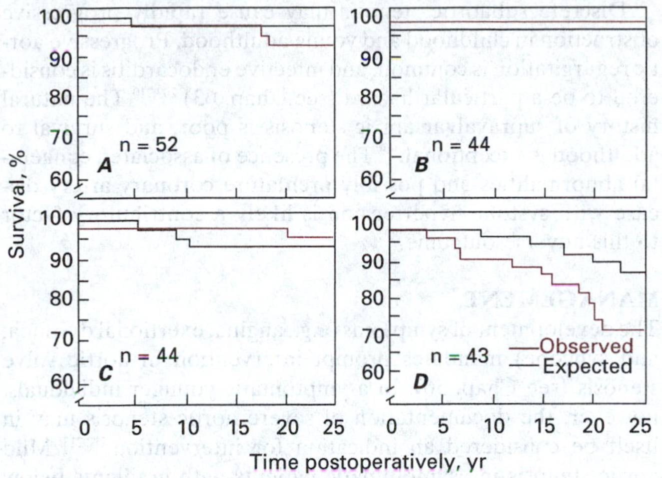

FIGURE 64-5 Long-term survival of perioperative survivors of surgical repair of pulmonary valve stenosis by age at time of operation. *A*. Ages 0 to 4 years. *B*. Ages 5 to 10 years. *C*. Ages 11 to 20 years. *D*. Ages 21 to 68 years. Expected is survival in an age- and sex-matched population. Values of *p* for comparison between the expected and observed survivals: .07, .34, .16, and <.002 for panels *A*, *B*, *C*, and *D*, respectively. (From Kopecky SL, Gersh BJ, McGoon MD, et al. Long-term outcome of patients undergoing surgical repair of isolated pulmonary valve stenosis: Follow-up at 20–30 years. *Circulation* 1988; 78:1150. Reproduced with permission from the publisher and authors.)

or in those with mild gradients after surgical or balloon valvotomy is low. Long-term follow-up is recommended to evaluate not only the right ventricular outflow tract gradient but also pulmonary regurgitation, right ventricular function, and exercise performance. In patients with good relief of pulmonary stenosis, no restriction of physical activities, including competitive sports, is required. In those with moderate residual obstruction or right ventricular dysfunction, exercise intensity should be reduced (see also Chap. 77).

Left Ventricular Outflow Tract Obstruction

Congenital left ventricular outflow tract obstruction may occur at valvar, subvalvar, and supravalvar levels (see Chap. 85). Aortic valve stenosis is a common abnormality in adults with congenital heart disease. It may either be an isolated defect or be associated with other lesions, such as coarctation or ventricular septal defect. It is usually due to a bicuspid aortic valve, which may be present in 1 to 2 percent of the total adult population and is three to four times more common in males than in females.[202] Unicuspid and tricuspid stenotic valves are less common.[162] Subvalvar stenosis encompasses a morphologic spectrum of fibrous or fibromuscular obstructions; it can be a discrete "membrane" below the aortic valve, a discrete fibromuscular ridge, or a diffuse narrowing extending well into the left ventricular cavity forming a "tunnel."[203] The condition occurs more commonly in patients with long and narrow left ventricular outflow tracts,[204] and perhaps this morphologic feature promotes turbulence and shear stresses that stimulate cellular proliferation.[205] Abnormal ventricular bands or chords may also contribute to obstruction, along with abnormal chordal attachments of the anterior mitral valve leaflet. A dynamic component of obstruction may also occur as left ventricular hypertrophy progresses. Common associated anomalies include ventricular septal defect and coarctation of the aorta. Supravalvar stenosis is the least common variety of left ventricular outflow tract obstruction in adolescents and adults, except in the context of Williams' syndrome.[206]

NATURAL HISTORY

The natural history of congenital valvar aortic stenosis in adults is variable but is characterized by progressive stenosis with time (Fig. 64-7; see Chap. 56).[159] By the age of 45 years, approximately half of all bicuspid aortic valves have some degree of narrowing. The severity of obstruction at the time of diagnosis correlates

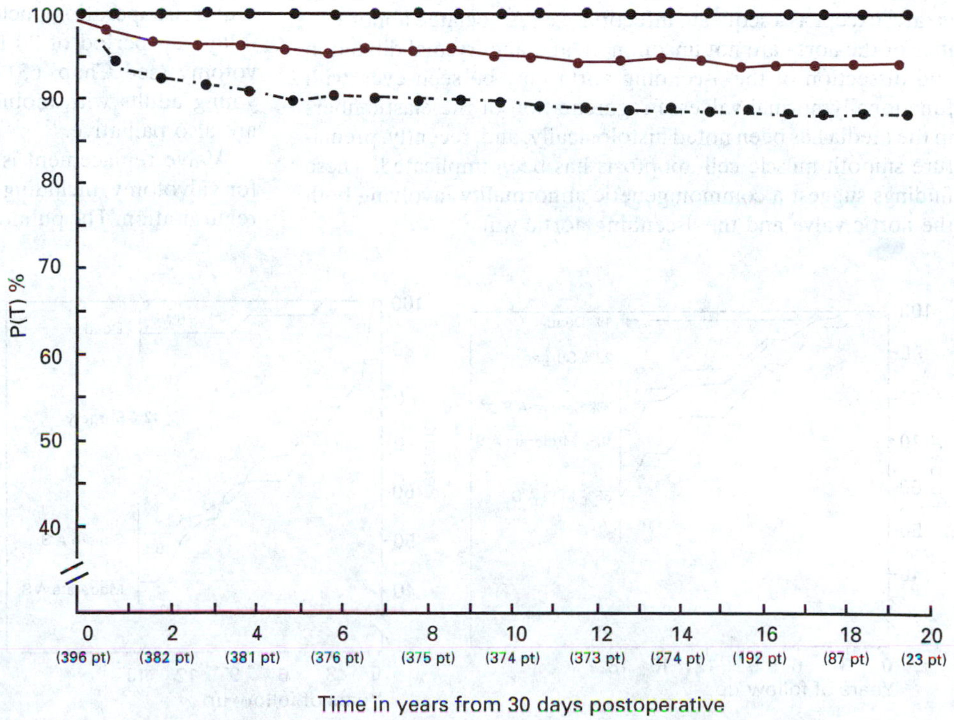

FIGURE 64-6 Probability of deterioration in operative survivors after repair of tetralogy of Fallot plotted against time in years. Time of deterioration is defined as the postoperative year in which late death (*middle curve*) or in which death, reoperation, or symptoms occurred (*bottom curve*). The top curve represents the controlled expected survival on the basis of an age- and sex-matched distribution. The number of patients at each follow-up interval is denoted in parentheses. (From Fuster V, McGoon DC, Kennedy M, et al. Long-term evaluation (12–22 years) of open-heart surgery for tetralogy of Fallot. *Am J Cardiol* 1980; 46:635. Reproduced with permission from the publisher and authors.)

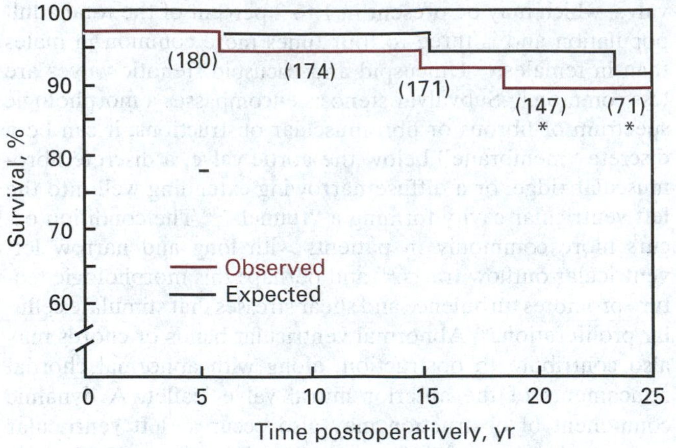

FIGURE 64-7 Long-term survival of perioperative survivors following surgical repair of isolated pulmonary stenosis and expected survival of age- and sex-matched control populations. Difference between expected and observed $p < .002$. (From Kopecky SL, Gersh BJ, McGoon MD, et al. Long-term outcome of patients undergoing surgical repair of isolated pulmonary valve stenosis: Follow-up at 20–30 years. *Circulation* 1988; 78:1150. Reproduced with permission from the American Heart Association and authors.)

with the pattern of progression (Fig. 64-8).[207] Bacterial endocarditis is relatively uncommon (1.8 to 2.7 cases per 100 patient-years),[208] but antibiotic prophylaxis is necessary, even for functionally normal valves. Slowly progressive aortic regurgitation is well recognized in young adulthood, but sudden deterioration is rare, except as a sequel to infection.[209,210] Associated abnormalities of the aorta are not uncommon, and aneurysmal dilatation and dissection of the ascending aorta may be seen even with functionally normal valves. Fragmentation of the elastic fibers in the media has been noted histologically, and, recently, premature smooth muscle cell apoptosis has been implicated. These findings suggest a common genetic abnormality involving both the aortic valve and the ascending aortic wall.[211]

Discrete subaortic stenosis may cause rapidly progressive obstruction in childhood and young adulthood. Progressive aortic regurgitation is common, and infective endocarditis is considered to be a particular hazard (see Chap. 63).[209,210] The natural history of supravalvar aortic stenosis is poor, and survival to adulthood is exceptional.[159] The presence of associated congenital abnormalities and possibly premature coronary artery disease with systolic hypertension is likely a contributory factor to this adverse outcome.

MANAGEMENT

The development of symptoms (e.g., angina, exertional dyspnea, and syncope) mandates prompt intervention in aortic valve stenosis (see Chap. 56). In asymptomatic younger individuals, however, the documentation of severe aortic stenosis may in itself be considered an indication for intervention.[212,213] Mild aortic stenosis in asymptomatic patients with gradients below 50 mmHg warrants careful surveillance. The management of patients in the intermediate group (gradients 50 to 75 mmHg) is more controversial, but evidence argues in favor of elective intervention. Calculation of aortic valve area is important, since left ventricular–aortic gradients may be misleading if there is reduced cardiac output.

Surgery in the young adult with congenital aortic stenosis must be considered palliative.[152,214] In the absence of calcification, young patients may be candidates for aortic valvotomy (see also Chaps. 56 and 63). Perioperative mortality rates in adolescents and adults are extremely low, and late survival is excellent. A large proportion (35 to 45 percent), however, will require reoperation, including aortic valve replacement, over a follow-up period of 20 to 25 years.[150,152] Catheter balloon valvotomy (see Chap. 63) has been utilized in adolescents and young adults with mobile noncalcified valves, but the results are also palliative.[215]

Valve replacement is the only option for valves unsuitable for valvotomy, including those with significant calcification and regurgitation. The pulmonary autograft (Ross) operation represents an attractive surgical alternative to prosthetic or homograft aortic valve replacement. The choice of operation is discussed elsewhere (see Chap. 56), but the age and size of the patient are major considerations, as are individual characteristics that determine the safety of anticoagulation, such as the desire for future pregnancies.

Subaortic stenosis is usually amenable to more definitive surgical repair. This fact, in conjunction with the potential for progressive aortic regurgitation, justifies a more aggressive approach even in asymptomatic patients with lesser gradients.[216,217] Excision of the obstructive membrane, together with a myectomy or myotomy, is usually required. Subaortic stenosis occasionally recurs, and persistent or progressive aortic regurgi-

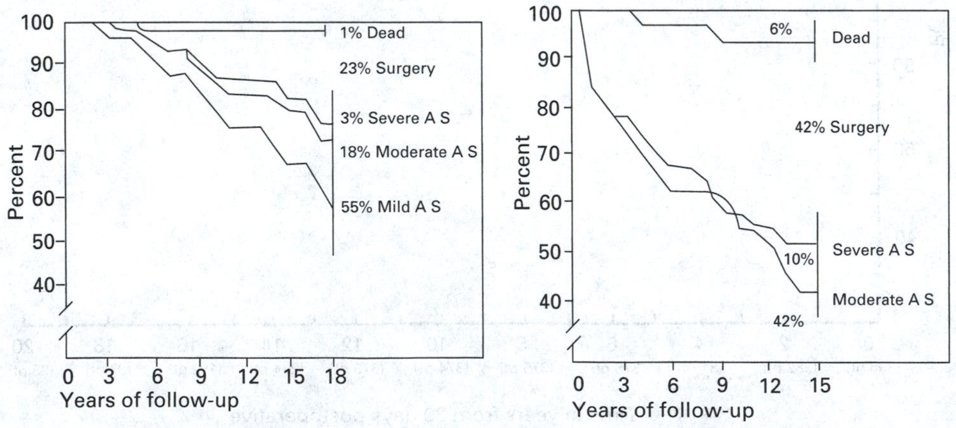

FIGURE 64-8 (*Left*) Cumulative actuarial curves of 153 patients presenting with *mild* aortic stenosis. Bars show ±1 standard error in age at presentation 6.5 years (range 1 to 25 years); mean follow-up was 8.8 years (range 1 to 26 years). (*Right*) Cumulative actuarial curves of 54 patients presenting with *moderate* aortic stenosis. Conventions are as in the left-hand figure. Mean age at presentation was 11.8 years (range 1 to 25 years). Mean follow-up was 8.5 years (range 1 to 24 years). (From Hossack KF, Neutze JM, Lowe JB, Barratt-Boyes BG. Congenital valvar aortic stenosis: Natural history and assessment for operation. *Br Heart J* 1980; 43:561. Reproduced with permission from the publisher and authors.)

tation may develop. Operative mortality rates are low, but the risks are greater in patients with "tunnel" forms of obstruction and in patients with obstruction at several levels. Such situations usually require a more aggressive surgical intervention with extensive myectomy, a Konno procedure, or modification thereof.[218]

Hospital mortality rates for repair of supravalvular aortic stenosis are low, and late morbidity and mortality rates are also excellent. Nevertheless, residual abnormality, such as aortic regurgitation or stenosis, may persist after aortoplasty.

Medical follow-up of patients who have undergone surgical or balloon valvotomy should focus on the development of restenosis, the severity and progression of aortic regurgitation, and the constant hazard of infective endocarditis. Echocardiography has facilitated serial evaluation of gradients, valve areas, ventricular dimensions, function, and mass. The acceptable level of physical activity in patients with left ventricular outflow tract obstruction remains very controversial. It is debatable whether any patient who has had significant obstruction should be allowed to participate in competitive sports. We consider a residual gradient greater than 20 mmHg or persistent left ventricular hypertrophy to be contraindications to vigorous physical activity. Before one approves strenuous activity in others, evaluation should include ECG monitoring and maximal exercise testing (see Chap. 14).

Coarctation of the Aorta

Although coarctation of the aorta is a congenital malformation, nearly 20 percent of the cases presenting at the Mayo Clinic over a 20-year period were diagnosed initially in adolescence or adulthood. Most commonly, coarctation diagnosed at ages beyond childhood was discovered in asymptomatic patients in whom a routine physical examination for athletic participation or employment disclosed upper limb hypertension with diminished or absent femoral pulses. Coarctation of the aorta may occur anywhere along the descending aorta, even below the diaphragm, but in more than 95 percent of cases it is located below the origin of the left subclavian artery, and may involve the origin of this vessel. Usually, there is a discrete infolding of the aortic wall, causing eccentric narrowing of the lumen. Frequently, there is secondary aortic dilatation proximal and distal to the coarcted area.

NATURAL HISTORY

Isolated, severe aortic coarctation may cause congestive heart failure as early as the neonatal period. More frequently, however, coarctation producing symptoms during early infancy is associated with other congenital cardiovascular abnormalities, such as ventricular septal defect, left ventricular outflow tract obstruction, or mitral valve abnormality. Many patients with undetected coarctation will remain symptom-free until adolescence or early adulthood, when symptoms such as headaches related to hypertension, leg fatigue, or leg cramps may develop. Occasionally, a major catastrophic event, such as a cerebrovascular accident, infective endocarditis, or even rupture of the aorta, is the first recognized symptom. A bicuspid aortic valve is found in approximately 25 to 50 percent of patients with coarctation, and these abnormal valves have a tendency to calcify in early or middle adult life, producing aortic stenosis. Aortic stenosis may be the presenting condition, and subsequent investigation may disclose an additional coarctation of the aorta. In the era before surgical intervention, approximately 50 percent of patients with coarctation died within the first three decades, and 75 percent were dead by age 50.[219] Death was most frequently caused by a complication of hypertension, such as stroke or aortic dissection, but other causes included endocarditis, endarteritis, and congestive heart failure.

MANAGEMENT

Infrequently, a mild degree of coarctation may be present that would not justify intervention. In the great majority of cases, however, symptoms or the presence of significant upper-body hypertension mandate surgical repair. On occasion, an asymptomatic adolescent or adult patient with a severe coarctation will be normotensive at rest because of well-developed collaterals around the coarctation site. Such patients have inappropriate hypertension with exercise, however, and should be repaired. There is evidence that residual hypertension and late complications are directly related to age at the time of repair.[220]

Surgery for coarctation has been available since 1945.[221] Various techniques have been used, including end-to-end anastomosis, patch grafting, and the use of the subclavian flap technique.[222] Aneurysmal or atherosclerotic changes in the aorta found in adolescents or adults may occasionally mandate the use of an interposition prosthetic graft. Surgery is performed without cardiopulmonary bypass, and the risk of death from operation is small, although it is higher in adults than in children. Serious morbidity is rare, but occasionally paraplegia secondary to spinal cord ischemia and bowel ischemia or infarction occur.[223] For patients who require concomitant surgical procedures, such as aortic valve replacement, an ascending-to-descending aortic bypass may be utilized through a median sternotomy.[224] Some patients require antihypertensive medication because of transient postoperative hypertension for a short period, whereas in others hypertension may persist, requiring long-term treatment.

Balloon angioplasty of native coarctation has been utilized, but the role of this technique remains controversial.[225] Immediate reduction of the degree of obstruction and gradient is usually possible but is achieved at the price of tearing both the aortic intima and media. Late aneurysm formation, presumably secondary to the disruption of the media, has been observed.[226] Currently, most centers do not perform catheter balloon angioplasty as the primary procedure for coarctation, reserving it for recoarctation, where it appears to have a much greater role.[227] Balloon-expandable stents have also been utilized recently with good results, although long-term follow-up data are not available.[228–231]

LATE RESULTS

The Mayo Clinic has published late results in 646 patients with coarctation operated upon between 1946 and 1981.[220] The median age at operation was 16 years (range 1 week to 72 years) with 72 patients (11 percent) over age 35 years of age. Although survival was good (91 percent at 10 years and 72 percent at 30 years), the mean age of death was 38 years, confirming the previous finding that life expectancy is reduced, even after repair. In this and other series reporting long-term follow-up, the most common cause of death was premature coronary artery disease with secondary myocardial infarction.[232,233] Other causes included congestive heart failure, stroke, and ruptured aortic aneurysm. Age at operation was a powerful prognostic factor.

The older the patient at the time of repair, the greater the probability of premature death, making it highly likely that the duration of preoperative obstruction and hypertension is important in the etiology of arterial disease and subsequent cardiovascular events.

The incidence of recoarctation with all surgical techniques is low for repairs performed after infancy, but surgery in later years for associated abnormalities, such as aortic and mitral valve disease, may be required. The majority of survivors are asymptomatic, but there is a high incidence of late hypertension, despite satisfactory early fall in blood pressure after surgery and good relief of obstruction. In one series, only 32 percent of patients were normotensive 30 years after repair, and 25 percent were significantly hypertensive.[233] Long-term blood pressure surveillance, including blood pressures with exercise, is therefore mandatory, since hypertension is directly related to many of the late vascular complications.[220,232,233] This incidence may decline significantly as more patients are diagnosed and repaired during infancy or early childhood. Long-term regular follow-up should also include surveillance of the repaired aorta (MRI imaging is very suitable), assessment of the aortic valve, and endocarditis prophylaxis.

Transposition of the Great Arteries

In complete transposition of the great arteries, the aorta arises from the right ventricle and the pulmonary artery from the left ventricle (discordant ventriculoarterial connection). As a result, the systemic and arterial circulations run "in parallel" rather than "in series," and predominantly desaturated blood enters the aorta. Oxygenation and survival depend on mixing between the systemic and pulmonary circulations at the atrial level in simple transposition (via a patent foramen ovale or atrial septal defect; see Chap. 63). In approximately half the cases, there are associated anomalies: ventricular septal defect (30 percent), left ventricular outflow tract obstruction (5 to 10 percent), ventricular septal defect with left ventricular outflow tract obstruction (10 percent), patent ductus arteriosus, and, more rarely, coarctation of the aorta or AV valve anomalies.[234] These associated conditions affect both the natural history and surgical management.

NATURAL HISTORY

Transposition of the great arteries is relatively common, but the natural history is so poor that very few patients survive past childhood without intervention. Death is usually due to profound hypoxia and its hematologic consequences. In transposition of the great arteries with large ventricular septal defect, severe hypoxia is rare, but patients do badly as a result of heart failure from excessive pulmonary flow and early pulmonary vascular disease.[129] Transposition with ventricular septal defect and left ventricular outflow tract obstruction presents with early hypoxia. Occasionally, prolonged survival into adult life may occur with a large atrial septal defect, ventricular septal defect, and/or patent ductus arteriosus, with the development of pulmonary vascular disease (Eisenmenger's syndrome) or with associated ventricular septal defect and left ventricular outflow tract obstruction.

MANAGEMENT

The outlook has been transformed by the use of catheter balloon atrial septostomy.[235] In the late 1950s and early 1960s, the Senning[236] and Mustard[237] operations, involving atrial redirection of the systemic and pulmonary venous returns, were introduced. These operations are usually performed between 3 and 12 months of age, with a trend over the years to earlier surgery. Both procedures have been undertaken with excellent early mortality rates (approximately 2 percent operative mortality rate and less than 10 percent for the whole early-management protocol). Long-term follow-up for both procedures is now available, with comparable late results, apart from a lower incidence of baffle obstruction after the Senning operation.[238] Follow-up now extends to 30 years in some patients.[239] A recent study reported actuarial survival rates of 90 percent, 80 percent, and 80 percent at 10, 20, and 28 years, respectively, after the Mustard repair.[240,241] Seventy-six percent of the survivors were in NYHA class I. Thus, cardiologists are likely to see patients who have undergone these types of atrial redirection. Late problems, however, are now recognized, with sudden death, arrhythmia, tricuspid regurgitation, and right (systemic) ventricular dysfunction being the major concerns.[240] These late complications have led to the increasing acceptance of the arterial switch operation as the operation of choice.[242] This procedure involves transection and reanastomosis of the great arteries (aorta to left ventricle and pulmonary artery to right ventricle) with coronary artery transfer. The mortality rate for this procedure has decreased, but the long-term results into adult life are not yet available. For transposition with ventricular septal defect, the mortality rate for atrial repair with ventricular septal defect closure has always been higher than for simple transposition, and arterial switch is the operation of choice. Transposition with ventricular septal defect and left ventricular outflow tract obstruction is usually palliated in infancy with a systemic-to-pulmonary shunt followed by repair by the Rastelli procedure in later childhood.[243] This operation involves closure of the ventricular septal defect to connect the left ventricle to the aorta and insertion of a valved conduit from the right ventricle to the pulmonary artery. Long-term results are good, but further surgery to replace the extracardiac conduit in adolescent and adult life is inevitable (see "Surgical Considerations," above).

LATE RESULTS

Two specific problems after atrial redirection have caused concern during long-term follow-up: arrhythmia and systemic ventricular dysfunction. Loss of sinus rhythm is progressive and has not been prevented by modification of surgical technique for either the Mustard or the Senning operation.[41,244] In most cases, it is asymptomatic, but occasionally profound bradycardia may necessitate pacemaker insertion. There appears, however, to be no relationship between loss of sinus rhythm and risk of sudden death. More worrisome is the development of atrial tachyarrhythmias, including atrial flutter. This arrhythmia has profound hemodynamic consequences after intraatrial repair and is a risk factor for sudden death, especially in the presence of right ventricular dysfunction. Deteriorating performance of the right ventricle supporting the systemic circulation has been reported in some patients, but the precise basis for this problem remains unclear.[9] Although a major concern, it is not yet known whether or not ventricular performance will inevitably deteriorate in the majority of patients and, if so, over what period.[9]

Risk stratification for sudden death remains a clinical challenge. Late death cannot be predicted merely from serial ECGs or ambulatory monitoring.[41] This difficulty underscores the need for a more sophisticated approach involving both electrophysiologic and hemodynamic measurements. Assessment should include evaluation of cardiac performance at rest and exercise, and evaluation of systemic and venous pathways. Transesophageal echocardiography is particularly useful in this situation. Heart transplantation should be considered in the patient who has severe right ventricular failure or disabling arrhythmias. An alternative approach is to perform pulmonary artery banding as preparation for conversion of the atrial repair to an arterial switch. Published results have indicated a significant surgical mortality rate for this approach. As a result, case selection and timing, as well as optimal surgical strategy, remain unclear.[245] The rather limited information after arterial switch operation suggests that electrophysiologic problems are much less prevalent.[246] More recent studies confirm the theoretical advantages of anatomic repair over atrial repair with respect to preservation of sinus node function and lower prevalence of clinically relevant tachyarrhythmias.[247] The systemic left ventricle after the switch is at risk from the surgical procedure itself, potential myocardial ischemia from coronary distortion, and aortic regurgitation. Early results, however, are encouraging, but few patients have yet reached adult life.[248] Because of the high incidence of observed and potential medical problems, all patients who have had both atrial and arterial repair of transposition of the great arteries should have lifelong follow-up by a cardiologist at a center specializing in adult congenital heart disease.

Congenitally Corrected Transposition (Atrioventricular and Ventriculoarterial Discordance)

In congenitally corrected transposition of the great arteries, there is a discordant AV connection (right atrium to left ventricle and left atrium to right ventricle) and a discordant ventriculoarterial connection (left ventricle to pulmonary artery and right ventricle to aorta). As a result of this "double discordance," the systemic and pulmonary venous returns flow to the appropriate great arteries, giving rise to the potentially confusing term *corrected transposition*.[249]

NATURAL HISTORY

In a small proportion of cases (approximately 10 percent in reported series, but this is probably an underestimate), there are no associated cardiac defects.[250,251] Such individuals are pink and asymptomatic, and survival to the ninth decade has been reported.[76] The only specific difference from normal hearts is the tendency to develop AV conduction problems and complete heart block. Complete heart block may be present from birth (approximately 10 percent of patients)[252] and is said to develop in about 2 percent of patients per year.[253] It is not clear whether the systemic right ventricle in patients with corrected transposition can maintain function over extended periods or whether this has an impact on outcome, since few studies have examined enough patients without associated defects over a long enough period. The majority of patients have a ventricular septal defect (90 percent) and/or pulmonary stenosis (80 percent).[250] The combination of these lesions may cause cyanosis. Abnormalities of the tricuspid valve (systemic AV valve) are common and may be due to an intrinsic tricuspid valve abnormality, such as Ebstein's malformation. These defects influence the natural history and surgical strategy required.

MANAGEMENT

Strategies and indications for surgery differ from those in patients with normal connections because of the potential for the operation to aggravate systemic ventricular dysfunction, systemic AV valve incompetence, or conduction problems. Palliative surgery in childhood is sometimes performed, since definitive repair may involve insertion of an extracardiac conduit. In a large retrospective study of 111 patients managed over a 20-year period, it was concluded that patients with symptomatic heart failure should be repaired before the systemic ventricle dilates and the tricuspid regurgitation becomes severe.[251] Patients with more than mild tricuspid regurgitation whose valves were not replaced did very poorly. In contrast, the patients with cyanosis did much better, and the timing of intracardiac surgery can be delayed and be determined by the patient's symptoms. In one recent series of surgical repair of 127 patients, 56 percent required reoperation within 20 years for AV valve regurgitation, pulmonary stenosis, or both.[254] Left AV valve regurgitation is common in adults with congenitally corrected transposition[255] and tends to be progressive.[256] It may be related to an Ebstein-like malformation of the left AV valve, but these valves, in contrast to Ebstein's anomaly of the right AV valve, cannot be repaired adequately and always need to be replaced. Left AV valve replacement should always be performed before there is compromise of systemic (morphologic right) ventricular function. In one series of 40 patients, left AV valve replacement was accomplished without surgically induced complete heart block, with an early mortality rate of 10 percent ($n = 4$) and 8 late deaths.[257] The principal cause of death in all 12 patients was systemic ventricular failure. Survival correlated with preoperative systemic ventricular ejection fraction of 44 percent or greater. It thus seems appropriate to refer these patients for valve replacement at the earliest signs of ventricular dysfunction.

Recently, alternative surgical strategies involving a "double switch" have been adopted by some units. These involve an atrial repair by a Mustard or Senning operation together with connection of the left ventricle to the aorta (via a patch through the ventricular septal defect) or an arterial switch.[258,259] The advantage of these approaches is that the morphologic left ventricle (with mitral valve) supports the systemic circulation. While this is an attractive option, it should be stressed that few patients who have received double-switch procedures have reached adolescence, and long-term follow-up data are not yet available for comparison with the conventional surgical approach.

LATE RESULTS

The long-term outcome for well-repaired patients is good, but those with severe symptomatic heart failure preoperatively do badly. Atrial arrhythmias are common in long-term follow-up and in one recent series occurred in 36 percent of survivors.[260] Since repairs may involve insertion of an extracardiac conduit, prosthetic AV valve, and pacemaker, careful long-term follow-up is mandatory.

Complex Lesions

A number of complex congenital heart defects involve structural abnormalities that preclude the creation of a biventricular circulation. The changing nomenclature and classification that have been applied to these defects over the years are a major source of confusion (see Chap. 63). This group of patients includes those with double-inlet ventricle (single ventricle), absent right or left AV connection (tricuspid or mitral atresia), some cases of pulmonary atresia/intact ventricular septum, and cases with straddling of an AV valve and hypoplastic left or right ventricles. The natural history of these defects is highly variable and depends to a large extent on the impact of the associated defects. In a recent report of 191 patients with double-inlet ventricle presenting in the first year of life, the actuarial survival rate before definitive repair for the whole group was 57 percent at 1 year and 42 percent at 10 years.[158] On multivariate analysis, pulmonary stenosis, balanced pulmonary flow, and older age at presentation were factors favoring survival, while right atrial isomerism, common AV orifice, pulmonary atresia, obstruction to systemic output, and anomalous pulmonary venous return were detrimental. Despite the complex morphologic defects, prolonged natural survival is possible, particularly if the physiology is well balanced.[261] The patients with double-inlet left ventricle with discordant ventriculoarterial connection and pulmonary stenosis with balanced pulmonary flow do best, with predicted actuarial survivals of 96 percent at 1 year and 91 percent at 10 years.

MANAGEMENT

For most patients with complex congenital heart disease, prolonged survival into adult life is possible only with one or more palliative operations (e.g., systemic to pulmonary shunt, Glenn shunt, pulmonary artery banding, and relief of systemic outflow obstruction) or after a Fontan-type procedure. With palliative surgery alone, clinical deterioration usually begins in the second decade of life and is often due to progressive ventricular dysfunction and/or AV valve regurgitation.[262–264]

TABLE 64-5 Indications for Hospitalizations after Fontan Procedure for 215 Surviving Patients Who Returned a Questionnaire

Indication	Patients Hospitalized (No.)[a]
Cardiac operation	62
Other	57
Arrhythmia	52
Pacemaker insertion or replacement	22
Heart failure	14
Abdominal swelling	10
Leg edema	9
Endocarditis	7
Protein-losing enteropathy	6
Hypoproteinemia	4
Stroke	4
Liver problems	1
Brain abscess	1

[a]A patient may have provided multiple indications for one hospitalization.

SOURCE: Driscoll DJ, Offord KP, Feldt RH, et al. Five- to fifteen-year follow-up after Fontan operation. *Circulation* 1992; 85:469–496. Reproduced with permission from the publisher and authors.

The goals of management during childhood have been to maintain suitable anatomy and physiology for the Fontan circulation. A number of modifications of Fontan's original operation have been introduced (Fig. 64-9).[265–268] The basic principle is to separate the systemic and pulmonary circuits by returning systemic venous blood to the pulmonary artery without incorporating a subpulmonary ventricle. This circulation is less "flexible" than one with two functioning ventricles; the operative risk and postoperative status are largely dependent on the patient's suitability. Most important are a low pulmonary vascular resistance and adequate ventricular function (both systolic and diastolic), allowing the circulation to operate with an acceptably low systemic venous pressure. Careful preoperative hemodynamic assessment is vital to optimize patient selection. The operative risk varies considerably among institutions.

LONG-TERM RESULTS

The early and medium-term results of the successful Fontan operation are excellent when compared to the preoperative status of the patients. Improvements in arterial saturation and exercise tolerance have been confirmed by objective testing.[268] The patients with the best hemodynamics can perform well at submaximal levels of exercise equivalent to most normal daily activities.[269] With longer follow-up, however, increasing problems develop (Table 64-5).[270,271] Fontan's own analysis of 334 patients revealed a premature decline in survival and functional status and a late rise in hazard for which no risk factors could be identified other than the Fontan state per se.[271] Arrhythmia

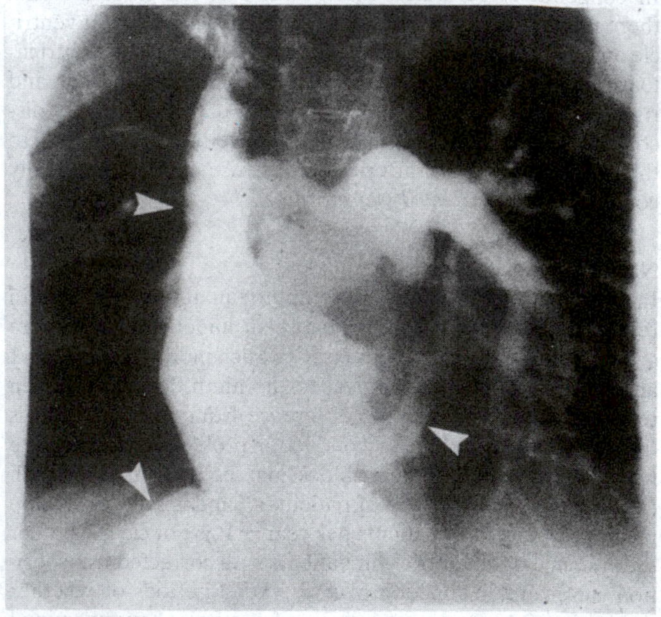

A

FIGURE 64-9 Angiograms. *A.* Fontan conduit from right atrium to pulmonary artery. There is dilatation of the right atrium with filling of the inferior vena cava, superior vena cava, and coronary sinus. *B.* Total cavopulmonary connection. The superior vena cava is connected to the right pulmonary artery ("bidirectional Glenn"), and the inferior vena cava is baffled to the pulmonary artery. (Courtesy of Dr. I. D. Sullivan, Great Ormond Street Hospital for Children, London.)

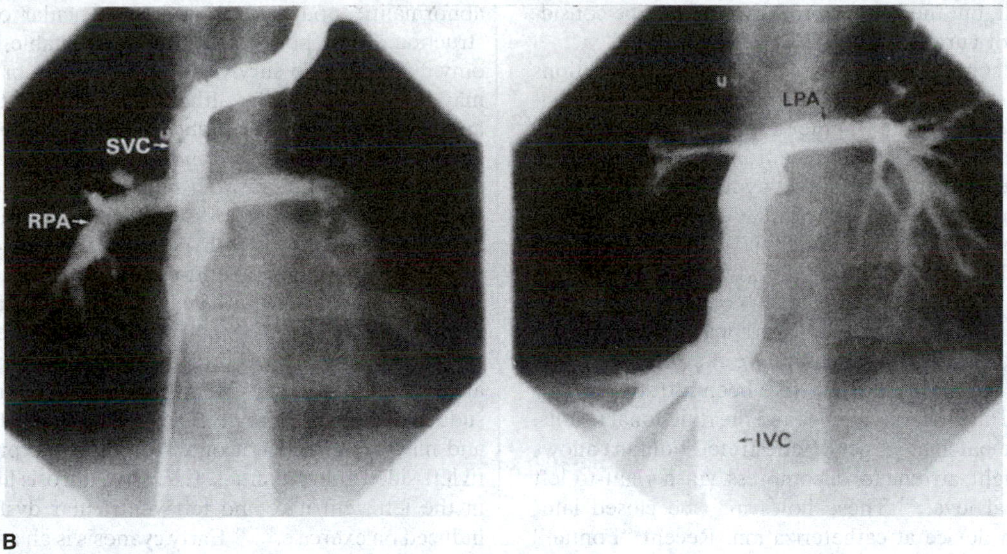

FIGURE 64-9 (*Continued*)

is a particularly common problem and occurs in approximately 20 percent at 10-year follow-up (Table 64-6).[270] Other problems include thrombus in the atria and declining ventricular function.[270–272] Anticoagulation policy differs widely even among specialist centers. The increasing concerns regarding stasis of blood in the right atrium and thrombus formation have led to wider routine use of long-term anticoagulants, but this is not standard practice. Patients with a history of documented atrial arrhythmias, a fenestration in the Fontan connection, and "smoke" in the right atrium on echocardiography have the strongest indications for anticoagulation. Protein-losing enteropathy (PLE) is another important complication and probably results from elevated systemic venous pressure, which subsequently causes lymphangiectasia. PLE is associated with fluid accumulation, such as pleural effusion, ascites, and peripheral edema. The diagnosis can be confirmed by quantifying gastrointestinal protein loss utilizing $alpha_1$ antitrypsin clearance. The cumulative risk for the development of PLE by 10 years in one reported large series was approximately 13 percent;[273] once this complication had developed, the 5-year survival rate was approximately 50 percent. Therapy includes sodium restriction, dietary modification, and anticongestive measures such as diuretics and afterload-reducing agents. Many patients require periodic albumin infusion, but medical management of PLE is usually only partially successful. Obstruction in the Fontan circuit should always be ruled out as a potential cause, since reoperation may result in resolution of the PLE. Chronic subcutaneous heparin therapy may also resolve the PLE,[274,275] as may percutaneous atrial fenestration.[265,276] Occasional reports suggest improvement with steroid therapy.[277] Cardiac transplantation appears to pose a high risk and does not always resolve the protein loss.[274] Other concerns are the effects of nonpulsatile pulmonary flow, favoring the development of pulmonary arteriovenous malformations, as seen after the Glenn anastomosis.[278] Extrapolation of these data to current

TABLE 64-6 Arrhythmias in 215 Survivors of the Fontan Operation

Results from Follow-up Questionnaire	5 Years Postop Patients No.	5 Years Postop Patients %	Current Patients No.	Current Patients %
Syncope	18	8	17	8
Rapid heart rate (tachycardia)	44	20	45	21
Slow heart rate (bradycardia)	17	8	15	7
Palpitations	51	24	60	28
Atrial flutter or fibrillation	26	12	41	19
Premature ventricular contractions	13	6	15	7
Ventricular tachycardia	9	4	13	6
Pacemaker	[b]	[b]	22	10
Number of antiarrhythmic medications[a]				
0	179	83	167	78
1	31	13	40	19
2	5	2	8	4

[a]Excluding digitalis.
[b]"Presence of a pacemaker" asked only for patient's current status.
SOURCE: From Driscoll DJ, Offord KP, Feldt RH, et al. Five-to-fifteen-year follow-up after Fontan operation. *Circulation* 1992; 85:469–496. Reproduced with permission from the publisher and authors.

practice is difficult, but the Fontan procedure should be considered palliative, not curative.

Despite these complications, more and more modifications of the Fontan operation are being performed, and more long-term data are necessary to see whether important complications can be reduced in this way. Much recent interest has involved conversion of the Fontan to a more "hydrodynamically efficient" circuit to improve atrial arrhythmias and PLE.[279] A high mortality rate, however, is associated with PLE surgery, and in one series only 50 percent of the survivors were cured.[274] Atrial arrhythmias may also persist after Fontan conversion[279,280] even though hydrodynamics are improved. Perhaps concomitant arrhythmia circuit cryoablation may improve the results.[281]

Some surgical modifications that have been introduced may improve early and late hemodynamics and the functional results. Perforation of the patch at surgery (fenestrated Fontan) allows a hypertensive right atrium to decompress via a right-to-left shunt at the atrial level.[282] These holes may be closed later with an occlusion device at catheterization. Recent "Fontan" operations have excluded the right atrium from the circulation, creating a total cavopulmonary connection (superior vena cava to right pulmonary artery via a bidirectional Glenn anastomosis and inferior vena cava blood channeled to the pulmonary artery).[283] Data suggest improved flow and energy characteristics compared to the standard atriopulmonary connection and fewer early supraventricular arrhythmias.[46] Other modifications have created an extracardiac Fontan connection using a tube graft in the hope of preventing atrial distention and atrial arrhythmias.[284,285]

All patients who have complex congenital heart defects palliated by systemic-to-pulmonary shunt, cavopulmonary anastomosis (bidirectional Glenn), or Fontan should have lifelong regular cardiac follow-up at a specialist center. Particular attention should be paid to ventricular function, detection of thrombus in the right atrium, residual shunts, systemic AV valve regurgitation, AV malformations in the lung, obstruction at the Fontan anastomosis (especially in early operations involving a right atrium-to-pulmonary artery conduit), and PLE (see above).

Ebstein's Anomaly of the Tricuspid Valve

Ebstein's anomaly is characterized by displacement of the proximal attachments of the tricuspid valve from the AV ring into the right ventricle (see Chap. 63). This structural abnormality divides the right ventricle into an "atrialized" portion and a distal "ventricularized" portion. The severity is variable and accounts for the broad clinical spectrum, from severe disease causing fetal or neonatal death to mild disease compatible with natural survival as late as the eighth decade of life.[286] Ebstein's anomaly is an uncommon defect occurring in less than 1 percent of patients with congenital heart disease, but it is disproportionately represented in the adult congenital heart disease population because of its favorable natural history.

The diagnosis of Ebstein's anomaly is now much easier with echocardiography, which has altered our understanding of the natural history. In a large collaborative study of Ebstein's anomaly reported in 1974, only 7 percent of patients were under 1 year of age.[286] It is not surprising that neonates presenting with Ebstein's anomaly represent the worst end of the spectrum, with a severe anatomic defect and a high incidence of associated abnormalities, particularly right ventricular outflow tract obstruction. Their poor outcome is predictable from their anatomy.[287] Those who survive this period with or without surgery may live into adult life, although there is continued morbidity and death throughout childhood. Many patients are minimally symptomatic in childhood and do not present until adolescence or adult life. Symptoms and signs, when they develop, include cyanosis due to right-to-left shunting at the atrial level, dyspnea and fatigue secondary to hypoxia and low cardiac output, and palpitation due to supraventricular arrhythmia. Ebstein's anomaly is often associated with ventricular preexcitation, which may involve one or more, usually right-sided, accessory pathways. Approximately 25 to 30 percent of adults will have symptomatic arrhythmias that may be difficult to treat and can result in sudden death.[288] Progressive heart failure may develop with time and may be related not only to right-sided problems but also to left-sided abnormalities. Excessive fibrosis has been reported in the left ventricle, and left ventricular dysfunction may be induced on exercise.[287,289] Early cyanosis is an adverse risk factor for survival, as is congestive cardiac failure.[290]

MANAGEMENT

Surgery may consist of repair or replacement of the tricuspid valve together with closure of the atrial septal defect to prevent cyanosis (Fig. 64-10).[291] In 189 patients aged 11 months to 64 years (mean 19.1 years), a tricuspid valve reconstruction was possible in 58.2 percent, and in 36.5 percent a prosthetic valve, usually a bioprosthesis, was inserted. In the occasional patient, the atrial septal defect may be responsible for a left-to-right shunt and can be closed as the sole procedure. In others, the functioning right ventricle is too small for a biventricular circulation, and a Fontan procedure may be the only option. Cross-sectional echocardiography is very useful in determining whether the tricuspid valve is amenable to repair, delineating the mobility or tethering of the elongated anterior leaflet and the presence or absence of fenestration. The results of surgery are affected by the presence of arrhythmia. Uncontrolled preoperative supraventricular arrhythmia is a risk factor for early postoperative rhythm problems that may have serious hemodynamic consequences.[288] It is usually recommended that division of an accessory pathway be performed at the time of tricuspid valve surgery. The pathways are usually in the posteroseptal or right free-wall position and may be multiple. An alternative approach is to perform catheter radiofrequency ablation of the accessory pathway (see Chap. 28) before surgery. Thus far, few such procedures have been performed in patients with Ebstein's anomaly. In hearts with marked enlargement of the right atrium, catheter ablation is challenging and, in the setting of an atrial communication, poses the additional risk of a paradoxical embolus and stroke. If there are no accessory pathways, a right-sided maze procedure at the time of tricuspid valve surgery may successfully control supraventricular arrhythmia.[169]

LATE RESULTS

The long-term outlook for well-repaired patients is good; reduction in heart size is usual (see Fig. 64-10), and atrial arrhythmias are reduced. Exercise capacity improves postoperatively, particularly in those who are cyanotic before surgery.[292] Of 149 patients receiving a porcine bioprosthesis in the Mayo Clinic series, the 10-year survival was 92.5 percent, and 92 percent of the survivors were NYHA class I or II. Bioprosthesis durability in the tricuspid position performs favorably, with freedom from bioprosthesis replacement being 80.6 percent at 10 and 15 years.[293]

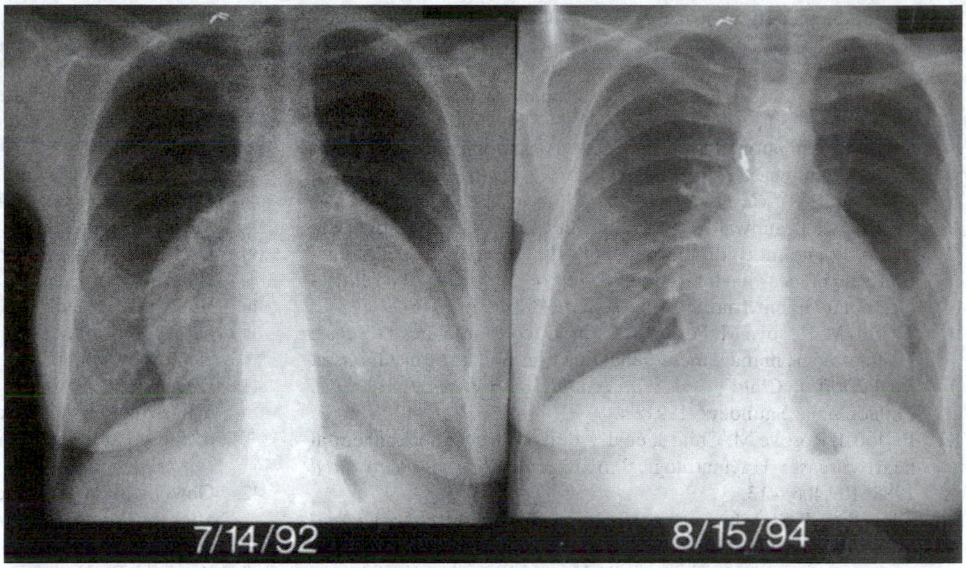

FIGURE 64-10 (*Left*). The chest radiograph shows severe cardiac enlargement associated with Ebstein's anomaly in a 32-year-old woman. She had had a right Blalock-Taussig shunt at age 12. (*Right*). Following tricuspid valve repair and closure of a secundum atrial septal defect, there has been dramatic reduction in the size of the heart.

Marfan's Syndrome

Although the autosomally dominant Marfan's syndrome is congenital in the sense that the patient is born with an abnormal gene or genes, the heart defect is usually acquired. Mutations of fibrillin 1, the main constituent of extracellular microfibrils, are the cause of the pleiotropic manifestations of Marfan's syndrome.[294] The typical phenotypic features—tall, thin stature; pectus deformities; arachnodactyly; and high-arched palate—by which the condition is currently diagnosed, may be obvious, subtle, or absent (see Fig. 10-7). Cardiovascular complications occur in 30 to 60 percent of patients and are the cause of a decreased life expectancy.[295] Mitral valve prolapse is the commonest finding in the pediatric population,[296] but aortic root dilation with a potential for aortic dissection or severe aortic valve regurgitation is the most serious later complication.[297] In a review of 257 patients seen between 1939 and 1972, the median age of death was reported to be about 45 years, with aortic root problems accounting for three-fourths of the deaths (see also Chap. 76).[295] By 1995, a multicenter study reported that the median survival had improved to 72 years.[298]

MANAGEMENT

The risk of dissection is broadly related to the degree of dilation of the aortic root. Dilation can be followed serially by regular cross-sectional echocardiography, which should be performed at least annually. Particularly close monitoring is necessary during puberty and the rapid-growth phase of adolescence. Treatment with beta blockade has been advocated for patients with evidence of aortic root enlargement. Elective aortic root replacement has a low operative mortality rate, but, in contrast, emergency repair, usually for acute aortic dissection, carries a much higher early mortality rate. In a recent multicenter study of 675 patients having aortic root replacement, the 30-day mortality rate was 1.5 percent for those having elective repair, 2.6 percent for those having urgent repair (within 7 days of a surgical consultation), and 11.7 percent for those having emergency repair (within 24 h of a surgical consultation).[297] Forty-six percent of the 158 patients with aortic dissection had an aneurysm with a diameter of 6.5 cm or less. Elective aortic root surgery, therefore, is generally recommended when the aorta exceeds 5.5 cm in diameter.[299] The aortic valve itself may also need to be replaced, although preliminary results from valve-sparing procedures, which eliminate the need for long-term anticoagulants necessary for conventional mechanical valve replacements, suggest cautious optimism.[297,300] It is important to note that more than 10 percent of patients in the multicenter study had problems with the residual aorta, emphasizing the need for continued vigilance of the aorta with MRI or computed tomographic scanning and meticulous control of blood pressure. Since regular, long-term follow-up visits are required, patients with Marfan's syndrome are not uncommon in adult congenital heart clinics. In addition to cardiac care, such patients need expert help with skeletal and ocular problems, genetic counseling, advice on physical activity (see above), and general psychosocial support.

References

1. Ferencz C, Rubin J, McCarter R, et al. Congenital heart disease: Prevalence at live birth. *Am J Epidemiol* 1985; 121:31–36.
2. MacMahon B, McKeown T, Record R. The incidence and life expectation of children with congenital heart disease. *Br Heart Jr* 1953; 15:121–129.
3. Gross R, Hubbard J. Surgical ligation of a persistent ductus arteriosus. *JAMA* 1939; 112:729–731.
4. Perloff J. Congenital heart disease in adults. In: Kelly W, ed. *Textbook of Internal Medicine*. Philadelphia: Lippincott; 1989:223.
5. Stark J. Do we really correct congenital heart defects? *J Thorac Cardiovasc Surg* 1989; 97:(1)1–9.
6. Warnes C. Establishing an adult congenital heart disease clinic. *Am J Card Imaging* 1995; 9:11–14.
7. *1996 Consensus Conference on Adult Congenital Heart Disease*. Montreal: Canadian Cardiovascular Society; 1996.
8. Skorton D, Cheitlin M, Freed M, et al. Training in the care of adult patients with congenital heart disease. *J Am Coll Cardiol* 1995; 25:1–34.
9. Graham T, Arwood G, Boucek R, et al. Abnormalities of right ventricular function following Mustard's operation for transposition of the great arteries. *Circulation* 1975; 52:678–684.
10. Penny D, Redington A. Angiographic demonstration of incoordinate motion of the ventricular wall after the Fontan operation. *Br Heart J* 1991; 66:456–459.
11. Redington A. Functional assessment of the heart after corrective surgery for complete transposition. *Cardio Young* 1991; 1:84–90.
12. Gewillig M, Lundstrom U, Deanfield J, et al. Impact of the Fontan

operation on left ventricular size and contractility. *Circulation* 1990; 81:118–127.
13. Packer M, O'Connor C, Ghali J, et al. Effect of amlodipine on morbidity and mortality in severe chronic heart failure. *N Engl J Med* 1996; 335:1107–1114.
14. CIBIS Investigators and Committees. A randomized trial of beta-blockade in heart failure: The Cardiac Insufficiency Bisprolol Study (CIBIS). *Circulation* 1994; 90:1765–1773.
15. Pfeffer M, Braunwald E, Moye L, et al. Effect of captopril on mortality and morbidity in patients with left ventricular dysfunction after myocardial infarction: Results of the survival and ventricular enlargement trial. *N Engl J Med* 1992; 327:669–677.
16. Territo M, Rosove M, Perloff J. Cyanotic congenital heart disease: Haematologic management, renal function, and urate metabolism. In: Perloff J, Child J, eds. *Congenital Heart Disease in Adults*. Philadelphia: Saunders; 1991:94.
17. Perloff J, Rosove M, Child J, et al. Adults with cyanotic congenital heart disease: Haematological management. *Ann Intern Med* 1988; 109:406–413.
18. Oldershaw P, St. John Sutton, M. Haemodynamic effects of haematocrit reduction in patients with polycythaemia secondary to cyanotic congenital heart disease. *Br Heart J* 1980; 44:584–588.
19. Rosove M, Hocking W, Canobbio M, et al. Chronic hypoxaemia and decompensated erythrocytosis in cyanotic congenital heart disease. *Lancet* 1986; 2:313–315.
20. Ammash N, Warnes CA. Cerebrovascular events in adult patients with cyanotic congenital heart disease. *J Am Coll Cardiol* 1996; 28:768–772.
21. Ross E, Perloff J, Danovitch G, et al. Renal function and urate metabolism in late survivors with cyanotic congenital heart disease. *Circulation* 1986; 73:396–400.
22. Dittrich S, Haas NA, Buhrer C, et al. Renal impairment in patients with long-standing cyanotic congenital heart disease. *Acta Paediatr* 1998; 87:949–954.
23. Harinck E, Hutter P, Hoorntje T, et al. Air travel and adults with cyanotic heart disease. *Circulation* 1996; 93:272–276.
24. Jordan C, White R Jr, Fischer K, et al. The scoliosis of congenital heart disease. *Am Heart J* 1972; 84:463–469.
25. Niwa K, Perloff J, Kaplan S, et al. Eisenmenger syndrome in adults: Ventricular septal defect, truncus arteriosus, univentricular heart. *J Am Coll Cardiol* 1999; 34:223–232.
26. Daliento L, Somerville J, Presbitero P, et al. Eisenmenger syndrome: Factors relating to deterioration and death. *Eur Heart J* 1998; 19:1845–1855.
27. Somerville J. How to manage the Eisenmenger syndrome. *Int J Card* 1997; 63:1–8.
28. Ammash N, Connolly H, Abel M, et al. Noncardiac surgery in Eisenmenger syndrome. *J Am Coll Cardiol* 1999; 33:222–227.
29. Rosenzweig EB, Kerstein D, Barst RJ. Long-term prostacyclin for pulmonary hypertension with associated congenital heart defects. *Circulation* 1999; 99:1858–1865.
30. Working Party of the British Society for Antimicrobial Chemo. The antibiotic prophylaxis of infective endocarditis. *Lancet* 1982; 2:1323–1326.
31. Dajani A, Talbert K, Wilson W, et al. Prevention of bacterial endocarditis. *JAMA* 1997; 277:1794–1801.
32. Sullivan N, Sutter V, Mims M, et al. Clinical aspects of bacteremia after manipulation of the genitourinary tract. *J Infect Dis* 1973; 127:49–55.
33. DeSwiet M, Ramsey I, Rees G. Bacterial endocarditis after insertion of intrauterine contraceptive device. *Br Med J* 1975; 2:76–77.
34. Cetta F, Graham LC, Lichtenberg RC, et al. Piercing and tattooing in patients with congenital heart disease: Patient and physician perspectives. *J Adolesc Health* 1999; 24:160–162.
35. Cetta F, Warnes CA. Adults with congenital heart disease: patient knowledge of endocarditis prophylaxis. *Mayo Clin Proc* 1995; 70:50–54.
36. Godman M, Roberts N, Izukawa T. Late postoperative conduction disturbances after repair of ventricular septal defect and tetralogy of Fallot. *Circulation* 1974; 49:214–221.
37. Vetter V, Horowitz L. Electrophysiologic residua and sequelae of surgery for congenital heart defects. *Am J Cardiol* 1982; 50:588–604.
38. Garson A Jr. Chronic postoperative arrhythmia. In: Gillette P, Garson A Jr, eds. *Pediatric Arrhythmia: Electrophysiology and Pacing*. Philadelphia: Saunders; 1990:667.
39. Dodo H, Gow R, Hamilton R, et al. Chaotic atrial rhythm in children. *Am Heart J* 1995; 129:990–995.
40. Boelens M, Friedli B. Sinus node function and conduction system before and after surgery for secundum atrial septal defect: An electrophysiologic study. *Am J Cardiol* 1984; 53:1415–1420.
41. Deanfield J, Camm J, Macartney F, et al. Arrhythmia and late mortality after Mustard and Senning operation for transposition of the great arteries: An eight year prospective study. *J Thorac Cardiovasc Surg* 1988; 96:569–576.
42. Gewillig M, Wyse R, de Leval M, et al. Early and late arrhythmia after the Fontan operation: Predisposing factors and clinical consequences. *Br Heart J* 1992; 67:72–79.
43. Warfield D, Hayes D, Hyberger L, et al. Permanent pacing in patients with univentricular heart. *PACE* 1999; 22:1193–1201.
44. Ward D, Clarke B, Schofield P, et al. Long-term transvenous ventricular pacing in adults with congenital abnormalities of the heart and great arteries. *Br Heart J* 1983; 50:325–329.
45. Stewart W, DiCola V, Hawthorne J. Doppler ultrasound measurement of cardiac output in patients with physiologic pacemakers: Effects of left ventricular function and retrograde ventriculoatrial conduction. *Am J Cardiol* 1984; 54:308–312.
46. Murphy J, Gersh B, Warnes C, et al. The late survival after surgical repair of isolated ventricular septal defect [abstract]. *Circulation* 1989; 80(suppl II):490.
47. Kulbertus H, Coyne J, Hallidie-Smith K. Conduction disturbances before and after surgical closure of ventricular septal defect. *Am Heart J* 1969; 77:123–131.
48. Deanfield J, McKenna W, Hallidie-Smith K. Detection of late arrhythmia and conduction disturbance after correction of tetralogy of Fallot. *Br Heart J* 1980; 44:577–583.
49. Wolff G, Rowland T, Ellison R. Surgically induced right bundle branch block with left anterior hemiblock. *Circulation* 1972; 46:587–594.
50. Deanfield J. Late ventricular arrhythmias occurring after tetralogy of Fallot: Do they matter? *Int J Cardiol* 1991; 30:143–150.
51. Silka MJ, Hardy BG, Menashe VD, et al. A population-based prospective evaluation of risk of sudden cardiac death after operation for common congenital heart defects. *J Am Coll Cardiol* 1998; 32:245–251.
52. Gewillig M, Cullen S, Mertens B, et al. Risk factors for arrhythmia and death after Mustard operation for simple transposition of the great arteries. *Circulation* 1991; 84(suppl IV):187–192.
53. Balaji S, Gewillig M, Bull C, et al. Arrhythmias after the Fontan procedure: Comparision of total cavopulmonary connection and atriopulmonary connection. *Circulation* 1991; 84(suppl IV): 162–167.
54. Gardiner H, Dhillon R, Bull C, et al. Prospective study of the incidence and determinants of arrhythmia after total cavopulmonary connection. *Circulation* 1996; 94(suppl II):II-17–II-21.
55. Garson A, Nihill M, McNamara D, et al. Status of the adult and adolescent after repair of tetralogy of Fallot. *Circulation* 1979; 59:1232–1240.
56. Kavey R, Blackman M, Sondheimer H. Incidence and severity of chronic ventricular dysrhythmia after repair of tetralogy of Fallot. *Am Heart J* 1982; 342–350.
57. Vaksmann G, Fournier A, Davignon A, et al. Frequency and prognosis of arrhythmias after operative "correction" of tetralogy of Fallot. *Am J Cardiol* 1990; 66:346–349.

58. Lucron H, Marcon F, Bosser G, et al. Induction of sustained ventricular tachycardia after surgical repair of tetralogy of Fallot. *Am J Cardiol* 1999; 83:1369–1373.
59. Marie P, Marcon F, Brunotte F, et al. Right ventricular overload and induced sustained ventricular tachycardia in operatively "repaired" tetralogy of Fallot. *Am J Cardiol* 1992; 69:785–789.
60. Deanfield J, McKenna W, Rowland E. Local abnormalities of right ventricular depolarization after repair of tetralogy of Fallot: A basis for ventricular arrhythmia. *Am J Cardiol* 1985; 55:522–526.
61. Deanfield J, McKenna W, Presbitero P, et al. Ventricular arrhythmia in unrepaired and repaired tetralogy of Fallot: Relation to age, timing of repair and haemodynamic status. *Br Heart J* 1984; 52:77–86.
62. Sullivan I, Presbitero P, Gooch V, et al. Is ventricular arrhythmia in repaired tetralogy of Fallot an effect of operation or a consequence of the course of the disease? *Br Heart J* 1987; 58:40–44.
63. Jones M, Ferrans V. Myocardial degeneration in congenital heart disease: Comparison of morphologic findings in young and old patients with congenital heart disease associated with muscular obstruction to right ventricular outflow. *Am J Cardiol* 1977; 39:1051–1063.
64. Walsh E, Rockenmacher S, Keane J, et al. Late results in patients with tetralogy of Fallot repaired during infancy. *Circulation* 1988; 77:1062–1067.
65. Kobayashi J, Hirose H, Nakano S, et al. Ambulatory electrocardiographic study of the frequency and cause of ventricular arrhythmia after correction of tetralogy of Fallot. *Am J Cardiol* 1984; 54:1310–1313.
66. Quattlebaum T, Varghese J, Neill C, et al. Sudden death among postoperative patients with tetralogy of Fallot: A follow-up study of 243 patients for an average of twelve years. *Circulation* 1976; 54:289–293.
67. Dunnigan A, Pritzker M, Benditt D, et al. Life-threatening ventricular tachycardias in later survivors of surgically corrected tetralogy of Fallot. *Br Heart J* 1984; 52:198–206.
68. Gatzoulis M, Clark A, Newman C, et al. Right ventricular diastolic function 15–35 years after repair of tetralogy of Fallot: Restrictive physiology predicts superior exercise performance. *Circulation* 1995; 91:1775–1781.
69. Gatzoulis M, Till J, Somerville J, et al. Mechanoelectrical interaction in tetralogy of Fallot: QRS prolongation relates to right ventricular size and predicts malignant ventricular arrhythmias and sudden death. *Circulation* 1995; 92:231–237.
70. Larson M, Warnes C. Repaired tetralogy of Fallot: ECG predictors of death and ventricular tachycardia [abstract]. *J Am Coll Cardiol* 1998; 31(suppl A):355A.
71. McLeod K, Hillis W, Houston A, et al. Reduced heart rate variability following repair of tetralogy of Fallot. *Heart* 1999; 81:656–660.
72. Roos-Hesselink J, Perlroth J, McGhie J, et al. Atrial arrhythmias in adults after repair of tetralogy of Fallot: Correlations with clinical, exercise, and echocardiographic findings. *Circulation* 1995; 91:2214–2219.
73. Rodefeld M, Gandhi S, Huddleston C, et al. Anatomically based ablation of atrial flutter in an acute canine model of the modified Fontan operation. *J Thorac Cardiovasc Surg* 1996; 112:898–907.
74. Kalman J, VanHare G, Olgin J, et al. Ablation of "incisional" reentrant atrial tachycardia complicating surgery for congenital heart disease: Use of entrainment to define a critical isthmus of conduction. *Circulation* 1996; 93:502–512.
75. Canobbio MM, Mair DD, van der Velde M, et al. Pregnancy outcomes after the Fontan repair. *J Am Coll Cardiol* 1996; 28:763–767.
76. Connolly HM, Grogan M, Warnes CA. Pregnancy among women with congenitally corrected transposition of the great arteries. *J Am Coll Cardiol* 1999; 33:1692–1695.
77. Connolly HM, Warnes CA. Outcome of pregnancy in patients with complex pulmonic valve atresia. *Am J Cardiol* 1997; 79:519–521.
78. Zuber M, Gautschi N, Oechslin E, et al. Outcome of pregnancy in women with congenital shunt lesions. *Heart* 1999; 81:271–275.
79. Genoni M, Jenni R, Hoerstrup SP, et al. Pregnancy after atrial repair for transposition of the great arteries. *Heart* 1999; 81:276–277.
80. Connolly HM, Warnes CA. Ebstein's anomaly: Outcome of pregnancy. *J Am Coll Cardiol* 1994; 23:1194–1198.
81. Warnes C. Cyanotic congenital heart disease, . In: Oakley C, eds. *Heart Disease in Pregnancy.* London: BMJ Publishing Group; 1997:83–96.
82. Warnes C, Elkayam U. Congenital heart disease and pregnancy. In: Elkayam U, Gleicher N, eds. *Cardiac Problems in Pregnancy.* New York: John Wiley and Associates; 1998; 39–53.
83. Neill C, Swanson S. Outcome of pregnancy in congenital heart disease [abstract]. *Circulation* 1961; 24:1003.
84. Presbitero P, Somerville J, Stone S, et al. Pregnancy in cyanotic congenital heart disease: Outcome of mother and fetus. *Circulation* 1994; 89:2673–2676.
85. Gleicher N, Midwall J, Hochberger D, et al. Eisenmenger's syndrome and pregnancy. *Obst Gynecol* 1975; 34:721–741.
86. Avila W, Grinberg M, Snitcowsky R, et al. Maternal and fetal outcome in pregnant women with Eisenmenger's syndrome. *Eur Heart J* 1995; 16:460–464.
87. Pitts J, Crosby W, Basta L. Eisenmenger's syndrome in pregnancy: Does heparin prophylaxis improve the maternal mortality rate? *Am Heart J* 1977; 93:321–326.
88. Rossiter J, Repke J, Morales A, et al. A prospective longitudinal evaluation of pregnancy in the Marfan syndrome. *Am J Obstet Gynecol* 1995; 173:1599–1606.
89. Elkayam U, Ostrzega E, Shotan A, et al. Cardiovascular problems in pregnant women with the Marfan syndrome. *Ann Intern Med* 1995; 123:117–122.
90. Siu SC, Sermer M, Harrison DA, et al. Risk and predictors for pregnancy-related complications in women with heart disease. *Circulation* 1997; 96:2789–2794.
91. Lao T, Sermer M, Magee L, et al. Congenital aortic stenosis and pregnancy: A reappraisal. *Am J Obstet Gynecol* 1993; 169:540–545.
92. Mendelson C. Pregnancy and coarctation of the aorta. *Am J Obstet Gynecol* 1940; 39:1014–1021.
93. Connolly H, Ammash N, Warnes C. Pregnancy in women with coarctation of the aorta [abstract]. *J Am Coll Cardiol* 1996; 27(suppl A):43A.
94. Hall J, Pauli R, Wilson K. Maternal and fetal sequelae of anticoagulation during pregnancy. *Am J Med*, 1980; 68:122–140.
95. Iturbe-Alessio I, Del Carmen Fonseca M, Mutchinik O, et al. Risks of anticoagulant therapy in pregnant women with artificial heart valves. *N Eng J Med* 1986; 315:1390–1393.
96. Salazar E, Izaguirre R, Verdejo J, et al. Failure of adjusted doses of subcutaneous heparin to prevent thromboembolic phenomena in pregnant patients with mechanical cardiac valve prostheses. *J Am Coll Cardiol* 1996; 27:1698–1703.
97. Sbarouni E, Oakley C. Pregnancy and prosthetic heart valves. *Br Heart J* 1994; 71:196–201.
98. Cotrufo M, deLuca T, Calabro R, et al. Coumadin anticoagulation during pregnancy in patients with mechanical valve prostheses. *Eur J Cardiothorac Surg* 1991; 5:300–305.
99. Elkayam U. Anticoagulation in pregnant women with prosthetic heart valves. *J Am Coll Cardiol* 1996; 27:1704–1706.
100. Nora J, Nora A. The evolution of specific genetic and environmental counseling in congenital heart disease. *Circulation* 1978; 57:205–213.
101. Burn J. The aetiology of congenital heart disease. In: Anderson R, Macartney F, Shinebourne E, et al., eds. *Paediatric Cardiology.* Edinburgh: Churchill Livingstone; 1987:15.
102. Allan L, Crawford D, Chita S, et al. Familial recurrence of congenital heart disease in a prospective series of mothers referred for fetal echocardiography. *Am J Cardiol* 1986; 58:334–337.

103. Driscoll D, Michels V, Gersony W, et al. Occurrence risk for congenital heart defects in relatives of patients with aortic stenosis, pulmonary stenosis, or ventricular septal defect. *Circulation* 1993; 87(suppl I):I-114–I-120.
104. Houston A, Hillis S, Lilley S, et al. Echocardiography in adult congenital heart disease. *Heart* 1998; 80 (suppl 1):12–26.
105. Tworetzky W, McElhinney DB, Brook MM, et al. Echocardiographic diagnosis alone for the complete repair of major congenital heart defects. *J Am Coll Cardiol* 1999; 33:228–33.
106. Stumper O. Imaging the heart in adult congenital heart disease [editorial]. *Heart* 1998; 80:535–536.
107. Ammash NM, Seward JB, Warnes CA, et al. Partial anomalous pulmonary venous connection: diagnosis by transesophageal echocardiography. *J Am Coll Cardiol* 1997; 29:1351–1358.
108. Choe YH, Ko JK, Lee HJ, et al. MR imaging of non-visualized pulmonary arteries at angiography in patients with congenital heart disease. *J Korean Med Sci* 1998; 13:597–602.
109. Hartnell GG, Notarianni M. MRI and echocardiography: How do they compare in adults? *Semin Roentgenol* 1998; 33:252–261.
110. Wimpfheimer O, Boxt LM. MR imaging of adult patients with congenital heart disease. *Radiol Clin North Am* 1999; 37:421–438.
111. Harrison D, McLaughlin P. Interventional cardiology for the adult patient with congenital heart disease: The Toronto Hospital experience. *Can J Cardiol* 1996; 12:965–971.
112. Gersony WM, Hayes CJ, Driscoll DJ, et al. Second natural history study of congenital heart defects. Quality of life of patients with aortic stenosis, pulmonary stenosis, or ventricular septal defect. *Circulation* 1993;87(suppl I): I-52–I-65.
113. Deanfield J. Adult congenital heart disease with special reference to the data on long-term follow-up of patients surviving to adulthood with or without surgical correction. *Eur Heart J* 1992; 13(suppl H):111–116.
114. Truesdell S, Skorton DJ, Lauer RM. Life insurance for children with cardiovascular disease. *Pediatrics* 1986; 77:687–691.
115. Celermajer D, Deanfield J. Employment and insurance for young adults with congenital heart disease. *Br Heart J* 1993; 69:539–543.
116. Garson A, Allen H, Gersony W, et al. Cost of congenital heart disease in children and adults: Sources of variation assessed by multicenter study [abstract]. *Circulation* 1991; 84(suppl II):II-385.
117. Mahoney L, Truesdell S, Hamburgen M, et al. Insurability, employability, and psychosocial considerations. In: Perloff J, Child J, eds. *Congenital Heart Disease in Adults*. Philadelphia: Saunders; 1991: 178.
118. Kellerman J, Zeltzer L, Ellenberg L, et al. Psychological effects of illness in adolescence: Anxiety, self-esteem, and perception of control. *J Pediatr* 1980; 97:126–131.
119. Brandhagen D, Feldt R, Williams D. Long-term psychologic implications of congenital heart disease: A 25-year follow-up. *Mayo Clin Proc* 1991; 66:474–479.
120. Utens EM, Bieman HJ, Verhulst FC, et al. Psychopathology in young adults with congenital heart disease. Follow-up results. *Eur Heart J* 1998; 19:647–651.
121. Zeltzer L, Kellerman J, Ellenberg L, et al. Psychologic effects of illness in adolescence: Impact of illness in adolescents—crucial issues and coping styles. *J Pediatr* 1980; 97:132–138.
122. Gupta S, Giuffre RM, Crawford S, et al. Covert fears, anxiety and depression in congenital heart disease. *Cardiol Young* 1998; 8:491–499.
123. Myers-Vando R, Steward M, Folkins C, et al. The effects of congenital heart disease on cognitive development, illness causality concepts, and vulnerability. *Am J Orthopsychiatr* 1979; 49:617–625.
124. Silbert A, Wolff P, Mayer B, et al. Cyanotic heart disease and psychological development. *Pediatrics* 1969; 43:192–200.
125. Aram D, Ekelman B, Ben-Shachae G, et al. Intelligence and hypoxemia in children with congenital heart disease. *J Am Coll Cardiol* 1985; 6:889–893.
126. Newburger J, Silbert A, Buckley L, et al. Cognitive function and age at repair of transposition of the great arteries in children. *N Engl J Med* 1984; 310:1495–1499.
127. Huffman J. Sex and the teenager. In: Huffman J, Dewhurst J, Capuaro V, eds. *The Gynecology of Childhood and Adolescence*. Philadelphia: Saunders; 1981:527.
128. Swan L, Hillis WS, Cameron A. Family planning requirements of adults with congenital heart disease [editorial]. *Heart* 1997; 78:9–11.
129. Bonnar J. Coagulation effects of oral contraception. *Am J Obstet Gynecol* 1987; 157:1042–1048.
130. Fraser I. Progestogens for contraception. *Austr Fam Phys* 1988; 17:882–885.
131. Whittemore R. Pregnancy and congenital heart disease. In: Adams F, Emmanoulides G, Riemenschneider T, eds. *Heart Disease in Infants, Children, and Adults*. Baltimore: Williams & Wilkins; 1989:684.
132. Rocchini A, Katch V, Anderson J, et al. Blood pressure in obese adolescents: Effects of weight loss. *Pediatrics* 1988; 82:16–23.
133. Powell K, Thompson P, Casperen C, et al. Physical activity and the incidence of coronary heart disease. *Annu Rev Public Health* 1987; 8:281–287.
134. 26th Bethesda Conference. Recommendations for determining eligibility for competition in athletes with cardiovascular abnormalities. *J Am Coll Cardiol* 1994; 24:845–899.
135. Stark J, Pacifico A, eds. *Reoperations in Cardiac Surgery*. Berlin: Springer-Verlag; 1989.
136. Dore A, Glancy DL, Stone S, et al. Cardiac surgery for grown-up congenital heart patients: Survey of 307 consecutive operations from 1991 to 1994. *Am J Cardiol* 1997; 80:906–913.
137. Jonas R, Freed M, Mayer J Jr, et al. Long-term follow-up of patients with synthetic right heart conduits. *Circulation* 1985; 72(suppl II):77–83.
138. Ross D, Somerville J. Correction of pulmonary atresia with a homograft aortic valve. *Lancet* 1966; 2:1446–1447.
139. Merin G, McGoon D. Reoperation after insertion of aortic homograft as a right ventricular outflow tract. *Ann Thorac Surg* 1973; 16:122–126.
140. Shabbo F, Wain W, Ross D. Right ventricular outflow reconstruction with aortic homograft conduit: Analysis of the long-term results. *Thorac Cardiovasc Surg* 1980; 28:21–25.
141. Di Carlo D, de Leval M, Stark J. "Fresh" antibiotic sterilized aortic homografts in extracardiac valved conduits. *Thorac Cardiovasc Surg* 1984; 32:10–14.
142. Cerfolio R, Danielson G, Warnes C, et al. Results of an autologous tissue reconstruction for replacement of obstructed extracardiac conduits. *J Thorac Cardiovasc Surg* 1995; 110:1359–1366.
143. Stark J. Reoperations in patients with extracardiac valved conduits. In: Stark J, Pacifico A, eds. *Reoperations in Cardiac Surgery*. Berlin: Springer-Verlag; 1989:271.
144. Studer M, Blackstone E, Kirklin J, et al. Determinants of early and late results of repair of atrioventricular septal (canal) defects. *J Thorac Cardiovasc Surg* 1982; 84:523–542.
145. Poirier R, McGoon D, Danielson G, et al. Late results after repair of tetralogy of Fallot. *J Thorac Cardiovasc Surg* 1977; 73: 900–908.
146. Zhao H, Miller D, Reitz B, et al. Surgical repair of tetralogy of Fallot: Long-term follow-up with particular emphasis on late death and reoperation. *J Thorac Cardiovasc Surg* 1985; 89:204–220.
147. Ebert P. Second operation for pulmonary stenosis or insufficiency after repair of tetralogy of Fallot. *Am J Cardiol* 1982; 50:637–640.
148. Wessel H, Cunningham W, Paul M, et al. Exercise performance in tetralogy of Fallot after intracardiac repair. *J Thorac Cardiovasc Surg* 1980; 80:582–593.
149. Yemets I, Williams W, Webb G, et al. Pulmonary valve replacement late after repair of tetralogy of Fallot. *Ann Thorac Surg* 1997; 64:526–530.
150. Presbitero P, Somerville J, Revel-Chion R, et al. Open aortic

valvotomy for congenital aortic stenosis: Late results. *Br Heart J* 1982; 47:26–34.
151. Stewart J, Paton B, Blunt S Jr, et al. Congenital aortic stenosis: Ten to twenty years after valvulotomy. *Arch Surg* 1978; 113:1248–1252.
152. Hsieh K, Keane J, Nadas A, et al. Long-term follow-up of valvulotomy before 1968 for congenital aortic stenosis. *Am J Cardiol* 1986; 58:338–341.
153. Puga F, Leoni F, Julsrud P, et al. Complete repair of pulmonary atresia, ventricular septal defect, and severe peripheral arborization abnormalities of the central pulmonary arteries: Experience with preliminary unifocalization procedures in 38 patients. *J Thorac Cardiovasc Surg* 1989; 6:1018–1029.
154. Sullivan I, Wren C, Stark J, et al. Surgical unifocalisation in pulmonary atresia and ventricular septal defect: A realistic goal? *Circulation* 1988; 78(suppl III):5–13.
155. Watterson K, Wilkinson J, Kari T, et al. Very small pulmonary arteries: The central end-to-side shunt. *Ann Thorac Surg* 1991; 52:1132–1137.
156. Speziali G, Driscoll DJ, Danielson GK, et al. Cardiac transplantation for end-stage congenital heart defects: The Mayo Clinic experience, Mayo Cardiothoracic Transplant Team [comments]. *Mayo Clin Proc* 1998; 73:923–928.
157. Mendeloff EN, Huddleston CB. Lung transplantation and repair of complex congenital heart lesions in patients with pulmonary hypertension. *Semin Thorac Cardiovasc Surg* 1998; 10:144–151.
158. Franklin R, Spiegelhalter D, Anderson R, et al. Double inlet ventricle presenting in infancy: Survival without definitive repair. *J Thorac Cardiovasc Surg* 1991; 101:767–776.
159. Child J, Perloff J. Natural survival patterns: A narrowing base. In: Child J, Perloff J, eds., *Congenital Heart Disease in Adults*. Philadelphia: Saunders; 1991:21.
160. Borow K, Braunwald E. Congenital heart disease in the adult. In: Braunwald E, eds. *Heart Disease*. Philadelphia: Saunders; 1988:976.
161. Warnes C, Fuster V, Driscoll D, et al. Atrial septal defect. In: Giuliani E, Fuster V, Gersh B, et al., eds. *Cardiology Fundamentals and Practice*. St. Louis: Mosby-Year Book; 1991:1622.
162. Kirklin J, Barratt-Boyes BG, eds. *Cardiac Surgery*. New York: Wiley; 1986.
163. Massumi R, Nutter D. The syndrome of familial defects of the heart and upper extremities (Holt-Oram syndrome). *Circulation* 1966; 34:65–76.
164. Nora J, McNamara D, Fraser F. Hereditary factors in atrial septal defect. *Circulation* 1967; 35:448–456.
165. Perloff J. Ostium secundum atrial septal defect: Survival for 87–94 years. *Am J Cardiol* 1984; 53:388–389.
166. Campbell M. Natural history of atrial septal defect. *Br Heart J* 1970; 32:820–826.
167. Shah D, Azhar M, Oakley C, et al. Natural history of secundum atrial septal defect in adults after medical or surgical treatment: A historical prospective study. *Br Heart* 1994; 71:224–228.
168. Konstantinides S, Geibel A, Olschewski M, et al. A comparison of surgical and medical therapy for atrial septal defects in adults. *N Engl J Med* 1995; 333:469–473.
169. Theodoro D, Danielson G, Porter C, et al. Right-sided maze procedure for right atrial arrhythmias in congenital heart disease. *Ann Thorac Surg* 1998; 65:149–154.
170. Lock J. The adult with congenital heart disease: Cardiac catheterization as a therapeutic intervention. *J Am Coll Cardiol* 1991; 18:330–331.
171. Hellenbrand W, Fahey J, McGowan F, et al. Transesophageal echocardiographic guidance of transcatheter closure of atrial septal defect. *Am J Cardiol* 1990; 66:207–213.
172. Banerjee A, Bengur AR, Li JS, et al. Echocardiographic characteristics of successful deployment of the Das AngelWings atrial septal defect closure device: Initial multicenter experience in the United States. *Am J Cardiol* 1999; 83:1236–1241.
173. Thanopoulos BD, Laskari CV, Tsaousis GS, et al. Closure of atrial septal defects with the Amplatzer occlusion device: Preliminary results [comments]. *J Am Coll Cardiol* 1998; 31:1110–1116.
174. Walsh KP, Tofeig M, Kitchiner DJ, et al. Comparison of the Sideris and Amplatzer septal occlusion devices. *Am J Cardiol* 1999; 83:933–936.
175. Murphy J, Gersh B, McGoon M, et al. Long-term outcome after surgical repair of isolated atrial septal defect. *N Engl J Med* 1990; 323:1645–1697.
176. Brandenburg R Jr, Holmes D Jr, Brandenburg R, et al. Clinical follow-up study of paroxysmal supraventricular arrhythmias after operative repair of a secundum type atrial septal defect in adults. *Am J Cardiol* 1983; 51:273–276.
177. St. John Sutton M, Tajik A, McGoon D. Atrial septal defect in patients aged 60 or older: Operative results and long-term postoperative follow-up. *Circulation* 1981; 64:402–409.
178. Engle M, Kline S, Borer J. Ventricular septal defect. In: Roberts W, ed. *Adult Congenital Heart Disease*. Philadelphia: Davis; 1987:409.
179. Wood P. The Eisenmenger syndrome or pulmonary hypertension with reversed central shunt. *Br Med J* 1958; 2:701–709.
180. Warnes C, Fuster V, Driscoll D, et al. Ventricular septal defect. In: Guiliani E, Fuster V, Gersh B, et al., eds. *Cardiology: Fundamentals and Practice*. St. Louis: Mosby-Year Book; 1991:1639.
181. Tatsuno K, Konno S, Sakakibara S. Ventricular septal defect with aortic insufficiency: Angiocardiographic aspects and a new classification. *Am Heart J* 1973; 85:13–21.
182. Cartmill T, DuShane J, McGoon D, et al. Results of repair of ventricular septal defect. *J Thorac Cardiovasc Surg* 1966; 52:486–499.
183. Blake R, Chung E, Wesley H, et al. Conduction defects, ventricular arrhythmias and late death after surgical closure of ventricular septal defect. *Br Heart J* 1982; 47:305–315.
184. Bridges N, Perry S, Keane J, et al. Preoperative transcatheter closure of congenital muscular ventricular septal defects. *N Engl J Med* 1991; 324:1312–1317.
185. Reeder G, Danielson G, Seward J, et al. Fixed subaortic stenosis in atrioventricular canal defect: A Doppler echocardiographic study. *J Am Coll Cardiol* 1992; 20:386–394.
186. Report of the New England Regional Infant Cardiac Program. *Pediatrics* 1980; 65(suppl):441–444.
187. Rastelli G, Ongley P, Kirklin J, et al. Surgical repair of the complete form of persistent common atrioventricular canal. *J Thorac Cardiovasc Surg* 1968; 55:299–308.
188. Bergin M, Warnes C, Tajik A, et al. Partial atrioventricular canal defect: Long-term follow-up after initial repair in patients greater than or equal to 40 years old. *J Am Coll Cardiol* 1995; 25:1189–1194.
189. Abraham K, Cherian G, Rao V, et al. Tetralogy of Fallot in adults: A report on 147 patients. *Am J Med* 1979; 66:811–816.
190. Phadke A, Phadke S, Handy M, et al. Acyanotic Fallot's tetralogy with survival to the age of 70 years: Case report. *Indian Heart J* 1977; 29:46–49.
191. Bertranou E, Blackstone E, Hazelrig J, et al. Life expectancy without surgery in tetralogy of Fallot. *Am J Cardiol* 1978; 42:458–466.
192. Deanfield J, Ho S, Anderson R, et al. Late sudden death after repair of tetralogy of Fallot: A clinicopathological study. *Circulation* 1983; 67:636–641.
193. Katz N, Blackstone E, Kirklin J, et al. Late survival and symptoms after repair of tetralogy of Fallot. *Circulation* 1982; 65:403–410.
194. Murphy J, Gersh B, Mair D, et al. Long-term outcome in patients undergoing surgical repair of tetralogy of Fallot. *N Engl J Med* 1993; 329:593–599.
195. Lillehei C, Varco R, Cohen M, et al. The first open heart corrections of tetralogy of Fallot: A 26–31 year follow-up of 106 patients. *Ann Surg* 1986; 204:490–501.
196. Wennevold A, Rygg I, Lauridsen P, et al. Fourteen- to nineteen-

year follow-up after corrective repair of tetralogy of Fallot. *Scand J Thorac Cardiovasc Surg* 1982; 16:41–45.
197. Dodds GA 3d, Warnes CA, Danielson GK. Aortic valve replacement after repair of pulmonary atresia and ventricular septal defect or tetralogy of Fallot. *Thorac Cardiovasc Surg* 1997; 113: 736–741.
198. Bjarke B. Oxygen uptake and cardiac output during submaximal and maximal exercise in adult subjects with totally corrected tetralogy of Fallot. *Acta Med Scand* 1975; 197:177–186.
199. Nugent E, Freedom R, Nora J, et al. Clinical course in pulmonary stenosis. *Circulation* 1977; 56(suppl I):I-38–I-47.
200. Kopecky S, Gersh B, McGoon M, et al. Long-term outcome of patients undergoing surgical repair of isolated pulmonary valve stenosis: Follow-up at 20 to 30 years. *Circulation* 1988; 78:1150–1156.
201. Mullins C, Latson L, Neches W, et al. Balloon dilatation of miscellaneous lesions: Results of Valvuloplasty and Angioplasty of Congenital Anomalies Registry. *Am J Cardiol* 1990; 65:802–803.
202. Friedman W, Johnson A. Congenital aortic stenosis. In: Roberts W, ed. *Adult Congenital Heart Disease*. Philadelphia: Davis; 1987:357.
203. Kelly D, Wulfsberg B, Rowe R. Discrete subaortic stenosis. *Circulation* 1972; 46:309–322.
204. Kleinert S, Geva T. Echocardiographic morphometry and geometry of the left ventricular outflow tract in fixed subaortic stenosis. *J Am Coll Cardiol* 1993; 22:1501–1508.
205. Freedom R. The long and short of it: Some thoughts about the fixed forms of left ventricular outflow tract obstruction. *J Am Coll Cardiol* 1997; 30:1843–1846.
206. Williams J, Barratt-Boyes B, Lowe J. Supravalvular aortic stenosis. *Circulation* 1961; 24:1311–1318.
207. Mills P, Leech G, Davies M, et al. The natural history of a nonstenotic bicuspid aortic valve. *Br Heart J* 1978; 40:951–957.
208. Gersony W, Hayes C. Bacterial endocarditis in patients with pulmonary stenosis, aortic stenosis, or ventricular septal defect. *Circulation* 1977; 56(suppl I):I-84–I-87.
209. Fontana R, Edwards J. *Congenital Cardiac Disease: A Review of 357 Cases Studied Pathologically*. Philadelphia: Saunders; 1962.
210. Muna W, Ferrans V, Pierce J, et al. Discrete subaortic stenosis in Newfoundland dogs: Association of infective endocarditis. *Am J Cardiol* 1978; 41:746–754.
211. Bonderman D, Gharehbaghi-Schnell E, Wollenek G, et al. Mechanisms underlying aortic dilatation in congenital aortic valve malformation. *Circulation* 1999; 99:2138–2143.
212. Cohen L, Friedman W, Braunwald E, et al. Natural history of mild congenital aortic stenosis elucidated by serial hemodynamic studies. *Am J Cardiol* 1972; 30:1–5.
213. Wagner H, Ellison R, Keane J, et al. Long-term follow-up of valvotomy before 1968 for congenital aortic stenosis. *Am J Cardiol* 1986; 58:338–341.
214. Kugelmeier J, Egloff L, Real F, et al. Congenital aortic stenosis: Early and late results of aortic valvotomy. *Thorac Cardiovasc Surg* 1982; 30:91–95.
215. Sandhu S, Lloyd T, Crowley D, et al. Effectiveness of balloon valvuloplasty in the young adult with congenital aortic stenosis. *Cathet Cardiovasc Diagn* 1995; 36:122–127.
216. Somerville J, Stone S, Ross D. Fate of patients with fixed subaortic stenosis after surgical removal. *Br Heart J* 1980; 43:629–647.
217. Brauner R, Laks H, Drinkwater D Jr, et al. Benefits of early surgical repair in fixed subaortic stenosis. *J Am Coll Cardiol* 1997; 30:1835–1842.
218. van Son J, Schaff H, Danielson G, et al. Surgical treatment of discrete and tunnel suboartic stenosis: Late survival and risk of reoperation. *Circulation* 1993; 88:II59–II69.
219. Campbell M. Natural history of coarctation of the aorta. *Br Heart J* 1970; 32:633–640.
220. Cohen M, Fuster V, Steele P. Coarctation of the aorta: Long-term follow-up and prediction of outcome after surgical correction. *Circulation* 1989; 80:840–845.
221. Gross R, Hufnagel C. Coarctation of the aorta: Experimental studies regarding its surgical correction. *N Engl J Med* 1945; 233:287–293.
222. Waldhausen J, Shitman V, Werner J, et al. Surgical intervention in infants with coarctation of the aorta. *J Thorac Cardiovasc Surg* 1981; 81:323–325.
223. Keen G. Spinal cord damage and operations for coarctation of the aorta: Aetiology, practice, and prospects. *Thorax* 1987; 42:11–18.
224. Morris R, Samuels L, Brockman S. Total simultaneous repair of coarctation and intracardiac pathology in adult patients. *Ann Thorac Surg* 1998; 65:1698–1702.
225. Sperling D, Dorsey T, Rowen M, et al. Percutaneous transluminal angioplasty of congenital coarctation of the aorta. *Am J Cardiol* 1983; 51:562–564.
226. Ritter S. Coarctation and balloons: Inflated or realistic? *J Am Coll Cardiol* 1989; 13:696–699.
227. Yetman AT, Nykanen D, McCrindle BW, et al. Balloon angioplasty of recurrent coarctation: A 12-year review. *J Am Coll Cardiol* 1997; 30:811–816.
228. Ebeid M, Prieto L, Latson L. Use of balloon-expandable stents for coarctation of the aorta: Initial results and intermediate-term follow-up. *J Am Coll Cardiol* 1997; 30:1847–1852.
229. Rao P, Thapar M, Wilson A, et al. Intermediate-term follow-up results of balloon aortic valvuloplasty in infants and children with special reference to causes of restenosis. *Am J Cardiol* 1989; 64:1356–1360.
230. Magee A, Brzezinska-Rajszys G, Qureshi S, et al. Stent implantation for aortic coarctation and recoarctation. *Heart* 1999; 82:600–606.
231. de Lezo J, Pan M, Romero M, et al. Immediate follow-up findings after stent treatment for severe coarctation of aorta. *Am J Cardiol* 1999; 83:400–406.
232. Maron B, Humphries J, Rowe R, et al. Prognosis of surgically corrected coarctation of the aorta: A 20-year postoperative appraisal. *Circulation* 1973; 47:119–126.
233. Presbitero P, Demarie D, Villani M, et al. Long-term results (15–30 years) of surgical repair of aortic coarctation. *Br Heart J* 1987; 57:462–467.
234. Fyler D. Report of the New England regional cardiac infant program. *Pediatrics* 1980; 65:375–460.
235. Rashkind W, Mille W. Creation of an atrial septal defect without thoracotomy: A palliative approach to complete transposition of the great arteries. *JAMA* 1966; 196:991–992.
236. Senning A. Surgical correction of transposition of the great vessels. *Surgery* 1959; 45:966–980.
237. Mustard W. Successful two-stage correction of transposition of the great vessels. *Surgery* 1964; 55:469–472.
238. Turina M, Seibenmann R, Segesser L, et al. Late functional deterioration after atrial correction for transposition of the great arteries. *Circulation* 1989; 80(suppl I):162–167.
239. Gelatt M, Hamilton R, McCrindle B, et al. Arrhythmia and mortality after the Mustard procedure: a 30-year single-center experience. *J Am Coll Cardiol* 1997; 29:194–201.
240. Wilson NJ, Clarkson PM, Barratt-Boyes BG, et al. Long-term outcome after the Mustard repair for simple transposition of the great arteries. 28-year follow-up. *J Am Coll Cardiol* 1998; 32:758–765.
241. Puley G, Siu S, Connelly M, et al. Arrhythmia and survival in patients 18 years of age after the Mustard procedure for complete transposition of the great arteries. *Am J Cardiol* 1999; 83:1080–1084.
242. Jatene A, Fontes V, Paulista P, et al. Successful anatomic correction of transposition of the great vessels: A preliminary report. *Arg Braz Cardiol* 1975; 28:461–464.
243. Rastelli G, Wallace R, Ongley P. Complete repair of transposition

of the great arteries with pulmonary stenosis: A review and report of a case corrected by using a new surgical technique. *Circulation* 1969; 39:83–95.

244. Flinn C, Wolff G, Dick M, et al. Cardiac rhythm after the Mustard operation for complete transposition of the great arteries. *N Engl J Med* 1984; 310:1635–1638.
245. Mee R. Two-stage repair: Pulmonary artery banding and switch. *J Thorac Cardiovasc Surg* 1986; 92:385–390.
246. Wernovsky G, Hougen T, Walsh E, et al. Mid-term results after the arterial switch operation for transposition of the great arteries with intact ventricular septum: Clinical, hemodynamic, echocardiographic, and electrophysiologic data. *Circulation* 1988; 77:1333–1344.
247. Rhodes L, Wernovsky C, Keane J, et al. Arrhythmias and intracardiac conduction after the arterial switch operation. *J Thorac Cardiovasc Surg* 1995; 19:303–310.
248. Colan S, Trowitzsch E, Wernovsky G, et al. Myocardial performance after arterial switch operation for transposition of the great arteries with intact ventricular septum. *Circulation* 1988; 78:132–141.
249. Warnes G. Congenitally corrected transposition: The uncorrected misnomer. *J Am Coll Cardiol* 1996; 27:1244–1245.
250. Allwork S, Bentall H, Becker A, et al. Congenitally corrected transposition of the great arteries: Morphologic study of 32 cases. *Am J Cardiol* 1976; 38:910–923.
251. Lundstrom U, Bull C, Wyse R, et al. The natural and "unnatural" history of congenitally corrected transposition. *Am J Cardiol* 1990; 65:1222–1229.
252. Friedberg D, Nadas A. Clinical profile with congenitally corrected transposition of the great arteries: A study of 60 cases. *N Engl J Med* 1970; 282:1053–1059.
253. Huhta J, Maloney J, Ritter D, et al. Complete atrioventricular block in patients with atrioventricular discordance. *Circulation* 1983; 67:1374–1377.
254. Yeh T, Connelly M, Coles J, et al. Atrioventricular discordance: Results of repair in 127 patients. *J Thorac Cardiovasc Surg* 1999; 117:1190–1203.
255. Prieto LR, Hordof AJ, Secic M, et al. Progressive tricuspid valve disease in patients with congenitally corrected transposition of the great arteries. *Circulation* 1998; 98:997–1005.
256. Voskuil M, Hazekamp MG, Kroft LJ, et al. Postsurgical course of patients with congenitally corrected transposition of the great arteries. *Am J Cardiol* 1999; 83:558–562.
257. van Son J, Danielson G, Huhta J, et al. Late results of systemic atrioventricular valve replacement in corrected transposition. *J Thorac Cardiovasc Surg* 1995; 109:642–653.
258. Yagihari T, Kishimoto H, Isobe F, et al. Double switch operation in cardiac anomalies with atrioventricular and ventriculoarterial discordance. *J Thorac Cardiovasc Surg* 1994; 107:351–358.
259. Ilbawi M, DeLeon S, Backer C, et al. An alternative approach to the surgical management of physiologically corrected transposition with ventricular septal defect and pulmonary stenosis or atresia. *J Thorac Cardiovasc Surg* 1990; 100:410–415.
260. Connelly M, Piu P, Williams W, et al. Congenitally corrected transposition in the adult: Functional status and complications. *J Am Coll Cardiol* 1996; 27:1238–1243.
261. Ammash N, Warnes C. Survival into adulthood of patients with unoperated single ventricle. *Am J Cardiol* 1996; 77:542–544.
262. LaCorte M, Dick M, Scheer G, et al. Left ventricular function in tricuspid atresia: Angiographic analysis in 28 patients. *Circulation* 1975; 52:996–1000.
263. Moodie D, Ritter D, Tajik A, et al. Long-term follow-up in the unoperated univentricular heart. *Am J Cardiol* 1984; 53:1124–1128.
264. Moodie D, Ritter D, Tajik A, et al. Long-term follow-up after palliative operation for univentricular heart. *Am J Cardiol* 1984; 53:1648–1651.
265. Warnes C, Feldt R, Hagler D. Protein-losing enteropathy after the Fontan operation: Successful treatment by percutaneous fenestration of the atrial septum. *Mayo Clin Proc* 1996; 71:378–379.
266. Fontan F, Baudet E. Surgical repair of tricuspid atresia. *Thorax* 1971; 26:240–248.
267. Choussat A, Fontan E, Besse P, et al. Selection criteria for Fontan's procedure. In: Anderson R, Shinebourne E, eds. *Paediatric Cardiology*. Edinburgh: Churchill Livingstone; 1977:559–566.
268. Fontan F, Deville C, Quagebeur J, et al. Repair of tricuspid atresia in 100 patients. *J Thorac Cardiovasc Surg* 1983; 85:647–660.
269. Gewillig M, Lundstrom U, Bull C, et al. Exercise responses in patients after Fontan repair: Patterns and determinants of performance. *J Am Coll Cardiol* 1990; 15:1424–1432.
270. Driscoll D, Offord K, Felot R, et al. Five to fifteen year follow-up after Fontan operation. *Circulation* 1992; 81:1520–1536.
271. Fontan F, Kirklin J, Fernandez G, et al. Outcome after a "perfect" Fontan operation. *Circulation* 1990; 81:152–1536.
272. Matsuda H, Kawashima Y, Kishimoto H, et al. Problems with the modified Fontan operation for univentricular heart of the right ventricular type. *Circulation* 1987; 76(suppl II):II-45–II-52.
273. Feldt R, Driscoll D, Offord K, et al. Protein-losing enteropathy after the Fontan operation. *J Thorac Cardiovasc Surg* 1991; 112:672–680.
274. Mertens L, Hagler DJ, Sauer U, et al. Protein-losing enteropathy after the Fontan operation: an international multicenter study: PLE study group. *J Thorac Cardiovasc Surg* 1998; 115:1063–1073.
275. Kelly AM, Feldt RH, Driscoll DJ, et al. Use of heparin in the treatment of protein-losing enteropathy after Fontan operation for complex congenital heart disease. *Mayo Clin Proc* 1998; 73:777–779.
276. Mertens L, Dumoulin M, Gewillig M. Effective percutaneous fenestration of the atrial septum in protein-losing enteropathy after the Fontan operation. *Br Heart J* 1994; 72:591–592.
277. Zellers T, Brown K. Protein-losing enteropathy after the modified Fontan operation: Oral prednisone treatment with biopsy and laboratory proved improvement. *Pediatr Cardiol* 1996; 17:115–117.
278. Mathur M, Glenn W. Long-term evaluation of cavopulmonary artery anastomosis. *Surgery* 1973; 74:889–916.
279. Kreutzer J, Keane J, Lock J, et al. Conversion of modified Fontan procedure to lateral atrial tunnel cavopulmonary anastomosis. *J Thorac Cardiovasc Surg* 1996; 111:1169–1176.
280. van Son J, Mohr F, Hambsch J, et al. Conversion of atriopulmonary or lateral atrial tunnel cavopulmonary anastomosis to extracardiac conduit Fontan modification. *European J C-T Surg* 1999; 15:150–157.
281. Deal B, Mavrousid C, Backer C, et al. Impact of arrhythmia circuit cryoablation during Fontan conversion for refractory atrial tachycardia. *Am J Cardiol* 1999; 83:563–568.
282. Bridges N, Lock J, Castaneda A. Baffle fenestration with subsequent transcatheter closure: Modifications of the Fontan operation for patients at higher risk. *Circulation* 1990; 82:1681–1689.
283. de Leval M, Kilner P, Gewillig M, et al. Total cavopulmonary connection: A logical alternative to atriopulmonary connection for complex Fontan operations. *J Thorac Cardiovasc Surg* 1988; 96:682–695.
284. Laschinger J, Redmond J, Cameron D, et al. Intermediate results of the extracardiac Fontan procedure. *Ann Thorac Surg* 1996; 62:1261–1267.
285. Petrossian E, Reddy V, McElhinney D, et al. Early results of the extracardiac conduit Fontan operation. *J Thorac Cardiovasc Surg* 1999; 117:688–696.
286. Watson H. Natural history of Ebstein's anomaly of the tricuspid valve in childhood and adolescence: An internation cooperative study of 505 cases. *Br Heart J* 1974; 36:417–427.
287. Celermajer D, Dodd S, Greenwald S, et al. Morbid anatomy in neonates with Ebstein's anomaly of the tricuspid valve: Pathophysiologic and clinical implications. *J Am Coll Cardiol* 1992; 19:1049–1053.

288. Till J, Celermajer D, Deanfield J. The natural history of arrhythmias in Ebstein's anomaly [abstract]. *J Am Coll Cardiol* 1992, 19(suppl A):273A.
289. Saxena A, Fong L, Tristram M, et al. Late noninvasive evaluation of cardiac performance in mildly symptomatic older patients with Ebstein's anomaly of the tricuspid valve: Role of radionuclide imaging. *J Am Coll Cardiol* 1991; 17:182–186.
290. Kumar A, Fyler D, Miettinen O, et al. Ebstein's anomaly: Clinical profile and natural history. *Am J Cardiol* 1981; 28:84–95.
291. Danielson G, Driscoll D, Mair D, et al. Operative treatment of Ebstein's anomaly. *J Thorac Cardiovasc Surg* 1992; 104:1195–1202.
292. MacLellan-Tobert S, Driscoll D, Mottram C, et al. Exercise tolerance in patients with Ebstein's anomaly. *J Am Coll Cardiol* 1997; 29:1615–1622.
293. Kiziltan H, Theodoro D, Warnes C, et al. Late results of bioprosthetic tricuspid valve replacement in Ebstein's anomaly. *Ann Thorac Surg* 1998; 66:1539–1545.
294. Ramirez F, Gayraud B, Pereira L. Marfan syndrome: New clues to genotype-phenotype correlations. *Ann Med* 1999; 31:202–207.
295. Murdoch J, Walker B, Halpern B, et al. Life expectancy and causes of death in the Marfan syndrome. *N Engl J Med* 1972; 286:804–808.
296. Pyeritz R, Wappel M. Mitral valve dysfunction in the Marfan syndrome. *Am J Med* 1983; 74:797–807.
297. Gott VL, Greene PS, Alejo DE, et al. Replacement of the aortic root in patients with Marfan's syndrome. *N Engl J Med* 1999; 340:1307–1313.
298. Silverman D, Burton K, Gray J, et al. Life expectancy in the Marfan syndrome. *Am J Cardiol* 1995; 75:157–160.
299. Coady M, Rizzo J, Hammond G, et al. What is the appropriate size criterion for resection of thoracic aortic aneurysms? *J Thorac Cardiovasc Surg* 1997; 113:476–491.
300. Yacoub M, Gehle P, Chandrasekaran V, et al. Late results of a valve-preserving operation in patients with aneurysms of the ascending aorta and root. *J Thorac Cardiovasc Surg* 1998; 115:1080–1090.

PART ELEVEN

CARDIOMYOPATHY AND SPECIFIC HEART MUSCLE DISEASES

CHAPTER 65

CLASSIFICATION OF CARDIOMYOPATHIES

Jay W. Mason

Despite controversy in classifying the cardiomyopathies, there is general agreement on the definition. Cardiomyopathy is a primary disorder of the heart muscle that causes abnormal myocardial performance and is not the result of disease or dysfunction of other cardiac structures. Thus, the term *cardiomyopathy* excludes cases of myocardial failure due to myocardial infarction (so-called ischemic cardiomyopathy, a misnomer), systemic arterial hypertension, and valvular stenosis or regurgitation. Although cardiomyopathy is easily defined, classification of its various forms is difficult. This difficulty results because the great majority of cases of cardiomyopathy are associated with generalized cardiac dilatation and ventricular systolic dysfunction, in which the etiology is unknown.

CLASSIFICATION SCIENCE

Physicians and biomedical scientists use classification schemes to draw relations and distinctions between diseases. This process promotes understanding and aids recollection. Even disorders we know little about can be understood if appropriately placed in a class with other disorders we do know about.

The science of classification requires that all items within the classified domain be included and that each item appear in only one class. Inability to make clear distinctions between biologic systems makes this latter requirement the most demanding. Classification must be based on those features of the individual units within the domain that are understood or recognizable and that permit a useful distinction between groups.

Thus, the classification of cardiomyopathies should be based on an extensive, current category of knowledge about heart diseases and should be as useful as possible to physicians and scientists.

CATEGORIES OF KNOWLEDGE ABOUT CARDIOMYOPATHIES

Knowledge about cardiomyopathies falls into several categories: Etiology, gross anatomy, histology, genetics, biochemistry, immunology, hemodynamic function, prognosis, treatment, and others. No single classification scheme can utilize all of these areas of knowledge because there is so much overlap between them.[1]

The best classifications use a single category of knowledge with which to separate items in the domain. However, the most useful knowledge category differs among users of the classification. A histologic classification will be useful to the pathologist, while a functional categorization is more valuable to the treating physician. If only one classification is to be used by both clinicians and scientists, etiologic categorization seems to be most successful. It must be recognized, however, that no single classification can serve all users and all purposes.

Several commonly employed classifications of cardiomyopathy are discussed below. For clarity, the primary categories of each classification are displayed in Tables 65-1 to 65-6, but only a few representative diseases are mentioned within each category. The exceptions are the etiologic classification (Table 65-3) and the *International Classification of Disease,* Ninth Revision (ICD-9) classification (Table 65-5), in which more nearly complete listings are provided.

THE WORLD HEALTH ORGANIZATION CLASSIFICATION

The only currently used clinical classification of cardiomyopathy that was developed by consensus is that of the *World Health Organization* (WHO) and the International Society and Federation of Cardiology.[2,3] This scheme is outlined in Table 65-1. Because it was developed by a panel of experts and has the implied backing of the WHO, it is widely recognized and frequently used. Although it has been in existence since 1980, it has not gained general acceptance.

The 1980 WHO committee[2] reserved the term *cardiomyopathy* for myocardial disease of unknown cause. This somewhat restricted usage has not been adopted widely and is not fully adhered to in this text. The more common usage includes all

TABLE 65-1 World Health Organization Classifications of Cardiomyopathies

- I. Former WHO classification[a]
  - A. Heart muscle diseases of unknown cause
    1. Dilated cardiomyopathy
    2. Hypertrophic cardiomyopathy
    3. Restrictive cardiomyopathy
    4. Unclassified cardiomyopathy
  - B. Specific heart muscle disease
    1. Infective
    2. Metabolic
       - a. Endocrine
       - b. Familial storage diseases and infiltrations
       - c. Deficiency
       - d. Amyloid
    3. General system disease
       - a. Connective tissue disorders
       - b. Infiltrations and granulomas
    4. Heredofamilial
       - a. Muscular dystrophies
       - b. Neuromuscular disorders
    5. Sensitivity and toxic reactions
- II. New WHO classification[b]
  - A. Functional classification of cardiomyopathy
    1. Dilated cardiomyopathy
    2. Hypertrophic cardiomyopathy
    3. Restrictive cardiomyopathy
    4. Arrhythmogenic right ventricular cardiomyopathy
    5. Unclassified cardiomyopathies
  - B. Specific cardiomyopathies
    1. Ischemic cardiomyopathy
    2. Valvular cardiomyopathy
    3. Hypertensive cardiomyopathy
    4. Inflammatory cardiomyopathy
       - a. Idiopathic
       - b. Autoimmune
       - c. Infectious
    5. Metabolic cardiomyopathy
       - a. Endocrine
       - b. Familial storage diseases and infiltrations
       - c. Deficiency
       - d. Amyloid
    6. General system disease
       - a. Connective tissue disorders
       - b. Infiltrations and granulomas
    7. Muscular dystrophies
    8. Neuromuscular disorders
    9. Sensitivity and toxic reactions
    10. Peripartal cardiomyopathy

[a]This dates from 1980; see reference 2.
[b]This dates from 1995; see reference 3.
NOTE: These are listings of major categories only; specific disorders are not listed.

TABLE 65-2 Functional Classification of Cardiomyopathies

- I. Cardiac dilatation
  - A. With systolic failure
    1. Idiopathic dilated cardiomyopathy
    2. Late cardiac amyloidosis
    3. Tachycardia-induced congestive failure
  - B. Without systolic failure
    1. High cardiac output state
    2. Bradycardia-induced congestive failure
- II. Cardiac hypertrophy
  - A. With obstruction
    1. Hypertrophic obstructive cardiomyopathy
  - B. Without obstruction
    1. Hypertrophic cardiomyopathy
    2. Left ventricular hypertrophy due to systemic hypertension
- III. Cardiac restriction
  - A. Early cardiac amyloidosis
  - B. Endomyocardial fibrosis

NOTE: This is a complete listing of primary categories, but only a few specific examples are provided for illustration.

forms of heart disease in which the myocardium is primarily involved, as defined at the start of this chapter, but excludes valvular heart disease, systemic arterial hypertension, and coronary atherosclerosis. In its 1995 classification, the WHO committee (entirely new except for one member) moved toward this more common usage, stating, "With increasing understanding of etiology and pathogenesis, the difference between cardiomyopathy and specific heart muscle disease has become indistinct."[3]

Examination of the 1980 and 1995 WHO classifications reveals that they are, in fact, somewhat awkward schemes that employ two separate categorizations in series, one based primarily on left ventricular morphology and function and the other based on etiology. A resultant disadvantage is that diseases are placed in two schema that overlap.

FUNCTIONAL CLASSIFICATION OF CARDIOMYOPATHIES

The most widely used functional classification of cardiomyopathy recognizes three disturbances of function: dilatation, hypertrophy, and restriction (Table 65-2). *Dilatation* is dominated by left ventricular cavity enlargement and systolic failure. *Hypertrophy* includes both obstructive and nonobstructive forms. *Restriction* is characterized by inadequate compliance causing restriction of diastolic filling. The value of this scheme is that virtually all cardiomyopathies are readily placed in one of the three categories, and the therapeutic approaches to each category are distinctly different. For example, left ventricular afterload reduction is a cornerstone of therapy for dilated cardiomyopathies with systolic failure, but is of little benefit in the restrictive forms. There are some shortcomings of the functional classification however. Many diseases are physiologically heterogeneous. Almost all hypertrophic conditions have an element of diastolic restriction. Most dilated ventricles display

TABLE 65-3 Etiologic Classification of Cardiomyopathies

I. Infective/inflammatory
- Idiopathic lymphocytic myocarditis
- Peripartum myocarditis
- Eosinophilic myocarditis
- Giant-cell myocarditis
- Viral myocarditis
- Rickettsial myocarditis
- Bacterial myocarditis
- Mycobacterial heart disease
- Spirochetal heart disease
- Fungal myocarditis
- Protozoal myocarditis
- Metazoal myocarditis
- Helminthic myocarditis
- Chemical or drug hypersensitivity
- Autoimmune myocarditis

II. Metabolic
- A. Endocrine
  - 1. Thyroid disease
    - Thyrotoxicosis
    - Hypothyroidism
  - 2. Pheochromocytoma
  - 3. Acromegaly
  - 4. Diabetes mellitus
  - 5. Carcinoid heart disease
- B. Uremia
- C. Hyperoxaluria
- D. Gout
- E. Storage diseases and infiltrative processes
  - 1. Lysosomal storage diseases
    - GM1 gangliosidosis
    - Tay-Sachs disease and variants
    - Sandhoff's disease
    - Niemann-Pick disease
    - Gaucher's disease
    - Fabry's disease
    - Farber's disease
    - Fucosidosis
    - Hurler's syndrome
    - Scheie's syndrome
    - Hunter's syndrome
    - Sanfilippo
    - Morquio
    - Moroteaux-Lamy
  - 2. Glycogen storage diseases
    - Pompe's disease
    - Cori's disease
    - Andersen's disease
    - Dominantly inherited cardioskeletal myopathy with lysosomal glycogen storage and normal acid maltase levels
  - 3. Refsum's syndrome
  - 4. Hand-Schüller-Christian
  - 5. Adipositos cordis
  - 6. Hemochromatosis
- F. Deficiencies
  - 1. Electrolyte
    - Hypocalcemia
    - Hypophosphatemia
  - 2. Nutritional
    - Kwashiorkor
    - Beriberi
    - Pellagra
    - Scurvy
    - Selenium
    - Carnitine

III. Amyloid
- AL (primary amyloid, myeloma-associated amyloid)
- AA (secondary amyloid, familial Mediterraneanfever-associated amyloid)
- AF (familial amyloid)
- SSA (senile cardiac amyloid, senile systemic amyloid)
- IAA (atrial amyloid)

IV. General system disorders
- A. Collagen vascular (connective tissue)
  - Systemic lupus erythematosus
  - Polyarteritis nodosa
  - Rheumatoid arthritis
  - Scleroderma
  - Dermatomyositis
  - Whipple's disease
  - Kawasaki's disease
- B. Sarcoidosis
- C. Neoplastic

V. Muscular dystrophies, myopathies, and neuromuscular disorders
- A. Muscular dystrophies
  - Duchenne's muscular dystrophy
  - Becker's muscular dystrophy
  - Myotonic dystrophy
  - Facioscapulohumeral muscular dystrophy
  - Limb girdle dystrophy
  - Scapuloperoneal dystrophy, including Emery-Dreifuss
  - Congenital muscular dystrophy
  - Distal muscular dystrophy
- B. Congenital myopathies
  - Central-core disease
  - Nemaline myopathy
  - Myotubular myopathy (centronuclear)
  - Congenital fiber-type disproportion
- C. Mitochondrial myopathies, including Kearns-Sayre syndrome
- D. Neuromuscular disorders, Friedreich's ataxia

VI. Toxicity, hypersensitivity, and physical agent effects
- A. Toxic effects
  - 1. Caused by drugs, heavy metals, and chemical agents
    - Alcohol (ethyl)
    - Amphetamine/methamphetamine
    - Anthracyclines
    - Antidepressants
    - Antimony
    - Arsenic
    - Arsine gas
    - Carbon monoxide
    - Catecholamines
    - Chloroquine
    - Cobalt
    - Cocaine
    - Cyclophosphamide
    - Emetine
    - 5-Fluorouracil
    - Hydrocarbons
    - Interferon
    - Lead
    - Lithium
    - Mercury
    - Methysergide
    - Paracetamol
    - Phenothiazines
    - Phosphorus
    - Reserpine
  - 2. Caused by scorpions, spiders, arthropods, and snakes
    - Scorpions
    - Arthropods
    - Black widow spider
    - Snakes
- B. Hypersensitivity reactions
  - Acetazolamide
  - Amitriptyline
  - Amphotericin B
  - Ampicillin
  - Carbamazepine
  - Chlorthalidone
  - Hydrochlorothiazide
  - Indomethacin
  - Isoniazid
  - Methyldopa
  - Oxyphenbutazone
  - Para-aminosalicylic acid
  - Penicillin
  - Phenindione
  - Phenylbutazone
  - Phenytoin
  - Streptomycin
  - Sulfadiazine
  - Sulfisoxazole
  - Sulfonylureas
  - Tetracycline
- C. Physical agents
  - Heat
  - Hypothermia
  - Radiation

VII. Miscellaneous
- Peripartum heart disease
- Tachycardia-induced cardiomyopathy
- Ectodermal dysplasia-associated cardiomyopathy
- Idiopathic endocardial fibrosis
- Endocardial fibroelastosis
- Infantile cardiomyopathy
- Arrhythmogenic right ventricular dysplasia

NOTE: This is an essentially complete listing of cardiomyopathies of known cause.

myocyte hypertrophy. Some diseases change from one category to another during their course; the best example is cardiac amyloidosis, which initially exhibits diastolic stiffness, with complete preservation of systolic performance, followed years later by dilatation and systolic failure.

The functional scheme also associates diseases that have vastly different causes, some of which require special therapeutic interventions. For example, the primary therapy for cardiac hemochromatosis, often an initially restrictive disease, is removal of excessive iron stores; this would not, of course, be

TABLE 65-4 Endomyocardial Biopsy Histology Classification of Cardiomyopathies

I. Inflammatory/immune cardiomyopathy
  - Lymphocytic myocarditis
  - Rheumatic carditis
  - Sarcoidosis
  - Giant cell myocarditis
  - Cardiac allograft rejection
  - Chagas' cardiomyopathy
  - Hypersensitivity myocarditis

II. Infectious cardiomyopathy
  - Toxoplasmosis
  - Lyme carditis
  - Cytomegalovirus

III. Infiltrative cardiomyopathy
  - Glycogen storage
  - Hemochromatosis
  - Right ventricular lipomatosis
  - Amyloidosis

IV. Cardiac tumors
  - Cardiac origin
  - Noncardiac origin

V. Miscellaneous specific cardiomyopathies
  - Anthracycline cardiotoxicity
  - Endocardial fibrosis
  - Endocardial fibroelastosis
  - Fabry's disease
  - Carcinoid disease
  - Irradiation injury
  - Kearns-Sayre syndrome
  - Henoch-Schönlein purpura
  - Chloroquine cardiomyopathy
  - Carnitine deficiency
  - Hypereosinophilic syndrome

VI. Nonspecific abnormalities
  - Idiopathic dilated cardiomyopathy
  - Other cardiomyopathies of unknown cause

VII. No histologic abnormality

NOTE: This represents a relatively complete listing of diagnoses that have been made by endomyocardial biopsy and reported in the literature.

TABLE 65-5 ICD-9 Classification of Heart Disease

ICD-9 Code	Description
402.00	Hypertensive heart disease, malignant, w/o CHF
402.01	Hypertensive heart disease, malignant, w CHF
402.10	Hypertensive heart disease, benign, w/o CHF
402.11	Hypertensive heart disease, benign, w CHF
402.90	Hypertensive heart disease, unspecified, w/o CHF
402.91	Hypertensive heart disease, unspecified, w CHF
422.90	Acute myocarditis, unspecified
422.91	Idiopathic myocarditis
425.0	Endomyocardial fibrosis
425.1	Hypertrophic obstructive cardiomyopathy
425.2	Obscure cardiomyopathy of Africa
425.3	Endomyocardial fibroelastosis
425.4	Idiopathic cardiomyopathy
425.5	Alcoholic cardiomyopathy
425.7	Nutritional and metabolic cardiomyopathy
425.8	Cardiomyopathy in other diseases classified elsewhere
425.9	Secondary cardiomyopathy, unspecified
428.0	Congestive heart failure
428.1	Left heart failure
428.9	Heart failure, unspecified
429.0	Myocarditis, unspecified
429.1	Myocardial degeneration
429.3	Cardiomegaly
429.82	Hyperkinetic heart disease
674.84	Postpartum cardiomyopathy

CHF = congestive heart failure.

effective treatment for other diseases similarly classified. Despite its shortcomings, the functional classification of cardiomyopathy remains the most popular among clinicians because it is based on easily understood physiology and is relevant to therapy.

ETIOLOGIC CLASSIFICATION

This scheme utilizes knowledge about cardiomyopathies more extensively than all the others. It has the most primary categories because there are numerous known causes that are not interrelated. Table 65-3 categorizes the diseases covered in Chaps. 69, 73 to 80, 85, 86, and 91 to 94. The general outline established by WHO in 1980 is followed roughly. In many cases the etiologic agent is poorly understood (e.g., uremic "cardiomyopathy"), or the cardiomyopathy is associated with another disease, but the mechanism responsible for heart failure is not known (e.g., cardiomyopathy of systemic neoplasia).

While this classification has the advantage of being inclusive, it has the disadvantage of being awkwardly long. It has 7 primary and 42 secondary categories. In addition, most similarly classified disorders are anatomically, physiologically, and therapeutically unrelated. Thus, this classification is not used routinely by clinicians. It has been used most frequently as an organizational scheme in textbooks and reviews concerning heart muscle disease and cardiomyopathy.

ENDOMYOCARDIAL BIOPSY CLASSIFICATION

Because the heart can be safely biopsied, antemortem histologic diagnosis can be used to classify cardiomyopathies. Dozens of specific myocardial diseases can be detected by biopsy (Table 65-4). The great strength of histologic diagnosis is that it is definitive and unequivocal when a specific disease is observed. In contrast, numerous deficiencies make this method of classification relatively restricted in use. The foremost problem is that, although the number of specific histologic diagnoses is large, they represent a small proportion of all cases—certainly fewer

TABLE 65-6 Therapeutic Classification of Cardiomyopathies

I. Reduce ventricular afterload
Idiopathic dilated cardiomyopathy
Late cardiac amyloidosis
II. Reduce ventricular preload
Endocardial fibrosis
Early cardiac amyloidosis
III. Increase ventricular compliance
Hypertrophic cardiomyopathy
IV. Relieve ventricular obstruction
Hypertrophic obstructive cardiomyopathy
V. Improve cardiac rhythm
Cardiomyopathy of persistent tachycardia
VI. Specific therapy
A. Replace deficiency
Carnitine deficiency cardiomyopathy
B. Remove toxic agent
Hemochromatosis
Hypersensitivity
C. Immunosuppression
Giant cell myocarditis
Lymphocyte myocarditis(?)
D. Correct systemic disease
Uremic cardiomyopathy
Cardiomyopathy of cancer
Systemic lupus erythematosus

NOTE: This is a complete listing of primary categories with a few specific examples for illustration.

than 15 percent. The histology in most patients with cardiomyopathy is nonspecific and nondiagnostic. Hypertrophy, or fiber attenuation, and fibrosis may be seen in varying degrees in almost any disorder and are the only findings in most cases of idiopathic dilated cardiomyopathy and hypertrophic cardiomyopathy (as well as in many instances of heart failure due to myocardial infarction and valvular dysfunction). Furthermore, completely normal histology may occasionally be seen on biopsy in cases of severe dilatation and systolic failure.

Myocardial biopsy samples can be subjected to several additional analytic techniques that expand the potential for classification using endomyocardial biopsy. While at present these analyses are only investigational and none can be generally applied, it is likely that one or more of them will become clinically useful in the future and could form the basis of a classification with wide appeal.

ICD-9 CLASSIFICATION

ICD-9-CM stands for *International Classification of Disease*, Ninth Revision, Clinical Modification. This system was developed by WHO in 1948 for registering disease incidences. In 1977, the United States National Center for Health Statistics modified the ICD-9 code to allow coding of medical records. That modification is the current ICD-9-CM. In 1989 it became mandatory for physicians in the United States to include an ICD-9-CM code on their Medicare claims. It is fascinating to see how utterly different a classification system intended for governmental statistics and claims payment is in comparison to those intended for scientific or clinical purposes. The code is a remarkable hodgepodge, combining multiple categories of knowledge into one classification system. Diseases are variously defined according to one or more features such as etiology, anatomy, physiology, comorbidity, symptoms, and even method and extent of diagnosis. It is no wonder that this code is impossible to remember and notoriously ambiguous and difficult to use. In Table 65-5, the codes describing cardiomyopathies have been extracted from the 1999 version of the ICD-9-CM, where they appear in several groups scattered throughout the listing. Relatively few—25—cardiomyopathy diagnoses are coded, and these represent only 9 specific entities. Some well-recognized myocardial diseases are completely ignored, such as arrhythmogenic right ventricular dysplasia. This classification system and the method of classification it represents are certainly not recommended to physicians and scientists. ICD-9-CM should remain in the bailiwick of bureaucrats and serve as a paragon of classification chaos.

THERAPEUTIC CLASSIFICATION

A classification based on specific therapies borrows heavily from the functional and the etiologic classifications of cardiomyopathy. This classification adds information regarding treatment that is not available in other schemes and therefore may be useful to clinicians.

Nevertheless, this classification has several shortcomings. First, often more than one class of therapy is appropriate for a disease. Therefore, the classification must categorize diseases on the basis of their *primary* therapy. This introduces some instability to the classification, since therapeutic preferences are subject to variance in opinion and to change with new research. The greatest fault of therapeutic categorization is that when new therapies are introduced, the existing classification becomes obsolete. The therapeutic classification shown in Table 65-6 illustrates the sensitivity of this approach to opinion. Some might argue, for example, that diuretic therapy remains the primary treatment for dilated cardiomyopathy.

Note that some commonly employed therapies, such as inotropic agents and cardiac transplantation, do not appear in Table 65-6 because they are often not the initial or primary therapies.

GENE-BASED CLASSIFICATION

Aside from traumatic, iatrogenic, infectious, and certain other secondary cardiac disorders, most heart diseases result from an abnormality of gene function. Many diseases caused by adverse gene behavior are due to inherited or acquired genetic mutations. Several diseases are now defined genetically, including hypertrophic cardiomyopathy, long QT syndrome, forms of dilated cardiomyopathy, muscular dystrophies involving the heart, and arrhythmogenic right ventricular dysplasia. A genetic classification of cardiomyopathies would specify the type of genetic disorder (chromosomal, single genic, polygenic, mitochondrial, or somatic cellular) and the mode of inheritance (autosomal or X-linked, and dominant or recessive), the chromosomes or chromosomal locations involved, and the genes involved. A complete genetic classification might also specify the specific mutation or the regional location of the mutation within the gene, since phenotype does and therapy might vary with each specific mutation or region of mutation. A classification system based upon genetic mutations is diagnostically and therapeutically useless unless the biochemical and resultant physiologic aberrations are understood. Thus, the classification should specify the affected protein products of the mutations, as well as the affected functions provided by the proteins.

In the future, many cardiac diseases will be shown to be due to genes functioning at the extremes of normal behavior, and these behavior abnormalities could be classified in much the same way as inherited mutations. Gene-based classification will become the best classification system for cardiomyopathies, because it will at once precisely and uniquely define the disease, and make evident the necessary diagnostic and therapeutic actions.[4]

SUMMARY

No single classification of cardiomyopathy is generally accepted within the biomedical community. An attempt to gain a consensus for one of the many classifications in current use is not likely to succeed because we are unable to subdivide meaningfully cases of idiopathic dilated cardiomyopathy, which constitute the large majority of all cases. At present, it seems best for the individual health practitioner or scientist to use the classification scheme that best serves his or her purpose. For clinicians, this will often be the functional classification.

In the future, a widely acceptable classification may develop that is based on the molecular genetics of myocardial disease. Although this field is only beginning to develop, it is the discipline most likely to contribute to the understanding of causes and the development of new treatments for myocardial disease.

References

1. Abelmann WH. Classification and natural history of primary myocardial disease. *Prog Cardiovasc Dis* 1984; 27:73–94.
2. Report of the WHO/ISFC task force on the definition and classification of cardiomyopathies. *Br Heart J* 1980; 44:672–673.
3. Richardson P, McKenna W, Bristow M, et al. Report of the 1995 World Health Organization/International Society and Federation of Cardiology task force on the definition and classification of cardiomyopathies. *Circulation* 1996; 93:841–842.
4. Keating MT, Sanguinetti MC. Molecular genetic insights into cardiovascular disease. *Science* 1996; 272:681–685.

CHAPTER 66

DILATED CARDIOMYOPATHIES

Michael R. Bristow / Luisa Mestroni / Teresa J. Bohlmeyer / Edward M. Gilbert

This chapter describes the phenotypic and clinical characteristics of the primary and secondary dilated cardiomyopathies, the most common cause of the clinical syndrome of chronic heart failure.[1] Heart failure is an enormously important clinical problem that, if not contained or solved, ultimately may overwhelm health care resources.[2] The clinical syndrome of heart failure is a complex process where the primary pathophysiology is quickly obscured by a variety of superimposed secondary adaptive, maladaptive, and counterregulatory processes (see also Chap. 20). Heart failure is best understood and approached from the vantage point of *myocardial failure,* most commonly associated with a dilated cardiomyopathy phenotype.[3] As an indication of the importance of the problems of cardiomyopathy and heart failure, the cardiomyopathies have been reclassified recently by a World Health Organization/International Society and Federation of Cardiology (WHO/ISFC) task force[3] (and elaborated on further below).

IMPORTANCE OF HEART FAILURE

Due to its high prevalence (1–1.5 percent of the adult population) and high morbidity, including frequent hospitalizations, the clinical syndrome of heart failure is among the most costly medical problems in the United States.[2] Despite improvements in the treatment of heart failure introduced in the last 10 years, including the general availability of cardiac transplantation and better medical treatment, clinical outcome following the onset of symptoms has not changed substantially.[1] That is, mortality remains high (median survival of 1.7 years for men and 3.2 years for women),[1] the natural history remains progressive,[1] the cost is excessive,[2] and disability[2] and morbidity[2,4] are among the highest of any disease or disease syndrome.

RELATIONSHIP OF MYOCARDIAL FAILURE AND DILATED CARDIOMYOPATHIES TO THE CLINICAL SYNDROME OF HEART FAILURE

The vast majority of the cases of heart failure are caused by heart muscle disease (cardiomyopathy). Within the WHO categorization[3] of cardiomyopathy (Table 66-1), the most common cause of the clinical syndrome of heart failure is a secondary (ischemic, valvular, hypertensive, etc.) or a primary (e.g., idiopathic or familial) *dilated cardiomyopathy,* defined as a ventricular chamber exhibiting increased diastolic and systolic volumes

TABLE 66-1 The World Health Organization/International Society and Federation of Cardiology Classification of the Cardiomyopathies[3]

Category	Definition
I. Dilated (DCM)	↑ EDV, ↑ ESV; low EF
1. Primary	
2. Secondary	
II. Restrictive (RCM)	↓ EDV, ↔ ESV; ↑ FP, ↔ EF
1. Primary	
2. Secondary	
III. Hypertrophic (HCM)	↑ ↑ Septal and ↑ posterior wall thickness, myofibrillar disarray Mutation in sarcomeric protein, autosomal dominant inheritance
IV. Arrhythmogenic RV Dysplasia (ARVC)	Fibrofatty replacement of RV myocardium Autosomal dominant (most) and recessive inheritance
V. Unclassified	Not meeting criteria for other categories
1. Primary	
2. Secondary	Features of > one category

ABBREVIATIONS: EDV = end-diastolic volume; ESV = end systolic volume; EF = LV ejection fraction; FP = LV filling pressure; CM = cardiomyopathy.

and a low (<40 percent) ejection fraction. The natural history of the clinical syndrome of heart failure depends on the course of myocardial failure, since (1) the most powerful single predictor of outcome is the degree of left ventricular (LV) dysfunction, as assessed by the LV ejection fraction,[5] (2) treatment that improves intrinsic ventricular function improves heart failure natural history,[6] and (3) treatment that ultimately worsens intrinsic function, such as many types of positive inotropic agents, is associated with an adverse effect on outcome.[6]

THE WHO/ISFC CLASSIFICATION OF CARDIOMYOPATHIES

The WHO/ISFC classification of cardiomyopathies was revised recently[3] to accommodate several rapidly emerging realities. The first was that the molecular genetic basis of previously unknown types of heart muscle disease is rapidly being elucidated, and so it really makes no sense to reserve the classification for "unknown etiologies" of cardiomyopathy.[7] The second consideration was that many of the mechanisms responsible for the natural history of myocardial dysfunction are qualitatively similar in primary versus secondary dilated cardiomyopathies,[8] which accurately predicted a qualitatively similar response to treatment targeted at these mechanisms.[9,10] This made the exclusion of secondary or "known cause"[7] cardiomyopathies gratuitous, and their inclusion in the new classification allows all cardiomyopathies to be classified under one scheme.

As shown in Table 66-1, the WHO/ISFC cardiomyopathy classification uses two separate methods to define the individual categories. The first is based on the global anatomic description of chamber dimensions in systole and diastole. Thus the dilated and restrictive categories have definitions based on LV dimensions or volume, which also define function via calculated ejection fraction (see Table 66-1). The justification for this is that these two groups have distinct natural histories and respond distinctly differently to medical treatment. The second method of creating individual categories within the WHO/ISFC classification is for cardiomyopathies that are genetically based, have unique myocardial phenotypic features, and do not exhibit extracardiac phenotypes. Thus hypertrophic cardiomyopathy (HCM), caused by mutations in contractile proteins manifesting as a unique phenotype, merits a separate category. The same is true for arrhythmogenic right ventricular dysplasia (ARVC), which also has a unique phenotype and likely will turn out to be completely genetic in basis, as has HCM. On the other hand, genetic cardiomyopathies without unique phenotypes, such as the dilated cardiomyopathy of Becker-Duchenne, are included as one form of the anatomic/chamber dimension category (category I).

The WHO/ISFC classification includes another assignment of nomenclature in "secondary" cardiomyopathies, i.e., those associated with known cardiac or systemic processes.[3] These are referred to as *specific cardiomyopathies,* named for the disease process with which they are associated. Thus an ischemic cardiomyopathy would be a specific cardiomyopathy related to previous myocardial infarction (MI) and the subsequent remodeling process, which usually would fall within the dilated class. On the other hand, a hypertensive cardiomyopathy might be classified as either dilated or restrictive depending on the chamber dimensions. Therefore, the correct term for these cardiomyopathies would be *ischemic dilated cardiomyopathy* and *hypertensive dilated* (or *restrictive*) *cardiomyopathy.*

MOLECULAR MECHANISMS IN CARDIOMYOPATHIES AND MYOCARDIAL FAILURE: DISEASE PHENOTYPE PRODUCED BY ALTERATIONS IN GENE EXPRESSION

As shown in Table 66-2, there are three general categories of mechanisms whereby altered gene expression can lead to a phenotypic change in cardiac myocytes.[11] These are (1) a single-gene defect, e.g., as present in β-myosin heavy-chain codon 403 in familial HCM[12] and in an analogous region of the α-myosin heavy chain in HCM transgenic mouse models,[13,14] (2) polymorphic variation in modifier genes, such as is present in many components of the renin-angiotensin system,[15–19] and (3) maladaptive regulated expression of completely normal genes, such as for the mechanisms responsible for progressive myocardial dysfunction and remodeling in secondary dilated cardiomyopathies.[6,11]

Genetic Causes of Cardiomyopathies in Humans and Animal Models

TABLE 66-2 Three General Mechanisms by Which Alterations in Gene Expression Can Influence the Development or Progression of a Dilated Cardiomyopathy

Type of Process	Examples
Gene mutation	Cardiac α-actin,[34] desmin,[35] dystrophin,[36,37] lamin[38,39]
Polymorphic variation in modifier genes	Angiotensin converting enzyme (ACE),[16,43,44] β_2-adrenergic receptor[46]
Altered expression of a completely normal, wild type gene	Decreased expression: β_1-adrenergic receptors,[8] α-MHC,[47,48] SERCA-2[49] Increased expression: ANP,[50] β-MHC,[47] ACE,[51,52] TNF-α,[53] endothelin,[54] βARK[55]

ABBREVIATIONS: MHC = myosin heavy chain; TNF = tumor necrosis factor; βARK = β-adrenergic receptor kinase; SERCA = sarcoplasmic reticulum calcium ATPase; ANP = atrial natriuretic peptide.

The ability to genetically manipulate the cardiovascular system has made it possible to investigate the role of a number of genes in the developing and adult mouse heart (for a review, see Robbins[20]). The discovery that mutations in sarcomeric proteins lead to HCM has made it possible to generate animal models for this disease.[13,14] In the case of myosin mutations, a single genetic defect initiates a pathway that ultimately leads to hypertrophy and then in males results in late decompensation and ventricular dilatation.[14] Multiple gene mutations have now been associated causally with familial dilated cardiomyopathies, as discussed later in this chapter.

A serendipitous genetic model of dilated cardiomyopathy and heart failure (*myf*5 mice) has been generated by activation of a skeletal muscle genetic program in the heart.[21] These mice have a dilated cardiomyopathy phenotype characterized by progressive myocardial dysfunction and dilatation. They develop the clinical syndrome of heart failure, and they have an extraordinarily high (>90 percent at 260 days) heart failure–related mortality.[21] Another serendipitous genetic model of dilated cardiomyopathy is the muscle LIM protein (MLP) knockout mouse.[22] MLP is a positive regulator of muscle differentiation that is ordinarily expressed at high levels in the heart and which may be involved in myofibrillar protein assembly along the actin-based cytoskeleton.[22] MLP knockout mice exhibit typical features of dilated cardiomyopathy, including decreased systolic and diastolic function and β-adrenergic receptor pathway desensitization.[22]

These characteristics make this model very useful in assessing the mechanisms that lead to the development and progression of myocardial failure. Thus, in transgenic mouse models, both altered expression of contractile proteins and perturbation of myocyte cytoarchitecture can lead to the dilated cardiomyopathy phenotype.

There are several additional transgenic mouse models of cardiomyopathy that may be more relevant to the production of a dilated phenotype in humans. Three of them involve overexpression of components of the adrenergic receptor pathway, the heterodimeric G-protein α_s subunit ($G\alpha_s$)[23,24] and the β_1-[25,26] and β_2-adrenergic receptors.[27] These β-adrenergic pathway transgenic mouse models exhibit similar histopathology consisting of myocyte hypertrophy and increased fibrosis, evidence of apoptosis, systolic and diastolic dysfunction, and ultimately, development of LV dilatation.[23-28]

Several transgenic models of concentric or symmetrical LV hypertrophy have now been reported, including overexpression of the protooncogenes *ras*[29] and *myc*,[30] α_1-adrenergic receptors,[31] the heterodimeric G-protein α subunit ($G\alpha_q$),[32] and protein kinase C (PKC).[33] The mechanisms for the induction of increased ventricular wall thickness are diverse, inasmuch as the *ras*, α_1-receptor, $G\alpha_q$, and PKC overexpressors exhibit true cellular hypertrophy with an increase in cell size,[29,31-33] whereas the *myc* animal exhibits cardiac myocyte hyperplasia.[30] The HCM phenotypes discussed earlier illustrate the principle that apparently diverse signals can culminate in the same phenotype, presumably by converging on final common pathways.

Multiple gene defects have been identified that can produce a dilated cardiomyopathy in humans, as discussed in more detail in the section on familial forms of dilated cardiomyopathy. As listed in Table 66-2, these include mutations in the cardiac α-actin,[34] desmin,[35] dystrophin,[36,37] and lamin[38,39] genes.

Polymorphic Variation in Modifier Genes

Genes exhibit polymorphic variation; i.e., normal variants of genes exist in the population that are of slightly different size or sequence.[40] Some gene polymorphisms are associated with differences in function of the expressed protein gene product, and some of these differences in function likely account for "biologic variation" routinely encountered in population studies of disease susceptibility or clinical response to treatment.

Examples of "modifier" genes that may have an impact on the natural history of a dilated cardiomyopathy (see Table 66-2) include the angiotensin-converting enzyme (ACE) *DD* genotype, where individuals are homozygous for the "deletion" variant, which is associated with increased circulating[15] and cardiac tissue[41] ACE activity. The *DD* genotype appears to increase the extent of hypertrophy in HCM[42] and may be a risk factor for early remodeling after MI[43] and for the development of end-stage ischemic or idiopathic dilated cardiomyopathy.[16,44] Other potentially important polymorphic variants that may influence the natural history of a cardiomyopathy involve the angiotensin AT_1 receptor[18,45] and β_2-adrenergic receptors.[46]

Altered, Maladaptive Expression of a Completely Normal Gene

The third way in which altered gene expression can contribute to the development of a cardiomyopathy is altered, maladaptive expression of a completely normal "wild type" gene.[11] This occurs most commonly in the context of progression of heart muscle disease and myocardial failure, which is the natural history of virtually all cardiomyopathies once they are established. Examples in this category (see Table 66-2) include downregulation of β_1-adrenergic receptors,[8] α-myosin heavy chain (α-MHC),[47,48] and sarcoplasmic reticulum Ca^{2+} ATPase[49] genes and upregulation in the atrial natriuretic peptide (ANP),[50] β-myosin heavy chain (β-MHC),[47] ACE,[51,52] tumor necrosis factor (TNF-α),[53] endothelin,[54] β-adrenergic receptor kinase (βARK)[55] genes. These concepts are discussed further below.

PATHOPHYSIOLOGIC PROCESSES INVOLVED IN MYOCARDIAL DYSFUNCTION, REMODELING, AND THEIR PROGRESSION

Tissue preparations and myocytes isolated from failing human hearts exhibit evidence of decreased contractile function.[56] Assuming that loading conditions and ischemia are not adversely affecting cardiac myocyte function, in the setting of chronic systolic dysfunction from a dilated cardiomyopathy, progressive myocardial failure is most likely caused by myocardial cell loss or changes in the gene expression of proteins that regulate or produce muscle contraction. Figures 66-1 and 66-2 summarize these general points and emphasize the central roles of the renin-angiotensin system (RAS) and the adrenergic nervous system (ANS) in promoting cell loss, growth and remodeling, and altered gene expression.[6]

Myocardial Dysfunction and Remodeling due to Altered Expression of Contractility Regulating Genes and Changes in Sarcomeric Assembly

Gene expression can be defined, broadly, as the expression of a fully or normally functioning protein gene product or, more narrowly (and commonly), as the steady-state abundance of a gene's mRNA transcript. Using either definition, numerous

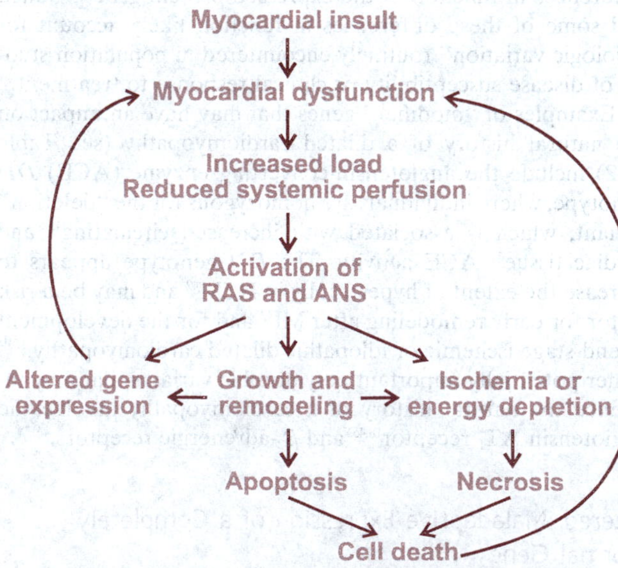

FIGURE 66-1 Relationship of neurohormonal activation and production of cardiac myocyte loss due to apoptosis and necrosis and altered gene expression. Cell loss and altered gene expression result in more myocardial dysfunction, and a vicious cycle is established. RAS = renin angiotensin system; ANS = adrenergic nervous system.

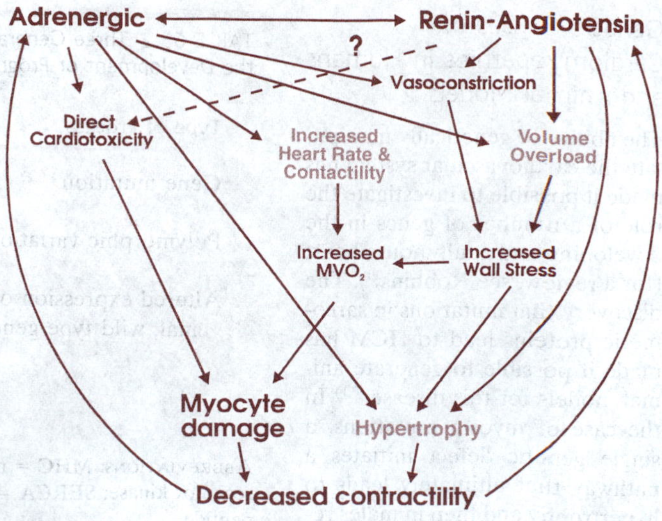

FIGURE 66-2 Heart failure compensatory mechanisms that are activated to support the failing heart. Light-colored areas indicate physiologic mechanisms that stabilize pump function.

abnormalities of gene expression of normal, wild-type genes have been demonstrated in the failing human heart, as discussed earlier, with examples listed in Table 66-2. In order to characterize the abnormalities that may account for progressive myocardial dysfunction and remodeling, it is useful to subdivide them into two general categories,[57] as shown in Table 66-3. The first category encompasses mechanisms that subserve *intrinsic* function, or the mechanisms responsible for contraction and relaxation of the heart in the basal or resting state. *Intrinsic function* is defined as myocardial contraction and relaxation in the absence of extrinsic influences, such as neurotransmitters or hormones. The second general category is *modulated* function, which comprises the mechanisms responsible for the remarkable ability of the heart to increase or decrease its performance dramatically (by 2- to 10-fold) and rapidly in response to various physiologic or physical stimuli. Other critical organs such as the brain, kidney, and liver do not exhibit this quality. *Modulated function* is defined as stimulation or inhibition of myocardial contraction or relaxation by endogenous bioactive compounds, including neurotransmitters, cytokines, autocrine/paracrine substances, and hormones.

In the failing human heart, changes are present in the expression of genes potentially responsible for both general types of myocardial function depicted in Table 66-2.[6,57] Abnormalities of intrinsic function include the factors responsible for an altered length-tension relation,[58–60] a blunted force-frequency response,[61,62] and/or the signals responsible for abnormal cellular and chamber remodeling.[63,64] In the case of the abnormal force-frequency and length-tension responses, the evidence favors abnormal contractile function of individual cardiac myocytes.[56] As shown in Table 66-3, these abnormalities likely reside in the contractile proteins or their regulatory elements,[47,48,65–67] mechanisms involved in excitation-contraction coupling,[49] or the cytoskeleton.[22,68–70] However, within these possibilities for altered intrinsic function, there is not currently a consensus as to which specific abnormalities are present in idiopathic dilated cardiomyopathy (IDC), the most common form of heart failure studied in humans. For cellular remodeling, in both human ventricles[71,72] and animal models,[64,73] the assembly of sarcomeres in series leads to a myocyte that is markedly increased in length but not in diameter, which contributes to remodeling at the chamber level. Such remodeling places the chamber and the myocyte at an energetic disadvantage because of the attendant increase in wall stress,[74] which is one of the major determinants of myocardial oxygen consumption. Inadequate myocyte energy production, particularly associated with key subcellular ion flux mechanisms or the myosin ATPase cycle,[75] in turn would contribute to myocyte contractile dysfunction. Moreover, the hypertrophy process itself leads to a qualitative change in contractile protein gene expression (induction of a "fetal" gene program) that reduces contractile function.[11,47,48,65] On the other hand, cardiac myocyte contractile dysfunction likely plays a role in the remodeling process, inasmuch as medical treatment that improves intrinsic myocardial function can reverse remodeling.[6] Thus contractile dysfunction and remodeling at the cellular level are intimately related to the progressive contractile dysfunction and chamber enlargement that define the natural history of myocardial failure.[76] These concepts are summarized in Fig. 66-3.

TABLE 66-3 General Categorization of Myocardial Function

Intrinsic (Function in the Absence of Neural or Hormonal Influence)	Modulated (Function that May Be Stimulated or Inhibited by Extrinsic Factors Including Neurotransmitters, Cytokines, or Hormone)
• Contractile proteins	• R-G-adenylyl cyclase pathways
• E-C coupling mechanisms	• R-G-phospholipase C pathways
• R-G-adenylyl cyclase pathways	
• Bioenergetics	
• Cytoskeleton	
• Sarcomere and cell remodeling	

ABBREVIATIONS: E-C = excitation-contraction; R-G = receptor–G-protein.

In contrast to abnormalities of intrinsic function, a consensus has been reached on several specific abnormalities in the stimulation component of modulated function. Most of these changes concern β-adrenergic signal transduction.[8,11,57] The ability of β-adrenergic stimulation to increase heart rate and contractility is markedly attenuated in the failing heart due to multiple changes at the level of receptors, G-proteins, and adenylyl cyclase. This produces a major abnormality in the stimulation component of modulated function. In addition, the inhibition component of modulated function is also abnormal in the failing heart, due to a reduction in parasympathetic drive.[77]

There is obviously overlap between the two major subdivisions of myocardial function. Recent data indicate that even in the absence of adrenergic stimulation, β-adrenergic receptors have intrinsic activity.[78–81] That is, a small number of receptors are in an activated state without agonist occupancy and as such can support intrinsic myocardial function.[79,80] Thus overexpression of human β_2-adrenergic receptors is able to markedly increase intrinsic myocardial function,[80] as is enhancement of sarcoplasmic reticulum calcium uptake and release by genetic ablation of the phospholamban gene.[82] The recent realization that active state, agonist-unoccupied β-adrenergic receptors can modulate intrinsic myocardial function is the reason why the "R-G-adenylyl cyclase" mechanism appears in both categories in Table 66-3.

Progressive Myocardial Dysfunction and Remodeling due to Loss of Cardiac Myocytes

The second general mechanism by which myocardial function may be adversely affected is by loss of cardiac myocytes, which also may play a role in the progression of ventricular dysfunction in dilated cardiomyopathies. Cardiac myocyte loss can occur via toxic mechanisms producing necrosis or by "programmed cell death" producing apoptosis. Apoptosis, which is likely due to a combination of growth signaling and cell cycle dysregulation, has been described in end-stage IDC,[83] as well as in the β_1-adrenergic receptor,[25] the $G\alpha_s$ overexpressor transgenic mice,[28] and in models of hypertrophy.[84] However, the human hearts with IDC or ischemic cardiomyopathy were taken from very late stage, literally dying patients maintained on multiple powerful intravenous inotropic medications,[83] and it is not clear if apoptosis plays a significant role in remodeling and/or chamber systolic dysfunction until this point in the natural history of the dilated cardiomyopathies.

IMPORTANCE OF "COMPENSATORY" MECHANISMS IN THE PROGRESSION OF MYOCARDIAL FAILURE

As depicted in Figs. 66-1 and 66-2, there is now a large body of information supporting the idea that *activation of the ANS and RAS compensatory mechanisms contributes to, or is responsible for, the progressive nature of both myocardial failure and the natural history of the heart failure clinical syndrome.*[6] This evidence includes the observations that activation of both these systems is associated with progression of myocardial dysfunction and the heart failure syndrome and clinical trial data that consistently demonstrate that inhibition of these systems can prevent deterioration in or improve myocardial function as well as reduce mortality.[6,10] Despite the fact that in human heart failure

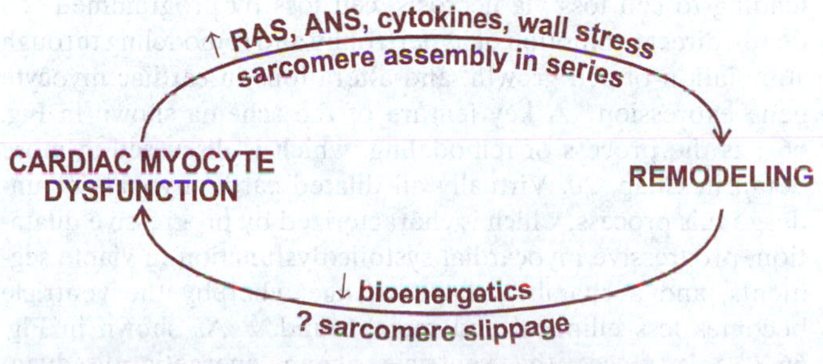

FIGURE 66-3 Relationship between progressive myocardial dysfunction and remodeling. RAS = renin angiotensin system; ANS = adrenergic nervous system.

we now know that chronic activation of the ANS and RAS contributes to the progressive nature of myocardial dysfunction, we know virtually nothing about how these systems adversely affect the biology of the cardiac myocyte. What we do know is that mechanisms within both general categories outlined in Table 66-3 must be involved in the adverse myocardial effects mediated by the ANS and RAS. This is so because modulated function may be improved by treatment with ACE inhibitors or β-blocking agents. Progressive myocardial dysfunction and remodeling are attenuated by both β-blocking agents and ACE inhibitors, and in cardiomyopathies, intrinsic myocardial function is improved and remodeling is reversed by chronic treatment with β-blocking agents.[6] Additionally, mortality in chronic heart failure is directly related to activation of the ANS[85,86] and RAS[87] and may be related to activation of other neurohormonal or autocrine/paracrine systems as well.

Regardless of the type or cause of dilated cardiomyopathy, an initial myocardial insult resulting in this phenotype exhibits common pathophysiologic features that are summarized in Fig. 66-1. That is, a myocardial insult that produces systolic dysfunction will be followed by the initiation of processes designed to temporarily stabilize pump function. The possible mechanisms available for such stabilization are in fact limited. As shown in Fig. 66-2, in chronological order of their action, they are an increase in heart rate and contractility mediated by an increase in cardiac β-adrenergic signaling (produced within seconds of the onset of pump dysfunction), volume expansion in order to use the Frank-Starling mechanism to increase stroke volume (evident within hours of the onset of pump dysfunction), and cardiac myocyte hypertrophy to increase the number of contractile elements (evident within days to weeks of the onset of pump dysfunction). As shown in Fig. 66-2, these compensatory adjustments are largely accomplished by activation of the RAS and ANS. However, despite the short-term (days to months) stability achieved via these mechanisms, they ultimately prove harmful.[6] The best evidence that chronic, continued activation of the RAS and ANS contributes to progressive myocardial dysfunction and remodeling comes from clinical trials where both inhibitors of the RAS (ACE inhibitors) and ANS (β-adrenergic receptor–blocking agents) prevent these two phenomena, and β-blocking agents actually may reverse remodeling and progressive systolic dysfunction,[6] as alluded to.

Much current work is focused on the precise pathophysiologic mechanisms by which activation of the RAS and ANS produces remodeling and adverse effects on myocardial function. Some of the possibilities are given in Fig. 66-1, and they include an exacerbation of ischemia and/or energy depletion leading to cell loss via necrosis, cell loss by programmed cell death, direct promotion of hypertrophy and remodeling through stimulation of cell growth, and alterations in cardiac myocyte gene expression.[6] A key feature of the schema shown in Fig. 66-1 is the process of remodeling, which is discussed in more detail in Chap. 20. Virtually all dilated cardiomyopathies undergo this process, which is characterized by progressive dilatation, progressive myocardial systolic dysfunction in viable segments, and a chamber shape change whereby the ventricle becomes less elliptical and more round.[6,63] As shown in Fig. 66-3, this places the ventricle at an energetic disadvantage,[6,63,74] which likely contributes to further myocardial dysfunction, which then contributes to progressive remodeling. The latter observation is based on data obtained with β-adrenergic blocking agents, which produce an improvement in systolic dysfunction that can be detected prior to a reversal in remodeling.[6] As emphasized by Fig. 66-3, each myocardial degenerative process likely begets the other, leading to an inexorably progressive deterioration in myocardial performance and clinical condition.

SCOPE OF DILATED CARDIOMYOPATHIES

The number of cardiac or systemic processes that can produce or are associated with a dilated cardiomyopathy are plentiful and remarkably varied, as shown in Table 66-4. The dilated phenotype is by far the most common form of cardiomyopathy, comprising over 90 percent of subjects referred to specialized centers.[88] In the United States, the most common dilated cardiomyopathy is ischemic dilated cardiomyopathy,[1] or the cardiomyopathy that follows MI. Other common secondary dilated cardiomyopathies are hypertensive and valvular dilated cardiomyopathies, both produced in part by chronically increased wall stress. The primary cardiomyopathy, IDC, is another relatively common dilated phenotype,[89,90] as discussed below.

SELECTED, COMMON TYPES OF DILATED CARDIOMYOPATHIES

Ischemic Cardiomyopathy

DEFINITION/DIAGNOSIS

Ischemic cardiomyopathy is defined as a dilated cardiomyopathy in a subject with a history of MI or evidence of clinically significant (i.e., ≥70 percent narrowing of a major epicardial artery) coronary artery disease, in whom the degree of myocardial dysfunction and ventricular dilatation is not explained solely by the extent of previous infarction or the degree of ongoing ischemia.[3] In other words, *an ischemic dilated cardiomyopathy is present when a post-MI left ventricle experiences remodeling and a drop in ejection fraction.*

DISTINCT PATHOPHYSIOLOGY

Dilatation of the left ventricle and a decrease in ejection fraction occurs in 15 to 40 percent of subjects within 12 to 24 months following an anterior MI[91,92] and in a smaller percentage of subjects following an inferior MI.[92] Based on limited data,[43] it is tempting to speculate that the subjects who undergo the remodeling process and develop an ischemic dilated cardiomyopathy are individuals with particularly heightened compensatory mechanisms (see Figs. 66-1 and 66-2), perhaps as a result in polymorphic variation in these systems.[16] As discussed earlier, the remodeling process is an attempt by the compromised ventricle to increase its performance by increasing stroke volume, but ultimately, it correlates with an adverse outcome[6,63] in the long term.

The gross pathology of ischemic cardiomyopathy includes transmural or subendocardial scarring, representing old MIs, that may comprise up to 50 percent of the LV chamber. The histopathology of the noninfarcted regions is similar to changes that occur in IDC,[71] as discussed below.

PROGNOSIS

Several studies have concluded that ischemic cardiomyopathy patients have a worse prognosis than subjects with a "non-

TABLE 66-4 Types of Dilated Cardiomyopathies

Ischemic insult (ischemic cardiomyopathy)	
Valvular disease (mitral regurgitation, aortic regurgitation, aortic stenosis) (valvular cardiomyopathy)	
Chronic hypertension (hypertensive cardiomyopathy)	
Tachyarrhythmias (supraventricular, ventricular, atrial flutter)	
Familial (autosomal dominant, X-linked)	
Idiopathic	
Toxins	
	Ethanol
	Chemotherapeutic agents (anthracyclines such as doxorubicin and daunorubicin)
	Cobalt
	Antiretroviral agents (zidovudine, didanosine, zalcitabine)
	Phenothiazines
	Carbon monoxide
	Lithium
	Lead
	Cocaine
	Mercury
Metabolic abnormalities	
	Nutritional deficiencies (thiamine, selenium, carnitine, protein)
	Endocrinologic disorders (hypothyroidism, acromegaly, thyrotoxicosis, Cushing's disease, pheochromocytoma, catecholamines, diabetes mellitus)
	Electrolyte disturbances (hypocalcemia, hypophosphatemia)
Infectious	
	Viral (coxsackie virus, cytomegalovirus, HIV)
	Rickettsial
	Bacterial
	Mycobacterial
	Spirochetal
	Fungal
	Parasitic (toxoplasmosis, trichinosis, Chagas' disease)
Systemic disorders	
	Systemic lupus erythematosis
	Juvenile rheumatoid arthritis
	Polyarteritis nodosa
	Kawasaki disease
	Collagen vascular disorders (scleroderma, lupus erythematosus, dermatomyositis)
	Hemochromatosis
	Amyloidosis
	Sarcoidosis
	Pseudoxanthoma elasticum
	Hypereosinophilic syndrome
Hypersensitivity myocarditis	
Peri/postpartum dysfunction	
Arrhythmogenic right ventricular dysplasia or cardiomyopathy	
Infantile histiocytoid	
Neuromuscular dystrophies	
	Becker or Duchenne's muscular dystrophy, X-linked cardioskeletal myopathy
Facioscapulohumoral muscular dystrophy	
Erb's limb-girdle dystrophy	
Myotonic dystrophy	
Friedreich's ataxia	
Emery-Dreifuss muscular dystrophy	
Inborn errors of metabolism	
Mitochondrial cardiomyopathies	
Keshan cardiomyopathy	

ischemic" dilated cardiomyopathy,[93,94] probably because the risk of ischemic events is added to the risk of having a dilated cardiomyopathy.

TREATMENT

The treatment of ischemic dilated cardiomyopathy and chronic heart failure is covered in detail in Chap. 21. In general, treatment consists of the use of ACE inhibitors in asymptomatic or symptomatic patients, the use of diuretics in volume-overloaded subjects, and the use of digoxin in subjects who remain symptomatic on the former medications. An emerging treatment strategy is the use of β-adrenergic blocking agents in mild to moderately symptomatic subjects,[6,10] whereas in both ischemic and nonischemic dilated cardiomyopathies,[9,10,95–97] second- and third-generation compounds improve LV function,[6,9–11] reduce hospitalizations,[9,10,95–97] and lower mortality.[9,10] Additionally, adjunctive therapy includes anticoagulation in subjects with lower LV ejection fractions to prevent thromboembolic complications, amiodarone to treat symptomatic arrhythmias, maintaining potassium levels in the high normal (4.3–5.0 meq/L) range to prevent sudden death, frequent clinic visits to adjust medications, and an aggressive approach to treating ischemia, including revascularization.

Hypertensive Cardiomyopathy

DEFINITION/DIAGNOSIS

A *hypertensive dilated cardiomyopathy* is diagnosed when myocardial systolic function is depressed out of proportion to the increase in wall stress. In other words, a subject presenting in heart failure with a hypertensive crisis would not carry this diagnosis unless ventricular dilatation and depressed systolic function remained after correction of the hypertension. In addition to producing a "pure" form of hypertensive cardiomyopathy, hypertension is a major risk factor for heart failure from any cause.[98] Within the WHO/ISFC classification, "hypertensive heart disease" may present in the "dilated," "restrictive," or "unclassified" categories.

DISTINCT PATHOPHYSIOLOGY

The most important pathophysiologic element in hypertension in dilated cardiomyopathy is sustained increased systolic wall stress. Interestingly, in both systolic pressure overloaded right and left ventricles, phenotypic expression is qualitatively variable[99,100] and can include dilatation and systolic dysfunction without increased wall thickness, increased wall thickness, concentric hypertrophy with or without systolic dysfunction, and systolic dysfunction without concentric hypertrophy. Other contributors to the pathophysiology of hypertensive cardiomyopathies are local neurohormonal mechanisms.[101]

PROGNOSIS

The prognosis depends on the presence of other comorbid conditions such as diabetes mellitus and coronary artery disease, as well as the extent of control of afterload. Compared with other forms of cardiomyopathy, in the absence of comorbid conditions, the prognosis of hypertensive cardiomyopathy in subjects whose afterload is controlled is probably better than for most other types of dilated cardiomyopathy.[102]

TREATMENT

The treatment is as for ischemic dilated cardiomyopathy, except that afterload must be vigorously controlled.[101] This consists of the addition of pure antihypertensive vasodilators such as amlodipine or α-blocking agents to standard heart failure therapy.

Valvular Cardiomyopathy

DEFINITION/DIAGNOSIS

A *valvular cardiomyopathy* occurs when a valvular abnormality is present and myocardial systolic function is depressed out of proportion to the increase in wall stress. This most commonly occurs with left-sided regurgitant lesions (mitral regurgitation and aortic regurgitation), less commonly occurs with aortic stenosis, and never occurs as a consequence of pure mitral stenosis.

DISTINCT PATHOPHYSIOLOGY

The classic explanation for the typical phenotypes observed in valvular cardiomyopathies relates to exposure to different types of wall stress.[103] Within this construct, the pattern of eccentric hypertrophy derives from increased diastolic wall stress.[103] Thus long-standing mitral regurgitation most commonly results in compensated eccentric hypertrophy that can progress to a dilated failing phenotype. Aortic regurgitation is a particularly poorly tolerated hemodynamic insult because wall stress is increased in both systole and diastole,[103] and when decompensation occurs, ventricular volume will be increased with or without increased wall thickness. Aortic stenosis classically results in compensated concentric hypertrophy, but when decompensation occurs, a variety of phenotypes can be observed that are similar to hypertensive cardiomyopathies. A disturbing and fairly commonly observed phenomenon is the development of a dilated cardiomyopathy after surgical correction of mitral and sometimes aortic valve disease in subjects who preoperatively had only mild LV dysfunction. These cases are likely due to the superimposition of myocardial damage resulting from open heart surgery and/or underlying dysfunction that was likely greater than appreciated preoperatively.

PROGNOSIS

The prognosis is variable and depends on the number of associated conditions, the nature and extent of the valvular abnormality, and most important, the severity of the cardiomyopathy at the time of surgical correction (see below). In general, *severely depressed myocardial function will not improve much with surgical repair of aortic regurgitation or mitral regurgitation, but the prognosis is likely to be improved because of elimination of some of the hemodynamic insult.* Replacement of the mitral valve should not be attempted in the majority of subjects with severe mitral regurgitation and LV ejection fractions less than 25 percent because of prohibitively high operative/perioperative mortality rates. On the other hand, there is no impairment of LV systolic function severe enough to preclude valve replacement of severe aortic stenosis, since function invariably will improve on relief of the hemodynamic insult, and the prognosis is relatively good.

TREATMENT

The treatment of a valvular dilated cardiomyopathy is surgical valve replacement or repair as soon as the cardiomyopathy is detected. Catheter valvuloplasty may be an option for severe aortic stenosis (AS) patients who are not good surgical candidates for reasons other than heart failure.[104] Medical treatment may be the only option in subjects with aortic insufficiency or mitral regurgitation whose LV function is severely impaired. The medical treatment of either disorder should be as mentioned earlier for ischemic cardiomyopathy plus aggressive afterload reduction, usually hydralazine/nitrates on top of ACE inhibitors. The calcium channel blocker amlodipine is another option for afterload reduction,[105] particularly for aortic insufficiency, where calcium channel blocker therapy has been shown to improve survival.[106]

Idiopathic Dilated Cardiomyopathy, Including Familial Forms

DEFINITION/DIAGNOSIS

IDC is diagnosed by excluding significant coronary artery disease, valvular abnormalities, and other causes. IDC is a relatively common cause of heart failure, with an estimated prevalence rate of 0.04 percent[89] and incidence rates varying from 0.005 to 0.006 percent.[89,90] The true incidence of IDC is undoubtedly higher, owing to the fact that subjects may remain asymptomatic until marked ventricular dysfunction has occurred. The incidence of IDC increases with age, and males are afflicted at a higher rate than are females.[89] As discussed below, histologic features are nonspecific and consist of myocardial cell hypertrophy and varying amounts of increased interstitial fibrosis. Although the diagnosis is not difficult, problems arise when an apparent IDC presents in someone with a history of hypertension or excessive alcohol intake. In such cases, it is best to reassign the etiology to alcohol only when the intake has exceeded 80 g/day for males and 40 g/day for females for more than 5 years and to hypertensive heart disease when blood pressure has been uncontrolled and high (>160/100 mmHg), as well as sustained (for years). All subjects with an unexplained dilated cardiomyopathy need a thyroid-stimulating hormone (TSH) determination done to exclude hypo- or hyperthyroidism, and subjects with diastolic dysfunction need to have an infiltrative process excluded. As discussed below, this is best done by performing an endomyocardial biopsy.

DISTINCT PATHOPHYSIOLOGY

IDC may be familial in as many as 35 to 50 percent of the patients when first-degree relatives are carefully screened.[107,108] The analysis of the phenotype identifies a wide range of clinical and pathologic forms indicating genetic heterogeneity. Accordingly, several chromosomal assignments for gene location have been made, and recently, as shown in Table 66-2, several genes have been identified.[34–39,109–118] The majority of familial patients present with autosomal dominant inheritance and a phenotype characterized by low and age-related penetrance (which is the proportion of carriers who manifest the disease). It is estimated that only 20 percent of gene carriers under the age of 20 display the disease phenotype.[119] Autosomal dominant dilated cardiomyopathy can be due to mutations of the cardiac actin[34] or desmin gene,[35] but in the majority of cases the disease gene is still unknown. The detection of an altered creatine kinase level can indicate the existence of a subclinical skeletal muscle disease. In these patients, an X-linked inheritance suggests mutations in the dystrophin gene,[36,37,120–122] whereas an autosomal dominant transmission and the presence of conduction defects and arrhythmia suggests mutations in the lamin A/C gene.[38,39] In *laminopathy,* the phenotype of the affected relatives can be very variable, from a pure IDC to a mild Emery-Dreifuss-like or limb-girdle-like muscle dystrophy[39] (see Chap. 62). Skeletal muscle and endomyocardial biopsy are diagnostic in X-linked dilated cardiomyopathy, showing abnormalities of dystrophin protein expression by immunocytochemistry.[123,124] Finally, autosomal recessive transmission of dilated cardiomyopathy occurs in mutations of sarcoglycan genes, which encode for dystrophin complex–associated proteins.[125]

Dystrophin, sarcoglycans, desmin, and lamin are cytoskeletal proteins. The contractile protein cardiac α-actin also has a force-transmission or cytoskeletal role.[34] Other data support the hypothesis that IDC could represent, in the majority of cases, a disease of the cytoskeleton; absence of the protein metavinculin in the myocardium was reported in one IDC patient,[70] and as discussed earlier, a dilated cardiomyopathy can be created in mice[22] or is present in a hamster line[126] related to mutations in cytoskeletal genes. However, as discussed earlier, it appears that other genetic abnormalities such as mutations in contractile proteins[14,21,34,127,128] and overexpression of β-adrenergic receptors[25–27] or $G\alpha_s$[24] also can produce a dilated phenotype.

In children, X-linked familial IDC suggests mutation in the G4.5 or tafazzin gene, particularly if associated with certain other signs (such as endocardial fibroelastosis, neutropenia, short stature, or skeletal muscle abnormalities).[116] The function of tafazzin is still unknown. In mitochondrial DNA (mtDNA) mutations, myocardial dysfunction usually is associated with multiorgan involvement (encephalopathy, lactic acidosis, skeletal muscle abnormalities, retinitis pigmentosa, etc.).[129] It is still unclear whether a mtDNA mutation can lead to an isolated IDC phenotype in adults.

Although still incomplete, new knowledge on the genetics of IDC has important clinical implications. The frequency of familial forms indicates the need of family screening in IDC, which can allow genetic counseling, an early detection of the disease, and early therapeutic interventions in affected relatives. The complexity of the phenotype requires an accurate skeletal muscle investigation, which can direct the diagnosis toward a specific type of familial myopathy. Finally, family investigations require more sensitive diagnostic criteria[130] that are able to detect minor cardiac abnormalities as initial signs of the disease. These include initial dilatation without marked systolic dysfunction, arrhythmia, and isolated wall and other abnormalities.[39,108,131]

The major morphologic feature of IDC on postmortem examination is dilatation of the cardiac chambers.[130,131] One ventricle (usually the left) may be more dilated than the other ventricle. The weight of the heart is increased in IDC, with a mean cardiac weight of 551 g for women and 632 g for men.[131] Although there is an increase in muscle mass and myocyte cell volume in IDC, LV wall thickness is usually not increased because of the marked dilatation of the ventricular cavities. Grossly visible scars may be present in either ventricle, and while most scars are small, some may be large and transmural. Scarring occurs in the absence of significant narrowing of the epicardial coronary arteries. In most cases, the degree of fibrosis does not appear to be extensive enough to cause changes in systolic or diastolic function. Intracardiac thrombi and mural endocardial plaques (from the organization of thrombi) are present at necropsy in more than 50 percent of patients with IDC.[132,133] The effect of anticoagulation on the incidence of thrombi has not been studied carefully, but systemic and pulmonary emboli are more frequent in patients with ventricular thrombi or plaques.[134]

The characteristic findings of IDC on microscopy are marked myocyte hypertrophy, very large, bizarrely shaped nuclei[135–137] (Fig. 66-4), increased interstitial fibrosis (see Fig. 66-4), myocyte atrophy, and myofilament loss.[133,138] In isolated cardiac myocytes, the major cellular phenotypic change is marked increase in cell length without a concomitant increase in diameter.[72] As described earlier, this cellular lengthening or remodeling contributes to the chamber remodeling/dilatation that characterizes IDC and other cardiomyopathies. These morphologic changes in IDC are not specific and are generally found in secondary cardiomyopathies such as in the noninfarcted regions of ischemic dilated cardiomyopathy.[71] Also, the morphometric changes in IDC do not correlate with the severity of illness.[137,138] Ultrastructural abnormalities such as mitochondrial changes, T-tubular dilatation, and intracellular lipid droplets may be observed in IDC but also can be observed in other forms of heart disease.[137] There may be interstitial parenchymal and perivascular focal infiltrates of small lymphocytes.[136–140] The lymphocytic infiltrates that are present on histologic examination in IDC are not associated with adjacent myocyte damage, in contrast to myocarditis where adjacent myocyte necrosis is observed. Fibrosis is nearly always present in IDC,[136–140] and its pattern is quite variable from a fine perimyocytic distribution to coarse scars indistinguishable from those present in chronic ischemia. However, small intramural arteries and capillaries are structurally normal in IDC.[137]

A number of immune regulatory abnormalities have been identified in IDC, including humoral and cellular autoimmune reactivity against myocytes,[141] decreased natural killer cell activity,[142] and abnormal suppressor cell activity.[143,144] These abnormalities suggest that immune defects may be important etiologic factors in the development of IDC. These findings, however, are not universally present in patients with IDC, and some abnormalities are also present in other types of heart muscle disease. For example, an increase in the cardioselective M7 antimitochondrial antibodies is found in both IDC and hypertrophic cardiomyopathy but not in heart failure from coronary artery disease.[145] The incidence of some autoreactive antibodies, such as antinuclear and antifibrillary antibodies, increases with the severity of heart failure.[146] It is likely that many of the antibodies detected in IDC and other myocardial diseases do not have pathogenic relevance, but rather are secondary to the primary degenerative process. However, it is possible that certain antibodies present in IDC may have important functional implications. For example, anti-β_1-adrenergic receptor antibodies[147,148] could modify β-adrenergic receptor activity[149] and produce chronic increases in signal transduction that are harmful to the failing heart. Disturbed energy metabolism from antibodies to the ADP/ATP carrier of the inner mitochondrial membrane is another potential pathogenetic autoimmune mechanism[150,151]; these antibodies are present in some individuals with IDC[150] and have been shown to impair metabolism and myocardial function.[151]

There has been great interest in histocompatibility locus antigens (HLAs) in IDC because these antigens are known to be associated with immune regulatory functions, and many autoimmune diseases are found to have positive HLA antigenic associations. HLA associations also have been identified in IDC; the frequency of HLA-B27, HLA-A2, HLA-DR4, and HLA-DQ4 is increased compared with controls, and the frequency of HLA-DRw6 is decreased compared with controls.[152] Genetic abnormalities in the HLA region potentially could alter immune response and thereby increase disease susceptibility to infectious agents such as enteroviruses. Thus the association in IDC with specific HLAs suggest a possible immunologic etiology for this disease. However, these specific HLAs are present in less than 50 percent of patients with IDC, and the heterogeneity of these antigens does not point to a unique site for a putative disease-associated gene. Thus, while the autoimmune hypothesis is an attractive candidate for the etiology of some cases of IDC, it remains unproved.

A clinical and pathologic syndrome that is similar to IDC may develop after resolution of viral myocarditis in animal models and biopsy-proven myocarditis in human subjects.[153] This has led to speculation that IDC may develop in some individuals as a result of subclinical viral myocarditis. Theoretically, an episode of myocarditis could initiate a number of autoimmune reactions that injure the myocardium and ultimately result in the development of IDC. The

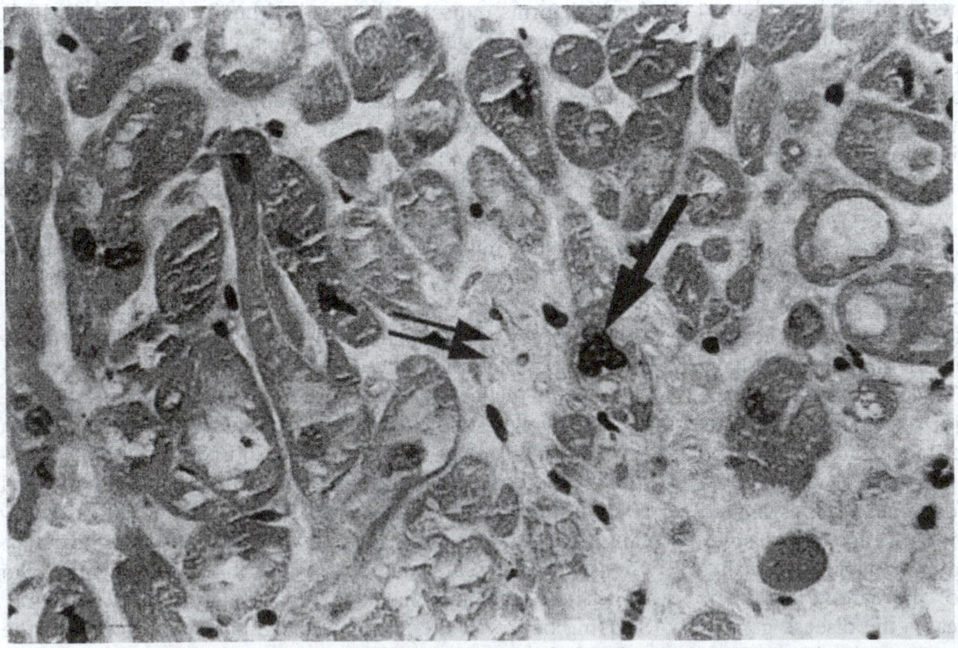

FIGURE 66-4 Right ventricular endomyocardial biopsy from a subject with IDC. Note the increased nuclear size (*arrow*) and the increased interstitial fibrosis.

abnormalities in immune regulation and the variety of antimyocardial antibodies present in IDC are consistent with this hypothesis. However, it is generally not possible to isolate an infectious virus or to demonstrate the presence of viral antigens in the myocardium of patients with IDC.[153,154] Enteroviral RNA sequences are found in heart biopsy samples in IDC, but only in approximately one-third of patients.[154–156] Furthermore, active myocardial inflammation is usually not detected in IDC.[139,140] However, in controlled trials, corticosteroid therapy of patients with IDC does not result in significant clinical improvements.[157] Importantly, recent experimental data have shown in vitro and in vivo that the enteroviral protease 2A is able to cleave dystrophin and disrupt the cytoskeleton in cardiac myocytes, providing a potential link between viral infection and a genetic model of the disease.[158] Furthermore, analysis of human viruses other than enteroviruses suggests that adenoviruses, herpesvirus, and cytomegalovirus also can cause myocarditis and potentially IDC, particularly in children and young subjects.[159,160] Further investigation will be necessary to understand the significance of these findings, particularly in the adult population.

As also discussed in Chap. 22, endomyocardial biopsy of the right or left ventricle may be a valuable diagnostic adjunct for diagnosing specific myocardial processes that can produce a dilated phenotype, such as myocarditis and infiltrative cardiomyopathies. Since several of these other dilated cardiomyopathies may have specific treatments and/or a different prognosis than IDC, endomyocardial biopsy may be warranted in many individuals presenting with a dilated cardiomyopathy. In the future, biopsy may be used more frequently to identify genetic disorders resulting in abnormal gene or protein expression,[50] such as now can be done to diagnose Becker-Duchenne cardiomyopathy.[123,124] Since special staining, electron microscopy, or molecular analysis of the biopsy material may be necessary, endomyocardial biopsy is best performed in specialized cardiomyopathy/heart failure centers.

PROGNOSIS

Several studies of the natural history of IDC have been conducted.[159,160] The prognosis is generally better than for ischemic cardiomyopathy,[93,94] and prior to the routine use of ACE inhibitors, survival was approximately 50 percent in 5 years.[161] The prognosis has been improved substantially since then,[162] inasmuch as ACE inhibition,[163] cardiac transplantation[164] and β-adrenergic blockade[10] are all effective treatments in this cardiomyopathy.

TREATMENT

The treatment of IDC is similar to that discussed earlier for ischemic cardiomyopathy, except that there is no issue of revascularization. The risk of thromboembolic complications may be higher than in ischemic cardiomyopathy, resulting in a lower threshhold for anticoagulation. β-Adrenergic blockade produces a quantitatively greater degree of improvement in LV function compared with ischemic cardiomyopathy[165,166] either because there is a greater degree of adrenergic activation[8] or there is more viable myocardium to work with in IDC. Approximately 10 percent of IDC subjects treated with β-adrenergic blockade will normalize their myocardial function, and this form of treatment should be offered to all IDC patients who do not have a contraindication before considering cardiac transplantation.[167]

SELECTED SPECIFIC DILATED CARDIOMYOPATHIES WITH UNIQUE MANAGEMENT ISSUES

Anthracycline Cardiomyopathy

DEFINITION/DIAGNOSIS

The commonly used and highly efficacious anthracycline antibiotic anticancer agents doxorubicin and daunorubicin produce a dose-related cardiomyopathy[168–173] that may limit their clinical application. Within the WHO/ISFC classification, an anthracycline cardiomyopathy would most likely be in the "dilated" category, but because the extent of dilatation initially may be minimal (see below), it also could be in the "unclassified" category. The cardiomyopathy produced by these agents depends on the total cumulative dose, and for the more widely used compound doxorubicin (Adriamycin), the incidence of heart failure due to cardiomyopathy dramatically increases above total cumulative doses of 450 mg/m^2 in subjects without underlying cardiac problems or other risk factors.[169] *Prior mediastinal radiation involving the heart is a powerful risk factor for anthracycline cardiomyopathy,*[170] *and the risk is also evident if radiation treatment follows chemotherapy.*[172,173] In subjects with risk factors, anthracycline cardiomyopathy can present at lower cumulative doses than 450 mg/m^2.[170–172]

Although the diagnosis of anthracycline cardiomyopathy can be made clinically, the definitive diagnosis depends on the demonstration of a substantial number of cardiac myocytes exhibiting the characteristic anthracycline effect.[168,170–173] Tissue sampling is best done by endomyocardial biopsy, which allows for "thin section" electron microscopic processing of the sample and more definitive resolution of the anthracycline effect with light microscopy.[168,170–173]

DISTINCT PATHOPHYSIOLOGY

In the absence of a tissue diagnosis, anthracycline cardiomyopathy may be diagnosed clinically by exclusion of other causes of cardiomyopathy in a subject who has had at least 350 mg/m^2 of doxorubicin or the equivalent amount of another anthracycline. As shown in Fig. 66-5, the anthracycline cardiac myocytic lesion consists of cell vacuolization progressing to cell dropout, and when 16 to 25 percent of the total number of sampled cells exhibit this morphology, myocardial dysfunction results.[170]

There are some distinguishing clinical features of anthracycline cardiomyopathy that may relate to its pathophysiology. These include a relative absence of hypertrophy and dilatation and a higher heart rate (110–130 beats per minute) than is usually encountered in ambulatory heart failure. The reasons for these features are that the onset of symptoms may be relatively acute (remodeling takes time to develop), and the anthracycline inhibits contractile protein synthesis,[174] reducing the amount of compensatory dilatation and remodeling. In this situation, the only option available for stabilizing cardiac output is increasing the heart rate, since increasing stroke volume via a larger end-diastolic volume has been precluded. The increased heart rate is produced by a greater than expected hyperadrener-

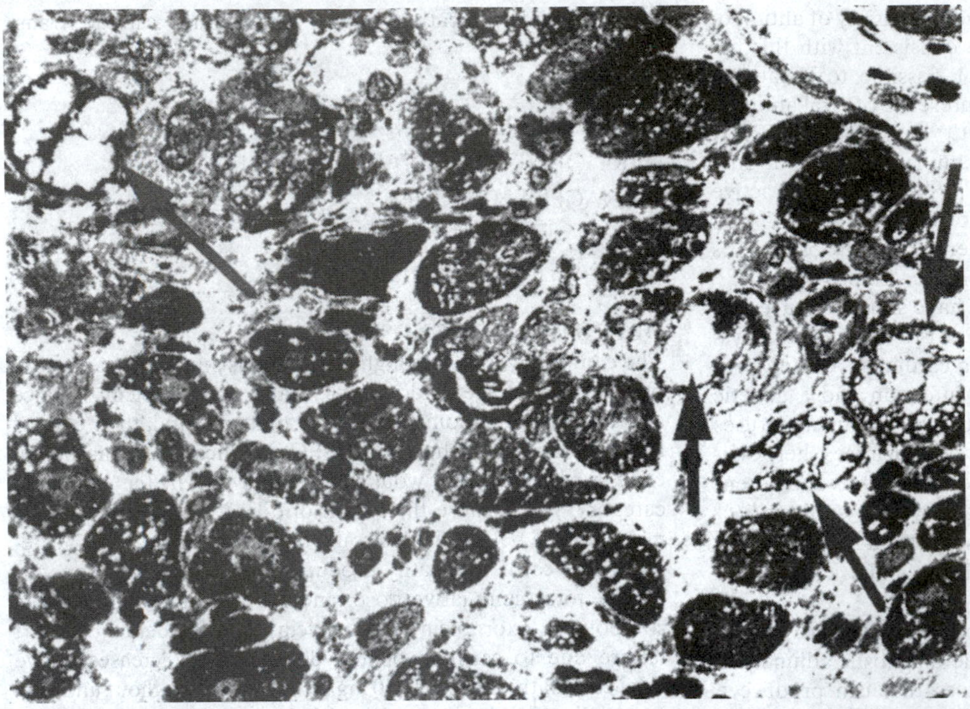

FIGURE 66-5 Cardiac myocyte vacuolization in cases of Adriamycin cardiomyopathy classified on endomyocardial biopsy as grade 3 by the Billingham classification.[170,171,178]

gic state, and so these subjects may be exceptionally dependent on adrenergic support.

PROGNOSIS

The prognosis of anthracycline cardiomyopathy is variable and depends on numerous factors, including the age and underlying prechemotherapy cardiac status of the patient and the time of presentation relative to the last dose of drug. Subjects who present late (several months) or very late (years) after the last dose have a better prognosis because the anthracycline myocardial effect takes at least 60 days to become fully manifest.[175] That is, subjects who develop heart failure within a few days of the last dose of drug have an additional cardiomyopathic burden to face, since the last one to two doses produce their full morphologic effect over the next 1 to 2 months.

TREATMENT/PREVENTION

Subjects who develop anthracycline cardiomyopathy should be treated aggressively with conventional heart failure treatment, since some degree of reversibility is likely. Conventional treatment consists of ACE inhibitors, digoxin, and diuretics. β-Adrenergic blockade has been used successfully in some subjects,[176,177] but because of the high adrenergic drive, it may be difficult to administer. On the other hand, the heightened adrenergic mechanism may be producing a commensurate amount of adverse effect on the myocardium, and so the potential for a favorable response may be even greater than in other kinds of cardiomyopathy. In severe refractory cases, cardiac transplantation may be performed provided that the patient's cancer is in complete remission and is not likely to recur ($\approx$70 percent chance of cure).

Several strategies have been shown to lower the risk of developing anthracycline cardiomyopathy without compromising the chemotherapy response rate. These include using endomyocardial biopsy and right-sided heart catheterization with exercise to assess risk, which virtually eliminates clinical cardiomyopathy and allows more anthracycline to be administered to less susceptible subjects[178]; using serial radionuclide angiography with[179] or without[180] exercise as a monitoring strategy, which may be somewhat helpful but because of a low specificity reduces the total amount of chemotherapy that can be administered safely to some subjects[178,179]; giving the agents as low-dose weekly[181] or as 48- to 72-h infusions[182] rather than as every 3- to 4-week boluses; using a liposomal formulation[183]; or concomitantly administering a second agent that reduces toxicity.[184] Unfortunately, none of these strategies completely eliminates the risk of developing a clinical cardiomyopathy.

Postpartum Cardiomyopathy

DEFINITION/DIAGNOSIS

Postpartum or *peripartum cardiomyopathy* is defined as the presentation of systolic dysfunction and clinical heart failure during the last trimester of pregnancy or within 6 months of delivery.[185] Given the extreme hemodynamic load produced by pregnancy, it is perhaps surprising that postpartum cardiomyopathy is not more common.

DISTINCT PATHOPHYSIOLOGY

Postpartum cardiomyopathy most likely will be classified within the "dilated" WHO/ISFC category but occasionally will be "unclassified" because dilatation and remodeling have not had time to occur. Postpartum cardiomyopathy is likely a heterogeneous group of disorders consisting of the addition of the hemodynamic load of pregnancy to a variety of underlying myocardial processes, including hypertensive heart disease, familial or idiopathic dilated cardiomyopathy, and myocarditis.[185,186]

PROGNOSIS

Approximately half of subjects who develop postpartum cardiomyopathy will recover completely,[187] and the majority of the rest will improve. Subjects who have developed a postpartum cardiomyopathy should never become pregnant again, even if myocardial function has recovered fully.

TREATMENT

Treatment should be aggressive and as for IDC. Cardiac transplantation may be required in severely compromised patients who do not improve.

Amyloid Cardiomyopathy

DEFINITION/DIAGNOSIS

As discussed in Chap. 68, amyloidosis is a group of diseases characterized by extracellular deposition of proteins characterized by their unique β-pleated sheet conformation and recognized electron microscopically as randomly arranged nonbranching fibers ranging from 8 to 14 nm in length. Amyloidosis is classified according to the type of amyloid protein involved.[188] Amyloidosis involving the heart is not rare and accounts for up to 10 percent of all nonischemic cardiomyopathies in autopsy studies.[189,190]

Amyloid cardiomyopathy may present in the WHO/ISFC "restrictive," "dilated," or "unclassified" categories. Most commonly it presents as a restrictive cardiomyopathy with conduction system abnormalities. In the setting of systemic amyloidosis (secondary or primary forms), the presence of increased wall thickness on echocardiogram plus low electrocardiographic voltage is highly suggestive of cardiac involvement.[191] In primary systemic amyloidosis, a monoclonal immunoglobulin spike is detectable in urine or serum in approximately 80 percent of subjects.[192] The definitive diagnosis of amyloid cardiomyopathy is made by tissue examination, ideally premortem by endomyocardial biopsy.[191] In systemic forms, the tissue diagnosis may be made by rectal, skin, or tongue biopsy of any abnormal tissue in these locations coupled with an unexplained myocardial process. As shown in Fig. 66-6, the characteristic histologic signature of amyloid is extracellular deposition of a fibrillar protein with a characteristic periodicity on electron microscopy.[193] Although a Congo Red stain can identify most cases, electron microscopy is more sensitive and specific and should be used routinely when amyloid is suspected.

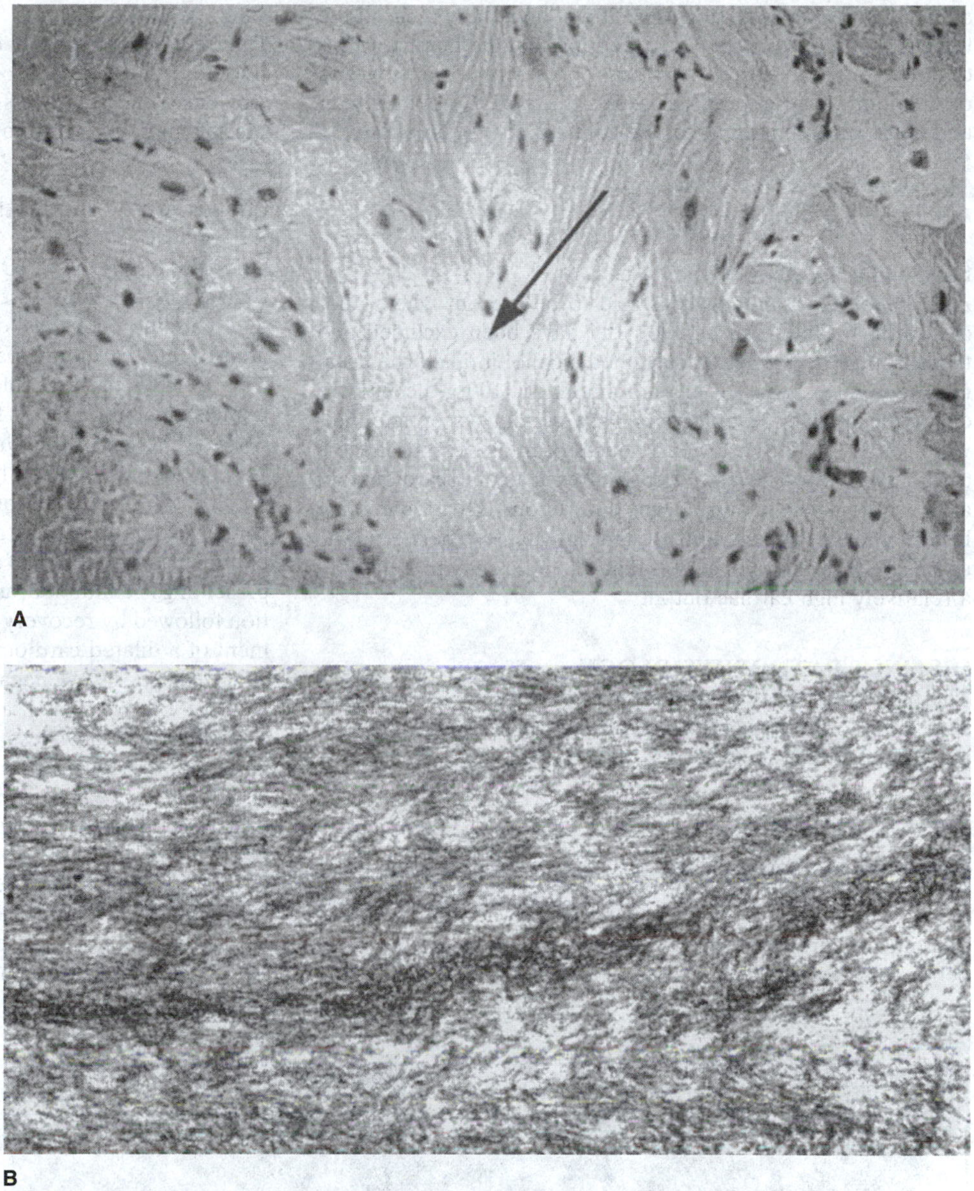

FIGURE 66-6 *A.* Right ventricular biopsy demonstrating interstitial amyloid deposition (H&E stain, ×100). *B.* Electron micrograph of the same biopsy specimen illustrating the characteristic 8- to 14-nm, nonbranching, randomly oriented amyloid fibrils.

DISTINCT PATHOPHYSIOLOGY

Although the source and chemical nature of amyloid protein differs among the various types of amyloidosis, the tissue/organ pathophysiology is the same, i.e., the slow destruction of the heart by the inexorable deposition of a β-pleated sheet fibril that is insoluble and impervious to proteolytic digestion.[190]

PROGNOSIS

The prognosis is uniformly bad regardless of the type of amyloidosis, and the majority of patients with amyloid cardiomyopathy are dead within 2 years of diagnosis.

TREATMENT

There is no definitive treatment of amyloid cardiomyopathy. Treatment is completely empirical and consists of diuretics when needed, pacemaker treatment of bradyarrhythmias, and the avoidance of digoxin, which may be arrhythmogenic in any infiltrative cardiomyopathy. There is limited evidence that chemotherapy directed at amyloid secretion by abnormal β-lymphocytes can produce favorable effects in some patients.[194] Cardiac transplantation should be avoided even in primary localized amyloid cardiomyopathy because it will invariably recur in the heart or in other organs. The exception may be familial forms of amyloidosis, where the abnormal protein is a transthyretin or prealbumin variant synthesized in the liver. Combined liver and heart transplantation can be curative in this situation.[195]

Alcohol Cardiomyopathy

DEFINITION/DIAGNOSIS

An *alcohol cardiomyopathy* is said to be present when other causes of a dilated cardiomyopathy have been excluded and there is a history of heavy, sustained alcohol intake. The usual requirement in terms of alcohol amount is 100 g alcohol per day, typically over several years. However, in susceptible individuals it is likely that lower amounts of intake can produce a cardiomyopathy. The histologic features of alcohol cardiomyopathy are nonspecific and do not differ from IDC. Other than history, the only potentially distinguishing feature between IDC and alcohol cardiomyopathy is that the latter may present with a relatively high cardiac output.

DISTINCT PATHOPHYSIOLOGY

The pathophysiology of alcohol cardiomyopathy is thought to be related to the toxic effects of alcohol, plus in some subjects nutritional components such as thiamine deficiency.

PROGNOSIS

The prognosis depends on the degree of impairment of myocardial function and the extent of abstinence from alcohol and, in an extremely compromised patient, the administration of thiamine. There is evidence that the prognosis is somewhat better for alcohol cardiomyopathy than for IDC.[196]

TREATMENT

The treatment of alcohol cardiomyopathy does not differ from IDC, except the inclusion of total abstinence from alcohol. Obviously, these subjects are not good candidates for cardiac transplantation because of the high relapse rate to alcoholism.

Chagas' Cardiomyopathy

DEFINITION/DIAGNOSIS

Chagas' disease is discussed in Chap. 69 as a cause of myocarditis. In addition, Chagas' disease is the most common cause of nonischemic cardiomyopathy in South and Central America, with over 10 million people afflicted.[197] It is caused by a parasite, the leishmanial or tissue form of the protozoan *Trypanosoma cruzi.* Although in the United States the vector (*Triatoma,* or kissing bug) is found only in the Southwest, Chagas' disease may be transmitted by blood transfusions, and as a result, it could become relatively more important in this country. The natural history consists of an initial myocarditis most commonly presenting in childhood, associated with acute myocardial infection followed by recovery and in some individuals the development of a dilated cardiomyopathy 10 to 30 years later.

The diagnosis of Chagas' cardiomyopathy is based on clinical (history, LV functional, and electrocardiographic) criteria and a positive serologic test for *T. cruzi.*[198] Electrocardiographic abnormalities consist of bundle-branch or hemiblocks (indeed, hemiblocks were first described by Rosenbaum et al.[199] in Chagas' afflicted hearts with discrete foci of involvement), LV hypertrophy, and first- or second-degree atrioventricular (AV) block.[200] The histologic lesion of chronic Chagas' consists of mononuclear infiltrates, fibrosis, and as shown in Fig. 66-7, foci of the leishmanial form of *T. cruzi* in myocardial fibers. The LV functional abnormalities initially may be segmental and may include an apical aneurysm but later become more global.[198,200]

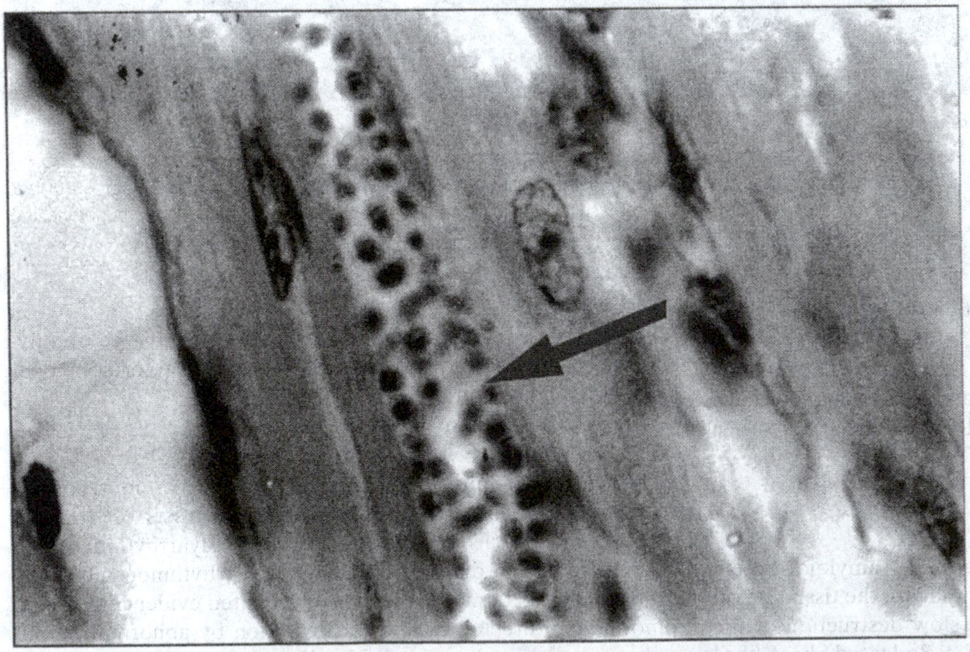

FIGURE 66-7 Leishmanial forms of *T. cruzi* within the swollen cytoplasm of a cardiac myocyte (Chagas' cardiomyopathy) (H&E stain, ×250). (Courtesy Dr. Elmer Koneman.)

DISTINCT PATHOPHYSIOLOGY

The basis for Chagas' cardiomyopathy is unknown but may be immunologic, whereby antibodies generated against *T. cruzi* cross-react with cardiac myocyte antigens including myosin.[201]

PROGNOSIS

The prognosis is relatively good for a dilated cardiomyopathy and similar to IDC; the 5-year survival in Chagas' cardiomyopathy with heart failure is around 50 percent.[198] Compared with IDC, death likely occurs more commonly due to an arrhythmic mechanism.[198] However, as for IDC and most other dilated cardiomyopathies, mortality risk depends directly on the degrees of ventricular dysfunction and exercise intolerance.[198]

TREATMENT

There is no definitive treatment for Chagas' cardiomyopathy, and nonspecific treatment includes pacemaker implantation for heart block and heart failure treatment as for IDC. The one exception may be the more frequent use of amiodarone, which appears to be particularly effective in treating arrhythmias associated with Chagas' cardiomyopathy and in one study reduced mortality compared with standard treatment.[202] The role of cardiac transplantation is still somewhat uncertain, but it can be done at acceptable risk,[203] especially when coupled with trypanocidal agents.[204]

SUMMARY

Dilated cardiomyopathies are important because they are the most common cause of heart failure, which is the single most costly medical problem in the adult U.S. population. Cardiomyopathies in general are a heterogeneous group of diseases, but they can be classified under a newly modified WHO/ISFC classification system, which, although imperfect, should be of great value in standardizing the terminology and encouraging systematic investigative and clinical approaches to diagnosis and treatment. Within this classification system, primary and secondary dilated cardiomyopathies comprise the single largest and most important group. Current diagnosis and treatment of dilated cardiomyopathies vary somewhat among the various types, but the cornerstones of medical management are similar in most cases.

Genetic causes and influences on the natural history of dilated cardiomyopathies are the new frontier in this field, and their elucidation is almost certain to lead to new therapeutic and diagnostic approaches. In the near future, molecular genetic testing will be done routinely for many cardiomyopathies that may have a single gene defect as the cause. As we learn more about the influence of polymorphic genetic variation on the natural history and selection of specific medical therapy, genetic testing will be performed in most patients with cardiomyopathies.

References

1. Ho KKL, Anderson KM, Kannel WB, et al. Survival after the onset of congestive heart failure in Framingham Heart Study subjects. *Circulation* 1993; 88:107–115.
2. O'Connell JB, Bristow MR. Economic impact of heart failure in the United States: Time for a different approach. *J Heart Lung Transplant* 1994; 13:S107–S112.
3. Richardson P, McKenna W, Bristow MR, et al. Report of the 1995 World Health Organization/International Society and Federation of Cardiology Task Force on the definition and classification of cardiomyopathies. *Circulation* 1996; 93:841–842.
4. Guccione AA, Felson DT, Anderson JJ, et al. The effects of specific medical conditions on the functional limitations of elders in the Framingham Study. *Am J Public Health* 1994; 84:351–358.
5. Cohn JN, Johnson GR, Shabetai R, et al, for the V-HeFT VA Cooperative Studies Group. Ejection fraction, peak exercise oxygen consumption, cardiothoracic ratio, ventricular arrhythmias, and plasma norepinephrine as determinants of prognosis in heart failure. *Circulation* 1993; 87(suppl VI):VI-5–VI-16.
6. Eichhorn EJ, Bristow MR. Medical therapy can improve the biologic properties of the chronically failing heart: A new era in the treatment of heart failure. *Circulation* 1996; 94:2285–2296.
7. WHO/ISFC Task Force on Cardiomyopathies. Report of the WHO/ISFC Task Force on the definition and classification of cardiomyopathies. *Br Heart J* 1980; 44:672–673.
8. Bristow MR, Anderson FL, Port JD, et al. Differences in β-adrenergic neuroeffector mechanisms in ischemic vs idiopathic dilated cardiomyopathy. *Circulation* 1991; 84:1024–1039.
9. Packer M, Bristow MR, Cohn JN, et al. Effect of carvedilol on morbidity and mortality in patients with chronic heart failure. *N Engl J Med* 1996; 334:1349–1355.
10. Bristow MR. β-Adrenergic receptor blockade in chronic heart failure. *Circulation* 2000; 101:558–569.
11. Bristow MR. Why does the myocardium fail? New insights from basic science. *Lancet* 1998; 352(suppl):8–14.
12. Geisterfer-Lawrence AA, Kass S, Tanigawa G, et al. A molecular basis for familial hypertrophic cardiomyopathy: A beta-cardiac myosin heavy chain missense mutation. *Cell* 1990; 62:999–1006.
13. Geisterfer-Lawrence AA, Christe M, Conner DA, et al. A mouse model of familial hypertrophic cardiomyopathy. *Science* 1996; 272:731–735.
14. Vikstrom KL, Factor SM, Leinwand LA. Mice expressing mutant myosin heavy chains are a model for familial hypertrophic cardiomyopathy. *Mol Med* 1996; 2:556–567.
15. Tiret L, Rigat B, Visvikis S, et al. Evidence, from combined segregation and linkage analysis, that a variant of the angiotensin I-converting enzyme (ACE) gene controls plasma ACE levels. *Am J Hum Genet* 1992; 51(1):197–205.
16. Raynolds MV, Bristow MR, Bush E, et al. Angiotensin-converting enzyme DD genotype in patients with ischæmic or idiopathic dilated cardiomyopathy. *Lancet* 1993; 342:1073–1075.
17. Jeunemaitre X, Charru A, Rigat B, et al. Sib-pair linkage analysis of renin gene haplotypes in human essential hypertension. *Hum Genet* 1992; 88:301–306.
18. Bonnardeaux A, Davies E, Jeunemaitre X, et al. Angiotensin II type 1 receptor gene polymorphisms in human essential hypertension. *Hypertension* 1994; 24:63–69.
19. Jeunemaitre X, Soubrier F, Kotelevtsev Y, et al. Molecular basis of human hypertension: Role of angiotensinogen. *Cell* 1992; 71:169–180.
20. Robbins, J. Gene targeting and animal models of cardiovascular disease. *Circ Res* 1993; 73:3–9.
21. Edwards JG, Lyons GE, Micales BK, et al. Cardiomyopathy in transgenic *myf*5 mice. *Circ Res* 1996; 78:379–387.
22. Arber S, Hunter JJ, Ross J Jr, et al. MLP-deficient mice exhibit a disruption of cardiac cytoarchitectural organization, dilated cardiomyopathy, and heart failure. *Cell* 1997; 88:393–403.
23. Iwase M, Bishop SP, Uechi M, et al. Adverse effects of chronic endogenous sympathetic drive induced by cardiac $G_{s\alpha}$ overexpression. *Circ Res* 1996; 78:517–524.
24. Iwase M, Uechi M, Vatner DE, et al. Dilated cardiomyopathy induced by cardiac Gs-alpha overexpression (abstract). *Circulation* 1996; 94:I-16.
25. Bisognano JD, Wenberger HD, Bohlmeyer TJ, et al. Myocardial-directed overexpression of the human beta1-adrenergic receptor in transgenic mice. *J Mol Cell Cardiol* 2000; 32:817–830.
26. Engelhardt S, Hein L, Wiesman F, Lohse MJ. Progressive hypertrophy and heart failure in β_1-adrenergic receptor transgenic mice. *Proc Natl Acad Sci USA* 1999; 96:7059–7064.
27. Liggett SB, Tepe NM, Lorenz JN, et al. Early and delayed consequences of β_2-adrenergic receptor overexpression in mouse hearts: Critical role for expression level. *Circulation* 2000; 101:1707–1714.
28. Geng Y-J, Ishikawa Y, Vatner DE, et al. Apoptosis of cardiac myocytes in $G_{s\alpha}$ transgenic mice. *Circ Res* 1999; 84(1):34–42.
29. Hunter JJ, Tanaka N, Rockman HA, et al. Ventricular expression of a MLC-2v-*ras* fusion gene induces cardiac hypertrophy and selective diastolic dysfunction in transgenic mice. *J Biol Chem* 1995; 270:23173–23178.
30. Robbins RJ, Swain JL. C-*myc* protooncogene modulates cardiac

hypertrophic growth in transgenic mice. *Am J Physiol* 1992; 62:H590–H597.
31. Milano CA, Dolber PC, Rockman HA, et al. Myocardial expression of a constitutively active α_{1B}-adrenergic receptor in transgenic mice induces cardiac hypertrophy. *Proc Natl Acad Sci USA* 1994; 91:10109–10113.
32. D'Angelo DD, Sakatra Y, Lorenz JN, et al. Transgenic Gαq overexpression induces cardiac contractile failure in mice. *Proc Natl Acad Sci USA* 1997; 94:8121–8126.
33. Wakasaki H, Koya D, Schoen FJ, et al. Targeted overexpression of protein kinase Cβ2 isoform in myocardium causes cardiomyopathy. *Proc Natl Acad Sci USA* 1997; 94(17):9320–9325.
34. Olson TM, Michels VV, Thibodeau SN, et al. Actin mutation in dilated cardiomyopathy, a heritable form of heart failure. *Science* 1998; 280:750–752.
35. Li D, Tapscoft T, Gonzalez O, et al. Desmin mutation responsible for idiopathic dilated cardiomyopathy. *Circulation* 1999; 100: 461–464.
36. Towbin JA, Hejtmancik F, Brink P, et al. X-linked cardiomyopathy (XLCM): Molecular genetic evidence of linkage to the Duchenne muscular dystrophy (dystrophin) gene at the Xp21 locus. *Circulation* 1993; 87:1854–1865.
37. Muntoni F, Cau M, Ganau A, et al. Deletion of the dystrophin muscle-promoter region associated with X-linked dilated cardiomyopathy. *N Engl J Med* 1993; 329:921–925.
38. Fatkin D. Missense mutations in the rod domain of the lamin A/C gene as causes of dilated cardiomyopathy and conduction system disease. *N Engl J Med* 1999; 341:1715–1724.
39. Brodsky GL, Muntoni F, Miocic S, et al. A lamin a/c gene mutation associated with dilated cardiomyopathy with skeletal muscle involvement. *Circulation* 2000; 101:1394–1399.
40. Lander ES, Schork NJ. Genetic dissection of complex traits. *Science* 1994; 265:2037–2048.
41. Jan Danser AH, Maarten ADH, Schalekamp MD, et al. Angiotensin-converting enzyme in the human heart: Effect of the deletion/insertion polymorphism. *Circulation* 1995; 92:1387–1388.
42. Lechin M, Quinones MA, Omran A, et al. Angiotensin I converting enzyme genotypes and left ventricular hypertrophy in patients with hypertrophic cardiomyopathy. *Circulation* 1995; 92:1808–1812.
43. Pinto YM, van Gilst WH, Kingma JH, Schunkert H, for the Captopril and Thrombolysis Study Investigators. Deletion-type allele of the angiotensin-converting enzyme gene is associated with progressive ventricular dilatation after anterior myocardial infarction. *J Am Coll Cardiol* 1995; 25:1622–1626.
44. Andersson B, Sylven C. The DD genotype of the angiotensin-converting enzyme gene is associated with increased mortality in idiopathic dilated cardiomyopathy. *J Am Coll Cardiol* 1996; 28:162–167.
45. Raynolds MV, Roden RL, Blain-Nelson P, et al. Association of genetic variants in the angiotensin II type 1 receptor and angiotensinogen with end-stage heart muscle disease. *J Am Coll Cardiol* 1996; 27A.
46. Liggett SB, Wagoner LE, Craft LL, et al. The Ile164 β_2-adrenergic receptor polymorphism adversely affects the outcome of congestive heart failure. *J Clin Invest* 1998; 102(8):1534–1539.
47. Lowes BD, Minobe WA, Abraham WT, et al. Changes in gene expression in the intact human heart: downregulation of α-myosin heavy chain in hypertrophied, failing ventricular myocardium. *J Clin Invest* 1997; 100:2315–2324.
48. Miyata S, Minobe WA, Bristow MR, Leinwand LA. Myosin isoform expression in the failing and non-failing human heart. *Circ Res* 2000; 86:386–390.
49. Mercadier JJ, Lompre AM, Duc P, et al. Altered sarcoplasmic reticulum Ca-ATPase gene expression in the human ventricle during end-stage heart failure. *J Clin Invest* 1990; 85:305–309.
50. Feldman AM, Ray PE, Silan CM, et al. Selective gene expression in failing human heart: Quantification of steady-state levels of messenger RNA in endomyocardial biopsies using the polymerase chain reaction. *Circulation* 1991; 83:1866–1872.
51. Studer R, Reinecke H, Muler B, et al. Increased angiotensin I converting enzyme gene expression in the failing human heart: Quantification by competitive RNA polymerase chain reaction. *J Clin Invest* 1994; 94:301–310.
52. Zisman LS, Asano K, Dutcher DL, et al. Differential regulation of cardiac angiotensin converting enzyme binding sites and AT1 receptor density in the failing human heart. *Circulation* 1998; 98:1735–1741.
53. Torre-Amione G, Kapadia S, Lee J, et al. Tumor necrosis factor-α and tumor necrosis factor receptors in the failing human heart. *Circulation* 1996; 93:704–711.
54. Zolk O, Quattek J, Sitzler G, et al. Expression of endothelin-1, endothelin-converting enzyme, and endothelin receptors in chronic heart failure. *Circulation* 1999; 99:2118–2123.
55. Ungerer M, Böhm M, Elce JS, et al. Altered expression of β-adrenergic receptor kinase and β_1-adrenergic receptors in the failing human heart. *Circulation* 1993; 87:454–463.
56. Davies CH, Davia K, Bennett JG, et al. Reduced contraction and altered frequency response of isolated ventricular myocytes from patients with heart failure. *Circulation* 1995; 92:2540–2549.
57. Bristow MR, Gilbert EM. Improvement in cardiac myocyte function by biologic effects of medical therapy: A new concept in the treatment of heart failure. *Eur Heart J* 1995; 16(suppl. F):20–31.
58. Ross J, Braunwald E. Studies on Starling's law of the heart: IX. The effects of impeding venous return on performance of the normal and failing ventricle. *Circulation* 1964; 30:719–727.
59. Schwinger RHG, Böhm M, Koch A, et al. The failing human heart is unable to use the Frank-Starling mechanism. *Circ Res* 1994; 74:959–969.
60. Holubarsch C, Thorsten R, Goldstein DJ, et al. Existence of the Frank-Starling mechanism in the failing human heart: Investigations on the organ, tissue, and sarcomere levels. *Circulation* 1996; 94:683–689.
61. Feldman MD, Gwathmey JK, Phillips P, et al. Reversal of the force-frequency relationship in working myocardium from patients with end-stage heart failure. *J Appl Cardiol* 1988; 3:273–283.
62. Muleiri LA, Hasenfuss G, Leavitt B, et al. Altered myocardial force-frequency relationship in the human heart failure. *Circulation* 1992; 85:1743–1750.
63. Cohn JN. Structural basis for heart failure: Ventricular remodeling and its pharmacological inhibition. *Circulation* 1995; 91:2504–2507.
64. Gerdes AM, Capasso JM. Structural remodeling and mechanical dysfunction of cardiac myocytes in heart failure. *J Mol Cell Cardiol* 1995; 27:849–856.
65. Nadal-Ginard B, Mahdavi V. Molecular basis of cardiac performance. *J Clin Invest* 1989; 84:1693–1700.
66. Hirzel HO, Tuchschmid CR, Schneider J, et al. Relationship between myosin isoenzyme composition, hemodynamics, and myocardial structure in various forms of human cardiac hypertrophy. *Circ Res* 1985; 57:729–740.
67. Anderson PAW, Malouf NN, Oakley A, et al. Troponin T isoform expression in humans: A comparison among normal and failing adult heart, fetal heart, and adult and fetal skeletal muscle. *Circ Res* 1991; 69:1226–1233.
68. Tsutsui H, Ishihara K, Cooper G IV. Cytoskeletal role in the contractile dysfunction of hypertrophied myocardium. *Science* 1993; 260:682–687.
69. Yoshida K, Ikeda S, Nakamura A, et al. Molecular analysis of the Duchenne muscular dystrophy gene in patients with Becker muscular dystrophy presenting with dilated cardiomyopathy. *Muscle Nerve* 1993; 16:1161–1166.
70. Maeda M, Holder E, Lowes B, et al. Dilated cardiomyopathy

associated with deficiency of the cytoskeletal protein metavinculin. *Circulation* 1997; 95(1):17–20.
71. Gerdes AM, Kellerman SE, Moore JA, et al. Structural remodeling of cardiac myocytes from patients with chronic ischemic heart disease. *Circulation* 1992; 86:426–430.
72. Gerdes AM, Kellerman SE, Schocken DD. Implications of cardiomyocyte remodeling in heart dysfunction. In: Dhalla NS, Beamish RE, Takeda N, Nagano N, eds. *The Failing Heart.* New York: Raven Press; 1995:197–205.
73. Gerdes AM, Odera T, Wang X, McCune SA. Myocyte remodeling during progression to failure in rats with hypertension. *Hypertension* 1996; 28(4):609–614.
74. Zhang J, McDonald KM. Bioenergetic consequences of left ventricular remodeling. *Circulation* 1995; 92:1011–1019.
75. Sata M, Sugiura S, Yamashita H, et al. Coupling between myosin ATPase cycle and creatine kinase cycle facilitates cardiac actomyosin sliding in vitro: A clue to mechanical dysfunction during myocardial ischemia. *Circulation* 1996; 93:310–317.
76. Cintron C, Johnson G, Francis G, et al. Prognostic significance of serial changes in left ventricular ejection fraction in patients with congestive heart failure. *Circulation* 1993; 87(suppl VI):VI-17–VI-23.
77. Binkley PF, Nunziata E, Haas GH, et al. Parasympathetic withdrawal is an integral component of autonomic imbalance in congestive heart failure: Demonstration in human subjects and verification in a paced canine model of ventricular failure. *J Am Coll Cardiol* 1991; 18:464–472.
78. Chidiac P, Hebert TE, Valiquette M, et al. Inverse agonist activity of β-adrenergic antagonists. *Mol Pharmacol* 1994; 45:490–499.
79. Mewes T, Dutz S, Ravens U, Jakobs KH. Activation of calcium currents in cardiac myocytes by empty β-adrenoceptors. *Circulation* 1993; 88:2916–2922.
80. Milano CA, Allen LF, Rockman HA, et al. Enhanced myocardial function in transgenic mice overexpressing the β_2-adrenergic receptor. *Science* 1994; 264:562–566.
81. Bond RA, Leff P, Johnson TD, et al. Physiological effects of inverse agonists in transgenic mice with myocardial overexpression of the β_2-adrenoceptor. *Nature* 1995; 374:272–276.
82. Luo W, Grupp IL, Harrer J, et al. Targeted ablation of the phospholamban gene is associated with markedly enhanced myocardial contractility and loss of β-agonist stimulation. *Circ Res* 1994; 75:401–409.
83. Narula J, Haider N, Virmani R, et al. Apoptosis in myocytes in end-stage heart failure. *N Engl J Med* 1996; 335:1182–1189.
84. Teiger E, Than VD, Richard L, et al. Apoptosis in pressure overload-induced heart hypertrophy in the rat. *J Clin Invest* 1996; 97:2891–2897.
85. Cohn JN, Levine TB, Olivari MT, et al. Plasma norepinephrine as a guide to prognosis in patients with chronic congestive heart failure. *N Engl J Med* 1984; 311:819–823.
86. Kaye DM, Lefkovits J, Jennings GL, et al. Adverse consequences of high sympathetic nervous activity in the failing human heart. *J Am Coll Cardiol* 1995; 26:1257–1263.
87. Swedberg K, Eneroth P, Kjekshus J, Wilhelmsen L. Hormones regulating cardiovascular function in patients with severe congestive heart failure and their relation to mortality. *Circulation* 1990; 82:1730–1736.
88. Bristow MR, O'Connell JB. Myocardial diseases. In: Kelley WN, ed. *Textbook of Internal Medicine,* 3d ed. Philadelphia: Lippincott; 1997:398–405.
89. Codd MB, Sugrue DD, Gersh BJ, Melton LJ. Epidemiology of idiopathic dilated and hypertrophic cardiomyopathy: A population based study in Olmstead County, MN, 1975–1984. *Circulation* 1989; 80:564–572.
90. Rakar S, Sinagra G, Di Lenarda A, et al. Epidemiology of dilated cardiomyopathy: A prospective post-mortem study of 5252 necropsies. *Eur Heart J* 1997; 18:117–123.
91. McKay RG, Pfeffer MA, Pasternak RC, et al. Left ventricular remodeling after myocardial infarction: A corollary to infarct expansion. *Circulation* 1986; 74:693–702.
92. Mitchell GF, Lamas GA, Vaughan DE, Pfeffer MA. Left ventricular remodeling in the year after myocardial infarction: A quantitative analysis of contractile segment lengths and ventricular shape. *J Am Coll Cardiol* 1992; 19:1136–1144.
93. Franciosa JA, Willen M, Ziesche S, Cohn JN. Survival in men with severe chronic left ventricular failure due to either coronary heart disease or idiopathic dilated cardiomyopathy. *Am J Cardiol* 1983; 51:831–836.
94. Likoff MJ, Chandler SL, Kay HR. Clinical determinants of mortality in chronic congestive heart failure secondary to idiopathic dilated or to ischemic cardiomyopathy. *Am J Cardiol* 1987; 59(6):634–638.
95. Bristow MR, Gilbert EM, Abraham WT, et al. Carvedilol produces dose-related improvements in left ventricular function and survival in subjects with chronic heart failure. *Circulation* 1996; 94:2807–2816.
96. MERIT-HF Study Group. Effect of metoprolol CR/XL in chronic heart failure: Metoprolol CR/XL Randomized Intervention Trial in Congestive Heart Failure (MERIT-HF). *Lancet* 1999; 353:2001–2006.
97. CIBIS-II Investigators and Committees. The cardiac insufficiency bisoprolol study II (CIBIS-II): A randomised trial. *Lancet* 1999; 353:9–13.
98. Levy D, Larson MG, Vasan RS, et al. The progression from hypertension to congestive heart failure. *JAMA* 1996; 275:1557–1562.
99. Quaife RA, Lynch D, Badesch DB, et al. Right ventricular phenotypic characteristics is subjects with primary pulmonary hypertension or idiopathic dilated cardiomyopathy. *J Cardiac Failure* 1999; 5:46–54.
100. Devereux RB, Roman MJ. Left ventricular hypertrophy in hypertension: Stimuli, patterns, and consequences. *Hypertens Res* 1999; 22(1):1–9.
101. Bristow MR. Mechanisms of development of heart failure in the hypertensive patient. *Cardiology* 1999; 92:3–6.
102. Nielsen I. The natural history of hypertensive heart disease as suggested by echocardiography. *Acta Med Scand Suppl* 1986; 714:165–169.
103. Grossman W. Cardiac hypertrophy: Useful adaptation or pathologic process? *Am J Med* 1980; 69:576–584.
104. Moreno PR, Jang IK, Block PC, Palacios IF. The role of percutaneous balloon valvuloplasty in patients with cardiogenic shock. *J Am Coll Cardiol* 1994; 23:1071–1075.
105. Packer M, O'Conner CM, Ghali JK, et al. Effect of Amlodipine on morbidity and mortality in severe chronic heart failure. *N Engl J Med* 1996; 335:1107–1114.
106. Scognamiglio R, Rahimtoola SH, Fasoli G, et al. Nifedipine in asymptomatic patients with severe aortic regurgitation and normal left ventricular function. *N Engl J Med* 1994; 331(11):689–694.
107. Grunig E, Tasman JA, Kucherer H, et al. Frequency and phenotypes of familial dilated cardiomyopathy. *J Am Coll Cardiol* 1998; 31:186–194.
108. Baig MK, Goldman JH, Caforio ALP, et al. Familial dilated cardiomyopathy: Cardiac abnormalities are common in asymptomatic relatives and may represent early disease. *J Am Coll Cardiol* 1998; 31:195–201.
109. Krajinovic M, Pinamonti B, Sinagra GF, et al. Linkage of familial idiopathic dilated cardiomyopathy to chromosome 9. *Am J Hum Genet* 1995; 57:846–852.
110. Durand J-B, Bachinski LL, Bieling LC, et al. Localization of a gene responsible for familial dilated cardiomyopathy to chromosome 1q32. *Circulation* 1995; 92:3387–3389.
111. Siu B, Niimura H, Osborne JA, et al. Familial dilated cardio-

myopathy locus maps to chromosome 2q31. *Circulation* 1999; 99:1022–1026.

112. Jung M, Poepping I, Perrot A, et al. Investigation of a family with autosomal dominant dilated cardiomyopathy defines a novel locus on chromosome 2q14-q22. *Am J Hum Genet* 1999; 65:1068–1077.
113. Bowles KL, Gajarski R, Porter P, et al. Gene mapping of familial autosomal dominant dilated cardiomyopathy to chromosome 10q21-23. *J Clin Invest* 1996; 98:1355–1360.
114. Kass S, MacRae C, Graber HL, et al. A gene defect that causes conduction system disease and dilated cardiomyopathy maps to chromosome 1p1-1q1. *Nature Genet* 1994; 7:546–551.
115. Olson TM, Keating MT. Mapping a cardiomyopathy locus to chromosome 3p22-p25. *J Clin Invest* 1996; 97:528–532.
116. D'Adamo P, Fassone L, Gedeon A, et al. The X-linked gene G4.5 is responsible for different infantile dilated cardiomyopathies. *Am J Hum Genet* 1997; 61:862–867.
117. van der Kooi AJ, van Meegen M, Ledderhof TM, et al. Genetic localization of a newly recognized autosomal dominat limb-girdle muscular dystrophy with cardiac involvement (LGMD1B) to chromosome 1q11-21. *Am J Hum Genet* 1997; 60:891–895.
118. Messina DN, Speer MC, Pericak-Vance MA, McNally EM. Linkage of familial dilated cardiomyopathy with conduction defect and muscular dystrophy to chromosome 6q23. *Am J Hum Genet* 1997; 61:909–917.
119. Mestroni L, Rocco C, Gregori D, et al. Familial dilated cardiomyopathy: Evidence for genetic and phenotypic heterogeneity. *J Am Coll Cardiol* 1999; 34:181–190.
120. Ortiz-Lopez R, Li M, Su J, et al. Evidence for a dystrophin missense mutation as a cause of X-linked dilated cardiomyopathy. *Circulation* 1997; 95:2434–2440.
121. Muntoni F, Di Lenarda A, Porcu M, et al. Dystrophin gene abnormalities in two patients with idiopathic dilated cardiomyopathy. *Heart* 1997; 78:608–612.
122. Milasin J, Muntoni F, Severini GM, et al. A point mutation in the 5′ splice site of the dystrophin gene first intron responsible for X-linked dilated cardiomyopathy. *Hum Mol Genet* 1996; 5:73–79.
123. Bies RD, Maeda M, Roberds SL, et al. A 5′ dystrophin duplication mutation causes membrane deficiency of alpha-dystroglyean in a family with X-linked cardiomyopathy. *J Mol Cell Cardiol* 1997; 29 (12):31175–31188.
124. Maeda M, Nakao S, Miyazato H, et al. Cardiac dystrophin abnormalities in Becker muscular dystrophy assessed by endomyocardial biopsy. *Am Heart J* 1995; 129:702–707.
125. Melacini P, Fanin M, Duggan DJ, et al. Heart involvement in muscular dystrophies due to sarcoglycan gene mutations. *Muscle Nerve* 1999; 22:473–479.
126. Nigro V, Okazaki Y, Belsito A, et al. Identification of the Syrian hamster cardiomyopathy gene. *Hum Mol Genet* 1997; 6:601–607.
127. Fatkin D, Christe ME, Aristizabal O, et al. Neonatal cardiomyopathy in mice homozygous for the Arg403Gln mutation in the alpha cardiac myosin heavy chain gene. *J Clin Invest* 1999; 103:147–153.
128. McConnell BK, Jones KA, Fatkin D, et al. Dilated cardiomyopathy in homozygous myosin-binding protein-C mutant mice. *J Clin Invest* 1999; 104:1235–1244.
129. Tiranti V, Jaksch M, Hofmann S, et al. Loss-of-function mutations of SURF-1 are specifically associated with Leigh syndrome with cytochrome c oxidase deficiency. *Ann Neurol* 1999; 46: 161–166.
130. Mestroni L, Maisch B, McKenna WJ, et al. Guidelines for the study of familial dilated cardiomyopathies. *Eur Heart J* 1999; 20:93–102.
131. Crispell KA, Wray A, Ni H, et al. Clinical profiles of four large pedigrees with familial dilated cardiomyopathy: Preliminary recommendations for clinical practice. *J Am Coll Cardiol* 1999; 34:837–847.
132. Silver MA. Anatomy of the failing heart in dilated cardiomyopathy. In: Engelmeier RS, O'Connell JB, eds. *Drug Therapy in Dilated Cardiomyopathy and Myocarditis*. New York: Marcel Dekker; 1988:1–12.
133. Roberts WC, Siegel RJ, McManus BM. Idiopathic dilated cardiomyopathy: Analysis of 152 necropsy patients. *Am J Cardiol* 1987; 60:1340–1355.
134. Falk RH, Foster E, Coats MH. Ventricular thrombi and thromboembolism in dilated cardiomyopathy: A prospective follow-up. *Am Heart J* 1992; 123:136–142.
135. Rowan R, Maesk MA, Billingham ME. Ultrastructural morphometric analysis of endomyocardial biopsies. *Am J Cardiovasc Pathol* 1988; 2:137–144.
136. Baandrup U, Olsen EG. Critical analysis of endomyocardial biopsies from patients suspected of having cardiomyopathy. *Br Heart J* 1981; 45:475–486.
137. Arbustini E, Pucci R, Pozzi R, et al. Ultrastructural changes in myocarditis and dilated cardiomyopathy. In: Baroldi G, Camerini F, Goodwin JF, eds. *Advances in Cardiomyopathies*. Berlin: Springer-Verlag; 1990:274–289.
138. Schwarz F, Mall G, Zebe H, et al. Determinants of survival in patients with congestive cardiomyopathy: Quantitative morphologic findings and left ventricular hemodynamics. *Circulation* 1984; 70:923–928.
139. Tazelaar HD, Billingham ME. Leukocytic infiltrates in idiopathic dilated cardiomyopathy. *Am J Surg Pathol* 1986; 10:405–412.
140. Hammond EH, Anderson JL, Menlove RL. Diagnostic and prognostic value of immunofluorescence and electron-microscopic findings in idiopathic dilated cardiomyopathy. In: Bavoldi G, Camerini F, Goodwin JF, eds. *Advances in Cardiomyopathies*, 1st ed. Berlin: Springer-Verlag; 1990:290–301.
141. Kawai C, Takatsu T. Clinical and experimental studies on cardiomyopathy. *N Engl J Med* 1975; 293:592–597.
142. Anderson JL, Carlquist JF, Hammond EH. Deficient natural killer cell activity in patients with idiopathic dilated cardiomyopathy. *Lancet* 1982; 2:1124–1127.
143. Fowles RE, Bieker CP, Stinson EB. Defective in vitro suppressor cell function in idiopathic congestive cardiomyopathy. *Circulation* 1979; 59:483–491.
144. Gerli R, Rambotti P, Spinozzi F, et al. Immunologic studies of peripheral blood from patients with idiopathic dilated cardiomyopathy. *Am Heart J* 1986; 112:350–355.
145. Klein R, Maisch B, Kochsiek K, Berg PA. Demonstration of organ specific antibodies against heart mitochondria (anti-M) in sera from patients with some forms of heart disease. *Clin Exp Immunol* 1984; 58:283–292.
146. Maisch B, Deeg P, Liebau G, Kichsiek K. Diagnostic relevance of humoral and cytotoxic immune reactions in primary and secondary dilated cardiomyopathy. *Am J Cardiol* 1983; 52:1071–1078.
147. Limas CJ, Goldenberg IF, Limas C. Autoantibodies against β-adrenoreceptors in human idiopathic dilated cardiomyopathy. *Circ Res* 1989; 64:97–103.
148. Magnusson Y, Marullo S, Hoyer S, et al. Mapping of a functional autoimmune epitope on the β_1-adrenergic receptor in patients with idiopathic dilated cardiomyopathy. *J Clin Invest* 1990; 86:1658–1663.
149. Magnusson Y, Wallukat G, Waagstein F, et al. Autoimmunity in idiopathic dilatated cardiomyopathy: Characterization of antibodies against the β_1-adrenoceptor with a positive chronotropic effect. *Circulation* 1994; 89:2760–2767.
150. Schultheiss H-P, Bolte HD. Immunological analysis of autoantibodies against the adenine nucleotide translocator in dilated cardiomyopathy. *J Mol Cell Cardiol* 1985; 17:603–617.
151. Schultheiss H-P. Disturbance of the myocardial energy metabolism in dilated cardiomyopathy due to autoimmunological mechanisms. *Circulation* 1993; 87(suppl IV):IV-43–IV-48.
152. Anderson JL, Carlquist JF, Lutz JR, et al. HLA A, B, and DR

typing in idiopathic dilated cardiomyopathy: A search for immune response function. *Am J Cardiol* 1984; 33:1326–1330.

153. Gilbert EM, Mason JW. Immunosuppressive therapy of myocarditis. In: Engelmeier RS, O'Connell JB, eds. *Drug Therapy in Dilated Cardiomyopathy and Myocarditis*. New York: Marcel Dekker; 1987:233–263.
154. Archard LC, Freeke CA, Richardson PJ, Olsen EGJ. Persistence of enterovirus RNA in dilated cardiomyopathy: A progression from myocarditis. In: Shultheiss H-P, ed. *New Concepts in Viral Heart Disease*. Berlin: Springer-Verlag; 1989:347–359.
155. Giacca M, Severini GM, Mestroni L, et al. Low frequency of detection by nested polymerase chain reaction of enterovirus ribonucleic acid in endomyocardial tissue of patients with idiopathic dilated cardiomyopathy. *J Am Coll Cardiol* 1994; 24:1033–1040.
156. Bowles NE, Richardson PJ, Olsen ECJ, Archard LC. Detection of Coxsackie-B virus specific RNA sequences in myocardial biopsy samples from patients with myocarditis and dilated cardiomyopathy. *Lancet* 1986; 1:1120–1128.
157. Parrillo JE, Cunnion RE, Epstein SE, et al. A prospective, randomized, controlled trial of prednisone for dilated cardiomyopathy. *N Engl J Med* 1989; 321:1061–1067.
158. Badorff C, Lee GH, Lamphear BJ, et al. Enteroviral protease 2A cleaves dystrophin: Evidence of cytoskeletal disruption in an acquired cardiomyopathy. *Nature Med* 1999; 5:320–326.
159. Pauschinger M, Doerner A, Kuehl U, et al. Enteroviral RNA replication in the myocardium of patients with left ventricular dysfunction and clinically suspected myocarditis. *Circulation* 1999; 99(7):889–895.
160. Martin AB, Webber S, Fricker FJ, et al. Acute myocarditis: Rapid diagnosis by PCR in children. *Circulation* 1994; 90(1):330–339.
161. Fuster V, Gersh BJ, Giuliani ER, et al. The natural history of idiopathic dilated cardiomyopathy. *Am J Cardiol* 1981; 47: 525–531.
162. Redfield MM, Gersh BJ, Bailey KR, et al. Natural history of idiopathic dilated cardiomyopathy: Effect of referral bias and secular trend. *J Am Coll Cardiol* 1993; 22:1921–1926.
163. The SOLVD Investigators. Effect of angiotensin converting enzyme inhibition with enalapril on survival in patients with reduced left ventricular ejection fraction and congestive heart failure: Results of the Treatment Trial of the Studies of Left Ventricular Dysfunction (SOLVD), a randomized double blind trial. *N Engl J Med* 1991; 325:293–302.
164. Hosenpud JD, Novick RJ, Bennett LE, et al. The Registry of the International Society for Heart and Lung Transplantation: Thirteenth official report (1996). *J Heart Lung Transplant* 1996; 15:655–674.
165. Woodley SL, Gilbert EM, Anderson JL, et al. β-Blockade with bucindolol in heart failure due to ischemic vs idiopathic dilated cardiomyopathy. *Circulation* 1991; 84:2426–2441.
166. Bristow MR, Colucci WS, Fowler MB, et al. Effect of carvedilol on survival and hospitalization in patients with ischemic or nonischemic cardiomyopathy (abstract). *Circulation* 1996; 94:I-338.
167. Waagstein F, Bristow MR, Swedberg K, et al. Beneficial effects of metoprolol in idiopathic dilated cardiomyopathy. *Lancet* 1993; 342:1441–1446.
168. Bristow MR, Mason JW, Billingham ME, Daniels JR. Doxorubicin cardiomyopathy: Evaluation by phonocardiography, endomyocardial biopsy, and cardiac catheterization. *Ann Intern Med* 1978; 88:168–175.
169. Von Hoff DD, Layard MW, Basa P, et al. Risk factors for doxorubicin-induced congestive heart failure. *Ann Intern Med* 1979; 91:710–717.
170. Bristow MR, Mason JW, Billingham ME, Daniels JR. Dose-effect and structure function relationships in doxorubicin cardiomyopathy. *Am Heart J* 1981; 102:709–718.
171. Bristow MR, Billingham ME, Mason JW, Daniels JR. The clinical spectrum of anthracycline antibiotic cardiotoxicity. *Cancer Treat Rep* 1978; 62:873–879.
172. Billingham ME, Bristow MR, Glatstein J, et al. Adriamycin cardiotoxicity: Endomyocardial biopsy evidence of enhancement by irradiation. *Am J Surg Pathol* 1977; 1:17–23.
173. Kantrowitz NE, Bristow MR. Cardiotoxicity of antitumor agents. *Prog Cardiovasc Dis* 1984; 27:195–200.
174. Lewis W, Kleinerman J, Puszkin S. Interaction of adriamycin in vitro with myofibrillar proteins. *Circ Res* 1982; 50:547–553.
175. Jaenke RS. Delayed and progressive myocardial lesions after Adriamycin administration in rabbits. *Cancer Res* 1976; 36:2958–2966.
176. Eiswirth CC, Bowden RE, Kazamias T, et al. Treatment of Adriamycin cardiomyopathy with metoprolol. *Circulation* 1986; 74(supp II):1236.
177. Shaddy RE, Olsen SL, Bristow MR, et al. Efficacy and safety of metoprolol in the treatment of doxorubicin-induced cardiomyopathy in pediatric patients. *Am Heart J* 1995; 129:197–199.
178. Bristow MR, Lopez MB, Mason JW, et al. Efficacy and cost of cardiac monitoring in patients receiving doxorubicin. *Cancer* 1982; 50(1):32–41.
179. McKillop JH, Bristow MR, Goris ML, et al. Sensitivity and specificity of radionuclide ejection fractions in doxorubicin cardiotoxicity. *Am Heart J* 1983; 105:1048–1056.
180. Alexander J, Dainiak N, Berger HJ, et al. Serial assessment of doxorubicin cardiotoxicity with quantitative radionuclide angiocardiography. *N Engl J Med* 1979; 300:278–283.
181. Torti FM, Bristow MR, Howes AE, et al. Endomyocardial biopsy evidence of reduced cardiotoxicity of doxorubicin delivered on a weekly schedule. *Ann Intern Med* 1983; 99:745–749.
182. Legha SS, Benjamin RS, Mackay B, et al. Reduction of doxorubicin cardiotoxicity by prolonged continuous intravenous infusion. *Ann Intern Med* 1982; 96:133–139.
183. Rahman A, More N, Schein PS. Doxorubicin-induced chronic cardiotoxicity and its prevention by liposomal administration. *Cancer Res* 1982; 42:1817–1825.
184. Speyer JL, Green MD, Kramer E, et al. Protective effect of the bispiperazinedione ICRF-187 against doxorubicin-induced cardiac toxicity in women with advanced breast cancer. *N Engl J Med* 1988; 319(12):745–752.
185. Julian DG, Szekely P. Peripartum cardiomyopathy. *Prog Cardiovasc Dis* 1985; 27:223–240.
186. Midei MG, DeMent SH, Feldman AM, et al. Peripartum myocarditis and cardiomyopathy. *Circulation* 1990; 81:922–928.
187. O'Connell JB, Costanzo-Nordin MR, Subramanian R, et al. Peripartum cardiomyopathy: Clinical, hemodynamic histologic and prognostic characteristics. *J Am Coll Cardiol* 1986; 8:52–56.
188. Jacobson DR, Busbaum JN. Genetic aspects of amyloidosis. *Adv Hum Genet* 1991; 20:69–75.
189. Kyle RA, Griepp PR. Amyloidosis (AL): Clinical and laboratory feature in 229 cases. *Mayo Clin Proc* 1983; 58:665–672.
190. Glenner GG. Amyloid deposits and amyloidosis. *N Engl J Med* 1980; 302:1283–1292.
191. Hamer JP, Janssen S, van Rijswik MH, Lie KI. Amyloid cardiomyopathy in systemic non-hereditary amyloidosis: Clinical, echocardiographic and electrocardiographic findings in 30 patients with AA and 24 patients with AL amyloidosis. *Eur Heart J* 1992; 13:623–627.
192. Stone MJ. Amyloidosis: A final common pathway for protein deposition in tissues. *Blood* 1990; 75:531–545.
193. Schroeder JS, Billingham ME, Rider AK. Cardiac amyloidosis: Diagnosis by transvenous endomyocardial biopsy. *Am J Med* 1975; 59:269–273.
194. Kyle RA, Gertz MA, Greipp PR, et al. A trial of three regimens for primary amyloidosis: Colchicine alone, melphalan and prednisone, and melphalan, prednisone, and colchicine. *N Engl J Med* 1997:336(17)1202–1207.

195. Holmgren G, Ericzon B-G, Groth C-G. Clinical improvement and amyloid regression after liver transplantation in hereditary transthyretin amyloidosis. *Lancet* 1993; 341:1113–1116.
196. Prazak P, Pfisterer M, Osswald S, et al. Differences of disease progression in congestive heart failure due to alcoholic as compared to idiopathic dilated cardiomyopathy. *Eur Heart J* 1996; 17(2):251–257.
197. World Health Organization Expert Committee Chagas' disease. *World Health Organ Tech Rep Ser* 1984; 697:50–55.
198. Mady C, Cardoso RHA, Barretto ACP, et al. Survival and predictors of survival in patients with congestive heart failure due to Chagas' cardiomyopathy. *Circulation* 1994; 90:3098–3102.
199. Rosenbaum MB. The hemiblocks: Diagnostic criteria and clinical significance. *Mod Concepts Cardiovasc Dis* 1970; 39:141–146.
200. Laranja FS, Dias E, Nobrega G, Miranda A. Chagas' disease: A clinical, epidemiological, and pathological study. *Circulation* 1956; 14:1035–1060.
201. Tibbetts RS, McCormick TS, Rowland EC, et al. Cardiac antigen-specific autoantibody production is associated with cardiomyopathy in *Trypanosoma cruzi*–infected mice. *J Immunol* 1994; 152(3):1493–1499.
202. Nul DR, Grancelli HO, Perrone SV, et al. Randomised trial of low-dose amiodarone in severe congestive heart failure. *Lancet* 1994; 344:493–498.
203. Bocchi EA, Bellotti G, Mocelin AO, et al. Heart Transplantation for chronic Chagas' heart disease. *Ann Thorac Surg* 1996; 61:1727–1733.
204. Blanche C, Aleksic I, Takkenberg JJM, et al. Heart transplantation for Chagas' cardiomyopathy. *Ann Thorac Surg* 1995; 60:1406–1409.

CHAPTER 67

HYPERTROPHIC CARDIOMYOPATHY

Barry J. Maron

Hypertrophic cardiomyopathy (HCM) is a genetically transmitted primary cardiac disease that has been of great interest to clinicians and laboratory scientists because of its particularly diverse clinical, morphologic, pathophysiologic, and molecular genetic manifestations.[1–22] Because of the broad and heterogeneous HCM disease spectrum as well as the relatively low prevalence in cardiologic practice, a measure of confusion and uncertainty has persisted regarding this condition.

HISTORICAL CONSIDERATIONS

There is some uncertainty regarding the first gross anatomic description of HCM. About 1900, French and German authors reported four patients at autopsy in whom striking hypertrophy involving the ventricular septum appeared to be responsible for obstruction to left ventricular ejection.[23,24] The first unequivocal description of HCM was the detailed pathologic report of Teare,[25] which stimulated widespread interest in this disease among cardiologists, pathologists, and surgeons. Teare described a condition in eight patients (seven of whom died suddenly) characterized by an asymmetric pattern of left ventricular wall thickening and nondilated ventricular cavities. The striking ventricular septal hypertrophy and bizarre arrangement of muscle bundles observed in these patients was initially thought to represent a benign tumor of the heart.

NOMENCLATURE AND PREVALENCE

Over the past 40 years, numerous studies have led to a dramatic evolution of our concepts concerning the clinical and pathologic spectrum of HCM; in the process, the disease has acquired a myriad of names[7] (Fig. 67-1). This multiplicity of descriptive terms largely reflects the enormous clinical, functional, and morphologic diversity of this disease. However, many of the terms that have been used to describe HCM are somewhat misleading by emphasizing the presence of left ventricular outflow obstruction at rest, a clinical feature that occurs in only a minority of HCM patients (about 20 to 25 percent).[1,3,5] The prevalence of HCM appears to be about 0.2 percent in the general population[26] and 1 percent in primary medical practice[27] based on identification of the disease phenotype with two-dimensional (2D) echocardiography. It is possible, however, that many individuals with HCM go undetected in the community because they manifest no or only mild symptoms and are not referred for echocardiographic studies.[28–31] Reports from a large number of diverse geographic areas suggest that HCM has extensive if not worldwide occurrence; there is also some evidence that the morphologic expression of the disease may differ in certain ethnic or racial groups (such as Japanese).[32–34]

DEFINITION AND CRITERIA FOR DIAGNOSIS

The clinical diagnosis of HCM is based on definition of the most characteristic morphologic feature of the disease—i.e., thickening of the left ventricular wall associated with a nondilated cavity in the absence of another cardiac or systemic disease capable of producing the magnitude of hypertrophy evident (e.g., systemic hypertension or aortic stenosis)[7] (Fig. 67-2). Because the nonobstructive form of HCM is predominant, the well-described clinical features of dynamic obstruction to left

Asymmetrical hypertrophic cardiomyopathy
Asymmetrical hypertrophy of the heart
Asymmetrical septal hypertrophy
Brock's disease
Diffuse muscular subaortic stenosis
Diffuse subvalvular aortic stenosis
Dynamic hypertrophic subaortic stenosis
Dynamic muscular subaortic stenosis
Familial hypertrophic cardiomyopathy
Familial hypertrophic subaortic stenosis
Familial muscular subaortic stenosis
Familial myocardial disease
Functional aortic stenosis
Functional hypertrophic subaortic stenosis
Functional obstructive cardiomyopathy
Functional obstruction of the left ventricle
Functional obstructive subvalvular aortic stenosis
Functional subaortic stenosis
Hereditary cardiovascular dysplasia
HYPERTROPHIC CARDIOMYOPATHY
Hypertrophic constrictive cardiomyopathy
Hypertrophic hyperkinetic cardiomyopathy
Hypertrophic infundibular aortic stenosis
Hypertrophic nonobstructive cardiomyopathy
Hypertrophic obstructive cardiomyopathy
Hypertrophic stenosing cardiomyopathy
Hypertrophic subaortic stenosis
Idiopathic hypertrophic cardiomyopathy
Idiopathic hypertrophic obstructive cardiomyopathy
Idiopathic hypertrophic subaortic stenosis
Idiopathic hypertrophic subvalvular stenosis
Idiopathic muscular hypertrophic subaortic stenosis
Idiopathic muscular stenosis of the left ventricle
Idiopathic myocardial hypertrophy
Idiopathic stenosis of the flushing chamber of the left ventricle
Idiopathic ventricular septal hypertrophy
Irregular hypertrophic cardiomyopathy
Left ventrical muscular stenosis
Low subvalvular aortic stenosis
Muscular aortic stenosis
Muscular hypertrophic stenosis of the left ventricle
Muscular stenosis of the left ventricle
Muscular subaortic stenosis
Muscular subvalvular aortic stenosis
Non-dilated cardiomyopathy
Nonobstructive hypertrophic cardiomyopathy
Obstructive cardiomyopathy
Obstructive hypertrophic aortic stenosis
Obstructive hypertrophic cardiomyopathy
Obstructive hypertrophic myocardiopathy
Obstructive myocardiopathy
Pseudoaortic stenosis
Stenosing hypertrophy of the left ventricle
Stenosis of the ejection chamber of the left ventricle
Subaortic hypertrophic stenosis
Subaortic idiopathic stenosis
Subaortic muscular stenosis
Subvalvular aortic stenosis of the muscular type
Teare's disease

FIGURE 67-1 The multitude of terms used to describe HCM.

ventricular outflow—such as systolic anterior motion of the mitral valve, partial premature closure of the aortic valve, and a loud systolic ejection murmur—are not required for diagnosis.[1] Also, not all individuals harboring a genetic abnormality capable of producing the clinical and morphologic abnormalities of HCM show left ventricular hypertrophy at all phases of life.[10,22,31,35–37] For example, some children with HCM will not have left ventricular wall thickening identifiable by 2D echocardiogram prior to about age 16[35] and a few adults with incomplete penetrance may also show little or no hypertrophy.[10,36,38–40]

MORPHOLOGIC CHARACTERISTICS

Gross Features

Left ventricular hypertrophy is the gross anatomic marker of HCM and the likely determinant of many of the clinical features identifiable in most patients with this disease[1–7,16–18] (Figs. 67-3 and 67-4). Since the left ventricular cavity is usually small or normal in size, the increased left ventricular mass is due almost entirely to an increase in wall thickness. Although a symmetric (concentric) pattern of left ventricular hypertrophy can be observed,[12,18,41] the distribution of hypertrophy is almost always asymmetric; i.e., with segments of the left ventricular wall thickened to a dissimilar degree, and with the ventricular septum showing disproportionate magnitude of hypertrophy.[12,18] Examination of the heart at necropsy also typically shows dilatation of the atria, enlargement and elongation of the mitral valve leaflets, and areas of replacement fibrosis (scarring) in the left ventricular wall.[16,17,20,42,43] In addition, most hearts show a characteristic fibrous plaque on the mural endocardium of the left ventricular outflow tract in apposition to the thickened anterior mitral leaflet, presumably resulting from systolic (or diastolic) contact between mitral valve and septum[16] (Fig. 67-3).

Based on both echocardiographic and necropsy analyses of large numbers of patients, it is apparent that the HCM disease spectrum is characterized by vast structural diversity with regard to the patterns and extent of left ventricular hypertrophy[12,18,41,43] (Figs. 67-5 and 67-6). Indeed, no single phenotypic expression can be considered "classic" or particularly typical of this disease. While maximal thickness of the left ventricular wall varies greatly, the average value in a population is usually 21 to 22 mm. Wall thickness is markedly increased in many patients, with some showing the most severe hypertrophy observed in any cardiac disease (60 mm is the most extreme dimension).[44,45] On the other hand, the HCM phenotype is not always expressed as a particularly thickened left ventricle;

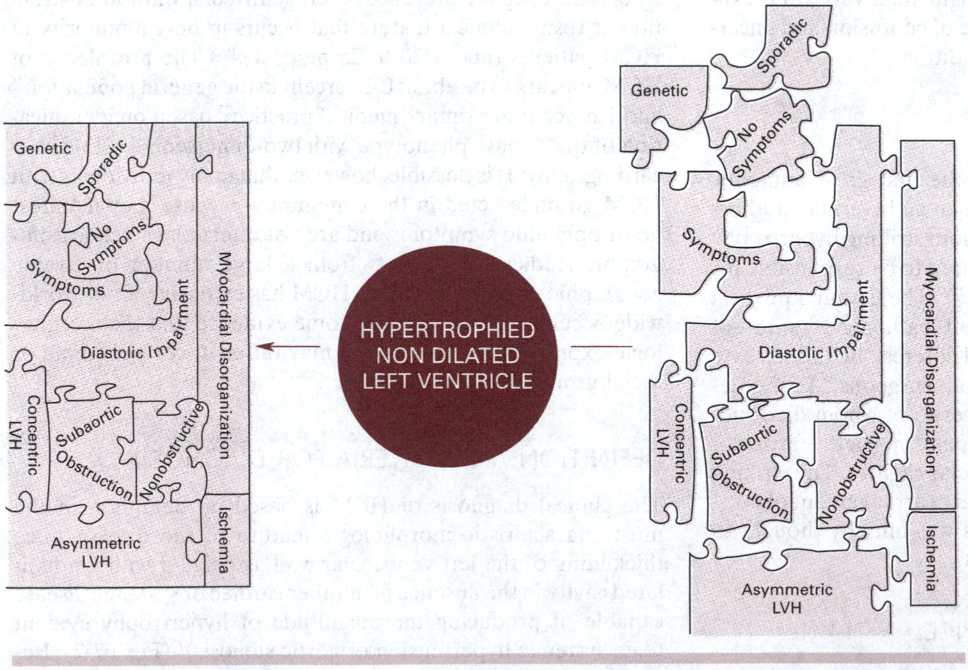

FIGURE 67-2 Diagrammatic representation of the basic morphologic definition of HCM (*dark circle*) as it unifies the clinical and morphologic diversity characteristic of the disease spectrum.

some patients may show only a mild increase of 15 to 18 mm, and a few genotyped affected individuals have been observed with normal thicknesses (≤12 mm).[10,36,40,46] Often the pattern of wall thickening is strikingly heterogeneous, involving noncontiguous segments of left ventricle (i.e., with areas of normal thickness evident in between), or with marked differences in wall thickness in adjacent segments of the wall. Transitions between thickened areas and regions of normal thickness are often sharp and abrupt, not infrequently creating right-angled contours of the wall.

In most patients the pattern of hypertrophy is diffuse, involving both septum and substantial portions of the lateral free wall, while the posterior segment of free wall is usually least affected by the hypertrophic process.[12,18] In others, hypertrophy involves only the ventricular septum while sparing the free wall. Of note, in an important proportion of patients (about one-third), wall thickening may be relatively mild and confined to a single segment of left ventricle.[12,13,18] Such segmental hypertrophy is usually localized to the anterior septum but may also be limited to the posterior septum,[12,18] anterolateral free wall,[12,18] posterior free wall,[47] or even the most apical portion of the left ventricle.[14,15,32,48–50] Therefore, the ventricular septum is usually, but not always, prominently involved in the hypertrophic process. Infiltrative and myocardial storage diseases such as cardiac amyloid and Fabry's disease may occasionally mimic HCM morphologically (Chap. 10).

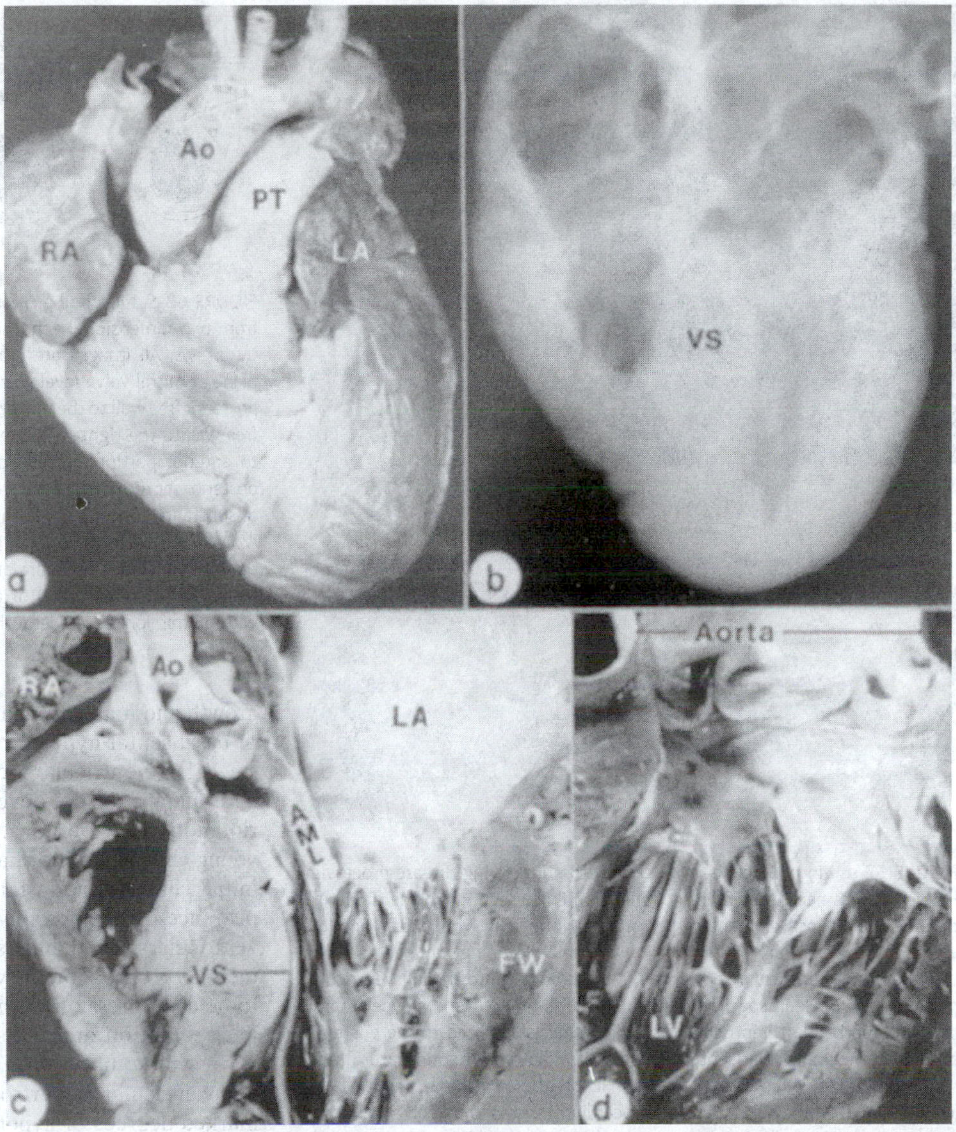

FIGURE 67-3 Anatomic features of HCM are demonstrated in the heart of a 26-year-old man. *A.* Exterior view; both right atrium (RA) and left atrium (LA) are dilated. Ao = aorta; PT = pulmonary trunk. *B.* Radiography of specimen showing asymmetric thickening of ventricular septum (VS). *C.* Coronal section; the septum is clearly thicker than left ventricular free wall (F); an endocardial mural contact plaque (*arrowhead*) is present in the left ventricular outflow tract in apposition to the anterior mitral leaflet (AML). *D.* Closer view of plaque and thickened anterior leaflet. (From Roberts WC et al.[16] with permission from the authors and publisher.)

Hypertrophy confined to the left ventricular apex ("apical HCM") has been reported most commonly by Japanese investigators,[32,34,49] who have described this subgroup of HCM patients to be clinically benign and with a "spade" deformity of the left ventricular cavity on angiography and a distinctive electrocardiographic (ECG) pattern of deep ("giant") T wave inversion. Reports from outside Asia would suggest, however, that apical hypertrophy is uncommonly accompanied by marked T-wave inversion and associated with adverse outcome in some patients.[14,15,48,50] This heterogeneous morphologic expression described for HCM is underlined by the fact that even first-degree relatives with the disease usually show great dissimilarity in the pattern of left ventricular wall thickening.[11]

In some young athletes, segmental hypertrophy of the anterior ventricular septum (wall thicknesses of 13 to 15 mm), consistent with a relatively mild morphologic expression of HCM, may often be difficult to distinguish from the physiologic left ventricular hypertrophy that can represent an adaptation to intense forms of athletic training.[51,52] In asymptomatic individuals within this morphologic "gray zone," the differential diagnosis between athlete's heart and nonobstructive HCM can often be resolved by clinical assessment and noninvasive testing[52] (Fig. 67-7).

HCM can represent a congenital heart malformation in which phenotypic expression in the form of left ventricular wall thickening begins during fetal development[53] and is evident at or shortly after birth.[54–56] Indeed, HCM has been reported in a small number of very young children, including a few infants under 6 months of age.[54–56] When HCM presents in infancy, the

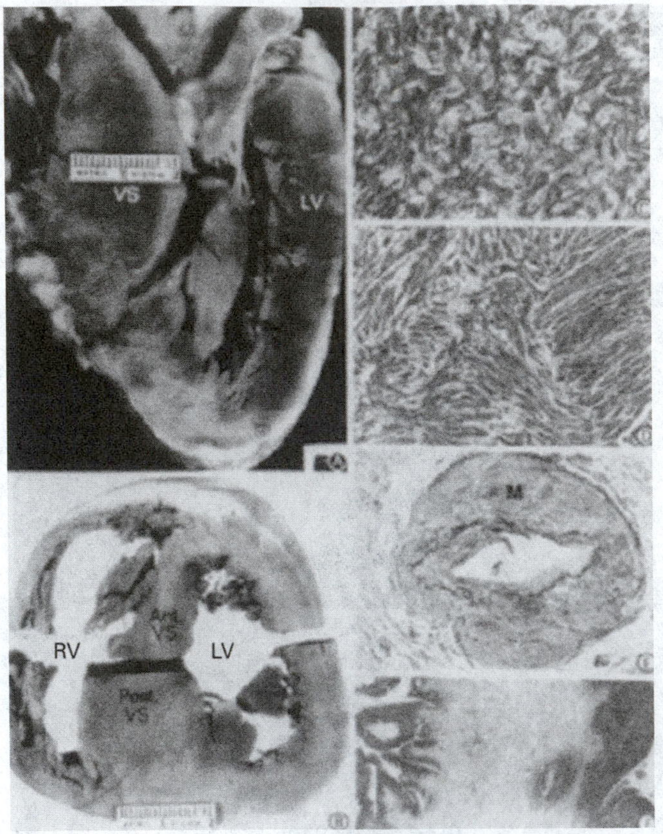

FIGURE 67-4 Morphologic components of the underlying disease process in HCM. *A.* Gross heart specimen sectioned in a cross-sectional plane similar to that of the echocardiographic (parasternal) long axis. The pattern of left ventricular hypertrophy is asymmetric, with wall thickening confined primarily to the anterior ventricular septum (VS), which bulges into the left ventricular outflow tract. *B.* Heart specimen illustrating a different pattern of hypertrophy, in which marked left ventricular wall thickening is localized to the posterior portion of the ventricular septum (Post. VS), while the anterior septum (Ant. VS) is only mildly thickened. *C* and *D.* Histopathology characteristic of the left ventricle in HCM. *C.* Septal myocardium shows markedly disordered architecture, with adjacent hypertrophied cardiac muscle cells arranged at perpendicular and oblique angles to each other. *D.* Bundles of hypertrophied cells show a disorganized, "interwoven" arrangement. *E.* Intramural coronary artery with apparently narrowed lumen and thickened wall due primarily to medial (M) hypertrophy. *F.* Extensive scarring of ventricular septum, which is transmural in distribution. LV = left ventricular free wall. (From Maron BJ et al.[3] with permission from the authors and publisher.)

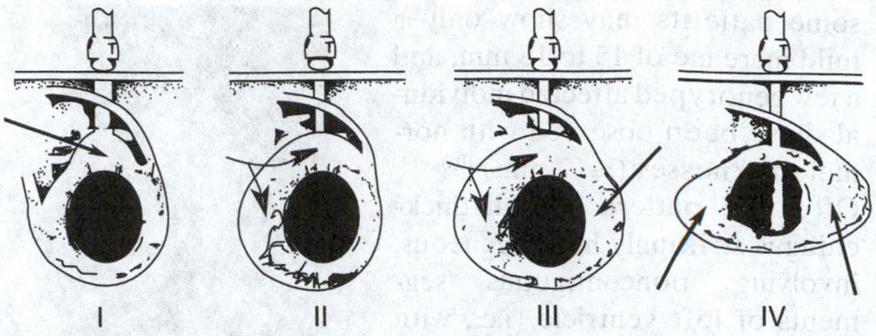

FIGURE 67-5 Morphologic variability in HCM, based on observations made from two-dimensional echocardiography; areas of hypertrophy are indicated by arrows. All images are drawn in the standard short-axis cross-sectional plane at mitral valve level with anterior chest wall and transducer to the top, posterior free wall to the bottom, posterior septum to the left, and anterolateral free wall to the right. *I.* Relatively mild left ventricular hypertrophy confined to anterior portion of ventricular septum. *II.* Hypertrophy of anterior and posterior septum in the absence of free wall thickening. *III.* Diffuse hypertrophy of substantial portions of both ventricular septum and anterolateral free wall. *IV.* Included are more unusual patterns of hypertrophy in which the thickened portions of left ventricle are present in the posterior septum or anterolateral free wall (as shown here) or at the left ventricular apex. (From Maron BJ[12] with permission from the author and publisher.)

disease is usually associated with marked septal hypertrophy as well as severe progressive congestive heart failure and biventricular outflow obstruction.[54,55,57] However, most cases of idiopathic left ventricular hypertrophy presenting in the first 2 years are not true HCM due to sarcomere protein mutations, but are often associated with other conditions such as Noonan syndrome.[57]

Later in childhood, serial echocardiographic investigations have shown prominent left ventricular remodeling. The morphologic expression of HCM is not usually complete until adulthood,[35,58] and during adolescence children often show striking spontaneous increases in wall thicknesses (i.e., of about 100 percent) and more widespread distribution of hypertrophy, including de novo development of wall thickening, when body growth and maturation are accelerated (Fig. 67-8). Progression of basal septal hypertrophy associated with a developmentally small left ventricular outflow tract appears to be the major determinant for the development of mitral valve systolic anterior motion and outflow obstruction during childhood.[59] In some young children, abnormalities on the 12-lead ECG may be the initial clinical manifestation of HCM, even preceding the appearance of hypertrophy on the echocardiogram.[31,60] Such left ventricular remodeling is usually not associated with development or progression of symptoms or sudden death and appears to be an expression of the genetically predetermined morphologic evolution of the disease.[35,61]

In symptomatic adult patients with HCM, the magnitude of left ventricular hypertrophy may *decrease* with aging.[62] Very marked degrees of hypertrophy (e.g., maximum wall thickness ≥30 mm) are largely limited to patients under age 40, while older patients over age 60 generally have more modest hypertrophy and rarely show wall thicknesses >25 mm. The explanation for this inverse relation between age and magnitude of hypertrophy could be a higher rate of premature death in younger patients with severe morphologic forms or, alternatively, to a process of wall thinning and remodeling occurring very gradually over long periods of time in many patients.[61]

Histologic Features

Several histologic features of left ventricular myocardium represent components of the primary cardiomyopathic disease process in HCM[1,3,42,63–73]: (1) disarray of cardiac muscle cells (myocytes) (Fig. 67-4*C* and *D*); (2) replacement fibrosis (Fig. 67-4*F*); (3) expansion of the interstitial (matrix) collagen compartment; and (4) abnormally small intramural coronary arteries (Fig. 67-4*E*). Marked distortion of cellular architecture with myocyte disarray, described prominently by Teare in his initial report of HCM,[25] is a characteristic feature of the left ventricle.[64–68,71] Many cardiac muscle cells in both the ventricular septum and left ventricular free wall show increased transverse diameter and

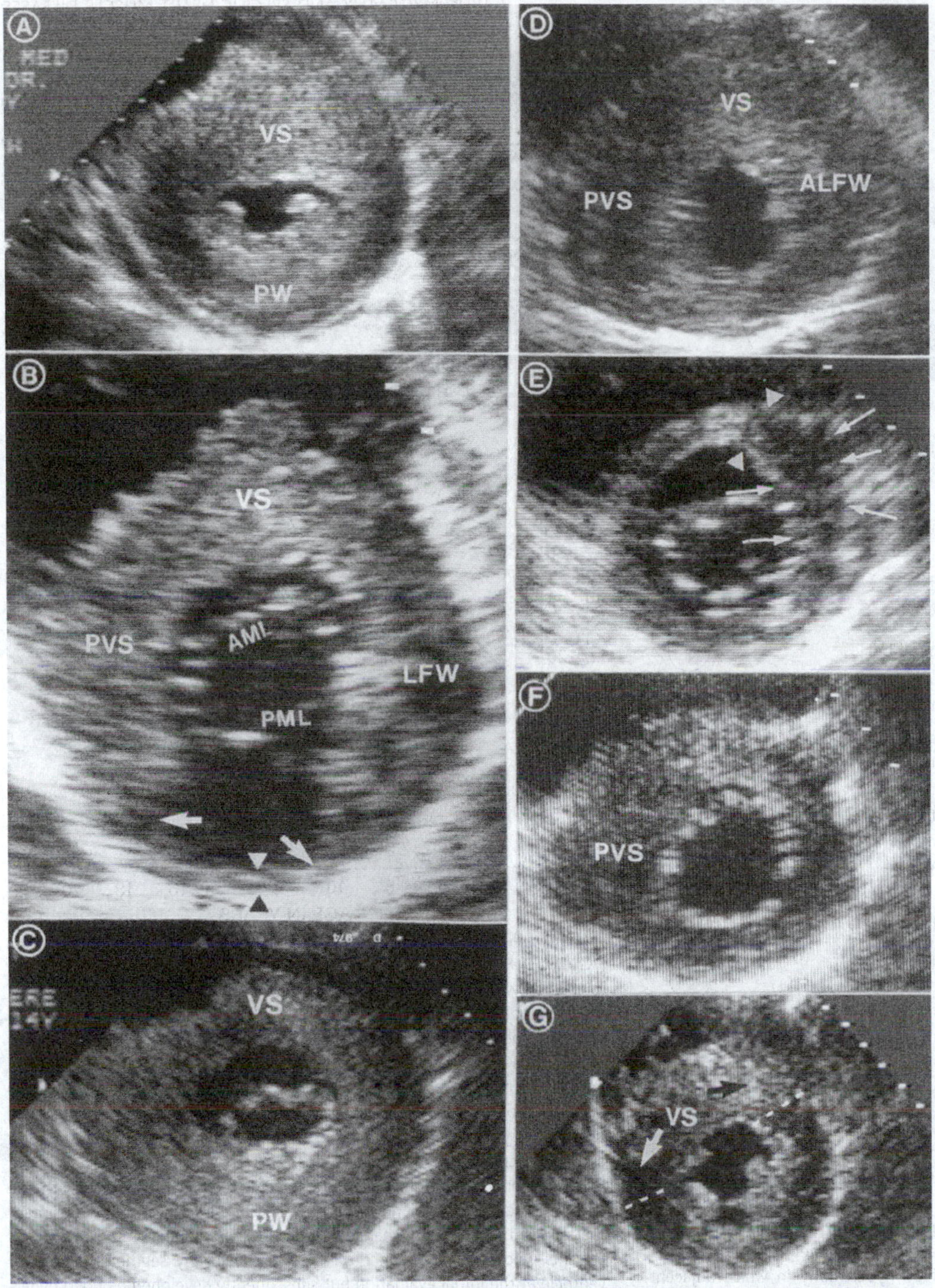

FIGURE 67-6 Variability of patterns of left ventricular hypertrophy in patients with hypertrophic cardiomyopathy, shown in a composite of diastolic stop-frame images in the parasternal short-axis plane. *A*, *B*, and *D*. Wall thickening is diffuse, involving substantial portions of ventricular septum and free wall. At the papillary muscle level (*A*), all segments of the left ventricular wall are hypertrophied, including the posterior free wall (PW), but the pattern of thickening is asymmetric, with the anterior portion of ventricular septum (VS) massive (i.e., 50 mm). *B*. Hypertrophy is diffuse, involving three segments of the left ventricle but with the posterior wall spared and thin (<10 mm) (*arrowheads*) and with particularly abrupt changes in wall thickness evident (*arrows*). *C*. Marked hypertrophy in a pattern distinctly different from that in *A*, *B*, and *D*, in which the thickening of the posterior wall is predominant and the ventricular septum is of nearly normal thickness. *D*. Diffuse distribution of hypertrophy involving three segments of the left ventricle similar to that in *B* but without sharp changes in the contour of the wall. *E*. Hypertrophy predominantly of lateral free wall (*arrows*) and only a small portion of the contiguous anterior septum (*arrowheads*). *F*. Hypertrophy predominantly of posterior ventricular septum (PVS) and, to a lesser extent, the contiguous portion of the anterior septum. *G*. Thickening of anterior and posterior septum to a similar degree but with sparing of the free wall. Calibration dots are 1 cm apart. AML = anterior mitral leaflet; LVW = lateral free wall; PML = posterior mitral leaflet. (From Klues HG et al.[18] with permission from the authors and publisher.)

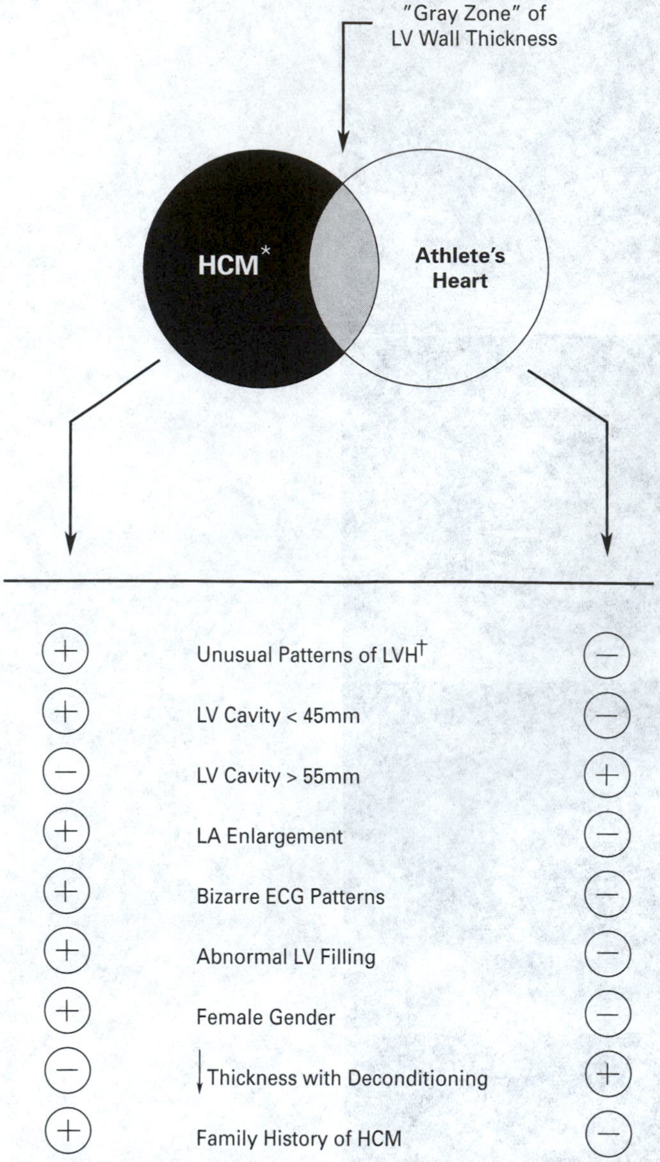

FIGURE 67-7 Criteria used to distinguish HCM from athlete's heart when left ventricular (LV) wall thickness is within the shaded gray zone of overlap, consistent with both diagnoses. *Assumed to be the nonobstructive form, since substantial mitral valve systolic anterior motion would confirm, per se, the diagnosis of HCM in an athlete. †May involve a variety of abnormalities, including heterogeneous distribution of LV hypertrophy in which adjacent regions may be of greatly different thicknesses, with sharp transitions evident between segments; also, asymmetric patterns in which anterior ventricular septum is spared from the hypertrophic process and the region of predominant thickening may be in the posterior septum or anterolateral or posterior free wall. ↓ = decreased; LA = left atrial. (From Maron BJ et al.[52] with permission from the authors and Williams & Wilkins.)

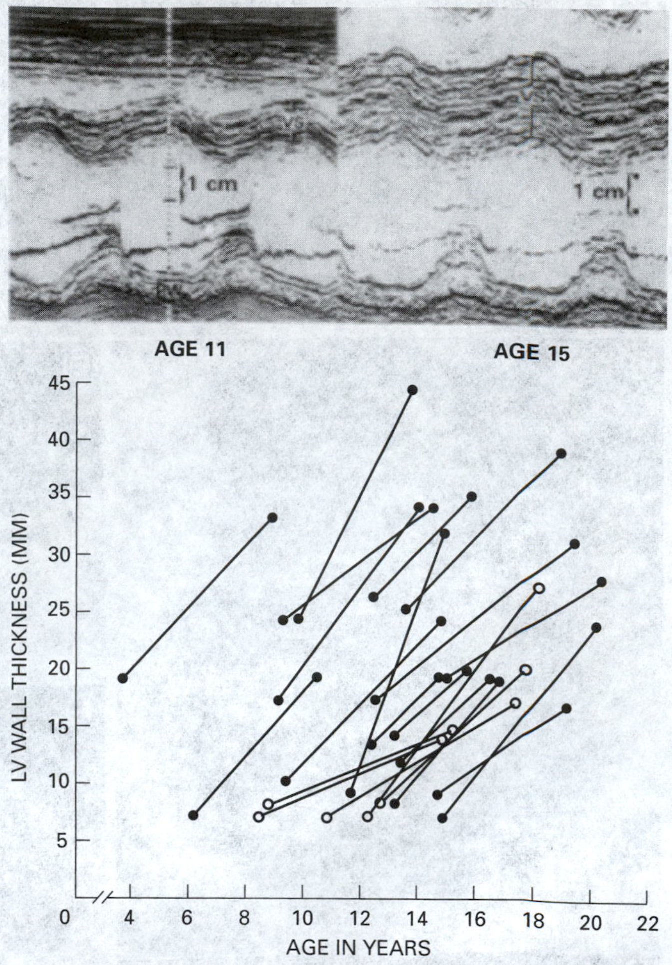

FIGURE 67-8 Development and progression of left ventricular hypertrophy in children with HCM. *Upper panel:* Development of marked hypertrophy of the anterior basal ventricular septum (VS). M-mode echocardiograms shown here were obtained at the same cross-sectional level in a girl with a family history of HCM. At age 11, ventricular septal thickness was at upper limit of normal (10 mm); at age 15, septal thickness had increased markedly (to 33 mm), and appearance of the echocardiogram is typical of HCM. The patient remained asymptomatic throughout this period of time but died suddenly and unexpectedly at age 17. PW = posterior left ventricular free wall. *Lower panel:* Dynamic, striking changes in left ventricular wall thickness with age in 22 children; each patient is represented by the left ventricular segment that showed the greatest change in wall thickness. Open symbols denote 5 patients who had no evidence of hypertrophy in any segment of the left ventricle at the initial evaluation but subsequently developed de novo hypertrophy typical of HCM. (From Maron BJ et al.[35] with permission of the authors and the Massachusetts Medical Society.)

bizarre shapes, maintain intercellular connections with several adjacent cells, and are arranged in a disorganized pattern at oblique and perpendicular angles to each other. This myocyte disarray is present in about 95 percent of patients dying of HCM and usually occupies substantial portions of both septum (i.e., about 33 percent) and left ventricular free wall (i.e., 25 percent) (see Fig. 74-4*C* and *D*). However, there is little correlation between absolute wall thickness and amount of disorganized myocardium in segments of the left ventricular wall.[71] Therefore areas of normal or only mildly increased left ventricular wall thickness may also show evidence of the cardiomyopathic process in HCM, in the form of cellular disarray.[71]

Dispersion of disorganized cardiac muscle cells throughout the left ventricular myocardium may impair intercellular transmission of normal electrophysiologic impulses, predispose to electrical instability, and thereby serve as an arrhythmogenic

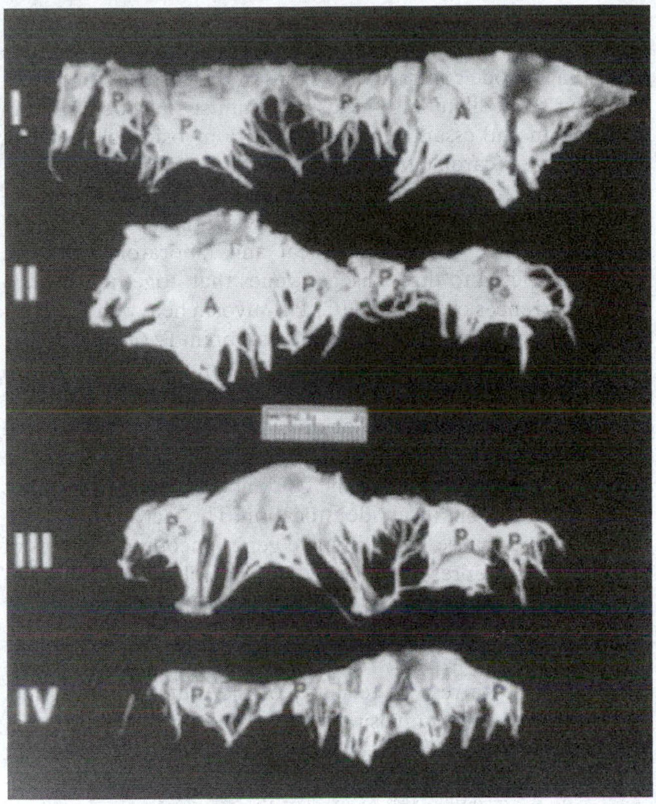

FIGURE 67-9 Mitral valves from three patients with obstructive HCM, aged 31, 29, and 60 years (I, II, and III), and from a normal control patient without cardiovascular disease (IV), showing variation in valvular size and structure present in HCM. Valves are opened with the circumference displayed in a horizontal orientation, exposing the atrial surface, with annular margin to top and chordal attachments to bottom. *I.* Large valve (area 22 cm^2) in which both the anterior (A) and posterior (P) leaflets are greatly elongated and increased in area. *II.* Large valve in which increased valve size (area 18 cm^2) is due primarily to elongation and enlargement of the anterior leaflet (A). *III.* Segmental elongation and increased area confined to a scallop of posterior leaflet. (From Klues HG et al.[20] with permission of the authors and Lippincott Williams & Wilkins.)

substrate responsible for the genesis of primary ventricular tachycardia/fibrillation.[74]

Patients with HCM (and without atherosclerotic coronary artery disease) often exhibit myocyte necrosis and replacement fibrosis in the left ventricle at necropsy.[42,63,69,72] A spectrum of severity and distribution is observed ranging from isolated small

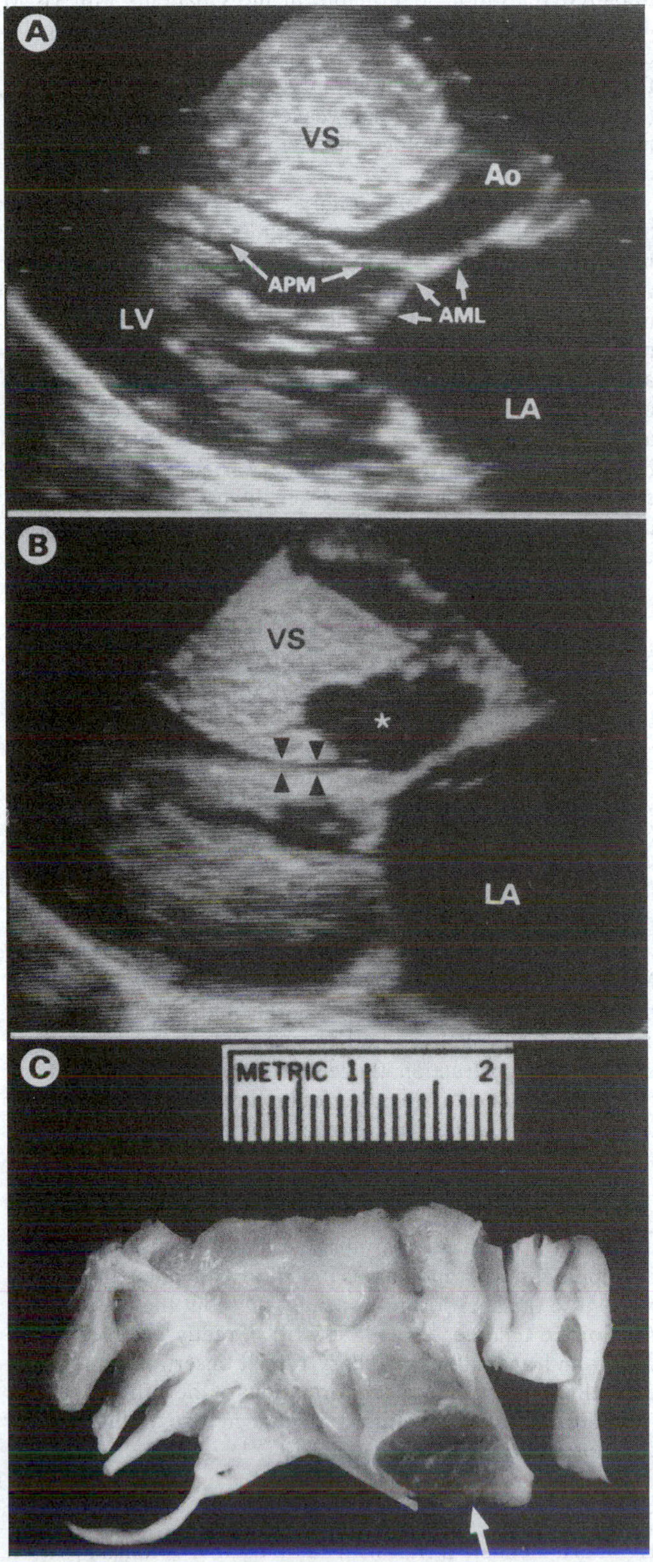

FIGURE IT Anomalous papillary muscle insertion directly into anterior mitral leaflet (*AML*) in patient with obstructive HCM. *A. Before myotomy-myectomy:* parasternal long-axis echocardiogram shows AML in direct continuity with the hypertrophied anomalous anterolateral papillary muscle (*APM*), which displaced anteriorly within the left ventricular cavity, producing a long area of midcavity muscular contact with the ventricular septum (VS) and outflow obstruction (*arrows*); tips of the mitral leaflets coapt in the usual position, and typical systolic anterior motion is absent (*small arrows*). *B. After myotomy-myectomy:* Long axis echocardiogram shows extensive muscular resection (*), extending from base of the septum to beyond the distal margins of the anterior mitral leaflet; nevertheless, a large area of direct muscular contact remains after operation between papillary muscle and ventricular septum (*arrowheads*), which is responsible for persistent and marked obstruction to left ventricular outflow. *C.* Mitral valve specimen excised at operation; a massively hypertrophied anterolateral anomalous papillary muscle (*arrow*) inserted directly into the body of the anterior leaflet. Ao = aorta; LA = left atrial; LV = left ventricle. (From Klues HG et al.[19] with permission of the authors and Lippincott Williams & Wilkins.)

scars to extensive, grossly visible replacement scarring that may even be transmural[42] (Fig. 67-4*F*). These areas of fibrosis, which likely result from repetitive bursts of myocardial ischemia or are related in some other way to the underlying cardiomyopathic disease process, can be identifiable during life as irreversible thallium-201 myocardial perfusion abnormalities[75] and may well contribute to the increased ventricular chamber stiffness and impaired relaxation identifiable in most patients with HCM as well as representing a nidus for the genesis of ventricular arrhythmias.[1,3,5,74] In addition, the interstitial collagen matrix of the left ventricle is substantially increased in size; its components (perimysial coils, pericellular weaves, and struts) are increased in number and morphologically abnormal, often showing a disorganized arrangement.[73]

Abnormal intramural coronary arteries are present in about 80 percent of patients with HCM studied at necropsy and are most commonly evident in the ventricular septum.[69,70] The walls of these arterioles are thickened (because of increased smooth muscle cells, collagen, elastic fibers, and mucoid deposits in the media and intima), and frequently the lumen appears narrowed and compromised (Fig. 67-4*E*). Increased numbers or clusters of abnormal intramural arteries are often observed within or at the margins of sizable areas of fibrosis.[42,69] This association between abnormal intramural coronary arteries and myocardial scarring suggests that a form of "small-vessel disease" present in patients with HCM may be responsible for myocardial ischemia and necrosis.[69]

Mitral Valve Abnormalities

Morphometric analysis of mitral valves removed at operation or necropsy from patients with outflow obstruction supports the concept that primary structural abnormalities of the mitral valve are also characteristic of many patients with HCM[20,43] (Fig. 67-9). About two-thirds of patients show alterations in mitral valve size and shape, with an increased mitral valve tissue area (up to twice normal) due primarily to leaflet elongation (but without evidence of myxomatous degeneration). These enlarged valves demonstrate considerable structural heterogeneity, either with both the anterior and posterior leaflets increased in size or asymmetric and segmental enlargement of one leaflet.[20] Mitral valve systolic anterior motion and outflow obstruction may occur both with normal or enlarged mitral valves but show age-related morphologic and functional features. In younger patients with obstruction, the leaflets are usually elongated and the valve is situated more posterior in the left ventricular outflow tract (at end-diastole), in contrast to elderly patients in whom the mitral valve is often normal-sized and situated much closer to the ventricular septum.[43]

In addition, other HCM patients show a congenital malformation of the mitral apparatus due to an arrest in embryonic development, with anomalous insertion of papillary muscle directly into the anterior mitral leaflet (without the interposition of chordae tendineae)[19] (Fig. 67-10). Greatly enlarged mitral valves and anomalous papillary muscle insertion represent a constellation of structural malformations of the mitral apparatus (in >50 percent of patients studied at necropsy) that expand the morphologic definition of HCM.[19,20,43]

ETIOLOGY AND GENETICS

HCM is a mendelian trait with an autosomal dominant pattern of familial inheritance.[1–5,8–11,22,38–40,76–83] Based on 10 years of molecular genetic studies, it is now known that HCM is genetically heterogeneous and caused by mutations in any one of nine genes that encode contractile proteins of the cardiac sarcomere, involving thick filaments (myosin subunits—i.e., beta-myosin heavy chain and essential and regulatory myosin light chains), thin filaments (cardiac troponin T, cardiac troponin I, α-tropomyosin, and α-actin), and—in the case of titin cardiac myosin-binding protein C—the structural network that joins thick and thin filaments.[5,8–11,22,38–40,76–83] Clinical and laboratory data are largely restricted to three disease genes that, together, explain most occurrences of familial HCM: β-myosin heavy chain, myosin-binding protein C, and cardiac troponin T. Overall, more than 100 individual disease-causing HCM mutations have been reported, either of the missense type (with the replacement of one amino acid by another) or mutations leading to truncated proteins. Indeed, most genotyped pedigrees show a mutation apparently unique to that family. Undoubtedly, numerous other genes and mutations await identification. The fact that all mutations known to cause HCM involve genes encoding proteins of the sarcomere represents a unifying principle that permits us to regard this heterogeneous condition as a single disease entity (and as a disease of the sarcomere).[5,8–10,84]

It has been suggested that the prognosis of HCM varies considerably with respect to many of the mutations reported. For example, some β-myosin heavy chain point mutations appear benign (e.g., Val606Met), whereas others are more virulent and associated with reduced survival (e.g., Arg403Gln, Arg453-Cys, and Arg719Trp).[8,9,22,76,82] In addition, cardiac troponin-T mutations may have malignant forms associated with reduced survival even though cardiac hypertrophy is often relatively mild.[5,22,38,39] Although, collectively, these observations suggest that genetic data may ultimately predict prognosis and influence clinical management, at present such a risk stratification strategy should be regarded as preliminary considering the relatively small number of genotyped families and the aforementioned genetic heterogeneity.

Occurrence of premature sudden cardiac death in a family should dictate a genetic and/or echocardiographic evaluation in surviving relatives, since the clinical expression of HCM may be particularly virulent in certain families (e.g., "malignant" HCM).[85] Also, because HCM is the most common cause of sudden unexpected death in young competitive athletes,[86] youthful family members should be screened for HCM prior to participation in intense athletic training. Because phenotypic (i.e., morphologic) expression of HCM may not be complete until 17 to 18 years of age,[35] a single screening echocardiogram during early childhood may not definitively exclude HCM. Therefore, children in families with HCM in whom left ventricular hypertrophy is absent on 2D echocardiography should continue to have examinations periodically until they achieve full growth and maturation. There now appears to be one clear exception to the tenet that development or progression of left ventricular hypertrophy does not occur in adulthood—i.e., myosin-binding protein-C mutations[10,46] (Fig. 67-11), which are associated with age-related penetrance; in some young adults, the HCM phenotype may not be evident on echocardiography, and is delayed until much later in life[10,46] (Fig. 67-12).

Routine echocardiographic screening at $\leq$12 years of age is usually unproductive, since phenotypic expression of the mutant gene is rarely present at that age.[31,35,59,77] Family screening can usually be deferred in young children until adolescence unless they are involved in intense sports programs (such as swimming

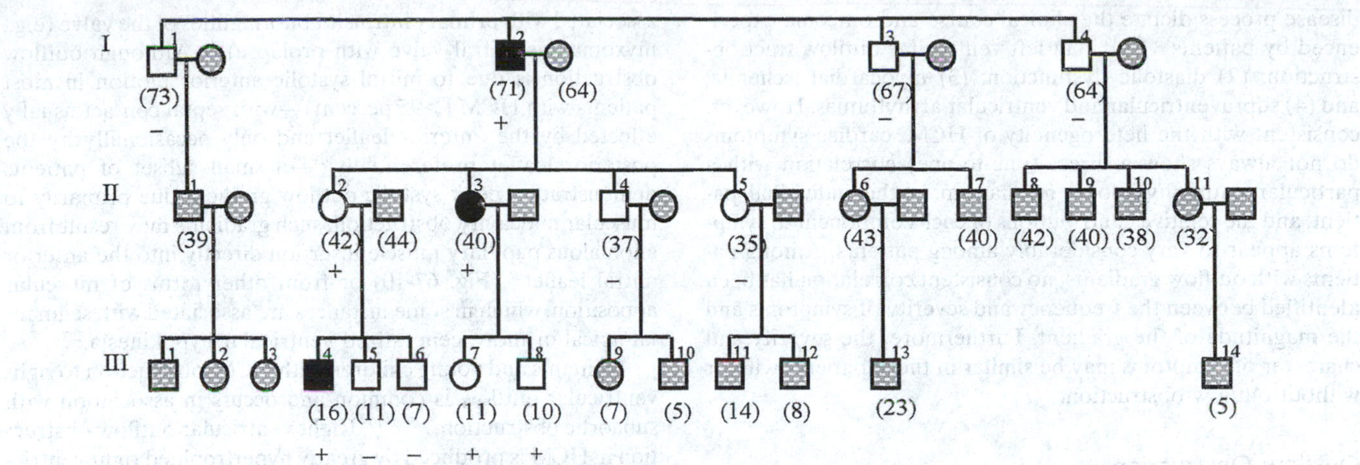

FIGURE 67-11 Pedigree of HCM family with a myosin-binding protein C mutation and variable penetrance. The genetically affected 42-year-old woman (II.2) is both the offspring of an affected parent (I.2), the mother of a 16-year-old affected child (III.4), and the sister of an affected 40-year-old sibling (II.3). In contrast to her father, child, and sister, this woman (II.2) showed no evidence of left ventricular hypertrophy and the HCM phenotype by two-dimensional echocardiography (or 12-lead ECG).

and tennis) or are members of families with HCM-related sudden deaths.[85]

With the advent of preclinical genetic diagnosis of HCM, a number of asymptomatic youthful family members have been identified as affected on the basis of a DNA diagnosis in the absence of typical phenotypic features of their disease (as assessed with echocardiography and electrocardiography).[5,10,22,31,36,37,40] The increasing availability of gene-based diagnosis will lead to the identification of greater numbers of children and adults with a preclinical diagnosis of HCM (i.e., who have a gene defect but no phenotypic manifestations of HCM).[5,10,22,31,36,37,40] At present, the clinical implications of such gene abnormalities and the appropriate management are largely unresolved issues, although—of note—very few such patients have been reported with adverse outcome.[87,88] Therefore there is not sufficient evidence available at present to preclude such individuals from competitive athletics in the absence of cardiac symptoms or risk factors such as family history of sudden cardiac death.[89] It should be emphasized that, at present, due to the substantial genetic heterogeneity of HCM and the complex, time-consuming, and expensive techniques required for genetic screening, DNA diagnosis is quite demanding, permits only research-oriented genotyping of selected pedigrees, and is not routinely available for clinical practice.[22]

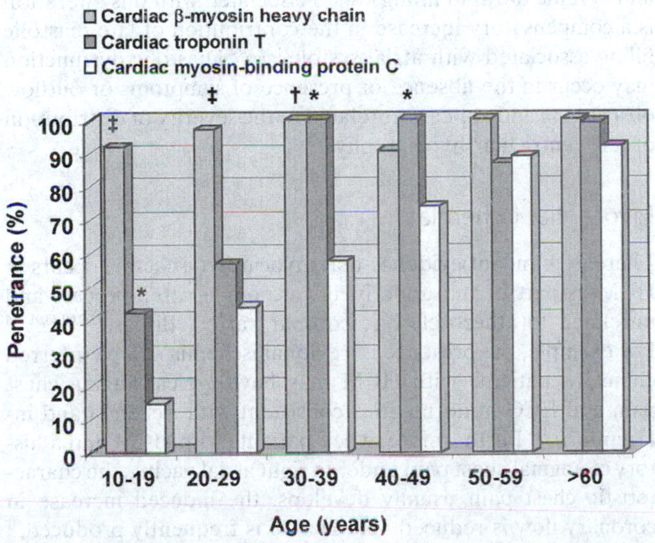

FIGURE 67-12 Age-related penetrance of familial HCM caused by mutations in the genes for cardiac myosin-binding protein C, cardiac troponin T, and cardiac β-myosin heavy chain. Solid bars denote the percentage of persons with both cardiac myosin-binding protein C mutations and left ventricular hypertrophy. Comparable clinical data for cardiac troponin T and β-myosin heavy chain are shown. Significant differences in the penetrance of familial HCM caused by cardiac myosin-binding protein C mutations and by mutations in cardiac troponin T or cardiac β-myosin heavy chain are indicated as follows: $* = p < 0.05$; $\nsim = p < 0.005$; $\neq = p < 0.001$. (From Niimura H et al.[10] with permission of the authors and the Massachusetts Medical Society.)

Although the reported sarcomeric protein mutations are regarded as disease-causing for HCM, many of the abnormal and primary structural features of this disease are not confined to protein abnormalities of the sarcomere but extend to alterations in connective tissue elements—e.g., mitral valve enlargement and elongation as well as other anomalies of the mitral apparatus,[19,20,43] abnormal small intramural coronary arteries,[69,70] and an expanded collagen matrix.[72,73] This fact, together with the observations that the patterns of left ventricular hypertrophy in closely related family members are usually dissimilar[11] and that hypertrophy is frequently confined to only a portion of the wall,[11–13,18] suggests that phenotypic expression is importantly influenced by genetic factors other than the causal mutation (e.g., by modifier genes)[90] or by undefined environmental influences.

PATHOPHYSIOLOGY

The symptoms of HCM are varied and include those of pulmonary congestion—such as exertional dyspnea, orthopnea, and paroxysmal nocturnal dyspnea—as well as fatigue, chest pain (which may be atypical of angina pectoris), palpitations, and impaired consciousness, including dizziness, near syncope, and syncope. The onset of symptoms is often in early adulthood between 20 and 40 years of age, although they can become evident at any age.

A number of pathophysiologic components of the HCM

disease process dictate the clinical course and outcome experienced by patients[1,3–5,91–101]: (1) left ventricular outflow tract obstruction; (2) diastolic dysfunction; (3) myocardial ischemia; and (4) supraventricular and ventricular arrhythmias. However, consistent with the heterogeneity of HCM, cardiac symptoms do not always show a direct (one-to-one) correlation with a particular pathophysiologic mechanism in the individual patient, and the relative contributions of each component to symptoms appear to vary considerably among patients. Among patients with outflow gradients, no consistent correlation has been identified between the frequency and severity of symptoms and the magnitude of the gradient. Furthermore, the severity and character of symptoms may be similar in those patients with or without outflow obstruction.

Outflow Obstruction

Obstruction to left ventricular outflow exhibited by patients with HCM (due to systolic anterior motion of the mitral valve and midsystolic contact with the ventricular septum)[4,6,94–97,102,104] is characteristically dynamic, showing spontaneous variability.[2] Interventions or circumstances that decrease myocardial contractility (e.g., beta-blocking drugs) or increase ventricular volume or arterial pressure (squatting or vasoconstrictor agents) have the effect of reducing or abolishing subaortic obstruction. Interventions or circumstances that increase contractility (exercise or infusion of isoproterenol) or decrease arterial pressure or ventricular volume (Valsalva maneuver or a hypotension-producing agent) will increase or provoke obstruction. Not uncommonly, patients with little or no obstruction to left ventricular outflow under basal conditions are capable of generating substantial labile gradients with physiologic or pharmacologic provocations[2–4] or just after the cessation of exercise.[98]

The increase in systolic intraventricular pressure associated with outflow obstruction may increase myocardial wall stress and oxygen demand. It is generally conceded that outflow obstruction in HCM can, in some patients, have long-term detrimental consequences on left ventricular function and be responsible for the genesis of symptoms.[1–6,95] The magnitude of the systolic pressure gradient can be reliably estimated noninvasively by the magnitude and duration of mitral valve systolic anterior motion on M-mode echocardiogram[4,6,94,95] or, more easily and quantitatively, by continuous-wave Doppler interrogation, obviating the necessity of performing serial cardiac catheterizations.[105] The combined use of color-coded, pulsed, and continuous-wave Doppler echocardiography allows assessment of the site and severity of outflow obstruction[104] (Chap. 13).

For the subaortic gradient to occur in HCM, several of the following morphologic and hemodynamic factors will be present: (1) reduced outflow tract dimension at end-diastole; (2) substantial hypertrophy involving the basal anterior ventricular septum; (3) displacement of mitral valve and papillary muscles anteriorly within the ventricular cavity; (4) increased length of the mitral leaflets; and (5) hyperdynamic left ventricular ejection, creating a high-velocity jet which streams through the narrowed outflow tract, pulling the mitral leaflets forward toward the septum (i.e., Venturi effect), or perhaps more likely due to drag (the hydrodynamic pushing force of flow) on the leaflets as they protrude into the outflow tract.[90] While mitral regurgitation due to outflow obstruction is usually mild-to-moderate in HCM, it may occasionally be much more severe when associated with primary intrinsic abnormalities of the valve (e.g., myxomatous mitral valve with prolapse).[106] Although outflow obstruction is due to mitral systolic anterior motion in most patients with HCM (>95 percent)—with septal contact usually effected by the anterior leaflet and only occasionally by the posterior leaflet preferentially[103]—a small subset of patients demonstrate a peak systolic outflow gradient due primarily to muscular midcavity obstruction; such gradients may result from anomalous papillary muscle insertion directly into the anterior mitral leaflet[19] (Fig. 67-10) or from other forms of muscular apposition, which in some instances are associated with segmental apical or more generalized ventricular hypokinesia.[107]

In infants and young children with HCM, obstruction to right ventricular outflow is common and occurs in association with subaortic obstruction.[54,55,95,108] Right ventricular outflow obstruction in HCM is produced by greatly hypertrophied right ventricular musculature (crista supraventricularis, moderator band, or trabeculae), reflecting an excessive hypertrophic process, and projecting into the relatively small outflow tract.[109]

Diastolic Dysfunction

Echocardiographic, Doppler, contrast, or radionuclide angiographic and hemodynamic studies of left ventricular diastolic function have identified characteristic abnormalities in relaxation and filling that are present in about 80 percent of patients with HCM[1,3,4,6,92,93,99,110–113] and are presumed to have an important role in the genesis of fatigue, exertional dyspnea, and angina pectoris. Therefore, considering the overall HCM disease spectrum, diastolic dysfunction is probably the single most important pathophysiologic mechanism responsible for symptoms. Prior studies have shown that the early filling phase of diastole is significantly prolonged and associated with a decreased rate and volume of rapid filling.[1,4,92,93] Associated with this alteration is a compensatory increase in the contribution of late diastolic filling associated with atrial systole.[1,4,92,93] Diastolic dysfunction may occur in the absence or presence of symptoms or outflow obstruction and appears unrelated to the severity or distribution of left ventricular hypertrophy.[92,113]

Myocardial Ischemia

There is abundant evidence that myocardial ischemia occurs in HCM as part of the underlying cardiomyopathic process and unrelated to atherosclerotic coronary artery disease.[1,3,69,70,91,114] For example, the presence of regional ischemia can be inferred clinically; patients with HCM may have typical angina chest pain and ECG abnormalities consistent with ischemia and infarction.[115,116] Furthermore, when patients with HCM and a history of anginal chest pain undergo right atrial pacing, the characteristic chest pain usually develops, the induced increase in coronary flow is reduced, and lactate is frequently produced.[91] Also, such patients may have fixed or exercise-induced reversible thallium-201 defects indistinguishable from those of patients with myocardial ischemia secondary to coronary artery disease.[75] Nevertheless, it has proven exceedingly difficult to measure or quantitate precisely the extent and location of such ischemia or to consistently derive clinical correlations or prognostic information for this finding.[110]

Myocardial ischemia and impaired vasodilator reserve in HCM may be due to several potential mechanisms: (1) compromised coronary blood flow to the left ventricular myocardium because of abnormal intramural coronary arteries (i.e., "small vessel disease"); (2) excessive myocardial oxygen demand that exceeds the capacity of the coronary system to deliver oxygen; or (3) prolonged diastolic relaxation, resulting in elevated myocardial wall tension.

ELECTROCARDIOGRAPHIC FEATURES

The 12-lead ECG is abnormal in about 90 percent of patients with HCM and shows a wide variety of patterns, often bizarre in appearance.[2,4,48–50,116] However, no particular ECG alteration is characteristic of most patients with HCM; common abnormalities are increased precordial voltages consistent with left ventricular hypertrophy, ST-segment changes and T-wave inversion, left atrial enlargement, abnormally deep Q waves, and diminished or absent R waves in the right precordial leads. Infants and young children often have the paradoxic finding of right ventricular hypertrophy on ECG, which may reflect obstruction to right ventricular outflow.

PREPARTICIPATION SCREENING FOR HCM IN ATHLETIC POPULATIONS

Detection of preexisting cardiovascular abnormalities (such as HCM) with the potential for significant morbidity or sudden death during intense physical activity is an important objective of the widespread practice of preparticipation screening of high school[117,118] and college-aged athletes.[119] In the United States, customary screening practice dictates a personal and family history and physical examination.[117–119] However, under the conditions of standard screening, it is difficult to identify or raise the suspicion of HCM, given that the vast majority of patients have the nonobstructive form of the disease with either no or only a soft systolic heart murmur, and that historical clues such as syncope or family history of sudden death are also uncommon.[1,118] Ideally, the detection of HCM would be enhanced by the incorporation of noninvasive testing during screening, such as 12-lead ECG[120] or echocardiography.[118] However, cost-efficacy and other considerations make the routine application of such tests impractical throughout the United States.[118] Echocardiographic screening for HCM is also limited by the frequency of borderline wall-thickness measurements (and the uncertainty and anxiety created by such findings), as well as the fact that the HCM phenotype may not always be detectable with echocardiography prior to about age 16.[35]

NATURAL HISTORY INCLUDING SUDDEN CARDIAC DEATH

HCM may be identified clinically at virtually any age, from infancy to old age (with even a few patients >90 years of age). Understanding the clinical course of HCM, particularly when viewed in the context of predicting outcome for individual patients, has for 40 years been constrained by three obstacles: (1) uncommon occurrence of the disease (i.e., 0.2 percent in the general population)[26]; (2) heterogeneity of disease expression[1–22,29,32–34,37–46,58–62,77–83,121]; and (3) tertiary center referral bias.[28,122,123]

Indeed, because much of the considerable published literature on HCM is based on studies performed at tertiary referral centers,[28,124–130] the overall clinical picture of HCM that has emerged is profoundly influenced by the biases created by highly selective patient referral patterns,[28,122,123] which has led to an overestimation of the overall risk for premature death and morbidity. This concept is substantiated by the fact that annual mortality figures from such referral centers are considerably higher (3 to 4 percent and up to 6 percent in children)[108,125,126,128,129] than those more recently reported in relatively unselected regional populations (about 1 percent per year).[122,131–136] Indeed, patient referral patterns are probably the strongest determinants of our prevailing perceptions regarding the clinical expression and impact of HCM.[122,123]

In general terms, it is reasonable to characterize HCM as a complex disorder capable of important clinical consequences, including causing premature death in some patients. However, the disease has a more favorable overall clinical course than previously thought, as many patients achieve normal life expectancy with little or no disability and often without the aid of therapeutic interventions. These observations emphasize the need to provide many HCM patients, including many children, with reassurance regarding their clinical outlook, as well as prudence concerning possible adverse consequences.

On the other hand, when HCM is viewed in terms of patient subgroups (rather than the overall disease), some individuals are clearly at much higher risk and may be subject to three modes of death: (1) sudden and unexpected, often in the young; (2) progressive heart failure in midlife; and (3) stroke associated with atrial fibrillation, largely in the elderly.

While frequent in children and young adults, sudden death is not confined to these age groups and may also occur in midlife and beyond, without a statistically significant predilection for any particular age group. Therefore the potential risk period in HCM is particularly long. However, reports of sudden death in infants and very young children are exceedingly rare. Sudden death in HCM usually occurs in previously asymptomatic (or only mildly symptomatic) patients, and such catastrophes are often the first clinical manifestation of the disease.[124] Although most patients die in the morning hours[137] while engaged in sedentary pursuits or during mild exertion, a substantial proportion collapse during or just after vigorous physical activity.[86,124] The latter observation—as well as the fact that HCM is the most common cause of sudden death among young competitive athletes[86] (Fig. 67-13)—supports the view that intense physical activity can act as a trigger for sudden death in the presence of underlying cardiovascular disease.[138] Therefore it is prudent to recommend the disqualification of young athletes with HCM from intense competitive sports, in accord with the standards of the 26th Bethesda Conference,[89] in an effort to decrease the risk of exercise-related sudden death.

Based on stored electrogram data from HCM patients experiencing appropriate implantable cardioverter-defibrillator discharges, ventricular tachycardia/fibrillation appears to be the primary mechanism most commonly responsible for sudden death in HCM,[74] although a number of other mechanisms may also be involved.[139–146] No particular symptom complex has been shown to be reliably associated with subsequent sudden death in HCM with the exception of recurrent or exertional syncope, particularly in the young.[5] Furthermore, patients with or without subaortic obstruction may die suddenly, and some patients appear to tolerate marked outflow obstruction for virtually their

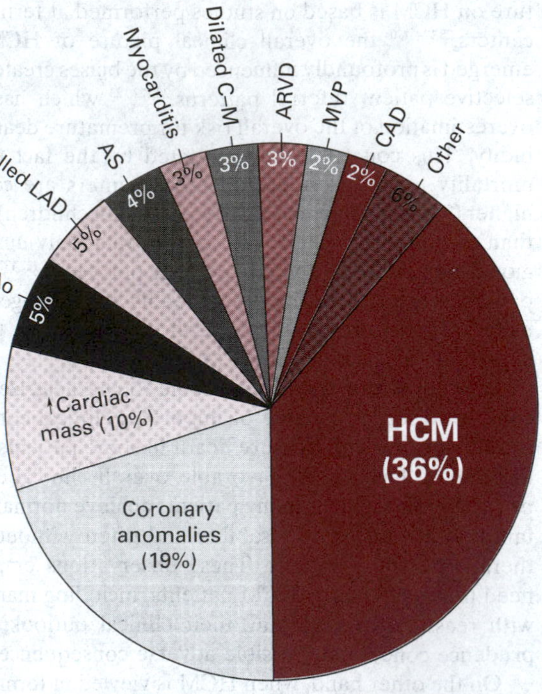

FIGURE 67-13 Causes of sudden cardiac death in young competitive athletes (median age, 17), based on systematic tracking of 158 athletes in the United States, 1985 to 1995. In an additional 2 percent, no evidence of cardiovascular disease sufficient to explain death was found at necropsy; ↑ (increased) cardiac mass = hearts with increased weight and some morphologic features consistent with (but not diagnostic of) HCM. Ao = aorta; LAD = left anterior descending coronary artery; AS = aortic stenosis; C-M = cardiomyopathy; ARVD = arrhythmogenic right ventricular dysplasia; MVP = mitral valve prolapse; CAD = coronary artery disease; HCM = hypertrophic cardiomyopathy. (Adapted from Maron BJ et al.[86] with permission of Lippincott Williams & Wilkins.)

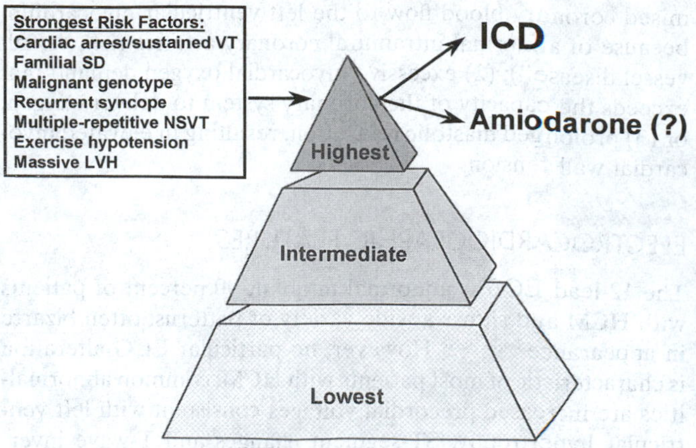

FIGURE 67-14 Assessment of risk for sudden cardiac death in HCM population. Treatment for the prevention for sudden death is limited to that small subset perceived to be at highest risk compared to all other patients with HCM, based on the presence of ≥1 of the risk factors shown. Patients regarded as low risk are asymptomatic with mild left ventricular hypertrophy and *without* either ventricular tachycardia on ambulatory Holter ECG, hypotensive blood pressure response to exercise, and family history of premature HCM-related death. ICD = implantable cardioverter-defibrillator; LVH = left ventricular hypertrophy; NSVT = nonsustained ventricular tachycardia; SD = sudden death; VT = ventricular tachycardia. (From Maron,[1] with permission of the author and *Lancet*.)

entire lives without adverse consequences.[122] Indeed, the presence or magnitude of the outflow gradient has not been independently associated with increased risk for sudden death, although an association with heart failure–related or total cardiovascular mortality has been cited.[122,136,148]

However, other disease variables have been associated with an increased likelihood of sudden death. The most important of these proposed risk factors include[1,5,8,9,22,38,74,82,85,145,147–149] (Fig. 67-14) the following: prior cardiac arrest or sustained ventricular tachycardia, "malignant" genotype or family history of premature HCM death, multiple-repetitive (or prolonged) bursts of nonsustained ventricular tachycardia on ambulatory ECGs, massive degree of left ventricular hypertrophy (wall thickness, ≥30 mm). A hypotensive blood pressure response to exercise may also be informative regarding risk but is encumbered by a low positive predictive accuracy and is much more powerful as a negative predictor of outcome.[139,140]

A recent retrospective analysis of children with HCM suggested that an intramural course of a segment of the proximal left anterior descending coronary artery (i.e., myocardial bridging) constitutes a risk factor for sudden cardiac arrest.[145] It was proposed that such muscular bridges could produce systolic coronary arterial narrowing, residual diastolic compression, and myocardial ischemia, thereby justifying surgical unroofing when detected.

The data available at this time do not provide convincing evidence that programmed electrical stimulation has a major role in risk stratification in HCM. Particularly aggressive programmed stimulation protocols with triple ventricular premature depolarizations seldom induce monomorphic ventricular tachycardia but frequently trigger polymorphic ventricular tachycardia or ventricular fibrillation in patients with HCM.[5,150] Based on experience in HCM as well as in coronary artery disease and dilated cardiomyopathy, these latter arrhythmias are generally regarded as nonspecific responses.[5]

END-STAGE PHASE

A final phase of disease evolution occurring in about 10 percent of symptomatic patients in a referral-based population has been variously referred to as the "end-stage," "burned-out," or "dilated" phase of HCM[61] (Fig. 67-15). This distinctive clinical course is characterized by progressive congestive symptoms with marked exercise limitation and atrial arrhythmias, associated with substantial left ventricular remodeling—i.e., enlarging left ventricular cavity size (occasionally with marked absolute dilatation), thinning of portions of the wall, systolic dysfunction, and—in a few patients—spontaneous reduction of the subaortic gradient. Therefore, the disease in end-stage patients is transformed from the typical morphologic and functional appearance of HCM (hyperdynamic, hypertrophied, and nondilated left ventricle) to a clinical state that is more suggestive of a dilated form of cardiomyopathy (Chap. 66) in which the thickness of the left ventricular wall may be virtually normal. Many such patients exhibit irreversible myocardial perfusion abnormalities, which undoubtedly represent areas of extensive myocardial scarring.[42,63,69,75]

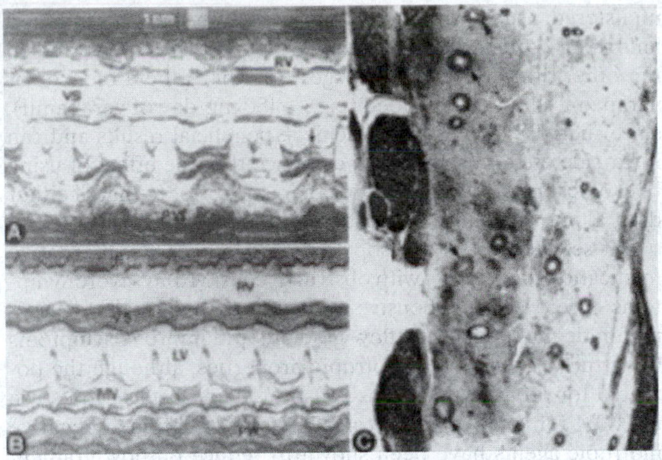

FIGURE 67-15 Studies in patients with HCM and normal extramural coronary arteries showing changes occurring in association with progressive congestive cardiac failure and transmural myocardial infarction (end-stage phase). *A.* Echocardiographic study from a 26-year-old patient with exertional chest pain and dyspnea. Ventricular septum (VS) is markedly thickened (23 mm) and pattern of hypertrophy is asymmetric. Left ventricular end-diastolic dimension is reduced (38 mm), and there is a trivial degree of mitral systolic anterior motion (*arrow*). PW = posterior wall; RV = right ventricle. *B.* From same patient at 30 years of age (9 months before death) after clinical deterioration with progressive cardiac failure, pulmonary edema associated with chronic atrial fibrillation, and cardiopulmonary collapse. Appearance of left ventricle has changed dramatically. Septum has thinned considerably (to 13 mm) and is about as thick as the posterior wall; left ventricular (LV) and right ventricular cavities have enlarged substantially. MV = mitral valve. *C.* Low-power photomicrograph of a specimen from a patient with a clinical course similar to that of the patient in *A* and *B* showing transmural scarring of the septum and numerous abnormal intramural coronary arteries, some with thickened walls and narrowed lumen (*arrows*) (Magnification ×6). (From Maron BJ et al.[3] with permission of the authors and the Massachusetts Medical Society.)

It is possible that the morphologic and functional changes that result in end-stage depression of left ventricular contractile function are due to impaired coronary blood flow and myocardial ischemia resulting from small-vessel coronary artery disease. Patients evolving into the end-stage phase of HCM or experiencing sudden and unexpected cardiac death may coexist in the same family (and share the identical disease-causing mutation).[151] Also, a few patients with aborted episodes of cardiac arrest have themselves died many years later in the end-stage phase.[152]

HYPERTROPHIC CARDIOMYOPATHY IN THE ELDERLY

Older patients (over age 60 to 65) with morphologic and clinical features consistent with HCM have been reported.[1,21,153,154] In certain of these patients, HCM may be well tolerated to particularly advanced ages (i.e., 80 to 90 years) and therefore should be regarded as a disease compatible with normal longevity. In an unselected HCM population, about 20 percent of patients had achieved the age of ≥75 years.[122] In other elderly patients, symptoms are not present early in life, but severe functional limitation and heart failure may intervene abruptly for the first time after age 60 to 65.[21,153,155] This prolonged period of symptomatic latency is notable for a disease usually expressed morphologically by age 20 and in which symptoms are usually evident by age 40 to 50.

Older patients with HCM differ in many respects from many younger patients with regard to certain morphologic features.[21,153–155,156] Older patients characteristically have relatively small hearts with only modestly increased left ventricular wall thickness (usually 20 mm)[21,62,122,155] and severely distorted outflow tract morphology, with greatly reduced size, and exaggerated anterior displacement of a normal-sized mitral valve. Substantial deposits of calcium in the mitral annular region are frequently present and may contribute to anterior displacement of the valve in some patients. Outflow obstruction often occurs in the presence of restricted mitral valve systolic anterior motion, with contact between ventricular septum and anterior mitral leaflet produced by a combination of anterior excursion of the mitral valve toward the septum and posterior movement of septum toward the mitral valve.[43] It is uncertain whether the HCM phenotype in such older patients always conveys the same genetic etiology as in younger patients; however, some older patients have been documented to carry the same mutant genes encoding sarcomeric proteins characteristic of other (younger) HCM patients.

MEDICAL TREATMENT

Asymptomatic Patients and Prevention of Sudden Cardiac Death

Those patients with clear evidence of high risk should be offered treatment for the prevention of sudden cardiac death.[1,5] The implantable cardioverter-defibrillator (ICD) has proved effective and reliable in relatively young and high-risk HCM patients by virtue of sensing ventricular tachycardia/fibrillation and restoring sinus rhythm by appropriate defibrillation shocks or antitachycardia pacing at an overall rate of 7 percent per year.[74] The ICD may be lifesaving,[74,157] both in the context of secondary prevention after cardiac arrest or in sustained ventricular tachycardia (11 percent per year) or for primary (prophylactic) prevention due to the perception of high risk based on ≥1 sudden death risk factors.[74] Alternatively, long-term prophylactic treatment with amiodarone[158] would seem less realistic in relatively young HCM patients, given the potential side effects and the long risk period in HCM as well as the paucity of data substantiating amiodarone as affording effective protection against sudden cardiac death specifically in this disease. Prophylactic and empiric administration of beta blockers or verapamil to asymptomatic patients for the primary purpose of reducing the risk for sudden death, for which there are no or little data, now seems outdated in view of the availability of more definitive therapeutic measures such as the ICD. Drug treatment to prevent or delay progression of congestive symptoms is empiric, with a complete lack of any controlled data.

Alleviation of Symptoms

Therapeutic strategies for symptomatic patients with HCM are summarized in Fig. 67-16. Responses of HCM patients to medical treatment are highly variable; consequently, therapy must often be tailored to the individual requirements of symptomatic patients.[1,5,159] Historically, beta-adrenergic blocking drugs (pro-

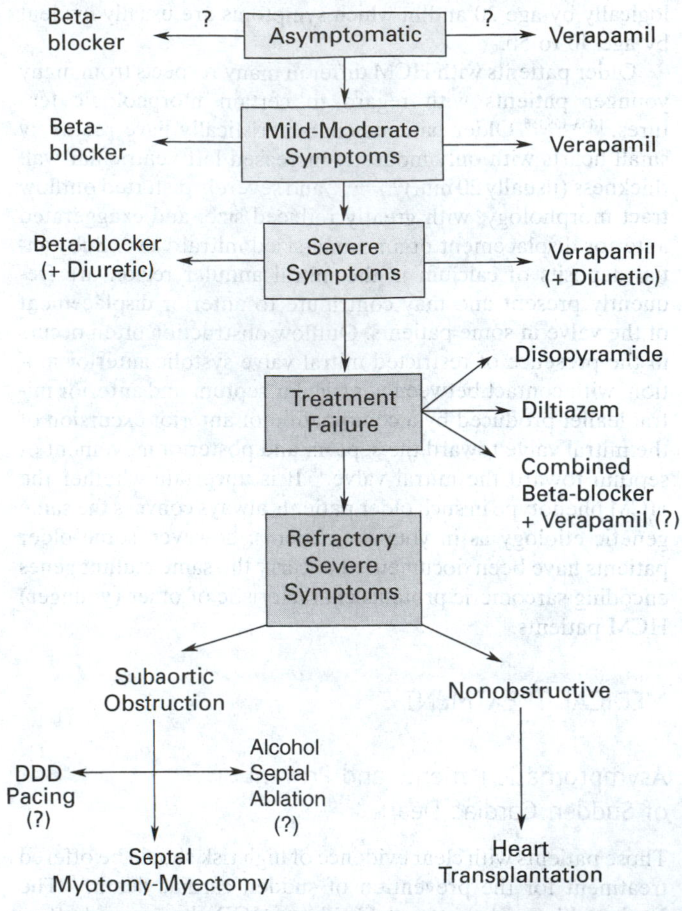

FIGURE 67-16 Therapeutic strategies for patients with HCM. Question marks indicate treatment recommendations that are largely unresolved.

pranolol or more cardioselective agents such as atenolol, metoprolol, or nadolol) have been utilized extensively to relieve symptoms in patients with either the obstructive or nonobstructive form of HCM.[1,3–6,159] The beneficial effects of beta blockers on symptoms (principally exertional dyspnea and chest pain) and exercise capacity appear to be due largely to decreased heart rate, with consequent prolongation of diastole, increased passive left ventricular filling, and decreased filling pressures. By reducing inotropic state, beta blockers may also lessen myocardial oxygen demand and decrease the left ventricular outflow gradient during exercise when sympathetic tone is increased.

Calcium channel blockers (principally verapamil) are also important therapeutic agents in the management of symptomatic patients with HCM.[1,160,161] Orally administered verapamil provides improvement in cardiac symptoms and exercise tolerance for many patients with HCM, including those who have failed to benefit from beta blockers. This symptomatic improvement with verapamil appears to be due largely to normalization of left ventricular filling parameters.[1,5]

Beta blockers and verapamil are usually administered empirically at the onset of symptoms by titrating drug dosage to the historical assessment of functional disability, although some investigators utilize exercise testing with or without measurement of oxygen consumption to gauge the effect of medications on symptoms. Furthermore, there is no consensus on the sequence with which beta blockers and verapamil should be administered; usually a trial with one or the other drug is initiated and should a benefit fail to result, the patient is converted to the other drug. Excessive dosages of either a beta blocker or verapamil should be avoided (e.g., >480 mg/day of verapamil), since such drug levels rarely achieve beneficial results and can incur side effects. There is no evidence that the effect of using beta blockers and verapamil together is superior to that of either drug alone, and this combination should be avoided.

At selected centers, disopyramide has been an alternative medication for patients with obstructive HCM and severe symptoms otherwise unresponsive to standard therapy.[6,162–164] Disopyramide may reduce outflow gradient and improve symptoms by virtue of its negative inotropic properties, although the potential for proarrhythmia has constituted an obstacle to its use in HCM for some investigators. The aforementioned negative inotropic agents have been shown to reduce outflow gradient in HCM by slowing left ventricular ejection acceleration.[164]

Some patients with particularly severe symptoms of heart failure despite treatment with beta blockers or verapamil may show symptomatic improvement with the judicious addition of diuretic agents.[3] The aforementioned therapeutic considerations apply to those patients with HCM in whom symptoms of congestive failure typically occur in the presence of normal or hyperdynamic systolic performance. Conversely, in the subgroup of patients experiencing congestive symptoms secondary to systolic dysfunction (i.e., end-stage HCM)[1,4–6,61,159] therapeutic strategy is similar to that employed for heart failure in other diseases with impaired systolic function, including the use of diuretics, angiotensin-converting enzyme inhibitors, and digitalis; ultimately, heart transplantation should be considered in this subgroup of patients[61,165] (see Chap. 22).

Prevention of Infective Endocarditis

Bacterial endocarditis, a recognized complication of HCM, is virtually confined to patients with the obstructive form of the disease (and mitral valve systolic anterior motion) with a prevalence of about 0.5 percent.[166] Vegetations most commonly involve the anterior mitral leaflet or septal endocardium at the site of mitral valve contact (likely a consequence of the high-velocity outflow jet) and less commonly the aortic valve.[166,167]

Atrial Fibrillation

Atrial fibrillation is a particularly important arrhythmia in HCM,[134,168,169] reportedly occurring in up to about 20 percent of patients followed longitudinally with this disease.[122,134] Atrial fibrillation is associated with an increased risk for systemic thromboembolism, heart failure, and death.[1,3–6] Of note, HCM patients with atrial fibrillation usually show substantial left atrial enlargement but, paradoxically, usually only relatively mild left ventricular hypertrophy.[168] Onset of atrial fibrillation may importantly impair the clinical course in HCM, probably because absence of the atrial systolic contribution to ventricular filling is critical to cardiac function in patients with such poorly compliant ventricles. In many patients, however, chronic atrial fibrillation appears to be reasonably well tolerated as long as ventricular rate is controlled.[169] Beta-adrenergic blocking agents or verapamil are usually efficacious in controlling heart rate in patients with chronic atrial fibrillation. Recurrent atrial fibrillation is managed by restoring sinus rhythm with electrical cardioversion, if necessary, or alternatively by drugs—with amiodarone probably the most effective antiarrhythmic agent for the prevention of recurrent atrial fibrillation. Because of the risk of peripheral embolism and stroke, anticoagulant therapy should be administered (and continued indefinitely) in most patients once atrial fibrillation has been documented.

SURGICAL TREATMENT

Operation is regarded as the standard treatment for those HCM patients with obstruction to left ventricular outflow under basal conditions (gradient ≥50 mmHg), and severe drug-refractory symptoms.[1,3–6,159,170–186] Therefore surgery is performed to relieve incapacitating symptoms and subaortic obstruction by normalizing the markedly increased systolic intraventricular pressures.[1,3–6,159,170–186] General agreement is lacking, however, as to whether symptomatic patients with marked outflow gradients—which are present solely or predominantly under provokable conditions such as exercise or with maneuvers in the catheterization laboratory (e.g., isoproterenol infusion, amyl nitrite inhalation, or Valsalva maneuver)—are appropriate operative candidates.[2,4,6,171,179]

Ventricular septal myotomy-myectomy (Morrow operation)[170] (Fig. 67-17) is the surgical procedure of choice; a small amount of muscle is removed from the basal anterior septum (usually about 2 to 6 g) through an aortotomy. However, mitral valve replacement has been employed[177,179,184] in selected patients when the operative site for muscular resection in the basal anterior portion of the septum is relatively thin (i.e., ≤18 mm) or when the distribution of septal hypertrophy is atypical.[179]

Occasionally, patients have outflow obstruction from a mechanism other than mitral valve systolic anterior motion. For example, anomalous papillary muscle insertion directly into anterior mitral leaflet without the interposition of the chordae tendineae (Fig. 67-10) producing muscular mid-ventricular obstruction[19] should always be contemplated prior to surgery, since the operative strategy may require a more extensive myectomy[186] or possibly mitral valve replacement.[19] Suture plication of the anterior mitral leaflet (in combination with myotomy-myectomy) has also been introduced in patients judged to have a greatly enlarged mitral valve, so as to reduce the likelihood that mitral valve systolic anterior motion will persist postoperatively.[185]

Intraoperative 2D echocardiography is an important guide to mapping the distribution and magnitude of septal hypertrophy [179,187,188] and determining how the muscle resection should be tailored to the distribution of septal hypertrophy in the individual patient to achieve the desired hemodynamic result and avoid iatrogenic complications such as ventricular septal defect. Transesophageal echocardiography (Chap. 13) may also be useful in assessing morphologic and functional abnormalities during surgery, particularly of the mitral valve.[187,188]

Results from a number of North American and European centers employing septal myotomy-myectomy over the past 40 years, in about 2000 patients, have demonstrated salutary hemodynamic as well as symptomatic effects.[1,3–6,159,170–183,189] Operative mortality at the most experienced centers has improved over the past several years and is presently less than 1 to 2 percent.[1,5] Older patients with associated cardiac lesions, such as coronary artery disease requiring bypass grafting, may be at greater operative risk.[190]

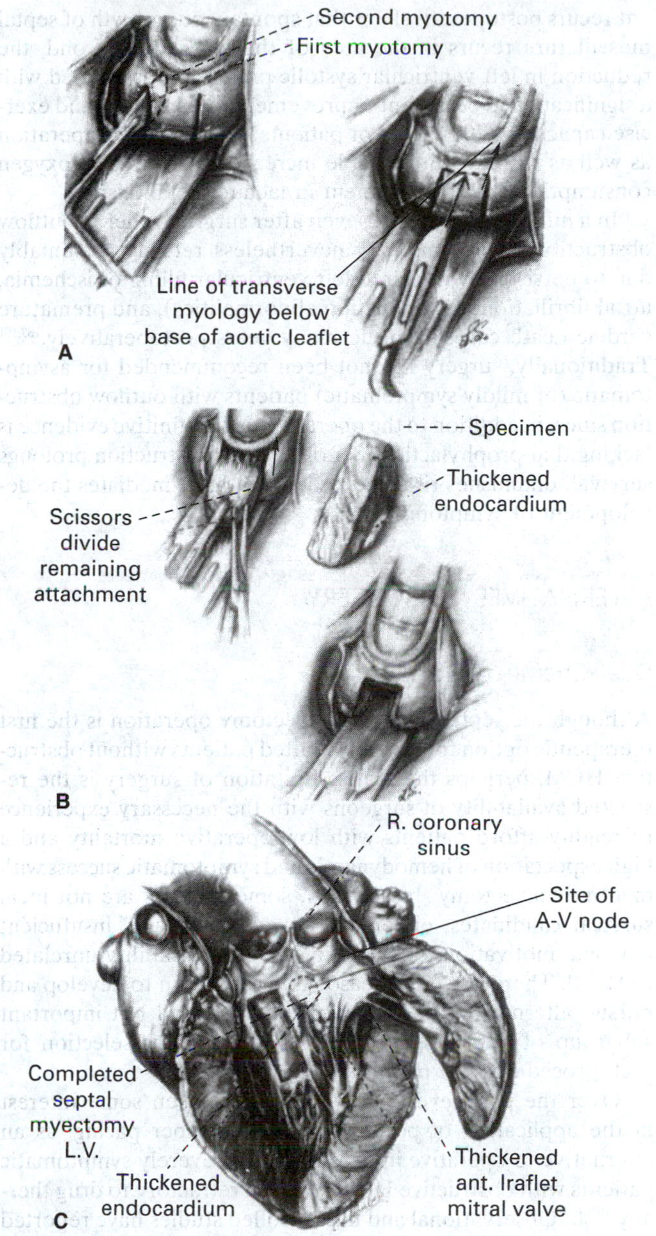

FIGURE 67-17 Illustration of ventricular septal myotomy-myectomy operation (Morrow procedure). *A.* Two vertical, parallel myotomies are made in the cephalad portion of the septum about 1 cm apart. Transverse incision is then made, connecting the two parallel myotomies. *B.* Attachments of the muscle bar to the septum are divided; this segment of muscle is isolated and then excised. *C.* After completion of the myotomy-myectomy, a rectangular channel about 4 cm long and 2 cm wide is evident extending from the aortic annulus to a point just distal to the caudal margins of the mitral leaflets. (From Maron BJ et al.[176] with permission from the authors and the *European Heart Journal.*)

Several important effects of operation have been defined in patients with HCM.[1,3–6,159,170–183,189] First, in more than 90 percent of patients, myotomy-myectomy (or mitral valve replacement) abolishes or substantially reduces the basal subaortic gradient and mitral valve systolic anterior motion without importantly compromising left ventricular function; this consequence of surgery appears to be permanent, with no evidence that the gradient recurs postoperatively or that spontaneous growth of septal musculature recurs in the area of the resection. Second, the reduction in left ventricular systolic pressure is associated with a significant and persistent improvement in symptoms and exercise capacity in 70 percent of patients ≥5 years after operation as well as with a demonstrable increase in myocardial oxygen consumption and improvement in lactate metabolism.[191]

In a minority of patients, even after surgical relief of outflow obstruction, symptoms may nevertheless return (presumably due to persistently impaired left ventricular filling or ischemia, atrial fibrillation, or conduction abnormalities), and premature cardiac death can still ensue many years postoperatively.[189,191] Traditionally, surgery has not been recommended for asymptomatic (or mildly symptomatic) patients with outflow obstruction since, in addition to the operative risk, definitive evidence is lacking that prophylactic relief of outflow obstruction prolongs survival, diminishes risk for sudden death, or mediates the development of symptoms.

ALTERNATIVES TO SURGERY

Dual-Chamber Pacing

Although the septal myotomy-myectomy operation is the first therapeutic option for severely limited patients without obstructive HCM, perhaps the major limitation of surgery is the restricted availability of surgeons with the necessary experience to readily afford patients with low operative mortality and a high expectation of hemodynamic and symptomatic success with myotomy-myectomy. In addition, some patients are not ideal surgical candidates, either due to advanced age, insufficient personal motivation, or a limiting medical disability unrelated to HCM. Therefore it is a reasonable aspiration to develop and pursue alternatives to operation for this small but important subgroup of patients. However, proper patient selection for such procedures is a paramount consideration.

Over the past several years there has been some interest in the application of permanent dual-chamber pacing, as an alternative to operative intervention, for severely symptomatic patients with obstructive HCM who are refractory to drug therapy.[192–194] Observational and uncontrolled studies have reported pacing to be associated with reduction in outflow gradient and amelioration of symptoms in many patients over relatively short time periods.[172–174] However, this reported symptomatic benefit has not been consistently accompanied by improved exercise tolerance documented by objective parameters (e.g., treadmill exercise duration and measured oxygen consumption). Randomized, double-blind, crossover pacing studies have shown that the subjectively perceived symptomatic improvement reported by patients is largely due to a placebo effect.[195–197] In addition, the effect of pacing on outflow gradient and symptoms is variable and reduction in obstruction is often much more modest than that achieved with surgery.[196,198] Other laboratory catheterization studies report dual-chamber pacing to have deleterious effects on left ventricular systolic and diastolic function.[199–201] For these reasons and because the underlying HCM disease process and the risk for sudden death do not appear to be altered by permanent dual-chamber pacing, this potential treatment modality cannot be regarded as a primary treatment for the diverse clinical and functional spectrum of HCM.[196] However, there may well be a therapeutic role for certain subsets of patients with this disease.[196,201] In one randomized study, those patients ≥65 years old showed the most convincing benefit from pacing.[196]

Alcohol Septal Ablation

A second, recently introduced potential alternative to surgery is alcohol septal ablation, in which about 2 mL of alcohol is injected directly into the first septal perforator coronary artery for the purpose of producing an MI, septal thinning, and reduced mitral valve systolic anterior motion.[202–205] This procedure is intended to mimic the morphologic and functional consequences of ventricular septal myotomy-myectomy. At present the septal ablation technique is associated with a risk similar to that of surgery but is capable of producing a substantial reduction in the basal gradient. As yet, there is little objective substantiation for the improvement in symptoms reported by many patients over short-term follow-up. This is of particular importance in assessing symptomatic and functional changes for a disease in which pathophysiology is complex and symptoms are variable, often difficult to assess by history, and subject to a placebo effect.[196] As is the case with pacing, alcohol ablation should not be regarded as a primary treatment for the disease or one capable of reducing the risk of sudden death. Indeed, there is concern[206,207] that this intervention could paradoxically increase the future long-term risk for life-threatening ventricular tachyarrhythmias and sudden death—a risk directly attributable to the intramyocardial scar produced by alcohol ablation (which is not present following myotomy-myectomy) in a patient population that already harbors an arrhythmogenic substrate and often a particularly long period of risk.

References

1. Maron BJ. Hypertrophic cardiomyopathy. *Lancet* 1997; 350: 127–133.
2. Braunwald E, Lambrew CT, Rockoff D, et al. Idiopathic hypertrophic subaortic stenosis: I. A description of the disease based upon an analysis of 64 patients. *Circulation* 1964; 30(suppl IV):3–217.
3. Maron BJ, Bonow RO, Cannon RO, et al. Hypertrophic cardiomyopathy: Interrelation of clinical manifestations, pathophysiology, and therapy. *N Engl J Med* 1987; 316:780–789, 844–852.
4. Wigle ED, Sasson Z, Henderson MA, et al. Hypertrophic cardiomyopathy: The importance of the site and extent of hypertrophy—A review. *Prog Cardiovasc Dis* 1985; 28:1–83.
5. Spirito P, Seidman CE, McKenna WJ, Maron BJ. Management of hypertrophic cardiomyopathy. *N Engl J Med* 1997; 30:775–785.
6. Wigle ED, Rakowski H, Kimball BP, et al. Hypertrophic cardiomyopathy: Clinical spectrum and treatment. *Circulation* 1995; 92:1680–1692.
7. Maron BJ, Epstein SE: Hypertrophic cardiomyopathy: A discussion of nomenclature. *Am J Cardiol* 1979; 43:1242–1244.
8. Marian AJ, Roberts R. Recent advances in the molecular genetics of hypertrophic cardiomyopathy. *Circulation* 1995; 92:1336–1347.
9. Schwartz K, Carrier L, Guicheney P, et al. Molecular basis of familial cardiomyopathies. *Circulation* 1995; 91:532–540.
10. Niimura H, Bachinski LL, Sangwatanaroj S, et al. Mutations in the gene for human cardiac myosin-binding protein C and late-onset familial hypertrophic cardiomyopathy. *N Engl J Med* 1998; 338:1248–1257.
11. Ciró E, Nichols PF, Maron BJ. Heterogeneous morphologic ex-

pression of genetically transmitted hypertrophic cardiomyopathy: Two-dimensional echocardiographic analysis. *Circulation* 1983; 67:1227–1233.
12. Maron BJ, Gottdiener JS, Epstein SE. Patterns and significance of distribution of left ventricular hypertrophy in hypertrophic cardiomyopathy: A wide-angle, two-dimensional echocardiographic study of 125 patients. *Am J Cardiol* 1981; 48:418–428.
13. Spirito P, Maron BJ, Bonow RO, et al. Severe functional limitation in patients with hypertrophic cardiomyopathy and only mild localized left ventricular hypertrophy. *J Am Coll Cardiol* 1979; 44:401–412.
14. Webb JG, Sasson Z, Rakowski H, et al. Apical hypertrophic cardiomyopathy: Clinical follow-up and diagnostic correlates. *J Am Coll Cardiol* 1990; 15:83–90.
15. Louie EK, Maron BJ. Apical hypertrophic cardiomyopathy: Clinical and two-dimensional echocardiographic assessment. *Ann Intern Med* 1987; 106:663–670.
16. Roberts CS, Roberts WC. Morphologic features. In: Zipes DP, Rowlands DJ, eds. *Progress in Cardiology 2/2.* Philadelphia: Lea & Febiger; 1989:3.
17. Olsen EG. Anatomic and light microscopic characterization of hypertrophic obstructive and non-obstructive cardiomyopathy. *Eur Heart J* 1983; 4 (suppl F):1–8.
18. Klues HG, Schiffers A, Maron BJ. Phenotypic spectrum and patterns of left ventricular hypertrophy in hypertrophic cardiomyopathy: Morphologic observations and significance as assessed by two-dimensional echocardiography in 600 patients. *J Am Coll Cardiol* 1995; 26:1699–1708.
19. Klues HG, Roberts WC, Maron BJ. Anomalous insertion of papillary muscle directly into anterior mitral leaflet in hypertrophic cardiomyopathy: Significance in producing left ventricular outflow obstruction. *Circulation* 1991; 84:1188–1197.
20. Klues HG, Maron BJ, Dollar AL, et al. Diversity of structural mitral valve alterations in hypertrophic cardiomyopathy. *Circulation* 1992; 85:1651–1660.
21. Lewis JF, Maron BJ. Elderly patients with hypertrophic cardiomyopathy: A subset with distinctive left ventricular morphology and progressive clinical course late in life. *J Am Coll Cardiol* 1989; 13:36–45.
22. Maron BJ, Moller JH, Seidman CE, et al. Impact of laboratory molecular diagnosis on contemporary diagnostic criteria for genetically transmitted cardiovascular diseases: Hypertrophic cardiomyopathy, long-QT syndrome, and Marfan syndrome. *Circulation* 1998; 98:1460–1471.
23. Liouville H. Rétrécissement ventriculo-aortique. *Gazette Med Paris* 1869; 24:161–163.
24. Schmincke A. Über linseitige muskulöse Conusstenosen. *Dtsch Med Wochenschr* 1907; 33:2082.
25. Teare D. Asymmetrical hypertrophy of the heart in young adults. *Br Heart J* 1958; 20:1–18.
26. Maron BJ, Gardin JM, Flack JM, et al. Prevalence of hypertrophic cardiomyopathy in a general population of young adults: Echocardiographic analysis of 4111 subjects in the CARDIA study. *Circulation* 1995; 92:785–789.
27. Maron BJ, Peterson EE, Maron MS, et al. Prevalence of hypertrophic cardiomyopathy in an outpatient population referred for echocardiographic study. *Am J Cardiol* 1994; 73:577–580.
28. Spirito P, Chiarella F, Carratino L, et al. Clinical course and prognosis of hypertrophic cardiomyopathy in an outpatient population. *N Engl J Med* 1989; 320:749–755.
29. Shapiro LM, Zezulka A. Hypertrophic cardiomyopathy: A common disease with a good prognosis: Five year experience of a district general hospital. *Br Heart J* 1983; 50:530–533.
30. Maron BJ, Mathenge R, Casey SA, et al. Clinical profile of hypertrophic cardiomyopathy identified de novo in rural communities. *J Am Coll Cardiol* 1999; 33:1590–1595.
31. Rosenzweig A, Watkins H, Hwang D-S, et al. Preclinical diagnosis of familial hypertrophic cardiomyopathy by genetic analysis of blood lymphocytes. *N Engl J Med* 1991; 325:1753–1760.
32. Yamaguchi H, Ishimura T, Nishiyama S, et al. Hypertrophic nonobstructive cardiomyopathy with giant negative T waves (apical hypertrophy): Ventriculographic and echocardiographic features in 30 patients. *Am J Cardiol* 1979; 44:401–412.
33. Ando H, Imaizumi T, Urabe Y, et al. Apical segmental dysfunction in hypertrophic cardiomyopathy: Subgroup with unique clinical features. *J Am Coll Cardiol* 1990; 16:1579–1588.
34. Koga Y, Itaya K-I, Toshima H. Prognosis of hypertrophic cardiomyopathy. *Am Heart J* 1984; 108:351–359.
35. Maron BJ, Spirito P, Wesley Y, et al. Development and progression of left ventricular hypertrophy in children with hypertrophic cardiomyopathy. *N Engl J Med* 1986; 315:610–614.
36. Charron P, Dubourg O, Desnos M, et al. Diagnostic value of electrocardiography and echocardiography for familial hypertrophic cardiomyopathy in a genotyped adult population. *Circulation* 1997; 96:214–219.
37. Charron P, Dubourg O, Desnos M, et al. Diagnostic value of electrocardiography and echocardiography for familial hypertrophic cardiomyopathy in genotyped children. *Eur Heart J* 1998; 19:1377–1382.
38. Watkins H, McKenna WJ, Thierfelder L, et al. The role of cardiac troponin T and α tropomyosin mutations in hypertrophic cardiomyopathy. *N Engl J Med* 1995; 332:1058–1064.
39. Moolman JC, Corfield VA, Posen B, et al. Sudden death due to troponin T mutations. *J Am Coll Cardiol* 1997; 29:549–555.
40. Maron BJ, Niimura H, Casey SA, et al. Hypertrophic cardiomyopathy in adult patients without left ventricular hypertrophy: Genotype–phenotype correlations for cardiac myosin binding protein-C mutations (abstr). *Circulation* 1998; 98(suppl I): I-596–I-597.
41. Shapiro LM, McKenna WJ. Distribution of left ventricular hypertrophy in hypertrophic cardiomyopathy: A two-dimensional echocardiographic study. *J Am Coll Cardiol* 1983; 2:437–444.
42. Maron BJ, Epstein SE, Roberts WC. Hypertrophic cardiomyopathy and transmural myocardial infarction without significant atherosclerosis of the extramural coronary arteries. *Am J Cardiol* 1979; 43:1086–1102.
43. Klues HG, Roberts WC, Maron BJ. Morphologic determinants of echocardiographic patterns of mitral valve systolic anterior motion in obstructive hypertrophic cardiomyopathy. *Circulation* 1993; 87:1570–1579.
44. Louie EK, Maron BJ. Hypertrophic cardiomyopathy with extreme increase in left ventricular wall thickness: Functional and morphologic features and clinical significance. *J Am Coll Cardiol* 1986; 8:57–65.
45. Maron BJ, Gross BJ, Stark SI. Extreme left ventricular hypertrophy. *Circulation* 1995; 92:2748.
46. Charron P, Dubourg O, Desnos M, et al. Clinical features and prognostic implications of familial hypertrophic cardiomyopathy related to the cardiac myosin-binding protein C gene. *Circulation* 1998; 97:2230–2236.
47. Lewis JF, Maron BJ. Hypertrophic cardiomyopathy characterized by marked hypertrophy of the posterior left ventricular free wall: Significance and clinical implications. *J Am Coll Cardiol* 1991; 18:421–428.
48. Alfonso F, Nihoyannopoulos P, Steward J, et al. Clinical significance of giant negative T waves in hypertrophic cardiomyopathy. *J Am Coll Cardiol* 1990; 15:965–971.
49. Sakamoto T, Tei C, Murayama M, et al. Giant T wave inversion as a manifestation of asymmetrical apical hypertrophy (AAH) of the left ventricle: Echocardiographic and ultrasono-cardiotomographic study. *Jpn Heart J* 1976; 17:611–616.
50. Maron BJ, Bonow RO, Seshagiri TN, et al. Hypertrophic cardiomyopathy with ventricular septal hypertrophy localized to the

apical region of the left ventricle (apical hypertrophic cardiomyopathy). *Am J Cardiol* 1982; 49:1838–1848.
51. Pelliccia A, Maron BJ, Spataro A, et al. The upper limit of physiologic cardiac hypertrophy in highly trained elite athletes. *N Engl J Med* 1991; 324:295–301.
52. Maron BJ, Pelliccia A, Spirito P. Cardiac disease in young trained athletes: Insights into methods for distinguishing athlete's heart from structural heart disease with particular emphasis on hypertrophic cardiomyopathy. *Circulation* 1995; 91:1596–1601.
53. Maron BJ, Verter J, Kapur S. Disproportionate ventricular septal thickening in the developing normal human heart. *Circulation* 1978; 57:520–526.
54. Skinner JR, Manzoor A, Hayes AM, et al. A regional study of presentation and outcome of hypertrophic cardiomyopathy in infants. *Heart* 1997; 77:229–223.
55. Maron BJ, Tajik AJ, Ruttenberg HD, et al. Hypertrophic cardiomyopathy in infants. Clinical features and natural history. *Circulation* 1982; 65:7–17.
56. Schaffer MS, Freedom RM, Rowe RD. Hypertrophic cardiomyopathy presenting before 2 years of age in 13 patients. *Ped Cardiol* 1983; 4:113–119.
57. Maron BJ. Hypertrophic cardiomyopathy. In: Allen HD, Gutgesell HP, Clark EB, Driscoll DJ, eds. *Moss and Adam's Heart Disease in Infants, Children and Adolescents,* 6th ed. Baltimore, MD: Lippincott Williams & Wilkins; in press.
58. Spirito P, Maron BJ. Absence of progression of left ventricular hypertrophy in adult patients with hypertrophic cardiomyopathy. *J Am Coll Cardiol* 1987; 9:1013–1017.
59. Panza JA, Maris TJ, Maron BJ. Development and determinants of dynamic obstruction to left ventricular outflow in young patients with hypertrophic cardiomyopathy. *Circulation* 1992; 85:1398–1405.
60. Panza JA, Maron BJ. Relation of electrocardiographic abnormalities to evolving left ventricular hypertrophy in hypertrophic cardiomyopathy. *Am J Cardiol* 1989; 63:1258–1265.
61. Maron BJ, Spirito P. Implications of left ventricular remodeling in hypertrophic cardiomyopathy. *Am J Cardiol* 1998; 81:1339–1344.
62. Spirito P, Maron BJ. Relation between extent of left ventricular hypertrophy and age in patients with hypertrophic cardiomyopathy. *J Am Coll Cardiol* 1989; 13:820–823.
63. Tanaka M, Fujiwara H, Onodera T, et al. Quantitative analysis of myocardial fibrosis in normals, hypertensive hearts, and hypertrophic cardiomyopathy. *Br Heart J* 1986; 55:575–581.
64. Ferrans VJ, Morrow AG, Roberts WC. Myocardial ultrastructure in idiopathic hypertrophic subaortic stenosis. A study of operatively excised left ventricular outflow tract muscle in 14 patients. *Circulation* 1972; 45:769–792.
65. Maron BJ, Roberts WC. Quantitative analysis of cardiac muscle cell disorganization in the ventricular septum of patients with hypertrophic cardiomyopathy. *Circulation* 1979; 59:689–706.
66. Maron BJ, Anan TJ, Roberts WC. Quantitative analysis of the distribution of cardiac muscle cell disorganization in the left ventricular wall of patients with hypertrophic cardiomyopathy. *Circulation* 1981; 63:882–894.
67. St. John Sutton MG, Lie JT, Anderson KR, et al. Histopathological specificity of hypertrophic obstructive cardiomyopathy. *Br Heart J* 1980; 44:433–443.
68. Fujiwara H, Kawai C, Hamashima Y. Myocardial fascicle and fiber disarray in 25 μ-thick sections. *Circulation* 1979; 59:1293–1298.
69. Maron BJ, Wolfson JK, Epstein SE, et al. Intramural ("small vessel") coronary artery disease in hypertrophic cardiomyopathy. *J Am Coll Cardiol* 1986; 8:545–557.
70. Tanaka M, Fujiwara H, Onodera T, et al. Quantitative analysis of narrowings of intramyocardial small arteries in normal hearts, hypertensive hearts, and hearts with hypertrophic cardiomyopathy. *Circulation* 1987; 75:1130–1139.
71. Maron BJ, Wolfson JK, Roberts WC. Relation between extent of cardiac muscle cell disorganization and left ventricular wall thickness in hypertrophic cardiomyopathy. *Am J Cardiol* 1992; 70:785–790.
72. Factor SM, Butany J, Sole MJ, et al. Pathologic fibrosis and matrix connective tissue in the subaortic myocardium of patients with hypertrophic cardiomyopathy. *J Am Coll Cardiol* 1991; 17:1343–1351.
73. Shirani J, Pick R, Roberts WC, et al. Morphology and significance of the left ventricular collagen network in young patients with hypertrophic cardiomyopathy and sudden cardiac death. *J Am Coll Cardiol.* 2000; 35:36–44.
74. Maron BJ, Shen W-K, Link MS, et al. Efficacy of implantable cardioverter-defibrillators for the prevention of sudden death in patients with hypertrophic cardiomyopathy. *N Engl J Med.* 2000; 342:365–373.
75. O'Gara PT, Bonow RO, Maron BJ, et al. Myocardial perfusion abnormalities in patients with hypertrophic cardiomyopathy: Assessment with thallium-201 emission computed tomography. *Circulation* 1987; 76:1214–1223.
76. Watkins H, Rosenzweig A, Hwang D-S, et al. Characteristics and prognostic implications of myosin missense mutations in familial hypertrophic cardiomyopathy. *N Engl J Med* 1992; 326:1108–1114.
77. Maron BJ, Nichols PF, Pickle LW, et al. Patterns of inheritance in hypertrophic cardiomyopathy: Assessment of M-mode and two-dimensional echocardiography. *Am J Cardiol* 1984; 53:1087–1094.
78. Coviello DA, Maron BJ, Spirito P, et al. Clinical features of hypertrophic cardiomyopathy caused by mutation of a "hot spot" in the alpha-tropomyosin gene. *J Am Coll Cardiol* 1997; 29:635–640.
79. Morgensen J, Klausen IbC, Pedersen AK, et al. α-Cardiac actin is a novel disease gene in familial hypertrophic cardiomyopathy. *J Clin Invest* 1999; 103:R39–R43.
80. Kimura A, Harada H, Park J-E, et al. Mutations in the cardiac troponin I gene associated with hypertrophic cardiomyopathy. *Nature Genet* 1997; 16:379–382.
81. Yamauchi-Takihara K, Nakajima-Taniguchi C, Matsui H, et al. Cardiomyopathy associated with mutations in the α-tropomyosin gene. *Heart* 1996; 76:63–65.
82. Anan R, Greve G, Thierfelder L, et al. Prognostic implications of novel β cardiac myosin heavy chain gene mutations that cause familial hypertrophic cardiomyopathy. *J Clin Invest* 1994; 93:280–285.
83. Flavigny J, Richard P, Isnard R, et al. Identification of two novel mutations in the ventricular regulatory myosin light chain gene (MYL2) associated with familial and classical forms of hypertrophic cardiomyopathy. *J Mol Med* 1998; 76:208–214.
84. Thierfelder L, Watkins H, MacRae C, et al. α-Tropomyosin and cardiac troponin T mutations cause familial hypertrophic cardiomyopathy: A disease of the sarcomere. *Cell* 1994; 77:701–712.
85. Maron BJ, Lipson LC, Roberts WC, et al. "Malignant" hypertrophic cardiomyopathy: Identification of a subgroup of families with unusually frequent premature death. *Am J Cardiol* 1978; 41:1133–1140.
86. Maron BJ, Shirani J, Poliac LC, et al. Sudden death in young competitive athletes: Clinical, demographic and pathological profiles. *JAMA* 1996; 276:199–204.
87. McKenna WJ, Stewart JT, Nihoyannopoulos P, et al. Hypertrophic cardiomyopathy without hypertrophy: Two families with myocardial disarray in the absence of increased myocardial mass. *Br Heart J* 1990; 63:287–290.
88. Maron BJ, Kragel AH, Roberts WC. Sudden death due to hypertrophic cardiomyopathy in the absence of increased left ventricular mass. *Br Heart J* 1990; 63:308–310.
89. Maron BJ, Isner JM, McKenna WJ. Hypertrophic cardiomyopa-

thy, myocarditis and other myopericardial disease, and mitral valve prolapse. Task Force 3. In: 26th Bethesda Conference. Recommendations for determining eligibility for competition in athletes with cardiovascular abnormalities. *J Am Coll Cardiol* 1994; 24:880–885.
90. Lechin M, Quiñones MA, Omran A, et al. Angiotensin-I converting enzyme genotypes and left ventricular hypertrophy in patients with hypertrophic cardiomyopathy. *Circulation* 1995; 92:1808–1812.
91. Cannon RO, Rosing DR, Maron BJ, et al. Myocardial ischemia in hypertrophic cardiomyopathy: Contribution of inadequate vasodilator reserve and elevated left ventricular filling pressures. *Circulation* 1985; 71:234–243.
92. Maron BJ, Spirito P, Green KJ, et al. Noninvasive assessment of left ventricular diastolic function by pulsed Doppler echocardiography in patients with hypertrophic cardiomyopathy. *J Am Coll Cardiol* 1987; 10:733–742.
93. Bonow RO, Fredrick TM, Bacharach SL, et al. Atrial systole and left ventricular filling in patients with hypertrophic cardiomyopathy: Effect of verapamil. *Am J Cardiol* 1983; 51:1386–1391.
94. Pollick C, Rakowski H, Wigle ED. Muscular subaortic stenosis: The quantitative relationship between systolic anterior motion and pressure gradient. *Circulation* 1984; 69:43–49.
95. Maron BJ, Epstein SE. Clinical significance and therapeutic implications of the left ventricular outflow tract pressure gradient in hypertrophic cardiomyopathy. *Am J Cardiol* 1986; 11:752–756.
96. Sherrid MV, Chu CK, Delia E, et al. An echocardiographic study of the fluid mechanics of obstruction in hypertrophic cardiomyopathy. *J Am Coll Cardiol* 1993; 22:816–825.
97. Cape EG, Simons D, Jimoh A, et al. Chordal geometry determines the shape and extent of systolic anterior motion. *J Am Coll Cardiol* 1989; 13:1438–1448.
98. Klues HG, Leuner C, Kuhn H. Hypertrophic obstructive cardiomyopathy: No increase of the gradient during exercise. *J Am Coll Cardiol* 1991; 19:527–533.
99. Briguori C, Betocchi S, Romano M, et al. Exercise capacity in hypertrophic cardiomyopathy depends on left ventricular diastolic function. *Am J Cardiol* 1999; 84:309–315.
100. Lazzeroni E, Picano E, Morozzi L, et al. Dipyridamole-induced ischemia as a prognostic marker of future adverse cardiac events in adult patients with hypertrophic cardiomypathy. *Circulation* 1997; 96:4268–4272.
101. Yamada M, Elliott PM, Kaski JC, et al. Dipyradimole stress thallium-201 perfusion abnormalities in patients with hypertrophic cardiomyopathy: Relationship to clinical presentation and outcome. *Eur Heart J* 1998; 19:500–507.
102. Spirito P, Maron BJ. Patterns of systolic anterior motin of the mitral valve in hypertrophic cardiomyopathy: Assessment by two-dimensional echocardiography. *Am J Cardiol* 1984; 54:1039–1046.
103. Maron BJ, Harding AM, Spirito P, et al. Systolic anterior motion of the posterior mitral leaflet: A previously unrecognized cause of dynamic subaortic obstruction in hypertrophic cardiomyopathy. *Circulation* 1983; 68:282–293.
104. Schwammenthal E, Block M, Schwartzkopff B, et al. Prediction of the site and severity of obstruction in hypertrophic cardiomyopathy by color flow mapping and continuous wave Doppler echocardiography. *J Am Coll Cardiol* 1992; 20:964–972.
105. Panza JA, Petrone RK, Fananapazir L, et al. Utility of continuous wave Doppler in noninvasive assessment of the left ventricular outflow tract reassure gradient in patients with hypertrophic cardiomyopathy. *J Am Coll Cardiol* 1992; 19:91–99.
106. Petrone RK, Klues HG, Panza JA, et al. Significance of the occurrence of mitral valve prolapse in patients with hypertrophic cardiomyopathy. *J Am Coll Cardiol* 1992; 20:55–61.
107. Fighali S, Krajcer Z, Edelman S, et al. Progression of hypertrophic cardiomyopathy into a hypokinetic left ventricle: Higher incidence in patients with midventricular obstruction. *J Am Coll Cardiol* 1987; 9:288–294.
108. Fiddler GI, Tajik AJ, Weidman WH, et al. Idiopathic hypertrophic subaortic stenosis in the young. *Am J Cardiol* 1978; 42:793–799.
109. Maron BJ, McIntosh CL, Klues HG, et al. Morphologic basis for obstruction to right ventricular outflow in hypertrophic cardiomyopathy. *Am J Cardiol* 1993; 71:1089–1094.
110. Lele SS, Thomson HL, Seo H, et al. Exercise capacity in hypertrophic cardiomyopathy: Role of stroke volume limitation, heart rate and diastolic filling characteristics. *Circulation* 1995; 92:2886–2894.
111. Frenneaux MP, Porter A, Caforio ALP, et al. Determinants of exercise capacity in hypertrophic cardiomyopathy. *J Am Coll Cardiol* 1992; 19:1521–1526.
112. Chikamori T, Counihan PJ, Doi YL, et al. Mechanisms of exercise limitations in hypertrophic cardiomyopathy. *J Am Coll Cardiol* 1992; 19:507–512.
113. Spirito P, Maron BJ. Relation between extent of left ventricular hypertrophy and diastolic filling abnormalities in hypertrophic cardiomyopathy. *J Am Coll Cardiol* 1990; 15:808–813.
114. Pasternac A, Noble J, Streulens Y, et al. Pathophysiology of chest pain in patients with cardiomyopathies and normal coronary arteries. *Circulation* 1982; 65:778–789.
115. Elliott PM, Kaski JC, Prasad K, et al. Chest pain during daily life in patients with hypertrophic cardiomyopathy: An ambulatory electrocardiographic study. *Eur Heart J* 1996; 17:1056–1064.
116. Maron BJ, Wolfson JK, Ciró E, et al. Relation of electrocardiographic abnormalities and patterns of left ventricular hypertrophy identified by two-dimensional echocardiography in patients with hypertrophic cardiomyopathy. *Am J Cardiol* 1983; 51:189–194.
117. Glover DW, Maron BJ. Profile of preparticipation cardiovascular screening for high school athletes. *JAMA* 1998; 279:1817–1819.
118. Maron BJ, Thompson PD, Puffer JC, et al. Cardiovascular preparticipation screening of competitive athletes. *Circulation* 1996; 94:850–856.
119. Pfister GC, Puffer JC, Maron BJ. Preparticipation cardiovascular screening for U.S. collegiate student-athletes. *JAMA* 2000; 283:1597–1599.
120. Corrado D, Basso C, Schiavon M, et al. Screening for hypertrophic cardiomyopathy in young athletes. *N Engl J Med* 1998; 339:364–369.
121. Kyriakidis M, Triposkiadis F, Anastassakis A, et al. Hypertrophic cardiomyopathy in Greece: Clinical course and outcome. *Chest* 1998; 114:1091–1096.
122. Maron BJ, Casey SA, Poliac LC, et al. Clinical course of hypertrophic cardiomyopathy in a regional United States cohort. *JAMA* 1999; 281:650–655.
123. Maron BJ, Spirito P. Impact of patient selection biases on the perception of hypertrophic cardiomyopathy and its natural history. *Am J Cardiol* 1993; 72:970–972.
124. Maron BJ, Roberts WC, Epstein SE. Sudden death in hypertrophic cardiomyopathy: A profile of 78 patients. *Circulation* 1982; 67:1388–1394.
125. McKenna WJ, Deanfield JE. Hypertrophic cardiomyopathy: An important cause of sudden death. *Arch Dis Child* 1984; 59:971–975.
126. Hecht GM, Panza JA, Maron BJ. Clinical course of middle-aged asymptomatic patients with hypertrophic cardiomyopathy. *Am J Cardiol* 1992; 69:935–940.
127. Adelman AG, Wigle ED, Ranganathan N, et al. The clinical course in muscular subaortic stenosis: A retrospective and prospective study of 60 hemodynamically proved cases. *Ann Intern Med* 1972; 77:515–525.
128. McKenna WJ, Deanfield JE, Faroqui A, et al. Prognosis in hypertrophic cardiomyopathy: Role of age and clinical electrocardio-

graphic and hemodynamic features. *Am J Cardiol* 1981; 47:532–538.

129. Shah PM, Adelman AG, Wigle ED, et al. The natural (and unnatural) history of hypertrophic obstructive cardiomyopathy. *Circ Res* 1973; 34,35 (suppl II):II-179–II-195.
130. Frank S, Braunwald E. Idiopathic hypertrophic subaortic stenosis: Clinical analysis of 126 patients with emphasis on the natural history. *Circulation* 1968; 37:759–788.
131. Kofflard MJ, Waldstein DJ, Vos J, et al. Prognosis in hypertrophic cardiomyopathy: A retrospective study. *Am J Cardiol* 1993; 72:939–943.
132. Spirito P, Rapezzi C, Autore C, et al. Prognosis in asymptomatic patients with hypertrophic cardiomyopathy and nonsustained ventricular tachycardia. *Circulation* 1994; 90:2743–2747.
133. Cannan CR, Reeder GS, Bailey KR, et al. Natural history of hypertrophic cardiomyopathy: A population-based study, 1976 through 1990. *Circulation* 1995; 92:2488–2499.
134. Cecchi F, Olivotto I, Montereggi A, et al. Hypertrophic cardiomyopathy in Tuscany: Clinical course and outcome in an unselected regional population. *J Am Coll Cardiol* 1995; 26:1529–1536.
135. Takagi E, Yamakado T, Nakano T. Prognosis of completely asymptomatic adult patients with hypertrophic cardiomyopathy. *J Am Coll Cardiol* 1999; 33:206–211.
136. Maki S, Ikeda H, Muro A, et al. Predictors of sudden cardiac death in hypertrophic cardiomyopathy. *Am J Cardiol* 1998; 82:774–778.
137. Maron BJ, Kogan J, Proschan MA, et al. Circadian variability in the occurrence of sudden cardiac death in patients with hypertrophic cardiomyopathy. *J Am Coll Cardiol* 1994; 23:1405–1409.
138. Maron BJ. Cardiovascular risks to young persons on the athletic field. *Ann Intern Med* 1998; 129:379–386.
139. Olivotto I, Maron BJ, Montereggi A, et al. Prognostic value of systemic blood pressure response during exercise in a community-based patient population with hypertrophic cardiomyopathy. *J Am Coll Cardiol* 1999; 33:2044–2051.
140. Sadoul N, Prasas L, Elliott PM, et al. Prospective diagnostic assessment of blood pressure response during exercise in patients with hypertrophic cardiomyopathy. *Circulation* 1997; 96:2987–2991.
141. Nicod P, Polikar R, Peterson KL. Hypertrophic cardiomyopathy and sudden death. *N Engl J Med* 1988; 318:1255–1257.
142. Stafford WJ, Trohman RG, Bilsker M, et al. Cardiac arrest in an adolescent with atrial fibrillation and hypertrophic cardiomyopathy. *J Am Coll Cardiol* 1985; 7:701–704.
143. Krikler DM, Davies MJ, Rowland E, et al. Sudden death in hypertrophic cardiomyopathy: Associated accessory atrioventricular pathways. *Br Heart J* 1980; 43:245–251.
144. Elliott PM, Sharma S, Varnava A, et al. Survival after cardiac arrest in patients with hypertrophic cardiomyopathy. *J Am Coll Cardiol* 1999; 33:1596–1601.
145. Yetman AT, McCrindle BW, MacDonald LC, et al. Myocardial bridging in children with hypertrophic cardiomyopathy—A risk factor for sudden death. *N Engl J Med* 1998; 339:1201–1209.
146. Maron BJ, Fananapazir L. Sudden cardiac death in hypertrophic cardiomyopathy. *Circulation* 1992; 85(suppl I):I-57–I-63.
147. Spirito P, Bellone P, Harris KM, et al. Magnitude of left ventricular hypertrophy predicts sudden death in hypertrophic cardiomyopathy. *N Engl J Med* 2000; 342:1778–1785.
148. Spirito P, Maron BJ. Relation between extent of left ventricular hypertrophy and occurrence of sudden cardiac death in hypertrophic cardiomyopathy. *J Am Coll Cardiol* 1990; 15:1521–2526.
149. Cecchi F, Maron BJ, Epstein SE. Long-term outcome of patients with hypertrophic cardiomyopathy successfully resuscitated after cardiac arrest. *J Am Coll Cardiol* 1989; 13:1283–1288.
150. Kuck K-H, Kunze KP, Schlueter M, et al. Programmed electrical stimulation in hypertrophic cardiomyopathy: Results in patients with and without cardiac arrest or syncope. *Eur Heart J* 1988; 9:177–185.
151. Hecht GM, Klues HG, Roberts WC, et al. Coexistence of sudden cardiac death and end-stage heart failure in familial hypertrophic cardiomyopathy. *J Am Coll Cardiol* 1993; 22:489–497.
152. Maron BJ, Hecht G, Klues HG, et al. Both aborted sudden cardiac death and end-stage phase in hypertrophic cardiomyopathy. *Am J Cardiol* 1993; 72:363–365.
153. Fay WP, Taliercio CP, Ilstrup DM, et al. Natural history of hypertrophic cardiomyopathy in the elderly. *J Am Coll Cardiol* 1990; 16:821–826.
154. Lever HM, Kuram RF, Currie PH, et al. Hypertrophic cardiomyopathy in the elderly: Distinctions from the young based on cardiac shape. *Circulation* 1989; 79:580–589.
155. Lewis JF, Maron BJ. Clinical and morphologic expression of hypertrophic cardiomyopathy in patients ≥65 years of age. *Am J Cardiol* 1994; 73:1105–1111.
156. Chikamori T, Doi YL, Yonezawa Y, et al. Comparison of clinical features in patients ≥60 years of age to those 40 years of age with hypertrophic cardiomyopathy. *Am J Cardiol* 1990; 66:875–877.
157. Silka MJ, Kron J, Dunnigan A, et al. Sudden cardiac death and the use of implantable cardioverter-defibrillators in pediatric patients. *Circulation* 1993; 87:800–807.
158. McKenna WJ, Oakley CM, Krikler DM, et al. Improved survival with amiodarone in patients with hypertrophic cardiomyopathy and ventricular tachycardia. *Br Heart J* 1985; 53:412–416.
159. Louie EK, Edwards LC. Hypertrophic cardiomyopathy. *Prog Cardiovasc Dis* 1994; 36:275–308.
160. Kaltenbach M, Hopf R, Kober G, et al. Treatment of hypertrophic obstructive cardiomyopathy with verapamil. *Br Heart J* 1979; 42:35–42.
161. Rosing DR, Condit JR, Maron BJ, et al. Verapamil therapy: A new approach to the pharmacologic treatment of hypertrophic cardiomyopathy: III. Effects of long-term administration. *Am J Cardiol* 1981; 48:545–553.
162. Sherrid M, Delia E, Dwyer E. Oral disopyramide therapy for obstructive hypertrophic cardiomyopathy. *Am J Cardiol* 1988; 62:1085–1088.
163. Pollick C. Muscular subaortic stenosis: Hemodynamic and clinical improvement after disopyramide. *N Engl J Med* 1982; 307: 997–999.
164. Sherrid MV, Pearle G, Gunsburg DZ. Mechanism of benefit of negative inotropes in obstructive hypertrophic cardiomyopathy. *Circulation* 1998; 97:41–47.
165. Shirani J, Maron BJ, Cannon RO, et al. Clinicopathologic features of hypertrophic cardiomyopathy managed by cardiac transplantation. *Am J Cardiol* 1993; 72:434–440.
166. Spirito P, Rapezzi C, Bellone P, et al. Infective endocarditis in hypertrophic cardiomyopathy: Prevalence, incidence and indications for antibiotic prophylaxis. *Circulation* 1999; 99:2132–2137.
167. Roberts WC, Kishel JC, McIntosh CL, et al. Severe mitral or aortic valve regurgitation, or both, requiring valve replacement for infective endocarditis complicating hypertrophic cardiomyopathy. *J Am Coll Cardiol* 1992; 19:365–377.
168. Spirito P, Lakatos E, Maron BJ. Degree of left ventricular hypertrophy in chronic atrial fibrillation in hypertrophic cardiomyopathy. *Am J Cardiol* 1992; 69:1217–1222.
169. Robinson KC, Frenneaux MP, Stockins B, et al. Atrial fibrillation in hypertrophic cardiomyopathy: A longitudinal study. *J Am Coll Cardiol* 1990; 15:1279–1285.
170. Morrow AG, Reitz BA, Epstein SE, et al. Operative treatment in hypertrophic subaortic stenosis: Techniques and the results of pre- and postoperative assessments in 83 patients. *Circulation* 1975; 52:88–102.
171. Williams WG, Wigle ED, Rakowski H, et al. Results of surgery for hypertrophic obstructive cardiomyopathy. *Circulation* 1987; 76(suppl V):104–108.

172. McCully RB, Nishimura RA, Tajik AJ, et al. Extent of clinical improvement after surgical treatment of hypertrophic obstructive cardiomyopathy. *Circulation* 1996; 94:467–471.
173. Robbins RC, Stinson EB. Long-term results of left ventricular myotomy and myectomy for obstructive hypertrophic cardiomyopathy. *J Thorac Cardiovasc Surg* 1996; 111:586–594.
174. Schoendube FA, Klues HG, Reigh S, et al. Long-term clinical and echocardiographic follow-up after surgical correction of hypertrophic obstructive cardiomyopathy with extended myectomy and reconstruction of the subvalvular mitral apparatus. *Circulation* 1995; 92(suppl II):II-122–II-127.
175. Schulte HD, Bircks WH, Loesse B, et al. Prognosis of patients with hypertrophic obstructive cardiomyopathy after transaortic myectomy: Late results up to twenty-five years. *J Thorac Cardiovasc Surg* 1993; 106:709–717.
176. Maron BJ, Epstein SE, Morrow AG. Symptomatic status and prognosis of patients after operation for hypertrophic obstructive cardiomyopathy: Efficacy of ventricular septal myotomy and myectomy. *Eur Heart J* 1983; 4(suppl F):175–185.
177. Krajcer Z, Leachman RD, Cooley DA, et al. Septal myotomy-myectomy versus mitral valve replacement in hypertrophic cardiomyopathy: Ten-year follow-up in 185 patients. *Circulation* 1989; 80(suppl I):I-57–I-64.
178. Mohr R, Schaff HV, Danielson GK, et al. The outcome of surgical treatment of hypertrophic obstructive cardiomyopathy: Experience over 15 years. *J Thorac Cardiovasc Surg* 1989; 97:666–674.
179. McIntosh CL, Maron BJ. Current operative treatment of obstructive hypertrophic cardiomyopathy. *Circulation* 1988; 78:487–495.
180. Cohn LH, Trehan H, Collin JJ. Long-term follow-up of patients undergoing myotomy-myectomy for obstructive hypertrophic cardiomyopathy. *Am J Cardiol* 1992; 70:657–660.
181. ten Berg JM, Maarten JS, Knaepen PJ, et al. Hypertrophic obstructive cardiomyopathy: Initial results and long-term follow-up after Morrow septal myectomy. *Circulation* 1994; 90:1781–1785.
182. Heric B, Lytle BW, Miller DP, et al. Surgical management of hypertrophic obstructive cardiomyopathy: Early and late results. *J Thorac Cardiovasc Surg* 1995; 110:195–208.
183. Theodoro DA, Danielson GK, Feldt RH, et al. Hypertrophic cardiomyopathy in pediatric patients: Results of surgical treatment. *J Thorac Cardiovasc Surg* 1996; 112:1589–1599.
184. McIntosh CL, Greenberg CJ, Maron BJ, et al. Clinical and hemodynamic results after mitral valve replacement in patients with obstructive hypertrophic cardiomyopathy. *Ann Thorac Surg* 1989; 47:236–246.
185. McIntosh CL, Maron BJ, Cannon RO, et al. Initial results of combined anterior mitral leaflet plication and ventricular septal myotomy-myectomy for relief of left ventricular outflow tract obstruction in patients with hypertrophic cardiomyopathy. *Circulation* 1992; 86:II-60–II-67.
186. Maron BJ, Nishimura RA, Danielson GK. Pitfalls in clinical recognition and a novel operative approach for hypertrophic cardiomyopathy with severe outflow obstruction due to anomalous papillary muscle. *Circulation* 1998; 98:2505–2508.
187. Marwick TH, Stewart WJ, Lever HM, et al. Benefits of intraoperative echocardiography in the surgical management of hypertrophic cardiomyopathy. *J Am Coll Cardiol* 1992; 20:1066–1072.
188. Grigg LE, Wigle ED, Williams WG, et al. Transesophageal Doppler echocardiography in obstructive hypertrophic cardiomyopathy: Clarification of pathophysiology and importance in intraoperative decision making. *J Am Coll Cardiol* 1992; 20:41–52.
189. Maron BJ, Merrill WH, Freier PA, et al. Long-term clinical course and symptomatic status of patients after operation for hypertrophic subaortic stenosis. *Circulation* 1978; 57:1205–1213.
190. Siegman IL, Maron BJ, Permut LC, et al. Results of operation for coexistent obstructive hypertrophic cardiomyopathy and coronary artery disease. *J Am Coll Cardiol* 1989; 13:1527–1533.
191. Cannon RO, McIntosh CL, Schenke WH, et al. Effect of surgical reduction of left ventricular outflow obstruction on hemodynamics, coronary flow, and myocardial metabolism in hypertrophic cardiomyopathy. *Circulation* 1989; 79:766–775.
192. Jeanrenaud X, Goy J-J, Kappenberger L. Effects of dual-chamber pacing in hypertrophic obstructive cardiomyopathy. *Lancet* 1992; 339:1318–1323.
193. Fananapazir L, Epstein ND, Curiel RV, et al. Long-term results of dual-chamber (DDD) pacing in obstructive hypertrophic cardiomyopathy: Evidence for progressive, symptomatic and hemodynamic improvement and reduction of left ventricular hypertrophy. *Circulation* 1994; 90:2731–2742.
194. Slade AKB, Sadoul N, Shapiro L, et al. DDD pacing in hypertrophic cardiomyopathy. A multicentre clinical experience. *Heart* 1996; 75:44–49.
195. Nishimura RA, Trusty JM, Hayes DL, et al. Dual-chamber pacing for hypertrophic cardiomyopathy: A randomized, double-blind, crossover trial. *J Am Coll Cardiol* 1997; 29:435–441.
196. Maron BJ, Nishimura RA, McKenna WJ, et al. Assessment of permanent dual-chamber pacing as a treatment for drug-refractory symptomatic patients with obstructive hypertrophic cardiomyopathy: A randomized, double-blind cross-over study (M-PATHY). *Circulation* 1999; 99:2927–2933.
197. Linde C, Gadler F, Kappenberger L, et al. Placebo effect of pacemaker implantation in obstructive hypertrophic cardiomyopathy. *Am J Cardiol* 1999; 83:903–907.
198. Ommen SR, Nishimura RA, Squires RW, et al. Comparison of dual-chamber pacing versus septal myectomy for the treatment of patients with hypertrophic obstructive cardiomyopathy: Early and late results. *J Thorac Cardiovasc Surg* 1995; 110:195–208.
199. Nishimura RA, Hayes DL, Holmes DR, et al. Effects of dual-chamber pacing on systolic and diastolic function in patients with hypertrophic cardiomyopathy: Acute Doppler echocardiographic and catheterization hemodynamic study. *J Am Coll Cardiol* 1996; 27:427–430.
200. Betocchi S, Losi M-A, Piscione F, et al. Effects of dual-chamber pacing in hypertrophic cardiomyopathy on left ventricular outflow tract obstruction and on diastolic function. *Am J Cardiol* 1996; 77:498–502.
201. Kappenberger L, Linde C, Daubert C, et al. Pacing in hypertrophic obstructive cardiomyopathy: A randomized crossover study. *Eur Heart J* 1997; 18:1249–1256.
202. Seggewiss H, Gleichman U, Faber L, et al. Percutaneous transluminal septal myocardial ablation in hypertrophic obstructive cardiomyopathy: Acute results and 3-month follow-up on 25 patients. *J Am Coll Cardiol* 1998; 31:252–258.
203. Knight C, Kurbaan AS, Seggwiss H, et al. Nonsurgical septal reduction for hypertrophic obstructive cardiomyopathy: Outcome in the first series of patients. *Circulation* 1997; 95:2075–2081.
204. Lakkis NM, Nagueh SF, Kleiman NS, et al. Echocardiography-guided ethanol septal reduction for hypertrophic obstructive cardiomyopathy. *Circulation* 1998; 98:1750–1755.
205. Geitzen FH, Leuner ChJ, Raute-Kreinsen U, et al. Acute and long-term results after transcoronary ablation of septal hypertrophy (TASH): Catheter interventional treatment for hypertrophic cardiomyopathy. *Eur Heart J* 1999; 20:1342–1354.
206. Maron BJ. New interventions for obstructive hypertrophic cardiomyopathy: Promise and prudence (editorial). *Eur Heart J* 1999; 20:1292–1294.
207. Spirito P, Maron BJ. Perspectives on the role of new treatment strategies in hypertrophic obstructive cardiomyopathy (editorial). *J Am Coll Cardiol* 1999; 33:1071–1075.

CHAPTER 68

RESTRICTIVE, OBLITERATIVE, AND INFILTRATIVE CARDIOMYOPATHIES

Brian D. Hoit

RESTRICTIVE CARDIOMYOPATHY

Definition of Restrictive Cardiomyopathy

The World Health Organization (WHO) and World Heart Foundation define cardiomyopathies as heart muscle diseases of unknown etiology and classify them according to hemodynamic and pathophysiologic criteria.[1] Although this definition differentiates primary cardiomyopathies from other pathologic processes that disturb myocardial function—such as ischemic, hypertensive, valvular, and congenital heart diseases—the WHO classification, despite recent modifications, remains controversial. The clinicopathologic classification scheme initially proposed by Goodwin is similar and includes dilated or congestive, hypertrophic, and restrictive forms.[2] *Restrictive cardiomyopathy* refers to either an idiopathic or systemic myocardial disorder characterized by restrictive filling, normal or reduced left ventricular (LV) and right ventricular (RV) volumes, and normal or nearly normal systolic (LV and RV) function. Thus, the clinical and hemodynamic picture thus simulates constrictive pericarditis and is characterized by elevated venous pressure with prominent X and Y descents, a small or normal sized LV, and pulmonary congestion. Restrictive cardiomyopathy may be noninfiltrative or infiltrative and occurs with or without obliteration; infiltration may be interstitial (e.g., amyloid, sarcoid) or cellular (e.g., hemochromatosis).

Restrictive cardiomyopathy has assumed importance in clinical cardiology for several reasons. First, these myocardial disorders epitomize diastolic heart failure; thus, abnormal ventricular diastolic compliance and impaired ventricular filling constitute their central pathophysiologic components and congestion and elevated diastolic pressure are their major clinical and hemodynamic manifestations. Second, the hemodynamic and clinical manifestations may mimic those produced by constrictive pericarditis, which, in contrast to restrictive cardiomyopathy, is a surgically curable disorder. Accordingly, its lack of recognition may have dire consequences. Third, restrictive cardiomyopathy may present with interventricular conduction delays, heart block, or skeletal muscle disease, often making the diagnosis difficult. Fourth, diagnostic criteria for restriction are not universally accepted, and the morphologic spectrum overlaps with hypertrophic cardiomyopathy challenges our traditional concepts of classification.[3] Finally, a comprehensive echo Doppler assessment has become an important, noninvasive means of detecting the pathophysiology, morphology, and prognosis of the restrictive cardiomyopathies.[4,5]

Clinical Features of Restrictive Cardiomyopathy

Involvement of the myocardium (or endomyocardium), and ventricular obliteration, may occur either in isolation or in the setting of systemic or iatrogenic disease (Table 68-1). Thus, in the strictest sense, restrictive cardiomyopathy is not necessarily a primary disease of heart muscle. Irrespective of the etiology, terminology, or the nature of myocardial process, the ventricles are small (generally $<110\ mL/m^2$), and stiff, restricting ventricular filling. Despite normal (or near normal) systolic function, ventricular diastolic, jugular, and pulmonary venous pressures are increased. Typically, LV filling pressures exceed RV filling pressures by more than 5 mmHg, but equalization of the diastolic pressures and a "square root" dip and plateau of early diastolic pressures of the RV and LV may be seen if the compliances of these chambers are similarly affected. Importantly, the hemodynamics of constrictive pericarditis may be simulated. Moreover, elevated atrial pressures produce symptoms of systemic and pulmonary venous congestion (dyspnea, orthopnea, edema, abdominal discomfort), and relatively underfilled ventricles are responsible for reduced cardiac output and fatigue. In patients with restrictive cardiomyopathy as part of a systemic disorder, cardiac symptoms may dominate or overshadow symptoms referable to other organ systems. Patients with constrictive cardiomyopathy generally have lower RV systolic pressures (<40 mmHg) and an RV end-diastolic pressure greater than one-third of the pressure RV systolic pressure as opposed to patients with restrictive cardiomyopathy but these differences are far from absolute.

Physical Findings

Physical examination reflects the elevated systemic and pulmonary venous pressure. Striking elevation of the jugular venous

TABLE 68-1 Classification of the Restrictive Cardiomyopathies

Myocardial
1. Noninfiltrative cardiomyopathies
Idiopathic
Familial
Pseudoxanthoma elasticum
Scleroderma
2. Infiltrative cardiomyopathies
Amyloidosis
Sarcoidosis
Gaucher's disease
3. Storage disease
Hemochromatosis
Fabry's disease
Glycogen storage diseases
Endomyocardial
1. Obliterative
Endomyocardial fibrosis
Hypereosinophilic syndrome
2. Nonobliterative
Carcinoid
Malignant infiltration
Iatrogenic (radiation, drugs)

pulse and prominent X and especially Y descents are characteristic (see Chap. 10). A *diastolic* arterial pulse, owing to a reduced stroke volume and tachycardia, may be seen in severe cases. The apical impulse is not displaced and systolic murmurs of atrioventricular regurgitation and filling sounds marking the abrupt cessation of rapid early diastolic filling may be present.

Diagnostic/Imaging Studies

Electrocardiographic (ECG) abnormalities such as abnormal voltage, atrial and ventricular arrhythmias, and conduction disturbances are frequent; when restrictive cardiomyopathy is due to amyloid infiltration, low voltage is usual (Fig. 68-1). The chest radiograph usually reveals normal-sized ventricles, although atrial enlargement and pericardial effusion may produce an enlarged cardiac silhouette. Pleural effusions and signs of pulmonary congestion may also be present. Echocardiographic findings are nonspecific but in many cases are useful to exculpate other, more common causes of heart failure.

DIFFERENTIATION FROM CONSTRICTIVE PERICARDITIS

Although several clinical, imaging, and hemodynamic features are helpful in distinguishing restrictive cardiomyopathy from constrictive pericarditis (Table 68-2), considerable overlap and diagnostic confusion exist. The pathophysiologic basis for this distinction includes (1) transmission of intrathoracic pressure to the ventricles (limited by the stiff pericardium in constrictive pericarditis but not in restrictive cardiomyopathy); (2) the principal determinant of the diastolic ventricular pressure-volume relation (ventricular versus pericardial compliance in restrictive cardiomyopathy as compared to constrictive pericarditis, itself); and (3) involvement of the ventricular septum in restrictive cardiomyopathy versus the capacity for ventricular interdependence in constrictive pericarditis.

Recently, Doppler techniques (spectral Doppler, color M-mode, and Doppler tissue imaging) have assumed an important role in characterizing the nature of transvalvular filling and in clinically distinguishing between constrictive pericarditis and restrictive cardiomyopathy (see also Chap. 13).[5-7] These Doppler flow patterns and the associated respiratory changes are illustrated in Fig. 68-2. In the *normal subject,* the early filling wave (E) of mitral flow is greater than the late, atrial systolic wave (A), and neither change significantly with respiration. In contrast, the E and A velocities of tricuspid valve flow increase slightly with inspiration. The deceleration time of the LV early diastolic wave ranges from 150 to 240 ms, and the LV isovolumic relaxation time ranges from 70 to 110 ms. Pulmonary venous flow is generally biphasic, with a dominant wave during systole (S) and a smaller wave during diastole (D); respiratory changes are minimal and atrial systolic reversals are generally small. Hepatic vein flow consists of a larger S and smaller D wave with small reversals (V_r and A_r) after each wave, respectively. With expiration, S and D waves decrease and V_r and A_r increase. Doppler tissue imaging (DTI) shows a prominent longitudinal axis velocity in early diastole (E_a >8 cm/s) and a smaller velocity after atrial contraction (A_a). The slope of early diastolic LV filling on color M-mode (Vp) is >45 cm/s. In the patient with *restrictive cardiomyopathy*, mitral valve flow shows an increased E/A ratio (≥2) with a short (<150 ms) deceleration time and a short (<70 ms) isovolumic relaxation time (a "restrictive" pattern of filling) without respiratory variation. The tricuspid valve flow shows an increased E/A ratio without respiratory variation, a shortened deceleration time, and a short isovolumic relaxation time that shortens further with inspiration. The S/D ratio of pulmonary venous flow is <1, atrial reversals are increased (not shown in Fig. 68-1), and there is little respiratory variation. The S/D ratio of hepatic venous flow is <1 and prominent reversals are seen during inspiration. Doppler tissue imaging shows a striking decrease in E_a (<8 cm/s) and the propagation velocity on color M-mode is <45 cm/s.

In *constrictive pericarditis*, mitral and tricuspid valve flows are also "restrictive," but unlike those in restrictive cardiomyopathy, they display marked respiratory variation. The isovolumic relaxation time shortens during expiration. The S/D of pulmonary venous flow is <1, with increased velocities (especially diastolic) in expiration, resulting in a further decrease in the S/D ratio. In contrast to restrictive cardiomyopathy, hepatic venous flow reversals occur in expiration, early diastolic tissue velocities (E_a) are normal on DTI, and the transmitral propagation velocity is >45 cm/s.

Despite the considerable interest and potential clinical value in the ability to discriminate restrictive cardiomyopathy from constrictive pericarditis, there is no uniform agreement regarding the characteristic features of the Doppler indices, especially those of venous flows. Moreover, rigorous studies of the sensitivity and specificity of these Doppler findings are lacking and relatively few patients have been examined. Thus, the diagnostic certainty is related to the number of "pathognomonic" findings in concert with clinical information and additional imaging studies.

One report suggested that radionuclide ventriculographic indices of LV diastolic function could differentiate constrictive pericarditis and restrictive cardiomyopathy.[8] However, measurements of LV filling—such as the peak filling rate, time to peak filling, and various filling fractions—require careful attention to technical detail. The need for stable heart rates, the lack of venous flows, and the inability to observe the influence of respiration on cardiac blood flows are important limitations of the radionuclide ventriculographic technique.

Magnetic resonance imaging (MRI) and computed tomography (CT) are useful for accurately assessing pericardial thickness (Fig. 68-3); a pericardium >4.0 mm thick can distinguish the two entities (see also Chap. 18A).[9] Recent preliminary data suggest that constrictive pericarditis is associated with severe autonomic dysfunction that involves all segments of the autonomic nervous system, whereas in restrictive cardiomyopathy the autonomic dysfunction is localized to the parasympathetic efferent pathway.[10] Invasive hemodynamics may be helpful (below), and occasionally a histologic diagnosis is necessary.

It is important to remember that clinical and laboratory testing, including imaging and pathologic studies, may produce results consistent with mixed constrictive pericarditis and restrictive cardiomyopathy; indeed, the two entities may coexist [for example, after mediastinal irradiation or after coronary artery bypass grafting (CABG)]. In these cases, a decision to treat conservatively or surgically explore a patient requires experienced clinical judgment.

Cardiac Catheterization

Most patients in whom restrictive cardiomyopathy is a serious consideration should undergo right- and left-sided heart catheterization to document the diagnosis, assess severity, and, in some patients, establish the etiology by means of endomyocardial biopsy. As in patients with constrictive pericarditis, extra care must be taken to obtain high-quality pressure recordings with appropriate gain and optimal damping conditions, and to attend to details such

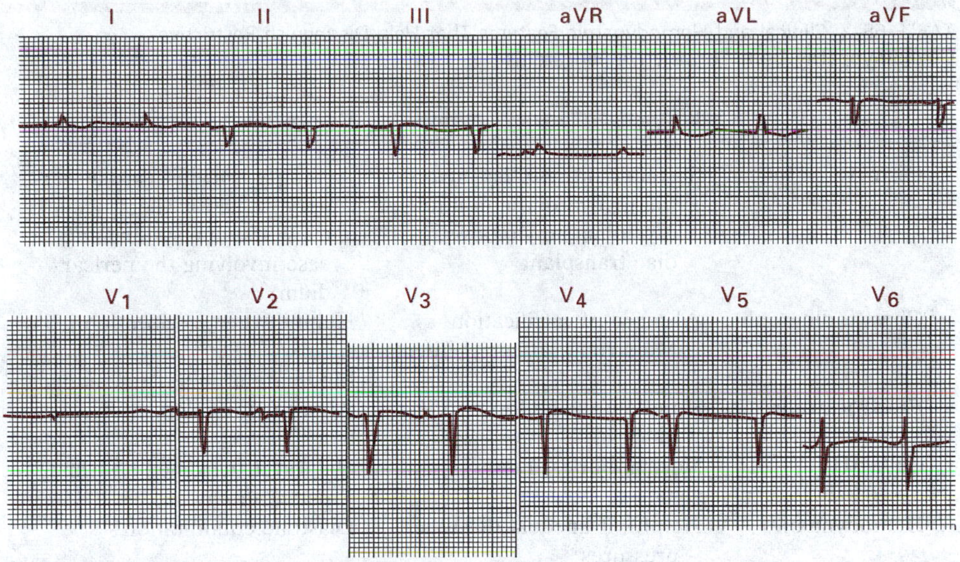

FIGURE 68-1 Electrocardiogram of a patient with amyloidosis. Note the low voltage, which is in striking contrast to the increased left ventricular wall thickness shown echocardiographically. (From Shabetai R. Restrictive, obliterative, and infiltrative cardiomyopathies. In: Alexander WA, Schlant R, Fuster V, et al., eds. *Hurst's The Heart*, 9th ed. New York: McGraw-Hill; 1998:2077. Reproduced with permission.)

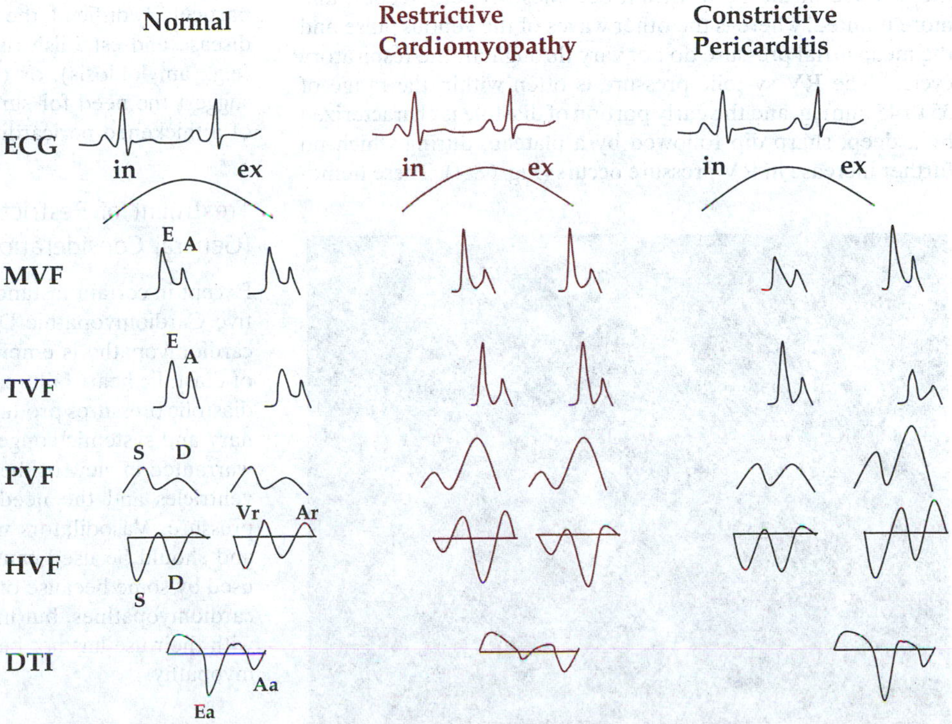

FIGURE 68-2 Schematic of Doppler flows during inspiration (in) and expiration (ex) in normals, restrictive cardiomyopathy, and constrictive pericarditis. See text for details. E, early diastolic filling; A, atrial systolic filling; S, systolic flow; D, diastolic flow; Vr, V-wave reversals; Ar, atrial systolic reversals; Ea, early diastolic tissue velocities; Aa, late diastolic tissue velocites; MVF, mitral valve flow; TVF, tricuspid valve flow; PVF, pulmonary venous flow; HVF, hepatic venous flow; DTI, Doppler tissue imaging. (From Hoit BD. Restrictive cardiomyopathy. In: Pohost G, O'Rourke R, Shah P, Berman D, eds. *Imaging in Cardiovascular Disease*. New York: Lippincott Williams & Wilkins; in press. Reproduced with permission.)

TABLE 68-2 Clinical and Hemodynamic Features That Help Distinguish Restrictive Cardiomyopathy from Constrictive Pericarditis

	Restrictive Cardiomyopathy	Constrictive Pericarditis
History	Systemic disease that involves the myocardium, multiple myeloma, amyloidosis, cardiac transplant	Acute pericarditis, cardiac surgery, radiation therapy, chest trauma, systemic disease involving the pericardium
Chest radiograph	Absence of calcification Massive atrial enlargement	Helpful when calcification persists Moderate atrial enlargement
Electrocardiogram	Bundle branch blocks, AV block	Abnormal repolarization
CT/MRI	Normal pericardium	Helpful if thickened (>4 mm) pericardium
Hemodynamics	Helpful if unequal diastolic pressures Concordant effect of respiration on diastolic pressures	Diastolic equilibration Dip and plateau
Biopsy	Fibrosis, hypertrophy, infiltration	Normal

as the transducer height and system calibration. The venous pressure is elevated and the deep and rapid fall of the right atrial Y descent is striking. During inspiration, the descent of the V wave in the right atrium becomes deeper, steeper, and more pointed, whereas the other waves of the venous pulse and the mean atrial pressure do not vary throughout the respiratory cycle.[11] The RV systolic pressure is often within the range of 35 to 45 mmHg, and the early portion of diastole is characterized by a deep, sharp dip followed by a plateau, during which no further increase in RV pressure occurs (Fig. 68-4). These hemodynamic features are identical to those of constrictive pericarditis and may cause diagnostic confusion. There is usually only modest pulmonary hypertension and the pulmonary arterial diastolic pressure is a few millimeters higher than the pulmonary wedge pressure, which is often quite elevated. It is not uncommon for the pulmonary wedge and the right atrial pressures to be identical and to simulate further the hemodynamics of constrictive pericarditis; however, a higher LV than RV filling pressure strongly favors the diagnosis of restrictive cardiomyopathy rather than constrictive pericarditis. LV systolic pressure is normal, while the LV diastolic pressure tracing shows the same abnormalities as those of the RV (Fig. 68-4).

Left ventriculography usually shows a normal ejection fraction and the absence of major regional wall motion abnormalities. Endomyocardial biopsy is an integral part of the workup of many patients with restrictive cardiomyopathy. When distinction from constrictive pericarditis is particularly difficult, the biopsy may furnish proof of myocardial disease and establish the cause of restrictive cardiomyopathy (e.g., amyloidosis), or (by virtue of unremarkable histology) suggest the need for surgical exploration, even in the absence of a thickened pericardium.

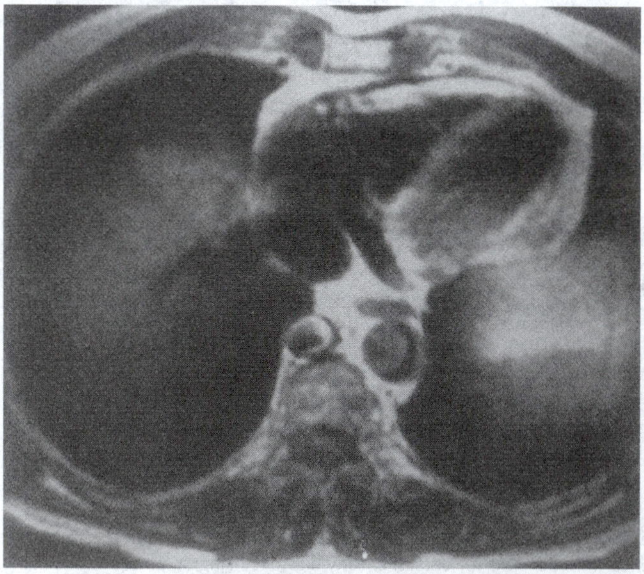

FIGURE 68-3 Magnetic resonance image showing normal pericardium as a low-intensity (*black*) line anterior to the right ventricle between high-intensity (*white*) epicardial and mediastinal fat. (From Hoit BD. Imaging the pericardium. *Cardiol Clin* 1990; 8:588. Reproduced with permission.)

Treatment of Restrictive Cardiomyopathy (General Considerations)

Except in certain instances described below ("Specific Restrictive Cardiomyopathic Diseases"), the treatment of restrictive cardiomyopathy is empiric and directed toward the treatment of diastolic heart failure. Reduction in the elevated ventricular diastolic pressures produces substantial improvement in pulmonary and systemic congestion, but judicious use of diuretics is warranted in view of the steep pressure-volume relation of the ventricles and the need to maintain a relatively high filling pressure. Vasodilators may also jeopardize ventricular filling and should be used cautiously. Calcium channel blockers are used by some because of their beneficial effect in hypertrophic cardiomyopathies, but improvement in ventricular compliance with their use has not been demonstrated in restrictive cardiomyopathy.

SPECIFIC RESTRICTIVE CARDIOMYOPATHIC DISEASES

A useful classification of the restrictive cardiopathies is shown in Table 68-1. This scheme is based upon the cardiac compartment predominantly involved (i.e., myocardial versus endomyocardial) and subdivides the myocardial diseases into the noninfil-

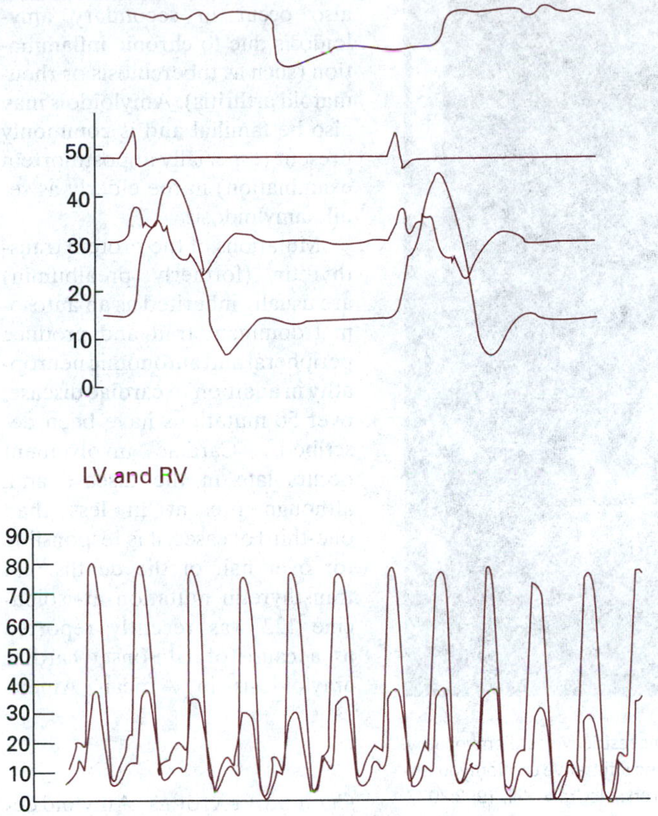

FIGURE 68-4 *Top:* Right-sided heart hemodynamic data from a patient with amyloidosis recorded with a high-fidelity catheter. From the top tracing down is a respirometer, electrocardiogram, right ventricular (RV) dP/dt, and RV pressure. Note the characteristic dip-and-plateau configuration. *Bottom:* Simultaneous RV and LV pressure tracings from another patient with cardiac amyloidosis. In this patient, the typical dip-and-plateau pattern was not present, but during inspiration LV and RV diastolic pressures equilibrated. (From Shabetai R. Restrictive, obliterative, and infiltrative cardiomyopathies. In: Alexander WA, Schlant R, Fuster V, et al., eds. *Hurst's The Heart*, 9th ed. New York: McGraw-Hill; 1998:2079. Reproduced with permission.)

trative, infiltrative, and storage and the endomyocardial diseases into obliterative (i.e., endomyocardial fibrosis and the hypereosinophilic syndrome), carcinoid, infiltrative, and iatrogenic.

Myocardial Diseases

NONINFILTRATIVE CARDIOMYOPATHIES

Idiopathic and Familial Restrictive Cardiomyopathy Recent data suggest that idiopathic restrictive cardiomyopathy may be an autosomal dominant disorder involving myocardium, conduction tissue, and skeletal muscle, with resultant restrictive ventricular filling and heart failure, AV block, and distal skeletal myopathy. Deposition of the intermediate filament desmin has been linked to this syndrome and may represent a distinct pathologic entity; accumulation of desmin immunoreactive material on heart biopsy may be confirmed ultrastructurally.[12,13] Changes in collagen subtypes and matrix metalloproteinase activity may play an important role in the genesis of increased LV stiffness.[14]

Myocyte hypertrophy and fibrosis on endomyocardial biopsy characterize idiopathic restrictive cardiomyopathy, and the absence of myocyte disarray is an important pathologic distinction from hypertrophic cardiomyopathy. However, overlap syndromes characterized by physiologic evidence of restriction and myocyte hypertrophy but without myocyte disarray or LV hypertrophy on echocardiography are reported.[15] Moreover, it was recently postulated that primary restrictive and hypertrophic cardiomyopathies may represent different phenotypic expressions of the same genetic disease.[16] An echocardiographic feature distinguishing primary restrictive cardiomyopathy from cardiac amyloidosis (in addition to the associated clinical features) is the increased LV wall thickness in the latter. In both disorders (and restrictive cardiomyopathies in general), ventricular dimensions are normal or reduced, systolic function is variable, and atrial dimensions are increased.

Two-dimensional and Doppler echocardiography are reliable, noninvasive techniques for diagnosing primary restrictive cardiomyopathy (see Chap. 13).[17] A dominant mitral early diastolic "E" velocity, an increased pulmonary venous atrial systolic "A" reversal velocity and duration, and shortened mitral deceleration time are present in both children and adults with primary restrictive cardiomyopathy (Fig. 68-5). On CT or MRI scans, evidence of restrictive filling (e.g., right atrial and caval enlargement) are common in both restrictive cardiomyopathy and constrictive pericarditis. MRI may differentiate primary restrictive cardiomyopathy from amyloidosis on the basis of tissue characterization.[18]

Pseudoxanthoma Elasticum Pseudoxanthoma elasticum is a rare, genetically heterogeneous disorder characterized by fragmentation and calcification of elastic fibers involving the skin, eyes, and gastrointestinal and cardiovascular systems. Although endocardial fibroelastosis uncommonly causes restrictive cardiomyopathy (Fig. 68-6), coronary artery disease with premature death is a major problem in these patients.[19]

Progressive Systmic Sclerosis Myocardial fibrosis, which may have a patchy distribution and be present in both ventricles, is found in the majority of patients with scleroderma at autopsy. On echocardiography, LV wall thickening in the absence of hypertension and evidence of LV dysfunction may be seen, but heart failure due to either restrictive or dilated cardiomyopathy is rare.[20] Pericardial involvement and electrocardiographic abnormalites (heart block, supraventricular and ventricular tachycardia, and pseudoinfarction patterns) are common. Pulmonary hypertension is a leading cause of morbidity and mortality in patients with scleroderma.

INFILTRATIVE CARDIOMYOPATHIES

Amyloidosis Amyloidosis is a systemic disorder characterized by interstitial deposition of linear, rigid, nonbranching amyloid protein fibrils in multiple organs (e.g., heart, kidney, liver, nerve). Although there are several types of amyloidosis, cardiac involvement is most common in primary amyloidosis (AL type), which is caused by plasma cell production of immunoglobulin light chains; the latter occurs often in association with multiple myeloma. Multiple myeloma is also reported to cause diastolic heart failure in the absence of amyloidosis.[18,21] Cardiac deposition of amyloid protein (protein A, a nonimmunoglobin) may

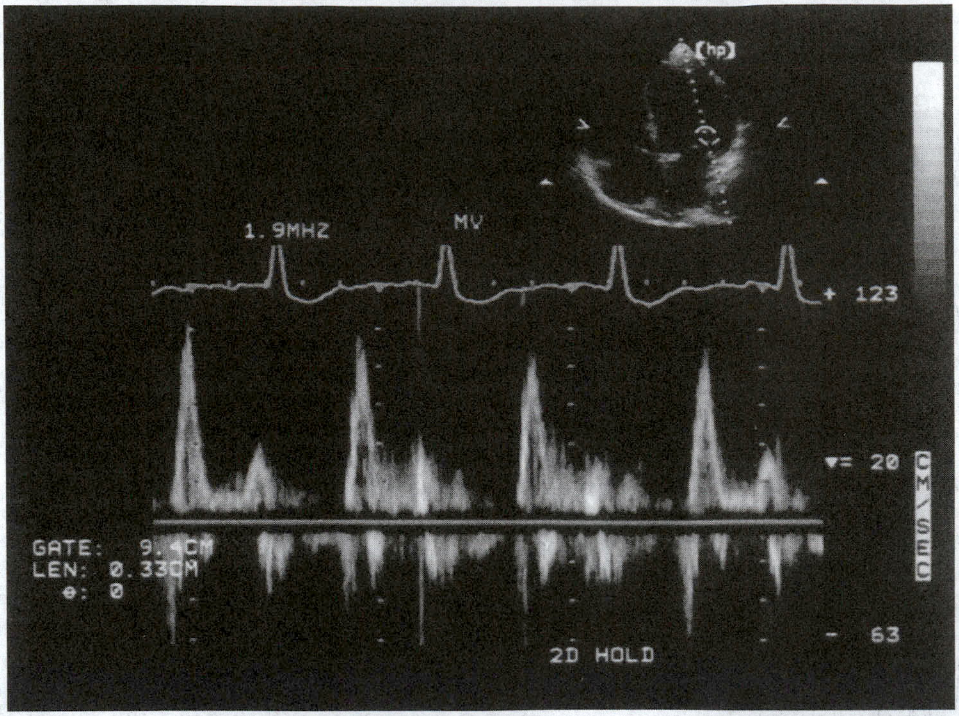

FIGURE 68-5 Doppler record of mitral inflow velocity from a patient with idiopathic restrictive cardiomyopathy. Note the dominant early diastolic wave. (From Shabetai R. Restrictive, obliterative, and infiltrative cardiomyopathies. In: Alexander WA, Schlant R, Fuster V, et al., eds. *Hurst's The Heart*, 9th ed. New York: McGraw-Hill; 1998:2077. Reproduced with permission.)

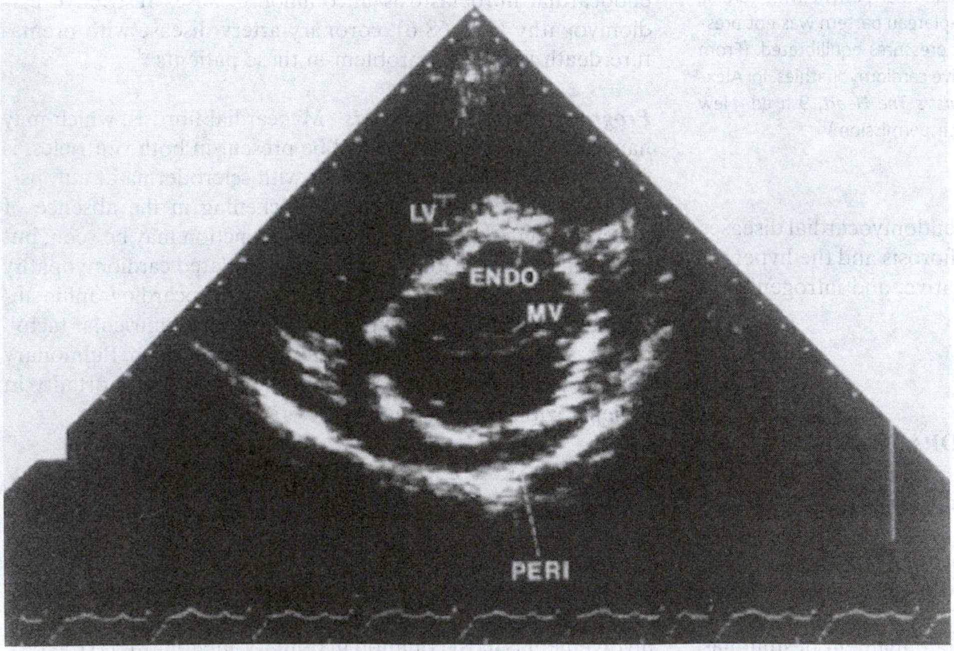

FIGURE 68-6 Short-axis view of the left ventricle (LV) at the mitral valve (MV) level in a patient with pseudoxanthoma elasticum. Note the calcified endomyocardium (ENDO) and echodense pericardium (PERI). The endocardial calcification was clearly visible by fluoroscopy. (From Shabetai R. Restrictive, obliterative, and infiltrative cardiomyopathies. In: Alexander WA, Schlant R, Fuster V, et al., eds. *Hurst's The Heart*, 9th ed. New York: McGraw-Hill; 1998:2085. Reproduced with permission.)

also occur in secondary amyloidosis due to chronic inflammation (such as tuberculosis or rheumatoid arthritis). Amyloidois may also be familial and is commonly present (especially at postmortem examination) in the elderly as senile amyloidosis.

Mutations of the protein transthyretin (formerly prealbumin) are usually inherited as an autosomal dominant trait and produce peripheral and autonomic neuropathy in addition to cardiac disease; over 50 mutations have been described.[22] Cardiac involvement occurs late in the disease and, although present in less than one-third of cases, it is responsible for over half of the deaths.[23] A transthyretin mutation at isoleucine 122 was recently reported as a cause of late-onset cardiac amyloidosis in African Americans.[24]

Clinical Features Amyloid deposits may be interstitial and widespread, resulting in restrictive cardiomyopathy, or localized to (1) conduction tissue, resulting in heart block and ventricular arrhythmias (especially familial amyloid); (2) the cardiac valves, causing valvular regurgitation; (3) the pericardium, producing constriction; and (4) the coronary arteries, resulting in ischemia. Amyloid may be isolated to the subendocardium in senile amyloid and amyloid secondary to chronic disease. Deposition of amyloid and atrial natriuretic factor (ANF) in the atria is frequent in aged hearts.[25] Despite sinus rhythm, atrial mechanical failure and thrombus formation may result due to electromechanical dissociation.[26] Atrial and brain natriuretic peptide are expressed in ventricular myocytes in patients with cardiac amyloidosis.[27] In some cases, the clinical picture is dominated by autonomic neuropathy (orthostatic hypotension, syncope, diarrhea, lack of sweating, and impotence) and nephropathy and cardiac involvement are unrecognized. Cardiac manifestations define a spectrum, often progressive through stages of severity, from the asymptomatic to biventricular failure.

Diagnostic/Imaging Studies The cardiac silhouette on the chest radiograph may be normal or moderately enlarged. The ECG typically shows decreased voltage, a pseudoinfarction pattern, left axis deviation; arrhythmias and conduction disturbances may predominate the clinical course.

The M-mode echocardiogram may reveal symmetrical wall thickness involving the right and left ventricles, a small or normal LV cavity, variable (but often depressed) systolic function, left atrial enlargement, and a small pericardial effusion (Fig. 68-7). Digitized M-mode tracings may reveal decreased rates of systolic wall thickening and diastolic wall thinning and increased isovolumic relaxation time,[28] especially in the early stages.

Two-dimensional echo findings include thickening of the ventricular myocardium, the interatrial septum and valves (especially the AV valves), enlarged papillary muscles, and dilated atria and inferior vena cava (Fig. 68-8). LV wall thickness is an important prognostic variable; in one study, patients with biopsy-proven amyloidosis having a mean wall thickness ≥15 mm had a median survival of 0.4 years, whereas patients with a mean wall thickness ≤12 mm had a median survival of 2.4 years.[29] Highly reflective echoes producing a granular or sparkling appearance and occurring in a patchy distribution are characteristic echocardiographic findings but are neither sensitive nor specific; concentric hypertrophy, as occurs in hypertension or aortic stenosis, may produce a uniformly speckled or echolucent appearance of the myocardium; and idiopathic hypertrophic cardiomyopathy may display a patchy, granular sparkling. Although they correlate with wall thickness, granular echoes may not be seen. Importantly, their recognition is subjective and is affected by ultrasound instrument settings. Thus, granular sparkling alone is an unreliable finding. The infiltrative pathology associated with amyloidosis may be detected by tissue characterization using MRI.[18] Amyloid cardiomyopathy may exist despite the absence of echocardiographic evidence of infiltration.[30]

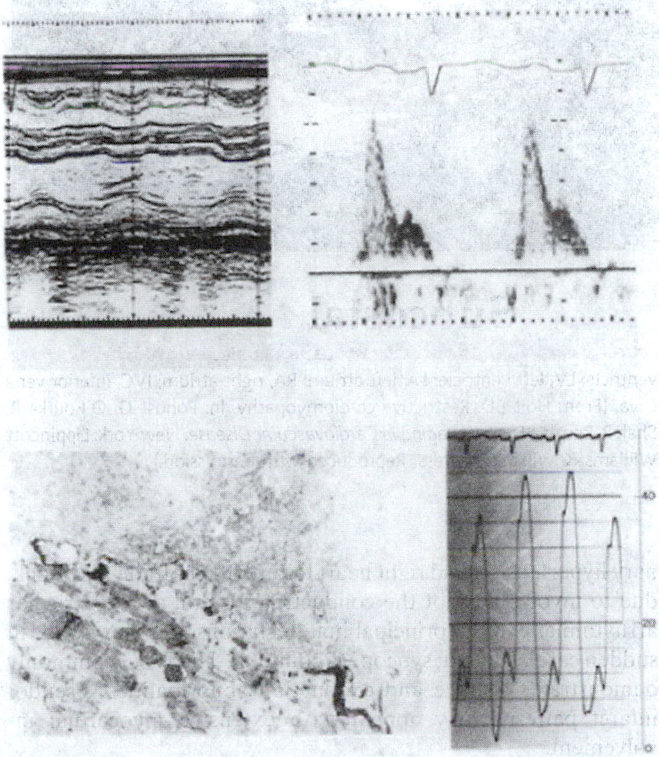

FIGURE 68-7 Amyloidosis. *Top left:* M-mode echocardiogram showing increased thickness of the left ventricular myocardium (calibration mark = 1 cm). *Top right:* Doppler tracing of mitral inflow velocity. Note that the atrial contribution to mitral blood flow velocity is markedly reduced (calibration mark = 20 cm/s). *Bottom left:* electromicrograph showing extensive replacement of myocardium by amyloid. *Bottom right:* Right ventricular pressure tracing. A diastolic dip-plateau pattern is absent because of tachycardia. (From Shabetai R. Restrictive, obliterative, and infiltrative cardiomyopathies. In: Alexander WA, Schlant R, Fuster V, et al., eds. *Hurst's The Heart*, 9th ed. New York: McGraw-Hill; 1998:2083. Reproduced with permission.)

Doppler studies may show the restrictive pattern of LV filling—i.e., a transmitral E/A ratio ≥2 without respiratory variation, transmitral diastolic deceleration time <150 ms, and an isovolumic relaxation time ≤70 ms (Fig. 68-7). The RV filling pattern is often abnormal. The systolic-to-diastolic pulmonary venous flow ratio is <1 and atrial reversals increase with inspiration in the pulmonary and hepatic veins. However, the *earliest sign* of amyloid cardiomyopathy is impaired LV relaxation, manifest by an E/A ratio <1, and increased isovolumic relaxation and transmitral diastolic deceleration times. The severity of combined systolic and diastolic abnormalities can be determined with an echo Doppler index using isovolumic contraction and relaxation and ejection times.[31] In addition, Doppler has shown utility in prognosis; a deceleration time <150 ms and an increased E/A transmitral ratio are strong predictors of cardiac death.[32]

Abnormalities of LV filling are also demonstrated with the LV time-activity curve from radionuclide ventriculography.[33] Moreover, radionuclide imaging using technetium-99m pyrophosphate or Indium-111 antimyosin may be useful in diagnosis. The variable clinical, diagnostic, and prognostic features reflect the location, nature, and extent of amyloid deposition and the temporal course of the disease. Serum and urine protein electrophoresis is diagnostic in most cases of primarily amyloidosis, but monoclonal protein is not secreted in 10 percent of cases.[23] Endomyocardial biopsy of the RV (most helpful if an abdominal fat aspirate is negative) provides the diagnosis, establishes the histochemistry, and quantifies myocardial damage and atrophy.[34]

Treatment of Amyloidosis The treatment of amyloidosis is unrewarding and symptomatic therapy is fraught with hazard; patients are sensitive to digoxin and calcium channel blockers, and hypotension with vasodilators and diuretics is a threat due to the steep LV pressure-volume relation. Immunosuppressive therapy with melphalan and prednisone is the established treatment regimen for primary (AL) amyloidosis. In a recent study, multiple alkylating agents failed to increase the response rate or survival time over this conventional regimen.[35] Orthotopic cardiac transplantation is generally not recommended because of the systemic nature of amyloidosis and the possibility of recurrence in the transplant, but successful cases have been reported.[36] Liver transplantation may be lifesaving in patients with familial amyloidosis,[37] since the liver is the site of transthyretin production.

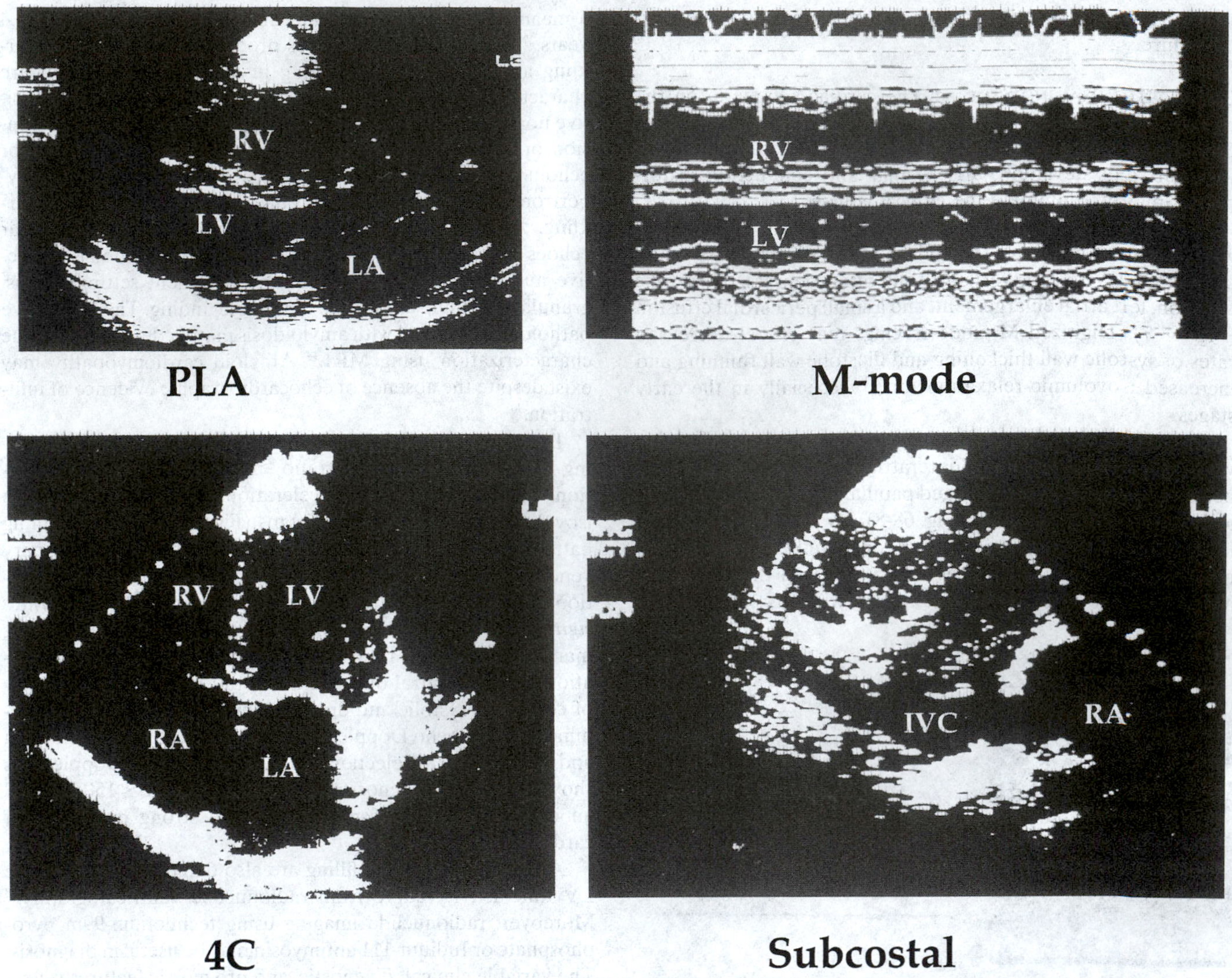

FIGURE 68-8 M-mode and two-dimensional echocardiogram from a patient with biopsy-proven amyloidosis causing hemodynamic restriction. The left ventricular systolic function is mildly impaired, and there is biatrial enlargement and vena cava plethora. Left ventricular hypertrophy is best seen in the M-mode study. PLA, parasternal long axis; 4C, four chamber view; RV, right ventricle; LV, left ventricle; LA, left atrium; RA, right atrium; IVC, inferior vena cava. (From Hoit BD. Restrictive cardiomyopathy. In: Pohost G, O'Rourke R, Shah P, Berman D, eds. *Imaging in Cardiovascular Disease*. New York: Lippincott Williams & Wilkins; in press. Reproduced with permission.)

Sarcoidosis Sarcoidosis is a disorder of unknown etiology characterized by the presence of noncaseating granulomas that involve many organs (e.g., lung, skin, lymph nodes, liver, spleen). Granulomas involve the heart in sarcoidosis in as many as 25 percent of patients but are frequently subclinical.[38] Nevertheless, in approximately half of the fatalities, cardiac involvement is responsible.[39] Rarely, sarcoid is confined to the heart. The combination of extracardiac manifestations and cardiac abnormalities favors a presumptive diagnosis of sarcoidosis without biopsy.

Interstitial granulomatous inflammation initially produces diastolic dysfunction, but later, when the disease is more extensive, it may produce systolic (at times focal) abnormalities. Localized thinning and dilatation of the basilar LV resembling ischemic heart disease are characteristic. Restrictive cardiomyopathy is uncommon. However, sarcoid pulmonary involvement is frequent and produces echo and Doppler findings of pulmonary hypertension and right heart failure. High-grade AV block, due to involvement of the conduction system, and ventricular arrhythmias are the principal manifestations and may result in sudden cardiac death; syncope is common. The ECG commonly demonstrates T-wave and conduction abnormalities. Pseudoinfarct patterns may appear with extensive myocardial involvement.

Echocardiographic findings include evidence of systolic and diastolic LV dysfunction, LV aneurysm formation, abnormal ventricular wall thickness, pericardial effusion, regional wall motion abnormalities in the basal septum with apical sparing, and evidence of cor pulmonale. Thallium 201 and gallium 67 have been used to indicate areas of myocardial involvement and serve to predict the response to corticosteroids. MRI may detect mass lesions due to sarcoid granuloma or scar.[40] Endomyocardial biopsy is useful but may be falsely negative. An important entity in the differential diagnosis is giant-cell myocarditis, which is characterized by a more aggressive and fatal course than cardiac sarcoid.[41]

Treatment with prednisone is warranted in highly suspicious or proven cases because the cardiac granuloma may be sensitive. In patients at high risk for sudden cardiac death, an automatic implantable cardioverter defibrillator (AICD) may be appropriate,[42] and cardiac transplantation is an appropriate consideration in some cases.[43]

Gaucher's Disease Gaucher's disease is due to an inherited deficiency of the enzyme β-glucocerebroside, which results in accumulation of cerebroside in the reticuloendothelial system, brain, and heart. Diffuse interstitial infiltration of the left ventricle occurs, with reduced LV wall compliance and cardiac output, but is often subclinical. LV and left-sided valvular thickening and pericardial effusion are seen on echo.[44]

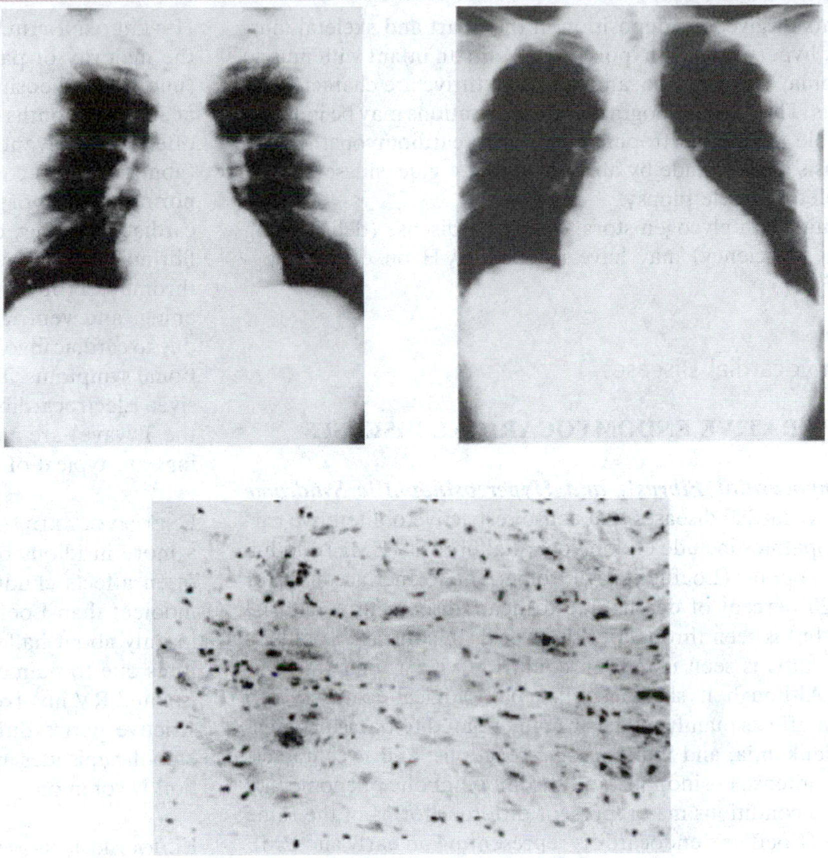

FIGURE 68-9 Chest radiograph of a patient with cardiac hemochromatosis before (*top right*) and after (*top left*) several months of treatment with phlebotomy. *Bottom:* Endomyocardial biopsy that established the diagnosis. (From Shabetai R. Restrictive, obliterative, and infiltrative cardiomyopathies. In: Alexander WA, Schlant R, Fuster V, et al., eds. *Hurst's The Heart*, 9th ed. New York: McGraw-Hill; 1998:2084. Reproduced with permission.)

STORAGE DISEASES

Hemochromatosis Primary hemochromatosis is an autosomal recessive iron-storage disease that involves the heart, pancreas, skin, liver, and gonads. Myocardial iron deposition in hemochromatosis, either primary or secondary (e.g., resulting from multiple transfusions, ineffective erythropoesis), usually produces dilated cardiomyopathy but may cause restrictive cardiomyopathy. Arrhythmia and conduction disturbances are common; indeed, congestive heart failure, conduction abnormalities, and supraventricular and ventricular arrhythmias occur in one-third of patients.[45] Interstitial fibrosis is variable and unrelated to the extent of iron deposition, which occurs in the myocyte; secondarily, myocardial fibrosis may develop. Bronze diabetes and hepatic dysfunction, reflecting iron deposition in the skin, pancreas and liver are frequent associated manifestations.

One report suggests that cardiac involvement progresses temporally from a small, concentrically hypertrophied LV with diastolic dysfunction to a dilated LV with systolic dysfunction.[46] However, this sequence of events is not universally accepted, and systolic abnormalities may require provocation.[47] Findings consistent with either dilated or restrictive cardiomyopathy may be seen; the presence of systolic dysfunction indicates a poor prognosis (Fig. 68-9). Granular sparkling and atrial enlargement may be observed, but these are nonspecific signs. Quantitative ultrasonic analysis of integrated backscatter has been used experimentally to detect changes in the echo reflectivity of the myocardium due to iron deposition in thalassemia major.[48] Computed tomography and magnetic resonance imaging may demonstrate subclinical cardiac involvement, and tissue characterization may be possible with MRI. Endomyocardial biopsy is confirmatory; in selected instances, it may be useful in excluding the diagnosis.

Repeated phlebotomy is recommended for primary hemochromatosis, and the chelating agent desferrioxamine is often beneficial in secondary hemochromatosis. Cardiac transplantation (with or without liver transplantation) may be considered in selected cases.

Fabry's Disease Fabry's disease is an X-linked, genetically heterogeneous disorder of glycosphingolipid metabolism caused by lysosomal ceramide (α-galactosidase) deficiency that leads to accumulation of glycolipid in the heart, skin, and kidneys. Glycolipid accumulation in the myocardium and vascular and valvular endothelium may present with either a restrictive, hypertrophic, or dilated cardiomyopathy, mitral regurgitation, ischemic heart disease, or aortic degeneration. Echocardiographic findings in restrictive cardiomyopathy mimic those seen in amyloid, and LV mass correlates with the severity of disease.[49] Hypertension, mitral valve prolapse, and heart failure are common clinical presentations. Definitive diagnosis may require endomyocardial biopsy.

Pompe's Disease Pompe's disease (glycogen storage type II) is due to an inherited (autosomal recessive) metabolic abnormality due to acid maltase deficiency that causes massive amounts of glycogen deposition in the heart and skeletal muscles. A hypertrophied, hypokinetic LV in an infant with muscle hypotonia, hyperreflexia, and failure to thrive are characteristic findings. The echocardiographic manifestations may be indistinguishable from hypertrophic obstructive cardiomyopathy. The diagnosis can be made by absence of α-1,4-glucosidase activity on skeletal muscle biopsy.

Adults with glycogen storage type III disease (debranching enzyme deficiency) may have marked LVH on echocardiography.[50]

Endomyocardial Diseases

OBLITERATIVE ENDOMYOCARDIAL DISEASES

Endomyocardial Fibrosis and Hypereosinophilic Syndrome Endomyocardial diseases that cause restrictive obliterative cardiomyopathies include endomyocardial fibrosis (EMF) and hypereosinophilic (Loeffler's) syndrome. The former accounts for 10 to 20 percent of deaths due to heart disease in equatorial Africa but is seen throughout the world. In contrast, Loeffler's endocarditis is seen mainly in countries with a temperate climate. Although it shares similar pathological features with EMF, it affects mainly men; is usually related to parasitic infections, leukemia, and immunologic reactions; and is characterized by intense eosinophila and thromboembolic phenomena.[51] The two conditions may represent different forms of the same disease (Loeffler's endocarditis representing an early and EMF an advanced stage), but considerable differences exist. Moreover, the endemic variety EMF may be related to high levels of cerium and low levels of magnesium; it may be pathophysiologically distinct from Loeffler's.[52]

HYPEREOSINOPHILIC SYNDROME Cardiac involvement occurs in the majority of patients with the hypereosinophilic syndrome (unexplained eosinophilia exceeding 1500 eosinophils/mm^3 for at least 6 months and symptoms of organ involvement) and often has a biventricular distribution. Cardiotoxic eosinophils (abnormal cells containing vacuoles and having fewer than the normal number of granules) are central to the pathogenesis. The cardiac pathology consists of an acute eosinophilic myocarditis, fibrinoid vasculitis of the intramural coronary arteries, mural thrombosis (often with eosinophils), fibrotic endocardial thickening, and ventricular obliteration. In addition to symptoms due to cardiac involvement, patients have skin rash and constitutional symptoms. The disease is aggressive and rapidly progressive. Electrocardiographic abnormalities (especially involving the T wave) are common but nonspecific. Hemodynamic findings are typical of restrictive cardiomyopathy.

ENDOMYOCARDIAL FIBROSIS In contrast to Loeffler's, EMF has a more insidious onset, has no gender predilection, and most often affects children and young adults. The disease is more indolent than Loeffler's, and biventricular involvement occurs in only about half the cases. LV involvement produces symptoms due to pulmonary congestion, whereas the less common isolated RV involvement (about 10 percent) may simulate constrictive pericarditis. Atrioventricular valve regurgitation and embolic episodes are frequent complications, and atrial fibrillation is common.

ECHOCARDIOGRAPHIC FEATURES Endomyocardial disease is characterized by endocardial fibrosis of the apex and subvalvular regions of one or both ventricles, resulting in restriction to inflow to the affected ventricle. Although their clinical presentations differ, the pathology, and therefore the cardiac imaging studies, are generally similar in the endomyocardial diseases. M-mode echo findings are nonspecific and digitized M-mode studies reveal a decreased peak filling rate and a decreased duration of the peak filling.[53] On two-dimensional echo, apical obliteration of the right and/or left ventricle, apical thrombus, preservation of ventricular systolic function with thickening of the posterior atrioventricular valve apparatus and posterobasilar LV wall, echo densities in the endocardium, and small ventricular and large atrial cavities are noted (Fig. 68-10).[54] Involvement of the posterior mitral and tricuspid valve leaflets results in mitral and tricuspid regurgitation; less commonly, restricted motion may produce stenosis. Sparing of the outflow tracts is characteristic. Doppler interrogation yields typical patterns of restriction (increased E/A, decreased IVRT, decreased deceleration time), mitral and tricuspid regurgitation, and, less often, stenosis. Not sur-

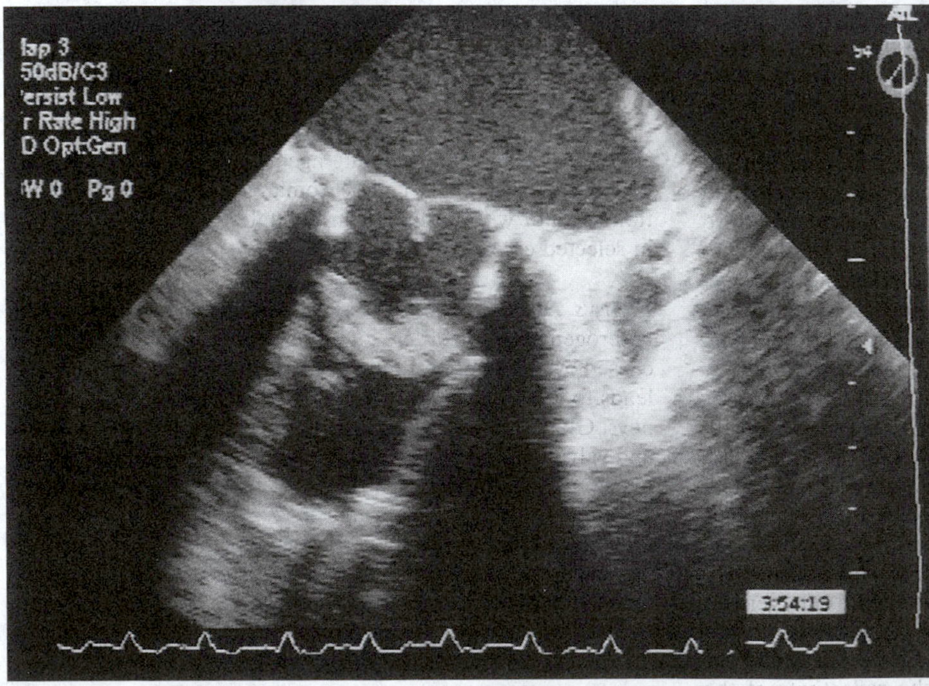

FIGURE 68-10 Transesophageal echocardiogram from a patient with eosinophilic endocarditis and prosthetic mitral valve replacement. Thrombus is noted below the valve struts, which at the the time of surgery was found to be adherent to the posterior LV wall. Note the apical obliteration and the apical endocardial thickening and calcification.

prisingly, the location, extent, and severity of involvement determine the clinical picture.

TREATMENT OF THE OBLITERATIVE RESTRICTIVE CARDIOMYOPATHIES

Medical therapy of Loeffler's is often ineffective and frustrating. Treatment consists of symptomatic relief, anticoagulants, corticosteroids, and hydroxyurea for myocarditis (interferon α has had some success[55]), and palliative surgery in the late, fibrotic stage. Surgical excision of fibrotic endocardium and valve replacement may offer symptomatic improvement, but at the expense of high (15 to 25 percent) operative mortality. The prognosis of advanced disease is grim (50 percent 2-year mortality), but it is considerably better in those with milder disease.

NONOBLITERATIVE ENDOMYOCARDIAL DISEASES

Carcinoid Syndrome Carcinoid syndrome results from metastatic carcinoid tumors (most commonly arising in the small bowel and appendix, but also the bronchus and other sites) and consists of cutaneous flushing, diarrhea, and bronchoconstriction; involvement of the heart occurs as a late complication of carcinoid syndrome in approximately 50 percent of patients. (see also Chaps. 59 and 77). Hepatic metastases produce serotonin, bradykinin, and other substances that affect right heart structures but are inactivated in the lungs. Thus, LV involvement is distinctly uncommon and its presence suggests a right-to-left intracardiac shunt.[56] Fibrous endocardial plaques comprising smooth muscle cells in a stroma of collagen and acid mucopolysaccharide on the tricuspid and pulmonic valves and right heart endocardium are characteristic. Although tricuspid and pulmonic stenosis and regurgitation dominate the clinical picture, restrictive cardiomyopathy may occur.

The chest radiograph is often normal, but cardiomegaly, pleural effusions, and nodules may be evident; unlike the case with congenital pulmonic stenosis, poststenotic dilatation of the pulmonary artery trunk does not occur.[57] Electrocardiographic abnormalities are common, but nonspecific. Two-dimensional echocardiography reveals thickened, retracted tricuspid and pulmonic valves and right atrial and ventricular enlargement; right atrial wall thickening may be seen on transesophageal echo. Low-velocity tricuspid and pulmonic regurgitation on Doppler indicates normal pulmonary arterial pressures, which is typical of carcinoid heart disease. In one series, echocardiographic findings were detected in two-thirds of patients with carcinoid.[58] In another study, cardiac involvement was associated with a reduced 3-year survival as compared with those without cardiac involvement.[57] Catheterization findings are usually those of tricuspid regurgitation and/or pulmonic stenosis. Therapy is symptomatic, and valvular replacement (mechanical) or repair is warranted in patients with severe valve dysfunction.

Malignant Infiltration Infiltrating tumors of the heart are generally metastatic (lung, breast, melanoma, lymphoma, leukemia) and rarely produce restriction to ventricular filling unless the pericardium is involved (see Chap. 77). Infiltration on echocardiography is suggested by a localized increase in wall thickness, often associated with abnormal wall motion and pericardial effusion. CT and MRI scans are also useful.

Iatrogenic Disease Pericardial disease frequently complicates radiation therapy to the chest and may produce constrictive pericarditis; however, endo- and myocardial involvement may produce restrictive cardiomyopathy, at times presenting years after radiation therapy has been completed.[59] Anthracyclines and methysergide can cause endomyocardial fibrosis. Oils containing L-tryptophan were withdrawn from the market when they were implicated in the genesis of the eosinophilia-myalgia syndrome; this syndrome was associated with restrictive cardiomyopathy.[60] Finally, a restrictive pattern of LV filling is common soon after orthotopic cardiac transplantation and may persist for at least 1 year in as many as 15 percent.[61]

References

1. WHO/ISFC Task Force. Definition and classification of cardiomyopathies. *Br Heart J* 1980; 44:672–673.
2. Goodwin J, Oakley C. The cardiomyopathies. *Br Heart J* 1972; 44:672–673.
3. Angelini A, Calzolari V, Thiene G, et al. Morphologic spectrum of primary restrictive cardiomyopathy. *Am J Cardiol* 1997; 80:1046–1050.
4. Appleton C, Hatle L, Popp R. Demonstration of restrictive ventricular physiology by Doppler echocardiography. *J Am Coll Cardiol* 1988; 11:757–768.
5. Klein A, Cohen G, Pietrolungo J, et al. Differentiation of constrictive pericarditis from restrictive cardiomyopathy by Doppler transesophageal echocardiographic measurements of respiratory variations in pulmonary venous flow. *J Am Coll Cardiol* 1993; 22:1935–1943.
6. Garcia M, Rodriguez L, Ares M, et al. Differentiation of constrictive pericarditis from restrictive cardiomyopathy: Assessment of left ventricular diastolic velocities in longitudinal axis by doppler tissue imaging. *J Am Coll Cardiol* 1996; 27:108–114.
7. Akasaka T, Yoshida K, Yamamuro A, et al. Phasic coronary flow characteristics in patients with constrictive pericarditis: Comparison with restrictive cardiomyopathy. *Circulation* 1997; 96:1874–1881.
8. Gerson M, Fowler N. Differentiation of constrictive pericarditis and restrictive cardiomyopathy by radionuclide ventriculography. *Am Heart J* 1989; 118:114–120.
9. Masui T, Finck S, Higgins C. Constrictive pericarditis and restrictive cardiomyopathy: Evaluation with MR imaging. *Radiology* 1992; 182:369–373.
10. Singh M, Juneja R, Bali HK, et al. Autonomic functions in restrictive cardiomyopathy and constrictive pericarditis: A comparison. *Am Heart J* 1998; 136:443–448.
11. Shabetai R, Fowler NO, Guntheroth WG. The hemodynamics of cardiac tamponade and constrictive pericarditis. *Am J Cardiol* 1970; 26:480–489.
12. Arbustini E, Morbini P, Grasso M, et al. Restrictive cardiomyopathy, atrioventricular block and mild to subclinical myopathy in patients with desmin-immunoreactive material deposits. *J Am Coll Cardiol* 1998; 31:645–653.
13. Zachara E, Bertini E, Lioy E, et al. Restrictive cardiomyopathy due to desmin accumulation in a family with evidence of autosomal dominant inheritance. *G Ital Cardiol* 1997; 27:436–442.
14. Hayashi T, Shimomura H, Terasaki F, et al. Collagen subtypes and matrix metalloproteinase in idiopathic restrictive cardiomyopathy. *Int J Cardiol* 1998; 64:109–116.
15. Cooke R, Chambers J, Curry P. Noonan's cardiomyopathy: A non-hypertrophic variant. *Br Heart J* 1994; 71:561–565.
16. Angelini A, Calzolari V, Thiene G, et al. Morphologic spectrum of primary restrictive cardiomyopathy. *Am J Cardiol* 1997; 80:1046–1050.
17. Cetta F, O'Leary P, Seward J, et al. Idiopathic restrictive cardiomyopathy in childhood: Diagnostic features and clinic course. *Mayo Clin Proc* 1995; 70:634–640.
18. Celetti F, Fattori R, Napoli G, et al. Assessment of restrictive

cardiomyopathy of amyloid or idiopathic etiology by magnetic resonance imaging. *Am J Cardiol* 1999; 83:798–801.

19. Navarro-Lopez F, Llorian A, Ferrer-Roca O, et al. Restrictive cardiomyopathy in psuedoxanthoma elasticum. *Chest* 1980; 78:113–115.
20. Botstein G, LeRoy E. Primary heart disease in systemic sclerosis (scleroderma): Advances in clinical and pathologic features, pathogenesis, and new therapeutic approaches. *Am Heart J* 1981; 102:913–919.
21. Schattner A, Epstein M, Berrebi A, et al. Case report: Multiple myeloma presenting as a diastolic heart failure with no evidence of amyloidosis. *Am J Med Sci* 1995; 310:256–257.
22. Saraiva MJ. Transthyretin mutations in health and disease. *Hum Mutat* 1995; 5:191–196.
23. Kyle RA. Amyloidosis. *Circulation* 1995; 91:1269–1271.
24. Jacobson DR, Pastore RD, Yaghoubian R, et al. Variant-sequence transthyretic (isoleucine 122) in late-onset cardiac amyloidosis in black Americans. *N Engl J Med* 1997; 336:466–473.
25. Kawamura S, Takahashi M, Ishihara T, et al. Incidence and distribution of isolated atrial amyloid: Histologic and immunohistochemical studies of 100 aging hearts. *Pathol Int* 1995; 45:335–342.
26. Dubrey S, Pollak A, Skinner M, et al. Atrial thrombi occurring during sinus rhythm in cardiac amyloidosis: Evidence for atrial electromechanical dissociation. *Br Heart J* 1995; 74:541–544.
27. Takemura G, Takatsu Y, Doyama K, et al. Expression of atrial and brain natriuretic peptides and their genes in hearts of patients with cardiac amyloidosis. *J Am Coll Cardiol* 1998; 4:754–765.
28. Sutton MSJ, Reichek N, Kastor J, et al. Computerized M-mode echocardiographic analysis of left ventricular dysfunction in cardiac amyloid. *Circulation* 1982; 66:790–799.
29. Cueto-Garcia L, Reeder G, Kyle R, et al. Echocardiographic findings in systemic amyloidosis: Spectrum of cardiac involvement and relation to survival. *J Am Coll Cardiol* 1985; 6:737–743.
30. Gertz MA, Grogan M, Kyle RA, et al. Endomyocardial biopsy-proven light chain amyloidosis (AL) without echocardiographic features of infiltrative cardiomyopathy. *Am J Cardiol* 1997; 80:93–95.
31. Tei C, Dujardin KS, Hodge DO, et al. Doppler index combining systolic and diastolic myocardial performance: Clinical value in cardiac amyloidosis. *J Am Coll Cardiol* 1996; 28:658–664.
32. Klein AL, Hatle LK, Taliercio CP, et al. Prognostic significance of Doppler measures of diastolic function in cardiac amyloidosis: A Doppler echocardiography study. *Circulation* 1991; 83:808–816.
33. Lenihan DJ, Gerson MC, Hoit BD, et al. Mechanisms, diagnosis, and treatment of diastolic heart failure. *Am Heart J* 1995; 130:153–166.
34. Arbustini E, Merlini G, Gavazzi A, et al. Cardiac immunocyte-derived (AL) amyloidosis: An endomyocardial biopsy study in 11 patients. *Am Heart J* 1995; 130:528–536.
35. Gertz MA, Lacy MQ, Lust JA, et al. Prospective randomized trial of melphalan and prednisone versus vincristine, carmustine, melphalan, cyclophosphamide, and prednisone in the treatment of primary systemic amyloidosis. *J Clin Oncol* 1999; 17:262–267.
36. Pelosi F Jr, Capehart J, Roberts WC. Effectiveness of cardiac transplantation for primary (AL) cardiac amyloidosis. *Am J Cardiol* 1997; 79:532–535.
37. Skinner M, Lewis WD, Jones LA, et al. Liver transplantation as a treatment for familial amyloidotic polyneuropathy. *Ann Intern Med* 1994; 15:133–134.
38. Gibbons W, Levy R, Nava S, et al. Subclinical cardiac dysfunction in sarcoidosis. *Chest* 1991; 100:44–50.
39. Perry A, Vuitch F. Causes of death in patients with sarcoidosis: A morphologic study of 38 autopsies with clinicopathologic correlations. *Arch Pathol Lab Med* 1995; 119:167–172.
40. Chandra M, Silverman ME, Oshinski J, et al. Diagnosis of cardiac sarcoidosis aided by MRI. *Chest* 1996; 110:562–565.
41. Cooper LH, Berry G, Rizeq M, et al. Giant cell myocarditis. *J Heart Lung Transplant* 1995; 14:394–401.
42. Okayama K, Kurata C, Tawarchara K, et al. Diagnostic and prognostic value of myocardial scintigraphy with thallium-201 and gallium-67 in cardiac sarcoidosis. *Chest* 1995; 107:330–334.
43. Valantine HA, Tazelaar H, Macoviak J, et al. Cardiac sarcoidosis: Response to steroids and transplantation. *J Heart Transplant* 1987; 5:244–250.
44. Saraclar M, Atalay S, Kocak N, et al. Gaucher's disease with mitral and aortic involvement: Echocardiographic findings. *Pediatr Cardiol* 1991; 13:56–58.
45. Hauser SC. Hemochromatosis and the heart. *Heart Dis Stroke* 1993; 2:487–491.
46. Arnett E, Nienhius A, Henry W, et al. Massive myocardial hemochromatosis: A structure-function conference at the National Heart and Lung Institute. *Am Heart J* 1975; 90:777–787.
47. Dabestani A, Child J, Henze E, et al. Primary hemochromatosis: Anatomic and physiologic characteristics of the cardiac ventricles and their response to phlebotomy. *Am J Cardiol* 1984; 54:153–159.
48. Lattanzi F, Bellotti P, Picano E, et al. Quantitative ultrasonic analysis of myocardium in patients with thalassemia major and iron overload. *Circulation* 1993; 87:748–754.
49. Goldman M, Cantor R, Schwartz M, et al. Echocardiographic abnormalities and disease severity in Fabry's disease. *J Am Coll Cardiol* 1986; 7:1157–1161.
50. Coleman R, Winter H, Wolf B, et al. Glycogen storage disease type III (glycogen debranching enzyme deficiency): Correlation of biochemical defects with myopathy and cardiomyopathy. *Ann Intern Med* 1992; 116:896–900.
51. Olsen E, Spry C. Relation between eosinophilia and endomyocardial disease. *Prog Cardiovasc Dis* 1985; 27:241–254.
52. Shaper A. What's new in endomyocardial fibrosis? *Lancet* 1993; 342:255–256.
53. Davies J, Gibson D, Foale R, et al. Echocardiographic features of eosinophilic endomyocardial disease. *Br Heart J* 1982; 48:434–440.
54. Gottdiener J, Maron B, Schooley R, et al. Two-dimensional echocardiographic assessment of the idiopathic hypereosinophilic syndrome: Anatomic basis of mitral regurgitation and peripheral embolization. *Circulation* 1983; 67:572–578.
55. Butterfield JH, Gleich GJ. Interferon-alpha treatment of six patients with the idiopathic hypereosinophilic syndrome. *Ann Intern Med* 1994; 121:648–653.
56. Lundin L, Norheim I, Landelius J, et al. Carcinoid heart disease: Relationship of circulating vasoactive substances to ultrasound-detectable cardiac abnormalities. *Circulation* 1988; 77:264–269.
57. Pellikka P, Tajik A, Khandheria B, et al. Carcinoid heart disease: Clinical and echocardiographic spectrum in 74 patients. *Circulation* 1993; 87:1188–1196.
58. Lundin L, Norheim I, Landelius J, et al. Carcinoid heart disease: Relation of circulating vasoactive substances to ultrasound-detectable cardiac abnormalities. *Circulation* 1988; 77:264–269.
59. Brosius FC III, Waller BF, Roberts WC, et al. Radiation heart disease: Analysis of 16 young (aged 15 to 33 years) necropsy patients who received over 3,500 rads to the heart. *Am J Med* 1981; 70:519–530.
60. Berger PB, Duffy J, Reeder GS, et al. Restrictive cardiomyopathy associated with eosinophilia-myalgia syndrome. *Mayo Clin Proc* 1994; 69:162–165.
61. Valantine HA, Fowler MB, Hunt SA, et al. Changes in Doppler echocardiographic indexes of left ventricular function as potential markers of acute cardiac rejection. *Circulation* 1987; 76:V86–V92.

CHAPTER 69

MYOCARDITIS AND SPECIFIC CARDIOMYOPATHIES—ENDOCRINE DISEASE AND ALCOHOL

Donna M. Mancini / Ainat Beniaminovitz

The diagnosis of cardiomyopathy encompasses a wide spectrum of diseases with widely divergent pathogenic mechanisms, that have as their final common pathway the syndrome of congestive heart failure. These heart muscle diseases may be primary or secondary—i.e., resulting from specific cardiac or systemic disorders. A list of etiologies associated with the development of cardiomyopathy is presented in Fig. 69-1.

Coronary artery disease, hypertension, valvular heart disease, and cardiomyopathy are the most common causes of heart failure for both sexes. Comparison of the Framingham[1] and SOLVD[2] (Study of Left Ventricular Dysfunction) registries demonstrates a shift in the predominant etiology of heart failure from hypertension to ischemic heart disease. This probably reflects recent intensified efforts to control high blood pressure.

Inflammatory cardiomyopathies, particularly viral myocarditis, have served as a model to understand the development of heart failure. More than 70 different specific cardiomyopathies associated with general systemic disease, neuromuscular disorders, sensitivity and toxic reactions, and the peripartum state have been described. When considered as a group, these disorders are infrequent; when considered individually, they are rare.

This chapter reviews the inflammatory cardiomyopathies and specific cardiomyopathies with an emphasis on endocrine and infiltrative disorders. Cardiac disorders caused by pulmonary hypertension and congenital cardiac anomalies are not addressed.

ISCHEMIC

Ischemic cardiomyopathy is defined as a dilated cardiomyopathy in a patient with known coronary disease, specifically a patient with a prior history of infarct or a greater than 70 percent narrowing of a major epicardial artery.

Compensatory mechanisms to improve stroke volume result in myocyte hypertrophy, ventricular dilatation, and activation of the sympathetic nervous system. Remodeling of the left ventricle and a decrease in ejection fraction occur in 15 to 40 percent of patients within 12 to 24 months following an anterior wall infarct[3] and in a smaller percentage following an inferior infarction.[4] In the Framingham study, 14 percent of men developed *congestive heart failure* (CHF) within 5 years of a first myocardial infarction[4] and half were dead within 5 years.[5] Prognosis in ischemic heart failure is known to be worse than in other forms of cardiomyopathy,[6,7] presumably due to the superimposed risk of ongoing ischemic events. Aggressive coronary revascularization in instances of significant heart failure may be justified and may achieve a survival benefit without necessarily affecting functional improvement[8] (see also Chaps. 40 and 48).

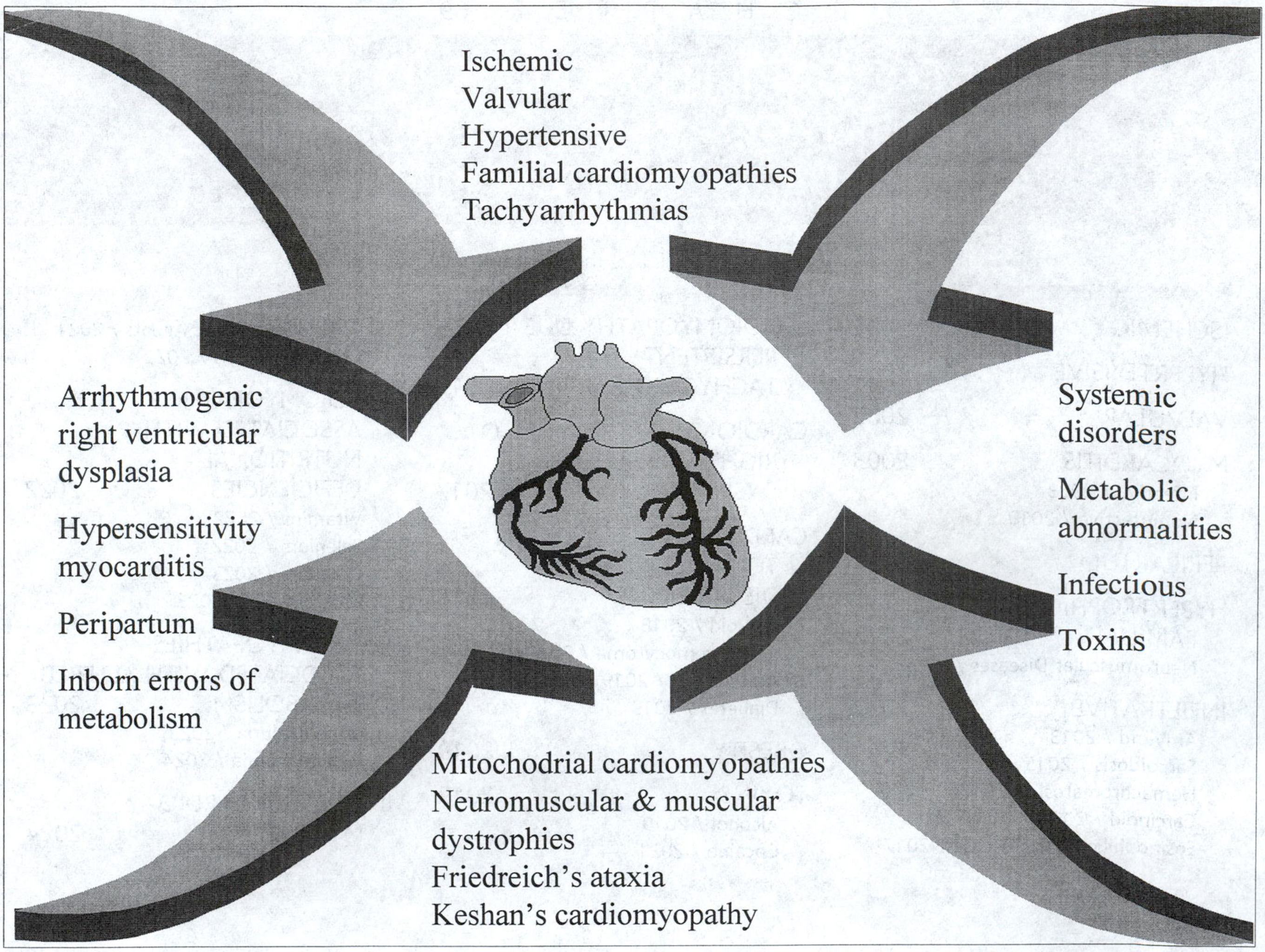

FIGURE 69-1 Various etiologies that can lead to cardiomyopathy.

HYPERTENSIVE

Cardiac hypertrophy due to long-standing arterial hypertension is associated with a high incidence of heart failure.[9] Initially, myocyte hypertrophy occurs to reduce wall stress and to accommodate the increased pressure load imposed on the heart.[10] This increase in myocyte wall thickness is accompanied by biochemical and molecular changes, such as a shift to fetal phenotype gene expression[11] and alterations in the intracellular handling of calcium.[12] Alterations in the nonmyocyte compartment—such as excessive myocardial fibrosis—also ensue.[13] In concert these changes lead to an altered contractile performance of the heart.[14]

Although the precise mechanisms that accelerate the progression from compensated hypertrophy to failure are not known, activation of the renin-angiotensin system has been postulated to play a major role.[15] In vivo, angiotensin II has been shown to increase left ventricular mass[16] and contributes to cardiac phenotype modulation independently from its effect on arterial pressure.[17] In vitro, studies have demonstrated that angiotensin II causes myocyte hypertrophy and promotes interstitial fibrosis.[18] A current clinical trial with the angiotensin-converting enzyme (ACE) inhibitor ramapril has demonstrated that blockade of the renin-angiotensin system in patients with normal left ventricular function but at high risk for cardiovascular events leads to a decrease in the combined end point of death from cardiovascular causes, myocardial infarction, and stroke.[19] This clinical prevention trial further confirms the deleterious effects of the renin-angiotensin axis on cardiac function.

The patient with hypertensive cardiomyopathy typically presents with left ventricular hypertrophy in association with features of dilated or restrictive cardiomyopathy. The prognosis is generally better than that of other forms of cardiomyopathy[20]; however, the prognosis is significantly worsened by the presence of comorbid conditions such as diabetes mellitus, coronary artery disease, and persistent hypertension[21] (see also Chap. 58).

Hypertensive cardiomyopathies are common in the elderly and may be related to an increased prevalence of hypertension due to central arterial stiffness and inherent myocardial changes that occur with normal aging. Recent advances in molecular biology and in echocardiographic and Doppler techniques have led to an improved understanding of the various distinct causes of hypertrophic heart disease in the elderly[22] and the realization that the process is not solely due to the changes associated with aging. Hypertrophic obstructive cardiomyopathy, once thought to be a familial disorder affecting primarily younger individuals, has been diagnosed in older individuals with increasing frequency.[23,24] As shown in Table 69-1, the clinical syndrome, prognosis, and echocardiographic/electrocardiographic findings are somewhat different in the elderly form of the disease.[25]

Similarly, hypertensive hypertrophic cardiomyopathy is another significantly unappreciated cause of hypertensive cardiomyopathy in the elderly.[26] In contrast to the hypertrophic obstructive form, there is a higher female predominance,[26] which is thought to be due to gender-specific differences in the degree of myocyte hypertrophy to intraventricular pressure-overload previously described in women with aortic stenosis.[27] There is no apparent familial component, and patients give a long history of isolated systolic hypertension. In comparison to the prevalence of hypertension in patients over age 65, which varies from 50 to 70 percent, hypertensive hypertrophic cardiomyopathy remains relatively rare, suggesting a unique and currently poorly understood pathophysiology.[28] Many postulate that in hypertensive hypertrophic cardiomyopathy, as in the hypertrophic obstructive form, the development of senescent hypertension may act influentially on an already genetically altered substrate to lead to the respective phenotypes.[29]

TABLE 69-1 Differences between Old and Young Patients with Hypertrophic Cardiomyopathy

Findings	Old	Young
Echocardiographic	Ovoid ventricle Large left atrium LVH diffuse Proximal septal bulge	Crescentic ventricle Small left atrium LVH anterior septum No septal bulge
Mutations	Gene for cardiac myosin-binding protein C	β-myosin heavy chain and cardiac troponin genes
Etiology	Sporadic, 40%	Primarily inherited
Symptoms	More severe	Less severe
Progression	Slower	Rapid
Prognosis	Better	Worse
Sudden death	Uncommon	Common

VALVULAR

Valvular cardiomyopathy is defined as systolic dysfunction out of proportion to the wall stress imposed by the initial valvular lesion.[30] It occurs most commonly with left-sided regurgitant (mitral and aortic insufficiency) rather than stenotic lesions (aortic and mitral stenosis). The prognosis depends on the nature and extent of the valvular abnormality but more importantly on the degree of left ventricular dysfunction at the time of the proposed surgical repair. Generally even severe left ventricular dysfunction due purely to aortic stenosis will have a favorable prognosis after surgical repair. This is in marked contrast to a surgical approach for similar degrees of left ventricular dysfunction due to mitral[31] or aortic regurgitation. Owing to high surgical risks, medical therapy with afterload reduction—and, if indicated, cardiac transplantation—are acceptable modes of therapy in these instances. Cardiac reduction surgery with valve repair has become an increasingly popular modality for treatment of these high-risk patients. No large-center randomized trial is currently available to evaluate the efficacy and safety of this approach.

MYOCARDITIS

Infective

VIRAL

As early as 1806, a relationship between infection and chronic heart disease (diphtheria) was postulated, but it was not until the 1970s, with the advent of endomyocardial biopsies, that diagnosis of myocarditis could be established during life. Multiple infectious etiologies (Table 69-2)[32] have been implicated as the cause of myocarditis, with the most common being viral, specifically, Coxsackie B.[33] In the majority of patients, active myocarditis remains unsuspected because the cardiac dysfunction is subclinical, asymptomatic, and self-limited. Histologic evidence of myocarditis following traumatic death is identified in 1 to 3 percent of autopsies,[34,35] suggesting that the frequency of myocarditis is underestimated by analyzing data only from symptomatic patients.

Pathogenesis Infection by cardiotropic viruses prompted the initial hypothesis that the viral infection was responsible for myocardial injury. However, several investigators noted that cardiac dysfunction increased after the eradication of the infective agent and speculated that the pathogenesis may be due to the immunologic responses initiated by the virus (Fig. 69-2). Support for this theory comes initially from the work of Woodruff, who noted that the histologic evidence of cardiac injury in Coxsackie B infection occurred only after the virus was no longer detectable in the myocardium.[36] Subsequently, demonstration of T-lymphocyte and macrophage infiltration,[37] perforin granules,[38] and a variety of cytokines known to depress myocardial contractility[39] in endomyocardial biopsies of patients with active carditis strengthened the concept of immune-mediated injury. Furthermore, immunosuppressive therapy in animal models attenuated inflammation—with improved survival, less cellular infiltrate, and less necrosis.

The specific immune responses that lead to the myocardial injury are incompletely defined. A murine model of myocarditis induced by coxsackie B3 has provided some insight into immunologic sequence of events. Following infection with coxsackie B3 virus, macrophages are present in the infiltrate until day 8.[40] After macrophage activity decreases, both effector (CD8) and helper (CD4) T cells are identified within myocardial lesions. At peak infiltration, some murine strains showed a predominance of CD8-positive cells while in others CD4 cells predominate, suggesting participation of both humoral- and cell-mediated immune responses.[41] In human subjects, T-lymphocyte and macrophage infiltration characterizes the immunohistochemical picture, whereas B lymphocytes and natural killer cells are absent.[37] T-lymphocyte subset analysis of human serum does not demonstrate consistency in dominance of CD4 or CD8 cells.

TABLE 69-2 Causes of Myocarditis

- Infectious
  - Viruses
    - Coxsackievirus, echovirus, HIV, Epstein-Barr virus, influenza, cytomegalovirus, adenovirus, hepatitis (A and B), mumps, poliovirus, rabies, respiratory synctial virus, rubella, vaccinia, varicella zoster, arbovirus
  - Bacteria
    - *Cornyebacterium diptheriae, Streptococcus pyogenes, Staphylococcus aureus, Haemophilus pneumoniae, Salmonella* spp., *Neisseria gonorrhoeae, Leptospira, Borrelia burgdorferi, Treponema pallidum, Brucella, Mycobacterium tuberculosis,* Actinomyces, *Chlamydia* spp., *Coxiella burnetti, Mycoplasma pneumoniae, Rickettsia* spp.
  - Fungi
    - *Candida* spp., *Aspergillus* spp., *Histoplasma, Blastomyces, Cryptococcus, Coccidioidomyces*
  - Parasites
    - *Trypanosoma cruzii, Toxoplasma, Schistosoma, Trichina*
- Noninfectious
  - Drugs causing hypersensitivity reactions
    - Antibiotics: sulfonamides, penicillins, chloramphenicol, amphotericin B, tetracycline, streptomycin
    - Antituberculous: isoniazid, para-aminosalicylic acid
    - Anticonvulsants: phenindione, phenytoin, carbemazepine
    - Anti-inflammatories: indomethacin, phenylbutazone
    - Diuretics: acetazolamide, chlorthalidone, hydrochlorothiazide, spironolactone
    - Others: amitriptyline, methyldopa, sulfonylureas
  - Drugs not causing hypersensitivity reactions
    - Cocaine, cyclophosphamide, lithium, interferon alpha
  - Nondrug causes
    - Radiation, giant-cell myocarditis

The mechanisms of injury when lymphocytes infiltrate the myocardium are unknown. In the murine model, messenger ribonucleic acid (m-RNA) of perforin, the pore-forming protein mediating cytotoxicity, was identified in cytoplasmic granules of infiltrating cells by in situ hybridization.[42] Similarly, biopsy samples from patients with active myocarditis contain perforin granules in infiltrating cells,[38] implying that direct cytotoxicity can occur. Alternatively, release of cytokines such as interleukin-1, interleukin-6, interleukin-8, and tumor necrosis factor alpha may cause reversible depression of myocardial contractility without resulting in cell death.[39] Therefore, the effect of T cell–mediated immune injury may be either irreversible as a result of cell death through cytotoxicity (perforin) or reversible as a result of injury mediated by cytokines. A marked reduction in myocardial cell damage is noted in T cell–depleted mice inoculated with encephalomyocarditis virus.

Antiheart antibodies in the serum of patients with myocarditis have been reported but may reflect nonspecific myocardial damage.[43] When serum from patients with myocarditis was screened for autoantibodies, high-titer immunoglobulin G (IgG) with cardiac specificity was detected in 59 percent of patients with myocarditis and in none of the normal samples.[44] Antibodies with specificity for contractile and energy-transport proteins have been identified. In sera from patients with active myocarditis, Western immunoblotting demonstrated reactivity of a fraction that includes antibody to the heavy chain of cardiac myosin.[44] In a murine myocarditis model, cardiac myosin antibodies are observed following coxsackie B virus infection.[45] Moreover, injection of cardiac antimyosin antibodies without infection results in myocarditis that is histologically similar to that seen following coxsackie B3 virus infection.[46,47]

The role of viral infection has been deemphasized following the popularization of the immune injury hypothesis. Viral infection is the trigger for the immune response that is deleterious. Attempts to culture virus from human myocardial tissue generally have been unsuccessful. Only a single case report of Coxsackievirus identified in a myocardial biopsy specimen in an adult has been described.[48] However, identification of viral genomic fragments in myocardial samples by in situ hybridization and polymerase chain reaction from patients with myocarditis and dilated cardiomyopathy have been reported.[49–66] These genomic fragments may not be capable of replicating as intact cardiotropic virus but probably serve as a persistent source of antigen to drive the deleterious immune responses.[67]

In addition to the tropism of the virus, host immune responses play an important role in determining the severity of the clinical disease. When quantitative peripheral T- and B-lymphocyte populations were analyzed in patients with dilated cardiomyopathy and myocarditis, no consistent changes were detected.[68,69] However, immunologic assays demonstrate a reduction in the function of natural killer cells, antibody-dependent cellular cytotoxic cells, and suppressor cells and an increase in circulating levels of interleukin-1 and tumor necrosis factor alpha.[69–72] These immunoregulatory defects may predispose the host with a high antigenic load to develop immune responses that are not modulated by the natural inhibitory immunoregulatory mechanisms.

In addition to chronic inflammatory immune mechanism or persistent viral infection, apoptotic cell death may be another mechanism by which myocarditis can result in cardiomyopathy. Several different viruses have been reported to be triggers for apoptosis.

The association between acute myocarditis and dilated cardiomyopathy has been recognized for the past two centuries. However, the link between these two diseases remains circumstantial. Autoreactive antibodies and interleukin-2 receptors are identified commonly in both patients with myocarditis and those with dilated cardiomyopathy. Serologic titers to cardiotropic viruses are more common in patients with cardiomyopathy than in normal subjects. Viral genomic material can be detected more frequently by polymerase chain reaction (PCR) in patients with dilated cardiomyopathy versus other cardiac diseases. Animal models of myocarditis can progress to dilated cardiomyopathy, as can patients with clinically suspected or biopsy-proven myocarditis. However, the percentage of patients with idiopathic dilated cardiomyopathy that represent the end stage of an active myocarditis is unknown.

Clinical Presentation The clinical manifestations of myocarditis are variable. Most patients have a self-limited disease, whereas others present in profound cardiogenic shock. The most obvious symptom suggesting myocarditis is an antecedent viral syndrome. Flu-like symptoms occur in approximately 60 percent of patients.[73] Chest pain may occur in up to 35 percent of patients and may be typically ischemic, somewhat atypical, or pericardial in character. Occasionally patients will present with a clinical syndrome identical to an acute myocardial infarction, with left ventricular asynergy, electrocardiographic evidence of injury or Q waves, and ischemic cardiac pain[74] (Fig. 69-3). In this syndrome, at autopsy, the coronary arteries are widely patent, although viral coronary arteritis has been reported.[75,76] Coronary vasospasm has also been associated with acute myocarditis.[77]

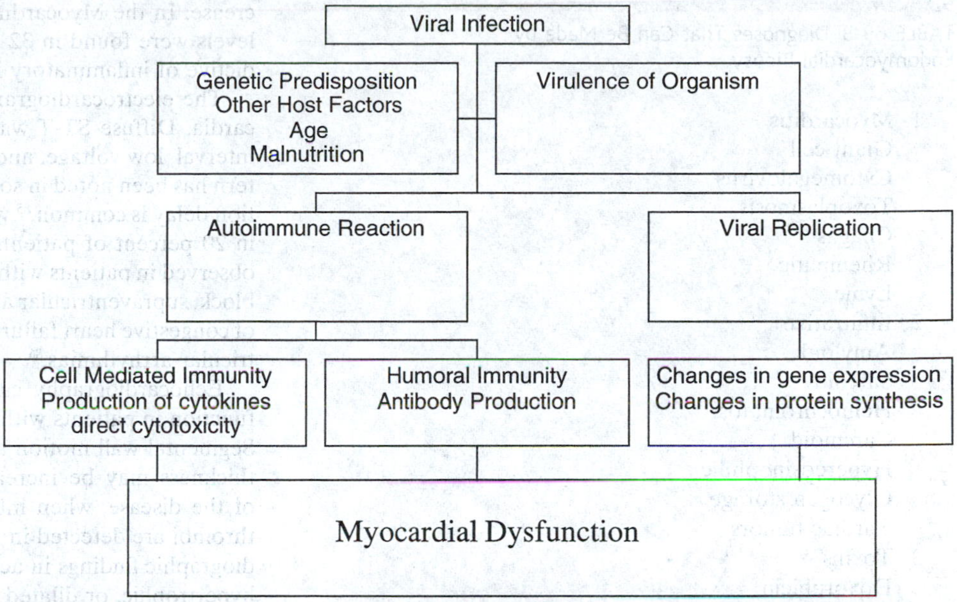

FIGURE 69-2 Flow diagram illustrating various factors that contribute to the development of myocardial dysfunction after viral infection.

Patients may present with syncope or palpitations with atrioventricular (AV) block or ventricular arrhythmia. Complete AV block is common with some patients presenting with Stokes-Adams attacks. The complete heart block is generally transient and rarely requires a permanent pacemaker.[78] Sudden cardiac death can be the initial presentation of myocarditis in some patients, presumably from complete heart block or ventricular tachycardia. In a 20-year review of sudden death among Air Force recruits, 20 percent had myocarditis documented at autopsy.[79] In some patients with refractory ventricular arrhythmias, endomyocardial biopsy or autopsy has revealed myocarditis. Systemic or pulmonary thromboembolic disease is also associated with myocarditis.[80,81]

A familial tendency for the development of myocarditis may be present. In one report, a suppressor cell defect was detected, predisposing to development of active myocarditis.[82] Patients with peripartum cardiomyopathy have a high frequency of myocarditis on endomyocardial biopsy.[83] The immunoregulatory changes during and following pregnancy may heighten susceptibility to viral myocarditis, and exposure to trophoblastic antigens may predispose to immune-mediated myocardial injury.

Patients with new-onset left ventricular dysfunction given the diagnosis of idiopathic dilated cardiomyopathy may actually have active myocarditis despite the absence of clinical signs and symptoms of acute infection.[84]

Diagnosis Laboratory findings are generally not diagnostic. Sixty percent of patients will have an elevated erythrocyte sedimentation rate and 25 percent an elevated white blood cell count.[73] Elevated titers to cardiotropic viruses may be present. However, a fourfold rise in IgG titer over a 4- to 6-week period is required to document acute infection. Elevated IgM antibody titer may denote an acute infection more specifically than a rise in IgG antibody titer. Unfortunately, a rise in antibody titer documents only the response to a recent viral infection and does not indicate active myocarditis.

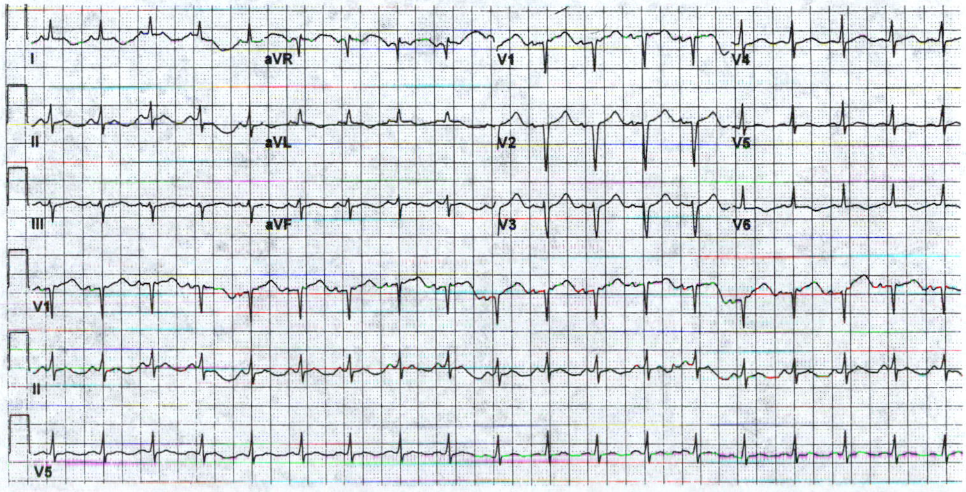

FIGURE 69-3 Electrocardiographic tracing consistent with an anteroseptal myocardial infarction and lateral ischemia in a patient with acute myocarditis and normal coronary arteries.

TABLE 69-3 Diagnoses That Can Be Made by Endomyocardial Biopsy

1. Myocarditis
   - Giant cell
   - Cytomegalovirus
   - Toxoplasmosis
   - Chagas
   - Rheumatic
   - Lyme
2. Infiltrative
   - Amyloid
   - Sarcoid
   - Hemochromatosis
   - Carcinoid
   - Hypereosinophilic
   - Glycogen storage
   - Cardiac tumors
3. Toxins
   - Doxorubicin
   - Chloroquine
   - Radiation injury
4. Genetic
   - Fabry
   - Kearns-Sayre syndrome
   - Right ventricular dysplasia

Abnormalities in peripheral T- and B-lymphocyte counts have been reported, but these findings have not been consistent and cannot be used as diagnostic adjuncts.

Increase in the MB band of CPK is observed in approximately 12 percent of patients.[73] Troponin levels may also increase. In the Myocarditis Treatment Trial, elevated troponin levels were found in 32 percent of the patients and were predictive of inflammatory involvement.

The electrocardiogram most frequently shows sinus tachycardia. Diffuse ST-T-wave changes, prolongation of the QTc interval, low voltage, and even an acute myocardial infarct pattern has been noted in some patients with myocarditis. Conduction delay is common,[85] with left bundle branch block identified in 20 percent of patients. Cardiac arrhythmias are frequently observed in patients with myocarditis, including complete heart block, supraventricular arrhythmias—especially in the presence of congestive heart failure or pericardial inflammation, and ventricular arrhythmias.[86]

Echocardiography can reveal left ventricular systolic dysfunction in patients with a normal-sized left ventricular cavity. Segmental wall motion abnormalities may be observed.[87] Wall thickness may be increased, particularly early in the course of the disease, when inflammation is fulminant.[88] Ventricular thrombi are detected in 15 percent of those studies.[89] Echocardiographic findings in active myocarditis can mimic restrictive, hypertrophic, or dilated cardiomyopathy.

Endomyocardial biopsy is the critical test to confirm the diagnosis. Endomyocardial biopsy techniques enable the repetitive sampling of the human myocardium with minimal discomfort and minor morbidity.[84,90,91] Right ventricular myocardial specimens can be obtained by accessing the right internal jugular or femoral vein. Intravascular biopsy of the left ventricle is infrequently performed due to the higher morbidity associated with this approach. The right ventricular bioptome is positioned under fluoroscopy or echocardiography to sample the interventricular septum.[90] As the myocarditis can be focal, a minimum of four to six fragments are obtained. Sampling error is reduced by less than 5 percent. Using the Stanford bioptome, typical samples are 2 to 3 mm in maximal diameter and 5 mg in wet weight. Samples are processed, paraffin-imbedded, sectioned, and stained with hematoxylin-eosin and trichrome. Special stains are employed if other diagnoses are considered. Diagnoses that can be made or confirmed by endomyocardial biopsy are listed in Table 69-3.

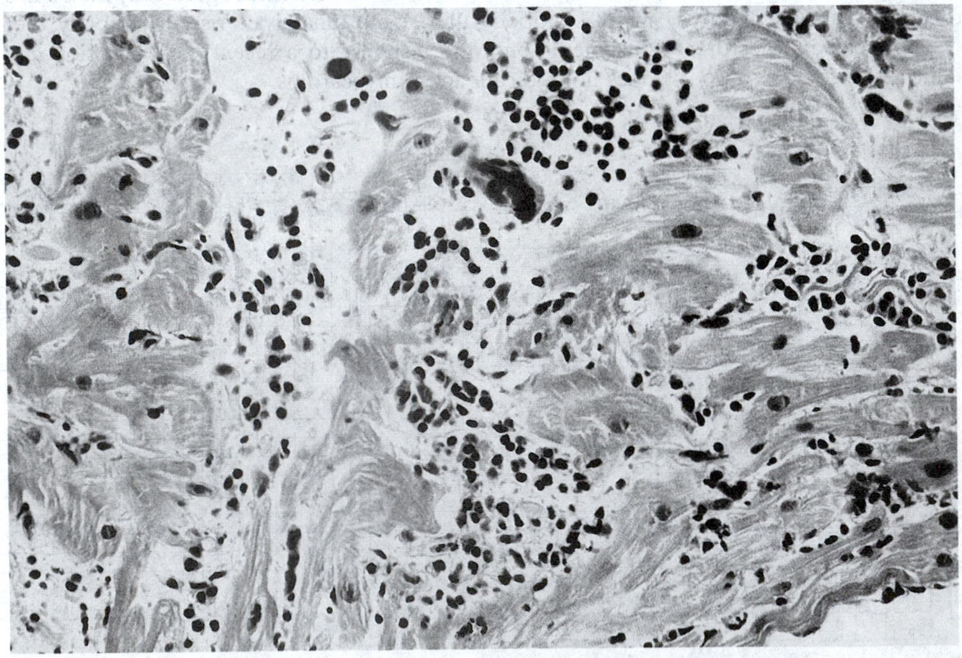

FIGURE 69-4 Photomicrograph showing extensive interstitial infiltrates of lymphocytes and myocytes with focal myocyte necrosis. (H&E, ×40.)

Several investigators have performed endomyocardial biopsies in patients with unexplained congestive heart failure and/or ventricular arrhythmia.[84,92–122] The percentage of patients with biopsies interpreted as myocarditis varied widely, primarily owing to the different diagnostic criteria for active myocarditis used by the investigators. This variability of endomyocardial biopsy criteria prompted a meeting of cardiac pathologists to reach a consensus on the pathologic definition of myocarditis, now known as "the Dallas criteria." Active myocarditis was defined as "an inflammatory infiltrate of the myocardium with necrosis and/or degeneration of adjacent myocytes not typical of the ischemic damage associated with coronary artery disease."[123] Examination of a minimum of four to six fragments from each patient is required for interpretation. The term *borderline* myocarditis is applied when the inflammatory infiltrate is too sparse or myocyte injury is not demonstrated. Repeat biopsy is then suggested. A high frequency of active myocarditis is confirmed by repeat biopsy in patients whose initial histologic samples demonstrated borderline myocarditis.[124] When right ventricular endomyocardial biopsy has failed to establish the diagnosis, sampling the left ventricle may improve diagnostic yield (Fig. 69-4).

Endomyocardial biopsy must be applied as quickly as possible to maximize the diagnostic yield. Biopsies in patients with peripartum cardiomyopathy have the highest yield when performed early after onset of symptoms.[83] Resolution of active myocarditis has been documented within 4 days of initial biopsy, with progressive clearing over several weeks on serial biopsy.[125] Progression of active myocarditis to dilated cardiomyopathy has been documented when serial biopsies are performed.[126]

Newer molecular biology techniques are being applied to the analysis of endomyocardial tissue for the detection of viral nucleic acid. The usefulness of PCR amplification of viral genomic material from endomyocardial tissue in children with suspected myocarditis was shown in a study that found PCR-amplified viral product in 67 percent of the children studied.

Noninvasive Studies Although technetium-99m-pyrophosphate scintigraphy has proved useful in the detection of myocarditis in a murine model, it has not been effective in diagnosing myocarditis in humans. Imaging with gallium 67, an inflammation-avid radioisotope, has shown promise as a screening method for active myocarditis, with a specificity and sensitivity of 83 percent and a negative predictive value of 98 percent in biopsy-proven myocarditis.[100] Indium 111–labeled antimyosin antibody scans can be used to detect myocyte necrosis. Application of this technique in patients with myocarditis has demonstrated a sensitivity of 83 percent, a specificity of 53 percent, and a positive predictive value of a normal scan of 92 percent.[124] In those patients who were antimyosin antibody–positive and biopsy-negative, the possibility of inflammation undetected by biopsy has been considered. Antimyosin imaging, however, detects myocyte injury independent of etiology, and noninflammatory causes of heart muscle injury in young patients may cause false-positive scans. The usefulness of scintigraphy in diagnosing myocarditis is limited by low specificiy, radiation exposure, and expense (see also Chap. 16).

Tissue alterations associated with myocarditis may be identifiable using magnetic resonance imaging (MRI).[127] Preliminary results suggest that myocardial inflammation may induce abnormal signal intensity of the myocardial walls. Use of T2-weighted images to visualize tissue edema has been described in several case reports of patients with active myocarditis. More recently, contrast media–enhanced MRI has been used to characterize myocardial changes in myocarditis. The MRI imaging contrast agent gadopentetate dimeglumine accumulates in inflammatory lesions (see Chap. 18A). It is a hydrophilic agent that accumulates in the extracellular space of water-containing tissues. Gadolinium increases the signal of T1-weighted images. A total of 19 patients with clinically suspected myocarditis and 18 normal subjects underwent contrast-enhanced MRI. Global relative enhancement was higher in patients than controls. Contrast MRI also visualized the area of inflammation and the extent of inflammation and may prove to be a valuable technique in both the diagnosis and monitoring of disease activity.

Despite the promise of noninvasive techniques, endomyocardial biopsy remains the diagnostic standard.

Treatment The immune injury hypothesis generated application of potential therapies, including immunosuppression. Anecdotal success with immunosuppression in active viral myocarditis[101,106] led to the large Multicenter Myocarditis Treatment Trial.[128] In this study, 111 patients with biopsy-proven myocarditis were randomized between conventional medical therapy versus steroid/azathioprine or steroid/cyclosporine immunosuppression. The primary end point of the study was change in ejection fraction over 28 weeks. For all patients, the average increase in ejection fraction over baseline was 9 percent. Treatment assignment was not predictive of improvement in left ventricular ejection fraction, attenuation of clinical disease, or mortality[129] (Fig. 69-5).

Recently, immune modulatory therapy with immune globulin has been shown to be an effective treatment for Kawasaki's disease and new-onset cardiomyopathy in pediatric patients.[130] Subsequently, a small open-label study was performed in 10 adult patients with new-onset heart failure.[131] Significant improvement in left ventricular function was observed in 9 of 10 patients. These findings formed the basis for a multicenter study investigating the use of this treatment modality. The IMAC trial (Intervention in Myocarditis and Acute Cardiomyopathy with immune globulin) used a single infusion of high-dose immunoglobulin (2 g/kg) to treat presumed inflammatory cardio-

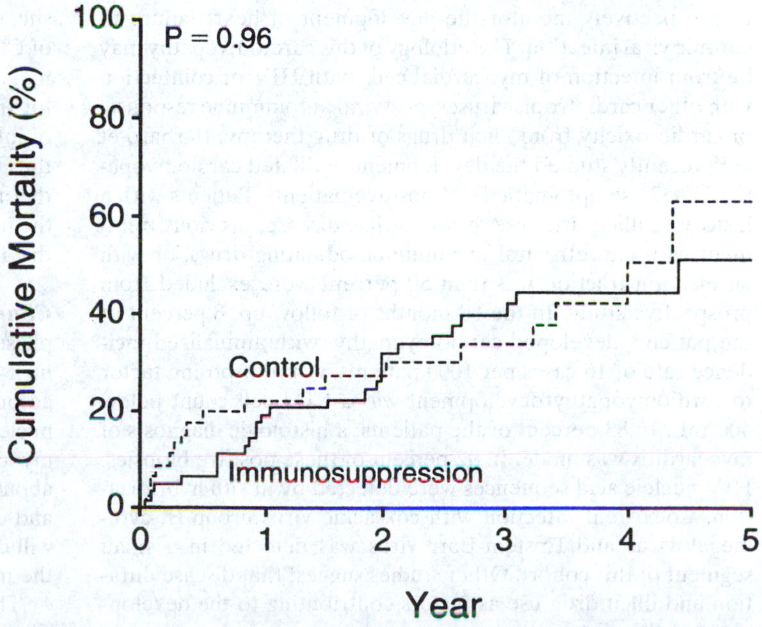

FIGURE 69-5 Actuarial mortality curves from the Myocarditis Treatment Trial illustrating no difference in survival between the treatment groups. (From Mason et al.,[129] with permission.)

myopathies. In this placebo-controlled 6-month trial, the improvement in left ventricular ejection fraction and symptoms was similar in both groups. Thus no benefit of immunomodulation could be demonstrated.

Despite the experimental data supporting the immune injury hypothesis, no randomized study has yet demonstrated the efficacy of immunosuppressive therapy in myocarditis. Immunosuppressive therapy is therefore not routinely recommended for infective myocarditis. Standard heart failure treatment remains the mainstay of therapy.

Prognosis About one-third of those who present with clinical carditis and recover will be left with some cardiac abnormality ranging from mild changes on electrocardiography (ECG) to significant heart failure. The multicenter myocarditis trial provided insight into the natural history of myocarditis with current treatment. The degree of left ventricular dysfunction at initial presentation was most predictive of recovery. Approximately 40 percent of patients fully recovered.[104] Other predictors of recovery included shorter duration of disease and less intensive conventional drug therapy. One-year survival in this study was 80 percent, with a 4-year survival of only 44 percent.

The prognosis of myocarditis depends to some extent on the causative agent, but if clinical heart failure develops, 5-year mortality rates are in the 50 to 60 percent range, comparable with figures seen in idiopathic cardiomyopathy.[132] Chronic inflammation, viral persistence, or both may affect disease progression and prognosis. Future therapies will need to identify the predominant factor to target treatment and hopefully improve survival.

Human Immunodeficiency Virus Human immunodeficiency virus (HIV) is increasingly recognized as a cause of dilated cardiomyopathy. In some inner-city hospitals, it may represent a very common diagnosis. The relatively recent emergence of this virus in the early 1980s has provided a unique opportunity to prospectively monitor the development of heart failure to chronic viral infection. The etiology of this cardiomyopathy may be from infection of myocardial cells with HIV or coinfection with other cardiotropic viruses, postviral autoimmune response, or cardiotoxicity from illicit drugs or drug therapy. Barbaro et al.[133] recently studied the development of dilated cardiomyopathy in 952 asymptomatic HIV-positive patients. Patients with a history of illicit drug use, prior cardiac disease, previous treatment with antiretroviral or immunomodulating drugs, or with an ejection fraction less than 50 percent were excluded from prospective study. In the 60 months of follow up, 8 percent of the patients developed cardiomyopathy, with annualized incidence rate of 16 cases per 1000 patients. A predisposing factor to cardiomyopathy development was a CD4 cell count below 400/mL. In 83 percent of the patients, a histologic diagnosis of myocarditis was made. In 92 percent of these positive biopsies, HIV nucleic acid sequences were detected by in situ hybridization. Coexistent infection with coxsackie virus group B, cytomegalovirus and Epstein-Barr virus was detected in a small segment of this cohort. Other studies suggest that disease duration and illicit drug use as factors contributing to the development of this disease.[134]

As the symptoms of heart failure and HIV can be very similar (i.e., fatigue, wasting, etc.), careful cardiologic follow-up of these patients is probably indicated to detect early development of left ventricular dysfunction. Conventional heart failure management can then be instituted to alleviate cardiac-related symptoms.

Cytomegalovirus Cytomegalovirus may lead to myocarditis in the general population, but ordinarily the myocarditis is self-limited and asymptomatic. In the cardiac transplant recipient, however, cytomegalovirus myocarditis may become a more serious disease resulting in cardiac dysfunction.[135] The treatment of cytomegalovirus myocarditis is intravenous ganciclovir, which effectively eradicates the virus. Early cytomegalovirus infection correlates with the development of allograft coronary artery disease, the major cause of death beyond the first year after cardiac transplantation. It is proposed that infection of either subintimal fibroblasts or endothelial cells results in immunologic injury that predisposes to this potentially fatal condition.

NONVIRAL

Chagas' Disease American trypanosomiasis, or Chagas' disease, is the most common cause of congestive heart failure in the world.[136] This condition results from the bite of the reduviid bug, leading to infection with *Trypanosoma cruzi,* and is endemic to rural South and Central America.

Pathogenesis The pathogenesis of chronic, chagasic cardiomyopathy is controversial because the parasite is rarely present in the myocardium. As in the viral cardiomyopathy model, the cardiac injury is thus thought to be immunologically mediated.[137] Both cellular and humoral immune responses have been implemented in the myocardial injury.[137] Myocardial biopsies demonstrate that the inflammatory infiltrate in chronic Chagas' disease consists mainly of CD8+ T cells, with a low number of CD4+ T cells.[138–140] This suggests some degree of immunologic depression in the host, since the activation of T-helper cells is known to be the most effective mechanism of defense against the parasites.[141] Some have postulated that the diminished expression of CD4+ T cells during acute *T. cruzi* infection may be related to a mechanism of tolerance induced by the parasite. Evidence for this comes from studies that have shown that the addition of interleukin-1 (IL-1) in vitro restores helper T-cell function, thus implementing a macrophage defect in this process.[142] Furthermore, IL-2 and the IL-2 receptor are absent or scarce in the inflammatory infiltrate,[143] attesting to the attenuated role of the T-helper subset in this disease.

Clinical Presentation This parasitic disease has an acute phase, where hematogenous spread of the parasite leads to invasion of various tissues and organ systems. The invasion is accompanied by an intense inflammatory reaction with mononuclear cells and is characterized by fever, sweating, myalgias, myocarditis, hepatosplenomegaly, and a case fatality rate of about 5 percent. Most patients recover from the acute illness and enter an asymptomatic latent phase, but 20 to 30 percent will develop a chronic form of the disease up to 20 years after the initial infection.

The chronic stage is a result of gradual tissue destruction. The gastrointestinal tract and the heart are the most common sites of involvement, with the primary cause of death being cardiac failure. In the gut, the destruction of the myenteric plexus is responsible for the development of megaesophagus and megacolon. In the heart, the myofibrils and the Purkinje fibers are replaced by fibrous tissue, leading to cardiomegaly, congestive heart failure, heart block, and arrhythmia. The microscopic findings are those of extensive fibrosis, but a chronic cellular infiltrate composed of lymphocytes, plasma cells, and macrophages is often present and parasites are found in about a quarter of the patients.

The diagnosis of the acute disease depends on the discovery of trypomastigotes in the blood of the infected individual. In chronic infection, direct diagnosis is less useful due to less circulating trypomastigotes. Xenodiagnosis (where the patient is bitten by reduviid bugs bred in the laboratory and subsequent identification of the parasites in the intestine of the insect) is the most useful test, which will detect infection in about half the patients. The complement-fixation test (Machado-Guerreiro test) also has high sensitivity and specificity for identification of chronic Chagas' disease. In the other lab tests, it is necessary to rely on positive serologic tests (such as the indirect immunofluorescent antibody, the enzyme-linked immunosorbent assay, and the hemagglutination tests) together with symptoms and signs compatible with Chagas' disease.

Endomyocardial biopsy may show active myocarditis using the Dallas criteria.[144] Noninvasive assessment commonly shows segmental wall motion abnormalities, specifically apical aneurysms. Electrocardiographic findings include complete heart block, atrioventricular block, or right bundle branch block with or without fascicular block in 11 percent of infected individuals.[145] Ventricular arrhythmias may require antiarrhythmic drugs, including amiodarone.[146]

The treatment of chronic Chagas' disease is symptomatic and includes a pacemaker for complete heart block, an implantable cardioverter-defibrillator for recurrent ventricular arrhythmia, and standard therapy for congestive heart failure as outlined for other forms of myocarditis. Antiparasitic agents such as Nifurtimox and benzimidazole eradicate parasitemia during the acute phase and are typically curative. They should be administered if the disease has not previously been treated and may be used as prophylaxis if there is a high likelihood of recurrence, such as following immunosuppressive therapy. The role of immunosuppression therapy for chagasic myocarditis is controversial, and heart transplantation is effective for end-stage refractory cardiac disease.

Lyme Carditis Lyme disease may result from infection with the spirochete *Borrelia burgdorferi,* introduced by a tick bite. The initial presenting symptom in patients with the disease who progress to cardiac involvement is frequently complete heart block. Left ventricular dysfunction may be seen but is unusual.[147] Endomyocardial biopsy may show active myocarditis. Rarely are spirochetes seen on biopsy. Corticosteroid administration is helpful in treating Lyme carditis following therapy with tetracycline.[148]

Among other infectious etiologies is *Toxoplasma gondii,* which is curable by pyrimethamine and sulfadiazine[149] and occurs most commonly in the immune-deficient host. Leptospirosis is yet another common cause in fatal cases of myocarditis. Fifty percent of cases have ST- and T-wave changes on electrocardiography.

Rheumatic Carditis One form of myocarditis that has declined dramatically in the latter half of the twentieth century is rheumatic carditis.[150] The availability of antibiotics and changes in the virulence and serotypes of group A streptococcus may explain the decreasing frequency of this disease.[151]

Acute rheumatic fever can occur in children and young adults. It generally follows a group A streptococcal pharyngitis, but only indirect evidence linking the two has been found. Rheumatic carditis may result from a direct toxic effect of some streptococcal product versus an immunologic mechanism.[152–154] Group A streptococci have a number of structural components similar to those of human tissue. Antibodies to streptococci cross-react with the glycoproteins of heart valves. The serum of patients with rheumatic fever contains autoantibodies to myosin and sarcolemma. The Aschoff body, pathognomic for this disorder, represents persistent focal inflammatory lesions in the myocardium. These nodules can persist for years after an acute attack. Macrophages containing myosin have been identified in these nodules.

Clinical diagnosis is made using the Jones criteria[155] (see also Chap. 55). The major manifestations are carditis, polyarthritis, chorea, erythema marginatum, subcutaneous nodules, and evidence of preceding streptococcal infection (i.e., positive throat culture, history of scarlet fever, elevated antistreptolysin titers). Minor criteria are nonspecific findings such as fever, arthralgia, previous rheumatic fever or rheumatic heart disease, elevated ESR or reactive protein, and prolonged PR interval. Diagnosis is made by the presence of two major criteria or one major and two minor criteria. Debate into whether the Jones criteria should be modified to incorporate Doppler-Echo indices are ongoing.[156,157]

Two-thirds of patients present with an antecedent pharyngitis, followed by the symptoms of rheumatic fever in 1 to 5 weeks, with a mean presentation of 18.6 days. Severe carditis resulting in death can occur but is unusual. CHF is observed in only 5 to 10 percent of cases. Usually the carditis is mild, with the predominant effect being scarring of the heart valves. Physical exam is notable for fever and heart murmurs reflecting the acute valvulitis. The mitral valve is involved three times as frequently as the aortic valve; therefore mitral murmurs are more common. Mitral regurgitation is the most common finding. A mid diastolic murmur over the apical area can frequently be heard. This

TABLE 69-4 Drug Causes of Eosinophilic Myocarditis

Drug	
Acetazolamide	Oxyphenylbutazone
Amitriptyline	Para-aminosalicylic acid
Amphotericin B	Penicillin
Ampicillin	Phenindione
Carbamazepine	Phenobarbital
Cefaclor	Phenylbutazone
Chloramphenicol	Phenytoin
Chlorthalidone	Spironolactone
Desipramine	Streptomycin
Hydrochlorothiazide	Sulfadiazine
Indomethacin	Sulfisoxazole
Interleukin-4	Sulfononylureas
Isoniazid	Tetanus toxoid
Methyldopa	Tetracycline

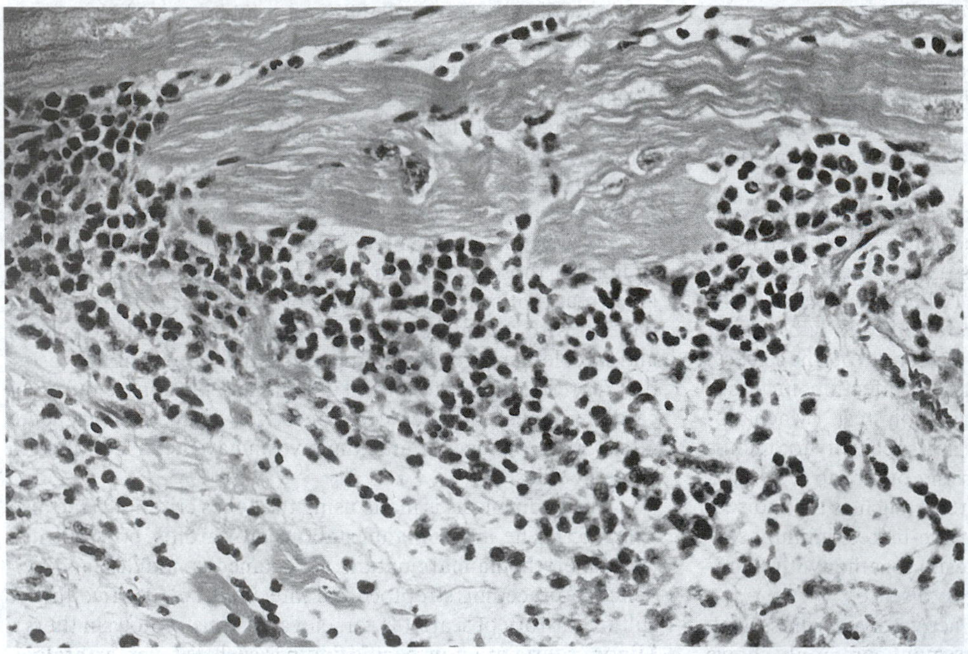

FIGURE 69-6 Photomicrograph showing interstitial infiltrates rich in eosinophils. (H&E, ×40.)

is called the Carey Coombs murmur, and its presence almost certainly confirms mitral valvulitis. Aortic insufficiency can be auscultated with aortic valvulitis.

There are no characteristic ECG findings through PR prolongation, and nonspecific ST-T-wave changes are frequently described. Endomyocardial biopsy demonstrates the Aschoff nodules as well as a diffuse cellular interstitial infiltrate including lymphocytes, polymorphonuclear cells, histiocytes, and eosinophils.

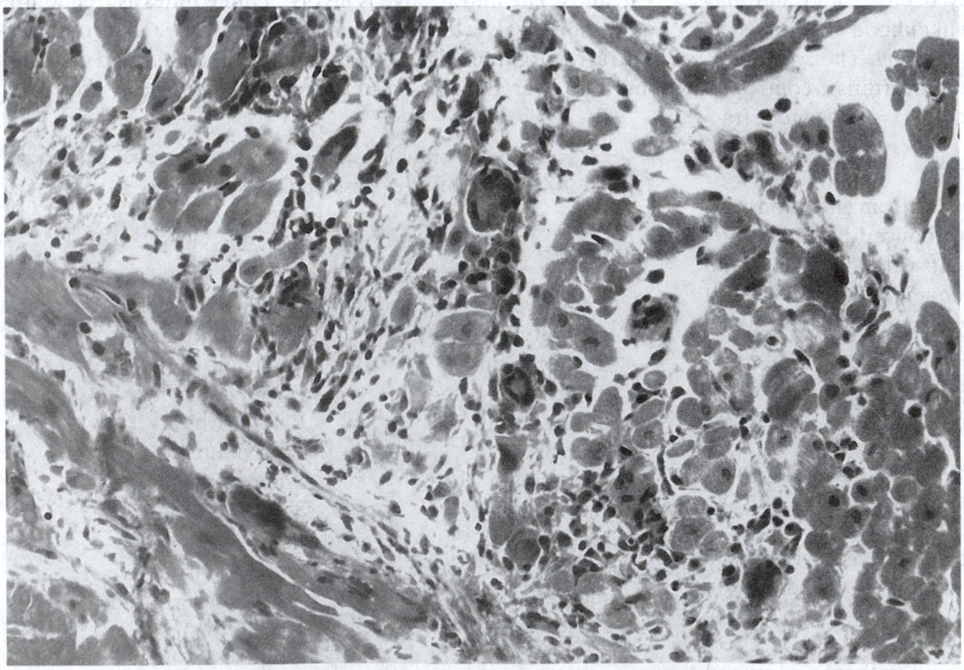

FIGURE 69-7 Photomicrograph showing extensive myocyte damage and infiltrates of mononuclear cells and numerous multinucleated giant cells. (H&E, ×60.)

Laboratory tests suggestive of rheumatic fever include antibodies to antistreptolysin O and anti-DNAase B, an elevated sedimentation rate, and elevated C-reactive protein. Extracardiac manifestations generally predominant with an acute migratory polyarthritis of the large joints. Aspirin and penicillin are the mainstays of therapy. Corticosteroids can also provide symptomatic relief. Once rheumatic fever is diagnosed, antibiotic prophylaxis is required to prevent recurrent episodes. The most effective method is a single monthly intramuscular injection of 1.2 million units of benzathine Penicillin G until age 21.

Noninfective

HYPERSENSITIVITY

Hypersensitivity myocarditis is an example of the early phase of eosinophilic myocarditis and is thought to be due to an allergic reaction to a variety drugs (Table 69-4). Methyldopa, the penicillins, sulfonamides, tetracycline, and the antituberculous drugs are the pharmaceuticals most commonly associated with this entity. It is characterized by peripheral eosinophilia and infiltration into the myocardium by eosinophils, multinucleated giant cells, and leukocytes (Fig. 69-6).[158] The major basic protein of the eosinophil granule may be detected in the presence of acute necrotizing myocarditis, suggesting toxicity of the granule contents.[159] Good success has been reported with stopping the offending agent and treatment with corticosteroids.[160] Unfortunately, the presence of this condition often goes unnoticed and the first manifestation of cardiac involvement is sudden death due to arrhythmia.

GIANT-CELL MYOCARDITIS

Giant-cell myocarditis is an extremely rare but aggressive form of myocarditis, typically progressive and unresponsive to medical therapy.[161] This disease is most prevalent in young adults, with a mean age at onset of 42 years (and a range of 16 to 69 years). Association with other autoimmune disorders is reported in approximately 20 percent of cases. Diagnosis is made by endomyocardial biopsy. Widespread or multifocal necrosis with a mixed inflammatory infiltrate including lymphocytes and

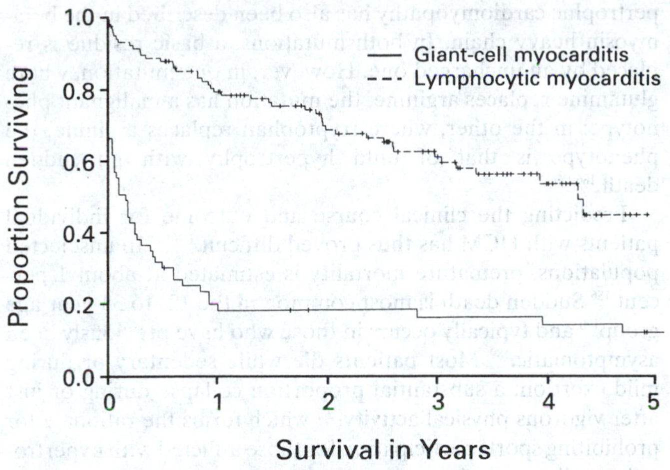

FIGURE 69-8 Kaplan Meier survival curves for patients with giant-cell myocarditis versus lymphocytic myocarditis. (From Cooper et al.,[161] with permission.)

histiocytes is required for histologic diagnosis. Eosinophils are frequently noted, as are multinucleated giant cells in the absence of granuloma (Fig. 69-7). Immunophenotyping of the cellular infiltrate has shown lymphocyte populations composed of T-helper or in some cases T-suppressor cells.

The clinical course is usually characterized by progressive CHF and is frequently associated with refractory ventricular arrhythmia.[162] It is almost uniformly and rapidly fatal. Comparison of survival of patients with giant-cell myocarditis with that of patients with lymphocytic myocarditis demonstrates significantly worse survival in those patients with giant-cell disease (Fig. 69-8). There have been rare reports of response to aggressive immunosuppressive regimens that include cyclosporine and azathioprine in addition to corticosteroids.[162,163] Use of immunosuppressive therapy in these patients appears to prolong survival. Cardiac transplantation represents the best treatment option, though most patients expire prior to identification of a suitable donor. Giant-cell myocarditis may recur following cardiac transplantation, but the frequency of recurrence is unknown. Giant cells can be detected on routine surveillance biopsies up to 9 years posttransplant. This cellular infiltrate may respond to an increase in immunosuppressive therapy.

PERIPARTUM

Peripartum cardiomyopathy is an uncommon form of CHF first described by Virchow in 1870.[164] Estimates of its incidence vary from 1 to 1300 to 1 in 15,000 pregnancies.[165] The disease occurs more commonly in obese multiparous black females over age 30.[166] Cesarean delivery, multiple gestations, preeclampsia, and chronic hypertension are other predisposing factors. Patients present with heart failure in the last trimester of pregnancy or in the first 5 months postpartum. Absence of a demonstrable cause of heart failure and structural heart disease is required to make the diagnosis. Indeed, the hemodynamic stress of pregnancy can frequently unmask previously unknown cardiac disease (see also Chap. 82).

PATHOGENESIS

The etiology of this disorder is unclear. Proposed mechanisms include nutritional deficiencies, genetic disorders, viral or autoimmune etiologies, hormonal problems, volume overload, alcohol, physiologic stress of pregnancy, or unmasking of latent idiopathic dilated cardiomyopathy. Several lines of evidence suggest that peripartum cardiomyopathy may be the result of myocarditis due to a viral illness or an autoimmune etiology.[167–172] Given the relatively immunosuppressed state of pregnancy, susceptibility to cardiotropic viruses is higher,[167] as is the viral load during infection.[168] Furthermore, studies have demonstrated that when cardiac output rises, as is the case in pregnancy, myocardial viral lesions worsen.[169] Additionally, several studies have demonstrated histologic evidence of myocarditis on endomyocardial biopsy samples obtained from patients with peripartum cardiomyopathy.[170–172] Other investigators have postulated an autoimmune etiology to peripartum cardiomyopathy, specifically immunologic responses to fetal and endometrial antigens that cross-react with the patient's myocytes. In one case report, a patient with peripartum cardiomyopathy had antibodies to smooth muscle and actin produced in response to actin and myosin released during uterine degeneration after delivery. These antibodies later cross-reacted with the myocardium and induced cardiomyopathy.[173]

CLINICAL PRESENTATION

The presentation is that of heart failure. Presenting symptoms include shortness of breath, dyspnea on exertion, edema, palpitations, syncope, sudden death, and thromboembolic phenomena. The incidence of thromboembolism is high due to the hypercoagulability of pregnancy. Physical findings are notable for S3, S4, tricuspid or mitral insufficiency murmurs, edema, rales, ascites, hepatomegaly, jugular venous distension. The ECG frequently shows left ventricular hypertrophy. Echocardiographic findings can range from single-chamber left ventricular enlargement to four-chamber dilatation. In a small percentage of patients, endomyocardial biopsy may reveal myocarditis, but generally the findings are nonspecific.

PROGNOSIS AND TREATMENT

Too few patients with peripartum cardiomyopathy have been studied to fully analyze the natural history of the disease. In a small series of 27 patients, left ventricular size was analyzed at 6 months; 14 patients (50 percent) had normal dimensions. None of these patients died of CHF—compared with 85 percent of those patients with persistent cardiomegaly, who died from CHF within 5 years.[174] The authors concluded, therefore, that if the congestive cardiomyopathy persists for more than 6 months, it is likely to be irreversible and to be associated with a worse prognosis. Similar findings were published in another series by O'Connell et al.[83] These authors also noted that those patients with higher ejection fractions and smaller ventricular diastolic dimensions at the time of diagnosis have a better long-term prognosis. Other prognostic studies suggest that those patients with persistent symptoms more than 2 weeks postpartum have a worse prognosis, raising the question as to whether this disorder has different etiologies.[175] The role of corticosteroids in the treatment of this disorder is controversial.[170,171] The incidence of thromboembolism is high due to the hypercoagulabilty of pregnancy; therefore anticoagulation is recommended.[175]

Patients with refractory heart failure referred for transplant have a survival posttransplant comparable with that of patients with idiopathic dilated cardiomyopathy, though higher early rejection rates are noted.

In patients with stable heart failure or recovery of left ventricular function, the possibility of subsequent pregnancy must be addressed. There are several case reports of patients with this diagnosis who went on to subsequent pregnancies. The outcomes of these patients are variable, with a few having uneventful pregnancies and others developing an exacerbation or recurrence of fulminant heart failure. Subsequent pregnancy should be viewed as high risk and all patients with this disorder should be counseled on birth control and even sterilization.

HYPERTROPHIC AND FAMILIAL

Hypertrophic cardiomyopathy is characterized by disproportionate hypertrophy primarily of the left ventricle (Fig. 69-9) and occasionally the right ventricle. It most typically involves the septum but can also be concentric[176] and occurs in the absence of a recognizable stimulus to hypertrophy. This has led many to postulate and subsequently demonstrate a genetic basis to this disease.[177] Inheritance is of an autosomal dominant pattern; however, the phenotypic expression of this disease as measured by echocardiography is highly variable and reflects the different genetic mutations and incomplete penetrance.[178–180] The identification of certain well-characterized genetic abnormalities offers some measure of prognostication. Several familial hypertrophic cardiomyopathy–causing mutations have been characterized in the genes encoding sarcomeric contractile proteins—namely, the beta-myosin heavy chain,[181] cardiac troponin T,[178] alpha tropomyosin,[178] and cardiac myosin–binding protein C.[182,183] Previous theories suggested that variations resulting in a change in charge of the substituted amino acid were associated with a poor survival index.[184,185] However, the genotypic-phenotypic correlation is not always preserved. For example, a cytosine-for-guanine mutation hot spot responsible for familial hypertrophic cardiomyopathy has also been described in the beta-myosin heavy chain. In both mutations, a basic residue is replaced by an uncharged one. However, in one mutation, where glutamine replaces arginine, the mutation has a malignant phenotype; in the other, where tryptophan replaces arginine, the phenotype is that of mild hypertrophy with no sudden death.[186,187]

Predicting the clinical course and outcome for individual patients with HCM has thus proved difficult.[188,189] In unselected populations, premature mortality is estimated at about 1 percent.[186] Sudden death is most common in the 12- to 35-year age group[190] and typically occurs in those who have previously been asymptomatic.[189] Most patients die while sedentary or during mild exertion; a substantial proportion collapse during or just after vigorous physical activity,[190] which forms the rationale for prohibiting sports participation for those afflicted with hypertrophic cardiomyopathy.

The mechanism of sudden death in hypertrophic cardiomyopathy is complex and probably multifactorial.[191] Recurrent syncope is the only symptom that has been shown to be reliably associated with subsequent sudden death.[192] Other proposed risk factors include prior cardiac arrest, sustained ventricular tachycardia, massive left ventricular hypertrophy, a malignant genotype or a previous family history of sudden premature death, repetitive salvos of nonsustained ventricular tachycardia on Holter monitoring, and early onset of symptoms in childhood.[193–196] The main forms of therapy have been primarily beta blockade, calcium channel blockers, amiodarone, and implantable cardioverter-defibrillators, with conflicting data on their impact on mortality.[197] Cardiac transplantation is pursued when significant symptomatic systolic dysfunction develops.[198]

As in the case of the myosin mutations noted in the hypertrophic cardiomyopathies, single genetic defects are presumed to underlie the dilated cardiomyopathies that have been described in several large families. There has been recent evidence that dilated cardiomyopathy is more frequently familial than generally realized.[199] In a single-center study of 96 patients with a diagnosis of idiopathic cardiomyopathy, approximately 20 percent had a familial basis.[200] Other studies have estimated a familial role in up to 50 percent of cases when first-degree relatives are carefully screened.[201] The influence of a preceding viral infection,[202] alcohol use,[203] or pregnancy[204] on the clinical manifestation of cardiomyopathy in familial situations remain unclear.

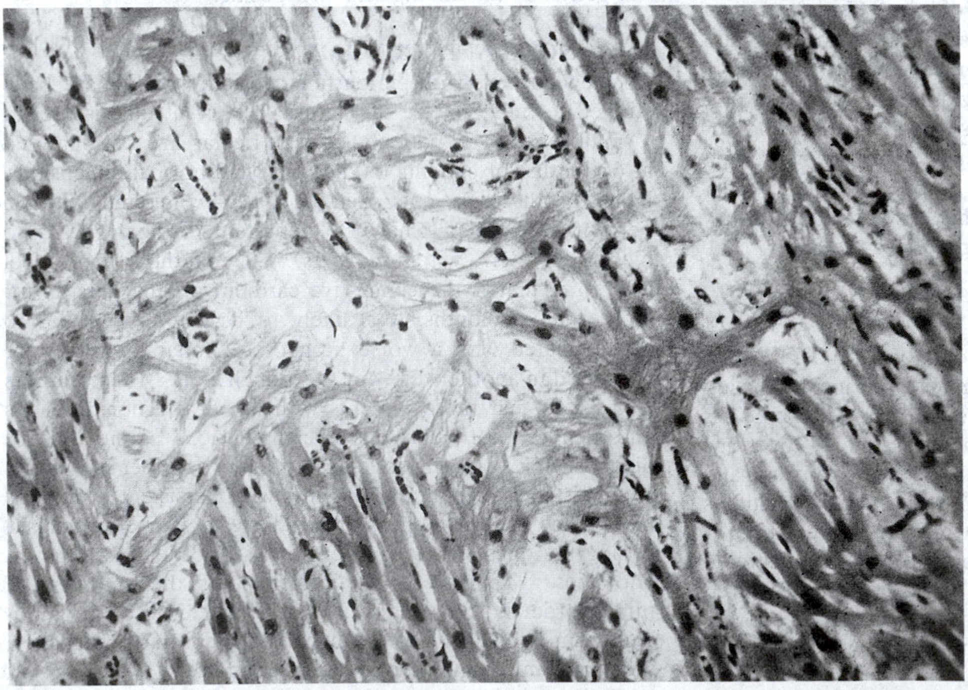

FIGURE 69-9 Photomicrograph showing significant myocyte disarray in hypertrophic cardiomyopathy. (H&E, ×40.)

Neuromuscular Diseases

Several heritable neuromuscular dystrophies may be associated with cardiomyopathy. Included in this category are diseases such as Beckel's, Duchenne's, and X-linked cardioskeletal myopathy, myotonic dystrophy (Stingert's disease), congenital myotonic dystrophy, limb-girdle muscular dystrophy (Erb's disease), familial centronuclear myopathy, Dugelberg-Welander syndrome, Friedreich's ataxia and Barth's syndrome. The myocardial involvement, natural history, and prognosis of each of these disorders are variable.

Duchenne's dystrophy is an X-linked disease with proximal muscle weakness and cardiomyopathy. A dystrophin gene mutation is responsible. Death usually results from respiratory and/or cardiorespiratory failure. Patients with myotonic dystrophy present between age 20 and 50 years, usually with arrhythmias.

Several mitochondrial myopathies have also been described.[177,205] Mitochondria are essential cellular organelles that convert oxygen to biochemically useful energy. Additionally, mitochondria function as calcium storage sites and modulators of cellular pH. As such, mitochondrial function affects muscle and ventricular function. Mitochondria are unique organelles with their own maternally inherited DNA, which encodes several respiratory chain proteins. Genetic defects in the mitochondrial respiratory chain enzymes—specifically complexes I, III, and IV—have been recognized as the cause in some cardiomyopathies. The presentation in mitochondrial myopathies is extremely heterogeneous, as each cell will contain a mixture of normal and mutant DNAs. Deletion mutations in DNA can occur and are frequently observed in these myopathies.

Mitochondrial myopathies include such disorders as Kearns-Sayre syndrome, chronic ophthalmoplegia, myoclonic epilepsy, ragged-red-fiber disease, and mitochondrial encephalomyopathy. The MELAS syndrome—mitochondrial encephalopathy, lactic acidosis, and stroke-like episodes—is associated with cardiomyopathy and generalized microangiopathy. Kearns-Sayre syndrome results from a deletion mutation in mitochondrial DNA. This ocular myopathic disease is associated with dilated or hypertrophic cardiomyopathy with cardiac conduction defects.

Defects in transport of molecules from the cytoplasm into the mitochondria have also been associated with cardiac and skeletal myopathy. One example is that of carnitine deficiency, discussed later in this chapter.

INFILTRATIVE

The infiltrative cardiomyopathies comprise several acquired and heritable conditions; these include amyloidosis, hemochromatosis, carcinoid, sarcoidosis, glycogen storage disease, endocardial fibroelastosis, and endomyocardial fibrosis due to hypereosinophilic syndromes or other collagen vascular disorders such as scleroderma or Churg-Strauss syndrome.

Amyloid

CLASSIFICATION AND PATHOGENESIS

The most commonly encountered of the infiltrative cardiomyopathies is amyloidosis, leading to an overproduction of a monoclonal immunoglobulin protein that is deposited throughout the body. Secondary amyloidosis results from the deposition of a protein other than immunoglobulin. Whereas primary amyloid has no associated systemic diseases, other chronic diseases are present in the secondary form. Secondary amyloidosis may result from familial, senile, or chronic inflammatory processes (rheumatoid arthritis, juvenile rheumatoid arthritis, ankylosing spondylitis, Crohn's disease, tuberculous paraplegia associated with decubitus ulcers, cystic fibrosis, and heroin use with chronically infected cutaneous injection sites). Familial Mediterranean fever is an autosomal recessive inherited disease of Sephardic Jews, Armenians, and other Mediterranean peoples associated with amyloid deposition. In the familial diseases, more than 40 different genetic mutations of the plasma protein transthyretin (prealbumin) have been associated with amyloid deposition. Inheritance is autosomal dominant, with the genetic defect being confined to a single amino acid substitution in the mature protein.[206,207]

The frequency of cardiac involvement varies with the different etiologies. Of patients with primary amyloid, one-third to one-half have cardiac involvement and more than one-fourth have symptomatic heart failure. Cardiac involvement in patients with secondary amyloidosis is much less frequent. Indeed, in amyloid due to chronic inflammatory processes, amyloid protein deposition is usually limited to the intima and media of arterioles and not the heart. Familial amyloidosis is the rarest form of systemic amyloidosis, affecting only about 4 percent of cases; however, cardiomyopathy is present in 68 percent of those affected. Familial amyloidosis can manifest initially with progressive neuropathy, cardiomyopathy, or renal involvement. In some of the families, cardiac amyloidosis is not even symptomatic, while in others cardiac symptoms predominate. Senile cardiac amyloidosis is common in the elderly but often does not lead to a clinical cardiac syndrome and is only detected postmortem.[208]

CLINICAL PRESENTATION

Amyloid fibrils are rigid and as such lead primarily to relaxation abnormalities and diastolic dysfunction; however, when myocardial replacement occurs, systolic dysfunction becomes a prominent feature.[209] The cardiomyopathy may be restrictive or congestive in nature. Systolic left ventricular function deteriorates late in the disease process only after marked amyloid deposition.[210–217] The clinical presentation is that of congestive heart failure, with a more frequent occurrence of right-sided symptoms. Sudden death and myocardial infarction may result from vascular involvement. Atrial arrhythmias, from infiltration of atrial tissue with amyloid, are not uncommon.

DIAGNOSIS

Diagnosis is made by characteristic echocardiographic features and endomyocardial biopsy.[218] Echocardiography can demonstrate symmetric thickening of the left ventricular wall with a diffuse hyper-refractile, granular sparkling appearance of the myocardium (Fig. 69-10*A*) (see also Chap. 13). Abnormal left ventricular diastolic filling manifested by reduction in the rate, in the volume of rapid diastolic filling with enhanced atrial contraction can be seen very early in cardiac amyloidosis.[219] The ECG typically demonstrates low voltage despite marked hypertrophy on echo (Fig. 69-10*B*). A pseudoinfarct or postinfarct anterior wall pattern is often present.[220] Cardiac involvement is generally present when mean left ventricular wall thickness on echocardiogram is greater than 11 mm in the absence of a history of hypertension or valvular heart disease, with unexplained low voltage (<0.5 mV) on the ECG. The majority of patients presenting with cardiac involvement have a mono-

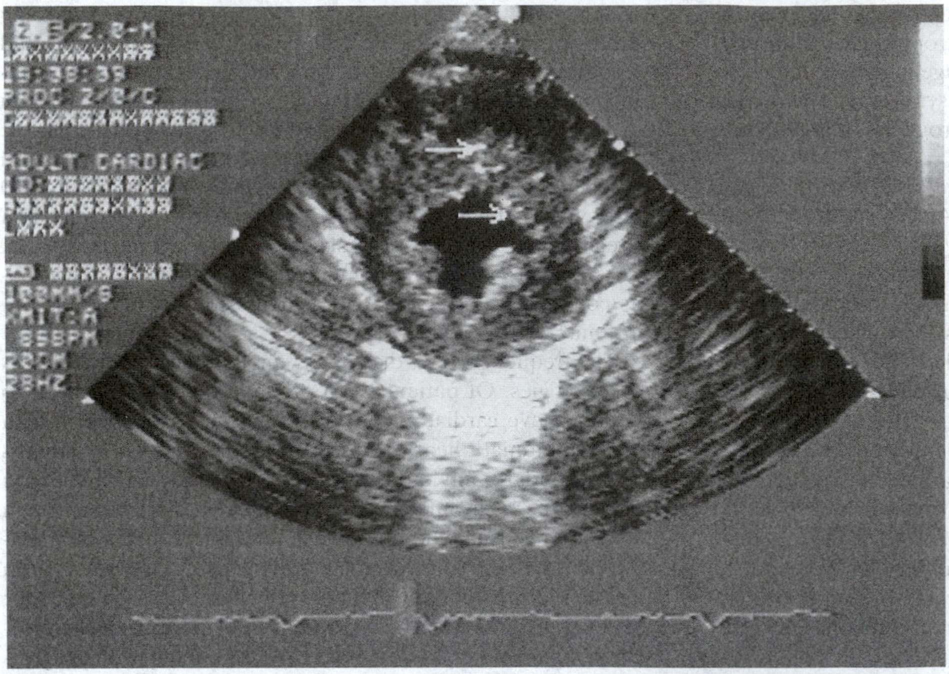

A

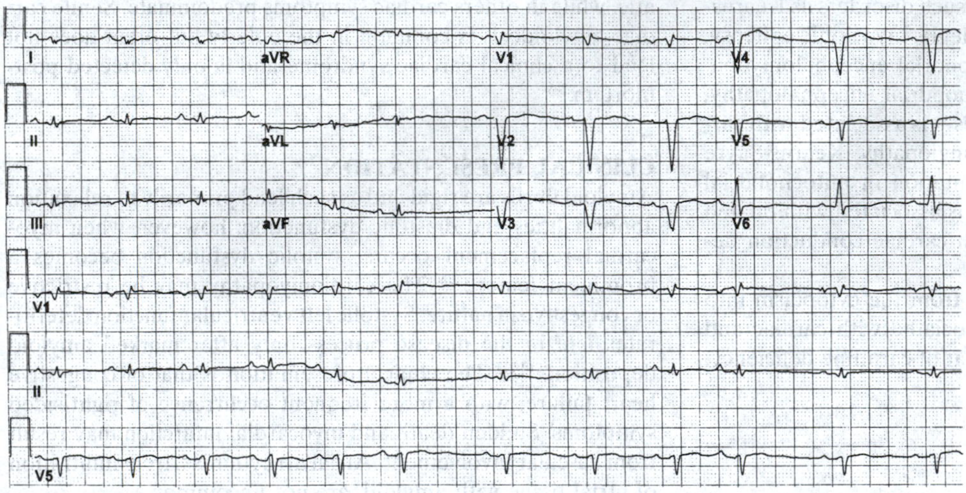

B

FIGURE 69-10 Cardiac amyloidosis. *A.* Two-dimensional echocardiographic parasternal short-axis view demonstrating symmetrical thickening of the left ventricular wall and granular sparkling appearance of the myocardium. *B.* 12-lead electrocardiogram demonstrating low voltage and a pseudoinfarct pattern. *C.* Photomicrograph showing diffuse interstitial accumulations of waxy homogeneous material. (H&E, ×60.) *D.* Electron microscopy of an amyloid deposit (asterisk) in a cardiac biopsy.

clonal protein spike in the serum or urine reflecting the primary nature of the disease.[210]

Amyloid is detected easily in endomyocardial biopsy specimens using Congo red staining and is seen in the interstitium in a pericellular or nodular pattern, in the endocardium, or in myocardial blood vessels. Sulfated alcian blue, methyl violet, and thioflavine T are other histochemical stains used to detect cardiac amyloid (Fig. 69-10*C*). Immunoperoxidase stains for kappa and lambda light chains and for prealbumin may categorize the type of cardiac amyloid. Electron microscopic examination of biopsy specimens is likely the most sensitive method of recognizing amyloidosis (Fig. 69-10*D*).

Radionuclide imaging using technetium-99m pyrophosphate and indium-111 antimyosin showing increased diffuse uptake can also be used to diagnose cardiac amyloidosis.

TREATMENT

Prognosis is typically poor and treatment ineffective.[221] Increased myocardial concentrations of digoxin may occur from binding of the drug to amyloid fibrils, thus increasing the propensity for digoxin toxicity. Digoxin should therefore be used with caution in these patients. Prognosis depends on the extent of myocardial involvement, but once heart failure is present, the prognosis is poor, with a 5-year survival less than 5 percent. Indeed, patients with primary amyloidosis who fall into New York Heart Association (NYHA) class 3 or have recurrent cardiac syncope rarely survive for more than 6 months. Echocardiography with Doppler assessment can provide prognostic information. A shortened deceleration time and an increased ratio of early diastolic filling velocity to the atrial filling velocity were more powerful predictors of mortality from cardiac causes than left ventricular wall thickness or fractional shortening.[222–224]

A recent clinical trial comparing colchicine to the combination of melphalan, prednisone, and colchicine failed to demonstrate any survival benefit in cases of cardiac amyloid. Stem-cell transplant as treatment for primary amyloidosis is now being investigated.

Because of recurrence in the transplanted heart, results following heart transplantation have proved disappointing.[225] The immediate and early postoperative outcomes are similar to those in patients undergoing transplantation for other cardiac diseases; however, late survival is reduced (39 percent at 48 months) owing to recurrence of the disease in the transplanted organ and progressive disease in other organ systems. With the continuing donor shortage, the outcome associated with primary amyloidosis is unacceptable to the majority of cardiac transplant centers. In the future, combined cardiac and bone marrow transplant may provide successful treatment.

Sarcoidosis

PATHOGENESIS

Sarcoidosis is a systemic granulomatous disease of unknown etiology characterized by enhanced cellular immune responses. The pathologic hallmark of this disease is the noncaseating granuloma (Fig. 69-11). The initial lesion is an inflammatory infiltrate consisting of activated helper-inducer T lymphocytes and abundant macrophages that secrete cytokines. The macrophages aggregate and differentiate into epithelioid and multinucleated giant cells. Fibroblasts, mast cells, collagen fibers, and proteoglycans encase the inflammatory cells into a ball-like cluster. The fibrotic response results in end-organ damage.

Clusters of cases have been observed, suggesting spread by person-to-person exposure or environmental agents/pathogens. Genetic factors may also play a role in the development of the disease, as an exaggerated cellular immune response and the formation of granulomas may develop in genetically predisposed hosts after exposure to the offending antigen.

CLINICAL PRESENTATION

The clinical manifestations of sarcoidosis are protean. The disease may be widespread or limited to a single organ. Virtually any organ except the adrenal gland may be involved. The lymphoid, pulmonary, cardiovascular, hepatobiliary, and hematologic systems are the most commonly involved, with the lungs being affected in over 90 percent of patients.[226–228]

Cardiac sarcoid is more common than previously recognized. In a recent autopsy study of 38 patients with sarcoidosis, 76 percent had cardiac involvement, accounting for 50 percent of the deaths. In other series, sarcoidosis affected the heart in 25 to 50 percent of autopsy cases with fatality in 50 percent of the cases with cardiac involvement.[229] Cardiac sarcoid is more likely fatal and less likely to be diagnosed antemortem than pulmonary sarcoid. Frequently the initial presentation is that of sudden death. Myocardial involvement peaks between the third and sixth decades of life. Less than 10 percent of patients with sarcoid have symptoms referable to the cardiovascular system.

In myocardial sarcoid, portions of the myocardial wall are replaced by sarcoid granulomas, which preferentially involve the cephalad portion of the ventricular septum or the left ven-

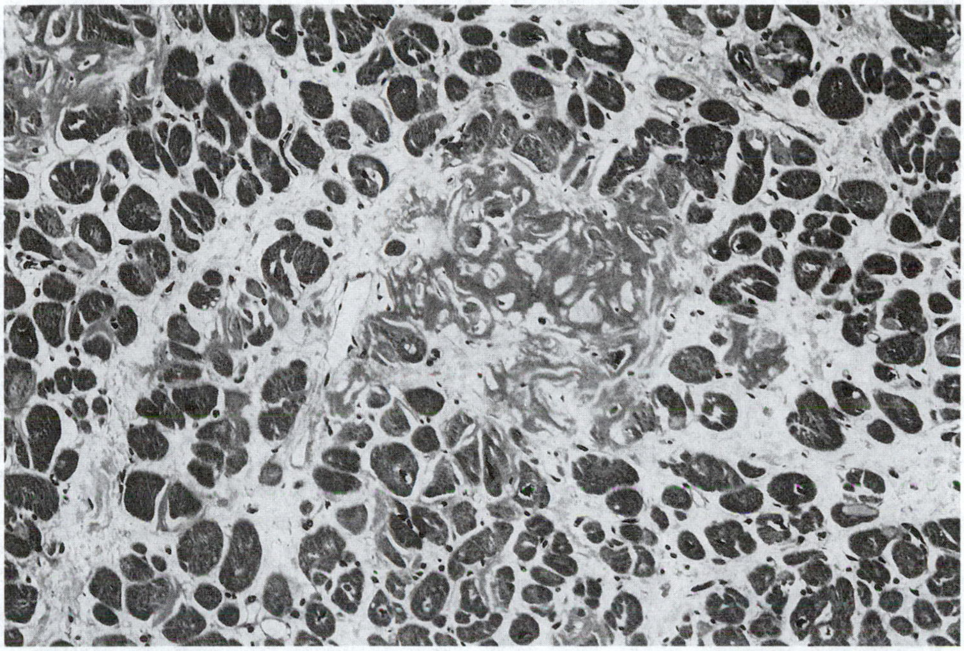

C

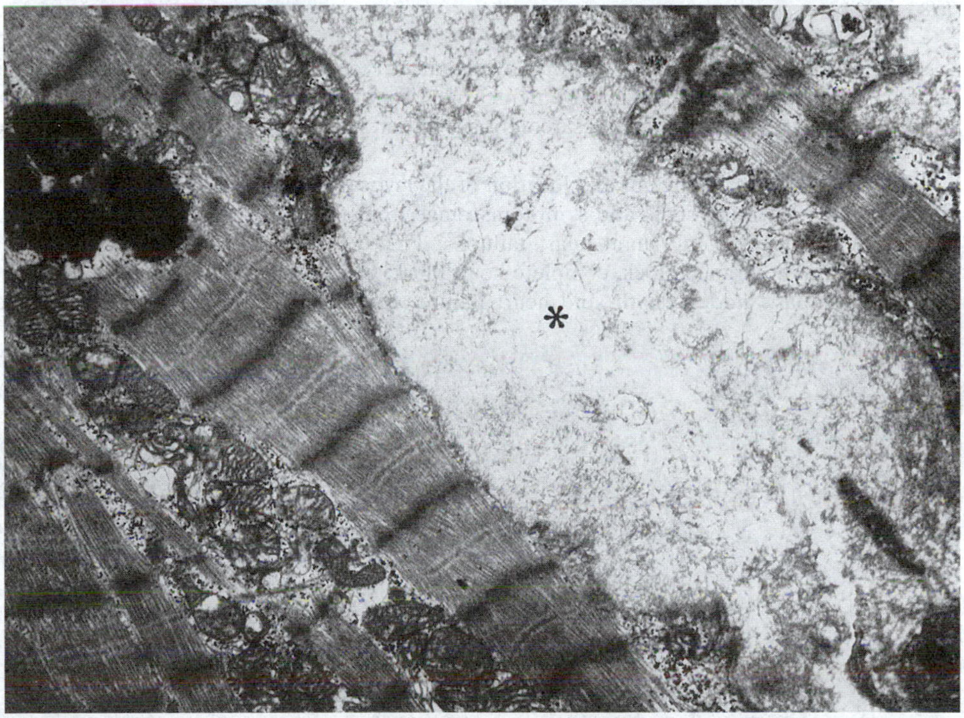

D

FIGURE 69-10 (*Continued*)

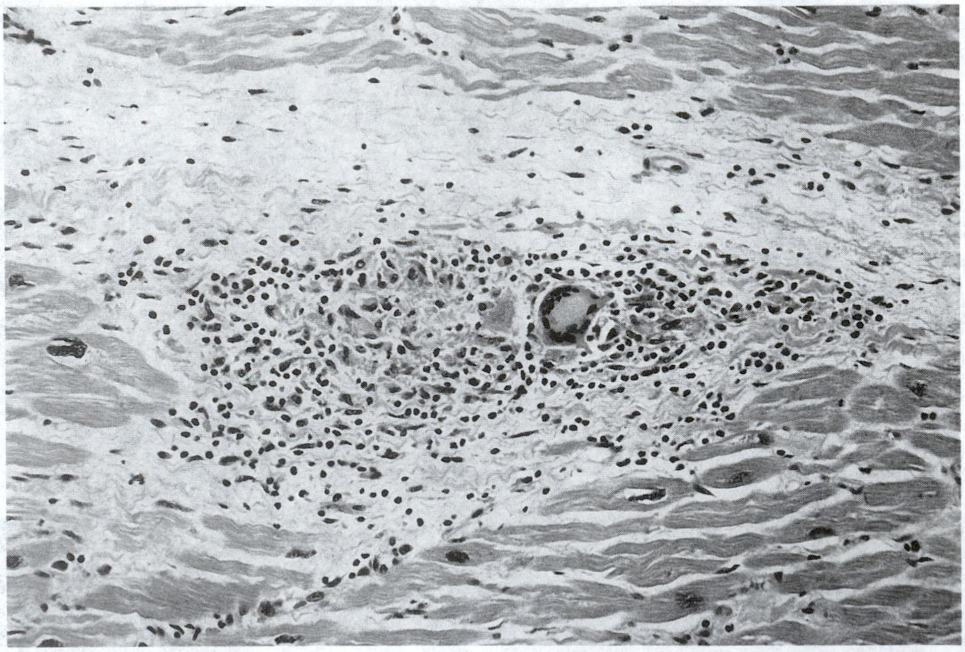

FIGURE 69-11 Photomicrograph showing interstitial noncaseating granulomas with a multinucleated giant cell. (H&E, ×40.)

tricular papillary muscles.[230] Myocardial involvement is much more common than pericardial involvement.[226,231-234] Cor pulmonale due to extensive pulmonary sarcoidosis with interstitial fibrosis may occur.

Because of the varied extent and location of the myocardial granulomas, presenting signs and symptoms range from first-degree heart block to fulminant heart failure.[235] First-degree AV block, bundle-branch block, complete heart block, ventricular arrhythmias, sudden death, and heart failure occur with a frequency of 10 to 20 percent.[235] Heart failure can present as a cardiomyopathy with restrictive hemodynamics or systolic dysfunction. Some 25 percent of the deaths due to cardiac sarcoid are from heart failure, while sudden death accounts for one-third to one-half of the deaths.

DIAGNOSIS

In diagnosing cardiac sarcoid, evidence of other organ system involvement including lymphadenopathy, hepatomegaly, splenomegaly, or pulmonary findings should be sought. In cases where the heart is involved to a much greater degree than are other organs, little or no evidence of extracardiac sarcoidosis may be found. Chest x-ray, ECG, and echocardiography findings will depend on the extent and location of involvement. Due to the scattered nature of the granulomas, endomyocardial biopsy lacks sensitivity and seldom makes the diagnosis despite high specificity. Magnetic resonance imaging has been useful in diagnosing scars or lesions in the myocardium due to sarcoid.[236]

TREATMENT

Although no controlled trials have been performed, high-dose corticosteroids are usually given in the hope that the course of disease may be altered. Administration of corticosteroids can improve cardiac symptoms and reverse ECG changes in over half of the treated patients.[237] Antiarrhythmic drugs should be used as necessary, although drug therapy of ventricular tachycardia in patients with sarcoidosis, even when guided with programmed ventricular stimulation, is associated with a high rate of arrhythmia recurrence or sudden death.[238] Automatic internal cardioverter-defibrillators have been advocated. Prognosis after the diagnosis of cardiac sarcoid is variable but can be poor.[227] In one series of 247 patients, survival was 41 percent at 5 years and 15 percent at 10 years.[226,239] Transplantation is also a successful treatment, as the recurrence of sarcoid in the allograft is low, possibly due to posttransplant steroid therapy.[240]

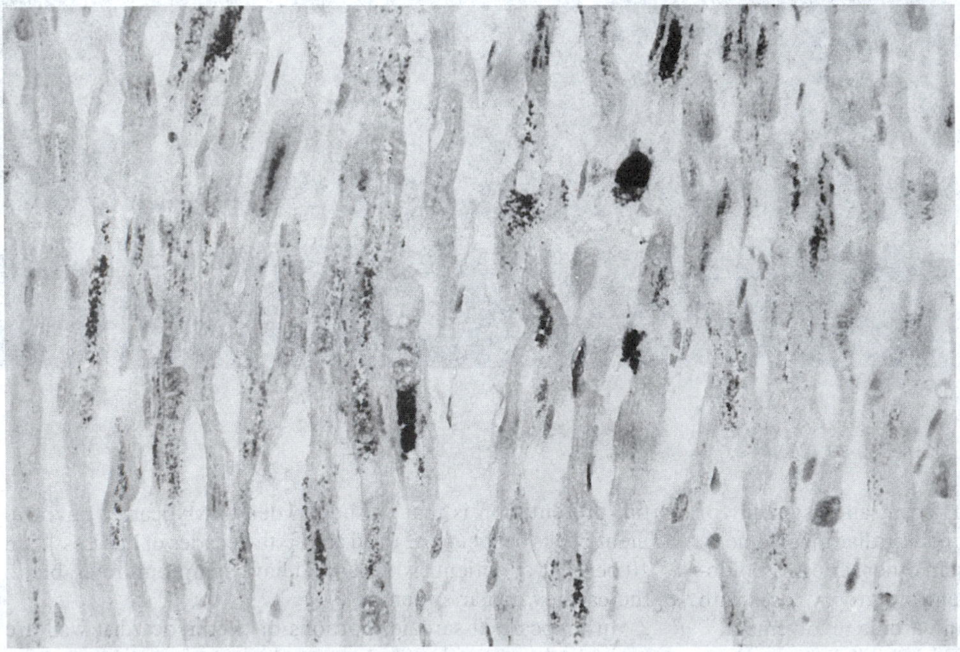

FIGURE 69-12 Photomicrograph showing Perls' stain of hemachromatosis with deposits scattered throughout the myocyte. (×100.)

Hemachromatosis

Primary hemachromatosis is an inborn error of metabolism leading to iron deposition in a variety of organs, including the heart, and resultant secondary myocardial fibrosis. Both restrictive and dilated presentations can occur.[241,242] In contrast to amyloidosis, treatment with phlebotomy[243] is highly effective. In the secondary forms of hemachromatosis due to multiple blood transfusions for blood dyscrasias, chelation therapy is highly effective. Diagnosis is made by symptom constellation in the presence of an elevated serum iron and ferritin. Endomyocardial biopsy is diagnostic (Fig. 69-12).

Carcinoid

Carcinoid heart disease typically leads to a restrictive pattern and often has asymmetrical involvement due to the predilection of the carcinoid for the tricuspid valve apparatus.[244,245] Diagnosis is generally made with right-sided heart findings in the setting of systemic features of carcinoid syndrome. Cardiac involvement responds favorably to control of the primary tumor with chemotherapy or catheter embolization.[244] Tricuspid valve replacement and/or pulmonary valvulotomy and outflow tract enlargement have been recommended when hemodynamically indicated.[244] Alternatively, balloon valvuloplasty for tricuspid or pulmonary stenoses has been used successfully[246] (see also Chaps. 59 and 77).

There are other heritable lesions leading to infiltrative cardiomyopathy. Pseudoxanthoma elasticum (also known as endocardial fibroelastosis) is an inherited disorder of elastic tissue metabolism that leads to a thickening and calcification of the endocardium.[247] Similarly, a number of metabolic inherited disorders cause massive infiltration of the myocardium in infancy and childhood. The best known is Pompe's disease, which is an autosomal recessive disorder caused by a deficiency of the enzyme α-glucosidase, leading to massive glycogen deposition in the cardiac and skeletal musculature. Interestingly, the pathophysiology resembles that of hypertrophic rather than restrictive cardiomyopathy.[248] Prognosis is poor, with no known therapy. Death typically ensues within the first year of life.

Eosinophilic Heart Disease

Eosinophilic heart disease was originally described several decades ago by Löffler,[249] who reported the observation of endocardial lesions, termed "endocarditis parietalis fibroplastica," in association with blood eosinophilia. Although initially thought to represent an isolated disease, Löffler's syndrome is now recognized to be only one manifestation of a spectrum of hypereosinophilic syndromes. Recently cases of isolated eosinophilic myocarditis without signs of endocardial involvement, with or without vasculitis, have been described.[250] Hypereosinophilic syndromes are characterized by peripheral eosinophilia and endocardial disease consisting of eosinophilic infiltration, fibrosis, and eventual occlusion of the ventricular cavity by scar and thrombus.[251] This leads to a very severe form of restrictive myocardial disease referred to as *obliterative myocardial disease.*[252]

PATHOGENESIS

Löffler's endomyocardial disease is considered to be an immunologic disorder caused by clones of abnormal eosinophils infiltrating both sides of the heart. This group of diseases may begin with myocarditis due to the direct toxic effects of the eosinophils and their granules.[253] Indeed, hypersensitivity myocarditis, discussed earlier in this chapter, may be an early variant of this disease. Chronic disease culminates in endomyocardial fibrosis after the disappearance of the initial eosinophilia.[254] The eosinophilic endocardial disease has since been well described[255,256] and is characterized by intense endocardial fibrotic thickening of the apex and subvalvular regions of one or both ventricles. These changes lead to inflow obstruction and restrictive physiology.

CLINICAL PRESENTATION

Löffler's syndrome was initially described primarily in men from temperate climates in their fourth decade of life with a hypereosinophilic syndrome. Diffuse organ involvement may be observed (lungs, bone marrow, brain), with cardiac involvement in more than 75 percent of patients. The typical clinical presentation includes weight loss, fever, cough, skin rash, and congestive heart failure. Overt cardiac dysfunction occurs in about half the patients and is the leading cause of death. Chest x-ray reveals cardiomegaly. ECG findings most commonly include nonspecific ST- and T-wave changes, atrial fibrillation, and right bundle-branch block. Echocardiography commonly demonstrates localized thickening of the left ventricle with valvular leaflet abnormalities[257] and atrial enlargement due to atrioventricular valvular regurgitation and restrictive physiology. In cases of advanced endomyocardial fibrosis, there may be apical obliteration by thrombus[253] but normal systolic function.

Diagnosis is easily established in the acute phase by endomyocardial biopsy and typical ECG images.[252] Variable degrees of acute inflammatory eosinophilic myocarditis are observed. Marked changes can be seen histologically in the coronary vessels, including inflammatory, fibrotic, and thrombotic changes typically containing eosinophils. Fibrotic thickening of up to several millimeters[253] can be observed. Mural thrombosis is common.

Medical therapy with corticosteroids and cytotoxic drugs[159,257,258] in the early stages of disease may substantially improve survival. Routine therapy for heart failure with digitalis, diuretics, afterload reduction, and anticoagulation are adjuncts in the management of these patients. Surgical therapy offers palliation once the later fibrotic stages have been reached.[259]

CARDIOMYOPATHY DUE TO PERSISTENT TACHYCARDIA

Incessant supraventricular or ventricular tachycardia can lead to severe dilated cardiomyopathy in both animals and humans.[260] Successful medical or surgical treatment of the tachyarrhythmia can lead to resolution of the myopathy. The mechanism between the sustained tachycardia and the development of cardiomyopathy is unknown but may be related to depletion of high-energy substrates.

CARDIOMYOPATHY DUE TO RIGHT VENTRICULAR DYSPLASIA

Right ventricular dysplasia is a cardiomyopathy predominantly of the right ventricle. Left ventricle involvement is usually of a lesser and variable degree. Several anomalies may be included under this general heading: Uhl's anomaly,[261] arrhythmogenic right ventricular dysplasia,[262] and right ventricular cardiomyopathy.[263] It is currently recognized as an important inherited cardiomyopathy and a cause of sudden death, especially in youth.[264] Its cause is unknown, although an autosomal dominant pattern with variable expression and penetrance has been suggested, since many cases show a strong familial tendency.[265]

Clinically patients typically present with recurrent ventricular tachycardia of left-bundle-branch-block morphology and, less commonly, CHF. Standard electrocardiography discloses incomplete or complete right-bundle-branch block in most patients or T-wave inversions in leads V_1-V_3 (Fig. 69-13*A*). These conduction or repolarization abnormalities are thought to be due to adipose infiltration of the myocardium. Clinical diagnosis is based on detection of predominantly right ventricular morphologic changes on imaging studies. Echocardiography is an effective tool to demonstrate the characteristic abnormal structure[266] of the right ventricle, including hypokinesis, massive dilatation, and a "parchment-thin" wall[267] (Fig. 69-13*B*). In addition, tricuspid regurgitation and paradoxic ventricular septal wall motion are common. Pathologically, there is variable infiltration or replacement of the right ventricular myocardium by adipose and fibrous tissue.[268]

The importance of right ventricular dysplasia is its association with sudden death, with an incidence of up to 20 percent in some series.[264] Therapy therefore is focused on the prevention of sudden death with implantation of automatic internal cardioverter-defibrillators.

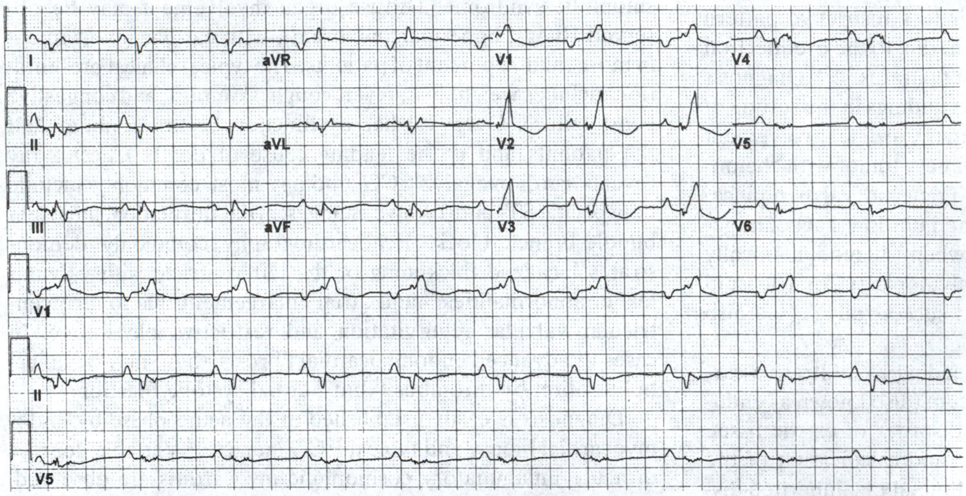

A

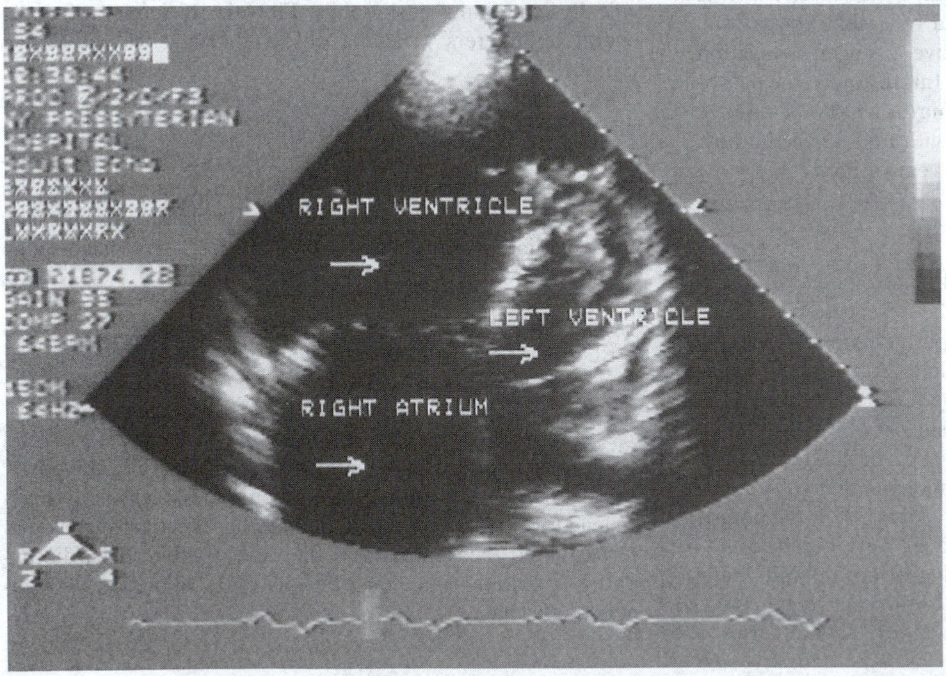

B

FIGURE 69-13 Uhls' anomaly. *A*. Twelve-lead electrocardiogram demonstrating characteristic right bundle branch block with T-wave inversions in leads V_1–V_3. *B*. Two-dimensional echocardiographic four-chamber view demonstrating massive right ventricular dilation with a "parchment-thin" wall.

CARDIOMYOPATHY DUE TO ENDOCRINE DISORDERS

Thyroid

Thyroid hormone has long been recognized to affect the heart and the peripheral vasculature.[269] Changes in cardiac function are mediated by T3 regulation of cardiac-specific genes.[270] Thyroid hormone metabolism is frequently abnormal in patients with CHF. In a study of 84 patients with advanced heart failure, T3 levels were found to be low.[271] Furthermore, a low T3/reverse T3 ratio was the only independent predictor of prognosis when a multivariate regression analysis was performed with known predictors of poor outcome such as ejection fraction, serum sodium, or hemodynamic variables. The low conversion to T3 was postulated to be an adaptive mechanism to decreased catabolism. In a subsequent study, Hamilton et al. studied the effects of intravenous T3 infusion to patients with class III or IV heart failure.[272] Cardiac output increased without a change in left ventricular ejection fraction or filling pressures. This was thought to be secondary to the effects of T3, causing vascular smooth muscle dilatation and therefore peripheral vasodilation. In another study of thyroid hormone replacement in heart failure, 20 patients with class II and III idiopathic dilated cardiomyopathy were given L-thyroxine orally.[273] Cardiac output improved, peripheral vascular resistance decreased, and exercise performance increased. The improved exercise performance was explained by a higher oxygen consumption at peak exercise due to improved oxygen uptake by skeletal muscle, increased perfusion of the musculature, or improved muscle metabolism by local action of L-thyroxine occurring during training. Similar results were obtained in a study by Moruzzi and colleagues.[274] In this series of 20 patients, ejection fraction, cardiac output, and left ventricular diastolic dimensions all increased. Functional capacity and peak exercise cardiac output also improved. The beneficial effects were sustained with the longer therapy regimen.

Like thyroid deficiency, thyroid toxicity can lead to the development of both high-output and low-output cardiac failure. A prolonged tachycardia and high-output state caused by thyrotoxicosis is thought eventually to produce left ventricular dilatation. A consequent progressive decline in systolic function leads to low-output heart failure. This process can often be reversed by reduction of excess hormone levels. In a study of 7 patients with a dilated cardiomyopathy and hyperthyroidism, Umpierrez et al. demonstrated echocardiographic normalization of left ventricular function after treatment with propylthiouracil or methimazole.[275]

Pheochromocytoma

Hypertension and its sequelae are the major cardiovascular manifestations of pheochromocytoma. However, there have been reports of a specific catecholamine-induced myocarditis[276] and/or cardiomyopathy.[277–279] Degenerative and fibrotic myocardial changes have been described in autopsy specimens of patients dying of suprarenal tumors.[276] Although progression to cardiac involvement is unusual, when the presentation of the tumor is aggressive, pheochromocytoma patients typically die of cardiovascular causes, most commonly congestive heart failure or malignant ventricular arrhythmias.[276,277] In the largest series, 15 of the 26 patients with proven pheochromocytomas had a pathologic diagnosis of myocarditis at autopsy.[276] Hemodynamic stabilization is generally obtained with alpha and beta blockers, and prompt adrenalectomy is required to eliminate catecholamine-induced cardiotoxicity. The cardiac abnormalities can be reversed with tumor resection[280,281] (see also Chap. 51).

Acromegaly

It is not clear whether acromegalic cardiomyopathy is a specific entity or is secondary to the hypertension or atherosclerosis associated with this condition. However, 10 to 20 percent of patients with acromegaly develop congestive heart failure.[282] The congestive heart failure that develops in these patients is particularly resistant to conventional therapy[283] owing to higher collagen content in the acromegalic heart.[282] Histopathologically, the myocytes display cellular hypertrophy, patchy fibrosis, and myofibrillar degeneration. Inflammatory and degenerative damage to the sinoatrial and AV nodes can lead to sudden death.[283] Surgery and irradiation remain the mainstays of therapy, but often the cardiopathic manifestations persist despite a fall in growth hormone levels.[284]

Diabetes

Analysis of the Framingham data showed that the risk of developing heart failure was substantially increased among diabetic patients. Even after exclusion of patients with prior coronary or rheumatic disease and controlling for age, hypertension, obesity, and hypercholesterolemia, the diabetic patients have a fivefold increased risk of developing congestive heart failure.[285] This increased incidence suggested that the metabolic abnormalities associated with diabetes may contribute to myocyte dysfunction and produce a diabetes-induced cardiomyopathy. Histologically, this cardiomyopathy shows no evidence of epicardial atherosclerotic disease or abnormalities in myocardial capillary basal lamina.[286,287] Typically, interstitial fibrosis and arteriolar hyalinization are present. Clinically both systolic and diastolic dysfunction can occur, and the severity of the dysfunction is related to the degree of metabolic control.[288]

OBESITY

Heart failure in the markedly obese is usually chronic. It often occurs due to reduction in left ventricular compliance due to the increases in left ventricular mass and resultant elevations of filling pressures. The chronic increases in cardiac work due to an increased myocardial output and arterial hypertension ultimately lead to systolic dysfunction. With exercise and weight reduction, left ventricular mass decreases[289] and function improves.[290] The improvement in function, however, seems limited to those patients whose obesity was of relatively short duration.[291]

TOXINS

Alcohol

Congestive cardiomyopathy as a result of chronic alcohol abuse accounts for up to 45 percent of all dilated cardiomyopathies.[292] The untoward effects of alcohol on cardiac function were initially described more than 100 years ago. As an estimated 10 percent of the adult population are heavy alcohol users, cardiac toxicity from alcohol is a major problem.

PATHOGENESIS

The cardiodepressant effects of alcohol have been demonstrated following acute and chronic ingestion in animal models and in normal and alcoholic human subjects. Chronic excessive alcohol use can result in congestive heart failure, hypertension, and arrhythmias. Cardiac damage results from direct toxic effects of alcohol or one of its metabolites. Nutritional deficiencies, toxic cofactors, sympathetic stimulation, or coexistent hypertension may also contribute to disease development.[293]

Orally ingested alcohol is converted in the liver to acetaldehyde by the alcohol dehydrogenase enzyme system. Acetaldehyde is then converted into acetic acid by oxidation via acetaldehyde dehydrogenase. The activity of these enzyme systems varies greatly between individuals and in particular between races. Thus, depending on individual enzyme system activity, there are varying levels of alcohol and acetaldehyde concentrations after ingestion of an alcoholic beverage. Alcohol and acetaldehyde are both potent vasodilators. Additionally, acetaldehyde results in marked catecholamine release. Both alcohol and acetaldehyde interfere with a variety of cellular metabolic functions, including calcium transport and binding, lipid metabolism and fatty acid composition of the sarcolemma, protein synthesis, myofibrillar ATPase, and mitochondrial respiration.[292,294] Though ethanol can interfere with a number of myocardial metabolic steps, no predominant factor has been identified. Recently a nonoxidative pathway for the metabolism of alcohol in several organ systems including the heart has been described.[295] Nonesterified fatty acids are esterified with ethanol to produce fatty acid ethyl esters (FAEE). These molecules can accumulate in mitochondria and impair cellular function. Fatty acid ethyl esters are synthesized at high rates in the heart owing to the lack of oxidative ethanol metabolism in this organ. Other studies have demonstrated interference with lipid metabolism leading to triglyceride accumulation and alteration of the fatty acid composition of the sarcolemma.[292] Increased levels of acyl-CoA from enhanced glycerol acyltransferase activity may lead to triglyceride accumulation. The cellular membrane shows reduced changes results in decreased calcium uptake by the sarcolemma. Alcohol also is found to be an inhibitor of the sodium-potassium ATPase.

For many years, alcoholic cardiomyopathy was believed to be due to nutritional deficiencies. The stereotypical malnourished skid-row derelict could have a variety of nutritional deficiencies. Indeed, those subjects with heavy beer consumption could develop thiamine deficiency. As beer contains no thiamine, the consumption of this high-calorie, high-carbohydrate beverage can exhaust existing thiamine stores, particularly in the presence of a deficient diet. Thus, a small percentage of patients with alcohol cardiomyopathy may have coexistent thiamine deficiency. However, the majority of patients develop this disease despite adequate diets.[293]

Contamination of alcoholic beverages with heavy metals has resulted in heart failure. In the nineteenth century, an epidemic of heart failure occurred in Manchester, England, following accidental contamination of the beer with arsenic. More recently, in the 1960s, a new variant of alcoholic cardiomyopathy was described.[296] Patients presented with massive pericardial effusion, low cardiac output, elevated venous pressure, and polycythemia. After considerable medical detective work, the syndrome was linked to cobaltous chloride that was added to the beer as a foaming agent to increase and stabilize the beer head. Removal of the additive resulted in the resolution of this miniepidemic.

CLINICAL PRESENTATION

Although approximately 10 percent of the adult population are heavy drinkers, the prevalence of cardiac disease in this group is low—significantly lower than the prevalence of liver disease in the same population. Although patients with alcoholic cirrhosis may have evidence of asymptomatic myocardial disease, the simultaneous presentation of overt alcoholic liver and cardiac disease is extremely rare.[297]

The disease is observed most frequently in males age 30 to 55 years with a greater than 10-year history of heavy alcohol use. The disease is extremely rare in premenopausal women. The amount and duration of alcohol use is frequently difficult to establish. Criteria used to define heavy chronic alcohol use have included such estimates as the use of 125 mL/day of alcohol and/or 30 to 50 percent of daily calories derived from alcohol for a minimum of 10 years. In a study of 50 asymptomatic alcoholic men, Rubin et al. demonstrated that cardiomyopathy, as well as abnormalities of skeletal muscle, are common among persons with chronic alcoholism, and that alcohol is toxic to striated muscle in a dose-dependent manner.[203]

Presenting symptoms include dyspnea on exertion, orthopnea, paroxysmal nocturnal dyspnea, fatigue, weakness, arrhythmias, or embolic phenomena. Atrial fibrillation is extremely common, followed by atrial flutter and ventricular premature contractions. Sudden death can be the initial presentation. ECG findings include first-degree heart block, left ventricular hypertrophy, nonspecific interventricular conduction defects, bundle-branch blocks and prolongation of the QT interval. The echocardiogram frequently shows left ventricular hypertrophy, single- to four-chamber enlargement, and mural thrombi.

In animal studies, left ventricular biopsies from dogs that developed alcoholic cardiomyopathy showed an accumulation of glucoprotein-like material in the interstitium on light microscopy as well as a dilatation of the intercalated discs on electron microscopic evaluation. These studies also demonstrated abnormalities of the sarcoplasmic reticulum and swelling of subsarcolemma regions.[298,299] The severity of these changes related to the duration and extent of alcohol use. Several histologic changes have been described on endomyocardial biopsies in alcoholic cardiomyopathy, but none of these changes are pathognomonic. Changes include myocyte loss, increased fibrosis, loss of sarcolemmal integrity, myofibrillar degeneration, mitochondrial swelling, intercellular edema and accumulation of fatty acids in particular triglycerides, and diminished levels of arachidonate in the cellular membrane.[300] Electron microscopy shows mitochondrial swelling with dense intramitochondrial inclusions, swollen vesiculated sarcoplasmic reticulum, and myofibrillar disruption.

TREATMENT

The mainstay of treatment is abstinence from alcohol. Alcohol withdrawal may have a remarkable impact on disease manifestation and progression, especially in the milder forms of the disease.[301–303] In animal models, following cessation of alcohol use, the hearts recover. In humans, the duration and extent of abuse is correlated with outcome.[304] Prognosis is extremely poor in those patients who continue to drink compared with patients who become abstinent. Ninety-one percent of patients who abstain from alcohol after the initial diagnosis are alive at 42 months, versus 43 percent of those who continue to drink.

Although early in the disease process abstinence can result in recovery, there is a point at which cessation of alcohol is no longer effective,[305] and this correlates with the development of structural histologic abnormalities.[301] Survival of patients with alcoholic dilated cardiomyopathy who are abstinent appears to be significantly better than the long-term survival of patients with a comparable class of CHF due to idiopathic cardiomyopathy.[301,306] In a series of 75 patients with CHF, 23 had alcoholic cardiomyopathy compared with 52 with an idiopathic etiology.[306] Mean left ventricular ejection fraction, diastolic volumes, and NYHA class were similar. Overall survival was measured at 1, 5, and 10 years, and was 100, 81, and 81 percent for patients with alcoholic cardiomyopathy, and 89, 48, and 30 percent for patients with idiopathic cardiomyopathy, respectively. In another series however, no mortality difference was found,[307] but this may be due to persistent alcohol use in that cohort despite the onset of CHF.

Cocaine

Myocardial ischemia, infarction, coronary spasm, cardiac arrhythmias, sudden death, myocarditis, and dilated cardiomyopathy are all reported cardiovascular complications of cocaine abuse.[308] Clinical and experimental evidence suggests a variety of theories for the cardiotoxic effects of cocaine (see also Chap. 71).

The pharmacologic effects of cocaine on the heart partly explain its toxic effects.[309] By blocking the reuptake of norepinephrine, cocaine induces tachycardia, vasoconstriction, hypertension, cardiomyopathy, and ventricular arrhythmias. Cardiomyopathy may then result from secondary changes in the heart due to tachycardia or sustained increased ventricular afterload.

Cocaine has also been shown to exert a direct toxic effect on the heart. In vitro studies with isolated rabbit ventricular tissue[310] or isolated blood-perfused dog preparations[311] showed that high-dose cocaine depressed myocardial contractile force. Acute ventricular dilatation and reversible systolic dysfunction after intravenous cocaine administration have been documented in vivo in dogs.[312]

The risks and manifestations of toxic effects of cocaine in any given individual are unpredictable. The duration or amount of cocaine use is not predictable of disease. For example, among Andean Indians, heart failure rarely occurs from the chewing of coca even though plasma levels of cocaine are comparable to those of intranasal cocaine abusers.[313] This raises the possibility of a genetic susceptibility or that a metabolite or contaminant and not cocaine itself may be the inciting factor for development of cardiac damage.

Dilated cardiomyopathy in the absence of coronary abnormalities and myocarditis has been reported.[314,315] In these cases, myocardial depression is global and is generally reversible; it is attributed to a direct myocardial depressant effect of cocaine.[316]

There are no clinical or histologic features specific for cocaine-induced myocardial damage. Endomyocardial biopsy[308] and autopsy studies[317] confirm the presence of myocyte necrosis and a diffuse inflammatory cellular infiltrate in cocaine users. "Contraction-band necrosis" has been seen in a patient presenting with a clinical course similar to that of catecholamine cardiomyopathy,[318] but this is not characteristic. Although eosinophilic infiltrates can be seen, cocaine is not included in the list of typical drugs associated with a hypersensitivity syndrome. Thus the diagnosis is usually presumptive and is one of exclusion. The treatment of cocaine-related myocarditis and cardiomyopathy is nonspecific and focuses on abstinence and heart failure therapy.

Chemotherapeutic Agents

Several chemotherapeutic agents can cause an acute and/or chronic cardiomyopathy. Among them, the anthracycline group (doxorubicin) and cyclophosphamide are the most common agents associated with heart failure.

Doxorubicin has been used as single or combination therapy for treatment of many different tumors including breast and esophageal tumors as well as sarcomas and lymphomas from the late 1960s. Its use is limited by its cardiotoxicity. The cause of the cardiotoxicity is unknown, but it is suspected to be due to increased oxidative stress from the generation of free radicals by doxorubicin. Moreover, endogenous antioxidants are reduced by treatment with doxorubicin. Increased oxidative stress results in the loss of myofibrils and cellular vacuolization, similar to what is observed with doxorubicin administration.[319]

Doxorubicin can be associated with early or late cardiotoxicity. Risk factors for the development of doxorubicin cardiomyopathy include age greater than 70 years, combination chemotherapy, mediastinal irradiation, prior cardiac disease, hypertension and liver disease. The early or acute cardiotoxicity manifests as a pericarditis-myocarditis syndrome[320] and is not dose-related. Left ventricular dysfunction is rarely seen, but arrhythmias, abnormalities of conduction, decreased QRS voltage, and nonspecific ST-segment and T-wave abnormalities are observed in up to 40 percent of patients.[321] The prognosis is good, with quick resolution of the abnormalities upon discontinuation of therapy.

In contrast, the late or chronic cardiotoxicity is due to the development of a dose-dependent degenerative cardiomyopathy[322] (Fig. 69-14). This syndrome generally occurs at doses above 550 mg/m^2. Serial assessment of nuclear ejection fractions is used clinically to monitor for adverse effects. However, histopathologic grading is most useful in delineating the safety of continued doxorubicin administration.[323] Cardiotoxicity may occur during therapy within a year of the last dose of anthracycline or as late as 6 to 10 years after its cessation. Therefore a course

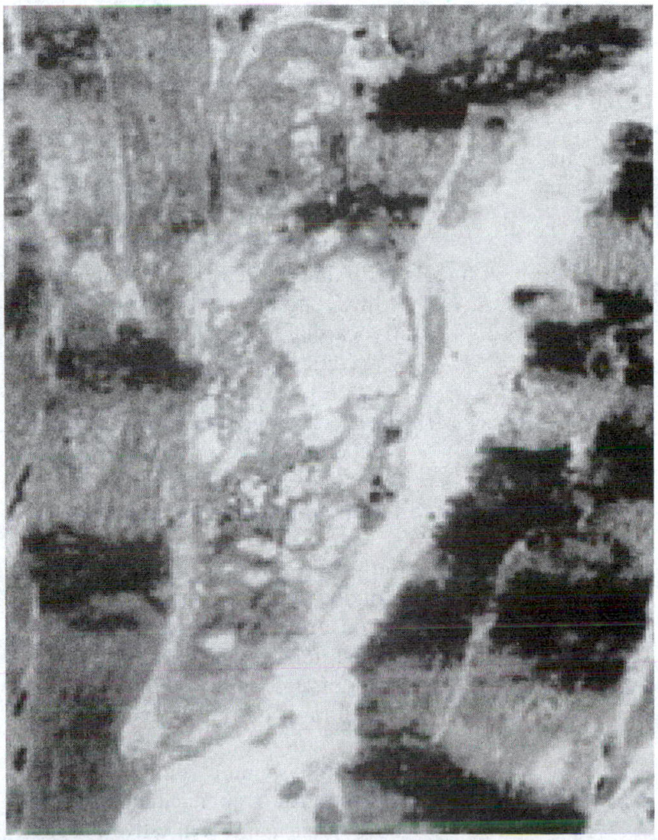

FIGURE 69-14 Loss of myofibrils and vacuolization of cytoplasm (toluidine blue stain, ×40) in a patient with doxorubicin cardiotoxicity. (From Singal et al.,[319] with permission.)

of this chemotherapy commits patients to prolonged cardiac surveillance.

Prognosis depends to some extent on the severity at time of presentation, but the incidence of death even in milder forms remains high.[324] The best management of anthracycline cardiotoxicity is prevention by limiting dosage. Lowering the peak blood levels of the drug by giving a continuous rather than bolus infusion also appears to significantly decrease drug-related damage.[325] Coadministration of doxorubicin with agents that would block free radical formation and not decrease its antineoplastic effects has been studied. Dexrazoxane, an iron chelating agent, has been used in clinical trials of patients with breast cancer or small-cell lung cancer to limit the cardiotoxicity of doxorubicin. The incidence of heart failure and the decrease in ejection fraction is less in those patients receiving combined therapy. Unfortunately, dexrazoxane is a potent myelosuppressive agent potentiating the effects of doxorubicin. It also may interfere with cancer therapy.

Heart failure due to doxorubicin has been very difficult to treat and is typically refractory to conventional therapy. In children with doxorubicin-induced cardiomyopathy, recent reports have described diminished symptoms and improved left ventricular function after treatment with beta blockers. Further studies on the use of these agents are needed.

In contrast to the anthracyclines, cyclophosphamide leads to an acute cardiotoxicity that is not related to cumulative dose.[326] Pericarditis, systolic dysfunction, arrhythmias, and myocardial edema make up the spectrum of cardiac abnormalities. Prior left ventricular dysfunction is a risk factor for development of significant cardiomyopathy with cyclophosphamide. Although mortality is not trivial, survivors exhibit no residual cardiac abnormalities.[327]

TABLE 69-5 Major Cardiovascular Complications of Chemical Toxins

Agent	Cardiac Toxicity
Cobalt	Congestive heart failure
Cocaine	Coronary abnormalities, arrhythmias, myocarditis, myocardial depression
Interferon alpha	Arrhythmias, dilated cardiomyopathy, congestive heart failure
Interleukin-2	Myocardial ischemia/infarct, arrhythmias, eosinophilic myocarditis
Phenothiazines	Electrocardiographic, arrhythmias, sudden death
Emetine	Mononuclear and histiocyte infiltration, electrocardiographic abnormalities
Methysergide	Left-sided valvular lesions, fibrotic endocardial and pericardial lesions, restriction and constriction
Chloroquine	Arrhythmias, cardiac dysfunction
Lithium	Arrhythmias, cardiac dilatation with myofibrillar degeneration
Hydrocarbons	Electrocardiographic changes, arrhythmias, and cardiomegaly
Lead	Electrocardiographic changes, arrhythmias, and congestive heart failure
Carbon monoxide	Arrhythmias and transient biventricular dysfunction

Chemical Toxins

A variety of compounds can lead to a spectrum of cardiotoxicity, including cardiomyopathy. They include interferon alpha,[328] IL-2,[329] phenothiazines,[330] emetine,[331] methysergide,[332] chloroquine,[333] lithium,[334] hydrocarbons,[335] lead,[336] and carbon monoxide.[337] A summary of the cardiotoxicity seen with each compound is outlined in Table 69-5.

CARDIOMYOPATHIES ASSOCIATED WITH NUTRITIONAL DEFICIENCIES

Vitamins

Thiamine deficiency, or beriberi, causes a high-output state, which leads to left ventricular dilatation and an elevated pulmonary capillary wedge pressure.[338] Vitamin D deficiency, or rickets, and vitamin D excess are associated with cardiovascular morbidity and mortality as well. There are about 25 reported cases of hypocalcemic cardiomyopathy in the adult population caused mostly by idiopathic hypoparathyroidism.[339] Similarly in children, cardiomyopathy has been documented in cases of hypocalcemia caused by vitamin D deficiency rickets.[340] Excess doses of vitamin D in humans have been associated with calcium deposition in the heart and QT shortening but not frank cardiomyopathy. Similarly, vitamin A, vitamin B_6, vitamin C, and niacin deficiency are not directly associated with overt cardiac dysfunction in humans but can be associated with ECG abnormalities.

Selenium

Interest in the role of selenium deficiency in cardiovascular diseases originated from observations of cardiomyopathy and sudden cardiac death in animals with dietary selenium deficiency.[341] Cardiomyopathy associated with inadequate dietary intake of selenium, termed Keshan's disease, has also been described in humans. This syndrome was discovered in regions of China with a low soil content of selenium.[342] Whether the cardiomyopathy results from the actual selenium deficiency or the selenium deficiency increases suspectibility to cardiotropic viruses is unclear. Coxsackievirus B3 (CVB 3/20), which causes no pathology in hearts of selenium-adequate mice, induces extensive myocarditis in selenium-deficient mice.[343] Furthermore, Coxsackievirus B3 recovered from the hearts of selenium-deficient mice and inoculated into selenium-adequate mice induced significant heart damage, suggesting mutation of the virus to a virulent genotype.[344] These findings may underlie the seasonal variation characteristic of Keshan's disease.

This disease is typically seen in children and pregnant women. Both acute and chronic forms of Keshan's disease exist.[345] In the acute form, cardiogenic shock, severe arrhythmias, and pulmonary edema are the manifestations of the systolic impairment. The chronic type shows a moderate to severe heart enlargement with varying degrees of cardiac insufficiency; often patients are asymptomatic. Its incidence is dramatically reduced with supplementation of sodium selenite.

Other than Keshan's disease, circumstantial evidence supports an association between selenium deficiency and cardiomyopathy. Congestive cardiomyopathy with low selenium levels has been reported in patients receiving total parenteral nutrition.[346] Patients with congestive cardiomyopathy have significantly lower serum selenium concentrations than healthy control subjects. Left ventricular ejection fraction is positively correlated with the selenium concentration in patients with cardiomyopathies.[346]

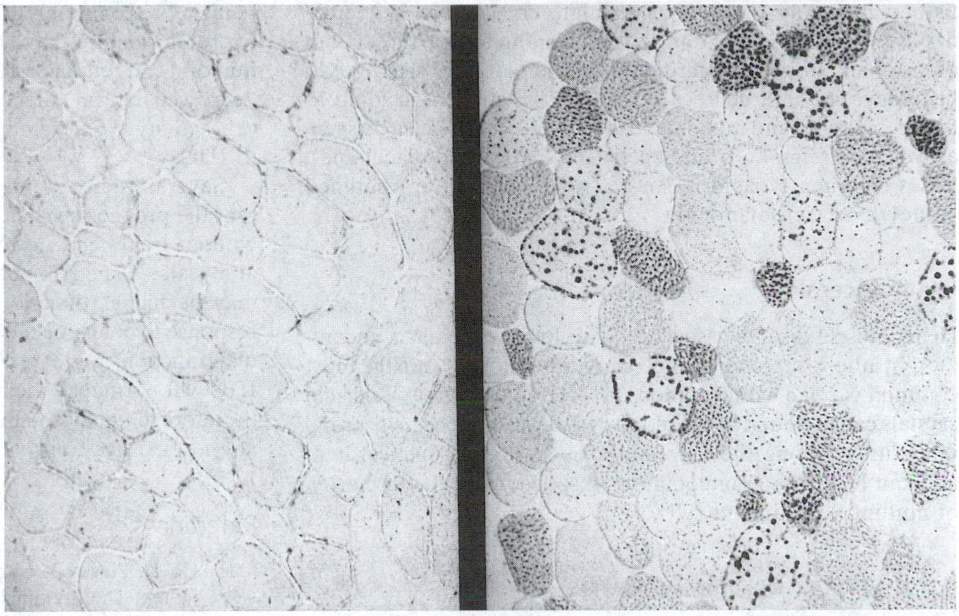

FIGURE 69-15 Photomicrograph of Oil red O stain demonstrating lipid deposits in type I and IIb fibers in normal (*right*) and carnitine-deficient (*left*) skeletal muscle.

Carnitine

L-Carnitine is an essential compound in the transport of long chain fatty acids into mitochondria, where they undergo beta oxidation. Since the normal heart obtains approximately 60 percent of its total energy production from fatty acid oxidation, this function of carnitine is thought to be of major importance.[347] Because of this function of carnitine and numerous case reports that have shown that some patients with carnitine deficiency exhibit cardiomyopathy,[348–350] it is believed that adequate levels of carnitine are required for normal energy metabolism and contractile function of the heart.[351] Interestingly, not all patients with carnitine deficiency exhibit cardiomyopathy. This may be explained perhaps by the degree of carnitine deficiency or by how cardiac performance is assessed.[352]

Deficiencies of carnitine can be either primary or secondary. Primary deficiencies arise from several genetic disorders involving carnitine synthesis or handling. These rare conditions are severe and are associated with muscle and plasma carnitine levels as low as 10 percent of normal (Fig. 69-15). Several case reports have established that primary carnitine deficiency is associated with cardiomyopathy.[353–355] The cardiomyopathy that ensues presents within 3 to 4 years of birth[356] and is profound; clinically, however, it responds to carnitine supplementation.

Secondary carnitine deficiencies are much more common and arise from a large number of genetic diseases associated with defects in acyl-CoA metabolism.[357] In patients with long-chain or short-chain acyl-CoA dehydrogenase deficiency, carnitine levels are reduced to 25 to 50 percent of normal and a depression in cardiac contractile performance has been found.[357,358] Secondary carnitine deficiencies can also be acquired as a result of liver disease, renal disease[359,360] (Fanconi's syndrome, renal tubular acidosis), dietary insufficiencies[361] (chronic total parenteral nutrition, malabsorption), diabetes mellitus, and heart failure.[362] Many of these types of secondary carnitine deficiency are often associated with cardiomyopathy.[355,363] In cases of secondary carnitine deficiency, however, it has been difficult to determine whether the symptoms are due to carnitine deficiency or to the underlying genetic metabolic disorder. Based on this observation and the inconsistent reports of cardiomyopathy with these secondary deficiencies, it appears that a clear and strong association can only be made between cardiomyopathy and primary carnitine deficiency.

Coenzyme Q

Coenzyme Q (2,3-dimethoxy-5 methyl-6-decapreyl-1,4-benzoquinone) is another important factor involved in oxidative phosphorylation in mitochondria of the heart.[364] It has been postulated that its depletion, when found in myocardial biopsies of patients with cardiomyopathy,[365] may contribute to heart failure.[366] Several studies have claimed subjective and objective improvement in patients with heart failure after oral therapy with coenzyme Q.[367–369] These studies were small, unblinded, and uncontrolled trials. Recently a placebo-controlled double-blinded randomized crossover trial of coenzyme Q was performed in 30 patients with heart failure stabilized on conventional vasodilator therapy.[370] In this study, treatment with 3 months of oral coenzyme Q failed to improve resting left ventricular systolic function or quality of life despite an increase in plasma levels of coenzyme Q to more than twice basal values. Thus, given the lack of convincing and consistent data, coenzyme Q supplementation is not included in the basic repertoire of heart failure medications.

CARDIOMYOPATHIES ASSOCIATED WITH ALTERED METABOLISM

Hyperoxaluria

Both primary and secondary oxalosis are characterized by excessive deposition of calcium oxalate crystals in various body tissues, including the heart.[371] Oxalate crystals are frequently deposited in the conduction system, leading to heart block and occasionally in the myocardium and the coronary arteries. On histology, variable degrees of cellular reaction—including fibrosis, necrosis, and mononuclear cell infiltration—can be seen, as well as foreign-body giant cells and myocardial granulomas. Cases of primary oxalosis can be treated with after combined kidney/liver transplantation.[372,373]

Hyperuricemia

Heart muscle disease associated with hyperuricemia is uncommon[374]; atherosclerosis and coronary artery disease are the most common cardiac manifestations associated with gout. Uric acid crystals can be found in the blood vessel walls, in the myocardial interstitium, along the valve surfaces, and in the pericardium and can lead to a granulomatous response with the formation of multinucleated giant cells.[373]

IDIOPATHIC CARDIOMYOPATHY

Idiopathic cardiomyopathy (IDC) is the term used to describe a group of myocardial diseases of unknown cause. Idiopathic dilated cardiomyopathy probably represents the end result of a number of disease processes involving myocyte dysfunction, myocyte loss, myocyte hypertrophy and fibrosis. It is a diagnosis of exclusion. As discussed earlier in this chapter, an idiopathic dilated cardiomyopathy may be the end result of an infectious myocarditis. Endocardial biopsy in patients with dilated cardiomyopathy may reveal an inflammatory infiltrate. Surreptitious alcohol use as well as undiagnosed and untreated hypertension probably represent other etiologies of cardiomyopathy in many of these cases. Familial factors have generally been more predominant in hypertrophic cardiomyopathies than in dilated congestive cardiomyopathy. However more and more data are accumulating to suggest that genetic factors contribute to these cases as well. When one is making the diagnosis of idiopathic dilated cardiomyopathy, it is most important to exclude potentially reversible etiologies (Table 69-6).

The incidence of IDC has been estimated at 0.005 to 0.006 percent,[375] with the incidence increasing with age and males being more commonly afflicted.[376] A number of immune regulatory abnormalities have been characterized in IDC and include humoral and cellular autoimmune reactivity against myocytes,[377] decreased natural killer cell activity,[378] and abnormal suppressor cell activity.[70] Such findings suggest an immunologic etiology to IDC.

TABLE 69-6 Potentially Reversible Dilated Cardiomyopathies

Ischemic with viable myocardium	Endocrine
Valvular without surgically correctable lesion	Hyperthyroidism
Inflammatory	Pheochromocytoma
CMV	Metabolic
Toxoplasmosis	Hypocalcemia
Mycoplasma	Hypophatemia
Lyme	Uremia
Toxic	Carnitine
Alcohol	Nutritional
Cocaine	Selenium
Cobalt	Thiamine
	Infiltrative
	Hemachromatosis
	Sarcoidosis
	Hypersensitivity

Several studies of the natural history of IDC have concluded that the prognosis is better than for ischemic cardiomyopathy[7]; without treatment, however, mortality approaches 50 percent at 5 years.[379] The risk of thromboembolic complications in IDC may be higher than for the ischemic group, but the clinical response to beta blockade as gauged by improvement in ventricular function is greater.[380] About 10 percent of patients with IDC will normalize their ejection fraction on beta blockade[381]; therefore, if tolerated, this therapy is warranted before consideration of cardiac transplantation.

References

1. Ho K, Pinsky J, Kannel W, et al. The epidemiology of heart failure: The Framingham study. *J Am Coll Cardiol.* 1993; 22:6.
2. Limacher M, Yusef G. Gender differences in presentation, morbidity and mortality in the Studies of Left Ventricular Dysfunction (SOLVD): A preliminary report. In: Wenger N, Sperpff L, Packard B, eds. *Cardiovascular Health and Disease in Women.* Greenwich, CT: Le Jacq Communications; 1993.
3. Mckay R, Pfeffer M, Pasternak R, et al. Left ventricular remodeling after myocardial infarction: A corollary to infarct expansion. *Circulation* 1986; 74:693.
4. Mitchell G, Lamas G, Vaughan D, et al. Left ventricular remodeling in the year after myocardial infarction: A quantitative analysis of contractile segment lengths and ventricular shape. *J Am Coll Cardiol* 1992; 19:1136.
5. Mckee P, Catelli W, McNamara P, et al. The natural history of congestive heart failure: The Framingham Study. *N Engl J Med* 1971; 285:1441.
6. Bristow M, Gilbert E, Abraham W, et al. Carvedilol produces dose-related improvements in left ventricular function and survival in subjects with chronic heart failure. *Circulation* 1996; 94:2807.
7. Likoff M, Chandler S, Kay H. Clinical determinants of mortality in chronic congestive heart failure secondary to idiopathic or dilated cardiomyopathy. *Am J Cardiol* 1987; 59:634.
8. Iskander S, Iskandarian A. Prognostic utility of myocardial viability assessment. *Am J Cardiol* 1999; 83(5):696.
9. Kannel W, Castelli W, McNamara P, et al. Role of blood pressure in the development of congestive heart failure in the Framingham study. *N Engl J Med* 1972; 287:781.
10. Grossman W, Jones D, McLaurin, KP. Wall stress and patterns of hypertrophy in the human left ventricle. *J Clin Invest* 1975; 58:56.
11. Lompre A, Schwartz K, d'Albis A, et al. Myosin isoenzyme redistribution in chronic heart overload. *Nature* 1979; 282:105.
12. Arai M, Matsui H, Periasamy M. Sarcoplasmic reticulum gene expression in cardiac hypertrophy and heart failure. *Circ Res* 1994; 74:555.
13. Jalil J, Doering C, Janicki J, et al. Fibrillar collagen and myocardial stiffness in the intact hypertrophied rat left ventricle. *Circ Res* 1989; 64:1041.
14. Lecarpentier Y, Waldenstrom A, Clergue M, et al. Major alterations in relaxation during cardiac hypertrophy induced by aortic stenosis in guinea pig. *Circ Res* 1987; 61:107.
15. Pfeffer J, Pfeffer M, Braunwald E. Influences of chronic captopril therapy on the infarcted left ventricle of the rat. *Circ Res* 1985; 57:84.
16. Khairallah P. Angiotensin and myocardial protein synthesis. In:

Tarazi RC, Dunbar J, Kanabus J, eds. *Perspective in Cardiovascular Research.* New York: Raven Press; 1983.

17. Kim S, Ohta K, Hamaguchi A, et al. Angiotensin II induces cardiac phenotypic modulation and remodeling in vivo in rats. *Hypertension* 1995; 25:1252.
18. Sadoshima JS. I: Molecular characterization of angiotensin II-induced hypertrophy of cardiac myocytes and hyperplasia of cardiac fibroblasts. *Circ Res* 1993; 73:413.
19. Yusuf S, Sleight P, Pogue J, et al. Effects of an angiotensin-converting-enzyme inhibitor, ramapril, on death from cardiovascular causes, myocardial infarction, and stroke in high-risk patients. *N Engl J Med* 2000; 342:145.
20. Nielsen I. The natural history of hypertensive heart disease as suggested by echocardiography. *Acta Med Scand* 1986; 714:165.
21. Levy D, Larson M, Vasan R, et al. The progression from hypertension to congestive heart failure. *JAMA* 1996; 275:1557.
22. Niimura H, Bachinski L, Sangwatanaroj S, et al. Mutations in the gene for cardiac myosin-binding protein C and late-onset familial hypertrophic cardiomyopathy. *N Engl J Med* 1998; 338: 1248.
23. Lewis J, Maron B. Elderly patients with hypertrophic cardiomyopathy: A subset with distinctive left ventricular morphology and progressive clinical course in late life. *J Am Coll Cardiol* 1989; 13:36.
24. Lewis J, Maron B. Clinical and morphological expression of hypertrophic cardiomyopathy in patients >65 years of age. *Am J Cardiol* 1994; 73:1105.
25. Zieman S, Fortuin N. Hypertrophic and restrictive cardiomyopathies in the elderly. *Cardiol Clin* 1999; 17:151.
26. Topol E, Traill T, Fortuin N. Hypertensive hypertrophic cardiomyopathy of the elderly. *N Engl J Med* 1985; 312:277.
27. Aurigemma G, Gaasch W. Gender differences in older patients with pressure-overload hypertrophy of the left ventricle. *Cardiology* 1995; 86:310.
28. Karam R, Lever H, Healy B. Hypertensive hypertrophic cardiomyopathy or hypertrophic cardiomyopathy with hypertension? A study of 78 patients. *J Am Coll Cardiol* 1989; 13:580.
29. Shapiro L. Hypertrophic cardiomyopathy in the elderly. *Br Heart J* 1990; 63:265.
30. Richardson P, McKenna W, Bristow M, et al. Report of the 1995 World Health Organization/International Society and Federation of Cardiology Task Force on the definition and classification of cardiomyopathies. *Circulation* 1996; 93:841.
31. Ramanathan K, Knowles J, Connor M, et al. Natural history of chronic mitral insufficiency: Relation of peak systolic pressure/end-systolic volume ratio to morbidity and mortality. *J Am Coll Cardiol* 1984; 3:1412.
32. Brodison A, Swann J. Myocarditis: A review. *J Infect* 1998; 3:99.
33. Keeling P, Lukaszyk A, Poloniecki J, et al. A prospective case controlled study of antibodies to coxsackie B virus in idiopathic dilated cardiomyopathy. *J Am Coll Cardiol* 1994; 23:593.
34. Stevens P, Underwood Ground K. Occurrence and significance of myocarditis in trauma. *Aerospace Med* 1970; 41:776.
35. Limas C, Goldenberg I, Limas C. Influence of anti-beta-receptor antibodies on cardiac adenylate cyclase in patients with idiopathic dilated cardiomyopathy. *Am Heart J* 1990; 119:1322.
36. Woodruff J. Viral myocarditis: A review. *Am J Pathol* 1980; 101: 427.
37. Chow L, Ye Y, Linder J, et al. Phenotypic analysis of infiltrating cells in human myocarditis. *Arch Pathol Lab Med* 1989; 113:1357.
38. Young L, Joag S, Zheng L-M, et al. Perforin-mediated myocardial damage in acute myocarditis. *Lancet* 1990; 336:1019.
39. Satoh M, Tamura G, Segawa I, et al. Expression of cytokine genes and presence of enteroviral genomic RNA in endomyocardial biopsy tissues of myocarditis and dilated cardiomyopathy. *Virchows Arch* 1996; 427:503.
40. Godeny E, Gauntt C. In situ immune autoradiographic identification of cells in heart tissues of mice with coxsackie virus B3-induced myocarditis. *Am J Pathol* 1987; 129:267.
41. Lodge P, Herzum M, Olszewski J, et al. Coxsackievirus B3 myocarditis. *Am J Pathol* 1987; 128:455.
42. Seko Y, Shinkai Y, Kawasaki A, et al. Expression of perforin in infiltrating cells in murine hearts with acute myocarditis caused by coxsackievirus B3. *Circulation* 1991; 84:788.
43. Camp T, Hess E, Conway G, et al. Immunologic findings in idiopathic cardiomyopathy. *Am Heart J* 1969; 77:610.
44. Neumann D, Burek C, Baughman K, et al. Circulating heart-reactive antibodies in patients with myocarditis or cardiomyopathy. *J Am Coll Cardiol* 1990; 16:839.
45. Neu N, Craig S, Rose N, et al. Coxsackievirus induced myocarditis in mice: Cardiac myosin autoantibodies do not cross-react with the virus. *Clin Exp Immunol* 1987; 69:566.
46. Neu N, Rose N, Beisel K, et al. Cardiac myosin induces myocarditis in genetically predisposed mice. *Immunology* 1987; 139:3630.
47. Pummerer C, Luze K, Grässl G, et al. Identification of cardiac myosin peptides capable of inducing autoimmune myocarditis in BALB/c mice. *J Clin Invest* 1996; 97:2057.
48. Sutton G, Harding H, Truehart L, et al. Coxsackie B4 myocarditis in an adult: Successful isolation of virus from ventricular myocardium. *Aerospace Med* 1967; 38:66.
49. Easton A, Eglin R. The detection of coxsackievirus RNA in cardiac tissue by in situ hybridization. *J Gen Virol* 1988; 69:285.
50. Kandolf R, Hofschneider P. Viral heart disease. *Springer Semin Immunopathol* 1989; 11:1.
51. Bowles N, Rose M, Taylor P, et al. End-stage dilated cardiomyopathy. *Circulation* 1989; 80:1128.
52. Tracy S, Chapman N, McManus B, et al. A molecular and serologic evaluation of enteroviral involvement in human myocarditis. *J Biol Cell Cardiol* 1990; 22:403.
53. Jin O, Sole M, Butany J, et al. Detection of enterovirus RNA in myocardial biopsies from patients with myocarditis and cardiomyopathy using gene amplification by polymerase chain reaction. *Circulation* 1990; 82:8.
54. Grasso M, Arbustini E, Silini E, et al. Search for coxsackievirus B3 RNA in idiopathic dilated cardiomyopathy using gene amplification by polymerase chain reaction. *Am J Cardiol* 1992; 69:658.
55. Weiss L, Movahed L, Billingham M, et al. Detection of coxsackievirus B3 RNA in myocardial tissues by the polymerase chain reaction. *Am J Pathol* 1991; 138:497.
56. Schwaiger A, Umlauft F, Weyrer K, et al. Detection of enteroviral ribonucleic acid in myocardial biopsies from patients with idiopathic dilated cardiomyopathy by polymerase chain reaction. *Am J Heart J* 1993; 126:406.
57. Petitjean J, Kopecka H, Freymuth F, et al. Detection of enteroviruses in endomyocardial biopsy by molecular approach. *J Med Virol* 1992; 37:76.
58. Keeling P, Jeffery S, Caforio A, et al. Similar prevalence of enteroviral genome within the myocardium from patients with idiopathic dilated cardiomyopathy and controls by the polymerase chain reaction. *Br Heart J* 1992; 68:554.
59. Katsuragi M, Yutani C, Mukai T, et al. Detection of enteroviral genome and its significance in cardiomyopathy. *Cardiology* 1993; 83:4.
60. Severini G, Mestroni L, Falaschi A, et al. Nested polymerase chain reaction for high-sensitivity detection of enteroviral RNA in biological samples. *J Clin Microbiol* 1993; 31:1345.
61. Liljeqvist J, Bergström T, Holmström S, et al. Failure to demonstrate enterovirus aetiology in Swedish patients with dilated cardiomyopathy. *J Med Virol* 1993; 39:6.
62. Satoh M, Tamura G, Segawa I. Enteroviral RNA in endomyocardial biopsy tissues of myocarditis and dilated cardiomyopathy. *Pathol Int* 1994; 44:345.
63. Nicholson F, Ajetunmobi J, Li M, et al. Molecular detection and

serotypic analysis of enterovirus RNA in archival specimens from patients with acute myocarditis. *Br Heart J* 1995; 74:522.
64. Ueno H, Yokota Y, Shiotani H, et al. Significance of detection of enterovirus RNA in myocardial tissues by reverse transcription-polymerase chain reaction. *Int J Cardiol* 1995; 51:157.
65. Fujioka S, Koide H, Kitaura Y, et al. Molecular detection and differentiation of enteroviruses in endomyocardial biopsies and pericardial effusions from dilated cardiomyopathy and myocarditis. *Am Heart J* 1996; 131:760.
66. Andreoletti L, Hober D, Decoene C, et al. Detection of enteroviral RNA by polymerase chain reaction in endomyocardial tissue of patients with chronic cardiac diseases. *J Med Virol* 1996; 48:53.
67. Gauntt C, Pallansch M. Coxsackievirus B3 clinical isolates and murine myocarditis. *Virus Res* 1996; 41:89.
68. Gerli R, Rambotti P, Spinozzi F, et al. Immunologic studies of peripheral blood from patients with idiopathic dilated cardiomyopathy. *Am Heart J* 1986; 112:350.
69. Huber K, Gersh B, Sugrue D, et al. T-lymphocyte subsets in patients with idiopathic dilated cardiomyopathy. *Int J Cardiol* 1989; 22:59.
70. Fowles R, Bieber C, Stinson E. Defective in vitro suppressor cell function in idiopathic congestive cardiomyopathy. *Circulation* 1979; 59:483.
71. Anderson J, Fowles R, Bieber C, et al. Idiopathic cardiomyopathy, age, and suppressor-cell dysfunction as risk determinants of lymphoma after cardiac transplantation. *Lancet* 1978; 2:1174.
72. Matumori A, Yamada T, Suzuki H, et al. Increased circulating cytokines in patients with myocarditis and cardiomyopathy. *Br Heart J* 1994; 72:561.
73. Investigators MTT. Incidence and clinical characteristics of myocarditis. *Circulation* 1991; 84:II-2.
74. Costanzo-Nordin M, O'Connell J, Subramanian R, et al. Myocarditis confirmed by biopsy presenting as acute myocardial infarction. *Br Heart J* 1985; 53:25.
75. Saffitz J, Schwartz D, Southworth W, et al. Coxsackie viral myocarditis causing transmural right and left ventricular infarction without coronary narrowing. *Am J Cardiol* 1983; 52:644.
76. Burch G, Shewey L. Viral coronary arteritis and myocardial infarction. *Am Heart J* 1976; 92:11.
77. Ferguson D, Farwell A, Bradley W, et al. Coronary artery vasospasm complicating acute myocarditis. *West J Med* 1988; 148:664.
78. Kimby A, Sodermark T, Volpe U, et al. Stokes-Adams attacks requiring pacemaker treatment in three patients with acute nonspecific myocarditis. *Acta Med Scand* 1980; 207:177.
79. Phillips M, Robinowitz M, Higgins J, et al. Sudden cardiac death in Air Force recruits: A 20-year review. *JAMA* 1986; 256:2696.
80. Tomioka N, Kishimoto C, Matsumori A, et al. Mural thrombus in experimental viral myocarditis in mice: Relation between thrombosis and congestive heart failure. *Cardiovasc Res* 1986; 20:665.
81. Kojima J, Miyazaki S, Fujiwara H, et al. Recurrent left ventricular mural thrombi in a patient with acute myocarditis. *Heart Vessels* 1988; 4:120.
82. O'Connell J, Fowles R, Robinson J, et al. Clinical and pathologic findings of myocarditis in two families with dilated cardiomyopathy. *Am Heart J* 1984; 107:127.
83. O'Connell J, Costanzo-Nordin M, Subramanian R, et al. Peripartum cardiomyopathy: Clinical, hemodynamic, histologic and prognostic characteristics. *J Am Coll Cardiol* 1986; 8:52.
84. Mason J, Billingham M, Ricci D. Treatment of acute inflammatory myocarditis assisted by endomyocardial biopsy. *Am J Cardiol* 1980; 45:1037.
85. Toshima H, Ohkita Y, Shingu M. Clinical features of acute coxsackie B viral myocarditis. *Jpn Circ J* 1979; 43:441.
86. Karjalainen J, Viitasalo M, Kala R, et al. 24-Hour electrocardiographic recordings in mild acute infectious myocarditis. *Ann Clin Res* 1984; 16:34.
87. Chandraratna P, Nimalasuriya A, Reid C, et al. Left ventricular asynergy in acute myocarditis. *JAMA* 1983; 250:1428.
88. Arvan S, Manalo E. Sudden increase in left ventricular mass secondary to acute myocarditis. *Am Heart J* 1988; 116:200.
89. Pinamonti B, Alberti E, Cigalotto A, et al. Echocardiographic findings in myocarditis. *Am J Cardiol* 1988; 62:285.
90. Miller L, Labovitz A, McBride L, et al. Echocardiography-guided endomyocardial biopsy. *Circulation* 1988; 78:III.
91. Caves P, Schultz W, Dong EJ, et al. New instrument for transvenous cardiac biopsy. *Am J Cardiol* 1974; 33:264.
92. Noda S. Histopathology of endomyocardial biopsies from patients with idiopathic cardiomyopathy: Quantitative evaluation based on multivariate statistical analysis. *Jpn Circ J* 1980; 44:95.
93. Baandrup V, Olsen E. Critical analysis of endomyocardial biopsies from patients suspected of having cardiomyopathy: I. Morphological and morphometric aspects. *Br Heart J* 1981; 45:475.
94. Das J, Rath B, Das S, et al. Study of endomyocardial biopsies in cardiomyopathy. *Indian Heart J* 1981; 18:18.
95. Nippoldt T, Edwards W, Holmes DJ, et al. Right ventricular endomyocardial biopsy. *Mayo Clin Proc* 1982; 57:407.
96. Fenoglio JJ, Ursell P, Kellogg C, et al. Diagnosis and classification of myocarditis by endomyocardial biopsy. *N Engl J Med* 1983; 308:12.
97. Unverferth D, Fetters J, Unverferth B, et al. Human myocardial histologic characteristics in congestive heart failure. *Circulation* 1983; 68:1194.
98. Parrillo J, Aretz H, Palacios I, et al. The results of transvenous endomyocardial biopsy can frequently be used to diagnose myocardial diseases in patients with idiopathic heart failure. *Circulation* 1984; 69:93.
99. Zee-Cheng C-S, Tsai C, Palmer D, et al. High incidence of myocarditis by endomyocardial biopsy in patients with idiopathic congestive cardiomyopathy. *J Am Coll Cardiol* 1984; 3:63.
100. O'Connell J, Henkin R, Robinson JA, et al. Gallium-67 imaging in patients with dilated cardiomyopathy and biopsy-proven myocarditis. *Circulation* 1984; 70:58.
101. Daly K, Richardson P, Olsen E, et al. Acute myocarditis: Role of histological and virological examination in the diagnosis and assessment of immunosuppressive treatment. *Br Heart J* 1984; 51:30.
102. Rose A, Fraser R, Beck W. Absence of evidence of myocarditis in endomyocardial biopsy specimens from patients with dilated (congestive) cardiomyopathy. *S Afr Med J* 1984; 66:871.
103. Regitz V, Olsen E, Rudolph W. Histologisch nachweisbare Myokarditis bei Patienten mit eingeschrankter linksventrikularer Funktion. *Herz* 1985; 10:27.
104. Dec G, Palacios I, Fallon J, et al. Active myocarditis in the spectrum of acute dilated cardiomyopathies: Clinical features, histologic correlates, and clinical outcomes. *N Engl J Med* 1985; 312:885.
105. Salvi A, Silvestri F, Gori D, et al. La biopsia endomiocardica: Un'esperienza relativa a 156 pazienti. *G Ital Cardiol* 1985; 15:251.
106. Mortensen S, Baandrup U, Buch J, et al. Immunosuppressive therapy of biopsy proven myocarditis: Experiences with corticosteroids and cyclosporin. *Int J Immunother* 1985; 1:35.
107. Hosenpud J, McAnulty J, Niles N. Lack of objective improvement in ventricular systolic function in patients with myocarditis treated with azathioprine and prednisone. *J Am Coll Cardiol* 1985; 6:797.
108. Cassling R, Linder J, Sears T, et al. Quantitative evaluation of inflammation in biopsy specimens from idiopathically failing or irritable hearts: Experience in 80 pediatric and adult patients. *Am Heart J* 1985; 110:713.
109. French W, Siegel R, Cohen A, et al. Yield of endomyocardial biopsy in patients with biventricular failure. *Chest* 1986; 90:181.
110. Hammond E, Menlove R, Anderson J. Predictive value of immunofluorescence and electron microscopic evaluation of endomyo-

cardial biopsies in the diagnosis and prognosis of myocarditis and idiopathic dilated cardiomyopathy. *Am Heart J* 1987; 114:1055.
111. Maisch B, Bauer E, Hufnagel G, et al. The use of endomyocardial biopsy in heart failure. *Eur Heart J* 1988; 9:59.
112. Chow L, Dittrich H, Shabetai R. Endomyocardial biopsy in patients with unexplained congestive heart failure. *Ann Intern Med* 1988; 109:535.
113. Leatherbury L, Chandra R, Shapiro S, et al. Value of endomyocardial biopsy in infants, children and adolescents with dilated or hypertrophic cardiomyopathy and myocarditis. *J Am Coll Cardiol* 1988; 12:1547.
114. Hobbs R, Pelegrin D, Ratliff N, et al. Lymphocytic myocarditis and dilated cardiomyopathy: Treatment with immunosuppressive agents. *Cleve Clin J Med* 1989; 56:628.
115. Latham R, Mulrow J, Virmani R, et al. Recently diagnosed idiopathic dilated cardiomyopathy: Incidence of myocarditis and efficacy of prednisone therapy. *Am Heart J* 1989; 117:876.
116. Popma J, Cigarroa R, Buja L, et al. Diagnostic and prognostic utility of right-sided catheterization and endomyocardial biopsy in idiopathic dilated cardiomyopathy. *Am J Cardiol* 1989; 63:955.
117. Vasiljevic J, Kanjuh V, Seferovic P, et al. The incidence of myocarditis in endomyocardial biopsy samples from patients with congestive heart failure. *Am Heart J* 1990; 120:1370.
118. Lieberman E, Hutchins G, Herskowitz A, et al. Clinicopathologic description of myocarditis. *J Am Coll Cardiol* 1991; 18:1617.
119. Strain J, Grose R, Factor S, et al. Results of endomyocardial biopsy in patients with spontaneous ventricular tachycardia but without apparent structural heart disease. *Circulation* 1983; 68:1171.
120. Sugrue D, Holmes DJ, Gersh B, et al. Cardiac histologic findings in patients with life-threatening ventricular arrhythmias of unknown origin. *J Am Coll Cardiol* 1984; 4:952.
121. Vignola P, Aonuma K, Swaye P, et al. Lymphocytic myocarditis presenting as unexplained ventricular arrhythmias: Diagnosis with endomyocardial biopsy and response to immunosuppression. *J Am Coll Cardiol* 1984; 4:812.
122. Hosenpud J, McAnulty J, Niles N. Unexpected myocardial disease in patients with life threatening arrhythmias. *Br Heart J* 1986; 56:55.
123. Aretz H, Billingham M, Edwards W, et al. Myocarditis: A histopathological definition. *Am J Cardiovasc Pathol* 1986; 1:3.
124. Dec G, Palacios I, Fallon J, et al. Antimyosin antibody cardiac imaging: Its role in the diagnosis of myocarditis. *J Am Coll Cardiol* 1990; 16:97.
125. Keogh A, Billingham M, Schroeder J. Rapid histological changes in endomyocardial biopsy specimens after myocarditis. *Br Heart J* 1990; 64:406.
126. Billingham M, Tazelaar H. The morphological progression of viral myocarditis. *Postgrad Med J* 1986; 62:581.
127. Gagliardi M, Bevilacqua M, Di Renzi P, et al. Usefulness of magnetic resonance imaging for diagnosis of acute myocarditis in infants and children, and comparison with endomyocardial biopsy. *Am J Cardiol* 1991; 68:1089.
128. Hahn E, Hartz V, Moon R, et al. The Myocarditis Treatment Trial: Design, methods and patient enrollment. *Eur Heart J* 1995; 16:162.
129. Mason J, O'Connell J, Herskowitz A, et al. A clinical trial of immunosuppressive therapy for myocarditis. *N Engl J Med* 1995; 333:269.
130. McNamara D, Rosenblum W, Janosko K, et al. Intravenous immune globulin in the therapy of myocarditis and acute cardiomyopathy. *Circulation* 1997; 95:2476.
131. McNamara D, Starling R, Dec W, et al. Intervention in myocarditis and acute cardiomyopathy with immune globulin: Results from the randomized placebo controlled IMAC trial (abstr). *Circulation* 1999; 100.
132. Grogan M, Redfield M, Baily K, et al. Long term outcome of patients with biopsy proven myocarditis: Comparison with idiopathic dilated cardiomyopathy. *J Am Coll Cardiol* 1995; 26:80.
133. Barbaro G, DiLorenzo G, Grisoris B, Barbarini G. Incidence of dilated cardiomyopathy and detection of HIV in myocardial cells of HIV-positive patients: Gruppo Italiano per lo Studio Cardiologico dei Pazienti Affetti da AIDS. *N Engl J Med* 1998; 339:1093.
134. Flotats A, Domingo P, Carrio I. Dilated Cardiomyopathy in HIV-infected patients. *N Engl J Med* 1999; 340:732.
135. Gonwa T, Capehart J, Pilcher J, et al. Cytomegalovirus myocarditis as a cause of cardiac dysfunction in a heart transplant recipient. *Transplantation* 1989; 47:197.
136. Marsden P. South American trypanosomiasis (Chagas' disease). *Int Rev Trop Med* 1971; 4:97.
137. Sadigursky M, von Kreuter B, Ling P-Y, et al. Association of elevated antisarcolemma, anti-idiotype antibody levels with the clinical and pathologic expression of chronic Chagas myocarditis. *Circulation* 1989; 80:1269.
138. D'Avila Reis D, Jones E, Tostes S, et al. Characterization of inflammatory infiltrate in chronic myocardial lesions: Presence of tumor necrosis factor-alpha+ cells and dominance of granzyme A+, CD8+ lymphocytes. *Am J Trop Med Hyg* 1993; 48:637.
139. Higuchi M, Reis M, Aiello V, et al. Association of an increase in CD8+ T cells with the presence of Trypanosoma cruzi antigens in chronic, human, chagasic myocarditis. *Am J Trop Med Hyg* 1997; 56:485.
140. Araujo F. Development of resistance to Trypanosoma cruzi in mice depends on a viable population of L3zt4+ (CD4+) T lymphocytes. *Infect Immun* 1989; 57:2246.
141. Sher A, Coffman R. Regulation of immunity to parasites by T cells and T cell-derived cytokines. *Annu Rev Immunol* 1992; 10:385.
142. Ribeiro-dos-Santos R, Pirmez A, Savino W. Role of autoreactive immunological mechanisms in chagasic carditis. *Res Immunol* 1991; 142:134.
143. Reis M, Higuchi MdL, Benvenuti L, et al. An in situ quantitative immunohistochemical study of cytokines and IL-2R+ in chronic, human, chagasic myocarditis: Correlation with the presence of myocardial *T. cruzi* antigens. *Clin Immunol Immunopathol* 1997; 83:165.
144. Higuchi M, De Morais C, Barreto A, et al. The role of active myocarditis in the development of heart failure in chronic Chagas' disease: A study based on endomyocardial biopsies. *Clin Cardiol* 1987; 10:665.
145. Maguire J, Mott K, Lehman J, et al. Relationship of electrocardiographic abnormalities and seropositivity to *Trypanosoma cruzi* within a rural community in northeast Brazil. *Am Heart J* 1983; 105:287.
146. Chiale P, Halpern M, Nau G, et al. Efficacy of amiodarone during long-term treatment of malignant ventricular arrhythmias in patients with chronic chagasic myocarditis. *Am Heart J* 1984; 107:656.
147. Steere A, Batsford W, Weinberg M, et al. Lyme carditis: Cardiac abnormalities of Lyme disease. *Ann Intern Med* 1980; 93:8.
148. Olson L, Okafor E, Clements I. Cardiac involvement in Lyme disease: Manifestations and management. *Mayo Clin Proc* 1986; 61:745.
149. Luft B, Billingham M, Remington J. Endomyocardial biopsy in the diagnosis of toxoplasmic myocarditis. *Transplant Proc* 1986; 18:1871.
150. Wallace M, Garst P, Papadimos T, et al. The return of acute rheumatic fever in young adults. *JAMA* 1989; 262:2557.
151. Massell B, Chute C, Walker A, et al. Penicillin and the marked decrease in morbidity and mortality from rheumatic fever in the United States. *N Engl J Med* 1988; 318:280.
152. Stollerman G. Rheumatogenic streptococci and autoimmunity. *Clin Immunol Immunopathol* 1991; 61:131.
153. Bessen D, Jones K, Fischetti V. Evidence for two distinct classes

of streptococcal M protein and their relationship to rheumatic fever. *J Exp Med* 1989; 169:269.
154. Krisher K, Cunningham M. Myosin: A link between streptococci and heart. *Science* 1985; 227:413.
155. Jones T. Diagnosis of rheumatic fever. *JAMA* 1944; 126:481.
156. Vasan R, Shrivastava S, Vijayakumar M, et al. Echocardiographic evaluation of patients with acute rheumatic fever and rheumatic carditis. *Circulation* 1996; 94:73.
157. Narula J, Rahimtoola S. Diagnosis of acute rheumatic carditis: The echoes of change. *Circulation* 1999; 100:1576.
158. Kounis N, Zavras G, Soufas G, et al. Hypersensitivity myocarditis. *Ann Allergy* 1989; 62:71.
159. Spry C, Tai P-C. The eosinophil in myocardial disease. *Eur Heart J* 1987; 8:81.
160. Kim C, Vlietstra R, Edwards W, et al. Steroid-responsive eosinophilic myocarditis: Diagnosis by endomyocardial biopsy. *Am J Cardiol* 1984; 53:1472.
161. Cooper L, Berry G, Shabetai R. Idiopathic giant-cell myocarditis—natural history and treatment. *N Engl J Med* 1997; 336:1860.
162. Zhang S, Kodama M, Hanawa H, et al. Effects of cyclosporine, prednisolone, and aspirin on rat autoimmune giant cell myocarditis. *J Am Coll Cardiol* 1993; 21:1254.
163. Davidoff R, Palacios I, Southern J, et al. Giant cell versus lymphocytic myocarditis: A comparison of their clinical features and long-term outcomes. *Circulation* 1991; 83:953.
164. Brown C, Bertlet B. Peripartum cardiomyopathy: A comprehensive review. *Am J Obstet Gynecol* 1998; 178:409.
165. Cunningham F, Pritchard J, Hankins G, et al. Peripartum heart failure: Idiopathic cardiomyopathy or compounding cardiovascular events? *Obstet Gynecol* 1986; 67:157.
166. Seftel H, Susser M. Maternity and myocardial failure in African women. *Br Heart J* 1961; 43.
167. Farber P, Glasgow L. Factors modulating host resistance to virus infection: II. Enhanced susceptibility of mice to encephalomyocarditis virus infection during pregnancy. *Am J Pathol* 1968; 53:463.
168. Farber P, Glasgow L. Viral myocarditis during pregnancy: Encephalomyocarditis virus infection in mice. *Am Heart J* 1970; 80:96.
169. Takatsu T, Kitamura Y, Morita H, et al. Viral myocarditis and cardiomyopathy. In: Sekigushi M, Olsen E, eds. *Cardiomyopathy*. Tokyo: University of Tokyo Press; 1978.
170. Midei M, Dement S, Feldman A, et al. Peripartum myocarditis and cardiomyopathy. *Circulation* 1990; 81:922.
171. Melvin K, Richardson P, Olson E, et al. Peripartum cardiomyopathy due to myocarditis. *N Engl J Med* 1982; 307:731.
172. Nizeq M, Rickenbocker P, Fowler M, et al. Incidence of myocarditis in peripartum cardiomyopathy. *Am J Cardiol* 1994; 74:74.
173. Knobel B, Melamud E, Kishon Y. Peripartum cardiomyopathy. *Isr J Med Sci* 1984; 20:1061.
174. Demakis J, Rahimtoola S, Sutton G, et al. Natural course of peripartum cardiomyopathy. *Circulation* 1971; 44:1053.
175. Carvalho A, Brandao A, Martinez E, et al. Prognosis in peripartum cardiomyopathy. *Am J Cardiol* 1989; 64:540.
176. Report of the WHO/ISGC Task Force on the Definition and Classification of the Cardiomyopathies. *Br Heart J* 1980; 44:672.
177. Marin-Garcia J, Goldenthal M. Cardiomyopathy and abnormal mitochondrial function. *Cardiovasc Res* 1994; 28:456.
178. Watkins H, McKenna W, Thierfelder L, et al. Mutations in the genes for cardiac troponin T and μ-tropomyosin in hypertrophic cardiomyopathy. *N Engl J Med* 1995; 332:1058.
179. Maron B, Spirito P, Wesley Y, et al. Development and progression of left ventricular hypertrophy in children with hypertrophic cardiomyopathy. *N Engl J Med* 1986; 315:610.
180. Solomon S, Wolff S, Watkins H, et al. Left ventricular hypertrophy and morphology in familial hypertrophic cardiomyopathy with mutations of the b-myosin heavy chain gene. *J Am Coll Cardiol* 1993; 22:498.
181. Schwartz K, Carrier L, Guicheney P, et al. Molecular basis of familial cardiomyopathies. *Circulation* 1995; 91:532.
182. Watkins H, Conner D, Thierfelder L, et al. Mutations in the cardiac myosin binding protein-C gene on chromosome 11 cause familial hypertrophic cardiomyopathy. *Nature Genet* 1995; 11:434.
183. Bonne G, Carrier L, Bercovici J, et al. A splice acceptor site mutation in the cardiac myosin binding protein-C gene causes familial hypertrophic cardiomyopathy. *Nature Genet* 1995; 11:438.
184. Watkins H, Rosenzweig A, Hwang D-S, et al. Characteristics and prognostic implications of myosin missense mutations in familial hypertrophic cardiomyopathy. *N Engl J Med* 1992; 326:1108.
185. Anan R, Greve G, Thierfelder L, et al. Prognostic implications of novel b-cardiac myosin heavy chain gene mutations that cause familial hypertrophic cardiomyopathy. *J Clin Invest* 1994; 93:280.
186. Posen B, Moolman J, Corfield V, et al. Clinical and prognostic evaluation of familial hypertrophic cardiomyopathy in two South African families with different cardiac b-myosin heavy chain gene mutations. *Br Heart J* 1995; 74:40.
187. Dausse E, Komadja M, Fetler L. Familial hypertrophic cardiomyopathy: Microsatellite haplotyping and identification of a hotspot for mutations in the b-myosin heavy chain gene. *J Clin Invest* 1993; 92:2807.
188. Newman H, Sugrue D, Oakley C, et al. Relation of left ventricular function and prognosis in hypertrophic cardiomyopathy: An angiographic study. *J Am Coll Cardiol* 1985; 5:1064.
189. Hecht G, Panza J, Maron B. Clinical course of middle-aged asymptomatic patients with hypertrophic cardiomyopathy. *Am J Cardiol* 1992; 69:935.
190. Maron B, Shirani J, Poliac L, et al. Sudden death in young competitive athletes: Clinical, demographic and pathologic profiles. *JAMA* 1996; 276:199.
191. Maron B, Roberts W, Epstein S. Sudden death in hypertrophic cardiomyopathy: A profile of 78 patients. *Circulation* 1982; 67: 1388.
192. Nicod B, Polikar R, Peterson K. Hypertrophic cardiomyopathy and sudden death. *N Engl J Med* 1988; 318:1255.
193. Mckenna W, Deanfield J, Faroqui A, et al. Prognosis in hypertrophic cardiomyopathy: Role of age and clinical electrocardiographic and hemodynamic features. *Am J Cardiol* 1981; 47:532.
194. Gilligan D, Nihoyannopoulos P, Chan W, et al. Investigation for a hemodynamic basis for syncope in hypertrophic cardiomyopathy: Use of a head-up tilt test. *Circulation* 1992; 85:2140.
195. Maron B, Cecchi F, McKenna W. Risk factors and stratification for sudden cardiac death in hypertrophic cardiomyopathy. *Br Heart J* 1994; 72:S13.
196. Spirito P, Maron B. Relation between extent of left ventricular hypertrophy and occurrence of sudden cardiac death in hypertrophic cardiomyopathy. *J Am Coll Cardiol* 1990; 15:1521.
197. Spirito P, Seidman C, McKenna W, et al. Management of hypertrophic cardiomyopathy. *N Engl J Med* 1997; 30:775.
198. Shirani J, Maron B, Cannon R, et al. Clinicopathologic features of hypertrophic cardiomyopathy managed by cardiac transplantation. *Am J Cardiol* 1993; 73:434.
199. Valentine H, Hunt S, Fowler M, et al. Frequency of familial nature of dilated cardiomyopathy and usefulness of cardiac transplantation in this subset. *Am J Cardiol* 1989; 63:959.
200. Michaels V, Moll P, Miller F, et al. The frequency of familial dilated cardiomyopathy in a series of patients with idiopathic cardiomyopathy. *N Engl J Med* 1992; 326:77.
201. Gregori D, Rocco C, DiLenarda A, et al. Estimating the frequency of familial dilated cardiomyopathy and the risk of misclassification errors (abstr). *Circulation* 1996; 94:I270.
202. Abelmann W, Lorell B. The challenge of cardiomyopathy. *J Am Coll Cardiol* 1989; 13:1219.

203. Rubin E. Alcoholic myopathy in heart and skeletal muscle. *N Engl J Med* 1979; 301:28.
204. Honey M. A case of fatal peripartum cardiomyopathy. *Br Heart J* 1986; 55:114.
205. Anan R, Nakagawa M, Miyata M, et al. Cardiac involvement in mitochondrial diseases. *Circulation* 1995; 91:955.
206. Kushwaha S, Fallon J, Fuster V. Medical progress: Restrictive cardiomyopathy. *N Engl J Med* 1997; 336:267.
207. Carrell R, Lomas D. Conformational disease. *Lancet* 1997; 350:134.
208. Hodkinson H, Pomerance A. The clinical significance of senile cardiac amyloidosis: A prospective clinico-pathological study. *Q J Med* 1977; 46:381.
209. Swanton R, Brooksby I, Davis M, et al. Systolic and diastolic ventricular function in cardiac amyloidosis: Studies in six cases diagnosed with endomyocardial biopsies. *Am J Cardiol* 1977; 39:658.
210. Cohen A. Amyloidosis. In: Wilson J, Braunwald E, Isselbacher K, et al., eds. *Harrison's Principles of Internal Medicine,* 12th ed. New York: McGraw-Hill; 1991.
211. Cohen A. Amyloidosis. *N Engl J Med* 1967; 277:522.
212. Kyle R, Greipp P. Amyloidosis (AL): Clinical and laboratory features in 229 cases. *Mayo Clin Proc* 1983; 58:665.
213. Roberts W, Waller B. Cardiac amyloidosis causing cardiac dysfunction: Analysis of 54 necropsy patients. *Am J Cardiol* 1983; 52:137.
214. Olson L, Gertz M, Edwards W, et al. Senile cardiac amyloidosis with myocardial dysfunction: Diagnosis by endomyocardial biopsy and immunohistochemistry. *N Engl J Med* 1987; 317:738.
215. Nichols W, Liepnieks J, Snyder E, et al. Senile cardiac amyloidosis associated with homozygosity for a transthyretin variant (ILE-122). *J Lab Clin Med* 1990; 117:175.
216. Nordlie M, Sletten K, Husby G, et al. A new prealbumin variant in familial amyloid cardiomyopathy of Danish origin. *Scand J Immunol* 1988; 27:119.
217. Gertz M, Kyle R, Greipp P. Response rates and survival in primary systemic amyloidosis. *Blood* 1991; 77:257.
218. Bhandari A, Nanda N. Myocardial texture characterization by two-dimensional echocardiography. *Am J Cardiol* 1982; 51:817.
219. Click R, Olson L, Edwards W, et al. Echocardiography and systemic diseases. *J Am Soc Echocardiogr* 1994; 7:201.
220. Gertz M, Kyle R. Primary systemic amyloidosis: A diagnostic primer. *Mayo Clin Proc* 1989; 64:1505.
221. Kyle R, Bayrd E. Amyloidosis: Review of 236 cases. *Medicine* 1975; 54:271.
222. Klein A, Hatle L, Taliercio C, et al. Prognostic significance of Doppler measures of diastolic function in cardiac amyloidosis: A Doppler echocardiography study. *Circulation* 1991; 83:808.
223. Klein A, Hatle L, Burstow D, et al. Comprehensive Doppler assessment of right ventricular diastolic function in cardiac amyloidosis. *J Am Coll Cardiol* 1990; 15:99.
224. Klein A, Hatle L, Taliercio C, et al. Serial Doppler echocardiographic follow-up of left ventricular diastolic function in cardiac amyloidosis. *J Am Coll Cardiol* 1990; 16:1135.
225. Hosenpud J, DeMarco T, Frazier O, et al. Progression of systemic disease and reduced long-termed in patients with cardiac amyloidosis undergoing heart transplantation: Follow-up results of a multicenter survey. *Circulation* 1991; 84:III.
226. Bascom R, Johns C. The natural history and management of sarcoidosis. *Adv Intern Med* 1986; 31:213.
227. Roberts W, McAllister H, Ferrans V. Sarcoidosis of the heart: A clinicopathologic study of 35 necropsy patients and review of 78 previously described necropsy patients. *Am J Med* 1977; 63:86.
228. Silverman K, Hutchins G, Bulkley B. Cardiac sarcoid: A clinicopathologic study of 84 unselected patients with systemic sarcoidosis. *Circulation* 1978; 58:1204.
229. Perry A, Vuitch F. Causes of death in patients with sarcoidosis: A morphologic study of 38 autopsies with clinicopathologic correlation. *Arch Pathol Lab Med* 1995; 119:167.
230. Wenger N, Ablemann W, Roberts W. Cardiomyopathy and specific heart muscle disease. In: Hurst J, Schlant R, Rackley C, Sonnenblick E, Wenger N, eds. *The Heart,* 7th ed. New York: McGraw-Hill; 1990.
231. *Tenth International Conference on Sarcoidosis and Other Granulomatous Disorders.* New York: New York Academy of Sciences; 1986.
232. Matsui Y, Iwai K, Tackibana T, et al. Clinicopathologic study of fatal cardiac sarcoidosis. *Ann NY Acad Sci* 1976; 278:455.
233. Stein E, Stimmel B, Siltzbach L. Clinical course of cardiac sarcoidosis. *Ann NY Acad Sci* 1976; 278:470.
234. Burstow D, Tajik J, Bailey K, et al. Two-dimensional echocardiographic findings in systemic sarcoidosis. *Am J Cardiol* 1989; 63:478.
235. Fleming H. Cardiac sarcoidosis. *Semin Respir Med* 1986; 8:65.
236. Fawcett F, Goldberg M. Heartblock resulting from myocardial sarcoidosis. *Br Heart J* 1974; 36:220.
237. Schaedel H, Kirsten D, Schmidt A, et al. Sarcoid heart disease: Results of follow-up investigations. *Eur Heart J* 1991; 12:26.
238. Winters S, Cohen M, Greenberg S, et al. Sustained ventricular tachycardia associated with sarcoidosis: Assessment of the underlying cardiac anatomy and the prospective utility of programmed ventricular stimulation, drug therapy and an implantable antitachycardia device. *J Am Coll Cardiol* 1991; 18:937.
239. Fleming H. Sarcoidosis heart disease. *BMJ* 1986; 292:1095.
240. Valentine H, Tazelaar H, Macoviak J, et al. Cardiac sarcoidosis: Response to steroids and transplantation. *J Heart Transplant* 1987; 5:244.
241. Skinner C, Kenmure C. Hemachromatosis presenting as congestive cardiomyopathy and responding to venesection. *Br Heart J* 1973; 35:466.
242. Short E, Winkle R, Billingham M. Myocardial involvement in idiopathic hemachromatosis, morphological and clinical improvement following venesection. *Am J Med* 1981; 70:1275.
243. Skinner M, Anderson J, Simms R, et al. Treatment of 100 patients with primary amyloidosis: A randomized trial of melphalan, prednisone, and colchicine versus colchicine only. *Am J Med* 1996; 100:290.
244. Strickman N, Hall R. Carcinoid heart disease. In: Kapoor A, Reynolds R, eds. *Cancer and the Heart.* New York: Springer-Verlag; 1986.
245. Pellikka P, Tajik A, Khandheria B, et al. Carcinoid heart disease: Clinical and echocardiographic spectrum in 74 patients. *Circulation* 1993; 87:1188.
246. Onate A, Alsibar J, Inguanzo R, et al. Balloon dilation of tricuspid and pulmonary valve in carcinoid heart disease. *Texas Heart Inst J* 1993; 20:115.
247. Rosenzweig B, Guarneri E, Kronzon I. Echocardiographic manifestations in a patient with pseudoxanthoma elasticum. *Ann Intern Med* 1993; 119:487.
248. Hwang B, Meng C, Lin C, et al. Clinical analysis of 5 infants with glycogen storage disease of the heart-Pompe's disease. *JPN Heart J* 1986; 27:25.
249. Löffler W. Endocarditis parietalis fibroplastica mit Bluteosinophilie, ein eigenartiges Krankheitsbild. *Schweiz Med Wochenschr* 1936; 66:817.
250. Galiuto L, Enriquez-Sarano M, Reeder G, et al. Eosinophilic myocarditis manifesting as myocardial infarction: Early diagnosis and successful treatment. *Mayo Clin Proc* 1997; 72:603.
251. Daves J, Spry C, Sapsford R, et al. Cardiovascular features of 11 patients with eosinophilic endomyocardial disease. *Q J Med* 1983; 52:23.
252. Acquatella H, Schiller N, Puigbo J, et al. Value of two-dimensional echocardiography in endomyocardial disease with and

without eosinophilia: Clinical and pathologic study. *Circulation* 1983; 67:1219.
253. Olsen E, Spry C. Relation between eosinophilia and endomyocardial disease. *Prog Cardiovasc Dis* 1985; 27:241.
254. Moodie D, Baum J, Gill C, et al. Endomyocardial fibrosis: Diagnosis and surgical treatment of two cases occurring in the United States. *Clevel Clin Q* 1986; 53:159.
255. Oakley C, Olsen E. Eosinophilia and heart disease (editorial). *Br Heart J* 1977; 39:233.
256. Solley G, Maldonado J, Gleich G, et al. Endomyocardiopathy with eosinophilia. *Mayo Clin Proc* 1976; 51:697.
257. Hendren W, Jones E, Smith M. Aortic and mitral valve replacement in idiopathic hypereosinophilic syndrome. *Ann Thorac Surg* 1988; 46:570.
258. Arnold M, McGuire L, Lee J. Löffler's fibroplastic endocarditis. *Pathology* 1988; 20:79.
259. Blake D, Palmer I, Olinger G. Mitral valve replacement in idiopathic hypereosinophilic syndrome. *J Thorac Cardiovasc Surg* 1985; 89:630.
260. Packer D, Bardy G, Worley S, et al. Tachycardia-induced cardiomyopathy: A reversible form of left ventricular dysfunction. *Am J Cardiol* 1986; 57:563.
261. Uhl H. A previously undescribed congenital malformation of the heart: Almost total absence of the myocardium of the right ventricle. *Bull Johns Hopkins Hosp* 1972; 91:197.
262. Marcus F, Fontaine G, Guiraudon G, et al. Right ventricular dysplasia: A report of 24 adult cases. *Circulation* 1982; 65:384.
263. Gerlis L, Schmidt-Ott S, Ho S, et al. Dysplastic conditions of the right ventricular myocardium: Uhl's anomaly v arrhythmogenic right ventricular dysplasia. *Br Heart J* 1993; 69:142.
264. Thiene G, Nava A, Corrado D, et al. Right ventricular cardiomyopathy and sudden death in young people. *N Engl J Med* 1988; 318:129.
265. Nava A, Thiene G, Canciani B, et al. Familial occurrence of right ventricular dysplasia: A study involving nine families. *J Am Coll Cardiol* 1988; 12:1222.
266. Kisslo J. Two-dimensional echocardiography in arrhythmogenic right ventricular dysplasia. *Eur Heart J* 1989; 10:22.
267. Segall H. Parchment heart (Osler). *Am Heart J* 1950; 40:948.
268. Hasumi M, Sekiguchi M, Hiroe M, et al. Endomyocardial biopsy approach to patients with ventricular tachycardia with special reference to arrhythmogenic right ventricular dysplasia. *Jpn Circ J* 1987; 51:242.
269. Maitland M, Frishman W. Thyroid hormone and cardiovascular disease. *Am Heart J* 1998; 135:187.
270. Dillman W. Biochemical basis of thyroid hormone action in the heart. *Am J Med* 1990; 88:626.
271. Hamilton M, Stevenson L, Luu M, et al. Altered thyroid hormone metabolism in advanced heart failure. *J Am Coll Cardiol* 1990; 16:91.
272. Hamilton M, Stevenson L. Thyroid hormone abnormalities in heart failure: Possibilities for therapy. *Thyroid* 1996; 6:527.
273. Moruzzi P, Doria E, Agostoni P, et al. Usefulness of L-thyoxine to improve cardiac and exercise performance in idiopathic dilated cardiomyopathy. *Am J Cardiol* 1994; 73:374.
274. Moruzzi P, Doria E, Agostoni P. Medium-term effectiveness of L-thyroxine treatment in idiopathic dilated cardiomyopathy. *Am J Med* 1996; 101:461.
275. Umpierrez G, Challapalli S, Patterson C. Congestive heart failure due to reversible cardiomyopathy in patients with hyperthyroidism. *Am J Med* Sci 1995; 310:99.
276. Van Vliet P, Rarchell H, Titus J. Focal myocarditis associated with pheochromocytoma. *N Engl J Med* 1966; 274:1102.
277. Imperato-McGinley J, Cautier T, Ehlers K, et al. Reversibility of catecholamine-induced dilated cardiomyopathy in a child with a pheochromocytoma. *N Engl J Med* 1987; 316:793.
278. Scott I, Parkes R, Cameron D. Pheochromocytoma and cardiomyopathy. *Med J Aust* 1988; 148:94.
279. Behrana A, Haselton P, Leen C, et al. Multiple extra-adrenal paragangliomas associated with catecholamine cardiomyopathy. *Eur Heart J* 1989; 10:182.
280. Lam J, Shub G, Sheps S. Reversible dilatation of hypertrophied left ventricle in pheochromocytoma: Serial two-dimensional echocardiographic observations. *Am Heart J* 1985; 109:613.
281. Salathe M, Wein P, Ritz R. Rapid reversal of heart failure in a patient with phaeochromocytoma and catecholamine-induced cardiomyopathy who was treated with captopril. *Br Heart J* 1992; 68:527.
282. Lie J, Grossman S. Pathology of the heart in acromegaly: Anatomic findings in 27 autopsied patients. *Am Heart J* 1980; 100:41.
283. Rossi L, Thiene G, Caregaro L, et al. Dysrhythmias and sudden death in acromegalic heart disease. A clinicopathologic study. *Chest* 1977; 72:495.
284. Baldwin A, Cundy T, Butler J, et al. Progression of cardiovascular disease in acromegalic patients treated by external pituitary irradiation. *Acta Endocrinol* 1985; 108:26.
285. Abbott R, Donahue R, Kannel W, et al. The impact of diabetes on survival following myocardial infarction in men vs women. The Framingham Study. *JAMA* 1988; 260:3456.
286. Zoneraich S. *Diabetes and the Heart.* Springfield, IL: Charles C Thomas; 1978.
287. Sutherland C, Fisher B, Frier B, et al. Endomyocardial biopsy pathology in insulin-dependent diabetic patients with abnormal ventricular function. *Histopathology* 1989; 14:593.
288. Hausdorf G, Rieger U, Koepp P. Cardiomyopathy in childhood diabetes mellitus: Incidence, time of onset, and relation to metabolic control. *Int J Cardiol* 1988; 19:225.
289. MacMahon S, Wilcken D, Macdonald G. The effect of weight reduction on left ventricular mass: A randomized controlled trial in young, overweight, hypertensive patients. *N Engl J Med* 1986; 314:334.
290. Alpert M, Terry B, Kelly D. Effect of weight loss on cardiac chamber size, wall thickness, and left ventricular function in morbid obesity. *Am J Cardiol* 1985; 55:783.
291. Backman L, Freyschuss U, Hallberg D, et al. Reversibility of cardiovascular changes in extreme obesity: Effects of weight reduction through jejunoileostomy. *Acta Med Scand* 1979; 205:367.
292. Waldenstrom A. Alcohol and congestive heart failure. *Alcohol Clin Exp Res* 1998; 22:315s.
293. McCall D. Alcohol and the cardiovascular system. *Curr Probl Cardiol* 1987; 12:351.
294. Richardson P, Patel V, Preedy V. Alcohol and the myocardium. *Novartis Foundation Symp* 1998; 216:35.
295. Beckemeier M, Bora P. Fatty acid ethyl esters: Potentially toxic products of myocardial ethanol metabolism. *J Mol Cell Cardiol* 1998; 30:2487.
296. Morin Y, Daniel P. Quebec's beer drinkers cardiomyopathy: Etiologic considerations. *Can Med Assoc J* 1967; 97:926.
297. Krelbrek H, Nielsen B, Eriksen J, et al. Left ventricular performance in alcoholic patients without chronic liver disease. *Br Heart J* 1987; 58:352.
298. Regan T, Khan M, Ettinger P, et al. Myocardial function and lipid metabolism in the chronic alcoholic animal. *J Clin Invest* 1974; 54:740.
299. Regan T, Levinson G, Oldewurtel H, et al. Ventricular function in noncardiacs with alcoholic fatty liver: The role of ethanol in the production of cardiomyopathy. *J Clin Invest* 1969; 48:397.
300. Reitz R, Helsabeck E, Mason D. Effects of chronic alcohol ingestion on the fatty acid composition of the heart. *Lipids* 1973; 8:80.
301. Demakis J, Proskey A, Rahimtoola S, et al. The natural course of alcoholic cardiomyopathy. *Ann Intern Med* 1974; 80:293.
302. Pravin D, Nicolosi G, Lestuzzi C, et al. Normalization of variables of left ventricular function in patients with alcoholic cardiomyop-

athy after cessation of excessive alcohol intake: An echocardiographic study. *Eur Heart J* 1987; 8:535.
303. Milani L, Bagolin E, Sanson A. Improvement of left ventricular function in chronic alcoholics following abstinence of ethanol. *Cardiology* 1989; 76:299.
304. Vecchia L, Bedogni F, Bozzola L, et al. Prediction of recovery after abstinence in alcoholic cardiomyopathy: Role of hemodynamic and morphometric parameters. *Clin Cardiol* 1995; 19:45.
305. Regan T. Alcoholic cardiomyopathy. *Progr Cardiovasc Dis* 1984; 27:141.
306. Prazak P, Pfistere M, Osswald S, et al. Differences of disease progression in congestive heart failure due to alcoholic as compared to idiopathic dilated cardiomyopathy. *Eur Heart J* 1996; 17:251.
307. Ikram H, Williamson H, Won M, et al. The course of idiopathic dilated cardiomyopathy in New Zealand. *Br Heart J* 1987; 57:521.
308. Isner J, Chokshi S. Cardiovascular complications of cocaine. *Curr Probl Cardiol* 1991; 16:538.
309. Waller B. Cocaine and the heart. *Ind Med* 1988; 81:956.
310. Hauge N, Perrault C, Morgan J. Effects of cocaine on intracellular Ca++ handling in mammalian myocardium (abstr). *Circulation* 1988; 78:359.
311. Herman E, Vlck J. A study of direct effect of cocaine on the heart (abstr). *Fed Proc* 1987; 46:1148.
312. Franker T, Temsey-Armos P, Brewster P, et al. Mechanisms of cocaine-induced myocardial depression in dogs. *Circulation* 1990; 81:1012.
313. Van Dyke C, Byck R. Cocaine. *Sci Am* 1982; 246:128.
314. Weiner R, Lockhart J, Schwartz R. Dilated cardiomyopathy and cocaine abuse. *Am J Med* 1986; 81:699.
315. Chakko S, Myerburg R. Cardiac complications of cocaine abuse. *Clin Cardiol* 1995; 18:67.
316. Hale S, Alker K, Rezkalla S, et al. Adverse effects of cocaine in cardiovascular dynamics, myocardial blood flow, and coronary artery diameter in an experimental model. *Am Heart J* 1989; 118:927.
317. Virmani R, Robinowitz M, Smialek J, et al. Cardiovascular effects of cocaine: An autopsy study of 40 patients. *Am Heart J* 1988; 115:1068.
318. Chokshi S, Moore R, Pandian N, et al. Reversible cardiomyopathy associated with cocaine intoxication. *Ann Intern Med* 1989; 111:1039.
319. Singal P, Iliskovic N. Current concepts: Doxorubicin-induced cardiomyopathy. *N Engl J Med* 1998; 339:900.
320. Bristow M, Billingham M, Mason J, et al. Clinical spectrum of anthracycline antibiotic cardiotoxicity. *Cancer Treat Rev* 1978; 873:62.
321. Lena L, Page J. Cardiotoxicity of Adriamycin and related anthracyclines. *Cancer Treat Rev* 1976; 3:111.
322. Lipshultz S, Colan S, Gelber R, et al. Late cardiac effects of doxorubicin therapy for acute lymphoblastic leukemia in childhood. *N Engl J Med* 1991; 324:808.
323. Fowles R. Cardiac catheterization and endomyocardial biopsy. In: Kapoor A, Reynolds R, eds. *Cancer and the Heart*. New York: Springer-Verlag; 1986.
324. Greene H, Reich S, Dalen J. How to minimize doxorubicin toxicity. *J Cardiovasc Med* 1982; 7:306.
325. Legla S, Benjamin R, MacKay B, et al. Reduction of doxorubicin cardiotoxicity by prolonged continuous intravenous infusion. *Ann Intern Med* 1982; 96:133.
326. Goldberg M, Antin J, Guinan E, et al. Cyclophosphamide cardiotoxicity: An analysis of dosing as a risk factor. *Chem Toxins* 1986; 68:1114.
327. Gottdiener J, Applebaum F, Ferrans V, et al. Cardiotoxicity associated with high dose cyclophosphamide therapy. *Arch Intern Med* 1981; 141:758.
328. Deyton L, Walker R, Kovacs J, et al. Reversible cardiac dysfunction associated with interferon alpha therapy in AIDS patients with Kaposi's Sarcoma. *N Engl J Med* 1989; 321:1246.
329. Schuchter L, Hendricks C, Holland K, et al. Eosinophilic myocarditis associated with high-dose interleukin-2 therapy. *Am J Med* 1990; 88:439.
330. Horowitz J. Drugs that induce heart problems: Which agents? What effects? *J Cardiovasc Med* 1983; 8:308.
331. Khan M, Haider B, Thind L. Emetine-induced cardiomyopathy in rabbits. *J Submicrosc Cytol* 1983; 15:495.
332. Harbin A, Gerson M, O'Connell J. Stimulation of acute myopericarditis by constrictive pericardial disease with endomyocardial fibrosis due to methylsergide therapy. *J Am Coll Cardiol* 1984; 4:196.
333. Ratliff N, Estes M, Myles J, et al. Diagnosis of chloroquine cardiomyopathy by endomyocardial biopsy. *N Engl J Med* 1987; 316:191.
334. Brafy H, Horgan J. Lithium and the heart: Unanswered questions. *Chest* 1988; 93:166.
335. Cunningham S, Dalzell G, McGirr P, et al. Myocardial infarction and primary ventricular fibrillation after glue sniffing. *BMJ* 1987; 294:739.
336. Kopp S, Barron J, Tow J. Cardiovascular actions of lead and relationship to hypertension: A review. *Environ Health Perspect* 1988; 78:91.
337. McMeekin J, Finegan B. Reversible myocardial dysfunction following carbon monoxide poisoning. *Can J Cardiol* 1987; 3:118.
338. Watson R. *Nutrition and Heart Disease II*. Boca Raton; FL: CRC Press; 1987.
339. Kudoh C, Tanaka S, Marusaki S, et al. Hypocalcemic cardiomyopathy in a patient with idiopathic hypoparathyroidism. *Intern Med* 1992; 31:561.
340. Mustafa A, Birgas J-L, McCrindle B. Dilated cardiomyopathy as a first sign of nutritional vitamin D deficiency rickets in infancy. *Can J Cardiol* 1999; 15:699.
341. Burk R. Selenium in nutrition. *World Rev Nutr Diet* 1978; 30:88.
342. Yang G. Keshan disease: An endemic selenium-related deficiency disease. In: Chandara R, ed. *Trace Elements in Nutrition of Children*. New York: Raven Press; 1985.
343. Beck M, Kolbeck P, Shi Q, et al. Increased virulence of a human enterovirus (Coxsackievirus B3) in selenium deficient mice. *J Infect Dis* 1994; 170:351.
344. Beck M, Shi Q, Morris V, et al. Rapid genomic evolution of a non-virulent Coxsackievirus B3 in selenium-deficient mice results in selection of identical virulent isolates. *Nature Med* 1995; 1:433.
345. Huttunen J. Selenium and cardiovascular disease—an update. *Biomed Environ Sci* 1997; 10:220.
346. Oster O, Prellwitz W. Selenium and cardiovascular disease. *Biol Trace Elem Res* 1990; 24:91.
347. Neely J, Morgan H. Relationship between carbohydrate metabolism and energy balance of heart muscle. *Annu Rev Physiol* 1974; 36:413.
348. Tripp M, Katcher M, Peters H, et al. Systemic carnitine deficiency presenting as familial endocardial fibroelastosis. *N Engl J Med* 1981; 305:385.
349. Waber L, Valle D, Neill C, et al. Carnitine deficiency presenting as familial cardiomyopathy: A treatable defect in carnitine transport. *J Pediatr* 1982; 101:700.
350. Christensen E, Virke-Jorgensen J. Six years experience with carnitine supplementation in a patient with an inherited defective carnitine transport system. *J Inherit Metab Dis* 1995; 18:233.
351. Rebouche C, Paulson D. Carnitine metabolism and functions in humans. *Ann Rev Nutr* 1986; 6:41.
352. Paulson D. Carnitine deficiency-induced cardiomyopathy. *Mol Cell Biochem* 1998; 180:33.
353. Famularo G, De Simone C. A new era for carnitine. *Immunol Today* 1995; 16:211.
354. Christensen E. Cardiomyopathy and abnormal carnitine metabolism. *J Pediatr* 1989; 114:903.

355. Scholte H, Rodriguez Pereira R, de Jonge P, et al. Primary carnitine deficiency. *J Clin Chem Clin Biochem* 1990; 28:351.
356. Stanley C. Carnitine disorders. *Adv Pediatr* 1993; 42:209.
357. Bennett M, Hale D, Pollitt R, et al. Endocardial fibroelastosis and primary carnitine deficiency due to a defect in the plasma membrane carnitine transport (clinical conference). *Clin Cardiol* 1996; 19:243.
358. Duran M, Loof N, Ketting D, et al. Secondary carnitine deficiencies. *J Clin Chem Clin Biochem* 1990; 28:359.
359. Gahl W, Bernardini I, Dalakas M, et al. Muscle carnitine repletion by long-term carnitine supplementation in nephrotic cystinosis. *Pediatr Res* 1993; 34:115.
360. Ahmad S, Robertson H, Golper T, et al. Multicenter trial of L-carnitine in maintenance hemodialysis patients: II. Clinical and biochemical effects. *Kidney Int* 1990; 38:912.
361. Heinonen O, Takala J. Carnitine status during prolonged total parenteral nutrition. *J Pediatr* 1993; 122:503.
362. Regitz V, Bossaller C, Strasser R, et al. Metabolic alterations in end-stage and less severe heart failure—Myocardial carnitine decrease. *J Clin Chem Clin Biochem* 1990; 28:611.
363. Paulson D, Sanjak M, Shug A. *Carnitine Deficiency and the Diabetic Heart.* Boca Raton; FL: CRC Press; 1992.
364. Crane F. Physiological coenzyme Q function and pharmacological reactions. In: Folkers K, Yamamura Y, eds. *Biomedical and Clinical Aspects of Coenzyme Q*. Amsterdam: Elsevier; 1986.
365. Kitamura N, Yamaguchi A, Otaki M, et al. Myocardial tissue level of coenzyme Q_{10} in patients with cardiac failure. In: Folkers K, Yamamura Y, eds. *Biomedical and Physical Aspects of Coenzyme Q*. Amsterdam, Elsevier; 1984.
366. Folkers K, Vadhanavikit S, Mortensen S. Biochemical rationale and myocardial tissue data on the effective therapy of cardiomyopathy with coenzyme Q_{10}. *Proc Natl Acad Sci USA* 1985; 82:901.
367. Langsjoen P, Langsjoen P, Folkers K. Long-term efficacy and safety of coenzyme Q_{10} therapy for idiopathic dilated cardiomyopathy. *Am J Cardiol* 1990; 65:521.
368. Morisco C, Trimarco B, Condorelli M. Effect of coenzyme Q_{10} therapy in patients with congestive cardiac failure: A long-term muticenter randomized study. *Clin Invest* 1993; 71:S134.
369. Lampertico M, Comis S. Italian muticenter study on the efficacy and safety of coenzyme Q_{10} as adjuvant therapy in heart failure. *Clin Invest* 1993; 71:S129.
370. Waton P, Scalia G, Galbraith A, et al. Lack of effect of coenzyme Q on left ventricular function in patients with congestive heart failure. *J Am Coll Cardiol* 1999; 33:1549.
371. Danpure C. Recent advances in the understanding, diagnosis, and treatment of primary hyperoxaluria type 1. *J Inherit Metab Dis* 1989; 12:210.
372. Rodby R, Tyszka T, Williams J. Reversal of cardiac dysfunction secondary to type 1 primary hyperoxaluria after combined liver-kidney transplantation. *Am J Med* 1991; 90:498.
373. Fyfe B, Israel D, Quish A, et al. Reversal of primary hyperoxaluria cardiomyopathy after combined liver and renal transplantation. *Am J Cardiol* 1995; 75:210.
374. Rosenberg A, Bergstrom L, Troost B, et al. Hyperuricemia and neurologic deficits: A family study. *N Engl J Med* 1970; 282:992.
375. Torp A. Incidence of congestive cardiomyopathy. *Postgrad Med J* 1978; 54:435.
376. Codd M, Sugrue D, Gersh B, et al. Epidemiology of idiopathic dilated and hypertrophic cardiomyopathy: A population based study in Olmstead County, MN 1975–1984. *Circulation* 1989; 80:564.
377. Kawai C, Takatsu T. Clinical and experimental studies on cardiomyopathy. *N Engl J Med* 1975; 293:592.
378. Anderson J, Carliquist J, Hammond E. Deficient natural killer cell activity in patients with idiopoathic dilated cardiomyopathy. *Lancet* 1982; 2:1124.
379. Fuster V, Gersh B, Giuliani E, et al. The natural history of idiopathic dilated cardiomyopathy. *Am J Cardiol* 1981; 47:525.
380. Woodley S, Gilbert E, Anderson J, et al. β-blockade with bucindilol in heart failure due to ischemic vs idiopathic dilated cardiomyopathy. *Circulation* 1991; 84:2426.
381. Waagstein F, Bristow M, Swedberg K, et al. Beneficial effects of metoprolol in idiopathic dilated cardiomyopathy. *Lancet* 1993; 342:1441.

C H A P T E R 70

AIDS AND THE CARDIOVASCULAR SYSTEM

Melvin D. Cheitlin

INTRODUCTION

The pandemic of acquired immunodeficiency syndrome (AIDS), after nearly 2 decades, has taken a tragic toll in lives in the United States and threatens a catastrophe in Africa and Southeast Asia. An estimated 10 million people worldwide are infected with the human immunodeficiency virus (HIV), and at least another 12 million have full-blown AIDS.[1] In the United States, over a million people are HIV positive, and about 2 million have been diagnosed with AIDS.[2,3]

In New York City, AIDS has become the most important cause of premature death among patients under age 65. In terms of years of potential life lost, AIDS advanced in rank order from the 8th leading cause of death in 1983 to the leading cause in 1994.[4]

AIDS is caused by infection with a virus of the family Retroviridae. This group of retroviruses comprises enveloped ribonucleic acid (RNA) viruses possessing an RNA-dependent deoxyribonucleic acid (DNA) polymerase (reverse transcriptase). There are two classes of AIDS viruses: HIV-1 and HIV-2.

The most specific definition of infection by HIV is by identification of the HIV organism in the host's tissues. Since isolation of the virus is not easily done and therefore lacks sensitivity, a patient with repeated positive screening test results for antibodies to HIV, as with an enzyme-linked immunosorbent assay (ELISA), confirmed by a supplemental test such as the Western blot immunofluorescence assay, should be considered to be infected by HIV.

The following classification system for the different stages of HIV infection as proposed by the United States Centers for Disease Control (CDC) is helpful[5]:

Group I: Acute infection
Group II: Asymptomatic infection
Group III: Persistent generalized lymphadenopathy (PGL)
Group IV: Chronic disease—AIDS with constitutional disease (such as unexplained diarrhea, weight loss, or fever over 1 month), neurologic disease, secondary infectious diseases, secondary cancers (Kaposi's sarcoma, non-Hodgkin's lymphoma, and primary lymphoma of the brain)

In January 1993, the CDC, together with other state and territorial health departments, broadened the surveillance definition for AIDS in adolescents and adults to add a measure of immunosuppression (a CD4+ T-lymphocyte count $<200/\mu L$ or a CD4+ percentage <14), as well as three additional clinical conditions: pulmonary tuberculosis, recurrent pneumonia (two or more episodes within a year), or invasive cervical cancer.[6]

Patients with HIV infection have also been divided into three clinical categories. Category A includes asymptomatic patients, those with acute HIV infection or progressive lymphadenopathy. Category B includes symptomatic patients without AIDS-defining conditions. Category C includes patients with 25 AIDS-defining conditions, including opportunistic infections, tumors, central nervous system abnormalities, wasting syndrome, pulmonary tuberculosis, invasive cervical carcinoma, and recurrent pneumonia.[6]

The recognition of human infection by HIV in 1981 represented the startling development of a modern epidemic with many of the aspects of epidemics of the past, such as those of poliomyelitis and the black plague. This infection is due to a retrovirus that invades the nucleus of certain cells containing a specific receptor on their cell membranes and incorporates the DNA copy of HIV in the host's genetic material or genome. After an asymptomatic latent period from infection of 2 to 6 weeks, most patients experience a primary HIV-1 infection that is a self-limited viral syndrome not unlike infectious mononucleosis, characterized by fever, fatigue, pharangitis, lymphadenopathy, and maculopapular rash.[7] Over 95 percent of the patients seroconvert to a positive HIV serology within 6 months, most within 6 to 12 weeks.[8] After an apparent incubation (dormant) period of a mean of 8 to 10 years, the virus can eventually express itself by releasing into the cytoplasm double-stranded DNA copies of the virus, thus killing the cell and invading other immune cells, usually T-helper lymphocytes, to the point that the host's immune defense mechanisms are compromised.[9]

Studies have demonstrated a high rate of viral replication in the lymph nodes during this quiescent period, indicating active progression of the disease, despite the low levels of infectious HIV in the plasma of some patients.[10]

A long-term prospective study showed the actuarial rate of progression from the time of infection to the appearance of AIDS to be 53 percent at 10 years and 68 percent at 14 years after infection, with an increasing progression after 5 years of infection.[11] About 30 percent of patients with PGL will progress to AIDS in 5 years.[12] A minority of patients have an accelerated course and develop full-blown AIDS in 1 or 2 years.[13] Small groups of patients have also been described who have had HIV infection for over 10 years without any symptoms.[14] At some point, there is a breakdown of the body's defense against certain neoplastic changes, resulting in the development of non-Hodgkin's lymphoma and Kaposi's sarcoma. These complications lead inevitably, at least in a very high percentage of cases, to death.

The average length of life after infection in the absence of treatment is approximately 10 years.[11] With the introduction of highly active antiviral therapy (HAART) including nucleocide reverse-transcriptase inhibitors and especially the protease-inhibitor drugs, elimination of the virus from the peripheral blood and prolongation of life have been demonstrated.[15] The impact of the new treatment with multiple drugs is seen in a fall in the rate of AIDS deaths by 12 percent in the United States in 1996 and by 47 percent in 1997.[16]

At the beginning of the epidemic in the United States, the HIV organism struck mainly at the male homosexual population. Later it was found to be transmitted not only through sexual intercourse but also through bloodborne contamination, soon affecting the population using intravenous drugs and other populations receiving blood products and blood transfusions, such as hemophiliacs. The disease is also transmitted perinatally, so that an increasing number of pediatric patients with AIDS are being seen. Although in the U.S. male-to-male sexual activity and intravenous drug users account for 75 percent of cases, in the developing world heterosexual transmission accounts for the majority of cases.[17]

From work with HIV-1, it has been found that the usual way in which the virus attacks cells is through interaction with a receptor on the surface membrane of the cell, the so-called CD4 receptor. This is present in T-helper lymphocytes. Macrophages, microglia, and Langerhans' cells may have specific receptors for HIV other than CD4. Other cells seem to lack an HIV receptor and therefore are much less often found to be sites of infection; the myocardial cell is one such cell.

From the beginning of the epidemic, it was recognized that the heart could be involved but that significant clinical involvement of the heart was unusual. Originally it was believed, through autopsy studies, that the heart was involved mainly because of pericarditis or metastatic Kaposi's sarcoma.[18,19] A few patients with nonbacterial thrombotic endocarditis (NBTE) were reported, but this could be nonspecific, since many of these patients have a wasting disease in which NBTE is not unusual.[20] On further review of autopsy series and clinical series and especially with the study of patients with AIDS who had echocardiography, it was apparent that abnormalities of the heart were seen frequently, even though clinical manifestations of heart disease still remained unusual.

AUTOPSY FINDINGS

The incidence of cardiac involvement at autopsy varies, depending on the definition of cardiac disease. In 15 autopsy series, the incidence of cardiac involvement varies from none to 70 percent of the hearts, depending on whether lymphocytic infiltration with or without myocardial necrosis is included.[18–26] The presence of autopsy-proven cardiac involvement in patients who, during life, had clinically significant cardiac involvement is less impressive, especially if one includes the patients with localized, isolated collections of myocardial lymphocytes.

In evaluating autopsy reports, it is often difficult to discern how many patients had clinically significant abnormalities during life. In the large series of consecutive autopsies of AIDS patients, between 5 and 20 percent appear to have had cardiac lesions of potential clinical importance. These include patients with myocarditis with clinical manifestations, mainly with known pathogens—such as toxoplasmosis, clinically evident pericarditis, or nonbacterial endocarditis—which can cause systemic emboli.[27]

The largest recent autopsy series is by Barbero et al., where 440 AIDS patients had an autopsy. Cardiac involvement was documented in 18.6 percent and dilated cardiomyopathy in 2.7 percent.[28]

More important are the relatively few patients in whom cardiac abnormality was listed as the cause of death. The most common cause of death is respiratory failure and infection.[24,26,29,30] Neoplasm, lymphoma, and encephalopathy are also frequent causes of death.[31] Of 858 autopsied patients with AIDS from 15 series in the literature, only 9 (1 percent) had the cause of death listed as cardiac. If the cases with a recognized etiology for heart disease are removed, only 0.5 percent of deaths were possibly due to HIV "myocarditis."

Right ventricular hypertrophy and/or dilatation was reported in 12 of 71 patients (16.9 percent)[25] and in 18 of 115 patients (15.7 percent).[24] Pericarditis varied in frequency from 3 of 41 (7.3 percent)[20] to 3 of 101 (3 percent).[22]

ECHOCARDIOGRAPHIC FINDINGS

Echocardiography in patients with either AIDS or PGL has been reported in a number of studies.[32–39] The prevalence of echocardiographic abnormalities varies from 15 to 60 percent and would be higher if the finding of mitral valve prolapse, an echocardiographic abnormality that may be related to cachexia, is included. The prevalence of left ventricular hypokinesis also varies from 12.5 to 41 percent in three large series.[33,34,36] In one series,[33] four of the eight patients had congestive heart failure; one died and at autopsy had a dilated cardiomyopathy without evidence of inflammatory myocarditis or cardiac opportunistic infections. Only in this study[33] was clinical congestive heart failure mentioned. Dilated cardiomyopathy was seen only in the hospitalized patients. In a large prospective echocardiographic study in 296 HIV-infected adults that was conducted over 4 years, Currie and colleagues found 13 (4 percent) with dilated cardiomyopathy.[37]

Cecchi and colleagues, from 1398 patients admitted for HIV infection, selected 127 (9 percent) with a clinical suspicion of cardiac disease and did echocardiograms on them: 92 (72 percent) had evidence of cardiac involvement, 6.5 percent of total

HIV patients; 38 (2.7 percent) had pericardial effusion, and 20 (1.4 percent) had dilated cardiomyopathy.[38]

The finding of pericardial effusion was common, varying from 20 to 40 percent.[34,36,38] The incidence of tamponade varies: In one series[34] of 18 patients with pericardial effusion, 5 (28 percent) had tamponade. In this report of 300 patients with AIDS, 16 (5 percent) had clinically apparent heart disease, due in most cases to opportunistic infection or tumor.[34] Over a period of 3 years at the San Francisco General Hospital, Rapaport found that, of 1171 patients hospitalized with AIDS, an echocardiogram was ordered for 88 (7.5 percent) because of suspicion of cardiac disease (personal communication). Of these echocardiograms, 52 (59 percent) showed at least one abnormality. Of the 88 echocardiograms, 16 (18 percent) showed either left ventricular dilatation and/or left ventricular hypokinesis, and 26 (30 percent) showed pericardial effusion. There were no control subjects.

Steffen and colleagues[39] reported the prospectively collected results of echocardiography in 151 HIV-seropositive patients, 92 percent of whom were men with a median age of 37 years, and 73 percent were homosexual men. Of these, 13 percent were intravenous drug users, of whom 74 percent were in Walter Reed stages IV to VI, a classification using counts of T4 helper cells and clinical data.[40] A total of 107 patients (71 percent) had normal echocardiograms. Echocardiographic abnormalities attributed to HIV infection were present in 31 patients (20 percent). There was an association of abnormal echocardiographic findings with advanced clinical stages of the disease. The mortality during follow-up was the same for those with normal echocardiograms (35 of 102) as for those with abnormal echocardiograms (12 of 29) ($p = .48$). Even in those with the most advanced clinical disease, there was no independent prognostic significance of the echocardiographic cardiac involvement, with 44 percent of both echo-normal and echo-abnormal patients dying. This study shows a remarkably low incidence of HIV-associated echocardiographic abnormalities, most often asymptomatic pericardial effusion.

These studies suggest that the prevalence of echocardiographic abnormalities in HIV-positive patients depends on the stage of their clinical illness, with the sickest patients having the most abnormalities.

PERICARDIAL INVOLVEMENT

In general, pericardial effusion and pericarditis constitute the most commonly recognized cardiac involvement in AIDS. At autopsy, Kaposi's sarcoma involvement and lymphoma may be clinically silent, accompanied by asymptomatic pericardial effusion, or they may be clinically important because of pericardial tamponade.[41] Pericarditis due to specific organisms has frequently been reported. These organisms are most commonly *Mycobacterium tuberculosis*[34,42,43] or *Mycobacterium avium–intracellulare*.[35,42,44] One study[34] reported pericardial tamponade in five patients and large pericardial effusions in six. Of the patients with clinical heart disease in this study, 22 percent had echocardiographic evidence of tamponade, and another 33 percent had large pericardial effusions.

In a review of 15 autopsy and echocardiographic studies involving 1139 patients with HIV disease, the incidence of pericardial disease was 21 percent. Most cases were asymptomatic without an identifiable etiology. In those that were symptomatic, about two-thirds were caused by infection or neoplasm and one-third were of undetermined etiology. In the 66 published cases of pericardial tamponade, 26 percent were caused by *M. tuberculosis*.[42]

At San Francisco General Hospital, experience has been similar. In a consecutive series of 88 in-hospital AIDS patients who had echocardiograms, 36 (41 percent) had normal echocardiograms, whereas the most common abnormality, seen in 26 (30 percent), was pericardial effusion. We have recognized a total of 25 patients with AIDS or PGL who have pericardial disease. Ten of these patients had pericardiocentesis, of whom eight (32 percent) presented with tamponade, two had pericardial windows, and one died and was autopsied. Another two patients, who had neither pericardiocentesis nor pericardial windows, died and were autopsied. No etiology was found on examination of either fluid or tissue in any of the 12 patients.

In a prospective echocardiographic study among 231 patients recruited over a 5-year period, the prevalence of pericardial effusion for AIDS patients entering into the study was 5 percent. Over the follow-up time, the incidence of pericardial effusion increased as the stage of the HIV progressed from 0 percent per year in asymptomatic HIV-infected patients to 11 percent per year in patients with AIDS; 80 percent of these effusions were small and asymptomatic.[45] The survival of the AIDS patients who developed pericardial effusion was significantly shorter than the survival of those who did not, 36 percent versus 93 percent at 6 months. This shortened survival period remained significant even after adjustment for lead-time bias and was independent of CD4+ T-cell count.[45] Since death was not due directly to the pericardial effusion, the development of pericardial effusion in the setting of HIV infection probably suggests end-stage HIV disease.

Flum and colleagues also reported that AIDS-associated pericardial effusion was a grave prognostic sign. They reported 29 patients who had surgical windows for large effusions; only in 2 patients did this result in a change in clinical management. The mortality was 69 percent at 8 weeks after pericardial window.[46] They concluded that pericardial biopsy for diagnosis provided little practical therapeutic information and that surgical windows were justified only to relieve tamponade.

The etiology of pericardial effusion or pericarditis is not obvious; it may be HIV infection or other opportunistic viral infections with Coxsackie virus, cytomegalovirus, or neoplastic.[45] Occasionally, pericarditis has been reported to be caused by common organisms such as *Staphylococcus*,[46] *Cryptococcus neoformans*,[47] or herpes simplex virus.[48]

MYOCARDIAL INVOLVEMENT

For a number of years, involvement of the pericardium and myocardium with both common and unusual opportunistic infections and neoplasms, such as Kaposi's sarcoma and lymphoma, has been recognized. At times, this involvement appears to be incidental and associated with the presence of organisms in many tissues, including the heart. Often, this involvement is not accompanied by signs of cell necrosis or even inflammation. At other times, the infection is accompanied by an intense myocarditis. Opportunistic infection has included viruses (herpes simplex, cytomegalovirus, and Coxsackie virus), bacteria, protozoa (*Toxoplasma gondii*), and fungi (*Candida albicans, C. neoformans,* and *Aspergillus fumigatus*).[49–51] These specific infections have been diagnosed at autopsy but also during life with myocardial biopsy. The importance of identifying a specific organism as the cause of the myocarditis rests in the potential for treatment[42,52]; for instance, amphotericin B and flucytosine may be used to treat cryptococcosis. Grange and colleagues[53] reported a case of *T. gondii* myocarditis in a 58-year-old man with AIDS who was treated successfully with pyrimethamine and clindamycin. A similar case was reported by Albrecht and colleagues.[54]

The most common neoplasms are Kaposi's sarcoma and lymphoma of the non-Hodgkin's type.[18,19,24] With Kaposi's sarcoma, the tumor involvement of the myocardium or pericardium is most frequently an incidental finding. On occasion, myocardial involvement by lymphoma is diagnosed by needle biopsy of the myocardium.

One study reported a collection of 21 cases of lymphoma in AIDS patients—3 Hodgkin's and 18 non-Hodgkin's lymphoma of various histologic types—almost all of which were in the high-grade categories.[55] Unfortunately, these tend to be histologically aggressive tumors involving many organs, and they respond poorly to treatment. At times, the patient presents with pericardial tamponade or even superior vena cava syndrome.[56–58] Echocardiography revealing infiltration into the myocardium and/or myocardial or pericardial masses is most helpful in establishing a diagnosis.

CARDIOMYOPATHY

In 1986, Cohen and colleagues reported three patients with AIDS who had clinical, echocardiographic, and morphologic findings of dilated cardiomyopathy.[59] All had a decreased ejection fraction, and two had congestive heart failure. All three died, and two had findings at autopsy compatible with myocarditis resulting in cardiomyopathy. Microscopic examination in both showed focal collections of inflammatory cells together with myofibrillar atrophy and myocardial necrosis. A subsequent report described 58 consecutively autopsied patients.[60] Seven (12 percent) had major clinical cardiovascular abnormalities, including four with congestive heart failure and others with ventricular tachycardia. All were late in the course of their disease. All patients with these major clinical cardiac abnormalities had focal myocarditis at autopsy. The etiology in these cases was not obvious but was believed to be viral myocarditis.

In another study of 71 patients with AIDS, 8 had left ventricular dilatation and decreased contractility and 4 had congestive heart failure.[33] In a similar echocardiographic study, none of 102 AIDS patients had congestive heart failure, although 41 percent had left ventricular hypokinesia.[36]

In autopsy studies reported in the literature, cardiac causes of death have been rare; clinically, the incidence of congestive heart failure has been extremely small, although microscopic focal myocarditis is frequently described. In 14 studies in the literature, 1009 patients with AIDS were reported. A total of eight died of cardiac involvement. One had cryptococcal myocarditis and one had toxoplasmic myocarditis; five came from one institution.[25]

Symptomatic cardiomyopathy in association with HIV-1 infection is uncommon; however, echocardiographic evidence of left ventricular dysfunction is more common, especially in patients who are the furthest along in the course of HIV disease. Individual reports of one to five cases of patients with either dilated left ventricle, hypokinetic left ventricle, or both have been frequent enough to require explanation.[59,61] Furthermore, the occurrence of cardiomyopathy in children, in whom a disease unrelated to HIV infection would be rare, further suggests a relationship between HIV disease and cardiomyopathy.[62]

Lipshultz and colleagues did a prospective study on 196 HIV-infected children, median age 2.1 years. Only two had congestive heart failure at enrollment. An echocardiogram done every 4 months revealed a 2-year accumulative incidence of cardiomyopathy of 4.7 percent (95 percent confidence interval, 1.5–7.9 percent).[63]

Prospective echocardiographic studies have been reported that show a high prevalence of myocardial dysfunction. DeCastro and colleagues did serial echocardiograms prospectively on 136 HIV-positive patients over a mean follow-up time of 415 ± 220 days. Seven AIDS patients developed clinical and echocardiographic findings of global left ventricular dysfunction. Of the six who died, five were autopsied: three had acute lymphocytic myocarditis, one had cryptococcal myocarditis, and one had myocardial fibrosis.[64]

Blanchard and colleagues did serial echocardiograms on 70 HIV-positive outpatients. Of the 50 patients with AIDS, 7 (14 percent) had echocardiographic evidence of left ventricular dysfunction. On repeat echocardiogram, three of the seven had improved left ventricular function, implying a transient problem that caused a transient decrease in left ventricular function.[65]

At San Francisco General Hospital, the cases of 74 AIDS outpatients were prospectively followed using serial quantitative Doppler echocardiography every 4 months. Control populations included HIV-positive patients without disease, HIV-positive patients with AIDS-related complex, and HIV-negative gay men. Over the follow-up period of 16.5 ± 12 months, no differences in left ventricular systolic or diastolic function were detected between the groups and no differences in mean values from the first to the last echocardiogram.[66]

The prospective study by Barbaro and colleagues reported 952 asymptomatic HIV-positive patients whose cases were followed clinically and by echocardiography for 60 ± 5.3 months.[67] By echocardiogram, dilated cardiomyopathy was diagnosed in 76 (8 percent) of patients—an incidence of 1.6 cases per 100 patients per year. A myocardial biopsy was done on all patients with cardiomyopathy, and a histologic diagnosis of myocarditis made in 83 percent. By in situ hybridization HIV nucleic acid sequences were found in 58 patients but only 36 (63 percent) had active myocarditis. Of these 36 patients, 25 percent had other cardiotropic virus infections with Coxsackie B virus in 6 (17 percent), cytomegalovirus in 2 (6 percent), and Epstein-Barr virus in 1 (3 percent). The authors concluded that dilated cardiomyopathy may be related either to direct HIV infection or to an autoimmune process induced by HIV, possibly in association with other cardiotropic viruses.

Possible Reasons for Cardiomyopathy

There are many theories on the etiology of congestive heart failure with a dilated, poorly contracting left ventricle found in the occasional patient. These explanations may well be related also to the more frequently observed echocardiographic reduction in left ventricular function with or without left ventricular dilatation. The most frequently mentioned etiology is that of myocarditis or postmyocarditis cardiomyopathy. There are occasional reports of virus being grown from cardiac muscle. In 1987, Calabrese and colleagues[68] were the first to report the culturing of HIV from a right ventricular myocardial biopsy from a patient with a hypokinetic right ventricle and a normal left ventricle.

There is some evidence that HIV itself invades the myocardial cell. The myocyte has no CD4+ receptors, which are the major way by which the virus enters the cell. Although there are other ways and possibly other receptors by which the virus could invade the cell, no one has convincingly shown the virus or a portion of the viral DNA or RNA within the genome of the myocardial cell.[69] One study reported detecting HIV nucleic acid sequences by in situ hybridization in cardiac tissue sections from 6 of 22 patients examined who had died of AIDS.[61] The hybridization target was thought to be myocytes, but this could not be proved by this technique. Furthermore, the myocardial cells showing the positive hybridization signal were sparse, comprising only one or a few cells per section; the myocardium was normal by light microscopy; and none of the patients had clinical evidence of cardiac disease. Still, the most compelling evidence for the ability of HIV virus to enter the myocardial cell comes from the previously mentioned study by Barbaro and colleagues.[67]

Other Theories for the Development of Cardiomyopathy

OPPORTUNISTIC INFECTIONS

Patients with AIDS are exposed to and susceptible to multiple bacterial, viral, mycotic, and protozoal infections. Epstein-Barr virus and cytomegalovirus are both known to cause myocarditis in AIDS patients.[67,70] *Cryptococcus neoformans* and *T. Gondii* myocarditis have been well described.[29,52,53,71] Myocarditis due to *M. avium–intracellulare* has been reported.[20] *Aspergillus* endocarditis and myocarditis have been reported.[72]

DILATED CARDIOMYOPATHY AS A POSTVIRAL DISORDER

The study of patients with myocarditis without AIDS has shown that the myocarditis can be precipitated by viral infection and that the inflammatory reaction can progress when the virus is no longer recoverable from either the heart or even the patient. The viral infection precipitates an immune reaction either to viral antigen that cross-reacts with a myocardial protein or to altered myocardial protein, which acts as a foreign antigen, thus precipitating the immune reactions that continue the myocardial necrosis and inflammatory cell infiltration[73] (see also Chap. 69).

The evidence that congestive cardiomyopathy is precipitated by a previous viral myocarditis includes the biopsy finding of inflammatory infiltrate in some patients with dilated cardiomyopathy[74,75] and detection of increased elevated viral antibody titers and viral-specific RNA sequences in myocardial biopsies.[76] Thus, the cardiomyopathy can result from a previous infection with a number of organisms that are no longer recoverable from the myocardium.

Herskowitz and colleagues[77] reported the histologic and immunopathologic results of 37 endomyocardial biopsy samples from patients infected with HIV-1 who developed unexplained global left ventricular dysfunction. Twenty-eight patients had New York Heart Association (NYHA) class III and IV congestive heart failure. Four patients had myocarditis secondary to known etiologies. Of the remaining 33 patients, 17 (51 percent) had histologic evidence of idiopathic active or borderline myocarditis. Specific hybridization within myocytes was abnormal in five patients with HIV-1 antisense riboprobe and in 16 of the 33 with cytomegalovirus immediate early (IE-2) antisense riboprobe. This study is compatible with the possibility that cardiotropic virus infection and myocarditis may be important in the pathogenesis of HIV-associated cardiomyopathy.[77]

IMPAIRMENT OF THE IMMUNE MECHANISM LEADING TO CARDIOMYOPATHY

Humorally mediated autoimmune reactions involving antimyosin antibodies may also be implicated in the development of cardiomyopathy.[78] Circulating cardiac autoantibodies have been identified in four of six AIDS patients with cardiomyopathy and in none of the HIV-positive patients without cardiomyopathy. In situ hybridization with genomic probes failed to show evidence of HIV or any other viruses within the heart muscle. Results of ELISA showed a high titer of immunoglobulin G antibody to myosin and to cardiac mitochondrial adenine nucleotide transporter. In this study, it was concluded that the cardiomyopathy may be related not to HIV infection of the heart but rather to autoimmunity. Apparent improvement of left ventricular function in children with AIDS by using intravenously administered immunoglobulin is also suggestive of an immunologic etiology for the left ventricular dysfunction.[79]

ROLE OF CYTOKINES IN MYOCARDITIS

Ho and colleagues[80] proposed a primary role for neuroglial cell damage from the cytolytic effect of release of substances termed *cytokines* from HIV-infected monocytes, the "innocent bystander" destruction mechanism. Cytokines are biologically active mediators and are soluble proteins released by immune cells. Reversible myocardial depression is well documented in human and canine septic shock.[81,82] This was subsequently demonstrated to be due to a "myocardial depressant factor."[83] The exact nature of this myocardial depressant factor is not agreed upon, but it could be related to a variety of mediators of sepsis such as endotoxin and the cytokine tumor necrosis factor (TNF) and interleukin 2.[84]

Other studies showed that the administration of endotoxin-released TNF caused depression of left ventricular function independent of left ventricular volume or loading conditions,[85] and elevated circulating levels of TNF have been noted in patients with severe chronic heart failure.[86] Increased circulating levels of TNF have been noted in patients with advanced HIV-1 infection.[87] This finding is consistent with a finding of increased production of the cytokine TNF by peripheral monocytes of patients with AIDS.[88]

Barbaro and colleagues[89] investigated the myocardial expression of TNF-α and inducible nitric oxide synthase (INOS) in endomyocardial biopsies in patients with HIV dilated cardiomyopathy and compared them with myocardium from patients with idiopathic dilated cardiomyopathy. The mean intensity of both TNF-α and INOS immunostaining was greater in the HIV patients compared with the idiopathic cardiomyopathy patients.

The staining intensity of both TNF-α and INOS was inversely correlated with the CD4 count.

The increased levels of cytokines—including TNF, interleukins 1 and 2, and α-interferon—may lead to myocardial dysfunction either acting locally in a paracrine fashion on adjacent myocardium or systemically causing a decrease in myocardial function.[90,91]

CACHEXIA

Many patients with AIDS have marked weight loss and cachexia. In patients with anorexia nervosa, wall motion as assessed by two-dimensional echo Doppler was found to be abnormal in 8 of 14 patients but not in control subjects; also, lower stroke volume was found in patients compared with controls, possibly because of decreased heart size.[92] Starvation and refeeding studies in animals have demonstrated myofibrillar atrophy and cardiac interstitial edema that are accompanied by a decrease in left ventricular compliance and decreased peak systolic force.[93] These changes are thought to be due to protein-calorie malnutrition. Congestive heart failure may occur, especially during refeeding and recovery.[94]

VITAMIN- AND SELENIUM-DEFICIENCY STATES

Cachectic people can have vitamin-deficiency states; it is doubtful that many patients with cardiomyopathy have this as a prime etiology. Selenium deficiency has been described, together with reduced cardiac selenium levels in AIDS, similar to the Keshan's disease seen in Chinese with selenium deficiency. In one study, 10 patients with AIDS who had decreased left ventricular fractional shortening on echocardiography received sodium selenite for 23 days.[95] Six of eight showed a return toward normal of left ventricular fractional shortening within 21 days. Selenium deficiency has been reported to be common in malnourished pediatric patients with AIDS.[96]

DRUG-INDUCED CARDIOMYOPATHY

The effect of drugs, both recreational and therapeutic, on myocardial function is not well delineated in patients with AIDS. In most patients with AIDS and cardiomyopathy, however, drugs do not seem to be the cause[61,97]; nevertheless, in patients with AIDS, drugs such as doxorubicin, α_2-interferon, and interleukin 2 have been shown to produce cardiomyopathy that is sometimes reversible. Recombinant α_2-interferon-related cardiomyopathy in patients treated for primary renal cancer has been reported.[98] One report described three cases of reversible cardiac dysfunction associated with α-interferon therapy in AIDS patients with Kaposi's sarcoma.[99]

Cocaine use has been associated with myocarditis and dilated cardiomyopathy, which occasionally has been reported to be reversible.[100,101] Pentamidine has been reported to cause ventricular tachycardia.[102] The most common currently used drug in AIDS, zidovudine (AZT), a nucleoside analog, is a drug that inhibits replication of HIV in vitro, probably by inhibiting the reverse-transcriptase enzyme, which is essential to the replication of the retrovirus. No adverse cardiac effects have been reported in phase 1 clinical trials, and one study failed to show cardiotoxicity[103]; however, a toxic mitochondrial myopathy caused by long-term AZT after 12.8 months of therapy has been reported.[104] This myopathy is characterized by abnormal mitochondria with paracrystalloid inclusions. AZT-induced cardiomyopathy in rats has been shown to be related to oxidative damage and activated ADP-ribosylation reactions damaging mitochondrial energy production.[105] Whether this can occur in cardiac muscle in some patients is not clear. Foscarnet therapy for the treatment of cytomegalovirus infection has also been reported to produce a reversible cardiomyopathy.[106]

Conclusions

Clinical heart muscle disease and heart failure in AIDS are unusual. When this condition occurs, there may be explanations other than direct infection with HIV. The exact incidence of heart muscle disease in AIDS is as yet unknown but must be small, and the mechanisms that can cause failure are probably multiple.

METABOLIC CARDIOVASCULAR COMPLICATIONS OF ANTIVIRAL DRUGS

With the introduction of protease inhibitors, a class of drugs that suppresses HIV replication, to the treatment of patients with HIV infection, metabolic abnormalities have been seen that have potential for development of cardiovascular disease. New-onset hyperglycemia similar to type II diabetes mellitus has been described, as well as worsening of preexisting diabetes in 1 to 6 percent of patients. This problem has been described with all of the protease inhibitors.[107] The cause of the hyperglycemia is not known, but it does respond to sulfonylureas, suggesting that the drug causes increased resistance to the peripheral effects of insulin although it is not possible to rule out a reduction in insulin secretion.[108] The treatment of hyperglycemia is similar to that of type II diabetes: diet and oral hypoglycemic drugs.

Lipid metabolic abnormalities have also been seen in patients taking protease inhibitors with extremely high triglyceride levels to over 1000 mg/dL,[109] which can occur within 2 weeks of starting therapy. In a study of ritonavir plus saquinavir, 11 percent of patients developed triglycerides above 1500 mg/dL. There were no instances of pancreatitis. There are also elevations in serum cholesterol.[110]

Although the mechanism by which this drug induces hyperlipidemia is unknown, there is a 60 percent homology of the catalytic region of the HIV-1 protease to which the drugs bind to two proteins regulating lipid metabolism: cytoplasmic retinoic acid-binding protein type I (CRABP-I) and low-density lipoprotein-receptor-related protein (LRP). Binding of the protease inhibitors to LRP would impair hepatic chylomicron uptake and triglyceride clearance.[108] The elevated triglycerides respond to gemfibrozil.

In 45 HIV-infected patients taking protease inhibitors who had abnormally elevated lipids, the National Cholesterol Education Program Guidelines were followed without disrupting the HIV therapy. Mean serum cholesterol prior to initiation of the protease inhibitors was 170 mg/dL. On the protease inhibitor, the mean cholesterol rose to 289 mg/dL, and triglycerides were 879 mg/dL. On diet, gemfibrozil alone, or with atorvastatin, the cholesterol fell to 201 mg/dL ($p = .01$) over a 10-month period.[111]

Finally, an abnormal redistribution of fat from the periphery centrally to the abdomen and thorax has been described. There is a loss of subcutaneous fat from the face and limbs (partial lipodystrophy), and the development of fat deposits in the abdomen ("protease pouch") and dorsocervical fat pad ("buffalo hump").[112–114] The abdominal fat may be either in the subcutaneous tissue or in the intraabdominal visceral fat.[112] The abnormal fat distribution appears to be associated with the use of ritonavir-saquinavir combinations rather than with indinavir and does not respond to dietary restriction or exercise. In patients with a buffalo hump, hypercortosolism has been ruled out as a cause, and half the patients with a buffalo hump had never been on protease inhibitors.[113] The relationship of these abnormalities to protease inhibitors is still not clear.

Since the protease inhibitors are such important drugs in the management of patients with HIV infection, every attempt must be made to control their metabolic side effects without stopping the drug. Diet and oral hypoglycemic drugs can control the hyperglycemia. Gemfibrozil and HMG-CoA reductase inhibitors decrease the elevated triglycerides, cholesterol, and low-density lipoproteins, as noted. A potential problem is that protease inhibitors are metabolized by the hepatic cytochrome P450 CYP4-A system, and these drugs can both induce and/or inhibit the system. Therefore, other drugs metabolized by the cytochrome P450 system can have their plasma levels either decreased or increased when used together with the protease inhibitors, resulting in an extensive list of drug interactions and possibly drug toxicity. The importance of treating the metabolic abnormalities, however, is seen in the increasing number of reports of premature, extensive coronary artery disease in patients taking protease inhibitors.[115]

CLINICAL WORKUP AND THERAPY

The workup of patients with AIDS and suspected cardiac involvement begins with the history and physical examination for symptoms and signs of cardiac disease. Since there is no therapeutic advantage to finding subclinical cardiovascular involvement, there is no justification for screening electrocardiograms or echocardiograms. If there are signs or symptoms suggesting cardiovascular disease—such as a friction rub, an S_3 gallop, or other evidence of congestive heart failure—an echocardiogram is useful in identifying pericardial effusion and in evaluating right and left ventricular function. Invasive diagnostic studies are rarely necessary.

If left ventricular dilatation and hypokinesis are found with or without clinical evidence of heart failure, consideration should be given to stopping all drugs that are not absolutely essential.[116] If, in a 2-week follow-up, echocardiography reveals improvement, the suspected drug should be eliminated.

The question of whether a myocardial biopsy is helpful is controversial. The finding of a treatable cause of biopsy-proved myocarditis is rare. Furthermore, there is no evidence that treating biopsy-proved focal myocarditis with steroids or antimetabolites is effective.[117] Therefore, by available evidence, myocardial biopsy is of little value.

The potential cardiotoxic roles of drugs for opportunistic infection as well as other known etiologies—such as hypertension, hypertrophic cardiomyopathy, and coronary artery disease—should be considered. The treatment of congestive heart failure is similar to that of the treatment of heart failure from other etiologies, e.g., diuretics, digoxin, and angiotensin-converting enzyme inhibitors (see Chap. 21).

CARDIOVASCULAR SURGERY IN AIDS PATIENTS

There has been an increased interest in the danger to AIDS health care workers of becoming infected or of infecting patients and in the possibility of accelerating the disease through surgery. The problem is illustrated by the following questions:

1. Are we performing an expensive procedure that will cause prolonged hospitalization and probably not affect the outcome in AIDS patients?
2. What is the risk of accelerating the disease by surgery?
3. What is the risk of HIV infection to health care workers?
4. What is the risk of getting HIV infection during open-heart surgery?

In general, it is not wise to perform expensive procedures with some degree of morbidity and mortality that result in prolonged hospitalization of patients with a limited life span due to their underlying disease. For this reason, patients with AIDS should not be subjected to surgery that will most probably not significantly affect their survival. Before protease inhibitors were available, probably 70 percent of patients found to have AIDS would die within 3 to 4 years of the diagnosis.[118] Now, with newer drugs, life has been markedly prolonged. Therefore, if patients with AIDS have medically uncontrollable symptoms, invasive procedures that can ameliorate these symptoms are indicated.

With infective endocarditis, the vast majority of HIV-infected patients are intravenous drug users, and the most common valve involved is the tricuspid valve, which almost always can be treated medically. The most frequent problem in which the question of cardiovascular surgery arises in a relatively young subgroup involves the intravenous drug user with infective endocarditis on the aortic and/or mitral valve and congestive heart failure. The presence of HIV disease in these patients, who overall have a high mortality and poor results from surgery, would suggest that they be treated medically for as long as possible.[119] If failure persists, valvular replacement should be done.

HIV-positive patients and patients with PGL who have not had an opportunistic infection or cancer can have a prolonged course over many years and, in general, should be treated like patients without HIV disease. In fact, life span might be prolonged after HIV infection by using combinations of drugs, including reverse-transcriptase inhibitors and the new protease inhibitors. In this subgroup, cardiovascular surgery should be considered for the usual indications.

The question of whether progression of the HIV disease is accelerated by the immunologic challenge that occurs from cardiopulmonary bypass is largely unanswered. Instances of HIV-positive patients who developed AIDS shortly after open-heart surgery have been reported. It is known that cardiopulmonary bypass temporaily depresses phagocytic function and immune globulin production.[120] Cardiopulmonary bypass per se in HIV-negative patients causes prolonged abnormalities in the CD4+/CD8+ T-cell ratio up to 6 days postoperatively.[121] There is, therefore, a basis for concern that cardiopulmonary bypass surgery could accelerate the progression of HIV disease, and this must be taken into consideration.

Whether all patients undergoing cardiovascular surgery or other invasive procedures should have HIV testing is a matter of heated debate. Although the risk to health care personnel is small, HIV infection is usually tantamount to fatal infection; fear is great among both health care workers and the public. On the other hand, AIDS is an emotional subject, and patients who are known to be HIV positive may be subjected to prejudice and discrimination. At present, HIV testing of both health care workers and patients is voluntary; however, there are proposed recommendations requiring disclosure to patients that a health care worker is HIV positive and informed consent from patients before any invasive procedure is done. At present, there is only one instance of transmission of disease by a health care worker, that of an HIV-positive dentist who is believed to have infected five patients, probably from reuse of inadequately sterilized instruments. This matter is still under considerable debate.

Because of this risk, some cardiovascular surgeons and cardiologists are refusing to operate on or catheterize an HIV-positive person or a patient who will not allow an HIV test to be done. In 1989, a survey was done of the attitudes of cardiac surgeons in the United States concerning operating on HIV-positive patients.[122] More than half responded, and two-thirds of these were reportedly willing to perform open-heart surgery on HIV-positive patients no matter how the patients had acquired their HIV infection. One-quarter of the surgeons would not operate no matter how the HIV infection was acquired, and the rest were uncertain. Once the patient has gone from the HIV-carrier state to AIDS, two-thirds of the cardiac surgeons would not operate. Of those responding, 90 percent want to be able to test all their patients for HIV status. Whether these attitudes have changed in the last decade is unknown.

A physician's fear of becoming infected with HIV is understandable, but as in the case of other professions that involved personal dangers, the profession of the physician requires performance. Both the American College of Physicians and the American Medical Association currently have standards stating that physicians may not ethically refuse to treat patients solely because the patients are HIV positive.

As of 1995, the literature has reported 49 health care workers in the United States who had no other risk factors and were known to be HIV negative at exposure who have seroconverted after exposure.[123] The danger to health care personnel is greatest when there is exposure to blood and the chance of accidental needle or knife perforation or blood splash into the eyes or mouth. In one prospective study of 1307 consecutive procedures, accumulated exposure, parenteral or cutaneous, occurred in only 84 procedures (6.4 percent).[124] Parenteral exposure occurred in 1.7 percent. Knowledge of the patient's HIV status or awareness of the patient's high-risk status for such infection did not appear to influence the rate of exposure, suggesting that preoperative testing for HIV infection would not decrease the frequency of accidental exposure to blood.

In combined data from 20 prospective studies of the risk of HIV-1 transmission to health care workers, there were 6498 parenteral exposures among 1948 subjects.[125] The chance of seroconversion was 0.32 percent per exposure (95 percent confidence interval, 0.18 to 0.46 percent); in 2885 mucous membrane exposures, there was one seroconversion (0.03 percent per exposure). The risk of a health care worker developing HIV seroconversion from work-related activities was very low: approximately one infection in 300 documented exposures to HIV-positive blood.

References

1. Chu SY, Berkelman RL, Curran JW. Epidemiology of HIV in the United States. In: De Vita VT, Hellman S, Rosenberg SA, eds. *AIDS: Etiology, Diagnosis, Treatment and Prevention*, 3d ed. Philadelphia: Lippincott; 1992:99–100.
2. Centers for Disease Control and Prevention. HIV/AIDS surveillance report. Atlanta: CDC 1994; 6(2):7.
3. Steele FR. A moving target: CDC still trying to evaluate HIV-1 prevalence. *J NIH Res* 1994; 6:25–26.
4. Obiri GU, Fordyce EJ, Singh TP, et al. Effect of HIV/AIDS versus other causes of death on premature mortality in New York City, 1983–1994. *Am J Epidemol* 1998; 147:840–845.
5. Centers for Disease Control. Classification system for human T-lymphotropic virus type III/lymphadenopathy-associated virus infections. *MMWR* 1986; 35:334–339.
6. Centers for Disease Control. 1993 Revised classification system for HIV infection and expanded surveillance case definition for AIDS among adolescents and adults. *MMWR* 1992; 41(RR-17):1–19.
7. Schacker T, Collier AC, Hughes J, et al. Clinical and epidemiologic features of primary HIV infection. *Ann Intern Med* 1996; 125:257–264.
8. Horsburgh CR Jr, Ou CY, Jason J, et al. Duration of human immunodeficiency virus infection before detection of antibody. *Lancet* 1989; 2:637–640.
9. Bacchetti P, Moss AR. Incubation period of AIDS in San Francisco [letter]. *Nature* 1989; 338:251–253.
10. Feinberg MB, Greene WC. Molecular insights into human immunodeficiency virus type 1 pathogenesis. *Curr Opin Immunol* 1992; 4:466–474.
11. Rutherford GW, Lifson AR, Hessol NA, et al. Course of HIV-1 infection in a cohort of homosexual and bisexual men: An 11 year follow-up study. *BMJ* 1990; 301:1183–1188.
12. Osmond D. Progression to AIDS in persons testing seropositive for antibody to HIV. In: Cohen PT, Sande MA, Volberding PA, eds. *The AIDS Knowledge Base.* Waltham, MA: Medical Publishing Group; 1990:1.1.6.
13. Piatak M Jr, Saag MS, Yang LC, et al. High levels of HIV-1 in plasma during all stages of infection determined by competitive PCR. *Science* 1993; 259:1749–1754.
14. Pantaleo G, Menzo S, Vaccarezza M, et al. Studies in subjects with long-term nonprogressive human immunodeficiency virus infection. *N Engl J Med* 1995; 332:209–216.
15. Deeks SG, Smith M, Holodniy M, et al. HIV-1 protease inhibitors: A review for clinicians. *JAMA* 1997; 277:145–153.
16. Palalla FJ, Delaney KM, Moorman AC, et al. The HIV outpatient study investigators. *N Engl J Med* 1998; 338:853–860.
17. Mann J, Ching , Piot P, et al. The international epidemiology of AIDS. *Sci Am* 1988; 259:82–89.
18. Silver MA, Macher AM, Reichert CM, et al. Cardiac involvement by Kaposi's sarcoma in acquired immune deficiency syndrome (AIDS). *Am J Cardiol* 1984; 53:983–985.
19. Welch K, Finkbeiner W, Alpers CE, et al. Autopsy findings in the acquired immune deficiency syndrome. *JAMA* 1984; 252:1152–1159.
20. Cammarosano C, Lewis W. Cardiac lesions in acquired immune deficiency syndrome (AIDS). *J Am Coll Cardiol* 1985; 5:703–706.
21. Roldan EO, Moskowitz L, Hensly GT. Pathology of the heart in acquired immunodeficiency syndrome. *Arch Pathol Lab Med* 1987; 111:943–946.
22. Wilkes MS, Fortin AH, Felix JC, et al. Value of necropsy in acquired immunodeficiency syndrome. *Lancet* 1988; 2:85–88.
23. Baroldi G, Corallo S, Moroni M, et al. Focal lymphocytic myocarditis in acquired immunodeficiency syndrome (AIDS): A correlative morphologic and clinical study in 26 consecutive fatal cases. *J Am Coll Cardiol* 1988; 12:463–469.

24. Lewis W. AIDS: Cardiac findings from 115 autopsies. *Prog Cardiovasc Dis* 1989; 32:207–215.
25. Anderson DW, Virmani R, Reilly JM, et al. Prevalent myocarditis at necropsy in the acquired immunodeficiency syndrome. *J Am Coll Cardiol* 1988; 11:792–799.
26. Magno J, Margaretten W, Cheitlin M. Myocardial involvement in acquired immunodeficiency syndrome: Incidence in a large autopsy study [abstr]. *Circulation* 1988; 78(suppl II):II-459.
27. Garcia I, Fainstein V, Rios A, et al. Nonbacterial thrombotic endocarditis in a male homosexual with Kaposi's sarcoma. *Arch Internal Med* 1983; 143:1243–1244.
28. Barbaro G, DiLorenzo G, Grisorio B, et al. Cardiac involvement in the acquired immunodeficiency syndrome: A multicenter clinical and pathological study. Gruppo Italiano par lo studio cardiologico dei pazienti affetti da AIDS Investigators. *AIDS Res Hum Retroviruses* 1998; 14:1071–1077.
29. Lanjewar DN, Katdare GA, Jain PP, et al. Pathology of the heart in acquired immunodeficiency syndrome. *Indian Heart J* 1998; 50:321–325.
30. Moskowitz L, Hensley GT, Chan JC, et al. Immediate causes of death in acquired immunodeficiency syndrome. *Arch Pathol Lab Med* 1985; 109:735–738.
31. Murray JF, Garay SM, Hopewell PC, et al. Pulmonary complications of the acquired immunodeficiency syndrome: An update—Report of the second National Heart, Lung and Blood Institute workshop. *Am Rev Respir Dis* 1987; 135:504–509.
32. Kinney EL, Brafman D, Wright RJ II. Echocardiographic findings in patients with acquired immunodeficiency syndrome (AIDS) and AIDS-related complex (ARC). *Cathet Cardiovasc Diagn* 1989; 16:182–185.
33. Himelman RB, Chung WS, Chernoff DN, et al. Cardiac manifestations of human immunodeficiency virus infection: A two-dimensional echocardiographic study. *J Am Coll Cardiol* 1989; 13:1030–1036.
34. Monsuez JJ, Kinney EL, Vittecoq D, et al. Comparison among acquired immune deficiency syndrome patients with and without clinical evidence of cardiac disease. *Am J Cardiol* 1988; 62:1311–1313.
35. Levy WS, Simon GL, Rios JC, et al. Prevalence of cardiac abnormalities in human immunodeficiency virus infection. *Am J Cardiol* 1989; 63:86–89.
36. Corallo S, Mutinelli MR, Moroni M, et al. Echocardiography detects myocardial damage in AIDS: Prospective study in 102 patients. *Eur Heart J* 1988; 9:887–892.
37. Currie PF, Jacob AJ, Foreman AR, et al. Heart muscle disease related to HIV infection: Prognostic implications. *BMJ* 1994; 309:1605–1607.
38. Cecchi E, Parrini I, Chinaglia A, et al. Cardiac complications in HIV infections. *G Ital Cardiol* 1997; 27:917–924.
39. Steffen HM, Muller R, Schrappe-Bächer M, et al. Prevalence of echocardiographic abnormalities in human immunodeficiency virus 1 infection. *Am J Noninvasive Cardiol* 1991; 5:280–284.
40. Redfield RR, Wright DC, Tramont EC. The Walter Reed staging classification for HTLV-III/LAV infection: Special report. *N Engl J Med* 1986; 314:131–132.
41. Chyu KY, Birnbaum Y, Naqvi T, et al. Echocardiographic detection of Kaposi's sarcoma causing cardiac tamponade in a patient with acquired immunodeficiency syndrome. *Clin Cardiol* 1998; 21:131–133.
42. Estok L, Wallach F. Cardiac tamponade in a patient with AIDS: A review of pericardial disease in patients with HIV infection. *Mt Sinai J Med* 1998; 65:33–39.
43. Heidenreich PA, Eisenberg MJ, Kee LL, et al. Pericardial effusion in AIDS: Incidence and survival. *Circulation* 1995; 92:3229–3234.
44. Flum DR, McGinn JT Jr, Tyras DH. The role of the "pericardial window" in AIDS. *Chest* 1995; 107:1522–1525.
45. Azrak EC, Kern MJ, Bach RG. Hemodynamics of cardiac tamponade in a patient with AIDS-related non-Hodgkin's lymphoma. *Cathet Cardiovasc Design* 1998; 45:287–291.
46. Decker CF, Tuazon CU. *Staphylococcus aureus* pericarditis in HIV-infected patients. *Chest* 1994; 105:615–616.
47. Zuger A, Louie E, Holzman RS, et al. Cryptococcal disease in patients with acquired immunodeficiency syndrome: Diagnostic features and outcome of treatment. *Ann Intern Med* 1986; 104:234–240.
48. Freedberg RS, Gindea AJ, Dieterich DT, et al. Herpes simplex pericarditis in AIDS. *NY State J Med* 1987; 87:304–306.
49. Francis CK. Cardiac involvement in AIDS. *Curr Probl Cardiol* 1990; 15:571–639.
50. Zuger A, Louie E, Holzman RS, et al. Cryptococcal disease in patients with the acquired immunodeficiency syndrome: Diagnostic features and outcome of treatment: Clinical review. *Ann Intern Med* 1986; 104:234–240.
51. Hofman P, Drici MD, Gibelin P, et al. Prevalence of toxoplasma myocarditis in patients with the acquired immunodeficiency syndrome. *Br Heart J* 1993; 70:376–381.
52. Kinney EL, Monsuez JJ, Kitzis M, et al. Treatment of AIDS-associated heart disease. *Angiology* 1989; 40:970–976.
53. Grange F, Kinney EL, Monsuez JJ, et al. Successful therapy for *Toxoplasma gondii* myocarditis in acquired immunodeficiency syndrome. *Am Heart J* 1990; 120:443–444.
54. Albrecht H, Stellbrink HJ, Fenske S, et al. Successful treatment of *Toxoplasma gondii* myocarditis in an AIDS patient. *Eur J Clin Microbiol Infect Dis* 1994; 13:500–504.
55. Ioachim HL, Cooper MC, Hellman GC. Lymphomas in men at high risk for acquired immune deficiency syndrome (AIDS): A study of 21 cases. *Cancer* 1985; 56:2831–2842.
56. Montalbetti L, Della Volpe A, Airughi ML, et al. Primary cardiac lymphoma: A case report and review. *Minerva Cardioangiol* 1999; 47:175–182.
57. Levitt LJ, Ault KA, Pinkus GS, et al. Pericarditis and early cardiac tamponade as a primary manifestation of lymphoscarcoma cell leukemia. *Am J Med* 1979; 67:719–723.
58. Golfarb A, King CL, Rosenzweig BP, et al. Cardiac lymphoma in the accquired immunodeficiency syndrome. *Am Heart J* 1989; 118:1340–1344.
59. Cohen IS, Anderson DW, Virmani R, et al. Congestive cardiomyopathy in association with the acquired immunodeficiency syndrome. *N Engl J Med* 1986; 315:628–630.
60. Reilly JM, Cunnion RE, Anderson DW, et al. Frequency of myocarditis, left ventricular dysfunction and ventricular tachycardia in the acquired immune deficiency syndrome. *Am J Cardiol* 1988; 62:789–793.
61. Kaminski HJ, Katzman M, Wiest PM, et al. Cardiomyopathy associated with the acquired immune deficiency syndrome. *J AIDS* 1988; 1:105–110.
62. Lipshultz SE, Orav EJ, Sanders SP, et al. Cardiac structure and function in children with human immunodeficiency virus infection treated with zidovudine. *N Engl J Med* 1992; 327:1260–1265.
63. Lipshultz SE, Easley KA, Orav EJ, et al. Left ventricle structure and function in children with human immunodeficiency virus: The prospective P2 C2 HIV Multicenter Study. Pediatric Pulmonary and Cardiac Complications of Vertically Transmitted HIV Infection (P2 C2 HIV) Study Group. *Circulation* 1998; 97:1246–1256.
64. DeCastro S, d'Amati G, Gallo P, et al. Frequency of development of acute global left ventricular dysfunction in human immunodeficiency virus infection. *J Am Coll Cardiol* 1994; 24:1018–1024.
65. Blanchard DG, Hagenhoff C, Chow LC, et al. Reversibility of cardiac abnormalities in human immunodeficiency virus (HIV)-infected individuals: A serial echocardiographic study. *J Am Coll Cardiol* 1991; 17:1270–1276.
66. Cheitlin MD. Cardiovascular complications of HIV infection. In:

Sande MA, Volberding PA, eds. *The Medical Management of AIDS,* 4th ed. Philadelphia: Saunders; 1995:332.
67. Barbaro G, Di Lorenzo G, Grisorio B, et al. Incidence of dilated cardiomyopathy and detection of HIV in myocardial cells of HIV-positive patients. Gruppo Italiano per lo Studio Cardilogico dei Pazianti Affetti, da AIDS. *N Engl J Med* 1998; 339:1093–1099.
68. Calabrese LH, Proffitt MR, Yen-Lieberman B, et al. Congestive cardiomyopathy and illness related to the acquired immunodeficiency syndrome (AIDS) associated with isolation of retrovirus from myocardium. *Ann Intern Med* 1987; 107:691–692.
69. Grody WW, Cheng L, Lewis W. Infection of the heart by the human immunodeficiency virus. *Am J Cardiol* 1990; 66:203–206.
70. Stewart JM, Kaul A, Gromisch DS, et al. Symptomatic cardiac dysfunction in children with human immunodeficiency virus infection. *Am Heart J* 1989; 117:140–144.
71. Acierno LJ. Cardiac complications in acquired immunodeficiency syndrome (AIDS): A review. *J Am Coll Cardiol* 1989; 13:1144–1154.
72. Cox JN, Di Dio F, Pizzolato GP, et al. *Aspergillus* endocarditis and myocarditis in a patient with the acquired immunodeficiency syndrome (AIDS): A review of the literature—Case report. *Virchows Arch* [*A*] 1990; 417:255–259.
73. Lowry PJ, Thompson RA, Littler WA. Cellular immunity in congestive cardiomyopathy: The normal cellular immune response. *Br Heart J* 1985; 53:394–399.
74. Zee-Cheng CS, Tsai CC, Palmer DC, et al. High incidence of myocarditis by endomyocardial biopsy in patients with idiopathic congestive cardiomyopathy. *J Am Coll Cardiol* 1984; 3:63–70.
75. Parrillo JE, Aretz HT, Palacios I, et al. The results of transvenous endomyocardial biopsy can frequently be used to diagnose myocardial disease in patients with idiopathic heart failure: Endomyocardial biopsy in 100 consecutive patients revealed a substantial incidence of myocarditis. *Circulation* 1984; 69:93–101.
76. Bowles NE, Richardson PJ, Olsen EGJ, et al. Detection of Coxsackie-B-virus-specific RNA sequences in myocardial biopsy samples from patients with myocarditis and dilated cardiomyopathy. *Lancet* 1984; 1:1120–1123.
77. Herskowitz A, WU T-C, Willoughby SB, et al. Myocarditis and cardiotrophic viral infection associated with severe left ventricular dysfunction in late-stage infection with human immunodeficiency virus. *J Am Coll Cardiol* 1994; 24:1025–1032.
78. Herskowitz A, Ansari AA, Neumann DA, et al. Cardiomyopathy in acquired immunodeficiency syndrome: Evidence for autoimmunity [abstr]. *Circulation* 1989; 80(suppl II):II-322.
79. Lipshultz SE, Orav J, Sanders SP, et al. Immunoglobulins and left ventricular structure and function in pediatric HIV infection. *Circulation* 1995; 92:2220–2225.
80. Ho DD, Pomerantz RJ, Kaplan JC. Pathogenesis of infection with human immunodeficiency virus. *N Engl J Med* 1987; 317:278–286.
81. Parker MM, Shelhamer JH, Bacharach SL, et al. Profound but reversible myocardial depression in patients with septic shock. *Ann Intern Med* 1984; 100:483–490.
82. Natanson C, Fink MP, Ballantyne HK, et al. Gram-negative bacteremia produces both severe systolic and diastolic cardiac dysfunction in a canine model that simulates human septic shock. *J Clin Invest* 1986; 78:259–270.
83. Parrillo JE, Burch C, Shelhamer JH, et al. A circulating myocardial depressant substance in humans with septic shock: Septic shock patients with a reduced ejection fraction have a circulating factor that depresses in vitro myocardial cell performance. *J Clin Invest* 1985; 76:1539–1553.
84. Cunnion RE, Parrillo JE. Myocardial dysfunction in sepsis: Recent insights [editorial]. *Chest* 1989; 95:941–945.
85. Suffredini AF, Fromm RE, Parker MM, et al. The cardiovascular response of normal humans to the administration of endotoxin. *N Engl J Med* 1989; 321:280–287.
86. Levine B, Kalman J, Mayer L, et al. Elevated circulating levels of tumor necrosis factor in severe chronic heart failure. *N Engl J Med* 1990; 323:236–241.
87. Lähdevirta J, Maury CPJ, Teppo AM, et al. Elevated levels of circulating cachectin/tumor necrosis factor in patients with acquired immunodeficiency syndrome. *Am J Med* 1988; 85:289–291.
88. Wright SC, Jewett A, Mitsuyasu R, et al. Spontaneous cytotoxicity and tumor necrosis factor production by peripheral blood monocytes from AIDS patients. *J Immunol* 1988; 141:99–104.
89. Barbaro G, Di Lorenzo G, Soldini M, et al. Intensity of myocardial expression of inducible nitric oxide synthase influences the clinical course of human immunodeficiency virus-associated cardiomyopathy. Gruppo Italiano per lo Studio Cardiologico dei pazienti affetti dei AIDS (GISCA). *Circulation* 1999; 100: 933–939.
90. Odeh M. The role of tumour necrosis factor-alpha in acquired immunodeficiency syndrome. *J Intern Med* 1990; 228:549–556.
91. Yamamoto N. The role of cytokines in the acquired immunodeficiency syndrome. *Int J Clin Lab Res* 1995; 25:29–34.
92. Goldberg SJ, Comerci GD, Feldman L. Cardiac output and regional myocardial contraction in anorexia nervosa. *J Adolesc Health Care* 1988; 9:15–21.
93. Abel RM, Grimes JB, Alonso D, et al. Adverse hemodynamic and ultrastructural changes in dog hearts subjected to protein-calorie malnutrition. *Am Heart J* 1979; 97:733–744.
94. Schocken DD, Holloway JD, Powers PS. Weight loss and the heart: Effects of anorexia nervosa and starvation. *Arch Intern Med* 1989; 149:877–881.
95. Dworkin BM, Antonecchia PP, Smith F, et al. Reduced cardiac selenium content in the acquired immunodeficiency syndrome. *J Parenter Enteral Nutr* 1989; 13:644–647.
96. Kavanaugh-McHugh AL, Ruff A, Perlman E, et al. Selenium deficiency and cardiomyopathy in acquired immunodeficiency syndrome. *J Parenter Enteral Nutr* 1991; 15:347–349.
97. Kaul S, Fishbein MC, Siegel RJ. Cardiac manifestations of acquired immune deficiency syndrome: A 1991 update. *Am Heart J* 1991; 122:535–544.
98. Cohen MC, Huberman MS, Nesto RW. Recombinant alpha$_2$ interferon-related cardiomyopathy. *Am J Med* 1988; 85:549–551.
99. Deyton LR, Walker RE, Kovacs JA, et al. Reversible cardiac dysfunction associated with interferon alpha therapy in AIDS patients with Kaposi's sarcoma. *N Engl J Med* 1989; 321:1246–1249.
100. Chokshi SK, Moore R, Pandian NG, et al. Reversible cardiomyopathy associated with cocaine intoxication. *Ann Intern Med* 1989; 111:1039–1040.
101. Brown J, Kind A, Francis CK. Cardiovascular effects of alcohol, cocaine, and acquired immune deficiency. *Cardiovasc Clin* 1991; 21:341–376.
102. Wharton JM, Demopulos PA, Goldschlager N. Torsade de pointes during administration of pentamidine isothionate. *Am J Med* 1987; 83:571–576.
103. Richman DD, Fischl MA, Grieco MH, et al. The toxicity of azidothymidine (AZT) in the treatment of patients with AIDS and AIDS-related complex: A double-blind, placebo-controlled trial. *N Engl J Med* 1987; 317:192–197.
104. Dalakas MC, Illa I, Pezeshkpour GH, et al. Mitochondrial myopathy caused by long-term zidovudine therapy. *N Engl J Med* 1990; 322:1098–1105.
105. Szabados E, Fischer GM, Toth K, et al. Role of reactive oxygen species and poly-ADP-ribose polymerase in the development of AZT-induced cardiomyopathy in rats. *Free Radic Biol Med* 1999; 26:302–317.
106. Brown DL, Sather S, Cheitlin MD. Reversible cardiac dysfunction associated with foscarnet therapy for cytomegalovirus esophagitis in an AIDS patient. *Am Heart J* 1993; 125:1439–1441.
107. Eastone JA, Decker CF. New onset diabetes mellitus associated with the use of protease inhibitors. *Ann Intern Med* 1997; 127:948.

108. Carr A, Samaras K, Chisholm DJ, et al. Pathogenesis of HIV-1 protease inhibitor-associated peripheral lipodystrophy, hyperlipidemia, and insulin resistance. *Lancet* 1998; 351:1881–1883.
109. Danner SA, Carr A, Leondard J, et al. Safety, pharmacokinetics and preliminary efficacy of ritonavir, an inhibitor of HIV-1 protease. *N Engl J Med* 1995; 333:1528–1533.
110. Cameron DW, Japour AJ, Xu Y, et al. Ritonavir and saquinavir combination therapy for the treatment of HIV infection. *AIDS* 1999; 13:213–224.
111. Melroe NH, Kopaczewski J, Henry K, et al. Intervention for hyperlipidemia associated with protease inhibitors. *J Assoc Nurses AIDS Care* 1999; 10:55–69.
112. Miller KD, Jones E, Janovsk JA, et al. Visceral abdominal fat accumulation associated with use of indinavir. *Lancet* 1998; 351:871–875.
113. Lo JC, Mullighan K, Tai VW, et al. Buffalo hump in men with HIV-1 infection. *Lancet* 1998; 351:867–870.
114. Carr A, Samaras K, Burton S, et al. A syndrome of peripheral lipodystrophy, hyperlipidemia and insulin resistance in patients receiving HIV protease inhibitors. *AIDS* 1998; 12:F51–F58.
115. Henry K, Melroe IT, Heubsch J, et al. Severe premature coronary artery disease with protease inhibitors [research letter]. *Lancet* 1998; 351:1321–1328.
116. Herskowitz A, Willouby SB, Baughman KL, et al. Cardiomyopathy associated with antiretroviral therapy in patients with HIV infection: A report of six cases. *Ann Intern Med* 1992; 116:311–313.
117. Mason JW, O'Connell JB, Herskowitz A, et al. A clinical trial of immunosuppressive therapy for myocarditis: The Myocarditis Treatment Trial Investigators. *N Engl J Med* 1995; 333:269–275.
118. Centers for Disease Control. Acquired immunodeficiency syndrome: United States—Update. *MMWR* 1986; 35:17–21.
119. Ribera E, Miro JM, Cortes E, et al. Influence of human immunodeficiency virus 1 and degree of immunosuppression in the clinical characteristics and outcome of infective endocarditis in intravenous drug users. *Arch Intern Med* 1998; 158:2043–2050.
120. Utley JR. The immune response. In: *Pathophysiology and Techniques of Cardiopulmonary Bypass I.* Baltimore: Williams and Wilkins; 1982:132–144.
121. Pollock R, Ames F, Rubio P, et al. Protracted severe immune dysregulation induced by cardiopulmonary bypass: A predisposing etiologic factor in blood transfusion-related AIDS? *J Clin Lab Immunol* 1987; 22:1–5.
122. Condit D, Frater RWM. Human immunodeficiency virus and the cardiac surgeon: A survey of attitudes. *Ann Thorac Surg* 1989; 47:182–186.
123. Heptonstall J, Porter K, Gill ON. *Occupational HIV: Summary of published reports.* London: Public Health Laboratory Services. Communicable Disease Surveillance Centre; Dec 1995.
124. Gerberding JL, Littell C, Tarkington A, et al. Risk of exposure of surgical personnel to patients' blood during surgery at San Francisco General Hospital. *N Engl J Med* 1990; 322:1788–1793.
125. Gerberding JL. Management of occupational exposures to blood-borne viruses. *N Engl J Med* 1995; 332:444–451.

CHAPTER 71

EFFECT OF NONCARDIAC DRUGS, ELECTRICITY, POISONS, AND RADIATION ON THE HEART

Andrew L. Smith / Wendy M. Book

This chapter details many deleterious side effects of treatments and environmental agents on the heart. Toxic effects may occur acutely and require emergent intervention or may be chronic and not be manifest until days or years after exposure.

NONCARDIAC DRUGS

Chemotherapeutic Agents

The use of chemotherapeutic agents may result in acute or chronic cardiovascular toxicity. The heart, composed of nonproliferating myocytes, was traditionally thought to be protected from the effects of drugs on rapidly dividing cells. A variety of agents are now recognized to cause cardiovascular complications, including cardiomyopathy, myocarditis, pericarditis, myocardial ischemia, arrhythmias, and peripheral hypotension or vasospasm (see Table 71-1).[1]

Cardiovascular alterations in the patient receiving chemotherapy may be the result of a specific drug or combination of drugs or be related to tumor-associated factors such as hypercoagulability or release of myocardial depressant factors. Correlating a specific therapy with a particular adverse event may be difficult; however, knowledge of side effects of each agent should be considered when prescribing therapy.

ANTHRACYCLINES

The anthracycline antineoplastics—doxorubicin, daunorubicin, and epirubicine—are the leading cause of chemotherapy-related heart disease. These agents may cause cardiac problems during therapy, weeks after completion of therapy, or, unexpectedly, years later.[2] During acute therapy, electrocardiographic (ECG) changes occur in approximately 30 percent of patients and usually regress within weeks. Findings include ST-T changes, decreased QRS voltage, prolongation of the QT interval, and atrial and ventricular ectopy. Sustained atrial or ventricular arrhythmias are rare. The occurrence of early ECG abnormalities does not predict cardiomyopathy and is not an indication to discontinue therapy.[1] The development of persistent sinus tachycardia (although nonspecific) in an otherwise stable oncology patient, however, may raise the suspicion of ventricular dysfunction and impending congestive heart failure.

Congestive heart failure is related to the cumulative dose of the anthracycline administered. The incidences of heart failure at specific doses of doxorubicin include 0.4 percent at 400 mg/m^2 of body surface area, 7 percent at 550 mg/m^2, and 18 percent at 700 mg/m^2 (see Fig. 71-1). Traditionally, the cardiac limiting dose has been described as 550 mg/m^2 because of the acute rise in heart failure seen above this dose. There is great individual variability, however, with reports of heart failure occurring with doses less than 100 mg/m^2 and, conversely, with some patients tolerating greater than 1000 mg/m^2 without cardiac compromise.[3,4] Risk factors for anthracycline-induced cardiomyopathy are debated but include prior chest radiation, age greater than 70, and preexisting heart disease.[3–5] Young women may be at particularly increased risk for late cardiac dysfunction.[5] Rapid infusion schedules associated with higher peak drug concentrations appear to result in greater cardiotoxicity. Combination therapy with cyclophosphamide is an additional risk factor.[1]

The pathogenesis of anthracycline-induced cardiotoxicity is not known. Theories generally implicate free-radical damage. One proposal is that enzymatic reduction of the anthracycline-quinone ring results in lipid peroxidation and cell membrane damage. Another theory involves the formation of an anthracycline-iron complex, which undergoes "redoxcycling" that results

TABLE 71-1 Chemotherapeutic Agents Commonly Associated with Cardiovascular Toxicity

Drug	Associated Toxicity
Anthracyclines	
Doxorubicin	Cardiomyopathy
Daunorubicin	
Epirubicin	
Idarubicin	
Mitoxantrone	
Alkylating agents	
Cyclophosphamide	Reversible systolic dysfunction, hemorrhagic myocarditis
Cisplatin	Raynaud's phenomenon
Antimetabolites	
5-Fluorouracil	Coronary vasospasm
Other	
Amsacrine	Arrhythmias
Paclitaxel	Arrhythmias
Interleukin 2	Hypotension, myocarditis
Interferon alpha	Hypotension, cardiomyopathy

in oxygen radicals and degradation of microsomal, mitochondrial, and membrane lipids. Disturbances of calcium exchange have also been noted.[6]

The average time to clinical development of heart failure symptoms is 1 month from the end of therapy, but it may occur anytime within 1 year. Patient presentation is similar to that for other dilated cardiomyopathies (see Chap. 66). Biventricular systolic dysfunction occurs, and restrictive hemodynamics have been described.[7] The clinical course varies from fulminant heart failure to gradually progressive deterioration. Some patients have reversibility of systolic dysfunction. Therapy, in addition to withholding further anthracycline dosing or other myocardial toxins, is generally considered the same as recommended for patients with heart failure from dilated cardiomyopathy (Chap. 21).

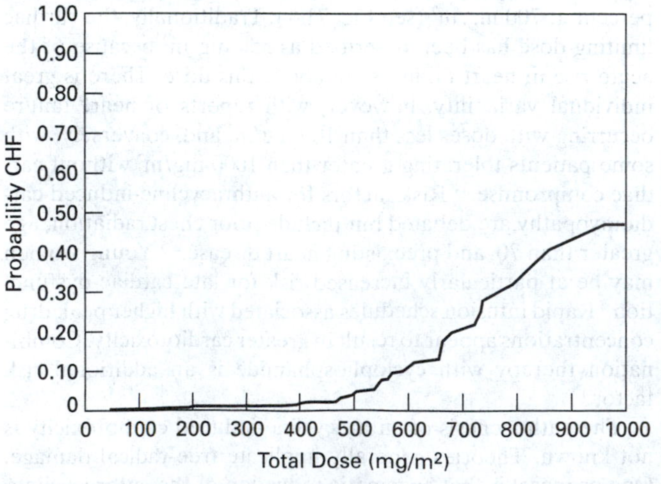

FIGURE 71-1 The development of doxorubicin-induced heart failure is related to cumulative dose. Toxicity may occur at any dose, but at 550 mg/m^2 the probability increases significantly. (From Von Hoff et al.,[3] with permission.)

Noninvasive assessment of left ventricular function has been utilized to guide anthracycline dosing and prevent cardiac toxicity. Serial echocardiography and/or radionuclide angiography (see Chaps. 13 and 16) are most commonly used.[8–10] Improved echocardiographic technologies are likely to increase the use of echocardiography in the adult population. The most commonly used parameter is resting left ventricular ejection fraction. Recognition that resting left ventricular ejection fraction is relatively insensitive for detecting early cardiotoxicity[2] has resulted in investigation of other variables (exercise or dobutamine echocardiography,[9] Doppler velocities, and systolic time intervals) in assessing this problem. These methods have generally been evaluated in small studies and have not gained widespread acceptance in current therapy guidelines. Adult guidelines for serial assessment have been developed. A drop in left ventricular ejection fraction greater than 10 percent (EF units) and to below a normal value of 50 percent is an indication to discontinue therapy. A baseline left ventricular ejection fraction less than 30 percent has generally been considered a contraindication to initiating anthracycline therapy.[10]

Compared with the noninvasive methods, endomyocardial biopsy is considered more specific and provides earlier sensitivity in detection of anthracycline cardiotoxicity. The Billingham score, which quantifies cytoplasmic changes and the percent of myocytes damaged, has been utilized to assess the risk of congestive heart failure.[11] Clinical utility has been limited because of the invasive nature of this procedure and the special expertise required in obtaining and reading the specimens. Additionally, variability of histologic changes and the potential for sampling error have been noted.[12]

There is growing recognition of the occurrence of cardiac dysfunction years after completion of anthracycline therapy. This is particularly of concern in children. One study reported a 23 percent incidence of late cardiac abnormalities (decreased systolic function by noninvasive testing) in survivors of pediatric malignancies treated with anthracycline therapy.[13] The incidence of abnormalities was higher in the patients with the longer elapsed times since therapy, with a 38 percent incidence in patients with a follow-up period greater than 10 years. This study, as well as others,[14] suggests that subclinical myocardial damage may not become clinically evident until years after therapy. Although fewer than 5 percent of these patients had developed clinical heart failure, the potentially progressive nature of systolic dysfunction raises the issue of need for long-term clinical follow-up. There are presently no accepted guidelines, however, in either the pediatric or adult population for chronic monitoring. Early treatment of systolic dysfunction with angiotensin-converting enzyme inhibitors may be warranted in asymptomatic patients.[2] Additionally, patients presenting late after anthracycline therapy with exertional fatigue and normal resting ejection fractions have been noted to have abnormalities on dobutamine echocardiography. This observation suggests abnormalities in cardiac reserve that may lead to symptoms.

Clinical strategies for preventing anthracycline cardiotoxicity have had to balance the need for antineoplastic efficacy. Lower clinical toxicity has been noted with prolonged infusions of doxorubicin over 48 to 96 h in order to avoid high peak concentrations.[15] Several antioxidants have been evaluated, but with inconclusive results.[6,16] *Dexrazoxane*,[17] an iron-chelating agent, reduces free-radical generation by anthracyclines and is approved for use in women with breast cancer after a cumulative dose of doxorubicin of 300 mg/m^2. Studies demonstrate a decrease in cardiotoxicity and most but not all trials have suggested preserved efficacy of antitumor activity. New anthracyclines, including epirubicine and idarubicin, appear to have diminished cardiotoxic effects, although long-term results cannot presently be assessed.[2]

OTHER CHEMOTHERAPEUTIC AGENTS

Mitoxantrone, an anthracendione lacking the amino sugar of anthracyclines, causes cardiotoxicity with features similar to anthracycline-induced cardiomyopathy.[1] This drug appears to have less cardiotoxicity than doxorubicin at equal myelotoxic doses. Cumulative doses above 160 mg/m^2 are associated with an increasing incidence of congestive heart failure.[18]

High-dose *cyclophosphamide* (120 to 240 mg/kg over several days) used in bone marrow transplantation may cause acute cardiac toxicity.[1,19] Symptomatic systolic dysfunction, usually reversible with drug discontinuation, is associated with decreased QRS voltage on the ECG. Pericardial effusions have been noted, and a hemorrhagic myocarditis may result in death. Necropsy data demonstrate endothelial injury with resultant interstitial fibrin deposition and capillary microthrombosis. The cardiotoxicity of cyclophosphamide is likely due to damage from its biologically active metabolites. Rapid metabolizers of cyclophosphamide appear to be prone to cardiotoxicity. The metabolites cause the toxic endothelial damage leading to muscle damage.[19] Cyclophosphamide may also potentiate the cardiotoxic effects of the anthracyclines.[1]

5-*Fluorouracil* may occasionally cause angina, ECG changes, and rarely myocardial infarction.[1,20] The majority of episodes occur during the first cycle of therapy and resolve spontaneously after discontinuation. Arrhythmias and systolic dysfunction have been observed. The understanding of 5-fluorouracil toxicity is complicated because combination chemotherapy is generally utilized, patients may be systemically ill, and many receiving this medication have preexisting coronary artery disease.[20] The incidence of cardiac toxicity is uncertain but ranges from 1 to 8 percent.[21] Patients with known coronary artery disease are at higher risk for serious cardiotoxicity. The mechanism of toxicity remains unclear, although coronary vasospasm has been suspected. Coronary catheterization has generally failed to demonstrate vasomotor hyperreactivity with 5-fluorouracil on ergonovine challenge.

Amsacrine (AMSA) has been associated with prolongation of the QT interval. Malignant ventricular arrhythmias may occur in 1 percent of patients and are exacerbated by hypokalemia.[22]

Paclitaxel (taxol) is being used with increased frequency for breast and ovarian cancer. The most common cardiovascular effect is the development of transient asymptomatic bradycardia, occurring in up to 30 percent of patients. Bradycardia with adverse consequences occurs in only 0.1 percent of patients. A possible relationship of paclitaxel to heart failure has been questioned, but confirmatory data are lacking.[23]

Herceptin (recombinant humanized anti-HER2 antibody) is a relatively new treatment for breast cancer that appears to have favorable antitumor effects when added to standard chemotherapy in selected patients. Unfortunately, cardiac toxicity may limit the use of this drug. In a breast cancer treatment trial, 27 percent of patients receiving doxorubicin, paclitaxel, and Herceptin had cardiac dysfunction compared with 6 percent receiving doxorubicin and paclitaxel without Herceptin. Close cardiac monitoring is warranted.[24]

Immunomodulating Agents

The biological response modifiers *interleukin-2* (IL-2) and *interferon alpha* have been associated with cardiovascular toxicity predominantly secondary to peripheral vasodilatation. IL-2 causes tachycardia, hypotension, and a capillary leak syndrome. Myocarditis has been reported in patients who died soon after initiation of therapy. IL-2 therapy requires pretreatment assessment of cardiovascular risks and close monitoring during drug administration. Interferon alpha may cause supraventricular tachyarrhythmias. A reversible cardiomyopathy has been described.[1,19,25]

Psychotropic Agents

Psychiatric illness, particularly depression, is common in patients with cardiovascular disease[43] (see Chap. 80). Morbidity and mortality following cardiac events are increased in patients with depression, particularly if untreated.[26,27] A variety of psychotropic agents have conduction or vascular effects (see Table 80-11). A thorough understanding of these therapeutic but potentially toxic agents is necessary in the treatment of patients with preexisting cardiac disease. Intentional overdose with these drugs may result in serious cardiac manifestations.

TRICYCLIC ANTIDEPRESSANTS

The tricyclic antidepressants, including the tertiary (amitryptyline, clomipramine, doxepin, imipramine, trimipramine) and secondary (desipramine, nortriptyline, protriptyline) amines, have potentially serious cardiovascular effects. These effects include increased heart rate, orthostatic hypotension, ECG changes, and possible depression of ventricular function. These drugs have electrophysiologic properties similar to the type IA antiarrhythmics. There is the potential for late proarrhythmia in patients with structural heart disease who are taking these agents.[28]

The tricyclic antidepressants have several properties that account for the majority of cardiovascular effects. These drugs inhibit uptake of both norepinephrine and serotonin, resulting in greater toxicity compared to the selective serotonin reuptake inhibitors (SSRIs). A hyperadrenergic state may result in tachycardia. Alpha blockade occurs at higher drug levels and may cause marked hypotension in the setting of overdose. The anticholinergic effects result in tachycardia, dry mouth, and constipation; in overdose they may delay gastrointestinal absorption of the drug. Sodium channel blockade, typical of the type IA antiarrhythmic compounds, results in conduction abnormalities[52] and the potential to suppress ventricular function.[29]

The most frequent side effect of tricyclic antidepressant treatment, orthostatic hypotension, is common in older patients and does not generally improve when doses are reduced to lower levels that will still maintain antidepressant effects. Orthostasis, mediated predominantly by alpha-1 adrenergic receptor blockade, may occur with all of these drugs but is less likely with nortriptyline.[29,30]

The most common ECG changes include nonspecific ST-T changes and prolongation of the QT interval, PR interval, and QRS duration. PR prolongation is due to prolonged infranodal conduction. Patients with preexisting conduction disease, particularly bundle branch block, are at increased risk of toxicity.[31] The type IA antiarrhythmic properties may potentially suppress ventricular ectopy. The results of recent antiarrhythmic studies, however, including those with type I agents, suggest the potential for a proarrhythmic effect for these drugs at therapeutic doses in patients with serious structural heart disease.[28,32] Tricyclic antidepressants are generally contraindicated in the recovery phase following myocardial infarction. Although tricyclic antidepressant therapy may be indicated in the treatment of severely depressed patients, the threshold for use should rise as the severity of heart disease increases or when there is QT prolongation.[28] These issues are discussed in detail in Chap. 80.

Tricyclic antidepressants may impair left ventricular function in patients with severe systolic dysfunction; however, decreases in left ventricular ejection fraction have generally not been noted in patients with moderately impaired function. Tricyclic antidepressant overdose carries a mortality of 2 to 3 percent, which is generally related to cardiac complications. Clinical status at initial presentation and serum drug levels are not predictive of prognosis. QRS prolongation is a sign of toxicity but may be absent in the patient with serious cardiac complications. Rightward deviation of the terminal 40 ms of the frontal plane QRS axis is a more sensitive marker. This finding, manifest by a terminal R wave in lead aV_R, has an 83 percent sensitivity and 63 percent specificity for toxicity.[33]

Aggressive support measures in tricyclic antidepressant overdose should be initiated immediately and include airway maintenance, gastric lavage, and repeated dosing of activated charcoal. Alkalinization with intravenous sodium bicarbonate decreases unbound drug and reverses cardiac and central nervous system conduction defects. Alkalinization is indicated in cardiac arrest, hypotension, arrhythmias, acidosis, and QRS prolongation. Hypotension refractory to volume loading and bicarbonate therapy should be treated with vasopressors, including norepinephrine and phenylephrine, and with vasopressor doses of dopamine. Type I antiarrhythmics (quinidine, procainamide, disopyramide) should not be used. Sodium bicarbonate is the initial therapy for ventricular dysrhythmias.[34]

The duration of monitoring after tricyclic overdose is controversial. Signs of major toxicity generally occur within 6 h of presentation in the emergency department. If clinical or ECG evidence of toxicity is absent and two doses of activated charcoal have been given, patients may not require admission for medical monitoring. Fluoxetine increases tricyclic antidepressant serum levels, and additional monitoring is recommended in patients receiving this medication. Patients with cardiac disease or other serious medical problems may require a longer period of observation.[35]

OTHER ANTIDEPRESSANTS

Selective serotonin reuptake inhibitors (SSRIs) have not been extensively studied in patients with cardiac disease.[36] Case reports of cardiac toxicity are rare, despite the increasing popularity of these agents in the treatment of depression. These agents have rarely been associated with orthostatic hypotension and with bradycardia. Cardiac function does not appear to be depressed by these agents.[37] The SSRIs may affect the cytochrome P450 system and may therefore alter the metabolism of a variety of drugs, including agents used in cardiovascular disease such as antiarrhythmic medications, beta blockers, calcium channel blockers, and warfarin (see Chap. 80).

The monoamine oxidase inhibitors (MAOIs) have little effect on cardiac conduction or myocardial contractility. Orthostatic hypotension is common, particularly in elderly patients. The major concern with these agents is interaction with other drugs or tyramine-containing substances, resulting in hypertensive crisis.[38]

Lithium, used commonly in the treatment of bipolar disorder, is generally well tolerated in patients with cardiac disease. Suppression of sinus node automaticity, resulting in bradycardias, is the most common complication.[39] In patients free of known heart disease, clinically significant sinus node dysfunction occurs in fewer than 1 percent and is reversible with discontinuation of lithium therapy. Preexisting sinus node disease or concomitant therapy with drugs altering sinus node function, however, may result in sinus bradycardia. Lithium-induced hypothyroidism may be a contributing factor.[40] Pacemaker therapy may be required to allow continuation of lithium therapy.

Lithium therapy has been associated with ECG changes simulating hypokalemia. T-wave inversion, prominent U waves, and QT prolongation may occur. PR prolongation, bundle branch block, and complete heart block are rare.[39] Overdose with lithium may result in severe bradycardias requiring temporary pacemaker therapy. A low anion gap may suggest the presence of lithium toxicity.[41]

ANTIPSYCHOTIC AGENTS

The phenothiazine antipsychotic agents have potential cardiac toxicity similar to that of the tricyclic antidepressants. These drugs may cause sinus tachycardia, PR and QT prolongation, and disturbances of intraventricular conduction. Chlorpromazine and thioridazine[42] are the most commonly implicated phenothiazines as causes of torsades de pointes. The butyrophenone haloperidol is also associated with torsades de pointes at high doses given intravenously.[43]

Noncardiac Drugs and Toxic Antidepressants Causing Torsades de Pointes

As discussed above, the tricyclic phenothiazine and other psychotropic agents may prolong the QT interval and induce torsades de pointes. A variety of antiarrhythmic agents, particularly the type I agents, are most strongly associated with this potentially fatal arrhythmia. Other toxic causes of torsades de pointes[44] are listed in Table 71-2.

TABLE 71-2 Noncardiac Drugs and Toxins Known to Cause Torsades de Pointes

Psychotropic agents	Antihistamines
Tricyclic antidepressants	Terfenadine
Tetracyclic antidepressants	Astemizole
Phenothiazines	Other
Haloperidol	Cisapride
Chloral hydrate	Pentamidine
Antibiotics	Probucol
Erythromycin	Arsenic
Trimethoprim-sulfamethoxazole	Organophosphates
	Liquid protein diets

The antibiotics erythromycin and trimethoprim-sulfamethoxazole[45,46] have only rarely been associated with torsades de pointes, the exception being the effect of erythromycin on the metabolism of terfenadine, astemizole, and cisapride. Liquid protein diets and starvation[47] may cause marked electrolyte and chemical disturbances, triggering QT prolongation. Probucol[48] may prolong the QT interval, resulting in torsades de pointes.

The QT prolongation and torsades de pointes reported with the antihistamines terfenadine and astemizole and with cisapride have been associated with high drug levels from excessive dosing or altered metabolism.[49,50] Prolongation of the QT interval induced by terfenadine, astemizole, and cisapride is due to the electrophysiologic activity of blocking HERG, the ion channel that is responsible for the rapid component of the delayed rectifier current for potassium(I_{kr}).[50] These drugs are metabolized by the cytochrome P450 3A isoenzyme.[51] A variety of agents inhibit this isoenzyme, including antifungals (ketoconazole, fluconazole, itraconazole), erythromycin or clarithromycin (not azithromycin), SSRIs (fluvoxamine, nefazodone, fluoxetine, sertaline), quinine, and grapefruit juice. Serious cardiac arrhythmias have been reported in patients taking terfenadine, astemizole, or cisapride with drugs that inhibit the cytochrome P450 3A isoenzyme. Patients with a history of prolonged QT interval or those with serious underlying cardiac disease are at higher risk for this problem. Some women appear to have slow metabolism of these drugs; thus female gender is a risk factor for drug-induced arrhythmias.[50]

Methylxanthines and Beta-Adrenergic Agonists

The methylxanthines caffeine and theophylline have pharmacologic actions of central nervous system stimulation, bronchial smooth muscle relaxation, and cardiac muscle stimulation and have diuretic effects on the kidneys. At therapeutic doses or those consumed in xanthine-containing beverages, these agents competitively inhibit adenosine receptors. At higher doses, they exhibit phosphodiesterase inhibition.[52] The effect of caffeine consumption on the cardiovascular system is variable and depends on chronicity of use, dose exposure, and individual responsiveness. Although elevations of catecholamines may occur with acute administration, this effect resolves with chronic usage. At higher concentrations, caffeine may cause tachycardia and dysrhythmias. Despite the concern that caffeine may be detrimental in patients predisposed to cardiac rhythm disturbances, it appears that moderate amounts of caffeine consumption may be well tolerated in patients with ventricular arrhythmias. The role of coffee, with or without caffeine, as a risk factor for coronary artery disease has been debated. While heavy coffee drinking (>4 cups a day) has been suggested as a potential risk factor for cardiovascular mortality, the data are inconclusive.[53,54]

Theophylline has the potential to cause a slight increase in heart rate with minimal effects on blood pressure. Patients with obstructive lung disease commonly have atrial and ventricular arrhythmias, which can be exacerbated by theophylline therapy. Theophylline toxicity is associated with sinus tachycardia, atrial and ventricular arrhythmias, and hypotension.[55] Hypokalemia, hypercalcemia, hyperglycemia, hypophosphatemia, and metabolic acidosis may occur. Esmolol may be useful in the management of refractory arrhythmias. Dialysis may be helpful in patients with refractory arrhythmias or hypotension.[56,57]

The beta-adrenergic agonists terbutaline and albuterol are commonly used to treat asthma and premature labor. Although adverse reactions are uncommon with aerosol therapy, these agents may cause tachycardia and atrial and ventricular arrhythmias and, rarely, may worsen angina pectoris.[58] Use of oral beta$_2$ agonists has been associated with the development of heart failure.[59] Intravenous therapy may cause hypokalemia and acidosis. Controversy exists over the safety of long-term aerosol therapy with beta-adrenergic agonists in asthma. These concerns, however, relate predominantly to airway hyperresponsiveness and not to direct cardiac toxicity.[60]

Antimigraine Drugs

Ergotamine The ergot alkaloids are commonly used in the treatment of migraine headaches. Ergotamine causes constriction of smooth muscle, and its effect on vascular smooth muscle may result in hypertension and increased peripheral vascular resistance.[61] Ergonovine maleate may be used in the catheterization laboratory to diagnose coronary artery spasm. Chronic use of ergotamine may result in variant angina or myocardial infarction.[61,62] Severe circulatory disturbances of the upper and lower extremities and abdominal arteries have been described.[62] Ergotamine and methysergide have similar chemical structures. Valvular heart disease has been reported with both agents. Either may cause pericardial, pleural, or peritoneal fibrosis or multivalvular heart disease. The occurrence of these side effects is less frequent with ergotamine.[63,64]

Methysergide Methysergide, used in treating vascular headaches, can cause retroperitoneal, pulmonary, and cardiac fibrosis. Cardiac involvement most commonly affects the valves but may affect the endocardium, myocardium, and rarely the aorta. Regurgitant valvular lesions are most common, affecting the mitral and aortic valves more commonly than the tricuspid and pulmonary valves.[65] Patients receiving methysergide therapy should be monitored for the development of murmurs. Therapy should be discontinued if a new murmur is detected. Regression of valvular lesions may occur, although valve replacement is occasionally required. Patients with known valvular disease should not be given methysergide.

Sumatriptan Sumatriptan, a selective serotonin type I agonist, may cause coronary artery vasospasm. Sumatriptan should not be taken within 24 h of treatment with ergotamine-like medications because of the risk of prolonged vasoconstriction.[66]

The antimigraine drugs ergotamine, methysergide, and sumatriptan are generally contraindicated in patients with obstructive coronary artery disease.[67]

Weight-Loss Medications

Dexfenfluramine and the combination of fenfluramine and phentermine may cause valvular heart disease (Chaps. 56, 57, and 59).[68–72] These agents had been prescribed for weight loss in obese patients, but dexfenfluramine and fenfluramine were withdrawn from the market in 1997 when up to 30 percent of users were reported to develop asymptomatic valve regurgitation.[69] Later reports suggested a lower incidence of problems, including reports of valvular regurgitation in approximately

7 percent of dexfenfluramine-treated patients versus 2 to 5 percent of controls.[70] The true incidence of valvular problems is uncertain and differences in reported cases may be secondary to differences in length of therapy, time from therapy to cardiac evaluation, and methods used to determine abnormalities. Mild aortic regurgitation is the most common finding. Abnormalities often improve with cessation of therapy.[71,72]

Histamine H_2-Receptor Antagonists

The histamine H_2-receptor antagonists have rarely been associated with cardiac effects. Episodes of severe bradycardia have been reported as well as hypotension, asystole, and ventricular arrhythmias. These complications have generally occurred with large doses given intravenously.[73] Electrophysiologic studies have not demonstrated any direct effect on sinus node function.[74]

Chloroquine

The antimalarial agent chloroquine is commonly used to treat collagen vascular and dermatologic disorders. Irreversible retinal damage is the primary concern with long-term or high-dose therapy. Skeletal myopathy and less commonly cardiomyopathy may occur. With cardiac involvement, features of restrictive cardiomyopathy are most common. Myocardial biopsy with analysis by electron microscopy showing curvilinear and myeloid bodies is diagnostic. These findings may be seen on skeletal muscle biopsy. The ECG may demonstrate T-wave changes and conduction abnormalities. Acute chloroquine poisoning results in hypotension, tachycardia, and prolongation of the QRS and is often fatal.[75,76]

Oral Contraceptive Agents

Epidemiologic studies prior to the 1980s demonstrated that women using oral contraceptives had an increased risk of cardiovascular disease, including venous thromboembolism, myocardial infarction, hypertension, and stroke.[128] Oral contraceptive formulations used in the 1960s and 1970s consisted of relatively high-dose estrogen. Although rare, the risk of myocardial infarction was increased approximately fourfold. Women smokers, particularly those older than age 35, had a dramatically increased risk of infarction. Coronary angiography done postinfarction not uncommonly demonstrated a discrete lesion in a single vessel or no obstructive lesions, suggesting acute thrombosis as a possible mechanism. The risk of venous thromboembolism was 4 to 10 times that of nonusers during this era.[77,80]

Recent formulations of oral contraceptives consist of less than 50 μg of ethinyl estradiol in combination with a low-dose progestin. Recent studies suggest that these second- and third-generation combined oral contraceptives are much safer in terms of cardiovascular complications.[77] The risks of venous thromboembolism and myocardial infarction are significantly reduced compared with the first-generation agents. Hypertension is rare, and the risk of stroke in otherwise healthy women is only minimally increased.[78]

Third-generation oral contraceptives that contain desogestrol or gestodene are reportedly associated with a 1.5 to 2.5 increased risk of venous thromboembolism compared with the second-generation agents. The significance of this finding has generated controversy, but generally, the cardiovascular risk profile of these agents is considered favorable. However, smokers greater than 35 years of age should use a nonestrogen contraceptive.[77–80]

Anabolic Steroids

Illicit use of androgens has been identified as a problem in competitive athletes and body builders. It is estimated that 300,000 persons in the United States have had recent steroid use and over 1 million have had prior use.[81–83] Anabolic steroids, including testosterone, stanozolol, and nandrolone, are frequently used in combination and at high doses for intermittent periods of several weeks to months. Doses commonly exceed 100 times the doses used for medical purposes.[81] Animal data indicate that these agents can cause abnormal lipids, left ventricular hypertrophy, increased blood volume, and hypertension. Data on human toxicity are limited but suggest similar toxicity.[84] Stanozolol and nandrolone reduce total high-density lipoprotein levels by over 50 percent and increase low-density lipoprotein levels by over 30 percent.[85] Isolated reports of young men (<age 35) developing severe coronary atherosclerosis, myocardial infarctions, or stroke exist in the literature.[81,86] Because of the secrecy surrounding the use of these agents, the full clinical significance of abuse is not known.

Cocaine

Cocaine is a common drug of abuse associated with potentially lethal cardiac toxicity. It is estimated that over 30 million Americans have used cocaine at least once and that 5 million use it regularly.[87] Cocaine may be swallowed, inhaled nasally, smoked, or injected intravenously. Cardiovascular toxicity is broad, ranging from sudden death to chronic cardiomyopathy.[88] A summary of the cardiovascular syndrome associated with illicit cocaine use is shown in Table 71-3. Use of cocaine with other drugs

TABLE 71-3 Cardiovascular Complications of Cocaine

Sudden death
Acute myocardial infarction
Chest pain without myocardial infarction
Accelerated coronary atherosclerosis
Intimal hyperplasia of coronary vessels
Electrocardiographic abnormalities
Sinus tachycardia
Premature ventricular complexes
Ventricular tachycardia
Torsades de pointes
Ventricular fibrillation
Prolongation of QT interval
Early repolarization (ST-segment changes)
Acute reversible myocarditis
Dilated cardiomyopathy
Acute severe hypertension
Acute aortic dissection, rupture
Pneumopericardium
Stroke
Subarachnoid hemorrhage
Endocarditis (intravenous use)

such as ethanol[89] or tobacco[90] may have combined detrimental effects. Cardiovascular susceptibility in an individual is difficult to predict due to the lack of dose-response relationship and the high degree of variability in the individual response to cocaine.[91]

Cocaine has a generalized sympathomimetic effect and has local anesthetic properties.[88] It blocks the reuptake of norepinephrine and dopamine on preganglionic sympathetic nerve terminals. This produces sympathetic stimulation both centrally and peripherally. These catecholamine effects acutely result in tachycardia, hypertension, increased myocardial contractility, and vascular constriction. The local anesthetic effect, occurring through blockade of the fast sodium channel, results in slowed conduction in myocardial tissues. This may result in ECG abnormalities, including prolongation of the PR, QRS, and QT intervals, similar to those seen with toxicity from type I antiarrhythmic agents. These effects increase the vulnerability to reentrant ventricular arrhythmias.[87,88,92]

Use of cocaine may result in increased thrombogenicity.[88,90] Platelet aggregation is enhanced and endothelial function is altered,[94] resulting in the potential for development of coronary thrombosis in the absence of coronary atherosclerosis. Chronic use of cocaine is associated with premature coronary atherosclerosis.[88,93] Cocaine indirectly causes constriction of both diseased and nondiseased coronary artery segments, but its effect is more marked in diseased vessels. Ethanol use and tobacco smoking may worsen the potential for vasospasm.[89,90] In up to one-third of reported cases, patients with cocaine-induced myocardial infarctions have normal coronary arteries.[88] The combined cardiac effects—including early coronary atherosclerosis, coronary vasospasm, increased thrombogenicity, increased myocardial oxygen demands, and proarrhythmic effects—make this drug a lethal threat to users of all ages.

Cocaine may produce direct or indirect myocardial toxicity. Animal studies suggest a direct negative inotropic effect on the heart, possibly related to its local anesthetic properties. Chronic dosing has demonstrated myocardial contraction bands, myofibrillar disorganization, interstitial edema, and mitochondrial swelling. Mononuclear infiltrates have been noted. Myocardial changes may mimic those seen with catecholamine excess, as in pheochromocytoma. Clinical case reports have described transient toxic cardiomyopathy, acute myocarditis, and permanently dilated cardiomyopathy.[88]

Chest pain is the most common reason for cocaine users to seek medical attention. Over 64,000 patients are evaluated annually for cocaine-related chest pain, of whom over half are admitted to the hospital.[95] The evaluation of cocaine-related chest pain is difficult. Prospective studies demonstrate that approximately 6 percent of patients presenting to an emergency department with cocaine-related chest pain have myocardial infarction. These patients are often young men without other risk factors for coronary artery disease except for tobacco smoking. The duration and quality of discomfort does not readily distinguish those eventually noted to have enzyme documentation of infarction. Many young patients have early repolarization patterns with ST elevation in leads V_1 to V_3, a normal variant that may be confused with acute infarction. Infarction has been noted in patients with normal or nonspecific ECGs. Because of the difficulty in excluding myocardial infarctions, patients are often monitored for a period of at least 12 h until enzymes have excluded infarction (Chaps. 40 and 42).[87]

Treatment strategies for cocaine-induced myocardial ischemia have been developed based on the known cardiac and nervous system toxicity of the drug.[87,92] Randomized prospective trials of therapy do not exist. Patients presenting with anxiety, tachycardia, or hypertension may respond well to benzodiazepines. Nitroglycerin may reverse coronary vasoconstriction induced by cocaine. Aspirin may prevent thrombus formation. Patients not responding to these measures may benefit from the alpha-adrenergic antagonist phentolamine or from calcium channel blocker therapy with verapamil.[87] Beta-adrenergic antagonists have been avoided because of the potential of enhanced coronary vasoconstriction and for unopposed alpha-mediated hypertensive crisis. Combined alpha and beta blockade with labetalol has been utilized to treat tachyarrhythmias but is not an accepted therapy for myocardial ischemia.[87] However, the bias against beta blockade is undergoing clinical reevaluation with recognition that beta blockers may block the hyperadrenergic effects that result in thrombosis and vasospasm.[96]

In documented myocardial infarction, thrombolytic therapy is highly effective; however, over 40 percent of patients without infarction will meet accepted ECG criteria for use of lytic therapy.[97] The early repolarization pattern common in young men makes diagnosis difficult, particularly when a prior ECG is not available. Thrombolytic therapy carries increased risk of hemorrhagic stroke in patients with recently uncontrolled hypertension. Therefore emergent coronary angiography may be necessary to document coronary occlusion as well as direct strategies such as primary angioplasty or thrombolysis[147] (see Chap. 42).

Management of supraventricular or ventricular tachyarrhythmias may be facilitated by administration of benzodiazepines. Rhythm disturbances may be exacerbated by acidosis or electrolyte disorders. Intravenous sodium bicarbonate and magnesium may be beneficial. Lidocaine should be used cautiously because of concerns of lowered seizure threshold and potential proarrhythmic effects following recent cocaine use.[92]

Patients with cocaine-associated chest pain not related to myocardial infarction have a favorable 1-year prognosis, particularly if cocaine use is discontinued. Urgent diagnostic cardiac evaluation is not generally recommended. Unfortunately, recurrent cocaine use after cocaine-associated chest pain occurs in over 60 percent of cases.[87]

Methamphetamines

The biologic effects of methamphetamines are similar to those of cocaine, but vasoconstriction is less. Cardiovascular toxicity is common and includes tachycardia, hypertension, and arrhythmias. Chest pain and myocardial infarction are less common than with cocaine.[98] Chronic use may result in a catecholamine-mediated dilated cardiomyopathy.

ELECTRICAL INJURY

Environmental Accidents

Accidental contact with electricity may occur in the home, where young children are particularly vulnerable.[100] Job-related electrical injuries are most common in construction and electrical workers but may also occur on any job in which electrical equipment is used, including the health care setting. Approximately 1200 deaths related to domestic electrical injury occur each year in the United States. There are two to three times as many serious injuries, including burns and neurologic complications.[101] Lightning kills at least 100 people per year in the United States, representing a 30 percent mortality rate in reported cases. Lightning injuries generally occur between May and September in the late afternoon hours, and affect predominantly young people involved in outdoor recreational activities.[102] Death following electrical shock is usually secondary to immediate cardiac rhythm disturbances, although later cardiac complications secondary to internal injury may occur.

PATHOPHYSIOLOGY

The degree of total body injury from electricity is determined by the amount of current delivered, tissue resistance, and duration of contact. Specific organs or tissues injured are in part determined by the path of the current. Electrical injuries are classified as high-voltage (>1000 V) or low-voltage (<1000 V). High-voltage electrical wires and household current (120 or 220 V) are alternating currents (AC) that may result in prolonged exposure due to tetatanic muscle contractions and inability of the victim to "let go." The frequencies of domestically generated AC (50 to 60 cycles per second) result in an increased risk for ventricular fibrillation even at household voltages.[101] Sources of domestic direct current (DC) are usually low-voltage (3 to 24 V), including batteries, appliance transformers, and portable emergency generators and are less likely to cause injury. Lightning is extremely high voltage direct current of brief duration.

Heat injury tissue necrosis is more severe with high-voltage AC. These burns are often internal and may mimic crush injuries. Tissue resistance to current flow is least in nervous and vascular tissues; therefore the heart and neurovascular bundles may serve as conduits for electrical current through the thorax. Arm-to-arm pathway of current is associated with greater risk for cardiac injury, followed by arm-to-leg pathways determined by entry and exit sites. A stride potential, leg to leg, is infrequently associated with cardiac effects.

CARDIOVASCULAR EFFECTS

Cardiac damage in electrical injury may occur as a result of contusion injury or myocardial necrosis or may be in part related to massive release of catecholamines. Typical symptoms or signs of myocardial damage may be absent. Lightning injuries result from brief, high-voltage direct current. Immediate death may be secondary to asystole or ventricular fibrillation or may result from apnea secondary to injury of the central respiratory centers. Lightning strikes may occur by a direct hit, side splash, or ground strike. Direct hits cause mechanical trauma to organs secondary to dissipated energy. Strikes to the chest can result in severe, often reversible global myocardial dysfunction or localized myocardial contusion. ECG abnormalities, including QT_c prolongation and ST-T abnormalities, may be the result of cardiac or neurologic injury. ST elevation has been noted with direct strikes. Conduction abnormalities, including right bundle branch block and complete heart block, have been noted. Pericardial effusions may develop following direct strikes. Elevated levels of CK-MB are generally noted.[102] Splash strikes in which a tree or other object is hit prior to the victim's being hit are associated with CK-MB release in less than two-thirds of patients. Severe myocardial injury is unlikely unless there is a short distance between the directly hit object and the victim. Ground strikes generally do not cause a significant cardiac injury but may be associated with nonspecific ST-T abnormalities.

Domestic alternating current accidents may cause myocardial necrosis and conduction abnormalities. An injury pattern mimicking infarction may be seen on the ECG but is generally related to direct myocardial injury and not from coronary thrombosis.[165] Household voltages (120 to 220 V) may cause sudden death, particularly when they involve arm-to-arm pathways or low skin resistance in a wet victim. Serious myocardial damage is rare.[100]

Treatment for cardiac arrest should be initiated immediately after the patient is disconnected from the current source. Resuscitation efforts should be continued for a prolonged period. In lightning strikes involving multiple victims, attention should be directed first to those who are "apparently dead." This is because there is a higher resuscitation rate for these individuals than for those with medical cardiac arrest. Of note, lightning victims with vital signs generally survive without immediate medical attention.[103]

Patients surviving high-voltage injuries generally require admission, usually for attention to neurologic complications and internal or external burn injuries and less commonly for cardiac monitoring. An initially normal ECG carries a favorable cardiac prognosis, leading some authors to question the need for 24-h ECG monitoring. Patients with arm-to-arm or arm-to-leg passage of current may be at risk for postadmission rhythm disturbances; a higher index of suspicion is required in such patients. Adults and children presenting to the emergency department following low-voltage shocks of less than 240 V have a low incidence of myocardial injury and most do not require further monitoring.[100]

Electroconvulsive Therapy

Electroconvulsive therapy (ECT) is accepted for the treatment of a variety of psychiatric illnesses including depression resistant to pharmacologic therapy, severe suicidal ideation with vegetative signs, acute mania, and depression with intolerance to medication side effects secondary to cardiac problems[104] (see also Chap. 80). ECT involves a brief unilateral or bilateral electrical stimulus to the brain while the patient is under short-acting anesthesia with a hypnotic drug and a muscle depolarizing agent.[105] The shock produces brief, intense stimulation of the central nervous system. Cardiovascular complications may result from this stimulation or from the drugs used to modify the response.[106,107]

Initially, the ECT stimulus activates the vagus nerve and may produce bradycardia, hypotension, and rarely asystole. Sympathetic discharge occurs, which is amplified by a 15-fold rise in epinephrine and 3-fold rise in norepinephrine levels, resulting in tachycardia and hypertension. Transient atrial and ventricular tachyarrhythmias may occur in approximately 10 percent of patients with known or suspected cardiovascular disease. Transient ECG alterations—including ST-T-wave changes, QRS changes, QT prolongation, and peaked T waves—may occur.[104–108]

The mortality rate of ECT is less than 3 in 10,000, and the complication rate is approximately 0.3 percent. Patients with severe heart disease may successfully undergo ECT with acceptable risk. Prior to ECT, electrolyte abnormalities should be

TABLE 71-4 Plants with Cardiac Glycoside Effects

Foxglove (*Digitalis purpurea, D. Lanata*)
Oleander (*Nerium oleander*)
Lily-of-the-valley (*Convallaria majolis*)
Christmas rose (*Helleborus niger*)
Wallflower (*Cheirina cheiri*)
Milkweed (*Asclepias* sp.)

corrected and systemic hypertension should be controlled. Patients with pulmonary disease require special evaluation, because hypoxia and respiratory acidosis may precipitate cardiovascular events.[104]

Following ECT, hypertension and tachycardia may be controlled with adrenergic blockade with intravenous labetalol[109] or esmolol.[107] Other antihypertensive agents such as clonidine or calcium channel blockers may be utilized. Sustained ventricular arrhythmias are treated with lidocaine, but pretreatment with lidocaine is not indicated.[104] Patients with cardiac pacemakers can safely undergo ECT.[110] Currently used pacemakers are not likely to be affected by ECT current. Although these newer devices have not been systematically studied, the 50 to 100 W delivered to the scalp during ECT are probably inadequate to reprogram current pacemakers.

Lithotripsy

Extracorporeal shock wave lithotripsy used to treat renal stones and gallstones has the potential to cause cardiac arrhythmias. Rhythm disturbances may be related to electrical stimulus from the shock wave or from enhanced vagal tone associated with the procedure. Electrocardiographic monitoring is recommended for patients with cardiac disease. Gating of the shock waves to the QRS cycle may be necessary in high-risk patients, although ungated lithotripsy with newer devices is reportedly safe in most patients.[111,112]

POISONS

Plants

A variety of plants contain active cardiac glycosides. Ingestion of these plants may result in a clinical presentation similar to that of digoxin toxicity, including gastrointestinal and visual disturbances as well as dysrhythmias. Plants with cardiac glycoside–like effects[113] are listed (Table 71-4).

Herbal Therapies

The use of herbal treatments and nonprescription remedies is increasing among patients. In one study, 38 percent of congestive heart failure patients questioned were using herbal products.[114] Herbal medicines may contain varying doses and contaminants and are not subject to regulations governing safety and efficacy. Serious adverse effects and drug interactions may therefore occur. The cardiac effects of some herbal remedies are listed in Table 71-5.[115–117]

Snakes and Scorpions

Snake bites cause fewer than 15 deaths per year in the United States but over 40,000 deaths per year worldwide. The majority of lethal snake bites occur in Asia, South America, and Africa. Snake venoms contain a variety of enzymes and toxins that may affect the nervous system, blood vessels, coagulation systems, or heart. The majority of deaths are from the elapids (cobra, mamba, coral snake, taipan), the bites of which cause severe neuromuscular toxicity. Cardiotoxins are present in variable amounts in snake venom. Cobra venoms may cause augmentation of myocardial contraction at low concentration and asystole at high concentration. Rattlesnake venom may affect myocardial sodium channels and depress myocardial contractility. These venoms may cause pulmonary hypertension.[118]

TABLE 71-5 Cardiac Effects of Common Herbal Therapies

Aconite (in Chinese herbal medicines)	Arrhythmias via QT prolongation
Adonis vernalis (pheasant's eye)	Sudden death
Caulophyllum thalictroides (blue cohosh)	Neonatal heart failure, contains cardiac glycosides
Cimicifuga (black cohosh)	Bradycardia
Corydalis racemosa (dl-tetrahydropalmatine)	Hypotension
Corynanthe johimbe (yohimbe)	Hypo- or hypertension, tachycardia
Danshen	Increased bleeding risk with warfarin
Delphinium (larkspur)	Myocardial depression, arrhythmias
Digitalis purpurea (foxglove)	Arrhythmias, heart block
Ephedra (ma huang)	Hypertension, arrhythmias, palpitations, death
Feverfew	Decreased platelet activity
Garlic	Increased bleeding risk with anticoagulants
Ginger	Increased bleeding risk with anticoagulants
Ginkgo	Decreased platelet activity
Hawthorne	Hypotension at high doses
Lingusticum wallichii	Inhibits platelet aggregation, hypotension
Licorice	Hypokalemia, arrhythmias, hypertension
Stephania tetrandra	Interferes with calcium channel blockers, myocardial depressant, hypotension
Tripterygium wilfordii (hook F)	Hypotension, circulatory collapse
Veratrum (hellebore)	Bradycardia, hypotension

SOURCE: From Ernst,[115] Vann,[116] and Yu et al.[117]

Scorpion stings are a common medical problem in areas including India, Southeast Asia, the southwestern United States, Mexico, and Israel. Venoms from different families have different toxicities. The *Buthidae* venoms, primarily neurotoxic, result in spontaneous sympathetic and parasympathetic depolarization. Massive catecholamine release may cause cardiac toxicity, including tachycardia, hypertension, arrhythmias, and myocardial impairment.[119,120]

Arthropods

Direct cardiac effects related to bee, hornet, and wasp stings are difficult to establish. Cardiac complications, including arrhythmias, are generally related to anaphylaxis or epinephrine administration. Animal studies of bee venom toxicity suggest direct cardiac effects.[121,122]

Marine Toxins

Exposure to marine toxins may have serious cardiovascular effects. The venom of scorpion fish can cause sympathetic and parasympathetic discharges. Rhythm disturbances and heart failure may result. Stingray venom contains phosphodiesterases and has rarely been associated with cardiac rhythm disturbances. Ingestion of sea cucumber, which contains holothurin, may result in cardiac glycoside toxicity. Ingestion of pufferfish, which contain tetrodotoxin, may result in vascular collapse and severe bradycardia.[118,123]

Halogenated Hydrocarbons

Halogenated hydrocarbons are used in fire extinguishers, solvents, and refrigerants and in the manufacture of pesticides and plastics. Heavy acute exposure to these compounds may result in cardiac arrhythmias and sudden death.[124] Direct cardiac effects include depression of myocardial contractility and sensitization to the arrhythmogenic effects of catecholamines. Indirect cardiotoxicity may result from hypoxia or central nervous system toxicity.[125]

Organophosphates

Organophosphates, used commercially in pesticides, are powerful inhibitors of acetylcholinesterase, and this inhibition can result in parasympathetic overstimulation. Suicide attempts account for the majority of fatalities associated with ingestion of large doses of organophosphates. Signs and symptoms of ingestion include respiratory depression, bronchospasm and secretion, and pulmonary edema. Deaths are generally related to respiratory failure. Cardiac toxicity is generally associated with QT prolongation. Torsades de pointes, atrioventricular conduction disturbances, and ST-T abnormalities have been noted. Cardiac arrhythmias have been noted up to 15 days after exposure. Direct myocardial toxicity has been postulated, in addition to cholinergic hyperactivity.[126] Treatment includes atropine administration at doses sufficient to dry mucous membranes and to increase heart rate to 100 beats per minute. Obidoxime therapy has also been studied in severe overdoses.[127]

Carbon Monoxide

Toxicity from carbon monoxide is related to tissue hypoxia. Carbon monoxide has a much higher affinity for hemoglobin than does oxygen, preventing adequate oxygen exchange. Carbon monoxide exposure worsens angina pectoris and increases the risk of myocardial infarction. Carbon monoxide poisoning results in ECG abnormalities, including sinus tachycardia, atrial fibrillation, atrioventricular block, and ST-T abnormalities. Cardiac enzyme elevation may occur. Severe exposure can result in myocardial necrosis and cardiomyopathy.[128] Transient evidence of cardiac toxicity, however, is not necessarily associated with long-term sequelae.[129]

RADIATION

Mediastinal radiation—commonly used to treat Hodgkin's disease, lung cancer, breast cancer, and seminoma—may result in acute or late cardiac sequelae. Prior to the 1960s, the heart was thought to be resistant to the effects of clinical radiation. It is now recognized that a variety of cardiac problems may result from radiation, including acute or chronic pericardial disease, coronary atherosclerosis, myocardial dysfunction, conduction defects, and, occasionally, valvular dysfunction (Table 71-6).[130,131]

The incidence of radiation-induced heart disease is influenced by several factors, including total radiation dose, fraction size, volume of heart irradiated, concomitant anthracycline use, and presence of mediastinal tumor.[130] Improved radiation techniques have diminished the occurrence of acute or chronic cardiac toxicity.[132] Cardiac injury has generally been associated with doses above 40 Gy.[130] Increased toxicity is associated with radiation for Hodgkin's disease, where larger volumes of the heart are irradiated, compared to the small cardiac exposure given as adjuvant treatment for breast carcinoma. Large doses per fraction and anterior-weighted fields result in greater toxicity.[133]

Pericardial disease is the most common manifestation of radiation toxicity to the heart. With the current techniques of subcarinal shielding, equal weighting of anterior and posterior ports, and limiting the dose to less than 30 Gy, the incidence of clinical pericarditis is approximately 2.5 percent.[132] Anatomic changes of the pericardium occur in the majority of patients but are clinically silent. Clinically apparent pericarditis is most frequent 4 to 6 months after therapy. Acute pericarditis, asymptomatic pericardial effusion, or pericardial tamponade may occur. Other etiologies of pericarditis should be considered,

TABLE 71-6 Radiation-induced Cardiac Disease

Pericardial
Acute pericarditis
Chronic pericarditis
Pericardial constriction
Coronary atherosclerosis
Restrictive cardiomyopathy
Dilated cardiomyopathy (concomitant anthracyclines)
Conduction disease
Valvular abnormalities

particularly malignant involvement of the pericardium. Pericarditis occurring during treatment of a mediastinal mass contiguous to the heart is generally secondary to tumor effects and does not correlate with late pericardial complications.[134,135]

Radiation may cause an exudative pericarditis. Cellular infiltrate is uncommon. Pericardial fibrosis may follow secondary to fibroblast proliferation and collagen deposition. The majority of patients with pericardial effusion recover spontaneously.[130] Constrictive pericarditis may occur months to years after pericardial effusion or may develop in patients without previously recognized pericardial disease.

The majority of patients with pericardial disease have a relatively benign course. Treatment is based on symptoms, including pericardiocentesis for tamponade and antipyretics for fever. Animal data suggest possible benefit from steroids.[130]

The surgical management of postirradiation constrictive pericarditis is difficult.[134] Extensive mediastinal and pericardial fibrosis make pericardiectomy technically challenging. Surgical morbidity and mortality are significant. Radiation-induced constriction is often associated with coronary atherosclerosis, myocardial dysfunction, or conduction and valvular abnormalities. Comorbid cardiac or general medical conditions should be considered when patients are selected for pericardiectomy.

Clinically important myocardial dysfunction related to radiation generally occurs in combination with pericardial disease. Asymptomatic patients may have varying degrees of myocardial fibrosis. The anterior right ventricle is most susceptible. Areas of fibrosis may be patchy or diffuse. Noninvasive techniques such as echocardiography may show mild impairment of systolic function; however, this is usually not clinically significant.[132] Diastolic abnormalities may occur due to fibrosis.

Restrictive cardiomyopathy has been reported but is rare.[130] Premature coronary artery disease may result from radiation therapy, particularly in patients who were irradiated in an era when cardioprotective techniques were not used. Several series have reported a significantly increased risk of coronary artery disease years following therapeutic radiation involving cardiac exposure.[135] The Stockholm Trial demonstrated increased mortality secondary to coronary artery disease in women receiving high-dose radiation to the heart as adjuvant therapy for carcinoma of the left breast.[135] A review of 635 patients at Stanford treated for Hodgkin's disease before age 21 between the years 1961 and 1991 showed a significantly increased risk for myocardial infarction.[136,137] It is not clear, however, whether present techniques of mediastinal radiation will result in a clinically significant increase in coronary events. Percutaneous angioplasty and coronary bypass surgery have been successful in selected patients. The commonly associated mediastinal and pericardial fibrosis, however, make surgical revascularization more difficult.[130]

Clinically significant valvular heart disease secondary to radiation is rare but, when present, usually involves the aortic or mitral valves.[130,131] Fibrous thickening of the cardiac valves has been noted at autopsy. This thickening often causes asymptomatic aortic or mitral regurgitation.[138] Coexisting pericardial disease is the rule. Symptoms related to valvular dysfunction have been noted to occur 15 to 40 years after radiation treatment. Surgical reports are rare and most commonly are for replacement of the aortic valve due to aortic stenosis.[131]

Radiation may result in fibrosis of the nodal and infranodal pathways. Complete atrioventricular block, right bundle branch block, and, less commonly, left bundle branch block may occur. Progression to complete heart block is rare.

References

1. Frishman WH, Sung HM, Yee HCM, et al. Cardiovascular toxicity with cancer chemotherapy. *Curr Probl Cardiol* 1996; 21:225–288.
2. Shan K, Lincoff AM, Young JB. Anthracycline-induced cardiomyopathy. *Ann Intern Med* 1996; 125:47–58.
3. Von Hoff DD, Layard MW, Basa P, et al. Risk factors for doxorubicin-induced congestive heart failure. *Ann Intern Med* 1979; 91:710–717.
4. Bristow MR, Mason JW, Billingham ME, Daniels JR. Doxorubicin cardiomyopathy: Evaluation of phonocardiography, endomyocardial biopsy, and cardiac catheterization. *Ann Intern Med* 1978; 88:168–175.
5. Lipschultz SE, Lipsitz SR, Mone SM, et al. Female sex and higher drug dose as risk factors for late cardiotoxic effects of doxorubicin therapy for childhood cancer. *N Engl J Med* 1995; 332:1738–1743.
6. Singal PK, Iliskovic N, Li T, Kumar D. Adriamycin cardiomyopathy: Pathophysiology and prevention. *FASEB J* 1997; 11:931–936.
7. Moreg JS, Oglon DJ. Outcomes of clinical congestive heart failure induced by anthracycline chemotherapy. *Cancer* 1992; 70:2637–2641.
8. Steinherz J, Graham T, Hurwitz R, et al. Guidelines for cardiac monitoring of children during and after anthracycline therapy: Report of the Cardiology Committee of the Children's Cancer Study Group. *Pediatrics* 1992; 89:942–949.
9. Weegner KM, Bledsoe M, Chauvenet A, Wofford M. Exercise echocardiography in the detection of anthracycline cardiotoxicity. *Cancer* 1991; 68:435–438.
10. Schwartz RG, McKenzie WB, Alexander J, et al. Congestive heart failure and left ventricular dysfunction complicating doxorubicin therapy: Seven-year experience using radionuclide angiocardiography. *Am J Med* 1987; 82:1109–1118.
11. McKillop JH, Bristow MR, Goris ML, et al. Sensitivity and specificity of radionuclide ejection fraction in doxorubicin cardiotoxicity. *Am Heart J* 1983; 106:1048–1056.
12. Isner JM, Ferrans VJ, Cohen SR, et al. Clinical and morphologic cardiac findings after anthracycline chemotherapy: Analysis of 64 patients studied at necropsy. *Am J Cardiol* 1983; 51:1167–1174.
13. Steinherz LJ, Steinherz PG, Tan CTC, et al. Cardiac toxicity 4 to 20 years after completing anthracycline therapy. *JAMA* 1991; 266:1672–1677.
14. Leandro J, Dyck J, Poppe D, et al. Cardiac dysfunction late after cardiotoxic therapy for childhood cancer. *Am J Cardiol* 1994; 74:1152–1156.
15. Legha SS, Benjamin RS, MacKay B, et al. Reduction of doxorubicin cardiotoxicity by prolonged continuous intravenous infusion. *Ann Intern Med* 1982; 89:133–139.
16. Siveski-Iliskovic N, Hill M, Chow DA, Signal PK. Probucol protects against adriamycin cardiomyopathy without interfering with its antitumor effect. *Circulation* 1995; 91:10–15.
17. Seifert CF, Nesser ME, Thompson DF. Dexrazoxane in the prevention of doxorubicin-induced cardiotoxicity. *Ann Pharmacother* 1994; 28:1063–1072.
18. Benjamin RS. Rationale for the use of mitoxantrone in the older patient: Cardiac toxicity. *Semin Oncol* 1995; 22:11–13.
19. Feenstra J, Grobbee DE, Remme WJ, Stricker BH. Drug induced heart failure. *J Am Coll Cardiol* 1999; 33:1152–1162.
20. Robben NC, Pippas AW, Moore JO. The syndrome of 5-fluorouracil cardiotoxicity: An elusive cardiopathy. *Cancer* 1993; 71:493–509.
21. Akhtar SS, Salim KP, Bano ZA. Symptomatic cardiotoxicity with

high dose 5-fluorouracil infusion: A prospective study. *Oncology* 1993; 50:441–445.

22. Weiss RB, Grillo-Lopez AJ, Marsoni S, et al. Amsacrine-associated cardiotoxicity: An analysis of 82 cases. *J Clin Oncol* 1986; 4:918–928.
23. Rowinsky EK, Donchower RC. Paclitaxel (taxol). *N Engl J Med* 1995; 332:1004–1014.
24. McNeil C. Herceptin raises its sights beyond advanced breast cancer. *J Natl Cancer Inst* 1998; 90:882–883.
25. DuBois JS, Udelson JE, Atkins B. Severe reversible, global and regional ventricular dysfunction associated with high-dose interleukin-2 immunotherapy. *J Immunother* 1995; 18:119–123.
26. Roose SP, Dalak GW. Treating the depressed patient with cardiovascular problems. *J Clin Psychiatry* 1992; 53(9, suppl):25–31.
27. Fraser-Smith N, Lesperance F, Talajic M. Depression following myocardial infarction: Impact on 6-month survival. *JAMA* 1993; 270:1819–1825.
28. Glassman AH, Roose SP, Bigger JT. The safety of tricyclic antidepressants in cardiac patients—Risk benefit reconsidered. *JAMA* 1993; 269:2673–2675.
29. Franco-Bronson K. The management of treatment-resistant depression in the medically ill. *Psychiatr Clin North Am* 1996; 19:329–348.
30. Glassman AH, Preud'home XA. Review of the cardiovascular effects of heterocyclic antidepressants. *J Clin Psychiatry* 1983; 54(2, suppl):16–22.
31. Roose SP, Glassman AH, Gardina EGV, et al. Tricyclic antidepressants in depressed patients with cardiac conduction disease. *Arch Gen Psychiatry* 1987; 44:273–275.
32. The Cardiac Arrhythmia Suppression Trial II Investigators. Effect of the antiarrhythmic agent moricizine on survival after myocardial infarction. *N Engl J Med* 1992; 327:227–233.
33. Wolfe TR, Caravati EM, Rollin DE. Terminal 40-ms frontal plane QRS axis as a marker for tricyclic antidepressant overdose. *Ann Emerg Med* 1989; 18:348–351.
34. Shanon M. Toxicology reviews: Targeted management strategies for cardiovascular toxicity from tricyclic antidepressant overdose: The pivotal role for alkalinization and sodium loading. *Pediatr Emerg Care* 1998; 14:293–298.
35. Ciraulo DA, Shader RI. Fluoxetine drug-drug interactions: I. Antidepressants and antipsychotics. *J Clin Psychopharmacol* 1990; 10:48–50.
36. Sheline YI, Freedland KE, Carney RM. How safe are serotonin reuptake inhibitors for depression in patients with coronary heart disease? *Am J Med* 1997; 102:54–59.
37. Strik JJMH, Honig A, Lousberg R, et al. Cardiac side effects to two selective serotonin reuptake inhibitors in middle-aged and elderly depressed patients. *Int Clin Psychopharmacol* 1998; 13:263–267.
38. Rudorfer MV, Manji HK, Potter WZ. Comparative tolerability profiles of the newer versus older antidepressants. *Drug Safety* 1994; 10:18–46.
39. Rosenqvist M, Bergfeldt L, Aili H, et al. Sinus node dysfunction during long-term lithium treatment. *Br Heart J* 1993; 70:371–375.
40. Numata T, Abe H, Terao T, et al. Possible involvement of hypothyroidism as a cause of lithium-induced sinus node dysfunction. *PACE* 1999; 22:954–957.
41. Simard M, Gumbiner B, Lee A, et al. Lithium carbonate intoxication: A case report and review of the literature. *Arch Intern Med* 1989; 149:36–46.
42. Kemper AJ, Dunlap R, Pietro DA. Thioridazine-induced torsade de pointes: Successful therapy with isoproterenol. *JAMA* 1983; 249:2931–2934.
43. Di Salvo TG, O'Gara PT. Torsades de pointes caused by high-dose intravenous haloperidol in cardiac patients. *Clin Cardiol* 1995; 18:285–290.
44. Haverkamp W, Shenasa M, Borggrefe M, Breithardt G. Torsades de pointes. In: Zipes DP, Jalife J, eds. *Cardiac Electrophysiology: From Cell to Bedside*, 2nd ed. Philadelphia: Saunders; 1995: 885–899.
45. Orban Z, MacDonald LL, Peters MA, Guslits B. Erythromycin-induced cardiac toxicity. *Am J Cardiol* 1995; 75:859–861.
46. Lopez JA, Harold JG, Rosenthal ML, et al. QT prolongation and torsades de pointes after administration of trimethoprim-sulfamethoxazole. *Am J Cardiol* 1987; 59:376–377.
47. Pringle TH, Scorbie IN, Murray RG, et al. Prolongation of the QT interval during therapeutic starvation: A substrate for malignant arrhythmias. *Int J Obesity* 1983; 7:253–261.
48. Reinoehl J, Frankovich D, Machado C, et al. Probucol-associated tachyarrhythmic events and QT prolongation: Importance of gender. *Am Heart J* 1996; 131:1184–1191.
49. Vitola J, Vukanovic J, Roden D. Cisapride-induced torsades de pointes. *J Cardiovasc Electrophysiol* 1998; 9:1109–1113.
50. Priori SG. Exploring the hidden danger of noncardiac drugs. *J Cardiovasc Electrophysiol* 1998; 9:1114–1116.
51. Nemeroff CB, DeVane CL, Pollack BG. Newer antidepressants and the cytochrome P450 system. *Am J Psychiatry* 1996; 153:311–320.
52. Chen TM, Benowitz NL. Caffeine and coffee: Effects on health and cardiovascular disease. *Comp Biochem Physiol* 1994; 109C:173–189.
53. Grayboys TB, Bedell SE. Caffeine ingestion: Yet another wake-up call? *Am Heart J* 1998; 136:574–575.
54. Swagemakers JJM, Gorgels, APM, Weijenberg MP, et al. Risk indications for out-of-hospital cardiac arrest in patients with coronary artery disease. *J Clin Epidemiol* 1999; 52:601–607.
55. Sessler CN, Cohen MD. Cardiac arrhythmias during theophylline toxicity: A prospective continuous electrocardiographic study. *Chest* 1990; 98:672–678.
56. Seneff M, Scott J, Friedman B, et al. Acute theophylline toxicity and the use of esmolol to reverse cardiovascular instability. *Ann Emerg Med* 1990; 19:671–673.
57. Greenberg A, Piraino BH, Kroboth PD, Weiss J. Severe theophylline toxicity: Role of conservative measures, antiarrhythmic agents and charcoal hemoperfusion. *Am J Med* 1984; 76:854–860.
58. Lee H, Izquierdo R, Evans HE. Cardiac response to oral and aerosol administration of beta agonists. *J Pediatr* 1983; 103:655–658.
59. Martin RM, Dunn NR, Freemantle SH, Mann RD. Risk of nonfatal cardiac failure and ischemic heart disease with long acting B_2 agonists. *Thorax* 1998; 53:558–562.
60. Taylor DR, Sears MR, Cockcroft DW. The beta-agonist controversy. *Med Clin North Am* 1996; 80:719–748.
61. Koh KK, Roe IH, Lee M, et al. Variant angina complicating ergot therapy of migraine. *Chest* 1994; 105:1259–1260.
62. Roithinger FX, Punzengruber C, Gremmel F, et al. Myocardial infarction after chronic ergotamine abuse. *Eur Heart J* 1993; 14:1579–1581.
63. Redfield MM, Nicholson WJ, Edwards WD, Tajik AJ. Valve disease associated with ergot alkaloid: Echocardiographic and pathologic correlations. *Ann Intern Med* 1992; 117:50–52.
64. Allen MB, Tosh G, Walters G, Muers MF. Pleural and pericardial fibrosis after ergotamine therapy. *Respir Med* 1994; 88:67–69.
65. Mason JW, Billingham ME, Friedman JP. Methysergide-induced heart disease: A case of multivalvular and myocardial fibrosis. *Circulation* 1977; 56:889–890.
66. Liston H, Bennett L, Usher B, Nappi, J. The association of the combination of sumtriptan and methysergide in myocardial infarction in a premenopausal woman. *Arch Intern Med* 1999; 159:511–513.
67. VanDenBrink AM, Reekers M, Bax W, et al. Coronary side-effect potential of current and prospective antimigraine drugs. *Circulation* 1998; 98:25–30.
68. Connolly HM, Crary JL, McGoon MD, et al. Valvular heart

disease associated with fenfluramine-phentermine [published correction appears in *N Engl J Med* 1997; 337:1783]. *N Engl J Med* 1997; 337:581–588.
69. Cardiac valvulopathy associated with exposure to fenfluramine or dexfenfluramine: US Department of Health and Human Services interim public health recommendations, Nov 1997. *MMWR* 1997; 46:1061–1066.
70. Weissman NJ, Tighe JF Jr, Gottdiener JS, Gwynne JT. An assessment of heart valve abnormalities in obese patients taking dexfenfluramine, sustained-release dexfenfluramine, or placebo. *N Engl J Med* 1998; 339:725–732.
71. Hensrud DD, Connolly HM, Grogan M, et al. Echocardiographic improvement over time after cessation of use of fenfluramine and phentermine. *Mayo Clin Proc* 1999; 74:1191–1197.
72. Shively BK, Roldan CA, Gill EA, et al. Prevalence and determinants of valvulopathy in patients treated with dexfenfluramine. *Circulation* 1999; 100:2161–2167.
73. MacMahon B, Bakshi M, Walsh MJ. Cardiac arrhythmias after intravenous cimetidine. *N Engl J Med* 1981; 305:832–833.
74. Gould L, Reddy CVR, Singh BK, Zen B. Electrophysiologic properties of cimetidine in man. *Pacing Clin Electrophysiol* 1981; 4:3–7.
75. Cubero GI, Reguero JJ, Ortega JM. Restrictive cardiomyopathy caused by chloroquine. *Br Heart J* 1993; 69:451–452.
76. Ratliff NB, Estes ML, Myles JL, et al. Diagnosis of chloroquine cardiomyopathy by endomyocardial biopsy. *N Engl J Med* 1987; 316:191–193.
77. Rosenberg L, Begaud B, Bergan U, et al. What are the risks of third generation oral contraceptives? *Hum Reprod* 1996; 11:687–693.
78. Jick H, Jick SS, Gurewich V, et al. Risk of idiopathic cardiovascular death and nonfatal venous thromboembolism in women using oral contraceptives with differing progestagen compounds. *Lancet* 1995; 346:1589–1593.
79. Schwingl PJ, Ory HW, Visness CM. Estimates of the risk of cardiovascular death attributable to low-dose oral contraceptives in the United States. *Am J Obstet Gynecol* 1999; 180: 241–249.
80. Consensus Conference on Combination Oral Contraceptives and Cardiovascular Disease. *Fertil Steril* 1999; 71:1S–6S.
81. Bagatell CJ, Brewner WJ. Androgens in men—Uses and abuses: *N Engl J Med* 1996; 334:707–714.
82. Yesalis CE, Kennedy NK, Kopstein AN, Bahrke MS. Anabolic-adrogenic steroid use in the United States. *JAMA* 1993; 270:1217–1221.
83. Nieminen MS, Ramo MP, Viitasalo M, et al. Serious cardiovascular side effects of large doses of anabolic steroids in weight lifters. *Eur Heart J* 1996; 17:1576–1583.
84. Blue JG, Lombardo JA. Steroids and steroid-like compounds. *Clin Sports Med* 1999; 18:667–689.
85. Glazer G. Atherogenic effects of anabolic steroids on serum lipid levels: A literature review. *Arch Intern Med* 1991; 151:1925–1933.
86. Mewis C, Spyridopulous I, Kuhlkamp V, Seipel L. Manifestation of severe coronary heart disease after anabolic drug abuse. *Clin Cardiol* 1996; 19:153–155.
87. Hollander JE. The management of cocaine-associated myocardial ischemia. *N Engl J Med* 1995; 333:1267–1272.
88. Kloner RA, Hale S, Alker Rezkalla S. The effects of acute and chronic cocaine use on the heart. *Circulation* 1992; 85:407–419.
89. Pirwitz MJ, Willard JE, Landau C, et al. Influence of cocaine, ethanol, or their combination on epicardial coronary arterial dimensions in humans. *Arch Intern Med* 1995; 155:1186–1191.
90. Moliterno DJ, Willard JE, Lange RA, et al. Coronary-artery vasoconstriction induced by cocaine, cigarette smoking, or both. *N Engl J Med* 1994; 330:454–459.
91. Knuepfer MM, Mueller PJ. Review of evidence for a novel model of cocaine-induced cardiovascular toxicity. *Pharmacol Biochem Behav* 1999; 63:489–500.
92. Om A, Ellahham S, Disciascio G. Management of cocaine-induced cardiovascular complications. *Am Heart J* 1993; 125: 469–475.
93. Hollander JE, Hoffman RS, Burstein JL, et al. Cocaine-associated myocardial infarction: Mortality and complications. *Arch Intern Med* 1995; 155:1081–1086.
94. Wilbert-Lampe U, Seliger C, Zilker R, et al. Cocaine increases the endothelial release of immunoreactive endothelin and its concentrations in human plasma and urine. *Circulation* 1998; 98:385–390.
95. Hollander JE, Hoffman RS, Gennis P, et al. Prospective multicenter evaluation of cocaine associated chest pain. *Ann Emerg Med* 1994; 1:330–339.
96. Leikin JB. Cocaine and B-adrenergic blockers: A remarriage after a decade-long divorce? *Crit Care Med* 1999; 27:688–689.
97. Gitter MJ, Goldsmith SR, Dunbar DN, Sharkey SW. Cocaine and chest pain: Clinical features and outcome of patients hospitalized to rule out myocardial infarction. *Ann Intern Med* 1991; 115:277–282.
98. Derlet RW, Rice P, Horowitz BZ, Lord RV. Amphetamine toxicity: Experiences with 127 cases. *J Emerg Med* 1989; 7:157–161.
99. Hong R, Matsuyama E, Nur K. Cardiomyopathy associated with the smoking of crystal amphetamine. *JAMA* 1991; 265:1152–1154.
100. Bailey B, Gaudreauh HP, Thivierge RL, et al. Cardiac monitoring of children with household electrical injuries. *Ann Emerg Med* 1995; 25:612–617.
101. Carleton SC. Cardiac problems associated with electrical injury. *Cardiol Clin* 1995; 13:263–277.
102. Lichtenberg R, Dries D, Ward K, et al. Cardiovascular effects of lightning strikes. *J Am Coll Cardiol* 1993; 21:531–536.
103. Jain S, Bandi V. Electrical and lightning injuries. *Crit Care Clin* 1999; 15:319–331.
104. Banazak DA. Electroconvulsive therapy: A guide for family physicians. *Am Fam Physician* 1996; 53:273–278.
105. Sackeim HA, Devanand DP, Prudie J. Stimulus intensity, seizure threshold, and seizure duration: Impact on the efficacy and safety of electroconvulsive therapy. *Psychiatr Clin North Am* 1991; 14:803–843.
106. Rice EH, Sombrotto LB, Markowitz JC, Leon AC. Cardiovascular morbidity in high-risk patients during ECT. *Am J Psychiatry* 1994; 151:1637–1641.
107. O'Connor CJ, Rothenberg DM, Soble JS, et al. The effect of esmolol pretreatment on the incidence of regional wall motion abnormalities during electroconvulsive therapy. *Anesth Analg* 1996; 82:143–147.
108. Graybar G, Goethe J, Levy T, et al. Transient large upright T-wave on the electrocardiogram during multiple monitored electroconvulsive therapy. *Anesthesiology* 1983; 59:467–469.
109. Leslie JB, Kalayjiam RW, Sirgo MA, et al. Intravenous labetolol for the treatment of postoperative hypertension. *Anesthesiology* 1987; 67:413–421.
110. Abiusa P, Dunkelman R, Proper M. Electroconvulsive therapy in patients with pacemakers. *JAMA* 1978; 240:2459–2462.
111. Greenstein A, Kaver I, Lechtman V, et al. Cardiac arrhythmias during nonsynchronized extracorporeal shock wave lithotripsy. *J Urol* 1995; 154:1321–1322.
112. Zeng ZR, Lindstedt E, Roijer A, et al. Arrhythmia during extracorporeal shock wave lithotripsy. *Br J Urol* 1993; 71:10–16.
113. Mashour NH, Lin GI, Frishman WH. Herbal Medicine for the treatment of cardiovascular disease. *Arch Intern Med* 1998; 158:2225–2234.
114. Ackman ML, Campbell JB, Buzak KA, et al. Use of nonprescrip-

tion medications by patients with congestive heart failure. *Ann Pharmacother* 1999; 33:674–679.
115. Ernst E. Harmless herbs? A review of the recent literature. *Am J Med* 1998; 104:170–178.
116. Vann A. The herbal medicine boom: Understanding what patients are taking. *Cleve Clin J Med* 1998; 65:12–13.
117. Yu CM, Chan JCN, Sanderson JE. Chinese herbs and warfarin potentiation by "Danshen." *J Intern Med* 1998; 241:337–339.
118. Karalliedde L. Animal toxins. *Br J Anaesth* 1995; 75:319–327.
119. Gueron M, Ilia R, Sofer S. The cardiovascular system after scorpion envenomation: A review. *Clin Toxicol* 1992; 30:245–258.
120. Blum A, Lubezki A, Sclarovsky S. Black scorpion envenomation: Two cases and review of the literature. *Clin Cardiol* 1992; 15:377–378.
121. Horen WP. Insect and scorpion sting. *JAMA* 1972; 221:894–898.
122. Lefer AM, Curtis MT. Cardiotoxicity of naturally occurring animal peptides. In: Van Stee EW, ed. *Cardiovascular Toxicology*. New York: Raven Press; 1982; 221–258.
123. Brown CK, Shepherd SM. Marine trauma, envenomations and intoxications. *Emerg Med Clin North Am* 1992; 10:385–408.
124. Weill H. Cardiorespiratory effects of inhalant occupational exposures. *Circulation* 1981; 63:250A–252A.
125. Zakhari S, Aviado DM. Cardiovascular toxicology of aerosol propellants, refrigerants, and related solvents. In: Van Stee EW, ed. *Cardiovascular Toxicology*. New York: Raven Press; 1982:281–314.
126. Roth A, Zellinger I, Arad M, Atsmon J. Organophosphates and the heart. *Chest* 1993; 103:576–578.
127. Thiermann H, Mast U, Klimmek R, et al. Cholinesterase status, pharmacokinetics and laboratory findings during obidoxime therapy in organophosphate poisoned patients. *Hum Exp Toxicol* 1997; 16:473–480.
128. Marius-Nunez AL. Myocardial infarction with normal coronary arteries after acute exposure to carbon monoxide. *Chest* 1990; 97:491–494.
129. Roberts JR, Bain M, Klachko MN, et al. Successful heart transplantation from a victim of carbon monoxide poisoning. *Ann Emerg Med* 1995; 26:652–655.
130. Stewart JR, Fajardo LF, Gillette SM, Constine LS. Radiation injury to the heart. *Int J Radiat Oncol Biol Phys* 1995; 31:1205–1211.
131. Mittal S, Berko B, Bavaria J, Herrmann HC. Radiation-induced cardiovascular dysfunction. *Am J Cardiol* 1996; 78:114–115.
132. Arsenian MA. Cardiovascular sequelae of therapeutic thoracic radiation. *Prog Cardiovasc Dis* 1991; 33:299–311.
133. Gustavsson A, Bendahl P, Cwikiel M, et al. No serious late cardiac effects after adjuvant radiotherapy following mastectomy in premenopausal women with early breast cancer. *Int J Radiation Oncol Biol Phys* 1999; 43:745–754.
134. Ni Y, Von Segesser LK, Turina M. Futility of pericardiectomy for postirradiation constrictive pericarditis. *Ann Thorac Surg* 1990; 49:445–448.
135. Shapiro CL, Hardenbergh PH, Gelman R, et al. Cardiac effects of adjuvant doxorubicin and radiation therapy in breast cancer patients. *J Clin Oncol* 1998; 16:3493–3501.
136. Hancock SL, Donaldson SS. Radiation-related heart disease: Risks after treatment of Hodgkin's disease during childhood and adolescence. In: Bricker JT, Green DM, D'Angio GJ, eds. *Cardiac Toxicity After Treatment for Childhood Cancer*. New York: Wiley-Liss; 1993:35–43.
137. Hancock SL, Donaldson SS, Hoppe RT. Heart disease after Hodgkin's treatment in children and adolescents. *J Clin Oncol* 1993; 11:1208–1215.
138. Carlson RG, Mayfield WR, Norman S, Alexander JA. Radiation-associated valvular disease. *Chest* 1991; 99:538–545.

P A R T   T W E L V E

PERICARDIAL DISEASES AND ENDOCARDITIS

C H A P T E R 72

DISEASES OF THE PERICARDIUM

Brian D. Hoit

INTRODUCTION

Anatomy of the Pericardium

The pericardium is composed of visceral and parietal components. The visceral pericardium is a mesothelial monolayer that adheres firmly to the epicardium, reflects over the origin of the great vessels, and, together with a tough, fibrous coat, envelops the heart as the parietal pericardium (Fig. 72-1). The pericardial space is enclosed between these two serosal layers and normally contains up to 50 mL of a plasma ultrafiltrate, the pericardial fluid. Pericardial reflections around the great vessels tether the pericardium superiorly and result in the formation of two potential spaces: the oblique and transverse sinuses. The left atrium is anterior to the oblique sinus and is therefore largely an extrapericardial chamber; this relationship explains why effusions generally are not seen behind the left atrium. Superior and inferior pericardiosternal and diaphragmatic ligaments limit displacement of the pericardium and its contents within the chest and neutralize the effects of respiration and change of body position. The phrenic nerves are embedded in the parietal pericardium and, for this reason, are vulnerable to injury during pericardial resection.

Histologically, the pericardium is composed predominantly of compact collagen layers interspersed with elastin fibers. The abundance and orientation of the collagen fibers are responsible for the characteristic viscoelastic mechanical properties of the pericardium. For example, the pressure-volume relation of the pericardium is nonlinear; i.e., the relation is initially flat (producing little to no change in pressure for large changes in volume) and develops a "bend" or "knee" at a critical pressure, which terminates in a steep slope (producing large changes in pressure for small changes in volume) (Fig. 72-2). In addition, the pericardium is anisotropic; i.e., it stretches more in the short axis than in the long axis.

Physiology of the Pericardium

The pericardium is not essential for life; no adverse consequences follow congenital absence or surgical removal of the pericardium. However, the pericardium serves many important (although subtle) functions (Table 72-1). The pericardium limits distention of the cardiac chambers and facilitates interaction and coupling of the ventricles and atria.[1] Thus, changes in pressure and volume on one side of the heart can influence pressure and volume on the other side. Limitation of cardiac filling vol-

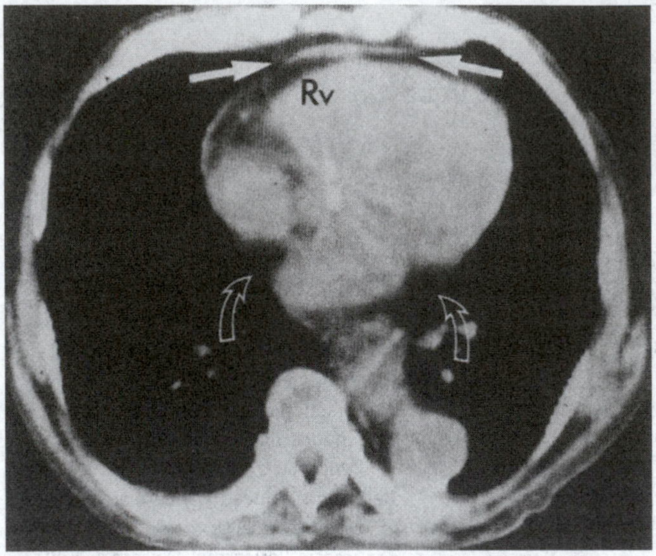

FIGURE 72-1 Computed tomographic (CT) scan shows the normal pericardium as a thin, curvilinear line (*open arrows*). The increased thickening over the anterior surface of the heart (*solid arrows*) is probably an artifact from transmitted right ventricular pulsations. (From Moncada R, Baker M. In: Higgins CB, ed. *CT of the Heart and Great Vessels*. Mt. Kisco, NY: Futura; 1983:292. Reproduced with permission.)

umes by the pericardium also may limit cardiac output and oxygen delivery during exercise.[2] The pericardium also influences quantitative and qualitative aspects of ventricular filling[3]; the thin-walled right ventricle (RV) and atrium are more subject to the influence of the pericardium than is the more resistant, thick-walled left ventricle (LV).[4]

Although the magnitude and importance of pericardial restraint of ventricular filling at physiologic cardiac volumes remain controversial, there is general agreement that pericardial reserve volume (i.e., the difference between unstressed pericardial volume and cardiac volume) is relatively small and that

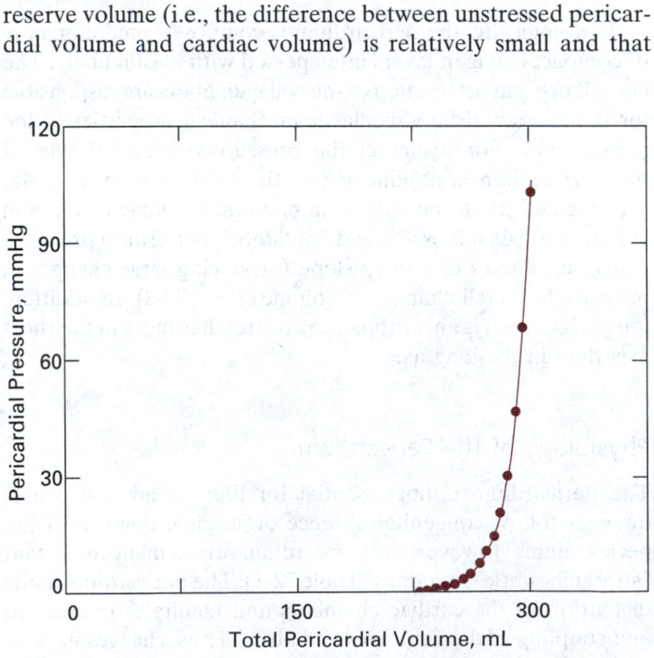

FIGURE 72-2 Pericardial pressure-volume relation in a dog. (From Holt JP. The normal pericardium. *Am J Cardiol* 1970; 26:455. Reproduced with permission.)

TABLE 72-1 Functions of the Pericardium

- Mechanical
  - Effects on chambers
    - Limits short-term cardiac distention
    - Facilitates cardiac chamber coupling and interaction
    - Maintains pressure-volume relation of and output from cardiac chambers
    - Maintains geometry of left ventricle
  - Effects on whole heart
    - Lubricates, minimizes friction
    - Equalizes gravitation, inertial, hydrostatic forces
    - Mechanical barrier to infection
- Immunologic
- Vasomotor
- Fibrinolytic
- Modulation of myocyte structure, function, and gene expression
- Vehicle for drug delivery and gene therapy

pericardial influences become significant when the reserve volume is exceeded. This may occur with rapid increases in blood volume and in disease states characterized by rapid increases in heart size (e.g., acute mitral and tricuspid regurgitation, pulmonary embolism, RV infarction). In contrast, chronic stretching of the pericardium results in "stress relaxation"; this explains why large but slowly developing effusions do not produce tamponade. In addition, the pericardium adapts to cardiac growth by "creep" (i.e., an increase in volume with constant stretch) and cellular hypertrophy. Pericardial thickening, which is characterized by mesothelial cell and matrix rearrangments, and the absence of diastolic abnormalities on echocardiography are features of vibroacoustic disease.[5]

The pericardium serves a variety of other important functions. It prevents excessive torsion and displacement of the heart, minimizes friction with surrounding structures, and is an anatomic barrier to the spread of infection from contiguous structures. The thin layer of pericardial fluid reduces friction on the epicardium and is thought to equalize gravitational forces over the surface of the heart; transmural cardiac pressures therefore do not change during acceleration or differ regionally within cardiac chambers. In addition, pericardial fluid equalizes inertial and hydrostatic forces. The pericardium also has immunologic, vasomotor, and fibrinolytic activity.[6] Epicardial mesothelial cells may modulate myocyte structure and function and gene expression.[7] Finally, the pericardial space has been used as a vehicle for drug delivery in gene therapy; studies using radiolabeled growth factors indicate that substances more consistently and reproducibly gain access to the coronary arteries via pericardial fluid than via endoluminal delivery.[8,9]

PERICARDIAL MICROPHYSIOLOGY

The pericardium is richly innervated; neuroreceptors in the epicardium and fibrosa, sympathetic afferents, stretch-sensitive mechanoreceptors, and phrenic afferents monitor dynamic changes in cardiac volume and tension.[10] Chemo- and mechanoreceptors with sympathetic afferents may be responsible for the transmission of pericardial pain.[11]

The mesothelium of the pericardium is metabolically active

and produces prostaglandin E_2, eicosanoids, and prostacylin; these substances modulate sympathetic neurotransmission and myocardial contractility and may influence epicardial coronary arterial tone. The concentration of angiogenic growth factors bFGF and VEGF increases in unstable angina,[12] suggesting a role for these factors in response to ischemia and injury. The level of brain natriuretic peptide (BNP) in the pericardial fluid is a more sensitive and accurate indicator of ventricular volume and pressure than is either plasma BNP or atrial natriuretic factor and may play an autocrine/paracrine role in heart failure.[13] In addition, levels of pericardial 8-iso-PGF2α (a marker of oxidant stress) increase directly with increasing ventricular dilatation and severity of heart failure, suggesting a role of oxidant stress in ventricular remodeling and the development of heart failure.[14]

Pericardial Pressure

Pericardial pressure measured by a fluid-filled catheter in the pericardial space is subatmospheric and is essentially equal to pleural pressure throughout the respiratory cycle. Small fluctuations related to the events of the cardiac cycle (pericardial pressure is lowest during ventricular ejection) are superimposed on the larger fluctuations related to the events of the respiratory cycle. Although much of the understanding of pericardial physiology is based on fluid pressure, pericardial restraint is a contact force, defined as fluid pressure plus deformational force (much like the force at the knee joint that, although considerable, is negligible when measured with a needle in the joint space). Pericardial contact pressure measured with flat balloons is considerably higher than liquid pressure and varies regionally.[3]

Balloon pressure is similar to the theoretical pericardial pressure that is calculated as the difference in LV diastolic pressure before and after pericardiectomy. This theoretical pressure has important implications for understanding the role of the pericardium in states of altered ventricular loading, such as pulmonary hypertension, aortic stenosis, and congestive heart failure, but does not explain pericardial influences on transmural pressure, for example, during acceleration and deceleration. When liquid versus contact pressure is more relevant is controversial among physiologists but is far less relevant to clinicians, who measure pericardial pressure only when there is a pericardial effusion.

Pathology of the Pericardium

In view of its simple structure, clinicopathologic processes involving the pericardium are understandably few; indeed, pericardial heart disease includes only pericarditis (an acute, subacute, or chronic fibrinous, "noneffusive," or exudative process) and its complications, tamponade and constriction (an acute, subacute, or chronic adhesive, fibrocalcific response), and congenital lesions. However, despite a limited number of clinical syndromes, the pericardium is affected by virtually every cate-

TABLE 72-2 Causes of Pericardial Heart Disease

- Idiopathic
- Infectious
  - Bacterial (pneumococcus, streptococcus, staphlococcus, *Haemophilus influenzae*, gram-negative rods, *B. melitensis, F. tularensis, Legionella pneumophilia, P. gonorrhoeae, N. meningitidis,* Lyme disease, myocoplasma)
  - Viral (coxsackie virus, echovirus, adenovirus, varicella, influenza, cytomegalovirus, HIV, hepatitis B, mumps, infectious mononucleosis)
  - Mycobacterial (*M. tuberculosis, M. avium-intracellulare*)
  - Fungal (histoplasmosis, coccidioidomycosis, blastomycosis, *Candida albicans, Nocardia,* actinomycosis)
  - Protozoal (toxoplasmosis, echinococcosis, amebiasis)
  - AIDS-associated
- Neoplastic
  - Primary (mesothelioma, fibrosarcoma)
  - Secondary (breast, lung, melanoma, lymphoma, leukemia)
- Immune/inflammatory
  - Connective tissue diseases (rheumatoid arthritis, systemic lupus erythematosis, scleroderma, acute rheumatic fever, dermatomyositis, mixed connective tissue disease, Wegener's granulomatosis)
  - Arteritis (temporal arteritis, polyarteritis nodosa, Takayasu's arteritis)
  - Acute myocardial infarction and post-MI (Dressler's syndrome)
  - Postcardiotomy
  - Posttraumatic
- Metabolic
  - Nephrogenic
  - Aortic dissection
  - Myxedema
  - Amyloidosis
- Iatrogenic
  - Radiation injury
  - Instrument/device trauma (implantable defibrillators, pacemakers, catheters)
  - Drugs (hydralazine, procainamide, daunorubicin, isoniazid, anticoagulants, cyclosporine, methysergide, phenytoin, dantrolene, mesalazine)
  - Cardiac resuscitation
- Traumatic
  - Blunt
  - Penetrating
  - Surgical
- Congenital
  - Pericardial cysts
  - Congenital absence of pericardium
  - Mulibrey nanism

gory of disease, including infections, neoplastic, immune/inflammatory, metabolic, iatrogenic, traumatic, and congenital etiologies. Thus, the physician is likely to encounter patients with pericardial disease in a variety of settings, either as an isolated phenomenon or as a complication of a variety of systemic disorders, trauma, or certain drugs.

Pericardial disease often remains clinically silent and may be detected only during the evaluation of unrelated complaints by the electrocardiogram (ECG), chest radiography, or echocardiography. Despite exhaustive etiologic lists (Table 72-2), the cause of pericardial heart disease often is never identified. Recently, an increased prevalence of pericarditis, (owing largely to therapeutic advances such as cardiovascular surgery, hemodialysis, and radiation therapy), pericardial involvement in AIDS, and advances in the recognition, diagnosis, and therapy of pericarditis and its complications have resulted in a resurgence of interest in pericardial heart disease. The remainder of this chapter reviews pericarditis and its sequelae, pericardial effusions, cardiac tamponade and constrictive pericarditis, and congenital diseases of the pericardium.

ACUTE PERICARDITIS

Acute fibrinous or dry pericarditis is a syndrome characterized by typical chest pain, a pathognomonic pericardial friction rub, and specific ECG changes. A variety of conditions are associated with acute pericarditis (Table 72-2). The following description refers to viral and idiopathic pericarditis without significant effusion. Specific forms of pericardial heart disease are reviewed later in the chapter.

History

Acute pericarditis typically produces sharp retrosternal pain that radiates to the trapezius ridge and is aggravated by lying down and relieved by sitting up; its onset frequently is heralded by a prodrome of fever, malaise, and myalgia (Fig. 72-3). The pain of pericarditis is often worse with inspiration and is difficult to distinguish from pleurisy; in some cases, the pain is indistinguishable from that of myocardial infarction. The quality, severity, and location of pain vary greatly, and chest pain may be absent in acute pericarditis, especially in early pericarditis complicating myocardial infarction or cardiac surgery and in uremic pericarditis.

Physical Findings

The hallmark of acute pericarditis is the pericardial friction rub; because of its superficial, creaky, or scratchy character, it often is likened to the sound of walking on dry snow or the squeak of a leather saddle (Fig. 72-3). Rubs are heard anywhere over the precordium but most often between the lower left sternal edge and the cardiac apex; they usually are heard best with the diaphragm of the stethoscope applied firmly and with respiration suspended. Most pericardial friction rubs are independent of the respiratory cycle, but on occasion they are louder during inspiration. The pericardial rub may be confined to ventricular systole but most often includes a component during atrial systole and occasionally during ventricular diastolic filling, resulting in biphasic and triphasic rubs, respectively. Biphasic rubs must be distinguished from murmurs of mixed aortic valve disease, and monophasic rubs often are mistaken for systolic murmurs. Frequent examinations are necessary to detect a rub because of its evanescent nature; pericardial fluid does not prevent a friction rub.

In uncomplicated pericarditis, the jugular venous pressure usually remains normal. Ventricular third and fourth heart sounds indicate coexisting myocardial disease. The history and physical examination are helpful also in recognizing complications and in identifying underlying diseases associated with pericarditis. Depending on the etiology, there may be fever and other signs of inflammation or systemic illness.

Electrocardiography

The ECG may either confirm the clinical suspicion of pericardial disease or first alert the clinician to the presence of pericarditis (Fig. 72-4). Serial tracings may be needed to distinguish the ST-segment elevations caused by acute pericarditis from those caused by acute myocardial infarction

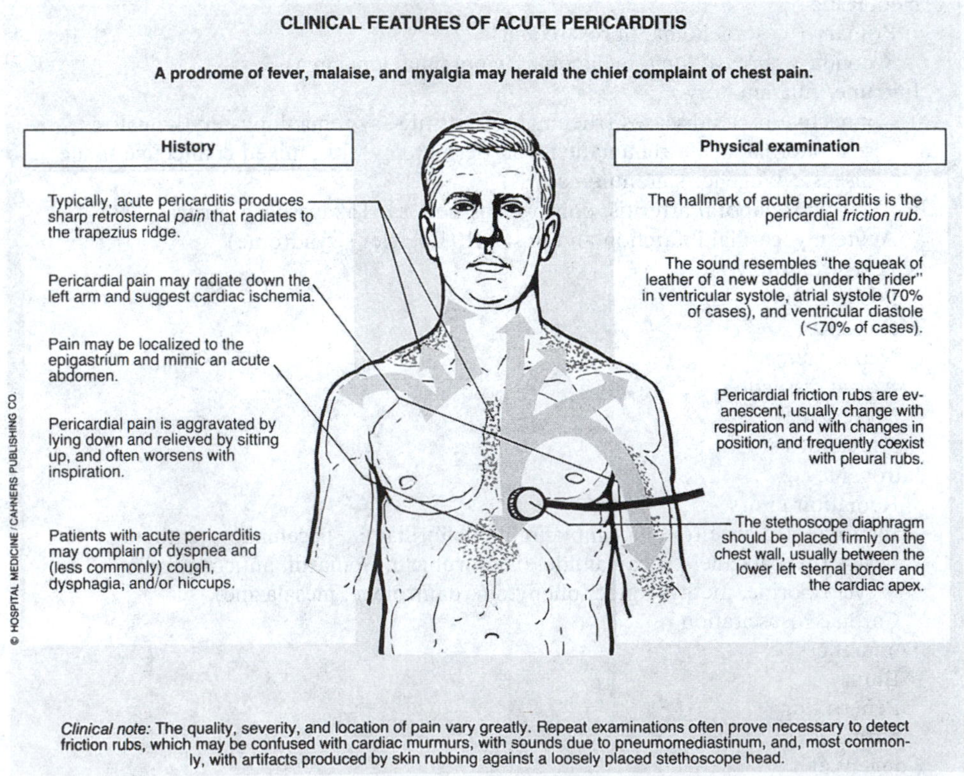
CLINICAL FEATURES OF ACUTE PERICARDITIS
A prodrome of fever, malaise, and myalgia may herald the chief complaint of chest pain.
History
Typically, acute pericarditis produces sharp retrosternal pain that radiates to the trapezius ridge.
Pericardial pain may radiate down the left arm and suggest cardiac ischemia.
Pain may be localized to the epigastrium and mimic an acute abdomen.
Pericardial pain is aggravated by lying down and relieved by sitting up, and often worsens with inspiration.
Patients with acute pericarditis may complain of dyspnea and (less commonly) cough, dysphagia, and/or hiccups.
Physical examination
The hallmark of acute pericarditis is the pericardial friction rub.
The sound resembles "the squeak of leather of a new saddle under the rider" in ventricular systole, atrial systole (70% of cases), and ventricular diastole (<70% of cases).
Pericardial friction rubs are evanescent, usually change with respiration and with changes in position, and frequently coexist with pleural rubs.
The stethoscope diaphragm should be placed firmly on the chest wall, usually between the lower left sternal border and the cardiac apex.
Clinical note: The quality, severity, and location of pain vary greatly. Repeat examinations often prove necessary to detect friction rubs, which may be confused with cardiac murmurs, with sounds due to pneumomediastinum, and, most commonly, with artifacts produced by skin rubbing against a loosely placed stethoscope head.
© HOSPITAL MEDICINE/CAHNERS PUBLISHING CO.

FIGURE 72-3 Clinical features of acute pericarditis: history and physical examination. (From Hoit BD. Acute pericarditis: Diagnosis and differential diagnosis. *Hosp Pract* 1991; 27:23–43. Reproduced with permission.)

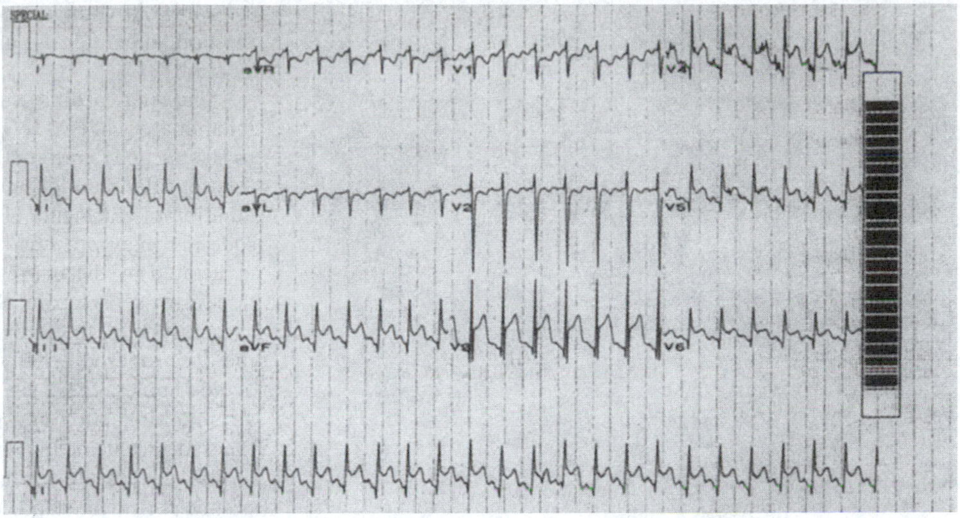

FIGURE 72-4 Twelve-lead electrocardiogram from a patient with acute pericarditis. (From Hoit BD. Pericardial disease and pericardial heart disease. In: O'Rourke RA, ed. *Stein's Internal Medicine*, 5th ed. St. Louis, Missouri: Mosby-Year Book; 1998:273. Reproduced with permission.)

(MI) or normal early repolarization. The ST-T wave changes in acute pericarditis are diffuse and have characteristic evolutionary changes. In the first stage, ST-segment elevations (which differ from ischemic ST elevations by their upward concavity and seldom exceed 5 mm in height) typically occur within a few hours of the onset of chest pain and persist for hours or days. Depression of the PR segment (except in lead aVR) may be seen in this stage and may differentiate acute pericarditis from early repolarization variants.[15] In the second stage, the ST segments return to baseline; at this point, the T waves may appear normal or exhibit a loss of amplitude. In the third stage, tracings show inversion of T waves. T-wave inversions may persist indefinitely, particularly with tuberculous, uremic, or neoplastic pericarditis. The ECG normalizes in the variably present fourth stage. In a typical case of acute pericarditis, the approximate time frame for these ECG changes is 2 weeks. However, only about half of patients with acute pericarditis display all four ECG stages, and variations are very common. Atrial arrhythmias complicate 5 to 10 percent of cases of acute pericarditis.[16]

The ST-segment elevation seen in acute pericarditis usually can be distinguished from that of acute MI by the absence of Q waves, the upwardly concave ST segments, and the absence of associated T-wave inversions. The acute ST-segment elevation of Prinzmetal's variant of angina is more transitory and is associated with ischemic pain. Although the ST-segment elevation in the early repolarization variant (common in young individuals, especially blacks, athletes, and psychiatric patients) may simulate the ECG of acute pericarditis, the former is distinguished by the absence of PR-segment depression and evolutionary ST-T wave changes.

Imaging and Laboratory Studies

In uncomplicated acute pericarditis, the chest radiograph is generally normal. However, an enlarged cardiac silhouette may be evident because of a moderate or large pericardial effusion (Fig. 72-5). The chest radiograph may provide evidence of tuberculosis, fungal disease, pneumonia, or neoplasm.

Echocardiographic identification of pericardial effusion confirms the clinical diagnosis of acute pericarditis (Fig. 72-6), but a patient with purely fibrinous acute pericarditis often has a normal echocardiogram. Echocardiography estimates the volume of pericardial fluid, identifies cardiac tamponade, suggests the basis of pericarditis, and documents associated acute myocarditis with congestive heart failure.

Although ^{99}technetium pyrophosphate scans may be positive in patients with pericarditis associated with epicarditis and gallium scans have proved useful in displaying the characteristics of purulent pericarditis, these tests rarely are used to diagnose acute pericarditis.

Nonspecific blood markers of inflammation, such as the erythrocyte sedimentation rate and the white blood cell count, usually increase in cases of acute pericarditis. Patients with extensive epicarditis occasionally have increases in serum cardiac isoenzymes suggestive of acute MI.

Therapy for Acute Pericarditis

Hospitalization is warranted for most patients who present with an initial episode of acute pericarditis to determine the etiology

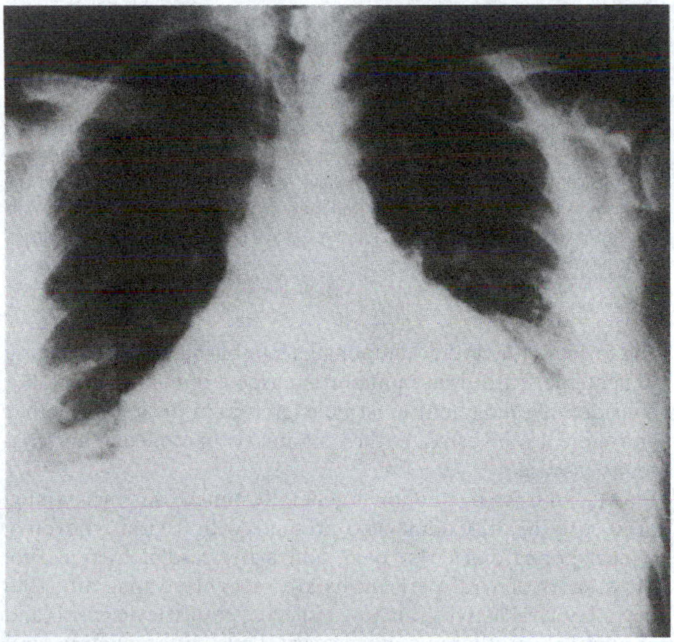

FIGURE 72-5 Chest radiograph from a patient with a large pericardial effusion. Note the "flask-shape" appearance of the cardiac silhouette. (From Hoit BD. Imaging the pericardium. *Cardiol Clin* 1990; 8:588. Reproduced with permission.)

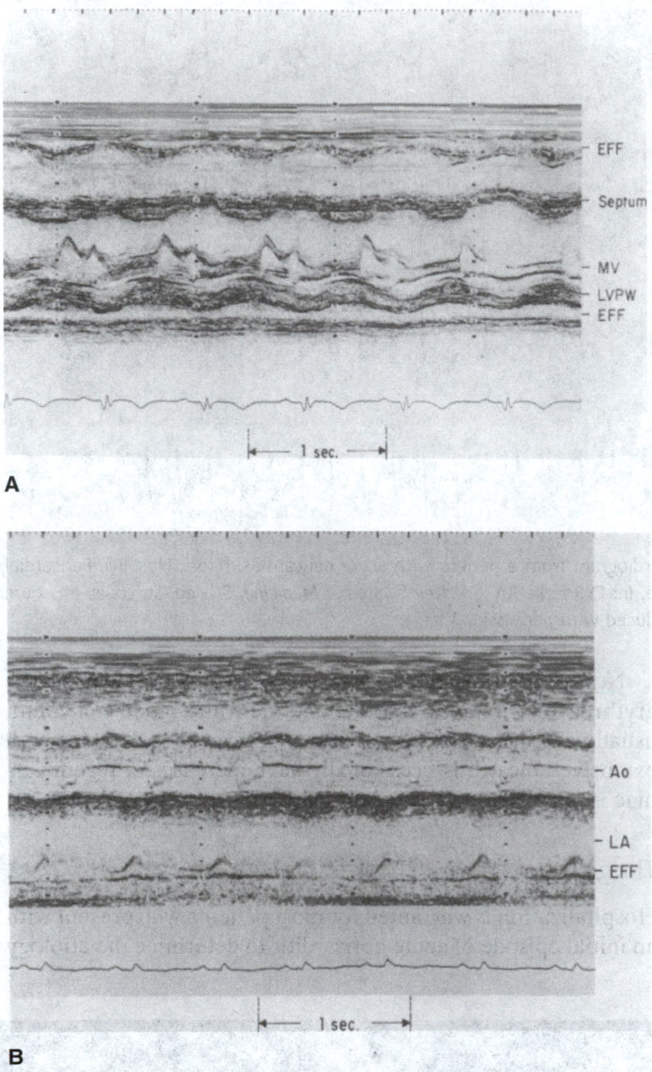

FIGURE 72-6 M-mode echocardiograms of pericardial effusion (EFF). *A.* The effusion appears as an echo-free space posterior to the left ventricular posterior wall (LVPW). Note that parietal pericardium has relatively flat motion throughout the cardiac cycle. MV = mitral valve. *B.* Pericardial effusion behind the left atrium (LA). Note the exaggerated motion of the posterior left atrial wall. (From Hoit BD. Imaging the pericardium. *Cardiol Clin* 1990; 8:588. Reproduced with permission.)

and observe for cardiac tamponade. Establishing the exact cause of acute pericarditis is an important aspect of management, but considerable judgment must be exercised in deciding whether and how to investigate the possibility of concomitant systemic disease.

An extensive evaluation is generally unnecessary in a young, previously healthy adult who presents with a viral syndrome, typical pericardial chest pain, and a pericardial friction rub. Most cases of viral pericarditis are recognized long after the period of viral activity, making a specific etiologic diagnosis and antiviral chemotherapy unnecessary. Thus, differentiating viral from idiopathic pericarditis is difficult, expensive, and generally of little practical importance. Depending on the history and symptoms at presentation, trauma, myocarditis, systemic lupus erythematosus (SLE), and/or purulent pericarditis require consideration in younger patients. In older adults, myocardial infarction, tuberculosis, and neoplastic disease should be considered.

Acute pericarditis usually responds to oral nonsteroidal anti-inflammatory agents (e.g., ASA 650 mg q3–4h or ibuprofen 600 to 800 mg q6h). Indomethacin reduces coronary blood flow and theoretically should be avoided. Some data suggest that the addition of colchicine (1 mg/day) is effective for an acute episode and may prevent recurrences.[17] The intensity of therapy is dictated by the distress of the patient; narcotics may be required for severe pain. Some cases necessitate steroid therapy (prednisone 60 to 80 mg/day) for a week to control pain, with the dose tapered rapidly thereafter. Corticosteroids should be avoided unless there is a specific indication. They may enhance viral multiplication and produce recurrences when the dose is tapered; colchicine may be useful in this situation. Nevertheless, corticosteroids are useful in acute pericarditis associated with uremic pericarditis and connective tissue diseases. Importantly, tuberculous and pyogenic pericarditis should be excluded before steroid therapy is initiated.

Patients in whom pericarditis represents one manifestation of systemic illness (such as sepsis, uremia, connective tissue disease, or neoplasia) should, in addition to palliative and supportive treatment, receive therapy directed toward the primary disorder.

RECURRENT PERICARDITIS

Recurrent or relapsing acute pericarditis is one of the most distressing disorders of the pericardium for both patient and physician; it may occur with or without pericardial effusion and occasionally is associated with pleural effusion or parenchymal pulmonary lesions. Recurrences occur with highly variable frequency over a course of many years. The reasons for relapse are unclear, but the phenomenon suggests that acute pericarditis itself may represent or generate an autoimmune process. Recurrences may be spontaneous but more commonly are associated with discontinuation or tapering doses of anti-inflammatory drugs. When associated with pericardial effusion, relapsing pericarditis can cause cardiac tamponade; however, this is unusual.

Painful recurrences of pericarditis may respond to nonsteroidal anti-inflammatory agents but commonly require corticosteroids. Once steroids are administered, dependency and the development of steroid-induced abnormalities are potential sequelae. Prednisone is begun at a high dose (60 to 80 mg/day), but rapid tapering should be initiated within a few days of clinical resolution. When necessary, the risks of long-term steroids should be minimized by using the lowest possible dose, alternate-day therapy, combinations with nonsteroidal drugs, or colchicine (1 to 2 mg/day).[18] In the most difficult cases, relapse occurs every time the dose of prednisone is reduced below 5 to 20 mg/day. When this occurs, the patient should be maintained for several weeks on the lowest suppressive dose before the next taper commences. Azathioprine (50 to 100 mg/day) also has been used to prevent recurrent episodes.[19] Although encouraging results have been reported in a series of patients who underwent pericardiectomy for recurrent pericarditis, pericardiectomy may simply abbreviate rather than terminate the painful recurrences. Thus, pericardiectomy should be considered only when repeated attempts at medical treatment have clearly failed.

PERICARDIAL EFFUSION

Etiology

Accumulation of transudate, exudate, or blood in the pericardial sac is a common complication of pericardial disease and should be sought in all patients with acute pericarditis.

Pericardial effusions are reported to be associated with heart failure, valvular disease, and myocardial infarction in 14, 21, and 15 percent of cases, respectively.[20] Hydropericardium results from elevated right atrial pressure and limited venous and lymphatic drainage from the pericardium. Although this is the usual explanation for effusions associated with heart failure and LV hypertrophy, recurrent bloody effusions that can be attributed only to congestive heart failure may occur.

Pericardial effusions are very common after cardiac surgery. In 122 consecutive patients studied before and serially after cardiac surgery, effusions were present in 103 patients; the majority appeared by postoperative day 2, reached their maximum size by postoperative day 10, and usually resolved without sequelae within the first postoperative month.[21] Symptoms and physical findings of significant postoperative pericardial effusions are frequently nonspecific, and echo-detection and echo-guided pericardiocentesis, when necessary, are safe and effective; prolonged catheter drainage reduces the recurrence rate.[22] Pericardial effusions in cardiac transplant patients are associated with an increased incidence of acute rejection.[23] Chronic effusive pericarditis is an entity of unknown etiology that may be associated with large, asymptomatic effusions. Many conditions that cause pericarditis (e.g., uremia, tuberculosis, neoplasia, connective tissue disease) produce chronic pericardial effusions.

Nature of the Pericardial Fluid

Characteristics of the pericardial fluid other than culture and cytology are usually too nonspecific to be of diagnostic value. However, in one retrospective series, one-fifth of the patients had a specific etiologic diagnosis that had implications for management and prognosis.[24] Moreover, in certain situations it is mandatory to determine the nature of the pericardial fluid. For example, in patients with neoplastic disease, it is important to determine whether pericardial effusion indicates invasion of the pericardium or a complication of radiation therapy. Cytologic examination of the fluid is also important in cases in which the primary tumor has not been identified clearly. In cases of bacterial or other nonviral infections, it becomes necessary to discover whether the pericardial effusion is exudative and to culture pericardial fluid; this is particularly important when tuberculous or fungal pericarditis is suspected. Transudative effusions (hydropericardium) occur in heart failure and other states associated with chronic salt and water retention (including pregnancy), and exudative effusions occur in a large number of the infectious and inflammatory causes of pericarditis. Although frank hemorrhagic effusions suggest recent intrapericardial bleeding, sanguineous and serosanguineous effusions occur in many infectious and inflammatory disorders. In certain disorders, the nature of the pericardial fluid has greater diagnostic value. For example, chylous pericarditis implies injury or obstruction to the thoracic duct, and cholesterol pericarditis is either idiopathic or associated with hypothyroidism, rheumatoid arthritis, or tuberculosis.

Diagnostic Studies

Specific diagnoses are possible using visual, cytologic, and immunologic analysis of the pericardial effusion and pericardioscopic-guided biopsy of the epicardium and pericardium.[20,25] Observations using these techniques have suggested that (1) fibrin strands and neovascularization are common in inflammatory pericardial diseases, (2) the etiology of viral pericarditis can be established by using a variety of methods, such as in situ hybridization, microneutralization, and polymerase chain reaction, (3) combined analysis of the cytology in the effusion and epicardial biopsy are most important, and pericardial biopsy is often inconclusive, and (4) viral and autoreactive effusions are associated with high titers of antimyolemmal and antisarcolemmal antibodies and in vitro cardiocytolysis of isolated rat heart cells. However, the clinical utility of these diagnostic methods and observations remains to be determined.

There are clinical situations in which it is unnecessary to obtain pericardial fluid for analysis. For example, when pericardial effusion is found in a patient with typical viral or idiopathic pericarditis, pericardiocentesis should not be considered unless the effusion fails to respond to anti-inflammatory treatment or cardiac tamponade develops. Similarly, when a patient undergoing chronic hemodialysis develops pericardial effusion, examination of pericardial fluid is needed only when the clinical course suggests a different etiology or when hemodynamic embarrassment is suspected.

IMAGING STUDIES

Echocardiography is the procedure of choice for the diagnosis of pericardial effusion. Although flask-shaped enlargement of the cardiac silhouette on chest radiography occurs with a moderate or large pericardial effusion (Fig. 72-5), differentiation of large effusions from cardiac dilatation often is difficult or impossible. In contrast, the relative contributions of cardiac enlargement and pericardial effusion to overall cardiac enlargement and the relative roles of tamponade and myocardial dysfunction to altered hemodynamics can be evaluated with echocardiography. Attention to technical detail results in excellent sensitivity and specificity. The diagnostic feature on M-mode echocardiography is the persistence of an echo-free space between parietal and visceral pericardium throughout the cardiac cycle (Fig. 72-6). Separations that are observed only in systole represent clinically insignificant accumulations. Two-dimensional (2-D) echocardiography (Fig. 72-7) has superior spatial orientation and allows delineation of the size and distribution of pericardial effusion as well as detection of loculated fluid. As the amount of pericardial fluid increases, fluid distributes from the posterobasilar LV apically and anteriorly and then laterally and posteriorly to the left atrium. Fluid adjacent to the right atrium is an early sign of pericardial effusion. Frondlike, bandlike, or shaggy intrapericardial echoes should alert one to the possibility of a difficult and potentially less therapeutic pericardiocentesis (Fig. 72-8) but have little value in identifying the cause of the effusion.

Pericardial effusions are easily detected by computed tomography (Fig. 72-9). The size, geometry, and distribution of pericardial effusions can be obtained with this technique, and the attenuation coefficients for blood, exudate, chyle, and serous fluid are generally sufficiently characteristic to identify the nature of the effusion. Computed tomography may be useful in identifying loculated and atypically loculated pericardial effu-

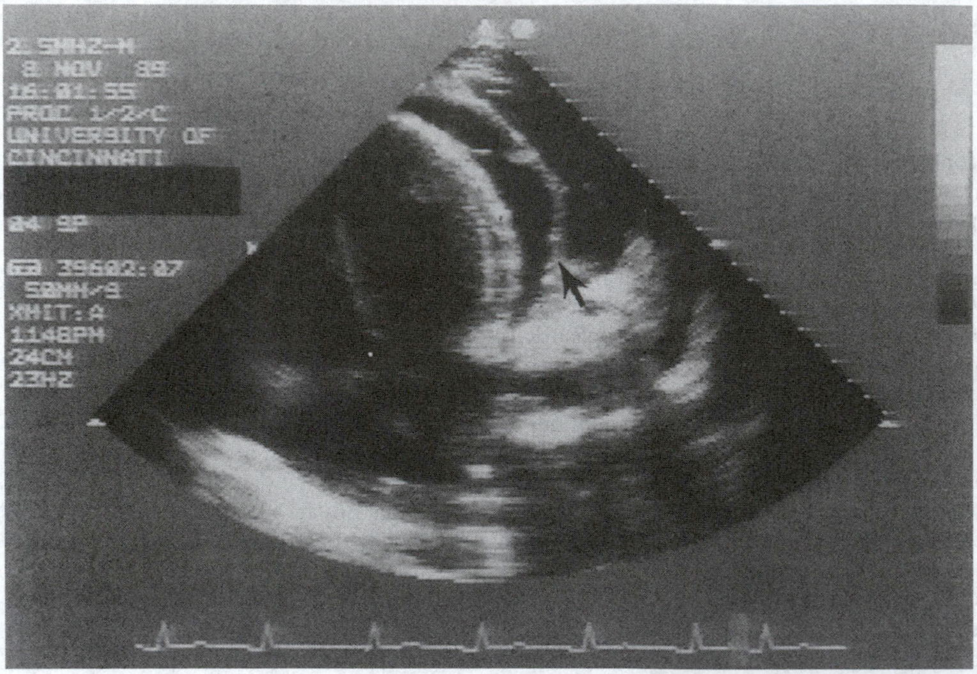

FIGURE 72-7 Two-dimensional echocardiogram from a patient with pleural and pericardial effusions. The thickness of the pericardium (*arrow*) can be appreciated in this patient. (From Hoit BD. Imaging the pericardium. *Cardiol Clin* 1990; 8:596. Reproduced with permission.)

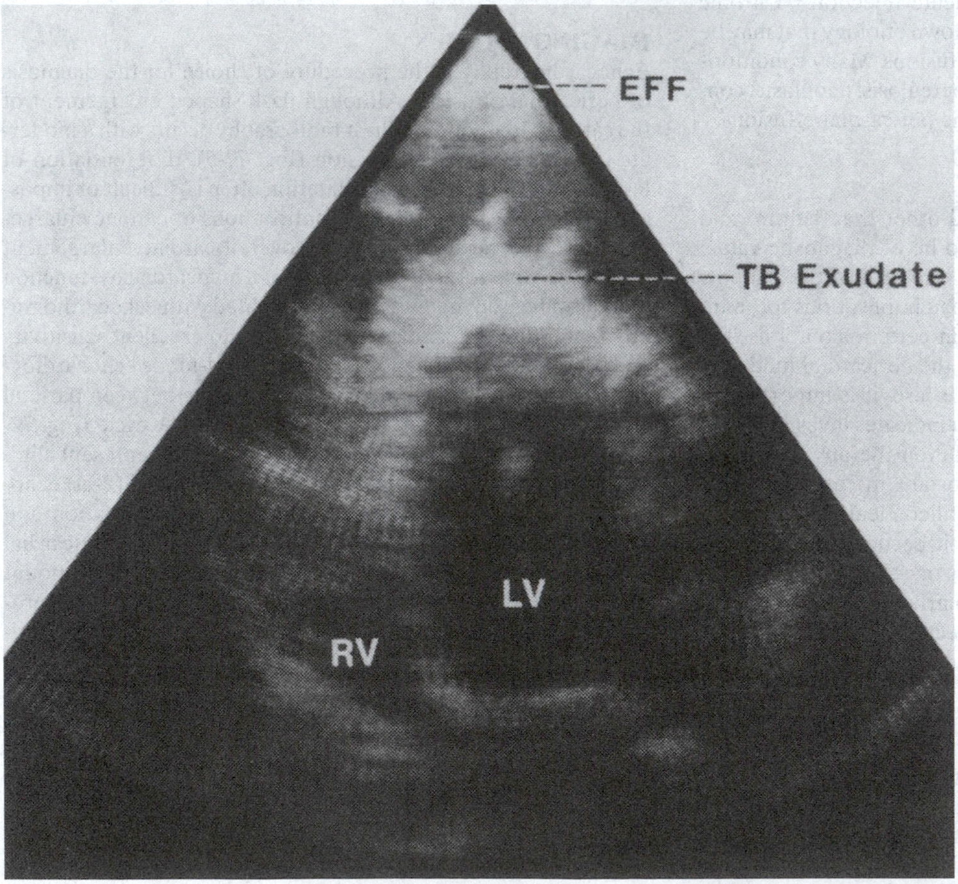

FIGURE 72-8 Two-dimensional echocardiogram from a patient with tuberculous pericarditis. Note the thickened pericardium with shaggy exudate that bridges a large pericardial effusion (EFF). (From Hoit BD. Imaging the pericardium. *Cardiol Clin* 1990; 8:590. Reproduced with permission.)

sions and in guiding pericardiocentesis. Loculated and recurrent pericardial effusions can be treated safely and effectively with video-assisted thoracoscopic pericardial fenestration.[26]

Magnetic resonance imaging (MRI) detects pericardial effusion with high sensitivity and provides an estimate of pericardial fluid volume; in addition, it effectively detects loculated pericardial effusion and pericardial thickening.[27] Inflamed pericardium and adhesions have a high signal intensity relative to pericardial fluid and myocardium, providing a potential means of identifying the nature of the effusion.

Treatment of Pericardial Effusion

Drainage of a pericardial effusion is usually unnecessary unless purulent pericarditis is suspected or cardiac tamponade supervenes, although on occasion, pericardiocentesis is needed to establish the etiology of a hemodynamically insignificant pericardial effusion. Persistent or progressive effusion, particularly when the cause is uncertain, also warrants pericardiocentesis. However, routine drainage of a large pericardial effusion without tamponade or suspected purulent pericarditis has a low diagnostic yield and no clear therapeutic benefit.[28] Anticoagulants should be discontinued temporarily if possible to reduce the risk of cardiac tamponade. In patients on chronic oral anticoagulation, heparin should be used, since its effect can be reversed rapidly. Large effusions may respond to nonsteroidal anti-inflammatory drugs, corticosteroids, or colchicine.[17] Specific treatment for pericardial effusion is considered below.

CARDIAC TAMPONADE

Cardiac tamponade is a hemodynamic condition characterized by equal elevation of atrial and pericardial pressures, an exaggerated inspiratory decrease in arterial systolic pressure (pulsus paradoxus), and arterial hypotension.

Arterial hypotension is generally a late sign in chronic effusions, and occasionally, a heightened sympathoadrenal state produces systemic hypertension. As intrapericardial pressure rises, venous pressures increase to maintain cardiac filling and prevent collapse of the cardiac chambers. Although the absolute intracardiac pressures are elevated, the transmural pressures—i.e., cavitary diastolic pressure minus pericardial pressure—are practically zero or even negative. The greatly reduced preload is responsible for the fall in cardiac output, and when compensatory mechanisms are exhausted, arterial pressure decreases.

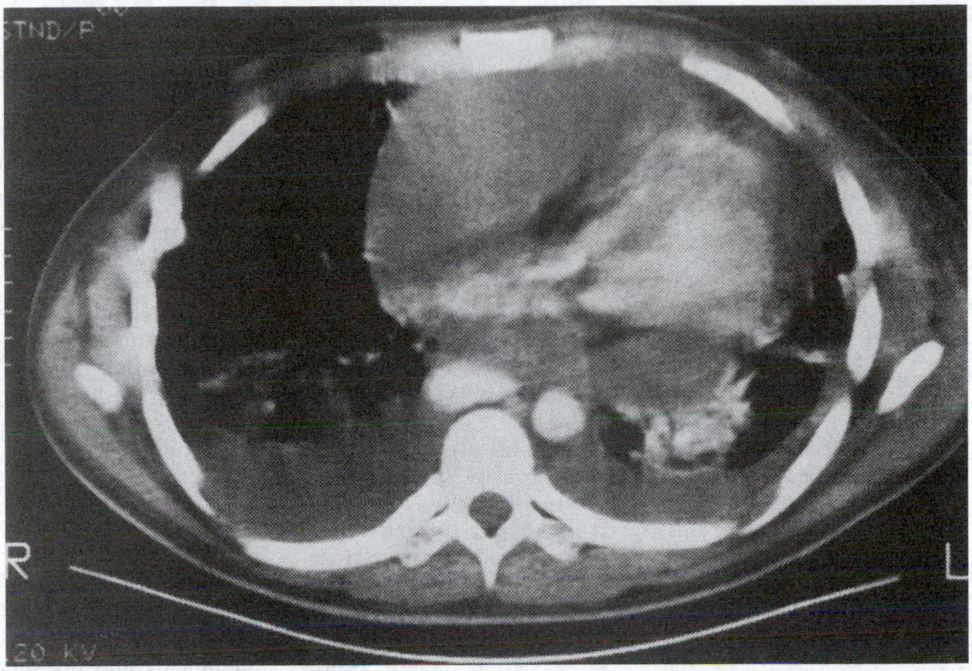

FIGURE 72-9 Computed tomographic scan from a patient with a large pericardial effusion. Note the compression of contrast-filled cardiac chambers. (From Hoit BD. Imaging the pericardium. *Cardiol Clin* 1990; 8:590. Reproduced with permission.)

Clinical Features

Cardiac tamponade may be acute or chronic and should be viewed hemodynamically as a continuum ranging from mild (pericardial pressure lower than 10 mmHg) to severe (pericardial pressure higher than 15 to 20 mmHg). Mild cardiac tamponade is frequently asymptomatic, whereas moderate tamponade and especially severe tamponade produce precordial discomfort and dyspnea.

Tamponade may be so sudden that the patient does not complain of symptoms; in less drastic circumstances, patients with acute cardiac tamponade may complain of severe shortness of breath accompanied by chest tightness and dizziness. The venous pressure is greatly elevated, and the systemic arterial pressure is severely depressed. Pulsus paradoxus usually can be appreciated but may be absent when hypotension is extreme. In striking contrast to the elevation of venous pressure, arterial hypotension, and pulsus paradoxus, cardiac pulsations often are impalpable (Beck's triad). In the most severe cases, consciousness may be impaired, and except for the raised venous pressure, such patients appear to be in hypovolemic shock.

When cardiac tamponade complicates a diagnostic procedure, vague discomfort, generalized uneasiness, and precordial pain are common. Fluoroscopy shows an enlarged cardiac silhouette and diminished pulsations.

Cardiac tamponade should be suspected in a victim of recent chest trauma who appears to be in shock, especially when the venous pressure is elevated. When circumstances are deemed life-threatening, an immediate therapeutic trial of rapid infusion of fluid and diagnostic pericardiocentesis should be attempted. Otherwise, pericardiocentesis should be delayed until the presence of significant pericardial fluid can be demonstrated by prompt echocardiography. An exception to this rule is when tamponade occurs in the diagnostic laboratory; in this instance, when pressures are being monitored and fluoroscopy is available, the diagnosis can be established safely without echocardiographic confirmation.

Other causes of acute tamponade are cardiac rupture complicating acute MI and rupture of a dissecting hematoma of the proximal aorta. Although successful pericardiocentesis may relieve aortic tamponade and increase hemorrhage, a limited pericardiocentesis is reasonable if cardiac tamponade is severe enough to be considered a threat to survival. Finally, after cardiac surgery, dyspnea and fatigue should raise the suspicion of tamponade; in these instances, the effusion is often loculated, and echocardiographic and hemodynamic findings may be unreliable.

A large number of diseases may be associated with more slowly developing cardiac tamponade. In these instances, symptoms may be due to the underlying illness, the culpable pericardial disease, and/or the tamponade itself. Many patients with inflammatory pericarditis give a history of prodromal fever, myalgia, and arthralgia, and patients with neoplastic disease may have symptoms associated with the neoplasm and its treatment. The symptoms of cardiac compression include rapidly progressive dyspnea accompanied by fullness or tightness in the chest, occasionally with dysphagia; pericardial pain is often absent. The course may be less rapid, allowing time for an increase in abdominal girth and the rapid onset and progression of edema.

Pathophysiology

Elevated intrapericardial pressure exerted on the heart throughout the cardiac cycle, with only slight momentary relief when intrapericardial pressure falls (owing to the decrease in cardiac volume during ventricular ejection), is responsible for the pathophysiologic findings of cardiac tamponade. To understand the relation between venous and pericardial pressures in cardiac tamponade, it is useful to review the normal biphasic pattern of venous return. A surge of venous return occurs at the onset

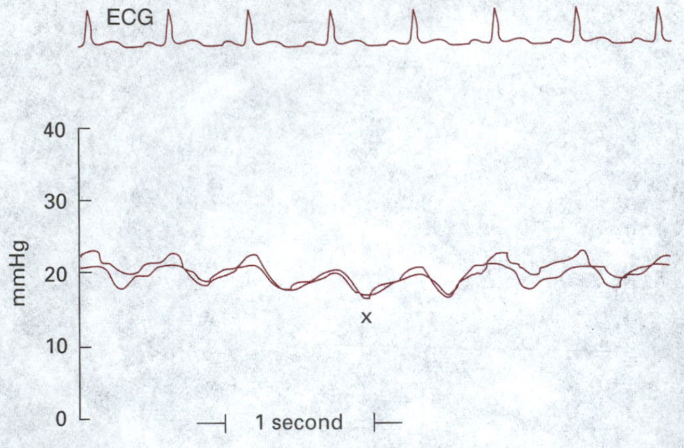

FIGURE 72-10 Simultaneous right atrial and pericardial pressures from a patient with severe cardiac tamponade. The pressures are elevated and equal to one another, and only the X descent on the right atrial tracing is present; the Y descent is absent. The pressures fall normally during inspiration. (From Shabetai R. Diseases of the pericardium. In: Alexander WA, Schlant R, Fuster V, et al., eds. *Hurst's The Heart*, 9th ed. New York: McGraw-Hill; 1998:2179. Reproduced with permission.)

of ventricular ejection and is accompanied by a small reduction in intrapericardial pressure. A second surge of venous return occurs in early diastole, when the tricuspid valve opens and atrial pressure decreases. In contrast, the venous return in cardiac tamponade is unimodal and is confined to ventricular systole, and in severe cardiac tamponade, venous return is halted in diastole, at a time when cardiac volume and intrapericardial pressure are maximal. Pericardial pressure and right atrial pressure are elevated above normal and are equal to each other (Fig. 72-10). The inspiratory fall in intrathoracic pressure is transmitted to the pericardial space and preserves the normal inspiratory increase in systemic venous return (Kussmaul's sign is absent).

Although systolic ventricular function is often supranormal, unrelieved extreme tamponade becomes fatal when venous pressure cannot increase to equal the pericardial pressure and maintain circulation. In severe cases, diminution of myocardial perfusion is aggravated by direct compression of the epicardial coronary arteries, abnormal transmyocardial distribution of blood flow, and, as a result, impaired ventricular systolic function.

PULSUS PARADOXUS

In healthy individuals, systolic blood pressure may decline by as much as 10 mmHg during quiet inspiration. Pulsus paradoxus is an exaggeration of this normal physiologic response. A number of normal and abnormal mechanisms combine to create pulsus paradoxus in cardiac tamponade. Inspiratory augmentation of systemic venous return in cardiac tamponade increases the volume of the right side of the heart at the expense of the left side. The volume of the left side of the heart is decreased, in part by bulging of the intraventricular septum from right to left (changing the size, shape, and compliance of the LV) and in part by increased transmural pericardial pressure (decreasing pulmonary venous return). However, the inspiratory expansion of the volume of the right side of the heart and the transit time of the resulting augmented right heart stroke volume are important in the genesis of pulsus paradoxus. In addition, the negative thoracic pressure produced by inspiration is transmitted to the aorta, increasing LV afterload and reducing stroke volume. LV stroke volume falls more sharply than normal in response to decreased ventricular filling in cardiac tamponade because the small ventricle is operating on the steep ascending limb of the Starling curve. Finally, inspiratory traction by the diaphragm on the taut pericardium, reflex changes in vascular resistance and cardiac contractility, and increased respiratory effort owing to pulmonary congestion contribute to the genesis of pulsus paradoxus.

Pulsus paradoxus appears when both ventricles fill against a common resistance. Therefore, when LV diastolic pressure is elevated by coexisting LV disease, pulsus paradoxus does not develop in cardiac tamponade.[29] Similarly, atrial septal defects and aortic regurgitation prevent reciprocal inspiratory changes in the filling of the two sides of the heart; therefore, in these conditions, cardiac tamponade can occur without pulsus paradoxus.[30]

Physical Findings

Physical findings are dictated by both the severity of cardiac tamponade and the time course of its development. Careful inspection of the jugular venous pulse waveform is essential for the diagnosis, although the venous pressure may be normal in early tamponade, whereas extreme elevations of venous pressure may go unrecognized in a recumbent or semirecumbent patient. Compression of the heart by pericardial fluid results in a characteristic loss of the atrial Y descent, but because of the decrease in intrapericardial pressure that occurs during ventricular ejection, the systolic atrial filling wave and the X descent are maintained. Kussmaul's sign, a failure of venous pressure to decrease during inspiration, is a sign of constriction and generally is not seen in pure cardiac tamponade.

An inspiratory decline of systolic arterial pressure exceeding 10 mmHg (pulsus paradoxus) may be detected with palpation of an arterial pulse, such as the femoral or brachial artery, and quantified by using sphygmomanometry by subtracting the pressure at which Korotkoff's sounds are heard only during expiration from the pressure at which sounds are heard through the respiratory cycle. The origin of the paradoxical pulse is complex and multifactorial, and pulsus paradoxus is neither sensitive nor specific for cardiac tamponade.[30] Nevertheless, in the appropriate clinical setting, pulsus paradoxus is a key finding that signifies cardiac tamponade, and its presence should be sought diligently.

Diagnostic and Imaging Studies

Low voltage on the ECG and/or electrical alternans should suggest cardiac tamponade. However, electrical alternans is insensitive, occurring in only about 20 percent of instances.[31] When effusion is massive, the heart swings freely within the pericardial sac and acquires a pendular, rotary motion that is associated with electrical alternans. When tamponade is suspected, an echocardiogram should be obtained unless even a brief delay might prove life-threatening. During inspiration, a greater than normal increase in RV dimension and a decrease in LV dimension occur in many cases of tamponade. These respiratory changes also accompany other conditions associated with pulsus paradoxus, such as chronic obstructive lung disease and pulmonary embolism.[32] Diastolic collapse of the RV, which is recognized as an abnormal posterior motion of the anterior RV wall during diastole (Fig. 72-11), signifies that pericardial pressure exceeds early diastolic RV pressure, i.e., that transmural RV diastolic pressure is negative (see also Chap. 13). Although this sign is a relatively sensitive and specific marker for tamponade, RV diastolic collapse is sensitive to alterations in ventricular loading conditions and may not be seen in the presence of RV hypertrophy. In addition, right heart chamber collapse occurs with smaller collections of fluid and higher pericardial pressures when there is coexisting LV dysfunction.[29] Late diastolic right atrial collapse is virtually 100 percent sensitive for tamponade but is less specific (Fig. 72-12). A duration of right atrial collapse exceeding one-third of the cardiac cycle increases specificity without sacrificing sensitivity.[33] Posterior loculated effusions after cardiac surgery have been reported to produce left atrial and LV diastolic collapse.[34,35] The value of transesophageal echocardiography has been recognized in the detection and treatment of unusual cases of cardiac tamponade.[36] In patients with unexplained hypotension who are undergoing transesophageal echo, a diagnosis of a nonventricular limitation to cardiac output was associated with improved survival in the intensive care unit compared with a diagnosis of ventricular disease or hypovolemia/low systemic vascular resistance.[37]

During cardiac tamponade, tricuspid and pulmonary flow velocities measured by Doppler echocardiography (Fig. 72-13) increase markedly with inspiration, and mitral and aortic valve flow velocities decrease significantly compared with normal control patients and patients with asymptomatic effusions.[38] Changes in the pattern of venous flow (reflecting the predominance of systolic flow) and exaggerated respiratory variations of venous flow velocities (Fig. 72-14) also are seen in cardiac tamponade.[39] Indeed, abnormal venous flow had a good correlation with clinical tamponade with greater sensitivity than RV diastolic collapse and greater specificity than right atrial collapse.[40]

Cardiac Catheterization

The diagnosis of cardiac tamponade is confirmed by right heart catheterization. The right atrial, pulmonary capillary wedge, and pulmonary artery diastolic pressures are elevated, usually between 10 and 30 mmHg, and are equal within 4 to 5 mmHg (Fig. 72-15). Pericardial pressure is elevated and is equal to right atrial pressure; the degree of elevation is related to both the severity of tamponade and the patient's intravascular volume status (Fig. 72-16). The right atrial and wedge pressure tracings reveal an attenuated or absent Y descent. Cardiac output is reduced, and systemic vascular resistance is elevated. Equal elevation of diastolic pressures also may be seen with dilated cardiomyopathy and with RV infarction. Neither Kussmaul's sign nor the early ventricular diastolic dip and plateau (i.e., the "square root" sign) characteristic of pericardial constriction is seen in tamponade.

Management of Cardiac Tamponade

Removal of small amounts of pericardial fluid (~50 mL) produces considerable symptomatic and hemodynamic improvement because of the steep pericardial pressure-volume relation. Unless there is concomitant cardiac disease or coexisting constriction (i.e., effusive-constrictive pericarditis), removal of all the pericardial fluid normalizes pericardial, atrial, ventricular diastolic, and arterial pressures and cardiac output.

Unless the situation is immediately life-threatening, pericardiocentesis should be performed by experienced staff in a facility equipped for hemodynamic monitoring. The advantages of needle pericardiocentesis include the ability to perform careful

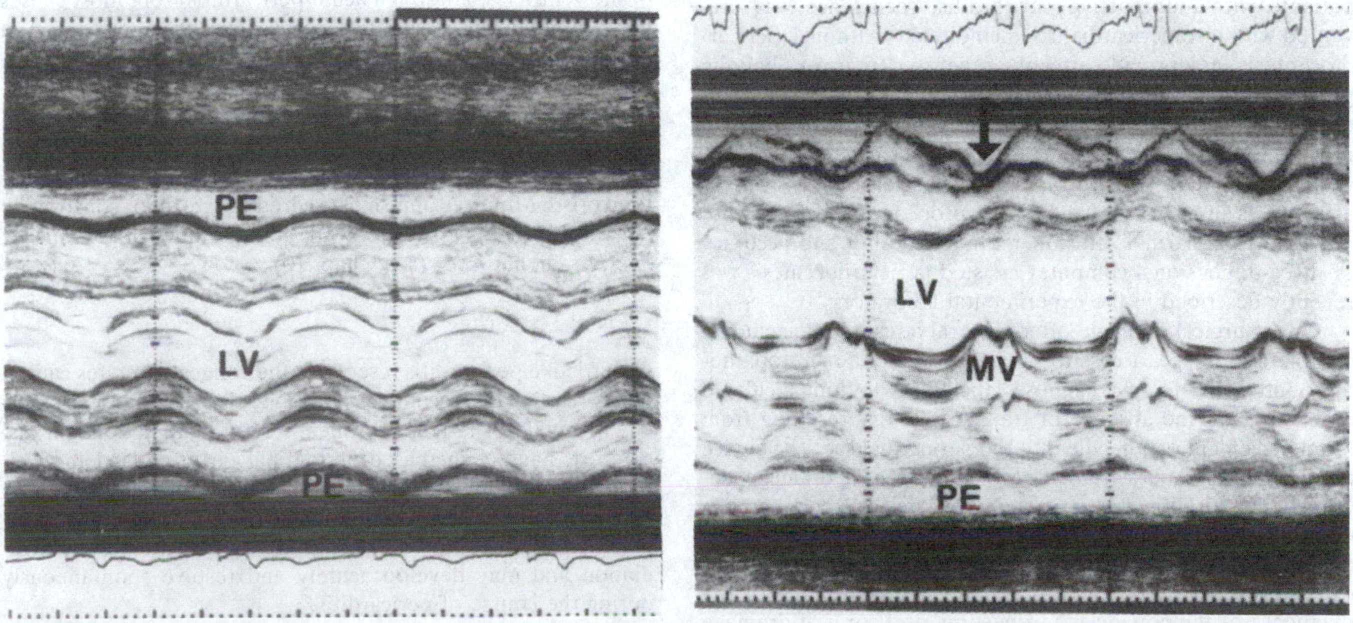

FIGURE 72-11 M-mode echocardiograms of pericardial effusion. The effusion (PE) appears as an echo-free space surrounding the heart. The effusion on the left does not cause cardiac compression. The effusion on the right demonstrates right ventricular diastolic collapse (*arrow*), evident as abnormal motion of the anterior free wall of the right ventricle that occurs after the mitral valve (MV) opens. LV-left ventricle. (From Hoit BD. Pericardial disease and pericardial heart disease. In: O' Rourke RA, ed. *Stein's Internal Medicine*, 5th ed. St. Louis, Missouri: Mosby-Year Book; 1998:273. Reproduced with permission.)

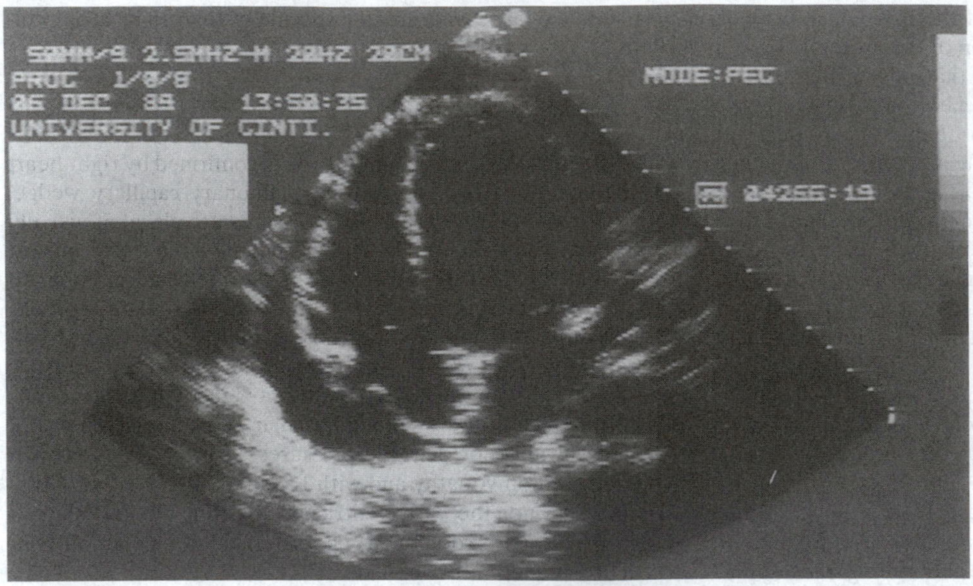

FIGURE 72-12 Two-dimensional echocardiogram in the apical four-chamber view. During late diastole, there is inversion of the lateral wall of the right atrium. (From Hoit BD. Imaging the pericardium. *Cardiol Clin* 1990; 8:593. Reproduced with permission.)

hemodynamic measurements and relatively simple logistic and personnel requirements. The safety of the procedure has been improved by using 2-D echo guidance.[41] A catheter can be advanced over a guidewire into the pericardial space and remain there for several days; sclerosing agents, steroids, urokinase, and specific chemotherapeutic agents may be given through the catheter.[42,43] In a pilot study, intrapericardial instillation of cisplatin for 24 hours prevented recurrence of a hemodynamically significant pericardial effusion after 6 to 12 months in 14 out of 15 patients with a neoplastic effusion; in 12 out of 14 patients with autoreactive pericarditis, recurrence was prevented with intrapericardial triamcinolone.[25] Although pericardiocentesis may provide effective relief, percutaneous balloon pericardiotomy, subxiphoid pericardiotomy, or the surgical creation of a pleuropericardial or peritoneal-pericardial window[44,45] may be required. Nevertheless, in one retrospective review, pericardiocentesis with intrapericardial sclerotherapy was as effective as an open surgical drainage procedure in patients with malignant pericardial effusion.[46] The feasibility and accuracy of three-dimensional computer-assisted pericardiocentesis was recently described in the experimental laboratory.[47]

Open surgical drainage offers several advantages, including complete drainage, access to pericardial tissue for histopathologic and microbiologic diagnoses, the ability to drain loculated effusions, and the absence of traumatic injury resulting from blind placement of a needle into the pericardial sac. The choice between needle pericardiocentesis and surgical drainage depends on institutional resources and physician experience, the etiology of the effusion, the need for diagnostic tissue samples, and the prognosis of the patient. Needle pericardiocentesis is often the best option when the etiology is known and/or the diagnoses of tamponade is in question, and surgical drainage is optimal when the presence of tamponade is certain but the etiology is unclear. It should be recognized that surgical approaches (subxiphoid pericardiotomy and thoracoscopic drainage) can be performed using local anesthesia with little attendant morbidity. Irrespective of the method of retrieval, pericardial fluid should be sent for smear, culture, and cytology.

Fluids should be given to patients with cardiac tamponade who are awaiting pericardial drainage in an effort to expand the intravascular volume. Dobutamine or nitroprusside may be used to increase cardiac output after the blood volume has been expanded, but only as a temporizing measure. Vagal reflexes complicating tamponade and pericardiocentesis are treated with atropine. Positive-pressure breathing should be avoided, and if present, metabolic acidosis should be corrected.

Recurrent effusions may be treated by repeat pericardiocentesis, sclerotherapy with tetracycline, surgical creation of a pericardial window, or pericardiectomy. A pericardial window usually is performed in patients with malignant effusions, and pericardiectomy may be required for recurrent effusions in dialysis patients. In critically ill patients, a pericardial window may be created percutaneously with a balloon catheter.[48,49]

CONSTRICTIVE PERICARDITIS

Constrictive pericarditis is a condition in which a thickened, scarred, and often calcified pericardium limits diastolic filling of the ventricles. Although acute pericarditis from most causes may eventuate in constrictive pericarditis, the most common antecedents are idiopathic conditions, cardiac trauma and surgery, tuberculosis and other infectious diseases, neoplasms (particularly lung and breast), radiation therapy, renal failure, and connective tissue diseases. Rare causes include Dressler's syndrome, sarcoidosis, Whipple's disease, amyloidosis, and dermatomyositis. Mulibrey nanism is a hereditary form of constrictive pericarditis that is associated with abnormalities of the *mu*scle, *li*ver, *br*ain, and *ey*es (see Chap. 10).

Clinical Features

Constrictive pericarditis resembles the congestive states caused by myocardial disease and chronic liver disease. Patients generally complain of fatigue, dyspnea, weight gain, abdominal discomfort, nausea, increased abdominal girth, and edema. Although symptoms usually develop over years, they progress over a period of months in patients with subacute constrictive pericarditis after trauma, cardiac surgery, and mediastinal irradiation and may develop acutely and resolve spontaneously during the course of pericarditis.[50]

Physical Findings

Physical findings include ascites, hepatosplenomegaly, edema, and, in long-standing cases, severe wasting. This general appearance often leads to an erroneous diagnosis of hepatic cirrhosis. However, misdiagnosis is avoided through a careful examination of the neck veins. In constrictive pericarditis, the venous pressure is elevated and displays deep Y and often deep X descents. The venous pressure fails to decrease with inspiration (Kussmaul's sign), but frank inspiratory swelling of the neck veins is uncommon. Kussmaul's sign lacks specificity, as it is seen also in cases of restrictive cardiomyopathy, RV failure and infarction, and tricuspid stenosis.[51] The heart is often normal-sized, and when it is not, enlargement is modest. A pericardial knock that is similar in timing to the third heart sound is pathognomonic but occurs infrequently.[51,52] Pulsus paradoxus may occur with associated pericardial effusion (effusive-constrictive pericarditis). Except in severe cases, the arterial blood pressure is normal.

Diagnostic and Imaging Studies

Low QRS voltage, nonspecific T-wave changes, and P mitrale are common, but the ECG findings are nonspecific (Fig. 72-17). Atrial fibrillation is seen in approximately one-third of cases, and atrial flutter is seen less often, although the exact percentage of atrial arrhythmias depends on the duration of constriction.

The cardiac silhouette may be normal or enlarged. Pericardial calcification is present in less than half the cases seen in the United States and Europe. Pericardial calcification may be seen with chronic adhesive pericarditis in the absence of constriction, but then it is usually less dense and has a more patchy distribution (Fig. 72-18).

Pericardial thickening and calcification and abnormal ventricular filling produce characteristic changes on the M-mode echocardiogram.[53] Increased pericardial thickness is suggested by parallel motion of the epicardium and parietal pericardium, which are sep-

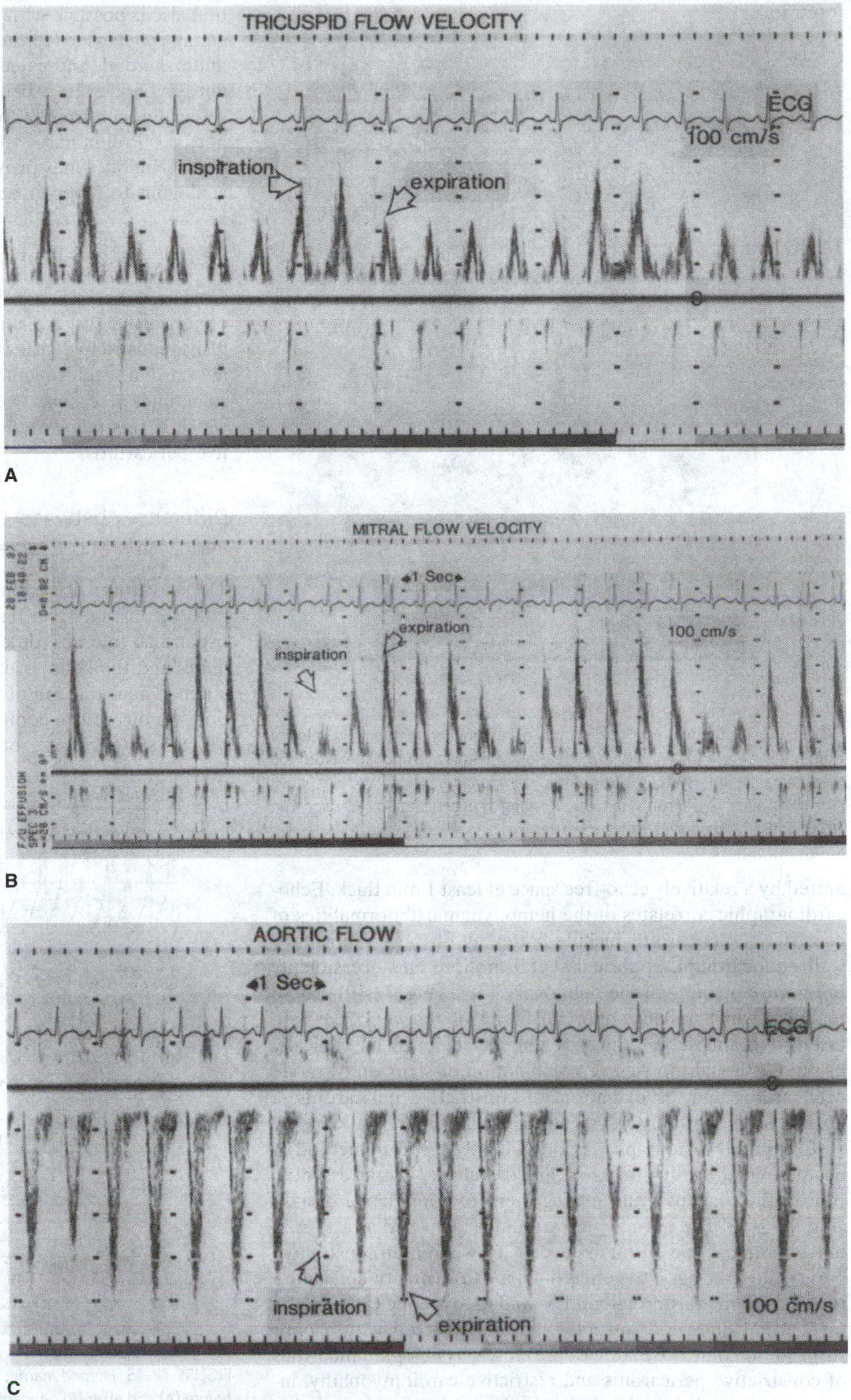

FIGURE 72-13 Doppler echocardiogram in a patient with cardiac tamponade. Note the inspiratory increase of tricuspid flow velocities (*A*) and the expiratory increase of mitral (*B*) and aortic (*C*) flow velocities. (From Hoit BD. Imaging the pericardium. *Cardiol Clin* 1990; 8:594. Reproduced with permission.)

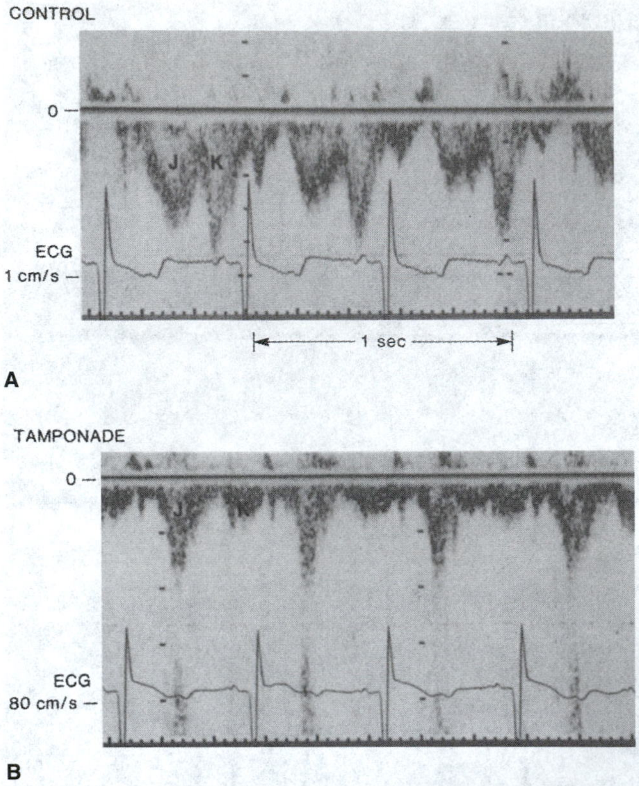

FIGURE 72-14 Doppler echocardiograms of pulmonary venous flow velocity from a dog before (*A*) and after (*B*) creation of cardiac tamponade. Note the predominance of systolic flow after tamponade. J = systolic flow; K = diastolic flow. (From Hoit BD. Imaging the pericardium. *Cardiol Clin* 1990; 8:595. Reproduced with permission.)

arated by a relatively echo-free space at least 1 mm thick. Echocardiographic correlates of the hemodynamic abnormalities of constrictive pericarditis include flattening of the LV posterior wall endocardium, abnormal septal motion, and occasionally premature opening of the pulmonary valve (Fig. 72-19). These findings, which reflect abnormal filling of the ventricles, are insensitive and subtle and lack the specificity to be clinically useful. Although no sign or combination of signs on M-mode echocardiography is diagnostic of constrictive pericarditis, a normal study virtually rules out the diagnosis.[53]

Computed tomography (CT) is a highly accurate method of evaluating pericardial thickness and therefore plays an essential role in the diagnosis and management of constrictive disease (Fig. 72-20).[54] The normal pericardium is identified as a 1- to 2-mm curvilinear line of soft tissue density, whereas in constrictive pericarditis, the parietal pericardium is 4 to 20 mm thick. Failure to visualize the posterolateral LV wall on dynamic CT suggests myocardial fibrosis or atrophy and is associated with a poor surgical outcome.[55] Because of the close physiologic similarities of constrictive pericarditis and restrictive cardiomyopathy, increased pericardial thickness detected by tomographic scanning is the most reliable means of distinguishing between the two disorders, as normal pericardial thickness excludes most cases of constrictive pericarditis. CT also is useful in planning pericardiectomy because of its ability to define the distribution of pericardial thickening.[56]

Accurate definition of pericardial thickness and its distribution also is possible with MRI (Fig. 72-21).[27,57] Unlike CT, ECG gating is necessary for adequate visualization, resolution is not quite as good, and calcification is difficult to distinguish from fibrosis. However, excellent diagnostic accuracy in identifying surgically confirmed constrictive pericarditis has been reported.[58] Preliminary studies suggest that phase velocity mapping techniques may provide additional diagnostic information, analogous to Doppler echo.

Cardiac Catheterization

Cardiac catheterization is used to confirm the clinical suspicion of pericardial disease, uncover occult constriction, diagnose effusive-constrictive disease, and identify associated coronary, myocardial, and valvular disease. Endomyocardial biopsy is sometimes necessary to exclude restrictive cardiomyopathy, which shares many hemodynamic abnormalities with constrictive pericarditis.

Differences between Constrictive Pericarditis and Cardiac Tamponade

The waveform of venous pressure in constrictive pericarditis differs from that in cardiac tamponade. In constrictive pericarditis, cardiac volume is determined by the thickened, rigid pericardium, and the heart is unable to exceed this volume, which is attained near the end of the first third of diastole. During ejection, venous return commences unimpeded, and therefore, the normal systolic surge of venous return is preserved. Cardiac

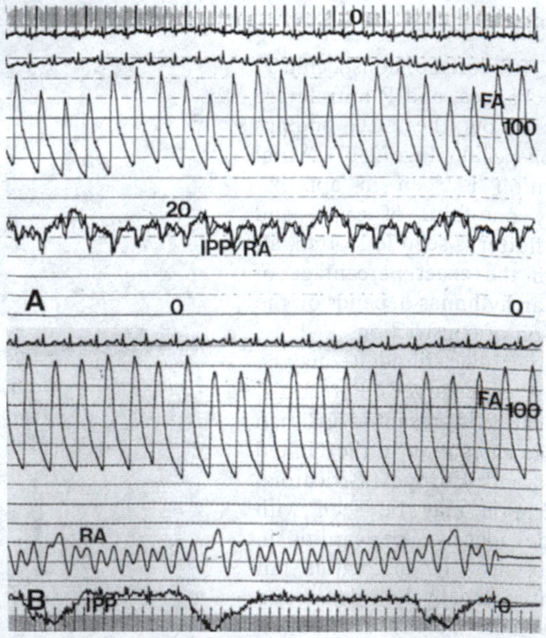

FIGURE 72-15 Hemodynamic record from a patient with cardiac tamponade before (*A*) and after (*B*) pericardiocentesis. *A*. Pulsus paradoxus is evident from the femoral artery (FA) pressure tracing. Note the absent Y descent on the right atrial (RA) tracing and the equal and elevated RA and pericardial (IPP) pressures. *B*. After removal of pericardial fluid, pericardial and right atrial pressures decrease and the pulsus paradoxus disappears. (Courtesy of Noble O Fowler, MD. From Hoit BD. Pericardial disease and pericardial heart disease. In: O'Rourke RA, ed. *Stein's Internal Medicine*, 5th ed. Mosby-Year Book;1998:273. Reproduced with permission.)

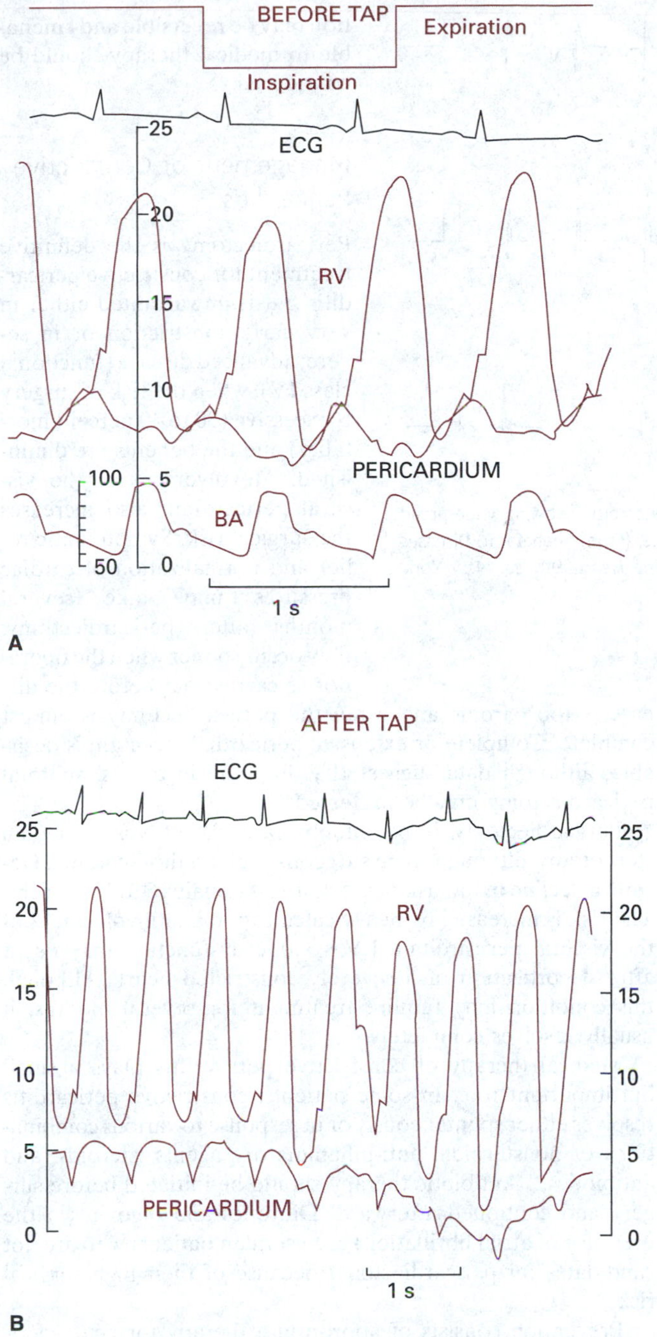

FIGURE 72-16 *A*. Low-pressure cardiac tamponade. Right ventricular (RV) diastolic pressure is only slightly elevated but is equal to pericardial pressure. Hypotension and pulsus paradoxus are absent. *B*. After pericardiocentesis, pericardial pressure is consistently lower than ventricular diastolic pressure. (From Shabetai R. Diseases of the pericardium. In Alexander WA, Schlant R, Fuster V, et al., eds. *Hurst's The Heart,* 9th ed. New York: McGraw-Hill; 1998:2185. Reproduced with permission.)

compression remains insignificant at end systole (unlike cardiac tamponade), so that when the tricuspid valve opens, blood fills the ventricles at a supranormal rate. Thus, in constrictive pericarditis, the venous return is biphasic, but with a diastolic component greater than or equal to the systolic component.

Unlike cardiac tamponade, the intrapericardial space is obliterated in constrictive pericarditis. As a result, during inspiration, the decreased intrathoracic pressure is not transmitted to the heart, venous pressure does not fall, and systemic venous return fails to increase. Another important distinction from cardiac tamponade is that early diastolic filling is faster than normal in constrictive pericarditis, and consequently, the ventricular diastolic pressure is characterized by a dip in early diastole (Fig. 72-22). By the end of the rapid filling phase, the ventricles are completely filled and the ventricular diastolic pressure remains unchanged and elevated for the remainder of diastole. The resultant pattern of ventricular diastolic pressure in constrictive pericarditis is referred to as the "dip-and-plateau pattern" or the "square-root sign."

In contrast to cardiac tamponade, early diastolic filling in constrictive pericarditis is unrestrained, and only at the end of the first third of diastole does the stiff pericardium abruptly restrict ventricular filling. As a result, ventricular pressure falls rapidly in early diastole and subsequently rises abruptly to an elevated level, where it remains until the next ventricular systole. End-diastolic ventricular pressures and mean atrial pressures are elevated and nearly equal (within 5 mmHg), and end-diastolic volumes and, consequently, stroke volume and cardiac output are reduced. These pathophysiologic changes are responsible for the hemodynamic and physical findings that characterize constrictive pericarditis.[51]

Pulsus paradoxus is much less common in constrictive pericarditis than it is in cardiac tamponade because in constrictive pericarditis, inspiratory increases in venous return and in the volume of the right side of the heart seldom occur, and the position of the ventricular septum relative to the two ventricles is not as dramatically altered.

Systolic LV function is usually unimpaired in both constrictive pericarditis and cardiac tamponade. Long-standing calcific constrictive pericarditis may invade the myocardium and coronary vessels, leading to conduction disturbances and impaired ventricular function.

Syndromes of Constrictive Pericarditis

Classic *chronic constrictive pericarditis* is encountered less frequently than it was in the past, whereas *subacute constrictive pericarditis* is becoming more common. In the latter syndrome, pericardial calcification is uncommon and the course may span a matter of weeks to a few years. *Postoperative constrictive pericarditis* is an important cause of constriction, with a reported incidence of 0.2 percent[59]; this incidence is surprisingly low considering that in these operations the pericardium is subject to cellular injury and is exposed to proinflammatory substances such as blood and local hypothermia.

Occult constrictive pericarditis requires a fluid challenge for detection.[60] In the first series reported, the patients complained of nondescript chest pain, for which they underwent cardiac catheterization and coronary arteriography. Although hemodynamic studies revealed normal basal atrial and ventricular pressures, the right atrial pressure waveform assumed the characteristics of constrictive pericarditis and the diastolic pressures in the two ventricles became equal after a rapid infusion (10 min) of approximately 1 L of saline solution. Histologic examination confirmed the surgical findings of a thickened and fibrosed pericardium. Rapid, large fluid challenges at cardiac catheterization should be administered with caution; furthermore, the induction of hemodynamic changes suggesting constrictive pericarditis by

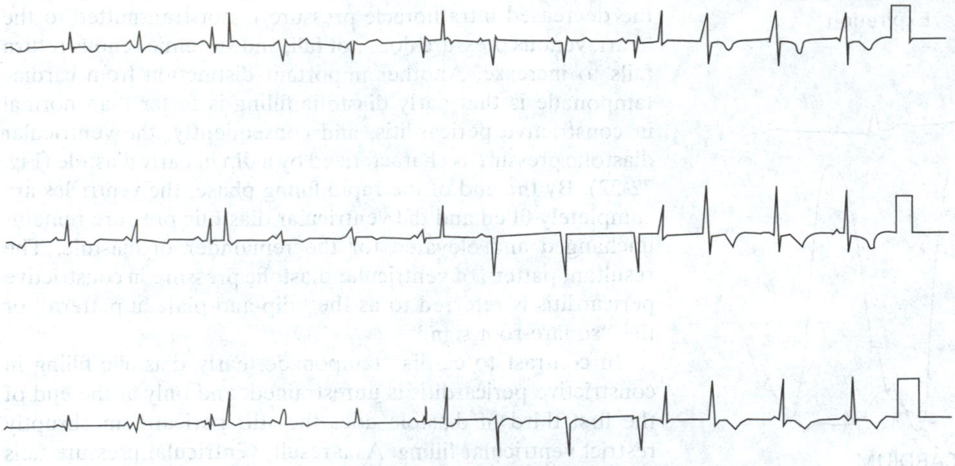

FIGURE 72-17 Electrocardiogram of a patient with tuberculous constrictive pericarditis showing widespread inversed polarity of the T waves. Leads are mounted in the conventional sequence. (From Shabetai R. Diseases of the pericardium. In Alexander WA, Schlant R, Fuster V, et al., eds. *Hurst's The Heart*, 9th ed. New York: McGraw-Hill; 1998:2188. Reproduced with permission.)

this technique should seldom, if ever, be taken alone as an indication for pericardiectomy.

Localized constrictive pericarditis is rare, but occasionally a localized band constricts the inflow or outflow region of one or more of the cardiac chambers. The clinical picture then simulates valve disease or venous obstruction. Evidence of *transient* (*acute*) *constriction* may occur in ~15 percent of patients with acute effusive pericarditis.[61] Therefore, before one proceeds with pericardiectomy, the possibility that pericardial constriction may be reversible and amenable to medical therapy should be considered.

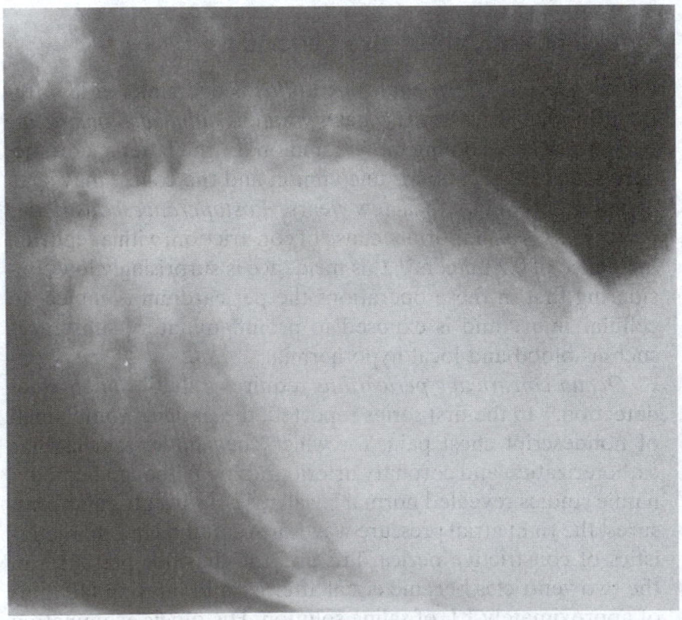

FIGURE 72-18 Calcification of the pericardium seen on a lateral chest radiograph in a patient with chronic constrictive pericarditis. (Courtesy of Ralph Shabetai, MD. From Hoit BD. Imaging the pericardium. *Cardiol Clin* 1990; 8:595. Reproduced with permission.)

Management of Constrictive Pericarditis

Pericardiectomy is the definitive treatment for constrictive pericarditis but is unwarranted either in very early constriction or in severe, advanced disease (functional class IV), when the risk of surgery is excessive (30 to 40 percent mortality) and the benefits are diminished.[62] Involvement of the visceral pericardium also increases the surgical risk. Symptomatic relief and normalization of cardiac pressures may take several months after pericardiectomy; they occur sooner when the operation is carried out before the disease is too chronic and when the pericardiectomy is almost complete. Complete or extensive pericardial resection is desirable, although data suggest that in some instances, subtotal pericardiectomy may be preferred.[63]

Pericardiectomy is commonly carried out via a median sternotomy, although some surgeons prefer a thoracotomy. Despite a decline in the risk of mortality, it remains 5 to 15 percent. The risk is increased by heavy calcification and involvement of the visceral pericardium. LV systolic dysfunction may occur after decortication of a severely constricted heart. Although this condition may require treatment for several months, it usually resolves completely.

Medical therapy of constrictive pericarditis plays a small but important role. In some patients, constrictive pericarditis resolves either spontaneously or in response to various combinations of nonsteroidal anti-inflammatory agents, steroids, and antibiotics.[50] Antibiotic therapy should be initiated before surgery and continued afterward. Diuretics and digoxin (in the presence of atrial fibrillation) are useful in patients who are not candidates for pericardiectomy because of their high surgical risk.

Prevention consists of appropriate therapy for acute pericarditis and adequate pericardial drainage. Although urokinase instillation is promising, corticosteroids are often ineffective.

EFFUSIVE-CONSTRICTIVE PERICARDITIS

Effusive-constrictive pericarditis occurs when pericardial fluid accumulates between the thickened, fibrotic parietal pericardium and visceral pericardium. Neoplasia, chest irradiation, infection, idiopathic pericarditis, and connective tissue diseases are common antecedents. Transient effusive-constrictive pericarditis may complicate chemotherapy.[64] The hemodynamic features are those of cardiac tamponade before, and constrictive pericarditis after, pericardiocentesis. Thus, removal of pericardial fluid fails to lower atrial and ventricular diastolic pressures, but the previously attenuated or absent atrial Y descent becomes prominent (Fig. 72-23).

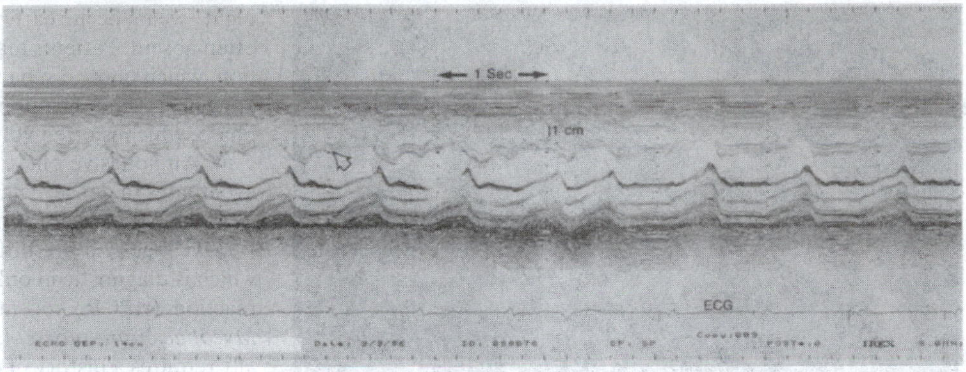

FIGURE 72-19 M-mode echocardiogram from a patient with constrictive pericarditis. An abrupt posterior motion of the septum begins after the onset of atrial systole. This atrial systolic notch is not seen on premature or paced beats. Note also the thickened pericardium and flat posterior wall in middle and late diastole. (From Tei C, Child JS, Tanaka H, et al. Atrial systolic notch on the interventricular septum echogram: An echocardiographic sign of constrictive pericarditis. *J Am Coll Cardiol* 1983; 1:908. Reproduced with permission.)

SPECIFIC FORMS OF PERICARDIAL HEART DISEASE

Idiopathic Pericarditis

Acute pericarditis is most often idiopathic and is typically a self-limited disease lasting 2 to 6 weeks.[65] Recurrence occurs in 25 percent of cases and occasionally proves resistant to therapy. Small pericardial effusions occur commonly, but cardiac tamponade is unusual. Heart failure caused by associated myocarditis and constrictive pericarditis are uncommon. These complications usually can be detected by clinical and echocardiographic evaluation. The clinical course and prognosis of individuals with pericarditis are otherwise determined largely by the presence and nature of any underlying disease.

Infectious Pericarditis

VIRAL PERICARDITIS

Viral pericarditis is the most common infectious type, although a definitive diagnosis from acute and convalescent (3 weeks) viral neutralizing antibodies is generally not helpful in a sporadic case of pericarditis. Viral isolation from pericardial fluid and in situ hybridization techniques have been used to identify a specific etiology.[20,66] However, viral infection often is presumed rather than proved, and many cases are classified as idiopathic. Epicardial biopsy via a pericardioscope is a promising investigative technique for establishing the etiology of acute pericarditis. Common viral infections causing acute pericarditis are those resulting from echovirus and coxsackie virus; however, a great many different viruses may cause pericarditis (Table 72-2).

BACTERIAL PERICARDITIS

Bacterial (purulent) pericarditis most often is caused by streptococci, staphylococci, and gram-negative rods; *Haemophilus influenzae* is an important cause in children.[67] The increasing frequency of cardiac surgery and instrumentation, selection-induced changes in the flora responsible for hospital-acquired infections, and the prolonged survival of immunocompromised hosts (HIV, steroids) have changed the incidence and bacterial spectrum of purulent pericarditis. Pericardial involvement often is unrecognized when it complicates systemic infection; unusually high fever and white blood cell counts are clues to the presence of pericarditis. Children and immunosuppressed patients of all ages are most vulnerable, and the characteristic features of acute pericarditis are frequently absent. The course of bacterial pericarditis is fulminant, often presenting with cardiac tamponade; adhesive and constrictive pericarditis are common sequelae in survivors and may develop suddenly and early.[67,68] However,

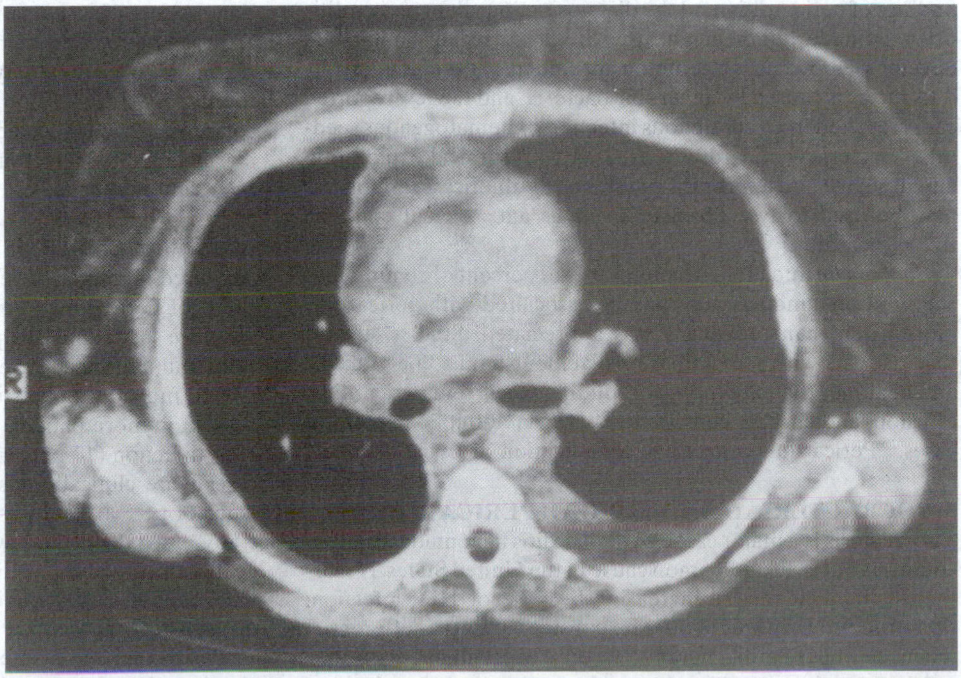

FIGURE 72-20 Computed tomogram from a patient with constrictive pericarditis. The diffusely thickened pericardium is bordered by low-intensity epicardial and mediastinal fat. (Courtesy of Dr. N. O. Fowler. From Hoit BD. Imaging the pericardium. *Cardiol Clin* 1990; 8:597. Reproduced with permission.)

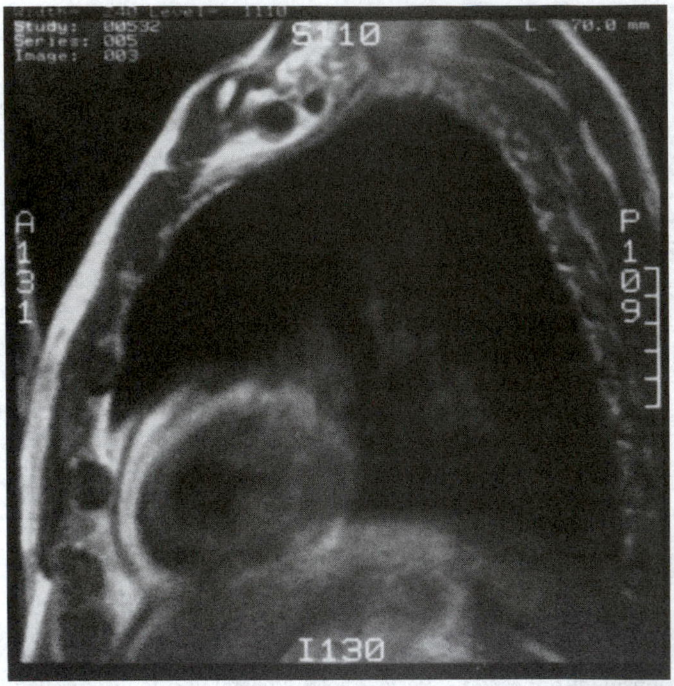

FIGURE 72-21 MRI scan (spin-echo image) from a patient with constrictive pericarditis. The pericardium is viewed as a line of low signal intensity (black) sandwiched between higher-intensity epicardial and pericardial fat (white). Note the regional variation of pericardial thickness, which is normally 1 to 2 mm. (From Hoit BD. Pericardial disease and pericardial heart disease. In: O'Rourke RA, ed. *Stein's Internal Medicine*, 5th ed. St. Louis, Missouri: Mosby-Year Book;1998:273. Reproduced with permission.)

pericarditis complicating systemic infection and sepsis may go unrecognized and misdiagnosed.[69] Many patients lack the typical findings of pericarditis, and the diagnosis of purulent pericarditis often is made either at autopsy or after cardiac tamponade develops; empyema is a common antecedent.[67] Purulent pericarditis rarely is caused by anaerobic bacteria, and the few reported cases resulted from contiguous infection or hematogenous seeding.[70] Bacterial pericarditis is treated with surgical exploration and drainage and appropriate systemic antibiotics. Fibrinolytics may be used to lyse fibrous adhesions and prevent constrictive pericarditis.[71–73]

Legionella infections account for ~10 percent of community-acquired pneumonias and may be associated with pericarditis more often than previously was appreciated. Studies suggest that patients with pericardial involvement tend to be younger and healthier than are those without it.[74] Recurrent pericarditis, effusion, and chronic constriction occur in about 20 percent of cases.[75] Pericarditis is an early complication of Lyme disease.[76]

MYOCBACTERIAL AND FUNGAL PERICARDITIS

Tuberculosis is a major cause of pericarditis in nonindustrialized countries but is an uncommon cause in the United States. Nevertheless, its incidence is increasing because of HIV infection; therefore, tuberculosis should be considered in the differential diagnosis of pericardial heart disease.[77] Tuberculous pericarditis results from hematogenous spread of primary tuberculosis or from the breakdown of infected mediastinal lymph nodes; therefore, affected individuals generally lack the typical symptoms and signs of pulmonary tuberculosis. Fever, weight loss, and night sweats occur early; pericardial pain and friction rubs are often absent. Patients may present with tamponade or constriction, which may be subacute. A fibrinous pericarditis with caseating necrosis and mononuclear infiltrate gives rise to an effusive phase, which is often voluminous and hemodynamically significant. An adhesive phase follows resolution of the effusion and eventuates in dense, calcific adhesions with clinical constriction in nearly 50 percent of patients.

Mycobacteria are difficult to culture from pericardial fluid, which is diagnostic in only one-third of cases; polymerase chain reaction (rtPCR) recently was used to amplify and identify *Mycobacterium tuberculosis.*[78] A presumptive diagnosis generally requires a history of contact and/or purified protein derivative conversion (although the latter lacks sensitivity and specificity). Gadolinium-enhanced MRI may be useful in early diagnosis.[79] Increased adenosine deaminase activity in pericardial fluid is supportive. However, the diagnosis of tuberculous pericarditis is based on (1) histologic identification, (2) culture of *M. tuberculosis,* (3) pericarditis with proven extracardiac tuberculosis, or (4) pericardial effusion responsive to antituberculosis therapy.

Early pericardiectomy has been recommended by some researchers in all cases of tuberculosis pericarditis, but the long-term (16 years) prognosis of patients without cardiac compression during the acute illness who are treated with medical therapy alone is excellent.[80] Multiple-drug therapy and corticosteroids are effective in tuberculous pericarditis, whereas atypical mycobacterial infections (especially *M. avium-intracellulare*) may be resistant to treatment. Patients with tuberculous pericarditis should receive triple-drug therapy (isoniazid, rifampin, and streptomycin or ethambutol) for a minimum of 9 months. Corticosteroids may be useful if pericardial effusion persists or recurs during therapy; pericardiectomy may be necessary for recurrent cardiac tamponade. Patients should be observed for constriction; up to half these patients will require pericardiectomy.[81] In contrast, pericarditis complicating deep fungal infection (histoplasmosis, coccidioidomyocosis) may be immunologic, resolve spontaneously, and not require specific therapy. Surgical decompression and specific antifungal therapy may be necessary for disseminated infection with *Candida, Aspergillus, Actinomycetes,* and *Nocardia.*

AIDS PERICARDITIS

Acquired immunodeficiency syndrome (AIDS) is an important cause of pericardial heart disease. Typically, pericardial effusions are small and asymptomatic in outpatients, but large effusions and tamponade are common in hospitalized patients with AIDS. Indeed, in one study, a moderate or large effusion was present in more patients with symptomatic than asymptomatic HIV infection (17 percent versus 2 percent), and most of these cases were clinically unsuspected.[82] The incidence and prevalence of pericardial effusion in a prospective, 5-year follow-up study of AIDS patients were high (11 percent/year and 5 percent, respectively).[83] A literature review of echocardiographic and autopsy series found an average incidence of pericardial disease of 21 percent.[84]

Pericardial involvement may be due to associated malignancies (e.g., lymphoma and Kaposi's sarcoma), viruses (including HIV) and opportunistic infections (e.g., mycobacteria, cytomegalovirus, *Nocardia,* and cryptococci) and, irrespective of its cause, predicts a poor prognosis in patients with HIV infection.[85]

Large, symptomatic pericardial effusion in patients with HIV infection should be aggressively investigated, as two-thirds of these cases have an identifiable cause.[84] Tamponade in patients with HIV is mycobacterial (*M. tuberculosis* or *avium-intracellulare*) in origin in approximately one-third of patients.[84]

In 68 patients with HIV infection prospectively admitted to the intensive care unit, only 5 had evidence of cardiac disease, but 35 had echocardiographic abnormalities (20 effusions, 2 with tamponade, 15 cases of left ventricular dysfunction, and 4 valvular abnormalities).[86] The presence of an effusion was associated with greater 6-month mortality in patients with AIDS (96 percent versus 36 percent); interestingly, an asymptomatic pericardial effusion may signal end-stage HIV disease, independent of the CD4 count and albumin level.[83]

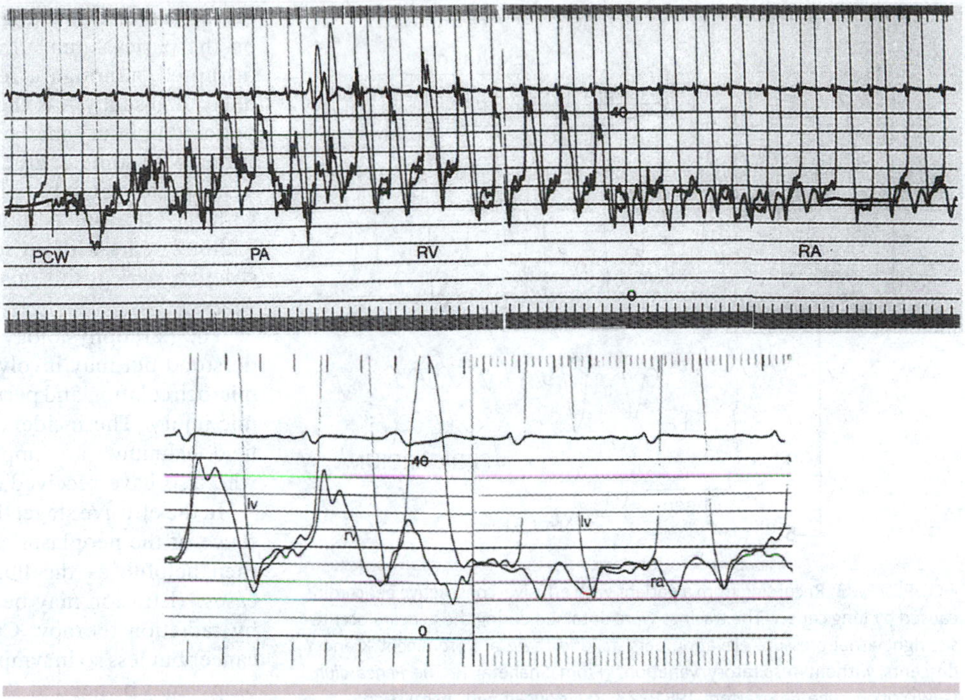

FIGURE 72-22 Hemodynamic record of a patient with surgically proven constrictive pericarditis. *Top*. Slow paper speed recording of high-gain left ventricular (LV) pressure and simultaneous right heart pullback from pulmonary capillary wedge (PCW) to pulmonary artery (PA), right ventricle (RV), and right atrium (RA). *Bottom*. Fast paper speed recording of LV and simultaneous RV and RA pressure tracings. Note the increased and equal atrial and diastolic pressures, the prominent X and Y descents on the RA tracing, and the dip and plateau on the RV and LV tracings during longer diastoles. (Courtesy of Peter J. Engel, MD. From Hoit BD. Pericardial disease and pericardial heart disease. In: O'Rourke RA, ed. *Stein's Internal Medicine*, 5th ed. St. Louis, Missouri: Mosby-Year Book; 1998:273. Reproduced with permission.)

Neoplastic Pericarditis

Metastatic neoplasia remains the leading cause of pericardial disease in hospitalized patients, most often in patients with lung or breast cancer, melanoma, lymphoma, and acute leukemia. Many cases are asymptomatic and are found only incidentally at autopsy, but others cause symptoms and may progress to cardiac tamponade. Primary cardiac tumors may invade the pericardium directly.

Primary mesothelioma of the pericardium is a rare and highly lethal tumor.[87] Signs and symptoms are nonspecific, and chest radiography and echocardiography are insensitive for its detection; CT and MRI are the most promising diagnostic tests. Other primary tumors of the pericardium are quite rare.

In patients with elevated jugular pressure and an intrathoracic mass, an important inclusion in the differential diagnosis is the superior vena cava syndrome. In this disorder, the characteristic pulsations of the jugular veins are not observed and pulsus paradoxus is not present. However, in a patient with respiratory distress, pulsus alternans, arrhythmia, and/or tachycardia, pulsus paradoxus may be obscured.

The pericardium may be thickened and cause constriction; less commonly, effusive-constrictive pericarditis occurs. Echocardiography rapidly and accurately detects pericardial effusion, identifies metastatic lesions, and provides evidence for cardiac compression. MRI is particularly useful in evaluating pericardial mass lesions. Neoplastic cells can be recovered from the pericardial fluid, which is usually bloody, in many cases. However, it is important to remember that more than half of pericardial effusions in cancer patients are due to causes other than metastatic disease, such as infections, radiation, and drug therapy; thus, the presence of pericarditis in cancer patients does not imply imminent death.[88]

Postmyocardial Infarction Pericarditis

Pericarditis is common in the first few days after an MI, occurring in as many as 28 to 43 percent of fatal infarctions, but is clinically apparent in as few as 7 percent of cases.[89] When friction rub is required for diagnosis, there is an underestimation of the incidence of postinfarction pericarditis. On average, pericarditis was diagnosed by rub alone in 14 percent compared with 25 percent when classic symptoms, a rub, or both were used as diagnostic criteria.[90] The detection of atypical T-wave evolution on ECG (i.e., either persistent positivity or temporally late positivity) may be a more sensitive and objective means of diagnosing postinfarction pericarditis.[91]

Pericardial involvement is related to infarct size and is associated with a poor prognosis.[92] An important clinical problem is the extent to which acute pericarditis in myocardial infarction influences management with anticoagulants. A pericardial friction rub occurring in the first 2 or 3 days without an associated pericardial effusion should not influence clinical decisions, but pericarditis occurring later in the course or accompanied by pericardial effusion or tamponade is a contraindication to anticoagulant therapy.

In a prospective, consecutive series of 174 patients with acute myocardial infarction, pericarditis occurred in 24 percent and was associated with anterior infarct location, heparin therapy,

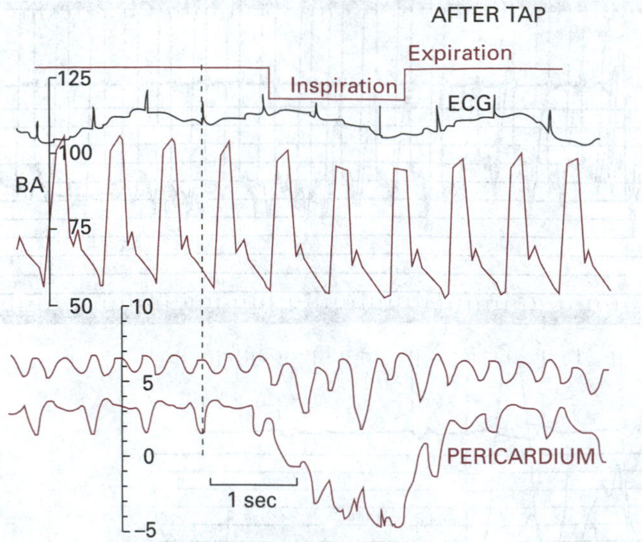

FIGURE 72-23 Recording from a patient with effusive-constrictive pericarditis caused by lung cancer. The tracings were obtained during the pericardiocentesis; right atrial pressure elevation persists, and there are prominent X and Y descents without respiratory variation. (From Shabetai R. *The Pericardium*. New York: Grune & Stratton; 1981:273. Reproduced with permission.)

and pericardial effusion.[93] Cardiac tamponade seldom occurs, except in patients who receive systemic anticoagulants or have cardiac rupture.

Thrombolytic therapy almost invariably precedes the development of pericarditis; therefore, clinical decision making usually is not affected. Surprisingly, thrombolytic therapy reduces the incidence of postinfarction pericarditis by approximately one-half.[94] However, when acute pericarditis is mistaken for acute myocardial infarction, thrombolytic therapy can have calamitous consequences. In patients treated mistakenly for myopericarditis with thrombolytics, the outcome was favorable.[95]

Dressler's syndrome (postmyocardial infarction syndrome) consists of pleuropericardial chest pain, friction rub, fever, leukocytosis, and pulmonary infiltrates. It usually occurs weeks or months (>10 days to 2 weeks) after the causative infarction. Dressler's syndrome may be caused by a combination of viral activation and myocardial antibodies and is clinically and pathogenetically similar to the postpericardiotomy syndrome. Cardiac tamponade of and late constriction may occur. For reasons that are not entirely clear, thrombolytic therapy has helped render post–myocardial infarction pericarditis nearly extinct.[96]

Radiation-Induced Pericardial Disease

Radiation injury to the pericardium is said to occur after exposure in excess of 4000 rads; the incidence also is dependent on the use of subcarinal blocks, the nature of the radiation source, and the duration and fractionation of the radiation regimen. For example, approximately 20 percent of Hodgkin's disease patients receiving ^{60}Co radiation with anterior weighting of the beam develop pericarditis, whereas the incidence of pericarditis after high-dose radiation for breast cancer (which includes less of the heart in the radiation field) is less than 5 percent.

Acute pericarditis occurring early during therapy is uncommon and most likely is a result of the radiation-induced effects on the tumor rather than a direct toxic effect of the radiation on the pericardium.[97] In this instance, therapy should not be disrupted, although a reduction in dose may be necessary. A delayed (usually less than 1 year but highly variable) form of pericardial injury may present as acute pericarditis or effusion (often with some degree of cardiac compression). The reaction of the pericardium to radiation is fibrinous inflammation,[98] often with an effusion. Although the acute lesion usually subsides within 2 years without sequelae, constrictive and effusive-constrictive pericarditis may become manifest only after many years.

The pathophysiology of radiation pericarditis is poorly understood but may involve extensive damage to the pericardial microcirculation and pericardial lymphatics with resultant ischemic injury. The incidence increases when anteriorly weighted field techniques are employed and is more common in patients who also have received adjunctive chemotherapy.

In the effusive stage, the differential diagnosis includes recurrence of the neoplasm, and examination of pericardial fluid is then helpful, as the fluid is positive in about 30 percent of cases.[99] Effusion may be due to the hypothyroid state induced by radiation therapy. Cytology is reliable in breast and lung cancer but less so in lymphoma and leukemia, where pericardial biopsy may be needed. Acute radiation-induced pericarditis can be managed symptomatically as acute idiopathic pericarditis. Hemodynamically insignificant pericardial effusion also can be managed conservatively, as spontaneous resolution is the rule; however, pericardiectomy should be offered to symptomatic patients with large, recurrent pericardial effusions. Constrictive pericarditis requires pericardiectomy unless the biopsy reveals significant endomyocardial fibrosis.

Traumatic Pericardial Disease

Blunt trauma and penetrating trauma are important causes of pericarditis, particularly among young men.[100] Chronic constrictive pericarditis, recurrent pericardial effusion, and recurrent acute pericarditis are well-recognized complications. Traumatic pericarditis may be life-threatening. The application of echocardiography in the trauma unit rapidly and accurately diagnoses hemopericardium in patients with potentially penetrating cardiac wounds.[101] Failure to repair the injury responsible for tamponade is associated with a poor clinical outcome.[102] Constrictive pericarditis occasionally occurs and may be delayed, presenting weeks or years after the injury.[103] Chylous pericardial effusions generally follow traumatic or surgical injury to the thoracic duct but may result from neoplastic obstruction of the thoracic duct or may be idiopathic.

Nephrogenic Pericardial Disease

Pericarditis complicates both uremia and dialytic therapy (hemo- and peritoneal dialysis) and may be clinically silent. The clinical manifestation of nephrogenic pericardial disease may be acute fibrinous pericarditis, pericardial effusion, or cardiac tamponade; classic constrictive pericarditis is rare.

The pathogenesis remains unknown. The etiology of pericarditis in dialyzed patients may be different from that in end-stage renal disease. The theory that uremic pericarditis is a chemical response to retained products of metabolism fails to account for a poor relationship between the blood urea nitrogen

(BUN) or other nitrogenous metabolites and the frequency of pericarditis. Since pericarditis is less common in patients undergoing peritoneal dialysis than in those receiving hemodialysis, there is a possible role for "middle molecules." Moreover, the hemorrhagic diathesis seen in the uremic syndrome may predispose to pericarditis; the resultant pericarditis is highly vascular, and consequently, the uremia or dialysis-related pericardial effusion is generally bloody. Renal insufficiency is associated with increased susceptibility to infection, and therefore, the possibility of viral, tuberculous, or even bacterial pericarditis must be considered. Immunologic abnormalities also have been implicated as a cause of pericardial disease in this setting. A presumptive diagnosis of dialysis-related pericarditis should be made only after other causes of pericardial heart disease (such as neoplasia and post-MI) that are common in this patient population have been excluded.

The clinical manifestations of cardiac tamponade may be atypical and difficult to distinguish from cardiovascular deterioration in patients undergoing hemodialysis. Cardiac tamponade remains one of the principal causes of hemodialysis-associated morbidity and terminates fatally in 20 percent of cases.

Although intensification of dialysis is an accepted treatment modality for hemodynamically insignificant disease, considerable controversy exists regarding the optimal management of large, persistent, or recurrent pericardial effusion and tamponade. Severe tamponade is an indication for pericardial drainage, but a conservative approach—intensification of dialysis and nonsteroidal anti-inflammatory agents—may suffice in less severe cases. The instillation of nonabsorbable steroids directly into the pericardial space has been advocated.[42] Dialysis-associated effusive pericarditis usually responds to an intensification of dialysis and regional heparinization or to a change to peritoneal dialysis. Pericardiectomy may be necessary for intractable effusions.

Myxedema Pericardial Disease

Pericarditis with effusion (sometimes containing cholesterol) occurs in about one-third of patients with myxedema. Effusions develop slowly and may reach a prodigious size; slow resolution usually follows the institution of thyroid replacement therapy. A case of hypothyroidism and viral pericarditis in a patient presenting to the emergency room with abdominal pain and shock was reported recently.[104]

Connective Tissue Disease–Related Pericardial Disease

Pericarditis may accompany virtually any connective tissue disease and may present as either acute or chronic pericarditis with or without an effusion.[105] Although tamponade, effusive-constrictive disease, and constrictive pericarditis are recognized complications, most cases are subclinical and in many instances are recognized only at autopsy.[106]

Rheumatoid pericardial disease is more common in middle-aged men in whom the onset of arthritis is acute. Serologic tests for rheumatoid disease are usually positive, and typical rheumatoid nodules are common. Rheumatoid arthritis is one of the causes of cholesterol pericarditis. Constrictive pericarditis is usually subacute and seldom is calcific. Pericardiectomy may be required within months of the first diagnosis of acute pericarditis and is almost always required within 5 years.[107,108]

Effusions are common in patients with SLE, and recurrent pericarditis, adhesion, and constriction may eventuate[109]; indeed, pericardial disease develops in nearly all patients with SLE when life is prolonged by steroid treatment. The pericardial fluid usually has a high protein content and a normal or slightly reduced glucose content; LE cells may be found. As in rheumatoid arthritis, the complement level is low.

Pericardial involvement may be found in systemic sclerosis (scleroderma), often in association with cardiomyopathy and diffuse scleroderma.[110] Dermatomyositis is not infrequently associated with pericardial involvement, including tamponade. Pericarditis is a rare complication in a wide variety of connective tissue disorders and arteritides (Table 72-2).

Iatrogenic Pericardial Disease

Iatrogenic pericardial disease results from both the calculated complications and the unanticipated misadventures of diagnostic and therapeutic procedures. Radiation pericarditis is one type of iatrogenic pericardial disease and was discussed earlier.

Postcardiotomy syndrome, which complicates 5 to 30 percent of cardiac operations, usually appears in the second or third week to 2 months after cardiac surgery; affected patients frequently have high titers of antiheart and antiviral antibodies and may develop cardiac tamponade.

Cardiac perforation complicating diagnostic cardiac catheterization and pacemaker insertion, complications of endoscopic sclerotherapy of esophageal varices, and automatic defibrillator electrode placement are other causes of iatrogenic pericardial disease. Pericardial abnormalities may develop in response to a number of drugs, of which the more important are hydralazine, procainamide, and daunorubicin, although these abnormalities have been reported with a number of agents (Table 72-2). Cardiac tamponade after thrombolysis with rtPA given for stroke has been reported.[111]

CONGENITAL PERICARDIAL HEART DISEASE

Absence and Partial Absence of the Pericardium

Congenital absence of the pericardium is an uncommon anomaly, usually involving a portion or the whole of the left parietal pericardium. Its presence usually is suspected from the chest radiogram, which shows a leftward shift of the cardiac silhouette, elongation of the left heart border, and radiolucencies between the aortic knob and the pulmonary artery and between the left hemidiaphragm and the base of the heart (Fig. 72-24). This anomaly may be associated with congenital malformations of the heart and lungs.[112]

Although most of these patients are asymptomatic, chest pain may result from torsion of the great vessels, and recurrent pulmonary infections may be a significant feature. Physical findings are not often helpful, but a conspicuous LV heave may be found when the deficiency is substantial. Systolic and diastolic murmurs have been described.

The ECG in patients with complete absence of the left side of the pericardium usually shows an incomplete right bundle branch block. Echocardiographic changes consist of RV enlargement and paradoxical septal motion. Contrast-enhanced CT and MRI detect lesions missed by chest radiography and

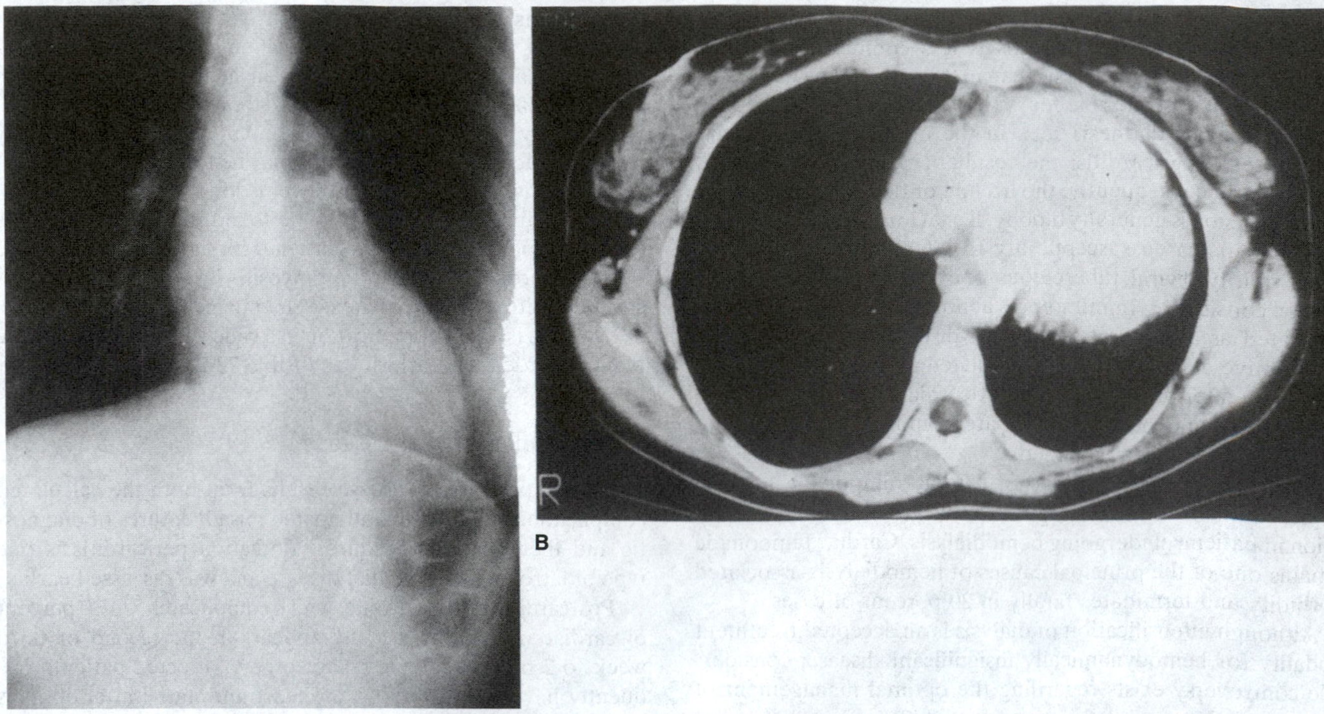

FIGURE 72-24 *A.* Posteroanterior chest radiogram of a patient with congenital absence of the pericardium. *B.* Computed tomography scan of the same patient. (Reproduced with permission from Hoit BD. Imaging the pericardium. *Cardiol Clin* 1990; 8:598.)

echocardiography and reliably establish the anatomy of the defect.[113]

Total and very small defects are not associated with pathophysiologic changes, whereas medium-size defects may allow herniation of the left atrium. Strangulation requires surgical closure or enlargement of the defect to reduce the herniation; this may be accomplished with a thoracoscope.

Pericardial Cysts

Pericardial cysts are rare remnants of defective embryologic development of the pericardium. Cysts usually present as a prominent round, sharply demarcated opacity seen on chest radiography in an asymptomatic patient. They vary greatly in size and most commonly are found in the right cardiophrenic angle, although hilar and mediastinal locations are observed occasionaly. Cysts are benign and produce no local or general symptoms; their importance lies in differentiation from neoplasm. Although they can be demonstrated on echocardiography, the nature of the lesion usually is confirmed by CT. A case of video-assisted surgical excision of a recurrent pericardial cyst has been reported.[114]

References

1. Shabetai R. The pericardium: An essay on some recent developments. *Am J Cardiol* 1978; 42(6):1036–1043.
2. Hammond HK, White FC, Bhargava V, et al. Heart size and maximal cardiac output are limited by the pericardium. *Am J Physiol* 1992; 263(6 part 2):H1675–H1681.
3. Hoit BD, Lew WY, LeWinter M. Regional variation in pericardial contact pressure in the canine ventricle. *Am J Physiol* 1988; 255(6 part 2):H1370–H1377.
4. Ditchey R, Engler RL, LeWinter MM, et al. The role of the right heart in acute cardiac tamponade in dogs. *Circ Res* 1981; 48:701–710.
5. Castelo Branco NA, Aguas AP, Sousa Pereira A, et al. The human pericardium in vibroacoustic disease. *Aviat Space Environ Med.* 1999; 70:A54–A62.
6. Spodick D. Macrophysiology, microphysiology, and anatomy of the pericardium: A synopsis. *Am Heart J* 1992; 124:1046–1051.
7. Eid H, Larson DM, Springhorn JP, et al. Role of epicardial mesothelial cells in the modification of phenotype and function of adult rat ventricular myocytes in primary coculture. *Circ Res* 1992; 71(1):40–50.
8. Laham RJ, Hung D, Simons M. Therapeutic myocardial angiogenesis using percutaneous intrapericardial drug delivery. *Clin Cardiol* 1999; 22:I-6–I-9.
9. Stoll HP, Carlson K, Keefer LK, et al. Pharmacokinetics and consistence of pericardial delivery directed to coronary arteries: Direct comparison with endoluminal delivery. *Clin Cardiol* 1999; 22:I-10–I-16.
10. Spodick DH. *The Pericardium: A Comprehensive Textbook.* New York: Marcel Dekker; 1997.
11. Kostreva DR, Pontus SP. Pericardial mechanoreceptors with phrenic afferents. *Am J Physiol* 1993; 264:H1836–H1846.
12. Fujita M, Ikemoto M, Kishishita M, et al. Elevated basic fibroblast growth factor in pericardial fluid of patients with unstable angina. *Circulation.* 1996; 94:610–613.
13. Tanaka T, Hasegawa K, Fujita M, et al. Marked elevation of brain natriuretic peptide levels in pericardial fluid is closely associated with left ventricular dysfunction. *J Am Coll Cardiol* 1998; 31(2):399–403.
14. Mallat Z, Philip I, Lebret M, et al. Elevated levels of 8-iso-prostaglandin F2alpha in pericardial fluid of patients with heart

failure: A potential role for in vivo oxidant stress in ventricular dilatation and progression to heart failure. *Circulation* 1998; 97(16):1536–1539.

15. Wanner WR, Schaal SF, Bashore TM, et al. Repolarization variant versus acute pericarditis: A prospective electrocardiographic and echocardiographic evaluation. *Chest* 1983; 83:180–184.
16. James JN. Pericarditis and the sinus node. *Arch Intern Med* 1962; 110:305–311.
17. Adler Y, Finkelstein Y, Guindo J, et al. Colchicine treatment for recurrent pericarditis: A decade of experience. *Circulation* 1998; 97(21):2183–2185.
18. Guindo J, Rodriguez de la Serna A, Ramio J, et al. Recurrent pericarditis: Relief with colchicine [see comments]. *Circulation* 1990; 82(4):1117–1120.
19. Marcolongo R, Russo R, Laveder F, et al. Immunosuppressive therapy prevents recurrent pericarditis. *J Am Coll Cardiol* 1995; 26(5):1276–1279.
20. Maisch B. Percardial diseases, with a focus on etiology, pathogenesis, pathophysiology, new diagnostic imaging methods, and treatment. *Curr Opin Cardiol* 1994; 9(3):379–388.
21. Weitzman LB, Tinker WP, Kronzon I, et al. The incidence and natural history of pericardial effusion after cardiac surgery—an echocardiographic study. *Circulation* 1984; 69:506–511.
22. Tsang TS, Barnes ME, Hayes SN, et al. Clinical and echocardiographic characteristics of significant pericardial effusions following cardiothoracic surgery and outcomes of echo-guided pericardiocentesis for management: Mayo Clinic experience, 1979–1998. *Chest* 1999; 116(2):322–331.
23. Ciliberto GR, Anjos MC, Gronda E. Significance of pericardial effusion after heart transplantation. *Am J Cardiol* 1995; 76: 297–300.
24. Mueller XM, Tevaearai HT, Hurni M, et al. Etiologic diagnosis of pericardial disease: The value of routine tests during surgical procedures. *J Am Coll Surg* 1997; 184(6):645–649.
25. Maisch B, Pankuweit S, Brilla C, et al. Intrapericardial treatment of inflammatory and neoplastic pericarditis guided by pericardioscopy and epicardial biopsy—results from a pilot study. *Clin Cardiol* 1999; 22(I suppl 1):I17–I22.
26. Geissbuhler K, Leiser A, Fuhrer J, et al. Video-assisted thoracoscopic pericardial fenestration for loculated or recurrent effusions. *Eur J Cardiothorac Surg* 1998; 14(4):403–408.
27. Sechtem U, Tsholakoff D, Higgins CB. MRI of the abnormal pericardium. *AJR* 1986; 147:245–252.
28. Merce J, Sagrista-Sauleda J, Permanyer-Miralda G, et al. Should pericardial drainage be performed routinely in patients who have a large pericardial effusion without tamponade? *Am J Med* 1998; 105(2):106–109.
29. Hoit BD, Gabel M, Fowler NO. Cardiac tamponade in left ventricular dysfunction. *Circulation* 1990; 82(4):1370–1376.
30. Hoit BD, Shaw D. The paradoxical pulse in tamponade: Mechanisms and echocardiographic correlates. *Echocardiography* 1994; 11:477–487.
31. Spodick DH. Electric alteration of the heart: Its relation to the kinetics and physiology of the heart during cardiac tamponade. *Am J Cardiol* 1962; 10:155–165.
32. Settle HP Jr, Engel PJ, Fowler NO, et al. Echocardiographic study of the paradoxical arterial pulse in chronic obstructive lung disease. *Circulation* 1980; 62(6):1297–1307.
33. Gillam LD, Guyer DE, Gibson TC, et al. Hydrodynamic compression of the right atrium: A new echocardiographic sign of cardiac tamponade. *Circulation* 1983; 68(2):294–301.
34. Chuttani K, Pandian NG, Mohanty PK. Left ventricular diastolic collapse: An echocardiographic sign of regional cardiac tamponade. *Circulation* 1991; 83:1999–2006.
35. Russo AM, O'Connor WH, Waxman HL. Atypical presentations and echocardiographic findings in patients with cardiac tamponade occurring early and late after cardiac surgery. *Chest* 1993; 104(1):71–78.
36. Golub RJ, McNulty CM, McClellan JR, et al. Usefulness of transesophageal Doppler echocardiography in the surgical drainage of a loculated purulent pericardial effusion. *Am Heart J* 1993; 126:724–727.
37. Heidenreich PA, Stainback RF, Redberg RF, et al. Transesophageal echocardiography predicts mortality in critically ill patients with unexplained hypotension. *J Am Coll Cardiol* 1995; 26(1): 152–158.
38. Appleton CP, Hatle LK, Popp RL. Relation of transmitral flow velocity patterns to left ventricular diastolic function: New insights from a combined hemodynamic and Doppler echocardiographic study. *J Am Coll Cardiol* 1988; 12:426–440.
39. Hoit BD, Ramrakhyani K. Pulmonary venous flow in cardiac tamponade: Influence of left ventricular dysfunction and the relation to pulsus paradoxus. *J Am Soc Echocardiogr* 1991; 4(6):559–570.
40. Merce J, Sagrista-Sauleda J, Permanyer-Miralda G, et al. Correlation between clinical and Doppler echocardiographic findings in patients with moderate and large pericardial effusion: Implications for the diagnosis of cardiac tamponade. *Am Heart J* 1999; 138(4):759–764.
41. Callahan JA, Seward JB, Nishimura RA, et al. Two-dimensional echocardiographically guided pericardiocentesis: Experience in 117 consecutive patients. *Am J Cardiol* 1985; 55(4):476–479.
42. Quigg RJ Jr, Idelson BA, Yoburn DC, et al. Local steroids in dialysis-associated pericardial effusion: A single intrapericardial administration of triamcinolone. *Arch Intern Med* 1985; 145(12): 2249–2450.
43. Shepherd FA, Morgan C, Evans WK, et al. Medical management of malignant pericardial effusion by tetracycline sclerosis. *Am J Cardiol* 1987; 60(14):1161–1166.
44. Olson JE, Ryan MB, Blumenstock DA. Eleven years' experience with pericardial-peritoneal window in the management of malignant and benign pericardial effusions. *Ann Surg Oncol* 1995; 2(2):165–169.
45. Allen KB, Faber LP, Warren WH, et al. Pericardial effusion: Subxiphoid pericardiostomy versus percutaneous catheter drainage. *Ann Thorac Surg* 1999; 67(2):437–440.
46. Girardi LN, Ginsberg RJ, Burt ME. Pericardiocentesis and intrapericardial sclerosis: Effective therapy for malignant pericardial effusions. *Ann Thorac Surg* 1997; 64(5):1427–1428.
47. Chavanon O, Barbe C, Troccas J, et al. Accurate guidance for percutaneous access to a specific target in soft tissue: Preclinical study of computer-assisted pericardiocentesis. *J Laparoendosc Adv Surg Tech* 1999; 9(3):259–266.
48. Ziskind AA, Pearce AC, Lemmon CC, et al. Percutaneous balloon pericardiotomy for the treatment of cardiac tamponade and large pericardial effusions: Description of technique and report of the first 50 cases. *J Am Coll Cardiol* 1993; 21(1):1–5.
49. Selig MB. Percutaneous transcatheter pericardial interventions: Aspiration, biopsy, and pericardioplasty. *Am Heart J* 1993; 125: 269–271.
50. Oh JK, Hatle LK, Mulvagh SL, Tajik AJ. Transient constrictive pericarditis: Diagnosis by two-dimensional Doppler echocardiography. *Mayo Clin Proc* 1993; 68(12):1158–1164.
51. Fowler NO. Constrictive pericarditis: Its history and current status. *Clin Cardiol* 1995; 18:341–350.
52. Schiavone WA. The changing etiology of constrictive pericarditis in a large referral center. *Am J Cardiol* 1986; 58:373–375.
53. Engel PJ, Fowler NO, Tei CW, et al. M-mode echocardiography in constrictive pericarditis. *J Am Coll Cardiol* 1985; 6:471–474.
54. Isner JM, Carter BL, Bankoff MS, et al. Differentiation of constrictive pericarditis from restrictive cardiomyopathy by computed tomographic imaging. *Am Heart J* 1983; 105:1019–1025.
55. Rienmuller R, Doppman JL, Lissner J, et al. Constrictive pericar-

dial disease: Prognostic significance of a nonvisualized left ventricular wall. *Radiology* 1985; 156(3):753–755.
56. Oren RM, Grover-McKay M, Stanford W, et al. Accurate preoperative diagnosis of pericardial constriction using cine computed tomography. *J Am Coll Cardiol* 1993; 22(3):832–838.
57. Sayad DE, Clarke GD, Peshock RM. Magnetic resonance imaging of the heart and its role in current cardiology. *Curr Opin Cardiol* 1995; 10(6):640–649.
58. Blackwell GG, Pohost GM. The usefulness of cardiovascular magnetic resonance imaging. *Curr Probl Cardiol* 1994; 19(3): 117–175.
59. Kutcher MA, King SB III, Alimurung BN, et al. Constrictive pericarditis as a complication of cardiac surgery: Recognition of an entity. *Am J Cardiol* 1982; 50:742–748.
60. Bush CA, Stang JM, Wooley CF, et al. Occult constrictive pericardial disease: Diagnosis by rapid volume expansion and correction by pericardiectomy. *Circulation* 1977; 56:924–930.
61. Sagrista-Sauleda J, Permanyer-Miralda G, Candell RJ, et al. Transient cardiac constriction: An unrecognized pattern of evolution in effusive acute idiopathic pericarditis. *Am J Cardiol* 1987; 59:961–966.
62. Seifert FC, Miller DC, Oesterle SN, et al. Surgical treatment of constrictive pericarditis: Analysis of outcome and diagnostic error. *Circulation* 1985; 72(3 part 2):II264–II273.
63. Nataf P, Cacouch P, Dorent R. Results of subtotal pericardiectomy for constrictive pericarditis. *Eur J Cardiothorac Surg* 1993; 7:252–256.
64. Woods T, Vidarsson B, Mosher D, et al. Transient effusive-constrictive pericarditis due to chemotherapy. *Clin Cardiol* 1999; 22(4):316–318.
65. Fowler NO, Harbin AD. Recurrent acute pericarditis: Follow-up study of 31 patients. *J Am Coll Cardiol* 1986; 7:300–305.
66. Maisch B, Drude L. Epi and pericardial biopsy by pericardioscopy. *Circulation* 1990; 82:III-417.
67. Sagrista-Sauleda J, Barrabes JA, Permanyer-Miralda G, et al. Purulent pericarditis: Review of a 20-year experience in a general hospital. *J Am Coll Cardiol* 1993; 22(6):1661–1665.
68. Klacsmann PG, Bulkey BH, Hutchins GM. The changed spectrum of purulent pericarditis: An 86-year autopsy experience in 200 patients. *Am J Med* 1977; 63:666–673.
69. Arsura EL, Kilgore WB, Strategos E. Purulent pericarditis misdiagnosed as septic shock. *South Med J* 1999; 92(3):285–288.
70. Skiest D, Steiner D, Werner M, et al. Anaerobic pericarditis: Case report and review. *Clin Infect Dis* 1994; 19:435–440.
71. Mann-Segal DD. The use of fibrinolytics in purulent pericarditis. *Intensive Care Med* 1999; 25(3):338–339.
72. Defouilloy C, Meyer G, Slama M, et al. Intrapericardial fibrinolysis: A useful treatment in the management of purulent pericarditis. *Intensive Care Med* 1997; 23(1):117–118.
73. Winkler WB, Karnik R, Slany J. Treatment of exudative fibrinous pericarditis with intrapericardial urokinase. *Lancet* 1994; 344: 1541–1542.
74. Puelo J, Matar F, McKeown P, et al. Legionella pericarditis diagnosed by direct fluorescent antibody staining. *Ann Thorac Surg* 1995; 60:444–446.
75. Nelson D, Rensimer E, Raffin T. Legionella pneumophilia pericarditis without pneumonia. *Arch Intern Med* 1985; 145:926.
76. Nagi KS, Joshi R, Thakur RK. Cardiac manifestations of Lyme disease: A review. *Can J Cardiol* 1996; 12(5):503–506.
77. Mastroianni A, Coronado O, Chiodo F. Tuberculous pericarditis and AIDS: Case reports and review. *Eur J Epidemiol* 1997; 13(7):755–759.
78. Rana BS, Jones RA, Simpson IA. Recurrent pericardial effusion: The value of polymerase chain reaction in the diagnosis of tuberculosis. *Heart* 1999; 82(2):246–247.
79. Hayashi H, Kawamata H, Machida M, et al. Tuberculous pericarditis: MRI features with contrast enhancement. *Br J Radiol* 1998; 71(846):680–682.
80. Long R, Younes M, Patton N, et al. Tuberculous pericarditis: Long-term outcome in patients who received medical therapy alone. *Am Heart J* 1989; 117(5):1133–1139.
81. Fowler N. Tuberculous pericarditis. *JAMA* 1991; 266:99–103.
82. Silva-Cardoso J, Moura B, Martins L, et al. Pericardial involvement in human immunodeficiency virus infection. *Chest* 1999; 115(2):418–422.
83. Heidenreich PA, Eisenberg MJ, Kee LL, et al. Pericardial effusion in AIDS: Incidence and survival [see comments]. *Circulation* 1995; 92(11):3229–3234.
84. Estok L, Wallach F. Cardiac tamponade in a patient with AIDS: A review of pericardial disease in patients with HIV infection. *Mt Sinai J Med.* 1998; 65(1):33–39.
85. Chen Y, Brennessel D, Walters J, et al. Human immunodeficiency virus-associated pericardial effusion: Report of 40 cases and review of the literature. *Am Heart J* 1999; 137(3):516–521.
86. Blanc P, Boussuges A, Souk-aloun J, et al. Echocardiography on HIV patients admitted to the ICU. *Intensive Care Med* 1997; 23(12):1279–1281.
87. Thomason R, Schlegel W, Luccam M. Primary malignant mesothelioma of the pericardium. *Tex Heart Inst* 1994; 21:170–174.
88. Wilkes JD, Fidias P, Vaickus L, et al. Malignancy-related pericardial effusion: 127 cases from the Roswell Park Cancer Institute. *Cancer* 1995; 76(8):1377–1387.
89. Widimsky P, Gregor P. Pericardial involvement during the course of myocardial infarction: A long-term clinical and echocardiographic study. *Chest* 1995; 108(1):89–93.
90. Fowler NO. *The Pericardium in Health and Disease.* Mt. Kisco, NY: Futura; 1985.
91. Oliva P, Hammill S, Edwards W. Electrocardiographic diagnosis of postinfarction regional pericarditis: Ancillary observations regarding the effect of reperfusion on the rapidity and amplitude of T wave inversion after acute myocardial infarction. *Circulation.* 1993; 88:896–904.
92. Correale E, Maggioni AP, Romano S, et al. Comparison of frequency, diagnostic and prognostic significance of pericardial involvement in acute myocardial infarction treated with and without thrombolytics: Gruppo Italiano per lo Studio della Sopravvivenza nell'Infarto Miocardico (GISSI). *Am J Cardiol* 1993; 71(16):1377–1381.
93. Madias J, Perdoncin R, Bartoszyk O. Pericarditis and pericardial effusion in patients with acute myocardial infarction. *Am J Noninvas Cardiol* 1994; 8:270–277.
94. Correale E, Maggioni AP, Romano S, et al. Pericardial involvement in acute myocardial infarction in the post-thrombolytic era: Clinical meaning and value. *Clin Cardiol* 1997; 20(4):327–331.
95. Millaire A, de Groote P, Decoulx E, et al. Outcome after thrombolytic therapy of nine cases of myopericarditis misdiagnosed as myocardia infarction. *Eur Heart J* 1995; 16(3):333–338.
96. Shahar A, Hod H, Barabash GM, et al. Disappearance of a syndrome: Dressler's syndrome in the era of thrombolysis. *Cardiology* 1994; 85(3–4):255–258.
97. Stewart J, Fajardo L. Radiation-induced heart disease: An update. *Prog Cardiovasc Dis* 1984; 27:173–194.
98. Benoff LJ, Schweitzer P. Radiation therapy-induced cardiac injury. *Am Heart J* 1995; 129(6):1193–1196.
99. King D, Nieberg R. The use of cytology to evaluate pericardial effusions. *Ann Clin Lab Sci* 1979; 9:18–23.
100. Liedtke JA, DeMuth WE. Nonpenetrating cardiac injuries: A collective review. *Am Heart J* 1973; 86:687–697.
101. Rozycki GS, Feliciano DV, Oshsner MG, et al. The role of ultrasound in patients with possible penetrating cardiac wounds: A prospective multicenter study. *J Trauma* 1999; 46(4):543–551.
102. Thakur RK, Aufderheide TP, Boughner DR. Emergency echo-

cardiographic evaluation of penetrating chest trauma. *Can J Cardiol* 1994; 10(3):374–376.

103. Meleca MJ, Hoit BD. Previously unrecognized intrapericardial hematoma leading to refractory abdominal ascites. *Chest* 1995; 108(6):1747–1748.

104. Gupta R, Munyak J, Haydock T, et al. Hypothyroidism presenting as acute cardiac tamponade with viral pericarditis. *Am J Emerg Med* 1999; 17(2):176–178.

105. Langley RL, Treadwell EL. Cardiac tamponade and pericardial disorders in connective tissue diseases: Case report and literature review. *J Natl Med Assoc* 1994; 86(2):149–153.

106. Spodick DH. Pericarditis in systemic diseases: Diseases of the pericardium. *Cardiol Clin* 1990; 8:709–715.

107. Hakala M, Pettersson T, Tarkka M, et al. Rheumatoid arthritis as a cause of cardiac compression: Favourable long-term outcome of pericardiectomy. *Clin Rheumatol* 1993; 12:199–203.

108. Thould A. Constrictive pericarditis in rheumatoid arthritis. *Ann Rheum Dis* 1986; 45:89–94.

109. Moder KG, Miller TD, Tazelaar HD. Cardiac involvement in systemic lupus erythematosus. *Mayo Clin Proc* 1999; 74(3): 275–284.

110. Thompson AE, Pope JE. A study of the frequency of pericardial and pleural effusions in scleroderma. *Br J Rheumatol* 1998; 37(12):1320–1321.

111. Kasner SE, Villar-Cordova CE, Tong D, et al. Hemopericardium and cardiac tamponade after thrombolysis for acute ischemic stroke. *Neurology* 1998; 50(6):1857–1859.

112. Nasser W. Congenital absence of the left pericardium. *Am J Cardiol* 1970; 26:466–478.

113. Gassner I, Judmaier W, Fink C, et al. Diagnosis of congenital pericardial defects, including a pathognomonic sign for dangerous apical ventricular herniation, on magnetic resonance imaging. *Br Heart J* 1995; 74:60–66.

114. Horita K, Sakao Y, Itoh T. Excision of a recurrent pericardial cyst using video-assisted thoracic surgery. *Chest* 1998; 114(4): 1203–1204.

CHAPTER 73

INFECTIVE ENDOCARDITIS

Merle A. Sande / Mrinka Kartalija / Jeff Anderson

Infective endocarditis is the disease caused by microbial infection of the endothelial lining of the heart. Its characteristic lesion is a *vegetation,* which usually develops on a heart valve but occasionally appears elsewhere on the endocardium. Sometimes a nidus of infection develops on the lining of a large artery, causing *infective endarteritis;* this variant can produce clinical findings that resemble those of infective endocarditis.

DEFINITIONS AND TERMINOLOGY

The following abbreviations for various forms of endocarditis will be used in this chapter:

- IE: Infective endocarditis
- SBE: Subacute bacterial endocarditis
- ABE: Acute bacterial endocarditis
- NVE: Native valve endocarditis
- PVE: Prosthetic valve endocarditis
- NBTE: Nonbacterial thrombotic endocarditis

The terms *subacute* and *acute bacterial endocarditis* (SBE and ABE) have descriptive value when accurately applied. SBE progresses over a period of weeks to months and is usually caused by organisms of low virulence such as viridans streptococci, which possess limited ability to infect other tissues.[1–4]

In contrast, ABE evolves over a period of days to 1 or 2 weeks; the clinical progress is rapidly changing, complications develop earlier, and the diagnosis is usually made in less than 2 weeks.[4–6] ABE is most often caused by primary pathogens such as *Staphylococcus aureus,* which are capable of causing invasive infection at many other sites in the body.

Infection of a heart valve that was either previously normal or damaged by congenital or acquired disease is termed *native valve endocarditis* (NVE). Infection of an artificial heart valve is termed *prosthetic valve endocarditis* (PVE). This infection was first arbitrarily defined as early PVE, when onset is within the first 2 months after surgery, and as late PVE thereafter.[6–11] Some authors have defined infections occurring between 2 months and 1 year of valve replacement as intermediate PVE,[11] while others consider any prosthetic valve infection beginning before 1 year as early PVE.

Sterile vegetations sometimes develop within the heart. The term *noninfective endocarditis* is a misnomer, because the lesions are primarily thrombotic rather than inflammatory.[12] Thus the term *nonbacterial thrombotic endocarditis* (NBTE) is used broadly to describe any sterile vegetation. This category includes a spectrum of lesions ranging from microscopic aggregates of platelets to the large vegetations of marantic endocarditis, which sometimes develop in patients with terminal malignancy or other chronic diseases.[13–15]

Infective endocarditis is designated best by naming the infecting organism, for example, "*Staph. aureus* endocarditis" or "*Candida albicans* PVE." This terminology is specific and informative, allowing useful inferences about the likely natural history, prognosis, and treatment of the case in question.

EARLY STUDIES

Riviere, Lancisi, and Morgagni each described patients who died with endocarditis in the seventeenth and eighteenth centuries.[16] Jean-Baptiste Bouillaud introduced the terms *endocardium* and *endocarditis* between 1824 and 1835. By 1846, Virchow recognized valvular vegetations at autopsy, but the microbial etiology of infective endocarditis was not fully appreciated until Virchow et al. independently demonstrated bacteria in vegetations between 1869 and 1872.[16]

William Osler studied the disease extensively, choosing infective endocarditis as the subject for his Goulstonian lectures of 1885.[17,18] Further major contributions to the knowledge of the natural history, pathogenesis, and pathology of the disease were made by Lenharz, Harbitz, and Schottmuller[16] in Germany; by Horder[19] in England; and by Blumer,[1] Thayer,[2] Allen,[20] Libman and Friedberg,[21] and Beeson et al.[22] in the United States. The technique of blood culture was introduced in Europe and the United States between 1890 and 1910.[3] In 1955, Kerr published a classic monograph summarizing the state of knowledge on subacute bacterial endocarditis to that date.[3]

Attempts to cure endocarditis before the advent of antimicrobial drugs were unsuccessful. In 1939, one patient with infective endarteritis involving a patent ductus arteriosus was cured by surgical closure of the ductus.[23] The first successes in the treatment of endocarditis are closely linked to the history of penicillin.[24] The first patient to receive parenteral penicillin was a young man with streptococcal endocarditis who was treated in 1940 at Columbia University in New York.[25] Although the patient did not receive enough penicillin to effect a cure, his treatment antedated the first administration of penicillin to a patient by Florey's team (Abraham et al.) in Oxford[26] by several months. After initial failures, by 1944 it had been established that penicillin,[27] unlike sulfonamides,[28] could cure most cases of streptococcal endocarditis. Subsequently, the antibiotic treatment of endocarditis was clearly established.[29–33] After antibiotics, the next great advance was cardiac valve replacement for treatment of endocarditis in 1965,[34] which provided an essential intervention to improve survival rates in selected patients.

EPIDEMIOLOGY

Incidence

The incidence of infective endocarditis can only be estimated, because it is not a reportable disease. Various studies in developed countries have estimated the incidence to be 1.6 to 6.0 cases per 100,000 person-years.[35–39] In the United States, this would result in 4000 to 15,000 new cases per year. In a study from the Delaware Valley, where the population includes a large number of intravenous drug users (IDU), the estimated rate was much higher: 11.6 cases per 100,000 per year.[40]

Evolution of the Clinical Syndrome

IE today is a different disease from that seen in the preantibiotic era, when its salient clinical features were exhaustively reported.[1–3] Since 1961, many authors have described the "changing face" of "modern endocarditis,"[41–47] identifying the following trends:

- Increased median age of patients
- Increased ratio of males to females
- Increased proportion of acute cases
- Reduced incidence of some of the classic physical signs of advanced SBE, such as Osler's nodes, finger clubbing, splenomegaly, or Roth's spots
- Decreased proportion of cases due to streptococci, with an increased incidence of staphylococci
- Lengthened list of etiologic organisms, with more reports of cases caused by gram-negative bacilli, fungi, and miscellaneous rare or unusual microbes
- Increased number of cases in IDU
- Increased number of prosthetic valve infections
- Increased incidence of concomitant human immunodeficiency virus (HIV) infection and endocarditis

Susceptible Populations

These striking changes in the clinical features and epidemiology of IE are due to changes in susceptible populations, to earlier diagnosis and treatment of patients with subacute disease and to the impact of antibiotic therapy.[45,48] The prevalence of rheumatic valvular disease, formerly the most common substrate for endocarditis, has steadily decreased; meanwhile, the number of children surviving with congenital heart disease has increased. The number of individuals using illicit drugs intravenously has increased markedly in the United States and Europe since the 1960s, and HIV has spread widely throughout this group as well.[49]

Effect of Antibiotics

Although the advent of antibiotics revolutionized treatment of endocarditis, the overall incidence of the disease has not changed strikingly. The availability of rapidly effective treatments for pneumococcal pneumonia and gonorrhea has probably been responsible for the striking decrease in the incidence of endocarditis caused by *Streptococcus pneumoniae* and *Neisseria gonorrhoeaea* since 1944, while the incidence of reported cases caused by miscellaneous unusual antibiotic-resistant organisms has increased during the antibiotic era.[48,50–53] Apart from these special cases, the widespread use of antimicrobial agents seems to have exerted considerably less influence than have alterations in the populations at risk on the changing epidemiology of endocarditis.[45] Prophylactic use of antibiotics before medical procedures that cause bacteremia has not reduced the incidence of endocarditis significantly; this is not surprising considering

TABLE 73-1 Approximate Frequency of Major Preexisting Cardiac Lesions in Patients with Infective Endocarditis in the United States

Lesion	Children under 2 years, %	Children 2–15 Years, %	Adults 15–50 Years, %	Adults >50 Years, %	Adults Who Are IV Drug Abusers, %
No known heart disease	50–70	10–15	10–20	10	50–60
Congenital heart disease[a]	30–50	70–80	25–35	15–25	10
Rheumatic heart disease	Rare	10	10–15	10–15	10
Degenerative heart disease	0	0	Rare	10–20	Rare
Previous cardiac surgery	5	10–15	10–20	10–20	10–20
Previous endocarditis	Rare	5	5–10	5–10	10–20

[a]Includes mitral valve prolapse.
SOURCE: Adapted from Refs. 35–51, 58–70, 81, 202.

that only a small proportion of all cases can be attributed to such procedures.[54–56] Also, startling studies question the effectiveness of prophylactic antibiotics during dental procedures to prevent endocarditis.[56,57]

Preexisting Heart Disease

Some patients develop endocarditis even though they have no known heart disease. This is most common in cases of ABE,[57] in children less than 2 years of age,[58–64] and in IDUs.[65–70] Most patients who develop IE, however, have a preexisting cardiac condition. Approximate figures for the frequency of the main predisposing factors in children, adults, and IDUs are given in Table 73-1.

The relative propensity of various cardiac lesions to become infected can be estimated by noting their frequency in published series of cases of IE, even though there is wide variation among individual studies (Table 73-2).

Mitral valve prolapse (MVP) can predispose to endocarditis.[71–78] (see Chap. 58). MVP underlies 15 to 30 percent or more of cases.[35,72,75,76,80] However, MVP is common and represents a broad spectrum of valvular and clinical disease. The annual percentage of patients with MVP that develop complications (including IE) is small, and the need for IE prophylaxis is controversial. Hence, American Heart Association recommendations include an algorithm to more clearly define when prophylaxis is recommended in MVP.[79] The risk of IE is primarily increased (five- to eightfold) when MVP is associated with regurgitation.[72,73,78] The use of prophylactic antibiotics is supported by cost-benefit analysis in those with auscultatory or Doppler evidence for mitral insufficiency.[79] In contrast, endocarditis risk is not increased in the absence of regurgitation and prophylaxis is not recommended[2,8,9,79] (see Chap. 58).[72,73] However, this remains controversial. Although commonly used to confirm diagnoses, routine use of echocardiography does not appear to be cost effective.[74]

Children

IE occurs at all ages but is relatively uncommon during childhood and rare during infancy,[58–64,81,82] although the incidence is increasing among smaller infants with cyanotic disease.[83] Males predominate—65 percent in one series.[84] Endocardial infection in children with no predisposing heart disease develops most often in association with infection elsewhere, often in infants and very young children.[85] Endocarditis in these settings is likely to be caused by invasive pathogens and follow an acute course. IE can occur as a rare complication of septicemia caused by staphylococci or group B streptococci or of pneumonia, other respiratory tract infections, osteomyelitis, and severe burns.[58,62]

TABLE 73-2 Estimates of the Relative Risk of Infective Endocarditis Posed by Various Cardiac Lesions

Relatively High Risk	Intermediate Risk	Very Low or Negligible Risk
Prosthetic heart valves	Mitral valve prolapse with regurgitation	Mitral valve prolapse without regurgitation
Previous infective endocarditis	Pure mitral stenosis	Trivial valvular regurgitation by echocardiography without structural abnormality
Cyanotic congenital heart disease	Tricuspid valve disease	Atrial septal defects, secundum type
Aortic valve disease	Pulmonary valve disease	Arteriosclerotic plaques
Mitral regurgitation	Asymmetric septal hypertrophy	Coronary artery disease
Mitral regurgitation and stenosis	Hyperalimentation or pressure-monitoring lines that reach the right atrium	Syphilitic aortitis
Patent ductus arteriosus	Nonvalvular intracardiac prosthetic implants	Cardiac pacemakers
Ventricular septal defect	Degenerative valvular disease in elderly patients	Surgically corrected cardiac lesions (without prosthetic implants, more than 6 months after operation)
Coarctation of the aorta		

SOURCE: Adapted from Refs. 36, 38, 39, 43, 50, 51, 71–81, 86, 116, 370.

Nosocomial cases associated with intravenous catheters are important.[85] Endocarditis complicating congenital or other preexisting heart lesions is more likely to occur in older children and present as a subacute disease without an obvious portal of entry.[85] Children with a systemic pulmonary shunt constructed surgically are most likely to have endocarditis caused by viridans streptococci.[84] *Haemophilus influenzae* type B endocarditis is very rare, even though this organism was a common cause of bacteremia in children prior to the introduction of conjugate vaccines.

The leading underlying cardiac lesions in children are tetralogy of Fallot and other forms of cyanotic congenital heart disease, ventricular septal defects, aortic stenosis, patent ductus arteriosus, pulmonary stenosis, and coarctation of the aorta. A high proportion of cases (77 percent of those with chronic heart disease) occur in children who have undergone palliative or corrective surgery for congenital cardiac defects.[62,84,86] Atrial septal defects of the ostium secundum type very rarely become infected (Chap. 64). Successful repair of ventricular septal defects and closure of patent ductus arteriosus appears to have greatly reduced the risk of endocarditis. In developed countries, preexisting rheumatic heart disease is now much less common than congenital disease. No underlying cardiac disease is found in about 15 percent of children with endocarditis, but the proportion is higher in those less than 2 years of age (Table 73-1).

A firm diagnosis of IE is more difficult to make in infants and small children than it is in adults. Signs and symptoms, however, are similar: fever occurs in 99 percent of pediatric cases, fatigue in 60 percent, arthralgias in 17 percent, petechiae in 21 percent, changing murmur in 21 percent, splenomegaly in 21 percent, and congenative heart failure in 9 percent. Blood cultures are positive in over 90 percent of the cases, which is also similar to adults. Viridans streptococci account for 38 percent of cases, *Staph. aureus* for 32 percent, enterococci for 7 percent, and a mixture of gram-positive cocci and gram-negative organisms for the rest.[84] Once the diagnosis is suspected, improved diagnostic criteria can help determine whether the child has endocarditis.[85] The clinical manifestations of acute rheumatic fever may mimic endocarditis (and vice versa), but fortunately the two conditions rarely coexist.

The choice of antibiotic treatment for children should be governed by the same principles as for adults, with appropriate 0dose adjustment for age. As in adults, valve replacement or other potentially curative surgical treatment should not be delayed if the child has heart failure that does not respond well to medical therapy.[87] Children with *Staph. aureus* endocarditis are most likely to have persistent fever bactermia, and complications, require surgery, and have a higher mortality rate than those who do not have *Staph. aureus*.[84,88]

The Elderly

With the increase in elderly people, endocarditis in this group has become more common.[89–92] The median age of patients with endocarditis has risen steadily for three decades, from about 30 to about 50 years. At present, approximately one-fourth of all patients are over age 60.[35,93] The annual risk for endocarditis is strongly age-related, being about 5 times higher in patients over age 80.[39] Male patients now outnumber females by approximately 1.5 to 1 overall, but by as much as 8 to 1 among patients over age 60.[33,94] Elderly patients are more likely to have underlying degenerative or calcific valve lesions.[90] Older patients (>70 years) had a higher proportion of bacteria from a gastrointestinal source (group D streptococci and enterococci accounted for 50 percent of cases in one series).[92] There is a higher mortality rate (28 versus 13 percent) for patients who are <70 years.[92]

Intravenous Drug Users

Illicit intravenous drug use poses a high risk for IE.[65–70,95] IDUs are 300 times more likely to die suddenly with IE than are nonusers.[96] Bacteremias related to parenteral drug abuse are common and arise either from direct intravenous injection of bacteria or from the skin flora and local infections at injection sites, including cellulitis, abscesses, or suppurative thrombophlebitis. Addicts seldom use sterile injection techniques, sometimes even taking water from toilet bowls to dissolve their drugs. Nevertheless, the organisms that cause drug-related endocarditis most frequently originate from the addict's skin and mucosal bacterial flora.[97] Strains of *Staph. aureus* cause more than 60 percent of cases of endocarditis among parenteral drug abusers, more than all other species combined.[50,70] Infections with gram-negative bacilli, especially *Pseudomonas* species[98,99] or yeasts and other fungi,[100] are notably more common than in nonaddicts (Table 73-3). *Candida parapsilosis* and other *Candida* species are the most common fungi causing drug-related endocarditis, but occasional infections with a wide range of other fungal species have been recorded.[100,101] Polymicrobial and culture-negative cases of endocarditis occur occasionally in IDUs, but together account for less than 5 percent of cases.[65,67,70,102]

Endocarditis in addicts frequently follows an acute course,[5,65,66,101] reflecting the high frequency of *Staph. aureus* infection. This finding partly explains the overall modest increase in the proportion of acute to subacute cases that has been observed over the past 25 years.[45]

The outstanding clinical feature of endocarditis in IDUs is the unusually high incidence of right-sided valvular infection. In various series, the tricuspid valve is involved in 60 to 70 percent of cases.[50,61,103] The aortic and/or mitral valves are involved in 30 to 40 percent.[50,103] More than one valve on either side of the heart may be infected simultaneously. Pulmonary valve infection is unusual even among IDUs, occurring in only some 2 percent of cases.

Tricuspid vegetations commonly embolize to the lungs, causing septic pulmonary infarcts, which result in multiple focal opacities on chest x-ray, sometimes with cavitation. In a drug addict with fever, this radiologic finding is a highly characteristic sign of acute right-sided endocarditis.[5,70] Mortality rates are much lower (4 percent) with endocarditis in IDUs than in other patient populations, even though the most common cause is *Staph. aureus*. This most likely reflects the benign nature of tricuspid valve involvement compared to left-sided disease.

Patients Infected with Human Immunodeficiency Virus

The primary risk factor for IE in HIV-infected people is the continued use of intravenous drugs, although IE is independently associated with HIV infection. Prior endocarditis, female sex, and skin abscesses are independent risk factors.[104] In one study, the adjusted odds ratio for HIV-infected IDUs with CD4 cell levels > 350 who developed endocarditis was 2.31 versus non-HIV-infected IDUs, but increased to an odds ratio of 8.31

TABLE 73-3 Frequency of Various Organisms Causing Infective Endocarditis[a]

Organism	NVE, %	IV Drug Abusers, %	Early PVE, %	Late PVE, %
Streptococci	60	15–25	5	35
Viridans, alpha-hemolytic	35	5–10	<5	25
Streptococcus bovis	10	<5	<5	<5
Enterococcus faecalis	10	10	<5	<5
Other streptococci	<5	<5	<5	<5
Staphylococci	25	50	50	30
Coagulase-positive	23	50	20	10
Coagulase-negative	<5	<5	30	20
Gram-negative aerobic bacilli	<5	5	20	10
Fungi	<5	<5	10	5
Miscellaneous bacteria	<5	5	5	5
Diphtheroids, propionibacteria	<1	<5	5	<5
Other anaerobes	<1	<1	<1	<1
Rickettsiae	<1	<1	<1	<1
Chlamydiae	<1	<1	<1	<1
Polymicrobial infection	<1	1–5	5	5
Culture-negative endocarditis	5–10	<5	<5	<5

[a]These are representative figures collated from the literature; wide local variations in frequency are to be expected. NVE = native valve endocarditis; PVE = prosthetic valve endocarditis; IV = intravenous.
SOURCE: Adapted from Refs. 43, 51, 65–70, 100–110, 115, 159.

when the CD4 cell count fell to < 350.[107] Several cases of *Bartonella* endocarditis have been reported in patients with acquired immunodeficiency syndrome (AIDS);[105] this appears to be a rare instance of true opportunistic infection of the endocardium. Patients in the earlier stages of HIV infection respond well to standard treatment for endocarditis, but mortality due to IE is high after the CD4+ T-cell count falls below 200 cells per cubic millimeter [49,106] (see also Chap. 70).

Post-Cardiac Surgery Patients

Intracardiac operations, especially valve replacements, have created a whole new population at risk for IE. In the 1950s, surgeons first noted that *Staph. epidermidis* endocarditis occurred fairly frequently after mitral valvotomy.[108] Subsequently, *Staph. epidermidis,* which rarely infects native valves, has become a common cause of both early and late PVE (Table 73-3).[8–11,95] Contamination of blood circulating through pump oxygenators with *Staph. epidermidis* or other organisms or from the operating room air can initiate infection at the time of operation, resulting in early PVE. In late PVE, the causative organisms usually originate from the normal flora of the skin or gastrointestinal tract, but their portal of entry largely remains unknown. Gram-negative bacilli and fungi infect prosthetic valves much more frequently than native valves, especially in early postoperative cases.[11,95,109] The spectrum of organisms causing late PVE more nearly resembles that of subacute native valve infection (Table 73-3).

Figure 73-1 shows the curve for incidence of PVE per month after valve replacement. The peak time of onset is 3 to 9 weeks after operation, with the risk falling quickly thereafter.[9] This important time relationship emphasizes that *Staph. epidermidis* and certain other organisms are often inoculated during or immediately after surgery, while streptococci infect the prosthesis during bacteremias that may occur at any time, unrelated to surgery.

The total number of cases of postsurgical endocarditis has increased along with the number of operations, even though the incidence per patient has decreased. This decrease reflects improved operative techniques and possibly the use of prophylactic antibiotics. Currently the rate is about 0.5 percent for early PVE, with a range of 0.3 to 1.2 percent.[8–11]

Patients with prosthetic valves now routinely survive for many years and remain at higher risk for late IE for the rest of their lives.[11,95,109,110] Late PVE occurs at a rate of about 0.3 to 0.5 percent per year.

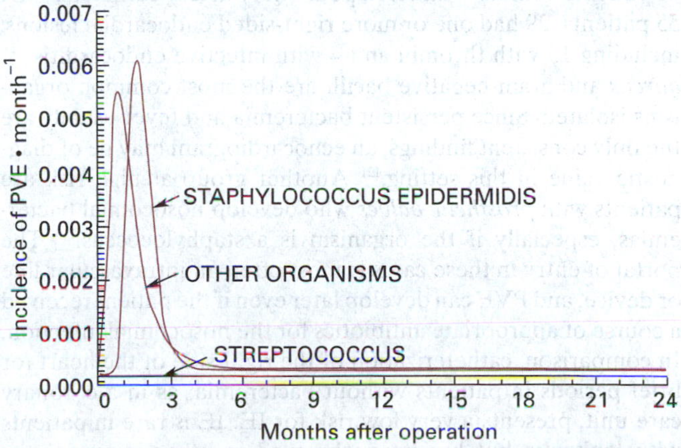

FIGURE 73-1 Incidence of prosthetic valve endocarditis (PVE) over 24 months after valve replacement. The hazard function has been stratified according to the infecting organisms. (From Ivert TSA, Dismukes WE, Cobbs CG, et al. Prosthetic valve endocarditis. *Circulation* 1984; 69:223. Reproduced with permission.)

Obstetric and Gynecologic Patients

Endocarditis occurring as a complication of pregnancy is most likely to develop at the time of delivery or in the puerperium.[111] Normal delivery presents a low risk of endocarditis, even in the presence of preexisting valvular disease,[112] but bacteremias associated with perinatal infective complications such as endometritis, parametritis, septic thrombophlebitis in pelvic veins, or urinary tract infection can seed the mother's endocardium.[111] Septic abortion or pelvic infection related to intrauterine contraceptive devices also can provide the portal of entry for bacteremia resulting in endocarditis.[113] The organisms most often involved are *Enterococcus faecalis,* group B streptococci, *Staph. aureus,* and occasionally gram-negative enteric bacilli or anaerobes.

Nosocomial Endocarditis

Hospital-acquired IE can involve either prosthetic or native valves.[114,115] This serious complication is not rare; one study[116] reported no fewer than 35 examples of probable nosocomial endocarditis among 125 cases (28 percent), and the rate may be rising.[114] Intensive medical care predisposes to endocarditis in several ways. Endocardial damage can be produced by surgery, by intracardiac catheters, and by intravascular devices such as hyperalimentation catheters and cerebrospinal fluid shunts if they reach into the right atrium. Portals of entry for microorganisms are provided by wounds, biopsy sites, pacemakers, intravenous and arterial catheters,[117] urinary catheters, and intratracheal airways. In one study, 75 percent of the suspected sources of infection were vascular access sites.[118] Nosocomial bacteremias arising from local infections are common in seriously ill patients. Up to two-thirds of patients with nosocomial endocarditis had no known predisposing cardiac abnormalities.[118]

Many of the previously mentioned factors coexist in *severely burned* patients. In one study, either NBTE or IE was found at autopsy in all of 6 burned patients who sustained repeated episodes of bacteremia while a pressure-monitoring catheter was maintained in the right side of the heart before death.[119] This observation has been confirmed in another autopsy study of patients with flow-directed pulmonary artery catheters.[120] Of 55 patients, 29 had one or more right-sided endocardial lesions, including 13 with thrombi and 4 with infective endocarditis. *S. aureus* and gram-negative bacilli are the most common organisms isolated. Since persistent bacteremia and fever usually are the only consistent findings, an echocardiogram may be of diagnostic value in this setting.[121] Another group at high risk are patients with *prosthetic valves* who develop nosocomial bacteremias, especially if the organism is a staphylococcus.[115] The portal of entry in these cases is most often an intravascular line or device, and PVE can develop later even if the patient received a course of appropriate antibiotics for the nosocomial infection. In comparison, catheterization of the right side of the heart for brief periods in patients without bacteremia, as in a coronary care unit, presents a very low risk for IE. IE is rare in patients with leukemia but has been observed in other immunocompromised patients—for example, after bone marrow transplantation[122] and heart transplantation.[123] In a report of 46 cases after solid organ transplantation, *Aspergillus fumigatus* and *Staph. aureus* were causative in 50 percent, whereas viridans streptococci were isolated in only 4 percent. Six of 10 cases that occurred within 30 days of transplantation were fungal. No predisposing cardiac abnormality was known to be present in 80 percent. Infected venous access devices and wounds were suspected portals of entry in three-fourths of the cases. The mortality rate was 57 percent, and most infections were not diagnosed prior to death.[124]

Overall, the leading organisms causing nosocomial endocarditis are staphylococci, enterococci, *Candida* species, and gram-negative bacilli. *Staph. aureus* is especially associated with wound infections, cellulitis, and cannula infections; *Staph. epidermidis* with ventriculoatrial shunts; and *C. albicans* with parenteral alimentation.

The prognosis for nosocomial native valve endocarditis is worse than for other forms of native valve infection (up to 50 percent mortality).[114,118] These patients often have serious underlying disease that may delay diagnosis of endocarditis by obscuring the symptoms and signs, while the organisms most commonly involved (staphylococci and enterococci) are more difficult to eradicate than viridans streptococci.

Hemodialysis

Creation of arteriovenous shunts for hemodialysis predisposes patients to develop IE by providing a ready portal of entry for bacteremias. Another possible factor is increased cardiac output. Dogs with high cardiac output due to surgically created arteriovenous fistulas are predisposed to develop not only infective endarteritis at the site of the shunt but endocarditis as well.[125] Therefore, it is not surprising that endocarditis has been reported in 2 to 6 percent of patients on long-term hemodialysis employing either arteriovenous fistulas or cannulas. *Staph. aureus* and *Staph. epidermidis* have been the most common etiologic organisms, followed by viridans streptococci and *E. faecalis.*[126] The diagnosis of endocarditis is difficult in these patients, partly because coexisting intravascular infection at the shunt site often confuses the clinical picture. Mortality is high (53 percent), and a high index of suspicion and use of an echocardiography followed by aggressive treatment of both shunt infections and endocarditis in dialysis patients are necessary to improve outcome.[126] In one study of 20 cases of IE in hemodialysis patients, vegetations were found in 50 percent by transthoracic echocardiogram (TTE) and 81 percent by transesophageal echocardiogram (TEE).[127] In 65 hemodialysis patients with *Staph. aureus* bacteremia, 8 (12 percent) were found to have IE by TEE (6 of whom had normal TTEs).[128]

Pacemaker Infective Endocarditis

The placement of permanent pacemaker leads into the right ventricle may result in endocardial lead infection in 0.2 to 7 percent of patients. These may occur early (6 weeks to 3 months after placement) and are caused by *Staph. epidermidis* in 90 percent, or late, when *Staph. epidermidis* or *Staph. aureus* each account for nearly 50 percent, with gram-negative bacilli causing the remaining few. The definitive diagnosis usually requires TEE, which will detect vegetations in or around the leads in >90 percent of cases. The chest x-ray is predictive in one-third for pulmonary emboli. Cure requires removal of the pacemaker generator and leads, and treatment with antibiotics.[129–132]

Infective Endarteritis

Focal intravascular infection located outside the heart itself can mimic most of the clinical manifestations of endocarditis, including vascular and immunologic phenomena.[50] In the past, about one-quarter of all patients with an uncorrected patent ductus arteriosus developed bacterial endarteritis.[3] Coarctations of the aorta also presented a significant risk, but endocarditis located on an associated bicuspid aortic valve was 3 times more common than was endarteritis with vegetations located in the coarctation. Endarteritis occasionally complicates traumatic arteriovenous fistulas, but arteriosclerotic aneurysms rarely become infected.[50] When bacterial endarteritis does occur within an aneurysm, the organisms usually grow in a multilayered thrombus in the lumen of the aneurysm rather than in vegetations.

The spectrum of organisms causing infective endarteritis is similar to that found in endocarditis except that there is a higher frequency of infection with salmonellae in arteriosclerotic abdominal aneurysms.[50,133] The pattern of embolization observed differs according to the site of infection. Thus, petechiae may occur on the skin of the lower extremities in a patient with an infected abdominal aneurysm, and infarctions may appear in the lungs of a patient with an infected dialysis fistula in the forearm.

Because many of the congenital and acquired vascular lesions that predispose to infective endarteritis can be corrected by modern surgery, endarteritis—except in arteriovenous shunts constructed for the purpose of hemodialysis—is uncommon today in developed countries.

ETIOLOGIC ORGANISMS

The range of microbial species that can cause infective endocarditis is extraordinarily wide, yet only a few species account for the great majority of cases. On native valves, streptococci and staphylococci together cause more than 80 percent of infections.[38,43,51,116] By comparison, NVE caused by *Staph. epidermidis,* enteric bacilli, and fungi are uncommon. Among IDUs and patients with prosthetic valves, the incidence of infection due to these organisms is higher. Table 73-3 offers representative data from the literature on the relative frequency of the major etiologic organisms on native valves, in drug addicts, and on prosthetic valves. It should be emphasized that the relative frequency with which various organisms cause endocarditis can vary widely between countries and between medical centers.

Streptococci

Streptococci cause more cases of endocarditis than any other group of organisms.[38,51,134–136] The alpha-hemolytic or viridans streptococci account for the majority of these cases, but have decreased in frequency when compared with others during the last 30 years. Viridans streptococci are ubiquitous (although outnumbered by anaerobes) in the oropharyngeal and gastrointestinal flora. They are usually low-grade pathogens (except for *Strep. milleri*), often recovered from clinical specimens in mixed culture with other organisms but seldom themselves causing disease. Their strong association with SBE is therefore determined by the frequency with which they enter the bloodstream and by their ability to adhere to endocardium rather than by their innate virulence.

The nomenclature of these organisms is complex and has been subject to repeated revisions.[134,137,138] The following species frequently cause SBE: *Strep. sanguis, Strep. mitis, Strep. oralis,* and *Strep. gordonii.* Many other species occasionally cause SBE; for example, the *Strep. milleri* group: *Strep. anginosus, Strep. intermedius,* and *Strep. constellatus.*[134,136,137] A few cases are caused by strains that require media supplemented with L-cysteine or pyridoxine for growth.[139–142] These strains are more difficult to isolate from blood and seem to be more difficult to eradicate with antibiotic treatment than the other viridans streptococci.

Group D streptococci are next in frequency among the streptococci as a cause of endocarditis.[94,143,144] The nonenterococcal group D species, *Strep. bovis*, accounts for about one-fifth of streptococcal cases. IE caused by *Strep. bovis* tends to occur in older patients, affect multiple valves, and require surgery more commonly than IE caused by other organisms.[145] Gastrointestinal lesions, especially colonic polyps and cancers, are present in >50 percent of patients who develop *Strep. bovis* bacteremia and/or endocarditis.[146,147] Hence, recovery of this species from blood cultures should prompt investigation for colonic disease, whether or not the patient has gastrointestinal symptoms.

Strains of *E. faecalis* (enterococci) cause about 10 percent of streptococcal cases. In the past it was said that this species caused endocarditis "in young women and old men," because it was found in association with infections of the genital and urinary tract in women of childbearing age and of the urinary tract in old men with prostatic disease. Today, enterococcal endocarditis is also likely to be found in drug addicts, in patients with nosocomial endocarditis, and in those with chronic renal failure.[94] Enterococci commonly cause urinary tract, wound, and intravenous line infections, which often give rise to nosocomial bacteremias.[148,149] Fewer than 2 percent of such patients have endocarditis, but if enterococcal bacteremia is community-acquired without a primary focus of infection, about one-third will have IE.[148] Antibiotic resistance, especially in strains of *E. faecium,* presents major difficulties in treatment of enterococcal endocarditis.[94,150–152]

Many other species and strains of streptococci occasionally cause endocarditis, but they are rare compared with the viridans and group D organisms. *Strep. pneumoniae* endocarditis has become uncommon since the advent of antibiotics. This species causes acute endocarditis,[153] affects primarily the aortic valve in patients without underlying valvular disease (15 of 16 in one series), and often requires immediate valve replacement for aortic insufficiency and cardiac failure (7 of 16).[154,155] In debilitated alcoholics, bacteremic pneumococcal pneumonia is occasionally complicated by the development of pneumococcal endocarditis and meningitis. This triad of simultaneous pneumococcal infections carries an extremely poor prognosis.[153] Beta-hemolytic streptococci rarely cause IE, but in a report of 31 cases, one-third had underlying diabetes mellitis, three-fourths had significant complications, and one-half required cardiac surgery.[156] In children, group A streptococcus may complicate varicella.[157] Group B streptococcal endocarditis is also rare, but may complicate obstetric or other surgical procedures (abortions) or injection drug use, and may involve the tricuspid valve.[158]

Staphylococci

Staph. aureus is the leading cause of acute bacterial endocarditis. Median duration of illness prior to hospitalization was 3 days in one series.[160] It is the predominant etiologic organism in IDUs with endocarditis[70] and frequently causes PVE.[95] *Staph. aureus* endocarditis is also a complication of diabetes mellitis (13 percent in one study), corticosteroid therapy (11 percent), cirrhosis (5 percent), malignancy (4 percent), and chronic renal failure (4 percent).[160] In nosocomial cases, infected intravascular devices were the most common portal of entry. Because it is an invasive primary pathogen, patients with staphylococcal ABE often develop disseminated disease with metastatic infections in skin and soft tissue, bone, joints, eye, or brain.[159–162] More than one-third of patients with *Staph. aureus* endocarditis will have central nervous system involvement.[160]

Only a minority of all patients with *Staph. aureus* bacteremia have endocarditis (6 to 15 percent), and it is often difficult to identify this subgroup clinically. However, use of TEE in this setting is highly effective in establishing the diagnosis of IE. Factors that increase the probability that such a patient has endocarditis are (1) community-acquired bacteremia, (2) absence of a primary focus of infection, and (3) presence of metastatic foci of staphylococcal infection. Up to two-thirds of patients with all 3 of these characteristics have endocarditis.[162] *Staph. epidermidis* is a rare cause of native valve infection (<5 percent), usually associated with an indolent subacute or chronic course.[163] However, serious complications, including systemic embolization, congestive heart failure, myocardial abscess, and valve destruction are common and mortality is high (up to 36 percent).[164] *Staph. lugdunensis,* a recently described species of coagulase negative staphylococcus, appears to be especially virulent and more likely to infect native cardiac valves than *Staph. epidermidis*.[165] In striking contrast, *Staph. epidermidis* is a common cause of PVE (40 to 50 percent), which may follow either an acute or subacute clinical course.[163,166]

Gram-Negative Bacteria

Although most of the species of gram-negative bacteria that colonize and/or infect humans have been reported to cause IE, they account for only a small proportion of cases of native valve infection. A significant subgroup of cases are caused by a group of nutritionally fastidious gram-negative bacilli: *Haemophilus* species, *Actinobacillus actinomycetemcomitans, Cardiobacterium hominis, Eikenella corrodens*, and *Kingella kingae*. These are often referred to by the acronym HACEK, which is derived from their initials,[167,168] and cause approximately 3 percent of cases of IE. In one report, most patients had symptoms between 2 weeks and 3 months and presented with fever, a new or changing murmur, splenomegaly, and emboli.[169] Blood cultures usually took 3 to 4 days to turn positive.[169] Prognosis with medical therapy and surgery, when necessary (one-fourth of patients), was good, with 87 percent overall survival.

Cases caused by *Haemophilus* predominate in this group. Endocarditis caused by this genus is usually due to *H. parainfluenza* (62 percent), *H. aphrophilus* (21 percent), *H. paraphrophilus* (10 percent), and only rarely to *H. influenzae*. *Haemophilus* endocarditis is characterized by large vegetations and arterial emboli (35 to 60 percent).[170]

The common aerobic enteric gram-negative bacilli seldom cause endocarditis. For example, cases of endocarditis caused by *Escherichia coli* and *Klebsiella* are notably rare,[99] even though these species frequently cause gram-negative bacteremia. The reasons for this striking disparity are probably multiple, including low adhesiveness of gram-negative enteric bacilli to heart valves[171] and fibrin[172] and susceptibility of many strains to complement-mediated bacteriolysis.[173] Despite these factors, two special populations are at increased risk of gram-negative endocarditis: IDUs and patients with prosthetic valves. Gram-negative bacilli account for about 5 percent of endocarditis in IDUs,[65,68–70] with *Pseudomonas* species, *Serratia,* and *Enterobacter* species predominating. Gram-negative bacilli cause 15 to 20 percent of early PVE and about 10 percent of late PVE.[11,95] Strains of gram-negative bacilli such as *Stenotrophomonas* (*Xanthomonas*) *multophilia,* which are resistant to most antibiotics, are becoming more common. They typically cause nosocomial IE (50 percent), occur on prosthetic heart valves (50 percent), and are associated with IDUs or indwelling vascular catheters (18.8 percent).[174]

Interesting but unusual cases caused by species of *Salmonella, Brucella, Acinetobacter,* and other gram-negative bacilli have been reported.[99] *Brucella* endocarditis is well known in the Mediterranean basin[175–177] but is rare in most other regions. Endocarditis caused by anaerobic bacteria is rare (1 percent or less of cases),[178,179] possibly because the oxygen tension in heart blood is too high to favor growth of these species on the endocardium.

N. gonorrhoeaea causes an acute form of the disease,[2] often involving the right side of the heart. Like the pneumococcus, *N. gonorrhoeaea* has become uncommon as a cause of endocarditis since the introduction of penicillin.[51,52]

Yeasts and Dimorphic Fungi

Although many species of yeasts and other fungi can infect the endocardium, only two genera account for the great majority: *Candida* and *Aspergillus*.[100,101,180,181] *Candida* causes native valve infections in IDUs and in patients receiving parenteral alimentation, while *Aspergillus* species often involve prosthetic valves. Fungal infection of native valves in nonaddicts is rare (Table 73-3).

Miscellaneous Organisms

Many less common organisms occasionally cause endocarditis; for example, *Coxiella burnetii* (Q fever) and *Chlamydia*. Q-fever endocarditis is a chronic, febrile systemic illness with prominent hepatic as well as cardiac valvular involvement.[182–188] Most cases have been reported from Europe, Canada, and Australia and occur in approximately 7 percent of cases of Q fever. Patients typically present with intermittent fever for months to years (91 percent) or with congestive heart failure (77 percent), and almost all have underlying valvular heart disease (97 percent). Diagnosis is difficult and usually based on serology or identification of the organism in cardiac tissue.[183] One report indicates that *Bartonella* may cause up to 3 percent of cases of IE[189]; in the past, most of these cases were listed as culture-negative, while some were misdiagnosed as chlamydial due to false-positive cross-reacting serologic tests.[189] When suspected on clinical and epidemiological grounds (homeless patient: *Bartonella quintana;* close association with cats: *Bartonella henselae*), PCR (polymerase chain reaction)-based genomic detection or antibody determination are considerably more sensitive than culture in identification of the organism.[190] Chlamydial endocarditis is rare; a few cases have been reported in bird fanciers.[191,192] In such cases, the etiologic diagnosis can be established only by specialized culture techniques, serologic studies, or examination of vegetations using immunofluorescent antibodies. More than 50 cases of *Listeria monocytogenes* endocarditis in both native and prosthetic valves have been reported with a high mortality rate (37 percent).[193] Many other unusual species occasionally infect prosthetic valves, including *Mycoplasma hominis*,[194] *Legionella* species,[53] and mycobacteria.[195] Some examples of rare or unusual organisms that have caused one or more cases of endocarditis are listed in Table 73-4.

Culture-Negative Endocarditis

The term, *culture-negative endocarditis*, refers to the active IE whose repeated blood cultures are all negative.[196–198] This syndrome was occasionally observed in the preantibiotic era,[199] usually in subacute cases of long duration (*Endocarditis lenta*). Today, most (but not all) culture-negative cases are caused by antibiotic treatment that is sufficient to suppress the bacteremia but not to sterilize the vegetation. In most such cases, organisms will eventually reappear in the blood after antibiotics are discontinued, usually within a few days. The blood cultures from a few patients with active endocarditis remain persistently culture-negative after antibiotics are stopped.[116]

Negative blood culture results should be expected from about one-fifth of patients with NVE or PVE caused by *Candida* or other yeasts,[101] and from four-fifths of patients with endocarditis caused by *Aspergillus* or other molds.[101,180,200,201]

The reported incidence of culture-negative endocarditis varies widely. Among large unselected series of cases collected from several hospitals, as much as 15 to 20 percent may be culture-negative.[51,196–198] Smaller series of patients studied by a single clinical and laboratory team that is experienced in evaluation of endocarditis usually show only about 5 percent culture-negative cases.[202,203] Thus, in a patient with suspected IE, other diagnoses should be meticulously excluded before a diagnosis of culture-negative endocarditis is accepted. When a patient appears to have IE but blood cultures are negative, the following checklist of possibilities should be considered:

- The patient has received some antibiotic therapy, commonly an oral drug such as ampicillin that was taken at home.
- The etiologic organism is slow-growing, requiring longer incubation of the blood culture for isolation, e.g., some nutritionally variant streptococci, some HACEK species, or mycobacteria.
- The etiologic organism is nutritionally fastidious, requiring special procedures or supplemented media for isolation, e.g., nutritionally variant streptococci, *C. burnetii* (Q fever), *Chlamydia, Mycoplasma, Bartonella,* and *Legionella.*
- The etiologic organism is a strict anaerobe, requiring anaerobic culture conditions.
- The etiologic organism is *Aspergillus* or another mold; these are rarely recovered from blood during the course of endocarditis (although they may be recovered from an arterial embolus removed at surgery).
- The etiologic organism is nonculturable, which is usually diagnosed by PCR on cardiac tissue during surgery for valve insufficiency. Few clinical cases are present as these patients may not have gastrointestinal symptoms, although most will have arthralgias.[200]
- The patient has an alternative diagnosis that simulates IE—e.g., rheumatic fever, tuberculosis, brucellosis, etc.
- The patient has NBTE or marantic endocarditis, associated with a major underlying disease such as malignancy or tuberculosis.
- The patient has Libman-Sacks endocarditis (a variant of NBTE), associated with antiphospholipid antibody syndrome and/or systemic lupus erythematosus.

In some cases, a working diagnosis of endocarditis based on clinical manifestations can be supported by the progress of the disease and good response to empiric antibiotic treatment. If blood culture results always remain negative, a definitive etiologic diagnosis can be made only by detecting organisms in an infected embolus or in vegetations excised during surgery or at autopsy.

TABLE 73-4 Some Unusual or Rare Causes of Infective Endocarditis

Bacteria	Fungi
Bacillus cereus	*Blastoschizomyces capitatus*
Bartonella elizabethae	*Conidiobolus* sp.
Bartonella henselae	*Curvularia lunata*
Corynebacterium diphtheriae biotype *gravis*	*Engyodontium album*
Corynebacterium jeikeium	*Fusarium oxysporum*
Corynebacterium pseudodiphtheriticum	*Histoplasma capsulatum*
Erysipelothrix rhusiopathiae	*Neosartorya fischeri*
Haemophilus influenzae type b	*Phialophora richardsiae*
Lactobacillus species	*Pseudallescheria boydii*
Legionella species	*Scedosporium inflatum*
Mycoplasma hominis	*Scedosporium apiospermum*
Rothia dentocariosa	*Thermomyces lanuginosus tsiklinsky*
Streptobacillus moniliformis	*Trichosporon beigelii*

PATHOGENESIS AND PATHOLOGY

A general concept of the pathogenesis of NBTE and SBE is presented in Fig. 73-2.

Noninfective Endocarditis

Sterile thrombotic lesions may develop on heart valves in a variety of clinical conditions.[204] Small aggregates of platelets can occasionally be found on normal valves, but they occur frequently on the surfaces of valves damaged by congenital, rheumatic, or granlomatous disease[205] or by IE. These could be considered as incipient vegetations or microvegetations.

The common factor leading to platelet deposition is endothelial damage. This exposes subendothelial connective tissue containing collagen, which activates platelets to adhere and aggregate at the site. These microscopic platelet thrombi may embolize away harmlessly, or they may be stabilized and grow by deposition of fibrin and more platelets to form vegetations of NBTE. This process can be duplicated experimentally by

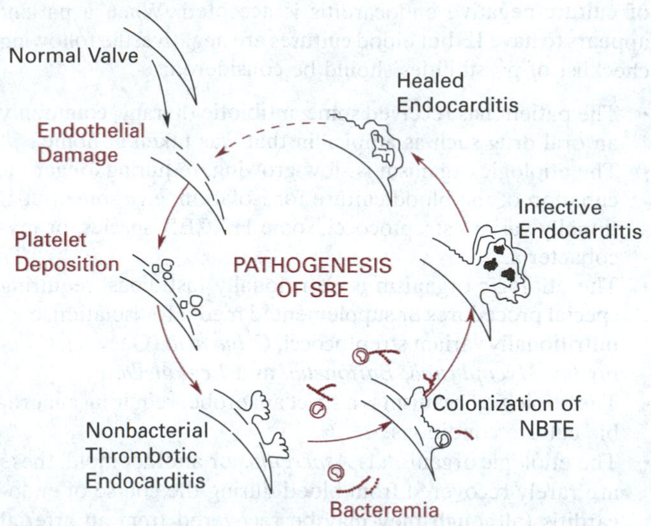

FIGURE 73-2 The main events in the pathogenesis of nonbacterial thrombotic endocarditis (NBTE) and subacute bacterial endocarditis (SBE).

catheter-induced endothelial damage in animals.[206] In humans, intracardiac pressure-monitoring catheters may produce identical lesions.[119,120] Both experimental[207] and human[119,122,204] NBTE can be colonized by circulating bacteria, resulting in IE.

The vegetations of marantic endocarditis occur most often in patients with advanced malignancy[13–15] but may also complicate other chronic wasting diseases, such as tuberculosis or uremia.

Sterile vegetations (termed *Libman-Sacks endocarditis*—see Chap. 76) sometimes develop in patients with systemic lupus erythematosus and/or antiphospholipid antibodies.[208] Typically, Libman-Sacks vegetations are small, sessile masses located on the ventricular surfaces of the mitral valve leaflets.

The vegetations of NBTE are friable white or tan masses, usually situated along the lines of valve closure (Fig. 73-3, Plate 101). These vary greatly in size; from tiny to large and exuberant, with a corresponding tendency to embolize to arteries supplying the myocardium, spleen, kidney, brain, mesentery, or extremities and causing infection. Since there is little inflammatory

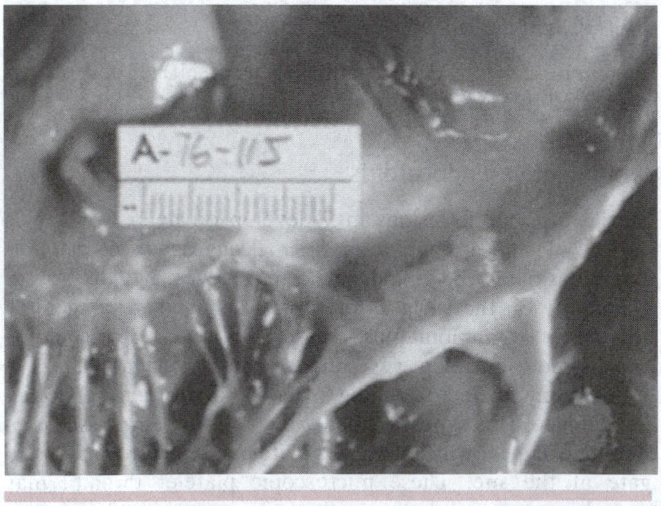

FIGURE 73-3 (Plate 101) Typical vegetation of nonbacterial thrombotic endocarditis found at necropsy in a cachectic patient who died with disseminated lung cancer.

reaction at the site of attachment, fresh vegetations can dislodge and embolize frequently.[204] Histologically, the vegetations of NBTE consist of degenerating platelets interwoven with strands of fibrin, forming a bland, eosinophilic mass, featureless except for a few trapped leukocytes.[204,206]

Pathogenesis of Infective Endocarditis

For IE to develop, two events are essential. First, microbes must attach to an endocardial surface. Second, the microbes must persist and multiply locally, eluding host defense mechanisms. In the case of SBE, which usually develops on previously abnormal valves, bacteria circulating in the bloodstream probably colonize preexisting platelet aggregates or NBTE.[204] It is not known whether ABE, which often affects apparently normal valves, develops in a like manner by colonization of microscopic sterile vegetations, or by direct microbial invasion of normal endothelium.

A critical initial step in the pathogenesis of IE is the attachment or adherence of the circulating microorganism to the disrupted cardiac valve endothelium that has deposits of fibrin and platelets (NBTE). The characteristic that gives the microbe selective adherence advantage to this surface are virulence factors for the development of IE. Early studies identified dextran production in viridans streptococci as an important adherence factor (it had been previously shown to be important in adherence to teeth and production of dental caries).[172] A host of other microbial factors have been described. These include a fibrinectin-binding protein,[377] enterococcal aggregation substance, and enterococcal binding substances (proteins that also mediate formation of mating aggregate between bacteria that cause horizontal transfer of plasmids encoding such things as antibiotic resistance[210] and FimA, a surface-associated protein found on oral streptoccci and enterococci, that, when used as an antigen (similar to other surface proteins of the Lral family) produce an antibody that reduces adherence to valve surfaces and reduces development of endocarditis in animal model.[209–212] Since FimA is found in 80 percent of streptococci and enterococci strains that produce endocarditis, a protective vaccine strategy is an intriguing probability. Binding to fibronectin appears to be an important property shared by many but not all of the bacterial species that commonly cause endocarditis.[50,209] Clumping factor produced by coagulase-positive staphylococci favors attachment to fibrinogen, adherence to platelet-fibrin clots, and ability to cause endocarditis in rats.[213] Extracellular slime production by coagulase-negative staphylococci may favor localization on prosthetic valves.[214] *Thus, microbial adherence, which can be mediated by a variety of different surface components and receptors, is a key virulance factor for colonization of the endocardium.*[50,209]

The role of the platelet in this postadherance event has been elucidated. First, adherence of *Staph. aureus* to platelets is an important virulance factor for development of experimental IE.[219–225] In addition, acetylsallicylic acid treatment reduces *Staph. aureus*-induced platelet aggregation and adherence to fibrin (with or without platelets) matrices in vitro and reduced vegetation size and embolic events in vivo.[224,225] When *Staph. aureus* (or enterococci) adhere to damaged valves in vivo, tissue thromboplastin is generated, which locally activates the clotting cascade, generating thrombin.[205,220] A vegetation is formed that provides a protected environment for unrestricted bacterial growth. However, thrombin also elicits the secretion from platelets of a low-molecular-weight cationic protein with potent antimicrobial properties (against *Staph. aureus, Staph. epidermidis,* viridans streptococci and *Candida*) termed *thrombin-induced platelet microbiocidal protein* (tPMP).[221] Strains of *Staph. aureus* that are resistant to tPMP are more likely to cause endocarditis in animals and humans.[222] In addition, strains that hypersecrete alpha toxin (a toxin known to lyse platelets and release tPMP) produced a less virulent form of IE, likely due to the antimicrobial action of tPMP.[223]

Therefore, once lodged on NBTE, bacteria must elude local defenses, including platelet microbicidal proteins[215] and leukocytes, if they are to survive. Microbes that cannot do this may die out quickly after adhering to the endocardium.[216] Those that can survive antimicrobial defense mechanisms multiply rapidly in the vegetation, soon reaching high numbers and then entering a stationary growth phase.[207] The vegetation provides an ideal supporting stroma for the growth of microbial colonies, into which essential nutrients can diffuse from the blood. The presence of bacteria is a powerful stimulus for further thrombosis,[217,218] which may be mediated by thromboplastin generated by leukocytes when they are exposed to fibrin.[218] New layers of fibrin are deposited around growing bacteria, causing the vegetations to enlarge.[206] Inflammatory cytokines are produced by monocytes[226] (and presumably other leukocytes) in response to endocardial infection and likely cause some of the patient's symptoms.

The location of vegetations is relevant to understanding and managing endocarditis. Approximate incidence of vegetations at various locations is given in Table 73-5. The frequency of involvement of each valve is directly proportional to the mean blood pressure upon it;[227] thus, the left side of the heart is involved much more often than the right. This rule does not hold true for acute endocarditis in IDUs, in whom tricuspid infection by *Staph. aureus* predominates (Table 73-5).

Vegetations are usually located on the downstream side of anatomic abnormalities in the heart or great vessels. Rodbard[228] developed the unifying concept that vegetations usually arise at a site where blood flows from a high-pressure source (e.g., the left ventricle) through a narrow orifice (e.g., a stenotic aortic valve) into a low-pressure sink (e.g., the aorta). Illustrative examples from human disease include aortic stenosis, ventricular septal defect, coarctation, and mitral regurgitation. Experimentally, Rodbard showed that bacteria carried in an aerosol flowing through a constricted tube into an area of low pressure were deposited on the walls of the tube immediately beyond the constriction due to Venturi pressure effects and turbulence.[228] These observations fit well with the actual location of vegetations found at autopsy in cases of endocarditis (Fig. 73-4). Vegetations also may develop on jet lesions, which are areas of

TABLE 73-5 Approximate Frequency of Anatomic Location of Vegetations in SBE, ABE, and Endocarditis Associated with IV Drug Abuse[a]

Location	SBE, %	ABE, %	Endocarditis in IV Drug Abusers, %
Left-sided valves	85	65	40
Aortic	15–26	18–25	15–20
Mitral	38–45	30–35	15–20
Aortic and mitral	23–30	15–20	13–20
Right-sided valves	5	20	50–70
Tricuspid	1–5	15	45–65
Pulmonary	1	Rare	2
Tricuspid and pulmonary	Rare	Rare	3
Left- and right-sided sites	Rare	5–10	5–10
Other sites (patent ductus, ventricular septal defect, coarctation, jet lesions)	10	5	5

[a]SBE = subacute bacterial endocarditis; ABE = acute bacterial endocarditis.
SOURCE: Adapted from Refs. 51, 65–70, 86, 116, 159, 227, 230.

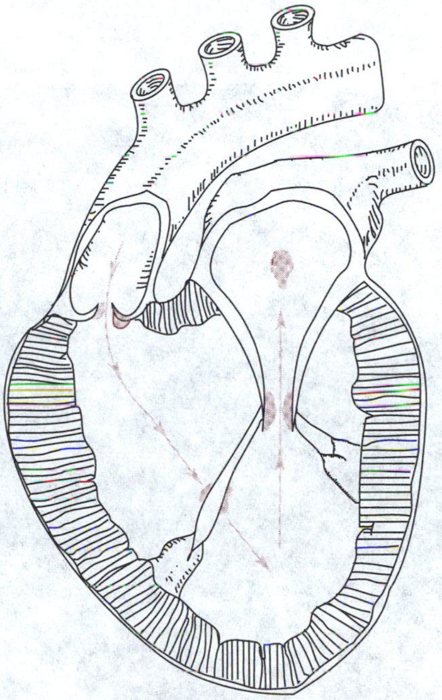

FIGURE 73-4 The sites where endocarditis occurs in aortic and mitral regurgitation. The arrows on the left indicate a high-velocity regurgitant stream passing through the orifice of an incompetent aortic valve into a low-pressure sink (left ventricle in diastole). Vegetations appear on the ventricular surface of the aortic valve. The regurgitant stream may cause a jet lesion on the chordae tendineae of the anterior leaflet of the mitral valve. The arrow on the right shows regurgitation from the high-pressure source of the left ventricle during systole into the left atrium, with vegetations developing on the atrial surface of the mitral valve. Vegetations also can occur on the jet lesion where the regurgitant stream through the mitral valve strikes the atrial endocardium, an area known as *MacCallum's patch.* (From Rodbard S. Blood velocity and endocarditis. *Circulation* 1963; 27:8. Reproduced with permission.)

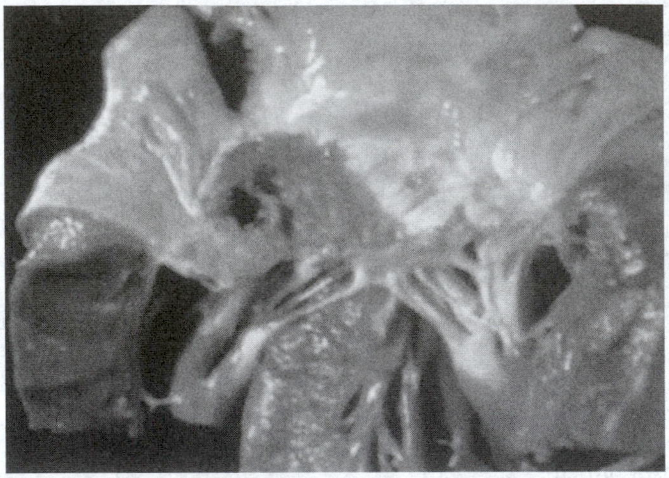

FIGURE 73-5 (Plate 102) Typical vegetation of bacterial endocarditis, complicated by perforation of the anterior mitral valve leaflet. Note that the valve shows preexisting chronic rheumatic disease, with thickening, deformity, and fusion of chordae tendineae.

endothelial roughening and reactive fibrosis at sites where a swift, turbulent regurgitant stream of blood strikes the endothelium.[229] *MacCallum's patch,* on the wall of the left atrium in some patients with mitral regurgitation, is an example of a jet lesion; an infected vegetation occasionally develops at this site (Fig. 73-4).

Vegetations of infective endocarditis vary greatly in size and morphology, from small (<1 mm), warty nodules to large (several centimeters), cauliflower-like polypoid masses. That may cause functional stenosis of valve orifices (Fig. 73-5, Plate 102). Fungal vegetations are often larger than bacterial ones, but otherwise the etiologic species does not correlate reliably with vegetation size. Their color also varies widely, from white to tan to greenish-gray.[67,230] Histologically, colonies of microorganisms are found embedded in a fibrin-platelet matrix.[206,207,231,232] The vegetation characteristically contain relatively few leukocytes that are prevented from reaching bacteria by layers of fibrin, which form protective barriers around colonies (Fig. 73-6).

Development of an abscess is one of the most important complications of valvular infection, and it occurs more frequently with ABE than it does with SBE.[229,231] Abscesses often develop by direct extension of active infection into the fibrous cardiac skeleton—that is, into the rings of supporting connective tissue around the valves. From there, abscesses can extend into the adjacent myocardium and rupture into the pericardium. Hematogenous seeding occasionally leads to development of abscesses elsewhere in the myocardium.

Abscesses are found in the majority of patients who die with active prosthetic valve infection, often spreading around the sewing ring of the prosthesis and causing partial dehiscence of the prosthetic valve.[11,95] Because these valve-ring abscesses are located close to the cardiac conduction system, conduction disturbances commonly result.[233]

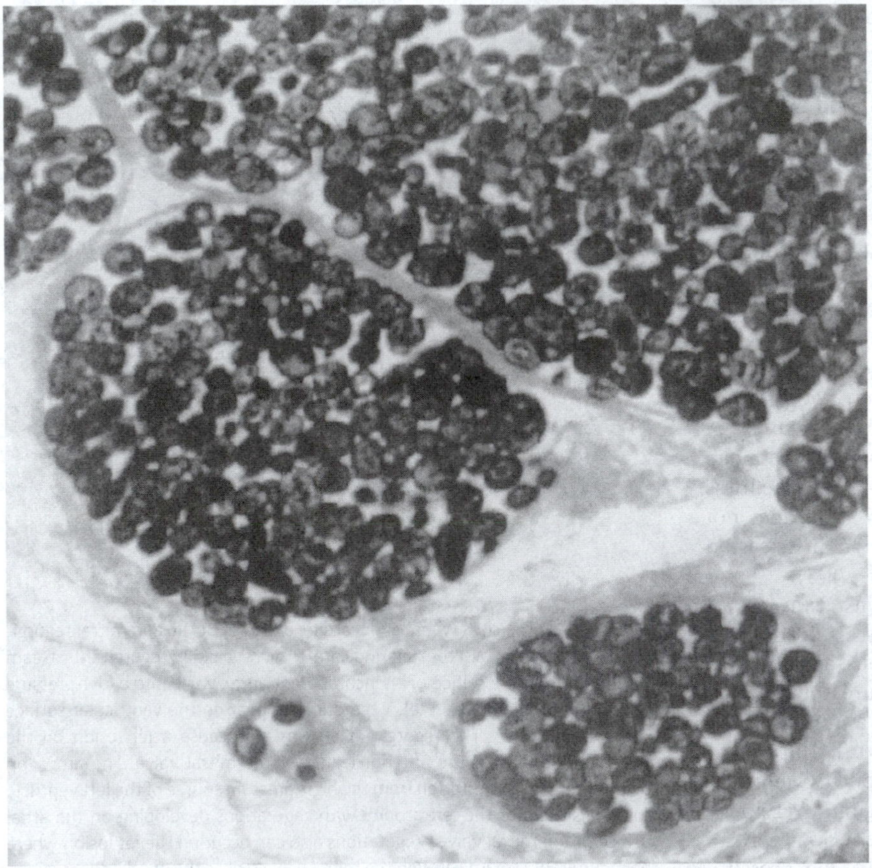

FIGURE 73-6 Electron micrograph of a vegetation of experimental streptococcal endocarditis (×7800). Note the very large number of cocci in colonies, the protective layers of fibrin, and the absence of leukocytes—all factors that may impede the efficacy of antimicrobial therapy. (From Durack DT. Experimental bacterial endocarditis: 4. Structure and evolution of very early lesions. *J Pathol* 1975; 115:81. Reproduced with permission.)

Immune Response

Presence of bacteria in endocardial vegetations stimulates the humoral immune system to produce nonspecific antibodies. This can result in a polyclonal increase in gamma globulins, positive rheumatoid factor, and, occasionally, false-positive serologic test results for syphilis.[234] Rheumatoid factor develops in 25 to 50 percent of patients with SBE present for >6 weeks and can provide a useful diagnostic clue; it reverts to negative after eradication of the organisms.[235–237] Antiendocardial and antisarcolemmal antibodies have been detected in 60 to 100 percent of cases;[238] they are more commonly found in SBE than they are in ABE.

Specific antibodies to many of the commensal organisms that cause SBE may be present in low titer before infection. Titers rise during active infection[3] and fall after treatment.

Hemolytic complement levels are low in about 30 percent of patients early in the course of endocarditis, rising later and returning to normal after treatment.[239–245] The lowest levels are found in patients with immune-complex glomerulonephritis.

Circulating immune complexes have been detected in 82 to 97 percent of patients with either ABE or SBE.[244–247] Higher concentrations are correlated with the presence of extracardiac manifestations such as arthritis, splenomegaly, and glomerulonephritis; with longer duration of illness; and with hypocomplementemia. Several studies confirm that glomerulonephritis in patients with endocarditis is mediated by immune complexes.[248,249] It is likely but unproven that arthritis and tenosynovitis—and possibly pericarditis, Osler's nodes, and Roth's spots[244,246,247]—also may represent inflammatory responses involving immune complexes. Antibodies to teichoic acids were found in the serum of 93 percent of patients with *Staph. aureus* endocarditis,[250] but this did not prove to be useful as a routine diagnostic test. Additional relevant information on experimental infective endocarditis is contained in References 251 to 254.

CLINICAL MANIFESTATIONS

Clinical and laboratory manifestations of infective endocarditis can be grouped under three headings (Table 73-6):

- Evidence of a systemic infection
- Evidence of an intravascular lesion
- Evidence of an immunologic reaction to infection

History

The symptoms of subacute endocarditis develop insidiously and with great variability.[3,43,51,116] Fevers, chills, rigors, and night sweats provide evidence of systemic infection. General malaise—with anorexia, fatigue, and weakness—is typical. Weight loss is common, along with headaches and musculoskeletal complaints, including myalgias, arthralgias, and back pains.[255] This symptom complex is often described by the patient or the physician as a "flu-like illness." Evidence of an intravascular lesion is provided by symptoms of left- or right-sided heart failure and by manifestations of embolization, such as focal neurologic injury, chest pain, flank pain, left-upper-quadrant pain, hematuria, or ischemia of an extremity. Symptoms usually persist and worsen intermittently over 4 to 8 weeks before the diagnosis is made.[256,257]

In the acute form of IE, the course is accelerated, and the symptoms are often accentuated in severity. Patients experience hectic fevers, rigors, and prostration, usually leading to hospital admission within a few days.[5,51,103,251,258]

Symptoms of cardiac failure may develop gradually or worsen suddenly in either acute or subacute disease due to mechanical complications such as perforation of a valve leaflet, rupture of one of the chordae tendineae, rupture of a sinus of Valsalva, or development of functional stenosis from obstruction of blood flow by large vegetations.[231,259] Alternatively, heart failure may develop insidiously, or preexisting chronic heart

TABLE 73-6 Summary of the Major Clinical Manifestations of Infective Endocarditis

Manifestation	History	Examination	Investigations
SYSTEMIC INFECTION	Fever, chills, rigors, sweats, malaise, weakness, lethargy, delirium, headache, anorexia, weight loss, backache, arthralgia, myalgia Portal of entry: oropharynx, skin, urinary tract, drug addiction, nosocomial bacteremia	Fever, pallor, weight loss, asthenia, splenomegaly	Anemia, leukocytosis (variable), raised erythrocyte sedimentation rate, positive blood culture, abnormal cerebrospinal fluid
INTRAVASCULAR LESION	Dyspnea, chest pain, focal weakness, stroke, abdominal pain, cold and painful extremities	Murmurs, signs of cardiac failure, petechiae (skin, eye, mucosae), Roth's spots, Osler's nodes, Janeway lesions, splinter hemorrhages, stroke, mycotic aneurysm, ischemia or infarction of viscera or extremities	Blood in urine, chest roentgenogram, echocardiography, arteriography, liver-spleen scan, lung scan, brain scan, CT scan, histology, culture of emboli
IMMUNOLOGIC REACTIONS	Arthralgia, myalgia, tenosynovitis	Arthritis, signs of uremia, vascular phenomena, finger clubbing	Proteinuria, hematuria, casts, uremia, acidosis, polyclonal increases in gamma globulins, rheumatoid factor, decreased complement, immune complexes in serum, antistaphylococcal teichoic acid antibodies

SOURCE: Adapted from Refs. 3–6, 43, 50, 51, 116.

failure may worsen due to progressive damage to the valves or associated structures. Myocarditis or myocardial infarction due to coronary artery embolism may contribute to heart failure.

Physical Examination

The physical exam in IE is a diagnosticians delight since the variety of unique physical findings often allows one to make the diagnosis at the bedside.

Patients with endocarditis may appear acutely or chronically ill. Intermittent chills, rigors, and sweating often provide evidence of a systemic infection. Asthenia and recent weight loss are often notable. Anemia is common,[85] especially in SBE, so many patients are pale. The skin of some patients with long-standing SBE shows the sallow hue of uremia.[3]

VASCULAR PHENOMENA

Patients with endocarditis may exhibit a variety of striking physical findings arising from vascular abnormalities.

Petechiae In both SBE and ABE, petechiae are common; they are rare in NBTE. In a few cases, the petechiae have a pale central spot. Most are due to microembolization to small vessels in the skin or mucous membranes. They are commonly found in crops in the conjunctival sac, on the hard palate, behind the ears and over the chest. But all areas of the trunk and extremities may be affected.

Splinter Hemorrhages Linear subungual hemorrhages, resembling tiny splinters of wood under the nails but not reaching the nail margin, are found in about 20 percent of patients with SBE. They are probably caused by microembolization to linear capillaries under the nail. Because splinter hemorrhages are found in some 5 to 8 percent of patients admitted to the hospital who do not have endocarditis, they are of limited diagnostic value when occuring alone.[260]

Osler's Nodes These are painful, tender, erythematous nodules in the skin of the extremities, usually in the pulp of the fingers[261] (Fig. 10-17, Plate 34; Fig. 10-18). Occasionally, the center of these pea-sized, red lesions is pale, but necrosis does not occur. Osler's nodes occur in 10 to 20 percent of patients with SBE and in fewer than 10 percent of patients with ABE.[261] They are probably caused by inflammation around the site of lodgment of small, infected emboli in distal arterioles, because the etiologic organism can be recovered from some of the lesions.[262] Inflammation due to focal immunologic reactions probably contributes to formation of Osler's nodes, especially in subacute cases.[247]

Janeway Lesions Janeway lesions are small (less than 5 mm), flat, nontender red spots, irregular in outline, found on the palms and soles of a few patients with SBE and ABE. Unlike petechiae, they are not hemorrhagic, and they blanch on pressure.[3,44]

Ocular Lesions Conjunctival petechiae show up as small, bright-red hemorrhages that are easily seen if the upper and lower eyelids are everted. These petechiae are not specific for endocarditis, being found sometimes after cardiac surgery and occasionally in septicemia (Fig. 73-7, Plate 103). Nevertheless, the discovery of conjunctival hemorrhages in a patient with unexplained fever and a heart murmur makes the diagnosis of endocarditis highly likely.

Retinal hemorrhages are found in 10 to 25 percent of cases of both SBE and ABE. They are quite variable in appearance. Some simply represent petechiae in the retina; their round or flame-shaped outline is determined by the layer of the retina in which they develop. Those with a white or yellow center surrounded by a bright-red, irregular halo are known as *Roth's spots,* which probably represent cytoid bodies and associated hemorrhage caused by microinfarction of retinal vessels. Roth's spot are not foci of bacterial infection and are nonspecific to IE.

Loss of vision during the course of endocarditis can occur from embolization to the brain or to the retinal artery, from optic neuritis, or from ophthalmitis. Endophthalmitis may occur in patients with *Candida* endocarditis and/or candidemia. The typical retinal lesions are rounded, white, cotton-like exudates with extension into the vitreous and overlying vitreous haze.[263] Panophthalmitis occurs in some patients with ABE due to hematogenous spread of virulent pathogens.

CLUBBING OF THE FINGERS

Previously common in SBE, finger clubbing is now found in less than 5 percent of cases (Fig. 10-16, Plate 33), presumably because endocarditis is now diagnosed and treated earlier. The pathogenesis of this reaction, which usually resolves after eradication of the infecting organism, is not understood.

SIGNS OF EMBOLIZATION

Decreased or absent arterial pulses in an extremity may signal occlusion of a large artery by a fragment of vegetation. Focal neurologic signs may develop transiently or progress to a completed stroke due to embolization to a cerebral artery (see "Complications," later). Infarctions of the spleen, kidney, or bowel can present with pain and tenderness on palpation of the abdomen, mimicking an acute abdominal event such as bowel obstruction or peritonitis. Myocardial infarction due to obstruction of a coronary artery can cause heart failure or death and is sometimes an unexpected finding at autopsy in patients who

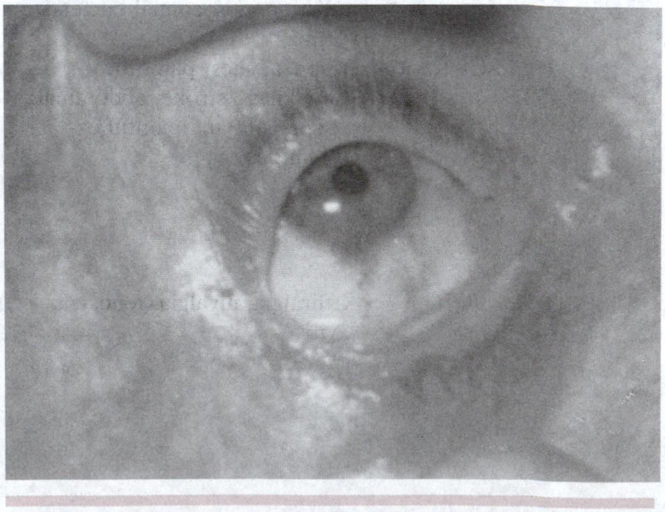

FIGURE 73-7 (Plate 103) Typical conjunctival petechiae in a patient with subacute bacterial endocarditis due to *Streptococcus sanguis.*

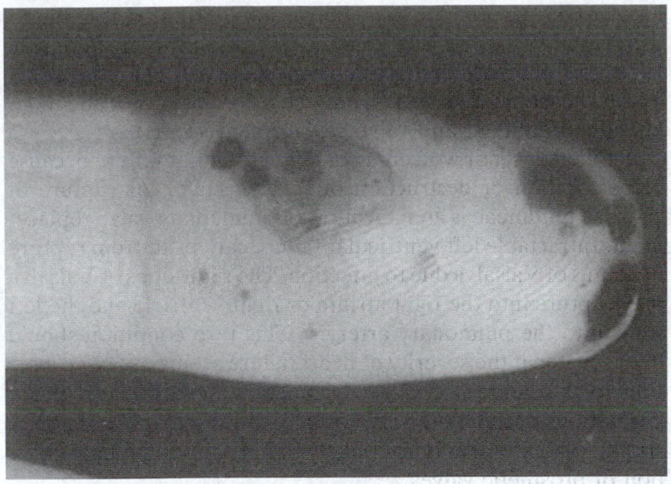

FIGURE 73-8 (Plate 104) Ischemic, hemorrhagic, and pustular lesions on the extremities in acute *Staphylococcus aureus* endocarditis.

die with active disease. These complications are illustrated in Figs. 73-8 to 73-13, Plates 104–109.

SPLENOMEGALY

Development of splenomegaly is common, occurring in about one-quarter of patients with ABE and one-half of those with SBE. The spleen is usually soft and only slightly tender except in the case of recent embolic infarction, when palpation may be very painful. Radionuclide scanning may reveal infarction or a splenic abscess.

CARDIAC EXAMINATION

The pulse is often rapid as a result of fever or congestive failure. Irregularities of conduction may indicate the presence of an abscess near the conducting system. Underlying or newly developed aortic regurgitation associated with IE may result in a collapsing pulse (Chaps. 10 and 56).

One or more murmurs are present in virtually all patients at some stage of the disease. Even though some of the classic findings of IE are less often seen today than they are formerly,

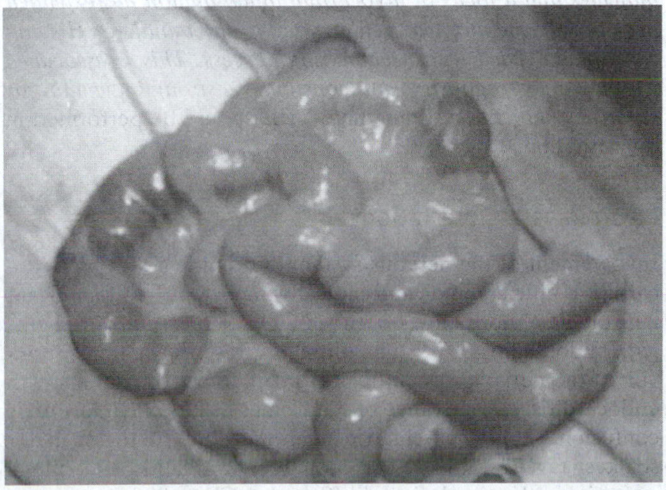

FIGURE 73-9 (Plate 105) Segmental ischemia and necrosis in the gut, presenting as acute abdomen.

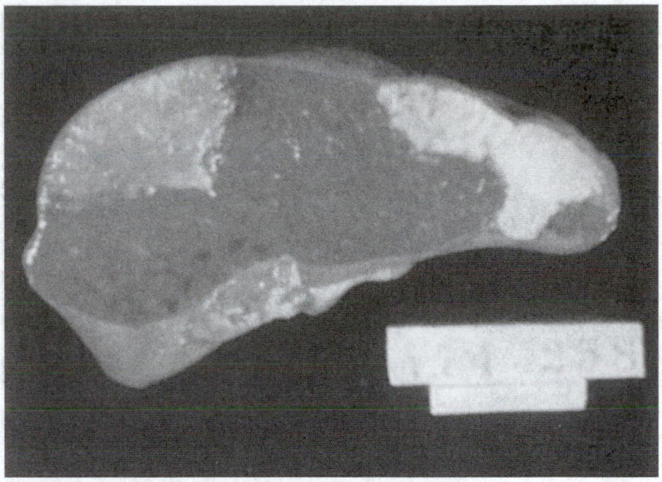

FIGURE 73-10 (Plate 106) Infarctions in the spleen.

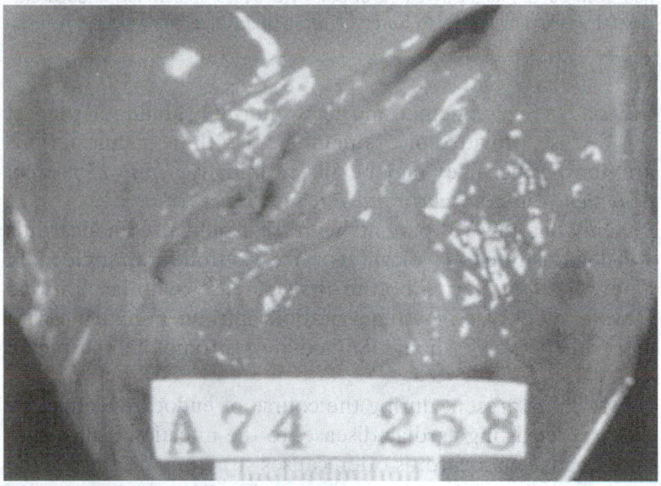

FIGURE 73-11 (Plate 107) An infected embolus in a coronary artery.

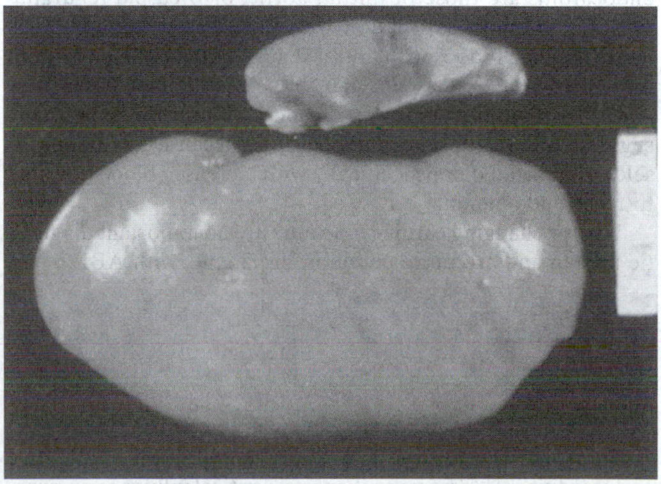

FIGURE 73-12 (Plate 108) Kidney from a patient with subacute bacterial endocarditis, showing two abnormalities: (1) typical ischemic infarctions due to emboli and (2) swelling and petechiae (flea-bitten kidney) due to immune-complex glomerulonephritis.

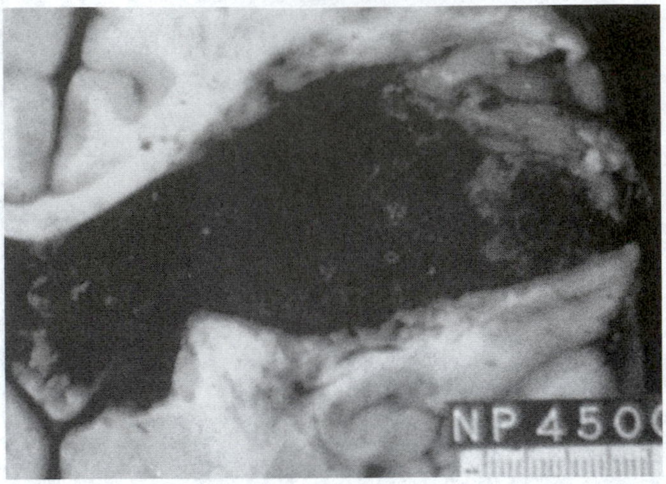

FIGURE 73-13 (Plate 109) Massive cerebral hemorrhage with intraventricular extension due to rupture of a small, peripheral mycotic aneurysm. The patient had been bacteriologically cured of *Staphylococcus epidermidis* endocarditis several weeks previously. Cultures of the blood, valve, and aneurysm taken at necropsy were negative.

the triad of fever, anemia, and a new murmur should still suggest this disease, provided one remembers that these manifestations are nonspecific. They may be absent initially. *Up to 15 percent of patients do not have a murmur when first seen.*

Only one-third of patients with tricuspid valve endocarditis will demonstrate the typical regurgitant systolic murmur located along the right sternal border that increases with inspiration.[5] Development of a new regurgitation murmur in patients with a prosthetic valve should immediately prompt the suspicion of PVE.

Murmurs present during the course of endocarditis may be due to preexisting cardiac disease, to the infection itself, or to both. Active endocarditis often causes structural damage to the valve, including deformities, tears, perforations, and rupture of chordae tendineae. Since these changes often lead to valvular insufficiency, the murmurs most often heard in association with endocarditis are those of mitral, aortic, or tricuspid regurgitation. IE occurs in association with pure mitral stenosis much less often than it does with mitral regurgitation (with or without associated stenosis) (see Chap. 57). Development of a new aortic regurgitation murmur during a febrile illness strongly suggests the diagnosis of endocarditis, because this finding is seldom associated nonspecifically with increased blood flow due to fever and anemia.

New or changing cardiac murmurs are an important diagnostic finding and are more common in patients with ABE.

COMPLICATIONS

Heart Failure

Heart failure is the most important complication of infective endocarditis,[51,264–266] because it exerts a critical influence on prognosis. In 1951, Cates and Christie[215] reported a death rate of 37 percent among 314 patients with SBE who had no heart failure and 85 percent death rate among 94 patients who had moderate or severe failure. In the past, congestive heart failure occurred in up to 55 percent of cases, being more common in patients with aortic valve disease (75 percent) than in those with mitral valve (50 percent) or tricuspid valve disease (19 percent).[265] Today, heart failure is less common because of earlier and more effective treatment and valve replacement surgery.

Sudden onset or worsening of left ventricular failure because of perforation or destruction of a valve leaflet or rupture of chordae tendineae is an indication for immediate valve replacement. Intractable left ventricular failure can result from rupture of a sinus of Valsalva due to infection. The right sinus of Valsalva may rupture into the right atrium or right ventricle and the left sinus into the pulmonary artery.[231] This rare condition should be suspected if the severity of heart failure seems out of proportion to the degree of valve dysfunction. Occasionally, bulky vegetations occlude the valve orifice, causing functional stenosis; this phenomenon is most likely to occur during fungal infection of prosthetic valves.[267,268]

Embolization

This important complication is recognized in 12 to 40 percent of patients during the course of SBE and in 40 to 60 percent of those with ABE, but autopsy findings indicate that many other arterial emboli go undetected. Pelletier and Petersdorf[116] reported a 50 percent incidence of major arterial emboli in 125 cases, affecting brain (25 cases), lung (17 cases), coronary artery (8 cases), spleen (8 cases), extremities (8 cases), gut (4 cases), and eye (3 cases). The presence of infection-related antiphospholipid antibodies has been found to be a major risk factor for embolic events.[269]

Conduction Abnormalities

A conduction abnormality is detected during the course of IE in 4 to 16 percent of patients, especially in association with aortic valve infection.[233,259,270] Types of abnormalities observed include first-degree atrioventricular block (45 percent), third-degree atrioventricular block (20 percent), second-degree atrioventricular block (15 percent), and isolated bundle branch blocks (15 percent).[233] *The development of a new, unstable, or changing conduction abnormality is important because it often indicates that a focus of myocardial inflammation has extended near or into the atrioventricular node or the bundle of His and can be associated with a valve-ring abscess. This is associated with a worse prognosis*[266] *and constitutes a strong indication for surgical intervention.* Immediate TEE should be performed in this situation.

Neurologic Manifestations

Involvement of the nervous system during the course of endocarditis is both common and clinically important.[271–274] Significant neurologic abnormalities occur in 29 to 50 percent of patients with endocarditis.[271,274,275] The initial or presenting complaint involves the nervous system in 10 to 15 percent of patients with endocarditis. A wide range of syndromes occurs, including toxic confusional states, psychiatric symptoms, and minor or major strokes (Fig. 73-13, Plate 00), meningoencephalitis, and cranial or peripheral nerve lesions.[274] (See also Chap. 89.)

Of 55 patients with cerebrovascular complications of endocarditis, four-fifths suffered infarction and one-fifth hemorrhage.[275] Infarction is usually due to embolism, most often to the middle cerebral arteries. In some series, neurologic complications approach or even surpass heart failure as the leading determinant of mortality.[274] Hemorrhage can be a complication of either emboli or mycotic aneurysms.[116,271–273,276,277]

A meningeal reaction cerebritis occurs in 7 to 15 percent of patients, especially those with staphylococcal ABE.[43,271,273–275] This reaction may be mistakenly diagnosed as acute bacterial meningitis because the cerebrospinal fluid contains polymorphonuclear leukocytes and may have a raised protein concentration. In a minority of such cases (up to 20 percent of those with acute staphylococcal infection) cerebrospinal fluid cultures yield the bacteria causing endocarditis. The glucose level, however, is usually normal; the results of cerebrospinal fluid culture are usually negative; and the abnormalities usually resolve without complications during treatment of the endocarditis. Thus, these cerebrospinal fluid abnormalities more often represent a perivascular cerebritis than true bacterial meningitis.

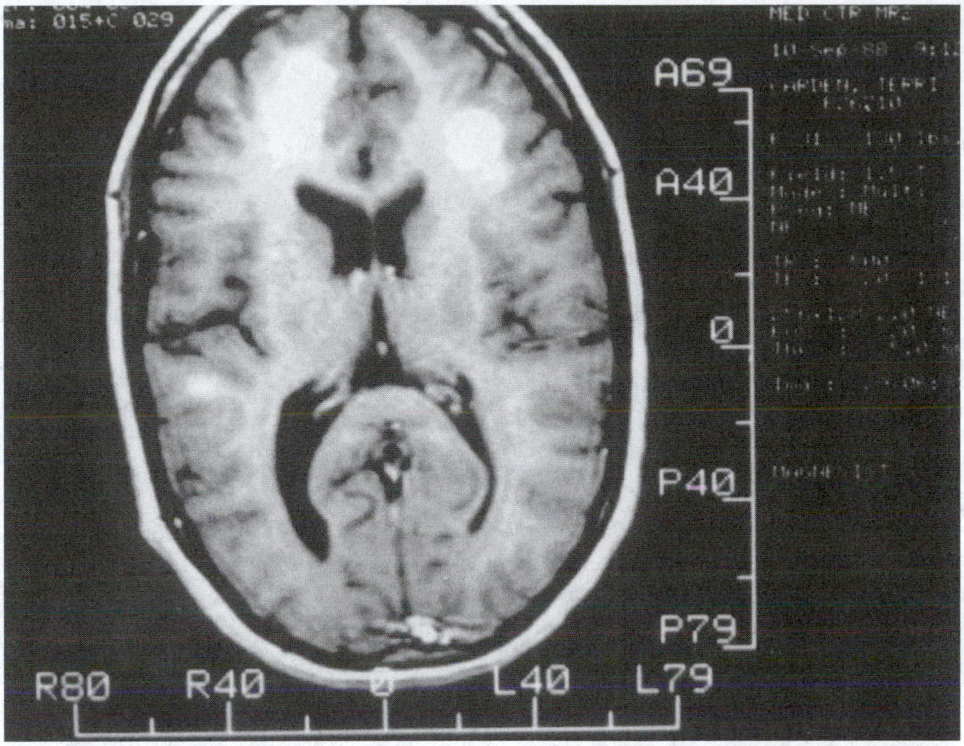

FIGURE 73-14 Magnetic resonance image of the brain in a patient with acute left-sided *Staphylococcus aureus* endocarditis, showing multiple areas of focal cerebritis. This patient had no focal central nervous system signs and recovered fully with antimicrobial therapy. (MRI by courtesy of the Department of Radiology, Duke University, Durham, NC.)

This cerebritis may develop in brain tissue surrounding small infected emboli lodged in cerebral vessels with associated meningoencephalitis.[274] Computed tomography and magnetic resonance imaging often reveal multiple areas of cerebritis, even in patients with no central nervous system symptoms (Fig. 73-14). In patients with ABE, this inflammatory reaction may progress to form a brain abscess, but more often cerebritis will resolve uneventfully during antibiotic treatment of the underlying disease. Brain abscesses are uncommon in patients with SBE.[274] Bacterial meningitis does occur in some patients with pneumococcal endocarditis.[153]

Mycotic Aneurysm

This complication develops in 3 to 15 percent of patients with IE, and the consequences of expansion and rupture of the aneurysm can be very serious, especially in the brain (Fig. 73-13, Plate 109). In order of frequency, the sites most often involved are the proximal aorta, including the sinuses of Valsalva (25 percent of cases), arteries to the viscera (24 percent), arteries to the extremities (22 percent), and arteries to the brain (15 percent).[276–278] Unfortunately, intracerebral aneurysms are often multiple.[277,278]

Mycotic aneurysms develop when the wall of an artery is damaged by the inflammatory response to microbes.[232,243,279,280] These microbes reach the arterial wall via microemboli to the vasa vasorum or by impaction of a larger infected embolus in the lumen. The arterial wall is apparently an unfavorable culture medium for bacteria because the organisms responsible for weakening the vessel often die out spontaneously, even if untreated. The mycotic aneurysm may continue to enlarge even when living organisms are no longer present, due to the physical effects of arterial blood pressure (Fig. 73-9, Plate 105).[276–278,281]

DIFFERENTIAL DIAGNOSIS

Because the clinical manifestations of endocarditis are numerous and often nonspecific, the differential diagnosis of this disease is very wide.[3,43,116,282] Of the many conditions that may be considered, only a few leading examples are listed here.

ABE shares many clinical features with nonendocarditic septicemias due to invasive bacterial pathogens such as *Staph. aureus, Neisseria,* pneumococci, and gram-negative bacilli. The differential diagnosis for a case of ABE might include sepsis, pneumonia, meningitis, brain abscess, stroke, malaria, acute pericarditis, vasculitis, and disseminated intravascular coagulation.

SBE must be considered during the workup of every patient with fever of unknown origin.[202,282,283] Its manifestations can mimic those of rheumatic fever, osteomyelitis, tuberculosis, meningitis, intraabdominal infections, salmonellosis, brucellosis, glomerulonephritis, myocardial infarction, stroke, endocardial thrombi, atrial myxoma, connective tissue diseases; arthrites of unkown etiology, vasculitis, occult malignancies (especially lymphomas), chronic cardiac failure, pericarditis, and even psychoneurosis.

TABLE 73-7 Criteria for Diagnosis of Infective Endocarditis

Definite Infective Endocarditis

PATHOLOGIC CRITERIA

Microorganisms: demonstrated by culture or histology in a vegetation, or in a vegetation that has embolized, or in an intracardiac abscess, *or*
Pathologic lesions: vegetation or intracardiac abscess present, confirmed by histology showing active endocarditis

CLINICAL CRITERIA, USING SPECIFIC DEFINITIONS LISTED IN TABLE 73-8

Two major criteria, *or*
One major and three minor criteria, *or*
Five minor criteria

Possible Infective Endocarditis

Findings consistent with infective endocarditis that fall short of "definite," but not "rejected"

Rejected

Firm alternate diagnosis for manifestations of endocarditis,
or
Resolution of manifestations of endocarditis, with antibiotic therapy for 4 days or less, *or*
No pathologic evidence of infective endocarditis at surgery or autopsy after antibiotic therapy for 4 days or less

SOURCE: From Durack et al.,[202] with permission.

Diagnostic Criteria

IE can be surprisingly difficult to diagnose with certainty.[202,284] In the course of clinical practice, the diagnosis is suspected much more often than it is confirmed. This is because the presenting symptoms and signs can be highly variable and consistent with many other possible diagnoses. Furthermore, the primary lesion (an endocardial vegetation) is inaccessible to direct inspection except at surgery or autopsy. Major and minor criteria have been defined[202]; they are analogous to the modified Jones criteria[285] (Chap. 55) for diagnosis of acute rheumatic fever[86,202,203] (Tables 73-7 and 73-8). Several diagnostic schemes have been developed to assist the clinician in working through a diagnostic workup, however, it is important to emphasize that while these may be useful guidelines, each patient must be considered on an individual basis. The so-called Duke criteria has received the most attention.[202]

Because the Duke criteria emphasize specificity[203,286] above sensitivity, they should not be used to guide urgent management decisions early in the course of a suspected case. To illustrate: a diagnosis of endocarditis made solely on the basis of presence of fever and a heart murmur would be very sensitive but very nonspecific. These findings alone might make a clinician suspect the diagnosis or begin treatment for endocarditis, but the vari-

TABLE 73-8 Definitions of Terminology Used in the Diagnostic Criteria for Endocarditis

Major Criteria

POSITIVE BLOOD CULTURE FOR INFECTIVE ENDOCARDITIS

Typical microorganism for infective endocarditis from two separate blood cultures: viridans streptococci,[a] *Strep. bovis,* HACEK group, or community-acquired *Staph. aureus* or enterococci, in the absence of a primary focus, *or*
Persistently positive blood culture, defined as recovery of a microorganism consistent with infective endocarditis from:

1. Blood cultures drawn more than 12 h apart *or*
2. All of three or a majority of four or more separate blood cultures, with first and last drawn at least 1 h apart

EVIDENCE OF ENDOCARDIAL INVOLVEMENT

Positive echocardiogram for infective endocarditis

1. Oscillating intracardiac mass, on valve or supporting structures, or in the path of regurgitant jet or on implanted material, in the absence of an alternative anatomic explanation, *or*
2. Abscess, *or*
3. New partial dehiscence of prosthetic valve, *or*
New valvular regurgitation (increase or change in preexisting murmur not sufficient)

Minor Criteria

- Predisposition: predisposing heart condition *or* intravenous drug use
- Fever: ≥38.0°C (100.4°F)
- Vascular phenomena: major arterial emboli, septic pulmonary infarcts, mycotic aneurysm, intracranial hemorrhage, conjunctival hemorrhages, Janeway lesions
- Immunologic phenomena: glomerulonephritis, Osler's nodes, Roth's spots, rheumatoid factor
- Microbiologic evidence: positive blood culture but not meeting major criterion as previously defined[b] *or* serologic evidence of active infection with oganism consistent with infective endocarditis[c]
- Echocardiogram: consistent with infective endocarditis but not meeting major criterion as previously defined

[a]Including nutritional variant strains.
[b]Excluding single positive cultures for coagulase-negative staphylococci or organisms that do not cause endocarditis.
[c]Positive serologies for *Coxiella* or *Bartonella* may be considered major criteria.[292]
HACEK = *Haemophilus* spp., *Actinobacillus actinomycetemcomitans, Cardiobacterium hominis, Eikenella* spp., and *Kingella kingae*
SOURCE: Adapted from Durack et al.,[202] with pemission.

ous diagnostic schemes might guide the clinician to make a final diagnosis, to decide on valve replacement, or to accept the diagnosis for the purpose of epidemiologic studies or clinical trials.

LABORATORY INVESTIGATIONS

Routine Laboratory Tests

Anemia usually develops during the course of SBE.[85,287] It is most often mild or moderate in degree and of the hypoproliferative type, with a normochromic, normocytic smear. Anemia occurs less often in ABE and may be due to hemolysis. Chronic low-grade hemolysis associated with a prosthetic valve may confuse interpretation of the blood picture in a patient with PVE. In addition, blood smear may show schistocytes and other red blood cell fragments. Leukocytosis is not a reliable manifestation of SBE.[85] A low-grade, variable elevation of the polymorphonuclear leukocyte count is characteristic, but in some cases the leukocyte count is normal. A high granulocyte count with an increase in band forms is commonly found in patients with ABE. These neutrophils often show toxic granulations. In a few cases of ABE, staphylococci can be identified inside neutrophils on examination of a gram-stained smear of the buffy coat of the peripheral blood.[288] In addition, abnormal histiocytes may be found in smears of peripheral blood in one-third of patients with SBE,[289] but these tests are not in routine use.

The erythrocyte sedimentation rate (ESR) is elevated in about 90 percent of cases of IE. The median ESR on admission is about 65 mm/h, but the range is wide and 10 percent are in the normal range. The median ESR may rise slightly during treatment and does not fall to normal until 3 to 6 months after diagnosis, so it is not useful as evidence of successful antibiotic therapy. The C-reactive protein is usually elevated (96 percent) and falls to normal more quickly than the ESR during successful treatment.[290] Cryoglobulins have also been reported.[291]

Urinalysis shows microscopic hematuria and/or slight proteinuria in >50 percent of cases, even in the absence of specific renal complications.[3,287] Red blood cell casts and heavy proteinuria are found in those patients who develop immune-complex glomerulonephritis, often in association with decreased total serum complement.[248] Gross hematuria suggests that renal infarction has occurred.

Serologic Tests

Nonspecific serologic abnormalities are common during the course of IE. A positive rheumatoid factor is found in >50 percent of cases of SBE,[235–237] with symptoms for longer than 6 weeks.[202] Rheumatoid factor is rarely positive in patients with ABE. A polyclonal increase in gammaglobulins is characteristic of active endocarditis. Occasional false-positive serologic test results for syphilis occur.[234]

Specific serologic tests are important for the diagnosis of IE caused by *Coxiella* (Q fever) and *Bartonella,* both species that are difficult or slow to grow from culture. In these special cases, positive serology (1:800 antiphase 1 IgG antibody titer for Q fever or positive microimmunofluorescence or PCR test for *Bartonella*) or a single positive blood culture may be added as major criteria for diagnosis of IE.[189,292]

Blood Cultures

Isolation of a typical organism or detection of persistent bacteremia constitutes the most important diagnostic test for endocarditis. Blood cultures should be drawn from all patients with undiagnosed fever and a heart murmur. Cultures should also be taken from patients with other symptoms or signs consistent with endocarditis if no other diagnosis has been made.

Bacteremia in SBE is usually continuous.[22] The number of organisms in venous blood varies widely but is usually between 1 and 200 bacteria per mL in subacute cases. Because most blood cultures in untreated patients will be positive, it is seldom necessary to draw more than 3 separate blood specimens to isolate the organism.[293] In one study, the etiologic organism was recovered from cultures taken on the first day of admission to the hospital in 93 percent of patients with culture-positive endocarditis.[294] In other studies, however, the rate of persistently positive blood cultures was lower, in the range of 62 to 68 percent.[116,202] Additional specimens obtained over a longer period may be needed to isolate the etiologic organism from patients who have received recent antibiotic therapy.

A practical approach for investigation of suspected SBE is to draw 3 separate samples of venous blood, each of 16 to 20 mL, on the first day, with at least 1 h between the first and last venipuncture. Half of each sample should be inoculated into an aerobic broth culture medium, and the other half into another broth (usually anaerobic) medium. These media should be capable of supporting growth of fastidious, nutritionally variant bacteria[139,295] and ideally should contain a resin to remove antibiotics. As soon as a culture turns positive, Gram's stain and subculture should be performed. If all 3 samples (6 bottles) are negative by the second or third day but the diagnosis of endocarditis still seems likely, two more samples of venous blood should be drawn for culture. If the patient had received previous antibiotic therapy, several further venous samples may be taken over the following weeks to identify a possible late recrudescence of bacteremia after partial treatment. For ABE, 3 venous blood samples are drawn for culture and empiric antibiotic therapy is begun at once, because in patients with acute endocarditis, treatment should not be delayed until culture results are available. In cases of *Staph. aureus* endocarditis, greater than 95 percent of blood culture would be positive, usually within 24 hours.[5]

Because *Staph.* epidermidis[251] and diphtheroids[296] can cause endocarditis, special care must be taken during venipuncture to avoid contamination of the specimen with these common skin organisms, which could result in diagnostic confusion. Since endocarditis usually produces continuous bacteremia, all cultures are usually positive; when only 1 of 3 grow a *Staph.* epidermidis or diphtheroid, contamination and not true bacteremia should be suspected! If the diagnosis of endocarditis remains likely, and cultures are negative, cultures should be incubated for 3 weeks and Gram's stains made at 5 days, 2 weeks, and 3 weeks even if no growth is apparent on inspection. The HACEK group of organisms, pyridoxyl requiring viridans streptococci, some fungi, *Bartonella,* and some others may take longer than the standard 3 to 5 days to grow.[297] A number of new seralogic and PCR-based techniques are under development and are desperately needed to clarify diagnosis in these culture-negative cases.[298–300]

Electrocardiography

Electrocardiographic studies should be performed initially and repeated at intervals according to progress during treatment. A disturbance of conduction or onset of myocardial irritability [↑ frequency of ventricular premature complexes (VPCs) or atrial premature complexes (APCs)] that develops during the course of endocarditis suggests extension of infection into the myocardium (see earlier). Such extension may be due to focal myocarditis or to an abscess located close to the conduction system.[110] Thus, development of a prolonged PR interval, if due to an abscess, can have major implications: a probable need for valve replacement and a worse prognosis.[87] Electrocardiograms can reveal evidence of silent myocardial infarction due to embolization of a vegetation to a coronary artery. Continuous electrocardiogram monitoring may be appropriate when conduction or rhythm changes are observed and disease progression is a concern.

Echocardiography

Echocardiographic studies are important in the diagnosis of IE.[301–305] Positive echocardiographic findings, properly defined, constitute an important criteria for the clinical diagnosis of endocarditis and, in the setting of positive blood cultures, essentially establishes the diagnosis of IE.[202] TTE combined with color-flow Doppler imaging (see Chap. 13) provides a wealth of information for both the diagnosis and the management of endocarditis, including the detection of vegetations, valvular perforations[306] and other abnormalities,[307] abscesses, and pericarditis, as well as the assessment of ventricular function (Fig. 73-15*A–D*).[302–304] Sensitivity for detection of vegetations, originally in the range of 33 to 63 percent, today is 50 to 75 percent.[307] Sensitivity can be improved to better than 95 percent by use of TEE (see Chap. 14) in selected cases.[270,302] Transesophageal studies also detect abscesses and valve perforation with much greater sensitivity.[304] TEE is markedly better than TTE for evaluation of prosthetic valve endocarditis, especially involving mitral valves.[308,309]

Echocardiography has some limitations.[301] It is not cost-effective as a means of excluding IE in patients with a low pretest probability of having the disease.[310,311] With higher prior probability, a negative study result has useful negative predictive value, especially if transesophageal studies have been performed, but it cannot totally exclude the diagnosis of endocarditis.[170,202,310,311] It is particularly useful in patients with *Staph. aureus* bacteremia. In one study, TTE identified vegetations in 7 of 26 patients with IE, while TEE revealed evidence of vegetations in all (100 percent).[311] These data suggest that a negative TEE allows the clinician to treat for bacteremia alone (usually antibiotic therapy for 2 weeks versus 4 to 6 weeks for IE). Sensitivity for detection of vegetations is somewhat lower on the right side (about 70 percent) than on the left (better than 95 percent).[270,301] The presence of a prosthetic valve sometimes interferes with detection of vegetations, but even in these patients echocardiographic findings are usually informative. Occasionally, the specificity of echocardiography is compromised by false-positive readings for "vegetations" that do not exist. Such readings are particularly common in patients with myxomatous degeneration of valve leaflets or other preexisting disease with focal pathology. This must be considered when surgery is contemplated.

Sequential echocardiograms performed during treatment can guide decisions on the need and timing for surgery by providing objective assessments of cardiac function. For example, premature mitral valve closure due to elevated end-diastolic pressure is a useful echocardiographic sign indicating severe aortic regurgitation, usually requiring urgent valve replacement (see Chap. 56).[270] Echocardiograms may detect development of an abscess, perforation of a valve, or rupture of an infected sinus of Valsalva,[231] all strong indications for surgical intervention. During successful antimicrobial treatment, vegetations may disappear, decrease in size, or even persist unchanged; therefore, serial echocardiograms should not be used as a "test of cure."[301] Significant enlargement of a vegetation during treatment, however, indicates possible treatment failure and constitutes a relative indication for surgical intervention. The valve of echocardiography to determine risk of embolization and/or death is controversial. A large meta-analysis concluded that the odds ratio for embolization was 2.8 ($p < 0.01$) when vegetations >10 mm were detected but did not predict death.[312] In another study of *Staph. aureus*, IE visualization of vegetation by TTE carried a higher risk of embolization or death (68 percent) than identified only by TEE (16 percent, $p < 0.01$).[313] Therefore, the value of echocardiography as a mechanism for predicting outcome remains unclear.[314,315]

Other Imaging Studies

The most important contribution of the chest x-ray in assessment of endocarditis is to provide evidence of early congestive heart failure, because this complication carries such important implications for both prognosis and management (see "Complications," earlier).

Various other x-ray findings can be helpful in assessing patients with endocarditis. The presence of multiple small, patchy infiltrates in the lungs of an IDU with fever strongly suggests the diagnosis of septic emboli arising from right-sided IE.[65–67] Valvular calcification may identify a previously abnormal valve, thus aiding the localization of presumed intravascular infection. Widening of the aorta may be caused by a mycotic aneurysm. Fluoroscopy can demonstrate abnormal motion of a prosthetic valve, indicating presence of a vegetation or partial dehiscence of the valve from the aortic root. This information often helps to decide whether or not valve replacement is needed during management of PVE.

Computed tomography (Chap. 17) and magnetic resonance imaging (Chap. 18)[274] can be helpful in defining the cause of focal neurologic lesions in patients with endocarditis, especially infarction, hemorrhage from a mycotic aneurysm, and brain abscess. The computed tomography scan is very effective for diagnosis of intracranial complications[316] and infected aortic aneurysms.[133] Magnetic resonance imaging adds additional useful information in some cases (Fig. 73-14).[317] In one study, Magnetic resonance imaging provided evidence of cerebral embolization in 12 patients with IE. Angiographic studies are usually used to demonstrate mycotic aneurysms in the brain or elsewhere.[277,278]

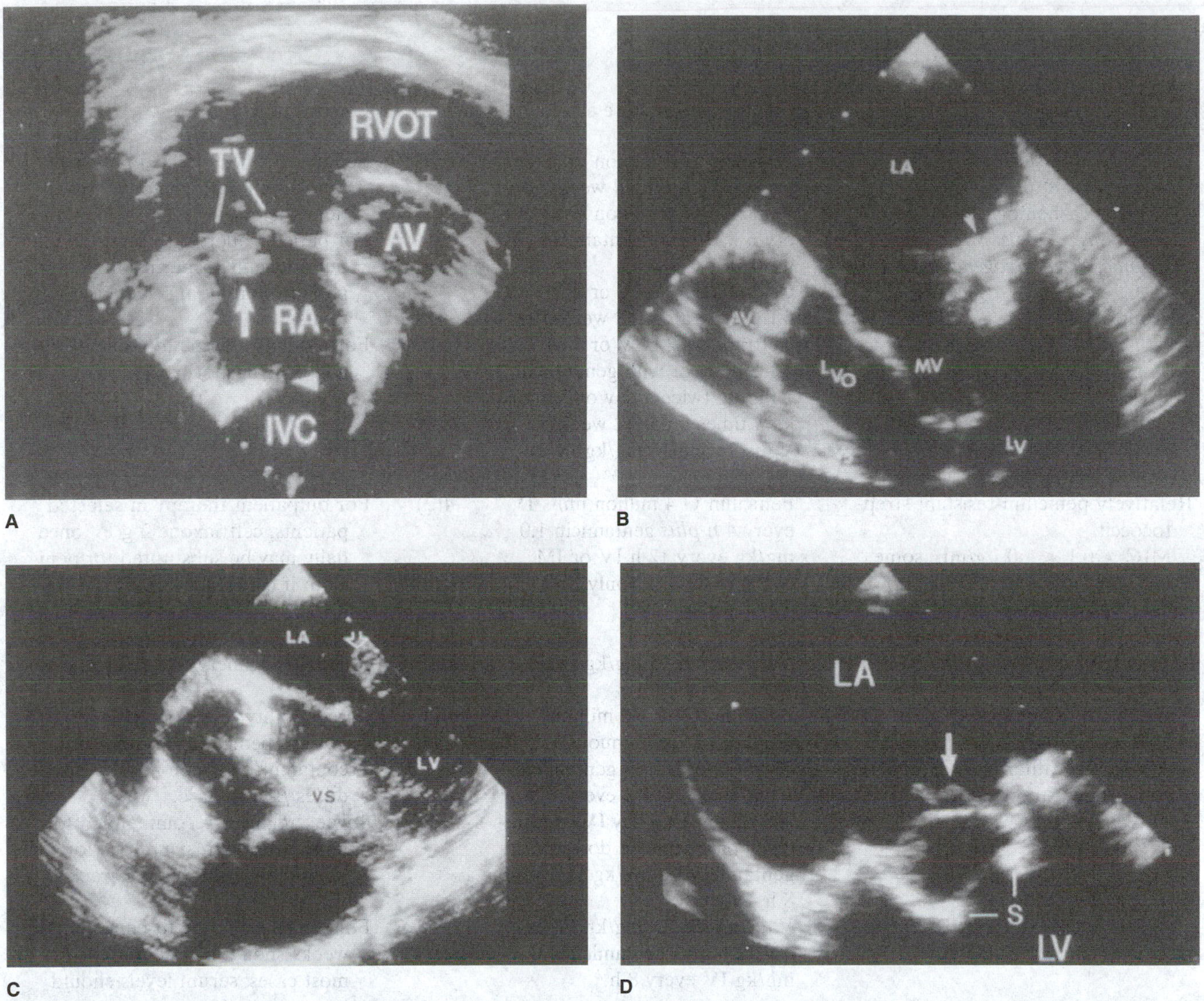

FIGURE 73-15 *A–D.* Echocardiograms from 4 patients with infective endocarditis showing vegetations located at different sites. *A.* Transesophageal echocardiogram (TEE) showing a large vegetation *(arrow)* on the tricuspid valve (TV). IVC = inferior vena cava; RA = right atrium; AV = aortic valve; RVOT = right ventricular outflow tract. *B.* Large vegetation *(arrowhead)* involving both the atrial and ventricular surfaces of the posterior mitral valve leaflet. LA = left atrium; MV = anterior leaflet of the mitral valve; LVO = left ventricular outflow tract; AV = aortic valve. *C.* TEE showing vegetations on both the mitral *(open arrow)* and aortic valve *(arrow)* in a patient with acute *Staphylococcus aureus* endocarditis. LA = left atrium; LV = left ventricle; VS = ventricular septum. *D.* TEE showing a vegetation on the cusp of a bioprosthetic valve *(arrow)*. LA = left atrium; LV = left ventricle; S = artificial valve struts. (Kindly provided by Dr. B. Khanderia and Dr. J. Steckelberg, Mayo Clinic, Rochester, Minn.)

Cardiac Catheterization with Cineangiography

This investigation is usually not necessary for patients who respond well to antimicrobial therapy without developing cardiac failure. When surgical intervention is considered, cardiac catheterization and cineangiography (Chap. 15) can extend and add to information provided by echocardiography. The condition of the coronary arteries should be assessed before valve replacement in adults over 40 years of age, because simultaneous coronary bypass may be indicated if the patient has coronary artery disease. Other relevant anatomic abnormalities such as valvular lesions, congenital defects, asymmetric septal hypertrophy, coarctation of the aorta, or mycotic aneurysm can be better defined. Occasionally, a previously unsuspected diagnosis, such as the presence of a sinus of Valsalva aneurysm, will be made. Physiologic measurements including cardiac output, pressures in the left and right sides of the heart, and the degree of aortic regurgitation may help to decide whether or not valve replacement is indicated and may influence the timing of the operation. Among 35 patients who underwent cardiac catheterization during active endocarditis, the clinical assessment was materially modified by catheterization in 23 patients, the diagnosis of the site of valve involvement was altered in 14, and in 6 valve-ring abscesses were revealed.[318] Surgery was postponed or canceled in 6 patients in whom catheterization revealed only mild hemodynamic abnormalities. There were no serious complications, indicating that catheterization should not be avoided for fear of dislodging emboli when a proper indication exists. In summary,

TABLE 73-9 Treatment Regimens for Infective Endocarditis[a,b]

Organism	Treatment Regimen: Dose and Route	Duration in Weeks	Comments
Fully penicillin-sensitive streptococci: MIC ≤ 0.1 μg/mL viridans (α-hemolytic) streptococci; *Strep. bovis; Strep. pneumoniae; Strep. pyogenes* group A, C, etc.; *Strep. agalactiae* group B	1. Penicillin G 4 million units every 6 h IV alone (4 weeks) *or*	4	Suitable for hospitalized patients but less convenient for outpatient therapy
	2. Penicillin G 4 million units every 6 h IV with gentamicin (2 weeks)	4	For patients allergic to penicillins but not cephalosporins or for outpatient therapy in selected patients
	3. Ceftriaxone 2 g IV or 1 M once daily alone (2 weeks) *or*		
	4. Ceftriaxone 2 g IV or 1 M once daily or with gentamicin 1 mg/kg twice a day or 3 mg/kg 4 times a day (2 weeks)	4	For patients allergic to penicillins and cephalosporins
	5. Vancomycin 15 mg/kg IV every 12 h (4 weeks)[a,b]		
Relatively penicillin-resistant streptococci: MIC > 0.1 < 1.0 μg/mL, some viridans (α-hemolytic) streptococci; some *Strep. pneumoniae;* etc.	1. Penicillin G 4 million units IV every 4 h *plus* gentamicin 1.0 mg/kg every 12 h IV or IM (for first 2 weeks only)[a] *or*	4(2)	For outpatient therapy in selected patients, ceftriaxone 2 g IV once daily may be substituted for penicillin if ceftriaxone MIC ≤ 4 μg/mL, *plus* gentamicin 2.0 mg/kg given once daily
	2. Vancomycin 15 mg/kg IV every 12 h[b]	4	For patients allergic to penicillins
Penicillin-resistant streptococci: MIC ≥ 1.0 μg/mL, *E. faecalis, E. faecium,* other enterococci; some other streptococci	1. Penicillin G 18–30 million units/day IV continuously or in divided doses *plus* gentamicin 1 mg/kg IV or IM every 8 h *or*	4–6	Susceptibility testing needed; do not use penicillin- or ampicillin-containing regimen if strain produces β-lactamase.
	2. Ampicillin 12 g/day IV continuously or in divided doses *plus* gentamicin 1.0 mg/kg IV every 8 h, *or*	4–6	4-week regimen recommended for most cases with symptoms for <3 months, otherwise 6 weeks
	3. Vancomycin 15 mg/kg IV every 12 h *plus* gentamicin 1.0 mg/kg IV every 8 h[a,b]	4–6	For patients allergic to penicillin; 4 weeks should be adequate for most cases; serum levels should be monitored
Staphylococci (in the absence of prosthetic material)	Methicillin-susceptible staphylococci:		
	1. Nafcillin 2 g IV every 4 h IV 4–6 wks *or*	4–6	β-lactam–containing regimens preferred over vancomycin unless patient is definitely hypersensitive to penicillins and cephalosporins; for patients with severe disseminated staphylococcal infection, antimicrobial synergy may be advantageous during early stages of treatment; therefore, gentamicin 1.0 mg/kg IV every 8 h for first 3–5 days only may be added to any of these regimens
	2. Nafcillin 2 g IV every 4 h IV × 4–6 wks plus gentamicin 1.0 mg/kg every 8 h IV × 3–5 days	4–6	
	3. Vancomycin 15 mg/kg IV every 12 h 4–6 wks[b]	4–6	
In right sided uncomplicated tricuspid endocarditis	Nafcillin 2 g IV every 4 h and gentamicin 1 mg/kg twice a day or 3 mg/kg 4 times a day	2	
	Methicillin-resistant staphylococci: Vancomycin 15 mg/kg IV every 12 h[b]	4–6	

TABLE 73-9 Treatment Regimens for Infective Endocarditis (*Continued*)

Organism	Treatment Regimen: Dose and Route	Duration in Weeks	Comments
Staphylococci (associated with prosthetic valve or other prosthetic material)	Methicillin-susceptible staphylococci: Nafcillin 2 g IV every 4 h *plus* gentamicin 1.0 mg/kg IV every 8 h[a] plus rifampin 600 mg orally 4 times a day	≥6	Cefazolin or vancomycin may be substituted for nafcillin if necessary due to drug hypersensitivity
	Methicillin-resistant staphylococci: Vancomycin 15 mg/kg IV every 12 h *plus* gentamicin 1.0 mg/kg IV or IM every 8 h *plus* rifampin 300 mg orally every 8 h[a,b]	≥6	
HACEK group organisms: *Haemophilus* species *Actinobacillus actinomycetemcomitans* *Cardiobacterium hominis* *Eikenella* species *Kingella kingae*	1. Ceftriaxone 2 g IV or IM once daily *or*	4	Other third-generation cephalosporins may be substituted, using appropriate dose adjustment
	2. Ampicillin 12 g/day IV continuously or in divided doses *plus* gentamicin 1.0 mg/kg every 12 h IV or IM[a]	4	Less convenient for outpatient therapy
Pseudomonas aeruginosa, other gram-negative bacilli	Extended-spectrum penicillin *or* third-generation cephalosporin *or* imipenem *plus* aminoglycoside	4–6	Combination therapy recommended; final choice of antibiotic regimen to be made after sensitivity results available
Neisseria species	1. Penicillin G 2 million units IV every 6 h *or*	3–4	Organisms often highly sensitive to penicillin, but must be tested for β-lactamase production; 3 weeks should be adequate for most patients without complications
	2. Ceftriaxone 1 g IV or IM once daily	3–4	

[a]All gentamicin- and vancomycin-containing regimens require monitoring for potential toxicity; monitoring of serum concentrations usually will be required.
[b]Vancomycin dose not to exceed 2.0 g per 24 h.
SOURCE: Adapted from Scheld and Sande[50] and from Wilson et al., and The Sanford Guide 2000.[323]

cardiac catheterization and cineangiography should be performed in most adults with IE who are over 40 years of age and in selected younger patients when surgery is considered.

Radionuclide Imaging

Liver-spleen imaging may reveal defects due to splenic infarction, which confirms embolization. In animals, experimental vegetations have been located by scanning for radiolabeled platelets deposited from the bloodstream onto a growing endocardial lesion.[319] Gallium 67 scans have shown increased uptake in the heart in some patients with endocarditis. Scintigraphic studies following injection of indium 111 labeled leukocytes have detected some intracardiac abscesses,[77,320] but no radionuclide imaging technique has sufficient sensitivity and specificity to justify routine use for detection of vegetations in IE. In selected cases, leukocyte scintigraphy using indium 111 labeled leukocytes can detect mycotic aneurysms and extracardiac foci of infection.[321] Single photon emission computed tomography immunoscintigraphy with antigranulocyte antibody has been described as a nuclear medicine option for diagnosis of IE.

TREATMENT

General Principles

Optimal management aims to eradicate the infecting organism as soon as possible, to operate with correct timing if surgical intervention should be required, and to treat complications. Because IE carries a significant risk of death even when well managed, it is important that treatment be continued long enough to ensure that relapse will not occur. In contrast, patients with the more easily cured forms of endocarditis should not be subjected to unnecessarily long, expensive, and potentially toxic treatment in a hospital.[322] This can happen when physicians treat on the basis of outdated rules, such as the one stating that "endocarditis should be treated for 6 weeks." In fact, many patients can be cured in 2[323–325] or 4 weeks,[326] while some require treatment for 6 weeks or longer.

Microbiologic Tests

To choose and regulate antibiotic therapy correctly, certain basic microbiologic information about the infecting organism is required. For group A streptococcal infection, nothing more than positive identification of the organism is necessary, because these organisms, with only rare exceptions, are still sensitive to low concentrations of penicillin. For other species of streptococci, staphylococci, and most other bacteria, the minimal inhibitory concentration (MIC) of relevant antibiotics should be determined. Some of these organisms are resistant to intermediate or high concentrations of penicillin.[327,328] Many strains are tolerant—that is, inhibited but not killed by antibiotic levels achievable in serum.[329,330] Because there is no definitive evidence that tolerance determines treatment outcome in humans, however, it is not necessary to measure minimal bactericidal concentrations (MBC) in most cases.

The serum bactericidal titer (SBT or Schlichter test) has been used frequently to monitor the treatment of endocarditis.[33,331] In this test, the infecting organism is exposed in vitro to the patient's serum, which is drawn while the patient is receiving antibiotic treatment to determine the maximal dilution of serum that will inhibit and kill the organism. On the basis of empirical clinical experience, it was said that the SBT should be 1:8 or higher at intervals during each day of treatment. For streptococcal endocarditis, this can usually be achieved without difficulty; SBTs are often high, in the range of 1:128 to 1:1024. The SBT is technically difficult to perform and to standardize, however, and after years of use, its clinical utility remains unproven.[331,332] Therefore, SBTs are now regarded as obsolete by most experts. Rarely, measurement of the SBT might be informative: in treating unusual organisms, in using unusual antibiotics, in using unusual regimens (such as oral treatment), or when treatment appears to be failing.

Dosage regimens that result in widely fluctuating antibiotic concentrations in serum are traditionally employed for treatment of endocarditis, and they are usually effective. Whether or not the maintenance of continuous serum antibiotic concentrations offers any therapeutic benefit over intermittent dosing regimens is not known; perhaps continuous infusion of antibiotic would be desirable for treatment of some gram-negative organisms, which regrow more rapidly than most gram-positive organisms when antibiotic levels fall below the minimal inhibitory concentration.

Choice of Antibiotics

Bactericidal antibiotics are generally chosen for treatment of endocarditis whenever possible.[33,326] This is not an absolute rule; some patients have been cured with bacteriostatic drugs such as sulfonamides, tetracycline, or chloramphenicol, but the results of treatment with these agents are unreliable.[28,333,334] Bactericidal action is presumably needed because host defense mechanisms are inadequate in the vegetation; relatively few phagocytes are present, and they are hampered by protective layers of fibrin around the colonies of bacteria (Figs. 73-2 and 73-6). To effect a cure, antibiotic therapy must eradicate organisms completely, without the help of phagocytes to eliminate the subpopulation of microbes that are relatively resistant to antibiotics because they are in the resting phase. In this important respect, IE differs strikingly from bacterial pneumonia in normal hosts, where phagocytes are plentiful and bacteriostatic antibiotics are usually effective. Nevertheless, in treating unusual organisms, it may occasionally be necessary to use a bacteriostatic antibiotic in combination with other drugs to achieve the optimal antibacterial effect. When treatment with unusual combinations of antibiotics is needed, in vitro laboratory tests can be performed to find out whether synergism, indifference, or antagonism exists between them.

For the common forms of bacterial endocarditis caused by gram-positive organisms, specific therapeutic regimens can be recommended with confidence based on extensive published experience.[323,335] Regimens for the more common forms of endocarditis are listed in Table 73-9.

Currently, increasing rates of antibiotic resistance threaten the efficacy of traditional treatment regimens. Penicillin resistance is increasing among viridans streptococci, the majority of which had previously been fully sensitive.[336,337] In 1996, 13 percent of blood culture isolates showed high-level resistance (MIC 4.0 mg/mL or greater) and 42 percent showed intermediate resistance (MIC 0.25 to 2.0 mg/mL).[337] Use of combined antibiotic regimens such as beta-lactam plus aminoglycoside or even vancomycin plus aminoglycoside should be considered for treatment of resistant strains.[336] Synergistic combinations of a beta-lactam and an aminoglycoside have been used successfully to treat enterococci for many years, but increasing resistance among enterococci, especially vancomycin-resistant enterococci, presents new problems for therapy.[338] The most resistant species is *Enterococcus faecium,* which may exhibit high-level resistance to vancomycin as well as intrinsic resistance to beta-lactam antibiotics and imipenem.[94] The optimal treatment for IE caused by these problem strains is not known. Several antibiotic combinations have been tried with some success often with adjunctive surgical valve replacement. These include high-dose ampicillin plus imipenem +/− a fluoroquinolone,[94,339] ampicillin plus imipenem plus vancomycin,[340] ampicillin plus a fluoroquinolone,[341] and quinupristin/dalfopristin plus doxycycline plus rifampin.[342] Since great variability exists between isolates as to sensitivity and whether drugs are cidal or static, in vitro testing with time-kill experiments and testing various drugs alone and in combination will help with selection. An infectious disease consultation is recommended.[94,339–344]

Staph. epidermidis PVE is difficult to eradicate with antibiotics alone.[166] These staphylococci are frequently resistant to semisynthetic penicillins, cephalosporins, and other antibiotics. A regimen combining vancomycin, rifampin, and an aminoglycoside chosen according to sensitivity tests is most likely to succeed. The organism may develop resistance to rifampin during treatment.

Treatment of endocarditis due to less common organisms must be chosen on the basis of more limited published experience,[50,51,108,326] together with the results of tests performed upon the infecting organism in the microbiology laboratory. Treatment must often be individualized. In general, one of the beta-lactam antibiotics should be included in the regimen whenever possible. Combinations of two or more antibiotics are often employed. The list of potentially useful regimens for these rarer forms of infective endocarditis is too long to detail here.

Empiric Therapy

When the etiologic organism is not known, the choice of empiric therapy should depend on whether the patient has acute or subacute disease. ABE requires broad-spectrum therapy that covers *Staph. aureus* as well as many species of streptococci and gram-negative bacilli. SBE requires a regimen that treats most streptococci, including *E. faecalis.* To meet these requirements, the following suggestions are offered:

- For ABE: nafcillin 2.0 g IV q 4 h plus ampicillin 2.0 g IV q 4 h plus gentamicin 1.5 mg/kg IV q 8 h. If methicillin-resistant *Staph. aureus* is considered likely (for example, in a hospital-acquired case), vancomycin 1.0 g IV q 12 h should be substituted for nafcillin in this regimen until the antibiotic sensitivity is known.
- For SBE: ampicillin 2.0 g IV q 4 h plus gentamicin 1.5 mg/kg IV q 8 h.

Treatment should be adjusted as appropriate when the etiologic organism is identified and again when antibiotic sensitivity is known. In those few cases where empiric therapy is administered as a therapeutic trial to help confirm a diagnosis, treatment should be continued without interruption or unnecessary changes for at least 2 weeks; otherwise, no useful diagnostic information will be gained.

Duration of Therapy

Extensive experience with treatment of the common forms of endocarditis provides the basis for recommendations on duration of therapy (Table 73-9). In the case of *Staph. aureus* endocarditis, the response to appropriate treatment can be variable; some patients recover swiftly without complications, especially young IDUs, who can often be cured within 2 weeks.[70,324] In contrast, some patients remain febrile for 10 to 14 days due to complications such as abscesses or other extracardiac manifestations of disseminated staphylococcal disease. Although 4 weeks of therapy is adequate in most cases, this should not be regarded as a rigid rule, because some patients with *Staph. aureus* endocarditis require treatment for 6 weeks or longer to achieve a cure. For *E. faecalis* endocarditis, 4 weeks of treatment is usually adequate. The relapse rate, however, seems to be higher in patients with mitral valve infection and in those who have had symptoms for more than 3 months,[143] where treatment should continue for 6 weeks.

Parenteral treatment can be completed in the patient's home or in the outpatient clinic in carefully selected cases. Availability of antibiotics with long half-lives, such as vancomycin or ceftriaxone, allows once-daily administration. Supervised parenteral treatment outside the hospital should be fully effective in achieving a microbiologic cure and offers obvious benefits: convenience for the patient and cost containment.[344–346] The risks posed by a possible late complication, such as an embolic stroke or the sudden onset of heart failure, must be balanced against these benefits in selecting candidates for home parenteral therapy. Further trials are needed to refine the criteria and proper applications for outpatient therapy for endocarditis, but current experience indicates that more than one-half of endocarditis patients could receive at least some of their treatment as outpatients.

In general, the less extensive the published experience with a particular organism and treatment regimen, the more one should lean toward prolonging treatment in order to provide a reasonable margin of safety. Guidelines for the duration of treatment of the more common etiologic organisms are listed in Table 73-9. For less common organisms, the optimal duration of treatment required may vary according to individual circumstances.

Role of Surgery

Optimal management of IE requires operative intervention during treatment for about one-third of patients.[87,347] Correct selection of this subgroup of patients and optimal timing of surgery are both critically important.[348]

Major indications for surgery are moderate or severe heart failure not responding to medical treatment, valvular obstruction, periannular or myocardial abscess, prosthetic valve dehiscence, persistent bacteremia despite appropriate antibiotics, and fungal infection. In most such cases, surgery should proceed promptly even if the infection is still active.

Relative indications for surgery include recurrent emboli; staphylococcal and gram-negative bacillary infections, especially involving prosthetic valves; persistent fever despite treatment; and vegetations that enlarge during treatment.[11,110,266,348]

Correct timing is the essence of good surgical management of endocarditis.[347] If surgery is undertaken too soon, the risks of operative mortality and the early and late morbidity associated with valve replacement may be inflicted on the patient unnecessarily, because some patients respond well to medical therapy, allowing surgery to be postponed indefinitely. If surgery can be delayed safely, antibiotic therapy should have eradicated or at least greatly reduced the number of organisms in the vegetation and in any sites of metastatic infection, thus increasing the chance of a successful outcome if surgery becomes necessary. If time is available for the effective treatment of complications such as septicemia, renal failure, pneumonia, myocarditis, and neurologic complications[316] before surgery, the operative risk should be lower. In comparison, if surgery is delayed too long, patients may die suddenly, or their hemodynamic status may deteriorate so seriously that surgery is no longer feasible. This would be a tragic error, because many authors have emphasized that both survival and long-term outcome can be improved by earlier operation for selected patients, even if the endocardial infection is still active.[266,349,350]

Careful, frequent reexamination of the patient, together with repeated echocardiographic studies and sometimes cardiac catheterization to confirm the clinical findings, is indicated in every case where operation might be needed. The decision to operate should also be influenced by knowledge of the natural history of the type of endocarditis being treated. For example, penicillin-sensitive streptococcal endocarditis can almost always be cured bacteriologically (Table 73-10), and the immediate prognosis is good provided that cardiac failure or other major complications do not develop. Therefore, surgery should usually be considered only for those patients with cardiac failure that does not respond well to medical treatment. Similarly, because young IDUs with acute staphylococcal endocarditis have a good prognosis,[5,324] surgery should usually be reserved for those who develop intrac-

TABLE 73-10 Estimate of Microbiologic Cure Rates for Various Forms of Endocarditis[a]

Native Valve Endocarditis	Antimicrobial Therapy Alone		Antimicrobial Therapy Plus Surgery	
Viridans streptococci, group A streptococci, *Strep. bovis,* pneumococci, gonococci	98		98	
Enterococcus faecalis	90		>90	
Staph. aureus (in young intravenous drug users)	90		>90	
Staph. aureus (in elderly patients with chronic underlying diseases)	50		70	
Gram-negative aerobic bacilli[b]	40		65	
Fungi	<5		50	
Prosthetic Valve Endocarditis	**Early PVE**	**Late PVE**	**Early PVE**	**Late PVE**
Viridans streptococci, group A streptococci, *Strep. bovis,* pneumococci, gonococci	*c*	80	*c*	90
Enterococcus faecalis	*c*	60	*c*	75
Staph. aureus	25	40	50	60
Staph. epidermidis	20	40	60	70
Gram-negative aerobic bacilli[b]	<10	20	40	50
Fungi	<1	<1	30	40

[a]Morbidity and mortality are significantly greater than these figures for microbiologic cure indicate.
[b]Excluding HACEK species.
[c]Insufficient data to estimate rates.
SOURCE: Adapted from Refs. 9, 11, 32, 33, 110, 116, 259, 323, 324, 350, 365.

table heart failure or definite signs of treatment failure. In contrast, the likelihood that fungal prosthetic valve endocarditis can be eradicated with antifungal drugs alone is negligible (Table 73-10). Such patients should usually undergo valve debridement or replacement early, without waiting to test the remote possibility that antifungal treatment could eradicate the infection.[351] The development of severe aortic regurgitation, especially when accompanied by heart failure, usually requires urgent surgery. Other examples of patients who are highly likely to require operation are those with early-onset PVE, valve-ring abscesses, or gram-negative bacillary infection of prosthetic valves.[11]

Over the past decade, surgical approaches have evolved toward increasingly radical debridement of infected tissue and more extensive use of reconstructive materials.[266,351] For example, an aortic root homograft instead of a standard prosthetic valve is now often inserted after debridement of a valve-ring abscess.[352] The Ross operation, transposing the patient's own pulmonary valve into the aortic position as an autograft after extensive debridement of infected tissue (replacing the pulmonary valve with a homograft) has been advocated as treatment for patients with complicated aortic root infections.[353,354]

In addition to valve replacement, several other surgical procedures may be available for the treatment of endocarditis.[348] Debridement of vegetations ("vegetectomy"), often combined with valvuloplasty, can cure the infection while sparing the native valve in selected patients.[267,268,355] This can be especially beneficial for young patients, women who wish to bear children, and patients who cannot or will not take anticoagulant therapy reliably.

Early consultation with the surgical service should be sought for most patients with endocarditis, so that an appropriate operation can be performed without delay if necessary. The sudden onset of aortic or mitral regurgitation with consequent acute left ventricular failure can occur without warning, even in the most favorable forms of endocarditis.

Anticoagulant Therapy

Even though the infected vegetation is essentially a thrombotic lesion, there is no evidence that anticoagulation has any useful therapeutic effect on the course of the endocarditis itself. On the contrary, early experience showed that simultaneous treatment with penicillin and heparin carried an increased risk of fatal intracerebral hemorrhage.[356] For this reason, anticoagulation was considered to be strongly contraindicated in patients with endocarditis, until further experience showed that warfarin could usually be given safely during the treatment of patients with prosthetic valve infections.[357–359] However in a series of 21 pH with PVE caused by *Staph. aureus,* 12 had CVS events including 6 intracranial hemorrhages and 5 ischemic strokes that had hemorrhagic transformation. All 11 died, and all had been on oral anticoagulants.[359] Currently available information suggests the following guidelines for patients with IE:

- Avoid use of heparin except for urgent indications, such as treatment of massive pulmonary embolism.
- Discontinue or avoid oral anticoagulants if possible, especially in patients with intracranial complications and if *Staph. aureus* is the cause of IE.
- Anticoagulate with warfarin if there is a clear-cut indication, such as a mechanical prosthetic heart valve, taking care to regulate the prothrombin time between International Normalized Ratio (INR) 2.5 and 3.5.

- Choose an antibiotic treatment regimen that does not require intramuscular injections if anticoagulation is instituted.

Thrombolytic agents theoretically could promote lysis or resolution of vegetations. Adjunctive treatment with recombinant tissue plasminogen activator decreased vegetation size and improved the results of short-term penicillin therapy in rabbits with fresh vegetations.[12] Similarly, aspirin therapy can reduce the size of experimental vegetations and improve rate of sterilization by antibiotics.[360] The potential value of antithrombotic agents, however, has not been demonstrated in human beings; thrombolytic therapy might not work on the older vegetations typical of SBE in human beings and could possibly cause serious hemorrhagic complications.

Management of Complications

HEART FAILURE

The development of moderate or severe cardiac failure due to structural valvular damage indicates the need for **prompt surgical intervention** in most patients with endocarditis, even if the intracardiac infection is still active.[347,349] In patients with mild heart failure, the decision should be individualized, always remembering that lives may be lost unnecessarily if cardiac function suddenly worsens, so that surgery becomes either hazardous or unfeasible.

EMBOLI

The occurrence of one or more significant arterial emboli during the treatment of endocarditis is a relative indication for surgery. The predictable early and long-term mortality and morbidity rates of valve replacement must be weighed against the highly unpredictable likelihood of further emboli. For this reason, embolization is a weaker indication for valve replacement than is cardiac failure.[348,349] In the author's opinion, operative intervention during antibiotic treatment should seldom be undertaken solely to prevent further emboli unless the patient has suffered more than one or two proved major emboli. Because the frequency of emboli falls rapidly after 1 to 2 weeks of antibiotic therapy,[361] the most logical time to operate for the purpose of preventing emboli would be early, within 1 week of diagnosis.

RENAL FAILURE

In the preantibiotic era, patients with SBE frequently developed chronic renal failure before they died.[3] Subsequently, both the incidence of renal failure and its importance as a cause of death have greatly diminished. In one series, up to one-third of 204 patients with IE developed evidence of acute renal failure, however. Risk factors for renal failure were increased age, hypertension, thrombocytopenia, IE caused by *Staph. aureus,* and PVE. While the earlier diagnosis and antibiotic treatment have forestalled the development of immune-complex glomerulonephritis, in those (about 5 to 10 percent) who still develop this complication of SBE, timely dialysis can maintain the patient until antibiotic treatment results in disappearance of the bacterial antigens that triggered immune-complex nephritis. Renal function usually normalizes smoothly once infection has been controlled, but recovery may take weeks or months. In a few cases, creatinine clearance worsens for a time despite effective antibacterial treatment, perhaps reflecting persistence of bacterial antigen in vegetations after bacteriologic cure. Corticosteroids may have been of value in a small number of cases.[362] Some patients with septicemia, shock, or disseminated intravascular coagulation associated with ABE develop acute renal failure and require dialysis as part of their intensive care.

MYCOTIC ANEURYSM

This complication is diagnosed in less than 5 percent of patients with IE, but the local consequences of aneurysm expansion and rupture can be very serious, especially in the brain (see Chap. 89).[276,278,279] Small aneurysms will often thrombose or resolve spontaneously during or after antibiotic therapy. Once aneurysms exceed 0.5 to 2 cm in diameter, they are likely to enlarge and eventually rupture despite eradication of the etiologic bacteria by antibiotic therapy.[281] Surgery is indicated for accessible aneurysms before this complication occurs.

Intracranial mycotic aneurysms are especially difficult to manage. They may present with headaches, subarachnoid hemorrhage, or stroke, but many are asymptomatic. Even small aneurysms may bleed at any time; they may be multiple and/or located in inaccessible sites. This presents a therapeutic dilemma: whether to treat conservatively with antibiotics and hope for resolution (risking serious or fatal hemorrhage) or to operate (risking neurologic damage and permanent sequelae). Symptoms or signs consistent with an intracranial aneurysm indicate the need for prompt imaging, using computed tomography and/or magnetic resonance imaging. Cerebral angiography may be needed if the findings are inconclusive. In general, large (over 0.5 cm in diameter) or expanding aneurysms or aneurysms that have already leaked or begun to bleed should be clipped if a surgical approach is feasible. An individualized decision must be made on whether or not to operate for smaller aneurysms that have not leaked or ruptured.

PROGNOSIS

IE is one of the few infectious diseases that are virtually always fatal if untreated. Spontaneous recovery was reported occasionally in the preantibiotic era,[3] but most of these patients probably had illnesses other than IE. The interval between the onset of symptoms and death in patients with untreated subacute disease varied widely, with a median time to death of about 6 months.[3] Almost all patients with acute IE died within less than 4 weeks.

Heart failure is the leading adverse prognostic factor.[264] Other adverse factors include central nervous system complications, renal failure, culture-negative disease, gram-negative bacillary or fungal infection, prosthetic valve infection, and development of abscesses in the valve ring or myocardium.[363] Survival 6 months after PVE in one series was only 54 percent.[364] Six-month survival after early-onset PVE (37 percent) was significantly worse than it was for late-onset PVE (65 percent). Because modern treatment methods, including valve replacement, are effective for treatment of heart failure, central nervous system complications have replaced heart failure as the most important adverse prognostic factor in some case studies.[274]

Favorable prognostic factors include youth, early diagnosis and treatment, infection involving a prolapsing mitral valve, and penicillin-sensitive streptococcal infection. The prognosis is good for young IDUs with *Staph. aureus* infection of the tricuspid valve.[5,335] With earlier diagnosis and appropriate therapy, including surgery, the prognosis for elderly patients can be substantially improved.[90] Eradication of the etiologic organisms (microbiological cure) can be achieved in a high proportion of all patients with bacterial endocarditis.[6,323,344,345] Both early and long-term mortality rates remain significant, however, due to any preexisting disease and added damage caused by endocarditis before the organisms were eradicated. Survival curves after admission with IE show a significant number of late deaths despite microbiologic cure.[9,365]

An analysis of experience over the past 25 years permits a reasonably accurate formulation of the prognosis for microbiologic cure among the various subgroups of patients with IE. Approximate figures are listed in Table 73-10.

RECURRENT ENDOCARDITIS

Recurrent endocarditis is a general term that includes both relapses and reinfections. The term *relapse* refers to recurrence of infection with the same organism because treatment failed. The frequency of relapse can be predicted from published experience for each of the various forms of IE (Table 73-10). Because relapses occasionally occur even after an optimal treatment regimen has been used, follow-up clinical evaluation should be meticulously performed during the first 2 months after treatment. Any clinical suspicion that relapse might have occurred indicates the need to draw blood cultures. Most relapses occur within a few weeks of ending treatment, but living organisms can persist in seemingly healed vegetations for many months and may occasionally cause late relapse.

The term *reinfection* refers to a new episode of endocarditis occurring after the cure of a previous episode.[366] Usually a different etiologic organism is involved, but if the new isolate appears similar to the initial etiologic organism, molecular typing techniques can be used to determine if the case is a relapse or an infection.

Patients remain permanently at risk of reinfection after cure of IE because of residual valve damage superimposed on the original predisposing lesion (see Tables 73-1 and 73-2). Recurrent episodes are fairly common, being recorded in from 2 to 31 percent of cases.[3,46,48,365,366] This wide variation in reported incidence is partly due to variable duration of follow-up. IDUs and patients with severe periodontitis are at highest risk for reinfection. Occasionally, a patient may suffer three or more separate episodes of IE.[366] Patients who have previously had NVE and have required valve replacement, are at high risk to develop prosthetic valve infection (often with a different organism) for reasons that are not yet understood.[9]

THE CHALLENGE OF PROPHYLAXIS

Because various invasive procedures induce bacteremias with bacterial species that often cause IE,[367–369] prophylactic antibiotics are frequently given to susceptible patients in an attempt to prevent bacterial endocarditis. Although antibiotics definitely can prevent endocarditis in experimental animals, its effectiveness in human beings has not been proved in prospective randomized clinical trials and likely never will be. Many relevant questions remain unanswered. These include the following:

- Is antibiotic prophylaxis effective?
- Does the prophylactic effect (benefit) outweigh the potential side effect of the drug cost and influence the emergence of drug-resistant bacteria?
- Which operations and diagnostic procedures should be covered?
- Which patients should receive antibiotics?
- What antibiotic regimens will be most effective?

Although the risk of infection has not been quantitated, it is sufficiently low that most of these questions cannot be answered by clinical trials; the number of susceptible patients required to provide significant results would be too large.[55,349]

Less than 15 percent of SBE cases and even fewer of ABE cases follow identifiable medical procedures that cause transient bacteremias[54,367,368,370]; therefore, the proportion of cases that is potentially preventable by antibiotics is vanishingly small.

Because endocarditis causes serious morbidity and mortality, the American Heart Association and the practicing medical community have accepted the practice of using antibiotic prophylaxis without evidence-based studies. It has been accepted that prevention of even a few cases could be worthwhile. For this reason, currently accepted standards of practice require that an antibiotic regimen be administered before certain dental and surgical procedures in patients with known heart lesions that pose a significant risk of endocarditis.

Because several hundred cases of streptococcal endocarditis following dental and genitourinary tract procedures have been recorded, the potential causative role of these procedures is certainly suggested.[367,368] A rather short "incubation period" for endocarditis is typical, in that most of these patients noticed symptoms within 2 weeks of the procedure.[256] It should be emphasized that the link between a case of endocarditis and a recent procedure causing bacteremia cannot be proved, because the infection could have been caused by one of the transient, asymptomatic, low-grade bacteremias that occur very commonly, induced by everyday events such as chewing and cleaning the teeth. In fact, when 273 cases of endocarditis are examined retrospect from 1, 2, and 3 months prior to endocarditis, no correlation to dental procedures were found.[56,367]

In the absence of prospective controlled trials, empirical recommendations[55,370,371] for prophylaxis of bacterial endocarditis have been made on the basis of indirect information. This information includes the reported frequency of bacteremia after various procedures (Table 73-11); the relative risk posed by the patient's cardiac lesion (Table 73-2); case reports of prophylaxis failures[75]; in vitro susceptibility studies on the relevant organisms, especially streptococci; experimental studies in laboratory animals[254,372]; and retrospective studies in human beings.[373–375]

Information from these sources indicates that experimental endocarditis in animals can be prevented by bactericidal antibiotics; that prevention is probably effective in human beings; that only a small proportion of total cases is potentially preventable by use of antibiotics[370,374]; and that the cost per prevented case would be very high.[76,374] Thus, prevention probably would not be cost-effective as a general strategy, but it might be effective for selected individuals (namely patients with previous IE and patients with prosthetic valves), especially for high-risk procedures such as tooth extractions.[370,376]

For the individual patient, the decision to administer prophylaxis should be made by assessing two main factors: the risk posed by the preexisting cardiac lesion and the risk posed by the procedure that might cause bacteremia. For example, if a patient with a prosthetic valve undergoes prostate resection, antibiotic prophylaxis is recommended because both factors present a significant risk of endocarditis. In contrast, if a patient with mitral valve prolapse is scheduled for gastroscopy, prophylaxis is not necessary because the risk for endocarditis in this setting is very low.[369] Such risk assessments may be difficult or inaccurate; in many situations uncertainties will remain. For these, there is no one "correct" answer; the patient's and the physician's attitudes and preferences may influence the decision to use prophylaxis. Updated consensus recommendations by the AHA may be useful in guiding decision making.[79]

These guidelines emphasize the following points:

1. Most cases are not attributable to an invasive procedure.
2. Cardiac conditions should be stratified into light, moderate, and negligible risk categories; these are primarily based on potential outcomes if endocarditis occurs.
3. There are procedures that may cause high grade bacteremia and for which prophylaxis is most likely to be effective.
4. There is an algorithm to use in deciding on prophylaxis in patients with mitral valve prolapse.
5. The initial dose of amoxicillin is reduced to 2 g for oral and dental procedures and a follow-up dose is no longer recommended; clindamycin (not erythromycin) is recommended as an alternative therapy in penicillin-allergic individuals.
6. Prophylactic recommendations in gastrointestinal and genitourinary procedures have been simplified.[79]

Attempted prophylaxis does not always succeed. Of 52 cases of apparent prophylaxis failure in one series, 42 involved patients with heart disease who received oral penicillin or erythromycin, usually to cover dental procedures.[75]

Surprisingly, in one series 12 of 16 patients with known cardiac abnormalities who developed IE with organisms of dental origin and who had a dental procedure within 3 months of onset of IE received prophylactic antibiotics according to AHA guidelines. In fact, only 10 percent of cases of IE in this study would qualify for prophylaxis according to the AHA standards. Even if a prophylaxis was 100 percent effective, it would reduce the incidence of IE by only 2.0 cases per 1,000,000 person-years.

The authors agree with Durack, that on the basis of existing data, it is most reasonable to use prophylaxis prior to dental extractions or gingival surgery including implant placement but not routine dental care, filling of cavities, root canal, cleaning and scaling of teeth, in patients with prosthetic valves or history of prior endocarditis. If any of the four conditions are present, antibiotic prophylaxis seems reasonable.[56]

Common errors in attempted prevention of endocarditis are starting antibiotics too early, continuing for too long, using low doses, covering tooth extractions but not lesser dental procedures, and confusing prevention of rheumatic fever (requiring long-term, low-dose antimicrobial drugs) with prevention of endocarditis (short-term, high-dose).[55]

TABLE 73-11 Representative Rates for Frequency of Bacteremia after Various Dental, Diagnostic, and Therapeutic Procedures

Procedure	% Bacteremia	% Range (if available)
None	0	(0–3)
Oral cavity		
Extraction of teeth	60	(18–85)
Periodontal surgery	88	(60–90)
Brushing teeth or irrigation	40	(7–50)
Tonsillectomy	35	(33–38)
Respiratory tract		
Tracheal intubation	<10	(0–16)
Nasotracheal suctioning	16	
Bronchoscopy (rigid bronchoscope)	15	
Bronchoscopy (flexible bronchoscope)	0	
Genitourinary tract		
Catheter insertion and removal	3	(0–26)
Prostatectomy (sterile urine)	12	(11–13)
Prostatectomy (infected urine)	60	(58–82)
Dilatation of strictures	28	(19–86)
Normal delivery	3	(1–5)
Intrauterine device insertion or removal	0	
Gastrointestinal tract		
Upper gastrointestinal endoscopy	4	(0–8)
Transesophageal echocardiography	1	(0–17)
Endoscopic retrograde cholangiopancreatography	5	(0–6)
Barium enema	10	(5–11)
Colonoscopy	5	(0–5)
Sigmoidoscopy (rigid sigmoidoscope)	5	
Sigmoidoscopy (flexible sigmoidoscope)	0	
Proctoscopy	2	
Hemorrhoidectomy	8	
Esophageal dilatation	45	
Vascular system		
Cardiac catheterization	2	(0–5)
Insufficient data		
Insertion and removal of tympanostomy tubes		
Cesarean section		

SOURCE: From Durack,[370] with permission.

TABLE 73-12 Suggested Regimens for Prophylaxis of Infective Endocarditis[a]

Standard Regimen	
For dental procedures and oral or upper respiratory tract surgery	Amoxicillin 2.0 g orally 1 h before procedure[b]
Special Regimens	
Parenteral regimen for high-risk patients; also for gastrointestinal (GI) or genitourinary (GU) tract procedures	Ampicillin 2.0 g IM or IV *plus* gentamicin 1.5 mg/kg IM or IV, 0.5 h before procedure,[b] 6 h later, ampicillin 1 g IM or IV or amoxicillin 1 g orally
Parenteral regimen for penicillin-allergic patients	Vancomycin 1.0 g IV *slowly* over 1–2 h; *plus* gentamicin 1.5 mg/kg IM or IV[b]; complete within 30 min of starting the procedure
Oral regimen for penicillin-allergic patients (oral and respiratory tract only)	Clindamycin 600 mg orally 1 h before procedure[b]
Oral regimen for minor GI or GU tract procedures	Amoxicillin 2.0 g orally 1 h before procedure[b]
Parenteral regimen for cardiac surgery including valve replacement	Cefazolin 2.0 g IV on induction of anesthesia, repeated 8 and 16 h later[c] *or*
	Vancomycin 1.0 g IV *slowly* over 1 h starting on induction of anesthesia, then 0.5 g IV 8 and 16 h later[c]

[a]Note that (1) these regimens are empiric suggestions, no regimen has been proved effective for prevention of endocarditis, and prevention failures may occur with any regimen; (2) these regimens are not intended to cover all clinical situations, and the practitioner should use his or her own judgment on safety and cost-benefit issues in each individual case; (3) one or two additional doses may be given if the period of risk for bacteremia is prolonged.

[b]Pediatric dosages: ampicillin 50 mg/kg; gentamicin 1.5 mg/kg; amoxicillin: for children who weigh more than 60 lb, use same as for adults; for children less than 60 lb, use one-half the adult dose; vancomycin 20 mg/kg; clindamycin 20 mg/kg; cefazolin 30 mg/kg. Do not exceed 2.0 g ampicillin, 120 mg gentamycin.

[c]Vancomycin is preferred if *Staph. epidermidis* is an important cause of postoperative infection in that hospital. Gentamicin 1.5 mg/kg IV or IM may be added to each dose, only if postoperative gram-negative infections have occurred with significant frequency.

SOURCE: Durack DT. Nine controversies in the management of infective endocarditis. In: Petersdorf RG, et al., eds. *Update V: Harrison's Principles of Internal Medicine*. New York: McGraw-Hill; 1984:35; and Dajani, et al. (*JAMA* 1997; 277:1794–1801).[371] Adapted and reproduced with permission of the publisher and author.

In the absence of pelvic infection, prophylaxis for endocarditis in patients with heart lesions is not recommended to cover normal delivery, therapeutic abortion, dilation and curettage, and insertion or removal of intrauterine contraceptive devices. Similarly, antibiotics are not recommended before many common procedures, such as cardiac catheterization, insertion of temporary pacemakers, endotracheal intubation, bronchoscopy, endoscopy, or radiographic contrast studies of the upper and lower gastrointestinal tract. In comparison, some physicians choose to cover even these low-risk procedures in patients with prosthetic valves because they are at higher risk for endocarditis than are patients with native valves. Specific regimens suggested for prophylaxis of endocarditis are listed in Table 73-12.

Cardiac surgeons currently administer antibiotics to virtually all patients undergoing cardiac surgery, attempting to prevent both wound infections and endocarditis, although the efficacy of prophylaxis in prevention of endocarditis has not been proved.[55] Current recommendations call for parenteral administration of an antistaphylococcal antibiotic just prior to operation, followed by 1 or 2 further doses (Table 73-12). The regimen may be modified if local experience shows that cases of early PVE caused by *Staph.* epidermidis or gram-negative bacilli have occurred with significant frequency (Table 73-12).

The paradigms that have been proposed by various expert bodies (including the AHA) for the use of antibiotics to prevent IE have developed over time and have been based on indirect evidence derived from studies in animals that demonstrated that prevention was possible, on case reports tying IE to various procedures known to cause bacteremia, and from a concern about the dire consequences of the disease. These recommendations have been accepted as "standard of care" and failure to follow them has taken on medicolegal implications. Various authors have questioned this practice and new information has emerged calling into question the clinical benefit of prophylactic antibiotics in this setting. This is especially important in an era where overuse of antimicrobials is fueling the dangerous epidemic of antibiotic-resistant bacteria. Therefore, it seems prudent for the various expert committees who write such recommendations to carefully weigh the apparent minimal benefits with the downsides of toxicity, cost, and resistance that has come with excessive use of antibiotics.

NOTE

This chapter is a modification of the original chapter by David Durack in previous editions of this book.

References

1. Blumer G. Subacute bacterial endocarditis. *Medicine* 1923; 2:105–170.

2. Thayer WS. Studies on bacterial (infective) endocarditis. *Johns Hopkins Hosp Rep* 1926; 22:1–185.
3. Kerr A Jr. *Subacute Bacterial Endocarditis.* Springfield, IL: Charles C Thomas; 1955.
4. Hermans PE. The clinical manifestations of infective endocarditis. *Mayo Clin Proc* 1982; 57:15–21.
5. Chambers HF, Korzeniowski OM, Sande MA, National Collaborative Endocarditis Study Group. *Staphylococcus aureus* endocarditis: Clinical manifestations in addicts and nonaddicts. *Medicine* 1983; 62:170–177.
6. Korzeniowski OM, Kaye D. Infective endocarditis. In: Braunwald E, ed. *The Heart: A Textbook of Cardiovascular Medicine,* 4th ed. Philadelphia: Saunders, 1992:1078–1105.
7. Sande MA, Johnson WD Jr, Hook EW, Kay D: Bacteremia associated with cardiac catheterization. *N Engl J Med* 1969; 281:1104–1106.
8. Baumgartner WA, Miller DC, Reitz BA, et al. Surgical treatment of prosthetic valve endocarditis. *Ann Thorac Surg* 1983; 35:87–104.
9. Ivert TSA, Dismukes WE, Cobbs CG, et al. Prosthetic valve endocarditis. *Circulation* 1984; 69:223–232.
10. Braimbridge MV, Eykyn SJ. Prosthetic valve endocarditis. *J Antimicrob Chemother* 1987; 20:173–180.
11. Douglas JL, Cobbs CG. Prosthetic valve endocarditis. In: Kaye D, ed. *Infective Endocarditis,* 2d ed. New York: Raven Press; 1992:375–396.
12. Meyer MW, Witt AR, Krishnan LK, et al. Therapeutic advantage of recombinant human plasminogen activator in endocarditis: Evidence from experiments in rabbits. *Thromb Haemost* 1995; 73:680–682.
13. MacDonald RA, Robbins SL. The significance of nonbacterial thrombotic endocarditis: An autopsy and clinical study of 78 cases. *Ann Intern Med* 1957; 46:255–273.
14. Barry WE, Scarpelli D. Nonbacterial thrombotic endocarditis. *Arch Intern Med* 1962; 109:79–84.
15. Bryan CS. Nonbacterial thrombotic endocarditis in patients with malignant tumors. *Am J Med* 1969; 46:787–793.
16. Major RM. Notes on the history of endocarditis. *Bull Hist Med* 1945; 17:351–359.
17. Osler W. Chronic infectious endocarditis. *Q J Med* 1909; 2:219–230.
18. Osler W. The Goulstonian lectures, on malignant endocarditis. *Br Med J* 1885; 1:467–579.
19. Horder TJ. Infective endocarditis: With an analysis of 150 cases and with special reference to the chronic form of the disease. *Q J Med* 1909; 2:289–329.
20. Allen AC. Nature of vegetations of bacterial endocarditis. *Arch Pathol* 1939; 27:661–671.
21. Libman E, Friedberg CK. *Subacute Bacterial Endocarditis.* New York: Oxford University Press; 1947.
22. Beeson PB, Brannon ES, Warren JV. Observations of the sites of removal of bacteria from the blood in patients with bacterial endocarditis. *J Exp Med* 1945; 81:9–23.
23. Touroff ASW, Vesell H. Subacute streptococcus viridans endocarditis complicating patent ductus arteriosus: Recovery following surgical treatment. *JAMA* 1940; 115:1270–1272.
24. Durack DT. Review of early experience in treatment of bacterial endocarditis, 1940–1955. In: Bisno AL, ed. *Treatment of Infective Endocarditis.* New York: Grune & Stratton; 1981:1–14.
25. Dawson MH, Hunter TH. The treatment of subacute bacterial endocarditis with penicillin: Results in twenty cases. *JAMA* 1945; 127:129–137.
26. Abraham EP, Chain E, Fletcher CM, et al. Further observations on penicillin. *Lancet* 1941; 2:177–189.
27. Loewe L, Rosenblatt P, Greene HJ, Russell M. Combined penicillin and heparin therapy of subacute bacterial endocarditis: Report of seven consecutive successfully treated patients. *JAMA* 1944; 124:144–149.
28. Galbreath WR, Hull E. Sulfonamide therapy of bacterial endocarditis: Results in 42 cases. *Ann Intern Med* 1943; 18:201–203.
29. Bloomfield AL, Armstrong CD, Kirby WMM. The treatment of subacute bacterial endocarditis with penicillin. *J Clin Invest* 1945; 24:251–267.
30. Hunter TH. The treatment of some bacterial infections of the heart and pericardium. *Bull NY Acad Med* 1952; 28:213–228.
31. Finland M. Treatment of bacterial endocarditis (concluded). *N Engl J Med* 1954; 250:419–428.
32. Geraci JE. The antibiotic therapy of infective endocarditis: Therapeutic data on 172 patients seen from 1951 through 1957: Additional observations on short-term therapy (two weeks) for penicillin-sensitive streptococcal endocarditis. *Med Clin North Am* 1958; 42:1101–1148.
33. Weinstein L, Schlesinger J. Treatment of infective endocarditis—1973. *Prog Cardiovasc Dis* 1973; 26:275–296.
34. Wallace AG, Young G Jr, Osterhout S. Treatment of acute bacterial endocarditis by valve excision and replacement. *Circulation* 1965; 31:450–453.
35. Harris SL. Definitions and demographic characteristics. In: Kaye D, ed. *Infective Endocarditis.* 2d ed. New York: Raven Press; 1992:1–18.
36. Steckelberg JM, Wilson WR. Risk factors for infective endocarditis. *Infect Dis Clin North Am* 1993; 7:9–19.
37. Smith RH, Radford DJ, Clark RA, Julian DG. Infective endocarditis: A survey of cases in the southeast of Scotland 1969–72. *Thorax* 1976;31:373–379.
38. Van Der Meer JTM, Thompson J, Valkenburg HA, Michel MF. Epidemiology of bacterial endocarditis in the Netherlands: 1. Patient characteristics. *Arch Intern Med* 1992; 152:1863–1868.
39. Hogevik H, Olaison L, Andersson R, et al. Epidemiologic aspects of infective endocarditis in an urban population: A 5-year prospective study. *Medicine* 1995; 74:324–339.
40. Berlin JA, Abrutyn E, Strom BL, et al. Incidence of infective endocarditis in the Delaware Valley, 1988–1990. *Am J Cardiol* 1995; 76:933–936.
41. Kaye D, McCormack RC, Hook EW. Bacterial endocarditis: The changing pattern since the introduction of penicillin therapy. *Antimicrob Agents Chemother* 1961; 37–46.
42. Uwaydah MM, Weinberg AN. Bacterial endocarditis—A changing pattern. *N Engl J Med* 1965; 273:1231–1235.
43. Lerner PI, Weinstein L. Infective endocarditis in the antibiotic era. *N Engl J Med* 1966; 274:199–206; 259–266; 323–331; 388–393.
44. Finland M, Barnes MW. Changing etiology of bacterial endocarditis in the antibiotic era: Experiences at the Boston City Hospital 1933–1965. *Ann Intern Med* 1970; 72:341–348.
45. Durack DT, Petersdorf RG. Changes in the epidemiology of endocarditis. In: Kaplan EL, Taranta AV, eds. *Infective Endocarditis: An American Heart Association Symposium.* Dallas: American Heart Association; 1977:3–8.
46. Baddour LM. Twelve-year review of recurrent native-valve infective endocarditis: A disease of the modern antibiotic era. *Rev Infect Dis* 1988; 10:1163–1170.
47. Dysson C, Infective endocarditis: An epidemiological review of 128 episodes. *J Infect* 1999; 38(2):87–93.
48. Garvey GJ, Neu HC. Infective endocarditis—An evolving disease: A review of endocarditis at the Columbia-Presbyterian Medical Center, 1968–1973. *Medicine* 1978; 57:105–127.
49. Pulvirenti JJ, Kerns E, Benson C, et al. Infective endocarditis in injection drug users: Importance of human immunodeficiency virus serostatus and degree of immunosuppression. *Clin Infect Dis* 1996; 22:40–45.
50. Scheld WM, Sande MA. Endocarditis and intravascular infections. In: Mandell GL, Douglas RG Jr, Dolin R, eds. *Principles*

and Practice of Infectious Diseases, 4th ed. New York: Churchill Livingstone; 1995:740–783.
51. Weinstein L, Rubin RH. Infective endocarditis—1973. *Prog Cardiovasc Dis* 1973; 16:239–273.
52. Tunkel AR, Mandell GL. Infecting microorganisms. In: Kaye D, ed. *Infective Endocarditis,* 2d ed. New York: Raven Press; 1992:85–97.
53. Tompkins LS, Roessler BJ, Redd SC. Legionella prosthetic-valve endocarditis. *N Engl J Med* 1988; 318:530–534.
54. Bayliss R, Clarke C, Oakley C, et al. The teeth and infective endocarditis. *Br Heart J* 1983; 50:506–512.
55. Durack DT. Prophylaxis of infective endocarditis. In: Mandell GL, Douglas RG Jr, Dolin R, eds. *Principles and Practice of Infectious Diseases,* 4th ed. NewYork: Churchill Livingstone; 1995:793–813.
56. Strom BL, et al. Dental and Cardiac Risk Factors for Infective Endocarditis. *Ann Intern Med* 1998; 129:761–769.
57. Mansur AJ, Grinberg M, da Luz PL, Bellotti G. The complications of infective endocarditis: A reappraisal in the 1980s (see comments). *Arch Intern Med* 1992; 152:2428–2432.
58. Johnson DH, Rosenthal A, Nadas AS. A forty-year review of bacterial endocarditis in infancy and childhood. *Circulation* 1975; 51:581–588.
59. Hansen D, Schmiegelow K, Jacobsen JR. Bacterial endocarditis in children: Trends in its diagnosis, course, and prognosis. *Pediatr Cardiol* 1993; 13:198–203.
60. Saiman L, Prince A, Gersony WM. Pediatric infective endocarditis in the modern era. *J Pediatr* 1993; 122:847–853.
61. Awadallah SM, Kavey RW, Byrum CJ, et al. The changing pattern of infective endocarditis in childhood. *Am J Cardiol* 1991; 68:90–94.
62. Stull TL, LiPuma JJ. Endocarditis in children. In: Kaye D, ed. *Infective Endocarditis,* 2d ed. New York: Raven Press; 1992:313–327.
63. Ifere OAS, Masokano KA. Infective endocarditis in children in the Guinea savannah of Nigeria. *Ann Trop Paediatr* 1991; 11:233–240.
64. Saitoh M, Hishi T, Tamura M, Komoshita S. Forty year review of bacterial endocarditis in infants and children. *Acta Paediatr Jpn* 1991; 33:613–616.
65. El-Khatib MR, Wilson FM, Lerner AM. Characteristics of bacterial endocarditis in heroin addicts in Detroit. *Am J Med Sci* 1976; 271:197–201.
66. Reisberg BE. Infective endocarditis in the narcotic addict. *Prog Cardiovasc Dis* 1979; 22:193–204.
67. Dressler FA, Roberts WC. Infective endocarditis in opiate addicts: Analysis of 80 cases studied at necropsy. *Am J Cardiol* 1989; 63:1240–1257.
68. Weisse AB, Heller DR, Schimenti RJ, et al. The febrile parenteral drug user: A prospective study in 121 patients. *Am J Med* 1993; 94:274–280.
69. Carrel T, Schaffner A, Vogt P, et al. Endocarditis in intravenous drug addicts and HIV infected patients: Possibilities and limitations of surgical treatment. *J Heart Valve Dis* 1993; 2:140–147.
70. Sande MA, Lee BL, Mills J, Chambers HF III. Endocarditis in intravenous drug users. In: Kaye D, ed. *Infective Endocarditis,* 2d ed. New York: Raven Press; 1992:345–359.
71. Corrigall D, Bolen J, Hancock EW, Popp RP. Mitral valve prolapse and infective endocarditis. *Am J Med* 1977; 63:215–222.
72. Clemens JD, Horwitz RI, Jaffe CC, et al. A controlled evaluation of the risk of bacterial endocarditis in persons with mitral-valve prolapse. *N Engl J Med* 1982; 307:776–781.
73. Beton DC, Brear SG, Edwards JD, Leonard JC. Mitral valve prolapse:An assessment of clinical features, associated conditions and prognosis. *Q J Med* 1983; 52:150–164.
74. Heidenreich PA. The clinical impact of echocardiography on antibiotic prophylaxis use in patients with suspected mitral valve prolapse. *Am J Med* 1997; 102(4): 337–343.
75. Durack DT, Kaplan EL, Bisno AL. Apparent failures of endocarditis prophylaxis: Analysis of 52 cases submitted to a national registry. *JAMA* 1983; 250:2318–2322.
76. Clemens JD, Ransohoff DF. A quantitative assessment of predental antibiotic prophylaxis for patients with mitral-valve prolapse. *J Chronic Dis* 1984; 37:531–544.
77. Devereux RB, Hawkins I, Kramer-Fox R, et al. Complications of mitral valve prolapse: Disproportionate occurrence in men and older patients. *Am J Med* 1986; 81:751–758.
78. MacMahon SW, Hickey AJ, Wilcken DEL, et al. Risk of infective endocarditis in mitral valve prolapse with and without precordial systolic murmurs. *Am J Cardiol* 1986; 58:105–108.
79. Dajani AS, Taubert KA, Wilson W, et al. *Prevention of Bacterial Endocarditis.* Dallas: American Heart Association Medical/ Scientific Statement; 1997; 71–0117.
80. MacMahon SW, Roberts K, Kramer-Fox R, et al. Mitral valve prolapse and infective endocarditis. *Am Heart J* 1987; 113:1291–1298.
81. Dhawan A, Grover A, Marwaha RK, et al. Infective endocarditis in children: Profile in a developing country. *Ann Trop Paediatr* 1993; 13:189–194.
82. Elward K, Hruby N, Christy C. Pneumococcal endocarditis in infants and children: Report of a case and review of the literature. *Pediatr Infect Dis J* 1990; 9:652–657.
83. Brook MM, Pediatric bacterial endocarditis: Treatment and prophylaxis. *Pediatr Clin North Am* 1999; 46(2):275–287.
84. Martin JM, Neches WH, Wald ER, et al. Infective endocarditis: 35 years of experience at a children's hospital. *Clin Infect Dis* 1997; 24(4):669–675.
85. Del Pont JM, De Cicco LT, Vartalitis C, et al. Infective endocarditis in children: Clinical analyses and evaluation of two diagnostic criteria. *Pediatr Infect Dis* 1995; 14:1079–1086.
86. Kaplan EL, Rich H, Gersony W, Manning J. A collaborative study of infective endocarditis in the 1970s: Emphasis on infections in patients who have undergone cardiovascular surgery. *Circulation* 1979; 59:327–335.
87. Jung JY, Saab SB, Almond CH. The case for early surgical treatment of left-sided primary infective endocarditis. *J Thorac Cardiovasc Surg* 1975; 70:509–518.
88. Picarelli D, Leone R, Duhagon P, et al. Active infective endocarditis in infants and childhood: Ten-year review of surgical therapy. *J Card Surg* 1997; 12(6):406–411.
89. Bayliss R, Clarke C, Oakley CM, et al. Incidence, mortality and prevention of infective endocarditis. *J R Coll Phys Lond* 1986; 20:15–20.
90. Werner GS, Schulz R, Fuchs FB, et al. Infective endocarditis in the elderly in the era of transesophageal echocardiography: Clinical features and prognosis compared with younger patients. *Am J Med* 1996; 100:90–97.
91. Felder RS, Nardone D, Palac R. Prevalence of predisposing factors for endocarditis among an elderly institutionalized population. *Oral Surg Oral Med Oral Pathol* 1992; 73:30–34.
92. Selton-Suty C, Hoen B, Grentzinger A, et al. Clinical and bacteriological characteristics of infective endocarditis in the elderly. *Heart* 1997; 77(3):260–263.
93. Steckelberg JM, Melton LJ, Ilstrup DM, et al. Influence of referral bias on the apparent clinical spectrum of infective endocarditis. *Am J Med* 1990; 88:582–588.
94. Eliopoulos GM. Enterococcal endocarditis. In: Kaye D, ed. *Infective Endocarditis,* 2d ed. New York: Raven Press; 1992:209–229.
95. Threlkeld MG, Cobbs CG. Infectious disorders of prosthetic valves and intravascular devices. In: Mandell GL, Bennett JE, Dolin R, eds. *Principles and Practice of Infectious Diseases,* 4th ed. New York: Churchill Livingstone; 1995:783–793.
96. Burke AP, Kalra P, Li L et al. Infectious endocarditis and sudden

unexpected death: incidence and morphology of lesions in intravenous addicts and non-drug abusers. *J Heart Valve Dis* 1997; 6(2):198–203.
97. Tuazon CU, Sheagren JN. Increased rate of carriage of *Staphylococcus aureus* among narcotic addicts. *J Infect Dis* 1974; 129:725–727.
98. Reyes MP, Lerner AM. Current problems in the treatment of infective endocarditis due to *Pseudomonas aeruginosa*. *Rev Infect Dis* 1983; 5:314–321.
99. Cohen PS, Maguire JH, Weinstein L. Infective endocarditis caused by gram-negative bacteria: A review of the literature, 1945–1977. *Prog Cardiovasc Dis* 1980; 22:205–242.
100. Rubinstein E, Noriega ER, Simberkoff MS, et al. Fungal endocarditis: Analysis of 24 cases and review of the literature. *Medicine* 1975; 54:331–344.
101. Moyer DV, Edwards JE Jr. Fungal endocarditis. In: Kaye D, ed. *Infective Endocarditis,* 2d ed. New York: Raven Press; 1992:299–312.
102. Baddour LM, Meyer J, Henry B. Polymicrobial infective endocarditis in the 1980s. *Rev Infect Dis* 1991; 13:963–970.
103. Faber M, Frimodt-Moller N, Espersen F, et al. *Staphylococcus aureus* endocarditis in Danish intravenous drug users: High proportion of left-sided endocarditis. *Scand J Infect Dis* 1995; 27:483–487.
104. Spijkerman IJ, van Ameijden EJ, Mientjes GH, et al. Human immunodeficiency virus infection and other risk factors for skin abscesses and endocarditis among injection drug users. *J Clin Epidemiol* 1996; 49(10):1149–1154.
105. Drancourt M, Birtles R, Chaumentin G, et al. New serotype of *Bartonella henselae* in endocarditis and cat-scratch disease. *Lancet* 1996; 347:441–443.
106. Ribera E, et al. Influence of human immunodeficiency virus 1 and degree of immunosuppression in the clinical characteristics and outcome of infective endocarditis in intravenous drug users. *Arch Intern Med* 1998; 158(18):2043–2050.
107. Manoff SB. Human immunodeficiency virus infection and infective endocarditis among injecting drug users. *Epidemiology* 1996; 7(6):566–570.
108. Resnekov L. Staphylococcal endocarditis following mitral valvotomy with special reference to coagulase-negative *Staphylococcus albus*. *Lancet* 1959; 2:597–600.
109. Watanakunakorn C. Prosthetic valve infective endocarditis. *Prog Cardiovasc Dis* 1979; 22:181–192.
110. Karchmer AW, Dismukes WE, Buckley MJ, Austen WG. Late prosthetic valve endocarditis: Clinical features influencing therapy. *Am J Med* 1978; 64:199–206.
111. Seaworth BJ, Durack DT. Infective endocarditis in obstetric and gynecologic practice. *Am J Obstet Gynecol* 1986; 154:180–188.
112. Sugrue D, Blake S, Troy P, MacDonald D. Antibiotic prophylaxis against infective endocarditis after normal delivery—Is it necessary? *Br Heart J* 1980; 44:499–502.
113. Cobbs CG. IUD and endocarditis. *Ann Intern Med* 1973; 78:451.
114. Fernandez-Guerrero ML, Verdejo C, Azofra J, de Gorgolas M. Hospital-acquired infectious endocarditis not associated with cardiac surgery: An emerging problem. *Clin Infect Dis* 1995; 20:16–23.
115. Fang G, Keys TF, Gentry LO, et al. Prosthetic valve endocarditis resulting from nosocomial bacteremia: A prospective, multicenter study. *Ann Intern Med* 1993; 119:560–567.
116. Pelletier LL, Petersdorf RG. Infective endocarditis: A review of 125 cases from the University of Washington Hospitals, 1963–72. *Medicine* 1977; 56:287–313.
117. Raad II, Bodey GP. Infectious complications of indwelling vascular catheters. *Clin Infect Dis* 1992; 15:197–210.
118. Lamas CC. Hospital acquired native valve endocarditis: analysis of 22 cases presenting over 11 years. *Heart* 1998; 79(5):442–447.
119. Ehrie M, Morgan AP, Moore FD, O'Connor NE. Endocarditis with the indwelling balloon-tipped pulmonary artery catheter in burn patients. *J Trauma* 1978; 18:665–666.
120. Rowley KM, Clubb KS, Smith GJW, Cabin HS. Right-sided infective endocarditis as a consequence of flow-directed pulmonary artery catheterization: A clinicopathological study of 55 autopsied patients. *N Engl J Med* 1984; 311:1152–1156.
121. Cartotto RC. Acute bacterial endocarditis following burns: Case report and review. *Burns* 1998; 24(4):369–373.
122. Martino P, Micozzi A, Venditti M, et al. Catheter-related right-sided endocarditis in bone marrow transplant recipients. *Rev Infect Dis* 1990; 12:250–257.
123. Khoo DE, Zebro TJ, English TAH. Bacterial endocarditis in a transplanted heart. *Pathol Res Pract* 1989; 185:445–447.
124. Paterson DL. Infective endocarditis in solid organ transplant recipients. *Clin Infect Dis* 1998; 26(3):689–694.
125. Lillehei CW, Bobb JRR, Visscher MB. The occurrence of endocarditis with valvular deformities in dogs with arteriovenous fistulas. *Ann Surg* 1950; 132:577–590.
126. Cross AS, Steigbigel RT. Infective endocarditis and access site infections in patients on hemodialysis. *Medicine* 1976; 55:453–465.
127. Robinson DL, Bacterial endocarditis in hemodialysis patients, *Am J Kidney Dis* 1997; 30(4):521–524.
128. Marr KA. Incidence and outcome of *Staphylococcus aureus* bacteremia in hemodialysis patients. *Kid Int* 1998; 54(5):1684–1689.
129. Klug D, Lacroix D, Savoye C, et al. Systemic infection related to endocarditis on pacemaker leads: Clinical presentation and management. *Circulation* 1997; 95(8):2098–2107.
130. Cacoub P. Pacemaker infective endocarditis. *Am J Cardiol* 1998; 82(4):480–484.
131. Victor F. Pacemaker lead infection: Echocardiographic features, management, and outcome. *Heart* 1999; 81(1):82–87.
132. Voet JG. Pacemaker lead infection: Report of three cases and review of the literature. *Heart* 1999; 81(1):88–91.
133. Gomes MN, Choyke PL, Wallace RB. Infected aortic aneurysms: A changing entity. *Ann Surg* 1992; 215:435–442.
134. Brennan RO, Durack DT. The viridans streptococci in perspective. In: Remington JS, Swartz MN, eds. *Current Clinical Topics in Infectious Diseases.* New York: McGraw-Hill; 1984:253–289.
135. Sussman JI, Baron EJ, Tenenbaum MJ, et al. Viridans streptococcal endocarditis: Clinical, microbiological, and echocardiographic correlations. *J Infect Dis* 1986; 154:597–603.
136. Watanakunakorn C, Pantelakis J. Alpha-hemolytic streptococcal bacteremia: A review of 203 episodes during 1980–1991. *Scand J Infect Dis* 1993; 25:403–408.
137. Facklam RR. Physiological differentiation of viridans streptococci. *J Clin Microbiol* 1977; 5:184–201.
138. Douglas CWI, Heath J, Hampton KK, Preston FE. Identity of viridans streptococci isolated from cases of infective endocarditis. *J Med Microbiol* 1993; 39:179–182.
139. Carey RB, Gross KC, Roberts RB. Vitamin B6-dependent *Streptococcus mitor (mitis)* isolated from patients with systemic infections. *J Infect Dis* 1975; 131:722–726.
140. Rouff KL. Nutritionally variant streptococci. *Clin Microbiol Rev* 1991; 4:184–190.
141. Bouvet A, Grimont F, Grimont PAD. *Streptococcus defectivus* sp. nov. and *Streptococcus adjacens* sp. nov., nutritionally variant streptococci from human clinical specimens. *Int J Syst Bacteriol* 1989; 39:290–294.
142. Bouvet A. Human endocarditis due to nutritionally variant streptococci: *Streptococcus adjacens* and *Streptococcus defectivus*. *Eur Heart J* 1995; 16(suppl B):24–27.
143. Wilson WR, Wilkowske CJ, Wright AJ, et al. Treatment of streptomycin-susceptible and streptomycin-resistant enterococcal endocarditis. *Ann Intern Med* 1984; 100:816–823.
144. Moellering RC Jr, Watson BK, Kunz LJ. Endocarditis due to group D streptococci: Comparison of disease caused by *Strepto-*

coccus bovis with that produced by the enterococci. *Am J Med* 1974; 57:239–250.
145. Kupferwasser I. Clinical and morphological characteristics in *Streptococcus bovis* endocarditis: A comparison with other causative microorganisms in 177 cases. *Heart* 1998; 80(3):276–280.
146. Murray HW, Roberts RB. *Streptococcus bovis* bacteremia and underlying gastrointestinal disease. *Arch Intern Med* 1978; 138:1097–1099.
147. Klein RS, Catalano MT, Edberg SC, et al. *Streptococcus bovis* septicemia and carcinoma of the colon. *Ann Intern Med* 1979; 91:560–562.
148. Maki DG, Agger WA. Enterococcal bacteremia: Clinical features, the risk of endocarditis, and management. *Medicine* 1988; 67:248–269.
149. Murray BE. The life and times of the enterococcus. *Clin Microbiol Rev* 1990; 3:46–65.
150. Megran DW. Enterococcal endocarditis. *Clin Infect Dis* 1992; 15:63–71.
151. Eliopoulos GM. Increasing problems in the therapy of enterococcal infections. *Eur J Clin Microbiol Infect Dis* 1993; 12:409–412.
152. Frieden TR, Munsiff SS, Low DE, et al. Emergence of vancomycin-resistant enterococci in New York City. *Lancet* 1993; 342:76–79.
153. Bruyn GAW, Thompson J, Van Der Meer JWM. Pneumococcal endocarditis in adult patients. A report of five cases and review of the literature. *Q J Med* 1990; 74:33–40.
154. Aronin SI. Review of pneumococcal endocarditis in adults in the penicillin era. *Clin Infect Dis* 1998; 26(1):1341–1342.
155. Lindberg J. Pneumococcal endocarditis is not just a disease of the past: An analysis of 16 cases diagnosed in Denmark 1986–1997. *Scand J Infect Dis* 1998; 30(5):469–472.
156. Baddour LM. Infective endocarditis caused by beta-hemolytic streptococci. The Infectious Diseases Society of America's Emerging Infections Network. *Clin Infect Dis* 1998; 26(1):66–71.
157. Winterbotham A. Endocarditis caused by group A beta-hemolytic streptococcus in an infant: Case report and review. *Clin Infect Dis* 1999; 29(1):196–198.
158. Azzam ZS. Group B streptococcal tricuspid valve endocarditis: A case report and review of literature. *Int J Cardiol* 1998; 64(3):259–263.
159. Pankey GA. Acute bacterial endocarditis at the University of Minnesota Hospitals, 1939–1959. *Am Heart J* 1962; 64:583–591.
160. Roder BL. Clinical features of *Staphylococcus aureus* endocarditis: A 10-year experience in Denmark. *Arch Intern Med* 1999; 159(5):462–469.
161. Watanakunakorn C, Tan JS, Phair JP. Some salient features of *Staphylococcus aureus* endocarditis. *Am J Med* 1973; 54:473–481.
162. Bayer AS, Lam K, Gintzon L, et al. *Staphylococcus aureus* bacteremia: Clinical, serologic, and echocardiographic findings in patients with and without endocarditis. *Arch Intern Med* 1987; 147:457–462.
163. Keys TF, Hewitt WL. Endocarditis due to micrococci and *Staphylococcus epidermidis*. *Arch Intern Med* 1973; 132:216–220.
164. Huebner J. Coagulase-negative staphylococci: Role as pathogens. *Ann Res Med* 1999; 50:223–236.
165. Borgert SJ. Destructive native valve endocarditis caused by *Staphylococcus lugdunensis*. *South Med J* 1999; 92(8):812–814.
166. Karchmer AW, Archer GL, Dismukes WE. *Staphylococcus epidermidis* causing prosthetic valve endocarditis: Microbiologic and clinical observations as guides to therapy. *Ann Intern Med* 1983; 98:447–455.
167. Chen YC, Chang SC, Luh KT, Hsieh WC. *Actinobacillus actinomycetemcomitans* endocarditis: A report of four cases and review of the literature. *Q J Med* 1992; 81:871–878.
168. Geraci JE, Wilson WR. Endocarditis due to gram-negative bacteria: Report of 56 cases. *Mayo Clin Proc* 1982; 57:145–148.
169. Badley AD. Infective endocarditis caused by HACEK microorganisms. *Ann Rev Med* 1997; 48:25–33.
170. Darras-Joly C. Haemophilus endocarditis: Report of 42 cases in adults and review: Haemophilus Endocarditis Study Group. *Clin Infect Dis* 1997; 24(6):1087–1094.
171. Gould K, Ramirez-Ronda CH, Holmes RK, Sanford JP. Adherence of bacteria to heart valves *in vitro*. *J Clin Invest* 1975; 56:1364–1370.
172. Scheld WM, Valone JA, Sande MA. Bacterial adherence in the pathogenesis of endocarditis: Interaction of bacterial dextran, platelets, and fibrin. *J Clin Invest* 1978; 61:1394–1404.
173. Durack DT, Beeson PB. Protective role of complement in experimental *E. coli* endocarditis. *Infect Immun* 1977; 16:213–217.
174. Gutierrez RF. Endocarditis caused by *Stenotrophomas maltophilia*: Case report and review. *Clin Infect Dis* 1996; 23(6):1261–1265.
175. Al-Kasab S, Al-Fagih MR, Al-Yousef S, et al. *Brucella* infective endocarditis: Successful combined medical and surgical therapy. *J Thorac Cardiovasc Surg* 1988; 95:862–867.
176. Delvecchio G, Fracassetti O, Lorenzi N. *Brucella* endocarditis. *Int J Cardiol* 1991; 33:328–329.
177. Uddin MJ. The role of aggressive medical therapy along with early surgical intervention in the cure of *Brucella endocarditis*. *Ann Thorac Cardiovasc Surg*. 1998; 4 (4):209–213.
178. Felner JM, Dowell VR. Anaerobic bacterial endocarditis. *N Engl J Med* 1970; 283:1188–1192.
179. Nastro LJ, Finegold SM. Endocarditis due to anaerobic gram-negative bacilli. *Am J Med* 1973; 54:482–496.
180. Kammer RB, Utz JP. *Aspergillus* species endocarditis: The new face of a not so rare disease. *Am J Med* 1974; 56:506–521.
181. Aspesberro F. Fungal endocarditis in critically ill children. *Eur J Pediatric* 1999; 158(4):275–280.
182. Turck WPG, Howitt G, Turnberg LA, et al. Chronic Q fever. *Q J Med* 1976; 45:193–217.
183. Siegman-Igra Y. Q fever endocarditis in Israel and a worldwide review. *Scand J Infect Dis* 1997; 29(1):41–49.
184. Kimbrough RC, Ormsbee RA, Peacock M, et al. Q fever endocarditis in the United States. *Ann Intern Med* 1979; 91:400–402.
185. Spelman DW. Q fever: A study of 111 consecutive cases. *Med J Aust* 1982; 1:547–553.
186. Falconer H, Terry SI, Spencer H. Cryptococcosis in the West Indies. *West Indian Med J* 1980; 29:142.
187. Raoult D, Marrie T. State of the art clinical article: Q fever. *Clin Infect Dis* 1995; 20:489–496.
188. Raoult D, Brouqui P, Marchou B, Gastaut JA. Acute and chronic Q fever in patients with cancer. *Clin Infect Dis* 1992; 14:127–130.
189. Raoult D, Fournier PE, Drancourt M, et al. Diagnosis of 22 new cases of *Bartonella* endocarditis. *Ann Intern Med* 1996; 125:646–652.
190. La Sacola B. Culture of *Vartonella quintana* and *Bartonella henselae* from human samples: A 5-year experience (1990 to 1998). *J Clin Micorobiol* 1999; 37(6): 1899–1905.
191. Ward C, Ward AM. Acquired valvular heart disease in patients who keep pet birds. *Lancet* 1974; 734–736.
192. van der Bel-Kahn J, Watanakunakorn C, Menefee MG, et al. *Chlamydia trachomatis* endocarditis. *Am Heart J* 1978; 95:627–636.
193. Spyrou N, Anderson M, Foale R. *Listeria* endocarditis: Current management and patient outcome—world literature review. *Heart* 1997; 77(4):380–383.
194. Cohen JI, Sloss LJ, Kundsin R, Golightly L. Prosthetic valve endocarditis caused by *Mycoplasma hominis*. *Am J Med* 1989; 86:819–821.
195. Malinverni R, Bille J, Glauser MP. Single-dose rifampin prophylaxis for experimental endocarditis induced by high bacterial inocula of *Viridans* streptococci. *J Infect Dis* 1987; 156:151–157.
196. Cannady PB Jr, Sanford JP. Negative blood cultures in infective endocarditis: A review. *South Med J* 1976; 69:1420–1424.

197. Pesanti EL, Smith IM. Infective endocarditis with negative blood cultures: An analysis of 52 cases. *Am J Med* 1979; 66:43–50.
198. Hoen B, Selton-Suty C, Lacassin F, et al. Infective endocarditis in patients with negative blood cultures: Analysis of 88 cases from a one-year nationwide survey in France. *Clin Infect Dis* 1995; 20:501–506.
199. Libman E. The clinical features of cases of subacute bacterial endocarditis that have spontaneously become bacteria-free. *Am J Med Sci* 1913; 146:626–645.
200. Gubler JG. Whipple endocarditis without overt gastrointestinal disease: Report of four cases. *Ann Intern Med* 1999; 131:144–146.
201. Roux JP, Koussa A, Cajot MA, et al. Primary *Aspergillus* endocarditis: Apropos of a case and review of the international literature. *Ann Chir* 1992; 46:110–115.
202. Durack DT, Bright DK, Lukes AS, Duke Endocarditis Service. New criteria for diagnosis of infective endocarditis: Utilization of specific echocardiographic findings. *Am J Med* 1994; 96:200–209.
203. Cecchi E, Parrini I, Chinaglia A, et al. New diagnostic criteria for infective endocarditis. A study of sensitivity and specificity. *Eur Heart J* 1997; 18:1149–1156.
204. Angrist A, Oka M, Nakao K. Vegetative endocarditis. *Pathol Annu* 1967; 2:155–212.
205. Grant RT, Wood JE Jr, Jones TD. Heart valve irregularities in relation to subacute bacterial endocarditis. *Am Heart J* 1928; 14:247–261.
206. Durack DT. Experimental bacterial endocarditis: IV. Structure and evolution of very early lesions. *J Pathol* 1975; 115:81–89.
207. Durack DT, Beeson PB. Experimental bacterial endocarditis: I. Colonization of a sterile vegetation. *Br J Exp Pathol* 1972; 53:44–49.
208. Hojnik M, George J, Ziporen L, Shoenfeld Y. Heart valve involvement (Libman-Sacks endocarditis) in the antiphospholipid syndrome. *Circulation* 1996; 93:1579–1587.
209. Livornese LL Jr, Korzeniowski O. Pathogenesis of infective endocarditis. In: Kaye D, ed. *Infective Endocarditis,* 2d ed. New York: Raven Press; 1992:19–35.
210. Schlievert PM. Aggregation and binding substances enhance pathogenicity in rabbit models of *Enterococcus faecalis* endocarditis. *Infect Immun* 1998; 66(1):218–223.
211. Burnette-Curley D, Wells V, Viscount H, et al. FimA, a major virulence factor associated with *Streptococcus parasanguis* endocarditis. *Infect Immun* 1995; 63:4669–4674.
212. Viscount HB, Munro CL, Burnette-Curley D, et al. Immunization with FimA protects against *Streptococcus parasanguis* endocarditis in rats. *Infect Immun* 1997; 65(3):994–1002.
213. Moreillon P, Entenza JM, Francioli P, et al. Role of *Staphylococcus aureus* coagulase and clumping factor in pathogenesis of experimental endocarditis. *Infect Immun* 1995; 63:4738–4743.
214. Baddour LM, Christensen GD, Hester MG, Bisno AL. Production of experimental endocarditis by coagulase-negative staphylococci: Variability in species virulence. *J Infect Dis* 1984; 150:721–727.
215. Yeaman MR, Puentes SM, Norman DC, Bayer AS. Partial characterization and staphylocidal activity of thrombin-induced platelet microbicidal protein. *Infect Immun* 1992; 60:1202–1209.
216. Dankert J, Hess J, Durack DT. Pathogenesis of viridans streptococcal endocarditis (VSE): Disappearance of adherent streptococci from vegetations. *26th Interscience Conference on Antimicrobial Agents and Chemotherapy* (abstr). 1986.
217. Drake TA, Rogers GM, Sande MA. Tissue factor is a major stimulus for vegetation formation in enterococcal endocarditis in rabbits. *J Clin Invest* 1984; 73:1750–1753.
218. van Ginkel CJW, Thorig L, Thompson J, et al. Enhancement of generation of monocyte tissue thromboplastin by bacterial phagocytosis: Possible pathway for fibrin formation on infected vegetations in bacterial endocarditis. *Infect Immun* 1979; 25:388–395.
219. Sullam PM. Diminished platelet binding in vitro by *Staphylococcus aureus* is associated with reduced virulence in a rabbit model of infective endocarditis. *Infert Immuon* 1996; 64(12):4915–4921.
220. Drake T, Pang M. *Staphylococcus aureus* induces tissue factor expression in cultured human cardiac valve endothelium. *J Infect Dis.* 1988; 66:3476–3479.
221. Dhawan VK, Yeaman MR, Cheung AL, et al. Phenotypic resistance to thrombin-induced platelet microbiocidal protein in vitro is correlated with enhanced virulence in experimental endocarditis due to *Staphylococcus aureus. Infect Immun* 1997; 65(8):3293–3299.
222. Dhawan VK, et al. In vitro resistance to thrombin-induced platelet microbicidal protein is associated with enhanced progression and hematogenous dissemination in experimental *Staphylococcus aureus* infective endocarditis. *Infect Immun* 1998; 66(7):3476–3479.
223. Bayer AS, Ramos MD, Menzies BE, et al. Hyperproduction of alpha-toxin by *Staphylococcus aureus* results in paradoxically reduced virulence in experimental endocarditis: A host defense role for platelet microbicidal proteins. *Infect Immun* 1997; 65(11):4652–4660.
224. Korzeniowski OM, Sande MA. Personal communication.
225. Kupferwasser LI, et al. Acetylsalicylic acid reduces vegetation bacterial density, hematogenous bacterial dissemination, and frequency of embolic events in experimental *Staphylococcus aureus* endocarditis through antiplatelet and antibacterial effects. *Circulation* 1999; 99(21):2791–2797.
226. Capo C, Zugun F, Stein A, et al. Upregulation of tumor necrosis factor alpha and Interleukin-1 beta in Q fever endocarditis. *Infect Immun* 1996; 64:1638–1642.
227. Lepeschkin E. On the relation between the site of valvular involvement in endocarditis and the blood pressure resting on the valve. *Am J Med Sci* 1952; 224:318–319.
228. Rodbard S. Blood velocity and endocarditis. *Circulation* 1963; 27:18–28.
229. Edwards JE, Burchell HB. Endocardial and intimal lesions (jet impact) as possible sites of origin of murmurs. *Circulation* 1958; 18:946–960.
230. Buchbinder NA, Roberts WC. Left-sided valvular active infective endocarditis: A study of forty-five necropsy patients. *Am J Med* 1972; 53:20–35.
231. Scully RE, Mark EJ, McNeely WF, McNeely BU. Case records of the Massachusetts General Hospital. *N Engl J Med* 1996; 334:105–111.
232. McFarland MM. Pathology of infective endocarditis. In: Kaye D, ed. *Infective Endocarditis,* 2d ed. New York: Raven Press; 1992:57–83.
233. DiNubile MJ, Calderwood SB, Steinhaus DM, Karchmer AW. Cardiac conduction abnormalities complicating native valve active endocarditis. *Am J Cardiol* 1986; 58:1213–1217.
234. Phair JP, Clarke J. Immunology of infective endocarditis. *Prog Cardiovasc Dis* 1977; 22:137–144.
235. Williams RC, Kunkel HG. Rheumatoid factor, complement, and conglutinin aberrations in patients with subacute bacterial endocarditis. *J Clin Invest* 1962; 41:666–675.
236. Messner RP, Laxdal T, Quie PG, Williams RC Jr. Rheumatoid factors in subacute bacterial endocarditis—Bacterium, duration of disease or genetic predisposition? *Ann Intern Med* 1968; 68:746–754.
237. Sheagren JN, Tuazon CU, Griffin C, Padmore N. Rheumatoid factor in acute bacterial endocarditis. *Arthritis Rheum* 1976; 19:887–890.
238. Maisch B, Eichstadt H, Kochsick K. Immune reactions in infective endocarditis: I. Clinical data and diagnostic relevance of antimyocardial antibodies. *Am Heart J* 1983; 106:329–337.
239. Weinstein L, Schlesinger JJ. Pathoanatomic, pathophysiologic

and clinical correlations in endocarditis. (First of two parts.) *N Engl J Med* 1974; 291:832–837.
240. Wadsworth AB. A study of the endocardial lesions developing during pneumococcus infection in horses. *J Med Res* 1919; 34:280–291.
241. Mair W. Pneumococcal endocarditis in rabbits. *J Pathol Bacteriol* 1923; 26:426–428.
242. Durack DT, Gilliland BC, Petersdorf RG. Effect of immunization on susceptibility to experimental *Streptococcus mutans* and *Streptococcus sanguis* endocarditis. *Infect Immun* 1978; 22:52–56.
243. Durack DT, Beeson PB. Pathogenesis of infective endocarditis. In: Rahimtoola SH, ed. *Infective Endocarditis.* New York: Grune & Stratton; 1978:1–53.
244. Bayer AS, Theofilopoulos AN, Eisenberg R, et al. Circulating immune complexes in infective endocarditis. *N Engl J Med* 1976; 295:1500–1505.
245. Bayer AS, Theofilopoulos AN, Tillman DB, et al. Use of circulating immune complex levels in the serodifferentiation of endocarditic and nonendocarditic septicemias. *Am J Med* 1979; 66:58–62.
246. Maisch B, Mayer E, Schubert U, et al. Immune reactions in infective endocarditis: II. Relevance of circulating immune complexes, serum inhibition factors, lymphocytotoxic reactions, and antibody-dependent cellular cytotoxicity against cardiac target cells. *Am Heart J* 1983; 106:338–344.
247. Cabane J, Godeau P, Hereeman A, et al. Fate of circulating immune complexes in infective endocarditis. *Am J Med* 1979; 66:277–282.
248. Gutman RA, Striker GE, Gilliland BC, Cutler RE. The immune complex glomerulonephritis of bacterial endocarditis. *Medicine* 1972; 51:1–25.
249. Levy RL, Hong R. The immune nature of subacute bacterial endocarditis (SBE) nephritis. *Am J Med* 1973; 54:645–652.
250. Nagel JG, Tuazon CU, Cardella TA, Sheagren JN. Teichoic acid serologic diagnosis of staphylococcal endocarditis: Use of gel diffusion and counterimmunoelectrophoretic methods. *Ann Intern Med* 1975; 82:13–17.
251. Freedman LR, Valone J Jr. Experimental infective endocarditis. *Prog Cardiovasc Dis* 1979; 22:169–180.
252. Contrepois A. Notes on the history of experimental endocarditis. *Clin Infect Dis* 1995; 20:461–466.
253. Durack DT, Beeson PB. Experimental bacterial endocarditis: II. Survival of bacteria in endocardial vegetations. *Br J Exp Pathol* 1972; 53:50–53.
254. Durack DT. Experience with prevention of experimental endocarditis. In: Kaplan EL, Taranta AV, eds. *Infective Endocarditis: An American Heart Association Symposium.* American Heart Association Monograph No. 52. Dallas: American Heart Association, 1977:28–32.
255. Churchill MA Jr, Geraci JE, Hunder GG. Musculoskeletal manifestations of bacterial endocarditis. *Ann Intern Med* 1977; 87:754–759.
256. Starkebaum MK, Durack DT, Beeson PB. The "incubation period" of subacute bacterial endocarditis. *Yale J Biol Med* 1977; 50:49–58.
257. Karchmer AW. Staphylococcal endocarditis. In: Kaye D, ed. *Infective Endocarditis,* 2d ed. New York: Raven Press; 1992:225–249.
258. Khan MY, Hall WH, Gerding DN. Infective endocarditis in narcotic addicts. *Minn Med* 1975; 83–84.
259. Steckelberg JM, Murphy JG, Wilson WR. Cure rates and long-term prognosis. In: Kaye D, ed. *Infective Endocarditis,* 2d ed. New York: Raven Press, 1992:435–453.
260. Kilpatrick ZM, Greenberg PA, Sanford JP. Splinter hemorrhages—Their clinical significance. *Arch Intern Med* 1965; 115:730–735.
261. Howard EJ. Osler's nodes. *Am Heart J* 1960; 59:633–634.
262. Alpert JS, Krous HF, Dalen JE, et al. Pathogenesis of Osler's nodes. *Ann Intern Med* 1976; 85:471–473.
263. Edwards JE Jr, Foos RY, Montgomerie JZ, Guze LB. Ocular manifestations of *Candida* septicemia: Review of seventy-six cases of hematogenous candida endophthalmitis. *Medicine* 1974; 53:47–75.
264. Cates JE, Christie RV. Subacute bacterial endocarditis: A review of 442 patients treated in 14 centres appointed by the Penicillin Trials Committee of Medical Research Council. *Q J Med* 1951; 20:93–130.
265. Mills J, Utley J, Abbott J. Heart failure in infective endocarditis. *Chest* 1974; 66:151–159.
266. Lytle BW, Priest BP, Taylor PC, et al. Surgical treatment of prosthetic valve endocarditis. *J Thorac Cardiovasc Surg* 1996; 111:198–207.
267. Tanaka M, Abe T, Hosokawa S, et al. Tricuspid valve *Candida* endocarditis cured by valve-sparing debridement. *Ann Thorac Surg* 1989; 48:857–858.
268. Pruett TL, Rotstein OD, Anderson RW, Simmons RL. Tricuspid valve endocarditis: Successful treatment with valve-sparing debridement and antifungal chemotherapy in a multiorgan transplant recipient. *Am J Med* 1986; 80:116–118.
269. Kupferwasser LI, Hafner G, Mohr-Kahaly S, et al. The presence of infection-related antiphospholipid antibodies in infective endocarditis determines a major risk factor for embolic events. *J Am Coll Cardiol* 1999; 33(5):1365–1371.
270. Sokil AB. Cardiac imaging in infective endocarditis. In: Kaye D, ed. *Infective Endocarditis,* 2d ed. New York: Raven Press; 1992:125–150.
271. Ziment I. Nervous system complications in bacterial endocarditis. *Am J Med* 1969; 47:593–607.
272. Pruitt AA, Rubin RH, Karchmer AW, Duncan GW. Neurologic complications of bacterial endocarditis. *Medicine* 1978; 57:329–343.
273. Jones HR Jr, Siekert RG. Neurological manifestations of infective endocarditis: Review of clinical and therapeutic challenges. *Brain* 1989; 112:1295–1315.
274. Francioli P. Central nervous system complications of infective endocarditis. In: Scheld WM, Whitley RJ, Durack DT, eds. *Infections of the Central Nervous System,* 2d ed. New York: Lippincott-Raven, 1997:523–553.
275. Jones HR, Siekert RG, Geraci JE. Neurologic manifestations of bacterial endocarditis. *Ann Intern Med* 1969; 71:21–28.
276. Stengel A, Wolferth CC. Mycotic (bacterial) aneurysms of intravascular origin. *Arch Intern Med* 1923; 31:527–554.
277. Brust JCM, Dickinson PCT, Hughes JEO, Holtzman RNN. The diagnosis and treatment of cerebral mycotic aneurysms. *Ann Neurol* 1990; 27:238–246.
278. Salgado AV, Furlan AJ, Keys TF. Mycotic aneurysm, subarachnoid hemorrhage, and indications for cerebral angiography in infective endocarditis. *Stroke* 1987; 18:1057–1060.
279. Nakata Y, Shionoya S, Kamiya K. Pathogenesis of mycotic aneurysm. *Angiology* 1968; 19:593–601.
280. Masuda J, Yutani C, Waki R, et al. Histopathological analysis of the mechanisms of intracranial hemorrhage complicating infective endocarditis. *Stroke* 1992; 23:843–850.
281. Bamford J, Hodges J, Warlow C. Late rupture of a mycotic aneurysm after "cure" of bacterial endocarditis. *J Neurol* 1986; 233:51–53.
282. Bush LM, Johnson CC. Clinical syndrome and diagnosis. In: Kaye D, ed. *Infective Endocarditis,* 2d ed. New York: Raven Press; 1992:99–115.
283. Durack DT, Street AC. Fever of unknown origin—Reexamined and redefined. *Curr Clin Top Infect Dis* 1991; 11:35–51.
284. von Reyn CF, Levy BS, Arbeit RD, et al. Infective endocarditis: An analysis based on strict case definitions. *Ann Intern Med* 1981; 94:505–517.

285. Dajani AS, Ayoub E, Bierman FZ, et al. Guidelines for the diagnosis of rheumatic fever: Jones criteria, 1992 update. *JAMA* 1992; 268:2069–2073.
286. Dodds GA, Sexton DJ, Durack DT, et al. Negative predictive value of the Duke criteria for infective endocarditis. *Am J Cardiol* 1996; 77:403–407.
287. Kaye MM, Kaye D. Laboratory findings including blood cultures. In: Kaye D, ed. *Infective Endocarditis,* 2d ed. New York: Raven Press; 1992:117–124.
288. Powers DL, Mandell GL. Intraleukocytic bacteria in endocarditis patients. *JAMA* 1974; 227:312–313.
289. Engle RL, Koprowska I. The appearance of histiocytes in blood in subacute bacterial endocarditis. *Am J Med* 1959; 26:965–973.
290. Hogevik H, Olaison L, Andersson R, et al. C-reactive protein is more sensitive than erythrocyte sedimentation rate for diagnosis of infective endocarditis. *Infection* 1997; 25(2):82–85.
291. Agarwal A, Clements J, Sedmak DD, et al. Subacute bacterial endocarditis masquerading as type III essential mixed cryoglobulinemia. *J Am Soc Nephrol,* 1997; 8(12):1971–1976.
292. Fournier PE, Casalta JP, Habib G, et al. Modification of the diagnostic criteria proposed by the Duke Endocarditis Service to permit improved diagnosis of Q fever endocarditis. *Am J Med* 1996; 100:629–633.
293. Belli J, Waisbren BA. The number of blood cultures necessary to diagnose most cases of bacterial endocarditis. *Am J Med Sci* 1956; 232:284–288.
294. Werner AS, Cobbs CG, Kaye D, Hook EW. Studies on the bacteremia of bacterial endocarditis. *JAMA* 1967; 202:127–131.
295. Ellner JJ, Rosenthal MS, Lerner PI, McHenry M. Infective endocarditis caused by slow-growing, fastidious, gram-negative bacteria. *Medicine* 1979; 58:145–158.
296. Gerry JL, Greenough WB. Diphtheroid endocarditis: Report of nine cases and review of the literature. *Johns Hopkins Med J* 1976; 139:61–68.
297. Zbinden R, Hany A, Luthy R, et al. Antibody response in six HACEK endocarditis cases under therapy. *APMIS* 1998; 106(5):547–552.
298. Patel R, Newell J, Procop GW, et al. Use of polymerase chain reaction for citrate synthase gene to diagnose Bartonella quintana endocarditis. *Am J Clin Path* 1999; 112(1):36–40.
299. Goldenberger D, Kunzli A, Vogt P, et al. Molecular diagnosis of bacterial endocarditis by broad-range PCR amplification and direct sequencing. *J Clin Microbiol* 1997; 35(11):2733–2739.
300. Das I, De Giovanni JV, Gray J. Endocarditis caused by *Haemophilus parainfluenzae* identified by 16s ribosomal RNA sequencing. *J Clin Path* 1997; 50(1):72–74.
301. Stewart JA, Silimperi D, Harris P, et al. Echocardiographic documentation of vegetative lesions in infective endocarditis: Clinical implications. *Circulation* 1980; 61:374–380.
302. Mugge A, Daniel WG, Frank G, Lichtlen PR. Echocardiography in infective endocarditis: Reassessment of prognostic implications of vegetation size determined by the transthoracic and transesophageal approach. *J Am Coll Cardiol* 1989; 14:631–638.
303. Pavlides GS, Hauser AM, Stewart JR, et al. Contribution of transesophageal echocardiography to patient diagnosis and treatment: A prospective analysis. *Am Heart J* 1990; 120:910–914.
304. Daniel WG, Mugge A, Martin RP, et al. Improvement in the diagnosis of abscesses associated with endocarditis by transesophageal echocardiography. *N Engl J Med* 1991; 324:795–800.
305. Dodds GAI, Durack DT. Criteria for the diagnosis of endocarditis and the role of echocardiography. *Echocardiography* 1995; 12:663–668.
306. De Castro S, d'Amati G, Cartoni D, et al. Valvular perforation in left-sided infective endocarditis: a prospective echocardiographic evaluation and clinical outcome. *Am Heart J* 1997; 134:656–664.
307. Aly AM, Simpson PM, Humes RA. The role of transthoracic echocardiography in the diagnosis of infective endocarditis in children [in process citation]. *Arch Pediatr Adoles Med* 1999; 153:950–954.
308. Morguet AJ, Werner GS, Andreas S, Kreuzer H. Diagnostic value of transesophageal compared with transthoracic echocardiography in suspected prosthetic valve endocarditis. *Herz* 1995; 20:390–398.
309. Lengyel M. The impact of transesophageal echocardiography on the management of prosthetic valve endocarditis: Experience of 31 cases and review of the literature. *J Heart Valv Dis* 1997; 6:204–211.
310. Lindner JR, Case RA, Dent JM, et al. Diagnostic value of echocardiography in suspected endocarditis: An evaluation based on the pretest probability of disease. *Circulation* 1996; 93:730–736.
311. Fowler VG, Li J, Corey GR, et al. Role of echocardiography in evaluation of patients with *Staphylococcus aureus* bacteremia: experience in 103 patients. *J Am Coll Cardiol* 1997; 30:1072–1078.
312. Tischler MD, Vaitkus PT, et al. The ability of vegetation size on echocardiography to predict clinical complications: A meta-analysis. *J Echocardiog* 1997; 10:562–568.
313. Fowler VG, Sanders LL, Kong LK, et al. Infective endocarditis due to *Staphylococcus aureus*: 59 prospectively identified cases with follow-up. *Clin Infec Dis* 1999; 28(1):106–114.
314. Lancellotti P, Galiuto L, Albert A, et al. Relative value of clinical and transesophageal echocardiographic variables for risk stratification in patients with infective endocarditis. *Clin Cardiol* 1998; 21(8):572–578.
315. De Castro S, Magni G, Beni S, et al. Role of transthoracic and transesophageal echocardiography in predicting embolic events in patients with active infective endocarditis involving native cardiac valves. *Am J Cardiol* 1997; 80(8):1030–1034.
316. Gillinov AM, Shah RV, Curtis WE, et al. Valve replacement in patients with endocarditis and acute neurologic deficit. *Ann Thorac Surg* 1996; 61:1125–1129.
317. Moriarty JA, Edelman RR, Tumeh SS. CT and MRI of mycotic aneurysms of the abdominal aorta. *J Comput Assist Tomogr* 1992; 16:941–943.
318. Welton DE, Young JB, Raizner AE, et al. Value and safety of cardiac catheterization during active infective endocarditis. *Am J Cardiol* 1979; 44:1306–1310.
319. Riba AL, Thakur ML, Gottschalk A, et al. Imaging experimental infective endocarditis with indium-111–labeled blood cellular components. *Circulation* 1979; 59:336–343.
320. Campeau RJ, Ingram C. Perivalvular abscess complicating infective endocarditis: Complementary role of echocardiography and Indium-111–Labeled leukocytes. *J Clin Nucl Med* 1998; 23:582–584.
321. Ben-Haim S, Seabold JE, Hawes DR, Rooholamini SA. Leukocyte scintigraphy in the diagnosis of mycotic aneurysm. *J Nuc Med* 1992; 33:1486–1493.
322. Olaison L, Belin L, Hogevik H, et al. Incidence of beta-lactam-induced delayed hypersensitivity and neutropenia during treatment of infective endocarditis. *Arch Intern Med* 1999; 159(6):607–615.
323. Wilson WR, Karchmer A, Dajani A, et al. Antibiotic treatment of adults with infective endocarditis due to viridans streptococci, enterococci, staphylococci and HACEK microorganisms. *JAMA* 1995; 274:1706–1713.
324. Chambers HF, Miller RT, Newman MD. Right sided Staphylococcus aureus endocarditis in intravenous drug abusers: Two-week combination therapy. *Ann Intern Med* 1988; 109:619–624.
325. Wilson WR, Geraci JE, Wilkowske CJ, Washington JA. Short-term intramuscular therapy with procaine penicillin plus streptomycin for infective endocarditis due to *Viridans* streptococci. *Circulation* 1978; 57:1158–1161.
326. Baldassare JS, Kaye D. Principles and overview of antibiotic therapy. In: Kaye D, ed. *Infective Endocarditis.* 2d ed. New York: Raven Press; 1992:169–190.

327. Blount JG. Bacterial endocarditis. *Am J Med* 1965; 38:909–922.
328. Pulliam L, Inokuchi S, Hadley WK, Mills J. Penicillin tolerance in experimental streptococcal endocarditis. *Lancet* 1979; 2:957.
329. Denny AE, Peterson LR, Gerding DN, Hall WH. Serious staphylococcal infections with strains tolerant to bactericidal antibiotics. *Arch Intern Med* 1979; 139:1026–1031.
330. Brennan RO, Durack DT. Therapeutic significance of penicillin tolerance in experimental streptococcal endocarditis. *Antimicrob Agents Chemother* 1983; 23:273–277.
331. Reller LB. The serum bactericidal test. *Rev Infect Dis* 1986; 8:803–808.
332. MacGowan A, McMullin C, James P, et al. External quality assessment of the serum bactericidal test: Results of a methodology/interpretation questionnaire. *J Antimicrob Chemother* 1997; 39(2):277–284.
333. Kane LW, Finn JJ. The treatment of subacute bacterial endocarditis with aureomycin and chloromycetin. *N Engl J Med* 1951; 244:623–628.
334. Schein J, Baehr G. Sulfonamide therapy of subacute bacterial endocarditis. *Am J Med* 1948; 4:66–72.
335. Korzeniowski O, Sande MA, National Collaborative Endocarditis Study Group. Combination antimicrobial therapy for *Staphylococcus aureus* endocarditis in patients addicted to parenteral drugs and in nonaddicts: A prospective study. *Ann Intern Med* 1982; 97:496–503.
336. Martinez F, Martin-Luengo F, Garcia A, Valdes M. Treatment with various antibiotics of experimental endocarditis caused by penicillin-resistant *Streptococcus sanguis*. *Eur Heart J* 1995; 16:687–691.
337. Doern GV, Ferraro MJ, Brueggmann AB, Ruoff KL. Emergence of high rates of antimicrobial resistance among viridans group streptococci in the United States. *Antimicrob Agents Chemother* 1996; 40:891–894.
338. Johnson AP, Warner M, Woodford N, et al. Antibiotic resistance among enterococci causing endocarditis in the UK: Analysis of isolates referred to a reference laboratory. *Br Med J* 1998; 317:629–630.
339. Brandt CM, Rouse MS, Laue NW, et al. Effective treatment of multidrug-resistant enterococcal experimental endocarditis with combinations of cell wall-active agents. *J Infect Dis* 1996; 173:909–913.
340. Antony SJ, Ladner J, Stratton CW, et al. High-level aminoglycoside-resistant enterococcus causing endocarditis successfully treated with a combination of ampicillin, imipenem and vancomycin. *Scand J Infec Dis* 1997; 29(6):628–630.
341. Tripodi MF, Locatelli A, Adinolfi LE, et al. Successful treatment with ampicillin and fluoroquinolones of human endocarditis due to high-level gentamicin-resistant enterococci. *Eur J Clin Microbiol Infect Dis* 1998; 17(10):734–736.
342. Matsumura S, Simor AE. Treatment of endocarditis due to vancomycin-resistant Enterococcus faecium with quinupristin/dalfopristin, doxycycline, and rifampin: A synergistic drug combination. *Clin Infect Dis* 1998; 27(6):1554–1556.
343. Landman D, Quale JM; Management of infections due to resistant enterococci: A review of therapeutic options. *J Antimicrob Chemother* 1997; 40(2):161–170.
344. Francioli P, Etienne J, Hoigne R, et al. Treatment of streptococcal endocarditis with a single daily dose of ceftriaxone sodium for 4 weeks: Efficacy and outpatient treatment feasibility. *JAMA* 1992; 267:264–267.
345. Stamboulian D, Bonvehi P, Arevalo C, et al. Antibiotic management of outpatients with endocarditis due to penicillin-susceptible streptococci. *Rev Infect Dis* 1991; 13:S160–S163.
346. Rehm SJ. Outpatient intravenous antibiotic therapy for endocarditis. *Infect Dis Clin N Am* 1998; 12(4):879–901.
347. Aranki SF, Adams DH, Rizzo RJ, et al. Determinants of early mortality and late survival in mitral valve endocarditis. *Circulation* 1995; 92:143–149.
348. Douglas JL, Dismukes WE. Surgical therapy of infective endocarditis on natural valves. In: Kaye D, ed. *Infective Endocarditis*, 2d ed. New York: Raven Press; 1992:397–411.
349. Durack DT. Nine controversies in the management of endocarditis. In: Petersdorf RG, ed. *Update V: Harrison's Principles of Internal Medicine*. New York: McGraw-Hill; 1984:35–45.
350. Vlessis AA, Hovaguimian H, Jaggers J, et al. Infective endocarditis: Ten year review of medical and surgical therapy. *Ann Thorac Surg* 1996; 61:1217–1222.
351. Muehrcke D, Lytle BW, Cosgrove DM III. Surgical and long-term antifungal therapy for fungal prosthetic valve endocarditis. *Ann Thorac Surg* 1996; 60:538–543.
352. Glazier JJ, Verwilghen J, Donaldson RM, Ross DN. Treatment of complicated prosthetic aortic valve endocarditis with annular abscess formation by homograft aortic root replacement. *J Am Coll Cardiol* 1991; 17:1177–1182.
353. Joyce F, Tingleff J, Pettersson G. Expanding indications for the Ross operation. *J Heart Valve Dis* 1995; 4:352–363.
354. Joyce F, Tingleff J, Pettersson G. The Ross operation: Results of early experience including treatment for endocarditis. *Eur J Cardiothorac Surg* 1989; 9:384–392.
355. Hughes CF, Noble N. Vegetectomy: An alternative surgical treatment for infective endocarditis of the atrioventricular valves in drug addicts. *J Thorac Cardiovasc Surg* 1988; 95:857–861.
356. Katz LN, Elek SR. Combined heparin and chemotherapy in subacute bacterial endocarditis. *JAMA* 1944; 124:149–152.
357. Wilson WR, Geraci JE, Danielson GK, et al. Anticoagulant therapy and central nervous system complications in patients with prosthetic valve endocarditis. *Circulation* 1978; 57:1004–1007.
358. Kanis JA. The use of anticoagulants in bacterial endocarditis. *Postgrad Med J* 1974; 50:312–313.
359. Tornos P, Almirante B, Mirabet S, et al. Infective endocarditis due to Staphylococcus aureus: Deleterious effect of anticoagulant therapy. *Arch Intern Med* 1999; 159(5):473–475.
360. Nicolau DP, Marangos MN, Nightingale CH, Quintiliani R. Influence of aspirin on development and treatment of experimental *Staphylococcus aureus* endocarditis. *Antimicrob Agents Chemother* 1995; 39:1748–1751.
361. Steckelberg JM, Murphy JG, Ballard D, et al. Emboli in infective endocarditis: The prognostic value of echocardiography. *Ann Intern Med* 1991; 114:635–640.
362. Conlon PJ, Jefferies F, Krigman HR, et al. Predictors of prognosis and risk of acute renal failure in bacterial endocarditis. *Clin Neph* 1998; 49(2):96–101.
363. Ahern H. Cellular responses to oxidative stress: Extensively studied bacterial systems provide insights into more complex systems and, potentially, human diseases. *ASM News* 1991; 57:627–630.
364. Lu VL, Fang GD, Keys TF, et al. Prosthetic valve endocarditis: Superiority of surgical valve replacement versus medical therapy only. *Ann Thorac Surg* 1994; 58:1073–1077.
365. Ormiston JA, Neutze JM, Agnew TM, et al. Infective endocarditis: A lethal disease. *Aust NZ J Med* 1981; 11:620–629.
366. Welton DE, Young JB, Gentry WO, et al. Recurrent infective endocarditis: Analysis of predisposing factors and clinical features. *Am J Med* 1979; 66:932–938.
367. Everett ED, Hirschmann JV. Transient bacteremia and endocarditis prophylaxis: A review. *Medicine* 1977; 56:61–77.
368. Sullivan NM, Sutter VL, Mims MM, et al. Clinical aspects of bacteremia after manipulation of the genitourinary tract. *J Infect Dis* 1973; 127:49–55.
369. Shorvon PJ, Eykyn SJ, Cotton PB. Gastrointestinal instrumentation, bacteraemia, and endocarditis. *Gut* 1983; 24:1078–1093.
370. Durack DT. Prevention of infective endocarditis. *N Engl J Med* 1995; 332:38–44.
371. Dajani AS, Taubert KA, Wilson WR, et al. Prevention of bacterial

endocarditis: Recommendations by the American Heart Association. *Circulation* 1997; 96:358–366. (*JAMA* 1997; 277:1794–1801)

372. Glauser MP, Francioli P. Relevance of animal models to the prophylaxis of infective endocarditis. *J Antimicrob Chemother* 1987; 20(suppl A):87–93.
373. Horstkotte D, Friedrichs W, Pippert H, Bircks W, Loogen F. Nutzen der Endokarditisprophylaxe bei Patienten mit prothetischen Herzklappen. *Z Kardiol* 1986; 75:8–11.
374. van der Meer JTM, Van Wijk W, Thompson J, et al. Efficacy of antibiotic prophylaxis for prevention of native-valve endocarditis. *Lancet* 1992; 339:135–140.
375. Imperiale TF, Horwitz RI. Does prophylaxis prevent postdental infective endocarditis? A controlled evaluation of protective efficacy. *Am J Med* 1990; 88:131–136.
376. Gould IM, Buckingham JK. Cost effectiveness of prophylaxis in dental practice to prevent infective endocarditis. *Br Heart J* 1993; 70:79–83.

PART THIRTEEN

THE HEART, ANESTHESIA, AND SURGERY

CHAPTER 74

PERIOPERATIVE EVALUATION AND MANAGEMENT OF PATIENTS WITH KNOWN OR SUSPECTED CARDIOVASCULAR DISEASE WHO UNDERGO NONCARDIAC SURGERY

David S. Bach / Kim A. Eagle

Each year in the United States, approximately 25 million patients undergo noncardiac surgery. Of these, approximately 50,000 patients suffer perioperative myocardial infarction, and more than half of 40,000 perioperative deaths are caused by cardiac events.[1-3] As the population of the United States continues to age over the next several decades, both the total number and the percentage of patients who are over 65 years of age will increase. These patients represent the largest group in whom surgeries are performed, a group in whom approximately a quarter of surgeries are associated with significant risk of cardiac morbidity and death, and a group at increased risk for the presence of cardiac disease. As such, an increasing number of patients with significant perioperative risk can be expected to undergo noncardiac surgery.

Most perioperative cardiac morbidity and deaths are related to myocardial ischemia, congestive heart failure, or arrhythmia. Therefore, preoperative evaluation and perioperative management to reduce morbidity and mortality rates emphasize the detection, characterization, and treatment of coronary artery disease, left ventricular systolic dysfunction, and significant arrhythmias. However, not all patients with underlying cardiac disease are at significantly increased perioperative risk of a morbid cardiac event. The goals of preoperative evaluation are therefore twofold: first, to identify patients at increased risk of an adverse perioperative cardiac event and, second, to identify patients with a poor long-term prognosis due to cardiovascular disease who come to medical attention only because of other disease leading to noncardiac surgery. In this sense, the preoperative evaluation represents an opportunity to identify and treat patients, thereby affecting long-term prognosis, even though their risk at the time of noncardiac surgery may not be prohibitive.

Preoperative evaluation can identify many patients at increased risk of an adverse cardiac event, and perioperative management can affect that risk. The internist and cardiologist, therefore, play a vital role in the evaluation and management of patients before and during noncardiac surgery. This chapter reviews available data and recommendations for the preoperative evaluation and perioperative management of patients with known or suspected cardiovascular disease undergoing noncardiac surgery. However, the nature of preoperative evaluation and perioperative management should be individualized to the patient and the clinical scenario surrounding surgery. Patients presenting with an acute surgical emergency mandate only a rapid preoperative assessment, with subsequent management directed at preventing or minimizing cardiac morbidity and death. Among such patients, a more thorough evaluation can often be performed after surgery. In contrast, patients undergoing an elective procedure with no surgical urgency can undergo a more thorough preoperative evaluation. Among patients presenting for cardiac evaluation prior to "same-day" elective surgery, perioperative risk to the patient must be weighed against the impact of additional testing and cancellation or delay of the surgical procedure.

CLINICAL DETERMINANTS OF PERIOPERATIVE CARDIOVASCULAR RISK

The majority of patients at increased risk of adverse perioperative cardiac events can be identified using simple, clinically assessable features. Specifically, a careful history, physical examination, and review of the resting 12-lead electrocardiogram (ECG) are usually sufficient to allow stratification of most patients into low, intermediate, or high risk for an adverse perioperative cardiac event. A number of investigators have established readily accessible clinical markers that predict increased perioperative risk of myocardial infarction, congestive heart failure, or death.[4–14] Some investigators have used a quantitative scoring system to rank the importance of individual risk factors.[4,12,14] The advantage of such systems rest with the observation that some clinical features are stronger predictors of perioperative risk than are others. At the time of this writing, current recommendations of the American College of Cardiology (ACC) and the American Heart Association (AHA)[15] designate risks factors as belonging to three groups: major, intermediate, and minor (Table 74-1). Using these guidelines, greater weight is given for active than for quiescent disease, and the severity of disease is used to modify its importance.

TABLE 74-1 Clinical Predictors of Increased Perioperative Cardiovascular Risk (Myocardial Infarction, Congestive Heart Failure, Death)

MAJOR
Unstable coronary syndromes
Recent myocardial infarction[a] with evidence of important ischemic risk by clinical symptoms or noninvasive study
Unstable or severe[b] angina (Canadian class III or IV)[c]
Decompensated congestive heart failure
Significant arrhythmias
High-grade atrioventricular block
Symptomatic ventricular arrhythmias in the presence of underlying heart disease
Supraventricular arrhythmias with uncontrolled ventricular rate
Severe valvular disease
INTERMEDIATE
Mild angina pectoris (Canadian class I or II)
Prior myocardial infarction by history or pathologic Q waves
Compensated or prior congestive heart failure
Diabetes mellitus
MINOR
Advanced age
Abnormal electrocardiogram (left ventricular hypertrophy, left bundle-branch block, ST-T abnormalities)
Rhythm other than sinus (e.g., atrial fibrillation)
Low functional capacity (e.g., inability to climb one flight of stairs with a bag of groceries)
History of stroke
Uncontrolled systemic hypertension

[a]The American College of Cardiology National Database Library defines recent MI as >7 days but ≤1 month (30 days).
[b]May include "stable" angina in patients who are unusually sedentary.
[c]Campeau L. Grading of angina pectoris. *Circulation* 1976:54:522–523

History

Historical features are important in the identification of patients at increased perioperative cardiac risk. Because most perioperative morbidity and deaths are related to myocardial ischemia, congestive heart failure, and arrhythmias, the assessment of historical risk factors relies heavily on the recognition of coronary artery disease, left ventricular dysfunction, and significant arrhythmias. Risk factors recognized as predictive of increased perioperative risk[15] include advanced age, poor functional capacity, and prior history of coronary artery disease, congestive heart failure, arrhythmia, valvular heart disease, diabetes mellitus, uncontrolled systemic hypertension, and stroke. Coronary artery disease is a major risk factor in the setting of recent myocardial infarction or unstable or severe angina pectoris, and an intermediate risk factor in the setting of mild stable angina pectoris or remote myocardial infarction. Similarly, congestive heart failure is a major risk factor if decompensated and an intermediate risk factor if compensated. A history of arrhythmias may be a major, intermediate, or minor risk factor, depending on the nature and severity of the arrhythmia as well as the presence of underlying heart disease.

A patient's preoperative functional capacity significantly influences the assessment of perioperative cardiac risk. Good functional capacity in an asymptomatic patient predicts low perioperative risk despite the presence of other risk factors. Impaired functional capacity is important in three regards in the assessment of perioperative cardiac risk. First, among patients with chronic coronary artery disease and among those following an acute cardiac event, poor functional capacity is associated with an increased risk of subsequent cardiac morbidity and death.[16] Second, many of the historical features that predict increased perioperative risk assume physical activity. Because most symptoms of cardiac disease are either associated exclusively with or exacerbated by increased physical activity, significant noncardiac limitations in physical capacity are associated with inherent problems in the ability to detect symptoms of and thereby diagnose underlying cardiac diseases. Finally, poor functional capacity is associated with impaired conditioning and therefore a lesser ability to accommodate the cardiovascular stresses that may accompany noncardiac surgery. Because the ability to perform tasks in daily activities correlates well with maximal oxygen uptake on treadmill testing, the assessment of functional capacity on preoperative history is an important feature in the assessment of perioperative risk.

Physical Examination

Features on physical examination may be useful in assessment of perioperative risk. Patients with uncontrolled systemic hypertension should be identified and treated. Because congestive heart failure[4,15,17] and valvular heart disease[4,15,17] are associated with increased risk, physical findings suggestive of these diagnoses should be sought. Elevated jugular venous pressure, pulmonary rales, positive hepatojugular reflux, or a third heart sound on physical examination identify patients with hypervolemia. Patients with aortic stenosis can be identified by a typical murmur with diminished and delayed upstroke of the carotid or brachial pulse. Other cardiac murmurs on physical examination may help identify patients with other forms of valvular heart disease. Patients with mitral stenosis, mitral regurgitation, or aortic regurgitation may be at increased perioperative risk of developing congestive heart failure in the setting of sufficiently severe disease, as well as increased risk of infective endocarditis. Finally, the presence of carotid or other vascular bruits helps identify patients at increased risk of occult coronary artery disease.

Comorbid Diseases

A patient's overall health affects perioperative cardiovascular risk; associated medical conditions may exacerbate risk or complicate perioperative cardiac management. Patients with diabetes mellitus have an increased risk of concomitant coronary artery disease, and the possibility of silent ischemia complicates both the preoperative recognition of coronary artery disease and the perioperative recognition of ischemia. Patients with either restrictive or obstructive pulmonary disease are at increased risk of perioperative respiratory complications, and the associated hypoxemia, hypercapnea, acidosis, and increased work of breathing can exacerbate cardiac stress and precipitate myocardial ischemia. Patients with preexisting renal dysfunction may be predisposed to volume retention in the perioperative period, and hypovolemia may lead to renal hypoperfusion and thereby exacerbate renal dysfunction. Patients with anemia of any cause are at increased risk of myocardial ischemia and congestive heart failure, mediated by increased cardiac stress and increased cardiac work. Optimization of management and control of noncardiac conditions may therefore reduce the risk of cardiac morbidity in the perioperative period.

Surgery-Specific Risks

Perioperative cardiac risk is related in two ways to the type of noncardiac surgery being performed. First, some types of noncardiac surgery identify a group of patients at increased risk for concomitant cardiac disease based on shared risk factors that predispose patients for both noncardiac and cardiac disease. The most notable example of this relationship is seen with peripheral vascular surgery and coronary artery disease. In this case, the same factors that result in clinical peripheral arterial occlusive disease also predispose to the development of coronary artery disease. Among such patients, coronary artery disease may be known or occult, with no symptoms because of the physical limitations associated with surgical peripheral vascular disease. Second, the nature of noncardiac surgery is such that different types of surgery are associated with variable degrees of cardiac stress, mediated by fluctuations in heart rate, blood pressure, intravascular volume, and oxygenation as well as the cardiac stresses associated with duration of the procedure, pain, and neurohumeral activation.[4,5,11,12,18–21] Emergency procedures are associated with a two- to fivefold increase in perioperative cardiac risk compared with elective procedures.[1,17] Other types of noncardiac surgery associated with high perioperative risk include aortic and peripheral vascular surgery, and prolonged abdominal, thoracic, or head and neck procedures with large fluid shifts. The ACC/AHA Task Force Report on Perioperative Cardiac Evaluation[15] stratifies noncardiac surgical procedures as high, intermediate, and low cardiac risk (Table 74-2).

TABLE 74-2 Cardiac Risk[a] Stratification For Noncardiac Surgical Procedures

High (Reported Cardiac Risk Often >5%)
Emergent major operations, particularly in the elderly
Aortic and other major vascular
Peripheral vascular
Anticipated prolonged surgical procedures associated with large fluid shifts and/or blood loss
Intermediate (Reported Cardiac Risk Generally <5%)
Carotid endarterectomy
Head and neck
Intraperitoneal and intrathoracic
Orthopedic
Prostate
Low[b] (Reported Cardiac Risk Generally <1%)
Endoscopic procedures
Superficial procedure
Cataract
Breast

[a] Combined incidence of cardiac death and nonfatal myocardial infarction.
[b] Do not generally require further preoperative cardiac testing.
SOURCE: Eagle et al.,[15] with permission.

The perioperative administration of anesthesia can affect the physiology of cardiac function and therefore may affect perioperative cardiac risk. Although there is no one best myocardial protective anesthetic technique,[22–26] differences in anesthetic techniques may favor the use of one over another for individual patients. Opioid-based general anesthesia generally does not affect cardiovascular function, although the commonly employed inhalational agents cause afterload reduction and decreased myocardial contractility. Spinal anesthesia results in sympathetic blockade, with decreases in both preload and afterload and the potential for shifts in both systemic blood pressure and intravascular volume. In general, hemodynamic affects are minimal when spinal anesthesia is used for infrainguinal procedures, whereas higher dermatomal levels of spinal anesthesia required for abdominal procedures may be associated with significant hemodynamic affects, including hypotension and reflex tachycardia. No study has clearly demonstrated any beneficial change in outcome from the use of pulmonary artery catheters, ST-segment monitoring, or transesophageal echocardiography. Decisions regarding specific anesthetic technique and intraoperative monitoring are therefore best left to the anesthesiologists involved in the patient's care.

Clinical Assessment of Perioperative Risk

Patients at very low risk and those at high risk of an adverse perioperative cardiac event typically can be identified using clinically available features described above. Patients at low risk generally require no additional testing prior to noncardiac surgery. Among patients undergoing elective noncardiac sur-

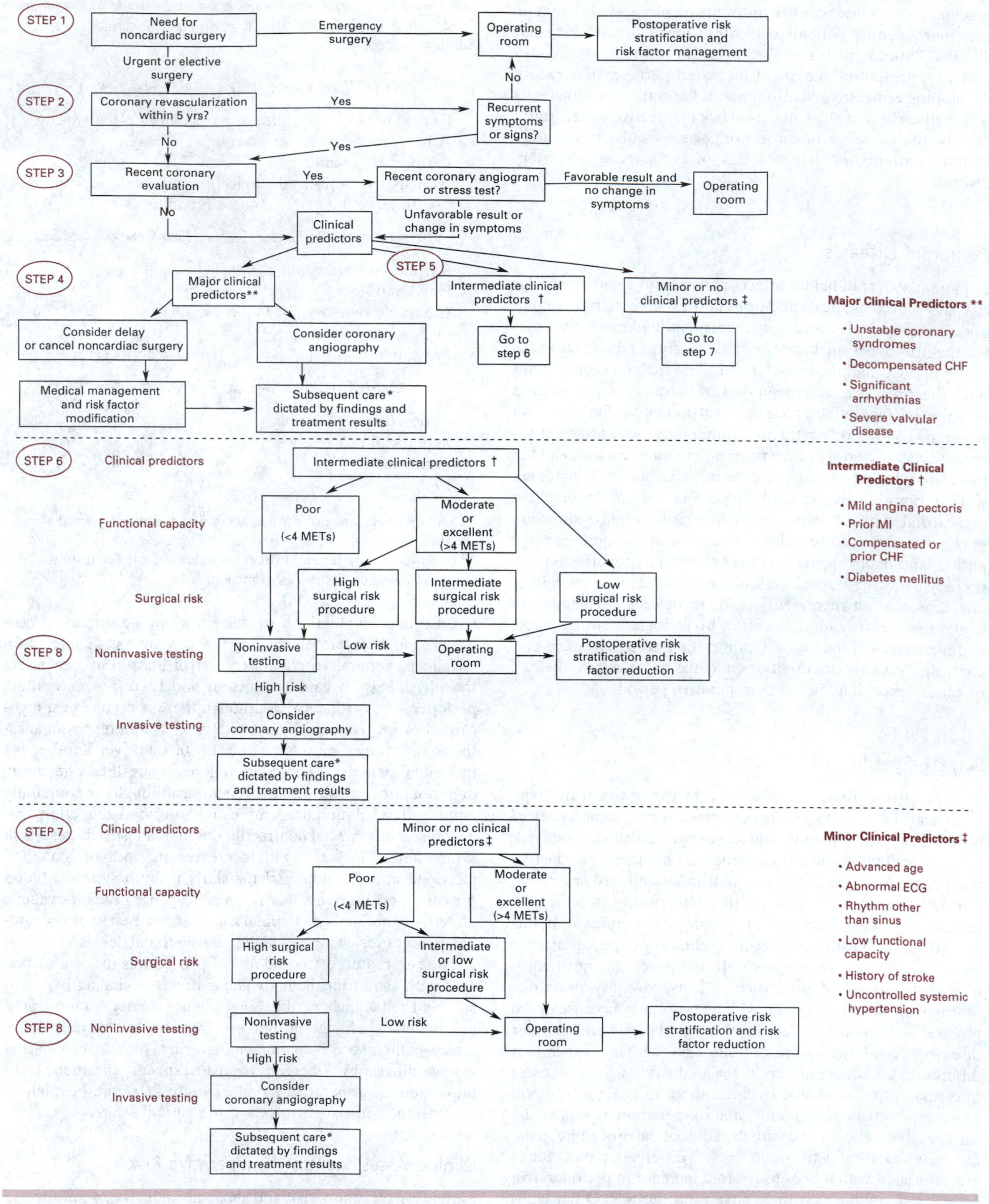

FIGURE 74-1 Stepwise approach to preoperative cardiac assessment. (From Eagle et al.[15] Reproduced with permission from the publisher and authors.) *Subsequent care may include cancellation or delay of surgery, coronary revascularization followed by noncardiac surgery, or intensified care.

gery in whom risk is determined to be intermediate or high, additional testing may be useful to better define risk.[15] It is useful to employ a stepwise approach to the preoperative assessment of cardiac risk (Fig. 74-1). Using this algorithm, the evaluating clinician first determines the urgency of noncardiac surgery. Then, a history of recent coronary revascularization or recent cardiac testing; clinical features, including the presence of major, intermediate, or minor risk factors; estimation of functional capacity; and the nature of the planned surgical procedure are used to determine whether additional testing may be helpful in further defining perioperative cardiac risk. Such testing may include coronary angiography or noninvasive testing to assess for the presence and significance of coronary artery disease.

PREOPERATIVE TESTING

Factors identifiable on history and physical examination and features inherent to a specific noncardiac surgical procedure are usually sufficient to identify patients at very low or at high risk of morbid perioperative cardiac events. Additional testing is useful to better stratify patients with intermediate cardiac risk and to help guide perioperative management in patients at high risk.

Resting Left Ventricular Function

Impaired left ventricular systolic or diastolic function is predictive of perioperative congestive heart failure. The greatest risk of complications occurs among patients with left ventricular ejection fraction of less than 35 percent; among critically ill patients, severely impaired left ventricular systolic function is associated with a higher risk of death. Preoperative left ventricular systolic function can be assessed noninvasively using radionuclide ventriculography or echocardiography, or invasively using contrast ventriculography. Unless recently defined, preoperative assessment of left ventricular systolic function should be performed among patients with poorly controlled congestive heart failure and should be considered among patients with prior congestive heart failure and among patients with dyspnea of unknown cause.

Functional Testing and Risk of Coronary Artery Disease

EXERCISE TESTING

Preoperative cardiac stress testing is useful in the objective assessment of functional capacity, to help identify patients at risk of perioperative myocardial ischemia or cardiac arrhythmias, and to aid in the assessment of long-term as well as perioperative prognosis. In general, poor functional capacity may be due to advanced age, deconditioning, myocardial ischemia or other causes of reduced cardiac reserve, or poor pulmonary reserve. Reduced functional capacity identifies patients at increased risk of subsequent cardiac morbidity and death.[16] Clinical history can be used to estimate functional capacity. In addition, preoperative exercise testing is a useful tool to objectively assess functional capacity as well as to assess hemodynamic response to stress and the potential for stress-induced myocardial ischemia or cardiac arrhythmias.

In a general population, the mean sensitivity and specificity of exercise electrocardiographic studies for the detection of coronary artery disease are 68 and 77 percent, respectively, with reported ranges of sensitivity from 23 to 100 percent and specificity from 17 to 100 percent.[27] The accuracy of exercise electrocardiographic studies for the detection of coronary artery disease is influenced by the prevalence of disease in the population studied, the degree of exercise achieved, and the number, location, and severity of diseased vessels. The mean sensitivity and specificity for the detection of multivessel disease is 81 and 66 percent, respectively.[28] In addition to assessment for the presence of coronary artery disease, exercise testing is useful for the assessment of prognosis. In a large cohort of 4083 medically treated patients in the Coronary Artery Surgery Study,[29] exercise testing was useful for identifying both high-risk and low-risk subgroups of patients. The mortality rate was 5 percent per year or more among a high-risk subset comprising 12 percent of the total population, who were able to achieve an exercise work load less than Bruce stage I and had an abnormal exercise electrocardiogram. In contrast, mortality was less than 1 percent per year among a low-risk subset comprising 34 percent of the total population, who were able to achieve at least Bruce stage III with a normal exercise electrocardiogram. Preoperative exercise testing has been shown to be useful in the prediction of perioperative cardiac risk among patients undergoing peripheral vascular surgery, abdominal aortic aneurysm repair, or other major noncardiac surgery.[30–40] In these published reports, the negative predictive value for perioperative death or myocardial infarction was 91 to 100 percent, with a positive predictive value of 0 to 81 percent.

NONEXERCISE STRESS TESTING

The ability to perform exercise testing for the assessment of coronary artery disease is limited among many patients undergoing preoperative evaluation for noncardiac surgery. Approximately 30 to 50 percent of patients undergoing noncardiac surgery are unable to achieve an adequate exercise work load for a diagnostic study. This is especially problematic among patients with peripheral vascular occlusive disease, in whom the same factors that cause peripheral disease predispose to coronary atherosclerosis; the surgical peripheral vascular disease severely limits exercise tolerance and therefore the ability to perform diagnostic exercise stress testing. For this reason, pharmacologic stress testing may offer advantages in the preoperative testing of some patients undergoing peripheral vascular surgery as well as other patients who are not able to perform adequate physical exercise due to noncardiac limitations in exercise or functional capacity.

Pharmacologic stress testing for the detection of coronary artery disease can be performed using one of two general methods. Infusion of the adrenergic agonist dobutamine results in increases in heart rate, myocardial contractility, and, to a lesser degree, blood pressure, resulting in increased myocardial oxygen demand. In the setting of a limited oxygen supply, increased demand causes myocardial ischemia. Dobutamine infusion is typically used in conjunction with echocardiographic imaging, whereby inducible ischemia is detected as a regional abnormality in left ventricular wall motion. Alternatively, pharmacological "stress" can be achieved using the coronary vasodilators dipyridamole or adenosine. Nuclear perfusion imaging, such as thallium scintigraphic imaging, is typically used in conjunction with dipyridamole and adenosine. Coronary artery disease is detected as abnormal coronary vasodilator reserve, with heterogeneity of perfusion in response to maximal coronary vasodilation.

Dipyridamole thallium scintigraphy has been extensively studied for the assessment of coronary artery disease and perioperative risk among patients undergoing vascular[11,41–56] and other noncardiac surgery.[57–62] Reports published between 1985 and 1994 found a uniformly high negative predictive value for perioperative morbidity associated with normal dipyridamole thallium scintigraphic results, with values ranging from 95 to 100 percent and an average value of approximately 99 percent. The positive predictive value of dipyridamole thallium redistribution for myocardial infarction or death from cardiac causes has been reported to be from 4 to 20 percent among studies including more than 100 patients. More recent studies have lower positive predictive values. However, this probably reflects changes in clinical practice, with alterations in clinical management made in response to the results of an abnormal scan leading to fewer total perioperative cardiac events. There is also important long-term prognostic value associated with preoperative nuclear perfusion imaging,[46,50,63] suggesting that late postoperative risk after uncomplicated noncardiac surgery can also be predicted by preoperative testing.

Although any abnormality on dipyridamole thallium scintigraphy is suggestive of coronary artery disease and is associated with a higher perioperative cardiac risk compared with patients with a normal scan, perioperative cardiac risk associated with a fixed perfusion defect is substantially lower than that associated with perfusion redistribution. In addition, the size of a perfusion defect is directly related to perioperative cardiac risk.[50,51,53] As such, the ability to predict perioperative cardiac risk is improved with the quantification of abnormalities on nuclear perfusion imaging.

Dobutamine stress echocardiography is well established for the noninvasive detection and characterization of coronary artery disease,[64–69] with an accuracy equivalent to that of dipyridamole thallium scintigraphy. Because the technique has evolved more recently than nuclear perfusion imaging, there are fewer studies that evaluate its utility in the assessment of perioperative cardiac risk. However, six studies published since 1991 have evaluated the utility of dobutamine stress echocardiography for preoperative assessment of patients undergoing vascular or other noncardiac surgery.[70–75] Negative predictive values for perioperative events ranged from 93 to 100 percent. Positive predictive values were 17 to 43 percent for any cardiac event and 7 to 23 percent for predicting myocardial infarction or death. As was seen with later studies using nuclear perfusion imaging, most studies of dobutamine stress echocardiography did not blind treating physicians to stress test results, and subsequent alteration of patient management based on abnormal noninvasive test results presumably contributed to a low event rate despite a positive test result. A meta-analysis of preoperative pharmacologic stress tests[76] demonstrated similar power of

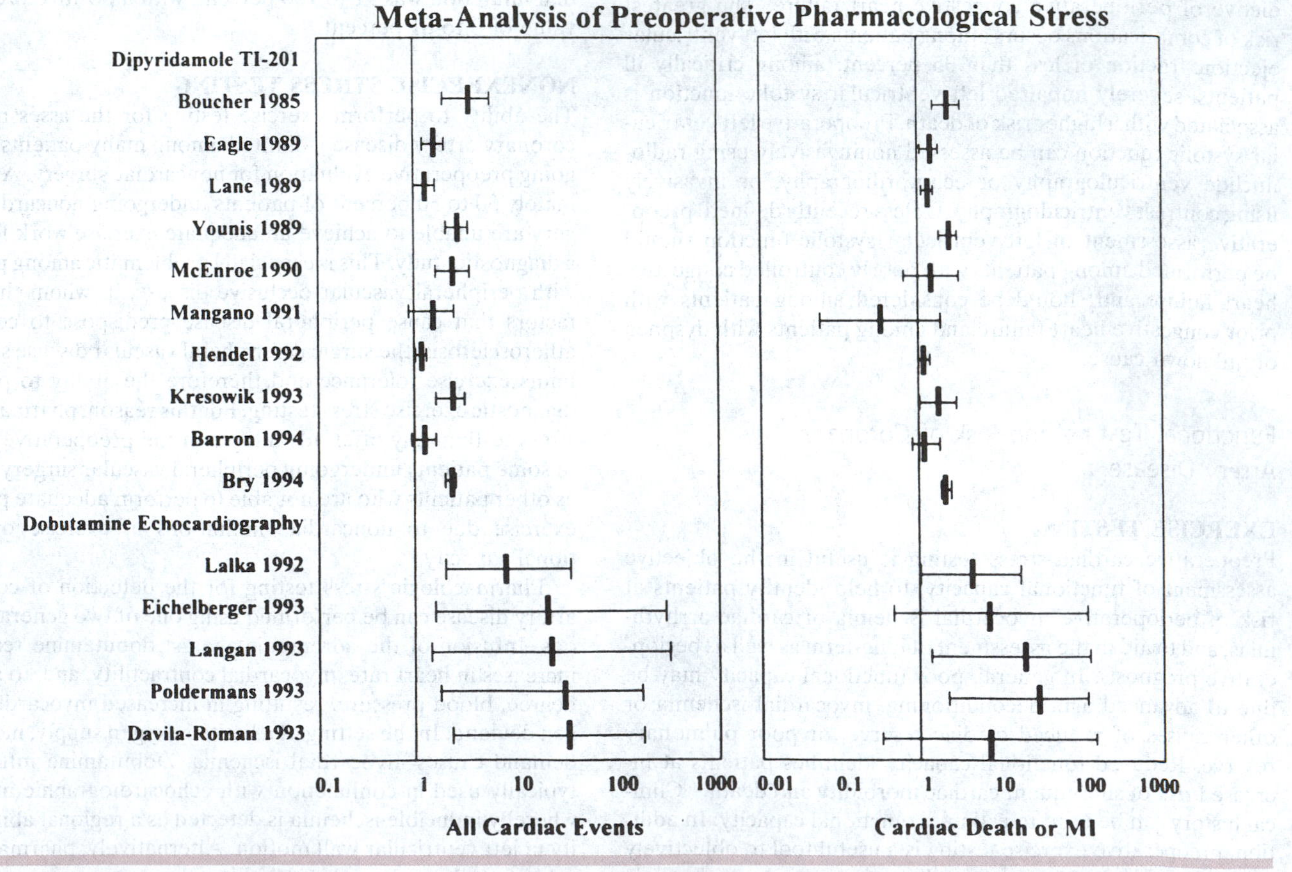

FIGURE 74-2 Univariate odds ratio for intravenous dipyridamole thallium 201 (Tl-201) myocardial perfusion and dobutamine stress echocardiography imaging. The odds ratio for any myocardial ischemic event is depicted on the left and that for cardiac death or nonfatal myocardial infarction on the right. (From Shaw et al.[76] Reproduced with permission from the publisher.)

dobutamine stress echocardiography and dipyridamole thallium scintigraphy in predicting adverse cardiac events after noncardiac surgery (Fig. 74-2).

Because clinical factors are usually able to identify patients at low or at high risk of an adverse cardiac event after noncardiac surgery,[15,21] preoperative stress testing typically has the greatest utility among patients at intermediate risk. Exercise electrocardiographic study allows assessment of functional capacity as well as evaluation for evidence of coronary artery disease based on ST-segment analysis and hemodynamics. Performance of exercise echocardiographic testing or exercise nuclear perfusion imaging should be considered in the presence of significant resting ECG abnormalities that preclude diagnostic testing for coronary artery disease, such as left bundle-branch block, left ventricular hypertrophy with strain, or digitalis effect. Nonexercise stress testing, such as dobutamine stress echocardiographic or dipyridamole thallium scintigraphic studies, should be considered among patients who are unable to perform adequate physical exercise.

FINANCIAL IMPLICATIONS OF NONINVASIVE TESTING

The performance of preoperative noninvasive testing should be based on an assessment of risk and benefit to the patient. In this setting, benefit is defined as the likelihood that testing may alter management and improve outcome because of an adverse perioperative or long-term prognosis. Risk to the patient should include risk associated with additional procedures precipitated by noninvasive testing as well as any risk associated with the noninvasive testing. Although the cost of testing should not play a determining role in the decision, cost must be considered in the present health care environment.

As noted above, clinical features can be used to identify patients at very low risk of an adverse perioperative cardiac event, including asymptomatic patients having undergone coronary revascularization within 5 years as well as those without specific clinical markers for increased risk. Additional testing of selected patients at intermediate or higher risk can potentially reduce the cost of testing without affecting patients' outcomes. Based on a previous study validating the use of selective noninvasive testing before major aortic surgery,[77] the cost implications of selective testing were assessed in the ACC/AHA Task Force report.[15] In the previous study, the application of a clinical algorithm resulted in only 29 percent of 201 patients undergoing noninvasive testing prior to aortic surgery, with an associated 0.5 percent perioperative cardiac mortality rate. Using estimated costs, the use of selected testing was associated with a total cost of $32,886 for 58 patients, compared with an estimated total cost of $113,967 if all 201 had undergone noninvasive screening. The low perioperative mortality rate associated with the use of a clinical algorithm and selected noninvasive testing suggests that substantial cost can be avoided without compromising patients' safety.

PREOPERATIVE THERAPY FOR CORONARY ARTERY DISEASE

Coronary artery disease is responsible for the majority of adverse perioperative cardiac events. Once recognized, specific therapy should be instituted to minimize the risk of perioperative myocardial ischemia, myocardial infarction, or death.

Coronary Revascularization

There are no prospective trials testing the impact of either preoperative coronary artery bypass grafting or percutaneous transluminal coronary angioplasty on perioperative cardiac morbidity and mortality rates. However, several retrospective studies suggest that patients having undergone previous successful surgical coronary revascularization have a low risk of perioperative cardiac events during noncardiac surgery and that the risk of death is comparable to that found among patients with no clinical indications suggestive of coronary artery disease.[78–81]

Although these data support the theory that coronary artery bypass surgery lowers the risk of adverse cardiac events associated with noncardiac surgery, they do not address the overall effect on morbidity and mortality rates associated with the surgical coronary revascularization. However, in the assessment of patients undergoing noncardiac surgery, the well-established long-term benefits of coronary artery bypass surgery should be considered, as should any impact on noncardiac surgical morbidity and mortality rates. There may be some patients for whom coronary artery bypass grafting should be performed prior to noncardiac surgery only because of an otherwise prohibitive perioperative cardiac risk. However, there are many more patients with advanced coronary artery disease who are candidates for surgical coronary revascularization based on long-term prognosis who are identified only during preoperative cardiac assessment. Among such patients, elective noncardiac surgery of intermediate or high risk should generally be postponed for the performance of coronary artery bypass surgery.

There are no prospective studies and few studies of any kind that evaluate the impact of preoperative percutaneous coronary angioplasty on perioperative cardiac morbidity and mortality rates. Three small, retrospective studies[82–84] have suggested that there is a low risk of perioperative myocardial infarction or death following preoperative coronary angioplasty. One study of 1049 noncardiac surgeries performed among 1829 patients enrolled in the Bypass Angioplasty Revascularization Investigation (BARI) trail demonstrated a low incidence of myocardial infarction or death among patients having undergone either coronary artery bypass surgery or percutaneous angioplasty, with events among 1.6 percent of patients in both groups.[85] The absence of any evident difference between groups suggests that previous percutaneous coronary angioplasty confers protection from perioperative cardiac events that is equivalent to that conferred by surgical revascularization. However, based on the limited data available, indications for percutaneous coronary angioplasty among patients undergoing preoperative evaluation should be considered the same as for the general population.[15]

The optimal timing of noncardiac surgery has not been defined for patients who undergo preoperative percutaneous coronary angioplasty. It may be prudent to delay elective noncardiac surgery for a few days following percutaneous coronary angioplasty, due to the early risks of arterial recoil and acute thrombosis. Ideally, elective surgery should be performed within 2 to 3 months of angioplasty, before restenosis can occur. However, patients of more than 6 months following percutaneous coronary angioplasty with no evidence of recurrent ischemia could be considered to have undergone successful revascularization, presumably with a low perioperative risk.

Medical Therapy for Coronary Artery Disease

Several nonrandomized studies have addressed the effect of anti-ischemic medical therapy on perioperative prognosis.[86–93] Although data are lacking to support the empiric use of nitroglycerin or calcium channel blockers, there is increasing evidence that the empiric use of perioperative beta blockers may reduce the risk of an adverse cardiac event. Three small, retrospective studies suggest that perioperative therapy with beta blockers may result in fewer episodes of myocardial ischemia detectable on ECG[91,92] and of acute myocardial infarction.[90] More recently, a randomized study among 112 high-risk patients undergoing vascular surgery demonstrated a reduction in risk of perioperative myocardial infarction or death from 34 to 3 percent with the use of empiric beta blocker therapy.[94] These data support the use of beta blockers therapy among high-risk patients undergoing intermediate or high-risk noncardiac surgery.

MANAGEMENT OF SPECIFIC CONDITIONS

Patients with a variety of medical conditions known to increase cardiovascular risk may require noncardiac surgery. For these patients, appropriate perioperative medical management may prevent the occurrence or minimize the impact of an adverse cardiovascular event. Factors that contribute to increased perioperative risk include interruptions in routine medical therapy as well as physical and mental stresses associated with the surgical procedure and convalescent period. As such, cardiovascular stresses include duress due to the disease for which surgery is planned and alteration in normal medications during the preoperative period; fluctuation in heart rate, blood pressure, intravascular volume, and oxygenation during surgery; dynamic fluid shifts; pain; and limitations in the use of oral medications in the postoperative period. It is important to note that the period of maximum cardiac risk appears to occur in the postoperative period.[95] Because cardiovascular risk is not limited to the intraoperative period, appropriate emphasis should be placed on the treatment of specific conditions throughout all phases of the perioperative period.

Coronary Artery Disease

Among patients with known coronary artery disease undergoing noncardiac surgery, perioperative management should include monitoring for evidence of myocardial ischemia, therapy to prevent and treat ischemia, and postoperative surveillance to ensure that the patient did not experience an ischemic event that could mandate alteration in therapy.

Monitoring can be accomplished with surveillance of ECG ST-segments,[9,95] transesophageal echocardiographic assessment of regional and global left ventricular wall motion,[49] and invasive measurement of pulmonary arterial and pulmonary capillary wedge pressures. Therapy to prevent ischemia should be individualized to the patient and the surgical procedure but in general can include nitroglycerin, beta-adrenergic antagonists, and calcium channel blocking agents alone or in combination. Among many patients with known coronary artery disease, the prevention of ischemia can involve the simple continuation of a routine anti-ischemic regimen or conversion of a regimen to a similar one available for topical or intravenous delivery during periods in which the patient is unable to take medications orally. Nitroglycerin compounds can be administered topically or via intravenous infusion. Several beta-adrenergic antagonists and calcium channel–blocking agents are available for administration via intravenous bolus or infusion. In addition, transdermal clonidine can be substituted for oral beta blockers. In some patients, oral medications can be crushed and delivered through a nasogastric tube that is then clamped for 30 min to allow absorption in the upper intestine. Because of the adverse effects associated with rapid withdrawal of beta-blocking medications as well as the demonstrated benefit associated with their perioperative use,[91,92,94,96–99] every effort should be made to continue these medications during the perioperative period among patients who receive them preoperatively.

At a minimum, an anti-ischemic regimen used prior to surgery should be continued during the perioperative period. Additional anti-ischemic medications can be used empirically and should be used in the event that ischemia is detected during the perioperative period. Intravenous nitroglycerin and/or beta blockers can be titrated to specific end points of heart rate or blood pressure or to resolution of the observed ischemia. In addition, pain relief and correction of any underlying anemia are helpful in reducing tendencies to postoperative ischemia.

Because patients with known coronary artery disease or risk factors for disease are at risk of acute myocardial infarction complicating noncardiac surgery, assessment for change in status is appropriate following a surgical procedure. A simple 12-lead ECG preoperatively, immediately postoperatively, and daily for 2 days is generally sufficient to evaluate for change if there has been no evidence of perioperative ischemia or infarction. Alternative means of assessing for perioperative infarction include assessment of serum creatine kinase (CPK), creatine kinase MB isoenzyme (CPK-MB) fractions, and troponin; echocardiographic assessment of left ventricular wall motion; and nuclear perfusion studies.

At the conclusion of the perioperative period, it is of obvious importance to resume anti-ischemic medications used by the patient prior to undergoing noncardiac surgery. In addition, antiplatelet agents, such as aspirin, which may have been temporarily discontinued prior to surgery, should be reinitiated when no longer contraindicated (see also Chap. 40).

Hypertension

Among patients who are treated for hypertension, preoperative evaluation should include review of present medications and any history of intolerance to previous antihypertensive medications, assessment for adequacy of antihypertensive therapy, and simple measures to evaluate for causes of secondary hypertension and for evidence of target organ damage or associated cardiovascular pathologic conditions. Brief evaluation for rare but potentially treatable causes of secondary hypertension should include assessment for an abdominal bruit, suggestive of renal artery stenosis; for radial-femoral delay, indicative of aortic coarctation; and for hypokalemia in the absence of diuretic use, which could suggest hyperaldosteronism.

Blood pressure should be well controlled prior to elective surgery,[96,97,99,100] and antihypertensive medications should be continued throughout the perioperative period. If there is a period in which the patient is unable to receive oral medications, topical or intravenous equivalents should be substituted. As noted above, rapid withdrawal of beta-blocking medications has associated adverse effects on heart rate and blood pressure, may precipitate myocardial ischemia, and should be avoided.

Mild or moderate preoperative hypertension in the absence of associated cardiovascular or metabolic abnormalities should not necessitate delay of surgery.[101] However, severe hypertension (e.g., diastolic blood pressure of 110 mmHg or greater) should be controlled prior to an elective surgical procedure. If surgery is urgent, then preoperative blood pressure control can usually be achieved rapidly with the use of intravenous beta blockers, calcium blockers, nitroglycerin, or nitroprusside. Finally, patients with preoperative hypertension appear to be predisposed to the development of intraoperative hypotension.[102] A potential for blood pressure lability, with associated ischemia and hypoperfusion, exists among patients with preoperative hypertension; therefore, blood pressure should be carefully monitored and treated if necessary.

Congestive Heart Failure

Congestive heart failure is associated with increased cardiovascular risk during noncardiac surgery.[4,5,9,12,14,103] A careful history and physical examination should include efforts to identify evidence of congestive heart failure, and every effort should be made to treat it prior to surgery.

Congestive heart failure may be the result of a variety of cardiac abnormalities, including left ventricular systolic dysfunction, diastolic dysfunction, and valvular heart disease. Similarly, left ventricular systolic dysfunction may be a harbinger of underlying coronary artery disease. Although congestive heart failure is an independent risk factor for adverse perioperative cardiac outcome, specific underlying causes of congestive heart failure may each be associated with specific independent risks, and the specific nature of the risk may be determined by the nature of the underlying disease. For these reasons, the cause of the underlying process responsible for congestive heart failure should be identified when possible. If left ventricular systolic function is not known, it is generally prudent to establish whether it is normal or abnormal prior to surgery. Similarly, evaluation for left ventricular diastolic dysfunction or valvular heart disease may help in perioperative management. If there are risk factors for coronary artery disease, further evaluation for coronary disease as a cause of left ventricular systolic dysfunction may be appropriate (see also Chap. 21).

Cardiomyopathy

Patients with dilated and hypertrophic cardiomyopathies are predisposed to develop congestive heart failure. Because perioperative management is affected by the nature of the underlying disease, effort should be undertaken to establish the responsible pathologic condition before surgery. Among patients with preoperative signs or symptoms of congestive heart failure, preoperative evaluation should include assessment of left ventricular systolic and diastolic function. Systolic function can be determined noninvasively using either echocardiographic or radionuclide techniques. Echocardiographic imaging offers additional information reflecting diastolic function and valvular function, which could also contribute to congestive heart failure. If not previously performed, preoperative echocardiographic imaging should be strongly considered among patients with congestive heart failure.

Patients with hypertrophic cardiomyopathy require special consideration during the perioperative period. Hypertrophic cardiomyopathy can affect hemodynamics by means of dynamic left ventricular outflow obstruction or may precipitate congestive heart failure mediated by diastolic dysfunction. Left ventricular noncompliance can make patients with hypertrophic cardiomyopathy extremely sensitive to even small amounts of excess intravascular volume, while an underfilled left ventricle can exacerbate dynamic left ventricular outflow obstruction, with a resulting decrease in stroke volume and systemic hypotension. Therefore, perioperative management should be directed at maintaining intravascular volume within a potentially narrow range, avoiding congestive heart failure and minimizing left ventricular outflow obstruction. Catecholamines as a class should be avoided because of their potential to exacerbate dynamic left ventricular outflow obstruction (see also Chap. 51).

Valvular Heart Disease

Most valvular heart disease in an adult population is acquired and therefore increasingly common among older patients undergoing noncardiac surgery. Organic valvular heart disease affects the use of prophylactic antibiotics and can require special consideration for hemodynamic monitoring and medical management in the perioperative period. Although most elective noncardiac surgery need not be delayed, some types of valvular heart disease can pose excessive risk to the patient and should be addressed prior to an elective surgical procedure.

Antibiotic prophylaxis should be used to reduce the risk of infective endocarditis among patients with organic valvular heart disease whenever noncardiac surgery involves a risk of bacteremia. Such procedures include oral, dental, gastrointestinal, and genitourologic procedures, in which normal bacterial flora may gain transient access to the bloodstream. Specific recommendations for prophylactic antibiotic regimens are published for specific types of noncardiac surgery in which there exists an increased risk of infective endocarditis.[104]

AORTIC STENOSIS

Severe aortic stenosis presents the greatest valve-associated cardiovascular risk for patients undergoing noncardiac surgery.[4] The presence of fixed obstruction to left ventricular outflow dramatically limits functional cardiac reserve and may be associated with intracavitary left ventricular pressures in excess of 300 mmHg. Accompanying left ventricular hypertrophy predisposes the patient to diastolic dysfunction and pulmonary congestion. It is important to note that the combination of left ventricular hypertrophy and left ventricular outflow obstruction with high intracavitary pressures predisposes to myocardial ischemia with or without concomitant coronary artery disease. In general, severe or symptomatic aortic stenosis should be addressed prior to the patient's undergoing elective noncardiac surgery. In most cases, aortic valve replacement is indicated as the definitive therapy of choice.[105–107] If cardiac surgery is contraindicated, percutaneous aortic balloon valvotomy can be used to mitigate left ventricular outflow obstruction, even if only as a temporizing measure (see Chap. 56).

MITRAL STENOSIS

The hemodynamic impact associated with mitral stenosis is affected by heart rate. Because increases in heart rate are associated with shortening of the diastolic portion of the cardiac cycle, left ventricular filling is adversely affected by increases in heart rate among patients with even mild or moderate mitral stenosis. As a result, pulmonary congestion can be precipitated by tachycardia of even moderate degree. For this reason, heart rate should be well controlled in the perioperative period among patients with mitral stenosis of any severity. Patients with severe mitral stenosis undergoing high-risk noncardiac surgery may benefit from surgical or percutaneous intervention.[108] The relative risks and benefits and the likelihood of success associated with percutaneous balloon mitral valvotomy, surgical commissurotomy, or mitral valve replacement must be weighed in the context of mitral valve anatomy and other patient-specific factors (see Chap. 57).

AORTIC REGURGITATION AND MITRAL REGURGITATION

Patients with significant aortic regurgitation are predisposed to volume overload in the perioperative period, and volume status should be carefully monitored to prevent pulmonary congestion. In addition, patients with severe aortic regurgitation may benefit from afterload reduction in the form of angiotensin-converting enzyme inhibitors, calcium channel blockers, nitroglycerin, or hydralazine. Just as patients with mitral stenosis are sensitive to tachycardia, patients with significant aortic regurgitation are sensitive to bradycardia. Prolongation of the diastolic interval associated with bradycardia increases the time during which aortic regurgitation occurs and increases total regurgitant volume.

Mitral regurgitation can be due to a variety of underlying causes. As for patients with congestive heart failure, establishing the cause of mitral regurgitation may help define other associated perioperative risks, especially if mitral regurgitation occurs as a manifestation of coronary artery disease. Patients with significant mitral regurgitation may develop volume overload and pulmonary congestion. Diuretics and afterload-reducing therapy should be used to optimize hemodynamic values preoperatively in patients with severe mitral regurgitation undergoing major noncardiac surgery.

Special attention should be paid to left ventricular function in patients with severe mitral regurgitation. The left atrium and pulmonary venous system serve as a low-impedance system that effectively "afterload-reduces" the left ventricle in the setting of significant mitral regurgitation. Because of this, even a mild decrease in left ventricular ejection fraction in the setting of severe mitral regurgitation should be taken as evidence of significant impairment in systolic function and reduced left ventricular functional reserve.

Among patients with mitral valve prolapse, appropriate antibiotic prophylaxis is warranted if there is evidence of regurgitation on either physical examination or echocardiographic Doppler imaging. In addition, antibiotic prophylaxis should be used in patients with mitral valve prolapse and evidence of leaflet thickening and/or leaflet redundancy on echocardiographic imaging[104] (see Chaps. 56 and 57).

PROSTHETIC HEART VALVES

Patients with either tissue or mechanical heart valve prostheses should receive appropriate antibiotic prophylaxis when undergoing noncardiac surgery with an accompanying potential for bacteremia.[104] Patients with mechanical heart valve prostheses also require careful management of anticoagulation in the perioperative period. As a general rule, anticoagulation can be discontinued when necessary for safe performance of noncardiac surgery and should be reinstituted when no longer contraindicated for hemostasis. The risk of valve thrombosis or thromboembolism is related to the location and type of valve prosthesis, the duration in which the patient is not fully anticoagulated, and the level of anticoagulation maintained during that period. A mechanical prosthesis in the mitral position is at greater risk of thrombus formation than is a similar valve in the aortic position, due to the larger cross-sectional area of the mitral prosthesis and associated lower velocities of flow. Similarly, anticoagulation titrated to a subtherapeutic level maintains more protection against thrombus formation than does no anticoagulation. Finally, the risk of thrombus formation is cumulative and increases with the time during which the patient receives less than therapeutic anticoagulation.

Patients who require minimally invasive procedures with a low hemorrhagic risk may be managed by allowing long-term anticoagulation to decrease to a subtherapeutic range and resuming the normal dose of warfarin immediately following the procedure.[109] Among patients with a mechanical heart valve undergoing major noncardiac surgery and in whom anticoagulation is contraindicated at the time of surgery, it is usually prudent to discontinue oral anticoagulation several days prior to surgery and administer intravenous heparin to maintain anticoagulation until the time of surgery. The short half-life of heparin allows the patient to safely undergo surgery within a few hours of its discontinuation. Reestablishing therapeutic anticoagulation usually requires several days after warfarin is initiated, and the patient should again receive heparin in the postoperative period until oral anticoagulation is fully therapeutic. Heparin should be reinitiated when the risk of bleeding is no longer prohibitive and may be started with either a bolus followed by intravenous infusion or with intravenous infusion alone, dictated by the risk of postoperative hemorrhage (see Chap. 60).

Arrhythmia and Conduction Disturbances

Supraventricular and ventricular arrhythmias typically do not represent a serious risk to the patient undergoing noncardiac surgery. However, the arrhythmia may herald the presence of underlying cardiopulmonary disease, and any increased perioperative risk associated with ventricular and supraventricular arrhythmias[4] is most likely due to the underlying disease. The finding of an arrhythmia in the perioperative period should prompt a search for underlying cardiopulmonary disease, drug toxicity, or metabolic derangement that could be both responsible for the arrhythmia and present a risk to the patient.

An otherwise benign arrhythmia can present risk if it unmasks an otherwise silent cardiac disease. For example, a rapid supraventricular tachycardia can provoke myocardial ischemia in the presence of minimal coronary artery disease and similarly can precipitate significant pulmonary congestion in the setting of only mild or moderate mitral stenosis. Ventricular ectopy, including isolated ventricular premature complexes, complex ectopy, and nonsustained ventricular tachycardia, usually do not require specific therapy unless there is evidence of associated hypoperfusion. Thus, hypotension or ongoing myocardial ischemia associated with an arrhythmia warrants therapy directed at the arrhythmia more than would the presence of the arrhythmia alone.

Perioperative atrial fibrillation is common, especially following intrathoracic surgical procedures, where there can be direct atrial irritation, as well as among patients with underlying cardiac or pulmonary diseases. Because of the high-catecholamine state early following major surgery, it may not be possible to establish and maintain normal sinus rhythm in the setting of postoperative atrial fibrillation, and therapy should be directed at rate control and anticoagulation when feasible. Cardioversion of atrial fibrillation in the early postoperative period should be limited to patients with evidence of hemodynamic compromise and hypoperfusion associated with the arrhythmia. For most patients, rate control can be accomplished with the use of beta-adrenergic antagonists or calcium channel–blocking agents administered orally or intravenously. Although digoxin can also be administered, it is typically not as effective for rate control in patients with a high-catecholamine state. Because of the risk of atrial thrombus formation and associated thromboembolic events, patients with atrial fibrillation, including postoperative atrial fibrillation, should be anticoagulated when feasible. Many patients with postoperative atrial fibrillation spontaneously revert to sinus rhythm when perioperative stresses have sufficiently decreased. If a patient does not spontaneously return to sinus rhythm, elective cardioversion should be performed prior to discharge. Any form of cardioversion from atrial fibrillation, whether chemical, electrical, or spontaneous, carries an associated risk of subsequent thromboembolism ascribed to a period of atrial mechanical dysfunction following cardioversion.[110,111] For this reason, patients should receive therapeutic anticoagulation for 3 to 4 weeks following successful cardioversion.

Patients with evidence of intraventricular conduction delay on ECG but without history of symptoms or electrical evidence of advanced heart block do not appear to be at substantial risk of progressing to complete heart block in the perioperative period. If high-grade conduction block develops, treatment can usually be managed in the short term with transthoracic pacing units. Special note should be made of the presence of a left bundle-branch block among patients undergoing right heart catheterization for hemodynamic monitoring. Because of the risk of inducing transient right bundle-branch block during catheter manipulation through the right ventricle, the possibility of complete heart block exists, and measures to provide temporary pacing should be available.

References

1. Mangano DT. Perioperative cardiac morbidity. *Anesthesiology* 1990; 72:153–184.
2. National Center for Health Statistics. *Vital Statistics of the United States: 1980*, vol 2, *Mortality*, part A. DHHS pub no (PHS) 85-1101. Hyattsville, MD: NCHS U.S. Public Health Services; 1985.
3. National Center for Health Statistics. *Vital Statistics of the United States: 1988*, vol 3. DHHS pub no (PHS) 89-1232. Washington, DC: NCHS U.S. Public Health Services; 1989:10–17, 66, 67, 100, 101.
4. Goldman L, Caldera DL, Nussbaum SR, et al. Multifactorial index of cardiac risk in noncardiac surgical procedures. *N Engl J Med* 1977; 297:845–850.
5. Ashton CM, Petersen NJ, Wray NP, et al. The incidence of perioperative myocardial infarction in men undergoing noncardiac surgery. *Ann Intern Med* 1993; 118:504–510.
6. Hollenberg M, Mangano DT, Browner WS, et al. Predictors of postoperative myocardial ischemia in patients undergoing noncardiac surgery: The study of perioperative ischemia research group. *JAMA* 1992; 268:205–209.
7. Hubbard BL, Gibbons RJ, Lapeyre AC III, et al. Identification of severe coronary artery disease using simple clinical parameters. *Arch Intern Med* 1992; 152:309–312.
8. Lette J, Waters D, Bernier H, et al. Preoperative and long-term cardiac risk assessment: Predictive value of 23 clinical descriptors, 7 multivariate scoring systems, and quantitative dipyridamole imaging in 350 patients. *Ann Surg* 1992; 216:192–204.
9. Mangano DT, Browner WS, Hollenberg M, et al. Association of perioperative myocardial ischemia with cardiac morbidity and mortality in men undergoing noncardiac surgery: The study of perioperative ischemia research group. *N Engl J Med* 1990; 323:1781–1788.
10. Michel LA, Jamart J, Bradpiece HA, et al. Prediction of risk in noncardiac operations after cardiac operations. *J Thorac Cardiovasc Surg* 1990; 100:595–605.
11. Eagle KA, Coley CM, Newell JB, et al. Combining clinical and thallium data optimizes preoperative assessment of cardiac risk before major vascular surgery. *Ann Intern Med* 1989; 110:859–866.
12. Detsky AS, Abrams HB, McLaughlin JR, et al. Predicting cardiac complications in patients undergoing non-cardiac surgery. *J Gen Intern Med* 1986; 1:211–219.
13. Foster ED, Davis KB, Carpenter JA, et al. Risk of noncardiac operation in patients with defined coronary disease: The coronary artery surgery study (CASS) registry experience. *Ann Thorac Surg* 1986; 41:42–50.
14. Cooperman M, Pflug B, Martin EW Jr, et al. Cardiovascular risk factors in patients with peripheral vascular disease. *Surgery* 1978; 84:505–509.
15. Eagle KA, Brundage BH, Chaitman BR, et al. Guidelines for perioperative cardiovascular evaluation for noncardiac surgery: Report of the American College of Cardiology/American Heart Association Task Force on Practice Guidelines. *Circulation* 1996; 93:1278–1317.
16. Morris CK, Ueshima K, Kawaguchi T, et al. The prognostic value of exercise capacity: A review of the literature. *Am Heart J* 1991; 122:1423–1431.
17. Detsky AS, Abrams HB, Forbath N, et al. Cardiac assessment for patients undergoing noncardiac surgery: A multifactorial clinical risk index. *Arch Intern Med* 1986; 146:2131–2134.
18. Tarhan S, Moffitt EA, Taylor WF, et al. Myocardial infarction after general anesthesia. *JAMA* 1972; 220:1451–1454.
19. Steen PA, Tinker JH, Tarhan S. Myocardial reinfarction after anesthesia and surgery. *JAMA* 1978; 239:2566–2570.
20. Rao TL, Jacobs KH, El-Etr AA. Reinfarction following anesthesia in patients with myocardial infarction. *Anesthesiology* 1983; 59:499–505.
21. Hertzer NR. Fatal myocardial infarction following peripheral vascular operations: A study of 951 patients followed 6 to 11 years postoperatively. *Cleveland Clin Q* 1982; 49:1–11.
22. Leung JM, Goehner P, O'Kelly BF, et al. Isoflurane anesthesia and myocardial ischemia: Comparative risk versus sufentanil anesthesia in patients undergoing coronary artery bypass graft surgery. The SPI (Study of Perioperative Ischemia) Research Group. *Anesthesiology* 1991; 74:838–847.
23. Baron JF, Bertrand M, Barre E, et al. Combined epidural and general anesthesia versus general anesthesia for abdominal aortic surgery. *Anesthesiology* 1991; 75:611–618.
24. Christopherson R, Beattie C, Frank SM, et al. Perioperative morbidity in patients randomized to epidural or general anesthesia for lower extremity vascular surgery: Perioperative Ischemia

Randomized Anesthesia Trial Study Group. *Anesthesiology* 1993; 79:422–434.
25. Slogoff S, Eeats AS. Randomized trial of primary anesthetic agents on outcome of coronary artery bypass operations. *Anesthesiology* 1989; 70:179–188.
26. Tuman KJ, McCarthy RJ, Spiess BD. Epidural anaesthesia and analgesia decreases postoperative hypercoagulability in high-risk vascular patients. *Anesth Analg* 1990; 70:S414.
27. Gianrossi R, Detrano R, Mulvihill D, et al. Exercise-induced ST depression in the diagnosis of coronary artery disease: A meta-analysis. *Circulation* 1989; 80:87–98.
28. Detrano R, Gianrossi R, Mulvihill D, et al. Exercise-induced ST segment depression in the diagnosis of multivessel coronary disease: A meta analysis. *J Am Coll Cardiol* 1989; 14:1501–1508.
29. Weiner DA, Ryan TJ, McCabe CH, et al. Prognostic importance of a clinical profile and exercise test in medically treated patients with coronary artery disease. *J Am Coll Cardiol* 1984; 3:772–779.
30. McCabe CJ, Reidy NC, Abbott WM, et al. The value of electrocardiogram monitoring during treadmill testing for peripheral vascular disease. *Surgery* 1981; 89:183–186.
31. Cutler BS, Wheeler HB, Paraskos JA, et al. Applicability and interpretation of electrocardiographic stress testing in patients with peripheral vascular disease. *Am J Surg* 1981; 141:501–506.
32. Arous EJ, Baum PL, Cutler BS, et al. The ischemic exercise test in patients with peripheral vascular disease: Implications for management. *Arch Surg* 1984; 119:780–783.
33. Gardine RL, McBride K, Greenberg H, et al. The value of cardiac monitoring during peripheral arterial stress testing in the surgical management of peripheral vascular disease. *J Cardiovasc Surg* (*Torino*) 1985; 26:258–261.
34. von Knorring J, Lepantalo M. Prediction of perioperative cardiac complications by electrocardiographic monitoring during treadmill exercise testing before peripheral vascular surgery. *Surgery* 1986; 99:610–613.
35. Leppo J, Plaja J, Gionet M, et al. Noninvasive evaluation of cardiac risk before elective vascular surgery. *J Am Coll Cardiol* 1987; 9:269–276.
36. Hanson P, Pease M, Berkoff H, et al. Arm exercise testing for coronary artery disease in patients with peripheral vascular disease. *Clin Cardiol* 1988; 11:70–74.
37. McPhail N, Calvin JE, Shariatmadar A, et al. The use of preoperative exercise testing to predict cardiac complications after arterial reconstruction. *J Vasc Surg* 1988; 7:60–68.
38. Carliner NH, Fisher ML, Plotnick GD, et al. Routine preoperative exercise testing in patients undergoing major noncardiac surgery. *Am J Cardiol* 1985; 56:51–58.
39. Kopecky SL, Gibbons RJ, Hollier LH. Preoperative supine exercise radionuclide angiogram predicts perioperative cardiovascular events in vascular surgery. *J Am Coll Cardiol* 1986; 7:226A.
40. Urbinati S, Di Pasquale G, Andreoli A, et al. Preoperative noninvasive coronary risk stratification in candidates for carotid endarterectomy. *Stroke* 1994; 25:2022–2027.
41. Boucher CA, Brewster DC, Darling RC, et al. Determination of cardiac risk by dipyridamole-thallium imaging before peripheral vascular surgery. *N Engl J Med* 1985; 312:389–394.
42. Cutler BS, Leppo JA. Dipyridamole thallium 201 scintigraphy to detect coronary artery disease before abdominal aortic surgery. *J Vasc Surg* 1987; 5:91–100.
43. Fletcher JP, Antico VF, Gruenewald S, et al. Dipyridamole-thallium scan for screening of coronary artery disease prior to vascular surgery. *J Cardiovasc Surg* (*Torino*) 1988; 29:666–669.
44. Sachs RN, Tellier P, Larmignat P, et al. Assessment by dipyridamole-thallium-201 myocardial scintigraphy of coronary risk before peripheral vascular surgery. *Surgery* 1988; 103:584–587.
45. McEnroe CS, O'Donnell RF Jr, Yeager A, et al. Comparison of ejection fraction and Goldman risk factor analysis of dipyridamole-thallium 201 studies in the evaluation of cardiac morbidity after aortic aneurysm surgery. *J Vasc Surg* 1990; 11:497–504.
46. Younis LT, Aguirre F, Byers S, et al. Perioperative and long-term prognostic value of intravenous dipyridamole thallium scintigraphy in patients with peripheral vascular disease. *Am Heart J* 1990; 119:1287–1292.
47. Mangano DT, London MJ, Tubau JF, et al. Dipyridamole thallium-201 scintigraphy as a preoperative screening test: A reexamination of its predictive potential. Study of Perioperative Ischemia Research Group. *Circulation* 1991; 84:493–502.
48. Strawn DJ, Guernsey JM. Dipyridamole thallium scanning in the evaluation of coronary artery disease in elective abdominal aortic surgery. *Arch Surg* 1991; 126:880–884.
49. Watters TA, Botvinick EH, Dae MW, et al. Comparison of the findings on preoperative dipyridamole perfusion scintigraphy and intraoperative transesophageal echocardiography: Implications regarding the identification of myocardium at ischemic risk. *J Am Coll Cardiol* 1991; 18:93–100.
50. Hendel RC, Whitfield SS, Villegas BJ, et al. Prediction of late cardiac events by dipyridamole thallium imaging in patients undergoing elective vascular surgery. *Am J Cardiol* 1992; 70:1243–1249.
51. Lette J, Waters D, Cerino M, et al. Preoperative coronary artery disease risk stratification based on dipyridamole imaging and a simple three-step, three-segment model for patients undergoing noncardiac vascular surgery or major general surgery. *Am J Cardiol* 1992; 69:1553–1558.
52. Madsen PV, Vissing M, Munck O, et al. A comparison of dipyridamole thallium 201 scintigraphy and clinical examination: I. The determination of cardiac risk before arterial reconstruction. *Angiology* 1992; 43:306–311.
53. Brown KA, Rowen M. Extent of jeopardized viable myocardium determined by myocardial perfusion imaging best predicts perioperative cardiac events in patients undergoing noncardiac surgery. *J Am Coll Cardiol* 1993; 21:325–330.
54. Kresowik TF, Bower TR, Garner SA, et al. Dipyridamole thallium imaging in patients being considered for vascular procedures. *Arch Surg* 1993; 128:299–302.
55. Baron JF, Mundler O, Bertrand M, et al. Dipyridamole-thallium scintigraphy and gated radionuclide angiography to assess cardiac risk before abdominal aortic surgery. *N Engl J Med* 1994; 330:663–669.
56. Bry JD, Belkin M, O'Donnell TF Jr, et al. An assessment of the positive predictive value and cost-effectiveness of dipyridamole myocardial scintigraphy in patients undergoing vascular surgery. *J Vasc Surg* 1994; 19:112–121.
57. Camp AD, Garvin PJ, Hoff J, et al. Prognostic value of intravenous dipyridamole thallium imaging in patients with diabetes mellitus considered for renal transplantation. *Am J Cardiol* 1990; 65:1459–1463.
58. Iqbal A, Gibbons RJ, McGoon MD, et al. Noninvasive assessment of cardiac risk in insulin dependent diabetic patients being evaluated for pancreatic transplantation using thallium-201 myocardial perfusion scintigraphy. *Transplant Proc* 1991; 23(part 2):1690–1691.
59. Coley CM, Field TS, Abraham SA, et al. Usefulness of dipyridamole-thallium scanning for preoperative evaluation of cardiac risk for nonvascular surgery. *Am J Cardiol* 1992; 69:1280–1285.
60. Shaw L, Miller DD, Kong BA, et al. Determination of perioperative cardiac risk by adenosine thallium-201 myocardial imaging. *Am Heart J* 1992; 124:861–869.
61. Takase B, Younis LT, Byers SL, et al. Comparative prognostic value of clinical risk indexes, resting two-dimensional echocardiography, and dipyridamole stress thallium-201 myocardial imaging for perioperative cardiac events in major nonvascular surgery patients. *Am Heart J* 1993; 126:1099–1106.
62. Younis L, Stratmann H, Takase B, et al. Preoperative clinical

assessment and dipyridamole thallium-201 scintigraphy for prediction and prevention of cardiac events in patients having major noncardiovascular surgery and known or suspected coronary artery disease. *Am J Cardiol* 1994; 47:311–317.
63. Stratmann H, Tamesis B, Wittry M, et al. Dipyridamole sestamibi tomography optimizes perioperative outcome and defines late prognosis in vascular surgery patients. *Circulation* 1993; 88:1–440.
64. Ritchie JL, Bateman TM, Bonow RO, et al. Guidelines for clinical use of cardiac radionuclide imaging: A report of the American College of Cardiology/American Heart Association Task Force on Assessment of Diagnostic and Therapeutic Cardiovascular Procedures (Committee on Radionuclide Imaging), developed in collaboration with the American Society of Nuclear Cardiology. *J Am Coll Cardiol* 1995; 25:521–547.
65. Berthe C, Pierard LA, Hiernaux M. Predicting the extent and location of coronary artery disease in acute myocardial infarction by echocardiography during dobutamine infusion. *Am J Cardiol* 1986; 58:1167–1172.
66. Cohen JL, Green TO, Ottenweller J, et al. Dobutamine digital echocardiography for detecting coronary artery disease. *Am J Cardiol* 1991; 67:1311–1318.
67. Sawada SG, Segar DS, Ryan T, et al. Echocardiographic detection of coronary artery disease during dobutamine infusion. *Circulation* 1991; 83:1605–1614.
68. Martin TW, Seaworth JF, Johns JP, et al. Comparison of adenosine, dipyridamole, and dobutamine in stress echocardiography. *Ann Intern Med* 1992; 116:190–196.
69. Marwick T, Willemart B, D'Hondt AM, et al. Selection of the optimal nonexercise stress for the evaluation of ischemic regional myocardial dysfunction and malperfusion: Comparison of dobutamine and adenosine using echocardiography and 99mTc-MIBI single photon emission computed tomography. *Circulation* 1993; 87:345–354.
70. Lane RT, Sawada SG, Segar DS, et al. Dobutamine stress echocardiography for assessment of cardiac risk before noncardiac surgery. *Am J Cardiol* 1991; 68:976–977.
71. Lalka SG, Sawada SG, Dalsing MC, et al. Dobutamine stress echocardiography as a predictor of cardiac events associated with aortic surgery. *J Vasc Surg* 1992; 15:831–840.
72. Poldermans D, Fioretti PM, Forster T, et al. Dobutamine stress echocardiography for assessment of perioperative cardiac risk in patients undergoing major vascular surgery. *Circulation* 1993; 87:1506–1512.
73. Eichelberger JP, Schwarz KQ, Black ER, et al. Predictive value of dobutamine echocardiography just before noncardiac vascular surgery. *Am J Cardiol* 1993; 72:602–607.
74. Langan EM III, Youkey JR, Franklin DP, et al. Dobutamine stress echocardiography for cardiac risk assessment before aortic surgery. *J Vasc Surg* 1993; 18:905–911.
75. Davila-Roman VG, Waggoner AD, Sicard GA, et al. Dobutamine stress echocardiography predicts surgical outcome in patients with an aortic aneurysm and peripheral vascular disease. *J Am Coll Cardiol* 1993; 21:957–963.
76. Shaw LJ, Eagle KA, Gersh BJ, et al. Meta-analysis of intravenous dipyridamole-thallium-201 imaging (1985 to 1994) and dobutamine echocardiography (1991 to 1994) for risk stratification before vascular surgery. *J Am Coll Cardiol* 1996; 27:787–798.
77. Cambria RP, Brewster DC, Abbott WM, et al. The impact of selective use of dipyridamole-thallium scans and surgical factors on the current morbidity of aortic surgery. *J Vasc Surg* 1992; 15:43–51.
78. Diehl JT, Cali RF, Hertzer NR, et al. Complications of abdominal aortic reconstruction: An analysis of perioperative risk factors in 557 patients. *Ann Surg* 1983; 197:49–56.
79. Crawford ES, Morris GC Jr, Howell JF, et al. Operative risk in patients with previous coronary artery bypass. *Ann Thorac Surg* 1978; 26:215–221.
80. Reul GJ Jr, Cooley DA, Duncan JM, et al. The effect of coronary bypass on the outcome of peripheral vascular operations in 1093 patients. *J Vasc Surg* 1986; 3:788–798.
81. Nielsen JL, Page CP, Mann C, et al. Risk of major elective operation after myocardial revascularization. *Am J Surg* 1992; 164:423–426.
82. Huber KC, Evans MA, Bresnahan JF, et al. Outcome of noncardiac operations in patients with severe coronary artery disease successfully treated preoperatively with coronary angioplasty. *Mayo Clin Proc* 1992; 67:15–21.
83. Elmore JR, Hallett JW Jr, Gibbons RJ, et al. Myocardial revascularization before abdominal aortic aneurysmorrhaphy: Effect of coronary angioplasty. *Mayo Clin Proc* 1993; 68:637–641.
84. Allen JR, Helling TS, Hartzler GO. Operative procedures not involving the heart after percutaneous transluminal coronary angioplasty. *Surg Gynecol Obstet* 1991; 173:285–288.
85. Hassan SA, Hlatky M, Boothroyd D, et al. Impact of prior coronary bypass surgery and angioplasty on peri-operative cardiac outcomes in patients undergoing non-cardiac surgery: Data from Bypass Angioplasty Revascularization Investigation (BARI) study [abstr]. *Circulation* 1999; 100(suppl I):I-529.
86. Coriat P, Daloz M, Bousseau D, et al. Prevention of intraoperative myocardial ischemia during noncardiac surgery with intravenous nitroglycerin. *Anesthesiology* 1984; 61:193–196.
87. Thomson IR, Mutch WA, Culligan JD. Failure of intravenous fentanyl-pancuronium anesthesia. *Anesthesiology* 1984; 61:385–393.
88. Gallagher JD, Moore RA, Jose AB, et al. Prophylactic nitroglycerin infusions during coronary artery bypass surgery. *Anesthesiology* 1986; 64:785–789.
89. Godet G, Coriat P, Baron JF, et al. Prevention of intraoperative myocardial ischemia during noncardiac surgery with intravenous diltiazem: A randomized trial versus placebo. *Anesthesiology* 1987; 66:241–245.
90. Pasternack PF, Imparato AM, Baumann FG, et al. The hemodynamics of beta-blockade in patients undergoing abdominal aortic aneurysm repair. *Circulation* 1987; 76(suppl 3, pt 2): III-1–III-7.
91. Stone JG, Foex P, Sear JW, et al. Myocardial ischemia in untreated hypertensive patients: Effect of a single small oral dose of a beta-adrenergic blocking agent. *Anesthesiology* 1988; 68:495–500.
92. Pasternack PF, Grossi EA, Baumann FG, et al. Beta blockade to decrease silent myocardial ischemia during peripheral vascular surgery. *Am J Surg* 1989; 158:113–116.
93. Dodds TM, Stone JG, Coromilas J, et al. Prophylactic nitroglycerin infusion during noncardiac surgery does not reduce perioperative ischemia. *Anesth Analg* 1993; 76:705–713.
94. Poldermans D, Boersma E, Bax JJ, et al. The effect of bisoprolol on perioperative mortality and myocardial infarction in high-risk patients undergoing vascular surgery. *N Engl J Med* 1999; 341:1789–1794.
95. Mangano DT, Hollenberg M, Fegert G, et al. Perioperative myocardial ischemia in patients undergoing noncardiac surgery: I. Incidence and severity during the 4 day perioperative period. *J Am Coll Cardiol* 1991; 17:843–850.
96. Stone JG, Foex P, Sear JW, et al. Risk of myocardial ischaemia during anesthesia in treated and untreated hypertensive patients. *Br J Anaesth* 1988; 61:675–679.
97. Prys-Roberts C, Meloche R, Foex P. Studies of anaesthesia in relation to hypertension: I. cardiovascular responses of treated and untreated patients. *Br J Anaesth* 1971; 43:122–137.
98. Cucchiara RF, Benefiel DJ, Matteo RS, et al. Evaluation of esmolol in controlling increases in heart rate and blood pressure during endotracheal intubation in patients undergoing carotid endarterectomy. *Anesthesiology* 1986; 65:528–531.

99. Magnusson J, Thulin T, Werner O, et al. Haemodynamic effects of pretreatment with metoprolol in hypertensive patients undergoing surgery. *Br J Anaesth* 1986; 58:251–260.
100. Goldman L, Caldera DL. Risks of general anesthesia and elective operation in the hypertensive patient. *Anesthesiology* 1979; 50:285–292.
101. Bedford RF, Feinstein B. Hospital admission blood pressure: A predictor for hypertension following endotracheal intubation. *Anesth Analg* 1980; 59:367–370.
102. Slogoff S, Keats AS. Does perioperative myocardial ischemia lead to postoperative myocardial infarction? *Anesthesiology* 1985; 62:107–114.
103. Gerson MC, Hurst JM, Hertzberg VS, et al. Cardiac prognosis in noncardiac geriatric surgery. *Ann Intern Med* 1985; 103:832–837.
104. Dajani AS, Bisno AL, Chung KJ, et al. Prevention of bacterial endocarditis: Recommendations by the American Heart Association. *JAMA* 1990; 264:2919–2922.
105. Bernard Y, Etievent J, Mourand JL, et al. Long-term percutaneous aortic valvuloplasty compared with aortic valve replacement in patients more than 75 years old. *J Am Coll Cardiol* 1992; 20:796–801.
106. Logeais Y, Langanay T, Roussin R, et al. Surgery for aortic stenosis in elderly patients: A study of surgical risk and predictive factors. *Circulation* 1994; 90:2891–2898.
107. Lieberman EB, Bashore TM, Hermiller JB, et al. Balloon aortic valvuloplasty in adults: Failure of procedure to improve long-term survival. *J Am Coll Cardiol* 1995; 26:1522–1528.
108. Reyes VP, Raju BS, Wynne J. Percutaneous balloon valvuloplasty compared with open surgical commissurotomy for mitral stenosis. *N Engl J Med* 1994; 331:961–967.
109. Stein PD, Alpert JS, Copeland J, et al. Antithrombotic therapy in patients with mechanical and biologic prosthetic heart valves. *Chest* 1992; 102(suppl):445S–455S.
110. Black IW, Fatkin D, Sagar KB, et al. Exclusion of atrial thrombus by transesophageal echocardiography does not preclude embolism after cardioversion of atrial fibrillation: A multicenter study. *Circulation* 1994; 89:2509–2513.
111. Fatkin D, Kuchar DL, Thorburn CW, et al. Transesophageal echocardiography before and during direct current cardioversion of atrial fibrillation: Evidence for "atrial stunning" as a mechanism of thromboembolic complications. *J Am Coll Cardiol* 1994; 23:307–316.

CHAPTER 75

ANESTHESIA AND THE PATIENT WITH CARDIOVASCULAR DISEASE

David L. Reich / Joel A. Kaplan

INTRODUCTION

Anesthetizing patients with cardiovascular disease is one of the most difficult challenges facing the anesthesiologist. The constellation of anesthetic drug effects, the physiologic stresses of surgery, and underlying cardiovascular diseases complicate and limit the choice of anesthetic techniques for any particular procedure. Generally speaking, the anesthesiologist's approach to the patient with cardiovascular disease is to select agents and techniques that would optimize the patient's cardiopulmonary function. The perioperative management of a patient with cardiovascular disease requires close cooperation between the cardiologist/internist and the anesthesiologist.[1] Each specialist has a unique knowledge base that complements the others. The approach should emphasize a continuum of care from the preoperative evaluation through the extended postoperative period.

PREOPERATIVE EVALUATION

The assessment of cardiac risk and preoperative optimization of the patient's cardiovascular status are the traditional goals of the preoperative evaluation of patients with cardiovascular disease. In 1977, Goldman et al. introduced the Cardiac Risk Index Score to guide more quantitatively the assignment of cardiac risk in patients undergoing noncardiac surgery.[2] This study had a major impact, because clinicians concluded that improvements in factors such as congestive heart failure symptomatology and general medical condition would decrease cardiac risk. While one major study does not support the predictive value of the Cardiac Risk Index Score or preoperative electrocardiographic ischemic changes in patients with coronary artery disease,[3] the emphasis on preoperative optimization continues and is supported by other studies.[4] This topic is reviewed in Chap. 83. The American College of Cardiology/American Heart Association Task Force on Practice Guidelines published, "Guidelines for Perioperative Cardiovascular Evaluation for Noncardiac Surgery."[5] The algorithmic approach to preoperative evaluation described in these guidelines and that advocated by Mangano and Goldman[6] are valuable in that more consistent clinical approaches should emerge.

The information derived from the cardiac evaluation that is of particular value to the anesthesiologist can be summarized by answers to the following questions:

1. Are further diagnostic studies required prior to elective surgery?
2. Will the patient derive benefit from delaying surgery in order to optimize preoperative medical therapy?
3. Will the patient derive benefit from preoperative myocardial revascularization (angioplasty or surgical revascularization)?
4. Should there be perioperative antithrombotic therapy?
5. What is the regimen of preoperative cardiovascular medications that should be continued through the perioperative period?

The accumulation of historical, clinical, laboratory, echocardiographic, radionuclide, and cardiac catheterization data in a cogent summary form comprises the ideal "medical clearance" consultation for the anesthesiologist. With the benefit of this information, the two specialties can make intelligent decisions regarding the patient's preoperative therapy and the optimal timing of surgery.[7]

PERIOPERATIVE MONITORING

Standards for basic intraoperative monitoring were established by the American Society of Anesthesiologists in 1986.[8] Accordingly, digital pulse oximetry and capnometry have been almost universally applied in the last several years. The indications for the use of more invasive monitors, such as intraarterial and central venous monitoring vary by institution and practitioner (Tables 75-1 and 75-2). The indications for pulmonary arterial catheters (PACs) are especially controversial. There are data from the intensive care setting suggesting that the PAC is harmful,[9] while other data indicate that it may provide prognostic information in the perioperative period.[10] Table 75-3 details specific indications for PAC that many practitioners accept.

The bispectral index is a parameter derived from a proprietary electroencephalographic analysis technology that has been shown to correlate with increasing sedation and loss of con-

TABLE 75-1 Indications for Intraarterial Monitoring

Major surgical procedures involving large fluid shifts and/or blood loss
Surgery requiring cardiopulmonary bypass
Surgery of the aorta
Patients with pulmonary disease requiring frequent arterial blood gases
Patients with recent myocardial infarctions, unstable angina, or severe coronary artery disease
Patients with decreased left ventricular function (congestive heart failure) or significant valvular heart disease
Patients in hypovolemic, cardiogenic, or septic shock, or with multiple organ failure
Procedures involving the use of deliberate hypotension or deliberate hypothermia
Massive trauma
Patients with right heart failure, chronic obstructive pulmonary disease, pulmonary hypertension, or pulmonary embolism
Patients requiring inotropes or intraaortic balloon counterpulsation
Patients undergoing surgery of the aorta requiring cross-clamping
Patients with massive ascites
Patients with electrolyte or metabolic disturbances requiring frequent blood samples
Inability to measure arterial pressure noninvasively (e.g., morbid obesity)

TABLE 75-2 Indications for Central Venous Line Placement

Major operative procedures involving large fluid shifts and/or blood loss in patients with good left ventricular function
Intravascular volume assessment when urine output is not reliable or unavailable (renal failure, urologic surgery)
Patients with tricuspid stenosis
Major trauma
Surgical procedures with a high risk of air embolism, such as sitting position craniotomies
Frequent blood sampling in patients who will not require an arterial line
Venous access for vasoactive or irritating drugs
Chronic drug administration
Inadequate peripheral intravenous access
Rapid infusion of intravenous fluids (using large cannulae)

sciousness.[11] While incomplete amnesia is rare with current anesthetic techniques, bispectral index use has been demonstrated to result in decreased propofol doses and faster recovery from propofol anesthesia.[12]

Transesophageal echocardiography is minimally/moderately invasive and has acquired a much larger role in intraoperative management. The availability of high-frequency transducers and color-flow Doppler mapping has enhanced the ability of anesthesiologists, cardiologists, and surgeons to make intraoperative diagnoses, evaluate hemodynamic aberrations, and assess the quality of cardiac surgical interventions inter alia. Practice guidelines for transesophageal echocardiography have been published by the American Society of Anesthesiologists.[13] Standardized intraoperative examination guidelines for multiplane transesophageal echocardiography have been published[14] and the National Board of Echocardiography has been formed to administer a certifying examination in perioperative transesophageal echocardiography. A list of indications for perioperative transesophageal echocardiography is presented in Table 75-4.

TABLE 75-3 Indications for Pulmonary Artery Catheter Monitoring

Major procedures involving large fluid shifts and/or blood loss in patients with severe coronary artery disease
Patients with recent myocardial infarctions or severely unstable angina
Patients with impaired left ventricular function (congestive heart failure) or significant mitral or aortic valvular pathology
Patients with pericardial tamponade
Patients in hypovolemic, cardiogenic, or septic shock, or with multiple organ failure
Massive trauma
Patients with right-sided heart failure, chronic obstructive pulmonary disease, pulmonary hypertension, or pulmonary embolism
Patients requiring high levels of positive end-expiratory pressure
Hemodynamically unstable patients requiring inotropes or intraaortic balloon counterpulsation
Patients undergoing surgery of the aorta requiring cross-clamping
Patients undergoing hepatic transplantation
Patients with massive ascites

CHOICE OF ANESTHETIC TECHNIQUE

The choice of anesthetic technique is inherently a difficult one because multiple factors must be considered. These include the desires of the patient, the requirements of the surgical procedure, and the patient's underlying medical condition. While a specific anesthetic technique is occasionally desirable for a particular procedure (e.g., spinal anesthesia for transurethral resection of prostate), it is extremely difficult to find scientific evidence that any particular anesthetic approach is superior to reasonable alternatives or that anesthetic technique per se influences patient outcome.[15,16]

There is controversy regarding the effects of regional anesthesia (with postoperative epidural analgesia) on cardiovascular morbidity/mortality in "high-risk" patients. Five prospective randomized trials have addressed this issue. Two reported reduced cardiac morbidity with epidural anesthesia[17,18] and three studies found no difference[19-21] (Table 75-5). *While some studies suggest that regional anesthesia and epidural analgesia have salutary effects in vascular surgical patients, the issue is unresolved due to the limited and conflicting clinical evidence. In addition,*

TABLE 75-4 Practice Guidelines for Perioperative Transesophageal Echocardiography

- Category I indications: Supported by the strongest evidence or expert opinion
  - Intraoperative evaluation of acute, persistent, and life-threatening hemodynamic disturbances in which ventricular function and its determinants are uncertain and have not responded to treatment
  - Intraoperative use in valve repair
  - Intraoperative use in congenital heart surgery for most lesions requiring cardiopulmonary bypass
  - Intraoperative use in repair of hypertrophic obstructive cardiomyopathy
  - Intraoperative use for endocarditis when preoperative testing was inadequate or extension of infection to perivalvular tissue is suspected
  - Preoperative use in unstable patients with suspected thoracic aortic aneurysms, dissection, or disruption who need to be evaluated quickly
  - Intraoperative assessment of aortic valve function in repair of aortic dissections with possible aortic valve involvement
  - Intraoperative evaluation of pericardial window procedures
  - Use in intensive care unit for unstable patients with unexplained hemodynamic disturbances, suspected valve disease, or thromboembolic problems
- Category II indications: Supported by weaker evidence and expert consensus
  - Perioperative use in patients with increased risk of myocardial ischemia or infarction
  - Perioperative use in patients with increased risk of hemodynamic disturbances
  - Intraoperative assessment of valve replacement
  - Intraoperative assessment of repair of cardiac aneurysms
  - Intraoperative evaluation of removal of cardiac tumors
  - Intraoperative detection of foreign bodies
  - Intraoperative detection of air emboli during cardiotomy, heart transplant operations, and upright neurosurgical procedures
  - Intraoperative use during intracardiac thrombectomy
  - Intraoperative use during pulmonary embolectomy
  - Intraoperative use for suspected cardiac trauma
  - Preoperative assessment of patients with suspected acute thoracic aortic dissections, aneurysms, or disruption
  - Intraoperative use during repair of thoracic aortic dissections without suspected aortic valve involvement
  - Intraoperative detection of aortic atheromatous disease or other sources or aortic emboli
  - Intraoperative evaluation of pericardiectomy, pericardial effusions, or evaluation of pericardial surgery
  - Intraoperative evaluation of anastomotic sites during heart and/or lung transplantation
  - Monitoring placement and function of assist devices
- Category III indications: Little current scientific or expert support
  - Intraoperative evaluation of myocardial perfusion, coronary artery anatomy, or graft patency
  - Intraoperative use during repair of cardiomyopathies other than hypertrophic obstructive cardiomyopathy
  - Intraoperative use for uncomplicated endocarditis during noncardiac surgery
  - Intraoperative monitoring for emboli during orthopedic procedures
  - Intraoperative assessment of repair of thoracic aortic injuries
  - Intraoperative use for uncomplicated pericarditis
  - Intraoperative evaluation of pleuropulmonary disease
  - Monitoring placement of intraaortic balloon pumps, automatic implantable cardiac defibrillators, or pulmonary artery catheters
  - Intraoperative monitoring of cardioplegia administration

SOURCE: Modified from American Society of Anesthesiologists. Practice guidelines for perioperative transesophageal echocardiography. *Anesthesiology* 1996; 84:986–1006, with permission.

there are no studies that clearly determine whether or not local anesthesia with intravenous sedation is advantageous compared with general or major regional anesthetic techniques.[5] Therefore, it is essential that the cardiologist/internist does not specifically exclude any anesthetic technique during a preoperative consultation.

Regional anesthetics are not infrequently converted to general anesthetics intraoperatively due to unexpectedly long surgery, patient discomfort, or changes in the surgical plan. No anesthesiologist can be certain that a particular technique will be adequate for the surgical procedure, given the unpredictability of the situation, and the anesthesiologist must have flexibility to alter the technique as needed.

Regional Anesthesia

The term *regional anesthesia* was coined by Cushing for operations where local anesthetics were used on localized areas of the body without loss of consciousness. The advantages of regional anesthesia include simplicity, low cost, and minimal equipment requirements. Many of the adverse effects of general anesthesia are avoided, such as myocardial and respiratory depression.

TABLE 75-5 Clinical Trials Evaluating Effects of Neuraxial Anesthesia on Cardiovascular Morbidity

Study	N	Population	Cardiac Morbidity	Vascular Graft Patency Rate
Yeager et al.[17]	53	Mixed	Reduced with epidural	Not reported
Tuman et al.[18]	80	Vascular surgery	Reduced with epidural	Improved with epidural
Baron et al.[19]	173	Aortic surgery	No difference	Not reported
Christopherson et al.[21]	100	Lower extremity Vascular surgery	No difference	Improved with epidural
Bode et al.[20]	423	Lower extremity Vascular surgery	No difference	Not reported

SOURCE: Modified from Christopherson R, Norris EJ: Regional versus general anesthesia. In: Reich DL, ed. *Anesthesiology Clinics of North America,* Vol. 15. Philadelphia, Saunders; 1997:37, with permission.

The disadvantages include patients' reluctance to be awake in the operating room, anesthetic agents of insufficient duration, and local anesthetic toxicity.

There is little evidence that regional or local anesthesia with intravenous sedation offers improved cardiac morbidity in high-risk patients.

The cardiovascular side effects of regional anesthesia vary depending on the technique chosen. Spinal and epidural anesthesia, for example, may cause major decreases in cardiac preload and afterload, while local anesthetic infiltration and axillary nerve blocks have almost no cardiovascular side effects. Regional anesthetics are contraindicated in anticoagulated patients and those with coagulopathies. Regional anesthesia may also be combined with general anesthesia in adults and children in order to decrease the requirements for the general anesthetic agents and for postoperative analgesia. The institution of analgesia prior to surgical stimulation (preemptive analgesia) may have salutary effects on postoperative pain control.

LOCAL ANESTHESIC AGENTS

The local anesthetics are classified on the basis of their chemical structure as esters or amides. The esters are hydrolyzed by esterases in the plasma, and the amides are metabolized in the liver. The duration of action of local anesthetic agents is affected by the protein-binding characteristics of the molecule and the addition of vasoconstrictors to the local anesthetic solution.[22] Toxic reactions to local anesthetics are generally characterized by central nervous system excitation (seizures), which may be followed by central nervous system depression and cardiovascular collapse.

Cocaine is the original ester local anesthetic. Its clinical use is mainly restricted to topical anesthesia of the nose and airway. It is the only local anesthetic agent that is intrinsically vasoconstrictive, an effect resulting from blockade of catecholamine reuptake at sympathetic nerve terminals. Cocaine's sympathomimetic effects result in central nervous system excitation, which increases requirements for general anesthetics. Cocaine toxicity has resulted in deaths from central nervous system toxicity and arrhythmias.[23] Cocaine can also elicit myocardial ischemia. The tachycardia associated with cocaine contraindicates its use in patients with coronary artery disease, mitral stenosis, or obstructive cardiomyopathy (see also Chap. 71).

Tetracaine is a long-acting ester local anesthetic used in spinal anesthesia. It is also used for topical anesthesia of the eye and airway, but may be toxic in the larger doses required for airway topical anesthesia. Chloroprocaine is a short-acting ester local anesthetic that is used in epidural anesthesia. This agent is rapidly metabolized by serum cholinesterase, leading to a low incidence of toxic reactions.

Compared to the esters, the amide local anesthetics are less rapidly metabolized (in the liver), and the potential for toxic reactions is somewhat greater. Some amide compounds (e.g., lidocaine) also have potent antiarrhythmic actions (see also Chap. 27). Lidocaine and mepivacaine are agents of intermediate duration of action that are commonly used in many types of regional blocks. Etidocaine and bupivacaine are agents of higher potency and longer duration of action that also exhibit more toxicity. Bupivacaine is particularly associated with cardiovascular collapse and arrhythmias upon inadvertent intravascular injection. Ropivacaine is the first new local anesthetic in two decades. It is similar in potency and duration to bupivacaine, but appears to have less cardiovascular toxicity and to cause less motor block.[24]

Epinephrine and phenylephrine may be added to local anesthetic solutions to prolong their duration of action by local vasoconstriction. Epinephrine is typically added in concentrations ranging from 2.5 μg/mL (1:400,000) to 10 μg/mL (1:100,000) for infiltration, nerve blocks, or epidural anesthesia. The systemic absorption of epinephrine occurs slowly and beta-adrenergic effects predominate, resulting in slight tachycardia and diastolic hypotension. In patients whose cardiovascular disease precludes the use of epinephrine, phenylephrine may be substituted at concentrations 10 times higher than that of epinephrine. Epinephrine may induce ventricular arrhythmias in patients anesthetized with halothane (see "Halothane" later).

SPINAL ANESTHESIA

The injection into the subarachnoid space of a relatively small dose of local anesthetic that produces profound motor and sensory blockade is known as spinal anesthesia. Spinal anesthesia also produces blockade of preganglionic sympathetic fibers, which usually results in hypotension. The level of spinal anesthesia is controlled by injection of a hyperbaric or hypobaric solution into the cerebrospinal fluid. The position of the patient is then manipulated to lateralize the blockade or to move the bolus of anesthetic in a more cephalad or caudad direction.

The level of sympathetic blockade is generally two dermatomal segments higher than that of the sensory dermatomal level.

The higher the level of sympathetic blockade, the more profound the arterial and venous vasodilation and postural hypotension. Intravenous hydration with crystalloid solutions is the primary treatment for hypotension. Intravenous boluses of ephedrine (5 to 10 mg) or phenylephrine (20 to 100 μg) are also used to temporarily increase the blood pressure during periods of relative hypovolemia. If the dermatomal level of sympathetic blockade reaches T1, then the patient is effectively sympathectomized. The loss of cardiac accelerator fiber function may lead to bradycardia. Complete sympathectomy always occurs with a "total spinal," which also produces respiratory insufficiency due to intercostal and phrenic nerve root blockade.

Spinal anesthesia must be undertaken cautiously, and with more intensive monitoring, in patients whose cardiovascular stability depends upon the maintenance of a high preload and afterload. Patients with any significant cardiac valvular disease, hypertrophic obstructive cardiomyopathy, or tetralogy of Fallot are prone to hemodynamic decompensation during spinal anesthesia. Patients with coronary artery disease usually tolerate spinal anesthesia well, so long as diastolic arterial pressure is maintained at an appropriate level to preserve coronary perfusion pressure.

EPIDURAL ANESTHESIA

The epidural space, which is filled with loose areolar tissue and a venous plexus, lies immediately external to the dura mater. An indwelling catheter is usually placed percutaneously for intermittent bolus injections or continuous infusions of local anesthetic and/or opioids. The epidural space may be entered by thoracic, lumbar, or caudal approaches. The advantages of epidural anesthesia are similar to those of spinal anesthesia and include moderate hypotension (which tends to decrease intraoperative blood loss) and contracted bowel loops during abdominal surgery. In addition, the ability to administer dilute local anesthetics and opioids through an indwelling epidural catheter is an effective means of postoperative analgesia.

The hemodynamic effects of epidural anesthesia are essentially similar to those of spinal anesthesia except that the onset of sympathetic blockade is more gradual. Thus, with appropriate monitoring, cautious administration of epidural anesthetics has been safely done in patients with mitral valvular disease, aortic stenosis, or hypertrophic obstructive cardiomyopathy. It should be emphasized, though, that intraarterial catheters and PACs may be required to monitor and treat changes in preload and afterload that occur with epidural anesthesia in patients with severe cardiovascular disease.

Generally, 10 to 15 times the volume of local anesthetic is required compared to spinal anesthesia. The potential for inadvertent intravascular injection of a toxic dose of local anesthetic is present. It is also possible inadvertently to inject a large volume into the subarachnoid space and cause a "total spinal" (see "Spinal Anesthesia" earlier).

The hemodynamic consequences of inadvertent intravenous injections of epinephrine-containing solutions may be significant for patients who cannot tolerate tachycardia. Epidural infusions of opioids for postoperative analgesia may be complicated by pruritus, urinary retention, somnolence, and respiratory depression. Thus, appropriate monitoring and nursing care are required.

COMBINED SPINAL-EPIDURAL ANESTHESIA

The injection of intrathecal anesthetic agents via a fine-bore needle through the epidural-introducing trocar followed by epidural catheter placement constitutes combined spinal-epidural anesthesia. The spinal anesthetic provides rapid onset and intense analgesia, while the epidural catheter permits the administration of agents for continued intraoperative anesthesia and postoperative analgesia.[25]

NERVE BLOCKS AND INFILTRATION OF LOCAL ANESTHETIC

Nerve blocks and local anesthetic infiltration may be performed to facilitate surgery of localized areas of the body. The brachial plexus may be blocked by interscalene, supraclavicular, or axillary approaches. The lower extremity may be anesthetized by blocking the femoral, obturator, and sciatic nerves. Local anesthetic infiltration is performed in regions such as the inguinal area to facilitate herniorrhaphies. These blocks, when properly performed, have minimal cardiovascular effects. They do require large volumes of local anesthetic solution, which result in toxic reactions if inadvertent intravascular injection occurs, however. Intercostal blocks are associated with high blood concentrations even without intravascular injection, because the neurovascular bundle enhances absorption of the local anesthetic and multiple blocks are required for clinical efficacy. Epinephrine is occasionally added to prolong the duration of block, but this may be contraindicated in certain patients with cardiovascular disease, such as those with mitral stenosis.

General Anesthesia

General anesthesia is defined as a reversible state consisting of amnesia, analgesia, immobility, and the prevention of undesirable reflexes. The general anesthetics include many drugs, almost all of which have cardiovascular side effects. Intravenous agents are nearly always used for the induction of anesthesia in adults. Anesthesia is maintained using inhalational agents, intravenous agents, or a combination of the two.

Neuromuscular blocking drugs (muscle relaxants) are commonly used to facilitate tracheal intubation and to lower the requirements for anesthetic agents (i.e., the dose of anesthetic that produces adequate amnesia and analgesia may not be sufficient to prevent movement or relax the abdominal musculature). In children, the induction of anesthesia is highly individualized according to patient needs, practitioner, and institution.

The physiologic consequences of general anesthesia have changed dramatically over the last several decades with the development of modern anesthetic agents. Ether and cyclopropane have sympathomimetic properties and were often used with spontaneous ventilation. Modern, nonexplosive inhalational anesthetic agents tend to be cardiac and respiratory depressants. With the exception of brief operations, most general anesthetics include tracheal intubation and mechanical ventilation. As an alternative to tracheal intubation, devices such as the laryngeal mask airway may be used to secure a patient's airway. The loss of consciousness is usually accompanied by a decrease in sympathetic tone. This, as well as the effects of positive pressure ventilation, causes a moderate decrease in cardiac output even when the anesthetic drugs are not myocardial depressants per se.

The patient with cardiovascular disease presents major concerns to the anesthesiologist. General anesthesia masks many of the symptoms of cardiovascular decompensation, such as angina, dyspnea, dizziness, and palpitations. Other signs of cardiovascular disease, such as tachycardia, are nonspecific and may be misinterpreted as hypovolemia or light anesthesia. Fluid shifts, obstructed venous return, and varying levels of noxious stimulation are other variables related to surgery that are unpredictable. It is for these reasons that appropriate monitoring and selection of anesthetic agents are vital to the intraoperative management of the patient with cardiovascular disease.

INTRAVENOUS ANESTHETICS

Intravenous anesthetic induction drugs are composed of lipophilic molecules that have an affinity for neuronal tissue or specific receptors. Their action is generally terminated by redistribution from the vessel-rich tissues (brain, heart, liver, and kidneys) to other tissues (muscle, fat, and skin). Elimination occurs via hepatic metabolism and takes place over several hours. Patients with diminished cardiac output secondary to cardiovascular disease will have prolonged effects from intravenous induction drugs.

Barbiturates Thiopental, an ultra-short-acting thiobarbiturate, is the prototype for agents of its class. It is quick, reliable, and pleasant for patients and does not have excitatory side effects. Its cardiovascular effects are marked by dose-dependent myocardial depression and dilation of venous capacitance vessels. The decrease in cardiac output is usually compensated for by arterial vasoconstriction, so that blood pressure is minimally decreased. Thiopental is a poor analgesic, however, and tachycardia and hypertension are common with tracheal intubation or any painful stimulus.

Standard doses of barbiturate for anesthetic induction are contraindicated in patients with preload-dependent cardiac lesions and/or severely impaired ventricular contractility. This includes patients with pericardial tamponade, mitral regurgitation, aortic regurgitation, mitral stenosis, and dilated cardiomyopathy. Reduced doses and slower injection of the drug will markedly decrease the cardiovascular effects.

Benzodiazepines Benzodiazepines may be used as premedication, to induce anesthesia, or as an adjunct to regional or general anesthesia. Their most useful therapeutic effects include sedation and amnesia. They tend to be unreliable in their rapidity of induction and occasionally fail to induce unconsciousness despite high doses. When used as sole agents, the benzodiazepines have minimal cardiovascular effects. When used in combination with other drugs such as opioids and potent volatile anesthetics, benzodiazepines produce hypotension, which may be due to myocardial depression or decreased systemic vascular resistance.

Opioids Synthetic opioids have assumed a major role in the anesthetic care of patients with cardiovascular disease. They can be used as premedication, as supplements to regional or inhalational anesthesia, as one of the main components of "nitrous-narcotic" anesthesia, or as the primary anesthetic agent (high-dose opioid anesthesia). They are often used as supplements during anesthesia induction to block the hemodynamic response to laryngoscopy and tracheal intubation. While opioids are excellent analgesics, they are unreliable amnesics, provide no muscle relaxation, and are associated with "breakthrough" hypertension and tachycardia intraoperatively.

A further problem with high doses of opioids is that they can produce truncal muscle rigidity, ocular movements, wrist flexion, and shoulder abduction—often referred to as "fentanyl seizures." These events, however, do not produce electroencephalographic changes characteristic of epileptiform activity.[26,27] The truncal rigidity does interfere with ventilation and requires the use of neuromuscular blockers. Ventilatory support is frequently continued postoperatively following high doses of opioids because the elimination half-lives of synthetic opioids are relatively long (1.5 to 4 h). The exception is remifentanil, a new synthetic opioid that is extremely short-acting due to ester hydrolysis. Continuous infusions of remifentanil are notable for the cardiovascular advantages of the synthetic opioids without the prolonged duration of effect.[28] The rapid offset of remifentanil's effect, however, must be counteracted by substituting another method of analgesia so as to avoid acute withdrawal of the opioid effect.

Despite the disadvantages noted earlier, high-dose synthetic (phenylpiperidine) opioid anesthesia does not depress myocardial contractility and is devoid of histamine release. It is therefore associated with markedly stable hemodynamics during anesthetic induction and maintenance in the majority of patients with cardiovascular disease. Nevertheless, patients with high resting sympathetic tone, congestive heart failure, and severe pulmonary hypertension are prone to transient hypotension during anesthetic induction. A mild bradycardia usually occurs on anesthetic induction due to an increase in vagal tone. The bradycardia is often advantageous in patients with diseases such as coronary artery disease or mitral stenosis. The bradycardia effect is reliably antagonized by atropine or pancuronium (see "Neuromuscular Blockade" later) in patients with conditions such as mitral regurgitation, which require faster heart rates. There is a trend to reduce the doses of opioids administered in cardiac anesthesia in order to facilitate more rapid tracheal extubation and discharge from the intensive care unit.[29]

Neither morphine nor meperidine is commonly used intraoperatively. Morphine is often used as premedication and for postoperative analgesia. With higher doses and rapid administration, morphine causes histamine release and is associated with hypotension and increased fluid requirements. It is also a venodilator. Meperidine produces tachycardia and histamine release, and it is a direct myocardial depressant. It has the lowest toxic:therapeutic dose ratio of the clinically relevant opioids.

Anesthesiologists only rarely administer naloxone or other opioid antagonists to reverse the effects of a systemic opioid in patients with cardiovascular disease. In surgical patients, complete reversal of the opioid effect results in the sudden onset of pain and surges in catecholamine levels. Naloxone administration has been complicated by pulmonary edema,[30] arrhythmias,[31] and cardiac arrest.[32] Low doses of intravenous naloxone have been safely used to reverse the pruritus and respiratory depression associated with epidural and intrathecal opioids without reversing the analgesia.[33]

Etomidate Etomidate is an imidazole anesthetic agent that enhances gamma-aminobutyric acid (GABA)-ergic transmission. It is associated with marked hemodynamic stability during bolus administration for anesthetic induction but does not blunt the hemodynamic response to laryngoscopy and tracheal intubation. This is one of the preferred agents for anesthetic induction in patients with valvular or ventricular dysfunction, hypovolemia, or pericardial effusion. Etomidate infusions are not used in the United States because of their association with adrenocortical insufficiency.

Propofol Propofol is a substituted phenol (diisopropylphenol) that may be used for anesthetic induction and maintenance. It is dissolved in a soybean oil and egg lecithin emulsion, which is mildly irritating on injection. Its main advantage is the rapid emergence and psychomotor recovery following termination of the drug infusion. Propofol may also be associated with reduced postoperative nausea and vomiting.[34] Propofol causes dose-dependent hypotension that appears to be due to a combination of myocardial depression and vasodilation. It is prudent to use reduced doses of propofol in patients with aortic or mitral valvular stenosis and cardiomyopathies. Propofol is used increasingly for sedation in intensive care units and to facilitate "fast-track" extubation following cardiac surgery.

Ketamine Ketamine is a cyclohexanone that is chemically related to phencyclidine. Its use as a sole anesthetic is limited by its indirect sympathomimetic effects and emergence delirium. Its sympathomimetic effects are advantageous, however, in certain groups of patients with cardiovascular disease. These include mainly those who are critically dependent on high resting sympathetic tone to maintain an adequate perfusion pressure: patients with pericardial tamponade, hypovolemia, and systemic-to-pulmonary arterial shunts. It is important to reduce the dose of ketamine in those with severe cardiac disease because ketamine is a direct myocardial depressant.[35] In patients who already have maximal sympathetic outflow, hypotension may ensue following ketamine due to an "unmasking" of its myocardial depressant effect. Ketamine is relatively contraindicated in patients who cannot tolerate tachycardia, such as those with coronary artery disease or mitral stenosis.[36]

Alpha$_2$-Adrenergic Agonists Clonidine and dexmedetomidine are alpha$_2$-adrenergic agonists that are sympatholytic, sedative-anxiolytic, antiarrhythmic, analgesic, and reversible.[37,38] Clonidine has also been demonstrated to reduce anesthetic requirements and improve hemodynamic stability during the intraoperative period. Once more convenient and specific compounds are developed, alpha$_2$-adrenergic agents may play a much larger role in the perioperative management of patients with cardiovascular disease.

INHALATIONAL ANESTHETICS

Inhalational anesthetics include nitrous oxide and the potent volatile agents. The study of the uptake and distribution of inhaled drugs with cerebral and cardiovascular effects is practically unique to anesthesiology, and cardiac output is a major determinant of uptake and distribution. The alveolar concentration of a drug is generally equal to the brain concentration. Thus, anything that hastens increases in the alveolar concentration of the drug will speed the onset of anesthesia. Two factors that speed the onset of anesthesia are a diminished cardiac output and an anesthetic agent with low solubility in the blood. Thus, patients with low cardiac output secondary to cardiovascular disease will have a more rapid onset of anesthesia. Intracardiac right-to-left shunting will decrease the onset of anesthesia, whereas left-to-right shunting has negligible effects.

Nitrous Oxide Nitrous oxide is an excellent analgesic but not a very potent anesthetic. Concentrations up to 75 percent may be given safely (so as to maintain an adequate $F_{I_{O_2}}$), but incomplete amnesia and movement in response to painful stimuli are likely. Thus, nitrous oxide is nearly always administered with other anesthetic agents, such as opioids or potent volatile agents, and neuromuscular blockers. It is also chosen because its relatively low solubility in the blood enhances the rapid onset and termination of its effects.

Nitrous oxide is a weak myocardial depressant, which mildly stimulates the sympathetic nervous system.[39] It does not exacerbate pulmonary hypertension in anesthetized patients with mitral valvular disease,[40] but is nevertheless avoided by most practitioners in patients with severe right ventricular dysfunction. As a sole agent, its cardiovascular effects are minimal, but cardiac output is lowered in the presence of opioids. It also accentuates the negative inotropic effects of potent volatile agents.[41]

Nitrous oxide rapidly diffuses into closed air spaces within the body due to its low blood solubility, high lipid solubility, and high concentrations required. Examples of closed air spaces include bowel gas, pneumothoraces, and air emboli. Once equilibrium is reached, 75% nitrous oxide will quadruple the size of any of these spaces. For this reason, nitrous oxide must be discontinued if a pneumothorax or air embolism is suspected. It is often avoided in cardiothoracic procedures, particularly in children prone to paradoxical embolization, or after cardiopulmonary bypass.

Potent Volatile Agents The use of inhalational anesthesia with potent volatile agents is the most common anesthetic technique because of its relatively low cost, reliable amnesia, and bronchodilation, as well as its low blood solubility and overall safety record. All agents are myocardial depressants and vasodilators and produce some degree of hypotension. The hypotension provides some indication of the depth of anesthesia, as does monitoring of end-tidal gas concentrations and possibly the bispectral index (see "Perioperative Monitoring" earlier).

The effect of these agents is rapidly changed when the inspiratory concentration is adjusted. The ability to titrate inhalational anesthesia is advantageous when compared to intravenous drugs, because the duration of surgical procedures and the degree of surgical stimulation are often unpredictable. For this reason, low doses of volatile anesthetics may be added as supplements to nitrous oxide- or intravenous-based anesthetic techniques for the control of hypertension and the prevention of awareness (incomplete amnesia).

The frequent production of nodal (junctional) rhythm is also common to these agents. The loss of atrial systole may be poorly tolerated, particularly in patients with aortic stenosis, hypertrophic cardiomyopathies, or mitral stenosis. All potent volatile agents have the potential for interactions with calcium channel blockers and beta-adrenergic blockers. Negative inotropic and conduction effects of these drugs may be augmented by the volatile anesthetic agents; however, all cardiac drugs should be continued until the time of surgery.

HALOTHANE Halothane represented a major advance in anesthesia when it was introduced in the 1950s, but its use is restricted by its cardiovascular effects and the small incidence of hepatotoxicity. Halothane depresses the myocardium and the sinoatrial node but is not a potent vasodilator. Thus, cardiac output and heart rate are depressed in a dose-dependent fashion. Blood pressure is not severely decreased, because the decrease in systemic vascular resistance is less than with the other volatile agents at equipotent dosages. This hemodynamic profile is beneficial in situations where myocardial contractility (and oxygen consumption) should be kept low and perfusion pressure maintained high. Examples include ischemic heart disease, hypertrophic obstructive cardiomyopathy, and, especially, tetralogy of Fallot.[42] Halothane is contraindicated in patients with dilated cardiomyopathy, congestive heart failure, aortic stenosis, aortic and mitral regurgitation, and pericardial tamponade.

Halothane lowers the threshold for epinephrine-induced ventricular arrhythmias more than do other volatile agents. As a practical matter, the initial epinephrine dose is restricted to 1.5 μg/kg during infiltration of local anesthetic solutions. If arrhythmias occur due to an inadvertent vascular injection, the halothane should be discontinued. Approximately five times the dose of epinephrine is required to induce ventricular arrhythmias in patients receiving enflurane and isoflurane.

ENFLURANE Enflurane is almost equal to halothane in its negative inotropic effect, but it is more vasodilating and less of a negative chronotrope. Thus, cardiac output is better maintained, but blood pressure is lower than with equipotent dosages of halothane. Enflurane is a reasonable choice as a supplement to intravenous anesthetic techniques when breakthrough hypertension occurs. Enflurane has been used less commonly in recent years for various reasons, including its cardiovascular effects, metabolism to inorganic fluoride, and the emergence of newer agents.

ISOFLURANE Isoflurane is somewhat less negatively inotropic than enflurane or halothane and is a potent arteriolar vasodilator, which tends to maintain cardiac output. Tachycardia frequently occurs at clinical dosages because the baroreceptor reflexes are not impaired. On the basis of its hemodynamic effects, isoflurane would be beneficial in patients with mitral or aortic regurgitation with good ventricular function. It is relatively contraindicated (as a sole agent) in patients with mitral or aortic stenosis, dilated and hypertrophic cardiomyopathies, and pericardial tamponade. Isoflurane is frequently used in patients with coronary artery disease, when it is often combined with opioids or beta-adrenergic blockers to prevent tachycardia and the dose is limited to preserve coronary perfusion pressure. The use of isoflurane remains controversial in patients with coronary artery anatomy that predisposes to coronary "steal."

The coronary steal phenomenon occurs when a zone of myocardium distal to a stenotic coronary artery derives its blood supply from collateral vessels that originate in a zone of myocardium with normal coronary arterial supply. The arterioles in the normal zone are partially constricted, while those in the collateral-dependent zone are maximally dilated due to the "upstream" coronary artery occlusion. This maintains the pressure gradient across the collateral vessels and the perfusion of the collateral-dependent zone. Some arteriolar vasodilators (e.g., adenosine, dipyridamole, and sodium nitroprusside) can dilate the arterioles in the normal myocardial zone, decrease the perfusion pressure across the collateral vessels, and precipitate myocardial ischemia due to coronary steal.

Isoflurane has been shown to induce myocardial ischemia with collateral-dependent myocardial blood flow in canine models[43] and in humans.[44] It remains controversial whether or not isoflurane should be used in patients with coronary artery disease, given the uncertainty regarding coronary artery anatomy in most patients. The tachycardia and hypotension associated with isoflurane, as well as evidence of maldistributed myocardial blood flow, might suggest that it should not be used. Nevertheless, a prospective clinical study in patients with "steal-prone anatomy"[45] and large outcome studies[15,16] have not found intraoperative myocardial ischemia or poorer outcome with isoflurane anesthesia. A reasonable conclusion would be that isoflurane should be used with caution and appropriate monitoring in patients suspected of having "steal-prone" coronary artery anatomy.[46]

DESFLURANE Desflurane is a volatile anesthetic that was introduced into clinical practice in 1992. It is much less soluble in blood than the volatile agents described earlier. Its blood:gas solubility coefficient is similar to that of nitrous oxide. Thus, more rapid induction and emergence would be expected. This is particularly advantageous in ambulatory procedures. Several studies have compared emergence from anesthesia with desflurane with that from other anesthetics and have demonstrated that initial psychomotor recovery is faster,[47] but that hospital discharge criteria occur at about the same time.[48] The coronary vascular effects of desflurane are similar to those of isoflurane, but desflurane is not associated with tachycardia at lower doses.[49] Despite desflurane's similarity to isoflurane with regard to myocardial depression and vasodilation, desflurane has a unique sympathomimetic effect. This effect is seen with rapid increases in end-tidal concentration in the absence of preanesthetic medication. The sympathomimetic action of desflurane can be blocked by fentanyl, esmolol, and clonidine.[50]

SEVOFLURANE The relatively low solubility and minimal airway irritation of sevoflurane make it a very useful anesthetic for the inhalation induction of anesthesia.[51] Its low solubility allows rapid alterations in alveolar concentration during the maintenance period of the anesthetic, thereby improving control of the depth of anesthesia. It is now achieving rapid acceptance in the United States despite initial concerns regarding the potential toxicity of compound A (a breakdown product created in the presence of alkaline carbon dioxide absorbing materials).[52] Biochemical markers of the transient nephrotoxicity of compound A have been measured in healthy volunteers.[53] High fresh gas flow rates are recommended to decrease the concentration of compound A, and it is prudent to avoid its prolonged use in patients with renal dysfunction.

The cardiovascular effects of sevoflurane are similar to those of isoflurane and desflurane except that sevoflurane is not associated with increases in heart rate. Sevoflurane progressively decreases blood pressure in a manner similar to the other volatile anesthetics. In animals, sevoflurane appears to be a slightly less potent coronary vasodilator than isoflurane and has not been associated with coronary steal. Myocardial contractility is depressed in a manner similar to that of equianesthetic concentrations of isoflurane and desflurane, and it does not potentiate epinephrine-induced cardiac arrhythmias. In several prospective, randomized, multicenter studies in which patients with coronary artery disease or risk factors for coronary artery disease received either sevoflurane or isoflurane, the incidence of adverse cardiac outcomes did not differ between treatment groups.[54]

NEUROMUSCULAR BLOCKADE

Benzylisoquinolinium Compounds The benzylisoquinolinium series of nondepolarizing neuromuscular blockers are all derivatives of the curare molecule. Most of these compounds have histamine-releasing properties that are dependent on the dose and rate of administration. *D*-Tubocurarine, metocurine, atracurium, and mivacurium are associated with clinically important histamine release following the administration of bolus doses to facilitate tracheal intubation. The newer agents, doxacurium and cisatracurium, are not associated with histamine release with large ("intubating") doses. While older agents, such as *D*-tubocurarine and metocurine, are mainly dependent upon renal elimination, atracurium and cisatracurium undergo a unique form of spontaneous degradation that is organ-independent (Hofmann elimination). Mivacurium undergoes enzyme-dependent ester hydrolysis.

Aminosteroid Compounds Pancuronium is the classic aminosteroid nondepolarizing neuromuscular blocking drug. The atropine-like molecular structure contains two quaternary nitrogen groups. The tachycardia and hypertension associated with pancuronium have been linked to myocardial ischemia during coronary artery bypass surgery.[55] The anticholinergic effects of pancuronium, however, can be useful (e.g., in patients with mitral regurgitation) for preventing the increase in vagal tone that occurs with high-dose opioid anesthetic inductions. Vecuronium and pipecuronium have minimal cardiovascular effects at usual clinical dosages. Rocuronium has a more rapid onset of action due to its lower potency than the others and has minimal cardiovascular side effects. While pancuronium elimination is almost entirely renal, the newer compounds are also degraded by the liver.

The newest aminosteroid compound is rapacuronium. Following bolus administration, it is characterized by rapid onset of action (due to its low potency) and relatively short duration of action.[56] The side effects include mild histamine release, hypotension, and bronchospasm, but the degree of hypotension did not correlate with histamine levels.[57] Based upon these data, it should be used with caution in patients with preload-dependent lesions and pulmonary hypertension. It is not recommended for infusion use in intensive care, and repeat dosing should be undertaken cautiously due to the presumed accumulation of active metabolites.

Succinylcholine Succinylcholine, essentially di-acetylcholine molecularly, is a depolarizing short-acting neuromuscular blocker that is still used because of its low cost, rapid onset, and short duration of action. Its cardiovascular effects depend on whether nicotinic or muscarinic receptor effects predominate in a given patient. Thus, tachycardia and hypertension or bradycardia and hypotension may occur. Vagal effects tend to predominate with repeated doses or in children. In patients with various disorders (including neuromuscular diseases, recent burns, and massive trauma), hyperkalemic cardiac arrest may occur with succinylcholine administration because of exaggerated release of intracellular potassium from myocytes.

THE POSTOPERATIVE PERIOD AND CARDIAC COMPLICATIONS

Emergence from anesthesia is frequently accompanied by hypertension and tachycardia, which is most often due to incomplete analgesia, but may also be related to withdrawal from antihypertensive drugs, hypoxemia, delirium, or bladder distension. If an underlying modifiable cause is not identified, then intravenous drugs—such as nitroglycerin, labetalol, or esmolol—are frequently used to control hemodynamics in patients with cardiovascular disease. Shivering is another phenomenon that may occur due to hypothermia or emergence from volatile anesthetics. Shivering results in severe increases in oxygen consumption, which may be poorly tolerated by patients with cardiovascular disease. Although the mechanism is unknown, low doses of meperidine decrease or eliminate shivering.[58]

In patients with risk factors, there is a high incidence of postoperative complications, such as myocardial infarction, pulmonary edema, malignant ventricular arrhythmia, and cardiac death.[3] Pain, high catecholamine levels, hypercoagulability, hypovolemia, anemia, intravascular volume shifts, drug effects, and a low level of monitoring all probably contribute to this phenomenon. Prospective trials suggest that prevention of hypothermia[59] and beta-adrenergic blockade during surgery and the postoperative hospitalization[60] may decrease the incidence of these complications in high-risk patients.

Traditionally, the anesthesiologist has not played a major role in postoperative management following discharge from the recovery room/post-anesthesia care unit. This situation has changed with the development of multidisciplinary pain services that administer epidural analgesia and patient-controlled analgesia. As noted earlier, it remains controversial whether or not regional anesthesia and intensive postoperative analgesia are capable of reducing morbidity and mortality. It is conceivable that more effective postoperative analgesia decreases the deleterious effects of the stress response. Future efforts to reduce perioperative risk likely will concentrate on assessing the effects of more intensive postoperative hemodynamic, analgesic, and anticoagulation management.

CONCLUSIONS

The optimal perioperative care of patients with cardiovascular disease is the joint responsibility of anesthesiologists, surgeons, and cardiologists/internists. Any anesthetic agent or technique has the potential for producing adverse effects, and the margin of safety is reduced in patients with cardiovascular disease. It is the anesthesiologist's role to acquire accurate and relevant information from the preoperative evaluation, to apply appropriate monitoring technology, to select an anesthetic technique that is suited to the planned procedure and the condition of the patient, and to manage hemodynamic alterations and analgesic requirements in the perioperative period. As cardiovascular disease continues to become more prevalent in the surgical population and preoperative testing and intraoperative monitoring become more sophisticated, the need for effective communication between the specialties of cardiology and anesthesiology will become even more important.

References

1. Wells PH, Kaplan JA. Optimal management of patients with ischemic heart disease for non-cardiac surgery by complementary anesthesia and cardiology intervention. *Am Heart J* 1981; 102:1030–1040.
2. Goldman L, Caldera DL, Nussbaum SR, et al. Multifactorial index of cardiac risk in noncardiac surgical procedures. *N Engl J Med* 1977; 297:845–850.
3. Mangano DT, Browner WS, Hollenberg M, et al. Association of perioperative myocardial ischemia with cardiac morbidity and mortality in men undergoing noncardiac surgery. *N Engl J Med* 1990; 323:1781–1788.
4. Goldman L. Multifactorial index of cardiac risk in non-cardiac surgery: Ten year status report. *J Cardiothorac Anesth* 1987; 1:237–244.
5. ACC/AHA Task Force on Practice Guidelines. Guidelines for perioperative cardiovascular evaluation for noncardiac surgery. *Circulation* 1996; 93:1278–1317.
6. Mangano DT, Goldman L. Preoperative assessment of patients with known or suspected coronary disease. *N Engl J Med* 1995; 333:1750–1756.
7. Kleinman B, Czinn E, Shah K, et al. The value to the anesthesia-surgical care team of the preoperative cardiac consultation. *J Cardiothorac Anesth* 1989; 3:682–687.
8. American Society of Anesthesiologists. *Standards for Basic Intraoperative Monitoring* (Approved by House of Delegates on October 21, 1986 and last amended on October 21, 1998). Park Ridge, IL: ASA; 1998.
9. Connors AF, Speroff T, Dawson NV, et al. The effectiveness of right heart catheterization in the initial care of critically ill patients. *JAMA* 1996; 276:889–897.
10. Reich DL, Bodian CA, Krol M, et al. Intraoperative hemodynamic predictors of mortality, stroke and myocardial infarction following coronary artery bypass surgery. *Anesth Analg* 1999; 88:814–822.
11. Glass PS, Bloom M, Kearse L, et al. Bispectral analysis measures sedation and memory effects of propofol, midazolam, isoflurane, and alfentanil in healthy volunteers. *Anesthesiology* 1997; 86:836–847.
12. Gan TJ, Glass PS, Windsor A, et al. Bispectral index monitoring allows faster emergence and improved recovery from propofol, alfentanil, and nitrous oxide anesthesia. BIS Utility Study Group. *Anesthesiology* 1997; 87:808–815.
13. American Society of Anesthesiologists. Practice guidelines for perioperative transesophageal echocardiography. *Anesthesiology* 1996; 84:986–1006.
14. Shanewise JS, Cheung AT, Aronson S, et al. ASE/SCA guidelines for performing a comprehensive intraoperative multiplane transesophageal echocardiography examination: Recommendations of the American Society of Echocardiography Council for Intraoperative Echocardiography and the Society of Cardiovascular Anesthesiologists Task Force for Certification in Perioperative Transesophageal Echocardiography. *Anesth Analg* 1999; 89:870–884.
15. Slogoff S, Keats AS. Randomized trial of primary anesthetic agents on outcome of coronary artery bypass operations. *Anesthesiology* 1989; 70:179–188.
16. Tuman KJ, McCarthy RJ, Spiess BD, et al. Does choice of anesthetic agent significantly affect outcome after coronary artery surgery? *Anesthesiology* 1989; 70:189–198.
17. Yeager MP, Glass DD, Neff RK, Brinck-Johnsen T. Epidural anesthesia and analgesia in high-risk surgical procedures. *Anesthesiology* 1987; 66:729–736.
18. Tuman KJ, McCarthy RJ, March RJ, et al. Effects of epidural anesthesia and analgesia on coagulation and outcome after major vascular surgery. *Anesth Analg* 1991; 73:696–704.
19. Baron JF, Bertrand M, Barre E, et al. Combined epidural and general anesthesia versus general anesthesia for abdominal aortic surgery. *Anesthesiology* 1991; 75:611–618.
20. Bode RH Jr, Lewis KP, Zarich SW, et al. Cardiac outcome after peripheral vascular surgery: Comparison of general and regional anesthesia. *Anesthesiology* 1996; 84:3–13.
21. Christopherson R, Beattie C, Frank SM, et al. Perioperative morbidity in patients randomized to epidural or general anesthesia for lower extremity vascular surgery. *Anesthesiology* 1993; 79:422–434.
22. Covino BG. Pharmacology of local anaesthetic agents. *Br J Anaesth* 1986; 58:701–716.
23. Fleming JA, Byck R, Barash PG. Pharmacology and therapeutic applications of cocaine. *Anesthesiology* 1990; 73:518–531.
24. McClure JH. Ropivacaine. *Br J Anaesth* 1996; 76:300–307.
25. Felsby S, Juelsgaard P. Combined spinal and epidural anesthesia. *Anesth Analg* 1995; 80:821–826.
26. Smith NT, Benthuysen JL, Bickford RG, et al. Seizures during opioid anesthetic induction—Are they opioid-induced rigidity? *Anesthesiology* 1989; 71:852–862.
27. Murkin JM, Moldenhauer CC, Hug CC Jr, Epstein CM. Absence of seizures during induction of anesthesia with high-dose fentanyl. *Anesth Analg* 1984; 63:489–494.
28. Dershwitz M, Randel GI, Rosow CE, et al. Initial clinical experience with remifentanil, a new opioid metabolized by esterases. *Anesth Analg* 1995; 81:619–623.
29. Cheng DCH. Fast track cardiac surgery pathways: Early extubation, process of care, and cost containment. *Anesthesiology* 1998; 88:1429–1433.
30. Prough DS, Roy R, Bumgarner J, Shannon G. Acute pulmonary edema in healthy teenagers following conservative doses of intravenous naloxone. *Anesthesiology* 1984; 60:485–486.
31. Azar I, Turndorf H. Severe hypertension and multiple atrial premature contractions following naloxone administration. *Anesth Analg* 1979; 58:524–525.
32. Andree RA. Sudden death following naloxone administration. *Anesth Analg* 1980; 59:782–784.
33. Bell SD, Seltzer JL. Postoperative pain management. In: Kaplan JA, ed. *Vascular Anesthesia.* New York: Churchill-Livingstone; 1991:565.
34. Ewalenko P, Janny S, Dejonckheere M, et al. Antiemetic effect of subhypnotic doses of propofol after thyroidectomy. *Br J Anaesth* 1996; 77:463–467.
35. Kunst G, Martin E, Graf BM, et al. Actions of ketamine and its isomers on contractility and calcium transients in human myocardium. *Anesthesiology* 1999; 90:1363–1371.
36. Reich DL, Silvay G. Ketamine: An update on the first 25 years of clinical experience. *Can J Anaesth* 1989; 36:186–197.
37. Flacke JW. Alpha2-adrenergic agonists in cardiovascular anesthesia. *J Cardiothorac Vasc Anesth* 1992; 6:344–359.
38. Maze M, Tranquilli W. Alpha2-agonists: Defining the role in clinical anesthesia. *Anesthesiology* 1991; 74:581–605.
39. Ebert TJ, Kampine JP. Nitrous oxide augments sympathetic outflow: Direct evidence from human peroneal nerve recordings. *Anesth Analg* 1989; 69:444–449.
40. Konstadt SN, Reich DL, Thys DM. Nitrous oxide does not exacerbate pulmonary hypertension or ventricular dysfunction in patients with mitral valvular disease. *Can J Anaesth* 1990; 37:613–617.
41. Stowe DF, Monroe SM, Marijic J, et al. Comparison of halothane, enflurane, and isoflurane with nitrous oxide on contractility and oxygen supply and demand in isolated hearts. *Anesthesiology* 1991; 75:1062–1074.
42. Samuelson PN, Lell WA. Tetralogy of Fallot. In: Lake CL, ed. *Pediatric Cardiac Anesthesia*, 3d ed. Stamford, CT: Appleton & Lange; 1998:303.

43. Buffington CW, Romson JL, Levine A, et al. Isoflurane induces coronary steal in a canine model of chronic coronary occlusion. *Anesthesiology* 1987; 66:280–292.
44. Reiz S, Balfors E, Sorensen MB, et al. Isoflurane: A powerful coronary vasodilator in patients with coronary artery disease. *Anesthesiology* 1983; 59:91–97.
45. Pulley DD, Kirvassilis GV, Kelermenos N, et al. Regional and global myocardial circulatory and metabolic effects of isoflurane and halothane in patients with steal-prone coronary anatomy. *Anesthesiology* 1991; 75:756–766.
46. Priebe HJ. Isoflurane and coronary hemodynamics. *Anesthesiology* 1989; 71:960–976.
47. Smiley RM, Ornstein E, Matteo RS, et al. Desflurane and isoflurane in surgical patients: Comparison of emergence time. *Anesthesiology* 1991; 74:425–428.
48. Apfelbaum JL, Lichtor JL, Lane BS, et al. Awakening, clinical recovery, and psychomotor effects after desflurane and propofol anesthesia. *Anesth Analg* 1996; 83:721–725.
49. Saidman LJ. The role of desflurane in the practice of anesthesia. *Anesthesiology* 1991; 74:399–401.
50. Weiskopf RB, Eger EI II, Noorani M, Daniel M. Fentanyl, esmolol, and clonidine blunt the transient cardiovascular stimulation induced by desflurane in humans. *Anesthesiology* 1994; 81:1350–1355.
51. Epstein RH, Stein AL, Marr AT, Lessin JB. High concentration versus incremental induction of anesthesia with sevoflurane in children: A comparison of induction times, vital signs, and complications. *J Clin Anesth* 1998; 10:41–45.
52. Smith I, Nathanson MH, White PF. The role of sevoflurane in outpatient anesthesia. *Anesth Analg* 1995; 81(6 suppl):S67–S72.
53. Goldberg ME, Cantillo J, Gratz I, et al. Dose of compound A, not sevoflurane, determines changes in the biochemical markers of renal injury in healthy volunteers. *Anesth Analg* 1999; 88:437–454.
54. Ebert TJ, Harkin CP, Muzi M. Cardiovascular responses to sevoflurane: A review. *Anesth Analg* 1995; 81(6 suppl):S11–S22.
55. Thomson IR, Putnins CL. Adverse effects of pancuronium during high-dose fentanyl anesthesia for coronary artery bypass grafting. *Anesthesiology* 1985; 62:708–713.
56. Wright PM, Brown R, Lau M, Fisher DM. A pharmacodynamic explanation for the rapid onset/offset of rapacuronium bromide. *Anesthesiology* 1999; 90:16–23.
57. Levy JH, Pitts M, Thanopoulos A, et al. The effects of rapacuronium on histamine release and hemodynamics in adult patients undergoing general anesthesia. *Anesth Analg* 1999; 89:290–295.
58. Guffin A, Girard D, Kaplan JA. Shivering following cardiac surgery: Hemodynamic changes and reversal. *J Cardiothorac Anesth* 1987; 1:24–28.
59. Frank SM, Fleisher LA, Breslow MJ, et al. Perioperative maintenance of normothermia reduces the incidence of morbid cardiac events: A randomized clinical trial. *JAMA* 1997; 277:1127–1134.
60. Mangano DT, Layug EL, Wallace A, Tateo I. Effect of atenolol on mortality and cardiovascular morbidity after noncardiac surgery: Multicenter Study of Perioperative Ischemia Research Group. *N Engl J Med* 1996; 335:1713–1720.

PART FOURTEEN

MISCELLANEOUS DISEASES AND CONDITIONS

C H A P T E R 76

THE CONNECTIVE TISSUE DISEASES AND THE CARDIOVASCULAR SYSTEM

Robert C. Schlant / William C. Roberts

The term *connective tissue disease* includes both a group of heritable conditions and a group of nonheritable acquired disorders. The heritable disorders of connective tissue associated with cardiovascular disease include Marfan's syndrome (MS), Ehlers-Danlos syndrome (EDS), pseudoxanthoma elasticum (PXE), osteogenesis imperfecta (OI), annuloaortic ectasia, and familial aneurysms.[1] The nonheritable disorders of connective tissue that may have major cardiovascular involvement include systemic lupus erythematosus (SLE), polyarteritis nodosa (PN), rheumatoid arthritis (RA), ankylosing spondylitis, systemic sclerosis (SS), polymyositis/dermatomyositis, giant-cell arteritis, the Churg-Strauss syndrome, the antiphospholipid syndrome, and possibly syphilis.

HERITABLE CONNECTIVE TISSUE DISEASES

Marfan's Syndrome

EPIDEMIOLOGY

The prevalence of the classic MS is about 5 per 100,000, without gender, racial, or ethnic predilection. Because of the great heterogeneity of the syndrome, the actual prevalence may be considerably greater, probably about 1 per 10,000.[2] MS has an autosomal dominant inheritance with high penetrance. In about 25 to 30 percent of patients, the disorder occurs without a positive family history and appears to be due to a new mutation.

MOLECULAR GENETICS

MS is associated with defects in the fibrillin-1 gene (FBN1) on chromosome 15, where 125 reported and unreported mutations (of several types) have been described[3–12] (see also Chap. 62). Nearly every genotyped family has a unique mutation in the fibrillin genes, with the most common single mutation identified in just four unrelated pedigrees. This intragenic heterogenicity and the large size of the gene have precluded the routine screening of mutations to establish the diagnosis of the MS.[9]

CLINICAL FEATURES

There is considerable variation in the clinical manifestations of MS, even within one family. The ocular, skeletal, and cardiovascular systems are characteristically involved. The four major manifestations include a positive family history, ectopia lentis, aortic root dilatation or dissection, and dural ectasia. Many of the other, relatively mild features of MS occur with a relatively high prevalence in the general population. These features include mitral valve prolapse, early myopia, scoliosis, and joint hypermobility. Other manifestations of MS include anterior chest deformity, especially asymmetric pectus excavatum or carinatum; long, thin extremities (dolichostenomelia) with arachnodactyly; tall stature with increased lower body height (Fig. 10-7); high, narrowly arched palate; myopia; fusiform ascending aortic aneurysm (*anuloaortic ectasia*) with aortic regurgitation (Fig. 76-1); aortic dissection; mitral regurgitation, which can result from a variety of causes, including mitral valve prolapse, dilatation of the mitral annulus, mitral annular calcium, dilatation of the left ventricular cavity, rupture of mitral chordae tendineae, papillary muscle dysfunction, or infective endocarditis; spontaneous pneumothorax; cutaneous striae; and inguinal hernia.[1,2]

In the absence of an unequivocally affected first-degree relative, requirements for the diagnosis include at least one major manifestation with involvement of the skeleton and at least two other systems.[12–14] In the presence of at least one unequivocally affected first-degree relative, there should be involvement of at least two systems; the presence of a major manifestation is still preferred, but this can vary depending on the family's phenotype.[12]

By echocardiogram, mitral valve prolapse occurs in nearly 60 percent of adults and aortic root enlargement in about 70

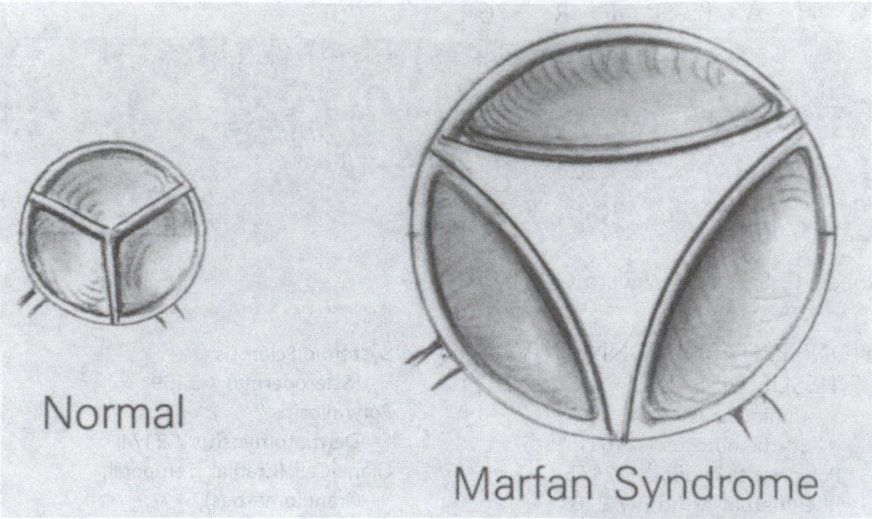

FIGURE 76-1 Mechanism of aortic regurgitation in Marfan's syndrome.

percent of adults with the MS.[15–17] It has been suggested that the MS and mitral valve prolapse are part of a phenotypic continuum.[17]

GENERAL EVALUATION

In addition to carefully recording the personal and family history and physical examination, the patient's height, arm span, and floor-to-pelvis distance should be measured. A slit-lamp ophthalmic examination and an electrocardiogram should be obtained. Patients with MS should be seen at least yearly, and a transthoracic echocardiogram should be obtained annually. Consideration should be given to obtaining a transesophageal echocardiogram or to magnetic resonance imaging (MRI).[18] If the diagnosis is definite or probable, consideration should be given to screening first-degree relatives by echocardiography. Genetic counseling should be offered to all patients. Psychiatric counseling also is often useful. If a patient develops suggestive widening of the proximal aorta, repeat transthoracic or, in some instances, transesophageal echocardiography should be performed more frequently. Patients with possible or definite MS and evidence of mitral valve abnormality should receive antibiotic prophylaxis prior to dental procedures (see Chap. 73).

MANAGEMENT

Patients with MS should avoid isometric, abrupt, or strenuous exertion; contact sports; scuba diving; and trauma. Patients with aortic dilatation and aortic or mitral regurgitation should avoid competitive sports.[19,20] Patients without aortic dilatation and aortic or mitral regurgitation should be allowed to perform low-to-moderate-intensity static and low-intensity dynamic sports, including bowling, golf, and archery.

β-Adrenergic blockade therapy should be used in all patients with MS to retard the rate of dilatation of the aortic root.[2,21,22] Although the optimal dose has not been established, some have suggested giving the largest dose that is clinically tolerated. Selective β_1-adrenergic blocking agents are preferred, although no randomized studies have been performed. Atenolol, which should be administered twice daily, appears to be the most widely used β-adrenergic blocker in this condition.

In asymptomatic patients, repair of aortic aneurysms has been recommended at different degrees of enlargement. Thus, some have advocated repair when the aortic diameter is 55 mm or greater,[23,24] at 60 mm or greater,[21,25–28] or when the aortic diameter increases to twice that of the uninvolved distal aorta.[29–32] Some patients develop aortic dissection with aortic root dimensions less than 50 to 55 mm.[33] Surgical repair is generally recommended when the diameter reaches 55 to 60 mm. Factors that encourage an earlier surgical intervention include a positive family history for aortic dissection or rupture,[34–36] severe aortic or mitral regurgitation, progressive dilatation of the aortic root on serial echocardiograms, the need for other major abdominal aortic or spinal surgical procedures, and planning for a pregnancy. In most patients, the ascending aorta and aortic valve are replaced, and the portion of the aorta containing the coronary ostia is reimplanted,[37] but there are exceptions.[38] Postoperatively annual assessment of the entire aorta by MRI may be useful.

In patients who require a mitral valve procedure, valve repair is usually preferred to replacement, although repair may not always be possible because of a large number of ruptured chordae tendineae, extensive annular calcium, or hugely dilated annuli.[38,39]

PROGNOSIS

While earlier studies indicated that the average lifetime is decreased about 35 percent,[2,40] beta-blocker therapy, antibiotic prophylaxis (against infective endocarditis), and aortic and valvular surgery have probably improved longevity. The most common causes of death of adolescents or adults with the MS are rupture of a fusiform aneurysm of the ascending aorta without longitudinal dissection (Fig. 76-2), ascending aortic dissection with rupture, or congestive heart failure from aortic and/or mitral regurgitation[33] (Fig. 76-3). The major histologic feature in the media of the wall of an aortic aneurysm is a massive loss of elastic fibers[33] (Fig. 76-4). Factors that can predispose to either aortic aneurysm or aortic dissection include systemic arterial hypertension, coarctation of the aorta, pregnancy, and trauma. In children with the MS, the most common cause of death is severe mitral regurgitation (Fig. 76-5).

PREGNANCY

Women with the MS should be counseled regarding the approximately 50 percent risk of transmission of the condition.[41] If the woman has moderate or severe aortic regurgitation or an aortic root diameter exceeding 40 mm, she should be advised that pregnancy greatly increases her risk of premature death. Women with an aortic root diameter of less than 40 mm usually tolerate pregnancy well, but nevertheless the chance of aortic dissection is increased by pregnancy.[42] β-Adrenergic blockers should be administered at least from the midtrimester onward.[43] There may be an advantage to the use of a selective β_1-adrenergic blocker.[44]

During pregnancy, transthoracic echocardiography should be performed every 6 to 10 weeks, depending on the initial findings. Using epidural anesthesia, vaginal delivery in the lat-

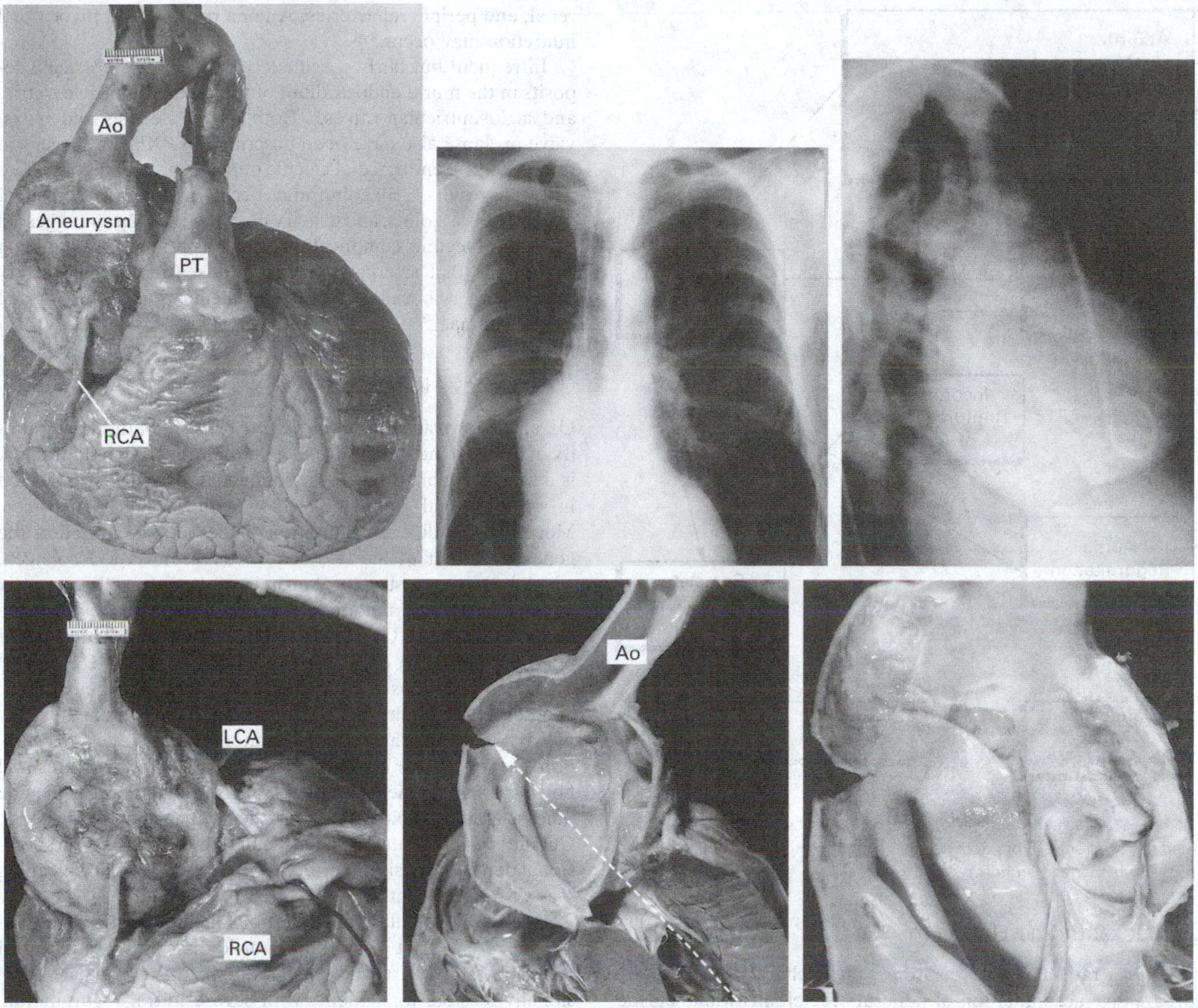

FIGURE 76-2 Heart and aorta of a 38-year-old man who was asymptomatic until exertional dyspnea appeared 5 months before death. *Top left:* Exterior view. Ao, ascending aorta; RCA, right coronary artery; PT, pulmonary trunk. *Bottom left:* Closer view of the massive aortic aneurysm after retracting the pulmonary trunk. LCA, left main coronary artery. The aneurysm does not involve the distal portion of the ascending aorta. *Bottom middle:* View of heart and aorta after removing their anterior half. Death resulted from rupture of the right lateral wall of the aorta at a point where blood ejected from left ventricle contacts the aortic wall (*arrow*). The aneurysmal bulge is mainly to the right. *Bottom right:* Close-up of the multiple healed tears in the ascending aorta. One of the previously incomplete tears ruptured through and through. Posteroanterior chest roentgenogram (*top middle*) and lateral aortogram (*top right*) show massive dilatation of the ascending aorta. (From Roberts and Honig.[33] Reproduced with permission of the publisher and authors.)

eral decubitus position is preferred, and forceps or vacuum delivery is recommended to shorten the second stage of labor. The increases in systemic blood pressure during uterine contractions should be prevented with beta-blocking agents. Postpartum hemorrhage should be anticipated. If fetal maturity can be confirmed in a patient who requires aortic surgery during pregnancy, a Cesarean section can be done before or concomitantly with thoracic surgery.[41,43,44]

Ehlers-Danlos Syndrome

EDS is a heterogeneous group of 14 or more disorders of connective tissue that are characterized primarily by skin fragility, easy bruising, "cigarette paper" scars, skin hyperextensibility, multiple ecchymoses, and joint hypermobility[1,45] (see Fig. 10-5). The numerous types of the EDS have different clinical manifestations, modes of inheritance, and natural history[45] (see also Chap. 62). In several types of the EDS, the heart, heart valves, great vessels, and larger conduit arteries may be involved. Some types of the EDS have spontaneous rupture of the aorta or large arteries, coronary or intracranial aneurysms, and arteriovenous fistulae. Other cardiovascular abnormalities in the EDS include mitral and tricuspid valve prolapse, dilatation of the aortic root, ectasia of the sinuses of Valsalva, aortic regurgitation, renal artery aneurysms, systemic arterial hypertension, and myocardial infarction.[46,47]

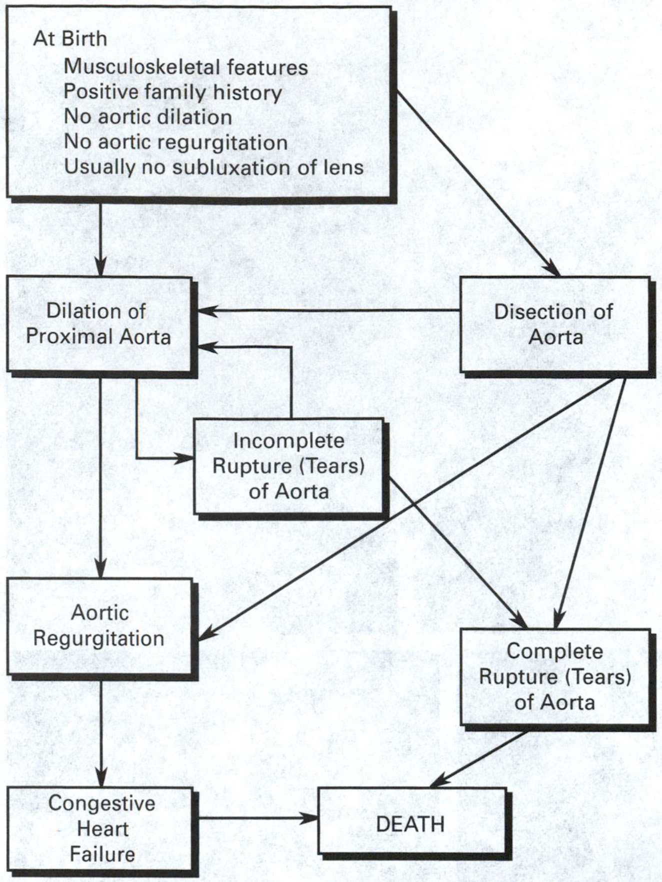

FIGURE 76-3 Scheme of development of cardiovascular complications in Marfan's syndrome. (From Roberts and Honig.[33] Reproduced with permission of the publisher and authors.)

Pseudoxanthoma Elasticum

PXE is a rare heritable disorder that is characterized by the progressive accumulation of mineral precipitants within elastic fibers, particularly those of the skin, Bruch's membrane, and blood vessels. It is transmitted either as an autosomal recessive or as an autosomal dominant trait.[1,48] The estimated prevalence is 1 in 160,000 (see also Chap. 62).

The elastic fiber changes cause skin, eye, gastrointestinal, and cardiovascular manifestations. The skin lesions have been described as resembling a "plucked chicken." Typically, there are yellow macules or papules that produce a rough, cobblestone texture and are maximal in the flexures of the lateral neck, axillae, antecubital fossae, groins, and popliteal spaces. They may form redundant folds of skin[1] (Fig. 10-6). The retinal changes include mottled *peau d'orange* hyperpigmentation, angioid streaks, and an increased incidence of retinal hemorrhage and disk drusen. Angioid streaks, which are breaks in Bruch's membrane behind the retina and are present in 85 percent of patients with PXE, usually develop after the second decade of life. They can be found in numerous other conditions, including MS, EDS, Paget's disease, and sickle cell anemia, although PXE is most common.[49]

There may be calcific deposits in the media of medium-sized arteries. Both vascular deposits similar to Mönckeberg's arteriosclerosis and intimal plaques similar to typical atherosclerotic plaques occur in the coronary, cerebral, gastrointestinal, renal, and peripheral arteries. Angina pectoris and myocardial infarction may occur.[50,51]

Infrequent but fairly specific lesions in PXE are calcific deposits in the mural endocardium of the cardiac ventricles, atria, and atrioventricular valves.[52] Both mitral stenosis and mitral valve prolapse also have been described in PXE.[53,54] Surgery to remove mural endocardial calcific deposits has been performed with fair results.[55] Bleeding may occur in the gastrointestinal system, uterus, joints, and urinary bladder. It has been suggested that some bleeding complications may be prevented by avoiding aspirin and that arterial grafts not be used in coronary artery bypass surgery because of possible calcification of the internal elastic laminae.[48]

Osteogenesis Imperfecta

OI, also known as *brittle bone disease* because of the susceptibility of affected individuals to sustain fractures from mild trauma, is a rare heritable disorder of connective tissue. It is inherited in an autosomal dominant fashion with variable penetrance. More than 80 different mutations have been identified in the genes for either of the two chains that from type I collagen, which is the major structural protein of the extracellular matrix of bone, skin, and tendon.[56] There is a wide variation in the clinical severity of OI, from some forms that are lethal in the perinatal period to other forms that may not be detected.[57–59] Most manifestations of OI are bony, ocular, otologic, cutaneous, and dental. The bony changes manifest themselves in a variety of ways, including short stature, in utero fractures, severe osteoporosis, and severe bone fragility, with repeated fractures and bowing of long bones. The ocular and otologic changes include blue sclerae, angioid streaks in the retina, and hearing loss. Cutaneous and dental changes result in easy bruising and occasional dentinogenesis imperfecta. An increased risk of bleeding may also be present.[59]

The cardiovascular manifestations include aortic regurgitation,[59–63] aortic root dilatation,[59] aortic dissection,[64] and mitral regurgitation.[65] Mitral valve repair and reconstruction are occasionally feasible for patients with severe mitral regurgitation, although most patients require valve replacement. Mitral valve replacement is difficult because of weakness and friability of the tissues and poor wound healing. In addition, some patients have increased bleeding despite normal preoperative coagulation tests and bleeding times.[59,60]

Annuloaortic Ectasia

Annuloaortic ectasia, a pear-shaped enlargement of the sinus and the proximal tubular portions of the ascending aorta, is often part of the MS, where it usually results in aortic regurgitation, partial or complete ascending aortic tears, or both. In some patients, annuloaortic ectasia is familial and no other stigmata of the MS are present.[66] The genetic and molecular changes in these patients are not established. Microscopically, there is severe loss of elastic fibers in the media of the ascending aorta.

Familial Aneurysms

Various types of familial aneurysms involving cardiovascular structures have been reported, including familial aortic dissection,[67] familial aneurysms of the ventricular septum,[68] familial aneurysms of the carotid arteries,[69] and familial intracranial aneurysms.[70] At this time, it is not established that these are heritable disorders of corrective tissue.

Homocystinuria

See Chapter 62.

NONHERITABLE CONNECTIVE TISSUE DISEASES

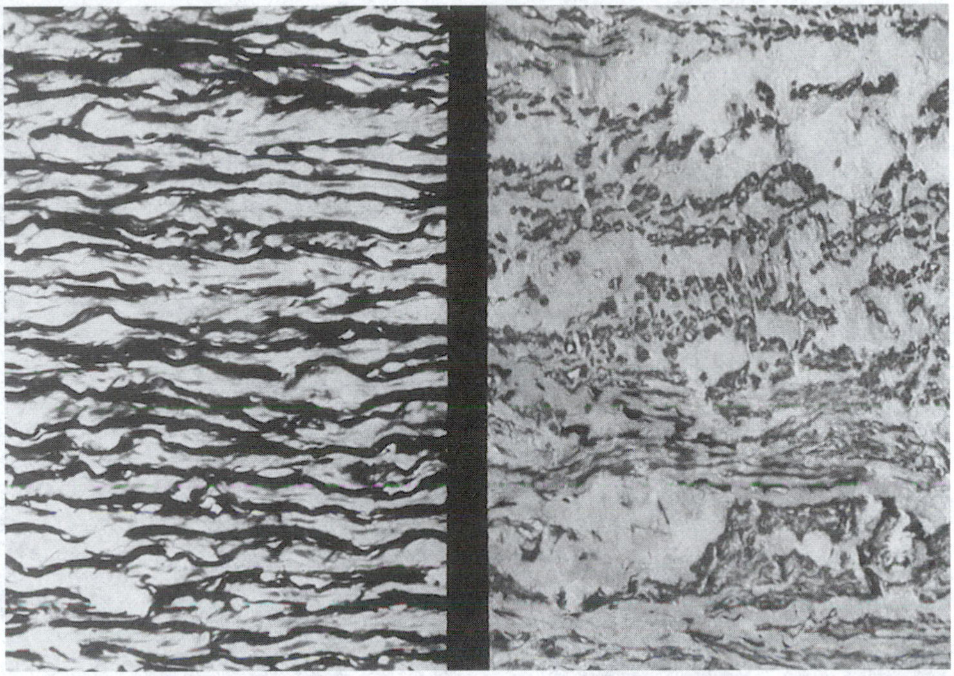

FIGURE 76-4 *Left:* Photomicrograph of the wall of the ascending aorta from a normal subject. *Right:* A similar histologic study (Movat stains) of the wall of an ascending aortic aneurysm in a 35-year-old woman with Marfan's syndrome. Note the virtual absence of elastic fibers. (From Roberts and Honig.[33] Reproduced with permission of the publisher and authors.)

The acquired or nonheritable autoimmune or connective tissue diseases represent a subset of the arthritides and rheumatic disorders. These disorders are systemic in nature, are commonly linked by a diffuse abnormality of vasculature, and are characterized by inflammatory lesions in skin, joints, muscles, and connective tissue linings such as pleura and pericardium. Involvement of the kidneys, brain, and heart is usually responsible for the fatal and most serious consequences. Specific acquired connective tissue diseases that may have major cardiac involvement include SLE, PN, giant-cell arteritis, RA, ankylosing spondylitis, polymyositis/dermatomyositis, SS, and, possibly, syphilis (Table 76-1). Although certain immunogenetic factors have been identified, their etiology remains uncertain.[71]

Systemic Lupus Erythematosus

SLE, which is one of the more common autoimmune diseases, is found worldwide and affects all races, is more common among blacks and females of childbearing age, and is usually more severe in blacks than in whites. SLE is much more frequent among females than among males; in patients less than 40 years of age, the female-male ratio is about 8:1. In the United States, the annual incidence of SLE is about 8 per 100,000 and the prevalence is approximately 1 per 2000. The following genes of the human major histocompatibility locus antigens are associated with an increased risk for SLE: HLA-B8, HLA-DR2, HLA-DR3, HLA-DR5, HLA-DR7, HLA-DQ, and null alleles at the C2 and/or C4 loci. Genetic deficiencies of the complement system—i.e., deficiencies of C1q, C2, C4, and C8—predispose individuals to SLE and SLE-like disorders.

The inflammatory process of SLE involves multiple organ systems, including skin, joints, kidneys, brain, heart, and virtually all serous membranes. Its clinical presentation is varied and depends on the organ system(s) involved. Fever, arthritis and arthralgias, skin rashes (Fig. 10-24), and pleuritis are common early signs of SLE.

The immunologic abnormalities of SLE have been well characterized and enable it to be diagnosed despite the diversity of clinical presentations. Typical serologic abnormalities include the presence of antinuclear antibodies (ANAs), positive serum anti-DNA antibodies, positive anti-Smith antibodies, positive anti-ribonucleoprotein (anti-RNP) antibodies, and hypocomplementemia, i.e., low serum C3 and C4. Less specific but frequently identified antibodies include anticytoplasmic antibodies, anticardiolipin (IgGaCL) antibodies, antiphospholipid (aPL) antibodies, and rheumatoid factor. Serum complement is decreased in most patients with SLE, and, insofar as serum complement is usually normal or elevated in other connective tissue disorders (such as RA, PN, SS, and disseminated infections), this serologic test may be useful in the diagnosis of SLE.[72] Certain patients with SLE are more likely to have elevated levels of aPL antibody, particularly those with recurrent venous thrombosis, thrombocytopenia, recurrent fetal loss, hemolytic anemia, livedo reticularis, leg ulcers, arterial occlusions, transverse myelitis, or pulmonary hypertension.[73] Cardiac abnormalities may occur more frequently in patients with increased aPL or anticardiolipin antibody titers compared with patients without increased levels.[71]

Although it may have an acute, fulminating course, SLE most often is characterized by a chronic course marked with exacerbations and remissions; the 10-year survival rate exceeds 80 percent. Nephritis and seizures decrease survival approximately twofold.[74] When patients die of SLE, it is most often in the setting of acute renal failure, central nervous system disease, associated infection, infective endocarditis, or coronary artery disease (see below).

CARDIAC INVOLVEMENT

Probably about 25 percent of patients with SLE have cardiac involvement.[75] In addition to the valvular thickening or verrucae and mitral or aortic valvular regurgitation (or occasional stenosis), there may be pericardial thickening and/or effusion, left ventricular regional or global systolic or diastolic dysfunction, or evidence of pulmonary hypertension.[75] Either valvular regur-

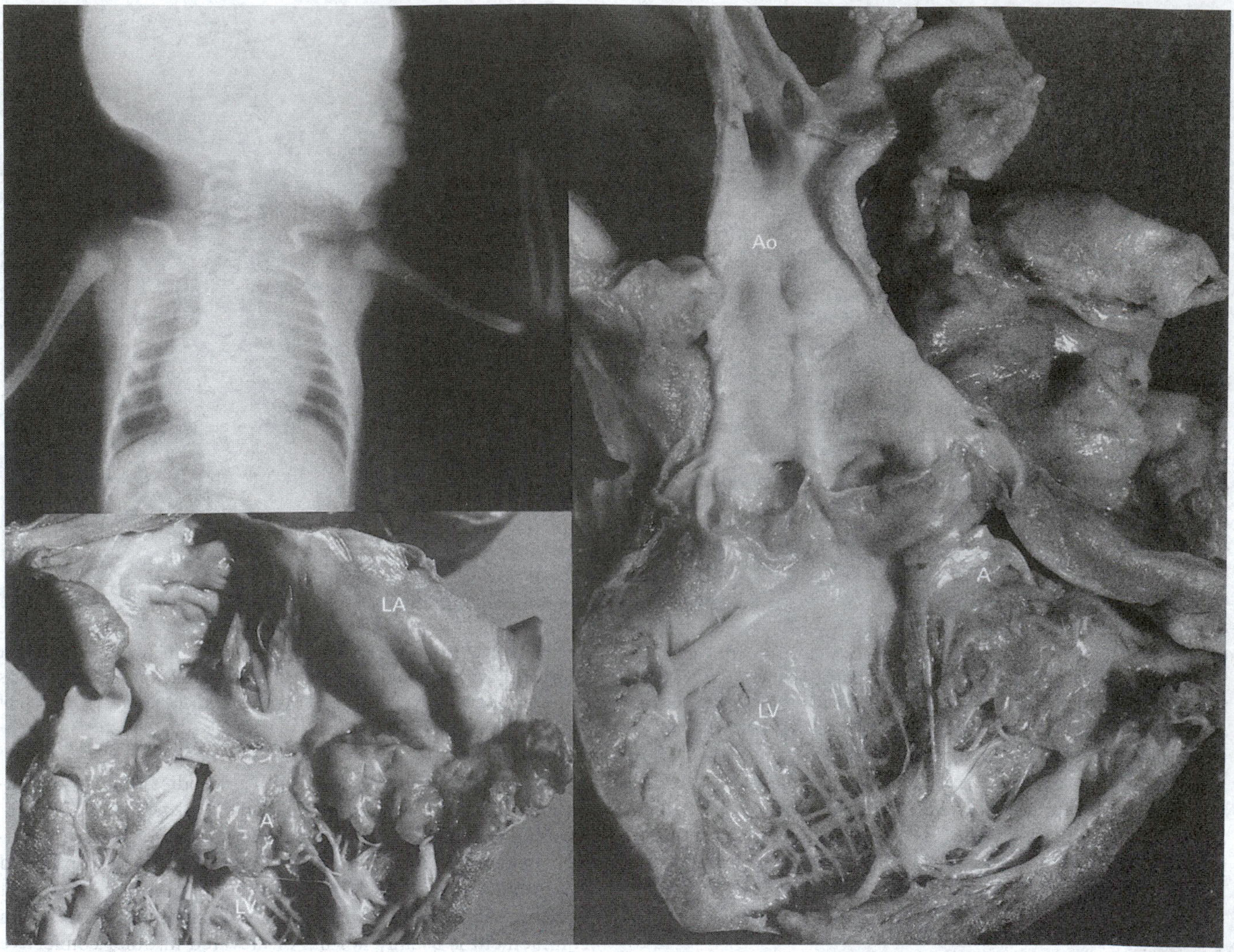

FIGURE 76-5 Congenital floppy mitral valve and floppy tricuspid valve in a 2-day-old boy who had long toes and fingers, a high-arched palate, and a grade 3/6 precordial systolic murmur typical of mitral regurgitation. The heart was enlarged (*top left*), and he died of congestive cardiac failure. At necropsy, the intima of the ascending aorta (Ao) was wrinkled (*right*), suggesting that the underlying media was abnormal at this early stage. Shown here are the opened aorta, aortic valve, and left ventricle (LV). A, anterior mitral leaflet. *Bottom left:* Opened left atrium (LA), mitral valve, and left ventricle (LV). The mitral leaflets are considerably elongated in both longitudinal and transverse dimensions. The left atrium is dilated. (From Roberts and Honig.[33] Reproduced with permission of the publisher and author.)

TABLE 76-1 Primary Cardiac Manifestations of the Nonhereditary Connective Tissue Diseases

Disease	Pericardium	Myocardium	Endocardium (Valves)	Coronary Arteries
Systemic lupus erythematosus	++	+	++	+/−
Systemic sclerosis	+	++	0	++
Polyarteritis nodosa	+/−	+	0	++
Ankylosing spondylitis	0	+/−	++	0
Rheumatoid arthritis	++	+	+	0
Polymyositis/dermatomyositis	++	++	+/−	+/−

NOTE: ++, major site of involvement; +, may be involved, but less frequently; +/−, rarely involved; 0, not involved.

gitation or stenosis due to SLE can require valve replacement.[75] It is unclear whether cardiac abnormalities are significantly more frequent in patients with elevated titers of aPL antibodies.[76-89] In general, valve disease in SLE is frequent but apparently independent of the presence or absence of aPL antibodies.

PERICARDITIS

SLE may cause a pancarditis with abnormalities of pericardium, endocardium, myocardium, and coronary arteries. Pericardial involvement is the most frequent, as observed clinically, by echocardiography, or at autopsy.[75] Pericardial effusions occur at some point in over half of the patients with active SLE. Signs of active or acute pericardial disease may precede (about 5%) the other clinical signs of SLE.[75] In most SLE patients, the pericardial involvement is clinically silent and, if manifest, runs a benign course. Pericardial tamponade may occur and should be considered in patients with unexplained signs of venous congestion.[75] On rare occasions, SLE pericardial disease may lead to pericardial constriction or to acute cardiac tamponade.[75,90] Although the size of the pericardial effusion usually is not sufficiently large to allow aspiration, serologic studies of the pericardial fluid can be useful in diagnosing pericardial effusions due to SLE.

The most common type of pericardial disease in SLE is the presence of diffuse or focal adhesions or fibrinous deposits.[75] The pericardial fluid usually contains mononuclear leukocytes and occasionally lupus erythematosus (LE) cells. In patients with long-standing SLE treated with anti-inflammatory agents, pericardial abnormalities appear to occur with the same frequency as in patients not receiving these agents, but at autopsy the involvement is less extensive and more likely to be fibrous rather than fibrinous. SLE patients with fibrinous pericardial disease, particularly those with severe debilitation or renal failure, are at increased risk for purulent pericarditis, which is usually fatal.[75]

ENDOCARDITIS AND VALVE DISEASE

The cardiovascular lesion of SLE that has received the most attention is the *atypical verrucous endocarditis* first described by Libman and Sacks in 1924,[91] long before SLE was recognized as a systemic disease. The lesions, as they were first described and subsequently attributed to SLE,[92] consist almost entirely of fibrin, and although they may occur on both surfaces of any of the four cardiac valves, they are now most frequently found on the left-sided valves, particularly the ventricular surface of the posterior mitral leaflet (Fig. 76-6).[75] These *verrucae* are similar histologically to those of nonbacterial thrombotic noninfective endocarditis, the valve lesion that occurs most frequently in patients with debilitating illnesses or cancer, except that occasionally hematoxylin bodies, considered the histologic counterpart of LE cells, may be found within Libman-Sacks lesions. While valvular verrucae in SLE (Libman-Sacks lesions) are usually clinically silent, they can be dislodged and embolize and can also become infected, producing infective endocarditis.[75,89] It is prudent to recommend antibiotic prophylaxis against infective endocarditis when patients with SLE undergo procedures that may be associated with bacteremia (see Chap. 73).

Echocardiographically, SLE has a characteristic appearance, with leaflet thickening and valve masses[75,89] (see also Chap. 13). The end-stage or healed form of the verrucous endocarditis of SLE is a fibrous plaque. In some instances, if the thrombotic lesions are extensive enough, their healing may be accompanied by focal scarring and deformity of the underlying valve tissue. This healed form of SLE "endocarditis" may cause valvular dysfunction, particularly mitral and/or aortic regurgitation.[75]

MYOCARDITIS

It is unclear whether infiltration of the myocardial interstitium with acute and/or chronic inflammatory cells and focal myocardial necrosis (i.e., myocarditis) occurs as a natural part of SLE, unassociated with anti-inflammatory drug therapy (glucocorticoid treatment).[75] Several reports have described clinical features consistent with myocarditis, but actual visualization of interstitial myocardial inflammatory cells with associated myofiber necrosis has not been demonstrated histologically. Hemodynamic and echocardiographic studies, however, have shown

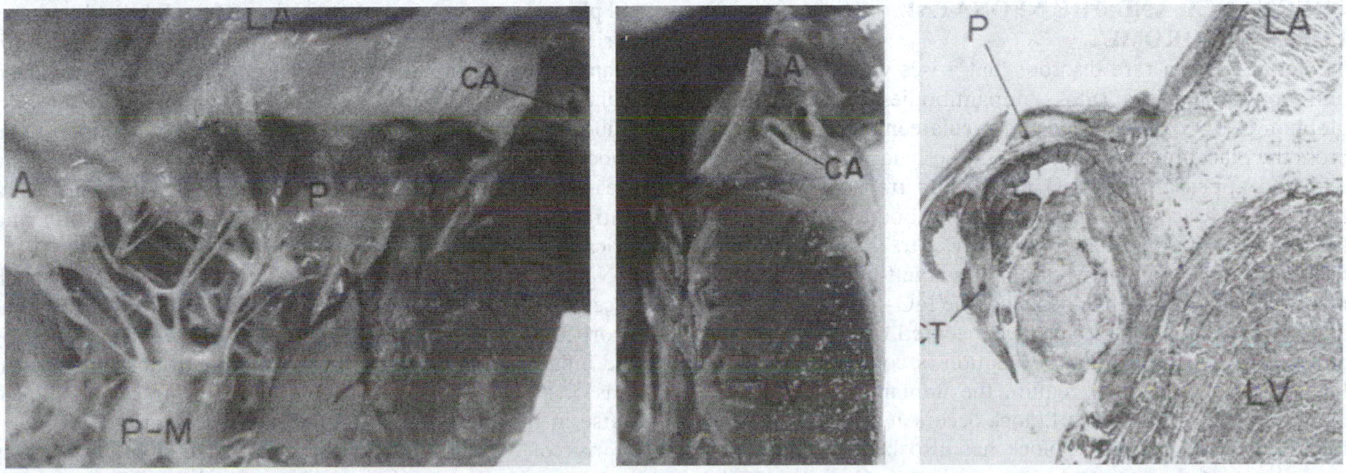

FIGURE 76-6 An example of Libman-Sacks endocarditis in systemic lupus erythematosus. *A* and *B*. The left atrium (LA) and left ventricle (LV) are open. *B* and *C*. Fibrofibrinous verrucae, present on the undersurface of the posterior leaflet (P) of the mitral valve, are often clinically silent. A, anterior leaflet of mitral valve; CA, left circumflex coronary artery; P-M, posteromedial papillary muscle; CT, chorda tendineae. H&E, ×8. (From Bulkley and Roberts.[87] Reproduced with permission from the publisher and author.)

abnormalities in both systolic and diastolic ventricular function in some SLE patients.[75] Whether these abnormalities result from an *autoimmune attack* on the myocardium or from the effects of systemic arterial hypertension, coronary artery disease, or coexisting pericardial disease is unclear (see below).

CORONARY ARTERY DISEASE

Both fatal and nonfatal acute myocardial infarction and sudden coronary death (without demonstrable infarction) from coronary artery disease may occur early in the course of SLE, particularly among young women. Studies of hearts in patients with fatal SLE have demonstrated a high incidence of coronary atherosclerosis in patients who received treatment with glucocorticoids for more than 2 years.[75,93,94] Accelerated coronary atherosclerosis is increasingly recognized as a leading cause of morbidity and mortality among young women patients with SLE who receive long-term glucocorticoid administration.[75,93] Although the causes of this premature coronary atherosclerosis are uncertain, glucocorticoid treatment as well as aPL antibodies have been incriminated. It has been speculated that SLE itself may induce an underlying vasculopathy or arteritis that may facilitate premature atherogenesis from long-term glucocorticoid treatment. Coronary disease in SLE was not described before glucocorticoid therapy was introduced.[75] In one study, the presence of elevated aPL antibodies in patients with SLE correlated with left ventricular (global or segmental) dysfunction, verrucous valvular (aortic or mitral) thickening, and global valvular (mitral or aortic) thickening and dysfunction, as well as mitral regurgitation and aortic regurgitation. Coronary thrombi may occur in patients with active lupus and an acute myocardial infarction in the presence of angiographically normal coronary arteries.[95] SLE also may cause coronary aneurysm;[96,97] aPL antibodies are known to promote platelet aggregation and to be associated with the presence of a clotting tendency, the so-called lupus anticoagulant syndrome.[76]

Inflammation (arteritis) of the wall of the sinus node artery in association with scarring of both sinus and atrioventricular nodes may account for some of the rhythm and conduction disturbances seen in these patients.[98]

PREGNANCY AND THE NEONATAL LUPUS SYNDROME

Neonatal LE is a rare disorder that arises when the so-called anti-Ro, or Sjögren's, (SSA) autoantibodies, mostly immunoglobulin G (IgG), are formed and circulate in pregnant patients, cross the placenta, and cause a lupuslike syndrome in newborns with the appearance of a skin rash and transient cytopenias from passively acquired maternal autoantibodies. Since the half-life of IgG antibodies is approximately 21 to 25 days, the neonatal lupus syndrome in newborn babies is self-limiting; it usually resolves in 3 to 6 months when all of the IgG-containing anti-Ro maternal autoantibodies have been cleared from the neonate's circulation. An unfortunate exception is complete congenital heart block, which may require the implantation of a pacemaker. Once complete heart block occurs, it is usually irreversible. Second-degree heart block has also been reported as a component of the neonatal lupus syndrome. One neonate has been described with first-degree heart block at birth that resolved 6 months later. Antibodies to the Ro (SSA) ribonucleoprotein complexes are present in over 85 percent of sera from mothers of infants with complete congenital heart block. In many patients, antibodies reactive to the La (SSB) antigen as well as the U1RNP protein particle are found in association with anti-Ro (SSA) antibodies.

In most cases, the neonatal lupus syndrome is a benign disorder, and most babies of mothers with anti-Ro (SSA), anti-La (SSB), or anti-U1RNP antibodies do not develop neonatal lupus. *A pregnant woman with SLE with positive anti-Ro, anti-La, or anti-RNP antibodies has a risk of less than 3 percent of having a child with neonatal lupus and congenital heart block. The risk that this patient might have an infant with the neonatal lupus syndrome but without congenital heart block may be as high as 1 in 3.* The neonatal lupus syndrome mediated by the presence of maternal anti-Ro antibodies can occur in babies of mothers who do not have overt SLE, who may or may not meet criteria for a diagnosis of SLE, and who may or may not have a positive test for antinuclear antibodies.

The neonatal lupus syndrome with congenital heart block can be diagnosed by the appearance of fetal bradycardia around week 23 of gestation.[99–101] The cardiac damage with conduction abnormalities in a neonate may result from binding of the passively transferred pathogenic anti-Ro antibodies to Ro (SSA)/La (SSB) antigens present in the fetal heart. It is not known whether these IgG anti-Ro antibodies represent *clinical markers* only or whether they are pathogenic. All mothers of neonates with complete congenital heart block have been HLA-DR3 positive. If a mother is HLA-DR3 positive and has circulating IgG anti-Ro antibodies, her neonate is at risk regardless of the neonate's HLA-DR status.

Other cardiac abnormalities reported in the neonatal lupus syndrome include right bundle branch block, second-degree atrioventricular block, 2:1 atrioventricular block, patent ductus arteriosus, patent foramen ovale, coarctation of the aorta, tetralogy of Fallot, atrial septal defect, hypoplastic right ventricle, ventricular septal defect, dysplastic pulmonic valve, mitral and tricuspid regurgitation, pericarditis, and myocarditis. Most of these patients eventually have a pacemaker inserted.

Pregnant women with SLE should have a serum anti-Ro (SSA) antibody determination as early in pregnancy as possible. Prenatal treatment of established congenital heart block has consisted of the administration of prednisone or dexamethasone and plasmapheresis from week 23 on, although heart block has persisted in most cases. It is unclear whether aggressive anti-inflammatory therapy in an effort to diminish the generalized fetal insult and to lower the titers of circulating anti-Ro (SSA) antibodies makes a difference in fetal cardiac outcome. Fetal echocardiography is useful in following the progression of the disease and also in helping to identify decreased left ventricular contractility, increased cardiac size, tricuspid regurgitation, and pericardial effusion.

Neither dexamethasone nor plasmapheresis has had much success in reversing intrauterine third-degree heart block. Glucocorticoids, however, may be helpful in suppressing an associated inflammatory response producing pleuropericardial effusions or ascites in the fetus. Close monitoring of the clinical course in the prospective mother is also essential because of the risk of exacerbation of the SLE. If fetal bradycardia is present, an *intrauterine therapeutic approach* for as long as possible is recommended to allow for fetal maturation to occur. Ultrasound images can be useful for assessing the degree of cardiac dysfunction present. Following delivery, the neonatologist should be prepared to have a cardiac pacemaker implanted.

Otherwise, all of the other clinical and laboratory features of the neonatal lupus syndrome (with the exception of complete heart block and/or similar severe cardiac fetal disease) should slowly and gradually disappear over the first few months of the baby's life. In one study, one-third of the children with autoantibody-associated congenital heart block died in the early neonatal period;[102] of those who survived, most required a pacemaker.

Women with SLE who are anti-Ro positive should be closely monitored during pregnancy, as should mothers of previous babies born with congenital complete heart block. Pregnant patients who are anti-Ro positive and whose babies have not had fetal bradycardia throughout most of the pregnancy should be reminded that congenital complete heart block is rare and that the neonatal cutaneous lupus syndrome is benign and transient. The long-term prognosis of the mothers of children born with congenital heart block is generally fairly good.[103] In these mothers, the risk of congenital heart block in children of subsequent pregnancies is low.[102] Newborns of mothers with SLE who have a normal pulse rate are unlikely to have significant abnormalities in atrioventricular conduction and do not need screening electrocardiograms at birth.[104]

A higher prevalence of clinical evidence of myocarditis and conduction defects is found in adult anti-Ro-positive patients with SLE than in patients who are anti-Ro negative or in healthy controls.[105] In general, clinical features consistent with myocarditis and conduction defects are relatively common in adults with SLE and seem associated with positive anti-Ro antibodies. Myocarditis at necropsy, however, is rare.[75] In most adults with SLE, positive anti-Ro antibodies have uncommonly been associated with complete heart block.[106] The role of the anti-Ro antibody in inducing heart blocks in adult patients with SLE is unclear.

SECONDARY EFFECTS ON THE HEART

Many, if not most, of the clinically significant cardiac problems occurring in patients with SLE are secondary. Systemic arterial hypertension is common in patients with SLE, particularly those with renal disease and long-standing glucocorticoid therapy, and is a major cause of cardiac enlargement and heart failure.[75] Pulmonary hypertension is also common, approaching 50 percent in a 5-year follow-up study.[107] Uremic pericarditis may occur, of course, in patients with severe renal failure. Premature or accelerated atherosclerosis has been increasingly recognized in young women with SLE receiving long-term glucocorticoid treatment.[75]

THERAPY

Therapy of cardiovascular SLE is the treatment of the underlying disease and includes nonsteroidal anti-inflammatory drugs, glucocorticoids, and, in severe cases, cytotoxic agents such as azathioprine and cyclophosphamide. Systemic arterial hypertension, congestive heart failure, and arrhythmias should be treated with standard therapeutic measures. SLE-induced valve disease can require valve replacement.[75,108,109] Pericardial tamponade may require either high-dose steroids, pericardiocentesis, or placement of a pericardial window, but recurrent effusions or pericardial thickening may develop. Premature cardiovascular events from accelerated atherosclerosis may result in sudden death or myocardial infarction.[75] The antimalarial agent hydroxychloroquine lowers serum cholesterol levels in patients with SLE[110] and may decrease myocardial ischemic damage.[111] An antimalarial such as hydroxychloroquine may be beneficial as a prophylactic agent to prevent premature or accelerated atherosclerosis in young women with SLE receiving long-term treatment with glucocorticoids. Although there are no studies documenting benefit, low-dose aspirin and hydroxychloroquine are often utilized in SLE patients receiving long-term glucocorticoid therapy.

Polyarteritis Nodosa

PN is characterized by segmental necrotizing inflammation of the medium- to small-sized arteries throughout the body, resulting in dysfunction of multiple organ systems. The commonly involved organs are the skin, kidneys, gastrointestinal tract, spleen and lymph nodes, central nervous and musculoskeletal systems, and heart. A variety of cutaneous lesions may be seen: livedo reticularis, palpable purpura, ulcerations, infarcts of distal digits, and nodules. Evidence of glomerulonephritis ranges from low-grade proteinuria to malignant hypertension and acute renal failure.

An association between PN and hepatitis B infection has been recognized for over a decade, and an association with hepatitis C virus infection has also been described;[112] hairy cell leukemia has been described in a few patients with PN. Although the erythrocyte sedimentation rate and serum gamma globulins may be elevated, and rheumatoid factor and antinuclear antibodies may be present, the final clinical diagnosis of PN rests on the combination of multisystem disease and biopsy evidence of active arteritis.[113] In PN, mesenteric vessel angiograms may show aneurysmal dilatation that mimics mycotic aneurysm in infective endocarditis. Since an inflammatory necrotizing arteritis may occur in a variety of disorders, other causes and types of arteritis must be excluded before the diagnosis of PN is made. Classed as separate entities are granulomatous or giant-cell arteritis, hypersensitivity angiitis, temporal arteritis, and arteritis involving the aorta and its major branches. The designation *microscopic polyangiitis* may more appropriately describe patients who have no arteritis, but who have small-vessel vasculitis affecting arterioles, venules, and capillaries. Also, arteritis associated with other connective tissue disorders, for example, rheumatoid vasculitis, is not thought to represent PN when arteritis is the major clinical disease presentation.[113]

CARDIAC INVOLVEMENT

The heart and the coronary arteries are frequent targets of PN. Most often this involvement is a vasculitis of the distal subepicardial coronary arteries just as they penetrate the myocardium (Fig. 76-7). The lesions are characterized by inflammatory infiltrates in the media and adventitia and occasionally by necrosis of the full thickness of the vessel wall, with prominent involvement of the surrounding perivascular connective tissue (Fig. 76-7). The lumens of the involved vessels may contain thrombi, and the walls may be aneurysmal. The latter is responsible for the nodular appearance of the arteries deemed characteristic of this disorder. An even later stage of the vasculitis process is evident as the lesions heal, first showing the formation of granulation tissue and subsequently fibrous tissue replacement of the original components of the artery. In this healing phase, intimal proliferation leading to coronary artery luminal narrowing is evident.[114]

The coronary arterial disease of PN may lead to myocardial

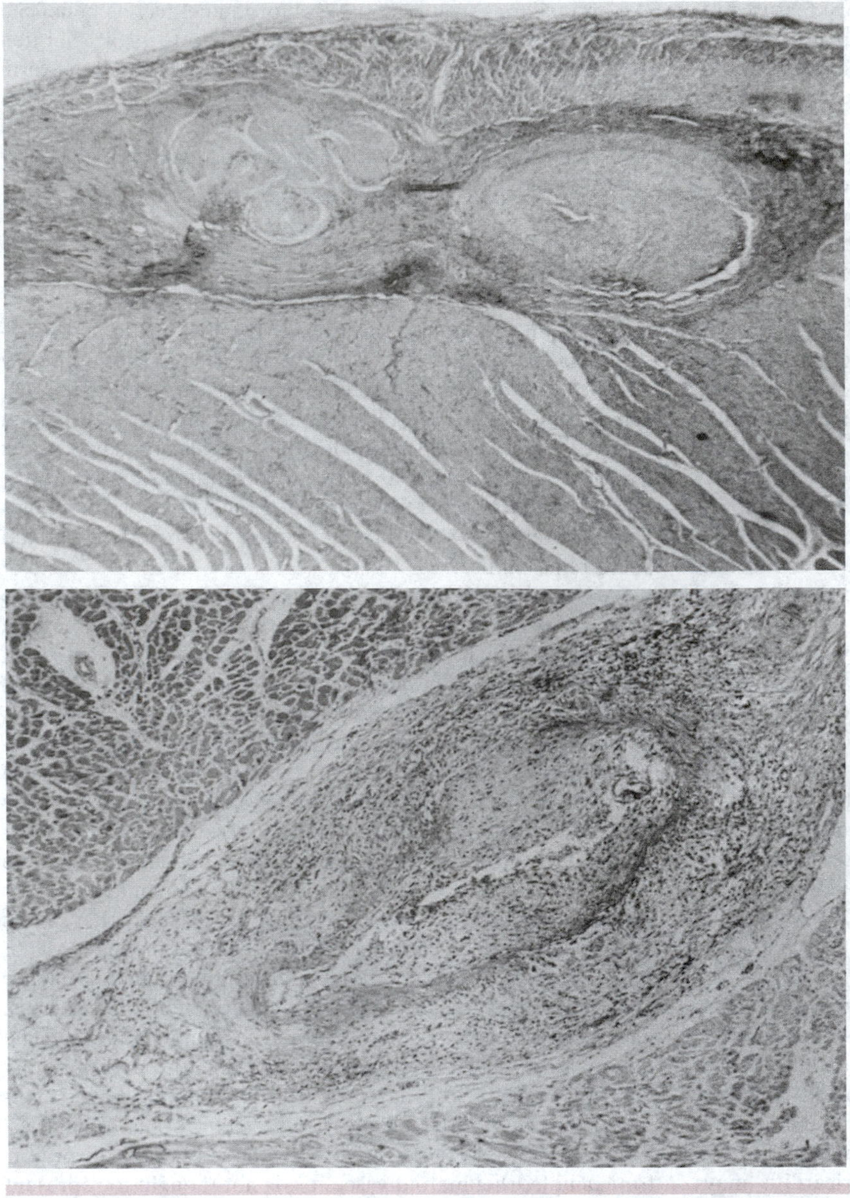

FIGURE 76-7 Polyarteritis nodosa. Examples of the necrotizing vasculitis affecting the extramural and intramural coronary arteries in polyarteritis. *Top:* Extramural coronary arteries. *Bottom:* Intramural coronary arteries. The intramural artery shows a necrotizing arteritis with inflammation involving the full thickness of the vessel. H&E, *top*, ×7; *bottom*, ×22.

infarction.[115] The myocardial necrosis and subsequent replacement fibrosis tend to be focal and patchy throughout the left ventricular wall. This is in contrast to the large areas of grossly visible, regional, subendocardial or transmural necrosis typically seen in the myocardial infarction caused by coronary artherosclerosis (see also Chap. 39).

Conduction system abnormalities have been identified in the heart of patients with PN. The size and location of the sinoatrial node and atrioventricular node arteries make them prime targets for polyarteritis.[116] Atrial and ventricular conduction disturbances may be a primary manifestation of PN, despite minimal involvement of vessels elsewhere in the heart.

Other cardiac abnormalities seen in patients with PN are those that are likely secondary to the underlying systemic arterial hypertension and renal disease. Cardiomegaly and left ventricular hypertrophy most often represent secondary cardiac manifestations of this disease. Similarly, pericardial disease may develop in a patient with PN, but this is most often due to renal insufficiency.

A new autoantibody identified in the serum of patients with systemic vasculitis, especially Wegener's granulomatosis, is the so-called antineutrophil cytoplasmic antibody (ANCA).[117] The ANCA test recognizes antibodies to azurophilic granules present in the cytoplasm of neutrophils. There are two types of ANCA: c-ANCA and p-ANCA. The antigen against which c-ANCA is directed is a 29-kDa serine proteinase. Approximately 90 percent of patients which Wegener's granulomatosis have positive c-ANCA antibodies, the *c* describing the cytoplasmic staining observed under fluorescent microscopy. In contrast, other vasculitides, including PN, tend to have a positive so-called p-ANCA antibody, the *p* describing the perinuclear staining observed in the immunofluorescent assay.

The antigen responsible for the p-ANCA antibody detection appears to be a myeloperoxidase. The detection of serum ANCA levels is a useful laboratory diagnostic marker in the evaluation of the systemic vasculitides, particularly c-ANCA for Wegener's granulomatosis. Serum p-ANCA positivity seems to be nonspecific. For instance, positive p-ANCA may be seen in other chronic inflammatory disorders such as Crohn's enteritis, Felty's syndrome, Kawasaki's vasculitis, leprosy, and tuberculosis. Therefore, the detection of a positive serum p-ANCA in a patient with the clinical picture suggestive of PN should not preclude the need for a biopsy or an angiogram.

CLINICAL MANIFESTATIONS OF CARDIAC DISEASE

Despite the dramatic involvement of coronary arteries that may accompany PN, the most frequent cardiovascular abnormalities seen in patients with PN are unrelated to the coronary arteries per se. Systemic arterial hypertension occurs in approximately 90 percent of these patients and, in combination with chronic renal failure, is the most likely cause of congestive heart failure, which may develop in up to 60 percent of patients.[113] Patients with PN also may develop acute myocardial infarction, which poses the diagnostic question of whether the myocardial injury is due to coronary arteritis with secondary thrombosis or to atherosclerosis, in a population that is typically middle-aged, male, steroid treated, and susceptible to atherosclerotic coronary artery disease as well.[115]

THERAPY

PN has a poor prognosis, especially when systemic arterial hypertension and renal disease are present. Treatment of the heart disease in PN is directed at the specific cardiac dysfunction, and glucocorticoid and other anti-inflammatory agents are administered for the underlying disease. Glucocorticoids are still the initial mainstay of therapy, although they can aggravate coexisting hypertension and even atherosclerosis. Often added to the treatment regimen are glucocorticoid-sparing agents such as cyclophosphamide, azathioprine, or methotrexate. The use of warfarin remains controversial; low-dose aspirin, however, is usually recommended.

Rheumatoid Arthritis

RA, the most common of the connective tissue diseases, is characterized by its deforming erosions of the joints; these erosions result from chronic synovial inflammation and proliferation. It tends to affect women twice as often as men and may run in families. Joint symptoms dominate its course, and symmetric involvement of the hands and wrists is most common. Other joints of the upper and lower extremities and the temporomandibular and sternoclavicular joints also may be affected. The most common systemic or extraarticular manifestations of RA include fever, weight loss, anemia, subcutaneous rheumatoid nodules, and lymphadenopathy. Less frequently, pleuritis and a diffuse, necrotizing vasculitis may occur.

PERICARDIAL INVOLVEMENT

Cardiac involvement is uncommon in RA but may take a variety of forms. A diffuse, nonspecific fibrofibrinous pericarditis occurs in about 50 percent of patients with RA; it is usually clinically silent and is overshadowed by pleuritis or joint pain.[118,119] The pericardial disease tends to be benign, but sizable effusions can occur and require pericardiocentesis, and pericardial constriction can rarely necessitate pericardiectomy. Constrictive pericarditis occurred in 4 of 47 patients with RA whose cases were followed over a 10-year period.[120] The histopathologic findings in all cases after pericardiectomy were consistent with chronic fibrosing pericardial disease. Another study reported on cardiac constriction from rheumatoid pericardial disease. These patients had disease longer, more severe disease, worse functional class, and more extraarticular features when compared with RA patients without cardiac constriction.[121] The presenting clinical features of cardiac constriction included dyspnea, edema, chest pain, and pulsus paradoxus. Chronic, symptomatic pericarditis may require glucocorticoid therapy. RA pericardial disease may shorten survival, especially in the older patients, and be associated with the presence of other cardiac disease, a greater number of extraarticular manifestations, jugular venous distension, and a lower mean systemic blood pressure.[122] Lymphocytic infiltrates of the CD8-positive type may occur in the pericardium of patients with rheumatoid pericardial disease, suggesting that these cells may play a role in the development of the pericardial disease[123] (see also Chap. 72).

MYOCARDIAL AND ENDOCARDIAL INVOLVEMENT

Rarely, rheumatoid nodules focally infiltrate the heart, including the myocardium and the four cardiac valves (Fig. 76-8).[118] These nodules may produce no symptoms, but, if extensive enough or strategically located, they can compromise cardiac function. A rheumatoid nodule may extend from the mural endocardium into a chamber to present as an intracavitary mass.[124] Rheumatoid nodules developing within the valve leaflets may result in mild valvular regurgitation; if the nodule becomes necrotic, perforation of the leaflet can occur and lead to severe valvular regurgitation. The incidence of such valvular infiltration has been estimated at 1 to 2 percent in autopsy studies of patients with RA. Although distinctly uncommon, arrhythmias and conduction disturbances, including complete heart block,[118] and congestive heart failure can also result from RA involvement of the heart. One echocardiographic study of 39 patients with RA detected left ventricular abnormalities in a quarter of the patients.[125] Acute myocardial infarction may be associated with RA.[126]

THERAPY

Since most of the cardiac lesions of RA are clinically silent, it is not certain that the specific therapies used in RA, including nonsteroid anti-inflammatory drugs (NSAIDs), methotrexate, penicillamine, gold, and glucocorticoids, affect the cardiac involvement. Treatment of cardiac constriction from rheuma-

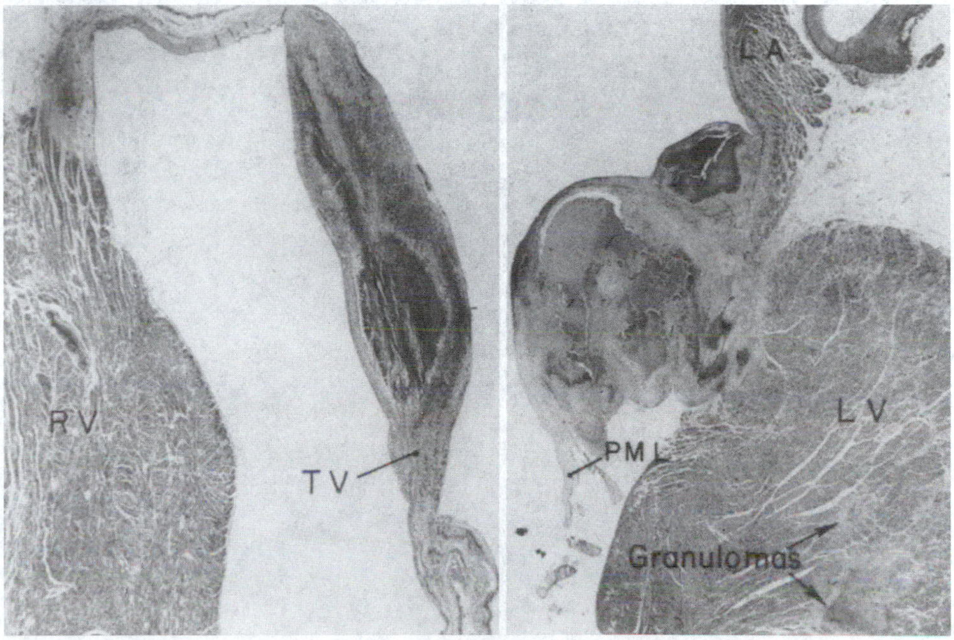

FIGURE 76-8 Rheumatoid arthritis. *A.* A tricuspid valve (TV) infiltrated by rheumatoid nodules. *B.* A mitral valve infiltrated by rheumatoid nodules. In addition, granulomas are present within the left ventricular (LV) wall. LA, left atrium; PML, posterior mitral leaflet; RV, right ventricle. H&E, *A*, ×12; *B*, ×65. (From Roberts WC, Dangel JC, and Bulkley BH.[118] Nonrheumatic valvular cardiac disease: A clinicopathologic survey of 27 different conditions causing valvular dysfunction. In: *Cardiovascular Clinics.* Copyright 1973 by F.A. Davis Company; used by permission of F.A. Davis Company.)

toid pericardial disease may include a trial of high-dose intravenous glucocorticoid (e.g., methylprednisolone) and/or surgical therapy. Pericardiocentesis should be performed only as a lifesaving procedure.[121]

Hydroxychloroquine and NSAIDs are often used. Both have an anticoagulant, antiplatelet effect, which may partially explain why thrombotic events such as deep vein thrombophlebitis as well as acute myocardial infarction are relatively uncommon in patients with RA. Otherwise, conventional treatments of pericarditis, arrhythmias, and conduction disturbances are utilized when these disorders produce clinical symptoms.

Ankylosing Spondylitis

Ankylosing spondylitis is the prototypical example within the group of the seronegative spondyloarthropathies. It is distinctly different from RA. Ankylosing spondylitis is characterized by a progressive inflammatory lesion of the spine, leading to chronic back pain, deforming dorsal kyphosis (Fig. 10-26), and, in its advanced stage, fusion of the costovertebral and sacroiliac joints with immobilization of the spine. This condition is much more frequent in men than in women (9:1), generally first occurring early in life but with a chronic progressive course of 20 to 30 years.[127] The HLA-B27 histocompatibility antigen is found in nearly all patients with ankylosing spondylitis. Other seronegative arthritides that have a high prevalence of this antigen include Reiter's syndrome, psoriatic arthritis, and juvenile arthritis.

CARDIAC INVOLVEMENT

Cardiovascular disease in ankylosing spondylitis takes the form of a sclerosing inflammatory lesion that is generally limited to the aortic root area. The inflammatory process, which extends immediately above and below the aortic valve, typically causes aortic regurgitation[128,129] (Fig. 76-9). As the inflammatory process extends below the aortic valve, it can infiltrate the basal portion of the mitral valve (which is contiguous with the aortic valve) and cause mitral regurgitation.[129] Extension of the inflammatory lesion into the cephalad portion of the ventricular septum, immediately caudal to the aortic valve, accounts for the associated conduction disturbances. Ventricular diastolic dysfunction may also occur.[130]

The major clinical manifestation of ankylosing spondylitis is aortic regurgitation, which occurs in about 5 percent of patients with this condition. Among patients with signs of spondylitis for 10 years, only 2 percent have clinical evidence of aortic regurgitation; by 30 years, that number increases fivefold.[128] Ankylosing spondylitis may be associated with aortic root inflammatory lesions, as may other seronegative spondyloarthropathies such as Reiter's syndrome and psoriatic arthropathy.[128]

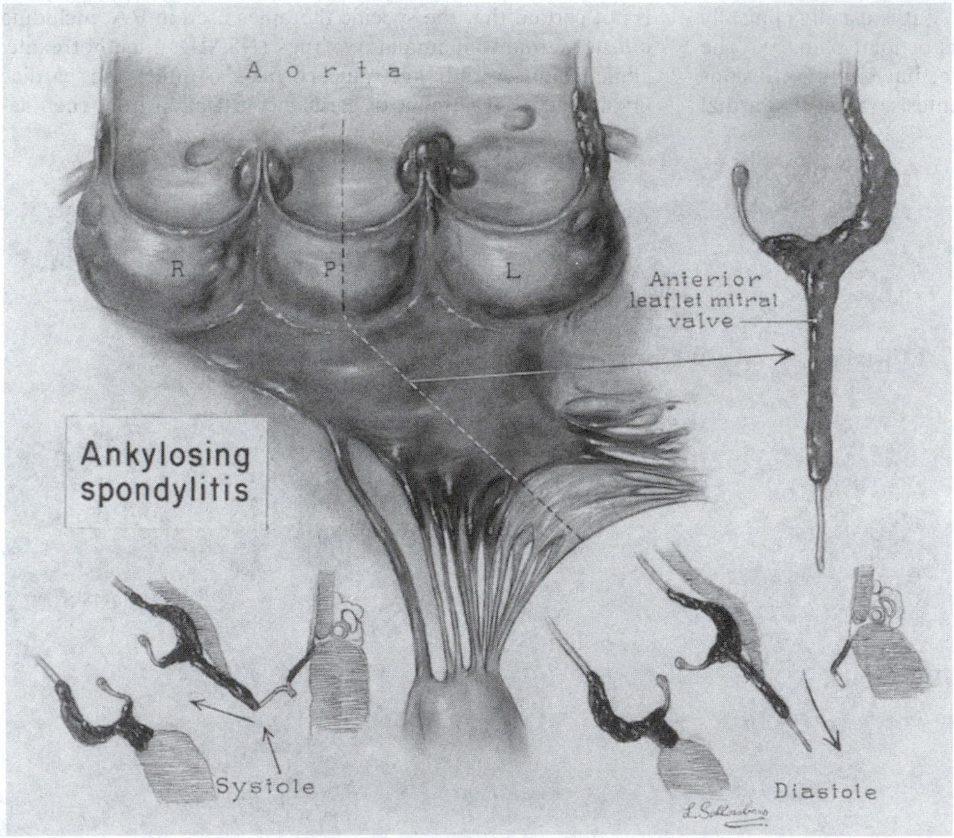

FIGURE 76-9 Diagram showing the characteristic features of ankylosing spondylitis of the heart. The aorta and aortic valve are opened, showing the thickening of the aorta in the vicinity of the aortic valve commissures and the thickening of the anterior mitral leaflet. The small diagrams at the *bottom* of the figure show the thickening in the wall of the aorta behind the sinuses extending below the aortic valve into the membranous ventricular septum and anterior mitral leaflet. In the patient whose heart was portrayed by this diagram, there was also some thickening in posterior mitral leaflet.

THERAPY

Drug therapy for ankylosing spondylitis is primarily directed at relief of the back pain and discomfort. This is accomplished with the use of NSAIDs, methotrexate, and sulfasalazine in addition to physical therapy; phenylbutazone is currently rarely used. Glucocorticoids are not used in this condition except for treatment of iritis. The inflammatory lesion of the heart generally runs a clinically silent course until aortic regurgitation develops. Not infrequently, however, the aortic regurgitation of ankylosing spondylitis may become severe enough to warrant aortic valve replacement[128,129] (see also Chap. 56).

Cardiovascular Syphilis

Although this condition has traditionally not been considered to be a connective tissue disorder, cardiovascular syphilis has histologic features nearly identical to those of ankylosing spondylitis, and spirochetes have never been identified in the aorta of a patient with cardiovascular syphilis. The distribution of the lesions, however, is distinctly different in these two conditions.[118] In cardiovascular syphilis, the process is usually limited to the tubular portion of ascending aorta, i.e., that portion up to the origin of the innominate artery. Because the process as a rule does not extend into the wall of aorta behind the sinuses of Valsalva, aortic regurgitation is infrequent in syphilis. Exactly what percentage of patients with cardiovascular syphilis develop aortic regurgitation is unclear, but it is probably no more than about 15 percent and only those patients in whom the process extends into the wall of aorta behind the sinuses of Valsalva. In syphilis, the process never involves the aortic valve cusps and never extends below (caudal to) the aortic valve. In contrast, in ankylosing spondylitis, the process always involves basal portions of the aortic valve cusps and always extends into the membranous ventricular septum, the basal portion of the anterior mitral leaflet, or both. Thus, because the process in syphilis never extends below the aortic valve, bundle branch or complete heart block and mitral regurgitation never develop in cardiovascular syphilis or, if they do, they are the result of a process other than syphilis. In contrast, heart block and mitral regurgitation are common in ankylosing spondylitis.

Cardiovascular syphilis characteristically involves the entire tubular portion of the aorta, which may become either diffusely or focally dilated. In contrast, in ankylosing spondylitis, the process involves only the proximal 1 cm of the tubular portion of the ascending aorta and then usually in the areas of the aortic valve commissures. Accordingly, aneurysms of the tubular portion of the ascending aorta do not occur in ankylosing spondylitis. Syphilitic aneurysms can become so large that they burrow into the sternum or compress adjacent structures such as the right atrium, superior vena cava, or pulmonary trunk. Rupture into the adjacent structures or into the pericardial sac may also occur.

Histologically, the aortic lesions in both cardiovascular syphilis and ankylosing spondylitis are similar. Both are characterized by extensive thickening by fibrous tissue of the adventitia, with collections of plasma cells and some lymphocytes within these tissues. The vasa vasora are larger than normal, their walls are thickened, and their lumens may be severely narrowed. The inflammatory infiltrates are located primarily in the perivascular locations. The media is thinner than normal and contains scars that are generally located transversely to the long axis of the aorta. Within the scars, elastic fibers may be absent. The overlying intima is thickened, and the intimal process has the "tree bark" appearance of typical atherosclerotic plaques. The intimal thickening is greater in syphilis than in ankylosing spondylitis, probably because the patients with cardiovascular syphilis are generally much older than the patients with ankylosing spondylitis. The average age of death among patients with ankylosing spondylitis and aortic regurgitation is 48 years, whereas the typical patient with cardiovascular syphilis, with or without associated aortic regurgitations, is usually in his or her 70s or 80s.

Systemic Sclerosis (Scleroderma)

SS, which was first identified over two centuries ago, is characterized by its striking skin manifestations; hence the name *scleroderma*. The systemic nature of this disease, and in particular its ability to affect the heart, became apparent much later. In 1943, Weiss and coworkers[131] described a pattern in the cardiac dysfunction of nine patients with scleroderma and correlated these changes with abnormalities in the heart at autopsy in two patients. Moreover, they recognized that the cardiac disease was a manifestation of an underlying primary vascular disorder.

SS is characterized by fibrous thickening of the skin (Fig. 10-22) and fibrous and degenerative alterations of the fingers and of certain target organs, particularly the esophagus, small and large bowels, kidneys, lung, and heart. Central to this degenerative process are diffuse vascular lesions. Functionally, the vascular disorder is characterized by Raynaud's phenomenon, which is a prominent feature of SS. Raynaud's disease of the digits is present in almost all patients with SS and is the first clinical symptom in most. Structurally, the vascular lesions show intimal and adventitial thickening of small- and medium-sized vessels, including arterioles. *The underlying pathophysiology of scleroderma that links structure and function is a Raynaud's-type phenomenon of visceral vasculature that leads to focal vascular lesions and parenchymal necrosis and fibrosis*. This concept is supported by findings in the heart as well as in the lungs and kidneys.[132] The underlying cause of the vascular disease in SS and the role of the immune system in its pathophysiology remain unclear. SS may be related to increased activity of endothelial cells, mast cells, and fibroblasts, perhaps under the influence of immigrant cells, such as T cells, macrophages, or platelets.[131]

Like most connective tissue diseases, SS may have a variable clinical expression. Some patients may have skin involvement predominantly; others have minimal skin abnormalities but severe visceral disease that may therefore evade diagnosis.[132] The CREST (*c*alcinosis, *R*aynaud's phenomenon, *e*sophageal dysmotility, *s*clerodactyly, *t*elangiectasia) syndrome is an SS variant that can be manifest as relatively mild skin changes limited to the face and fingers, but severe lung disease with a primary pulmonary hypertension picture can occur.[133] *Overlap syndromes* are seen when a patient with typical features of SS also has features of SLE or RA. Although SS may run a long and benign course, *malignant* renal, lung, or cardiac disease can occur, with rapid deterioration and death at a young age.

THE CARDIOVASCULAR SYSTEM

Cardiovascular disease in patients with SS can be due to either a primary involvement of the heart by the sclerosing disease or a secondary involvement from disease of the kidney or lungs.

Primary Systemic Sclerosis of the Heart Myocardial involvement is a principal determinant of survival in SS. When the heart is involved directly by scleroderma, a myocardial fibrosis occurs that bears no direct relation to large- or small-vessel occlusions or other anatomic abnormalities. The fibrosis tends to be patchy, involving all levels of the myocardium unpredictably and the right ventricle as often as the left. Focal patchy myocardial cell necrosis may also be evident, and at autopsy over three-quarters of patients with myocardial SS have foci of necrosis.[132] The type of necrosis is myofibrillar degeneration, or contraction-band necrosis (Fig. 76-10). This lesion is characteristic of myocardium that is subjected to transient occlusion followed by reperfusion. This could occur with vascular spasm and also may be induced experimentally by exposing myocardium to high concentrations of catecholamine. Thus, the morphologic characteristics of the myocardial lesions of primary cardiac SS are consistent with a Raynaud's phenomenon of the heart. There is also suggestive evidence that a Raynaud's phenomenon of the pulmonary arterioles may be responsible for the *primary* pulmonary hypertension-type lesion that may occur in CREST

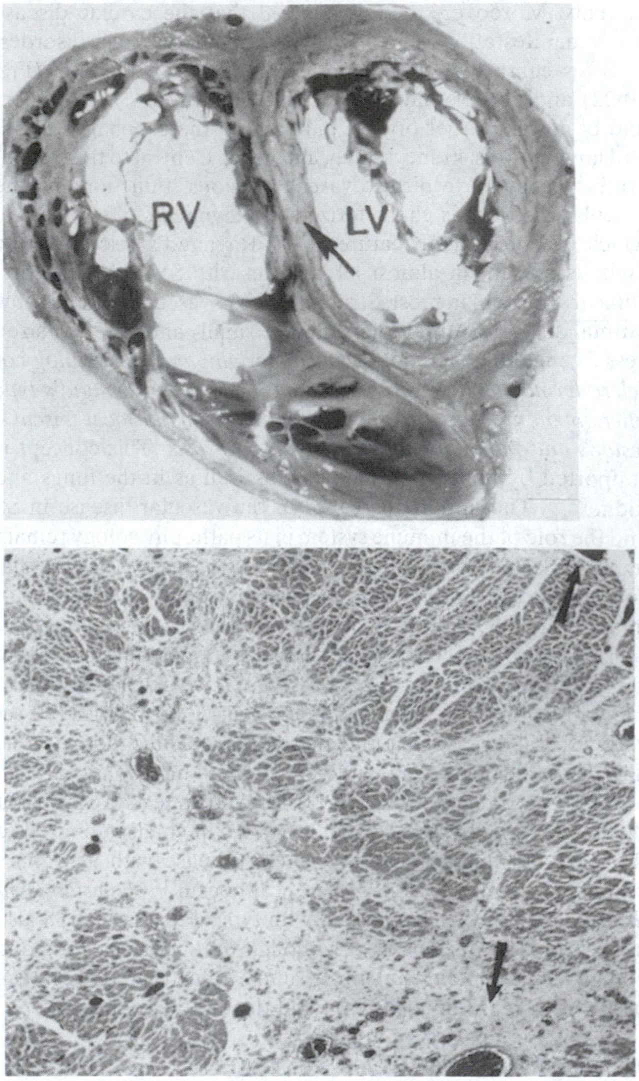

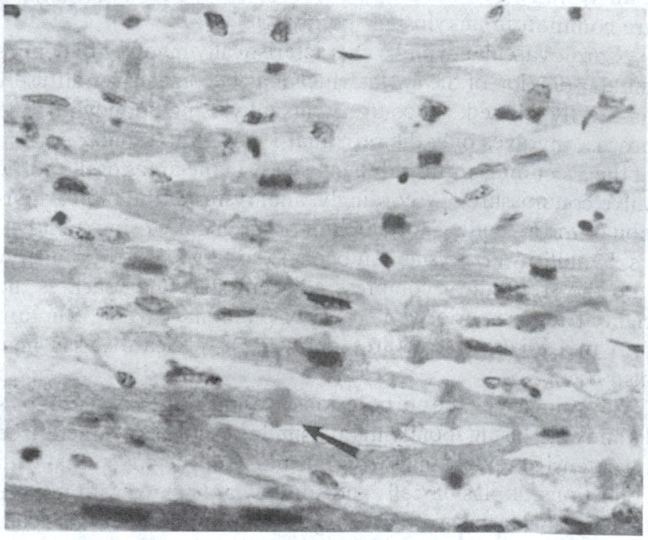

FIGURE 76-10 Systemic sclerosis (SS). *Top:* Cross section through the dilated right (RV) and left (LV) ventricle of a patient with cardiac SS. Marked fibrous scarring of both ventricles is especially evident in the interventricular septum (*arrow*). *Bottom left:* Photomicrograph of myocardium showing replacement fibrosis with patent intramural coronary arteries (*arrows*). *Bottom right:* Higher-power magnification showing contraction-band necrosis of many fibers surrounding the areas of scar. H&E, ×45 and ×60. (From Bulkley.[176] Reproduced with permission form the publisher and author.)

syndrome, and the kidneys in SS can also manifest a Raynaud's-type phenomenon. Some patients with SS have renal Raynaud's phenomenon when digital Raynaud's phenomenon is induced by cold-water immersion.[134] Thus, it is likely that the major visceral manifestations of SS in the heart, lungs, and kidneys are related to the vascular spasm that is evident and readily detectable in the digits. Changes that are comparable to the necrosis and scarring of the fingertips can also develop in the viscera.

The cause of the myocardial necrosis and fibrosis that develop in the setting of patent extramural and intramural vessels is unclear. That the myocardial disease relates in part to immunologic abnormalities or to primary and unrestrained fibrous tissue proliferation remains a possibility. The present evidence, however, suggests that the vascular system—and particularly the smaller arteries and arterioles—is the primary target organ of SS and that the cardiac sclerosis of scleroderma may be a consequence of focal, intermittent, and progressive ischemic injury.

Several functional studies have also suggested that microvascular spasm occurs in patients with cardiac scleroderma. Transient perfusion defects identified by thallium-201 radionuclide imaging in the setting of patent coronary arteries have also been identified in patients with SS and symptomatic cardiac disease.[135] Some patients with SS have reversible cold-induced myocardial perfusion defects as well as cold-induced acute and reversible left ventricular dysfunction.[136]

Clinical Manifestations The clinical features of myocardial SS include biventricular congestive heart failure, atrial and ventricular arrhythmias, myocardial infarction, angina pectoris, and sudden cardiac death.[137,138] These clinical manifestations reflect the underlying conditions of myocardial necrosis and fibrosis and may at times mimic ischemic heart disease due to coronary atherosclerosis. If the myocardial injury is extensive enough, leading to dilated hypodynamic ventricles, a syndrome resembling idiopathic dilated cardiomyopathy (Chap. 66) may be simulated.

Patients with SS may have cardiac involvement but no cardiac symptoms.[137,138] One study[139] examined 18 SS patients by electrocardiography, ambulatory electrocardiography, radionuclide ventriculography, myocardial scintigraphy, and echocardiography and found a high rate of cardiac abnormalities, including ventricular tachycardia in one patient, nonsustained ventricular tachycardia in five, supraventricular tachycardia in six, decreased left ventricular ejection fraction in two, decreased right ventricular ejection fraction in eight, and stress-induced reversible myocardial perfusion abnormalities in six. In other studies of patients with limited scleroderma, noninvasive cardiac techniques such as Doppler echocardiography and thallium-201 perfusion scintigraphy after a cold-stress test or radionuclide ventriculography[140] have found a number of cardiovascular abnormalities, such as mild mitral regurgitation, thickening of papillary muscles, abnormal left and right diastolic function, and systolic pulmonary arterial hypertension. A Japanese study of 13 patients with full-blown SS concluded that patients with SS frequently have deterioration of left ventricular diastolic function, especially those with left ventricular wall thickening out of proportion to left ventricular end-diastolic dimensions.[141]

Other investigators[142] have used electrocardiography and echocardiography to devise a simple *cardiac score* to improve the prediction of prognosis in patients with SS. Skeletal muscle myositis can complicate SS, and such patients may have an increased likelihood of developing myocarditis, heart failure, and symptomatic arrhythmias, and die suddenly.[143] Accordingly, it has been suggested that serum creatine kinase with MB fractionation and studies of left ventricular function be undertaken in patients with SS who have skeletal myositis. Autopsy studies have suggested that up to 50 percent of patients with SS have increased myocardial scar tissue and that up 30 percent of patients have extensive lesions.[144] Some clinical cardiac abnormalities, including symptoms of heart failure or abnormal rhythm with conduction disturbances, may occur in about 40 percent of patients with SS. The cardiac disorder in approximately one-half of patients has been attributed by some researchers to a primary myocardial scleroderma.

Pericardial and Endocardial Disease Pericardial involvement may occur in about 20 percent of patients with SS. Although the pericardial involvement is due to renal failure in as many as two-thirds of patients, some develop a fibrofibrinous or fibrous pericarditis for which no other cause is evident. Exudative pericardial effusions may accompany scleroderma pericardial disease and can be massive.[145] Pericardial tamponade may occur and may precede cutaneous thickening.[146] Rarely, constrictive pericardial disease may result from the pericardial sclerosis. Mitral regurgitation is common in patients with SS.[147] Tricuspid regurgitation occurs in patients with very dilated right ventricular cavities.

Secondary Cardiovascular Disease Since scleroderma most frequently manifests itself as renal and pulmonary parenchymal disease with pulmonary and systemic arterial hypertension, secondary cardiovascular disease is common. Left ventricular hypertrophy and congestive heart failure may be associated with long-standing systemic arterial hypertension and renal disease. Uremic pericarditis may occur. Cor pulmonale with marked right ventricular hypertrophy and right-sided heart failure may result from long-standing severe pulmonary scleroderma.

PULMONARY HYPERTENSIVE DISEASE

Although the pulmonary fibrosis of scleroderma had been known for years, the recognition of a *primary* pulmonary hypertensive lesion independent of parenchymal disease evolved later. Patients with this primary pulmonary vascular lesion tend to develop rapidly progressive dyspnea and right-sided congestive heart failure in the setting of clear lungs. Pulmonary pressures reach the systemic level and are refractory to treatment. Morphologically, the pulmonary arterial lesions show the range of advanced alterations (medial and intimal thickening and plexiform lesions) as seen in Eisenmenger's syndrome and primary pulmonary hypertension. Arterial vasospasm is believed to be a major component of SS primary pulmonary hypertension, and the association is supported by angiographic studies. On occasion, vasodilators such as tolazoline may induce partial lowering of pressure, but the fixed pulmonary lesions and focal thrombotic occlusions of the advanced stages make restoration of normal pressures unlikely. The fact that Raynaud's phenomenon of the digits accompanies idiopathic primary pulmonary hypertension in about one-third of patients[148] suggests that vascular hyperreactivity may be a common link between this disease and scleroderma (see also Chap. 52).

Although uncommon in scleroderma, severe pulmonary hypertension carries a grave prognosis. Sudden unexpected death occurs, and hypotension and death can occur precipitously in the setting of what would appear to be relatively benign procedures such as pericardiocentesis or cardiac catheterization.

TREATMENT

There is no uniformly effective therapy for the cardiovascular disease of SS.[149] Treatment consists of standard therapy for congestive heart failure and arrhythmias. Malignant ventricular arrhythmias in SS have responded seemingly well to insertion of an implantable cardioverter defibrillator[150] (see Chap. 30). Thrombolysis may provide improvement in the Raynaud's phenomenon, cutaneous sclerosis, and digital ulcerations.[151] A pilot study of antithymocyte gamma-globulin (ATGAM) appeared ineffective in improving the skin and pulmonary features of the disease.[152] Nifedipine may improve myocardial perfusion abnormalities as well as systemic and pulmonary hemodynamics in patients with pulmonary hypertension due to SS.[153] Nifedipine and amlodipine may also improve Raynaud's events involving the fingers. Captopril has been shown to improve myocardial perfusion.[154] Potential therapeutic value for SS cardiac disease has been attributed to *D*-penicillamine. No therapy, however, has proved effective for either the systemic disease or its cardiac manifestations.

Polymyositis/Dermatomyositis

These idiopathic autoimmune inflammatory myopathies are rare in the United States, with an estimated annual incidence of about 5 to 10 new patients per million. The clinical features include a typical heliotrope rash in dermatomyositis (DM), with periorbital edema and proximal muscle weakness present in both polymyositis (PM) and DM. PM is basically the same disease except for the absence of a skin rash.[155] Typical laboratory findings include an elevated serum creatine kinase level and elevation of other muscle enzymes such as a serum aldolase, reflecting the presence of muscle breakdown from the inflammatory process. The so-called anti-Jo-1 antibody, detectable in the serum of some patients with PM/DM, has been correlated with inflammatory arthritis, Raynaud's phenomenon, interstitial lung disease, and excess mortality, mostly due to respiratory failure. Typical changes in the electromyogram include short-wave potentials, low-amplitude polyphasic units, and increased spontaneous activity with muscle fibrillation. A positive skeletal muscle biopsy of a proximal muscle such as the deltoid is often confirmatory.[155]

In addition to skeletal muscle involvement, up to 40 percent of patients may have cardiac abnormalities, including atrioventricular conduction defects, tachyarrhythmias, pericarditis with effusion, and a dilated, poorly contracting left ventricle. Myocarditis leading to congestive heart failure has been found in autopsy studies.[156] Rarely, coronary arteritis has been reported in PM/DM. Accordingly, the evaluation of a middle-aged man with known PM/DM who presents with chest pain, or even classic angina with an elevated serum creatine kinase, poses a diagnostic challenge, and the differential diagnosis includes inflammatory myocarditis and coronary arteritis. An increase in cardiac creatine kinase-MB may be "buried" in the marked elevation of skeletal creatine kinase-MB. If coronary angiography is suggestive of coronary vasculitis rather than typical atheromatous plaques, oral high-dose prednisone, 40 to 60 mg daily, is appropriate. This is also the usual initial therapeutic approach in patients with PM/DM even when no cardiac involvement is apparent. There are no clinical studies available comparing the efficacy of glucocorticoid treatment with other immunosuppressive agents such as azathioprine (Imuran), methotrexate, chlorambucil, and cyclophosphamide (Cytoxan).

Most rheumatologists initially use a trial of glucocorticoid therapy in patients with PM/DM. If the response is suboptimal, treatment is instituted with methotrexate, azathioprine (Imuran), chlorambucil, and cyclophosphamide (Cytoxan), in that order. The response to steroids in PM/DM is unpredictable. Some patients do very well on oral prednisone therapy, whereas others fail to respond to any agents. A subset of patients with PM/DM who have the so-called inclusion body myositis are particularly intractable to anti-inflammatory treatment. This is also true for patients who have a rare autoantibody called the anti-signal-recognition-particle (anti-SRP) antibody. Because some patients with PM/DM benefit significantly from an initial trial of high-dose oral or intravenous glucocorticoid therapy, this therapy is usually used first. Intravenous immunoglobulin appears promising in the treatment of PM/DM.[157] Finally, myopathies can arise iatrogenically from commonly used drugs such as cholesterol-lowering agents, statins, and niacin, as well as from colchicine, zidovudine, and methylphenidate hydrochloride (Ritalin).

Giant-Cell (Cranial, Temporal, Granulomatous) Arteritis

Temporal arteritis is a systemic inflammatory vasculitis of unknown etiology that primarily involves extracranial vessels, especially branches of the external carotid artery, but can involve almost any artery in the body, as well as some veins. Giant-cell arteritis occurs almost exclusively in patients over 55 years of age. Common symptoms include headaches, scalp tenderness, jaw claudication, visual disturbances including blindness, diplopia, weight loss, anemia, and, in about 50 percent of patients, musculoskeletal symptoms attributable to polymyalgia rheumatica. Uncommon presentations of giant-cell arteritis include fever of unknown origin, chest pain from aortitis or myocardial infarction, aortic aneurysm,[158,159] coma, peripheral gangrene, peripheral neuropathies, and large-vessel involvement with limb claudication, aortic regurgitation, or stroke. Typical physical findings include tenderness of the temporal or occipital arteries, nodulations of the artery, a pulseless artery, and a tender scalp.

Most giant-cell arteritis patients have a greatly elevated erythrocyte sedimentation rate. The only specific diagnostic test is a temporal artery biopsy that demonstrates granulomatous arterial inflammation with disruption of the internal elastica lamina. Gaint cells need not be present. Unfortunately, the positive yield for giant-cell arteritis in unilateral temporal artery biopsies is no greater than 60 percent, and a contralateral biopsy may be necessary.

Since the occurrence of *skip* lesions in histologic samples is well known in giant-cell arteritis, ideally a 5-cm section of artery should be examined. Angiography is generally not helpful in diagnosis or in selecting a biopsy site. High-dose prednisone therapy is indicated to prevent blindness or to suppress inflammation in the presence of systemic involvement.

Churg-Strauss Vasculitis

Churg-Strauss syndrome, or allergic granulomatosis and angiitis, is a systemic vasculitis that develops in the setting of allergic rhinitis, asthma, and eosinophilia. Sinusitis and pulmonary infiltrates may cause confusion with Wegener's granulomatosis; the absence of cavitating pulmonary nodules or the presence of gastrointestinal involvement is often a helpful distinguishing feature. Peripheral neuropathy, cutaneous involvement, and renal disease are common clinical findings.

Pathologic studies show inflammatory lesions rich in eosinophils with intra- and extravascular granuloma formation. The major morbidity and mortality of Churg-Strauss vasculitis result from cardiac involvement. This may be associated with left ventricular dilatation and a reduced ejection fraction, as well as mitral regurgitation, which may require valve replacement.[158] Left ventricular systolic function may improve significantly with glucocorticoid therapy.[159]

Antiphospholipid Antibody Syndrome

The aPL antibody syndrome has been identified by the presence of aPL antibodies, usually in high titer, or the *lupus anticoagulant,* and any or all of the following clinical events:[160–173] recurrent arterial or venous thromboses, recurrent fetal losses, and thrombocytopenia. Livedo reticularis is also frequently present, and nonhealing leg ulcers and Coombs'-positive hemolytic anemia may be also. Clincally, the terms *anticardiolipin syndrome, antiphospholipid syndrome,* and *lupus anticoagulant syndrome* are usually considered to be equivalent, although some individuals may have one antibody but not the other. A false-positive Venereal Disease Research Laboratory test may also be detected in patients with aPL antibody syndrome; aPL antibodies, however, may be present in asymptomatic individuals. Often, anticardiolipin antibodies cross-react with β_2-glycoprotein 1 (B2GP1) antibodies. The mechanism(s) whereby anticardiolipin or aPL antibodies promote intravascular thrombosis remain(s) uncertain. These antibodies may react with lipid antigens on endothelial cells and/or platelets. The precise nature of the antigen recognized by B2GP1-dependent anticardiolipin antibodies is under active investigation. SLE is frequently present in patients with aPL antibody syndrome. The presence of anticardiolipin antibodies in patients with SLE may be associated with prolonged activated partial thromboplastin time, thrombocytopenia, and positive Coombs' test but not with the lupus anticoagulant (or the aPL) syndrome;[160] the presence of a prolonged activated partial thromboplastin time is strongly associated with venous and arterial thrombosis.

Therapy depends on the clinical setting. Patients with positive aPL antibodies but without evidence of thrombosis or recurrent fetal loss should not be treated. Patients with aPL antibody syndrome who have had thrombotic events or habitual abortions should be treated. Anticoagulation and antithrombotic therapy in these patients has included heparin, warfarin, low-dose aspirin, and the antimalarial agent hydroxychloroquine.[161] Although there is no convincing evidence of benefit, some advocate low-dose aspirin or heparin, with or without low-dose prednisone, alone or in combination to prevent fetal loss. An increased incidence of aortic or mitral regurgitation in association with the *primary* aPL antibody syndrome has been reported as well in patients with SLE who have aPL antibodies. Heart valve involvement, although frequent, appears unrelated to the presence or absence of aPL antibodies. The aPL antibody syndrome is frequently manifest by spontaneous small- and large-vessel arterial thrombosis in the cerebral and ocular circulations.[174] In healthy men, positive anticardiolipin antibody levels are a risk factor for deep venous thrombosis or pulmonary embolus but not for ischemic stroke.[174]

Although there are no controlled trials of therapy to prevent arterial occlusion, low-dose aspirin is often used. Therapy has often included aspirin and warfarin or heparin, as well as low-dose glucocorticoids.[175]

References

1. Beighton P, ed. *McKusick's Heritable Disorders of Connective Tissue,* 5th ed. St Louis: Mosby-Year Book; 1993.
2. Pyeritz PE, McKusick VA. The Marfan syndrome: Diagnosis and management. *N Engl J Med* 1979; 300:772–777.
3. Kainulainen K, Pulkkinen L, Savolainen A, et al. Location of chromosome 15 of the gene defect causing Marfan syndrome. *N Engl J Med* 1990; 323:935–939.
4. Hollister DW, Godfrey M, Sakai LY, Pyeritz RE. Immunohistologic abnormalities of the microfibrillar-fiber system in the Marfan syndrome. *N Engl J Med* 1990; 323:935–939.
5. Lee B, Godfrey M, Vitale E, et al. Linkage of Marfan syndrome and a phenotypically related disorder to two different fibrillin genes. *Nature* 1991; 352:330–334.
6. Maslen CL, Corson GM, Maddox BK, et al. Partial sequence of a candidate gene for the Marfan syndrome. *Nature* 1991; 352: 334–337.
7. Dietz HC, Curring GR, Pyeritz RE, et al. Marfan syndrome caused by a de novo missense mutation in the fibrillin gene. *Nature* 1991; 352:337–339.
8. Dietz HC, Valle D, Francomano CA, et al. The skipping of constitutive exons in vivo induced by nonsense mutations. *Science* 1993; 259:680–683.
9. Dietz HC, McIntosh I, Sakai LY, et al. Four novel FBN1 mutations: Significance for mutant transcript level and EGF-like domain calcium binding in the pathogenesis of Marfan syndrome. *Genomics* 1993; 17:468–475.
10. Dietz HC, Pyeritz RE. Mutations in the human gene for fibrillin-1 (FBN1) in the Marfan syndrome and related disorders. *Hum Mol Genet* 1995; 4:1799–1809.
11. Ramirez F. Fibrillin mutations in Marfan syndrome and related phenotypes. *Curr Opin Genet Dev* 1996; 6:309–315.
12. Burn J, Camm J, Davies MJ, et al. The phenotype/genotype relation and the current status of genetic screening in hypertrophic cardiomyopathy, Marfan syndrome, and the long QT syndrome. *Heart* 1997; 78:110–116.
13. Maron BJ, Moller JH, Seidman CE, et al. Impact of laboratory molecular diagnosis on contemporary diagnostic criteria for genetically transmitted cardiovascular diseases: Hypertrophic cardiomyopathy, long-QT syndrome, and Marfan syndrome. A statement for healthcare professionals from the Councils on Clinical Cardiology, Cardiovascular Disease in the Young, and Basic Science, American Heart Association. *Circulation* 1998; 98:1460–1471.
14. De Paepe A, Devereus RB, Dietz HC, et al. Revised diagnostic criteria for the Marfan syndrome. *Am J Med Genet* 1996; 62: 417–426.
15. Come PC, Fortuin NJ, White RI Jr, McKusick VA. Echocardiographic assessment of cardiovascular abnormalities in the Marfan syndrome: Comparison with clinical findings and with roentgenographic estimation of aortic root size. *Am J Med* 1983; 74:465–474.
16. Roman MJ, Devereus RB, Kramer-Fox R, Spitzer MC. Comparison of cardiovascular and skeletal features of primary valve prolapse and Marfan syndrome. *J Cardiol* 1989; 63:317–321.
17. Glesby MJ, Pyeritz RE. Association of mitral valve prolapse and systemic abnormalities of connective tissue: A phenotypic continuum. *JAMA* 1989; 262:523–518.
18. Wexler L, Higgins CB. The use of magnetic resonance imaging in adult congenital heart disease. *Am J Cardiac Imaging* 1995; 9:15–28.
19. Maron BJ. Heart disease and other causes of sudden death in young athletes. *Curr Probl Cardiol* 1998; 23:477–529.
20. Braverman AC. Exercise and the Marfan syndrome. *Med Sci Sports Exerc* 1998; 30(suppl 10):S387–S395.
21. Salim MA, Alpert BS, Ward JC, Pyeritz RE. Effect of beta-adrenergic blockade on aortic root rate of dilation in the Marfan syndrome. *Am J Cardiol* 1994; 74:629–633.
22. Shores J, Berger KR, Murphy EA, Pyeritz RE. Progression of aortic dilation and the benefit of long-term β-adrenergic blockade in Marfan's syndrome. *N Engl J Med* 1994; 30:1335–1341.
23. Treasure T. Elective replacement of the aortic root in Marfan's syndrome. *Br Heart J* 1993; 69:101–103.
24. Gott VL, Gillinov M, Pyeritz RE, et al. Aortic root replacement: Risk factor analysis of a seventeen-year experience with 270 patients. *J Thorac Cardiovasc Surg* 1995; 109:536–545.
25. Donaldson RM, Emanuel RW, Olsen EG, Ross DN. Management of cardiovascular complications in Marfan syndrome. *Lancet* 1980; 2:1178–1181.
26. Gott VL, Pyeritz RE, McGovern GJ, et al. Surgical treatment of aneurysms of the ascending aorta in the Marfan syndrome: Results of composite-graft repair in 50 patients. *N Engl J Med* 1986; 314:1070–1074.
27. Marsalese DL, Moodie DS, Vacante M, et al. Marfan's syndrome: Natural history and long-term follow-up of cardiovascular involvement. *J Am Coll Cardiol* 1989; 14:422–428.
28. Gott VL, Pyeritz RE, Cameron DE, et al. Composite graft repair in Marfan aneurysm of the ascending aorta: Results in 100 patients. *Ann Thorac Surg* 1991; 52:38–45.
29. Svensson LG, Crawford ES, Coseli JS, et al. Impact of cardiovascular operation on survival in the Marfan patient. *Circulation* 1989; 80(suppl I):I233–I242.
30. Svensson LG, Crawford ES, Hess KR, et al. Dissection of the aorta and dissecting aortic aneurysms: Improving early and long-term surgical results. *Circulation* 1990; 82(suppl IV):IV24–IV38.
31. Pyeritz RE. Marfan syndrome: Current and future clinical and genetic management of cardiovascular manifestations. *Semin Thorac Cardiovasc Surg* 1993; 5:11–16.
32. Smith JA, Fann JI, Miller C, et al. Surgical management of aortic dissection in patients with the Marfan syndrome. *Circulation* 1994; 90(part 2):II235–II242.
33. Roberts WC, Honig HS. The spectrum of cardiovascular disease

in the Marfan syndrome: A clinico-morphologic study of 18 necropsy patients and comparison to 151 previously reported necropsy patients. *Am Heart J* 1982; 104:115–135.
34. Silverman DI, Gray J, Roman MJ, et al. Family history of cardiovascular disease in the Marfan syndrome is associated with increased aortic diameter and decreased survival. *J Am Coll Cardiol* 1995; 26:1062–1067.
35. Hayashi J, Moro H, Namura O, et al. Surgical implication of aortic dissection on long-term outcome in Marfan patients. *Surg Today* 1996; 26:980–984.
36. Bachet J, Goudot B, Dreyfus G, et al. The proper use of glue: A 20-year experience with the GRF glue in acute aortic dissection. *J Card Surg* 1997; 12(suppl 2):243–253.
37. LeMaire SA, Coselli JS. Aortic root surgery in Marfan syndrome: Current practice and evolving techniques. *J Cardvasc Surg* 1997; 12(suppl 2):137–141.
38. David TE. Current practice in Marfan's aortic root surgery: Reconstruction with aortic valve preservation or replacement? What to do with the mitral valve. *J Cardvasc Surg* 1997; 12(suppl 2):147–150.
39. Gillinov AM, Hulyalkar A, Cameron DE, et al. Mitral valve operation in patients with the Marfan syndrome. *J Thorac Cardiovasc Surg* 1994; 107:724–731.
40. Murdoch JL, Walker BA, Halpern BL, et al. Life expectancy and causes of death in the Marfan syndrome. *N Engl J Med* 1972; 286:804–808.
41. Pyeritz RE. Maternal and fetal complications of pregnancy in the Marfan syndrome. *Am J Med* 1981; 71:784–790.
42. Santucci JJ, Katz S, Pogo GJ, Boxer R. Peripartum acute myocardial infarction in Marfan's syndrome, *Am Hear J* 1994; 127:1404–1407.
43. Rossiter JP, Repke JT, Morales AJ, et al. A prospective longitudinal evaluation of pregnancy in the Marfan syndrome. *Am J Obstet Gynecol* 1995; 173:1599–1606.
44. Ulkayan U, Ostrzega E, Shotan A, Mehra A. Cardiovascular problems in pregnant women with Marfan syndrome. *Ann Intern Med* 1995; 123:117–122.
45. Steinmann B, Royce PM, Superti-Furga A. The Ehlers Danlos syndrome. In: Royce PM, Steinmann B, eds. *Connective Tissue and its Heritable Disorders: Molecular, Genetic, and Medical Aspects*. New York: Wiley-Liss; 1993:351.
46. Takahashi T, Koide T, Yamaguchi H, et al. Ehlers-Danlos syndrome *Ann Thorac Surg* 1994; 58:1180–1182.
47. Hamano K, Minami Y, Fujimura Y, et al. Emergency operation for thoracic aortic aneurysm caused by the Ehler-Danlos syndrome. *Ann Thorac Surg* 1994; 58:1180–1182.
48. Lebwohl M, Halperin J, Phelps RG. Occult pseudoxanthoma elasticum in patients with premature cardiovascular disease. *N Engl J Med* 1993; 329:1237–1239.
49. Coleman K, Ross MH, McCabe M, et al. Disk drusen and angioid streaks in pseudoxanthoma elasticum. *Am J Ophthalmol* 1991; 112:166–170.
50. Slade AKB, John RM, Swanton RH. Pseudoxanthoma elasticum presenting with myocardial infarction. *Br Heart J* 1990; 63:372–373.
51. Kevorkian JP, Masquet C, Kural-Menasche S, et al. New report of severe coronary artery disease in an eighteen-year-old girl with pseudoxanthoma elasticum. *Angiology* 1997; 48:735–741.
52. Rosenzweig BP, Guarneri E, Kronzon I. Echocardiographic manifestations in a patient with pseudoxanthoma elasticum. *Ann Intern Med* 1993; 119:487–491.
53. Lebwohl MG, Distefano D, Prioleau PC, et al. Pseudoxanthoma elasticum and mitral valve prolapse. *N Engl J Med* 1982; 307:228–231.
54. Fukuda K, Uno K, Fujii T, et al. Mitral stenosis in pseudoxanthoma elasticum. *Chest* 1992; 101:1706–1707.
55. Challenor VF, Conway N, Monro JL. The surgical treatment of restrictive cardiomyopathy in pseudoxanthoma elasticum. *Br Heart J* 1988; 59:266–269.
56. Stover ML, Primorac D, Liu SC, et al. Defective splicing of mRNA from one COL1A1 allele of type I collagen in nondeforming (type I) osteogenesis imperfecta. *J Clin Invest* 1993; 92:1994–2002.
57. Byers PH. Osteogenesis imperfecta. In: Royce PM, Steinmann B, eds. *Connective Tissue and Its Heritable Disorders: Molecular, Genetic and Medical Aspects*. New York: Wiley-Liss; 1993:317.
58. Marini JC, Gerber NL. Osteogenesis imperfecta rehabilitation and prospects for gene therapy. *JAMA* 1997; 277:746–750.
59. Wong RS, Follis FM, Shively BK, Wenly JA. Osteogenesis imperfecta and cardiovascular diseases. *Ann Thorac Surg* 1995; 60:1439–1443.
60. Hortop J, Tsipouras P, Hanley JA, et al. Cardiovascular involvement in osteogenesis imperfecta *Circulation* 1986; 73:54–61.
61. Almassi GH, Hughes GR, Bartlett J. Combined valve replacement and coronary bypass grafting in osteogenesis imperfecta. *Ann Thorac Surg* 1995; 60:1395–1397.
62. Wood SJ, Thomas J, Braimbridge MV. Mitral valve disease and open heart surgery in osteogenesis imperfecta tarda. *Br Heart J* 1973; 35:103–106.
63. Zegdi R, D'Attellis N, Fornes P, et al. Aortic valve surgery in osteogenesis imperfecta: Report of two cases and review of the literature. *J Heart Valve Dis* 1998; 7:510–514.
64. Moriyama Y, Nishida T, Toyohira H, et al. Acute aortic dissection in a patient with osteogenesis imperfecta. *Ann Thorac Surg* 1995; 60:1397–1399.
65. Fowler NO, Van der Bel-Kahn JM. Indications for surgical replacement of the mitral valve with particular reference to common and uncommon causes of mitral regurgitation. *Am J Cardiol* 1979; 44:148–156.
66. Roman MJ, Devereus RB. Heritable aortic disease. In: Lindsay J, ed. *Diseases of the Aorta*. Philadelphia: Lea & Febiger; 1994:5.
67. Pascal N, Bloor C, Godfrey M, et al. Familial aortic dissecting aneurysm. *J Am Coll Cardiol* 1989; 13:811–819.
68. Chen M, Rigby ML, Redington AN. Familial aneurysms of the interventricular septum. *Br Heart J* 1991; 65:104–106.
69. Jaksche VH. Familiäre Aneurysmen: Vier Karotisaneurysmen aus einer zehnköpfigen Familie. *Zentralbl Neurochir* 1986; 47:351–353.
70. Elshunnar KS, Whittle IR. Familial intracranial aneurysms: Report of five families. *Br J Neurosurg* 1990; 4:181–186.
71. Boumpas DT, Fessler BJ, Austin HA III, et al. Systemic lupus erythematosus: Emerging concepts. Part 2: Dermatologic and joint disease, the antiphospholipid antibody syndrome, pregnancy and hormonal therapy, morbidity and mortality, and pathogenesis. *Ann Intern Med* 1995; 123:42–53.
72. Wallace DJ, Hahn BH, eds. *Dubois' Lupus Erythematosus*, 4th ed. Philadelphia: Lea and Febiger; 1993.
73. Moder KG, Miller TD, Tazelaar HD. Cardiac involvement in systemic lupus erythematosus. *Mayo Clin Proc* 1999; 74:275–284.
74. Ward MM, Pyun E, Studenski S. Mortality risks associated with specific clinical manifestations of systemic lupus erythematosus. *Arch Intern Med* 1996; 156:1337–1344.
75. Roberts WC, High ST. The heart in systemic lupus erythematosus. *Curr Probl Cardiol* 1999; 24:1–56.
76. Alarcon-Segovia D, Deleze M, Oria CV, et al. Antiphospholipid antibodies and the antiphospholipid syndrome in systemic lupus erythematosus: A prospective analysis of 500 consecutive patients. *Medicine (Baltimore)* 1989; 68:353–365.
77. Leung W-H, Wong K-L, Lau C-P, et al. Association between antiphospholipid antibodies and cardiac abnormalities in patients with systemic lupus erythematosus. *Am J Med* 1990; 89:411–419.
78. Khamashta MA, Cervera R, Asherson RA, et al. Association of antibodies against phospholipids with heart valve disease in systemic lupus erythematosus. *Lancet* 1990; 335:1541–1544.

79. Nihoyannopoulous P, Gomez PM, Joshi J, et al. Cardiac abnormalities in systemic lupus erythematosus. *Circulation* 1990; 82:369–375.
80. O'Rourke RA. Antiphospholipid antibodies: A marker of lupus carditis? *Circulation* 1990; 82:636–638.
81. Leung WH, Wong KL, Lau C-P, et al. Cardiac abnormalities in systemic lupus erythematosus: A prospective M-mode, cross-sectional and Doppler echocardiographic study. *Int J Cardiol* 1990; 27:367–375.
82. Sturfelt G, Eskilsson J, Nived O, et al. Cardiovascular disease in systemic lupus erythematosus: A study of 75 patients from a defined population. *Medicine* (*Baltimore*) 1992; 71:216–223.
83. Ong ML, Veerapen K, Chambers JB, et al. Cardiac abnormalities in systemic lupus erythematosus: Prevalence and relationship to disease activity. *Int J Cardiol* 1992; 34:69–74.
84. Kaplan SD, Chartash EK, Pizzarello RA, Furie RA. Cardiac manifestations of the antiphospholipid syndrome. *Am Heart J* 1992; 124:1331–1337.
85. Gleason CB, Stoddard MF, Wagner SG, et al. A comparison of cardiac valvular involvement in the primary antiphospholipid syndrome versus anticardiolipin-negative systemic lupus erythematosus. *Am Heart J* 1993; 125:1123–1129.
86. Khamashta MA, Hughes GRV. Antiphospholipid antibodies and valve disease in patients with systemic lupus erythematosus. *J Am Coll Cardiol* 1993; 22:1268–1271.
87. Bulkley BH, Roberts WC. The heart in systemic lupus erythematosus and the changes induced in it by corticosteroid therapy: A study of 36 necropsy patients. *Am J Med* 1975; 58:243–264.
88. Gabrielli F, Alcini E, Di Prima MA, et al. Cardiac valve involvement in systemic lupus erythematosus and primary antiphospholipid syndrome: Lack of correlation with antiphospholipid antibodies. *Int J Cardiol* 1995; 51:117–126.
89. Roldan CA, Shively BK, Crawford MH. An echocardiographic study of valvular heart disease associated with systemic lupus erythematosus. *N Engl J Med* 1996; 335:1424–1430.
90. Kahl LE. The spectrum of pericardial tamponade in systemic lupus erythematosus: Report of ten patients. *Arthritis Rheum* 1992; 35:1343–1349.
91. Libman E, Sacks B. A hitherto undescribed form of valvular and mural endocarditis. *Arch Intern Med* 1924; 33:701–737.
92. Gross L. The cardiac lesion in Libman-Sacks disease with a consideration of its relationship to acute diffuse lupus erythematosus. *Am J Pathol* 1940; 16:375–407.
93. Sturfelt G, Eskilsson J, Nived O, et al. Cardiovascular disease in systemic disease in systemic lupus erythematosus: A study from a defined population. *Medicine* (*Baltimore*) 1992; 71:216–223.
94. Petri M, Spence D, Bone LR, Hochberg MC. Coronary risk factors in the Johns Hopkins lupus cohort: Prevalence by patients, and preventive practices. *Medicine* (*Baltimore*) 1992; 71:291–302.
95. Kutom AH, Gibbs HR. Myocardial infarction due to thrombi without significant coronary artery disease in systemic erythematosus. *Chest* 1991; 100:571–572.
96. Wilson VE, Eck SL, Bates ER. Evaluation and treatment of myocardial infarction complicating systemic lupus erythematosus. *Chest* 1991; 100:571–572.
97. Sumino H, Kanda T, Saski T, et al. Myocardial infarction secondary to coronary aneurysm in systemic lupus erythematosus: An autopsy case. *Angiology* 1995; 46:527–530.
98. James TN, Rupe CE, Monto RW. Pathology of the cardiac conduction system in systemic lupus erythematosus. *Ann Intern Med* 1965; 63:402–410.
99. McCauliffe DP. Neonatal lupus erythematosus: A transplacentally acquired autoimmune disorder. *Sem in Dermol* 1995; 14:47–53.
100. Brucato A, Franceschini F, Buyon JP. Neonatal lupus: Long-term outcomes of mothers and children and recurrence rate. *Clin Exp Rheumatol* 1997; 15:467–473.
101. Rabinerson D, Gruber A, Kaplan B, et al. Isolated persistent fetal bradycardia in complete A-V block: A conservative approach is appropriate—A case report and a review of the literature. *Am J Perinatol* 1997; 14:317–320.
102. Waltuck J, Buyon JP. Autoantibody-associated congenital heart block: Outcome in mothers and children. *Ann Intern Med* 1994; 120:544–551.
103. Press J, Uziel Y, Laxer RM, et al. Long-term outcome of mothers of children with complete congenital heart block. *Am J Med* 1996; 100:328–332.
104. Gobel MM, Dick M II, McCune WJ, et al. Atrioventricular conduction in children of women with systemic lupus erythematosus. *Am J Cardiol* 1993; 71:94–98.
105. Logar D, Kveder T, Rozman B, Pobovisek J. Possible association between anti-Ro antibodies and myocarditis or cardiac conduction defects in adults with systemic lupus erythematosus. *Ann Rheum Dis* 1990; 49:627–629.
106. Martinez-Costa X, Ordi J, Barbera J, et al. High-grade atrioventricular heart block in 2 adults with systemic lupus erythematosus. *J Rheumol* 1991; 18:1926–1928.
107. Winslow TM, Ossipov MA, Fazio GP, et al. Five-year follow up study of the prevalence and progression of pulmonary hypertension in systemic lupus erythematosus. *Am Heart J* 1995; 129:510–515.
108. Kalangos A, Panos A, Sezerman O. Mitral valve repair in lupus valvulitis: Report of a case and review of the literature. *J Heart Valve Dis* 1995; 4:202–207.
109. Morin AM, Boyer JC, Nataf P, Gandjbakhch I. Mitral insufficiency caused by systemic lupus erythematosus requiring valve replacement: Three case reports and a review of the literature. *Thorac Cardiovasc Surg* 1996; 44:313–316.
110. Petri M, Lakatta C, Madger L, Goldman D. Effect of prednisone and hydroxychloroquine on coronary artery disease risk factors in systemic lupus erythematosus: A longitudinal data analysis. *Am J Med* 1994; 96:254–259.
111. Chiariello M, Ambrosio G, Capelli-Bigazzi M, et al. Reduction in infarct size by the phospholipase inhibitor quinacrine in dogs with coronary artery occlusion. *Am Heart J* 1990; 120:801–807.
112. Cacoub P, Lunel-Fabiani F, Le-Thi Huong CLT. Polyarteritis nodosa and hepatitis C virus infection. *Ann Intern Med* 1992; 116:605–606.
113. Alarcon-Segovia D. The necrotizing vasculitides: A new pathogenetic classification. *Symp Rheumatol Dis* 1977; 61:241–260.
114. Schrader ML, Hochman JS, Bulkley BH. The heart in polyarteritis nodosa: A clinicopathologic study. *Am Heart J* 1985; 109:1353–1359.
115. Chu KH, Menapace FU, Blankenship JC, et al. Polyarteritis nodosa presenting as acute myocardial infarction with coronary dissection. *Cathet Cardiovasc Diagn* 1998; 44:320–324.
116. Thiene G, Valente M, Rossi L. Involvement of the cardiac conducting system in panarteritis nodosa. *Am Heart J* 1978; 95:716–724.
117. Charles LA, Jennette JC, Falk RJ. The role of HLGO cells in the detection of antineutrophil cytoplasmic autoantibodies. *J Rheumatol* 1991; 18:491–494.
118. Roberts WC, Dangel JC, Bulkley BH. Nonrheumatic valvular cardiac disease: A clinicopathologic survey of 27 different conditions causing valvular dysfunction. *Cardiovasc Clin* 1973; 4:333–446.
119. Bacon PA, Gibson DG. Cardiac involvement in rheumatoid arthritis: An echocardiographic study. *Ann Rheum Dis* 1974; 33:20–24.
120. Hakala M, Pettersson T, Tarkka M, et al. Rheumatoid arthritis as a cause of cardiac compression: Favourable long-term outcome of pericardiectomy. *Clin Rheumatol* 1993; 12:199–203.
121. Escalante A, Kaufman RL, Quismorio FP Jr, Beardmore TD.

Cardiac compression in rheumatoid pericarditis. *Semin Arthritis Rheum* 1990; 20:148–163.
122. Hara KS, Ballard DJ, Illstrup DM, et al. Rheumatoid pericarditis: Clinical features and survival. *Medicine (Baltimore)* 1990; 69: 81–91.
123. Travaglio-Encinoza A, Anaya JM, Dupuy D, et al. Rheumatoid pericarditis: New immunopathological aspects. *Clin Exp Rheumatol* 1994; 12:313–316.
124. Suriani RJ, Lansman S, Konstadt S. Intracardiac rheumatoid nodule presenting as a left atrial mass. *Am Heart J* 1994; 127: 463–465.
125. Maione S, Valentini G, Giunta A, et al. Cardiac involvement in rheumatoid arthritis: An echocardiographic study. *Cardiology* 1993; 83:234–239.
126. Kotha P, McGreevy MJ, Kotha A, et al. Early deaths with thrombolytic therapy for acute myocardial infarction in corticosteroid-dependent rheumatoid arthritis. *Clin Cardiol* 1998; 21:853–856.
127. Julkunen H. Rheumatoid spondylitis: Clinical and laboratory study of 149 cases compared with 182 cases of rheumatoid arthritis. *Acta Rheumatol Scand* 1962; 172(suppl 4):1–116.
128. Bulkley BH, Roberts WC. Ankylosing spondylitis and aortic regurgitation: Description of the characteristic cardiovascular lesion from study of eight necropsy patients. *Circulation* 1973; 48:1014–1027.
129. Roberts WC, Hollingsworth JR, Bulkley BH, et al. Combined mitral and aortic regurgitation in ankylosing spondylitis: Angiographic and anatomic features. *Am J Med* 1974; 56:237–243.
130. Gould BA, Turner J, Keeling DH, et al. Myocardial dysfunction in ankylosing spondylitis. *Ann Rheum Dis* 1992; 51:227–232.
131. Weiss S, Stead EA, Warren JV, Bailey OT. Scleroderma heart disease: With a consideration of certain other visceral manifestations of scleroderma. *Arch Intern Med* 1943; 71:749–776.
132. Bulkley BH, Klacsmann PG, Hutchins GM. Angina pectoris, myocardial infarction and sudden death with normal coronary arteries: A clinicopathologic study of 9 patients with progressive systemic sclerosis. *Am Heart J* 1978; 95:563–569.
133. Salerni R, Rodnan GP, Leon DR, Shaver JA. Pulmonary hypertension in the CREST syndrome variant of progressive systemic sclerosis (scleroderma). *Ann Intern Med* 1977; 86:394–399.
134. Cannon PJ, Hassar M, Case DB, et al. The relationship of hypertension and renal failure in scleroderma (progressive systemic sclerosis) to structural and functional abnormalities of the renal cortical circulation. *Medicine (Baltimore)* 1974; 53:1–46.
135. Follansbee WP, Curtiss EI, Medsger TA Jr, et al. Physiologic abnormalities of cardiac function in progressive systemic sclerosis with diffuse scleroderma. *N Engl J Med* 1984; 310:142–148.
136. Alexander EL, Firestein GS, Weiss JL, et al. Reversible cold-induced abnormalities in myocardial perfusion and function in systemic sclerosis. *Ann Intern Med* 1986; 105:661–668.
137. Clements PJ, Furst DE. Heart involvement in systemic sclerosis. *Clin Dermatol* 1994; 12:267–275.
138. Deswal A, Follansbee WP. Cardiac involvement in scleroderma. *Rheum Dis Clin North Am* 1996; 22:841–860.
139. Anvari A, Graninger W, Schneider B, et al. Cardiac involvement in systemic sclerosis. *Arthritis Rheum* 1992; 35:1356–1361.
140. Candell-Riera J, Armandans-Gil L, Simeon CP, et al. Comprehensive noninvasive assessment of cardiac involvement in limited systemic sclerosis. *Arthritis Rheum* 1996; 39:1138–1145.
141. Fujimoto S, Kagoshima T, Nakajima T, Dohi K. Doppler echocardiographic assessment of left ventricular diastolic function in patients with progressive systemic sclerosis. *Cardiology* 1993; 83:217–227.
142. Clements PJ, Lachenbruch PA, Furst DE, et al. Cardiac score: A semiquantitative measure of cardiac involvement that improves prediction of prognosis in systemic sclerosis. *Arthritis Rheum* 1991; 34:1371–1380.
143. Follansbee WP, Zerbe TR, Medsger TA Jr. Cardiac and skeletal muscle disease in systemic sclerosis (scleroderma): A high-risk association. *Am Heart J* 1993; 125:194–203.
144. D' Angelo WA, Fries JR, Masi AT, Shulman LE. Pathologic observations in systemic sclerosis (scleroderma): A study of fifty-eight autopsy cases and fifty-eight matched controls. *Am J Med* 1969; 46:428–440.
145. Satoh M, Tokuhira M, Hama N, et al. Massive pericardial effusion in scleroderma: A review of five cases. *Br J Rheumatol* 1995; 34:564–567.
146. Perez-Bocanegra C, Fonollosa V, Simeon CP, et al. Pericardial tamponade preceding cutaneous involvement in systemic sclerosis. *Ann Rheum Dis* 1995; 54:687–688.
147. Kazzam E, Caidahl K, Hallgren R, et al. Mitral regurgitation and diastolic flow profile in systemic sclerosis. *Int J Cardiol* 1990; 29:357–363.
148. Walcott G, Burchell HB, Brown AL. Primary pulmonary hypertension. *Am J Med* 1970; 71:70–79.
149. Pope JE. Treatment of systemic sclerosis. *Rheum Dis Clin North Am* 1996; 22:893–907.
150. Martinez-Taboada V, Olalla J, Blanco R, et al. Malignant ventricular arrhythmia in systemic sclerosis controlled with an implantable cardioverter defibrillator. *J Rheumatol* 1994; 21:2166–2167.
151. Fritzler MJ, Hart DA. Prolonged improvement of Raynaud's phenomenon and scleroderma after recombinant tissue plasminogen activator therapy. *Arthritis Rheum* 1990; 33:274–276.
152. Matteson EL, Shbeeb MI, McCarthy TG, et al. Pilot study of antithymocyte globulin in systemic sclerosis. *Arthritis Rheum* 1996; 39:1132–1137.
153. Alpert MA, Pressly TA, Mukerji V, et al. Acute and long-term effects of infedipine on pulmonary and systemic hemodynamics in patients with pulmonary hypertension associated with diffuse systemic sclerosis, the CREST syndrome and mixed connective tissue disease. *Am J Cardiol* 1991; 68:1687–1690.
154. Kazzam E, Caidahl K, Hällgren R, et al. Noninvasive evaluation of long-term cardiac effects of captopril in system sclerosis. *J Intern Med* 1991; 230:203–212.
155. Plotz PH, Dalakias M, Leff RL, et al. Current concepts in idiopathic inflammatory myopathies: Polymyositis, dermatomyositis, and related disorders. *Ann Intern Med* 1989; 111:143–157.
156. Dalakas MC. Polymyositis, dermatomyositis, and inclusion-body myositis. *N Engl J Med* 1991; 325:1487–1489.
157. Dalakas M, Illa I, Dambrosia JM, et al. A controlled trial of high-dose intravenous immune globulin as treatment for dermatomyositis. *N Engl J Med* 1993; 329:1993–2000.
158. Gonzales EB, Varner WT, Lisse JR, et al. Giant-cell arteritis in the southern United States: An 11-year retrospective study from the Texas Gulf coast. *Arch Intern Med* 1989; 149:1561–1565.
159. Hasley PB, Follansbee WP, Coulehan JL. Cardiac manifestations of Churg-Strauss syndrome: Report of a case and review of the literature. *Am Heart J* 1990; 120:996–999.
160. Abu-Shakra M, Gladman DD, Urowitz MB, Farewell V. Anticardiolipin antibodies in systemic lupus erythematosus: Clinical and laboratory correlations. *Am J Med* 1995; 99:624–628.
161. Khamashta MA, Cudrado MJ, Mujic F, et al. The management of thrombosis in the antiphospholipid-antibody syndrome. *N Engl J Med* 1995; 332:993–997.
162. Brenner B, Blumenfeld Z, Markiewicz W, Reisner SA. Cardiac involvement in patients with primary antiphospholipid syndrome. *J Am Coll Cardiol* 1991; 18:931–936.
163. Beynon HLC, Walport MJ. Antiphospholipid antibodies and cardiovascular disease. *Br Heart J* 1992; 67:281–284.
164. Soler J. Valvular heart disease in the primary antiphospholipid syndrome. *Ann Intern Med* 1992; 116:293–298.
165. Vianna JL, Khamashta MA, Ordi-Ros J, et al. Comparison of the primary and secondary antiphospholipid syndrome: A European multicenter study of 114 patients. *Am J Med* 1994; 96:3–9.

166. Cervera R, Asherson RA, Lie JT. Clinicopathologic correlations of the antiphospholipid syndrome. *Semin Arthritis Rheum* 1995; 24:262–277.
167. Violi F, Ferro D, Quintarelli C. Antiphospholipid antibodies, hypercoagulability and thrombosis. *Haematologica* 1995; 80(suppl 2):131–135.
168. Hojnik M, George J, Ziporen L, Shoenfeld Y. Heart valve involvement (Libman-Sacks endocarditis) in the antiphospholipid syndrome. *Circulation* 1996; 93:1579–1987.
169. Nesher G, Ilany J, Rosenmann D, Abraham AS. Valvular dysfunction in antiphospholipid syndrome: Prevalence, clinical features, and treatment. *Semin Arthritis Rheum* 1997; 27:27–35.
170. Ben-Chetrit E. Anti Ro/La antibodies and their clinical association. *Isr J Med Sci* 1997; 33:251–253.
171. Specker C, Perniok A, Brauckmann U, et al. Detection of cerebral microemboli in APS: Introducing a novel investigation method and implications of analogies with carotid artery disease. *Lupus* 1998; 7(suppl 2):S75–S80.
172. Asherson RA, Cervera R, Piette JC, et al. Catastrophic antiphospholipid syndrome: Clinical and laboratory features of 50 patients. *Medicine* (*Baltimore*) 1998; 77:195–207.
173. Matsuura E, Kobayashi K, Yasuda T, Koike T. Antiphospholipid antibodies and atherosclerosis. *Lupus* 1998; 7(suppl 2):S135–S139.
174. Ginsburg KS, Liang MH, Newcomer L, et al. Anticardiolipin antibodies and the risk for ischemic stroke and venous thrombosis. *Ann Intern Med* 1992; 117:997–1002.
175. Rosove MH, Brewer PMC. Antiphospholipid thrombosis: Clinical course after the first thrombotic event in 70 patients. *Ann Intern Med* 1992; 117:303–308.
176. Bulkley BH. Progressive systemic sclerosis: Cardiac involvement. *Clin Rheum Dis* 1979; 5–131.

C H A P T E R 77

NEOPLASTIC HEART DISEASE

Robert J. Hall / Denton A. Cooley / Hugh A. McAllister, Jr. / O. Howard Frazier / Susan Wilansky

Tumors of the heart, while uncommon, present in protean ways and have challenged the acumen of physicians since the seventeenth century. Antemortem diagnosis, however, was rare. Intracardiac myxoma was first diagnosed, with the aid of angiography, in 1952, with a subsequent attempt to remove the tumor surgically. The first such successful removal with the use of cardiopulmonary bypass was performed in 1954; the patient, then a 40-year-old woman, was still alive 38 years later.[1] Subsequently, increased clinical awareness coupled with angiographic and noninvasive diagnostic techniques led to more frequent correct diagnoses.[2]

The heart may be the site of a primary tumor or may be invaded secondarily by malignancies that arise in adjacent or remote organs. Whether the tumors are primary or secondary, neoplastic heart disease can be expressed in only limited ways (Table 77-1). In the presence of neoplastic disease, pericardial pain, effusion, tamponade, constriction, rapid increase in heart size, new heart murmurs, electrocardiographic changes, atrial or ventricular arrhythmias, atrioventricular (AV) block, and unexplained heart failure are suggestive of secondary invasion of the heart. The triad of obstruction, embolization, and constitutional manifestations characterizes intracavitary tumors, especially myxomas.

PRIMARY TUMORS OF THE HEART

Although less common than other heart tumors, primary tumors of the heart are far more challenging to both the physician and the surgeon. These tumors usually present as intracavitary lesions, and more than 75 percent are benign.[3] Current surgical techniques permit removal and potential "cure" in many patients with primary heart tumors, thus necessitating an awareness of their clinical and hemodynamic presentation.[4]

Primary tumors of the heart and pericardium are rare, with a frequency of 0.001 to 0.28 percent in reported or collected postmortem series.[3] Myxomas constitute nearly 50 percent of all histologically benign tumors of the heart. The frequency of occurrence and classification of 533 primary tumors and cysts of the heart and pericardium collected by the Armed Forces Institute of Pathology are presented in Table 77-2.[5]

Cardiac Myxomas

Intracardiac myxoma is the most frequent benign tumor of the heart. While most (75 percent) are located in the left atrium (LA), myxomas are also found in the right atrium (RA; 18 percent), right ventricle (RV; 4 percent), and left ventricle (LV; 4 percent).[5–7] Cardiac myxomas usually originate from the region of the fossa ovalis but may arise from a variety of locations within the atria.[5] Although myxomas have been reported as originating from the mitral annulus, the mitral valve itself, the aortic valve, and the inferior vena cava, it is likely that true myxomas only arise from the mural endocardium.[6]

PATHOLOGY

Attached to the endocardium by a broad base, myxomas are usually pedunculated, polypoid, and friable, although some may have a smooth surface and be rounded.[8–10] A myxoma appears as a soft, gelatinous, mucoid, usually gray-white mass, often with areas of hemorrhage or thrombosis. They vary from 1 to 15 cm in diameter, with most measuring 5 to 6 cm (Fig. 77-1*A*, *B*, and *C*).[5]

On microscopic examination, the myxoma is composed of an acid mucopolysaccharide myxoid matrix in which polygonal cells and occasional blood vessels are embedded. Channels, often filled with red blood cells, communicate from the surface to deep within the tumor and are lined by endothelial-like cells resembling multipurpose mesenchymal cells, from which the tumor is purported to arise. Similar endothelial cells line the surface of the tumor; however, fibrin, erythrocytes, and organized thrombi also may be present on the surface. Cystic areas; focal or gross hemorrhage; calcification; glandular elements; rarely, bone formation; and even hematopoietic tissue constitute the multiple, although uncommon, variations.[5]

A neoplastic origin of myxomas is supported by the ultrastructural characteristics of the tumor,[14] the results of biochemical analyses,[12] the cultural properties of the tumor cell,[5] and DNA analysis of the tumor. [6] Although myxomas can recur because of their incomplete removal[13] and distant growth of embolic myxomatous material has been observed,[13] the existence of a true malignant cardiac myxoma remains doubtful.[3] The occurrence of multiple tumors within the LA, bilaterally

TABLE 77-1 General Manifestations of Neoplastic Heart Disease

- Pericardial involvement
  - Pericarditis and pain
  - Pericardial effusion
  - Radiographic enlargement
  - Arrhythmia, predominantly atrial
  - Tamponade
  - Constriction
- Myocardial involvement
  - Arrhythmias, ventricular and atrial
  - Electrocardiographic changes
  - Radiographic enlargement
    - Generalized
    - Localized
  - Conduction disturbances and heart block
  - Congestive heart failure
  - Coronary involvement
    - Angina, infarction
- Intracavitary tumor
  - Cavity obliteration
  - Valve obstruction and valve damage
  - Embolic phenomena: systemic, neurologic, and coronary
  - Constitutional manifestations

TABLE 77-2 Tumors and Cysts of the Heart and Pericardium

Type	Number	Percentage
BENIGN		
Myxoma	130	24.4
Lipoma	45	8.4
Papillary fibroelastoma	42	7.9
Rhabdomyoma	36	6.8
Fibroma	17	3.2
Hemangioma	15	2.8
Teratoma	14	2.6
Mesothelioma of the AV node	12	2.3
Granular cell tumor	3	
Neurofibroma	3	
Lymphangioma	2	
Subtotal	319	59.8
Pericardial cyst	82	15.4
Bronchogenic cyst	7	1.3
Subtotal	89	16.7
MALIGNANT		
Angiosarcoma	39	7.3
Rhabdomyosarcoma	26	4.9
Mesothelioma	19	3.6
Fibrosarcoma	14	2.6
Malignant lymphoma	7	1.3
Extraskeletal osteosarcoma	5	
Neurogenic sarcoma	4	
Malignant teratoma	4	
Thymoma	4	
Leiomyosarcoma	1	
Liposarcoma	1	
Synovial sarcoma	1	
Subtotal	125	23.5
Total	533	100.0

SOURCE: McAllister and Fenoglio,[5] with permission.

in each atrium,[14] or simultaneously in the atrium and ventricle[15] raises the possibility of multicentric origin rather than metastasis of the tumor.

AGE, GENDER, AND FAMILIAL OCCURRENCE

Most patients with myxomas are 30 to 60 years of age,[2] although myxomas have been discovered in children, infants, neonates,[16,23] and the elderly.[17] Children have a higher incidence of ventricular myxomas than do adults. A higher incidence in females has characterized most series. Familial occurrence has been reported,[18,19] more frequently in males. Tumors are divided equally on both sides of the heart, and opposite atria are usually involved in afflicted members. Familial cases are associated with a younger age at presentation and a higher recurrence rate.[18,19]

GENERAL OR CONSTITUTIONAL MANIFESTATIONS

While asymptomatic patients with myxoma (Fig. 77-1*C*) have been reported, most present with one or more effects of a triad of constitutional, embolic, and obstructive manifestations.[2] Cardiac myxomas provoke systemic manifestations in 90 percent of the patients, characterized by weight loss, fatigue, fever, anemia (often hemolytic), elevated sedimentation rate, and elevated serum immunoglobulin concentration formed in response to tumor embolization, degenerative changes within the tumor, or overproduction of interleukin-6 by the tumor.[20] The globulin fraction most frequently elevated is immunoglobulin G (IgG), and immunoglobulin A is involved only rarely.[2] Cases involving coexisting cardiac myxoma and IgG multiple myeloma,[21] and systemic AL-amyloidosis have been reported.[22] Less common findings are leukocytosis, thrombocytopenia, clubbing, Raynaud's phenomenon, and breast fibroadenomas.[2] Polycythemia may result from tumor production of erythropoietin.[23] Patients with hemolytic anemia have features of intravascular mechanical destruction. Hemolytic anemia is more likely to occur in patients with calcified myxomas, which are found more commonly in the RA. The protracted multisystemic symptoms produced by myxomas may mimic connective tissue disease and polyarteritis nodosa.[24]

"Syndrome myxoma," or Carney's complex, characterizes a subset of patients with cardiac myxoma, associated with spotty skin pigmentation and peripheral and endocrine neoplasms. These patients, in contrast to those with "sporadic myxoma," are usually younger, have a high frequency of familial myxoma, and more frequently have multiple and recurrent tumors.[25–27]

Infected Myxoma Rarely, an intracavitary myxoma becomes infected, and blood cultures have demonstrated a variety of organisms.[27] Most patients with infected myxomas experience major neurologic embolic events. Thus, surgical resection should be carried out promptly before complications occur.

Embolization Systemic tumor embolization, more commonly from myxomas with irregular, papillary, frondlike surfaces,[8–10]

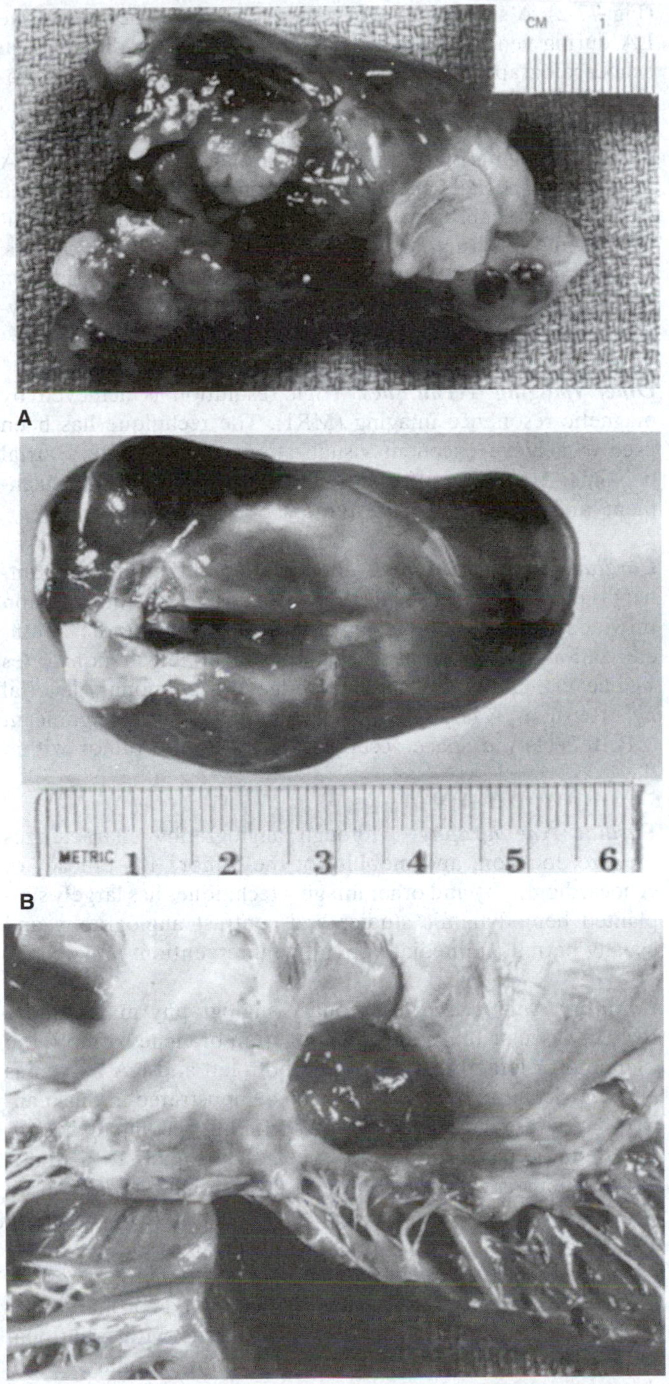

FIGURE 77-1 LA myxomas. *A.* More polypoid and irregular. *B.* Smooth-surfaced and rounded. Attachment to a portion of the atrial septum is seen on each tumor. *C.* An asymptomatic sessile myxoma attached above the posterior leaflet of the mitral valve was found coincidentally at necropsy.

occurs in 40 to 50 percent of patients with LA myxoma,[2] with tumor fragments or surface clots embolizing to arteries in the brain, kidneys, and extremities.[28,29] Rarely, a complete LA myxoma becomes detached and lodges in the aortic bifurcation.[30] The size and consistency of such an embolus may require direct exploration of the aortic bifurcation. Histologic examination of emboli recovered at operation from a peripheral artery can aid in diagnosing an otherwise unsuspected intracardiac myxoma.[3] Systemic embolization, especially in a young patient with sinus rhythm, should arouse suspicion of a myxoma once bacterial endocarditis has been ruled out.

Tumor embolization of the central nervous system constitutes about 50 percent of embolic events caused by LA myxomas, may represent the first symptomatic manifestation, is more common in the left hemisphere, and may be multiple and massive.[31] Embolization may be to the extracranial or intracranial cerebral vessels, with the former being amenable to surgical removal. Onset of the neurologic deficit may be gradual or sudden.

Intracranial arterial aneurysms secondary to myxomatous emboli have been demonstrated angiographically. Late rupture with intracranial hemorrhage has been reported. Care must be taken to avoid embolization during surgical removal of an intracardiac myxoma, not only because of the immediate consequences of an embolic phenomenon, but also because viable metastatic foci may cause symptoms years later. As a consequence, the patient who has sustained cerebral emboli is not necessarily "cured" after the primary tumor is surgically removed.[32]

Retinal artery embolism can occur with transient or permanent visual impairment, confirmed by ophthalmoscopic and histopathologic evidence of particulate embolic matter in the retinal artery.[33] Only rarely has occlusion of the retinal artery occurred in the absence of multifocal neurologic manifestations.

Coronary artery embolism associated with myxoma has been documented by both angiography in living patients and histology at postmortem study.[3] Myocardial infarction occasionally is the first manifestation of a myxoma.[34]

General Features Constitutional manifestations and embolic potential are common to varying degrees in patients with myxoma in any intracavitary location. The cardiac manifestations, symptoms, and physical findings are the consequence of the intracavitary mass and the particular location of the tumor. Myxomas of the LA may obstruct either the mitral or pulmonary venous orifices and produce pulmonary venous hypertension, secondary pulmonary hypertension, and right-sided heart failure. The clinical symptoms include dyspnea on exertion, orthopnea, paroxysmal nocturnal dyspnea, acute pulmonary edema, cough, and hemoptysis, along with palpitations, chest pain, fatigue, and peripheral edema. Episodes of syncope or dizziness are frequent, and sudden death may occur. A marked effect of the severity of any symptom caused by a change in position of the patient, especially if recumbency relieves dyspnea,[2] is suggestive of myxoma.

Physical Examination On physical examination, the first heart sound is loud and frequently split, with the second component corresponding to the tumor expulsion from the mitral orifice (see Chap. 10). P_2 is accentuated, and an early diastolic sound, the "tumor plop," is usually heard 80 to 120 ms after the aortic closure sound,[2] resembling an opening snap. The tumor plop may be confused with either an opening snap of the mitral valve or a third heart sound and follows A_2 at an intermediate interval between these events (Fig. 77-2).

An apical diastolic or systolic murmur or both are present in many patients. The auscultatory findings may vary with a change in position of the patient.[2] Features of pulmonary hyper-

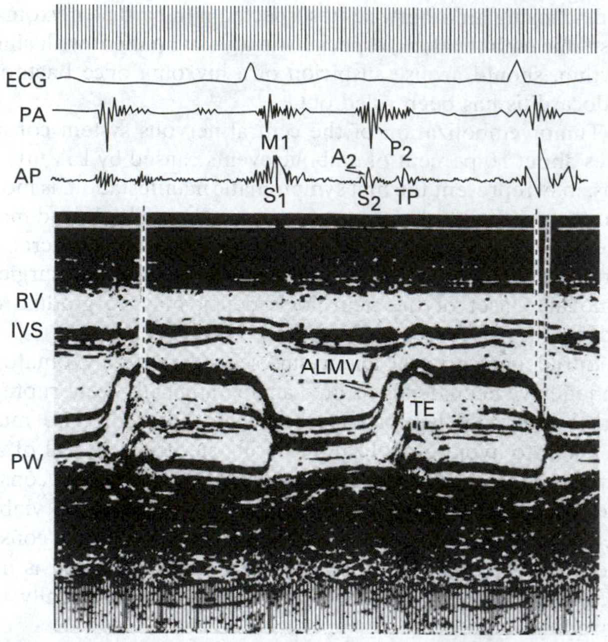

FIGURE 77-2 Recordings of a patient with a cystic LA myxoma, including (*top*) the electrocardiogram, (*middle*) phonocardiograms from the pulmonary area (PA) at high frequency and from the apex (AP) at medium frequency, and (*bottom*) the M-mode echocardiogram at the level of the mitral valve. Time lines equal 0.01-s intervals. The RV, septum (IVS), and posterior wall (PW) of the left ventricle are identified. The loud component of the first sound (M_1) is delayed (Q to M_1 = 0.09 s). The pulmonic second sound (P_2) is accentuated. Multiple linear tumor echoes (TE) are seen behind the anterior leaflet to the mitral valve (ALMV), first appearing at the mitral level 0.04 s after onset of mitral opening and completing the forward movement 0.09 s after onset of mitral opening, at which point the "tumor plop" (TP) is recorded. The A_2–TP interval measures 0.010 s.

tension are frequent and may result in a murmur of tricuspid regurgitation.

Electrocardiogram and Chest X-ray Results of electrocardiographic examination are nonspecific, reflecting hemodynamic alterations similar to those of mitral valvular disease; however, sinus rhythm is generally the rule. The chest roentgenogram reveals LA enlargement and the characteristic changes of pulmonary venous congestion and pulmonary hypertension. The absence of mitral valve calcification and the presence of a LA smaller than might be expected with presumed rheumatic mitral disease are helpful differentiating clues. Calcification may be evident in the tumor even on routine chest film,[35] but this is better visualized and motion is better appreciated on fluoroscopy. The "wrecking-ball" effect of a calcified mobile myxoma may cause destruction of the mitral valve or rupture of the chordae tendineae and may produce severe mitral regurgitation (MR).

Echocardiography The value of ultrasound in the noninvasive diagnosis of intracavitary tumors has been well documented.[2,10] M-mode recordings in patients with a prolapsing LA myxoma typically demonstrate a diminished EF slope of the anterior leaflet of the mitral valve, behind which a dense array of wavy tumor echoes is seen (see Chap. 13). The tumor plop coincides with the completion of this anterior movement of tumor echoes (Fig. 77-2). A similar array of tumor echoes may be seen in the LA during ventricular systole. Transthoracic two-dimensional echocardiography (TTE) and transesophageal echocardiography (TEE) identify the size, shape, point of attachment, and motion characteristics of LA atrial myxomas.[36] TEE permits superior imaging of the posterior cardiac structures and LA myxomas, especially their point of attachment (Fig. 77-3; see Chap. 13). Visualization of all four chambers permits recognition of multiple tumors or tumors in less common locations. Doppler assessment of mitral valve and pulmonary vein flow patterns provides further information regarding the hemodynamic consequences of LA myxomas.

Other Imaging Techniques High resolution is achieved by magnetic resonance imaging (MRI). The technique has been used to achieve excellent visualization of intracavitary atrial myxomas, providing information about the size, shape, attachment, and mobility of these tumors.[37–39]

Cardiac Catheterization Catheterization of the cardiac chambers is currently infrequently performed, since the information provided is readily obtained by echocardiographic studies. Catheterization of the right heart chambers invariably demonstrates significant pulmonary capillary wedge and pulmonary arterial hypertension.[2] A large *v* wave, even in the absence of significant MR, reflects the space-occupying effect of the tumor within the LA.

Cardiac Angiography Although angiography characterizes the size, location, and mobility of the tumor,[2] the efficacy of echocardiography and other imaging techniques has largely supplanted hemodynamic studies and contrast angiography and usually permits immediate operative intervention.

Coronary Angiography Coronary angiography may demonstrate a vascular blush in the tumor from branches of both the right and/or left coronary arteries; both left and RA myxomas and ventricular myxomas have been demonstrated in this manner.[8,55] Neovascularization of a LA thrombus accompanying mitral stenosis may produce an appearance similar to a tumor blush. Aneurysms and occlusion of the coronary artery caused by tumor emboli have also been demonstrated by coronary angiography. Myocardial infarction in myxoma patients with normal coronary arteries has been ascribed to cytokine secretion by the tumor.[40] Cardiac catheterization and coronary angiography are indicated primarily for patients with additional heart disease and to rule out concomitant coronary artery disease.[4]

Differential Diagnosis LA myxomas most often present as, and must be differentiated from, mitral valvular disease.[4] At our institution, intracavitary myxomas were discovered in a ratio of approximately 1 per 100 patients presenting for mitral valve surgery.[2] Characteristically, the clinical course is relatively recent in origin; however, it may occasionally span many years. Fever, constitutional symptoms, and embolic phenomena mimic infective endocarditis[4]; on rare occasions the myxoma itself may be infected. Muscle pain, skin rash, and Raynaud's phenomenon may simulate peripheral vasculitis.[41] Multiple systemic arterial aneurysms secondary to myxomatous embolization have mimicked polyarteritis nodosa.[24] Similarly, coronary artery aneurysmal dilatation and myocardial infarction have been attributed to coronary myxoma embolization. The correct diagnosis will be suspected if the physician maintains a high index of clinical suspicion in patients with diverse and protean features, especially when cardiac, embolic, and constitutional manifestations coexist. Echocardiographic imaging of the heart has greatly facilitated the recognition of intracavitary tumors and results in detection in some patients who are asymptomatic.[15] Intracavitary thrombi may at times mimic intracardiac tumor masses (Fig. 77-4).

RIGHT ATRIAL MYXOMA

Myxomas in the RA cavity constitute about one-fifth of all myxomas and tend to be more solid, have a wider attachment, and involve a greater amount of the atrial wall or septum than those in the LA. They originate from a variety of locations within the RA, including the inferior margin of the foramen ovale, the tricuspid valve, and the eustachian valve,[6,42,43] and characteristically produce tricuspid valve or vena cava obstruction. A myxoma arising from the inferior vena cava has been reported.[8]

Clinical Manifestations Clinicaly, symptoms of low cardiac output and manifestations of systemic venous hypertension are present, with a prominent jugular venous *a* wave, hepatomegaly, ascites, edema, and cyanosis,[6] which may be episodic and vary with the position of the patient. Persistence of sinus rhythm is common. Intermittent episodes of syncope and abrupt onset of dyspnea, features never seen with rheumatic tricuspid stenosis, are reported in one-third of these patients.[6] The pendular action of a prolapsing RA myxoma (wrecking-ball effect),[44] especially when it is calcified, may damage or destroy the tricuspid valve and produce severe tricuspid regurgitation.[38]

Pulmonary Emboli While embolic tumor phenomena occur less frequently with RA than with LA

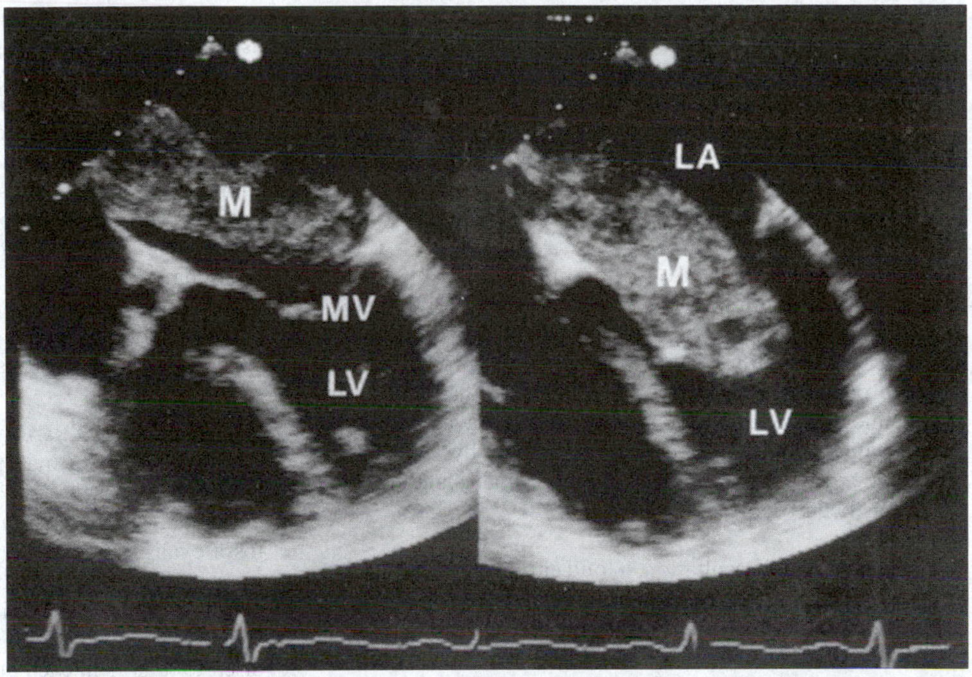

FIGURE 77-3 Transesophageal echocardiogram in the four-chamber view from a 50-year-old man who presented with exertional dyspnea and syncope. A large LA myxoma (M) attached to the interatrial septum is seen prolapsing across the mitral valve (MV) into the LV in diastole (*right panel*). (Courtesy of Susan Wilansky, M.D., Medical Director, Noninvasive Imaging, St. Luke's Episcopal Hospital, Houston, Texas, and Bernardo Triestman, M.D.)

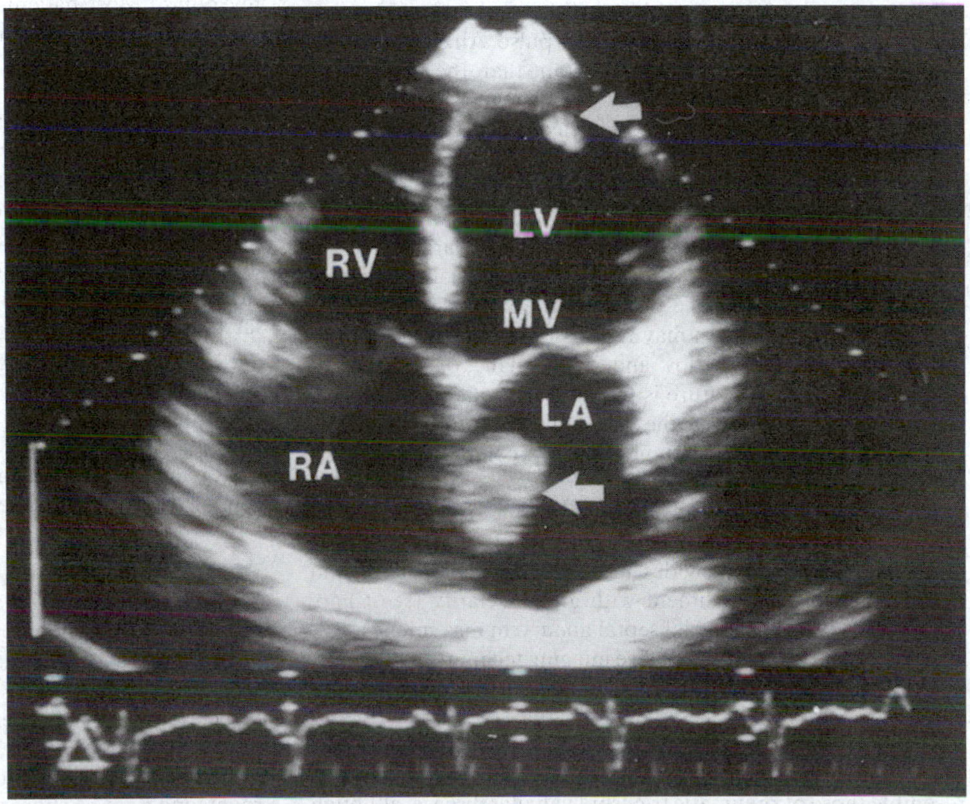

FIGURE 77-4 Two-dimensional echocardiogram, apical four-chamber view, of a patient with advanced congestive cardiomyopathy. Intracavitary masses (arrows), proved at autopsy to be thrombi, are present in the LA attached to the atrial septum (AS) and in the apex of the LV. The latter masses are both sessile and peduncalated. MV, mitral valve. (Courtesy of Carlos de Castro, Department of Cardiology, St. Luke's Episcopal Hospital, Houston, Texas.)

myxomas, pulmonary emboli have been reported,[6] at times are extensive,[44] and may produce irreversible pulmonary hypertension.[45] RA myxoma has been incorrectly diagnosed as recurrent pulmonary thromboembolism.[46]

Wide dissemination of myxomatous embolization to the pulmonary arteries has been reported, with active infiltration of the media[13] and formation of aneurysms.[6] Paradoxical embolization may occur if an interatrial communication exists.

Systemic Manifestations Constitutional symptoms are less frequent in patients with a RA myxoma.[2] Anemia, polycythemia,[2] and cyanosis have been reported. Polycythemia and cyanosis may be caused by either right-to-left shunting through a patent foramen ovale or atrial septal defect, low cardiac output and hypoxemic stimulation of the bone marrow, intravascular hemoconcentration, or erythropoietin production by the tumor.[23] Mesenteric vasculitis of a nonembolic, probably autoimmune, origin has been reported.[47]

Auscultation On auscultation, a loud early systolic sound may be heard. This sound occurs as late as 80 ms after the mitral component of the first sound and results from expulsion of the tumor from the right ventricle. A palpable tumor shock may coincide with this loud sound.[48] A crescendo murmur with inspiratory augmentation preceding this loud tumor expulsion sound is probably caused by early systolic tricuspid regurgitation (see Chap. 10). There may be a long diastolic murmur or, more commonly, only a late diastolic rumble, augmented by inspiration, accompanying atrial systole. If major injury to the tricuspid valve occurs, the murmur of TR will be present, and large *v* waves will be seen in the jugular venous pulse. An early diastolic sound may be heard but is less constant than the tumor plop that accompanies a LA myxoma. The changing quality of the sound and murmurs may mimic a pericardial rub. Such sounds have been called endocardial friction rubs (see Chap. 10).

Electrocardiogram and Chest X-ray The results of electrocardiography are often normal, although RA enlargement frequently is suggested.[6] Low-voltage, right-axis deviation and varying degrees of right bundle-branch block have been reported.[6] The chest roentgenogram may reveal some prominence or enlargement of the RA shadow and, occasionally, of the RV. An important radiologic feature is the mild or moderate degree of cardiomegaly, considering the severe clinical state of the patients. Calcification in the tumor is more common in patients with myxomas in the right atrium.[2]

Echocardiography TTE and TEE provide excellent images of the RA.[49] The latter provides more detail of the tumor and defines the site of attachment with greater clarity (see Chap. 13). A large prolapsing atrial septal aneurysm may mimic a RA tumor.[50] With current noninvasive imaging techniques, catheterization and angiography of the right-sided heart chambers are rarely necessary.

Differential Diagnosis The clinical features of RA myxoma resemble those of rheumatic tricuspid valvular disease, although the latter is always accompanied by significant mitral and, frequently, aortic valve disease. There are many similarities to constrictive pericarditis and Ebstein's anomaly of the tricuspid valve. Episodic dyspnea, sudden syncope, and variability of symptoms and findings with position of the patient may serve as helpful clues. Changing murmurs, along with fever and anemia, may suggest infective endocarditis. Tricuspid stenosis and regurgitation are prominent in patients with carcinoid syndrome, but involvement of the pulmonary valve and other features of a carcinoid tumor will usually serve to distinguish it from a RA myxoma. Obstruction of the right ventricular (RV) outflow tract may resemble a RA tumor. Pulmonary embolization of other diverse etiologies, with secondary thromboembolic pulmonary hypertension and right-sided heart failure, may be mimicked by RA myxoma. An awareness of the protean manifestations combined with echocardiographic findings usually facilitates a correct diagnosis.

BILATERAL ATRIAL MYXOMA

An atrial myxoma may pass through the foramen ovale and be present in both atria.[51] The tumor is usually shaped like a dumbbell, with the common stalk attached to the margin of the fossa ovalis. Surgery has been successful most often when the correct diagnosis was made preoperatively, emphasizing the importance of echographic exploration of all chambers.[14] Similar echocardiographic findings have been reported in patients with discrete tumors in each atrium. Multichambered cardiac myxomas occasionally involve chambers other than the usual biatrial combination and are more often familial.[6]

LEFT VENTRICULAR MYXOMA

A myxoma originates from the LV in 2.5 to 4 percent of reported myxomas.[3] Most patients are under 30 years of age. Women are affected three times more often than are men, and a short duration of symptoms is also characteristic. Systemic emboli, mostly cerebral,[52] occur in two-thirds of the patients, and constitutional symptoms are usually absent. Attacks of syncope occur in nearly half of the reviewed cases. Symptoms and physical findings are suggestive of aortic or subaortic obstruction. The location and movement of the tumor mass are demonstrated particularly well by TTE and by TEE (Chap. 13).[6] Echoes from an intracavitary LV myxoma must be differentiated from LV thrombi, which are usually apical but occasionally are pedunculated, and from ventricular septal rhabdomyomas. LV and RV myxomas have been identified by MRI (Chap. 18).[53] Planning for surgical excision can be based upon noninvasive imaging without resorting to cardiac catheterization and angiography unless coexistent cardiac or coronary disease is possible.[53,54] The tumor can be removed through a LA approach with mobilization of the anterior leaflet of the mitral valve.[55]

RIGHT VENTRICULAR MYXOMA

Myxomas of the RV are as infrequent as those of the LV. The patient will have symptoms and manifestations of right-sided heart failure, syncope, unexplained fever, and a murmur consistent with pulmonic stenosis. Pulmonary emboli may occur. An "ejection sound" has been reported, as well as delayed closure of the pulmonic valve. A right-sided tumor plop may be heard in diastole.[6] Calcium in the tumor may be recognized on the roentgenogram. Echocardiographic imaging, both TTE and TEE, will detect most RV myxomas.[56] A RV myxoma has been diagnosed in a neonate and has been successfully removed surgically. Other tumors, producing similar outflow tract obstruction, rarely occur within the RV.[6]

SURGERY FOR INTRACAVITARY MYXOMA

Surgical resection of a myxoma is the only acceptable therapy and, in view of the dangers of embolization and sudden death, should be performed promptly.[57] For complete removal of LA myxoma, we use a biatrial approach, excising a full thickness of interatrial septum if the tumor is attached to the region of the fossa ovalis.[58,59] RA myxomas are commonly attached to the fossa ovalis, and, with right-sided tumors, a full thickness of atrial septum also should be resected. If a large portion of the septum is removed, a patch of knitted Dacron cloth should be used for repair to avoid distortion, dysrhythmia, or possible atrial septal defect. We usually induce ventricular standstill with cardioplegia solution before manipulating the heart, to reduce the possibility of fragmentation of the gelatinous tumor. LA myxomas have been removed successfully during pregnancy, utilizing cardiopulmonary bypass, with subsequent uncomplicated completion of a full-term pregnancy. Surgical removal of a RV myxoma in a neonate has been reported.[60]

By its movement within the heart, a myxoma, especially when calcified, may traumatize either AV valve, which may require replacement or repair by annuloplasty.[2] Recurrences of atrial myxomas are rare and usually occur within a 48-month period.[6]

Other Benign Primary Cardiac Tumors

RHABDOMYOMA

The most frequent cardiac tumor in infants and children[3] is a rhabdomyoma, which is probably a hamartoma rather than a true neoplasm.[61] These tumors are usually multiple, usually involve the ventricular myocardium, and project into the cavity or move freely as a pedunculated mass.[62] Associated tuberous sclerosis is present in one-third of the patients.[63] Presenting manifestations may be caused by cardiac obstructive phenomena or by arrhythmias, AV block, pericardial effusion, ventricular preexcitation,[64] and even sudden death. These tumors can mimic pulmonary stenosis and produce hypoxic spells like those seen with tetralogy of Fallot. Ventricular outlet gradients,[64] angiographic abnormalities, echocardiography (Chap. 13), and MRI [65] can lead to demonstration of the tumor and successful surgical resection or heart transplantation.[66] Pedunculated rhabdomyomas that arise from the LA and cause mitral stenosis have been reported. Discrete and multiple myocardial hamartomas and rhabdomyomas have caused incessant ventricular tachycardia in infants and have been successfully removed surgically.[67] Rhabdomyomas are the tumors most frequently found at fetal echocardiography, constituting 17 of 19 fetal tumors found in 14,000 fetal echocardiograms.[68]

FIBROMA

Fibromas are usually ventricular and intramural. Although reported cases have occurred in the age range from newborn to 65 years, most occur in infants and children.[69] Calcification is common. Sudden death, occurring in nearly one-third of the patients, likely is due to involvement of the conduction system, production of arrhythmias, or obstruction of the LV outflow tract.[70] Two-dimensional echocardiography accurately delineates intramural ventricular tumors.[71] Left-axis deviation may occur as an interesting electrocardiographic feature. Total or partial resection of the tumor to relieve obstruction has been reported, with excellent probability of long-term survival. Cardiac transplantation has been used in the management of a young adult with a nonresectable (1030-g) LV fibroma.[72]

PAPILLARY FIBROELASTOMA

Also referred to as papillomas or papillary fibromas, papillary fibroelastomas arise from the cardiac valves[73,74] or occasionally from the ventricular endocardium, are most commonly seen in patients over age 50, and until recently have been a coincidental finding at surgery or postmortem examination. Grossly, these tumors resemble a sea anemone, with multiple papillary fronds attached to the endothelium by a short pedicle. There is a predilection for involvement of the aortic valve,[75] where angina, infarction, or sudden death may result from coronary embolization or ostial occlusion caused by the villous tumor.[3,76,77] Cerebral and ocular emboli from these lesions are being reported with increasing frequency.[103] Origin on right-sided cardiac valves is rare.[78,79] Obstruction of the RV outflow tract has been reported in a patient with a papillary tumor of the tricuspid valve. The tumor is histologically different from Lambl's excrescences, which are degenerative in origin and usually situated on the ventricular aspect of the semilunar valve along the line of closure.[3] Papillary fibroelastomas are being discovered with increasing frequency by echocardiographic (TTE and TEE) imaging of the heart, and because of their potential for cerebral and coronary embolization, surgical excision is recommended for even small papillary fibroelastomas.[80,81] Papillary fibroelastomas may mimic vegetations and bacterial endocarditis.

LIPOMA

Lipomas may occur throughout the heart,[82] including the pericardium. They may be massive. Intrapericardial lipomas may cause pericardial effusion, be mistaken for a pericardial cyst, or present as asymptomatic cardiac or mediastinal enlargement. Intramyocardial lipomas are encapsulated and usually are small.[3] Occasionally, a lipoma arising from the mitral or tricuspid valve may resemble an atrial myxoma on echocardiographic examination[83] and must also be differentiated from a cyst or lymphangioma of the mitral valve.[84] Surgical excision of lipomas yields excellent long-term results. Tissue characterization by MRI permits preoperative identification of these fatty tumors (see Chap. 18).

Lipomatous hypertrophy of the atrial septum is a nonencapsulated hyperplasia of adipose tissue and may not represent a true tumor. Varying in size from 2 to 8 cm, the tumescence may bulge into the atrial cavity or superior vena cava orifice and become a consideration in the differential diagnosis of intracavitary masses.[85] Although often found coincidentally at postmortem study, lipomatous hypertrophy of the atrial septum can be associated with unexplained supraventricular rhythm and conduction disturbances, recurrent pericardial effusion, and sudden death.[3,5] Features of both TTE and TEE are distinctive and include atrial septal thickening with a bilobed appearance due to sparing of the area of the fossa ovalis. Computed tomographic (CT) scanning and MRI provide noninvasive tissue characterization of lipomas that echocardiography does not provide.[86,87] The diagnosis may be confirmed by percutaneous transvenous biopsy.

CYSTIC TUMORS OF THE ATRIOVENTRICULAR NODE

Cystic tumors of the AV node most likely originate from either mesothelial or endodermal rests and are always benign.[6] Patients with these tumors tend to have partial or complete AV block, usually of long duration, and often die of complete heart block or ventricular fibrillation. These tumors are the smallest ones capable of causing sudden death.[6] Reported ages in patients have ranged from the newborn period to the ninth decade of life, with a strong female preponderance. These cystic tumors have also been referred to as mesotheliomas, lymphangioepitheliomas, and congenital polycystic tumors of the AV node.[6] Aside from chance intraoperative finding of this tumor,[88] in vivo recognition has not been reported, although the cystic structure may exceed 3 cm in size. The tumor is usually large enough to be recognized grossly at postmortem examination and should be suspected in all cases of sudden death without apparent cause, especially in children and young adults.[6] Most patients with these cystic tumors of the AV node have demonstrated complete AV block and have recurrent attacks of syncope. Even with complete AV block, a narrow QRS complex is common, and these patients may pursue a stable course for years. Electrophysiologic study discloses a block proximal to the His bundle.[6] Electronic pacing should aid in maintaining an adequate cardiac rate, but examples of electrical instability and sudden death reflect a special hazard in these patients, even during diagnostic electrophysiologic studies and after initiation of effective ventricular pacing. The presence of an accessory bypass tract and intermittent preexcitation has been reported.[89]

VASOFORMATIVE TUMORS

Hemangiomas[90] are rare cardiac tumors usually discovered at postmortem study. Coronary angiography yields a characteristic tumor blush.[6] Spontaneous resolution without treatment of a large cavernous hemangioma of the RV has been reported. Lymphangiomas and vascular hamartomas are rare primary tumors of the heart that usually present as diffuse proliferations rather than as distinct tumors. Therefore, total excision is often not practical.[91] Cardiac transplantation may be considered as an alternative in these cases.

INTRAPERICARDIAL PARAGANGLIOMA

Paragangliomas (pheochromocytomas and chemodectomas) may rarely be localized within the pericardium. Although these tumors may be found overlying or within any cardiac chamber, they most commonly occur over the base of the heart in the major region of vagus nerve distribution.[92] Improved detection and localization to the mediastinum have been provided by iodine-131 metaiodobenzylguanidine nuclear scanning. MRI can further localize cardiac paragangliomas and provide detailed information for guidance of surgical excision.[93] Since these tumors are highly vascular, adherent, and difficult to resect, management with cardiac transplantation may be necessary.[94] Human cardiac explantation and autotransplantation has also been applied to a patient with a large cardiac pheochromocytoma.[95]

MISCELLANEOUS BENIGN TUMORS

The right side of the ventricular septum is rarely the site of a congenital benign thyroid rest. Enlargement results in right ventricular outflow obstruction. Complete resection is indicated, and the condition is curable. Rarely, benign teratomas occur in the ventricular myocardium and may result in sudden death.[96]

Malignant Primary Tumors of the Heart

ANGIOSARCOMA (HEMANGIOSARCOMA)

Almost all primary malignant cardiac tumors are sarcomas,[97] most frequently angiosarcomas, and they usually originate in the RA or pericardium.[98] Intense vascularity may produce a continuous murmur. One-fourth of all angiosarcomas are partially intracavitary, with valvular or vena caval[99] obstruction, and characteristically manifest right-sided heart failure and pericardial tamponade with hemorrhagic fluid. Cardiac rupture due to a RA angiosarcoma has been reported.[6] Atrial angiosarcomas exhibit highly variable histologic patterns, which may overlap those of Kaposi's sarcoma. Echocardiography, angiography, CT, or MRI are helpful in the diagnosis (Fig. 77-5*A*).[100] Coronary angiography may demonstrate angiomatous vessels in the tumor area. The course is rapid, and widespread metastases often make surgery impractical, although tumor excision, radiation, and chemotherapy may offer some relief of symptoms and palliation.[3] An iatrogenic hemangiopericytoma of the right ventricle has been reported following intense radiotherapy to the cardiac area.[101]

RHABDOMYOSARCOMA

Rhabdomyosarcoma is the second most frequent primary sarcoma of the heart and, like angiosarcoma, is prevalent in males. There is no single chamber predilection; multiple sites are common, and significant obstruction of at least one valve is present in half of the patients.[102] Excision of the main tumor mass combined with radiation and chemotherapy has been advocated as the treatment for patients with primary malignant tumor of the heart, but in general the prognosis is poor and survival is short.[3]

OTHER MALIGNANT PRIMARY TUMORS

Fibrosarcoma,[103] liposarcoma,[104] primary malignant lymphoma,[105] and occasionally sarcomas of other basic cell types constitute the remaining but infrequent primary malignant cardiac tumors.[3] The fibrous histiocytoma has a predilection for the LA and rarely involves right-sided cardiac chambers.[106]

Malignant primary cardiac tumors may obstruct cardiac chambers or valves[6] or result in peripheral embolic phenomena.

Surgery for Primary Cardiac Tumors

Effective palliation and local control of the disease can be achieved with extensive resection of malignant primary tumors.[107,108] Echocardiography (see Chap. 13), MRI (see Chap. 18), and CT scanning (see Chap. 52) are all helpful in planning operative resection of cardiac tumors because these tests provide three-dimensional information (Fig. 77-5*B* and *C*).[109] Intraoperative echocardiography may be useful in guiding surgical resection.[110] Adjuvant chemotherapy and radiation therapy are necessary to improve long-term prognosis,[111] and the response to therapy can be assessed by MRI.[6] Cardiac transplantation has been utilized to completely resect an "inoperable" benign tumor and an unresectable malignant primary cardiac neoplasm.[112,113] Cardiac explantation and auto-

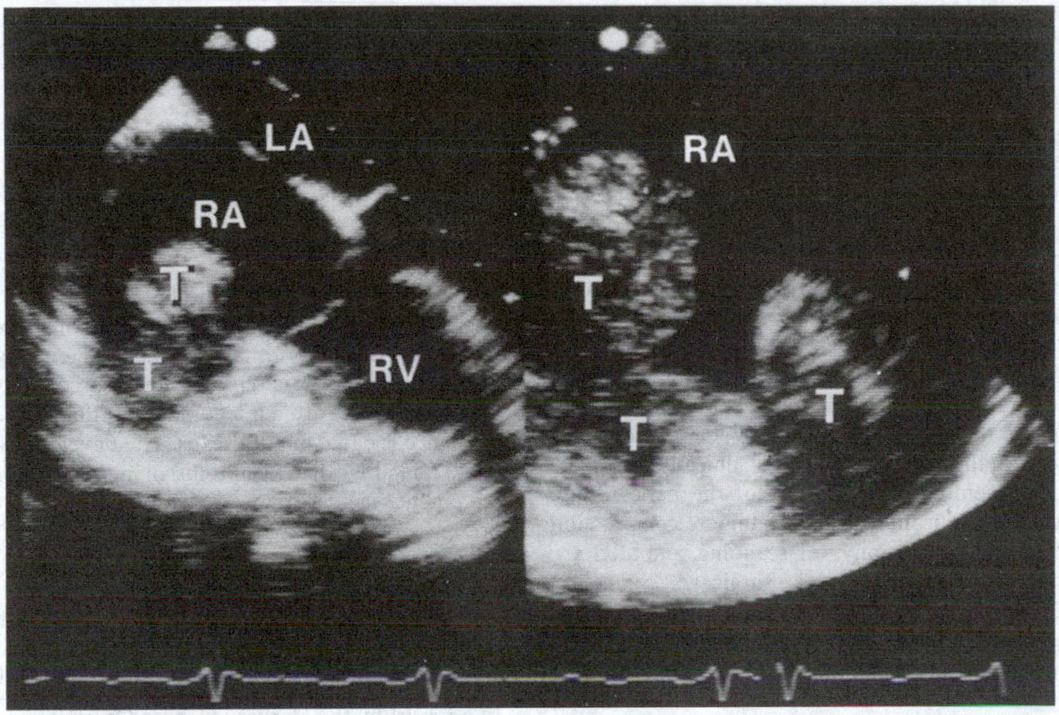

A

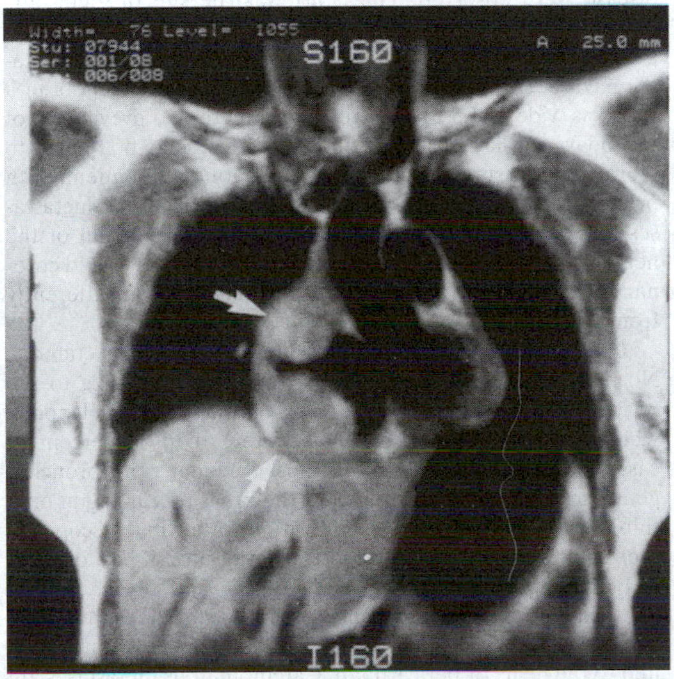

B

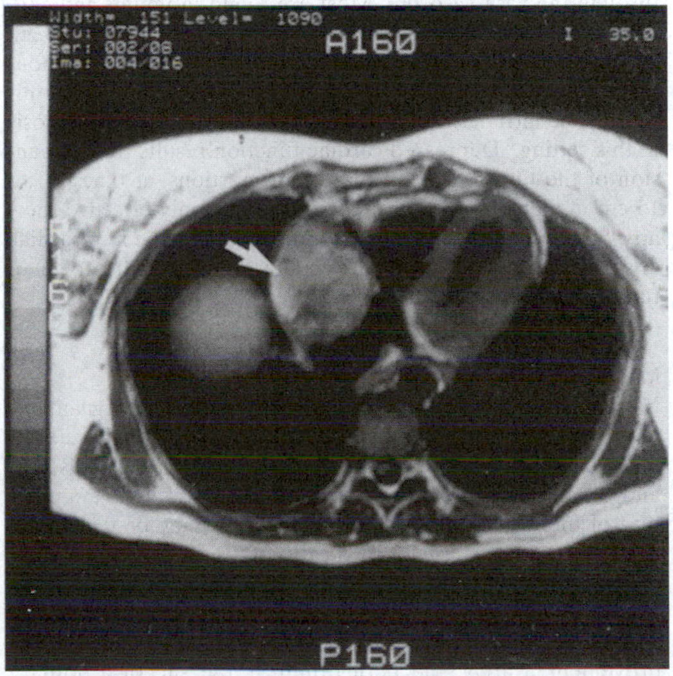

C

FIGURE 77-5 *A.* Biplane transesophageal echocardiogram from a 35-year-old woman who presented with shock of unknown cause. The horizontal plane (*left*) shows a tumor (T) in the RA. The vertical plane (*right*) shows a large, bilobular tumor (T) adherent to the RA wall. Histologic examination proved this to be an angiosarcoma. (Courtesy of Susan Wilansky, M.D., Medical Director, Noninvasive Imaging, St. Luke's Episcopal Hospital, Houston, Texas.) *B* and *C.* Magnetic resonance images. Arrowheads (*B* and *C*) denote a dumbbell-shaped, RA tumor of intermediate signal intensity, which is shown to abut the aorta in the coronal T1-weighted view and the tricuspid valve in the axial T1- weighted view. Note the loss of the usual high–signal-intensity margin (fat) along the right lateral aspect of the aorta in the coronal plane. This raises concern for malignant invasion of the aortic wall. (Courtesy of Clark L. Carrol, M.D., St. Luke's Episcopal Hospital, Texas Children's Hospital, and Texas Heart Institute, Houston, Texas.)

transplantation may facilitate resection of some cardiac tumors (Chap. 22).[114,115]

Tumors of the Pericardium

PERICARDIAL CYSTS

Pericardial, or mesothelial, cysts are the most frequent benign "tumors" of the pericardium. They are usually found coincidentally on a routine roentgenogram. However, 25 to 30 percent of the patients will have chest pain, dyspnea, cough, or paroxysmal tachycardia. Pericardial cysts occur most frequently in the third or fourth decade of life and equally among men and women. The right costophrenic location is the most common, although they may present in the upper mediastinum.[116] Only rarely does the cyst connect with the pericardial cavity. Clinically and radiographically, they resemble other tumors of the pericardium. Hemodynamically significant cardiac-chamber compression rarely results.[117] Echocardiography, CT scanning, and MRI are most helpful in the differential diagnosis. Surgical excision completely relieves symptoms and confirms the diagnosis;[3,6] however, percutaneous aspiration of the cystic contents is an attractive alternative to surgical resection.

TERATOMA

Most teratomas are extracardiac yet intrapericardial and receive their blood supply from the aortic root or pulmonary artery through the vasa vasorum. Most are found in infants and children, with a strong female preponderance.[3] Diagnosis has been established in utero by fetal echocardiography. Recurrent, nonbloody pericardial effusion is common in children with this tumor, and intrapericardial teratoma is the most likely diagnosis in this setting.[6] Depressed cardiac function results from expansion of the tumor to considerable proportions, at times up to 15 cm in diameter. Surgical excision is the only effective therapy[118] and is curative. It is rare for a teratoma to be intracardiac and arise from the interventricular septum, but this type of tumor can be successfully excised.[6]

MESOTHELIOMA

Mesothelioma ranks third in frequency among malignant tumors of the heart and pericardium.[5] The clinical manifestations resemble those of pericarditis, constrictive pericardial disease, and vena cava obstruction. Aspiration and histologic examination of the usually bloody pericardial fluid may be diagnostic. Males outnumber females by a ratio of 2:1, with the peak incidence in the third to fifth decades. The prognosis is poor, surgical excision is usually impossible, and treatment with radiation and chemotherapy generally produces only temporary improvement. Rarely, the pericardium is the site of a primary sarcoma.[119]

Primary Tumors of the Aorta

Primary tumors of the aorta are rare. Most frequently they are malignant sarcomas. Presentation may mimic aortic dissection, coarctation, atherosclerotic occlusive disease, and malignancies in other organs. All portions of the aorta may be involved, and distal metastases are common. Surgical extirpation will relieve the obstructive phenomena, but distant metastases usually lead to disease progression.[120]

SECONDARY TUMORS OF THE HEART

General Considerations

Metastatic tumors involve the heart, the pericardium, or both from a primary origin in some other organ 20 to 40 times more frequently than do primary tumors.[6] These secondary tumors are more frequently carcinomas than sarcomas. Cardiac metastases occur most often in people older than 50 years of age; the incidence is equal in both sexes. The development of otherwise unexplained cardiac symptoms or manifestations, cardiac enlargement, tachycardia, arrhythmias, or heart failure in the presence of neoplastic disease is suggestive of cardiac metastases.

Frequency and Origin of Secondary Tumors

In a report by the Harvard Cancer Commission of 4375 autopsies of patients who died of cancer, myocardial metastases were present in 146 patients (3.4 percent).[121] In a series of 2547 performed at Walter Reed General Hospital, 980 cases of malignant disease were observed. The heart was the site of metastatic tumor in 5.7 percent of the cases and the heart, including the pericardium, in 13.9 percent.[122] In other series, cardiac metastases have been present in patients with malignant tumors in a range as wide as 1.5 to 21 percent. An increased prevalence of secondary cardiac neoplasms in recent years may be related to more vigorous surgical and radiation treatment of patients with primary neoplasms. The relative infrequency of cardiac metastases has been attributed to the strong kneading action of the heart, the metabolic peculiarities of striated muscle, rapid coronary blood flow, and lymphatic connections that drain afferently from the heart.[121]

Cardiac metastases occur with all types of primary tumors. No malignant tumor tends particularly to metastasize to the heart, with the possible exception of malignant melanoma, which involves the myocardium in more than 50 percent of cases.[123] Cardiac metastases are most frequent, with bronchogenic carcinoma and carcinoma of the breast occurring in one-third of the cases.[6] Cardiac infiltration, often macroscopic, is seen in one-half of cases of leukemia and in one-sixth of cases of lymphoma.

Cardiac metastases are encountered with widespread systemic tumor dissemination; only rarely is metastatic tumor limited to the heart or pericardium. Carcinomatous metastases are generally grossly visible, multiple, discrete, small, white, firm nodules; microscopically, they resemble the primary tumor and the metastases in other organs. Diffuse infiltration is characteristic of sarcomatous metastases.

Metastatic tumors are classically thought to reach the heart by embolic hematogenous spread, lymphatic spread, or direct invasion, in descending order of frequency. Lymphatic spread of tumors is particularly frequent with carcinoma of the bronchus and the breast; the proximity of the heart to major mediastinal lymphatic channels seems to explain the high incidence of cardiac metastases from mediastinal tumors.

Manifestations

Secondary tumor involvement of the heart is more often symptomatic, and on rare occasions it may be the first or only expression of a remote primary tumor. At times, as with rapidly developing tamponade, recognition and appropriate therapy must be undertaken promptly. Secondary tumors of the heart may involve the pericardium, myocardium, endocardium, valves, and coronary arteries. Direct invasion of the heart through the venae cavae[124] or pulmonary veins[125] or through an expanding myocardial implant can produce an intracavitary tumor mass and result in obstruction to flow or cause valvular obstruction (Fig. 77-6). Depending on the character and location of the cardiac lesion, a variety of manifestations may serve to identify cardiac involvement.

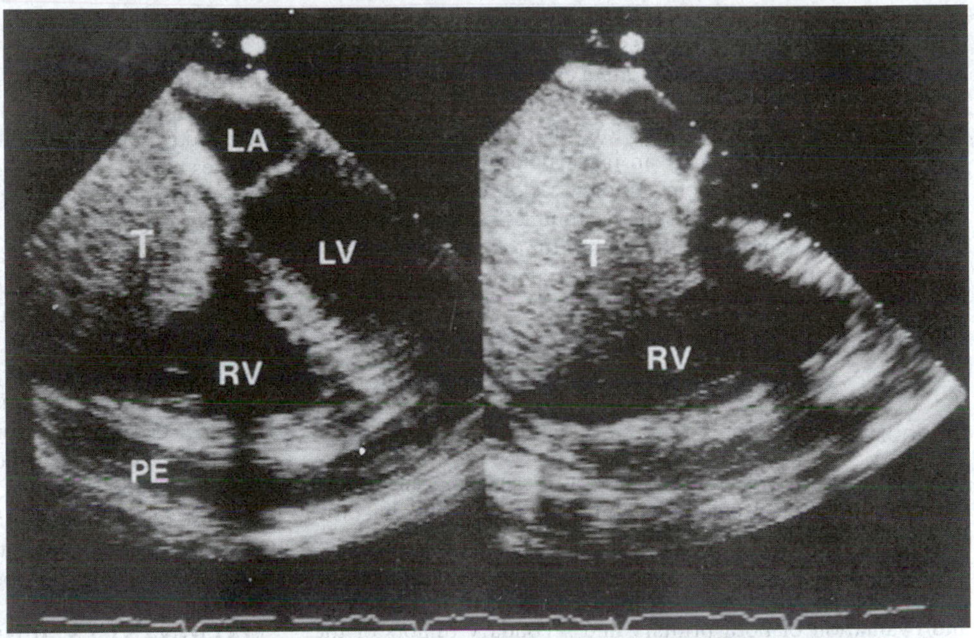

FIGURE 77-6 Transesophageal echocardiogram in a 55-year-old woman who presented with adenocarcinoma of the lung and obstructed superior vena caval syndrome. A large tumor (T) is seen in the RV in systole (*left panel*) and diastole (*right panel*). Subsequent images revealed that it originated from an obstructed superior vena cava. The echo-free space anterior to the RV represented pericardial effusion (PE). (Courtesy of Susan Wilansky, M.D., Medical Director, Noninvasive Imaging, St. Luke's Episcopal Hospital, Houston, Texas.)

PERICARDIAL INVOLVEMENT

Pericardial involvement is often first manifested by chest pain, aggravated by inspiration, and a pericardial friction rub. Accumulation of fluid within the pericardium, often but not always bloody, may result in progressive cardiac enlargement on roentgenogram, with symptoms and signs of cardiac tamponade, and may be the first manifestation of a cardiac malignancy (see Chap. 72). Clinically, the jugular venous pressure is increased, the arterial pressure is reduced, and "pulsus paradoxus" may be present (see Chap. 72). Reduced electrocardiographic QRS voltage can be expected. Electrical alternation, which is generally seen in patients with large effusions and serious tamponade, may indicate the need for prompt pericardiocentesis. The echocardiogram demonstrates pericardial fluid and may demonstrate features of hemodynamic tamponade, diastolic collapse of the RA and RV,[126] inferior vena caval plethora with a blunted inspiratory response, and altered inspiratory intracardiac Doppler flow velocities (see Chap. 72). Pericardial effusion and tamponade may be the first manifestations of cardiac involvement by a malignancy. The association of large quantities of pericardial fluid with tumor encasing the heart frequently results in persistent cardiac constriction, even after pericardiocentesis. Echocardiography and CT imaging are both useful for detecting pericardial metastases. Pericardioscopy performed during surgical drainage procedures has enabled visual diagnoses and guided biopsies of suspicious areas.[127]

MYOCARDIAL INVOLVEMENT

Atrial flutter and fibrillation are frequent, and a patient with either one may be unusually resistant to conventional therapy. Ventricular extrasystoles and serious ventricular arrhythmias[128] may accompany invasion of a tumor into the myocardium. Conduction disturbances and complete AV block also occur. Widespread muscle involvement by tumor invasion or obstruction of the cardiac lymphatic drainage system may cause congestive failure. Rarely, a pedunculated secondary tumor mass may produce a loud murmur and palpable thrill. Myocardial damage and heart failure also may result from some of the chemotherapeutic agents used in the treatment of patients with neoplastic diseases, and combined radiotherapy and chemotherapy may synergistically increase cardiac damage (see Chap. 81). The most frequent electrocardiographic abnormalities seen in patients with neoplastic heart disease are nonspecific changes of the ST segment and the T wave due to myocardial or pericardial involvement by the tumor. Pronounced and prolonged ST-segment elevation in the absence of myocardial infarction may occur with tumor invasion of the heart.[6]

CORONARY ARTERY INVOLVEMENT

In patients with malignant tumor, angina or myocardial infarction may result from concomitant atherosclerosis, coronary occlusion by tumor embolization, or external coronary compression by the tumor as well as from coronary fibrosis or accelerated atherogenesis in patients who have received radiation to the mediastinum.[6,129] The ECG pattern of myocardial infarction also can result from massive invasion of the myocardium by a tumor or from a large pericardial effusion.

INTRACAVITARY TUMOR

Extensions of tumors such as renal cell carcinoma,[130] hepatocellular carcinoma,[131] and uterine leiomyomatosis,[132] along the inferior vena cava and into the RA can present as an intracavitary obstructive mass. Leiomyosarcoma may be primary in the vena cava, most often the inferior, and extend directly into the heart.[133] Intracavitary metastases or an expanding myocardial tumor may progressively obliterate a cardiac chamber or result in a valvular obstruction and, rarely, produce fever of unknown origin. Successful surgical resection has been reported.[134] RA and tricuspid obstruction by an intracavitary mass can mimic pericardial constriction from tumor invasion or from previous intensive radiotherapy to the mediastinum. Systemic or pulmonary emboli, so common with primary tumors of the heart, are uncommon with secondary tumors. Right-sided intracavitary thrombi may mimic primary or secondary tumors on echographic imaging of the heart.[6]

Diagnostic Studies

Echocardiography, TTE and TEE, CT scanning, and, more recently, ultrafast CT facilitate identification of pericardial effusion and intracavitary and pericardial masses (Fig. 77-6)[6] (see also Chaps. 13, 17, and 18A). MRI provides a global view of cardiac anatomy and plays an important role in the diagnosis and evaluation of both primary and secondary tumors of the heart, providing information about the location, extent, and attachment of the tumor.[231] Pericardiocentesis may afford prompt symptomatic relief from pericardial tamponade and often provides a definitive cytologic diagnosis.[135] Ultrasound and fluoroscopic guidance aid in safe pericardial catheter placement (see Chap. 82). The results of endomyocardial biopsy may contribute to the diagnosis in some cases. Bone formation in metastatic osteogenic sarcoma occasionally may be visible radiographically.

Treatment

Malignant pericardial effusion usually recurs rapidly after pericardiocentesis. Depending on the cytologic type and radiosensitivity of the tumor, radiation to the cardiac area with or without systemic chemotherapy is the treatment of choice.[6] The heart can tolerate 20 to 40 Gy, beyond which the risk of radiation-induced pericardial, myocardial, and valvular[136] damage is increased. Patients with malignant pericardial effusions have responded to systemic chemotherapy and to intrapericardial administration of fluorouracil, radioactive gold (nitrogen mustard), and tetracycline.[137] Persistent reaccumulation of fluid may require surgical creation of a pericardial "window."[138] A pericardial-pleural "window" has also been produced with a percutaneous balloon catheter without surgery.[139] Patients with myocardial infiltration by tumor also respond to radiation therapy and systemic chemotherapy. Recurrent ventricular tachycardia has responded to administration of amiodarone.[140] Heart block is treated with temporary or permanent electronic pacing. Surgical removal of intracavitary, obstructing secondary tumors may ameliorate symptoms and prolong survival,[141] as may chemotherapy occasionally. Documentation of tumor regression is possible with echocardiographic imaging. MRI plays an important role in characterizing the three-dimensional extent and attachment of cardiac tumors. This information is of particular importance in planning a surgical approach aimed at either complete removal or palliative debulking of a tumor mass (see Chap. 82).[142]

Special Considerations

LEUKEMIA

Leukemic infiltration of the heart is usually found at postmortem study.[143] Cardiac infiltrates are found in most postmortem studies of patients with acute leukemia, with most having pericardial involvement. Cardiac symptoms are unusual. Chronic lymphocytic leukemia reportedly has caused myocardial infiltration in some patients, as well as mitral valve dysfunction and congestive heart failure.[6] Myocardial rupture has been reported as an early manifestation of acute myeloblastic leukemia.[144] Massive pericardial effusion, often hemorrhagic, and pericardial tamponade have been reported, but overt pericardial effusion is rare.[6] Management consists of pericardiocentesis and chemotherapy; occasionally, surgical decompression of the pericardium is necessitated by recurrent tamponade. Infective endocarditis, commonly fungal, may complicate acute leukemia. Because of advances in treatment and improved long-term remission in patients with acute lymphoblastic leukemia, complicating endocarditis has been managed by valve replacement.

MALIGNANT LYMPHOMA

Involvement of the heart in patients with malignant lymphoma is common, although it is infrequently detected before death. Cardiac or pericardial metastases occur with both Hodgkin's and non-Hodgkin's lymphoma and result from lymphatic and hematogenous spread as well as direct extension from other intrathoracic masses, resulting in predominantly epicardial and pericardial involvement.[3] Cardiac involvement may occasionally be the direct cause of death, but antemortem detection is infrequent.

ACQUIRED IMMUNODEFICIENCY SYNDROME AND HEART NEOPLASMS

Two varieties of malignancies involving the heart have been described in patients with acquired immunodeficiency syndrome (AIDS): Kaposi's sarcoma and, less commonly, malignant lymphoma.[145] Involvement of the heart by Kaposi's sarcoma may be primary or part of a widely disseminated process. The epicardium is a common location, with involvement of the underlying myocardium. Clinical cardiac dysfunction is minimal, although fatal pericardial tamponade has been reported (see Chap. 70).

Lymphomas, usually of high-grade malignant characteristics, occur with increased frequency in patients with AIDS and other immunosuppressed states (Chap. 70). Both primary and, more commonly, secondary lymphomas involve the heart either as a diffuse infiltrative process or as focal nodules in any layer of the heart. Clinical features may be absent in approximately 50 percent of patients. When present, they include cardiomegaly, pericardial effusion and tamponade, congestive failure, atrial arrhythmias, and progressive heart block.[146-149] Echocardiography is useful and demonstrates pericardial effusion, mass lesions, and wall-motion abnormalities. Transvenous biopsy can be useful in making the diagnosis. There is limited experience with heart surgery in this group of patients.

CARCINOID HEART DISEASE

While carcinoid tumors are never primary in the heart and only rarely metastasize to the heart and pericardium, products of the tumor produce a distinctive endocardial and valvular pathologic pattern.[150–153] Tumors producing the carcinoid syndrome most commonly arise in the gastrointestinal tract, but they may also arise in the bronchus, biliary tract, pancreas, and testis.[6,154] Appendiceal carcinoids rarely metastasize or produce the carcinoid syndrome. Ileal carcinoids, containing cytoplasmic granules that take up and reduce silver salts, frequently metastasize to the liver and produce the carcinoid syndrome. These carcinoids contain a high concentration of 5-hydroxytryptamine (5-HT), which is excreted mainly as 5-hydroxyindoleacetic acid (5-HIAA) in the urine. Bronchial, pancreatic, and gastric carcinoid tumors differ morphologically and histochemically, have a worse prognosis, and metastasize more widely than do ileal tumors. They also produce 5-HT and excrete 5-HIAA in the urine; however, the clinical picture may be atypical. Although they bear no morphologic or histochemical relation to the more typical carcinoid tumor, carcinomas of the bronchus, pancreas, or thyroid may occasionally secrete humoral substances that produce the carcinoid syndrome. In gastrointestinal carcinoid disease, the syndrome is produced by secretion of tumor products into the systemic circulation, and its recognition is delayed until after liver metastases. The carcinoid syndrome, which results from the systemic effect of circulating vasoactive amines, consists of cutaneous flushing, intestinal hypermobility, bronchial constriction, edema, and cardiac lesions. Among patients with carcinoid, those with carcinoid heart disease demonstrate strikingly higher plasma serotonin and 5-HIAA levels.[155]

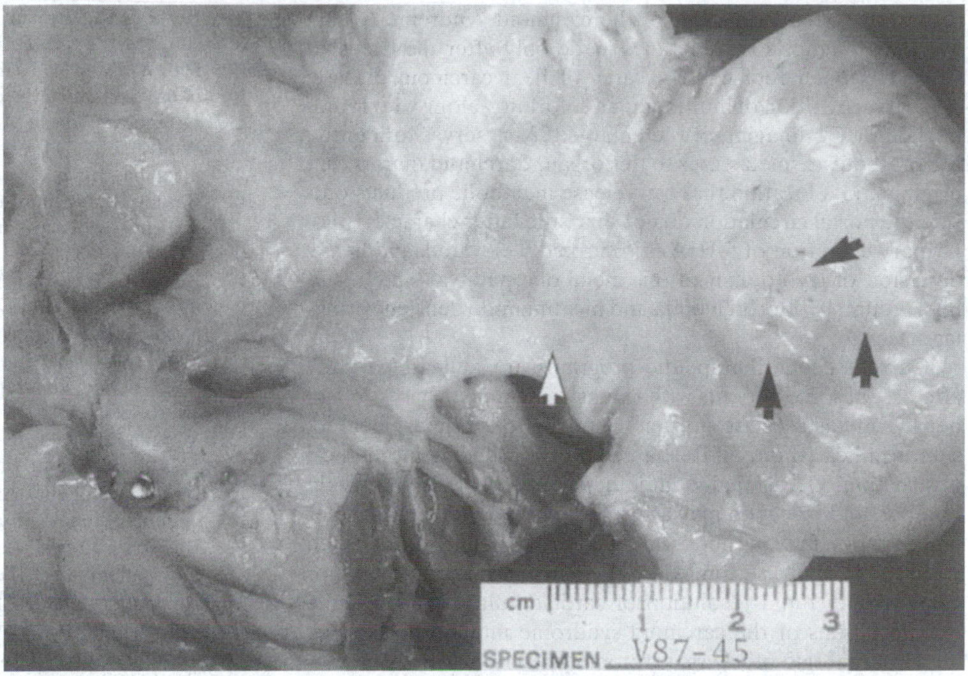

FIGURE 77-7 Carcinoid heart disease. The RA from a patient with carcinoid heart disease and combined tricuspid regurgitation and tricuspid stenosis. Note raised white plaques (black arrow) or the endocardial surface of the dilated RA and tricuspid valve (white arrow). Carcinoid heart disease occurs in 19 to 55 percent of patients with carcinoid.

Cardiac lesions are more commonly found in the right side of the heart than in the left (Fig. 77-6). Left-sided involvement occurs with bronchial tumors, in the presence of an intraatrial communication, or, in the absence of such a communication, when there is extensive right-sided heart involvement. Grossly glistening, white-yellow deposits are found on the pulmonary and tricuspid valves and, to varying degrees, on the RA and RV endocardium (see Chap. 59). Contraction of these deposits leads to tricuspid and pulmonary valve regurgitation and stenosis and occasionally may produce a restrictive type of myopathy.[156] Mitral valve involvement may result in both stenosis and regurgitation. On microscopic examination, the endocardial lesions consist of superficial deposits of fibrous tissue beneath a normal endothelium.[157] Metastatic lesions may be found in the myocardium. Serotonin, 5-HT, and bradykinin have been implicated in the pathogenesis of the cardiac lesions. Transforming growth factor β (TGF-β) has been shown to be produced by the fibroblasts in the carcinoid plaque and may play a critical role in progressive deposition of matrix proteins. The application of antibodies against TGF-β may potentially suppress the plaque progress.

Carcinoid heart disease cannot be recognized clinically until cardiac murmurs and signs of right-sided heart failure develop, especially elevated jugular venous pressure with inspiratory augmentation of the *v* wave, which is characteristic of tricuspid regurgitation (TR). A harsh, holosystolic, lower sternal border murmur with inspiratory accentuation is common, frequently followed by an early diastolic filling sound and diastolic rumble (see Chap. 58). A left upper sternal midsystolic murmur of pulmonic stenosis (PS) may or may not be identified separately. Murmurs of concomitant left-sided heart valvular involvement are rarely identified. There may be a parasternal heave and systolic pulsation of the liver, although enlargement and multinodular irregularity of the liver, ascites, and edema may be features of hepatic metastases without cardiac involvement (Fig. 77-7).

Roentgenographic examination of the chest will show the lung fields to be clear and the pulmonary trunk to be normal in size; the heart may be normal in size or show evidence of RV and RA enlargement. The electrocardiogram may show evidence of RA enlargement, but RV hypertrophy is rare.

Echocardiographic imaging reveals RV volume overload and abnormal right-sided valves. The tricuspid valve is typically thickened, retracted, and fixed in a semiopen position. Doming of the tricuspid valve may be present when the valve is predominantly stenotic. Color-flow Doppler will identify moderate to severe TR in the majority of patients. Pulmonary valve abnormalities are present in one-half of the patients, with pulmonic regurgitation more frequent than PS. Left-sided valvular involvement—mitral more often than aortic—is infrequent (7 percent).

Diagnosis of carcinoid heart disease depends on clinical recognition of the characteristic right-sided heart findings in the setting of systemic features of the carcinoid syndrome (Chap. 59). The diagnosis is sometimes made only after the tricuspid valve has been replaced. In cases of ileal carcinoid disease, clinical recognition of multinodular deformity, along with radionuclide or CT imaging of the enlarged liver, serves to identify the prerequisite metastases to this organ. Carcinoid tumors that originate in a location that can release metabolic products outside the portal circulation do not share the latter characteristics. Urinary excretion of 5-HIAA is markedly elevated, and heavy diversion of tryptophan to this metabolic pathway may result in profound hypoproteinemia and nicotinamide deficiency (pellagra).

Current chemotherapeutic programs are at least partially effective in some patients with extensive liver metastases. When hepatic metastases are present, removing the primary ileal lesion is indicated only if it is large and is producing mechanical obstruction. Occasionally, large hepatic metastases are few in number, and resection may afford symptomatic relief. Catheter embolization may permit segmental hepatic ablation in selected patients. In contrast, removal of an extraportal primary tumor can result in rapid resolution of cardiac failure. Some of the manifestations of the carcinoid syndrome may be blocked by alpha-adrenergic blockers, serotonin antagonists, and somatostatin analogs.[158]

Because heart failure is a frequent cause of disability and death when carcinoid heart disease complicates the carcinoid syndrome, tricuspid valve replacement and pulmonary valvotomy, with outflow tract enlargement if necessary, have been recommended when hemodynamically indicated. Implantation of a bioprosthetic valve[159,160] has generally been discouraged, although a review of reported cases of tricuspid valve replacement showed no significant difference in survival between patients with a bioprosthesis and those with a mechanical valve. Carcinoid plaque extending onto bioprosthetic valves early after surgery has been reported. Surgical mortality rates have been reported from 30 to 60 percent,[161–163] and only a small number of patients have undergone valve surgery. With proper care and planning, general anesthesia can be conducted with minimal risk.[164,165] Balloon valvuloplasty for tricuspid and pulmonary stenoses caused by carcinoid heart disease has been reported.[166]

References

1. Chitwood WR Jr. Clarence Crafoord and the first successful resection of a cardiac myxoma. *Ann Thorac Surg* 1992; 54:997–998.
2. Peters MN, Hall RJ, Cooley DA, et al. The clinical syndrome of atrial myxoma. *JAMA* 1974; 230:695–701.
3. McAllister HA Jr. Primary tumors and cysts of the heart and pericardium. *Curr Probl Cardiol* 1979; 4:1–51.
4. Reynen K. Cardiac myxomas [comments]. *N Engl J Med* 1995; 333:1610–1617.
5. McAllister HA, Fenoglio JJ. *Tumors of the Cardiovascular System*. Washington, DC: Armed Forces; 1978.
6. McAllister H, Hall R, Cooley D. Tumors of the heart and pericardiun. *Curr Probl Cardiol* 1999; 24:57–116.
7. Burke A, Virmani R. Tumors of the heart and great vessels. In: Rosai J, Sobin LH, eds. *Atlas of Tumor Pathology*, Vol 3d ser, fascicle 16. Washington, DC: Armed Forces Institute of Pathology; 1996:231.
8. Shimono T, Makino S, Kanamori Y, et al. Left atrial myxomas: Using gross anatomic tumor types to determine clinical features and coronary angiographic findings. *Chest* 1995; 107:674–679.
9. Burke AP, Virmani R. Cardiac myxoma: A clinicopathologic study. *Am J Clin Pathol* 1993; 100:671–680.
10. Ha JW, Kang WC, Chung N, et al. Echocardiographic and morphologic characteristics of left atrial myxoma and their relation to systemic embolism. *Am J Cardiol* 1999; 83(suppl A8):1579–1582.
11. Wold LE, Lie JT. Scanning electron microscopy of intracardiac myxoma. *Mayo Clin Proc* 1981; 56:198–200.
12. Bashey RI, Nochumson S: Cardiac myxoma. Biochemical analyses and evidence for its neoplastic nature. *NY State J Med* 1979; 79:29–32.
13. Read RC, White HJ, Murphy ML, et al. The malignant potentiality of left atrial myxoma. *J Thorac Cardiovasc Surg* 1974; 68:857–868.
14. Dashkoff N, Boersma RB, Nanda NC, et al. Bilateral atrial myxomas: Echocardiographic considerations. *Am J Med* 1978; 65:361–366.
15. Morgan DL, Palazola J, Reed W, et al. Left heart myxomas. *Am J Cardiol* 1977; 40: 611–614.
16. Balsara RK, Pelias AJ. Myxoma of right ventricle presenting as pulmonic stenosis in a neonate. *Chest* 1983; 83:145–146.
17. Davison ET, et al. Left atrial myxoma in the elderly: Report of four patients over the age of 70 and review of the literature. *J Am Geriatr Soc* 1977; 34:229–233.
18. van Gelder HM, O'Brien DJ, Staples ED, et al. Familial cardiac myxoma. *Ann Thorac Surg* 1992; 53:419–424.
19. Farah MG. Familial cardiac myxoma: A study of relatives of patients with myxoma. *Chest* 1994; 105:65–68.
20. Mochizuki Y, Okamura Y, Iida H, et al. Interleukin-6 and "complex" cardiac myxoma. *Ann Thorac Surg* 1998; 66:931–933.
21. Graham SL, Sellers AL. Atrial myxoma with multiple myeloma. *Arch Intern Med* 1979; 139:116–117.
22. Molstad P, Smith G, Aukrust P. Left atrial myxoma and systemic AL-amyloidosis. *Eur Heart J* 1992; 13:143–144.
23. Burns ER, Schulman IC, Murphy MJ Jr. Hematologic manifestations and etiology of atrial myxoma. *Am J Med Sci* 1982; 284:17–22.
24. Boussen K, Moalla M, Blondeau P, et al. Embolization of cardiac myxomas masquerading as polyarteritis nodosa. *J Rheumatol* 1991; 18:283–285.
25. Carney JA. Carney complex: The complex of myxomas, spotty pigmentation, endocrine overactivity, and schwannomas. *Semin Dermatol* 1995; 14:90–98.
26. Casey M, Mah C, Merliss AD, et al. Identification of a novel genetic locus for familial cardiac myxomas and Carney complex. *Circulation* 1998; 98:2560–2566.
27. Revankar SG, Clark RA. Infected cardiac myxoma: Case report and literature review. *Medicine (Baltimore)* 1998; 77:337–344.
28. Diflo T, Cantelmo NL, Haudenschild CC, et al. Atrial myxoma with remote metastasis: Case report and review of the literature. *Surgery* 1992; 111:352–356.
29. Misago N, Tanaka T, Hoshii T, et al. Erythematous papules in a patient with cardiac myxoma: A case report and review of the literature. *J Dermatol*, 1995. 22:600–605.
30. McMullin GM, Lane R. A rare cause of acute aortic occlusion. *Aust N Z J Surg* 1993; 63:65–68.
31. Browne WT, Wijdicks EF, Parisi JE, et al. Fulminant brain necrosis from atrial myxoma showers. *Stroke* 1993; 24:1090–1102.
32. Furuya K, Sasaki T, Yoshimoto Y, et al. Histologically verified cerebral aneurysm formation secondary to embolism from cardiac myxoma: Case report. *J Neurosurg* 1995; 83:170–173.
33. Rafuse PE, Nicolle DA, Hutnick CM, et al. Left atrial myxoma causing ophthalmic artery occlusion. *Eye* 1997; 11:25–29.
34. Cheitlin MD, McAllister HA, de Castro CM. Myocardial infarction without atherosclerosis. *JAMA* 1975; 231:951–959.
35. Sharratt GP, Grover ML, Monro JL. Calcified left atrial myxoma with floppy mitral valve. *Br Heart J* 1979; 42:608–610.
36. Tighe DA, Rousou JA, Kenia S, et al. Transesophageal echocardi-

ography in the management of mitral valve myxoma. *Am Heart J* 1995; 130:627–629.
37. Matsuoka H, Hamada M, Honda T, et al. Morphologic and histologic characterization of cardiac myxomas by magnetic resonance imaging. *Angiology* 1996; 47:693–698.
38. Kamata J, Yoshioka K, Nasu M, et al. Myxoma of the mitral valve detected by echocardiography and magnetic resonance imaging. *Eur Heart J* 1995; 16:1435–1438.
39. Rittoo D, Cotter L. Detection of a small left atrial myxoma: Value and limitations of four imaging modalities. *J Am Soc Echocardiogr* 1997; 10:874–876.
40. Isobe N, Kanda T, Sakamoto H, et al. Myocardial infarction in myxoma patients with normal coronary arteries: Case reports. *Angiology* 1996; 47:819–823.
41. Huston KA, Combs JJ Jr, Lie JT, et al. Left atrial myxoma simulating peripheral vasculitis. *Mayo Clin Proc* 1978; 53: 752–756.
42. Kuroda H, Nitta K, Ashida Y, et al. Right atrial myxoma originating from the tricuspid valve. *J Thorac Cardiovasc Surg* 1995; 109:1249–1250.
43. Teoh KH, Mulji A, Tomlinson CW, et al. Right atrial myxoma originating from the eustachian valve. *Can J Cardiol* 1993; 9:441–443.
44. Hickie JB, Gibson H, Windsor HM. "The wrecking ball": Right atrial myxoma. *Med J Aust* 1970; 2:82–86.
45. Heck HA Jr, Gross CM, Houghton JL. Long-term severe pulmonary hypertension associated with right atrial myxoma. *Chest* 1992; 102:301–303.
46. Jardine DL, Lamont DL. Right atrial myxoma mistaken for recurrent pulmonary thromboembolism. *Heart* 1997; 78:512–514.
47. Park JM, Garcia RR, Patrick JK, et al. Right atrial myxoma with a nonembolic intestinal manifestation. *Pediatr Cardiol* 1990; 11:164–166.
48. Massumi R. Bedside diagnosis of right heart myxomas through detection of palpable tumor shocks and audible plops. *Am Heart J* 1983; 105:303–310.
49. Lyons SV, McCord J, Smith S. Asymptomatic giant right atrial myxoma: Role of transesophageal echocardiography in management. *Am Heart J* 1991; 121:1555–1558.
50. Angelini P, Wilansky S, Gaos C, et al. Prolapsing large aneurysm of the atrial septum simulating a right atrial mass. *Cathet Cardiovasc Diagn* 1992; 26:122–126.
51. Peachell JL, Mullen JC, Bentley MJ, et al. Biatrial myxoma: A rare cardiac tumor. *Ann Thorac Surg* 1998; 65:1768–1769.
52. Abo-Auda WS, Chidambaram BS, Baker K, et al. Ventricular myxoma presenting as acute visual loss. *Tenn Med* 1998; 91:391–392.
53. Camesas AM, Lichtstein E, Kramer J, et al. Complementary use of two-dimensional echocardiography and magnetic resonance imaging in the diagnosis of ventricular myxoma. *Am Heart J* 1987; 114:440–442.
54. Gulbins H, Reichenspurner H, Wintersperger BJ, et al. Minimally invasive extirpation of a left-ventricular myxoma. *Thorac Cardiovasc Surg* 1999; 47:129–130.
55. Talwalkar NG, Livesay JJ, Treistman B, et al. Mobilization of the anterior mitral leaflet for excision of a left ventricular myxoma. *Ann Thorac Surg* 1999; 67:1476–1478.
56. Nass PC, Niemeyer MG, Brutal de la Riviere A, et al. Left atrial and right ventricular cardiac myxoma: A case report. *Eur J Cardiothorac Surg* 1989; 3:468–470.
57. Jones DR, Warden HE, Murray GF, Hill RC, et al. Biatrial approach to cardiac myxomas: A 30-year clinical experience [comments]. *Ann Thorac Surg* 1995; 59:851–856.
58. Cooley DA. Surgical management of cardiac tumors. In: Kapoor AS, Reynolds RD, eds. Cancer and the Heart. New York: Springer-Verlag; 1977: 126.
59. Massetti M, Babatasi G, Le Page O, et al. Modified biatrial approach for the extensive resection of left atrial myxomas. *Ann Thorac Surg* 1998; 66:275–276.
60. Abushaban L, Denham B, Duff D. 10 year review of cardiac tumours in childhood [comments]. *Br Heart J* 1993; 70:166–169.
61. Fenoglio JJ Jr, McAllister HA, Ferrans VJ. Cardiac rhabdomyoma: A clinicopathologic and electron microscopic study. *Am J Cardiol* 1976; 38:241–251.
62. Howanitz EP, Teske DW, Qualman SJ, et al. Pedunculated left ventricular rhabdomyoma. *Ann Thorac Surg* 1977; 41:443–445.
63. Guereta LG, Burgueros M, Elonza MD, et al. Cardiac rhabdomyoma presenting as fetal hydrops. *Pediatr Cardiol* 1977; 7:171–174.
64. Mehta AV. Rhabdomyoma and ventricular preexcitation syndrome: A report of two cases and review of literature. *Am J Dis Child* 1993; 147:669–671.
65. Boxer RA, La Corte MA, Singh S, et al. Diagnosis of cardiac tumors in infants by magnetic resonance imaging. *Am J Cardiol* 1985; 56:831–832.
66. Demkow M, Sorensen K, Whitehead BF, et al. Heart transplantation in an infant with rhabdomyoma. *Pediatr Cardiol* 1995; 16:204–206.
67. Garson A Jr, Smith RI Jr, Moak JP, et al. Incessant ventricular tachycardia in infants: Myocardial hamartomas and surgical cure. *J Am Coll Cardiol* 1987; 10:619–626.
68. Holley DG, Martin GR, Brenner JI, et al. Diagnosis and management of fetal cardiac tumors: A multicenter experience and review of published reports [comments]. *J Am Coll Cardiol* 1995; 26:516–520.
69. Busch U, Kampmann C, Meyer R, et al. Removal of a giant cardiac fibroma from a 4-year-old child. *Tex Heart Inst J* 1995; 22:261–264.
70. Williams DB, Danielson GK, McGoon DC, et al. Cardiac fibroma: Long-term survival after excision. *J Thorac Cardiovasc Surg* 1982; 84:230–236.
71. Biancaniello TM, Meyer RA, Gaum WE, et al. Primary benign intramural ventricular tumors in children: Pre- and postoperative electrocardiographic, echocardiographic, and angiocardiographic evaluation. *Am Heart J* 1982; 103: 852–857.
72. Jamieson SW, Gaudiani VA, Reitz BA, et al. Operative treatment of an unresectable tumor of the left ventricle. *J Thorac Cardiovasc Surg* 1981; 81:797–799.
73. Ryan PE Jr, Obeid AI, Parker FB Jr. Primary cardiac valve tumors. *J Heart Valve Dis* 1995; 4:222–226.
74. al-Mohammad A, Pambakian H, Young C. Fibroelastoma: Case report and review of the literature. *Heart* 1998; 79:301–304.
75. Grote J, Mugge A, Schafers HJ, et al. Multiplane transoesophageal echocardiography detection of a papillary fibroelastoma of the aortic valve causing myocardial infarction. *Eur Heart J* 1995; 16:426–429.
76. Eckstein FS, Schafers HJ, Grote J, et al. Papillary fibroelastoma of the aortic valve presenting with myocardial infarction. *Ann Thorac Surg* 1995; 60:206–208.
77. Prahlow JA, Barnard JJ. Sudden death due to obstruction of coronary artery ostium by aortic valve papillary fibroelastoma. *Am J Forensic Med Pathol* 1998; 19:162–165.
78. Lee CC, Celik C, Lajos TZ. Excision of papillary fibroelastoma arising from the septal leaflet of the tricuspid valve. *J Card Surg* 1995; 10:589–591.
79. Paelinck B, Vermeersch P, Kockx M. Calcified papillary fibroelastoma of the tricuspid valve. *Acta Cardiol* 1998; 53:165–167.
80. Brown RD Jr, Khandheria BK, Edwards WD. Cardiac papillary fibroelastoma: A treatable cause of transient ischemic attack and ischemic stroke detected by transesophageal echocardiography. *Mayo Clin Proc* 1995; 70:773–778.
81. Grinda JM, Couetil JP, Chauvaud S, et al. Cardiac valve papillary fibroelastoma: Surgical excision for revealed or potential embolization. *J Thorac Cardiovasc Surg* 1999; 117:106–110.
82. Sankar NM, Thiruchelvam T, Thirunavukkaarasu K, et al. Symp-

tomatic lipoma in the right atrial free wall: A case report. *Tex Heart Inst J* 1998; 25:152–154.
83. Barberger-Gateau P, Paquet M, Desaulniers D, et al. Fibrolipoma of the mitral valve in a child: Clinical and echocardiographic features. *Circulation* 1978; 58:955–958.
84. Leatherman L, Leachman RD, Hallman GL, et al. Cyst of the mitral valve. *Am J Cardiol* 1968; 21:428–430.
85. Basu S, Folliguet T, Anselmo M, et al. Lipomatous hypertrophy of the interatrial septum. *Cardiovasc Surg* 1994; 2:229–231.
86. Mortele KJ, Mergo PJ, Williams WF. Lipomatous hypertrophy of the atrial septum: Diagnosis with fat suppressed MR imaging. *J Magn Reson Imaging* 1998; 8:1172–1174.
87. Meaney JF, Kazerooni EA, Jamadar DA, et al. CT appearance of lipomatous hypertrophy of the interatrial septum. *AJR* 1997; 168:1081–1084.
88. Balasundaram S, Halees SA, Duran C. Mesothelioma of the atrioventricular node: First successful follow-up after excision. *Eur Heart J* 1992; 13:718–719.
89. Bharati S, Bauernfeind R, Josephson M. Intermittent preexcitation and mesothelioma of the atrioventricular node: A hitherto undescribed entity. *J Cardiovasc Electrophysiol* 1995; 6:823–831.
90. Pigato JB, Subramanian VA, McCaba JC. Cardiac hemangioma: A case report and discussion. *Tex Heart Inst J* 1998; 25:83–85.
91. Trout HHD, McAllister HA Jr, Giordano JM, et al. Vascular malformations. *Surgery* 1985; 97:36–41.
92. Dresler C, Cremer J, Logemann F, et al. Intrapericardial pheochromocytoma. *Thorac Cardiovasc Surg* 1998; 46:100–102.
93. Hamilton BH, Francis IR, Gross BH, et al. Intrapericardial paragangliomas (pheochromocytomas): Imaging features. *AJR Am J Roentgenol* 1997; 168:109–113.
94. Jeevanandam V, Oz MC, Shapiro B, et al. Surgical management of cardiac pheochromocytoma: Resection versus transplantation. *Ann Surg* 1995; 221:415–419.
95. Cooley DA, Frazier OH, Angelini P. Human cardiac explantation and autotransplantation: Application in a patient with a large cardiac pheochromocytoma. *Tex Heart Inst J* 1985; 12:171–176.
96. Swalwell CI. Benign intracardiac teratoma: A case of sudden death. *Arch Pathol Lab Med* 1993; 117:739–742.
97. Raaf HN, Raaf JH. Sarcomas related to the heart and vasculature. *Semin Surg Oncol* 1994; 10:374–382.
98. Adachi K, Tanaka H, Toshima H, et al. Right atrial angiosarcoma diagnosed by cardiac biopsy. *Am Heart J* 1988; 115: 482–485.
99. Uchita S, Hata T, Sushima Y, et al. Primary cardiac angiosarcoma with superior vena caval syndrome: Review of surgical resection and interventional management of venous inflow obstruction. *Can J Cardiol* 1998; 14:1283–1285.
100. Herrmann MA, Shankerman RA, Edwards WD, et al. Primary cardiac angiosarcoma: A clinicopathologic study of six cases. *J Thorac Cardiovasc Surg* 1992; 103:655–664.
101. Schmid KW, Thurner J Jr, Gruenewald K. Hemangiopericytoma of the heart following treatment of Hodgkin's disease: A case report. *Virchows Arch A Pathol Anat Histopathol* 1987; 411:485–488.
102. Schmaltz AA, and Apitz J. Primary rhabdomyosarcoma of the heart. *Pediatr Cardiol* 1982; 2:73–75.
103. Knobel B, Rosman P, Kishon Y, et al. Intracardiac primary fibrosarcoma: Case report and literature review. *Thorac Cardiovasc Surg* 1992; 40:227–230.
104. Cafferty LL, Epstein JI. Primary liposarcoma of the right atrium. *Hum Pathol* 1987; 18:408–410.
105. Cairns P, Butany J, Fulop J, et al. Cardiac presentation of non-Hodgkin's lymphoma. *Arch Pathol Lab Med* 1987; 111:80–83.
106. Teramoto N, Hayashi K, Miyatani K, et al. Malignant fibrous histiocytoma of the right ventricle of the heart. *Pathol Int* 1995; 45:315–319.
107. Putnam JB Jr, Sweeney MS, Colon R, et al. Primary cardiac sarcomas. *Ann Thorac Surg* 1991; 51:906–910.
108. Turner A, Batrick N. Primary cardiac sarcomas: A report of three cases and a review of the current literature. *Int J Cardiol* 1993; 40:115–119.
109. Rienmuller R, Tiling R. MR and CT for detection of cardiac tumors. *J Thorac Cardiovasc Surg* 1990; 38 (suppl 2):168–172.
110. Mora F, Mindich BP, Guarino T, et al. Improved surgical approach to cardiac tumors with intraoperative two-dimensional echocardiography. *Chest* 1987; 91:142–144.
111. Burke AP, Cowan D, Virmani R. Primary sarcomas of the heart. *Cancer* 1992; 69:387–395.
112. Goldstein DJ, Oz MC, Rose EA, et al. Experience with heart transplantation for cardiac tumors. *J Heart Lung Transplant* 1995; 14:382–386.
113. Harlamert HA, Moulton JS, Lewis W. Images in cardiovascular medicine: Primary malignant fibrous histiocytoma of the heart treated with orthotopic heart transplantation. *Circulation* 1998; 97:703–704.
114. Reardon MJ, DeFelice CA, Sheinbaum R, et al. Cardiac autotransplant for surgical treatment of a malignant neoplasm. *Ann Thorac Surg* 1999; 67:1793–1795.
115. Wagner S, Hutchisson B, Baird MG. Cardiac explantation and autotransplantation. *AORN J* 1999; 70:99–100, 102, 104–112.
116. Stoller JK, Shaw C, Matthay RA. Enlarging, atypically located pericardial cyst: Recent experience and literature review. *Chest* 1977; 89:402–406.
117. Ng AF, Olak J. Pericardial cyst causing right ventricular outflow tract obstruction [comments]. *Ann Thorac Surg* 1997; 63:1147–1148.
118. MacDonald S, Fay JE, Lynn RB. Intrapericardial teratoma: A continuing challenge. *Can J Surg* 1983; 26:81–82.
119. Lazoglu AH, DaSilva MM, Iwahara M, et al. Primary pericardial sarcoma. *Am Heart J* 1994; 127:453–458.
120. Neri E, Miracco C, Luzi P, et al. Intimal-type primary sarcoma of the thoracic aorta presenting as a saccular false aneurysm: Report of a case with evidence of rhabdomyosarcomatous differentiation. *J Thorac Cardiovasc Surg* 1999; 118:371–372.
121. Prichard RW. Tumors of the heart: Review of the subject and report of one hundred and fifty cases. *Arch Pathol* 1951; 51:98–128.
122. DeLoach JF, Haynes JW. Secondary tumors of the heart and pericardium: Review of the subject and report of one hundred thirty-seven cases. *Arch Int Med* 1953; 91:224–249.
123. Emmot WW, Vacek JL, Agee K, et al. Metastatic malignant melanoma presenting clinically as obstruction of the right ventricular inflow and outflow tracts: Characterization by magnetic resonance imaging. *Chest* 1987; 92:362–364.
124. Hayashi J, Ohzeki H, Tsuchida S, et al. Surgery for cavoatrial extension of malignant tumors. *Thorac Cardiovasc Surg* 1995; 43:161–164.
125. Hussain R, Neligan MC. Metastatic malignant schwannoma in the heart. *Ann Thorac Surg* 1993; 56:374–375.
126. Levine MJ, Lorell BH, Diver DJ, et al. Implications of echocardiographically assisted diagnosis of pericardial tamponade in contemporary medical patients: Detection before hemodynamic embarrassment. *J Am Coll Cardiol* 1991; 17:59–65.
127. Millaire A, Wurtz A, de Groote P, et al. Malignant pericardial effusions: Usefulness of pericardioscopy. *Am Heart J* 1992; 124:1030–1034.
128. Sheldon R, Isaac D. Metastatic melanoma to the heart presenting with ventricular tachycardia. *Chest* 1991; 99:1296–1298.
129. Virmani R, Khedekar RR, Robinowitz M, et al. Tumor embolization in coronary artery causing myocardial infarction. *Arch Pathol Lab Med* 1983; 107:243–245.
130. Chatterjee T, Muller MF, Carrel T, et al. Images in cardiovascular medicine: Renal cell carcinoma with tumor thrombus extending through the inferior vena cava into the right cardiac cavities. *Circulation* 1997; 96:2729–2730.

131. Fujisaki M, Kurihara E, Kikuchi K, et al. Hepatocellular carcinoma with tumor thrombus extending into the right atrium: Report of a successful resection with the use of cardiopulmonary bypass. *Surgery* 1991; 109:214–219.
132. Nakayama Y, Kitamura S, Kawachi K, et al. Intravenous leiomyomatosis extending into the right atrium. *Cardiovasc Surg* 1994; 2:642–645.
133. Peh WC, Cheung DL, Ngan H. Smooth muscle tumors of the inferior vena cava and right heart. *Clin Imaging* 1993; 17:117–123.
134. Luck SR, DeLeon S, Shkolnik A, et al. Intracardiac Wilms' tumor: Diagnosis and management. *J Pediatr Surg* 1982; 17:551–554.
135. Salcedo EE, Cohen GI, White RD, et al. Cardiac tumors: Diagnosis and management. *Curr Probl Cardiol* 1992; 17:73–137.
136. McAllister HA, Hall RJ. Iatrogenic heart disease. In: Cheng TO, ed. *The International Textbook of Cardiology*. New York: Pergamon Press; 1977:871.
137. Primrose WR, Clee MD, Johnston RN. Malignant pericardial effusion managed with vinblastine. *Clin Oncol* 1983; 9:67–70.
138. Chan A, Rischin D, Clarke CP, et al. Subxiphoid partial pericardiectomy with or without sclerosant instillation in the treatment of symptomatic pericardial effusions in patients with malignancy. *Cancer* 1991; 68:1021–1025.
139. Palacios IF, Tuzcu EM, Ziskind AA, et al. Percutaneous balloon pericardial window for patients with malignant pericardial effusion and tamponade [comments]. *Cathet Cardiovasc Diagn* 1991; 22:244–249.
140. Leak D. Amiodarone for control of recurrent ventricular tachycardia secondary to cardiac metastasis. *Tex Heart Inst J* 1998; 25:198–200.
141. Chen RH, Gaos CM, Frazier OH. Complete resection of a right atrial intracavitary metastatic melanoma [comments]. *Ann Thorac Surg* 1996; 61:1255–1257.
142. Lynch M, Balk MA, Lee RB, et al. Role of transesophageal echocardiography in the management of patients with bronchogenic carcinoma invading the left atrium. *Am J Cardiol* 1995; 76:1101–1102.
143. Terry LN Jr, Kligerman MM. Pericardial and myocardial involvement by lymphomas and leukemias: The role of radiotherapy. *Cancer* 1970; 25:1003–1008.
144. Bjorkholm M, Ost A, Biberfeld P. Myocardial rupture with cardiac tamponade as a lethal early manifestation of acute myeloblastic leukemia. *Cancer* 1982; 50:1777–1779.
145. Lewis W. AIDS: Cardiac findings from 115 autopsies. *Prog Cardiovasc Dis* 1989; 32:207–215.
146. Aboulafia DM, Bush R, Picozzi VJ. Cardiac tamponade due to primary pericardial lymphoma in a patient with AIDS. *Chest*, 1994; 106:1295–1299.
147. Chyu KY, Birnbaum Y, Naqvi T, et al. Echocardiographic detection of Kaposi's sarcoma causing cardiac tamponade in a patient with acquired immunodeficiency syndrome. *Clin Cardiol* 1998; 21:131–133.
148. Azrak EC, Kern MJ, Bach RG. Hemodynamics of cardiac tamponade in a patient with AIDS-related non-Hodgkin's lymphoma. *Cathet Cardiovasc Diagn* 1998; 45:287–291.
149. Estok L, Wallach F. Cardiac tamponade in a patient with AIDS: A review of pericardial disease in patients with HIV infection. *Mt Sinai J Med* 1998; 65:33–39.
150. Schiller VI, Fishbein MC, Siegel RJ. Unusual cardiac involvement in carcinoid syndrome. *Am Heart J* 1986; 112:1322–1323.
151. Le Metayer P, Constans J, Bernard N, et al. Carcinoid heart disease: Two cases of left heart involvement diagnosed by transthoracic and transoesophageal echocardiography. *Eur Heart J* 1993; 14:1721–1723.
152. Pelikka PA, Tajik AJ, Khandheria BK, et al. Carcinoid heart disease: Clinical and echocardiographic spectrum in 74 patients. *Circulation* 1993; 87:1188–1196.
153. Strickman NE, Hall RJ. Carcinoid heart disease. In: Kapoor AS, Reynolds RD, eds. *Cancer and the Heart*. New York: Springer-Verlag; 1986:135.
154. Koch CA, Azumi N, Furlong MA, et al. Carcinoid syndrome caused by an atypical carcinoid of the uterine cervix. *J Clin Endocrinol Metab* 1999; 84:4209–4213.
155. Robiolio PA, Rigolin VH, Wilson JS, et al. Carcinoid heart disease: Correlation of high serotonin levels with valvular abnormalities detected by cardiac catheterization and echocardiography. *Circulation* 1995; 92:790–795.
156. Johnston SD, Johnston PW, O'Rourke D. Carcinoid constrictive pericarditis. *Heart* 1999; 82:641–643.
157. McAllister HA Jr. Endocrine diseases and the cardiovascular system. In: Silver MD, ed. *Cardiovascular Pathology*, 2d ed. New York: Churchill Livingstone; 1991:1181.
158. Oates JA. The carcinoid syndrome. *N Engl J Med* 1986; 315:702–704.
159. Ridker PM, Chertow GM, Karlson EW, et al. Bioprosthetic tricuspid valve stenosis associated with extensive plaque deposition in carcinoid heart disease. *AM Heart J* 1991; 121:1835–1838.
160. Ohri SK, Schofield JB, Hodgson H, et al. Carcinoid heart disease: Early failure of an allograft valve replacement. *Ann Thorac Surg* 1994; 58:1161–1163.
161. Knott-Craig CJ, Schaff HV, Mullany CJ, et al. Carcinoid disease of the heart: Surgical management of ten patients. *J Thorac Cardiovasc Surg* 1992; 104:475–481.
162. Robiolio PA, Rigolin VH, Harrison JK, et al. Predictors of outcome of tricuspid valve replacement in carcinoid heart disease. *Am J Cardiol* 1995; 75:485–488.
163. Connolly HM, Nishimura RA, Smith HC, et al. Outcome of cardiac surgery for carcinoid heart disease. *J Am Coll Cardiol* 1995; 25:410–416.
164. Propst JW, Siegel LC, Stover EP. Anesthetic considerations for valve replacement surgery in a patient with carcinoid syndrome. *J Cardiothorac Vasc Anesth* 1994; 8:209–212.
165. Neustein SM, Cohen E. Anesthesia for aortic and mitral valve replacement in a patient with carcinoid heart disease. *Anesthesiology* 1995; 82:1067–1070.
166. Onate A, Alcibar J, Inguanzo R, et al. Balloon dilation of tricuspid and pulmonary valves in carcinoid heart disease. *Tex Heart Inst J* 1993; 20:115–119.

CHAPTER 78

DIABETES AND CARDIOVASCULAR DISEASE

Michael E. Farkouh / Elliot J. Rayfield / Valentin Fuster

INTRODUCTION

Diabetes mellitus, whether type 1 or type 2, is a very strong risk factor for the development of coronary artery disease (CAD) and stroke[1,2] (Table 78-1). Eighty percent of all deaths among diabetic patients are due to atherosclerosis, compared with about 30 percent among nondiabetic persons. A large National Institutes of Health (NIH) cohort study revealed that heart disease mortality in the general U.S. population is declining at a much greater rate than it is in diabetic subjects. In fact, diabetic women suffered an increase in heart disease mortality over that period.[3] Among all hospitalizations for diabetic complications, more than 75 percent are due to atherosclerosis. An increase in the prevalence of diabetes has been noted, which in part can be attributed to the aging of the population and an increase in the rate of obesity and the sedentary lifestyle in the United States.

Diabetes accelerates the natural course of atherosclerosis in all groups of patients and involves a greater number of coronary vessels with more diffuse atherosclerotic lesions[4–7] (Fig. 78-1). Cardiac catheterizations in diabetic patients have shown significantly more severe proximal and distal CAD.[8–11] In addition, plaque ulceration and thrombosis have been found to be significantly higher in diabetic patients.[12,13] Cardiovascular complications include CAD, peripheral artery disease, nephropathy, retinopathy, cardiomyopathy, and possible neuropathy (involvement of vasa vasorum). These observations underscore the heightened risks of a diabetic patient to develop vascular disease and compel the physician to correct all the metabolic abnormalities. By understanding the mechanisms underlying all these risks, physicians will be poised to prevent them.

CLINICAL PRESENTATIONS OF DIABETES MELLITUS

The risk factors for the development of diabetes are well established (Table 78-2). About 80 percent of all diabetic patients have type 2 diabetes mellitus, which characteristically occurs after age 40 years. The metabolic mechanisms of type 2 diabetes are the combination of insulin resistance and a genetically programmed defect in the pancreatic beta-cell secretion of insulin. Insulin resistance precedes the onset of type 2 diabetes by about 8 to 10 years and is associated with other cardiovascular risk factors: dyslipidemia, hypertension, and a procoagulant state.[14,15] The combination of these risk factors has been called syndrome X, the metabolic syndrome, and the cardiovascular dysmetabolic syndrome. Many patients with the metabolic syndrome exhibit either impaired fasting glucose (IFG) or impaired glucose tolerance (IGT) for many years before they develop frank diabetes.[16,17]

There are new criteria for the diagnosis of diabetes.[16] The cutoff for the diagnosis of diabetes has been lowered from 140 mg/dL to 126 mg/dL. The upper threshold for normoglycemia has been lowered from 115 mg/dL to 110 mg/dL. A fasting plasma glucose of 110 to 125 mg/dL is now referred to as IFG. These changes eliminate the need for oral glucose tolerance testing for the diagnosis of diabetes, which now rests on an elevation of the fasting plasma glucose level.

In contrast to type 2 diabetes, type 1 diabetes (10 percent of the diabetic population) usually is induced by immunologic destruction of pancreatic beta cells.[18] Type 1 diabetes classically has two peaks (at 4 years and 13 years of age) but can occur at any age. It typically produces microvascular disease (nephropathy, retinopathy) but also results in CAD.

TABLE 78-1 Clinical Evaluation of Risk Factors for the Development of Cardiovascular Disease in Diabetic Patients

Cigarette smoking
- Assess pack-years

Blood pressure
- Duration (if known), current and previous medications, assess presence of orthostatic hypertension.

Serum lipids and lipoproteins
- Dietary habits, alcohol intake, amount of exercise and whether aerobic
- Family history of dyslipidemia, eruptive xanthoma, lipemia, retinalis, xanthelasma, thyroid function tests
- LDL, HDL, cholesterol, fasting triglycerides.

Spot albumin/creatinine ratio (in micro- and macroalbuminuria)
- Serum creatinine
- Don't rely on dipstick protein, since negative results may reflect lack of sensitivity of test

Glycemic status
- Duration of diabetes; family history of diabetes; vascular, renal, and retinal complications
- Laboratory: fasting plasma glucose (FPG), hemoglobin A1c q 3 months: Dx FPG > 126 × 2: impaired fasting glucose 110–126 × 2; when in doubt, have patient undergo 2-h oral glucose tolerance test

TABLE 78-2 Assessment of Predisposing Risk Factors in Diabetic Patients

Body weight and fat distribution
- *History*
  - Age of onset of overweight, family history of obesity
- *Physical examination*
  - Measure body weight (kg), height (m); calculate body mass index (BMI, kg/m^2), BMI of 25–29.9 = overweight, >30.0 = obese, BMI >27 in a diabetic patient should be treated as high risk; measure waist circumference (abdominal obesity is >40 in. in men and >36 in. in women)
- *Physical activity*
  - History: job, activity in sports, walking, aerobics; in women, child care, housework
  - Physical examination: assess level of cardiovascular fitness in cardiac rehabilitation facility
- *Family history*
  - History of heart disease, sudden death, elevated cholesterol level, cigarette smoking; hypertension; diabetes, especially in first-degree relatives
- *Laboratory*
  - Measure fasting glucose and lipids in first-degree relatives

Stroke

Compared to nondiabetic subjects, the mortality from stroke in diabetic patients is almost threefold higher.[19] The small paramedial penetrating arteries are the most common site of cerebrovascular disease. In addition, diabetes increases the likelihood of severe carotid atherosclerosis.[20,21] Diabetic patients are likely to suffer increased brain damage with carotid emboli that would result in a transient ischemic attack in a nondiabetic individual.

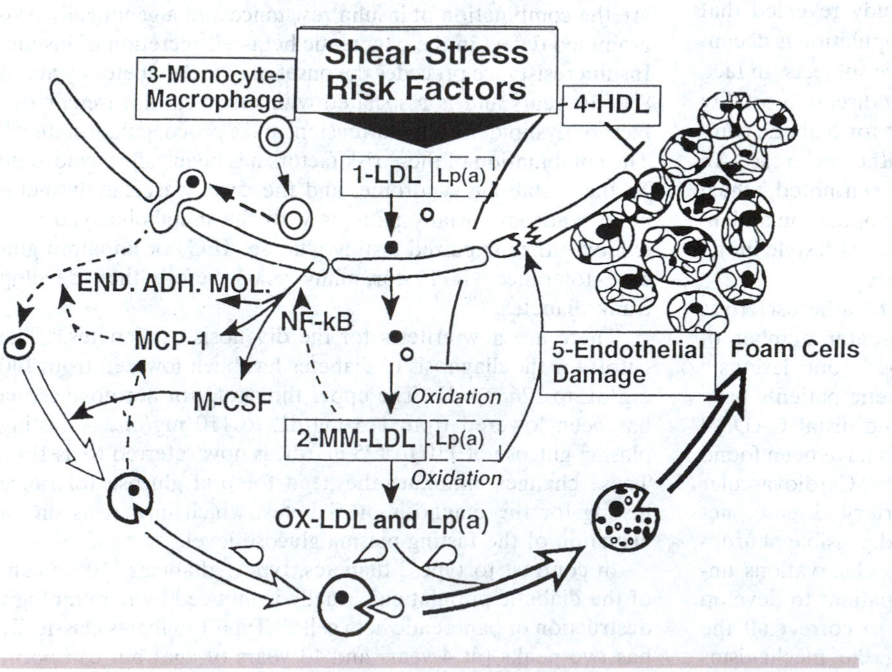

FIGURE 78-1 Schematic of staging (phases and lesion morphology of the progression of coronary atherosclerosis according to the gross pathologic and clinical findings). See text for more details.

Renal Disease

Nephropathy occurs in 40 percent of patients with type 1 and type 2 diabetes. Risk factors include poor glycemic control, hypertension, and ethnicity (blacks, Mexicans, Pima Indians).[22] Table 78-3 summarizes the key points for the assessment of renal status in a diabetic patient. The earliest clinical finding of diabetic kidney disease is microalbuminuria, which may occur at a time when renal histology is essentially normal.[23,24] The Diabetes Control and Complications Trial (DCCT) and the United Kingdom Prospective Diabetes Study group trial (UKPDS) showed that the development and progression of microalbuminuria can be prevented through strict glycemic control. Even once dipstick-positive proteinuria has developed, preliminary data from pancreatic transplant patients show improvement in glomerular pathology at 10 years.[25]

The UKPDS in type 2 diabetics and studies in patients with type 1 diabetes[26] using captopril have shown that control of hypertension slows the progression of nephropathy. The blood pressure should be maintained at <130/85, and angiotensin-converting enzyme (ACE) inhibitors are

TABLE 78-3 Evaluation of Renal Status

Urine albumin and protein
Yearly screen for microalbumin in type 1 and type 2 diabetes; microalbumin/creatinine ratio collected in a spot urine, ideally first morning urine specimen (normal <30 mg/g creatinine); must rule out other diseases that cause proteinuria
If urine albumin/creatinine is >300 mg/g in first morning specimen, macroalbuminuria is present and is usually not reversible with ACE inhibitors; nephrology consult
Nephrotic syndrome: urine protein >3 g/day; nephrology consult
Other reasons to consult nephrologists are diabetic patients with increasing creatinine from 1.4 to over 2.0, elevated creatinine and symptoms of uremia, microalbuminuria not responding to ACE inhibitor
Urinalysis
Red cells, pyuria, casts require nephrology consult
Blood pressure evaluation
If hypertension is present, exclude secondary causes, including with advancing renal insufficiency
Treatment with an ACE inhibitor is preferred first choice even in African-Americans (except if precluded by hyperkalemia or other complications)
Blood urea nitrogen, serum creatinine, and glomerular filtration rate
Yearly creatinine clearance should be obtained with 24-h urine collection and serum creatinine; most accurate way to estimate kidney function without using a radioisotope

the preferred antihypertensive agents.[27,28] The UKPDS, however, showed no difference in blood pressure control with captopril versus atenolol. The benefit of antihypertensive therapy with an ACE inhibitor in type 1 diabetes can be shown early in the course of disease, when microalbuminuria is the only abnormality.[29–31]

There is insufficient evidence to recommend ACE inhibitors in normotensive patients without microalbuminuria.[32] Although screening for microalbuminuria is not as useful in type 2 diabetes patients in predicting the progression to overt nephropathy as it is in type 1 diabetes patients, once microalbuminuria develops, the rate of loss of the glomerular filtration rate (GFR) is equivalent to that in type 1 diabetes.[33,34] Nonetheless, physicians should still recommend screening on at least a yearly basis, since the risk/benefit ratio of diagnosing microalbuminuria justifies treatment with an ACE inhibitor, if not for renal disease alone,[35,36] then for reducing the incidence of myocardial infarction.[37,38]

Patients on ACE inhibitors should be monitored for potassium, since they may develop hyperkalemia in the presence of a type 4 renal tubular acidosis.[27] Sodium restriction will reduce hypertension and therefore is advised. Dietary protein should be adjusted to 0.8 g/kg per day to decrease intraglomerular pressure.[27]

An optimal approach toward diabetic nephropathy combines control of hypertension, preferably with an ACE inhibitor; glycemic control; sodium restriction; and adjustment of protein intake.

Type 2 Diabetes and Coronary Artery Disease

Coronary artery disease is strongly associated with type 2 diabetes mellitus and is the leading cause of death regardless of the duration of disease. There is a twofold to fourfold increase in the relative risk ratio of cardiovascular disease in type 2 diabetes patients compared to the general population.[2,39–43] This increase is particularly disproportionate in diabetic women compared with diabetic men.[39,41,44] The protection that premenopausal women have against CAD is not seen if they suffer from diabetes.[45,46]

The degree and duration of hyperglycemia are a strong risk factor for the development of microvascular complications,[47] but in type 2 diabetes, macrovascular complications have not been documented to be associated with the length or severity of a patient's diabetes.[5,40,43,48] Even impaired glucose tolerance increases cardiovascular risk even though there is minimal hyperglycemia.[41,49–51]

The first detectable sign of a problem in people genetically prone to develop type 2 diabetes is insulin resistance, which can be seen as long as 15 to 25 years before the onset of diabetes.[52] Several atherogenic factors are associated with insulin resistance,[53–59] which can start the atherosclerotic process years before clinical hyperglycemia ensues.[60,61] It is unclear whether the compensatory hyperinsulinemia plays a role in atherosclerosis generation in insulin-resistant patients. A number of prospective studies have shown an association between fasting or postprandial hyperinsulinemia and the future development of CAD.[62–64] However, this association has been demonstrated in middle-aged white men[62–64] but not in women[65] or in other ethnic groups.[66,67]

Hyperglycemia itself plays an important role in enhancing the progression of atherosclerosis in type 2 diabetes. The threshold above which hyperglycemia becomes atherogenic is not known but may be in the range defined as impaired glucose tolerance (i.e., fasting plasma glucose level <126 mg/dL with 30-, 60-, or 90-min plasma glucose concentrations >200 mg/dL and a 2-h plasma glucose level of 140 to 200 mg/dL during an oral glucose tolerance test).[68] Despite the role played by all these factors, population-based studies show that the degree of hyperglycemia increases the risk for CAD and cardiovascular events.[69–71]

Type 1 Diabetes and Coronary Artery Disease

In contrast to type 2 diabetes, cardiovascular risk factors can be examined in relation to hyperglycemia in type 1 diabetes patients. Long-term follow-up of these patients has shown that the incidence of cardiovascular mortality rises after age 30.[72] There is evidence that diabetes accelerates the process of early atherosclerosis that occurs at a young age in the general population. The coronary mortality rate in type 1 diabetes is markedly accelerated, and one-third of these patients will die of CAD by age 55.[72] The protective effect of the premenopausal state is lost for females with type 1 diabetes.

It has been demonstrated that diabetic nephropathy dramatically increases the prevalence of CAD. Diabetic nephropathy is defined by proteinuria, a reduced GFR, and hypertension.

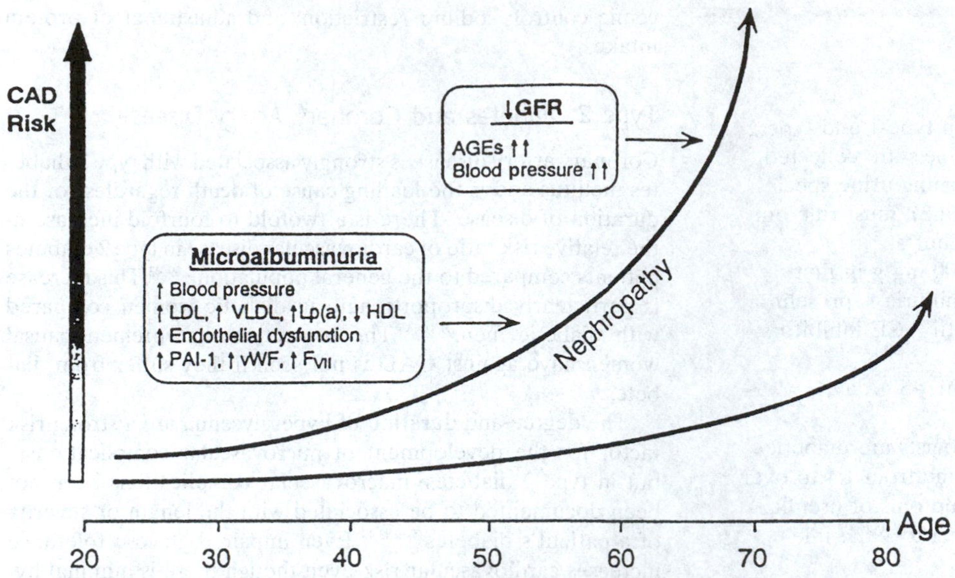

FIGURE 78-2 CAD risk in patients with diabetes mellitus. A subset of genetically predisposed patients develop diabetic nephropathy. In these patients, the risk for CAD increases dramatically. (From Aronson and Rayfield,[138] with permission.)

Patients with proteinuria can be divided into two groups: those with macroalbuminuria (greater than 300 mg/day) and those with microalbuminuria (30 to 300 mg/day). The presence of overt proteinuria increases the risk of cardiovascular mortality almost tenfold compared with the risk in patients without proteinuria.[73] In another cohort, the risk of developing CAD was almost 15 times greater in patients with proteinuria than it was in those without diabetic nephropathy.[72] Since this risk of developing CAD morbidity and mortality has been demonstrated for both macro- and microalbuminuria patients, both must be considered vital in the cardiovascular evaluation of a diabetic patient (Fig. 78-2).

DIABETES AND MECHANISMS OF CARDIOVASCULAR RISKS

Lipoprotein Disorders

Lipid disorders constitute one of the cornerstones in the cardiovascular management of diabetic patients. Many factors influence the lipid profile in these patients, including glycemic control, whether the diabetes is type 1 or type 2, and the presence of diabetic nephropathy.

TYPE OF DIABETES

In type 1 diabetes mellitus, the major determinant in the lipid profile is the level of glycemic control. Low-density lipoprotein (LDL) is moderately increased, triglycerides are markedly increased, and high-density lipoprotein (HDL) is decreased when the level of glycemic control is impaired. For patients with type 2 diabetes, lipid abnormalities are related not only to hyperglycemia but also to the interplay of the insulin-resistant state. Patients with type 2 diabetes may have normal LDL levels but elevated levels of the very low density lipoprotein (VLDL) triglycerides moiety and reduced HDL levels. The expected elevation in VLDL triglyceride is usually no more than 100 percent.

LDL Although LDL levels in patients with controlled type 1 or type 2 diabetes are normal, the atherogenic properties of LDL are increased. There is glycosylation of both apoprotein B[74] and the phospholipid component of LDL,[75] which changes LDL clearance and susceptibility to oxidative modifications. Glycosylation of apoprotein B occurs mainly in the LDL receptor–binding area[74] and is directly related to glucose levels. As a result, there is impairment in the LDL receptor–mediated uptake and therefore clearance of LDL.[76,77] Glycosylation also makes LDL more susceptible to oxidative modification. The product generated by the combined glycosylation and oxidation of LDL is more atherogenic than is either glycosylated or oxidized LDL alone.[78] Such LDL molecules are taken up more easily by the aortic intimal cells and macrophages, resulting in the formation of foam cells.[79–81]

Type 2 diabetic patients with insulin resistance have LDL particles that are small and rich with triglycerides but have little cholesterol in them (small, dense LDL).[82,83] These LDL particles increase the risk of CAD independent of the total LDL level, probably because of their increased susceptibility to oxidative modification. Therefore, even though LDL levels may be normal in these patients, high levels of small, dense LDL may contribute to the increased risk of CAD in such patients.[84]

VLDL Diabetic patients have elevated levels of VLDL as a result of increased free fatty acid mobilization and high glucose levels. There is an increase in triglyceride production by the liver, which results in large, triglyceride-rich VLDL particles.[85] The size of these VLDL particles, which is dependent primarily on the amount of triglycerides available, is an important factor in determining their eventual fate. The conversion of large VLDL particles to LDL is not efficient[86]; therefore, they are cleared from circulation by other pathways. Since the removal of VLDL by lipoprotein lipase also is affected, the level of VLDL triglyceride rises. Furthermore, the abundance of large triglyceride-rich VLDL is associated with an increase in small, dense, atherogenic LDL particles.[87] Numerous studies have shown that elevated triglyceride levels are associated with increased risk for CAD in diabetic patients.[44,88–90] In contrast, elevated triglycerides are not associated with CAD risk in nondiabetic patients.

HDL Low HDL level is a strong risk factor for the development of CAD in both diabetic and nondiabetic patients. There is decreased production and increased catabolism of HDL in diabetes. The decreased HDL production is a result of decreased lipoprotein lipase (LPL) activity. The failure of LPL to efficiently catabolize VLDL results in reduced availability of surface components for HDL production. By contrast, increased catabolism of HDL results from the hypertriglyceridemia of diabetes, producing triglyceride-rich HDL_2 that is prone to catabolism by liver enzymes.[91,92]

MANAGEMENT OF LIPID DISORDERS

Consistent with the National Cholesterol Education Program, the American Diabetes Association has published its consensus document concerning the management of lipid disorders.[93] For the most part, the cornerstone of therapy in diabetes revolves around dietary modifications, weight loss, physical exercise, and maximization of glycemic control.

Type of Diabetes As was previously mentioned, the management of lipid disorders in type 1 diabetes is closely coupled to glycemic control. For type 1 patients, the front-line strategy begins with glycemic control.

In type 1 diabetes, glycemic control can lead to marked reductions in triglyceride levels, but with little or no impact on HDL levels. In type 2, pharmacotherapy is often required sooner than later, given the modest impact of nonpharmacologic strategies.[93]

Medical therapy for hyperlipidemia is similar in diabetic and nondiabetic patients, but diabetic patients require certain considerations.

The hypertriglyceridemia of diabetes can be treated effectively with fibric acid derivatives[94,95] without an adverse effect on glucose metabolism. Type 2 diabetic patients experience a reduction in cardiovascular event rate when treated with gemfibrozil.[96] These drugs cause a 5 to 15 percent drop in LDL levels in patients with normal triglyceride levels, but in patients with hypertriglyceridemia, LDL levels go up. This elevation probably is due to the catabolism of atherogenic LDL particle, resulting in less atherogenic LDL.[97]

Although nicotinic acid lowers both cholesterol and triglyceride levels while raising HDL levels, it generally is not indicated in diabetes. It has an adverse effect on glycemic control[98] that results from the induction of insulin resistance.

Hydroxymethylglutaryl coenzyme A (HMG-CoA) reductase inhibitors are another group of drugs that are useful in lowering cholesterol levels in type 2 diabetes patients without having an adverse effect on glycemic control.[99] In a study assessing the effectiveness of a cholesterol-lowering drug for secondary prevention of morbidity and mortality in patients with angina or prior myocardial infarction, simvastatin was found to be more efficacious in diabetic patients than it was in the overall group.[100]

Bile acid resins can decrease the levels of LDL in diabetic patients,[101] but they can cause a significant rise in triglyceride levels, especially if VLDL levels are already high or if the diabetes is poorly controlled. In patients with high levels of both LDL and VLDL, bile acid resins can be used in low doses in combination with fibric acid derivatives.

Thrombosis and Diabetes

Diabetes mellitus is widely recognized as being perhaps the most significant risk factor for the development of acute coronary syndromes. The relationship between diabetes and acute coronary thrombosis is multifactorial, with the interaction of plaque disruption and the interplay of local and systemic thrombogenic factors playing the primary roles.

PLAQUE DISRUPTION

The inciting role of acute plaque disruption in the development of acute coronary thrombosis is well described. Although the lipid-rich core in plaque is felt to be causative in this process, more aggressive medical management of diabetes can have a favorable impact by decreasing plaque rupture and improving the clinical outcome.[102]

It is well described that not all disruptions of atherosclerotic plaques lead to clinical events. The complex interaction of local and systemic thrombogenic factors is an important determinant of whether clinically significant thrombus formation will occur.

PROTHROMBOSIS

Patients with diabetes demonstrate enhanced platelet aggregation[103,104] that correlates with increased cardiovascular events.[105] Diabetic patients have been shown to have platelets that are hypersensitive to agonists of aggregation.[106,107] The major mechanism is felt to be increased thromboxane production.[108,109] An increased incidence of cardiovascular events in diabetic patients has been shown to be correlated with platelet hyperaggregation.[105]

Diabetic patients have elevated levels of von Willebrand factor that correlate with vascular complications.[110,111] In addition, a relationship has been shown between the insulin resistance syndrome and elevated plasma von Willebrand levels.[112] Similarly, diabetic patients often demonstrate elevated fibrinogen levels, which are also predictive of cardiovascular complications.[113–115] Fibrinogen levels mirror glycemic control.

Factor V, VII, X, XI, and XII levels also are elevated in diabetic patients.[116–118] Factor VII levels correlate directly with fasting plasma glucose levels.[118] Evidence exists linking activation of the coagulation cascade with hyperglycemia. Since antithrombin III activity is decreased with hyperglycemia, glycemic control may play the pivotal role in limiting thrombosis and thrombosis-related complications in diabetic patients.[119]

The insulin resistance syndrome is marked by increased plasminogen-activator inhibitor-1 (PAI-1) levels. Impaired plasma fibrinolytic activity therefore can increase the risk for myocardial infarction.[120] Fasting plasma insulin levels have been shown to be directly correlated to the concentration of PAI-1. Glucose has a direct effect on PAI-1–producing tissues, leading to another explanation for the presence of impaired fibrinolysis in diabetic patients. Even when insulin resistance is adjusted for, serum triglyceride levels have been closely linked to impaired fibrinolysis.[121–123]

Endothelial Dysfunction

Hyperglycemia induces the expression of adhesion molecules such as VCAM-1, ICAM-1, and E-selectin[124] (Fig. 78-3). The binding of advanced glycosylation end products to their receptor results in oxidative stress and the transcription factor NF-κB[125,126] and VCAM-1.[127] These early stages in diabetic atherosclerosis may be the consequence of increased adhesive interactions of monocytes and the endothelial cell surface. Hyperglycemia-induced endothelial dysfunction is believed to result primarily from increased generation of oxygen free radicals that inactivate endothelium-derived relaxing factor (EDRF).[128,129] Enhanced levels of free radicals in the setting of sustained hyperglycemia result in the autoxidation of glucose,[130] the oxidation of lipids,[131] and the metabolism of AGEs.[132] AGEs rapidly inactivate nitric oxide and result in a reduction of endothelium-dependent vaso-

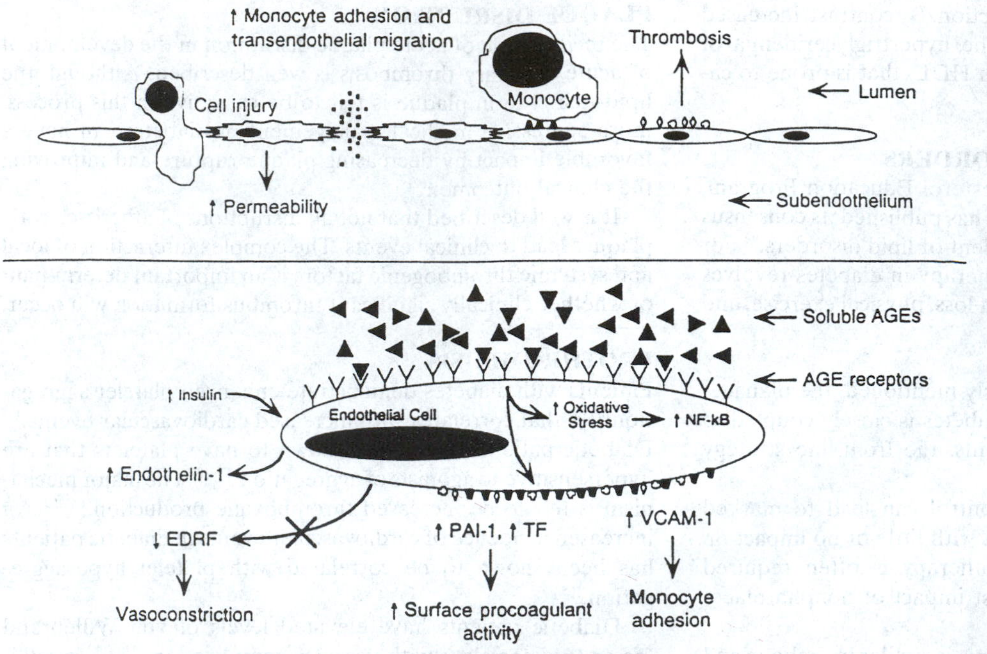

FIGURE 78-3 Generation of a dysfunctional endothelium caused by diabetes. (From Aronson and Rayfield,[138] with permission.)

dilatation.[133] Endothelial dysfunction is measured clinically by the vasodilatory response of forearm resistance vessels to endothelium-dependent agents such as acetylcholine. It recently has been determined that in vivo endothelial dysfunction occurs in subjects whose fasting plasma glucose concentrations fall in the range of IGF = 110 to 126 mg.[134]

Advanced Glycosylation End Products

AGEs are formed by nonenzymatic glucose-protein and lipoprotein interactions, with subsequent cross-linking on vascular tissues.[135,136] In the setting of aging and diabetes, AGEs form at a rate determined by the glucose concentration and the length of exposure.[137] AGEs accelerate atherogenesis by multiple mechanisms that can be classified as receptor-mediated or non-receptor-mediated.[138] AGE deposits have been demonstrated in atherosclerotic plaques and myocardium by immunohistochemistry in patients with diabetes and atherosclerosis.[139] In addition, serum levels of AGEs are significantly increased in type 2 diabetes patients with CAD in contrast to those without CAD.[140] Serum levels of AGEs correlate positively with isovolumetric relaxation time (IVRT) and left ventricular diameter during diastole in type 1 diabetic patients.[141] The systolic parameters did not correlate with serum levels of AGEs.[141]

AGEs can be prevented from forming by pharmacologic means. Aminoguanidines prevent the earlier nonenzymatic Amadori products from progressing to AGEs,[142] and cross-link breakers can break up AGEs in vascular tissues that are already formed.[143]

The cellular interactions for AGE are via a specific receptor for AGE determinants on the cell membrane.[144] Indeed, AGE receptors are present on all cells participating in atherogenesis, such as the monocyte-derieved macrophages, endothelial cells (ECs), and smooth muscle cells (SMCs)[144,145] (Table 78-4). When AGE binds to its receptor, monocytes undergo chemotaxis,[160] followed by mononuclear infiltration through an intact endothelial monolayer.[147,148] Pathologic studies of human atherosclerotic plaques showed infiltration of cells with AGE receptors in a thickened intima.[145] Monocyte-macrophage interactions with AGEs promote several mediators, including interleukin-1 (IL-1), tumor necrosis factor-alpha (TNFα), platelet-derived growth factor (PDGF), and insulin-like growth factor-1 (IGF-1).[146,147,149]

In smooth muscle cells, in the binding of AGE-modified proteins to the AGE receptor by cultured rat SMCs, there is increased cellular proliferation.[161] One can speculate that the response is induced by cytokines or growth factors. In summary, enhanced AGE formation involves receptor-mediated interaction of AGE protein

TABLE 78-4 Atherosclerosis-Promoting Effects of Advanced Glycosylation End Products

Promoting inflammation
*Secretion of cytokines (TNFα, IL-1)[146]
*Chemotactic stimulus for monocytes-macrophages[147,148]
Induction of cellular proliferation
*Stimulation of PDGF[147] and IGF-1[149] secretion from monocyte and (?) SMCs
Endothelial cells
*Increased permeability of EC monolayers[150,151]
*Increased procoagulant activity[150]
*Increased expression of adhesion molecules[152]
*Increased intracellular oxidative stress[153,154]
Extracellular matrix
Collagen cross-linking[155]
Enhanced synthesis of extracellular matrix components[156]
Trapping of LDL in subendothelium[157]
Glycosylated subendothelium matrix quenches NO[158]
Lipoprotein modifications
Glycosylated LDL
Reduced LDL recognition by cellular LDL receptors[76,77]
Increased susceptibility of LDL to oxidative modification[75,78,159]

NOTE: Asterisks indicate receptor-mediated events, whereas lack of an asterisk signifies non-receptor-mediated processes. TNFα: tumor necrosis factor-alpha; IL-1: interleukin-1; PDGF: platelet-derived growth factor; IGF-1: insulin-like growth factor-1; SMC: smooth muscle cells; EC: endothelial cells; LDL: low-density lipoproteins; NO: nitric oxide.

TABLE 78-5 Hyperlipidemia

Trial	Treatment	Outcome	Events Control Group	Events Treatment Group	Relative Risk Reduction, %	Number Needed to Treat	*p*
4S[162] (secondary prevention) n = 4444 202 DM[a]	Simvastatin	Death, nonfatal MI, revascularization	44/97 (45%)	24/105 (23%)	49	5	<.05
CARE[163] (primary prevention) n = 4159 586 DM	Pravastatin	Death, nonfatal MI, revascularization	112/304 (37%)	81/282 (29%)	21	12	.05
Helsinki Heart Study (primary prevention) n = 4081 135 DM	Gemfibrozil	Death, nonfatal MI, revascularization	8/76 (10.5%)	2/59 (3.4%)	67	14	<.02

[a]n = total number of patients; DM = diabetes mellitus patients.

with vascular wall cells, with subsequent migration of inflammatory cells into the lesion and the elaboration of growth factors and cytokines.

NON-RECEPTOR-MEDIATED MECHANISMS

Glycosylated modification of proteins and lipoproteins can interfere with their normal function (Table 78-4). Glycosylation of matrix components such as type IV collagen, laminen, and vitronectin decreases the binding of anionic heparin sulfate (HS), promoting a greater turnover of HS. The absence of HS may induce a compensatory overproduction of other matrix components by means of altered partitioning of growth factors between matrix-bound proteoglycans and cells.[156] Modification of the cell-binding domain of type IV collagen results in decreased endothelial cell adhesion.[156]

CLINICAL IMPLICATIONS

Lipid Disorders

The management of diabetic patients with lipid abnormalities is a unique challenge to the cardiologist. Important evidence from large randomized trials of lipid-lowering therapies is based on subgroup analyses in which diabetic patients represented less than 10 percent of all the patients enrolled. Two hundred two diabetic patients with a prior history of coronary artery disease were enrolled in the 4S study.[162] Although this number was too small, the comparison of simvastatin with placebo showed almost a 50 percent reduction in coronary events in favor of simvastatin (45 percent versus 23 percent, p = not significant). Similar trends were observed in the CARE trial, which compared pravastatin with placebo in secondary prevention.[163] In the CARE trial, the baseline mean LDL concentration in diabetic patients was 136 mg/dL. LDL was reduced 27 percent in the group receiving pravastatin, which translated into a 25 percent reduction in coronary events over 5 years compared with the control group.[164] Table 78-5 demonstrates the relatively low number needed to treat (NNT) to prevent a major cardiovascular complication in three of the main lipid-lowering trials. These therapies are the cornerstone of diabetic management in the current era.

In the trials of statin therapy in hyperlipidemia, the relative benefit appears similar between diabetic patients and nondiabetic patients. The concern for the clinician is that larger trials focusing on the diabetic population have to be carried out before the magnitude of the benefit of lipid-lowering therapy in reducing cardiovascular events can be determined.

Glycemic Control

The pathophysiology of type 2 diabetes is a consequence of peripheral resistance to insulin action (in muscle and fat cells), increased hepatic glucose production, and decreased secretion of insulin by pancreatic beta cells. About 80 percent of people with type 2 diabetes are obese.

Diet and exercise remain the cornerstone in the management of type 2 diabetes. Pharmacologic agents available to treat type 2 diabetes are insulin, insulin secretagogues (sulfonylureas, repaglinide), alpha glucosidase inhibitors (acarbose, miglitol), and insulin sensitizers (biguanides, thiazolidinediones). Each of these agents targets a different mechanism responsible for the hyperglycemia. Figure 78-4 shows each of these agents and the target organs involved in its mode of action.

The standards of care in patients with diabetes (American Diabetes Associations) are preprandial glucose levels of 80 to

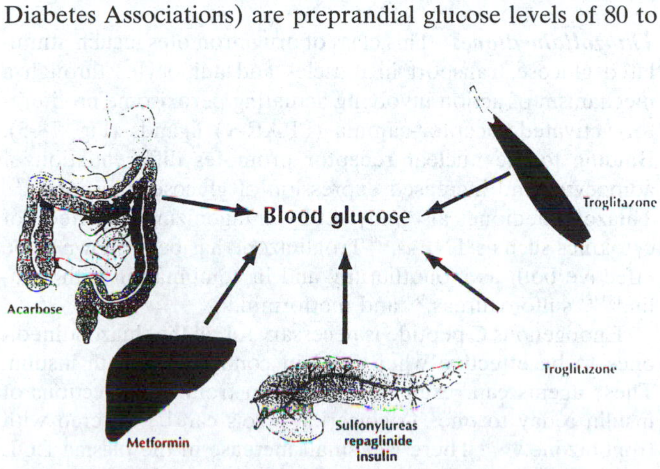

FIGURE 78-4 Mechanism of action of hypoglycemic agents.

120, bedtime glucose levels of 100 to 140, and hemoglobin A1c (Hb-A1c) below 7 percent.[165]

Plasma Hb-A1c reflects the average glucose level of the previous 8 weeks and allows a uniform measure for achieving a target as well as comparing the efficacies of different therapies.

PHARMACOLOGIC MANAGEMENT

Sulfonylureas Sulfonylureas are the typical therapy for lean type 2 diabetics and are used in combinations with other agents in obese type 2 patients. Sulfonylureas bind to a receptor on the beta cells and inhibit the Na-ATP channel; an increase in intracellular calcium results in insulin exocytosis.

Some experts point to a possible risk of increased myocardial damage in patients with known coronary artery disease who use sulfonylureas at the time of an ischemic event.[166] Prevention of protective ischemic preconditioning of the heart by inhibition of the K-ATP channel is the putative mechanism.[167] The UKPDS data do not support this concern. The authors agree and use sulfonylureas in appropriate patients with CAD.

Repaglinide This newer insulin secretagogue binds to a different receptor site than do the sulfonylureas on the K-ATP channel.[168] The half-life of this agent is 3.7 h, which makes it effective for postprandial rather than preprandial hyperglycemia, for use in the elderly, and for diabetic patients with chronic renal failure.[168]

Metformin Metformin is a biguanide drug that has been in use in Europe for over 30 years and was approved in the United States in 1995.[169] The main mode of action of metformin is decreasing hepatic glucose output primarily by inhibiting gluconeogenesis,[170] typically without hypoglycemia.[169]

Metformin is effective alone[171] or in combination with insulin,[172] sulfonylureas,[173] and thiazolidinediones.[174] The drug usually results in weight loss as a result of decreased appetite for up to 1 year after the initiation of therapy.

Significant decreases in LDL cholesterol and triglycerides occur.[173,175] The incidence of lactic acidosis with metformin is 9 per 100,000 person-years.[176] Contraindications to its use include an elevated creatinine (>1.4 in women, >1.5 in men), congestive heart failure, severe pulmonary disease, or any hypoxic state.[177]

Thiazolidinediones This class of drug promotes insulin-stimulated glucose transport in muscles and adipocytes through a mechanism of action involving actuating peroxisome proliferator activated receptor-gamma (PPAR-γ) ligands (Fig. 78-5). Binding to the nuclear receptor promotes differentiation of adipocytes and increased expression of glucose transporter.[178] Thiazolidinediones also may act by antagonizing the effects of cytokines such as TNF-α.[179] Troglitazone has been shown to be effective both as monotherapy and in combination with insulin,[180,181] sulfonylureas,[182] and metformin.[174]

Endogenous C peptide is necessary for all the thiazolidinediones to be effective when used in combination with insulin. These agents can result in a reduction from two injections of insulin a day to one. Triglyceride levels can be lowered with troglitazone.[183,184] There is a small increase in the plasma LDL concentration, along with a favorable increase in the ratio of the buoyant LDL to the more atherogenic small dense LDL.[185]

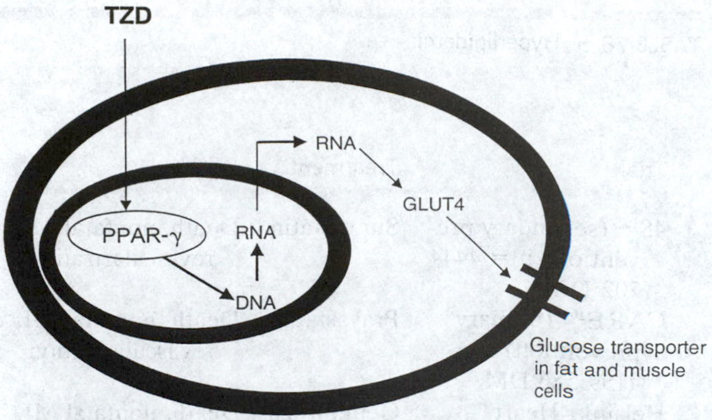

FIGURE 78-5 Mechanism of action of thiazolidinediones.

The thiazolidinediones are associated with weight gain partly resulting from improvement in glycemic control. With troglitazone, monitoring of liver function should be done monthly for the first year and quarterly thereafter.

Troglitazone has resulted in fulminant hepatic failure in about 1 in 60,000 patients on the medication; this is felt to be an idiosyncratic reaction. Patients with a history of liver

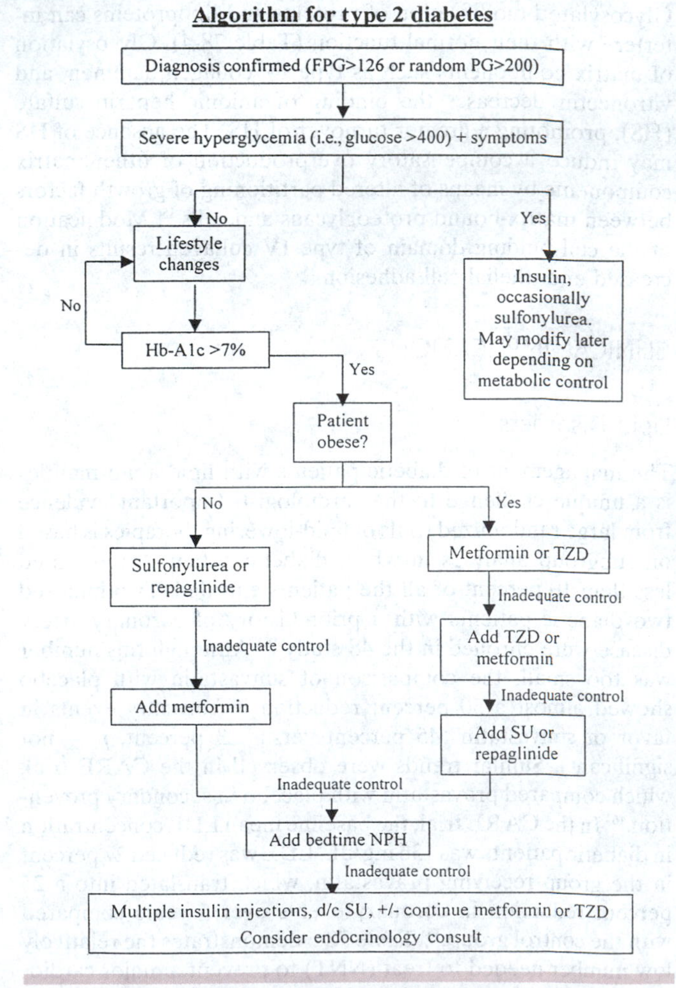

FIGURE 78-6 Algorithm for type 2 diabetes. Note: Acarbose or miglitol can be added anywhere along the treatment pathway. SU = sulfonylurea; TZD = thiazolidinedione.

disease, possibly including hepatitis C (depending on severity), and those who ingest more than a moderate amount of alcohol should not be started on this agent. Because of the potential for liver disease, troglitazone no longer is used as monotherapy unless the patient has been on combination therapy first and has achieved good glycemic control with troglitazone alone.

Two other drugs in this class were approved by the U.S. Food and Drug Administration (FDA) in mid-1999, and the data to date support equal efficacy with less hepatotoxicity. No head-to-head studies of these agents are available. Monitoring of liver function tests with rosiglitazone and pioglitazone is recommended every 2 months for the first year and periodically thereafter, since it has not been determined that serious liver events with troglitazone are a class effect of the thiazolidinediones or are specific to troglitazone.

Rosiglitazone monotherapy results in a decrease of Hgb-A1c of 0.8 to 1.5 percent greater than that seen with placebo, with the greatest reduction seen when it was given in two divided doses.[186,187] Combination studies of rosiglitazone with metformin for 26 weeks resulted in a 1.0 to 1.2 percent placebo-adjusted decrease in Hgb-A1c.[188] Although rosiglitazone is currently approved for use as monotherapy and in combination therapy with metformin, it also is expected to be efficacious with sulfonylureas or insulin. Rosiglitazone has been reported to result in an increase in LDL and HDL cholesterol concentrations between 12 percent and 19 percent, with changes in serum triglycerides similar to those seen with placebo.[189]

Pioglitazone, the newest thiazolidinedione, has been approved for use as monotherapy and in combination with metformins, sulfonylureas, and insulin. In three randomized, double-blind placebo-controlled trials of 16 to 26 weeks' duration, changes in Hgb-A1c were 1.0 to 1.4 percent.[190] Increases in ALT occurred in 0.26 percent of treated patients, a result that was not different from that with placebo.[190] Patients treated with pioglitazone showed a decrease in serum triglyceride (9.3 to 9.6 percent), increases in HDL (12.2 to 19.1 percent), and increases in LDL (5.2 to 6.0 percent) with the 30- to 45-mg doses, respectively.[190]

Alpha-Glucosidase Inhibitors Acarbose and miglitol work in the intestine to reversibly inhibit brush border alpha-glucosidases, resulting in a delay in carbohydrate absorption. Only about 1 percent of the drug is absorbed from the gastrointestinal tract. These drugs cause a 30 percent decrease in postprandial glucose in contrast to a 10 percent decrease in fasting glucose levels. They are adjuncts to other oral agents and rarely are potent enough to be used as monotherapy.

Insulin The natural history of type 2 diabetes is one of progressive beta-cell failure. Therefore, after approximately 10 years of the use of oral hypoglycemic agents, insulin will be required either in combination with oral agents or as the sole therapy. Although endogenous hyperinsulinemia is clearly associated with atherogenesis, there is no compelling evidence of increased risk of cardiovascular disease or increased mortality from exogenous insulin therapy.

Diabetes clinics nationwide have strived to optimize the glycemic control of patients with a view to minimizing the development of coronary and other vascular disease. Figure 78-6 shows an algorithm that is reasonable to use in the management of patients with type 2 diabetes. Table 78-6 shows the clinical trial evidence supporting intensive glycemic control.

TABLE 78-6 Glycemic Control

Trial	Treatment	Outcome	Events Control Group	Events Treatment Group	Relative Risk Reduction, %	Number Needed to Treat	*p*
Type 1 DM							
DCCT[198] n = 1441 patients[a] free of cardiac disease, HTN, and dyslipidemia	Intensive glycemic control versus conventional therapy	Macrovascular events	40/730 (5.5%)	23/711 (3.2%)	42	43	.08
Type 2 DM							
UKPDS[193–196] In newly diagnosed diabetes mellitus n = 3867	Sulfonylurea or insulin versus conventional therapy	Diabetes-related outcomes	438/1138 (38.4%)	963/2729 (35.2%)	8.3	31	.029
Steno[136] n = 160	Intensive comprehensive (includes hypertension (HTN), dyslipidemia, and glycemic control) therapy versus standard therapy	Macrovascular events Death MI Stroke Vascular ischemia	42/78 (53.8%)	26/77 (33.7%)	37.3	5	.03

[a]n = total number of patients.

TYPE 2 DIABETES: UNITED KINGDOM PROSPECTIVE DIABETES STUDY GROUP TRIAL

A number of important trials have evaluated the effects of glycemic control in cardiac patients with type 2 diabetes. Before the publication of the UKPDS, there was a great deal of controversy about the benefit of intensive glycemic control in type 2 patients. Both the University Group Diabetes Program study and other reports have questioned whether sulfonylureas adversely affect the heart by blocking the ATP-dependent potassium channels.[191,192] Two small, randomized trials suggested that intensive glycemic control with insulin for type 2 diabetics is effective in reducing cardiovascular events. The UKPDS trial is the largest and best conducted study of glycemic control in type 2 diabetic patients. It addresses the issue of the influence of tight glycemic control in reducing micro- and macroangiopathy in newly diagnosed patients with type 2 diabetes mellitus.[193,194] In this multicenter randomized controlled trial, 5102 patients in 23 centers in the United Kingdom were studied between 1977 and 1991. A hypertension study was included to assess whether treating high blood pressure in patients with type 2 diabetes could reduce the risk of diabetic complications.[195]

The first study compared the effects of intensive blood glucose control with either sulfonylurea or insulin and conventional treatment on the risk of micro- and macrovascular complications in type 2 diabetes patients. Intensive glycemic control was defined as a fasting plasma glucose (FPG) level of <108 mg/dL. Over a 10-year period, Hb-A1c was 7.0 percent in the intensive group compared with 7.9 percent in the conventional group. There was a 25 percent risk reduction in microvascular end points in the intensively treated group. No difference existed between the three agents used for intensive glycemic control (chlorpropamide, glibenclimide, and insulin). Patients in the intensive group had more hypoglycemic episodes than did those in the conventional group ($p < .0001$). Finally, none of the individual agents had an adverse effect on cardiovascular outcomes.

UKPDS 34, the second arm of the study, assessed whether intensive glucose control with metformin had any specific advantage or disadvantage. Mean Hb-A1c was 7.4 percent in the metformin group compared with 8.0 percent in the conventional group. Given that intensive glycemic control with metformin appears to decrease the risk of diabetes-related end points in overweight diabetes patients and is associated with less weight gain and fewer hypoglycemic attacks than insulin or sulfonylureas, the authors suggested that metformin may be the first-line pharmacologic therapy of choice in these patients. It should be noted that the UKPDS was conducted before the clinical availability of the thiazolidinediones as well as the statins (although the study did not address the issue of cholesterol reduction in diabetic patients).

A noteworthy finding in the UKPDS was a decrease in the risk of myocardial infarction of 16 percent.[193] The decrease was not statistically significant but demonstrated a trend toward fewer macrovascular events. The approximately 8-year time lag before type 2 diabetes is diagnosed may account for the inability of the UKPDS study to link hyperglycemia with macrovascular events.

UKPDS determined whether intensive blood pressure control prevents micro- and macrovascular complications in patients with type 2 diabetes. Tight blood pressure control was defined as <150/85. The angiotensin-converting enzyme inhibitor (ACE-I) captopril and the beta blocker atenolol were the drugs used to achieve the tight control. Reductions in risk in the group assigned to tight blood pressure control compared with the control group were 24 percent in diabetes-related end points, 32 percent in death from diabetic complications, 44 percent in strokes, and 37 percent in microvascular disease (almost all of which were statistically significant). There was a nonsignificant reduction in all-cause mortality.[193]

UKPDS 39 investigated whether tight blood pressure control with either a beta blocker (atenolol) or an ACE-I (captopril) has a specific advantage in terms of preventing the macro- and microvascular complications of type 2 diabetes. This study involving 1148 hypertensive patients showed that each agent was equally efficacious in reducing blood pressure, the risk of macrovascular end points, and deterioration of retinopathy.[196] Using these two classes of antihypertensive agents, the investigators showed that the blood pressure reduction per se was more important than was the treatment used.

The current strategy for type 2 diabetes mellitus is to optimize Hb-A1c levels with sulfonylureas, insulin-sensitizing agents, or insulin when necessary (see the previous discussion).

TYPE 1 DIABETES: DIABETES CONTROL AND COMPLICATIONS TRIAL

Intensive diabetes control versus standard therapy was evaluated in the DCCT.[197,198] The primary outcome was the development and progression of microvascular disease, but patients were followed for over 6 years so that cardiac events did ensue. There was almost a doubling of the cardiac event rate in patients treated in a conventional manner (40 versus 23 events), but this did not reach statistical significance. Since the patients in this study were between ages 13 and 39 and did not have diabetes for a long enough period, a nearly significant reduction in cardiovascular events is not surprising. Diabetic renal disease is a strong predictor of subsequent cardiovascular events, and therefore, the promising result of reduced proteinuria with intensive therapy in DCCT may translate into a cardioprotective effect in the long term. The current strategy for type 1 diabetes is to optimize glycemic control with multiple injections of insulin or with an insulin pump. Such patients should have a concomitant consultation with an endocrinologist.

Early Detection of Diabetes

Because of the significant increase in major microvascular complications and the risk of premature death, it is important to begin to screen for diabetes at a younger age than 45 years, the current recommendation.[199] Selecting populations at the highest risk for developing diabetes for aggressive screening strategies probably will occur in the next 10 years.

Current measures of cardiovascular surveillance for CAD in asymptomatic diabetic patients focus on routine stress testing in accordance with the American College of Cardiology/American Heart Association (ACC/AHA) guidelines[200] (Table 78-7). Exercise testing in diabetic patients is more likely to be accurate when combined with echocardiography or radionuclide imaging. Diabetic patients are less likely to have an appropriate blood pressure and heart rate response to exercise and less likely to experience any pain corresponding to ST-segment changes caused in part by autonomic dysfunction. The AHA

TABLE 78-7 Detection of Clinical and Subclinical Cardiovascular Disease in Diabetic Patients

A. Stress testing for coronary heart disease
- Consult AHA guidelines for exercise treadmill testing
- *Considerations for testing in diabetic patients*
  - Blunting of heart rate and blood pressure responses
  - Painless ST-segment depression common in diabetic patients (autonomic neuropathy)
  - Diagnostic specificity of ST-segment depression may be reduced (previous silent myocardial infarction, etc.)
  - Exercise or pharmacologic testing (^{99}Tc) perfusion scintography favorable for exercise testing in diabetic patients
  - Ambulatory ECG monitoring may be helpful in special instances in diabetic patients to diagnose silent ischemia, but not routinely

B. Noninvasive evaluation of cardiac function
- *Echocardiography (Doppler) and radionuclide ventriculography issues in diabetic patients*
  - Diastolic function common and often precedes systolic dysfunction
  - Left ventricular wall motion abnormalities suggest diabetic cardiomyopathy

C. Evaluation of autonomic dysfunction
- *In bedside evaluation two or more of these tests are abnormal*
  - Resting heart rate (supine), 100
  - Excess diastolic blood pressure response to handgrip exercise
  - Abnormal expiratory/inspiratory RR-interval ratio
  - Postural hypotension
- *Significance of autonomic dysfunction in diabetic patients*
  - 50% 5-year mortality
  - Sudden death common; consider electrophysiologic study
  - Greater complications after elective surgery
  - Increased danger with general anesthesia

D. Diagnosis of subclinical cardiovascular disease
- *History:* symptoms of claudication, angina, dyspnea on exertion, cerebrovascular disease
- *Physical examination:* routine checkup with evaluation of carotid and femoral bruits, peripheral arterial pulses, ratio of ankle to brachial artery systolic blood pressure (marker of subclinical peripheral vascular disease)
- *Laboratory:* urinary creatinine/albumin ratio (Table 78-1)
- *ECG:* left ventricular hypertrophy a strong predictor of CAD morbidity and mortality
- *Electron beam CT:* coronary calcium score highly correlated with total coronary atherosclerosis burden
- *Carotid ultrasound:* detects subclinical carotid atherosclerosis.

recommends that the finding of subclinical CAD should prompt clinicians to initiate more aggressive preventative measures[201] (Table 78-7).

Hypertension and Nephropathy

To date, there have been no randomized trials primarily evaluating the role of hypertension treatment with nephropathy as the end point in type 1 diabetic patients without microalbuminuria. Hypertensive diabetic patients are treated primarily with ACE inhibitors.

Compared with nondiabetic subjects, diabetic patients in the SHEP (Systolic Hypertension in the Elderly Program cooperative research group) study experienced a more pronounced benefit from treatment with clorthalidone. The 5-year rates of major cardiovascular events are illustrated in Fig. 78-7.[202]

The UKPDS demonstrated no advantage of captopril over atenolol in reducing macrovascular complications.[198] Clearly, this illustrates the significant role lowering of blood pressure plays in reducing adverse events independent of the agent used. The role of further blood pressure reduction even when high-risk patients such as diabetic patients are in the normal range needs to be delineated further. The Hypertension Optimal Treatment (HOT) study showed that the risk of major cardiovascular events in diabetic patients was halved if they had a target diastolic pressure ≤80 mmHg compared with those with a diastolic pressure ≤90 mmHg (p for trend = .005).[203] There was a lower but still significant decrease in the risk of silent myocardial infarction and about a 30 percent risk reduction in

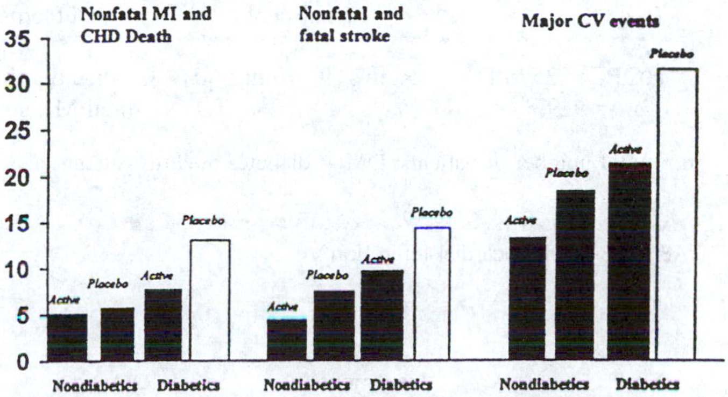

FIGURE 78-7 Five-year rates of nonfatal myocardial infarction (MI) and coronary heart disease (CHD) death, stroke, and major cardiovascular (CV) events by diabetes status and treatment (chlorthalidone vs placebo) in the Systolic Hypertension in the Elderly Program. (Data from Curb et al.[202] and from Furberg CD. Hypertension and diabetes: Current issues. *Am Heart J* 1999; 138:5401, with permission.)

TABLE 78-8 Hypertension

Trial	Treatment	Outcome	Control Group	Treatment Group	Relative Risk Reduction, %	p
CAPPP[204] n = 10985 572 DM[a]	Captopril versus conventional therapy	Cardiac death, nonfatal MI, stroke	263	309	33	.03

[a]n = total number of patients; DM = diabetes mellitus patients.

the rate of stroke in the ≤80 mmHg group compared with the ≤90 mmHg group.

The CAPPP trial showed significant lowering of cardiovascular events in hypertensive patients treated with captopril instead of standard therapy with beta blockers or diuretics (Table 78-8).[204] Approximately 5 percent of the patients were diabetic in this trial, and in these patients, similar trends in favor of captopril were observed. The Appropriate Blood pressure Control in Diabetics (ABCD) study also observed a benefit of ACE-I compared with conventional therapy in the treatment of hypertension in diabetic patients.[205]

HOPE

The HOPE trial evaluated over 9000 high-risk patients with evidence of vascular disease or diabetes in a randomized trial comparing ramipril with placebo over a 5-year period. A total of 3578 of these patients were diabetic. This study demonstrated a 22 percent reduction in primary cardiovascular end points of death, myocardial infarction, and stroke in favor of ramipril. The beneficial effect of ramipril was observed over all predefined subgroups. Interestingly, there was a 30 percent reduction in the diagnosis of new diabetic patients in the ramipril-treated arm. This result also was observed in the CAPPP study. Ramipril lowered systolic blood pressure by a mean of only 6 mmHg. This would account for only approximately 40 percent of the reduction in the rate of stroke and about a 25 percent reduction in the rate of myocardial infarction. Therefore, there is some benefit of ramipril independent of the blood pressure–lowering effect that accounts for the impressive cardiovascular protective effect. HOPE provides level 1 evidence supporting the front-line use of ACE-I in the treatment of diabetic patients at risk for cardiovascular events regardless of whether they are hypertensive. In the diabetic subgroup there was even a greater relative risk reduction in primary cardiovascular events (25 percent) (Table 78-9).

Acute Coronary Syndromes

Diabetic patients represent a high-risk group for developing and surviving acute myocardial infarction.[206] In particular, patients with type 1 diabetes have a worse outcome than do patients with type 2 disease, and diabetic women have almost twice the risk of mortality compared with diabetic men.[8,207–209]

Reperfusion therapy is the cornerstone of the management of acute myocardial infarction. In a meta-analysis of all major thrombolytic trials, diabetic patients had a nonsignificant trend toward increased reductions in 35-day mortality rates compared with nondiabetic patients.[210] The potential advantage of angi-

TABLE 78-9 Prevention Study

Trial	Treatment	Outcome	Events Control Group	Events Treatment Group	Relative Risk Reduction, %	Number Needed to Treat	p
HOPE[137] 3578 DM n = 9297[a]	Ramipril (10 mg qd)	Cardiac death, nonfatal MI, stroke	351/1769 (19.8%)	277/1808 (15.3%)	25	22	.0004

[a]n = total number of patients; DM = diabetes mellitus patients.

TABLE 78-10 Myocardial Infarction

Trial	Treatment	Outcome	Events Control Group	Events Treatment Group	Relative Risk Reduction, %	Number Needed to Treat	p
DIGAMI[211] After MI n = 620[a]	Standard therapy with glucose-insulin infusion versus standard therapy	Long-term (3.4 years) all cause mortality	138/314 (43.9%)	102/306 (33.3%)	24	9	.011

[a]n = total number of patients.

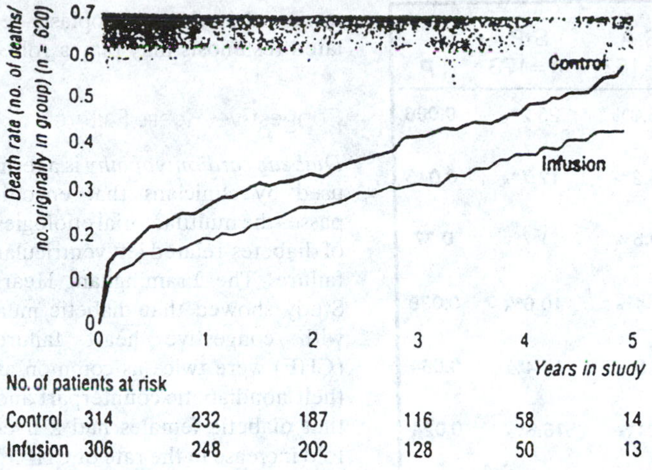

FIGURE 78-8 Actuarial mortality curves during long-term follow-up in patients receiving insulin-glucose infusion and in control group among total DIGAMI cohort. Absolute reduction in risk was 11 percent; relative risk was 0.72 (0.55 to 0.92); p = .011. (From Malmberg K for the DIGAMI Study group,[211] with permission.)

oplasty over thrombolytic therapy has not been addressed in the diabetic population.

Besides the use of aspirin and beta blockers, other new treatment strategies are emerging. The utilization of insulin and glucose infusion for at least 24 h after admission followed by intensive long-term insulin, was compared with usual care in the DIGAMI trial (Fig. 78-8 and Table 78-10). A total of 620 diabetic patients were randomized, and the trial demonstrated a 30 percent reduction in mortality at 12 months for the group treated under the intensive program.[211] A new trial is under way to evaluate whether this benefit was the result of acute therapy or the intensive posthospital therapy (Smith and colleagues, unpublished). This new trial also will evaluate the role of changing the diabetic regimen in type 2 diabetes from a sulfonylurea program to a nonsulfonylurea strategy.

Chronic Coronary Artery Disease

The association between CAD and diabetes is strong and has led to screening strategies in diabetic patients even before they are symptomatic. In addition, diabetic patients often are unaware of myocardial ischemic pain, and so silent myocardial infarction and ischemia is markedly increased in this population.[212] There is a heightened concern for the development of sudden cardiac death in diabetics.

Therapeutic modalities in diabetics with CAD revolve around standard therapy with aspirin, beta blockers, calcium channel blockers, and nitrates.

Epidemiologic evidence from the Bezafibrate Infarction Prevention Study registry shows almost a 50 percent reduction in mortality for type 2 patients with chronic CAD who were treated with beta blockers compared with controls.[213] Other randomized trial evidence has demonstrated that diabetes is a strong predictor of death and that diabetic patients may benefit more from beta blocker therapy than do nondiabetics.[214] In general, beta blockers are extremely well tolerated, and masking or prolonging of hypoglycemic symptoms appears to be highly infrequent, particularly with cardioselective beta blockers.

Coronary Revascularization

The high prevalence of CAD in diabetic patients necessitates the frequent use of revascularization procedures in these patients. Both coronary artery bypass grafting and coronary angioplasty are effective in diabetic patients, but the high rate of restenosis diabetic patients experience in the first 6 months after the procedure raises concerns about the long-term benefits of angioplasty.

TABLE 78-11 Coronary Revascularization

Trial	Treatment	Outcome	Events Control Group	Events Treatment Group	Relative Risk Reduction, %	Number Needed to Treat	p
BARI[227] Multivessel CAD n = 1829[a]	CABG vs. PTCA	Mortality from all causes	PTCA 131/915 (14.3%)	CABG 111/914 (12.1%)	15.3	45	.19
Diabetics n = 353 CABG 180 PTCA 173	Same	Same	34.5%	19.4%	43.7	7	.003
EPISTENT[226] n = 2399							
Diabetics (491) n = 335	Stent + abciximab versus Stent + placebo	Death and nonfatal MI at 6 months	Stent + placebo 22/173 (12.7%)	Stent + abciximab 10/162 (6.2%)	51.2	15	.041
n = 318	Stent + abciximab versus PTCA + abciximab	Same	PTCA + abciximab 12/156 (7.8%)	Stent + abciximab 10/162 (6.2%)	20.5	62	.13

[a]n = total number of patients.

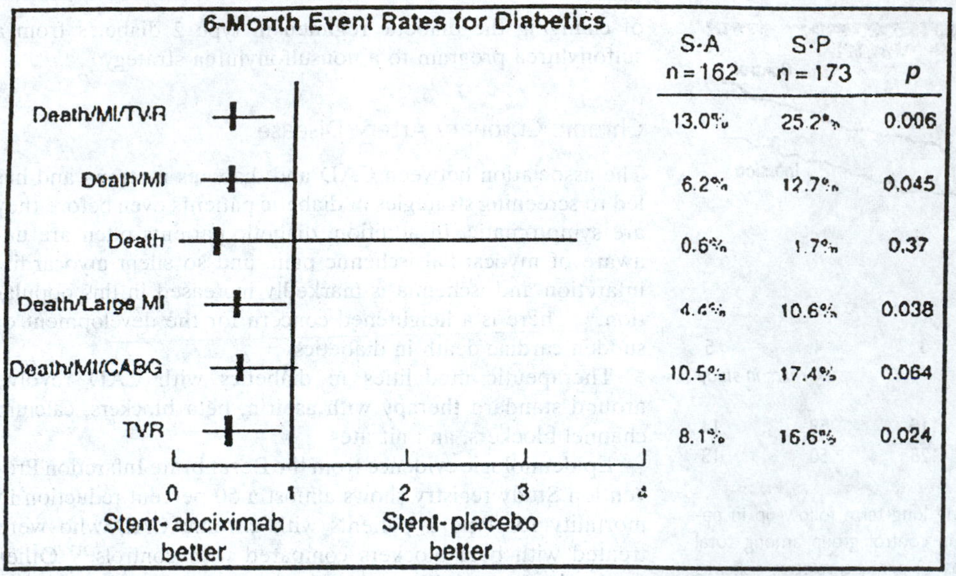

FIGURE 78-9 Absolute percentage of events, 95 percent confidence limits, and point estimates of listed end points for diabetic patients randomized to stenting-abciximab (S-A) or stentin-placebo (S-P). (From Marso SP, Michael A, Lincoff AM, et al. Optimising the percutaneous intervention outcomes for patients with diabetes mellitus. *Circulation* 1999; 100(25):2477, with permission.)

Before the use of stents and IIb-IIIa antagonists, the rate of restenosis after angioplasty in diabetic patients was shown to be as high as 47 to 71 percent.[215–223] The mechanism of restenosis is believed to be related to neointimal hyperplasia, which is tightly linked to the interplay between platelet-thrombus deposition, various growth factors present after injury, and endothelial dysfunction.[224,225]

The best evidence from randomized trials supportive of the utility of stents and abciximab comes from the EPISTENT trial.[226] Among the 2399 patients randomized, 20 percent (491 atients) had diabetes. Patients were assigned to a strategy of stent implantation and placebo, stent implantation and abciximab, or angioplasty and abciximab. For diabetic patients receiving stent and reopro, compared with stent alone, there was a >50 percent reduction in death and nonfatal myocardial infarction at 6 months (Table 78-11). A 6 months, diabetic patients were less likely to require repeat target organ revascularization if they received stent and abciximab (8.1 percent) compared with either stent and placebo (16.6 percent, $p = .02$) or angioplasty and abciximab (18.4 percent, $p = .008$). It appears that the effect of abciximab is linked to stent implantation, since elastic recoil and related adverse remodeling are significantly diminished with successful stent deployment, leaving neointimal hyperplasia as the main mode for restenosis. Because of the results of the EPISTENT trial, clinicians are more comfortable recommending percutaneous intervention (Fig. 78-9).

The largest randomized trial comparing angioplasty with bypass surgery in patients with multivessel CAD, the BARI trial, was a landmark study that highlighted the marked benefit of bypass over angioplasty in diabetic patients as opposed to nondiabetic subjects[227] (Fig. 78-10). In the diabetic subgroup, the 5-year mortality was reduced from 34 percent to 19 percent with surgical revascularization, translating into a number needed to treat to prevent one death of only seven (Table 78-11). The most marked difference between the two groups occurred after the first year of follow-up, suggesting that mechanisms other than angioplasty-related restenosis may play a role.

Congestive Heart Failure

Diabetic cardiomyopathy is a term used by clinicians that encompasses the multifactorial etiologies of diabetes-related left ventricular failure. The Framingham Heart Study showed that diabetic men with congestive heart failure (CHF) were twice as common as their nondiabetic counterpart and that diabetic females had a five-fold increase in the rate of CHF.[228] The spectrum of heart failure ranges from asymptomatic to overt systolic failure. Diabetes complicated by hypertension represents a particularly high-risk group for the development of CHF.[229,230] Diastolic dysfunction is exceedingly common (>50 percent prevalence in some studies) and may be linked to diabetes without the presence of concomitant hypertension.[231,232–234]

Given the prominence of the diabetic subgroup in randomized trials of ACE-I in CHF, much emphasis has been placed

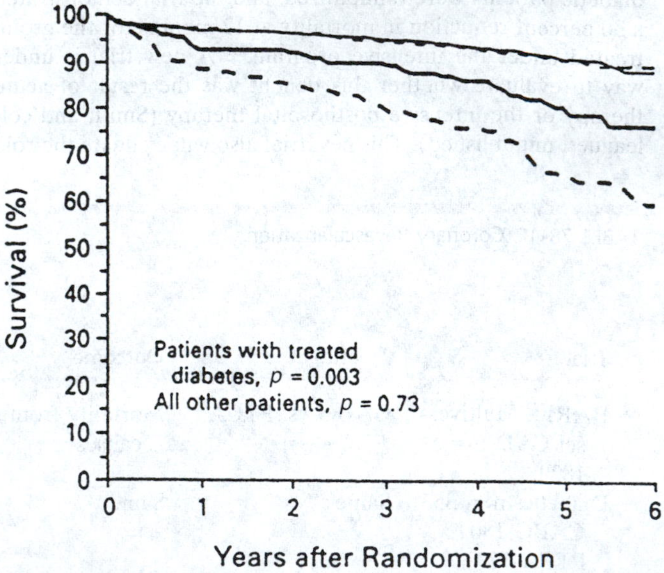

Patients with Treated Diabetes			
CABG	180	161	93
PTCA	173	139	69
All Other Patients			
CABG	734	696	449
PTCA	742	701	468

FIGURE 78-10 Survival among patients who were being treated for diabetes at baseline (heavy lines) and all other patients (light lines). Patients assigned to CABG are indicated by solid lines, and those assigned to PTCA by dashed lines. The numbers of patients at risk are shown below the graph at baseline, 3 years, and 5 years. [From the Bypass Angioplasty Revascularization Investigation (BARI) Investigators,[227] with permission.]

TABLE 78-12 Guide to Comprehensive Risk Reduction for Patients with Coronary and Other Vascular Disease who have Diabetes

<table>
<tr><th>Risk Intervention</th><th colspan="4">Recommendations</th></tr>
<tr><td>Smoking
Goal: complete cessation</td><td colspan="4">Urge smoking cessation
Try nicoderm patches or xyban; enroll in smoking cessation program</td></tr>
<tr><td>Blood pressure control
Goal: <135/85 mmHg</td><td colspan="4">Initiate lifestyle modification; weight reduction, increased physical activity; alcohol moderation; sodium restriction in all patients with blood pressure >135/85
Add blood pressure medication if BP not below above goal</td></tr>
<tr><td rowspan="5">Lipid management
Primary goal: LDL≤100 mg/dL
Secondary goals: HDL>35 mg/dL
TG<200 mg/dL</td><td colspan="4">Start AHA Step II Diet in all patients: ≤30% fat, <7% saturated fat, <200 mg/dL cholesterol
Assess fasting lipid profile. Immediately start cholesterol-lowering drugs when baseline LDL>130 mg/dL</td></tr>
<tr><td rowspan="4">LDL<100 mg/dL
No drug therapy</td><td>LDL 100–129 mg/dL
Consider adding drug therapy to diet as follows</td><td>LDL≥130 mg/dL
Add drug therapy as follows</td><td rowspan="4">HDL<35 mg/dL
Weight management, physical activity, and smoking cessation</td></tr>
<tr><td colspan="2">↘ Suggested drug therapy ↙</td></tr>
<tr><td>TG<200 mg/dL</td><td>TG 200–400 mg/dL</td></tr>
<tr><td>Statin resin</td><td>Statin fibrate</td></tr>
<tr><td></td><td colspan="4">TG>400 mg/dL: Consider combined drug therapy (statin + fibrate)</td></tr>
<tr><td>Glucose control
Goal: nearly normal fasting glucose
Goal: Hb-A 1c ≤1% above normal</td><td colspan="4">First-step therapy: lifestyle modifications
Second-step therapy: oral hypoglycemic agents (see algorithm)
Third-step therapy: insulin therapy (see algorithm)</td></tr>
<tr><td>Physical activity
Goal: minimum 30 minutes, 3–4 times a week</td><td colspan="4">Assess risk, preferably with exercise test, to guide prescription
Encourage minimum of 30–60 min of moderate-intensity activity 3–4 times weekly (walking, jogging, cycling, etc.) supplemented by an increase in daily lifestyle activities (e.g., walking breaks at work, using stairs, household work)
Maximum benefit 5 to 6 h a week
Advise medically supervised programs for moderate- to high-risk patients</td></tr>
<tr><td>Weight management</td><td colspan="4">Start intensive dietary therapy and appropriate physical activity, as outlined above, in patients whose BMI is ≥25 kg/m²
Particularly emphasize need for weight loss in patients with hypertension, elevated triglycerides, or elevated glucose levels</td></tr>
<tr><td>Antiplatelet agents/ anticoagulants</td><td colspan="4">Start aspirin 325 mg/day if not contraindicated
Manage warfarin to INR of 2–3.5 for post-MI patients not able to take aspirin</td></tr>
<tr><td>ACE inhibitors in post-MI patients</td><td colspan="4">Start early post-MI in stable high-risk patients [anterior MI, previous MI, Killip class II (S3 gallop, rales, radiographic congestive heart failure)]
Continue indefinitely for all with LV dysfunction (ejection fraction ≤40%) or symptoms of failure
Use as needed to manage blood pressure or symptoms in all other patients</td></tr>
<tr><td>Beta blockers</td><td colspan="4">Start in high-risk post-MI patients (arrhythmia, LV dysfunction, inducible ischemia) at 5 to 28 days; continue 6 months minimum; observe usual contraindications; appropriate use of beta-blockers not contraindicated in patients with diabetes; use as needed to manage angina, rhythm, or blood pressure in all other patients</td></tr>
<tr><td>Estrogen</td><td colspan="4">Observational studies (but not clinical trials) suggest benefit in regard to osteoporosis but not CAD; individualize recommendation consistent with other health risks</td></tr>
</table>

on initiating ACE-I therapy as soon as left ventricular dysfunction is noted, regardless of symptomatology.[235] The results of the HOPE trial probably will translate into even earlier initiation of ACE inhibition in patients without clinical LV dysfunction.

Summary of Clinical Guidelines

Table 78-12 summarizes the AHA recommendations for the indications for risk interventions in diabetic patients with atherosclerotic vascular disease.

FUTURE DIRECTIONS

On the clinical front, there are still many challenges in the prevention and management of diabetic cardiovascular complications. Given the findings of the HOPE trial, the potential for an expanded role for ACE inhibitors in the prevention of cardiovascular and renal disease in all diabetic patients needs to be explored. Glycemic control appears to be the mainstay of long-term diabetes management. Thus, development of better therapies and devices (e.g., closed-loop pumps, islet and pancreatic transplants) for achieving and maintaining Hb-A1c at not only <7 percent but in the normal range of <6 percent will be a primary goal in the next decade. The advent of stenting and the IIb-IIIa antagonist during coronary percutaneous revascularization has led to a reevaluation of the need for coronary bypass surgery in multivessel disease. Confirmation of the results of small trials demonstrating a benefit of intravenous glucose-insulin infusion during acute myocardial infarction is needed before this therapy can be adopted. Finally, the role of gene therapy in the management of diabetic atherosclerotic vascular disease needs to be addressed within the context of all other advances.

References

1. Schwartz CJ, Valente AJ, Sprague EA, et al. Pathogenesis of the atherosclerotic lesion: Implications for diabetes mellitus. *Diabetes Care* 1992; 15:1156–1167.
2. Stamler J, Vaccaro O, Neaton JD, Wentworth D. Diabetes, other risk factors and 12-year cardiovascular mortality for men screened in the multiple risk factor intervention trial. *Diabetes Care* 1993; 16:434–444.
3. Gu K, Cowie CC, Harris MI. Diabetes and decline in heart disease mortality in US adults. *JAMA* 1999; 281:1291–1297.
4. Kawate R, Yamakido M, Nishimoto Y, et al. Diabetes mellitus and its vascular complications in Japanese migrants on the island of Hawaii. *Diabetes Care* 1979; 2:161–170.
5. Head J, Fuller JH. International variations in mortality among diabetic patients: The WHO Multinational Study of Vascular Disease in Diabetics. *Diabetologia* 1990; 33:447–481.
6. Vigorita VJ, Morre GW, Hutchens GM. Absence of correlation between coronary arterial atherosclerosis and severity or duration of diabetes mellitus of adult onset. *Am J Cardiol* 1980; 46:535–542.
7. Waller BF, Palumbo PJ, Lie JT, Roberts WC. Status of the coronary arteries at necropsy in diabetes mellitus after age 30 years: Analysis of 229 diabetic patients with and without evidence of coronary heart disease and comparison to 183 control subjects. *Am J Med* 1980; 69:498–506.
8. Granger CB, Califf RM, Young S, et al. Outcome of patients with diabetes mellitus and acute myocardial infarction treated with thrombolytic agents: The Thrombolysis and Angioplasty in Myocardial Infarction (TAMI) Study Group. *J Am Coll Cardiol* 1993; 21:920–925.
9. Mueller HS, Cohen LS, Braunwald E, et al., for the TIMI investigators. Predictors of early mortality and morbidity after thrombolytic therapy of acute myocardial infarction. *Circulation* 1992; 85:1254–1264.
10. Stein B, Weintraub WS, Gebhart SSP, et al. Influence of diabetes mellitus on early and late outcome after percutaneous transluminal coronary angioplasty. *Circulation* 1995; 91:979–989.
11. Barzilay JI, Kronmal RA, Bittner V, et al. Coronary artery disease and coronary artery bypass grafting in diabetic patients aged >65 years (Report from the coronary artery surgery study [CASS] registry). *Am J Cardiol* 1994; 74:334–339.
12. Davis M, Bland J, Hangartner J, et al. Factors influencing the presence or absence of acute coronary artery thrombi in sudden ischemic death. *Eur Heart J* 1989; 10:203–208.
13. Silva JA, Escobar A, Collins TJ, et al. Unstable angina: A comparison between diabetic and non-diabetic patients. *Circulation* 1995; 92:1731–1736.
14. Hopkins PN, Hunt SC, Wu LL, et al. Hypertension, dyslipidemia, and insulin resistance: Links in a chain or spokes on a wheel? *Curr Opin Lipidol* 1996; 7:241–253.
15. Gray RS, Fabsitz RR, Cowan LD, et al. Risk factor clustering in the insulin resistance syndrome: The Strong Heart Study. *Am J Epidemiol* 1998; 148:869–878.
16. The Expert Committee on the Diagnosis and Classification of Diabetes Mellitus. Report of the Expert Committee on the Diagnosis and Classification of Diabetes Mellitus. *Diabetes Care* 1997; 20:1183–1202.
17. Haffner SM, Stern MP, Hazuda HP, et al. Cardiovascular risk factors in confirmed prediabetic individuals: Does the clock for coronary heart disease start ticking before the onset of clinical diabetes? *JAMA* 1990; 263:2893–2898.
18. Unger RH, Foster DW. Diabetes mellitus. In: Wilson JD, Foster DW, Kronenberg HM, Larsen PR, eds. *Williams Textbook of Endocrinology*. Philadelphia: Saunders; 1998:973.
19. Stamler J, Vaccaro O, Neaton JD, Wentworth D. Diabetes, other risk factors, and 12-year cardiovascular mortality for men screened in the Multiple Risk Factor Intervention Trial (MRFIT). *Diabetes Care* 1993; 16:434–444.
20. Folsom AR, Eckfeldt JH, Weitzman S, et al. Atherosclerosis Risk in Communities Study Investigators. Relation of carotid artery wall thickness in diabetes mellitus, fasting glucose and insulin, body size and physical activity. *Stroke* 1994; 25:66–73.
21. O'Leary DH, Polak JF, Kronmal RA, et al. Distribution and correlates of sonographically detected carotid artery disease in the Cardiovascular Health Study. *Stroke* 1992; 23:1752–1760.
22. Cooper ME. Pathogenesis, prevention, and treatment of diabetic nephropathy. *Lancet* 1998; 352:213–219.
23. Chavers BM, Bilous RW, Ellis EN, et al. Glomerular lesions and urinary albumin excretion in type I diabetes without overt proteinuria. *N Engl J Med* 1989; 320:966–970.
24. Ismail N, Becker B, Strzelczyk P, Ritz E. Renal disease and hypertension in non-insulin-dependent diabetes mellitus. *Kidney Int* 1999; 55:1–28.
25. Lebovitz HE, Wiegmann TB, Cnaan A, et al. Renal protective effects of enalapril in hypertensive NIDDM: Role of baseline albuminuria. *Kidney Int* 1994; 45:S150–S155.
26. Lewis EJ, Hunsicker LG, Bain RP, Rohde RD. The effect of angiotensin-converting-enzyme inhibition on diabetic nephropathy: The Collaborative Study Group. *N Engl J Med* 1993; 329:1456–1462.
27. Grundy SM, Benjamin IJ, Burke GL, et al. Diabetes and cardiovascular disease: A statement for healthcare professionals from the American Heart Association. *Circulation* 1999; 100:1134–1146.

28. Rose BD. Treatment of diabetic nephropathy. Up to Date Computer CD, Feb. 24, 1999.
29. Viberti G, Mogensen CE, Groop LC, Pauls JF. Effect of captopril on progression to clinical proteinuria in patients with insulin-dependent diabetes mellitus and microalbuminuria: European Microalbuminuria Captopril Study Group. *JAMA* 1994; 271:275–279.
30. The Microalbuminuria Captopril Study Group. Captopril reduces the risk of nephropathy in IDDM patients with microalbuminuria. *Diabetologia* 1996; 39:587–593.
31. Ravid M, Savin H, Jutrin I, et al. Long-term stabilizing effect of angiotensin-converting enzyme inhibition on plasma creatinine and on proteinuria in normotensive type II diabetic patients. *Ann Intern Med* 1993; 118:577–581.
32. Golan L, Birkmeyer JD, Welch HG. The cost-effectiveness of treating all patients with type 2 diabetes with angiotensin-converting enzyme inhibitors. *Ann Intern Med* 1999; 131:660–667.
33. Gaber L, Walton C, Brown S, Bakris G. Effects of different antihypertensive treatments on morphologic progression of diabetic nephropathy in uninephrectomized dogs. *Kidney Int* 1994; 46:161–169.
34. Ritz E, Stefanski A. Diabetic nephropathy in type II diabetes. *Am J Kidney Dis* 1996; 27:167–194.
35. Berkman J, Rifkin H. Unilateral nodular diabetic glomerulosclerosis (Kimmelstiel-Wilson): Report of a case. *Metabolism* 1973; 22:715–722.
36. Austin SM, Lieberman JS, Newton LD, et al. Slope of serial glomerular filtration rate and the progression of diabetic glomerular disease. *J Am Soc Nephrol* 1993; 3:1358–1370.
37. Bohlen L, de Courten M, Weidmann P. Comparative study of the effect of ACE-inhibitors and other antihypertensive agents on proteinuria in diabetic patients. *Am J Hypertens* 1994; 7:84S–92S.
38. Tatti P, Pahor M, Byington RP, et al. Outcome results of the Fosinopril versus Amlodipine Cardiovascular Events Randomized Trial (FACET) in patients with hypertension and NIDDM. *Diabetes Care* 1998; 21:597–603.
39. Kannel W, McGee D. Diabetes and glucose tolerance as risk factors for cardiovascular disease: The Framingham Study. *Diabetes Care* 1979; 2:120–126.
40. Jarrett RJ, Shipley MJ. Type 2 (non-insulin dependent) diabetes mellitus and cardiovascular disease—putative association via common antecedents: Further evidence from the Whitehall Study. *Diabetologia* 1988; 31:737–740.
41. Jarrett RJ, McCarthney P, Keen H. The Bedford Study: Ten-year mortality rates in newly diagnosed diabetics, borderline diabetics and normoglycemic controls and the risk indices for coronary heart disease in borderline diabetics. *Diabetologia* 1982; 22:79–84.
42. Fontbonne A, Eschwege E, Cambien F, et al. Hypertriglyceridemia as a risk factor for coronary heart disease mortality in subjects with impaired glucose tolerance or diabetes: Results from the 11-year follow-up of the Paris Prospective Study. *Diabetologia* 1989; 32:300–304.
43. Donahue RP, Orchard TG. Diabetes mellitus and macrovascular complications: An epidemiological perspective. *Diabetes Care* 1992; 15:1141–1155.
44. Barrett-Connor E, Cohn B, Wingard D, Edelstein SL. Why is diabetes mellitus a stronger risk factor for fatal ischemic heart disease in women than in men? The Rancho Bernardo Study. *JAMA* 1991; 256:627–631.
45. Barrett-Connor E, Wingard DL. Sex differential in ischemic heart disease mortality in diabetics: A prospective population-based study. *Am J Epidemiol* 1983; 118:489–496.
46. Nathan DM. Long-term complications of diabetes mellitus. *N Engl J Med* 1993; 328:1676–1685.
47. The Diabetes Control and Complication Trial Research Group. The effect of intensive treatment of diabetes on the development and progression of long-term complications in insulin-dependent diabetes mellitus. *N Engl J Med* 1993; 329:977–986.
48. American Diabetes Association. Consensus statement: Role of cardiovascular risk factors in prevention and treatment of macrovascular disease in diabetes. *Diabetes Care* 1993; 16:72–78.
49. Fuller JH, Shipley MJ, Rose G, et al. Coronary heart disease and impaired glucose tolerance: The Whitehall Study. *Lancet* 1980; 1:1373–1376.
50. Yamasaki Y, Kawamori R, Matsushima H, et al. Asymptomatic hyperglycemia is associated with increased intimal plus medial thickness of the carotid artery. *Diabetologia* 1995; 38:585–591.
51. Crub JD, Rodriguez BL, Burchfiel CM, et al. Sudden death, impaired glucose tolerance and diabetes in Japanese American men. *Circulation* 1995; 91:2591–2595.
52. Kahn CR. Insulin action, diabetogenes and the cause of type II diabetes. *Diabetes* 1994; 43:1066–1084.
53. Ferrannini E, Buzzigoli G, Bonadonna R, et al. Insulin resistance in essential hypertension. *N Engl J Med* 1987; 317:350–357.
54. Zavaroni I, Bonora E, Pagliara M, et al. Risk factors for coronary artery disease in healthy persons with hyperinsulinemia and normal glucose tolerance. *N Engl J Med* 1989; 320:702–706.
55. Larsson B, Savardsudd K, Welin L, et al. Abdominal adipose tissue distribution, obesity and risk of cardiovascular disease and death: 13-year follow-up of participants in the study of men born in 1913. *Br Med J* 1984; 288:1401–1404.
56. Peiris AN, Sothmann MS, Hoffman RG, et al. Adiposity, fat distribution and cardiovascular risk. *Ann Intern Med* 1989; 110:867–872.
57. Laakso M, Barrett-Connor E. Asymptomatic hyperglycemia is associated with lipid and lipoprotein changes favoring atherosclerosis. *Atherosclerosis* 1989; 9:665–672.
58. Modan M, Halkin H, Luskyn A, et al. Hyperinsulinemia is characterized by jointly disturbed plasma VLDL, LDL, and HDL levels. *Arteriosclerosis* 1988; 8:227–236.
59. Laws A, King AC, Haskell WL, Reaven GM. Relation of fasting plasma insulin concentrations to high-density lipoprotein cholesterol and triglyceride concentration in men. *Arterioscler Thromb* 1991; 11:1636–1642.
60. Reaven GM. Role of insulin resistance in human disease (syndrome X): An expanded definition. *Annu Rev Med* 1993; 44:121–131.
61. Reaven GM, Laws A. Insulin resistance, compensatory hyperinsulinemia and coronary heart disease. *Diabetologia* 1994; 37: 948–952.
62. Fontbonne A, Charles MA, Thibult N, et al. Hyperinsulinemia as a predictor of coronary heart disease mortality in a healthy population: The Paris Prospective Study, 15-year follow-up. *Diabetologia* 1991; 34:356–361.
63. Pyorala K, Savolainen E, Kaukola S, Haapakoski J. Plasma insulin as coronary heart disease risk factor: Relationship to other risk factors and predictive value over 9.5 year follow-up of the Helsinki Policeman Study population. *Acta Med Scand* 1985; 701(suppl):38–52.
64. Despres J-P, Lamarche B, Mauriege P, et al. Hyperinsulinemia is an independent risk factor for ischemic heart disease. *N Engl J Med* 1996; 334:952–957.
65. Modan M, Or J, Karasik A, et al. Hyperinsulinemia, sex and risk of atherosclerotic cardiovascular disease. *Circulation* 1991; 84:1165–1175.
66. Liu QZ, Knowler WC, Nelson RG, et al. Insulin treatment, endogenous insulin concentration and ECG abnormalities in diabetic Pima Indians: Cross sectional and prospective analysis. *Diabetes* 1992; 41:1141–1150.
67. Ferrara A, Barrett-Connor E, Edelstein SL. Hyperinsulinemia does not increase the risk of fatal cardiovascular disease in elderly men and women without diabetes: The Rancho Bernardo Study, 1984 to 1991. *Am J Epidemiol* 1994; 140:857–869.

68. Gerstein HC, Yusuf S. Dysglycemia and risk of cardiovascular disease. *Lancet* 1996; 347:949–950.
69. Singer DE, Nathan DM, Anderson KM, et al. Association of HbA1c with prevalent cardiovascular disease in the original cohort of the Framingham Heart Study. *Diabetes* 1992; 41:202–208.
70. Kuusisto J, Makkanen L, Pyorala K, Laakso M. NIDDM and its metabolic control predicts coronary heart disease in elderly subjects. *Diabetes* 1994; 43:960–967.
71. Uusitupa MI, Niskanen LK, Siitonen O, et al. Ten-year cardiovascular mortality in relation to risk factors and abnormalities in lipoprotein composition in type 2 (non-insulin-dependent) diabetic and nondiabetic subjects. *Diabetologia* 1993; 36:1175–1184.
72. Krolewski AS, Kosinki EJ, Warram JH, et al. Magnitude and determinants of coronary artery disease in juvenile-onset, insulin-dependent diabetes mellitus. *Am J Cardiol* 1987; 59:750–755.
73. Borch-Johnsen K, Kreiner S. Proteinuria: Value as predictor of cardiovascular mortality in insulin-dependent diabetes mellitus. *Br Med J* 1987; 294:1651–1654.
74. Bucala R, Mitchell R, Arnold K, et al. Identification of the major site of apolipoprotein B modification by advanced glycosylation end products blocking uptake by the low density lipoprotein receptor. *J Biol Chem* 1995; 270:10828–10832.
75. Bucala R, Makita Z, Koschinsky T, et al. Lipid advanced glycosylation: Pathway for lipid oxidation in vivo. *Proc Natl Acad Sci USA* 1993; 90:6434–6438.
76. Bucala R, Makita Z, Vega G, et al. Modification of low-density lipoprotein by advanced glycosylation end products contributes to the dyslipidemia of diabetes and renal insufficiency. *Proc Natl Acad Sci USA* 1994; 91:9441–9445.
77. Steinbrecher UP, Witztum JL. Glycosylation of low density lipoproteins to an extent comparable to that seen in diabetics slows their catabolism. *Diabetes* 1984; 33:130–134.
78. Lyons TJ. Glycation and oxidation: A role in the pathogenesis of atherosclerosis. *Am J Cardiol* 1993; 71:26B–31B.
79. Sobenin IA, Tertov VV, Koschinsky T, et al. Modified low-density lipoprotein from diabetic patients causes cholesterol accumulation in human intimal aortic cells. *Atherosclerosis* 1993; 100:41–54.
80. Lyons TJ, Klein R, Baynes JW, et al. Stimulation of cholesterol-ester synthesis in human monocyte-derived macrophages by low-density lipoproteins from type I (insulin-dependent) diabetic patients: The influence of nonenzymatic glycosylation of low-density lipoprotein. *Diabetologia* 1987; 30:916–923.
81. Klein RL, Laimins M, Lopes-Varella MF. Isolation, characterization and metabolism of the glycated and nonglycated subfractions of low-density lipoproteins isolated from type I diabetic patients and nondiabetic subjects. *Diabetes* 1995; 44:1093–1098.
82. Fiengold KR, Grunfeld C, Pang M, et al. LDL subclass phenotype and triglyceride metabolism in non-insulin-dependent diabetes. *Arterioscler Throm* 1992; 12:1496–1502.
83. Stewart MW, Laker MF, Dyer RG, et al. Lipoprotein compositional abnormalities and insulin resistance in type II diabetic patients with mild hyperlipidemia. *Arterioscler Throm* 1993; 13:1046–1052.
84. Austin MA, Mykkanen L, Kuusisto J, et al. Prospective study of small LDLs as a risk factor for non-insulin-dependent diabetes mellitus in elderly men and women. *Circulation* 1995; 92:1770–1778.
85. Howard BV, Abbott WF, Beltz WF, et al. The effect of non-insulin-dependent diabetes on very low density lipoprotein and low density lipoprotein metabolism in men. *Metabolism* 1987; 36:870–877.
86. Packard CJ, Munro A, Lorimer AR, et al. Metabolism of apolipoprotein B in large triglyceride-rich very low density lipoproteins of normal and hypertriglyceridemic subjects. *J Clin Invest* 1984; 84:2178–2192.
87. Austin MA, King MC, Vranizan KM, Krauss RM. Atherogenic lipoprotein phenotype: A proposed genetic marker for coronary heart disease risk. *Circulation* 1990; 82:495–506.
88. West KM, Ahuja MMS, Bennett PH, et al. The role of circulation glucose and triglyceride concentration and their interaction with other "risk factors" as determinants of arterial disease in nine diabetic population samples from the WHO multinational study. *Diabetes Care* 1983; 6:361–369.
89. Goldschmid MG, Barrett-Connor E, Edelstein SL, et al. Dyslipidemia and ischemic heart disease mortality among men and women with diabetes. *Circulation* 1994; 89:991–997.
90. Laasko M, Lehto S, Penttila I, Pyorala K. Lipids and lipoproteins predicting coronary heart disease mortality and morbidity in patients with non-insulin-dependent diabetes. *Circulation* 1993; 88:1421–1430.
91. Ginsberg HN. Diabetic dyslipidemia: Basic mechanisms underlying the common hypertriglyceridemia and low HDL cholesterol levels. *Diabetes* 1996; 45(suppl):27S–30S.
92. Patsch JR, Prasad S, Gotto AM, et al. High density lipoprotein 2: Relationship of the plasma levels of this lipoprotein species to its composition, to the magnitude of postprandial lipemia, and to the activities of lipoprotein lipase and hepatic lipase. *J Clin Invest* 1984; 80:341–347.
93. American Diabetes Association, Consensus statement: Detection and management of lipid disorders in diabetes. *Diabetes Care* 1993; 16:828–839.
94. Vinik AI, Colwell JA. Effects of gemfibrozil on triglyceride levels in patients with NIDDM. *Diabetes Care* 1993; 16:37–44.
95. Vega GL, Grundy SM. Gemfibrozil therapy in primary hypertriglyceridemia associated with coronary heart disease: Effect on metabolism of low-density lipoproteins. *JAMA* 1985; 253:2398–2403.
96. Koskinen P, Manttrai M, Manninen V, et al. Coronary heart disease incidence in NIDDM patients in the Helsinki Heart Study. *Diabetes Care* 1992; 15:820–825.
97. Lahdenpera S, Tilly-Kiesi M, Vuorinen-Markkola H, et al. Effects of gemfibrozil on low-density lipoprotein size, density distribution and composition in patients with type II diabetes. *Diabetes Care* 1993; 16:584–592.
98. Garg A, Grundy SM. Nicotinic acid as therapy for dyslipidemia in non-insulin-dependent diabetes mellitus. *JAMA* 1990; 264:723–726.
99. Garg A, Grundy SM. Lovastatin for lowering cholesterol levels in non-insulin dependent diabetes mellitus. *N Engl J Med* 1988; 318:81–86.
100. Scandinavian Simvastatin Survival Study Group. Randomized trial of cholesterol lowering in 4444 patients with coronary heart disease: Scandinavian Simvastatin Survival Study (4S). *Lancet* 1994; 344:1383–1389.
101. Garg A, Grundy SM. Cholestyramine therapy for dyslipidemia in non-insulin-dependent diabetes mellitus. *Ann Intern Med* 1994; 121:416–422.
102. Hope investigators. Effects of an angiotensin converting enzyme inhibitor, ramipril, on cardiovascular events in high-risk patients. *N Engl J Med* 2000; 342:145–153.
103. Winocour PD. Platelet abnormalities in diabetes mellitus. *Diabetes* 1992; 41(suppl 2):26–31.
104. Tschoepe D, Rosen P, Schwippert B, Gries FA. Platelets in diabetes: The role of the hemostatic regulation in atherosclerosis. *Semin Thromb Hemost* 1993; 19:122–128.
105. Breddin H, Krzywanek H, Althoff P, et al. Platelet aggregation as a risk factor in diabetes. *Horm Metab Res Suppl* 1985; 15:63–68.
106. Winocour PD. Platelet abnormalities in diabetes mellitus. *Diabetes* 1992; 41(suppl 2):26–31.
107. Winocour PD. Platelet turnover in advanced diabetes. *Eur J Clin Invest* 1994; 24(suppl 1):34–37.
108. Janero DR. Malondialdehyde and thiobarbituric acid-reactivity

as diagnostic indices of lipid peroxidation and peroxidative tissue injury. *Free Radic Biol Med* 1990; 9:515–540.
109. Davi G, Catalano I, Averna M, et al. Thromboxane biosynthesis and platelet function in type II diabetes mellitus. *N Engl J Med* 1990; 322:1769–1774.
110. Stehouwer CDA, Nauta JJP, Zeldenrust GC, et al. Urinary albumin excretion, cardiovascular disease and endothelial dysfunction in non-insulin-dependent diabetes mellitus. *Lancet* 1992; 340: 319–323.
111. Stehouwer CDA, Donker AJM. Urinary albumin excretion and cardiovascular disease in diabetes mellitus: Is endothelial dysfunction the missing link? *J Nephrol* 1993; 6:72–92.
112. Conlan MG, Folsom AR, Finch A, et al. Associations of factor VII and von-Willebrand factor with age, race, sex and risk factors for atherosclerosis: The atherosclerosis in communities (ARIC) study. *Thromb Haemost* 1993; 70:380–385.
113. Ganda OP, Arkin CF. Hyperfibrinogenemia: An important risk factor for vascular complications in diabetes. *Diabetes Care* 1992; 15:1245–1250.
114. Kannel WB, D'Agostino RB, Wilson RB, et al. Diabetes, fibrinogen and risk of cardiovascular disease: The Framingham experience. *Am Heart J* 1990; 120:672–676.
115. De Feo P, Gaisano GM, Haymond MW. Differential effects of insulin deficiency on albumin and fibrinogen synthesis in humans. *J Clin Invest* 1991; 88:833–840.
116. Garcia Frade LJ, de la Calle H, Alava I, et al. Diabetes mellitus as a hypercoagulable state: Its relationship with fibrin fragments and vascular damage. *Thromb Res* 1987; 47:533–540.
117. Landgraf-Leurs MM, Ladik T, Smolka B, et al. Increased thromboplastic potential in diabetes: A multifactorial phenomenon. *Klin Wochenschr* 1987; 65:600–606.
118. Ceriello A. Coagulation activation in diabetes mellitus: The role of hyperglycaemia and therapeutic prospects. *Diabetologia* 1993; 36:1119–1125.
119. Husted SE, Nielsen HK, Bak JF, Beck-Nielsen H. Antithrombin III activity, von Willebrand factor antigen and platelet function in young diabetic patients treated with multiple insulin injections versus insulin pump treatment. *Eur J Clin Invest* 1989; 19:90–94.
120. Hamsten A, de Faire U, Walldius G, et al. Plasminogen activator inhibitor in plasma: Risk factor for recurrent myocardial infarction. *Lancet* 1987; 2:3–9.
121. Mussoni L, Mannucci L, Sirtori M, et al. Hypertriglyceridemia and regulation of fibrinolytic activity. *Arterioscler Thromb* 1992; 12:19–27.
122. Mehta J, Mehta P, Lawson D, Saldeen T. Plasma tissue plasminogen activator inhibitor levels in coronary artery disease: Correlation with age and serum triglyceride concentrations. *J Am Coll Cardiol* 1987; 9:263–268.
123. Grant PJ, Kruithof EK, Felley CP, et al. Short-term infusions of insulin, triacylglycerol and glucose do not cause acute increases in plasminogen activator inhibitor-1 concentrations in man. *Clin Sci* 1990; 79:513–516.
124. Richardson M, Hadcock SJ, DeReske M, Cybulsky MI. Increased expression in vivo of VCAM-1 and E-selectin by the aortic endothelium of normolipemic and hyperlipemic diabetic rabbits. *Arterioscler Thromb* 1994; 14:760–769.
125. Yan SD, Schmidt AM, Anderson GM, et al. Enhanced cellular oxidant stress by the interaction of advanced glycation end products with their receptors/binding proteins. *J Biol Chem* 1994; 269:9889–9897.
126. Wautier JL, Wautier MP, Schmidt AM, et al. Advanced glycation end products (AGEs) on the surface of diabetic erythrocytes bind to the vessel wall via a specific receptor inducing oxidant stress in the vasculature: A link between surface-associated AGEs and diabetic complications. *Proc Natl Acad Sci USA* 1994; 91:7742–7746.
127. Schmidt AM, Hori O, Chen JX, et al. Advanced glycation end products interacting with their endothelial receptor induce expression of vascular cell adhesion molecule-1 (VCAM-1) in cultured human endothelial cells and in mice. A potential mechanism for the accelerated vasculopathy of diabetes. *J Clin Invest* 1995; 96:1395–1403.
128. Keegan A, Walbank H, Cotter MA, Cameron NE. Chronic vitamin E treatment prevents defective endothelium-dependent relaxation in diabetic rat aorta. *Diabetologia* 1995; 38:1475–1478.
129. Ting HH, Timimi FK, Boles KS, et al. Vitamin C improves endothelium-dependent vasodilation in patients with non-insulin-dependent diabetes mellitus. *J Clin Invest* 1996; 97:22–28.
130. Hunt JV, Dean RT, Wolff SP. Hydroxyl radical production and autoxidative glycosylation: Glucose autoxidation as the cause of protein damage in the experimental glycation model of diabetes mellitus and ageing. *Biochem J* 1988; 256:205–212.
131. Hunt JV, Smith CC, Wolff SP. Autoxidative glycosylation and possible involvement of peroxides and free radicals in LDL modification by glucose. *Diabetes* 1990; 39:1420–1424.
132. Mullarkey CJ, Edelstein D, Brownlee M. Free radical generation by early glycation products: A mechanism for accelerated atherogenesis in diabetes. *Biochem Biophys Res Commun* 1990; 173:932–939.
133. Bucala R, Tracey KJ, Cerami A. Advanced glycosylation products quench nitric oxide and mediate defective endothelium-dependent vasodilation in experimental diabetes. *J Clin Invest* 1991; 87:432–438.
134. Vehkavaara S, Seppala-Lindroos A, Westerbacka J, et al. In vivo endothelial dysfunction characterizes patients with impaired fasting glucose. *Diabetes Care* 1999; 22:2055–2060.
135. Vlassara H. Advanced glycation end-products and atherosclerosis. *Ann Med* 1996; 28:419–426.
136. Stitt AW, Bucala R, Vlassara H. Atherogenesis and advanced glycation: Promotion, progression and prevention. *Ann NY Acad Sci* 1997; 811:115–129.
137. Brownlee M, Cerami A, Vlassara H. Advanced glycation endproducts in tissue and the biochemical basis of diabetic complications. *N Engl J Med* 1988; 318:1315–1321.
138. Aronson D, Rayfield EJ. Diabetes. In: Topol E, ed. *Textbook of Cardiovascular Medicine.* Philadelphia: Lippincott-Raven; 1998: 171.
139. Nakamura Y, Horii Y, Nishino T, et al. Immunohistochemical localization of advanced glycosylation end products in coronary atheroma and cardiac tissue in diabetes mellitus. *Am J Pathol* 1993; 143:1649–1656.
140. Kilhovd BK, Berg TJ, Birkeland KI, et al. Serum levels of advanced glycation end products are increased in patients with type 2 diabetes and coronary heart disease. *Diabetes Care* 1999; 22:1543–1548.
141. Berg TJ, Snorgaard O, Faber J, et al. Serum levels of advanced glycation end products are associated with left ventricular diastolic function in patients with type-1 diabetes. *Diabetes Care* 1999; 22:1186–1190.
142. Brownlee M, Vlassara H, Kooney A, et al. Aminoguanidine prevents diabetes-induced arterial wall protein cross-linking. *Science* 1986; 232:1629–1632.
143. Vasan S, Zhang X, Zhang X, et al. An agent cleaving glucose-derived protein crosslinks in vitro and in vivo. *Nature* 1996; 382:275–278.
144. Schmidt AM, Hori O, Brett J, et al. Cellular receptors for advanced glycation end-products: Implications for induction of oxidant stress and cellular dysfunction in the pathogenesis of vascular lesions. *Arterioscler Thromb* 1994; 14:1521–1528.
145. Brett J, Schmidt AM, Yan SD, et al. Survey of the distribution of a newly characterized receptor for advanced glycation end-products in tissues. *Am J Pathol* 1993; 143:1699–1712.
146. Vlassara H, Brownlee M, Manogue KR, et al. Cachetin/TNF and

IL-1 induced by glucose modified proteins: Role in normal tissue remodelling. *Science* 1988; 240:1546–1548.

147. Kirstein M, Brett J, Radoff S, et al. Advanced protein glycosylation induces selective transendothelial human monocyte chemotaxis and secretion of PDGF: Role in vascular diseases of diabetes and aging. *Proc Natl Acad Sci USA* 1990; 87:9010–9014.
148. Vlassara H, Fuh H, Makita Z, et al. Exogenous advanced glycosylation end products induce complex vascular dysfunction in normal animal: A model for diabetic and aging complications. *Proc Natl Acad Sci USA* 1992; 89:12043–12047.
149. Kirstein M, Aston C, Hintz R, Vlassara H. Receptor-specific induction of insulin-like growth factor-1 (IGF-1) in human monocytes by advanced glycosylation end product-modified proteins. *J Clin Invest* 1992; 90:439–446.
150. Esposito C, Gerlach H, Brett J, et al. Endothelial receptor-mediated binding of glucose-modified albumin is associated with increased monolayer permeability and modulation of cell surface procoagulant properties. *J Exp Med* 1989; 170:1378–1407.
151. Wautier JL, Zoukourian C, Chappey O, et al. Receptor-mediated endothelial cell dysfunction in diabetic vasculopathy: Soluble receptor for advance glycation end-products blocks hyperpermeability in diabetic rats. *J Clin Invest* 1996; 97:238–243.
152. Schmidt AM, Osamu H, Chen JX, et al. Advanced glycation end-products interacting with their endothelial receptors induce expression of vascular cell adhesion molecule-1 (VCAM-1) in cultured human endothelial cells in mice. *J Clin Invest* 1995; 96:1395–1403.
153. Yan SD, Schmidt AM, Anderson GM, Zhang J, et al. Enhanced cellular oxidant stress by the interaction of advanced glycation end products with their receptors/binding proteins. *J Biol Chem* 1994; 269:9889–9897.
154. Wautier JL, Wautier MP, Schmidt AM, et al. Advanced glycation end products (AGEs) on the surface of diabetic erythrocytes bind to the vessel wall via a specific receptor inducing oxidant stress in the vasculature: A link between surface-associated AGEs and diabetic complications. *Proc Natl Acad Sci USA* 1994; 91:7742–7746.
155. Brownlee M, Vlassara H, Kooney A, et al. Aminoguanidine prevents diabetes-induced arterial wall protein cross-linking. *Science* 1986; 232:1629–1632.
156. Brownlee M. Glycation and diabetic complications. *Diabetes* 1994; 43:836–841.
157. Brownlee M, Vlassara H, Cerami A. Nonenzymatic glycosylation products on collagen covalently trap low-density lipoprotein. *Diabetes* 1985; 34:938–941.
158. Bucala R, Tracey KJ, Cerami A. Advanced glycosylation products quench nitric oxide and mediate defective endothelium-dependent vasodilatation in experimental diabetes. *J Clin Invest* 1991; 87:432–438.
159. Bowie A, Owens D, Collins P, et al. Glycosylated low density lipoprotein is more sensitive to oxidation: Implications for the diabetic patient? *Atherosclerosis* 1993; 102:63–67.
160. Schmidt AM, Yan SD, Brett J, et al. Regulation of human mononuclear phagocyte migration by cell surface-binding proteins for advanced glycation end-products. *J Clin Invest* 1993; 91:2155–2168.
161. Vlassara H, Bucala R, Striker L. Pathogenic effects of advanced glycosylation: Biochemical, biologic, and clinical implications for diabetes and aging. *Lab Invest* 1994; 70:138–151.
162. Pyorala K, Pedersen DR, Kjekshus J, et al. Cholesterol lowering with simvastatin improves prognosis of diabetic patients with coronary heart disease. *Diabetes Care* 1997; 20:614–620.
163. Sacks FM, Pfeffer MA, Moye LA, et al. The effect of pravastatin on coronary events after myocardial infarction in patients with average cholesterol levels. *N Engl J Med* 1996; 335:1001–1009.
164. CARE Circulation: Goldberg RB, Mellies MJ, Sacks FM, et al. Cardiovascular events and their reduction with pravastatin in diabetic and glucose-intolerant myocardial infarction survivors with average cholesterol levels: Subgroup analyses in the cholesterol and recurrent events (CARE) trial: The Care investigators. *Circulation* 1998; 98:2513–2519.
165. American Diabetes Association: Standard of medical care for patients with diabetes mellitus. *Diabetes Care* 2000; 23(suppl 1): S532–S542.
166. Muhlhauser I, Sawicki PT, Berger M. Possible risk of sulfonylureas in the treatment of non-insulin-dependent diabetes mellitus and coronary artery disease. *Diabetologia* 1997; 40:1492–1496.
167. Cleveland JC, Meldrum DR, Cain BS, et al. Oral sulfonylurea hypoglycemic agents prevent ischemic preconditioning in human myocardium. *Circulation* 1997; 96(1):29–32.
168. Owens DR. Repaglinide—prandial glucose regulator: A new class of oral antidiabetic drugs. *Diabetes Med* 1998; 15(suppl 4): S28–S36.
169. Metformin for non-insulin-dependent diabetes mellitus. *Med Lett Drugs Ther* 1995; 37(948):41–42.
170. Stumvoll M, Nurjhan N, Perriello G, et al. Metabolic effects of metformin in non-insulin-dependent diabetes mellitus. *N Engl J Med* 1995; 333(9):550–554.
171. Garber AJ, Duncan TG, Goodman AM, et al. Efficacy of metformin in type II diabetes: Results of a double-blind, placebo-controlled, dose-response trial. *Am J Med* 1997; 102:491–497.
172. Giugliano D, Quatraro A, Consoli G, et al. Metformin for obese, insulin-treated, diabetic patients: Improvement in glycemic control and reduction of metabolic risk factors. *Eur J Clin Pharmacol* 1993; 44:107–112.
173. DeFronzo RA, Goodman AM, and the Multicenter Metformin Study Group. Efficacy of metformin in patients with non-insulin-dependent diabetes mellitus. *N Engl J Med* 1995; 333:541–549.
174. Inzucchi SE, Maggs DG, Spollett GR, et al. Efficacy and metabolic effects of metformin and troglitazone in type II diabetes mellitus. *N Engl J Med* 1998; 338:867–872.
175. Robinson AC, Burke J, Robinson S, et al. The effects of metformin on glycemic control and serum lipids in insulin-treated NIDDM patients with suboptimal metabolic control. *Diabetes Care* 1998; 21(5):701–705.
176. Stang MR, Wysowski DK, Butler-Jones D. Incidence of lactic acidosis in metformin users. *Diabetes Care* 1999; 22:925–927.
177. *Physician Desk Reference,* ed. 52. Montvale, NJ: Medical Economics Company. 1998; 795–800.
178. Tafuri SR. Troglitazone enhances differentiation, basal-glucose uptake and Glut 1 protein levels in 3T3-L1 adipocytes. *Endocrinology* 1996; 137:4706–4712.
179. Miles PDG, Romeo OM, Higo K, et al. TNF-α-induced insulin resistance in vivo and its prevention by troglitazone. *Diabetes* 1997; 46:1678–1683.
180. Schwartz S, Raskin P, Fonseca V, Graveline JF, for the Troglitazone and Exogenous Insulin Study Group. Effect of troglitazone in insulin-treated patients with type II diabetes mellitus. *N Engl J Med* 1998; 338:861–866.
181. Buse JB, Gumbiner B, Mathias NP, et al. The Troglitazone Insulin Study Group: Troglitazone use in insulin-treated type II diabetic patients. *Diabetes Care* 1998; 21:1455–1461.
182. Horton ES, Whitehouse F, Ghazzi MN, et al. The Troglitazone Study Group: Troglitazone in combination with sulfonylurea restores glycemic control in patients with type II diabetes. *Diabetes Care* 1998; 21:1462–1469.
183. Ghazzi MN, Perez JE, Antonucci TK, et al. The Triglitazone Study Group, Whitcomb RW. Cardiac and glycemic benefits of troglitazone treatment in NIDDM. *Diabetes* 1997; 46:433–439.
184. Maggs DG, Buchanan TA, Burant CF, et al. Metabolic effects of troglitazone monotherapy in type 2 diabetes mellitus. *Ann Intern Med* 1998; 128:176–185.
185. Tack CJJ, Smits P, Demacker PNM, Stalenhoff AFH. Troglitazone decreases the proportion of small, dense LDL and increases

the resistance of LDL to oxidation in obese subjects. *Diabetes Care* 1998; 21:796–797.

186. Patel J, Miller E, Patwardhan R, the Rosiglitazone Study Group. Rosiglitazone improves glycemic control when used as monotherapy in type 2 diabetic patients. *Diabetic Medicine* 1998; 15(suppl 2):S38.
187. Grunberger G, Weston WM, Patwardhan R, Rappaport EB. Rosiglitazone once or twice daily improves the glycemic control in patients with type 2 diabetes. *Diabetes* 1998; 48(suppl 1):A102.
188. Fonesca V, Biswas N, Salzman A. Once-daily rosiglitazone in combination with metformin effectively reduces hyperglycemia in patients with type 2 diabetes. *Diabetes* 1999; 48(suppl 1):A100.
189. Package insert. SmithKline Beecham Pharmaceuticals, Philadelphia.
190. Package insert. Takeda Pharmaceuticals, Lincolnshire, IL.
191. University Group Diabetes Program. A study of the effects of hypoglycemic agents on vascular complications in patients with adult onset diabetes. *Diabetes* 1976; 25:1129–1153.
192. Garratt KN, Hassinger N, Grill DE, et al. Sulfonylurea drug use is associated with increased early mortality during direct coronary angioplasty for acute myocardial infarction among diabetic patients. *J Am Coll Cardiol* 1997; 29:493A (Abstr).
193. UK Prospective Diabetes Study Group. Intensive blood glucose control with sulfonylureas or insulin compared with conventional treatment and risk of complications in patients with type-2 diabetes. UKPDS 33. *Lancet* 1998; 352:837–853.
194. UK Prospective Diabetes Study Group. Effect of intensive blood glucose control with metformin on complications in overweight patients with type-2 diabetes. UKPDS 34. *Lancet* 1998; 352: 854–865.
195. UK Prospective Diabetes Study Group. Tight blood pressure control and risk of macrovascular and microvascular complications in type-2 diabetes. UKPDS 38. *BMJ* 1998; 317:703–713.
196. UK Prospective Diabetes Study Group. Efficacy of atenolol and captopril in reducing risk of macrovascular and microvascular complications in type 2 diabetes. UKPDS 39. *BMJ* 1998; 317: 713–720.
197. The Diabetes Control and Complications Trial Research Group. The effect of intensive treatment of diabetes on the development and progression of long-term complications in insulin-dependent diabetes mellitus. *N Engl J Med* 1993; 329:977–986.
198. The Diabetes Control and Complications Trial Research Group. Effect of intensive diabetes management on macrovascular events and risk factors in the Diabetes Control and Complications Trial. *Am J Cardiol* 1995; 75:894–903.
199. The cost-effectiveness of screening for type 2 diabetes. CDC Diabetes Cost-Effectiveness Study Group, Centers for Disease Control and Prevention. *JAMA* 1998; 280:1757–1763.
200. Gibbons RJ, Balady GJ, Beasley JW, et al. ACC/AHA guidelines for exercise testing: Executive summary: A report of the American College of Cardiology/American Heart Association Task Force on Practice Guidelines (Committee on Exercise Testing). *Circulation* 1997; 96:345–354.
201. Grundy SM, Benjamin IJ, Burke GL, et al. Diabetes and cardiovascular disease: A statement for healthcare professionals from the American Heart Association. *Circulation* 1999; 100:1134–1146.
202. Curb JD, Pressel SL, Cutler JA, et al. Effect of diuretic-based antihypertensive treatment on cardiovascular disease risk in older diabetic patients with isolated systolic hypertension: Systolic Hypertension in the Elderly Program Cooperative Research Group. *JAMA* 1996; 276:1886–1892.
203. Hansson L, Zanchetti A, Carruthers SG, et al., for the HOT Study Group. Effects of intensive blood-pressure lowering and low-dose aspirin in patients with hypertension: Principal results of Hypertension Optimal Treatment (HOT) randomized trial. *Lancet* 1998; 351:1755–1762.
204. Hansson L, Lindholm LH, Niskanen L, et al., for the Captopril Prevention Projects (CAPPP) study group. Effect of angiotensin-converting-enzyme inhibition compared with conventional therapy on cardiovascular morbidity and mortality in hypertension: The Captopril Prevention Project (CAPPP) randomised trial. *Lancet* 1999; 353:611–616.
205. Estacio RO, Jeffers BW, Hiatt WR, et al. The effect of nisoldipine as compared with enalapril on cardiovascular outcomes in patients with non-insulin-dependent diabetes and hypertension. *N Engl J Med* 1998; 338:645–652.
206. Woodfield SL, Lundergan CF, Reiner JS, et al. Angiographic findings and outcome in diabetic patients treated with thrombolytic therapy for acute myocardial infarction: the GUSTO-1 experience. *J Am Coll Cardiol* 1996; 28:1661–1669.
207. Jaffe AS, Spadaro JJ, Schechtman K, et al. Increased congestive heart failure after myocardial infarction of modest extent in patients with diabetes mellitus. *Am Heart J* 1984; 108:31–37.
208. Savage MP, Krolewski AS, Kenien GG, et al. Acute myocardial infarction in diabetes mellitus and significance of congestive heart failure as a prognostic factor. *Am J Cardiol* 1988; 62:665–669.
209. Stone PH, Muller JE, Hartwell T, et al., for the MILIS Study Group. The effect of diabetes mellitus on prognosis and serial left ventricular function after acute myocardial infarction: Contribution of both coronary disease and left ventricular dysfunction to the adverse prognosis. *J Am Coll Cardiol* 1989; 14:49–57.
210. Fibrinolytic Therapy Trialists (FTT) Collaborative Group. Indications for fibrinolytic therapy in suspected acute myocardial infarction: Collaborative overview of early mortality and major morbidity results from all randomized trials of more than 1000 patients. *Lancet* 1994; 343:311–322.
211. Malmberg K, for the DIGAMI Study Group. Prospective randomised study of intensive insulin treatment on long-term survival after acute myocardial infarction in patients with diabetes mellitus. *BMJ* 1997; 314:1512–1515.
212. Zarich S, Waxman S, Freeman RT, et al. Effect of autonomic nervous system dysfunction on the circadian pattern of myocardial ischaemia in diabetes mellitus. *J Am Coll Cardiol* 1994; 24:956–962.
213. Jonas M, Reicher-Reiss H, Boyko V, et al. Usefulness of beta-blocker therapy in patients with non-insulin-dependent diabetes mellitus and coronary heart disease. *Am J Cardiol* 1996; 77:1273–1277.
214. Kendall MJ, Lynch KP, Hjalmarson A, Kjekshus J. Beta-blockers and sudden cardiac death. *Ann Intern Med* 1995; 123:358–367.
215. Holmes DR Jr, Vietstra RE, Smith HC, et al. Restenosis after percutaneous transluminal coronary angioplasty (PTCA): A report from the PTCA Registry of the National Heart, Lung and Blood Institute. *Am J Cardiol* 1984; 53:77C–81C.
216. Weintraub WS, Kosinski AS, Brown CL, King SB. Can restenosis after coronary angioplasty be predicted from clinical variables? *J Am Coll Cardiol* 1993; 21:6–14.
217. Vandormael MG, Deligonul U, Kern MJ, et al. Multilesion coronary angioplasty: Clinical and angiographic outcome. *J Am Coll Cardiol* 1987; 10:246–252.
218. Quigley PJ, Hlatky MA, Hinohara T, et al. Repeat percutaneous transluminal coronary angioplasty and predictors of recurrent restenosis. *Am J Cardiol* 1989; 63:409–413.
219. Lambert M, Bonan R, Cote G, et al. Multiple coronary angioplasty: A model to discriminate systemic and procedural factors related to restenosis. *J Am Coll Cardiol* 1988; 12:310–314.
220. Galan KM, Hollman JL. Recurrence of stenosis after coronary angioplasty. *Heart Lung* 1986; 15:585–587.
221. Rensing BJ, Hermans RM, Vos J, et al. Luminal narrowing after percutaneous transluminal coronary angioplasty. *Circulation* 1993; 88:975–985.
222. Wong SC, Baim DS, Schatz RA, et al. Immediate results and late outcomes after stent implantation in saphenous vein graft

lesions: The multicenter US Palmaz-Schatz stane experience: The Palmaz-Schatz Stent Study Group. *J Am Coll Cardiol* 1995; 26:704–712.

223. Bach R, Jung F, Kohsiek I, et al. Factors affecting the restenosis rate after percutaneous transluminal coronary angioplasty. *Thromb Haemost* 1994; 74(suppl 1):55S–77S.

224. Kornowski R, Mintz GS, Kent KM, et al. Increased restenosis in diabetes mellitus after coronary interventions is due to exaggerated intimal hyperplasia. *Circulation* 1997; 95:1366–1369.

225. Aronson D, Bloomgarden Z, Rayfield EJ. Potential mechanisms promoting restenosis in diabetes mellitus. *J Am Coll Cardiol* 1996; 27:528–535.

226. Lincoff AM, Califf RM, Moliterno DJ, et al., for the Evaluation of Platelet IIb/IIIa Inhibition in Stenting Investigators (EPISTENT). Complementary clinical benefits of coronary artery stenting and blockade of platelet glycoprotein IIb/IIIa receptors. *N Engl J Med* 1999; 341:319–327.

227. The Bypass Angioplasty Revascularization Investigation (BARI) Investigators. Comparison of bypass surgery with angioplasty in patients with multivessel disease. *N Engl J Med* 1996; 335: 217–225.

228. Kannel WB, Hjortland M, Castelli WP. Role of diabetes in congestive heart failure: The Framingham Study. *Am J Cardiol* 1974; 34:29–34.

229. Van Hoeven KH, Factor SM. A comparison of the pathological spectrum of hypertensive, diabetic, and hypertensive-diabetic heart disease. *Circulation* 1990; 82:848–855.

230. Jain A, Avendaro G, Dharamsey S, et al. Left ventricular diastolic dysfunction in hypertension and role of plasma glucose and insulin: Comparison with diabetic heart. *Circulation* 1996; 93:1396–1402.

231. Zarich SW, Arbuckle BE, Cohen LR, et al. Diastolic abnormalities in young asymptomatic diabetic patients assessed by pulse Doppler echocardiography. *J Am Coll Cardiol* 1988; 12:114–120.

232. Raev DC. Which left ventricular function is impaired earlier in the evolution of diabetic cardiomyopathy? An echocardiographic study of young type I diabetic patients. *Diabetes Care* 1994; 17:633–639.

233. Paillole C, Dahan M, Payche F, et al. Prevalence and significance of left ventricular filling abnormalities determined by Doppler echocardiography in young type I (insulin-dependent) diabetic patients. *Am J Cardiol* 1990; 64:1010–1016.

234. Mildenerger RR, Bar-Shlomo B, Druck MN, et al. Clinically unrecognized ventricular dysfunction in young diabetic patients. *J Am Coll Cardiol* 1984; 4:234–238.

235. Shindler DM, Kostis JB, Yusuf S, et al. Diabetes mellitus: A predictor of morbidity and mortality in the Studies of Left Ventricular Dysfunction (SOLVD) trials and registry. *Am J Cardiol* 1996; 77:1017–1020.

236. Gaede P, Vedel P, Parving HH, Pedersen O. Intensified multifactorial intervention in patients with type 2 diabetes mellitus and microalbuminuria: The Steno type 2 randomised study. *Lancet* 1999; 353:617–622.

237. Heart Outcomes Prevention Evaluation Study Investigators. Effects of ramipril on cardiovascular and microvascular outcomes in people with diabetes mellitus: Results of the HOPE study and MICRO-HOPE sub-study. *Lancet* 2000; 355:253–259.

CHAPTER 79

TRAUMATIC HEART DISEASE

Panagiotis N. Symbas

Accidental or intentional trauma is the leading cause of death, hospitalization, and loss of working days in American society, particularly among young people.[1-3] Cardiac and great vessel injuries are a major contributor to this mortality and morbidity.[4] The heart and/or great vessels may be injured from penetrating and nonpenetrating trauma. Since the diagnostic and therapeutic modalities for the management of heart diseases have become more complex and more invasive, mechanical injuries to the heart caused by iatrogenic trauma have become increasingly important. These injuries result from the complications of various diagnostic, therapeutic, and resuscitative procedures, including cardiac catheterization, percutaneous coronary angioplasty,[5,6] percutaneous aortic or mitral valvuloplasty,[7,8] insertion of pacemaker leads[9] or Swan-Ganz catheters,[10] closed- and open-chest cardiac massage, and electric defibrillation.[11,12] The increasing use of invasive catheters has led to the more frequent migration of these catheters to the heart and the pulmonary vascular beds[13-15] and to nonbacterial thrombotic endocarditis and bacterial endocarditis.

Two other types of cardiac trauma that are not due to mechanical injury warrant separate classification. The first type includes injury to the heart from ionizing radiation, which predominantly causes pericarditis but also may result in myocardial injury.[16-18] The second includes the group of cardiac injuries caused by an electric current,[19,20] which may cause asystole, ventricular fibrillation, other arrhythmias, and myocardial injury (see also Chap. 71).

Many nonpenetrating injuries and an occasional penetrating injury of the heart are well tolerated. Thus, many of these lesions are diagnosed infrequently, since their initial clinical manifestations may be absent or relatively mild, and a lesion may be overlooked unless a high index of suspicion is maintained and specific studies are obtained.[21,22] Frequently, these cardiac injuries are overshadowed by the more overt manifestations of cerebral, abdominal, or musculoskeletal trauma. For these reasons and because only the more severe injuries are reflected in autopsy studies, the actual incidence of traumatic heart disease remains obscure.

PENETRATING INJURIES

Penetrating injuries usually are observed with wounds of the precordium but also may be associated with wounds elsewhere in the chest, neck, or upper abdomen. They usually are due to missile or knife wounds but occasionally are caused by a missile embolus reaching the heart through the venous system or by a needle migrating through the esophagus.

Penetrating Cardiac Trauma

Although penetrating cardiac trauma frequently involves only the free cardiac wall, injury to cardiac valves, chordae tendineae, papillary muscles, the atrial or ventricular septum, coronary arteries, and the conduction system may occur. The multiplicity of heart and great vessel lesions that may be produced by penetrating wounds is indicated in Table 79-1.

The relative frequency of a single penetrating wound of the free cardiac wall is due to its area of exposure on the anterior chest wall. In decreasing order of frequency, the structures affected are the right ventricle, left ventricle, right atrium, and left atrium.[23] Cardiac wounds may be single or multiple; the latter more commonly are caused by missiles.[23,24] Over 50 percent of victims with penetrating cardiac trauma succumb shortly after injury.[25] The remainder survive for varying periods; many can recover completely if treated immediately.

The pathophysiologic consequences and clinical manifestations of penetrating injuries to the heart depend on the size and site of the wound, the mode of injury, and especially the state of the pericardial wound. When the pericardial wound remains open and bleeding occurs freely into the pleural space, there are signs and symptoms of hemothorax and loss of circulating blood volume. When there is intrapericardial hemorrhage with a sealed pericardial wound, cardiac tamponade (see Chap. 72) is the presenting clinical picture. The diagnosis of cardiac injury should be suspected in a patient with chest, lower neck, epigastric, or especially precordial penetrating wounds and with symptoms and signs of cardiac tamponade and/or hemothorax and loss of circulating blood volume. The management of penetrating wounds of the heart consists of immediate thoracotomy and cardiorrhaphy.[23,25-30] When this cannot be done or while appropriate arrangements are being made for thoracotomy, the patient's blood volume should be expanded; pericardiocentesis is performed only to provide time for a safe operation.[23,31]

Although the management of symptomatic patients with a suspected penetrating cardiac wound is clearly defined, the man-

TABLE 79-1 Penetrating Wounds of the Heart

I. Pericardial damage
  A. Laceration or perforation
  B. Hemopericardium with or without cardiac tamponade
  C. Serofibrinous or suppurative pericarditis
  D. Pneumopericardium
  E. Constrictive pericarditis
II. Myocardial damage
  A. Laceration
  B. Penetration or perforation
  C. Retained foreign body
  D. Structural defects
    1. Aneurysm formation
    2. Septal defects
    3. Aorticocardiac fistula
III. Valvular injury
  A. Leaflet or cusp injury
  B. Papillary muscle or chordae tendineae laceration
IV. Coronary artery injury
  A. Laceration or thrombosis with or without myocardial infarction
  B. Arteriovenous fistula
  C. Aneurysm
V. Embolism
  A. Foreign body
  B. Thrombus (septic or sterile)
VI. Infective endocarditis
VII. Rhythm or conduction disturbances

SOURCE: Prepared by Loren F. Parmley, MD, and Thomas W. Mattingly, and modified with permission.

agement of the asymptomatic patients with a penetrating precordial wound presented a considerable dilemma in the past, when the options were either exploratory surgery or observation. Currently, the use of echocardiography by a cardiologist or preferably an immediately available and specially trained trauma surgeon facilitates and makes the treatment of these patients safer by avoiding unnecessary surgery or observation, with its accompanying risk of sudden deterioration and even death.[32]

Residual or Delayed Sequelae of Penetrating Cardiac Trauma

Patients with penetrating cardiac wounds should be observed closely immediately postoperatively and after discharge for the clinical manifestations of residual or delayed sequelae from their penetrating cardiac wounds. Such sequelae may include (1) ventricular or atrial septal defect, (2) injury of the valve cups, leaflets, or chordae tendineae, (3) aortocardiac or aortopulmonary communication, or communication from the coronary artery to the coronary vein or the cardiac chamber, (4) ventricular aneurysms, (5) posttraumatic or postoperative pericarditis, and (6) electrocardiographic abnormalities.[33,34] When symptoms and signs of a structural defect are detected, echocardiography and/or cardiac catheterization should be performed to define the lesion and its hemodynamic significance and determine the proper mode of therapy.[33,35]

Posttraumatic pericarditis, which is similar to the postcardiotomy syndrome seen after cardiac surgery, occurs in approximately 20 percent of all cases of penetrating heart wounds. Symptomatic management is the treatment of choice for this syndrome unless cardiac tamponade or other sequelae, such as purulent or constrictive pericarditis, require surgical intervention.

Missile wounds also may result in the presence of a projectile within the heart after either a direct injury to the heart or an injury to a systemic vein with subsequent migration of the missile to the heart. The missile or the thrombus associated with it may embolize into the systemic or pulmonary arteries.[36–38] Bacterial endocarditis also may occur if the projectile is not completely embedded in the myocardium.[39,40] Rarely, a patient with a projectile in the heart may develop cardiac neurosis, with an almost maniacal desire for removal of the foreign body.[41] In many patients, however, the retained missile in the heart results in no ill effects over a long period of observation.[42,43] Therefore, treatment for missiles in the heart should be individualized according to the patient's clinical course and the location, size, and shape of the missile.[42,43] Missiles that cause symptoms should be removed. Similarly, missiles that are free or partially protruding into a left cardiac chamber should be removed, because their embolization to the systemic arterial system may have serious consequences.[42,43] Missiles in the right side of the heart may be removed or left to embolize to the pulmonary vascular bed, from which they can be retrieved easily.[37] Intramyocardial and intrapericardial bullets and pellets are generally well tolerated and may be left in place.

A missile that has embolized to the systemic arterial bed should be removed surgically without delay unless it has resulted in a significant neurologic deficit.[38] Projectiles adjacent to or embedded within the wall of one of the great or coronary arteries should be extracted to prevent subsequent erosion and bleeding.

Coronary Artery Penetrating Trauma

Coronary artery injuries can result in cardiac tamponade and varying degrees of myocardial ischemia or myocardial infarction. The management of these wounds is dependent on the amount of myocardium at risk. Wounds of major branches of the coronary arterial system are repaired or bypassed, whereas small terminal vessels are ligated. Coronary artery aneurysms and arteriovenous fistulas are rare sequelae of injury, and their treatment should be individualized.[44]

Penetrating Trauma of the Aorta and Great Vessels

The pathophysiology of penetrating wounds to the great vessels is quite similar to that of penetrating wounds to the heart and depends on whether the site of the wound is intra- or extrapericardial.[45,46] In addition to the obvious results of immediate or delayed hemorrhage, a penetrating wound of a great vessel may result in the formation of a false aneurysm, with possible subsequent rupture, or an arteriovenous fistula, producing immediate or latent signs and symptoms of congestive heart failure.[47] Traumatic arteriovenous fistulas occasionally are complicated by the development of bacterial endarteritis and endocarditis.[48] These traumatic vascular lesions should be detected and repaired as soon as possible.

NONPENETRATING INJURIES

The vast majority of blunt injuries to the heart are due to automobile accidents, although other forms of trauma from contact sports, altercations, falls, and so on also may result in this type of injury. The cardiac injury usually is caused by direct compressing or decelerating forces delivered to the chest or rarely by an indirect force delivered to the abdomen or even to the extremities that results in a marked increase in intravascular pressures. A wide variety of injuries are produced by nonpenetrating trauma (Table 79-2).

Cardiac Contusion

Contusion of the heart usually refers to blunt injury to the heart that causes identifiable histopathologic changes within the myocardium. The pathologic lesions of myocardial contusion vary considerably in extent and character, ranging from small areas of petechiae or ecchymosis, which may be either subepicardial or subendocardial, to contusion of the full thickness of the myocardial wall with or without rupture of the heart.[1]

Histologically, various degrees of subepicardial or intramyocardial hemorrhage or disruption of the myocardial fibers and leukocyte infiltration and edema may be present.[1] The forces that produce nonpenetrating lesions of the heart are such that external evidence of chest injury may be meager or undetectable in almost one-third of traumatized patients. This lack of evidence of chest wall injury and the frequent absence of symptoms from the cardiac injury, along with the common presence of other, more obvious injuries to the body, may impede the early diagnosis of cardiac contusion.

TABLE 79-2 Nonpenetrating Trauma of the Heart

1. Pericardial injury
   a. Hemopericardium
   b. Rupture or laceration
   c. Serofibrinous pericarditis
   d. Constrictive pericarditis
2. Myocardial injury
   a. Contusion
   b. Rupture of free cardiac wall, early or delayed
   c. Rupture of septum
   d. Aneurysm
   e. Laceration
3. Disturbances of rhythm or conduction
4. Valve injury
   a. Rupture of valve leaflets, cusp, or chordae tendineae
   b. Contusion of papillary muscle
5. Coronary artery injury
   a. Thrombosis with or without myocardial infarction
   b. Arteriovenous fistula
   c. Laceration with or without myocardial infarction
6. Great vessel injury
   a. Rupture
   b. Aneurysm formation
   c. Aorta-cardiac chamber fistula
   d. Thrombotic occlusion

Patients with contusions of the heart are commonly asymptomatic, but they may complain of pain that is identical in character, location, and radiation to the pain of myocardial ischemia and/or myocardial infarction.[49] The pain is usually transient unless there is concomitant coronary artery injury or occult atherosclerotic coronary heart disease.[50] Coronary thrombosis can result from nonpenetrating trauma, but this is rare and usually is associated with existing atherosclerotic coronary artery disease.[51] In 546 necropsy cases of nonpenetrating cardiac trauma, no instance of coronary thrombosis was found. Dyspnea and hypotension also may be presenting symptoms. In mild or moderate myocardial contusion, these signs may be transient and are usually absent. Cardiac failure is relatively rare; when it is present, the possibility of an associated cardiac injury, such as rupture of the ventricular septum or of one of the cardiac valves, is high. Hemopericardium with or without the signs and symptoms of cardiac tamponade may be associated with myocardial contusion. Laceration of a coronary artery from a nonpenetrating injury also may occur rarely, producing cardiac tamponade or a coronary artery fistula.[52]

The diagnosis of cardiac contusion should be suspected in all patients with significant blunt trauma, particularly to the precordium. Unfortunately, none of the currently available diagnostic tests for myocardial contusion can conclusively establish the diagnosis in all patients. The appropriate use and interpretation of the available tests, however, can assist in the diagnosis of myocardial contusion with reasonable accuracy.

Electrocardiography has been the most widely used test for the diagnosis of contusion of the heart. Various electrocardiographic abnormalities have been considered suggestive of cardiac contusion, such as nonspecific ST-T or Q-wave changes, supraventricular tachyarrhythmias, and ventricular arrhythmias, including fibrillation, which is usually the cause of death at the time of the traumatic impact.[53–55] However, a variety of other clinical conditions[56–59] that are frequently present in traumatized patients (i.e., pain, anxiety, hemorrhage, hypoxia, hypokalemia, head trauma, alcohol or cocaine toxicity) may cause many of these abnormalities. Therefore, the presence of these other causes must be excluded before the electrocardiographic abnormalities are attributed to contusion of the heart.[60–62]

Elevation of the serum level of the MB fraction of creatinine kinase (CK) has been extrapolated from its use in acute myocardial infarction as a diagnostic aid in patients with cardiac contusion. Other clinical conditions that cause elevation in the level of this enzyme—i.e., tachyarrhythmias and skeletal muscle diseases, including trauma (see Chap. 42)—must be excluded before an abnormal level is ascribed to contusion of the heart.[60–62]

Radioisotope imaging of the heart in dogs with experimentally produced cardiac contusion has identified the area of injury only in animals with a full-thickness contusion.[63] Therefore, this is of diagnostic value in only a limited number of patients, since the incidence of full-thickness contusion is low in patients who survive the initial traumatic impact.

Two-dimensional transthoracic and transesophageal echocardiography (TTE and TEE) are useful in the diagnosis of cardiac contusion, particularly of the structural lesions associated with cardiac contusion.[64,65] The sensitivity and specificity of these tests for diagnosing contusion of the heart, however, have not been clearly defined (see Chap. 13).

Circulating cardiac troponin I was measured in a limited number of blunt trauma victims. It was concluded that this test is accurate for diagnosing cardiac contusion.[66] However additional studies are needed to determine its absolute accuracy.

The treatment of myocardial contusion is symptomatic. Appropriate limitation of activity and prevention and early treatment of arrhythmias are the most important therapeutic measures. The possible increased sensitivity of the heart to medications also must be considered when one is deciding what drugs to use in a patient with recent trauma.

Anticoagulants immediately after an injury should be avoided if possible because they may cause bleeding within the myocardium or pericardial space. Congestive heart failure should be treated with angiotensin-converting enzyme (ACE) inhibitors, and antiarrhythmic agents should be used to control ectopic rhythms as appropriate (see Chap. 24). If the myocardial contusion is severe, support with inotropic drugs (see Chap. 23) may be necessary. When all these measures fail, balloon counterpulsation[67] or even a left ventricular assist device[68] may be utilized.

Cardiac Rupture

Although minor, insignificant myocardial contusion of the right ventricle is the most common blunt cardiac injury; the most fatal lesion is rupture of the heart. The rupture may occur in the free cardiac wall or the ventricular septum. Rupture of the free cardiac wall is extremely difficult to diagnose and treat in a timely manner because of the frequently rapid demise of the patient and because traumatic cardiac rupture is often only one of many severe bodily injuries. As a result, rupture of the heart frequently has not been amenable to therapy. Readily available echocardiography in some emergency rooms, however, may increase the number of successfully treated patients.[69] The surgical repair of interventricular septal rupture is accomplished optimally after the patient has been stablized with medical therapy.

Residual or Delayed Sequelae of Blunt Injury to the Heart

Contusion of the heart usually heals with little or no obvious scarring or impairment of cardiac function. Large contusions, however, may cause a decrease in cardiac output, and extensive necrosis may lead to rupture or, rarely, congestive heart failure and the formation of a true or false aneurysm.[70] Cardiac aneurysms may cause arrhythmias, congestive heart failure, rupture, and mural thrombosis with embolism. Because of these complications, surgical repair of a traumatic aneurysm is usually advisable. Localized areas of necrosis and hemorrhage involving the cardiac conduction system may produce varying degrees of atrioventricular block or any of the different types of intraventricular conduction defects.

The most commonly injured valve in surviving patients is the aortic valve, with aortic regurgitation characteristically causing the rapid development of congestive heart failure. Injury of the atrioventricular valves is an uncommon result of nonpenetrating cardiac injury and usually occurs in the presence of severe cardiac trauma, resulting in death. Rupture of the mitral valve leaflet can have hemodynamic consequences somewhat similar to those of aortic valve injury but rarely is encountered clinically. In contrast, tricuspid valve injury may be tolerated for years before surgical correction is required.[71]

Rupture of the papillary muscle or chordae tendineae occurs more frequently than does rupture of valve leaflets. Cardiac contusion also may cause papillary muscle dysfunction with secondary mitral or tricuspid regurgitation.[72] The clinical outcome depends on whether the structures involved are on the right side of the heart, where the lesion may be well tolerated, or the left side, where the high-pressure system can lead to more serious hemodynamic sequelae. The murmurs produced by these lesions are generally typical of valvular regurgitation, but unusual high-pitched systolic and diastolic murmurs of variable loudness also may result (see Chap. 10). Traumatic tricuspid regurgitation may be present despite the absence of detectable murmur.[73] Prompt and correct diagnosis by echocardiographic, hemodynamic, and angiographic studies is important. Patients with hemodynamically significant valvular injury should undergo valvuloplasty or valve replacement.

Pericardial lesions often are overlooked and frequently heal without incident. Hemopericardium may occur but usually is due to the coexisting myocardial injury. When the hemorrhage is severe, cardiac tamponade occurs rapidly. When the oozing of blood or serum into the pericardium is slow, however, dilatation of the pericardial sac can develop over an extended period.

Posttraumatic pericarditis, which is similar to the post–myocardial infarction syndrome, develops less frequently with blunt than with penetrating cardiac injuries. The symptoms and signs of posttraumatic pericarditis are similar to those of pericarditis produced by a wide variety of causes (see Chap. 72). When hemopericardium or hydropericardium is suspected, echocardiography can confirm the diagnosis. Pericardial laceration usually is well tolerated, but herniation of the heart may occur, leading to more serious consequences and death.[74,75]

Aortic Rupture

Rupture of the aorta is the most common blunt injury of the great vessels. Rupture or avulsion of the innominate, carotid, or left subclavian arteries or the venae cavae also has been observed. Because of the variety of mechanical forces produced by blunt trauma (Fig. 79-1), combined with anatomic factors, the most common sites of rupture of the aorta from blunt injury

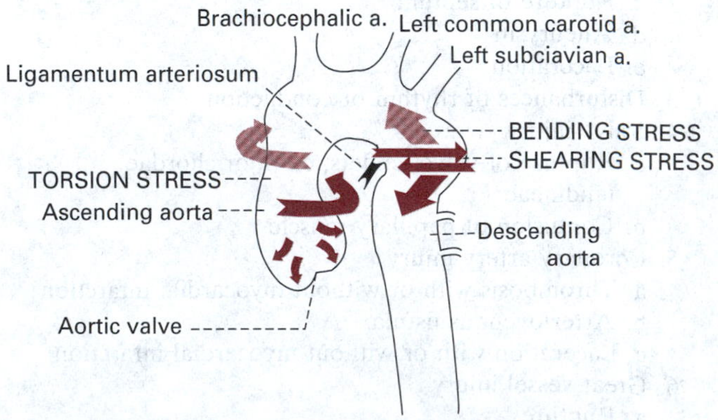

FIGURE 79-1 Diagrammatic illustration of the forces acting on the aortic wall during rupture of the aorta from blunt trauma. (From Symbas PN. *Traumatic Injuries of the Heart and Great Vessels*. Springfield, IL: Charles C Thomas; 1971:153. Courtesy of Charles C Thomas, Publisher, Springfield, Illinois.)

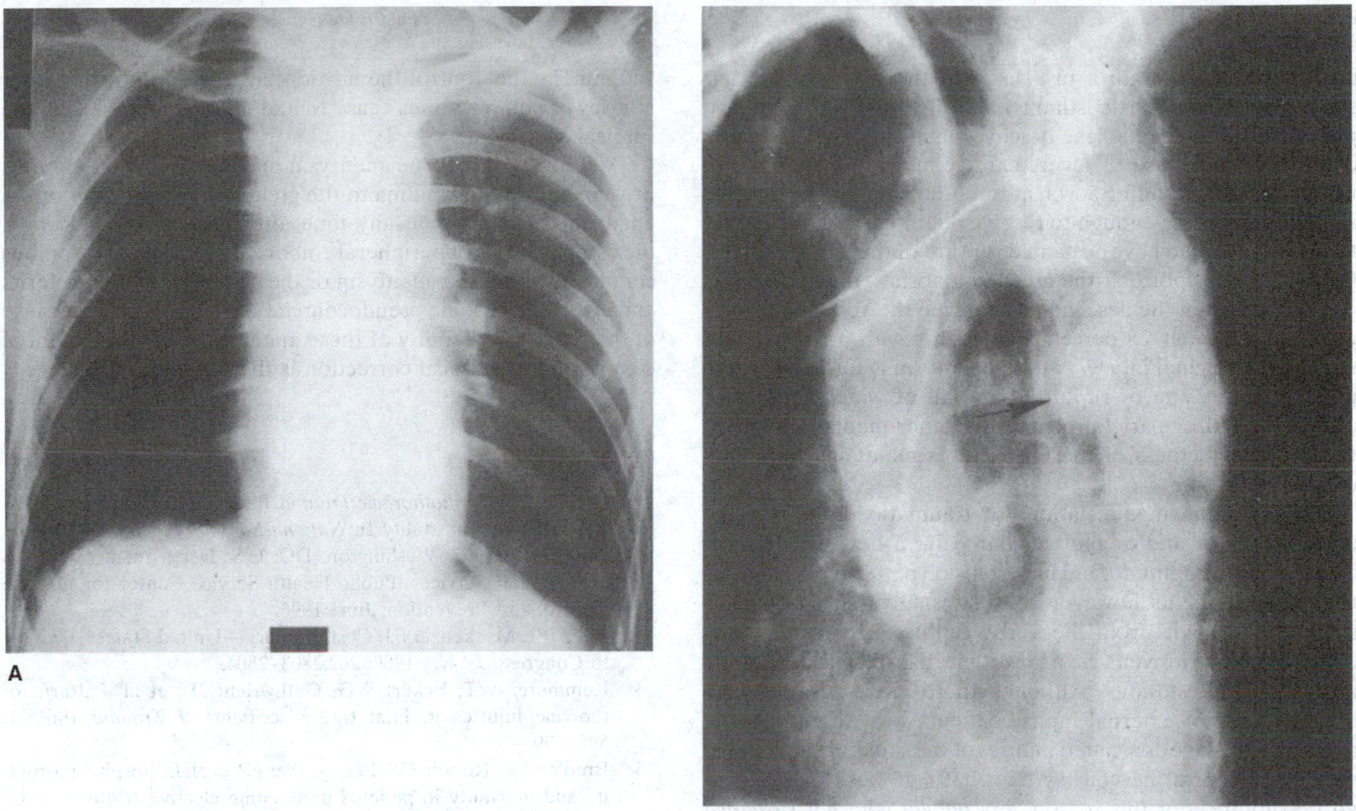

A

B

FIGURE 79-2 *A.* Chest roentgenogram of a young man who shortly before admission was involved in an automobile accident. Note the mediastinal widening. *B.* Aortogram the same day showing a false aneurysm distal to the origin of the left subclavian artery and two filling defects, one proximal and one distal to the aneurysm.

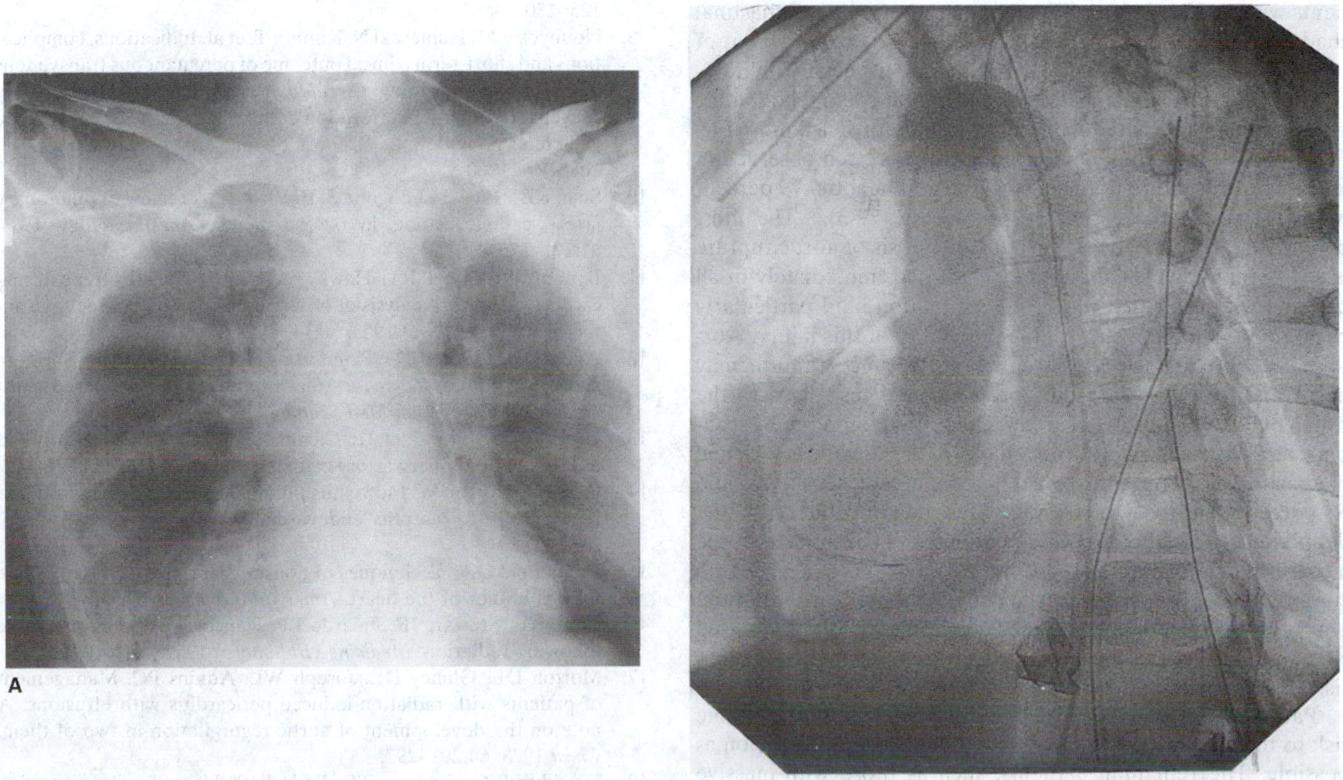

A

B

FIGURE 79-3 *A.* Chest roentgenogram of a young man shortly after a vehicular accident. *B.* Aortogram showing rupture of the ascending aorta.

are the descending aorta just distal to the origin of the left subclavian artery (aortic isthmus) and the ascending aorta just proximal to the origin of the brachycephalic artery.[76,77] Because of the high incidence of severe cardiac injury in patients with rupture of the ascending aorta, most of the patients who survive aortic rupture long enough to receive definitive surgical correction are those who have sustained rupture of the aortic isthmus. Occasionally, rupture at the ascending aorta,[78] the aortic arch, and other sites of the descending and even the abdominal aorta may occur. About 20 percent of patients with aortic rupture survive the original injury. A false aneurysm is formed in these patients at the site of rupture, the wall of which consists of adventitia and/or parietal pleura and other mediastinal structures. The intactness of these structures maintains continuity of the circulation.

The common manifestations of traumatic rupture of the aorta are chest and/or midscapular pain, a new murmur, increased pulse amplitude, and hypertension of the upper extremities.[79] Some patients, however, are surprisingly free of any major symptoms or signs from the aortic rupture. Hoarseness, evidence of a superior vena cava syndrome, paraplegia, and anuria are rare manifestations. Although there are occasionally no obvious signs of external injury, patients with rupture of the aorta usually have associated injuries of the skeleton, abdominal viscera, or central nervous system that can mask the signs of aortic rupture. For this reason, *any patient who has sustained severe blunt trauma or has been exposed to major deceleration forces should be suspected of having aortic rupture if there is an increased pulse pressure, upper extremity hypertension, and especially widening of the upper mediastinal silhouette.*

Chest roentgenography is of great diagnostic value in patients with aortic rupture. Widening of the superior mediastinal shadow, depression of the left main bronchus, displacement of the trachea and esophagus to the right, and especially obliteration of the aortic knob shadow are common roentgenographic abnormalities associated with injury at the aortic isthmus (Fig. 79-2). Widening of the mediastinum also has been observed in all cases with rupture of the aortic arch and in about 79 percent with rupture of the ascending aorta (Fig. 79-3).[78] The most definitive procedure to establish the diagnosis of aortic rupture is aortography, which should be performed immediately in all patients whose history, physical examination, and particularly chest roentgenogram suggest the possibility of this injury. Aortography should include the entire aorta, since rupture may occur at sites other than the aortic segment just distal to the origin of the left subclavian artery. Computed tomography scanning also is used widely to evaluate patients with a widened mediastinum.[80] The approximately 55 percent sensitivity and 65 percent sensitivity of this test limit its contribution to the definitive management of these patients.[81] TEE appears to be a useful diagnostic test[66] (see Chap. 13), but there has been no comprehensive study of its diagnostic value for aortic rupture. Until further experience is gained, caution should be exercised when it is used as the sole technique for establishing the diagnosis. Treatment should be undertaken as soon as possible.

Patients with no other organ injuries that add unacceptable risk to the surgical treatment should be operated on as soon as possible. The remaining patients, such as those with massive pulmonary injury, major central nervous injury, or retroperitoneal bleeding, may be treated medically with vasodilators or beta blockers to maintain the systemic blood pressure below 140 mmHg and control the aortic wall tension until the other injuries or complications cease to add unacceptable risk to the surgical treatment.[82]

A chronic false aortic aneurysm may be discovered months or years after blunt trauma to the great vessels. Rupture of the aneurysm may occur at any time after its formation. Rarely, the complications of peripheral embolization from the thrombus contained within the aneurysm or the development of bacterial endaortitis or chronic pseudocoarctation may occur.[83] Because of the relative instability of these aneurysms and the potential complications, surgical correction is the treatment of choice.

References

1. Symbas PN. *Cardiothoracic Trauma.* Philadelphia: Saunders; 1989.
2. James S. Injury mortality. In: *National Summary of Injury Mortality Data, 1987–1993.* Washington, DC: U.S. Department of Health and Human Services, Public Health Service Center for Disease Control and Prevention; June 1996.
3. Price PR, Mackenzie EJ. Cost of injury—United States: A report to Congress. *JAMA* 1989; 262:2803–2804.
4. Kemmerer WT, Eckert WG, Gathwright JB, et al. Patterns of thoracic injuries in fatal traffic accidents. *J Trauma* 1961; 1: 595–599.
5. Bredlau CE, Roubin GS, Leimgruber PP, et al. In-hospital morbidity and mortality in patients undergoing elective coronary angioplasty. *Circulation* 1985; 72:1044–1052.
6. Gaul G, Hollman J, Simpendorfer C, Franco I. Acute occlusion in multiple lesion coronary angioplasty: Frequency and management. *J Am Coll Cardiol* 1989; 13:283–288.
7. Safian RD, Berman AD, Diver DJ, et al. Balloon aortic valvuloplasty in 170 consecutive patients. *N Engl J Med* 1988; 319: 125–130.
8. Nobuyoshi M, Hamasaki N, Kimura T, et al. Indications, complications and short-term clinical outcome of percutaneous transvenous mitral commissurotomy. *Circulation* 1989; 80:782–792.
9. Meyer JA, Millar K. Perforation of the right ventricle by electrode catheters: A review and report of nine cases. *Ann Surg* 1968; 168:1048–1060.
10. Shah KB, Rao TL, Laughlin S, El Etr AA. A review of pulmonary artery catheterization in 6245 patients. *Anesthesiology* 1984; 61:271–275.
11. Bynum WR, Conell RM, Hawk WA. Causes of death after external cardiac massage: Analysis of observations on fifty consecutive autopsies. *Cleve Clin Q* 1963; 30:147–151.
12. Agdal N, Jorgensen TG. Penetrating laceration of the pericardium and myocardium and myocardial rupture following closed chest cardiac massage. *Acta Med Scand* 1973; 194:477–479.
13. Greene JF Jr, Fitzwater JE, Clemmer TP. Septic endocarditis and indwelling pulmonary artery catheters. *JAMA* 1975; 233:891–892.
14. Pace NL, Horton W. Indwelling pulmonary artery catheters: Their relationship to aseptic endocardial vegetation. *JAMA* 1975; 233:893–894.
15. Bloomfield DA. Techniques of nonsurgical retrieval of iatrogenic foreign bodies of the heart. *Am J Cardiol* 1971; 27:538–545.
16. Cohn KE, Stewart JR, Fajardo LF, Hancock EW. Heart disease following radiation. *Medicine* (*Baltimore*) 1967; 46:281–298.
17. Morton DL, Glancy DL, Joseph WL, Adkins PC. Management of patients with radiation-induced pericarditis with effusions: A note on the development of aortic regurgitation in two of them. *Chest* 1973; 64:291–297.
18. De Silva RA, Graboys TB, Podrid PJ, Lown B. Cardioversion and defibrillation. *Am Heart J* 1980; 100:881–895.
19. Bernstein T. Effects of electricity and lightning on man and animals. *J Forensic Sci* 1973; 18:3–11.

20. Jackson SH, Parry DJ. Lightning and the heart. *Br Heart J* 1980; 43:454–527.
21. Moritz AR, Atkins JP. Cardiac contusions: An experimental and pathologic study. *Arch Pathol* 1938; 25:445–462.
22. Samson PC. Battle wounds and injuries of the heart and pericardium: Experiences in forward hospitals. *Ann Surg* 1948; 127:1127–1149.
23. Symbas PN, Harlaftis N, Waldo WJ. Penetrating wounds: A comparison of different therapeutic methods. *Ann Surg* 1976; 183:377–381.
24. Symbas PN. *Cardiothoracic Trauma: Current Problems in Surgery.* St. Louis: Mosby Year Book; 1991:742.
25. Thourani VH, Filiciano DV, Cooper WA, et al. Penetrating cardiac trauma at an urban trauma center: A 22-year experience. *Am Surg* 1999; 65: 811–818.
26. Trinkle JK, Toon RS, Franz JL, et al. Affairs of the wounded heart: Penetrating cardiac wounds. *J Trauma* 1979; 19:467–472.
27. Ivatury RR, Rohman M, Steichen FM, et al. Penetrating cardiac injuries: Twenty-year experience. *Am Surg* 1987; 53:310–317.
28. Attar S, Suter CM, Hankins JR, et al. Penetrating cardiac injuries. *Ann Thorac Surg* 1991; 51:711–716.
29. Knott-Craig CJ, Dalton RP, Rossouw GJ, Barnard PM. Penetrating cardiac trauma: Management strategy based on 129 surgical emergencies over 2 years. *Ann Thorac Surg* 1992; 53:1006–1009.
30. Mitchell ME, Muakkassa FF, Poole GV, et al. Surgical approach of choice for penetrating cardiac wounds. *J Trauma* 1993; 34:17–20.
31. Cooper FW Jr, Stead EA Jr, Warren JV. The beneficial effect of intravenous infusions in acute cardiac tamponade. *Ann Surg* 1944; 120:822–825.
32. Rozycki GS, Feliciano DV, Schmidt JA, et al. The role of surgeon-performed ultrasound in patients with possible cardiac wounds. *Ann Surg* 1996; 224:1–8.
33. Symbas PN, DiOrio DA, Tyras DH, et al. Penetrating cardiac wounds: Significant residual and delayed sequelae. *J Thorac Cardiovasc Surg* 1973; 6:526–532.
34. Symbas PN. *Traumatic Heart Disease: Current Problems in Cardiology.* St Louis: Mosby Year Book; 1991:539.
35. Whisennand HH, Van Pelt SA, Beall AC Jr, et al. Surgical management of traumatic intracardiac injuries. *Ann Thorac Surg* 1979; 28:530–536.
36. Bland EF, Beebe GW. Missles in the heart: A 20-year follow-up report of world war cases. *N Engl J Med* 1966; 274:1039–1046.
37. Symbas PN, Hatcher CR Jr, Mansour KA. Projectile embolus of the lung. *J Thorac Cardiovasc Surg* 1968; 56:97–103.
38. Symbas PN, Harlaftis N. Bullet emboli in the pulmonary and systemic arteries. *Ann Surg* 1977; 185:318–320.
39. Decker HR. Foreign bodies in the heart and pericardium: Should they be removed? *J Thorac Surg* 1939; 9:62.
40. Harken DE. Experiments in intracardiac surgery: I. Bacterial endocarditis. *J Thorac Surg* 1942; 11:656–670.
41. Turner GG. Bullets in the heart for 23 years. *Surgery* 1942; 9:832–852.
42. Symbas PN, Picone AL, Hatcher CR Jr, Vlasis SE. Cardiac missles: A review of the literature and personal experience. *Ann Surg* 1990; 211:639–648.
43. Symbas PN, Vlasis SE, Picone AL, Hatcher CR Jr. Missles in the heart. *Ann Thorac Surg* 1989; 48:192–194.
44. Konecke LL, Spitzer S, Mason D, et al. Traumatic aneurysm of the left coronary artery. *Am J Cardiol* 1971; 27:221–223.
45. Symbas PN, Sehdava JS. Penetrating wounds of the thoracic aorta. *Ann Surg* 1970; 171:441–450.
46. Symbas PN, Kourias E, Tyras DH, Hatcher CR Jr. Penetrating wounds of the great vessels. *Ann Surg* 1974; 179:757–762.
47. Symbas PN, Schlant RC, Logan WD Jr, et al. Traumatic aorticopulmonary fistula complicated by postoperative low cardiac output treated with dopamine. *Ann Surg* 1967; 165:614–619.
48. Parmley LF Jr, Orbison JA, Hughes CW, Mattingly TW. Acquired arteriovenous fistulas complicated by endarteritis and endocarditis lenta due to *Streptococcus faecalis. N Engl J Med* 1954; 250: 305–309.
49. Kissane RW. Traumatic heart diseases, especially myocardial contusion. *Postgrad Med* 1954; 15:114–119.
50. Stern T, Wolf RY, Reichart B, et al. Coronary artery occlusion resulting from blunt trauma. *JAMA* 1974; 230:1308–1309.
51. Levy H. Traumatic coronary thrombosis with myocardial infarction: Postmortem study. *Arch Intern Med* 1949; 84:261–276.
52. Forker AD, Morgan JR. Acquired coronary artery fistula from nonpenetrating chest injury. *JAMA* 1971; 215:289–291.
53. Louhimo I. Heart injury after blunt thoracic trauma: An experimental study on rabbits. *Acta Chir Scand Suppl* 1968; 380:1–60.
54. Dolara A, Morando P, Pampaloni M. Electrocardiographic findings in 98 consecutive nonpenetrating chest injuries. *Dis Chest* 1967; 52:50–56.
55. Jones FL Jr. Transmural myocardial necrosis after nonpenetrating cardiac trauma. *Am J Cardiol* 1970; 26:419–422.
56. Potkin RT, Werner JA, Trobaugh GB, et al. Evaluation of noninvasive tests of cardiac damage in suspected cardiac contusion. *Circulation* 1982; 66:627–631.
57. Hoffman B. The genesis of cardiac arrhythmias. *Prog Cardiovasc Dis* 1966; 8:319–329.
58. Marriott HJ, Nizet PM. Physiologic stimuli simulating ischemic heart disease. *JAMA* 1967; 200:715.
59. Tindall GT, Iwata K, McGraw CP, Vanderveer RW. Cardiorespiratory changes associated with intracranial pressure waves: Evaluation of these changes in 27 patients with head injuries. *South Med J* 1975; 68:407–412.
60. Rapaport E. Serum enzymes and isoenzymes in the diagnosis of acute myocardial infarction. *Mod Concepts Cardiovasc Dis* 1977; 46:43–46.
61. Manor A, Alpan G. Specificity of creatine kinase MB isoenzyme for myocardial injury. *Clin Chem* 1978; 24:2206.
62. Snow N, Richardson JD, Flynt LM Jr. Myocardial contusion: Implication for patients with multiple traumatic injuries. *Surgery* 1982; 92:744–750.
63. Gonzalez AC, Harlaftis N, Gravanis M, Symbas PN. Imaging of experimental myocardial contusion: Observations and pathologic correlations. *AJR* 1977; 128:1039–1040.
64. Miller FA Jr, Seward JB, Gersh BJ, et al. Two-dimensional echocardiographic findings in cardiac trauma. *Am J Cardiol* 1982; 50:1022–1027.
65. Shapiro NG, Yanofsky SD, Trapp I, et al. Cardiovascular evaluation in thoracic blunt trauma using transesophageal echocardiography (TEE). *J Trauma* 1991; 131:835–839.
66. Adams JE III, Davila-Roman VG, Bessey PQ, et al. Improved detection of cardiac contusion with cardiac troponin I. *Am Heart J* 1996; 131:308–312.
67. Snow N, Luca AE, Richardson JD. Intra-aortic balloon counterpulsation for cardiogenic shock from cardiac contusion. *J Trauma* 1982; 22:426–429.
68. Chavanon O, Dutheil V, Hacini R, et al. Treatment of severe cardiac contusion with a left ventricular assist device in a patient with multiple trauma. *J Thorac Cardivasc Surg* 1999; 118:189–190.
69. Symbas NP, Bongiorno PF, Symbas PN. Blunt cardiac rupture: The utility of emergency department ultrasound. *Ann Thorac Surg* 1999; 67:1274–1276.
70. Singh R, Nolan SP, Schrank JP. Traumatic left ventricular aneurysm: Two cases with normal coronary angiograms. *JAMA* 1975; 234:412–414.
71. Liu S, Sako Y, Alexander CS. Traumatic tricuspid insufficiency. *Am J Cardiol* 1970; 26:200–204.
72. Schroeder JS, Stinson EB, Bieber CP, et al. Papillary muscle dysfunction due to nonpenetrating chest trauma, recognition in a potential cardiac donor. *Br Heart J* 1972; 34:645–647.

73. Marvin RF, Schrank JP, Nolan SP. Traumatic tricuspid insufficiency. *Am J Cardiol* 1973; 32:723–726.
74. Munchow OBG, Carter R, Vannix RS, Anderson FS. Cardiac arrest due to ventricular herniation: Report of a case of two successful cardiac resuscitations. *JAMA* 1960; 173:1350–1351.
75. Anderson M, Fredens M, Olesson KH. Traumatic rupture of the pericardium. *Am J Cardiol* 1971; 27:566–569.
76. Feczko JD, Lynch L, Pless JE, et al. An autopsy case review of 142 nonpenetrating (blunt) injuries of the aorta. *J Trauma* 1992; 33:846–849.
77. Symbas PN, Tyras DH, Ware RE, DiOrio DA. Traumatic rupture of the aorta. *Ann Surg* 1973; 178:6–12.
78. Symbas PJ, Horsley SW, Symbas PN. Rupture of the ascending aorta caused by blunt trauma. *Ann Thorac Surg* 1998; 66:113–117.
79. Symbas PN, Tyras DH, Ware RE, Hatcher CR Jr. Rupture of the aorta: A diagnostic triad. *Ann Thorac Surg* 1973; 15:405–410.
80. Fenner MN, Fisher KS, Sergel NL, et al. Evaluation of possible traumatic thoracic aortic injury using aortography and CT. *Am Surg* 1990; 56:497–499.
81. Miller FB, Richardson JD, Thomas HA, et al. Role of CT in diagnosis of major arterial injury after blunt thoracic trauma. *Surgery* 1989; 106:596–603.
82. Galli R, Pacini O, Di Bartolomeo R, et al. Surgical indication and timing of repair of traumatic ruptures of the aorta. *Ann Thorac Surg* 1998; 65:461–464.
83. Kinley CE, Chandler BM. Traumatic aneurysm of thoracic aorta: A case presenting as coarctation. *Can Med Assoc J* 96:279, 1967.

CHAPTER 80

EFFECTS OF MOOD AND ANXIETY DISORDERS ON THE CARDIOVASCULAR SYSTEM

Dominique L. Musselman / William McDonald / Charles B. Nemeroff

And now here's my secret, a very simple secret: It is only with the heart that one can see rightly; what is essential is invisible to the eye. (Antoine de Saint-Exupery, *The Little Prince,* 1943)

INTRODUCTION: DEPRESSION AND COMORBID MEDICAL ILLNESS

The interactions of personality traits, psychiatric symptoms and syndromes, and environmental stressors with the cardiovascular system have long intrigued investigators interested in the factors that contribute to the development and progression of atherosclerotic heart disease. Differences in rates of ischemic heart disease (IHD) remain substantially unexplained even after surveillance of the well-established risk factors. Although the type A personality pattern has been studied intensely as a risk factor for coronary artery disease (CAD),[1] lack of a consistent association between type A behavior and the subsequent development of IHD has stimulated questions about the contributions of the psychological concept of hostility as well as the syndrome of major depression.[2] Increasing evidence is accumulating suggesting that major depression (Table 80-1),[3] a mood disorder, is associated with drastically elevated morbidity and mortality after an index myocardial infarction (MI) and also acts as an independent risk factor in the development of atherosclerotic heart disease.

Depressive syndromes and major depression are exceedingly common. The most recent comprehensive study done in the United States, the National Comorbidity Study, reported lifetime prevalence rates of major depression and dysthymia of 13 percent and 5 percent, respectively.[4] Point prevalence rates of major depression in primary care outpatients range from 2 to 16 percent and 9 to 20 percent for all depressive disorders[5–9] and are even higher among medical inpatients: 8 percent for major depression and 15 to 36 percent for all depressive disorders.[10,11]

Minor depressive disorder (depressive symptoms subthreshold in severity compared with major depression and dysthymia) is also common in the community[12–15] and in primary care clinics.[6,7,16,17] The Epidemiologic Catchment Area Study of over 18,500 individuals reported the lifetime prevalence rate of subthreshold depressive symptoms to be 23 percent in comparison to 6 percent, the sum of the prevalence rates of major depression and dysthymia.[15] Although depression in patients with CAD is diagnosed infrequently by primary care physicians and cardiologists,[18–22] recognition and treatment of major depression is crucial, especially for patients after an MI. Not only do depressed patients experience great difficulties in problem solving and coping with challenges, depression adversely effects compliance with medical therapy[23] and rehabilitation[24,25] and increases medical comorbidity.[24] Minor depressive disorder also is associated with significant functional impairment and substantial increases in health care utilization.[14,15,26,27]

In patients with CAD, depression predicts future cardiac events[20,28,29] and hastens mortality.[22,30,31] Since the 1960s, multiple cross-sectional and longitudinal studies have scrutinized the association of cardiovascular disease (CVD), especially CAD and congestive heart failure (CHF), with depressive symptoms as well as major depression.

TABLE 80-1 DSM-IV Diagnostic Criteria for Depressive Disorders

Major Depressive Disorder

A. Five or more of the following symptoms have been present during the same 2-week period and represent a change from previous functioning; at least one of the symptoms is either (1) depressed mood or (2) loss of interest or pleasure.
   1. Depressed mood
   2. Markedly diminished interest or pleasure
   3. Significant weight loss or weight gain or decrease or increase in appetite
   4. Insomnia or hypersomnia
   5. Psychomotor agitation or retardation (observable by others)
   6. Fatigue or loss of energy nearly every day
   7. Feelings of worthlessness or excessive or inappropriate guilt
   8. Diminished concentration or indecisiveness
   9. Recurrent thoughts of death (not just fear of dying) or suicide

B. The symptoms cause clinically significant distress or impairment in social, occupation, or other important areas of functioning.

C. The symptoms are not due to the direct physiologic effects of a substance or a general medical condition.

D. The symptoms are not better accounted for by bereavement.

Dysthymic Disorder

A. Depressed mood for most of the day, for more days than not, for at least 2 years

B. Presence, while depressed, of two or more of the following:
   1. Poor appetite or overeating
   2. Insomnia or hypersomnia
   3. Low energy or fatigue
   4. Low self-esteem
   5. Poor concentration or difficulty making decisions
   6. Feelings of hopelessness

C. The disturbance is not better accounted for by a chronic major depressive disorder.

Source: Reprinted with permission from the *Diagnostic and Statistical Manual of Mental Disorders*, 4th ed. Copyright 1994, American Psychiatric Association.

EPIDEMIOLOGY

Depression and Cardiovascular Disease

Early studies reported the prevalence of depression to be 18 to 60 percent in patients with CAD.[18,24,31-34] Later studies reported relatively consistent prevalence rates of depression in patients with CVD (patients with CAD) ranging from 16 to 23 percent (mean, 19 percent; median, 18 percent) despite the potential methodologic weaknesses of some of the studies listed in Table 80-2 (such as the use of unmodified psychiatric diagnostic instruments to determine the prevalence of depression, excluding patients because of the severity of CVD, and measuring depressive symptoms at different times after hospital admission) and methodologic differences among the studies (dissimilar patient populations, different diagnostic instruments, different hospitalization status, unspecified type of heart disease).

Although the prevalence of major depressive symptoms in patients hospitalized for CHF has not been as well studied, preliminary evidence indicates that these patients have equally high or even higher rates of major depression.[37,39] However, although severity of physical illness is one of the most important variables associated with depression in patients with other medical illnesses, studies of patients with CVD do not always document a higher prevalence rate of depression in patients with measures of more advanced CVD or a greater level of disability.[20-22,31]

Depression as a Risk Factor for Ischemic Heart Disease

The notion that having a psychiatric illness such as major depression increases one's risk for developing ischemic heart disease remains controversial and often has been "explained" intuitively by the hypothesis that persons with psychiatric disorders generally have other risk factors for the development of CAD.[1] Table 80-3 describes the studies with the most rigorous methods: Those studies have been prospective in design, have used structured clinical interviews or diagnostic instruments, have included other risk factors for CVD in their analyses (such as hypertension, hypercholesterolemia, nicotine and other substance abuse, and physical inactivity), and have been controlled for demographic factors (such as age, sex, and socioeconomic status).

Nearly all the recent studies in Table 80-3 document increased cardiovascular morbidity and mortality in patients with depressive symptoms or major depression, implicating depression *as an independent risk factor* in the pathophysiologic progression of CVD rather than merely as a secondary emotional response to cardiovascular illness. Such large epidemiologic studies may use self-report instruments rather than clinical interviews to evaluate the importance of psychological factors in predicting CVD. Assessments of this type typically are added to large, multiple-risk-factor studies in which population-based samples are followed up prospectively.[1] The advantage of using "dimensional" measures of depression (rather than a categorical diagnosis of major depression) lies in the increased statistical power that allows these studies to detect smaller "effects." However, such epidemiologic data are not equivalent to clinical data. A relatively large clinical study supporting depression as an independent risk factor for CVD observed that patients with major depression experienced elevated mortality rates after an MI. Frasure-Smith and colleagues[22,31] found depression to be a significant predictor of mortality ($p < .001$) in 222 patients 6 months after an MI. Depression remained a significant predictor of mortality ($p = .01$) even after multivariate statistical methodology was used to factor out the effects of left ventricular dysfunction and previous MI. Multiple logistic regression analyses revealed that depression was significantly related to 18-month cardiac mortality even after controlling for other significant multivariate predictors of mortality [previous MI, Killip class,

TABLE 80-2 Prevalence of Major Depression in Patients with Cardiovascular Disease

Study	No./Type of Patients	Diagnostic Method	Prevalence, %
Carney et al., 1988[28]	52 CAD patients undergoing elective cardiac catheterization	DIS[35]	18
Schleifer et al., 1989[21]	283 patients hospitalized with MI	SADS[36]	18
Freedland et al., 1991[37]	60 patients hospitalized for CHF	Modified DIS[35]	17
Frasure-Smith et al., 1993[22]	222 patients hospitalized with MI	DIS[35]	16
Gonzalez et al., 1996[38]	99 hospitalized patients with CAD	DIS[35]	23
Koenig et al., 1998[39]	107 patients hospitalized with primary or secondary diagnosis of CHF	Expanded DIS[35]	37

ABBREVATIONS: CAD = coronary artery disease; MI = myocardial infarction; DIS = Diagnostic Interview Schedule, Version III; SADS = Schedule for Affective Disorders and Schizophrenia.

SOURCE: Adapted from and reprinted with permission from *Archives of General Psychiatry* 55:580–592, July 1998. Copyrighted 1998, American Medical Association.

frequency of premature ventricular contractions (PVCs)] (p = .003).

PATHOPHYSIOLOGY

Hypothalamic-Pituitary-Adrenocortical and Sympathomedullary Hyperactivity

Recent advances in biological psychiatry have included the discovery of numerous neurochemical, neuroendocrine, and neuroanatomic alterations in unipolar depression. Often proposed as important adjuncts in the diagnosis of depressed subjects, some of these biological markers may reflect important pathophysiologic alterations that contribute to the increased vulnerability of depressed patients to CVD. These markers include sympathoadrenal hyperactivity, diminished heart rate variability (HRV), alterations in platelet receptors and/or reactivity, and ventricular instability and myocardial ischemia in reaction to mental stress (Fig. 80-1, Plate 110).

Two primary components that are central to the "fight or flight" stress response observed by Cannon in 1911[62] and the "general adaptation syndrome" described by Selye in 1956[63] are the hypothalamic-pituitary-adrenocortical axis and the sympathoadrenal system. In response to stress, hypothalamic neurons containing corticotropin-releasing factor (CRF) increase the synthesis and release of corticotropin (ACTH), β-endorphin, and other pro-opiomelanocortin (POMC) products from the anterior pituitary gland. Many studies have documented evidence of hypothalamic-pituitary-adrenocortical axis hyperactivity in medication-free patients with major depression, i.e., elevated CRF concentrations in cerebrospinal fluid,[64–69] blunting of the ACTH response to CRF administration, nonsuppression of cortisol secretion after dexamethasone administration, hypercortisolemia, and pituitary and adrenal gland enlargement, as well as direct evidence of increased numbers of hypothalamic CRF neurons in postmortem brain tissue from depressed patients compared with controls.[70,71] Administered corticosteroids have long been known to induce hypercholesterolemia, hypertriglyceridemia, and hypertension. Other atherosclerosis-inducing actions of steroids include injury to vascular endothelial cells[72] and intima[73–75] and the inhibition of normal healing.[76] Indeed, elevated morning plasma cortisol concentrations have been significantly correlated with moderate to severe coronary atherosclerosis in young and middle-aged men.[77]

Many patients with major depression also exhibit dysregulation of the sympathoadrenal system. The adrenal medulla and sympathetic nervous system (SNS) together constitute the sympathoadrenal system. Although central nervous system (CNS) regulation of the sympathoadrenal system has been only partially characterized, hypothalamic CRF-containing neurons provide stimulatory input to several autonomic centers that are involved in regulating sympathetic activity.[78–80] Nerve impulses from regulatory centers in the CNS control catecholamine release from the sympathoadrenal system. Physiologic and pathologic conditions causing sympathoadrenal activation include physical activity, coronary artery ischemia, heart failure, and mental stress. Epinephrine in plasma is derived from the adrenal medulla, whereas plasma norepinephrine (NE) concentrations reflect the secretion of NE largely from sympathetic nerve terminals, with the remaining NE provided by the adrenal medulla and extraadrenal chromaffin cells. Peripheral plasma NE concentrations are determined not only by the rate of release from sympathetic nervous system nerve terminals but also by reuptake into presynaptic terminals, local metabolic degradation, and redistribution into multiple physiologic compartments. Hypersecretion of NE in unipolar depression has been documented by elevated plasma NE and NE metabolite concentrations[81–84] and elevated urinary concentrations of NE and its metabolites. Not only do depressed patients exhibit higher basal plasma concentrations of NE, those with melancholia exhibit even greater elevations in plasma NE concentrations when subjected to orthostatic challenge than do normal control subjects and depressed patients *without* melancholia.[85] Furthermore, depressed patients who are dexamethasone (DST) nonsuppressors exhibit significantly higher basal and cold-stimulated plasma concentrations of NE than do depressed patients who are DST suppressors.[85] After treatment with tricyclic antidepressants (TCAs), urinary excretion of NE and its metabolites diminishes together with plasma NE concentrations,[86–91] although Veith and colleagues[84] reported that chronic treatment with desipramine increased plasma concentrations of NE. Thus, sympathoadrenal hyperactivity seems to represent a state rather than a state or

TABLE 80-3 Antecedent Depression and Subsequent Risk of Cardiovascular Disease

Source	No./Type of Patients	Diagnostic Method	Relative Risk (RR) of Major Depression or Depressive Symptoms for Cardiac Disease or Cardiac Disease–Related Death
Ostfeld et al., 1964[40]	1990 male patients Western Electric Employees	MMPI[41] 16 PF[42]	None
Brozek et al., 1966[43]	258 men	MMPI[41]	None
Goldberg et al., 1979[44]	82 pairs (male and female) of case-control subjects randomly selected from two communities	CES-D Scale[45] and four other depression scales	None
Murphy et al., 1987[46]	1003 male and female subjects from the community	DPAX algorithm[47]	For cardiovascular disease-related death: Men 2.5 Women 1.5
Anda et al., 1993[48]	2832 men and women (age 45–77)	Depression subscale of GWS[49]	For IHD-related death: Depressed affect 1.5 [95% confidence interval (CI): 1.0–2.3] Severe hopelessness 2.1 (95% CI: 1.1–3.9)
Aromaa et al., 1994[29]	5355 men and women (age 40–64)	PSE[50]	For MI: Men 2.62 Women 1.90
Vogt et al., 1994[51]	1187 men and 1386 women (age 18 and older) in an HMO	Depression scale[52]	Depressive symptoms *not* related to incidence of CVD
Simonsick et al., 1995[53]	1063 men and 2398 women (age 65 years and older with hypertension)	CES-D Scale[45]	Elevated rates of CVD-related death in women with high scores on depressive symptoms
Everson et al., 1996[54]	2428 men (age 42–60)	Hopelessness self-report questionnaire	For CVD-related death: RH: 2.52 (95% CI: 1.52–4.17) (moderate hopelessness score) RH: 3.90 (95% CI: 2.14–7.11) (high hopelessness score)
Barefoot and Schroll, 1996[55]	409 men and 321 women (all born in 1914)	MMPI[56]	For MI: 1.7 (95% CI: 1.23–2.34)
Pratt et al., 1996[57]	1551 men and women	DIS	For MI: OR: 2.07 (95% CI: 1.16–3.71) (hx of dysphoria) OR: 4.54 (95% CI: 1.65–12.44) (hx of MDE)
Wassertheil-Smoller et al., 1996[58]	4736 men and women over age 60 with hypertension	CES-D[45]	Baseline CES-D score ≥16 did *not* predict future MI RR of future MI per 5-unit increase in CES-D score: women 1.25 (95% CI: 1.15–1.36)
Callahan et al., 1998[59]	3767 men and women 60 years and older	CES-D[45]	None
Mendes de Leon et al., 1998[60]	2812 men and women 65 years and older	CES-D[45]	None
Ford et al., 1998[61]	1190 men 55 years and older	Depression questionnaire	For MI: RR: 2.12 (95% CI: 1.11–4.06)

ABBREVIATIONS: RH = relative hazard; IHD = ischemic heart disease; MI = myocardial infarction; hx = history; MDE = episode of major depression; OR = odds ratio; CI = confidence interval.

SOURCE: Adapted from and reprinted with permission from *Archives of General Psychiatry* 55:580–592, July 1998. Copyright 1998, American Medical Association.

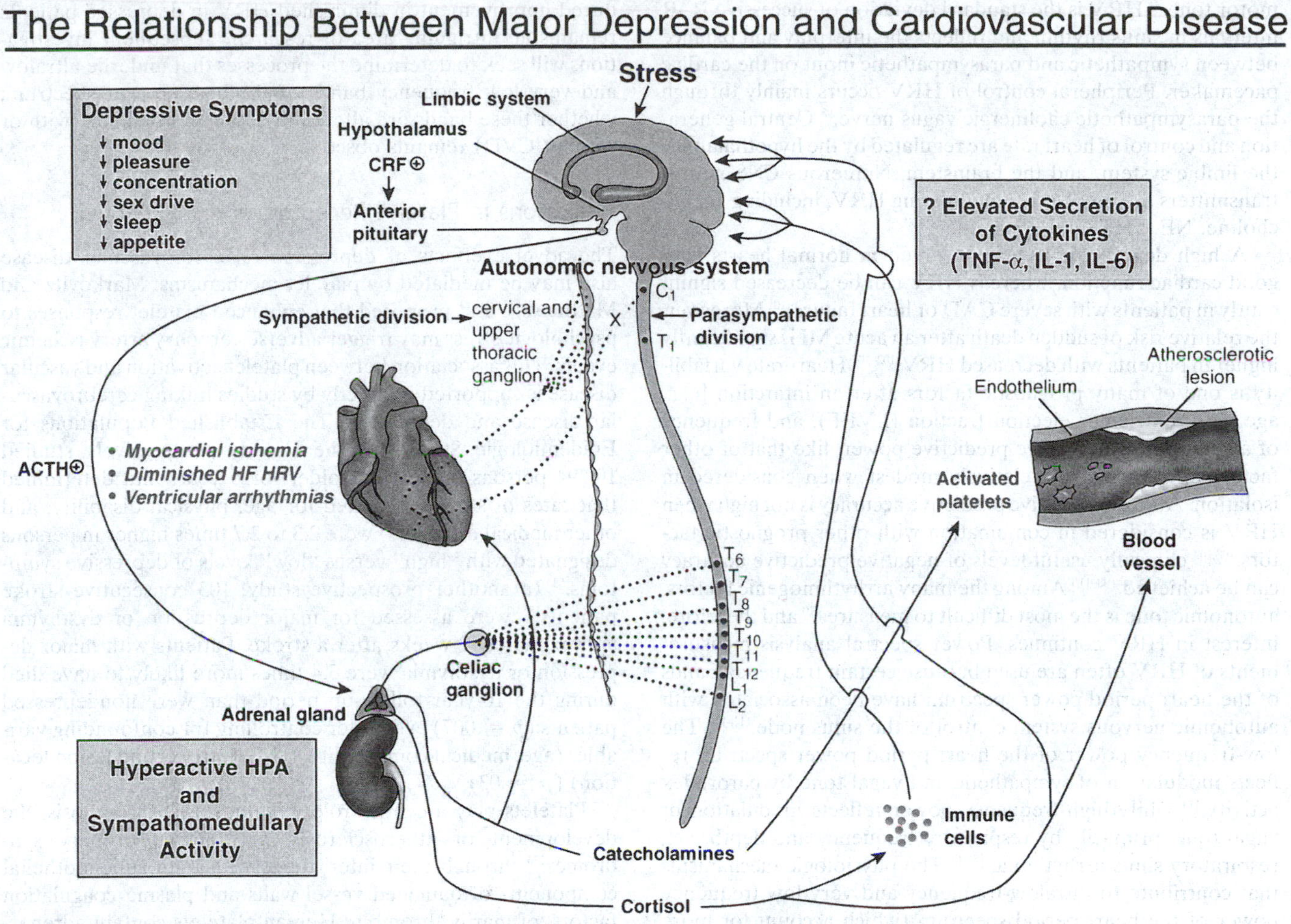

FIGURE 80-1 (Plate 110) Hypothetical schema of pathophysiologic findings associated with depression that probably contribute to increased susceptibility to cardiovascular disease. Autonomic nervous system innervation of the heart via the parasympathetic vagus (X) nerve and sympathetic (postganglionic efferents from the cervical and upper thoracic paravertebral ganglia) nerves is shown. CRF = corticotropin-releasing factor; ACTH = corticotropin; TNF-α = tumor necrosis factor α; IL-1 = interleukin-1; IL-6 = interleukin-6; HRV = heart rate variability; HPA = hypothalamic-pituitary-adrenocortical axis.

trait marker of depression, possibly reflecting increased CRF release within the CNS.

Sympathoadrenal hyperactivity contributes to the development of CVD through effects of catecholamines on the heart, blood vessels, and platelets. Sympathoadrenal activation modifies the function of circulating platelets through direct effects on platelets, catecholamine-induced changes in hemodynamic factors (increased shear stress), circulating lipids, and inhibition of vascular eicosanoid synthesis.[92] Arachidonic acid metabolites such as prostaglandins and leukotrienes contribute to diverse circulatory and hemostatic functions, including inhibition of platelet aggregation, and vascular contractility and permeability.[93] Elevations of plasma NE levels are found most frequently in young hypertensive patients[94] and in subjects with high-cardiac-output borderline hypertension who later proceed to established high-resistance hypertension.[95] Even normotensive depressed patients have been found to exhibit greater heart rates at rest, after orthostasis, and after exercise in comparison with normal controls. These depressed patients also exhibited increased plasma concentrations of NE and serotonin (5HT) at rest.[96] Thus, the sympathoadrenal hyperactivity observed in many patients with major depression may contribute to the development of CVD through the effects of catecholamines on cardiac function and platelets.

Diminished Heart Rate Variability

Alterations in autonomic nervous system activity, as demonstrated by reduced HRV, represent another mechanism that potentially contributes to the diminished survival of depressed patients with CVD. It is believed that the beat-to-beat fluctuations in hemodynamic parameters reflect the dynamic response of cardiovascular control systems to a myriad of naturally occurring physiologic perturbations, such as fluctuations in heart rate associated with respiration. Therefore, HRV may provide a sensitive measure of the functioning of the rapidly reacting sympathetic, parasympathetic, and renin-angiotensin systems. Cardiovascular homeostasis is maintained by the parasympathetic and sympathetic nervous systems through afferent pressor receptors and chemoreceptors and efferents that alter heart rate, atrioventricular conduction, and contractility, and impinge on the peripheral vasculature, altering arterial and venous vasomotor tone.[97] HRV is the standard deviation of successive R–R intervals in sinus rhythm and reflects the interplay and balance between sympathetic and parasympathetic input on the cardiac pacemaker. Peripheral control of HRV occurs mainly through the parasympathetic cholinergic vagus nerve.[98] Central generation and control of heart rate are regulated by the hypothalamus, the limbic system, and the brainstem. Numerous CNS neurotransmitters are involved in modulating HRV, including acetylcholine, NE, 5HT, and dopamine.[99,100]

A high degree of HRV is observed in normal hearts with good cardiac function, whereas HRV can be decreased significantly in patients with severe CAD or heart failure.[101] Moreover, the relative risk of sudden death after an acute MI is significantly higher in patients with decreased HRV.[102–107] Heart rate variability is one of many prognostic factors after an infarction [e.g., age, left ventricular ejection fraction (LVEF), and frequency of arrythmias]. Its positive predictive power, like that of other factors after an MI, is relatively modest when considered in isolation. Although positive predictive accuracy is not high when HRV is considered in combination with other prognostic factors,[108,109] clinically useful levels of negative predictive accuracy can be achieved.[108–110] Among the many arrhythmogenic factors, autonomic tone is the most difficult to measure,[110] and therefore, interest in HRV continues. Power spectral analysis measurements of HRV often are used because certain frequency bands of the heart period power spectrum have been associated with autonomic nervous system control of the sinus node.[111–113] The low-frequency power of the heart period power spectrum reflects modulation of sympathetic and vagal tone by baroreflex activity,[114] while high-frequency power reflects modulation of vagal tone, primarily by respiratory frequency and depth, i.e., respiratory sinus arrhythmia.[115,116] The physiologic mechanisms that contribute to ultralow-frequency and very low frequency power of the heart period spectrum (which account for more than 90 percent of the total power in a 24-h period) remain obscure. In a study of 715 patients after MI, certain frequency bands (total, ultralow, and very low frequencies) of the heart period power spectrum were strongly associated with mortality during 4 years of follow-up even after adjustment for other major risk factors. Indeed, very low frequency power was most strongly associated with death secondary to arrhythmia.[117]

Reduced high-frequency HRV has been observed in depressed patients in comparison with nondepressed groups,[101,118] although discrepant reports exist.[119,120] In patients with angiographically confirmed CAD, diminished HRV during 24-h Holter monitoring was significantly more common in depressed patients than in matched nondepressed patients.[121] Diminished high-frequency HRV is thought to reflect decreased parasympathetic tone, possibly predisposing patients to ventricular arrhythmias and perhaps to the excessive cardiovascular mortality found in CVD patients with a comorbid major depressive disorder.[122] Diminished HRV in patients with major depression also may be contributed to by a deficiency of omega-3 fatty acids[123] in this patient population. Not only have multiple studies documented a deficiency of omega-3 fatty acids in patients with major depression,[124–126] these polyunsaturated lipids possess antiarrhythmic properties and reduce the risk of ventricular arrhythmias.[127–132]

One study (without a placebo control group) revealed normalization of reduced HRV in depressed patients after effective treatment.[133] The prognostic importance of antidepressant-induced improvement in diminished HRV in depressed patients remains an intriguing area of research. Subsequent investigations will seek to determine the processes that underlie ultralow and very low frequency bands of the heart power spectrum; whether these bands are altered in depressed patients (with or without CVD) remains obscure.

Alterations in Platelet Receptors and/or Reactivity

The adverse effects of depression on cardiovascular disease also may be mediated by platelet mechanisms. Markovitz and Matthews[134] first proposed that enhanced platelet responses to psychologic stress may trigger adverse coronary artery ischemic events. This association between platelet activation and vascular disease is supported indirectly by studies linking cerebrovascular disease and depression. The Established Populations for Epidemiologic Studies of the Elderly prospectively studied 10,294 persons age 65 and older for 6 years and determined that rates of stroke (adjusted for age, physical disability, and other medical disorders) were 2.3 to 2.7 times higher in persons designated with "high" versus "low" levels of depressive symptoms.[53] In another prospective study, 103 consecutive stroke patients[135] were assessed for major depression or dysthymia approximately 2 weeks after a stroke. Patients with major depression or dysthymia were 3.4 times more likely to have died during the 10-year follow-up period than were nondepressed patients ($p = .007$) even after controlling for confounding variables (age, medical comorbidity, type of stroke, and lesion location) ($p = .03$).

Platelets play a central role in hemostasis, thrombosis, the development of atherosclerosis, and acute coronary syndromes[136] through their interactions with both subendothelial components of damaged vessel walls and plasma coagulation factors, primarily thrombin. Human platelets contain adrenergic, serotonergic, and dopaminergic receptors. Through activation of platelet alpha$_2$ adrenoceptors, increases in circulating catecholamines (>4 nmol/L) potentiate the effects of other agonists and, at higher concentrations, initiate platelet thrombotic responses, including secretion, aggregation, and activation of the arachidonate pathway. After injury to vessel endothelium, platelets and circulating leukocytes attach to the newly exposed subendothelial layer. Platelets adhere to collagen (and other components of the subendothelial matrix) exposed within a denuded area of the vascular endothelium. Thrombin stimulates platelet activation, converting platelet membrane GPIIb/IIIa complexes into functional receptors for fibrinogen. Activation also is accompanied by extrusion or secretion of platelet storage granule contents into the extracellular environment. Platelets activated at the site of an injury to the vessel wall accelerate the local formation of thrombin and release a variety of products from their storage granules, including chemotactic and mitogenic factors, inducing leukocyte migration from the bloodstream and vascular cell proliferation. These secreted platelet products, e.g., platelet factor 4, β-thromboglobulin (β-TG), and 5HT, stimulate and recruit other platelets and cause irreversible platelet-platelet aggregation, ultimately leading to the formation of a fused platelet thrombus. Platelets also contribute to vascular damage by stimulating lipoprotein uptake by macrophages and mediating vasoconstriction through the production and/or release of substances such as thromboxane A_2, platelet-activating factor, and 5HT.[92] Clinical trials have confirmed the importance of platelets in vascular damage; antiaggregating medications are useful in secondary prevention,[137–139] delay the progression of atherosclerotic lesions,[140] and improve post-MI outcomes.[141,142]

The authors sought to determine whether heightened susceptibility to platelet activation might be a mechanism by which depression in physically healthy young volunteers acts as a significant risk factor for cardiovascular and cerebrovascular disease and/or increased mortality after MI. Utilizing fluorescence-activated flow cytometric analysis, the authors discovered that in comparison with 8 normal controls, 12 depressed patients as a group exhibited enhanced baseline platelet activation as well as increased platelet responsiveness.[143]

In one study, 21 elderly patients suffering from comorbid CVD and major depression exhibited increased platelet activation as measured by markedly elevated plasma concentrations of the platelet secretion products PF4 and β-TG compared with 17 healthy control subjects and 8 *non*depressed age-matched patients with CVD.[144] Although the mechanism or mechanisms responsible remain unknown, the authors believe that heightened susceptibility to platelet activation and secretion underlies, at least in part, the increased vulnerability of depressed patients to CVD and/or mortality after an MI.

Serotonin secreted by platelets induces both platelet aggregation and coronary vasoconstriction, both of which are mediated by $5HT_2$ receptors. Vasoconstriction occurs especially when normal endothelial cell counterregulatory mechanisms of vascular relaxation are defective, as often occurs in patients with CAD.[144–146] Indeed, essential hypertension, elevated plasma cholesterol levels, older age, and smoking, which are well-known predisposing factors for the development of CVD, all contribute to 5HT-mediated platelet activation. Moreover, alterations in platelet 5HT-mediated activation also have been described in affective disorders, most notably major depression. Considerable evidence has accrued in the last two decades that supports the hypothesis that alterations in CNS and platelet serotonergic function occur in depressed patients.[147]

Serotonin-mediated platelet activation can contribute to the development of atherosclerosis, thrombosis, and vasoconstriction. Even though 5HT is a weak platelet agonist, it markedly amplifies platelet reactions to a variety of other agonists such as adenosine diphosphate (ADP), thromboxane A_2, catecholamines, and thrombin. Through an action on $5HT_2$ receptors, serotonin enhances platelet aggregation and the release of intragranular products and arachidonic acid metabolites in response to otherwise ineffective agonist concentrations.[146] This 5HT-induced platelet amplification occurs at the low concentrations attained when indoleamine is released from seeping platelets subjected to shear stresses[148] and from platelet activation by contact with an arterial wall lesion.[149,150] Several investigators have reported *increases* in platelet $5HT_2$ binding density in depressed patients.[151–155] Moreover, the changes appear to be state-dependent in that $5HT_2$ binding-site density returned to control values only in patients who showed clinical improvement. Depressed patients have been found to exhibit significant *reductions* in the number of platelet and brain 5HT transporter sites as detected by [^{3}H] imipramine binding[68,156–158] as well as by the more selective ligand [^{3}H] paroxetine.[147,159] The increased $5HT_2$ receptor binding density and decreased 5HT transporter sites suggest that depressed patients may be particularly susceptible to 5HT-mediated platelet activation and coronary artery vasoconstriction. Decreased numbers of platelet 5HT transporters would potentially hinder the uptake and storage of periplatelet serotonin, exposing the increased numbers of $5HT_2$ receptors to 5HT.[160]

Platelets from depressed patients exhibit significantly increased elevations of intracellular free calcium concentration, $[Ca^{2+}]i$, after 5HT-induced stimulation in comparison to controls.[161–164] Even functionally trivial increases in intraplatelet calcium "prime" the platelet secretion and aggregation response to stimulation by even a "weak" agonist such as 5HT[165] or in response to increased blood flow. Thus, platelets with elevated $[Ca^{2+}]i$, as are observed in depressed patients, probably would exhibit increased activation in comparison with normal comparison subjects under basal conditions or in response to shear-induced aggregation (e.g., after an orthostatic challenge). Future investigations will attempt to confirm and connect the pathophysiologic mechanisms of sympathoadrenal hyperactivity, exaggerated platelet reactivity, and alterations in the platelet 5HT system in depressed patients to the propensity of those patients for the development of CVD.

Myocardial Ischemia and Ventricular Instability in Reaction to Mental Stress

The combination of a vulnerable myocardium after MI, acute ischemia, and negative emotional arousal is thought to trigger fatal ventricular arrythmias.[166] The interplay of these factors in patients with CAD is being scrutinized. Jiang and colleagues[167] longitudinally assessed 126 patients with CAD over a 5-year period. Mental stress–induced myocardial ischemia at baseline in CAD patients was associated with significantly higher rates of subsequent fatal and nonfatal cardiac events independently of age, baseline LVEF, and previous MI. This study proposed that the relation between psychological stress and adverse cardiac events is mediated by myocardial ischemia. Although myocardial ischemia probably is the most significant factor in predisposition to ventricular instability, other factors also contribute. CNS control mechanisms can significantly decrease the threshold for ventricular fibrillation.[168] Ventricular fibrillation is believed to be the mechanism underlying sudden cardiac death, the most common cause of fatality among patients with CAD.[169] Indeed, psychological stress predisposes to abnormal ventricular activity by lowering the ventricular vulnerable-period threshold even to the point of fibrillation. The vagus nerve, however, exerts antiarrthymic activity through a direct action on the ventricular myocardium and interference with sympathetic activity.[170] Increased parasympathetic activity has a protective effect on myocardium electrically destabilized by increased adrenergic tone.[169]

Psychological and physical events can elicit a stress response, which usually is defined as the reaction of an organism to deleterious forces that disturb physiologic homeostasis.[171,172] Psychological stress in humans with CAD increases ventricular ectopic activity and increases the risk of ventricular fibrillation.[173,174] There are several similarities between the stress response and major depression: both can be characterized by increased blood pressure and heart rate as well as increased arousal and increased mobilization of energy stores.[175] Particularly relevant to both the stress response and depression are the critical brain structures the locus coeruleus and the central nucleus of the amygdala, which both are innervated by CRF-containing nerve terminals.[176,177] The stress response and major depression differ in some respects, however. In depression, some aspects of the normal stress response seem to escalate to a pathologic state[178] that fails to respond appropriately to usual counterregulatory responses, resulting in a sustained version of a usually transient phenomenon, i.e., hyperactivity of the hypothalamic-pituitary-adrenocortical (HPA) axis or the sympathoadrenal system. Although many studies have linked stressful life events to the onset of major depression,[179,180] some depressions are clearly endogeneous—i.e., they have no obvious environmental precipitant—although in most of these studies the role of early adverse events that are now known to be of paramount importance was not assessed.

Frasure-Smith and colleagues[31] proposed that depression worsens the prognosis after an MI through another mechanism: PVCs. The risk of sudden cardiac death associated with significant depressive symptoms (Beck Depression Inventory score ≥10) was greatest among patients with 10 or more PVCs per hour (60 percent of these patients died within 18 months), suggesting arrythymia as the link between depression and sudden cardiac death.[31] Depressed patients with CAD are not more likely to have arrhythmias than are nondepressed patients with CAD, but the risk associated with depression is confined largely to patients with PVCs. Patients who were *not* depressed experienced little increase in risk associated with PVCs even in the presence of a low LVEF.[31] Thus, the prognostic impact of PVCs may be related more to depression than to PVCs per se. In the Cardiac Arrhythmia Suppression Trial (CAST),[181] suppression of PVC frequency in post-MI patients did not reduce but actually increased mortality even though PVCs are associated with increased mortality after an MI. Treatment of depression may be necessary to improve survival in depressed patients with PVCs.[182]

ANXIETY DISORDERS AND CARDIOVASCULAR DISEASE

Epidemiology

Anxiety disorders are the most prevalent psychiatric disorders in the United States (Table 80-4), with simple phobias being the most common (9 percent) and social phobia (8 percent) being the most often observed (Tables 80-5 and 80-6). A survey of adult primary care patients (n = 637) enrolled in a health maintenance organization revealed that 10 percent had untreated anxiety disorders.[183]

TABLE 80-4 12-Month Prevalence of DSM-III-R Disorders in the National Comorbidity Survey

Disorder	Percent
Any anxiety disorder	19.3
Any addictive disorder	11.3
Any mood disorder	11.3
Nonaffective psychosis	0.3
Any National Comorbidity Survey disorder	30.9

SOURCE: From Kessler et al.[4]

TABLE 80-5 12-Month Prevalence of Diagnosed Anxiety Disorders in the National Comorbidity Survey

Disorder	Percent
Simple phobia	8.8
Social phobia	7.9
Posttraumatic stress disorder	3.9
Generalized anxiety disorder	3.1
Agoraphobia	2.8
Panic disorder	2.3
Obsessive-compulsive disorder	<1.0
Any anxiety disorder	19.3

SOURCE: From Kessler et al.[4]

Unfortunately, anxiety disorders, though common, remain largely undiagnosed and undertreated.[183,184] Stereotyped as the "worried well," patients with anxiety disorders such as phobias, panic disorder, and generalized anxiety disorder have substantially higher rates of health service utilization, increased social and role disability, diminished quality of life, and poor health outcomes.[183,185–189] Moreover, the comorbidity of anxiety and affective disorders is substantial. Nearly 60 percent of patients with major depression in the National Comorbidity Survey suffered from a comorbid anxiety disorder.[4] Indeed, patients with mixed anxiety and depressive symptoms (or comorbid anxiety and depressive syndromes) suffer increased emotional disability as well as poorer social and role function in comparison to patients with either condition alone.[183,188] *After elective catheterization, the physical disability of patients with CAD at 1 year of follow-up was associated with the severity of these patients' anxiety and depressive symptoms at catheterization,* not *with the number of main coronary vessels stenosed.*[184]

The prevalence of anxiety disorders in patients with CVD has been largely understudied, with most studies focusing on patients with mitral valve prolapse or individuals referred for evaluation of chest pain. Substantial numbers of patients each year who undergo coronary angiography because of symptoms of chest pain (yet have normal coronary arteries) are thought to have anxiety disorders such as panic disorder (Table 80-7). Subsequently categorized as having "atypical chest pain," these patients may suffer chest pain in response to anxiety and/or hyperventilation.[190–193]

However, a large, multicity survey of 875 primary care outpatients revealed that patients with CHF or MI exhibited a point prevalence rate of at least one anxiety disorder (panic disorder, phobia, or generalized anxiety disorder) of 18 percent[189] (Table 80-8). Whether the prevalence of anxiety disorders is elevated in patients who are hospitalized for CAD (e.g., elective coronary catheterization, post-MI, or unstable angina) remains to be determined.

A small number of prospective epidemiologic studies (which control for many of the commonly accepted risk factors for IHD) indicate an increased relative risk of nonfatal and fatal CVD events in patients with anxiety symptoms, even among individuals who have "simple" phobias, e.g., claustrophobia and fear of illness, heights, crowds, or going out alone (Table 80-9).

Moreover, an ancillary study of 348 CAST and CAST II participants who had asymptomatic ventricular arrhythmias

TABLE 80-6 Diagnostic Criteria for the Most Common DSM-IV Anxiety Disorders

DSM-IV Criteria for Simple Phobia

Marked and persistent fear that is excessive or unreasonable, cued by the presence or anticipation of a specific object or situation (e.g., flying, heights, animals, receiving an injection, seeing blood).

Exposure to the phobic stimulus almost invariably provokes an immediate anxiety response, which may take the form of a situationally bound or situationally predisposed panic attack.

The person (adults only) recognizes that the feature is excessive or unreasonable.

The phobic situation is avoided or is endured with intense anxiety or distress.

The avoidance, anxious anticipation, or distress in the feared situations interferes significantly with the person's normal routine, occupational (or academic) functioning or social activities or relationships or there is marked distress about having the phobia.

DSM-IV Diagnostic Criteria for Social Phobia

Marked fear of being focus of attention; avoidance of meeting unfamiliar people and close scrutiny by others

Fear of behaving in embarassing or humiliating way

Extreme anticipatory anxiety which may manifest as a panic attack

DSM-IV Diagnostic Criteria for Posttraumatic Stress Disorder

Experience of a traumatic event

Reexperienced by intrusive and distressing recollection, dreams, flashbacks, distress in similar situations

Persistent avoidance of stimuli associated with trauma

Persistent symptoms of increased arousal

Duration of disturbance of at least 1 month

DSM-IV Diagnostic Criteria for Panic Disorder

Recurrent and unexpected panic attacks plus one or more of the following:

- Persistent concern about having additional attacks (anticipatory anxiety)
- Worry about the consequences of the attacks
- A significant change in behavior related to the attacks (phobic avoidance)

Not due to a substance, medical condition, or mental illness

At least two unexpected panic attacks for diagnosis

Definition of Panic Attack

A period of intense fear or discomfort in which at least four of the following symptoms develop suddenly

—Palpitations or increased heart rate
—Sweating
—Trembling or shaking
—Sensations of shortness of breath or smothering
—Feeling of choking
—Nausea or abdominal distress
—Chest pain or discomfort
—Dizziness, light-headedness, or faintness
—Derealization or depersonalization
—Fear of losing control or going crazy
—Chills or hot flashes
—Paresthesia (numbness or tingling)
—Fear of dying

DSM-IV Criteria for Generalized Anxiety Disorder

Excessive anxiety and worry for more days than not for past 6 months

Difficulty controlling worry

Functional impairment and/or distress

Symptoms not attributable to other causes

- Physical symptoms
  - Restlessness or feeling keyed up/on edge
  - Fatigue
  - Muscle tension
- Psychological symptoms
  - Excessive anxiety or worry
  - Difficulty controlling worry
  - Irritability
  - Difficulty concentrating or mind going blank
  - Sleep disturbance

Source: Reprinted with permission from the *Diagnostic and Statistical Manual of Mental Disorders*, 4th ed. Copyright 1994, American Psychiatric Association.

TABLE 80-7 Prevalence of Anxiety Disorders in Patients Referred for Cardiologic Evaluation

Study	No./Type of Patients	Prevalence	Diagnostic Method
Bass and Wade, 1984[194]	99 patients without history of CAD referred for coronary arteriography due to CP	Of 31 patients without CAD: 29% with "anxiety neurosis"	Clinical Interview Schedule[195]
Cormier et al., 1988[196]	98 patients without history of CAD referred for coronary arteriography or ECG exercise tolerance testing due to CP	Of 49 patients without CAD: 47% with panic disorder 39% with major depression 43% with two or more phobias	DIS[35]

ABBREVIATIONS: CAD = coronary artery disease; CP = chest pain; Hx = history.

TABLE 80-8 Prevalence of Comorbid Anxiety Disorders in Primary Care Outpatients*

	Major Depression, %	Hypertension, %	Diabetes, %	Heart Disease, %
Panic disorder	9.4	0.9†	1.1†	1.2†
Phobia	22.7	5.5†	4.8†	9.2†
Generalized anxiety disorder	54.1	10.4†	11.9†	12.4†
Any anxiety disorder	66.3	14.6†	15.5†	17.8†

*Diagnosis of congestive heart failure or myocardial infarction within the previous year, adjusted for patient age, sex, race, education, marital status, income, study site, and each of the other medical or psychiatric conditions.
†Value significantly different from that of patients with current depression ($p \leq .05$), based on regression coefficients.
SOURCE: Sherbourne et al.[189]

TABLE 80-9 Antecedent Anxiety and Subsequent Risk of Cardiovascular Disease

Source	No./Type of Patients	Diagnostic Method	Relative Risk (RR) of Anxiety or Anxiety Symptoms for Cardiac Disease or Cardiac Disease–Related Death
Haines et al., 1987[197]	1457 men (age 40–62)	Crown-Crisp Index	For fatal MI: 3.77 (95% CI: 1.64–8.64)
Eaker et al., 1992[198]	749 women (age 45–64)	Somatic strain scale	For myocardial infarction and fatal CAD: 7.8 (95% CI: 1.9–32.3)
Kawachi et al., 1994[199]	33,999 men (age 42–77)	Crown-Crisp Index	For fatal MI: 2.45 (95% CI: 1.00–5.96) for men with "highest" phobic anxiety
Kawachi et al., 1994[200]	2271 men (age 21–80)	5-item anxiety scale from Cornell Medical Index	For CVD-related sudden death, OR: 4.5 (95% CI: 0.92–21.6)

ABBREVIATIONS: MI = myocardial infarction; CAD = coronary artery disease; CVD = cardiovascular disease; CI = confidence interval; OR = odds ratio.

after MI and were treated with placebo revealed that stressful life events during the initial 4 months of participation in CAST trial and higher anxiety were predictive of mortality independently of the effects of physiologic variables such as diabetes and ejection fraction.[182]

PATHOPHYSIOLOGY OF ANXIETY

The neurocircuitry of anxiety has been postulated to arise from the amygdala, the brain area that registers the emotional significance of environmental stimuli and stores emotional memories. The efferent pathways from the central nucleus of the amygdala travel to a multiplicity of critical brain structures, including the parabrachial nucleus (resulting in dyspnea and hyperventilation), the dorsomedial nucleus of the vagus nerve and nucleus ambiguous (activating the parasympathetic nervous system), and the lateral hypothalamus (resulting in SNS activation).[201] Through reciprocal neuronal pathways connecting the amygdala to the medial prefrontal cortex, cognitive experience of the specific anxiety disorder differs, although fear symptoms may overlap. During panic attacks the fear is of imminent death; in social phobia, the fear is of embarassment; in postraumatic stress disorder, the traumatic memory is remembered or reexperienced; in obsessive-compulsive disorder, obsessional ideas recur and intrude; and in generalized anxiety disorder, anxiety is "free-floating," i.e., not conditioned to specific situations or triggers.[202]

Described in the past with terms such as *cardiac neurosis, irritable heart syndrome, battle fatigue,* and *soldier's heart, panic disorder is the anxiety disorder most often associated with cardiovascular symptoms of chest pain, tachycardia, and dyspnea.* Discrete panic attacks can be induced in the laboratory setting, especially in patients with panic disorder, by a variety of stimuli: sodium lactate, caffeine, isoproterenol, the serotonin receptor agonist m-chlorophenylpiperazine (m-CPP), cholecystokinin tetrapeptide (CCK_4), inhalation of CO_2-enriched air, and voluntary acute hyperventilation of room air. The common element among these disparate inducers may be their ability to stimulate the respiratory rate with the induction of an accompanying subjective sense of breathlessness.[203] Although some researchers have proposed that patients with panic disorder have only a heightened sensitivity to and develop a learned intolerance of tachypnea,[204,205] the higher concordance rate of panic disorder observed in monozygotic compared with dizygotic twins[206] and evidence of altered respiratory rhythym during sleep[207,208] provide evidence of a genetic diathesis and a biological abnormality, respectively, underlying the phenotype of panic disorder.[203]

PATHOPHYSIOLOGY OF ANXIETY DISORDERS: A FOCUS ON THE CARDIOVASCULAR SYSTEM

Although the neurobiology of specific anxiety disorders has not been explored as fully as that of unipolar depression, potential neurochemical, neuroendocrine, and neuroanatomic alterations have not only been identified but increasingly scrutinized. Patients with major depression or anxiety disorders may experience common symptoms, e.g., alterations in psychomotor activity, impairment of sleep, increased appetite, and reduced concentration. Moreover, there are several shared neurobiological findings between patients with certain common syndromal anxiety disorders and those with depression, although differences also exist. The neurobiology of patients with certain anxiety disorders is reviewed below, with attention to mechanisms that contribute to the development of cardiovascular disease and/or cardiac-related mortality: HPA axis activity, sympathomedullary activity, diminished HRV, and alterations in platelet receptor number or function.

The only anxiety disorder in which alterations of HPA axis activity have been documented repeatedly is posttraumatic stress disorder (PTSD). In nearly all controlled studies of PTSD patients, alterations of HPA axis hyperactivity have been documented, including elevations of cerebrospinal fluid (CSF) CRF concentrations[209,210] and blunting of the ACTH response to CRF stimulation.[211] In comparison to control subjects, however, PTSD patients generally exhibit reduced plasma cortisol concentrations, diminished 24-h urinary cortisol concentrations, and a greater suppression of plasma cortisol concentrations in response to low doses (e.g., 0.5 mg) of dexamethasone.[212–216] However the two studies that measured CSF CRF concentrations in PTSD[209,210] found results identical to those repeatedly reported in depression: elevated CSF CRF concentrations. Whether patients with PTSD experience an increased (or decreased) relative risk of CVD is not known. Potential confounds in those studies include the very high rate of comorbid substance abuse and alcoholism as well as tobacco abuse in PTSD patients. Patients with panic disorder do not appear to exhibit alterations in HPA axis function consistently; scrutiny continues of patients with social phobia, generalized anxiety disorder, and obsessive-compulsive disorder.

Sympathomedullary function has been investigated intensively in patients with panic disorder. As was discussed previously, plasma concentrations of catecholamines are determined by the rate of release, local metabolic degradation, synaptic reuptake, and redistribution into other extravascular spaces.[217] To examine systemic as well as regional sympathomedullary kinetics, investigators infuse intravenous trace amounts of radiolabeled NE and epinephrine (EPI). Arterial or "arterialized venous" samples of endogenous catecholamines are then obtained, and a "compartmental analysis" is performed to mathematically fit the data into a two-compartment ("whole-body" versus "cardiac" or "extravascular" versus "vascular"/plasma compartments) model. Whole-body NE "spillover" (the rate of NE appearance in plasma), a sensitive measure of systemic SNS activity, is similar under basal conditions in panic patients and control subjects[218,219] and increases to a similar degree in both groups under laboratory mental stress.[219] Panic patients do, however, exhibit significantly higher cardiac spillover rates of coronary sinus (cardiac-derived) EPI under basal conditions, increased whole-body EPI secretion during laboratory mental stress, and surges of EPI whole-body spillover during panic attacks. Such increases in EPI in panic patients presumably are due to "loading" of sympathetic neuronal stores by uptake from plasma during surges of EPI secretion during panic attacks.[219] Further investigation of cardiac and/or systemic sympathomedullary activation during spontaneous or pharmacologically provoked panic attacks is needed to confirm these findings, along with prospective investigations of the cardiac-related risk of patients with panic disorder.[220,221] However, multiple prospective cohort studies (which control for other accepted risk factors for IHD) report that increasing severity of anxiety is associated with an increased risk for developing elevated systolic blood pressure[222] or hypertension.[223,224] However, given the comorbidity between anxiety and depressive symptoms and syndromes, further studies are required to determine whether the evidence of increased risk for the development of CAD (or hypertension) in anxiety disorder patients is independent of the contribution of depression.[225]

Another area awaiting investigation in patients with anxiety disorders is platelet receptor function, particularly the receptors most integral to thrombovascular repair and disease. Psychobiological studies of patients with panic disorder, in contrast to reports of patients with major depression, have not detected alterations of platelet 5HT transporters and platelet $5HT_2$ receptors. In comparison to control subjects, however, patients with panic attacks have been reported, like those with depression, to exhibit increased plasma concentrations of PF4 and β-TG, providing evidence of increased platelet secretion. Moreover, after treatment of panic patients with alprazolam, plasma concentrations of these alpha granule–specific proteins were reduced significantly.[226] The presence of anxiety disorders has been hypothesized to trigger coronary events through atherosclerotic plaque rupture, coronary vasospasm, ventricular arrhythmias, or atrial arrhthymias.[225] Panic-induced hyperventilation is a well-known precipitant of coronary spasm,[227,228] which in turn may induce ventricular arrhythmias and MI.[200,229,230]

The most compelling evidence regarding the association of anxiety disorders and cardiovascular dysfunction comes from reports of abnormal cardiac autonomic control.[225] Examination of HRV in patients with anxiety disorders has revealed that patients with panic disorder[231–234] and patients with generalized anxiety disorder[235] exhibit reductions in high-frequency HRV.[236] As was noted above, diminished HRV increases the risk of arrhythmias and sudden cardiac death. Indeed, patients with panic disorder or agoraphobia exhibit a higher density of PVCs in comparison to patients with other anxiety disorders[237] and normal comparison subjects.[238,239] Whether patients with panic disorder (or other anxiety disorders) exhibit increased rates of sudden cardiac death remains to be determined.

Although so-called mental disorders may produce effects on cardiovascular function, perhaps less well understood are the cardiovascular contributions to certain anxiety disorders. Whether cardiovascular abnormalities or dysfunction reliably produces symptoms of anxiety is an intriguing area of investigation; e.g., is worsening of CHF associated with an increased incidence of panic attacks? In comparison to gender- and age-matched controls, individuals with cardiac arrhythmias exhibited significantly higher self-reported anxiety scores.[240] Whether a causal biological mechanism exists between PVCs and anxiety symptoms or disorders or there is merely an association remains to be determined.[171,241–243]

Emergency room physicians and cardiologists are well acquainted with the challenges of evaluating patients with an acute onset of chest discomfort, combined with painful and overwhelming anxiety symptoms, which may or may not be associated with clinically significant cardiovascular disease (Table 80-10).

Certainly, the impact of anxiety disorders on the development of and worsening of CVD should be more completely discriminated from the contributions of depressive symptoms or syndromes.[225] Such knowledge carries the promise of anxiety symptom reduction and improved quality of life and the potential for new treatment modalities to enhance cardiovascular function in patients with CVD who have comorbid anxiety disorders.

TABLE 80-10 Medical Conditions Associated with Anxiety Symptoms

Cardiovascular disorders: mitral valve prolapse, coronary artery disease, paroxysmal tachycardia, hypertension, hypotension
Endocrinopathies: hyperthyroidism, hypothyroidism, diabetes, hypoglycemia, hypocalcemia, porphyria, endocrine tumors
Neurologic disorders: migraine headaches, transient ischemic attacks, temporal lobe seizures
Pulmonary disease: asthma, chronic obstructive pulmonary disease, pulmonary embolus
Vestibular dysfunction: Meniere's disease
Infectious diseases: tuberculosis, brucellosis, HIV/AIDS
Drug effects: cocaine abuse, alcohol or sedative withdrawal, sympathomimetics, caffeine, monosodium glutamate, akathesia

Treatment of Major Depression and Anxiety Disorders in Patients with Cardiovascular Disease

As with other medical disorders, effective treatment of major psychiatric illnesses such as major depression and panic disorder and prototype mood and anxiety disorders, respectively, require patient access to informed health care practioners, accurate diagnosis, affordable treatment, and safe, effective treatment modalities. Factors hampering well-conducted psychiatric (psychotherapeutic or psychopharmacologic/somatic) treatment include patient reluctance, social stigma regarding psychiatric treatment, managed care restrictions, and a dearth of psychiatrists and psychologists, particularly in rural areas. However, the evidence of the adverse impact of affective and anxiety disorders on relatively young and physically healthy individuals as well as medically ill patients heralds an opportunity and an accompanying incentive to prevent or limit the personal suffering, economic cost, and social disability associated with mental disorders. Although the safety and efficacy of anxiolytic and antidepressant treatment in patients with cardiovascular disease remain to be truly established in randomized clinical trials, these agents, particularly the newly introduced ones, are prescribed routinely to patients with heart disease. This seems appropriate given the drastic reduction in psychosocial function associated with anxiety or depressive disorders and the extant literature demonstrating the safety, and efficacy of these psychotropic agents in generally healthy populations, some data from psychopharmacologic treatment of medically ill patients, and the paucity of psychiatric practitioners available to patients with severe CVD.

Many heart patients believe that their persistent "worry," "lack of enjoyment of life," or "loss of interest" constitutes an understandable (and untreatable) condition. However, given the prevalence of major depression in patients with heart disease, the astute clinician's index of suspicion should always be heightened. Third-party information (particularly from a spouse or other caregiver) is often more revealing of the true extent of a patient's symptoms (e.g., irritability, social isolation, or listlessness), including attempts to "self-medicate" through abuse of alcohol, prescription medication, or illicit substances. A thorough evaluation of anxiety, panic attacks (if any), and depressive symptoms should be performed, including queries regarding feelings of pessimism, hopelessness, and the wish not to continue living. While the preferences of cardiac patients, as with any medical disorder, should be respected, cardiac patients and their families should always be gently apprised of the risks of untreated depression (CVD-related morbidity and mortality) versus the options of psychotherapeutic and/or psychopharmacologic treatment. Consultation with a knowledgeable mental health provider can assist in the discrimination of depressive disorders from complicated or pathologic grief, delirium, ascertainment of coexisting anxiety disorders (such as generalized anxiety disorder or social phobia), detection of intoxication or withdrawal syndromes, and appropriate emotional reactions.

The efficacy (and safety) of psychotherapeutic treatment of post-MI patients with comorbid major depression or any of the anxiety disorders is not known. However, the Enhancing Recovering in Coronary Heart Disease (ENRICHD) Patients Study, a multicenter, randomized clinical trial sponsored by the National Heart, Lung, and Blood Institute, is under way. ENRICHD is the first large-scale, randomized clinical trial to utilize psychotherapy as an initial intervention targeting post-MI patients with major depression (and/or low social support), proceeding to antidepressant treatment if depressive symptoms do not improve. Psychological interventions with post-MI patients[244–248] targeted to diminish "psychological distress"[246,249] or alter type A personality traits[245] have been studied previously on a more limited scale.

With the introduction of fluoxetine (Prozac) in the United States and citalopram (Celexa) in Europe in 1989, just over a decade of clinical information has been gleaned regarding the selective serotonin reuptake inhibitors (SSRIs) class of antidepressants. Furthermore, during the 1990s, these SSRIs and more recently the 5HT and NE reuptake inhibitor (SSNRI) venlafaxine superseded the benzodiazepines as the first-line treatment of choice for anxiety disorders. These newer antidepressants provide significant reduction of anxiety symptoms in approximately 60 percent of medically healthy patients without having a potential for addiction. SSRIs and SSNRIs have been approved by U.S. Food and Drug Agency for the treatment of panic disorder [paroxetine (Paxil) and sertraline (Zoloft)], social anxiety disorder (social phobia) (paroxetine), obsessive-compulsive disorder [aroxetine, sertraline, fluoxetine and fluvoxamine (Luvox)], and generalized anxiety disorder [venlafaxine (Effexor)] (Table 80-11). It is important to note that the SSRIs, although they all are potent 5HT reuptake inhibitors, also exert unique effects on other neurotransmitter systems. Thus, paroxetine is a very potent inhibitor of NE reuptake, whereas sertraline is a potent inhibitor of dopamine (DA) reuptake. The clinical sequelae of these pharmacologic properties remain obscure.

During the time (often 6 to 8 weeks) before the onset of an antidepressant's anxiolytic effect, benzodiazepines such as lorazepam, alprazolam, and clonazepam may be utilized. These agents are rapidly effective but should be used only for short-term treatment (6- to 8-week duration) of disabling anxiety symptoms. Benzodiazepines are sedating, produce gait instability, impair memory, may induce behavioral disinhibition, are ineffective in the treatment of coexisting depressive syndromes, and place patients at risk of physiologic (and psychological) dependence.

Psychotherapeutic and/or psychopharmacologic treatment of the 15 to 23 percent of post-MI patients who fulfill the criteria for major depression, particularly depressed patients with a comorbid anxiety disorder or subsyndromal anxiety, may have a significant effect (positive or negative) on both medical morbidity and mortality. Because of advances in the medical management of CVD patients, therapeutic trials determining improvement in survival must be quite large[249]; for example, the 22-month CAST trial included 1489 subjects.[181] Such past experience cautions against the raising of hopes for demonstrating improving cardiac outcome through antidepressant treatment of depression and anxiety disorders in patients with CVD. Nevertheless, awaiting the completion of a large-scale mortality trial similar to CAST may not be appropriate in light of the interpersonal, social, and medical burden of depression and early indications of SSRI efficacy in depressed patients with CVD.[250,251]

The use of tricyclic and structurally related antidepressants should be limited in patients with CVD because of the myriad side effects of these drugs on the cardiovascular system, including orthostatic hypotension, tachycardia, reduction in HRV, and slowing of intraventricular conduction (as a result of quinidine-like effects) (Table 80-11). These antidepressants should never be prescribed for patients with bifascicular and left fascicular block.[252,253] Monoamine oxidase inhibitors and trazodone are generally free of effects on cardiac conduction but, like the TCAs, may cause postural hypotension.[254] Because of their fewer potential adverse effects on the cardiovascular system and the lack of lethality from an overdose, pharmacotherapeutic treatment with SSRIs, the SSNRI venlafaxine, or other "atypical" antidepressants (such as bupropion, nefazodone, and mirtazapine) may offer significant advantages in depressed or anxious patients with CVD.

The only known cardiac effect of SSRIs is severe sinus node slowing, which to date has been reported in only a few cases.[262,263] Because 5HT has been implicated in both platelet aggregation and coronary artery vasoconstriction, the SSRIs, which are widely used to treat major depression, may produce effects on platelet function. There have been some reports of alterations of hemostasis[264–266] and platelet aggregation[267] after treatment with fluoxetine.

Because of inhibition of some cytochrome P450 isoenzymes, certain SSRIs may alter the metabolism of medications often used in patients with heart disease. The SSRIs that inhibit the P450 2D6 isoenzyme (fluoxetine, paroxetine, fluvoxamine, and higher doses of sertraline) should be used with caution in patients receiving medications metabolized by the P450 2D6 (e.g., lipophilic beta-blockers and type 1C antiarrhythmics: flecainide, mexiletine, propafenone). SSRIs that inhibit the P450 3A4 isoenzyme (fluoxetine, fluvoxamine, nefazodone) may increase the plasma concentrations of calcium channel blockers and warfarin.[268] Although the antidepressants venlafaxine, bupropion, citalopram, and mirtazapine exhibit minimal hepatic P450 enzyme inhibition, their safety remains to be established in patients with CVD who have comorbid depression or anxiety disorders.

After short-term treatment with buproprion,[269] fluoxetine,[270] paroxetine, fluvoxamine,[120] or paroxetine,[250] depressed patients exhibit no changes in HRV. A recent randomized, double-blind multicenter study compared the efficacy of nortriptyline and

TABLE 80-11 Cardiac-Related Side Effects of Psychotropic Agents Commonly Utilized for Treatment of Anxiety or Depression

Class	Cardiovascular Side Effect(s)	Likely Mechanism of Side Effect	Other Effects/Benefits*
Tricyclic and related cyclic antidepressants Nortriptyline (Pamelor) Imipramine (Tofranil) Amitriptyline (Elavil)	Orthostatic hypotension	Postsynaptic alpha$_1$-receptor blockade	Nortriptyline has lowest incidence of orthostatic hypotension[255,256]
Desipramine (Norpramin) Clomipramine (Anafranil)	Tachycardia	Secondary to hypotension	
Doxepin (Sinequan) Trimipramine (Surmontil)	Decreased heart rate variability	Postsynaptic cholinergic receptor blockade	Urinary retention, dry mouth, constipation, confusion, exacerbation of narrow-angle glaucoma
Protriptyline (Vivactil)	Slowing of intraventricular conduction	Quinidine-like effects	Avoid in patients with: bifascicular block, left bundle branch block, QTc > 44 ms, QRS > 11 ms Fatal in overdose
Monoamine oxidase inhibitors Phenelzine (Nardil) Tranylcypromine (Parnate) Isocarboxizide (Marplan)	Orthostatic hypotension Hypertensive crisis	Inhibition of metabolism of serotonin and catecholamines	Requires adherence to tyramine-free diet and avoidance of other antidepressants, and sympathomimetics Fatal in overdose
Selective serotonin reuptake inhibitors (SSRIs)		Postsynaptic serotonin receptor blockade	Typical SSRI side effects: nausea, insomnia, sexual dysfunction, nervousness
Fluoxetine (Prozac)	Sinus bradycardia[257]	Unknown	Requires 8 weeks for complete washout Inhibitor of CYP-450 IID6 and CYP-450 IIIA4 enzymes Also FDA-approved for treatment of adult obsessive-compulsive disorder (OCD)
Paroxetine (Paxil)	Clinically insignificant decreases in heart rate[250]	Unknown	Inhibitor of CYP-450 IID6 enzyme Also FDA-approved for treatment of social phobia, panic disorder, OCD
Sertraline (Zoloft)	None known		In high doses, inhibitor of CYP-450 IID6 enzyme Also FDA-approved for treatment of panic disorder, adult and pediatric OCD
Fluvoxamine (Luvox)	None known		Potent inhibitor of *multiple* CYP-450 enzymes Also FDA-approved for treatment of adult and pediatric OCD
Citalopram (Celexa)	None known		SSRI with most selective binding to serotonin transporter

TABLE 80-11 Cardiac-Related Side Effects of Psychotropic Agents Commonly Utilized for Treatment of Anxiety or Depression (*Continued*)

Class	Cardiovascular Side Effect(s)	Likely Mechanism of Side Effect	Other Effects/Benefits*
Selective serotonin-norepinephrine reuptake inhibitor (SNRI)			
Venlafaxine (Effexor)	Arrhythmia or cardiac block in overdose[260]	Unknown	No significant inhibition of CYP-450 enzymes
	Increased diastolic blood pressure in doses >300 mg per day[261]	Presynaptic inhibition of norepinephrine reuptake	FDA-approved for treatment of generalized anxiety disorder, major depression Side effect profile similar to SSRIs
Presynaptic Alpha$_2$-Receptor Antagonist			
Mirtazapine (Remeron)	None known	Postsynaptic histamine$_1$ receptor blockade	Very sedating in low doses Weight gain Minimal sexual side effects No significant inhibition of CYP-450 enzymes
Lithium*	Sinus node dysfunction Sinoatrial block T-wave inversion or flattening, particularly in patients >60 years of age Arrythmias and sudden death in patients with cardiac disease	Unknown	Narrow therapeutic index (.6–1.2 mmol/L) Many medications alter lithium plasma levels Fatal in overdose Mood stabilizer for patients with bipolar disorder Yearly ECG in patients over 50
Dopamine and norepinephrine reuptake inhibitor			
Bupropion (Wellbutrin; Zyban)	Significant increases in blood pressure in patients with preexisting hypertension[255]	Presynaptic inhibition of norepinephrine reuptake	No significant inhibition of CYP-450 enzymes Minimal sexual side effects Not proven effective in treatment of anxiety disorders FDA-approved for treatment of nicotine dependence
"Atypical" serotonergic agents			
Trazodone (Desyrel)	Orthostatic hypotension	Postsynaptic alpha$_1$-receptor blockade	Sedation, confusion, dizziness
	Cardiac arrhythmias rare[258]	Unknown	
		Unknown	Rare cases of priapism
Nefazodone (Serzone)	Sinus bradycardia[259]	Unknown	Similar side effect profile as trazodone (except without priapism) Minimal sexual side effects Potent inhibitor of *multiple* CYP-450 enzymes
Psychostimulants			
Dextroamphetamine (Dexedrine) Methylphenidate (Ritalin)	Rarely increases blood pressure or induces tachycardia in therapeutic doses	Release of dopamine and catecholamines	Avoid in patients with hyperthyroidism, severe hypertension, severe angina, tachyarrythmias

TABLE 80-11 Cardiac-Related Side Effects of Psychotropic Agents Commonly Utilized for Treatment of Anxiety or Depression (*Continued*)

Class	Cardiovascular Side Effect(s)	Likely Mechanism of Side Effect	Other Effects/Benefits*
Benzodiazepines Alprazolam (Xanax)		Allosteric alteration of $GABA_A$ receptors	Rapid relief of anxiety symptoms Can cause fatigue, ataxia, drowsiness, amnesia, and behavioral dyscontrol Relatively safe in overdose Physiologic and psychological dependence; withdrawal symptoms without gradual taper of dose
Clonazepam (Klonopin) Lorazepam (Ativan) Oxazepam (Serax)	Hypotension	Muscle relaxation via $GABA_A$ spinal cord receptors	
Partial $5HT_{1A}$-Receptor Agonist Buspirone (Buspar)	None known		FDA-approved for treatment of generalized anxiety disorder Nonaddictive
$Omega_1$ receptor Agonist Zolpidem (Ambien) Zalepelon (Sonata)	None known None known	Potentiation of $GABA_A$ receptor	Sedating Nonaddictive

*Medications that increase lithium levels: nonsteroidal anti-inflammatory drugs, diuretics (thiazides, ethacrynic acid, spironolactone, triamterene), angiotensin-converting enzyme inhibitors, metronidazole, tetracycline. Medications that decrease lithium levels: acetazolamide, theophylline, aminophylline, caffeine, osmotic diuretics.
ABBREVIATION: CYP-450 = cytochrome P-450.

paroxetine in depressed patients with IHD.[250] Both antidepressants were effective in the treatment of depression, but not surprisingly, there were more dropouts because of side effects and more cardiac-related effects with the TCA. Unfortunately, the safety of SSRIs remains to be established in large-scale, randomized treatment trials of post-MI patients with comorbid major depression.[271] The recently completed SADHART study, a randomized, multicenter, double-blind trial of sertraline versus placebo in the treatment of post-MI patients with comorbid major depression, attempted to determine the efficacy and safety of this SSRI in depressed patients with unstable angina and those who are post-MI. Any of the available oral antidepressants usually will produce a clinical therapeutic response (an improvement in depressive symptoms by 50 percent or more) in comparison to pretreatment severity of depressive symptoms in 60 to 70 percent of medically healthy patients provided that the antidepressant is administered in sufficient dosage over a treatment duration of 5 to 6 weeks.

Another somatic treatment modality, electroconvulsive therapy (ECT), is effective in up to 80 percent of patients with either unipolar or bipolar depression[272] over a relatively brief (2- to 3-week) treatment duration. ECT is the initial treatment of choice in depressed patients who are severely ill (e.g., at nutritional risk from severe calorie loss or dehydration) and require a rapid clinical response. ECT also should be considered for patients who have experienced a previous positive response to ECT, do not respond to oral antidepressants, cannot tolerate the associated side effects of antidepressants, or experience depression with psychotic symptoms (hallucinations, delusions, paranoia).

Electroconvulsive therapy produces a seizure by providing a brief pulse (approximately 1 to 2 s in duration) of electrical charge over the scalp in the area of the right parietal lobe (right unilateral ECT) or over both temples (bilateral ECT). This pulse elicits a generalized convulsive seizure that lasts approximately 30 to 60 s. The patient is anesthetized during the procedure with a short-acting barbiturate (e.g., methohexital) and paralyzed with a muscle relaxant such as succinylcholine. Respirations are controlled by masked ventilation, and intubation is not required unless there have been recurrent episodes of aspiration. The morbidity and mortality associated with ECT have decreased dramatically over the past 60 years. The introduction of curare and later succinylcholine decreased the incidence of orthopedic complications from almost 20 percent of cases to being a rare complication. Complications related to cognitive dysfunction, such as delirium and amnesia, also have been decreased through the use of brief pulse (versus sine wave) and unilateral (versus bilateral) ECT. Structural brain studies using magnetic resonance images have shown no evidence of brain damage secondary to ECT.[273] Moreover, most studies of memory problems associated with ECT have reported that patients have transient amnesia and that memory returns to the pre-ECT level of function within 6 months.

Until recently, however, the cardiac complications from ECT resulted in the most serious adverse events. As recently as the 1980s, deaths from ECT were estimated to be approximately 1 per 10,000 treatments (most patients receive 6 to 10 treatments per ECT trial), primarily as a result of cardiac complications. Two major cardiac complications occur in relation to the ECT stimulus: an initial asystole secondary to vagal nerve stimulation followed closely by the release of EPI with tachycardia and hypertension. Although the patient is paralyzed, the ECT electrode that conducts up to 100 J of energy to stimulate the seizure also produces a direct stimulus of the masseter muscles (a bite block is kept in place during the treatments) and the vagus nerve. The stimulation of the vagus can subsequently cause asystole. Within seconds of the vagal stimulation, an adrenergic discharge related to the onset of a generalized seizure causes the release of EPI with tachycardia, hypertension, and the potential for myocardial ischemia or arrhythmias. The tachycardia is relatively brief (1 to 2 min).

Although no absolute contraindications to ECT exist, certain clinical situations increase the risk of complications from a course of ECT, i.e., diseases that affect the CNS and/or the cardiothrombovascular system: a cerebral vascular accident (CVA) during the previous 6 months, any illness that increases intracranial pressure (e.g., brain tumor), medical disorders that disrupt the blood-brain barrier (e.g., meningitis), a cerebral or aortic aneurysm, MI, severe valvular heart disease, a high-grade atrioventricular block, symptomatic ventricular arrhythmias, supraventricular arrhythmias with uncontrolled ventricular rate, and coagulation or bleeding disorders.[274] Implanted cardiac pacemakers and defibrillators are usually not problematic during ECT.[275,276] Some practitioners choose to convert a demand pacemaker to a fixed mode, and an electrophysiologist should be consulted to determine whether the defibrillator's function should be inhibited during each ECT treatment. Electroconvulsive therapy also is tolerated by cardiac transplant patients who have normal cardiac function.[277]

Electroconvulsive therapy can be conceptualized as a cardiac stress test; however, because of the general anesthesia, the patient cannot report symptoms such as chest pain, and the seizure stimulating the tachycardia cannot be terminated abruptly. Therefore, the pre-ECT workup should include a complete review of systems and a screen for exercise intolerance, angina, evidence of congestive heart failure (patients will receive approximately 1 L of fluid per ECT treatment) or diabetes, extent of smoking history, cholesterol level, and other cardiac risk factors. The basic pre-ECT screening includes measurement of serum electrolytes (with particular attention to hydration status and potassium) and hemoglobin and the obtaining of an electrocardiogram (ECG). Chest x-rays are obtained in case of evidence of CHF or pulmonary disease. Patients with a history of back pain are evaluated with spine films; neuroimaging is used to determine whether there has been a recent CVA or increased intracranial pressure in patients with neurologic dysfunction. Although "beta blockers" are used during ECT treatment (see below), cardiovascular screening should determine whether the patient can tolerate transient tachycardia and hypertension. Additional cardiac screening includes a stress test in individuals at significant risk for CAD.

Modern ECT suites are equipped with continuous ECG and blood pressure and heart rate monitors as well as pulse oximetry and an electroencephalograph to record seizure activity. Patients should continue their pulmonary (except theophylline) and cardiac (except lidocaine) medications during a course of ECT treatment. Theophylline and lidocaine are discontinued because of prolongation and reduction of seizure duration, respectively. As a result of the increase in intraocular pressure during an ECT-induced seizure, glaucoma medications generally are continued, except for acetylcholinesterases. Hypoglycemic agents should not be administered the morning of ECT to prevent hypoglycemia in diabetic patients. Patients must not ingest food or fluids before ECT treatments but may receive intravenous fluids as tolerated. In addition to usual ECT medications (methohexital 1 mg/kg and succinylcholine 0.75–1.50 mg/kg), patients with hypertension, CAD, valvular heart disease, and CHF routinely receive prophylactic medication to prevent cardiac complications from the transient hypertension and tachycardia induced by ECT.[278] Such a "cardiac-modified" ECT protocol[279,280] should be utilized for elderly patients and those with cardiac disease. Usually either of two beta blockers, labetalol or esmolol, is utilized to reduce maximal heart rate, mean arterial pressure, and arrhythmia frequency during ECT. Labetalol (selective alpha$_1$- and nonselective beta-adrenergic receptor blockade and elimination half-life of 5 to 8 h) may induce significant hypotension.[281] Esmolol (beta$_1$-selective at the usual doses, rapid onset, and an elimination half-life of 9 min) may replace labetolol if labetolol induces prolonged bradycardia and hypotension. Esmolol, however, has been associated with shortened seizure duration during ECT. If elderly patients pretreated with a beta blocker continue to exhibit transient increases in blood pressure, a calcium channel blocker may be added. Nicardepine has replaced nifedipine as the calcium channel blocker of choice because nicardepine may be administered intravenously and has a shorter duration of action. The ECT protocol also involves adequate hydration before ECT, discontinuation of psychotropic medication whenever possible, and provision of anticholinergic medication (0.4 to 0.8 mg intravenous atropine or 0.2 mg of glycopyrrolate) to decrease oropharyngeal secretions and prevent bradycardias whenever beta blockers are used.[282] Continuous blood pressure monitoring and ECG monitoring should be performed during all treatments, along with monitoring for shortness of breath or chest pain.

The third most common cardiac complication is orthostatic hypotension, which usually occurs in the recovery room, particularly in elderly debilitated patients and patients with medical conditions associated with autonomic dysfunction (e.g., Parkinson's disease). As was noted above, consideration should be given to the utilization of shorter-acting beta blockers that have less alpha-adrenoreceptor blockade (esmolol for labetolol) and/or shorter-acting calcium channel blockers (nicardepine for nifedipine). After each ECT treatment, patients recover for over an hour in a setting similar to an outpatient surgical suite. Patients remain on a cardiac monitor with intravenous fluids and supplemental oxygen provided until they are oriented and exhibit no orthostatic hypotension (approximately 20 to 30 min). They are then dressed and asked to be seated upright in a chair until they are fully alert and able to ingest fluids orally (approximately 20 to 30 min in duration).

In summary, the magnitude of the risks associated with ECT are approximately equivalent to those of general anesthesia. The incidence of delirium during ECT can be reduced to less than 5 percent in elderly patients through the administration of twice-weekly ECT treatments and the use of unilateral electrode placement on the right temporal area in patients at risk (patients with structural brain changes, concomitant medical illness, Alzheimer's disease, Parkinson's disease, advanced age, and concomitant administration of psychotropic medications).[282] Cardiac complications are not uncommon with ECT but are reduced significantly with a cardiac ECT protocol. Although generally a safe and effective treatment, ECT in elderly patients with cardiovascular disease requires a multispecialty coordinated effort among a specially trained ECT-nursing service, psychiatrist, anesthesiologist, and cardiologist.

FUTURE DIRECTIONS FOR RESEARCH

Usually underdiagnosed and undertreated, major depression and anxiety disorders are encountered commonly in patients with CAD and patients referred for evaluation of chest pain. However, a burgeoning literature on the importance of major depression and anxiety disorders in patients with heart disease has accumulated over the past two decades. Several studies have shown depression and its associated symptoms to be a major risk factor in both the development of CVD and death after an index MI. Further evidence is accumulating regarding the increased risk of patients with anxiety disorders or anxiety symptoms for the development of IHD, although currently there is a dearth of information about the prevalence of anxiety disorders in patients with CAD or CHF. An intriguing area of investigation involves the possible effects of anxiety disorders on the thrombovascular system and the "reciprocal" cardiovascular contributions to anxiety symptoms or anxiety syndromes, such as panic disorder. Although treatment of depression in many patients with CVD improves their dysphoria and other signs and symptoms of depression, are these agents safe and effective in the treatment of anxiety disorders as well? One of many important questions to be answered is whether aggressive and consistent treatment of anxiety and depressive syndromes in patients with CVD not only improves their quality of life but diminishes cardiovascular-related morbidity and improves survival. Which treatment modalities (psychotherapeutic versus psychopharmacologic or a combination) will be most effective in patients with recurrent or more severe depression remains to be determined. Treatment studies also may assess the relation between depression and subsequent compliance with medication and modification of risk factors for CVD.[31] Future studies undoubtedly should include women to assess whether there are gender-specific psychiatric and psychobiological differences in the response to treatment[198,283–285] because women are more vulnerable to depression and because CVD is the leading cause of death among adult women in the United States.

The associations between diseases of the CNS (anxiety and depressive disorders) and disorders of peripheral "end organs" such as the heart raise intriguing questions regarding what is "cardiovascular" or "psychiatric." Illumination of the interplay between anxiety disorders, depressive syndromes, and the thrombovascular system, particularly in patients with CVD, undoubtedly will lead to the development of new treatment modalities that not only will improve patients' quality of life but potentially will decrease their morbidity and improve long-term survival rates.

ACKNOWLEDGMENTS

This research was supported by grants MH-01399, NIMH 156617-03, MH-42088, MH-49523, and RR-00039 from the National Institutes of Health, Bethesda, MD, an Established Investigator Award from the National Alliance for Research on Schizophrenia and Depression (Dr. Nemeroff), and a Research Award from the Dana Foundation (Dr. Musselman).

References

1. Hayward C. Psychiatric illness and cardiovascular disease risk. *Epidemiol Rev* 1995; 17:129–138.
2. Dimsdale JE. A perspective on Type A behavior and coronary disease. *N Engl J Med* 1988; 318:110–112.
3. American Psychiatric Association. *Diagnostic and Statistical Manual of Mental Disorders,* 4th ed. Washington, DC: American Psychiatric Association; 1994.
4. Kessler RC, McGonagle KA, Zhao S, et al. Lifetime and 12-month prevalence of DSM-III-R psychiatric disorders in the United States. *Arch Gen Psychiatry* 1994; 51:8–19.
5. Leeper J, Badger L, Milo T. Mental disorders among physical disability determination patients. *Am J Public Health* 1985; 75: 78–79.
6. Blacker CVR, Clare AW. Depressive disorder in primary care. *Br J Psychiatry* 1987; 150:737–751.
7. Barrett JE, Barrett JA, Oxman TE, Gerber PD. The prevalence of psychiatric disorders in a primary care practice. *Arch Gen Psychiatry* 1988; 45:1100–1106.
8. Von Korff M, Shapiro S, Burke JD, et al. Anxiety and depression in a primary care clinic: Comparison of Diagnostic Interview Schedule, General Health Questionnaire, and practitioner assessments. *Arch Gen Psychiatry* 1987; 44:152–156.
9. Cohen-Cole SA, Kaufman KG. Major depression in physical illness: Diagnosis, prevalence, and antidepressant treatment (a ten year review: 1982–1992). *Depression* 1993; 1:181–204.
10. Magni G, Schifano F, DeLeo D. Assessment of depression in an elderly medical population. *J Affect Disord* 1986; 11:121–124.
11. Feldman E, Mayou R, Hawton K, et al. Psychiatric disorder in medical inpatients. *Q J Med* 1987; 63:405–412.
12. Blazer D, Swartz M, Woodbury M, et al. Depressive symptoms and depressive diagnoses in a community population: Use of a new procedure for analysis of psychiatric classification. *Arch Gen Psychiatr* 1988; 45:1078–1084.
13. Bebbington P, Katz R, McGuffin P, et al. The risk of minor depression before age 65: Results from a community survey. *Psychol Med* 1989; 19:393–400.
14. Broadhead WE, Blazer DG, George LK, Tse CK. Depression, disability days, and days lost from work in a prospective epidemiologic survey. *JAMA* 1990; 264:2524–2528.
15. Johnson J, Weissman MM, Klerman GL. Service utilization and social morbidity associated with depressive symptoms in the community. *JAMA* 1992; 267:1478–1483.
16. Kessler LG, Cleary PD, Burke JD Jr. Psychiatric disorders in primary care: Results of a follow-up study. *Arch Gen Psychiatry* 1985; 42:583–587.
17. Ormel J, Koeter MWJ, van den Brink W, van de Willige G. Recognition, management, and course of anxiety and depression in general practice. *Arch Gen Psychiatry* 1991; 48:700–706.
18. Kurosawa H, Shimizu Y, Nishimatsu Y, et al. The relationship between mental disorders and physical severities in patients with acute myocardial infarction. *Jpn Circ J* 1983; 47:723–725.
19. Mayou R, Foster A, Williamson B. Medical care after myocardial infarction. *J Psychos Res* 1979; 23:23–26.
20. Carney RM, Rich MW, teVelde A, et al. Major depressive disorder in coronary artery disease. *Am J Cardiol* 1987; 60:1273–1275.

21. Schlelfer SJ, Macarini-Hinson MM, Coyle DA, et al. The nature and course of depression following myocardial infarction. *Arch Intern Med* 1989; 149:1785–1789.
22. Frasure-Smith N, Lesperance F, Talajic M. Depression following myocardial infarction: Impact on 6-month survival. *JAMA* 1993; 270:1819–1861.
23. Blumenthal JA, Williams RS, Wallace AG, et al. Physiological and psychological variables predict compliance to prescribed exercise therapy in patients recovering from myocardial infarction. *Psychosom Med* 1982; 44:519–527.
24. Stern JJ, Pascale L, Ackerman A. Life adjustment postmyocardial infarction: Determine predictive variables. *Arch Intern Med* 1977; 137:1680–1685.
25. Mayou R, Foster A, Williamson B. Psychosocial adjustment in patients one year after myocardial infarction. *J Psychosom Res* 1978; 22:447–453.
26. Skodol AE, Schwartz S, Dohrenwend BP, et al. Minor depression in a cohort of young adults in Israel. *Arch Gen Psychiatry* 1994; 51:542–551.
27. Wells KB, Stewart A, Hayes RD, et al. The functioning and well-being of depressed patients: Results of the Medical Outcomes Study. *JAMA* 1989; 262:914–919.
28. Carney RM, Rich MW, Freedland KE, Saini J. Major depressive disorder predicts cardiac events in patients with coronary artery disease. *Psychosom Med* 1988; 50:627–633.
29. Aromaa A, Raitasalo R, Reunanen A, et al. Depression and cardiovascular diseases. *Acta Psychiatr Scand* 1994; 377:77–82.
30. Ahern DK, Gorkin L, Anderson JL, et al. Biobehavioral variables and mortality or cardiac arrest in the Cardiac Arrhythmia Pilot Study (CAPS). *Am J Cardiol* 1990; 66:59–62.
31. Frasure-Smith N, Lesperance F, Talajic M. Depression and 18-month prognosis after myocardial infarction. *Circulation* 1995; 91:999–1005.
32. Wynn A. Unwarranted emotional distress in men with ischaemic heart disease. *Med J Aust* 1967; 2:847–851.
33. Hackett TP, Cassem NH, Wishnie HA. The coronary-care unit: An appraisal of its psychologic hazards. *N Engl J Med* 1968; 279:1365–1370.
34. Cay EL, Vetter N, Philip AE, Dugard P. Psychological status during recovery from an acute heart attack. *J Psychosom Res* 1972; 16:425–435.
35. Robins LN, Helzer JE, Croughan JL, et al. The NIMH Diagnostic Interview Schedule, Version III. Washington DC: Public Health Service (HSS), ADM-T-42-3 (5-81, 8-81); 1981.
36. Endicott J, Spitzer RL. A diagnostic interview: The Schedule for Affective Disorders and Schizophrenia. *Arch Gen Psychiatry* 1978; 35:837–844.
37. Freedland KE, Carney RM, Rich MW, et al. Depression in elderly patients with heart failure. *J Geriatr Psychiatry* 1991; 24: 59–71.
38. Gonzalez MB, Snyderman TB, Colket JT, et al. Depression in patients with coronary artery disease. *Depression* 1996; 4:57–62.
39. Koenig HG. Depression in hospitalized older patients with congestive heart failure. *Gen Hosp Psychiatry* 1998; 20:29–43.
40. Ostfeld AM, Lebovits BZ, Shekelle RB, Paul O. A prospective study of the relationship between personality and coronary heart disease. *J Chronic Dis* 1964; 17:265–276.
41. Hathaway SR, McKinley JC. *Minnesota Multiphasic Personality Inventory Manual*, rev. ed. New York: Psychological Corporation; 1951.
42. Cattell RB, Saunders DR, Stice G. *Handbook for the Sixteen Personality Factor Questionnaire.* Champaign, IL: Institute for Personality and Ability Testing; 1957.
43. Brozek J, Keyes A, Blackburn H. Personality differences between potential coronary and noncoronary subjects. *Ann NY Acad Sci* 1966; 134:1057–1064.
44. Goldberg EL, Comstock GW, Hornstra RK. Depressed mood and subsequent physical illness. *Am J Psychiatry* 1979; 136: 530–534.
45. Radloff LS. The CES-D scale: A self-report depression scale for research in the general population. *J Appl Psychol Meas* 1977; 1:385–401.
46. Murphy JM, Monson RR, Olivier DC, et al. Affective disorders and mortality. *Arch Gen Psychiatry* 1987; 44:473–480.
47. Murphy JM, Neff RK, Sobol AM, et al. Computer diagnosis of depression and anxiety: The Stirling County Study. *Psychol Med* 1985; 15:99–112.
48. Anda R, Williamson D, Jones D, et al. Depressed affect, hopelessness, and the risk of ischemic heart disease in a cohort of U.S. adults. *Epidemiology* 1993; 4:285–294.
49. Dupuy HJ. A concurrent validational study of the NCHS General Well-Being Schedule. *Vital Health Stat* 1977; 73.
50. Wing JK, Cooper JE, Sartorius N. *The Measurement and Classification of Psychiatric Symptoms.* London: Cambridge University Press; 1974.
51. Vogt T, Pope C, Mullooly JJH. Mental health status as a predictor of morbidity and mortality: A 15-year follow-up of members of a health maintenance organization. *Am J Public Health* 1994; 84:227–231.
52. McFarland BH, Freeborn DK, Mullooly JP, Pope CR. Utilization patterns among long-term enrollees in a prepaid group practice health maintenance organization. *Med Care* 1985; 23:1221–1233.
53. Simonsick EM, Wallace RB, Blazer DG, Berkman LF: Depressive symptomatology and hypertension-associated morbidity and mortality in older adults. *Psychosom Med* 1995; 57:427–435.
54. Everson SA, Goldberg DE, Kaplan GA, et al. Hopelessness and risk of mortality and incidence of myocardial infarction and cancer. *Psychosom Med* 1996; 58:113–121.
55. Barefoot JC, Schroll M. Symptoms of depression, acute myocardial infarction, and total mortality in a community sample. *Circulation* 1996; 93:1976–1980.
56. Greene RL. *The MMPI-2/MMPI: An Interpretive Manual.* Boston: Allyn and Bacon; 1991.
57. Pratt LA, Ford DE, Crum RM, et al. Depression, psychotropic medication, and risk of myocardial infarction: Prospective data from the Baltimore ECA follow-up. *Circulation* 1996; 94:3123–3129.
58. Wassertheil-Smoller S, Applegate WB, Berge K, et al. Change in depression as a precursor of cardiovascular events. *Arch Intern Med* 1996; 156:553–561.
59. Callahan CM, Wolinsky FD, Stump TE, et al. Mortality, symptoms, and functional impairment in late-life depression. *J Gen Intern Med* 1998; 13:746–752.
60. Mendes de Leon CF, Krumholz HM, Seeman TS, et al. Depression and risk of coronary heart disease in elderly men and women: New Haven EPESE, 1982–1991. *Arch Intern Med* 1998; 158:2341–2348.
61. Ford DE, Mead LA, Chang PP, et al. Depression is a risk factor for coronary artery disease in men: The Precursors Study. *Arch Intern Med* 1998; 158:1422–1426.
62. Vingerhoets A. *Psychosocial Stress: An Experimental Approach.* Groningen, Netherlands: Swets & Zeitlinger; 1985.
63. Selye H. *The Stress of Life.* New York: McGraw Hill; 1956.
64. Nemeroff CB, Widerlov E, Bissette G, et al. Elevated concentrations of CSF corticotropin-releasing factor-like immunoreactivity in depressed patients. *Science* 1984; 226:1342–1344.
65. Arato M, Banki CM, Nemeroff CB, Bissette G. Hypothalamic-pituitary-adrenal axis and suicide. *Ann NY Acad Sci* 1986; 487: 263–270.
66. Banki CM, Bissette G, Arato M, et al. Cerebrospinal fluid corticotropin-releasing factor-like immunoreactivity in depression and schizophrenia. *Am J Psychiatry* 1987; 144:873–877.
67. Banki CM, Karmasci L, Bissette G, Nemeroff CB. CSF corticotropin-releasing and somatostatin in major depression: Response to

antidepressant treatment and relapse. *Eur Neuropsychopharmacol* 1992; 2:107–113.
68. France RD, Urban B, Krishnan KRR, et al. CSF corticotropin-releasing factor-like immunoreactivity in chronic pain patients with and without major depression. *Biol Psychiatry* 1988; 23: 86–88.
69. Risch SC, Lewine RJ, Kalin NH, et al. Limbic-hypothalamic-pituitary-adrenal axis activity and ventricular-to-brain ratio studies in affective illness and schizophrenia. *Neuropsychopharmacology* 1992; 6:95–100.
70. Raadsheer FC, Hoogendijk WJG, Stam FC, et al. Increased numbers of corticotropin-releasing hormone expressing neurons in the hypothalamic paraventricular nucleus of depressed patients. *Neuroendocrinology* 1994; 60:436–444.
71. Raadsheer FC, van Heerikhuize JJ, Lucassen PJ, et al. Corticotropin-releasing hormone mRNA levels in the paraventricular nucleus of patients with Alzheimer's disease and depression. *Am J Psychiatry* 1995; 152:1372–1376.
72. Bjorkerud S. Effect of adrenocortical hormones on the integrity of rat aortic endothelium. In: Schettler G, Weizel A, eds. *Proceedings of the 3rd International Symposium on Atherosclerosis III*. Berlin: Springer-Verlag; 1973:245.
73. Nahas GG, Brunson JG, King WM, Cavert HM. Functional and morphologic changes in heart lung preparations following administration of adrenal hormones. *Am J Clin Pathol* 1958; 34: 717–729.
74. Valigorsky JM. Metaplastic transformation of aortic smooth muscle cells in cortisone-induced dissecting aneurysms in hamsters. *Fed Proc* 1969; 28:802.
75. Kemper JW, Baggenstoss AH, Slocumb CH. The relationship of therapy with cortisone to the incidence of vascular lesions in rheumatoid arthritis. *Ann Intern Med* 1957; 46:831–851.
76. Ross R, Harker L. Hyperlipidemia and atherosclerosis. *Science* 1976; 193:1094–1100.
77. Troxler RG, Sprague EA, Albanese RA, et al. The association of elevated plasma cortisol and early atherosclerosis as demonstrated by coronary angiography. *Atherosclerosis* 1977; 26: 151–162.
78. Swanson LW, Sawchenko PE. Organization of ovine corticotropin-releasing factor immunoreactive cells and fibers in the rat brain: An immunohistochemical study. *Neuroendocrinology* 1983; 36:165–186.
79. Merchenthaler I, Vigh S, Petruscz P, Schally AV. Immunocytochemical localization of corticotropin-releasing factor (CRF) in the rat brain. *Am J Anat* 1982; 165:385–396.
80. Cummings S, Elde R, Ellis J, Lindall A. Corticotropin-releasing factor immunoreactivity is widely distributed with the central nervous system of the rat: An immunohistochemical study. *J Neurosci* 1983; 8:1355–1368.
81. Wyatt RJ, Portnoy B, Kupfer DJ, et al. Resting plasma catecholamine concentrations in patients with depression and anxiety. *Arch Gen Psychiatry* 1971; 24:24:65–70.
82. Louis WJ, Doyle AE, Anavekar SN. Plasma noradrenaline concentration and blood pressure in essential hypertension, phaeochromocytoma and depression. *Clin Soc* 1975; 48:239S–242S.
83. Roy A, Pickar D, DeJong J, et al. Norepinephrine and its metabolites in cerebrospinal fluid, plasma and urine: Relationship to hypothalamic-pituitary-adrenal axis function in depression. *Arch Gen Psychiatry* 1988; 45:849–857.
84. Veith RC, Lewis L, Linares OA, et al. Sympathetic nervous system activity in major depression: Basal and desipramine-induced alterations in plasma NE kinetics. *Arch Gen Psychiatry* 1994; 51:411–422.
85. Roy A, Guthrie S, Pickar D, Linnoila M. Plasma NE responses to cold challenge in depressed patients and normal controls. *Psychiatry Res* 1987; 21:161–168.
86. Charney DS, Menkes DB, Henninger GR. Receptor sensitivity and the mechanism of action of antidepressant treatment. *Arch Gen Psychiatry* 1981; 38:1160–1180.
87. Golden RN, Markey SP, Risby ED, et al. Antidepressants reduce whole-body norepinephrine turnover while enhancing 6-hydroxymelatonin output. *Arch Gen Psychiatry* 1988; 45:150–154.
88. Linnoila M, Karoum F, Calil HM, et al. Alteration of NE metabolism with desipramine and zimelidine in depressed patients. *Arch Gen Psychiatry* 1982; 39:1025–1028.
89. Linnoila M, Guthrie S, Lane EA, et al. Clinical studies on NE metabolism: How to interpret the numbers. *Psychiatry Res* 1986; 17:229–239.
90. Scubee-Moreau JJ, Dresse AE. Effect of various antidepressant drugs on the spontaneous firing rate of locus coeruleus and raphe dorsalis neurons of the rat. *Euro J Pharmacol* 1979; 57:219–225.
91. Sulser F, Vetulani J, Mobley PL. Mode of action on antidepressant drugs. *Biochem Pharmacol* 1978; 27:257–261.
92. Anfossi G, Trovati M. Role of catecholamines in platelet function: Pathophysiological and clinical significance. *Euro J Clin Invest* 1996; 26:353–370.
93. Gerritsen ME. Physiological and pathophysiological roles of eicosanoids in the microcirculation. *Cardiovas Res* 1996; 32:720–732.
94. Goldstein DS. Plasma catecholamines and essential hypertension: An analytical review. *Hypertension* 1983; 5:86–99.
95. Lund-Johansen P. Hemodynamic alterations in early essential hypertension: Recent advances. In: Gross F, Strasser T, eds. *Mild Hypertension: Recent Advances*. New York: Raven Press; 1983:237.
96. Lechin F, van der Dijs B, Orozco B, et al. Plasma neurotransmitters, blood pressure, and heart rate during supine-resting, orthostasis, and moderate exercise conditions in major depressed patients. *Biol Psychiatry* 1995; 38:166–173.
97. Akselrod S, Gordon D, Ubel FA, et al. Power spectrum analysis of heart rate fluctuation: A quantitative probe of beat-to-beat cardiovascular control. *Science* 1981; 213:220–222.
98. Low PA. Autonomic nervous system function. *J Clin Neurophysiol* 1993; 10:14–27.
99. Spyer KM. Central nervous system control of the cardiovascular system. In: Bannister R, ed. *Autonomic Failure: A Textbook of Clinical Disorders of the Autonomic Nervous System*. Oxford, UK: Oxford University Press; 1988:56.
100. Shields RW. Functional anatomy of the autonomic nervous system. *J Clin Neurophysiol* 1993; 10:2–13.
101. Dalack GW, Roose SP. Perspectives on the relationship between cardiovascular disease and affective disorder. *J Clin Psychiatry* 1990; 51(suppl 7):4–9, 10–11.
102. Wolf M, Varigos G, Hunt D, Sloman JG. Sinus arrhythmia in acute myocardial infarction. *Med J Aust* 1978; 2:52–53.
103. Billman GE, Schwartz PJ, Stone HL. Baroreceptor reflex control of heart rate: A predictor of sudden cardiac death. *Circulation* 1982; 66:874–880.
104. Kleiger RE, Miller PJ, Bigger TJ, et al. Decreased heart rate variability and its association with increased mortality after acute myocardial infarction. *Am J Cardiol* 1987; 39:256–262.
105. Bigger JT, Kleiger RE, Fleiss JL, et al. Components of HR variability measured during healing of acute myocardial infarction. *Am J Cardiol* 1988; 61:208–215.
106. LaRovere MT, Specchia G, Mortana A, Schwartz PJ. Baroreflex sensitivity, clinical correlates, and cardiovascular mortality among patients with a first myocardial infarction: A prospective study. *Circ* 1988; 78:816–824.
107. Cripps T, Malik M, Farrell T, Camm AJ. Prognostic value of reduced heart rate variability after myocardial infarction: Clinical evaluation of a new analysis method. *Br Heart J* 1991; 65:14–19.
108. Viskin S, Belhassen B. Noninvasive and invasive strategies for the prevention of sudden death after myocardial infarction: Value, limitations and implications for therapy. *Drugs* 1992; 44:336–355.
109. Araya-Gomez V, Gonzalez-Hermosillo J, Casanova-Garces J, et

al. Identification of patients at risk of malignant arrythmia in the 1st year after myocardial infarction. *Arch Inst Cardiol Mex* 1994; 64:145–159.

110. Campbell RWF. Can analysis of heart rate variability predict arrhythmias and antiarrhythmic effects? In: Oto AM, ed. *Practice and Progress in Cardiac Pacing and Electrophysiology*. Dordrecht, Netherlands: Kluwer; 1996:63.

111. Sayers BM. Analysis of heart rate variability. *Ergonomics*. 1973; 16:17–32.

112. Pomeranz B, Macaulay RJB, Caudill MA, et al. Assessment of autonomic function in humans by heart rate spectral analysis. *Am J Physiol* 1985; 248:H151–H153.

113. Pagani M, Lombardi F, Guzzetti S, et al. Power spectral analysis of heart rate and arterial pressure variabilities as a marker of sympathovagal interaction in man and conscious dog. *Circ Res* 1986; 59:178–193.

114. Koizumi K, Terui N, Kollai M. Effect of cardiac vagal and sympathetic nerve activity on heart rate in rhythmic fluctuations. *J Auton Nerv Sys* 1985; 12:251–259.

115. Katona PG, Jih F. Respiratory sinus arrhythmia: Noninvasive measure of the parasympathetic cardiac control. *J Appl Physiol* 1975; 39:801–805.

116. Fouad FM, Tarazzi RC, Gerrario CM, et al. Assessment of parasympathetic control of heart rate by a noninvasive method. *Am J Physiol* 1984; 246:H838–H842.

117. Bigger TJJ, Fleiss JL, Steinman RC, et al. Frequency domain measures of heart period variability and mortality after myocardial infarction. *Circulation* 1992; 85:164–171.

118. Miyawaki E, Salzman C. Autonomic nervous system tests in psychiatry: Implications and potential uses of heart rate variability. *Integr Psychiatry* 1991; 7:21–28.

119. Yeragani VK, Pohl R, Ramesh C, et al. Effect of imipramine treatment on heart rate variability measures. *Neuropsychobiology* 1992; 26:27–32.

120. Rechlin T, Weis MDC. Heart rate variability in depressed patients and differential effects of paroxetine and amitriptyline on cardiovascular autonomic functions. *Pharmacopsychiatry* 1994; 27:124–128.

121. Carney RM, Saunders RD, Freedland KE, et al. Association of depression with reduced heart rate variability in coronary artery disease. *Am J Cardiol* 1995; 76:562–564.

122. Roose SP, Glassman AH, Dalack GW. Depression, heart disease, and tricyclic antidepressants. *J Clin Psychiatry* 1989; 50(suppl 7):12–16.

123. Severus WE, Ahrens B, Stoll AL. Omega-3 fatty acids—the missing link? (letter). *Arch Gen Psychiatry* 1999; 56:380–381.

124. Edwards R, Peet M, Shay J, Horrobin D. Omega-3 polyunsaturated fatty acid levels in the diet and in red blood cell membranes of depressed patients. *J Affect Dis* 1998; 48:149–155.

125. Adams PB, Lawson S, Sanigorski A, Sinclair AJ. Arachidonic acid to eicosapentaenoic acid ratio in blood correlates positively with clinical symptoms of depression. *Lipids* 1996; 31:S157–S161.

126. Maes M, Smith R, Christophe A, et al. Fatty acid composition in major depression: Decreased omega 3 fractions in cholesteryl esters and increased C20:4 omega-6/C20:5 omega-3 ratio in cholesteryl esters and phospholipids. *J Affect Dis* 1996; 38: 35–46.

127. Albert CM, Hennekens CH, O'Donnell CJ, et al. Fish consumption and risk of sudden cardiac death. *JAMA* 1998; 279:23–28.

128. Siscovick DS, Raghunathan TE, King I, et al. Dietary intake and cell membrane levels of long-chain n-3 polyunsaturated fatty acids and the risk of primary cardiac arrest. *JAMA* 1995; 274:1363–1367.

129. Burr ML, Fehily AM, Gilbert JF, et al. Effects of changes in fat, fish and fibre intake on death and myocardial reinfarction: Diet and reinfarction trial. *Lancet* 1989; 2:757–761.

130. Sellmayer A, Witzgall H, Lorenz RL, Weber PC. Effects of dietary fish oil on ventricular premature complexes. *Am J Cardiol* 1995; 76:974–977.

131. Christensen JH, Gustenhoff P, Korup E, et al. Effect of fish oil on heart rate variability in survivors of myocardial infarction: A double blind randomised controlled trial. *Brit Med J* 1996; 312:677–678.

132. Christensen JH, Korup E, Aaroe J, et al. Fish consumption, n-3 fatty acids in cell membranes, and heart rate variability in survivors of myocardial infarction with left ventricular dysfunction. *Am J Cardiol* 1997; 79:1670–1673.

133. Balogh S, Fitzpatrick DF, Hendricks SE, Paige SR. Increases in heart rate variability with successful treatment in patients with major depressive disorder. *Psychopharmacol Bull* 1993; 29:201–206.

134. Markovitz JH, Matthews KA. Platelets and coronary heart disease: Potential psychophysiologic mechanism. *Psychosom Med* 1991; 53:643–668.

135. Morris PLP, Robsin RG, Andrzejewski P, et al. Association of depression with 10-year poststroke mortality. *Am J Psychiatry* 1993; 150:124–129.

136. Lefkovits J, Plow EF, Topol EJ. Platelet glycoprotein IIb/IIIa receptors in cardiovascular medicine. *N Engl J Med* 1995; 332:1553–1559.

137. Hess H, Mietaschk A, Deichsel G. Drug-induced inhibition of platelet function delays progression of peripheral occlusive arterial disease: A prospective double-blind arteriographically controlled trial. *Lancet* 1985; 1:415–419.

138. Antiplatelet Trialists' Collaboration. Secondary prevention of vascular disease by prolonged antiplatelet treatment. *Brit Med J (Clinical Research Edition)* 1988; 296:320–331.

139. Verstraete M. Risk factors, interventions and therapeutic agents in the prevention of atherosclerosis-related ischaemic diseases. *Drugs* 1991; 42(suppl 5):22–38.

140. Ridker PM, Manson JE, Burning JE, et al. The effect of chronic platelet inhibition with low-dose aspirin on atherosclerotic progression and acute thrombosis: Clinical evidence from the Physicians' Health Study. *Am Heart J* 1991; 122:1588–1592.

141. Second International Trial of Infarct Survival Collaborative Group. Randomized trial of intravenous streptokinase, oral aspirin, both, or neither among 17,187 cases of suspected acute myocardial infarction: ISIS-2. *Lancet* 1988; 2:349–360.

142. Antiplatelet Trialists' Collaboration. Collaborative overview of randomized trials of antiplatelet therapy: I. Prevention of death, myocardial infarction, and stroke by prolonged antiplatelet therapy in various categories of patients. *Brit Med J* 1994; 308: 81–106.

143. Musselman DL, Tomer A, Manatunga AK, et al. Exaggerated platelet reactivity in major depression. *Am J Psychiatry* 1996; 153:1313–1317.

144. Laghrissi-Thode F, Wagner WR, Pollock BG, et al. Elevated platelet factor 4 and β-thromboglobulin plasma levels in depressed patients with ischemic heart disease. *Biol Psychiatry* 1997; 42:290–295.

145. Weyrich AS, Solis GA, Li KS, et al. Platelet amplification of vasospasm. *Am J Physiol* 1992; 263:H349–H358.

146. DeClerck F. Effects of serotonin on platelets and blood vessels. *J Cardiovasc Pharmacol* 1991; 17(suppl 5):S1–S5.

147. Owens MJ, Nemeroff CB. Role of serotonin in the pathophysiology of depression: Focus on the serotonin transporter. *Clin Chem* 1994; 40:288–295.

148. Osim EE, Wyllie JH. Evidence for loss of 5-hydroxytryptamine from circulating platelets. *J Physiol (Lond)* 1982; 326:25P–26P.

149. Ashton JH, Benedict CR, Fitzgerald C, et al. Serotonin as a mediator of cyclic flow variations in stenosed canine coronary arteries. *Circulation* 1986; 73:572–578.

150. Ashton JH, Ogletree ML, Michel IM, et al. Cooperative mediation by serotonin S2 and thromboxane S2/prostaglandin H2 receptor

activation of cyclic flow variation in dogs with severe coronary artery stenosis. *Circulation* 1987; 76:952–959.
151. Biegon A, Weizman A, Karp L, et al. Serotonin 5-HT2 receptor binding on blood platelets—a peripheral marker for depression? *Life Sci* 1987; 41:2485–2492.
152. Biegon A, Grinspoon A, Blumenfelt B, et al. Increased serotonin 5-HT2 receptor binding on blood platelets on suicidal men. *Psychopharmacology* 1990; 100:165–167.
153. Biegon A, Essar N, Israeli M, et al. Serotonin 5-HT2 receptor binding on blood platelets as a state dependent marker in major affective disorder. *Psychopharmacology* 1990; 102:73–75.
154. Arora RC, Meltzer HY. Increased serotonin (5-HT2) receptor binding as measured by 3H-LSD in the blood platelets of depressed patients. *Life Sci* 1989; 44:725–734.
155. Pandey GN, Pandey SC, Janicak PG. Platelet serotonin-2 binding sites in depression and suicide. *Biol Psychiatry* 1990; 28:215–222.
156. Briley MS, Langer SZ, Raisman R, et al. Tritiated imipramine binding sites are decreased in platelets of untreated depressed patients. *Science* 1980; 209:303–305.
157. Langer SZ, Arifian E, Briley MS, et al. High-affinity binding of 3H-imipramine in brain and platelets and its relevance to the biochemistry of affective disorders. *Life Sci* 1981; 29:211–218.
158. Paul SM, Rehavi M, Skolnick P, et al. Depressed patients have decreased binding of tritiated imipramine to platelet serotonin "transporter." *Arch Gen Psychiatry* 1981; 38:1315–1317.
159. Nemeroff CB, Knight DL, Franks J, et al. Further studies on platelet transporter binding in depression. *Am J Psychiatry* 1994; 151:1623–1625.
160. Cerrito F, Lazzaro MP, Gaudio E, et al. 5HT2-receptors and serotonin release: Their role in human platelet aggregation. *Life Sci* 1993; 53:209–215.
161. Kusumi I, Koyama T, Yamashita I. Serotonin-stimulated Ca^{2+} response is increased in the blood platelets of depressed patients. *Biol Psychiatry* 1991; 30:310–312.
162. Mikuni M, Kusumi I, Kagaya A, et al. Increased 5-HT2 receptor function as measured by serotonin-stimulated phosphoinositide hydrolysis in platelets of depressed patients. *Prog Neuropsychopharmacol Biol Psychiatry* 1991; 15:49–61.
163. Eckert A, Gann H, Riemann D, et al. Elevated intracellular calcium levels after 5-HT2 receptor stimulation in platelets of depressed patients. *Biol Psychiatry* 1993; 34:565–568.
164. Plein H, Berk M, Eppel S, Butkow N. Augmented platelet calcium uptake in response to serotonin stimulation in patients with major depression measured using Mn^{2+} influx and $^{45}CA^{2+}$ uptake. *Life Sci* 1999; 66:425–431.
165. Ware JA, Smith M, Salzman EW. Synergism of platelet aggregating agents: Role of elevation of cytoplasmic calcium. *J Clin Invest* 1987; 80:267–271.
166. Verrier RL. Behavioral stress, myocardial ischemia, and arrhythmias. In: Zipes DP, Jalife J, eds. *Cardiac Electrophysiology from Cell to Bedside.* Toronto: Saunders; 1990:343.
167. Jiang W, Babyak M, Krantz DS, et al. Mental stress-induced myocardial ischemia and cardiac events. *JAMA* 1996; 21:1651–1656.
168. Lown B, DeSilva RA, Reich P, Murawski BJ. Psychophysiologic factors in sudden cardiac death. *Am J Psychiatry* 1980; 137:1325–1335.
169. Lown B, Verrier RL. Neural activity and ventricular fibrillation. *N Engl J Med* 1976; 294:1165–1170.
170. Zaza A, Schwartz PJ. Role of the autonomic nervous system in the genesis of early ischemic arrhythmias. *J Cardiovasc Pharmacol* 1985; 7(suppl 5):S8–S12.
171. *Stedman's Medical Dictionary.* Baltimore: Williams & Wilkins; 1982.
172. Heit S, Owens MJ, Plotsky P, Nemeroff CB. Corticotropin-releasing factor, stress, and depression. *Neuroscientist* 1997; 3:186–194.
173. Tavazzi L, Zotti AM, Rondanelli R. The role of psychologic stress in the genesis of lethal arrhythmias in patients with coronary artery disease. *Eur Heart J* 1986; 7(suppl A):99–106.
174. Follick MJ, Gorkin L, Capone RJ, et al. Psychological distress as a predictor of ventricular arrhythmias in a post-myocardial infarct population. *Am Heart J* 1988; 116:32–36.
175. Gold PW, Goodwin FK, Chrousos GP. Clinical and biochemical manifestations of depression: Relation to the neurobiology of stress. *N Engl J Med* 1988; 319:413–420.
176. Valentino RJ, Foote SL, Page ME. The locus coeruleus as a site for integrating corticotropin-releasing factor and noradrenergic mediation of stress responses. *Ann NY Acad Sci* 1993; 697: 173–188.
177. Curtis AL, Pavcovich LA, Grigoriadis DE, Valentino RJ. Previous stress alters corticotropin-releasing factor neurotransmission in the locus coeruleus. *Neuroscience* 1995; 65:541–550.
178. Chrousos GP, Gold PW. The concepts of stress and stress system disorders: Overview of physical and behavioral homeostasis. *JAMA* 1992; 267:1244–1252.
179. Paykel E. Causal relationships between clinical depression and life events. In: Barrett JE, ed. *Stress and Mental Disorder.* New York: Raven Press; 1979.
180. Kendler KS, Kessler RC, Neale MC, et al. The prediction of major depression in women: Toward an integrated etiologic model. *Am J Psychiatry* 1993; 150:1139–1148.
181. Echt DS, Liebson PR, Mitchell LB, et al. Mortality and morbidity in patients receiving encainide, flecainide or placebo: The Cardiac Arrythmia Suppression Trial. *N Engl J Med* 1991; 324: 781–788.
182. Thomas SA, Friedmann E, Wimbush F, Shron E. Psychosocial factors and survival in the Cardiac Arrhythmia Suppression Trial (CAST): A reexamination. *Am J Crit Care* 1997; 6:116–126.
183. Fifer SK, Mathias SD, Patrick DL, et al. Untreated anxiety among adult primary care patients in a health maintenance organization. *Arch Gen Psychiatry* 1994; 51:740–750.
184. Sullivan MD, LaCroix AZ, Baum C, et al. Functional status in coronary artery disease: A one-year prospective study of the role of anxiety and depression. *Am J Med* 1997; 103:348–356.
185. Boyd JH. Use of mental health services for the treatment of panic disorder. *Am J Psychiatry* 1986; 143:1569–1574.
186. Klerman G, Weissman MM, Ouellette R, et al. Panic attacks in the community: Social morbidity and health care utilization. *JAMA* 1991; 265:742–746.
187. Markowitz JS, Weissman MM, Ouellette R, et al. Quality of life in panic disorder. *Arch Gen Psychiatry* 1989; 46:984–992.
188. Noyes R. The comorbidity and mortality of panic disorder. *Psychiatr Med* 1990; 8:41–66.
189. Sherbourne CD, Jackson CA, Meredith LS, et al. Prevalence of comorbid anxiety disorders in primary care outpatients. *Arch Family Med* 1996; 5:27–34.
190. Lum LC. Hyperventilation syndrome in medicine and psychiatry: A review. *J R Soc Med* 1987; 80:229–231.
191. Beck JG, Berisford MA, Taegtmeyer H. The effects of voluntary hyperventilation on patients with chest pain without coronary artery disease. *Behav Res Ther* 1991; 29:611–621.
192. Bass CM. Functional and cardiorespiratory symptoms. In: Bass CM, ed. *Somatization: Physiological and Psychologic Illness.* London: Blackwell; 1990:171.
193. Lynch P, Bakal DA, Whitelaw W, Fung T. Chest muscle activity and panic anxiety: A preliminary investigation. *Psychosom Med* 1991; 53:80–89.
194. Bass C, Wade C. Chest pain in normal coronary arteries: A comparative study of psychiatric and social morbidity. *Psychol Med* 1984; 14:51–61.
195. Goldberg DP, Cooper B, Eastwood MR, et al. A standardised psychiatric interview for use in community surveys. *Br J Prevent Social Med* 1970; 24:18–23.
196. Katon W, Hall ML, Russo J, et al. Chest pain: Relationship of psy-

chiatric illness to coronary arteriographic results. *Am J Med* 1988; 84:1–9.

197. Haines AP, Imeson JD, Meade TW. Phobic anxiety and ischaemic heart disease. *Brit M J* (*Clinical Research Edition*) 1987; 295: 297–299.
198. Eaker ED, Pinsky J, Castelli WP. Myocardial infarction and coronary death among women: Psychosocial predictors from a 20-year follow-up women in the Framingham Study. *Am J Epidemiol* 1992; 135:854–864.
199. Kawachi I, Colitz GA, Ascherio A. Prospective study of phobic anxiety and risk of coronary heart disease in men. *Circulation* 1994; 89:1992–1997.
200. Kawachi I, Sparrow D, Vokonas PS, et al. Symptoms of anxiety and risk of coronary heart disease: The normative aging study. *Circulation* 1994; 90:2225–2229.
201. Davis M. The role of the amygdala in fear-potentiated startle: Implications for animal models of anxiety. *Trends Pharmacol Sci* 1992; 13:35–41.
202. Ninan PT. The functional anatomy, neurochemistry, and pharmacology of anxiety. *J Clin Psychiatry* 1999; 60(suppl 22):12–17.
203. Stein MB, Uhde TW. Biology of anxiety disorders. In: Schatzberg AF, Nemeroff CB, eds. *The American Psychiatric Association Textbook of Psychopharmacology*, 2d ed. Washington, DC: American Psychiatric Association; 1998:609.
204. Klein DF. False suffocation alarms, spontaneous panics, and related conditions: An integrative hypothesis. *Arch Gen Psychiatry* 1993; 50:306–317.
205. McNally RJ, Eke M. Anxiety sensitivity, suffocation fear, and breath-holding duration as predictors of response to carbon dioxide challenge. *J Abnorm Psychol* 1996; 105:146–149.
206. Torgersen S. Twin studies in panic disorder. In: Ballenger J, ed. *Neurobiology of Panic Disorder*. New York: Liss; 1990:51.
207. Stein MB, Millar TW, Larsen DK, et al. Irregular breathing during sleep in patients with panic disorder. *Am J Psychiatry* 1995; 152:1168–1173.
208. Martinez JM, Papp LA, Coplan JD, et al. Ambulatory monitoring of respiration during anxiety. *Anxiety* 1996; 2:296–302.
209. Bremner JD, Licinio J, Darnell A, et al. Elevated CSF corticotropin-releasing factor concentrations in posttraumatic stress disorder. *Am J Psychiatry* 1997; 154:624–629.
210. Baker DG, West SA, Nicholson WE, et al. Serial CSF corticotropin-releasing hormone levels and adrenocortical activity in combat veterans with posttraumatic stress disorder. *Am J Psychiatry* 1999; 156:585–588.
211. Smith MA, Davidson J, Ritchie JC, et al. The corticotropin-releasing hormone test in patients with posttraumatic stress disorder. *Biol Psychiatry* 1989; 26:349–355.
212. Yehuda R, Southwick SM, Nussbaum G, et al. Low urinary cortisol excretion in PTSD. *J Nerv Ment Dis* 1990; 178:366–369.
213. Yehuda R, Teicher MH, Levengood RA, et al. Low urinary cortisol excretion in Holocaust survivors with posttraumatic stress disorder. *Am J Psychiatry* 1995; 152:982–986.
214. Yehuda R, Boisoneau D, Lowy MT, et al. Dose-response changes in plasma cortisol and lymphocyte glucocorticoid receptors following dexamethasone administration in combat veterans with and without posttraumatic stress disorder. *Arch Gen Psychiatry* 1995; 52:583–593.
215. Boscarino JA. Posttraumatic stress disorder, exposure to combat, and lower plasma cortisol among Vietnam veterans: Findings and clinical implications. *J Consultat Clin Psychol* 1996; 64: 191–201.
216. Stein MB, Yehuda R, Koverola C, et al. Enhanced dexamethasone suppression of plasma cortisol in adult women traumatized by childhood sexual abuse. *Biol Psychiatry* 1997; 42:680–686.
217. Linares OA, Zech LA, Jacquez JA, et al. Effect of sodium-restricted diet and posture on norepinephrine kinetics in humans. *Am J Physiol* 1988; 254:E222–E230.
218. Villacres EC, Hollifield M, Katon WJ, et al. Sympathetic nervous system activity in panic disorder. *Psychiatry Res* 1987; 21:313–321.
219. Wilkinson DJC, Thompson JM, Lambert GW, et al. Sympathetic activity in patients with panic disorder at rest, under laboratory mental stress, and during panic attacks. *Arch Gen Psychiatry* 1998; 55:511–520.
220. Weissman MM, Markowitz JS, Ouellette R, et al. Panic disorder and cardiovascular/cerebrovascular problems: Results from a community survey. *Am J Psychiatry* 1990; 147:1504–1508.
221. Coryell W, Noyes R, Clancy J. Excess mortality in panic disorder: A comparison with primary unipolar depression. *Arch Gen Psychiatry* 1982; 39:701–703.
222. Markovitz JH, Matthews KA, Wing RR, et al. Psychological, biological and health behavior predictors of blood pressure changes in middle-aged women. *J Hypertens* 1991; 9:399–406.
223. Markovitz JH, Matthews KA, Kannel WB, et al. Psychological predictors of hypertension in the Framingham Study: Is there tension in hypertension? [see comments]. *JAMA* 1993; 270:2439–2443.
224. Jonas BS, Franks P, Ingram DD. Are symptoms of anxiety and depression risk factors for hypertension? Longitudinal evidence from the national Health and Nutrition Examination Survey I Epidemiologic Follow-Up Study. *Arch Family Med* 1997; 6:43–49.
225. Kubzansky LD, Kawachi I, Weiss ST, Sparrow D. Anxiety and coronary heart disease: A synthesis of epidemiological, psychological, and experimental evidence. *Ann Behav Med* 1998; 20:47–58.
226. Sheehan DV, Coleman JH, Greenblatt DJ, et al. Some biochemical correlates of panic attacks with agoraphobia and their response to a new treatment. *J Clin Psychopharmacol* 1984; 4:66–75.
227. Girotti LA, Crosatto JR, Messuti H, et al. The hyperventilation test as a method for developing successful therapy in Prinzmetal angina. *Am J Cardiol* 1982; 49:834–841.
228. Freeman IJ, Nixon PGF. Are coronary artery spasm and progressive damage to the heart associated with the hyperventilation syndrome? *Brit Med J* 1985; 291:851–852.
229. Rasmussen K, Ravnsbaek J, Funch-Jensen P, et al. Oesophageal spasm in patients with coronary artery spasm. *Lancet* 1986; 1:174–176.
230. Myerburg RJ, Kessler KM, Mallon SM, et al. Life-threatening ventricular arrhythmias in patients with silent myocardial ischemia due to coronary artery spasm. *N Engl J Med* 1992; 326:1451–1455.
231. Friedman BH, Thayer JF. Heart rate variability and anxiety: Excess lability or flexibility? [Abstract]. *Psychophysiology* 1993; 30:S10.
232. Thayer JF, Friedman BH. Assessment of anxiety using heart rate nonlinear dynamics. In: Ditto W, ed. *Chaos in Biology and Medicine: SPIE Proceedings*. Bellingham, Washington: Society of Photo-optical Instrumentation Engineers; 1993:42–48.
233. Yeragani VK, Balon R, Pohl R, et al. Decreased R-R variance in panic disorder patients. *Acta Psychiatr Scand* 1990; 81:554–559.
234. Yeragani VK, Pohl R, Berger R, et al. Decreased heart rate variability in panic disorder patients: A study of power-spectral analysis of heart rate. *Psychiatry Res* 1993; 46:89–103.
235. Lyonsfield JD. An examination of image and thought processes in generalized anxiety. Association for the Advancement of Behavior Therapy. New York; 1991.
236. Thayer JF, Friedman BH, Borkovec TD. Autonomic characteristics of generalized anxiety disorder and worry. *Biol Psychiatry* 1996; 39:255–266.
237. Shear MK, Kligfield P, Harshfield G, et al. Cardiac rate and rhythm in panic patients. *Am J Psychiatry* 1987; 144:633–637.
238. Chignon J-M, Lepine J-P, Ades J. Panic disorder in cardiac outpatients. *Am J Psychiatry* 1993; 150:780–785.
239. Winkle RA. The relationship between ventricular ectopic beat frequency and heart rate. *Circulation* 1982; 66:633–637.
240. Katz C, Martin RD, Landa B, Chadda KD. Relationship of psychologic factors to frequent symptomatic ventricular arrhythmia. *Am J Med* 1985; 78:589–594.

241. Orth-Gomer K, Edwards ME, Erhardt L, et al. Relation between ventricular arrhythmias and psychological profile. *Acta Med Scand* 1980; 207:31–36.
242. Freeman AM, Cohen-Cole S, Fleece L, et al. Psychiatric symptoms, Type A behavior and arrhythmias following coronary bypass. *Psychosomatics* 1984; 25:586–589.
243. Follick MJ, Ahern DK, Gorkin L, et al. Relation of psychosocial and stress reactivity variables to ventricular arrhythmias in the Cardiac Arrhythmia Pilot Study (CAPS). *Am J Cardiol* 1990; 66:63–67.
244. Frasure-Smith N, Prince R. The ischemic heart disease life stress monitoring program: Impact on mortality. *Psychosom Med* 1984; 47:431–445.
245. Friedman M, Thoresen CE, Gill JJ, et al. Alteration of type A behavior and its effect on cardiac recurrences in postmyocardial infarction patients: Summary results of the recurrent coronary prevention project. *Am Heart J* 1986; 112:653–665.
246. Frasure-Smith N. In-hospital symptoms of psychological stress as predictors of long-term outcome after acute myocardial infarction in men. *Am J Cardiol* 1991; 67:121–127.
247. Frasure-Smith N, Lesperance F, Juneau M. Differential long-term impact of in-hospital symptoms of psychological stress after non-Q-wave and Q-wave myocardial infarction. *Am J Cardiol* 1992; 69:1128–1134.
248. Jones DA, West RR. Psychological rehabilitation after myocardial infarction: Multicentre randomised controlled trial. *Brit Med J* 1996; 313:1517–1521.
249. Frasure-Smith N, Lesperance F, Prince RH, et al. Randomised trial of home-based psychosocial nursing intervention for patients recovering from myocardial infarction. *Lancet* 1997; 350:473–479.
250. Roose SP, Laghriss-Thode F, Kennedy JS, et al. Comparison of paroxetine and nortriptyline in depressed patients with ischemic heart disease. *JAMA* 1998; 279:287–291.
251. Shapiro PA, Lesperance F, Frasure-Smith N, et al. An open-label preliminary trial for the treatment of major depression after acute-myocardial infarction (the SADHAT Trial). *Am Heart J* 1999; 137:1100–1106.
252. Muskin PR, Glassman AH. The use of tricyclic antidepressants in a medical setting. In: Finkel JB, ed. *Consultation-Liaison Psychiatry: Current Trends and Future Perspectives.* New York: Grune & Stratton; 1983:137.
253. Roose SP, Dalack GW. Treating the depressed patient with cardiovascular problems. *J Clin Psychiatry* 1992; 53:25–31.
254. Arana GW, Hyman SE. *Handbook of Psychiatric Drug Therapy.* 2d ed. Boston: Little, Brown; 1995:61.
255. Roose SP, Glassman AH, Siris SG, et al. Comparison of imipramine- and nortriptyline-induced orthostatic hypotension: A meaningful difference. *J Clin Psychopharmacol* 1981; 1:316–319.
256. Thayssen P, Bjerre M, Kragh-Sorensen P, et al. Cardiovascular effects of imipramine and nortriptyline in elderly patients. *Psychopharmacology (Berl)* 1981; 74:360–364.
257. Feder R. Bradycardia and syncope induced by fluoxetine (letter). *J Clin Psychiatry* 1991; 52:139.
258. Hyman SE, Arana GW, Rosenbaum JF. *Handbook of Psychiatric Drug Therapy.* Boston: Little, Brown; 1995.
259. Robinson DS, Roberts DL, Smith JM, et al. The safety profile of nefazodone. *J Clin Psychiatry* 1996; 57(suppl 2):31–38.
260. Franco-Brunson K. The management of treatment-resistant depression in the medically ill. *Psychiatr Clin North Am* 1996; 19:329–350.
261. Feighner JP. Cardiovascular safety in depressed patients: Focus on venlafaxine. *J Clin Psychiatry* 1995; 56:574–579.
262. Ellison JM, Milofsky JE, Ely E. Fluoxetine-induced bradycardia and syncope in two patients. *J Clin Psychiatry* 1990; 51:385–386.
263. Enemark B. The importance of ECG monitoring in antidepressant treatment. *Nordic J Psychiatry* 1993; 47(suppl 30):57–65.
264. Humphries JE, Wheby MS, VandenBerg SR. Fluoxetine and the bleeding time. *Arch Pathol Lab Med* 1990; 114:727–728.
265. Evans TG, Buys SS, Rodgers GM. Letter to the editor. *N Engl J Med* 1991; 324:1671.
266. Yaryura-Tobias JA, Kirschen H, Ninan P, Mosberg HF. Fluoxetine and bleeding in obsessive-compulsive disorder (letter). *Am J Psychiatry* 1991; 148:949.
267. Alderman CP, Moritz CK, Ben-Tovim DI. Abnormal platelet aggregation associated with fluoxetine therapy. *Ann Pharmacother* 1992; 26:1517–1519.
268. Callahan AM, Marangell LB, Ketter TA. Evaluating the clinical significance of drug interactions: A systematic approach. *Harvard Rev Psychiatry* 1996; 4:153–158.
269. Roose SP, Dalack GW, Glassman AH, et al. Cardiovascular effects of buproprion in depressed patients with heart disease. *Am J Psychiatry* 1991; 148:512–516.
270. Roose SP, Glassman AH, Attia E, et al. Cardiovascular effects of fluoxetine in depressed patients with heart disease. *Am J Psychiatry* 1998; 155:660–665.
271. Roose SP, Glassman AH, Attia E, Woodring S. Comparative efficacy of selective serotonin reuptake inhibitors and tricyclics in the treatment of melancholia. *Am J Psychiatry* 1994; 151:1735–1739.
272. American Psychiatric Association Task Force on Electroconvulsive Therapy. *The Practice of Electroconvulsive Therapy.* Washington, DC: American Psychiatric Association Press; 1990.
273. Weiner RD. Does electroconvulsive therapy cause brain damage? *Behav Brain Sci* 1984; 7:1–53.
274. Applegate RJ. Diagnosis and management of ischemic heart disease in the patient scheduled to undergo electroconvulsive therapy. *Convulsive Ther* 1997; 13:128–144.
275. Alexopoulos GS, Shamoian CJ, Lucas J, et al. Medical problems of geriatric psychiatric patients and younger controls during electroconvulsive therapy. *J Am Geriatr Soc* 1994; 32:651–654.
276. Pornnoppadol C, Isenberg K. ECT and the implantable converter defibrillator. *J Electroconvuls Ther* 1998; 14:124–126.
277. Block M, Admon D, Bonne O, Lerer B. Electroconvulsive therapy in depressed cardiac transplant patients. *Convuls Ther* 1992; 8:290–293.
278. Maneksha FR. Hypertension and tachycardia during electroconvulsive therapy: To treat or not to treat. *Convuls Ther* 1991; 70:28–35.
279. Figiel GS, deLeo B, Zorumski CF, et al. Combined use of labetalol and nifedipine in controlling the cardiovascular response from ECT. *J Geriatr Psychiatry Neurol* 1993; 6:20–24.
280. Figiel GD, McDonald L, LaPlante R. Cardiac modified ECT in the elderly (letter). *Am J Psychiatry* 1994; 151:790–791.
281. Stoudemire A, Knos G, Gladson M, et al. Labetalol in the control of cardiovascular responses to electroconvulsive therapy in high-risk depressed medical patients. *J Clin Psychiatry* 1990; 51:508–512.
282. Figiel G, McDonald WM, McCall WV, Zorumpski C. Electroconvulsive therapy. In: Schatzberg AF, Nemeroff CB, eds. *American Psychiatric Association Textbook of Psychopharmacology.* 2d ed. Washington, DC: American Psychiatric Association; 1998:523.
283. Lesperance F, Frasure-Smith N, Talajic M. Major depression before and after myocardial infarction: Its nature and consequences. *Psychosom Med* 1996; 58:99–110.
284. Grodstein F, Stampfer MJ. The epidemiology of coronary heart disease and estrogen replacement in postmenopausal women. *Progr Cardiovasc Dis* 1995; 38:199–210.
285. Kon Koh K, Mincemoyer R, Bui MN, et al. Effects of hormone-replacement therapy on fibrinolysis in postmenopausal women. *N Engl J Med* 1997; 336:683–690.

CHAPTER 81

ADVERSE CARDIOVASCULAR DRUG INTERACTIONS AND COMPLICATIONS

Lionel H. Opie / William H. Frishman

Toxicities from drug interactions have been shown to be a cause of morbidity and death in patients,[1] and these interactions often are associated with the loss of individual drug efficacy.[2] Recent technologies have resulted in an explosion of information concerning the cytochrome P450 isoenzyme system involved in the metabolism of cardiovascular drugs.[3–10] In addition to the isoenzyme inhibition and induction by various drugs, microsomal drug metabolism is affected by genetic polymorphisms,[9] age, nutrition, gender,[6] and hepatic diseases.[3,4,7] P-glycoprotein, which mediates the transcellular transport of many drugs, may also play an important role in clinically significant drug-drug interactions.[5]

Today, a knowledge of cardiovascular drug interactions is regarded as basic to our understanding of the pharmacologic properties of cardiovascular drugs. Such interactions can be either pharmacokinetic, whereby one agent interferes with the metabolism of another, or pharmacodynamic, whereby the hemodynamic properties of one agent are additive or subtractive to those of another (Fig. 81-1). An example of pharmacokinetic interaction is the decreased rate of hepatic metabolism of lidocaine during cimetidine therapy, with a possible risk of lidocaine toxicity. An example of a pharmacodynamic interaction arises when nifedipine is added to beta-adrenergic blockade in the therapy of severe angina, sometimes with excess hypotension as a side effect.

This chapter includes discussions of the drug interactions of the major classes of cardiovascular drugs, following an established sequence of these drugs.[11,12]

BETA-ADRENERGIC–BLOCKING DRUGS

Beta-adrenergic blockers demonstrate relatively few serious drug interactions (Table 81-1). An example of a pharmacokinetic interaction is that with cimetidine,[13] which reduces hepatic metabolism and therefore increases blood levels of carvedilol, propranolol, labetalol, and metoprolol, which are metabolized in the liver by the cytochrome oxidase system (Fig. 81-2). However, there is no interaction of cimetidine with beta blockers

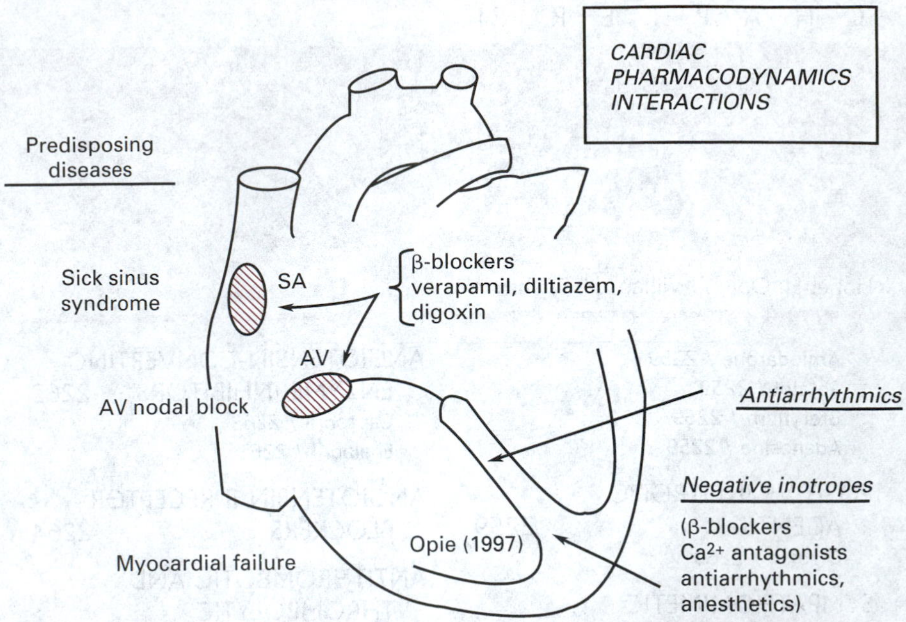

FIGURE 81-1 Cardiac pharmacodynamic interactions at the levels of the SA node, AV node, conduction system, and myocardium. The predisposing disease conditions are shown on the left. (Figure copyrighted by LH Opie.)

such as atenolol, sotalol, and nadolol, which are not metabolized in the liver. Another pharmacokinetic interaction is when verapamil raises blood levels of metoprolol through a hepatic interaction[14]; presumably, other beta blockers metabolized by the liver may be subject to a similar interaction.

Now used with increasing frequency in the acute phase of myocardial infarction, beta blockers may depress hepatic blood flow, thereby decreasing the hepatic inactivation of lidocaine.[15] Thus, beta blockade increases lidocaine blood levels, with an enhanced risk of toxicity. An example of a pharmacodynamic interaction with beta blockers is that seen with nonsteroidal anti-inflammatory drugs (NSAIDs), including indomethacin, which may attenuate the antihypertensive effects of beta blockers, possibly by decreasing the formation of vasodilatory prostaglandins.[16]

NITRATES

The chief drug interactions of nitrates are pharmacodynamic (Table 81-2). For example, during triple therapy of angina pectoris (nitrates, beta blockers, and calcium antagonists), the overall efficacy of the combination may be lessened because each drug can predispose patients to excess hypotension.[17] Even two components of triple therapy, such as diltiazem and nitrates, may interact adversely to cause moderate hypotension.[18] Nonetheless, high doses of diltiazem can improve persistent effort angina when added to maximum doses of propranolol and isosorbide dinitrate without any report of significant hypotension.[19] Therefore, individual patients vary greatly in their susceptibility to the hypotension of triple therapy. A dangerous drug-drug interaction is that of nitrates with sildenafil, an anti-impotence drug that can intensify the hypotensive effects of nitrates.[20] Sildenafil should not be used within 24 h of nitrate use. There is a reported beneficial interaction between nitrates and hydralazine whereby the latter drug appears to lessen nitrate tolerance.[21]

Unexpectedly, high doses of nitroglycerin may induce heparin resistance by altering the activity of antithrombin III.[22] Nitroglycerin can also lessen the therapeutic effects of the tissue plasminogen activator alteplase.

CALCIUM ANTAGONISTS

Many of the interactions of calcium antagonists are pharmacodynamic (Table 81-2),[23,24] such as added effects on the atrioventricular (AV) or sinus nodes (verapamil or diltiazem plus beta blockers, excess digitalis, or amiodarone), or on the systemic vascular resistance (e.g., nifedipine plus beta blockers causing excess hypotension). However, it is now increasingly recognized that verapamil and diltiazem (but probably not nifedipine) inhibit the hepatic oxidation of some drugs, the blood levels of which consequently increase. Such agents include cyclosporine (diltiazem), the antiepileptic carbamazepine (verapamil), prazosin (verapamil), lovastatin, atorvastatin and simvastatin (diltiazem), theophylline (verapamil), some HIV protease inhibitors (diltiazem), and quinidine (verapamil). In addition, nifedipine especially and also verapamil tend to increase hepatic blood flow, potentially leading to enhanced first-pass metabolism of agents such as propranolol, resulting in decreased beta blocker blood levels.[7] The effects of some dihydropyridine calcium channel blockers (e.g., felodipine and nifedipine) are potentiated by concomitant grapefruit juice ingestion.[25] The number of potentially toxic drug–drug interactions with bepridil are so great that it is used only as a last resort.[26,27]

Verapamil and Beta Blockers

Intravenous verapamil added to beta-adrenergic blockade has the additional risk of added hypotension or added nodal inhibition.[28,29] In patients with angina pectoris already receiving beta blockers, verapamil given intravenously[30] or orally[31] can reduce myocardial contractility,[31] increase heart size,[32] and cause sinus bradycardia.[33] By a hepatic pharmacokinetic interaction,[7,34] verapamil may raise blood levels of the beta blockers metabolized by the liver. Despite such hepatic interactions (e.g., verapamil with propranolol) in normal subjects, pharmacodynamic changes are more important.[35] The combination of verapamil and beta blockade in the therapy of angina pectoris must be used with care with preexisting depression of the sinoatrial (SA) or AV nodes and clinically detectable myocardial failure. The combination of verapamil and beta blockers improves myocardial function during exercise more than either agent alone.[36] Verapamil plus a beta blocker may have an additive therapeutic effect in hypertension, but with a small risk of excess inhibition of sinus rate, AV conduction, or left ventricular function.[37]

TABLE 81-1 Drug Interactions of Beta-Adrenergic–Blocking Agents

Cardiac Drug	Interacting Drugs	Mechanism	Consequence	Prophylaxis
		HEMODYNAMIC INTERACTIONS		
All beta blockers	Calcium antagonists, especially nifedipine	Added hypotension	Risk of myocardial ischemia	Blood pressure control, adjust doses
	Verapamil or diltiazem	Added negative inotropic effect	Risk of myocardial failure	Check for CHF, adjust doses
	Flecainide		Hypotension	Check LV function flecainide levels
	Sympathomimetics (S)	Opposing effects	Loss of clinical benefit	Avoid S
		ELECTROPHYSIOLOGICAL INTERACTIONS		
All beta blockers	Verapamil	Added inhibition of SA, AV nodes	Bradycardia, asystole, complete heart block	Exclude "sick-sinus" syndrome, AV nodal disease; adjust dose, exclude predrug LV failure
	Diltiazem	Added negative inotropic effect	Excess hypotension	
		HEPATIC INTERACTIONS		
Propranolol (P)	Cimetidine (C)	C decreases P metabolism	Excess propranolol effects	Reduce both drug doses
	Lidocaine	Low hepatic blood flow	Excess lidocaine effects	Reduce lidocaine dose
Metoprolol (M)	Verapamil (V)	V decreases M metabolism	Excess M effects	Reduce M dose
	Cimetidine (C)	C decreases M metabolism	Excess M effects	Reduce both drug doses
Labetalol (L)	Cimetidine (C)	C decreases L metabolism	Excess L and C effects	Reduce both drug doses
Carvedilol (CV)	Cimetidine (C)	C decreases CV metabolism	Excess CV effects	Reduce both drug doses
		ANTIHYPERTENSIVE INTERACTIONS		
Beta blockers	Indomethacin (I), NSAIDs	I inhibits vasodilatory prostaglandins	Decreased antihypertensive effect	Omit indomethacin; use alternative drugs
		IMMUNE INTERACTING DRUGS		
Acebutolol	Other drugs altering immune status: procainamide, hydralazine, captopril	Theoretical risk of additive immune effects	Theoretical risk of lupus or neutropenia	Check antinuclear factors and neutrophils; low doses during cotherapy

ABBREVIATION: LV = left ventricular.

Verapamil and Digoxin

Verapamil can increase blood digoxin levels by over 50 percent.[38] The dose of digoxin must be cut to about half, and blood levels of digoxin must then be rechecked. In digitalis toxicity, rapid intravenous verapamil is absolutely contraindicated because the sum of the inhibitory effects of these two agents on the AV node can be fatal. Experimentally, verapamil can inhibit the calcium-dependent delayed afterdepolarizations, which cause the ventricular automaticity found in digitalis toxicity. Oral verapamil and digitalis can, however, be combined in the absence of digitalis toxicity or AV block, because their pharmacologic sites of action are different; nevertheless, the digoxin level needs monitoring. The combination is often used for the management of supraventricular tachycardias.

Verapamil and Prazosin

The combination of verapamil with prazosin for hypertension provides added and synergistic activities.[39] A hepatic pharmacokinetic interaction with enhanced bioavailability of prazosin may explain these effects.[40,41]

Verapamil and Quinidine

Verapamil and quinidine may interact to cause excess hypotension,[42] either by combined inhibition of peripheral receptors or

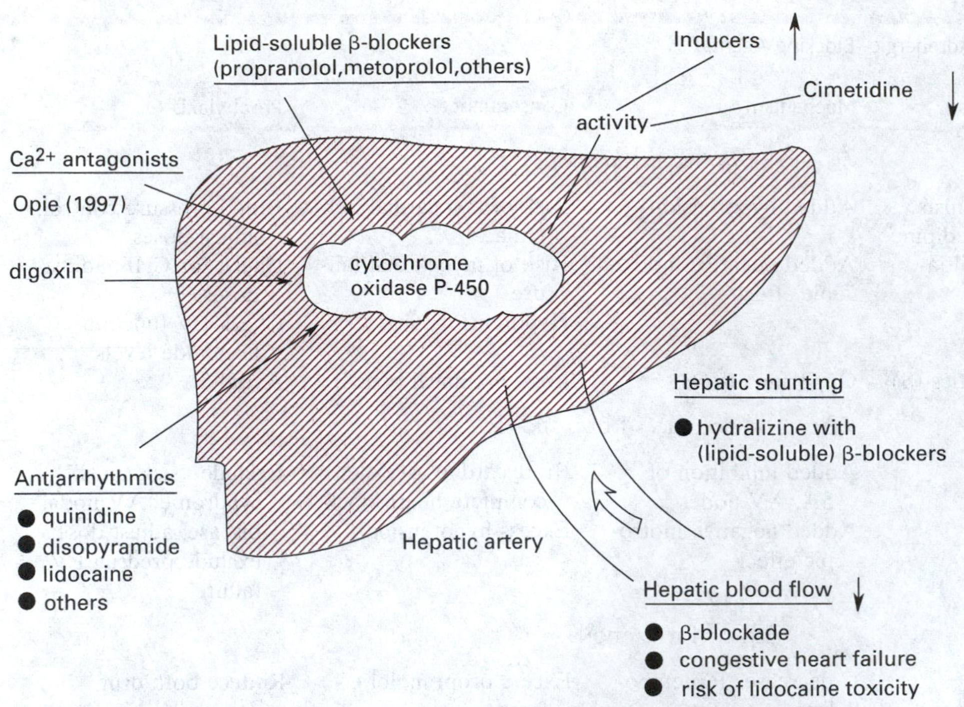

FIGURE 81-2 Potential hepatic pharmacokinetic interactions at the level of cytochrome oxidase P450 and potential pharmacodynamic interactions due to altered hepatic blood flow. (Figure copyrighted by LH Opie.)

by increase of quinidine levels.[43] The latter may be a hepatic interaction.

Verapamil and Disopyramide

Both verapamil and disopyramide are powerful negative inotropes. Thus, the combination can only be given when left ventricular function is good prior to initiation of therapy and can be closely monitored.

Verapamil and Theophylline

Verapamil may inhibit the hepatic metabolism of theophylline and lead to increased blood theophylline levels.[44]

Verapamil and Protease Inhibitors

Verapamil may inhibit the hepatic metabolism of the human immunodeficiency virus (HIV) protease inhibitors, causing decreased drug clearance of these agents and increased exposure to active drug.[24] No known toxicity has been observed at this time.[24]

Nifedipine

The combination of nifedipine with beta blockade is generally well tolerated except for the risk of hypotension.[45] Nifedipine and propranolol may have a pharmacokinetic interaction whereby blood levels of propranolol are increased; it is thought that nifedipine increases the hepatic blood flow so that propranolol breakdown in the liver is increased.[46] Although nifedipine is an afterload reducer, it also has a direct negative inotropic effect. Hence, combination with beta blockers, disopyramide, or any other negative inotropic agent should be undertaken with caution. Nifedipine combined with prazosin hydrochloride may cause excess hypotension[47]; thus, low initial additive doses are recommended (see "Prazosin, Doxazosin, and Terazosin," below).

Diltiazem

Diltiazem, like verapamil, may increase blood digoxin levels; however, the rise is likely to be much less, and some studies report no increase at all. Diltiazem plus long-acting nitrates occasionally causes excess hypotension.[18] Similar effects have been seen when diltiazem is combined with nifedipine.[48] The combination of high-dose diltiazem with beta blockade may cause bradycardia or hypotension.[49] Relatively few life-threatening interactions have been described for intravenous diltiazem. However, it can be expected to produce a spectrum of drug interactions similar to that of intravenous verapamil. As diltiazem is metabolized by the liver, it interacts with both cyclosporine and cilostazol, resulting in increased blood levels of both drugs.[50,51] Blood levels of some statins increase (Table 81-2).

ANTIARRHYTHMIC AGENTS

During antiarrhythmic therapy, numerous drug interactions are possible that are sometimes serious (Table 81-3).[52,53] Patients with serious ventricular arrhythmias frequently have associated angina pectoris (potentially necessitating treatment with calcium antagonists or beta blockers) or heart failure (requiring digitalis and diuretics). Nausea, a common symptom of patients with chronic cardiac conditions, may require cimetidine, with a risk of hepatic interactions (Table 81-3). The most frequent antiarrhythmic drug interactions are with digoxin (the levels of which increase with quinidine and verapamil), with diuretics (there is risk of ECG QT prolongation with antiarrhythmics, such as quinidine, disopyramide, amiodarone, and sotalol, which prolong duration of the action potential), and at the level of hepatic enzyme induction (cimetidine decreases hepatic metabolism of quinidine[54]; phenytoin and barbiturates have an opposite effect). There is also the risk of antiarrhythmic drug–drug interactions. Thus, amiodarone, when added to quinidine, enhances the risk of QT prolongation, while quinidine levels increase, so that quinidine toxicity is also more likely.[53] The combination of arrhythmic drugs, such as amiodarone and beta blockers, can also lead to life-threatening bradycardia. Type I antiarrhythmic drugs should not be used with certain macrolide antibiotics (erythromycin) because both drugs can prolong the QT interval, precipitating torsades de pointes, especially in

TABLE 81-2 Drug Interactions of Nitrates and Calcium Channel Blocking Agents

Cardiac Drug	Interacting Drugs	Mechanism	Consequence	Prophylaxis
		HEMODYNAMIC INTERACTIONS		
All nitrates	Calcium antagonists	Excess vasodilation	Syncope, dizziness	Monitor BP
	Prazosin (PZ)	Excess vasodilation	Syncope, dizziness	Check BP, low initial PZ doses
	Sildenafil (S)	Excess vasodilation	Syncope, dizziness	Avoid S
		CALCIUM ANTAGONIST DRUGS		
Verapamil (V)	Beta blockers	SA and AV nodal inhibition; myocardial failure	Added nodal and negative inotropic effects	Care during cotherapy Check ECG, BP, heart size
	Cimetidine	Hepatic metabolic interaction	Blood V rises	Adjust dose
	Digitalis poisoning	Added SA and AV nodal inhibition	Asystole; complete heart block after IV V	Avoid IV V in digitalis poisoning
	Digoxin (D)	Decreased digoxin clearance	Risk of D toxicity	Halve D dose; blood D level
	Disopyramide	Pharmacodynamic	Hypotension, constipation	Check BP, LV, and gut
	Flecainide (F)	Added negative inotropic effect	Hypotension	Check LV, F levels
	Prazosin	Hepatic interaction	Excess hypotension	Check BP during cotherapy
	Quinidine (Q)	Added alpha-receptor inhibition; V decreases Q clearance	Hypotension; increased Q levels	Check Q levels and BP
	Theophylline (T)	Inhibition of hepatic metabolism	Increased blood T levels	Reduce T, check levels
Nifedipine (N)	Beta blockers	Added negative inotropism	Excess hypotension	Check BP, use test dose of N
	Cimetidine	Hepatic metabolic interaction	Increased blood N levels	Decreased N dosage by 40%
	Digoxin (D)	Minor/modest changes in digoxin	Increased digoxin levels	Check D levels
	Prazosin (PZ)	PZ blocks alpha reflex to N	Postural hypotension	Test dose of N or PZ
	Propranolol (P)	N and P have opposite effects on blood liver flow	N decreases P levels; P increases N levels	Readjust P and N doses if needed
	Quinidine (Q)	N improves poor LV function; Q clearance faster	Decreased Q effect	Check Q levels
	Diltiazem	Hepatic metabolism of N inhibited	Increased hypotension	Decrease N levels
Diltiazem (D)	Beta blockers	Added SA nodal inhibition; negative inotropism	Bradycardia, hypotension	Check ECG and LV function
	Cimetidine	Hepatic metabolic interaction	Increased D levels	Reduce D dose by one-third
	Cyclosporine (C)	Hepatic metabolism of C inhibited	Increased blood C levels	Decrease C dose
	Digoxin (D)	Some fall in D clearance	Only in renal failure	Check D levels
	Flecainide (F)	Added negative inotropic effect	Hypotension	Check LV; F levels
	Cilostazol (Ci)	Hepatic metabolism of Ci inhibited	Increased Ci levels	Decrease Ci dose
	Simvastatin (Si) Lovastatin (L) Atorvastatin (A)	Hepatic metabolism of L inhibited	Increased L levels	Decrease Si, L, and A doses
Nicardipine (see also nifedipine)	Cyclosporine (C)	Hepatic metabolism of C inhibited	Increased blood C levels	Decrease C dose
	Digoxin (D)	Decreased D clearance	Blood D doubles	Decrease D, D levels

ABBREVIATIONS: BP = blood pressure; ECG = electrocardiogram; IV = intravenous; LV = left ventricle.

TABLE 81-3 Drug Interactions of Antiarrhythmic Drugs

Cardiac Drug	Interacting Drugs	Mechanism	Consequence	Prophylaxis
		CLASS 1A		
Quinidine (Q)	Amiodarone	Added QT effects; blood O rises	Torsades de pointes	Check QT, potassium
	Antibiotics (some)	Quinidine inhibits muscarinic receptors	Increased antibiotic-induced muscular weakness	Clinical care, drug levels
	Anticholinesterases	Quinidine inhibits muscarinic receptors	Decreased Ach efficacy in myasthenia gravis	Avoid Q if possible
	Antihypertensive agents Beta blockers	Added hypotensive and added SA nodal effects	Hypotension, excess bradycardia	Regulate BP Check BP ECG
	Cimetidine (C)	C inhibits oxidative metabolism of Q	Increased Q levels, risk of toxicity	Q levels, consider ranitidine
	Coumarin anticoagulants	Hepatic interaction with Q	Bleeding	Check prothrombin time
	Digoxin (Dig)	Decreased Dig clearance	Risk of Dig toxicity	Check Dig dose levels
	Diltiazem	Added inhibition of SA node	Excess bradycardia	Check ECG, heart rate
	Disopyramide	Added QT prolongation	Torsades de pointes	Check QT, potassium
	Diuretic, potassium losing	Hypokalemia and QT prolongation	Torsades de pointes	Check QT, potassium
	Hepatic enzyme inducers (phenytoin, barbiturates, rifampin)	Increased Q hepatic metabolism	Decreased Q levels	Q levels, doses
	Nifedipine	Increased Q clearance	Decreased Q levels	Q levels, doses
	Sotalol	Added QT prolongation	Torsades de pointes	Check QT, potassium
	Verapamil	Decreased Q clearance	Excess bradycardia	Check ECG, Q levels
	Warfarin	Hepatic interaction with Q	Bleeding	Check prothrombin time
Procainamide (P)	Captopril	Combined immune effects	Theoretical risk of neutropenia	Cotherapy with care
	Cimetidine	Decreased renal P clearance	Prolonged P half-life, excess P effect	Reduce P dose; consider ranitidine
Disopyramide (D)	Agents prolonging APD (quinidine, amiodarone, sotalol)	Added QT prolongation, especially if hypokalemic	Torsades de pointes	Check QT, potassium
	Beta blockers	Combined negative inotropism	Hypotension	Low doses
	Cimetidine	Hepatic D metabolism falls	Increased blood D levels	
	Digitalis toxicity	Added SA, AV nodal depression	SA, AV block	Avoid D in digitalis toxicity
	Hepatic enzyme inducers (phenytoin, rifampin, barbiturates)	Enhanced D hepatic metabolism	Blood D levels fall; readjust D dose	Readjust D dose

TABLE 81-3 Drug Interactions of Antiarrhythmic Drugs (*Continued*)

Cardiac Drug	Interacting Drugs	Mechanism	Consequence	Prophylaxis
	Drugs inhibiting SA or AV nodes/conduction system (quinidine, beta blockers, methyldopa, digoxin)	Pharmacodynamic additive effects	SA, AV block; conduction block	Check ECG; decrease doses
	Pyridostigmine (Py)	Inhibition of cholinesterase activity	Beneficial effect of Py on D; harmful effect of D on P	In myasthenia gravis, avoid D
		CLASS 1B		
Lidocaine (L)	Verapamil (V), Diltiazem (Di)	Combined negative inotropism	Hypotension	Avoid IV Di or V cotherapy
	Cimetidine	Decreased hepatic metabolism	Increased L levels	Decrease L infusion rate
	Halothane	Decreased hepatic blood flow	Increased L levels	Decrease L infusion rate
	Propranolol	Decreased hepatic blood flow	Increased L levels	Decrease L infusion rate
	Other beta blockers	Decreased hepatic blood flow	Increased L levels	Decrease L infusion rate
Mexiletine (M)	Hepatic enzyme inducers (phenytoin, barbiturates, rifampin)	Increased hepatic metabolism	Decreased plasma M levels	Increase M dose
		CLASS 1C		
Flecainide (F)	Amiodarone	Unknown	Blood F rises, added effect on nodes, myocardium	Decrease F dose
	Digoxin (Dig)	Decreased Dig clearance	Blood Dig rises slightly	Check Dig level
	Drugs inhibiting SA or AV nodes, IV conduction or myocardial function	Pharmacodynamic additive effects	SA, AV block; conduction block, cardiogenic shock	Avoid combinations Decrease doses
	Cimetidine	Decreased hepatic F loss	Blood F rises	Check F dose
Propafenone	Digoxin (Dig)	Pharmacokinetic	Increased Dig level	Decrease Dig dose
Moricizine (Mo)	Cimetidine	Decreased Mo metabolism	Blood Mo rises	Decrease Mo dose
		CLASS III		
Amiodarone (A)	Drugs prolonging QT interval (quinidine, disopyramide, phenothiazines, tricyclic antidepressants, thiazide diuretics, sotalol)	Pharmacodynamic additive effects	Torsades de pointes	Avoid low K^+; avoid combinations
	Quinidine (Q)	Pharmacokinetic	Blood Q rises	Check Q levels
	Procainamide (P)	Pharmacokinetic	Blood P rises	Check P dose
Sotalol	Procainamide	Hypokalemia plus class III action	Torsades de pointes	Exclude low K^+; use K^+-retaining diuretic

ABBREVIATIONS: Ach = acetylcholine; APD = action potential duration; BP = blood pressure; ECG = electrocardiogram; IV = intravenous.

women.[55-57] Other drugs that prolong the QT interval are shown in Fig. 81-2.

Quinidine

Because quinidine increases blood digoxin levels, the dose of quinidine must be decreased and blood digoxin levels checked.[58] Quinidine may enhance the effects of other hypotensive agents, including verapamil,[42] or of agents inhibiting the sinus node (beta blockers, verapamil, diltiazem, and methyldopa). Quinidine increases the effects of coumarin anticoagulants by a hepatic interaction.[59] When hepatic enzymes are induced by drugs such as phenytoin, phenobarbital, and rifampin (rifampicin), the hepatic metabolism of quinidine may markedly increase, with decreased steady-state concentrations of quinidine.[60,61] Conversely, cimetidine can inhibit hepatic enzymes to decrease the metabolism of quinidine with opposite effects. It appears that ranitidine has no such effects.[62] Verapamil may increase quinidine levels. Conversely, nifedipine may lower plasma quinidine levels, probably by improving left ventricular systolic function.[62-64]

Hypokalemia decreases the antiarrhythmic effect of quinidine and predisposes to QT prolongation by quinidine. When quinidine is combined with other drugs that also prolong the QT interval, such as amiodarone, sotalol, or thiazide diuretics, careful monitoring of the QT interval is required.[65]

Quinidine is a vagolytic drug and reduces the effects of procedures that enhance vagal activity, such as carotid sinus massage. Quinidine also inhibits muscarinic receptors to reduce the effects of anticholinesterases in myasthenia gravis.

Procainamide

Cimetidine inhibits the renal clearance of procainamide. Since the elimination half-life lengthens, the dose of procainamide needs reduction.[66]

Disopyramide

Since disopyramide is negatively inotropic, there is a potential danger of reduction of the cardiac output in patients already receiving other negative inotropes, such as the calcium antagonists—verapamil,[67] beta blockers, or flecainide—and in patients with preexisting myocardial failure. It is also potentially dangerous to combine disopyramide with other drugs likely to depress nodal or conduction tissues, such as quinidine, digoxin, beta blockers, and methyldopa. Disopyramide is ineffective in digitalis toxicity and should be avoided. There is no interaction between disopyramide and lidocaine. The concomitant use of disopyramide with other type I antiarrhythmic agents or beta blockers should be reserved for life-threatening arrhythmias because of a risk of bradycardia and hypotension. The risk of QT prolongation requires that disopyramide not be combined with other drugs prolonging the QT interval, such as the tricyclic antidepressants, and certain other antiarrhythmic agents, such as amiodarone or sotalol. Phenytoin[68] and other inducers of hepatic enzymes (e.g., barbiturates and rifampin) may lower disopyramide plasma levels. Pyridostigmine bromide may interact beneficially with disopyramide by inhibiting cholinesterase activity, reducing the anticholinergic side effects of disopyramide.[69]

Lidocaine

In patients receiving cimetidine,[70] propranolol,[15] or halothane,[71] the hepatic clearance of lidocaine is reduced, and toxicity may occur more readily. Lidocaine may cause SA arrest, especially during coadministration of other agents potentially depressing nodal function,[72] including beta blockers.

Tocainide

There are currently no known adverse drug interactions involving tocainide.

Dofetilide and Ibutilide

There are presently no known adverse drug interactions involving dofetilide or ibutilide. However, drugs known to directly prolong the QT interval and induce torsades de pointes (e.g., tricyclic antidepressants, antiarrhythmics, cisapride, astemizole, erythromycin, haloperidol, and protease inhibitors) should be avoided.[73]

Mexiletine

Narcotics delay the gastrointestinal absorption of mexiletine. Rifampin, barbiturates, and phenytoin all induce hepatic enzymes, reducing the plasma levels of mexiletine. Cimetidine inhibits the CYD 26 hepatic isoform that breaks down mexilitine. It should, but does not, increase plasma levels of mexiletine.[74] Rather, cimetidine has a beneficial side effect of decreasing the gastrointestinal symptoms associated with mexiletine. Disopyramide and mexiletine given together may predispose to a negative inotropic effect.[75] Mexiletine may, however, be combined with quinidine,[76,77] beta-adrenergic blockers,[78] and amiodarone,[79] provided that the appropriate contraindications for each drug are observed and the patient is closely monitored for heart failure.

Flecainide

Since flecainide inhibits the sinus and AV nodal function, its combination with beta blockers, verapamil, diltiazem, and digitalis can cause bradycardia and requires care. Flecainide also has additive negative inotropic effects that may exaggerate those of beta blockers,[80] verapamil, or disopyramide. Combined inhibitory effects on His-Purkinje conduction may arise during cotherapy with quinidine or procainamide and to a lesser extent with disopyramide. Flecainide blood levels are increased by amiodarone; when both of these drugs are used, the flecainide dose should be decreased by about one-third.[81] Studies of healthy volunteers suggest that (1) cimetidine delays the clearance of flecainide[82] and (2) flecainide increases blood digoxin levels.[80]

Propafenone

Propafenone is a class IC antiarrhythmic drug; therefore, it may interact adversely with other drugs, depressing nodal function, intraventricular conduction, or the inotropic state. Nonetheless, propafenone can be combined with quinidine or procainamide at reduced doses of both drugs.[74] Propafenone substantially increases serum digoxin levels.[83]

Amiodarone

The most serious interaction of amiodarone[65] is the potential for an additive proarrhythmic effect with other drugs that prolong the QT interval, such as class IA antiarrhythmic agents, sotalol, phenothiazines, tricyclic antidepressants, and thiazide diuretics. Amiodarone does not normally depress the sinus node, but it may do so when it is combined with beta blockers or calcium antagonists such as verapamil or diltiazem.[23] In patients receiving warfarin, amiodarone further prolongs the prothrombin time and, if not monitored closely, can lead to excessive bleeding.[84] Amiodarone may double digoxin levels (Table 81-3).

Sotalol

Cotherapy with any other agents that may cause hypokalemia (e.g., diuretics) or prolong the action potential duration (e.g., quinidine, disopyramide, amiodarone, tricyclic antidepressants, or probucol) may precipitate torsades de pointes.

Bretylium

Experimentally, bretylium may worsen digitalis-induced ventricular tachycardia.[85] Nonetheless, the drug may be lifesaving for patients with ventricular fibrillation thought to be induced by digitalis.[86]

Adenosine

Adenosine has an indirect effect, similar to that of the calcium antagonist verapamil, by enhancing the flow of the current $I_{k(ACh)}$. Aminophylline or theophylline, by competing with adenosine for the receptor sites, completely inhibits the adenosine-induced effect on AV conduction. Dipyridamole, on the other hand, inhibits the breakdown of adenosine and/or its uptake into the tissues, so that the amount of adenosine available for the antiarrhythmic effect is enhanced.[12] Effective doses of adenosine in patients receiving sustained dipyridamole therapy may only be one-quarter to one-eighth of the normal doses.

POSITIVE INOTROPIC AGENTS

Drug interactions of digitalis and other positive inotropic agents are shown in Table 81-4.

TABLE 81-4 Drug Interactions of Digitalis and Other Positive Inotropic Agents

Cardiac Drug	Interacting Drugs	Mechanism	Consequence	Prophylaxis
		POSITIVE INOTROPIC AGENTS		
Digitoxin	Verapamil	Nonrenal clearance of digitoxin falls	Digitoxin levels up by one-third	Check digitoxin levels
	Other drugs interacting with digoxin	Altered digitoxin clearance (?)	Digitoxin levels increase (?)	Check digitoxin levels
Digoxin (D)	Amiodarone	Reduced renal clearance of D	D level may double	Check D level; halve dose
	Captopril	Reduced D clearance	Blood D increases	Check D dose
	Diltiazem	Variable decrease of D clearance	Variable blood D increases	Check D level
	Diuretics; potassium-sparing amiloride/ triamterene, spironolactone (S)	Reduced extrarenal D clearance S reduces renal D clearance	D levels up by 20% D levels increase	Check D level Complex effects; check D levels
	Nifedipine	Variable fall of D clearance	Variable blood D rises	Check D level
	Nitrendipine	Reduced D clearance	Blood D doubles	Check D level; halve dose
	Prazosin (PZ)	PZ displaces D from binding sites	Blood D rises	Needs confirmation in humans
	Propafenone	Not defined	D level increases	Check D level
	Quinidine, quinine	Reduced D clearance	Blood D doubles	Check D level; halve dose
	Verapamil	Reduced D clearance	Blood D doubles or more	Check D level; halve dose
		SYMPATHOMIMETIC INOTROPES		
Dobutamine Amrinone Milrinone	Thiazide diuretics	Additive hypokalemic effects	Arrhythmias	Check blood potassium

Digoxin

The quinidine-digoxin interaction is best known (Fig. 81-3). Quinidine approximately doubles the blood digoxin levels, decreasing both renal and extrarenal clearance.[38,86–88] The previous dose of digoxin should be halved and the plasma digoxin rechecked. Quinine given for muscle cramps acts likewise. Recent evidence indicates that quinidine inhibits digoxin transport across epithelial cell membranes (especially in the kidney) owing to its high affinity for p-glycoprotein on the ATP-dependent efflux pump encoded by the *mdrla* gene.[88–90]

The verapamil-digoxin interaction is equally significant; digoxin levels increase by 60 to 90 percent.[38,91] The other calcium antagonists, nifedipine and diltiazem, increase digoxin levels much less than does verapamil.[87,92,93] Adjustment of the digoxin dose with these agents is usually not necessary except in the presence of renal failure (which decreases digoxin excretion). Nicardipine causes only a modest rise of digoxin levels.[94] Nitrendipine, however, resembles verapamil in approximately doubling the digoxin levels.[94] Thus, there are no simple rules to explain which class of calcium antagonists or which specific agent is likely to increase digoxin levels significantly.

Among other vasodilators, prazosin increases digoxin levels in dogs by reduction of plasma and tissue binding.[95] Among antiarrhythmics other than quinidine or verapamil, amiodarone and propafenone[83] also elevate serum digoxin levels. Other antiarrhythmics, including procainamide and mexiletine, have no interaction with digoxin except for a relatively small rise of digoxin levels with flecainide.[80] When cotherapy elevates digoxin levels, the features of digitalis toxicity may depend on the agent added. With quinidine, tachyarrhythmias become more likely; amiodarone and verapamil seem to repress the ventricular arrhythmias of digitalis toxicity, making bradycardia and AV block more likely.[96]

Diuretics may indirectly precipitate digitalis toxicity by causing hypokalemia, which, when really severe (plasma potassium below 2 to 3 meq/L), may stop the tubular secretion of digoxin. Potassium-sparing diuretics (amiloride, triamterene, and spironolactone)[97] as well as captopril decrease digoxin clearance by about 20 to 30 percent and may also elevate serum K^+ levels. When these combinations with digoxin are used in the therapy of congestive heart failure, the blood digoxin level must be watched. Unexpectedly, spironolactone and its metabolite canrenone may decrease features of digitalis toxicity,[98] probably through increased K^+ levels resulting from aldosterone inhibition. Nonetheless, the combination digoxin-quinidine-spironolactone markedly elevates digoxin levels.[99]

The gastrointestinal absorption of digoxin may be decreased by cholestyramine, probably because of the binding of digoxin to the resin; digoxin should therefore be given several hours before the resin, or else digoxin capsules may be used (Lanoxicaps; 0.2 mg = 0.25 mg of digoxin). Digoxin capsules also decrease interaction with kaolin pectate and acarbose,[100] which reduces digoxin absorption, and with erythromycin and tetracycline, which inhibit gastrointestinal flora that inactivate digoxin and thereby increase digoxin blood levels. Cancer chemotherapeutic agents may damage intestinal mucosa to depress digoxin absorption. NSAIDs decrease the renal clearance of digoxin, thereby increasing plasma digoxin levels. Rifampin and phenobarbital, through hepatic enzyme induction, can reduce plasma digoxin levels.[90]

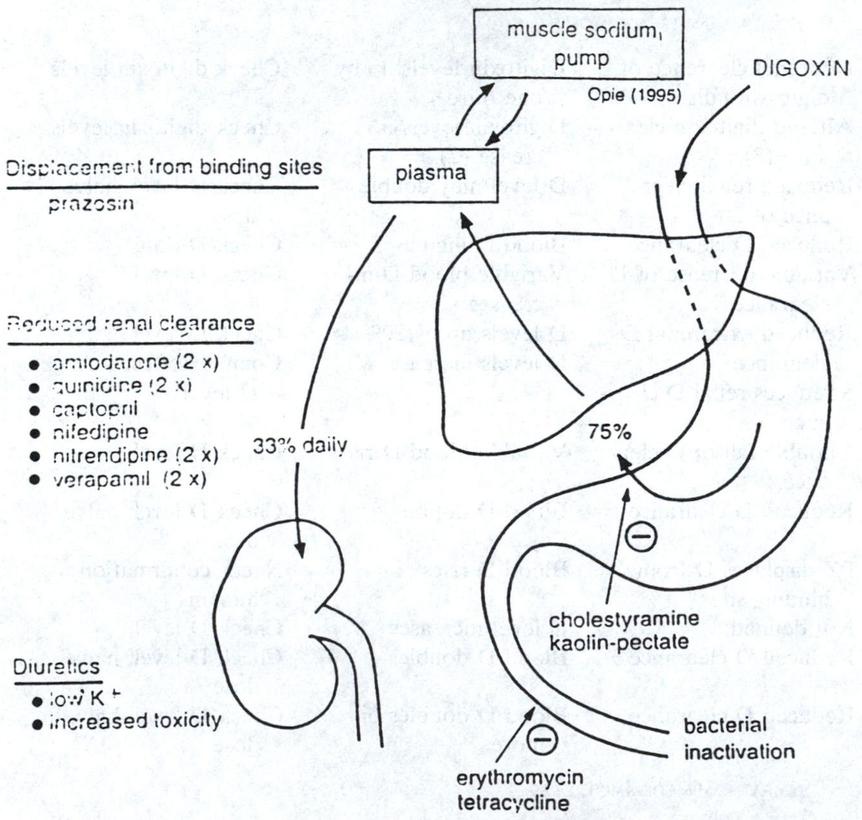

FIGURE 81-3 Potential site of digoxin interactions. Note the importance of reduced renal clearance. 2× means that an approximate doubling of digoxin blood levels has been reported. (Figure copyrighted by LH Opie.)

SYMPATHOMIMETIC AGENTS

Dopamine

Dopamine is contraindicated during the use of cyclopropane or halogenated hydrocarbon anesthetics (enhanced risk of arrhythmias). Monoamine oxidase inhibitors decrease the rate of dopamine metabolism by the tissues; the dose of dopamine should therefore be cut to one-tenth of usual.

Dobutamine

Dobutamine decreases plasma potassium levels and should be given with care together with diuretics, especially intravenous loop diuretics.

PHOSPHODIESTERASE INHIBITORS

Amrinone and Milrinone

Amrinone and milrinone are phosphodiesterase inhibitors that can also provoke arrhythmias. During diuretic therapy, plasma potassium levels need monitoring. When these drugs are combined with digitalis, the digoxin level does not change, but digoxin toxicity should be guarded against because of multiple mechanisms for arrhythmia development.

DIURETICS

Drug interactions with diuretics are summarized in Table 81-5.

Loop Diuretics

Hypokalemia, which may occur when loop diuretics are given acutely and intravenously, may precipitate digitalis toxicity. An interesting and complex set of interactions between furosemide and captopril has emerged. On the one hand, captopril decreases the renal excretion of furosemide, which is required for the diuretic effect of the latter. This may explain why captopril reduces furosemide-induced natriuresis to less than half.[101] This effect of captopril in altering furosemide excretion seems not to be shared by other angiotensin-converting enzyme (ACE) inhibitors.[102] There is an important pharmacodynamic interaction between captopril and furosemide. Both agents are able to dilate the postglomerular efferent arterioles. When captopril is given in a standard dose of 25 mg, furosemide has little or no diuretic effect. On the other hand, only minute doses of captopril, such as 1 mg, enhance the diuretic effect of furosemide.[103] The proposed mechanism is that the very low dose of captopril still allows sufficient circulating angiotensin II to maintain efferent arteriolar tone and thereby to keep the glomerular filtration rate sufficiently high for the furosemide to act. Both of these pharmacokinetic and pharmacodynamic interactions, therefore, argue for a low-dose captopril combination with furosemide. In patients with a low serum sodium level, which is an indirect indicator of a high-renin state, it is the high aldosterone level that retains sodium and stimulates vasopressin secretion, the latter causing the hyponatremia. Therapy of such patients by furosemide alone is ineffective, and the addition of captopril in a standard dose may achieve improvement.[12]

Quite apart from the complex interactions described above, it is generally regarded as a wise precaution to reduce the diuretic dose of patients with congestive heart failure (CHF) before adding an ACE inhibitor. The aim of this procedure is to lessen excessive first-dose hypotension. Overdiuresis tends to result in activation of the renin-angiotensin system and greater sensitivity to ACE inhibition.

Thiazide Diuretics

Steroids, estrogens, and indomethacin and other NSAIDs lessen the antihypertensive effect of thiazide diuretics and may worsen congestive heart failure.[104,105] ACE inhibitors tend to be potassium-retaining and may cause hyperkalemia if combined with other potassium retainers. The angiotensin II receptor blockers may have a weaker potassium-conserving effect. Diuretic-induced hypokalemia may predispose to ventricular arrhythmias, including torsades de pointes; when that happens, usually an antiarrhythmic agent, such as sotalol,[106] quinidine, or amiodarone (all of which may prolong the QT interval), is being used. Probenecid interferes with the urinary excretion of thiazide and loop diuretics, reducing diuretic efficacy. Since diuretics may impair the renal clearance of lithium, the blood level of lithium rises, with a risk of lithium toxicity.[107]

Potassium-Sparing Diuretics

Drugs that conserve potassium (e.g., ACE inhibitors, angiotensin II receptor blockers, and trimethoprim)[108,109] may potentiate hyperkalemia when used with potassium-sparing diuretics.

VASODILATORS

Drug interactions of vasodilators, ACE inhibitors, and angiotensin II receptor blockers are given in Table 81-6.

Nitroprusside and Hydralazine

Nitroprusside and hydralazine may decrease digoxin levels, possibly as a result of increased tubular excretion, by improving CHF, renal plasma flow, and renal excretion of digoxin.[110] Hy-

TABLE 81-5 Drug Interactions of Diuretics

Cardiac Drug	Interacting Drugs	Mechanism	Consequence	Prophylaxis
Loop and thiazide diuretics	Indomethacin and other NSAIDs	Pharmacodynamic	Decreased antihypertensive effect	Adjust diuretic dose or add another agent
	Probenecid	Decreased intratubular secretion of diuretic	Decreased diuretic effect	Increase diuretic dose
	ACE inhibitors	Excess diuretics, high renins	Excess hypotension; prerenal uremia	Lower diuretic dose; test dose ACE inhibitor
Furosemide (F)	Captopril	Possible interference with tubular secretion of F; added efferent arteriolar vasodilator	Loss of diuretic efficacy of F; decreased glomerular flow; diuretic effect of F less	Increase F dose (?); ultra low-dose captopril (?); Avoid Captopril (?)
K^+-retaining diuretics	ACE inhibitors AII receptor blockers	Added K^+ retention	Hyperkalemia	Check K^+ levels

ABBREVIATION: A II = angiotensin II.

TABLE 81-6 Drug Interactions of Vasodilators, Angiotensin Converting Enzyme Inhibitors, and Angiotensin II Receptor Blockers

Cardiac Drug	Interacting Drugs	Mechanism	Consequence	Prophylaxis
		VASODILATORS		
Hydralazine	Beta blockers (BB) (hepatic metabolized)	Hepatic shunting	BB metabolism ↓ Blood levels ↑	Propranolol, metoprolol dose ↓ (beneficial)
Hydralazine	Nitrates (N)	Renal blood flow ↑	Less N tolerance	
Hydralazine/ nitroprusside	Digoxin (D)	Increased renal D excretion	Decreased D levels	Check D levels
Prazosin (P)	Nifedipine (Nif)	Pharmacodynamic	Excess hypotension	Test dose of Nif
	Nitrates	Pharmacodynamic	Syncope, hypotension	Decrease P dose
	Verapamil	Hepatic metabolism	Synergistic antihypertensive effect	Adjust doses
Cilostazol (Ci)	Diltiazem	↓ hepatic metabolism	Increased Ci levels	Lower Ci dose
		ANGIOTENSIN-CONVERTING ENZYME INHIBITORS (ACEI)		
ACEI (class effect)	Diuretics	High renin levels in overdiuresed patients	"First" dose hypotension; risk of renal failure	Low test dose
ACEI (class effect)	Potassium-sparing diuretics	Added potassium retention	Hyperkalemia	Avoid combination
ACEI (class effect)	Indomethacin	Less vasodilation	Less BP ↓; less antifailure effects	Avoid if possible
ACEI (class effect ?)	Aspirin	Less vasodilation	Less antifailure effects	Low-dose aspirin
Captopril	Loop diuretic	Possible interference with tubular secretion	Lessened diuretic effect of furosemide	Consider alternate ACE inhibitor drug
Captopril	Immunosuppressive drugs, procainamide, hydralazine, possibly acebutolol	Added immune effects	Increased risk of neutropenia	Avoid combination; check neutrophils
	Probenecid (P)	P inhibits tubular secretion of C	Small risk in C levels	Decrease dose of C
		ANGIOTENSIN II RECEPTOR BLOCKERS (ARBs)		
ARBs (class effect)	Diuretics	High renin levels in overdiuresed patients	First dose hypotension, risk of renal failure	Low test dose
	Potassium sparing diuretics	Added potassium retention	Hyperkalemia	Avoid combination

ABBREVIATION: BP = blood pressure.

dralazine, by creating hepatic shunts, may substantially increase the blood levels of those beta blockers that undergo hepatic metabolism, such as propranolol and metoprolol.[111] Hydralazine interacts beneficially with nitrates, helping to lessen nitrate tolerance.[21]

Prazosin, Doxazosin, and Terazosin

There is an interaction between prazosin and the calcium antagonists verapamil and nifedipine, resulting in excessive hypotension. In the case of verapamil, part of the effect may be explained by a pharmacokinetic hepatic interaction. Both nitrates and prazosin may cause syncope, and these agents should be combined with care. Experimentally, prazosin may increase the plasma digoxin level. Similar interactions may hold for the other agents in this group.

ANGIOTENSIN-CONVERTING ENZYME INHIBITORS

In general, ACE inhibitors have few drug interactions (Table 81-6). In patients with CHF, excessive first-dose hypotension should be avoided to lessen the risk of renal impairment, which may lead to accumulation and interaction of renal-excreted drugs.

Because of potential hyperkalemia with potassium-sparing

TABLE 81-7 Drug Interactions of Antithrombotic Agents

Cardiac Drug	Interacting Drugs	Mechanism	Consequence	Prophylaxis
Aspirin (A)	ACE inhibitors	Vasodilation ↓	Less antifailure effect	Very low A dose
	Hepatic enzyme inducers (barbiturates, phenyton, rifampin)	Increased A metabolism	Decreased A effect	Adjust A dose; check A side effects
	Sulfinpyrazone (S), probenecid (P)	A decreases urate excretion	Decreased uricosuric effect of S or P	Increase dose of S or P
	Thiazide diuretics	A decreases urate excretion	Hyperuricemia	Check blood urate
	Warfarin	A is antithrombotic	Excess bleeding	Check INR or prothrombin time
Sulfinpyrazone (S)	Warfarin (W)	S displaces W from plasma proteins	Excess bleeding	Check INR or prothrombin time
Warfarin	Potentiating drugs			
	Allopurinol	Mechanism unknown	Excess bleeding	Check INR or prothrombin time
	Amiodarone	Mechanism unknown	Sensitizes to W for months	Avoid combination
	Aspirin	Added bleeding tendency	Excess bleeding	Check INR or prothrombin time
	Cimetidine	Decreased W degradation	Excess bleeding	Check INR or prothrombin time
	Quinidine	Hepatic interaction	Excess bleeding	Check INR or prothrombin time
	Statins	Hepatic interaction (?)	Excess bleeding	Check INR or prothrombin time
	Sulfinpyrazone	Displaces W from plasma proteins	Excess bleeding	Check INR or prothrombin time
	Acetaminophen	Hepatic interaction	Excess bleeding	Check INR or prothrombin time
	Inhibitory drugs			
	Cholestyramine, colestipol	Decrease absorption of W	Decreased W effect	Check INR or prothrombin time
Alteplase, tPA	Nitrates	Decreased tPA effect	Less thrombolytic benefit	Avoid; ? increase tPA dose

ABBREVIATION: INR = international normalized ratio.

diuretics, the ideal combination with an ACE inhibitor is a thiazide diuretic or furosemide, but without a potassium-retaining component.[12] In patients receiving NSAIDs, which tend to decrease renal plasma flow in their own right, addition of an ACE inhibitor can further decrease the glomerular filtration rate, with an added risk of hyperkalemia.[12] Captopril may interact with probenecid, which inhibits its tubular excretion, and, as mentioned earlier, there is a serious interaction with the loop diuretic furosemide.[101]

In patients with severe CHF, the acute combination of aspirin and an ACE inhibitor decreases the peripheral vasodilatation,[112] an effect not seen with ticlopidine.[113–115] Lower aspirin doses seem to have little or no hemodynamic interference,[116,117] but there are no true dose-response or chronic studies. It is best to keep the dose of aspirin as low as possible when combined with ACE inhibitors.

Captopril

Cotherapy of high-dose captopril with other drugs that alter or impair the immune status (e.g., hydralazine and procainamide) may predispose to neutropenia. Probenecid inhibits the renal tubular excretion of captopril, thereby increasing blood captopril levels[118]; doses of captopril may need downward adjustment. Captopril may decrease digoxin clearance by 20 to 30 percent.[97]

Enalapril

Drug interactions of enalapril are similar to those of captopril, except that the risk of neutropenia is less. It must be considered that enalapril has a longer duration of action; adverse hypotensive interactions with diuretics are therefore potentially more serious.

ANGIOTENSIN II RECEPTOR BLOCKERS

No significant drug–drug pharmacokinetic interactions have been found in interaction studies with hydrochlorothiazide, digoxin, warfarin, cimetidine, and phenobarbital (Table 81-6).[119] Moreover, in vitro studies show significant inhibition of the formation of the active metabolites by inhibitors of P450,3A4 or 2C9. Potent inhibitors of cytochrome P450,3A4 and 2C9 have been studied in patients, with no interaction with angiotensin II blockers observed.[120]

As with other drugs that block angiotensin II or its effects, concomitant use of potassium-sparing diuretics, potassium supplements, or salt substitutes containing potassium may lead to increases in serum potassium levels.

ANTITHROMBOTIC AND THROMBOLYTIC AGENTS

Table 81-7 summarizes the drug interactions of antithrombotic agents.

Aspirin

Since blood levels of uric acid may be increased by both aspirin and thiazide diuretics, special care is required in patients with a history of gout.[121] Conversely, aspirin may decrease the uricosuric effects of sulfinpyrazone and probenecid. Aspirin has some effects similar to those of the NSAIDs, inhibiting the effects of vasodilatory prostaglandins (Fig. 81-4). Thus, aspirin can reduce the natriuretic effect of spironolactone and some of the benefits of ACE inhibitors in CHF. Aspirin-induced gastrointestinal bleeding may be a greater hazard in patients receiving other NSAIDs or corticosteroid therapy. Antacids, by altering the pH of the stomach, may decrease the efficacy of enteric-coated preparations.

Inducers of the hepatic cytochrome oxidase system (e.g., barbiturates, phenytoin, and rifampin) increase aspirin breakdown. Aspirin tends to cause hypoglycemia in patients receiving oral hypoglycemics or insulin. Aspirin, especially in high doses, may exaggerate a bleeding tendency and anticoagulant-induced bleeding.[122] The dipyridamole-warfarin combination causes less bleeding than the aspirin-warfarin combination in patients who have undergone bypass surgery.[123] All these drug interactions should be less intense if the aspirin doses are kept low, as is the current trend.

Sulfinpyrazone

Sulfinpyrazone is highly bound to plasma proteins (98 to 99 percent) and may displace warfarin to precipitate bleeding. Like aspirin, sulfinpyrazone may sensitize patients who are given sulfonylureas and insulin to hypoglycemia.

Dipyridamole

Dipyridamole is a potent vasodilator. Thus, care is required when it is used in combination with other vasodilators. Note the interaction with adenosine, as discussed above.

Ticlopidine

Ticlopidine is an antiplatelet drug that interferes with ATP-induced platelet aggregation and does not appear to interfere with the vasodilating activity of ACE inhibitor drugs.[115]

Warfarin

Warfarin may be subject to many (up to 80) drug interactions.[12] A good rule is to suspect interactions unless one can be sure. The safest rule is to tell patients having oral anticoagulation not to use any new or over-the-counter drugs without consultation and for the physician to carefully check out any added compounds. More frequent measurements of the prothrombin time and dose adjustments are required when potentially interfering drugs are added.

Interfering drugs include those that reduce absorption of vitamin K or warfarin, such as cholestyramine.[12] Sulfinpyrazone increases warfarin levels by displacing it from plasma proteins. Other interfering drugs are inducers of the hepatic cytochrome oxidase system, which increase the rate of warfarin metabolism in the liver.

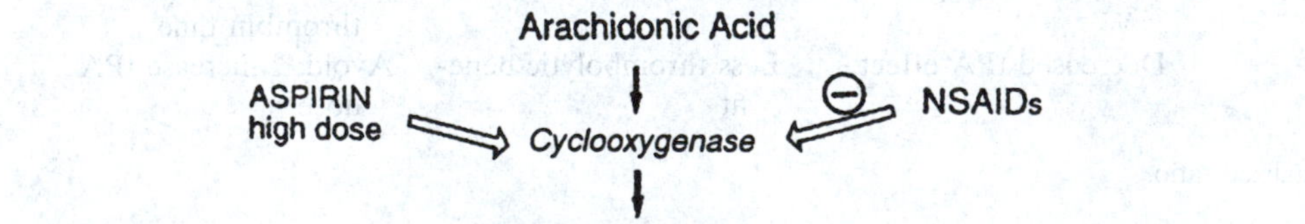

FIGURE 81-4 Possible mechanism whereby NSAIDs and aspirin block the cyclooxygenase pathway and thereby inhibit formation of vasodilatory prostaglandins. The resultant salt and water retention may decrease the effects of almost all antihypertensives, including ACE inhibitors. In addition, NSAIDs decrease renin and aldosterone through an entirely different mechanism, which would tend to lessen salt and water retention. (Adapted from Houston MC: Nonsteroidal anti-inflammatory drugs and antihypertensives. *Am J Med* 1991; 90(suppl 5A):42S–47S. Reproduced with permission from the publisher and authors.)

TABLE 81-8 Drug Interactions of Lipid-Lowering Agents

Cardiac Drug	Interacting Drugs	Mechanism	Consequence	Prophylaxis
Fibric acids (gemfibrozil, clofibrate, bezafibrate, fenofibrate)	Warfarin	Hepatic interference	Risk of bleeding	Check prothrombin time
Bile acid sequestrants (cholestyramine, colestipol)	Warfarin (W)	Decreased absorption	Decreased W effect	Check prothrombin time
HMG-CoA reductase inhibitors (statins) (lovastatin, simvastatin, pravastatin) atorvastatin, cerivastatin, fluvastatin	Fibrates, cyclosporine, erythromycin, niacin, antifungal azoles	Added damage to muscle with myositis	Rhabdomyolysis and risk of renal failure	Check creatine phosphokinase levels
Statins	Warfarin	Hepatic interaction	Increased risk of bleeding	Check INR or prothrombin time (beneficial)
Pravastatin	Cyclosporine	Hepatic interaction (?)	Enhanced immunosuppression	

Yet, other drugs decrease the hepatic degradation of warfarin to increase the anticoagulant effect, including antibiotics, such as metronidazole and cotrimoxazole. Cimetidine likewise inhibits hepatic degradation. Ranitidine does not do likewise. Other potentiating cardiovascular agents are allopurinol, clofibrate, quinidine, and amiodarone.[12,124] Amiodarone is especially dangerous because its very long half-life means a very long potentiation of warfarin. Heparin or aspirin may potentiate bleeding, although there are large interindividual variations.[125] Very high doses of aspirin impair synthesis of clotting factors.

It must be reemphasized that sulfinpyrazone has a powerful effect in displacing warfarin from blood proteins; thus, the dose of warfarin required may be reduced to only 1 mg.[103]

Heparins

Physically, heparin, including the low-molecular-weight heparins, is incompatible in a water solution with certain substances, including antibiotics, antihistamines, phenothiazides, and hydrocortisone.

TABLE 81-9 Herbal Medicines Associated with Drug Interactions

Anticoagulants		
Angelica	Fenugreek	Lungwort
Black haw	Garlic	Pau d'arco
Bogbean	Ginger	Poplar
Buchu	Gingko	Prickly ash
Cat's claw	Horse chestnut	Red clover
Chamomile	Irish moss	Tonkas bean
Chondroitin	Kelp	Wintergreen
Dong quai	Khella	Yarrow
Antihypertensives		
Arnica	Dandelion	
Betony	Goldenseal	
Black cohosh	Kelp	
Blue cohosh	Khella	
Capsicum	Queen Ann's lace	
Cat's claw	Yarrow	
Specific Drugs		
Broom (and beta blockers)		Fumitory (and digoxin)
Fumitory (and beta blockers)		Goldenseal (and digoxin)
Cowslip (and diuretics)		Aloe (and digoxin)
Cucumber (and diuretics)		St. John's wort (and digoxin)
Horsetail (and diuretics)		Queen Ann's lace (and digoxin)
Licorice (and diuretics)		
Dandelion (and diuretics)		

However, direct pharmacokinetic or pharmacodynamic drug interactions have not been described, except for a controversial interaction with nitrates.[126]

Tissue-Type Plasminogen Activator

Concurrent use of intravenous nitroglycerin diminishes the efficacy of recombinant tissue-type plasminogen activator (tPA or alteplase), possibly because of increased hepatic blood flow and enhanced catabolism of tPA.[127]

LIPID-LOWERING AGENTS

There are not many serious interactions with lipid-lowering agents (Table 81-8). A number of lipid-lowering agents may interact with warfarin, either by decreased absorption (cholestyramine) or by hepatic interference (clofibrate, bezafibrate, fenofibrate, or gemfibrozil). The precise mechanism is not clear. Clofibrate, fenofibrate, gemfibrozil, and many of the statins increase the effects of warfarin.

Simvastatin, lovastatin, and atorvastatin are metabolized by cytochrome P450,3A4. Clinical experience has shown that the risk of myopathy with these statins is increased substantially by concomitant use of the few drugs that substantially inhibit P450,3A4, including cyclosporine and erythromycin.[128] Calcium channel blockers and grapefruit juice are weak inhibitors of P450,3A4.[129]

Probucol, in the presence of additional agents, such as thiazide diuretics or group IA or III antiarrhythmics, may prolong the QT interval and theoretically precipitate torsades de pointes. The hydroxymethylglutaryl coenzyme A (HMG-CoA) reductase inhibitors, such as atorvastatin, cerivastatin, lovastatin, simvastatin, pravastatin, and fluvastatin, should ideally not be combined with the fibrates because of the higher risk of myositis with rhabdomyolysis and possible renal failure. Likewise, concurrent therapy with niacin, cyclosporine, or erythromycin may also carry a small risk of rhabdomyolysis. Adding an antifungal azole (a group that includes ketoconazole, used in transplantation) has precipitated myolysis in a patient already receiving a statin and niacin.[130] Yet, in clinical practice, the advantages of better lipid control with combined therapy seems to outweigh these risks. Furthermore, a positive interaction of pravastatin with cyclosporine is reported, whereby there appears to be increased immunosuppression.[131] Serum creatine kinase levels should be checked periodically, especially after increasing doses or after starting combination therapy.

ANTIHYPERTENSIVE DRUGS

Interactions for diuretics, beta-adrenergic blockers, calcium antagonists, ACE inhibitors, and alpha$_1$-adrenergic blockers have already been considered. In general, NSAIDs interfere severely with the antihypertensive efficacy of all antihypertensives.[132,133] An exception is nifedipine (and, presumably, other dihydropyridines).[134] Unlike other NSAIDs, aspirin[16] and sulindac may give relative protection from the negative interaction.[132] When calcium antagonists are used as antihypertensives, part of their effect is by natriuresis; thus, adding a diuretic is often relatively ineffective.[135]

HERBAL MEDICINE

Herbal supplements are commonly used by patients for various cardiac conditions.[136] Many of the herbs cause cardiac toxicity or can interact unfavorably with known cardiac drugs (Table 81-9).

Chamomile has antispasmodic actions and warfarin-like effects. Feverfew, garlic, and ginger have antiplatelet actions and can pose safety problems in patients taking warfarin. Gingko and ginseng should be avoided in patients receiving warfarin and heparin. Herbal acquertics can inhibit the activity of diuretics or other antihypertensive therapy. Gossypol and licorice are associated with renal loss of potassium and should not be used with thiazide and loop diuretics or digoxin. Plantain and hawthorn berries can mimic or potentiate digitalis toxicity. Kelp can interfere with the antiarrhythmic effects of amiodarone. St. John's wort can lower serum digoxin levels by reducing digoxin absorption, possibly by inducing p-glycoprotein in the gut.[137,138]

References

1. Doucet J, Chassagne P, Trivalle C, et al. Drug-drug interactions related to hospital admissions in older adults: A prospective study of 1000 patients. *J Am Geriatr Soc* 1996; 44:944–948.
2. Lacombe PS, Garcia Vicente JA, Costa Pagès J, Morselli PL: Causes and problems of nonresponse or poor response to drugs. *Drugs* 1996; 51:552–570.
3. Michalets EL. Update: Clinically significant cytochrome P-450 drug interactions. *Pharmacotherapy* 1998; 18:84–112.
4. Cheng JWM. Cytochrome P450 mediated cardiovascular drug interactions. *Heart Dis* 2000; 2:254–258.
5. Yu DK. The contribution of p-glycoprotein to pharmacokinetic drug-drug interactions. *J Clin Pharmacol* 1999; 39:1203–1211.
6. Tran C, Knowles SR, Liu BA, Shear NH. Gender differences in adverse drug reactions. *J Clin Pharmacol* 1998; 38:1003–1009.
7. Sokol SI, Cheng-Lai A, Frishman WH, Kaza CS. Cardiovascular drug therapy in patients with hepatic diseases and patients with congestive heart failure. *J Clin Pharmacol* 2000; 40:11–30.
8. Be alert for interactions between prescription and OTC drugs. *Drugs Ther Perspect* 1996; 7:12–14.
9. Huang J-D, Chuang S-K, Cheng C-L, Lai M-L. Pharmacokinetics of metoprolol enantiomers in Chinese subjects of major CYP2D6 genotypes. *Clin Pharmacol Ther* 1999; 65:402–407.
10. Strayhorn VA, Baciewicz AM, Self TH. Update on rifampin drug interactions: III. *Arch Intern Med* 1997; 157:2453–2458.
11. Opie LH, ed. *Drugs for the Heart,* 4th ed. Philadelphia: Saunders; 1995.
12. Opie LH. Cardiovascular drug interactions. In: Frishman WH, Sonnenblick EH, eds. *Cardiovascular Pharmacotherapeutics.* New York: McGraw Hill; 1997:1383.
13. Kirch W, Spahn H, Kohler H, Mutschler E. Influence of β-receptor antagonists on pharmacokinetics of cimetidine. *Drugs* 1983; 25(suppl 2):127–130.
14. McLean AJ, Knight R, Harrison PM, Harper RW. Clearance-based oral drug interaction between verapamil and metoprolol and comparison with atenolol. *Am J Cardiol* 1985; 55:1628–1629.
15. Ochs HR, Carstens G, Greenblatt DJ. Reduction in lidocaine clearance during continuous infusion and by coadministration of propranolol. *N Engl J Med* 1980; 303:373–377.
16. Webster J. Interactions of NSAIDs with diuretics and β-blockers: Mechanism and clinical implications. *Drugs* 1985; 30:32–41.

17. Tolins M, Weir K, Chesler E, Pierpont GL. "Maximal" drug therapy is not necessarily optimal in chronic angina pectoris. *J Am Coll Cardiol* 1984; 3:1051–1057.
18. Bruce RA, Hossack KF, Kusumi F, et al. Excessive reduction in peripheral resistance during exercise and risk of orthostatic symptoms with sustained-release nitroglycerin and diltiazem treatment of angina. *Am Heart J* 1985; 109:1020–1026.
19. Boden WE, Bough EW, Reichman MJ, et al. Beneficial effects of high-dose diltiazem in patients with persistent effort angina on β-blockers and nitrates: A randomized, double-blind, placebo-controlled, cross-over study. *Circulation* 1985; 71:1197–1205.
20. Cheitlin MD, Hutter AM Jr, Brindis RG, et al. ACC/AHA Expert Consensus Document: Use of sildenafil (Viagra) in patients with cardiovascular disease. *J Am Coll Cardiol* 1999; 33:273–282.
21. Gogia H, Mehra A, Parikh S, et al. Prevention of tolerance to hemodynamic effects of nitrates with concomitant use of hydralazine in patients with chronic heart failure. *J Am Cardiol* 1995; 26:1575–1580.
22. Becker RC, Corrao JM, Bovill EG, et al. Intravenous nitroglycerin-induced heparin resistance: A qualitative antithrombin III abnormality. *Am Heart J* 1990; 119:1254–1261.
23. Reicher-Reiss H, Neufeld HN, Ebner FX. Calcium antagonists: Adverse drug interactions. *Cardiovasc Drug Ther* 1987; 1: 403–409.
24. Abernethy DR, Schwartz JB. Calcium antagonist drugs. *N Engl J Med* 1999; 341:1447–1457.
25. Abernethy DR. Grapefruits and drugs: When is statistically significant clinically significant? *J Clin Invest* 1997; 10:2297–2298.
26. Frishman WH. Comparative efficacy and concomitant use of bepridil and beta blockers in the management of angina pectoris. *Am J Cardiol* 1992; 69(suppl):50D–60D.
27. Mullins ME, Horowitz Z, Linden DHJ, et al. Life-threatening interaction of mibefradil and β blockers with dihydropyridine calcium channel blockers. *JAMA* 1998; 280:157–158.
28. Yeh R, Gulamhusein SS, Klein GJ. Combined verapamil and propranolol for supraventricular tachycardia. *Am J Cardiol* 1984; 53:757–763.
29. Ellrodt AG, Ault MJ, Riedinger MS, Murati GH. Efficacy and safety of sublingual nifedipine in hypertensive emergencies. *Am J Med* 1985; 79(suppl 4A):19–25.
30. Kieval J, Kirsten EB, Kessler KM, et al. The effects of intravenous verapamil on hemodynamic status of patients with coronary artery disease receiving propranolol. *Circulation* 1982; 65:653–659.
31. Packer M, Meller J, Medina N, et al. Hemodynamic consequences of combined beta-adrenergic and slow calcium channel blockade in man. *Circulation* 1982; 65:660–668.
32. Johnston DL, Lesoway R, Humen DP, Kostuk WJ. Clinical and hemodynamic evaluation of propranolol in combination with verapamil, nifedipine and diltiazem in exertional angina pectoris: A placebo-controlled, double-blind, randomized, cross-over study. *Am J Cardiol* 1985; 55:680–687.
33. Winniford MD, Fulton KL, Corbett JR, et al. Propranolol-verapamil versus propranolol-nifedipine in severe angina pectoris of effort: A randomized, double-blind, cross-over study. *Am J Cardiol* 1985; 55:281–285.
34. Hamann SR, Kaltenborn KE, Vore M, et al. Cardiovascular pharmacokinetic consequences of combined administration of verapamil and propranolol in dogs. *Am J Cardiol* 1985; 56:147–156.
35. Murdoch DL, Thomson GD, Thompson GG, et al. Evaluation of potential pharmacodynamic and pharmacokinetic interactions between verapamil and propranolol in normal subjects. *Br J Clin Pharmacol* 1991; 31:323–332.
36. Johnston DL, Gebhardt VA, Donald A, Kostuk WJ. Comparative effects of propranolol and verapamil alone and in combination on left ventricular function in patients with chronic exertional angina: A double-blind, placebo-controlled, randomized, cross-over study with radionuclide ventriculography. *Circulation* 1983; 68:1280–1289.
37. McInnes GT, Findlay IN, Murray G, et al. Cardiovascular responses to verapamil and propranolol in hypertensive patients. *J Hypertens* 1985; 3(suppl 3):S219–S221.
38. Pedersen KE. Digoxin interactions: The influence of quinidine and verapamil on the pharmacokinetics and receptor binding of digitalis glycosides. *Acta Med Scand* 1985; 697(suppl):12–40.
39. Elliott HL, Pasanisi F, Meredith PA, Reid JL. Acute hypotensive response to nifedipine added to prazosin. *Br Med J* 1984; 288:238.
40. Pasanisi F, Elliott HL, Meredith PA, et al. Combined alpha-adrenoceptor antagonism and calcium channel blockade in normal subjects. *Clin Pharmacol Ther* 1984; 36:716–723.
41. Reid JL, Meredith PA, Pasanisi F. Clinical pharmacological aspects of calcium antagonists and their therapeutic role in hypertension. *J Cardiovasc Pharmacol* 1985; 7(suppl 4):S18–S20.
42. Maisel AS, Motulsky HJ, Insel PA. Hypotension after quinidine plus verapamil: Possible additive competition at alpha-adrenergic receptors. *N Engl J Med* 1985; 312:167–171.
43. Trohman RG, Estes DM, Castellanos A, et al. Increased quinidine plasma concentrations during administration of verapamil: A new quinidine-verapamil interaction. *Am J Cardiol* 1986; 57:706–707.
44. Hansten PD, Horn JR. Calcium channel blocker-induced drug interactions: Evidence for metabolic inhibition. *Drug Interact Newsl* 1986; 6:35–40.
45. Opie LH, White DA. Adverse interaction between nifedipine and beta blockade. *Br Med J* 1980; 281:1462–1464.
46. Kleinbloesem CH, van Brummelen P, Sandberg TH, et al. Kinetic and haemodynamic interactions between nifedipine and propranolol in healthy subjects utilizing controlled rates of drug input. In: Kleinbloesem CH, ed. *Nifedipine: Clinical Pharmacokinetics and Haemodynamic Effects.* The Hague: Drukkerij JH Pasmans BV; 1985:151.
47. Kiss I, Farsang C. Nifedipine-prazosin interaction in patients with essential hypertension. *Cardiovasc Drugs Ther* 1989; 3:413–415.
48. Frishman WH, Charlap S, Kimmel B, et al: Diltiazem compared to nifedipine and combination treatment with stable angina: Effects on angina, exercise tolerance and the ambulatory ECG. *Circulation* 1988; 77:774–786.
49. Hung J, Lamb IH, Connolly SJ, et al. The effect of diltiazem and propranolol, alone and in combination, on exercise performance and left ventricular function in patients with stable effort angina: A double-blind, randomized, and placebo-controlled study. *Circulation* 1983; 68:560–567.
50. Grino JM, Sabate I, Castelao AM, Alsina J. Influence of diltiazem on cyclosporin clearance. *Lancet* 1986; 2:1387.
51. Cheng JWM. Cilostazol. *Heart Dis* 1999; 1:182–186.
52. Bigger JT, Giardina EG. Drug interactions in antiarrhythmic therapy. *Ann NY Acad Sci* 1984; 427:140–161.
53. Jaillon P. Antiarrhythmic drug interactions: Are they important? *Eur Heart J* 1987; 8(suppl A):127–132.
54. Hardy BG, Zador IT, Golden L, et al. Effects of cimetidine on the pharmacokinetics of quinidine. *Am J Cardiol* 1983; 52:172–175.
55. Drici M-D, Knollman BC, Wang W-X, Woosley RL. Cardiac actions of erythromycin: Influence of female sex. *JAMA* 1998; 280:1774–1776.
56. Mishra A, Friedman HS, Sinha AK. The effects of erythromycin on the electrocardiogram. *Chest* 1999; 115:983–986.
57. Lee KL, Jim M-H, Tang SC, Tai Y-T. QT prolongation and Torsades de Pointes associated with clarithromycin. *Am J Med* 1998; 104:395–396.
58. Hager WD, Fenster P, Mayersohn M, et al. Digoxin-quinidine interaction: Pharmacokinetic evaluation. *N Engl J Med* 1979; 300:1238–1241.
59. Koch-Weser J. Quinidine-induced hypoprothrombinemic hemor-

rhage in patients on chronic warfarin therapy. *Ann Intern Med* 1968; 68:511–517.
60. Dada JL, Wilkinson GR, Nies AJ. Interaction of quinidine with anticonvulsant drugs. *N Engl J Med* 1976; 294:699–702.
61. Twum-Barima Y, Carruthers SG. Quinidine-rifampicin. *N Engl J Med* 1981; 304:1466–1469.
62. Farringer JA, McWay-Hess K, Clementi WA. Cimetidine-quinidine interaction. *Clin Pharmacol* 1984; 3:81–83.
63. Green JA, Clementi WA, Porter C, Stigelman W. Nifedipine-quinidine interaction. *Clin Pharmacol* 1983; 2:461–465.
64. Van Lith RM, Appleby DH. Quinidine-nifedipine interaction. *Drug Intell Clin Pharm* 1985; 19:829–830.
65. Marcus FI. Drug interactions with amiodarone. *Am Heart J* 1983; 106:924–930.
66. Christian CO, Meredith CG, Speeg KV. Cimetidine inhibits procainamide clearance. *Clin Pharmacol Ther* 1984; 36:221–227.
67. Lee JT, Davy JM, Kates RE. Evaluation of combined administration of verapamil and disopyramide in dogs. *J Cardiovasc Pharmacol* 1985; 7:501–507.
68. Kapil RP, Axelson JE, Mansfield IL, et al. Disopyramide pharmacokinetics and metabolism: Effect of inducers. *Br J Clin Pharmacol* 1987; 24:781–791.
69. Teichman SL, Fisher JD, Matos JA, Kim SG. Disopyramide-pyridostigmine: Report of a beneficial drug interaction. *J Cardiovasc Pharmacol* 1985; 7:108–113.
70. Feely J, Wilkinson GR, McAllister CB, Wood AJ. Increased toxicity and reduced clearance of lidocaine by cimetidine. *Ann Intern Med* 1982; 96:592–594.
71. Boyce JR, Cervenko FW, Wright FJ. Effects of halothane on the pharmacokinetics of lidocaine in digitalis-toxic dogs. *Can Anaesth Soc J* 1978; 25:323–328.
72. Jeresaty RM, Kahn AH, Landry AB. Sinoatrial arrest due to lidocaine in a patient receiving quinidine. *Chest* 1972; 61:683–685.
73. Frishman WH, Cheng-Lai A, Chen J, eds. Antiarrhythmic agents. In: *Current Cardiovascular Drugs,* 3d ed. Philadelphia: Current Medicine; 2000:54.
74. Klein R, Huang SK, Group Southwest Cardiology Research. Combination therapy of propafenone with quinidine or procainamide: Enhanced efficacy and reduced side-effects [abstr]. *J Am Coll Cardiol* 1985; 5:423.
75. Breithardt G, Selpel L, Abendroth RR. Comparative cross-over study of the effects of disopyramide and mexiletine on stimulus-induced ventricular tachycardia [abstr]. *Circulation* 1980; 62(suppl 3):153.
76. Duff HJ, Roden D, Primm RK, et al. Mexiletine in the treatment of resistant ventricular arrhythmias: Enhancement of efficacy and reduction of dose-related side-effects by combination with quinidine. *Circulation* 1983; 67:1124–1128.
77. Greenspan AM, Spielman SR, Webb CR, et al. Efficacy of combination therapy with mexiletine and a type 1A agent for inducible ventricular tachyarrhythmias secondary to coronary artery disease. *Am J Cardiol* 1985; 56:277–284.
78. Leahey EB, Heissenbuttel RH, Giardina EG, Bigger JT. Combined mexiletine and propranolol treatment of refractory ventricular tachycardia. *Br Med J* 1980; 2:357–358.
79. Waleffe A, Mary-Rabine L, Legrand V, et al. Combined mexiletine and amiodarone treatment of refractory recurrent ventricular tachycardia. *Am Heart J* 1980; 100:788–793.
80. Lewis GP, Holtzman JL. Interaction of flecainide with digoxin and propranolol. *Am J Cardiol* 1984; 53:52B–57B.
81. Shea P, Lal R, Kim SS, et al. Flecainide and amiodarone interaction. *J Am Coll Cardiol* 1986; 7:1127–1130.
82. Maga TB, Verbesselt R, Van Hecken A, et al. Oral flecainide elimination kinetics: Effects of cimetidine [abstr]. *Circulation* 1983; 68(suppl 3):416.
83. Hodges M, Salerno D, Granrud G. Double-blind placebo-controlled evaluation of propafenone in suppressing ventricular ectropic activity. *Am J Cardiol* 1984; 54:45D–50D.
84. Martinowitz U, Rabinovich J, Goldfarb D, et al. Interaction between warfarin sodium and amiodarone. *N Engl J Med* 1981; 304:671–672.
85. Gillis RA, Clancy MM, Anderson RJ. Deleterious effects of bretylium in cats with digitalis-induced ventricular tachycardia. *Circulation* 1973; 47:974–983.
86. Vincent JL, Dufaye P, Berre J, Kahn RJ. Bretylium in severe ventricular arrhythmias associated with digitalis intoxication. *Am J Emerg Med* 1984; 2:504–506.
87. Peipho RW, Culbertson VL, Rhodes RS. Drug interactions with the calcium-entry blockers. *Circulation* 1987; 75:181–194.
88. Hauptman PJ, Kelley RA. Digitalis. *Circulation* 1999; 99:1265–1270.
89. Greiner B, Eichelbaum M, Fritz P, et al. The role of intestinal p-glycoprotein in the interaction of digoxin and rifampin. *J Clin Invest* 1999; 104:147–153.
90. Haas GJ. How best to use digoxin in the treatment of CHF: Strategies and practical tips learned from clinical trials. *J Crit Illness* 1999; 14:484–491.
91. Lessem J, Bellinetto A. Interaction between digoxin and the calcium antagonists nicardipine and tiapamil. *Clin Ther* 1983; 5:595–602.
92. Kirch W, Hutt HJ, Dylewicz P, Ohnhaus EE. Dose-dependence of the nifedipine–digoxin interaction. *Clin Pharmacol Ther* 1986; 39:35–39.
93. Lessem JN. Interaction between Ca^{2+} antagonists and digitalis. *Cardiovasc Drugs Ther* 1988; 1:441–446.
94. Kirch W, Hutt HJ, Heidemann H, et al. Drug interactions with nitrendipine. *J Cardiovasc Pharmacol* 1984; 6:S982–S985.
95. Plunkett LM, Gokhale RD, Vallner JJ, Tackett RL. Prazosin alters free and total plasma digoxin levels in dogs. *Am Heart J* 1985; 109:847–851.
96. Marcus FI. Pharmacokinetic interactions between digoxin and other drugs. *J Am Cardiol* 1985; 5:82A–90A.
97. Waldorff S, Andersen JD, Heeboil-Nielsen N, et al. Spironolactone-induced changes in digoxin kinetics. *Clin Pharmacol Ther* 1978; 24:162–167.
98. Waldorff S, Hansen PB, Egeblad H, et al. Interactions between digoxin and potassium-sparing diuretics. *Clin Pharmacol Ther* 1983; 33:418–423.
99. Fenster PE, Hager WD, Goodman MM. Digoxin-quinidine-spironolactone interaction. *Clin Pharmacol Ther* 1984; 36:70–73.
100. Miura T, Ueno K, Tanaka K, et al. Impairment of absorption of digoxin by acarbose. *J Clin Pharmacol* 1998; 38:654–657.
101. McLay JS, McMurray JJ, Bridges AB, et al. Acute effects of captopril on the renal actions of furosemide in patients with chronic heart failure. *Am Heart J* 1993; 126:879–886.
102. Van Hecken AM, Verbresselt R, Buntinx A, et al. Absence of a pharmacokinetic interaction between enalapril and furosemide. *Br J Clin Pharmacol* 1987; 23:84.
103. Motwani JG, Fenwick MK, Morton JJ, Struthers AD: Furosemide-induced natriuresis is augmented by ultra-low-dose captopril but not by standard dose of captopril in chronic heart failure. *Circulation* 1992; 86:439.
104. Dzau VJ, Packer M, Lilly LS, et al. Prostaglandins in severe congestive heart failure: Relation to activation of the renin-angiotensin system and hyponatremia. *N Engl J Med* 1984; 310:347–352.
105. Heerdink ER, Leufkens HG, Herings RMC, et al. NSAIDs associated with increased risk of congestive heart failure in elderly patients taking diuretics. *Arch Intern Med* 1998; 158:1108–1112.
106. McKibbin JK, Pocock WA, Barlow JB, et al. Sotalol, hypokalaemia, syncope, and torsades de pointes. *Br Heart J* 1984; 51:157–162.
107. Jefferson JW, Kalin NH. Serum lithium levels and long-term diuretic use. *JAMA* 1979; 241:1134–1136.

108. Ruddy MC, Kostis JB, Frishman WH. Drugs that affect the renin-angiotensin system. In: Frishman WH, Sonnenblick EH, eds. *Cardiovascular Pharmacotherapeutics.* New York: McGraw-Hill; 1997:131.
109. Perazella MA. Trimethoprim is a potassium-sparing diuretic like amiloride and causes hyperkalemia in high-risk patients. *Am J Ther* 1997; 4:343–348.
110. Cogan JJ, Humphreys MH, Carlson CJ, et al. Acute vasodilator therapy increases renal clearance of digoxin in patients with congestive heart failure. *Circulation* 1981; 64:973–976.
111. Schneck DW, Vary JE. Mechanism by which hydralazine increases propranolol bioavailability. *Clin Pharmacol Ther* 1984; 35:447–453.
112. Hall D, Zeitler H, Rudolph W. Counteraction of the vasodilator effects of enalapril by aspirin in severe heart failure. *J Am Coll Cardiol* 1992; 20:1549–1555.
113. Teerlink JR, Massie BM. The interaction of ACE inhibitors and aspirin in heart failure: Torn between two lovers [editorial]. *Am Heart J* 1999; 138:193–197.
114. Guazzi M, Pontone G, Agostoni P. Aspirin worsens exercise performance and pulmonary gas exchange in patients with heart failure who are taking angiotensin-converting enzyme inhibitors. *Am Heart J* 1999; 138:254–260.
115. Spaulding C, Charbonnier B, Cohen-Solal A, et al. Acute hemodynamic interaction of aspirin and ticlopidine with enalapril: Results of a double-blind, randomized comparative trial. *Circulation* 1998; 98:757–765.
116. Van Wijngaarden J, Smit AJ, deGraeff PA, et al. Effects of acetylsalicylic acid on peripheral hemodynamics in patients with chronic heart failure treated with angiotensin-converting enzyme inhibitors. *J Cardiovasc Pharmacol* 1994; 23:240–245.
117. Baur LHB, Schipperheyn JJ, van der Laarse A, et al. Combining salicylate and enalapril in patients with coronary artery disease and heart failure. *Br Heart J* 1995; 73:227–236.
118. Singhvi SM, Duchin KL, Willard DA, et al. Renal handling of captopril: Effect of probenicid. *Clin Pharmacol Ther* 1982; 32:182–189.
119. Kazierad DJ, Martin DE, Ilson B, et al. Eprosartan does not affect the pharmacodynamics of warfarin. *J Clin Pharmacol* 1998; 38:649–653.
120. Meadowcroft AM, Williamson KM, Patterson H, et al. The effects of fluvastatin, a CYP2C9 inhibitor, on losartan pharmacokinetics in healthy volunteers. *J Clin Pharmacol* 1999; 39:418–424.
121. Grayzel AI, Liddle L, Seegmiller JE. Diagnostic significance of hyperuricemia in arthritis. *N Engl J Med* 1961; 265:763–768.
122. Moroz L. Increased blood fibrinolytic activity after aspirin ingestion. *N Engl J Med* 1977; 296:525–529.
123. Chesebro JH, Fuster V, Elveback LR, et al. Trial of combined warfarin plus dipyridamole or aspirin therapy in prosthetic heart valve replacement: Danger of aspirin compared with dipyridamole. *Am J Cardiol* 1983; 51:1537–1541.
124. Lin JC, Ito MK, Stolley SN, et al. The effect of converting from pravastatin to simvastatin on the pharmacodynamics of warfarin. *J Clin Pharmacol* 1999; 39:86–90.
125. O'Reilly RA, Sahud MA, Aggeler PM. Impact of aspirin and chlorthalidone on the pharmacodynamics of oral anticoagulant drugs in man. *Ann NY Acad Sci* 1971; 179:173–186.
126. Koh KK, Park GS, Song JH, Moon TH. Interaction of intravenous heparin and organic nitrates in acute ischemic syndromes. *Am J Cardiol* 1995; 76:706–709.
127. Romeo F, Rosano GM, Martuscelli E, De Luca F. Concurrent nitroglycerin administration reduces the efficacy of recombinant tissue-type plasminogen activator in patients with acute anterior wall myocardial infarction. *Am Heart J* 1995; 130:692–697.
128. Gruer PJK, Vega JM, Mercuri MF, et al. Concomitant use of cytochrome P450, 3A4 inhibitors and simvastatin. *Am J Cardiol* 1999; 84:811–815.
129. Rogers JD, Zhao J, Liu L, et al. Grapefruit juice has minimal effects on plasma concentrations of lovastatin-derived 3-hydroxy-3-methylglutaryl coenzyme A reductase inhibitors. *Clin Pharmacol Ther* 1999; 66:358–366.
130. Lees RS, Lees AM. Rhabdomyolysis from the coadministration of lovastatin and the antifungal agent itraconazole. *N Engl J Med* 1995; 333:664–665.
131. Keogh A, Spratt P, McCosker C, et al. Ketoconazole to reduce the need for cyclosporine after cardiac transplantation. *N Engl J Med* 1995; 333:628–633.
132. Houston MC. Nonsteroidal anti-inflammatory drugs and antihypertensives. *Am J Med* 1991; 90(suppl 5A):42S–47S.
133. NSAIDs and hypertension: Is it clinically important? *Drugs Ther Perspect* 1998; 11:14–16.
134. Salvetti A, Magagna A, Abdel-Haq B, et al. Nifedipine interactions in hypertensive patients. *Cardiovasc Drugs Ther* 1990; 4:963–968.
135. Weinberger MH. The relationship of sodium balance and concomitant diuretic therapy to blood pressure response with calcium channel entry blockers. *Am J Med* 1991; 90(suppl 5A):15S–20S.
136. Lin GI, Frishman WH. Use of alternative medications in treating cardiovascular disease. In: Frishman WH, Sonnenblick EH, eds. *Cardiovascular Pharmacotherapeutics.* New York: McGraw-Hill; 1997:989.
137. Johne A, Brockmöller Bauer S, Maurer A, et al. Pharmacokinetic interaction of digoxin with an herbal extract from St. John's wort (*Hypericum perforatum*). *Clin Pharmacol Ther* 1999; 66: 338–345.
138. Yu DK. The contribution of p-glycoprotein to pharmacokinetic drug–drug interactions. *J Clin Pharmacol* 1999; 39:1203–1211.

CHAPTER 82

HEART DISEASE AND PREGNANCY

John H. McAnulty / James Metcalfe / Kent Ueland

INTRODUCTION

The remarkable decrease in maternal morbidity and mortality over the last century is a high achievement. At the beginning of the twenty-first, cardiovascular disease still has significant consequences. This chapter describes how pregnancy affects the cardiovascular system and how the heart and heart disease affect pregnancy. Even if there were no heart disease, an understanding of the cardiovascular changes of a normal pregnancy is important for optimal care. But pregnancy in patients with heart disease is becoming more common. This is not because of a failure of health care. Rather, treatment of heart disease during childhood, usually with surgery, has led an increasing number of women with treated heart disease to survive to the age of childbearing and to be able to conceive. Because of this and because failure to treat heart disease may adversely affect both the mother and the child, the person caring for a pregnant woman must recognize heart disease and direct care accordingly.

HEART DISEASE ISSUES UNIQUE TO PREGNANCY

In the case of a woman with heart disease during pregnancy, some issues are always important. These are outlined below.

Health Priorities

Mother and child—the health of one importantly influences that of the other. The well-being of the fetus should be considered, but the safety of the mother is always the highest priority. Ideally, treatment of the mother with drugs, diagnostic studies, or surgery should be avoided. If required for maternal safety, however, they should be used.

Maternal Fragility

Despite advances in the recognition and management of heart disease, pregnancy puts the mother at risk. The normal hemodynamic changes of pregnancy may result in disability or death. The risk[1] is so great with some cardiovascular abnormalities that a recommendation of avoidance or interruption of pregnancy is supportable (Table 82-1).[2] Emotional stability is also threatened by pregnancy in the woman with heart disease. Misconceptions and apprehension are common. The following previously described case provides one example of the need to keep a pregnant woman and her family informed and comfortable:[3]

> A cardiac care unit nurse for 10 years, always logical and calm, and 7 months into her second pregnancy—could she be this frightened? She is, and it's about what the pregnancy will do to her heart and what her heart will

TABLE 82-1 Cardiovascular Abnormalities Placing a Mother and Infant at Extremely High Risk

Advise *avoidance* or *interruption of pregnancy*
Pulmonary hypertension
Dilated cardiomyopathy with congestive failure
Marfan's syndrome with dilated aortic root
Cyanotic congenital heart disease
Pregnancy counseling and close clinical follow-up required
Prosthetic valve
Coarctation of the aorta
Marfan's syndrome
Dilated cardiomyopathy in asymptomatic women
Obstructive lesions

SOURCE: Modified from McAnulty JH, et al.[2] Reproduced with permission from the publisher and authors.

do to her pregnancy. She, of course, knows too much. She has heard of a peripartum cardiomyopathy and is for some reason convinced that her labor will cause it. She is wrong about that (we believe), but she still is an appropriate representative of a prospective parent—easily worried about the effects of pregnancy on her health and worried about the baby. She knows about her ventricular ectopy. It has to be bad for the baby! She's probably wrong, but again, this is an example of how pregnancy raises issues that we ordinarily do not consider when taking care of a patient: an example of the apprehension that surrounds heart disease and pregnancy.

Fetal Vulnerability

The fetus depends on its mother for a continuous supply of oxygen and adequate nutrients. The mother must also remove the products of fetal metabolism, including heat. The maternal commitment to the fetus is exceptional, but if the mother requires a redistribution of volume for her own safety, blood is preferentially diverted away from the uterus. In the woman with a normal cardiovascular system, blood flow to the fetus seems to be adequate, even during periods of physical and emotional stress. In the woman with heart disease, however, where uterine blood flow may already be compromised, the chance of inadequate uterine perfusion increases. Treatment of maternal heart disease may also jeopardize the fetus. Diagnostic studies, drugs, or surgery may increase fetal loss, result in teratogenicity, or alter fetal growth.

Newborn Infant Vulnerability

The health of a newborn infant is a concern when the mother has heart disease. This fragility may be due to a marginal uterine blood flow during pregnancy or to lingering effects of the medications used to treat the mother. Additionally, the live-born infant of a parent with congenital heart disease will have an increased incidence of congenital heart disease (Table 82-2). Early infant nourishment may be jeopardized if maternal heart disease is severe enough to interfere with breast-feeding. Even if the mother is capable of breast-feeding, cardiovascular medications may be transmitted to the infant in breast milk. Finally, the infant is at risk of losing a parent, since life expectancy with many forms of heart disease is significantly less than normal.

Maternal Heart Disease May Not Be "Typical"

Many women with heart disease who become pregnant have a form of heart disease that is relatively new, having existed for less than 50 years. They have mechanically "altered" heart disease. Although much has been learned about hearts that have been altered by surgery (or a catheter), there is still much that is unknown. It is best not to consider a previous lesion mechanically "corrected," because there is always some residual disease. In some cases, the residual disease (a shunt, ventricular dysfunction, an arrhythmia redisposition, or persistent obstruc-

TABLE 82-2 Congenital Heart Disease in the Offspring of a Parent with Congenital Heart Disease

Congenital Heart Defect in a Parent	Risk of Congenital Heart Disease in Offspring If One Parent Is Affected,[a,b] Percentage
Intracardiac shunts	
Atrial septal defect	3–11
Ventricular septal defect	4–22
Patent ductus arteriosus	4–11
Obstruction to flow	
Left-sided obstruction[c]	3–26
Right-sided obstruction	3–22
Complex abnormalities	
Tetralogy of Fallot	4–15
Ebstein's anomaly	Uncertain
Transposition of the great arteries	Uncertain
Hypertrophic cardiomyopathy with asymmetric septal hypertrophy	50
Marfan's syndrome	50

[a]The higher number in each range comes from one large series.[159,162] The incidence of congenital heart disease in the offspring tends to be closer to the lower number for most other reported series.[155,156]
[b]The risk in obstructive lesions is decreased by corrective surgery prior to pregnancy.[160]
[c]Includes coarctation, aortic stenosis, discrete subaortic stenosis, supravalvular stenosis.
SOURCE: Modified from McAnulty JH, Metcalfe J, Ueland K: Cardiovascular disease. In: Burrow GN, Ferris TF, eds. *Medical Complication during Pregnancy*. Philadelphia: Saunders; 1988. Reproduced with permission from the publisher and authors.

tion) may adversely affect the mother and, in turn, may harm the fetus.

CARDIOVASCULAR ADJUSTMENTS DURING A NORMAL PREGNANCY

Maternal adaptation to pregnancy includes remarkable cardiovascular changes. These explain in part why some cardiac abnormalities are not well tolerated during pregnancy (see Table 82-1) and may result in symptoms and signs, even in a normal pregnancy, that are difficult to distinguish from those occurring with heart disease.

Hemodynamic Changes at Rest

Resting cardiac output increases by over 40 percent during pregnancy. The increase begins early, with the cardiac output reaching its highest levels by the 20th week.

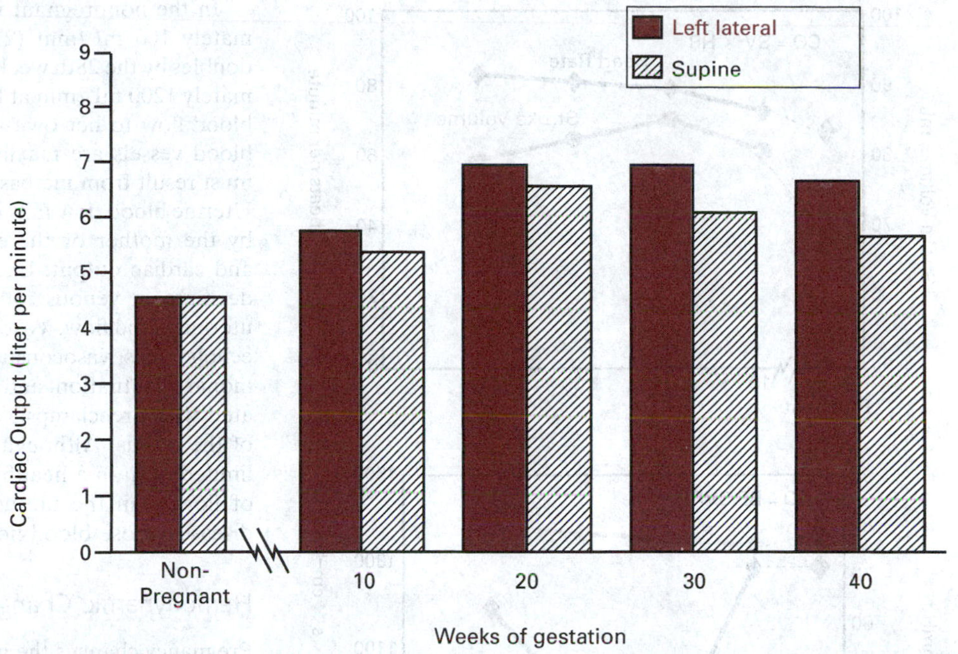

FIGURE 82-1 Cardiac output values during normal pregnancy when measured in the supine and left lateral positions. The values are derived from measurements made in many studies.[5-10] (From Neill and Swanson.[167] Reproduced with permission from the publisher and authors.)

In the last half of pregnancy, cardiac output is significantly affected by body position (Fig. 82-1), as the enlarged uterus diminishes venous return from the lower extremities.[4-9] Compared with measurements made near term, when the woman is in the left lateral position, cardiac output is lower by an average of 0.6 L/min when a woman is supine and by 1.2 L/min when she assumes the upright position.[8] In general, this results in few or no symptoms, but in some women, maintenance of the supine position may result in symptomatic hypotension, possibly in those whose collateral vessels are not well developed.[9-11] Symptoms of this "supine hypotensive syndrome of pregnancy" can be corrected by having the woman turn onto her side.

The hemodynamic changes associated with or causing the variation in cardiac output also change dramatically (Fig. 82-2). Cardiac output is the product of heart rate times stroke volume. Its early rise is due mainly to an increase in stroke volume.[4,7] By the 20th week, stroke volume gradually begins to fall because of obstruction of the vena cava by the enlarged uterus and increased dilation of the venous bed. The heart rate increases gradually throughout pregnancy, reaching a level that is approximately 25 percent above the nonpregnant levels by the time of delivery.

Cardiac output is also directly related to the mean blood pressure and inversely related to the systemic vascular resistance. There is a fall in blood pressure early in pregnancy, with a gradual return to nonpregnant levels by term. The fall in systemic vascular resistance is more marked, decreasing to two-thirds of resting nonpregnant values at about the 20th week of pregnancy and then gradually rising through the remainder of pregnancy, although not achieving nonpregnant levels until a few weeks after delivery.[4,7]

Finally, the cardiac output is equal to the oxygen consumption divided by the systemic arterial venous oxygen difference. The mother's oxygen consumption (which includes that of her fetus) increases by 20 percent within the first 20 weeks of pregnancy and increases steadily to a level that is approximately 30 percent above the nonpregnant levels by the time of delivery.[7] This increase is due both to the metabolic needs of the fetus and the increased metabolic needs of the mother. The increase in cardiac output occurs earlier than the rise in oxygen consumption; thus the arteriovenous oxygen difference narrows early in pregnancy with a gradual increase in oxygen extraction throughout pregnancy, so that by term, the systemic arteriovenous oxygen difference exceeds nonpregnant values.

At the beginning of labor, cardiac output measured in the supine position increases to over 7 L/min (Fig. 82-3). With each uterine contraction, this rises by still another 34 percent as a result of increases in heart rate as well as an increment in stroke volume resulting from extrusion of approximately 500 mL of blood into the central venous system with each contraction. Thus, at these times, the cardiac output can be as great as 9 L/min.[12] Administration of epidural anesthesia reduces this cardiac output to about 8 L/min, and the use of general anesthesia reduces it still further. Following delivery, there is a transient, marked elevation in cardiac output that approaches 10 L/min[12] (7 to 8 L/min with cesarean section),[13] with the cardiac output falling rapidly to near-normal, nonpregnant values within a few weeks after delivery, although there is a slight elevation that can persist for as long as a year.[14]

The increase in maternal cardiac output in women with twins or triplets is slightly greater than that in women with single pregnancies.[15]

The distribution of blood flow is not fully understood; it is affected by changes in local vascular resistance[16] (Fig. 82-4). Renal blood flow increases by approximately 30 percent in the first trimester and stays at about that level or declines slightly

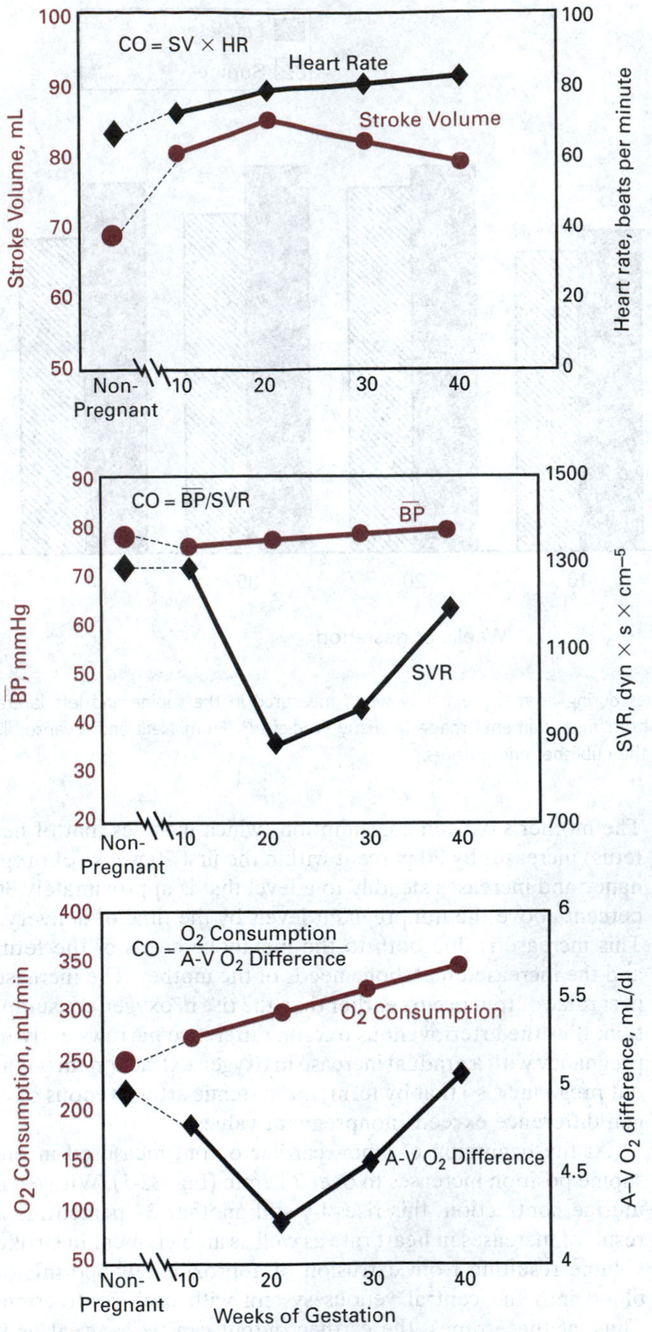

FIGURE 82-2 The cardiac output (CO) can be determined from other parameters in at least 3 ways: CO = heart rate (HR) × stroke volume (SV); CO = mean arterial pressure (BP) minus the RA pressure/systemic vascular resistance (SVR); CO = oxygen (O_2) consumption/arteriovenous (AV) O_2 difference. The expected values for these parameters measured in the supine position during pregnancy are based on information acquired from many studies.[5–8] (From Neill and Swanson.[167] Reproduced with permission from the publisher and authors.)

throughout the pregnancy. Nonpregnant mammary blood flow is usually less than 1 percent of the cardiac output but can be approximately 2 percent of the cardiac output at term. Blood flow to the skin increases by 40 to 50 percent—a mechanism for heat dissipation.

In the nonpregnant woman, uterine blood flow is approximately 100 mL/min (2 percent of the cardiac output). This doubles by the 28th week of pregnancy and increases to approximately 1200 mL/min at term, a value approaching the mother's blood flow to her own kidneys.[17–19] During pregnancy, uterine blood vessels are maximally dilated; flow can increase, but it must result from increased maternal arterial pressure and flow. Uterine blood flow falls if redistribution of total flow is required by the mother or there is a fall in maternal blood pressure and cardiac output. Excitement, heat, anxiety,[20] exercise, and decrease in venous return have all been shown to decrease uterine blood flow. Vasoconstriction caused by endogenous catecholamines, vasoconstrictive drugs, maternal mechanical pulmonary ventilation, and some anesthetics as well as that associated with preeclampsia and eclampsia can decrease perfusion of the uterus. Although uterine blood flow can potentially be limited even in a healthy woman, the concern about diversion of flow from the uterus is greater in the mother with heart disease, whose blood flow may already be compromised.

Hemodynamic Changes with Exercise

Pregnancy changes the hemodynamic response to exercise. For any given level of exercise in the sitting position, the cardiac output is greater than in nonpregnant women, and maximum cardiac output is reached at lower exercise levels. The increase in cardiac output is relatively greater than the increase in oxygen consumption, so the arteriovenous oxygen difference is wider than that produced by the same exercise in the nonpregnant woman. This suggests that oxygen delivery to the periphery is somewhat less efficient during pregnancy.[21] In a nonpregnant woman, training or conditioning results in a greater increase in stroke volume and a smaller increment in heart rate with exercise than would occur in an untrained individual. During pregnancy, this training effect is not seen—possibly because the increase in stroke volume is limited as a result of compression of the inferior vena cava or the increased venous distensibility.[22]

Exercise during pregnancy is not clearly any more dangerous or beneficial to the mother with heart disease than it would be when she was not pregnant. It does affect the fetus. In animal models, maternal exercise has been associated with a fall in uterine blood flow. In humans, it is known that the type of exercise affects maternal hemodynamics and uterine perfusion.[23,24] As an example, maximal exercise by swimming causes less fetal bradycardia (a marker of uterine blood flow) than the same level of cycling.[25] Additionally, regular aerobic endurance exercise during pregnancy has been associated with a reduction in birth weight. Since most of the reduction is due to a decrease in neonatal fat mass, it is not clear if this is detrimental.[26]

Infants born to mothers who work in a standing position may be abnormally small at birth.[27] Although the long-term effects of this are not clear, the implications in relation to exercise and work in the upright position would seem to be greater for women with heart disease.[28,29] This question, relating to exercise and the effect on the fetus, has become more important with an increasing enthusiasm for recreational exercise in the United States. Although there is not enough evidence available to suggest that the healthy pregnant woman should avoid recreational exercise, an argument can be made for advising the woman with heart disease to keep the exercise level below that which causes symptoms.

Mechanisms for Hemodynamic Changes

The mechanisms evoking the hemodynamic adaptation to pregnancy are not fully understood. They may in part be due to volume changes. Total body water increases steadily throughout pregnancy by 6 to 8 L (most is extracellular).[30] Sodium retention results in an excess accumulation of 500 to 900 meq by the time of delivery. As early as 6 weeks after conception, plasma volume increases, approaching its maximum of $1\frac{1}{2}$ times normal by the second trimester, where it stays throughout the pregnancy.[31] The red blood cell mass also increases, but not to the same degree as the increase in plasma volume. As a result, the hematocrit falls, though rarely to less than 30 percent. Peak hemodilution occurs at 24 to 26 weeks; then the hematocrit gradually increases.

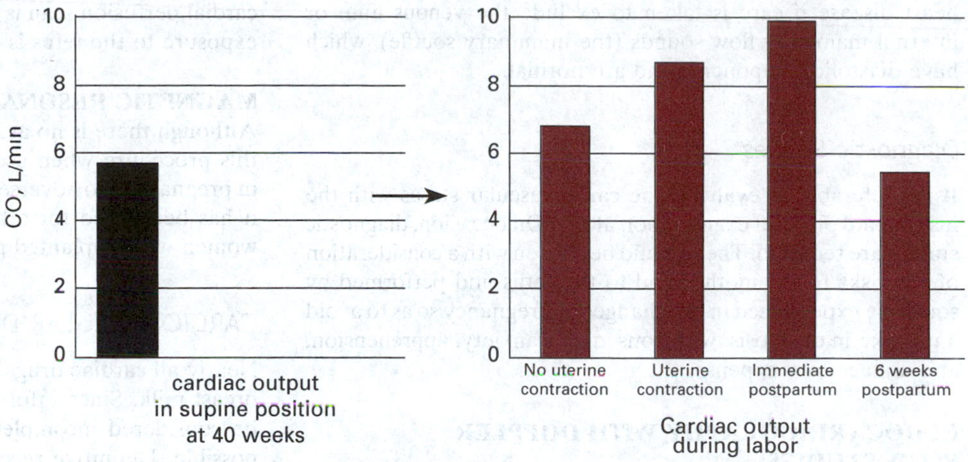

FIGURE 82-3 Cardiac output measured in the supine position is high at 40 weeks (*A*), increased during labor (*B*), particularly with contractions, and even higher in the minutes to hours following a vaginal delivery.[13,15] (From Neill and Swanson.[167] Reproduced with permission from the publisher and authors.)

Vascular alterations also contribute to the hemodynamic changes of pregnancy. Arterial compliance is increased,[32,33] and there is an increase in venous vascular capacitance.[33–35] These changes are advantageous in maintaining the hemodynamics of a normal pregnancy. There may be disadvantages as well. The arterial changes are associated with increased fragility; vascular accidents, when they occur in women, frequently do so during pregnancy.[36–40] The venous changes may explain in part the increase in thromboemboli during pregnancy.[41]

Intrinsic cardiac changes can also explain some of the hemodynamic changes.[42–44] The stroke volume increases by approximately 25 percent. The ejection fraction does not change; thus the heart has to enlarge (since the ejection fraction is the stroke volume divided by the end-diastolic volume). Since the increases in left ventricular end-diastolic and systolic volumes are small and not adequate to explain the constant ejection fraction, the heart must become reconfigured as well. If so, this occurs with only a 10 to 15 percent increase in myocardial mass during pregnancy.[45]

The ultimate cause (or causes) for these recognized changes is uncertain. Complex interactions of the renin-angiotensin-aldosterone system, the reproductive hormones, prostaglandins, and atrial natriuretic factor contribute to the fluid and sodium changes.[46,47] At the present time, the effects of the increased level of circulating steroid hormones seem to explain the vascular and myocardial changes satisfactorily.

DIAGNOSIS OF HEART DISEASE

Clinical Evaluation

The recognition and definition of heart disease are difficult at any time. This is particularly true during pregnancy. Symptoms suggesting heart disease—fatigue, dyspnea, orthopnea, pedal edema, and chest discomfort—occur commonly in pregnant women with normal hearts. Although they should alert a caregiver to the possibility of heart disease, the concern should increase if the dyspnea or orthopnea is progressive and limiting or if a woman develops hemoptysis, syncope with exertion, or chest pain clearly related to effort. Common examination features of a normal pregnancy include pedal edema, basilar pulmonary rales, a third heart sound, a systolic murmur, and visible neck vein pulsations. However, cyanosis or clubbing, a loud systolic murmur ($\geq 3/6$), cardiomegaly, a "fixed split" second heart sound, or evidence for pulmonary hypertension (a left parasternal lift and loud P_2) do not occur as part of a normal pregnancy and deserve attention. A diastolic murmur is unusual enough during pregnancy that its presence is an indication of

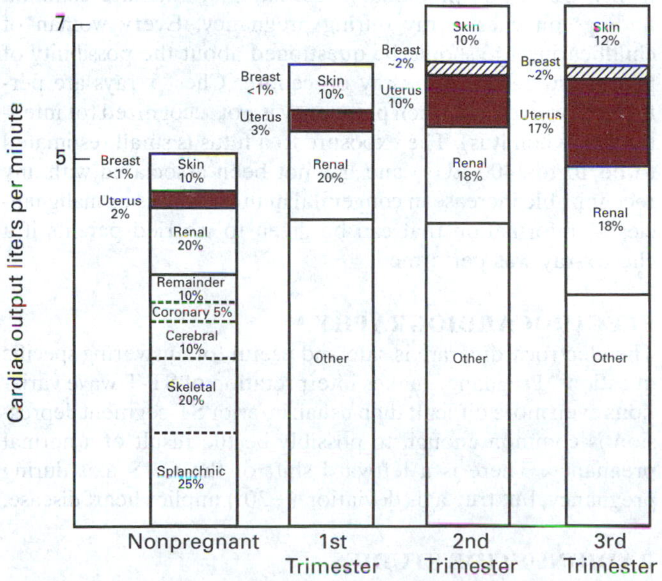

FIGURE 82-4 The changes in cardiac output and its distribution at rest in nonpregnant and pregnant women are depicted. Data used in this graph are fragmentary, especially early in pregnancy. (From Neill and Swanson.[167] Reproduced with permission from the publisher and authors.)

heart disease if care is taken to exclude the venous hum or internal mammary flow sounds (the mammary souffle), which have diastolic components and are normal.

Diagnostic Studies

It is preferable to evaluate the cardiovascular status with the history and physical examination alone. On occasion, diagnostic studies are required. They should be chosen with a consideration of the risks to the mother and to the fetus and performed by someone experienced in the changes of pregnancy so as to avoid a mistake in diagnosis, with consequent anxiety, apprehension, and unnecessary expense.

ECHOCARDIOGRAPHY WITH DOPPLER FLOW STUDIES

Echocardiography with evaluation of flow by Doppler is so safe, with no known risk to the mother or fetus, and is so diagnostically useful that overuse is the only significant concern (Chap. 13). Expense and potential misinterpretation are reasons to consider its use only when required to answer a specific question. The safety of transesophageal echocardiography has not been assessed in pregnancy. The use of anesthetic agents during the procedure would seem to create the greatest risk, and this is minor.

RADIOGRAPHIC PROCEDURES

All x-ray procedures should generally be avoided, particularly early in pregnancy. They increase the risk of abnormal fetal organogenesis or of a subsequent malignancy in the child, particularly leukemia. If a study is required, it should be delayed to as late in pregnancy as possible, the radiation dose should be kept to a minimum, and shielding of the fetus should be optimal. Interpretation should take into consideration the changes expected in a normal pregnancy. As an example, some increase in heart size and pulmonary vascular markings are common findings on chest x-ray during pregnancy. Every woman of childbearing age should be questioned about the possibility of pregnancy before any x-ray procedure. Chest x-rays are performed on occasion when pregnancy is not recognized (or intentionally when it is). The exposure to a fetus is small (estimated to be 10 to 1400 μGy) and has not been associated with any recognizable increase in congenital malformations or malignancies[48]—information that can be given to worried parents if a chest x-ray was performed.

ELECTROCARDIOGRAPHY

The electrocardiogram is safe and useful for answering specific questions. Pregnancy makes interpretation of ST-T wave variations even more difficult than usual; inferior ST-segment depression is common enough to possibly be the result of a normal pregnancy. There is a leftward shift of the QRS axis during pregnancy, but true axis deviation ($-30°$) implies heart disease.

RADIONUCLIDE STUDIES

Although many radionuclides should attach to albumin and thus not reach the fetus, separation can occur and fetal exposure is possible. It is preferable to avoid these studies. On occasion, a pulmonary ventilation/perfusion scan or even a thallium myocardial perfusion scan is required during pregnancy. Estimated exposure to the fetus is low (400 μGy).[41]

MAGNETIC RESONANCE IMAGING

Although there is no available information about the safety of this procedure when used for the evaluation of heart disease in pregnancy, no adverse fetal effects have been reported when it has been used for other purposes. It should be avoided in women with implanted pacemakers or defibrillators.

CARDIOVASCULAR DRUGS AND PREGNANCY

Nearly all cardiac drugs cross the placenta and are secreted in breast milk. Since information about the use of any drug can be considered incomplete, it is best to avoid their use when possible. Definitive recommendations about the use of drugs in pregnancy is difficult, but if required for maternal safety, they should not be withheld.[49,50]

Diuretics

Diuretics can and should be used for treatment of congestive heart failure that is uncontrolled by sodium restriction, and they remain front-line therapy for the treatment of hypertension. No one agent is clearly contraindicated—experience is greatest with the thiazide diuretics and with furosemide.[50,51] Diuretics should not be used for prophylaxis against toxemia or for treatment of pedal edema.

Inotropic Agents

The indications for the use of digitalis are not changed by pregnancy. Digoxin and digitoxin cross the placenta, and fetal serum levels approximate those in the mother. The same dose of digoxin in general will yield lower maternal serum levels during pregnancy than in the nonpregnant state.[52] If the desired clinical effect is not achieved, it may be helpful to measure levels (if the assay used is not affected by an immunoreactive substance of pregnancy).[53] Digitalis may shorten the duration of gestation and labor due to an effect on the myometrium similar to the inotropic effect on the myocardium.

When intravenous inotropic or vasopressor agents are required, the standard agents (dopamine, dobutamine, and norepinephrine) may be used, but the fetus is jeopardized because all result in decreased uterine blood flow and may stimulate uterine contractions. Ephedrine is an appropriate initial vasopressor drug as, at least in animal models, it does not adversely affect uterine blood flow.

There is no available information about the efficacy or safety of the phosphodiesterase inhibitors (amrinone, milrinone).

Adrenergic Receptor Blocking Agents

Observations that beta blockers may decrease umbilical blood flow, initiate premature labor, and result in a small and infarcted placenta with the potential for low-birth-weight infants have led to concerns about their use.[54] Large studies have not confirmed these concerns, however, and beta-blocking drugs have been used in a large number of pregnant women without adverse effects. Their use for the usual clinical indications is reasonable.[54–56] All the available beta-blocking agents cross the placenta, are present in human breast milk, and can reach significant levels in the fetus or the newborn. Recent concerns about low birth weights from maternal use of atenolol early in pregnancy[57,58] make use of alternative $beta_1$-selective agents preferable. If these agents are used during pregnancy, it is appropriate to monitor fetal heart rate as well as the newborn infant's heart rate, blood sugar, and respiratory status immediately after delivery.

Experience with the alpha-blocking agents phenoxybenzamine and phentolamine is sparse. Clonidine, prazosin, and labetalol, with their mixed alpha- and beta-blocking effects, have been used for treatment of hypertension without clear detrimental effects.[59]

Calcium Channel Blocking Drugs

Nifedipine, verapamil, diltiazem, nicardipine, and isradipine have been used to treat hypertension and arrhythmias without an adverse effect on the fetus or newborn infant.[50,60] The drugs cause relaxation of the uterus; nifedipine has been used for this purpose.

Antiarrhythmic Agents

Atrioventricular (AV) node blockade is occasionally required during pregnancy. This can be achieved with digoxin, beta blockers, and calcium blockers. Early reports suggest that adenosine can also be safely used as a node-blocking agent.[61]

As a general rule, it is preferable to avoid the standard antiarrhythmic drugs in any patient. This is true during pregnancy as well. When essential for recurrent arrhythmias or for maternal safety, they should be used; however, there is insufficient accumulated information to know whether or not these drugs increase the risk to the fetus or child.[50,62,63] If intravenous drug therapy is required, lidocaine is reasonable first-line therapy. There has been demonstration of transient neonatal depression when the neonate's blood level exceeds 2.5 μg/L, a reason to recommend keeping maternal blood levels below 4 μg/L (since fetal levels are 60 percent of maternal levels).[50,64] Intravenous procainamide and quinidine may cause hypotension; there is no available information about intravenous amiodarone. Based on its effects on maternal blood pressure, bretylium would seem likely to decrease uterine perfusion.

If oral antiarrhythmic therapy is necessary, it may still be appropriate to begin with quinidine since, given its long-term availability, it has been most frequently used without clear adverse fetal effects.[50,54,65] There is some information about procainamide,[66] disopyramide,[67] mexiletine,[68] flecainide,[69,70] and sotalol,[71] but it is insufficient to recommend their use unless it would be essential for the mother. The early available information concerning amiodarone would suggest an increased likelihood of fetal loss and deformity.[72–74]

Vasodilator Agents

When needed for a hypertensive crisis or emergency afterload and preload reduction, nitroprusside is the vasodilator drug of choice. Despite a paucity of information about its use during pregnancy, this controversial recommendation is made because the drug is highly effective, works instantly, and is easily tolerated; moreover, its effects dissipate immediately when the drug is stopped. The concern about the use of this drug is that its metabolite, cyanide, can be detected in the fetus, but this has not been demonstrated to be a significant problem in humans.[75,76] This metabolite is a reason to limit the duration of use of this drug whenever possible. Intravenous hydralazine, nitroglycerin, or labetalol are options for parenteral therapy.

Chronic afterload reduction to treat hypertension, aortic or mitral regurgitation, or ventricular dysfunction during pregnancy has been achieved with the calcium blocking drugs, hydralazine, and methyldopa.[59,77] Adverse fetal effects have not been reported. The *angiotension-converting enzyme* (ACE) inhibitors are contraindicated in pregnancy.[59,77,78] They increase the risk of abnormalities in fetal renal development. There are no data available on losartin and valsartin, the new angiotensin II blockers.

Antithrombotic Agents

The chronic use of warfarin is associated with a 1 to 5 percent chance per year of significant bleeding. More importantly, in considering its use during pregnancy, one must keep in mind that warfarin crosses the placenta, and fetal exposure during the first 3 months is associated with a 5 to 25 percent incidence of malformations that comprise the "warfarin embryopathy syndrome" (facial abnormalities, optic atrophy, digital abnormalities, epithelial changes, and mental impairment).[75–81] Women receiving the drug during the 7th to 12th week of gestation are particularly prone to having children with this syndrome.[82,83] The syndrome may be dose-related, with one study suggesting that it occurs only with doses greater than 5 mg per day.[84] Warfarin use at any time during pregnancy increases the risk of fetal bleeding or maternal uterine hemorrhage.

In women who require anticoagulation, heparin is preferable to warfarin. Self-administered subcutaneous high-dose heparin (16,000 to 24,000 units per day) has been proven feasible and efficacious.[85–88] This drug does not cross the placenta. Accumulating data suggest that low-molecular-weight heparin, while currently more expensive, is effective, easier to use (once or twice daily without the need to follow serial blood tests), and as safe as standard heparin therapy. Although evaluated for venous thrombosis prophylaxis,[89,90] its value in preventing thromboemboli in patients with mechanical prostheses has not been proven. (See Chap. Chap. 61.)

When anticoagulation is required, some have advocated using heparin for the first trimester and warfarin for the next 5 months, with a return to heparin prior to labor and delivery. Although successful pregnancy has been achieved with this approach, the authors favor avoidance of warfarin during pregnancy.

Antiplatelet agents increase the chance of maternal bleeding and they cross the placenta. The most commonly used, aspirin, has some observed and theoretical disadvantages.[91] It is associated with an increased incidence of abortion and fetal growth retardation, and its inhibition of prostaglandin synthesis may result in closure of the ductus arteriosis during fetal life.[92] Still, it has been frequently used and even recommended by some for specific indications and as prophylaxis against preeclampsia.[93]

These trade-offs are difficult to evaluate; thus aspirin should be avoided unless necessary. There are no data available on the effects of clopidogrel or ticlopidine during pregnancy.

Obstetric Drugs and Anesthetic Agents Used During Pregnancy

Drugs used specifically for pregnancy can cause hemodynamic alterations. Although there is some question as to their value,[94] beta-sympathetic amines are used to stop premature labor. All cause maternal tachycardia. Ritodrine and terbutaline have been associated with pulmonary edema, usually when glucocorticoids are being administered concurrently to promote fetal lung maturation. This pulmonary edema responds abruptly to cessation of the drugs and initiation of diuretic therapy. On other occasions, prostaglandins E_2 and F_2 are used to induce labor and have no significant hemodynamic effects.

Synthetic oxytocin (pitocin) is given to minimize blood loss after delivery. The synthetic preparation prevents vasoconstriction, but it has been associated, in turn, with transient hypotension.

Anesthesia for surgery during pregnancy and at the time of labor and delivery can adversely affect a woman with heart disease. In most cases, lumbar epidural anesthesia with a pudendal nerve block to minimize pain is effective and least likely to result in hemodynamic compromise.[95]

MANAGEMENT OF CARDIOVASCULAR SYNDROMES

Cardiovascular complications can occur with any form of heart disease. Management of each patient has to be individualized, but some recommendations are applicable in most cases.

Low-Cardiac-Output Syndrome

A low cardiac output is an ominous sign in any patient, and this is particularly true in pregnancy. It results in signs of poor perfusion (mental obtundation, peripheral vascular constriction, low urine output, and often a low blood pressure). Although potentially treatable causes such as tamponade or severe valvular stenosis should be considered, it is most often due to intravascular volume depletion. This should be prevented when possible and corrected when recognized. Although it is a concern in any pregnant woman, volume depletion is particularly dangerous in those with lesions that limit blood flow, such as pulmonary hypertension, aortic or pulmonic valve stenosis, hypertrophic cardiomyopathy, or mitral stenosis. Measures to prevent or treat a fall in central blood volume are outlined in Table 82-3.

TABLE 82-3 Measures to Protect Against a Fall in Central Blood Volume

- Position
  - 45–60° left lateral
  - 10° Trendelenburg
- Full-leg stockings
- Volume preloading for surgery and delivery 1500 mL of glucose-free normal saline
- Drugs
  - Avoid vasodilator drugs
  - Ephedrine for hypotension unresponsive to fluid replacement
  - Anesthetics (if required)
    - Regional: serial small boluses
    - General: emphasis on benzodiazepines and narcotics, low-dose inhalation agents

Congestive Heart Failure

Management of congestive heart failure during pregnancy should not differ greatly from that at other times. Attention to reduction in salt intake and limitation of activity to a level below that which causes symptoms are appropriate. In a woman with significant symptoms or pulmonary edema, standard therapy can be used with the concerns about the drugs as outlined earlier (remembering particularly that ACE inhibitors should be avoided). Congestive heart failure is one situation where maintaining a woman in the supine position may be beneficial by causing preload reduction with obstruction of return of blood from the inferior vena cava to the heart.

Thromboembolic Complications

The risk of venous thromboemboli increases fivefold during and immediately after pregnancy,[41,96,97] and there is arguably an increase in arterial emboli as well.[98,99] Both may be the result of a woman's hypercoagulable status during pregnancy, and the likelihood of venous thrombosis is increased by venous stasis. Prevention is optimal, and prophylactic full-dose heparin or low-molecular-weight heparin[100] is indicated in those at high risk of a thromboembolic complication, including women with thromboemboli during a previous pregnancy (a risk of 4 to 15 percent), antithrombin III deficiency (a risk of 70 percent), protein C deficiency (a risk of 33 percent), protein S deficiency (17 percent), and the anticardiolipin antibody syndrome.[41] Prothrombin gene mutations and factor V mutation resulting in the resistance to activated protein C (found in 3 to 5 percent of the population) may eventually be shown to be a reason for prophylaxis as well.[101,102]

If a thrombus or embolus is identified, 5 to 10 days of intravenous heparin therapy followed by full-dose subcutaneous heparin is recommended.[41] If a thromboembolus is life-threatening (e.g., a massive pulmonary embolus or a thrombosed prosthetic valve), thrombolytic therapy can be used.[103]

Hypertension

Hypertension can be present before pregnancy (in 1 to 5 percent) and persist throughout pregnancy, or it can develop with pregnancy.[59,104] When normotensive women become pregnant, 5 to 7 percent will develop hypertension. Because of the marked early fall in systemic vascular resistance, this often does not occur until the second half of pregnancy. It has been called *pregnancy-induced* or *gestational hypertension* or *toxemia.* When associated with proteinuria, pedal edema, central nervous system (CNS) irritability, elevation of liver enzymes, and coagulation disturbances, the hypertension syndrome is called *preeclampsia.* If convulsions occur, the diagnosis is *eclampsia.* It is not clear that hypertension alone puts the mother or fetus at risk during pregnancy, but preeclampsia increases maternal risk (approximately 1 to 2 percent chance of CNS bleed, convulsions, or other severe systemic illness) and may cause fetal growth retardation (10 to 15 percent). Maternal and fetal morbidity and mortality increase still further with eclampsia.

Guidelines for the level of blood pressure control are not well established. Until more is known, an argument can be made for keeping the systolic pressure below 160 mmHg and the diastolic pressure below 100 mmHg. This may provide a margin of safety against severe hypertensive episodes and possibly will improve fetal survival. Nonpharmacologic therapy is preferable when possible, although it is not clearly defined. While strict bed rest may achieve blood pressure lowering, it is not generally recommended, although limitation of activity and reduction of stress is commonly advised.[77,104] Unless the patient has previously demonstrated salt-sensitive hypertension, sodium restriction is generally inadvisable, since pregnant women with hypertension have lower plasma volumes than normotensive women. If drug treatment is required, experience is greatest with methyldopa.[59,105,106] This otherwise infrequently used antihypertensive agent has been demonstrated to promote fetal survival and to result in children with normal mental and physical development. It may be that other drugs will achieve the same goal, but they have not been studied adequately. Initial therapy could also include a β_1 selective beta blocker or a diuretic. Calcium channel blockers have been proven to be effective.[60] As mentioned earlier, ACE inhibitors should not be used, and the safety of angiotension II blocking agents is undefined.

Pulmonary Hypertension

Whether pulmonary hypertension (Chap. 52) is primary or secondary to prolonged left-to-right shunting (Eisenmenger's syndrome), drug abuse, a primary vascular disease syndrome, or recurrent pulmonary emboli, maternal mortality ranges from 30 to 70 percent.[107,108] Even with maternal survival, fetal loss exceeds 40 percent. Maternal death can occur at any time during pregnancy, but the mother is most vulnerable during the time of labor and delivery and in the first postpartum week. If recognized early in pregnancy, interruption is advised. If this is declined, or if the pulmonary hypertension is recognized late in pregnancy, close follow-up is required. Intravascular volume depletion puts these patients at greatest risk. For this group in particular, the measures outlined in Table 82-3 are important. Systemic vascular resistance and pressure must be maintained in patients with pulmonary hypertension who have a right-to-left shunt (to minimize still further shunting), and meticulous attention to avoidance of air or thrombus emboli from intravenous catheters is essential to avoid systemic emboli in these patients. At the time of labor and delivery, a central venous line allows adequate fluid administration, and a radial artery catheter makes determinations of blood pressure and oxygen saturation easier. These lines should be used for 48 to 72 h postdelivery.

Arrhythmias

In the woman with dizziness, palpitations, and light-headedness, pregnancy offers many other explanations, but arrhythmias should be considered as a possible cause (Chap. 24). The rules for treatment should be the same as in the nonpregnant patient with the possible exception that a rhythm causing hemodynamic instability should be treated somewhat more rapidly and aggressively because of the concern about diversion of blood flow away from the uterus. As always, if a potentially reversible cause can be identified, it should be corrected. If treatment is required, it should never be instituted without electrocardiographic documentation of the rhythm.

Tachyarrhythmias are as frequent during pregnancy as at other times. As always, the presence of *atrial* or *ventricular premature beats* or of *sinus tachycardia* is a reason to look for and to correct the cause but not a reason to institute specific treatment for arrhythmias.

Paroxysmal supraventricular tachycardia may occur somewhat more frequently during pregnancy than in the nonpregnant state, whether because of the mechanism of AV node reentry ("dual AV node mechanism") or owing to atrial ventricular reentry ("accessory pathway mechanism").[109–111] This is the most common sustained abnormal rhythm occurring with pregnancy. Initial treatment with vagal maneuvers is as appropriate as at other times. If medical treatment is required, intravenous adenosine or verapamil is effective. Cardioversion can be used if required, remembering that the rule "never cardiovert an awake patient" is just as applicable during pregnancy as at any other time.[112] If recurrent episodes require a chronic day-to-day drug, verapamil or a beta blocker would seem to be an optimal choice; digoxin may be effective, although it should be avoided if the patient has preexcitation. Management of *atrial fibrillation* and *flutter* should be as in the nonpregnant woman. If these rhythms occur in a woman with mitral stenosis, severe left ventricular dysfunction, or a previous thromboembolic event, antithrombotic therapy with heparin is indicated.

Ventricular tachycardia may occur during pregnancy.[113,114] If it is suggestive of a right ventricular outflow tract tachycardia (a left bundle branch block with vertical axis morphology), beta-blocker therapy may be effective. If a fascicular ventricular tachycardia (often with a right bundle branch block and left axis deviation), verapamil or diltiazem may be effective treatment. Emergency management of rapid ventricular tachycardia or ventricular fibrillation should be as recommended for the nonpregnant woman.[115,116] If possible, the pelvis should be rolled to the left to enhance blood return from the lower extremities. If pregnancy has proceeded beyond 24 weeks and maternal survival is in question, emergency cesarean section could be considered.

A prolonged QT-interval syndrome can be diagnosed first during pregnancy.[117,118] If this is recognized and it is an acquired form (of course, almost always from drugs), the offending cause should be eliminated. If the syndrome is congenital, beta-blocker therapy during pregnancy is warranted. Implantable defibrillators have been used with recurrent ventricular arrhythmias, but their value remains unproven in this syndrome, even when it is unrelated to pregnancy. In patients with a congenital syndrome, transmission with autosomal dominance can affect the child.

Bradyarrhythmias may also occur during pregnancy. Although they are a reason to look for a reversible cause, treatment is generally not required unless the patient has clear hemodynamic compromise. Complete heart block, which in this age group is most likely to be congenital in origin, is consistent with a successful pregnancy.[119] If required, a permanent pacemaker can be inserted.

Loss-of-Consciousness Spells

Pregnancy makes an assessment of a loss-of-consciousness spell even more difficult than usual. If a seizure disorder cannot be excluded as a cause, appropriate evaluation with electroencephalography is indicated. If a seizure is unlikely or excluded, the syndrome of syncope should include a consideration of the usual causes.

Endocarditis

Infective endocarditis can occur during pregnancy in women without a recognized heart abnormality, but structural abnormalities place individuals at much greater risk (Chap. 73). The clinical presentation of endocarditis is the same during pregnancy as at other times.[120,121] *Streptococcus* is the most common cause. Intravenous drug abusers are more likely to have staphylococcal infections, and women with genitourinary tract infections are more likely to have gram-negative infections, most commonly due to *Escherichia coli*. Optimal management includes prevention. Although it is not the recommendation of the American Heart Association committee addressing this issue,[122] most physicians caring for women with heart disease recommend antibiotic prophylaxis at the time of dental or surgical procedures or at labor and delivery. If endocarditis does occur, it should be treated aggressively with medical therapy, and the usual indications for surgery are appropriate during pregnancy. If open-heart surgery is required late in pregnancy, simultaneous cesarean section should be considered.

Surgery

Although not exactly a complication of pregnancy, pregnant women with recent disease have the same 0.5 to 2.0 percent chance of requiring surgery as in those who are not pregnant. A number of rules are appropriate to consider. Venous return must be maintained, and, when possible, surgery should be performed in the left lateral position. Unless there is severe congestive heart failure, volume loading with 1500 mL of normal saline prior to surgery or labor and delivery is important. This fluid should not include glucose at the time of labor and delivery, because it can cause subsequent hypoglycemia in the newborn. In the woman who requires assisted ventilation, hyperventilation should be avoided, as it decreases venous return. Pain relief should be assured to minimize the rise in catecholamine levels that would, in turn, decrease uterine blood flow. Fetal monitoring should be performed. If it is essential to perform heart surgery during pregnancy, the risks are greater than in the nonpregnant woman and fetal risk is high.[123]

SPECIFIC FORMS OF HEART DISEASE

Other sections of this book discuss each of the following cardiovascular abnormalities in detail. The remainder of this chapter relates the specific abnormalities to pregnancy and considers the potential problems during pregnancy, the demonstrated risk to the mother and fetus, and the management of both mother and fetus during pregnancy. As discussed earlier, with each abnormality, antibiotic prophylaxis against endocarditis with dental or surgical procedures is as appropriate during pregnancy as at other times[122] and is recommended at labor and delivery.

Rheumatic Heart Disease

Worldwide, rheumatic fever remains a common and virulent disease (see Chap. 55). The resultant valve and myocardial disease is probably the most common cause of heart disease during pregnancy.[123] In the United States, clinically recognized rheumatic fever is uncommon and, when it does occur, appears to be associated with less severe heart disease.[124] Still, even in this country, there are regions where its incidence is increasing.[125] In a woman presenting with myocarditis, rheumatic fever as a cause should be considered, particularly if it is associated with fever, joint discomfort, subcutaneous nodules, erythema marginatum, or chorea and if there is evidence of a group A streptococcal infection.[126] Rheumatic fever is the cause of almost all mitral stenosis; of some isolated mitral, aortic, or tricuspid regurgitation; and of some double- and triple-valve disease. Definition of valve morphology by echocardiography can help to clarify the etiology. Recognition of rheumatic fever as the cause of heart disease is important because it identifies those who need antibiotic prophylaxis to prevent recurrence of the disease; people at highest risk of developing rheumatic fever are those who have had it in the past. Twice-daily penicillin is the treatment regimen of choice, and this should be continued throughout pregnancy.[127]

Valve Disease

MITRAL STENOSIS

When present, mitral stenosis is caused almost exclusively by rheumatic fever, and the lesion is more common in women than in men (Chap. 57). The increased cardiac output, tachycardia, and fluid retention of pregnancy may double the resting pressure gradient across a stenotic mitral valve.[128] Symptoms attributable to an increase in left atrial pressure, with associated pulmonary vascular congestion and bronchial vein distention, occur in up to 25 percent of patients with mitral stenosis during pregnancy.[129,130] They usually become apparent by the 20th week and may be aggravated still further at the time of labor and delivery, with the associated increases in heart rate and cardiac output. Maternal death is rare when there is careful attention to the management of congestive heart failure. Although potentially at risk from the elevated left atrial pressure, the patient with mitral stenosis also depends on this pressure to fill the left ventricle and maintain cardiac output. Because the pregnant woman is especially liable to sudden shifts in the distribution of blood volume, preservation of an adequate intravascular volume is essential to prevent a dramatic fall in cardiac output.

If a woman contemplating pregnancy has symptomatic mitral valve stenosis, balloon dilation or valve surgery is appropriate before conception. If mitral stenosis is first recognized during pregnancy and symptoms develop, standard medical therapy is appropriate. If this does not control symptoms, balloon valvuloplasty can be performed (with appropriate radiation shielding of the fetus).[131,132] Mitral valve surgical commissurotomy or valve replacement has been performed, but fetal loss exceeds 30 percent.[123,133,134] Atrial fibrillation is of particular concern during pregnancy. The usual rapid ventricular response further compromises diastolic flow time and can result in pulmonary edema. Emergency treatment should include intravenous verapamil or cardioversion.

MITRAL REGURGITATION

Mitral regurgitation may be due to rheumatic fever, but unlike mitral stenosis, the majority of cases are due to other causes. Whatever the cause, in general it is well tolerated during pregnancy. If symptoms do occur, fatigue or dyspnea is most common. Treatment for congestive heart failure should be as described earlier. Afterload reduction is an important component of this therapy, remembering that ACE inhibitors should not be used. One cause of mitral regurgitation is *mitral valve prolapse* (Chap. 58). This deserves discussion not because it carries any particular risk during pregnancy but because it is so common, occurring in 5 to 10 percent of young adults. The volume and pressure changes of pregnancy may alter examination findings in a woman with mitral valve prolapse. Associated arrhythmias, endocarditis, cerebral emboli, and hemodynamically significant regurgitation may be rare complications and are no more likely to occur during pregnancy than at other times.[135–138] The physical examination is sufficient for diagnosis—diagnostic studies, including an echocardiogram, do little to benefit the patient. Antibiotic prophylaxis at the time of labor and delivery is recommended in those with a heart murmur.

AORTIC STENOSIS

More common in males, aortic valve stenosis is an unusual finding in pregnancy, but it does occur. The diagnostic criteria are the same during pregnancy as at other times. Concerns from an early review indicating high maternal and fetal mortality rates[139] should be tempered by more recent information (although still involving only small numbers) demonstrating that pregnancy can be carried through with little or no maternal mortality and with no clear increase in fetal loss.[140–143] The offspring can have as high as a 20 percent incidence of congenital heart disease, a value that interestingly can potentially be halved by correcting the outflow tract obstruction prior to pregnancy.[144]

If severe stenosis is recognized before pregnancy, balloon valvotomy or a surgical commissurotomy is recommended prior to conception (Chap. 56). If pregnancy does occur in the presence of severe aortic stenosis, measures to avoid hypovolemia are particularly important (see Table 82-3). If congestive heart failure develops, it can be treated as previously described, with emphasis, again, on the need to avoid excessive diuresis. If severe symptoms persist, a balloon valvuloplasty or aortic valve surgery can be performed during pregnancy,[123,145,146] the latter being associated with increased fetal loss.

AORTIC REGURGITATION

Unlike aortic stenosis, which is almost always congenital in etiology, aortic regurgitation has other causes and is encountered more frequently during pregnancy. These causes include rheumatic fever, endocarditis, dilation of the aortic root, or, more ominously, aortic dissection. A dilated root or dissection should raise the consideration of Marfan's syndrome as a cause. Aortic regurgitation is generally well tolerated during pregnancy. Congestive heart failure may occur but responds to treatment, with an emphasis on afterload reduction—again with a warning to avoid ACE inhibitors. If endocarditis should occur and the infection is not rapidly controlled, mortality with medical therapy is high and surgical therapy is indicated. If this occurs late in pregnancy, consideration of associated cesarean section is appropriate.

PULMONIC VALVE DISEASE

Many women with pulmonic valve disease will have had previous valve comissurotomy or balloon valvuloplasty for valve stenosis or as part of the correction of tetralogy of Fallot. The residual stenosis and invariable regurgitation are potential concerns but in general do not adversely affect the outcome of pregnancy. The occasional patient with significant pulmonic valve stenosis who has not been treated appears to tolerate pregnancy well. Intravascular volume depletion should be avoided. If severe symptoms (recurrent syncope, uncontrolled dyspnea, and chest pain) occur, balloon valvuloplasty can be performed.

TRICUSPID VALVE DISEASE

Significant tricuspid valve disease is also uncommon during pregnancy (Chap. 54). The incidence of regurgitation has increased because of intravenous drug use, with its resultant right-sided endocarditis. This regurgitation requires no specific therapy during pregnancy. Tricuspid stenosis is rare. If it is encountered, avoidance of intravascular volume depletion would seem to be important.

PROSTHETIC VALVE DISEASE

An artificial valve can perhaps be considered the ultimate form of valve disease. Although many have benefited from these valves, all are left with "prosthetic heart valve disease." One or more of its major associated complications—thromboemboli, bleeding (from anticoagulation), endocarditis, valve dysfunction, reoperation, or death—affects patients at a rate of greater than 5 percent per year throughout their lives.[147,148] Pregnancy increases the risk of each of these complications, and the prosthetic valve and its treatment can adversely affect the fetus.[88,149–153] All these are reasons that a prosthetic valve is a relative contraindication to pregnancy. Still, women with prosthetic valves often become pregnant. Anticoagulation is required in those with a *mechanical* prosthesis. Although some clinicians have suggested that warfarin is acceptable anticoagulation,[151] most would advise avoidance, particularly in the first and third trimesters.[153] Full-dose subcutaneous heparin is the therapy of choice, maintaining anticoagulation at the "high therapeutic level" by following levels of factor Xa; partial thromboplastin levels are unreliable during pregnancy. Low-molecular-weight heparin once a day may be a reasonable alternative but has not been evaluated in patients with prosthetic valves and thus cannot be recommended. A *heterograft* or *homograft* prosthesis is an alternative to a mechanical prosthesis. Because of the inherently lower thromboembolic rates associated with these tissue prostheses, anticoagulation is not needed. This opportunity to avoid anticoagulation therapy is a logical argument for using these prostheses in young women who are contemplating pregnancy. However, these valves do not completely eliminate the concern about thromboemboli, and the rate of heterograft degeneration is high in young women, resulting in the need for early valve replacement[154] (see Chap. 61).

Congenital Heart Disease

Congenital heart disease is now the most common heart disease encountered in women of childbearing age in the United States. In most, it has been altered by surgery (Chap. 64). Each abnormality is unique, but there are some issues that should be considered with all of them. First, some abnormalities significantly increase the risk of maternal morbidity and mortality during pregnancy (see Table 82-1). Second, there is an increased risk of fetal death, which increases with the severity of the maternal lesions. Third, the presence of a congenital cardiac abnormality in either parent or in a sibling increases the risk of cardiac and other congenital abnormalities in the fetus. Congenital heart disease is recognized in 0.8 percent of all live births in the United States.[155,156] Its presence in a parent increases this risk to 2 to 15 percent (see Table 82-2).[156–163] Although some have shown that the risk is two to three times greater if it is the mother rather than the father who has congenital heart disease,[161,163] this finding has not been universal.[162] Actually, the risk that a child will have heart disease can reach 50 percent when the abnormality is transmitted as an autosomal dominant trait, as in the case of Marfan's syndrome, the congenital long-QT syndrome, or hypertrophic cardiomyopathy. When recognized, maternal congenital heart disease should be corrected prior to surgery. In some cases, this will make the pregnancy safer for the mother and may provide a better intrauterine environment for fetal development. Fourth, the implications of residual or inoperable lesions must be clearly understood before pregnancy is undertaken. Finally, as with valve disease, antibiotic prophylaxis against endocarditis is as appropriate during pregnancy as at other times in patients with lesions that render them susceptible to this complication.

LEFT-TO-RIGHT SHUNTS

Some women with left-to-right shunts reach adulthood and become pregnant often without previous recognition of their disease. Although left-to-right shunting increases the chances of pulmonary hypertension, right ventricular failure, arrhythmias, and emboli, it is not clear that these complications are made more likely by a pregnancy. The degree of shunting is affected by the relative resistances of the systemic and pulmonary vascular circuits, both of which fall to a similar degree during pregnancy.[164] In general, there is no significant alteration in the degree of shunting with pregnancy. The right ventricular volume overload associated with the shunts is generally well tolerated during pregnancy.

In the United States, most patients with left-to-right shunts will have undergone surgical correction prior to pregnancy. If anything, this surgery makes pregnancy safer, and there is no clear increase in mortality in these patients with pregnancy as compared with women who have normal hearts.[165] The surgery does not influence the incidence of congenital heart disease in the offspring.

Atrial Septal Defect The symptoms and signs of an atrial septal defect can be subtle and the abnormality may not be recognized before pregnancy. In women with an ostium secundum defect, pregnancy is generally well tolerated by the mother and the fetus. When either parent has an atrial septal defect, 5 to 10 percent of their children will have congenital heart disease. This is not affected by corrective surgery in the mother.[161,162] Ostium primum defects are equally well tolerated during pregnancy unless they are associated with other significant congenital cardiovascular abnormalities.

Ventricular Septal Defect Over half of ventricular septal defects close in childhood, and since the murmur is usually detected in those in whom the lesion persists, an unrecognized defect at the time of pregnancy is uncommon. If such a defect is present, however, pregnancy is generally well tolerated. The occasional congestive heart failure or arrhythmias developing during pregnancy can be managed as described previously. If there is no associated pulmonary hypertension, there is no increase in maternal mortality with pregnancy. Fetal loss in women with uncorrected lesions may approach 20 percent. The child of such a mother has a 5 to 8 percent chance of being born with a cardiac defect; again, this incidence is not altered by previous surgical correction of the defect.[164]

Patent Ductus Arteriosus Like the other left-to-right shunts, a patent ductus is tolerated well during pregnancy. On occasion, congestive heart failure can occur, but standard treatment is effective. Antibiotic prophylaxis against endocarditis is recommended. Fetal loss is not clearly greater than that occurring in women without heart disease.

RIGHT-TO-LEFT SHUNT ("CYANOTIC" HEART DISEASE)

Right-to-left shunting can occur through an atrial or ventricular septal defect or a patent ductus arteriosus when pulmonary vascular resistance exceeds systemic vascular resistance or when there is an obstruction to right ventricular outflow and pulmonary vascular resistance is normal. All are forms of "cyanotic" heart disease. The presence of cyanosis, especially when sufficient to result in elevated hemoglobin levels, is associated with high fetal loss, prematurity, and reduced infant birth weights (see Fig. 82-5).[144,166,167] The situation of elevated pulmonary vascular resistance, or Eisenmenger's syndrome, has been discussed earlier under "Pulmonary Hypertension," but it is worth repeating that with this problem it is advisable to avoid or interrupt pregnancy. When the cyanosis is not due to Eisenmenger's syndrome, maternal mortality is less, but women are at increased risk of heart failure (approximately 15 percent) from thromboemboli, arrhythmias, and endocarditis (4.5 percent).[166]

Tetralogy of Fallot This is the most common form of right-to-left shunting resulting from obstruction to pulmonary flow when pulmonary vascular resistance is normal. If it is uncorrected, successful pregnancy can be achieved, but maternal mortality is high and fetal loss can exceed 50 percent. After surgical correction of the defect, maternal mortality does not clearly exceed that of a woman without heart disease;[165,168] the offspring have a 5 to 10 percent chance of having congenital heart disease.

OBSTRUCTIVE LESIONS

Two recommendations apply in women with obstructive cardiac lesions. First, volume depletion should be avoided, since it can result in a significant fall in cardiac output whether the obstruction is on the left or right side of the heart. Second, surgical or catheter treatment for the obstructive lesion is recommended prior to pregnancy, not only to increase maternal safety but

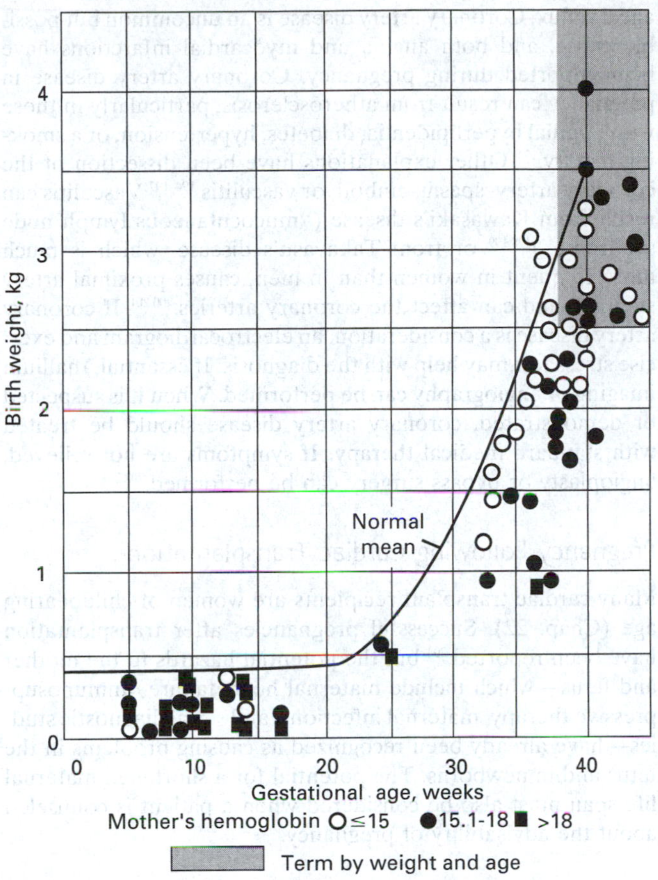

FIGURE 82-5 This figure shows that the severity of maternal cyanosis as manifest by the hemoglobin level relates directly to fetal loss (gestational age <20), prematurity, and infant birth weight. (From Neill and Swanson.[167] Reproduced with permission from the publisher and authors.)

also to decrease the chance of congenital heart disease in the offspring.[160]

Obstruction to flow from the *right ventricle* is preferably corrected prior to pregnancy. This approach will decrease maternal morbidity and may decrease the incidence of congenital heart disease in the offspring.[160] If an obstructive lesion persists into pregnancy, prevention of intravascular volume depletion is important.

Obstructive lesions to the left side of the heart include aortic valve stenosis, described previously. There is very little experience with isolated supravalvular aortic stenosis, bands or with subvalvular bands, but the approach recommended for aortic valve stenosis would seem applicable. Two other left ventricular obstructive disease processes warrant some discussion: coarctation of the aorta and hypertrophic obstructive cardiomyopathy.

Coarctation of the Aorta This condition is more common in men but may occur in women and, as in men, may be associated with a bicuspic aortic valve (Chap. 64). Affected individuals may reach childbearing age and may conceive. Maternal mortality rates range from 3 to 8 percent.[169] Surgical correction prior to pregnancy reduces the risk of aortic dissection or rupture—and thus death—to less than 1 percent.[170,171] If pregnancy occurs in a woman with a coarctation, blood pressure control, as described previously, is appropriate. Antibiotic prophylaxis is needed because of the associated bicuspic aortic valve. The effects of catheter dilation of a coarctation on subsequent pregnancies are uncertain, but it would seem that they are as likely to decrease the risks associated with pregnancy as the surgical procedure. It is not clear whether mechanical treatment decreases the rate of rupture of associated intracranial aneurisms.

Hypertrophic Obstructive Cardiomyopathy *Hypertrophic obstructive cardiomyopathy* (HOCM) (also called idiopathic hypertrophic subaortic stenosis, or IHSS) is inherited as an autosomal dominant trait with variable penetrance; thus offspring have a 50 percent chance of having the same abnormality (see Chaps. 4 and 67). The fall in peripheral vascular resistance and peripheral pooling of blood can cause hypotension, and the intermittent high catecholamine state of pregnancy can increase left ventricular outflow tract obstruction. An increase in the symptoms of dyspnea, chest discomfort, and palpitations has been noted during pregnancy.[172,173] It is not clear that pregnancy increases the approximately 1 to 3 percent chance per year of sudden death, although a death has been reported with this syndrome during pregnancy.[174] This is another obstructive lesion where it is important to avoid hypovolemia. Beta-blocker therapy has been recommended at the time of labor and delivery; the concept makes sense, although it is of unproven value.

COMPLEX CONGENITAL LESIONS

Predicting the outcome of pregnancy becomes more difficult as maternal abnormalities become more complex. In general, maternal and fetal morbidity and mortality are high, particularly when the abnormality results in maternal cyanosis. Still, surgery has made pregnancy a consideration, even in women with the most severe disease, such as a functional single-ventricle or tricuspid atresia.[175]

Transposition of the Great Vessels Women with d-transposition of the great arteries (some with single ventricles) may become pregnant. The little available information available indicates a very poor maternal and fetal outcome.[176] Partial or complete surgical correction of the lesion prior to pregnancy improves the outcome for the mother as well as the fetus.[176,178] If l-transposition ("corrected" transposition) is not complicated by cyanosis, ventricular dysfunction, or heart block, pregnancy should be well tolerated.[179]

Ebstein's Anomaly of the Tricuspid Valve This condition may be mild and unrecognized during pregnancy. Increasing problems of right ventricular dysfunction, obstruction to right-sided heart flow, and right-to-left shunting resulting in cyanosis increase the risk to the woman during pregnancy. Maternal morbidity and mortality are low if the patient does not have severe disease, and fetal loss is approximately 25 percent: significant right-to-left shunting is a reason to avoid pregnancy.[180,181]

Marfan's Syndrome It may be difficult to make the diagnosis of Marfan's syndrome, but it is important to do so because pregnancy is particularly dangerous for affected women. First, the risk of death from aortic rupture or dissection is high during pregnancy, particularly if the aortic root is enlarged (greater than 40 mm by echocardiography).[40,182,183] Second, the expected life span of the woman with Marfan's syndrome is reduced to about half of normal, implying that her years of motherhood will be limited. Third, half of the offspring will be affected with the syndrome. These are reasons that women with Marfan's syndrome should be advised to avoid pregnancy. The risks are sufficient to recommend interruption if pregnancy has occurred. Should the parents elect to continue the pregnancy, activity should be restricted and hypertension prevented. Beta blockade has not yet been clearly proved to be of value when used on a prophylactic basis, but its use in pregnant patients with Marfan's syndrome seems reasonable. This is the one cardiovascular syndrome where cesarean delivery is recommended in order to avoid the hemodynamic stresses of labor.

Myocardial Disease

HYPERTROPHIC CARDIOMYOPATHY

The hypertrophic cardiomyopathies are characterized as "concentric" or "asymmetric (Chap. 67)." The asymmetric form [hypertrophic obstructive cardiomyopathy" (or HOCM)] has been discussed as an obstructive lesion. A concentric hypertrophic cardiomyopathy may be the result of aortic stenosis or hypertension. When *not* due to either of these, the cause, prognosis, and management are often unclear, even unrelated to pregnancy. If congestive heart failure or abnormal rhythms occur, standard therapy is appropriate. Again, hypovolemia should be avoided.

DILATED CARDIOMYOPATHY

The cause of a dilated cardiomyopathy is often unclear, but up to 30 to 50 percent of these cases are familial.[184,185] Its occurence is a reason to suggest that pregnancy should be avoided. This strong recommendation is not supported by data from prospective trials but is given because myocardial dysfunction is the feature associated with increased maternal and fetal mortality in many forms of heart disease. It also comes from the observations of those who develop this problem as a result of pregnancy. This *peripartum cardiomyopathy* may simply be a dilated cardiomyopathy occurring in pregnancy, but the fact that it seems to occur almost exclusively in the third trimester or in the first 6 postpartum weeks suggests that it may be a unique entity.[186–189] Case reports have suggested that myocarditis may be a part of this disease and that, when it is proven by endomyocardial biopsy, treatment with anti-inflammatory drugs may affect outcome favorably.[190] It is not clear, however, that myocarditis is more common in this form of cardiomyopathy,[191] and a large prospective trial in other myocarditis situations has failed to support the value of treatment.[192] Small studies have suggested a possible role for treatment with immune globulin.[193] In the woman with a dilated cardiomyopathy during pregnancy, standard treatment for heart failure, thromboemboli, and arrhythmias is appropriate.

If ventricular function does not return to normal after pregnancy, subsequent pregnancies have been associated with maternal mortality rates approaching 50 percent (Chap. 66). When ventricular function returns to normal, a subsequent pregnancy is possible, but maternal mortality still approaches 10 percent.[188–190,193]

Coronary Artery Disease

Chest discomfort is common during a normal pregnancy and for the most part is due to abdominal distension or gastroesophageal reflux. Coronary artery disease is an uncommon but possible cause, and both angina and myocardial infarctions have been reported during pregnancy. Coronary artery disease in pregnancy can result from atherosclerosis, particularly in those with familial hyperlipidemia, diabetes, hypertension, or a smoking history.[194] Other explanations have been dissection of the coronary artery, spasm, emboli, or vasculitis.[194–197] Vasculitis can result from Kawasaki's disease ("mucocutaneous lymph node syndrome")[198,199] or from Takayasu's disease, which is much more frequent in women than in men, causes proximal artery stenosis, and can affect the coronary arteries.[200,201] If coronary artery disease is a consideration, an electrocardiogram and exercise stress test may help with the diagnosis. If essential, thallium imaging or angiography can be performed. When it is suspected or demonstrated, coronary artery disease should be treated with standard medical therapy. If symptoms are not relieved, angioplasty or bypass surgery can be performed.[202,203]

Pregnancy Following Cardiac Transplantation

Many cardiac transplant recipients are women of childbearing age (Chap. 22). Successful pregnancies after transplantation have been reported,[204] but the potential hazards to the mother and fetus—which include maternal heart failure, immunosuppressive therapy, maternal infections, and serial diagnostic studies—have already been recognized as causing problems in the fetus and in newborns. The potential for a shortened maternal life span must also be considered when a patient is counseled about the advisability of pregnancy.

References

1. Siu SC, Sermer M, Harrison DA, et al. Risk and predictors for pregnancy-related complications in women with heart disease. *Circulation* 1997; 96:2789–2794.
2. McAnulty JH, Morton MJ, Ueland K. The heart and pregnancy. *Curr Probl Cardiol* 1988; 13:589–665.
3. McAnulty JH. Heart diseases in pregnancy. In: Kloner RA, ed. *Guide to Cardiology*. New York: LeJacq Communications; 1995.
4. Ueland K, Novy MJ, Peterson EN, Metcalfe J. Maternal cardiovascular dynamics: IV. The influence of gestational age on the maternal cardiovascular response to posture and exercise. *Am J Obstet Gynecol* 1969; 104:856–864.
5. Capeless EL, Clapp JF. Cardiovascular changes in early phase of pregnancy. *Am J Obstet Gynecol* 1989; 161:1449–1453.
6. Easterling TR, Benedetti TJ, Schmucher BC, Millard SP. Maternal hemodynamics in normal and preeclamptic pregnancies: A longitudinal study. *Obstet Gynecol* 1990; 76:1061–1069.
7. Robson SC, Hunter S, Boys RJ, Dunlop W. Serial study of factors influencing changes in cardiac output during human pregnancy. *Am J Physiol* 1989; 256:H1060–H1065.
8. Clark SL, Cotton DB, Pivarnik JM, et al. Position change and central hemodynamic profile during normal third-trimester pregnancy and postpartum. *Am J Obstet Gynecol* 1991; 164:883–887.
9. Sady MA, Haydon BB, Sady SP, et al. Cardiovascular response to maximal cycle exercise during pregnancy and at two and seven months postpartum. *Am J Obstet Gynecol* 1990; 162:1181–1185.
10. Kerr MG. The mechanical effects of the gravid uterus in late pregnancy. *J Obstet Gynaecol Br Commonw* 1965; 72:513–529.
11. Kinsella SM, Lohmann G. Supine hypotensive syndrome (review). *Obstet Gynecol* 1994; 83:774–788.
12. Robson S, Dunop W, Boys R, Hunter S. Cardiac output during labor. *BMJ* 1987; 295:1169–1172.
13. James C, Banner T, Caton D. Cardiac output in women undergo-

ing cesarean section with epidural or general anesthesia. *Am J Obstet Gynecol* 1989; 160:1178–1183.
14. Clapp JF III, Capeless E. Cardiovascular function before, during, and after the first and subsequent pregnancies. *Am J Cardiol* 1997; 80:1469–1473.
15. Rovinsky JJ, Jaffin H. Cardiovascular hemodynamics in pregnancy: II. Cardiac output and left ventricular work in multiple pregnancy. *Am J Obstet Gynecol* 1966; 95:781–784.
16. Metcalfe J, McAnulty JH, Ueland K. *Heart Disease in Pregnancy: Physiology and Management.* Boston: Little, Brown; 1986:1–54.
17. Thoresen M, Wesche J. Doppler measurements of changes in human mammary and uterine blood flow during pregnancy and lactation. *Acta Obstet Gynecol Scand* 1988; 67:741–745.
18. Lunell NO, Nylund LE, Lewlander R, Sarby B. Uteroplacental blood flow in preeclampsia, measurement with indium-113m and a computer-linked gamma camera. *Clin Exp Hypertens (B)* 1982; 1:105–117.
19. Thaler I, Manor D, Itskovitz J, et al. Changes in uterine blood flow during human pregnancy. *Am J Obstet Gynecol* 1990; 162:121–125.
20. Teixerira JM, Fisk NM, Glover V. Association between maternal anxiety in pregnancy and increased uterine artery resistance index: Cohort based study. *BMJ* 1999; 318:1288–1289.
21. Guzman CA, Caplan R. Cardiorespiratory response to exercise during pregnancy. *Am J Obstet Gynecol* 1970; 108:600–607.
22. Morton MJ, Paul MS, Campos GR, et al. Exercise dynamics in late gestation: Effects of physical training. *Am J Obstet Gynecol* 1985; 152:91–97.
23. Veille JC, Hellerstein HK, Bacevice AE. Maternal left ventricular performance during bicycle exercise. *Am J Cardiol* 1992; 69:1506–1508.
24. Rauramo I, Forss M. Effect of exercise on maternal hemodynamics and placental blood flow in healthy women. *Acta Obstet Gynecol Scand* 1988; 67:21–25.
25. Watson WJ, Katz VL, Hackney AC, et al. Fetal responses to maximal swimming and cycling exercise during pregnancy. *Obstet Gynecol* 1991; 77:382–386.
26. Clapp JF III, Capeless EL. Neonatal morphometrics after endurance exercise during pregnancy. *Am J Obstet Gynecol* 1990; 163:1805–1811.
27. Naeye RL, Peters EC. Working during pregnancy: Effects on the fetus. *Pediatrics* 1982; 69:724–727.
28. Clapp JF III. Pregnancy outcome: Physical activities inside versus outside the workplace. *Semin Perinatol* 1996; 20(1):70–76.
29. Sternfeld B. Physical activity and pregnancy outcome: Review and recommendations. *Sports Med* 1997; 23(1):33–47.
30. Lindheimer MC, Katz AL. Sodium and diuretics in pregnancy. *N Engl J Med* 1973; 299:891–894.
31. Chesley LC. Plasma and red cell volumes during pregnancy. *Am J Obstet Gynecol* 1972; 112:440–450.
32. Hart MV, Morton MJ, Hosenpud JD, Metcalfe J. Aortic function during normal human pregnancy. *Am J Obstet Gynecol* 1986; 154:887–891.
33. Poppas A, Shroff SG, Korcarz CE, et al. Serial assessment of the cardiovascular system in normal pregnancy: Role of arterial compliance and pulsatile arterial load. *Circulation* 1997; 95:2407–2415.
34. Rovinsky JJ, Jaffin H. Cardiovascular hemodynamics in pregnancy: III. Cardiac rate, stroke volume, total peripheral resistance, and central blood volume in multiple pregnancy. Synthesis of results. *Am J Obstet Gynecol* 1966; 95:784–787.
35. Clark-Pearson DL, Jelovsek RD. Alterations of occlusive cuff impedance plethysmography results in the obstetric patient. *Surgery* 1981; 89:594–598.
36. Barrett JM, Vanhooydonk JD, Bochm FH. Pregnancy related rupture of arterial aneurysms. *Obstet Gynecol Surv* 1982; 37:557–566.
37. Anderson RA, Fineron PW. Aortic dissection in pregnancy: Importance of pregnancy-induced changes in the vessel wall and bicuspid aortic valve in pathogenesis. *Br J Obstet Gynaecol* 1994; 101:1085–1088.
38. Nolte JE, Rutherford RB, Nawaz S, et al. Arterial dissections associated with pregnancy (review). *J Vasc Surg* 1995; 21:515–520.
39. Elkayam U, Ostrzega E, Shotan A, Mehra A. Cardiovascular problems in pregnant women with the Marfan syndrome (review). *Ann Intern Med* 1995; 123:117–122.
40. Lipscomb KJ, Smith JC, Clarke B, et al. Outcome of pregnancy in women with Marfan's syndrome. *Br J Obstet Gynecol* 1997; 104(2):201–206.
41. Toglia MR, Weg JH. Venous thromboembolism during pregnancy. *N Engl J Med* 1996; 335:108–113.
42. Rubler S, Damani PM, Pinto ER. Cardiac size and performance during pregnancy estimated with echocardiography. *Am J Cardiol* 1977; 50:534–540.
43. Katz R, Karliner JS, Resnik R. Effects of a natural volume overload state (pregnancy) on left ventricular performance in normal human subjects. *Circulation* 1978; 58:434–441.
44. Sadaniantz A, Kocheril AG, Emans SP, et al. Cardiovascular changes in pregnancy evaluated by two-dimensional and Doppler echocardiography. *J Am Soc Echo* 1992; 5:253–258.
45. Morton MJ, Tsang H, Hohimer AR, et al. Left ventricular size, output and structure during guinea pig pregnancy. *Am J Physiol* 1984; 246:R40–R48.
46. Milsom I, Hedner J, Hedner T. Plasma atrial natriuretic peptide (ANP) and maternal hemodynamic changes during normal pregnancy. *Acta Obstet Gynecol Scand* 1988; 67:717–722.
47. Schrier RW. Pathogenesis of sodium and water retention in high-output and low-output cardiac failure, nephrotic syndrome, cirrhosis and pregnancy. *N Engl J Med* 1988; 319:1065–1072.
48. Ginsberg JS, Hirsh J, Rainbow AG, Coastes G. Risks to the fetus of radiographic procedures used in the diagnosis of maternal venous thromboembolic disease. *Thromb Haemost* 1989; 61: 189–196.
49. Committee on Drugs, American Academy of Pediatrics. The transfer of drugs and other chemicals into human breast milk. *Pediatrics* 1994; 93:137.
50. Cox JL, Gardner MJ. Cardiovascular drugs in pregnancy and lactation. In: Gleicher N, Gall SA, Sibai BM, et al, eds. *Principles and Practice of Medical Therapy in Pregnancy*, 3rd ed. Norwalk, CT: Appleton & Lange; 1998:911–926.
51. Collins R, Yusuf S, Peto R. Overview of randomized trials of diuretics in pregnancy. *BMJ* 1985; 290:17–23.
52. Rogers MC, Willerson JT, Goldblatt A, Smith TW. Serum digoxin concentrations in the human fetus, neonate and infant. *N Engl J Med* 1972; 287:1010–1013.
53. Gonzalez AR, Phelps EJ, Cochran EB, Sibai BM. Digoxin-like immunoreactive substance in pregnancy. *Am J Obstet Gynecol* 1987; 157:660–664.
54. Ueland K, McAnulty JH, Ueland FR. Special considerations in the use of cardiovascular drugs. *Clin Obstet Gynecol* 1981; 24:809–823.
55. Rubin PC. Beta blockers in pregnancy. *N Engl J Med* 1982; 305:1323–1326.
56. Frishman WH, Chesner M. Beta-andrenergic blockers in pregnancy. *Am Heart J* 1988; 115:147–152.
57. Lip GY, Beevers M, Churchill D, Shaffer LM, Beevers DG. Effect of atenolol on birth weight. *Am J Cardiol* 1997; 79:1436–1438.
58. Lydakis C, Lip GY, Beevers M, Beevers DG. Atenolol and fetal growth in pregnancies complicated by hypertension. *Am J Hypertension* 1999; 12:541–547.
59. Sibai BM. Treatment of hypertension in pregnant women (review). *N Engl J Med* 1996; 335:257–265.
60. Wide-Swensson DH, Ingemarsson I, Lunell NO, et al. Calcium channel blockade (isradipine) in treatment of hypertension in

pregnancy: A randomized placebo-controlled study. *Am J Obstet Gynecol* 1995; 173:872–878.
61. Elkayam U, Goodwin TM. Adenosine therapy for supraventricular tachycardia during pregnancy. *Am J Cardiol* 1995; 75:521–523.
62. Cox JL, Gardner JM. Treatment of cardiac arrhythmias during pregnancy. *Prog Cardiovasc Dis* 1993; 36:137–178.
63. Page RL. Treatment of arrhythmias during pregnancy (review). *Am Heart J* 1995; 130:871–876.
64. Juneja MM, Ackerman WE, Kaczorowski DM, et al. Continuous epidural lidocaine infusion in the parturient with paroxysmal ventricular tachycardia. *Anesthesiology* 1989; 71:305–308.
65. Hill LM, Malkasian GD Jr. The use of quinidine sulfate throughout pregnancy. *Obstet Gynecol* 1979; 54:366.
66. Allen NM, Page RL. Procainamide administration during pregnancy. *Clin Pharm* 1993; 12:58–60.
67. Leonard RF, Braun TE, Levy AM. Initiation of uterine contractions by disopyramide during pregnancy. *N Engl J Med* 1978; 299:84.
68. Lownes HE, Ives TJ. Mexiletine use in pregnancy and lactation. *Am J Obstet Gynecol* 1987; 157:446–447.
69. Perry JC, Ayres NA, Carpenter RJ Jr. Fetal supraventricular tachycardia treated by flecainide acetate. *J Pediatr* 1991; 118: 303–305.
70. Connaughton M, Jenkins BS. Successful use of flecainide to treat new onset maternal ventricular tachycardia in pregnancy. *Br Heart J* 1994; 72:297.
71. Wagner X, Jouglard J, Moulin M, et al. Coadministration of flecainide acetate and sotalol during pregnancy. *Am Heart J* 1990; 119:700–702.
72. Foster CJ, Love HG. Amiodarone in pregnancy: Case report and review of the literature. *Int J Cardiol* 1988; 20:307–316.
73. Ovadin M, Brito M, Hoyer GL, Marcus FI. Human experience with amiodarone in the embryonic period. *Am J Cardiol* 1994; 73:316–317.
74. Magee LA, Downar E, Sermer M, et al. Pregnancy outcome after gestational exposure to amiodarone in Canada. *Am J Obstet Gynecol* 1995; 172:1307–1311.
75. Stempel JE, O'Grady JP, Morton MJ, Johnson KA. Use of sodium nitroprusside in complications of gestational hypertension. *Obstet Gynecol* 1982; 60:533–538.
76. Shoemaker CT, Meyers M. Sodium nitroprusside for control of severe hypertensive disease of pregnancy: A case report and discussion of potential toxicity. *Am J Obstet Gynecol* 1984; 149:171–173.
77. Cunningham FG, Lindheimer MD. Hypertension in pregnancy. *N Engl J Med* 1992; 326:927–932.
78. Hanssens M, Keirse MJ, Vankelecom F, et al. Fetal and neonatal effects of treatment with angiotensin converting enzyme inhibitors in pregnancy. *Obstet Gynecol* 1991; 78:128–135.
79. Fillmore SJ, McDevitt E. Effects of coumarin compounds on the fetus. *Ann Intern Med* 1970; 73:731–735.
80. Hall JT, Pauli RM, Wilson KM. Maternal and fetal sequelae of anticoagulation during pregnancy. *Am J Med* 1980; 68:122.
81. Stevenson RE, Burton M, Frelauto GH, Taylor HA. Hazards of oral anticoagulants during pregnancy. *JAMA* 1985; 243:1549–1551.
82. Iturbe-Alessio I, Fonseca MC, Mutchinik O, et al. Risks of anticoagulant therapy in pregnant women with artificial heart valves. *N Engl J Med* 1986; 315:1390–1393.
83. Brabeck MC. Ambulatory management of thromboembolic diseases during pregnancy with continuous infusion of heparin. *JAMA* 1987; 257:1790–1791.
84. Vitale N, De Feo M, De Santo LS, et al. Dose-dependent fetal complications of warfarin in pregnant women with mechanical heart valves. *J Am Coll Cardiol* 1999; 33:1637–1641.
85. Ginsberg JS, Hirsh J. Use of antithrombotic agents during pregnancy: A series of eight cases. *Can J Anaesth* 1994; 41:502–512.
86. Ginsbert JS, Kowalchuk G, Hirsh J, et al. Heparin therapy during pregnancy. *Arch Intern Med* 1989; 149:2233–2236.
87. Anderson DR, Ginsburg JS, Brill-Edwards P, et al. The use of an indwelling Teflon catheter for subcutaneous heparin administration during pregnancy. *Arch Intern Med* 1993; 153:841–844.
88. Elkayam U. Anticoagulation in pregnant women with prosthetic heart valves: A double jeopardy (editorial). *J Am Coll Cardiol* 1996; 27:1704–1706.
89. Nelson-Piercy C, Letsky EA, De Sweit M. Low-molecular weight heparin for obstetric thromboprophylaxis: Experience of sixty-nine pregnancies in sixty-one women at high risk. *Am J Obstet Gynecol* 1997; 176:1062–1068.
90. Sanson BJ, Lensing AW, Prins MH, et al. Safety of low-molecular weight heparin in pregnancy: A systematic review. *Thromb Hemost* 1999; 81:668–672.
91. Corby DG. Aspirin in pregnancy and fetal effects. *Pediatrics* 1978; 62:930–937.
92. Werler MM, Mitchell AA, Shapiro S. The relation of aspirin use during the first trimester of pregnancy to congenital cardiac defects. *N Engl J Med* 1989; 321:1639–1642.
93. DuBard MB, Cutter GR. Low-dose aspirin therapy to prevent preeclampsia. *Am J Obstet Gynecol* 1993; 168:1083–1091.
94. The Canadian Preterm Labor Investigators Group. Treatment of preterm labor with the beta-adrenergic agonist ritodrine. *N Engl J Med* 1992; 327:308–312.
95. McAnulty JH. Anesthesia during pregnancy in the patient with heart disease. In: Bonica JJ, McDonald JS, eds. *Principles and Practice of Obstetric Analgesia and Anesthesia*. Philadelphia: Lea & Febiger; 1994:1013–1039.
96. Haemostatis and Thrombosis Task Force. Guidelines on the prevention, investigation and management of thrombosis associated with pregnancy: Maternal and neonatal haemostasis working papers of the Haemostasis and Thrombosis Task Force. *J Clin Pathol* 1993; 46:489–496.
97. Greer IA. Thrombosis in pregnancy: Maternal and fetal issues. *Lancet* 1999; 353:1258–1265.
98. Kittner SJ, Stern BJ, Feeser BR, et al. Pregnancy and the risk of stroke. *N Engl J Med* 1996; 335:768–774.
99. Donaldson JO, Lee NS. Arterial and venous stroke associated with pregnancy. *Neurol Clin* 1994; 12:583–599.
100. Sturridge F, de Swiet M, Letsky E. The use of low molecular weight heparin for thrombophylaxis in pregnancy. *Br J Obstet Gynaecol* 1994; 101:69–71.
101. Hellgren M, Svensson PJ, Dahlback B. Resistance to activated protein C as a basis for venous thromboembolism associated with pregnancy and oral contraceptives. *Am J Obstet Gynecol* 1995; 173:210–213.
102. Gerhart A, Scharf RE, Beckmann MW, et al. Prothrombin and factor V mutations in women with a history of thrombosis during pregnancy and the puerperium. *N Engl J Med* 2000; 342:374–380.
103. Turrentine MA, Braems G, Ramirez MM. Use of thrombolytics for the treatment of thromboembolic disease during pregnancy (review). *Obstet Gynecol Surv* 1995; 50:534–541.
104. National High Blood Pressure Education Program. Working Group report on high blood pressure in pregnancy. *Am J Obstet Gynecol* 1990; 163:1691–1712.
105. Rey E, LeLorier J, Burgess E, et al. Report of the Canadian Hypertension Society Consensus Conference: 3. Pharmacologic treatment of hypertensive disorders in pregnancy. *Can Med Assoc J* 1997; 157:1245–1254.
106. Witlin AG, Sibai BM. Hypertension. *Clin Obstet Gynecol* 1998; 41:533–544.
107. Avila S, Grinberg M, Snitcowsky R, et al. Maternal and fetal outcome in pregnant women with Eisenmenger's syndrome. *Eur Heart J* 1995; 16:460–464.
108. Weiss BM, Hess OM. Pulmonary vascular disease and pregnancy:

Current controversies, management strategies, and perspectives. *Eur Heart J* 2000; 21:104–115.
109. Widerhorn J, Woderhorn AL, Rahimtoola SH, Elkayam U. WPW syndrome during pregnancy: Increased incidence of supraventricular arrhythmias. *Am Heart J* 1992; 123:796–798.
110. Tawam M, Levine J, Mendelson M, et al. Effect of pregnancy on paroxysmal supraventricular tachycardia. *Am J Cardiol* 1993; 72:838–840.
111. Lee SH, Chan SA, Wu TJ, et al. Effects of pregnancy on first onset and symptoms of paroxysmal supraventricular tachycardia. *Am J Cardiol* 1995; 76:675–678.
112. Rosemond RL. Cardioversion during pregnancy. *JAMA* 1993; 269:3167.
113. Brodsky M, Doria R, Allen V, Sato D. New onset ventricular tachycardia during pregnancy. *Am Heart J* 1992; 123:933–941.
114. Varon ME, Sherer DM, Abramowicz JS, Akiyama T. Maternal ventricular tachycardia associated with hypomagnesemia. *Am J Obstet Gynecol* 1992; 167:1352–1355.
115. Lee RV, Rodgers BD, Shite LM, Harvey RC. Cardiopulmonary resuscitation of pregnant women. *Am J Med* 1986; 81:311–318.
116. Dildy GA, Clark SL. Cardiac arrest during pregnancy. *Obstet Gynecol Clin North Am* 1995; 22:303–314.
117. Nakazato Y, Nakata Y, Tokano T, et al. Long-term follow-up study of three patients with the long QT syndrome. *Jpn Circ J* 1992; 56:1025–1031.
118. McCurdy CM, Rutherford SE, Coddington CC. Syncope and sudden arrhythmic death complicating pregnancy: A case report of Ramano-Ward syndrome. *J Reprod Med* 1993; 38:233–234.
119. Dalvi BV, Chaudhuri A, Kulkarni HL, Kale PA. Therapeutic guidelines for congenital complete heart block presenting in pregnancy. *Obstet Gynecol* 1994; 79:802–804.
120. Seaworth BJ, Durack DT. Infective endocarditis in obstetric and gynecologic practice. *Am J Obstet Gynecol* 1986; 154:180–188.
121. Ebrahimi R, Leung CY, Elkayam U, Reid CL. Infective endocarditis. In: Gleicher N, ed. *Principles and Practice of Medical Therapy in Pregnancy*, 2d ed. Norwalk, CT: Appleton & Lange; 1992:795–801.
122. Dajani AS, Taubert KA, Wilson W, et al. Prevention of bacterial endocarditis—Recommendations by the American Heart Association. *JAMA* 1997; 277:1794–1801.
123. McAnulty JH. Rheumatic heart disease. In: Gleicher N, Gall SA, Sibai BM, et al, eds. *Principles and Practice of Medical Therapy in Pregnancy*, 2d ed. Norwalk, CT: Appleton & Lange; 1992:783–788.
124. Massell BF, Chute CG, Walker AM, Kurland GS. Penicillin and the marked decrease in morbidity and mortality from rheumatic fever in the United States. *N Engl J Med* 1988; 318:280–286.
125. Veasy LG, Widemeier SE, Orsmond GS, et al. Resurgence of acute rheumatic fever in the intermountain area of the United States. *N Engl J Med* 1987; 316:421–427.
126. Special Writing Group of the Committee on Rheumatic Fever, Endocarditis, and Kawasaki Disease of the Council on Cardiovascular Disease in the Young of the American Heart Association. Guidelines for the diagnosis of rheumatic fever: Jones criteria, 1992 update. *JAMA* 1992; 268:2069–2073.
127. Dajani AS, Bisno AL, Chung KJ, et al. Prevention of rheumatic fever. *Circulation* 1988; 78:1082–1086.
128. Bryg RJ, Gordon PR, Kudesia VS, Bhatia RK. Effect of pregnancy on pressure gradient in mitral stenosis. *Am J Cardiol* 1989; 63:384–386.
129. Ueland K, Metcalfe J. Acute rheumatic fever in pregnancy. *Am J Obstet Gynecol* 1966; 95:586–587.
130. Stephen SJ. Changing patterns of mitral stenosis in childhood and pregnancy in Sri Lanka. *J Am Coll Cardiol* 1992; 19:1276–1284.
131. Gupta A, Lokhandwala YY, Satoskar PR, Salvi VS. Balloon mitral valvotomy in pregnancy: Maternal and fetal outcomes. *J Am Coll Surg* 1998; 187:409–415.
132. Martinez-Reding J, Cordero A, Kuri J, et al. Treatment of severe mitral stenosis with percutaneous balloon valvotomy in pregnant patients. *Clin Cardiol* 1998; 21:659–663.
133. Commerford PJ, Hastie T, Beck W. Closed mitral valvotomy: Actuarial analysis of results in 654 patients over 12 years and analysis of preoperative predictors of long-term survival. *Ann Thorac Surg* 1982; 33:473–479.
134. Chambers CE, Clark SL. Cardiac surgery during pregnancy (review). *Clin Obstet Gynecol* 1994; 37:316–323.
135. Shapiro EP, Trible EL, Robinson JC, et al. Safety of labor and delivery in women with mitral valve prolapse. *Am J Cardiol* 1985; 56:806–807.
136. Degani S, Abinader EG, Scharf M. Mitral valve prolapse and pregnancy: A review. *Obstet Gynecol Surv* 1989; 72:113–118.
137. Cowles T, Gonik B. Mitral valve prolapse in pregnancy. *Semin Perinatol* 1990; 14:34–41.
138. Nishimura RA, McGoon MD. Perspectives on mitral-valve prolapse. *N Engl J Med* 1999; 341(1):48–59.
139. Arias F, Pineda J. Aortic stenosis and pregnancy. *J Reprod Med* 1978; 20:229–232.
140. Easterling TR, Chadwick HS, Otto CM, Benedetti TJ. Aortic stenosis in pregnancy. *Obstet Gynecol* 1988; 72:113–118.
141. Lao TT, Sermer M, McGee L, et al. Congenital aortic stenosis and pregnancy—A reappraisal (review). *Am J Obstet Gynecol* 1993; 169:540–545.
142. Banning AP, Pearson JF, Hall RJ. Role of balloon dilatation of the aortic valve in pregnant patients with severe aortic stenosis. *Br Heart J* 1993; 70:544–545.
143. American College of Cardiology/American Heart Association Task Force on Practice Guidelines (Committee on Management of Patients with Valvular Heart Disease). ACC/AHA Guidelines for the management of patients with valvular heart disease. *J Am Coll Cardiol* 1998; 32:1486–1588.
144. Whittemore R, Hobbins JC, Engle MA. Pregnancy and its outcome in women with and without surgical treatment of congenital heart disease. *Am J Cardiol* 1982; 50:641–651.
145. Lao TT, Adelman AG, Sermer M, Colman JM. Balloon valvuloplasty for congenital aortic stenosis in pregnancy. *Br J Obstet Gynaecol* 1993; 100:1141–1142.
146. Sullivan HJ. Valvular heart surgery during pregnancy (review). *Surg Clin North Am* 1995; 75:59–75.
147. Bloomfield P, Wheatley DJ, Prescott RJ, Miller HC. Twelve-year comparison of a Bjork-Shirley mechanical heart valve with porcine bioprostheses. *N Engl J Med* 1991; 324:573–579.
148. Hammermeister KE, Sethi GK, Henderson WG, et al. A comparison of outcomes in men 11 years after heart-valve replacement with a mechanical valve or bioprosthesis. *N Engl J Med* 1993; 328:1289–1296.
149. Sareli P, England MJ, Berk MR, et al. Maternal and fetal sequelae of anticoagulation during pregnancy in patients with mechanical heart valve prostheses. *Am J Cardiol* 1989; 63:1462–1465.
150. Born D, Martinez EE, Almeida PA, et al. Pregnancy in patients with prosthetic heart valves: The effects of anticoagulation on mother, fetus, and neonate. *Am Heart J* 1992; 124:413–417.
151. Salazar E, Izaguirre R, Verdejo J, Mutchinick O. Failure of adjusted doses of subcutaneous heparin to prevent thromboembolic phenomena in pregnant patients with mechanical cardiac valve prostheses. *J Am Coll Cardiol* 1996; 27:1698–1703.
152. North RA, Sadler L, Stewart AW, et al. Long-term survival and valve-related complications in young women with cardiac valve replacements. *Circulation* 1999; 99:2669–2676.
153. Elkayam U. Pregnancy through a prosthetic valve. *J Am Coll Cardiol* 1999; 33:1643–1645.
154. Jamieson WR, Miller DC, Akins CW, et al. Pregnancy and bioprostheses: Influence on structural valve deterioration. *Ann Thorac Surg* 1995; 60:S282–S286.
155. Mitchell SC, Korones SB, Berendes HW. Congenital heart dis-

ease in 56,109 births: Incidence and natural history. *Circulation* 1971; 43:323–332.
156. Nora JJ, Nora AH. The evolution of specific genetic and environmental counseling in congenital heart disease. *Circulation* 1978; 57:205–213.
157. Roberts N. A predictive study of congenital heart disease and need for care. *West J Med* 1978; 120:19–25.
158. McFaul PB, Dornan JC, Lamki H, Boyle D. Pregnancy complicated by maternal heart disease: A review of 519 women. *Br J Obset Gynaecol* 1988; 95:861–867.
159. Nora JJ, Nora AH. Maternal transmission of congenital heart diseases: New recurrence risk figures and the questions of cytoplasmic inheritance and vulnerability to teratogens. *Am J Cardiol* 1987; 59:459–463.
160. Whittemore R, Hobbins JC, Engle MA. Pregnancy and its outcome in women with and without surgical treatment of congenital heart disease. *Am J Cardiol* 1982; 50:641–651.
161. Morris CD, Menashe VD. Evidence for maternal transmission of congenital heart defects. *Circulation* 1993; 88(suppl):1–98.
162. Whittemore R, Wells JA, Castellsagne X. A second-generation study of 427 probands with congenital heart defects and their 837 children. *J Am Coll Cardiol* 1994; 23:1459–1467.
163. Nora J. From generational studies to a multilevel genetic-environmental interaction (editorial). *J Am Coll Cardiol* 1994; 23:1468–1471.
164. Metcalfe J, Ueland K. Maternal cardiovascular adjustments to pregnancy. *Prog Cardiovasc Dis* 1974; 16:363–374.
165. Morris CD, Manashe VD. 25-year mortality after surgical repair of congenital heart defect in childhood: A population-based cohort study. *JAMA* 1991; 266:3447–3452.
166. Presbytero P, Sommerville J, Stone S, et al. Pregnancy and cyanotic congenital heart disease, outcome of mother and fetus. *Circulation* 1994; 89:2673–2676.
167. Neill CA, Swanson S. Outcome of pregnancy in congenital heart disease. *Circulation* 1961; 24:1003–1011.
168. Zellers TM, Driscoll DJ, Michaels VV. Prevalence of significant congenital heart defects in children of parents with Fallot's tetralogy. *Am J Cardiol* 1990; 65:523–526.
169. Deal D, Wooley CF. Coarctation of the aorta and pregnancy. *Ann Intern Med* 1973; 78:706–710.
170. Connolly HM, Ammash NM, Warnes CA. Pregnancy in women with coarctation of the aorta (abstr). *J Am Coll Cardiol* 1996; 27(suppl A):43A.
171. Pitkin RM, Perloff JK, Koos BJ, Beall MH. Pregnancy and congenital heart disease. *Ann Intern Med* 1990; 112:445–454.
172. Oakley GD, McGarry K, Limb DG, Oakley CM. Management of pregnancy in patients with hypertrophic cardiomyopathy. *BMJ* 1979; 1:1749–1750.
173. Piacenza JM, Kirkorian G, Audra PH, Mellier G. Hypertrophic cardiomyopathy and pregnancy. *Eur J Obstet Gynecol Reprod Biol* 1998; 80(1):17–23.
174. Shah DM, Sunderji SG. Hypertrophic cardiomyopathy and pregnancy: Report of a maternal mortality and review of literature. *Obstet Gynecol Surv* 1985; 40:444–448.
175. Conobbio MM, Mair DD, Velde M, Koos BJ. Pregnancy outcomes after the Fontan repair. *J Am Coll Cardiol* 1996; 28: 763–767.
176. Patton DE, Lee W, Cotton DB, et al. Cyanotic maternal heart disease in pregnancy. *Obstet Gynecol Surv* 1990; 45:594–600.
177. Clarkson PM, Wilson NJ, Neutze JM, et al. Outcome of pregnancy after the Mustard operation for transposition of the great arteries with intact ventricular septum. *J Am Coll Cardiol* 1994; 24: 190–193.
178. Perloff JK. Pregnancy and congenital heart disease. *J Am Coll Cardiol* 1991; 18:340–342.
179. Connolly H, Grogan M, Warnes CA. Pregnancy among women with congenitally corrected transposition of great arteries. *J Am Coll Cardiol* 1999; 33:1692–1695.
180. Wooley CF, Sparks EH. Congenital heart disease, heritable cardiovascular disease, and pregnancy. *Prog Cardiovasc Dis* 1992; 35:41–60.
181. Connolly HM, Warnes CA. Ebstein's anomaly: Outcome of pregnancy. *J Am Coll Cardiol* 1994; 23:1194–1198.
182. Mor-Yosef S, Younis J, Granat M, et al. Marfan's syndrome in pregnancy. *Obstet Gynecol Surv* 1988; 43:382–385.
183. Pyeritz RE. Maternal and fetal complications of pregnancy in the Marfan syndrome. *Am J Med* 1981; 71:784–790.
184. Grunig E, Tasman JA, Kucherer H, et al. Frequency and phenotypes of familial dilated cardiomyopathy. *J Am Coll Cardiol* 1998; 31:86–94.
185. Olson TM, Michels VV, Thibodeau SN, et al. Actin mutations in dilated cardiomyopathy, a heritable form of heart failure. *Science* 1998; 280:750–752.
186. Damakil JG, Rahimtoola SH, Sutton GC, et al. Natural course of peripartum cardiomyopathy. *Circulation* 1971; 44:1053–1061.
187. O'Connell JB, Costanzo-Mordin MR, Surbranian R, et al. Peripartum cardiomyopathy: Clinical, hemodynamic, histologic and prognostic characteristics. *J Am Coll Cardiol* 1986; 8:52–56.
188. Lampert MB, Lang RM. Peripartum cardiomyopathy. *Am Heart J* 1995; 130:860–870.
189. Heider AL, Kuller JA, Strauss RA, Wells SR. Peripartum cardiomyopathy: A review of the literature. *Obstet Gynecol Surv* 1999; 54: 526–531.
190. Melvin KR, Richardson PJ, Olsen EG, et al. Peripartum cardiomyopathy due to myocarditis. *N Engl J Med* 1982; 308:731–734.
191. Rizeq MN, Rickenbacher PR, Fowler MB, Billingham ME. Incidence of myocarditis in peripartum cardiomyopathy. *Am J Cardiol* 1994; 74:474–477.
192. Parrilo JE, Cunnion RE, Epstein SE, et al. A prospective, randomized, controlled trial of prednisone for dilated cardiomyopathy. *N Engl J Med* 1989; 321:1061–1068.
193. Sutton MS, Cole P, Plappert M, et al. Effects of subsequent pregnancy on left ventricular function in peripartum cardiomyopathy. *Am Heart J* 1991; 121:1776–1778.
194. Roth A, Elkayam U. Acute myocardial infarction associated with pregnancy. *Ann Intern Med* 1996; 125:751–762.
195. Ciraulo DA, Markovitz A. Myocardial infarction in pregnancy associated with a coronary artery thrombus. *Arch Intern Med* 1979; 139:1046–1047.
196. Ahronheim JH. Isolated coronary periarteritis: Report of a case of unexpected death in a young pregnant woman. *Am J Cardiol* 1977; 40:287–290.
197. Jewett J. Two dissecting coronary-artery aneurysms post partum. *N Engl J Med* 1978; 298:1255–1256.
198. Nolan TE, Savage RW. Peripartum myocardial infarction from presumed Kawasaki's disease. *South Med J* 1990; 83:360–361.
199. Taubert KA, Rowley AH, Shulman ST. Nationwide survey of Kawasaki disease and acute rheumatic fever. *J Pediatr* 1991; 119:279–282.
200. Ishikawa A, Matsura S. Occlusive thromboaortopathy (Takayasu's disease) and pregnancy. *Am J Cardiol* 1982; 50:1293–1300.
201. Railton A, Allen DG. Takayasu's arteritis in pregnancy: A report of 4 cases. *S Afr Med J* 1988; 73:123–127.
202. Cowan NC, de Belder MA, Rothman MT. Coronary angioplasty in pregnancy. *Br Heart J* 1988; 59:588–592.
203. Garry D, Leikin E, Fleisher AG, Tejani N. Acute myocardial infarction in pregnancy with subsequent medical and surgical management. *Obstet Gynecol* 1996; 87(5 pt 2):802–804.
204. Morini A, Spina V, Aleandri V, et al. Pregnancy after heart transplant: Update and case report. *Hum Reprod* 1998; 13: 749–757.

CHAPTER 83

THE HEART AND OBESITY

Paul Poirier / Robert H. Eckel

INTRODUCTION

> Very fat people were apt to die earlier than those who were slender.
>
> Hippocrates (Aphorism 44)

Populations in industrialized countries are becoming more overweight as a result of changes in lifestyle. Both overweight and obesity must be regarded as serious current medical problems. Increased body fat is associated with an increased risk of heart disease, stroke, hypertension, dyslipidemia, type 2 diabetes mellitus, gallbladder disease, osteoarthritis, sleep apnea and respiratory problems, and endometrial, breast, prostate, and colon cancers.[1,2] Moreover, obesity is associated with reduced life expectancy.[3] The incidence of obesity in the United States has increased progressively since 1960, and the prevalence of obesity is three times higher in the United States than it is in France and one and a half times higher than in Great Britain.[4]

After a follow-up of 26 years, the Framingham Heart Study and the Manitoba Study have documented that obesity represents an independent predictor of cardiovascular disease, particularly among women.[5,6] Cardiovascular disease was defined as an incidence of coronary disease, coronary death, and congestive heart failure. This relation was independent of age, cholesterol, systolic blood pressure, cigarette smoking, left ventricular hypertrophy (LVH), and glucose intolerance. It is noteworthy that this association was more pronounced in individuals younger than age 50 years. These data have led the American Heart Association to state that obesity is a major modifiable risk factor for heart disease.[7,8] A regulatory system that maintains constant energy storage is likely to involve complex interactions among humoral, neural, metabolic, and psychological factors, among others. Thus, overweight/obesity is a complex multifactorial chronic disorder that develops from an interaction between genotype and the environment.[2,9] Because weight reduction is difficult to achieve and maintain, obesity is a self-perpetuating condition in which homeostatic mechanisms restrain further weight loss.

There are several definitions of overweight and obesity.[10] Although body weight that exceeds ideal standards as determined by age, sex, and height may be accounted for by greater muscle mass or bone mass, most individuals who weigh over their calculated ideal body weights have excessive adipose tissue mass. Because body mass index (BMI) is an assessment of total fat content that does not derive from frame size and gender, it has replaced relative weight as an index of body composition.[2] From a clinical viewpoint, overweight is defined as a body mass index (weight in kilograms divided by the square of height in meters) of 25 to 29.9 kg/m^2 and obesity as a BMI ≥30 kg/m^2 [2] (Table 83-1). Importantly, the number of overweight and obese individuals has risen since 1960; in the last decade, the percentage of people in these categories has increased to over 50 percent of adults age 20 years and older. Currently, all overweight and obese adults (age >18 years with a BMI ≥25 kg/m^2) are considered at risk for developing comorbidities such as hypertension, dyslipidemia, type 2 diabetes mellitus, and coronary heart disease.

Adipose tissue should not be regarded as merely a passive storehouse for fat but instead as a diffuse vascular organ in which the synthesis of a variety of molecules important to cardiovascular medicine is carried out. Although activated leukocytes, fibroblasts, and endothelial cells are assumed widely to be the major source of circulating interleukin-6 (IL-6), it has been estimated that in vivo, ~30 percent of total circulating

TABLE 83-1 Classification of Overweight and Obesity by Percentage of Body Fat, Body Mass Index (BMI), Waist Circumference, and Associated Disease Risk

		Disease Risk[a] Relative to Normal Weight and Waist Circumference	
	BMI, kg/m^2	Men, ≤102 cm Women, ≤88 cm	Men, >102 cm Women, >88 cm
Underweight	<18.5		
Normal	18.5–24.9		
Overweight	25.0–29.9	Increased	High
Obesity, class			
I	30.0–34.9	High	Very high
II	35.0–39.9	Very high	Very high
III (extreme obesity)	≥40	Extremely high	Extremely high

[a]Disease risk for type 2 diabetes, hypertension, and cardiovascular disease.
SOURCE: From Clinical Guidelines on the Identification, Evaluation, and Treatment of Overweight and Obesity in Adults.[2]

concentrations of IL-6 originate from adipose tissue.[11,12] This is important since IL-6 modulates the production of C-reactive protein in the liver and that protein may be an independent predictor of cardiovascular disease events.[13] Also, adipose tissue is a major source of tumor necrosis factor-alpha (TNF-alpha)[14,15] and plasminogen activator inhibitor-1 (PAI-1),[16] and circulating concentrations of PAI-1, angiotensin II, C-reactive protein, fibrinogen, and TNF-alpha are all related to BMI.[11,17] This is important because PAI-1 levels parallel the concentration of triglycerides, cytokines are implicated in endothelial cell dysfunction, and increases in angiotensin II may contribute to hypertension and heart failure, which are seen more often in obese persons.

ADAPTATION OF THE CARDIOVASCULAR SYSTEM IN OBESITY

Adipose Tissue Circulation

From morphologic studies, it has been shown that an extensive capillary network surrounds adipose tissue. The adipocytes are located close to vessels with the highest permeability, the lowest hydrostatic pressure, and the shortest distance for transport of molecules from adipocytes.[18] Resting blood flow is usually between 2 and 3 mL/min per 100 grams of adipose tissue,[19,20] whereas maximal blood flow amounts to only 25 to 30 mL/min per 100 grams of adipose tissue compared with 50 to 75 mL/min in skeletal muscle.[21] The interstitial space of adipose tissue accounts for approximately 10 percent of tissue wet weight.[22] Since a large part of body weight consists of adipose tissue, significant quantities of fluid are present in the interstitial space of adipose tissue and could be important in the regulation of blood volume if mobilized into the blood. For example, in a 100-kg person with 25 to 30 percent of body fat, 2 to 3 L of fluid may be present in this compartment. Clinically, this can have important repercussions in cardiologically compromised individuals if the extra volume is repartitioned in the circulation.

The function of adipose tissue is more severely impaired by hypovolemia, i.e., hemorrhagic shock, than is that of most other tissues. Interestingly, the beta-adrenoceptors that mediate vasodilatation in adipose tissue are mainly the beta$_1$ type, in contrast to those of skeletal muscle, which are mainly beta$_2$. This explains why during hemorrhagic shock increased epinephrine levels decrease blood flow much more in adipose tissue than they do in skeletal muscle.[18] More specifically, blood flow in subcutaneous adipose tissue is reduced to about 10 percent of resting blood flow, whereas in skeletal muscle, liver, myocardium, and hypothalamus, blood flow falls to about 60 percent of resting flow and renal cortical flow falls to about 40 percent.[18] As a consequence of this dramatic decrease in blood flow in adipose tissue, the fluid present in the interstitial compartment is not readily accessible to restore volemia.

While there are differences between blood flow in adipose tissue and that in other organs, the increment in blood flow with increasing adiposity is not proportional to the increment in adipose tissue mass; therefore, perfusion per unit of adipose tissue decreases significantly with increasing obesity, i.e., from 2.36 mL/min per 100 grams to 1.53 mL/min of adipose tissue in patients who have 15 to 26 percent body fat to >36 percent body fat, respectively.[20] Thus, increases in total body fat result in higher total blood flow secondary to the enlarged vascular bed, but the adipose tissue is less vascularized than lean tissue with increasing obesity. Thus, the increase in systemic blood flow seen in obesity[23] cannot be explained solely by increased requirements resulting from adipose tissue perfusion but most probably is caused by the concomitant increase in lean body mass in these individuals.

Cardiac Output

Any increase in body mass from adipose tissue or muscular tissue requires a higher cardiac output and expanded intravascular volume to meet the higher metabolic demand. Because of the need to move excess body weight, at any given level of activity, the cardiac workload is greater for obese subjects than it is for nonobese individuals. Thus, obese subjects are known to have higher cardiac output and a lower total peripheral resistance.[23] The high cardiac output is attributable to increased stroke volume, while heart rate is usually unchanged.[24] The increase in blood volume and cardiac output in obesity is in proportion to the amount of excess body weight and the duration of obesity. In the setting of this increase in cardiac output, cerebral blood flow, oxygen uptake, and cerebral arteriovenous O_2 difference did not differ from those in nonobese individuals.[25] This implies that the fraction of the cardiac output distributed to the brain is lower than normal in obesity.[25] In the same study, renal blood flow was normal or slightly reduced in obesity.

Thus, the percentage of total cardiac output to the kidney was about 20 percent lower than that in the splanchnic vascular flow bed, which approximated normal.[25] The increase in splanchnic flow was not sufficient to account for the observed increases in cardiac output. Also, in obesity, left ventricular filling pressure and volume increase, shifting left ventricular function to the left on the Frank-Starling curve and inducing chamber dilatation. The volume of the dilated chamber increases inappropriately to the stress on the left ventricular wall. Thus, the myocardium adapts by increasing contractile elements and subsequently myocardial mass. The end product is left ventricular hypertrophy, often of the eccentric type.[26,27] If this hemodynamic burden is sustained, premature impairment of left ventricular contractile function may result. Left atrial enlargement is also common in normotensive obese individuals and is associated with increased left ventricular mass. Importantly, left atrial enlargement is not necessarily mediated through impairment of left ventricular diastolic function and may simply reflect a physiologic adaptation to the expanded blood volume.[28]

If arterial pressure does not change, the increase in cardiac output is associated with a decrease in vascular resistance. Therefore, for any given level of arterial pressure, cardiac output is higher and vascular resistance is lower in an obese person than it is in a nonobese individual. However, obesity and hypertension often are associated. When both are present, obesity increases preload and hypertension increases postload. The heart of an obese hypertensive individual is now confronted with a double burden, and this may result in early left ventricular dysfunction and premature heart failure.

To examine the impact of obesity on the circulation, data have been obtained before and after surgically induced weight reduction at rest and during exercise by using right heart catheterization.[29] Resting oxygen consumption and cardiac output fell in proportion to weight loss.[29,30] Stroke volume fell in parallel to the decrease in blood volume and heart volume. Systemic arterial pressure declined, while systemic arterial resistance did not change. Left ventricular stroke work diminished. Filling pressures of the right and left sides of the heart decreased but were still higher in relation to cardiac output than they were in normal-weight subjects. Left ventricular dysfunction persisted, as evidenced by reduced myocardial wall compliance.[29] Right ventricular systolic pressure was lowered by 5 mmHg, and pulmonary arterial pressures by about 6 mmHg, but wedge pressure did not change.[29] At any given cardiac output, all pressures in the right ventricle, pulmonary artery, and pulmonary capillary venous position were higher than they were in normal-weight subjects,[29] with relative increases in left ventricular end-diastolic pressure.[24]

Obesity also is associated with persistence of elevated cardiac filling pressures during exercise.[29,31] Moreover, the average left ventricular filling pressure rose with exercise similarly (~20 mmHg) after weight loss. The average resting left ventricular filling pressure is within the upper limits of normal but is increased abnormally with increased venous return of passive leg raising and is increased further with exercise.[24] This is consistent with centralization of the circulating volume. With the increased venous return of passive leg raising, small increments of central blood volume were associated with a significant increase in left ventricular end-diastolic pressure. Normally, this intervention in healthy individuals would not cause any increase in diastolic filling pressures or would cause only a minimal change of 1 to 2 mmHg. This is consistent with a reduced distensibility of the central circulation in these patients. A decrease in central blood volume accompanies weight reduction, and when present, relief of edema and dyspnea accompanies this improvement.[24] However, myocardial hypertrophy and reduced ventricular compliance characterized by left ventricular diastolic dysfunction during exercise did not always regress with weight loss.[29,31]

FREQUENTLY PERFORMED PROCEDURES IN CARDIOLOGY AND OBESITY

Physical Examination

Fat mass is distributed differently in men and in women. The android, or male, pattern is characterized by fat distributed predominantly in the upper body above the waist, whereas the gynecoid, or female, pattern is characterized by fat predominantly in the lower body, that is, the lower abdomen, buttocks, hips, and thighs.

Although obesity often is described as an endocrine disease, fewer than 1 percent of obese patients have any significant endocrine dysfunction; hypothalamic (inflammation, trauma, tumor), pituitary (Cushing's disease), thyroid (hypothyroidism), adrenal (Cushing's syndrome), and ovarian (polycystic ovarian syndrome) dysfunctions have all been related to obesity. Obesity is the most common manifestation of Cushing's disease/syndrome, and weight gain is usually the initial symptom. Obesity is classically central, affecting mainly the face (moon facies), neck (buffalo hump), trunk, and abdomen, with relative sparing of the extremities. Hypogonadism also is associated with redistribution of body fat characterized by a lower abdominal–pelvic girdle fat distribution in patients who develop androgen deficiency.

In some ways, the presence of obesity may limit the accuracy of the physical examination. Jugular venous pulse often is not seen, and heart sounds are usually distant. A common finding in massive obesity is pedal edema, which can occur in part as a consequence of elevated ventricular filling pressure despite an elevation in cardiac output.[32,33] Obese individuals also can have increases in the demand for ventilation and breathing workload, especially in the supine position. At one time it was thought that Cheyne-Stokes breathing was pathognomonic of the cardiomyopathy of obesity.[34] Accurate blood pressure measurement is crucial, since many obese patients are hypertensive. A small cuff size can cause considerable increases in blood pressure.[35] This could result in incorrect classification of up to 35 percent of normotensive individuals as hypertensive in the presence of obesity.[35] When the bladder within the cuff is not long enough to encircle at least 80 percent of the arm, a wider cuff should be used. However, if the cuff is too wide, the pressure may be underestimated. One should always evaluate the presence of cor pulmonale when examining an obese individual. In the majority of individuals, splitting of the S_2 sound is most often heard at the second or third left interspace parasternally. However, in obese patients, the split S_2, when either inaudible or very poorly defined in the second interspace, often is best heard at the first left interspace.[36] Therefore, an increase in the intensity of P_2 suggestive of pulmonary hypertension may be missed at the bedside.

Surface Electrocardiogram

Obesity has the potential to affect the electrocardiogram (ECG) in several ways: (1) displacing the heart by elevating the diaphragm in the supine position, (2) increasing the cardiac workload, and (3) increasing the distance between the heart and the recording electrodes.

The voltage of the QRS complexes is attenuated by its passage through a fat-laden chest wall and is related to several factors, including the anatomy of the thorax, the degree of fatty infiltration of the heart, the degree of associated chronic lung disease, the increase in left ventricular muscle mass, and, most important, the selection of the ECG leads for measuring voltage. Overall, the effect of weight loss in obese patients on the QRS voltage is a source of controversy in the literature; studies have reported a decrease,[37–39] no change, [40] or an increase in the QRS amplitude after weight reduction.[41,42] Several factors, probably acting in different directions, are responsible for the ECG changes associated with weight reduction. In some instances, low QRS voltage after drastic weight loss could be secondary to lean mass loss and myocardial atrophy.[39,43,44] One must bear in mind that weight loss with modifications in the anatomy of the thorax (decrease in the amount of fat mass) may counterbalance a real decrease in left ventricular mass. These factors acting in opposite directions may affect the resultant QRS amplitudes differently.

In a study of over 1000 obese individuals, the heart rate, PR interval, QRS interval, QRS voltage, and QTc interval all showed an increase with increasing obesity.[45] Although the prolongation of the PR interval and the QRS interval probably was not clinically important, it is noteworthy that 8 percent of these patients presented with a QTc >0.44 s. Although the QRS axis also tended to shift leftward, fewer than 1 percent of the patients displayed an abnormal axis deviation. Interestingly, only 4 percent of this population had low QRS voltage and 19 percent presented with bradycardia.[45] Weight loss induced a rightward shift of the QRS axis.[41]

One study reported an increased incidence of false-positive criteria for inferior myocardial infarction in both obese individuals and women in the final trimester of pregnancy, presumably because of diaphragmatic elevation.[46] Several studies have documented nonspecific flattening of the T wave in the inferolateral leads in obese subjects.[42,47] In contrast, most conduction intervals, i.e., duration of the P wave, QRS complex, and the PQ interval in lead II, are not affected by weight loss.[41]

Since LVH is strongly associated with cardiac morbidity and mortality,[48] better ECG detection of LVH is mandatory in obese individuals. As left ventricular mass increases, electrical forces usually become more posteriorly oriented, and the S wave in lead V_3 may be the most representative voltage for evaluating posterior forces. In addition, it has been shown that with increasing LVH, the heart is oriented more horizontally, and this may explain the usefulness of the R wave in aV_L as an important determinant of LVH. Thus, it was proposed that for men at all ages, LVH is present by QRS voltage alone when the amplitude of the R wave in lead aV_L and the S wave in lead V_3 are >35 mm. For women of all ages, the same criteria were set at >25 mm.[49] When slightly different ECG voltage criteria in the same leads were compared with left ventricular mass estimated by echocardiography, a sensitivity of 49 percent, a specificity of 93 percent, and an overall accuracy of 76 percent were revealed. These percentages are higher than most widely used criteria, such as the Romhilt-Estes point score and the Sokolow-Lyon voltage (Table 83-2). Additionally, another study suggested that for simple LVH detection criteria, Sokolow-Lyon voltage should be avoided in obese hypertensive patients and replaced by the Cornell voltage criteria, which seems to be influenced less by the presence of obesity.[50]

TABLE 83-2 Detection of Left Ventricular Hypertrophy by QRS Voltage in Obesity

	Sensitivity in Obesity, %	Specificity in Obesity, %	Accuracy in Obesity, %
Sokolow-Lyon	20	93	65
Romhilt-Estes point score ≥4	31	83	63
Cornell	49	93	76

Sokolow-Lyon voltage criteria: R in V_5 or V_6 plus S in V_1 >35 mm.
Romhilt-Estes point score; *Am Heart J* 1968; 75:752–758.
Cornell voltage criteria: R in aV_L plus S in V_3 >28 mm in men, >20 mm in women.
SOURCE: Adapted from Casale et al.[49]

Radiology

In obesity, the chest x-ray generally shows an elevated diaphragm with a widened heart in a horizontal direction, with the apex displaced outward to the left.[47] The heart appears enlarged and the left ventricle hypertrophied, based on the criteria of a total transverse diameter of the heart more than half the maximum internal thoracic diameter (Fig. 83-1). This is often discordant with the findings on the surface ECG (see above). The apex or the lower portion of the left border of the heart may be hazy in outline owing to the presence of apical pericardial fat.[47] Moreover, portable bedside radiographs are usually of very poor quality in obese patients, limiting the value of this important diagnostic tool in an emergency situation. Also, many computed tomography (CT) scan tables have weight restrictions (about 160 kg) that prohibit imaging of severely obese patients.

Echocardiography

Transthoracic echocardiography can be technically difficult in obese patients, and obtaining a good echocardiographic window is often difficult. This is important in evaluating the presence of left ventricular diastolic dysfunction. Although the evaluation of the presence of left ventricular diastolic dysfunction is important in obese subjects, complete echocardiogram studies are feasible in only 10 to 50 percent of patients.[51–53] Pulmonary venous Doppler evaluation may be used, but if it is not technically accessible, transmitral Doppler imaging with the use of the Valsalva maneuver may properly evaluate the presence of left ventricular diastolic dysfunction.[54,55]

Another feature of the echocardiographic assessment in obese

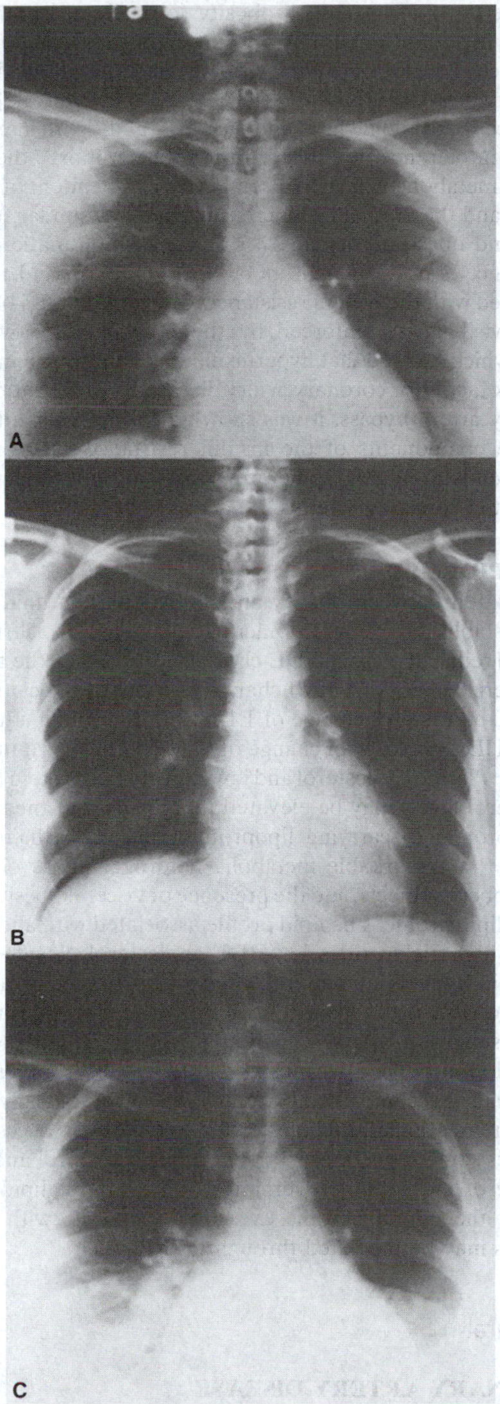

FIGURE 83-1 Chest films of a woman first presenting with severe pulmonary and systemic congestion. *A*. At age 20, weight is 184 kg. *B*. At age 31, weight reduction to 157 kg was associated with decrements in heart size as well as pulmonary congestion. *C*. Recurrence of cardiomegaly and pulmonary congestion attended regained weight at age 37. At age 43, weight 195 kg, echocardiogram demonstrated normal left ventricular systolic performance, with ejection fraction 64 percent, mean velocity of circumferential fiber shortening 1.36 cir/s. Left ventricular septal and posterior wall thickness were increased to 1.7 and 2.0 cm, respectively, and E-F slope was reduced to 30 mm/s, suggesting reduced left ventricular compliance. Left atrial dimension was enlarged to 5.2 cm. By age 48, atrial fibrillation had developed. (From Alexander JK. The cardiomyopathy of obesity. *Prog Cardiovasc Dis* 1985; 27:325–334. Reproduced with permission from Grune & Stratton, Inc., and the author.)

patients is the differentiation between subepicardial adipose tissue and pericardial effusion, which at times can be difficult. Epicardial adipose tissue is known to be a common cause of pseudopericardial effusion, and this adipose tissue depot may cause an underestimation of the amount of pericardial fluid.[56] Another issue is the presence of fat within the heart. Fat can accumulate in a variety of places, but the predominant site tends to be the interatrial septum. Lipomatous hypertrophy of the interatrial septum should be suspected in the presence of a dumb-bell-shaped appearance of the septum with thick echogenic tissue surrounding a thin echo at the level of the fossa ovalis.[57] In addition, an accumulation of fat may simulate a mass.

In the evaluation of the presence of LVH, it is customary to correct left ventricular mass by body surface area, and this is widely done clinically. However, even if indexation of left ventricular mass by body surface area is well adapted in nonobese subjects, evaluation of LVH prevalence in obesity, using a threshold equivalent to the one applied to the nonobese, would underestimate obesity as a predictor of increased left ventricular mass. To avoid this problem, some investigators have proposed that it is preferable to adjust left ventricular mass for height, height$^{2.13}$ or height$^{2.7}$.[58,59] This may reduce the variability in left ventricular mass associated with body size and sex. Of clinical importance, the application of different echocardiographic indexation methods to assess left ventricular mass did not modify the performance of the ECG criteria of Cornell.[50]

It is possible that these indexations may be more adapted for evaluating left ventricular mass in obese persons than is normalization for body surface area or even height.[60,61] Another potential way to normalize the left ventricular mass is with lean body mass.[62] Interestingly, after this indexation, there were no gender differences in left ventricular mass and the relative effects of adiposity and blood pressure on left ventricular mass were of similar amplitude.[62] Undoubtedly, the adiposity status has an impact on heart size, but the best indexation criteria to define LVH after an echocardiographic study in obese individual need to be refined and confirmed.

Nuclear Medicine

Cardiac function can be assessed adequately in severely obese subjects by using nuclear cardiology imaging techniques.[63–65] Because of the obvious limitations, a dipyridamole thallium-201 or technetium-99m perfusion scan may be used instead of exercise testing in very obese patients to evaluate the presence of ischemic heart disease. In spite of the attenuation factor caused by obesity, prolonged transmission scanning with thallium-201 is not required in obese compared with normal-size patients,[66] and triple-head simultaneous emission transmission tomography using technetium-99m is also accurate in obesity.[67]

Cardiac Catheterization

Obese individuals may have several limitations in the catheterization laboratory. The catheterization laboratory table usually does not accommodate subjects weighing more than 160 kg. Moreover, vascular access to the femoral vein and artery may be difficult. The percutaneous radial approach has advantages in very obese patients, in whom the percutaneous femoral technique may be technically difficult and bleeding may be hard to control after catheter removal. Indeed, the frequency of complications with the use of the percutaneous radial technique is very low and should be contemplated when the evaluation of extremely obese individuals is necessary in the catherization laboratory.[68]

OBESITY AND CARDIOVASCULAR DISEASE

Metabolic

VISCERAL OBESITY

Accumulation of intraabdominal (visceral) fat, located in the mesenterium and omentum, is associated with type 2 diabetes mellitus, hypertension, and coronary artery disease (Table 83-1). There is ample evidence to suggest that increased cardiovascular risk is at least partly accounted for by the metabolic and hemodynamic abnormalities associated with excessive abdominal fat distribution.[69] Indeed, disturbances in lipoprotein metabolism and plasma insulin-glucose homeostasis and elevations of blood pressure, which are risk factors for cardiac disease, have been reported in subjects with an excessive deposition of adipose tissue in the abdomen.[17,70] In addition, abdominal distribution of body fat is associated with increased plasma levels of fibrinogen, factor VII, and factor VIIIc coagulant activities and tissue plasminogen activator (TPA) antigen and PAI-1 antigen and activity.[17,70–72] This hypercoagulable state that accompanies excessive central fat deposition also may be associated with left ventricular dysfunction.[72] There is a beneficial impact of weight loss on plasma PAI-1 activity and other hemostatic factors in overweight individuals;[70,71] however, exercise seems to confer no additional benefit of the weight loss regimen on hemostatic factors.[70]

The presence of excess fat in the abdomen in proportion to total body fat is an independent predictor of coronary heart disease (CHD). Waist circumference is positively correlated with abdominal fat content and is the most practical anthropometric measurement for assessing a patient's abdominal fat content.[73] The waist circumference cutoffs lose their incremental predictive power in patients with a BMI ≥ 35 kg/m^2.[2] When obese subjects are matched for their levels of total body fat, subjects with high levels of visceral fat have dyslipidemia.[74] This further implicates visceral fat as a deleterious atherogenic factor.

BLOOD GLUCOSE AND HYPERINSULINEMIA

The increased risk of diabetes mellitus as weight increases has been shown in prospective studies in numerous countries.[75–77] The development of type 2 diabetes has been found to be associated with weight gain after age 18 in both men and women. The relative risk of diabetes increases approximately 25 percent for each additional unit of BMI over 22 kg/m^2.[78] Moreover cross-sectional and longitudinal studies have shown that abdominal obesity is a major risk factor for type 2 diabetes.[69,79,80] There is strong evidence that weight loss reduces blood glucose levels and hemoglobin A_{1c} levels in patients with type 2 diabetes, and it has been reported in three European cohorts (>17,000 men) followed for over 20 years that nondiabetic men with higher blood glucose had a significantly higher risk of death from cardiovascular and coronary heart disease.[81] In addition, it was demonstrated in the Framingham offspring cohort that metabolic factors associated with obesity (overall and central), including hypertension, low levels of high-density lipoprotein (HDL)-cholesterol, and increased levels of triglycerides and insulin, worsen continuously across the spectrum of glucose tolerance.[82] Although BMI increased steadily with increasing glucose intolerance, the association between most other measures of metabolic risk and glycemia was independent of overall obesity and the gradient of increasing risk was similar for nonobese and obese participants.[82,83] Thus, asymptomatic glucose intolerance is not a benign metabolic condition, and features associated with the insulin resistance syndrome should be taken seriously. This is reinforced by the Quebec Cardiovascular Study, which showed that hyperinsulinemia may be an independent risk factor for coronary artery disease.[84] Furthermore, after coronary artery bypass, it was shown after a 5-year follow-up that the components of the insulin resistance syndrome are associated with angiographic progression of atherosclerosis in nongrafted coronary arteries.[85]

DYSLIPIDEMIA

The relation between obesity and altered plasma lipid profile is well established. Generally, increased fasting plasma triglycerides and reduced plasma HDL-cholesterol levels on the average characterize obesity. A BMI change of 1 unit is associated with an HDL-cholesterol change of 1.1 mg/dL for young adult men and an HDL-cholesterol change of 0.69 mg/dL for young adult women.[2] Plasma cholesterol and low-density lipoprotein (LDL)-cholesterol levels may be elevated marginally, but the number of apoprotein B–carrying lipoproteins usually is increased.[74] However, a remarkable metabolic heterogeneity is observed among obese subjects, and the presence of visceral obesity worsens the lipid profile. The lipid profile associated with abdominal obesity, high triglycerides, low HDL-cholesterol, elevated apolipoprotein B levels, and an increased proportion of small dense LDL probably is the main contributor to the increase in CHD in this subgroup of obese patients.[74] There is evidence that weight loss produced by lifestyle modifications in overweight individuals is accompanied by reductions in serum triglycerides and increases in HDL-cholesterol.[86] Weight loss occasionally produces some reductions in serum total cholesterol and LDL-cholesterol levels.[87] Moreover, improvement in the lipid profile through the use of aerobic exercise in subjects with type 2 diabetes may be mediated through fat loss.[88]

Structural

CORONARY ARTERY DISEASE

Obesity may be an independent risk factor for ischemic heart disease. However, numerous studies have not been able to confirm this because of the short time period of observation. Indeed, the association between obesity and ischemic heart disease seems evident only after two decades of follow-up.[6] This relation was also stronger in younger individuals.[5,6] A high BMI was significantly associated with the development of myocardial infarction, coronary insufficiency, and sudden death, and among those adverse events, the association was strongest with sudden death.[6] In the Nurses Health Study, weight gains of 5 to 8 kg increased CHD risk (nonfatal myocardial infarction and CHD death) 25 percent and weight gains of ≥ 20 kg increased that risk more than 2.5 times in comparison with women whose weight was stable within a range of 5 kg.[89] In British men, an increase of 1 BMI unit was associated with a 10 percent increase in the rate of coronary events.[90] Although, obesity per se is considered a major modifiable risk factor for ischemic heart disease,[8] it is important to remember that overweight individuals present a cluster of other traditional and nontraditional risk factors, i.e., dyslipidemia, hypertension, type 2 diabetes mellitus, the prothrombotic state, hyperinsulinemia, hypertriglyceridemia, and elevated apolipoprotein B, that are all potentially deleterious. In the ECAT angina pectoris study, there was a strong relation between obesity and the fibrinolytic system even after adjusting for total triglycerides, cholesterol, age, and sex.[91] Thus, the detrimental impact of overweight/obesity as a risk factor for ischemic heart disease involves multiple mechanisms that accompany the obese state.

HYPERTENSION

The majority of patients with high blood pressure are overweight, and hypertension is about six times more common in obese than it is in lean subjects.[92] Not only is hypertension more common in obese subjects, weight gain in young people is an important risk factor for the subsequent development of hypertension. A 10-kg higher body weight is associated with a 3.0 mmHg higher systolic and a 2.3 mmHg higher diastolic blood pressure. These increases translate into an estimated 12 percent increase in risk for CHD and a 24 percent increase in risk for stroke.[2]

In the Framingham Heart Study, obesity was significantly correlated with increased left ventricular mass,[93] and it has been shown that a 10 percent reduction in weight in obese hypertensive patients not only reduced blood pressure but also decreased left ventricular wall thickness and left ventricular mass.[94] The effect on left ventricular mass was seen in both hypertensive[94] and nonhypertensive patients.[51] Moreover, it has been shown that weight reduction using modest amounts of exercise and a hypocaloric intake decreases left ventricular mass regardless of blood pressure level in obese subjects.[95] There is strong and consistent evidence from lifestyle trials in overweight hypertensive and nonhypertensive patients that weight loss produced by lifestyle modifications reduces blood pressure levels. Weight reduction is one of the rare antihypertensive strategies that decrease blood pressure in normotensive as well as hypertensive persons.[2,96]

Some investigators have suggested that reductions in blood pressure are attributable to reductions in salt intake concomitant with caloric restriction, but it has been established that reductions in blood pressure do not necessarily result from the reduction in salt intake.[95,97] Although the pathophysiologic mechanisms in the lowering of blood pressure with weight loss are not clear, numerous factors probably are involved. The reduction in blood pressure also could be attributable to reductions in total circulating and cardiopulmonary blood volume as well as reductions in sympathetic nervous system activity.[97] The reduction in plasma catecholamines and plasma renin activity that is associated with decreased sympathetic activity, also probably plays a role.[98,99]

Although both normotensive and hypertensive individuals have elevated cardiac output and blood volume compared with nonobese subjects,[100] normotensive obese patients have diminished vascular resistance whereas hypertensive obese patients have normal vascular resistance. However, estimates of cardiac output could be misleading in obesity. Cardiac output probably is better expressed in actual values rather than being related to body surface area (cardiac index) because when cardiac output (rather than cardiac index) is used to calculate total peripheral resistance, it is often normal or reduced in hypertensive obese patients.[101,102] Therefore, peripheral resistance and intravascular volume may be normal in mildly hypertensive obese patients because of the mutually opposing effects of the increase in arterial pressure and the increase in body weight.

LEFT VENTRICULAR DIASTOLIC DYSFUNCTION

A longer duration of obesity is associated with higher left ventricular mass, poorer left ventricular systolic function, and greater impairment of left ventricular diastolic function.[103] Obese subjects often present with abnormal left ventricular diastolic filling with a greater peak atrial velocity and a longer late diastolic flow time compared with nonobese subjects.[27] It has been shown by echocardiography that the eccentric left ventricular hypertrophy in obese subjects causes an abnormal left ventricular diastolic filling pattern similar to concentric left ventricular hypertrophy of hypertension. However, the increased intravascular volume in obesity may mask the Doppler-derived abnormalities of diastolic filling. It is interesting to note that the abnormal filling patterns seen in obese subjects are present despite hemodynamics that are unfavorable for detection.

Left ventricular diastolic dysfunction and increased left ventricular mass may be attributable to a disproportionate accumulation of collagen in the interstitial space of the hypertrophied left ventricle, a consequence that is secondary to pressure overload. However, in normotensive obese persons, the increase in left ventricular mass is not always accompanied by myocardial fibrosis,[104] and normal diastolic function is commonly found.[53] In addition, it was reported that only obese subjects with increased left ventricular mass appeared to have impaired left ventricular diastolic dysfunction, and that group of subjects had improvements in left ventricular function after weight lost.[53,105] Substantial weight loss may improve the abnormal pattern of ventricular filling and increased left ventricular dimension in diastole.[53] In another study involving hypertensive obese subjects, weight loss was associated with a greater decrease in ventricular and posterior wall thickness and left ventricular mass than was seen in subjects treated with metoprolol, suggesting that changes in weight, independent of changes in blood pressure, were directly associated with changes in left ventricular mass.[94]

LEFT VENTRICULAR HYPERTROPHY AND CONGESTIVE HEART FAILURE

As was stated previously, cardiac adaptation to obesity results in cardiac hypertrophy of the concentric[106,107] or eccentric type.[108] Pathologically, there is a proportionality between heart weight and body weight[106,109] (Fig. 83-2), and echocardiographic studies have shown that left ventricular end-diastolic dimension and septal and posterior wall dimensions are greater in obese subjects.[27] Possible explanations are that the reduction in left ventricular mass may be secondary to the reduction in blood pressure associated with weight loss or simply to the reduction in body weight. Indeed, 14 to 25 percent of the reduction in left ventricular mass could be explained by the change in body weight.[94,95] Work by Messerli and associates[108] suggests that the

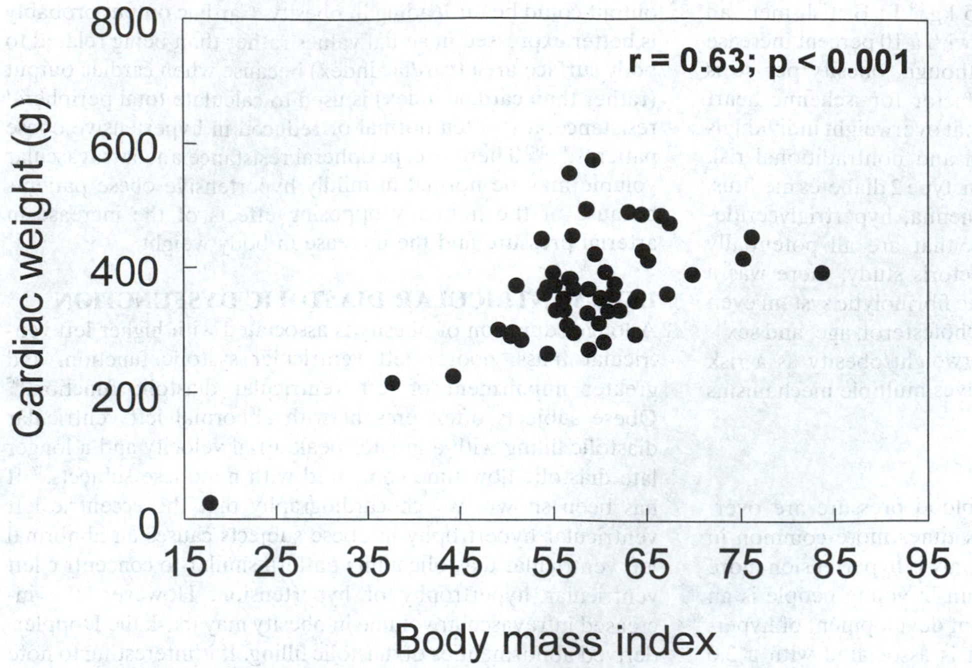

FIGURE 83-2 Relation between cardiac weight (g) and body mass index (BMI) from autopsies of 52 cases of obesity without demonstrable evidence of heart disease. (Adapted from Smith and Willius.[109])

combination of obesity and hypertension results in myocardial hypertrophy with left ventricular dilatation. Premature ventricular complex increases with body weight and is 30 times higher in obese patients with eccentric left ventricular hypertrophy than it is in lean subjects.[23] This could be one of the mechanisms that explain the importance of left ventricular hypertrophy as a parameter associated with cardiac morbidity and mortality in this population. Of note, the combination of obesity and hypertension burdens the heart with high preload and high afterload, greatly enhancing the risk of congestive heart failure. Sympathetic mechanisms have been implicated in the development of LVH,[48] and weight reduction in obese subjects reduces indexes of sympathetic activity such as plasma norepinephrine, urinary norepinephrine excretion, and resting heart rate. The renin-angiotensin system also may be involved in the pathogenesis of LVH, and weight reduction may decrease plasma renin activity and aldosterone levels.[98] The improvement in hyperinsulinemia also may contribute to the reduction in left ventricular mass in hypertensive obese subjects, since insulin resistance is an important independent contributing factor to left ventricular mass in normotensive nondiabetic obese subjects.[110] Nevertheless, the role of all these neurohumoral factors in the regression of cardiac hypertrophy associated with weight reduction merits further investigation.

OBSTRUCTIVE SLEEP APNEA, HYPOVENTILATION, PULMONARY HYPERTENSION, RIGHT VENTRICULAR FAILURE

There are numerous respiratory complications of obesity, including an increased breathing workload, respiratory muscle inefficiency, decreased functional reserve capacity and expiratory reserve volume, and closure of peripheral lung units. These complications often result in a ventilation-perfusion mismatch, especially in the supine position. Obesity is a classic cause of alveolar hypoventilation. Historically, the obesity-hypoventilation syndrome has been described as the "pickwickian" syndrome, and obstructive apnea was first observed in patients with severe obesity. Sleep apnea is defined as repeated episodes of obstructive apnea and hypopnea during sleep, together with daytime somnolence and/or altered cardiopulmonary function.[111] The prevalence of sleep-disordered breathing and sleep disturbances rises dramatically in obese subjects,[112] and obesity is by far the most important modifiable risk factor in sleep-disordered breathing.[113,114] It has been estimated that 40 million Americans suffer from sleep disorders and that the vast majority of these patients remain undiagnosed.[113,114]

Despite careful screening by history and physical examination, sleep apnea is revealed only by polysomnography in most patients.[115] Although, some clinical features could be useful in screening for sleep apnea, the diagnostic accuracy is inadequate.[116]

Patients with sleep apnea have an increased risk of diurnal hypertension, nocturnal dysrhythmias, pulmonary hypertension, right and left ventricular failure, myocardial infarction, stroke, and mortality.[117] The prevalence of pulmonary hypertension in subjects with obstructive sleep apnea is 15 to 20 percent; however, pulmonary hypertension rarely is observed in the absence of daytime hypoxemia.[118,119] According to Kessler and colleagues,[118] the extent of pulmonary hypertension in patients with obstructive sleep apnea is generally mild to moderate (pulmonary artery pressures ranging between 20 and 35 mmHg) and does not necessitate specific treatment.

Although there is a link between sleep apnea and systemic hypertension, the association of obesity with both disorders confounds the relationship. A physician who evaluates an obese patient who has been referred for hypertension should address related symptoms such as habitual snoring, nocturnal gasping or choking, witnessed episodes of apnea, and daytime sleepiness.[113,114,120] It is important to remember, however, that the clinical and ECG signs of cor pulmonale appear later than do those of pulmonary hypertension (assessed by right heart catheterization). Numerous treatments are available for sleep apnea, but weight loss in obese patients should always be advocated.[111]

AUTONOMIC NERVOUS SYSTEM ACTIVITY

The autonomic nervous system, an important contributor to the regulation of both the cardiovascular system and energy expenditure, is assumed to play a role in the pathophysiology of obesity and related complications.[121] Numerous techniques, e.g., heart rate variability, microneurography, and catecholamine turnover, have been used to examine the variation in the autonomic nervous system induced by diet and weight change in humans. However, the exact role of the sympathetic and parasympathetic nervous systems in obesity and weight loss is unclear. According to Peterson and coworkers,[121] both parasympathetic activity and sympathetic activity decrease as the percentage of body fat increases. This is in contrast to the findings of others who have used more invasive techniques to demonstrate that obesity is associated with predominantly sympathetic activation.[122] A 10 percent increase in body weight is associated with a decline in parasympathetic tone accompanied by a rise in mean heart rate, but heart rate declines during weight reduction.[123] Such reductions in vagal activity with increments in weight may be one mechanism for the arrhythmia and other cardiac abnormalities that accompany obesity. Discrepancies between studies of the impact of the autonomic nervous system in obesity can be explained in part by the techniques used to evaluate that system.[124] In addition, confounding conditions such as obstructive sleep apnea may be important.[114] In sleep apnea patients, sympathetic activity is increased,[115,125] and using microneurography, obesity per se (in the absence of obstructive sleep apnea) was not accompanied by increased sympathetic activity.[115]

ARRHYTHMIA, SUDDEN DEATH, AND QT INTERVAL

Hippocrates presumably stated, "Sudden death is more common in those who are naturally fat than in the lean." Obese subjects, even without dieting, have an increased risk of arrhythmias and sudden death in the absence of cardiac dysfunction.[23,126] In the Framingham study, the risk of sudden cardiac death with increasing weight was seen in both sexes.[6] Hence, the annual sudden cardiac mortality rate in obese men and women has been estimated to be 65 per 100,000 patients, about 40 times higher than the rate of unexplained cardiac arrest in a matched nonobese population.[127] In severely obese men age 25 to 34 years, a 12-fold excess mortality rate was seen, whereas in men age 35 to 44 years, a substantial risk with a sixfold excess mortality rate was demonstrated.[3]

Prolongation of the QTc interval is a risk factor for ventricular arrhythmias and sudden death. Importantly, there is a correlation between BMI and QTc, with longer intervals observed in obese subjects.[128] The relation between fatness and the QTc interval persisted even after absolute QT intervals were adjusted for heart rate using different formulas (Bazett, Framingham, Fridericia) and by multiple regression analysis.[128] Therefore, a prolonged QT interval is observed in a relatively high percentage of obese subjects, and the association between abnormal QTc and BMI is most evident in the severely obese.[40,128] Weight loss through starvation,[37,39] liquid protein diets,[43,44] very low calorie diets, or even obesity surgery[107] can be associated with prolongation of the QTc interval. To some extent, this occurs irrespective of the biological value of the constituent protein or the addition of mineral and trace supplements.[43] In addition, it has been shown that liquid protein diets frequently are associated with potentially life-threatening arrhythmias, a relationship documented by 24-h Holter recording but not in a study using routine ECG.[129] Ventricular tachycardia (torsades de pointes) and fibrillation often have been documented in subjects who died under observation.[43,130] Drug treatment with lidocaine, propranolol, phenytoin, mexiletine, disopyramide, and procainamide is usually ineffective.[37,43] Infusion of potassium, calcium, magnesium, bicarbonate, or glucagon and even ventricular overdrive pacing or open chest cardiac massage are ineffective in controlling the refractory arrhythmia.[43,107,130]

ECG changes in the course of weight loss in obese patients appear to be common. However, histologic findings in the hearts of those dying while ingesting liquid modified protein diets and a group of cachectic patients dying from malignant disease were similar[44] despite a lack of ECG abnormalities in the latter and QT prolongation in the former. Thus, the underlying mechanism and, in particular, the clinical significance of obesity-associated QT prolongation remain speculative. Also, a variety of arrhythmogenic factors have been implicated; acute heart failure with stretching of the myocardium that decreases the electric threshold in myocytes and facilitates spontaneous depolarization, myocyte hypertrophy, and multiple intercalated disks may facilitate the current flow and cause reentrant arrhythmias, and increased myocardial oxygen demand and impaired vasodilatory reserve may cause acute myocardial ischemia in the absence of coronary artery disease. Fatty infiltration of the myocardium is unlikely to be involved in the majority of cases. Because extremely obese patients often have a dilated cardiomyopathy, fatal arrhythmias may be the most common cause of death in those patients.[23,108]

CARDIAC SURGERY

Health care professionals often cite obesity as a risk factor for perioperative morbidity and mortality. The presence of hypertension, coronary artery disease, dyslipidemia, and type 2 diabetes mellitus and the technical difficulties inherent in the surgical and postsurgical care of the obese patients probably contribute to this perception. In contrast, obesity is not associated with increased mortality or postoperative cerebrovascular accidents after coronary artery bypass surgery.[131] However, sternal wound infection is increased in obese patients.[131] The large and poorly vascularized panniculus, the higher incidence of hyperglycemia in the obese, and the difficulty in wound surveillance may predispose to wound infections.[131]

Obesity also has been identified as a risk factor for superficial wound infection, saphenous vein harvest site infection, and atrial dysrhythmias.[132] These complications increase with increasing BMI. In accordance, obesity (defined by a BMI $>30\ kg/m^2$) was not associated with an increase risk of operative mortality, stroke, renal failure, acquired respiratory distress syndrome, prolonged mechanical ventilation, pneumonia, sepsis, pulmonary embolism, or ventricular arrhythmias.[132] In contrast to other findings, the risk of mediastinitis was not increased.[131] Strangely, despite well-documented alterations in respiratory physiology in obese patients, pulmonary complications were comparable to those seen in nonobese patients.[131,132] Obese patients have been shown to have a higher incidence of postoperative thromboembolic disease in noncardiac surgery.[133] The discrepancy between these results may reflect different treatment attitudes in the postoperative period, with more vigorous pulmonary cleansing being performed by the nursing staff or more vigilance being taken in enforcing postoperative use of incentive spirometry and early ambulation in patients undergoing cardiac surgery. Nevertheless, the high risk of thromboembolic disease in obese patients may warrant an aggressive approach to deep venous thrombosis prophylaxis.[133] Although major unanticipated problems with ventilation are relatively rare in the postanesthesia period, obesity is a risk factor for this complication.[134]

VASCULAR ACCESS

Poor peripheral venous access in obese patients may necessitate more frequent use of central venous lines. A short stubby neck, loss of physical landmarks, and a greater skin–blood vessel distance make internal jugular and subclavian vein cannulation in the coronary care unit technically more difficult.[133] This could result in multiple skin punctures and a higher incidence of catheter malpositioning. Femoral access may not be possible not only because of the volume of adipose tissue but also because of the presence of intertrigo.

CARDIOMYOPATHY OF OBESITY (ADIPOSITAS CORDIS)

Cardiomyopathy associated with obesity without evidence of other heart disease was recognized as early as 1818.[34] This case is of historical interest not only because it is a carefully recorded documentation of a fatty heart but also because it was the first reported case in which a specific type of respiration, now recognized as Cheyne-Stokes respiration, was described.[34] Subsequently, Smith and Willius[109] described excess epicardial fat and fatty infiltration of the myocardium in the hearts of obese subjects that might have interfered with cardiac function. Other groups have demonstrated the same findings showing increased fat in the atrioventricular sulci and the atrial septum.[135] Characteristically, the thickness of the atrial septum is increased (lipomatous hypertrophy). Of interest, myocardial fatty infiltration also has been described without a relationship to obesity.[136]

Myocardial fat infiltration is an uncommon autopsy finding, with an incidence of approximately 3 percent.[137] This condition is more prevalent in women.[137,138] The presence of excess adipose tissue on the surface of the right ventricle represents an exaggeration of the normal architecture. Thus, at least at first, the fatty heart is probably not an infiltrative process but most likely a metaplastic phenomenon.

With time, fat can infiltrate between muscle fibers and/or result in myocyte degeneration. With progressive disease, fatty heart can result in cardiac conduction defects.[139,140] Associated with fat infiltration of the right ventricle, there can be extensive fatty replacement of the sinus node musculature and, to a lesser degree, infiltration of the atrioventricular node and the right bundle branch[139] while the entire myocardium of the atrioventricular region is replaced by fat.[140] Fatty heart also can result in a restrictive cardiomyopathy.[136,141] Here, small irregular aggregates and bands of adipose tissue separate myocardial cells. The fibers often are reduced in diameter, presumably as a result of pressure-induced atrophy from the intervening fat.[141] In general, the right ventricle is more likely to be involved than is the left ventricle and the anterior wall is involved to a greater extent than is the posterior wall. Most of the time, cardiac hypertrophy is a direct reflection of BMI and the hypertrophy results from myocyte change, not from excessive fat infiltration or fibrosis.[104]

TREATMENT

The general goals of weight loss and management are at a minimum to prevent further weight gain, reduce body weight, and maintain a lower body weight indefinitely. Patients should have their BMI and levels of abdominal fat measured with the goal of weight reduction established to favorably affect outcomes, including cardiovascular health. Obesity management and treatment include counseling,[96] diet,[142] exercise,[142,143] drugs,[144] and surgery.[145]

Lifestyle Modifications

BEHAVIORAL

Behavioral strategies to reinforce changes in diet and physical activity in obese adults can produce weight loss in the range of 10 percent over a period of 6 months.[96] Although no single behaviorial therapy appears superior to any other in general, a combination of strategies appears to work best and interventions with the greatest intensity appear to be associated with the greatest benefit. Weight loss programs that result in slow but steady weight reduction, e.g., 1 to 2 lb/week, may be more effective than are those which result in rapid weight loss.[146] Long-term follow-up results in patients undergoing behavior therapy show a return to baseline weight for the majority of subjects in the absence of continued behavior intervention.[147–149] In obese patients who smoke, smoking cessation is mandatory. However, a major obstacle to cessation has been the attendant weight gain observed in about 80 percent of quitters.[150–152] Weight gain that accompanies smoking cessation has been quite resistant to most dietary, behavioral, and physical activity interventions. Importantly, the weight gain with smoking cessation is less likely to produce negative health consequences than is continued smoking.[96]

DIET

Weight reduction depends on an energy intake less than it does on energy expenditure. Here, energy density of the diet is important. In general, foods high in fat (9 kcal/g) and sugar are energy-dense. Thus, diets for weight reduction should be restricted not only in total calories but also in fat and sugar. Approximately 1 lb per week can be lost with no change in physical activity if 500 kcal/day is eliminated. Such diets would continue to include foods that are low in saturated fat and cholesterol but enriched in nutrients that are associated with a reduced risk for cardiovascular disease, e.g., fruits, vegetables, legumes, and whole-grain products.[153] Although diets high in fat and protein have become popular, there is concern about the long-term efficacy and safety of these diets. Unquestionably, weight reduction occurs and can be rapid on such carbohydrate-restricted diets.[154] Nevertheless, no evidence suggests that these diets are any more effective than are fat-restricted diets months to years after intervention, and some of these diets raise questions about enhanced atherogenesis and renal and skeletal complications if they are sustained.

EXERCISE

Aerobic exercise alone produces a modest weight reduction, generally 2 to 3 percent; however, it is extremely important to sustain the weight-reduced state.[155–157] Fat loss through dieting and/or exercise produces comparable and favorable changes in HDL-cholesterol and its subfractions HDL_2 and HDL_3 and triglycerides.[86,142] Furthermore, long-term aerobic exercise training can normalize the metabolic profile of obese subjects even if those subjects remain very obese at the end of the program (41 percent of body fat).[143] Even if weight loss is minimal, physically fit obese individuals are less prone to mortality from cardiovascular disease than are lean subjects who are not physically fit.[158] Initially, moderate levels of physical activity for 30 to 45 min, 3 to 5 days a week, should be encouraged. Thereafter, all adults should set a long-term goal of doing 30 min or more of moderate-intensity physical activity on most, and preferably all, days of the week.[159]

A combined intervention of behavior therapy, a low-calorie diet, and increased physical activity provides the most successful therapy for weight loss and weight maintenance. In overweight/obese patients who are psychologically ready for weight loss, this approach should be emphasized and sustained for at least 6 months before pharmacotherapy is considered.

Drugs

Weight loss drugs can be useful adjuncts to dietary therapy and physical activity for some patients, i.e., those with a BMI ≥30 kg/m^2 with or without concomitant comorbidities, and for patients with a BMI ≥27 kg/m^2 with concomitant risk factors or diseases.[2,96] The comorbidities considered sufficiently important to warrant pharmacotherapy at a BMI of 27 to 29.9 kg/m^2 are hypertension (≥140/90 mmHg), dyslipidemia (LDL ≥160 mg/dl, HDL <35 mg/dL), coronary artery disease, type 2 diabetes, and obstructive sleep apnea.[2,96] The two main categories of obesity drugs are anorectics that act centrally in the brain on adrenergic or serotonergic pathways and nutrient absorption inhibitors that decrease macronutrient absorption from the gastrointestinal tract.

Fenfluramine and dexfenfluramine, which reduce appetite by enhancing serotonin at nerve terminals in the hypothalamus, were removed from the marketplace in the United States after reports of cardiac valve disorders,[160] particularly aortic and mitral insufficiency. An increased risk of primary pulmonary hypertension also was associated with these agents.[161–164] The valvular abnormalities produced by fenfluramine and dexfenfluramine were histopathologically similar to those noted in patients with the carcinoid syndrome.[165,166] Of importance, the development of valvulopathy was correlated with the duration of exposure.[167] There were no cases reported of cardiac valve abnormalities associated with the use of phentermine alone,[168] and regression of valvular disease after the cessation of fenfluramine or dexfenfluramine is possible.[169] Unlike fenfluramine or dexfenfluramine, phentermine is a sympathomimetic drug that reduces food intake through its effects on adrenergic receptors in the hypothalamus.

Sibutramine hydrochloride promotes a sense of satiety by blocking the reuptake of both norepinephrine and serotonin in nerve terminals. Sibutramine also has a moderate effect on energy expenditure by attenuating the decrease in energy output during rest.[170] This drug has been approved for long-term use. It has limited but definite effects on weight loss and can facilitate weight loss maintenance.[170] In one study, the prevalence of cardiac valve dysfunction was not increased in 133 obese patients who were treated with sibutramine for an average of 7.6 months.[171] Increases in blood pressure and heart rate may occur with the use of this drug.[144] Like phentermine, sibutramine should not be used in patients with untreated hypertension, coronary heart disease, congestive heart failure, arrhythmias, or stroke.[170]

Orlistat reduces the absorption of dietary fat (approximately 30 percent reduction) by binding to pancreatic lipase in the intestinal lumen and inhibiting its action. Orlistat has an advantage over drugs that act on the central nervous system because it is not absorbed.[144,172] The major side effect is symptoms associated with steatorrhea. With long-term use, fat-soluble vitamins may need to be replaced.[173]

Surgery

Weight loss surgery that includes gastric plication and gastric bypass with a Roux-en-Y anastomosis is an option in a limited number of patients with extreme obesity, i.e., BMI ≥40 kg/m^2 or BMI ≥35 kg/m^2, with comorbid conditions. [2] Weight loss surgery should be reserved for patients who have extreme obesity in whom efforts at medical therapy have failed. An acceptable operative risk also must be present. Furthermore, lifelong medical surveillance after surgery is necessary.

CONCLUSIONS

Obesity is a chronic metabolic disorder that is associated with cardiovascular disease and increased morbidity and mortality. When the BMI is ≥30 kg/m^2, mortality rates from all causes, especially cardiovascular disease, are increased 50 to 100 percent. There is strong evidence that weight loss in overweight and obese individuals reduces risk factors for diabetes and cardiovascular disease. Additional evidence indicates that weight loss and the associated diuresis reduce blood pressure in overweight hypertensive and nonhypertensive individuals, reduce serum triglyceride levels, and increase high-density lipoprotein cholesterol (HDL-C) levels, and may produce some reduction in low-density lipoprotein cholesterol (LDL-C) levels. Weight loss also reduces blood glucose levels and hemoglobin A_{1c} levels in patients with type 2 diabetes, signs and symptoms of left ventricular failure, and obstructive sleep apnea. Although no prospective trials have convincingly shown changes in mortality with weight loss in obese patients, reductions in risk factors at least would predict a reduced incidence of cardiovascular disease and perhaps cardiovascular disease–related mortality.

References

1. Calle EE, Thun MJ, Petrelli JM, et al. Body-mass index and mortality in a prospective cohort of U.S. adults. *N Engl J Med* 1999; 341:1097–1105.
2. Clinical Guidelines on the Identification, Evaluation, and Treatment of Overweight and Obesity in Adults—The Evidence Report: National Institutes of Health. *Obes Res* 1998; (suppl 2):51S–209S.
3. Drenick EJ, Bale GS, Seltzer F, Johnson DG. Excessive mortality and causes of death in morbidly obese men. *JAMA* 1980; 243:443–445.
4. Vanltallie TB. Prevalence of obesity. *Endocrinol Metab Clin North Am* 1996; 25:887–905.
5. Hubert HB, Feinleib M, McNamara PM, Castelli WP. Obesity as an independent risk factor for cardiovascular disease: A 26-year follow-up of participants in the Framingham Heart Study. *Circulation* 1983; 67:968–977.
6. Rabkin SW, Mathewson FA, Hsu PH. Relation of body weight to development of ischemic heart disease in a cohort of young North American men after a 26 year observation period: The Manitoba Study. *Am J Cardiol* 1977; 39:452–458.
7. Eckel RH. Obesity and heart disease: A statement for healthcare

professionals from the Nutrition Committee, American Heart Association. *Circulation* 1997; 96:3248–3250.
8. Eckel RH, Krauss RM. American Heart Association call to action: Obesity as a major risk factor for coronary heart disease: AHA Nutrition Committee. *Circulation* 1998; 97:2099–2100.
9. Bouchard C, Després JP, Mauriège P. Genetic and nongenetic determinants of regional fat distribution. *Endocr Rev* 1993; 14:72–93.
10. Bray GA, Bouchard C, James WPT. *Handbook of Obesity*. New York: Marcel Dekker; 1998:31.
11. Yudkin JS, Stehouwer CD, Emeis JJ, Coppack SW. C-reactive protein in healthy subjects: Associations with obesity, insulin resistance, and endothelial dysfunction: A potential role for cytokines originating from adipose tissue? *Arterioscler Thromb Vasc Biol* 1999; 19:972–978.
12. Mohamed-Ali V, Goodrick S, Rawesh A, et al. Subcutaneous adipose tissue releases interleukin-6, but not tumor necrosis factor-alpha, in vivo. *J Clin Endocrinol Metab* 1997; 82:4196–4200.
13. Ridker PM. Novel risk factors and markers for coronary disease. *Adv Intern Med* 2000; 45:391–418
14. Kern PA, Saghizadeh M, Ong JM, et al. The expression of tumor necrosis factor in human adipose tissue: Regulation by obesity, weight loss, and relationship to lipoprotein lipase. *J Clin Invest* 1995; 95:2111–2119.
15. Hotamisligil GS, Arner P, Caro JF, et al. Increased adipose tissue expression of tumor necrosis factor-alpha in human obesity and insulin resistance. *J Clin Invest* 1995; 95:2409–2415.
16. Lundgren CH, Brown SL, Nordt TK, et al. Elaboration of type-1 plasminogen activator inhibitor from adipocytes: A potential pathogenetic link between obesity and cardiovascular disease. *Circulation* 1996; 93:106–110.
17. Cigolini M, Targher G, Bergamo AI, et al. Visceral fat accumulation and its relation to plasma hemostatic factors in healthy men. *Arterioscler Thromb Vasc Biol* 1996; 16:368–374.
18. Rosell S, Belfrage E. Blood circulation in adipose tissue. *Physiol Rev* 1979; 59:1078–1104.
19. Larsen OA, Lassen NA, Quaade F. Blood flow through human adipose tissue determined with radioactive xenon. *Acta Physiol Scand* 1966; 66:337–345.
20. Lesser GT, Deutsch S. Measurement of adipose tissue blood flow and perfusion in man by uptake of 85Kr. *J Appl Physiol* 1967; 23:621–630.
21. Oberg B, Rosell S. Sympathetic control of consecutive vascular sections in canine subcutaneous adipose tissue. *Acta Physiol Scand* 1967; 71:47–56.
22. Linde B, Chisolm G. The interstitial space of adipose tissue as determined by single injection and equilibration techniques. *Acta Physiol Scand* 1975; 95:383–390.
23. Messerli FH, Nunez BD, Ventura HO, Snyder DW. Overweight and sudden death: Increased ventricular ectopy in cardiopathy of obesity. *Arch Intern Med* 1987; 147:1725–1728.
24. Kaltman AJ, Goldring RM. Role of circulatory congestion in the cardiorespiratory failure of obesity. *Am J Med* 1976; 60:645–653.
25. Alexander JK, Dennis EW, Smith WG, et al. Blood volume, cardiac output, and distribution of systemic blood flow in extreme obesity. *Cardiovasc Res Cent Bull* 1963; 1:39–44.
26. Messerli FH. Cardiopathy of obesity—A not-so-Victorian disease. *N Engl J Med* 1986; 314:378–380.
27. Ku CS, Lin SL, Wang DJ, et al. Left ventricular filling in young normotensive obese adults. *Am J Cardiol* 1994; 73:613–615.
28. Sasson Z, Rasooly Y, Gupta R, Rasooly I. Left atrial enlargement in healthy obese: Prevalence and relation to left ventricular mass and diastolic function. *Can J Cardiol* 1996; 12:257–263.
29. Backman L, Freyschuss U, Hallberg D, Melcher A. Reversibility of cardiovascular changes in extreme obesity: Effects of weight reduction through jejunoileostomy. *Acta Med Scand* 1979; 205:367–373.
30. Backman L, Freyschuss U, Hallberg D, Melcher A. Cardiovascular function in extreme obesity. *Acta Med Scand* 1973; 193: 437–446.
31. Alexander JK, Peterson KL. Cardiovascular effects of weight reduction. *Circulation* 1972; 45:310–318.
32. De Divitiis O, Fazio S, Petitto M, et al. Obesity and cardiac function. *Circulation* 1981; 64:477–482.
33. Nakajima T, Fujioka S, Tokunaga K, et al. Correlation of intraabdominal fat accumulation and left ventricular performance in obesity. *Am J Cardiol* 1989; 64:369–373.
34. Cheyne J. A case of apoplexy in which the fleshy part of the heart was converted into fat. *Dublin Hosp Rep* 1818; 2:216–223.
35. Maxwell MH, Waks AU, Schroth PC, et al. Error in blood-pressure measurement due to incorrect cuff size in obese patients. *Lancet* 1982; 2:33–36.
36. Nelson WP, North RL. Splitting of the second heart sound in adults forty years and older. *Am J Med Sci* 1967; 254:805–807.
37. Pringle TH, Scobie IN, Murray RG, et al. Prolongation of the QT interval during therapeutic starvation: A substrate for malignant arrhythmias. *Int J Obes* 1983; 7:253–261.
38. Sandhofer F, Dienstl F, Bolzano K, Schwingshackl H. Severe cardiovascular complication associated with prolonged starvation. *Br Med J* 1973; 1:462–463.
39. Garnett ES, Barnard DL, Ford J, et al. Gross fragmentation of cardiac myofibrils after therapeutic starvation for obesity. *Lancet* 1969; 1:914–916.
40. Rasmussen LH, Andersen T. The relationship between QTc changes and nutrition during weight loss after gastroplasty. *Acta Med Scand* 1985; 217:271–275.
41. Pidlich J, Pfeffel F, Zwiauer K, et al. The effect of weight reduction on the surface electrocardiogram: A prospective trial in obese children and adolescents. *Int J Obes Relat Metab Disord* 1997; 21:1018–1023.
42. Eisenstein I, Edelstein J, Sarma R, et al. The electrocardiogram in obesity. *J Electrocardiol* 1982; 15:115–118.
43. Sours HE, Frattali VP, Brand CD, et al. Sudden death associated with very low calorie weight reduction regimens. *Am J Clin Nutr* 1981; 34:453–461.
44. Isner JM, Sours HE, Paris AL, et al. Sudden, unexpected death in avid dieters using the liquid-protein-modified-fast diet: Observations in 17 patients and the role of the prolonged QT interval. *Circulation* 1979; 60:1401–1412.
45. Frank S, Colliver JA, Frank A. The electrocardiogram in obesity: Statistical analysis of 1,029 patients. *J Am Coll Cardiol* 1986; 7:295–299.
46. Starr JW, Wagner GS, Behar VS, et al. Vectorcardiographic criteria for the diagnosis of inferior myocardial infarction. *Circulation* 1974; 49:829–836.
47. Master AM, Oppenheimer ET. A study of obesity: Circulatory, roentgen-ray and electrocardiographic investigations. *JAMA* 1929; 92:1652–1656.
48. Benjamin EJ, Levy D. Why is left ventricular hypertrophy so predictive of morbidity and mortality? *Am J Med Sci* 1999; 317:168–175.
49. Casale PN, Devereux RB, Kligfield P, et al. Electrocardiographic detection of left ventricular hypertrophy: Development and prospective validation of improved criteria. *J Am Coll Cardiol* 1985; 6:572–580.
50. Abergel E, Tase M, Menard J, Chatellier G. Influence of obesity on the diagnostic value of electrocardiographic criteria for detecting left ventricular hypertrophy. *Am J Cardiol* 1996; 77: 739–744.
51. Alpert MA, Lambert CR, Terry BE, et al. Effect of weight loss on left ventricular mass in nonhypertensive morbidly obese patients. *Am J Cardiol* 1994; 73:918–921.
52. Chakko S, Mayor M, Allison MD, et al. Abnormal left ventricular

diastolic filling in eccentric left ventricular hypertrophy of obesity. *Am J Cardiol* 1991; 68:95–98.

53. Alpert MA, Lambert CR, Terry BE, et al. Effect of weight loss on left ventricular diastolic filling in morbid obesity. *Am J Cardiol* 1995; 76:1198–1201.
54. Rakowski H, Appleton C, Chan KL, et al. Canadian consensus recommendations for the measurement and reporting of diastolic dysfunction by echocardiography: From the Investigators of Consensus on Diastolic Dysfunction by Echocardiography. *J Am Soc Echocardiogr* 1996; 9:736–760.
55. Dumesnil JG, Gaudreault G, Honos GN, Kingma JG Jr. Use of Valsalva maneuver to unmask left ventricular diastolic function abnormalities by Doppler echocardiography in patients with coronary artery disease or systemic hypertension. *Am J Cardiol* 1991; 68:515–519.
56. House AA, Walley VM. Right heart failure due to ventricular adiposity: "Adipositas cordis"—An old diagnosis revisited. *Can J Cardiol* 1996; 12:485–489.
57. Jornet A, Batalla J, Uson M, et al. Lipomatous hypertrophy of the interatrial septum. *Echocardiography* 1992; 9:501–503.
58. Levy D, Savage DD, Garrison RJ, et al. Echocardiographic criteria for left ventricular hypertrophy: The Framingham Heart Study. *Am J Cardiol* 1987; 59:956–960.
59. Levy D, Anderson KM, Savage DD, et al. Echocardiographically detected left ventricular hypertrophy: Prevalence and risk factors: The Framingham Heart Study. *Ann Intern Med* 1988; 108:7–13.
60. De Simone G, Daniels SR, Devereux RB, et al. Left ventricular mass and body size in normotensive children and adults: Assessment of allometric relations and impact of overweight. *J Am Coll Cardiol* 1992; 20:1251–1260.
61. Lauer MS, Anderson KM, Larson MG, Levy D. A new method for indexing left ventricular mass for differences in body size. *Am J Cardiol* 1994; 74:487–491.
62. Hense HW, Gneiting B, Muscholl M, et al. The associations of body size and body composition with left ventricular mass: Impacts for indexation in adults. *J Am Coll Cardiol* 1998; 32:451–457.
63. Alaud-din A, Meterissian S, Lisbona R, et al. Assessment of cardiac function in patients who were morbidly obese. *Surgery* 1990; 108:809–818.
64. Gal RA, Gunasekera J, Massardo T, et al. Long-term prognostic value of a normal dipyridamole thallium-201 perfusion scan. *Clin Cardiol* 1991; 14:971–974.
65. Ferraro S, Perrone-Filardi P, Desiderio A, et al. Left ventricular systolic and diastolic function in severe obesity: A radionuclide study. *Cardiology* 1996; 87:347–353.
66. Prvulovich EM, Lonn AH, Bomanji JB, et al. Transmission scanning for attenuation correction of myocardial 201TI images in obese patients. *Nucl Med Commun* 1997; 18:207–218.
67. Barnden LR, Ong PL, Rowe CC. Simultaneous emission transmission tomography using technetium-99m for both emission and transmission. *Eur J Nucl Med* 1997; 24:1390–1397.
68. Barbeau GR, Gleeton O, Juneau C, et al. Transradial approach for coronary angiography and interventions: Procedural results and vascular complications from a series of 7049 procedures. *Circulation* 1999; 100:I-306.
69. Lemieux S, Després JP. Metabolic complications of visceral obesity: Contribution to the aetiology of type 2 diabetes and implications for prevention and treatment. *Diabetes Metab* 1994; 20:375–393.
70. Svendsen OL, Hassager C, Christiansen C, et al. Plasminogen activator inhibitor-1, tissue-type plasminogen activator, and fibrinogen: Effect of dieting with or without exercise in overweight postmenopausal women. *Arterioscler Thromb Vasc Biol* 1996; 16:381–385.
71. Folsom AR, Qamhieh HT, Wing RR, et al. Impact of weight loss on plasminogen activator inhibitor (PAI-1), factor VII, and other hemostatic factors in moderately overweight adults. *Arterioscler Thromb* 1993; 13:162–169.
72. Licata G, Scaglione R, Avellone G, et al. Hemostatic function in young subjects with central obesity: Relationship with left ventricular function. *Metabolism* 1995; 44:1417–1421.
73. Pouliot MC, Després JP, Lemieux S, et al. Waist circumference and abdominal sagittal diameter: Best simple anthropometric indexes of abdominal visceral adipose tissue accumulation and related cardiovascular risk in men and women. *Am J Cardiol* 1994; 73:460–468.
74. Després JP. Dyslipidaemia and obesity. *Baillieres Clin Endocrinol Metab* 1994; 8:629–660.
75. Westlund K, Nicolaysen R. Ten-year mortality and morbidity related to serum cholesterol: A follow-up of 3751 men aged 40–49. *Scand J Clin Lab Invest* 1972; 127:1–24.
76. Lew EA, Garfinkel L. Variations in mortality by weight among 750,000 men and women. *J Chronic Dis* 1979; 32:563–576.
77. Larsson B, Bjorntorp P, Tibblin G. The health consequences of moderate obesity. *Int J Obes* 1981; 5:97–116.
78. Colditz GA, Willett WC, Rotnitzky A, Manson JE. Weight gain as a risk factor for clinical diabetes mellitus in women. *Ann Intern Med* 1995; 122:481–486.
79. Chan JM, Rimm EB, Colditz GA, et al. Obesity, fat distribution, and weight gain as risk factors for clinical diabetes in men. *Diabetes Care* 1994; 17:961–969.
80. Sparrow D, Borkan GA, Gerzof SG, et al. Relationship of fat distribution to glucose tolerance: Results of computed tomography in male participants of the Normative Aging Study. *Diabetes* 1986; 35:411–415.
81. Balkau B, Shipley M, Jarrett RJ, et al. High blood glucose concentration is a risk factor for mortality in middle-aged nondiabetic men: 20-year follow-up in the Whitehall Study, the Paris Prospective Study, and the Helsinki Policemen Study. *Diabetes Care* 1998; 21:360–367.
82. Meigs JB, Nathan DM, Wilson PW, et al. Metabolic risk factors worsen continuously across the spectrum of nondiabetic glucose tolerance: The Framingham Offspring Study. *Ann Intern Med* 1998; 128:524–533.
83. Fuller JH, Shipley MJ, Rose G, et al. Mortality from coronary heart disease and stroke in relation to degree of glycaemia: The Whitehall study. *Br Med J* 1983; 287:867–870.
84. Després JP, Lamarche B, Mauriège P, et al. Hyperinsulinemia as an independent risk factor for ischemic heart disease. *N Engl J Med* 1996; 334:952–957.
85. Korpilahti K, Syvanne M, Engblom E, et al. Components of the insulin resistance syndrome are associated with progression of atherosclerosis in non-grafted arteries 5 years after coronary artery bypass surgery. *Eur Heart J* 1998; 19:711–719.
86. Eckel RH, Yost TJ. HDL subfractions and adipose tissue metabolism in the reduced-obese state. *Am J Physiol* 1989; 256:E740–E746.
87. Eckel RH. The importance of timing and accurate interpretation of the benefits of weight reduction on plasma lipids. *Obes Res* 1999; 7:170–178.
88. Poirier P, Catellier C, Tremblay A, Nadeau A. Role of body fat loss in the exercise-induced improvement of the plasma lipid profile in non-insulin-dependent diabetes mellitus. *Metabolism* 1996; 45:1383–1387.
89. Willett WC, Manson JE, Stampfer MJ, et al. Weight, weight change, and coronary heart disease in women: Risk within the "normal" weight range. *JAMA* 1995; 273:461–465.
90. Shaper AG, Wannamethee SG, Walker M. Body weight: Implications for the prevention of coronary heart disease, stroke and diabetes mellitus in a cohort study of middle aged men. *Br Med J* 1997; 314:1311–1317.
91. ECAT angina pectoris study: Baseline associations of haemostatic factors with extent of coronary arteriosclerosis and other

coronary risk factors in 3000 patients with angina pectoris undergoing coronary angiography. *Eur Heart J* 1993; 14:8–17.
92. Stamler R, Stamler J, Riedlinger WF, et al. Weight and blood pressure: Findings in hypertension screening of 1 million Americans. *JAMA* 1978; 240:1607–1610.
93. Lauer MS, Anderson KM, Kannel WB, Levy D. The impact of obesity on left ventricular mass and geometry: The Framingham Heart Study. *JAMA* 1991; 266:231–236.
94. MacMahon SW, Wilcken DE, Macdonald GJ. The effect of weight reduction on left ventricular mass: A randomized controlled trial in young, overweight hypertensive patients. *N Engl J Med* 1986; 314:334–339.
95. Himeno E, Nishino K, Nakashima Y, et al. Weight reduction regresses left ventricular mass regardless of blood pressure level in obese subjects. *Am Heart J* 1996; 131:313–319.
96. Executive summary of the clinical guidelines on the identification, evaluation, and treatment of overweight and obesity in adults. *Arch Intern Med* 1998; 158:1855–1867.
97. Reisin E, Frohlich ED, Messerli FH, et al. Cardiovascular changes after weight reduction in obesity hypertension. *Ann Intern Med* 1983; 98:315–319.
98. Tuck ML, Sowers J, Dornfeld L, et al. The effect of weight reduction on blood pressure, plasma renin activity, and plasma aldosterone levels in obese patients. *N Engl J Med* 1981; 304:930–933.
99. Tuck ML, Sowers JR, Dornfeld L, et al. Reductions in plasma catecholamines and blood pressure during weight loss in obese subjects. *Acta Endocrinol* (*Copenh*) 1983; 102:252–257.
100. Alexander JK. Obesity and the circulation. *Mod Concepts Cardiovasc Dis* 1963; 32:799–803.
101. Frohlich ED, Messerli FH, Reisin E, Dunn FG. The problem of obesity and hypertension. *Hypertension* 1983; 5:III71–III78.
102. Messerli FH. Cardiovascular effects of obesity and hypertension. *Lancet* 1982; 1:1165–1168.
103. Alpert MA, Lambert CR, Panayiotou H, et al. Relation of duration of morbid obesity to left ventricular mass, systolic function, and diastolic filling, and effect of weight loss. *Am J Cardiol* 1995; 76:1194–1197.
104. Duflou J, Virmani R, Rabin I, et al. Sudden death as a result of heart disease in morbid obesity. *Am Heart J* 1995; 130:306–313.
105. Caviezel F, Margonato A, Slaviero G, et al. Early improvement of left ventricular function during caloric restriction in obesity. *Int J Obes* 1986; 10:421–426.
106. Amad KH, Brennan JC, Alexander JK. The cardiac pathology of chronic exogenous obesity. *Circulation* 1965; 32:740–745.
107. Drenick EJ, Fisler JS. Sudden cardiac arrest in morbidly obese surgical patients unexplained after autopsy. *Am J Surg* 1988; 155:720–726.
108. Messerli FH, Sundgaard-Riise K, Reisin ED, et al. Dimorphic cardiac adaptation to obesity and arterial hypertension. *Ann Intern Med* 1983; 99:757–761.
109. Smith HL, Willius FA. Adiposity of the heart: A clinical and pathologic study of one hundred and thirty-six obese patients. *Arch Intern Med* 1933; 52:911–931.
110. Sasson Z, Rasooly Y, Bhesania T, Rasooly I. Insulin resistance is an important determinant of left ventricular mass in the obese. *Circulation* 1993; 88:1431–1436.
111. Strollo PJJ, Rogers RM. Obstructive sleep apnea. *N Engl J Med* 1996; 334:99–104.
112. Vgontzas AN, Tan TL, Bixler EO, et al. Sleep apnea and sleep disruption in obese patients. *Arch Intern Med* 1994; 154:1705–1711.
113. Bearpark H, Elliott L, Grunstein R, et al. Snoring and sleep apnea: A population study in Australian men. *Am J Respir Crit Care Med* 1995; 151:1459–1465.
114. Young T, Palta M, Dempsey J, et al. The occurrence of sleep-disordered breathing among middle-aged adults. *N Engl J Med* 1993; 328:1230–1235.
115. Narkiewicz K, van de Borne PJ, Cooley RL, et al. Sympathetic activity in obese subjects with and without obstructive sleep apnea. *Circulation* 1998; 98:772–776.
116. Viner S, Szalai JP, Hoffstein V. Are history and physical examination a good screening test for sleep apnea? *Ann Intern Med* 1991; 115:356–359.
117. Partinen M, Jamieson A, Guilleminault C. Long-term outcome for obstructive sleep apnea syndrome patients: Mortality. *Chest* 1988; 94:1200–1204.
118. Kessler R, Chaouat A, Weitzenblum E, et al. Pulmonary hypertension in the obstructive sleep apnoea syndrome: Prevalence, causes and therapeutic consequences. *Eur Respir J* 1996; 9:787–794.
119. Laaban JP, Cassuto D, Orvoen-Frija E, et al. Cardiorespiratory consequences of sleep apnoea syndrome in patients with massive obesity. *Eur Respir J* 1998; 11:20–27.
120. Phillipson EA. Sleep apnea—A major public health problem. *N Engl J Med* 1993; 328:1271–1273.
121. Peterson HR, Rothschild M, Weinberg CR, et al. Body fat and the activity of the autonomic nervous system. *N Engl J Med* 1988; 318:1077–1083.
122. Scherrer U, Randin D, Tappy L, et al. Body fat and sympathetic nerve activity in healthy subjects. *Circulation* 1994; 89:2634–2640.
123. Hirsch J, Leibel RL, Mackintosh R, Aguirre A. Heart rate variability as a measure of autonomic function during weight change in humans. *Am J Physiol* 1991; 261:R1418–R1423.
124. Vaz M, Jennings G, Turner A, et al. Regional sympathetic nervous activity and oxygen consumption in obese normotensive human subjects. *Circulation* 1997; 96:3423–3429.
125. Carlson JT, Hedner J, Elam M, et al. Augmented resting sympathetic activity in awake patients with obstructive sleep apnea. *Chest* 1993; 103:1763–1768.
126. Kannel WB, Plehn JF, Cupples LA. Cardiac failure and sudden death in the Framingham Study. *Am Heart J* 1988; 115:869–875.
127. Alexander JK. The cardiomyopathy of obesity. *Prog Cardiovasc Dis* 1985; 27:325–334.
128. El-Gamal A, Gallagher D, Nawras A, et al. Effects of obesity on QT, RR, and QTc intervals. *Am J Cardiol* 1995; 75:956–959.
129. Lantigua RA, Amatruda JM, Biddle TL, et al. Cardiac arrhythmias associated with a liquid protein diet for the treatment of obesity. *N Engl J Med* 1980; 303:735–738.
130. Singh BN, Gaarder TD, Kanegae T, et al. Liquid protein diets and torsade de pointes. *JAMA* 1978; 240:115–119.
131. Birkmeyer NJ, Charlesworth DC, Hernandez F, et al. Obesity and risk of adverse outcomes associated with coronary artery bypass surgery: Northern New England Cardiovascular Disease Study Group. *Circulation* 1998; 97:1689–1694.
132. Moulton MJ, Creswell LL, Mackey ME, et al. Obesity is not a risk factor for significant adverse outcomes after cardiac surgery. *Circulation* 1996; 94:II87–II92.
133. Marik P, Varon J. The obese patient in the ICU. *Chest* 1998; 113:492–498.
134. Rose DK, Cohen MM, Wigglesworth DF, DeBoer DP. Critical respiratory events in the postanesthesia care unit: Patient, surgical, and anesthetic factors. *Anesthesiology* 1994; 81:410–418.
135. Roberts WC, Roberts JD. The floating heart or the heart too fat to sink: Analysis of 55 necropsy patients. *Am J Cardiol* 1983; 52:1286–1289.
136. De Scheerder I, Cuvelier C, Verhaaren R, et al. Restrictive cardiomyopathy caused by adipositas cordis. *Eur Heart J* 1987; 8:661–663.
137. Carpenter CL. Myocardial fat infiltration. *Am Heart J* 1962; 63:491–496.
138. Saphir O, Corrigan M. Fatty infiltration of the myocardium. *Arch Intern Med* 1933; 52:410–428.

139. Balsaver AM, Morales AR, Whitehouse FW. Fat infiltration of myocardium as a cause of cardiac conduction defect. *Am J Cardiol* 1967; 19:261–265.
140. Spain DM, Cathcart RT. Heart block caused by fat infiltration of the interventricular septum (cor adiposum). *Am Heart J* 1946; 32:659–664.
141. Dervan JP, Ilercil A, Kane PB, Anagnostopoulos C. Fatty infiltration: Another restrictive cardiomyopathic pattern. *Cathet Cardiovasc Diagn* 1991; 22:184–189.
142. Wood PD, Stefanick ML, Dreon DM, et al. Changes in plasma lipids and lipoproteins in overweight men during weight loss through dieting as compared with exercise. *N Engl J Med* 1988; 319:1173–1179.
143. Tremblay A, Després JP, Maheux J, et al. Normalization of the metabolic profile in obese women by exercise and a low fat diet. *Med Sci Sports Exerc* 1991; 23:1326–1331.
144. Atkinson RL. Use of drugs in the treatment of obesity. *Annu Rev Nutr* 1997; 17:383–403.
145. Marceau P, Hould FS, Potvin M, et al. Biliopancreatic diversion (doudenal switch procedure). *Eur J Gastroenterol Hepatol* 1999; 11:99–103.
146. Wadden TA, Foster GD, Letizia KA. One-year behavioral treatment of obesity: Comparison of moderate and severe caloric restriction and the effects of weight maintenance therapy. *J Consult Clin Psychol* 1994; 62:165–171.
147. Wadden TA, Sternberg JA, Letizia KA, et al. Treatment of obesity by very low calorie diet, behavior therapy, and their combination: A five-year perspective. *Int J Obes* 1989; 13:39–46.
148. Wadden TA, Stunkard AJ. Controlled trial of very low calorie diet, behavior therapy, and their combination in the treatment of obesity. *J Consult Clin Psychol* 1986; 54:482–488.
149. Perri MG, Nezu AM, Patti ET, McCann KL. Effect of length of treatment on weight loss. *J Consult Clin Psychol* 1989; 57:450–452.
150. Gerace TA, Hollis J, Ockene JK, Svendsen K. Smoking cessation and change in diastolic blood pressure, body weight, and plasma lipids: MRFIT Research Group. *Prev Med* 1991; 20:602–620.
151. Klesges RC, Meyers AW, Klesges LM, La Vasque ME. Smoking, body weight, and their effects on smoking behavior: A comprehensive review of the literature. *Psychol Bull* 1989; 106:204–230.
152. Williamson DF, Madans J, Anda RF, et al. Smoking cessation and severity of weight gain in a national cohort. *N Engl J Med* 1991; 324:739–745.
153. Krauss RM, Deckelbaum RJ, Ernst N, et al. AHA Dietary guidelines for healthy American adults. *Circulation* 1996; 94:1795–1800.
154. Cahill GFJ. Starvation in man. *Clin Endocrinol Metab* 1976; 2:397–415.
155. McGuire MT, Wing RR, Klem ML, Hill JO. Behavioral strategies of individuals who have maintained long-term weight losses. *Obes Res* 1999; 4:334–341.
156. Doucet E, Imbeault P, Almeras N, Tremblay A. Physical activity and low-fat diet: Is it enough to maintain weight stability in the reduced-obese individual following weight loss by drug therapy and energy restriction? *Obes Res* 1999; 4:323–333.
157. Tremblay A, Doucet E, Imbeault P, et al. Metabolic fitness in active reduced-obese individuals. *Obes Res* 1999; 6:556–563.
158. Lee CD, Blair SN, Jackson AS. Cardiorespiratory fitness, body composition, and all-cause and cardiovascular disease mortality in men. *Am J Clin Nutr* 1999; 69:373–380.
159. Pate RR, Pratt M, Blair SN, et al. Physical activity and public health: A recommendation from the Centers for Disease Control and Prevention and the American College of Sports Medicine. *JAMA* 1995; 273:402–407.
160. From the Centers for Disease Control and Prevention. Cardiac valvulopathy associated with exposure to fenfluramine or dexfenfluramine: US Department of Health and Human Services interim public health recommendations. *JAMA* 1997; 278:1729–1731.
161. Connolly HM, Crary JL, McGoon MD, et al. Valvular heart disease associated with fenfluramine-phentermine. *N Engl J Med* 1997; 337:581–588.
162. Weissman NJ, Tighe JFJ, Gottdiener JS, Gwynne JT. An assessment of heart-valve abnormalities in obese patients taking dexfenfluramine, sustained-release dexfenfluramine, or placebo: Sustained-Release Dexfenfluramine Study Group. *N Engl J Med* 1998; 339:725–732.
163. Khan MA, Herzog CA, St Peter JV, et al. The prevalence of cardiac valvular insufficiency assessed by transthoracic echocardiography in obese patients treated with appetite-suppressant drugs. *N Engl J Med* 1998; 339:713–718.
164. Abenhaim L, Moride Y, Brenot F, et al. Appetite-suppressant drugs and the risk of primary pulmonary hypertension: International Primary Pulmonary Hypertension Study Group. *N Engl J Med* 1996; 335:609–616.
165. Robiolio PA, Rigolin VH, Wilson JS, et al. Carcinoid heart disease: Correlation of high serotonin levels with valvular abnormalities detected by cardiac catheterization and echocardiography. *Circulation* 1995; 92:790–795.
166. Redfield MM, Nicholson WJ, Edwards WD, Tajik AJ. Valve disease associated with ergot alkaloid use: Echocardiographic and pathologic correlations. *Ann Intern Med* 1992; 117:50–52.
167. Ryan DH, Bray GA, Helmcke F, et al. Serial echocardiographic and clinical evaluation of valvular regurgitation before, during, and after treatment with fenfluramine or dexfenfluramine and mazindol or phentermine. *Obes Res* 1999; 7:313–322.
168. Jick H, Vasilakis C, Weinrauch LA, et al. A population-based study of appetite-suppressant drugs and the risk of cardiac-valve regurgitation. *N Engl J Med* 1998; 339:719–724.
169. Cannistra LB, Cannistra AJ. Regression of multivalvular regurgitation after the cessation of fenfluramine and phentermine treatment. *N Engl J Med* 1998; 339:771.
170. McNeely W, Goa KL. Sibutramine: A review of its contribution to the management of obesity. *Drugs* 1998; 5:1093–1244.
171. Bach DS, Rissanen AM, Mendel CM, et al. Absence of cardiac valve dysfunction in obese patients treated with sibutramine. *Obes Res* 1999; 7:363–369.
172. Zhi J, Mulligan TE, Hauptman JB. Long-term systemic exposure of orlistat, a lipase inhibitor, and its metabolites in obese patients. *J Clin Pharmacol* 1999; 39:41–46.
173. Melia AT, Koss-Twardy SG, Zhi J. The effect of orlistat, an inhibitor of dietary fat absorption, on the absorption of vitamins A and E in healthy volunteers. *J Clin Pharmacol* 1996; 36:647–653.

CHAPTER 84

THE HEART AND KIDNEY DISEASE

Stephen O. Pastan / William E. Mitch

Almost half of deaths in end-stage renal disease (ESRD) patients treated with chronic dialysis in the United States are caused by cardiovascular disease; acute myocardial infarctions cause 20.8 deaths per 1000 patient-years.[1,2] The cardiovascular mortality rate in ESRD patients on dialysis is approximately 10 to 20 times higher than it is in the general population (see Fig. 84-1).[3]

Specific risk factors for coronary artery disease and cardiovascular morbidity in dialysis patients include the high prevalence of hypertension and diabetes mellitus, hyperlipidemia, hypotension during hemodialysis, and abnormalities in calcium and phosphate metabolism causing hyperparathyroidism with vascular calcification. Pericardial disease, infective endocarditis, and fluid and electrolyte disturbances can also contribute significantly to cardiac dysfunction in ESRD.

CARDIOVASCULAR RISK FACTORS IN CHRONICALLY UREMIC PATIENTS

Systemic Arterial Hypertension

Some 60 to 90 percent of patients with progressive chronic renal failure develop systemic hypertension before beginning dialysis therapy.[4] Both an expanded extracellular fluid volume (ECV)[5,6] and vasoconstriction, mediated by sympathetic overactivity and by the renin-angiotensin axis,[6–9] play roles in the pathogenesis of hypertension in patients with kidney disease, including those with ESRD.

Hypertension due to sodium retention with ECV expansion in kidney disease (and especially, ESRD) is associated with an increased cardiac output and generally an increased total peripheral vascular resistance.[10] This differs from the situation in hypertensive subjects with normal renal function, who usually have a normal cardiac output and a high peripheral resistance (see Chap. 51). The difference may be related to anemia, which causes a secondary increase in cardiac output. Echocardiographic evidence of left ventricular hypertrophy, which results from hypertension and a contribution from anemia, is found in over 50 percent of dialysis patients.

Direct evidence that ECV expansion plays a critical role in the hypertension of chronic renal failure is found in studies demonstrating rapid resolution of hypertension in most patients when the ECV is reduced by diuretics or vigorous dialysis.[6,7,11] This is not the sole cause, because a small group (10 to 20 percent) of ESRD patients exhibit dialysis-resistant hypertension with high levels of plasma renin activity. Control of their hypertension requires drugs inhibiting the renin-angiotensin axis, but some patients may require bilateral nephrectomy.[6,12]

The mechanisms for arterial vasoconstriction may be more complicated than activation of the renin system alone. It has been proposed that circulating inhibitors of Na^+-K^+-ATPase increase peripheral vascular resistance by causing an increase in intracellular sodium, resulting in an increase in intracellular calcium and, hence, contraction of vascular smooth muscle cells.[13,14] Overactivity of the sympathetic nervous system has also been observed in chronic renal failure. This increase in activity is reversed by nephrectomy,[15] suggesting it is mediated by an afferent signal from the kidneys. Enalapril was shown to reduce sympathetic hyperactivity in patients with chronic renal failure,[8] implying this afferent signal is mediated by the renin-angiotensin system, possibly through activation of cerebral circumventricular receptors by angiotensin II.[16] Other proposed mechanisms causing hypertension in patients with chronic renal failure include a decrease in the production of vasodilator prostaglandins[17] or nitric oxide, an increase in the levels of plasma endothelin, a vasoconstrictor,[18] and hyperparathyroidism.[19]

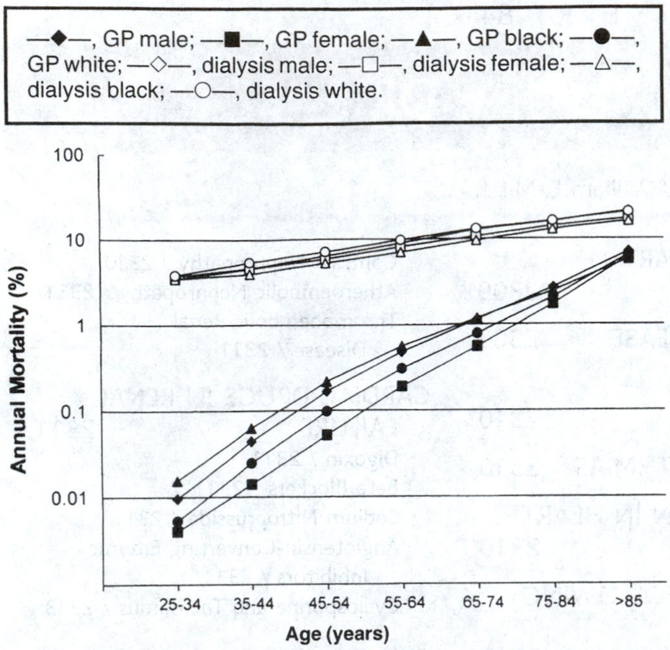

FIGURE 84-1 Cardiovascular mortality defined by death due to arrhythmias, cardiomyopathy, cardiac arrest, myocardial infarction, atherosclerotic heart disease, and pulmonary edema in the general population (GP) compared to ESRD treated by dialysis. Data is stratified by age, race, and gender. [Reproduced with permission from the *American Journal of Kidney Diseases* 1998; 32(5):(Suppl 3):S115, Fig. 1; Copyright © 1998 by the National Kidney Foundation.]

The use of recombinant human erythropoietin (EPO) to correct the anemia associated with ESRD worsens hypertension in approximately 20 to 30 percent of dialysis patients.[20] The proposed mechanism is that increasing hemoglobin is associated with a decline in cardiac output and an increase in peripheral vascular resistance; there may also be an increase in blood viscosity.[21]

The most common reason for *dialysis-resistant* hypertension is ECV expansion because of inadequate fluid removal by dialysis and ultrafiltration. Consequently, the cornerstone of managing hypertension in dialysis patients must be a reduction in the ECV to obtain a true "dry weight." The dry weight of a dialysis patient is defined as that weight at which there is no ECV expansion (e.g., edema or effusions), but there is a normal blood pressure. Unfortunately, this goal is difficult to achieve because patients become symptomatically hypotensive or develop leg cramps before the dry weight is achieved. Consequently, antihypertensive drugs are often required.

In patients who have persistent hypertension despite ECV depletion, antihypertensive medications that inhibit the renin-angiotensin axis [beta blockers or angiotensin converting enzyme (ACE) inhibitors] are the logical choice because of their "cardioprotective" properties. If these are ineffective, calcium channel blockers, clonidine or minoxidil, can be used but only after the ECV has been reduced. The dosage of antihypertensive drugs should be adjusted for the degree of renal failure: generally, antihypertensive drugs are withheld on the day of hemodialysis to prevent hypotension from occurring. Bilateral nephrectomy is occassionally used to treat dialysis-resistant hypertension.[22]

Diabetes Mellitus

Approximately 30 percent of all patients who begin maintenance dialysis therapy have diabetes. They have a significantly higher mortality rate than age-matched patients who do not have diabetes. The most significant factor contributing to their high death rate is coronary artery disease[2] (see also Chap. 78).

Hyperlipidemia

Hyperlipidemia is more common in patients with chronic renal failure than it is in the general population, but the types of abnormalities vary.[23] An elevated low density lipoprotein is common in nephrotic patients, as well as in those treated with chronic ambulatory peritoneal dialysis (CAPD) or patients with a renal transplant and the degree of LDL elevation is correlated with the tendency for cardiovascular disease. Hypertriglyceridemia is the most common lipid abnormality in patients with chronic renal failure or ESRD patients and is often found in association with a low HDL (but may occur in the absence of an elevated LDL).[23] Impaired degradation of very low density lipoprotein by lipoprotein lipase appears to be the major mechanism causing hypertriglyceridemia.[24] In patients treated with chronic ambulatory peritoneal dialysis, the high concentration of glucose in the dialysate worsens the serum triglyceride level because glucose increases the production of triglycerides.[25] About 50 to 80 percent of patients undergoing renal transplantation develop hypercholesterolemia.[23]

Other factors that may contribute to hyperlipidemia in patients with chronic renal failure or ESRD patients include the use of diuretics and beta blockers,[26,27] and possibly carnitine deficiency.[28] Heparin, given to prevent clotting within the dialyzer cartridge, will cause a transient fall in serum triglycerides by increasing the activity of lipoprotein lipase.[29] In order to standardize the measurement of plasma lipids, the blood sample should be obtained after a 12-h fast and before the patient is given heparin for dialysis.

At present, there is no definite evidence that lowering plasma triglycerides improves survival.[30] Strategies for lowering triglycerides and LDL cholesterol include restricting dietary fat, exercise, giving fish-oil supplements, and avoiding alcohol or treatment with beta blockers or diuretics[26,27,31-33] (see Chap. 38). The 3-hydroxy-3-methylglutaryl coenzyme A (HMG-CoA) reductase inhibitors are the preferred agents for drug therapy of triglycerides and LDL-cholesterol. They appear to be safe in ESRD patients but the dose must be reduced for patients taking cyclosporine or tacrolimus after renal transplantation. Clofibrate or gemfibrozil may be effective, but their use has been associated with an increased incidence of myositis and hepatotoxicity in dialysis patients (see Chap 38). Again, it is particularly important to adjust the dosage for the degree of renal failure; for instance, clofibrate should be reduced to 25 to 50 percent of the usual dose. Although definitive evidence that drug treatment prevents atherosclerosis in dialysis patients is lacking, attempts at treatment seem prudent.[31] The National Cholesterol Education Program Adult Treatment Panel guidelines are recommended for classifying and treating lipid abnormalities in patients with chronic renal disease.[34]

Homocysteine

Plasma levels of homocysteine are often elevated in patients with chronic renal failure (see Fig. 84-2). The exact mechanism

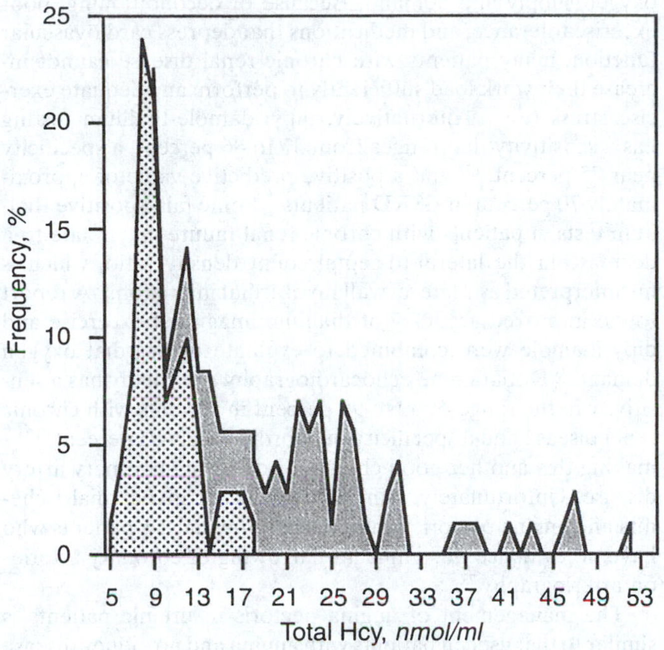

FIGURE 84-2 Distributions of fasting total homocysteine levels in ($N = 71$) dialysis-dependent ESRD patients; and ($N = 71$) age, sex, and race matched Framingham Offspring/Omni Study controls free of renal disease with serum creatinine levels <1.5 mg/dL. Symbols are: (▦) control; (■) ESRD. [Reproduced with permission from *Kidney International* 1997; 52(1):13, Fig. 2; Copyright © 1997 by the International Society of Nephrology.]

of homocysteine elevation is unknown, although reduced renal clearance appears to play a role.[35–37] Preliminary studies indicate that homocysteine is a risk factor for cardiovascular morbidity and mortality in patients with ESRD,[38] but larger studies that take into account the influence of other comorbid conditions are needed for confirmation.[36] Supplementation of patients with kidney diseases using folic acid (5 mg per day), vitamin B_{12} (0.4 mg per day) and vitamin B_6 (50 mg per day) can lower homocysteine levels by about 25 percent.[35,36] Such treatments may normalize levels in patients with chronic renal failure, but not in most ESRD patients on dialysis. The benefit of this type of vitamin supplementation on cardiovascular outcomes is not known.

Hemodialysis-Associated Hypotension

Clinically significant hypotension occurs in approximately 25 percent of hemodialysis sessions.[39] Usually, the consequences are minor, but acute myocardial and cerebral ischemia can occur. Excessive ultrafiltration and ECV depletion is the most common cause of hypotension during dialysis due to reduced cardiac output.[40] Rapid lowering of plasma osmolality during the removal of urea and other molecules also causes a shift of fluid from the ECV to the intracellular compartment, as these molecules do not move out of cells as rapidly as dialysis removes them from blood.[41,42] Finally, diffusion of acetate from an acetate-based dialysate into the patient can cause vasodilatation that interferes with the hemodynamic vasoconstriction that should occur when ECV is reduced.

The concentration of sodium in the dialysate is an important factor governing changes in plasma osmolality. Dialyzers currently in use can achieve high rates of fluid removal (i.e., ultrafiltration) but even so, a higher concentration of sodium in the dialysate can reduce the number of hypotensive episodes by removing more fluid from the intracellular compartment.[43]

Hypotension can occur when complement is activated by the dialyzer membranes leading to intrapulmonary shunting of blood and hypoxemia. This response is most often observed with cuprophane dialyzer membranes[44]; newer dialysis membranes cause less activation of the complement cascade.[45] Hypersensitivity to ethylene oxide, which is used to sterilize dialyzers, can also cause hypotension and, rarely, anaphylaxis.[46] Finally, ACE inhibitors may be associated with profound hypotension when polyacrylonitrile dialysis membranes are used because this membrane has a high negative surface charge that stabilizes enzymes that generate bradykinin.[47] Since ACE inhibitors block kininases, the high levels of bradykinin cause anaphylactoid reactions.

Other factors favoring hypotension during hemodialysis include (1) cardiac dysfunction from long-standing hypertension, ischemic or valvular heart disease, cardiomyopathy, or pericardial tamponade; (2) a rapid reduction in serum potassium and calcium depressing cardiac contractility; (3) autonomic neuropathy (particularly in diabetic patients); (4) sepsis; (5) occult hemorrhage (e.g., retroperitoneal hemorrhage after femoral vein catheterization to place a dialysis access catheter); (6) eating prior to or during dialysis resulting in splanchnic vasodilation; and (7) use of antihypertensive medications on the day of dialysis. Rarely a patient may develop a paradoxical withdrawal of sympathetic nervous system activity during hemodialysis resulting in a slowing of heart rate and a reduction in systemic vascular resistance and profound hypotension.[48]

To reduce the incidence of hypotension, a high-sodium and bicarbonate-buffered (rather than acetate-buffered) dialysate should be used and the rate and extent of ultrafiltration monitored carefully; antihypertensive medications should be avoided on hemodialysis days. "Sodium Modeling," the practice of lowering an initially hypertonic dialysis solution to isotonic levels during the dialysis session, may reduce the frequency of hypotensive events by offsetting fluid shifts from the ECV (see above).[49] Management of hypotension includes reducing the ultrafiltration rate, placing the patient in the Trendelenburg position, and administering saline through the arteriovenous access. Oxygen administration may be useful in patients with ischemic heart disease. Lowering the dialysate temperature can also reduce the incidence of hypotension in patients who have this reaction repeatedly.[50]

Hyperparathyroidism

Secondary hyperparathyroidism is virtually universal in dialysis patients.[51] Hyperphosphatemia due to the failure to excrete phosphate plays a major role in the pathogenesis of secondary hyperparathyroidism. Hyperphosphatemia reduces the plasma-ionized calcium concentration by direct complexing of calcium with phosphates which stimulates parathyroid hormone secretion. Hyperphosphatemia and the loss of kidney tissue also decrease the activity of 1 -hydroxylase in proximal tubule cells, leading to limited production of 1,25-dihydroxyvitamin D_3, the most active vitamin D analogue.[51,52] Finally, reduced levels of both the vitamin D and calcium receptors have been found in patients with uremic hyperparathyroidism, particularly in areas of nodular hyperplasia.[53,54] Receptor downregulation is likely to play an important role in the abnormal patterns of parathyroid hormone secretion and cellular growth.

All of these factors reduce the level of ionized calcium, which stimulates parathyroid hormone secretion. A deficiency of 1,25-dihydroxyvitamin D_3 also limits the ability of ionized calcium to suppress parathyroid hormone secretion.[55,56]

It is often taught that a high calcium × phosphate product (>60 mg^2/dL^2) is an independent risk factor for mortality and morbidity,[62] but it is almost certain that the pathophysiologic mechanism is due solely to a high serum phosphorus level. When the serum phosphorous level is high, the risk of vascular and soft tissue calcification rises sharply.[57,58] Calcification can occur in coronary and peripheral arteries[59] and in the myocardium.[60] Extensive valvular calcification can also impair native or prosthetic valve function.[61] Finally, it has been proposed that parathyroid hormone itself can directly impair myocardial function,[62] but not all investigators agree.[63]

Prevention or treatment of secondary hyperparathyroidism must be based on correcting hyperphosphatemia. This can be accomplished only if patients adhere to a diet containing less than 1 g of phosphorus per day. But even with compliance, many patients will need to take phosphate binders after meals. Calcium carbonate or calcium acetate are the preferred agents, because they also increase calcium intake and avoid the risk of aluminum toxicity (including aluminum-induced osteomalacia, anemia, and encephalopathy). Another agent, RenaGel, a non-calcium non-aluminum containing phosphorus binder, shows promise for the management of hyperphosphatemia.[64] If hypocalcemia persists and serum phosphorus is normal (especially if there is evidence of secondary hyperparathyroidism) intravenous administration of 1,25-dihydroxyvitamin D_3 (calcitriol) can be useful therapeutically. Vitamin D can also be given orally, but with somewhat greater risk of hypercalcemia. Vitamin D analogues, such as 19-Nor-1,25-dihydroxyvitamin D_2 (paricalcitol) have more specificity for parathyroid tissue and should result in fewer complications of hypercalcemia or worsening hyperphosphatemia.[65] Just as it is rarely necessary to perform bilateral nephrectomy to manage hypertension, subtotal parathyroidectomy should also be rare since severe hyperparathyroidism can be avoided. Prevention of hyperphosphatemia, hypocalcemia, and hyperparathyroidism is critical because hypocalcemia after parathyroidectomy is serious and requires that a patient take many calcium and vitamin D tablets.

ISCHEMIC HEART DISEASE

The prevalence of coronary artery disease approaches 40 percent in ESRD patients.[66] At autopsy, acute myocardial infarctions were noted in about 25 percent of dialysis patients.[67,68] Risk factors for coronary artery disease include smoking, hypertension, left ventricular hypertrophy, insulin-dependent or non-insulin-dependent diabetes mellitus, hyperlipidemia, and hyperparathyroidism[6,23,69] (see also Chap. 38). Factors increasing the risk of myocardial infarction include hypertension, ECV overload, anemia, hypotension and hypoxia during hemodialysis, and increased blood flow through the arteriovenous fistula.[70] These factors adversely affect the balance between myocardial oxygen supply and demand. Because of deconditioning, poor excerise tolerance, and medications that depress cardiovascular function, many patients with chronic renal disease cannot increase their work load sufficiently to perform an adequate exercise stress test.[71] Alternatively, dipyridamole-thallium testing has a sensitivity that ranges from 37 to 86 percent, a specificity near 75 percent,[71,72] and a positive predictive value of approximately 70 percent in ESRD patients.[73] Some false-positive thallium tests in patients with chronic renal failure may relate to a decrease in the lateral-to-septal count density ratio, which is misinterpreted as a lateral wall myocardial infarction.[74] A report found improved accuracy of thallium imaging if excercise and dipyridamole were combined to evaluate myocardial oxygen demand.[75] Dobutamine echocardiography reportedly has a sensitivity in the range of 69 to 95 percent in patients with chronic renal disease and a specificity of approximately 95 percent,[71,76,77] making this another good choice for detecting coronary artery disease. Unfortunately, clinically significant myocardial ischemia and angina pectoris can occur in some dialysis patients who have no evidence of significant narrowing of coronary arteries on arteriography.[78]

The management of angina pectoris in uremic patients is similar to that used in patients with angina and no kidney disease except that drug dosages often have to be reduced (see Chap. 40). Nitrates, beta blockers, and calcium channel blockers are well tolerated but usually are withheld before dialysis to avoid hypotension during the procedure. Exercise tolerance has been shown to improve in hemodialysis patients with coronary artery disease if anemia is corrected with erythropoietin: for this reason, the hematocrit should be maintained above 30 percent.[79] When using erythropoetin, attention must be paid to repleting iron stores and to hypertension as well as ECV overload. Hyperparathyroidism should be prevented for optimal control of coronary artery disease.

Treatment of angina pectoris that develops during hemodialysis includes (1) stopping ultrafiltration to avoid ECV depletion; (2) reducing blood flow through the dialyzer; and (3) administering oxygen. If there is hypotension, the patient should be placed in the Trendelenburg position and saline infused through the venous line before administering sublingual nitroglycerin (which could cause further hypotension). If there is no hypotension, nitroglycerin can be administered immediately but the blood pressure must be monitored repeatedly. Finally, it should be emphasized that changes in serum potassium and ionized calcium during dialysis and between dialysis treatments may complicate interpretation of the ECG. Electrocardiograms obtained during angina while on dialysis can differ from prior tracings taken between dialysis sessions.

In ESRD patients, acute and long-term management of myocardial infarction is similar to that in nonuremic patients except that controlling the degree of changes in ECV is more critical and requires restriction of salt and fluid intake plus judicious ultrafiltration to prevent hemodynamic instability. Hypertension and anemia should be managed as discussed. The concentration of potassium in the dialysate is generally 2 meq/L, but can be raised to 3 to 3.5 meq/L to stabilize serum potassium or prevent arrhythmias in patients receiving digoxin. Dietary potassium must be restricted in all dialysis patients, and potassium infusions must be avoided to prevent hyperkalemia. Patients with kidney disease are particularly prone to developing hyperkalemia and unnecessary dialysis treatments with the cardiovascular stress required should be avoided. The use of antiarrhythmic drugs should be carefully monitored by measuring serum levels.

The decision to perform coronary arteriography is based upon the same criteria as for patients without kidney disease (see Chaps. 40 to 42). However, the dose of contrast dye for kidney patients should be minimized and means taken to prevent loss of residual renal function. This is especially true for diabetic patients or patients with proteinuria. It is not necessary to dialyze patients immediately after arteriography unless there is concern about the consequences of excess fluid or heart failure.

Coronary artery bypass grafting has a mortality rate of approximately 10 percent in dialysis patients,[71,80] as well as an increased perioperative morbidity.[81] These data emphasize the importance of ensuring that there will be improved quality of life after coronary artery bypass grafting before recommending this operation for a dialysis patient. Dialysis should be performed just before cardiac surgery to optimize ECV status and avoid hyperkalemia. Interestingly, percutaneous transluminal coronary angioplasty has an unacceptably high rate of restenosis despite good initial angiographic success.[71,82,83] Therefore it should be reserved for dialysis patients who are not candidates for coronary artery bypass grafting. Preliminary data suggest that coronary stenting may improve coronary patency and survival compared with angioplasty alone.[83]

CONGESTIVE HEART FAILURE

Congestive heart failure accounts for 20 to 30 percent of the mortality occurring in ESRD patients.[3,84] Echocardiograms reveal a high prevalence of "hypertrophic cardiomyopathy" characterized by left ventricular hypertrophy, asymmetric septal hypertrophy, and/or impaired contractility,[85–87] as well as dilated cardiomyopathy.[88] Concentric left ventricular hypertrophy occurs in patients with current or previous systemic hypertension.[89] Risk factors for myocardial failure in dialysis patients include hypertension, persistent ECV expansion, anemia, arteriovenous fistula,[70] ischemic heart disease, metabolic acidosis, electrolyte disturbances (hyperkalemia, hypocalcemia), hyperparathyroidism,[90] and possibly the uremic state itself. Hemodialysis can improve cardiac function dramatically,[91–93] presumably by controlling hypertension, correcting volume overload, removing uremic toxins, and normalizing blood pH and electrolyte levels (particularly, ionized calcium[94] and potassium[95]).

In uremic patients who develop pulmonary edema, the pulmonary capillary pressure is lower than it is in nonuremic patients and is less than the plasma oncotic pressure. Thus, pulmonary capillary permeability must be increased, further complicating management.[96]

The prevention of heart failure in dialysis patients requires strict control of ECV and hypertension. Salt and fluid restriction must be combined with adequate fluid removal by diuretics or dialysis to maintain the patient's weight as close as possible to the estimated "dry weight." Reasons for an erroneous assessment of dry weight include an unsuspected loss of muscle mass (e.g., catabolic weight loss) that is unrecognized because the measured body weight does not change if fluid is retained. Finally, the adverse influence of the arteriovenous fistula can be tested by occluding it and determining whether or not the heart rate slows (Branham's sign). When this occurs, revision of the fistula may be required to decrease excessive blood flow and oxygen demands of the heart.[97]

Management of heart failure includes bed rest and oxygen therapy plus removal of excess fluid by ultrafiltration while excluding other causes of heart failure such as myocardial infarction, arrhythmias, or infective endocarditis. If digitalis is used, appropriate adjustment of dosage and frequent monitoring of plasma levels are necessary.

Left ventricular hypertrophy has been found to improve after using recombinant human erythropoietin to correct anemia in dialysis patients. Left ventricular muscle mass can decrease by an average of 18 percent over 45 weeks as the hematocrit increases to 32 percent.[20] Complete normalization of left ventricular hypertrophy is, however, uncommon, and it is unknown whether a decrease in left ventricular wall thickness will result in improved patient survival.[21,98]

PERICARDIAL DISEASE

Before dialysis was widely available, pericarditis was regarded as a preterminal event in uremic patients. The current incidence of clinically apparent pericarditis has decreased from 50 percent to 5 to 20 percent since the predialysis era.[99,100] The cause of pericarditis in dialysis patients is unknown but may be related to inadequate removal of uremic toxins; coincident diseases such as viral infections,[101] tuberculosis, systemic lupus erythematosus; or to drugs such as minoxidil.[102] Pericarditis appears to occur less frequently in peritoneal dialysis patients than it does in hemodialysis patients. This difference has been attributed to a higher clearance of "middle molecules" by peritoneal dialysis.[103]

The primary treatment for dialysis-associated pericarditis is intensive dialysis (e.g., daily hemodialysis for 1 to 2 weeks) and elimination of heparin in order to avoid pericardial hemorrhage and tamponade. Unfortunately, intensive dialysis for pericarditis can cause hypokalemia, hypophosphatemia, and volume depletion. Besides intensive dialysis, oral or intrapericardial administration of corticosteroids[104,105,112] and indomethacin[106] have been tried. The efficacy of indomethacin is questionable; results from a prospective, double-blind study led to the conclusion that the predominant effect of indomethacin is to reduce fever.[107]

Pericardial effusion frequently complicates pericarditis, but cardiac tamponade is rare; the exact frequency is unknown. An important clue to the development of cardiac tamponade is severe hypotension during dialysis, especially in the absence of volume depletion. Small pericardial effusions are found in 15 to 20 percent of stable, asymptomatic dialysis patients.[108] It is unclear whether or not daily dialysis is beneficial in these patients, but frequent evaluation of the size and hemodynamic importance of the effusion is prudent. Treatment of a large pericardial effusion by intensification of dialysis may result in improvement,[100,101] but if there is no improvement, or if hemodynamic compromise occurs, surgical drainage[100,109–111] of the pericardial effusion by subxiphoid pericardiotomy and creation of a pericardial "window" is the preferred procedure. This can be performed under local anesthesia,[112] and it is usually well tolerated (see Chap. 72). Although pericardiectomy is the definitive treatment for patients with pericarditis and clinically significant effusion, this more invasive procedure is not usually necessary.[100]

Constrictive pericarditis is rare in dialysis patients, even those with pericarditis.[113] It should be suspected when there is intractable right-sided heart failure in patients with a normal-sized or small heart. Cardiac catheterization will verify the diagnosis, and pericardiectomy is the definitive treatment (see Chap. 72).

INFECTIVE ENDOCARDITIS

Bacteremia occurs in approximately 10 to 20 percent of hemodialysis patients;[114–116] the incidence of *Staphylococcus aureus* bacteremia is about 1.2 episodes per 100 patient months.[115] *Staph. aureus* is the most frequent organism causing endocarditis,[114,117,118,125,126] although other microbes, including *Staph. epidermidis, Streptococcus viridans,* enterococci, and gram-negative organisms are also reported. Several factors predispose dialysis patients to infective endocarditis, which can have an incidence of 3 to 5 percent.[114,117,118] These include uremia-associated immunocompromise,[119,120] repeated puncture of the arteriovenous fistula, or an indwelling dialysis catheter. Other factors are aortic valve calcifications, found in 28 to 55 percent, and mitral valve calcifications in 10 to 40 percent of dialysis patients.[59,61,121,122] Calcified valves may serve as a nidus for infection; in this case, the aortic valve is involved in over 80 percent of cases.[114]

The diagnosis of infective endocarditis may be difficult in uremic patients because of the frequency of bacteremia and because systolic and diastolic murmurs are common (see also Chap. 73). Repeated blood cultures, physical examination, and an echocardiographic assessment are mandatory when infective endocarditis is suspected. Treatment of infective endocarditis consists of 4 to 6 weeks of parenteral antibiotics (see Chap. 73). Survival of hemodialysis patients undergoing valve replacement for endocarditis is poor.[123]

CARDIAC ARRHYTHMIAS

Risk factors for cardiac arrhythmias in dialysis patients include ischemic heart disease, calcification of the conduction system from secondary hyperparathyroidism and/or pericarditis, hemodialysis-associated hypotension, dialysis-induced acid-base and electrolyte disturbances (hyper- and hypokalemia, hyper- and hypocalcemia, and hypermagnesemia), and hypoxemia. Fortunately, serious arrhythmias are uncommon except in patients with underlying heart disease, those receiving digitalis, or those with severe hypokalemia.[124–126] Dialysis patients receiving digitalis have an excessive risk for atrial and ventricular arrhythmias during dialysis because of rapid shifts of potassium. Therefore, digitalis should be used only when necessary and in the lowest dosage. While the potassium concentration in the dialysate can be raised to decrease the risk of digitalis-toxic arrhythmias, there also must be strict restriction of dietary potassium to prevent hyperkalemia between dialyses. Hyperkalemia is believed to be responsible for a significant fraction of the 10 percent death rate from cardiac arrest in dialysis patients.

RENAL FUNCTION IN HEART FAILURE

In heart failure, enhanced sympathetic activity and activation of the renin-angiotensin-aldosterone axis enhance salt reabsorption by the kidney. Excess vasopressin release and increases in aquaporin-2 water channels augment water retention.[127,128] These responses expand the ECV and plasma volume leading to increased end-diastolic volume plus edema.[129] Circulating atrial natriuretic peptide levels are increased in heart failure[127,130]; possibly, atrial natriuretic peptide modulates the antinatriuretic effects caused by sympathetic and renin system activation. Excessive vasopressin-induced water reabsorption, coupled with increased water intake (possibly related to angiotensin-II-stimulated central thirst receptors) can cause hyponatremia. Hyponatremia is an important indicator of a poor prognosis.[131]

Renal vasoconstriction in heart failure patients can be sufficiently severe to cause prerenal azotemia, characterized by a blood urea nitrogen-creatinine ratio that is greater than the expected, normal of 10:1. Renal vasoconstriction causes a selective decrease in urea clearance resulting from enhanced sodium reabsorption and a secondary increase in urea reabsorption in the proximal tubule. The increase in salt and water reabsorption both reduces urine flow and causes a low urinary sodium excretion, as well as a high urine specific gravity and osmolality. In terms of diagnosis, the urinalysis is normal and there are no cellular or granular casts indicating kidney damage. Diuretic therapy can mask these characteristics by increasing urine flow and sodium excretion, thereby reducing the urine specific gravity and osmolality and diluting the presence of cellular or granular casts. Factors that can precipitate or exacerbate renal failure include excessive diuresis, use of ACE inhibitors or nonsteroidal anti-inflammatory drugs, and worsening cardiac function. The basis for renal insufficiency in these cases is that renal perfusion is reduced by heart failure. Consequently, the glomerular filtration rate becomes dependent on angiotensin-II-induced efferent glomerular arteriolar constriction. By blocking this response, ACE inhibitors can markedly decrease the glomerular filtration rate.[132] Non-steroidal anti-inflammatory drugs reduce the glomerular filtration rate by blocking the release of prostaglandins, which in turn, reduce activation of the renin-angiotensin system.[133] The ACE inhibitors and other antihypertensive agents (e.g., hydralazine) can also reduce glomerular filtration by causing systemic hypotension and reducing renal perfusion pressure.

The management of renal insufficiency in heart failure patients is aimed primarily at improving cardiac function (see Chap. 21). Non-steroidal anti-inflammatory drugs should be avoided, and diuretics should be used judiciously because excessive diuresis can predispose the patient to any factor that lowers blood pressure or that interrupts the glomerular efferent arteriolar vasoconstriction (e.g., an ACE inhibitor). Careful attention to changes in the blood urea nitrogen relative to serum creatinine and potassium is mandatory to avoid these problems. It should be emphasized that ACE inhibitor therapy may sharply reduce renal clearance (i.e., cause a sharp rise in serum creatinine) in heart failure patients that have an activation of the renin system. Often, this is a transient physiologic response and the serum creatinine will return to pretreatment values. If it does not, the drug should be withdrawn and a diagnosis of renal artery stenosis considered.

RENAL FAILURE FOLLOWING CARDIAC CATHETERIZATION

Contrast Nephropathy

The risk of renal damage following radiocontrast dye is high in patients with diabetes mellitus, multiple myeloma, preexisting renal failure, and, especially, proteinuria, volume depletion, heart failure, and with large amounts of contrast dye.[134–136] Renal failure after contrast dye is typically brief (approximately 5 to 7 days) unless there is preexisting renal damage. Interestingly, renal insufficiency in contrast-dye nephropathy can be associated with excessive edema (from reduced urinary sodium excretion) and hyperkalemia.[137] In high-risk patients, contrast dye studies should be avoided and noninvasive studies used to assess ventricular function and anatomy; at the very least, the amount of contrast dye should be minimized. Extracellular fluid volume expansion with saline prior to the studies reduces the incidence of contrast nephropathy to approximately 10 percent.[138]

Atheroembolic Nephropathy

This complication usually occurs in elderly patients with erosive aortic atherosclerosis. They develop cholesterol emboli to the kidneys, and this is most commonly detected after arterial catheterization.[134,139] Serum creatinine rises progressively and usually does not return to basal levels, and often renal insufficiency progresses to ESRD. Hypertension due to activation of the renin-angiotensin system may be present.[140] The urinalysis typically does not contain cellular or granular casts (the signs of acute tubular damage). Atheroembolization to other organs such as the eyes (cholesterol plaques seen by fundoscopy), pancreas (pancreatitis), and skin (livedo reticularis or gangrene) may be present, suggesting the diagnosis.[141] Occasionally, immunologic activation may occur yielding an "active" urinary sediment with hematuria and cellular casts, hypocomplementemia, eosinophilia, and a high sedimentation rate.[142–144] Biopsy of an affected organ (e.g., skin or kidney) can help establish the diagnosis, but the absence of atheroemboli in a kidney biopsy does not exclude the diagnosis since the affected vessels may be missed. There is no specific treatment.

Thromboembolic Renal Disease

In contrast to atheroembolic renal disease, thromboembolic renal arterial disease (e.g., in patients with atrial fibrillation or after myocardial infarction) can cause renal infarction. Such patients may present with flank pain, proteinuria, and hematuria; the serum lactate dehydrogenase level is increased and renal failure leads to an increased serum creatinine, particularly if both kidneys are affected.[145–147] A radioisotope scan or renal arteriography may confirm the diagnosis. Therapy includes anticoagulation, thrombolysis, and possibly surgical intervention.

CARDIAC DRUGS IN RENAL FAILURE

Many drugs used in the treatment of cardiovascular diseases are eliminated (i.e., cleared) by the kidneys. In order to avoid toxic side effects, the doses of these drugs must be modified depending on the level of the patient's glomerular filtration rate (see also Chap. 81). Dosing guidelines for commonly prescribed cardiovascular drugs in patients with diminished renal function are listed in Table 84-1. Specific drugs are discussed in more detail later.

Digoxin

The volume of distribution of digoxin is reduced 30 to 50 percent in ESRD patients; therefore the loading dose of digoxin should be reduced. The maintenance dosage should also be decreased because the primary route of elimination is by glomerular filtration of unmetabolized digoxin. Because of individual variation in digoxin pharmacokinetics, only general guidelines for maintenance dosages are available: 0.0625 to 0.125 mg every other day can result in a therapeutic plasma level but regular monitoring of the plasma digoxin level is still required. If a loading dose is not administered or if adjustments are made in the maintenance dose, the time required to attain a new steady state can be prolonged to approximately 3 weeks because of the longer half-life of digoxin in renal failure (4.4 days versus 1.6 days in normal subjects[148]). Concomitant administration of quinidine or verapamil can increase plasma digoxin levels and produce clinical toxicity.

Beta Blockers

Since atenolol (Tenormin) and nadolol (Corgard) are eliminated primarily by the kidneys, a dose reduction of 50 to 70 percent is necessary for patients with chronic renal failure.[149] These drugs should be withheld on the morning of a hemodialysis treatment because a significant fraction is removed by the dialysis procedure. The usual dose is then given after dialysis (Table 84-1).

Sodium Nitroprusside

In dialysis or predialysis patients, thiocyanate will accumulate when sodium nitroprusside is infused.[150] Thiocyanate can cause neurologic toxicity such as confusion, hyperreflexia, and seizures. Therefore the dose of nitroprusside for patients with chronic renal failure should be minimized and the drug given for as short a period as possible. Both the cyanide and thiocyanate levels in plasma should be monitored to avoid toxicity. Fenoldopam, a dopamine$_1$ recepter agonist, increases renal blood flow and glomerular filtration rate; this agent may be a good alternative to nitroprusside for the treatment of severe hypertension in patients with renal disease.[151]

Angiotensin-Converting Enzyme Inhibitors

The doses of ACE inhibitors should be reduced by approximately 50 percent in dialysis patients because they and their metabolites are excreted by the kidney. Accumulation of converting enzyme inhibitors can cause hematologic toxicity. These drugs have two other types of toxic effects in predialysis patients. First, in patients who are not treated by dialysis, they can cause hyperkalemia by blocking angiotensin-stimulated aldosterone release, resulting in decreased potassium excretion and hyperkalemia. Second, they can cause rapid loss of renal function in patients with renal artery stenosis or other conditions associated with activation of the renin-angiotensin system, including congestive heart failure.[132] The mechanism for the decrease in glomerular filtration rate is inhibition of angiotensin-induced constriction of the efferent glomerular arterioles. The resulting dilation leads to a decrease in the hydrostatic pressure across the glomerular capillary wall. These drugs, like other antihypertensive agents, should be withheld on the morning of a hemodialysis treatment to avoid hypotension.

TABLE 84-1 Dosing of Selected Cardiovascular Drugs in Renal Failure

Drug	Method of Modification	GFR >50	GFR 10–50	GFR <10	Supplemental Dose after Hemodialysis
Adrenergic Agents					
Clonidine	D	100%	100%	100%	No
Doxazosin	D	100%	100%	100%	No
Methyldopa	I	q8h	q8–q12h	q12–q24h	250 mg
Prazosin	D	100%	100%	100%	No
Terazosin	D	100%	100%	100%	?
Angiotensin-Converting Enzyme Inhibitors					
Benazepril	D	100%	75–100%	50%	No
Captopril	D	100%	75%	50%	25–30%
Cilazapril	D	75%	50%	10–25%	No
	I	q24h	q24–48h	q72h	
Enalapril	D	100%	75–100%	50%	20–25%
Fosinopril	D	100%	100%	75%	No
Lisinopril	D	100%	50–75%	25–50%	20%
Pentopril	D	100%	50–75%	50%	?
Perindopril	D	100%	75%	50%	25–50%
Quinapril	D	100%	75–100%	50%	25%
Ramapril	D	100%	50–75%	25–50%	20%
Angiotensin-II-Receptor Antagonists					
Losartan	D	100%	100%	100%	?
Valsartan	D	100%	100%	50%	?
Antiarrhythmics					
Amiodarone	D	100%	100%	100%	No
Bretylium	D	100%	25–50%	25%	No
Disopyramide	I	q8h	q12–24h	q24–48h	No
Flecainide	D	100%	100%	50–75%	No
Lidocaine	D	100%	100%	100%	No
Mexiletine	D	100%	100%	50–75%	No
N-Acetyl-procainamide	D	100%	50%	25%	No
	I	q6–8h	q8–q12h	q12–q18h	
Procainamide	I	q4h	q6–12h	q8–24h	200 mg
Propafenone	D	100%	100%	100%	No
Quinidine	D	100%	100%	75%	100–200 mg
Tocainide	D	100%	100%	50%	200 mg
Beta Blockers					
Acebutolol	D	100%	50%	30–50%	No
Atenolol	D	100%	50%	30–50%	25–50 mg
	I	q24h	q48h	q96h	
Betaxolol	D	100%	100%	50%	No
Bisoprolol	D	100%	75%	50%	?
Carvedilol	D	100%	100%	100%	No
Labetalol	D	100%	100%	100%	No
Metoprolol	D	100%	100%	100%	50 mg
Nadolol	D	100%	50%	25%	40 mg
Pindolol	D	100%	100%	100%	No
Propranolol	D	100%	100%	100%	No
Sotalol	D	100%	30%	15–30%	80 mg
Timolol	D	100%	100%	100%	No

TABLE 84-1 Dosing of Selected Cardiovascular Drugs in Renal Failure (*Continued*)

Drug	Method of Modification	GFR >50	GFR 10–50	GFR <10	Supplemental Dose after Hemodialysis
CALCIUM CHANNEL BLOCKERS—NO ADJUSTMENT NECESSARY					
CARDIAC GLYCOSIDES					
Digitoxin	D	100%	100%	50–75%	No
Digoxin	D	100%	25–75%	10–25%	No
	I	q24h	q36h	q48h	
IONOTROPIC AGENTS					
Amrinone	D	100%	100%	50–75%	?
Dobutamine	D	100%	100%	100%	?
Milrinone	D	100%	100%	50–75%	?
VASODILATORS					
Hydralazine	I	q8h	q8h	q16h	No
Fenoldopam	D	100%	100%	100%	No
Minoxidil	D	100%	100%	50–75%	No
Nitroprusside	D	100%	100%	50–75%	No

ABBREVIATIONS: GFR = glomerular filtration rate; D = Dose; I = interval; ? = unknown.
SOURCE: Adapted from Aronoff GR, Berns JS, Brier ME, et al. *Drug Prescribing in Renal Failure: Dosing Guidelines for Adults*, 4th ed. Philadelphia: American College of Physicians: 1999.

Cyclosporine and Tacrolimus

The use of cyclosporine A and tacrolimus in heart transplant recipients is often associated with acute reduction in renal function, which progresses to chronic renal failure in some patients[152] (see also Chap. 22). These agents constrict both afferent and efferent glomerular arterioles, resulting in a reduced blood flow and, ultimately, the glomerular filtration rate. Proximal tubular injury—with vacuolar changes, inclusion bodies, and giant mitochondria—has also been noted. Hyperkalemia and renal tubular acidosis can occur, but these acute effects are usually reversible if the dose is reduced or the drug is discontinued. Chronic irreversible nephrotoxicity associated with tubulointerstitial fibrosis, tubular atrophy, hyaline arteriolar degeneration, and glomerular sclerosis results in long-term renal damage with chronic renal failure. Although chronic renal failure remains stable in many patients, approximately 7 percent of heart transplant patients treated with cyclosporine A progress to ESRD.[153] Hemolytic uremic syndrome, presumably due to endothelial cell damage, has also been described with these agents but this is uncommon.[154]

References

1. Levey AS. Controlling the epidemic of cardiovascular disease in chronic renal disease: Where do we start? *Am J Kidney Dis* 1998; 32(Suppl 3):S5.
2. Causes of Death. United States Renal Data System 1999 Annual Report. *Am J Kidney Dis* 1999; 34(Suppl 1):S87.
3. Foley RN, Parfrey PS, Sarnak MJ. Clinical epidemiology of cardiovascular disease in chronic renal disease. *Am J Kidney Dis* 1998; 32(Suppl 3):S112.
4. Mailloux LU, Levey AS. Hypertension in patients with chronic renal disease. *Am J Kidney Dis* 1998; 32(Suppl 3):S120.
5. Ritz E, Charra B, Leunissen KML, et al. How important is volume excess in the etiology of hypertension in dialysis patients? *Sem Dialysis* 1999; 12:296.
6. Vertes V, Cangiano JL, Berman LB, et al. Hypertension in end-stage renal disease. *N Engl J Med* 1991; 280:978.
7. Weidmann P, Maxwell MH, Lupu AN, et al. Plasma renin activity and blood pressure in terminal renal failure. *N Engl J Med* 1991; 285:757.
8. Ligtenberg G, Blankestijn PJ, Oey PL, et al. Reduction of sympathetic hyperactivity by enalapril in patients with chronic renal failure. *N Engl J Med* 1999; 340:1321.
9. Kim KE, Onesti G, Schwartz AB, et al. Hemodynamics of hypertension in chronic end-stage renal disease. *Circulation* 1972; 46:452.
10. Kim KE, Onesti G, DelGuercio ET, et al. Sequential hemodynamic changes in end-stage renal disease and the anephric state during volume expansion. *Hypertension* 1991; 2:102.
11. Charra B, Calemarad E, Ruffet M, et al. Survival as an index of adequacy of dialysis. *Kidney Int* 1992; 41:1286.
12. Vaughan ED, Carey RM, Ayers CR, et al. Hemodialysis-resistant hypertension: Control with an orally active inhibitor of angiotensin-converting enzyme. *J Clin Endocrinol Metab* 1991; 48:869.
13. Kelly RA, O'Hara DS, Mitch WE, et al. Endogenous digitalis-like factors in hypertension and chronic renal insufficiency. *Kidney Int* 1986; 30:723.
14. Glatter KA, Graves SW, Hollenberg NK, et al. Sustained volume expansion and (Na-K) ATPase inhibition in chronic renal failure. *Am J Hypertension* 1994; 7:1016.
15. Converse RL Jr, Jacobsen TN, Toto RD, et al. Sympathetic overactivity in patients with chronic renal failure. *N Engl J Med* 1992; 327:1912.
16. Remuzzi, G. Sympathetic overactivity in hypertension patients with chronic renal disease. *N Engl J Med* 1999; 340:1360.
17. Cinotti GA, Pugliese F. Prostaglandins in blood pressure regulation. *Kidney Int* 1988; 35(suppl 25):57.
18. Shichiri M, Hirata Y, Ando K, et al. Plasma endothelin levels in patients with uremia. *Hypertension* 1990; 15:493.

19. Goldsmith DJA, Covic AA, Venning MC, et al. Blood pressure reduction after parathyroidectomy for secondary hyperparathyroidism: Further evidence implicating calcium homeostasis in blood pressure regulation. *Am J Kidney Dis* 1996; 27:819.
20. Radermacher J, Koch KM. Treatment of renal anemia by erythropoietin substitution: The effects on the cardiovascular system. *Clin Nephrol* 1995; 44(suppl 1):S56.
21. Mann JFE. Hypertension and cardiovascular effects–Long-term safety and potential long-term benefits of r-HuEPO. *Nephrol Dial Transplant* 1995; 10(suppl 2):80.
22. Zazgornik J, Biesenbach G, Janko O, et al. Bilateral nephrectomy: The best, but often overlooked, treatment for refractory hypertension in hemodialysis patients. *Am J Hypertension* 1998; 11:1364.
23. Kaski BL. Hyperlipidemia in patients with chronic renal disease. *Am J Kidney Dis* 1998; 32(Suppl 3):S142.
24. Chan MK, Persaud J, Varghese Z, et al. Pathogenic roles of post-heparin lipases in lipid abnormalities in hemodialysis patients. *Kidney Int* 1991; 25:812.
25. Lindholm B, Norbeck HE. Serum lipids and lipoproteins during continuous ambulatory peritoneal dialysis. *Acta Med Scand* 1986; 220:143.
26. Ames RP, Hill P. Elevation of serum lipid levels during diuretic therapy of hypertension. *Am J Med* 1976; 61:748.
27. Tanaka N, Sakaguchi S, Oshige K, et al. Effect of chronic administration of propranolol on lipoprotein composition. *Metabolism* 1976; 25:1071.
28. Lacour B, Chanard J, Haguet M, et al. Carnitine improves lipid anomalies in haemodialysis patients. *Lancet* 1980; 2:763.
29. Wessel-Aas T, Blomhoff JP, Wideroe T-E, et al. The effect of systemic heparinization on plasma lipoproteins and toxicity in patients on hemodialysis and continuous ambulatory peritoneal dialysis. *Acta Med Scand* 1984; 216:85.
30. Ritz E, Augustin J, Bommer J, et al. Should hyperlipemia of renal failure be treated? *Kidney Int* 1985; 28:S-84.
31. Golper TA. Therapy for uremic hyperlipidemia. *Nephron* 1991; 38:217.
32. Goldberg AP, Hagberg JM, Delez JA, et al. Metabolic effects of exercise training in hemodialysis patients. *Kidney Int* 1980; 18:754.
33. Hamazaki T, Nakazawa R, Tateno S, et al. Effects of fish oil rich in eicosapentaenoic acid on serum lipid in hyperlipidemic hemodialysis patients. *Kidney Int* 1984; 26:81.
34. Expert panel on detection evaluation and treatment of high blood cholesterol in adults: Summary of the second report of the National Cholesterol Education Program (NCEP) (Adult treatment panel II). JAMA 1993; 269:3015.
35. Bostom AG, Lathrop L. Hyperhomocysteinemia in end-stage renal disease: Prevalence, etiology, and potential relationship to arteriosclerotic outcomes. *Kidney Int* 1997; 52:10.
36. Beto JA, Bansal VK. Interventions for other risk factors: tobacco use, physical inactivity, menopause, and homocysteine. *Am J Kidney Dis* 1998; 32(Suppl 3):S172.
37. Guttormsen AB, Ueland PM, Svarstad E, et al. Kinetic basis of hyperhomocysteinemia in patients with chronic renal failure. *Kidney Int* 1997; 52:495.
38. Moustapha A, Naso A, Nahlawi M, et al. Prospective study of hyperhomocysteinemia as an adverse cardiovascular risk factor in end-stage renal disease [published erratum appears in *Circulation* 1998; 97:711]. *Circulation* 1998; 97:138.
39. Passaver J, Bussemaker E, Gross P. Dialysis hypotension: Do we see light at the end of the tunnel? *Nephrol Dial Transp* 1999; 13:3024.
40. Daugirdas JT. Dialysis-induced hypotension: A fresh look at pathophysiology. *Kidney Int* 1991; 39:233.
41. Rosa AA, Shideman J, McHugh R, et al. The importance of osmolality fall and ultrafiltration rate on hemodialysis side effects. *Nephron* 1981; 27:134.
42. Keshaviah P, Shapiro F. A critical examination of dialysis-induced hypotension. *Am J Kidney Dis* 1982; 2:290.
43. Henrich WL, Woodard TD, McPhaul JJ Jr. The chronic efficacy and safety of high sodium dialysate: Double-blind, crossover study. *Am J Kidney Dis* 1982; 2:349.
44. Hakim RM, Breillatt J, Lazarus JM, et al. Complement activation and hypersensitivity reactions to dialysis membranes. *N Engl J Med* 1984; 311:878.
45. Pastan S, Bailey J. Dialysis therapy. *N Eng J Med* 1998; 338:1428.
46. Dolovich J, Marshall CP, Smith EKM, et al. Allergy to ethylene oxide in chronic hemodialysis patients. *Artif Organs* 1984; 8:334.
47. Verresen L, Fiink E, Lemke HD, et al. Bradykinin is a moderator of anaphylactoid reactions during hemodialysis with AN69 membranes. *Kidney Int* 1994; 45:1497.
48. Converse RL Jr, Jacobsen TN, Jost CMT, et al. Paradoxical withdrawal of reflex vasoconstriction as a cause of hemodialysis-induced hypotension. *J Clin Invest* 1992; 90:1657.
49. Sang GL, Kovithavongs C, Ulan R, et al. Sodium ramping in hemodialysis: A study of beneficial and adverse effects. *Am J Kidney Dis* 1997; 29:669.
50. Cruz DN, Mahnesmith RL, Brickle HM, et al. Midrodrine and cool dialysate are effective therapies for symptomatic intradialytic hypotension. *Am J Kidney Dis* 1997; 33:920.
51. Felsenfeld AJ. Considerations for the treatment of secondary hyperparathyroidism in renal failure. *J Am Soc Nephrol* 1997; 8:993.
52. Portale AA, Halloran BP, Murphy MM, et al. Oral intake of phosphorus can determine the serum concentration of 1,25-dihydroxyvitamin D by determining its production rate in humans. *J Clin Invest* 1986; 77:7.
53. Fukuda N, Tanaka H, Tominaga Y, et al. Decreased 1,25-dihydroxyvitamin D3 receptor density is associated with a more severe form of parathyroid hyperplasia in chronic uremic patients. *J Clin Invest* 1993; 92:1436.
54. Gogusev J, Duchambon P, Hory B, et al. Depressed expression of calcium receptor in parathyroid gland tissue of patients with hyperparathyroidism. *Kidney Int* 1997; 51:328.
55. Delmez JA, Tindira C, Grooms P, et al. Parathyroid hormone suppression by intravenous 1,25-dihydroxyvitamin D. *J Clin Invest* 1991; 83:1349.
56. Silver J, Russell J, Sherwood LM. Regulation by vitamin D metabolites of messenger ribonucleic acid for preproparathyroid hormone in isolated bovine parathyroid cells. *Proc Natl Acad Sci USA* 1985; 82:4270.
57. Kuzda DC, Huffer WE, Conger JD, et al. Soft tissue calcification in chronic dialysis patients. *Am J Pathol* 1977; 86:403.
58. Goldsmith DG, Covic A, Sambrook PA, et al. Vascular calcification in long-term hemodialysis patients in a single unit: A retrospective analysis. *Nephron* 1977; 77:37.
59. Braun J, Oldendorf N, Moshage W, et al. Electron beam computed tomography in the evaluation of cardiac calcification in chronic dialysis patients. *Am Journal Kidney Dis* 1996; 27:394.
60. Llach F. Cardiac calcification: dealing with another risk factor in patients with kidney failure. *Sem Dial* 1999; 12:293.
61. Ribeiro S, Ramos A, Brandao A, et al. Cardiac valve calcification in haemodialysis patients: Role of calcium-phosphate metabolism. *Nephrol Dial Transplant* 1998; 13:2037.
62. McGonigle RJS, Fowler MB, Timmis AB, et al. Uremic cardiomyopathy: Potential role of vitamin D and parathyroid hormone. *Nephron* 1984; 36:94.
63. Gafter U, Battler A, Eldar M, et al. Effect of hyperparathyroidism on cardiac function in patients with end-stage renal disease. *Nephron* 1985; 41:30.
64. Slatopolsky EA, Burke SK, Dillon MA. RenaGel, a nonabsorbed calcium- and aluminum-free phosphate binder, lowers serum phosphorus and parathyroid hormone. The RenaGel Study Group. *Kidney Int* 1999; 55:299.

65. Llach F, Slatopolsky E, eds. New vitamin D analogues in the treatment of secondary hyperparathyroidism. *Am J Kid Dis* 1998; 32(Suppl 2):S1.
66. U.S. Renal Data System 1992, Annual Report. IV. Comorbid conditions and correlations with mortality risk among 3,399 incident hemodialysis patients. *Am J Kidney Dis* 1992; 20(Suppl 2):S32.
67. Ansari A, Kaupke CJ, Vaziri ND, et al. Cardiac pathology in patients with end-stage renal disease maintained on hemodialysis. *Int J Artif Organs* 1993; 64:560.
68. Wing AJ, Brunner FP, Brynger H, et al. Cardiovascular-related causes of death and the fate of patients with renovascular disease. *Contrib Nephrol* 1984; 41:306.
69. Manske CL. Hyperglycemia and intensive glycemic control in diabetic patients with chronic renal disease. *Am J Kidney Dis* 1998; 32(Suppl 3):S159.
70. Ori Y, Korets A, Katz M, et al. Hemodialysis arteriovenous access—A prospective hemodynamic evaluation. *Nephrol Dial Transplant* 1996; 14(Suppl 1):94.
71. Murphy SW, Foley RN, Parfrey PS. Screening and treatment for cardiovascular disease in patients with chronic renal disease. *Am J Kidney Dis* 1998; 32(Suppl 3):S184.
72. Dahan M, Lagallicier B, Himbert D, et al. Diagnostic value of myocardial thallium stress scintigraphy in the selection of CAD in patients undergoing chronic hemodialysis. *Arch Mal Coeur* 1995; 88:1121.
73. Brown JH, Vites NP, Testa HJ, et al. Value of thallium myocardial imaging in the prediction of future cardiovascular events in patients with end-stage renal failure. *Nephrol Dial Transplant* 1993; 8:433.
74. DePuey EG, Guertler-Krawczynska E, Perkins JV, et al. Alterations in myocardial thallium-201 distribution in patients with chronic systemic hypertension undergoing single-photon emission computed tomography. *Am J Cardiol* 1988; 62:234.
75. Dahan M, Viron BM, Faraggi M, et al. Diagnostic accuracy and prognostic value of combined dipyridamole-exercise thallium imaging in hemodialysis patients. *Kidney Int* 1998; 54:255.
76. Resis G, Marcovitz PA, Leichtman AB, et al. Usefulness of dobutamine stress echocardiography in detecting CAD in end-stage renal disease. *Am J Cardiol* 1995; 75:707.
77. Bates JR, Sawada SG, Segar DS, et al. Evaluation using dobutamine stress echocardiography in patients with insulin dependent diabetes mellitus before kidney and/or pancreas transplant. *Am J Cardiol* 1996; 77:175.
78. Roig E, Betriu A, Castaner A, et al. Disabling angina pectoris with normal coronary arteries in patients undergoing long-term hemodialysis. *Am J Med* 1981; 71:431.
79. Wizemann V, Kaufmann J, Kramer W. Effect of erythropoietin on ischemia tolerance in anemic hemodialysis patients with confirmed coronary artery disease. *Nephron* 1992; 62:161.
80. Francis GS, Sharma B, Collins AJ, et al. Coronary-artery surgery in patients with end-stage renal disease. *Ann Intern Med* 1980; 92:499.
81. Batiuk TD, Kurtz SB, Oh JK, et al. Coronary artery bypass operation in dialysis patients. *Mayo Clin Proc* 1991; 66:45.
82. Schoebel FC, Gradaus F, Ivens K, et al. Restenosis after elective coronary balloon angioplasty in patients with end-stage renal disease: A case-control study using quantitative coronary angiog raphy. *Heart* 1997; 78:337.
83. Herzog CA, Ma JZ, Collins AJ. Long-term survival of dialysis patients in the United States after coronary artery bypass surgery, coronary angioplasty, and coronary stenting. *J Am Soc Nephrol* 1999; 10:166A.
84. Harnett JD, Foley RN, Kent GM, et al. Congestive heart failure in dialysis patients: Prevalence, incidence, prognosis and risk factors. *Kidney Int* 1995; 47:884.
85. Bernardi D, Bernini L, Cini G, et al. Asymmetric septal hypertrophy and sympathetic overactivity in normotensive hemodialyzed patients. *Am Heart J* 1985; 109:539.
86. Levin A, Singer J, Thompson CR, et al. Prevelant left ventricular hypertrophy in the predialysis population: Identifying opportunities for intervention. *Am J Kid Dis* 1996; 27:347.
87. Wizemann V, Blank S, Kramer W. Diastolic dysfunction of the left ventricle in dialysis patients. *Contrib Nephrol* 1994; 106:106.
88. Foley RN, Parfrey PS, Kent GM, et al. Long-term evolution of cardiomyopathy in dialysis patients. *Kidney Int* 1998; 54:1720.
89. Tucker B, Fabbian F, Giles M, et al. Left ventricular hypertrophy and ambulatory blood pressure monitoring in chronic renal failure. *Nephrol Dial Transplant* 1997; 12:724.
90. London GM, De Vernejoul M-C, Fabiani F, et al. Secondary hyperparathyroidism and cardiac hypertrophy in hemodialysis patients. *Kidney Int* 1987; 32:900.
91. Nixon JV, Mitchell JH, McPhaul JJ Jr, et al. Effect of hemodialysis on left ventricular function. *J Clin Invest* 1983; 71:377.
92. Hung J, Harris PJ, Uren RF, et al. Uremic cardiomyopathy—Effect of hemodialysis on left ventricular function in end-stage renal failure. *N Engl J Med* 1980; 230:547.
93. Madsen BR, Alpert MA, Whiting RB, et al. Effect of hemodialysis on left ventricular performance. *Am J Nephrol* 1984; 4:86.
94. Van der Sande FM, Cheriex EC, van Kuijk WH, et al. Effect of dialysate calcium concentration on intradialytic blood pressure course in cardiac-compromised patients. *Am J Kid Dis* 1998; 32:125.
95. Chaignon M, Chen W-T, Tarazi RC, et al. Acute effects of hemodialysis on echographic-determined cardiac performance: Improved contractility resulting from serum increased calcium with reduced potassium despite hypovolemic-reduced cardiac output. *Am Heart J* 1982; 103:374.
96. Rackow EC, Fein IA, Sprung C, et al. Uremic pulmonary edema. *Am J Med* 1978; 64:1084.
97. Young PR Jr, Rohr MS, Marterre WF Jr. High output cardiac failure secondary to brachiocephalic arteriovenous hemodialysis fistula: Two cases. *Am Surg* 1998; 64:239.
98. Eckardt K. Cardiovascular consequences of renal anemia and erythropoietin therapy. *Nephrol Dial Transplant* 1999; 14:1317.
99. Wacker J, Merrill JP. Uremic pericarditis in acute and chronic renal failure. *JAMA* 1954; 156:764.
100. Rostand SG, Rutsky EA. Pericarditis in end-stage renal disease. *Cardiol Clin* 1990; 8:701.
101. Osanloo E, Shalhoub RJ, Cioffi RF, et al. Viral pericarditis in patients receiving hemodialysis. *Arch Intern Med* 1979; 139:301.
102. Houston MC, McChesney JA, Chatterjee K. Pericardial effusion associated with minoxidil therapy. *Arch Intern Med* 1981; 141:69.
103. Silverberg S, Oreopoulos DG, Wise DJ, et al. Pericarditis in patients undergoing long-term hemodialysis and peritoneal dialysis. *Am J Med* 1977; 63:874.
104. Eliasson G, Murphy JF. Steroid therapy in uremic pericarditis. *JAMA* 1974; 229:1634.
105. Buselmeier TJ, Simmons RL, Najarian JS, et al. Uremic pericardial effusion. *Nephron* 1976; 16:371.
106. Minuth NW, Nottebohm GA, Eknoyan G, et al. Indomethacin treatment of pericarditis in chronic hemodialysis patients. *Arch Intern Med* 1975; 135:807.
107. Spector D, Alfred H, Siedlecki M, et al. A controlled study of the effect of indomethacin in uremic pericarditis. *Kidney Int* 1983; 24:663.
108. Goldberg M, Lazarus JM, Gottlieb MN, et al. Treatment of uremic pericardial effusion. *Proc Clin Dial Transplant Forum* 1975; 5:20.
109. Luft FC, Kleit SA, Smith RN, et al. Management of uremic pericarditis with tamponade. *Arch Intern Med* 1974; 134:488.
110. Daugirdas JT, Leehey DJ, Popli S, et al. Subxiphoid pericardiostomy for hemodialysis-associated pericardial effusion. *Arch Intern Med* 1986; 146:1113.

111. Peraino RA. Pericardial effusion in patients treated with maintenance dialysis. *Am J Nephrol* 1983; 3:319.
112. Figueroa W, Alankar S, Pai N, et al. Subxiphoid pericardial window for pericardial effusion in end-stage renal disease. *Am J Kidney Dis* 1996; 27:664.
113. Moraski RE, Bousvaros G. Constrictive pericarditis due to chronic uremia. *N Engl J Med* 1969; 281:542.
114. Robinson DL, Fowler VG, Sexton DJ, et al. Bacterial endocarditis in hemodialysis patients. *Am J Kidney Dis* 1997; 30:521.
115. Marr KA, Kong L, Fowler VG, et al. Incidence and outcome of *Staphylococcus aureus* bacteremia in hemodialysis patients. *Kidney Int* 1998; 54:1684.
116. Nsouli KA, Lazarus JM, Schoenbaum SC, et al. Bacteremic infection in hemodialysis. *Arch Intern Med* 1979; 139:1255.
117. Leonard A, Raij L, Shapiro FL. Bacterial endocarditis in regularly dialyzed patients. *Kidney Int* 1973; 4:407.
118. Cross AS, Steigbigel RT. Infective endocarditis and access site infections in patients on hemodialysis. *Medicine* 1976; 55:453.
119. Haag-Weber M, Horl WH. Uremia and infection: Mechanisms of impaired cellular host defense. *Nephron* 1993; 63:125.
120. Ruiz P, Gomez F, Schrieber AD. Impaired function of macrophage Fc gamma receptors in end-stage renal disease. *N Engl J Med* 1990; 322:717.
121. Forman MB, Virmani R, Robertson RM, et al. Mitral annular calcification in chronic renal failure. *Chest* 1984; 85:367.
122. Straumann E, Meyer B, Mastroli M, et al. Aortic and mitral valve disease in patients with end-stage renal failure on hemodialysis. *Br Heart J* 1992; 67:236.
123. Baglin A, Hanslik T, Vaillant JN, et al. Severe valvular heart disease in patients on chronic dialysis: A five-year multicenter French survey. *Ann Med Int* 1997; 148:521.
124. Kyriakidis M, Voudiclaris S, Kremastinos D, et al. Cardiac arrhythmias in chronic renal failure. *Nephron* 1984; 38:26.
125. Weber H, Schwarzer C, Stummvoll HK, et al. Chronic hemodialysis: High risk patients for arrhythmias? *Nephron* 1984; 37:180.
126. Wizeman V, Kramer W, Funke T, et al. Dialysis-induced cardiac arrhythmias: Fact or fiction? *Nephron* 1985; 39:356.
127. Dzau VJ. Renal and circulatory mechanisms in congestive heart failure. *Kidney Int* 1987; 31:1402.
128. Xu DL, Martin PY, Ohara M, et al. Upregulation of aquaporin-2 water channel expression in chronic heart failure rat. *J Clin Invest* 1997; 99:1500.
129. Schrier RW, Abraham WT. Hormones and hemodynamics in heart failure. *N Engl J Med* 1999; 341:577.
130. Abraham WT. Natriuretic peptides in heart failure. *Congestive Heart Fail* 1998; 4:23.
131. Lee WH, Packer M. Prognostic importance of serum sodium concentration and its modification by converting-enzyme inhibition in patients with severe chronic heart failure. *Circulation* 1986; 73:257.
132. Suki WN. Renal hemodynamic consequences of angiotensin-converting enzyme inhibition in congestive heart failure. *Arch Intern Med* 1989; 149:669.
133. Dzau VJ, Packer M, Lilly LS, et al. Prostaglandins in severe congestive heart failure. *N Engl J Med* 1984; 310:347.
134. Rudnick MR. Nephrotoxic risks of renal angiography: Contrast media-associated nephrotoxicity and atheroembolism—A critical review. *Am J Kidney Dis* 1994; 24:713.
135. Taliercio CP, Vlietstra RE, Fisher LD, et al. Risks for renal dysfunction with cardiac angiography. *Ann Intern Med* 1986; 104:501.
136. Solomon R. Contrast-medium-induced acute renal failure. *Kidney Int* 1998; 53:230.
137. Fang LST, Sirota RA, Ebert TH, et al. Low fractional excretion of sodium with contrast media-induced acute renal failure. *Arch Intern Med* 1980; 140:531.
138. Solomon R, Werner C, Mann D, et al. Effects of saline, mannitol, and furosemide on acute decreases in renal function induced by radiocontrast agents. *N Engl J Med* 1994; 331:1416.
139. Thadhani RI, Camargo CA Jr. Atheroembolic renal failure after invasive procedures: Natural history based on 52 histologically proven cases. *Medicine* 1995; 74:350.
140. Dalakos TG, Streeten DHP, Jones D, et al. "Malignant" hypertension resulting from atheromatous embolization predominantly of one kidney. *Am J Med* 1974; 57:135.
141. McGowan JA, Greenberg A. Cholesterol atheroembolic renal disease. *Am J Nephrol* 1986; 6:135.
142. Richards AM, Eliot RS, Kanjuh VI, et al. Cholesterol embolism: A multiple-system disease masquerading as polyarteritis nodosa. *Am J Cardiol* 1965; 15:696.
143. Scully RE, Mark EJ, McNeely BU. Case records of the Massachusetts General Hospital. *N Engl J Med* 1986; 315:308.
144. Cosio FG, Zager RA, Sharma HM. Atheroembolic renal disease causes hypocomplementaemia. *Lancet* 1985; 2:118.
145. Lessman RK, Johnson SF, Coburn JW. Renal artery embolism. *Ann Intern Med* 1978; 89:477.
146. Winzelberg GG, Hull JD, Agar JWM, et al. Elevation of serum lactate dehydrogenase levels in renal infarction. *JAMA* 1979; 242:268.
147. London IL, Hoffstein P, Perkoff GT, et al. Renal infarction. *Arch Intern Med* 1968; 121:87.
148. Jelliffe RW. An improved method of digoxin therapy. *Ann Intern Med* 1968; 69:703.
149. Kirch W, Gorg ER. Clinical pharmacokinetics of atenolol–A review. *Eur J Drug Metab Pharmacokinet* 1982; 7:81.
150. Cohn JN, Burke LP. Nitroprusside. *Ann Intern Med* 1979; 91:752.
151. Oparil S, Aronson S, Deeb GM, et al. Fenoldopam: A new parenteral antihypertensive: consensus roundtable on the management of perioperative hypertension and hypertensive crises. *Am J Hypertension* 1999; 12:653.
152. Ader JL, Rostaing L. Cyclosporin nephrotoxicity: Pathophysiology and comparison with FK-506. *Curr Opin Nephrol Hypertension* 1998; 7:539.
153. Goldstein DJ, Zuech N, Sehgal V, et al. Cyclosporin-associated end-stage nephropathy after cardiac transplantation. *Transplantation* 1997; 63:664.
154. De Mattos AM, Olyaei AJ, Bennett WM. Pharmacology of immunosuppressive medications used in renal diseases and transplantation. *Am J Kid Dis* 1996; 28:631.

C H A P T E R 85

EXERCISE AND THE CARDIOVASCULAR SYSTEM: ACUTE HEMODYNAMICS, CONDITIONING TRAINING, THE ATHLETE'S HEART, AND SUDDEN DEATH

Gerald F. Fletcher / Thomas R. Flipse

Exercise for the cardiovascular system has evolved in recent years as an important component of preventive and maintenance health care. Exercise, defined as properly prescribed physical activity, can provide health benefits for asymptomatic, healthy individuals as well as for those who are at high risk for or have established cardiovascular disease. This chapter addresses the topics of acute hemodynamics, conditioning training and implementation, the athlete's heart, and sudden death with exercise.

ACUTE HEMODYNAMICS

During physical activity, body energy expenditure increases, requiring appropriate adjustments in blood flow that affect the entire cardiovascular system. These changes are the result of a combination and integration of neural, chemical, and other physiologic factors.

The cardiovascular "control center" is believed to be in the ventrolateral medulla of the brain and receives input that modulates its activity. Central impulses are provided by the somatomotor centers of the brain. Peripheral impulses are generated by the mechanoreceptors found in muscles, joints, and the vascular system; the chemoreceptors from the muscles and vascular system; and the vascular baroreceptors. These impulses arrive at the control center through autonomic afferent fibers. The control center regulates the output of blood from the heart and its preferential distribution to other organs and tissues in need.

The "feed-forward" command system, located in the higher areas of the brain, provides a coordinated and rapid response of the cardiovascular system to optimize tissue perfusion and maintain central blood pressure in relation to motor cortex activity. The central command provides the greatest control over heart rate during exercise[1] and is also involved in the preexercise anticipatory period.[2] The effect of the stimulating input from the higher command centers is an alteration of the autonomic tone. The involvement of the central command in cardiovascular regulation may explain in part the influence of one's emotional state on the cardiovascular response.

The cardiovascular control center also receives input from peripheral receptors in muscles, joints, and blood vessels. Stretch and tension of muscular and articular mechanoreceptors trigger afferent impulses. Impulses triggered by the stimulation of muscle chemoreceptors resulting from products of metabolism influence the control center as well. This reflex neural input, termed the exercise pressor reflex, provides rapid feedback that modifies the parasympathetic or sympathetic outflow to adjust the cardiovascular response to physical activity.[3] Input from mechanoreceptors in the muscles and joints is important in the regulation of the circulatory response during dynamic exercise.[4]

Baroreceptors are located in the aortic arch and carotid sinuses and respond to changes in arterial blood pressure, and regulate heart rate by reciprocal changes in activity of the two divisions of the autonomic nervous system. The arterial baroreceptors protect the cardiovascular system against relatively short-term changes in blood pressure, as seen during physical exercise. The cardiopulmonary mechanoreceptors in the atria, ventricles, and pulmonary vessels are tonically active and participate in the regulation of the circulatory responses through the autonomic nervous system. An increase in blood pressure results in a reflex slowing of the heart, and the converse applies during hypotension. During physical activity, this feedback mechanism is "reset" so that blood pressure is permitted to rise to the higher levels observed during exercise. The aortic and carotid bodies contain chemoreceptors sensitive to arterial oxygen, carbon dioxide, and hydrogen ion concentrations—indices that may be altered during physical activity. Decreased arterial oxygen levels cause an increase in the arterial pressure, while changes in carbon dioxide and hydrogen ion concentration have a relatively small effect by this pathway.

Circulatory Adjustments with Exercise

The circulatory response to exercise involves a complex series of adjustments resulting in an increase in cardiac output (CO) that is proportional to the increased metabolic demands placed on the body. These changes ensure that the metabolic needs of exercising muscles are met, that hyperthermia does not occur, and that blood flow to essential organs is protected. Certain major changes occur during exercise that provide blood flow required by the muscles. These are the increase in CO and the redistribution of blood flow, with a relative increase in flow to the exercising muscles. (CO is defined as the product of stroke volume and heart rate. The average CO at rest is about 5 L/min for both trained and untrained men. In women the value is usually 25 percent lower.)

Resting CO increases immediately before the onset of physical exercise as a result of anticipatory changes in the autonomic nervous system resulting in tachycardia and increased venous return. After the onset of exercise, CO may increase rapidly until steady-rate exercise is reached; this is followed by a gradual rise until a plateau is achieved. The magnitude of the hemodynamic response during physical activity depends on the intensity of exercise and the muscle mass involved. In sedentary individuals, the CO during maximal exercise increases approximately four times, to an average of 20 to 22 L/min. In elite-class athletes, however, the CO may rise eightfold, to values of 35 to 40 L/min.

HEART RATE RESPONSE TO EXERCISE

At the transition from rest to strenuous exercise, the heart rate increases rapidly to levels of 160 to 180 beats per minute. During short periods of maximal exercise, rates of 240 beats per minute have been recorded. The initial rapid increase is believed to be the result of central command influences or a rapid reflex from muscle mechanoreceptors. The almost instant acceleration in heart rate is due more to vagal withdrawal than to an increase in sympathetic tone. Later increases result from reflex activation of the pulmonary stretch receptors, which trigger increased sympathetic tone and more parasympathetic withdrawal. Increased circulating catecholamines play a role as well. It has been shown that during exercise the heart rate increase accounts for a greater percentage of the increase in CO than does the increase in stroke volume. For instance, the stroke volume normally reaches its maximum when the CO has increased to only one-half of its maximum. Any further increase in CO occurs by an increase in the heart rate.

STROKE VOLUME CHANGES WITH EXERCISE

Two physiologic mechanisms influence the stroke volume of the heart. The first is intrinsic to the myocardium and involves enhanced cardiac filling in diastole secondary to increased venous return followed by a more forceful systolic contraction. The second mechanism involves normal ventricular filling with a forceful contraction secondary to neurohormonal influences, which leads to more complete emptying.

ENHANCED DIASTOLIC FILLING

Greater ventricular filling during diastole, or preload, is caused by factors that slow heart rate and increase venous return. Increased end-diastolic volume stretches myocardial fibers and causes a greater contraction with a larger stroke volume. As myocardial fibers stretch, there is a more optimal arrangement of the myofilaments of the sarcomere, which results in enhanced contractility. It is believed that this mechanism is responsible for the increased stroke volume during transition from rest to exercise or from the upright to the supine position. CO and stroke volume are the highest in the supine position. In this position, the stroke volume is nearly maximal at rest and increases only slightly during exercise. In the upright position, at rest, the venous return to the heart is diminished, resulting in a smaller stroke volume and CO. During upright exercise, however, stroke volume can increase to the point where it approaches the maximum stroke volume observed in the recumbent position, usually without an increase in ventricular diastolic dimensions.[5]

IMPROVED SYSTOLIC EMPTYING

Although experimental findings are not always consistent, it seems that increases in stroke volume during upright exercise occur through the combined effect of enhanced diastolic filling and a more complete emptying during systole. The improved myocardial inotropy during exercise is the result of the increased levels of catecholamines. In the normal supine individual, increased CO with exercise results predominantly from an increase in heart rate, with little improvement of stroke volume. In the upright position, in the early phase of exercise CO rises due to a simultaneous increase in stroke volume and heart rate. In the later phases of exercise, the increase in heart rate is primarily responsible for the further increase in CO.

DISTRIBUTION OF CARDIAC OUTPUT DURING EXERCISE

Blood flow to various tissues is generally proportional to metabolic activity, but certain organs have blood flow variations with the metabolic demands of exercising muscle. At rest, about 20 percent of the 5 L/min CO is distributed to the skeletal muscle. This accounts for approximately 4 to 7 mL of blood delivered each minute to every 100 g of muscle. During physical activity, regional blood flow depends on the type of exercise, environmental conditions, and level of fatigue. Still, the majority (up to 85 percent) of the increased CO is diverted to the working muscles. This represents about 50 to 75 mL blood every minute per 100 g of muscle. Even within active muscle, the increased blood flow is highly regulated, so that the greatest amount is delivered to the oxidative portions of the muscle at the expense of the tissue with high glycolytic capacity.

Two factors are responsible for the increased muscle flow during exercise: increased CO and redistribution of blood flow. Local metabolic conditions and neural and hormonal vascular regulation control the shunting of blood from various tissues to active muscles. The local response is due primarily to the buildup of vasodilatory metabolites in the exercising muscle, the increase in skeletal muscle flow being directly proportional to the increase in body oxygen consumption ($\dot{V}O_2$).

During exertion, parasympathetic activity is withdrawn and sympathetic discharge is maximal. These changes result in increased release of norepinephrine from the sympathetic postganglionic nerve endings. Plasma epinephrine levels are also increased. As a result, the majority of the vascular beds of the body are constricted, except those in exercising muscles and in the coronary and cerebral circulation. Blood flow to the skin increases during light and moderate exercise, favoring body cooling. Further increases in workload cause a progressive decrease in skin flow as the rising cutaneous sympathetic vascular tone overcomes the thermoregulatory vasodilatory response.[2] The kidneys and splanchnic tissues use only 10 to 25 percent of the oxygen available in the blood supply. Consequently,

TABLE 85-1 Types of Exercise

	Isotonic	Isometric	Resistance
Alternative terminology	Dynamic	Static	Resistive
Example	Running	Static hand grip	Weight lifting
Oxygen uptake	Greatest	Least	Intermediate
CO	Greatest	Least	Intermediate
Peripheral resistance	Greatest decrease	Least decrease	Intermediate
Blood pressure	Decreases	Increases	Increases

ABBREVIATION: CO = cardiac output.

considerable reductions in blood flow to these tissues can be tolerated because of increased extraction of oxygen from the available blood supply.[6] Some tissues cannot, however, compromise their blood supply. At rest, the heart extracts about 75 percent of the oxygen in the coronary blood flow. Because of a limited margin of reserve, increased myocardial demands during exercise are met mainly by a fourfold increase in coronary blood flow. Cerebral blood flow also increases during exercise by approximately 25 to 30 percent compared to the resting flow.[7] During maximal exercise, however, cerebral flow may also decrease in association with hyperventilaton and respiratory alkalosis.

On cessation of exercise, there is an abrupt decrease in heart rate and CO secondary to removal of the sympathetic drive and reactivation of vagal activity. In contrast, systemic vascular resistance remains lower for some time due to persistent vasodilatation in the muscles. As a result, arterial pressure falls, often below preexercise levels, for periods up to 12 h into recovery.[8] Blood pressure is then stabilized at normal levels by the baroreceptor reflexes.

Exercise Type and Cardiovascular Response

Different types of exercise impose various loads on the cardiovascular system. Isotonic (dynamic) exercise is defined as muscular contraction of large muscle groups resulting in movement. It primarily induces a volume load to the heart. Isometric (static) exercise is defined as a constant muscular contraction of smaller muscle group without movement. It provokes more pressure than volume load to the heart. Significant increases in both CO and oxygen consumption and a fall in systemic vascular resistance characterize the acute load posed by isotonic exercise. In contrast, isometric exercise increases systemic vascular resistance while producing only minimal changes in CO and oxygen consumption.[9] A third type of exercise is resistance exercise. This is a combination of isometric and isotonic exercise evoked by using muscular contraction with movement, as in free-weight lifting. Most activities, such as sports or employment-related activities, usually combine all three types of exercise (see Table 85-1).

ISOTONIC (DYNAMIC) EXERCISE

The acute cardiovascular response to isotonic exercise is accomplished through both central and peripheral adaptations that result in increased oxygen delivery to and extraction by the exercising muscles. In normal sedentary individuals, $\dot{V}O_2$ typically increases tenfold from rest to maximal exertion,[10] while in world-class athletes the increase can be even greater. Maximal $\dot{V}O_2$ is considered an indicator of the level or degree of exercise training.[11]

During acute isotonic exercise, such as running, total peripheral vascular resistance falls as a result of marked vasodilatation of vessels in the exercising muscles, which overcomes the vasoconstriction of the splanchnic and renal vessels. This effect is pronounced at minimal levels of exercise, with little further change as exercise increases. As a result, afterload decreases and CO is redistributed mainly to the active muscles. These changes result from local autoregulation and are mediated by local factors related to the level of tissue metabolism (hypoxia, acidic pH, and increased local temperature), stimulation of sympathetic vasodilatory nerve endings, and the effects of circulating catecholamines.

During prolonged dynamic exercise, skeletal muscle metabolism is primarily aerobic and requires a significant increase in oxygen supply to meet the increased demand for adenosine triphosphate generation. The increased oxygen requirements are met by an augmentation of the local blood flow and improved oxygen extraction.

ISOMETRIC (STATIC) EXERCISE

The acute cardiovascular responses to isometric exercise are different from the responses to isotonic exercise. The oxygen requirements needed to sustain the contraction of a smaller muscle group without performing external work are lower.

With isometric exercise, the necessary $\dot{V}O_2$ is maintained with a smaller increase in CO. An increase in regional blood flow is limited because local vasodilatation is impeded by the mechanical compression of the blood vessels during the sustained muscular contraction.[12] Actually, regional blood flow may decrease. In order to maintain regional perfusion, a pressor response is evoked, which is thought to be, at least in part, mediated locally by reflexes originating in the muscles.[13] The amplitude of the increase in blood pressure is proportional both to the relative muscle tension and the mass of the muscle groups involved.

As a result of the increase in blood pressure and in the absence of an increase in venous return, stroke volume usually declines. In its "pure state," static exercise represents a pressure, or systolic, load. In order to maintain the higher CO, the heart rate must increase, often out of proportion to the metabolic needs of the active muscle groups.

RESISTANCE (RESISTIVE) EXERCISE

Resistance exercises are activities that use low or moderate repetition movements against a resistance, generating a rise in muscle tension. The acute cardiovascular response to resistance exercise is determined by the extent of both the isotonic and isometric components.

Weight lifting is considered the prototype resistance exercise and is thought to have a high isometric component. Blood pressure and heart rate responses during weight lifting are proportional to the relative intensity of muscle contraction, the mass of the muscle groups involved, and the duration of the contraction.[14] Weight-training exercises have been shown to cause an acute increase in blood pressure.[15] This is thought to be the result of the restricted muscle blood flow and a centrally mediated pressor response caused by increased muscle tension. The heart rate response during maximal upper body resistance exercise is lower than that seen during maximal isotonic exercise.[16] This is believed to be one of the factors to explain why the heart rate–blood pressure product during maximal resistance exercise is lower than that observed during maximal dynamic exercise.

Previous concerns regarding the safety of resistance training have been rebutted by several reports that reveal that moderate resistance training programs are safe even in subjects with cardiac disease.[17,18] At this time, it is believed that resistance training is useful for promoting muscle strength and flexibility but probably contributes less significantly than isotonic exercise to overall cardiovascular health.

CONDITIONING TRAINING

Physical conditioning or exercise training affects the cardiovascular and skeletal muscle systems in a variety of ways that improve work performance or exercise capacity. The response of the cardiovascular system to regular exercise is an increase in its capacity to deliver oxygen to active muscle. Physical training also improves the ability of the muscles to utilize oxygen. It is believed that, through conditioning induced by repetitive periods of dynamic exercise, the maximal $\dot{V}O_2$ may increase to two- to threefold. About half of this increase is due to increased CO and half to peripheral adaptations that improve oxygen extraction.[19] Through physical training, an individual can increase maximal exercise intensity and duration and achieve submaximal work loads with less cardiovascular effort. This aspect of exercise conditioning has the broadest therapeutic impact.

With conditioning, cardiac stroke volume increases, with exercise secondary to alterations in cardiac structure and function. At rest, CO, however, is similar for both trained and untrained individuals. Endurance training induces an increase in the resting parasympathetic tone, associated with a concomitant reduction in resting sympathetic activity. The effect is a bradycardia, with recorded heart rates averaging about 50 beats per minute, although values below 30 beats per minute have been recorded for healthy athletes. The CO is maintained by an increase in stroke volume. The underlying physiologic mechanisms are not fully understood, but it is believed that increased blood volume associated with training and intrinsic myocardial factors are responsible (Table 85-2). During exercise, trained individuals achieve a larger maximal CO than do sedentary persons. In the untrained person, there is only a small increase in stroke volume during the transition from rest to exercise, while the major augmentation in CO is induced by tachycardia. The improved cardiac performance after conditioning is secondary to both the Frank-Starling mechanism and augmented myocardial contraction and relaxation.

It has been shown that, in previously sedentary individuals, 8 weeks of aerobic training will increase stroke volume. This change results from increased end-diastolic dimensions of the ventricular cavity with preservation or even reduction of the end-systolic size.[20] The values are, however, much lower than those of well-trained athletes.[21] It is not known whether this is the result of prolonged training, genetic factors, or a combination of both. After cessation of training, these changes largely regress within 3 weeks.

Several factors contribute to the chronic adaptations seen with training. An increased parasympathetic tone induces bradycardia, which prolongs diastolic filling time, resulting in ventricular dilatation. In trained individuals, there is an increased preload, attributed to an expanded plasma volume in response to aerobic training.[22] Some studies have shown that endurance training results in increased compliance of the left ventricle.[23] This is probably due to enhanced early diastolic filling and increased peak myocardial lengthening during exercise.[24,25] These findings are in contrast to those in pressure overload conditions, when peak shortening and relaxation rates are diminished (Table 85-2).

These physiologic changes are accompanied by biochemical and ultrastructural alterations of the myocardial fibers, which have been demonstrated in the hearts of physically conditioned animals. There is an increase in lactic dehydrogenase and pyruvate kinase activity, which enhances the respiratory capacity of the cardiac myocytes. The size of the myocardial cells increases, as well as the number of mitochondria and myofibrils. In addition, changes in the sarcolemma and sarcoplasmic reticulum have been noted. These cellular organelles are implicated in the utilization of intracellular calcium, and the associated changes may explain the improved diastolic function of the conditioned heart.

It has been demonstrated that the cross-sectional area of the epicardial coronary arteries increases in response to exercise. Alterations in the microcirculation have been identified in animal studies, revealing an increased capillary density with an increased capillary-to-fiber ratio and a decrease in the diffusion distance between the capillaries and the mitochondria of myocytes.[26] Some data suggest that conditioning can promote coronary collateral formation to a potentially ischemic vascular bed.[27] These adaptations may enable the heart to better tolerate and recover from transient episodes of ischemia and to function at a lower percentage of its total oxidative capacity during exercise.[28] It is therefore likely that training-induced myocardial adaptations can provide protection from myocardial ischemia of coronary artery disease.

Skeletal muscle also undergoes adaptations with training that favor enhanced oxygen extraction. With long-term training, capillary density and capillary-to-fiber ratio in skeletal muscles increase.[29] The number of mitochondria increases, as do the oxidative enzyme levels in the mitochondria. It appears that other cellular adaptations occur with physical conditioning, including increases in myoglobin levels, in the levels of enzymes

TABLE 85-2 Clinical Effects of Exercise Training

Increase in oxygen consumption
Increase in cardiac stroke volume
Increase in maximal exercise CO
Increase in resting parasympathetic tone
Decrease in resting sympathetic tone
Decrease in resting heart rate

ABBREVIATION: CO = cardiac output.

involved in lipid metabolism, and in ATPase activity with physical conditioning.[30] It is estimated that improved peripheral oxygen extraction accounts for approximately 50 percent of the increased maximal $\dot{V}O_2$ observed during exercise. The proportion may be even higher when CO has a limited capability to increase, which is of practical benefit for individuals with a limited cardiac reserve.

Gender Differences

Few studies have assessed the physiologic responses of women to exercise, but the qualitative aspects of these responses are similar to those seen in men, and basically the same physiologic changes occur in response to acute dynamic or static exercise. There have been some basic quantitative differences, in that teenage girls have a 5 to 10 percent greater CO at any level of submaximal oxygen uptake than do boys.[31] This is likely explained by the 10 percent lower hemoglobin concentration in women than in men. In order to deliver the same amount of oxygen, there is a compensatory proportionate increase in CO. The maximal aerobic capacity in women is approximately 50 percent lower than in men.[32] If adjusted to lean body mass, the difference is reduced to about 10 to 15 percent, which probably represents a true gender-specific difference.

The absolute number of muscle fibers and the fiber-type distribution are similar in women and men.[33] For reasons that are unclear, muscle fibers in men are hypertrophied, resulting in a cross-sectional muscle mass that is higher than in women. The increased muscle mass in men explains the greater isometric strength, while strength adjusted to cross-sectional muscle area is similar.[34]

Another gender difference with potentially significant clinical implications is the mechanism through which stroke volume is increased during acute dynamic exercise. In men there is a progressive increase in ejection fraction with little or no increase in end-diastolic volume. In contrast, women tend to increase end-diastolic volume without a significant increase in ejection fraction,[35] which results in a plateau of ejection fraction during stress testing compared to the continued increase in men.

Aging Differences

Aging results in changes in cardiovascular structure and function and varies significantly among individuals. An increased frequency of acquired heart disease occurs during aging, and there needs to be a differentiation between normal aging and the interplay of aging and disease.

Left ventricular hypertrophy and prolongation of the isovolumic relaxation period in aging can cause a decrease in early left ventricular diastolic compliance similar to the changes seen in the hypertensive heart.[36] An augmented atrial contraction ensures enhanced ventricular filling later in diastole.[37] As a result, left ventricular end-diastolic volume does not decrease with age; the end-diastolic pressure is often higher in older subjects.[38] The resting ejection fraction remains stable in healthy subjects with aging,[39] while the resting CO decreases or remains unchanged.[40] Exercise-induced alterations in cardiovascular function of the elderly may be attributed in part to the effect of age on intrinsic cellular mechanisms or to the autonomic modulation of these mechanisms.[41]

It has been noted that exercise capacity and maximal $\dot{V}O_2$ decrease with aging.[42] When adjusted for lean body mass, however, the age difference in maximal $\dot{V}O_2$ is minimized.[43] Measurements of CO during exercise have failed to substantiate that a failure of CO to increase limits peak $\dot{V}O_2$ or work capacity in older subjects. There is no clear explanation for the decline in maximal work performance and reduced maximal $\dot{V}O_2$, with aging; however, there are several mechanisms that have been proposed to influence this process. These proposed mechanisms include skeletal muscle fatigue, increased work of breathing or overall decrease in pulmonary function, differences in muscle mass, reduced blood flow to skeletal muscle, decreased oxygen extraction, or psychological factors. These age-related changes can be overcome to some extent through physical conditioning. Healthy elderly individuals undergoing 1 year of conditioning have shown a significant rise in maximum $\dot{V}O_2$.[44] Potential mechanisms for this improvement include an improved beta-adrenergic sensitivity and/or a decrease in afterload.

With regard to the effect of exercise on the cardiovascular system in the elderly, there are certain significant changes. In the elderly there is a decrease in the maximal heart rate response during exercise at any work load, and this observation is likely explained by a decreased sympathetic response. The end-systolic volume, also fails to decrease with exercise, as it does in youth. This is thought to represent a diminished cardiac inotropy and increased impedance to ejection. These alterations are not attributable to decreased circulating catecholamine production, since the plasma levels of catecholamines in the elderly are actually higher during exercise.[45] Another difference from younger individuals is a greater increase in end-diastolic volume. The stroke volume is augmented secondary to utilization of the Frank-Starling mechanism. These changes result in a similar CO in elderly and younger individuals at any specific exercise load. However, the mechanisms for achieving the augmented CO differ markedly. While in young individuals CO is augmented by utilizing adrenergically mediated responses (increased heart rate, decreased end-systolic volume, and decreased impedance to left ventricle ejection), the elderly rely mainly on the effective utilization of the Frank-Starling mechanism, which compensates for the age-related decrease in beta-adrenergic responsiveness.

The ejection fraction at rest and during exercise is used clinically in the identification of heart disease and in assessing its severity and prognosis. Ejection fraction at rest is unchanged with age and increases during exercise in both young and old healthy subjects. This increase is less in older individuals due to a smaller decrease in end-systolic volume. In all individuals, however, a decrease in ejection fraction during exercise is abnormal and suggestive of a pathologic condition.

Implementation of Exercise Training

The type of activity, frequency, duration, intensity, and progression are important variables that influence the benefit obtained from different types of physical activity. The epidemiologic literature suggests that moderate-intensity activities, such as brisk walking, performed on a regular basis confer cardioprotection.[46–48] More vigorous activity and higher levels of conditioning may confer greater cardioprotection,[49] but this issue has not been clearly resolved. High-intensity exercise programs are often associated with poor compliance rates and more musculoskeletal injuries. For these reasons, a highly structured program of vigorous exercise, especially in the elderly, is not generally recommended. Health benefits can be gained by performing moderate-intensity activity in less formal settings.

Current guidelines recommend that persons of all ages perform exercise of moderate intensity for 30 to 60 min, four to six times weekly or at least 30 min of moderate-intensity physical activity on a near-daily basis.[50–53] At the present, only 10 to 20 percent of the population meets this recommendation.[51,54] Since only a small percentage of the population is employed in a physically demanding occupation, most need to perform this activity in their leisure time. Examples of recommended activities include brisk walking, cycling, swimming, and yard work. Daily activity does not need to be continuous. The duration of any period of activity should be at least 10 min, and the accumulated daily duration should be at least 30 min. Those who are sedentary should be encouraged to initially perform a duration of activity that is comfortable and to gradually increase to 30 to 60 min of daily activity. People who meet these daily standards and who wish to increase their activity further should be encouraged to do so. Figure 85-1 displays an exercise training model protocol for beginning and maintaining an effective training program. Resistance exercises can be added to the activity program to increase muscle strength. Resistance training using 8 to 10 different exercise sets with 10 to 15 repetitions each (arms, shoulders, chest, trunk, back, hips, and legs) performed at a moderate to high intensity (e.g., 10 to 15 pounds of free weight) for a minimum of 2 days per week is recommended.

Physicians and other health professionals should encourage the general public and their patients to follow these guidelines. Many physicians believe they lack adequate training in physical activity counseling, and implementation of preventive services into medical practice can be difficult due to time and financial constraints. To address these issues, the Centers for Disease Control and Prevention developed the Physician-Based Assessment and Counseling for Exercise (PACE) project.[55] This system includes a simple discussion of physical activity counseling

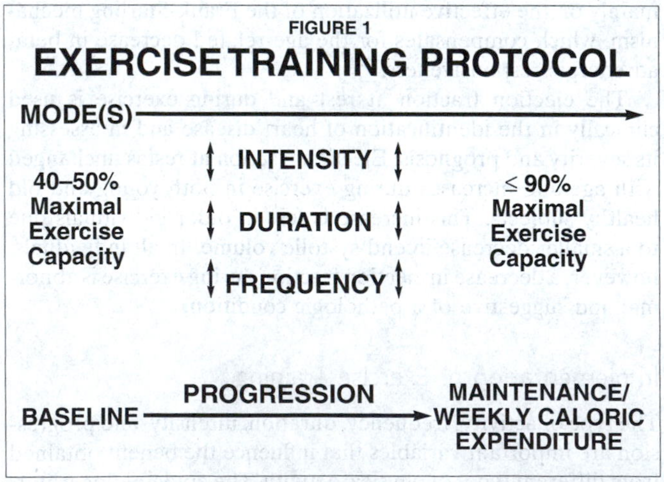

FIGURE 85-1 Exercise training model protocol. *Mode* refers to the type of exercise, such as walking, jogging, swimming, or biking. *Maximal exercise capacity* refers to that achieved at peak exercise testing and can be expressed in terms of oxygen consumption, metabolic units, heart rate, caloric expenditure, or perceived exertion. Intensity, duration, and frequency are each increased or decreased appropriately to ultimately achieve a maintenance level of total weekly caloric expenditure.

and illustrates how a clinician can efficiently incorporate physical activity counseling into a busy clinical practice through the use of paramedical personnel, such as nurses.

THE ATHLETE'S HEART

The structural characteristics of the hearts of apparently healthy, highly trained athletes differ considerably from those of normal individuals. Regardless of age, exercise training is followed by an increase in heart size, and this cardiac hypertrophy is viewed as a normal biologic response to an increased workload.

The duration of training affects cardiac size and structure. Short-term training is not associated with changes in cardiac dimensions, even though there is an improvement in maximal $\dot{V}O_2$ and submaximal heart response.[56,57] Prolonged endurance training is followed by left ventricular enlargement, which regresses to a pretraining level after cessation of the exercise training program. This involution is not apparently associated with any deleterious effects.[58] There is considerable variability among individuals in terms of the structural response of the heart to various forms of training. It is apparent that the structural and dimensional differences among the hearts of athletes reflect specific training demands.[59]

Isotonically trained athletes undergo an eccentric hypertrophy characterized by a slight increase in wall thickness and an increased end-diastolic volume with a normal ratio of volume to thickness. Endurance athletes have a higher prevalence of multivalvular regurgitation. The cause is not entirely clear but may reflect higher end-systolic annuli sizes of the tricuspid and mitral valves in these athlete's hearts.[60] In contrast, athletes involved in isometric training show a concentric hypertrophy defined by symmetrically thickened intraventricular septum and ventricular wall and little difference in end-diastolic volume compared to sedentary persons. The concentric hypertrophy with isometric training is not associated with changes in ventricular compliance.[61] It is interesting to note that measurements of diastolic filling in isometrically trained athletes who used anabolic steroids are significantly abnormal.[61,62] These studies suggest that anabolic steroids alter the normal physiologic hypertrophy, leading to increased myocardial stiffness.

The implications of these changes for myocardial blood flow and long-term cardiovascular health are unknown. The functional hypertrophy that occurs in response to exercise training is different from the pathologic hypertrophy secondary to chronic disease states. During exercise training, the myocardial overload is only temporary, allowing for a "recuperative period" between exercise sessions. The cardiac hypertrophy associated with training is not accompanied by "weakening" of the left ventricle, which is usually seen with chronic pathologic pressure loads. Even though the hearts of elite athletes are larger than the hearts of sedentary control subjects, the size is usually within the upper range of normal limits in relation to body size or to the increased end-diastolic volume. One study of highly trained athletes[63] revealed that left ventricular cavity dimension varied widely but was increased to a degree compatible with dilated cardiomyopathy in almost 15 percent of subjects. Because of the absence of systolic dysfunction, this cavitary enlargement is most likely the result of an extreme physiologic adaptation, of which the long-term consequences and significance are not known. At this time, there is no compelling scientific evidence to indicate that specific forms of exercise training can "harm" a normal heart. To the contrary, the cardiac functional capacity of the athlete is much greater, in terms of stroke volume and maximal CO, than that of healthy sedentary individuals.

The cardiovascular examination results for an athlete have distinctive features. There is resting bradycardia, with pulse rates as low as 30 to 40 beats per minute, and an exaggerated normal respiratory variation in heart rate. The bradycardia is due to increased vagal tone associated with conditioning and represents a physiologic adaptation requiring no specific intervention if the athlete is otherwise asymptomatic. The apical impulse may be slightly displaced due to left ventricular enlargement, but wide displacements suggest concurrent cardiac pathology. Both ventricular and atrial "gallop sounds" are not uncommonly encountered in athletes, especially in the supine position, but are considered normal. Short systolic murmurs are also relatively common, reflecting a larger stroke volume or functional regurgitation due to enlarged annuli of the atrioventricular valves.

Electrocardiographic abnormalities are often seen in the highly trained athlete (Table 85-3). These include sinus bradycardia with sinus arrhythmia, sinus pauses with occasional junctional escape beats, first-degree atrioventricular block, and even periods of Möbitz type I second-degree atrioventricular block.[64] These are likely vagally mediated and disappear with exercise or atropine administration. Morphologic P-wave changes are frequently noticed as a result of atrial enlargement. QRS voltage changes suggesting ventricular hypertrophy are often seen associated with T-wave inversion in the inferior leads. Juvenile T-wave pattern (T-wave inversions in the anterior leads) and elevated early "takeoff" of the T-wave are seen frequently. "Strain" patterns, with downsloping ST-T changes indicating abnormal repolarization, are not common but can be seen in athletes who perform isometric exercise.[65]

Chest roentgenograms may reveal symmetric globular cardiomegaly with a cardiothoracic ratio between 0.5 and 0.6. Such findings are not considered pathologic.

Echocardiography is the best tool for assessing cardiac hypertrophy associated with physical conditioning and is useful in differentiating functional hypertrophy from hypertrophic cardiomyopathy. At times, left ventricular wall thickness of greater than 13 mm or asymmetric septal hypertrophy (both rare occurrences in physiologic hypertrophy) pose diagnostic challenges. The distinction is important because hypertrophic cardiomyopathy may confer a risk of sudden death during exercise. In these cases, screening of relatives and/or a period of deconditioning, which would induce a regression of hypertrophy in cases of physiologic hypertrophy, may be indicated. The clinician's role is to recognize the physiologic adaptation to the conditioned state and distinguish such adaptation from pathologic conditions, which occur in athletes in the same frequency as in the general population.

TABLE 85-3 Electrocardiographic Changes Seen in Highly Trained Athletes

Sinus bradycardia and sinus pauses
Atrioventricular block
First degree
Type I second degree
Morphologic P-wave changes
QRS voltage of left ventricular hypertrophy
T-wave changes

SUDDEN DEATH

Sudden death in the athlete occurs rarely but invariably captures public attention, especially when the victim is young, vigorous, and apparently healthy. Through the efforts of the American Heart Association and similar organizations, regular exercise has been encouraged as part of a healthy lifestyle. Consequently, physicians and other health care workers may be asked to defend their recommendations in the face of media attention, and may find themselves addressing the anxieties of athletes, parents, and coaches when sudden death occurs. Fortunately, sudden death with exercise is a rare phenomenon; accidents, homicides, and illicit drug use among adolescents and young adults puts them at much greater risk.[66]

One of the earliest reports of sudden death during exercise dates back to 490 B.C. when Phidippides died after running the 26 miles from Marathon to Athens to report the defeat of the Persian army. The number of modern-day reports of sudden death in exercise is small. Each year there are approximately 4 million competitive high school athletes, 500,000 collegiate athletes, and 5000 professional athletes participating in sports.[67] In one review,[68] Maron reported 134 deaths in young competitive athletes over a 10-year period. While the number of reported cases of sudden death in young athletes is probably less than the actual figure, it remains a rare event. It is estimated that sudden death from cardiovascular disease in the high school and college athlete occurs in 1:200,000 to 1:300,000 individual athletes per academic year, and 1:70,000 over a 3-year high school career.[66]

The incidence of sudden death during exercise in older athletes (over 35 years of age) is higher. In one review in Seattle, 11 percent of 316 consecutive victims of sudden death died during or immediately after exercise, and, in Miami, 17 percent of 150 patients had exertion-related sudden death.[69] The majority of these victims had coronary artery disease. In Rhode Island, the incidence of sudden death while jogging for middle-aged men was 13 deaths per 100,000 joggers per year.[70] Nationally, the frequency of sudden death in apparently healthy men is 1:15,000 joggers, and 1:50,000 marathoners.[67] There appears to be a causal relationship between exertion and sudden death. When reexamined, the same data from Rhode Island revealed 1 death per 396,000 h of jogging, while the death rate for nonvigorous activity was 1 death per 3 million person-hours.[69]

There may be an association between sudden death and the intensity of exercise. In Seattle, the incidence of exercise-related sudden death is estimated at 5.4 per 100,000, but during vigorous activity the incidence is 5 times higher for men who exercise frequently and 56 times higher for men who exercise infrequently.[71] Among men who participate regularly in high-intensity exercise, the increase in risk during athletic training and competition is outweighed by a decrease in risk of sudden cardiac death at other times; therefore, their overall risk of sudden death was lower.[72]

Gender differences are present when evaluating the incidence of sudden death. Approximately 10 percent of events occur in women athletes, and several potential explanations exist. In the past, women have been less likely to participate in high school and college sports and have been subjected to less intensive training demands than men, although these trends are changing. At present, women do not participate as frequently as men in sports associated with the greatest risk for sudden cardiac death, and they less commonly have hypertrophic cardiomyopathy.[66] Racial differences also exist, which may be due to differences in access to health care. Hypertrophic cardiomyopathy is a significant cause of sudden death in African-American men, yet this finding is comparatively underreported in this subset of the population.[66]

In Maron's series of 134 athletes with sudden death, 52 percent were white, 44 percent were African-American, and the majority of events occurred during high school years, with a median age of 17 years. Basketball, football, and track were the most common sports associated with sudden death, and 63 percent of all cases of sudden death occurred between 3 P.M. and 9 P.M., coinciding with the peak participation time for these sports.[68] Ninety percent of victims collapse during or immediately after a training session. A prodromal complaint, such as chest pain, shortness of breath, or lightheadedness, was present in 90 percent of victims immediately prior to the event, and 18 percent had symptoms in the 3 years before their death.[68]

Sudden cardiac death may be due to mechanical abnormalities, but the majority of cases are due to dysrhythmias, namely, ventricular fibrillation. The healthy heart does not appear to be vulnerable to exercise-induced ventricular arrhythmias, except in cases of significant electrolyte abnormalities, drug use, heat stroke, or blunt trauma to the chest wall.[73] The proper substrate is needed, and this is usually a heart with a structural abnormality. An ill-timed ventricular ectopic beat is usually the trigger for a ventricular fibrillation, but exercise is believed to have significant influence on the development of ventricular fibrillation, and this may be due to transient myocardial ischemia. Other factors that may exert an influence include hypoxia due to an increase in myocardial oxygen demand in the setting of a shortened diastolic period and reduced coronary perfusion time. Alterations in autonomic tone, enhanced coagulability, and release of coronary vasoconstrictor substances, including thromboxane A_2, may play a role. Acidosis, electrolyte derangements, a rise in body temperature, and elevated circulating free fatty acid levels may also be responsible.[73] Finally, medications may play a role in some instances.

The most frequent cause of sudden death in athletes over 35 is coronary artery disease. The majority of these victims at necropsy do not have any evidence of acute thrombi, suggesting that transient myocardial ischemia may result from myocardial oxygen demands not being met during exercise during a fixed obstruction or perhaps due to coronary vasospasm.[73] Coronary artery thrombi are seen in only 25 percent of victims with coronary artery disease.[74] The true incidence may be greater. Plaque rupture may occur due to twisting of epicardial arteries as a result of exaggerated changes in systolic and diastolic dimensions during exercise, or the rise in systolic blood pressure may cause an increase in shear forces. Catecholamine-induced platelet aggregation may also play a role.[71] The majority of exercise-related sudden death due to coronary artery disease occurs in victims who had risk factors for this condition or prodromal symptoms, including chest pain.[70,74,75] This suggests that efforts directed at screening and counseling patients on symptoms may be effective at preventing sudden death in this patient population of patients.

For younger athletes (under 35 years of age), coronary artery disease is a very rare cause of exercise-induced sudden death. The majority of these deaths are due to congenital cardiac anomalies, and hypertrophic cardiomyopathy is the most common cause in this age group. It is present in 0.2 percent of the general population but accounts for 36 percent of the cases of sudden death in this subgroup.[66,68] Patients with this condition have a propensity for malignant ventricular arrhythmias, and exercise-induced alterations in circulating catecholamines, blood volume, and electrolytes contribute to the risk of sudden death with exertion.[66] Sudden cardiac death with exercise may be more likely if there is a family history of sudden death, a systolic pressure gradient greater than 50 mmHg, marked left ventricular hypertrophy, ventricular or atrial arrhythmias, or a history of syncope.[73] However, the heterogeneity of this disorder makes accurate stratification of the risk of sudden death difficult.[66] Therefore, the Twenty-Sixth Bethesda Conference report recommended that athletes with a diagnosis of hypertrophic cardiomyopathy avoid intense athletic training and competition.[76] (For a list of conditions associated with sudden cardiac death, see Table 85-4.)

Screening young athletes for sudden death is difficult because it is an infrequent event, with only a very few participants in sports at risk. Cardiac abnormalities known to cause sudden death in this age range occur infrequently in the general population,[67] and large-scale screening strategies must be designed with this in mind. In Italy, government legislation mandates that all persons between 12 to 35 years of age participating in sports must have annual medical clearance. In addition to a history and physical examination, an electrocardiogram, exercise test, and pulmonary function test are required. Echocardiograms are required in selected professional sports.[66] In the United States, there are no accepted standards for screening high school and college athletes. Five states do not require an examination, and 11 states do not have a standard medical form.[67] In addition to nurses and physician assistants, some states allow chiropractors and "naturopathic" clinicians to per-

TABLE 85-4 Cardiovascular Abnormalities Associated with Sudden Death

Coronary artery disease
Congenital malformations of the coronary arteries
Myocardial bridging of coronary arteries
Idiopathic left ventricular hypertrophy
Idiopathic dilated cardiomyopathy
Hypertrophic cardiomyopathy
Mitral valve prolapse
Aortic stenosis
Marfan syndrome
Coarctation of the aorta
Long-QT syndrome
Wolff-Parkinson-White syndrome
Idiopathic ventricular tachycardia
Arrhythmogenic right ventricular dysplasia
Sarcoidosis
Kawasaki's disease
Commotio cordis
Drug-related morphologic changes
Myocarditis

form preparticipation examinations.[66] The American Heart Association has recommended a national standard for preparticipation evaluations and that they be performed by a physician or, in select instances, a registered nurse or physician assistant. In any cases, the individual performing the evaluation should have the training and skills to perform the history and physical examination and to recognize potential heart disease.[67]

The American Heart Association has also recommended that a screening history and physical examination be performed on everyone before participating in high school and collegiate sports. In high school, the screening should be repeated every 2 years, with an interim history obtained in the intervening years. For collegiate athletes, an interim history and blood pressure measurement should be obtained in the third or fourth year, but repeated screening is not necessary.[67,77] The cardiovascular history should inquire about chest pain, syncope, unexplained shortness of breath, or diminished exercise tolerance. The athlete should be asked about a history of heart murmur or hypertension and any family history of premature death or significant cardiovascular conditions. At a minimum, the cardiovascular examination should include brachial blood pressure in the sitting position, assessment of femoral pulses to exclude coarctation of the aorta, recognition of the physical stigmata of Marfan syndrome, and precordial auscultation in supine and standing positions to identify a murmur associated with dynamic left ventricular outflow obstruction.[67] If a cardiovascular abnormality is suspected, the athlete should be referred to a cardiologist for evaluation.

The routine use of diagnostic tests as part of preparticipation screening evaluations is limited by low specificity and cost considerations. The electrocardiogram is abnormal in hypertrophic cardiomyopathy in approximately 95 percent of cases, and it proved useful in helping to identify this condition in a large series from Italy.[78] It is often abnormal in athletes with coronary anomalies and may identify the long-QT syndrome. However, it has a low specificity in the athletic population because of an increased frequency of ECG changes due to the physiologic adaptations of training (see Table 85-3).[67] The routine use of exercise testing to detect coronary artery disease in older athletes is not justified because of its low specificity as well. However, for an athlete with an intermediate pretest probability of coronary artery disease, exercise testing is useful. Echocardiograms are very accurate in the detection of hypertrophic cardiomyopathy, valvular heart disease, aortic root dilation, and left ventricular dysfunction. Although the routine use of the electrocardiogram, the echocardiogram, and other diagnostic testing would improve the diagnosis of hypertrophic cardiomyopathy and other cardiovascular abnormalities, the practical application on a national scale is limited by the cost of screening such a large number of athletes and by the infrequent occurrence of these cardiovascular abnormalities in the general population. The potential for false-positive test results, unnecessary disqualification from athletic participation, and heightened anxiety should be considered as well.

There are inherent limits to large-scale screening efforts, due to the nature of the cardiovascular abnormalities involved and the size of the athletic population in the United States. In retrospective studies, cardiovascular abnormalities were suspected by screening history and physical examinations in only 3 percent of athletes who died suddenly of cardiovascular abnormalities.[66] Even with the addition of noninvasive testing, it would not be possible to identify all athletes at risk. However, a uniform screening process such as the one outlined by the American Heart Association would be expcected to identify more cardiovascular abnormalities in athletes and, by disqualifying such individuals from intense athletic activity, may decrease the incidence of sudden death.[66]

References

1. Williamson JW, Nobrega AC, Garcia JA, et al. Cardiovascular responses at the onset of static exercise in patients with dual-chamber pacemakers. *J Appl Physiol* 1995; 79:1668–1672.
2. Rowell LB. *Human Cardiovascular Control*. New York: Oxford University Press; 1993:xv, 500.
3. Rowell LB, O'Leary DS. Reflex control of the circulation during exercise: Chemoreflexes and mechanoreflexes. *J Appl Physiol* 1990; 69:407–418.
4. Strange S, Secher NH, Pawelczyk JA, et al. Neural control of cardiovascular responses and of ventilation during dynamic exercise in man. *J Physiol* (*Lond*) 1993; 470:693–704.
5. Bevegard S, Holmgren A, Jonsson B. Circulatory studies in well-trained athletes at rest and during heavy exercise, with special reference to stroke volume and the influence of body position. *Acta Physiol Scand* 1963; 57:26–50.
6. Musch TI, Haidet GC, Ordway GA, et al. Training effects on regional blood flow response to maximal exercise in foxhounds. *J Appl Physiol* 1987; 62:1724–1732.
7. Thomas SN, Schroeder T, Secher NH, Mitchell JH. Cerebral blood flow during submaximal and maximal dynamic exercise in humans. *J Appl Physiol* 1989; 67:744–748.
8. Pescatello LS, Fargo AE, Leach CN Jr, Scherzer HH. Short-term effect of dynamic exercise on arterial blood pressure. *Circulation* 1991; 83:1557–1561.
9. Bechuza GR, Lenser MC, Hanson PG, Nagle FJ. Comparison of hemodynamic responses to static and dynamic exercise. *J Appl Physiol* 1982; 53:1589–1593.
10. Bruce RA, Kusumi F, Hosmer D. Maximal oxygen intake and normographic assessment of functional aerobic impairment in cardiovascular disease. *Am Heart J* 1973; 85:546–562.
11. Saltin B, Astrand PO. Maximal oxygen uptake in athletes. *J Appl Physiol* 1967; 23:353–358.
12. Asmussen E. Similarities and dissimilarities between static and dynamic exercise. *Circ Res* 1981; 48:I3–I10.
13. Hanson P, Nagle F. Isometric exercise: Cardiovascular responses in normal and cardiac populations. In: Hanson P, ed. *Exercise and the Heart: Cardiology Clinics*. Philadelphia: Saunders; 1987:157.
14. Seals DR, Washburn RA, Hanson PG, et al. Increased cardiovascular response to static contraction of large muscle groups. *J Appl Physiol* 1983; 54:434–437.
15. Wescott W, Howeff B. Blood pressure response during weight training exercises. *NSCA J* 1983; 5:67–71.
16. DeBusk RF, Valdez R, Houston N, Haskell W. Cardiovascular responses to dynamic and static effort soon after myocardial infarction: Application to occupational work assessment. *Circulation* 1978; 58:368–375.
17. Ghilarducci LE, Holly RG, Amsterdam EA. Effects of high resistance training in coronary artery disease. *Am J Cardiol* 1989; 64:866–870.
18. Sparling PB, Cantwell JD, Dolan CM, Niederman RK. Strength training in a cardiac rehabilitation program: A six-month follow-up. *Arch Phys Med Rehabil* 1990; 171:148–152.
19. Rowell LB. Human cardiovascular adjustments to exercise and thermal stress. *Physiol Rev* 1974; 54:75–159.
20. Ehsani AA, Hagberg JM, Hickson RC. Rapid changes in ventricular dimensions and mass in response to physical conditioning and deconditioning. *Am J Cardiol* 1972; 42:52–56.

21. Saltin B. Physiologic effects on physical conditioning. *Med Sci Sports* 1969; 1:50–56.
22. Convertino VA. Blood volume: Its adaptation to endurance training. *Med Sci Sports Exerc* 1991; 23:1338–1348.
23. Levy WC, Cerqueira MD, Abrass IB, et al. Endurance exercise training augments diastolic filling at rest and during exercise in healthy young and older men. *Circulation* 1993; 88:116–126.
24. Matsuda M, Sugishita Y, Koseki S, et al. Effect of exercise on left ventricular diastolic filling in athletes and nonathletes. *J Appl Physiol* 1983; 55:323–328.
25. Granger CB, Karimeddini MK, Smith VE, et al. Rapid ventricular filling in left ventricular hypertrophy: I. Physiologic hypertrophy. *J Am Coll Cardiol* 1985; 5:862–868.
26. Anversa P, Levicky V, Beghi C, et al. Morphometry of exercise-induced right ventricular hypertrophy in the rat. *Circ Res* 1983; 52:57–64.
27. Froelicher V, Jensen D, Atwood JE, et al. Cardiac rehabilitation: Evidence for improvement in myocardial perfusion and function. *Arch Phys Med Rehabil* 1980; 61:517–522.
28. Starnes JW, Bowles DK. Role of exercise in the cause and prevention of cardiac dysfunction. *Exerc Sport Sci Rev* 1995; 23:349–373.
29. Hermansen L, Wachtlova M. Capillary density of skeletal muscle in well-trained and untrained men. *J Appl Physiol* 1971; 30: 860–863.
30. Holloszy JO, Booth FW. Biochemical adaptations to endurance exercise in muscle. *Annu Rev Physiol* 1976; 38:273–291.
31. Bar-Or O, Shephard RJ, Allen CL. Cardiac output of 10- to 13-year-old boys and girls during submaximal exercise. *J Appl Physiol* 1971; 30:219–223.
32. Drinkwater BL. Women and exercise: Physiological aspects. *Exerc Sport Sci Rev* 1984; 12:21–51.
33. Costill DL, Daniels J, Evans W, et al. Skeletal muscle enzymes and fiber composition in male and female track athletes. *J Appl Physiol* 1976; 40:149–154.
34. Astrand PO, Rodahl K. *Textbook of work physiology: Physiological basis of exercise*. New York: McGraw-Hill; 1986:756.
35. Higginbotham MB, Morris KG, Coleman RE, Cobb FR. Sex-related differences in the normal cardiac response to upright exercise. *Circulation* 1984; 70:357–366.
36. Lakatta EG. Do hypertension and aging have a similar effect on the myocardium? *Circulation* 1987; 75:I69–I77.
37. Miyatake K, Okamoto M, Kinoshita N, et al. Augmentation of atrial contribution to left ventricular inflow with aging as assessed by intracardiac Doppler flowmetry. *Am J Cardiol* 1984; 53:586–589.
38. Nixon JV, Hallmark H, Page K, et al. Ventricular performance in human hearts aged 61 to 73 years. *Am J Cardiol* 1985; 56:932–937.
39. Gerstenblith G, Frederiksen J, Yin FC, et al. Echocardiographic assessment of a normal adult aging population. *Circulation* 1977; 56:273–278.
40. Raven PB, Mitchell J. The effect of aging on the cardiovascular response to dynamic and static exercise. *Aging* 1980; 12:269–296.
41. Lakatta EG. Health, disease and cardiovascular aging. In: Committee on an Aging Society, Institute of Medicine and National Research Council, ed. *Health in an Older Society*. Washington: National Academy Press; 1985:73–104
42. Bruce RA, Hornsten TR. Exercise stress testing in evaluation of patients with ischemic heart disease. *Prog Cardiovasc Dis* 1969; 11:371–390.
43. Fleg JL, Lakatta EG. Role of muscle loss in the age-associated reduction in $\dot{V}O_2$ max. *J Appl Physiol* 1988; 65:1147–1151.
44. Ehsani AA, Ogawa T, Miller TR, et al. Exercise training improves left ventricular systolic function in older men. *Circulation* 1991; 83:96–103.
45. Fleg JL, Tzankoff SP, Lakatta EG. Age-related augmentation of plasma catecholamines during dynamic exercise in healthy males. *J Appl Physiol* 1985; 59:1033–1039.
46. Powell KE, Thompson PD, Caspersen CJ, Kendrick JS. Physical activity and the incidence of coronary heart disease. *Annu Rev Public Health* 1987; 8:253–287.
47. Berlin JA, Colditz GA. A meta-analysis of physical activity in the prevention of coronary heart disease. *Am J Epidemiol* 1990; 132:612–628.
48. O'Connor GT, Buring JE, Yusuf S, et al. An overview of randomized trials of rehabilitation with exercise after myocardial infarction. *Circulation* 1989; 80:234–244.
49. Lee IM, Hsieh CC, Paffenbarger RS Jr. Exercise intensity and longevity in men: The Harvard Alumni Health Study. *JAMA* 1995; 273:1179–1184.
50. Fletcher GF, Balady G, Blair SN, et al. Statement on exercise: Benefits and recommendations for physical activity programs for all Americans, a statement for health professionals by the Committee on Exercise and Cardiac Rehabilitation of the Council on Clinical Cardiology, American Heart Association. *Circulation* 1996; 94:857–862.
51. U.S. Department of Health and Human Services, National Center for Chronic Disease Prevention and Health Promotion. *Physical Activity and Health: A Report of the Surgeon General*. Pittsburgh: President's Council on Physical Fitness and Sports; 1996:278.
52. Pate RR, Pratt M, Blair SN, et al. Physical activity and public health: A recommendation from the Centers for Disease Control and Prevention and the American College of Sports Medicine. *JAMA* 1995; 273:402–407.
53. NIH Consensus Development Panel: Physical activity and cardiovascular health. *JAMA* 1996; 276:241–246.
54. Caspersen CJ, Christenson GM, Pollard RA. Status of the 1990 physical fitness and exercise objectives: Evidence from NHIS 1985. Public Health Report 1986; 101:587–592.
55. Patrick K, Calfas KJ, Sallis JF, Long B. Basic principles of physical activity counseling: Project PACE. In: Thomas R, ed. *The Heart and Exercise*. New York: Igaku-Shoin; 1996:33.
56. Ricci G, Lajoie D, Petitclerc R, et al. Left ventricular size following endurance, sprint, and strength training. *Med Sci Sports Exerc* 1982; 14:344–347.
57. Thompson PD, Lewis S, Varady A, et al. Cardiac dimensions and performance after either arm or leg endurance training. *Med Sci Sports Exerc* 1981; 13:303–309.
58. Dickhuth HH, Horstmann T, Staiger J, et al. The long-term involution of physiological cardiomegaly and cardiac hypertrophy. *Med Sci Sports Exerc* 1989; 21:244–249.
59. Maron BJ. Structural features of the athlete heart as defined by echocardiography. *J Am Coll Cardiol* 1986; 7:190–203.
60. Douglas PS, Berman GO, O'Toole ML, et al. Prevalence of multivalvular regurgitation in athletes. *Am J Cardiol* 1989; 64:209–212.
61. Pearson AC, Schiff M, Mrosek D, et al. Left ventricular diastolic function in weight lifters. *Am J Cardiol* 1986; 58:1254–1259.
62. Urhausen A, Holpes R, Kindermann W. One- and two-dimensional echocardiography in bodybuilders using anabolic steroids. *Eur J Appl Physiol* 1989; 58:633–640.
63. Pelliccia A, Culasso F, Di Paolo FM, Maron BJ. Physiologic left ventricular cavity dilatation in elite athletes. *Ann Intern Med* 1999; 130:23–31.
64. Zehender M, Meinertz T, Keul J, Just H. ECG variants and cardiac arrhythmias in athletes: Clinical relevance and prognostic importance. *Am Heart J* 1990; 119:1378–1391.
65. Buttrick PM, Scheuer J. Exercise and the heart: Acute hemodynamics, conditioning training, the athlete's heart, and sudden death. In: Schlant RC, Alexander RW, eds. *Hurst's the Heart*, 8th ed. New York: McGraw-Hill; 1994:2057.
66. Maron BJ. Cardiovascular risks to young persons on the athletic field. *Ann Intern Med* 1998; 129:379–386.
67. Maron BJ, Thompson PD, Puffer JC, et al. Cardiovascular preparticipation screening of competitive athletes: A statement for health professionals from the Sudden Death Committee (clinical cardiology) and Congenital Cardiac Defects Committee (cardiovascular

disease in the young), American Heart Association. *Circulation* 1996; 94:850–856.
68. Maron BJ, Shirani J, Poliac LC, et al. Sudden death in young competitive athletes: Clinical, demographic, and pathological profiles. *JAMA* 1996; 276:199–204.
69. Cobb LA, Weaver WD. Exercise: A risk for sudden death in patients with coronary heart disease. *J Am Coll Cardiol* 1986; 7:215–219.
70. Thompson PD, Funk EJ, Carleton RA, Sturner WQ. Incidence of death during jogging in Rhode Island from 1975 through 1980. *JAMA* 1982; 247:2535–2538.
71. Thompson PD. The cardiovascular complications of vigorous physical activity. *Arch Intern Med* 1996; 156:2297–2302.
72. Siscovick DS, Weiss NS, Fletcher RH, Lasky T. The incidence of primary cardiac arrest during vigorous exercise. *N Engl J Med* 1984; 311:874–877.
73. Franklin BA, Fletcher GF, Gordon NF, et al. Cardiovascular evaluation of the athlete: Issues regarding performance, screening and sudden cardiac death. *Sports Med* 1997; 24:97–119.
74. Virmani R, Burke AP, Farb A, Kark JA. Causes of sudden death in young and middle-aged competitive athletes. *Cardiol Clin* 1997; 15:439–466.
75. Northcote RJ, Ballantyne D. Sudden cardiac death in sport. *Br Med J* (*Clin Res Ed*) 1983; 287:1357–1359.
76. Maron BJ, Mitchell JH. 26th Bethesda Conference: Recommendations for determining eligibility for competition in athletes with cardiovascular abnormalities. *J Am Coll Cardiol* 1994; 24:845–899.
77. Maron BJ, Thompson PD, Puffer JC, et al. Cardiovascular preparticipation screening of competitive athletes: An addendum to a statement for health professionals from the Sudden Death Committee (Council on Clinical Cardiology) and the Congenital Cardiac Defects Committee (Council on Cardiovascular Disease in the Young), American Heart Association. *Circulation* 1998; 97: 2294.
78. Corrado D, Basso C, Schiavon M, Thiene G. Screening for hypertrophic cardiomyopathy in young athletes. *N Engl J Med* 1998; 339:364–369.

CHAPTER 86

CARDIOVASCULAR AGING IN HEALTH AND THERAPEUTIC CONSIDERATIONS IN OLDER PATIENTS WITH CARDIOVASCULAR DISEASES

Edward G. Lakatta / Steven P. Schulman / Gary Gerstenblith

CARDIOVASCULAR AGING IN HEALTH

Introduction

The proportion of older persons that constitute populations worldwide is increasing. It is estimated that, by the year 2035, nearly one in four individuals will be 65 years of age or older. Cardiovascular diseases, such as coronary arterial atherosclerosis and hypertension, and resultant chronic heart failure reach epidemic proportions among older persons. The clinical manifestations and prognosis of these diseases as well as heart failure also worsen with increasing age. It is hypothesized that one reason for this is that specific pathophysiologic mechanisms causing clinical disorders in older persons become superimposed on heart and vascular substrates that are modified by the aging process per se. In this regard, quantitative information on age-associated alterations in cardiovascular structure and function in health is essential to define and target the specific characteristics of cardiovascular aging that render it such a major risk factor for cardiovascular diseases. Such information is also required to differentiate between the limitations of an elderly person that relate to disease and those that are within expected normal limits.

During the past two decades, a sustained effort has been applied to characterize the effects of aging in health on multiple aspects of cardiovascular structure and function in a single study population. In the Baltimore Longitudinal Study on Aging (BLSA), community-dwelling volunteers are rigorously screened to detect both clinical and occult cardiovascular disease and are characterized with respect to lifestyle (e.g., exercise habits) in an attempt to clarify the interactions of these factors and those changes that result from aging, per se. Perspectives gleaned from these studies will be emphasized throughout this section of the chapter, as will relevant information from studies in animal models.

Cardiovascular Structure

CARDIAC STRUCTURE

Cross-sectional studies of sedentary BLSA volunteer subjects without cardiovascular disease indicate that the left ventricular (LV) wall thickness, measured via M-mode (one-dimensional) echocardiography, increases progressively with age in both sexes (Fig. 86-1*A*).[1] This is mostly due to an increase in average myocyte size. In older, hospitalized patients without apparent cardiovascular disease, autopsy overall LV mass decreased with age, and cardiac myocyte enlargement was observed concurrently with an estimated decrease in myocyte number.[2] The observed frequency of apoptotic myocytes is higher in older male than female hearts.[3] An increase in the amount and a change in the physical properties of collagen (purportedly due to nonenzymatic cross-linking) also occur within the myocardium with aging. However, the cardiac myocyte-to-collagen ratio in the older heart either remains constant or increases.

There is an increase in elastic and collagenous tissue in all parts of the conduction system with advancing age. Fat accumulates around the sinoatrial node, sometimes producing a partial or complete separation of the node from the atrial musculature. There may be a pronounced decrease in the number of pace-

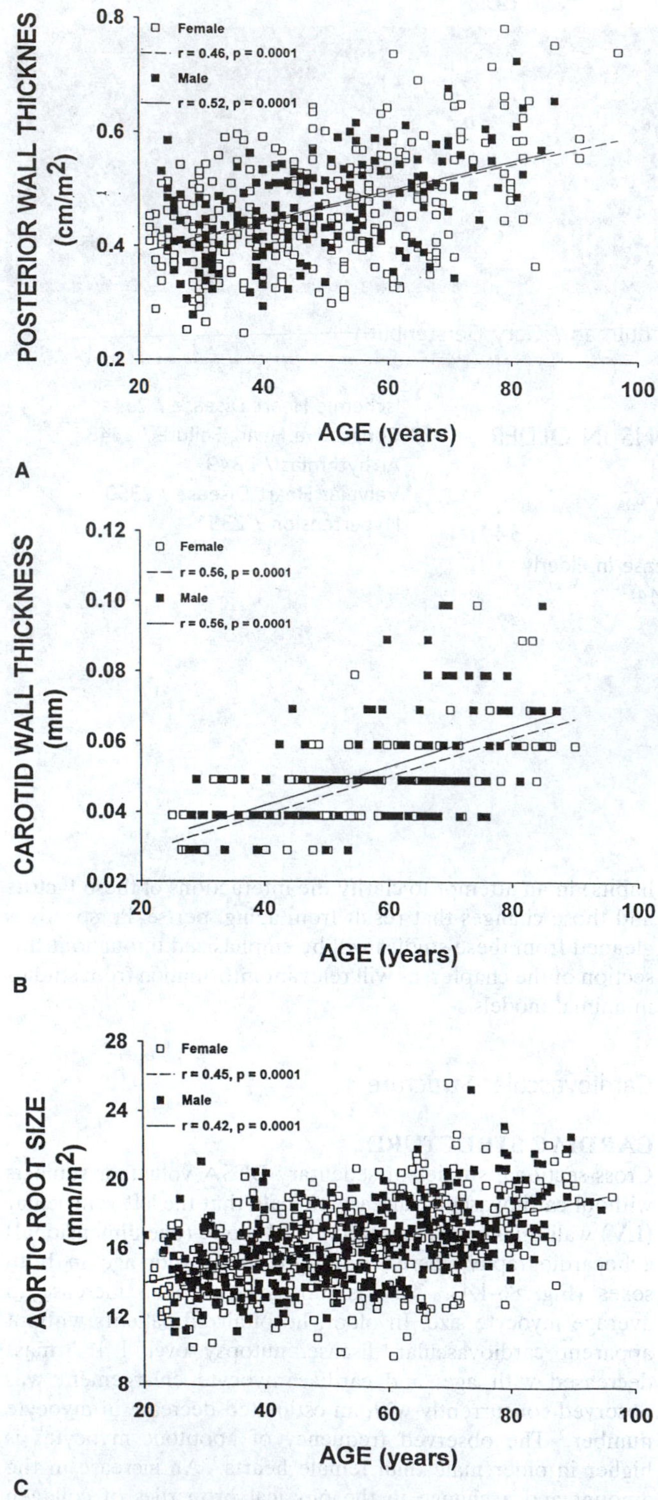

FIGURE 86-1 *A.* Aortic root diameter, measured via M-mode echocardiography. (From *Circulation* 1997; 56:273. Reproduced with permission from the publisher and authors.) *B.* Carotid intimal-medial wall thickness measured via echo Doppler techniques. (From *Circulation* 1998; 98: 1504. Reproduced with permission from the publisher and authors.) *C.* Left ventricular posterior wall thickness, measured by M-mode echocardiography, increases with age in healthy men and women from the Baltimore Longitudinal Study on Aging. (From *Circulation* 1997; 56:273, 1997. Reproduced with permission from the publisher and authors.)

maker cells in the sinoatrial node beginning at age 60, and by age 75 less than 10 percent of the cell number found in the young adult remains. A variable degree of calcification of the left side of the cardiac skeleton, which includes the aortic and mitral annuli, the central fibrous body, and the summit of the interventricular septum, also occurs with aging. Because of their proximity to these structures, the atrioventricular (AV) node, AV bundle, bifurcation, and proximal left and right bundle branches may be affected by this process.

The altered cardiac structural phenotype with aging in rodents in addition to an increase in LV mass, due to enlargement of myocyte size,[4] includes proliferation of the matrix in which the myocytes reside, which is focal in nature and may be linked to an altered cardiac fibroblast number or function.

With advancing age in rodents, the number of cardiac myocytes, which are postmitotic, terminally differentiated cells, also becomes reduced.[5] Putative stimuli for cardiac cell growth enlargement with aging in rodents are an age-associated increased vascular load, due to arterial stiffening (see below), and an additional load due to stretching of cells caused by dropout of neighboring myocytes. The reduction in myocyte number may be attributable to apoptosis as well as necrosis.[6] In fact, stretch, per se, is linked to cardiac myocyte apoptosis.[7] Stretch of cardiac myocytes and fibroblasts releases growth factors, one of which is angiotensin II, which in addition to modulating cell growth and matrix collagen production and, therefore, cell size, also leads to apoptosis.[8] Enhanced secretion of molecules like atrial natriuretic[9] and opioid[10] peptides, molecules that are usually produced in response to stress, is also observed in the senescent rodent heart.

VASCULAR STRUCTURE

With advancing age in healthy humans, the large arteries dilate (Fig. 86-1*A*), their walls, particularly the intima, become thickened (Fig. 86-1*B*), and changes occur within the vascular intima that appear to resemble those that occur during early atherosclerosis. Collagen content increases, and elastin becomes frayed. An increased elastase activity with aging may contribute to both elastin fragmentation and a reduction in its content with aging.[11]

Whereas the macroscopic changes in vascular cells and the matrix of large vessels in humans are well described, the specific molecular mechanisms that lead to vascular stiffening and a thickened intima remain to be elucidated. In general, changes in resistance vessels with aging in healthy individuals are less well studied but are apparently less marked than those in conduit arteries.

Age-associated macroscopic changes within large blood vessels in rodents are similar in many ways to those that occur in humans. Arterial remodeling with adult aging in rodents consists of dilation, medial thickening, and formation of an intima.[12–15] Chronic morphologic and biochemical modifications in the aortic intima of aging rats, i.e., fragmentation of the internal elastic membrane and intimal thickening, and localized increases in growth factors and collagenase activity appear as a muted version of alterations associated with chronic hypertension. Vascular smooth muscle (VSM) and endothelial cells are not terminally differentiated. VSM cells are subject to phenotypic modulation during which they revert to a proliferative, secretory and migratory mode. This *modulated* VSM phenotype repairs vascular damage and participates in vascular pathologies such as hypertension and atherosclerosis.

The thickened intima in older rats is composed of matrix molecules, including collagen and proteoglycan, and VSM cells and contains markedly higher levels of the matrix metalloproteinase, MMP-2, than do younger vessels.[16] The metalloproteinases can mediate tissue breakdown and remodeling. The intimal growth occurring during aging resembles, in some ways, neointimal formation in response to arterial balloon catheter-induced injury. In fact, neointimal growth in response to endothelial injury is markedly enhanced in old versus young rats, and this response is due to factors intrinsic to the vessel wall.[17] Ample evidence indicates the occurrence of discontinuities of the internal elastic lamina in the aorta with advancing age, in the absence of externally imposed experimental injury. Degradation of elastin by elastases and gelatinases (e.g., MMP-2 and MMP-9) may be implicated in elastic membrane breaks.[18]

The cytokine, transforming growth factor β (TGF-β), accumulates in the same regions of intima of old rats, as does MMP-2. TGF-β, which suppresses protease activity and activates tissue inhibitors of MMP,[19] is a potent factor for the synthesis of extracellular matrix proteins[13,20,21] and its expression can lead to excessive fibrosis.[19] Accumulation of TGF-β in the aortic wall of aged rats occurs with adult aging and may account for the concomitant increase in fibronectin.[16,22] There is some evidence to indicate that the collagenolytic[23] and antiproliferative actions of TGF-β decrease with aging.[24] Both fibronectin and TGF-β expression are regulated by angiotensin II,[25] and chronic administration of an angiotensin-converting enzyme inhibitor substantially reduces and delays the matrix and intimal changes associated with aging or hypertension.[12] This suggests that *age-associated changes in local vascular angiotensin regulation may have a role in the age-associated changes observed in TGF-β, fibronectin, and collagen deposition.*

Cardiovascular Function

CARDIAC VOLUMES AND EJECTION

Left Ventricular Filling and Preload Factors that determine ventricular volume (i.e., fiber stretch, end-diastolic blood volume, and filling pressure) are sometimes referred to as *preload*, which is a preexcitation determinant of myocardial function and pump performance, determined, in part, by ventricular filling characteristics. The latter are determined by the diastolic AV pressure gradient, one determinant of which is LV compliance (inverse of stiffness). Contrary to much that has been written on the subject, a reduction in ventricular compliance with age remains unproven because its measurement requires the simultaneous determination of pressure and volume, which have not been characterized in healthy younger and older persons. The early diastolic filling rate progressively slows after the age of 20 years, however, so that, by 80 years, the rate is reduced up to 50 percent (Fig. 86-2). This reduction in filling rate (demonstrated by echocardiography,[26] radionuclide angiography,[27] and Doppler ultrasonography[28] is likely attributable either to structural (fibrous) changes within the LV myocardium or to residual myofilament Ca^{2+} activation from the preceding systole (see below).

Despite the slowing of LV filling early in diastole, more filling occurs in late diastole, due, in part, to a more vigorous atrial contraction.[27] The augmented atrial contraction is accompanied by atrial enlargement and is manifested on auscultation as a fourth heart sound (atrial gallop).

Despite the age-associated changes in the diastolic filling pattern in older men, their LV end-diastolic volume index—i.e., normalized for body surface area (EDVI)—in the supine position, does not substantially differ from those in their younger counterparts (Fig. 86-3*A*). The acute reserve capacity of specific functions (e.g., EDV) that determine cardiac performance can be conveniently illustrated by depicting these over a wide range of demand for blood flow and pressure regulation, e.g., assumption of the sitting posture and during submaximal and exhaustive (max) upright exercise (Figs. 86-2*A* and 86-3). The lines depicted in these figures are the least-square linear regression on age of a given function in the steady state at different levels of effort in healthy, sedentary BLSA males. The overall magnitude of the acute, dynamic range of reserve of a given function in younger versus older subjects can quickly be gleaned from the length of the brackets depicted at the extremes of the regression lines.

Assumption of the sitting position reduces EDVI in younger but not in older individuals (Fig. 86-3*A*); during submaximal cycle-seated exercise EDVI increases equivalently at all ages, but during exhaustive exercise EDVI drops to the seated rest level in young men but remains elevated in older men (Fig. 86-3*A*). Thus, for EDVI, the average, acute, dynamic EDV reserve range during the postural change and during graded upright exercise is moderately *greater* at 85 than at 20 years. This does not support the widely held concept that the dynamic range of filling volumes is compromised in older hearts despite a reduction in LV early diastolic filling rate (Fig. 86-2*A*). In fact, during vigorous exercise (max), the LV at end diastole becomes acutely dilated in healthy, older but not younger persons. The interindividual variation of EDVI within the age-associated patterns depicted during exhaustive exercise (max) by the regression line for men in Fig. 86-3*A* is illustrated for both men and women in Fig. 86-4*A*.

Whether the capacity for *further* acute dilation of the LV of older persons beyond that observed in Figs. 86-1 to 86-3*A* and 86-4*A* is compromised cannot be readily determined either. In older BLSA persons with occult silent coronary disease, however, as evident by both ECG evidence and thallium scan perfusion deficits during exhaustive exercise, but not at rest, the LV EDVI at maximum exercise is greater than that in healthy age-matched subjects [as is the increase in LV end-systolic volume index (ESVI) and reduction in ejection fraction[28]]. Thus, at least in older patients with silent ischemia, the capacity exists for further acute EDVI dilation during exercise than that observed in healthy individuals.

Left Ventricular Ejection Figure 86-3*B* illustrates a remarkable age-associated reduction in the range of reserve in the ESVI: in younger men, the ESVI becomes progressively reduced with increasing demands for cardiovascular perfusion from supine rest to maximum upright exercise, but the range of acute ESV reserve at age 85 is only about a fifth of that at age 20. The age-associated failure in ESV regulation across the various levels of demand depicted in Fig. 86-3*B* causes a similar age-associated loss of ejection fraction regulation (Fig. 86-3*C*). See Fig. 86-4*B* and *C* for interindividual variations in ESVI and ejection fraction at max exercise in both males and females.

As a result of the age-associated changes in EDVI and ESVI

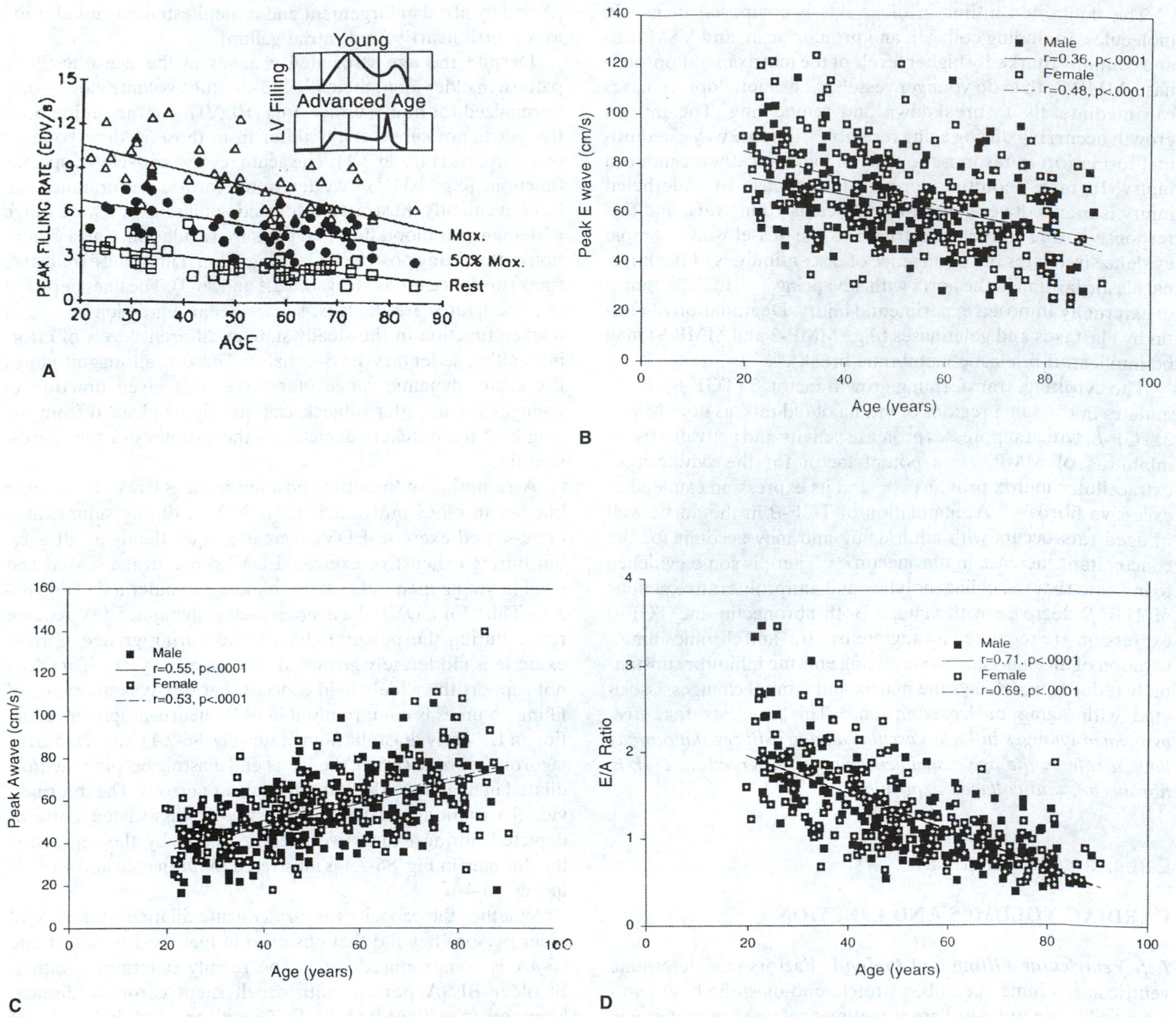

FIGURE 86-2 *A.* Maximum left ventricular filling rate assessed via equilibrium gated blood-pool scans in healthy volunteers from the Baltimore Longitudinal Study on Aging. (From *Am J Physiol* 1992; 263:H1932. Reproduced with permission from the publisher and authors.) Age-associated changes in the early diastolic left ventricular filling rate, E (*B*), the atrial contribution to filling, A (*C*), and the ratio of early to atrial filling rates (*D*). EDV = end-diastolic volume. (From *Am J Cardiol* 1992; 69: 823. Reproduced with permission from the publisher and authors.)

FIGURE 86-3 Least-squares linear regression on age of left ventricular values, ejection fraction (EF), heart rate (HR), and cardiac index (CI), at rest and during graded cycle exercise in 149 healthy males from the Baltimore Longitudinal Study on Aging (BLSA), who exercised to at least a 100-W workload. The *asterisk* indicates that regression on age is statistically significant. The overall magnitude of the acute, dynamic range of reserve of a given function in younger compared with older subjects can quickly be gleaned from the length of the *brackets* depicted at the extremes of the regression lines. For end-diastolic volume index (EDVI), the average, acute, dynamic EDV reserve range during the postural change and during graded upright exercise is moderately *greater* at 85 than at 20 years. (*A*) There is a remarkable age-associated reduction in the range of reserve in the end-systolic volume index (ESVI) (*B*) which causes a similar age-associated loss of EF regulation (*C*). The stroke volume index (SVI) is preserved in older persons over a wide range of performance (*D*). During progressive exhaustive exercise, however, when in older men the failure to reduce ESVI (*B*) impairs the EF (*C*), SVI is not augmented in older compared with younger men, as would be anticipated on the basis of their augmented EDVI. The maximum acute dynamic reserve range of HR is reduced by about one-third between 20 and 85 years of age (*E*). The loss of acute cardiac output reserve from seated rest to exhaustive, seated cycle exercise averages about 30 percent in healthy, community-dwelling BLSA volunteer men (*F*). This reduction is entirely due to a reduction in HR reserve, as SVI at max exercise is preserved. At max exercise, the age-associated increase in EDVI is of borderline statistical significance in women, but the change in EDVI from rest to max exercise in a given individual (not shown) significantly increases with age and is nearly identical in both men and women. (From *J Appl Physiol* 1995; 78:890. Reproduced with permission from the publisher and authors.)

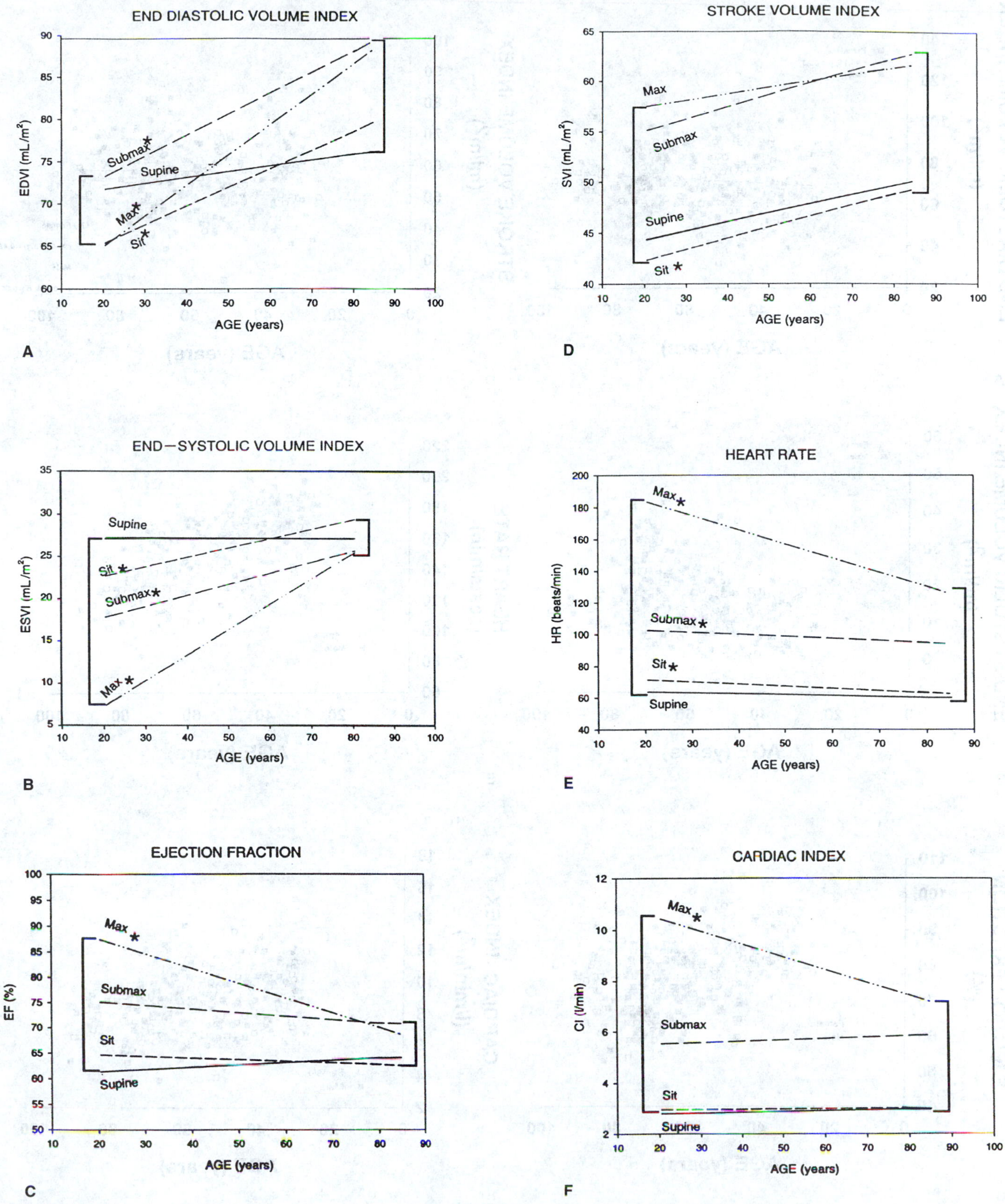
END DIASTOLIC VOLUME INDEX
EDVI (mL/m²)
Submax*
Supine
Max*
Sit*
AGE (years)
A
STROKE VOLUME INDEX
SVI (mL/m²)
Max
Submax
Supine
Sit *
AGE (years)
D
END—SYSTOLIC VOLUME INDEX
ESVI (mL/m²)
Supine
Sit *
Submax*
Max *
AGE (years)
B
HEART RATE
HR (beats/min)
Max*
Submax*
Sit*
Supine
AGE (years)
E
EJECTION FRACTION
EF (%)
Max *
Submax
Sit
Supine
AGE (years)
C
CARDIAC INDEX
CI (l/min)
Max*
Submax
Sit
Supine
AGE (years)
F

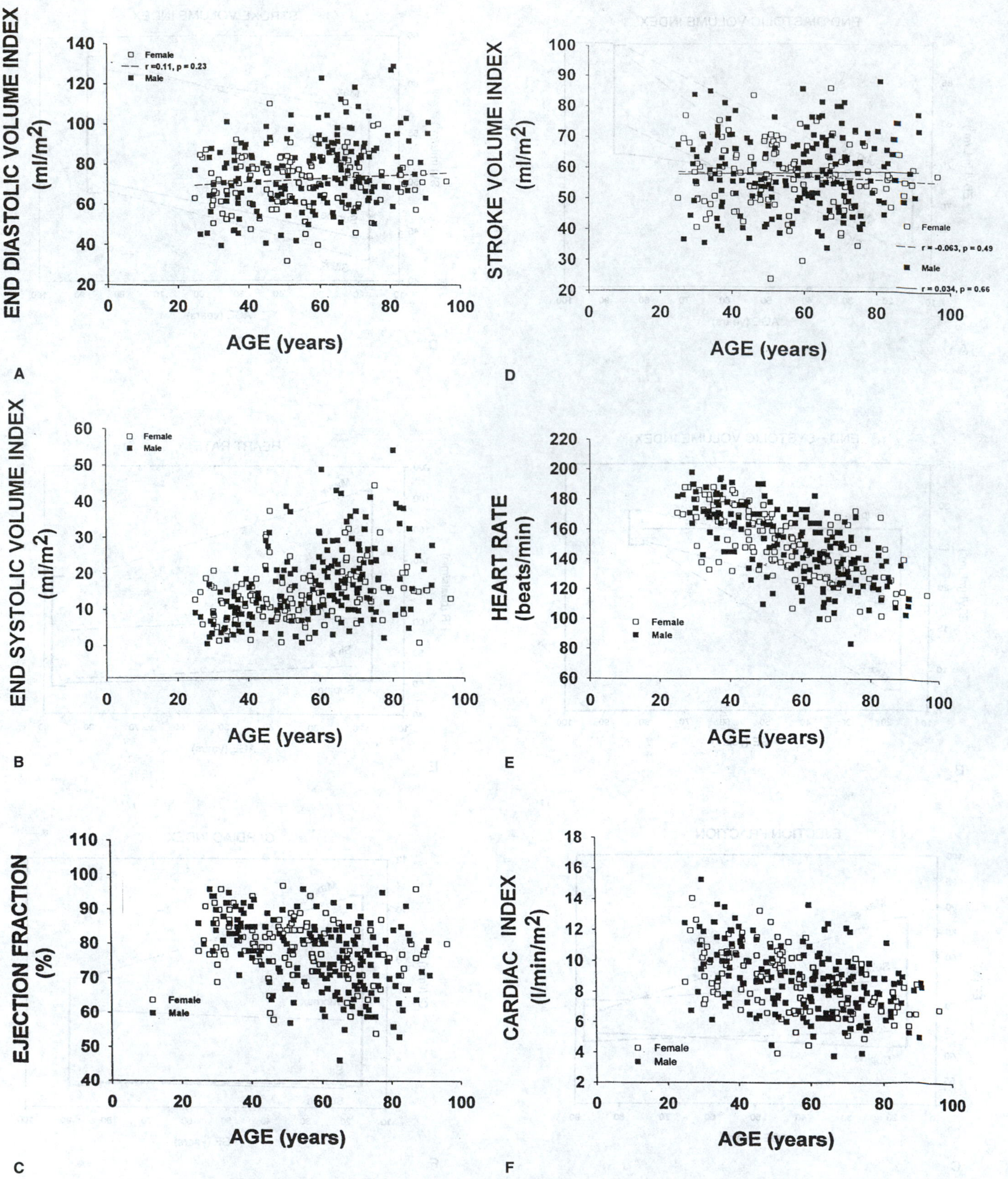

FIGURE 86-4 Scatter plots of heart rate and cardiac volumes, ejection fraction, and cardiac index in healthy sedentary men from the Baltimore Longitudinal Study on Aging (BLSA) depicted in Fig. 86-3 and for 113 BLSA women who exercised to a 75-W workload. Illustrated is the heterogeneity among individuals at a given age. In some instances (e.g., end-systolic volume index and ejection fraction), the heterogeneity increases with age. (From *J Appl Physiol* 1995; 78:80. Reproduced with permission from the publisher and authors.)

regulation depicted in Fig. 86-3*A* and *B*, the stroke volume index (SVI) is preserved in older persons over a wide range of performance (Fig. 86-3*D*). Specifically, the Frank-Starling mechanism is utilized in older men with the assumption of an upright, seated posture at rest (Fig. 86-3*A*) to produce a modest age-associated increase in SVI (Fig. 86-3*D*). During progressive exhaustive exercise, however, when in older men the failure to reduce ESVI (Fig. 86-3*B*) impairs the ejection fraction (Fig. 86-3*C*), SVI is not augmented in older compared with younger men, as would be anticipated on the basis of their augmented EDVI. In other words, *while healthy older persons utilize the Frank-Starling mechanism during vigorous exercise, this mechanism is impaired due to impaired LV ejection.* See Fig. 86-4*D* for interindividual variation of SVI in both men and women at maximum effort.

HEART RATE

In the supine position at rest, the heart rate in healthy BLSA men is not age related (Fig. 86-3*E*). In other populations, a reduction in the spontaneous and respiratory variations in resting heart rate is observed and reflects altered autonomic modulation with aging (see below). With assumption of the seated resting position, heart rate increases slightly less in older than in younger men (Fig. 86-3*E*). The magnitude of this age-associated reduction increases progressively during exercise. The net result is that maximum acute dynamic reserve range of heart rate is reduced by about one-third between 20 and 85 years of age. See Fig. 86-4*E* for individual variation in heart rate in both men and women at maximum effort.

CARDIAC OUTPUT

The *cardiac index,* as expected from the behavior of the SVI and heart rate functions in Fig. 86-3*D* and *E*, does not vary with age in either posture at rest (Fig. 86-3*E*), but *is reduced at max exercise in older men due to the age-associated decline in max heart rate.* The loss of acute cardiac output reserve from seated rest to exhaustive, seated cycle exercise averages about 30 percent in healthy, community-dwelling BLSA volunteer men. This reduction is entirely due to a reduction in heart rate reserve, as SVI at max exercise is preserved in healthy men rigorously screened to exclude occult coronary disease at older age. Alternatively stated, *subjects at the older end of the age range can augment their cardiac index 2.5-fold over seated rest, whereas those at the younger end of the spectrum can increase their cardiac index 3.5-fold.*

The hemodynamic patterns measured across the range of demands as illustrated in Fig. 86-3 for males are nearly identical in females. Exceptions are that, at seated rest, females do not exhibit a modest age-associated increase in EDVI because, unlike males, assumption of the upright posture does not produce a greater reduction in EDVI in younger than in older women. Due to the absence in women of an age-associated increase in EDVI in the seated position, the SVI does not increase with age at seated rest, and, in contrast to males, the calculated cardiac index at seated rest decreases modestly with age in women. At max exercise, the age-associated increase of EDVI is of borderline statistical significance in women. However, the change in EDVI from rest to max exercise in a given individual (not shown) significantly increases with age and is nearly identical, in both men and women.[29]

In summary, Figs. 86-3 and 86-4 illustrate that when cardiovascular function in adult volunteer community-dwelling subjects ranging in age from 20 to 85 years is compared, *impaired LV ejection reserve capacity is the most dramatic change in cardiac pump function with aging in health,* as indicated by the failure of older persons to regulate ESV (Figs. 86-3*B* and 86-4*B*) as effectively as younger ones do. *This impaired ESV regulation is accompanied by diminished cardioacceleration, LV dilation at end diastole* (Figs. 86-3 and 86-4*A* and *D*) *and an altered diastolic filling pattern* (Fig. 86-2). See Fig. 86-4 for interindividual variation in the maximum cardiac output in both BLSA men and women.

AEROBIC CAPACITY

The peak (max) upright, seated cycle aerobic capacity estimated by either peak oxygen consumption or work capacity (accompanying the hemodynamic pattern in Figs. 86-3 and 86-4) declines approximately 50 percent. Thus, in this study population, *the age-associated reduction in the cardiac component accounts for roughly half of the age-associated decline in aerobic capacity, the remainder being attributable to age-associated differences in oxygen utilization.* Such reductions in O_2 utilization during vigorous exercise result from age-associated reduction in muscle mass[30] and from a reduction in the shunting of blood from viscera to working muscles during exercise,[31] and the amount of O_2 consumed per unit of working muscle mass per amount of O_2 delivered to the muscle. The extent to which the maximum aerobic capacity declines with aging, and its suspected underlying mechanisms, vary among studies (see Lakatta[32] for a review).

Mechanisms of Deficient Cardiovascular Regulation with Aging in Otherwise Healthy Persons

The ESV is regulated across the range of demands for blood flow encountered in Fig. 86-3 by changes in intrinsic myocardial contractility, afterload, and autonomic modulation of both, with parasympathetic influences diminishing and sympathetic influences becoming more predominant with increasing demands for cardiovascular performance. The max heart rate is regulated, in large part, by the effectiveness of sympathetic modulation. The EDV is regulated by the venous return, by determinants of the AV pressure gradient, including distensibly characteristics of the LV, during exercise, by the filling time, and by the strength of the atrial contraction. Neither the AV pressure gradient nor the end-diastolic pressure either at rest or during the other demand levels depicted in Fig. 86-3 have been measured in a sufficient number of individuals of any study population due to experimental constraints in healthy volunteers.

MYOCARDIAL CONTRACTILITY

In humans, information as to how aging affects factors that regulate intrinsic myocardial contractility is incomplete because the effectiveness of intrinsic myocardial contractility in the intact circulation is difficult to separate from loading and autonomic modulatory influences on contractility. A deficit in maximal intrinsic contractility of older persons might be expected on the basis of the reduced maximum heart rate, as the heart rate, per se, is a determinant of the myocardial contractile state. Additional supporting evidence for reduced LV contractility with aging comes from studies in which the LV of older but not younger healthy BLSA men in the presence of β-adrenergic blockade dilates at end diastole in response to a given increase in afterload.[33]

The most reliable estimate of myocardial contractility, the slope of the ESP/ESV coordinates measured across a range of EDVs at rest, has not been estimated in a homogeneous, healthy study population across a broad age range, and by convention cannot be accessed during exercise. A single point, depicting ESP/ESV as a *contractility* index at each overall cardiovascular level of performance in Fig. 86-3, provides an age-associated pattern of myocardial contractile reserve that is nearly indentical to the ejection fraction in Fig. 86-3*C*.[29]

Most of our current information regarding age-associated changes in factors that regulate cardiac muscle or myocyte function is derived from studies in rodents. Coordinated changes in gene expression or in protein function that modify several key steps of cardiac muscle excitation-Ca^{2+} release-contraction relaxation coupling occur in rodent hearts with aging and result in a prolonged action potential, a prolonged Ca_i transient, and a prolonged contraction. A twofold prolongation of the action potential in cardiac muscle isolated from senescent 24-month rats, compared with that in myocardium of younger adult 6- to 8-month rats, is not due to an age-associated increase in the L-type sarcolemmal Ca^{2+} current density; however, the L-type current inactivates more slowly, and this could account, in part, for the prolonged action potential.[34] It is likely that reductions in outwardly directed K^+ currents with aging also substantially contribute to prolongation of the action potential.[34] The rate of Ca^{2+} sequestration by the sarcoplasmic reticulum decreases in senescent myocardium and may, in part, explain the prolonged Ca_i transient.[35] An age associated reduction in the transcription of the gene coding for the sarcoplasmic reticulum Ca^{2+} pump, Serca2,[36] could account for a decrease in the sarcoplasmic reticulum pump site density.[37] The cardiac Na^+-Ca^{2+} exchanger (NCX1) serves as the main transsarcolemmal Ca^{2+} extrustion mechanism. It has been suggested that the Na^+-Ca^{2+} exchanger is more active in ejecting Ca^{2+} from cells of older than younger hearts during diastole, and an increased NCX1 expression may compensate partly for a reduced sarcoplasmic reticulum pump function. The supporting evidence is that the abundance of cardiac Na^+-Ca^{2+} exchanger transcripts increases about 50 percent in senescent (24 month) compared with the young adult (6 month) rat heart.[38]

The contractile force of isolated cardiac muscle generated by a given increase in cell Ca^{2+} at low rates of electrical stimulation is not altered by age. In rodents, however, marked shifts occur in the myosin heavy-chain isoforms, i.e., the β isoform becomes predominant in senescence rats.[37,39] The myosin Ca^{2+}-ATPase activity declines with the decline in α myosin heavy chain (αMHC) content.[39,40] The altered cellular profile, which results in a contraction that exhibits reduced velocity and a prolonged time course, can be considered to be adaptive rather than degenerative, because the reduced velocity is energy efficient and a prolonged contraction permits continued ejection for a longer period into the stiffened vasculature that accompanies advancing age (vide infra).

Aggregate, age-associated alterations in the kinetics of the cytosolic Ca^{2+} transient, the Na-Ca exchanger,[41] Na-K pump, and the sarcoplasmic reticulum Ca^{2+} pump function, possibly in conjunction with nonspecific changes in sarcolemmal membrane composition ionic permeability,[42] may predispose senescent myocardium to altered cell Ca^{2+} homeostasis. Intriguingly, aged myocardium (and also that of young rodents chronically exposed to pressure overload) is more susceptible to Ca^{2+} overload and spontaneous sarcoplasmic reticulum Ca^{2+} release than is young adult myocardium.[43] Specifically, aged myocardium demonstrates a reduced threshold for Ca^{2+}-dependent diastolic aftercontractions and afterdepolarizations and for ventricular fibrillation during situations that increase cell Ca^{2+} loading[43] as well as the likelihood for the occurrence of spontaneous oscillatory sarcoplasmic reticulum Ca^{2+} release.[44] During higher pacing rates in older but not in younger hearts or cardiac myocytes[45] temporally summated, asynchronous spontaneous Ca^{2+} release occurring within and among cells, or a steady increase in diastolic Ca^{2+} within the cytosol, leads to incomplete diastolic myofilament relaxation and contributes to an increase in diastolic tone.

Many of the multiple changes in cardiac excitation, myofilament activation, contraction mechanisms, and gene expression that occur with aging can be interpreted as adaptive in nature, because they also occur in the hypertrophied myocardium of younger animals adapted to experimentally induced chronic hypertension.[32] Evidence suggests that the adaptive response to chronic pressure loading is reduced in older animals, possibly because some of the adaptive capacity of the heart is used as a response to the aging process.[32]

AFTERLOAD

Cardiac afterload has two components, one generated by the heart itself and the other by the vasculature. The cardiac component of afterload can be expected to increase as a function of ventricular volume, e.g., it increases acutely as the heart size increases during the various maneuvers listed in Figs. 86-3 and 86-4. Considerable evidence indicates that at rest the vascular load on the LV increases with age. The vascular load on the heart has four components: conduit artery compliance characteristics, reflected pulse waves, inertance, and resistance.

FIGURE 86-5 Considerable evidence indicates that at rest the vascular load on the left ventricle increases with age. The age-associated structural changes in compliance arteries (Fig. 86-1*A* and *B*) lead to a reduction in arterial compliance with aging. One manifestation of this is increased pulse-wave velocity (*A*), which causes reflected pulse waves to reach the base of aorta earlier (i.e., prior to closure of the aortic value), producing a late-systolic augmentation of the central pressure pulse contour (*B*). Early reflected pulse waves in conjunction with a resetting of the baroflex lead to an increase in the resting systolic pressure with aging, which by definition, in normotensives, occurs within the clinically normal range (*E*). On average, the diastolic pressure does not increase after middle age (*F*) and, in many older persons, becomes reduced, due to the reduced conduit artery compliance and early reflected pulse waves occurring centrally in late systole rather than in diastole. *The net result is a dramatic increase in pulse pressure with increasing older age.* Thus, the pulse pressure/stroke volume index (PP/SVI), an index of large-vessel stiffness, increases with aging (*D*). The total systemic vascular resistance calculated from the resting mean arterial pressure and cardiac output increases modestly or does not appreciably change at rest with aging in otherwise healthy persons (*C*). (*A* and *B* from *Circulation* 1993; 88:1456; *C* and *D* from *J Appl Physiol* 1995; 78:890; *E* and *F* from *J Gerontol* 1997; 52:M177. Each is reproduced with permission from the publisher and authors.)

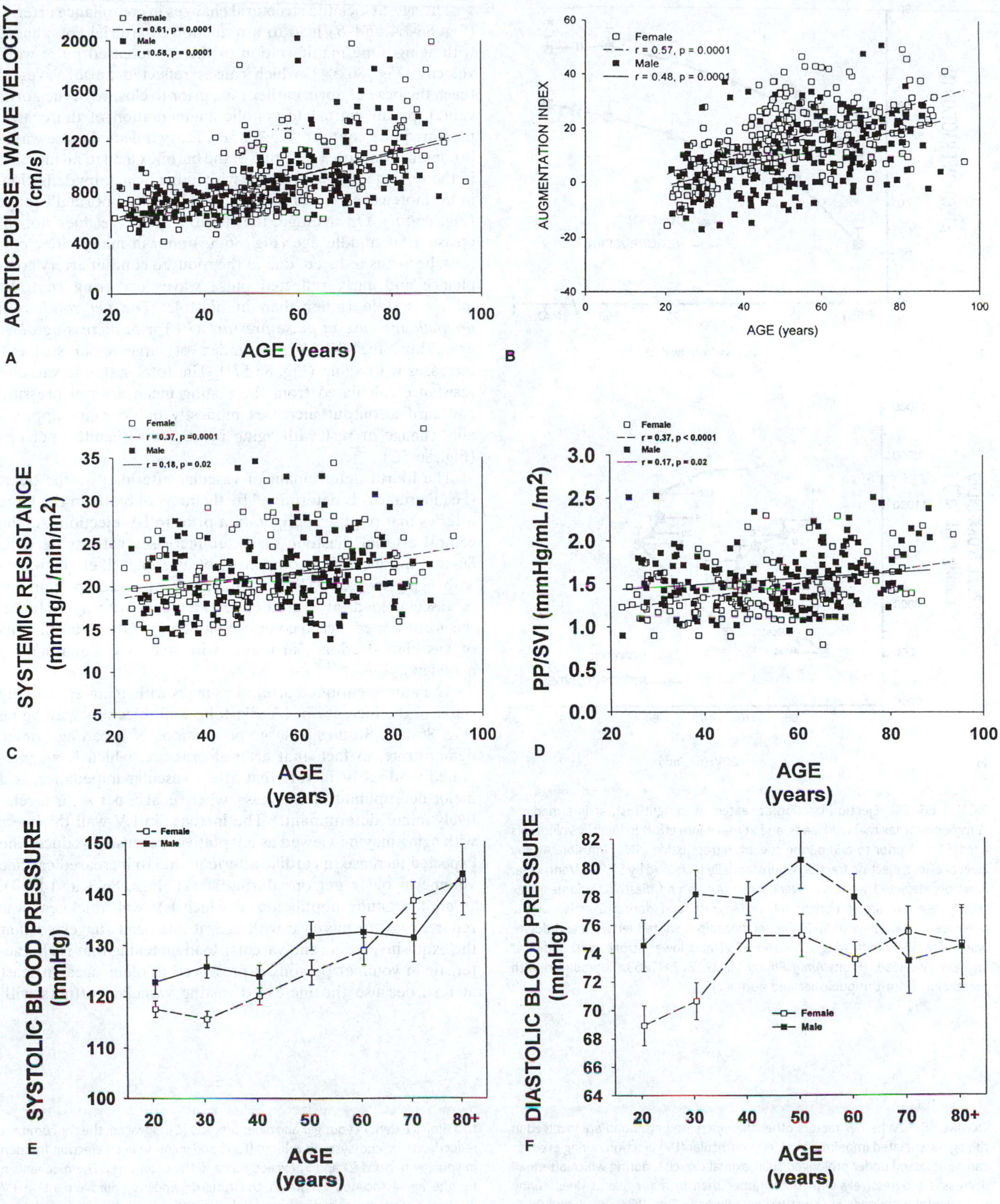
Female
r = 0.61, p = 0.0001
Male
r = 0.58, p = 0.0001
AORTIC PULSE – WAVE VELOCITY (cm/s)
AGE (years)
A
Female
r = 0.57, p = 0.0001
Male
r = 0.48, p = 0.0001
AUGMENTATION INDEX
AGE (years)
B
Female
r = 0.37, p = 0.0001
Male
r = 0.18, p = 0.02
SYSTEMIC RESISTANCE (mmHg/L/min/m2)
AGE (years)
C
Female
r = 0.37, p < 0.0001
Male
r = 0.17, p = 0.02
PP/SVI (mmHg/mL/m2)
AGE (years)
D
Female
Male
SYSTOLIC BLOOD PRESSURE (mmHg)
AGE (years)
E
Female
Male
DIASTOLIC BLOOD PRESSURE (mmHg)
AGE (years)
F

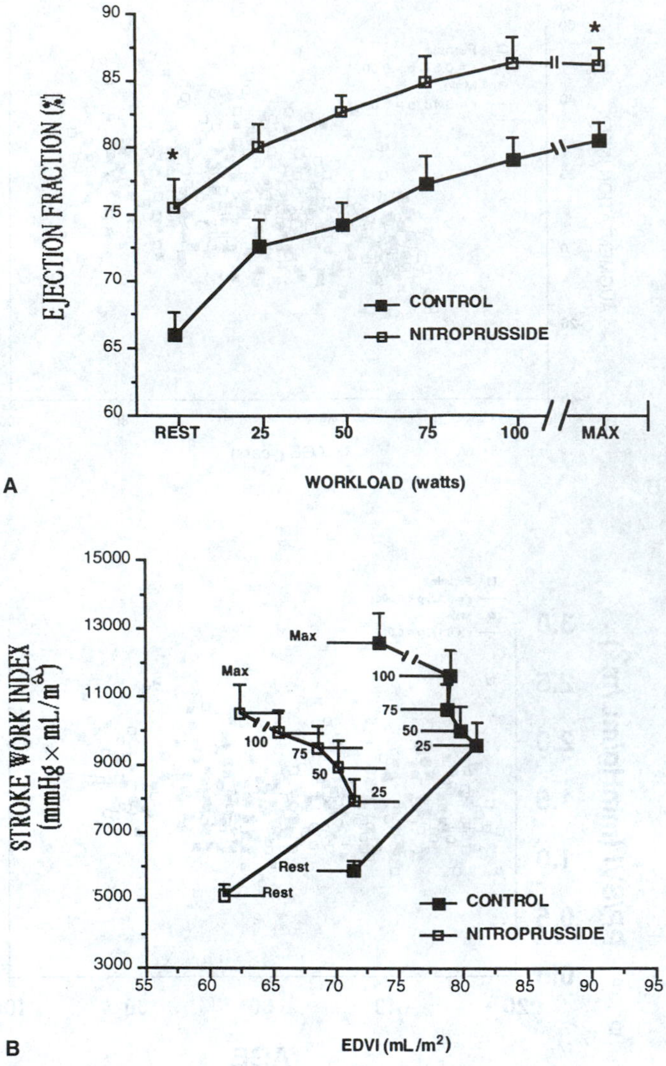

FIGURE 86-6 *A.* Ejection fraction at seated, at upright rest, at intermediate common submaximal workloads, and at maximum effort in healthy volunteers aged 71 ± 7 prior to and during sodium nitroprusside (SNP) infusion. At any level of effort, ejection fraction is substantially increased by SNP. *B.* Ventricular function, depicted as stroke work index versus end-diastolic volume index (EDVI) relationship at upright, at seated rest, and during exercise in the presence and absence of SNP. The relationship is shifted leftward and downward with SNP, indicating a smaller EDVI and lower stroke work index at any exercise load. (From *Am J Physiol* 1999; 277:H1863. Reproduced with permission from the publisher and authors.)

The age-associated structural changes in compliance arteries (Fig. 86-1*A* and *B*) lead to a reduction in arterial compliance with aging. One manifestation of this is increased pulse-wave velocity (Fig. 86-5*A*), which causes reflected pulse waves to reach the base of aorta earlier (i.e., prior to closure of the aortic value), producing a late systolic augmentation of the central pressure pulse contour (Fig. 86-5*B*). Early reflected pulse waves in conjunction with a resetting of the baroflex lead to an increase in the resting systolic pressure with aging, which by definition, in normotensives, occurs within the clinically "normal" range (Fig. 86-5*E*). On average, the diastolic pressure does not increase after middle age (Fig. 86-5*F*) and, in many older persons, becomes reduced, due to the reduced conduit artery compliance and early reflected pulse waves occurring centrally in late systole rather than in diastole. *The net result is a dramatic increase in pulse pressure (PP) with increasing older age.* Thus, the PP/SVI, an index of large-vessel stiffness, increases with aging (Fig. 86-5*D*). The total systemic vascular resistance calculated from the resting mean arterial pressure and cardiac output increases modestly or does not appreciably change at rest with aging in otherwise healthy persons (Fig. 86-5*C*).

The fourth determinant of vascular afterload on the heart (i.e., inertance) is determined by the mass of blood in the large arteries that requires acceleration prior to LV ejection. As the central arterial diastolic diameter increases with aging (Fig. 86-1*C*), the inertance component of afterload likely increases with aging as well. Thus, each of the pulsatile components of vascular load, measured at rest, increase with age. Hence, the aortic impedance, a composite function of the determinants of vascular afterload, increases with age (see Lakatta[32] for a review).

The aforementioned arterial changes with aging are a likely cause of the increase in LV diastolic wall thickness with aging (Fig. 86-1*C*). Studies in large populations of broad age range demonstrate, in fact, that arterial pressure, which is an integrated readout of factors that affect vascular impedance, is a major determinant of LV mass, whereas age, per se, is a relatively minor determinant.[46] The increase in LV wall thickness with aging may be viewed as adaptative, because it reduces the expected increase in cardiac afterload due to increased cardiac volume in older persons during stress (Figs. 86-3 and 86-4). In another study population in which LV wall thickness was reported not to increase with age, it has been suggested that the exquisite cardiac and vascular load matching that is characteristic in younger persons is preserved at older ages, at least at rest, because the increased resting vascular stiffness with

FIGURE 86-7 Whether factors other than increased afterload are involved in the age-associated impairment of left ventricular (LV) ejection during exercise can be assessed under prolonged submaximal exercise, during which afterload decreases progressively with time, rather than increasing as it does during incremental workloads in the study paradigms in Figs. 86-3, 86-4, and 86-6. When individuals exercise at a constant submaximal work rate (50 percent of age-matched VO_2 max) for prolonged times (i.e., 60 min or longer), arterial pressure drops with time (*A* and *B*), and the estimate of arterial stiffness—pulse pressure/stroke volume index (PP/SVI)—decreases with time, both changing to a similar extent in younger and older subjects (*C*). However, the concomitant reduction in LV end-systolic volume (ESV) and increase in LV ejection fraction in younger persons (*D* and *E*) exceed those in the older ones. The mechanism for the age-associated failure in the time-dependent improvement in LV ejection during prolonged submaximal exercise cannot be attributed to a failure of afterload reduction to occur with time, and thus other mechanisms limit the acute LVESV reserve in these healthy, older persons (From *Circ Suppl* 1999; 100:I-141. Reproduced with permission from the publisher and authors.)

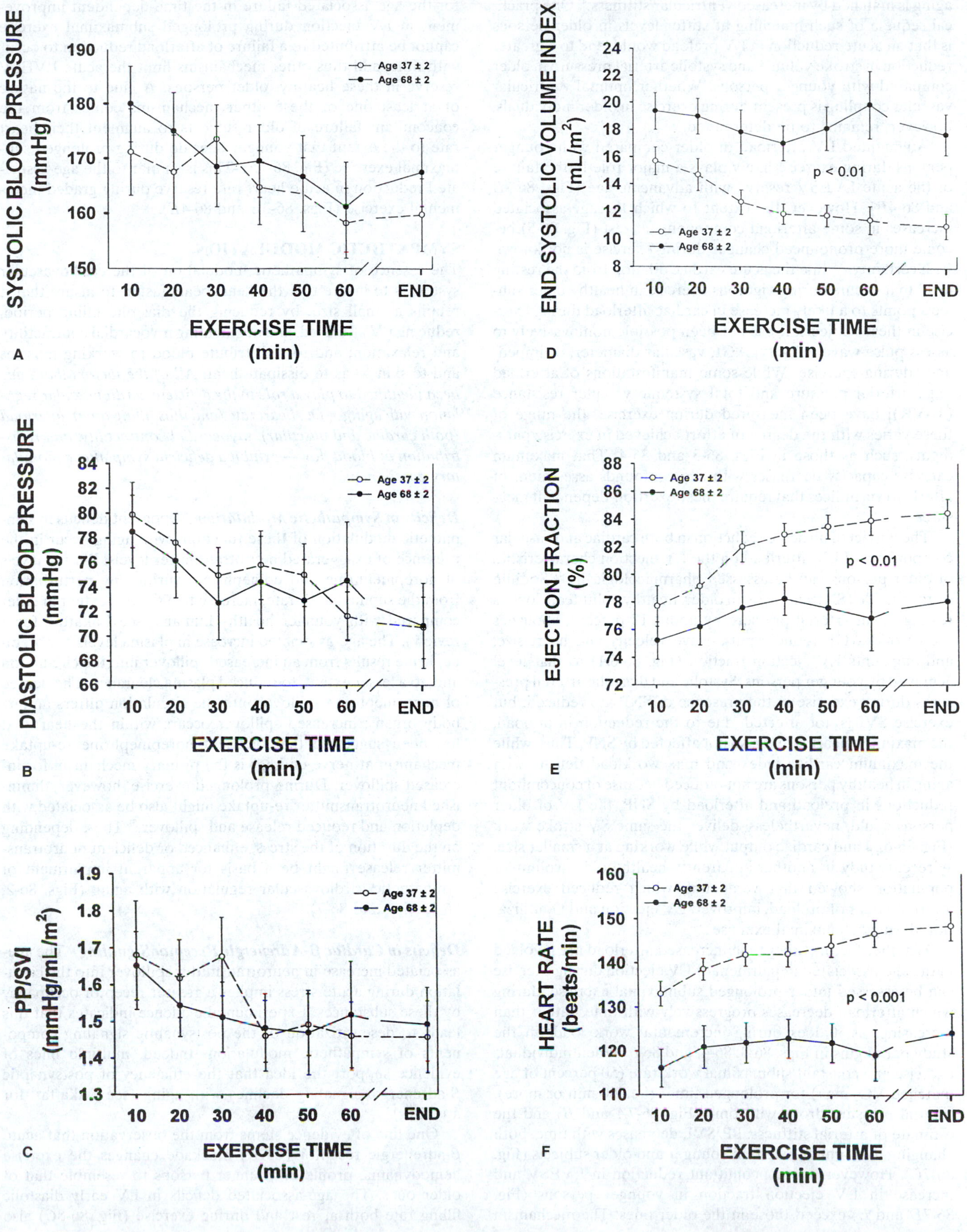
SYSTOLIC BLOOD PRESSURE (mmHg)
Age 37 ± 2
Age 68 ± 2
EXERCISE TIME (min)
A
END SYSTOLIC VOLUME INDEX (mL/m²)
p < 0.01
D
DIASTOLIC BLOOD PRESSURE (mmHg)
B
EJECTION FRACTION (%)
E
PP/SVI (mmHg/mL/m²)
C
HEART RATE (beats/min)
p < 0.001
F
10 20 30 40 50 60 END

aging is matched by increased ventricular stiffness.[45] One practical sequela of such matching at stiffer levels in older persons is that an acute reduction in LV preload would lead to a greater reduction in stroke volume and systolic arterial pressure in older compared with younger persons. Whether optimal ventricular vascular coupling is present during exercise in older individuals, however, remains to be determined.

Augmented LV afterload in older compared with younger persons during exercise likely plays a major role in the failure of the acute LVESV reserve with advancing age (Figs. 86-3*B* and 86-4*B*). However, the extent to which the age-associated increases in some afterload components at rest (Fig. 86-5) become more pronounced changes during exercise is not known with certainty. While the acute cardiac dilation from the resting level that occurs during vigorous exercise in healthy older subjects points to a likely increase in cardiac afterload during exercise in these subjects, it has not been possible noninvasively to assess pulse-wave velocity, AGI, vascular diameter, or impedance during exercise. While some manifestations of afterload [e.g., arterial pressure and total systemic vascular resistance (TSVR)] have been measured during exercise, the range of these varies with the degree of effort achieved in exercise paradigms, such as those in Figs. 86-3 and 86-4. That maximum exercise capacity decreases with age confounds assessment of afterload via indices that require these exertion-dependent measures.

The impact of an acute reduction in both cardiac and vascular components of LV afterload on the LV ejection characteristics of older persons can be assessed pharmacologically.[47] Sodium nitroprusside (SNP) infusion in older, healthy volunteers lowers resting mean arterial pressure by about 12 percent, abolishes the carotid AGI, reduces pulse-wave velocity and heart size, and augments LV ejection fraction (Fig. 86-6*A*) to that level achieved by younger persons. Systolic and diastolic arterial pressures during exercise in the presence of SNP are reduced, but exercise SVI is not affected, due to the reduction in preload; the maximum heart rate is also not affected by SNP. Thus, while the maximum cardiac index and max workload deficits with aging in healthy persons are not reduced because of concomitant reductions in preload and afterload by SNP, the LV of older persons could, nevertheless, deliver the same SV stroke work (Fig. 86-6*B*) and cardiac output while working at a smaller size. A recent study in another apparently healthy older volunteer population showed that verapamil, which reduced exercise afterload but not preload, improved LV ejection and O_2 utilization during submaximal exercise.[48]

Whether factors other than increased afterload are involved in the age-associated impairment of LV ejection during exercise can be assessed under prolonged submaximal exercise, during which afterload decreases progressively with time, rather than increasing, as it does during incremental work loads in the study paradigms in Figs. 86-3, 86-4, and 86-6. When individuals exercise at a constant submaximal work rate (50 percent of age matched VO_2 max) for prolonged times (i.e., 60 min or more), arterial pressure drops with time (Fig. 86-7*A* and *B*) and the estimate of arterial stiffness, PP/SVI, decreases with time, both changing to a similar extent in younger and older subjects (Fig. 86-7*C*). However, the concomittant reduction in LVESV and increase in LV ejection fraction in younger persons (Fig. 86-7*D* and *E*) exceed those in the older ones. The mechanism for the age-associated failure in the time-dependent improvement in LV ejection during prolonged submaximal exercise cannot be attributed to a failure of afterload reduction to occur with time, and thus other mechanisms limit the acute LVESV reserve in these healthy, older persons. A clue to the nature of at least one of these other mechanisms comes from the concomitant failure of older subjects to augment their heart rate to the extent that younger ones do during prolonged submaximal exercise (Fig. 86-7*F*). This is similar to the age-associated reduction in acute heart rate reserve during graded incremental exercise (Figs. 86-3*E* and 86-4*E*).

SYMPATHETIC MODULATION

The essence of sympathetic modulation of the cardiovascular system is to insure that the heart beats faster; to insure that it retains a small size, by reducing the diastolic filling period, reducing LV afterload, and augmenting myocardial contractility and relaxation; and to redistribute blood to working muscles and to skin so as to dissipate heat. *All of the factors that have been identified to play a role in the deficient cardiovascular regulation with aging—i.e., heart rate (and thus filling time), afterload (both cardiac and vascular), myocardial contractility, and redistribution of blood flow—exhibit a deficient sympathetic modulatory component.*

Deficits in Sympathetic Modulation Apparent deficits in sympathetic modulation of these functions with aging occur in the presence of exaggerated neurotransmitter levels. Plasma levels of norepinephrine and epinephrine, during any perturbation from the supine basal state, increase to a greater extent in older compared with younger healthy humans (see Lakatta[49] for a review). The age-associated increase in plasma levels of norepinephrine results from an increased spillover into the circulation and, to a lesser extent, to reduced plasma clearance. The degree of norepinephrine spillover into the circulation differs among body organs; increased spillover occurs within the heart.[50] It has been suggested that deficient norepinephrine re-uptake mechanism at nerve endings is the primary mechanism for increased spillover. During prolonged exercise, however, diminished neurotransmitter re-uptake might also be associated with depletion and reduced release and spillover.[51] Thus, depending on the duration of the stress, enhanced or deficient neurotransmitter release might be a basis for apparent impairment of sympathetic cardiovascular regulation with aging (Figs. 86-2, 86-3, 86-4, and 86-7).

Deficits in Cardiac β-Adrenergic Receptor Signaling The age-associated increase in neurotransmitter spillover into the circulation during acute stress implies a greater receptor occupancy by these substances. Experimental evidence indicates that this leads to desensitization of the postsynaptic signaling components of sympathetic modulation. Indeed, multiple lines of evidence support the idea that the efficiency of postsynaptic β-adrenergic signaling declines with aging (see Lakatta[49] for a review).

One line of evidence stems from the observation that acute β-adrenergic receptor (βAR) blockade changes the exercise hemodynamic profile of younger persons to resemble that of older ones. The age-associated deficits in LV early diastolic filling rate both at rest and during exercise (Fig. 86-8*C*) also

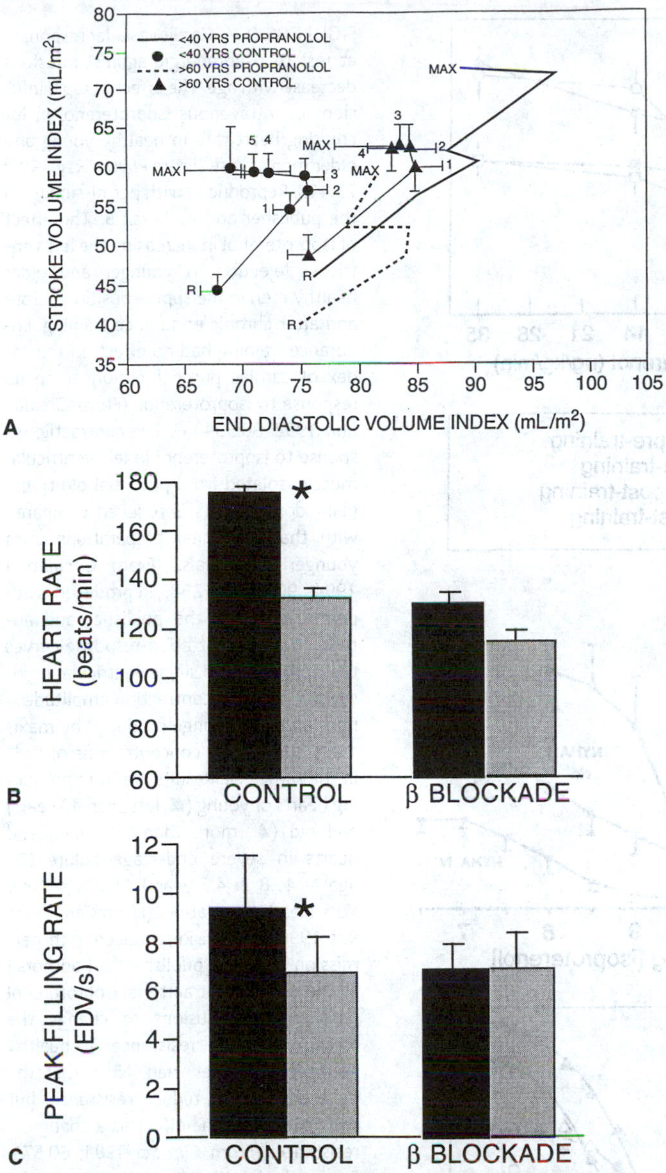

FIGURE 86-8 *A.* Stroke volume index as a function of end-diastolic volume (EDV) index at rest (R) and during graded cycle workloads in the upright seated position in healthy men from the Baltimore Longitudinal Study on Aging (BLSA), in the presence and absence (dashed line) of β-adrenergic blockade. R = seated rest; 1–4 or 5 = graded submaximal workloads on cycle ergometer; max = maximum effort. Stroke volume/end-diastolic functions with symbols are those measured in the absence of propranolol; *dashed and solid line* functions without symbols are the stroke volume compared with end-diastolic function measured in the presence of propranolol. Note that, in the absence of propranolol, the stroke volume versus EDV relation in older persons (▲) is shifted rightward from that in younger ones (●). This indicates that the left ventricle of older persons in the sitting position compared with that of younger ones operates from a greater preload both at rest and during submaximal and max exercise. Propranolol markedly shifts the stroke volume/EDV relationship in younger persons (*solid line without points*) rightward but does not markedly offset the curve in older persons (*dashed line without points*). Thus, with respect to this assessment of ventricular function curve, β-adrenergic blockade with propranolol makes younger men appear like older ones. The abolition of the age-associated differences in the left ventricular (LV) function curve after propranolol are accompanied by a reduction or abolition of the age-associated reduction in heart rate, which, at max, is shown in *B*. Note, however, that β-adrenergic blockade in younger individuals in this figure causes stroke volume index to increase to a greater extent than during β blockade in older ones, suggesting that mechanisms other than deficient β-adrenergic regulation compromise LV ejection. One potential mechanism is an age-associated decrease in *maximum intrinsic* myocardial contractility. Another likely mechanism is enhanced vascular afterload, due to the structural changes in compliance arteries noted above and possibly also to impaired vasorelaxation during exercise. (From *Circulation* 1994; 90:2333. Reproduced with permission from the publisher and authors.) *B.* Peak exercise heart rate in the same subjects as in *A* in the presence and absence of acute β-adrenergic blockade by propranolol. *C.* The age-associated reduction in peak LV diastolic filling rate at max exercise in healthy BLSA subjects is abolished during exercise in the presence of β-adrenergic blockade with propranolol. Solid = less than 40 years; light = more than 60 years. (From *Am J Physiol* 1992; 73:H1932. Reproduced with permission from the publisher and authors.)

are abolished by acute β-adrenergic blockade.[52] The heart rate reduction during exercise in the presence of acute β-adrenergic blockade is greater in younger than in older subjects (Fig. 86-8*B*), and significant β blockade-induced LV dilatation occurs only in younger subjects (Fig. 86-8*A*). Note, however, that β-adrenergic blockade in younger individuals in Fig. 86-8 causes SVI to increase to a greater extent than in β blockade in older ones, suggesting that mechanisms other than deficient β-adrenergic regulation compromise LV ejection. One potential mechanism is an age-associated decrease in *maximum intrinsic* myocardial contractility. Another likely mechanism is enhanced vascular afterload due to the structural changes in compliance arteries noted above and possibly also to impaired vasorelaxation during exercise. In this regard, it has been observed that the increase in impedance during exercise in old dogs is abolished by β-adrenergic blockade.[53]

The second type of evidence for a diminished efficacy of synaptic βAR signaling is that cardiovascular responses at rest to β-adrenergic agonist infusions decrease with age (Fig. 86-9). Cellular mechanisms for the deficiency in βAR signaling in humans include a reduction in receptor number, and affinity and coupling to adenyl cyclase via G_s proteins. There is evidence that other G protein-coupled receptor signaling may also deteriorate in humans with aging (see Lakatta[49] for a review). The efficacy of βAR (i.e., β_1 vs. β_2 vs. β_3) signaling has not yet been studied in humans. Studies in rodent models have delineated additional age-associated deficits in the β-adrenergic signaling cascade. A reduced contractile response to both β_1AR and β_2AR stimulation occurs with aging in rodent isolated LV muscle and in individual rat ventricular cardiocytes.[54,55] This is due to failure of βAR stimulation to augment the intracellular Ca^{2+} transient to the same extent in cells of senescent hearts to which it does in cells from younger adult hearts.[54] The blunted increase in the Ca^{2+} transient following βAR stimulation in cells from older compared with younger adult hearts is attributable to a decrease in the ability of either β_1AR and β_2AR stimulation to increase L-type sarcolemmal Ca^{2+} channel availability and thus to a lesser increase in Ca^{2+} influx via these channels during the action potential. The richly documented age-associated reduction in the postsynaptic response of myocardial cells to β_1AR stimulation appears to be due to multiple changes in molecular and biochemical receptor coupling and postreceptor mechanisms. However, the major limiting modification of this signaling

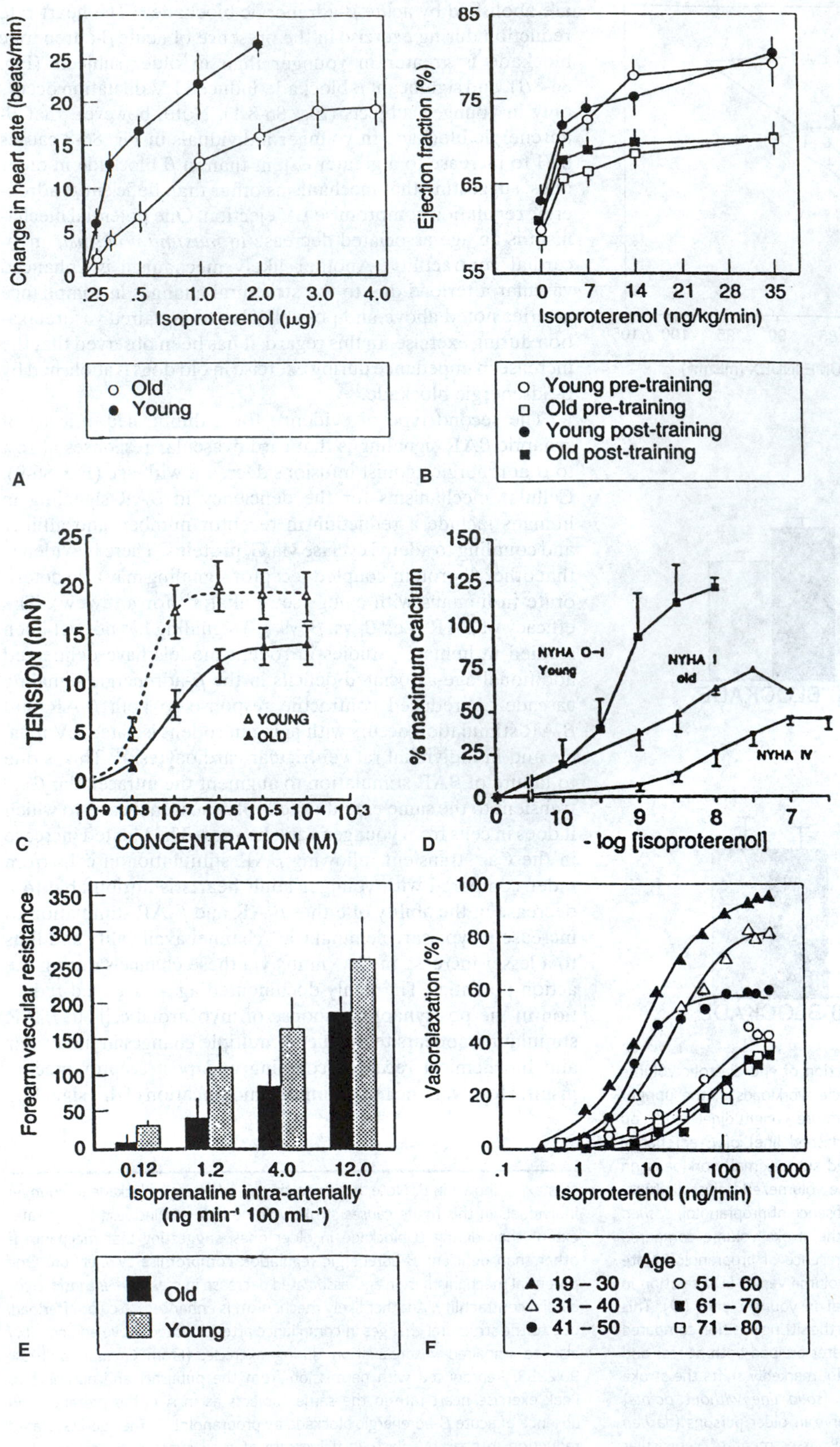

FIGURE 86-9 *A.* Cardiovascular responses at rest to β-adrenergic agonist infusions decrease with age. The effect of rapid infusions of intravenous isoproterenol in increasing heart rate in healthy young and older men at rest. (From *Physiol Rev* 1993; 73:413. Reproduced with permission from the publisher and authors.) *B.* The effect of isoproterenol in increasing the left ventricular ejection in younger and older healthy men in the supine position before and after chronic endurance training. Endurance training had no effect on this index of cardiac pump function or on its response to isoproterenol. (From *Circulation* 1992; 86:504.) *C.* The contractile response to isoproterenol in left ventricular muscle isolated from potential old transplant donor hearts is reduced compared with that in similar preparations from younger individuals. (From *Circulation* 1994; 90:1225–1238. Reproduced with permission from the publisher and authors.) *D.* Concentration-response curves to isoproterenol in single ventricular myocytes. Change in contraction amplitude is normalized to change produced by maximally stimulating concentrations of Ca^{2+} in the same cell. Results are from nonfailing hearts of young (■, less than 40 years) and old (▲, more than 50 years) and hearts in severe end-stage failure (▼, age = 45.8 ± 4.7 years). NYHA = New York Heart Association. (From *Cardiovasc Res* 1996; 31:152. Reproduced with permission from the publisher and authors.) *E.* The effect of intraarterial isoproterenol (isoprenaline) infusions to change the forearm vascular resistance in healthy younger and older men. Note that the drug effect is to reduce resistance, but the figure plots the effect as a change in resistance. (From *Clin Sci* 1981; 60:571. Reproduced with permission from the publisher and authors.) *F.* The effect of intravenous arterial infusion of isoproterenol in relaxing dorsal hand veins, previously constricted by phenylephrine, in men of varying ages. (From *J Pharmacol Exp Ther* 1986; 239:802. Reproduced with permission from the publisher and authors.)

pathway with advancing age appears to be at the coupling of the β-adrenergic receptor to adenyl cyclase via the G_s protein[55] and to changes in adenyl cyclase protein, per se, leading to a reduction in the ability to augment cell cAMP sufficiently to drive the phosphorylation of key proteins[56] that is required to alter protein function and augment cardiac contractility. The apparent desensitization of β_1AR and β_2AR signaling with aging is not mediated via increased β-adrenergic receptor kinase or increased G_i activity.[55]

PHYSICAL DECONDITIONING

A marked reduction in physical activity accompanies advancing age in a majority of adults. Thus, it may be hypothesized that a reduction in physical *conditioning* might be implicated as a factor in the reduced cardiovascular reserve of older, healthy sedentary individuals, as discussed. Alternatively, the issue arises as to whether physical conditioning via aerobic training of sedentary older persons can affect deficits in cardiovascular reserve capacity due to an *aging process,* per se.

It has been amply documented that physical conditioning of older persons can substantially increase their maximum aerobic work capacity and peak oxygen consumption. The extent to which this conditioning effect results from enhanced central cardiac performance or from augmented peripheral circulatory and O_2 utilization mechanisms, including changes in skeletal muscle mass, varies with the type and degree of conditioning achieved, gender, body position during study (see Lakatta[32] for a review), and likely genetic factors. A longitudinal study of older males in the upright position indicates that an enhanced physical conditioning status increases O_2 consumption and work capacity, in part by increases in the maximum CO by increasing the maximum SV, and in part by increasing the estimated total body (AV) O_2 utilization.[57] The augmentation of maximum SVI is due to an augmented reduction of LVESV (Fig. 86-10*A*) and, thus, a concomitant increase in LV ejection fraction, as the effect of conditioning status to increase LVEDI exercise is minimal (recall that LVEDI during acute vigorous exercise is already appreciably increased in older, sedentary, preconditioned men). This minor effect of physical conditioning on LVEDVI in older persons is in contrast to the effect of physical conditioning in younger persons, which substantially increases EDVI and SVI on the basis of the Frank-Starling mechanism, as well as via an enhanced LV ejection fraction. In contrast to the improved LV ejection, the max heart rate of older persons did not vary with physical conditioning status (Fig. 86-10*A*). *There is no strong evidence at hand that physical conditioning of older persons can offset the deficiency in sympathetic modulation.* Rather, conditioning effects to increase LV ejection appear to relate to the reduction in vascular afterload, as reflected in a reduced carotid AGI in older athletes compared with sedentary controls (Fig. 86-10*B*), and possibly to an augmentation of the maximum *intrinsic* myocardial contractility. In animal models, some, but not all, studied determinants of the latter are affected by physical conditioning status (see Lakatta[32] for a review).

Summary

In summary, an age-associated increase in vascular afterload on the heart is due to arterial stiffening and is reflected in the age-associated modest increase in systolic blood pressure at rest. In healthy individuals, these vascular changes are compen-

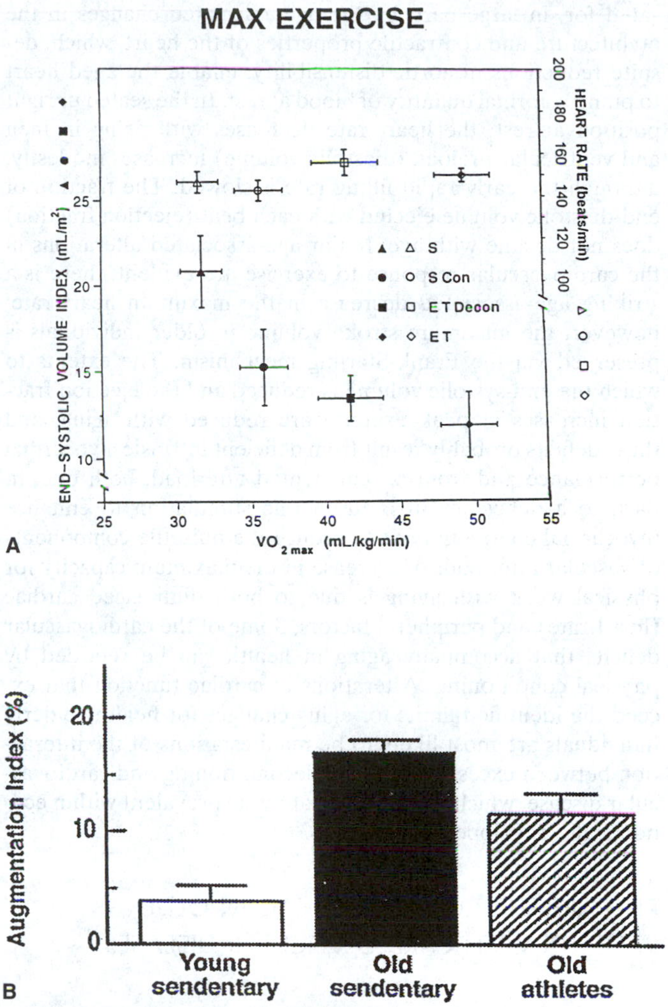

FIGURE 86-10 *A.* Heart rate and end-systolic volume during peak seated, upright exercise on a cycle ergometer across a broad range of aerobic capacity in healthy males who have been exercise conditioned or deconditioned. S = sedentary; ET = exercise trained; SCon = sedentary men after conditioning; ET Decon = men who had been exercise trained but stopped their training for the study to become detrained or deconditioned (DeCon). The figure shows that the extent to which the left ventricle empties, as manifest by the end-systolic volume, varies with the level of aerobic capacity (VO_2 max), which was varied among the four groups by either conditioning or deconditioning protocols. In contrast, the peak heart rate achieved does not vary with aerobic capacity. (From *Circulation* 1996; 94:359. Reproduced with permission from the publisher and authors.) *B.* With increasing age, the carotid pressure pulse exhibits a late peak, often observed as a second component. This is due to early reflected waves from peripheral sites, which, in part, are attributable to a reduced aortic compliance that causes the pulse-wave velocity to increase. The ratio of amplitude of the late component of the pressure pulse to the amplitude of the total pressure pulse is defined as an *augmentation index.* The increase in carotid augmentation index in highly trained older men (aged 60 to 85 years) is only about half of that expected on the basis of age. Thus, physical conditioning has an effect to alter the reflected waves in these older men. The effect may occur via a reduction in aortic stiffness, as the pulse-wave velocity is also reduced by conditioning (not shown). (From *Circulation* 1993; 881456. Reproduced with permission from the publisher and authors.)

sated for, in large part, by the age-associated changes in the architecture and contractile properties of the heart, which, despite reductions in aortic distensibility, enable the aged heart to pump a normal quantity of blood at rest. In the seated upright position at rest, the heart rate decreases with aging in men and ventricular preload (diastolic volume) increases modestly, although the early rapid filling rate is slowed. The fraction of end-diastolic volume ejected with each beat (ejection fraction) does not decline with age. Major age-associated alterations in the cardiovascular response to exercise are evident: there is a striking age-associated decrease in the maximum heart rate; however, the maximum stroke volume in older individuals is preserved via the Frank-Starling mechanism. The extents to which the end-systolic volume is reduced and the ejection fraction increases at peak exercise are reduced with aging, and these deficits probably result from deficient intrinsic myocardial performance and from an augmented afterload, both due, in part, to a deficiency in β-adrenergic stimulation to enhance myocardial contractility or to reduce the pulsatile components of vascular afterload. A decrease in the maximum capacity for physical work with aging is due to both diminished cardiac (heart rate) and peripheral factors. Some of the cardiovascular deficits that accompany aging in health can be retarded by physical conditioning. Alterations in cardiac function that exceed the identified limits for aging changes for healthy elderly individuals are most likely to be manifestations of the interaction between excessive physical deconditioning and cardiovascular disease, which are, unfortunately, so prevalent within economically developed populations.

THERAPEUTIC CONSIDERATIONS IN OLDER PATIENTS WITH CARDIOVASCULAR DISEASES

Cardiovascular Disease in Elderly Individuals

More successful recognition and treatment of cardiovascular risk factors and diseases continue to decrease age-adjusted cardiovascular mortality[58] and to increase the number and proportion of the cardiac patient population who are considered elderly. In the United States, cardiovascular disease is the leading cause of mortality, accounting for over 40 percent of deaths in those aged 65 years and older. Over 80 percent of all cardiovascular deaths occur in the same age group.[59] These data indicate that *age is the major risk factor for cardiovascular disease.*

One way to conceptualize why the clinical manifestations and the prognosis of these diseases worsen with age is that in older individuals the specific pathophysiologic mechanisms that cause clinical disorders are superimposed on heart and vascular substrates that are modified by aging per se (Fig. 86-11). The horizontal line separating the lower and upper parts of Fig. 86-11 represents the clinical practice *threshold* for disease recognition. Thus, entities above the line are presently classified as *diseases* that lead to heart and brain failure. The vascular and cardiac changes presently thought to occur as a result of the *normal* or *physiologic* aging process (i.e., those addressed in the previous sections) are depicted below the line. These age-associated changes in cardiac and vascular properties alter the substrate upon which cardiovascular disease is superimposed in several ways (Table 86-1). First, they lower the extent of disease severity required to cross the threshold that results in clinically significant signs and symptoms. For example, a mild degree of ischemia-induced relaxation abnormalities that may be asymptomatic in a younger individual may cause dyspnea in an older individual, who, by virtue of age alone, has preexisting slowed and delayed early diastolic relaxation.

Age-associated changes may also alter the manifestations and presentation of common cardiac diseases. This usually occurs in patients with acute infarction in whom the diagnosis is delayed because of atypical symptoms resulting in increased time to onset of therapy. Age-associated changes, including those in β-adrenergic responsiveness and in vascular stiffness also influence the response to and therefore the selection of different therapeutic inventions in older individuals with cardiovascular disease. Thus, in one sense, those processes below the line in Fig. 86-11 ought not to be considered to reflect normal or physiologic aging. Rather, they might be construed as specific risk factors for the diseases that they relate to, and thus might be targets of interventions designed to decrease the occurrence and/or manifestations of cardiovascular disease at later ages. Such a strategy would thus advocate treating "normal" aging. However, additional studies of the specific risks of each "normal" age-associated change and the effectiveness of treatment regimens to delay or prevent each change are required for this strategy to be put into practice. In the following section, the question of how aging influences the presentation and approach to the treatment of common cardiovascular diseases is considered, focusing on the influence and impact of the age-associated changes described previously.

Ischemic Heart Disease

In general, advancing age is associated with increasingly severe, diffuse atherosclerosis and with damage to the left ventricle. Therefore, almost all clinical manifestations of ischemic heart disease have a higher mortality rate and a worse outcome in the older population. The clinical assessment of elderly patients with coronary artery disease is often limited by the coexistence of diseases that make interpretation of symptoms difficult.[60] Thus, in the elderly, a high clinical index of suspicion plus the use of objective parameters such as stress test results are important in assessing and diagnosing ischemic heart disease. Treadmill testing is also useful to detect silent ischemia, which occurs with increasing frequency in the elderly and is a strong risk factor for the development of future symptomatic cardiac disease.[61]

ACUTE CORONARY SYNDROMES

Older patients with acute myocardial infarction are more likely to be female, have a preexisting history of angina and experience a non-Q-wave myocardial infarction[62,63] (see Chap. 42). Older patients are also more likely to present with atypical symptoms of acute myocardial ischemia and infarction, such as shortness of breath, confusion, and failure to thrive.[64] Furthermore, nearly one-half of myocardial infarctions in the elderly are unrecognized clinically.[64] Age is a powerful independent predictor of short-term and long-term mortality in patients with an acute myocardial infarction.[63–66] In patients admitted with a first ST-segment elevation myocardial infarction and treated with thrombolytic therapy, in-hospital mortality increases exponentially as a function of age from 1.9 percent among patients 40

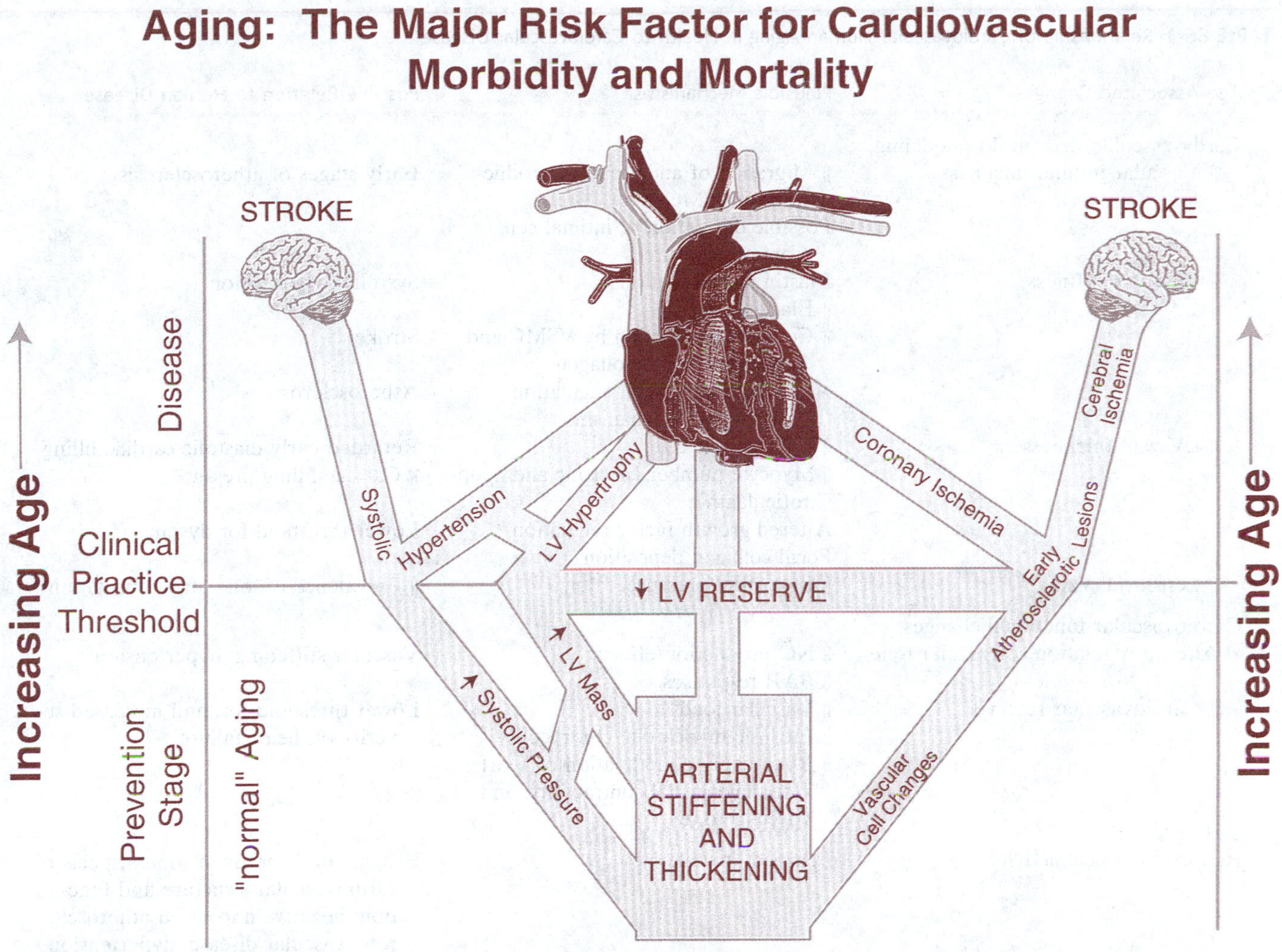

FIGURE 86-11 Changes in the vasculature and heart with aging in health may also be construed as risk factors for cardiovascular disease leading to heart and brain disorders in older age (see the text for details). LV = left ventricular. (From E. Braunwald, ed. *Heart Disease: A Textbook of Cardiovascular Medicine*, 5th ed. New York: WB Saunders; 1996:1687. Reproduced with permission from the publisher and authors.)

years or younger to 31.9 percent among patients older than 80 years.[65] Similarly, in the Global Utilization of Streptokinase and Tissue Plasminogen Activator for Occluded Arteries (GUSTO-1) Trial, 30-day mortality following a ST-segment elevation myocardial infarction increased from 3 percent in patients under 65 years of age to 19.6 percent in patient 75 to 85 years of age and to 30.3 percent in patients over 85 years of age.[67] *Age was the most powerful predictor of in-hospital and 30-day mortality in this trial.* Age is also a powerful predictor of recurrent ischemia and 30-day mortality in patients with non-ST-segment elevation acute coronary syndromes.[68] Hospital volume for acute coronary syndromes also influences outcome in the elderly.[69] Older patients admitted to hospitals with larger patient volumes for acute myocardial infarction have improved survival compared with lower-volume hospitals.

Elderly acute infarct patients experience a much greater incidence of heart failure and cardiogenic shock even though indices of infarct size, such as creatinine phosphokinase levels and QRS scores, do not change with age.[63,65] The risks of heart failure and shock increase three- to fourfold in patients older than 85 compared with those younger than 65.[67] The higher incidences of heart failure and shock may result from age-related changes in diastolic filling, aortic compliance, and decreased sensitivity to catecholamine stimulation, resulting in diminished cardiac reserve and afterload mismatch following ischemic damage. Mortality in older patients with myocardial infarction is less likely to result from ventricular fibrillation compared with younger patients but is much more likely to result from electromechanical dissociation and a finding of cardiac rupture on autopsy. The risk of death following hospital discharge also increases exponentially with increasing age, by almost 6 percent per year.[65]

The high morbidity and mortality associated with acute ischemic syndromes in the elderly dictate an aggressive management approach. Thrombolytic therapy in acute myocardial infarction reduces mortality, and data suggest a possible benefit in the elderly. In a meta-analysis of large randomized trials of thrombolytic therapy, subset analyses of the nearly 5800 patients older than 74 years showed a nonsignificant trend toward thrombolytic benefit, with a net saving of 1.0 life per 100 patients treated at 35 days after infarction. Although the percent decrease in mortality is less in older compared with younger pa-

TABLE 86-1 Relationship of Cardiovascular Human Aging in Health to Cardiovascular Disease

Age-Associated Changes	Plausible Mechanisms	Possible Relation to Human Disease
Cardiovascular structural remodeling		
⇑ Vascular intimal thickness	⇑ Migration of and ⇑ matrix production by VSMC	Early stages of atherosclerosis
	Possible derivation of intimal cells from other sources	
⇑ Vascular stiffness	Elastin fragmentation	Systolic hypertension
	⇑ Elastase activity	
	⇑ Collagen production by VSMC and ⇑ cross-linking of collagen	Stroke
	Altered growth factor regulation/tissue repair mechanisms	Atherosclerosis
⇑ LV wall thickness	⇑ LV myocyte size	Retarded early diastolic cardiac filling
	⇓ Myocyte number (necrotic and apoptotic death)	⇑ Cardiac filling pressure
	Altered growth factor regulation	Lower threshold for dyspnea
	Focal collagen deposition	
⇑ Left atrial size	⇑ Left atrial pressure/volume	⇑ Prevalence of lone atrial fibrillation
Cardiovascular functional changes		
Altered regulation of vascular tone	⇓ NO production/effects	Vascular stiffening; hypertension
	⇓ βAR responses	
⇓ Cardiovascular reserve	⇑ Vascular load	Lower threshold for, and increased severity of, heart failure
	⇓ Intrinsic myocardial contractility	
	⇓ β-Adrenergic modulation of heart rate, myocardial contractility, and vascular tone	
Reduced physical activity	Learned lifestyle	Exaggerated age Δs in some aspects of cardiovascular structure and function; negative impact on atherosclerotic vascular disease, hypertension, and heart failure

ABBREVIATIONS: VSMC = vascular smooth muscle cell; LV = left ventricular; NO = nitric oxide; βAR = β-adrenergic receptor.

tients treated with thrombolytics, the absolute benefit in terms of number of lives saved with treatment is similar.[70] In the GUSTO-1 trial,[67,71] subgroup analysis of 3655 patients over 75 years of age showed a similar absolute benefit compared with younger patients for accelerated dosed tissue plasminogen activator compared with steptokinase for the end point of death and nonfatal disabling stroke, although this subgroup comparison was not statistically significant. The use of accelerated tissue plasminogen activator appears relatively cost effective in the elderly.[72] In spite of these data, large registry data in the United States indicate that thrombolytic-eligible patients older than 75 are significantly less likely to receive reperfusion therapy than are patients younger than 65, with an odds ratio of 0.4.[73] Part of the reluctance of physicians to use thrombolytic agents in this age group arises from the concerns about intracranial hemorrhage. Age is an important predictor of hemorrhagic stroke with thrombolytic therapy and occurs more frequently with tissue plasminogen activator than with streptokinase.[67,74] Other comorbid conditions, such as cerebral vascular disease, hypertension, and body weight, must be considered, and age alone is not a criterion to exclude a patient from receiving thrombolytic therapy.[74]

Primary angioplasty is compared with thrombolytic therapy in several trials and may have beneficial effects on mortality, recurrent myocardial infarction, and recurrent ischemia.[75,76] Data from meta-analyses suggest a decrease in short-term death and nonfatal reinfarction in patients with ST-segment elevation myocardial infarction treated with primary angioplasty compared with thrombolytic therapy, with a particular benefit in the elderly.[77] Patients treated with direct angioplasty have a lower overall stroke and hemorrhagic stroke risk compared with thrombolytic-treated patients. Caveats from these studies include the short follow-up, operator expertise, and the importance of time delay prior to treatment; the delay is usually significantly longer with angioplasty than with thrombolytic therapy. Although elderly subjects treated with thrombolytic therapy will more often have multivessel coronary disease than will younger subjects, routine angioplasty following thrombolytic therapy does not decrease rates of death or recurrent myocardial infarction.[78] Angioplasty can be very effective, however, in relieving ischemia in elderly patients with postinfarction angina and unstable angina.[79,80]

In the Cooperative Cardiovascular Project, investigators reviewed records of approximately 200,000 Medicare beneficiaries who suffered a myocardial infarction. Only 34 percent of this elderly cohort were discharged home on a β-blockade.[81] Paradoxically, patients leaving hospital without β-blockade therapy have comorbidities that place them at the highest mortality risk. All subgroups of patients in this data base had a large survival advantage (approximately 40 percent reduction in 2-year mortality rate) with β-blockade therapy. Similarly, aspirin therapy decreases mortality rates in elderly infarct subjects and reduces recurrent ischemic pain in older unstable angina patients.[82] Nevertheless, among 10,000 Medicare beneficiaries with an acute myocardial infarction with no contraindication to aspirin therapy, only 61 percent of those received it within the first 2 hospital days.[83] Aspirin therapy in this large group of elderly infarct patients was independently associated with a lower 30-day mortality rate. Furthermore, only 76 percent of elderly subjects without any contraindications were discharged home on aspirin therapy after a myocardial infarction.[84] Aspirin use is independently associated with improved 6-month outcomes in this group. Angiotensin-converting enzyme (ACE) inhibitor therapy following acute myocardial infarction was evaluated in two groups of patients. First, patients with myocardial infarction started within 24 h of symptom onset and, second, in high-risk patients (LV dysfunction or congestive heart failure) with initiation of ACE inhibitor therapy 3 to 16 days after the infarction. A recent meta-analysis of the four large randomized placebo and open controlled trials evaluating the effects of ACE inhibitor therapy on early postinfarction mortality in approximately 100,000 patients[85] recently reported that 30-day mortality rate was significantly lower among the ACE inhibitor-treated patients (7.11 versus 7.59 percent). Thirty percent of the population was aged 65 to 74 years and 15 percent aged 75 years and older. Thirty-day mortality was 10.8 percent lower in the former group of patients treated with an ACE inhibitor as compared with the cohort not treated with ACE inhibitor. In patients 75 years of age and older, 30-day mortality was not reduced compared with the control group. In the trials that involved high-risk patients with LV dysfunction or clinical congestive heart failure, there is a large survival benefit among patients randomized to ACE inhibitor therapy.[86,87] In the Acute Infarction Ramipril Efficacy Study, in which ramipril was compared with placebo in 2006 postinfarction patients with clinical congestive heart failure, the mean age of the population was 65 years.[86] Treatment was initiated between days 3 and 10 after myocardial infarction. After an average of 15 months' follow-up, mortality was reduced from 23 percent in the placebo group to 17 percent in the ramipril group. Patients over 65 years of age had a larger survival advantage with the ACE inhibitor than did those under 65 years of age. In the 1749 postinfarct patients (mean age, 67.7 years) with echocardiographic evidence of LV dysfunction and randomized to the ACE inhibitor trandolapril versus placebo, long-term survival was significantly improved with ACE inhibitor therapy.[87] The 1121 patients at least 65 years of age had a relative risk of death of 0.83 with trandolapril compared with placebo. Therefore, *older patients with large infarctions, LV dysfunction, or clinical heart failure have a large survival advantage with long-term ACE inhibitor therapy.* For lower-risk elderly patients, the benefits are clearly less, and individualized treatment because of risk of hypotension and renal insufficiency, should be considered in this lower-risk, less benefiting group. Finally, lipid-lowering therapy also reduces morbidity and mortality among older patients after acute myocardial infarction. In the Cholesterol and Recurrent Events Trial evaluating either 40 mg of pravastatin or placebo over 5 years in 4159 patients with a myocardial infarction who had total cholesterol levels below 240 mg/dL and low-density lipoprotein levels between 115 and 174 mg/dL, 1283 patients were aged 65 to 75 years of age.[88] In this group, lipid-lowering therapy reduced the primary end point of cardiac death or nonfatal myocardial infarction by 39 percent. The individual secondary end points of cardiac death, nonfatal reinfarction, stroke, and need for coronary artery bypass surgery, were also reduced.

In patients with unstable angina or non-Q-wave myocardial infarction, recent studies show that the addition of a parenteral glycoprotein (GP) IIb/IIIa inhibitor to standard anti-ischemic therapy including aspirin and heparin reduces short-term risks of death, myocardial infarction, and refractory angina[89–125] (see Chap. 41). In a large randomized trial evaluating the GPIIb/IIIa inhibitor eptifibatide,[90] the mean age of the patient population was 64 years. In this nearly 11,000-patient trial, 30-day risk of death or nonfatal myocardial infarction was reduced from 15.7 percent in the placebo group to 14.2 percent in the eptifibatide-treated patients. In the subgroup of patients at least 65 years of age, there was no benefit for this GPIIb/IIIa inhibitor compared with placebo. In the randomized trial evaluating the GPIIb/IIIa inhibitor tirofiban compared with placebo,[91] patients treated with this GPIIb/IIIa inhibitor also benefited compared with aspirin and heparin alone, with the main end point of death, myocardial infarction, or refractory ischemia reduced from 17.9 percent to 12.9 percent at 7 days. In this 1915-patient trial, the mean age of the patients was 63 years. Both patients younger and older than 65 years of age benefited from GPIIb/IIIa inhibitor therapy: The composite event rate in the older group was reduced from 23.5 percent in the placebo group to 17.8 percent in the tirofiban group. Although bleeding is more common with GPIIb/IIIa inhibitor therapy than with placebo, bleeding is generally mild, with no increase in stroke rate or risk of intracranial hemorrhage. Therefore, *age should not exclude the addition of a GPIIb/IIIa inhibitor to standard anti-ischemic therapy in patients with unstable angina or non-Q-wave myocardial infarction.*

CHRONIC CORONARY DISEASE

The use of percutaneous transluminal angioplasty or coronary artery bypass surgery as therapy for chronic ischemic heart disease in the elderly has increased significantly over the last decade.[92] Revascularized Medicare patients are increasingly older, with a greater number of comorbid conditions. Nevertheless, 30-day and 1-year mortality rates have decreased significantly from 1987 to 1990 for both revascularization procedures in the elderly. The improved mortality rate likely represents improved technical approaches with angioplasty and bypass surgery, including increased use of internal mammary grafts.

Use of bypass surgery has also increased in the very elderly, increasing 67 percent in octogenarians from 1987 to 1990.[93] Thirty-day and 1-year mortality rates averaged 11.5 and 19.2 percent, respectively, both 2.5-fold greater than the corresponding operative mortality rate in the 65 to 70 year olds. Independent predictors of short-term and long-term mortality rates included increasing age, female gender, admission with acute myocardial infarction, congestive heart failure, cerebral or peripheral vascular disease, and chronic renal disease. Increasing age is also a significant independent predictor of stroke, which occurs in about 8 percent of the very elderly who undergo bypass surgery.[94] In spite of the high short-term morbidity and mortality rates, the 3-year mortality rate of this group was similar to that of the general octogenarian population. No randomized trial of medicine compared with bypass surgery has included the elderly, although significant improvement in quality of life with relief of medically refractory angina is achieved in many elderly bypass patients.[95,96] Therefore, the risk and benefits of bypass surgery should be assessed carefully, including consideration of comorbid conditions.

Angioplasty techniques and results have improved as well over the last several years.[97] Compared with prior data bases, elderly patients receiving the procedure more recently are older, with a more frequent history of a myocardial infarction, prior bypass surgery, and diabetes mellitus. In spite of the greater age and comorbidities, the procedural success rate has improved significantly in the elderly, to 93.5 percent, with a significant reduction in procedural complications, including death and myocardial infarction. The most dramatic decrease in complications was in the need for emergent bypass surgery, dropping to 0.65 percent, likely because of the introduction of coronary stents.[97] Although no trial randomized elderly subjects with multivessel disease to angioplasty compared with bypass surgery, the number of vessels with critical coronary artery disease and completeness of revascularization are powerful predictors of both short-term and long-term event-free survival in elderly patients after angioplasty and should be an important factor in deciding between angioplasty and bypass surgery.[98,99]

Cholesterol lowering is beneficial for elderly patients with chronic coronary artery disease. The Scandinavian Simvastatin Survival Study (4S) included 1848 patients 65 to 70 years of age with chronic coronary artery disease and an elevated baseline total cholesterol.[100] After 5.4 years of follow-up, cholesterol lowering with simvastatin resulted in significant decreases in total mortality, coronary heart disease mortality, major coronary events, and revascularization procedures. Therefore, *lipid-lowering therapy should be a goal in elderly patients with established coronary disease and elevated total cholesterol and low-density lipoprotein cholesterol.* Finally, observational data suggest that postmenopausal women benefit from the addition of hormone replacement therapy, with large reductions in future cardiovascular morbidity and mortality rates. This benefit was hypothesized to be due to not only the lipid-lowering effects of hormone replacement therapy, but also to the direct effects of estrogen on the coronary endothelium, likely via an increase in nitric oxide.[101] In a randomized, placebo-controlled trial evaluating premarin plus progesterone, however, there was no decrease in coronary death or nonfatal myocardial infarction among women with established coronary artery disease randomized to hormone therapy.[102] There are several potential explanations of why this was a negative trial, including data suggesting that, with increasing age and with atherosclerosis, there is less vascular expression of the estrogen receptor, likely due to methylation of the estrogen gene.[103,104] Further studies are in progress to determine whether there is a role for hormone replacement therapy in older women with coronary artery disease. Currently, *initiation of estrogen therapy is not recommended for the treatment of coronary artery disease in postmenopausal women.*

Congestive Heart Failure

In contrast to other cardiovascular disorders, the prevalence of chronic heart failure (CHF) is dramatically increasing. Approximately 4.7 million Americans have CHF, and each year 400,000 new cases are diagnosed.[105] The incidence of heart failure doubles with each decade of life, and the prevalence rises from 2 to 5 percent of those 70 to 79 years of age, and to almost 10 percent of those older than 80 years.[106] This is, in part, because heart failure represents a final common pathway for most other cardiac disorders and, in part, because of the more successful treatments of acute ischemic disease. These successes increase the numbers surviving, albeit with, or at increased risk for, heart failure. Although the etiology of CHF is ischemic in most patients, hypertension is also a common etiology, especially among African-Americans.[107]

CHF is also a highly lethal condition, with significant mortality, morbidity, and associated costs. Framingham investigators report a median survival of 1.66 years among men and 3.17 years among women in the community setting.[106] More than 90 percent of CHF deaths occur among adults older than 65 years.[108] CHF is also the leading cause of hospitalization in Medicare beneficiaries,[109] and hospitalization of these patients is itself a major risk factor for subsequent rehospitalization, mortality, and functional decline[110] (see also Chaps. 20 and 21).

The importance of the individual patient's role as a partner in his or her care and of individualizing treatment and monitoring plans cannot be overemphasized. Although patients may carry the same heart failure diagnosis, they differ markedly in terms of disease severity and complexity, associated comorbidities, social support, education, ingrained habits, access to medical personnel and knowledge, and understanding of health care information and directions. Noncompliance with medications or diet is often cited as a major factor contributing to hospitalization in heart failure patients. In a study of 7,247 elderly outpatients with CHF who were newly prescribed digoxin, only 10 percent filled enough prescriptions to have daily digoxin available for an entire year.[111] In 161 prospectively studied patients 70 years or older admitted with heart failure, 47 percent were readmitted within 90 days, and 38 percent of these readmissions were felt to have been possibly preventable.[112] The most common factors contributing to possibly preventable readmissions were noncompliance, failure to seek help promptly, and poor social support.

Age-associated biologic factors themselves are unlikely to result in heart failure but increase the likelihood for the development of symptoms in the presence of ischemic or hypertensive disease. Increased vascular load due to increased central vascular stiffness[113] and decreased endothelium-dependent vasodilatation[114] increase the likelihood of progressive LV dysfunction, adverse clinical outcomes, and a more variable and complicated response to conventional therapeutic interventions in older individuals with ischemic or hypertensive-induced LV damage.[115–117] In addition, the age-associated decrease in sympathetic responsiveness limits the ability of older people to augment heart rate and cardiac function in the presence of superimposed heart disease, particularly in the setting of acute depression of LV function. Finally, the decrease in early LV filling and the presumptive increase in LV filling pressures during exercise may worsen heart failure symptoms, especially in association with diseases that also impair LV filling, such as coronary artery disease and systemic arterial hypertension.

Evaluation of older patients with heart failure symptoms should include a noninvasive study to determine whether the primary problem is systolic dysfunction. *Up to 40 percent of older individuals with heart failure have normal systolic function.*[118] If ischemic, hypertensive, or valvular disease is responsible for failure, they should be specifically treated. Otherwise, *diuretics are particularly useful in patients with increased vascular stiffness presenting with acute congestive symptoms, since significant reductions in pressure occur with relatively small changes in intravascular volume.* Digitalis may improve signs and symptoms of heart failure without affecting overall survival in patients with systolic dysfunction and sinus rhythm.[119] However, the maintenance dose should be reduced to 0.125 mg/day because of the age-associated decreased volume of distribution and creatinine clearance. ACE inhibitors are a cornerstone of therapy in patients with systolic dysfunction, and their benefit extends to the elderly, as well.[120] Recent studies indicating the value of the β-blockades carvedilol[121] and metoprolol,[122] as well as aldosterone inhibition[123] in patients with continued symptoms despite ACE-I therapy, probably extend to the older population. It is possible to predict which older heart failure patients are at increased risk for early readmission. In this group, Rich et al.[124] and Stewart et al.[125] demonstrated that a multidisciplinary team approach including simplification of the medical regimen, close monitoring, and intensive patient education can decrease hospital admission and improve quality of life.

Arrhythmias

Supraventricular and ventricular arrhythmias increase in frequency with aging,[126] probably due to age-associated changes in the impulse formation and conduction system, including loss of pacemaker and conducting cell and fibrosis,[127] as well as increased incidence of mitral annular and aortic calcification, hypertension, and ischemic disease. Other illnesses may frequently present with arrhythmias in the elderly as well, including hyperthyroidism, anemia, hypoxia, electrolyte imbalance, infections, and hypotension or hypertension. Evaluation of older patients with symptomatic or asymptomatic arrhythmias, therefore, should include a search for these illnesses as well as other presenting triggers such as chest pain, exercise, smoking, caffeine, and medicine and alcohol ingestion (see Chap. 24). Long-term ambulatory electrocardiographic monitoring during the patient's normal activities is most likely to determine the nature and severity of the arrhythmia. Loop recorders, which enable continuous monitoring and recording when activated, may be particularly useful. These devices may be activated by the patient, which depends on the arrhythmia not being severe enough to preclude patient activation, or activated by the presence of the arrhythmia itself, which depends on the ability and reliability of the detection device. Invasive electrophysiology studies can be used to not only diagnose the arrhythmia but also to determine its mechanism, obtain prognostic information, and determine the suitability of different therapeutic approaches. The prognostic significance of an arrhythmia depends on the ventricular rate, the presence of atrial/ventricular synchrony, the duration of the arrhythmia, and the underlying cardiovascular substrate. Age-associated changes in both passive-state and active-state diastolic properties, as well as decreased systolic reserve (see above), may increase the likelihood that an older individual will develop hemodynamic compromise and/or ischemia during an arrhythmic episode.

Atrial fibrillation is common among the elderly. In the population-based Cardiovascular Health Study of 5201 men and women aged older than 65 years, 4.8 percent of women and 6.2 percent of men had atrial fibrillation.[128] In five randomized trials of anticoagulation for the prevention of stroke in atrial fibrillation, the mean age of enrolled patients was 69 years, with 25 percent over age 75.[129] Atrial fibrillation in this elderly cohort was associated with increasing age, heart failure, valvular heart disease, stroke, diabetes, and hypertension. Older individuals are more likely to experience hemodynamic compromise resulting from the increased ventricular rate and loss of atrial/ventricular synchrony accompanying the arrhythmia, because of the age-associated changes in relaxation properties and increased dependence on atrial contribution. Because of the increased likelihood of coronary disease, the higher rate is also more likely to be associated with myocardial ischemia. Atrial fibrillation may also result in atrial remodeling, which increases the likelihood of maintenance of the arrhythmia,[130] and lower output related to the irregularity of the rhythm.[131] The risk of embolic stroke in atrial fibrillation also increases with age. The Framingham Study reported that the risk of stroke attributed to atrial fibrillation rose from 7.3 percent in those 60 to 69 years of age to 30.8 percent in those aged 80 to 89 years.[132]

Therapeutic goals in patients with atrial fibrillation include stroke prevention, rate control, and possibly rhythm control. In randomized trials of anticoagulation versus placebo for the prevention of embolic strokes in atrial fibrillation, a significant reduction is seen generally with anticoagulation therapy, as well as in patients over 75 years of age.[133] This benefit of anticoagulation is greater than treatment with aspirin in the elderly, although there is a higher rate of intracranial hemorrhage.[134] Careful monitoring of the international normalized ratio (INR) is important, as most embolic strokes in the elderly occur when the ratio is under 2.0 and most cerebral hemorrhages occur when the ratio is above 3.0. Although the benefits of aspirin are less significant, it can be used in older patients who have a contraindication to warfarin therapy, including an inability to monitor the INR carefully. Rate control in patients without systolic dysfunction may be attempted with diltiazem, verapamil, and β-blockades; in patients with systolic dysfunction, β-blockades and digitalis may be used. In a recent randomized trial, the combination of atenolol and digitalis was found to be most effective in controlling both rest and exercise heart rates in atrial fibrillation patients.[135] If patients are intolerant of medical therapy, or if medical therapy is ineffective, AV node ablation and pacemaker insertion is highly safe and effective.[136] Cardioversion should be attempted in patients who are hemodynamically compromised, in acute atrial fibrillation, and for those who are at low likelihood of reversion to atrial fibrillation if conversion does occur. This can be attempted with electrical or pharmacologic[137] approaches (see also Chap. 24). Otherwise, the value of attempted conversion to sinus rhythm is not clear. If attempted, flecanide and propafenone are generally well tolerated by patients without ischemic or structural heart disease. Those with suspected tachycardia/bradycardiac syndrome, however, should be monitored for bradycardiac side effects. In patients with ischemic disease and preserved ventricular function, sotalol may be used. In patients with structural heart disease, the probability of pro-arrythmic effects is increased with all drugs. Potential side effects require close monitoring, therefore, when instituting agents other than amiodarone in these patients. In patients with heart failure, dofetilide, under careful monitoring conditions, was recently demonstrated to increase the likelihood of conversion to, and maintenance of, sinus rhythm[138] without the increase in mortality associated with some other antiarrhythmic agents in patients with heart failure. Experimental approaches include the Maze surgical procedure,[139] catheter ablation of atrial foci,[140] and the use of implantable defibrillators[141] to terminate atrial fibrillation. A more detailed discussion of the management of atrial fibrillation is presented in Chap. 24.

The use of programmable pacemakers to time atrial and ventricular systole appropriately may be particularly useful in older patients because diastolic filling and cardiac output are more dependent on atrial contribution. In the Medicare population, dual-chamber pacing was associated with improved 1- and 2-year survival, when compared with single-chamber pacing, after adjustment for confounding patient characteristics.[142]

Ventricular arrhythmias in the elderly are to be approached in the same fashion as in younger individuals, i.e., those that are asymptomatic and those unassociated with evidence of cardiac disease can be viewed as less serious than ventricular arrhythmias associated with evidence of LV dysfunction and/or ischemia. Both older and younger postmyocardial infarction patients benefit from β-blockade therapy, with a reduction in the rate of sudden death.[81] Life-threatening ventricular arrhythmias are common among elderly patients with severe coronary disease and LV dysfunction. As in younger subjects, aggressive management of elderly survivors of cardiac arrest or of those with hypotensive ventricular tachycardia is justified.[143] Antiarrhythmic therapy selected with electrophysiologic testing and/or placement of the implantable cardioverter defibrillator are well tolerated by the elderly and lead to improved survival.[144] Ventricular arrhythmias are discussed in detail in Chap. 24.

Valvular Heart Disease

The most frequent clinically significant valvular heart disease in the elderly is calcific aortic stenosis.[145] The development of clinically significant aortic stenosis may be very rapid in this age group (6 to 18 months), as calcification and severe scarring occur rather abruptly. Also, animal studies show that there is less compensatory hypertrophy in response to increased impedance to LV ejection in the elderly, which could also contribute to the development of heart failure.[146]

Clinical recognition of valvular aortic stenosis may be difficult in the elderly, and the features differ from those of isolated aortic stenosis in younger subjects (Table 86-2).[147] Aortic stenosis should be suspected in elderly patients presenting with congestive heart failure. By far, the most helpful study one can perform in screening an elderly subject for significant aortic stenosis is a Doppler echocardiogram looking for severe aortic valve calcification with decreased mobility, a small aortic valve area, and a significant transvalvular gradient. The presence of LV hypertrophy can be assessed as well as LV function. It appears that the condition of asymptomatic elderly patients with significant aortic stenosis by echocardiography can be followed carefully without surgical intervention until the first symptoms appear.[148] It should be noted, however, that if other disease (e.g., arthritis) limits an older patient, he or she might not be able to exercise to the point where symptoms occur, despite the presence of significant disease requiring surgery. These issues are complex and are discussed in greater detail in Chap. 56. To assess the need for bypass grafting at the time of the operation, coronary angiography should be performed in older individuals prior to aortic valve surgery. Aortic valve replacement often results in marked improvement in symptoms and LV function, as well as expected survival in older and even in very old patients.[149,150] Predictors of surgical mortality with aortic valve replacement include low ejection fraction and congestive heart failure, atrial fibrillation, associated surgical procedures, and an emergency procedure, suggesting that aortic valve replacement for symptomatic aortic stenosis should not be delayed merely because a patient is elderly.[151] Percutaneous aortic valvuloplasty in the elderly is associated with poor outcomes, including early restenosis, aortic regurgitation, stroke, high mortality rate, and heart failure.[152] It is useful only for palliation and as a "bridge" to valve replacement in very ill patients.[153]

Chronic aortic regurgitation may occur in elderly individuals secondary to aortic root dilatation. Symptoms include angina, even in patients without significant coronary disease, and congestive heart failure. It is important to recognize, however, that symptoms may not occur until significant LV dysfunction is present; therefore, the onset of dysfunction is enough to prompt surgery, rather than await the occurrence of symptoms. Vasodilator therapy in asymptomatic individuals with normal LV function may be helpful. In a randomized trial, nifedipine was shown to reduce LV volume and mass, increase ejection fraction, and delay the occurrence of systolic dysfunction.[154] Best operative results occur in individuals with no or minimal symptoms, mild to moderate ventricular dysfunction and a brief duration of left ventricular dysfunction[155] (see Chap. 56).

The most common cause of mi-

TABLE 86-2 Frequent Characteristics of Aortic Stenosis

	Older than 65 years	Younger than 65 years
Structure	Tricuspid	Bicuspid
Origin	Degeneration—calcium deposits in sinuses inhibit opening	Congenital bicuspid or deformed cusps—fusion of commissures
Exam	Murmur has a musical component at apex—may mimic mitral regurgitation	Murmur harsh at base
	Carotids may be normal	Carotid upstroke delayed
Gender	Women equal in frequency to men	Men predominate
Presentation	Congestive heart failure	Angina, syncope, and/or congestive heart failure
Rhythm	Atrial fibrillation common	Atrial fibrillation uncommon

tral stenosis in the elderly is rheumatic disease, which at times may not result in symptoms until the patient reaches old age. The diagnosis may be more difficult in the elderly because calcification of the valve may decrease the intensity of the first heart sound and the opening sound, and diminished cardiac output may decrease the intensity of the diastolic rumble. Doppler echocardiography is very useful in diagnosing the presence of significant disease. If symptoms are more than mild, or if pulmonary hypertension develops, surgery or balloon mitral valvuloplasty should be considered. Atrial fibrillation often triggers functional deterioration in older individuals because the dependence of filling on atrial contribution is exaggerated in the presence of mitral stenosis. Balloon mitral valvuloplasty compares favorably with open surgical commissurotomy in appropriate candidates—i.e., those with minimal calcification, good mobility, little subvalvular disease, and only mild mitral regurgitation[156]—and should be considered for elderly patients with symptomatic mitral stenosis.[156,157]

Mitral regurgitation in the elderly is most often related to ischemic heart disease and myxomatous degeneration of the mitral valve. As is true for aortic insufficiency, symptoms may be recognized only after significant LV dysfunction has occurred, and intervention should be considered on the basis of dysfunction, rather than await symptom onset. It should also be remembered that favorable unloading conditions will raise the ejection fraction in the presence of significant mitral regurgitation. Therefore, an ejection fraction of under 0.60 should be considered abnormal and is associated with a poorer postsurgical prognosis.[158] For elderly patients with mitral regurgitation, mitral valve repair is associated with a lower operative mortality and improved late outcomes, eliminates the need for anticoagulation in patients without atrial fibrillation, and results in excellent long-term results.[159,160] Thus, repair, rather than replacement, should be performed, if possible.

For elderly patients requiring valve replacement, the choice of a mechanical valve with the bleeding risk of lifelong anticoagulation must be balanced against a bioprosthetic valve and risk of structural deterioration. Additional factors in the choice include candidacy for anticoagulation and other requirements for anticoagulation, such as atrial fibrillation, age, and valve position. In a series of elderly subjects receiving aortic or mitral mechanical valve replacements, freedom from major anticoagulant-related hemorrhage was 76 percent at 10 years.[161] A bioprosthetic valve in the mitral position deteriorates more rapidly than in the aortic position. In a large series of elderly patients receiving porcine bioprostheses, freedom from structural deterioration at 10 years for the aortic valve bioprostheses was 98 percent and for the mitral valve bioprosthesis was 79 percent, with excellent long-term survival free of major morbidity[162] (see also Chap. 60).

Hypertension

Systolic pressure rises progressively with age, whereas diastolic pressure tends to plateau and even decline after 60 years, as noted. The consequent rise in pulse pressure, due primarily to an increase in central vascular stiffness, is a strong and independent risk factor for cardiovascular events,[163] for adverse consequences following an infarction,[164] and for the development of heart failure.[116] Numerous trials demonstrate the value of antihypertensive therapy in even mild diastolic hypertension in the elderly population.[165] Isolated systolic hypertension is more common in the elderly, and prospective randomized trials demonstrate that diuretic[166] and long-acting dihydropyridine calcium antagonist[167] therapy decrease the risk of stroke, congestive heart failure, and myocardial infarction or death among older patients with this entity. Although the general blood pressure goal is 140/90, lower goals are indicated in the presence of diabetes, target organ damage, or clinical cardiovascular disease.[168] Nonpharmacologic therapy, consisting of restricted salt intake and weight reduction, decreases blood pressure in many elderly hypertensives.[169] The selection of pharmacologic therapy should be based on prospective randomized trials; the presence of associated comorbidities (e.g., ischemia, renal insufficiency, systolic or nonsystolic dysfunction), and the duration of action and side-effect profile of the agent. Despite the widespread choice and effectiveness of proven therapies, the vast majority of hypertensive patients are not at the appropriate blood pressure goal.[168] Many patients require combination therapy to achieve satisfactory blood pressure control, particularly in the presence of diabetes and/or renal insufficiency (see also Chap. 51).

ACKNOWLEDGMENTS

The secretarial assistance of Christina R. Link and Spring Metcalf is greatly appreciated in preparing this chapter.

References

1. Lakatta EG. Cardiovascular aging research: The next horizons [Review]. *J Am Geriatr Soc* 1999; 47:613.
2. Olivetti G, Melissari M, Capasso JM, et al. Cardiomyopathy of the aging human heart: Myocyte loss and reactive cellular hypertrophy. *Circ Res* 1991; 68:1560.
3. Olivetti G, Giordano G, Corradi D, et al. Gender differences and aging: Effects in the human heart. *J Am Coll Cardiol* 1995; 26:1068.
4. Fraticelli A, Josephson R, Danziger R, et al. Morphological and contractile characteristics of rat cardiac myocytes from maturation to senescence. *Am J Physiol* 1989; 257:H259.
5. Anversa P, Palackal T, Sonnenblick EH, et al. Myocyte cell loss and myocyte cellular hyperplasia in the hypertrophied aging rat heart. *Circ Res* 1990; 67:671.
6. Kajstura J, Cheng W, Sarangarajan R, et al. Necrotic and apoptotic myocyte cell death in the aging heart of Fischer 344 rats. *Am J Physiol* 1996; 271:H1215.
7. Cheng W, Li B, Kajstura J, et al. Stretch-induced programmed myocyte cell death. *J Clin Invest* 1995; 96:2247.
8. Cigola E, Kastura J, Li B, et al. Angiotensin II activates programmed myocyte cell death in vitro. *Exp Cell Res* 1997; 231:363.
9. Esler MD, Turner AG, Kaye DM, et al. Ageing effects on human sympathetic neuronal function. *Am J Physiol* 1995; 268:R278.
10. Lakatta EG. Deficient neuroendocrine regulation of the cardiovascular system with advancing age in healthy humans [Point of view] *Circulation* 1993; 87:631.
11. Robert L. Aging of the vascular wall and atherogenesis: Role of the elastin-laminin receptor. *Atherosclerosis* 1996; 123:169.
12. Michel JB, Heudes D, Michel O, et al. Effect of chronic ANGI-converting enzyme inhibition on aging processes: II. Large arteries. *Am J Physiol* 1994; 267(1 pt 2):R124.
13. Fornieri C, Quaglino D, Mori G. Role of the extracellular matrix in age-related modifications of the rat aorta. *Arterioscler Thromb* 1992; 12:1008.
14. Haudenschild CC, Prescott MF, Chobanian AV. Aortic endothe-

lial and subendothelial cells in experimental hypertension and aging. *Hypertension* 1981; 3(suppl I):I-148.
15. Guyton JR, Lindsay KL, Dao DT. Comparison of aortic intima and inner media in young adult versus aging rats. *Am J Pathol* 1983; 111:234.
16. Li Z, Froehlich J, Galis ZS, et al. Increased expression of matrix metalloproteinase-2 in the thickened intima of aged rats. *Hypertension* 1999; 33:116.
17. Hariri RJ, Alonso DR, Hajjar DP, et al. Aging and atherosclerosis: I Development of myointimal hyperplasia after endothelial cell injury. *J Exp Med* 1986; 164:1171.
18. Senior RM, Griffin GL, Fliszar CJ, et al. Human 92- and 72-kilodalton type IV collagenase are elastases. *J Biol Chem* 1991; 266:7870.
19. Border WA, Ruoslahti E. Transforming growth factor-β in disease: The dark side of tissue repair. *J Clin Invest* 1992; 90:1.
20. Majesky MW, Lindner V, Twardzik DR, et al. Production of transforming growth factor β_1 during repair of arterial injury. *J Clin Invest* 1991; 88:904.
21. Battegay EJ, Raines EW, Seifert RA, et al. TGF-β induces bimodal proliferation of connective tissue cells via complex control of an autocrine PDGF loop. *Cell* 1990; 63:515.
22. Takasaki I, Chobanian AV, Sarzani R, et al. Effect of hypertension on fibronectin expression in the rat aorta. *J Biol Chem* 1990; 265:21,935.
23. Millis AJT, Hoyle M, McCue HM, et al. Differential expression of metalloproteinase and tissue inhibitor of metaproteinase genes in aged human fibroblasts. *Exp Cell Res* 1992; 201:373.
24. McCaffrey TA, Falcon DJ. Evidence for an age-associated dysfunction in the antiproliferative response to transforming growth factor-β in vascular smooth muscle cells. *Mol Biol Cell* 1993; 4:315.
25. Crawford DC, Chobanian AV, Brecher P. Angiotensin II induces fibronectin expression associated with cardiac fibrosis in the rat. *Circ Res* 1994; 74:727.
26. Gerstenblith G, Fredricksen J, Yin FCP, et al. Echocardiographic assessment of a normal adult aging population. *Circulation* 1977; 56:273.
27. Swinne CJ, Shapiro EP, Lima SD, et al. Age-associated changes in left ventricular diastolic performance during isometric exercise in normal subjects. *Am J Cardiol* 1992; 69:823.
28. Fleg JL, Schulman SP, Gerstenblith G, et al. Additive effects of age and silent myocardial ischemia on the left ventricular response to upright cycle exercise. *J Appl Physiol* 1993; 75:499.
29. Fleg JL, O'Connor FC, Gerstenblith G, et al. Impact of age on the cardiovascular response to dynamic upright exercise in healthy men and women. *J Appl Physiol* 1995; 78:890.
30. Fleg JL, Lakatta EG. Role of muscle loss in the age-associated reduction in VO_2 max. *J Appl Physiol* 1988; 65:1147.
31. Kenney WL, Ho CW. Age alters regional distribution of blood flow during moderate-intensity exercise. *J Appl Physiol* 1995; 79:1112.
32. Lakatta EG. Cardiovascular regulatory mechanisms in advanced age. *Physiol Rev* 1993; 73:413.
33. Yin FCP, Raizes GS, Guarnieri T, et al. Age-associated decrease in ventricular response to haemodynamic stress during beta-adrenergic blockade. *Br Heart J* 1978; 40:1349.
34. Walker KE, Lakatta EG, Houser SR. Age associated changes in membrane currents in rat ventricular myocytes. *Cardiovasc Res* 1993; 27:1968.
35. Orchard CH, Lakatta EG. Intracellular calcium transients and developed tensions in rat heart muscle: A mechanism for the negative interval-strength relationship. *J Gen Physiol* 1985; 86:637.
36. Lompre AM, Lambert F, Lakatta EG, et al. Expression of sarcoplasmic reticulum Ca^{2+}-ATPase and calsequestrin genes in rat heart during ontogenic development and aging. *Circ Res* 1991; 69:1380.
37. Tate CA, Taffet GE, Hudson EK, et al. Enhanced calcium uptake of cardiac sarcoplasmic reticulum in exercise-trained old rats. *Am J Physiol* 1990; 258:H431.
38. Koban MU, Moorman AFM, Holtz J, et al. Expressional analysis of the cardiac Na/Ca exchanger in rat development and senescence. *Cardiovasc Res* 1998; 37:405.
39. Effron MB, Bhatnagar GM, Spurgeon HA, et al. Changes in myosin isoenzymes, ATPase activity and contraction duration in rat cardiac muscle with aging can be modulated by thyroxine. *Circ Res* 1987; 60:238.
40. Bhatnagar GM, Walford GD, Beard ES, et al. ATPase activity and force production in myofibrils and twitch characteristics in intact muscle from neonatal, adult, and senescent rat myocardium. *J Mol Cell Cardiol* 1984; 16:203.
41. Koban MU, Moorman AFM, Holtz J, et al. Expressional analysis of the cardiac Na-Ca exchanger in rat development and senescence. *Cardiovasc Res* 1998; 37:405.
42. Pepe S, Tsuchiya N, Lakatta EG, et al. PUFA and aging modulate cardiac mitochondrial membrane lipid composition and Ca^{2+} activation of PDH. *Am J Physiol* 1999; 276 (*Heart Circ Physiol.* 45):H149.
43. Hano O, Bogdanov KY, Sakai M, et al. Reduced threshold for myocardial cell calcium intolerance in the rat heart with aging. *Am J Physiol* 1995; 269:H1607.
44. Lakatta EG. Chaotic behavior of myocardial cells: Possible implications regarding the pathophysiology of heart failure. *Perspect Biol Med* 1989; 32:421.
45. Chen C-H, Nakayama M, Nevo E, et al. Coupled systolic-ventricular and vascular stiffening with age implications for pressure regulation and cardiac reserve in the elderly. *J Am Coll Cardiol* 1998; 32:1221.
46. Chen C-H, Ting C-T, Lin S-J, et al. Which arterial and cardiac parameters best predict left ventricular mass? *Circulation* 1998; 98:422.
47. Nussbacher A, Gerstenblith G, O'Connor F, et al. Hemodynamic effects of unloading the old heart. *Am J Physiol* 1999; 277: H1863.
48. Chen C-H, Nakayama M, Talbot M, et al. Verapamil acutely reduces ventricular-vascular stiffening and improves aerobic exercise performance in elderly individuals. *J Am Coll Cardiol* 1999; 33:1602.
49. Lakatta EG. Deficient neuroendocrine regulation of the cardiovascular system with advancing age in healthy humans [Point of view]. *Circulation* 1993; 87:631.
50. Esler MD, Turner AG, Kaye DM, et al. Aging effects on human sympathetic neuronal function. *Am J Physiol* 1995; 268:R278.
51. Seals DR, Dempsey JA. Aging, exercise and cardiopulmonary function. In: Lamb DR, Gisolfi CV, Nadel E, eds. *Perspectives in Exercise Science and Sports Medicine,* vol 8. 1995:237.
52. Fleg JL, Schulman S, O'Connor F, et al. Effects of acute β-adrenergic receptor blockade on age-associated changes in cardiovascular performance during dynamic exercise. *Circulation* 1994; 90:2333.
53. Yin FCP, Weisfeldt ML, Milnor WR. Role of aortic input impedance in the decreased cardiovascular response to exercise with aging in dogs. *J Clin Invest* 1981; 68:28.
54. Xiao R-P, Spurgeon HA, O'Connor F, et al. Age-associated changes in β-adrenergic modulation on rat cardiac excitation-contraction coupling. *J Clin Invest* 1994; 94:2051.
55. Xiao R-P, Tomhave ED, Xiangwu J, et al. Age-associated reductions in cardiac β_1- and β_2-adrenoceptor responses without changes in inhibitory G proteins or receptor kinases. *J Clin Invest* 1998; 101:1273.
56. Jiang MT, Moffat MP, Narayanan N. Age-related alterations in the phosphorylation of sarcoplasmic reticulum and myofibrillar proteins and diminished contractile response to isoproterenol in intact rat ventricle. *Circ Res* 1993; 72:102.
57. Schulman SP, Fleg JL, Goldberg AP, et al. Continuum of cardio-

vascular performance across a broad range of fitness levels in healthy older men. *Circulation* 1996; 94:359.
58. Gillum RF. Trends in acute myocardial infarction and coronary heart disease death in the United States. *J Am Coll Cardiol* 1993; 23:1271.
59. National Center for Health Statistics. *Vital Statistics of the United States, 1988,* vol 2: *Mortality,* part A, tables 1-27, 1-129. Rockville, MD: National Center for Health Statistics; 1991.
60. Frishman WH, DeMaria AN, Ewy GA. Clinical assessment. *J Am Coll Cardiol* 1987; 10(abstr):48A.
61. Fleg JL, Gerstenblith G, Zonderman AB, et al. Prevalence and prognostic significance of exercise-induced silent myocardial ischemia detected by thallium scintigraphy and electrocardiography in asymptomatic volunteers. *Circulation* 1990; 81:428.
62. Nicod P, Gilpin E, Dittrich H, et al. Short- and long-term clinical outcome after Q wave and non-Q wave myocardial infarction in a large population. *Circulation* 1989; 79:528.
63. Goldberg RJ, Gore JM, Gurwitz JH, et al. The impact of age on the incidence and prognosis of initial acute myocardial infarction: The Worcester Heart Attack Study. *Am Heart J* 1989; 117:543.
64. Nadelmann J, Frishman WH, Ooi WL, et al. Prevalence, incidence and prognosis of recognized and unrecognized myocardial infarction in persons aged 75 years or older: The Bronx aging study. *Am J Cardiol* 1990; 66:533.
65. Maggioni AP, Maseri A, Fresco C, et al. Age-related increase in mortality among patients with first myocardial infarctions treated with thrombolysis. *N Engl J Med* 1993; 329:1442.
66. Keller NM, Feit F. Atherosclerotic heart disease in the elderly. *Curr Opin Cardiol* 1995; 10:427.
67. GUSTO Investigators. An international randomized trial comparing four thrombolytic strategies for acute myocardial infarction. *N Engl J Med* 1993; 329:673.
68. Armstrong PW, Fu Yuling, Chang W-C, et al. Acute coronary syndromes in the GUSTO-IIb trial. *Circulation* 1998; 98:1860.
69. Thiemann DR, Coresh J, Oetgen WJ, et al. Association between hospital volume and survival after acute myocardial infarction in the elderly. *N Engl J Med* 1999; 340:1640.
70. Fibrinolytic Therapy Trialists' Collaborative Group. Indications for fibrinolytic therapy in suspected acute myocardial infarction: Collaborative overview of early mortality and major morbidity results from all randomized trials of more than 1000 patients. *Lancet* 1994; 343:311.
71. White HD. Selecting a thrombolytic agent. *Cardiol Clin* 1995; 13:347.
72. Mark DB, Hlatky MA, Califf RM, et al. Cost effectiveness of thrombolytic therapy with tissue plasminogen activator as compared with streptokinase for acute myocardial infarction. *N Engl J Med* 1995; 332:1418.
73. Barron HV, Bowlby LJ, Breen T, et al. Use of reperfusion therapy for acute myocardial infarction in the United States: Data from the National Registry of Myocardial Infarction 2. *Circulation* 1998; 97:1150.
74. Gore JM, Granger CB, Simoons ML, et al. Stroke after thrombolysis: Mortality and functional outcomes in the GUSTO-I Trial. *Circulation* 1995; 92:2811.
75. Grines CL, Browne KF, Marco J, et al. A comparison of immediate angioplasty with thrombolytic therapy for acute myocardial infarction. *N Engl J Med* 1993; 328:672.
76. Zijlstra F, Hoorntje JCA, De Boer M-J, et al. Long-term benefit of primary angioplasty as compared with thrombolytic therapy for acute myocardial infarction. *N Engl J Med* 1999; 341:1413.
77. Weaver WD, Simes RJ, Betriu A, et al. Comparison of primary coronary angioplasty and intravenous thrombolytic therapy for acute myocardial infarction. *JAMA* 1997; 278:2093.
78. Aguirre FV, McMahon RP, Mueller H, et al. Impact of age on clinical outcome and postlytic management strategies in patients treated with thrombolytic therapy: Results from the TIMI II Study. *Circulation* 1994; 90:78.
79. Iniguez A, Macaya C, Hernandez R, et al. Long-term outcome of coronary angioplasty in elderly patients with post-infarction angina. *Eur Heart J* 1994; 15:489.
80. TIMI IIIB Investigators. Effects of tissue plasminogen activator and a comparison of early invasive and conservative strategies in unstable angina and non-Q-wave myocardial infarction: Results of the TIMI IIIB Trial. *Circulation* 1994; 89:1545.
81. Gottlieb SS, McCarter RJ, Vogel RA. Effect of beta-blockade on mortality among high-risk and low-risk patients after myocardial infarction. *N Engl J Med* 1993; 339:489.
82. Forman DE, Bernal JLG, Wei JY. Management of acute myocardial infarction in the very elderly. *Am J Med* 1992; 93:315.
83. Krumholz HM, Radford MJ, Ellerbeck EF, et al. Aspirin in the treatment of acute myocardial infarction in elderly Medicare beneficiaries: Patterns of use and outcomes. *Circulation* 1995; 92:2841.
84. Krumholz HM, Radford MJ, Ellerbeck EF, et al. Aspirin for secondary prevention after acute myocardial infarction in the elderly: Prescribed use and outcomes. *Ann Intern Med* 1996; 124:292.
85. ACE Inhibitor Myocardial Infarction Collaborative Group. Indications for ACE inhibitors in the early treatment of acute myocardial infarction. *Circulation* 1998; 97:2202.
86. Acute Infarction Ramipril Efficacy (AIRE) Study Investigators. Effect of ramipril on mortality and morbidity of survivors of acute myocardial infarction with clinical evidence of heart failure. *Lancet* 1993; 342:821.
87. Kober L, Torp-Pedersen C, Carlsen JE, et al., for the Trandolapril Cardiac Evaluation (TRACE) Study Group. A clinical trial of the angiotensin-converting-enzyme inhibitor trandolapril in patients with left ventricular dysfunction after myocardial infarction. *N Engl J Med* 1995; 333:1670.
88. Lewis SJ, Moye LA, Sacks FM, et al., for the CARE Investigators. Effect of pravastatin on cardiovascular events in older patients with myocardial infarction and cholesterol levels in the average range. *Ann Intern Med* 1998; 129:681.
89. Kong DF, Califf RM, Miller DP, et al. Clinical outcomes of therapeutic agents that block the platelet glycoprotein IIb/IIIa integrin in ischemic heart disease. *Circulation* 1998; 98:2829.
90. Platelet Receptor Inhibition in Ischemic Syndrome Management in Patients Limited by Unstable Signs and Symptoms (PRISM-PLUS) Study Investigators. Inhibition of the platelet glycoprotein IIb/IIIa receptor with tirofiban in unstable angina and non-Q wave myocardial infarction. *N Engl J Med* 1998; 338:1488.
91. PURSUIT Trial Investigators. Inhibition of platelet glycoprotein IIb/IIIa with eptifibatide in patients with acute coronary syndromes. *N Engl J Med* 1998; 339:436.
92. Peterson ED, Jollis JG, Bebchuk MS, et al. Changes in mortality after myocardial revascularization in the elderly: The National Medicare experience. *Ann Intern Med* 1994; 121:919.
93. Peterson ED, Cowper PA, Jollis JG, et al. Outcomes of coronary artery bypass graft surgery in 24461 patients aged 80 years or older. *Circulation* 1995; 92(suppl II):II-85.
94. Freeman WK, Schaff HV, O'Brien PC, et al. Cardiac surgery in the octogenarian: Perioperative outcome and clinical follow-up. *J Am Coll Cardiol* 1991; 18:29.
95. Ko W, Gold JP, Lazzaro R, et al. Survival analysis of octogenarian patients with coronary artery disease managed by elective coronary artery bypass surgery versus conventional medical treatment. *Circulation* 1992; 86(suppl II):II-191.
96. Glower DD, Christopher TD, Milano CA, et al. Performance status and outcome after coronary artery bypass grafting in persons aged 80 to 93 years. *Am J Cardiol* 1992; 70:567.
97. Thompson RC, Holmes DR, Grill DE, et al. Changing outcome of angioplasty in the elderly. *J Am Coll Cardiol* 1996; 27:8.

98. O'Keefe JH, Sutton MB, McCallister BD, et al. Coronary angioplasty versus bypass surgery in patients >70 years old matched for ventricular function. *J Am Coll Cardiol* 1994; 24:425.
99. Thompson RC, Holmes DR, Gersh BJ, et al. Predicting early and intermediate-term outcome of coronary angioplasty in the elderly. *Circulation* 1993; 88:1579.
100. Miettinen TA, Pyorala K, Olsson AG, et al., for the Scandinavian Simvastatin Study Group. Cholesterol-lowering therapy in women and elderly patients with myocardial infarction or angina pectoris. *Circulation* 1997; 96:4211.
101. Mendelsohn ME, Karas RH. The protective effects of estrogen on the cardiovascular system. *N Engl J Med* 1999; 340:1801.
102. Hulley S, Grady D, Bush T, et al., for the Heart and Estrogen/Progestin Replacement (HERS) Study Research Group. Randomized trial of estrogen plus progestin for secondary prevention of coronary heart disease in postmenopausal women. *JAMA* 1998; 280:605.
103. Losordo DW, Kearney M, Kim EA, et al. Variable expression of the estrogen receptor in normal and atherosclerotic coronary arteries of premenopausal women. *Circulation* 1994; 89:1501.
104. Post WS, Goldschmidt-Clermont PJ, Wilhide CC, et al. Methylation of the estrogen receptor gene is associated with aging and atherosclerosis in the cardiovascular system. *Cardiovasc Res* 1999; 43:985.
105. Massie BM, Shah NH. Evolving trends in the epidemiologic factors of heart failure: Rationale for preventive strategies and comprehensive disease management. *Am Heart J* 1997; 133:703.
106. Ho KK, Pinsky JL, Kannel WB, et al. The epidemiology of heart failure: The Framingham Study. *J Am Coll Cardiol* 1993; 22(suppl):6A.
107. Bourassa MG, Gurne O, Bangiwala SI, et al. Natural history and patterns of current practice in heart failure. *J Am Coll Cardiol* 1993; 22(suppl):14A.
108. Centers for Disease Control and Prevention. Changes in mortality from heart failure: United States, 1980–1995. *JAMA* 1998; 280:874.
109. Graves EJ. National hospital discharge survey: Annual summary, 1988. *Vital Health Stat* 1991; 13:1.
110. Wolinsky FD, Smith DM, Stump TE, et al. The sequelae of hospitalization for congestive heart failure among older adults. *J Am Geriatr Soc* 1997; 45:558.
111. Monane M, Bohn RZ, Gurwitz JH, et al. Noncompliance with congestive heart failure therapy in the elderly. *Arch Intern Med* 1994; 154:433.
112. Krumholz HM, Wang Y, Purent EM, et al. Quality of care for elderly patients hospitalized with heart failure. *Arch Intern Med* 1997; 157:2242.
113. Yin FCP. The aging vasculature and its effect on the heart. In: Weisfeldt ML, ed. *The Aging Heart.* New York: Raven; 1980:137.
114. Taddei S, Virdis A, Mattei P, et al. Aging and endothelial function in normotensive subjects and patients with essential hypertension. *Circulation* 1995; 91:1981.
115. Domanski MJ, Nitchell GF, Norman JE, et al. Independent prognostic information provided by sphygmomanometrically determined pulse pressure and mean arterial pressure in patients with left ventricular dysfunction. *J Am Coll Cardiol* 1999; 33:951.
116. Chae CU, Pfeffer MA, Glynn RJ, et al. Increased pulse pressure and risk of heart failure in the elderly. *JAMA* 1999; 281:634.
117. Chen CH, Nakayama M, Nevo E, et al. Coupled systolic-ventricular and vascular stiffening with age: Implications for pressure regulation and cardiac reserve in the elderly. *J Am Coll Cardiol* 1998; 32:1221.
118. Wong WF, Gold S, Fukuyama O, et al. Diastolic dysfunction in elderly patients with congestive heart failure. *Am J Cardiol* 1989; 63:1526.
119. Digitalis Investigation Group. The effect of digoxin on mortality and morbidity in patients with heart failure. *N Engl J Med* 1997; 336:525.
120. CONSENSUS Trial Study Group. Effects of enalapril on mortality in severe congestive heart failure. *N Engl J Med* 1987; 316:1429.
121. Packer M, Bristow MR, Cohn JN, et al. The effect of carvedilol on morbidity and mortality in patients with congestive heart failure. *N Engl J Med* 1996; 334:1349.
122. MERIT-HF Study Group. Effect of metoprolol CR/XL in chronic heart failure: Metoprolol CR/XL randomized intervention trial in congestive heart failure (MERIT-HF). *Lancet* 1999; 353:2001.
123. Pitt B, Zannad F, Remme WJ, et al., for the Randomized Aldactone Study Investigators. The effect of spironolactone on morbidity and mortality in patients with severe heart failure. *N Engl J Med* 1999; 341:709.
124. Rich MW, Beckham V, Wittenberg C, et al. A multidisciplinary intervention to prevent the readmission of elderly patients with congestive heart failure. *N Engl J Med* 1995; 333:1190.
125. Stewart S, Pearson S, Horowitz JD. Effects of a home-based intervention among patients with congestive heart failure discharged from acute hospital care. *Arch Intern Med* 1998; 158:1067.
126. Fleg JL, Kennedy HL. Cardiac arrhythmias in a healthy elderly population: Detection by 24-hour ambulatory electrocardiography. *Chest* 1982; 81:301.
127. Lev M. The pathology of complete atrioventricular block. *Prog Cardiovasc Dis* 1964; 6:31.
128. Furberg CD, Psaty BM, Manolio TA, et al. Prevalence of atrial fibrillation in elderly subjects (the Cardiovascular Health Study). *Am J Cardiol* 1994; 74:236.
129. Alberts GW. Atrial fibrillation and stroke. *Arch Intern Med* 1994; 154:1443.
130. Goette A, Honeycutt C, Langberg JJ. Electrical remodeling in atrial fibrillation: Time course and mechanisms. *Circulation* 1996; 94:2968.
131. Daoud EG, Weiss R, Bahu M, et al. Effect of an irregular ventricular rhythm on cardiac output. *Am J Cardiol* 1996; 78:1433.
132. Wolf PA, Abbott RD, Kannel WB. Atrial fibrillation: A major contributor to stroke in the elderly. *Arch Intern Med* 1987; 147:1561.
133. Atrial Fibrillation Investigators. Risk factors for stroke and efficacy of anti-thrombotic therapy in atrial fibrillation: Analysis of pooled data from five randomized trials. *Arch Intern Med* 1994; 154:1449.
134. Stroke Prevention in Atrial Fibrillation Investigators. Warfarin versus aspirin for prevention of thromboembolism in atrial fibrillation. Stroke Prevention in Atrial Fibrillation II Study. *Lancet* 1994; 343:687.
135. Rosenquist M, Lee MA, Mouliner L, et al. Long-term follow-up of patients after transcatheter direct current ablation of the atrioventricular junction. *J Am Coll Cardiol* 1990; 6:1467.
136. Morady F, Hasse C, Strickberger SA, et al. Long-term follow-up after radiofrequency modification of the atrioventricular node in patients with atrial fibrillation. *J Am Coll Cardiol* 1997; 27:113.
137. Ellenbogen KA, Stambler BS, Wood MA, et al. Efficacy of intravenous ibutilide for rapid termination of atrial fibrillation and atrial flutter: A dose-response study. *J Am Coll Cardiol* 1996; 28:120.
138. Torp-Pedersen C, Moller M, Bloch-Thomsen PE, et al., for the Danish Investigations of Arrhythmia and Mortality on Dofetilide Study Group. Dofetilide in patients with congestive heart failure and left ventricular dysfunction. *N Engl J Med* 1999; 341:857.
139. Cox JL, Schuessler RB, Lappas DG, et al. An 8 1/2 year experience with surgery for atrial fibrillation. *Ann Surg* 1996; 224:267.
140. Jais P, Haissaguerre M, Shah DC, et al. A focal source of atrial fibrillation treated by discrete radiofrequency ablation. *Circulation* 1997; 95:572.
141. Lau C-P, Tse H-F, Lok N-S, et al. Initial clinical experience with an implantable human atrial defibrillator. *PACE* 1997; 20:221.

142. Lamas GA, Pashos CL, Norman SLT, et al. Permanent pacemaker selection and subsequent survival in elderly Medicare pacemaker recipients. *Circulation* 1995; 91:1063.
143. Tresh DD, Platia EV, Guarnier T, et al. Refractory symptomatic ventricular tachycardia and ventricular fibrillation in elderly patients. *Am J Med* 1987; 83:399.
144. Tresh DD, Trouop PH, Thakur RK, et al. Comparison of efficacy of automatic implantable cardioverter defibrillator in patients older and younger than 65 years of age. *Am J Med* 1991; 90:717.
145. Seltzer A. Changing aspects of the natural history of valvular aortic stenosis. *N Engl J Med* 1987; 317:91.
146. Isoyama S, Wei JY, Izumo S, et al. The effect of age on the development of cardiac hypertrophy produced by aortic constriction in the rat. *Circ Res* 1987; 61:337.
147. Roberts WC, Perloff JK, Costantino T. Severe valvular aortic stenosis in patients over 65 years of age. *Am J Cardiol* 1971; 27:497.
148. Pellikka PA, Nushimura RA, Bailey KR, et al. The natural history of adults with asymptomatic hemodynamically significant aortic stenosis. *J Am Coll Cardiol* 1990; 15:1012.
149. Wong JB, Salem DN, Pauker SG. You're never too old. *N Engl J Med* 1993; 328:971.
150. Lindblom D, Lindblom U, Qvist J, Lundstrom H. Long-term relative survival rates after heart valve replacement. *J Am Coll Cardiol* 1990; 15:566.
151. Logeais Y, Langanay T, Roussin R, et al. Surgery for aortic stenosis in elderly patients: A study of surgical risk and predictive factors. *Circulation* 1994; 90:2891.
152. Bernard Y, Etievent J, Mourand JL, et al. Long-term results of percutaneous aortic valvuloplasty compared with aortic valve replacement in patients more than 75 years old. *J Am Coll Cardiol* 1992; 20:792.
153. Carabello BA, Crawford FA. Medical progress: Valvular heart disease. *N Engl J Med* 1997; 337:32.
154. Scognamiglio R, Rahimtoola SH, Fasoli G, et al. Nifedipine in asymptomatic patients with severe aortic regurgitation and normal left ventricular function. *N Engl J Med* 1994; 331:689.
155. Bonow RO. Management of chronic aortic regurgitation. *N Engl J Med* 1994; 331:736.
156. Reyes VP, Raju S, Wynne J, et al. Percutaneous balloon valvuloplasty compared with open surgical commissurotomy for mitral stenosis. *N Engl J Med* 1994; 331:961.
157. Tuzcu EM, Block PC, Griffin BP, et al. Immediate and long-term outcome of percutaneous mitral valvotomy in patients 65 years and older. *Circulation* 1992; 85:963.
158. Enriquez-Sarano M, Tajik AJ, Schaff HV, et al. Echocardiographic prediction of survival after surgical correction of organic mitral regurgitation. *Circulation* 1994; 90:830.
159. Jebara VA, Dervanian P, Acar C, et al. Mitral valve repair using Carpentier techniques in patients more than 70 years old: Early and late results. *Circulation* 1992; 86(suppl II):II-53.
160. Enriquez-Sarano M, Schaff HV, Orsazulak TA, et al. Valve repair improves the outcome of surgery for mitral regurgitation: A multivariate analysis. *Circulation* 1995; 91:1022.
161. Holper K, Ottke M, Lewe T, et al. Bioprosthetic and mechanical valves in the elderly: Benefits and risks. *Ann Thorac Surg* 1995; 60(suppl):S443.
162. Burr LH, Jamieson RE, Munro AI, et al. Porcine bioprostheses in the elderly: Clinical performance by age groups and valve positions. *Ann Thorac Surg* 1995; 60:S264.
163. Franklin SS, Khan SA, Wong ND, et al. Is pulse pressure useful in predicting risk for coronary heart disease? The Framingham Heart Study. *Circulation* 1999; 100:354.
164. Mitchell GF, Moyce LA, Braunwald E, et al. Sphygmomanometrically determined pulse pressure is a powerful independent predictor of recurrent events after myocardial infarction in patients with impaired left ventricular function. *Circulation* 1997; 96:4254.
165. Management Committee of the Australian Therapeutic Trial in Mild Hypertension. Treatment of mild hypertension in the elderly. *Med J Aust* 1981; 2:398.
166. SHEP Cooperative Research Group. Prevention of stroke by antihypertensive drug treatment in older persons with isolated systolic hypertension. *JAMA* 1991; 265:3255.
167. Staessen JA, Fagard R, Thijs L, et al. Randomized double-blind comparison of placebo and active treatment for older patients with isolated systolic hypertension. *Lancet* 1997; 350:757.
168. Sixth Report of the Joint National Committee on Prevention, Detection, Evaluation, and Treatment of High Blood Pressure. Bethesda, MD: National Institutes of Health, National Heart, Lung, and Blood Institute, National High Blood Pressure Education Program. NIH Publ 98-4080; November 1997.
169. Whelton PK, Appel LJ, Espeland MA, et al. Sodium reduction and weight loss in the treatment of hypertension in older persons: A randomized controlled trial of nonpharmacologic interventions in the elderly. *JAMA* 1998; 279:839.

CHAPTER 87

WOMEN AND CORONARY ARTERY DISEASE

Pamela Charney

INTRODUCTION

Only recently has coronary artery disease (CAD) been perceived as a major contributor of morbidity and mortality in women.[1] National acceptance by the public and physicians of the importance of CAD in women has yet to adequately evolve. In a national telephone survey of American women, 58 percent ". . . believed they were as likely or more likely to die of breast cancer than CAD."[2] In this telephone survey, although 86 percent of the women surveyed saw a doctor regularly, almost half of the women reported their physicians had "never talked to them about heart disease."

The increasing focus on women and CAD reflects both greater attention to older populations and enthusiasm for improving women's health. The initial CAD research focus was on middle-aged populations, where middle-aged men have a dramatically higher rate of CAD than middle-aged women. In middle-aged populations around the world, there is a consistent ratio of male-to-female CAD deaths varying from 2.5 to 4.5.[3] The etiology of this excess CAD mortality in men has not been determined, although the variable differences between countries suggest that "sex is not destiny with regard to CHD [coronary heart disease]."[3] Research has only recently included elderly subjects, where differences in mortality rates between women and men are smaller (Fig. 87-1).

In this chapter, prevention, diagnosis and management of women with coronary artery disease are addressed. More detailed discussions can be found in *Coronary Artery Disease in Women: Prevention, Diagnosis and Management*.[1] The section on prevention reviews clinically important gender differences in specific CAD risk factors. The section on diagnosis begins with discussion of the ways that CAD presents in asymptomatic women and then reviews models to assess CAD risk with attention to gender. Finally, symptomatic CAD in women is discussed, including the management of the women with angina and myocardial infarction. The chapter closes with an update on gender differences in sudden death.

PREVENTION: GENDER-SPECIFIC ISSUES

It is especially important to identify women at high risk for CAD for possible primary prevention. Young women with coronary artery mortality[4] are more likely to have a history of tobacco exposure, obesity, hypertension, diabetes, early menopause, or, less often, cocaine abuse.[5] These risk factors are also important in predicting nonfatal myocardial infarction.[1] Gender differences are reviewed in terms of tobacco use and cessation, diabetes, hypertension, lipids, obesity, physical activity and exercise, menopause and hormonal replacement therapy, psychosocial risk factors, and race.

Tobacco

Tobacco is the single most important coronary artery risk factor for women and men, as noted elsewhere.[1,6,7] Cigarette smoking has been associated with an earlier age of first myocardial infarction (see also Chap. 38).[8] The risk of myocardial infarction (fatal and nonfatal) increases 2.5-fold for women who smoke one to four cigarettes daily.[9] Since middle-aged women experience less symptomatic CAD than middle-aged men, the increased risk related to tobacco use on the incidence rates of myocardial infarction and sudden death is greater for women than men. Tobacco use also lowers the age of reported menopause.[10]

Tobacco exposure can occur not only through personal use

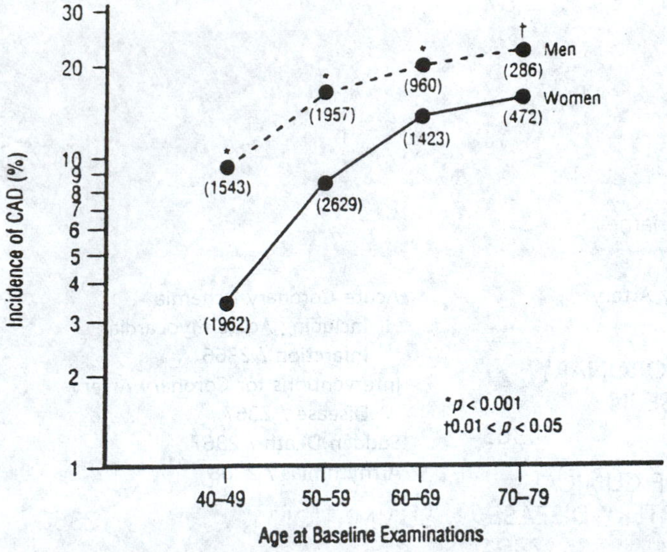

FIGURE 87-1 Framingham data: 10-year incidence of coronary artery disease (angina, myocardial infarction, coronary insufficiency, or death) among women and men by age. (From Eaker ED, Castelli WP. Coronary heart disease and its risk factors among women in the Framingham study. In: Eaker ED, Packard B, Wenger NK, et al., eds. *Coronary Heart Disease in Women: Proceedings of an NIH Workshop*. New York: Haymark Doyma; 1987:122–130. Future directions. In: Charney P, ed. *Coronary Artery Disease in Women*. Philadelphia: American College of Physicians; 576, with permission.)

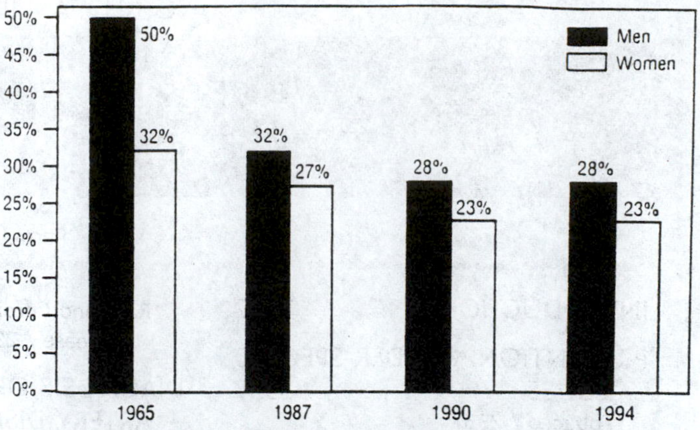

FIGURE 87-2 Prevalence of smoking among men and women in the United States. (Data from the U.S. Department of Health and Human Services. Centers for Disease Control and Prevention, Office of Smoking and Health. *MMWR Morb Mort Wkly Rep* 1995; 45:588–590. In: Ockene JK, Bonollo DP, Adams A. Smoking. In: Charney P, ed. *Coronary Artery Disease in Women*. Philadelphia: American College of Physicians; 1999:42).

of tobacco products but also by inhaling secondhand smoke. In epidemiologic studies, secondhand exposure is also related to an increased risk of CAD events.[7] For both women and men, the relative risks were similar (1.25; 95 percent CI 1.17–1.32). There was a dose-response curve when exposure to more than one package of cigarettes daily was compared with less than one pack cigarettes per day and when number of years of exposure was considered.

Over the last several decades, American women's personal use of cigarettes has not decreased dramatically as has occurred among men (Fig. 87-2). The prevalence of cigarette use among women reflects both higher initiation rates and greater difficulty stopping cigarette use.[6] By the year 2000, it is predicted that 23 percent of women will smoke, compared with 20 percent of men. Of all age and race groups, young white women currently have the highest tobacco initiation rates and are consuming more cigarettes, on average, than men of the same age.[11] Women smokers are more likely than men to report that smoking cigarettes aids in dealing with emotional stress.

Women have more difficulty quitting cigarette use, both initially and in the long term, although successful tobacco cessation for women as for men dramatically decreases the risk of further coronary events.[6] Only recently has exploration of gender and racial differences in tobacco cessation efforts focused on different responses to potential weight gain, social pressures, and physiologic withdrawal symptoms. For women, the frequent weight gain with tobacco cessation is often a substantial barrier to trying to stop smoking cigarettes. An increase in weight is a common consequence of efforts to stop smoking.[6] Smokers who stop cigarettes gain, on average, 7 to 10 lb. Fewer than 10 percent of those who stop smoking gain more than 20 lb. Weight gain tends to be higher among women, blacks, and smokers who inhale more than 25 cigarettes per day. Yet women smokers report that they are unwilling to experience any or minimal weight increase as a result of stopping smoking.[6]

To avoid weight gain with tobacco cessation, several types of interventions have been recommended.[6] It is often helpful for the physician to aid in the development of realistic expectations, encourage exercise, careful choice of snacks, and appropriate pharmacotherapy. Increasing physical activity or participating in exercise programs can increase calories expended and also aid in dealing with emotional stress. Minimizing excess calories is easier to achieve when low-sugar snacks are available to deal with cravings for sweets. Asking patients to begin a weight-reduction program while simultaneously stopping cigarettes is usually not realistic.

Multiple pharmacologic therapies have been explored, including the use of bupropion and nicotine gum, which has been reported to minimize weight gain.[6,12] Bupropion hydrocholorothiazide has been effective in smokers who are not depressed. It is contraindicated in patients with a history of seizures (since it lowers the seizure threshold with a 0.1 percent risk) and similarly in those who have experienced head trauma or are heavy consumers of alcohol. Bupropion can exacerbate symptoms related to anorexia and bulimia and should be avoided with recent use of an monoamine oxidase (MAO) inhibitor.

While social pressures to be thin hinder women's tobacco cessation efforts, social pressures from others are also noted to be an important stimulus for women to stop smoking. Social pressure to stop smoking cigarettes is reported twice as often by women as by men. The source of social pressure also is different, with women reporting pressure from children, while men report pressure from coworkers and friends.[13] Women have been observed in some studies to experience greater withdrawal symptoms than men.[14] In addition, it has been observed that black smokers may have more trouble stopping than white smokers.[15]

Physiologic issues affecting tobacco use and cessation are under exploration. Comparing black and white smokers with similar amounts of tobacco consumption, black smokers had higher cotinine levels than white smokers.[15] Physiologic addiction may have been underestimated previously in black smokers, resulting in undertreatment of nicotine addiction. Descriptions of physiologic symptoms must be considered, not just the number of cigarettes consumed. With improved pharmacologic agents to aid in tobacco cessation, aggressive management of tobacco cessation symptoms is possible.

Physicians are still identifying smoking status at only 67 percent of visits and counseling 50 percent of smokers about cessation, with specialists providing counseling substantially less often than primary care physicians (30 versus 12 percent of visits sampled in 1995).[16] These low physician identification and intervention rates are concerning, especially since surveys reveal that physicians can have a powerful effect on smoking cessation, even with minimal efforts.[6,17] Unfortunately, most programs to aid smokers with CAD have not focused on women's special issues. Programs that promote activities to minimize weight gain, including encouraging exercise and stressing social support may be more effective for women. Additional research is needed. In the meantime "Simple advice by one's physician to stop smoking is more effective than no advice at all, and as the physician-delivered smoking intervention becomes more intensive, the effects are greater."[17]

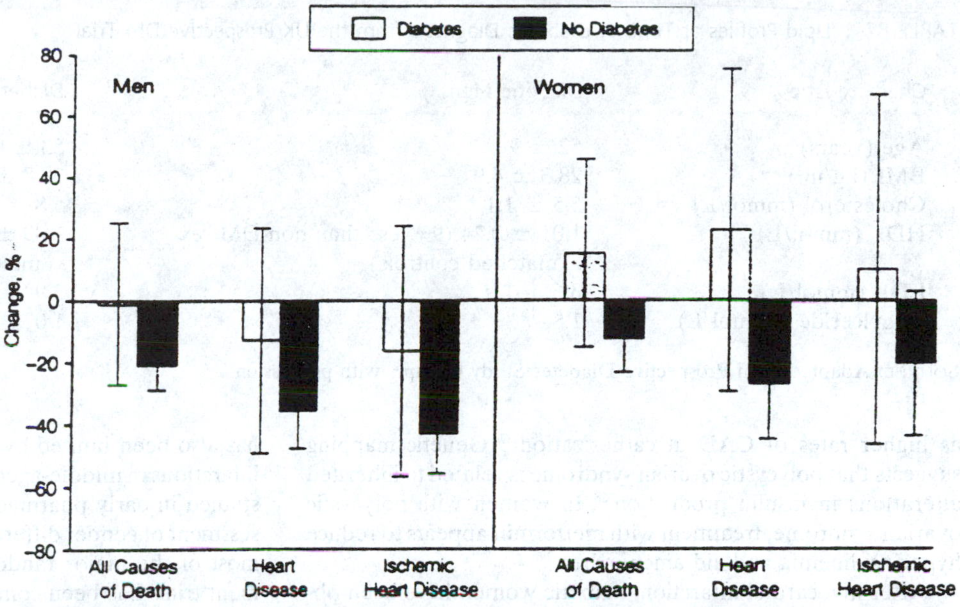

FIGURE 87-3 Change in mortality rates in women and men diabetics compared with nondiabetics. Cohort 1 was defined in 1971–1975 and followed up through 1982–1984, while Cohort 2 was defined in 1982–1984 and followed through 1992–1993. (From Gu K et al.,[20] with permission.)

Diabetes

Diabetic individuals have higher mortality rates from coronary artery disease than nondiabetics[18,19] (see also Chap. 78). Data from two of the National Health and Nutrition Examination Surveys elucidate some important gender differences.[20] The mortality rates from CAD have increased among diabetic women while decreasing among diabetic men (Fig. 87-3). Further research is required to determine whether these observations reflect gender differences in risk factors or natural history or less aggressive CAD prevention in diabetic women.

Diabetic women and men with hypertension have especially high rates of CAD.[18] This is common, since the prevalence of both diseases increases with advancing age. There is substantial variation in prevalence among different populations. Native Americans, Mexican Americans, and black populations have a higher prevalence of both of these disorders than American white populations.[11] Women and men generally have similar incidence rates of diabetes, although with increasing age, more women become hypertensive.

Women at risk for developing diabetes include obese women and those who have experienced gestational diabetes (compared with women who have had a pregnancy without glucose intolerance).[21] Obesity is increasingly common, and with increasing weight there is greater insulin resistance as well as a higher rate of glucose intolerance. For women at risk, regular physical activity[22] and avoiding gaining weight may decrease the chances of developing diabetes. Regular exercise not only decreases the risk of developing

Once a woman is diagnosed with diabetes, her "female advantage" in relation to the risk of CAD is lost.[20,23] Unlike the nondiabetic population, diabetic women have CAD rates similar to those of diabetic men. Diabetic women compared with nondiabetic women are at substantially greater risk of CAD.[18] For example, the 1-year mortality after a first hospitalization with myocardial infarction in a subgroup analysis of the WHO MONICA Project (World Health Organization Multinational Monitoring of Trends and Determinants of Cardiovascular Disease), from Finland, was 44.2 percent in diabetic men, 32.6 percent in nondiabetic men, 36.9 percent in diabetic women, and 20.2 percent in nondiabetic women.[24] The mechanisms for these observations are not fully elucidated and are suspected to be a least partially related to lipid abnormalities as well as insulin resistance.

Lipid abnormalities are common in diabetic patients. At the time of diagnosis of type II diabetes, women have substantially lower high-density lipoprotein (HDL) cholesterol than age-matched diabetic men or nondiabetic women[25] (Table 87-1). Other lipid abnormalities are also present, including elevated triglycerides. Subgroup analysis of diabetic patients treated with HMG-CoA reductase inhibitors within the larger Scandinavian Simvastatin Survival Study (4S) revealed improved lipoprotein patterns with treatment and less CAD events.[26] Larger studies including more women diabetics are in progress.

Insulin resistance is characterized by elevated levels of circulating insulin and is associated with glucose intolerance, higher levels of free fatty acid, central obesity, and hypertension. The relationship between elevated insulin levels and cardiovascular events has been under active investigation.[23] One clinical example is polycystic ovarian syndrome, where increased androgens, lower HDL, and higher triglycerides have been noted as well

TABLE 87-1 Lipid Profiles at Time of Diabetes Diagnosis from the UK Prospective DM Trial

Characteristic	Diabetic Men	Diabetic Women
Age (years)	52 ± 9	53 ± 9
BMI (kg/m^2)	28.3 ± 4.9	30.8 ± 6.7
Cholesterol (mmol/L)	5.5 ± 1.1	5.8 ± 1.2
HDL (mmol/L)	1.01 ± 0.24 (9% less than non-DM sex-matched controls)	1.09 ± 0.25 (23% less than non-DM sex-matched controls)
LDL (mmol/L)	3.6 ± 1.0	3.9 ± 1.1
Trigylcerides (mmol/L)	1.8	1.07

SOURCE: Adapted from Prospective Diabetes Study Group,[25] with permission.

as higher rates of CAD at catherization.[27] Genetic mapping suggests that polycystic ovarian syndrome is related to inherited alterations in insulin production.[28] In women with polycystic ovarian syndrome, treatment with metformin appears to reduce hyperinsulinemia and aid amenorrhea.[29]

After myocardial infarction, diabetic women have been observed to have a higher risk of death and congestive heart failure than diabetic men.[19,23] Treatment trials to prevent CAD and its complications in diabetic patients are in progress. The recently completed United Kingdom prospective diabetes study revealed that control of hypertension to below a blood pressure (BP) of 150 systolic as well as maximizing glucose control decreased coronary artery disease events.[29]

Therefore, diabetic women should be considered at high risk for coronary artery disease. Aggressive management of lipoprotein abnormalities[23,26] and hypertension,[29] if present, is beneficial. There is some evidence that glucose control decreases vascular disease. Regular exercise can also improve glucose control[22] and insulin resistance.[30]

Hypertension

The prevalence of hypertension also increases with advancing age, and—since life expectancy is greater for women than men—there are more elderly women with hypertension.[31] At all ages, black women and men have about double the incidence of hypertension as their white counterparts. Generally, women are more likely to have controlled (BP) than men. Both in epidemiologic studies of blood pressure and in treatment trials, lower blood pressure is associated with lower rates of CAD events.

Both systolic and diastolic blood pressures have been found in population and cohort studies to predict coronary events. Framingham data revealed that with a systolic BP greater than 180, the annual incidence of coronary heart disease (angina, coronary insufficiency, myocardial infarction, or death from these diagnoses) in women over 65 years of age is greater than 30 percent, while for older men above age 65, it is about 50 percent.[32] In other epidemiologic studies, higher diastolic blood pressure also predicts greater rates of clinical coronary artery disease.[33]

While treatment trials have also documented that lower blood pressure decreases the incidence of a first myocardial infarction and sudden death, this effect has been less dramatic than the decrease in stroke occurrence with blood pressure control. Analysis of myocardial infarction prevention in women has also been limited by the lower number of first myocardial infarctions in middle-aged women, the age group predominantly studied in early pharmacologic treatment trials.[34] Post hoc assessment of gender differences with individual patient data from most of the major randomized controlled hypertensive treatment trials has been completed.[34] These major treatment trials initiated pharmacologic therapy with thiazides and/or beta blockers versus placebo. Because most participants were middle-aged, the number of coronary events observed among women was smaller than the number of events among men. Since blood pressure control has only a limited impact on the prevention of myocardial infarction, the power to detect a treatment effect on coronary events for women was compromised. In contrast, with a greater reduction in stroke occurrence with treatment, the number of strokes for women and men was equal and adequate in number to reveal a treatment effect, which was similar for women and men. After reviewing the early studies, several authors have stressed the particular importance of identifying and treating hypertension in black women to prevent coronary artery disease events and stroke.[31,35]

Once older subjects were studied in clinical trials, the benefit of treating hypertension to prevent coronary events received greater recognition.[36,37] The number needed to treat (NNT) to prevent one myocardial infarction in representative trials in older and middle-aged women and men are compared in Table 87-2.[38] As Kannel states, ". . . coronary disease is the most common and lethal sequela of hypertension, equaling in incidence all the other cardiovascular outcomes combined."[39]

Gender-specific information about thiazide diuretics and angiotensin-converting enzyme (ACE) inhibitors for the pharmacologic therapy of hypertension is available. Thiazide diuretics are a reasonable first choice in the treatment of hypertension in women as well as men.[40] In epidemiologic studies, thiazide diuretics use has been associated with a lower incidence of hip fracture. In a meta-analysis of several cohort studies, current thiazide use, especially if long-term, was associated with as much as a 20 percent reduction of risk of hip fracture.[41] Evaluation of biochemical variables has suggested potential mechanisms.[42] No prospective treatment trials have explored this relationship. Although ACE drugs are effective in treating hypertension and congestive heart failure as well as preventing the progression of renal disease, these agents should be cautiously utilized in women of reproductive age because they are potentially teratogenic.[43] Cough, a common side effect of first-generation ACE inhibitors, occurs substantially more frequently in women than in men.[44]

Lipids

There are important gender differences in lipoprotein profiles.[45] Total cholesterol peaks in women from age 55 to 64 and in men at around age 50. HDL is usually greater in women than in men, with HDL levels remaining similar with increasing age. Many experts consider HDL more predictive for women than any other lipoprotein component, with the strongest correlation between low HDL levels and CAD events. Low-density lipoprotein (LDL) levels increase with increasing age for both women and men and are especially predictive of events in men. Triglyceride levels may be important in women but have not been shown to be independently important in men.

Many of the initial pharmacologic therapies for hyperlipidemia decreased LDL most effectively and were tested in middle-aged populations. Because women, on average, develop clinical CAD 10 years later than men, there was often inadequate power in primary prevention trials to determine the efficacy of treatment for women. Further data have become available, with older populations being studied and newer agents—such as the HMG-CoA reductase inhibitors, which simultaneously decrease LDL and increase HDL—being used. Secondary prevention studies in a variety of populations, including women, reveal benefit with treatment. Yet these agents are underprescribed after myocardial infarction and target treatment levels are not reached.[46] Most studies have found older age a barrier to prescribing and some researchers have found women less likely to receive treatment than men.[5,19,46]

There has only been adequate power to determine that secondary prevention with pharmacologic treatment of hyperlipidemia decreases CAD events in women. Primary prevention studies have had inadequate power for women because of the small number of observed CAD events. A recent meta-analysis combined primary and secondary treatment trials to reach adequate power for a secondary analysis by gender.[47] Results were dominated by secondary prevention trials. Women at high risk, such as women with diabetes, should be considered candidates for primary prevention with aggressive treatment of lipid abnormalities. There is controversy about aggressive treatment in the woman at low risk for vascular disease while results of further primary prevention clinical trials are pending.

Treatment of hyperlipidemia is discussed in detail in Chap. 38. The choice of agents for the treatment of hyperlipidemia in women includes hormonal therapy. In short-term studies of hyperlipidemia treatment, the HMG-CoA reductase inhibitors have been compared with hormonal replacement therapy regimens.[48,49] Although, both types of agents improve HDL, the HMG-CoA reductase inhibitors are more effective in improving LDL than hormonal therapy. In addition, triglyceride levels often increase with hormonal therapy and decrease with the HMG-CoA reductase inhibitors.[48,49] In a subsequent section, "Menopause and Hormonal Replacement Therapy," the risks and potential benefits of hormonal therapy are further discussed.

TABLE 87-2 Numbers Needed to Treat (NNT) to Prevent One Coronary Artery Event in Women and Men from Three Clinical Treatment Trials

		NNT to Prevent One CAD Event	
Treatment Study	Age of Subjects	Women	Men
STOP (25 month)	70–84 years	83	77
SHEP (5 years)	>age 59	50	111
HDFP (5 years)	30–51 years	143	59

Abbreviations: STOP = Swedish Trial in Older Patients with Hypertension; SHEP = Systolic Hypertension in the Elderly Program; HDFP = Hypertension Detection and Follow-up Program.
Source: From Cohen E, Swiderski D, Wheat ME, Charney P. Hypertension. In: Charney P, ed. *Coronary Artery Disease in Women.* Philadelphia: American College of Physicians; 1999:169.

Obesity

The prevalence of obesity has been increasing. Over 30 percent of white women and 50 percent of black or Mexican-American women are obese. In a recent third National Health and Nutrition Examination Survey, significantly more of the black and Mexican-American women were obese, with an elevated body mass index (BMI), than the white women (mean BMI for black women was 29.2 kg/m^2, 28.6 for Mexican-American women, and 26.3 kg/m^2 for white women).[50] Racial differences in BMI as well as glycosylated hemoglobin start in childhood, with black and Mexican-American girls having less favorable profiles than white girls.[11]

Obesity is linked to multiple cardiac risk factors (including insulin resistance, diabetes, hypertension, and hyperlipidemia), although it is has not clearly been documented to be independently associated with coronary artery event rates.[51] However, the pattern of weight distribution is predictive of coronary events.[51,52] The "apple" shape, with a greater central or abdominal girth, has been compared with the "pear" shape, with more weight on hips and buttocks. In the Nurses Health Study, both larger waist circumference and waist-hip ratio were independently associated with higher rates of CAD events.[52]

Increasingly, the relationship between greater weight and less physical activity has been elucidated. A study of obese twins revealed that lack of physical activity correlated with which twin was more obese.[53] This is particularly important, since even limited weight loss is associated with a lower risk of CAD events,[54,55] as is increased physical activity (see next section).

Behavioral interventions to decrease weight have been most successful when there is an exercise component.[51,56] One innovative trial for 40 obese women (mean weight 89.2 kg and BMI 32.9 kg) compared a 16-week program with instruction on a low-fat 1200-calorie diet and either training to increase daily physical exertion or addition of an aerobics class.[56] Compared with enrollment, all participants lost weight during the intensive program at the 1-year follow up. Women who had increased their activities of daily living most successfully sustained weight reduction. While new pharmacologic treatments for obesity have been developed, many have been documented to be hazardous.[57]

Physical Activity and Exercise

Gender differences in physiologic response to exercise have been studied.[58] Generally, women have smaller hearts, so cardiac output is increased by raising heart rate. Men, in comparison, accomplish an increase in cardiac output by increasing stroke volume. Women have a smaller work capacity and lower oxygen uptake. There are substantial limitations about what is known about women and physical activity, since—historically—studies have not collected data on housework and child care. Therefore, data about physical exertion in women may underestimate the actual amount of energy expended daily.

Yet in national surveys, sedentary lifestyles are reported by as many as 70 percent of adult women, with higher rates among black and hispanic women and those with less education or lower income.[50] Most studies on physical activity have focused on leisure activities and not included estimates of the energy required for housework or walking.[59] One community survey assessing change in physical activity from 1987 to 1991 found women more likely to exercise regularly if they had prior success with weight loss and exercise and received encouragement from their school-age children.[60] The women were less likely to begin or continue exercising if they worked outside the home. Especially for women, encouraging increased activity during daily activities of living is probably more important than counseling on initiating an exercise program. Recent programs to increase physical activity are cited in the section on obesity, above.

It is well known that overall mortality, CAD, and cancer mortality are inversely related to increasing levels of exercise. Physical activity is also important as secondary prevention. Both women and men are found to benefit from referral to cardiac rehabilitation programs after myocardial infarction.[61] However, fewer women than men are referred (6.9 percent women versus 13.3 percent men).[62]

Menopause and Hormonal Replacement Therapy

The importance of menopause as a risk factor for CAD in women is not fully defined. Women who have experienced early menopause after gynecologic surgery have been considered at higher risk for CAD and osteoporosis on the basis of less years of hormonal exposure.[63] However, a 1999 analysis from the Nurse's Health Study found only women smokers with a younger age of menopause to have a greater risk of CAD.[64]

Medical opinion on the potential benefits and risks of hormonal replacement therapy (HRT) after menopause has been evolving, as discussed elsewhere in this volume (Chaps. 38 and 86). Although population surveys have suggested that hormonal replacement therapy may decrease the risk of coronary artery disease, there are substantial differences between women who chose to take hormones and those who do not. Hormone users have tended to be healthier and wealthier, with less reported tobacco exposure and greater levels of exercise and access to medical care.[65] All these factors decrease the risk of CAD.

Although both retrospective and prospective epidemiologic evidence has suggested that users of hormonal therapy have substantially lower rates of CAD, results from clinical trials have not been confirmatory. The Heart & Estrogen/Progestin Replacement Study (HERS) is the only completed secondary prevention clinical trial of hormonal therapy.[66] Subjects were postmenopausal women with evidence of CAD [myocardial infarction (MI), coronary artery bypass graft (CABG), percutaneous transluminal coronary angioplasty (PTCA) for occlusion greater than 50 percent, or angiography with more than one major coronary artery] who were randomized to conjugated estrogen 0.625 mg plus medroxyprogesterone 2.5 mg or placebo and followed for 4 years. However, recruitment proceeded slowly and there were fewer coronary events than predicted as well as a higher crossover between treatment arms than expected. Results included no overall reduction in CAD events but substantially more venous thrombotic events and gallbladder disease in the group receiving hormonal therapy. Because of these risks, hormonal replacement therapy should be avoided in the setting of acute coronary ischemia. Assessment of hormonal replacement therapy for primary CAD prevention is currently in progress in the Women's Health Initiative.[65]

Multiple potential risks related to HRT have been described; they include increased thrombotic events, as noted in both epidemiologic trials and the HERS Study.[65,66] An increased risk of breast cancer with long-term use (greater than 5 years) is based on a worldwide review of the epidemiologic literature.[67] Other risks of HRT include higher rates of gallbladder disease[66] and elevated triglyceride levels. Vaginal bleeding frequently occurs with HRT and is a common reason why women chose to discontinue treatment.

Although there is controversy about the use of HRT to prevent CAD, there is clearer evidence for control of menopausal symptoms and a decreased rate of hip fracture with long-term use. Data from the Women's Health Initiative will provide evidence from a prospective double-blinded clinical trial. With the current limitations of medical knowledge, it is not surprising that utilization of HRT varies substantially among women potentially eligible for the treatment. In a 1995 national telephone survey of U.S. women, rates of hormonal treatment were shown to vary by geographic region and educational level rather than by medical condition.[68]

Psychosocial Risk Factors

Both socioeconomic and psychological factors affect the prevalence and outcome of CAD.[69] The effect of socioeconomic status on the incidence of CAD has been explored with increasing sophistication in the past decade. Coronary disease morbidity and mortality are greater among those of lower socioeconomic status (SES). Markers for SES have included years of formal education,[70] owning a car,[71] income defined by absolute[72] or relative amount,[73] and parental status.[71] More recently SES has also been defined independently of race.[11,50]

The importance of SES has been considered in a study from the Duke catherization population (consecutive patients with ≥75 percent stenosis of at least one coronary artery at catherization). The most important prognostic factor for CAD was the extent of coronary disease and ejection fraction at catherization, regardless of gender, with a 9-year median follow-up. However, SES and social support were independent risk factors and explained about 12 percent of the prognosis for individual women and men. Those with incomes below $10,000 per year were almost twice as likely to die as those with annual incomes ≥$40,000 within 5 years of follow-up.[72]

Women and men of lower SES from several United Kingdom studies were at increased risk for symptomatic CAD compared to those of a higher SES from the same area.[74–76] Lower SES has also been related to higher rates of tobacco use and higher inpatient mortality after MI.[74] Differences in event rates were greater for women than for men between different socioeconomic classes.

Among the many psychological issues with gender differences that affect outcomes in CAD, there is depression, which is diagnosed twice as often in women as in men.[77] Prospective data from the Baltimore Epidemiologic Catchment Area Study correlated a history of dysphoria or a major depressive episode with an increased risk of myocardial infarction for both women and men.[78] A positive response to a single question was central: "In your lifetime, have you ever had 2 weeks or more during which you felt sad, blue, depressed, or when you lost all interest and pleasure in things that you usually cared about or enjoyed?" The positive answer was associated with a 2.07 odds ratio of self-reporting an MI infarction at 13 years follow-up, compared with those giving a negative response. This odds ratio was independent of other coronary risk factors. Depression diagnosed with a patient interview 5 to 15 days after MI was a significant predictor of mortality at 6 months.[79] Although less women than men agreed to participate in this observation study, depression was more common in women than in men. Subsequent studies have revealed that depression after MI also predicts greater morbidity as well as higher subsequent mortality in women than in men.[80] As early as 1991, the question of whether higher rates of depression in women after MI correlate with sex differences in prognosis was raised;[81] the answer is still unavailable. Although a pharmacologic interventional trial of depression diagnosed after MI has not yet been reported, the selective serotonin reuptake inhibitors are probably safe in the presence of cardiac disease.[80]

Race and Coronary Artery Disease

Race and socioeconomic issues, in addition to traditional CAD risk factors, are important in understanding variations in black and white CAD mortality rates from the limited literature on these issues.[82–84] Social factors particularly important for black women are income, education, occupational status, and place of birth. Combined analysis of data from the 1986 National Mortality Feedback Survey, the 1985 National Health Interview Survey, and the U.S. Bureau of the Census revealed that young black women (age <55) had more than twice the rate of CAD mortality (sudden and nonsudden) than young white Americans.[83] CAD death rates for young black women in this study exceeded rates for young men and white women (Fig. 87-4). Importantly, family income, educational level, and occupational status accounted for more of this observed difference than traditional coronary risk factors.[83] In the Multicenter Investigation of the Limitation of Infarct Size study, black women ($n = 63$ of 985 randomized subjects) had a higher cumulative 4-year mortality after myocardial infarction than other sex and race groups.[82] The importance of birthplace for black New Yorkers rather than current geographic location has been described.[85,86]

Racial differences in physiology have also begun to be considered. Differences among electrocardiographic findings among black and white healthy subjects was detailed in 1998.[87] Differences in tobacco metabolism—such as slower cotinine clearance and higher serum cotinine levels—are seen in black smokers compared with white[88] and Hispanic smokers.[15]

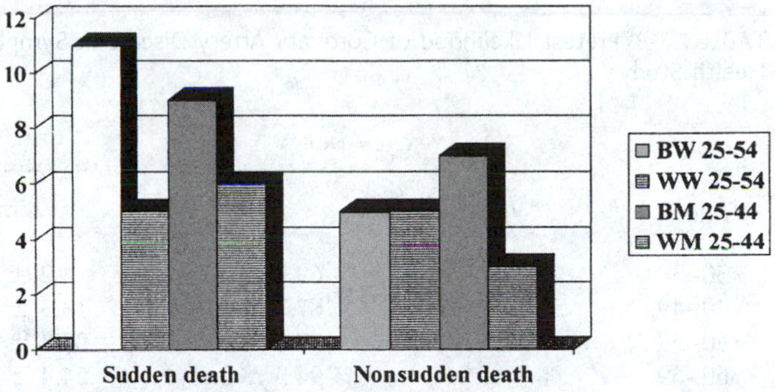

FIGURE 87-4 Coronary artery disease death rates for young adults (women age 25–54 years, men age 25–44 years) by race and gender. BW = black women; WW = white women; BM = black men; WM = white men. (Adapted from Escobedo LG, Giles WH, Anda RF. Socioeconomic status, race and death from coronary heart disease. *Am J Prev Med* 1997; 13:12–130, with permission.)

In summary, many important gender differences in specific cardiovascular risk factors have been briefly reviewed. More extensive discussions are available in other individual chapters and in *Coronary Artery Disease in Women*.[1] Models incorporating individual risk factors have been developed to aid in identifying women at higher risk for future CAD events. These models for risk stratification of individual women are discussed in the subsequent section on the management of CAD.

DIAGNOSIS OF CORONARY ARTERY DISEASE IN WOMEN

The biases that affect the diagnosis of CAD in women are explored below. Then, gender differences in noninvasive testing for CAD is discussed. Patterns of referral for coronary catherization are considered, followed by gender differences in cardiac catheterization results.

CAD is often diagnosed clinically by a careful history. The listener's preconceived biases can affect his or her perceptions of risk for CAD. In one study, where an actress portrayed a woman twice with the same script but different clothes and affect, physicians who reviewed the video where the actress described chest pain with "exaggerated emotional presentation style" predicted less CAD than when the same script was presented with a "businesslike affect."[89] More recently, physicians were recruited to view a video of different actors (black and white women and men) accompanied by the same written information. The black woman was least likely to be referred for cardiac catherization.[90] Since the clinical history is essential for the diagnosis of angina and acute coronary syndromes, provider assumptions affect the diagnosis of CAD. If the diagnosis is not considered, then evaluation and management will not occur. The clinical history typical for angina and acute coronary syndromes is reviewed at the beginning of the appropriate sections below as well as elsewhere in this textbook (Chaps. 40–42).

Once CAD is considered as a diagnosis, further evaluation is possible to assess disease presence and severity. Noninvasive stress testing can help to determine which patients with an intermediate risk for CAD will benefit from further interven-

TABLE 87-3 Pretest Likelihood of Coronary Artery Disease in Symptomatic Patients According to Age and Sex from the Cardiovascular Health Study

	Typical Angina		Atypical Angina		Nonanginal Chest Pain	
Age	Women	Men	Women	Men	Women	Men
30–39	25.8 ± 6.6%	69.7 ± 3.2%	4.2 ± 1.3%	21.8 ± 2.4%	0.8 ± 0.3%	5.2 ± 0.8%
40–49	55.2 ± 6.5	87.3 ± 1.0	13.3 ± 2.9	46.1 ± 1.8	2.8 ± 0.7	14.1 ± 1.3
50–59	79.4 ± 2.4	92.0 ± 0.6	32.4 ± 3.0	58.9 ± 1.5	8.4 ± 1.2	21.5 ± 1.7
60–69	90.1 ± 1.0	94.3 ± 0.4	54.4 ± 2.4	67.1 ± 1.3	18.6 ± 1.9	28.1 ± 1.9

Source: From Recommendations of the Task Force of the European Society of Cardiology: Management of stable angina pectoris. *Eur Heart J* 1997:398, with permission.

tions and to assess disease control.[91] Although a more extensive discussion can be found in Chap. 14, potential gender differences in noninvasive testing are discussed briefly here. Unfortunately, each of the noninvasive techniques has limitations in women.[92,93]

Exercise stress testing is the oldest way of assessing CAD risk noninvasively. However, if a completed exercise stress test reveals ST changes and depression greater than 1 mm, especially in younger women (where the prevalence of ST depression is less), this may indicate significant CAD.[94] In comparison, a negative exercise stress test with adequate exertion is often helpful because it decreases the need to consider cardiac catherization.[94] Gender-specific criteria have been proposed to compensate for the generally smaller ST changes seen in women.[95]

As a rule, stress imaging techniques are favored in assessing a woman for possible CAD or staging the severity of disease. Local expertise is an important consideration in deciding whether to use nuclear medicine or echocardiography techniques. Nuclear stress perfusion testing in women can be potentially hindered by soft tissue attenuation from breast tissue with the use of thallium, so technetium may be preferred. Stress echocardiography is highly dependent on operator expertise and may be technically difficult in obese patients. Many authors prefer stress imaging tests with lower false-positive rates than an exercise stress test for women.[94]

Patterns of referral to cardiac catherization may vary by gender, with some appropriate differences.[96,97] Because cardiac catherization is less likely to reveal CAD in women, many clinicians initially evaluate women at intermediate risk with stress imaging techniques. For example, anginal symptoms in women are less predictive of abnormal coronary anatomy than in men (Table 87-3). In the Coronary Artery Surgery Study (CASS), coronary artery disease was diagnosed by cardiac catherization in 63 percent of women with definitive angina, 40 percent in women with probable angina, and 4 percent in women with nonischemic pain.[98] Direct referral to cardiac catherization should occur with a high suspicion of significant CAD that might benefit from intervention or after an abnormal noninvasive stress test.

MANAGEMENT OF CLINICAL CORONARY ARTERY DISEASE IN WOMEN

Physicians have generally not appreciated some of the gender differences in CAD presentation and management. In a Gallup Survey completed in 1996 in Washington, D.C., "nearly two-thirds of the primary care physicians surveyed (256 internists and family practitioners) said that there is no difference between men and women in the symptoms, signs, or diagnosis of heart disease."[2] Meanwhile, research on CAD is extending our understanding of significant gender differences.[1]

The spectrum of presentations of CAD ranges from an asymptomatic disease phase to chronic angina and acute coronary syndromes including unstable angina, MI, and finally arrhythmia and sudden death. Both women and men may have silent or asymptomatic CAD for many years. Then, as described from Framingham data, the first presentation of symptomatic CAD is typically angina in women and MI in men.[99]

In this section, the entire spectrum of clinical CAD is reviewed, with attention to what is known in relation to caring for women patients. First, the asymptomatic women are considered, for whom coronary artery risk-assessment models have been developed. Then, angina and acute coronary syndromes are discussed. In addition, issues for women related to coronary artery bypass surgery and angioplasty are highlighted. Finally, considerations related to arrhythmias and sudden death are explored. Since women more frequently have atypical symptoms than men, women are more likely to present with occult CAD.

Asymptomatic Women

Some individuals are truly asymptomatic with respect to CAD. Others may have had atypical symptoms that have not yet been diagnosed as possible CAD. When Framingham researchers interviewed patients who had developed evidence of an interim myocardial infarction by electrocardiography (ECG) (25% of all myocardial infarctions), almost 50 percent, in retrospect, reported some symptoms.[100]

For truly asymptomatic women, national guidelines for prevention have been increasingly developed.[101] Important risk factors for both women and men include tobacco use, hypertension, physical inactivity, diabetes, obesity, and hyperlipidemia.[102] Counseling of asymptomatic women about CAD should include a review of the common risk factors, encouragement for implementing a healthy lifestyle, and an outline of the symptoms of CAD. The single most important intervention is avoiding exposure to tobacco.[1,6,7]

Tools to assess CAD risk are receiving increasing attention. Prospective cohort studies have been used to develop models predicting the impact of one or more risk factors on the likelihood of future coronary artery events.[50,103,104] When multiple individual risk factors are present, the cumulative risk of CAD is greater than the sum of its parts.[50,103,105] The prevalence and impact of risk factors are reviewed below—with data on women from the Third National Health and Nutrition Examination Survey,[50] the Chicago Heart Association Detection Project in Industry,[103,105] and the Framingham Heart Study.[104,106]

The Third National Health and Nutrition Examination Survey (NHANES III) explored the intersection between race, SES, and the prevalence of cardiovascular risk factors.[50] Among women, systolic blood pressure, tobacco use, BMI, leisure-time activity, non–high density lipoprotein cholesterol, and the presence of non-insulin-dependent diabetes were assessed in black (n = 1762), Mexican-American (n = 1481), and white women (n = 2023) age 25 to 64 years old. Participants completed both a home questionnaire and a physical examination in a mobile examination center. SES status was defined by the highest educational level attained, and a poverty income ratio was derived from family income and size. Compared with prior studies in which comparisons were attempted, more low-SES white women were included.

Results from NHANES III stressed the importance of race even when SES was included in a CAD risk model. As expected, increasing age was associated with a greater prevalence of all risk factors. However, there were substantial racial variations. Black and Mexican-American women had a higher BMI and systolic blood pressure, more diabetes, and reported more leisure-time activity (as well as lower tobacco use) than white women of a similar SES. With increasing age, black and Mexican-American women had greater prevalence rates of hypertension than white women. In contrast, smoking rates were more stable with increasing age for black and Mexican-American women, while they decreased for white women. Other large cohort studies, including the Chicago Heart Association Detection Project in Industry and cohorts from Framingham and the Lipid Research Clinics, have focused on white populations.

The prevalence and impact of individual and multiple risk factors in the Chicago Heart Association Detection Project in Industry were explored.[103] Employed participants age 40 to 64 years in the Chicago area were surveyed. Smoking status, hypertension, hyperlipidemia, and their relative importance in predicting CAD was assessed among 8686 women and 10,503 men, almost all white, who were followed for 22 years. At the time of enrollment, history of current tobacco use was obtained, a single BP was recorded, and a serum cholesterol was determined. Current tobacco use was reported by 35 percent of women (40 percent of men). Hypertension, defined as BP systolic ≥140, was noted in 53 percent of women (64 percent of men). Hypercholesteremia, defined as cholesterol ≥240 mg/dL, was present in 30 percent of women (22 percent of men). About 80 percent of participants in the Chicago Heart Association Detection Project in Industry had at least one of these risk factors initially. Two risk factors were found in about 34 percent of women and 38 percent of men. Less than 7 percent had all three risk factors. When coronary mortality was considered, those with the most risk factors were at the greatest risk of death. Tobacco use was a significantly more important predictor of mortality in women than in men (RR 2.85 versus 1.68, $p < 0.001$, comparing current smokers with nonsmokers). In a subsequent analysis, the number of risk factors present at screening also directly correlated with the eventual size of Medicare reimbursements.[105] Those without risk factors had the lowest number of Medicare claims.

Similarly, the cardiac risk profile for asymptomatic 50-years-olds in the Framingham cohort was used to predict who would be alive at age 75. For women, survival was associated with lower daily cigarette use and lower systolic blood pressure. In addition, a higher forced vital capacity and parental survival to age 75 were predictive of survival.[104]

Clustering of risk factors was also important on examination in the Framingham Offspring Study (age 30 to 74 years at enrollment) with 16 years of follow-up for coronary artery events (MI or sudden death).[54] On evaluation, 17 percent of all participants had three of the six risk factors (lowest quintile HDL cholesterol, highest quintile cholesterol, BMI, systolic blood pressure, triglycerides, and glucose). There were 79 first coronary artery events among the 1818 women who were initially free of symptomatic CAD, compared with 229 events among the 1759 men. However, CAD events were associated with three or more risk factors for 48 percent of the CAD events in women and 20 percent of the CAD events in men. When Framingham offspring where assessed 8 years apart, weight gain correlated most significantly with changes in blood pressure and lipoproteins for women and men.[106]

A more recent review has considered long-term cardiovascular outcomes among those with a low risk-factor profile, including data on women from the Chicago Heart Association Detection Project in Industry.[107] A low risk-factor profile was defined as follows: not a current smoker, BP ≤120/80, total cholesterol <200, no history of diabetes or MI, and no ECG abnormalities. Only 6.8 percent of the cohort age 40 to 59 years at entry met these criteria. These women had substantially lower CAD mortality with a mean follow up of 22 years (3.5 compared with 14.5 age-adjusted mortality rate per 10,000 person-years, RR 0.21, 95%; CI 0.05 to 0.84).

In summary, these studies indicate that risk factors are additive and that women without traditional cardiovascular risk factors (tobacco, hypertension, high cholesterol, diabetes, physical inactivity, family history, and old age) are at relatively low risk for coronary events. The largest benefit is derived from aggressive preventive measures in women with multiple risk factors or prior coronary events[108–110] (see also Chap. 40).

Angina

The clinical diagnosis of angina can be challenging. Women generally visit physicians more often than men and report more symptoms, including chest pain. In assessing chest symptoms to determine whether angina is the most probable diagnosis, attention to the type and duration of symptoms and their impact on activities of daily living often provide important clues. The chest pain associated with angina classically may be a heavy pressure or squeezing but may also be described as a burning, aching, or stabbing. Typically duration varies between 10 and 20 min, with MI more likely after 30 min of sustained pressure or pain. Often angina is precipitated by exertion. Women compared with men with angina more frequently report angina with emotional or mental stress.[111] Too often older women ascribe their decreased ability to complete housework or walk to "getting old." Therefore regular exploration of a patient's exercise tolerance and consideration of coronary artery disease in the differential when there is a decrease in exercise tolerance are essential.

As discussed under "Diagnosis of Coronary Heart Disease in Women," managing angina in women is complicated by the observation that anginal symptoms in women are less predictive of abnormal coronary anatomy than in men. In CASS, CAD was diagnosed by cardiac catherization in 63 percent of women with definitive angina, 40 percent in women with probable angina, and 4 percent in women with nonischemic pain[98] (Table 87-3). Data on women with unstable angina are discussed below and also reveal lower rates of CAD at cardiac catheterization.

Chronic angina has a generally favorable prognosis in women, with mortality rates of about 2 or 3 percent annually.[112] The management of women with chronic angina requires therapies effective for the prevention of MI in addition to symptom management. Most clinicians begin secondary prevention with the diagnosis of angina, although secondary prevention trials have begun after an MI, not usually after the diagnosis of angina. Secondary prevention treatment goals include tobacco avoidance (both smoking cessation and avoiding secondhand smoke); control of blood pressure, glucose, weight, and emotional stress; and the initiation or continuation of regular physical exercise or exertion.[112] Pharmacologic therapies include the use of aspirin, anti-ischemic agents, and lipid-lowering agents. Most clinicians would hesitate to begin HRT since the recent HERS study, discussed previously.

Potential gender differences in vasospastic responses have been a focus of research. When patients with both a history of chest pain and angiography indicating no more than slight coronary artery abnormalities received acetylcholine by intracoronary infusion, substantial gender differences were noted.[113] Of the 117 patients studied, large-artery spasm (n = 63) occurred predominantly in men (40 men versus 23 women), while microvascular spasm (n = 29) occurred more often in women (20 women versus 9 men). Patients with microvascular spasm had less coronary artery constriction after acetylcholine infusion, although angina (93 percent) and ischemic changes on ECG (83 percent) were often noted. Lactate levels in the coronary sinus were higher after acetylcholine infusion in patients with microvascular spasm (82 percent) than in those with large-artery spasm (53 percent). These types of studies have suggested that patterns of ischemia may vary by gender. More recent reviews of acute coronary syndromes have also suggested clinically important gender differences.

Acute Coronary Ischemia Including Acute Myocardial Infarction

Acute coronary ischemia includes unstable angina and MI; there are substantial gender differences in the presentation and natural history of each. Some differences may be physiologic and others are related to differences in management. Extensive general discussions of acute coronary ischemia syndromes can be found in other chapters within this volume. This section focuses on gender differences in presentation, prognosis, and management.

Gender differences in acute ischemia at the time of presentation and during short-term follow-up have been explored.[114–117] In a recent review of data from the National Registry of Myocardial Infarction–I, women had a higher mortality during the index hospitalization.[114] As in earlier studies, women arrived longer for evaluation after symptoms began; they also received less thrombolytic treatment (e.g., aspirin, beta blockers) as well as less invasive interventions (catherization, PTCA, and CABG). Women had higher mortality rates than men, even at similar ages or after similar interventions, from cardiogenic shock, sudden death, arrhythmias, myocardial rupture, and electromechanical dissociation (in descending order). Complementary results were noted in a Spanish registry of patients less than 80 years of age experiencing a first MI.[115] As well as a later presentation for care, women had higher mortality during hospitalization and within 6 months. Women more often developed acute pulmonary edema or cardiogenic shock (25 percent of women versus 11 percent of men) and less often developed at least one episode of ventricular fibrillation or sustained ventricular tachycardia requiring immediate medical care (15 percent of women versus 24 percent of men).

Prospective subgroup gender analysis of patients enrolled in Global Use of Strategies to Open Occluded Coronary Arteries in Acute Coronary Syndromes (GUSTO IIb) compared initial presentations, evaluation, and 30-day mortality.[116] Although most subjects enrolled had had an acute MI (53.8 percent of women and 67 percent of men), substantial numbers of participants had unstable angina (Table 87-4). At presentation, women were more often diagnosed with unstable angina than men (45.9 versus 35.6 percent, $p < 0.001$; odds ratio 1.51, 95 percent CI 1.34 to 1.69). Women subjects with acute coronary ischemia were older and had more comorbid conditions (diabetes, hypertension, angina, congestive heart failure) than the men, who were more likely to be smokers or have a prior MI, angioplasty, or CABG surgery. With MI, the initial entry ECG in women compared with men was less likely to have ST elevation (27.2 versus 37.0 percent, $p < 0.001$).

In GUSTO IIb, after cardiac catherization (completed in 53 percent of women and 59 percent of men), women were about twice as likely to demonstrate no vessels with CAD compared with men with unstable angina (30.5 versus 13.9 percent, $p < 0.001$), after MI with ST-segment elevation (10.2 versus 6.8 percent, $p < 0.02$) or

TABLE 87-4 Clinical Presentation of Consecutive Enrollees in GUSTO IIb

	Number of Women (Percentage of Women)	Number of Men (Percentage of Men)
MI with ST elevation	997 (27.2)	3134 (37.0)
MI without ST elevation	974 (26.6)	2544 (30.0)
Unstable angina	1690 (46.2)	2801 (33.0)
TOTAL	3661	8479

SOURCE: Adapted from Hochman JS, Tamis JE, Thompson TD. Sex, clinical presentation, and outcome in patients with acute coronary syndromes. *N Engl J Med* 1999; 341:226–232, with permission.

MI without ST-segment elevation (9.1 versus 4.2 percent, $p < 0.001$). These results are similar to those from the National Registry of Myocardial Infarction–II (MITI-II).[117]

Mortality by gender within 30 days after MI has been further elucidated by the GUSTO IIb and MITI-II reports.[116,117] Overall in GUSTO IIb, within 30 days, mortality for women was higher than for men (6.0 versus 4.0 percent, $p < 0.001$) despite similar reinfarction rates (6.2 percent for women, 5.6 percent for men, $p = 0.19$), with the difference explained by baseline variables such as older age and more comorbid conditions.[116] Among those with unstable angina, women had less mortality and reinfarction within 30 days than did men (odds ratio 0.65, 95 percent CI 0.49 to 0.87, $p = 0.003$). Bleeding complications were more common in women, but data analysis could not assess the role of revascularization procedures.

The interaction of gender and age was considered with data available from the National Registry of Myocardial Infarction–II.[117] Women with MI are often older and have more comorbid conditions than do men. Although overall there was a 14 percent early mortality in women after hospitalization for MI compared with 10 percent in men, when age was further considered, the picture became more complex. Upon analysis of the interaction of gender and age, the 30-day mortality after MI was about twice as great for women age 30 to 50 compared with men of the same age and progressively decreased with increasing age until reaching unity at age 75 (Fig. 87-5).

MI can also present as sudden death or without painful symptoms (silent MI). Sudden death is discussed further on, but a high percentage of first MIs are lethal in women. In the Framingham Heart Study, at 30 years of follow-up, the first presentation of MI resulted in death among 39 percent women and 31 percent of men.[100] Silent MI in the Framingham data was common, representing 25 percent of MI when diagnosed on the basis of new Q waves on screening ECG. Despite obtaining further history, almost half of the subjects had no symptoms. Silent MI is more common in women than in men (35 versus 28 percent).[100] The prognosis of silent MI has not been adequately studied. However, sudden death is one possible sequela.[118,119]

In long-term follow-up after MI, women have more symptoms than men, although long-term mortality is better or similar.[120] Women tend to have more angina and congestive heart failure despite better systolic left ventricular function.[120] Women as well as men most often develop congestive heart failure from ischemic heart disease.[58]

Finally, there has been a substantial lag in translating results of secondary treatment trials for MI into clinical practice. Therapies that are efficacious in women as well as men are often not prescribed—i.e., aspirin and agents to lower cholesterol.[46,104,114,121] Furthermore, treatment goals have often not been met (like achieving an elevated HDL and lower LDL and total cholesterol).[46] Rehabilitation is less often recommended for women, although it is equally effective.[61] To improve the prognosis of women after MI, it is essential to encourage less tobacco exposure (secondary as well as primary exposure) and the use of medications documented to decrease mortality and morbidity (beta blockers, angiotensin-converting enzyme inhibitors, aspirin, etc.) and to address other risk factors.

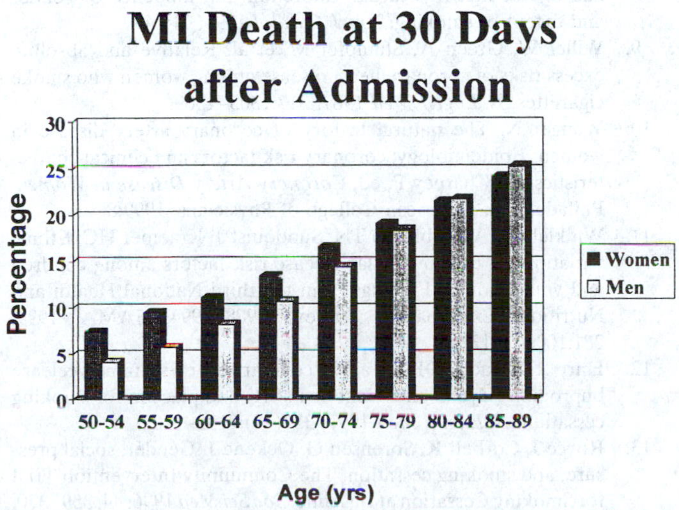

FIGURE 87-5 Mortality after myocardial infarction: Sex differences by age. (From Vaccarino V, Horowitz RI, Meehan TP, et al. Sex differences in mortality after myocardial infarction: Evidence for a sex-age interaction. *Arch Intern Med* 1998; 158:2054–2062, with permission.)

Interventions for Coronary Artery Disease

Gender differences in the prevalence and complications of angioplasty and CABG surgery are evolving. Both procedures are utilized less in women than in men, and there has been controversy as to whether women are undertreated or men overtreated.[122] Angioplasty initially was associated with a higher complication rate in women. However, with the development of smaller coronary artery catheters, outcomes and complications are similar for women and men.[123]

CABG surgery is more commonly performed in men than women. In the Thoracic Surgeon's National Cardiac Database as in other observational data, about one-quarter of the CABG procedures are completed on women patients.[124] The conduit selected is less often the internal mammary artery in women than in men, although this graft is associated with the best short- and long-term results. Reasons for this might include higher rates of diabetes in women undergoing CABG and the decreased use of internal mammary artery grafting in the setting of osteoporosis.[125] Since women compared to men undergoing CABG tend to be older and have more comorbid conditions, a higher postoperative complication rate, including slower postoperative recovery[126] and higher rates of depression,[127] is not unexpected. Gender differences are less apparent with follow-up after several years.[124]

Sudden Death

In the Framingham study, sudden death was common in both women and men.[100] Within 10 years of an MI, men more often experienced sudden death than did women (12 versus 5 percent).[100] The proportion of sudden death occurring in those without previously documented CAD was greater among women than among men (67 versus 55 percent).[100] Cardiac risk factors for sudden death in one epidemiologic case-controlled study revealed risk factors in white and black women similar to those for MI.[128]

Insights into the pathophysiology of sudden death are revealed in an autopsy study of women's hearts[119] comparing autopsies after sudden death ($n = 51$) and after trauma ($n = 15$). Death was witnessed for many of the women with sudden death and significant coronary artery pathology ($n = 36$, 71 percent). Reported symptoms included chest pain ($n = 8$), dizziness ($n = 3$), back pain ($n = 2$), shortness of breath ($n = 1$), left shoulder tingling ($n = 1$), fatigue ($n = 1$), malaise ($n = 1$), stomach distention ($n = 1$), nausea and vomiting ($n = 1$), and fever and chills ($n = 1$). Tobacco use was noted in 58 percent of those experiencing sudden death, compared with 50 percent of the controls. Chronic medical problems of the women who experienced sudden death included hypertension ($n = 11$), history of heart disease ($n = 9$), and medication for diabetes ($n = 5$).

On autopsy, healed prior MI was found in 35 percent. Pathologic examination revealed eroded plaque with acute thrombus ($n = 18$), stable plaque with healed infarct ($n = 18$), ruptured plaque with acute thrombus ($n = 8$), and stable plaque without infarction ($n = 7$). The acute thrombus associated with plaque erosion (often noted in early atherosclerosis) occurred more often in younger women smokers without obesity, high cholesterol, or elevated glycohemoglobin.[119] In comparison, plaque rupture was more often found in older women with elevated cholesterol. Further assessment of women dying with stable plaque without infarction revealed no association with known cardiac risk factors. Although sudden death is rare, tobacco use in young women is an important risk factor. Although only 2 of 51 women had a documented prior MI, on autopsy 35 percent of the sample had evidence of a prior MI. The relationship between sudden death and prior silent MI requires further elucidation.

Arrhythmias

Gender differences in arrhythmia identification, natural history, and management are just beginning to be explored. It is generally known that torsades de pointes occurs more commonly in women.[129,130] Preliminary small studies have considered heart rate variability[131] and QT duration[132] as potential contributors to the development of torsades de pointes. Heart rate variability is different in younger (33 ± 4 years) women and men but similar in more mature (67 ± 3 years) women and men.[131]

Palpitations were reported more commonly by women (17 percent) than men (12 percent) in a Norway population survey.[133] Gender differences were noted among American patients presenting to an emergency department with palpitations.[134] Men were more likely to have irregular beats (57 versus 40 percent) and to have symptoms that lasted more than 5 min (77 versus 61 percent). Although cardiac etiologies for palpitations were most common, psychiatric diagnoses (predominantly panic attacks) were a close second (43 versus 31 percent). After MI, women are more likely to have atrial fibrillation,[116] yet they die less often of arrhythmia than do men.[20] Finally, a German pacemaker registry retrospective review (with 31,913 entries) found that when pacemakers are implanted, women are more likely to receive a single-chamber pacer while men are more likely to receive a dual-chamber pacer.[135]

SUMMATION

Over the past few decades significant differences in individual patient factors that affect diagnosis and management have begun to be futher defined. How differences in sex, race, and SES might affect the care of individual patients is beginning to be explored. With increasing attention to physiologic and social issues, both women and men can receive more appropriate care.

At this juncture it is important to focus on primary and secondary prevention for both women and men, to consider the diagnosis of CAD in women with typical or atypical symptoms, and to manage CAD aggressively in both women and men with an otherwise good prognosis.

References

1. Charney P, ed. *Coronary Artery Disease in Women: Prevention, Diagnosis and Management.* Philadelphia: American College of Physicians; 1999.
2. Legato MJ, Padus E, Slaughter E. Women's perceptions of their general health, with special reference of their risk of coronary artery disease: Results of a national telephone survey. *J Women's Health* 1997; 6(2):189–198.
3. Barrett-Connor E. Sex differences in coronary heart disease: Why are women so superior? The 1995 Ancel Keys Lecture. *Circulation* 1997; 95:252–264.
4. Kreuger DE, Ellenberg SS, Bloom S, et al. Risk factors for fatal heart attack in young women. *Am J Epidemiol* 1981; 113(4):357–370.
5. Collins LJ, Douglas PS. Acute coronary syndromes. In: Charney P, ed. *Coronary Artery Disease in Women.* Philadelphia: American College of Physicians; 1999:403–406.
6. Ockene JK, Bonollo DP, Adams A. Smoking. In: Charney P, ed. *Coronary Artery Disease in Women.* 1999. Philadelphia: American College of Physicians; 1999.
7. He J, Vupputuri S, Allen K, et al. Passive smoking and the risk of coronary heart disease—A meta-analysis of epidemiologic studies. *N Engl J Med* 1999; 340:920–926.
8. Hansen EF, Andersen LT, Von Eyben FE. Cigarette smoking and age at first myocardial infarction and influence of gender and extent of smoking. *Am J Cardiol* 1993; 71:1439.
9. Willet W, Green A, Stampfer M, et al. Relative and absolute excess risks of coronary heart disease among women who smoke cigarettes. *N Engl J Med* 1987; 317:1303–1309.
10. Wenger N. The natural history of coronary artery disease in women: Epidemiology; coronary risk factors and clinical characteristics. In: Charney P, ed, *Coronary Artery Disease in Women.* Philadelphia: American College of Physicians; 1999:8.
11. Winkleby MA, Robinson TN, Sundquist J, Kraemer HC. Ethnic variations in cardiovascular disease risk factors among children and young adults: Findings from the third National Health and Nutrition Examination Survey, 1988–1994. JAMA 1999; 281:1006–1013.
12. Hurt RD, Sachs DP, et al. A comparison of sustained-release bupropion (Zyban and Wellbutrin SR) and placebo for smoking cessation. *N Engl J Med* 1997; 337(17):1195–1202.
13. Royce J, Corbett K, Sorensen G, Ockene J. Gender, social pressure, and smoking cessation: The Community Intervention Trial for Smoking Cessation at Baseline. *Soc Sci Med* 1996; 44: 359–370.
14. Bjoranson W, Rand C, Connett J, et al. Gender differences in smoking cessation after three years in the Lung Health Study. *Am J Public Health* 1995; 85(2):223–230.
15. Carballo RS, Giovino GA, Perchaeck TF, et al. Racial and ethnic differences in serum cotinine levels for cigarette smokers: Third

National Health and Nutrition Examination Survey, 1988–1991. *JAMA* 1998; 280:135–139.
16. Thorndike AN, Rigotti NA, Stafford RS, Singer DE. National patterns in the treatment of smokers by physicians. *JAMA* 1998; 279(8):604–608.
17. Fiore M, Bailey W, Cohen S, et al. *Smoking Cessation: Clinical Practice Guidelines No. 18.* Publication 96-0692. Rockville, MD: USDHHS, PHS, AHCPR; 1996.
18. Sowers JR. Diabetes mellitus and cardiovascular disease in women. *Arch Intern Med* 1998; 158:617–621.
19. Miettinen H, Lehto S, Salomaa V, Mahonen M, et al. Impact of diabetes on mortality after the first myocardial infarction. *Diabetes Care* 1998; 21(1):69–75.
20. Gu K, Cowie CC, Harris MI. Diabetes and decline in heart disease mortality in US adults. *JAMA* 1999; 281:1291–1297.
21. Sullivan M. Criteria for the oral glucose tolerance test in pregnancy. *Diabetes* 1964; 13(13):278–285.
22. Manson JE, Rimm EB, Stampfer MJ, et al. Physical activity and the incidence of non-insulin-dependent diabetes in women. *Lancet* 1991; 338:774–778.
23. Laws A. Diabetes and insulin resistance. In: Charney P, ed. *Coronary Artery Disease in Women.* Philadelphia: American College of Physicians; 1999:70–100.
24. Baldeweg S, Yudkin JS. Implications of the United Kingdom Prospective Diabetes Study. *Primary Care* 1999; 26(4): 809–827.
25. Prospective Diabetes Study Group. United Kingdom Prospective diabetes study 27: Plasma lipids and lipoproteins at diagnosis of NIDDM by age and sex, UK. *Diabetes Care* 1997; 20(11):1683–1687.
26. Pyorala K, Pedersen TR, Kjekshus J, et al. for the Scandinavian Simvastatin Survival Study (4S) Group. Cholesterol lowering with simvastatin improves prognosis of diabetic patients with coronary heart diease: A subgroup analysis of the Scandinavian Simvastatin Survival Study (4S). *Diabetes Care* 1997; 20(4):614–620.
27. Birdall MA, Farquhar CM, White HD. Association between polycystic ovaries and extent of coronary artery disease in women having cardiac catherization. *Ann Intern Med* 1997; 126:32–35.
28. Waterworth DM, Bennett ST, et al. Linkage and association of insulin gene VNTR reglatory polymorphism with polycystic ovarian syndrome. *Lancet* 1997; 349:968–990.
29. Velasquez EM, Mendoza S, Hamer T, et al. Metformin therapy in polycystic ovarian syndrome reduces hyperinsulinemia, insulin resistance, hyperandrogenemia, and systolic blood pressure, while facilitating normal menses and pregnancy. *Metabolism* 1994; 43:647–654.
30. Mayer-Davis EJ, D'Agostino R, Karter AJ, Haffner SM, et al. Intensity and amount of physical activity in relation to insulin sensitivity: The Insulin Resistance Atherosclerosis Study. *JAMA* 1998; 279:669–674.
31. The Women's Caucus, Working Group on Women's Health of the Society of General Internal Medicine. Hypertension in women: What is really known? *Ann Intern Med* 1991; 115:287–293.
32. Sagie A. The natural history of borderline isolated systolic hypertension. *N Engl J Med* 1993; 329:1912–1917.
33. Stamler J, Stamler R, Neaton JD, et al. Blood pressure, systolic and diastolic, and cardiovascular risks: US population data. *Arch Intern Med* 1993; 153:598–615.
34. Gueyffier F, Boutitie F, Boissel Jean-Pierre, et al. Effect of antihypertensive drug treatment on cardiovascular outcomes in women and men: A meta-analysis of individual patient data from randomized, controlled trials. *Am Coll Phys* 1997; 126:761–767.
35. Quan A, Kerlikowske K, Gueyffier F, et al. Efficacy of treating hypertension in women. *J Gen Intern Med* 1999; 14:718–729.
36. SHEP Cooperative Research Group. Prevention of stroke by antihypertensive drug treatment in older persons with isolated systolic hypertension: Final results of the Systolic Hypertension in the Elderly Program (SHEP). *JAMA* 1991; 265(24):3255–3264.
37. Dahlof B, Lindholm LH, Hansson L, et al. Morbidity and mortality in the Swedish Trial in Old Patients with Hypertension (STOP-Hypertension). *Lancet* 1991; 338:1281–1285.
38. Cohen E, Swiderski DM, Wheat ME, Charney P. Hypertension. In: Charney P, ed. *Coronary Artery Disease in Women.* Philadelphia: American College of Physicians; 1999:169.
39. Kannel WB. Blood pressure as a cardiovascular risk factor: Prevention and treatment. *JAMA* 1996; 275:1571–1576.
40. Joint National Committee on Prevention, Detection, Evaluation and Treatment of High Blood Pressure. The Sixth Report of the Joint National Committee on Prevention, Detection, Evaluation and Treatment of High Blood Pressure. *Arch Intern Med* 1997; 157:2413–2446.
41. Jones G, Nguyen T, Sambrook PN, Eismann JA. Thiazide diuretics and fractures: Can meta-analysis help? *J Bone Min Res* 1995; 10:106–111.
42. Peh CA, Horowitz M, Wishart JM, et al. The effect of chorothiazide on bone-related biochemical variables in normal post-menopausal women. *J Am Geriatr Soc* 1995; 41:513–516.
43. Feldkamp M, Jones KL, Ornoy A, et al. Postmarketing surveillance for angiotensin-converting enzyme inhibitor use during the first trimester of pregnancy—United States, Canada and Israel, 1987–1995. *MMWR* 1997; 46:240–242.
44. Os I, Bratland B, Dahlof B, et al. Female sex as an important determinant of lisinopril-induced cough (letter). *Lancet* 1992; 339:372.
45. Walsh ME. Lipids: Natural history and pharmacologic management. In: Charney P, ed. *Coronary Artery Disease in Women.* Philadelphia: American College of Physicians; 1999:101–128.
46. Majumdar SR, Gurwitz JH, Soumerai SB. Undertreatment of hyperlipidemia in the secondary prevention of coronary artery disease. *J Gen Intern Med* 1999; 14:711–717.
47. LaRosa JC, He J, Vupputuri S. Effect of statins on risk of coronary disease: A meta-analysis of randomized controlled trials. *JAMA* 1999; 282:2340–2346.
48. Davidson MH, Testolin LM, Maki KC, et al. A comparison of estrogen replacement, pravastatin, and combined treatment for the management of hypercholesterolemia in postmenopausal women. *Arch Intern Med* 1997; 157:1186–1192.
49. Darling GM, Johns JA, McCloud PI, Davis SR. Estrogen and progestin compared with simvastatin for hypercholesterolemia in postmenopausal women. *N Engl J Med* 1997; 337:595–601.
50. Winkleby M, Kraemer HC, Ahn DK, Varady AN. Ethnic and socioeconomic differences in cardiovascular disease risk factors: Findings for women from the Third National Health and Nutrition Examination Survey, 1988–1994. *JAMA* 1998; 280:356–362.
51. Berenson GS, Charney P, Ramachandaran S, et al. Obesity and other cardiovascular risk factors in young women. In: Charney P, ed. *Coronary Artery Disease in Women: Prevention, Diagnosis and Management.* Philadelphia: American College of Physicians; 1999:188–189.
52. Hennekens CH, Walters EE, Colditz GA, et al. Abdominal adiposity and coronary heart disease in women. *JAMA* 1998; 280 (21):1843–1848.
53. Samaras K, Kelly PJ, Chiano MN, et al. Genetic and environmental influences on total-body and central abdominal fat: The effect of physical activity in female twins. *Ann Intern Med* 1999; 130:873–882.
54. Wilson PWF, Kannel WB, Silbershatz H, D'Agostino RB. Clustering of metabolic factors and coronary heart disease. *Arch Intern Med* 1999; 159:1104–1109.
55. Rexrode KM, Carey VJ, Hennekens CH, Walters EE, et al. Abdominal adiposity and coronary heart disease in women. *JAMA* 1998; 280(21):1843–1848.

56. Andersen RD, Wadden TA, Bartlett SJ, et al. Effects of lifestyle activity vs. structured aerobic exercise in obese women. *JAMA* 1999; 381(4):335–340.
57. Jick H, Vasilakis C, Weinrauch LA, et al. A population-based study of appetite-suppressant drugs and the risk of cardiac-valve regurgitation. *N Engl J Med* 1998; 339(11):719–724.
58. Beniaminovitz A, Mancini D. Congestive heart failure. In: Charney P, ed. *Coronary Artery Disease in Women: Prevention, Diagnosis and Management*. Philadelphia: American College of Physicians; 1999:476–495.
59. Masse LC, Ainsworth BE, Tortolero S, et al. Measuring physical activity in midlife and older and minority women: Issues from an expert panel. *J Women's Health* 1998; 7:57–67.
60. Eaton CB, Reynes J, Assaf AR, et al. Predicting physical activity change in men and women in two New England communities. *Am J Prev Med* 1993; 9:209–219.
61. Fair JM, Berra K, King AC. Excercise as primary and secondary prevention in Charney P, ed. *Coronary Artery Disease in Women: Prevention, Diagnosis and Management*. Philadelphia: American College of Physicians; 1999:209–235.
62. Thomas RJ, Houston Miller N, Lamendola C, et al. National survey on gender differences in cardiac rehabilitation programs. *J Cardiopulm Rehabil* 1996; 16:402–412.
63. Oliver MF, Boyd GS. Effect of bilateral ovariectomy on coronary artery disease and serum lipid levels. *Lancet* 1959; 2:690.
64. Hu FB, Grodstein F, Hennekens CH, et al. Age at natural menopause and risk of cardiovascular disease. *Arch Intern Med* 1999; 159:1061–1066.
65. Blumenthal RS, Bush TL. Hormone replacement therapy and the prevention of coronary artery disease. In: Charney P, ed. *Coronary Artery Disease in Women: Prevention, Diagnosis and Management*. Philadelphia: American College of Physicians; 1999:264–288.
66. Hulley S, Grady D, Bush T, et al. Randomized trial of estrogen plus progestin for secondary prevention of coronary heart disease in postmenopausal women. *JAMA* 1998; 280(7):605–613.
67. Collaborative Group on Hormonal Factors in Breast Cancer. Breast cancer and hormone replacement therapy: Collaborative re-analysis of data from 51 epidemiological studies of 52,705 women with breast cancer and 108,411 women without breast cancer. *Lancet* 1997; 350:1047–1059.
68. Keating NL, Cleary PD, Rossi AS, et al. Use of hormonal replacement therapy by postmenopausal women in the United States. *Ann Intern Med* 1999; 130:545–553.
69. Jacobs SC, Stone PH. Psychosocial isses. In: Charney P, ed. *Coronary Artery Disease in Women*. Philadelphia: American College of Physicians; 1999:496–534.
70. Case RB, Moss AJ, Case N, et al. Living alone after myocardial infarction: Impact on prognosis. *JAMA* 1992; 267(4):515–519.
71. Smith GD, Hart C, Blane D, et al. Lifetime socioeconomic position and mortality: Prospective observational study. *BMJ* 1997; 314:547–552.
72. Williams RB, Barefoot JC, Califf RM, et al. Prognostic importance of social and economic resources among medically treated patients with angiographically documented coronary artery disease. *JAMA* 1992; 267:520–524.
73. Wilkinson RG. *Socioeconomic determinants of health*—Health inequalities: relative or absolute material standards? *BMJ* 1997; 314:591–595.
74. Morrison C, Woodward M, Leslie W, Turnstall-Pedoe H. Effect of socioeconomic group on incidence of, management of, and survival after myocardial infarction and coronary death: Analysis of community coronary event register. *BMJ* 1997; 314:541–546.
75. Bosma H, Marmot MG, Hemingway H, et al. Low job control and risk of coronary heart disease in Whitehall II (prospective cohort) study. *BMJ* 1997; 314:558–565.
76. Marmot MG, Bosma H, Hemingway H, et al. Contribution of job control and other risk factors to social variations in coronary heart disease incidence. *Lancet* 1997; 350:235–239.
77. Jacobs SC, Stone PH. Psychosocial issues. In: Charney P, ed. *Coronary Artery Disease in Women*. Philadelphia: American College of Physicians; 1999:508.
78. Pratt LA, Ford DE, Crum RM, et al. Depression, psychotropic medication, and risk of myocardial infarction: Prospective data from the Baltimore ECA follow-up. *Circulation* 1996; 94:3123–3129.
79. Frasure-Smith N, Lesperance F. Depression following myocardial infarction: Impact on 6-month survival. *JAMA* 1993; 270:1819–1825.
80. Creed F. The importance of depression following myocardial infarction. *Heart* 1999; 82:406–408.
81. Carney RM, Freedland KE, Smith L, et al. Relation of depression and mortality after myocardial infarction in women (letter). *Circulation* 1991; 84(4):1876–1877.
82. Toiler GO, Stone PH, Muller JE, et al. Effects of gender and race on prognosis after myocardial infarction: Adverse prognosis for women, particularly black women. *J Am Coll Cardiol* 1987; 9:473–482.
83. Escobedo LG, Giles WH, Anda RF. Socioeconomic status, race, and death from coronary heart disease. *Am J Prev Med* 1997; 13:123–130.
84. Charney P. Future directions. In: Charney P, ed. *Coronary Artery Disease in Women: Prevention, Diagnosis and Management*. Philadelphia: American College of Physicians; 1999:575–593.
85. Fang J, Madhavan S, Alderman MH. The association between birthplace and mortality from cardiovascular causes among black and white residents of New York City. *N Engl J Med* 1996; 335(21):1545–1551.
86. Shaukat N, Lear J, Lowy A, et al. First myocardial infarction in patients of Indian subcontinent and European origin: Comparison of risk factors, management, and long term outcome. *BMJ* 1997; 314:639–642.
87. Vitelli LL, Crow RS, Shahar E, et al. Electrocardiographic findings in a healthy biracial population. *Am J Cardiol* 1998; 81:453–459.
88. Perez-Stable EJ, Herrera B, Jacob P, Benowitz NL. Nicotene metabolism and intake in black and white smokers. *JAMA* 1998; 280:152–156.
89. Birdwell BG, Herbers JE, Kroenke K. Evaluating chest pain: The patient's presentation style alters the physician's diagnostic approach. *Arch Intern Med* 1993; 153:1991–1995.
90. Schulman KA, Berlin JA, Harless W, et al. The effect of race and sex on physician's recommendations for cardiac catherization. *N Engl J Med* 1999; 340:618–626.
91. Douglas PS, Ginsburg GS. The evaluation of chest pain in women. *N Engl J Med* 1996; 334:1311–1315.
92. Shaw LJ, Peterson ED, Johnson LL. Noninvasive testing techniques for diagnosis and prognosis. In: Charney P, ed. *Coronary Artery Disease in Women*. Philadelphia: American College of Physicians; 1999: 327–350.
93. Kwok Y, Kim C, Grady D, et al. Meta-analysis of excercise testing to detect coronary artery disease in women. *Am J Cardiol* 1999; 83:660–663.
94. Shaw LJ, Peterson ED, Johnson LL. Noninvasive testing techniques for diagnosis and prognosis. In: Charney P, ed. *Coronary Artery Disease in Women*. Philadelphia: American College of Physicians; 1999:327–350.
95. Okin PM, Kligfield P. Gender-specific criteria and performance of the exercise electrocardiogram. *Circulation* 1995; 92(5):1209–1216.
96. Shaw LJ, Peterson ED, Johnson LL. Noninvasive testing techniques for diagnosis and prognosis. In: Charney P, ed. *Coronary Artery Disease in Women*. Philadelphia: American College of Physicians; 1999:341–345.

97. Marwick TH, Miller DD. Influence of gender on the referral of patients to and from coronary angiography. In: Charney P, ed. *Coronary Artery Disease in Women*. Philadelphia: American College of Physicians; 1999:354–356.
98. Weiner DA, Ryan TJ, McCabe CH, et al. Exercise stress testing: Correlations among history of angina, ST segment response and prevalence of coronary artery disease in the Coronary Artery Surgery Study (CASS). *N Engl J Med* 1979; 301:230–235.
99. Lerner DS, Kannel W. Patterns of heart disease morbidity and mortality in the sexes: A 26-year follow-up of the Framingham population. *Am Heart J* 1986; 111:383–390.
100. Kannel WB, Abbott RD. Incidence and prognosis of myocardial infarction in women: The Framingham study. In: Eaker ED, Packard B, Wenger NK, et al., eds. *Coronary Heart Disease in Women: Proceedings of an NIH Workshop*. New York: Haymark Doyma; 1987:208–214.
101. Mosca L, Grundy SM, Judelson D, et al. Guide to preventive cardiology for women. *Circulation* 1999; 99:2480–2484.
102. Turnstall-Pedoe H, Woodward M, Tavendale R, et al. Comparison of the prediction by 27 different factors of coronary heart disease and death in men and women of the Scottish heart health study: A cohort study. *BMJ* 1997; 315:722–729.
103. Lowe LP, Greenland P, Ruth RJ, et al. Impact of major cardiovascular disease risk factors, particularly in combination, on 22-year mortality in women and men. *Arch Intern Med* 1988; 158:2007–2014.
104. Goldberg RJ, Larson M, Levy D. Factors associated with survival to 75 years of age in middle-aged men and women. *Arch Intern Med* 1996; 156:505–509.
105. Daviglus ML, Kiang L, Greenland P, et al. Benefit of a favorable cardiovascular risk-factor profile in middle age with respect to medicare costs. *N Engl J Med* 1998; 339:1122–1129.
106. Hubert HB, Eaker ED, Garrison R, Castelli WP. Life-style correlates of risk factor change in young adults: An eight-year study of coronary heart disease risk factors in the Framingham offspring. *Am J Epdemiol* 1987; 125(5):812–831.
107. Stamler J, Stamler R, Neaton JD, et al. Low risk-factor profile and long-term cardiovascular and noncardiovascular mortality and life expectancy: Findings for 5 large cohorts of young adults and middle-aged men and women. *JAMA* 1999; 282:2012–2018.
108. Grover SA, Paquet S, Levinton C, et al. Estimating the benefits of modifying risk factors of cardiovascular disease: A comparison of primary and secondary prevention. *Arch Intern Med* 1998; 158:655–662.
109. Perlman JA, Wolf PH, Ray R, Lieberknecht G. Cardiovascular risk factors, premature heart disease, and all-cause mortality in a cohort of Northern California women. *Am J Obstet Gynecol* 1988; 158:1568–1574.
110. Newnham HH, Silberberg J. Women's hearts are hard to break. *Lancet* 1997; 349:sl3–sl16.
111. Pepine CJ, Abrams J, Marks RG, et al. Characteristics of a contemporary population with angina pectoris: TIDES investigators. *Am J Cardiol* 1994; 74:226–231.
112. Del Valle N, Frishman WH, Charney P. Angina pectoris. In: Charney P, ed. *Coronary Artery Disease in Women*. Philadelphia: American College of Physicians; 1999:373–400.
113. Mohri M, Koyanagi M, Egashira K, et al. Angina pectoris caused by coronary microvascular spasm. *Lancet* 1998; 351:1165–1169.
114. Chandra NC, Ziegelstein RC, Rogers WJ, et al. Observations of the treatment of women in the United States with myocardial infarction: A report from the National Registry of Myocardial Infarction–I. *Arch Intern Med* 1998; 158:981–988.
115. Marrugat JM, Sala J, Masia R, et al. Mortality differences between men and women following first myocardial infarction. *JAMA* 1998; 280:1405–1409.
116. Hochman JS, Tamis J, Thompson TD, et al. Sex, clinical presentation, and outcome in patients with acute coronary syndromes. *N Engl J Med* 1999; 341:226–232.
117. Vaccarino V, Parsons L, Every NR, et al. Sex-based differences in early mortality after myocardial infarction. *N Engl J Med* 1999; 341:217–225.
118. Burke AP, Farb A, Malcolm GT, et al. Effect of risk factors on the mechanism of acute thrombosis and sudden death in women. *Circulation* 1998; 97:2110–2116.
119. Oparil S. Pathophysiology of sudden coronary death in women: Implications for prevention. *Circulation* 1998: 97:2103–2104.
120. Collins LJ, Douglas PS. Acute coronary syndromes. In: Charney P, ed. *Coronary Artery Disease in Women*. Philadelphia: American College of Physicians; 1999:407–413.
121. Collins LJ, Douglas PS. Acute coronary syndromes. In: Charney P, ed. *Coronary Artery Disease in Women*. Philadelphia: American College of Physicians; 1999:420–422.
122. Bickell NA, Pieper KS, Lee KL, et al. Referral patterns for coronary artery disease treatment: Gender bias or good clinical judgement. *Ann Intern Med* 1992; 116:791–797.
123. Ommen SR, Holmes DR Jr, Bell MR. Percutaneous transluminal coronary angioplasty. In: Charney P, ed. *Coronary Artery Disease in Women*. Philadelphia: American College of Physicians; 1999:463–475.
124. Hartz RS, Charney P. Coronary artery bypass grafting: Is it worth the risk? In: Charney P, ed. *Coronary Artery Disease in Women*. Philadelphia: American College of Physicians; 1999:438–462.
125. Mickleborough L, Takagi Y, Murayama H, et al. Is sex a factor in determining operative risk for aortocoronary bypass? *Circulation* 1995; 90(suppl II):80–84.
126. Moore S. A comparison of women's and men's symptoms during home recovery after coronary artery bypass surgery. *Heart Lung* 1995; 24:495–501.
127. Ai AL, Peterson C, Dunkle RE, et al. How gender affects psychological adjustment one year after coronary artery bypass surgery. *Womens Health* 1997; 26:45–65.
128. Krueger DE, Ellenberg SS, Bloom S, et al. Risk factors for fatal heart attack in young women. *Am J Epidemiol* 1981; 113(4): 357–370.
129. Makkar RR, Fromm BS, Steinman RT, et al. Female gender as a risk factor for torsades de pointes associated with cardiovascular drugs. *JAMA* 1993; 270:2590–2597.
130. Drici D, Knollmann BC, Wang W-X, Woosley RL. Cardiac actions of erythromycin: Influence of female sex. *JAMA* 1998; 280:1774–1776.
131. Stein PK, Kleiger RE, Rottman JN. Differing effects of age on heart rate variability in men and women. *Am J Cardiol* 1997; 80:302–305.
132. Burke JH, Ehlert FA, Kruse JT, et al. Gender-specific differences in the QT interval and the effect of autonomic tone and menstrual cycle in healthy adults. *Am J Cardiol* 1997; 79:178–181.
133. Lochen ML, Snaprud T, Zhang W, Rasmussen K. Arrhythmias in subjects with and without a history of palpitations: The Tromso study. *Eur Heart J* 1994; 15:345–349.
134. Weber BE, Kapoor WN. Evaluation and outcomes of patients with palpitations. *Am J Med* 1996; 100(2):138–148.
135. Schuppel R, Buchele G, Batz L, Koenig W. Sex differences in selection of pacemakers: Retrospective observation study. *BMJ* 1988; 316:492–495.

PART FIFTEEN

DISEASES OF THE GREAT VESSELS AND PERIPHERAL VESSELS

C H A P T E R 88

DIAGNOSIS AND TREATMENT OF DISEASES OF THE AORTA

Joseph Lindsay, Jr.

Structurally a simple conduit, the aorta can manifest disease in only a limited number of ways. When weakened by disease, its wall may dilate, producing an aneurysm, or it may split in its long axis, producing dissection. In either case, fatal rupture may result. Moreover, like all pipes, it may become obstructed. More often than narrowing of the main trunk, however, obstruction at the origin of a main branch is encountered. In contrast to these relatively few clinical manifestations, an array of disease processes can involve the aorta. Not surprisingly, there is considerable overlap in the clinical presentation of these disorders.

This chapter will first discuss the various diseases that involve the aorta together with their pathogenetic mechanisms, characteristic pathologic features, and typical clinical findings. A description of the common clinical manifestations of aortic disease for which there may be several etiologies or for which the etiology is unknown will follow.

ETIOLOGIC AND PATHOGENETIC CONSIDERATIONS IN AORTIC DISEASE

Medial Changes of Aging

Circumferential plates or lamellae of elastin fibers constitute the most conspicuous feature of the aortic media when it is examined histologically. Dispersed between the circular elastic fibers are longitudinally oriented smooth muscle cells, collagen fibers, microfibrils, and ground substance.[1]

Clinicians have long recognized dilatation and elongation of the aorta in the elderly. Characteristic alterations in the structure of the aortic wall accompany these changes. Schlatmann and Becker[2] identified these as fragmentation of elastic fibers and loss of smooth muscle cell nuclei, so-called medionecrosis. Moreover, collagenous tissue and basophilic ground substance deposits are a feature of the aging aorta.[3]

Aortic Atherosclerosis

PATHOLOGIC ANATOMY

By middle life, aortic atherosclerosis is nearly universal in the Western world. Its severity varies from individual to individual. Diabetes, hypercholesterolemia, smoking, and hypertension are among the factors promoting it. The pathology of atherosclerosis is discussed in Chap. 35.

Advanced atherosclerotic changes display a characteristic distribution, and involvement is most severe below the renal arteries in the abdominal aorta, is common but less severe in the descending thoracic segment, and is least severe in the ascending segment.[4] With diabetes mellitus, however, disease is frequently severe throughout. Individuals with familial hypercholesterolemia are a second exception to the rule that the ascending aorta is spared.[5] Also, the aortic root and aortic valve may be severely involved in familial cholesterolemia. Both supravalvular and valvular aortic stenosis may develop.[6] Finally, syphilitic ascending aortitis promotes severe atherosclerosis.

CLINICAL MANIFESTATIONS

Aortic atherosclerosis is manifest as aneurysm, obstruction of the infrarenal aorta, embolization from atheromatous plaques to distal arterial beds, and medial dissection initiated by penetration of a plaque into the media.

Aneurysm Aneurysm of the abdominal aorta has long been presumed to result from penetration into and weakening of the media by atherosclerosis. Thus abdominal aortic aneurysms characteristically appear in individuals with the most severe aortic atherosclerosis in nonaneurysmal segments.[7]

Recent recognition of familial clustering of patients with abdominal aortic aneurysm,[8] the identification of genetic defects in collagen in a family with multiple aneurysms,[9] and the detection of abnormal collagenase and elastase in tissue from aortic aneurysms resected at operation have led some to the assumption that atherosclerosis is invariably the underlying pathophysiologic mechanism. These findings suggest that atherosclerosis represents a secondary response to dilatation of the aorta resulting from medial weakness.[10] This debate will be discussed in greater detail below. Aneurysm of the descending thoracic aorta also traditionally has been attributed to atherosclerosis, since such lesions are commonly accompanied by an infrarenal aneurysm.

Obstruction of the Terminal Aorta. Obstruction of the main aortic channel most often develops in the infrarenal aorta and may extend into the proximal iliac arteries. Obstruction of branch arteries is more common than aortic obstruction.

Atheroembolism The luminal surface of a severely diseased aortic segment is often rough and covered with thrombus. Embolization of plaque material and thrombus from these surfaces now appears to be far more common than was once appreciated.[11–14] Emboli to the brain, the lower extremities, and the coronary, renal, or visceral circulations have been reported.

Transesophageal echocardiography now provides rather startling views of pedunculated thrombus or other atherosclerotic material waving in the aortic blood flow[12] (Fig. 88-1). Aortas with ulcerated plaques, pedunculated or mobile thrombi, or spontaneous echo contrast are more apt to embolize than are those with flat, layered atherosclerosis.[13] Anticoagulant therapy may be protective against future events.[14]

A variation on the theme, the clinical syndrome labeled *cholesterol embolization,* with small atherosclerotic particles obstructing small arteries, is a rare complication of severe aortic atherosclerosis. Clinical signs include mottled skin and "purple toes" in the lower extremities together with renal insufficiency and visceral ischemia in more severe cases.[15] This rarely recognized condition may be spontaneous but is more commonly encountered as a complication of intraaortic catheter manipulation. Because eosinophilia is frequent in the initial phases of this event, an immune reaction to the free particles has been suggested.

Penetrating Atherosclerotic Ulcers Atherosclerotic plaque penetration into the media predisposes to formation of an intramural hematoma.[16] Extension circumferentially and in the long axis of the media may produce a limited medial dissection (Fig. 88-2). Radial extension results in pseudoaneurysm or rupture. Penetrating ulcers are most commonly recognized in the descending thoracic aorta.

The clinical picture resembles that of aortic dissection or of expansion/rupture of a preexisting aneurysm. Sudden onset of severe back pain in a hypertensive patient or one known to have atherosclerosis is typical. Many are identified in the course of imaging for suspected aortic dissection. Since they are more limited in axial length than typical dissection, and since they are located in the descending thoracic aorta, aortic regurgitation and altered pulses are not characteristic features. Surgical treatment is often indicated, although some patients survive without operation.[16]

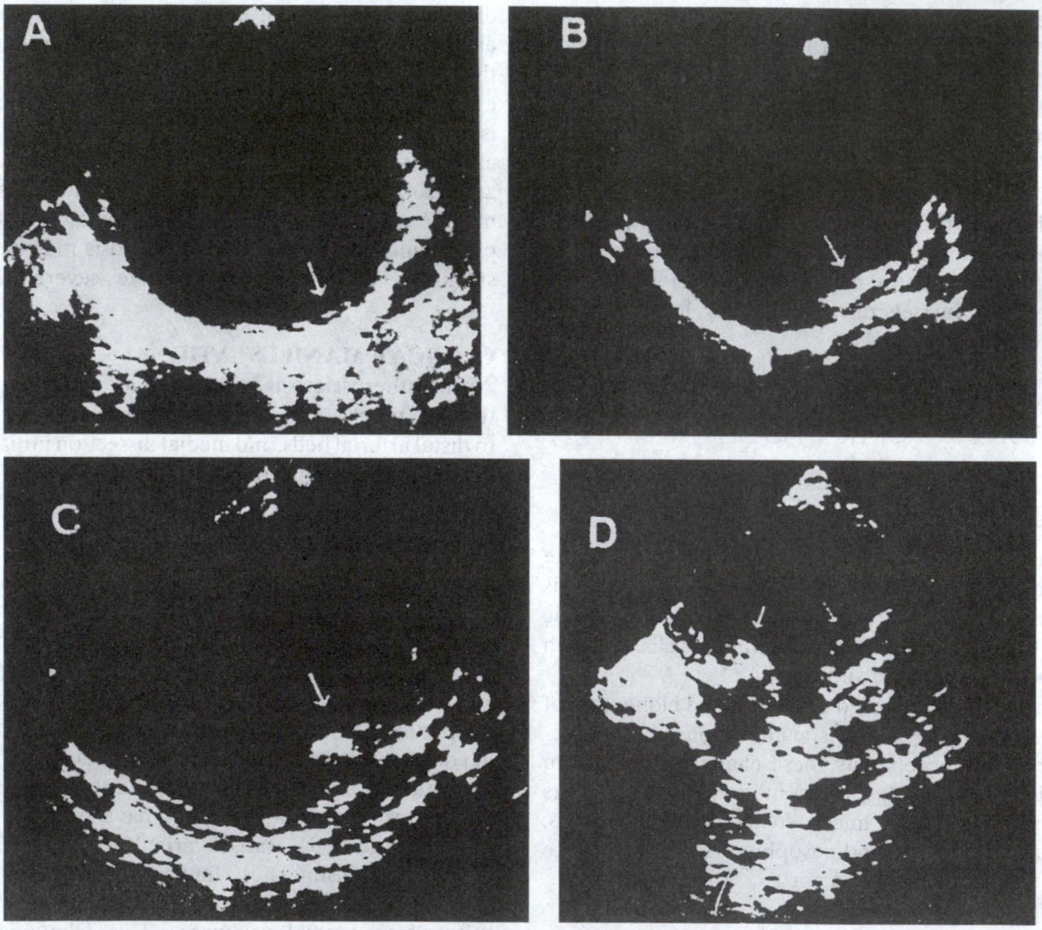

FIGURE 88-1 Panels from transesophageal echocardiographic examinations of the descending thoracic aorta in four patients. Varying degrees of atherosclerotic plaquing are illustrated. A minimal degree is shown in *A* (*upper left*) and a more severe but still moderate degree in *B* (*upper right*). *C* and *D* demonstrate protruding plaques, the configuration with the most serious threat of embolization. (From Lindsay J Jr et al. Diseases of the aorta. In: Schlant RC, Alexander AW, Lipton MJ, eds. *Diagnostic Atlas of the Heart*. New York: McGraw-Hill, 1996:319. Reproduced with permission from the publisher and authors.)

Abnormalities of the Aortic Media

The occurrence of aneurysm and medial dissection reflects a defective aortic media. Although often a component of an acquired process such as atherosclerosis or panaortitis, medial weakness may be genetically determined. Such is the case in aortic disease in a variety of congenital syndromes (e.g., bicuspid aortic valve, coarctation of the aorta) and in heritable disorders of connective tissue (e.g., Marfan's syndrome, polycystic kidney disease, Turner's syndrome, and Ehlers-Danlos syndrome).[17]

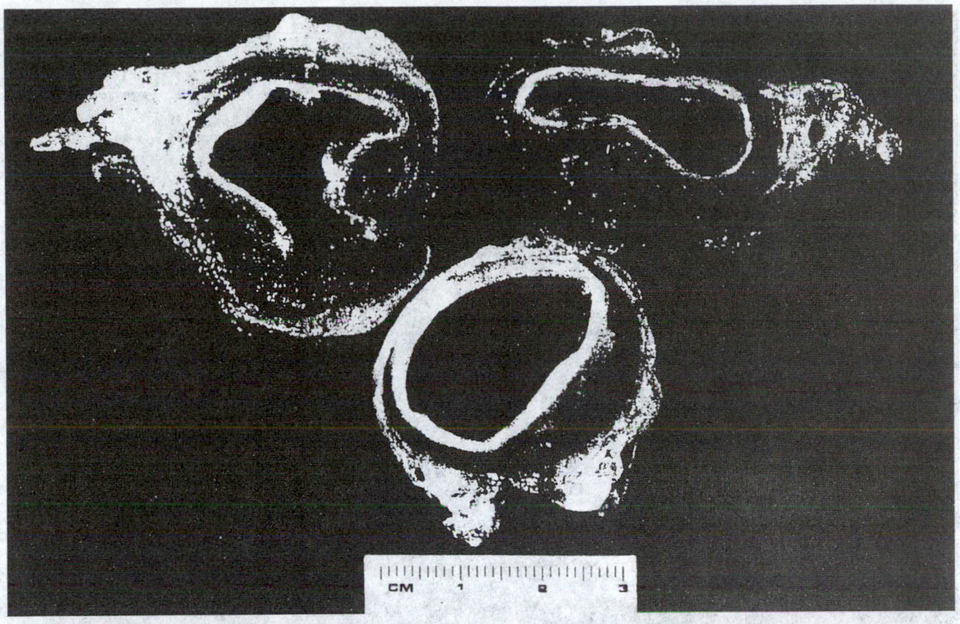

FIGURE 88-2 A necropsy specimen from an elderly woman who died suddenly after having severe back pain suspicious of aortic dissection. It demonstrates a penetrating atherosclerotic plaque (*upper left*) providing communication from the aortic lumen to an adjacent medial hematoma (*bottom*). An aortogram had been negative for dissection, but transesophageal echocardiography revealed the medial hematoma. (From Lindsay J Jr et al. Diseases of the aorta. In: Schlant RC, Alexander AW, Lipton MJ, eds. *Diagnostic Atlas of the Heart*. New York: McGraw-Hill, 1996:321. Reproduced with permission from the publisher and authors.)

CYSTIC MEDIAL DEGENERATION

Microscopic changes in the aortic media, termed *cystic medial necrosis* by Erdheim, were long thought to be diagnostic of medial degeneration. They were identified in Marfan's syndrome, in other instances of aortic aneurysm or dissection,[18,19] and in a variety of familial or congenital syndromes.[17] The features include fragmentation of elastic fibers, disappearance of the nuclei of smooth muscle cells, increase in collagenous fibers, and most characteristically, replacement of the degenerated tissue with interstitial collections ("cysts") of basophilic-staining ground substance.

The fundamental nature of this lesion has been questioned. Hirst and Gore[20] pointed out that the lesion was neither cystic nor necrotic. Recent detailed histologic studies of the media in aortic dissection have failed to demonstrate a close association with this marker of medial degeneration.[21] Schlatmann and Becker[2,19] suggest that qualitatively similar lesions are common with aging, albeit more common and more severe in patients with Marfan's syndrome, with dilatation of the aorta from any cause, or with aortic dissection. They proposed that the observed changes reflect hemodynamic stress. It is noteworthy that the presence of this lesion has been reported in aortas with coarctation of the aorta.[22] Thus, although clearly defective in many cases of aortic aneurysm or dissection, the aortic media often reveals no specific histologic lesion, and the focus now is on subcellular and molecular abnormalities.[17,23] A defect in a microfibrillar constituent of the matrix protein, fibrillin, has been identified in the Marfan's syndrome, and the responsible gene has been identified.[24]

CLINICAL MANIFESTATIONS

Marfan's Syndrome A characteristic aneurysm of the proximal aorta is the cardiovascular hallmark of Marfan's syndrome.[17,18] Aneurysmal dilatation of the ascending aorta extends proximally into the aortic sinuses and ends distally just short of the innominate artery. The result is a "Florence flask" or "onion bulb" deformity. The descriptive term *anuloaortic ectasia* has been applied.[18] Rupture of such aneurysms or the hemodynamic effects of aortic regurgitation, from aortic root dilatation, are responsible for most of the premature deaths from this disorder. Localized or extensive medial dissection is another calamitous complication.

In the most complete presentation of Marfan's syndrome, skeletal, ocular, and cardiovascular anomalies are present, and a family history of similar abnormalities exists[17,18] (see Chaps. 10 and 76). Long extremities, particularly long, thin, hands and feet (arachnodactyly), and sparse muscle mass are typical. Subluxed or frankly dislocated lenses attributable to lax supporting ligaments are characteristic. In addition, myxomatous transformation of the aortic and mitral valves may produce valvular incompetence. Exceptionally, medial degeneration severe enough to result in aneurysm, rupture, or dissection is found in the main pulmonary arteries or in the aorta distal to the ascending segment.

Medial Degeneration Associated with Congenital Aortic or Aortic Valvular Deformity Ascending aortic aneurysm, often in the form of anuloaortic ectasia, and aortic dissection are reported frequently in patients with congenitally deformed aortic valves. The risk of aortic dissection has been estimated to be increased ninefold in subjects with bicuspid or unicuspid valves.[25] There is echocardiographic evidence for increased prevalence of dilatation of the aortic root and ascending aorta in subjects with a biscupid aortic valve[26] (Fig. 88-3). Patients with coarctation are at risk for aortic aneurysm, dissection, and rupture.[17] The strong association of bicuspid aortic valve with

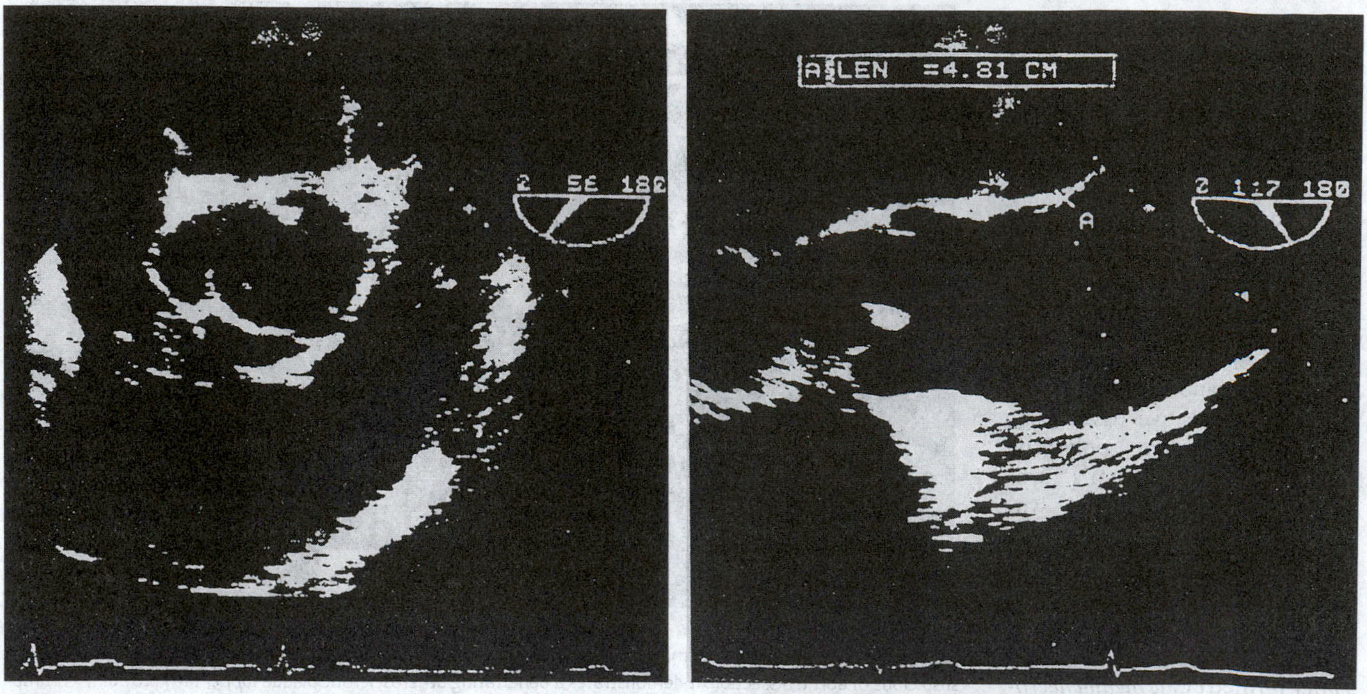

FIGURE 88-3 Transesophageal echocardiographic examination from a patient with bicuspid aortic valve (*left panel*) demonstrating the commonly associated dilatation of the aortic root. (From Lindsay J Jr. Diseases of the aortic root. *Heart Dis Stroke* 1994; 3:377. Reproduced with permission from the publisher and author.)

coarctation, together with clinical observations, is a foundation for the hypothesis that there may be a specific, perhaps genetic medial defect in this spectrum of disease.[27] The fact that Turner's syndrome, with which bicuspid aortic valve, coarctation of the aorta, and aortic dissection are strongly associated bolsters this possibility.[28]

Medial Degeneration in Heritable Disorders of Connective Tissue Reports linking polycystic kidney disease,[29,30] Ehlers-Danlos syndrome,[31] and osteogenesis imperfecta[32] with aortic aneurysm and dissection further support the idea that medial degeneration may have a genetic basis.

Isolated Anuloaortic Ectasia While dilatation of the aortic root and ascending aorta occurs in association with a variety of heritable disorders, it is far more often encountered in individuals with no other manifest disease.[18,33] Isolated anuloaortic ectasia is the most frequent cause of aortic regurgitation requiring valve replacement[34] and is responsible for significant numbers of fatal ruptures or dissections. The finding of fibrillin gene mutations in three patients with anuloaortic ectasia without complete Marfan phenotype suggests that genetic defects of the media may underlie many of these cases.[35]

Infectious Aortitis

A variety of bacterial, mycobacterial, and fungal organisms may infect the walls of the aorta. Microorganisms may gain a foothold through several mechanisms: (1) seeding of the vasa vasorum during hematogenous spread, (2) direct invasion of the wall from the aortic lumen (usually in previously diseased segments or at prosthetic grafts), (3) septic emboli (usually from infective endocarditis) that lodge at a branch point, (4) spread of infection from contiguous structures (e.g., infected cardiac valves or tuberculous periaortic nodes), and (5) traumatic aortic injury with subsequent infection.[36]

SYPHILITIC AORTITIS

Epidemiology Alone among the infectious aortic diseases, treponemal infection produces a chronic aortitis. Clinically evident involvement of the cardiovascular system occurs in about 10 percent of patients with untreated tertiary syphilis of long duration and is the primary cause of death in about the same percentage.[37] Autopsy evidence of the process is more frequent. About half of patients with untreated syphilis for more than 10 years have autopsy evidence of cardiovascular involvement.[37]

Pathology During the spirochetemic phase of primary syphilis, *Treponema pallidum* organisms lodge in the adventitia of the vasa vasorum and initiate an inflammatory response, characteristically a perivascular lymphocytic and plasma cell infiltrate. Later, an obliterative endarteritis develops, resulting in patchy medial necrosis and elastic fiber fragmentation and leading to weakening of the aortic wall and predisposition to aneurysm formation. The intima of the aorta has a characteristic wrinkled appearance, with atherosclerotic plaques frequently superimposed, obscuring the wrinkling and giving the so-called tree bark appearance. Because the infection is seeded through the vasa vasorum, the process is most severe in the ascending aorta and the arch, where vasa density is highest.

Clinical Manifestations *Syphilitic aortitis may present in four ways:*[37] *asymptomatic aortitis, aortic regurgitation, coronary ostial stenosis, and aortic aneurysm.* Asymptomatic aortitis may be unrecognized until necropsy but sometimes can be identified from chest x-ray by linear calcium deposits in the ascending aorta. Aortic regurgitation, present in about 20 to 30 percent of patients with syphilitic aortitis,[37] results primarily from dilatation of the aortic root. Coronary arterial ostial stenosis occurs in 25 to 30 percent of syphilitic aortitis patients, and as many as 85 percent have associated aortic regurgitation.[37] Interestingly, while angina is common in patients with syphilitic ostial stenosis, myocardial infarction is rare.

Aneurysm, the least common manifestation of syphilitic aortitis, is present in 5 to 10 percent of affected patients.[37] About 75 percent are saccular and 25 percent are fusiform. Half are located in the ascending aorta, 30 to 40 percent in the transverse arch, 10 to 15 percent in the proximal descending thoracic aorta, and fewer than 5 percent in the abdominal aorta. Rarely, syphilis causes aneurysm of a sinus of Valsalva. When not treated surgically, syphilitic aortic aneurysms are associated with a 2-year mortality of 80 percent.[37] Thus operation is warranted in patients with large syphilitic aortic aneurysms.

Although antibiotics are indicated for all patients with cardiovascular syphilis, it is unclear if treatment slows progression of syphilitic aortic disease.

Diagnosis The diagnosis of cardiovascular syphilis may be difficult, especially in patients over age 50, when many of the effects of syphilis are mimicked by hypertensive and atherosclerotic disease. Serology can be helpful. Between 40 and 95 percent of patients with cardiovascular syphilis have an elevated venereal disease research laboratory (VDRL) titer, and nearly all have a positive fluorescent treponemal antibody absorption (FTA-ABS) test.[37] Rare, untreated patients have no serologic evidence of the disease. *Thus cardiovascular syphilis must be considered in patients with aortic regurgitation and dilatation of the aortic root, aneurysms of the thoracic aorta, and ostial coronary arterial narrowing (especially when accompanied by aortic regurgitation).* Fortunately, the frequency of cardiovascular syphilis has fallen dramatically over recent decades due to early identification and treatment of the disease.

BACTERIAL AORTITIS COMPLICATING BLOOD-BORNE INFECTIONS

Bacterial aortitis most often presents as an infection of a preexisting aneurysm. Less frequently, the infection may be responsible for initiating an aneurysm or a false aneurysm.

Salmonella species and *Staphylococcus aureus* are the most frequent of a wide spectrum of invading organisms.[38,39] Infections of prosthetic graft material result from agents similar to those causing infective endocarditis (see Chap. 73).

Salmonella organisms have a strong proclivity for invading vascular endothelium. Cohen et al.[40] found a 25 percent prevalence of endothelial infection (arteritis or endocarditis) in patients over age 50 with nontyphoidal *Salmonella* bacteremia. Endothelial invasion was uncommon in patients under age 50 probably because of a lower prevalence of atherosclerosis to serve as a nidus. Thus antibiotic treatment has been recommended for acute *Salmonella* gastroenteritis in patients over age 50.[40]

Clinical Manifestations and Diagnosis Diagnosis of infectious aortitis or aneurysm can be elusive and relies heavily on clinical suspicion prompting further evaluation.[41,42] Symptoms are nonspecific. In abdominal aortic infections, abdominal, back, or flank pain is prominent, whereas chest or shoulder pain is more characteristic of thoracic aortic infections.[43] Physical findings include fever in nearly all patients[44] and a pulsatile abdominal mass in nearly half. Leukocytosis is very common,[44] as are positive blood cultures. In patients with *Salmonella* aortic infection, 83 percent had positive blood cultures and 74 percent had positive stool cultures, even though only a third had gastroenteritis.[43]

There are no specific diagnostic studies for aortic infection. Abdominal ultrasound and computed tomography (CT) are useful to identify an aneurysm and occasionally to show periaortic inflammation or mass. Noncalcified aneurysms and aneurysms with smooth walls seen on aortography or CT scanning are characteristic of an infectious process.[36] Often the diagnosis requires surgery and even at operation may be questionable.

Thus the diagnosis of aortic infection is made most often on the basis of a compatible clinical picture and supporting, if not conclusive, diagnostic tests. Unexplained fever, leukocytosis, and bacteremia (especially Salmonella species) in a patient with a high likelihood of having atherosclerosis should prompt a thorough search for evidence of aortic infection and may be sufficient reason for operative exploration.

Treatment *Infections of the aorta almost always lead to fatal aortic rupture unless treated surgically.* Antibiotics alone are not sufficient. The specific surgical approach is dictated primarily by the extent of involvement of periaortic tissue. If the aortic bed is relatively clean, excision and simple interposition grafting is acceptable. If periaortic infection is widespread, then extraanatomic grafting (e.g., axillobifemoral, thoracic aortobifemoral) is necessary.[41] Some have recommended that essentially all patients with aortic infection be treated, at least initially, with extraanatomic grafting.[36]

INFECTIOUS AORTITIS RESULTING FROM CONTIGUOUS SPREAD

Tuberculous aortitis most often results from spread from infected periaortic nodes. False aneurysm, perforation, or aortoenteric fistula[45,46] may result.

An infection of the aortic valve may invade the valve ring and adjacent structures, producing a perivalvular abscess (sometimes called a *valve ring abscess*). This complication of aortic valvular endocarditis is frequent, especially when infecting organisms are virulent or when patients with prosthetic valves are affected.[47,48] Perivalvular abscesses may compress adjacent structures or rupture into the pericardial space. If the abscess drains into the aortic lumen, a false aneurysm of a sinus of Valsalva may result.[49] Moreover, abscesses may disrupt attachment of the aortic media to the fibrous skeleton of the heart, producing fistulous communications.[48,49]

Nonspecific Aortitis

Narrowing of an aortic segment or of one of its branches, aneurysm formation, or aortic regurgitation may be produced by an arteritis for which no specific etiology can been found. It may occur as an isolated abnormality or be associated with noninfectious inflammatory involvement of other organs as in, for example, lupus erythematosus or rheumatoid arthritis.

TAKAYASU'S DISEASE

The prototypical nonspecific aortitis, Takayasu's arteritis, was named for the Japanese ophthalmologist who first called attention to the funduscopic findings of the disease.[50] Because of its predilection for the brachiocephalic vessels, this arteritis has been labeled *pulseless disease* and *aortic arch syndrome.* The classic form occurs with the greatest frequency in the Orient; however, patients with a similar nonspecific aortitis are encountered worldwide.[51] Whether they represent similar or identical diseases is uncertain.

The description to follow will focus on the prototypical illness described in the Orient. The reader may infer that variations on the theme will be encountered elsewhere.[52]

Etiology The etiology of Takayasu's arteritis is unknown. No infectious agent has been identified, but data support the presence of an "autoimmune" process.[53] Antiendothelial antibodies were identified recently in 18 of 19 patients.[54] A genetic predisposition has been postulated because of clustering of the disorder and of similar histocompatability antigens.[55]

Pathology Histologic examination discloses a granulomatous arteritis during active stages of the disease that is similar to giant cell arteritis and to the aortitis associated with seronegative spondylitis. In later stages, medial degeneration, fibrous scarring, intimal proliferation, and thrombosis result in narrowing of the vessel. Aneurysm formation is observed less commonly than are stenosis and aortic rupture or dissection.

Distribution of stenoses has been defined angiographically.[52] The left subclavian artery, particularly in its midportion, is narrowed in about 90 percent of patients. The right subclavian, the left carotid, and the brachiocephalic trunk follow closely in frequency of stenosis. Thoracic aortic lesions are seen in two-thirds of patients,[52] whereas the abdominal aorta is involved in half, and aortoiliac involvement is present in only 12 percent. Pulmonary arteritis is present in about half of patients. Pulmonary hypertension may be found at catheterization.

Clinical Features Manifestations of the illness appear during the second or third decade in 70 to 80 percent of instances, but it has been reported in childhood and in middle life. Women are eight or nine times more often affected than men.[50–52]

During the early or "prepulseless" period of the illness, constitutional manifestations (e.g., fever, night sweats, malaise, nausea and vomiting, weight loss, arthralgia, and skin rash) are encountered frequently. The patient may experience Raynaud's phenomenon, and splenomegaly may be found on examination. Laboratory study may disclose an elevated erythrocyte sedimentation rate, anemia, and serum protein abnormalities.[50–52]

Claudication or numbness of an upper extremity due to subclavian artery narrowing and evidence of ischemia of the central nervous system occur frequently. Postural dizziness or frank syncope usually reflects cerebral ischemia due to narrowing of the brachiocephalic arteries.[50–52,56]

Hypertension, observed in more than half of aortitis patients, is usually associated with narrowing of the renal arteries or of the aorta proximal to those branches. Difficulty may be encountered in accurately measuring arterial pressure because of arch vessel stenosis.

Cardiac manifestations may result from aortic regurgitation, coronary artery narrowing, or severe hypertension. Dilatation of the aortic root commonly accompanies the aortic valve incompetence. Angina pectoris, heart failure, and myocardial infarction are reported. Pericarditis has been observed clinically, but more commonly healed pericarditis is noted at necropsy.

The retinopathy to which Takayasu first directed attention is believed to result from ischemia of the retina. Ocular ischemia also may be manifested by transient loss of vision, cataracts, corneal opacity, and iridial atrophy. Blindness is a common complication.

Involvement of the visceral arteries occasionally results in splanchnic ischemia, and intermittent claudication due to aortoiliac obstruction may occur.

Recently, attention has been directed toward the special problems that may arise during pregnancy in patients with this disorder.[57] Hypertension is frequent. Good outcomes can result with meticulous obstetrical care.

Diagnosis The American College of Rheumatology has identified *six major criteria for the diagnosis of Takayasu's arteritis.*[58] *Onset of illness by the age of 40 years* was recommended as an obligatory criterion to avoid overlap with patients having giant cell arteritis. Others include *upper extremity claudication, diminished brachial pulses, a 10-mmHg or more difference between the systolic blood pressure in the two arms, a subclavian or aortic bruit, and identification of narrowing of the aorta or a major branch. Identification in a patient of three of these six criteria is associated with high diagnostic sensitivity and specificity.*

Prognosis One-third to one-quarter of patients with severe aortitis at diagnosis will have a significant event or will die within 5 years. Those with few or no ischemic complications at the time of diagnosis fare better and have a good 5- and 10-year outlook. Severe hypertension or cardiac involvement predicts a shortened life expectancy.[56]

Cerebrovascular accidents and blindness are the most common major events. Congestive heart failure and aortic rupture or dissection are less frequent.

Management Adrenocorticoids appear to be effective in suppressing the inflammation of the active phase.[59,60] Immunosuppressive therapy also has been used. Operative treatment may relieve symptoms from arterial obstruction, and percutaneous angioplasty has been used with favorable initial results.[61]

GIANT CELL ARTERITIS

Giant cell arteritis (temporal arteritis, polymyalgia rheumatica) involves extracranial arteries, including the aorta in 10 to 13 percent of cases. Its peak incidence in late life seems to set it apart from other varieties of nonspecific arteritis. Like them, it may produce narrowing of the brachiocephalic arteries, aneurysm of the ascending aorta, aortic regurgitation, and aortic dissection.[62] Unlike Takayasu's arteritis, giant cell arteritis rarely involves the descending thoracic or abdominal aorta.

AORTITIS IN HLA-B27–ASSOCIATED SPONDYLOARTHROPATHIES

Although the etiology of neither ankylosing spondylitis nor Reiter's syndrome is known, more than 90 percent of afflicted individuals have the histocompatibility antigen HLA-B27, which is infrequent in the general population. This observation may provide a clue to a common pathogenetic mechanism.[63]

Aortitis has been demonstrated to accompany a sizable minority of patients with these disorders,[64] especially in those with spondylitis of long duration, in those with peripheral joint complaints in addition to spondylitis, and in patients with associated iritis. Aortitis may be present in some patients with HLA-B27 who are not afflicted with spondyloarthropathy and manifests as lone aortic regurgitation or conduction abnormalities,[63] findings reasonably attributable to inflammation of the aortic root and surrounding regions.

Histologically, the inflammatory aortic lesion in this setting resembles that of syphilis. Focal destruction of the medial elastic tissue is seen. The intima and adventitia, but not the media, are thickened. An obliterative arteritis of the vasa vasorum may be detected.[64]

Unlike syphilis, the process is largely limited to the aortic wall behind and immediately above the sinuses of Valsalva and may extend below the aortic valve to involve the membranous ventricular septum and the base of the anterior leaflet of the mitral valve.[64] The aortic valve cusps are thickened and retracted and their edges rolled. Transesophageal echocardiography shows more thickening of the aortic wall than dilatation.[65]

As in syphilis, aortic regurgitation is the most frequent clinical manifestation of these forms of aortitis. Extension into the interventricular septum occasionally results in atrioventricular conduction abnormalities. Either condition may be severe and life-threatening.

Congenital Anomalies of the Aorta

Aortic arch anomalies and the complex congenital conditions manifest in infancy or early childhood are discussed in Chap. 63. Coarctation of the aorta and sinus of Valsalva aneurysms are discussed below.

CLINICAL MANIFESTATIONS OF AORTIC DISEASE

Aortic Aneurysm

Aneurysms, areas of focal or diffuse dilatation of the aorta, develop at sites of congenital or acquired medial weakness. Hypertension may expose weakness that might otherwise not be manifest. Once begun, aneurysm formation is progressive because, for any level of intraluminal pressure, tangential wall tension increases with the square of the radius. Thus expansion and rupture are nearly inevitable unless the patient succumbs to intercurrent disease before this can occur.[66]

Fusiform and *saccular* aneurysms are described. In the former, circumferential dilatation, the result of a diffuse area of weakness, produces a spindle-shaped deformity. In the latter, balloon-like dilatation occurs, beginning at a relatively narrow neck. Many aneurysms are not pure examples of either. In both varieties, by the time the aortic wall has been stretched to aneurysmal size, little or no recognizable medial tissue remains; the wall of the aneurysmal sack is composed almost entirely of fibrous tissue.[67]

The lumen of an aneurysm virtually always contains laminated thrombus, which may fill a saccular aneurysm or cover the circumference of a fusiform one. Thus angiographic opacification of the aortic lumen often does not clearly delineate the size or extent of an aneurysm.

Aneurysms may result from a variety of causes. Heritable medial weakness as a basis for aortic dilatation has been discussed. With the declining incidence of syphilis, aneurysms resulting from aortitis, either infectious or nonspecific, are uncommon. Saccular aneurysms are often encountered in regions of the aorta weakened by aortic dissection.[68] Despite alternative etiologic possibilities, the great majority of aortic aneurysms, particularly those of the descending thoracic or abdominal aorta, are generally assumed to be "atherosclerotic"[66] because of the frequent presence of atherosclerosis elsewhere and of its risk factors.

The assumption that atherosclerosis alone is sufficient to produce aneurysm has been challenged.[67] Among other reasons, strong family clustering of abdominal aneurysms, as well as their association with aneurysmal dilatation of other arteries, provides reason to suspect that an underlying genetically determined defect may play an important role in this process, as alluded to earlier.[69–71] It appears likely that both genetically influenced factors and atherosclerosis are involved, perhaps with varying contributions in a given individual.

SINUS OF VALSALVA ANEURYSM

Congenital failure of fusion of the aortic media with the fibrous skeleton of the heart at the aortic valve ring provides a point of weakness through which a sinus of Valsalva aneurysm may develop.[72] Aneurysm of the right coronary sinus is most frequent. Most of the rest protrude from the noncoronary sinus. Congenital aneurysms of the left coronary sinus are rare. In that location, infectious endocarditis is a more frequent cause.

Because the root of the aorta is nearly surrounded by cardiac chambers, sinus of Valsalva aneurysms may intrude on and may rupture into one of them. Those of the right coronary sinus protrude into the right ventricular outflow tract. When they rupture, a fistulous connection between the aorta and right ventricle results. Similarly, an aneurysm of the noncoronary sinus, located posteriorly and to the right of the anterior sinus, typically protrudes into the right atrium and usually ruptures into that structure. The rare aneurysms of the left coronary sinus protrude into the pericardial space from beneath the left main coronary artery.

Some defects in the right coronary sinus are extensive enough to produce undermining of the aortic valve and incompetence of that valve, and some are associated with incomplete closure of the membranous ventricular septum and an interventricular shunt.

Rarely recognized prior to rupture, sinus of Valsalva aneurysm may be detected on imaging of a patient for some other purpose. Rarely, the mass of the unruptured aneurysm may obstruct the right ventricular outflow tract or the left coronary artery.[73] Heart block or other conduction abnormalities may be produced from protrusion into the interventricular septum.

Rupture of a sinus of Valsalva aneurysm usually results in a large shunt from the aorta to the right heart chambers.[73] The patient presents with a continuous murmur and bounding arterial pulses. Often severe heart failure is present. The diagnosis is readily made from the clinical picture and echocardiography. Surgical correction is indicated.

THORACIC AORTIC ANEURYSM

Etiology and Pathologic Anatomy Anuloaortic ectasia, the typical aneurysm resulting from medial degeneration, has its greatest diameter in the proximal ascending aorta, including the aortic sinuses. The diameter quickly tapers, approaching a normal dimension before the takeoff of the innominate artery. Limited or extensive medial dissection may complicate this aneurysm.[17,18,74] The hallmark aortic manifestation of Marfan's syndrome, such lesions are often encountered in individuals with no musculoskeletal or ocular manifestations of that disorder.

Syphilitic aneurysms are still encountered occasionally. They are typically saccular. The ascending aorta and arch are most often affected, but the aortic dilatation often extends into the aortic sinuses and into the descending aortic segment. The abdominal aorta is rarely affected.

Saccular aneurysms of the thoracic aorta frequently follow aortic dissection when operative repair is not carried out. Moreover, they may develop in the descending thoracic aorta even after successful operative repair of a dissection involving the ascending aorta.[68] Such aneurysms may expand gradually over time and require operative treatment months or years after the acute dissection.

About equal in frequency to thoracic aneurysms following dissection are those which have in the past been assumed to be atherosclerotic in origin. They are, however, far less common than infrarenal abdominal aneurysms. Unlike anuloaortic ectasia, these are typically located in the descending thoracic segment and are usually, but not invariably, fusiform. When they extend proximally into the arch or distally into the abdomen, they present a particularly challenging surgical problem. An aneurysm of the abdominal aorta is quite frequently associated and should be sought whenever a thoracic aneurysm is encountered.[75,76]

Clinical Features Aneurysms limited to the ascending aorta rarely produce symptoms directly unless they are undergoing active expansion or rupture. They are commonly recognized in the course of evaluation of a patient with the murmur of aortic regurgitation. Since the aortic root is located within the cardiac silhouette and the entire ascending aorta within the pericardial space, dilatation may not be readily appreciated on a chest radiograph.

Like aneurysms of the ascending aorta, those of the arch and descending segments are often asymptomatic and are detected fortuitously in the course of an incidental imaging study. Those of the arch, however, are more likely than those in other locations to produce symptoms. The arch is fixed by the brachiocephalic arteries, and aneurysms of that segment may compress a variety of mediastinal structures as well as the thoracic spine. Compression of the tracheobronchial tree may be attended by cough or dyspnea. Tracheal deviation or "tug" may be detected on physical examination. Pressure on the esophagus may result in dysphagia, rarely severe. Hoarseness may result from compression of the recurrent laryngeal nerve. Adjacent vascular structures may be compressed, resulting in pulmonary arterial stenosis or superior vena caval obstruction.

Chest pain, described as deep and aching or throbbing, has been the most frequent symptom reported in patients with thoracic aneurysm. Pain may be associated with erosion of the rib cage or vertebrae. The appearance of pain clearly related to an aneurysm must be regarded as a signal of expansion and threatened rupture.[76] It is not unusual for expansion or rupture to be the initial manifestation of a thoracic aneurysm. Massive, usually fatal hemorrhage into the mediastinum, pleural space, esophagus, or tracheobronchial tree ensues. Rupture of an aneurysm of the ascending aorta, because of the intrapericardial location of that structure, results in acute hemopericardium and cardiac tamponade. Hemoptysis may precede by days or weeks fatal hemorrhage in descending thoracic aneurysms that have become adherent to adjacent lung. Rarely, aneurysms may rupture into adjacent vascular structures, producing aortovenous or aortopulmonary fistulas.

Diagnosis The aorta may be imaged by a variety of modalities. Of these, chest x-ray and transthoracic echocardiography are the most readily available and thus most useful for screening purposes. Aortography, computed tomography, magnetic resonance imaging/angiography, and transesophageal echocardiography all provide detailed information regarding the aorta's anatomy.[77]

Natural History and Prognosis Most of the data concerning the natural history of thoracic aortic aneurysms come from retrospective, somewhat dated reports of hospital experience.[75,76] If anuloaortic ectasia and aortic dissection are excluded, the vast majority of cases studied have involved the descending aortic segment. Joyce's classic review[75] suggests a 50 percent 5-year and a 70 percent 10-year mortality. A 5-year mortality of 44 percent was reported more recently.[78]

One-third to one-half of deaths result from rupture of the aneurysm; most of the remainder result from other vascular diseases. The location of the aneurysm does not influence the mortality rate, but advanced age, size more than 6 cm, hypertension, and presence of other cardiovascular disease all increase risk. Symptoms related to the aneurysm itself portend an unfavorable outcome.

To the extent that mortality data in patients with Marfan's syndrome apply to all patients with anuloaortic ectasia, their outlook appears to be worse than for those with aneurysm of the descending aorta. In one early series, 52 of 56 patients with Marfan's syndrome died as a consequence of aortic disease at an average age of 32 years.[79] More recently, the mean age of death in Marfan's patients was found to be 41 years.[80] This improvement may be attributable to advances in surgery or to improved medical therapy (including the use of β-receptor blocking drugs), but different methods of data handling make comparison difficult

Management Until very recently, surgical repair was the only known effective treatment for thoracic aneurysms. The introduction of stent-graft stents offers promise of a less morbid intervention, but experience with this technique is still limited.[81]

Operative intervention is urgently indicated in patients if symptoms suggest expansion or compression of an adjacent structure. Cardiac failure from aortic regurgitation or aortocameral fistula also may necessitate early operative treatment. Available data suggest that in asymptomatic patients, the larger the aneurysm and the more rapid its increase in size, the more likely rupture will occur.[82–84] It is generally agreed that a diameter of 6 cm represents a point at which an operation should be considered.[82–84] For aneurysms in Marfan's patients, a somewhat lower threshold (5 cm) is recommended by some experts. As is true of other aortic aneurysms, the presence of chronic obstructive lung disease is associated with an increased risk of rupture.[85] Compared with the patient who has no other disease, the individual with associated coronary or cerebrovascular disease has a greater operative risk and a smaller risk of dying from rupture of the aneurysm before succumbing to the associated vascular disease.

Traditional surgical treatment consists of replacing the resected aneurysmal segment with a graft attached to relatively normal aorta proximally and distally. Specific surgical procedures vary with the site of the aneurysm and the need for maintaining circulation to distal body parts during aortic occlusion. Accordingly, the surgeon divides thoracic aneurysms into those affecting (1) the ascending aorta, (2) the arch of the aorta containing origins of the brachiocephalic vessels, (3) the descending thoracic aorta arising just distal to the origin of the left subclavian artery, and (4) thoracoabdominal aneurysms, i.e., those arising in the descending thoracic aorta and extending into the abdominal aorta.

For aneurysms of the ascending aorta, total cardiopulmonary bypass is required. The myocardium is protected by cold cardioplegia while the coronary ostia are exposed. The aneurysm is opened, and a graft is sutured in place from within. Finally, the aneurysm is trimmed and sutured around the graft. If the aneurysm is associated with aortic valve incompetence, the leaflets are excised, and a composite graft including a prosthetic valve is sutured in place. The coronary ostia are sutured to an appropriate opening made in the composite graft or to a smaller Dacron graft that is sutured side-to-side to the composite graft.

For aneurysms of the transverse arch of the aorta, total cardiopulmonary bypass is also required, and profound hypothermia is used to protect the brain. A graft is sutured to relatively normal aorta proximally and distally from within the aneurysm, and the brachiocephalic, left common carotid, and left subclavian arteries are attached individually to appropriate openings in the graft. It is often possible to preserve the relatively normal aortic wall segment from which these vessels arise. This segment can be attached to an appropriate opening made in the graft.

For aneurysms arising distal to the left common carotid artery, it is usually desirable to employ atrial-femoral bypass, femoral-femoral partial cardiopulmonary bypass, or various types of shunts during the period of aortic occlusion. Although many techniques to prevent spinal cord ischemia are being studied, there is not as yet convincing evidence that any predictably reduce the incidence of paraparesis associated with these procedures.

The surgical mortality rate for aneurysms of the ascending aorta is about 3 percent.[84] For descending thoracic aortic aneurysms, the rate is approximately 6 percent.[84] It is somewhat higher for those affecting the transverse arch and origins of the brachiocephalic vessels. Late deaths are usually due to associated diseases or other causes, although aneurysms occasionally may develop in other parts of the aorta and require surgical treatment.

Thoracoabdominal aneurysms arise in the descending thoracic aorta and extend distally for varying distances into the abdominal aorta as far as the bifurcation and occasionally into the common iliac arteries. They present a particular challenge to the surgeon because the arteries supplying blood to the abdominal organs arise from this portion of the aorta.

The surgeon must expose the aorta in both the thorax and the abdomen. A left intercostal incision is made and extended down the midline of the abdomen, after which the diaphragm is incised, and the abdominal structures are mobilized retroperitoneally to expose the entire aneurysm. A graft is interposed. In most cases, it is possible to attach the segment of the aorta from which arise the celiac, superior mesenteric, and renal arteries to an opening in the graft and thus avoid the need to use individual grafts to each artery. Occasionally, however, it may be necessary to use a separate graft for one or more of these arteries.

An operative mortality rate of 7 to 11 percent is reported from experienced centers.[84] As in aneurysms of the descending thoracic aorta, paresis or paraplegia is a potential complication.

ABDOMINAL AORTIC ANEURYSM

Rupture of an abdominal aortic aneurysm is the tenth leading cause of death (15,000 annually) for men 55 years of age and older in the United States. Moreover, 40,000 aneurysmectomies are performed each year. In contrast to the well-known decline in age-adjusted deaths from coronary atherosclerosis, the incidence of abdominal aneurysms is increasing.[86] This lesion is particularly treacherous because it is often clinically silent until rupture occurs.

Etiology Until recently, virtually all abdominal aneurysms have been attributed to atherosclerosis,[86] an assumption that is being challenged, as noted earlier. In addition, an occasional traumatic, congenital, or mycotic abdominal aneurysm is encountered, and one is occasionally found as a residual of aortic dissection or in patients with Marfan's syndrome.

Pathologic Anatomy Abdominal aneurysms are, as a rule, fusiform but may be saccular and usually are located distal to the renal arteries but may extend to the aortic bifurcation and involve the iliac arteries. Exceptionally, they extend above the renal arteries. In this case, the origins of not only the renal arteries but also the major visceral arteries may be involved, complicating operative management.[66,86]

Between 5 and 10 percent of abdominal aneurysms are accompanied by an intense inflammatory and fibrotic reaction in the anterior and lateral periaortic tissue,[87,88] a process histologically similar to retroperitoneal fibrosis. These *inflammatory aneurysms* may result from a hypersensitivity reaction to an antigen or antigens in the atherosclerotic plaque. Systemic manifestations, such as weight loss, abdominal pain, and an elevated erythrocyte sedimentation rate, may reflect the inflammatory response. The difficulty of operative repair is increased.

Clinical Features Men are three or four times more likely to have an abdominal aortic aneurysm than women. The typical patient is in the seventh or eighth decade. Most are asymptomatic and are detected in the course of an examination directed at unrelated symptoms.[66,86]

Pain attributable to the aneurysm, especially if it is of recent onset, should be viewed as threatened rupture. Characteristically constant and located in the midabdomen, lumbar region, or pelvis, the pain may be severe and have a boring quality. Detection of an aneurysm that is tender to palpation carries much the same threat of rupture.[87] Because they present with abdominal pain and often a tender abdominal mass, inflammatory aneurysms may mimic threatened rupture.[87,88]

Unless the patient is obese, physical examination almost always discloses an abdominal mass in the epigastrium, slightly to the left of the midline. If definite expansile movement can be detected, the diagnosis of abdominal aneurysm is reasonably secure. Bruits may be audible, and femoral pulses are reduced in some patients.

Rupture may be the initial manifestation. Rapid exsanguination may result from free rupture into the peritoneal cavity. Fortunately, more often the rupture is directed into the retroperitoneal space, where hemorrhage may be retarded. Abdominal pain and evidence of occult blood loss may persist for hours or days, allowing time for diagnosis and operative treatment. Rarely, the rupture is confined for several days to a few weeks. In such instances, the patient may present a puzzling diagnostic picture consisting of abdominal pain, fever, and slight to moderate blood loss.[87,88] Recognition of the nature of the illness can be lifesaving because secondary rupture always ensues.

Rarely, rupture occurs into an adjacent retroperitoneal structure. When a communication develops with the vena cavae or other large vein, a loud continuous murmur in the abdomen and high-output congestive heart failure may ensue.[88] Rupture into the duodenum results in gastrointestinal bleeding,[88] but aortoduodenal fistulas are more common after graft replacement of the infrarenal aorta.

An unruptured aneurysm also may produce serious complications. Acute thrombosis may mimic saddle embolism. Furthermore, embolization of thrombus or atherosclerotic debris from aneurysms (and indeed from severely atherosclerotic, nonaneurysmal segments) to the lower extremities is far more frequent than is generally appreciated.[88,89] Secondary bacterial infection of an aortic aneurysm gives rise to fever, leukocytosis, and abdominal pain and may lead to rupture.

Diagnostic Studies Anteroposterior or cross-table lateral radiographs of the abdomen often confirm the presence of aneurysm by demonstrating the characteristic "egg-shell" calcification of its wall. Imaging with ultrasound provides reproducible measurements of the dimensions of the aneurysm, and computed tomography or magnetic resonance imaging provides more definitive confirmation of the diagnosis. Aortography can be reserved for instances in which additional information regarding the extent of the aneurysm or the degree of involvement of branch arteries is required. The aortogram, a depiction of the luminal contour, may be misleading as to the size of the aneurysm because its lumen is characteristically filled or lined with thrombus.[90]

Management Because of the threat of fatal rupture, frequently in a previously asymptomatic patient, screening of at-risk populations by means of abdominal ultrasound has been proposed. Fewer than 5 percent of those older than age 65 were found to have abdominal aneurysm, and in fewer than 1 percent did it exceed 4 cm in diameter,[91] leading to questioning of the cost-effectiveness of such an approach. The cost-effectiveness of screening could be enhanced by limiting the screening to patients with a family history of aneurysmal disease or patients with atherosclerotic disease in other arteries.[92]

Abdominal aneurysms detected in asymptomatic patients during screening present a sometimes difficult management choice.[93] The risk of fatal rupture must be balanced against the risk of aneurysmectomy, a situation that has spurred efforts to define features predicting high risk for rupture.[66,86,94–96] The larger the aneurysm is, the greater is the risk of rupture. Therefore, when discovered in a patient who is a reasonable operative risk, *aneurysms 5 cm or more in size should be resected, whereas those smaller than 4 cm may be followed safely pending an increase in size.* Aneurysms more than 4 cm but less than 5 cm in size fall into a gray zone in which there is lack of agreement. *The recently reported randomized UK Small Aneurysm Trial, however, suggests that aneurysms smaller than 5.5 cm may be followed safely with serial ultrasound examinations.*[97] In addition to aneurysm size, systemic hypertension and chronic obstructive lung disease are independent predictors of increased risk.

Patients with abdominal aneurysms commonly have coronary and cerebrovascular disease and are more likely to die from these diseases than of rupture and have an increased operative risk for aneurysmectomy.[98] With appropriate preoperative screening for and treatment of coronary disease, the risk of aneurysmectomy is acceptable in experienced centers.[66,99,100]

Symptomatic aneurysms require urgent surgical treatment because early rupture can be confidently predicted.[101] A ruptured abdominal aneurysm is a surgical emergency. Surgery for an abdominal aortic aneurysm does not require maintenance of the distal circulation. The aorta is clamped proximally between the aneurysm and the renal arteries, the iliac arteries are clamped distally, and the aneurysm is opened. From within, the graft is sutured proximally to normal aorta and distally to the aortic bifurcation or individually to the iliac arteries. Finally, the aneurysmal walls are trimmed and sutured over the graft. Operative mortality is less than 5 percent.[66]

Active investigation of the use of endovascular stent-grafts to isolate the aneurysm from the aortic lumen is underway in several centers. Early results suggest that this is both feasible and less morbid than the standard operative approach. Long-term results are not yet available.[102,103]

Aortic Dissection

Aortic dissection is an even more common potentially fatal aortic disease than even rupture of an abdominal aneurysm.[104–106] Every busy general hospital will encounter several each year. *Because fundamental differences exist between the pathogenesis, clinical presentation, and treatment of dissections and those of aneurysms, the confusing term* dissecting aneurysm *should be discarded.*

PATHOLOGIC ANATOMY

Cleavage of the aortic media in its long axis by a column of blood characterizes aortic dissection. The split in the media typically occupies about half the circumference of the aorta and may extend through its entire length. The plane of dissection often follows the greater curvature of the ascending aorta and the arch. In the descending aorta, the path of the dissection is most often located lateral to the true lumen, but it may be medial and may spiral "barber pole" fashion about the long axis.[107]

In classic aortic dissection, the "false channel" created by this medial hematoma communicates with the "true lumen" through an intimal tear located near its proximal end. Such tears typically are single and transverse in orientation, but exceptions are frequent. Multiple secondary ("reentry") tears, located more distally along the false channel, are common.

Two patterns predominate. In about two-thirds of instances the false channel originates in the ascending aorta and the proximal ("entry") tear is located a few centimeters above the aortic valve. The false channel frequently extends to the aortoiliac bifurcation (Fig. 88-4). Dissections that do not involve the ascending aorta account for about a quarter of all cases. In them, the proximal tear most often lies just distal to the left subclavian artery. The medial hematoma begins in proximity to the origin of the left subclavian artery and extends distally for varying distances[104–107] (Fig. 88-5).

The most widely applied nomenclature is that of DeBakey.[104–106] In this classification, dissections involving the ascending aorta are type I, whereas those originating beyond the arch are type III. Type II is limited to the ascending aorta. Apart from length, many type II dissections are indistinguishable from type I, but others originate within chronic fusiform dilatation of the ascending aorta. The Stanford classification applies type A to any dissection involving the ascending aorta and type B to those which do not[106] (Fig. 88-6).

Many medial dissections do not follow these classic patterns. In some, the hematoma is short and limited to the arch or to the descending thoracic or abdominal segments. In another rather frequently encountered variation, an entry tear is located just beyond the left subclavian artery, but the dissection extends proximally into the ascending aorta.

There is a subset of patients with the clinical syndrome of aortic dissection resulting from a medial hematoma but no intimal tear,[108] as demonstrated by computed tomography, transesophageal echocardiography, or magnetic resonance imaging.[109–111] They are now included under the rubric *intramural hematoma.* In one series of patients with medial

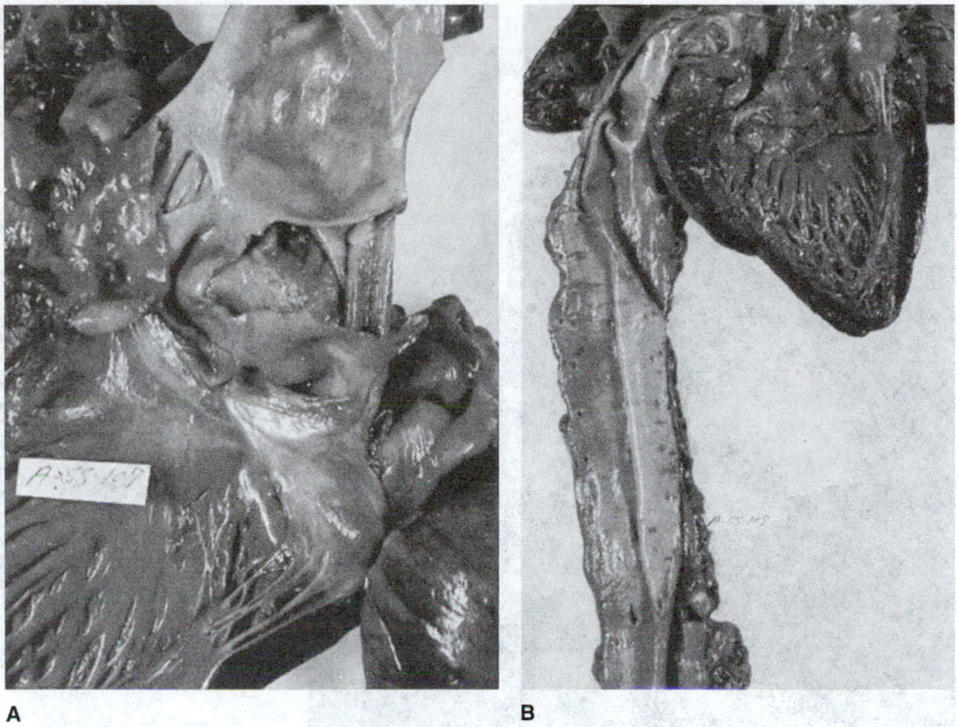

FIGURE 88-4 Necropsy specimen demonstrating the features of a typical proximal aortic dissection. *A*. The large intimal rent may be seen a few centimeters above the aortic cusps. *B*. The false channel created by the dissecting hematoma is shown. Notice the cleanly sheared layers of media.

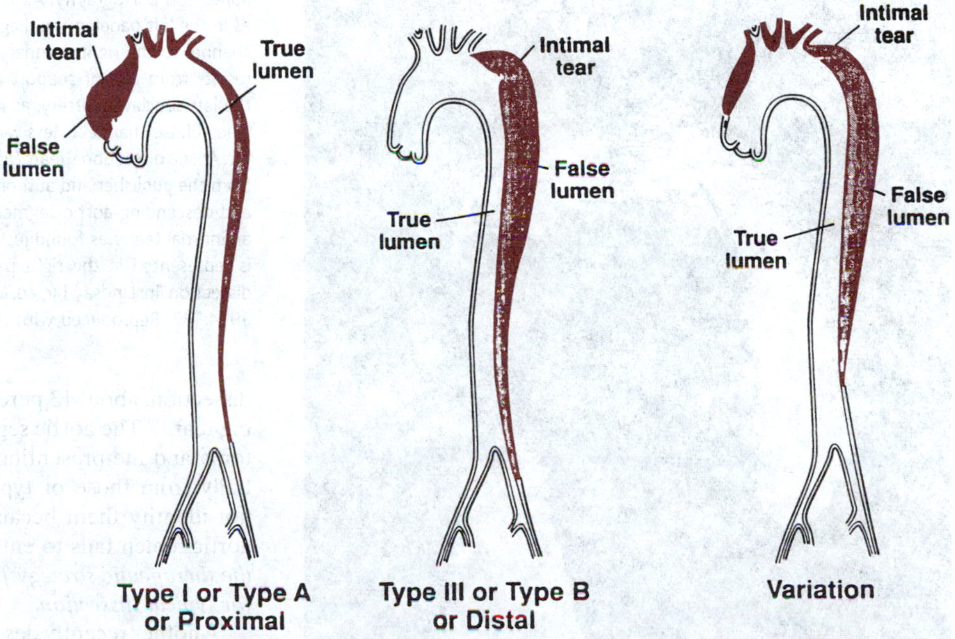

FIGURE 88-5 Artist's depiction of the three major anatomic patterns of aortic dissection. The left panel illustrates the most common variety, in which an intimal tear is located just above the aortic valve, and the medial cleavage plane extends in the long axis for a varying distance, often to the bifurcation. The center panel depicts the second most common variety. An intimal tear is found just beyond the left subclavian artery, and the medial dissection extends distally. The right panel depicts an important, but uncommon, variation. From an intimal tear just distal to the left subclavian artery, the medial dissection extends both antegrade down the thoracic aorta and retrograde into the descending segment. (From Lindsay J Jr. Aortic dissection. *Heart Dis Stroke* 1992; 1:69. Reproduced with permission from the publisher and author.)

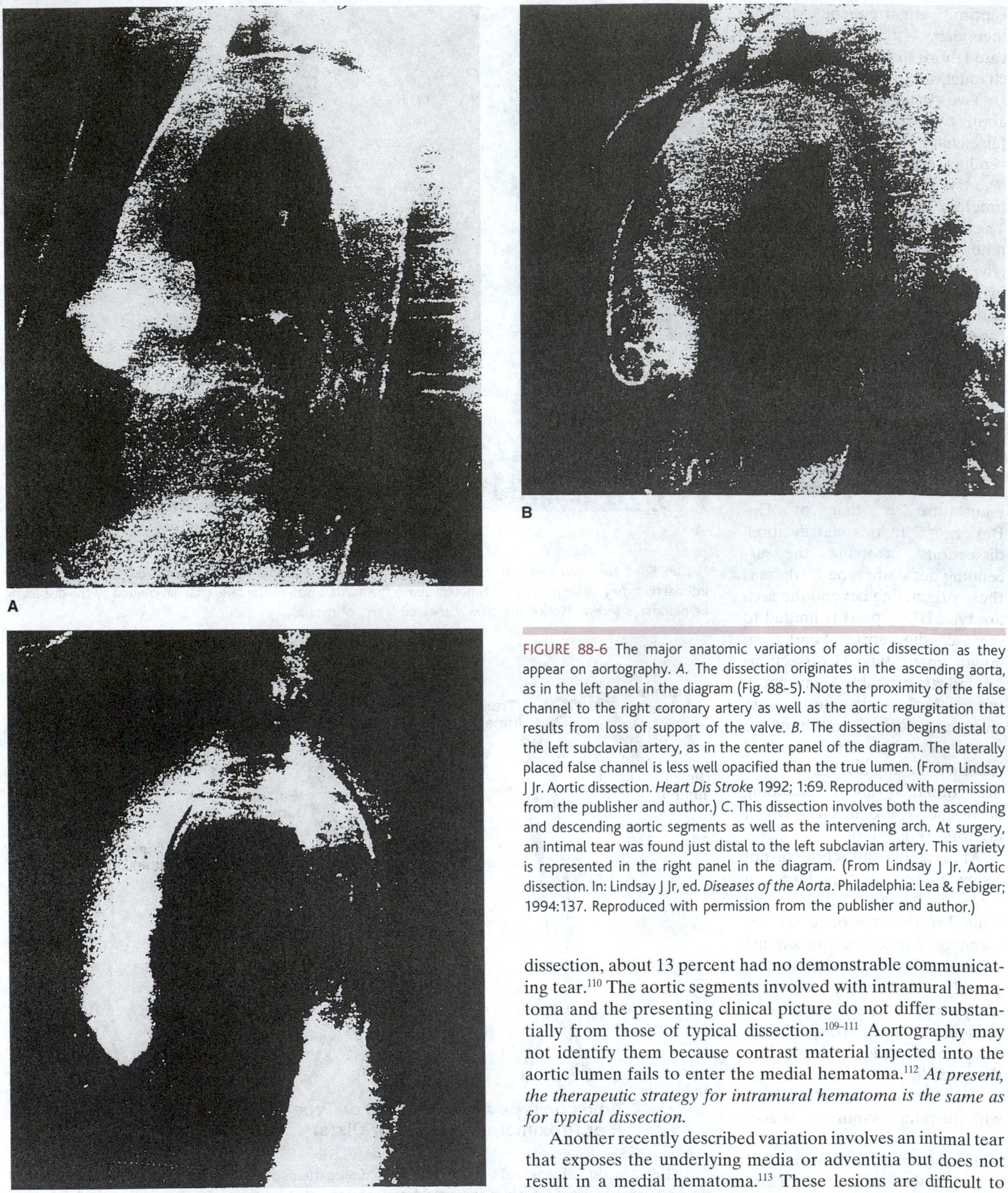

A

B

C

FIGURE 88-6 The major anatomic variations of aortic dissection as they appear on aortography. *A.* The dissection originates in the ascending aorta, as in the left panel in the diagram (Fig. 88-5). Note the proximity of the false channel to the right coronary artery as well as the aortic regurgitation that results from loss of support of the valve. *B.* The dissection begins distal to the left subclavian artery, as in the center panel of the diagram. The laterally placed false channel is less well opacified than the true lumen. (From Lindsay J Jr. Aortic dissection. *Heart Dis Stroke* 1992; 1:69. Reproduced with permission from the publisher and author.) *C.* This dissection involves both the ascending and descending aortic segments as well as the intervening arch. At surgery, an intimal tear was found just distal to the left subclavian artery. This variety is represented in the right panel in the diagram. (From Lindsay J Jr. Aortic dissection. In: Lindsay J Jr, ed. *Diseases of the Aorta*. Philadelphia: Lea & Febiger; 1994:137. Reproduced with permission from the publisher and author.)

dissection, about 13 percent had no demonstrable communicating tear.[110] The aortic segments involved with intramural hematoma and the presenting clinical picture do not differ substantially from those of typical dissection.[109–111] Aortography may not identify them because contrast material injected into the aortic lumen fails to enter the medial hematoma.[112] *At present, the therapeutic strategy for intramural hematoma is the same as for typical dissection.*

Another recently described variation involves an intimal tear that exposes the underlying media or adventitia but does not result in a medial hematoma.[113] These lesions are difficult to detect with available imaging techniques.

One additional variety of medial hematoma was described in the section on aortic atherosclerosis. Penetrating atherosclerotic ulcers that have disrupted the aortic media have been demonstrated by imaging techniques and may create a potential for rupture, false aneurysm formation, or dissection by hematoma.[16]

These lesions appear almost exclusively in the middle and distal descending thoracic aorta. Exceptionally, major branch vessels are threatened. The initial presentation of a complication of a penetrating plaque (whether partial rupture or medial dissection) may mimic typical aortic dissection. Surgery may be indicated in selected patients because external rupture is a hazard.[16]

Death from aortic dissection most often occurs from disruption of the outer wall of the false channel opposite the entrance tear.[104–108] Rupture of proximal dissection therefore produces abrupt hemopericardium and cardiac tamponade. Hemorrhage into the mediastinum or either pleural space may occur, whereas external rupture of distal dissection often results in a left hemothorax. Death from external rupture, often abrupt, may be delayed by temporary cessation of hemorrhage attributable to falling arterial pressure and increasing tension in the periaortic tissue. Dramatic clinical syndromes result in those rare instances in which the false channel ruptures into the right heart chambers producing a large left-to-right shunt.[114]

In approximately half of patients with proximal dissection, medial hematoma undermines the support of the aortic valve leaflets, rendering the valve incompetent. Fortunately, very serious hemodynamic consequences of aortic regurgitation appear infrequently during the acute phase.[104–106]

One or more branch vessels of the aorta become obstructed by dissection in about half of patients with type I and in fewer with type III dissection.[104–106] The results may be catastrophic, particularly in patients with type I, in whom the coronary and cerebral circulations are jeopardized. Obstruction by the dissection of the orifice of one of the coronary arteries rarely may produce an acute myocardial infarction. Failure to recognize the underlying process may result in thrombolytic therapy with disastrous results.[115] Obstruction of renal or splanchnic arteries may produce life-threatening complications such as severe hypertension and acute renal failure. The iliac arteries are the branch arteries most frequently compromised. Although not immediately life-threatening, narrowing of these arteries may produce dramatic, painful ischemia of the lower extremities.[116]

The aortic wall containing the medial hematoma is weakened. If it does not rupture during the acute dissection, it is often the site of subsequent aneurysm formation. Rupture of these constitutes a major threat to the survivor of the initial illness.[68,117]

PATHOGENESIS

Arterial hypertension is a major factor in causing aortic dissection in 80 percent of patients.[104–108] In most patients, no conclusive evidence of an underlying medial defect can be identified. Increased arterial pressure must certainly expose any existing weakness of the aortic wall and may, in addition, accentuate medial degeneration.

The frequency with which dissecting hematoma is noted in Marfan's syndrome,[17,18] in certain other congenital and heritable conditions,[17,18] and in experimental lathyrism provides a strong argument for the importance of an underlying medial defect in at least some individuals with this disorder. Indeed, histologic evidence of degeneration of elastin or of smooth muscle cells in the aortic media of such patients has long been noted. As noted previously, considerable doubt on the specificity of the classic histologic findings has been raised. Such findings are frequently absent in patients with dissection and are remarkably similar to changes encountered in older patients without dissection.[21] It seems likely that any fundamental medial defect or defects may be unrecognizable by light microscopy.

The role of the intimal ("entry") tear in the genesis of medial dissection is debated. Many investigators feel that it exposes the media to blood under luminal pressure and that the resulting shear forces initiate and propagate the medial cleavage. Others propose that medial weakness leads to hemorrhage from the vasa vasorum. The resulting intramural hematoma splits the medial layers.[104–108] In this hypothesis the intimal tears are secondary. Instances of medial hematoma in which no intimal tear can be identified support the existence of this mechanism.

CLINICAL FEATURES

Most common in the fifth through the seventh decades of life, aortic dissection has been reported in children as well as the very old. Men are affected at least twice as commonly as women.[104–108]

Predisposing Conditions Certain congenital lesions (e.g., coarctation and bicuspid aortic valve) are associated with increased frequency of dissection.[26] A greater-than-expected incidence is encountered in patients with aortic stenosis even after aortic valve replacement. The same is true with certain heritable disorders such as Marfan's and Turner's syndromes.[17]

Iatrogenic vascular trauma, a complication of cardiac catheterization, coronary bypass surgery, cardiopulmonary bypass, or intraaortic balloon counterpulsation, may produce extensive aortic dissection.

Pregnancy, either because of its effects on the aortic wall or because of attendant hemodynamic stress, has been reported to predispose to medial dissection.[118] This conclusion has been based on the fact that half or more of the reports of aortic dissection in women younger than 40 years have occurred during pregnancy. Since the total number reported is relatively small (certainly in relation to the frequency of pregnancy), and since most reports concern one or a few cases, it is possible that selective reporting accounts for this association.[119]

History Sudden, excruciating pain, presumably attributable to the progress of the medial cleavage, announces the onset of dissection in 90 percent of instances. Patients may describe the pain as "cutting," "ripping," or "tearing," but such vivid descriptors cannot always be elicited.[104–106] Patients will most commonly locate the discomfort in the anterior chest, somewhat less frequently in the interscapular area, in the epigastrium, or in the lumbar region. Since these locations often are the site of pain related to more common processes (e.g., myocardial infarction or cholecystitis), the examiner must be alert to the possibility of aortic dissection in any patient with pain in these sites in whom the more common diagnoses are not immediately obvious.

Two features of the pain of dissection help to separate it from that of other conditions. *The discomfort of dissection typically is at its most intense from its inception and does not build in intensity, as is the case with other disorders producing severe pain in the trunk. Moreover, it often is located either simultaneously or sequentially in more than one of the four sites mentioned earlier.* Suspicion should be aroused particularly by pain occurring both above and below the diaphragm.[104–106]

When pain is not a prominent feature, it is usually because

a sudden neurologic episode has diminished the patient's ability to perceive or report pain. Syncope is the most frequent neurologic event and a particularly ominous sign. It seems always to reflect external rupture, almost always of the ascending aorta into the pericardial space. Less frequently, focal neurologic signs reflect arterial occlusion of the cerebral or spinal circulation.

Unusually, aortic dissection is nearly painless even in the absence of a neurologic event. For example, occlusion of the femoral or the subclavian artery may be the predominant clinical feature, and arterial embolism may be simulated.[104–106] Rarely, the acute episode goes entirely unrecognized by the patient. In such instances, diagnostic study of patients who have an abnormal chest x-ray, aortic regurgitation or obstruction of an arterial branch of the aorta uncovers chronic dissection.

Physical Examination Although none are diagnostic of dissection, physical findings that greatly increase the probability of its presence often can be detected. *The murmur of aortic regurgitation can be heard in about half of all patients with acute type I dissection. Loss or diminution of an arterial pulse also may be detected in half. One or both of these cardinal findings is present in all but a small minority of that subgroup.* In contrast, patients with dissection limited to the descending aorta less frequently have pulse deficits and uncommonly have a murmur of aortic regurgitation.

The frequency with which hypertension underlies aortic dissection has been mentioned. Even those with neither a definitive history of hypertension nor a measurable blood pressure elevation will on examination have left ventricular hypertrophy or vascular changes in the optic fundi indicating a hypotensive history. Extraordinarily high readings can be encountered, particularly in those with type III dissection. Renal ischemia, a consequence of renal artery involvement, has been invoked to explain diastolic blood pressures that may reach 140 to 160 mmHg or more.[104–106]

Twenty percent of patients with dissection involving the ascending aorta present with hypotension. Such a presentation requires immediate consideration of operative treatment because external rupture almost always is responsible.

Diagnostic Studies Of the routine studies, only the chest x-ray provides diagnostic information of much value. The aortic shadow is abnormal in 80 to 90 percent of patients but also may be abnormal in many instances in patients who do not have dissection. Dilatation of the ascending aorta, reflected by protrusion of its shadow from the right side of the mediastinum, is a characteristic finding in proximal dissection. Dilatation of the aortic knob and descending thoracic aorta is typical of distal disease. Certain other findings, e.g., progressive widening of the aortic silhouette on serial films, a lobulated or serrated margin of the aortic shadow, or a "double lumen" effect created by a less radiopaque false channel, are uncommon but more specific. The same may be said for detection of intimal calcification more than 6 mm inside the margin of the aorta.[90]

For confirmation of the diagnosis, either computed tomography after intravenous contrast material or transesophageal echocardiography may be employed. Both have high sensitivity and specificity. Some believe that magnetic resonance imaging is even more accurate; however, its value is limited in acutely ill patients because of the longer imaging time and the relative inaccessibility of patients during the imaging process.[90,120–122]

An aortogram is occasionally required to provide details of branch vessel involvement. Two aortic channels usually can be identified because of the variation in intensity and timing of their opacification (see Fig. 88-6). Moreover, the aortogram may identify a linear lucency representing the aortic intima and media separating the two channels. At times the false channel is not opacified because of thrombosis or because it does not communicate with the true lumen. In such cases, the true lumen may appear to be compressed and to lie at a distance from the margins of the aortic shadow. The resulting appearance of a thickened aortic wall also can be produced by thrombosis within an aneurysm, aortitis, or mediastinal hematoma or tumor. These usually, but not invariably, can be distinguished from dissection because in these the aortic lumen is not significantly compressed.

NATURAL HISTORY AND PROGNOSIS

Older reports of aortic dissection must be used to provide information about its natural history because virtually all patients in the past 30 years have been operated on and/or had aggressive antihypertensive treatment. Thirty-five percent of untreated patients succumb within the initial 24 hours, and 50 percent die within 48 hours, 70 percent by 1 week, and 80 percent by 2 weeks.[108,123]

Certain subgroups with widely differing natural histories can be identified. Hypotension (systolic blood pressure <100 mmHg) usually indicates aortic rupture and nearly certain early death. Almost all such patients have involvement of the ascending aorta; one-quarter of those with such involvement present in this way. Those with distal (type III or type B) dissection are at the other end of the spectrum with regard to their natural history. Older reports indicate that about half survive the acute phase without aggressive treatment. Absent modern therapeutic intervention, the mortality rate of patients with proximal dissection who are hypertensive or normotensive is intermediate between these extremes.

Patients who survive the first 2 weeks continue to experience a high mortality rate in the first year. About half the survivors die within 3 months, and an additional 10 percent die within 1 year of the onset of their illness. The few who pass the first anniversary may expect reasonable longevity. Late deaths may be due to cerebrovascular complications of hypertension, heart failure from severe aortic regurgitation, or rupture of a saccular aneurysm of the residual false channel.[124]

MANAGEMENT

The life-threatening complications of acute aortic dissection include very severe hypertension, cardiac tamponade, massive hemorrhage, severe aortic regurgitation, or ischemic injury to the myocardium, the central nervous system, and kidneys. Optimal management requires close surveillance of vascular pressures, urine flow, mental status, and neurologic signs in an intensive care unit. Pain relief can be difficult even with potent narcotics but usually can be obtained with drug therapy to reduce arterial pressure.[104–106]

A successful outcome requires that progression of the medial cleavage be halted and that external rupture of the weakened aortic wall be prevented. In as much as the aortic defect is structural, operative treatment represents the most effective long-term remedy. Aggressive antihypertensive treatment lessens the stress on the aortic wall and thus the likelihood of progression of the dissection and of rupture. Such therapy is widely employed prior to and, in selected instances, as an alternative to surgical management.[104–106]

In the acute phase, one of several drug regimens may be employed to reduce arterial pressure and its rate of rise. *Aggressive use of a β-blocking agent may be adequate in patients who present with relatively modest levels of hypertension. With more severe hypertension, intravenous nitroprusside combined with a β-blocking agent may be required. Drug therapy should aim to lower systolic arterial pressure to 100 to 120 mmHg. Optimal blood pressure reduction may not be possible if oliguria (<25 mL/h) or mental confusion appears.*

Our intensivists currently prefer *intravenous esmolol as the β-blocking regimen for acute dissection.* Because of its short half-life (9 min), it can be readily titrated in these often unstable patients. *An initial loading dose of 0.5 mg/kg administered over 1 min is followed by an infusion of 0.05 mg/kg per minute. The infusion rate can be increased at 4-min intervals by 0.05 mg/kg per minute. Rates beyond 0.2 mg/kg per minute have not been shown to provide added therapeutic benefit. The substantial amounts of fluid required to maintain this infusion limit the usefulness of this agent in some patients. If there is concern for volume excess, labetalol may be employed. This adrenergic-receptor blocking agent affects both nonselective β and α_1 receptors. A bolus infusion of 0.25 mg/kg over 2 min is recommended. Additional boluses of 0.25 to 0.5 mg/kg may be given every 15 min to effect. A cumulative dose of 300 mg should not be exceeded. A continuous infusion may result in drug accumulation because the half-life of this agent is 5.5 h.* Appropriate oral doses of β-blocking agents can be given for long-term maintenance after the need for acute β blockade has passed.

The ability of *intravenous nitroprusside* to reduce arterial pressure promptly and consistently and the ease with which its hypotensive effects can be titrated recommend it as the *current drug of choice for the patient whose blood pressure does not respond to β blockade. As little as 0.5 μg kg per minute may produce the desired result. Occasionally, as much as 5 μg/kg per minute is necessary. A dose of 10 μg/kg per minute should not be exceeded. A β-blocking agent nearly always should be used in conjunction with nitroprusside* because animal data suggest that when used alone, it does not reduce and may, through reflex mechanisms, enhance the rate of rise of arterial pressure.

Many potent antihypertensive agents (e.g., hydralazine, minoxidil, and diazoxide) cannot be recommended because they produce reflex stimulation of the left ventricle and consequently an increase in the rate of rise of aortic pressure.

Not all patients with acute aortic dissection have elevated blood pressure. Hypotension, it has been noted, may reflect aortic rupture and dictates emergency operation. Some individuals have pressures only slightly higher than the 100- to 120-mmHg target level, and pharmacologic treatment is of dubious value, although β-adrenergic blockade may be tried to reduce the rate of rise of aortic pressure.

As noted earlier, operative treatment must be considered in all patients, but certain subgroups can be recognized whose clinical presentation dictates the timing of the surgery. At one extreme are those who are hypotensive on admission and require emergency operation, as noted. On the other hand, operative treatment may never be an option in those with severe comorbid illness. Further, it may not be justified in those with severe neurologic injury from the dissection. In these inoperable individuals, antihypertensive therapy is continued indefinitely by converting the drug regimen to an oral one that avoids vasodilators.

The appropriateness and urgency of surgery for aortic dissection depend on its location and the clinical picture. *In cases involving the ascending aorta, operative repair should be undertaken as soon as the patient can be stabilized and appropriate diagnostic information compiled.* By contrast, for those with *uncomplicated type III (type B) dissection, it is now believed that operation during the acute phase does not appear to improve survival beyond that achieved with drug treatment unless there is intractable pain, uncontrollable hypertension, or serious organ malperfusion.*[104,106] Those who are relatively good operative risks may benefit from operation in the subacute or chronic phase to protect them from rupture of a residual saccular aneurysm. Risk factors (e.g., age, the presence of chronic obstructive lung disease, size of aneurysms, and its rate of expansion) for such late rupture are similar to those of degenerative thoracic aneurysms.[125]

The surgical technique for aortic dissection varies with the origin and extent of the dissection. The surgeons's *primary goal is always to remove the proximal (i.e., "entry") tear and to close the false channel at that site.* External rupture is most frequent just across from the entrance tear, as noted. For ascending aortic dissection, the procedure consists in transection of the ascending aorta with use of cardiopulmonary bypass, obliteration of the false lumen by approximation of the inner and outer walls of the false channel, and end-to-end anastomosis of the transected aorta. It is usually necessary to restore vascular continuity by means of a patch or tube graft. Aortic valve incompetence secondary to loss of commissural support of the valve leaflets may be corrected when this repair effectively resuspends the valve. Other patients may require prosthetic valve replacement or the use of a composite graft. Surgical mortality approaches 15 to 20 percent but varies with the location and extent of the disease as well as age and comorbid conditions.

Surgical treatment for dissection beginning in the arch or beyond requires much the same operative approach as has been described for aneurysms in these locations. The segment containing the entrance tear is resected, the false channel obliterated by suture closure of the inner and outer layers, and excised segment replaced with a graft. The morbidity and mortality of operative repair of the arch and descending aorta are somewhat greater than when the ascending aorta is treated.

Placement of a stent-graft through an endoluminal approach is being investigated in several centers as a less morbid approach to the treatment of distal dissection.[126]

Aortic Obstruction

COARCTATION OF THE AORTA

In its most common form, aortic coarctation consists of hemodynamically significant narrowing of the aortic isthmus, that segment lying between the left subclavian artery and the insertion of the ductus arteriosus. A common congenital abnormality, it accounts for about 9 percent of all congenital heart disease in children and is the fourth leading cause of symptomatic congenital heart disease in infancy.[127,128] Heart failure in an infant typically announces its presence. Associated, complex cardiac anomalies are frequent contributing factors (see Chaps. 63 and 64). A less complex and often asymptomatic abnormality, bicus-

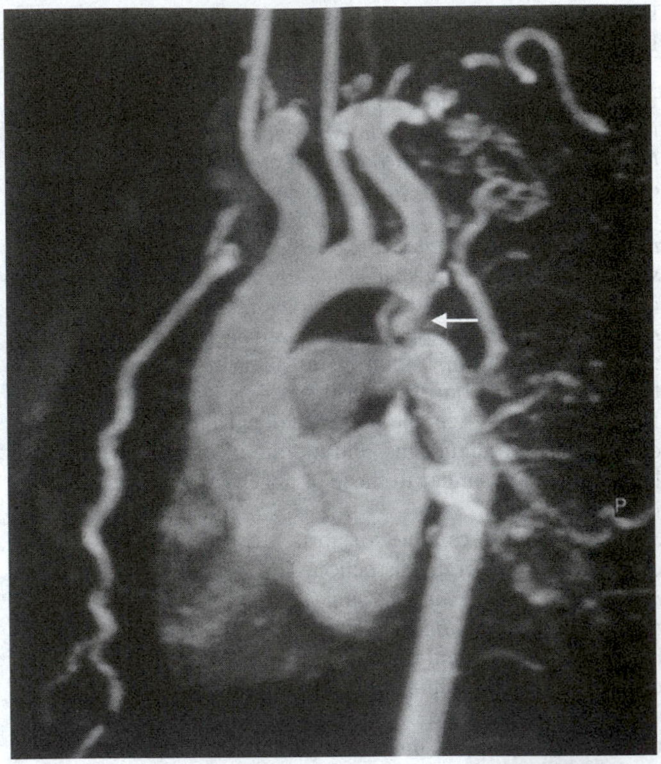

FIGURE 88-7 Magnetic resonance angiographic study from an adult with coarctation of the aorta. The tightly coarcted segment is indicated with an arrow. The collateral circulation is dramatically demonstrated. The left subclavian and innominate arteries, the source of these collaterals, are markedly dilated. (Courtesy of Dr. Karen Kuehl.)

pid aortic valve, is the most frequent associated anomaly. It is present in half or more of patients. Absent the appearance of heart failure in infancy, coarctation may be detected as upper extremity hypertension in an older child or young adult.

Large, tortuous collateral arteries develop in response to the aortic obstruction. These connections between branches of the subclavian and the intercostal arteries deliver blood to the distal aorta (Fig. 88-7). They enlarge, often to near aneurysmal proportions, gradually eroding the undersides of the ribs, producing the characteristic rib notching found on chest x-ray. Flow through these collaterals often produces recognizable bruits over the rib cage.

The natural history of this lesion is grim. Untreated, many patients die in childhood, and 80 percent die by age 50.[127,128] In the older patients, death is precipitated by cerebral hemorrhage (at least in part due to an association with berry aneurysm), aortic dissection or rupture, and infectious endocarditis.

Management Relief of the obstruction is the treatment of choice. Operative repair was first performed in 1945.[129] Currently, resection and end-to-end anastomosis, patch angioplasty, or subclavian flap angioplasty are employed. Catheter-based balloon dilatation or stenting is gaining acceptance as a less morbid option.[130–132]

Resection of the coarcted segment has not been as curative as expected. Persistent hypertension has been a significant problem, and the formation of aneurysms accompanied by dissection or rupture is well known.[129]

PSEUDOCOARCTATION OF THE AORTA

Congenital kinking, so-called pseudocoarctation of the aorta, may be detected during the investigation of a mediastinal mass or of a systolic murmur. An abnormally elongated thoracic aorta tethered to the ligamentum arteriosum produces a silhouette shaped like an S or a 3 on the chest x-ray, resembling true coarctation; however, rib notching is not present. Exclusion of hemodynamically significant coarctation may require sophisticated imaging or the demonstration that no pressure difference exists between the upper and the lower aortic segments. True coarctation may coexist, and congenital cardiovascular anomalies similar to those found in true coarctation may be associated.

Some authorities believe the abnormality to be a sharp downward angulation of the aorta at the attachment of the ligamentum arteriosum as a result of elongation of the fourth aortic arch. Others consider the embryologic defect to be the same as for typical isthmic coarctation, but in these cases the narrowing is not severe enough to result in significant obstruction.[133]

ABDOMINAL AORTIC COARCTATION (MIDDLE AORTIC SYNDROME)

Although rare, hemodynamically significant narrowing of the descending thoracic or abdominal aorta often produces life-threatening hypertension that is surgically correctable.[134–136] Although it often appears to be a congenital lesion, it may result from healed aortitis.[137] For this reason, some writers prefer to avoid the term *coarctation* and label it *middle aortic syndrome.*

Although the narrowed aortic segment typically is focal, diffuse hypoplasia of the abdominal aorta involving the branch arteries may occur. The renal arteries may be stenosed, hypoplastic, or thrombosed, resulting in severe hypertension. Visceral artery narrowing may result in bowel ischemia. Intermittent claudication from involvement of the iliac arteries is more frequent than in patients with typical coarctation.

On examination, upper extremity hypertension will be present together with feeble pulses and hypotension in the legs, findings similar to those of the more common postductal coarctation. Attention may be directed to the unusual location of the stenosis by a bruit in the lumbar or umbilical area.

Operative treatment usually is required because severe hypertension significantly shortens the life expectancy of patients.

CHRONIC OBSTRUCTION OF THE TERMINAL AORTA

Etiology and Pathogenesis Atherosclerosis of the aortoiliac bifurcation is the most common cause of chronic obstruction of the infrarenal aorta.[135,138] Many patients with symptomatic femoropopliteal atherosclerosis also have aortoiliac narrowing. Rarely, infrarenal coarctation, aortitis, clinically silent embolism, or in situ thrombosis produce this situation.

Rupture of atherosclerotic plaques sets the stage for mural thrombus and gradual progression of luminal narrowing and, in many instances, complete occlusion of the terminal aorta. Collateral vessels develop concomitantly, connecting the lumbar and inferior mesenteric arteries to branches of the internal iliac and common femoral arteries. Thus the symptoms of lower extremity ischemia typically progress over months or years, and progression to complete occlusion may not be marked by a clinical event. This indolent course, however, may be punctuated by an abrupt acceleration of symptoms, the result of a sudden increase in the size of the obstructing thrombus or its extension to a significant collateral.[135,138]

Aortoiliac atherosclerosis frequently has unusual features in that patients with aortoiliac narrowing may be younger and have a shorter duration of symptoms than do patients with femoropopliteal obstruction.[135,139] The predilection of atherosclerosis for the terminal aorta may be enhanced in some individuals because they have anatomic variations of the aortoiliac bifurcation that produce an "impedance mismatch." For example, an iliac bifurcation angle more acute than normal has been observed in some patients,[140] and in others, the aorta and iliac arteries are smaller than average.[141]

Clinical Features Men are affected far more often than women. The mean age of patients in most series falls in the sixth decade, but some are much younger. The usual risk factors for atherosclerosis are found frequently.

The original description of the clinical features of distal aortoiliac narrowing by René Leriche[142] (hence the Leriche syndrome) still applies, but variations on the theme are more frequent than the full-blown syndrome. Pain and tiredness in the lower back, buttocks, or thighs produced by exertion and relieved by brief periods of rest are hallmarks. Claudication may occur in the calf or foot in association with the more proximal distress and can be the sole complaint. Men often complain of inability to maintain a penile erection.

Absence of, or reduction in, the femoral pulse is typical. More distal pulses in the legs are reduced or absent, and bruits are commonly audible over femoral arteries and in the midline of the abdomen near the umbilicus. Low skin temperature, diminished hair growth, atrophy of the skin and subcutaneous tissue, and diminished muscle bulk in the lower limbs are common but not universal signs. Frank gangrene is infrequent, and amputation for ischemia is therefore seldom required.[136,139]

The findings in patients with aortoiliac obstruction overlap those in patients with femoropopliteal narrowing. A firm identification of involvement of the aortoiliac segment may be difficult on clinical grounds, and in many patients, obstructing lesions are present at both levels. Modern imaging techniques have made diagnosticians less dependent on clinical findings for the localization of the level of arterial obstruction.[135,138]

Natural History and Prognosis The survival rate for patients with the Leriche syndrome appears to be lower than for those in a control population matched for age and sex, but death rarely results from aortoiliac disease. Coronary and cerebrovascular atherosclerosis are largely responsible for the higher death rate. Significant morbidity or death occasionally follows occlusion of the renal arteries by proximal extension of the thrombotic process.[135,138]

Management End-to-side bypass with a flexible, knitted bifurcation graft is the preferable method of treatment. In the absence of femoropopliteal occlusive disease, this approach is usually successful in restoring normal distal circulation. Even when there is combined aortoiliac and femoropopliteal disease, bypass of the aortoiliac occlusion alone may increase lower extremity flow sufficiently to relieve symptoms.

Percutaneous transluminal angioplasty is being used with increasing frequency in the treatment of iliac and femoropopliteal obstructive atherosclerotic disease. The early success rate appears to be satisfactory, but the long-term patency rate remains to be determined.

ACUTE OBSTRUCTION OF THE TERMINAL AORTA

Etiology Sudden occlusion of the terminal aorta may result from a large ("saddle") embolus, trauma, medial dissection, or in situ thrombosis superimposed on an aneurysm or severe atherosclerosis. With either dissection or trauma, the etiology is usually obvious.[143,144]

Most emboli large enough to occlude the terminal aorta come from the heart, and embolus must be considered in acute aortoiliac occlusion in patients with mitral stenosis, atrial fibrillation, or recent myocardial infarction. Rarely, embolization of a vegetation from fungal endocarditis may be large enough to occlude the aortic bifurcation.[143,144]

In situ thrombosis of an aneurysm or of a severely atherosclerotic aorta may develop when blood flow through these vessels is considerably reduced, as may be the case in shock or congestive heart failure.

Clinical Features Unlike gradually progressive obstruction, abrupt total or near-total interruption of flow through the terminal aorta or common iliac arteries poses an immediate threat to life and limb. Although the clinical picture varies depending on the presence of preexisting collaterals, the full-blown syndrome is characterized by the abrupt onset of pain, typically severe and located in the lumbar area, the buttocks, the perineum, the abdomen, and the legs. Numbness, paresthesia, dysesthesia, and finally paralysis of the affected limb dominate the picture. Pulses are absent in the legs, although at times faint femoral pulsations may be detected. The legs are cold and pale. Unless circulation is restored promptly, massive muscle necrosis may produce myoglobinuria, renal failure, acidosis, and hyperkalemia.

Management In contrast to chronic aortoiliac occlusion, acute obstruction to blood flow does not allow for the formation of collateral circulation. Immediate revascularization is necessary for survival. The procedure used depends on the cause of the occlusion. Moreover, consideration must be given to treatment of the source of the embolus (e.g., mitral stenosis or left ventricular mural thrombus), in order to prevent recurrent embolization to such vital organs as the brain.

Aortoiliac embolectomy may be performed directly through an incision in the distal aorta or proximal iliac arteries but requires laparotomy in a severely ill patient and does not provide the means for removing more distally lodged embolic material. The preferable approach is to expose both common femoral arteries in the groins and, through transverse arteriotomies, to remove, with balloon-tipped Fogarty catheters, the embolic material lodged proximally and distally. Even large amounts of embolic material in the distal aorta itself can be removed safely in this manner. Good circulation usually is restored. Subsequent mortality rates, however, remain high because of the underlying disease.

References

1. Wolinsky H, Glagov S. A lamellar unit of aortic medial structure and function in mammals. *Circulation* 1976; 20:99–111.
2. Schlatmann TJ, Becker AE. Histologic changes in the normal aging aorta: Implications for dissecting aortic aneurysm. *Am J Cardiol* 1977; 39:13–20.
3. Cornwell GG III, Westermark P, Murdoch W, et al. Senile aortic amyloid: A third distinctive type of age-related cardiovascular amyloid. *Am J Pathol* 1982; 108:135–140.
4. Khoury Z, Gottlieb S, Stern S, et al. Frequency and distribution of atherosclerotic plaques in the thoracic aorta as determined by transesophageal echocardiography in patients with coronary artery disease. *Am J Cardiol* 1997; 79:23–27.
5. Kawaguchi A, Miyatake K, Yutani C, et al. Characteristic cardiovascular manifestation in homozygous and heterozygous familial hypercholesterolemia. *Am Heart J* 1999; 137:410–418.
6. Summers RM, Andrasko-Bourgeois J, Feuerstein IM, et al. Evaluation of the aortic root by MRI: Insights from patients with homozygous familial hypercholesterolemia. *Circulation* 1998; 98:509–518.
7. Reed D, Reed C, Stemmermann G, et al. Are aortic aneurysms caused by atherosclerosis? *Circulation* 1992; 85:205–211.
8. Bengtsson H, Norrgard O, Angquist KA, et al. Ultrasonographic screening of the abdominal aorta among siblings of patients with abdominal aortic aneurysms. *Br J Surg* 1989; 76:589–591.
9. Kontusaari S, Tromp G, Kuivaniemi H, et al. A mutation in the gene for type iii procollagen (*COL3A1*) in a family with aortic aneurysms. *J Clin Invest* 1990; 80:1465–1473.
10. Tilson MD. Aortic aneurysms and atherosclerosis. *Circulation* 1992; 85:378–379.
11. Khatibzadeh M, Mitusch R, Stierle U, et al. Aortic atherosclerotic plaques as a source of systemic embolism. *J Am Coll Cardiol* 1996; 27:664–669.
12. Davila-Roman VG, Murphy SF, Nickerson NJ, et al. Atherosclerosis of the ascending aorta is an independent predictor of long-term neurologic events and mortality. *J Am Coll Cardiol* 1999; 33:1308–1316.
13. Finkelhor RS, Youssefi ME, Lamont WE, et al. Embolic risk based on aortic atherosclerotic morphologic features and aortic spontaneous echocardiographic contrast. *Am Heart J* 1999; 137:1088–1093.
14. Ferrari E, Vidal R, Chevallier T, et al. Atherosclerosis of the thoracic aorta and aortic debris as a marker of poor prognosis: Benefit of oral anticoagulants. *J Am Coll Cardiol* 1999; 33:1317–1322.
15. Om A, Ellahham S, DiSciascio G. Cholesterol embolism: An underdiagnosed clinical entity. *Am Heart J* 1992; 124:1321–1326.
16. Vilacosta I, San Roman JA, Aragoncillo P, et al. Penetrating atherosclerotic ulcer: Documentation by transesophageal echocardiography. *J Am Coll Cardiol* 1998; 32:83–89.
17. Roman MJ, Devereux RB. Heritable aortic disease. In: Lindsay J Jr, ed. *Diseases of the Aorta*. Philadelphia: Lea and Febiger; 1994:55–74.
18. Savunen T. Annulo-aortic ectasia: A clinical, structural and biochemical study. *Scand J Thorac Cardiovasc Surg Suppl* 1986; 37:1–45.
19. Schlatmann TJ, Becker AE. Pathogenesis of dissecting aneurysm of the aorta: Comparative histopathologic study of significance of medial changes. *Am J Cardiol* 1977; 39:21–26.
20. Hirst AE, Gore I. Is cystic medionecrosis the cause of dissecting aortic aneurysm? *Circulation* 1976; 53:915–916.
21. Nakashima Y, Kurozumi T, Sueishi K, et al. Dissecting aneurysm: A clinicopathologic and histopathologic study of 111 autopsied cases. *Hum Pathol* 1990; 21:291–296.
22. Isner JM, Donaldson RF, Fulton D, et al. Cystic medial necrosis in coarctation of the aorta. *Circulation* 1987; 75:689–695.
23. Bonderman D, Gharehbaghi-Schnell E, Wollenek G, et al. Mechanisms underlying aortic dilatation in congenital aortic valve malformation. *Circulation* 1999; 99:2138–2143.
24. Tsipouras P, Del Mastro R, Sarfarazi M, et al. Genetic linkage of the Marfan syndrome, ectopia lentis, and congenital contractural arachnodactyly to the fibrillin genes on chromosomes 15 and 5. *N Engl J Med* 1992; 326:905–909.
25. Roberts CS, Roberts WC. Dissection of the aorta associated with congenital malformation of the aortic valve. *J Am Coll Cardiol* 1991; 17:712–716.
26. Nistri S, Sorbo MD, Marin M, et al. Aortic root dilatation in young men with normally functioning bicuspid valves. *Heart* 1999; 82:19–22.
27. Lindsay J Jr. Coarctation of the aorta, bicuspid aortic valve and abnormal ascending aortic wall. *Am J Cardiol* 1988; 61:182–184.
28. Subramaniam PN. Turner's syndrome and cardiovascular abnormalities: A case report and review of the literature. *Am J Med Sci* 1989; 297:260–262.
29. Nunez L, O'Connor LF, Pinto AG, et al. Annuloaortic ectasia and adult polycystic kidney: A frequent association. *Chest* 1986; 90:299–300.
30. Biagini A, Maffei S, Baroni M, et al. Familial clustering of aortic dissection in polycystic kidney disease. *Am J Cardiol* 1993; 72:741–742.
31. Leier CV, Call TD, Fulkerson PK, et al. The spectrum of defects in the Ehlers-Danlos syndrome, types I and III. *Ann Intern Med* 1980; 92:171–178.
32. Hortop J, Tsipouras P, Hanley JA, et al. Cardiovascular involvement in osteogenesis imperfecta. *Circulation* 1986; 73:54–61.
33. Marsalese DL, Moodie DS, Lytle BW, et al. Cystic medial necrosis of the aorta in patients without Marfan's syndrome: Surgical outcome and long-term follow-up. *J Am Coll Cardiol* 1990; 16:68–73.
34. Roman MJ, Devereux RB, Niles NW, et al. Aortic root dilatation as a cause of isolated, severe aortic regurgitation. *Ann Intern Med* 1987; 106:800–807.
35. Milewicz DM, Michael K, Fisher N, et al. Fibrillin-1 (*FBN1*) mutations in patients with thoracic aortic aneurysms. *Circulation* 1996; 94:2708–2711.
36. Ewart JM, Burke ML, Bunt TJ. Spontaneous abdominal aortic infections: Essentials of diagnosis and management. *Am Surg* 1983; 49:37–50.
37. Jackman JD, Radolf JD. Cardiovascular syphilis. *Am J Med* 1989; 87:425–433.
38. Atnip RG. Mycotic aneurysms of the suprarenal abdominal aorta: Prolonged survival after in situ aortic and visceral reconstruction. *J Vasc Surg* 1989; 10:635–641.
39. Oz MC, McNicholas KW, Serra AJS, et al. Review of *Salmonella* mycotic aneurysms of the thoracic aorta. *J Cardiovasc Surg* 1989; 30:99–103.
40. Cohen PS, O'Brien TF, Schoenbaum SC, Medeiros AA. The risk of endothelial infection in adults with salmonella bacteremia. *Ann Intern Med* 1978; 89:931–932.
41. Johansen K, Devin J. Mycotic aortic aneurysms: A reappraisal. *Arch Surg* 1983; 118:583–641.
42. Sessa C, Farah I, Voirin L, et al. Infected aneurysms of the infrarenal abdominal aorta: Diagnostic criteria and therapeutic strategy. *Ann Vasc Surg* 1997; 11:453–463.
43. Oskoui R, Davis WA, Gomes MN. *Salmonella* aortitis: A report of a successfully treated case with a comprehensive review of the literature. *Arch Intern Med* 1993; 153:517–525.
44. Bennett DE. Primary mycotic aneurysms of the aorta. *Arch Surg* 1967; 94:758–765.
45. Allins AD, Wagner WH, Cossman DV, et al. Tuberculous infection of the descending thoracic and abdominal aorta: Case report and literature review. *Ann Vasc Surg* 1999; 13:439–444.
46. Golzarian J, Cheng J, Giron F, et al. Tuberculous pseudoaneu-

rysm of the descending thoracic aorta. *Tex Heart Inst J* 1999; 26:232–235.
47. Arnett EN, Roberts WC. Valve ring abscess in active infective endocarditis: Frequency, location, and clues to clinical diagnosis from the study of 95 necropsy patients. *Circulation* 1976; 54:140–145.
48. Daniel WG, Mugge A, Martin RP, et al. Improvement in the diagnosis of abscesses associated with endocarditis by transesophageal echocardiography. *N Engl J Med* 1991; 324:795–800.
49. Feigl D, Feigl A, Edwards JE. Mycotic aneurysms of the aortic root: A pathologic study of 20 cases. *Chest* 1986; 90:553–557.
50. Ito I. Aortitis syndrome (Takayasu's arteritis): A historical perspective. *Jpn Heart J* 1995; 36:273–281.
51. Kerr GS, Hallahan CW, Giordano J, et al. Takayasu Arteritis. *Ann Intern Med* 1994; 120:919–929.
52. Ishikawa K. Diagnostic approach and proposed criteria for the clinical diagnosis of Takayasu's arteriopathy. *J Am Coll Cardiol* 1988; 12:964–972.
53. Noris M, Daina E, Gamba S, et al. Interleukin-6 and RANTES in Takayasu's arteritis: A guide for therapeutic decisions. *Circulation* 1999; 100:55–60.
54. Eichorn J, Sima D, Thiele B, et al. Anti-endothelial cell antibodies in Takayasu's arteritis. *Circulation* 1996; 94:2396–2401.
55. Takeuchi Y, Matsuki K, Saito Y, et al. HLA-D region genomic polymorphism associated with Takayasu's arteritis. *Angiology* 1990; 41:421–426.
56. Ishikawa K, Maetani S. Long-term outcome for 120 Japanese patients with Takayasu's disease. *Circulation* 1994; 90:1855–1860.
57. Wong VCW, Wang RYC, Tse TF. Pregnancy and Takayasu's arteritis. *Am J Med* 1983; 75:597–601.
58. Arend WP, Michel BA, Bloch DA, et al. The American College of Rheumatology 1990 criteria for the classification of Takayasu arteritis. *Arthritis Rheum* 1990; 33:1129–1134.
59. Ishikawa K. Effects of prednisolone therapy on arterial angiographic features in Takayasu's disease. *Am J Cardiol* 1991; 68:410–413.
60. Fraga A, Mintz G, Valle L, et al. Takayasu's arteritis: Frequency of systemic manifestations (study of 22 patients) and favorable response to maintenance corticosteroid therapy with adrenocorticosteroids (12 patients). *Arthritis Rheum* 1972; 15:617–624.
61. Tyagi S, Singh B, Kaul UA, et al. Balloon angioplasty for renovascular hypertension in Takayasu's arteritis. *Am Heart J* 1993; 125:1386–1393.
62. Evans JM, O'Fallon WM, Hunder GG. Increased incidence of aortic aneurysm and dissection in giant cell (temporal) arteritis. *Ann Intern Med* 1995; 122:502–507.
63. Bergfeldt L, Insulander P, Lindblom D, et al. HLA-B27: An important genetic risk factor for lone aortic regurgitation and severe conduction system abnormalities. *Am J Med* 1988; 85:12–18.
64. Bulkley BH, Roberts WC. Ankylosing spondylitis and aortic regurgitation: Description of the characteristic cardiovascular lesion from study of eight necropsy patients. *Circulation* 1973; 48:1014–1027.
65. Roldan CA, Chavez J, Wiest PW, et al. Aortic root disease and valve disease associated with ankylosing spondylitis. *J Am Coll Cardiol* 1998; 32:1397–1404.
66. Kent KC, Boyce SW. Aneurysms of the aorta. In: Lindsay J Jr, ed. *Diseases of the Aorta*. Philadelphia: Lea and Febiger; 1994:109–125.
67. Patel MI, Hardman DTA, Fisher CM. Current views on the pathogenesis of abdominal aortic aneurysms. *J Am Coll Surg* 1995; 181:371–382.
68. Heinemann M, Laas J, Karck M, et al. Thoracic aortic aneurysm after acute type A aortic dissection: Necessity for follow-up. *Ann Thorac Surg* 1990; 49:580–584.
69. Verloes A, Sakalihasan N, Koulischer L, et al. Aneurysms of the abdominal aorta: Familial and genetic aspects in three hundred thirteen pedigrees. *J Vasc Surg* 1995; 21:646–655.
70. Salo JA, Soisalon-Soininen S, Bondestam S, et al. Familial occurrence of abdominal aneurysm. *Ann Intern Med* 1999; 130: 637–642.
71. Davies MJ. Aortic aneurysm formation. *Circulation* 1998; 98:193–195.
72. Sakakibara S, Konno S. Congenital aneurysm of the sinus of Valsalva: Anatomy and classification. *Am Heart J* 1962; 63:405–424.
73. Lindsay J Jr. Anatomic and pathogenetic bases for some uncommon clinical syndromes from aortic disease. In: Lindsay J Jr, ed. *Diseases of the Aorta*. Philadelphia: Lea and Febiger; 1994:165–177.
74. Smith JA, Fann JI, Miller DC, et al. Surgical management of aortic dissection in patients with the Marfan syndrome. *Circulation* 1994; 90(2):II235–II242.
75. Joyce JW, Fairbairn JF II, Kincaid OW, et al. Aneurysms of the thoracic aorta: A clinical study with special reference to prognosis. *Circulation* 1964; 29:176–181.
76. Pressler V, McNamara JJ. Thoracic aortic aneurysm: Natural history and treatment. *J Thorac Cardiovasc Surg* 1980; 79:489–498.
77. Goldstein SA, Lindsay J Jr. Thoracic aortic aneurysms: Role of echocardiography. *Echocardiography* 1996; 13:213–232.
78. Clouse WD, Hallett JW Jr, Schaff HV, et al. Improved prognosis of thoracic aortic aneurysms. *JAMA* 1998; 280:1926–1929.
79. Murdoch JL, Walker BA, Halpern BL, et al. Life expectancy and causes of death in the Marfan syndrome. *N Engl J Med* 1972; 286:804–808.
80. Silverman DI, Burton KJ, Gray J, et al. Life expectancy in the Marfan Syndrome. *Am J Cardiol* 1995; 75:157–160.
81. Dake MD, Miller DC, Mitchell RS, et al. The "first generation" of endovascular stent-grafts for patients with aneurysms of the descending thoracic aorta. *J Thorac Cardiovasc Surg* 1998; 116:689–704.
82. Dapunt OE, Galla JD, Sadeghi AM, et al. The natural history of thoracic aortic aneurysms. *J Thorac Cardiovasc Surg* 1994; 107:1323–1333.
83. Kouchoukos NT, Dougenis D. Surgery of the thoracic aorta. *N Engl J Med* 1997; 336:1876–1888.
84. Coady MA, Rizzo JA, Hammond GL, et al. What is the appropriate size criterion for resection of thoracic aortic aneurysms? *J Thorac Cardiovasc Surg* 1997; 113:476–491.
85. Juvonen T, Ergin MA, Galla JD, et al. Prospective study of the natural history of thoracic aortic aneurysms. *Ann Thorac Surg* 1997; 63:1533–1545.
86. Ernst CB. Abdominal aortic aneurysm. *N Engl J Med* 1993; 328:1167–1172.
87. Sterpetti AV, Hunter WJ, Feldhaus RJ, et al. Inflammatory aneurysms of the abdominal aorta: Incidence, pathologic, and etiologic considerations. *J Vasc Surg* 1989; 9:643–650.
88. Leseche G, Schaetz A, Arrive L, et al. Diagnosis and management of 17 consecutive patients with inflammatory abdominal aortic aneurysms. *Am J Surg* 1992; 164:39–44.
88a. Sullivan CA, Rohrer MJ, Cutler BS. Clinical management of the symptomatic but unruptured abdominal aortic aneurysm. *J Vasc Surg* 1990; 11:799–803.
88b. Bower TC, Cherry KJ Jr, Pairolero PC. Unusual manifestations of abdominal aortic aneurysms. *Surg Clin North Am* 1989; 69:745–754.
89. Keen RR, McCarthy WJ, Shireman PK, et al. Surgical management of atheroembolization. *J Vasc Surg* 1995; 21:773–781.
90. Dolmatch BL, Gray RJ, Horton KM, et al. Diagnostic imaging in the evaluation of aortic disease. In: Lindsay J Jr, ed. *Diseases of the Aorta*. Philadelphia: Lea and Febiger; 1994:197–250.
91. Scott RAP, Wilson NM, Ashton HA, et al. Is surgery necessary

for abdominal aneurysm less than 6 cm in diameter? *Lancet* 1993; 342:1395–1396.

92. Vazquez C, Sakalihasan N, D'Harcour J-B, et al. Routine ultrasound screening for abdominal aortic aneurysm among 65- and 75-year-old men in a city of 200,000 inhabitants. *Ann Vasc Surg* 1998; 12:544–549.
93. Lederle FA. Management of small abdominal aortic aneurysms. *Ann Intern Med* 1990; 113:731–732.
94. Nevitt MP, Ballard DJ, Hallett JW Jr. Prognosis of abdominal aortic aneurysm: A population-based study. *N Engl J Med* 1989; 321:1009–1014.
95. Guiruis EM, Barber GG. The natural history of abdominal aortic aneurysms. *Am J Surg* 1991; 162:481–483.
96. Nehler MR, Taylor LM Jr, Moneta GL, et al. Indications for operation for infrarenal abdominal aneurysms: Current guidelines. *Semin Vasc Surg* 1995; 8:108–114.
97. UK Small Aneurysm Trial Participants. Mortality results for randomised controlled trial of early elective surgery or ultrasonographic surveillance for small abdominal aortic aneurysms. *Lancet* 1998; 352:1649–1655.
98. Roger VL, Ballard DJ, Hallett JW Jr, et al. Influence of coronary artery disease on morbidity and mortality after abdominal aortic aneurysmectomy: A population-based study, 1971–1987. *J Am Coll Cardiol* 1989; 14:1245–1252.
99. Graor RA. Preoperative evaluation and management of coronary and carotid artery occlusive disease in patients with abdominal aortic aneurysms. *Surg Clin North Am* 1989; 69:737–743.
100. Cambria RP, Eagle K. Cardiac screening before abdominal aortic aneurysm surgery: A reassessment. *Semin Vasc Surg* 1995; 8:93–102.
101. Koskas F, Kieffer E, for the AURC. Surgery for ruptured abdominal aortic aneurysm: Early and late results of a prospective study by the AURC in 1989. *Ann Vasc Surg* 1997; 11:473–481.
102. Zarins CK, White RA, Schwarten D, et al. Aneux stent graft versus open surgical repair of abdominal aortic aneurysms: Multicenter prospective trials. *J Vasc Surg* 1999; 29:292–308.
103. Seelig MH, Oldenburg WA, Hakaim AG, et al. Endovascular repair of abdominal aortic aneurysms: Where do we stand? *Mayo Clin Proc* 1999; 74:999–1010.
104. Spittell PC, Spittell JA Jr, Joyce JW, et al. Clinical features and differential diagnosis of aortic dissection: Experience with 236 cases (1980–1990). *Mayo Clin Proc* 1993; 68:642–651.
105. Crawford ES. The diagnosis and management of aortic dissection. *JAMA* 1990; 264:2537–2541.
106. Lindsay J Jr. Aortic dissection. In: Lindsay J Jr, ed. *Diseases of the Aorta*. Philadelphia: Lea and Febiger; 1999:127–142.
107. Roberts WC. Aortic dissection: Anatomy, consequences, and causes. *Am Heart J* 1981; 101:195–214.
108. Hirst AE Jr, Johns VJ Jr, Kime SW Jr. Dissecting aneurysms of the aorta: A review of 505 cases. *Medicine* 1958; 37:217–279.
109. Mohr-Kahaly S, Erbel R, Kearney P, et al. Aortic intramural hemorrhage visualized by transesophageal echocardiography: Findings and prognostic implications. *J Am Coll Cardiol* 1994; 23:658–664.
110. Nienaber CA, von Kodolitsch Y, Peterson B, et al. Intramural hemorrhage of the thoracic aorta: Diagnostic and therapeutic implications. *Circulation* 1995; 92:1465–1472.
111. Harris KM, Braverman AC, Gutierrez FR, et al. Transesophageal echocardiographic and clinical features of aortic intramural hematoma. *J Thorac Cardiovasc Surg* 1997; 114:619–626.
112. Bansal RC, Chandrasekaran K, Ayala K, et al. Frequency and explanation of false negative diagnosis of aortic dissection by aortography and transesophageal echocardiography. *J Am Coll Cardiol* 1995; 25:1393–1401.
113. Svensson LG, Labib SB, Eisenhauer AC, et al. Intimal tear without hematoma: An important variant of aortic dissection that can elude current imaging techniques. *Circulation* 1999; 99:1331–1336.
114. Lindsay J Jr. Aortocameral fistula: A rare complication of aortic dissection. *Am Heart J* 1993; 126:441–443.
115. Kamp TJ, Goldschmidt-Clermont PJ, Brinker JA, et al. Myocardial infarction, aortic dissection, and thrombolytic therapy. *Am Heart J* 1994; 128:1234–1237.
116. Hughes JD, Bacha EA, Dodson TF, et al. Peripheral vascular complications of aortic dissection. *Am J Surg* 1995; 170:209–212.
117. Moore NR, Parry AJ, Trottman-Dickenson B, et al. Fate of the native aorta after repair of acute type A dissection: A magnetic resonance imaging study. *Heart* 1996; 75:62–66.
118. Williams GM, Gott VL, Brawley RK, et al. Aortic disease associated with pregnancy. *J Vasc Surg* 1988; 8:470–475.
119. Oskoui R, Lindsay J Jr. Aortic dissection in women less than 40 years of age and the unimportance of pregnancy. *Am J Cardiol* 1994; 73:821–822.
120. Keren A, Kim CB, Hu BS, et al. Accuracy of biplane and multiplane transesophageal echocardiography in diagnosis of typical acute aortic dissection and intramural hematoma. *J Am Coll Cardiol* 1996; 28:627–636.
121. Cigarroa JE, Isselbacher EM, DeSanctis RW, et al. Diagnostic imaging in the evaluation of suspected aortic dissection. *N Engl J Med* 1993; 328:35–43.
122. Armstrong WF, Bach DS, Carey LM, et al. Clinical and echocardiographic findings in patients with suspected acute aortic dissection. *Am Heart J* 1998; 136:1051–1060.
123. Lindsay J Jr, Hurst JW. Clinical features and prognosis in dissecting aneurysm of the aorta: A reappraisal. *Circulation* 1967; 35:880–888.
124. Doroghazi RM, Slater EE, DeSanctis RW, et al. Long-term survival of patients with treated aortic dissection. *J Am Coll Cardiol* 1984; 3:1026–1034.
125. Juvonen T, Ergin MA, Galla JD, et al. Risk factors for rupture of chronic type-B dissections. *J Thorac Cardiovasc Surg* 1999; 117:776–786.
126. Nienaber CA, Fattori R, Lund G, et al. Nonsurgical reconstruction of thoracic aortic dissection by stent-graft placement. *N Engl J Med* 1999; 340:1539–1545.
127. Reifenstein GH, Levine SA, Gross RE. Coarctation of the aorta. *Am Heart J* 1947; 33:146–168.
128. Liberthson RR, Pennington DG, Jacobs ML, et al. Coarctation of the aorta: Review of 234 patients and clarification of management problems. *Am J Cardiol* 1979; 43:835–840.
129. Maron BJ, Humphries JO, Rowe RD, et al. Prognosis of surgically corrected coarctation of the aorta: A 20-year postoperative appraisal. *Circulation* 1973; 47:119–126.
130. McCrindle BW, Jones TK, Morrow WR, et al. Acute results of balloon angioplasty of native coarctation versus recurrent aortic obstruction are equivalent. *J Am Coll Cardiol* 1996; 28:1810–1817.
131. Eid Fawzy M, SivanandamV, Galal O, et al. One- to ten-year follow-up results of balloon angioplasty of native coarctation of the aorta in adolescents and adults. *J Am Coll Cardiol* 1997; 30:1542–1546.
132. Ebeid MR, Prieto LR, Latson LA. Use of balloon-expandable stents for coarctation of the aorta: Initial results and intermediate-term follow-up. *J Am Coll Cardiol* 1997; 30:1847–1852.
133. Hoeffel JC, Henry M, Mentre B, et al. Pseudocoarctation or congenital kinking of the aorta: Radiologic considerations. *Am Heart J* 1975; 89:428–436.
134. Bergamini TM, Bernard JD, Mavroudis C, et al. Coarctation of the abdominal aorta. *Ann Vasc Surg* 1995; 9:352–356.
135. Lindsay J Jr. Acquired obstructive disease of the aorta. In: Lindsay J Jr, ed. *Diseases of the Aorta*. Philadelphia: Lea and Febiger; 1994:145–156.
136. Mickley V, Fleiter T. Coarctations of the descending and abdomi-

nal aorta: Long-term results of surgical therapy. *J Vasc Surg* 1998; 28:206–214.

137. Lande A. Takayasu's arteritis and congenital coarctation of the descending thoracic and abdominal aorta: A critical review. *AJR* 1976; 127:227–233.
138. Brewster DC. Clinical and anatomical considerations for surgery in aortoiliac disease and results of surgical treatment. *Circulation* 1991; 83(suppl I):I-42–52.
139. Stubbs DH, Kasulke RJ, Kapsch DN, et al. Populations with the Leriche syndrome. *Surgery* 1981; 89:612–616.
140. Sharp WV, Donovan DL, Teague PC, et al. Arterial occlusive disease: A function of vessel bifurcation angle. *Surgery* 1982; 91:680–685.
141. Palmaz JC, Carson SN, Hunter G, et al. Male hypoplastic infrarenal aorta and premature atherosclerosis. *Surgery* 1983; 94: 91–94.
142. Leriche R, Morel A. The syndrome of thrombotic obliteration of the aortic bifurcation. *Ann Surg* 1948; 127:193–204.
143. Busuttil RW, Keehn G, Milliken J, et al. Aortic saddle embolus: A twenty-year experience. *Ann Surg* 1983; 197:698–706.
144. Webb KH, Jacocks MA. Acute aortic occlusion. *Am J Surg* 1988; 155:405–407.

CHAPTER 89

CEREBROVASCULAR DISEASE AND NEUROLOGIC MANIFESTATIONS OF HEART DISEASE

Louis R. Caplan

Most vascular diseases affect both the heart and the brain. Heart diseases often lead to lesions and dysfunction within the brain, and central nervous system (CNS) diseases influence the heart and its function.

BRAIN AND CEREBROVASCULAR COMPLICATIONS OF HEART DISEASE

Cerebral complications occur when (1) the heart pumps unwanted materials into the circulation that reach the brain (embolism), (2) pump function fails and the brain is hypoperfused, and (3) drugs given to treat cardiac disease have neurologic side effects.

Cardiogenic Brain Embolism

ETIOLOGY

The diagnostic criteria for cardiogenic embolism were formerly very restrictive. Embolism was diagnosed when sudden focal neurologic signs, maximal at onset, developed in patients with peripheral systemic embolism and recent myocardial infarction or rheumatic mitral stenosis.[1] With the use of these criteria, cardiogenic embolism was diagnosed in only 3 to 8 percent of stroke patients.[2–5] None of these criteria are secure. In various stroke registries, about 10 to 20 percent of patients did not have maximal symptoms at onset.[5–7] Many other cardiac lesions are now well-accepted sources of emboli, e.g., atrial fibrillation. Only about 2 percent of patients with a cardiogenic brain embolism have clinically recognized peripheral emboli. In necropsy studies of patients with brain embolism, however, infarcts are found commonly in the spleen and kidneys and in other organs. The symptoms of peripheral embolism are often so minor and nonspecific (transient abdominal discomfort, leg cramp, etc.) that they seldom are diagnosed correctly.

Before the advent of echocardiography, 30 percent of stroke patients were considered likely to have a cardiogenic embolism.[5,6] Later studies using stricter criteria attributed up to 22 percent[8] of strokes to a cardiogenic embolism. With more advanced diagnostic techniques, more cardiac abnormalities are recognized; in the Lausanne Stroke Registry, 23 percent of patients with a first stroke had a potential cardiac source of embolism.[9] Because many patients have coexisting cardiac and extracranial vascular disease,[9] criteria for the diagnosis of cardiac embolism remain controversial.

Cardiac sources can be divided into three groups:[1] (1) *cardiac wall and chamber abnormalities*, e.g., cardiomyopathies, hypokinetic and akinetic ventricular regions after myocardial infarction, atrial septal aneurysms, ventricular aneurysms, atrial myxomas, papillary fibroelastomas and other tumors, septal defects, and patent foramen ovale, (2) *valve disorders*, e.g., rheumatic mitral and aortic disease, prosthetic valves, bacterial endocarditis, fibrous and fibrinous endocardial lesions, mitral valve prolapse, and mitral annulus calcification, and (3) *arrhythmias*, especially atrial fibrillation and "sick-sinus" syndrome.

Some cardiac sources have much higher rates of initial and

recurrent embolism. The Stroke Data Bank[10] divided potential sources into *strong sources* (prosthetic valves, atrial fibrillation, sick-sinus syndrome, ventricular aneurysm, akinetic segments, mural thrombi, cardiomyopathy, diffuse ventricular hypokinesia) and *weak sources* (myocardial infarct over 6 months old, aortic and mitral stenosis and regurgitation, congestive failure, mitral valve prolapse, mitral annulus calcification, hypokinetic ventricular segments).

The risk of embolism varies within individual cardiac abnormalities, depending on many factors. For example, in patients with atrial fibrillation, associated heart disease, patient age, duration, chronic versus intermittent fibrillation, and atrial size all influence embolic risk. The presence of a potential cardiac source of embolism does not mean that a stroke was caused by an embolus from the heart. Coexistent occlusive cerebrovascular disease is common. In the Lausanne registry, among patients with potential cardiac embolic sources, 11 percent had severe cervicocranial vascular occlusive disease (>75 percent stenosis) and 40 percent had mild to moderate stenosis proximal to brain infarcts.[9]

Mitral valve prolapse (MVP) as a source of embolism continues to be controversial[1] (see Chap. 58). Clinical studies indicate that MVP is associated with stroke.[11,12] Morphologic lesions such as thrombi and fibrous lesions clearly suggest embolism;[13] fibrin-platelet depositions on the surfaces of the mitral leaflets have been noted,[13] as well as thrombi in the angle between the posterior mitral valve leaflet and the left atrial wall.[12,14] Patients with MVP also have other disorders, such as atrial fibrillation, syncope, and migraine. The rate of recurrence of stroke in patients with MVP as the only known cause is very low.[11,12] In light of the very high incidence of MVP, the frequency of MVP-related stroke is extremely low.[12,14,15] Most neurologists feel that warfarin anticoagulants ordinarily are not indicated in prophylaxis of patients with MVP even after an initial stroke. Aspirin prophylaxis (80 to 325 mg/day) is, however, advisable. Demonstration of an intracardiac thrombus by echocardiography would change that recommendation to warfarin.

Mitral annulus calcification (MAC) is an important and often unrecognized cause of embolism. Ulceration and extrusion of calcium through overlapping cusps have been seen at necropsy,[16] thrombi have been found on valves attached to the ulcerative process,[17] and calcific emboli have been seen in surgical embolectomies.[12,16] Several series have shown a convincing relationship between MAC and brain emboli and stroke.[1,18,19] Bacterial endocarditis also can develop on a MAC.

More patients have cardiogenic embolism than are diagnosed. Clinical features and brain investigations such as computed tomography (CT), magnetic resonance imaging (MRI), and angiography (CT, MRI, and digital subtraction) may suggest emboli, but often a source is not identified. These cases, which are termed *infarcts of unknown causes* (IUC) in the Stroke Data Bank,[6,20] include as many as 40 percent of patients.

Some disorders are associated with *fibrous and fibrinous lesions of the heart valves and endocardium*.[1] Similar valve lesions occur in patients with systemic lupus erythematosus (Libman-Sachs endocarditis[21]), the antiphospholipid antibody syndrome,[22] and cancer and other debilitating diseases (nonbacterial thrombotic endocarditis). Mobile fibrous strands also are found frequently during echocardiography.[1,23,24] Fibrin-platelet aggregates may attach to these fibrous and fibrinous lesions. Warfarin anticoagulants are ineffective in preventing embolism in these conditions.

Embolic complications are common in patients who have *infective endocarditis*.[1,25] Mycotic aneurysms can cause fatal subarachnoid bleeding. Bleeding also can result from vascular necrosis caused by an infected embolus.[25] Embolization usually stops when infection is controlled.[25] Warfarin does not prevent embolization and probably is contraindicated unless there are other important lesions, such as prosthetic valves and life-threatening pulmonary embolism (see Chap. 73). In children and young adults with congenital heart defects, especially those with right-to-left shunts and polycythemia, brain abscess is an important complication (see Chap. 63).

Emboli often arise from sources other than the heart, such as the aorta, proximal arteries (intraarterial or so-called local embolism), leg veins (paradoxical emboli), fat in the liver or bones (fat embolism), and materials introduced by the patient or physician (drug particles or air).[1] The type of embolic material also varies (Table 89-1).[1,26] *Atheromatous plaques in the aortic arch and ascending aorta are a very important and previously neglected source of embolism to the brain* (Figs. 89-1 and 89-2). Ulcerated atheromatous plaques often are found at necropsy in patients with ischemic strokes, especially patients in whom the stroke etiology was not determined during life.[27] Transesophageal echocardiography (TEE) often shows these atheromas, but technical factors limit visualization of the entire arch (see Chap. 13). The aorta also can be insonated by B-mode ultrasound probes placed in the supraclavicular fossa on each side.[28] *Large (>4 mm), protruding mobile aortic atheromas are especially likely to cause embolic strokes and are associated with a high rate of recurrent strokes.*[29]

CLINICAL FINDINGS

Anterior Circulation Recipient Sites Balloons placed into the circulation tend to follow the same flow patterns;[30] anterior circulation material reaches the middle cerebral arteries (MCA) and their branches.[30] The most common sites are the mainstem MCA, the upper or lower divisions of the MCA, and their branches. The upper division of the MCA supplies the frontal and parietal lobes above the sylvian fissure, and the lower division supplies the convexal temporal and inferior parietal lobes. Resultant neurologic deficits include the following.

MCA Upper Division Contralateral hemiparesis, hemisensory loss; aphasia (left hemisphere); lack of awareness of deficit, neglect of the left visual space, and motor impersistence[31] (right hemisphere).

MCA Inferior Division Wernicke-type fluent aphasia, agitation, right-upper-quadrantanopia (left hemisphere); agitation and hyperactivity, left neglect, poor drawing and copying (right hemisphere).[32]

MCA Mainstem Findings include features of both upper and lower division infarcts.

Posterior Circulation Recipient Sites Vertebrobasilar territory symptoms usually are attributed to local disease within that circulation without consideration of a possible cardiogenic

TABLE 89-1 Embolic Materials

Cardiac	Intraarterial
1. Red fibrin-dependent thrombi	1. Red fibrin-dependent thrombi
2. White platelet-fibrin nidi	2. White platelet-fibrin nidi
3. Material from marantic endocarditis	3. Combined fibrin-platelet and fibrin-dependent clots
4. Bacteria from vegetations	4. Cholesterol crystals
5. Calcium from valves and mitral annulus calcification	5. Atheromatous plaque debris
6. Myxoma cells and debris	6. Calcium from vascular calcifications
	7. Air
	8. Mucin from tumors
	9. Talc or microcrystalline cellulose from injected drugs

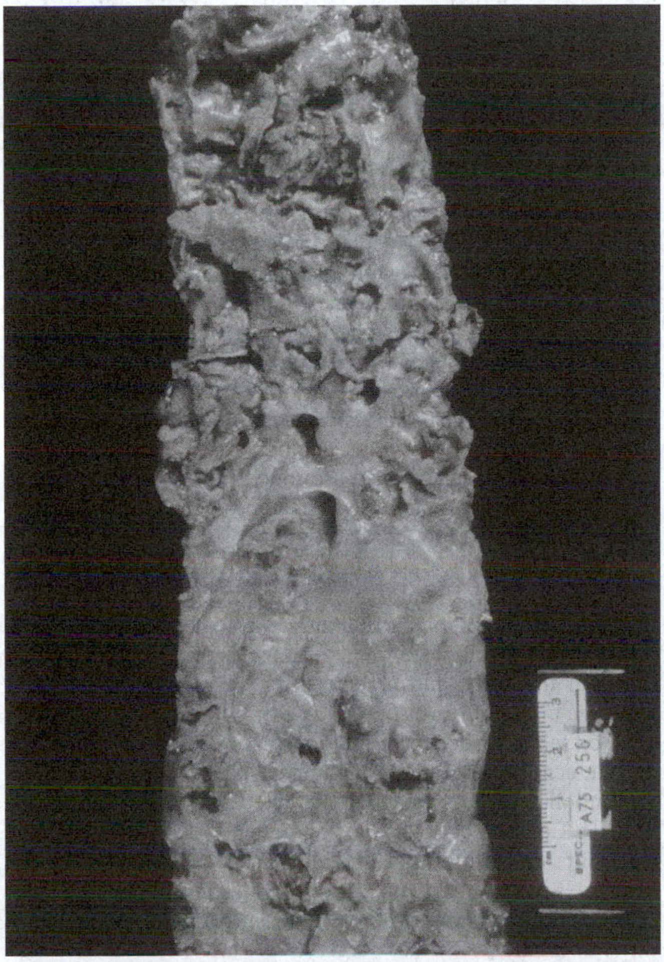

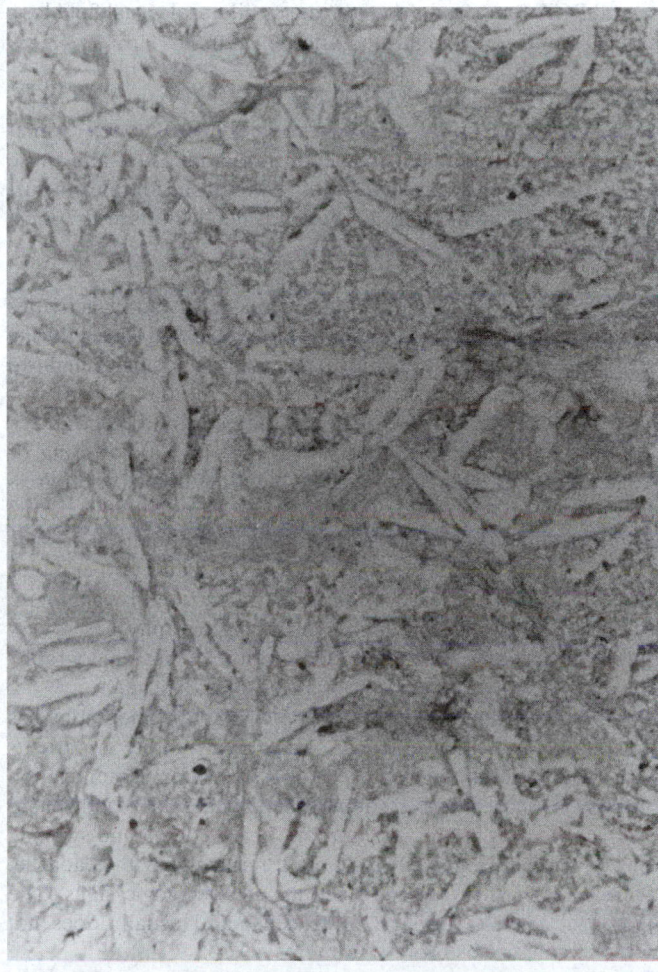

FIGURE 89-1 Descending aorta at necropsy from a patient in whom TEE before surgery showed severe disease of the ascending aorta and aortic arch with mobile protruding plaques. This patient died after CAB surgery, having never awakened after the procedure. Submitted by Dr. Denise Barbut. (From Caplan LR. *Stroke: A Clinical Approach*, 3d ed. Boston: Butterworth-Heinemann; 2000, with permission.)

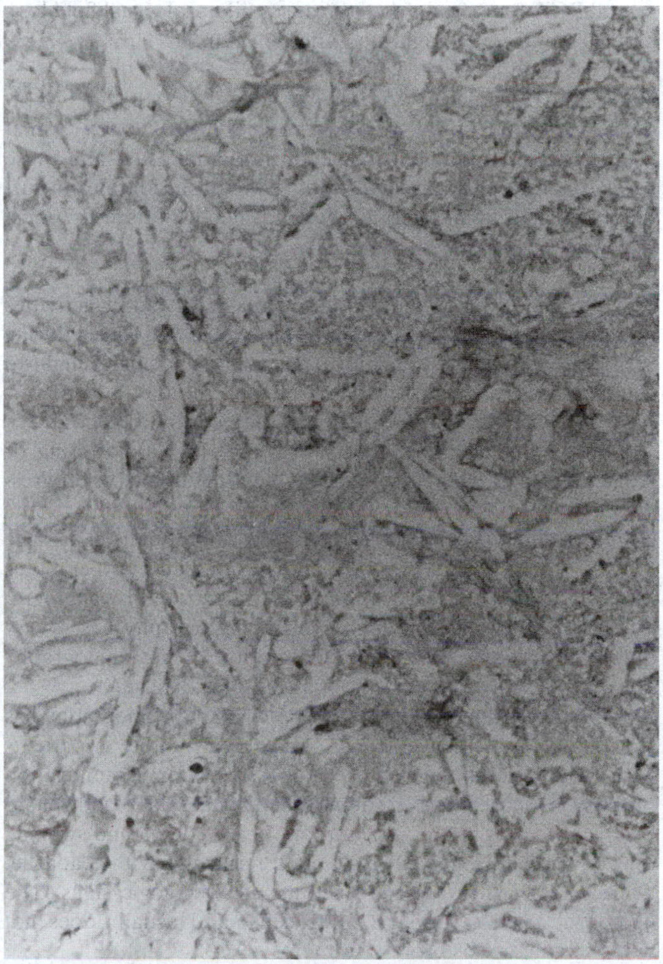

FIGURE 89-2 Cholesterol crystals and other particulate debris are caught in a filter placed in the aorta at the time when aortic clamps are removed. Submitted by Dr. Denise Barbut. (From Caplan LR. *Stroke: A Clinical Approach*, 3d ed. Boston: Butterworth-Heinemann; 2000, with permission.)

embolism. In the major stroke registries,[1,5,9] however, about 20 percent of emboli of cardiac origin go to the posterior circulation. Twenty percent is expected, as about one-fifth of cerebral blood flow goes to this circulation. In the posterior circulation, certain recipient sites are favored.

Posterior Cerebral Artery (PCA)[33,34] Particles and clots go to the most distal part of the system; the PCA is the terminal vessel in the vertebrobasilar circuit. The hallmark of PCA lesions is hemianopia and/or hemisensory loss contralateral to the infarct. Patients with left-PCA territory infarcts also often cannot read or name colors but retain the ability to write and spell. Amnesia is sometimes prominent and may last up to 6 months. Right-PCA territory infarction often is associated with left visual neglect.

Top of the Basilar Artery[35] The major clinical features are apathy and sleepiness; abnormal vertical gaze; and hallucinations, unusual reports, and other behavioral abnormalities. Bilateral PCA territory infarction causes bilateral visual field loss, amnesia, and severe agitation and delirium.

Vertebral Artery (VA) Intracranially and Its Posterior Inferior Cerebellar Artery (PICA) Branch Somewhat larger emboli may occlude an intracranial VA and cause cerebellar infarction involving mostly the posterior inferior surface.[36] Ataxia, vomiting, and occipital headache are the most common signs.

Onset and Course Most embolic events occur during activities of daily living, but some embolic strokes have their onset during rest or sleep. Sudden coughing, sneezing, or arising at night to urinate can precipitate an embolism.[1,5] Although the deficit is most often maximal at the outset, 11 percent of embolic stroke patients in the Harvard Stroke Registry had a stuttering or stepwise course, whereas 10 percent had fluctuations or progressive deficits. Later progression, if it develops, usually occurs within the first 48 h. Progression usually is due to distal passage of emboli. "Nonsudden embolism" is explained by an embolus moving from its initial location, as demonstrated by angiography, to a more distal branch.[1] Early angiography has a very high rate of showing intracranial emboli,[6,37] but angiography after 48 h shows a much lower rate of blockage.

More recently, transcranial Doppler (TCD) sonography has shown a high incidence of MCA blockage acutely in patients with sudden-onset hemispheric strokes, but later, recanalization of the MCA and normalization of the intracranial blood velocities occur.[1,38] As in all large infarcts, brain edema and swelling may develop during the 24 to 72 h after a stroke, with headache, decreased alertness, and worsening of neurologic signs. The edema is often cytotoxic (inside cells) and usually does not respond to corticosteroid treatment.

DIAGNOSTIC TESTING

Emboli usually cause occlusion of distal branches and produce surface infarcts that are roughly triangular, with the apex of the triangle pointing inward. CT and MRI findings can suggest the presence of embolism by the location and shape of the lesion,[39] the presence of superficial wedge-shaped infarcts in multiple different vascular territories, hemorrhagic infarction, and visualization of thrombi within arteries. Among 60 patients with cardiogenic sources of embolism studied by CT in whom occlusive atherosclerotic cerebrovascular disease had been excluded, 56 had superficial large or small cortical or subcortical infarcts and only 4 had deep infarcts.[39] Emboli can block the MCA and occasionally cause solely deep infarcts because the superficial territory has good collateral flow; these infarcts are called *striatocapsular* because they involve the internal capsule and the adjacent basal ganglia, which are supplied by lenticulostriate branches of the MCA.[1,5,40] Tiny emboli may cause small deep or superficial infarcts.

MRI is more sensitive for the detection of brain infarcts than is CT and is also superior in detecting hemorrhagic infarction by imaging hemosiderin. Hemorrhagic infarction has long been considered characteristic of embolism, especially when the artery leading to the infarct is patent.[41] The mechanism of hemorrhagic infarction is reperfusion of ischemic zones, which occurs with spontaneous passage of the embolus, after iatrogenic opening of an occluded artery (e.g., endarterectomy, fibrinolytic treatment), or after restoration of the circulation after a period of systemic hypoperfusion. Hemorrhage occurs into proximal reperfused regions of brain infarcts.[1,5,42] At times, it is also possible to image the acute embolus on CT.[1,43]

In unselected series of stroke patients, transthoracic echocardiography (TTE) (see Chap. 13) has been variably useful in detecting sources.[1,44,45] TTE is useful in patients with known cardiac disease to clarify potential embolic sources and heart function,[5] young patients without stroke risk factors, and stroke patients who do not have lacunar infarction or ultrasound evidence of intrinsic atherostenosis of a major extracranial and intracranial artery. TEE (see Chap. 13) provides much better visualization of the aorta, atria, cardiac valves, and septal regions. Reports of TEE suggest that the diagnostic yield is 2 to 10 times that of TTE.[46,47] Aortic plaques, atrial septal aneurysms, and atrial septal defects also are much better seen with TEE (Fig. 89-3). The use of an echo-enhancing agent such as agitated saline helps detect intracardiac shunts.

Echocardiography has definite limitations. Particles as small as 2 mm can block major brain arteries but are beyond the imaging resolution of current echocardiographic technology. Also, thromboembolism is a dynamic process. When a clot forms in the heart and embolizes, there may be no residual evidence until it re-forms.[1,26] Cardiac thrombi are imaged differently on sequential echocardiograms;[1,48] even large thrombi seen on one echocardiogram can disappear later.[48]

Embolic signals are now detected by monitoring with TCD.[1,49] Embolic particles passing under TCD probes produce transient, short-duration, high-intensity signals referred to as high-intensity transient signals (HITS). Examples of HITS are show in Figs. 89-4 and 89-5. TCD monitoring of patients with atrial fibrillation,[50] cardiac surgery,[51] prosthetic valves, left ventricular assist devices, carotid artery disease, and carotid endarterectomy have shown a relatively high frequency of embolic signals. In the future, monitoring of emboli with TCD will become an important diagnostic modality to guide treatment.

PREVENTION AND TREATMENT

Early studies showed that warfarin is effective in preventing brain embolism in patients with rheumatic mitral stenosis and atrial fibrillation (AF). Previously, the intensity of anticoagulation was higher than that currently used, and brain hemorrhages and other bleeding complications were common. Trials have now shown that low-dose warfarin [International Normalized Ratio (INR) 2.0 to 3.0] is also effective in preventing brain emboli in patients with nonrheumatic AF.

In the Copenhagen Atrial Fibrillation Aspirin Anticoagulation (AFASAK) study, 1007 patients (median age, 74.2 years) with chronic, nonrheumatic AF were assigned to warfarin (INR 2.8 to 4.2), aspirin (75 mg/day), or placebo.[52] The study was halted prematurely when an analysis of effectiveness reached a predetermined level of significance in favor of warfarin treatment. The principal outcome was the composite of ischemic or hemorrhagic stroke, transient ischemic attack (TIA), and systemic embolism. The observed reduction for warfarin compared to placebo was 64 percent, an absolute risk reduction of 3.5 percent per year. An analysis by intention to treat, which excluded TIA and minor stroke, indicated a risk reduction of about 50 percent ($p < .05$) and an absolute reduction of about 1.5 percent per year.

The Stroke Prevention in Atrial Fibrillation (SPAF) study investigators evaluated warfarin and aspirin in patients with nonrheumatic AF.[53] The study evaluated two groups of patients on the basis of their eligibility for warfarin. In the first group, 627 patients who were judged eligible for warfarin were randomized to open-label warfarin (INR, 2.8 to 4.5; prothrombin time, 1.3 to 1.8 times control) or were double-blinded to either aspirin (325 mg daily, enteric-coated) or matching placebo. In the second group, 703 patients ineligible for warfarin were randomized (double-blind) to aspirin (325 mg daily, enteric-coated) or placebo. The principal outcome, a composite of ischemic stroke and systemic embolism, was decreased significantly during a mean follow-up of 1.3 years. The outcome of disabling ischemic stroke or vascular death was reduced by warfarin by 54 percent ($p = .11$), an absolute reduction of 2.6 percent per year. Aspirin also decreased the principal outcome in both study

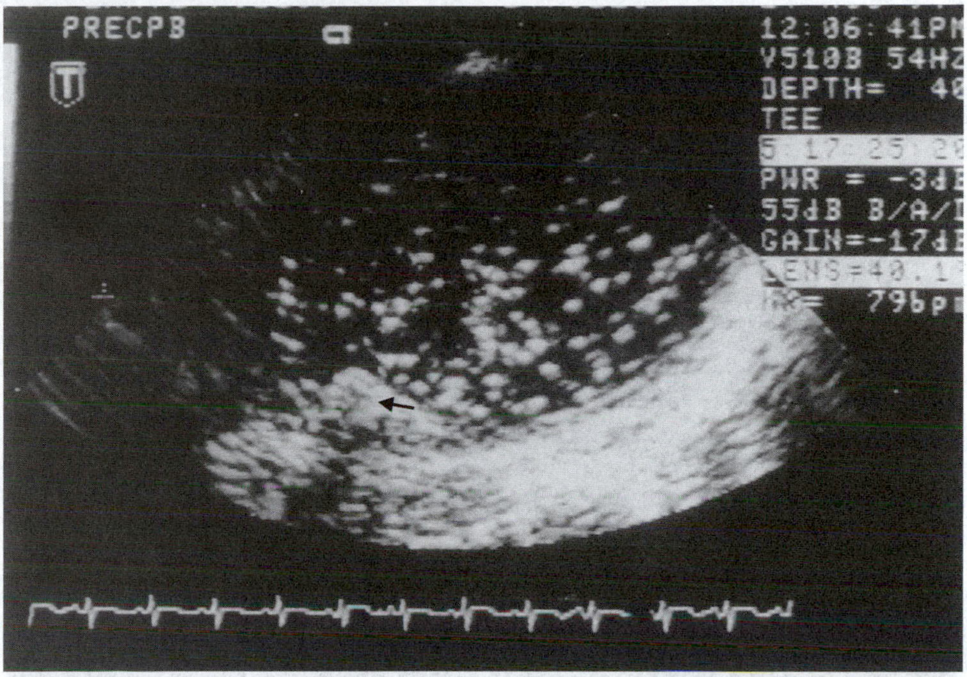

FIGURE 89-3 TEE recording during cardiac surgery from the aorta at the level of the origin of the left subclavian artery. A mobile plaque is seen protruding into the aortic lumen (small black arrow). This recording was taken after the release of aortic clamps and shows a "shower" of emboli within the aortic lumen beyond the area where the aorta was previously clamped. Submitted by Dr. Denise Barbut. (From Caplan LR. *Stroke: A Clinical Approach*, 3d ed. Boston: Butterworth-Heinemann; 2000, with permission.)

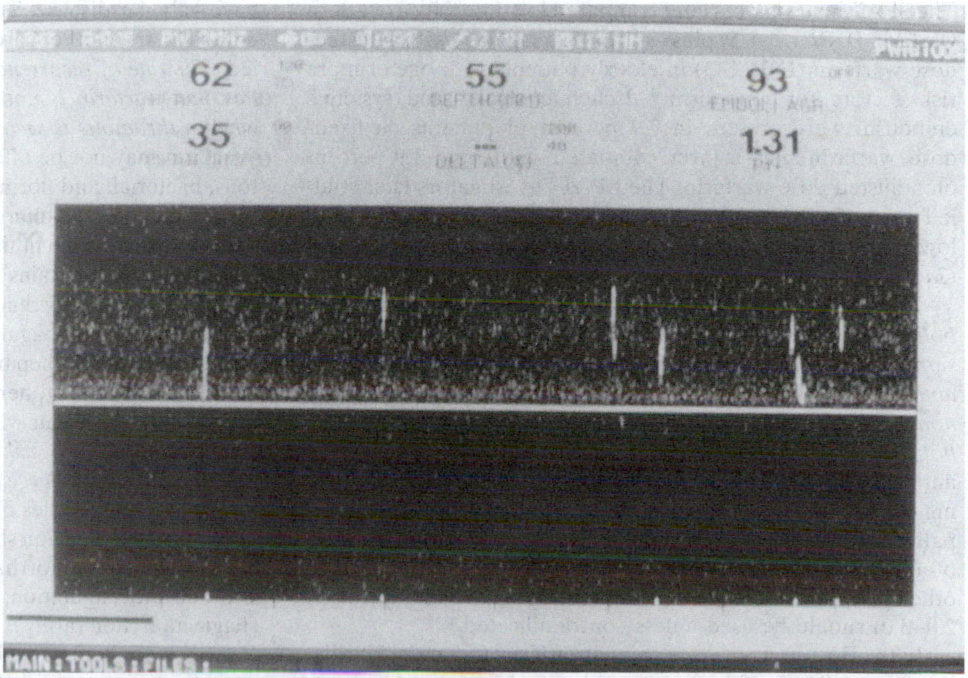

FIGURE 89-4 TCD recording from the MCA during steady-state cardiac bypass surgery at a time when the aorta was being manipulated. The white streaks represent microemboli. Submitted by Dr. Denise Barbut. (From Caplan LR. *Stroke: A Clinical Approach*, 3d ed. Boston: Butterworth-Heinemann; 2000, with permission.)

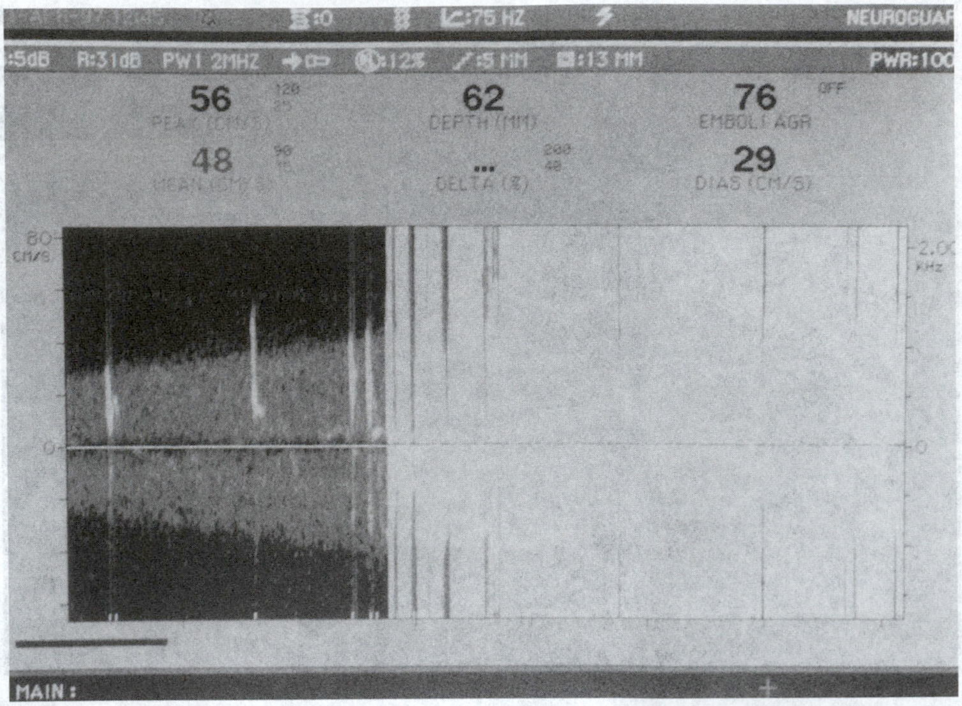

FIGURE 89-5 TCD recording from the MCA during cardiac bypass surgery. A few distinct emboli (white streaks in the left side of the figure) are followed by a massive shower of emboli ("whiteout") at the time of the release of aortic clamps. Submitted by Dr. Denise Barbut. (From Caplan LR. *Stroke: A Clinical Approach*, 3d ed. Boston: Butterworth-Heinemann; 2000, with permission.)

groups. The risk reduction was 42 percent (p = .02), and the absolute reduction was 2.7 percent per year. The outcome of disabling stroke or death was reduced 22 percent by aspirin (p = .33), an absolute reduction of about 1 percent per year. The SPAF investigators later compared low-intensity fixed-dose warfarin (INR 1.2–1.5) plus aspirin (325 mg/day) with adjusted-dose warfarin (INR 2–3) in elderly patients with one or more risk factors for embolism.[54] Ischemic stroke and systemic embolism were present in 7.9 percent of patients on fixed-dose warfarin plus aspirin compared with only 1.9 percent on adjusted-dose warfarin. The SPAF investigators later studied the effectiveness of 325 mg of aspirin in patients with low risk and found that the rate of ischemic stroke was low (2 percent per year).[55]

The SPAF study identified three risk factors for thromboembolism—recent congestive heart failure, a history of hypertension, and previous thromboembolism[56,57]*—and suggested that anticoagulation with warfarin is not indicated in patients with none of the three risk factors who are at low risk for thromboembolism (2.5 percent per year).* In such patients the dangers of anticoagulant therapy may outweigh its benefits. Aspirin (325 mg daily) probably constitutes reasonable and safe therapy for patients with lone, nonrheumatic AF who are under 60 years of age and have none of the three identified risk factors.[56–58] In other patients with AF, long-term oral warfarin therapy (INR 2.0–3.0) should be used unless contraindicated.[55,58]

In the Boston Area Anticoagulation Trial for Atrial Fibrillation (BAATAF), 420 patients with nonrheumatic AF, mean age 68 years, were randomized unblinded to warfarin (target prothrombin time ratio, 1.2 to 1.5 × control, INR 1.5 to 2.7) or to a control group whose members were allowed to take aspirin.[59] The principal outcome was ischemic stroke or systemic embolism, and the mean follow-up was 2.2 years. The incidence of stroke was reduced 86 percent in the warfarin group compared with control (p = .002), equivalent to an absolute risk reduction of 2.6 percent per year. There was no demonstrable benefit of aspirin, but the study was not designed to test aspirin.

The European Atrial Fibrillation Trial (EAFT) study group addressed the question of the optimal level of anticoagulation by reviewing the results of its own trial.[60] *No treatment effect was found with anticoagulation responses below INRs of 2.0.* The rate of thromboembolic events was lowest at INRs from 2 to 3.9; most major hemorrhages occurred at INRs of 5.0 and above. The EAFT group recommended a target of 3.0 with a range of 2 to 5.0.[60] Fixed-dose warfarin with a target of INR 1.3 to 1.5 was not as effective as standard adjusted-dose warfarin at an average INR of 2.4 even when aspirin 325 mg/day was added to the low fixed-dose warfarin in another study.

Warfarin is about 50 percent more effective than aspirin in preventing stroke in patients with atrial fibrillation who do not have valvular disease. The effectiveness of anticoagulation on embolism from other cardiac conditions has not been well studied. *The rate of recurrence of stroke in patients with MVP is so low that warfarin is not recommended for prophylaxis except when a thrombus is seen on echocardiography* (see Chap. 58). Warfarin may not be effective in preventing calcific, myxomatous, bacterial, and fibrin-platelet emboli and has been posited to worsen cholesterol crystal embolization.[61]

The timing of the initiation of warfarin anticoagulation after embolic stroke remains controversial. Embolic brain infarcts often become hemorrhagic, and serious brain hemorrhage has occurred after anticoagulation.[62–65] Large infarcts, hypertension, large bolus doses of heparin, and excessive anticoagulation have been associated with hemorrhage. Because most hemorrhagic transformations occur within 48 h, the *recommendations of the Cerebral Embolism Task Force were to avoid early anticoagulation in patients with large infarcts or hemorrhagic transformation on repeat CT.*[66] Studies of patients with cerebral and cerebellar hemorrhagic infarction show that in the vast majority, the cause is embolic, that hemorrhagic infarction occurs equally with and without anticoagulation, and that the development of hemorrhagic infarction rarely is accompanied by clinical worsening.[67,68] Patients with hemorrhagic transformation who were continued on anticoagulants did not worsen. The risk of reembolism must be balanced against the small but definite risk of important bleeding. *If the patient has a large brain infarct, heparin should be delayed and bolus heparin infusions should be avoided. If the risk of reembolism is high, immediate heparinization is advisable, whereas if the risk seems low, it is prudent to delay anticoagulants for at least 48 h.* A recent study showed that *patients with atrial fibrillation with embolic strokes who were treated with well-controlled heparin anticoagulation soon after a stroke onset fared better than did patients who were treated later.*[68,69]

Paradoxical Embolism

While once considered rare, emboli entering the systemic circulation through right-to-left shunting of blood are now often recognized with the use of newer diagnostic technologies. By far the most common potential intracardiac shunt is a residual patent foramen ovale (PFO). The high frequency of PFOs in the normal adult population has made it difficult to be certain in an individual stroke patient with a PFO whether paradoxical embolism through the PFO was the cause of the stroke or whether the PFO was merely an incidental finding. Autopsy series have shown that about 30 percent of adults have a probe-patent foramen ovale at necropsy.[70] Hagen and associates studied 956 patients with clinically and pathologically normal hearts and found a PFO in 27.3 percent.[70] The frequency of PFOs declined with age: 34.3 percent during the first three decades of life, 25.4 percent during the fourth through eighth decades, and 20.2 percent during the ninth and tenth decades. The average diameter of PFOs was 4.9 mm, and the size tended to increase with age.[70] Echocardiographic studies have shown that PFOs are more common in patients with an undetermined cause of stroke than in those in whom another etiology has been defined.[71,72]

A review of series of patients with paradoxical embolism[73] through a PFO and the author's experience allow the derivation of five criteria that, when four or more are met, establish with a high degree of certainty the presence of a paradoxical embolism.[1] The findings are (1) *a situation that promotes thrombosis of leg or pelvic veins*, e.g., long sitting in one position or recent surgery, (2) *increased coagulability*, e.g., the use of oral contraceptives, the presence of Leiden factor with resistance to activated protein C, dehydration, (3) *the sudden onset of stroke during sexual intercourse, straining at stool, or another activity that includes a Valsalva maneuver* or promotes right-to-left shunting of blood, (4) *a pulmonary embolism* within a short time before or after the neurologic ischemic event, and (5) *the absence of other putative causes of stroke after thorough evaluation.*

Brain Hypoperfusion Resulting from Cardiac Pump Failure

After cardiopulmonary resuscitation (CPR), the heart often recovers in individuals in whom the brain has been irreversibly harmed by ischemic-anoxic damage.[74] Cardiologists must be familiar with the pathology, signs, and prognosis of brain dysfunction after periods of circulatory failure.

Different brain regions have selective vulnerability to hypoxic-ischemic damage. The regions that are most remote and at the edges of a major vascular supply are more liable to injury. These zones usually have been referred to as "border zones" or "watersheds."

The cerebral cortex is most vulnerable to injury. Damage may be diffuse or "laminar," involving layers of the cortex. The hippocampus is one of the most vulnerable areas.[75,76] In the brain, the border zone regions are between the anterior cerebral artery (ACA) and the MCA and between the MCA and the PCA. Damage is usually most severe in the posterior parietotemporooccipital region and in the frontal areas most remote from the heart, which thus are called *distal fields*. A similar border zone exists in the cerebellum between the cerebellar arteries and in the brainstem between the medial and lateral penetrating arteries. The basal ganglia and thalamus are most involved if hypoxia is severe but some circulation is preserved. This situation applies most to hanging, strangulation, drowning, and carbon monoxide exposure.[77] Cerebellar neurons, especially Purkinje's cells, also may be selectively injured.

When circulatory arrest is complete and abrupt, brainstem nuclei are especially vulnerable to necrosis, especially in young humans and experimental animals.[78] When hypoxia and ischemia are especially severe, the spinal cord also may be damaged.[79] When cortical damage is very severe and protracted, cytotoxic edema causes massive brain swelling, with cessation of blood flow and brain death.

CLINICAL FINDINGS

Very severe damage leads to mortal injury to the cortex and brainstem, irreversible coma, and brain death. When initially examined, such patients have no brainstem reflexes (pupillary, corneal, and oculovestibular and oculocephalic reflexes) and no response to stimuli except perhaps a decerebration response. These findings do not improve, and respiratory control is absent or lost.

When cerebral cortical damage is very severe but brainstem ischemic changes are reversible, brainstem reflexes are preserved but there is no meaningful response to the environment. Automatic facial movements such as blinking, tongue protrusion, and yawning usually persist. The eyes may rest slightly up and move from side to side. When this state does not improve, it is referred to as the *persistent vegetative state*[74,75,80] or "wakefulness without awareness." Laminar cortical necrosis causes seizures. These seizures are often multifocal myoclonic twitches or jerks of the facial and limb muscles that are difficult to control with anticonvulsants; oversedation should be avoided.

With severe border-zone injury, there is weakness of the arms and proximal lower extremities with preservation of face, leg, and foot movement (the "man in a barrel" syndrome). With less severe ischemia, the symptoms and signs are predominantly visual. Patients describe difficulty seeing and cannot integrate the features of large objects or scenes despite a retained ability to see small objects in some parts of their visual fields. Reading is impossible. There are features of Balint's syndrome,[74] including asimultagnosia (seeing things piecemeal or sequentially), optic ataxia (poor eye-hand coordination), and optic apraxia (difficulty in directing gaze). Apathy and inertia are also common and are due to damage to the frontal lobe. Amnesia is also very common. These patients cannot form new memories and have patchy, retrograde amnesia for events during and before hospitalization. This Korsakoff-type syndrome is due to hippocampal damage and may not be fully reversible. Amnesia may be accompanied by visual abnormalities, apathy, and confusion or may be isolated.

PROGNOSIS

Shortly after resuscitation or arrest, patients with less severe cerebral injuries show some reactivity to the environment. Eye opening and restless limb movements develop. The eyes may fixate on objects. Noise, a flashlight, or a gentle pinch arouses patients to avoid or react to stimuli. Soon these patients awaken fully and may begin to speak. Cognitive and behavioral abnormalities may be detected after the patient awakens, depending on the degree of injury.

Prognostic signs and variables have been extensively studied.[74,81,82] The initial neurologic findings and their course are helpful in predicting the outcome. Among patients who have meaningful responses to pain at 1 h, almost all survivors have preserved intellectual function. Patients who do not respond to pain by 24 h either die or remain in a vegetative state. Being comatose predicts a poor prognosis.[82] *Thus, two simple observations—the presence or absence of coma and the response to pain—predict the neurologic outcome very early.*[82]

In a study in Seattle of out-of-hospital cardiac arrests, patients who did not awaken died on average 3.5 days after arrest.[83] Of 459 patients, 183 never awakened (39 percent). Among those who did awaken, 91 (32 percent) had persistent neurologic deficits.[84] Prognosis could be made by analyzing pupillary light reflexes, eye movements, and motor responses.[84] Bystander initiation of CPR was not significantly related to awakening,[84] in contrast to another study that found that outcome was better if CPR was started by bystanders before the emergency team arrived.[85] Patients awake on admission were included in one study[85] but excluded in the other.[84] After in-hospital CPR, pneumonia, hypotension, renal failure, cancer, and a housebound state before hospitalization were significantly related to death in the hospital (see Chap. 34).[86]

DIAGNOSTIC TESTING

Neurologic imaging and other tests have proved to be relatively unhelpful, in contrast to a neurologic examination.[74] CT is used to exclude other causes of coma, such as brain hemorrhage. Electroencephalography (EEG) is helpful in studying cortical activity in unresponsive patients and assessing brain death. Similarly, the absence of responses to visual and somatosensory stimuli is a poor prognostic sign. TCD may be helpful in the evaluation of brain death.[87]

TREATMENT

Other than maintaining adequate circulation and oxygenation, treatment has not been helpful in improving outcome. Increased blood sugar correlates with a poor outcome,[88] and experimental animals subjected to circulatory arrest do worse if they have been fed glucose before the arrest. Blood calcium and the presence of free radicals and excitatory neurotoxins have all been postulated to affect neuronal cell death.[89] A multifaceted approach to therapy has been most successful.[90]

Neurologic Effects of Cardiac Drugs and Cardiac Encephalopathy

Drugs given to patients with cardiac disease often have neurologic side effects[91] (see Chap. 81). Digitalis can cause visual hallucinations, yellow vision, and general confusion.[92] Digitalis levels need not be elevated excessively; the symptoms disappear with cessation of the drug. Quinidine can cause confusion with delirium, seizures and coma, vertigo, tinnitus, and visual blurring.[93] Chronic cognitive and behavioral changes and "quinidine dementia" are less well known.[93] Similar toxicity has been seen with lithium. Patients may become acutely comatose while being treated with intravenous lidocaine. This effect has been associated with the accidental administration of very large doses; more common CNS effects of less extreme toxicity include sedation, irritability, and twitching. The twitching may progress to seizures accompanied by respiratory depression. Amiodarone often causes ataxia, weakness, tremors, paresthesias, visual symptoms, and a parkinsonian-like syndrome and occasionally causes delirium.[91]

Patients with congestive heart failure often develop an encephalopathy characterized by decreased alertness, sleepiness, a decrease in all intellectual functions, asterixis, and variability of alertness and cognitive functions from minute to minute and hour to hour.[91] These patients may not have pulmonary, liver, or renal failure or electrolyte abnormalities. This cardiac encephalopathy is probably multifactoral. Posited explanations include decreased brain perfusion resulting from low cardiac output and high central venous pressure, intracranial fluid effusion similar in etiology to pericardial and pleural effusions and ascites, and side effects of cardiac and other drugs.[91]

NEUROLOGIC AND CEREBROVASCULAR COMPLICATIONS OF CARDIAC SURGERY

The frequency of abnormalities of intellectual function and behavior after cardiac surgery is quite high.[94] Fortunately, most changes are reversible with time. The reported incidence of neurologic complications after cardiac surgery varies widely from 7 to 61 percent for transient complications and from 1.6 to 23 percent for permanent complications.[95,96]

Prospectively, transient complications have been noted in 61 percent of patients.[97] In one series, 16.8 percent of patients had stroke or encephalopathy after coronary artery bypass surgery (CABS); the encephalopathies usually cleared, and only 2 percent of these patients had severe strokes.[98]

Atherothrombotic Hemodynamically Mediated Brain Infarcts

A major concern has been that the hemodynamic and circulatory stress of heart surgery will lead to underperfusion of areas supplied by already stenosed or occluded arteries, leading to brain infarcts. This concern underlies neck auscultation for bruits, ultrasound carotid artery testing, and cerebral angiography before CABS. However, hemodynamically induced infarction related to preexisting atherosclerotic occlusive cervicocranial arterial disease is a rare complication of heart surgery. Embolism arising from cardiac and aortic sources is much more common and a much greater concern.[94] *Patients with carotid bruits have a very low rate of stroke after elective surgery.*[99] *In a retrospective study of CABS patients with known carotid disease, ipsilateral strokes occurred in 1.1 percent of arteries with 50 to 90 percent stenosis, 6.2 percent of arteries with >90 percent stenosis, and only 2 percent of vessels with carotid occlusion.*[100,101] Stroke rates vary greatly in those undergoing combined as opposed to staged procedures.[102] Definitive management of combined cerebral and coronary artery disease awaits the outcome of clinical trials. Intracranial flow and velocity do not show significant changes in patients with high-grade carotid stenosis during CABS.[103]

Most studies have relied on clinical localization of focal deficits and inference about their mechanisms. A neuroradiology study reviewed neuroimaging results from 30 patients with acute strokes in relation to CABS.[104] Only one had evidence of a hemodynamic atherostenotic mechanism. Thromboembolic infarction often occurs in the days after surgery, when cessation of anticoagulation and the activation of coagulation factors promote hypercoagulability.

Brain Embolism

A strong argument against a hemodynamic cause of many strokes is their timing. Strokes occur more frequently *after* recovery from the anesthetic. If the mechanism of stroke were hemodynamic, the major circulatory stress would be intraoperative and patients would awaken with the deficit. In two studies in which the authors recorded the timing of CABS-related strokes, only 16 percent[105] and 17 percent,[106] respectively, of patients had deficits noted immediately postoperatively. The distribution of infarcts and their multiplicity on neuroimaging scans were most consistent with embolism. Embolic infarcts may involve either the anterior or the posterior circulation.[94,98,104,105] In a series of postoperative posterior circulation strokes, the majority were embolic and followed cardiac surgery.[106]

Emboli may arise from preexisting cardiac abnormalities such as hypofunctioning ventricles and dilated atria and from aortic atheromas or postoperative arrhythmias.[94] *Mounting evidence links operative and postoperative embolism to aortic ulcerative atherosclerotic lesions. Cross-clamping of the ascending aorta and aortotomy liberate cholesterol or calcific plaque debris.*[94,107] Figure 89-1 shows the aorta of a patient who died having never awakened after CABS. Figure 89-2 shows cholesterol crystals and other debris trapped within a filter placed in the aorta at the time of unclamping.

In a series in which embolic signals were monitored during CABS surgery, 34 percent of those signals were detected as the aortic cross-clamps were removed, and another 24 percent as aortic partial occlusion clamps were removed.[107] The number of microemboli detected correlates with abnormalities of cognitive function studied after surgery.[94,108] Figure 89-3 shows microemboli within the aorta shown by TEE after the release of aortic clamps. Figures 89-4 and 89-5 show TCD recordings during manipulation of the aorta and after the release of aortic clamps.

Necropsy examination of patients dying after cardiac surgery have shown severe bilateral, predominantly border-zone infarcts.[109] The small arteries of the brain and other viscera (heart, kidney, spleen, pancreas) may be packed with birefringent cholesterol crystal emboli.[109] TEE makes it possible to detect protruding ulcerative plaques in the aorta preoperatively and intraoperatively.[94,110] Intraaortic atherosclerotic debris identified by TEE has been found to be associated with embolic events.[110] Intraoperative B-mode ultrasonography with the probe placed on the aorta also has been used to detect severe aortic atherosclerotic plaques.[111] Ultrasonic imaging showed aortic atheromas in 58 percent of patients, whereas visual examination and palpation detected plaques in only 24 percent.[111] *Atherosclerosis of the ascending aorta is a very important risk factor for post-CABS stroke.*[94] *In patients who are scheduled to undergo elective cardiac surgery, consideration should be given to having TEEs performed before surgery to evaluate cardiac lesions and thrombi, cardiac function, and aortic atheromas.*

In some patients, hypercoagulability related to surgery can precipitate occlusive thrombosis in atherostenotic arteries, and the newly formed thrombus can lead to intraarterial embolism. *Cardiac, aortic, and intraarterial embolism accounts for the vast majority of cardiac surgery–related focal neurologic deficits.*

Encephalopathy

Gilman described a diffuse CNS disorder after open heart surgery—characterized by altered levels of consciousness and activity and confusion[112]—that is now referred to as *encephalopathy.* Clinical and imaging studies usually do not show important focal neurologic signs or large focal infarcts. The incidence of encephalopathy varies.[96] In one series, 57 of 1669 (3.4 percent) CABS patients had postoperative changes in mental state, including delirium and encephalopathy.[113] In the Cleveland Clinic prospective series, 11.6 percent were "encephalopathic" on the fourth postoperative day.[98]

Encephalopathy has multiple causes. Embolization of particulate matter was considered the leading cause, and this led to technical improvements, including the introduction of membrane rather than bubble oxygenators and on-line filtration.[96] These technical advances have led to a decrease in the risk of macroemboli (>25 mm) as a cause, but they do not provide protection against microemboli of air, fat, or particles.[96]

Necropsy studies of patients who died after cardiopulmonary bypass or angiography have awakened interest in this subject.[96,114] Focal, small capillary and arteriolar dilatations (SCADs) were commonly found in the brain.[114] About one-half of SCADs show birefringent crystalline material within the dilated capillaries. SCADs could, at least in part, explain the decreased cerebral blood flow found during cardiopulmonary bypass. SCADs are iatrogenically generated microemboli, but their origin is unknown. Their morphology is most consistent with air or fat.

Other causes of encephalopathy are common. Hypoxic-ischemic insults caused by hypotension and hypoperfusion do occur. *Drugs are a very common cause of encephalopathy in the postoperative period. Particularly important are haloperidol, narcotics, and sedatives.* Morphine sometimes is used heavily intraoperatively, and opiate withdrawal with restlessness and hyperactivity can result. Agitation and restlessness are often early signs of organic encephalopathy and may lead to the administration of haloperidol, barbiturates, phenothiazines, or benzodiazepines for calming and sedation. When these drugs wear off and the patient begins to awaken, agitation may occur and more sedatives may be given. Haloperidol causes rigidity, restlessness, agitation, hallucinations, and confusion. In experimental animals, haloperidol delays recovery from strokes by months, and its use is not advised.[115] Phenothiazines and sedatives are also problematic; *in general, the use of sedatives and narcotics should be minimized and the doses should be tapered as soon as possible.*

Intracranial Hemorrhage after Cardiac Surgery

Intracerebral or subarachnoid hemorrhages after cardiac surgery have been reported occasionally, most commonly in children who had repair of congenital heart disease[116] or after cardiac transplantation.[117] The postulated mechanism involves an abrupt increase in brain blood flow with rupture of small intracranial arteries that are not prepared for the new load. Usually, there is a prolonged period when cardiac output is low, and this output is increased suddenly by the surgery. Abrupt increases in brain blood flow and pressure in other situations also have been associated with intracerebral hemorrhage.[118]

Peripheral Nerve Complications

Brachial plexus and peripheral nerve lesions frequently develop after cardiac surgery and can be confused with CNS complications.[119] In one series, new peripheral nervous system deficits occurred in 13 percent of patients.[119] The most common deficit is a unilateral brachial plexopathy characterized by shoulder pain and usually weakness and numbness in one hand. It probably is caused by the positioning of the arm during surgery, with traction on the lower trunk of the brachial plexus. Ulnar, peroneal, and saphenous nerve injuries also are common and also are related to positioning. Diaphragmatic and vocal cord paralyses probably are related to local effects of cardiac surgery on the recurrent laryngeal and phrenic nerves.

CARDIAC EFFECTS OF BRAIN LESIONS

Information is beginning to emerge on cardiac muscle changes (myocytolysis), arrhythmias, pulmonary edema, ECG changes, and sudden death resulting from brain disease and sudden emotional stresses.[120]

Cardiac Lesions

The two lesions found most commonly in the hearts of patients dying with acute CNS lesions are patchy regions of myocardial necrosis and subendocardial hemorrhage. The abnormalities range from eosinophilic staining of cells with preserved striations to transformation of myocardial cells into dense eosinophilic contraction bands. These changes have been referred to as *myocytolysis*.[120] Subendocardial petechiae and frank hemorrhages also are noted. These lesions were described in the 1950s but were considered rare.[121,122] One study found a very high incidence of myocardial abnormalities in patients dying of brain lesions that increase intracranial pressure rapidly.[123] Stress-related release of catecholamines and possibly corticosteroids may be responsible, at least in part, for the cardiac lesions found in patients with CNS lesions.[120,124–127]

Electrocardiographic and Enzyme Changes

In stroke patients, especially those with subarachnoid hemorrhage, electrocardiograms (ECGs) may show a prolonged QT interval; giant, wide, roller-coaster inverted T waves; and U waves.[128] These changes often are called *cerebral T waves*. Patients with stroke who have continuous ECG monitoring have a high incidence of T-wave and ST-segment changes, various arrhythmias, and cardiac enzyme abnormalities. ECG changes may include a prolonged QT interval, depressed ST segments, flat or inverted T waves, and U waves.[120,128–130] Less often, tall, peaked T waves and elevated ST segments are noted (see Chap. 11).

Cardiac and skeletal muscle enzymes, including the MB isoenzyme of creatine kinase (MB-CK), are often abnormal in stroke patients.[131–133] During the 4 to 7 days after a stroke, there is usually a slow rise and later a fall in serum MB-CK levels, a pattern quite different from that found in acute myocardial infarction (see Chap. 42); the temporal pattern of cardiac isoenzyme release is more compatible with smoldering low-grade necrosis, such as patchy, focal myocytolysis.[121] The ST-segment and T-wave abnormalities and cardiac arrhythmias correlate significantly with raised levels of MB-CK in stroke patients.[121]

Arrhythmias

Various cardiac arrhythmias have been found in stroke patients, most frequently sinus bradycardia and tachycardia and premature ventricular contractions.[120,129,130] Some arrhythmias are manifestations of primary cardiac problems, but others are undoubtedly secondary to the brain lesions. The incidence of sinus tachycardia and bradycardia is maximal on the first day after intracerebral hemorrhage.[134] Ventricular bigeminy, atrioventricular dissociation and block, ventricular tachycardia, atrial fibrillation, and bundle branch blocks are found less often.[134] All arrhythmias are more common in patients who have primary brainstem lesions or brainstem compression.

Pulmonary Edema

Acute pulmonary edema may complicate strokes, especially subarachnoid hemorrhage (SAH) and posterior circulation ischemia and hemorrhage.[121] Pulmonary edema has been found in 70 percent of patients with fatal SAH and correlates with the severity and suddenness of the development of raised intracranial pressure.[135]

Centrally mediated sympathetic discharges such as those caused by increased intracranial pressure produce intense systemic vasoconstriction.[136] Blood shifts from the high-resistance systemic circulation to the lower-resistance pulmonary circulation. Increased pulmonary capillary pressure leads to pulmonary hypertension and rupture of pulmonary vessels, with lung hemorrhage. The pulmonary edema fluid has a high protein content and can develop despite normal cardiac function.[121,136]

Sudden Death

Sudden death associated with stressful situations, including so-called voodoo death, must involve CNS mechanisms.[127,137,138] Ventricular fibrillation, the presumed mechanism of sudden death, can be elicited reliably by stimulation of cardiac sympathetic nerves in both normal and ischemic hearts.[139] Ischemia reduces the threshold for ventricular fibrillation.[121,140] Stress must cause CNS stimulation that triggers autonomic activation.[127] Sudden vagotonic stimulation can cause bradycardia and cardiac standstill. The effects of vagal stimulation on the development of ventricular arrhythmias are uncertain.[139] Patients with lateral medullary and lateral pontine infarcts that affect reticular formation structures die unexpectedly; these patients have a high incidence of various types of autonomic dysregulation, such as labile blood pressure, syncope, tachycardia, and flushing, as well as a failure of automatic respiration.

COEXISTENT VASCULAR DISEASES AFFECTING BOTH HEART AND BRAIN

Atherosclerosis

The most common and important vascular disease that affects both the brain and the heart is atherosclerosis. The most common cause of death in stroke patients is coronary artery disease,[141] and extra- and intracranial arterial atherosclerosis[142] is common in patients with coronary artery disease.

PATHOLOGY AND PREDOMINANT SITES OF DISEASE

In white men, the predominant atherosclerotic lesions involve the origins of the internal carotid artery (ICA) and the VA origins in the neck.[5,143] Fatty streaks and flat plaques first affect the posterior wall of the common carotid artery (CCA) opposite the flow divider between the ICA and the external carotid artery (ECA), a region of low shear stress.[144] Atherosclerotic plaques at this site do not differ from plaques in the aorta or coronary arteries (see Chap. 36). At first, plaques expand gradually and encroach on the lumen of the ICA and sometimes the CCA (Fig. 89-6). Atheromatous plaques often develop concurrently at the VA origin or spread from the parent subclavian artery to involve the VA origin.[145] When plaques reach a critical size, they affect the turbulence, flow, and motion of the arteries, causing complications to develop within the plaques. Cracking, ulcerations, and mural thrombi develop, and the overlying endothelium is damaged with the development of occlusive thrombi.[146] Fresh thrombi that are loosely adherent to vascular walls rapidly propagate and embolize. Because the ICA has no nuchal branches, a clot often propagates cranially, usually extending as far as the first branch of the ophthalmic artery, which arises from the intracranial siphon portion of the ICA. In the VA, collateral channels from the ECA and the thyrocervical trunk usually provide collateral channels that reconstitute the VA in the neck and limit the propagation of thrombi. During 2 to 3 weeks after the development of an occlusive thrombus, a clot gradually organizes and is much less likely to propagate or embolize. The reduction in cranial blood flow caused by severe stenosis or occlusion of the ICA or VA stimulates the development of collateral circulation that usually becomes adequate.

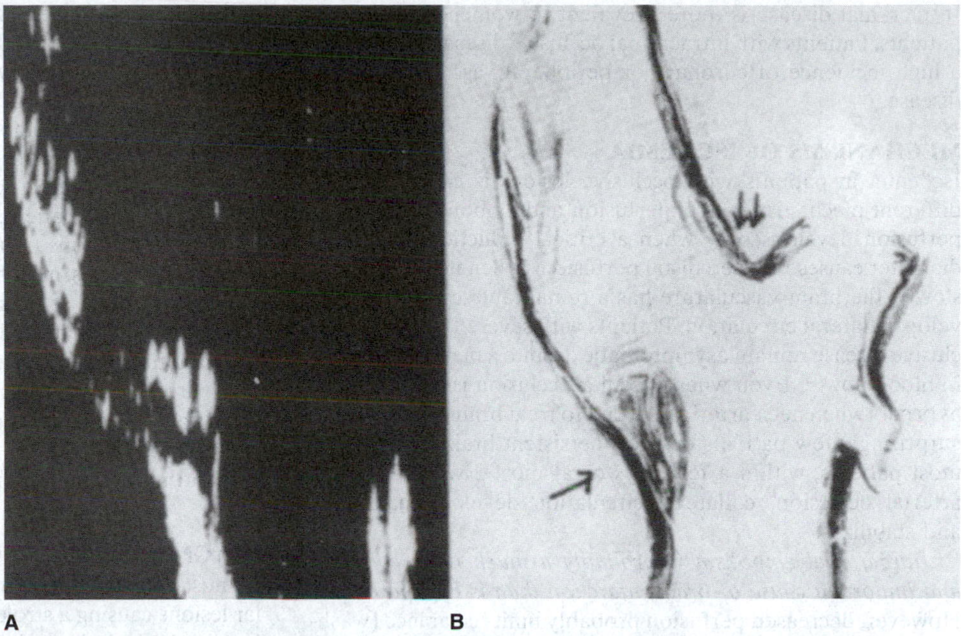

FIGURE 89-6 *A.* B-mode ultrasonic image showing plaque at internal carotid artery origin. *B.* A carotid specimen. The plaque (single arrow) is opposite the flow divider between the internal and external carotid arteries (two arrows). [From Hennerici M, Steinke W. Abbildende Ultraschallverfahren (B-scan) in duplex system. In: *Durchblutungsstorungen des Gehirns—Neue Diagnostischen Möglichkeiten*. Gutersloh: Bertelsmann; 1987, with permission.]

Figure 89-7 shows diagrammatically the sites of predilection for the development of atherosclerosis in the cervicocranial circulation. Note the concentration of these sites at branch points and flow dividers. There are important race and sex differences in the distribution of cerebral atherosclerosis.[147–149] White men usually develop lesions of the ICA and VA origins. Patients with ICA-origin disease have a high frequency of hypercholesterolemia, coronary artery disease, and peripheral vascular occlusive disease. With the exception of the basilar artery (BA) and the ICA siphon, intracranial occlusive disease develops only after extracranial disease is well established in this group. Blacks and individuals of Chinese, Japanese, and Thai ancestry have a much higher incidence of intracranial occlusive disease and a rather low frequency of extracranial disease.[147,149,150]

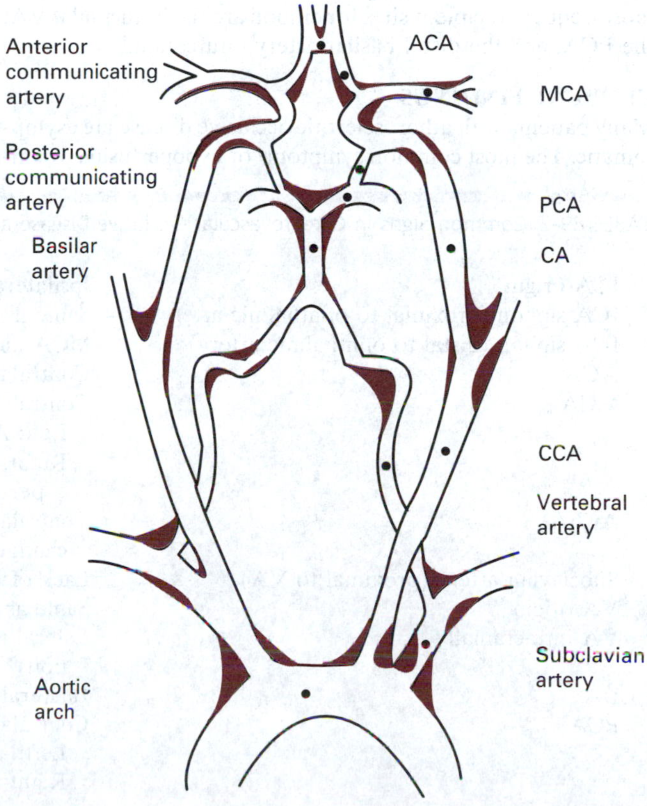

FIGURE 89-7 Sites of predilection for atherosclerotic narrowing. Dark areas represent plaques. (From Caplan LR. *Stroke: A Clinical Approach*, 3d ed. Boston: Butterworth-Heinemann; 2000, with permission.)

Intracranial disease is more prevalent in women and diabetic patients. Patients with intracranial occlusive disease do not have a high incidence of coronary or peripheral vascular occlusive disease.

MECHANISMS OF ISCHEMIA

Ischemia in patients with occlusive lesions is caused by two different mechanisms: hypoperfusion and embolism.[5,151] Hypoperfusion develops only when a critical reduction in luminal diameter causes reduced distal perfusion. When flow is reduced slowly, the brain vasculature has a remarkable capacity to develop collateral circulation. Patients with severe ICA-origin occlusive disease remain asymptomatic despite a marked decrease in blood flow.[152] Even when vascular occlusion is abrupt—e.g., as occurs when neck arteries are tied to treat brain aneurysms—surprisingly few patients develop persistent brain ischemia. In most patients, within a few days or at most 2 weeks after an arterial occlusion, collateral circulation develops maximally and stabilizes.

Intraarterial embolism is probably a much more common and important cause of brain infarction than is hypoperfusion. However, decreased perfusion probably limits clearance (washout) of emboli.[151] In patients with anterior circulation infarcts, angiography shows a very high frequency of intraarterial intracranial emboli distal to an ICA thrombosis.[153] These emboli most often involve the MCA and its branches. If angiography is repeated or performed later than 48 h after a stroke, MCA occlusion is usually not present.[5,6] Intraarterial emboli often fragment and move distally. Intraarterial embolism is also very common in the posterior circulation, where the most common donor sites are the VA origin and the intracranial VA and the most frequent recipient sites for emboli are the intracranial VA, the PCA, and the distal basilar artery bifurcation.[154]

CLINICAL FINDINGS

Many patients with atherosclerotic occlusive disease are asymptomatic. The most common symptoms of hypoperfusion or embolism are headache, TIAs, and neurologic signs related to brain infarction. Headaches are due to vascular distention or brain swelling secondary to infarction. Unaccustomed headaches often precede strokes.[5,155] TIAs are caused by hypoperfusion or intraarterial emboli. Frequent, very brief stereotyped spells precipitated by postural changes suggest a hemodynamic mechanism. In contrast, emboli cause longer, less frequent attacks.[156] In many patients with clinical TIAs—i.e., TIAs with no lasting symptoms or signs—neuroimaging tests show brain infarcts.[157] Strokes may have various temporal features, such as being maximal at outset, fluctuating, stepwise, or gradually progressive. The pattern is related to the adequacy of collateral circulation and the propagation and embolization of thrombi.

Neurologic symptoms and signs depend on the region of brain that is ischemic. Table 89-2 outlines the most common clinical patterns resulting from occlusions of the major extracranial and intracranial arteries.[5,143]

DIAGNOSTIC TESTING

In most patients, the nature and severity of the brain and vascular lesions causing a stroke can be defined. CT and MRI should localize brain lesions, distinguish between infarcts and hemorrhages, and determine the location, extent, and size of the processes. CT or MRI is usually the first test in patients with suspected stroke because the information allows clinicians to exclude nonvascular disease such as tumor or abscess, differentiate hemorrhage from ischemia and show subdural hematomas, identify the vascular territory involved, and define the extent of brain already damaged.

The vascular territory involved should be inferred by the nature of the neurologic symptoms and signs and the location of brain lesions on CT or MRI. Echocardiography, especially TEE, has dramatically improved the ability to detect potential cardiac sources of emboli (see Chap. 13).

Ultrasound techniques can be used to screen for obstructive lesions in the major extracranial and intracranial arteries in both

TABLE 89-2 Common Signs in Cerebrovascular Occlusive Disease at Various Sites

ICA origin	Ipsilateral transient monocular blindness; MCA and ACA signs
ICA siphon (proximal to ophthalmic artery)	Same as ICA origin
ICA siphon (distal to ophthalmic artery)	MCA and ACA signs
ACA	Contralateral weakness of the lower limb and shoulder shrug
MCA	Contralateral motor, sensory, and visual loss Left: Aphasia Right: Neglect of left space, lack of awareness of deficit, apathy, impersistence
AChA	Contralateral motor, sensory, and visual loss, usually without cognitive changes
Subclavian artery (proximal to VA)	Lack of arm stamina, cool hand, transient dizziness, veering, diplopia
VA origin	Same as subclavian, but no ipsilateral arm or hand findings
VA intracranially	Lateral medullary syndrome; staggering and veering (cerebellar infarction)
BA	Bilateral motor weakness; ophthalmoplegia and diplopia
PCA	Contralateral hemianopia and hemisensory loss Left: alexia with agraphia Right: neglect of left visual space

ABBREVIATIONS: ICA = internal carotid artery; ACA = anterior cerebral artery; MCA = middle cerebral artery; AChA = anterior choroidal artery; VA = vertebral artery; BA = basilar artery; PCA = posterior cerebral artery.

anterior (carotid) and posterior (vertebrobasilar) circulation arteries. For extracranial use, the two most important are *B-mode scans* and *Doppler spectra*, both pulsed and continuous-wave (CW) Doppler. The anatomy of the carotid bifurcation (the CCA, proximal ICA, and ECA) and the proximal VAs can be imaged by high-frequency, 5- to 10-MHz B-mode ultrasound systems, which provide images of the vessels in real time both longitudinally and in cross section (Fig. 89-8). Plaque calcifications and clots are often difficult to image. Pulsed Doppler registers frequency shifts from moving columns of blood. Doppler analysis can show the direction and velocity of blood flow. Multigated Doppler and B-mode scanning are now used together in so-called duplex systems.[5,158] The duplex system is probably more than 90 percent effective in separating arteries that are normal or minimally narrowed from those which have moderate disease (30 to 70 percent narrowing) and those with severe narrowing (>70 percent stenosis). B-mode scanning sometimes suggests the presence of ulceration or hemorrhage in plaques that show heterogeneous images.[158] CW Doppler uses a movable probe to measure flow velocities along the carotid and vertebral arteries; the technique is less time-consuming and expensive than the duplex system and in expert hands is very accurate in detecting high-grade stenosis.[159] Ultrasound techniques cannot reliably separate complete occlusion from very high degrees of stenosis. Color-flow and power Doppler can show turbulence and altered flow dynamics.

TCD ultrasound is used to analyze the presence of intracranial arterial stenoses and provide information about the intracranial effects of extracranial occlusive lesions. The technique takes advantage of the soft spots in the temporal bones and natural foramina (the orbit and the foramen magnum) that provide windows for ultrasound recording. The depth and angle of the probe recording can be varied, allowing the recording of velocities and sound spectra from all the major intracranial arteries.[5,87,160] Major obstructive lesions are shown reliably by both extracranial ultrasound and TCD. Continuous recording of intracranial arteries with TCD is a very sensitive and accurate method of detecting emboli passing under the probes.[94,107,161] Examples of microembolic signals are shown in Figs. 89-4 and 89-5.

Magnetic resonance angiography (MRA) (see Chap. 18) provides an additional method of imaging both the extracranial and intracranial arteries for areas of stenosis and occlusion.[5,150,162] CT angiography (CTA), using a spiral (helical) CT machine and dye injected intravenously, also can image the major large craniocervical arteries.[163] Standard catheter angiography is warranted when ultrasound and CTA or MRA have not sufficiently defined the vascular lesion and treatment is clinically feasible.[5,150]

TREATMENT

For rational treatment, the following should be known: the location, nature, and severity of the occlusive lesion; the location, extent, and reversibility of the brain lesion; and the blood constituents and coagulability.[5,164] Treatment should *not* be guided solely by the temporal pattern of the symptoms, such as TIA, progressing stroke, or so-called completed stroke.[5,164] These time courses do not predict the cause and mechanism of ischemia, do not indicate whether an infarct is present, and do not identify patients who will have further or recurrent ischemia.

Physicians should first decide whether any specific therapy is indicated. Very severe neurologic deficits, serious intercurrent illnesses (dementia, cancer, etc.), and psychosocioeconomic considerations may make patients unsuitable for specific treatments. If treatment is feasible, the next questions to be considered are what brain tissue is at risk for further ischemia and what the benefit/risk ratio of specific treatments may be. To determine the tissue at risk, clinicians consider the cause and the deficit. For example, a man with a slight hemiplegia caused

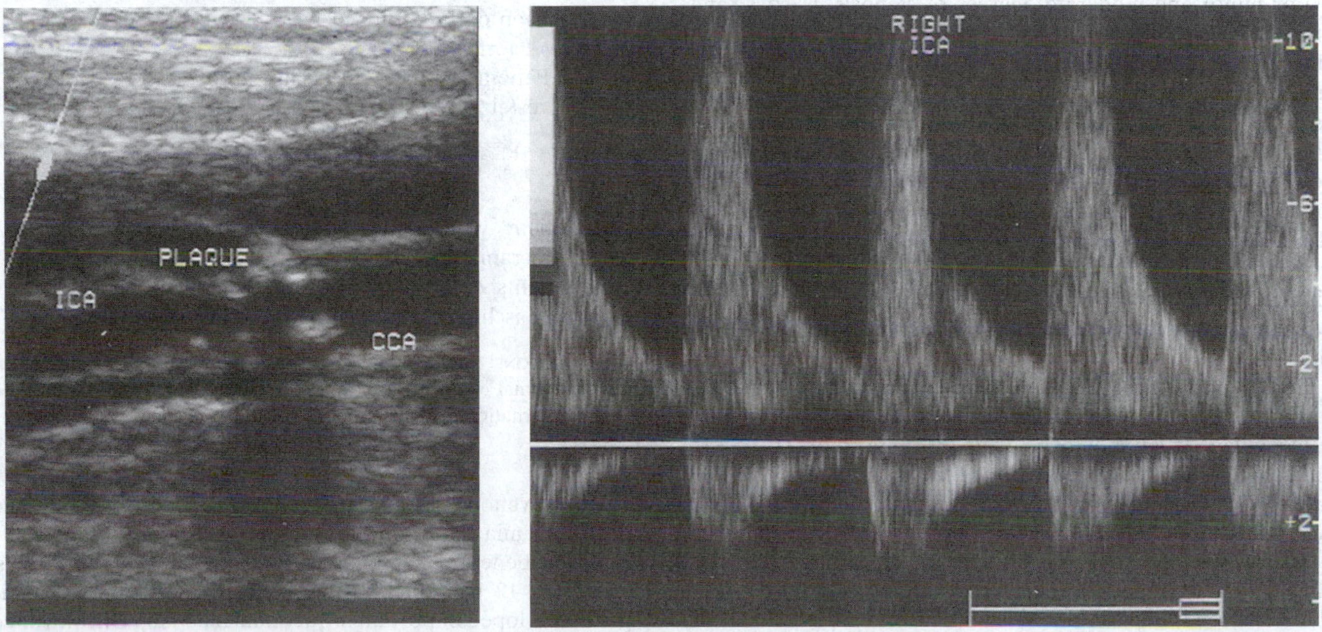

A B

FIGURE 89-8 Duplex scan of carotid artery plaque. *A.* B-mode ultrasonic image showing plaque protruding into internal carotid artery (ICA) lumen. *B.* Doppler spectra at level of plaque showing high voltage related to stenosis.

by a small lacunar infarct in the anterior limb of the internal capsule may have infarcted the entire tissue supplied by an occluded small artery. In that case, treatment consists of controlling hypertension, the cause of the microvasculopathy. If, however, that patient has a small cortical infarct in the precentral gyrus resulting from ICA disease, the rest of the ICA territory is at risk for further ischemia and aggressive treatment is warranted. Suppose a patient has a moderate-size MCA infarct. If the patient is a Chinese woman with intrinsic atherosclerotic disease of that MCA, she may have little tissue at risk for further ischemia. No aggressive treatment should be given. If that woman's infarct is due to cardiogenic embolism, the whole remainder of the brain will be at risk for further damage from another embolus. Newer MRI techniques—diffusion-weighted and perfusion MRI—along with MRA, can show, even very soon after the symptoms begin, brain that is already infarcted and brain tissue that is underperfused but not yet infarcted.[5,163,165,166]

Patients who have little tissue at risk are not candidates for specific therapy. If there is considerable residual at-risk tissue, the guidelines for the use of anticoagulants and antiplatelet agents given in Table 89-3 are used to direct treatment, which depends on the location and severity of the causative vascular lesions. Carotid endarterectomy (CEN) has been shown to be effective in symptomatic patients with severe ICA stenosis (>70 percent).[167–170]

The Asymptomatic Carotid Artery Study (ACAS) suggested that carotid endarterectomy is slightly better than medical therapy in asymptomatic patients with severe carotid stenosis when the operation is executed by surgeons who have a record of very low surgical morbidity and mortality.[171] For CEN to be effective, the operative mortality and morbidity must not be greater than 2 to 4 percent.[167–171] Surgery is also feasible on the extracranial vertebral artery in selected patients with an intraarterial embolism from that site or with intractable posterior circulation hemodynamic ischemia, a rare occurrence.[172]

For minor and moderate degrees of stenosis in extra- and intracranial arteries, agents that alter platelet aggregation and adhesion are recommended. The most likely mechanism of ischemia in these patients is "white clot"—platelet fibrin emboli. Aspirin,[173,174] ticlopidine,[175,176] clopidogrel,[177] and a tablet containing 25 mg aspirin and 200 mg of modified-release dipyridamole given two times a day[178] have all proved effective in randomized trials that contained large numbers in patients with TIAs and minor strokes. Many nonsteroidal anti-inflammatory drugs have antiplatelet effects, as do the omega-3 fish oils containing eicosapentanoic acid. Clopidogrel is as effective as ticlopidine and has fewer serious hematologic complications[177] (see Chap. 44).

For patients with severe stenosis of large intracranial arteries, warfarin is recommended if there are no contraindications. The anticoagulant level should be kept at an INR of 2.0 to 3.0. Anticoagulation should be continued for at least 2 months. The state of the intracranial arteries can be monitored by using TCD and/or MRA or CTA.[163] The same regimen is used for patients with severe extracranial stenosis who are not operative candidates or refuse surgery. For patients with complete occlusions when first seen, heparin and then warfarin are prescribed for 2 to 3 months.[5]

Thrombolytic drugs, especially recombinant tissue-type plasminogen activator (rt-PA) and streptokinase, have been given intravenously and intraarterially in patients with acute brain ischemia. In a study in which the arterial lesions were not defined, intravenous therapy with rt-PA given within 90 min and 3 h of ischemia onset, in the aggregate provided a statistically significant benefit.[179] Unfortunately, in this and other studies, about 6 to 12 percent of patients treated with thrombolytic agents developed important intracranial bleeding. Uncontrolled studies have shown that patients with distal intracranial arterial embolic occlusions do well with intravenous thrombolytic therapy.[180–182] Patients with ICA occlusions in the neck and intracranially rarely reperfuse after intravenous thrombolytic therapy, especially if collateral circulation is poor. Intraarterially admin-

TABLE 89-3 Suggested Use of Anticoagulants and Platelet Antiaggregants

Heparin (Standard Dose)

Short term, 2–4 weeks. Usually given by intravenous infusion, keeping APTT between 60 and 100 s (1.5–2 × control APTT).

1. Immediate therapy for definite cardiac-origin cerebral embolism (large cerebral infarct, hypertension, bacterial endocarditis, or sepsis would delay or contraindicate this use).
2. Patients with severe stenosis or occlusion of the ICA origin, ICA siphon, MCA, vertebral artery, or basilar artery with less than a large clinical deficit. Subsequent treatment could consist of warfarin or surgery.

Heparin (Subcutaneous Minidose)

For prophylaxis of deep vein occlusion in patients immobilized by stroke (unless contraindicated) (see Chap. 60).

Warfarin

Usually overlapped with heparin; keeping prothrombin time around INR of 2.0–3.0 (approximately 1.3–1.5 × control).

1. Long term (>3 months)
   a. Patients with cardiogenic cerebral embolization and rheumatic heart disease, atrial fibrillation with large atria or prior cerebral embolism, prosthetic valves, and some hypercoagulable states.
   b. Patients with severe stenosis of the ICA origin, ICA siphon, MCA stem, vertebral artery, and basilar artery. Used until studies show artery has been occluded for at least 3 weeks.
2. Short term (3–6 weeks)
   a. Patients with recent occlusion of the ICA, MCA, vertebral, or basilar arteries.

Platelet Antiaggregants (Aspirin, Ticlopidine, Clopidogrel)

1. Patients with plaque disease of the extracranial and intracranial arteries without severe stenosis.
2. Patients with polycythemia or thrombocytosis and related ischemic attacks.

Abbreviations: APTT = activated partial thromboplastin time; ICA = internal carotid artery; MCA =55 middle cerebral artery; INR = International Normalized Ratio.

istered prourokinase thrombolysis also has been proved to be very effective in opening blocked intracranial arteries within the anterior circulation.[183] Patients with in situ thrombosis superimposed on preexisting severe atherostenosis do less well than do patients with embolism. The dose, timing, mode of delivery, and target group for therapy remain unsettled. The author believes that vascular imaging should precede the administration of thrombolytic agents. Brain and vascular imaging can give physicians guidance in selecting who should receive thrombolytics and by what route.[184]

Because all patients with atherosclerosis are at risk of developing more lesions, control of risk factors is very important and should be begun in the hospital. Risk factors include smoking, hyperlipidemia, obesity, inactivity, and hypertension (see Chap. 38). Blood pressure should not be lowered excessively during the acute ischemic period, as this may decrease flow in collateral arteries. Blood pressure control can be instituted 3 to 4 weeks after the stroke. Rehabilitation also must begin early.

Management of Coexisting Coronary and Cerebrovascular Disease

Many patients have both coronary and cerebrovascular occlusive disease. In candidates for both CABS and CEN, controversy surrounds which surgery should be done first or whether both procedures should be done together under the same anesthetic. *In general, the most symptomatic system should be operated on first.* Thus, if a patient has severe coronary disease with active cardiac ischemia but asymptomatic severe extracranial occlusive disease, he or she should have a CABS procedure, and CEN can be considered later.[5] By contrast, if a patient has active cerebrovascular symptoms (recent TIAs or a nondisabling stroke within the last 3 months) and minor or stable coronary symptoms, a CEN will be in order without a CABS. If the patient has active coronary and cerebrovascular symptoms, the CEN and CABS should be performed together.[185–187] The reasons for this view are as follows: (1) The morbidity and mortality of the two procedures done together are considerably higher than those of either alone. The stroke risk is especially high.[187] (2) Patients with asymptomatic bruits and even severe stenosis have a very low rate of stroke resulting from hemodynamic changes during CABS or other surgery. Most operative and postoperative strokes are cardioembolic. (3) With good medical care, the risk of myocardial infarction during CEN in patients with stable coronary disease is relatively low (see Chap. 91).

In patients considered for cardiac surgery who have symptoms of brain ischemia, it is important to define the extent of cerebrovascular disease preoperatively by noninvasive means (ultrasound and/or MRA) as well as to define cardiac and coronary artery anatomy and function. Staged surgical procedures sometimes are warranted. In some patients with excessive surgical risks, anticoagulation represents an alternative treatment. Clearly, optimal medical therapy should be instituted preoperatively and continued after surgery.

Systemic Arterial Hypertension

High blood pressure, both acute and chronic, damages deep, penetrating small intracranial arteries; accelerates the development of atherosclerosis in the extracranial and large intracranial arteries; and results in ischemic syndromes of lacunar infarction,[5,188,189] diffuse ischemic changes in white matter and basal gray matter structures (Binswanger's disease[5,190]), and intracerebral hemorrhage. Hypertension is also common in patients with aneurysmal SAH and may contribute to enlargement and rupture of aneurysms.

Hypertension especially damages the deep arteries that penetrate perpendicularly from the major intracranial arteries (Fig. 89-9) (see Chap. 51). Serial sections of these arteries in patients with hypertension show characteristic abnormalities consisting of focal microaneurysmal enlargements and small hemorrhagic extravasations through the arterial walls. Subintimal foam cells may obliterate the lumen, and pink-staining amorphous fibrinoid material is found within the walls of thickened arteries. In places, the vessels often are replaced by whorls, tangles, and wisps of connective tissue that completely obliterate the usual vascular layers, causing segmental arterial disorganization as a consequence of *lipohyalinosis* and *fibrinoid degeneration*.[5,191] Microaneurysms are common in patients with hypertensive intracerebral hemorrhages and in hypertensive older patients.[192–194]

The two major patterns of brain ischemia in patients with hypertension are *discrete lacunar infarcts* and a more *diffuse patchy white and gray matter degeneration with gliosis*. Both are caused by sclerotic changes in deep intracerebral arteries and arterioles. The term *lacunae* (hole) refers to a small, deep infarct caused by lipohyalinosis of the penetrating artery that feeds the ischemic brain tissue.[191] Other vascular pathologic processes, such as microdissections and tiny emboli, occasionally also cause lacunes.[191] Some patients are normotensive and have miniature atherosclerotic lesions (so-called microatheromas) at the orifices of the branches or within the parent arteries blocking or extending into the branches.[5,188] Amyloid angiopathy also can cause small, deep infarcts in normotensive and hypertensive patients. Single lacunes cause discrete clinical syndromes.[5,195,196] The most common syndromes are pure motor hemiparesis,[197] pure sensory stroke,[198] ataxic hemiparesis,[199] and the dysarthria–clumsy hand syndrome[200] (see Chap. 51).

Since the advent of CT and MRI, it has become widely

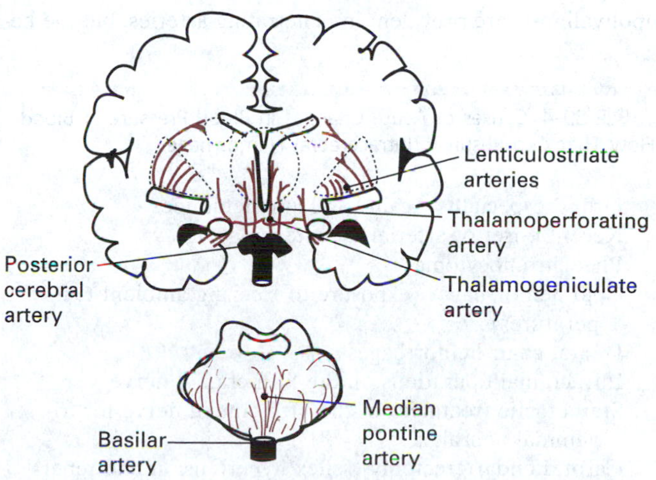

FIGURE 89-9 Deep penetrating arteries prone to the development of lipohyalinosis and microaneurysms (dark blue). Occlusion of these arteries causes lacunar infarcts, and their rupture causes intracerebral hemorrhage. (From Caplan LR. *Stroke: A Clinical Approach*, 3d ed. Boston: Butterworth-Heinemann; 2000, with permission.)

appreciated that hypertensive patients with lacunes often have more diffuse changes in the white matter of the brain that are referred to as *leuko-araiosis*.[190,201] The clinical picture consists of acute strokes; subacute progression of neurologic signs; dementia, especially the frontal lobe apathetic type; slow shuffling gait disorder; and parkinsonian, pyramidal, and pseudobulbar signs.[190,202,203] The clinical signs and gross pathology are identical to those partially described by Otto Binswanger in 1894 and 1895 and by his students Alzheimer and Nissl.[202] The deep arteries are thickened and hyalinized and show lipohyalinosis and sometimes amyloid angiopathy in regions of white matter atrophy and gliosis. Invariably, lacunar infarcts also are found. The pathogenesis most likely is related to diffuse vascular narrowing in deep arteries and altered microvascular flow and perfusion. Some studies suggest altered hemorrheology and increased blood viscosity, and some patients have had polycythemia.[190] The diagnosis is made on the basis of the clinical findings, the CT and MRI abnormalities, and the absence of cortical infarcts, larger artery occlusive disease, or cardioembolic sources.

HYPERTENSIVE INTRACEREBRAL HEMORRHAGE

Intracerebral hemorrhage (ICH) accounts for about 10 percent of all strokes.[5,6] Head trauma, vascular malformations, bleeding diatheses, drugs (especially amphetamines and cocaine), amyloid angiopathy, and intracranial aneurysms account for some cases.[192,204] Traditionally, spontaneous ICH usually has been equated with hypertensive hemorrhage. Many of these patients, however, have no history of hypertension and no associated changes of hypertensive vasculopathy at necropsy.[118,192,205,206] Acute elevations of blood pressure and/or blood flow to the brain (Table 89-4) can cause ICH through the sudden increase in blood pressure, causing breakage of capillaries and arterioles.[118,192]

Hypertensive ICH issues from the deep penetrating arteries, and so the locations parallel the distribution of those arteries. Hematomas develop in the same sites as lacunes; the most common locations are the putamen/internal capsule (30 to 40 percent), caudate nucleus (8 percent), lobar white matter (20 percent), thalamus (15 percent), pons (10 percent), and cerebellum (10 percent).[192] In fatal hematomas, microaneurysms and lipohyalinosis are prevalent in penetrating arteries, but the hematomas obscure findings in the middle of the lesions.[207] Along the outside, circumferentially, fibrin globules represent rupture sites.[207] Arterioles or capillaries rupture in the center of the lesion, suddenly increasing local tissue pressure and leading to pressure on adjacent capillaries, which then rupture. As the hematoma gradually grows on its periphery (Fig. 89-10), local tissue pressure and finally intracranial pressure increase until the hematoma is contained. Alternatively, the pressure is decompressed by the lesion emptying into the ventricular system or into the subarachnoid space on the brain surface.[5]

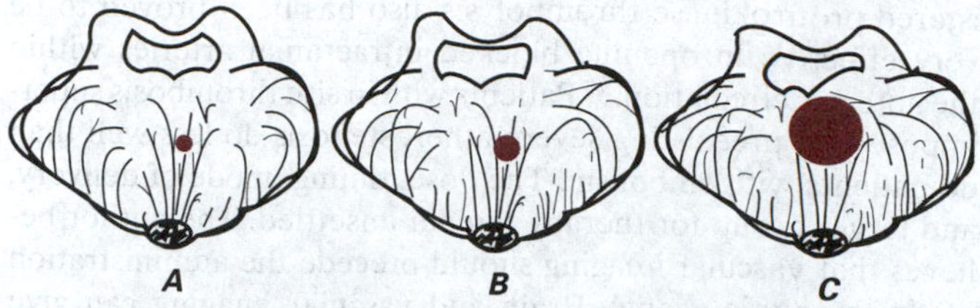

FIGURE 89-10 Gradual evolution of a hypertensive pontine intracerebral hematoma. *A.* The earliest leakage of blood from a paramedian penetrating artery. *B* and *C.* The hematoma has grown. (From Caplan LR. *Stroke: A Clinical Approach*, 3d ed. Boston: Butterworth-Heinemann; 2000, with permission.)

TABLE 89-4 Causes of Acute Changes in Blood Pressure or Blood Flow That Can Result in Intracerebral Hemorrhage

Drugs, especially cocaine and amphetamines
Recent onset of arterial hypertension
Pheochromocytoma
Cold hemorrhages (exposure to freezing ambient temperatures)
Dental chair hemorrhages
Intracranial operations on the fifth cranial nerve
Stereotactic treatment of the fifth cranial nerve for trigeminal neuralgia
Carotid endarterectomy (reflex hypertension and reperfusion)
Cardiac transplantation, especially in children
Surgical repair of congenital heart disease in children
Migraine

Clinical Findings Patients with ICH most often have a gradual evolution of neurologic signs; symptoms do not begin abruptly, as they do in SAH.[192] The first neurologic signs are related to the bleeding site; e.g., left putaminal hematoma patients may first notice right arm weakness or numbness, whereas cerebellar hematoma patients stagger and feel off balance. As the hematoma grows, the focal signs worsen. When and if the hematoma increases sufficiently in size to increase intracranial pressure, headache, vomiting, and decreased levels of alertness develop.[192] In the presence of small, restricted hemorrhages, headache is absent and the patient remains alert. The course and findings mimic so-called progressing ischemic stroke. Headache is absent or not a very prominent symptom in more than half of patients with ICH. Loss of consciousness is also not invariable but is a bad prognostic sign when present. Clinical localization of the hematoma rests on an analysis of pupillary responses, eye movements, and the presence and distribution of motor signs.

Diagnosis CT accurately shows the location, size, shape, and extent of hematomas. Also shown is the presence of ventricular and surface drainage, surrounding edema, and pressure shifts in surrounding tissues. MRI in a patient with an acute hematoma is more difficult to interpret, but old hematomas are more readily shown by imaging hemosiderin-containing cavities. Susceptibility-weighted images acquired on echo-planar machines can show even very acute intracerebral hemorrhages.[208] MRI is superior to CT in imaging arteriovenous malformations and cavernous angiomas. Lumbar puncture seldom is warranted. An atypical location, an absence of hypertension, and abnormal vascular echoes on MRI are indications for angiography.

Prognosis and Treatment Coma, increased intracranial pressure, and large hematoma size (>3 cm in one dimension on CT) all indicate a poor prognosis.[192,209] Ordinarily, severe systemic hypertension should be reduced, but not excessively. The hematoma causes increased intracranial pressure, and the spinal fluid pressure and the pressure in the dural sinuses increase pari passu. Patients with ICH can die from raised intracranial pressure. To perfuse the brain and maintain an arteriovenous pressure gradient, the systemic arterial pressure must rise. Overzealous reduction of systemic blood pressure can cause clinical deterioration. The patient's state of alertness and neurologic signs should be monitored carefully, together with the blood pressure.

Recent hematomas in the cerebral lobes, cerebellum, and right putamen sometimes are drained surgically without leaving a major deficit, at times by using stereotactic equipment with CT guidance. The indications for drainage are increased intracranial pressure and the presence of lesions that require removal (tumor, arteriovenous malformation, aneurysm).[192] When hematomas resolve, they leave a cavity, disconnecting but not destroying the overlying cortex.

Small hematomas usually resolve well without specific therapy except blood pressure control, whereas massive hematomas usually kill or maim patients before they can be treated. Medium-size hematomas (2 to 4 cm), which increase intracranial pressure and cause worsening signs or decreased consciousness while patients are under observation, are indications for drainage if they are favorably located.

Subarachnoid Hemorrhage

SAH is not caused directly by hypertension in most cases, although an abrupt increase in blood pressure (e.g., resulting from cocaine or amphetamines) sometimes can lead to SAH, as can a bleeding diathesis, trauma, and amyloid angiopathy. *The most common lesions causing SAH are abnormal vessels such as aneurysms and vascular malformations on or near the surface of the brain.* SAH involves bleeding directly into the subarachnoid space with rapid dissemination into the cerebrospinal fluid (CSF) pathways. Usually blood is released suddenly under systemic arterial pressure, causing an abrupt rise in intracranial pressure and producing headache, vomiting, and interruption of conscious behavior and memory, at least temporarily.[5,210] In some patients, the jet and spread of blood cause neck ache, backache, or sciatica instead of headache. These patients usually are agitated and restless or sleepy and have a stiff neck.

The most common cause of SAH is leakage from a berry aneurysm. Often there has been a past history of a "warning leak," that is, a sudden-onset headache unusual for the patient that lasts days and usually prevents normal daily activities.[210,211] Aneurysms most often are located at bifurcations of major intracranial arteries. The most common sites are the ICA–posterior communicating artery junction, the ACA–anterior communicating artery junction, and the MCA bifurcation. CT often can suggest the site of rupture if blood is pooled locally near a typical site.[212] Large aneurysms are occasionally visible on contrast-enhanced CT or MRI. CTA and MRA are useful tests for screening for aneurysms.[163] Lumbar puncture is very important in the diagnosis of SAH.[213] The absence of blood in the CSF effectively excludes the diagnosis of SAH if the fluid is examined within 24 h of the onset of the headache, although bleeds that are very small in volume or older than 72 h can be missed. The CSF pressure, the presence of xanthochromia, and quantification of the hemoglobin and bilirubin content of the CSF by spectrophotometry can help establish and date the bleeding and document increased intracranial pressure.[213]

The two most important complications of aneurysmal SAH are rebleeding and brain ischemia caused by vasoconstriction (so-called vasospasm). Once an aneurysm has ruptured, either a tiny cap of platelets and fibrin seals the point of rupture or continued bleeding leads to death. Lysis of the fibrin cap initiates rebleeding. Surgical clipping of the aneurysmal sac or obliteration of the aneurysm by endovascular use of balloons or other devices should be attempted before rebleeding occurs.

Vasoconstriction of arteries is thought to be due to blood or blood products that bathe the adventitia of arteries.[214–217] In the presence of a large accumulation of blood, there is a much higher incidence of arterial vasoconstriction and resultant brain ischemia and infarction. Delayed ischemia also can develop after surgery, as manipulation of vessels can precipitate or potentiate vasoconstriction. The clinical findings in patients with vasoconstriction confirmed by angiography are often those of diffuse brain swelling, such as headache, decreased alertness, and confusion. When vasoconstriction is focal or multifocal, the clinical findings are those of focal ischemia, such as hemiparesis, aphasia, and hemianopia. Vasoconstriction usually has its onset 3 to 5 days after a hemorrhage. The peak time for constriction is days 5 to 9; vasoconstriction usually improves after the second week unless rebleeding occurs.[218]

Vasoconstriction is detected by angiography in 30 to 70 percent of patients with SAH, depending on the timing of the study.[218,219] Severe vasoconstriction is manifested by a lumen size of <0.5 mm, delayed anterograde flow, and evidence of collateral filling distal to the vasoconstricted vessel. TCD is effective in monitoring for the presence of vasoconstriction, which increases blood flow velocities.[220] Single-photon emission computed tomography (SPECT) also can show regions of poor perfusion and document the presence of delayed ischemia.[221]

Many treatments have been tried to prevent or treat vasoconstriction after SAH.[217] These treatments include removal of blood by lumbar puncture and at the time of early surgery, pharmacologic agents such as calcium channel blockers to minimize contraction of the arterial wall, and hypervolemia to prevent ischemia by maintaining perfusion. At present, the most popular approaches are early surgery, nimodipine (a calcium channel blocker), and hypervolemic therapy, especially after aneurysmal clipping. Hypovolemia is common after SAH, as is hyponatremia. Hypervolemia does not reverse the vasoconstriction but helps maintain brain perfusion.

Coagulopathies

Hypercoagulability and bleeding caused by decreased coagulability affect most body organs, including the brain and heart. An increased tendency toward clotting can be caused by abnormalities of the formed blood elements or serologic factors.[222–224] Increased numbers of red blood cells and platelets and qualitative abnormalities such as sickle cell disease can cause intravascular clotting, especially in the presence of dehydration and reduced plasma volume. Excessive platelet activation, or so-called sticky platelets, also can explain increased coagulability but has proved hard to measure reliably in vitro.[225] The level of beta-thromboglobulin is a good marker for platelet activation (see Chap. 44). Serologic abnormalities may be congenital or acquired. Decreased amounts of natural anticoagulants (antithrombin III, protein C, and protein S), resistance to activated protein C, and prothrombin gene mutations can cause hypercoagulability.[222–224,226] These proteins may be decreased in patients with hypoproteinemia, especially that resulting from the nephrotic syndrome and urinary protein loss. Fibrinogen levels and the levels of various coagulation factors, such as factors VIII and XI, also may be high in patients with a prothrombotic state (see Chap. 44). In many of these patients—e.g., those on high-dose estrogen birth control pills, pregnant women, and patients with cancer—serologic and standard coagulation tests (in vitro) do not clarify the mechanism of the excessive clotting in vivo. Stroke patients may have serologic evidence of platelet activation and increased fibrin formation but decreased natural fibrinolytic and anticoagulant activity.[223,226]

Recently, measurement of various serum antiphospholipid antibodies has elicited considerable interest. The substances that usually are measured are the so-called lupus anticoagulant[227–229] and anticardiolipin antibodies. Increased activity of antiphospholipid antibodies (APLAs) is found in patients with systemic lupus erythematosus, acquired immunodeficiency syndrome (AIDS), giant-cell arteritis, and Sneddon's syndrome[229–232] (livedo reticularis and strokes) as well as in association with the use of some drugs (e.g., phenytoin, phenothiazines, procainamide, hydralazine, and quinidine). When the APLAs are not associated with other conditions and the patient has clinical evidence of excess clotting, the disorder is considered primary and is referred to as the *primary APLA syndrome*.[232–235] Patients with APLAs have an increased incidence of spontaneous abortions, venous occlusive disease of the legs and pulmonary embolism, brain infarcts (often multiple), thrombocytopenia, and false-positive syphilis serologic tests. Older patients with APLAs often also have important risk factors for stroke.[232–235]

Patients with systemic illnesses often have an elevated erythrocyte sedimentation rate, and strokes and pulmonary emboli often follow and complicate myocardial infarction (see Chap. 42). Customarily, such brain infarcts have been attributed to cardiogenic embolism, but some undoubtedly are related to thromboses precipitated by increased levels of acute-phase reactant coagulation proteins. Cancer, especially mucinous adenocarcinoma, has been associated with multiple vascular occlusions, large and tiny brain infarcts, and venous and arterial occlusions.[236]

Deficient coagulability can lead to serious intracranial bleeding. The hemorrhage can be into the brain (ICH), the CSF (SAH), or the subdural and epidural compartments. Thrombocytopenia, hemophilia, and leukemia are conditions that commonly lead to intracranial hemorrhage. The most common iatrogenic cause of bleeding is anticoagulation with heparin or warfarin.[192,237] Brain hemorrhage also has been described after fibrinolytic treatment of patients with coronary artery disease[238] and after rt-PA infusion to treat cerebrovascular occlusive disease[179–184] (see Chaps. 42 and 44).

Anticoagulant-related ICH, a catastrophic complication with high morbidity and mortality, is relatively rare considering the frequency of anticoagulant use. Anticoagulant-related hemorrhages develop more insidiously and evolve more slowly and more often than do other causes of ICH.[237] Many are erroneously attributed to brain ischemia, especially when anticoagulants have been prescribed to treat TIAs. Any patient taking anticoagulants who develops CNS symptoms should be considered to have anticoagulant-related ICH until CT or MRI excludes that diagnosis. The hematoma grows slowly and insidiously increases intracranial pressure. Many patients require surgical drainage of their hematomas to ensure survival. Anticoagulants should be stopped immediately, and their effect reversed by fresh frozen plasma or vitamin K. It is probably safe to resume anticoagulation with heparin 7 days to 2 weeks after the ICH if indicated, e.g., for prophylaxis in patients with artificial heart valves.[239] In patients treated with fibrinolytic agents, hemorrhages are most often lobar or cerebellar and may be multiple. ICH is more common when there is a past stroke, when heparin or other agents that affect coagulation are given with or after fibrinolytic agents, and when there is a hemostatic defect secondary to treatment.[239]

Arterial Dissections

Aortic dissections involving the innominate or carotid arteries (see Chap. 88) are a well-known cause of stroke and other manifestations of brain ischemia. Less well known are the syndromes produced by dissections of the extracranial and intracranial arteries, which are especially likely to occur in young, active individuals without risk factors for atherosclerosis or stroke but after trauma or chiropractic or other neck manipulations. They also are associated with fibromuscular dysplasia, Marfan's syndrome, pseudoxanthoma elasticum, and migraine.

Dissections start with a tear in the media and spread longitudinally (Fig. 89-11), often disrupting adventitial fibers or even rupturing through the adventitia to produce an extravascular hematoma and a false aneurysm or pseudoaneurysm within muscle and connective tissue. Intracranially, such a rupture can produce SAH. Other dissections cause arterial obstruction and secondary thrombosis of the narrowed vascular lumen. Most cerebrovascular dissections occur in the extracranial vessels, particularly the pharyngeal portion of the ICA and the nuchal vertebral arteries.[5,240–243]

Extracranial dissections produce sharp pain and throbbing headache; brain and retinal ischemic episodes, which may occur in rapid-fire attacks ("carotid allegro"[243]); and pressure on adjacent structures, especially cranial nerves X through XII, which exit at the skull base. Strokes, usually from embolization of

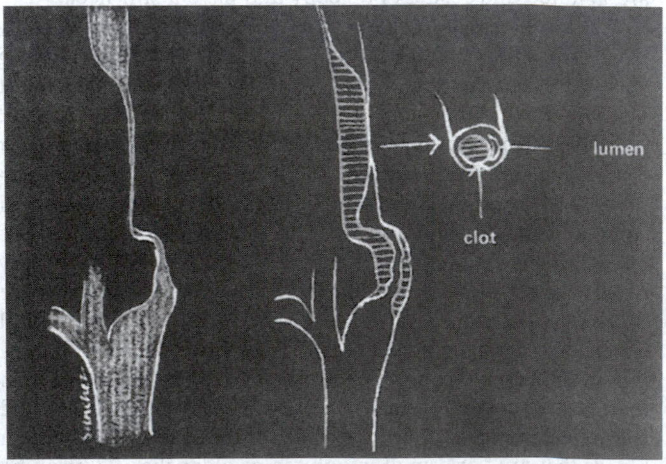

FIGURE 89-11 Diagrams of a carotid artery dissection. *A*. The lumen encroached on by the intramural clot. *B*. The dissection (cross-hatched). (From Caplan LR. *Stroke: A Clinical Approach*, 3d ed. Boston: Butterworth-Heinemann; 2000, with permission.)

clots, are common but may have a benign course. Intracranial dissections have a worse prognosis, often with vascular rupture and SAH. The diagnosis is confirmed by angiography, CT, or MRI. Ultrasound studies can be helpful in suggesting the diagnosis of dissection in the neck.[244]

Treatment consists of the use of heparin acutely, followed by warfarin. In patients in whom the dissected artery is initially occluded and remains occluded, warfarin can be stopped after 6 to 12 weeks. The author continues warfarin in other patients until there no longer is severe luminal narrowing, monitoring the dissected arteries by using noninvasive techniques (ultrasound, CTA, or MRA). Intracranial dissections with SAH have been treated surgically.[241,245]

References

1. Caplan LR. Brain embolism. In: Caplan LR, Hurst JW, Chimowitz MI. *Clinical Neurocardiology*. New York: Marcel Dekker, 1999; 35–185.
2. Aring C, Merritt H. Differential diagnosis between cerebral hemorrhage and cerebral thrombosis. *Arch Intern Med* 1935; 56: 435–456.
3. Whisnant J, Fitzgibbons J, Kurland L, Sayre GP. Natural history of stroke in Rochester, Minnesota, 1945–1954. *Stroke* 1971; 2:11–22.
4. Matsumoto N, Whisnant J, Kurland L, Okazaki H. Natural history of stroke in Rochester, Minnesota, 1955–1969. *Stroke* 1973; 4:2–29.
5. Caplan LR. *Stroke: A Clinical Approach*, 3d ed. Boston: Butterworth-Heinemann; 2000.
6. Mohr J, Caplan LR, Melski J, et al. The Harvard Cooperative Stroke registry: A prospective study. *Neurology* 1978; 28:754–762.
7. Foulkes MA, Wolf PA, Price TR, et al. The Stroke Data Bank: Design, methods, and baseline characteristics. *Stroke* 1988; 19: 547–554.
8. Kunitz S, Gross C, Heyman A, et al. The Pilot Stroke Data Bank: Definition, design and data. *Stroke* 1984; 15:740–746.
9. Bogousslavsky J, Cachin C, Regli F, et al. Cardiac sources of embolism and cerebral infarction—clinical consequences and vascular concomitants: The Lausanne Stroke Registry. *Neurology* 1991; 41:855–859.
10. Kittner SJ, Sharkness CM, Sloan M, et al. Infarcts with a cardiac source of embolism in the NINDS Stroke Data Bank: Neurologic examination. *Neurology* 1992; 42:299–302.
11. Sandok BA, Giuliani ER. Cerebral ischemic events in patients with mitral valve prolapse. *Stroke* 1982; 13:448–450.
12. Lauzier S, Barnett HJM. Cerebral ischemia with mitral valve prolapse and mitral annulus calcification. In: Furlan AJ, ed. *The Heart and Stroke*. London: Springer-Verlag; 1987:63.
13. Pomerance A, Davies MJ. Strokes: A complication of mitral leaflet prolapse. *Lancet* 1977; 2:1186.
14. Hanson MR, Conomy JP, Hodgman JR. Brain events associated with mitral valve prolapse. *Stroke* 1980; 11:499–506.
15. Jones HR, Naggar CZ, Selyan MP, et al. Mitral valve prolapse and cerebral ischemic events: A comparison between a neurology population with stroke and a cardiology population with mitral valve prolapse observed for 5 years. *Stroke* 1982; 13:451–453.
16. Pomerance A. Pathological and clinical study of calcification in the mitral valve ring. *J Clin Pathol* 1970; 23:354–361.
17. Stein JH, Soble JS. Thrombus associated with mitral valve calcification. *Stroke* 1995; 26:1697–1699.
18. DeBono DP, Warlow CP. Mitral-annulus calcification and cerebral or retinal ischemia. *Lancet* 1979; 2:383–385.
19. Benjamin EJ, Plehn JF, D'Agostino RB, et al. Mitral annular calcification and the risk of stroke in an elderly cohort. *N Engl J Med* 1992; 327:374–379.
20. Sacco RL, Ellenberg JH, Mohr JP, et al. Infarcts of undetermined cause: The NINCDS Stroke Data Bank. *Ann Neurol* 1989; 25: 382–390.
21. Galve E, Candell-Riera J, Pigrau C, et al. Prevalence, morphology, types and evaluation of cardiac valvular disease in systemic lupus erythematosus. *N Engl J Med* 1988; 319:817–823.
22. Barbut D, Borer JS, Wallerson D, et al. Anticardiolipin antibody and stroke: Possible relation of valvular heart disease and embolic events. *Cardiology* 1991; 79:99–109.
23. Cohen A, Tzourio C, Chauvel C, et al. Mitral valve strands and the risk of ischemic stroke in elderly patients. *Stroke* 1997; 28: 1574–1578.
24. Caplan LR. Mitral valve strands: What are they and what is their relation to stroke? *Neurol Network Comment* 1998; 2:11–14.
25. Kanter MC, Hart RG. Neurologic complications of infective endocarditis. *Neurology* 1991; 41:1015–1020.
26. Caplan LR. Of birds and nests and brain emboli. *Rev Neurol (Paris)* 1991; 147:265–273.
27. Amarenco P, Duyckaerts C, Tzourio C, et al. The prevalence of ulcerated plaques in the aortic arch in patients with stroke. *N Engl J Med* 1992; 326:221–225.
28. Weinberger J, Azhar S, Danisi F, et al. A new noninvasive technique for imaging atherosclerotic plaque in the aortic arch of stroke patients by transcutaneous real-time B-mode ultrasonography. *Stroke* 1998; 29:673–676.
29. The French Study of Aortic Plaques in Stroke Group. Atherosclerotic disease of the aortic arch as a risk factor for recurrent ischemic stroke. *N Engl J Med* 1996; 334:1216–1221.
30. Gacs G, Merel MD, Bodosi M. Balloon catheter as a model of cerebral emboli in humans. *Stroke* 1982; 13:39–42.
31. Fisher CM. Left hemiplegia and motor impersistence. *J Nerv Ment Dis* 1956; 123:201–218.
32. Caplan LR, Kelly M, Kase CS, et al. Infarcts of the inferior division of the right middle cerebral artery: Mirror image of Wernicke's aphasia. *Neurology* 1986; 36:1015–1020.
33. Caplan LR. Posterior cerebral artery. In: Bogousslavsky J, Caplan LR, eds. *Stroke Syndromes*. New York: Cambridge University Press; 1995:290.
34. Yammamoto Y, Georgiadis AL, Chang H-M, et al. Posterior cerebral artery territory infarcts in the New England Medical Center Posterior Circulation Registry. *Arch Neurol* 1999; 56: 824–832.
35. Mehler MF. The rostral basilar artery syndrome: Diagnosis, etiology, prognosis. *Neurology* 1989; 39:9–16.
36. Amarenco P. The spectrum of cerebellar infarctions. *Neurology* 1991; 41:973–979.
37. Fieschi C, Argentino C, Lenzi GL, et al. Clinical and instrumental evaluation of patients with ischemic stroke within the first six hours. *J Neurol Sci* 1989; 91:311–322.
38. Kushner MJ, Zanotte EM, Bastianiello S, et al. Transcranial Doppler in acute hemispheric brain infarction. *Neurology* 1991; 41:109–113.
39. Ringlestein EB, Koschorke S, Holling A, et al. Computed tomographic patterns of proven embolic brain infarcts. *Ann Neurol* 1989; 26:759–765.
40. Bladin PF, Berkovic SF. Striatocapsular infarction. *Neurology* 1984; 34:1423–1430.
41. Fisher CM, Adams RD. Observations on brain embolism. *J Neuropathol Exp Neurol* 1951; 10:92–94.
42. Fisher CM, Adams RD. Observations on brain embolism with special reference to hemorrhagic infarction. In: Furlan AJ, ed. *The Heart and Stroke*. London: Springer-Verlag; 1987:17.
43. Tomsick T, Brott T, Barsan W, et al. Thrombus localization with emergency cerebral computed tomography. *Stroke* 1990; 21:180.

44. Bergeron GA, Shah PM. Echocardiography unwarranted in patients with cerebral ischemic events. *N Engl J Med* 1981; 304:489.
45. Greenland P, Knopman D, Mikell F, et al. Echocardiography in diagnostic assessment of stroke. *Ann Intern Med* 1981; 95:51–54.
46. Tegeler CH, Downes TR. Cardiac imaging in stroke. *Stroke* 1991; 22:1206–1211.
47. Cohen A, Chauvel C. Transesophageal echocardiography in the management of transient ischemic attack and ischemic stroke. *Cerebrovasc Dis* 1996; 6(suppl 1):15–25.
48. DeWitt LD, Pessin MS, Pandian NG, et al. Benign disappearance of ventricular thrombus after embolic stroke: A case report. *Stroke* 1988; 19:393–396.
49. Markus HS, Harrison MJ. Microembolic signal detection using ultrasound. *Stroke* 1995; 26:1517–1519.
50. Tong DC, Bolger A, Albers GW. Incidence of transcranial Doppler-detected cerebral microemboli in patients referred for echocardiography. *Stroke* 1994; 25:2138–2141.
51. Barbut D, Hinton RB, Szatrowski TP, et al. Cerebral emboli detected during bypass surgery are associated with clamp removal. *Stroke* 1994; 25:2398–2402.
52. Petersen P, Boysen G, Godtfredsen J, et al. Placebo-controlled, randomized trial of warfarin and aspirin for prevention of thromboembolic complications in chronic atrial fibrillation: The Copenhagen AFASAK Study. *Lancet* 1989; 1:175–179.
53. Stroke Prevention in Atrial Fibrillation Investigators. The stroke prevention in atrial fibrillation trial: Final results. *Circulation* 1991; 84:527–539.
54. Stroke Prevention in Atrial Fibrillation Investigators. Adjusted-dose warfarin versus low-intensity fixed-dose warfarin plus aspirin for high-risk patients with atrial fibrillation: Stroke Prevention in Atrial Fibrillation III randomized clinical trial. *Lancet* 1996: 348:633–638.
55. Stroke Prevention in Atrial Fibrillation Investigators. Prospective identification of patients with nonvalvular atrial fibrillation at low risk during treatment with aspirin: Stroke prevention in Atrial Fibrillation III Study. *Circulation* 1997; 96(suppl):I-28 (Abstract).
56. The Stroke Prevention in Atrial Fibrillation Investigators. Predictors of thromboembolism in atrial fibrillation: I. Clinical features of patients at risk. *Ann Intern Med* 1992; 116:1–5.
57. The Stroke Prevention in Atrial Fibrillation Investigators. Predictors of thromboembolism in atrial fibrillation: II. Echocardiographic features of patients at risk. *Ann Intern Med* 1992; 116: 6–12.
58. Pritchett ELC. Management of atrial fibrillation. *N Engl J Med* 1992; 326:1264–1271.
59. The Boston Area Anticoagulation Trial for Atrial Fibrillation Investigators. The effect of low-dose warfarin on the risk of stroke in patients with nonrheumatic atrial fibrillation. *N Engl J Med* 1990; 323:1505–1511.
60. European Atrial Fibrillation Trial Study Group. Optimal oral anticoagulation therapy in patients with nonrheumatic atrial fibrillation and recent cerebral ischemia. *N Engl J Med* 1995; 333: 5–10.
61. Moldveen-Geronimus M, Merriam JC. Cholesterol embolization: From pathologic curiosity to clinical entity. *Circulation* 1967; 35: 946–953.
62. Shields RW Jr, Laureno R, Lachman T, et al. Anticoagulant-related hemorrhage in acute cerebral embolism. *Stroke* 1984; 15: 426–437.
63. Cerebral Embolism Study Group. Immediate anticoagulation of embolic stroke: A randomized trial. *Stroke* 1983; 13:668–676.
64. Toni D, Fiorelli M, Bastianello S, et al. Hemorrhagic transformation of brain infarct. *Neurology* 1996; 46:341–345.
65. Cerebral Embolism Task Force. Cardiogenic brain embolism: The second report of the Cerebral Embolism Task Force. *Arch Neurol* 1989; 46:727–743.
66. Pessin MS, Estol CJ, Lafranchise F, et al. Safety of anticoagulation after hemorrhagic infarction. *Neurology* 1993; 43:1298–1303.
67. Chaves CJ, Pessin MS, Caplan LR, et al. Cerebellar hemorrhagic infarction. *Neurology* 1996; 46:346–349.
68. Chamorro A, Vila N, Ascaso C, Blanc R. Heparin in acute stroke with atrial fibrillation: Clinical relevance of very early treatment. *Arch Neurol* 1999; 56:1098–1102.
69. Caplan LR. When should heparin be given to patients with atrial fibrillation-related brain infarcts? *Arch Neurol* 1999; 56:1059–1060.
70. Hagen PT, Scholz DG, Edwards WD. Incidence and size of patent foramen ovale during the first 10 decades of life: An autopsy study of 965 normal hearts. *Mayo Clin Proc* 1984; 59:17–20.
71. Lechat PH, Mas JL, Lascault G, et al. Prevalence of patent foramen ovale in patients with stroke. *N Engl J Med* 1988; 318:1148–1152.
72. Petty GW, Khanderia BK, Chu C-P, et al. Patent foramen ovale in patients with cerebral infarction: A transesophageal echocardiographic study. *Arch Neurol* 1997; 54:819–822.
73. Gautier JC, Durr A, Koussa S, et al. Paradoxical cerebral embolism with a patent foramen ovale: A report of 29 patients. *Cerebrovasc Dis* 1991; 1:193–202.
74. Caplan LR. Cardiac arrest and other hypoxic-ischemic insults. In: Caplan LR, Hurst JW, Chimowitz MI, eds. *Clinical Neurocardiology*. New York: Marcel Dekker, 1999; 1–34.
75. Dougherty JH, Rawlinson DG, Levy DE, et al. Hypoxic-ischemic brain injury and the vegetative state: Clinical and neuropathologic correlation. *Neurology* 1981; 31:991–997.
76. Cummings JL, Tomiyasu U, Read S, et al. Amnesia with hippocampal lesions after cardiopulmonary arrest. *Neurology* 1984; 34: 679–681.
77. Dooling E, Richardson EP. Delayed encephalopathy after strangling. *Arch Neurol* 1976; 33:196–199.
78. Gilles F. Hypotensive brainstem necrosis. *Arch Pathol* 1969; 88: 32–41.
79. Caronna JJ, Finkelstein S. Neurological syndromes after cardiac arrest. *Stroke* 1978; 9:517–520.
80. Levy DE, Knill-Jones RP, Plum F. The vegetative state and its prognosis following non-traumatic coma. *Ann NY Acad Sci* 1978; 315:293–306.
81. Willoughby J, Leach B. Relation of neurological findings after cardiac arrest to outcome. *Br Med J* 1974; 3:437–439.
82. Levy D, Carrona JJ, Singer BH, et al. Predicting outcome from hypoxic-ischemic coma. *JAMA* 1985; 253:1420–1426.
83. Longstreth WT, Inui TS, Cobb LA, et al. Neurologic recovery after out-of-hospital cardiac arrest. *Ann Intern Med* 1983; 38: 588–592.
84. Longstreth WT, Diehr P, Inui TS. Prediction of awakening after out-of-hospital cardiac arrest. *N Engl J Med* 1983; 308:1378–1382.
85. Thompson RG, Hallstrom AP, Cobb LA. Bystander-initiated cardiopulmonary resuscitation in the management of ventricular fibrillation. *Ann Intern Med* 1979; 90:737–740.
86. Bedell SE, Delbanco TG, Cook EF, Epstein FH. Survival after cardiopulmonary resuscitation in the hospital. *N Engl J Med* 1983; 309:569–576.
87. Caplan LR, Brass LM, DeWitt LD, et al. Transcranial Doppler ultrasound: Present status. *Neurology* 1990; 40:696–700.
88. Longstreth WT, Inui TS. High blood glucose level on hospital admission and poor neurological recovery after cardiac arrest. *Ann Neurol* 1984; 15:59–63.
89. Collins RC, Dobkin BH, Choi DW. Selective vulnerability of the brain: New insights into the pathophysiology of stroke. *Ann Intern Med* 1989; 110:992–1000.
90. Giswold S, Safar P, Rao G, et al. Multifaceted therapy after global brain ischemia in monkeys. *Stroke* 1984; 15:803–812.
91. Caplan LR. Encephalopathies and neurological effects of drugs used in cardiac patients. In: Caplan LR, Hurst JW, Chimowitz

MI, eds. *Clinical Neurocardiology*. New York: Marcel Dekker; 1999:186.

92. Closson RG. Visual hallucinations as the earliest symptom of digoxin intoxication. *Arch Neurol* 1983; 40:386.
93. Gilbert GJ. Quinidine dementia. *JAMA* 1977; 237:2093–2094.
94. Barbut D, Caplan LR. Brain complications of cardiac surgery. *Curr Probl Cardiol* 1997; 22:455–476.
95. Slogoff S, Girgis KZ, Keats AS. Etiologic factors in neuropsychiatric complications associated with cardiopulmonary bypass. *Anesth Analg* 1982; 61:903–911.
96. Gilman S. Neurological complications of open heart surgery. *Ann Neurol* 1990; 28:475–476.
97. Shaw PJ, Bates D, Cartlidge NEF, et al. Early neurological complications of coronary artery bypass surgery. *Br Med J* 1985; 291: 1384–1387.
98. Breuer AC, Furlan AJ, Hanson MR, et al. Central nervous system complications of coronary artery bypass graft surgery: Prospective analysis of 421 patients. *Stroke* 1983; 14:682–687.
99. Ropper AH, Wechsler LR, Wilson LS. Carotid bruit and the risk of stroke in elective surgery. *N Engl J Med* 1982; 307:1388–1390.
100. Furlan AJ, Craciun AR. Risk of stroke during coronary artery bypass graft surgery in patients with internal carotid artery disease documented by angiography. *Stroke* 1985; 16:797–799.
101. Sila C. Neuroimaging of cerebral infarction associated with coronary revascularization. *AJNR* 1991; 12:817–818.
102. Hertzer NR, Loop FD, Beven EG, et al. Surgical staging for simultaneous coronary and carotid disease: A study including prospective randomization. *Vasc Surg* 1989; 9:455–463.
103. VonReutern G-M, Hetzel A, Birnbaum D, et al. Transcranial Doppler ultrasound during cardiopulmonary bypass in patients with internal carotid artery disease documented by angiography. *Stroke* 1988; 19:674–680.
104. Hise JH, Nippu ML, Schnitker JC. Stroke associated with coronary artery bypass surgery. *AJNR* 1991; 12:811–814.
105. Wijdicks EFM, Jack CR. Coronary artery bypass grafting-associated stroke. *J Neuroimag* 1996; 6:20–22.
106. Tettenborn B, Caplan LR, Sloan MA, et al. Postoperative brainstem cerebellar infarcts. *Neurology* 1993; 43:471–477.
107. Barbut D, Hinton RB, Szatrowski TP, et al. Cerebral emboli detected during bypass surgery are associated with clamp removal. *Stroke* 1994; 25:2398–2402.
108. Pugsley W, Paschalis C, Treasure T, et al. The impact of microemboli during cardiopulmonary bypass on neuropsychological functioning. *Stroke* 1994; 25:1393–1399.
109. Price DL, Harris J. Cholesterol emboli in cerebral arteries are a complication of retrograde aortic perfusion during cardiac surgery. *Neurology* 1970; 20:1207–1214.
110. Karalis DG, Chandrasekaran K, Victor MF, et al. Recognition and embolic potential of intraaortic atherosclerotic debris. *J Am Coll Cardiol* 1991; 17:73–78.
111. Marshall JNG, Barzilai B, Kouchoukos N, Saffitz J. Intraoperative ultrasonic imaging of the ascending aorta. *Ann Thorac Surg* 1989; 48:339–344.
112. Gilman S. Cerebral disorders after open-heart operations. *N Engl J Med* 1965; 272:489–498.
113. Coffey CE, Massey EW, Roberts KB, et al. Natural history of cerebral complications of coronary artery bypass graft surgery. *Neurology* 1983; 33:1416–1421.
114. Moody DM, Bell MA, Challa VR, et al. Brain microemboli during cardiac surgery or aortography. *Ann Neurol* 1990; 28:477–486.
115. Feeney DM, Gonzalez A, Law WA. Amphetamine, haloperidol and experience interact to affect the rate of recovery after motor cortex injury. *Science* 1982; 217:855–857.
116. Humphreys RP, Hoffman JH, Mustard WT, Trusler GA. Cerebral hemorrhage following heart surgery. *J Neurosurg* 1975; 43: 671–675.
117. Sila CA. Spectrum of neurologic events following cardiac transplantation. *Stroke* 1989; 20:1586–1589.
118. Caplan LR. Intracerebral hemorrhage revisited. *Neurology* 1988; 38:624–627.
119. Lederman RJ, Breuer AC, Hanson MR, et al. Peripheral nervous system complications of coronary artery bypass graft surgery. *Ann Neurol* 1982; 12:297–301.
120. Caplan LR, Hurst JW. Cardiac and cardiovascular findings in patients with nervous system disease—strokes. In: Caplan LR, Hurst JW, Chimowitz MI, eds. *Clinical Neurocardiology*. New York: Marcel Dekker; 1999:303.
121. Norris JW, Hachinski V. Cardiac dysfunction following stroke. In: Furlan AJ, ed. *The Heart and Stroke*. London: Springer-Verlag; 1987:171.
122. Smith RP, Tomlinson BE. Subendocardial hemorrhages associated with intracranial lesions. *J Pathol Bacteriol* 1954; 68:327–334.
123. Kolin A, Norris JW. Myocardial damage from acute cerebral lesions. *Stroke* 1984; 15:990–993.
124. Samuels MA. Electrocardiographic manifestations of neurologic disease. *Semin Neurol* 1984; 4:453–459.
125. Myers MG, Norris JW, Hachinski V, Sole MJ. Plasma norepinephrine in stroke. *Stroke* 1981; 12:200–204.
126. Marion DW, Segal R, Thompson ME. Subarachnoid hemorrhage and the heart. *Rev Neurosurg* 1986; 18:101–106.
127. Samuels M. "Voodoo" death revisited: The modern lessons of neurocardiology. *Neurologist* 1997; 3:293–304.
128. Burch GE, Myers R, Abildskov JA. A new electrocardiographic pattern observed in cerebrovascular accidents. *Circulation* 1954; 9:719–723.
129. Dimant J, Grob D. Electrocardiographic changes and myocardial damage in patients with acute cerebrovascular accidents. *Stroke* 1977; 8:448–455.
130. Rolak LA, Rokey R. Electrocardiographic features: In: Rolak LA, Rokey R, eds. *Coronary and Cerebral Vascular Disease*. Mt. Kisco, NY: Futura; 1990:139–197.
131. Fabinyi G, Hunt D, McKinley L. Myocardial creatine kinase isoenzyme in serum after subarachnoid hemorrhage. *J Neurol Neurosurg Psychiatry* 1977; 40:818–820.
132. Neil-Dwyer G, Cruickshank J, Stratton C. Beta-blockers, plasma total creatine kinase and creatine kinase myocardial isoenzyme, and the prognosis of subarachnoid hemorrhage. *Surg Neurol* 1986; 25:163–168.
133. Myers MG, Norris JW, Hachinsky VC, et al. Cardiac sequelae of acute strokes. *Stroke* 1982; 13:838–842.
134. Stober T, Sen S, Anstatt T, Bette L. Correlation of cardiac arrhythmias with brainstem compression in patients with intracerebral hemorrhage. *Stroke* 1988; 19:688–692.
135. Wier BK. Pulmonary edema following fatal aneurysmal rupture. *J Neurosurg* 1978; 49:502–507.
136. Theodore J, Robin ED. Pathogenesis of neurogenic pulmonary edema. *Lancet* 1975; 2:749–751.
137. Engel GL. Psychologic factors in instantaneous cardiac death. *N Engl J Med* 1976; 294:664–665.
138. Lown B, Temte JV, Reich P, et al. Basis for recurring ventricular fibrillation in the absence of coronary heart disease and its management. *N Engl J Med* 1976; 294:623–629.
139. Talman WT. Cardiovascular regulation and lesions of the central nervous system. *Ann Neurol* 1985; 18:1–12.
140. Schwartz PJ, Stone HL, Brown AM. Effects of unilateral stellate ganglion blockage on the arrhythmias associated with coronary occlusion. *Am Heart J* 1976; 92:589–599.
141. Adams H, Kassell N, Mazuz H. The patients with transient ischemic attacks: Is this the time for a new therapeutic approach? *Stroke* 1984; 15:371–375.
142. Hennerici M, Aulich A, Sandmann W, Freund HJ. Incidence of asymptomatic extracranial arterial disease. *Stroke* 1981; 12: 750–758.

143. Caplan LR. Cerebrovascular disease: Large artery occlusive disease. In: Appel S, ed. *Current Neurology*, vol 87. Chicago: Year Book; 1988:179–226.
144. Zarins CK, Giddins DP, Bharadvaj BK, et al. Carotid bifurcation atherosclerosis. *Circ Res* 1983; 53:502–514.
145. Hutchinson EC, Yates DO. The cervical portion of the vertebral artery: A clinicopathologic study. *Brain* 1956; 79:319–331.
146. Fisher CM, Ojemann RG. A clinico-pathologic study of carotid endarterectomy plaques. *Rev Neurol (Paris)* 1986; 142:573–589.
147. Caplan LR, Gorelick PB, Hier DB. Race, sex, and occlusive vascular disease: A review. *Stroke* 1986; 17:648–655.
148. Gorelick PB, Caplan LR, Hier DB, et al. Racial differences in the distribution of posterior circulation occlusive disease. *Stroke* 1985; 16:785–790.
149. Feldmann E, Daneault N, Kwan E, et al. Chinese-white differences in the distribution of occlusive cerebrovascular disease. *Neurology* 1990; 40:1541–1545.
150. Caplan LR, Wolpert SM. Angiography in patients with occlusive cerebrovascular disease: Views of a stroke neurologist and neuroradiologist. *AJNR* 1991; 12:593–601.
151. Caplan LR, Hennerici M. Impaired clearance of emboli is an important link between hypoperfusion, embolism, and ischemic stroke. *Arch Neurol* 1998; 55:1475–1482.
152. Chambers BR, Norris JW. Outcome in patients with asymptomatic neck bruits. *N Engl J Med* 1986; 315:860–865.
153. Ringelstein EB, Zeumer H, Angelou D. The pathogenesis of strokes from internal carotid artery occlusion: Diagnostic and therapeutical implications. *Stroke* 1983; 14:867–875.
154. Caplan LR, Tettenborn B. Vertebrobasilar occlusive disease: Review of selected aspects. 2: Posterior circulation embolism. *Cerebrovasc Dis* 1992; 2:320–326.
155. Gorelick PB, Hier DB, Caplan LR, Langenberg P. Headache in acute cerebrovascular disease. *Neurology* 1986; 36:1445–1450.
156. Pessin MS, Hinton RC, Davis KR, et al. Mechanism of acute carotid stroke. *Ann Neurol* 1979; 6:245–252.
157. Caplan LR. Significance of unexpected (silent) brain infarcts. In: Caplan LR, Shifrin EG, Nicolaides AN, Moore WS, eds. *Cerebrovascular Ischaemia: Investigation and Management*. London: Med-Orion; 1996:423–433.
158. O'Donnell TF, Erdoes L, Mackey WC, et al. Correlation of B-mode ultrasound imaging and arteriography with pathologic findings at carotid endarterectomy. *Arch Surg* 1985; 120:443–449.
159. Zwiebel WJ, Zagzebski JA, Crummy AB, Hirscher M. Correlation of peak Doppler frequency with lumen narrowing in carotid stenosis. *Stroke* 1982; 13:386–391.
160. Hennerici M, Rautenberg W, Sitzer G, Schwartz A. Transcranial Doppler ultrasound for the assessment of intracranial arterial flow velocity: I. Examination technique and normal values. *Surg Neurol* 1986; 315:860–865.
161. Spencer MP, Thomas GI, Nicholls SC, et al. Detection of middle cerebral artery emboli during carotid endarterectomy using transcranial Doppler ultrasonography. *Stroke* 1990; 21:415–423.
162. Edelman RR, Mattle HP, Atkinson DJ, Hoogewoud HM. MR angiography. *AJR* 1990; 154:937–946.
163. Caplan LR, DeWitt LD, Breen JC. Neuroimaging in patients with cerebrovascular disease In: Greenberg J, ed. *Neuroimaging: A Companion to Adams and Victor's Principles of Neurology*. New York: McGraw-Hill; 1999:493–520.
164. Caplan LR. Treatment of cerebral ischemia: Where are we headed? *Stroke* 1984; 15:571–574.
165. Warach S, Gaa J, Siewert B, et al. Acute human stroke studied by whole brain echo planar diffusion-weighted magnetic resonance imaging. *Ann Neurol* 1995; 37:231–241.
166. Sorensen AG, Buonanno F, Gonzalez RG, et al. Hyperacute stroke: Evaluation with combined multisection diffusion-weighted and hemodynamically weighted echo-planar MR imaging. *Radiology* 1996; 199:391–401.
167. North American Symptomatic Carotid Endarterectomy Trial (NASCET) Collaborators. Beneficial effect of carotid endarterectomy in symptomatic patients with high-grade carotid stenosis. *N Engl J Med* 1991; 325:445–453.
168. Barnett HJM, Taylor DW, Eliasziw M, et al for the North American Symptomatic Carotid Endarterectomy Trial Collaborators. Benefit of carotid endarterectomy in patients with symptomatic moderate or severe stenosis. *N Engl J Med* 1998; 339:1415–1425.
169. European Carotid Surgery Trialist's Collaborative Group. MRC European Carotid Surgery Trial: Interim results for symptomatic patients with severe (70–99 percent) or with mild (0–29 percent) carotid stenosis. *Lancet* 1991; 1:1235–1243.
170. European Carotid Surgery Trialist's Collaborative Group. Randomised trial of endarterectomy for recently symptomatic carotid stenosis: Final results of the MRC European Carotid Surgery Trial (ECST). *Lancet* 1998; 351:1379–1387.
171. Executive Committee for the Asymptomatic Carotid Atherosclerosis Study. Endarterectomy for asymptomatic carotid artery stenosis. *JAMA* 1995; 273:1421–1428.
172. Berguer R, Caplan LR, eds. *Vertebrobasilar Arterial Disease*. St Louis: Quality Medical Publishers; 1991:201–261.
173. Fields WS, Lemak NA, Frankowski RF, Hardy RJ. Controlled trial of aspirin in cerebral ischemia. *Stroke* 1977; 8:301–314.
174. Antiplatelet Trialists' Collaboration. Collaborative overview of randomised trials of antiplatelet therapy. 1: Prevention of death, myocardial infarction, and stroke by prolonged antiplatelet therapy in various categories of patients. *Br Med J* 1994; 308:81–106.
175. Hass WK, Easton JD, Adams HP, et al. A randomized trial comparing ticlopidine hydrochloride with aspirin for the prevention of stroke in high risk patients. *N Engl J Med* 1989; 321:501–507.
176. Warlow CP. Ticlopidine, a new antithrombotic drug: But is it better than aspirin for long term use? *J Neurol Neurosurg Psychiatry* 1990; 53:185–187.
177. CAPRIE Steering Committee. A randomised, blinded, trial of clopidogrel versus aspirin in patients at risk of ischaemic events. *Lancet* 1996; 348:1329–1339.
178. Diener HC, Cunha L, Forbes C, et al. European Stroke Prevention Study: 2. Dipyridamole and acetylsalicylic acid in the secondary prevention of stroke. *J Neurol Sci* 1996; 143:1–13.
179. The National Institute of Neurological Disorders and Stroke rt-PA Study Group. Tissue plasminogen activator for acute ischemic stroke. *N Engl J Med* 1995; 333:1581–1587.
180. del Zoppo GJ, Poeck K, Pessin MS, et al. Recombinant tissue plasminogen activator in acute thrombotic and embolic stroke. *Ann Neurol* 1992; 32:78–86.
181. Wolpert SM, Bruckmann H, Greenlee R, et al. Neuroradiologic evaluation of patients with acute stroke treated with recombinant tissue plasminogen activator. *AJNR* 1993; 14:3–13.
182. Pessin MS, del Zoppo GJ, Furlan AJ. Thrombolytic treatment in acute stroke: Review and update of selected topics. In: Moskowitz MA, Caplan LR, eds. *Cerebrovascular Diseases: Nineteenth Princeton Stroke Conference*. Boston: Butterworth-Heinemann; 1995:409–418.
183. Furlan A, Higashida R, Wechsler L, et al. A randomized trial of intra-arterial prourokinase for acute ischemic stroke of less than 6 hours duration due to middle cerebral artery occlusion. *JAMA* 1999; 282:2003–2011.
184. Caplan LR, Mohr JP, Kistler JP, et al. Should thrombolytic therapy be the first-line treatment for acute ischemic stroke? Thrombolysis—Not a panacea for ischemic stroke. *N Engl J Med* 1997; 337:1309–1310.
185. Pettigrew LC. Surgical considerations. In: Rolak L, Rokey R,

eds. *Coronary and Cerebral Vascular Disease*. Mt Kisco, NY: Futura; 1990:349–377.

186. Hertzer NR, Loop FD, Beven EG. Management of coexistent carotid and coronary artery disease: A surgical viewpoint. In: Furlan A, ed. *The Heart and Stroke*. London: Springer-Verlag; 1987:305–318.
187. Easton JD, Hart RG. Asymptomatic carotid artery disease in patients undergoing open heart surgery: A neurologic viewpoint. In: Furlan A, ed. *The Heart and Stroke*. London: Springer-Verlag; 1987:319–327.
188. Caplan LR. Intracranial branch atheromatous disease. *Neurology* 1989; 39:1246–1250.
189. Caplan LR. Lacunar infarction: A neglected concept. *Geriatrics* 1976; 31:71–75.
190. Caplan LR. Binswanger's disease revisited. *Neurology* 1995; 45: 626–633.
191. Fisher CM. The arterial lesions underlying lacunes. *Acta Neuropathol* 1969; 12:1–15.
192. Kase CS, Caplan LR. *Intracerebral Hemorrhage*. Boston: Butterworth-Heinemann; 1994.
193. Rosenblum WI. Miliary aneurysms and "fibrinoid" degeneration of cerebral blood vessels. *Hum Pathol* 1977; 8:133–139.
194. Fisher CM. Pathological observations in hypertensive cerebral hemorrhage. *J Neuropathol Exp Neurol* 1971; 30:536–550.
195. Mohr JP. Lacunes. *Stroke* 1982; 13:3–11.
196. Fisher CM. Lacunar strokes and infarcts: A review. *Neurology* 1982; 32:871–876.
197. Fisher CM. Pure motor hemiplegia of vascular origin. *Arch Neurol* 1965; 13:30–44.
198. Fisher CM. Pure sensory stroke and allied conditions. *Stroke* 1982; 13:434–447.
199. Fisher CW. Ataxic hemiparesis. *Arch Neurol* 1978; 35:126–128.
200. Fisher CM. A lacunar stroke, the dysarthric-clumsy hand syndrome. *Neurology* 1967; 17:614–617.
201. Hachinski VC, Potter P, Merskey H. Leuko-araiosis. *Arch Neurol* 1987; 44:21–23.
202. Caplan LR, Schoene W. Subcortical arteriosclerotic encephalopathy (Binswanger disease): Clinical features. *Neurology* 1978; 28: 1206–1219.
203. Babikian V, Ropper AH. Binswanger's disease: A review. *Stroke* 1987; 18:2–12.
204. Kase CS. Intracerebral hemorrhage: Non-hypertensive causes. *Stroke* 1986; 17:590–594.
205. Bahemuka M. Primary intracerebral hemorrhage and heart weight: A clinicopathological case-control review of 218 patients. *Stroke* 1987; 18:531–536.
206. Brott T, Thalinger K, Hertzberg V. Hypertension as a risk factor for spontaneous intracerebral hemorrhage. *Stroke* 1986; 17:1078–1083.
207. Fisher CM. Pathological observations in hypertensive cerebral hemorrhages. *J Neuropathol Exp Neurol* 1971; 30:536–550.
208. Linfante I, Linas RH, Caplan LR, Warach S. MRI features of intracerebral hemorrhage within 2 hours from symptoms onset. *Stroke* 1999; 30:2263–2267.
209. Tuhrim S, Dambrosia JM, Price TR, et al. Prediction of intracerebral hemorrhage survival. *Ann Neurol* 1988; 24:258–263.
210. Adams HP, Jergenson DD, Kassell NF, Sahs AL. Pitfalls in the recognition of subarachnoid hemorrhage. *JAMA* 1980; 244: 794–796.
211. Ostergaard JR. Warning leaks in subarachnoid hemorrhage. *Br Med J* 1990; 301:190–191.
212. Weisberg L. Computed tomography in aneurysmal subarachnoid hemorrhage. *Neurology* 1979; 29:802–808.
213. Caplan LR, Flamm ES, Mohr JP, et al. Lumbar puncture and stroke. *Stroke* 1987; 18:540A–544A.
214. Heros R, Zervas NT, Varsos V. Cerebral vasospasm after subarachnoid hemorrhage: An update. *Ann Neurol* 1983; 14:599–608.
215. Kassell N, Sasaki T, Colohan A, Nazar G. Cerebral vasospasm following aneurysmal subarachnoid hemorrhage. *Stroke* 1985; 16: 562–572.
216. MacDonald RL, Weir BK. A review of hemoglobin and the pathogenesis of cerebral vasospasm. *Stroke* 1991; 22:971–982.
217. Wilkins RH. Attempts at prevention or treatment of intracranial arterial spasm: An update. *Neurosurgery* 1986; 18:808–825.
218. Weir B, Grace M, Hansen J, Rothberg C. Time course of vasospasm in man. *J Neurosurg* 1978; 48:173–178.
219. Kwak R, Niizuma H, Ohi T, Suzuki J. Angiographic study of cerebral vasospasm following rupture of intracranial aneurysms: I. Time of the appearance. *Surg Neurol* 1979; 11:257–262.
220. Sloan MA, Haley EC, Kassell NF, et al. Sensitivity and specificity of transcranial Doppler ultrasonography in the diagnosis of vasospasm following subarachnoid hemorrhage. *Neurology* 1989; 39: 1514–1518.
221. Davis S, Andrews J, Lichtenstein M, et al. A single-photon emission computed tomography study of hypoperfusion after subarachnoid hemorrhage. *Stroke* 1990; 21:252–259.
222. Hart RG, Kanter MC. Hematologic disorders and ischemic stroke: A selective review. *Stroke* 1990; 20:1111–1121.
223. Coull BM, Goodnight SH. Current concepts of cerebrovascular disease and stroke: Antiphospholipid antibodies, prothrombotic states and stroke. *Stroke* 1990; 21:1370–1374.
224. Feinberg WM, Bruck DC, Ring ME. Hemostatic markers in acute stroke. *Stroke* 1989; 20:592–597.
225. Wu K, Hoak J. Increased platelet aggregation in patients with transient ischemic attacks. *Stroke* 1975; 6:521–524.
226. Feinberg WM. Coagulation. In: Caplan LR, ed. *Brain Ischemia: Basic Concepts and Clinical Relevance*. London: Springer-Verlag; 1995:85–96.
227. Hart R, Miller V, Coull B, Bril V. Cerebral infarction associated with lupus anticoagulants: Preliminary report. *Stroke* 1984; 15: 114–118.
228. Levine SR, Welch KMA. The spectrum of neurologic disease associated with antiphospholipid antibodies, lupus anticoagulants, and anticardiolipin antibodies. *Arch Neurol* 1987; 44: 876–883.
229. Kushner M, Simonian N. Lupus anticoagulant, anticardiolipin antibodies and cerebral ischemia. *Stroke* 1989; 20:225–229.
230. Levine SR, Langer SL, Albers JW, Welch KMA. Sneddon's syndrome: An antiphospholipid antibody syndrome. *Neurology* 1988; 38:798–800.
231. Rebollo M, Vol JF, Garijil F, et al. Livedo reticularis and cerebrovascular lesions (Sneddon's syndrome): Clinical, radiologic, and pathologic features in eight cases. *Brain* 1983; 106:965–979.
232. Antiphospholipid Antibodies in Stroke Study Group (APASS). Clinical and laboratory findings in patients with antiphospholipid antibodies and cerebral ischemia. *Stroke* 1990; 21:1268–1273.
233. DeWitt LD, Caplan LR. Antiphospholipid antibodies and stroke. *AJNR* 1991; 12:454–456.
234. Asherson RA. A "primary antiphospholipid syndrome"? (editorial). *J Rheumatol* 1988; 15:1742–1746.
235. Coull BM, Boudette DN, Goodnight SH, et al. Multiple cerebral infarction and dementia associated with anticardiolipin antibodies. *Stroke* 1987; 18:1107–1112.
236. Amico L, Caplan LR, Thomas C. Cerebrovascular complications of mucinous cancers. *Neurology* 1989; 39:522–526.
237. Kase C, Robinson R, Stein R, et al. Anticoagulant-related intracerebral hemorrhage. *Neurology* 1985; 35:943–948.
238. Bovill EG, Terrin ML, Stump DC, et al. Hemorrhagic events during therapy with recombinant tissue-type plasminogen activator, heparin, and aspirin for acute myocardial infarction. *Ann Intern Med* 1991; 115:256–265.
239. Babikian V, Kase C, Pessin M, et al. Resumption of anticoagulation after intracranial bleeding in patients with prosthetic valves. *Stroke* 1988; 19:407–408.

240. Hart RG, Easton JD. Dissections of cervical and cerebral arteries. *Neurol Clin North Am* 1983; 1:255–282.
241. Anson J, Crowell RM. Cervicocranial arterial dissection. *Neurosurgery* 1991; 29:89–96.
242. Mokri B, Houser W, Sandok B, Piepgras D. Spontaneous dissections of the vertebral arteries. *Neurology* 1988; 38:880–885.
243. Ojemann RG, Fisher CM, Rich JC. Spontaneous dissecting aneurysms of the internal carotid artery. *Stroke* 1972; 3:434–440.
244. Hennerici M, Steinke W, Rautenberg W. High-resistance Doppler flow pattern in extracranial carotid dissection. *Arch Neurol* 1989; 46:670–672.
245. Berger MS, Wilson CB. Intracranial dissecting aneurysms of the posterior circulation. *J Neurosurg* 1984; 61:882–894.

CHAPTER 90

DIAGNOSIS AND MANAGEMENT OF DISEASES OF THE PERIPHERAL ARTERIES AND VEINS

Paul W. Wennberg / Thom W. Rooke

INTRODUCTION

Peripheral vascular disease (PVD) is common in the adult population.[1,2] Arterial disease, which affects 10 to 15 percent of the adult population in developed countries, is seen commonly in cardiology practices, but venous and lymphatic disease must not be ignored. The natural history of each disease, regardless of the underlying etiology, may include ischemia, pain, swelling, and ultimately ulceration. Despite its high prevalence, few individuals receive formal PVD training in internal medicine or cardiology training programs. Despite or because of this, cardiologists often are consulted on patients with peripheral atherosclerosis, deep vein thrombosis, peripheral vasculitis, and many other PVDs. Fortunately, the history and physical examination often make the diagnosis relatively straightforward. Well-defined invasive and noninvasive testing methods are available that can provide confirmation, quantification, and in some instances clarification of the diagnosis.

This chapter provides an introduction to PVD. History, physical examination, and noninvasive laboratory testing are emphasized, followed by brief discussions of specific disease entities commonly seen in cardiovascular practice. Aortic disease, cerebrovascular diseases, vascular surgery, and percutaneous interventions are discussed elsewhere (Chaps. 56, 89, 91, and 93).

ASSESSMENT OF ARTERIAL DISEASE

History

General information, including the age, gender, associated medical problems (including prior trauma, vascular and orthopedic procedures, and past or current medication use), and risk factors for atherosclerosis, should be obtained. Symptoms, including onset, progression, and aggravating or alleviating factors, should be clarified. Claudication, ischemic rest pain, and skin ulceration are the usual presenting complaints of occlusive arterial disease. The description of symptoms may be quite different from patient to patient.

Claudication

Claudication ("limping") is a stereotypical, reproducible distress in single or multiple muscle groups of the lower extremity brought on in a predictable manner by sustained exercise and relieved by rest. The distress may be described as numbness, weakness, giving way, aching, cramping, or pain. It may change in character and/or location as the causative lesion or lesions progress. Claudication occurs at a predictable distance or time, but when the workload is increased by a rapid pace, a burden, or walking uphill or over rough terrain, the distance or time shortens. When the distance to claudication abruptly decreases, one must consider thrombosis in situ or an embolic event. Claudication often worsens after a period of inactivity such as hospitalization but usually returns to baseline with reconditioning.

Claudication occurs in muscle groups rather than joints. Relief with rest is independent of position and is timely, usually within 5 to 10 min. When these criteria are not met, musculoskeletal or neurologic disorders should be suspected. While lifestyle limitation and changes in quality of life should be an integral part of the history, quantitation of disease severity by history alone is unreliable. Variability in pace, workload, and estimates of distance all are based on the patient's perception. Standardized treadmill testing utilizing ankle/brachial indexes at rest and after the completion of an exercise protocol confirms the diagnosis, determines the severity, and documents claudication distance for future follow-up.

Variants of Claudication

There are many causes of claudication, but four specific variants merit mention here (Table 90-1). In the first, a classic claudication history is obtained, but on examination, the pulses are normal and no bruits are noted. After exercise, the pedal pulses disappear, the feet become pale, proximal bruits are noted, and the ankle/brachial indexes drop. The symptoms and findings normalize within minutes of rest. Initially, this was thought to be *vasospastic claudication*,[3] but arteriography has shown occlusive disease in proximal vessels, usually of atherosclerotic origin,[4] that is subcritical at rest. During exercise, blood is shunted into collateral arterial muscular beds, depriving downstream arteries of flow. Popliteal entrapment or adventitial cystic disease of the popliteal artery also can cause this syndrome.[5]

A second variant is *pseudoclaudication*, which may be of neurogenic or muscular origin. A patient with neurogenic claudication will describe exercise-induced distress with a dysesthetic quality that clears slowly or requires a specific posture for relief, usually with the hips in flexion. Clumsiness may develop as walking progresses. Symptoms occur with prolonged standing or in fixed positions such as being seated or lying. A history of back injury should be sought. Compression of the distal spinal cord by hypertrophic bone, disk protrusion, or tumor may be the cause.[6] Arterial and neurogenic disease may coexist. In this situation, the dominant lesion can be identified by observing symptoms and measuring the arterial indexes after exercise.[7]

Muscular distress induced by exercise is common in patients with amyotrophic lateral sclerosis, muscular dystrophy, McArdle's syndrome, and other myopathies. The muscular deficits are apparent on examination. Exercise testing clarifies the status of the arterial system.

Venous claudication is described as a congestive, often "bursting" distress of the thighs and calves induced by standing, running, and sometimes walking. Relief with rest is slow and is accelerated notably when the patient reclines and elevates the legs. This type occurs with significant iliocaval obstruction. Signs of venous hypertension of the legs and lower abdomen often are noted and should be apparent during the examination.

TABLE 90-1 Differential Diagnosis of Claudication

Atherosclerosis obliterans
Arteritis (Takayasu's, giant cell)
Embolic disease/acute arterial occlusion
Degenerative joint disease (hip, back, knee)
Spinal stenosis
Myopathy
Thromboangiitis obliterans
Popliteal entrapment
Venous claudication/varicosities
Baker's cyst
Deconditioning
Aortic dissection
Aortic coarctation
Retroperitoneal fibrosis

Ischemic Distress

With severe perfusion deficits, patients can experience persistent distress of two types: rest pain and ischemic neuropathy. Rest pain is constant and agonizing in quality and is confined to the affected digits, foot, or hand and less commonly the entire limb. It may localize to sites of infarction, ulceration, or infection. Small, localized areas of ischemic pain can occur with vasculitis, microembolization, or thrombosis but more often are caused by trauma to an area with poor perfusion as a result of chronic occlusive disease. It is important to inquire about new shoes, recent trimming of callus or nails, and other potential sources of trauma. Rest pain is noted commonly at night and is relieved by dependency, i.e., hanging the limb off the bed or sleeping in a chair, or, paradoxically, with walking. Pain later becomes constant, interrupting sleep, suppressing appetite, inducing weight loss, and requiring large doses of analgesics. The area is sensitive to touch by clothing and bedding. Depression is often present. Eventually, muscular atrophy and contractures at the ankle, knee, or hip may result as the limb is passively or actively protected and held immobile.

Ischemic neuropathy is a constant distress described as aching, throbbing, burning, pulling, or tearing. It is diffuse and often affects the entire lower leg or forearm. Shifting or lancinating pain often is experienced. Exacerbation of pain may occur spontaneously, often accompanied by diffuse cyanosis and coolness of the skin.

ARTERIAL EXAMINATION

The aorta and the radial, ulnar, subclavian, carotid, femoral, popliteal, posterior tibial, and dorsalis pedis arteries are accessible to palpation, although the dorsalis pedis artery may be congenitally absent. The temporal and occipital arteries are also accessible and should be palpated when temporal arteritis is suspected. Pulses are graded on a scale of 0 to 5; 0 being absence, 4 normal, and 5 aneurysmal. When a pulse is not present, a Doppler examination should be performed to establish whether the pulse is absent, obscured by overlying tissue or edema, or simply below the level of detection by palpation. Typically, when the arterial pressure is below 60 mmHg or an ankle brachial index (ABI) is below 0.6, pedal pulses are not palpable.

Auscultation of the femoral, iliac, aortic, carotid, and subclavian areas should be performed routinely.

The abdominal aorta is best examined with the patient supine on a firm surface, with the knees flexed and the arms at the side. Examination begins with the gentle pressure of eight fingers spread across the epigastrium in an effort to appreciate diffuse pulsation. Two or three fingers of each hand gradually are brought deeper on either side of the aorta until its pulsation and dimensions are defined. Alternatively, the fingers may occupy one side, and the thumbs the opposite side. It is helpful to coach the patient to breathe and relax, penetrating deeper with each expiration and warning that modest discomfort may be felt.

The popliteal artery is more difficult to examine, especially when musculoskeletal structures are prominent or relaxation is poor. It is best approached with the patient supine with the knee relaxed and "cradled" into the fingers. The pulse sometimes may be located by palpating distally between the heads of the gastrocnemius muscle. Popliteal examination routinely should include both of these sites as well as the adductor muscle mass distal to the adductor. Aneurysms can occur at any of these three locations (Fig. 90-1).

The radial pulse is quite accessible, but the ulnar artery is subject to variation and frequently is obscured by tendons. It is a particularly important vessel because of the relatively high incidence of trauma to this artery as it crosses the wrist. Deep and superficial palmar arches connect these two arteries into an arcade that supplies the digits. The *Allen test* ascertains arch patency. This test depends on the integrity of the radial, ulnar, and palmar arch arteries. It is performed by occluding the radial and ulnar artery with firm digital pressure and having the patient exsanguinate the hand by making a fist. The hand is relaxed and partially opened when the radial or ulnar artery is released. It is imperative that the wrist be relaxed to avoid false-positive results caused by ligamentous compression.[8] The procedure then is repeated for the other artery. If the noncompressed artery is patent, flushing of the entire hand will occur within 3 s after release. Delayed refilling is diagnostic of occlusive disease in the noncompressed vessel. Digital or microcirculatory deficits are suggested if refilling is slow or absent in isolated digits.[9]

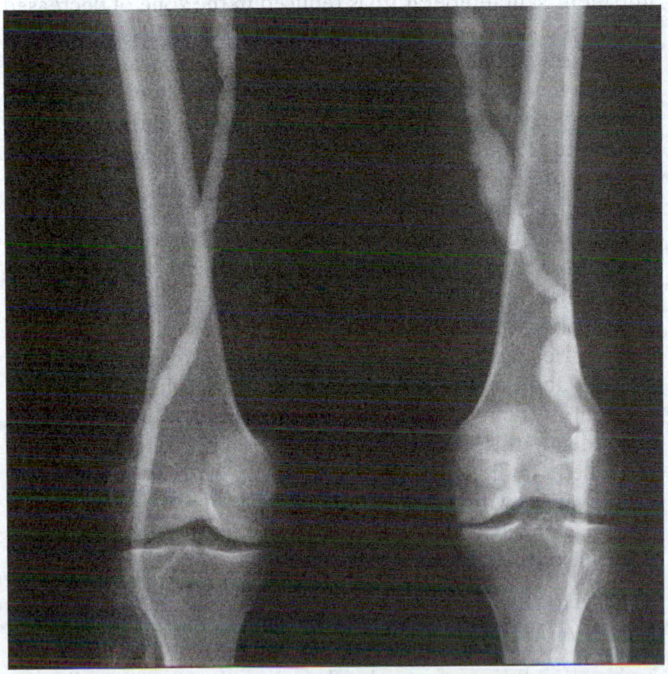

FIGURE 90-1 Popliteal artery aneurysms located at multiple levels on the left, starting at the adductor hiatus. Diffuse arteriomegaly is present on the left.

Aneurysms

Arterial aneurysms are a major cause of death and disability. Early detection allows definitive repair. The three most common aneurysms are accessible to examination, including 40 to 60 percent of abdominal aortic aneurysms and almost all popliteal and femoral aneurysms.[10-13] It should be noted that aneurysms tend to occur concurrently at multiple sites. Therefore, when a popliteal aneurysm is found, a careful search for iliac, femoral, and aortic aneurysms should be performed. The size and pulsatility of paired arteries are normally of similar magnitude. Ectasia is suspected when a pulse is larger or more forceful than expected. *Aneurysm* is defined as a focal enlargement one and one half or more times larger than the usual diameter of the artery. Arteriomegaly is present when the artery is widened, usually over a long distance, but is not yet aneurysmal (Fig. 90-1). The diagnosis is suspected when a palpable, often visible pulsation is transmitted to the fingers on each side of an enlarged vessel. Tortuosity of the carotids, abdominal aorta, and subclavian arteries can mimic an aneurysm. Ultrasound or angiographic studies may be needed to clarify the diagnosis when the examination is unclear.

Many abdominal aortic aneurysms are detected by palpation. They present as a pulsating mass below the xiphoid and above the umbilicus, often filling the epigastrium. Most aneurysms are centered to the left of the midline, but tortuosity occasionally may result in lateralization, commonly to the right. Slight discomfort is usual during examination, but significant tenderness suggests an inflammatory aneurysm, recent expansion, or a contained rupture. When the mass extends below the umbilicus, it may represent either extension into the iliac arteries or a large, overlapping aortic aneurysm. Isolated iliac aneurysms usually are hidden in the pelvis, and less than a fifth can be detected by abdominal examination or digital examination of the rectum or pelvis. Most are found incidentally on an imaging study or after the onset of symptoms.[14] Femoral aneurysms often are first noted by the patient. Popliteal lesions are easily overlooked unless the popliteal space is examined routinely at all three sites described above. Femoral and popliteal aneurysms often are first detected after acute thrombosis, distal micro- or macroembolization, or edema from perianeurysm venous compression or thrombosis.[12,13]

Most thoracic and thoracoabdominal aneurysms are diagnosed incidentally on imaging procedures but may present with pain, cough, dysphagia, hemoptysis, or dysphonia. Physical signs are late manifestations of thoracic aneurysms and may include aortic valve incompetence, unilateral or bilateral jugular venous distention, and pulsatility in the upper intercostal spaces of the precordium. Carotid and axillosubclavian aneurysms are easily diagnosed by palpation, and some present with local pain, thrombosis, or distal embolic complications.[15,16] Visceral aneurysms are rarely large enough to be palpated; 3 to 5 percent present as rupture, and the majority are found incidentally at surgery or during imaging.[17,18]

Bruits

Bruits extending into diastole suggest a high-grade stenosis. However, bruits may disappear when a critical narrowing is reached. A continuous bruit throughout systole and diastole is pathognomonic of an underlying arteriovenous fistula. Bruits may be found at an acquired fistula of paired arteries and veins (Fig. 90-2); over multiple congenital fistulas of the liver, lung, soft tissue, or skull; and over areas of tumor necrosis or prior biopsies. A supraclavicular bruit that disappears with shoulder hyperabduction may be found in young patients.[19] Finally, an epigastric bruit may represent compression of the celiac artery rather than visceral or renal artery stenosis, especially in the young, if asymptomatic, or in the absence of other vascular disease.[20]

Extensions of the Arterial Examination

The value of the Allen test in establishing patency of the radial, ulnar, and digital arteries was discussed above. Pedal perfusion traditionally has been tested by timing elevation pallor and venous refilling (Table 90-2). With the patient supine, both feet are elevated to 60° for 1 min. If no pallor is seen, perfusion is judged to be normal. The appearance of pallor within 15 s suggests poor healing capacity, and pallor without elevation is indicative of severe ischemia. The patient then sits upright, and refilling of the pedal veins is timed. Normal filling occurs in less than 15 s, filling between 30 and 45 s suggests slow healing, and values beyond 60 s confirm severe ischemia. Venous incompetence invalidates venous filling times, and the test is not practical in the presence of significant edema or obesity. Several maneuvers are used to screen for arterial, venous, and neurogenic compression syndromes of the thoracic outlet. Because these tests are frequently abnormal in the normal population and because of the complexity of the syndromes, the reader is referred to detailed reviews.[21,22]

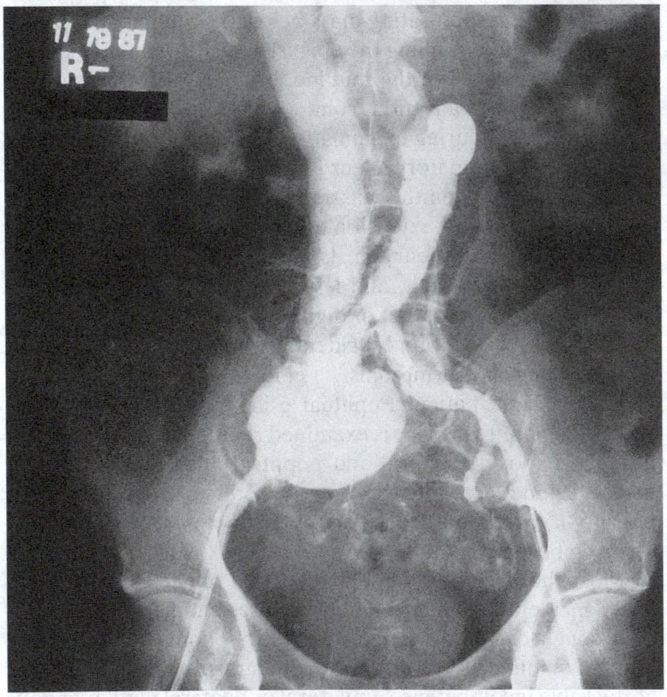

FIGURE 90-2 An aortogram in a 72-year-old who presented with worsening dyspnea over several months and a continuous bruit over the right lower quadrant. A right iliac aneurysm has ruptured, creating a fistula into the right iliac vein. Immediate contrast accumulation is seen in the inferior vena cava. After repair, the patient's symptoms from high-output cardiac failure resolved.

TABLE 90-2 Elevation Pallor and Venous Refilling

ELEVATION PALLOR[a]	
Grade	Pallor Onset
Normal	None
I	>60 s
II	<60 s
III	<30 s
IV	Without elevation
VENOUS REFILLING[b]	
Severity	Venous Refill
Normal	<15 s
Moderate	20–30 s
Severe	>40 s

[a]Feet held passively at 60° while supine.
[b]Upon sitting after elevation.

The Skin

Occlusive arterial disease can alter skin temperature, color, and nutrition. Skin temperature is reduced in the zone of decreased perfusion caused by acute or chronic occlusive disease. Differences are best felt with the dorsum of the fingers, and comparisons to the contralateral or proximal limb should be made. Profound coolness suggests severe ischemia. Chronically cool hands and feet reflect the basic vasomotor tone of some patients, not the presence of poor circulation. Limbs with neurologic damage, immobility, or reflex sympathetic dystrophy are often cool. Edema can accompany these states, obscuring pulses and therefore mimicking arterial disease. Ankle/brachial indexes differentiate occlusive disease from these vasomotor changes (see "Laboratory Assessment: Arterial Disease," below). Skin color varies with blood flow and therefore with temperature, activity, and emotional stimuli. A red or purplish color of the forefoot is common with chronic ischemia and increases with dependency; this is due to chronic arteriolar dilation in response to inadequate flow. Pallor can be seen with acute ischemia or on elevation with chronic ischemia. Skin that is chronically deprived of blood becomes thin, translucent, and shiny. Nails may thicken, and calluses may develop.

LABORATORY ASSESSMENT: ARTERIAL DISEASE

Testing usually is performed to document the severity of disease. However, confirmation or clarification of the diagnosis, monitoring of disease progression, and assessment of outcome after intervention are all appropriate indications for vascular testing. Vascular tests generally are classified as invasive (such as angiography) or noninvasive. This section focuses on noninvasive testing. Noninvasive testing of the arterial system is divided into three broad categories, depending on the type of information generated.

Anatomic Studies

Imaging techniques, including two-dimensional ultrasound, magnetic resonance imaging, computed tomography, and angiography, provide anatomic information. The presence or absence of aneurysms, dissections, stenoses, or occlusions is determined readily by these tests (Chaps. 13, 16, 17, and 18).

Hemodynamic Studies

These techniques provide information about the hemodynamic significance of a vascular lesion. These tests measure a pressure drop or an increase in flow velocity across a lesion, providing information about the hemodynamic impact of the stenosis.

Functional Studies

The information obtained by anatomic or hemodynamic testing may be insufficient to explain the symptoms or degree of impairment described by the patient. In this case, a functional vascular test can be helpful. Functional studies often involve some form of "stress testing." For example, treadmill testing is the most commonly used test to assess claudication.

CONTINUOUS-WAVE DOPPLER

The most widely used continuous-wave (CW) Doppler devices are simple hand-held units that can be purchased for a few hundred dollars and are easily carried in a coat pocket. The Doppler detects blood motion and may be used alone as a means of screening for vascular disease,[23,24] or it may be an integral part of other tests, such as segmental pressure determination (described below).

In a normal artery, the waveform is triphasic. During cardiac systole, there is forward flow in the arteries. During early diastole, the flow reverses direction (because of the elastic recoil of the peripheral arteries). Finally, during middle to late diastole, there is a return of forward flow as arterial blood runs off through the distal vessels.[25] The normal triphasic signal becomes altered by a hemodynamically significant stenosis. If the degree of stenosis is minimal, subtle changes such as dampening of the signal and/or loss of the mid-diastolic forward flow component may be noted distal to the lesion, resulting in a biphasic signal. As the severity of the stenosis worsens, the signal eventually becomes monophasic as only systolic flow is present and then is absent with occlusion. The location of a stenosis may be estimated by assessing the Doppler signal at multiple sites along the limb. CW Doppler is inexpensive and may be performed at the bedside as an extension of the vascular examination. It requires training and practice for effective use, and the information obtained may be limited by the fact that this is a "blind" technique. Duplicated vessels, anatomic variations, and obesity may reduce its accuracy.

SEGMENTAL PRESSURES AND EXERCISE TESTING

Segmental pressures are measured by placing inflatable cuffs around the limb at multiple levels and sequentially inflating and deflating them to determine the arterial pressure at each site.[25] Pneumatic cuffs typically are placed around the thigh, calf, ankle, upper or lower arm, or digits. A CW Doppler (see above) is positioned over the artery at a site distal to the pressure cuff or cuffs and is used to determine the systolic pressure at which arterial flow resumes as the cuff is deflated. The limb pressures typically are divided by a reference arterial pressure (the brachial artery systolic pressure) to create an index. The most commonly reported segmental pressure is the ABI. Severity of disease is determined by the ABI (Table 90-3).

Segmental pressures provide a simple, reproducible, inexpensive, and accurate method of determining whether arterial obstruction is present, the severity of the obstruction, and the approximate location of the obstruction or obstructions. The stress or exercise ABI identifies arterial lesions that are too minor to produce pressure changes at rest. The subject is placed on a treadmill and ambulated according to a standardized protocol. Protocols may be "fixed" (for example, 2 miles/h at a 12 percent incline for a maximum of 5 min) or utilize "graded" exercise similar to that used in cardiac exercise studies.[26] Elements of the lower extremity study (i.e., ABIs or CW Doppler analysis) are performed before and after exercise. Exercise studies can be used to identify parameters such as the minimum walking distance that will produce claudication, the walking distance at which a patient normally would stop, and the maximum walking distance.

The major disadvantage of segmental pressure measurement is that it cannot be used in patients whose blood vessels are noncompressible or poorly compressible because of calcification of the arterial wall.[27] This occurs most commonly in diabetic patients. When vessels are stiff, the cuff cannot produce sufficient pressure to obliterate blood flow and the arterial pressure cannot be determined. Even when the large vessels of the limb are noncompressible, however, the digital vessels in the toes and fingers often remain uncalcified and can be used to estimate pressure if an appropriate cuff is available. Many groups utilize the great toe index in such situations.

TABLE 90-3 The Ankle/Brachial Index

	Preexercise	Postexercise	Claudication	Walking Time, min
Normal	>0.95	>0.95	None	5
Minimal	>0.95	<0.95	None	5
Mild	>0.80	>0.50	Present late	5
Moderate	<0.80	<0.50	Present, limiting	<5
Severe	<0.50	<0.15	Early, limiting	<3

ABI is the systolic blood pressure of the higher arm/systolic blood pressure at the ankle measured in the supine position. Postexercise values are after 5 min at a 10 percent grade at 2 mph (the authors' laboratory protocol; other protocols may be used). Speed may be varied if needed.

PULSE VOLUME RECORDING

Pulse volume recording (PVR) is used to assess the arterial pulsatility of the limb.[28] A pneumatic pressure cuff is placed around the limb at a given level. The cuff is filled with air to a low pressure (typically 40 to 60 mmHg) and is connected by a flexible hose to a pressure transducer. The blood ejected from the left ventricle during cardiac systole causes a transient distention of the limb, which in turn produces a transient rise in cuff pressure. The cyclic changes in cuff pressure with each heartbeat provide an index of arterial "pulsatility." Measurements typically are made at multiple levels along the limb (as is done with segmental pressures), and the tracings are analyzed to determine whether there is a particular level at which the waveform changes shape or pulse dampening occurs.[29] When an altered pulse volume waveform is present, it can be inferred that there is a hemodynamically signficant lesion proximal to the site of the cuff.

TRANSCUTANEOUS OXIMETRY

Transcutaneous oxygen (Tcp_{O_2}) measurement is used to evaluate skin blood flow.[30] Oxygen-sensing electrodes are attached to the skin by means of adhesive rings that create an airtight seal. The seal ensures that the only oxygen that reaches the electrode has diffused from the skin. The surface temperature of the electrode is maintained at a relatively high temperature (43 to 45°C) so that the small vessels underlying the electrode are maximally dilated. Cutaneous blood flow is determined in part by the patency of the proximal arteries.[31] The amount of oxygen that diffuses out of the skin depends on numerous factors, including the arterial partial pressure of oxygen, the cutaneous blood flow, and the rate of oxygen consumption by the skin. When cutaneous blood flow is high (relative to the metabolic rate of the skin), Tcp_{O_2} may approach arterial O_2. In contrast, when cutaneous blood flow is low, Tcp_{O_2} is reduced. Tcp_{O_2} is not so much a measurement of skin blood flow as a measurement of the adequacy of cutaneous oxygen delivery. Transcutaneous oximetry has been shown to be useful in a number of situations, including evaluation of critical ischemia. It may be difficult to determine the functional severity of arterial occlusive disease solely on the basis of historical or clinical findings even when basic noninvasive testing is available. This difficulty is especially relevant when the clinician is attempting to determine whether limb revascularization is required for pain relief, ulcer healing, or limb salvage. Tcp_{O_2} can be used to predict whether the cutaneous perfusion is adequate for healing at a given amputation site (Table 90-4). Values above 40 mmHg are typically sufficient for healing, while those below 20 mmHg are not likely to heal.[32]

TABLE 90-4 Interpretation of Tcp_{O_2} Values

	Rest	Elevation
Normal	45	<10
Mild	40–45	<10
Moderate	20–39	<10
Severe	20–39 or <20	>10 any
Critical	0	

Tcp_{O_2} values in mmHg at rest and after 30° elevation. A fall greater than 10 mmHg with elevation increases the degree of severity by one grade. Values less than 20 have poor potential for healing; values of 20–30 have a variable potential for healing.

Certain disease states may affect the small vessels or microcirculation without involving larger arteries. When this occurs, techniques such as CW Doppler, segmental pressures, and PVR will not detect a significant abnormality. In contrast, Tcp_{O_2} measurements usually demonstrate the inadequacy of circulation when it is due to small vessel occlusive disease. Tcp_{O_2} determination is often valuable in the assessment of patients with diabetes (when noncompressible or poorly compressible vessels are present) and/or small vessel disease.[33] Although Tcp_{O_2} measurement is an accurate way to assess the severity of cutaneous ischemia, it has several limitations. These limitations include its inability to localize the occlusive disease to a particular segment or vessel and the fact that each laboratory must standardize and validate the technique before the results can be relied on for diagnostic and therapeutic decisions.[34,35]

Imaging Techniques

Imaging modalities such as two-dimensional (2D) real-time ultrasound, computed tomography (CT), and magnetic resonance imaging (MRI) are described in greater detail elsewhere (see Chaps. 13, 17, and 18). They increasingly are being used in place of angiography, especially for the evaluation of aneurysm, dissection, and arterial rupture. New acquisition and processing techniques are enabling CT and MR angiography (MRA) to replace conventional angiography as a means of identifying arterial stenoses and occlusions. Indeed, in diabetic patients and others at high risk of renal damage from contrast, MRA should be strongly considered if it is available and has sufficient resolution to plan surgical intervention. Continued technological advances in these noninvasive modalities may allow CT and MRI to compete with conventional angiography in all but a few selected circumstances.

ARTERIAL DISEASES OF THE LOWER EXTREMITY

Arterial Occlusive Disease

Arteriosclerosis obliterans (ASO) is the most common cause of lower extremity ischemic syndromes in western societies regardless of age.[36] The presentation varies greatly with the time course of progression, the presence and extent of collateral vessels, comorbidities, and activity of the patient. If the patient is active, intermittent claudication is the usual presenting complaint; if inactive, rest pain, ulceration, dependent rubor with edema secondary to compensatory dependency, or gangrene may be the presenting complaint.

In general, symptoms occur distal to the level of stenosis. Superficial femoral disease causes claudication of the entire calf. Both thigh and calf symptoms occur with common femoral and external iliac lesions, hip and buttock claudication alone suggests an internal iliac stenosis, and foot and calf claudication suggests popliteal or infrapopliteal disease. Impotence suggests aortoiliac disease.

PREVALENCE AND NATURAL HISTORY

There is a relatively high prevalence of ASO that increases with age.[1,36,37] The Framingham Study estimated the annual incidence of symptomatic disease at 0.3 percent and 0.1 percent for men and women, respectively.[38,39] The prevalence of intermittent claudication increases with age: 1.8 percent under age 60, 3.7 percent age 60 to 70, and just over 5 percent at age 70 and above. Risk factors for ASO reflect those for coronary disease.[40] Diabetes increases the risk of ASO threefold (higher if asymptomatic ASO is included).[41] In a hypertensive elderly population, the incidence of ASO as defined by an ABI <0.90 was slightly higher than 25 percent. The risk of death, usually from a cardiovascular event, increases dramatically as the ABI decreases.[42,43] The 5-year mortality of an ABI less than 0.85 is 10 percent; if ABI is less than 0.40, it approaches 50 percent.

The rate of progression of symptoms or the need for revascularization is slow.[44] Symptoms that have worsened at 5 years occur in approximately 20 percent of these patients.[45] The requirement for revascularization because of imminent tissue or limb loss or rest pain approaches 5 percent per year. Amputation rates are similarly low, around 1 percent per year. However, up to 15 percent of those who continue smoking undergo amputation within 5 years. Diabetic patients have an amputation rate of 25 percent over 9 years.[46–49]

TREATMENT

Aggressive *risk factor modification* should be the cornerstone of therapy in all patients. The slow rate of progression and the high incidence of vascular comorbidities indicate an optimum role for modifying the underlying atherosclerotic process. Smoking cessation is a must. Control of diabetes should be emphasized since the risk for amputation is increased in this population, although the benefit has not been documented in large arteries. Lipid lowering has a beneficial role in patients with ASO.[50,51] The goals are similar to those for patients with coronary artery disease.[52] Hypertension control should be optimized (see Chap. 51).

A *walking program* should be initiated in all patients. Bicycling and other forms of exercise used for cardiovascular conditioning unfortunately do not provide the same benefit that walking provides. The effectiveness of a structured walking program has been well demonstrated.[53–55] Twenty to 30 min 4 to 5 days per week improves exercise capacity and increases total and absolute walking distance from 50 to 300 percent. The mechanism of this improvement is not clear, but increased collateral formation or recruitment, muscle training, improved oxygen uptake, and improved mechanics of walking are all plausible.[56] Diligent foot care and protection must be emphasized, particularly in diabetic patients and those with severe reductions in ABI or Tcp_{O_2} values. Footwear must be supportive and protective, and nail care should be performed regularly by professionals.

Medical therapy for peripheral artery disease has been slow to develop. Pentoxyfilline has proved effective in some patients with ASO,[57] but stomach irritation limits its use in others. Recently, cilostazol has been approved for use for patients with claudication. It is effective in increasing walking distance, but the effect is lost when the drug is stopped. Several other medications are currently in development. Direct vasodilators have proved ineffective, although verapamil increased walking distance in one study.[58] Beta blockade has long been believed to be contraindicated for patients with ASO, but two studies have refuted this idea.[54,59] In light of the beneficial effects of beta blockade in patients with coronary artery disease, these agents should not be withheld from patients with peripheral ASO.

Revascularization should be considered in patients with rest pain, impending tissue loss, or significant limitation of lifestyle. Surgical revascularization has been available for years. Large vessel bypass surgery with synthetic graft material is well established and durable. More recently, in situ distal bypass utilizing reversed or intact saphenous vein has shown promising long-term patency. Percutaneous balloon angioplasty with or without stent placement is often useful for lesions of the proximal renal and iliac arteries. There is decreasing long-term effectiveness at more distal vessels because of the reduction in both artery size and flow rates. However, for patients at high risk for limb loss (deemed poor surgical candidates or technically unfeasible for revascularization), it is reasonable to consider angioplasty for limb salvage.

Acute Arterial Occlusion

PRESENTATION

Acute arterial occlusion presents as a clinical pentad of pain, pallor, paresthesia, paralysis, and pulselessness. The limb also may be cold. Some or all of these findings may be present. The limb is at risk if flow is not restored quickly. Distal changes caused by microembolisation also may be seen. There are two exceptions to the usual presentation of acute arterial occlusion. The first is branch vessel occlusion in the setting of acute aortic dissection. Variability may be present on examination. The pulse deficit and the area affected may migrate, causing discrepancies between examiners as the dissection progresses. The second is ergot toxicity, which usually is diagnosed only after a direct question about its use is asked.[60]

ETIOLOGY

The etiology of acute arterial occlusions is classified into three groups: trauma and dissection, thrombosis in situ, and embolism. Attention to arterial integrity is of prime importance in dealing with injuries caused by penetration (including medical interventions), crush or fracture, and deceleration injuries. In situ thrombosis occurs with both occlusive and aneurysmal disease. Any of the lesions listed in Table 90-1, aneurysms, clotting disorders, but predominantly atherosclerosis with its multiple manifestations and risk factors can be the substrate of thrombosis.

A small percentage of acute emboli come from proximal occlusive or aneurysmal arterial lesions, but the majority originate from the heart. Both the left ventricle and the left atrium may harbor a thrombus.[61] Emboli tend to be multiple and recurrent and to distribute randomly, mostly to the legs but with a significant incidence of cerebral, renal, visceral, and arm events.[62] Venous thrombi from the right side of the heart or limbs can pass across cardiac septal defects or patent foramina ovali and cause arterial events.[63]

MANAGEMENT

Immediate measures are needed to protect the limb and restore blood flow. Heparin is given to prevent clot propagation and treat the embolic source or sources.[64,65] Angiography is required to plan repair when there is preexisting occlusive or aneurysmal disease or when the etiology is uncertain. Many surgeons perform balloon embolectomy without angiography when an embolic source is certain and the vessel was previously normal. Ideally, all acute occlusions warrant repair, although the urgency is governed by the degree of ischemia. Severe ischemia is suggested by pallor at rest, profound coolness, tender or hard muscles, and loss of motor and sensory function. When severe ischemia is present, repair must occur within hours to salvage the limb. Additional time may be taken to address ancillary problems in patients with lesser degrees of ischemia, and sometimes no repair is elected when the occlusion has a minimal impact on the patient's lifestyle. If acute cardiac events create prohibitive risks for surgery, the heart may be stabilized over a few hours before embolectomy or revascularization is performed under local anesthesia.[66,67] When indicated, lysis of acute occlusion can be effective.[68–70]

PREVENTION

Acute arterial occlusion is often preventable, and conditions known to cause occlusion warrant treatment. Aneurysms, adventitial cystic disease, popliteal entrapment syndromes, and atrial myxoma are treated surgically. Treatable medical disorders include vasculitis, hematologic disorders, and thyrotoxicosis. Atrial or ventricular thrombi, atrial fibrillation, acute myocardial infarction, congestive failure, severe cardiomyopathy, and prosthetic valves all warrant chronic antithrombotic therapy to prevent thrombus formation.

Unusual Causes

Leg claudication and ischemia result from numerous disorders (Table 90-1). Many are suggested by the history (acute arterial occlusion, aortic dissection, temporal and Takayasu's arteritis, radiation therapy, ergot use, and competitive cycling), some by physical findings (coarctation, pseudoxanthoma elasticum, occluded aneurysms), and others only through imaging.

THROMBOANGIITIS OBLITERANS

Thromboangiitis obliterans (TAO), or Buerger's disease, is the most common of these disorders.[21,71–73] Buerger first described this inflammatory vasculopathy with a characteristic, highly cellular intraluminal thrombus that affects small and medium-size arteries and veins. TAO always is associated with tobacco use and may be an autoimmune response to it. TAO is seen predominantly in males in the second through fifth decades, although the incidence in women is rising. Clinically, TAO differs from atherosclerosis in that concurrent involvement of the upper extremity is common. The initial involvement is in digital, pedal, and hand vessels; progression to the calf, thigh, and forearm is brisk and occurs over a few months or years. One-third of these patients report Raynaud's phenomenon. Recurrent episodes of superficial phlebitis of the calves or forearms are seen frequently. Biopsy of acute lesions, particularly accessible veins, is diagnostic, and angiographic features are characteristic. Rare manifestations include coronary, cerebral, or visceral artery lesions. Progressive tissue loss is inevitable until tobacco exposure is stopped. Stability or improvement is variable but is possible only after all exposure to tobacco ceases.[74] Surgical sympathectomy and intravenous prostacyclin analogs can accelerate healing of ischemic lesions,[75] but amputation of damaged digits and limbs often is required.

POPLITEAL ENTRAPMENT SYNDROME

Popliteal entrapment syndrome occurs when the popliteal artery is trapped by the medial gastrocnemius or various muscular and ligamentous bands during passive dorsiflexion or active plantar flexion. The entrapment may cause claudication and (later) occlusion. It usually is seen in relatively young, healthy individuals and typically occurs with significant exertion. Surgical repair is the treatment of choice.[76] Although uncommon, entrapment syndromes can be seen at other sites.

ADVENTITIAL CYSTIC DISEASE

Adventitial cystic disease is a slowly enlarging growth in the popliteal (or occasionally common femoral) artery that is analogous in structure and content to a ganglion or mucoid cyst. It may cause claudication and subsequent occlusion. Surgical repair is the treatment of choice.[77]

TAKAYASU'S AND GIANT CELL ARTERITIS

Takayasu's arteritis and giant-cell (temporal) arteritis (GCA) are similar in pathologic process but affect different age groups. In general, Takayasu's arteritis involves arteries below the neck, and GCA involves arteries above the neck. However, involvement of the aorta and great vessels, subclavian and axillary arteries, renal and iliofemoral, profunda femoral, and superficial femoral arteries has been described with each one. Disease is usually bilateral and results in claudication that progresses briskly over a few months. Ischemia is rare. Both have characteristic clinical and laboratory findings, including an elevated sedimentation rate and typical arteriographic features. These diseases are unique among arteriopathies in that acute stenotic lesions significantly improve with steroid therapy. Adjunctive cytotoxic drugs are also useful.[78–80]

ERGOT

Ergot compounds can induce Raynaud's phenomenon, claudication, acute ischemia, and tissue infarction. These problems usually are seen in those using ergot to treat migraine headaches. Intravenous nitroprusside infusion may help acute ischemia.[60] The incidence of ergot toxicity is decreasing as alternatives for migraine treatment become available, but it should be considered in patients with ischemia and few, if any, risk factors.

FIBROMUSCULAR DYSPLASIA

Fibromuscular dysplasia has been described in almost all arteries. It usually affects women in the middle years. Renal artery disease is the most common, but carotid, mesenteric, and both upper and lower extremity diseases may be seen.

Aneurysmal Disease

Abdominal aneurysms are found in 15 percent of men over age 65 screened by ultrasound,[81] and a familial tendency for aneurysms in both males and females has been identified.[82] Effective repair of aneurysms has been available for several decades. An appreciation of three general characteristics of aneurysms allows a logical approach to management. First, aneurysms caused by degenerative etiologies progressively enlarge over years. Second, aneurysms caused by infectious or traumatic etiologies expand over days to months. Third, aneurysms tend to be multiple. Five to 10 percent of patients with an aortic aneurysm and 50 percent or more with peripheral aneurysms will have aneurysms elsewhere.[83,84] Rupture is the primary worry with thoracic, abdominal, iliac, and visceral artery aneurysms, whereas thrombosis and embolism are typical of carotid and peripheral aneurysms. Aneurysms may cause dysfunction of adjacent structures by compression or fistula formation with those structures (Fig. 90-2). Ascending thoracic aorta aneurysms may contribute to aortic valve regurgitation or dissection, particularly when caused by cystic medial necrosis or congenital defects of the arterial wall.

These patients should be screened for aneurysmal disease during examination. Further imaging should be considered if an aneurysm is found elsewhere or in the setting of unexplained occlusion of a distal artery, microembolic syndromes, limb edema (possibly caused by aneurysm compression), fistula, and any continuous bruit. Aneurysms should be sought in the setting of diseases known to cause them, including syphilis, heritable disorders of collagen, several of the vasculitides, and atherosclerosis. Hypertension, smoking, and age predispose to aneurysm formation.

Microcirculatory Disorders

There are many etiologies that produce microcirculatory disease (Table 90-5). Digital and microcirculatory ischemia may present as focal digital cyanosis, petechiae, splinter hemorrhages, ulcer, infarction, or gangrene and may be accompanied by livedo reticularis and Raynaud's phenomenon. Skin findings may be single or multiple and are usually acute. Most initial lesions heal spontaneously with little or no tissue loss. Recurrences are common and can result in loss of digits or large areas of skin (Fig. 90-3). Most etiologies are diagnosed by clinical features and selective tests. Vasculitic syndromes respond to steroids and/or cytotoxic agents. Anticoagulants are given for associated circulating anticoagulant or antiphospholipid syndromes.[85] Myeloproliferative disease and dysproteinemias are treated with chemotherapy, sometimes enhanced by plasmapheresis. Clotting syndromes are controlled with anticoagulants. Culture-sensitive antibiotics are essential for treating endocarditis, and infected prosthetic valves usually must be removed. Digital ischemia with advanced malignancy is rare and may be idiopathic or associated with coagulopathy, dysproteinemia, or marantic endocarditis.

TABLE 90-5 Etiology of Microcirculatory Disease

Embolism
Arteriosclerosis obliterans
Anticoagulation
Trauma, instrumentation
Surgery
Vasculitis
Endocarditis
Ergot toxicity
Cold injury
Malignancy
Hepatitis
Hematologic
Polycythemia vera
Thrombocytosis
Dysproteinemia
Cryoglobulinemia
Cold agglutinins
Circulating anticoagulants
Antiphospholipid antibodies
Thrombotic cytopenic purpura
Heparin-induced thrombocytopenia

Microembolism

Microembolism usually originates from an ulcerative plaque or aneurysm and only rarely from the heart. Solitary lesions showering atheroemboli are readily treated surgically.[86] When lesions are found at several levels, surgical choices are more difficult. Suprarenal sources can cause progressive azotemia or intestinal ischemia and require a formidable repair.[87] Thromboulcerative disease of the entire aorta can shower emboli randomly to the brain, viscera, kidneys, skin, and muscle. Anemia, leukocytosis, azotemia, an elevated sedimentation rate, and abnormal urinary sediment usually are noted. This syndrome of diffuse microembolization often requires biopsy for differentiation from vasculitis.[88] Microembolic events may be spontaneous or can be precipitated by surgery, instrumentation, or anticoagulant therapy.[87] Antiplatelet agents may prevent recurrences when surgery is not feasible; however, efficacy is poorly documented.[89]

Vasospastic Disorders

The color and warmth of the acral parts vary considerably from person to person in a normal population, reflecting individual vasomotor tone. Livedo reticularis, acrocyanosis, and Raynaud's phenomenon are distinctive clinical syndromes manifested by abnormal color and temperature changes of the skin. These syndromes are induced or intensified as a result of stimuli from cold, emotion, or drugs. They cause spasm in digital arteries, arterioles, and perhaps venules. These disorders are usually benign, lifelong primary processes, but all three syndromes can have important secondary causes. Careful clinical examination and selective testing usually will confirm the specific etiology and define the prognosis and the direction of therapy.

LIVEDO RETICULARIS

Livedo reticularis is characterized by a persistent, symmetric, bluish lacy pattern on the extremities and sometimes the trunk that is variable in extent and intensity. It is most apparent after stimulation by cold or emotion and fades with warmth and exercise. It is first seen in childhood or at puberty and is more common in women and fair-skinned individuals. It is so common in its milder form that it often is overlooked or considered a variant of normal skin. It has been postulated that spasm of the cutaneous arterioles (with secondary dilation of the capillaries and venules) causes slow flow, increased oxygen uptake, and reduced oxyhemoglobin, producing color change. Primary livedo reticularis often is seen with acrocyanosis and primary Raynaud's disease. Treatment is rarely needed.

Secondary livedo reticularis is patchy, focal, or asymmetric in distribution and relatively late in onset; it may be complicated by local infarction or ulceration. The lesions may be elevated or tender when caused by vasculitis. Therapy is directed at the

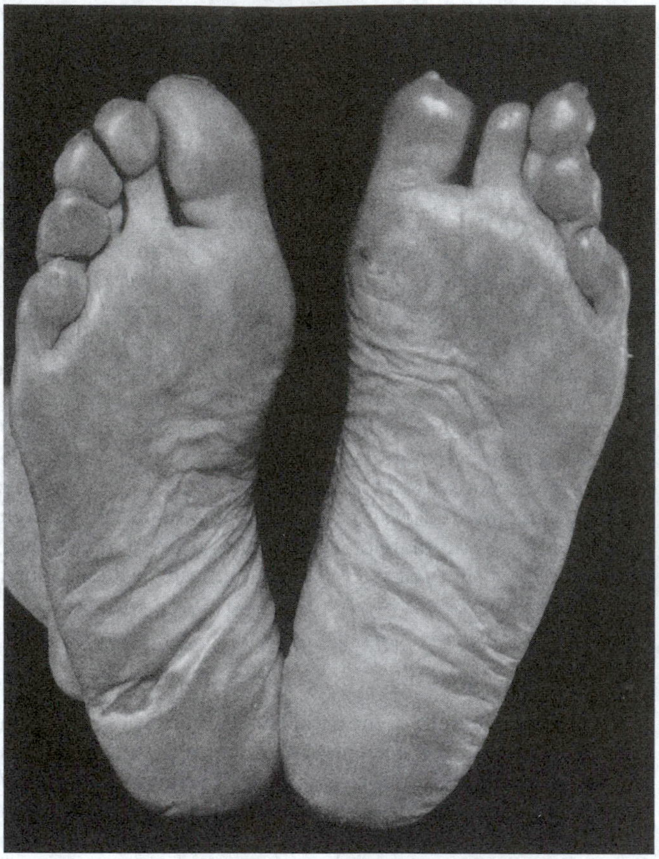

A

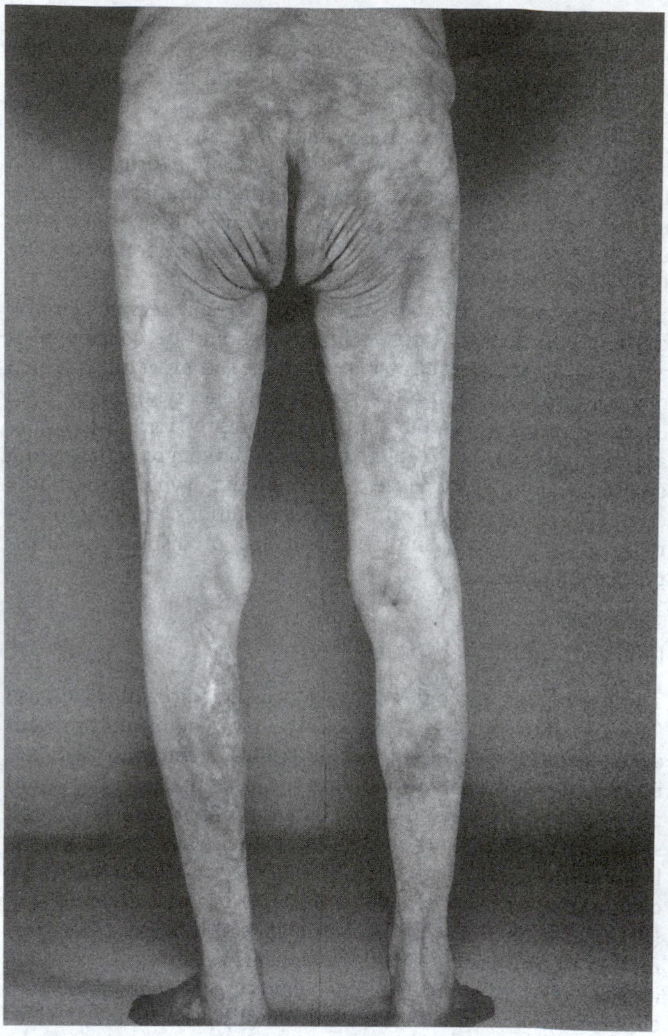

B

FIGURE 90-3 Two photographs of skin changes caused by microemboli. *A.* Cyanotic toe pads and livedo reticularis over the plantar aspect of both feet. *B.* Extensive livido reticularis in the same patient. A previously unknown 7-cm aortic aneurysm was found and repaired.

underlying cause (Table 90-6). Vasodilators and sympathectomy are of unpredictable, anecdotal value for healing painful ulcers. Hemosiderin deposition can occur in secondary and, on occasion, primary livedo reticularis. Erythema ab igne can be confused with livedo reticularis. This is a focal, well-defined lesion with broader bands of fixed red color, often with a hemosiderin stain. It is a reaction to chronic, local heat exposure such as a heating pad or fireplace.

TABLE 90-6 Etiologies of Livido Reticularis

Environmental (cold)	Reflex sympathetic dystrophy
Atheroembolism (cholesterol)	Myeloproliferative diseases
Connective tissue disease	Vasculitis
Cutaneous vasculitis	Thrombocytosis
Amantidine HCl	

ACROCYANOSIS

Acrocyanosis is a benign, persistent cyanotic discoloration and coolness of the hands (or fingers or sometimes the feet) that is seen more commonly in women. Cold and emotion intensify, whereas warmth and exercise ameliorate, the findings. Mild local edema is not uncommon and is not bothersome; associated hyperhidrosis may require treatment. Acrocyanosis is painless and does not ulcerate, but it is a bothersome cosmetic problem for some. Calcium entry blockers or $alpha_1$ antagonists often reduce the symptoms. A modest degree of acrocyanosis sometimes is seen in limbs immobilized by neurogenic deficits. Rarely, beta-blockade will induce the syndrome.

RAYNAUD'S PHENOMENON

Raynaud's phenomenon is diagnosed from history alone. It is difficult to demonstrate even with ice immersion, as generalized cooling usually is needed to bring out the findings. The syndrome is defined as episodes of blue or white color changes of the digits, often followed by reactive hyperemia during recov-

TABLE 90-7 Raynaud's Phenomenon: Secondary Causes

Collagen vascular disease	Medications
Scleroderma	Beta blockers
Mixed connective tissue disease	Ergotamine
	Methysergide
Rheumatoid arthritis	Vinblastine, bleomycin
Myositis	Estrogens
Sjögren's syndrome	Imipramine
Necrotizing vasculitis	Microcirculatory diseases
Hematologic disorders	Beurger's disease
Neurogenic	Hypothenar hammer syndrome
Thoracic outlet irritation	
Carpal tunnel syndrome	Environmental
Neuropathy	Cold injury
Myxedema	Vibration syndrome
Acromegaly	Vinyl chloride disease
Pulmonary hypertension	

ery. It is induced by cold or emotional stimuli. Many patients describe the white phase (some describe blue changing to white, and a few blue only), but most note the subsequent hyperemia. A dead, numb feeling (but rarely pain) accompanies the ischemic phase, and a dysesthetic, throbbing, or painful sensation is common during recovery. Fingers are involved more often than are toes, initially the distal digits and later the entire digit but rarely the palm. The thumbs often are spared. Recovery time is 3 to 10 min but can exceed 1 h in advanced cases, usually of secondary origin. Allen and Brown[90] defined primary Raynaud's as episodes of bilateral color changes induced by cold or emotion without evidence of ischemia or other disease for 2 years. Later development of secondary disease was noted in 2 to 5 percent of patients.[91–93] A prospective study confirmed that patients without laboratory evidence of digital occlusive, clotting, or serologic abnormalities have a benign course, with only 2 percent showing secondary causes in the subsequent decade.[94]

The causes of secondary Raynaud's phenomenon are diverse (Table 90-7). Most can be defined by history and examination, knowledge of their natural behavior, vascular laboratory measurements of digital obstruction, and clotting or serologic tests. Arteriography (from the arch through the digits) is reserved for unusual problems or for planning surgery when needed. Trophic skin changes and ischemic lesions usually reflect occlusive etiologies, while a unilateral Raynaud's suggests a secondary process.[93,95]

Most patients with primary Raynaud's phenomenon require no therapy and quickly learn to keep not only the hands but the whole body warm. Treatment of secondary forms is directed at the underlying cause when feasible. Calcium channel blockers and non-beta-adrenergic blocking sympatholytics, alone or in combination, can suppress the episodes in some patients, but drugs and sympathectomy have little impact on ischemic complications. These complications are best treated with local debridement and control of infection and pain.

UPPER EXTREMITY ARTERIAL DISEASE

Upper extremity arterial occlusive disease is less common but more varied in etiology than disease of the lower extremity. Associated vasospastic and microcirculatory disorders are more common. The origin of the brachiocephalic artery, the axillosubclavian area, and the arteries of the hand account for the majority of stenotic lesions. Problems arising in the muscular portion of the arm are less common. Causes include embolic occlusion, trauma, vasculitis, fibromuscular dysplasia, and infections. Arterial testing of the upper extremity should be performed to document the level and severity of disease, especially when lesions are progressive or symptomatic or when tissue loss is occurring or is imminent. Noninvasive testing should survey the entire limb, including the digits. Angiography should include the aortic arch and extend through the hand, with vasodilation of the digital arteries to differentiate "fixed" occlusions from vasospasm.

Chronic atherosclerotic occlusive disease is seen predominantly at the origin of the innominate or, more commonly, the left subclavian artery. Claudication is uncommon or modest because arm use is more intermittent and because the upper extremity has excellent collateral circulation. Radiologic or ultrasound evidence of flow reversal or "steal" from the vertebral artery is not uncommon, but any neurologic symptoms most often are explained by associated carotid disease rather than the subclavian lesion.[96] Acute macroemboli to the arm come predominantly from the heart and only occasionally from proximal aneurysmal or stenotic lesions. Most acute occlusions in situ reflect direct or iatrogenic trauma, thrombosis in or from an aneurysm, or a clotting disorder.

Acute or chronic microcirculatory disease of the hands may be due to numerous mechanisms (Table 90-5). Connective tissue diseases, hematologic disorders, and occupational trauma may result in microvascular disease. Raynaud's phenomenon (see above) can accompany any acute or chronic occlusive process. It also may reflect direct neural irritation at the thoracic outlet or represent a response to medications or the environment. Women who present with Raynaud's phenomenon, digital ulceration, and telangectasias over the facies should be fully evaluated for connective tissue disease, particularly scleroderma or a variant of scleroderma. In such cases, peripheral alpha blockers or calcium channel inhibitors may prove effective.[97]

Aneurysmal disease of the upper extremity is rare. When it is present, the usual location is the proximal brachiocephalic or axillosubclavian arteries. Atherosclerosis, trauma, and thoracic outlet syndrome are the most common etiologies. Thrombosis, distal micro- or macroemboli, and a painful mass are the expected presentations. Rupture is rare unless there is infection.[98]

Several specific entities should be remembered. TAO may present initially with Raynaud's phenomenon or hand ischemia. If it presents late, digital necrosis may be present. It is usually bilateral and may be associated with lower extremity involvement of ischemia, claudication, or superficial thrombophlebitis.[99] Takayasu's syndrome nearly always presents with upper extremity claudication or ischemia. Additionally, 10 percent of patients with temporal arteritis have disease of the great vessels or the proximal arm arteries. Limiting arm claudication progresses rapidly in these patients over just a few months. The process can be halted or improved with steroid therapy.[79,80]

Thoracic Outlet Syndrome

Thoracic outlet syndrome usually results from an osseous lesion (commonly a cervical rib) that causes an aneurysm or stenosis of the subclavian artery. Symptoms may be variable. This reflects the anatomy in that the artery, vein, and nervous bundle all pass through a small, dynamic space. The usual mechanism of damage is the clavicle and a cervical rib (or the first rib) impinging on the subclavian artery like a scissors. This predisposes to thrombosis and Raynaud's phenomenon (Fig. 90-4). Venous and neurogenic complaints may be present. The patient is usually young and active with progressive and frequently puzzling complaints of arm fatigue, swelling, or paresthesia.

The presence of positive thoracic outlet maneuvers does not make the diagnosis of thoracic outlet syndrome. Imaging for the presence of a functional stenosis with duplex ultrasound, the vascular laboratory, or arteriography can be used to document the presence of a functional hemodynamic change. Clinical correlation is required for the diagnosis. Resection of a cervical rib or first rib frequently is required.[100] However, improvement of symptoms is variable, particularly if they are neurogenic in origin.

Hammer Hand Syndrome

Hammer hand syndrome results from trauma to the hypothenar area caused by using the hand as a hammer or by repetitive force on levers or other devices. These activities may produce occlusion or aneurysm formation of the ulnar artery, usually at the level of the hammate bone. Digital ischemia and Raynaud's phenomenon of one or more digits can result from emboli. Improvement follows if the trauma is stopped, but continued problems require surgical treatment.[101] Vibratory tools such as chain saws, grinders, and jackhammers can induce hand dysesthesias and Raynaud's phenomenon when used for several years. Symptoms initially occur during use and later become chronic. Ischemia is a rare and late occurrence.[102]

CLINICAL ASSESSMENT: VENOUS DISEASE

Disease of the venous system is a rapidly changing area of vascular medicine. Anticoagulation therapy is undergoing refinements, surgical management of deep venous obstruction and incompetence is evolving, and new imaging techniques are enhancing diagnosis.[103,104]

Varicose Veins

Varicosities of the superficial veins begin with the incompetence of one or more valves. When proximal valves fail, the column of blood supported by the distal valves increases. As more valves become incompetent, the vein dilates and becomes tortuous. *Primary varicosities* are often a familial trait; their symptoms are exacerbated by prolonged standing, obesity, and pregnancy. *Secondary varicosities* may reflect underlying perforator and deep venous obstruction and/or incompetence, which shifts venous return to the superficial veins. Common secondary causes of varicosities include extrinsic venous compression, prior deep vein thrombosis, congenital lesions, arteriovenous fistulas, and right-sided heart disease. Edema and venous stasis changes rarely are caused by primary varicosities and usually signal the presence of an underlying secondary process. The history, examination, and (when necessary) laboratory evaluation of the deep venous system usually allow the physician to differentiate primary from secondary varicosities.

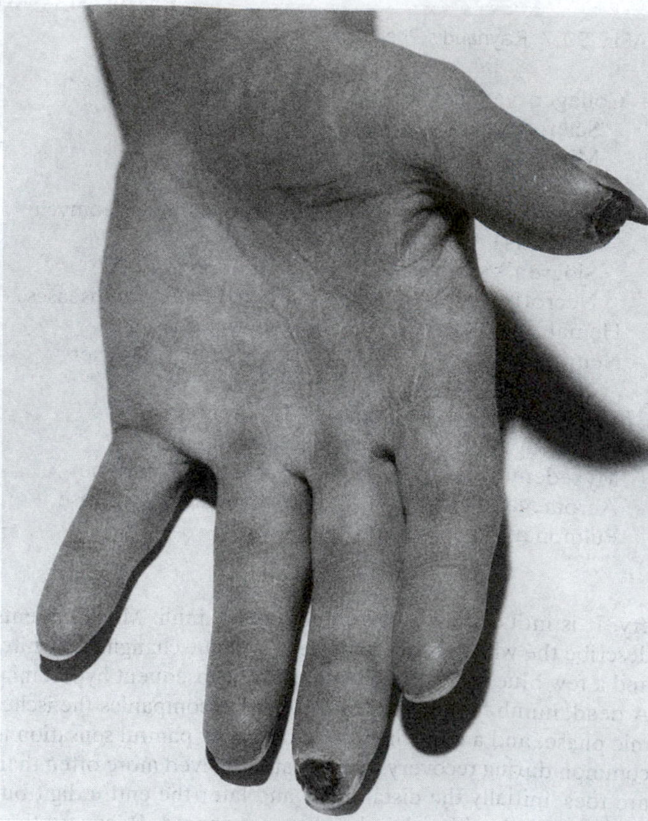

A

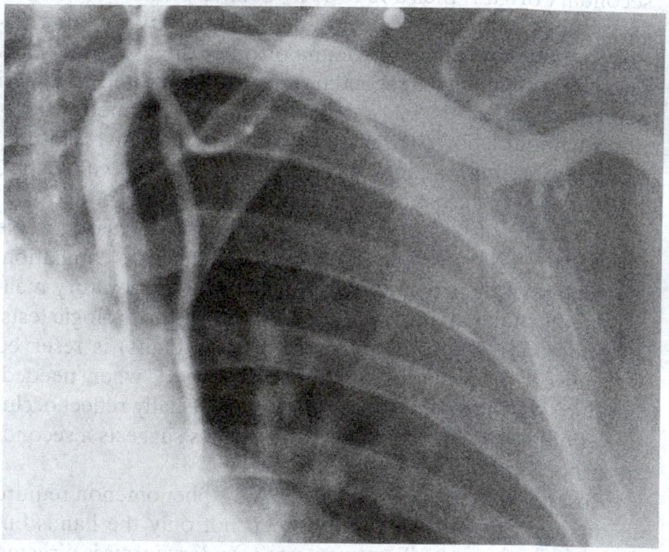

B

FIGURE 90-4 *A*. Photograph of a 24-year-old male who presented with left hand rest pain and ischemic ulcers of digits 1 and 3. He worked as a painter, during which time he experienced arm claudication. Raynaud's phenomenon was present for about 9 months. Thoracic outlet maneuvers were positive bilaterally. *B*. Selective angiography of the left subclavian artery reveals a poststenotic aneurysm with faint shadowing suggestive of thrombus. Cervical ribs were present and were resected.

Varicose veins may ache or burn with standing or prolonged sitting (especially with the legs in a dependent position). Enlargement usually occurs over time, and superficial thrombophlebitis may occur. Rarely, veins may bleed; this bleeding is often brisk despite the venous source because venous pressure is elevated when the limb is dependent. Control of bleeding therefore must include pressure and limb elevation. Both symptoms and progression can be ameliorated by the use of graduated compression hose of 20 to 30 mmHg or more. Ablation of the vein should be considered if complications or discomfort interferes with occupation or lifestyle. Sclerotherapy is effective for certain varicosities and cutaneous "spiders." Surgical removal is indicated for longer segments of proximal varicosities, especially if perforator or saphenofemoral incompetence is present.

Superficial Thrombophlebitis

The presence of a warm, tender, erythematous, and indurated linear lesion in the anatomic course of a superficial vein suggests superficial thrombophlebitis. Ultrasound can differentiate thrombophlebitis from lymphangitic streaks, erythema nodosum, and other lesions. Thrombophlebitis often occurs in a varix or at sites of indwelling catheters or needles. Active infection may be associated with needle use or with the use of illicit street drugs. In such cases, appropriate antibiotics should be used. Infected or suppurative thrombophlebitis often requires surgical removal for the infection to clear. Lesions occurring in a previously normal vein, whether single or migratory, can be idiopathic but may be associated with malignancy, thromboangiitis obliterans, or vasculitis. The lesions of the latter two conditions may be nodular rather than linear and require diagnostic biopsy.[105] An age-appropriate evaluation for underlying diseases that can predispose to clotting should be performed. Superficial thrombophlebitis is usually self-limited, but recovery can be accelerated by rest, topical warmth, and anti-inflammatory agents. Systemic anticoagulation is appropriate for lesions that progress despite conservative care and those located where the lesser or greater saphenous veins enter the deep system.[106]

Deep Vein Thrombosis

The morbidity and mortality of deep vein thrombosis (DVT) remain high. Risk factors for DVT and pulmonary embolism have been well defined in several studies (Table 90-8).[107] The manifestations of DVT are a prominent superficial venous pattern, edema, muscle turgidity, and discomfort. However, these findings may be absent or subtle. For this reason, objective testing to confirm and define the extent of DVT should be obtained whenever it is suspected. Definitive testing also establishes the need for anticoagulation and provides the means to assess clot propagation. A confirmed diagnosis facilitates treatment choices when anticoagulation is relatively or absolutely contraindicated. If the diagnosis is disproved, the cost of treatment and the risks of hemorrhage, heparin-induced thrombocytopenia, and warfarin necrosis are avoided.[108,109]

A wide spectrum of diseases can mimic DVT (Table 90-9). They are diagnosed by their clinical findings and confirmed by appropriate testing (see "Laboratory Assessment: Venous Disease," below) Less than half of patients considered to have DVT have the diagnosis confirmed when tested objectively.[110–112]

Treatment with heparin acutely and warfarin for 12 to 16 weeks is highly effective in preventing clot propagation and pulmonary embolism (see Chap. 53). The recent literature suggests treatment for a minimum of 6 to 12 months in patients with spontaneous DVT.[113] Heparin-induced thrombocytopenia

TABLE 90-8 Risk Factors for Deep Vein Thrombosis

Age	Prior superficial vein thrombosis
Immobility	Hospitalization
Recent surgery	Malignancy
Progesterone therapy	Trauma
Residency in care facility	
Prior deep vein thrombosis	

TABLE 90-9 Etiology of Edema

	One Limb	Multiple Limbs
Decreased Outflow	Deep vein thrombosis	Proximal DVT (IVC)
	Deep vein insufficiency	Bilateral DVT
	Lymphedema	Lymphedema
	Superficial varicosities	Central venous compression
	Extrinsic compression	Pregnancy
	Baker's cyst	Pelvic mass
	May-Thurner syndrome	Obesity
	Pelvic mass	Dependency/immobility
	Factitial	Renal failure
	Arterial aneurysms	Congestive heart failure
		Pulmonary hypertension
Increased Inflow	AV malformations	Pregnancy
	Klippel-Trenaunay syndrome	Drug-induced
	Orthopedic	Cushing's syndrome
	Fracture	
	Osteomyelitis	
	Charcot joint	
	Gastrocnemius or popliteal muscle rupture	
Other	Low oncotic pressure	
	Anemia	
	Hypoalbuminemia	
	Lipedema	
	Hypothyroidism	

is detected by monitoring platelets at 2- to 3-day intervals, and warfarin necrosis is avoided by overlapping heparin with warfarin for 4 to 5 days.[108,109] Low-molecular-weight heparin (adjusted for weight) has shown promise in treating uncomplicated DVT while coumadin is taking effect.[114–116] The risk of major hemorrhage from anticoagulation is 1 to 2 percent when control is strict and attention is paid to drugs that alter warfarin's effect.[117] The international normalized ratio (INR) should be followed to ensure consistency between laboratories.

Thrombus isolated to the calf is less dangerous than thrombus in the thigh, but upward of 20 percent of such thrombi can extend proximally and 10 percent embolize. Laboratory surveillance of the lesion is required if anticoagulants are not used.[118] Caval occlusive procedures (primarily percutaneously placed filters) are used when anticoagulants are contraindicated or have failed to prevent a large pulmonary embolism. If a caval filter is placed and the contraindication to anticoagulation resolves, long-term anticoagulation should be considered since the filter itself may be thrombogenic. Thrombolytic therapy[119] that is given early accelerates recovery and may reduce the incidence or severity of postphlebitic syndrome. However, well-defined indications for thrombolytic therapy in DVT have not been established. Long-term use of compression stockings to the knee (or above, if tolerated) drastically reduces the incidence of postphlebitic syndrome, venous stasis changes, and venous ulceration.[120]

PHLEGMASIA CERULEA DOLENS

Phlegmasia cerulea dolens is a rare complication of DVT that is characterized by rapid and massive edema, severe pain, and cyanosis. This most commonly occurs in the setting of extensive iliofemoral thrombosis. A third of these patients die of pulmonary embolism, and half develop distal gangrene. It is seen most commonly with advanced malignancy or severe infections but can follow surgery, fractures, and other common precipitants of thrombosis.[121] Urgent treatment, including placement of a caval filter, heparinization, and sometimes debulking of the clot by thrombectomy or thrombolysis, is essential to minimize loss of life or limb.

There are numerous causes of limb pain and swelling that clinically mimic acute DVT. Objective testing may be indicated in many cases. D-dimer,[122] duplex ultrasound, or venography will confirm acute thrombosis in about one-third of suspicious episodes.[123] Patients who have *chronic deep venous insufficiency* are most likely to be symptomatic from other conditions. These patients may have acute episodes of pain and swelling that mimic new thrombosis, especially if they are not compliant in using elastic support hose or if the limb is stressed by prolonged dependency, travel, hot weather, or increased sodium intake.

Prophylactic anticoagulation is warranted in patients with prior venous thromboembolism or known clotting disorders who are traumatized or undergo medical or surgical illness with prolonged bed rest.[104,105,124] If anticoagulation must be interrupted for a surgical procedure, baseline duplex ultrasound and postoperative surveillance ultrasound (on or about day 2) may be obtained. With this approach, new clot can be detected even when old clot is present or symptoms are masked by analgesia. When thromboembolic events occur without a recognized risk factor for venous stasis or injury, a search for venous compression, inherited or acquired clotting abnormalities, or systemic disease is appropriate. Even when the results are negative, such screening is valuable in planning the duration of therapy and establishing the prognosis.

CENTRAL VENOUS THROMBOSIS

Occlusion of the superior vena cava (SVC) or inferior vena cava (IVC) may be an acute thrombotic event or may occur gradually from extrinsic compression or extension of distal thrombosis. The acute syndromes produce massive regional swelling and discomfort. Venous collaterals are prominent in chronic occlusion. The presence of superficial collateral veins in IVC syndrome is best appreciated with the patient upright. Malignancy is the cause of over 80 percent of SVC obstructions and about half of IVC obstructions. Relatively benign causes of the SVC syndrome include indwelling catheters (common) and fibrosing mediastinitis (rarely).[125] Inferior vena caval clots often extend from leg thrombosis. Both syndromes may be the initial manifestation of a primary clotting abnormality. Thrombolytic therapy may clear thrombosis if given early, and bypass surgery is effective and durable in selected instances of either syndrome.[126]

THROMBOSIS IN OTHER VEINS

Acute and chronic hepatic vein thrombosis presents with varying degrees of hepatic failure and ascites. Clotting disorders, tumors, and congenital venous anomalies are the most common causes.[127] Acute axillosubclavian thrombosis often is attributed to unusual effort or positioning. There is often evidence of thoracic outlet obstruction. Compression by tumor or aneurysm, indwelling catheters, and clotting defects are other causes. Thrombolytic therapy can be effective when given early and should be followed by anticoagulation. Some patients with local lesions can be further improved by balloon dilatation or surgery.[128]

Chronic Venous Insufficiency

Chronic deep venous incompetence or obstruction (causing venous hypertension in the upright position) may produce chronic venous insufficiency. This is characterized by leg edema, venous dilation, and intradermal deposition of proteins and hemosiderin. Cutaneous changes of fibrosis, lichenification, cellulitis, and ulceration may follow. Edema of the foot (with sparing of the toes) differentiates edema of chronic venous insufficiency from lymphedema. Symptoms include heavy congested limbs, venous claudication, pruritus, and skin ulceration that is often painless. Prior deep venous thrombosis, chronic right-sided heart disease, and an arteriovenous fistula also may produce this syndrome. Increased ambulatory pressure can be confirmed by direct measurement or plethysmography. Both incompetence and obstruction can be documented by bidirectional Doppler, ultrasound, duplex ultrasound, or venography.[129] Once ulceration has occurred, successful management is staged. Reduction of the edema must occur first, followed by healing of the ulcer and finally lifelong control of venous hypertension utilizing rigid or elastic support at 30 to 40 mmHg of compression (or more if required). Repair or replacement of incompetent proximal valves and bypass of iliocaval obstruction are promising in only a very select subset of these patients. The initial durability of these operations is encouraging.[130,131]

LABORATORY ASSESSMENT: VENOUS DISEASE

As with arterial testing, the indications for peripheral venous testing include objective documentation and diagnosis of venous disease, assessment of severity, and monitoring of progression or regression. Venous tests may be invasive (such as venography) or noninvasive, and the information they provide may be anatomic, hemodynamic, or functional.

Anatomic Studies

Duplex ultrasound, CT, MRI/MRA, and venography are the anatomic methods available for evaluation of the venous system. Venography is considered the "gold standard" for the determination of DVT. Venous duplex ultrasound is the most commonly used method, although it has the potential advantage of differentiating acute thrombus from old thrombus on the basis of the presence or absence of distention (common with acute clot) and increased echogenicity (common with chronic clot). It is less sensitive than venography above the groin and below the knee.

Physiologic Studies

CONTINUOUS-WAVE DOPPLER

Continuous-wave Doppler detects the movement of blood. CW Doppler provides qualitative (but not quantitative) information about the presence of hemodynamically significant reflux or obstruction. When the limb is interrogated at multiple levels, localization of the abnormality may be estimated (specificity 88 percent, sensitivity 85 percent).[132] However, this is a poor technique for evaluating partially obstructing thrombus or calf DVT. Although it is relatively sensitive for detecting areas of hemodynamically significant valvular incompetence, it cannot determine the functional significance of venous incompetence. In contrast to the triphasic arterial signal, the venous signal is much more complex. The components of venous flow evaluated by CW Doppler include the following.

Spontaneity When the Doppler is placed over a large vein, a spontaneous venous flow signal should be heard. Minor repositioning should be all that is necessary to obtain a detectable flow signal in most veins. If more extraordinary measures are needed, such as elevating, compressing, or another manipulation of the limb, this suggests an abnormality in venous flow.

Phasicity Venous return varies with the respiratory cycle. Above the diaphragm, there is an increase in venous return during inspiration. Below the diaphragm, venous return decreases during inspiration because increased intraabdominal pressure during inspiration opposes venous return. A loss of phasicity with respiration suggests venous obstruction.

Augmentation If a Doppler is placed over a vein in the proximal limb (for example, the femoral vein) and a distal portion of the limb (for example, the calf) is compressed, there should be an increase in venous return. This phenomenon, which is called augmentation, occurs only if the vein is patent between the site of compression and the site of Doppler interrogation.

Competency If a normal limb is compressed proximally (for example, over the thigh) or if a Valsalva maneuver is performed, the Doppler flow signal obtained distally (for example, over the popliteal vein) should cease temporarily as flow is stopped by the closure of venous valves. If the valves are incompetent, a retrograde flow signal will be noted.

Pulsatility Unlike arterial flow, venous flow is not necessarily pulsatile. When significant pulsatility is noted, one must consider the possibility of tricuspid regurgitation, right-sided heart failure, pulmonary hypertension, volume overload, an arteriovenous fistula, or other causes of increased venous pressure with pulsatility.

Venous Plethysmography

Many plethysmographic techniques have been developed to measure the changes in limb volume that occur when venous return is enhanced or impeded. The most popular techniques are strain gauge plethysmography, air plethysmography, and impedance plethysmography. A fourth modality, photoplethysmography,[133] is not truly a plethysmographic technique but instead estimates the amount of blood in the limb by reflecting infrared light off red blood cells flowing through the cutaneous vasculature.

PLETHYSMOGRAPHY FOR VENOUS INCOMPETENCE

Venous incompetence can be diagnosed and quantified by using plethysmography.[134,135] The patient is placed in an upright position (sitting or standing), and an air cuff or strain gauge is positioned around the lower portion of the limb. Once a steady volume measurement is obtained, the patient is tipped back and the legs are elevated to drain them of blood. The plethysmographic reading falls as blood drains from the veins and the limb becomes smaller. Once the blood has been emptied, the patient is returned to the upright position and the veins refill. If the valves are competent, refilling must occur in an antegrade fashion through the arteries and capillaries. In normal individuals, this may take a minute or more. If there is venous incompetence, the veins refill quickly and the leg volume returns to baseline more rapidly than normal. The next question is whether the incompetence is superficial or deep. If the incompetence is primarily superficial, placing tourniquets around the leg and/or directly compressing the incompetent superficial vein with a finger will normalize the refilling time.

EXERCISE VENOUS PLETHYSMOGRAPHY

This approach is used to assess the function of the "muscle pump" that normally compresses the veins and ejects blood out of the limb whenever muscular contraction occurs.[134,135] As was described above, the plethysmograph is placed around the lower limb or ankle while the patient is upright (sitting or standing). Once a stable baseline volume measurement is achieved, the patient exercises the leg by a series of toe or heel raises or deep knee bends. If a treadmill is available, the patient may walk. In patients with normal venous pump function, the leg volume decreases during exercise. At the end of exercise, the volume returns to baseline as the veins refill. Legs with impaired venous pump function (caused by venous obstruction, valvular incompetence, or primary pump failure) do not decrease their plethysmographic volume normally during exercise.

OUTFLOW PLETHYSMOGRAPHY

Plethysmographic techniques also can be used to evaluate limbs for the venous obstruction seen with acute or chronic DVT. Impedance plethysmography (IPG) is the best studied and most widely employed technique.[136–138] Unlike "anatomic" tests such as venography and ultrasound scanning (i.e., tests that directly image the thrombus), functional tests such as IPG identify the presence of venous thrombi by detecting the hemodynamic abnormalities they produce. Because IPG relies on indirect evidence of venous obstruction, it may be subject to more false positives and negatives than are imaging tests. Nevertheless, the ease of performance, low cost, and reasonable overall accuracy of IPG continue to make it a useful screening tool in appropriate settings.

The basic principles that underlie IPG are simple. A high-frequency, low-intensity electrical current that is too weak to be felt by the subject is passed between two electrodes that encircle the lower limb. Between the electrodes are two other electrodes across which voltage measurements are made. The voltage difference between the "measuring" electrodes is dependent on the electrical impedance of the underlying limb. Electrical impedance is dependent on the volume of blood (or other fluid) within the limb. The rate of change in limb volume is dependent on the rate of flow, which is reflected in the rate of change in electrical impedance.

To test for the presence of DVT, the patient lies supine with the legs slightly flexed and elevated. A pneumatic compression cuff is placed around the thigh and inflated to a pressure above venous pressure but below arterial pressure (typically 40 to 50 mmHg), producing venous occlusion. As blood becomes trapped beyond the cuff, the volume of the lower leg increases and the electrical impedance and voltage change. After an inflation period of 1 to 2 min, the cuff is deflated rapidly and venous flow resumes. As blood drains from the limb, the volume and voltage change rapidly. Values for the increase in leg volume produced by cuff inflation and the decrease in leg volume 3 s after cuff deflation are plotted on a standard diagram, and the presence or absence of obstruction consistent with DVT is determined.

CLINICAL APPLICATION

The accuracy of IPG as a means of detecting proximal DVT has been studied extensively, with generally impressive results. One analysis that compared IPG with venography in 2561 limbs demonstrated a sensitivity of 93 percent, a specificity of 94 percent, and an overall accuracy of 94 percent.[132] False positives occur when conditions other than acute DVT cause and mimic venous obstruction. The most common examples include elevated venous pressure from congestive heart failure, extrinsic vein compression, and "old" nonrecanalized venous thrombi. In contrast, false-negative tests usually are due to below-the-knee thrombi or nonoccluding proximal thrombi. As one would predict, the accuracy of IPG is variable and depends on the subgroup of patients being studied. Although there is ample documentation that the test is useful when applied to symptomatic patients, concern has been raised about its reliability as a tool for screening high-risk, asymptomatic patients. Other pitfalls of testing include unsuitable body habitus (such as morbid obesity or severe limb edema) and inability on the part of the patient to cooperate during the examination. Despite these caveats, IPG offers considerable prognostic information about the likelihood of a subsequent pulmonary embolism in patients suspected of having DVT. In one report involving short-term follow-up on 1074 patients with bilaterally negative IPG, there were no fatal pulmonary emboli and only a 1 percent incidence of clinical suspicion for nonfatal pulmonary emboli.[139] Other plethysmographic techniques have demonstrated similar results. IPG is best suited for use with cooperative, anatomically suitable patients in whom there is either a clinical suspicion of acute proximal DVT or a need to demonstrate that a patient is not at high risk for pulmonary embolism.

LYMPHEDEMA

The lymphatic vessels contain valves that are similar to those in veins but even more fragile. Trauma to a lymph vessel may easily damage these valves. There are multiple lymphatic vessels or channels (deep and superficial) in each limb. In contrast to the venous system, the superficial lymphatic vessels carry the large majority of flow. These systems coalesce at the inguinal lymph nodes and continue as the iliac and paraaortic lymphatic channels, which finally empty into the thoracic duct at the left subclavian vein.

Etiology

Lymphedema is the collection of lymphatic fluid in the dermal and subcutaneous tissues and may be primary or secondary. *Primary* lymphedema may be present at birth as an isolated occurrence or as part of a congenital familial syndrome. Onset of lymphedema in the teens or early twenties is called *lymphedema praecox* (Fig. 90-5) and is seen more often in females (usually at menarche). Rarely, primary lymphedema with onset in later years is called *lymphedema tarda.* This is a diagnosis of exclusion since a secondary cause is much more likely in this age group.

Secondary lymphedema is much more common than primary. Trauma, recurrent infection, obstruction by mass, infiltrative processes, or direct damage to the lymphatic system by radiation can cause lymphatic vessel destruction. Lymphedema of an upper extremity may occur after a radical or modified radical mastectomy. Recurrent cellulitis is common in patients with lymphedema. Streptococcus, which can enter the skin through a crack in the toe webs caused by trychophytosis, further inflames and damages the lymphatic channels and the connecting lymph nodes. Repeated infection damages and eventually obliterates the vessel; preventing these infections is therefore a cornerstone of treatment.

Diagnosis

History and physical examination allow the diagnosis in the majority of cases.[140] Unlike edema and lipedema, lymphedema involves the toes. The skin is thickened and takes on a consistency termed *peau d'orange* (literally, "an orange peel"). Dependent edema also spares the toes since footwear does not allow the swelling to occur. Lipedema, which is caused by excess fatty deposits that usually are increased at the time of menarche,

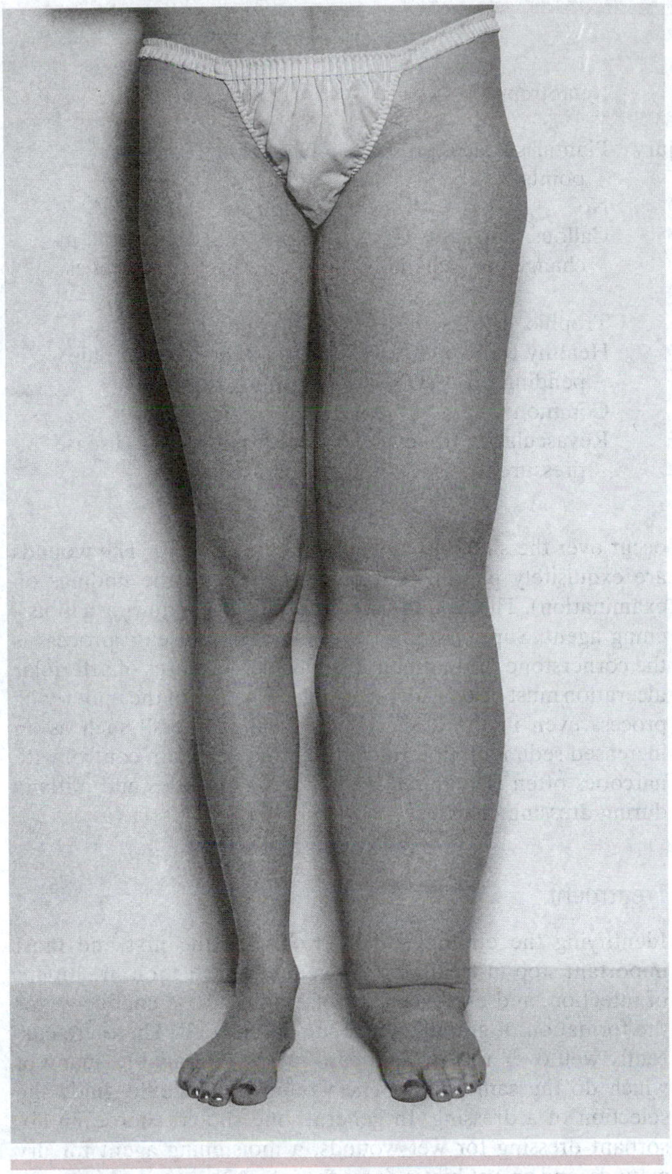

FIGURE 90-5 Photograph of a young woman with lymphedema praecox. Note the asymmetry and note that the toes are affected. The leg was reduced with elevation and compression.

is more difficult to differentiate. These fatty deposits may be asymmetric and may run in families. In lipedema, the toes are spared and there is often a ridge or fold overhanging the ankle. Lipedema and lymphedema may coexist. Laboratory testing may help differentiate the two.

Testing

Lymphangiography and lymphoscintigraphy are the two techniques currently available for direct imaging of the lymphatic system. Lymphangiography is more difficult to perform and carries a risk of lymphangitis. However, anatomic features are obtained and differentiation between primary (absence of lymphatic structures) and secondary (obstruction at a level by a mass, an injury, or lymph node hypertrophy caused by lymphoma) lymphedema often can be determined. The lymphoscintogram is based on the uptake and movement of ^{99}Tc-labeled antimony trisulfide colloid after injection between the web spaces of digits. It is easier to perform this lymphangiography and has a significantly lower risk of lymphangitis. While it has good ability to differentiate lymphedema from other causes of edema, it cannot reliably distinguish primary from secondary lymphedema.

Treatment

The mainstay of treatment for lymphedema is compression. First the leg must be reduced in size by elevation, mechanical pumping, or manual massage. Wrapping of the distal-to-proximal portion of the affected limb or limbs is required whenever the patient is up and also should be encouraged when the patient is supine. Once the leg volume has decreased, a compression garment of 40 to 50 mmHg should be worn daily and replaced two to four times per year as needed. Early and aggressive treatment of cellulitis and fungal infections helps prevent worsening.

ULCERATION

Lower and upper extremity ulceration of vascular etiology is common. However, nonvascular etiologies are also common and must be kept in mind when a properly treated ulcer does not respond to therapy. Dermatologic, oncologic, hematologic, infectious, and factitious causes must be considered in such circumstances. Ulceration caused by a vascular etiology can be classified into four categories: arterial, arteriolar, venous, and neurotrophic (Table 90-10). Multifactorial ulcerations are common, particularly in diabetic patients and immunosuppressed persons. It is beyond the scope of this section to detail the diagnosis and treatment of each, but general principals will be discussed.

Arterial Ulcers

Arterial ulcers generally are located on the distal portion of the lower extremities but may occur anywhere. A traumatic event or surgical procedure such as vein harvesting or toenail trimming often initiates the ulcer. A dense black eschar can form over a dry base. Findings of arterial insufficiency are common. The wound may be tender, and infection can occur. Healing is often problematic until oxygen delivery is increased. In such cases, revascularization is indicated. If this is not possible, external compression devices may be successful, although they are not widely available.

Venous Ulcers

Venous ulcers are relatively painless. They typically develop above the malleoli, usually after years of deep venous insufficiency. Skin changes include thickening, hemosiderin deposits, and edema. The ulcer base is wet and frequently has secondary infection. Varicose veins may cause local venous ulcers after trauma. The natural history is an enlarging ulcer that appears deep because of associated edema. Treatment requires compression and elevation. The edema must be driven out of the leg to create an environment for granulation. Compression with elastic wraps (and foam pads over the ulcer sites to provide

TABLE 90-10 Recognition of Ulcers of Vascular Etiology

Type	Venous	Arterial	Neurotrophic	Arteriolar
Location	Above medial and lateral malleoli	Shins, toes, sites of injury	Plantar surface, pressure points	Shin, calf
Pain	No, unless infected	Yes	No	Exquisite
Skin	Stasis pigmentation Thickening with lipodermatosclerosis	Shiny, pale decreased hair; may see livido	Callous, normal to changes of ischemia	Normal or "satellite" ulcers in various stages
Edges	Clean	Smooth	Trophic, calloused	Serpiginous
Base	Wet, weeping, healthy granulation	Dry, pale with eschar	Healthy to pale depending on ASO	Dry, punched-out, pale, thin eschar
Cellulitis	Common	Often	Common	No
Treatment	Compression	Revascularize	Revascularize, relieve pressure	Treat underlying disease and pain

added compression) is the treatment method of choice. If there is infection, a short course of antibiotics may be required.

Neurotrophic Ulcers

Neurotrophic ulceration is seen in all adult medical specialties. Diabetes, peripheral neuropathies, spinal cord injuries, and other causes of decreased sensation may be present. External pressure by a shoe, a brace, or a foreign body embedded in the foot may start the ulcer. The wound edges develop callus that can mask undermining. The edges must be probed bluntly to determine the extent or presence of fistula tracts. Infection is common, particularly when the decreased sensation masks the pain that infection normally causes. *Osteomyelitis* is frequently present, especially when the ulcer has been present for months and has been treated with short courses of oral antibiotics. Treatment includes relief of the pressure and debridement of the callus. Infection must be treated aggressively, and the presence of osteomyelitis must be excluded. In diabetic patients, arterial occlusive disease also may be present. Revascularization, bony debridement, or amputation often is required to prevent sepsis or achieve healing.

Arteriolar Ulcers

Arteriolar ulcers are caused by occlusion of dermal arterioles that vertically penetrate the dermal layer. This anatomy leads to the characteristic "cookie cutter" appearance and serpiginous edge seen in these ulcers. Islands or satellites of ulcers often occur over the shin, but any area can be affected. The wounds are exquisitely painful (out of proportion to the findings on examination). The wound base is usually dry, requiring a moistening agent. Suppression of the underlying disease process is the cornerstone of treatment (Table 90-11). Flares of arteriolar ulceration must be considered an exacerbation of the underlying process even in the absence of "usual markers" such as an increased sedimentation rate and antibodies. Pain control with narcotics often is required during acute episodes and initially during dressing changes.

TABLE 90-11 Etiologies of Arteriolar Ulcers

Connective tissue diseases
Rheumatoid arthritis
Scleroderma
Mixed connective tissue diseases
Lupus erythematosus
Vasculitis
Malignancy
Myeloproliferative disorders
Inflammatory bowel disease

Treatment

Identifying the etiology of the wound is the first and most important step in treatment. In general, protection, treatment of infection, and establishment of an ulcer base conducive for the formation of granulation tissue are needed. There are currently well over 1000 wound care products available, many of which do the same thing. The wound base should guide the selection of a dressing. In general, one should choose an absorbant dressing for wet wounds, a moistening agent for dry wounds, and an antibiotic agent for infected wounds. Moisture-neutral dressings are also available. Debridement using wet-to-dry gauze or nonstick products to prevent irritation often is required. Blunt or sharp manual debridement also may be necessary.

References

1. Stoffers H, Rinkens P, Kester A, et al. The prevalence of asymptomatic and unrecognized peripheral arterial occlusive disease. *Int J Epidemiol* 1996; 25:282.
2. Elhadd T, Jung R, Newton R, et al. Incidence of asymptomatic peripheral arterial occlusive disease in diabetic patients attending a hospital clinic. *Adv Exp Med Biol* 1997; 428:45.
3. Leary W, Allen E. Intermittent claudication as a result of arterial spasm induced by walking. *Am Heart J* 1941; 22:719–725.
4. DeWesse J. Pedal pulses disappearing with exercise. *N Engl J Med* 1960; 262:1214.
5. Barnett A, Dugdale L, Ferguson I. Disappearing pulse syndrome due to myxomatous degeneration of the popliteal artery. *Med J Aus* 1966; 2:355.
6. Kavanaugh G, Svein H, Holman C, Johnson R. "Pseudoclaudica-

tion" syndrome produced by compression of the cauda equina. *JAMA* 1968; 206:2477.
7. Goodreau J, Creasy J, Flanigan D, et al. Rational approach to the differentiation of vascular and neurogenic claudication. *Surgery* 1978; 84:749.
8. Kamienski R, Barnes R. Critique of the Allen test for continuity of the palmar arch assessment by Doppler ultrasound. *Surg Gynecol Obstet* 1976; 142:861.
9. Allen E. Thromboangiitis obliterans: Methods of diagnosis of chronic occlusive arterial lesions distal to the wrist with illustrative cases. *Am J Med Sci* 1929; 178:237.
10. Lederle F, Walker J, Reinke D. Selective screening for abdominal aortic aneurysms with physical examination and ultrasound. *Arch Intern Med* 1988; 148:1753.
11. Littooy F, Stefan G, Greisler H, et al. Use of sequential B-mode ultrasonography to manage abdominal aortic aneurysms. *Arch Surg* 1989; 124:419.
12. Wychulis A, Spittell JJ, Wallace R. Popliteal aneurysms. *Surgery* 1970; 68:942.
13. Pappas C, James J, Bernatz P, Schirger A. Femoral aneurysms: Review of surgical management. *JAMA* 1964; 190:489.
14. McCready R, Pairolero P, Gilmore J, et al. Isolated iliac artery aneurysms. *Surgery* 1983; 94:688.
15. Zwolak R, Whitehouse W, Knake J, et al. Atherosclerotic extracranial carotid artery aneurysms. *J Vasc Surg* 1985; 1:415.
16. Pairolero P, Walls J, Payne W, et al. Subclavian-axillary artery aneurysms. *Surgery* 1981; 90:757.
17. Stanley J, Thompson N, Fry W. Splanchnic artery aneurysms. *Arch Surg* 1970; 101:689.
18. Trastek V, Pairolero P, Joyce J, et al. Splenic artery aneurysms. *Surgery* 1982; 91:649.
19. Perloff J. *Physical Examination of the Heart and Circulation*. Philadelphia: Saunders; 1982.
20. McLaughlin M, Colapinto R, Hobbs B. Abdominal bruits: Clinical and angiographic correlation. *JAMA* 1975; 232:1238.
21. Beven E. Thoracic outlet syndromes. In: Young JR, Graor RA, Olin JW, et al, eds. *Peripheral Vascular Diseases*. St. Louis: Mosby–Year Book; 1991:497.
22. Stoney R, Cheng S. Neurogenic thoracic outlet syndrome. In: Rutherford RB, ed. *Vascular Surgery*, 4th ed. Philadelphia: Saunders; 1995:976.
23. Strandness DJ, McCutcheon E, Rushmer R. Application of transcutaneous Doppler flowmeter in evaluation of occlusive arterial disease. *Surg Gynecol Obstet* 1966; 122:1039.
24. Strandness DJ, Schultz R, Sumner D, Rushmer R. Ultrasound flow detection: A useful technic in the evaluation of peripheral vascular disease. *Am J Surg* 1967; 113:311.
25. Johnston K. Processing continuous wave Doppler signals and analysis of peripheral arterial waveform. In: Bernstein EF, ed. *Vascular Diagnosis Problems and Solutions*, 4th ed. St. Louis: Mosby; 1993:149.
26. Regensteiner J. Exercise rehabilitation for patients with peripheral arterial disease. *Exerc Sport Sci Rev* 1995; 23:1.
27. Hobbs J, Yao J. A limitation of the Doppler ultrasound method of measuring ankle systolic pressure. *Vasa* 1974; 3:160.
28. Darling R, Raines J. Quantitative segmental pulse volume recorder: A clinical tool. *Surgery* 1973; 72:873.
29. Symes J, Graham A, Mousseau M. Doppler waveform analysis versus segmental pressure and pulse-volume recording: Assessment of occlusive disease in the lower extremity. *Can J Surg* 1984; 27:345.
30. Rooke T. The use of transcutaneous oximetry in the noninvasive vascular laboratory. *Int Angiol* 1992; 11:36.
31. Rooke T, Hollier L, Osmundson P. The influence of sympathetic nerves on transcutaneous oxygen tension in normal and ischemic lower extremities. *Angiology* 1987; 38:400.
32. Bacharach J, Rooke T, Osmundson P, et al. Predictive value of transcutaneous oxygen pressure and amputation success by use of supine and elevation measurements. *J Vasc Surg* 1992; 15:558.
33. Rooke T, Osmundson P. The influence of age, sex, smoking, and diabetes on lower limb transcutaneous oxygen tension in patients with arterial occlusive disease. *Arch Intern Med* 1990; 150:129.
34. Rooke T, Osmundson P. Variability and reproducibility of transcutaneous oxygen tension measurements in the assessment of peripheral vascular disease. *Angiology* 1989; 40:695.
35. Rooke T, Heser J, Hallett J, et al. Hemodynamic changes following the surgical revascularization of lower limbs in patients with arterial occlusive disease: A comparison of six methods. *J Vasc Technol* 1993; 17:27.
36. Criqui M, Denenberg J, Langer R, et al. The epidemiology of peripheral arterial disease: Importance of identifying the population at risk. *Vasc Med* 1997; 2:221.
37. Stoffers H, Rinkens P, Kester A, et al. The prevalence of asymptomatic and unrecognized peripheral arterial occlusive disease. *Int J Epidemiol* 1996; 2:282.
38. Kannel W, McGee D. Update on some epidemiologic features of intermittent claudication: The Framingham Study. *J Am Geriatr Soc* 1985; 33:13.
39. Brand F, Kannel W, Evans J, et al. Glucose intolerance, physical signs of peripheral arterial disease, and risk of cardiovascular events: The Framingham Study. *Am Heart J* 1998; 136:919.
40. Hooi J, Stoffers H, Kester A, et al. Risk factors and cardiovascular diseases associated with asymptomatic peripheral arterial occlusive disease: The Limburg PAOD Study: Peripheral Arterial Occlusive Disease. *Scand J Prim Health Care* 1998; 16:177.
41. Brand F, Abbott R, Kannel W. Diabetes, intermittent claudication, and risk of cardiovascular disease: The Framingham Study. *Diabetes* 1989; 38:504.
42. Criqui M, Deneberg J. The generalized nature of atherosclerosis: How peripheral arterial disease may predict adverse events from coronary artery disease. *Vasc Med* 1998; 3:241.
43. McKenna M, Wolfson S, Kuller L. The ratio of ankle and arm blood pressure as an independent risk factor of mortality. *Athero* 1991; 87:119.
44. McDaniel M, Cronenwett J. Basic data related to the natural history of intermittent claudication. *Ann Vasc Surg* 1989; 3:273.
45. Boyd A. The natural course of arteriosclerosis of the lower extremities. *Proc R Soc Med* 1962; 55:591.
46. Juergens J, Barker N, Hines EJ: Arteriosclerosis obliterans: Review of 520 cases with special reference to pathogenic and prognostic factors. *Circulation* 1960; 21:188.
47. Schadt D, Hines AJ, Juergens J, et al. Chronic atherosclerotic occlusion of the femoral artery. *JAMA* 1961; 175:937.
48. Moss SEM, Klein RM. The 14-year incidence of lower extremity amputation in a diabetic population: The Wisconsin Epidemiologic Study of Diabetic Retinopathy. *Diabetes Care* 1999; 22:951.
49. Adler A, Boyko E, Ahroni J, et al. Lower extremity amputation in diabetes: The independent effects of peripheral vascular disease. *Diabetes Care* 1999; 22:1029.
50. Hamalainen H, Ronnemaa T, Halonen J, et al. Factors predicting lower extremity amputations in patients with type 1 or type 2 diabetes mellitus: A population-based 7-year follow-up study. *J Intern Med* 1999; 246:97.
51. Migdalis I, Dimakopoulos N, Kourti A, et al. The prevalence of peripheral vascular disease in type 2 diabetic patients with and without proteinuria. *Int Angiol* 1994; 13:229.
52. Barndt R, Blankenhorn D, Crawford D, et al. Regression and progression of early femoral atherosclerosis in treated hyperlipoproteinemic patients. *Ann Intern Med* 1977; 86:139.
53. Hiatt W. Benefit of exercise conditioning for patients with peripheral arterial disease. *Circulation* 1990; 81:602.
54. Hiatt W, Stoll S, Nies A. Effect of beta-adrenergic blockers in the peripheral circulation in patients with peripheral arterial disease. *Circulation* 1985; 72:1226.

55. Lundgren F, Dahlloff A, Lundholm K, et al. Intermittent claudication—surgical reconstruction or physical training? A prospective randomized trial of treatment efficiency. *Ann Surg* 1989; 209:346.
56. Dahloff A, Bjorntorp P, Holm J, et al. Metabolic activity of skeletal muscle in patients with peripheral arterial insufficiency: Effect of physical training. *Eur J Clin Invest* 1974; 4:9.
57. Hood S, Moher D, Barber G. Management of intermittent claudication with pentoxyfilline: Meta-analysis of randomized controlled trials. *Can Med Assoc J* 1996; 155:1053.
58. Bagger J, Helligose P, Randsbaek F, et al. Effect of verapamil in intermittent claudication: A randomized, double-blind, placebo-controlled, cross-over study after individual dose response assessment. *Circulation* 1997; 95:422.
59. Radack K, Wyderski R: β-Adrenergic blocker therapy does not worsen intermittent claudication in subjects with peripheral arterial disease: A meta-analysis of randomized controlled trials. *Arch Intern Med* 1991; 151:1769.
60. Shepherd R. Ergotism. In: White RA, Hollier LH, eds. *Vascular Surgery: Basic Science and Clinical Correlations*. Philadelphia: Lippincott; 1994:177.
61. Hight D, Tilney N, Couch N. Changing clinical trends in patients with peripheral arterial emboli. *Surgery* 1976; 79:171.
62. Darling R, Austen W, Linton R. Arterial embolism. *Surg Gynecol Obstet* 1967; 124:106.
63. Meister S, Grossman W, Dexter L, Dalen J. Paradoxical embolism: Diagnosis during life. *Am J Med* 1972; 53:292.
64. Holm J, Schersten T. Anticoagulant treatment during and after embolectomy. *Acta Chir Scand* 1972; 138:683.
65. Green R, DeWeese J, Rob C. Arterial embolectomy before and after the Fogarty catheter. *Surgery* 1975; 77:24.
66. Fogarty T, Cranley J, Krause R, et al. A method for extraction of arterial emboli and thrombi. *Surg Gynecol Obstet* 1963; 116:241.
67. Thompson J, Weston A, Aigler L, et al. Arterial embolectomy after acute myocardial infarction: A study of 31 patients. *Ann Surg* 1970; 171:979.
68. McNamara T, Fischer J. Thrombolysis of peripheral arterial and graft occlusions: Improved results using high-dose urokinase. *AJR* 1985; 144:769.
69. Ouriel K, Veith F, Sasahara A. Thrombolysis or peripheral arterial surgery: Phase I results. *J Vasc Surg* 1996; 23:64.
70. Ouriel K, Vieth F, Sasahara A. Thrombolysis of Peripheral Arterial Surgery (TOPAS) investigators. A comparison of recombinant urokinase with vascular surgery as initial treatment for acute arterial occlusion of the legs. *N Engl J Med* 1998; 338:1105.
71. Lie J. The rise and fall and resurgence of thromboangiitis obliterans (Buerger's disease). *Acta Pathol Jpn* 1989; 39:153.
72. Mills J, Taylor LJ, Porter J. Buerger's disease in the modern era. *Am J Surg* 1987; 154:123.
73. Olin J, Young J, Graor R, et al. The changing clinical spectrum of thromboangiitis obliterans (Buerger's disease). *Circulation* 1990; 82:3.
74. Shigematsu H, Shigematsu K. Factors affecting the long-term outcome of Buerger's disease (thromboangiitis obliterans). *Int Angiol* 1999; 18:58.
75. Fiessinger J, Schafter M. Trial of iloprost versus aspirin treatment for critical limb ischaemia of thromboangiitis obliterans. *Lancet* 1990; 335:555.
76. Collins P, McDonald P, Lim R. Popliteal artery entrapment: An evolving syndrome. *J Vasc Surg* 1989; 10:484.
77. Ishikawa K. Cystic adventitial disease of the popliteal artery and of other stem vessels in the extremities. *Jpn J Surg* 1987; 17:221.
78. Klein R, Hunder G, Stanson A, et al. Large artery involvement in giant cell (temporal) arteritis. *Ann Intern Med* 1975; 83:806.
79. Hall S, Barr W, Lie J, et al. Takayasu arteritis: A study of 32 North American patients. *Medicine (Baltimore)* 1985; 64:89.
80. Kerr G, Hallahan C, Giordano J, et al. Takayasu arteritis. *Ann Intern Med* 1994; 120:919.
81. Bergqvist D, Bengtsson J, Sternby N. Associated atherosclerotic manifestations. In: Greenhalgh RM, Mannick JA, eds. *The Cause and Management of Aneurysms*, vol 47. London: Saunders; 1990:47.
82. Johansen K, Koepsell T. Familial tendency for abdominal aortic aneurysms. *JAMA* 1986; 256:1934.
83. Dent T, Lindenauer M, Ernst C, et al. Multiple arteriosclerotic aneurysms. *Arch Surg* 1972; 105:338.
84. Joyce J, Fairbairn JI, Kincaid O, et al. Aneurysms of the thoracic aorta: A clinical study with special reference to prognosis. *Circulation* 1964; 29:176.
85. Gastineau D, Kazmier F, Nichols W, et al. Lupus anticoagulant: An analysis of the clinical and laboratory features of 219 cases. *Am J Hematol* 1985; 19:265.
86. Karmody A, Powers S, Monaco V, et al. "Blue toe" syndrome: An indication for limb salvage surgery. *Arch Surg* 1976; 111:1263.
87. Hollier L, Kazmier F, Ochsner J, et al. "Shaggy" aorta syndrome with atheromatous embolization to visceral vessels. *Ann Vasc Surg* 1991; 5:439.
88. Richards A, Eliot R, Kanjuh V, et al. Cholesterol embolism: A multiple-system disease masquerading as polyarteritis nodosa. *Am J Cardiol* 1965; 15:696.
89. Kaufman J, Shah D, Leather R. Atheroembolism and microembolic syndromes (blue toe syndrome and disseminated atheroembolism). In: Rutherford RB, ed. *Vascular Surgery*, 4th ed. Philadelphia: Saunders; 1995:669.
90. Allen E, Brown G. Raynaud's disease: A critical review of minimal requisites for diagnosis. *Am J Med Sci* 1932; 183:187.
91. DeTakats G, Fowler E. Raynaud's phenomenon. *JAMA* 1962; 179:99.
92. Priollet P, Vayssairat M, Housset E. How to classify Raynaud's phenomenon: Long-term follow-up study of 73 cases. *Am J Med* 1987; 87:494.
93. Gifford RJ, Hines EJ. Raynaud's disease among women and girls. *Circulation* 1957; 16:1012.
94. Landry G, Edwards J, McLafferty R, et al. Long-term outcome of Raynaud's syndrome in a prospectively analyzed patient cohort. *J Vasc Surg* 1996; 23:76.
95. Coffman J. *Raynaud's Phenomenon*. New York: Oxford University Press; 1989.
96. Walker P, Paley D, Harris K. What determines the symptoms associated with subclavian artery occlusive disease? *J Vasc Surg* 1985; 2:154.
97. Rose N, Leskovsek N. Scleroderma: Immunopathogenesis and treatment. *Immunol Today* 1998; 19:499.
98. Bower T, Pairolero P, Hallet JJ, et al. Brachiocephalic aneurysms: The case for early recognition and repair. *Ann Vasc Surg* 1991; 5:125.
99. Hirai M, Shionaya S. Arterial obstruction of the upper limb in Buerger's disease: Its incidence and primary lesion. *Br J Surg* 1979; 66:124.
100. Kieffer E, Ruotolo C. Arterial complications of thoracic outlet compression. In: Rutherford RB, ed. *Vascular Surgery*, 4th ed. Philadelphia: Saunders; 1995:992.
101. Conn JJ, Bergan J, Bell J. Hypothenar hammer syndrome: Post-traumatic digital ischemia. *Surgery* 1970; 68:1122.
102. *Vibration Syndrome: Current Intelligence Bulletin 38*. Washington, DC: National Institute of Occupational Safety and Health; 1982.
103. Hirsh J, Hull R. *Venous Thromboembolism: Natural History, Diagnosis and Management*. Boca Raton, FL: CRC Press; 1987.
104. LeClerc J. *Venous Thromboembolic Disorders*. Philadelphia: Lea & Febiger; 1991.
105. Zimran A, Shilo S, Herskro C. Chronic cutaneous polyarteritis

nodosa simulating recurrent thrombophlebitis. *Isr J Med Sci* 1985; 21:154.

106. Plate G, Eklof B, Jensen R, et al. Deep venous thrombosis, pulmonary embolism, and acute surgery in thrombophlebitis of the long saphenous vein. *Acta Chir Scand* 1985; 151:242.
107. O'Fallon W, Heit J, Mohr D, et al. Predictors of recurrence after deep vein thrombosis and pulmonary embolism: A population-based cohort study. *Blood* 1998; 10:560a.
108. Ansell J, Deykin D. Heparin-induced thrombocytopenia and recurrent thromboembolism. *Am J Hematol* 1980; 8:325.
109. Colp M, Minifee P, Wolma F. Coumadin necrosis: A review of the literature. *Surgery* 1988; 103:271.
110. Haeger K. Problems of acute deep vein thrombosis: The interpretation of signs and symptoms. *Angiology* 1969; 20:219.
111. Barnes R, Wu K, Hoak J. Fallibility of the clinical diagnosis of venous thrombosis. *JAMA* 1975; 234:605.
112. Ouriel K, Whitehouse WJ, Zarins C. Combined use of Doppler ultrasound and phlebography in suspected deep venous thrombosis. *Surg Gynecol Obstet* 1984; 159:242.
113. Kearon C, Gent M, Hirsh J, et al. A comparison of three months of anticoagulation with extended anticoagulation for a first episode of idiopathic venous thrombosis. *N Engl J Med* 1999; 340:901.
114. Litin S, Heit J, Mees K. Use of low-molecular-weight heparin in the treatment of venous thromboembolic disease: Answers to frequently asked questions. *Mayo Clin Proc* 1998; 73:545.
115. Lensing A, Prins M, Davidson B, et al. Treatment of deep venous thrombosis with low-molecular-weight heparins. *Arch Intern Med* 1995; 155:601.
116. Green D, Hirsh J, Heit J, et al. Low molecular weight heparin: A critical analysis of clinical trials. *Pharmacol Rev* 1994; 46:89.
117. Robitaille P, LeClerc J, Brave G. Treatment of venous thromboembolism. In: LeClerc J, ed. *Venous Thromboembolic Disorders*. Philadelphia: Lea & Febiger; 1991:267.
118. Kakkar V, Howe C, Nicholaides A, et al. Deep vein thrombosis of the leg: Is there a higher risk group? *Am J Surg* 1970; 120:527.
119. Comerota A. Venous thromboembolism. In: Rutherford RB, ed. *Vascular Surgery*, 4th ed. Philadelphia: Saunders; 1995:1995.
120. Prandoni P, Lensing A, Cogo A, et al. The long-term clinical course of acute deep venous thrombosis. *Ann Intern Med* 1996; 125:1.
121. Brockman S, Vasko J. Phlegmasia cerulea dolens. *Surg Gynecol Obstet* 1965; 121:1347.
122. Heit J, Minor T, Andrews J, et al. Determinates of plasma D-dimer sensitivity for acute pulmonary embolism as defined by pulmonary angiography. *Arch Pathol Lab Med* 1999; 123:235.
123. LeClerc J, Jay R, Hull R. Recurrent leg symptoms following deep vein thrombosis: A diagnostic challenge. *Arch Intern Med* 1985; 145:1867.
124. Hyers T, Hull R, Weg J. Antithrombosis therapy for venous thromboembolic disease. *Chest* 1989; 95:S375.
125. Parish B, Marschke RJ, Dines D, et al. Etiologic considerations in superior vena cava syndromes. *Mayo Clin Proc* 1981; 56:407.
126. Lockridge S, Kibbe W, Doty D. Obstruction of the superior vena cava. *Surgery* 1979; 85:14.
127. Lillimoe K, Cameron J. The Budd-Chiari syndrome. In: Rutherford RB, ed. *Vascular Surgery*, 4th ed. Philadelphia: Saunders; 1995:1195.
128. Machleder H. Evaluation of a new treatment strategy for Paget-Schroetter syndrome: Spontaneous thrombosis of the axillary-subclavian vein. *J Vasc Surg* 1993; 17:305.
129. Nicholaides A, Christopoulos D, Vasdekis S. Progress in the investigation of chronic venous insufficiency. *Ann Vasc Surg* 1989; 3:278.
130. Kistner R, Ferris E. Technique of surgical reconstruction of femoral vein valve. In: Bergan JJ, Yao JST, eds. *Operative Techniques of Vascular Surgery*. New York: Grune & Stratton; 1980:291.
131. Lalka S. Management of chronic obstructive venous disease of the lower extremity. In: Rutherford RB, ed. *Vascular Surgery*, 4th ed. Philadelphia: Saunders; 1995:1862.
132. Wheeler H, Anderson FJ. Use of noninvasive tests as the basis for treatment of deep vein thrombosis. In: Rutherford RB, ed. *Vascular Diagnosis*, 4th ed. St. Louis: Mosby; 1993:862.
133. Abramowitz H, Queral L, Flinn W, et al. The use of photoplethysmography in the assessment of venous insufficiency: A comparison to venous pressure measurements. *Surgery* 1979; 86:434.
134. Katz M, Comerota A, Kerr R. Air plethysmography (APG): A new technique to evaluate patients with chronic venous insufficiency. *J Vasc Technol* 1991; 15:23.
135. Rooke T, Heser JL, Osmonson PJ. Exercise strain-gauge venous plethysmography: Evaluation of a "new" device for assessing lower limb venous incompetence. *Angiology* 1987; 43:219.
136. Brown J, Ward P, Wilkinson A, et al. Impedance plethysmography: A screening procedure to detect deep vein thrombosis. *J Bone Joint Surg* 1987; 69:264.
137. Huisman M, Buller H, TenCate J, et al. Serial impedance plethysmography for suspected deep venous thrombosis in outpatients: The Amsterdam General Practitioner Study. *N Engl J Med* 1986; 314:823.
138. Patterson R, Fowl R, Keller J, et al. The limitations of impedance plethysmography in the diagnosis of acute deep venous thrombosis. *J Vasc Surg* 1989; 9:725.
139. Wheeler H, Anderson FJ, Cardullo P, et al. Suspected deep vein thrombosis: Management by impedance plethysmography. *Arch Surg* 1982; 117:1296.
140. Campisi C. Lymphoedema: Modern diagnostic and therapeutic aspects. *Int Angiol* 1999; 18:14.

C H A P T E R 91

SURGICAL TREATMENT OF PERIPHERAL VASCULAR DISEASE

Thomas F. Dodson / Robert B. Smith III

The emergence of managed care and the advent of minimally invasive procedures have wrought an evolutionary upheaval in the field of vascular surgery, and the pace of change has accelerated, with new technology and new discoveries carrying the field into the twenty-first century. In a recent editorial, a leading medical journal[1] looked back over the most important medical developments of the past 1000 years, and the advances the editors chose to highlight were not surprising. The discovery of cells and their structures, the development of anesthesia, the elucidation of the role of microbes in disease, the development of body imaging, and the discovery of antimicrobial agents were cited, along with several others.

Vascular surgery is a relatively new entrant in the field of medicine and surgery. Its modern origins date back only about 50 years, with the first femoral-to-popliteal bypass being done in 1948 and the first abdominal aortic aneurysm being repaired in 1951.[2] The past 50 years have brought remarkable progress to this young discipline. New technologies currently being evaluated include minimally invasive surgery,[3] gene therapy,[4] the role of computers and the internet,[5-7] tissue engineering,[8] and telemedicine,[9,10] to mention just a few.

This chapter is divided into three sections: (1) carotid endarterectomy, (2) upper and lower extremity revascularization, and (3) upper and lower extremity venous thrombosis. While vascular surgery remains only a "palliative" therapy for people with atherosclerotic and venous disease, "curative" therapies no doubt await insightful and determined investigators. The scalpel will clearly yield to the gene in the days to come.[11]

CAROTID ENDARTERECTOMY

Stroke continues to be the third leading cause of death in the United States, outranked only by heart disease and cancer. There are nearly 500,000 cases of stroke each year in this country, with approximately one-third of patients dying as a result.[12] However, there has been a decline over the past four decades in both the incidence of stroke and the mortality resulting from it. In the past several years, however, evidence has suggested that this long decline in stroke mortality and morbidity may have plateaued in the Minneapolis-St. Paul area.[12] Ironically, recent data from the Mayo Clinic in Rochester, Minnesota, noted that, in the period 1985 to 1989, there was a continuance of an earlier "leveling off" of incidence rates and a suggestion that stroke rates have actually increased over the past 10 years.[13,14] While it has been suggested that "environmental factors" influence the risk of stroke, certainly, better control of hypertension, a gradual reduction in the percentage of individuals who smoke cigarettes, an increased awareness of the benefits of a physically active lifestyle, greater attention to cholesterol reduction and dietary modification, and greater use of anticoagulants in patients with atrial fibrillation have probably all contributed to the decline in stroke deaths in the United States.

In terms of who should undergo operation for carotid artery disease, we are finally on relatively firm ground. There have been six prospective randomized trials published on this topic since 1991, five of which have shown a benefit for surgery in preventing cerebral ischemia.[15-20] Data continue to come from these randomized prospective studies, and Barnett and colleagues recently reported that, based on a further review of the North American Symptomatic Carotid Endarterectomy Trial (NASCET) data, carotid endarterectomy in symptomatic patients with 50 to 69 percent stenosis produced only a "moderate" reduction in the risk of further stroke.[21] An analysis of this information noted an absolute risk reduction of 10.1 percent at 5 years for those symptomatic patients with carotid stenoses of 50 to 69 percent but also noted no benefit for patients with symptomatic stenoses of less than 50 percent. The authors further suggested that decision making regarding these patients with a moderate degree of stenosis could be aided by a full evaluation of underlying risk factors, but that their analysis did not justify a "large" increase in the rate of carotid endarterectomy. As pointed out in an editorial commenting on Barnett's paper, the accumulation of scientific data about carotid endarterectomy is "virtually unmatched in clinical surgical research,"[22] and internists and surgeons alike have embraced this information: the number of carotid endarterectomies performed in 1996—130,000—doubled the number performed in 1991.[23]

TABLE 91-1 Treatment Plan for Patients with Carotid Disease

Category of Patient	Treatment
Patients with Symptomatic Carotid Stenoses	
>80% stenosis of internal carotid artery	CEA indicated
50–79% stenosis of carotid artery but with vascular laboratory data suggesting closer to 79%	CEA probably indicated; assess risk factors
50–79% stenosis of carotid artery but with vascular laboratory data suggesting closer to 50%	CEA may be indicated; assess risk factors
<50% stenosis of carotid artery	Trial of medical therapy
Patients with Asymptomatic Carotid Stenoses	
>80% stenosis of carotid artery	CEA indicated
50–79% stenosis of carotid artery but with vascular laboratory data suggesting closer to 79%	CEA may be indicated; assess risk factors
50–79% stenosis of carotid artery but with vascular laboratory data suggesting closer to 50%	CEA not indicated
<50% stenosis of carotid artery	CEA not indicated

ABBREVIATION: CEA = carotid endarterectomy.

Our current decision making process for patients with carotid disease is outlined in Table 91-1.

With respect to preoperative imaging of patients with carotid disease, the "gold standard," cerebral arteriography, is being utilized less in an effort to reduce both the risk and the cost of the overall procedure. As noted in the previous edition of this text, the Asymptomatic Carotid Atherosclerosis Study (ACAS) and the NASCET study had 1.2 percent and 0.7 percent morbidity rates, respectively from cerebral angiography. A recent evaluation of "silent embolism" after cerebral angiography by Bendszus and colleagues from Germany raised this issue anew. By using sophisticated techniques [diffusion-weighted magnetic resonance imaging (MRI)] both before and after angiography, they were able to demonstrate 42 "bright lesions" in 23 patients (of 100 patients total) after 23 procedures.[24] It is interesting to note that no new neurologic deficits were observed in any of these patients, and the authors suggested that these changes were silent because they were located in "noneloquent brain areas." The frequency of the lesions was correlated with the amount of contrast medium, the amount of time used for fluoroscopy, the number of vessels that proved difficult to probe, and the number of catheters used.

Over the last several years, a number of papers have addressed the issue of carotid endarterectomy without angiography.[25–28] The consensus of opinion is that, with a dedicated vascular laboratory, the great majority of patients (perhaps as many as 90 percent) can be safely evaluated with an ultrasound only. Indications suggesting the need for arteriography include: (1) uncertainty about the accuracy or reliability of the vascular laboratory; (2) uncertainty about possible complete occlusion of the internal carotid artery in a patient with ongoing localizing symptoms; (3) concern about proximal or intrathoracic disease; (4) patients with "technically difficult" studies due to variant arterial anatomy; and (5) patients with symptoms and an indeterminate study.[27]

The great majority of our patients have their carotid endarterectomies done under local anesthesia with light sedation given by the anesthesiologist.[29] Others have utilized cervical block anesthesia with similarly good results.[30,31] We feel that these techniques are safer than a general anesthetic and provide moment-to-moment assessment of the patient's neurologic condition, avoiding the necessity of concern at the end of the case as the patient awakens from general anesthetic. We also shunt the patient routinely (Fig. 91-1), realizing, however, that approximately 80 percent of patients can undergo operation safely without the use of a shunt.

One change that we have made in recent years in our technique of carotid endarterectomy is an increased tendency to patch the carotid after endarterectomy. In years past, our indications for use of the patch were (1) female gender and (2) recurrent stenoses and the necessity for reoperation. Two papers that have been influential in this regard are the work of Moore and colleagues reporting on results of the ACAS study,[32] and the work of AbuRahma and colleagues reporting on a randomized prospective trial of primary closure versus patching.[33] In the former study, the authors were able

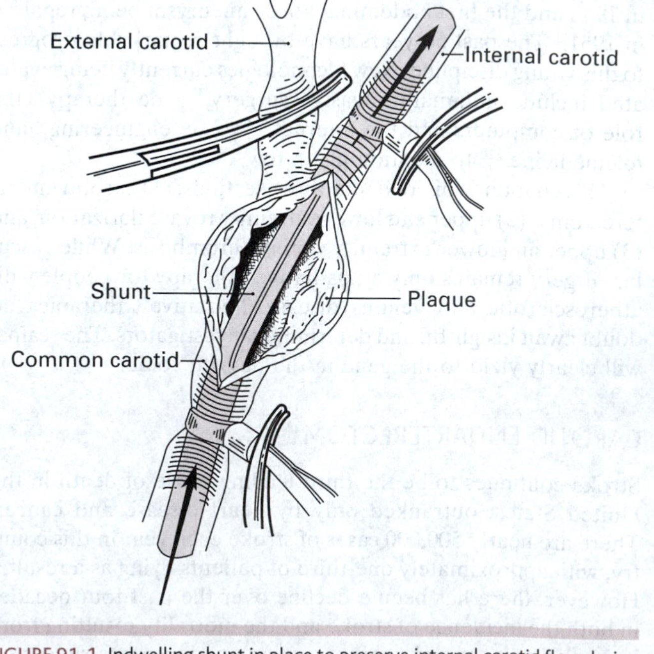

FIGURE 91-1 Indwelling shunt in place to preserve internal carotid flow during the endarterectomy.

to show an overall incidence of recurrent carotid stenosis of 4.5 percent in patients who underwent patch angioplasty, compared with an incidence of 16.9 percent in patients undergoing primary arterial repair. The second report, from West Virginia University, looked at 74 patients undergoing bilateral carotid endarterectomies with primary closure on one side and patch angioplasty on the other. Not only did patch angioplasty have a lower incidence of recurrent stenosis (1 versus 22 percent), but the total internal carotid occlusion rate was lower as well (0 versus 8 percent with primary closure). Addition of a patch adds only a few minutes to the operation, with no increase in perioperative morbidity or mortality rates.

A carotid endarterectomy performed under local anesthesia with intraoperative sedation imposes a low degree of surgical stress on the patient, with only a rare need for blood transfusion. The risk of operation rises with increases in the patient's symptoms: the asymptomatic patient has the lowest risk, about 1 percent perioperative morbidity and mortality rates; the patient with transient ischemic attacks has a perioperative risk of about 3 percent, with a doubling of the yearly stroke risk from 1 percent (in the asymptomatic patient) to 2 percent; the patient who has had a completed stroke has a perioperative risk of about 5 percent, with a yearly stroke risk of 4 percent.[34] For the past several years, we have adopted a clinical pathway for patients undergoing carotid endarterectomy that utilizes the postanesthesia care unit (PACU) for several hours after operation, with subsequent transfer to the vascular surgery ward rather than to the intensive care unit (ICU). Only patients with complications, with coexistent carotid and coronary disease awaiting cardiac surgery, or with instability are admitted to the ICU. While the majority of our patients are discharged on the second postoperative day, other groups have demonstrated the safety and cost reductions possible with discharge within 24 h of operation.[35,36]

The treatment of carotid artery disease represents a benchmark for many other common vascular problems. Large randomized studies were performed to answer difficult questions. The economic milieu made a search for more cost-effective and efficient care a necessity, and we have responded by diminishing invasive preoperative testing and markedly shortening hospital stay, both of which were accomplished without sacrifice of quality of care.[37] Other questions remain to be answered in a similar fashion.

In discussing the "best evidence-based surgical procedure for the prevention of occlusive stroke,"[38] it is important to note that all the questions about carotid disease are not settled, and certainly they never will be. The use of balloon angioplasty for the treatment of vascular stenoses has been a mainstay in the armamentarium of cardiologists and interventional radiologists since Gruentzig's work nearly three decades ago. It is no wonder that lesions in the carotid territory have beckoned to those physicians with catheter-based skills. Surgical investigators, in many cases vascular surgeons worried both about the potential for harm to their patients and about the potential loss of revenue, have expressed concern,[39] have embraced the new technology,[40] or have worked to compare the two competing methods of treatment of carotid disease.[41] One of a series of articles from the University of Alabama in Birmingham by Jordan and his colleagues on this topic showed that percutaneous transluminal angioplasty—in a retrospective review—carried a "significantly higher" neurologic risk than did carotid endarterectomy performed under regional anesthesia. In another study appearing at about the same time,[42] Naylor and colleagues reported on a prospective randomized trial of CEA versus carotid angioplasty in which the trial was stopped because of an increased number of complications in the angioplasty arm. Reporting on only 17 patients, they suspended the trial when 5 of the 7 patients who had carotid angioplasty had a stroke. None of the 10 patients who had carotid endarterectomy had complications.

To address concerns about the potential increased risk of embolic events during percutaneous angioplasty and stenting, some investigators have been evaluating filter devices that could be positioned downstream from the carotid stenosis prior to angioplasty and stenting. One such device was reported on by Ohki and colleagues recently,[43] and their data indicated that 88 percent of the particles liberated during the procedure were captured by their device. This experiment utilized carotid bifurcation plaques obtained from patients after carotid endarterectomy and subjected them to a perfusion circuit with continuous flow through the plaque. Human trials were suggested as the next step.

A statement on this important topic was issued by an American Heart Association Science Advisory group in 1998.[44] They concluded that carotid angioplasty and carotid stenting should, "with rare and infrequent exception," be undertaken only as part of a prospective, randomized trial. In that regard, after a great deal of debate, study, and discussion, our vascular center has decided to enter the Carotid Revascularization Endarterectomy versus Stent Trial (CREST) study.[45] For further discussion of this subject, please see Chap. 92.

UPPER AND LOWER EXTREMITY REVASCULARIZATION

Upper Extremity Revascularization

Chronic arterial insufficiency of the upper extremity is most often due to occlusive disease of the aortic arch branches near their origin, either the subclavian artery or the brachiocephalic trunk. Symptoms may either be limited to ischemic manifestations of the arm and hand or may include posterior circulation insufficiency of the brain due to subclavian steal syndrome. Selection of patients for surgical intervention is extremely important in this group of disorders, since many patients have few or no symptoms and should not be subjected to an operative procedure simply for the correction of an anatomic or radiologic finding.[46,47] Individuals who are significantly limited by arm claudication or those who have symptomatic subclavian steal syndrome should be thoroughly evaluated by vascular examination and complete angiography. Since the patterns of occlusive lesions are extremely variable, any surgical procedure must be carefully planned. Generally, extrathoracic bypass procedures are preferred if a normal donor artery is available; otherwise, a transthoracic procedure may be required to originate a prosthetic bypass from the aortic arch itself. A recent large series of patients with symptomatic atherosclerotic occlusive disease of the innominate artery was presented by Azakie and colleagues, from the University of California at San Francisco.[48] They operated upon 94 patients between 1960 and 1997, performing innominate endarterectomies in 72 patients and bypass grafting in 22 patients. Although there were three perioperative deaths and four strokes (three of which resolved), their long-term results were very good, with freedom from recurrence requiring operation of 99 percent at 5 years and an actuarial survival rate of 85 percent at 5 years. If an extrathoracic bypass is feasible, the operation imposes a low degree of surgical stress, and there is little likelihood of a need for blood transfusions. General anesthesia is preferred, but selected operations for poor-risk patients can be performed with local anesthesia if necessary.

Atheromatous occlusive disease of the subclavian artery is the most common lesion involving the proximal branches of the aortic arch. Extrathoracic revascularization of this vessel can be achieved by one of several techniques, depending on the pattern of obstruction and the relationship of the artery in question to a patent donor vessel. When the ipsilateral common carotid artery is patent and has minimal or no disease, it is frequently chosen as the site of arterial inflow. Perler and colleagues performed carotid-subclavian bypasses or transposition procedures on 31 individuals for a variety of conditions between 1979 and 1989. They achieved relief of symptoms in 30 patients (97 percent), with a symptom-free survival rate of 89 percent at 1 year and 84 percent at 2 years.[49]

Vein grafts are often utilized to improve flow to the upper arm or forearm. Since the demonstration of this technique in 1965 by Garrett, et al.,[50] others have published series of bypass grafts for upper limb ischemia.[51,52] In the largest such series, comprising 74 patients who underwent 95 separate operations over a 15-year period, there were no operative deaths and only a single major amputation. The survival rate was 86 percent at 5 years, with an overall patency rate of 61 percent at that time. Vein grafts were superior at all sites to prostheses.[53] A third alternative (after transthoracic or transsternal operations and extraanatomic bypasses) to improve perfusion to the upper extremity is the utilization of endovascular techniques for aortic arch lesions. A multidisciplinary approach utilizing endovascular techniques for treatment of lesions of the subclavian, innominate, and common carotid arteries was presented by the group from the Cleveland Clinic.[54] In a series of 83 patients, initial technical success was achieved in 82 of 87 procedures (94 percent), but complications occurred in 18 of 87 procedures (20.7 percent), and the 30-day mortality rate for the entire group was 4.8 percent (4 of 83 patients). The investigators acknowledged that there is "no reliable way, short of angiography, to assess anatomic patency" of the vessels that were angioplastied and stented. They also concluded that the results, particularly when complete occlusions were included in the patients being considered for intervention, "seem to favor" surgical treatment.

A more optimistic report, but involving fewer patients, was submitted recently by the cardiology group from the Lahey Clinic. They reported on 18 patients with symptomatic aortic arch vessel stenosis or occlusion.[55] This group of patients represented all patients referred to their practice over a period of 4 years, and all were treated with percutaneous techniques utilizing Palmaz stents. Primary patency was 100 percent with *no* major complications, and, at a mean follow-up of 17 months, all patients were asymptomatic, again, with, 100 percent primary patency (determined by noninvasive studies). The authors concluded by stating that percutaneous stenting should become the "preferred" therapy for the treatment of aortic arch atherosclerotic disease.

Lower Extremity Revascularization

Just as patients with asymptomatic carotid bruits have a higher risk of a cardiac ischemic event than of a stroke,[56] patients with peripheral vascular disease have an increased risk of death from cardiovascular causes. In a study of 565 men and women who were evaluated for the presence of large-vessel peripheral arterial disease (abnormal segment-to-arm blood pressure ratios or abnormal flow velocities), 67 subjects with peripheral arterial disease were identified. During a follow-up of 10 years, 21 of the 34 men (61.8 percent) and 11 of the 33 women (33.3 percent) died. In patients without evidence of arterial disease, the death rates were 16.9 percent for the men and 11.6 percent for the women.[57] The same conclusion was found by Vogt and colleagues, who demonstrated that patients with a diminished ankle-arm blood pressure index of 0.9 or less had a crude overall mortality rate about fivefold greater than that of patients with a higher value of this index.[58] Unfortunately, utilization of the ankle-brachial index (ABI) to follow the progression of lower extremity atherosclerotic disease has been found to be unreliable. In a study of 193 extremities in 114 patients with a mean follow-up of 3.3 years,[59] Porter and colleagues from Portland, Oregon, found that the ABI had a sensitivity of only 41 percent in determining the progression of disease. While the ABI was stated to be "poor" at identifying a *worsening* of vascular disease, it remains an important and easily performed screening test.

Patients with Claudication

A conservative approach to patients with claudication is generally appropriate. This conservatism is based on the fact that the outcome of local disease in the leg is relatively benign, while the outcome for the individual patient is increasingly malignant. A recent article by a TransAtlantic Inter-Society study group[60] noted that, of 100 patients presenting to a physician with claudication, 75 patients would have stability or improvement in the leg over 5 years. Of the 25 whose condition would deteriorate over this period of time, only 5 patients would require an intervention, and only 2 would require amputation. With respect to "systemic outcome," the outlook is not so sanguine. Thirty of the patients will die within 5 years, and 5 to 10 of the individuals will have a nonfatal cardiovascular event within this period of time. The majority of the deaths will be due, of course, to cardiac events.

Given that the symptom of claudication is such an ominous predictor of widespread vascular disease, risk-factor modification is the first step in the treatment of such patients. Of the four factors that are involved in patients with claudication—smoking, diabetes, dyslipidemia, and hypertension—*tobacco use is the single most important factor*.[61] In fact, patients who continue to smoke have double (60 percent) the 5-year mortality rate of patients who are able to stop smoking. Likewise, tight control of diabetes, utilization of statin agents to treat hyperlipidemia, and treatment of hypertension are all directed toward reducing further atherosclerosis, particularly in the cerebral and coronary beds.

After control of risk factors, an exercise program is the next step in the effective treatment of the claudicant. In an interesting study carried out by both the Department of Surgery and the Department of Psychiatry and Behavioral Medicine at Brown

University,[62] Patterson and colleagues found that both patients who exercised at home and those who exercised under supervision improved after a 12-week period of time. The degree of improvement was more marked in those patients who were supervised (280 percent increase) than in those who exercised at home (170 percent increase). Depending upon the degree of limitation imposed by the claudication, either type of program may be of benefit.

The next concern in the treatment of patients with claudication is the consideration of pharmacologic therapy. Pentoxifylline (Trental) was the first drug approved for treatment of claudication in the United States, but we have largely discontinued using this agent because of its cost as well as its limited clinical benefit. A relatively new drug, cilostazol (Pletal) has now been approved for use in patients with claudication, and it seems to have real potential. In a multicenter, randomized, double-blind placebo controlled trial conducted by Money and colleagues, it was found that cilostazol "significantly increased" absolute claudication distance at all measured time points.[63] Because cilostazol is a phosphodiesterase inhibitor, it should not, however, be administered in patients with congestive heart failure (see also Chap. 90).

The final issue in the evaluation of patients with claudication is that of potential intervention with an operative or endovascular approach to the underlying atherosclerotic lesion. This has been and remains a controversial topic, perhaps even more so in light of the increasing interest in catheter-based therapies. Two recent papers have addressed the topic of operative intervention. The first, from Charleston, West Virginia,[64] was an interesting study that compared patients with bilateral claudication who had saphenous vein grafts placed on one side and polytetrafluoroethylene (PTFE) grafts on the other. These were really "ideal" patients, since they were required to have two- to three-vessel runoff before entry into the study. There were no operative deaths or perioperative amputations for either procedure, and both grafts were found to have "comparable" patencies with identical limb salvage (98 percent) at 72 months. The second paper, from Shah and colleagues at Albany,[65] evaluated 409 infrainguinal reconstructions for claudication and was designed to answer the rhetorical question, "Is it worth the risk?" In this large series, they had only one limb lost due to embolization and no operative deaths. Their conclusions, even acknowledging that 18 percent of their interventions required second procedures, were that infrainguinal bypass grafting procedures were "valid treatment options" in selected patients with claudication. Contradicting what we stated earlier about the poor long-term survival in patients with claudication, they had a 93 percent cumulative patient survival rate at 4 years, compared with a 65 percent cumulative patient survival rate when operative intervention was required for limb salvage.

Percutaneous transluminal angioplasty (PTA) in patients with claudication was addressed by Whyman and colleagues in a randomized controlled trial.[66] Sixty-two patients with short femoral artery stenoses or occlusions and iliac stenoses were randomized to either PTA plus medical therapy or to medical therapy alone. At 2 years of follow-up, the PTA group and the control group "did not differ significantly" in the four categories analyzed. They concluded by stating that the addition of angioplasty to conventional medical treatment "does not confer a measurable benefit in the patient's perceived or measured walking ability after 2 years." They also acknowledged that a large randomized trial would be needed in order to settle the issue of which, if any, patients might benefit from angioplasty.

A recent paper by Golledge and colleagues, from London, looked directly at the outcomes of femoropopliteal angioplasty in 43 patients with intermittent claudication, 4 with rest pain, and 27 patients with tissue loss.[67] Although "technical success" was achieved in 67 patients (91 percent), failure of the procedure occurred in the remaining 7 patients. With respect to the 43 patients with claudication, 9 of the 43 patients with intermittent claudication still had symptoms at 1 year. Seven other patients with claudication required another intervention. In 27 of the 43 patients (63 percent), the claudication had resolved. Considering all patients, symptomatic improvement was found in only 51 percent of patients 1 year from the time of angioplasty, although approximately two-thirds of patients with intermittent claudication were symptom free at 12 months. The authors suggested that a longer period of follow-up would be required to assess durability of the angioplasty procedure.

TABLE 91-2 Outcome after Lower Extremity Revascularization

Author	Study Size	Study Methods	Results
Nicoloff et al. 1998[71]	112 patients	112 consecutive patients who underwent bypass surgery for limb salvage	7 deaths (6%); 75 patients (67%) ambulatory and 30 (27%) nonambulatory at last follow-up; ideal results felt to be "infrequent"
Pomposelli et al. 1998[69]	262 patients	262 patients, 80 years old or older, who had 299 lower extremity bypass operations; limb salvage was the indication in 96%	Limb salvage rate at 5 years 92%; patient survival 44%; patients with poor levels of ambulatory status preoperatively more likely to end up nonambulatory or to require nursing home care
Seabrook et al. 1999[70]	70 patients	70 patients who had successful in situ saphenous vein bypasses for limb-threatening ischemia	37 of 69 patients (53%) reporting no problems with revascularized limb; a significant proportion requiring the assistance of a cane, walker, or wheelchair for mobility

Patients with Rest Pain

Ischemic rest pain is frequently an intolerable symptom and implies potential loss of the foot or limb. Whereas patients with claudication are generally managed in a conservative or nonoperative manner, patients with rest pain or a nonhealing lesion are evaluated for a potential operation, frequently as outpatients in the increasingly cost-conscious environment. The question of amputation versus revascularization for rest pain or a nonhealing lesion arises, especially in the elderly.

In the previous edition of this text, we stated that about 95 percent of patients with rest pain should have an attempt at revascularization, while the remaining 5 percent, for reasons of their moribund condition, little chance of functional recovery, or irretrievable limb ischemia, should undergo amputation. We still feel that this is the correct approach, but our outlook on this aggressive approach has been colored by information gained from a number of centers in this country. The data are summarized in Table 91-2.[68–70] Basically, all the studies suggest that operation for limb salvage is a major operative intervention, and that many of these patients have "functional disabilities" that mandate continued close observation and care. One of the authors stated that "it is abundantly clear that limb-threatening ischemia is a manifestation of atherosclerosis that occurs in patients who are approaching the end of life, at a time when functional status is frequently declining rapidly and interval survival is short."[71] In an attempt to better delineate who might benefit from lower extremity bypass procedures, Kalman and colleagues, from Toronto, looked at 358 consecutive in-situ distal leg bypass procedures from 1986 to 1995.[72] They asserted that four significant variables were associated with a late lower survival rate: male gender, diabetes, chronic renal insufficiency, and a history of cerebrovascular disease. When all four variables were present, the predicted 5-year survival rate was reduced to 2 percent. The paper concluded that these variables *were* predictive of lower late survival rates and that they might be used in the decision for either revascularization or amputation.

As noted earlier, we are in a period of transition in terms of the imaging of carotid artery disease, and approaches to imaging of the vasculature of the extremities are also evolving. We continue to order arteriograms to assess the vasculature of the arms and legs, but magnetic resonance angiography (MRA) with contrast agent enhancement may ultimately supplant contrast arteriography (Fig. 91-2).[73,74] MRA has also been utilized in graft surveillance, with an accuracy of 95 percent when combined with color-flow duplex imaging.[75] We currently utilize MRA to identify runoff vessels in patients who are otherwise candidates for revascularization but in whom contrast angiography has been of poor quality or has failed to demonstrate patent runoff vessels. The utility of MRA in this setting has been confirmed by investigators who noted a limb-salvage rate of 78 percent in patients with angiographically occult runoff vessels that were detectable by MRA.[76]

Although we prefer to utilize the greater saphenous vein as a conduit in almost all infrainguinal bypasses, there are a number of alternatives. In situations where there is inadequate autogenous material available for bypass, utilization of PTFE below the knee, in one recent series, yielded a 2-year patency of 52 percent with a limb-salvage rate of 62 percent.[77] While most investigators acknowledge the relatively poor long-term results with PTFE bypasses to infrapopliteal arteries, some authors still recommend its utilization in the above-knee position.[78,79]

Other options include the use of arm and lesser saphenous vein grafts[80]; composite sequential bypass utilizing vein sewn to PTFE[81]; use of an anastomotic vein patch, as popularized by Taylor and colleagues[82]; umbilical vein grafts[83];

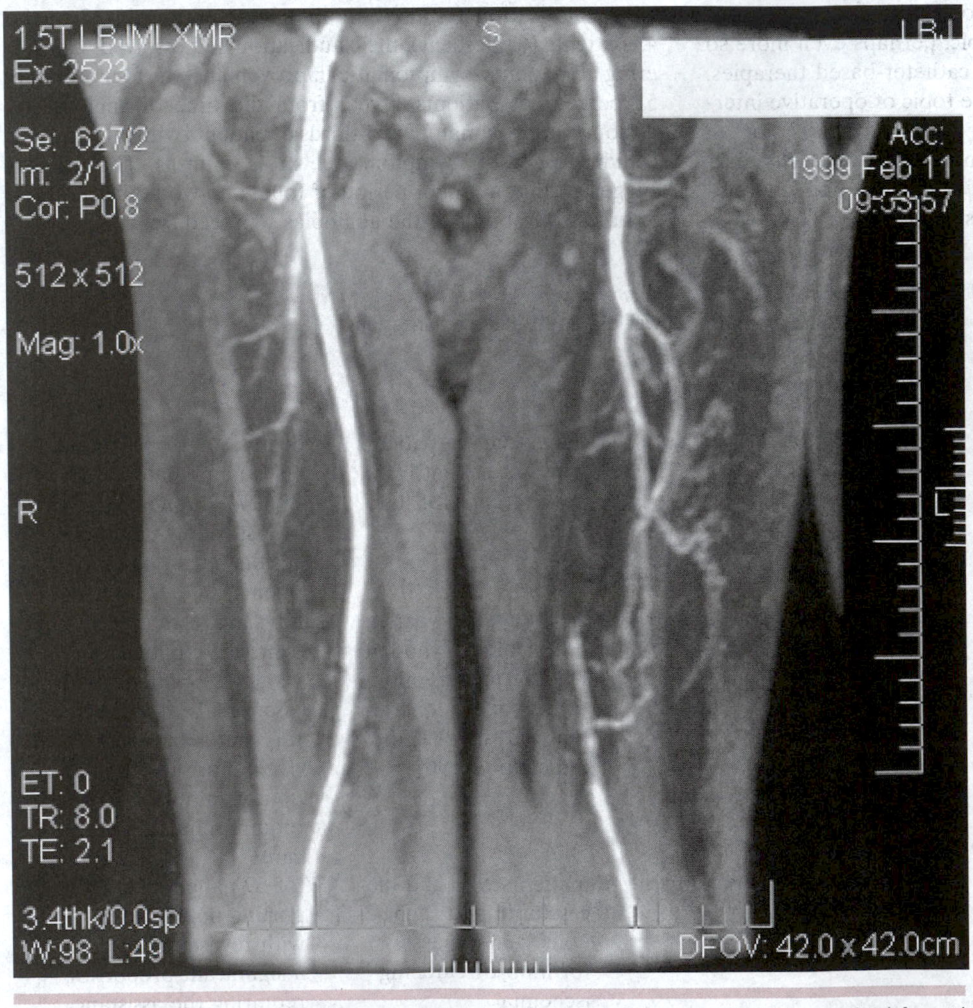

FIGURE 91-2 Magnetic resonance angiogram with gadolinium enhancement, showing left superficial femoral artery (SFA) occlusion in a patient with rest pain.

distal venous arterialization,[84] and cryopreserved vein allografts.[85,86] With respect to the latter, Carpenter and colleagues have documented a primary graft patency at 1 year of 13 percent and a limb-salvage rate of 42 percent. In his more recent paper, he endeavored to define the immune response to allograft bypass and concluded that the allografts are immunogenic and prompt a T cell–mediated response. He suggested that it may be possible to modify the factor of rejection by the use of immunosuppressive medication. In a recent report by Castier, he and his colleagues, from Clichy, France, used cryopreserved *arterial* allografts in 32 patients with limb-threatening ischemia between 1993 and 1997.[87] While arterial dilatation occurred in two patent grafts (requiring replacement), the overall primary patency was 57 percent at 12 months and 39 percent at 18 months. This work remains investigational.

In the largest series on long-term results of in-situ saphenous vein bypass grafts, Shah et al. documented a cumulative secondary patency rate of 91 and 81 percent at 1 and 5 years, respectively, and a limb-salvage rate of 97 and 95 percent at 1 and 5 years, respectively.[88] These results continue to set the standard for infrainguinal reconstruction performed today. It has also been shown in a prospective, randomized, multicenter study that a comparison of in-situ (Fig. 91-3) and reversed saphenous vein bypasses revealed "no significant differences" in overall patency rates.[89] The authors concluded that surgeons should therefore be adept at both procedures. We are increasingly utilizing "vein mapping" to help locate acceptable venous conduits preoperatively; these veins include the accessory ipsilateral greater saphenous vein, the contralateral greater saphenous vein, the lesser saphenous vein, and arm veins. Again, Shah et al. have shown that utilization of "spliced" excised vein segments will yield a primary patency rate of 72 percent at 1 year and 45 percent at 4 years.[90] At present, there seem to be few fundamental impediments to the ability of vascular surgeons to operate on distal extremity vasculature. Intensive surveillance, involving utilization of duplex scanning of vein grafts at 1 month, 3 months, 6 months, and every 6 months thereafter, seems to aid in detecting graft-threatening lesions, although it also adds to cost.[91]

We have also learned, since the publication of the last edition of this text, that the addition of anticoagulation to patients in a high-risk setting after infrainguinal bypass grafting may be beneficial in promoting graft patency. In a randomized prospective trial carried out by Sarac and colleagues, from the University of Florida, the authors were able to show that, while perioperative therapy with heparin increased the wound hematoma rate, long-term anticoagulation with warfarin improved both the patency rate and the limb-salvage rate in patients at high risk for graft thrombosis.[92] A recent meta-analysis confirmed this finding and also suggested that platelet inhibitors reduced the risk of graft occlusion after infrainguinal bypass surgery.[93]

Angioplasty of the femoral, popliteal, and even tibioperoneal vessels has been recommended by some investigators.[94–99] Randomized controlled trials are needed to determine the efficacy of these approaches.[100] Endovascular techniques such as stent placement[101] and percutaneous femoropopliteal graft placement[102,103] are also being evaluated in patients with femoral and popliteal artery disease. Cost-effective analyses of femoropopliteal revascularization procedures are now available, and more are to follow.[104,105]

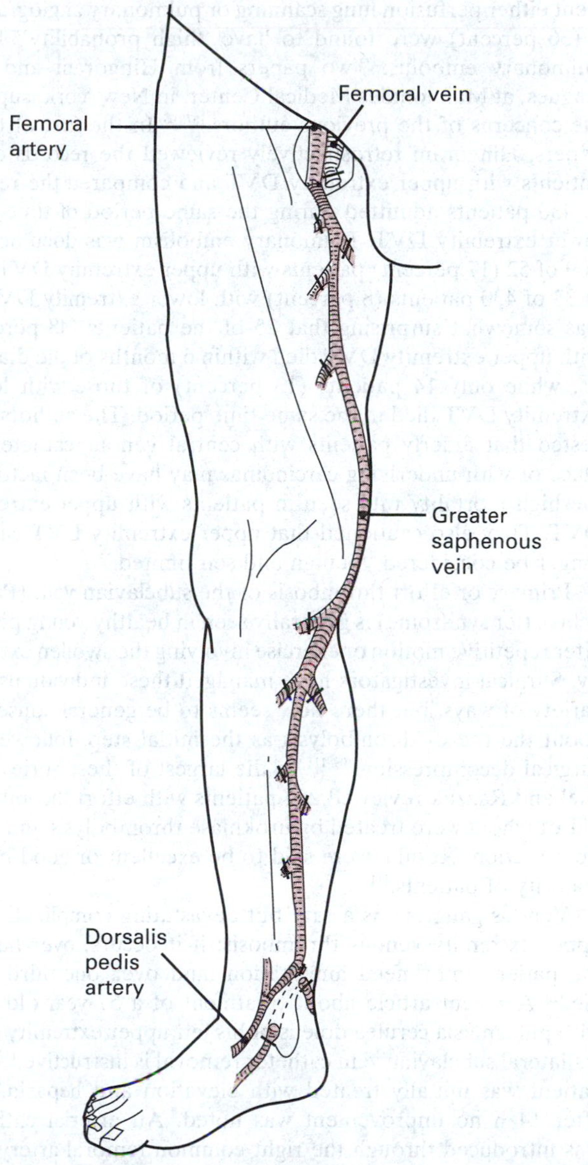

FIGURE 91-3 In-situ bypass from femoral artery to dorsalis pedis artery.

UPPER AND LOWER EXTREMITY VENOUS THROMBOSIS

Upper Extremity Venous Thrombosis

Deep venous thrombosis (DVT) of the upper extremity was thought in the past to be a rare event and to have a relatively benign outcome. However, recent information from both the United States and other countries challenges these assumptions. In a report from Padua, Italy, Prandoni and colleagues evaluated 58 patients suspected of having upper extremity DVT in the years 1990 to 1994.[106] Their evaluations revealed that 27 of the 58 patients (47 percent) had thrombosis and that central venous catheters, "thrombophilic states," and previous lower extremity thromboses were all associated with the development of upper extremity thrombosis. Of the 22 patients who underwent either perfusion lung scanning or pulmonary angiography, 8 (36 percent) were found to have "high probability" for a pulmonary embolus. Two papers from Hingorani and colleagues, at Maimonides Medical Center, in New York, support the concerns of the previous authors.[107,108] In the first of these papers, Hingorani retrospectively reviewed the records of 52 patients with upper extremity DVT and compared the results to 430 patients admitted during the same period of time with lower extremity DVT. Pulmonary embolism was documented in 9 of 52 (17 percent) patients with upper extremity DVT and in 33 of 430 patients (8 percent) with lower extremity DVT. It was somewhat surprising that 25 of the patients (48 percent) with upper extremity DVT died within 6 months of the diagnosis, while only 14 patients (13 percent) of those with lower extremity DVT died in the same time period. The authors suggested that elderly patients with central venous catheters in place or with underlying carcinomas may have been factors in the high mortality rate seen in patients with upper extremity DVT. They also cautioned that upper extremity DVT can no longer be considered "benign and self-limited."

Primary or effort thrombosis of the subclavian vein (Paget-Schroetter syndrome) is generally seen in healthy young people after repetitive motion or exercise involving the swollen extremity. Surgical investigators have managed these individuals in a variety of ways, but there now seems to be general consensus about the use of thrombolysis as the initial step, followed by surgical decompression.[109–111] In the largest of these series, Urchel and Razzuk reviewed 264 patients with effort thrombosis, 211 of whom were treated by urokinase thrombolysis and first-rib resection. Results were said to be excellent or good in the majority of patients.[111]

Venous gangrene is a rare but devastating complication of upper extremity venous thrombosis; if it occurs, over half of the patients may need amputation, and over one-third may die.[112] A recent article about treatment of a 57-year-old man with phlegmasia cerulea dolens of his left upper extremity after ipsilateral subclavian vein catheter removal is instructive.[113] The patient was initially treated with elevation and heparin, and after 14 h no improvement was noted. An arterial catheter was introduced through the right common femoral artery and positioned in the left brachial artery, and an infusion of urokinase was started. After 12 h the extremity was improved, and within 4 days the extremity appeared normal. While urokinase is not currently available, this case does illustrate the potential limb-saving ability of this and other thrombolytic agents.

Patients who develop upper extremity DVT and have contraindications to or unsuccessful use of anticoagulation have been a significant source of concern. A recent paper by Spence and associates, from Cleveland,[114] showed that superior vena cava filters can be successfully placed without undue difficulty, and, in their series of 41 patients, using four different types of filters, they had no complications and no clinical evidence of pulmonary embolism or superior vena cava syndrome.

Lower Extremity Venous Thrombosis

DVT (see also Chap. 90) of the lower extremities is an insidious and potentially lethal problem in hospitalized patients. It has been estimated that there are approximately 600,000 cases of venous thromboembolism in the United States each year.[115] Risk factors have been detailed in multiple publications and include age above 40, past history of DVT, general anesthesia, operations, pregnancy, malignant disease, hypercoagulable states, and trauma.[115] With respect to patients with cancer, an important nationwide study of patients with DVT was undertaken in Denmark to look at the potential association of primary venous thrombosis and the subsequent diagnosis of cancer.[116] Although they found the expected "strong associations" with cancers of the pancreas, ovary, liver, and brain, they concluded that an "aggressive search" for a hidden malignancy in a patient with a primary DVT was not cost effective and was therefore not indicated. Hypercoagulable states (Fig. 91-4) have received renewed attention in recent years.[115–121] A relatively new addition to abnormalities in coagulation occurred with the discovery of factor V Leiden, and this abnormality has been found in about one-fifth of patients with venous thrombosis. In an attempt to look at the risk of recurrent venous thrombosis in patients who carried the mutation, Simioni and colleagues searched for factor V Leiden in 251 unselected patients who had had a first episode of symptomatic DVT diagnosed by venography.[122] They found the mutation in 41 of the patients (16.3 percent), and, after a follow-up of 8 years, approximately 40 percent of patients had had recurrent venous thrombosis, compared to an incidence of recurrence of 18 percent in patients who did not have this mutation.

In a more recent attempt to clarify the risk of recurrent DVT in patients with and without genetic mutations, De Stefano and colleagues looked at a retrospective cohort of 624 patients who had had a first episode of DVT.[123] They looked at patients who were heterozygous carriers of factor V Leiden, patients who were heterozygous for both factor V Leiden and a prothrombin mutation, and patients who had neither mutation. In contradistinction to the previous study, they found that the risk of recurrent DVT was similar among carriers of factor V Leiden and patients without the mutation. Carriers of both factor V Leiden

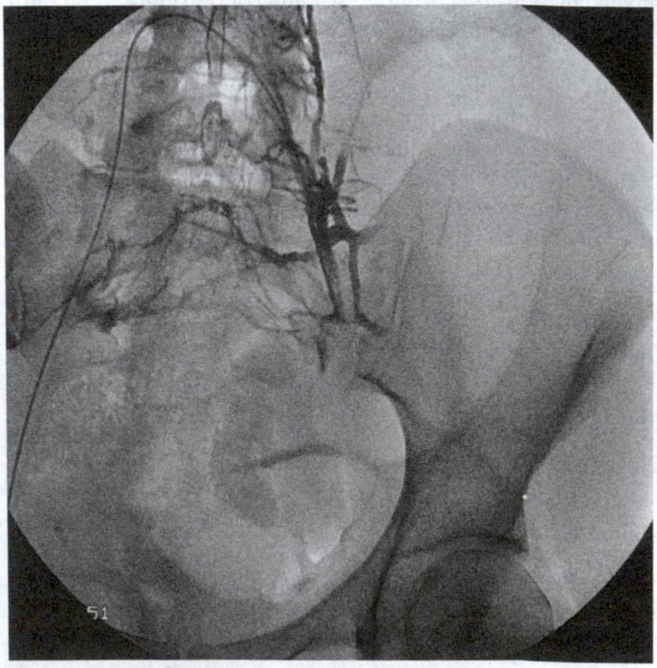

FIGURE 91-4 Venogram in a 31-year-old woman with a swollen leg, hypercoagulable state, and left iliac vein occlusion.

and the prothrombin mutation were, however, at an increased risk of recurrent DVT, and they recommended consideration of lifelong anticoagulation. Studies have documented DVT in 58 percent of trauma patients,[124] 11 percent of patients undergoing lower extremity amputation,[125] and 33 percent of patients in a medical ICU.[126] An excellent overview of the multifactoral nature of venous thrombosis was recently provided by Rosendaal, from Leiden University Medical Center, in the Netherlands.[127]

Patients with DVT are effectively treated by heparin given either by continuous intravenous infusion or by subcutaneous injection. The past decade has brought a number of changes in the therapeutic approach to patients with clot in major lower extremity veins: a 5-day course of heparin has been shown to be as effective as a 10-day course[128]; 6 months of oral anticoagulant therapy has been shown to have a lower recurrence rate than the same dose given for 6 weeks[129]; and low-molecular-weight heparin has been found effective in treating patients at home with proximal DVT.[130,131] Low-molecular-weight heparin has also been shown to be efficacious in reducing the risk of venous thromboembolism in patients with acute medical illnesses,[132] and in a recent head-to-head comparison between enoxaparin and coumadin, enoxaparin-treated patients had a lower recurrence rate of symptomatic venous thromboembolism as well as a lower incidence of bleeding.[133] A review of low-molecular-weight heparins and a look at "new" antithrombotic agents have been provided by Hirsh and colleagues, from Hamilton, Ontario.[134,135]

In recent years, there has been some enthusiasm for lytic therapy in patients with DVT. The reasoning has been that lytic therapy could lyse the clot, restore normalcy to the leg and, more importantly perhaps, to the valves of the affected leg, thereby reducing the long-term sequelae of DVT, primarily the postphlebitic syndrome, which manifests as edema, hyperpigmentation, and ulceration and occurs in up to one-third of patients (Fig. 91-5).[136] The obvious issue is weighing the risks of lytic therapy against the chronic problems of the postphlebitic syndrome. In an attempt to assemble data from a large number of patients who have undergone thrombolytic therapy for lower

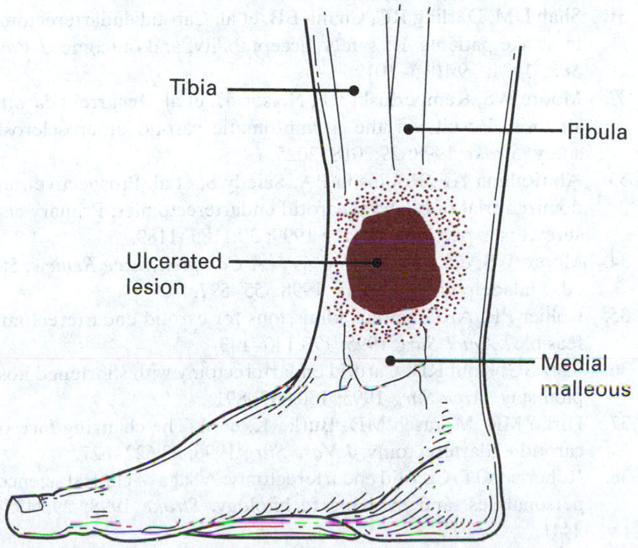

FIGURE 91-5 Venous stasis ulceration of the lower extremity after an episode of deep venous thrombosis.

extremity DVT, Mewissen and colleagues formed a venous registry and collected data from 63 centers.[137] After 312 urokinase infusions in 303 limbs of 287 patients, they found that complete lysis was achieved in 96 infusions (31 percent) and that "major" bleeding complications, most often at the puncture site, occurred in 54 patients (11 percent). Six of the patients (1 percent) developed pulmonary emboli, and there were two deaths, one from an intracranial hemorrhage and one from a pulmonary embolus. While the authors concluded that catheter-directed therapy is "safe and effective," there is currently little unanimity of opinion on this topic.

This issue was also addressed by O'Meara et al., who used decision analysis after estimating the probabilities of various adverse outcomes of treatment and found that all 36 patients interviewed were unwilling to accept an increased risk of death from lytic therapy in order to avoid the postphlebitic syndrome. In other words, in this study, all the patients selected heparin when presented with the data.[138] A recent report describing a spontaneous spinal epidural hematoma with subsequent paraplegia in an 18-year-old female after heparin and urokinase therapy for DVT lends credence to their decision.[139]

The two ends of the spectrum in patients with DVT are represented by patients with clot in their calf veins or clot in the superficial veins of the leg and patients with near total venous occlusion. While patients with clot in their calf veins and patients with clot in the superficial veins are often viewed as having benign problems, data collected over the past decade have suggested that this may be a false assumption. In one study conducted at the beginning of the last decade, investigators showed that 24 (32 percent) of 75 patients with lower extremity calf vein thrombi had propagation of their thrombi, and 11 of those 24 (46 percent) had propagation into the popliteal or larger veins of the thigh.[140] Three recent papers that looked at patients with superficial thrombophlebitis documented a high incidence of hypercoagulability in such patients,[141] extension into the common femoral vein in 9 percent of cases with pulmonary emboli in 10 percent of that group,[142] and an unexpectedly high incidence of pulmonary emboli (33 percent) in 7 of 21 patients with superficial thrombophlebitis studied by perfusion lung scanning.[143] Observations such as these would suggest that calf vein thrombi and superficial thrombi are not benign problems.

Patients with extensive clot in the lower extremities may go on to phlegmasia cerulea dolens or acute iliofemoral venous thrombosis. This condition, which is characterized by near total venous occlusion, may lead to total venous occlusion and venous gangrene. Venous thrombectomy for this condition has received renewed enthusiasm in the surgical literature,[144,145] but lytic therapy[146,147] and nonoperative therapy[148] also have their proponents.

While heparin and warfarin sodium are excellent therapy for the majority of patients with DVT, not all patients can tolerate the complications of these agents. Such patients include individuals with recent trauma, active bleeding, or hemolysis; those with complications of heparin therapy; and those with inferior vena caval clot or iliofemoral venous thrombosis.

For these patients, the treatment of choice is often the placement of a vena cava filter. In a review of their 20-year experience, Greenfield and colleagues noted a caval patency rate of 96 percent, with a rate of recurrent emboli of 4 percent.[149] There was no procedural mortality rate, and the morbidity rate was minimal. In an attempt to answer some of the questions surrounding the use of vena cava filters, Decousus and colleagues randomly assigned 400 patients with proximal DVT who were at risk for pulmonary emboli to receive a vena cava filter (200 patients) or no filter (200 patients), and, in a second aspect of the study, patients were also assigned to receive low-molecular-weight heparin or unfractionated heparin.[150] While the patients who received vena cava filters had a lower incidence of pulmonary emboli by day 12 (1.1 percent versus 4.8 percent for those who did not receive filters), there was an increased incidence of recurrent DVT in the patients receiving filters. There were no significant differences in mortality rates or other outcomes. Low-molecular-weight heparin produced a better outcome in terms of the incidence of symptomatic or asymptomatic pulmonary embolism at day 12 and also for recurrent venous thrombosis, but the results were not statistically significant. In a follow-up editorial on this subject, Haire suggested that only "well-designed comparative trials" could give us the necessary information on which to base our clinical decisions about the proper use of vena cava filters.[151]

References

1. Editors. Looking back on the millennium in medicine. *N Engl J Med* 2000; 342:42–49.
2. Friedman S. *A History of Vascular Surgery*. New York: Futura; 1989.
3. Rattner DW. Future directions in innovative minimally invasive surgery. *Lancet* 1999; 353(suppl I):12–15.
4. Hollingsworth SJ, Barker SGE. Gene therapy: Into the future of surgery. *Lancet* 1999; 353(suppl I):19–20.
5. Schneider JR, Lindsay TF. The internet and vascular surgery: A brief description of the internet, the world wide web, and some of the vascular surgical resources available. *Vasc Surg* 1997; 31:605–613.
6. Soot LC, Moneta GL, Edwards JM. Vascular surgery and the internet: A poor source of patient-oriented information. *J Vasc Surg* 1999; 30:84–91.
7. Veldenz HC, Dennis JW. The internet and education in surgery. *Am Surgeon* 1998; 64:877–880.
8. Kaihara S, Vacanti JP. Tissue engineering: Toward new solutions for transplantation and reconstructive surgery. *Arch Surg* 1999; 134:1184–1188.
9. Deaton DH, Balch D, Kesler C, et al. Telemedicine and endovascular aortic grafting. *Am J Surg* 1999; 177:75–77.
10. Wirthlin DJ, Buradagunta S, Edwards RA, et al. Telemedicine in vascular surgery: Feasibility of digital imaging for remote management of wounds. *J Vasc Surg* 1998; 27:1089–1100.
11. Isner JM, Baumgartner I, Rauh G, et al. Treatment of thromboangiitis obliterans (Buerger's disease) by intramuscular gene transfer of vascular endothelial growth factor: Preliminary clinical results. *J Vasc Surg* 1998; 28:964–975.
12. Bronner LL, Kanter DS, Manson JE. Primary prevention of stroke. *N Engl J Med* 1995; 333:1392–1400.
13. Brown RD, Whisnant JP, Sicks JD, et al. Stroke incidence, prevalence, and survival: Secular trends in Rochester, Minnesota, through 1989. *Stroke* 1996; 27:373–380.
14. Bonita R, Beaglehole R. The enigma of the decline in stroke deaths in the United States: The search for an explanation. *Stroke* 1996; 27:370–372.
15. The CASANOVA Study Group. Carotid surgery versus medical therapy in asymptomatic carotid stenosis. *Stroke* 1991; 22:1229–1235.
16. Hobson RW II, Weiss DG, Fields WS, et al. Efficacy of carotid endarterectomy for asymptomatic carotid stenosis. *N Engl J Med* 1993; 328:221–279.
17. Executive Committee for the Asymptomatic Carotid Atherosclerosis Study. Endarterectomy for asymptomatic carotid artery stenosis. *JAMA* 1995; 273:1421–1428.
18. Mayberg MR, Wilson SE, Yatsu F, et al. Carotid endarterectomy and prevention of cerebral ischemia in symptomatic carotid stenosis. *JAMA* 1991; 266:3289–3294.
19. European Carotid Surgery Trialists' Collaborative Group. MRC European carotid surgery trial: Interim results for symptomatic patients with severe (70–99%) or with mild (0–29%) carotid stenosis. *Lancet* 1991; 337:1235–1243.
20. North American Symptomatic Carotid Endarterectomy Trial Collaborators. Beneficial effect of carotid endarterectomy in symptomatic patients with high-grade carotid stenosis. *N Engl J Med* 1991; 325:445–453.
21. Barnett HJM, Taylor DW, Eliasziw M, et al. Benefit of carotid endarterectomy in patients with symptomatic moderate or severe stenosis. *N Engl J Med* 1998; 339:1415–1425.
22. Chassin MR. Appropriate use of carotid endarterectomy. *N Engl J Med* 1998; 339:1468–1471.
23. Barnett HJM, Taylor DW, Eliasziw M, et al. Benefit of carotid endarterectomy in patients with symptomatic moderate or severe stenosis. *N Engl J Med* 1998; 339:1415–1425.
24. Bendszus M, Koltzenburg MY, Burger R, et al. Silent embolism in diagnostic cerebral angiography and neurointerventional procedures: A prospective study. *Lancet* 1999; 354:1594–1597.
25. Zwolak RM. Carotid endarterectomy without angiography: Are we ready? *Vasc Surg* 1997; 31:1–9.
26. Elmore JR, Franklin DP, Thomas DD, et al. Carotid Endarterectomy: The mandate for high quality duplex. *Ann Vasc Surg* 1998; 12:156–162.
27. Collier PE. Changing trends in the use of preoperative carotid arteriography: The community experience. *Cardiovasc Surg* 1998; 6:485–489.
28. Ballotta E, Da Giau G, Abbruzzese E, et al. Carotid endarterectomy without angiography: Can clinical evaluation and duplex ultrasonographic scanning alone replace traditional arteriography for carotid surgery workup? *Surg* 1999; 126:20–27.
29. Chaikof EL Dodson TF, Thomas BL, et al. Four steps to local anesthesia for endarterectomy of the carotid artery. *Surg Gynecol Obstet* 1993; 177:308–310.
30. Allen BT, Anderson CB, Rubin VG, et al. The influence of anesthetic technique on perioperative complications after carotid endarterectomy. *J Vasc Surg* 1994; 19:834–843.
31. Shah DM, Darling RC, Chang BB, et al. Carotid endarterectomy in awake patients: Its safety, acceptability, and outcome. *J Vasc Surg* 1994; 19:1015–1019.
32. Moore WS, Kempczinski RF, Nelson JJ, et al. Recurrent carotid stenosis: Results of the asymptomatic carotid atherosclerosis study. *Stroke* 1998; 29:2018–2025.
33. AbuRahma AF, Robinson PA, Saiedy S, et al. Prospective randomized trial of bilateral carotid endarterectomies: Primary closure versus patching. *Stroke* 1999; 30:1185–1189.
34. Moore WS, ed. *Vascular Surgery: A Comprehensive Review*, 5th ed. Philadelphia: Saunders; 1998:555–597.
35. Collier PE. Are one-day admissions for carotid endarterectomy feasible? *Am J Surg* 1995; 170:140–143.
36. Katz SG, Kohl RD. Carotid endarterectomy with shortened hospital stay. *Arch Surg* 1995; 130:887–891.
37. Hirko MK, Morasch MD, Burke K. et al. The changing face of carotid endarterectomy. *J Vasc Surg* 1996; 23:622–627.
38. Robertson JT. Carotid endarterectomy: A saga of clinical science, personalities, and evolving technology. *Stroke* 1998; 29:2435–2441.
39. Beebe HG. The carotid angioplasty premise. *Vasc Surg* 1996; 30:269–273.
40. Criado FJ, Wellons E, Clark NS, et al. Evolving indication for

and early results of carotid artery stenting. *Am J Surg* 1997; 174:111–114.
41. Jordan WD Jr, Voellinger DC, Fisher WS, et al. A comparison of carotid angioplasty with stenting versus endarterectomy with regional anesthesia. *J Vasc Surg* 1998; 28:397–403.
42. Naylor AR, Bolia A, Abbott RJ, et al. Randomized study of carotid angioplasty and stenting versus carotid endarterectomy: A stopped trial. *J Vasc Surg* 1998; 28:326–334.
43. Ohki T, Roubin GS, Veith FJ, et al. Efficacy of a filter device in the prevention of embolic events during carotid angioplasty and stenting: An ex vivo analysis. *J Vasc Surg* 1999; 30:1034–1044.
44. Bettmann MA, Katzen BT, Whisnant J, et al. Carotid stenting and angioplasty: A statement for health care professionals from the Councils on Cardiovascular Radiology, Stroke, Cardiothoracic and Vascular Surgery, Epidemiology and Prevention, and Clinical Cardiology, American Heart Association. *Stroke* 1998; 29:336–338.
45. Hobson RW II, Brott T, Ferguson R, et al. CREST: Carotid revascularization endarterectomy versus stent trial. *Cardiovasc Surg* 1997; 5:457–458.
46. Fields WS, Lemak NA. Joint study of extracranial arterial occlusion. *JAMA* 1972; 222:1139–1143.
47. Hafner CD. Subclavian steal syndrome. *Arch Surg* 1976; 111:1074–1080.
48. Azakie A, McElhinney DB, Higashima R, et al. Innominate artery reconstruction: Over 3 decades of experience. *Ann Surg* 1998; 228:402–410.
49. Perler BA, Williams GM. Carotid-subclavian bypass: A decade of experience. *J Vasc Surg* 1990; 12:716–723.
50. Garrett ED, Morris GC, Howell JF, et al. Revascularization of upper extremity with autogenous vein bypass graft. *Arch Surg* 1965; 91:751–757.
51. McCarthy WJ, Flinn WR, Yao JST, et al. Result of bypass grafting for upper limb ischemia. *J Vasc Surg* 1986; 3:741–746.
52. Katz SG, Kohl RD. Direct revascularization for the treatment of forearm and hand ischemia. *Am J Surg* 1993; 165:313–316.
53. Mesh CL, McCarthy WJ, Pearce WH, et al. Upper extremity bypass grafting: A 15-year experience. *Arch Surg* 1993; 128: 795–802.
54. Sullivan TM, Gray BH, Bacharach M, et al. Angioplasty and primary stenting of the subclavian, innominate, and common carotid arteries in 83 patients. *J Vasc Surg* 1998; 28:1059–1065.
55. Hadjipetrou P, Cox S, Piemonte T, et al. Percutaneous revascularization of atherosclerotic obstruction of aortic arch vessels. *J Am Coll Cardiol* 1999; 33:1238–1245.
56. Chambers BR, Norris JW. Outcome in patients with asymptomatic neck bruits. *N Engl J Med* 1986; 9:860–865.
57. Criqui MH, Langer RD, Fronek A, et al. Mortality over a period of 10 years in patients with peripheral arterial disease. *N Engl J Med* 1992; 326:381–386.
58. Vogt MT, Cauley JA, Newman AB, et al. Decreased ankle/arm blood pressure index and mortality in elderly women. *JAMA* 1993; 270:465–469.
59. McLafferty RB, Moneta GL, Taylor LM. et al. Ability of ankle-brachial index to detect lower-extremity atherosclerotic disease progression. *Arch Surg* 1997; 132:836–841.
60. TransAtlantic Inter-Society Consensus. Management of peripheral arterial disease. *J Vasc Surg* 2000; 31:S1–S34.
61. Hiatt WR, ed. Morbidity of PAD: Medical approaches to claudication, in Hirsch AT, ed: An office-based approach to the diagnosis and treatment of peripheral arterial disease: IV. *Excerpta Medi,* 1999; 6–15.
62. Patterson RB, Pinto B, Marcus B, et al. Value of a supervised exercise program for the therapy of arterial claudication. *J Vasc Surg* 1997; 25:312–319.
63. Money SR, Heard JA, Isaacsohn JL, et al. Effect of cilostazol on walking distances in patients with intermittent claudication caused by peripheral vascular disease. *J Vasc Surg* 1998; 27:267–275.
64. AbuRahma AF, Robinson PA, Holt SM. Prospective controlled study of polytetrafluoroethylene versus saphenous vein in claudicant patients with bilateral above knee femoropopliteal bypasses. *Surg* 1999; 126:594–602.
65. Byrne J, Darling RC III, Chang BB, et al. Infrainguinal arterial reconstruction for claudication: Is it worth the risk? An analysis of 409 procedures. *J Vasc Surg* 1999; 29:259–269.
66. Whyman MR, Fowkes FGR, Kerracher EMG, et al. Is intermittent claudication improved by percutaneous transluminal angioplasty? A randomized controlled trial. *J Vasc Surg* 1997; 26:551–557.
67. Golledge J, Ferguson K, Ellis M, et al. Outcome of femoropopliteal angioplasty. *Ann Surg* 1999; 229:146–153.
68. Nicoloff AD, Taylor LM, McLafferty RB, et al. Patient recovery after infrainguinal bypass grafting for limb salvage. *J Vasc Surg* 1998; 27:256–266.
69. Pomposelli FB Jr, Arora S, Gibbons GW, et al. Lower extremity arterial reconstruction in the very elderly: Successful outcome preserves not only the limb but also residential status and ambulatory function. *J Vasc Surg* 1998; 28:215–225.
70. Seabrook GR, Cambria RA, Freischlag JA, et al. Health-related quality of life and functional outcome following arterial reconstruction for limb salvage. *Cardiovasc Surg* 1999; 7:279–286.
71. Nicoloff AD, Taylor LM, McLafferty RB, et al. Patient recovery after infrainguinal bypass grafting for limb salvage. *J Vasc Surg* 1998; 27:261.
72. Kalman PG, Johnston KW. Predictors of long-term patient survival after in situ vein leg bypass. *J Vasc Surg* 1997; 25:899–904.
73. Link J, Steffens JC, Brossmann J, et al. Iliofemoral arterial occlusive disease: Contrast-enhanced MR angiography for preinterventional evaluation and follow-up after stent placement. *Radiology* 1999; 212:371–377.
74. Sueyoshi E, Sakamoto U, Matsuoka Y, et al. Aortoiliac and lower extremity arteries: Comparison of three-dimensional dynamic contrast-enhanced subtraction MR angiography and conventional angiography. *Radiology* 1999; 210:683–688.
75. Turnipseed WD, Sproat IA. A preliminary experience with use of magnetic resonance angiography in assessment of failing lower extremity bypass grafts. *Surgery* 1992; 112:664–669.
76. Carpenter JP, Golden MA, Barker CF, et al. The fate of bypass grafts to angiographically occult runoff vessels detected by magnetic resonance angiography. *J Vasc Surg* 1996; 23:483–489.
77. Eagleton MJ, Ouriel K, Shortell C, et al. Femoral-infrapopliteal bypass with prosthetic grafts. *Surgery* 1999; 126:759–765.
78. Prendiville EJ, Yeager AN, O'Donnell TF, et al. Long-term results with the above-knee popliteal expanded polytetrafluoroethylene graft. *J Vasc Surg* 1990; 11:517–524.
79. O'Riordain DS, Buckley DJ, O'Donnell JA. Polytetrafluoroethylene in above-knee arterial bypass surgery for critical ischemia. *Am J Surg* 1992; 164:129–131.
80. Calligaro KD, Syrek JR, Dougherty MJ, et al. Use of arm and lesser saphenous vein compared with prosthetic grafts for infrapopliteal arterial bypass: Are they worth the effort. *J Vasc Surg* 1997; 26:919–927.
81. Oppat WF, Pearce WH, McMillan WD, et al. Natural history of composite sequential bypass: Ten years' experience. *Arch Surg* 1999; 134:754 758.
82. Taylor RS, Loh A, McFarland RJ, et al. Improved technique for polytetrafluoroethylene bypass grafting: Long-term results using anastomotic vein patches. *Br J Surg* 1992; 79:348–354.
83. Dardik H, Miller N, Dardik A, et al. A decade of experience with the glutaraldehyde-tanned human umbilical cord vein graft for revascularization of the lower limb. *J Vasc Surg* 1988; 7:336–346.
84. Taylor RS, Belli A, Jacob S. Distal venous arterialisation for

salvage of critically ischaemic inoperable limbs. *Lancet* 1999; 354:1962–1965.
85. Carpenter JP, Tomaszewski JE. Immunosuppression for human saphenous vein allograft bypass surgery: A prospective randomized trial. *J Vasc Surg* 1997; 26:32–42.
86. Carpenter JP, Tomaszewski JE. Human saphenous vein allograft bypass grafts: Immune response. *J Vasc Surg* 1998; 27:492–499.
87. Castier Y, Leseche G, Palombi T, et al. Early experience with cryopreserved arterial allografts in below-knee revascularization for limb salvage. *Am J Surg* 1999; 177:197–202.
88. Shah DM, Darling RC, Chang BB, et al. Long-term results of in situ saphenous vein bypass: Analysis of 2058 cases. *Ann Surg* 1995; 222:438–448.
89. Wengerter K, Veith FJ, Gupta SK, et al. Prospective randomized multicenter comparison of in situ and reversed vein infrapopliteal bypasses. *J Vasc Surg* 1991; 13:189–199.
90. Chang BB, Darling RC, Bock DEM, et al. The use of spliced vein bypasses for infrainguinal arterial reconstruction. *J Vasc Surg* 1995; 21:403–412.
91. Bergamini TM, George SM, Massey HT, et al. Intensive surveillance of femoropopliteal-tibial autogenous vein bypasses improves long-term graft patency and limb salvage. *Ann Surg* 1995; 221:507–516.
92. Sarac TP, Huber TS, Back MR, et al. Warfarin improves the outcome of infrainguinal vein bypass grafting at high risk for failure. *J Vasc Surg* 1998; 28:446–457.
93. Tangelder MJD, Lawson JA, Algra A, et al. Systematic review of randomized controlled trials of aspirin and oral anticoagulants in the prevention of graft occlusion and ischemic events after infrainguinal bypass surgery. *J Vasc Surg* 1999; 30:701–709.
94. Polak J. Femoropopliteal angioplasty with US guidance: An example of a niche market. *Radiology* 1996; 199:317–318.
95. Bakal CW, Cynamon J, Sprayregen S. Infrapopliteal percutaneous transluminal angioplasty: What we know. *Radiology* 1996; 200:36–43.
96. Fraser SCA, Al-Kutoubi MA, Wolfe JHN. Percutaneous transluminal angioplasty of the infrapopliteal vessels: The evidence. *Radiology* 1996; 200:33–36.
97. Kalman PG, Johnston KW, Sniderman KW. Indications and results of balloon angioplasty for arterial occlusive lesions. *World J Surg* 1996; 20:630–634.
98. Treiman GS, Treiman RL, Ichikawa L, et al. Should percutaneous transluminal angioplasty be recommended for treatment of infrageniculate popliteal artery or tibioperoneal trunk stenosis? *J Vasc Surg* 1995; 22:457–463.
99. Stanley B, Teague B, Raptis S, et al. Efficacy of balloon angioplasty of the superficial femoral artery and popliteal artery in the relief of leg ischemia. *J Vasc Surg* 1996; 23:679–685.
100. Bradbury AW, Ruckle CV. Angioplasty for lower-limb ischemia: Time for randomized controlled trials. *Lancet* 1996; 347:277–278.
101. White GH, Liew SC, Waugh RC, et al. Early outcome and intermediate follow-up of vascular stents in the femoral and popliteal arteries without long-term anticoagulation. *J Vasc Surg* 1995; 21:270–281.
102. Cragg AH, Dake MD. Percutaneous femoropopliteal graft placement. *Radiology* 1993; 187:643–648.
103. Shapiro MJ, Levin DC. Percutaneous femoropopliteal graft placement: Is this the next step? *Radiology* 1993; 187:618–619.
104. Hunink MGM, Cullen KA, Donaldson MC. Hospital costs of revascularization procedures for femoropopliteal arterial disease. *J Vasc Surg* 1994; 19:632–641.
105. Hunink MGM, Wong JB, Donaldson MC, et al. Revascularization for femoropopliteal disease: A decision and cost-effectiveness analysis. *JAMA* 1995; 274:165–171.
106. Prandoni P, Polistena P, Bernardi E, et al. Upper-extremity deep vein thrombosis. *Arch Intern Med* 1997; 157:57–62.
107. Hingorani A, Ascher E, Hanson J, et al. Upper extremity versus lower extremity deep venous thrombosis. *Am J Surg* 1997; 174:214–217.
108. Hingorani A, Ascher E, Lorenson E, et al. Upper extremity deep venous thrombosis and its impact on morbidity and mortality rates in a hospital-based population. *J Vasc Surg* 1997; 26:853–860.
109. Azakie A, McElhinney DB, Thompson RW, et al. Surgical management of subclavian-vein effort thrombosis as a result of thoracic outlet compression. *J Vasc Surg* 1998; 28:777–786.
110. Lee MC, Grassi CJ, Belkin M, et al. Early operative intervention after thrombolytic therapy for primary subclavian vein thrombosis: An effective treatment approach. *J Vasc Surg* 1998; 27:1101–1108.
111. Urschel HC, Razzuk MA. Neurovascular compression in the thoracic outlet: Changing management over 50 years. *Ann Surg* 1998; 228:609–617.
112. Smith BM, Shield GW, Riddell DH, et al. Venous gangrene of the upper extremity. *Ann Surg* 1985; 201:511–519.
113. Gagne PJ, Martinez JM. Treatment of upper-extremity phlegmasia cerulea dolens with intra-arterial thrombolysis. *Vasc Surg* 1999; 33:633–639.
114. Spence LD, Gironta MG, Malde HM, et al. Acute upper extremity deep venous thrombosis: Safety and effectiveness of superior vena caval filters. *Radiology* 1999; 53–58.
115. Weinmann EE, Salzman EW. Deep-vein thrombosis. *N Engl J Med* 1994; 331:1630–1641.
116. Sorensen HT, Mellemkjaer L, Steffensen FH, et al. The risk of a diagnosis of cancer after primary deep venous thrombosis or pulmonary embolism. *N Engl J Med* 1998; 338:1169–1173.
117. Svensson PJ, Dahlback B. Resistance to activated protein C as a basis for venous thrombosis. *N Engl J Med* 1994; 330:517–522.
118. Ridker PM, Hennekens CH, Lindpaintner K, et al. Mutation in the gene coding for coagulation factor V and the risk of myocardial infarction, stroke, and venous thrombosis in apparently healthy men. *N Engl J Med* 1995; 332:912–917.
119. Khamashta MA, Cuadrado MJ, Mujic F, et al. The management of thrombosis in the antiphospholipid-antibody syndrome. *N Engl J Med* 1995; 332:993–997.
120. Mandel H, Brenner B, Berant M, et al. Coexistence of hereditary homocystinuria and factor V Leiden: Effect on thrombosis. *N Engl J Med* 1996; 334:763–768.
121. Den Heijer M, Koster T, Blom HJ, et al. Hyperhomocysteinemia as a risk factor for deep-vein thrombosis. *N Engl J Med* 1996; 334:759–762.
122. Simioni P, Prandoni P, Lensing AWA, et al. The risk of recurrent venous thromboembolism in patients with an $Arg^{506}\rightarrow Gln$ mutation in the gene for factor V (factor V Leiden). *N Engl J Med* 1997; 336:399–403.
123. De Stefano V, Martinelli I, Mannucci PM, et al. The risk of recurrent deep venous thrombosis among heterozygous carriers of both factor V Leiden and the G20210A prothrombin mutation. *N Engl J Med* 1999; 341:801–806.
124. Geerts WH, Code KI, Jay RM, et al. A prospective study of venous thromboembolism after major trauma. *N Engl J Med* 1994; 331:1601–1606.
125. Yeager RA, Moneta GL, Edwards JM, et al. Deep vein thrombosis associated with lower extremity amputation. *J Vasc Surg* 1995; 22:612–615.
126. Hirsch DR, Ingenito EP, Goldhaber SZ. Prevalence of deep venous thrombosis among patients in medical intensive care. *JAMA* 1995; 274:335–337.
127. Rosendaal FR. Venous thrombosis: A multicausal disease. *Lancet* 1993; 353:1167–1173.
128. Hull RD, Raskob GE, Rosenblood D, et al. Heparin for 5 days as compared with 10 days in the initial treatment of proximal venous thrombosis. *N Engl J Med* 1990; 332:1260–1264.
129. Schulman S, Rhedin AS, Lindmarker P, et al. A comparison of

six weeks with six months of oral anticoagulant therapy after a first episode of venous thromboembolism. *N Engl J Med* 1995;332:1661–1665.

130. Levine M, Gent M, Hirsh J, et al. A comparison of low-molecular-weight heparin administered primarily at home with unfractionated heparin administered in the hospital for proximal deep-vein thrombosis. *N Engl J Med* 1996; 334:677–681.
131. Koopman MMW, Prandoni P, Piovella F, et al. Treatment of venous thrombosis with intravenous unfractionated heparin administered in the hospital as compared with subcutaneous low-molecular-weight heparin administered at home. *N Engl J Med* 1996; 334:682–687.
132. Samama MM, Cohen AT, Darmon J, et al. A comparison of enoxaparin with placebo for the prevention of venous thromboembolism in acutely ill medical patients. *N Engl J Med* 1999; 341:793–800.
133. Gonzalez-Fajardo JA, Arreba E, Castrodeza J, et al. Venographic comparison of subcutaneous low-molecular weight heparin with oral anticoagulant therapy in the long-term treatment of deep venous thrombosis. *J Vasc Surg* 1999; 30:283–292.
134. Wood AJJ. Low-molecular-weight heparins. *N Engl J Med* 1997; 337:688–698.
135. Hirsh J, Weitz JI. New antithrombotic agents. *Lancet* 1999; 353:1431–1436.
136. Prandoni P, Lensing AWA, Cogo A, et al. The long–term clinical course of acute deep venous thrombosis. *Ann Intern Med* 1996; 125:1–7.
137. Mewissen MW, Seabrook GR, Meissner MH, et al. Catheter-directed thrombolysis for lower extremity deep venous thrombosis: Report of a national multicenter registry. *Radiology* 1999; 211:39–49.
138. O'Meara JJ, McNutt RA, Evans AT, et al. A decision analysis of streptokinase plus heparin as compared with heparin alone for deep-vein thrombosis. *N Engl J Med* 1994; 330:1864–1869.
139. Krieger NR, Mehigan JT. Spontaneous spinal epidural hematoma after combined urokinase and heparin thrombolytic therapy for deep venous thrombosis. *Vasc Surg* 1996; 30:67–70.
140. Lohr JM, Kerr TM, Lutter KS, et al. Lower extremity calf thrombosis: To treat or not to treat? *J Vasc Surg* 1999; 14:618–623.
141. Hanson JN, Ascher E, DePippo P, et al. Saphenous vein thrombophlebitis (SVT): A deceptively benign disease. *J Vasc Surg* 1998; 27:677–680.
142. Blumberg RM, Barton E, Gelfand ML, et al. Occult deep venous thrombosis complicating superficial thrombophlebitis. *J Vasc Surg* 1998; 27:338–343.
143. Verlato F, Zucchetta P, Prandoni P, et al. An unexpectedly high rate of pulmonary embolism in patients with superficial thrombophlebitis of the thigh. *J Vasc Surg* 1999; 30:1113–1115.
144. Juhan CM, Alimi YS, Barthelmey PJ, et al. Late results of iliofemoral venous thrombectomy. *J Vasc Surg* 1997; 25:417–422.
145. Juhan C, Alimi Y, de Mauro P, et al. Surgical venous thrombectomy. *Cardiovasc Surg* 1999; 7:586–590.
146. Elliot MS, Immelman EJ, Jeffrey P, et al. The role of thrombolytic therapy in the management of phlegmasia caerulea dolens. *Br J Surg* 1979; 66:422–424.
147. Hood DB, Weaver FA, Modrall JG, et al. Advances in the treatment of phlegmasia cerulea dolens. *Am J Surg* 1993; 166:206–210.
148. Patel KR, Paidas CN. Phlegmasia cerulea dolens: The role of nonoperative therapy. *Cardiovasc Surg* 1993; 1:518–523.
149. Greenfield LJ, Proctor MC. Twenty-year clinical experience with the Greenfield Filter. *Cardiovasc Surg* 1995; 3:199–205.
150. Decousus H, Leizorovicz A, Parent F, et al. A clinical trial of vena caval filters in the prevention of pulmonary embolism in patients with proximal deep-vein thrombosis. *N Engl J Med* 1998; 338:409–415.
151. Haire WD. Vena caval filters for the prevention of pulmonary embolism. *N Engl J Med* 1998; 338:463–464.

CHAPTER 92

NONSURGICAL INTERVENTIONS FOR CAROTID DISEASE

Samir R. Kapadia / Sanjay S. Yadav

INTRODUCTION

Stroke remains a major public health problem, and carotid artery atherosclerotic disease causes a substantial portion of all strokes. Cardiologists are frequently involved in the care of patients with carotid stenosis because many of them have either occult or symptomatic coronary artery disease. Compared to endarterectomy, carotid stenting is a less invasive procedure that provides an attractive treatment alternative for some patients, particularly those with severe cardiac comorbidities. The feasibility and safety of carotid stenting procedure as a treatment for severe carotid stenosis has improved with technological advances. This chapter outlines salient features of atherosclerotic carotid artery disease and the current status of nonsurgical treatment.

EPIDEMIOLOGY

Prevalence

Stroke killed approximately 160,000 people in 1996, accounting for approximately 1 of every 14.5 deaths in the United States.[1] Stroke ranks as the third leading cause of death, behind heart disease and cancer. More importantly, stroke is a leading cause of serious long-term disability. According to the data from the Health Care Financing Administration (HCFA), in 1995 $3.7 billion was paid to Medicare beneficiaries for stroke. The total economic burden is estimated to be $20 billion every year due to health care costs and lost productivity. Each year about 600,000 people suffer a new or recurrent stroke. About 500,000 of these are first attacks, and 100,000 are recurrent attacks. This incidence of stroke in the United States may be underestimated because of incomplete inclusion of minority populations.[2]

Atheroembolic events leading to ischemic stroke account for almost 85 percent of the acute strokes and almost two-thirds of these can be attributed to a large-vessel stenosis.[3–5] Depending upon the population studied, intracranial occlusive disease is present in 5 to 15 percent of the patients with acute ischemic strokes, whereas extracranial carotid artery disease is present in 30 to 40 percent. Although the association between carotid artery disease and neurologic sequelae dates back to ancient Greece, C. Miller Fisher was the first to clearly suggest a causal relation between extracranial carotid atherosclerosis and stroke in the modern era.[6,7]

Risk Factors

Presence and severity of carotid atherosclerosis correlates with the presence and severity of coronary atherosclerosis and peripheral vascular disease.[8–13] The risk factors for coronary atherosclerosis are also associated with carotid atherosclerosis.[14–17] The incidence of severe carotid disease increases with age in men and women. One-half of men over 75 years are found to have some carotid atherosclerosis by ultrasonography, but greater than 50 percent stenosis is present only in 5 percent.[18,19] There may be substantial racial differences in the severity and distribution of carotid atherosclerosis. Caucasian patients have predominantly extracranial carotid artery atherosclerosis, whereas African-Americans, Japanese, and Chinese have predominantly intracranial vascular lesions.[20,21] Smoking is the most important risk factor for prediction of carotid atherosclerotic disease, followed by hypertension, diabetes, male gender, and elevated systolic blood pressure.[22] Association of hypercholesterolemia with stroke has been clouded by the fact that many epidemiologic studies failed to separate ischemic and hemorrhagic strokes for analysis. Therefore, hypercholesterolemia did not always pan out to be a risk factor for "stroke."[23] Multiple studies have, however, associated increased total cholesterol, increased low-density lipoprotein cholesterol, increased triglycerides, and decreased high-density lipoprotein cholesterol with carotid atherosclerosis.[17,24–26] In patients with coronary disease, even low levels of high-density lipoprotein cholesterol without elevated levels of low-density lipoprotein or total cholesterol have been associated with carotid disease.[27] Meta-analyses with clinical trials of HMG-CoA inhibitors have further added support to the association between hypercholesterolemia and ischemic stroke.[28–30]

Natural History

The risk of stroke in asymptomatic patients with ultrasound-proven carotid atherosclerosis has been studied in observational trials. These studies have demonstrated that the % stenosis, progression of atherosclerosis between examination intervals and presence or absence of ulceration affects the outcome.[31,32] The annual risk of stroke for stenosis that is <75 percent is <1 percent, but this risk increases to 2 to 5 percent with stenosis >75 percent.[33–36] The evidence of silent brain infarction or embolization may also increase the risk for future symptomatic strokes.[37] Patients who continue to remain asymptomatic in the first year of observation have significantly lower risk of subsequent stroke than are those who are symptomatic. The majority of patients who develop stroke during the observation of an asymptomatic lesion have no warning symptoms.[31,33,35,38–42]

In symptomatic patients, the risk of subsequent neurologic events is much higher than in those asymptomatic. The risk of stroke in patients with transient ischemic attacks (TIAs) from severe carotid stenosis is approximately 10 percent within the first year, with a cumulative stroke risk of approximately 30 to 35 percent at the end of 5 years. Presence of hemispheric TIAs, recent TIA, increasing frequency of TIA, or high-grade stenosis identifies the high-risk patient population.[43]

ANATOMY

In approximately 70 percent of patients, the great vessels originate from the aortic arch with three separate ostia for the innominate, left common carotid, and left subclavian arteries. The most common anomaly is origin of the left common carotid artery from the innominate artery, which is seen in approximately 20 percent of patients—the so-called bovine arch. The common carotid artery divides into the internal and external carotid arteries at the C4–C5 intervertebral space. The internal carotid artery is posterior and lateral to the external carotid artery and ascends without branching until it enters the subarachnoid space, where it gives rise to the ophthalmic artery before dividing into the anterior and middle cerebral arteries. The carotid artery can be divided into the cervical, petrous, precavernous, cavernous, paraclenoid, and supraclenoid segments from its origin to the terminal bifurcation. The diameter of the carotid sinus is approximately 7 mm, and the diameter of the distal internal carotid at the level of the siphon is approximately 4 mm.[44] Pressure on the carotid sinus stimulates mechanoreceptors in the media and adventitia that are responsible for the carotid sinus reflex leading to bradycardia and hypotension.

The brain has an extensive collateral circulation. The most significant collaterals are provided by the circle of Willis, which consists of the anterior communicating artery uniting the right and left anterior cerebral arteries and posterior communicating arteries uniting the middle cerebral and posterior cerebral arteries. A symmetrical and normal circle of Willis is present in less than one-third of individuals.[45]

MORPHOLOGY OF DISEASE

As in other arterial beds, there is a predilection for lesions at branch points and bends. The most common site of cerebrovascular atherosclerotic disease is the carotid bifurcation affecting the outer wall of the carotid sinus and extending into the distal common carotid artery.

It was thought that atherosclerotic plaques become highly vascularized with time, and these vessels rupture, either spontaneously or as a result of trauma.[46] Plaque hemorrhage may lead to immediate obstruction of the artery but this mechanism is not as frequent as previously thought.[47] More commonly, ulceration and subsequent luminal thrombosis followed by embolism leads to symptoms.[48] Ulcers are noted much more commonly in surgical specimens than at angiography, being present in up to one-third of the plaques removed at endarterectomy.[49] In the North American Symptomatic Carotid Endarterectomy Trial (NASCET), plaque ulceration more than doubled the risk for stroke.[50] Using conventional cut-film angiography, the ulcer size can be defined by multiplying the length and width of the ulcer in millimeters. The presence of a large (>40 mm) ulcer independent of associated carotid stenosis identifies a group of patients who are at risk of stroke at the rate of 7.5 percent per year.[31,32]

Several investigators have proposed the use of noninvasive diagnostic imaging techniques, such as B-mode ultrasonography, to characterize plaque composition and to identify the high-risk, unstable carotid lesion.[51–53] An attempt has been made to characterize plaque according to the relative contribution of echogenic (high-intensity) and echolucent (low-intensity) material using the classification by Gray-Weale et al.[54] Another method is to subjectively classify the plaques as either homogeneous or heterogeneous.[55] However, these distinctions are neither reliable nor reproducible.[56] Reproducible grading of ultrasound images is not consistently achievable among experienced observers, and within-observer agreement may vary with time. Helical computed tomography has been used for studying detailed plaque morphology and composition, and studies are being performed to correlate plaque anatomy with clinical outcome.[57]

Magnetic resonance imaging is the first noninvasive imaging technique that allows reliable discrimination of lipid cores, fibrous caps, calcifications, normal media, and adventitia in human atheromatous plaques in vivo. This technique also characterizes intraplaque hemorrhage and acute thrombosis. Further investigations of plaque progression, stabilization, and rupture in human atherosclerosis are currently being conducted.[58,59]

CLINICAL PRESENTATION

Transient ischemic attack is the initial symptom of carotid stenosis in the majority of the patients with symptomatic carotid disease. If no therapy is instituted, 30 to 40 percent of these patients subsequently develop stroke. The diagnosis of TIA is based on careful history taking. By definition, symptoms resolve within 24 h of onset. The symptoms of vertebrobasilar insufficiency have to be differentiated from those of carotid artery related TIAs. The motor and sensory changes from carotid disease usually involve the contralateral face and body, whereas posterior circulation events often have bilateral or crossed deficits. Dysphasia, dysarthria, contralateral visual field loss, and amaurosis fugax are manifestations of carotid disease. Vertebrobasilar insufficiency can present with ataxia, dysarthria, diplopia, or bilateral visual field loss. Hemicranial headache can occur with TIA from carotid stenosis and occipital headaches are seen with vertebrobasilar insufficiency.

DIAGNOSIS

Ultrasonography

The standard method of studying carotid arteries is with duplex ultrasonography, which is a combination of Doppler ultrasonography and B-mode imaging with a single instrument and transducer. This allows for visualization of the vessel along with the angle of ultrasound interrogation, leading to more accurate calculations of blood flow velocity. When performed by trained sonographers using a standard protocol and with ongoing quality assurance, this method can approach 90 percent sensitivity and specificity for identification of important carotid stenosis.[60–62]

Ultrasonography of the carotid artery, particularly the intimal–medial thickness (IMT), has been used as a surrogate end point in many trials examining risk factor modification, and the severity of IMT has been found to correlate well with the degree of coronary artery disease.[11,16] Moreover, the plaque morphology and progression of disease in carotid atherosclerotic lesions have correlation with the behavior of coronary atherosclerosis lesions.[9,13,63]

Magnetic Resonance Angiography

Magnetic resonance angiography (MRA) is useful in the study of carotid bifurcation, as anatomically this is a relatively motionless, sizable, and superficial structure. The newer MRA techniques allow reliable imaging of the carotid arteries from the origin of the aortic arch to the intracranial branches.

Several MRA techniques have been proposed to assess carotid bifurcation, including 2D and 3D time-of-flight (TOF) MRA and first-pass gadolinium-enhanced MRA. Several blinded-reader studies have been published comparing MRA with conventional angiography. The results based mostly on 2D TOF MRA indicate high sensitivity (>90 percent) and high negative predictive value (>90 percent) for detecting narrowing of >70 percent by NASCET criteria. The specificity of MRA is approximately 70 percent due to artifacts from tortuous vessels, turbulence of blood flow, and other technical reasons. Combining 2D TOF with single-slab 3D TOF technique through stenotic segments may yield better sensitivity and specificity.[64–67] MRA generally overestimates the degree of stenosis and is particularly poor at distinguishing between subtotal and total occlusions. However, the combination of ultrasound and MRA may raise sensitivity and specificity to a significantly high level, reducing the need for diagnostic angiography.

Angiography

Angiography is the gold standard for diagnosis of carotid stenosis. It allows accurate measurement of luminal stenosis of the entire vessel from its origin to the intracranial branches. The plaque morphology, lesion length, and reference diameter of the vessel can be accurately determined by angiography. In patients with symptomatic carotid disease, angiography identifies intracranial stenosis in a significant number of patients.[68] It is an invasive procedure with some risk of complications such as embolization and dissection, which are rare, however.[69] Currently, angiography is used in patients where noninvasive tests give uncertain results or when percutaneous therapy is considered.

NONSURGICAL MANAGEMENT

Pharmacologic Management

Antiplatelet, anticoagulant, and antihyperlipidemic agents are the potential modes of therapy in carotid stenosis. Although there are multiple studies of these agents in therapy of stroke, few have focused on the management of carotid artery disease. In the following paragraphs the available data are briefly reviewed.

ANTIPLATELET AGENTS

A number of trials have studied the role of various antiplatelet agents or their combinations in the management of stroke. Most of these studies did not specifically investigate the patients with carotid stenosis, or did they carefully exclude patients with cardioembolic stroke. The Antiplatelet Trialists' Collaboration performed a meta-analysis of 164 randomized trials of antiplatelet drugs including over 100,000 patients to analyze the effectiveness of different antiplatelet therapies in prevention of vascular events.[70] Among primary prevention recipients there was approximately a 30 percent reduction in nonfatal myocardial infarction, but there was no reduction in the incidence of stroke. In the group with a prior stroke or TIA ($n = 7850$), the incidence of subsequent ischemic nonhemorrhagic stroke was reduced from 12.2 percent in patients receiving a placebo to 9.7 percent with antiplatelet therapy ($p < 0.01$). Interestingly, there was no difference in effectiveness between different aspirin dosages or combination regimens.

Newer antiplatelet agents, the thienopyridine derivatives ticlopidine and clopidogrel, have gained widespread use in management of cardiovascular disease. The efficacy of these agents in preventing cardiovascular events has been compared to aspirin in randomized trials. In the Ticlopidine Aspirin Stroke Study, 3069 patients with noncardiogenic TIAs or minor strokes were randomized to ticlopidine or aspirin (650 mg twice a day). There was a trend in favor of ticlopidine for preventing nonfatal stroke or death at 3 years (17 versus 19 percent; $p = 0.048$).[71] The incidence of serious adverse side effects with ticlopidine, including neutropenia and thrombotic thrombocytopenic purpura, decreases the clinical usefulness of this drug.

Clopidogrel appears to have an effectiveness similar to ticlopidine with a better side effect profile and convenient pharmacokinetics. Clopidogrel was assessed in the Clopidogrel versus Aspirin in Patients at Risk of Ischemic Events trial. This trial randomized 19,185 patients with various forms of cardiovascular disease including recent ischemic stroke to clopidogrel or aspirin.[72] The combined incidence of ischemic stroke, myocardial infarction, and vascular death at approximately 2 years favored clopidogrel (5.3 versus 5.8 percent; $p = 0.043$), although the absolute reduction in events was small (0.27 percent per year). In this study, a total of 6431 patients were randomized after an ischemic stroke from atherothrombosis (59 percent) or lacunar infarction (40 percent). The outcome of the patients receiving clopidogrel was similar to that receiving aspirin (9.7 versus 10.6 percent). Therefore, clopidogrel has at least equal efficacy compared to aspirin in preventing vascular events. Whether clopidogrel plus aspirin offers an advantage over either agent alone has not been addressed.

The best data regarding outcomes of patients with significant carotid artery stenosis treated with antiplatelet therapy are derived from the medical intervention arms of the carotid endarterectomy randomized trials.[33,73–79] In the Asymptomatic Carotid Atherosclerosis Study (ACAS), 834 patients with >60 percent stenosis were randomized to 325 mg of aspirin daily plus risk factor modification.[80] The annual risk for ipsilateral stroke or any perioperative stroke or death in patients treated with aspirin alone was extremely low, only 2.2 percent per year. Moreover, aspirin is important in these patients due to their high cardiovascular risk as highlighted in the Mayo Asymptomatic Carotid Endarterectomy Study.[77] This study did not require and even discouraged the use of aspirin or any other antiplatelet drug in the surgical cohort. After randomizing only 71 patients, the trial was prematurely terminated due to an excessive rate of myocardial infarctions in the surgical group (carotid endarterectomy 22 versus aspirin 0 percent; $p = 0.0037$). Limited data exist regarding antiplatelet treatment compared to placebo in patients with documented asymptomatic carotid artery stenosis. The impact of aspirin in preventing ipsilateral TIAs or strokes from a 50 percent carotid artery stenosis in initially asymptomatic patients was analyzed from the medical arm of the VA Cooperative Study on Asymptomatic Carotid Stenosis.[81] In the original study, 233 patients were initially randomized to aspirin, but 37 (16 percent) did not actually take any aspirin because of intolerance or noncompliance. At about 4-year follow-up, incidence of ipsilateral TIA or stroke was 37.8 percent in patients not receiving aspirin compared to only 17.4 percent in the group taking aspirin ($p = 0.005$).

In symptomatic patients, however, antiplatelet drugs appear less effective for preventing recurrent stroke. In the NASCET, 331 patients with symptomatic 70 to 99 percent carotid artery stenosis were randomized to 1300 mg aspirin daily or lower doses if the high dose was not well tolerated.[74] Despite high compliance (94 percent) with aspirin therapy, 26 percent of these patients suffered an ipsilateral stroke at 2 years of follow-up. In the European Carotid Surgery Trial (ECST), the annual risk for a major ipsilateral stroke with severe symptomatic carotid stenosis was more than 5 percent.[78]

ANTICOAGULANTS

The role of anticoagulation in patients with known carotid disease has not been adequately studied. In a meta-analysis of 16 randomized studies of anticoagulant therapy after cerebral or retinal ischemia or infarction, anticoagulant therapy was shown to be ineffective in management of these patients.[82] The Stroke Prevention in Reversible Ischemia Trial study randomized 1243 patients with prior TIA or minor stroke of noncardiac origin to aspirin 30 mg daily or anticoagulant drugs with a target International Normalized Ratio (INR) of 3.0 to 4.5.[83] The combined primary end point of vascular death, stroke, myocardial infarction, or major bleeding complication was more than twice as common in the anticoagulant group ($p < 0.05$) because of excess bleeding events. The available data do not support the use of anticoagulant therapy in the management of carotid artery disease.[44]

ANTIHYPERLIPIDEMIC AGENTS

Although earlier studies using clofibrate failed to show reduction in stroke rate,[84,85] meta-analyses from HMG-CoA reductase inhibitors (statins) have conclusively shown the efficacy of antihyperlipidemic therapy in stroke reduction.[28–30] The effect of statins on atherosclerotic plaque has been carefully studied in patients with documented carotid atherosclerosis. These trials have meticulously assessed the effects of statins on the rate of change in carotid IMT using serial ultrasound measurements. In almost every study plaque regression was observed, although the magnitude of the change was small.[86–88]

Although the primary end points of these small and other larger studies were coronary events and mortality, 3 meta-analyses [28–30] focused on the effects on stroke of cholesterol reduction by statins. The first was an overview of 16 trials, which included about 29,000 patients treated and followed-up for an average of 3.3 years.[29] The average reductions in total and low-density lipoprotein-cholesterol were large, 22 and 30 percent, respectively. Patients assigned to statins had a 29 percent reduction in risk of stroke and a 22 percent reduction in risk of total mortality. There was no evidence of any increased risk in noncardiovascular mortality or cancer. Another similar analysis by Blauw et al. from 20,438 patients concluded that approximately 4 strokes could be prevented per 1000 patients treated with statins.[30] Bucher et al. have gone further and reviewed all randomized controlled trials of any cholesterol-lowering therapy that provided data on nonfatal and fatal strokes.[28] Twenty-eight trials were included in this meta-analysis, with over 49,000 and 56,000 in the intervention and control groups, respectively. The statins had a 24 percent reduction in risk of nonfatal and fatal stroke. By contrast, the risk ratios with fibrates, resins, and dietary modification had no effect on the incidence of stroke.[28] With this quite compelling evidence, patients with hypercholesterolemia and moderate-to-high risk of coronary or cerebrovascular events should be offered intensive lipid-lowering treatment with statins.

Percutaneous Intervention

Percutaneous transcatheter techniques have been used extensively in various vascular distributions. Although carotid angioplasty had been first attempted as early as in 1977, the enthusiasm for this procedure has been limited by the fear of cerebral embolism.[89] There has been a rapid growth and invigorated interest in this procedure due to the technological advances in endovascular procedures. Percutaneous intervention of the carotid arteries, when performed safely, has many advantages over surgical treatment. The potential risks of general anesthesia and the local surgical complications of endarterectomy, such as neck hematoma, infection, cervical strain, and cranial nerve damage can be completely eliminated. Furthermore, this treatment approach is particularly appealing for patients with coexistent coronary, myocardial, or valvular heart disease.

BALLOON ANGIOPLASTY

Carotid angioplasty is of historical interest only as it has been almost completely replaced by stenting, which is a safer and more dependable procedure. Angioplasty was first reported by Mathias in 1977[90] and, in 1980, both Kerber et al.[91] and Mullan et al.[92] published case reports of successful carotid angioplasty during carotid endarterectomy. Since then, multiple case reports and observational series of angioplasty of the brachiocephalic vessels have been published, but these reports lack detailed outcome assessment and are of only historical value.[93–100] Procedural success ranged from 79 to 98 percent. Strokes occurred in 4 to 6 percent of patients, with no reported deaths during follow-up.

CAROTID STENTING

In 1994, Marks et al.[101] and Mathias[102] published the first reports of stent use in patients with high cervical carotid artery dissection and stenosis. Since then, several observational series reporting promising results of carotid stenting as a treatment option for carotid stenosis have been published.

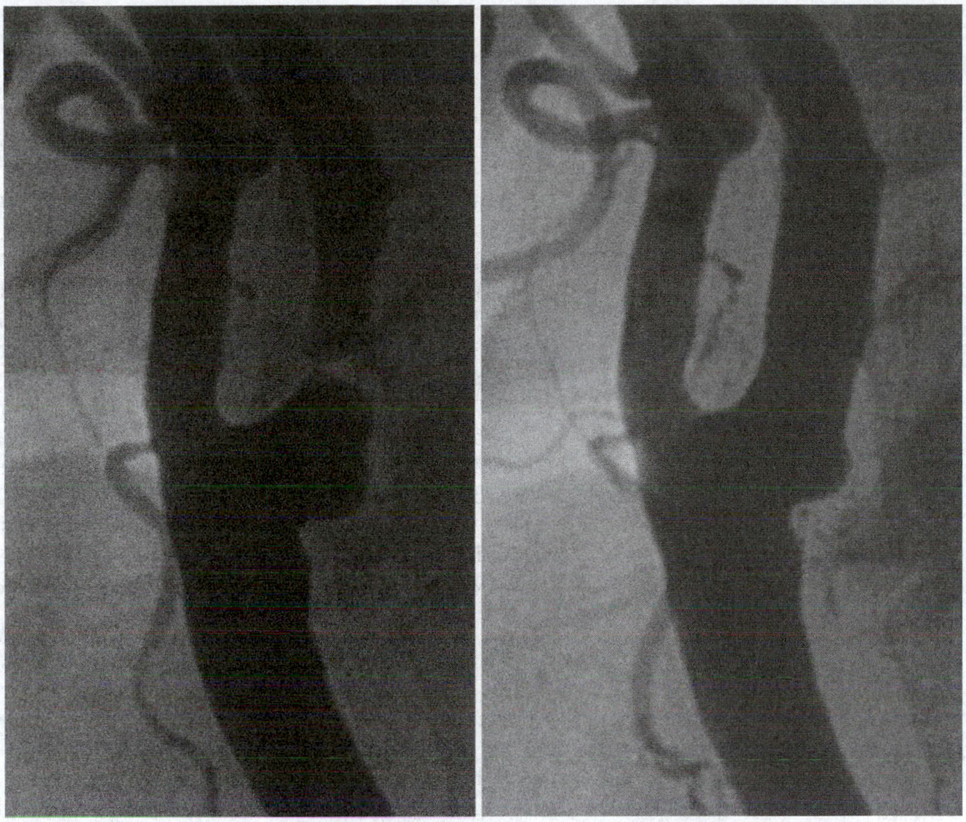

FIGURE 92-1 *A.* Severe stenosis of internal carotid artery. *B, C.* Angiogram after placement of the self-expanding SMART stent (Cordis).

Procedure Slightly different techniques of carotid stenting with similar basic principles have been reported. The goal is to access the carotid arteries with minimal manipulation of catheters, cross the lesion with least possible trauma, gently predilate the lesion, place a self-expandable stent to cover the lesion, and gently postdilate the stent to achieve an acceptable lumen. A technique utilizing a telescoping apparatus with a long sheath is popular in the United States. Various self-expandable stents are being investigated for this specific use (Fig. 92-1).[104–111] Safety and efficacy of adjuvant pharmacologic therapy for platelet inhibition is also being actively studied.

Bradycardia and hypotension are not uncommon during carotid artery stenting procedures but are typically transient. Management of more prolonged hemodynamic alterations may involve temporary transvenous pacing and/or vasoactive medications.[103] In patients with severe left ventricular systolic dysfunction or valvular heart diseases, intraprocedural hemodynamic monitoring with a pulmonary artery catheter is helpful.

Outcome Several reports of carotid stenting have been published.[104–110] Wholey and Eles reviewed carotid artery stenting data from major interventional centers in Europe, South America, and North America[111] (Table 92-1). The data were collected from surveys of the operators from various centers and also from the review of published case series. The survey included questions on patient characteristics, procedural techniques, and the results of carotid stenting. This series reported on a total of 3129 carotid artery stent placement procedures as of October 1998, 46 percent of which were performed at "high-volume" carotid stent centers in Europe and North America. One-third (37 percent) of the patients were asymptomatic. Technical success, defined as less than 30 percent residual stenosis covering a region no longer than the original lesion without any alteration of intracranial arterial anatomy, was achieved in 98.8 percent of patients. Various different stents were used depending on availability and operator preference. Stent deformation as detected by x-rays was seen in 28 instances (2 percent of all Palmaz stents), exclusively occurring with the balloon expandable Palmaz stent (Cordis, Johnson and Johnson Interventional Systems; Warren, NJ). Procedural and 30-day events were recorded. There were 74 (2.4 percent) reported TIAs. Minor strokes were defined as a new neurologic event that resulted in slight functional impairment that either completely resolved within 7 days or caused an increase in the National Institutes of Health (NIH) stroke scale of less than 4. Minor stroke rates ranged from 0 to 7 percent in different centers with a total event rate of 78 (2.49 percent). Major stroke was defined as a new neurologic deficit that persisted after 7 days and increased the NIH stroke scale by 4 or more. Major strokes were reported in 43 patients with an event rate of 1.4 percent (range 0–8 percent). Procedure-related mortality at 30 days occurred in 30 (0.96 percent) patients. Postprocedure neurologic sequelae occurred in 14 (0.79 percent) cases. Ultrasound studies were performed at 1 and 6 months poststent placement at all high-

TABLE 92-1 Results of Carotid Stenting

Study	Lesions (n)	Technical Success	30-Day Outcome: Stroke	MI	Death	Mean Follow-up	Stroke After 30 Days	Restenosis
Diethrich et al.[110]	117	116 (99.1%)	10 (8.3%)	0 (0.0%)	1 (0.9%)	7.6 Months	2 (1.7%)	2 (1.7%)
Henry et al.[106]	174	173 (99.4%)	5 (2.9%)	0 (0.0%)	0 (0%)	12.7 Months	0 (0.0%)	4 (2.3%)
Laborde et al.[107]	87	87 (100%)	4 (5.3%)	0 (0.0%)	1 (1.1%)	8.7 Months	1 (1.1%)	2 (5.2%)
Wholey et al.[109]	114	108 (95%)	4 (3.5%)	1 (0.9%)	2 (1.9%)	6 Months	0 (0.0%)	1 (1.0%)
Shawl et al.[105]	96	96 (100%)	3 (3.1%)	0 (0.0%)	0 (0.0%)	8 Months	0 (0.0%)	1 (1.4%)
Yadav et al.[108]	126	126 (100%)	8 (6.3%)	0 (0.0%)	1 (0.8%)	6 Months	0 (0.0%)	4 (4.9%)
Global Experience[111]	3129	3091 (98.8%)	121 (3.9%)	—	61 (2.0%)	6 Months	14 (0.79%)	68 (2.3%)

MI = myocardial infarction.

volume centers. Restenosis defined as diameter stenosis of >50 percent was approximately 2.5 percent.

The series reported by Yadav et al., Diethrich et al., and Wholey et al. have provided the most rigorous detail of carotid stenting techniques, procedural success, and patient outcomes.[108–110] Yadav et al.[108] published their initial experience of carotid stenting in 107 consecutive patients. All procedures were successful. Patients had independent neurologic examinations before and after the procedure. Periprocedural complications included 1 stent thrombosis, 6 minor strokes, and 1 major stroke. Clinical follow-up at 30 days showed 1 additional minor stroke, 1 major stroke, 1 myocardial infarction, and 1 death not due to cerebrovascular disease. The incidence of combined end point of all strokes and death was 7.9 percent with 1.6 percent ipsilateral major stroke and death. A total of 81 (76 percent) patients underwent angiography or ultrasound evaluation 6 months after stenting. Four (4.9 percent) of these 81 patients had asymptomatic restenosis. Five asymptomatic patients had repeat intervention, with angioplasty for restenosis in 2, angioplasty for stent deformation in another 2, and endarterectomy for restenosis in 1. On 6-month follow-up, there were no strokes or deaths from cerebrovascular disease. The University of Alabama group extended their experience to 146 procedures with similar results.[112] It is important to recognize that these results were obtained in a high-risk cohort and represent the initial learning curve for carotid stenting. Of the patients treated with stenting in this series, 77 percent would have been ineligible for carotid endarterectomy on the basis of the ACAS and NASCET exclusion criteria.[74,80] The other major carotid stent series have included patients with a similar high-risk profile.

Diethrich and colleagues[110] reported their experience in 110 patients with severe carotid stenosis. Stenting was successful in 99 percent of patients. There were 7 (6.4 percent) strokes (2 major, 5 minor), 5 (4.5 percent) TIAs, and 2 asymptomatic stent occlusions in the first 30 days after the procedure. Overall, 89 percent (98) of patients had successful procedures and were free from death, surgical intervention, stroke, or stent occlusion at 30 days. During a mean of 7.6 months of follow-up, no additional neurologic events were reported.

Wholey et al. reported 114 lesions in 108 consecutive patients (58 men, mean age 70.1 years) with ≥70 percent carotid stenosis treated with percutaneous stent implantation.[111] Of these, 44 percent were asymptomatic. Stents were successfully placed in 108 (95 percent) lesions. Of the 6 technical failures, 5 were access related and 1 was due to seizures during balloon dilation. Two major (1.8 percent) and 2 minor (1.8 percent) strokes occurred, all in symptomatic patients, 1 of whom died. There were 5 (4.4 percent) TIAs and 2 (1.8 percent) brief seizure episodes during dilation. The total stroke or death rate was 5.3 percent. In the mean 6-month follow-up, there was 1 restenosis (1.0 percent) from a stent compression, which was successfully dilated. There were no neurologic sequelae, cranial palsies, or cases of stent or vessel thrombosis on follow-up.

Henry et al. reported their experience of 174 stenting procedures in 163 patients.[106] This series differs from the others as a cerebral emboli protection device was used in a small subset ($n = 32$, 18 percent). The majority (65 percent, 106 patients) of the patients were asymptomatic. Immediate technical success was achieved in all but 1 (99.4 percent) patient. Eight (4.6 percent) neurologic complications occurred in the periprocedural period: 3 TIA, 2 minor strokes, and 3 major strokes. Two major complications developed despite cerebral protection. Over a mean follow-up of 1 year, no ipsilateral neurologic complications were seen. Palmaz stent compression was seen in 1 patient and 4 (2.5 percent) patients were identified with restenosis.

Due to relatively small sample size and infrequent events in each series, independent predictors for procedural strokes have not been well studied. Like surgical trials, symptom status appears to correlate with the frequency of adverse neurologic outcomes after carotid stenting. This was seen in the series reported by Yadav et al., where 8 (11 percent) ipsilateral neurologic deficits or deaths were encountered after 74 procedures for symptomatic carotid stenosis and only 2 (4 percent) after 52 procedures in asymptomatic patients.[108] Similarly, Wholey et al. observed a higher stroke rate in symptomatic patients[109] than in asymptomatic patients. In a multivariate analysis of 271 carotid procedures in 231 patients, however, Mathur et al. found advanced age and long or multiple stenoses to be the independent predictors of procedural stroke.[113]

Restenosis, a long-term complication after carotid stenting, is fortunately rare. In the major carotid stent series, 33 (5 percent) of 655 carotid artery procedures were complicated by restenosis when systematically studied with either angiography or ultrasound follow-up evaluations. Stent deformation occurred in 10 (1.5 percent) patients, all occurring with the Palmaz stent. Even though only 4 (0.6 percent) cases of restenosis or stent deformation were symptomatic, 16 (24.4 percent) underwent treatment with repeat dilatation, repeat stenting, endarterectomy, or bypass grafting. As balloon-expandable stents are replaced by self-expanding stents, stent deformation has become clinically irrelevant.

The field of carotid stenting is rapidly evolving with the advent of pharmacologic and technological advances. Availability of better, tailor-made instruments, emboli protection devices, and advanced pharmacologic adjuvant therapies will make carotid stenting a more attractive procedure.

Emboli Protection Devices The major cause of stroke during carotid endarterectomy and percutaneous carotid intervention is the procedural embolization of plaque debris along with platelet and thrombin aggregates into the cerebral circulation. Transcranial Doppler monitoring, a noninvasive method to detect echogenic microemboli, has demonstrated frequent embolization during carotid endarterectomy and stenting.[114–117] Although data are limited, there appears to be a correlation between the number of emboli and neurologic outcome after endarterectomy.[116,117] Consequently, various mechanical and pharmacologic approaches to prevent distal embolization are currently under investigation to improve the safety of carotid stenting.

Various mechanical devices to prevent embolization are under investigation.[118–120] Henry et al. reported their experience in 58 carotid artery stent procedures using a prototype cerebral protection device and compared the results to 212 other patients treated without the emboli protection device.[120] This cerebral protection catheter is a low-profile, balloon-tipped device designed to block cerebral emboli when positioned in the internal carotid artery distal to the target lesion. Conceptually, the protection balloon occludes the run-off circulation to the brain, trapping any particles dislodged following balloon angioplasty or stent delivery so that they can subsequently be extracted via aspiration into the guiding catheter. In this series, there was 1 immediate neurologic complication (0.5 percent) compared to 11 (5.2 percent) in the group treated without the device. Feasibility of transient carotid occlusion without consequences and potential endothelial injury and embolization from the occlusion balloon itself, however, are important concerns that need further evaluation. An alternative mechanical embolization device that allows continued perfusion while capturing emboli has been developed (Figs. 92-2 and 92-3). This filter-type device has been tested in carotid, coronary, and peripheral interventions and should be available in the near future for rigorous randomized trials.[118]

Adjuvant Pharmacologic Therapy Pharmacologic protection against embolization is based on randomized clinical trials utilizing platelet glycoprotein IIb/IIIa inhibitors during coronary interventions. Various Gp IIb/IIIa inhibitors, especially abciximab, have been shown to be effective in reducing the ischemic complications of death, myocardial infarction, or urgent repeat revascularization after percutaneous coronary interventional procedures.[121–123]

The coronary experience has been extended to selected patients in 22 carotid stent procedures involving visible thrombus, total occlusion, or acute stroke. The preliminary data from these high-risk patients suggested relatively high bleeding complications with 2 (9 percent) central nervous system bleeding, one hemorrhagic transformation of a previously ischemic stroke and one other subarachnoid hemorrhage from a ruptured aneurysm.[124] Periprocedural glycoprotein IIb/IIIa receptor inhibition may be safer and more effective when used in a routine prophylactic manner. This approach is being currently evaluated.[124a] Other potential therapies including low molecular weight heparin or direct thrombin inhibitors have not been studied in carotid stenting procedures. Only preliminary information on the efficacy and safety of clopidogrel therapy has been available.[125]

ENDARTERECTOMY VERSUS NONSURGICAL THERAPY

Randomized trials have compared surgical therapy with medical management in symptomatic and asymptomatic carotid stenosis; however, there is no randomized trial comparing surgical therapy with contemporary carotid stenting procedure. Preliminary results from one randomized trial comparing surgery to carotid angioplasty have been reported.[73] A brief summary of these comparative trials is provided here.

Surgery versus Medical Therapy

SYMPTOMATIC DISEASE

Three pivotal studies in patients with symptomatic carotid disease have been completed and have documented improved outcomes with endarterectomy in patients with symptomatic severe carotid stenosis.

The ECST was a multicenter, randomized trial in which patients with nondisabling stroke, TIA, or retinal infarction within the preceding 6 months were randomly assigned to carotid endarterectomy or medical therapy.[78] The rate of perioperative stroke, defined as a stroke within 30 days of carotid endarterectomy or death was 7.0 percent irrespective of the stenosis severity. Patients with severe stenosis (>70 percent) assigned to surgical intervention had significant reduction in surgical death or any stroke at 3-year follow-up (12.3 versus 21.9 percent; $p < 0.01$).[76] The risk of surgical death or ipsilateral stroke by 3 years was 10.3 percent in patients assigned surgical intervention compared with 16.8 percent in patients assigned medical therapy. Patients with mild and moderate stenosis did not have an observed benefit with surgery.

The NASCET enrolled patients with 30 to 99 percent carotid artery stenosis who had experienced TIAs or nondisabling stroke within 4 months of randomization.[74] This study was undertaken in surgical centers with a documented <6 percent stroke or death rate within 30 days of carotid endarterectomy

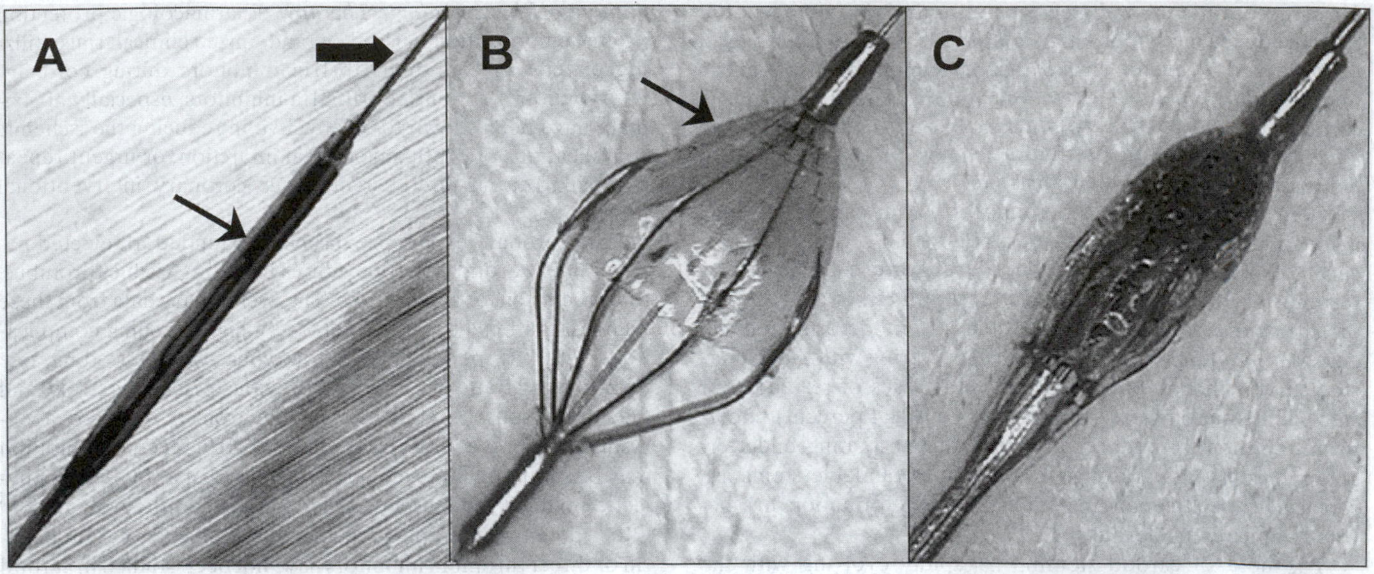

FIGURE 92-2 *A*. An emboli protection device (Angioguard, Cordis) in closed state. The bold arrow represents 0.014 in. wire that leads the device (4 French) shown by the smaller arrow. *B*. Open device with a filter with 100 μM pore size. *C*. Closed filter with captured embolic debris.

in 50 consecutive procedures performed within the preceding 24 months. Patients were stratified according to the degree of carotid stenosis (30–69 percent or 70–99 percent).

The study results from 662 patients with 70 to 99 percent stenosis were published initially.[74] The primary end point was the occurrence of nonfatal or fatal ipsilateral stroke. All patients were examined by neurologists 1, 3, 6, 9, and 12 months after entry and then every 4 months. Stroke or death occurred in 3.8 percent of patients within 30 days of surgery. The life-table estimate of the risk for ipsilateral stroke by 24-month follow-up was 9 percent in the patients treated with carotid endarterectomy compared to 26 percent in the patients treated medically (absolute risk reduction 17 percent; $p < 0.001$). The risk for any stroke (12.6 versus 27.6 percent; $p < 0.001$) and the risk for major stroke or death (8.0 versus 18.1 percent; $p < 0.01$) were also significantly reduced in patients treated with carotid endarterectomy. Review of survival curves for the occurrence of ipsilateral stroke, any stroke, any stroke or death, and other subgroups showed that the early hazard associated with surgery dissipated by 3 to 4 months and that there was persistent benefit with surgery during long-term follow-up. Subgroup analysis by the extent of carotid artery stenosis show the greatest benefit in absolute reduction of ipsilateral stroke during long-term follow-up in patients with more severe carotid disease (26 percent in the 90–99 percent group; 18 percent in the 80–89 percent group; and 12 percent in the 70–79 percent group).

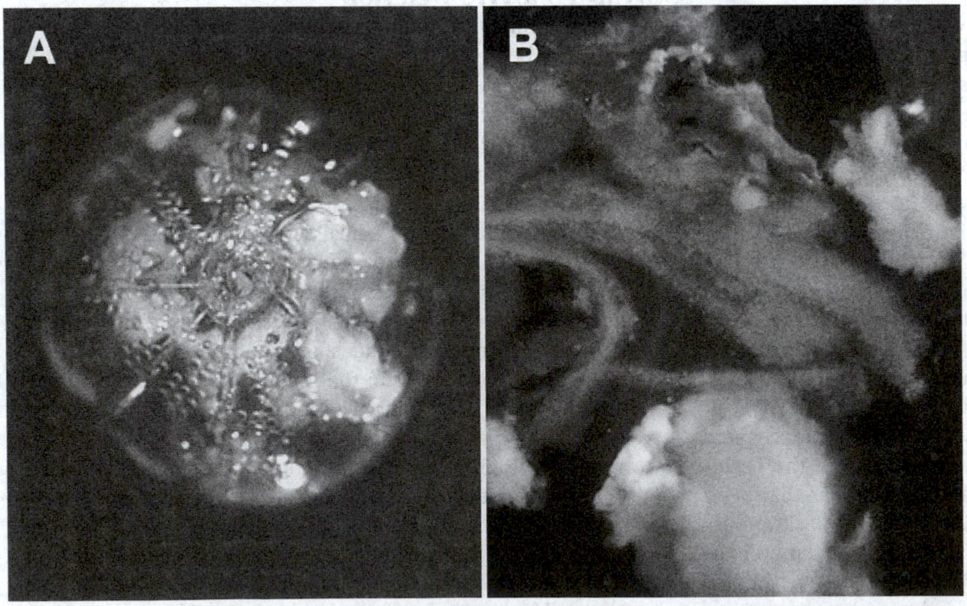

FIGURE 92-3 *A*. Filter with atheromatous embolic debris. *B*. Magnified view of typical atheromatous embolic particles retrieved during intervention.

A total of 2267 patients with <70 percent stenosis were also randomized to medical therapy or endarterectomy in the NASCET trial.[75] Post hoc analyses divided patients into groups with 50 to 69 percent stenosis and those with <50 percent stenosis. In patients with 50 to 69 percent stenosis, a 6.5 percent reduction in the primary end point of any ipsilateral stroke was observed by 5-year follow-up (15.7 versus 22.2 percent; $p = 0.045$). In the group with <50 percent stenosis, a nonsignificant absolute reduction of 3.8 percent was observed (14.9 versus 18.7 percent; $p = 0.16$). The risk for any stroke or death was significantly reduced in the surgical group at 5-year follow-up for patients with 50 to 69 percent stenosis (33.2 versus

43.3 percent; $p = 0.005$), but no reduction was observed with surgery in patients with <50 percent stenosis (36.2 versus 37 percent; $p = 0.97$).

The Veterans Affairs Cooperative Studies Program Trialist Group randomly assigned 189 men from a total of 5000 screened patients to medical therapy or endarterectomy.[79] All patients had >50 percent stenosis of the internal carotid artery ipsilateral to the presenting symptoms. Patients with TIA, transient monocular blindness, or recent small, completed strokes within last 4 months were enrolled. At a mean follow-up of 11.9 months, a significant reduction in stroke or crescendo TIAs in patients assigned to carotid endarterectomy compared with patients assigned to medical treatment was observed (7.7 versus 19.4 percent; absolute risk reduction, 11.7 percent; $p = 0.011$). The benefit of surgery was more profound in patients with internal carotid artery stenosis >70 percent (absolute risk reduction, 17.7 percent; $p = .004$). Perioperative complications (stroke or death) within 30 days of randomization occurred in 6 of 91 (6.6 percent) patients with endarterectomy (3 strokes and 3 deaths).

ASYMPTOMATIC DISEASE

The efficacy of carotid endarterectomy for patients with asymptomatic carotid artery disease is less well defined. The ACAS trial enrolled 1659 patients between 1983 and 1993 with asymptomatic carotid stenosis of ≥60 percent.[80] There was an impressively low perioperative stroke or death rate of 2.3 percent and the median follow-up of 2.7 years. The aggregate risk over 5 years for ipsilateral stroke and any perioperative stroke or death was estimated to be 5.1 percent for surgical patients and 11.0 percent for patients treated medically with aggregate risk reduction of 53 percent ($p = 0.004$). The low surgical complication rate was due in part to stringent selection criteria for participating centers, which required <3 percent incidence of stroke in the preceding 50 consecutive operations in asymptomatic patients.[126] The low rate of perioperative complications leads to the questioning of the broader application of the results to other surgical centers that may not be able to reproduce such low complication rates.[127]

The Veteran Affairs Asymptomatic Carotid Stenosis study tested endarterectomy versus aspirin treatment strategies in a randomized multicenter trial.[33] A total of 444 patients with asymptomatic carotid stenosis of ≥50 percent were randomly assigned to optimal medical treatment including antiplatelet medication (aspirin) plus carotid endarterectomy ($n = 211$) or optimal medical treatment alone ($n = 233$). Mean follow-up was approximately 4 years. The combined incidence of ipsilateral neurologic events was 8.0 percent in the surgical group and 20.6 percent in the medical group ($p = 0.001$). The incidence of ipsilateral stroke alone was high in the surgical group (4.7 percent), but was higher (9.4 percent) in the medically managed group. These differences did not reach statistical significance, however.

Operation Versus Aspirin (CASANOVA) trial randomized asymptomatic patients with 50 to 90 percent stenosis.[73] Altogether, 334 carotid endarterectomies were performed. Patients undergoing unilateral or bilateral surgery ($n = 206$) were compared with a medically treated group ($n = 160$) having either unilateral stenosis with no surgery or bilateral stenosis and surgery on the more affected side. Statistical analysis found no significant difference in the number of neurologic deficits and deaths between the two groups. However, this trial is difficult to interpret because of an almost 50 percent crossover rate from the medical to the surgical arm and the exclusion of patients with stenosis >90 percent. Another trial of patients with asymptomatic carotid artery disease is ongoing.[128]

Surgery versus Percutaneous Intervention

One randomized trial, CAVATAS, which compared surgery to percutaneous intervention, has been reported.[129] This study evaluated the safety and efficacy of percutaneous angioplasty versus endarterectomy of the carotid artery. Symptomatic patients with 70 percent stenosis were randomly assigned to angioplasty or surgery, or (if the patient was unsuitable for surgery) to angioplasty or best medical treatment. Preliminary data indicate that 253 patients were randomized to carotid endarterectomy and 251 to carotid angioplasty (of whom 25 percent received stents). A major periprocedural complication was observed in 6.3 percent of patients in both groups (M. Brown, personal communication).[44] CAVATAS-2, with a larger sample size, should provide more insights into the role of percutaneous carotid intervention.

Two important trials comparing carotid artery stenting with endarterectomy have been planned. The Carotid Revascularization Endarterectomy versus Stent Trial will randomize patients who are at low surgical risk to stenting or surgery. The primary end points for this trial are (1) any stroke, myocardial infarction, or death within 30 days, and (2) ipsilateral stroke after 30 days. This trial is planning to recruit 2500 patients, as event rate is likely to be low. A clinical events committee will adjudicate all events. The secondary end points for this study include comparisons of 30-day morbidity and mortality, long-term morbidity and mortality, restenosis rates, quality of life, and cost effectiveness for the two treatment alternatives. Multivariate analysis to identify subgroups of patients at differential risk for the two procedures will be performed.

The Stenting and Angioplasty with Protection in Patients at High Risk for Endarterectomy Trial will randomize patients at high surgical risk to carotid endarterectomy or carotid artery stenting. The high-risk patient population is defined as patients with severe cardiac comorbidities (unstable angina, valvular heart disease, or severe congestive heart failure), previous neck radiation, previous radical neck dissections, restenosis after endarterectomy, or presence of contralateral occlusion. Both de novo and restenotic lesions will be treated in symptomatic (>70 percent stenosis) or asymptomatic (>80 percent stenosis) patients. A total of 720 patients at 24 sites will be enrolled, and a parallel stent and surgical registries will be maintained for the nonrandomized patients. The primary end point is a 30-day composite of any stroke, death, or myocardial infarction. The secondary end point is 1-year ipsilateral stroke and death rate. This trial will utilize the Cordis nitinol carotid stent and Cordis Angioguard, an emboli protection device.

SUMMARY

Stroke is the leading cause of long-term serious disability in the United States, a substantial portion of which is caused by atherosclerotic carotid artery disease. The conventional risk factors for coronary atherosclerosis are also responsible for carotid atherosclerosis. Carotid stenosis is encountered in medical practice in either a symptomatic or asymptomatic state. In symptomatic patients, medical management with antiplatelet agents does not provide adequate protection against stroke. Carotid endarterectomy can help to reduce risk of subsequent stroke. Asymptomatic patients with severe carotid stenosis can benefit from surgical intervention if endarterectomy can be performed at a low operative risk.

Percutaneous carotid stenting using self-expanding stents is becoming popular for the treatment of carotid stenosis. Although this initial experience has been reported from the high-risk patient population, the results are encouraging with acceptable periprocedural stroke rates. Moreover, emboli protection devices, modern adjuvant pharmacotherapy, and modern self-expanding stents were not utilized in these studies. With rapidly expanding technology and advances in the interventional pharmacology, improvement in clinical outcome is likely. At this stage, randomized trials to compare endarterectomy with carotid stenting are warranted and are currently underway. Cautious optimism is necessary until the optimal equipment, emboli protection devices, and adjuvant pharmacotherapies are fully investigated. Until then, carotid stenting should be restricted to high-risk candidates for carotid endarterectomy including patients with severe cardiac comorbidities, previous neck surgeries or radiation or other technical contraindications for surgery.

References

1. American Heart Association. Heart and Stroke Statistical Update. *Dallas: American Heart Association.* 1999.
2. Oddone EZ, Horner RD, Sloane R, et al. Race, presenting signs and symptoms, use of carotid artery imaging, and appropriateness of carotid endarterectomy. *Stroke* 1999; 30:1350–1356.
3. Fields WS, Maslenikov V, Meyer JS, et al. Joint study of extracranial arterial occlusion. V. Progress report of prognosis following surgery or nonsurgical treatment for transient cerebral ischemic attacks and cervical carotid artery lesions. *JAMA* 1970; 211:1993–2003.
4. Hass WK, Fields WS, North RR, et al. Joint study of extracranial arterial occlusion. II. Arteriography, techniques, sites, and complications. *JAMA* 1968; 203:961–968.
5. Bamford J, Dennis M, Sandercock P, et al. The frequency, causes and timing of death within 30 days of a first stroke: The Oxfordshire Community Stroke Project. *J Neurol Neurosurg Psych* 1990; 53:824–829.
6. Fisher C. Occlusion of the carotid arteries. *Arch Neurol Psychol* 1954; 72:187–204.
7. Fisher C. Occlusion of internal carotid artery. *Arch Neurol Psychol* 1951; 65:364–377.
8. von Kemp K, van den Brande P, Peterson T, et al. Screening for concomitant diseases in peripheral vascular patients. Results of a systematic approach. *Intern Angiol* 1997; 16:114–122.
9. Saito D, Shiraki T, Oka T, et al. Morphologic correlation between atherosclerotic lesions of the carotid and coronary arteries in patients with angina pectoris. *Japan Circ J* 1999; 63:522–526.
10. Hulthe J, Wikstrand J, Emanuelsson H, et al. Atherosclerotic changes in the carotid artery bulb as measured by B-mode ultrasound are associated with the extent of coronary atherosclerosis. *Stroke* 1997; 28:1189–1194.
11. Crouse JR III, Craven TE, Hagaman AP, et al. Association of coronary disease with segment-specific intimal-medial thickening of the extracranial carotid artery. *Circulation* 1995; 92:1141–1147.
12. Wofford JL, Kahl FR, Howard GR, et al. Relation of extent of extracranial carotid artery atherosclerosis as measured by B-mode ultrasound to the extent of coronary atherosclerosis. *Arterioscler Thromb* 1991; 11:1786–1794.
13. O'Leary DH, Polak JF, Kronmal RA, et al. Carotid-artery intima and media thickness as a risk factor for myocardial infarction and stroke in older adults. Cardiovascular Health Study Collaborative Research Group. *N Engl J Med* 1999; 340:14–22.
14. Crouse JR, Toole JF, McKinney WM, et al. Risk factors for extracranial carotid artery atherosclerosis. *Stroke* 1987; 18: 990–996.
15. Howard G, Wagenknecht LE, Burke GL, et al. Cigarette smoking and progression of atherosclerosis: The Atherosclerosis Risk in Communities (ARIC) Study. *JAMA* 1998; 279:119–124.
16. Kallikazaros I, Tsioufis C, Sideris S, et al. Carotid artery disease as a marker for the presence of severe coronary artery disease in patients evaluated for chest pain. *Stroke* 1999; 30:1002–1007.
17. Salonen JT, Seppanen K, Rauramaa R, et al. Risk factors for carotid atherosclerosis: The Kuopio Ischaemic Heart Disease Risk Factor Study. *Ann Med* 1989; 21:227–229.
18. Colgan MP, Strode GR, Sommer JD, et al. Prevalence of asymptomatic carotid disease: Results of duplex scanning in 348 unselected volunteers. *J Vasc Surg* 1988; 8:674–678.
19. Josse MO, Touboul PJ, Mas JL, et al. Prevalence of asymptomatic internal carotid artery stenosis. *Neuroepidemiol* 1987; 6:150–152.
20. Heyman A, Fields WS, Keating RD. Joint study of extracranial arterial occlusion. VI. Racial differences in hospitalized patients with ischemic stroke. *JAMA* 1972; 222:285–289.
21. Leung SY, Ng TH, Yuen ST, et al. Pattern of cerebral atherosclerosis in Hong Kong Chinese: Severity in intracranial and extracranial vessels. *Stroke* 1993; 24:779–786.
22. Whisnant JP, Homer D, Ingall TJ, et al. Duration of cigarette smoking is the strongest predictor of severe extracranial carotid artery atherosclerosis. *Stroke* 1990; 21:707–714.
23. Cholesterol, diastolic blood pressure, and stroke: 13,000 strokes in 450,000 people in 45 prospective cohorts. Prospective studies collaboration. *Lancet* 1995; 346:1647–1653.
24. Salonen R, Seppanen K, Rauramaa R, et al. Prevalence of carotid atherosclerosis and serum cholesterol levels in eastern Finland. *Arteriosclerosis* 1988; 8:788–792.
25. Bonithon-Kopp C, Touboul PJ, Berr C, et al. Factors of carotid arterial enlargement in a population aged 59 to 71 years: The EVA study. *Stroke* 1996; 27:654–660.
26. Bonithon-Kopp C, Scarabin PY, Taquet A, et al. Risk factors for early carotid atherosclerosis in middle-aged French women. *Arterioscler Thromb* 1991; 11:966–972.
27. Wilt TJ, Rubins HB, Robins SJ, et al. Carotid atherosclerosis in men with low levels of HDL cholesterol. *Stroke* 1997; 28:1919–1925.
28. Bucher HC, Griffith LE, Guyatt GH. Effect of HMGcoA reductase inhibitors on stroke. A meta-analysis of randomized, controlled trials. *Ann Intern Med* 1998; 128:89–95.
29. Hebert PR, Gaziano JM, Chan KS, et al. Cholesterol lowering with statin drugs, risk of stroke, and total mortality. An overview of randomized trials. *JAMA* 1997; 278:313–321.
30. Blauw GJ, Lagaay AM, Smelt AH, et al. Stroke, statins, and cholesterol. A meta-analysis of randomized, placebo-controlled, double-blind trials with HMG-CoA reductase inhibitors. *Stroke* 1997; 28:946–950.
31. Hennerici M, Hulsbomer HB, Hefter H, et al. Natural history of asymptomatic extracranial arterial disease. Results of a long-term prospective study. *Brain* 1987; 110:777–791.
32. Autret A, Pourcelot L, Saudeau D, et al. Stroke risk in patients with carotid stenosis. *Lancet* 1987; 1:888–890.
33. Hobson RWD, Weiss DG, Fields WS, et al. Efficacy of carotid endarterectomy for asymptomatic carotid stenosis. The Veterans Affairs Cooperative Study Group. *N Engl J Med* 1993; 328: 221–227.

34. Hertzer NR, Flanagan RA Jr, Beven EG, et al. Surgical versus nonoperative treatment of symptomatic carotid stenosis: 211 patients documented by intravenous angiography. *Ann Surg* 1986; 204:154–162.
35. Hertzer NR, Flanagan RA Jr, Beven EG, et al. Surgical versus nonoperative treatment of asymptomatic carotid stenosis: 290 patients documented by intravenous angiography. *Ann Surg* 1986; 204:163–171.
36. Mansour MA, Littooy FN, Watson WC, et al. Outcome of moderate carotid artery stenosis in patients who are asymptomatic. *J Vasc Surg* 1999; 29:217–225; (discussion) 225–227.
37. Meissner I, Wiebers DO, Whisnant JP, et al. The natural history of asymptomatic carotid artery occlusive lesions. *JAMA* 1987; 258:2704–2707.
38. Chambers BR, Norris JW. Outcome in patients with asymptomatic neck bruits. *N Engl J Med* 1986; 315:860–865.
39. Chambers BR, Norris JW. The case against surgery for asymptomatic carotid stenosis. *Stroke* 1984; 15:964–967.
40. Olin JW, Fonseca C, Childs MB, et al. The natural history of asymptomatic moderate internal carotid artery stenosis by duplex ultrasound. *Vasc Med* 1998; 3:101–108.
41. Roederer GO, Langlois YE, Jager KA, et al. The natural history of carotid arterial disease in asymptomatic patients with cervical bruits. *Stroke* 1984; 15:605–613.
42. Roederer GO, Langlois YE, Lusiani L, et al. Natural history of carotid artery disease on the side contralateral to endarterectomy. *J Vasc Surg* 1984; 1:62–72.
43. Dennis M, Bamford J, Sandercock P, et al. Prognosis of transient ischemic attacks in the Oxfordshire Community Stroke Project. *Stroke* 1990; 21:848–853.
44. Mendelsohn FO, Mahaffey KW, Yadav JS. Management of atherosclerotic carotid disease: Medical, surgical and interventional aspects. In: Topol EJ, ed. *Textbook of Cardiovascular Medicine,* vol 2. NJ: Lippincott Williams & Wilkins Healthcare; 1999:1.
45. Riggs HE, Rupp C. Variation in form of the circle of Willis. The relation of variation to collateral circulation: Anatomic analysis. *Arch Neurol* 1963; 8:24–30.
46. Lusby RJ, Ferrell LD, Ehrenfeld WK, et al. Carotid plaque hemorrhage. Its role in production of cerebral ischemia. *Arch Surg* 1982; 117:1479–1488.
47. Lennihan L, Kupsky WJ, Mohr JP, et al. Lack of association between carotid plaque hematoma and ischemic cerebral symptoms. *Stroke* 1987; 18:879–881.
48. Sitzer M, Muller W, Siebler M, et al. Plaque ulceration and lumen thrombus are the main sources of cerebral microemboli in high-grade internal carotid artery stenosis. *Stroke* 1995; 26:1231–1233.
49. Imparato AM, Riles TS, Gorstein F. The carotid bifurcation plaque: Pathologic findings associated with cerebral ischemia. *Stroke* 1979; 10:238–245.
50. Eliasziw M, Streifler JY, Fox AJ, et al. Significance of plaque ulceration in symptomatic patients with high-grade carotid stenosis. North American Symptomatic Carotid Endarterectomy Trial. *Stroke* 1994; 25:304–308.
51. Reilly LM, Lusby RJ, Hughes L, et al. Carotid plaque histology using real-time ultrasonography. Clinical and therapeutic implications. *Am J Surg* 1983; 146:188–193.
52. O'Donnell TF Jr, Erdoes L, Mackey WC, et al. Correlation of B-mode ultrasound imaging and arteriography with pathologic findings at carotid endarterectomy. *Arch Surg* 1985; 120:443–449.
53. Geroulakos G, Ramaswami G, Nicolaides A, et al. Characterization of symptomatic and asymptomatic carotid plaques using high-resolution real-time ultrasonography. *Br J Surg* 1993; 80:1274–1277.
54. Gray-Weale AC, Graham JC, Burnett JR, et al. Carotid artery atheroma: Comparison of preoperative B-mode ultrasound appearance with carotid endarterectomy specimen pathology. *J Cardiovasc Surg* (*Torino*) 1988; 29:676–681.
55. Leahy AL, McCollum PT, Feeley TM, et al. Duplex ultrasonography and selection of patients for carotid endarterectomy: Plaque morphology or luminal narrowing? *J Vasc Surg* 1988; 8:558–562.
56. Arnold JA, Modaresi KB, Thomas N, et al. Carotid plaque characterization by duplex scanning: Observer error may undermine current clinical trials. *Stroke* 1999; 30:61–65.
57. Estes JM, Quist WC, Lo Gerfo FW, et al. Noninvasive characterization of plaque morphology using helical computed tomography. *J Cardiovasc Surg* (*Torino*) 1998; 39:527–534.
58. Toussaint JF, LaMuraglia GM, Southern JF, et al. Magnetic resonance images lipid, fibrous, calcified, hemorrhagic, and thrombotic components of human atherosclerosis in vivo. *Circulation* 1996; 94:932–938.
59. Shinnar M, Fallon JT, Wehrli S, et al. The diagnostic accuracy of ex vivo MRI for human atherosclerotic plaque characterization. *Arterioscler Thromb Vasc Biol* 1999; 19:2756–2761.
60. Beebe HG, Salles-Cunha SX, Scissons RP, et al. Carotid arterial ultrasound scan imaging: A direct approach to stenosis measurement. *J Vasc Surg* 1999; 29:838–844.
61. Alexandrov AV, Vital D, Brodie DS, et al. Grading carotid stenosis with ultrasound. An interlaboratory comparison. *Stroke* 1997; 28:1208–1210.
62. Alexandrov AV, Brodie DS, McLean A, et al. Correlation of peak systolic velocity and angiographic measurement of carotid stenosis revisited. *Stroke* 1997; 28:339–342.
63. Salonen JT, Salonen R. Ultrasound B-mode imaging in observational studies of atherosclerotic progression. *Circulation* 1993; 87:II56–II65.
64. Anderson CM, Saloner D, Lee RE, et al. Assessment of carotid artery stenosis by MR angiography: Comparison with x-ray angiography and color-coded Doppler ultrasound. *AJNR Am J Neuroradiol* 1992; 13:989–1003; (discussion) 1005–1008.
65. Mittl RL Jr, Broderick M, Carpenter JP, et al. Blinded-reader comparison of magnetic resonance angiography and duplex ultrasonography for carotid artery bifurcation stenosis. *Stroke* 1994; 25:4–10.
66. Pan XM, Anderson CM, Reilly LM, et al. Magnetic resonance angiography of the carotid artery combining two- and three-dimensional acquisitions. *J Vasc Surg* 1992; 16:609–615; (discussion) 615–618.
67. Pan XM, Saloner D, Reilly LM, et al. Assessment of carotid artery stenosis by ultrasonography, conventional angiography, and magnetic resonance angiography: Correlation with ex vivo measurement of plaque stenosis. *J Vasc Surg* 1995; 21:82–88; (discussion) 88–89.
68. Kappelle LJ, Eliasziw M, Fox AJ, et al. Importance of intracranial atherosclerotic disease in patients with symptomatic stenosis of the internal carotid artery. The North American Symptomatic Carotid Endarterectomy Trial. *Stroke* 1999; 30:282–286.
69. Wholey MH. Do the benefits of angiography outweigh the risks in the treatment of patients with carotid artery occlusive disease? (editorial). *Cardiovasc Intervent Radiol* 1999; 22:183–184.
70. Collaborative overview of randomised trials of antiplatelet therapy—I: Prevention of death, myocardial infarction, and stroke by prolonged antiplatelet therapy in various categories of patients. Antiplatelet Trialists' Collaboration (published erratum appears in *Br Med J* 1994; 308(6943):1540). *Br Med J* 1994; 308:81–106.
71. Bellavance A. Efficacy of ticlopidine and aspirin for prevention of reversible cerebrovascular ischemic events. The Ticlopidine Aspirin Stroke Study. *Stroke* 1993; 24:1452–1457.
72. CAPRIE Steering Committee. A randomised, blinded trial of clopidogrel versus aspirin in patients at risk of ischaemic events (CAPRIE). *Lancet* 1996; 348:1329–1339.

73. The CASANOVA Study Group. Carotid surgery versus medical therapy in asymptomatic carotid stenosis. *Stroke* 1991; 22:1229–1235.
74. North American Symptomatic Carotid Endarterectomy Trial Collaborators. Beneficial effect of carotid endarterectomy in symptomatic patients with high-grade carotid stenosis. *N Engl J Med* 1991; 325:445–453.
75. Barnett HJ, Taylor DW, Eliasziw M, et al. Benefit of carotid endarterectomy in patients with symptomatic moderate or severe stenosis. North American Symptomatic Carotid Endarterectomy Trial Collaborators. *N Engl J Med* 1998; 339:1415–1425.
76. European Carotid Surgery Trialists' Collaborative Group. MRC European Carotid Surgery Trial: Interim results for symptomatic patients with severe (70–99%) or with mild (0–29%) carotid stenosis. *Lancet* 1991; 337:1235–1243.
77. Mayo Asymptomatic Carotid Endarterectomy Study Group. Results of a randomized controlled trial of carotid endarterectomy for asymptomatic carotid stenosis. *Mayo Clin Proc* 1992; 67:513–518.
78. European Carotid Surgery Trialists' Collaborative Group. Randomised trial of endarterectomy for recently symptomatic carotid stenosis: Final results of the MRC European Carotid Surgery Trial (ECST). *Lancet* 1998; 351:1379–1387.
79. Mayberg MR, Wilson SE, Yatsu F, et al. Carotid endarterectomy and prevention of cerebral ischemia in symptomatic carotid stenosis. Veterans Affairs Cooperative Studies Program 309 Trialist Group. *JAMA* 1991; 266:3289–3294.
80. Executive Committee for the Asymptomatic Carotid Atherosclerosis Study. Endarterectomy for asymptomatic carotid artery stenosis. *JAMA* 1995; 273:1421–1428.
81. Hobson RWD, Krupski WC, Weiss DG. Influence of aspirin in the management of asymptomatic carotid artery stenosis. VA Cooperative Study Group on Asymptomatic Carotid Stenosis. *J Vasc Surg* 1993; 17:257–263; (discussion) 263–265.
82. Jonas S. Anticoagulant therapy in cerebrovascular disease: Review and meta-analysis (published erratum appears in *Stroke* 1989; 20(4):562). *Stroke* 1988; 19:1043–1048.
83. The Stroke Prevention in Reversible Ischemia Trial (SPIRIT) Study Group. A randomized trial of anticoagulants versus aspirin after cerebral ischemia of presumed arterial origin. *Ann Neurol* 1997; 42:857–865.
84. Acheson J, Hutchinson EC. Controlled trial of clofibrate in cerebral vascular disease. *Atherosclerosis* 1972; 15:177–183.
85. The treatment of cerebrovascular disease with clofibrate. Final report of the Veterans Administration Cooperative Study of Atherosclerosis, Neurology Section. *Stroke* 1973; 4:684–693.
86. Crouse JR III, Byington RP, Bond MG, et al. Pravastatin, lipids, and atherosclerosis in the carotid arteries (PLAC-II) (published erratum appears in *Am J Cardiol* 1995; 75(12):862). *Am J Cardiol* 1995; 75:455–459.
87. Furberg CD, Adams HP Jr, Applegate WB, et al. Effect of lovastatin on early carotid atherosclerosis and cardiovascular events. Asymptomatic Carotid Artery Progression Study (ACAPS) Research Group. *Circulation* 1994; 90:1679–1687.
88. MacMahon S, Sharpe N, Gamble G, et al. Effects of lowering average of below-average cholesterol levels on the progression of carotid atherosclerosis: Results of the LIPID Atherosclerosis Substudy. LIPID Trial Research Group (published erratum appears in *Circulation* 1996; 97(24):2479). *Circulation* 1998; 97:1784–1790.
89. Beebe HG, Archie JP, Baker WH, et al. Concern about safety of carotid angioplasty (editorial). *Stroke* 1996; 27:197–198.
90. Mathias K. A new catheter system for percutaneous transluminal angioplasty (PTA) of carotid artery stenoses. *Fortschr Med* 1977; 95:1007–1011.
91. Kerber CW, Cromwell LD, Loehden OL. Catheter dilatation of proximal carotid stenosis during distal bifurcation endarterectomy. *Am J Neuroradiol* 1980; 1:348–349.
92. Mullan S, Duda EE, Patronas NJ. Some examples of balloon technology in neurosurgery. *J Neurosurg* 1980; 52:321–329.
93. Brown MM, Butler P, Gibbs J, et al. Feasibility of percutaneous transluminal angioplasty for carotid artery stenosis. *J Neurol Neurosurg Psych* 1990; 53:238–243.
94. Kachel R, Basche S, Heerklotz I, et al. Percutaneous transluminal angioplasty (PTA) of supra-aortic arteries especially the internal carotid artery. *Neuroradiology* 1991; 33:191–194.
95. Tsai FY, Matovich V, Hieshima G, et al. Percutaneous transluminal angioplasty of the carotid artery. *Am J Neuroradiol* 1986; 7:349–358.
96. Higashida RT, Tsai FY, Halbach VV, et al. Cerebral percutaneous transluminal angioplasty. *Heart Dis Stroke* 1993; 2:497–502.
97. Bergeron P, Chambran P, Hartung O, et al. Cervical carotid artery stenosis: Which technique, balloon angioplasty or surgery? *J Cardiovasc Surg (Torino)* 1996; 37:73–75.
98. Kachel R. Results of balloon angioplasty in the carotid arteries. *J Endovasc Surg* 1996; 3:22–30.
99. Gil-Peralta A, Mayol A, Marcos JR, et al. Percutaneous transluminal angioplasty of the symptomatic atherosclerotic carotid arteries: Results, complications, and follow-up. *Stroke* 1996; 27:2271–2273.
100. Motarjeme A, Keifer JW, Zuska AJ. Percutaneous transluminal angioplasty of the brachiocephalic arteries. *Am J Roentgenol* 1982; 138:457–462.
101. Marks MP, Dake MD, Steinberg GK, et al. Stent placement for arterial and venous cerebrovascular disease: Preliminary experience. *Radiology* 1994; 191:441–446.
102. Mathias K. Stent placement in arteriosclerotic disease of the internal carotid artery. In: Adam A, Dondelinger RF, Mueller PR, eds. *Textbook of Metallic Stents.* Oxford: Isis Medical Media; 1997:189.
103. Mendelsohn FO, Weissman NJ, Lederman RJ, et al. Acute hemodynamic changes during carotid artery stenting. *Am J Cardiol* 1998; 82:1077–1081.
104. Theron JG, Payelle GG, Coskun O, et al. Carotid artery stenosis: Treatment with protected balloon angioplasty and stent placement. *Radiology* 1996; 201:627–636.
105. Shawl FA, Efstratiou A, Lapetina FL, et al. Stent supported carotid angioplasty (SSCA) in patients with symptomatic coronary artery disease: Acute and long term results. *J Am Coll Cardiol* 1998; 31(suppl):454A.
106. Henry M, Amor M, Masson I, et al. Angioplasty and stenting of the extracranial carotid arteries. *J Endovasc Surg* 1998; 5:293–304.
107. Laborde JC, Fajadet J, Cassagneau B, et al. Carotid stenting in patients at risk for surgery: Immediate and long-term results. *J Am Coll Cardiol* 1998; 31(suppl):63A.
108. Yadav JS, Roubin GS, Iyer S, et al. Elective stenting of the extracranial carotid arteries. *Circulation* 1997; 95:376–381.
109. Wholey MH, Jarmolowski CR, Eles G, et al. Endovascular stents for carotid artery occlusive disease. *J Endovasc Surg* 1997; 4:326–338.
110. Diethrich EB, Ndiaye M, Reid DB. Stenting in the carotid artery: Initial experience in 110 patients. *J Endovasc Surg* 1996; 3:42–62.
111. Wholey MH, Eles G. Cervical carotid artery stent placement. *Semin Interv Cardiol* 1998; 3:105–115.
112. Roubin GS, Yadav S, Iyer SS, et al. Carotid stent-supported angioplasty: A neurovascular intervention to prevent stroke. *Am J Cardiol* 1996; 78:8–12.
113. Mathur A, Roubin GS, Iyer SS, et al. Predictors of stroke complicating carotid artery stenting. *Circulation* 1998; 97:1239–1245.
114. McCleary AJ, Nelson M, Dearden NM, et al. Cerebral haemodynamics and embolization during carotid angioplasty in high-risk patients. *Br J Surg* 1998; 85:771–774.

115. Markus HS, Clifton A, Buckenham T, et al. Carotid angioplasty. Detection of embolic signals during and after the procedure. *Stroke* 1994; 25:2403–2406.
116. Gaunt ME, Martin PJ, Smith JL, et al. Clinical relevance of intraoperative embolization detected by transcranial Doppler ultrasonography during carotid endarterectomy: A prospective study of 100 patients. *Br J Surg* 1994; 81:1435–1439.
117. Ackerstaff RG, Jansen C, Moll FL, et al. The significance of microemboli detection by means of transcranial Doppler ultrasonography monitoring in carotid endarterectomy. *J Vasc Surg* 1995; 21:963–969.
118. Yadav JS, Grube E, Rowold S, et al. Detection and characterization of emboli during coronary intervention. *Circulation* 1999; 100:I780.
119. Whitlow PL, Lylyk P, Parodi P. Protected carotid stenting: Preliminary results of a multicenter trial. *Circulation* 1999; 100:I436.
120. Henry M, Amor M, Henry I, et al. Carotid angioplasty and stenting with a new cerebral protection device: The percusurge guardwire device. *Circulation* 1999; 100:I674.
121. The EPISTENT Investigators. Randomised placebo-controlled and balloon-angioplasty-controlled trial to assess safety of coronary stenting with use of platelet glycoprotein-IIb/IIIa blockade. Evaluation of platelet IIb/IIIa inhibitor for stenting. *Lancet* 1998; 352:87–92.
122. The EPILOG Investigators. Platelet glycoprotein IIb/IIIa receptor blockade and low-dose heparin during percutaneous coronary revascularization. *N Engl J Med* 1997; 336:1689–1696.
123. Tcheng JE. Glycoprotein IIb/IIIa receptor inhibitors: Putting the EPIC, IMPACT II, RESTORE, and EPILOG trials into perspective. *Am J Cardiol* 1996; 78:35–40.
124. Chastain HDI, Mt Wong P, Mathur A, et al. Does abciximab reduce complications of cerebral vascular stenting in high risk lesions? *Circulation* 1997; 96:I283.
124a. Kapadia SR, Bajzer CT, Ziada KM, et al. Initial experience of glycoprotein IIb/IIIa inhibition with abciximab during carotid stenting: A safe adjunctive therapy. *J Am Coll Cardiol* 2000; 35:86A.
125. Bajzer CT, Kapadia SR, Yadav JS. Clopidogrel use in carotid artery stenting. *Am J Cardiol* 1999; Sept 22 (abstr 15):7P.
126. Moore WS, Vescera CL, Robertson JT, et al. Selection process for surgeons in the Asymptomatic Carotid Atherosclerosis Study. *Stroke* 1991; 22:1353–1357.
127. Moore WS, Young B, Baker WH, et al. Surgical results: A justification of the surgeon selection process for the ACAS trial. The ACAS Investigators. *J Vasc Surg* 1996; 23:323–328.
128. Halliday AW, Thomas D, Mansfield A. The Asymptomatic Carotid Surgery Trial (ACST). Rationale and design. Steering Committee. *Eur J Vasc Surg* 1994; 8:703–710.
129. Sivaguru A, Venables GS, Beard JD, et al. European carotid angioplasty trial. *J Endovasc Surg* 1996; 3:16–20.

CHAPTER 93

ADVANCES IN THE MINIMALLY INVASIVE TREATMENT OF PERIPHERAL VASCULAR DISEASE

Michael L. Marin / Larry H. Hollier / Michael Poon / Valentin Fuster

INTRODUCTION

The treatment of peripheral vascular disease (PVD) is actively changing, largely as a result of an enhanced understanding of the natural history of clinically significant disease and advances in new therapeutic technologies. The recognition that the individual symptoms of PVD are frequently only a part of the broader problem of diffuse atherosclerosis continues to refocus management of patients with peripheral occlusive disease and arterial aneurysms toward more conservative therapies and the use of less invasive technology.

The use of minimally invasive approaches to PVD has exploded in the past 10 years, following similar advances in the treatment of coronary artery disease. The potential advantages to patients and in turn to the health care system are being realized in the form of reduced morbidity, shorter lengths of stay in the hospital, and a reduction in the total cost of care.

However, these advances must not proceed without clearly defined treatment benefits and acceptable long-term therapeutic durability. This chapter reviews current advances in the least invasive therapies for the treatment of occlusive and aneurysmal disease of peripheral arteries and explores the value and limitations of these approaches.

PERIPHERAL ARTERY OCCLUSIVE DISEASES

Occlusive disease of peripheral arteries includes atherosclerosis within all vessels except the intracerebral and coronary vasculature. Minimally invasive or endovascular therapy has been attempted in almost all these vascular beds; however, the success of these procedures varies. Therapeutic approaches have included atherosclerotic plaque ablation (atherectomy), thrombolytic therapy, balloon angioplasty, intravascular stents, and stented grafts.[1]

Occlusive Disease of Aortic Arch Vessels

The advantages of treating symptomatic occlusive lesions of branch vessels of the aortic arch with catheter-based techniques can be quite dramatic, with the restoration of normal circulation without the need for intrathoracic surgery. The proximal innominate, carotid, and subclavian arteries may be accessed readily through a transfemoral catheter-based approach.[2] Luminal restoration may be achieved by using several endovascular modalities, including ballon angioplasty with or without intravascular stent placement, which appears to provide the most favorable results (Fig. 93-1 and Table 93-1). Along with the potential for primary lesion restenosis, distal arterial dissections, vessel rupture, and embolization to the cerebral circulation are complications that fortunately are uncommon after endovascular treatment of occlusive lesions of proximal arch vessels.[3,4]

Internal carotid bifurcation occlusive disease is a more common lesion that has become an important and controversial area for treatment with minimally invasive endoluminal techniques (Fig. 93-2).[5] The excellent results achieved with conventional surgical procedures to correct these extracavitary lesions and a distinct tendency of these lesions to be friable and embolize with catheter manipulations have created significant concern about the future of this approach to stroke prevention.[6] However, good results have been achieved at several centers with internal carotid artery stenting, and the potential for distal em-

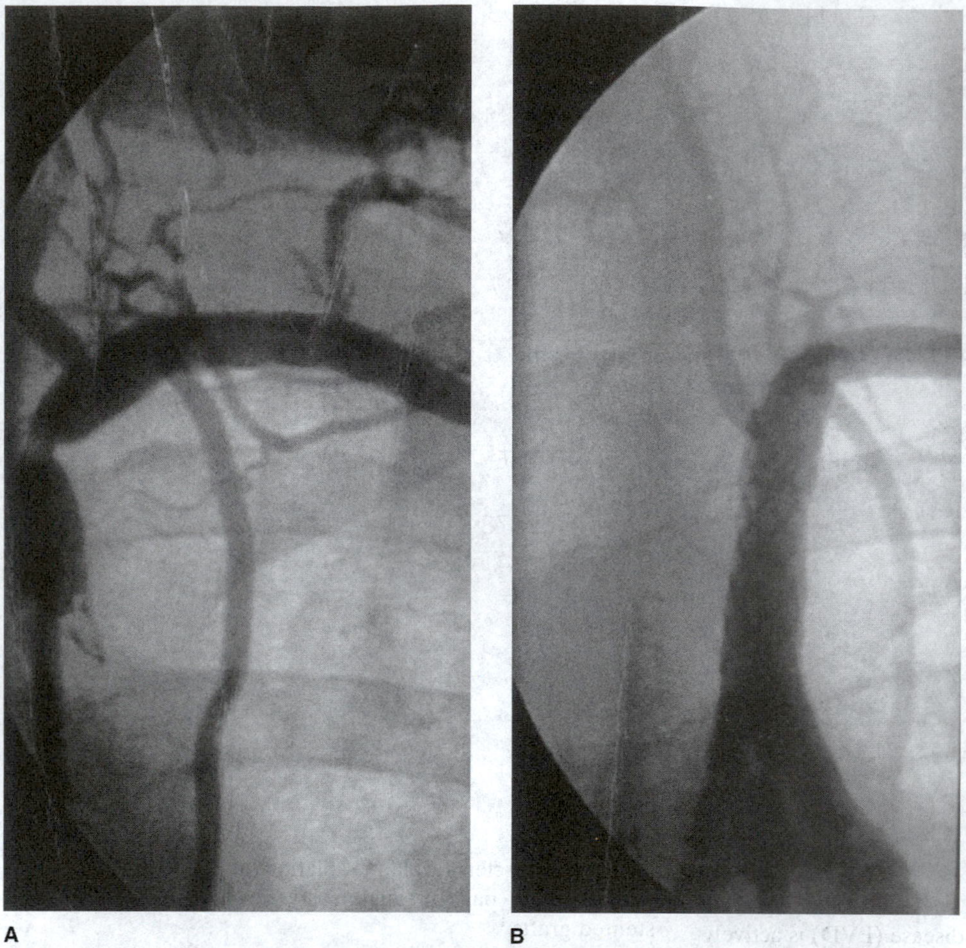

FIGURE 93-1 *A.* Aortic arch angiogram of a 63-year-old woman with left upper extremity claudication. *B.* After angioplasty with a 6-mm balloon, a residual intralesion stenosis and a vessel wall dissection prompted placement of a Palmaz balloon-expandable stent.

bolization "protection devices" to prevent thromboembolic complications may further expand the use of these procedures.[5]

Occlusive Disease of the Visceral Segment

Treatment of occlusive disease of the celiac, superior mesenteric and renal arteries can be accomplished successfully with full resolution of the underlying hemodynamically significant lesions and clinical improvement. Chronic intestinal ischemia secondary to celiac, superior, or inferior mesenteric artery occlusion and/or stenosis can have profound clinical results in select patients.[7,8] Both proximal and distal superior mesenteric artery lesions have been treated with isolated balloon angioplasty and more recently with the insertion of intravascular stents (Fig. 93-3 and Table 93-2). Despite sporadic reports of successful treatment of chronic mesenteric ischemia with endovascular treatments, comparative studies with standard surgical revascularization have not been performed.

The endoluminal treatment of renal artery stenosis has received considerable attention, particularly as improved stent technology has become available (Fig. 93-4). Early work with balloon dilatation of renal artery stenoses was limited by vessel dissections and early restenosis after treatment. This was especially true for ostial renal lesions, which probably are primarily of aortic atherosclerotic plaque origin. Recently, several careful prospective studies have demonstrated the technical effectiveness of renal stenting; however, questions remain about whether endovascular intervention for renal artery stenoses will positively affect the control of hypertension or the prevention of renal failure[9–13] (Table 93-3). Several ongoing trials may soon shed additional light on this area.[14]

Occlusive Disease of the Iliac, Femoral, Popliteal, and Tibial Arteries

Occlusive disease of the lower extremities represents a significant health problem, limiting function (ambulation) and creating significant risks for limb loss. Endovascular therapy of the iliac vessels, particularly the common iliac artery, has evolved to become standard treatment for this clinically significant problem.[15–19] Percutaneous transluminal angioplasty (PTA) with the use of supplemental stents can provide full relief of clinically

TABLE 93-1 Subclavian Artery Intervention

Type of Study	Reference	No. Vessels	Type of Lesion	Angioplasty (A) versus Stenting (S)	Technical Success, %	Follow-up, Months
Retrospective	2	43	Stenosis	A	84	15
Retrospective	3	55	Stenosis, arteritis	A	92.8	43
Retrospective	4	36	Stenosis	A	94	—

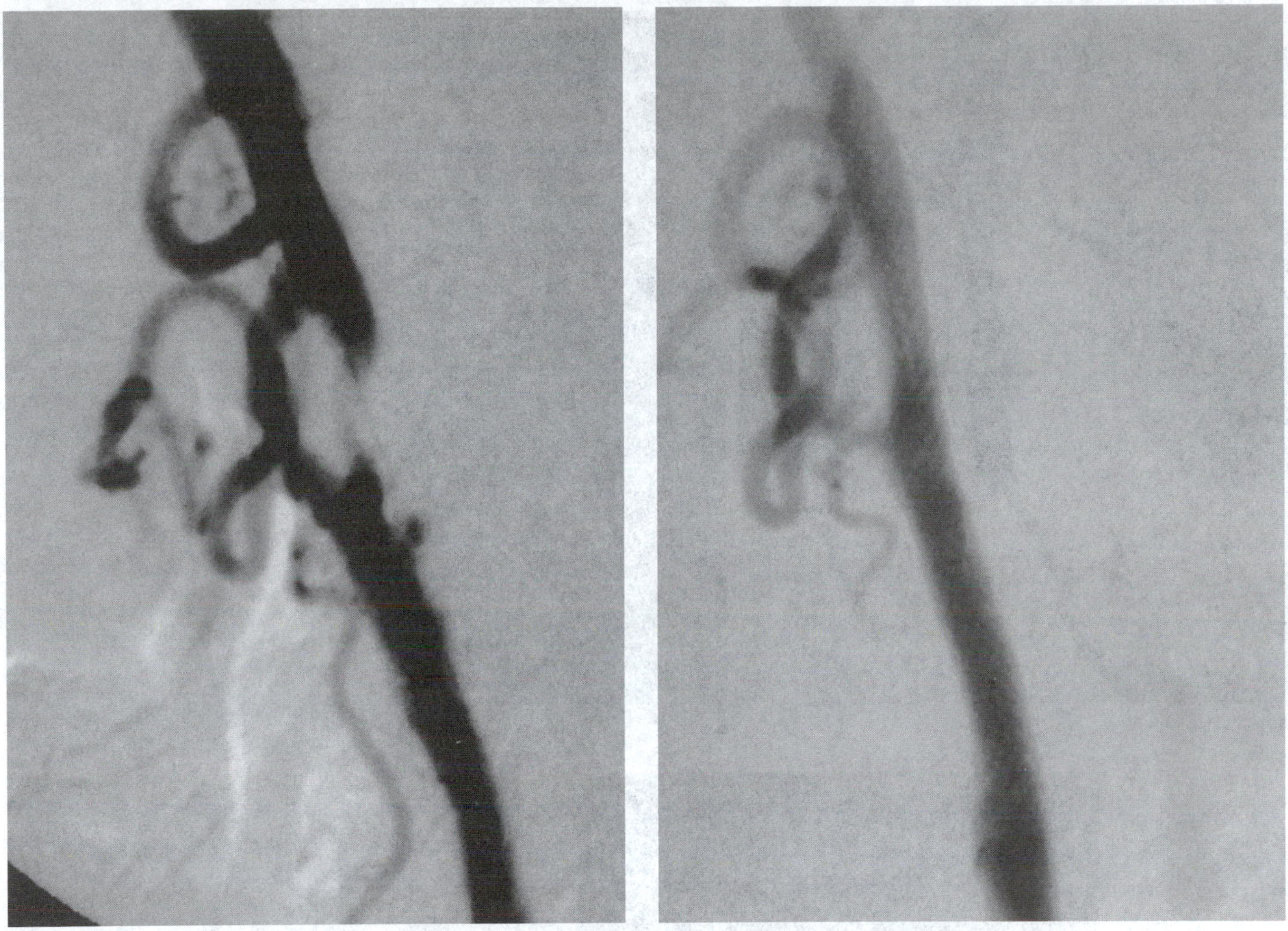

FIGURE 93-2 *A.* Carotid angiogram of an asymptomatic, high-grade left internal carotid artery stenosis. *B.* The lesion is corrected after treatment with balloon angioplasty and the implantation of a Wallstent.

important common iliac artery stenoses with good patency and relief of symptoms (Fig. 93-5 and Table 93-4).

The same results have not been fully achieved within the femoropopliteal segment of the vasculature. These regions tend to contain diffuse occlusive disease, and intervention in one isolated area of the superficial femoral or popliteal arteries often does not provide sufficient pressure gradient resolution to achieve symptomatic relief. When isolated focal lesions are present, angioplasty and occasionally stent implantation may give acceptable results (Fig. 93-6 and Table 93-5).[20–23] However, immediate successful endovascular treatment of the superficial femoral and popliteal arteries has commonly resulted in lesion restenosis or occlusion with the return of ischemic symptoms.

Some data suggest efficacy of PTA in select patients with tibial artery occlusive disease under the premise that limb salvage may be achieved, with even short-term restoration of the pedal circulation achieving the clearance of sepsis and the healing of wounds.[24–26] In select circumstances, extremities will remain healed and free from ischemic ulcers despite failure at the site of intervention (Table 93-6).

TABLE 93-2 Mesenteric Artery Intervention

Type of Study	Reference	No. Vessels	Type of Lesion	Angioplasty (A) versus Stenting (S)	Technical Success, %	Follow-up, Months
Retrospective	8	41	Stenosis	A	88	27
Retrospective	9	20	Stenosis	A	83	25

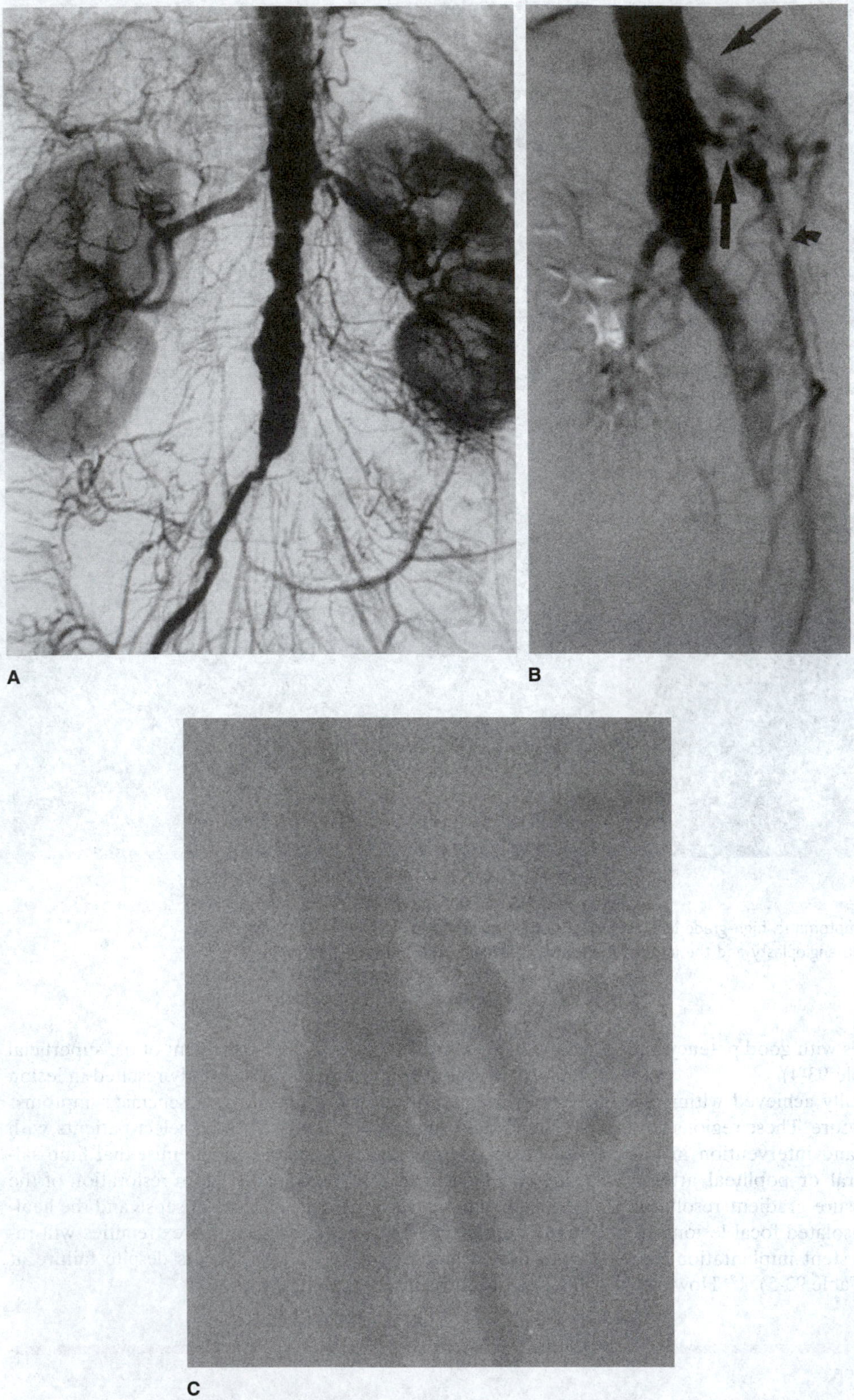

FIGURE 93-3 *A.* Mesenteric angiogram in a 69-year-old woman with a 40-lb weight loss over 16 months and severe postprandial abdominal pain. *B.* Proximal (*arrow*) and midsuperior mesenteric artery (*small arrow*) and celiac artery (*arrow*) stenoses are corrected by balloon angioplasty and Palmaz stent placement. *C.* Full resolution of abdominal symptoms and reestablishment of normal weight parameters accompanied recovery over a 4-month period after treatment.

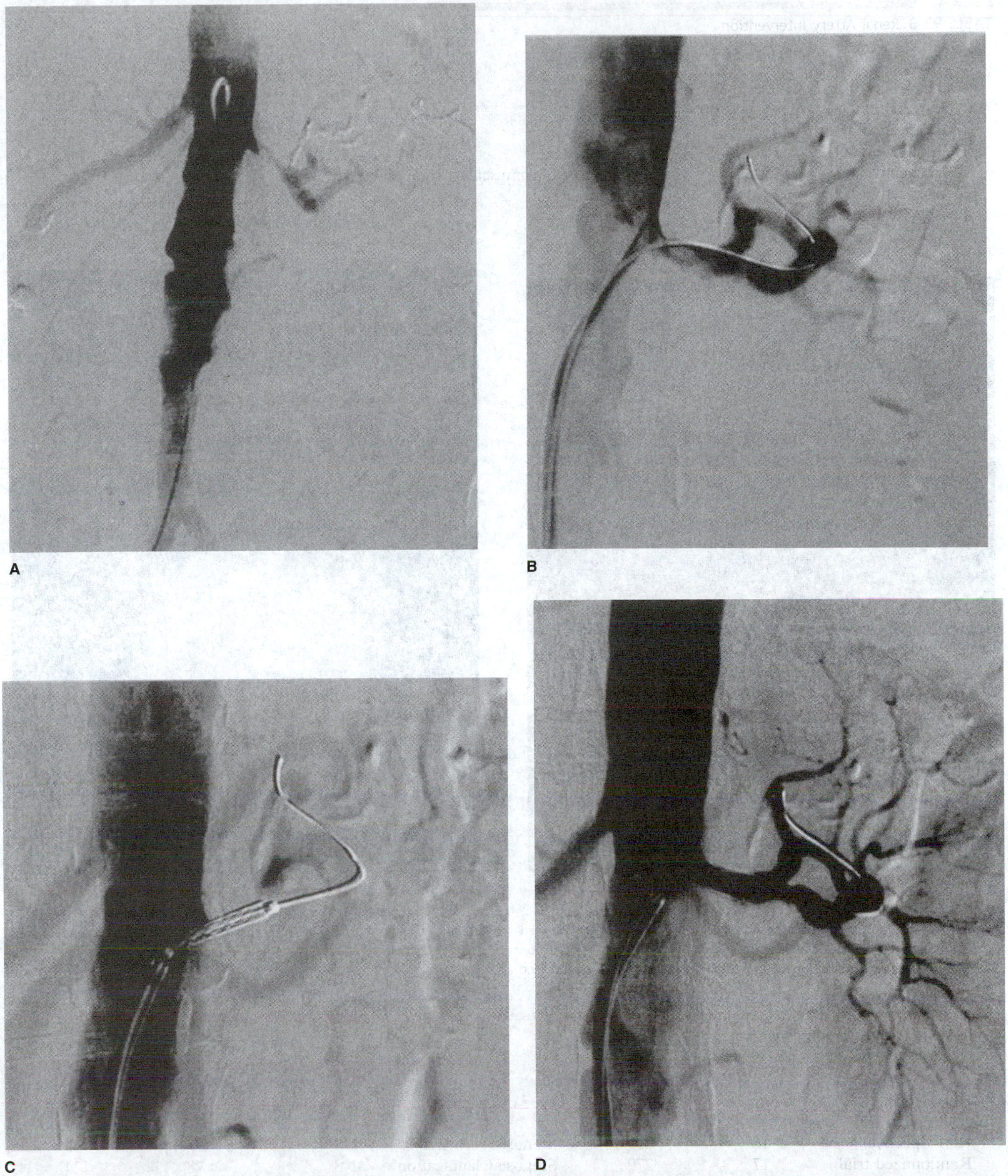

FIGURE 93-4 *A*. Aortogram demonstrating an isolated left renal artery stenosis in a 71-year-old woman with poorly controlled hypertension and normal renal function. *B*. Balloon angioplasty produced local dissection with residual stenosis. *C* and *D*. After implantation of an AVE stent in accordance with the SOAR trial protocol, full resolution of the hemodynamically significant lesion was achieved. The patient continues to require two medications to control her hypertension. (From Becquemin JP, Cavillon A, Haiduc F. Surgical transluminal femoropopliteal angioplasty: Multivariate analysis outcome. *J Vasc Surg* 1994; 19:495–502. Reproduced with permission from the publisher and authors.)

TABLE 93-3 Renal Artery Intervention

Type of Study	Reference	No. Vessels	Type of Lesion	Angioplasty (A) versus Stenting (S)	Technical Success, %	Follow-up, Months
Multicenter trial	10	120	Stenosis	A and S	98	8
Randomized trial	11	43	Stenosis	A and S	88	12
Retrospective	12	591	Stenosis, fibromuscular dysplasia	A	92	—
Retrospective	13	163	Stenosis	A and S	100	48
Prospective	14	74	Stenosis	A and S	100	27

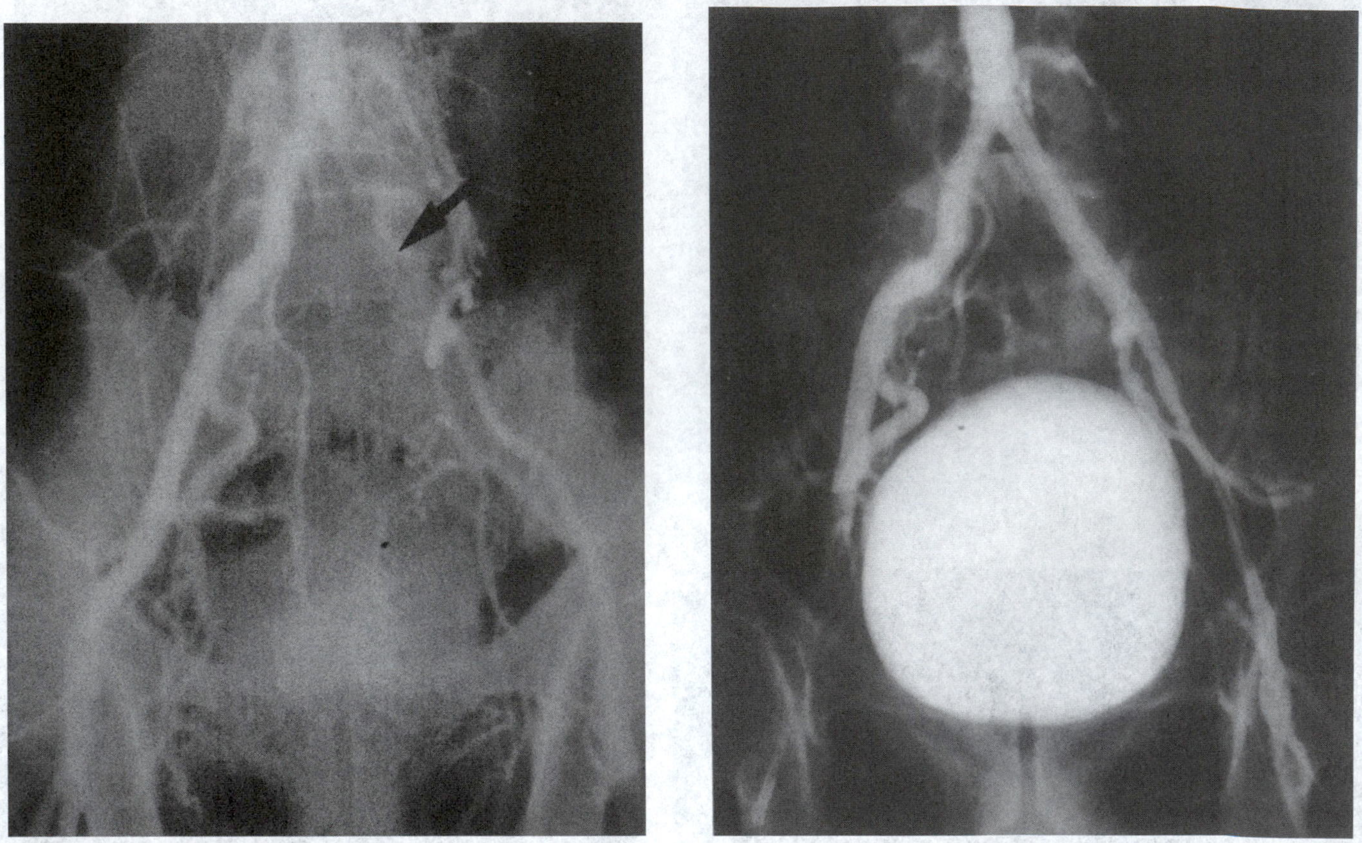

A B

FIGURE 93-5 *A.* Aortogram with pelvic runoff views of a 61-year-old man with left thigh and buttock claudication and common iliac artery occlusion (*arrow*). *B.* After recannalization of the totally occluded left common iliac artery (*arrow*), normal flow was reestablished to the left leg with percutaneous balloon angioplasty and the placement of an iliac stent.

TABLE 93-4 Iliac Artery Intervention

Type of Study	Reference	No. Patients	Type of Lesion	Stent versus Angioplasty	Patency, %	Follow-up, Months
Retrospective	16	235	Stenosis/occlusive	NS*	75.4	60
Randomized trial	17	279	Stenosis/claudication	NS	78	24
Meta-analysis	18	2416†	Stenosis/claudication	NS	53	48
Multicenter trial	19	140	Stenosis/occlusive	Wallstent	71	24
Retrospective	20	238	Stenosis/occlusive	Palmaz	86	48

*NS = no significance.
†2416 patients from 14 different studies.

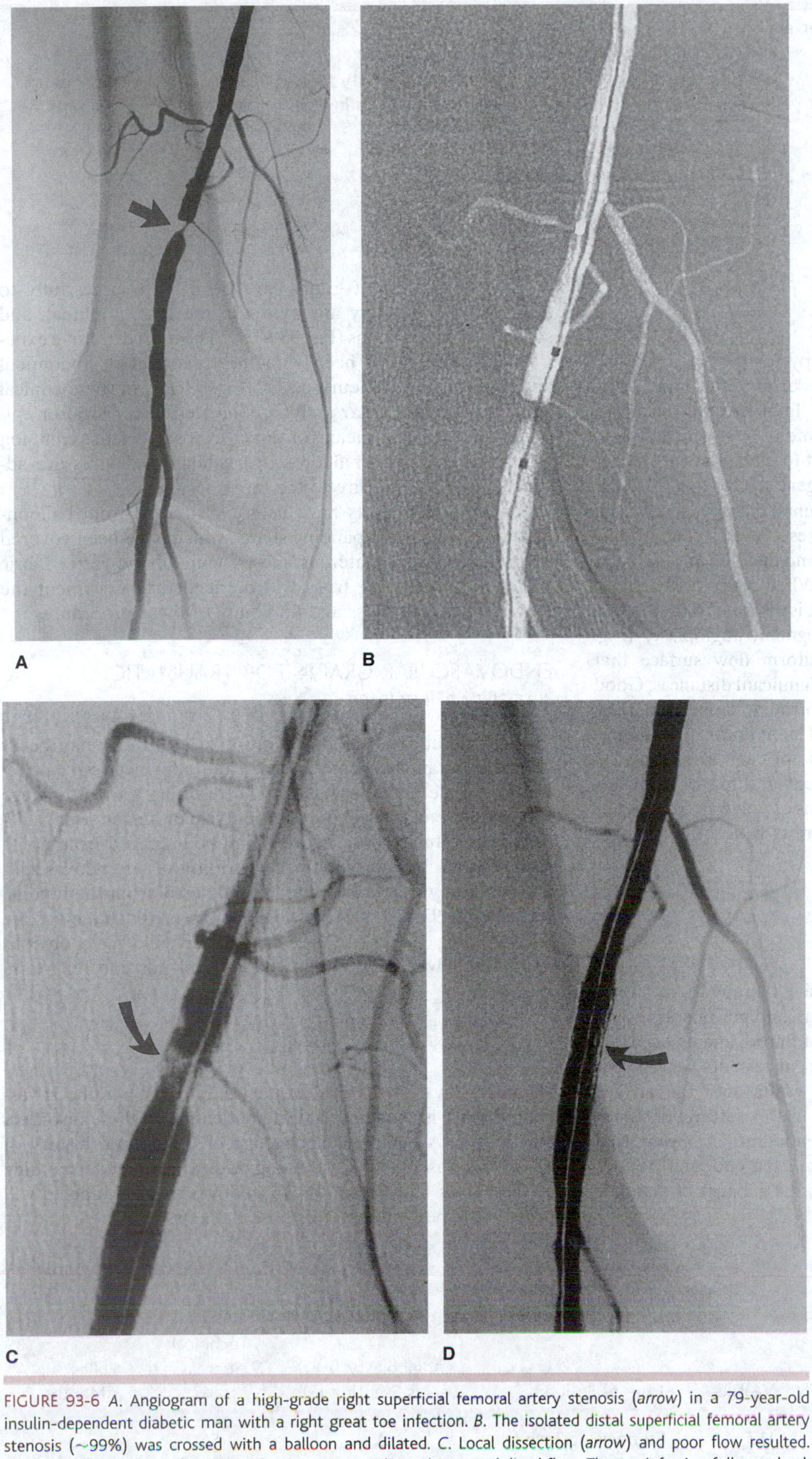

FIGURE 93-6 *A.* Angiogram of a high-grade right superficial femoral artery stenosis (*arrow*) in a 79-year-old insulin-dependent diabetic man with a right great toe infection. *B.* The isolated distal superficial femoral artery stenosis (~99%) was crossed with a balloon and dilated. *C.* Local dissection (*arrow*) and poor flow resulted. *D.* A Palmaz stent (*arrow*) repaired the dissection, with resulting good distal flow. The toe infection fully resolved; however, instent restenosis was demonstrated by ultrasonography at 6 months.

TABLE 93-5 Femoropopliteal Artery Intervention

Type of Study	Reference	No. Patients	Type of Lesion	Angioplasty (A) versus Stenting (S)	Patency, %	Follow-up, Months
Retrospective	21	96	Stenosis/occlusive	A	49	18
Retrospective	22	106	Stenosis/claudication	A	42	36
Multivariate	23	103	Stenosis	A	51	24
Retrospective	24	254	Stenosis/occlusive	A	35	72

Endovascular Stent Grafts for the Treatment of Occlusive Disease

The limitations of endoluminal therapy for treating occlusive disease occur when lesions are diffuse or multifocal, including extensive regions of the vasculature. In these circumstances, endovascular interventions are commonly not successful in achieving a durable repair. In an effort to blend the advantages of durable conventional bypass surgery employing vascular grafts with the unique traits of endoluminal therapy, endovascular stent grafts were developed.[27,28] These devices combine the unique properties of prosthetic grafts and metallic intravascular stents into a catheter-based system. When used for the treatment of occlusive disease, an endograft is inserted to completely reline a diseased vessel after long-segment angioplasty (Fig. 93-7). The endograft provides a uniform flow surface that may be extended endoluminally over significant distances. Good results have been achieved in the aortoiliac circulation (Fig. 93-8).[30] However, long-term patency of stent grafts in the superficial femoral or popliteal arteries has not been achieved.[30]

The different devices used for stent grafting of occlusive disease all employ varying combinations of polyester or polytetrafluoroethylene (PTFE) prosthetic grafts with self-expanding or balloon-expandable metallic stents.

ANEURYSMAL DISEASE OF THE AORTA AND PERIPHERAL ARTERIES

Clinical application of minimally invasive therapy for the treatment of aneurysmal disease of the aorta and peripheral vessels began in 1990 with the seminal work of Parodi and associates.[31] Expansion of the potential of intravascular stents was accomplished by the fixation of prosthetic grafts onto the surface of the metallic stent support system. In this setting, the stent functions to fix or "anastomose" the "endograft" to the internal surface of the vessel wall. By doing this, the endograft relines the vessel, assuming responsibility for the support of systemic blood pressure.

Endovascular stent grafts have been used successfully to treat peripheral artery aneurysms in the iliac, popliteal, and subclavian distributions (Fig. 93-9).[32–34] The most extensive experience, however, has been with the treatment of abdominal and thoracic aortic aneurysms[35–38] (Fig. 93-10). In these clinical situations, endovascular grafts are inserted under local or epidural anesthesia by means of direct exposure of the common femoral artery. Under fluoroscopic guidance, devices are advanced over a guidewire to the target lesion.

Endovascular grafts have been constructed from balloon-expandable or self-expanding stents, which have been covered by prosthetic graft materials, most commonly polyester fabric (Fig. 93-11). Ongoing trials will be needed to document the long-term effectiveness and durability of these procedures.

ENDOVASCULAR GRAFTS FOR TRAUMATIC VASCULAR INJURIES

The complication of a direct injury to an artery may occur secondary to an iatrogenic cause or, alternatively, from a penetrating missile or knife wound. The resulting arterial damage may produce an arterial pseudoaneurysm or an abnormal arteriovenous fistula. These injuries may be managed from a site remote from the injury with the insertion of an endovascular graft device, which relines the injured vessel from the luminal surface (Fig. 93-12).[39,40] Repairing the vessels from a remote site and avoiding surgery in the traumatized field have obvious important advantages for immediate and possible long-term success.

SUMMARY

Minimally invasive therapy for the treatment of peripheral vascular disease is changing the way patients with these disorders are treated. A complete knowledge of the natural history of peripheral vascular disease along with a clear understanding of the values and limitations of endovascular treatments will provide the best therapy for those patients.

TABLE 93-6 Tibial Artery Intervention

Type of Study	Reference	No. Vessels	Type of Lesion	Angioplasty (A) versus Stenting (S)	Technical Success, %	Follow-up, Months
Retrospective	25	417	Stenosis/occlusive	A	86	—
Retrospective	26	40	Stenosis	A	59	24
Retrospective	27	25	Stenosis	A	20	36

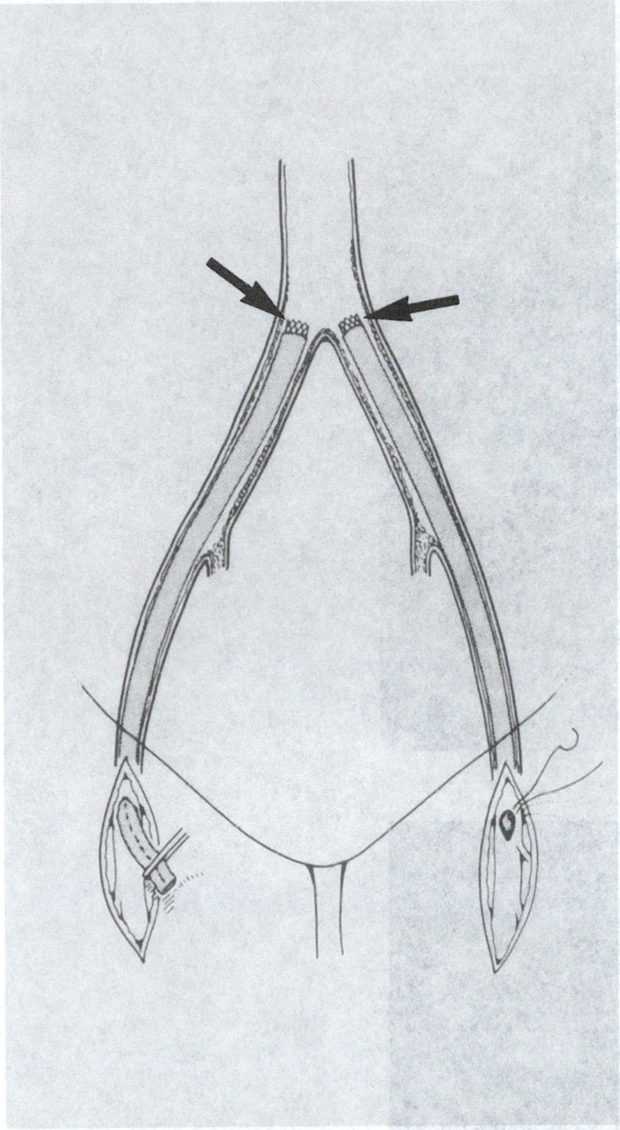

FIGURE 93-7 Artist's drawing of the technique for endovascular stent grafting of long-segment iliac artery occlusive disease. The diseased segment is recanalized with a hydrophilic guidewire. The entire diseased segment is dilated with a balloon angioplasty catheter. An endovascular stent graft is inserted to reline the diseased segment. The endograft is fixed ("anastomosed") to the proximal inflow artery with a metallic stent (*arrows*).

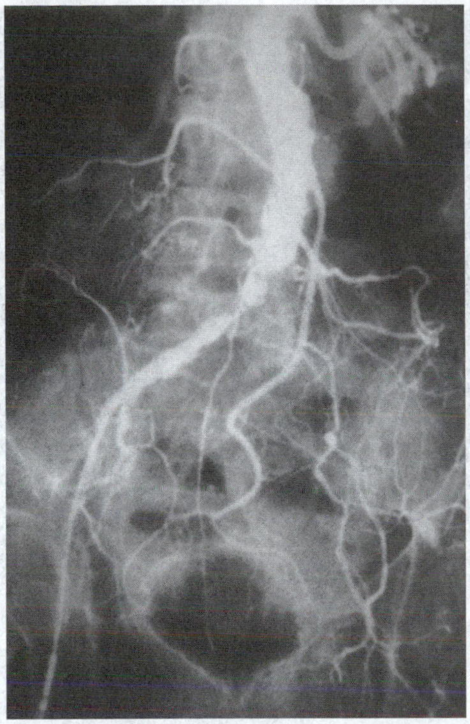

A

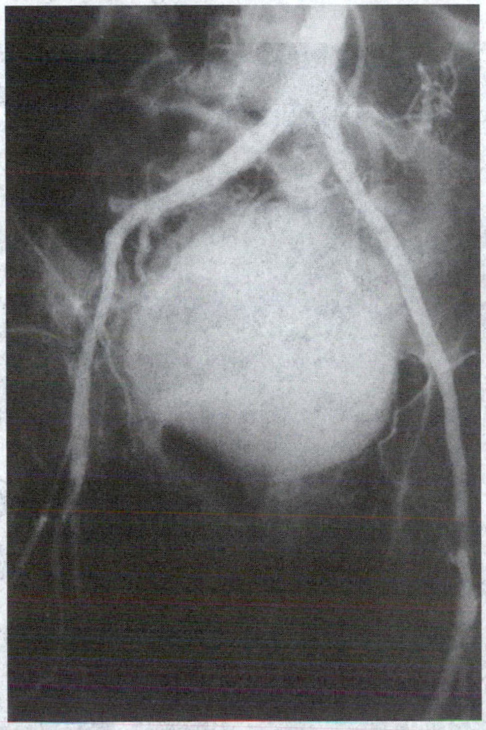

B

FIGURE 93-8 *A*. Aortogram from an 83-year-old diabetic man with limb-threatening ischemia of the left leg. Total left iliac occlusion is seen. *B*. Endovascular iliac stent graft insertion reestablished the circulation to the left leg. The right iliac stenoses were treated by balloon angioplasty.

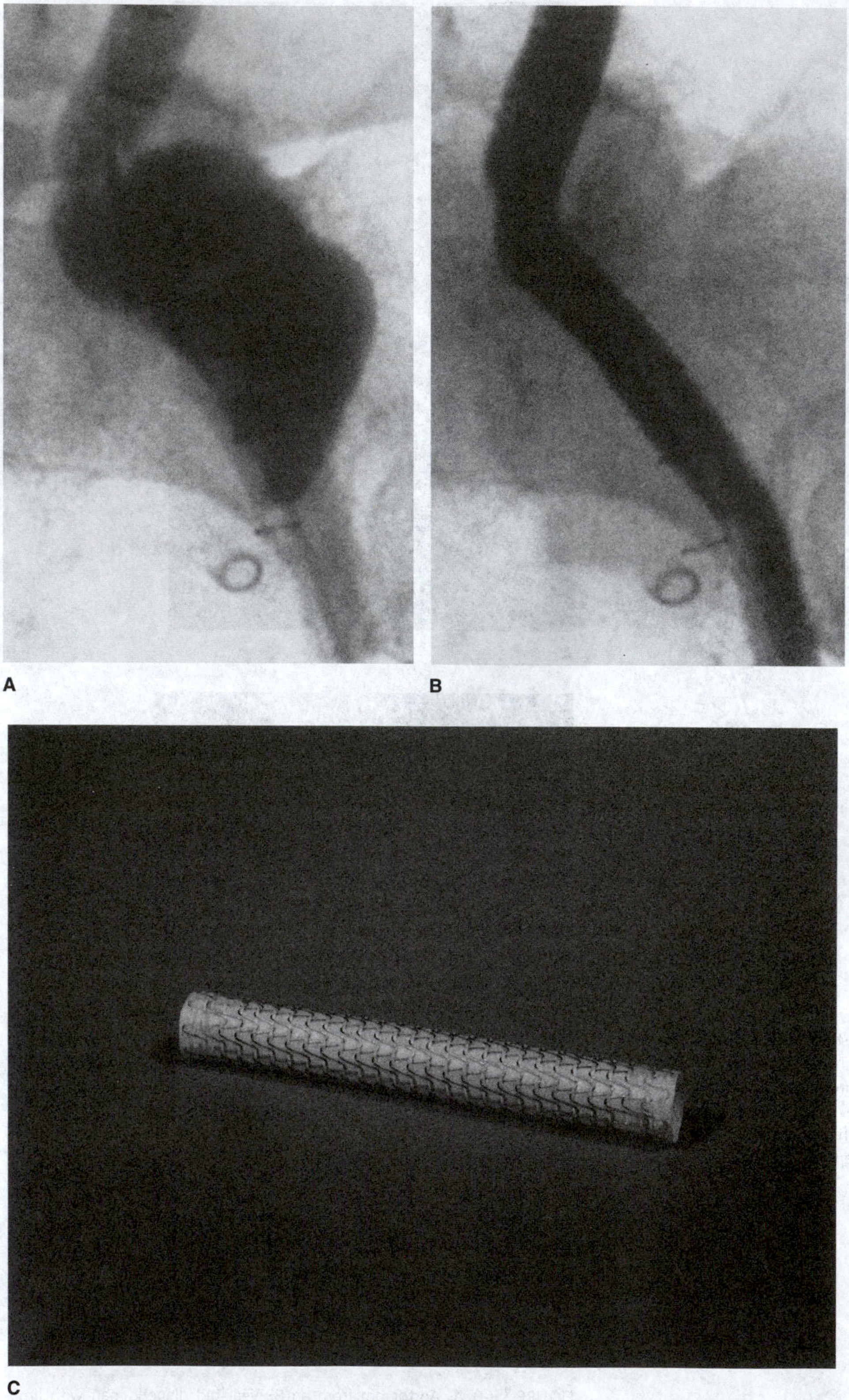

FIGURE 93-9 *A.* Angiogram of a 76-year-old man with an asymptomatic left common iliac artery aneurysm. *B.* After insertion of an endovascular stent graft, the aneurysm is fully excluded from the circulation. *C.* An example of an iliac endograft constructed from nitinol and ePTFE.

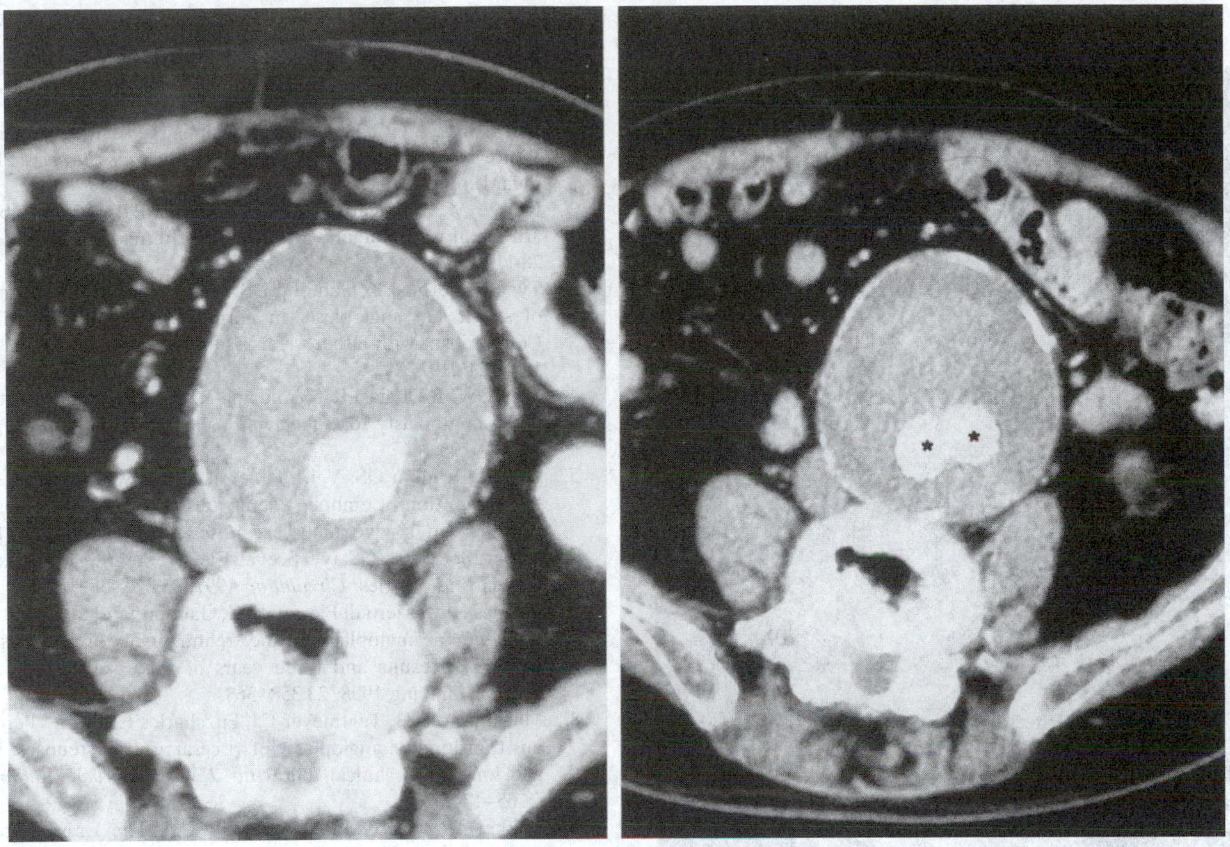

A B

FIGURE 93-10 *A.* Computed tomography scan of a 73-year-old man demonstrated a 7-cm infrarenal abdominal aortic aneurysm. *B.* After insertion of an endovascular bifurcated stent graft, the aortic aneurysm is excluded. The two limbs of the graft are denoted with an asterisk.

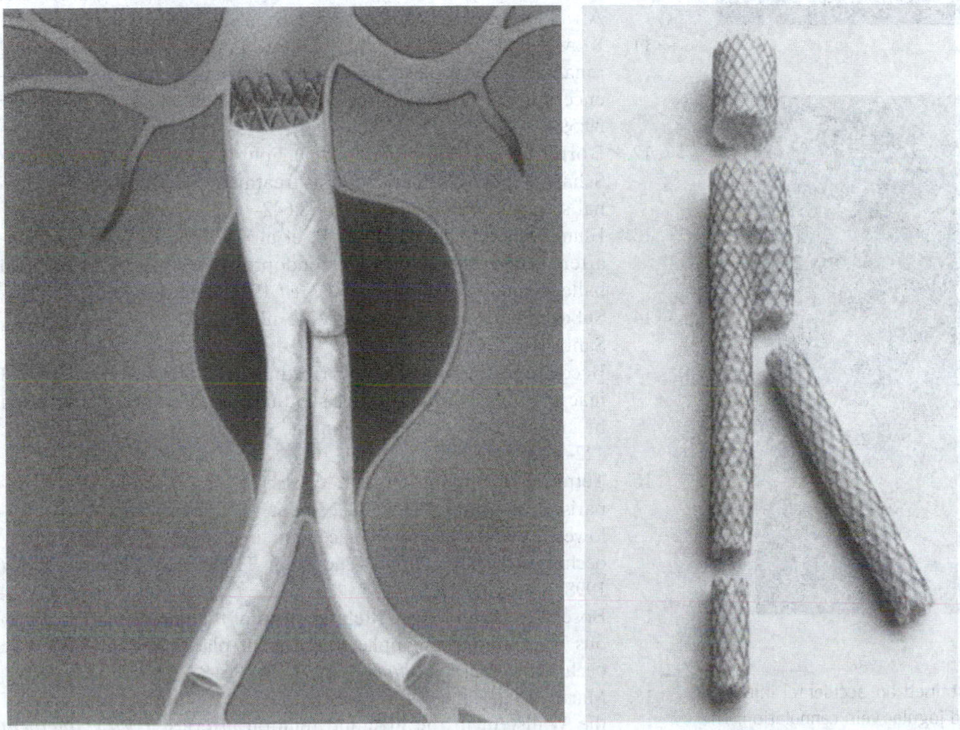

A B

FIGURE 93-11 *A.* Photograph demonstrating the endovascular bifurcated graft technique for the treatment of abdominal aortic aneurysms. *B.* AneuRx bifurcated graft. This device combines polyester vascular graft material with a nitinol stent. Several modular pieces may be inserted to complete the reconstruction.

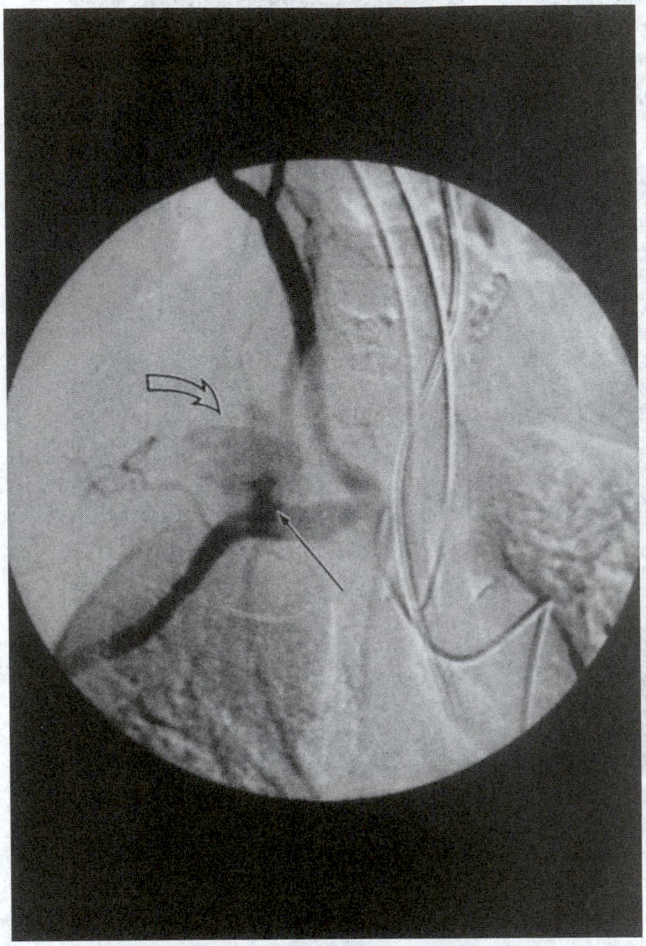

A

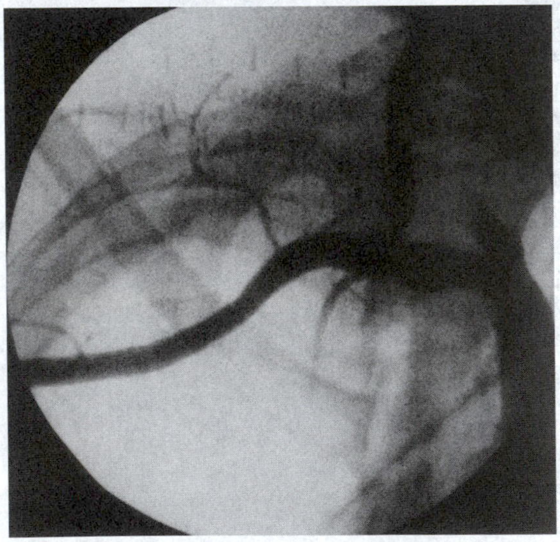

B

FIGURE 93-12 *A.* An 87-year-old woman sustained an accidental injury to the right subclavian artery during an attempted jugular vein cannulation. The site of injury (*arrow*) and the pseudoaneurysm (*open arrow*) are seen. *B.* After the insertion of a covered stent graft, the vessel injury is repaired.

References

1. Marin ML, Veith FJ. Endovascular surgery. In: Kerstein MD, White JV, eds. *Alternatives to Open Vascular Surgery*. Philadelphia: Lippincott; 1995:352.
2. Korner M, Baumgartner I, Do DD, et al. PTA of the subclavian artery and innominate arteries: Long-term results. *Vasa* 1999; 28:117–122.
3. Tyagi S, Verma PK, Gambhir DS, et al. Early and long-term results of subclavian angioplasty in aortoarteritis (Takayasu disease): Comparison with atherosclerosis. *Cardiovasc Intervent Radiol* 1998; 21:219–224.
4. Bogey WM, Demasi RJ, Vithalana R, et al. Percutaneous transluminal angioplasty for subclavian artery stenosis. *Am Surg* 1994; 60:103–106.
5. Ohki T, Roubin GS, Veith FJ, et al. Efficacy of a filter device in the prevention of embolic events during carotid angioplasty and stenting: An ex-vivo analysis. *J Vasc Surg* 1999; 30:1034–1044.
6. Yadar JS, Roubin GS, Iyer S, et al. Elective stenting of the extracranial carotid arteries. *Circulation* 1997; 95:376–381.
7. Maspes F, Mazzetti di Pietralata G, Gandini R, et al. Percutaneous transluminal angioplasty in the treatment of chronic mesenteric ischemia: Results and three years of follow-up in 23 patients. *Abdom Imaging* 1998; 23:358–363.
8. Matsumoto AH, Tegtmeyer CJ, Fitzcharles EK, et al. Percutaneous transluminal angioplasty of visceral arterial stenoses: Results and long-term, clinical follow-up. *J Vasc Intervent Radiol* 1995; 6:165–174.
9. Bakker J, Goffette PP, Henry M, et al. The Erasme study: A multicenter study on the safety and clinical results of the Palmaz stent used for the treatment of atherosclerotic ostial renal artery stenosis. *Cardiovasc Intervent Radiol* 1999; 22:468–474.
10. Van de Veb PJ, Kaatee R, Beutler JJ, et al. Arterial stenting and balloon angioplasty in ostial atherosclerotic renovascular disease: A randomized trial. *Lancet* 1999; 353:282–286.
11. Klow NE, Paulsen D, Vatne K, et al. Percutaneous transluminal renal artery angioplasty using coaxial technique: Ten years experience from 591 procedures in 419 patients. *Acta Radiol* 1998; 39:594–603.
12. Dorros G, Jaff M, Mathiak L, et al. Four year follow-up of Palmaz-Schatz stent revascularization as treatment for atherosclerotic renal stenosis. *Circulation* 1998; 98:642–647.
13. Blum U, Krumme B, Flugel P, et al. Treatment of ostial renal-artery stenoses with vascular endoprostheses after unsuccessful balloon angioplasty. *N Engl J Med* 1997; 336:459–465.
14. Suboptimal Renal Angioplasty Results (SOAR) Trial. AVE Inc., Santa Rosa, CA.
15. Becquemin JP, Allaire E, Qvarfordt P, et al. Surgical transluminal iliac angioplasty with selective stenting: Long-term results assessed by means of duplex scanning. *J Vasc Surg* 1999; 29(3): 422–429.
16. Tetteroo E, Van der Graaf Y, Bosch JL, et al. Randomized comparison of primary stent placement vs. primary angioplasty followed by selective stent placement in patients with iliac-artery occlusive disease: Dutch Iliac Stent Trial Study Group. *Lancet* 1998; 351:1153–1159.
17. Bosch JL, Hunink MG. Meta-analysis of the results of percutaneous transluminal angioplasty and stent placement for aortoiliac occlusive disease. *Radiology* 1997; 204:96–97.
18. Martin EC, Katzen BT, Benenati JF, et al. Multicenter trial of the Wallstent in the iliac and femoral arteries. *J Vasc Intervent Radiol* 1995; 6:843–849.
19. Henry M, Amor M, Ethevenot G, et al. Palmaz stent placement in iliac and femoropopliteal arteries: Primary and secondary patency in 310 patients with 2–4 year follow-up. *Radiology* 1995; 197:167–174.

20. O'Donohoe MK, Sultan S, Colgan MP, et al. Outcome of the first 100 femoropopliteal angioplasties performed in the operating theatre. *Eur J Vasc Endovasc Surg* 1999; 17:66–71.
21. Matsi PJ, Manninen HI. Impact of different patency criteria on long-term results of femoropopliteal angioplasty: Analysis of 106 consecutive patients with claudication. *J Vasc Intervent Radiol* 1995; 6:159–163.
22. Becquemin JP, Cavillon A, Haiduc F. Surgical transluminal femoropopliteal angioplasty: Multivariate analysis outcome. *J Vasc Surg* 1994; 19:495–502.
23. Johnston KW. Femoral and popliteal arteries: Reanalysis of results of balloon angioplasty. *Radiology* 1992; 183:767–771.
24. Dorros G, Jaff MR, Murphy KJ, et al. The acute outcome of tibioperoneal vessel angioplasty in 417 cases with claudication and critical limb ischemia. *Cathet Cardiovasc Diagn* 1998; 45:251–256.
25. Varty K, Bolia A, Naylor AR, et al. Infrapopliteal percutaneous transluminal angioplasty: A safe and successful procedure. *Eur J Vasc Endovasc Surg* 1995; 9:341–345.
26. Treiman GS, Treiman RL, Ichikawa L, et al. Should percutaneous transluminal angioplasty be recommended for the treatment of infrageniculate popliteal artery or tibioperoneal trunk stenosis? *J Vasc Surg* 1995; 22:457–463.
27. Marin ML, Veith FJ, Panetta TF, et al. Transfemoral stented graft treatment of occlusive arterial disease for limb salvage: A preliminary report. *Circulation* 1993; 88(4):1.
28. Cragg AH, Dake MD. Percutaneous femoropopliteal grafting: Report of a new technique (abstract). *J Vasc Intervent Radiol* 1993; 4:64.
29. Marin ML, Veith FJ, Sanchez LS, et al. Endovascular repair of aorto-iliac occlusive disease. *World J Surg* 1996; 20:679–686.
30. Cragg AH, Dake MD. Percutaneous femoropopliteal graft placement. *Radiology* 1993; 187:643–648.
31. Parodi JC, Palmaz JC, Barone HD. Transfemoral intraluminal graft implantation for abdominal aortic aneurysms. *Ann Vasc Surg* 1991; 5:491–499.
32. Marin ML, Veith FJ, Panetta TF, et al. Transfemoral endoluminal stented graft repair of a popliteal artery aneurysm. *Am J Surg* 1994; 19:754–757.
33. Marin ML, Veith FJ, Lyon RT, et al. Transfemoral endovascular repair of iliac artery aneurysms. *Am J Surg* 1995; 170:179–182.
34. Parsons RE, Marin ML, Veith FJ, et al. Midterm results of endovascular stented grafts for the treatment of isolated iliac artery aneurysms. *J Vasc Surg* 1999; 30:915–921.
35. Blum U, Voshage G, Lanmer J, et al. Endoluminal stent grafts for infrarenal abdominal aortic aneurysms. *N Engl J Med* 1997; 336:13–20.
36. Marin ML, Veith FJ, Cynamon J, et al. Initial experience with transluminally placed endovascular grafts for the treatment of complex vascular lesions. *Ann Surg* 1999; 222:449–469.
37. Dake MD, Miller DC, Semba CP, et al. Transluminal placement of endovascular stent grafts for the treatment of descending thoracic aortic aneurysms. *N Engl J Med* 1994; 331:1729–1734.
38. Temudom T, D'Ayala M, Marin ML, et al. Endovascular grafts in the treatment of thoracic aortic aneurysms and pseudoaneurysms. *Ann Vasc Surg*, 2000; 14:230–238.
39. Marin ML, Veith FJ, Panetta TF, et al. Percutaneous transfemoral insertion of a stented graft to repair a traumatic femoral arteriovenous fistula. *J Vasc Surg* 1993; 18:299–302.
40. Marin ML, Veith FJ, Panetta TF, et al. Transluminally placed endovascular stented graft repair for arterial trauma. *J Vasc Surg* 1994; 20:466–473.

PART SIXTEEN

COST-EFFECTIVE STRATEGIES, INSURANCE, AND LEGAL PROBLEMS

C H A P T E R 94

COST-EFFECTIVE STRATEGIES IN CARDIOLOGY

William S. Weintraub / Harlan Krumholz

A SOCIETAL PERSPECTIVE

How do society and individuals decide to allocate resources or spend money? In capitalist societies, the invisible hand of the market guides resource use, and in principle, regulators, generally governmental agencies, ensure a "level playing field" and prevent various forms of abuse but otherwise try to stay out of the way. Free markets are guided by a principle called *willingness to pay,* which economists define as that price, governed by supply and demand, which consumers are willing to pay for a service.[1] Services in society that are deemed a "right," such as education, are not governed by free markets, since society may view that all people have a right to such services, independent of their ability to pay. Medicine is largely, although not entirely, in the class of a "right," more like education than a good governed by willingness to pay such as automobiles. When a service is not priced by willingness to pay, naturally there will be concern over how to fairly price or value it and how much of it to buy. The *value* of a service can be defined as its fair cost. The concern for value in medicine is a major societal issue. We can define *value* in health care as good care at a fair price. Whether society is achieving value in health care is a major issue all over the world.

Health care expenditures in the United States have risen dramatically in the last half of the twentieth century. Between 1960 and 1997, federal health care expenditures rose from $2.9 billion to $367 billion, and total national expenditures rose from $28.65 billion to $1.09 trillion[2] (Fig. 94-1). This represents an increase in percentage of gross national product over this period from 5.1 to 13.5 percent. This unprecedented and unparalleled increase in expense for one sector of the American economy is placing American medicine in considerable peril. The Health Care Financing Agency (HCFA) expects expenditures to double in the next 10 years, reaching 16.2 percent of the gross domestic product. The Hospital Insurance (HI) program, or Medicare Part A, pays for hospital, home health, skilled nursing, and hospice care for the aged and disabled, insuring about 39 million people in 1998. The HI program, financed primarily by

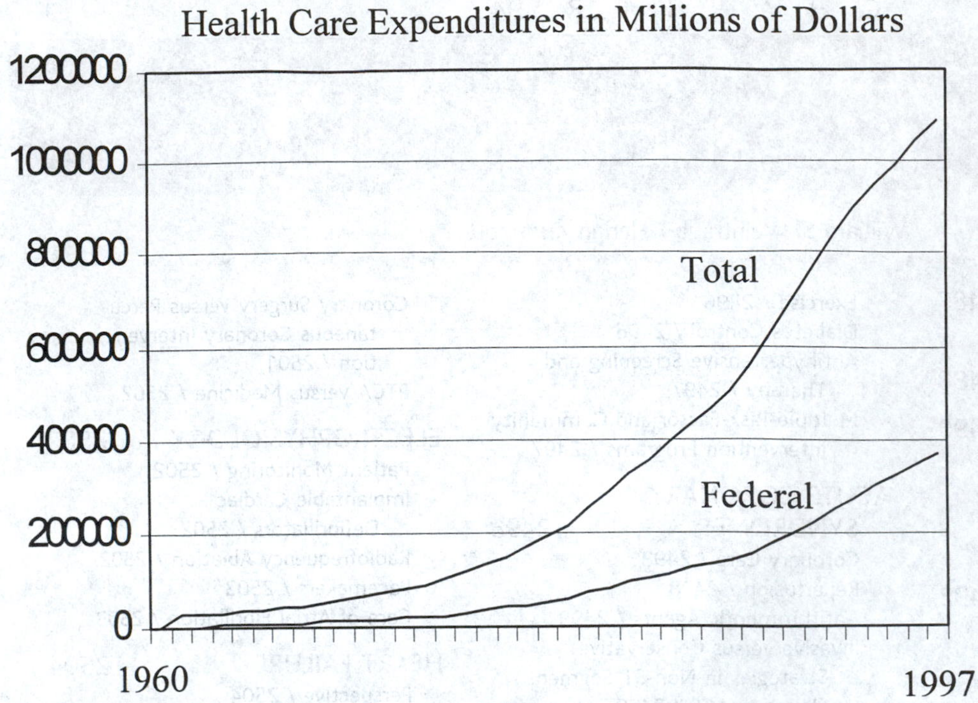

FIGURE 94-1 Increasing costs of medical services over time.

payroll taxes, mainly pays benefits for current beneficiaries, with leftover income held in a trust fund invested in U.S. Treasury securities.

A board of trustees, created by Congress, oversees annual reports on the financial status of the HI trust fund. As of 1999, income exceeds expenditures and is expected to do so for 8 more years, and by drawing down on the trust fund, benefits could continue for several years. However, given current assumptions, the HI trust fund will be depleted in 2015. In addition, there will be relatively fewer people paying and more people consuming HI resources as the population ages. It is expected that there will be 3.6 workers per HI beneficiary when the baby boom generation begins to reach age 65 in 2010, declining to 2.3 by 2030 as the last of the baby boomers reaches age 65. Current public policy has not adequately addressed how to manage the future financial status of Medicare in the United States.

Cardiovascular disease consumes substantial societal resources in economically advantaged countries and thus is responsible for a considerable part of the projected economic challenges in the future. In the United States alone, the American Heart Association estimates that the cost of cardiovascular disease in 1999 will total $286.5 billion[3] (Table 94-1). Of this total, $178.2 billion will be related to direct consumption of medical resources, and an additional $108.3 billion will be related to lost productivity due to early death and disability. Costs related to coronary artery disease (CAD) lead the other categories at $99.8 billion, but this is just a little over a third of the total. Given its magnitude, there is a strong societal interest that the $178.2 billion in direct costs is spent wisely and that the $108.3 billion in lost productivity is minimized. The field of health care economics has developed to address these societal issues.

BACKGROUND ON ECONOMIC ANALYSES

In an environment of limited resources, different societal needs compete for resources. If resources were not limited, then medical care could be provided based on clinical outcome alone, no matter how small the benefit. In such a world of inexhaustible resources, it would be reasonable to provide a treatment that benefited only 1 of every million or 10 million or 100 million individuals screened or treated. Since this is no longer and perhaps never was entirely the case, new forms of diagnostic testing and therapies, as well as existing ones, have to be justified on both an effectiveness and an economic basis. The problems of assessment of costs and comparison with outcome are especially relevant and complicated when expensive forms of therapy are used commonly and have multiple complex and interrelating indices of their effectiveness. Within medicine, these issues are perhaps most relevant to cardiovascular care because of the vast array of diagnostic and therapeutic strategies, as well as the high cost and the diversity of outcome measures.

Frequently, costs are compared between competing forms of therapeutic or diagnostic strategies. This comparison can involve performing a simulation in which costs and outcome are estimated from the literature, nonrandomized comparisons, and randomized trials. Even within randomized trials, an economic analysis can range from a simulation to a very detailed component of the trial with extensive primary data collection. For any of these designs, the simplest type of economic study is a comparison of costs, or a cost-minimization study. Such a study is useful when it is reasonable to assume that two treatment or diagnostic arms offer similar outcomes to one another.

There are three related forms of economic analyses that can be used to study relative efficacies and relative costs: cost-effectiveness, cost-utility, and cost-benefit. *Cost-effectiveness analysis measures the cost per unit of effectiveness.*[4] This form of analysis assumes that there is one overall measure of effectiveness, often survival. This method breaks down when there are multiple measures of effectiveness. For instance, one form of therapy may increase the risk of death but offer improved symptomatic status. This may, in principle, be addressed through *cost-utility analysis, in which all measures of effectiveness are incorporated into one measure called utility.*[4] Utility, however, is a very difficult parameter to measure, as will be discussed below. A third and somewhat less popular form of analysis is *cost-benefit analysis, in which measures of both cost and effectiveness are reduced to a single measure, generally dollars (or other currency).*[4] While cost-benefit analysis has not been popular in medicine due to the inherent difficulty of expressing

TABLE 94-1 Estimated Direct and Indirect Costs of Cardiovascular Diseases and Stroke, United States, 1999

	Heart Disease†	Coronary Heart Disease	Stroke	Hypertensive Disease	Congestive Heart Failure	Total Cardiovascular Disease*
Direct Costs						
Hospital/nursing home	$76.4	$40.7	$24.2	$7.1	$15.0	$124.3
Physicians/other professionals	13.8	7.7	2.2	7.7	1.4	26.8
Drugs	6.6	3.2	0.3	8.1	1.0	16.0
Home health/other medical durables	5.0	1.5	2.8	1.5	2.1	11.1
Total expenditures*	$101.8	$53.1	$29.5	$24.5	$19.6	$178.2
Indirect Costs						
Lost productivity/morbidity	16.5	6.9	5.4	5.0	NA	26.5
Lost productivity/mortality	64.8	39.8	10.4	3.8	1.4	81.8
Grand total*	$183.1	$99.8	$45.3	$33.3	$21.0	$286.5

*Totals may not add up due to rounding and overlap.
†This category includes coronary heart disease, congestive heart failure, and part of hypertensive disease as well as other "heart" diseases.
SOURCE: Direct costs were extrapolated from estimates for 1997 by Thomas A. Hodgson, chief economist and acting director, Division of Health and Utilization Analysis, OAEHP, CDC/NCHS. Estimates of indirect costs were made by Thomas J. Thom, statistician in the division of Epidemiology and Clinical Applications, NHLBI.

clinical outcome in monetary terms, it is, at least in theory, the most generalizable of these methods.

We can begin to understand the approach of cost-effectiveness analysis by considering two competing therapies (or tests), A and B, to treat (or diagnose) the same condition, as considered in Fig. 94-2. In the upper left-hand corner in panel 1, therapy A is more effective and less expensive than therapy B. In this setting, A is said to dominate B. Similarly in panel 4, A is less effective and more expensive than B. In this setting, B would dominate A. Commonly, however, the more effective therapy or test is also more expensive. Thus in panel 2, A is more effective but also more expensive. Similarly, in panel 3, B is more effective but also more expensive. In such a common

1: Therapy A vs B More Effective, Less Expensive	2: Therapy A vs B More Effective, More Expensive
3: Therapy A vs B Less Effective, Less Expensive	4: Therapy A vs B Less Effective, More Expensive

FIGURE 94-2 Decision matrix.

clinical situation, where a form of therapy or a test is both more effective and more expensive than a competing therapy or test, cost-effectiveness analysis can help society decide whether to allocate resources to the more effective service.

The perspective in these analyses can have an important impact on their structure and outcome. An analysis from a hospital's perspective may not include the long-term consequences of a particular clinical strategy, whereas this issue may be most important to the patient and the payer. Also, different stakeholders place different values on the outcomes and costs of medical care. For instance, physicians and patients traditionally have been more concerned about effectiveness, whereas employers and insurance companies have been more concerned about costs.

The perspective of all the various stakeholders may be viewed in aggregate as "society." To be most useful in serving societal goals, cost and cost-effectiveness analyses should be performed from a societal perspective. From a societal perspective, an economic analysis should attempt to measure all the costs and measures of outcome associated with a particular treatment. These costs should include those incurred by the patient, the costs of medical resources that could have been used for other patients, and any loss of income that the patient sustained because of poor health. Outcome should include events, quality of life, and survival. By looking at the sum of all these costs in relation to outcome, a policymaker could decide, for example, whether the public good benefited more by allocating limited health care resources to a lipid screening program or to coronary revascularization.

While it is possible, in theory, to line up the cost-effectiveness of multiple procedures into what are called *league tables,* limitations in data quality and variability in study design limit the wide applicability of such efforts.[5] An effort to create league tables was attempted in Oregon, with cost-effectiveness used to guide whether a form of therapy or a test would be funded.

This experiment was criticized and finally abandoned because of the limited amount and quality of data available, as well as concern over whether the approach was appropriate.[6] Far more common are cost-effectiveness analyses that compare two alternative treatments for a single medical condition, e.g., percutaneous transluminal angioplasty (PTCA) and coronary artery bypass grafting (CABG) for symptomatic angina. Such analyses examine the incremental cost-effectiveness of CABG compared with PTCA. In addition to focusing on a single clinical condition, the analyses most commonly limit the measured costs to direct and some portion of indirect medical costs. The purpose of these analyses is not to dictate a decision but to inform the decision-making process.

DETERMINING COSTS

Taxonomy for Costs

When considering a procedure or form of therapy, it is common to ask what it costs. An economic perspective on cost is more theoretical.[7] Economists are more concerned with how society chooses to allocate limited resources rather than with what something costs per se. Cost may be used to sum resource use when a procedure or test uses resources of several types and to permit comparison of costs between services. To accomplish the end of summarizing resource use to arrive at cost, accounting methods are used. Cost accounting has a particular taxonomy, as shown in Table 94-2.

Costs must be considered from one of several possible perspectives.[8] Thus, for a hospital, the cost is the expenses to provide a service. For payers, the cost is what the providers charge, plus their administrative expenses. In principle, cost studies often seek to determine societal costs, which should be used in cost-effectiveness analyses to gain the widest perspective. However, societal costs are never directly measurable, and thus combinations of cost proxies from one or several stakeholders, where measurable, often are used as estimates.

Costs are classified as direct or indirect.[9] Definitions of indirect costs may lead to uncertainty categorizing a particular cost. Theoretically, *direct costs* are those incurred by a stakeholder for a therapy or test, and *indirect costs* are those incurred by other societal groups. Generally, direct costs relate to the provision of medical care, whereas indirect costs are other societal costs.

Medical costs for a procedure such as coronary surgery can be divided into three components: in-hospital direct costs, follow-up direct costs, and indirect costs. In-patient costs comprise hospital costs (e.g., room, laboratory testing, pharmacy, etc.) and physician professional billings. Follow-up direct costs include physician office visits, outpatient testing, medications, home health providers, and additional hospitalizations. Indirect costs reflect lost patient or business opportunity or productivity costs and may be referred to as *productivity costs*.[10]

A final way of thinking about costs is that direct costs are realistically linked to a particular service, whereas indirect costs are not. This type of indirect cost is also called *overhead*.[11]

The appropriate length of time over which to measure costs depends on the procedures being studied and outcomes being measured. Thus the cost of angioplasty could be considered to be the costs of the initial hospitalization and over the first 6 months when restenosis commonly would occur. Alternatively, the cost of angioplasty could be considered the initial hospitalization alone, and the costs during the initial 6 months could be considered follow-up or induced costs, which are those generated beyond the specific time of service delivery.[12] Induced costs also could be a savings. For instance, there may be savings for stents relative to balloon angioplasty in follow-up due to less additional revascularization.

Typically, in the United States, hospital costs are used as a proxy for societal costs. What a hospital charges for a service is not its cost.[13] Measuring hospital cost is difficult and has been approached using what is called either *top-down* or *bottom-up accounting*.[14] Top-down costing involves dividing all the money spent on a hospitalization or procedure by the number of episodes of care of the particular type performed. A payer perspective would be the amount the payer pays the provider for the service. In contrast, a bottom-up approach involves individually costing all resources used for a service, i.e., supplies, equipment depreciation and facilities, salaries, etc. All methods involve a set of assumptions and limitations. When considering the cost of a specific procedure using top-down costing, it must be assumed that costs in the department in which the procedure is provided can be separated from costs in other departments. For instance, it is not clear that the cardiac catheterization laboratory costs can be clearly separated from hospital maintenance costs. There also may be variability within a department. Therefore, using identical methods to calculate the costs of angioplasty and diagnostic catheterization may not be appropriate if angioplasty consumes more resources in a period of time, such as technician time. Bottom-up methods also are limited by the ability to account for all resources consumed and to appropriately apply costs.

Another issue in measuring hospital costs is average versus marginal or incremental cost.[15] Average cost is calculated by dividing all costs for a therapy or test by the number of that particular type. In contrast, the marginal cost is the cost of the next similar procedure. Average costs include all resources used, including overhead, whose costs would not be decreased if not used. Marginal costing accepts fixed costs as a given and focuses only on variable costs or those additional resources consumed

TABLE 94-2 Summary of Taxonomy for Costs

Cost perspective
Provider, i.e., hospital or professional
Payer, i.e., insurance carrier
Patient
Cost category
Direct costs
Indirect costs
Accounting method
Top-down
Bottom-up
Costs per service
Average cost
Marginal (incremental) cost

by each additional patient. Variable costs are separated analytically from fixed costs by establishing the perspective and time frame as fixed. For instance, facilities' cost is commonly considered fixed, but how should marginal personnel costs be assigned? If coronary surgery decreases as angioplasty becomes more common, do the operating room nurses remain on staff in the operating room, or will they be assigned to other duties? Because of these difficulties, most cost and cost-effectiveness studies use average costs.

Cost Measurement

Commonly used at nonfederal hospitals in the United States, there is a particularly detailed approach to top-down costing that is based on the UB92 summary of charges.[16] The UB92 is a uniform billing statement used by all third-party carriers. Charges are available for, but not limited to, such services as the surgical suite, cardiac catheterization laboratory, intensive care unit, postoperative or postprocedural floor care, respiratory therapy, supplies, electrocardiogram (ECG), telemetry, social services, etc. While hospitals will set their charges to maximize insurance reimbursements, the relationship between costs and charges, in the form global specific cost-to-charge ratios, must be developed using American Hospital Association guidelines and then filed annually with HCFA in the form of a hospital cost report, which is in the public domain.

An alternative approach is to use bottom-up cost accounting and assign cost weights to each type of resource used.[17] The sum of resources times their cost weights yields total cost. However, the methods are sufficiently laborious that they are rarely used.

Another approach is to use a payer perspective.[18] In the United States, Medicare diagnosis-related group (DRG) reimbursement rates could be used to define cost. Similar methods are available in other countries. The use of DRGs to assign cost does not account for variation in cost within that DRG and may not even reflect average resource use. While it is an excellent measure of cost from the point of view of governmental agencies, it probably does not represent as meaningful a proxy for societal cost as do provider level hospital costs.

Assessing professional medical costs is challenging. It is not sufficient to consider physicians' fees alone, since other professionals provide services.[19,20] The goal must be to capture all the professional services for a procedure. For coronary surgery, this may include such fees as the surgeon and assistants; the consultant cardiologist; and anesthesia, radiology, clinical pathology, professional components of any other testing, and any other consultants or ancillary services.[21] There is no cost-to-charge ratio, analogous to the situation for the hospital, available for physician fees to convert their charges to costs.

In the United States, there has been an effort to rationalize physician payments by developing a set of scales for services.[22] This system, the resource-based relative value scale (RBRVS), was developed over time to try to assess the relative time, physical, and cognitive efforts associated with physician services.[22] Each service is assigned a number called the relative value unit (RVU). If the profile of physician services for a procedure or hospitalization is known, then RVUs for each service may be used to develop a proxy for the physician costs. The total RVUs may be converted to a dollar figure by a conversion factor. HCFA, the federal agency that administers Medicare and Medicaid, has a standard conversion factor. The appeal of the RBRVS is that it is a relative weighting system that assigns unique weights for physician work and practice costs for each physician service by Current Procedural Terminology (CPT) code. As a result, after assigning a conversion factor, standardized estimates of the costs can be calculated and used as a gauge of physician costs. While there are still some problems with this approach, especially for the practice cost values in the RBRVS, it holds considerable promise and overcomes some of the major drawbacks of physician charge data.

Determining the costs of outpatient services presents different challenges in determining patient services use, including direct and indirect medical costs. Direct costs include physician office visits, medications, procedures and testing, rehabilitation, nursing home stays, and home health services, as well as patient out-of-pocket expenses, including travel. Assessment of these costs is difficult and complicated by insurance, since patients cannot be expected to reliably respond to how much they paid out of pocket for services and how much the insurance company paid for services. Unless there is access to a comprehensive insurance claims database, the most reasonable approach is to have patients identify the services they have received. Costs can then be attributed to the individual services and medications. Office visits and other medical services costs may be similarly estimated. Professional services can be estimated using the Medicare fee schedule, as discussed earlier. Medication costs can be estimated from compiled prices by sampling pharmacies or using published wholesale pharmaceutical prices. Using these cost estimates, a partial simulation of postdischarge direct costs may be determined.

Indirect productivity costs include missed time from work by the patient or family members. Follow-up indirect costs probably are the most difficult to determine and often are excluded as immeasurable. In any case, it is not possible to directly measure all the indirect costs. For instance, if an executive in a company has coronary surgery and is out of work for 6 weeks, there may or may not be loss of pay, but the effect on the business cannot be determined readily. Indirect costs, if measured at all, often are confined to family loss of income, and the numbers must be examined with both interest and skepticism.

Over a long time horizon, inflation must be considered. Costs must be inflated or deflated by multiplying by a constant to convert from any one year to another, based on the medical inflation rate.[23] Future costs also should be discounted to reflect the opportunity costs of current dollars, or future costs should be expressed at their present value.[24] For instance, if a policymaker were given the alternative of spending $1000 now or $1000 in 5 years to treat a given condition and obtain the same outcome, the decision would always be the latter. Costs generally are discounted at a rate of 3 percent per year.[24]

Variation in Cost

Variation in cost for a service arises from either differences in the type of measurement, as discussed earlier, or differences in resource use. Table 94-3 presents a framework for considering variation in medical costs, according to quality of care, patient, and geographic levels. These levels do not separate clearly, providing a somewhat confusing picture of the sources of variation.

TABLE 94-3 Sources of Variation in Cost

Quality of care
1. Process: Access, appropriateness, management
2. Structure: Facilities, supplies, staffing
3. Outcome: Iatrogenic complications, patients' health status

Patient level
1. Demographic: Age, sex, race
2. Disease severity: Extent of left ventricular dysfunction or severity of coronary atherosclerosis
3. Comorbidity: Cardiac or noncardiac
4. Outcome: Noniatrogenic complications, patients' health status

Geographic and non-medical economic factors
1. Facilities
2. Supplies
3. Labor

Quality of care is often broken down into the subunits of process, structure, and outcome.[25] These components of quality also may be viewed as reflecting variation in cost. For process measures of access and appropriateness, the effect on cost may be less on the individual service and more at the societal level for provision of that service. Thus, if access to coronary surgery is inadequate, the initial cost to society of coronary surgery may fall as fewer surgeries are performed, but costs may rise due to induced costs or productivity costs of failing to perform necessary surgery. However, if access to adequate diabetes care is inadequate, there may be an increase in the cost to society of inadequately treated diabetes. Similarly, if inappropriate angioplasty is being performed, then the societal cost will rise, even if the individual service is little affected. Management, on the other hand, will affect the individual service. Accordingly, if a service is handled efficiently with care maps to decrease unnecessary resource use of an overall service, such as excessive blood drawing after coronary surgery and an organized and early discharge, then costs can be decreased. Variation in management will cause variation in cost; thus, if there is variation of use of major services, such as cardiac catheterization after hospitalization for unstable angina, then costs will vary accordingly. While it may be appropriate to either perform or not perform a catheterization, the choice will affect cost. Clearly, management and appropriateness issues overlap.

Structure is related to cost. Facilities and supplies vary considerably in cost even within a single geographic location. Staffing also may vary in intensity, with some institutions having more patients being cared for by a nurse than others. Outcome also may vary with quality of care. Complications may be iatrogenic and relate to quality of care and generally increase the cost of a service. Similarly, a patient's health status may vary with quality, which will affect induced productivity costs. Thus, if there is variation in relief from angina after revascularization due to variation in quality of care, then there may be variation in ability to return to work.

Patient-level factors, such as age, gender, and race, may affect cost as much as, or perhaps more than, quality of care. Age may be thought of as similar to comorbidity, potentially raising cost. Disease severity or acuteness, however measured, also may affect costs. Thus it may cost more to perform coronary surgery or coronary angioplasty on patients with a recent acute myocardial infarction (MI) than without one.[26-28] Similarly, comorbidity may increase costs. *However, complications generally have a greater effect on costs than comorbidity or severity.*[26-28] Complications and health status outcomes related to patient-level factors do not separate cleanly from complications and heath status outcomes related to quality of care.

Finally, variation in cost may be influenced by geographic and nonmedical economic factors such as land and construction costs, cost of living, and personnel availability.[29] Also, there may be variation in cost that is independent of both quality and geography. Thus buying cooperatives of hospitals may be able to purchase supplies at greater discounts than single providers may.

Thus variation in cost of service is complicated and limits the ability to explain it. Correlates of cost variability often are studied using multivariate regression techniques.[26] While elegant, these models have significant limitations. First, studies from one or similar institutions may not be generalizable. Second, the correlates cannot always be neatly categorized, since a procedural complication may be at either the patient or provider level. Next, comorbidity, disease severity, and provider-level factors may themselves induce complications. Thus models should be developed in which patient and provider factors are correlated with outcome variables and where cost is correlated with preservice and pre- and postservice variables. Finally, cost often is not normally distributed. The distribution can be normalized to some extent by using its logarithm. However, correlating variables with the logarithm of cost is not as informative as correlating variables with cost itself.

Thus determining the specific cost of any service is difficult and, therefore, limits generalizing estimate costs outside the bounds of a particular study. In the same sense that effect sizes are considered subject to confidence intervals, cost estimates must be recognized as "estimates." This limitation also applies to using cost measurements in cost-effectiveness analyses and in constructing league tables in which several cost-effectiveness analyses are compared.

COMPARING COSTS WITH OUTCOME

Determining therapeutic or diagnostic costs independently of patient outcome is not particularly helpful for clinical decision making or setting policy. Measuring costs without considering outcomes would preclude judgments about the value of allocating resources in the health care system. The most extreme cost-minimization approach would be to stop offering medical services. However, the goal of the health care system is to maximize patient outcomes within the resource constraints. Consequently, costs and outcomes need to be considered. While it is possible to relate cost to any measure of outcome, the most generalizable approach in medicine is cost-utility analysis based on patient preference.[30]

Determination of Patient Utility and Quality-Adjusted Life Years

In the treatment of coronary artery disease, it is unusual for one measurement of outcome to be of sufficient clinical importance that all other outcome measures may be ignored in clinical decision making. While death overwhelms other outcome measures in importance, it is relatively infrequent over short periods of time for most conditions. Consequently, it is also important to consider other outcomes such as MI, unstable angina, revascularization procedures, measures of quality of life, and return to work and weigh them together. In trials comparing percutaneous coronary intervention with coronary surgery, there was no difference in mortality.[31–36] While surgery relieved angina somewhat better[31–36] at higher cost,[33,36–40] it was a disadvantage to the patient to have to undergo the surgery in the first place. Without some method to integrate various measures of outcome, it may be difficult to make an informed choice. In principle, this task may be accomplished through the determination of patient utility.

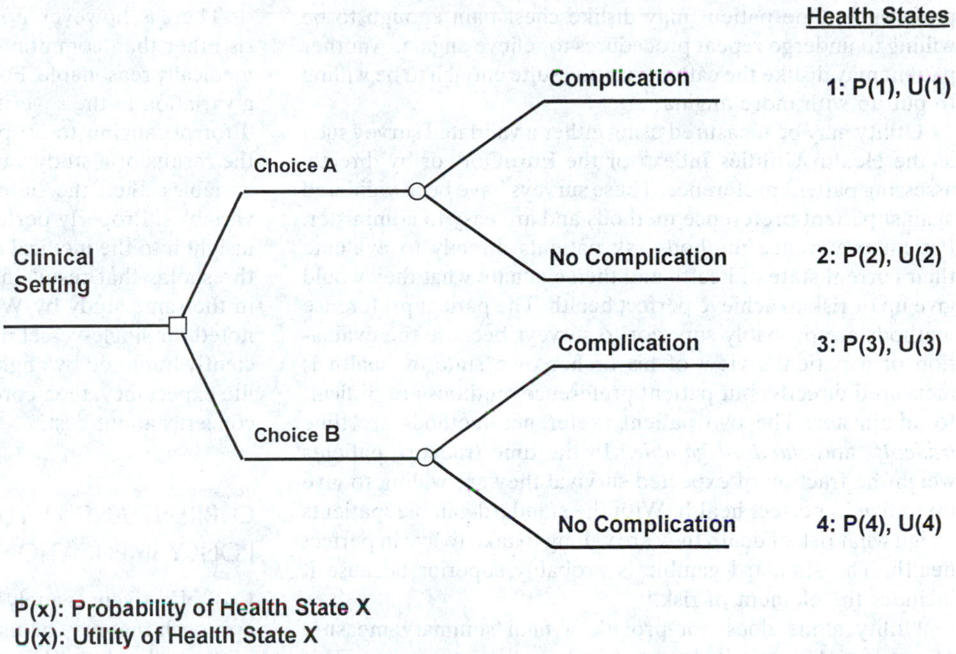

FIGURE 94-3 Idealized decision tree for a decision on diagnostic strategy or therapeutic choice.

The utility of a therapy or test is the sum of benefits, both positive and negative, that accrues to a patient over time as a result of the procedure.[41] It is, in principle, all-encompassing. We may consider the assessment of utility beginning with a decision tree (Fig. 94-3). A decision tree takes a patient at a specific point and then considers, in principal, all possible events up to some point in the future. In this model, branch points or nodes with squares represent choices and nodes with circles represent chance events. In the simplified model shown, a single choice is made, and for each choice, there are two possible outcomes. Each outcome is called a *health state*. Each health state has a utility and a probability of occurrence. The utility of choice A in Fig. 94-3 is the sum of the utility of health state 1 times its probability plus the utility of health state 2 times its probability. If choices were this easy, then the ability to determine utility of diagnostic or therapeutic strategies would be simple. However, decision trees are almost never this simple. The decision trees for diagnostic tests tend to be much more complicated than for therapeutics because a test can lead to additional tests or to a range of therapeutic alternatives. For any one treatment, there may be multiple possible health states, and the paucity of literature may make it difficult to determine the probability of different ones, much less the utility associated with each.

Utility changes over time. We may compare the utility after coronary angioplasty if a patient either does or does not suffer restenosis in Fig. 94-4. After successful angioplasty, the patient feels well and utility rises, but then the patient may suffer restenosis and utility falls. After successful redilation, utility rises again. After angioplasty not complicated by restenosis, utility gradually rises. Ultimately, the patients get to the same point, but the patient who has the episode of restenosis suffers a period of decreased utility. Utility measurement should involve patient

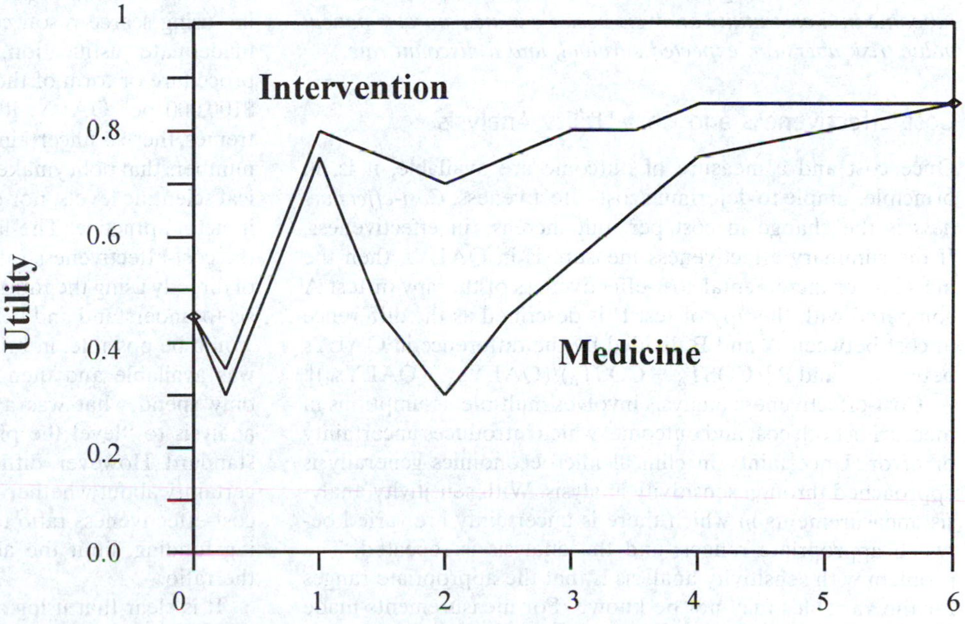

FIGURE 94-4 Theoretical time course of utility after coronary angioplasty in a patient who does not suffer restenosis (*top line*) and a patient who does suffer restenosis (*bottom line*).

preference. One patient may dislike chest pain enough to be willing to undergo repeat procedures to relieve angina. Another patient may dislike the catheterization suite enough to be willing to put up with more angina.

Utility may be measured using either a validated survey such as the Health Utilities Index[42] or the EuroQol[43] or by directly assessing patient preference. These surveys have been validated against patient preference methods and are easy to administer. Patient preference methods ask patients directly to evaluate their current state of health and then evaluate what they would give up or risk to achieve perfect health. The patient preference methods are probably superior to surveys because the evaluation of a patient's view of his or her own state of health is measured directly, but patient preference methods are difficult to administer. The two patient preference methods are time *tradeoff*[4] and *standard gamble.*[4] In the time tradeoff, patients weigh the fraction of expected survival they are willing to give up to live in perfect health. With the standard gamble, patients weigh what risk of death they are willing to take to live in perfect health. The standard gamble is probably superior because it includes the element of risk.[4]

Utility alone does not provide a final summary measure of outcome because it does not include life expectancy. This summary measure can be determined using quality-adjusted life years (QALYs), which are calculated by combining utility and survival.[44] Median or mean survival must be estimated from either the data set under consideration or from the literature. Survival, as with cost presented earlier, generally is discounted, which means that patients value a year of survival at the present time more than a year of survival in the future. The "true" discount rate for survival is unknown. Values in the literature for the discount rate have varied from 2 to 10 percent, with 3 percent being the most popular.[24] Thus, with a discount rate of 3 percent, next year's survival is 3 percent less important than this year's survival. *QALYs is the best summary measure of outcome in a cost-utility analysis because it incorporates patient value, risk aversion, expected survival, and a discount rate.*

Cost-Effectiveness and Cost-Utility Analysis

Once cost and a measure of outcome are available, it is, in principle, simple to determine cost-effectiveness. *Cost-effectiveness* is the change in cost per unit increase in effectiveness. If the summary effectiveness measure is in QALYs, then the marginal or incremental cost-effectiveness of therapy or test A compared with therapy or test B is described as the difference in cost between A and B divided by the difference in QALYs between A and B $[(COST_A - COST_B)/(QALYs_A - QALYs_B)]$.

Cost-effectiveness analysis involves multiple assumptions in measuring both cost and outcome, which introduces uncertainty or error. Uncertainty in clinical microeconomics generally is approached through sensitivity analysis. With sensitivity analysis, measurements in which there is uncertainty are varied between appropriate ranges, and the analysis is repeated. The problem with sensitivity analysis is that the appropriate ranges for the variables may not be known. For measurements made using several different scales, such as the multiple models for calculating marginal costs, these different scales may be used to perform the sensitivity analysis. For measurements that are continuous, such as professional charges, one standard deviation may be appropriate.

There is, however, no absolute standard for sensitivity analysis other than common sense and an intuitive feel for what is medically reasonable. For instance, Weinstein and Stason[45] used a variation in the severity of angina to decrease QALYs from 0 for no angina to 50 percent for severe disabling angina. If the results of a study vary significantly with changes in certain variables, then the outcome is said to be sensitive for those variables. Properly performed, sensitivity analyses should give insight into the medical decision-making process by identifying thresholds that result in changes in the process. For instance, in the same study by Weinstein and Stason,[45] a threshold was noted for single-vessel disease such that if a patient were sufficiently bothered by angina to be willing to give up 8 percent of life expectancy, then coronary surgery was indicated, excluding concerns about cost.

CURRENT AND FUTURE TRENDS AND POLICY IMPLICATIONS

Cost-effectiveness analysis in clinical medicine offers a powerful approach that may be used to help guide clinical decision making as well as for policy. To date, most cost-effectiveness analyses have been simulations. The formidable difficulties in determining cost and utility have limited the use of these tools in medical care. As the methods and science of cost-effectiveness analyses improve, these analyses should be integrated increasingly into clinical trials and applied routinely to observational databases. With the current changes in health care, accountability and cost are increasingly important, and we can expect to see more studies using these methods and greater incorporation of cost-effectiveness analysis into the medical care delivery system.

The cost-effectiveness ratio, expressed in dollars per QALY, can be used, at least in principle, to affect societal choice regarding using scarce resources. A number that is often used, with inadequate justification, is that below $50,000 per QALY, a procedure or form of therapy is cost-effective, whereas at over $100,000 per QALY, it is too expensive. Between these extremes, there is uncertainty. However, these are relatively rough numbers that policymakers may use and do not represent empirical scientific levels, nor do they reflect thresholds for decisions in actual practice. The lack of an empirical standard to which the cost-effectiveness ratio may be compared reveals the limits of directly using the ratio as opposed to cost-effectiveness analysis to understand and help inform the policymaking process. It would be possible, in principle, to figure out how much money was available and then set the limit on cost-effectiveness to only spend what was available, thus using cost-effectiveness analysis to "level the playing field" and providing a uniform standard. However, difficulties in measurement, as well as uncertainty about whether the appropriateness of using the single cost-effectiveness ratio uniformly for all major policy concerning funding, limit the ability of policymakers to directly use the ratio.

It is clear that using a single number for policymaking purposes is inappropriate because cost-effectiveness methods can vary considerably, despite recent efforts to create standards,[46] leading to different numbers. In addition, the cost-effectiveness ratio may not reflect the difference perspective of small changes made for many people with an inexpensive form of therapy versus a big change for the few for expensive therapy. Finally, cost-effectiveness analysis does not adequately reflect the variability of patient populations. Policy planners, representing society, may choose to lower the threshold for a form of therapy for the young compared with the elderly, even though the impact of age is already included in the calculation of the ratio. Thus cost-effectiveness is not designed to be used for policymaking purposes in the absence of other information but rather should help guide both clinical decision making and public policy. All this being said, the cost-effectiveness of most well established medical therapies compares well with the cost-effectiveness of other health choices, such as airbags in cars, asbestos abatement, or toxic waste control.[46]

COST-EFFECTIVENESS IN PREVENTION, DIAGNOSIS, AND THERAPY

Hyperlipidemia

Until recently, estimates of the cost-effectiveness of lipid lowering were based on decision-analytic models,[2,3,47–50] with data coming from epidemiologic studies, such as Framingham.[51] The models incorporated assumptions concerning the relationship of lipid lowering to subsequent prevention of cardiovascular events. The models also had to make assumptions concerning resource use. More recently, there have been a series of randomized trials that have shown the benefit of lipid lowering and also have included cost-effectiveness analyses (see also Chap. 38).

Education concerning lipid lowering will be inexpensive for each patient but may be quite expensive in the aggregate. A population-wide program was studied by Tosteson et al.[48] using a decision-analytic approach. A population-wide program with a cost of $4.95 per person per year and cholesterol-lowering effects on average of 2 percent reduction would prolong life at an estimated cost of only $3200 per year of life saved.

A cautionary note also was sounded by Goldman et al.[49] Using a decision-analytic model in high-risk patients, therapy with HMG-CoA reductase inhibitor was shown to dominate no therapy. However, in lower-risk populations, therapy has became much less cost-effective and is perhaps not warranted in younger patients with isolated elevation of serum lipids.

Recently, a series of clinical trials in the United States and Europe has established and more clearly defined the benefit of lipid lowering. In the Scandinavian Simvastatin Survival Study (4S),[52] 4444 men and women with a prior MI or episode of unstable angina and with total serum cholesterol between 213 and 309 mg/dL (5.5 and 8.0 mmol/L) were randomized to a low-cholesterol diet and to either placebo or simvastatin. At 5.4 years of mean follow-up, active therapy was associated with reduced all-cause mortality (30 percent; 11.5 versus 8.2 percent), reduced cardiac mortality (42 percent; 8.5 versus 5.0 percent), reduced major coronary events (34 percent; 22.6 versus 15.9 percent), and reduced cardiovascular accidents/transient ischemic attacks (37 percent; 4.3 versus 2.7 percent). Coronary revascularization procedures were reduced by 32 percent (411 versus 278), and cardiac hospitalizations were reduced by 26 percent (acute MI, 37 percent, 630 versus 395; angina, 22 percent, 401 versus 312; stroke/transient ischemic attack, 27 percent, 110 versus 80). A cost-effectiveness analysis was developed from the 4S resource clinical and resource use data, with costs attributed to these resources.[53,54] In 4S, estimated direct medical costs ranged from approximately $4000 to $30,000 per year of life gained, with therapy most cost-effective in older men with the highest baseline cholesterol and least cost-effective in younger women with the lowest baseline cholesterol. When indirect costs were included in the analyses, the estimated cost per year of life gained decreased further, with estimated net savings in the youngest patients and a cost of approximately $13,000 per year of life gained in elderly women with baseline cholesterol of 213 mg/dL.

In the West of Scotland Coronary Prevention Study (WOSCOPS), 6595 Scottish men aged 45 to 64 with moderate hypercholesterolemia [mean cholesterol 272 mg/dL (7 mmol/L) and low-density lipoprotein cholesterol >155 mg/dL (4 mmol/L)] and no history or evidence of MI were randomized to placebo or 40 mg/day pravastatin, with a mean follow-up of 4.9 years.[55] Active therapy reduced all-cause mortality by 22 percent from 4.1 to 3.2 percent, reduced cardiac mortality rates (28 percent; 1.7 versus 1.2 percent), and reduced major coronary events (31 percent; 7.9 versus 5.5 percent). No statistical difference was found in stroke (1.6 percent in placebo and pravastatin groups; 51 versus 46). Coronary revascularization procedures were reduced by 37 percent (2.5 versus 1.7 percent). Data on cardiac hospitalizations are not available. A cost-effectiveness analysis was constructed, based on the outcomes data and resource use. Cost per year of life gained (discounted at 3 to 6 percent annually) was estimated as $25,000 to $40,000, depending on risk group and model assumptions.[56]

Using data from the Pravastatin Limitation of Atherosclerosis in the Coronary Arteries[57] (PLAC I) study and the Pravastatin, Lipids, and Atherosclerosis in the Carotids (PLAC II) study and survival estimates 10 years after MI from Framingham, the Markov decision-analytic model was used to estimate the cost-effectiveness of lipid lowering in secondary prevention. Depending on specific patient risk, cost per life-year saved varied from $7124 to $12,665.

In high-risk groups, such as those with elevated low-density lipoprotein (LDL) cholesterol noted after acute MI, therapy with statins is clearly cost-effective. However, there remains considerable uncertainty as to the cost-effectiveness of therapy in lower-risk populations. Several populations, including the elderly and young groups without a prior event and moderate elevations of lipids, cannot be well assessed from present data. Furthermore, there have been no trials with lipid lowering that included patient preference or any attempt to construct QALYs.

Smoking Cessation

Cigarette smoking remains a potent and prevalent risk factor for premature death and disability. In the United States, approximately one-quarter of the men and one-fifth of the women are current cigarette smokers.[58] These 50 million individuals who annually purchase 24 billion packages of cigarettes[59] have a markedly elevated risk of cancer, pulmonary disease, and vascular disease.[60] As a result, it is estimated that about 400,000 premature deaths occur in the United States each year as a result of cigarette smoking (see also Chap. 38).

The direct medical costs attributed to cigarette smoking are substantial. The Centers for Disease Control and Prevention (CDC) conservatively estimate that medical care expenditures attributable to cigarette smoking in 1993 were $50.0 billion.

These costs included $26.9 billion for hospital expenditures, $15.5 billion for physician expenditures, $4.9 billion for nursing home expenditures, $1.8 billion for prescription drugs, and $900 million for home health services. For each pack of cigarettes sold, more than $2 was spent on medical care attributable to smoking. Of note, for each pack sold, about 90 cents of public funds was spent on medical care attributable to smoking. These estimates do not include the full range of harms caused by smoking, such as injuries from smoking-related fires or complications from premature births.

Cigarette smoking also accounts for important indirect costs such as days lost from work or disability days. Smokers reportedly are absent from work about 7 more days per year than nonsmokers. This loss in productivity associated with the health consequences of smoking is estimated to cost $47 billion.[61]

The benefit of smoking cessation is most likely to be achieved in the short term. These short-term benefits are not inconsequential. Lightwood and Glantz[62] specifically examined the short-term economic benefits of smoking cessation as a result of the rapid decline in the risk of acute MI and stroke. They estimated that a 7-year program that produced a 1 percent annual reduction in smoking prevalence would reduce the number of acute MI hospitalizations by 63,840 and the number of stroke hospitalizations by 34,261. The resulting savings would be $3.2 billion, with the prevention of about 13,000 deaths.

If all smokers quit, however, society would not realize a long-term economic benefit. Costs attributed to smoking would diminish gradually, and in the short-run, costs would be lower. However, over time, the higher survival rate as a result of smoking cessation will lead to a larger number of older individuals who will incur health care costs. As a result, the elimination of smoking would, in the long run, produce a net increase in health care costs. These increased costs would be associated with added years of life and healthier years. *Consequently, we can understand successful smoking-cessation strategies as potentially cost-effective but probably not cost saving in the long run.*

Several studies have examined the cost-effectiveness of interventions to assist smokers to quit.[63,64] These studies have overwhelmingly found effective smoking-cessation programs to be cost-effective relative to other medical interventions. Cromwell et al.[65] evaluated the cost-effectiveness of the clinical recommendations in the Agency for Health Care Policy and Research Clinical Practice Guideline on Smoking Cessation. The guideline included 15 recommended smoking-cessation interventions. The cost per smoker who successfully quit among the counseling interventions that did not include pharmacotherapy ranged from $2186 for group intensive counseling to $7922 for minimal counseling. The cost per QALY ranged from $1108 for group intensive counseling to $4015 for minimal counseling. The addition of pharmacotherapy increased the cost of the intervention but also the effectiveness. With transdermal nicotine as an adjunct therapy, the cost per QALY ranged from $1171 for group intensive counseling to $2405 for minimal counseling. With nicotine gum, it ranged from $1822 for group intensive counseling to $4542 for minimal counseling. These estimates are based on patients presenting to a primary care clinic.

Smoking-cessation programs may be even more cost-effective relative to other interventions for patients with cardiovascular disease because of their high risk of future events. Krumholz et al.[66] evaluated the cost-effectiveness of a nurse-based educational intervention for patients who had survived an acute MI. The cost-effectiveness of the program was estimated to be $220 per year of life saved. The value of these types of programs was illuminated in the sensitivity analysis. A smoking-cessation program after acute MI would remain less than $20,000 per year of life saved even if the program only produced 3 additional ex-smokers for every 1000 (baseline assumption 26 per 100) enrolled or if the program cost as much as $8840 per smoker (baseline assumption $100). Similar favorable estimates of the value of these interventions would be expected in other high-risk groups with cardiovascular disease.

Exercise

There is strikingly little information on exercise to prevent coronary artery disease. Nevertheless, the cost-effectiveness of exercise was investigated using a decision-analytic model by Jones and Eaton.[67] These investigators constructed hypothetical cohorts of sedentary men and women aged 35 to 74 years. Assuming a relative risk of 1.9 for heart disease associated with sedentary behavior, $5.6 billion would be saved annually if 10 percent of adults began a regular walking program. Alternatively, $4.3 billion could be saved if the entire sedentary population began walking regularly, accounting for costs in individuals who dislike exercising. Using the baseline assumptions, walking was found to be economically beneficial for men aged 35 to 64 years and women aged 55 to 64 years. The threshold of relative risk at which economic benefit is found for walking overall was estimated at 1.7, and for those who walk voluntarily, most adults would benefit even at a relative risk of just 1.15.

Diabetes Control

Diabetes is a common and important risk factor for cardiovascular disease. Glycemic control is related to the risk of subsequent complications.[68] As a consequence, the HbA1c level is considered an indicator of the quality of care for an organization, with recommendations for the level to be less than 7 percent.[69] Nevertheless, many diabetics do not reach this level of glycemic control (see also Chaps. 38 and Chap. 78).[70]

In economic terms, glycemic control is also important. The level of glycemic control of adult diabetics is associated with medical care expenditures. An observational study of adults with diabetes enrolled in a large health maintenance organization reported that medical care charges were strongly related to HbA1c levels.[71] An increase of 1 percent in the HbA1c level was associated with a 7 percent increase in charges. Because these patients tend to require many medical services, the impact on health care expenditures can be substantial. For example, among the patients with hypertension and heart disease, in addition to diabetes, a difference in the HbA1c level of from 9 to 10 percent was associated with a difference in costs of more than $4000 over 3 years—even after adjustment for age, sex, and other chronic conditions.

Interventions that improve glycemic control can result in fewer microvascular complications.[71,72] The resources required to produce this benefit are substantial because the interventions may include closer monitoring, increased patient education, frequent telephone contact, more clinical visits, and higher drug costs.

For type I diabetes, the Diabetes Control and Complications Trial (DCCT) may best demonstrate the benefit of these interventions.[72] This trial showed that an intensive treatment regimen decreased the risk of development or progression of retinopathy, nephropathy, and neuropathy by 50 to 75 percent. An economic analysis of the DCCT revealed that the intensive intervention was more expensive than conventional therapy by about $30,000 over the lifetime of each patient.[73] However, considering what is achieved by this investment, the cost-effectiveness of this intervention has been calculated to be $28,661 per year of life saved. With adjustments for quality of life, the intensive intervention costs $19,987 per QALY.

For type II diabetes, the United Kingdom Prospective Diabetes Study (UKPDS), the largest and longest study of this topic, demonstrated that improved blood glucose control reduces the risk of developing retinopathy and nephropathy and possibly reduces neuropathy.[74] This study and others modeled the economic impact of interventions to improve glycemic control for type II diabetes.[75] The intensive treatment doubled the cost of medical care for these patients, which was partially offset by a reduction in the number of complications. The cost-effectiveness of an intensive program was calculated to be $16,002 per QALY.

Antihypertensive Screening and Therapy

Hypertension is a risk factor for stroke, ischemic heart disease, heart failure, and end-stage renal disease (see also Chaps. 38 and Chap. 51). The Sixth Report of the Joint National Committee details our current knowledge about prevention, detection, evaluation, and treatment of hypertension.[76] The screening and treatment of hypertension in the United States, based on 1995 dollars, was estimated to cost $23.7 billion, including $6.7 billion in indirect costs for lost wages and lowered productivity.[77] The costs of the complications of hypertension would be considerably higher. The reduction in vascular events provided by screening and treating hypertension partially offsets their cost, producing a favorable cost-effectiveness ratio.

Investigators from Stanford demonstrated the value of screening in an article that was published about a decade ago.[78] The results suggest that screening is economically attractive in men and women of all ages. The ratios compared favorably with other common interventions in medicine. Men and older adults have more favorable ratios because they are more likely to have high blood pressure. In 1990 dollars, screening has a cost-effectiveness ratio of $8374 per QALY for men age 60. Screening for hypertension had the least favorable cost-effectiveness ratio, with $44,412 per QALY for 20-year-old women. In the sensitivity analysis, the ratio became less favorable as the benefit of the therapy decreased and as the cost of the medication increased.

Other investigators have examined the cost-effectiveness of treatment once a patient with hypertension is identified. A classic study in this area used a computer simulation, the CHD Policy Model, to estimate the cost-effectiveness of various antihypertensive treatments.[79] The antihypertensive and cholesterol effects of each of the medications were derived from a meta-analysis of trials that evaluated the efficacy of these agents. The CHD Policy Model, based on estimates derived from the Framingham Heart Study, calculated the effects of these changes in blood pressure and cholesterol on the incidence of coronary heart disease. They focused specifically on various antihypertensive medications in persons aged 35 through 64 years with a diastolic blood pressure of 95 mmHg or greater and no known coronary heart disease. In 1987 dollars and compared with no treatment, the cost per year of life saved was estimated to be $10,900 for propranolol, $16,400 for hydrochlorothiazide, $61,900 for prazosin hydrochloride, and $72,100 for captopril. Studies of older patients also have found that the treatment of hypertension is economically attractive.[80]

Since the publication of this study, the options for treatment have expanded. The abundance of antihypertensive strategies presents a challenge to these studies in selecting a comparison group. A strategy that is only more expensive than a competing treatment without evidence of incremental benefit will always be dominated in the analysis. The incremental advantage of many of our current treatments for hypertension over the inexpensive option of using low-dose hydrochlorothiazide is speculative and has led some observers to speculate that substantial resources are being squandered in the treatment of this condition.[81] The Sixth Joint National Committee report does recommend diuretics or beta blockers as first-line agents for managing essential hypertension. A recent economic analysis of the Joint National Committee guidelines concurred that a diuretic or beta blocker is much less expensive to achieve and maintain blood pressure control compared with a calcium-channel blocker or angiotensin-converting enzyme (ACE) inhibitor.[82]

Multiple-Risk-Factor and Community Intervention Programs

The Stanford Coronary Risk Intervention Project (SCRIP) tested the hypothesis that intensive multiple-risk-factor reduction would reduce progression of atherosclerosis in the coronary arteries of men and women compared with subjects randomly assigned to usual care.[83] Patients in the risk-reduction arm were provided individualized programs of a low-fat and low-cholesterol diet, exercise, weight loss, smoking cessation, and lipid-lowering medications. Intensive risk reduction resulted in improvements in various risk factors, including serum lipids, weight, exercise capacity, and diet, compared with relatively small changes with usual care. The risk-reduction group showed a rate of narrowing of diseased coronary artery segments 47 percent less than usual care group. There were 25 hospitalizations in the risk-reduction group for cardiac events compared with 44 with usual care. Based on data from the SCRIP program, Superko[84] estimated that when the cost savings of the reduced number of events is balanced against the cost of treatment, the prevention program would cost on average $1500 per patient per year, with a range of costing $2273 to a cost savings of $901 per patient per year.

DeBusk et al.[85] evaluated a physician-directed, nurse-managed, home-based case-management system for coronary risk-factor modification in a randomized trial during the first year after acute MI. In the hospital, specially trained nurses initiated interventions for smoking cessation, exercise training, and diet and drug therapy for hyperlipidemia. Intervention after discharge was conducted primarily by telephone and mail. In the special intervention, there was greater smoking cessation and lipid lowering as well as improved exercise performance compared with usual care. Superko[84] estimated the cost of the program at $550 per year. While a true cost-effectiveness analysis is not available, this type of program may be more attractive than other, more resource-intensive approaches.

There have been multiple studies of primary prevention programs. The 10-year results of the North Karelia project showed a 28 percent decrease in smoking, 3 percent decrease in serum cholesterol, and 3 percent decrease for systolic blood pressure.[86] In the Pawtucket Heart Health Program, citizens of all ages participated in multilevel education, screening, and counseling programs.[87] Projected cardiovascular disease rates were 16 percent lower during the education program but lessened to 8 percent after education. The Pawtucket investigators concluded that greater risk-factor control would require a sustained community effort along with state and national efforts. Modest effects of a community intervention also were noted in the Stanford Five-City Project, with the investigators concluding that better design for intervention was needed.[88] Similarly disappointing results were noted in the Minnesota Heart Health Program.[89] In a pooled analysis of the three American programs, trends were estimated for cigarette smoking, blood pressure, total cholesterol, body mass index, and coronary heart disease mortality risk for women and men, with estimates of intervention effect in the expected direction in 9 of 12 comparisons; however, none was statistically significant.[90] Kottke et al.[91] conducted a simulation based on clinical trial data, which suggested that only a population approach can prevent the majority of deaths from cardiovascular disease. However, the implementation of such programs to date has not been entirely satisfactory, and it is difficult to draw any conclusions concerning cost-effectiveness. Well-designed programs with control or resources and adequate data to conduct cost-effectiveness studies would appear to still be needed.

ACUTE CORONARY SYNDROMES

Coronary Care

Patients with an acute MI often suffer life-threatening complications that require rapid, high-level intervention. Consequently, the standard of care is to admit patients with an acute MI to a coronary care unit. Admission to these units is costly, and relatively few patients benefit from the units' advanced capabilities. The value of this triage for specific groups of patients can be illuminated through an economic analysis (see also Chap. 42).

To address this issue, Tosteson et al.[92] made use of clinical and resource use data from 12,139 emergency department patients who presented with acute chest pain. They compared a coronary care unit with admission to an intermediate care facility with central electrocardiographic monitoring and personnel to detect and treat in-hospital complications. Information on the effectiveness of coronary care units is sparse, particularly in this setting of alternatives with some of the same capabilities. Based on data from the Multicenter Chest Pain Study, the authors estimated that mortality for patients with an acute MI would be 15 percent higher for admission to an intermediate care unit compared with a coronary care unit.[93] Using this assumption, the value of admission to a coronary care unit varied depending on the age of the patient and the initial probability of an acute MI. In 1992 dollars, for patients who were 55 to 64 years old and had a 1 percent probability of MI, admission to a coronary care unit had a cost-effectiveness ratio of $1.4 million per year of life saved, whereas the same aged patients with a 99 percent probability of an MI had a cost-effectiveness ratio of $15,000 per year of life saved. The cost-effectiveness ratio was less than $75,000 per year of life saved if the probability of MI exceeded 20 percent. The cost-effectiveness of coronary care units was less favorable for younger patients because of their higher underlying risk of a life-threatening complication.

Reperfusion

With the advent of information about the efficacy of thrombolytic therapy for the treatment of patients with suspected acute MI, interest turned to the economic value of this intervention. Since the two largest and earliest trials of thrombolytic therapy used streptokinase, the early economic evaluations focused on this agent.[94–98]

A cost-effectiveness analysis published in 1992 examined the use of streptokinase compared with no treatment.[94] The investigators focused on the treatment of elderly patients with suspected acute MI, a group for which there is less enthusiasm about using thrombolytic therapy. Based on data available from GISSI-1 and ISIS-2, the relative benefit of thrombolytic therapy was assumed to be lower in elderly patients and the risk of thrombolytic therapy was assumed to be higher, but the absolute risk of an acute MI was much higher compared with younger patients. The smaller relative reduction in the higher risk associated with MI offset the higher risk of complications. Thus the decision analysis suggested that thrombolytic therapy was economically attractive over a broad range of assumptions about the risks and benefits. After considering the costs of the treatment, complications, and long-term health care of survivors, the authors estimated that the cost-effectiveness ratio of streptokinase compared with conventional medical therapy was $21,200 per year of life saved for an 80-year-old patient. The authors calculated similar estimates for younger patients. Several studies have found similar results. One analysis has even suggested that thrombolytic therapy could be cost saving because of its impact on reducing rehospitalization[98] (see also Chap. 42).

With the emergence of tissue-type plasminogen activator (tPA) as a more expensive and more effective alternative to streptokinase, studies addressed whether the incremental benefit was large enough to justify the incremental cost. The GUSTO trial investigators performed a substudy to address this issue specifically.[99] The investigators collected detailed information about resource consumption in a subgroup of the GUSTO subjects. They found that both treatment groups were similar in their use of resources in the year after enrollment. The treatment groups had a mean length of hospital stay of 8 days, including an average of 3.5 days in the intensive care unit. During the initial hospitalization, the treatment groups had a similar rate of CABG (13 percent) and PCTA (31 percent). Overall, the 1-year health costs, excluding the difference in the cost of the thrombolytic agent, were $24,990 per patient treated with tPA and $24,575 per patient treated with streptokinase. The major difference in the cost of the therapies was the cost of the drugs: $2750 for tPA and $320 for streptokinase. The primary analysis assumed no increase in costs for the tPA group after the first year. Based on the GUSTO results and an estimate of the patients' life expectancy, the additional life expectancy per patient treated with tPA was estimated to be 0.14 years.

Based on these estimates, the authors concluded that the cost-effectiveness ratio of using tPA instead of streptokinase was $32,678 per year of life saved. This ratio varied considerably based on the infarction site and the age of the patient. In general, the younger and lower-risk patients had higher cost-effectiveness ratios. For example, the cost-effectiveness ratio for tPA in a patient aged 40 years or younger with an inferior MI was $203,071 per year of life saved compared with $13,410 per year of life saved for a person aged 75 years or older with an anterior MI. An analysis conducted independent of the GUSTO trial reached similar conclusions.[100] Comparisons with other new agents await strong evidence of their superiority to tPA.

Mechanical approaches to reperfusion have been employed with increasing frequency. The clinical or economic advantage of primary angioplasty remains controversial.[101–103] Several studies have suggested a substantial advantage of primary angioplasty.[104–106] Economic analyses based on early studies suggested that primary angioplasty is associated with a reduction in mortality without increasing cost.[107,108] Other recent clinical studies of actual practice, however, have provided less impressive results associated with the use of primary angioplasty,[103,109] making estimates of the effectiveness more difficult.

A fundamental problem in this area is that the field is moving rapidly. Changes in costs and techniques require rapid access to recent data in order to develop relevant economic models. For example, stents, initially considered to be contraindicated in acute MI because of concerns that they would incite thrombus formation, are becoming the standard for primary mechanical reperfusion therapy. As evidence of the efficacy of stents accumulates, there will be a need to examine their economic impact compared with balloon angioplasty and thrombolytic therapy. Also, as more rapid discharge protocols evolve for patients who receive reperfusion therapy, the balance of costs and effectiveness may shift.[110]

Antithrombotic Agents

Aspirin reduces mortality and morbidity for patients with acute coronary syndromes. As a result of the marked benefit and the minimal cost of the therapy, no formal economic analysis of aspirin for the treatment of acute coronary syndromes has been published in the mainstream journals. The ISIS-2 trial found that aspirin avoided 25 deaths for every 1000 patients with suspected acute MI.[111] In addition, the 1 month of aspirin therapy in ISIS-2 was associated with halving the risk of stroke or reinfarction. Aspirin avoided about 10 reinfarctions and 3 strokes for every 1000 patients treated. The avoidance of complications would likely translate into cost savings, leading aspirin to be considered a "strongly dominant" therapy.

Heparin for the treatment of acute MI also has not been formally evaluated in an economic analysis because it has not been shown to provide a strong benefit for acute MI in the aspirin era.[112] In addition, while aspirin plus heparin is the standard of care for patients hospitalized with unstable angina, a metaanalysis of the unstable angina studies found only borderline significant results in favor of heparin.[113] Given the uncertainty about its effectiveness, heparin would only be a favored therapy if there were evidence that heparin reduces cost. No studies have revealed an economic advantage to heparin therapy in this setting.

New agents are emerging with increasing frequency. For example, low-molecular-weight heparin is emerging as an effective therapy for unstable angina.[114] The greater cost and benefit of this new treatment make it ideal for economic analyses. Mark et al.[115] performed an economic analysis for a subset of patients enrolled in the Efficacy and Safety of Subcutaneous Enoxaparin in Non-Q-Wave Coronary Events Study Group (ESSENCE).[115] Patients treated with enoxaparin had lower resource use during the initial hospitalization, and this benefit persisted at 30 days, with a cumulative cost savings associated with enoxaparin of $1172 ($p = 0.04$). The investigators concluded that enoxaparin both improves important clinical outcomes and saves money relative to therapy with standard unfractionated heparin, making it a strongly dominant therapy.

The use of a monoclonal antibody fragment against the platelet receptor glycoprotein IIb/beta IIIa inhibitors is growing. Treatment of high-risk patients undergoing coronary revascularization reduces the short-term risk of death, MI, or coronary revascularization.[116] An economic analysis of the EPIC trial found that the use of this therapy for high-risk patients was associated with a cost savings of $622 per patient during the initial hospitalization from reduced acute ischemic events.[117] During the 6-month follow-up, the therapy decreased repeat hospitalization rates by 23 percent ($p = 0.004$) and repeat revascularization by 22 percent ($p = 0.04$), producing a mean $1270 savings per patient (exclusive of drug cost) ($p = 0.018$). If the cost of the drug were less than $1270, then the strategy would be effective and cost saving.

The Randomized Efficacy Study of Tirofiban for Outcomes and Restenosis (RESTORE) trial found that in patients undergoing coronary angioplasty for acute coronary syndromes, tirofiban protects against early adverse cardiac events related to abrupt closure.[118] A subsequent economic analysis reported that the use of tirofiban (including drug costs) was not associated with an increase in health care costs.[119]

Neither of these studies directly examined the use of this agent in patients with acute ischemic syndromes. Future studies (with economic substudies), such as the TACTICS (Treat Angina with Aggrastat and Determine Cost of Therapy with Invasive or Conservative Therapy)–TIMI 18 trial will address this issue.[120]

Invasive versus Conservative Strategies in Non-ST-Segment Elevation Acute Coronary Syndromes

The relative value of an invasive strategy with early catheterization and possible revascularization compared with a conservative strategy with exercise testing in patients with unstable angina or non-ST-segment elevation acute MI has been studied in several clinical trials with equivocal results to date.[121–123] None of these trials included an economic component. An invasive versus a conservative strategy for non-ST-segment acute coronary syndromes is currently being studied in the TACTICS–TIMI 18 trial. It will be the first trial in this area with a formal cost and cost-effectiveness analysis built into the structure of the trial.[120,124]

Beta-Blocker Therapy

Beta-blocker therapy has been shown to reduce mortality following an acute MI.[125] Goldman et al.[126] conducted the most widely cited economic analysis of the costs and effectiveness of beta-blocker therapy. Using data from the literature, they estimated that beta-blocker therapy produced a relative reduction in mortality of 25 percent in years 1 to 3 after an MI and a 7 percent reduction for years 4 to 6. They evaluated the cost-effectiveness of the therapy under the assumption that the benefit did not persist after year 6. Costs were calculated using 1987 dollars. The investigators stratified potential patients by their estimated mortality into low, medium, and high risk: 1.5, 7.5, and 13 percent, respectively, in the first year. The cost-effectiveness ratio was strongly associated with the underlying risk of the patient. For a 45 year-old man with low risk, the cost-effectiveness ratio was $23,457, with medium risk it was $5890, and with high risk it was $3623.

ACE Inhibition

Several large randomized trials have demonstrated a reduction in acute MI for patients with left ventricular dysfunction after an acute MI who are treated with an ACE inhibitor.[127] Tsevat et al.[128] examined the cost-effectiveness of this intervention using resource use, survival, and health-related quality of life information from the Survival and Ventricular Enlargement (SAVE) trial, a randomized trial of captopril for survivors of an anterior MI with an ejection fraction of 40 percent or less. The investigators conservatively estimated that the benefit of captopril did not persist beyond 4 years. The trial found that captopril improved survival at 3.5 years by about 20 percent. Costs were calculated in 1991 dollars. The cost-effectiveness ranged from $60,800 per QALY for 50-year-old patients to $3600 for 80-year-old patients. McMurray et al.[129] also found that ACE inhibitors are an economically attractive intervention after MI.

Rehabilitation

In a decision-analytic model, Ades et al.[130] studied the cost-effectiveness of cardiac rehabilitation to coordinate exercise training and secondary prevention after acute MI. The cost-effectiveness of cardiac rehabilitation, in dollars per year of life saved, was calculated by combining published results of randomized trials of cardiac rehabilitation on mortality rates, epidemiologic studies of long-term survival in the overall postinfarction population, and studies of patient charges for rehabilitation services and averted medical expenses for hospitalizations after rehabilitation. Cardiac rehabilitation participants had an incremental life expectancy of 0.202 years. In 1988, the average cost of rehabilitation and exercise testing was $1485, partially offset by averted cardiac rehospitalizations of $850 per patient. A cost-effectiveness value of $2130 per year of life saved was determined for the late 1980s, projected to a value of $4950 per year of life saved in 1995. A sensitivity analysis was conducted to support these findings.

REVASCULARIZATION

Societal Burden

Revascularization, either by CABG or PTCA, represents an expensive form of therapy for the treatment of angina pectoris and, in some patients, the prolongation of life. The societal burden is substantial with over 367,000 CABG and over 482,000 PTCA procedures performed in 1996.[3] These numbers represent a 227 percent increase in CABG since 1979 and a 213 percent increase in PTCA since 1987. Given the difficulties in estimating cost, all cost figures across multiple institutions and health care systems must be considered "best guess" estimates. Nonetheless, the American Heart Association estimates the average cost of coronary surgery at $44,820 and of percutaneous coronary intervention of $20,370 in 1995. These costs may be too low if estimation of in-hospital costs is too high or too low or if induced and productivity costs are not accounted for adequately. If these numbers are accurate, the cost of coronary surgery is approximately $16 billion and angioplasty $10 billion.

Variation in Costs

The variation in costs of revascularization has been investigated in a number of studies. Within institutions, only a fraction of the variation in costs of coronary surgery or coronary angioplasty can be accounted for by either patient-level or procedural-level factors.[23,26–28,131] Complications predict variation to a greater extent. A study from Emory University, for instance, found that the hospital component of the cost of coronary surgery in 1990 dollars was $16,776 if there were no complications, $17,794 with one complication, $23,624 with three complications, and $50,609 with five or more complications.[26] In a study from Duke University, the surgeon was found to be responsible for much of the variability in cost of coronary surgery.[28] Data from the Cleveland Clinic, Emory University, and others have shown that complications also account for more of the variability in cost of angioplasty than preprocedural or procedural data.[26–28] The need for emergent bypass surgery has been shown to be a strong determinant of hospital costs after coronary angioplasty.[27,131] However, the ability to account for variation in cost is best described when length of stay is added to the models.[23,26,131]

Length of stay represents a summary variable that may include multiple unmeasured or unidentified variables and, when studied in models with other variables, may confound or obscure the effect of clinical variables on cost. This problem is apparent within single institutions. Considering broader groups of institutions in different geographic regions will result in even greater variation. Medicare data suggest that hospital-level variables account for some of the variability in hospital costs of coronary surgery, whereas geographic and other provider factors also account for additional variability in the angioplasty costs.[29,132] However, the ability to account for variation in cost across multiple institutions is modest.[132]

The evaluation of cost as well as cost-effectiveness of these procedures is complicated by technological improvements and changes in the delivery of health care. In addition, care maps and other efforts to improve efficiency have dramatically decreased the incidence of complications, shortened length of stay, and cut costs.[131,132] Just as these improvements may not be reflected in published clinical trials concerning outcomes, the available cost-effectiveness analyses also will not entirely reflect either technologic improvements nor increased efficiency in health care delivery.

Coronary surgery has improved in recent years with greater use of arterial grafts, improved anesthesia and cardioplegia, and the introduction of less invasive coronary surgery. In this regard, outcome and costs in 1996 dollars in 12,266 patients undergoing coronary bypass surgery between 1988 and 1996 at Emory University were evaluated.[23] The patients became sicker, especially with more hypertension, diabetes, prior MIs, and a decrease in ejection fraction over the period. Mortality tended to decrease from 4.7 to 2.7 percent ($p = 0.07$). After accounting for increasing indices of severity of disease over the period, there was a significant decrease in mortality (odds ratio 0.90 per year; $p = 0.0001$). The Q-wave MI rate fell from 4.1 to 1.3 percent ($p < 0.0001$). Mean hospital cost decreased from $22,689 to $15,987, and postoperative length of stay decreased from 9.2 to 5.9 days. After accounting for other variables, cost decreased by $1118 per year and length of stay by 0.55 days per year.

PTCA also has improved with technological improvements, especially coronary stents. Stent procedures have improved with better deployment and less need for full anticoagulation. Thus, in the era of stents plus ticlopidine or clopidogrel, stents do not add as much to the cost of intervention as during the era of full anticoagulation. In this regard, Peterson et al.[133] showed that the in-hospital cost of balloon angioplasty in 109 patients studied between 1995 and 1996 was $10,219. In 64 patients from 1993 to 1995, the cost of PTCA with stenting plus warfarin was $15,793, and in 217 patients undergoing PTCA with stenting plus ticlopidine the cost was $13,065. Improvements in PTCA services between 1990 and 1997 in 1997 dollars were investigated in 17,399 patients undergoing PTCA at Emory University.[131] Mortality changed little from 0.63 to 0.88 percent ($p = 0.84$). The Q-wave MI rate fell from 0.68 to 0.24 percent ($p = 0.036$). Emergent coronary surgery fell from 3.50 to 1.56 percent ($p < 0.0001$). Mean hospital cost decreased from $9816 to $7442 ($p < 0.0001$), and the length of stay after the procedure decreased from 2.81 to 2.00 days ($p < 0.0001$).

Some technologic improvements have been specifically subjected to economic analyses. The use of stents was compared with balloon angioplasty in the STRESS trial.[134] In this relatively early evaluation of stents, there was less additional revascularization and less restenosis with stents but no difference in survival. Costs were higher with stents, due to the prolonged hospitalization and full anticoagulation. Stents ultimately may dominate balloon angioplasty, since hospital stay is now likely to be similar, as stent costs decline while additional procedures continue to be avoided. In both the EPIC and RESTORE trials, the costs of PTCA with and without glycoprotein IIb/IIIa antagonists during balloon angioplasty in the setting of unstable angina or non-Q-wave MI was studied.[135,136] In both studies, there was improved outcome with glycoprotein IIb/IIIa blockade, with little or no increase in costs. A formal cost-effectiveness analysis of glycoprotein IIb/IIIa blockade for balloon angioplasty has been published in preliminary form.[137] Finally, a purely theoretical paper has suggested that a therapy costing in the range of $1000 that decreases restenosis after coronary angioplasty by 50 percent could offer a cost-effectiveness ratio of $16,000 per QALY.[138]

Coronary Surgery versus Medicine

Coronary surgery has been compared with medicine in three major clinical trials conducted in the 1970s and early 1980s (see Chap. 48). None of these trials incorporated cost assessment or cost-effectiveness analyses in their designs. However, the cost-effectiveness of coronary surgery was studied in a relatively early, although detailed decision-analytic study by Weinstein and Stason.[45] Costs included those of surgery, medical management of angina, and treatment of future MIs. CABG was shown to increase unadjusted life expectancy by 0.6 year in patients with two-vessel disease and 6.9 years in patients with left main coronary disease. With one-vessel disease, a gain in quality-adjusted life expectancy may be noted, due to less angina after surgery. For patients with severe angina, the cost-effectiveness of CABG ranged from $3800 per QALY gained in left main disease to $30,000 in one-vessel disease.

Coronary Surgery versus Percutaneous Coronary Intervention

The cost-effectiveness of CABG versus PTCA was first assessed using a decision-analytic model by Wong et al.[139] 8 years after the Weinstein and Stason article.[45] This article was published after PTCA was more established but before the era of stents and before results of randomized trials comparing PTCA with CABG. The model predicted that patients treated with PTCA would have more additional revascularization procedures than patients treated with CABG but that cost would be similar in the long term. In patients with angiographically suitable two-vessel disease, PTCA was found to be a reasonable alternative to CABG. Even in patients with three-vessel disease, bypass surgery was only slightly better than angioplasty.

CABG versus PTCA as an initial revascularization strategy has been compared in a series of six randomized trials from the late 1980s and early 1990s.[31–36] These trials showed little difference in death or MI except in the subgroup with treated diabetes, for which several trials showed a benefit to coronary surgery.[32,140] However, there generally was less angina and less need for additional revascularization procedures after coronary surgery. Cost analyses were performed in the EAST and BARI trials in the United States, ERACI in Argentina, RITA in the United Kingdom, and GABI in Germany.[36–40]

In the EAST trial, Weintraub et al.[37] examined the in-hospital and 3-year costs of patients randomized to revascularization with coronary surgery or coronary angioplasty. While the in-hospital costs of surgery were higher than those of angioplasty, there was little difference in 3-year costs. This was due to the need for additional procedures in many of the angioplasty patients.

BARI[32] was a multicenter trial with 1829 patients and included prospective information on economic costs and quality of life in 934. The initial cost of angioplasty was $21,113 and coronary surgery was $32,247 ($p < 0.001$). However, by 5 years, the costs were much closer, $56,225 for angioplasty and $58,889 for surgery ($p = 0.047$). The costs were surprisingly and disturbingly high in both treatment arms, and there was considerable overlap. The BARI trial showed that CABG dominated PTCA for treated diabetics with three-vessel disease.

Two European randomized trials of PTCA and CABG have included economic end points: the RITA trial[36,38] of 1011 patients and the GABI trial[33] of 358 patients. In the GABI trial, the initial procedural costs were $16,562 for CABG and $5000 for PTCA. After 1 year, the authors found that there was little increase in cumulative costs in the CABG group, whereas the cumulative costs for the PTCA group were $11,250.[33] Similar results were found in the RITA trial, where initially there were much higher costs in the CABG group, but by 2 years the cumulative costs in the PTCA group were 80 percent of those for the CABG group.[38] Cost at 3 years in the ERACI trial also was higher in the CABG group than in the PTCA group but had narrowed from in-hospital costs.[40]

Other than for treated diabetics in the BARI trial, there are inadequate data to perform a cost-effectiveness analysis comparing PTCA with CABG from any of the trials to date because the difference in symptomatic status makes it necessary to include utility assessment. This is essential because if there is no difference in survival, and life years alone were the measure of outcome, then the decision could be made on the basis of cost alone. There are three more contemporary trials comparing PTCA with CABG. There is ARTS in Europe and Israel and ERACI II in Argentina. Preliminary data from ERACI II suggest that PTCA with stenting may dominate CABG, but this is a small trial with only preliminary data in late 1999.[141] There is an ongoing trial in the United Kingdom, continental Europe, and Canada, SoS, which is comparing contemporary coronary intervention with stents with coronary bypass surgery. SoS will incorporate a formal cost-effectiveness analysis with utility assessment (see also Chap. 45).

PTCA versus Medicine

The cost-effectiveness of PTCA compared with medicine also was assessed as part of the now somewhat historical paper by Wong et al.[139] referred to earlier concerning the comparison of PTCA with CABG. This study suggested that in patients with severe angina or documented ischemia, angioplasty was cost-effective for single-vessel disease. PTCA has been compared with medicine in three randomized trials, ACME,[142] AVERT,[143] and RITA II.[144] All showed less angina with PTCA. AVERT and RITA II found more cardiovascular events with angioplasty. However, these trials have been small, underpowered to examine hard end points, and have largely included low-risk patients. None included a formal cost or cost-effectiveness analysis. In the ongoing COURAGE trial, a larger cohort of 3260 higher-risk patients, all treated with the best available medical therapy, are being randomized to PTCA with medicine versus medicine alone. COURAGE includes a formal cost-effectiveness analysis with utility assessment by direct patient preference.

ELECTROPHYSIOLOGY

Patient Monitoring

Monitoring involves multiple areas, including Holter monitoring, cardiac event recording, and monitoring in the hospital. Event recorders were compared with a 48-h monitor in a randomized trial by Kinlay et al.[145] using a randomized crossover trial design in 43 patients with palpitations. Event monitors were twice as likely to provide a diagnostic rhythm strip ECG during symptoms as the 48-h monitor. Event monitors dominated continuous monitors with cost savings.

Implantable Cardiac Defibrillators

Implantable cardiac defibrillators (ICDs) have become widely used to prevent sudden cardiac death in patients at high risk (see also Chap. 31). The cost-effectiveness of this therapy has been investigated with decision-analytic models as well as within the context of randomized trials. Kupersmith et al.[146] investigated the cost-effectiveness of ICD implantation using a decision-analytic model. These investigators based their model on a patient population of 218 well-characterized patients for whom the time of first appropriate discharge was determined.[147] All patients underwent electrophysiologic testing. The authors assumed that the time of first appropriate shock would have been the time of death without the ICD, which was compared with observed mortality. Costs were based on the Medicare fee schedule. Cost-effectiveness was $31,100 per year of life saved. At an ejection fraction of less than 25 percent and greater than or equal to 25 percent, cost-effectiveness was $44,000 and $27,200 per year of life saved. Endocardial ICDs became popular at the time of this study and decreased the cost-effectiveness ratio to $25,700 per year of life saved.

Owens et al.[148] also developed a decision-analytic model, but with a different construction and a somewhat different question. Specifically, ICDs were compared with amiodarone in patients at high or intermediate risk using a highly detailed model with event rates from the literature and costs estimated from published cost rates in California.[149] In high-risk patients, if an ICD reduces total mortality by 20 percent, the marginal cost-effectiveness of an ICD relative to amiodarone was $74,400 per QALY saved. If an ICD reduces mortality by 40 percent, the cost-effectiveness of ICD use was $37,300 per QALY saved, with the results sensitive to assumptions about quality of life. Decision-analytic models were noted by Larsen et al.[149] and Kupermann et al.[150] In these studies, the cost-effectiveness of treatment with an ICD was better than that noted by Owens et al.[148] at $30,500[150] and $47,700[149] per life year saved, adjusted to 1995 dollars. However, the study by Owens et al.[148] considered the more superior antiarrhythmic agent amiodarone.

In a small, randomized trial conducted by Wever et al.,[151] 60 consecutive postinfarct survivors of sudden cardiac death were randomly assigned either ICD as first choice or antiarrhythmic drugs and guided by electrophysiologic testing. Fifteen patients died, 4 in the early ICD group and 11 in the electrophysiologic testing-guided strategy group ($p = 0.07$). The cost-effectiveness of ICD compared with drug therapy was $11,315 per life year saved by early ICD implantation. If quality-of-life measures are taken into account, the cost-effectiveness of early ICD implantation was even more favorable.

Cost-effectiveness of ICD compared with conventional therapy from the MADIT trial was reported by Mushlin et al.,[152] based on 181 patients randomized in the United States. Hospital costs were estimated from the UB92 formulation of the hospital bill and converted to costs using hospital-specific cost-to-charge ratios. Corresponding physician costs were based on a national study of Medicare claims that calculated the ratio of physician to hospital costs for each DRG.[153] Additional professional costs were calculated from payment rates in the Medicare RBRVS. MADIT included epicardial implants in the beginning of the trial and endocardial implants later on. The discounted survival was 3.46 years for the ICD group and 2.66 years for the conventional therapy group to 4 years of follow-up and was associated with an incremental cost-effectiveness ratio of $27,000 (95 percent confidence interval, $200 to $68,200) per life year saved. The results probably would have been more favorable if all patients were treated with endocardial implants. These results probably offer the strongest argument for the cost-effectiveness of ICDs.

Radiofrequency Ablation

Radiofrequency ablation (RFA) can be curative of supraventricular arrhythmias and offers the potential for dominating older forms of therapy (see also Chap. 28). This was studied in a small group of patients by Kalbfleisch et al.[154] The authors determined charges for radiofrequency catheter modification of the atrioventricular (AV) node in 15 patients with symptomatic AV node reentrant tachycardia despite pharmacologic therapy and compared these charges with the estimated health care charges by the same patients before the catheter procedure was performed. The duration and frequency of symptoms were 16 ± 9 years and 4.5 ± 6 episodes per month, respectively. Fourteen of the 15 patients required only one procedure for diagnosis and cure of AV node reentrant tachycardia, and 1 patient required two sessions; all underwent electrophysiologic study before discharge from the hospital to confirm the short-term efficacy of the procedure. The mean duration of the hospital stay was 3 ± 1.5 days, with a charge per patient in 1991 dollars of $15,893 ± $3338, including hospital and physician components. All patients had a successful outcome and required no additional antiarrhythmic therapy. The estimated cost of health care utilization for these 15 patients before cure of AV node reentrant tachycardia was $7651 per patient per year. While small in scale, and with less than optimal costing methods, this study reflects dominance of RFA. A similar costing study from Australia of RFA compared with continued medical therapy also showed dominance of the procedure.[155] RFA in 20 patients was compared with surgical treatment in 20 patients and medical therapy in 12 patients in the nonrandomized comparison. RFA dominated medical therapy. Surgical therapy was slightly more efficacious, but at much higher cost.[156]

A more sophisticated decision-analytic model was created by Hogenhuis et al.[157] In four groups of patients with Wolff-Parkinson-White syndrome, those with (1) prior cardiac arrest, (2) paroxysmal supraventricular tachycardia or atrial fibrillation (PSVT/AF) with hemodynamic compromise, (3) PSVT/AF without hemodynamic compromise, and (4) no symptoms, the authors developed a cost-effectiveness analysis examining five clinical management strategies: (1) observation, (2) observation until a cardiac arrest dictates the need for therapy, (3) initial drug therapy guided by noninvasive monitoring, (4) initial RFA, and (5) initial surgical ablation. A model was developed that included the risks of cardiac arrest, PSVT/AF, drug side effects, procedure-related complications and mortality, the efficacy of drugs and RFA, and cost. RFA was assumed to have an overall efficacy of 92 percent in preventing cardiac arrest and arrhythmias. The model predicted that RFA would yield life expectancy greater than or equal to other strategies. In cardiac arrest survivors and patients who have had PSVT/AF with hemodynamic compromise, the model suggested that RFA would prolong survival at a lower cost. For patients with PSVT/AF without hemodynamic compromise, the marginal cost-effectiveness of attempted RFA ranged from $6600 for 20-year-olds to $19,000 for 60-year-olds per QALY gained. However, for asymptomatic patients, RFA costs ranged from $174,000 for 20-year-olds to $540,000 for 60-year-olds per QALY gained.

Pacemakers

There is a paucity of cost-effectiveness data concerning pacemakers. This may be so because in the classic indication of heart block they are so clearly life-saving that even if they do not dominate no therapy, there can be little doubt about their cost-effectiveness (see also Chap. 31). Some effort has gone into resource utilization issues. Stamato et al.[158] performed a cost-minimization study in which they showed that charges and probably costs will be lower with implantation in a catheterization laboratory as opposed to the operating room. The cost-effectiveness of dual-chamber DDD pacing compared with single-chamber VVI pacing was studied using a decision-analytic model by Sutton and Bourgeois.[159]

Over a 10-year period, a computer model calculated the incidence and prevalence of atrial fibrillation, stroke, permanent disability, heart failure, and mortality in six patient categories: sick sinus syndrome paced VVI, sick sinus syndrome and atrioventricular block upgraded to DDD, sick sinus syndrome paced DDD from the outset, atrioventricular block paced VVI and those upgraded to DDD, and atrioventricular block paced initially DDD. Survival and functional capacity were improved with DDD pacing both for sick sinus syndrome and for atrioventricular block. DDD pacing also was less expensive in the long term, with health care costs in follow-up being a number of times more expensive than the pacemaker. In appropriate patients, DDD pacing dominates VVI pacing. Other efforts have gone into establishing guidelines to ensure the appropriate use of pacemakers.[160–163]

Care of Atrial Fibrillation

The major risk of atrial fibrillation is embolic stroke. The cost-effectiveness of anticoagulation was considered using a decision-analytic model by Gage et al.[164] The authors obtained the probabilities of adverse outcomes from trials involving anticoagulation for nonvalvular atrial fibrillation. They noted a 22 percent reduction in ischemic stroke with aspirin therapy from a metaanalysis[165] and a 68 percent reduction with warfarin therapy from the atrial fibrillation investigators' collaborative analysis of five clinical trials.[166] The authors obtained utility estimates by interviewing 74 patients with atrial fibrillation, using the time tradeoff method for three degrees of severity of stroke and for daily therapy with aspirin or warfarin. Costs were estimated, based on the literature. For patients at medium risk of stroke (i.e., patients with atrial fibrillation and one additional stroke risk factor, including a history of stroke, transient ischemic attack, hypertension, diabetes, or heart disease), the cost-effectiveness of warfarin therapy as compared with aspirin therapy was $8000 (range, $200 to $30,000) per QALY. Both warfarin and aspirin dominated no therapy. For patients at low risk of stroke (i.e., isolated atrial fibrillation), quality-adjusted life expectancy was 6.70 years with warfarin therapy, 6.69 years with aspirin therapy, and 6.51 years with no therapy. The marginal cost-effectiveness of warfarin over aspirin was $370,000 per QALY saved in the base case. If the annual rate of stroke were 0.5 percent higher in low-risk patients, warfarin treatment would cost $66,000 per QALY. Aspirin dominated no therapy.

In a decision-analytic model from Sweden, Gustafsson et al.[167] found that anticoagulation dominated no therapy, and in a decision-analytic model from the United Kingdom, Lightowlers and McGuire[168] found anticoagulation to be cost-effective and dominate no therapy in higher-risk patients.

Recent efforts have focused on strategies for managing cardioversion, antiarrhythmic therapy, and anticoagulation. Eckman et al.[169] constructed a decision-analytic model considering the base case of a 65-year-old man with nonvalvular atrial fibrillation. Cardioversion followed by a combination of amiodarone and warfarin was the most effective strategy, yielding a gain of 2.3 QALYs compared with no therapy. The marginal cost-effectiveness ratio of cardioversion followed by aspirin with amiodarone was $33,800 per QALY and without amiodarone was $10,800 per QALY. Cardioversion followed by amiodarone and warfarin had a marginal cost-effectiveness ratio of $92,400 per QALY compared with amiodarone and aspirin.

Catherwood[170] constructed a similar decision-analytic model considering multiple strategies involving cardioversion followed by aspirin, amiodarone, and warfarin. Strategies involving cardioversion dominated no cardioversion. For patients at high risk of stroke (5.3 percent per year), cardioversion alone followed by repeated cardioversion plus amiodarone therapy on relapse was cost-effective at $9300 per QALY compared with cardioversion alone followed by warfarin therapy on relapse. This strategy also was preferred for moderate-risk patients (3.6 percent per year), but with a higher cost-effectiveness ratio of $18,900 per QALY. In the lowest-risk patients (1.6 percent per year), cardioversion alone followed by aspirin therapy on relapse was preferred.

Another issue concerning the care of patients with atrial fibrillation is the role of transesophageal echocardiography in avoiding prolonged anticoagulation prior to cardioversion. This was investigated using a decision-analytic model by Seto et al.[171] The authors studied the cost-effectiveness of three strategies: (1) conventional therapy with transthoracic echocardiography and warfarin therapy for 1 month before cardioversion, (2) initial transthoracic echo followed by transesophageal echo and early cardioversion if no thrombus was detected, and (3) initial transesophageal echo with early cardioversion if no thrombus is detected. With strategies 2 and 3, if a thrombus was seen, a follow-up transesophageal echo was performed. If no thrombus was seen, cardioversion was performed. All strategies used anticoagulation before and extending for 1 month after cardioversion. Life expectancy, utilities, event probabilities, and cost were ascertained from the literature. Strategy 3 (cost, $2774; QALYS, 8.49) dominated strategy 2 (cost, $3106; QALYs, 8.48) and conventional therapy (cost, $3070; QALYs, 8.48). The study demonstrated that transesophageal echo-guided cardioversion dominated conventional therapy if the risk of stroke after transesophageal echo negative for atrial thrombus is slightly less than that after conventional therapy. However, the issue of the best way to facilitate cardioversion to minimize periprocedural stroke is not yet certain.

HEART FAILURE

Perspective

Heart failure is a major medical problem in economically advantaged countries. In the United States, the approximate prevalence of congestive heart failure is 4.6 million, with an incidence of 400,000 new cases a year and approximately 870,000 hospitalizations a year. Furthermore, hospitalizations for heart failure have increased by 130.8 percent between 1979 and 1996.[3] In 1995, the Health Care Financing Agency paid $3.4 billion to Medicare beneficiaries for heart failure, and it is the single most common cause of hospitalizations over the age of 65.[2] The American Heart Association estimates the total annual direct and indirect care costs of heart failure at $21 billion dollars.[3]

Heart failure differs from other areas of consideration in this chapter because it is a disease process rather than a single form of therapy or service. Thus the economics of heart failure and cost-effectiveness strategies must approach it as a process and then consider breaking the process down. Heart failure must be considered a process in which patients have a baseline health state, with associated baseline continuing costs for medication and office visits as well as productivity costs. The patient may then decompensate, resulting in a hospitalization, presumably with a somewhat worse health state and associated costs. Efforts will then be made to return the patient to his or her baseline health state and maintain him or her there. Finally, patients may be considered for transplantation to try to reverse or partially reverse heart failure, also with associated cost (see also Chaps. 21 and Chap. 22).

Digoxin

Despite over 200 years of experience, the role of digoxin in the treatment of congestive heart failure remains uncertain. In the absence of adequate clinical data, the cost-effectiveness data similarly will be limited. Nonetheless, Ward et al.[172] developed a decision-analytic model concerning digoxin withdrawal in patients with stable heart failure. The clinical sequelae of digoxin withdrawal came from the Prospective Randomized Study of Ventricular Failure and Efficacy of Digoxin (PROVED) and Randomized Assessment of Digoxin and Inhibitors of Angiotensin-Converting Enzyme (RADIANCE) trials.[173,174] Costs were estimated from hospital and Medicare data. Outcomes included treatment failures, digoxin toxicity, and health care costs. Continuation of digoxin therapy in patients with heart failure nationally would avoid 185,000 office visits, 27,000 emergency visits, and 137,000 hospital admissions for heart failure, but with 12,500 cases of digoxin toxicity. The net annual savings would be $406 million (90 percent confidence interval, $106 to $822 million). Sensitivity analysis showed that digoxin is cost saving if the incidence of digoxin toxicity is 33 percent or less. Thus digoxin therapy was found to dominate withdrawal of digoxin in stable heart failure.

In a large randomized trial study, the effect of digoxin on mortality and hospitalization in patients with heart failure and left ventricular ejection fractions of 0.45 or less were randomly assigned to digoxin (3397 patients) or placebo (3403 patients) in addition to diuretics and ACE inhibitors.[175] While there was no effect on mortality, there were 26.8 percent hospitalizations in the digoxin groups versus 34.7 percent in the placebo group ($p < 0.001$). Although no formal cost-effectiveness analysis is available, Mark estimated that the digoxin therapy is at least cost neutral and probably cost saving.[176]

ACE Inhibition

The efficacy of ACE inhibition in preserving left ventricular size and in prolonging survival in patients with heart failure has been established in a series of clinical trials. In a meta-analysis of 32 trials totaling 7105 patients, the mortality rate in patients randomized to ACE inhibitor was 15.8 percent compared with 21.9 percent for placebo (odds ratio, 0.77; 95 percent confidence interval, 0.67 to 0.88).[177] None of these trials included prospective economic evaluations. However, there have been several decision-analytic analyses based on these trials.

Tsevat et al.[128] studied the effectiveness of ACE inhibition after MI, and the results are reviewed in that section. Glick et al.[178,179] developed a decision-analytic model based on the SOLVD trial. SOLVD was an 83-center trial in which 2569 patients with symptomatic heart failure and ejection fractions of 35 percent or less received either the ACE inhibitor enalapril or placebo. At 41.4 months of follow-up, enalapril decreased mortality and hospitalization by 16 and 26 percent, respectively. Costs were estimated based on HCFA reimbursement rates in 1992 dollars. For patients with heart failure, enalapril dominates placebo in the short term and is highly economically attractive in the long term. Enalapril saved approximately $717 per patient over the period of the SOLVD treatment trial. When trial data were projected over a patient's lifetime, therapy with enalapril produced a cost utility ratio of $115 per QALY. As pointed out by Boyko et al.,[180] there is variation in the cost of ACE inhibitors, and as these agents become less expensive, their cost-effectiveness ratio may become even more attractive.

Somewhat more general in the treatment of heart failure is the Paul et al.[181] decision-analytic model based on the SOLVD and VheFt I and II trials. These trials considered the strategies of (1) standard therapy (digoxin and diuretics) with no vasodilator agents, (2) hydralazine hydrochloride-isosorbide dinitrate combination, and (3) ACE inhibition with enalapril. Using data from three major randomized, controlled trials to estimate treatment efficacy, mortality rates, and hospitalization rates, the cost was $5600 per year of life gained with hydralazine–isosorbide dinitrate compared with standard therapy. Compared with the hydralazine–isosorbide dinitrate combination therapy, the incremental cost-effectiveness ratio for enalapril therapy was $9700 per year of life saved.

The cost-effectiveness of ACE inhibition also has been studied in Europe using decision-analytic techniques. In mild heart failure, Kleber[182] found ACE inhibition to be cost-effective but not cost saving. However, in the Netherlands, van Hout et al.[183] found ACE inhibition to dominate not using ACE. Similarly, in a study from the United Kingdom based on SOLVD, Hart et al.[184] found that ACE therapy potentially could dominate not using ACE therapy.

Beta Blockade

Recently, beta blockade, especially with carvedilol, has been added to the therapeutic armamentarium for heart failure. There have been four randomized trials in 1094 patients with New York Heart Association class II to IV symptoms and left ventricular ejection fraction of 0.35 or less.[185] The series of trials was terminated early, based on a finding of a 65 percent mortality reduction in patients receiving carvedilol (95 percent confidence interval, 39 to 82 percent). Delea, et al.[186] constructed a decision-analytic model estimating life expectancy and health care costs for patients with heart failure receiving carvedilol plus conventional therapy (digoxin, diuretics, and ACE inhibitors) or conventional therapy alone. Benefit estimates were based on the carvedilol trial results, assuming either "limited benefits" persisting for 6 months, the average duration of follow-up in the clinical trials, or "extended benefits" persisting for 6 months and then declining gradually over 3 years. For conventional therapy alone, estimated life expectancy was 6.67 years, and for carvedilol it was 6.98 and 7.62 years, assuming limited and extended benefits, respectively. Expected lifetime costs of heart failure–related care were estimated at $28,756 for conventional therapy and $36,420 and $38,867 for carvedilol, assuming limited and extended benefits, respectively. Cost per life year saved for carvedilol was $29,477 and $12,799 under limited and extended benefits assumptions, respectively. Thus the cost-effectiveness of cardvedilol remains in a reasonable range but is not as attractive as ACE inhibition.

Disease Management Strategies

Heart failure is particularly well suited to developing strategies, such as the development of heart failure clinics, to improve management. Evaluating treatment strategies is difficult because (1) it is difficult to construct randomized trials logistically, (2) there may be contamination in which the management strategy is used to some extent in the control arm, (3) there may be differences between programs that are inherent in different medical centers that make collaboration for multisite efforts difficult, and (4) different health care systems may vary substantially. These variations also may limit generalizability. The difficulties in mounting trials to evaluate outcome of management strategies is a similar limitation for randomized trials. Nonetheless, several small efforts have been made.

Rich et al.[187] conducted a randomized trial using a nurse-directed, multidisciplinary intervention on readmission rate within 90 days of hospital discharge, quality of life, and costs for elderly patients admitted to the hospital with heart failure. The intervention was comprised of educating the patient and family, diet, early discharge planning, reviewing medications, and intensive follow-up. Survival for 90 days without readmission was achieved in 91 of the 142 patients in the treatment group versus 75 of the 140 patients with conventional care ($p = 0.09$). There were 53 readmissions in the treatment group versus 94 in the control group (risk ratio, 0.56; $p = 0.02$). The number of readmissions for heart failure was reduced by 56.2 percent in the treatment group (54 versus 24 in the control group; $p = 0.04$). In the control group, 23 patients (16.4 percent) had more than one readmission versus 9 (6.3 percent) in the treatment group (risk ratio, 0.39; $p = 0.01$). In a subgroup of 126 patients, quality-of-life scores at 90 days improved more from baseline in the treatment group ($p = 0.001$). Because of the reduction in hospital admissions, the total cost of care was $460 less per patient in 1994 dollars in the treatment group, confirming strong dominance for the management strategy.

Weinberger et al.[188] studied 1396 patients hospitalized with chronic diseases, half of whom had congestive heart failure, who were randomized to intensive medical management versus usual care. There were more repeat hospitalizations in the specialized care group. This seemingly contradictory finding[188] reveals that disease management is not easily subjected to scientific scrutiny.

West et al.[189] and Kornowski et al.[190] studied a disease management strategy based on outpatient care rather than focusing on patients being discharged. In a study in Israel, Kornowski et al.[190] analyzed outcome of 42 patients aged 78 ± 8 years with New York Heart Association congestive heart failure class III or IV who were examined at home weekly by local internists and a trained paramedical team. The year before, entry to the home-care program was compared with the first year of home surveillance. Functional status (ability to perform daily activities on a 1 to 4 scale) improved from 1.4 ± 0.9 to 2.3 ± 0.7 ($p < 0.001$). The total hospitalization rate fell from 3.2 ± 1.5 to 1.2 ± 1.6 hospitalizations per year and length of stay from 26 ± 14 to 6 ± 7 days per year ($p < 0.001$ for both). Cardiovascular admissions fell from 2.9 ± 1.5 to 0.8 ± 1.1 hospitalizations per year and stay from 23 ± 13 to 4 ± 4 days per year ($p < 0.001$). This study showed improved outcome but at an uncertain tradeoff in resource use between increased home visits and decreased hospitalizations for the intervention.

West et al.[189] used a strategy of physician-led but nurse-managed, home-based heart failure management not involving home visits. Nurses directed the implementation of guidelines for pharmacologic and dietary therapy by frequent telephone contact of 51 patients with heart failure for 138 ± 44 days. Compared with the period before enrollment, sodium intake fell by 38 percent ($p = 0.0001$), vasodilator doses increased ($p = 0.01$), and functional status and exercise capacity improved significantly ($p = 0.01$). Compared with the 6 months before enrollment, general medical and cardiology visits declined by 23 and 31 percent, respectively (both $p < 0.03$), and emergency room visits for heart failure and for all causes declined 67 and 53 percent, respectively (both $p < 0.001$). Compared with 1 year before enrollment, hospitalization rates for heart failure and for all causes declined 87 and 74 percent ($p = 0.001$). Thus this strategy improved clinical outcome for heart failure while reducing resource use, again suggesting strong dominance.

Rich[191] and Philbin[192] have both reviewed disease management programs. Between 1983 to 1998, 16 studies, 10 observational and 6 randomized trials, of multidisciplinary heart failure disease management programs were published in the English language literature. All studies reported reduced hospitalization, and several studies reported improved quality of life, functional capacity, patient satisfaction, and compliance. All studies that included a cost analysis found the disease management programs to be cost-effective. Rich[191] suggested that current data are limited by generalizability to the more heterogeneous population of patients with heart failure, and the feasibility of translating specific disease management programs into diverse practice environments, and how to individualize the programs for each patient. While the impact of heart failure disease management programs on survival is also unknown, these programs appear to be cost-effective at reducing morbidity and improving quality of life in selected patients with heart failure.

Heart Transplantation

Heart transplantation remains sufficiently infrequent, with just 2290 in the United States in 1997, that its overall impact on cost from a public health standpoint is small (see also Chap. 22). The American Heart Association estimates the average cost of transplants at $253,200, with an annual follow-up cost of $21,200.[3] Cardiac transplantation has not been subjected to rigorous cost-effectiveness analysis, perhaps because of inadequate natural history data with which to compare transplant patients. Although cardiac transplantation is certainly expensive, these patients generally would have a life expectancy of a few weeks to months in the absence of the transplant. In a somewhat preliminary, and now dated study, Evans[193] showed that overall cost-effectiveness of heart transplant was estimated at $44,300 per year of life saved.

DIAGNOSIS

Establishing the cost-effectiveness of diagnostic testing is considerably more difficult than it is for therapeutics because diagnostics by themselves rarely affect outcome. Rather, diagnostics generally lead to a range of choices of therapeutic options with the potential for very different outcomes. Thus decision-analytic models with diagnostics tend to be more complicated than with therapeutics, and consequently, the uncertainty is much greater. Randomized trials with diagnostics are also quite unusual. Thus such cost-effectiveness analyses as exist are essentially all decision-analytic simulations.

Testing for CAD

Garber and Solomon[194] evaluated the cost-effectiveness of noninvasive and direct coronary angiography in the diagnosis of CAD. The tests evaluated included treadmill exercise ECG, planar thallium imaging, single-photon-emission computed tomography, stress echocardiography, and positron-emission tomography, all followed by coronary angiography, if positive, and finally, direct coronary angiography. Survival was based on the medically or surgically treated patients in the CASS study. How survival after angioplasty was calculated is not clear. Based on a metaanalysis of trials comparing angioplasty with medicine, surgery was assumed to have 1.6 times the ability of angioplasty to relieve symptoms. Sensitivities and specificities of testing were developed from a metaanalysis of the literature. Positron-emission tomography (PET) was the most sensitive noninvasive test and exercise testing the least sensitive. Single-photon emission computed tomography (SPECT) was nearly as sensitive as and somewhat less specific than PET (specificity, 0.77 for SPECT and 0.82 for PET). Stress echocardiography is more specific than PET (0.88 compared with 0.82) but less sensitive (0.76 compared with 0.91). There were no published data on the sensitivity of PET for detecting severe (left main and three-vessel) coronary disease, but planar thallium imaging, SPECT, and echocardiography are highly sensitive for detecting severe disease. These figures are based on studies that included small numbers of patients. Exercise testing is not as sensitive (see also Chap. 40).

Little difference in life expectancy was noted with the various strategies, but somewhat more variation to QALYs because the calculation of QALYS gives credit to strategies that improve symptoms rapidly. Nonetheless, the differences amounted to a couple of weeks over approximately 12 years in men and 14 years in women. Costing was based on Medicare payments.

Single-photon emission computed tomography (SPECT) had higher QALYs at higher cost than stress echocardiography with a marginal cost-effectiveness ratio of $64,000 in 65-year-old men to nearly $150,000 in 45-year-old women. Positron emission tomography (PET) generally produced slightly better outcomes than SPECT but at much greater cost. While immediate angiography dominated PET in every group, immediate angiography was more expensive than SPECT with a margin from about $80,000 in 65-year-old men to nearly $200,000 in 45-year-old women.

Strategies in which patients are neither tested nor treated initially are not no-cost strategies, since patients may experience an MI and undergo medical or surgical treatment in the future.

Thus the cost-effectiveness of stress echocardiography compared with no testing ranges from $31,000 per QALY in 65-year-old men to $98,000 per QALY in 45-year-old women.

At a different prevalence of disease, the ranking of tests changes somewhat. For 55-year-old men with a 75 percent pretest risk for disease, initial angiography becomes more attractive (it will be chosen whenever a cost-effectiveness ratio of $45,000 is acceptable), and stress echocardiography remains preferable to exercise testing (with a cost-effectiveness ratio of $22,000 per QALY. At a 25 percent prevalence of disease, echocardiography seems to be the most attractive test under most circumstances; single-photon-emission computed tomography (SPECT) would be chosen over echocardiography only if a cost-effectiveness ratio of $110,000 is considered acceptable, and immediate angiography would be chosen over SPECT only at a cost-effectiveness ratio of $355,000. Thus stress echocardiography remains a cost-effective strategy at a wide range of prevalence of disease, whereas immediate angiography is a cost-effective choice when the pretest probability of disease is high.

Somewhat similar analyses have been offered by Kim et al.[195] and Kuntz et al.[196] The study by Kim et al.[195] specifically studied women. In a 55-year-old woman with definite angina, direct angiography was found to be appropriate, with a marginal cost-effectiveness of $17,000 per QALY. This figure rises as the probability of angina falls, and in the midrange of probabilities, echocardiography was felt to be preferable. In the study by Kuntz et al.,[196] the incremental cost-effectiveness of direct coronary angiography compared with exercise echocardiography was $36,400 per QALY in a 55-year-old man. For 55-year-old men with atypical angina, exercise echocardiography compared with exercise electrocardiography at a cost of $41,900 per QALY. If exercise echocardiography was not available, exercise single-photon-emission computed tomography (SPECT) cost $54,800 per QALY saved compared with exercise electrocardiography. For a 55-year-old man with nonspecific chest pain, the cost-effectiveness of exercise electrocardiography compared with no testing was $57,700 per QALY.

These studies can be criticized easily for making multiple assumptions. However, the end result is quite reasonable. *In patients with chest pain in the intermediate range of probabilities, a test that includes myocardial imaging, either echocardiography or single-photon-emission computed tomography (SPECT), is appropriate, with echo more appropriate in the lower probability range and SPECT in the higher probability range.* Immediate angiography is appropriate as the probability of disease rises. In lower-risk populations, a treadmill exercise test is probably appropriate, and ultimately, in very low-risk populations, in the single digits of pretest probability, reassurance and watchful waiting would be the strategy of choice.

Triage after MI

The proper evaluation of patients after acute MI in terms of assessment of residual ischemia has remained uncertain. The alternatives are to do nothing and follow patients clinically, to obtain an exercise ECG, to obtain an exercise ECG along with an imaging test, or to perform cardiac catheterization. There are no adequate randomized trials in this area and certainly none that include a cost-effectiveness analysis.

Thus this area has been explored exclusively with decision-analytic models. Dittis et al.[197] developed a model with the options of exercise ECG, exercise thallium scintigraphy, and coronary angiography, followed by CABG surgery for patients with left main coronary disease only or patients with left main disease, three-vessel disease, or single- or double-vessel disease and a significant amount of myocardium in jeopardy. Proceeding directly to angiography for risk stratification was the most effective approach, lowering expected mortality from 8 percent to approximately 3 percent. However, the marginal costs for this strategy were high. The most cost-effective approach was to screen patients initially with exercise ECG.

The approach of using the exercise ECG as a screen after MI was studied by Kuntz et al.,[198] who developed a decision-analytic model for representative patient subgroups based on relevant clinical characteristics. The model estimates QALYs and direct lifetime costs for two strategies: coronary angiography and treatment guided by its results versus initial medical therapy without angiography. Decision-tree chance-node probabilities were estimated from pooled data of randomized clinical trials, and additional relevant literature costs were estimated with the use of the Medicare Part A database; quality-of-life adjustments were derived from a survey of 1051 patients who had had a recent acute MI. The incremental cost-effectiveness ratios for coronary angiography and treatment guided by its result, compared with initial medical therapy without angiography, varied from $17,000 to over $1 million per QALY gained. Patient subgroups with severe postinfarction angina or a strongly positive exercise tolerance test typically had cost-effectiveness ratios of less than $50,000 per QALY gained. In addition, most patient subgroups with a prior MI had cost-effectiveness ratios of less than $50,000 per QALY of life gained, even with a negative exercise test result.

CONCLUSIONS

Health care economics offer a powerful set of tools for establishing cost and overall measures of outcome and relating cost to outcome. These tools have been used increasingly in cardiovascular medicine for the purposes of gaining greater insight to facilitate improved patient management but also to help guide public policy. These tools have been applied widely now in cardiovascular medicine, with peer-reviewed literature on cost and often cost-effectiveness analysis, in most areas of cardiovascular medicine. However, the methods of measurement and analysis have varied widely, limiting the ability to compare studies and thus generalize the findings. A recent effort in the United States[24] should provide a guide to investigators performing cost-effectiveness analyses to perform them in a more standard manner. The quality of data available in many areas probably poses a greater problem. Over time, however, the quality of data and of scholarship should increase, making economic studies ever more meaningful and relevant to the practice of medicine.

ACKNOWLEDGMENT

We thank Lesley Wood for her careful editorial review.

References

1. Allenet B, Sailly J-C. Willingness of pay as a measure of benefit in health. *J D'Econ Med* 1999; 17:301–326.

2. *http://www.hcfa.gov.*
3. *1999 Heart and Stroke Statistical Update*. Dallas: American Heart Association; 1998.
4. Drummond MF, Stoddart GL, Torrance GW. *Methods for the Economic Evaluation of Health Care Programmes*. Oxford, England: Oxford University Press; 1990:74–167.
5. Kupersmith J, Holmes-Rovner M, Hogan A, et al. Cost-effectiveness analysis in heart disease: II. Preventive therapies. *Prog Cardiovasc Dis* 1995; 37:243–271.
6. Borna S, Sundaram S. An approach to allocating limited health resources. *J Health Soc Behav* 1999; 11:85–94.
7. Schlander M. Rational resource allocation in the health care system: I. Why rationing may become inevitable. *Med Welt* 1999; 50:36–41.
8. Weintraub WS, Warner CD, Mauldin PD, et al. Economic winners and losers after introduction of an effective new therapy depend on the type of payment system. *Am J Managed Care* 1997; 3:743–749.
9. Weintraub WS. Microeconomic methods in cardiovascular care. In: Talley JD, Mauldin PD, Becker ER, eds. *Cost-Effective Diagnosis and Treatment of Coronary Artery Disease*. Baltimore: Williams & Wilkins; 1999:17–29.
10. Rothermich EA, Pathak DS. Productivity-cost controversies in cost-effectiveness analysis: Review and research agenda. *Clin Ther* 1999; 21:255–267.
11. Evans DB. Principles involved in costing. *Med J Aust* 1990; 153:S10–S12.
12. Hlatky MA. Analysis of costs associated with CABG and PTCA. *Ann Thorac Surg* 1996; 61:S30–S32.
13. Finkler SA. The distinction between costs and charges. *Ann Intern Med* 1982; 96:102–109.
14. Finkler SA, Ward DM. *Essentials of Cost Accounting for Health Care Organizations*, 2d ed. Rockville, MD: Aspen Publications; 1999:11–43.
15. Hlatky MA, Lipscomb J, Nelson C, et al. Resource use and cost of initial coronary revascularization: coronary angioplasty versus coronary bypass surgery. *Circulation* 1990; 82(suppl IV):IV-208–IV-213.
16. Weintraub WS, Mauldin PD, Talley JD, et al. Determinants of hospital costs in acute myocardial infarction. *Am J Managed Care* 1996; 2:977–986.
17. Lefebvre C, Van Der Perre T. Activity based costing. *Acta Hospital* 1994; 34:5–16.
18. Coulam RF, Gaumer GL. Medicare's prospective payment system: A critical appraisal. *Health Care Financ Rev* 1991; 13:45–77.
19. Becker ER, Mauldin PD, Weintraub WS. CABG and PTCA physician practice profiles using the resource-based relative value scale (RBRVS): Better methods for explaining the variation. *Clin Res* 1994; 42:225A.
20. Becker ER, Mauldin PD, Bernadino ME. Using physician work RVUs to profile surgical packages: methods and results for kidney transplant surgery. *Best Pract Benchmark Healthcare* 1996; 3:140–146.
21. Becker ER, Mauldin PD, Culler SD, et al. Applying the resource-based relative-value scale to the Emory Angioplasty versus Surgery Trial. *Am J Cardiol* 2000; 85:685–691.
22. Hsiao WC, Braun P, Yntema D, et al. Estimating physicians' work for a resource-based relative value scale. *N Engl J Med* 1998; 319:835–841.
23. Weintraub WS, Craver JM, Jones EL, et al. Improving cost and outcome of coronary surgery. *Circulation* 1998; 98:23–28.
24. Gold MR, Siegel JE, Russell LB, et al. *Cost-Effectiveness in Health and Medicine*. New York: Oxford University Press; 1996.
25. Quality of Care and Outcomes Research in CVD and Stroke Working Groups. Measuring and improving quality of care: A report from the American Heart Association/American College of Cardiology First Scientific Forum on Assessment of Healthcare Quality in Cardiovascular Disease and Stroke. *Circulation* 2000; 101:1483–1493.
26. Mauldin PD, Weintraub WS, Becker E. Predicting hospital charges and costs for coronary surgery from pre-operative and post-operative variables. *Am J Cardiol* 1994; 74:772–775.
27. Ellis SG, Miller DP, Brown KJ, et al. In-hospital costs of percutaneous coronary revascularization: Critical determinants and implications. *Circulation* 1995; 92:741–747.
28. Mark DB, Gardner LH, Nelson CL, et al. Long-term costs of therapy for CAD: A prospective comparison of coronary angioplasty, coronary bypass surgery and medical therapy in 2258 patients. *Circulation* 1993; 88(2):I-480.
29. Topol EJ, Ellis SG, Cosgrove DM, et al. Analysis of coronary angioplasty practice in the United States with an insurance-claims database. *Circulation* 1993; 87:1489–1497.
30. Harris RA. Nease RF Jr. The importance of patient preferences for comorbidities in cost-effectiveness analyses. *J Health Econ* 1997; 16:113–119.
31. King SB III, Lembo NJ, Weintraub WS, for the EAST Investigators. A randomized trial comparing coronary angioplasty with coronary bypass surgery. *N Engl J Med* 1994; 331:1044–1050.
32. The BARI Investigators. Comparison of coronary bypass surgery with angioplasty in patients with multivessel disease. *N Engl J Med* 1996; 335:217–225.
33. Hamm CW, Reimers J, Ischinger T, et al. A randomized study of coronary angioplasty compared with bypass surgery in patients with symptomatic multivessel coronary artery disease. *N Engl J Med* 1994; 331:1037–1043.
34. CABRI Trial Participants. First-year results of CABRI (Coronary Angioplasty versus Bypass Revascularization Investigation). *Lancet* 1995; 346:1179–1184.
35. Rodriguez A, Boullon F, Perez-Balino N, et al. Argentine randomized trial of percutaneous transluminal coronary angioplasty versus coronary artery bypass surgery in multivessel disease (ERACI): In-hospital results and 1-year follow-up. *J Am Coll Cardiol* 1993; 22:1060–1067.
36. The RITA Investigators. Coronary angioplasty versus coronary artery bypass surgery: the Randomized Intervention Treatment of Angina (RITA) trial. *Lancet* 1993; 341:573–580.
37. Weintraub WS, Mauldin PD, Becker E, et al. A comparison of the costs of and quality of life after coronary angioplasty or coronary surgery for multivessel coronary artery disease: Results from the Emory Angioplasty versus Surgery Trial (EAST). *Circulation* 1995; 92:2831–2840.
38. Hlatky MA, Rogers WJ, Johnstone I, et al. Medical care costs and quality of life after randomization to coronary angioplasty or coronary bypass surgery. *N Engl J Med* 1997; 336:92–99.
39. Sculpher MJ, Seed P, Henderson RA, et al. Health service costs of coronary angioplasty and coronary artery bypass surgery: The Randomized Intervention Treatment of Angina (RITA) trial. *Lancet* 1994; 344:927–930.
40. Rodriguez A, Mele E, Peyregne E, et al. Three-year follow-up of the Argentine Randomized Trial of Percutaneous Transluminal Coronary Angioplasty versus Coronary Artery Bypass Surgery in Multivessel Disease (ERACI). *J Am Coll Cardiol* 1996; 27:1178–1184.
41. Alchian A. The meaning of utility measurement. *Am Econ Rev* 1953; 143:26–50.
42. Feeny DH, Torrance GW, Furlong WJ. Health utilities index. In: Spilker B, ed. *Quality of Life and Pharmacoeconomics in Clinical Trials*. Philadelphia: Lippincott-Raven; 1996:239–252.
43. Cook TA, O'Regan M, Galland RB. Quality of life following percutaneous transluminal angioplasty for claudication. *Eur J Vasc Endovasc Surg* 1996; 11:191–194.
44. Loomes G, McKenzie L. The use of QALYs in health care decision making. *Soc Sci Med* 1989; 28:299–308.

45. Weinstein MC, Stason WB. Cost effectiveness of coronary artery bypass surgery. *Circulation* 1982; 66(suppl III):56–65.
46. Tengs TO, Adams ME, Pliskin JS, et al. Five-hundred life-saving interventions and their cost-effectiveness. *Risk Anal* 1995; 15:369–390.
47. Schulman KA, Kinosian B, Jacobson TA, et al. Reducing high blood cholesterol level with drugs: Cost-effectiveness of pharmacologic management. *JAMA* 1990; 264:3025–3033.
48. Tosteson AN, Weinstein MC, Hunink MG, et al. Cost-effectiveness of populationwide educational approaches to reduce serum cholesterol levels. *Circulation* 1997; 95:24–30.
49. Goldman L, Weinstein MC, Goldman PA, et al. Cost-effectiveness of HMG-CoA reductase inhibition for primary and secondary prevention of coronary heart disease. *JAMA* 1991; 265:1145–1151.
50. Garber AM, Browner WS, Hulley SB. Cholesterol screening in asymptomatic adults, revisited. *Ann Intern Med* 1996; 124: 518–531.
51. Abbott RD, McGee D, Kannel WB, et al. The probability of developing certain cardiovascular disease in eight years at specified values of some characteristics. In: Kannel WB, Wolf PA, Garrison RJ, eds. *The Framingham Study: An Epidemiological Investigation of Cardiovascular Disease* (publication no. NIH 87:2284). Bethesda: US Department of Health, Education & Welfare; 1987:sec 37.
52. Randomized trial of cholesterol lowering in 4444 patients with coronary heart disease: The Scandinavian Simvastatin Survival Study. *Lancet* 1994; 344:1383–1389.
53. Pedersen TR, Kjekshus J, Berg K, et al. Cholesterol lowering and the use of healthcare resources: Results of the Scandinavian Simvastatin Survival Study. *Circulation* 1996; 93:1796–1802.
54. Johannesson M, Jonsson B, Kjekshus J, et al. Cost effectiveness of simvastatin treatment to lower cholesterol levels in patients with coronary heart disease. *N Engl J Med* 1997; 336:332–336.
55. Shepherd J, Cobbe SM, Ford I, et al. Prevention of coronary heart disease with pravastatin in men with hypercholesterolemia. *N Engl J Med* 1995; 333:1301–1307.
56. Caro J, Klittich W, McGwire A, et al. The West of Scotland Coronary Prevention Study: Economic benefit analysis of primary prevention with pravastatin. *Br Med J* 1997; 315:1577–1582.
57. Ashraf T, Hay JW, Pitt B, et al. Cost-effectiveness of pravastatin in secondary prevention of coronary artery disease. *Am J Cardiol* 1996; 78:409–414.
58. State-specific prevalence among adults of current cigarette smoking and smokeless tobacco use and per capita tax-paid sales of cigarettes—United States, 1997. *MMWR* 1998; 47:922–926.
59. US Department of Agriculture. *Tobacco Situation and Outlook Report* (publication no. TBS-227). Washington: US Department of Agriculture, Economic Research Service, Commodity Economics Division; June 1994.
60. US Department of Health and Human Services. *Reducing the Health Consequences of Smoking: 25 Years of Progress*. A Report of the Surgeon General (DSS Publication No. CDC89;8411). U.S. Department of Health and Human Services, Public Health Service, Centers for Disease Control, Center for Chronic Disease Prevention and Health Promotion, Office on Smoking and Health; 1989.
61. MacKenzie TD, Bartecchi CF, Schrier RW. The human costs of tobacco use. *N Engl J Med* 1994; 330:975–980.
62. Lightwood JM, Glantz SA. Short-term economic and health benefits of smoking cessation. *Circulation* 1997; 96:1089–1096.
63. Warner KE. Cost effectiveness of smoking-cessation therapies: Interpretation of the evidence—and implications for coverage. *Pharmacoeconomics* 1997; 11:538–549.
64. Meenan RT, Stevens VJ, Hornbrook MC, et al. Cost-effectiveness of a hospital-based smoking cessation intervention. *Med Care* 1998; 36:670–678.
65. Cromwell J, Bartosch WJ, Fiore MC, et al. Cost-effectiveness of the clinical practice recommendations in the AHCPR guideline for smoking cessation. *JAMA* 1997; 278:1759–1766.
66. Krumholz HM, Chen BJ, Tsevat J, et al. Cost-effectiveness of a smoking cessation program after myocardial infarction. *J Am Coll Cardiol* 1993; 22:1703–1705.
67. Jones TF, Eaton CB. Cost-benefit analysis of walking to prevent coronary heart disease. *Arch Farm Med* 1994; 3:703–710.
68. Moss SE, Klein R, Klein BEK, et al. The association of glycemia and cause-specific mortality in a diabetic population. *Arch Intern Med* 1994; 154:2473–2479.
69. American Diabetes Association. Standards of medical care for patients with diabetes mellitus. *Diabetes Care* 1997; 20(suppl 1):S5–S13.
70. Hayward RA, Manning WG, Kaplan SH, et al. Starting insulin therapy in patients with type 2 diabetes: Effectiveness, complications and resource utilization. *JAMA* 1997; 278:1663–1669.
71. Gilmer TP, O'Connor PJ, Manning W, et al. The cost to health plans of poor glycemic control. *Diabetes Care* 1997; 20:1847–1853.
72. The Diabetes Control and Complications Trial Research Group. Intensive diabetes treatment and complications in IDDM. *N Engl J Med* 1993; 329:977–986.
73. The Diabetes Control and Complications Trial Research Group. Lifetime benefits and costs of intensive therapy as practiced in the diabetes control and complications trial. *JAMA* 1996; 276: 1409–1415.
74. UK Prospective Diabetes Study Group. Intensive blood-glucose control with sulphonylureas or insulin compared with conventional treatment and risk of complications in patients with type 2 diabetes. *Lancet* 1998; 352:837–853.
75. Eastman RC, Javitt JC, Herman WH, et al. Model of complications of NIDDM: II. Analysis of the health benefits and cost-effectiveness of treating NIDDM with the goal of normoglycemia. *Diabetes Care* 1997; 20:735–744.
76. The sixth report of the joint national committee on prevention, detection, evaluation, and treatment of high blood pressure. *Arch Intern Med* 1997; 157:2413–2446.
77. Dustan HP, Roccella EJ, Garrison HH. Controlling hypertension: A research success story. *Arch Intern Med* 1996; 156:1926–1935.
78. Littenberg B, Garber AM, Sox HC Jr. Screening for hypertension. *Ann Intern Med* 1990; 112:192–202.
79. Edelson JT, Weinstein MC, Tosteson AN, et al. Long-term cost-effectiveness of various initial monotherapies for mild to moderate hypertension. *JAMA* 1990; 263:407–413.
80. Johannesson M, Dahlof B, Lindholm LH, et al. The cost-effectiveness of treating hypertension in elderly people: An analysis of the Swedish Trial in Old Patients with Hypertension (STOP Hypertension). *J Intern Med* 1993; 234:317–323.
81. Moser M. Why are physicians not prescribing diuretics more frequently in the management of hypertension? *JAMA* 1998; 279:1813–1816.
82. Ramsey SD, Neil N, Sullivan SD, et al. An economic evaluation of the JNC hypertension guidelines using data from a randomized controlled trial. Joint National Committee. *J Am Board Fam Pract* 1999; 12:105–114.
83. Haskell WL, Alderman EL, Fair JM, et al. Effects of intensive multiple risk factor reduction on coronary atherosclerosis and clinical cardiac events in men and women with coronary artery disease: The Stanford Coronary Risk Intervention Project (SCRIP). *Circulation* 1994; 89:975–990.
84. Superko HR. Sophisticated primary and secondary atherosclerosis prevention is cost effective. *Can J Cardiol* 11(suppl C): 35C–40C.
85. DeBusk RF, Miller NH, Superko HR, et al. A case-management system for coronary risk factor modification after acute myocardial infarction. *Ann Intern Med* 1994; 120:721–729.

86. Puska P, Tuomilehto J, Nissinen A, et al. Ten years of the North Karelia project. *Acta Med Scand* 1985; 701(suppl):66–71.
87. Carleton RA, Lasater TM, Assaf AR, et al. The Pawtucket Heart Health Program: Community changes in cardiovascular risk factors and projected disease risk. *Am J Public Health* 1995; 85:777–785.
88. Winkleby MA, Taylor CB, Jatulis D, et al. The long-term effects of a cardiovascular disease prevention trial: The Stanford five-city project. *Am J Public Health* 1996; 86:1773–1779.
89. Luepker RV, Rastam L, Hannan PJ, et al. Community education for cardiovascular disease prevention: Morbidity and mortality results from the Minnesota Heart Health Program. *Am J Epidemiol* 1996; 144:351–362.
90. Winkleby MA, Feldman HA, Murray DM. Joint analysis of three U.S. community intervention trials for reduction of cardiovascular disease risk. *J Clin Epidemiol* 1997; 50:645–658.
91. Kottke TE, Puska P, Salonen JT. et al. Projected effects of high-risk versus population-based prevention strategies in coronary heart disease. *Am J Epidemiol* 1985; 121:697–704.
92. Tosteson AN, Goldman L, Udvarhelyi IS, et al. Cost-effectiveness of a coronary care unit versus an intermediate care unit for emergency department patients with chest pain. *Circulation* 1996; 94:143–150.
93. Beamer AD, Lee TH, Cook EF, et al. Diagnostic implications for myocardial ischemia of the circadian variation of the onset of chest pain. *Am J Cardiol* 1987; 60:998–1002.
94. Krumholz HM, Pasternak RC, Weinstein MC, et al. Cost effectiveness of thrombolytic therapy with streptokinase in elderly patients with suspected acute myocardial infarction. *N Engl J Med* 1992; 327:7–13.
95. Laffel GL, Fineberg HV, Braunwald E. A cost-effectiveness model for coronary thrombolysis/reperfusion therapy. *J Am Coll Cardiol* 1987; 5(suppl B):79B–90B.
96. Simoons ML, Vos J, Martens LL. Cost-utility analysis of thrombolytic therapy. *Eur Heart J* 1991; 12:694–699.
97. Midgette AS, Wong JB, Beshansky JR, et al. Cost-effectiveness of streptokinase for acute myocardial infarction: A combined meta-analysis and decision analysis of the effects of infarct location and of likelihood of infarction. *Med Decis Making* 1994; 14:108–117.
98. Herve C, Castiel D, Gaillard M, et al. Cost-benefit analysis of thrombolytic therapy. *Eur Heart J* 1990; 11:1006–1010.
99. Mark DB, Hlatky MA, Califf RM, et al. Cost effectiveness of thrombolytic therapy with tissue plasminogen activator as compared with streptokinase for acute myocardial infarction. *N Engl J Med* 1995; 332:1418–1424.
100. Kalish SC, Gurwitz JH, Krumholz HM, et al. A cost-effectiveness model of thrombolytic therapy for acute myocardial infarction. *J Gen Intern Med* 1995; 10:321–330.
101. Lange RA, Hillis LD. Should thrombolysis or primary angioplasty be the treatment of choice for acute myocardial infarction? Thrombolysis—the preferred treatment. *N Engl J Med* 1996; 335:1311–1312.
102. Grines CL. Should thrombolysis or primary angioplasty be the treatment of choice for acute myocardial infarction? Primary angioplasty—the strategy of choice. *N Engl J Med* 1996; 335(17):1313–1316.
103. Berger AK, Schulman KA, Gersh BJ, et al. Primary coronary angioplasty versus thrombolysis for the management of acute myocardial infarction in elderly patients. *JAMA* 1999; 282: 341–348.
104. Grines CL, Browne KF, Marco J, et al. A comparison of immediate angioplasty with thrombolytic therapy for acute myocardial infarction. The Primary Angioplasty in Myocardial Infarction Study Group. *N Engl J Med* 1993; 328:673–679.
105. Gibbons RJ, Holmes DR, Reeder GS, et al. Immediate angioplasty compared with the administration of a thrombolytic agent followed by conservative treatment for myocardial infarction. The Mayo Coronary Care Unit and Catheterization Laboratory Groups. *N Engl J Med* 1993; 328:685–691.
106. Zijlstra F, de Boer MJ, Hoorntje JC, et al. A comparison of immediate coronary angioplasty with intravenous streptokinase in acute myocardial infarction. *N Engl J Med* 1993; 328:680–684.
107. Reeder GS, Bailey KR, Gersh BJ, et al. Cost comparison of immediate angioplasty versus thrombolysis followed by conservative therapy for acute myocardial infarction: A randomized prospective trial. Mayo Coronary Care Unit and Catheterization Laboratory Groups. *Mayo Clin Proc* 1994; 69:5–12.
108. The PAMI Trial Investigators. Analysis of the relative costs and effectiveness of primary angioplasty versus tissue-type plasminogen activator: The Primary Angioplasty in Myocardial Infarction (PAMI) trial. *J Am Coll Cardiol* 1997; 29:901–907.
109. Every NR, Parsons LS, Hlatky M, et al. A comparison of thrombolytic therapy with primary coronary angioplasty for acute myocardial infarction: Myocardial Infarction Triage and Intervention Investigators. *N Engl J Med* 1996; 335:1253–1260.
110. Grines CL, Marsalese DL, Brodie B, et al. Safety and cost-effectiveness of early discharge after primary angioplasty in low risk patients with acute myocardial infarction. PAMI-II Investigators: Primary Angioplasty in Myocardial Infarction. *J Am Coll Cardiol* 1998; 31:967–972.
111. Randomised trial of intravenous streptokinase, oral aspirin, both, or neither among 17,187 cases of suspected acute myocardial infarction: ISIS-2. ISIS-2 (Second International Study of Infarct Survival) Collaborative Group. *Lancet* 1988; 2:349360.
112. Collins R, Peto R, Baigent C, et al. Aspirin, heparin, and fibrinolytic therapy in suspected acute myocardial infarction. *N Engl J Med* 1997; 336:847–860.
113. Oler A, Whooley MA, Oler J, et al. Adding heparin to aspirin reduces the incidence of myocardial infarction and death in patients with unstable angina. *JAMA* 1996; 276:811–815.
114. Cohen M, Demers C, Gurfinkel EP, et al. A comparison of low-molecular-weight heparin with unfractionated heparin for unstable coronary artery disease: Efficacy and Safety of Subcutaneous Enoxaparin in Non-Q-Wave Coronary Events Study Group (ESSENCE). *N Engl J Med* 1997; 337:447–452.
115. Mark DB, Cowper PA, Berkowitz SD, et al. Economic assessment of low-molecular-weight heparin (enoxaparin) versus unfractionated heparin in acute coronary syndrome patients: Results from the ESSENCE randomized trial. Efficacy and Safety of Subcutaneous Enoxaparin in Non-Q wave Coronary Events (unstable angina or non-Q-wave myocardial infarction). *Circulation* 1998; 97:1702–1707.
116. Topol EJ, Califf RM, Weisman HF, et al. Randomised trial of coronary intervention with antibody against platelet IIb/IIIa integrin for reduction of clinical restenosis: Results at six months. The EPIC Investigators. *Lancet* 1994; 343:881–886.
117. Mark DB, Talley JD, Topol EJ, et al. Economic assessment of platelet glycoprotein IIb/IIIa inhibition for prevention of ischemic complications of high-risk coronary angioplasty. The EPIC Investigators. *Circulation* 1996; 94:629–635.
118. Topol EJ, Ferguson JF, Weisman HF, et al. Long-term protection from myocardial ischemic events in a randomized trial of brief integrin beta-3 blockade with percutaneous coronary intervention. *JAMA* 1997; 278:479–484.
119. Weintraub WS, Culler S, Boccuzzi SJ, et al. Economic impact of GPIIB/IIIA blockade after high-risk angioplasty: Results from the RESTORE trial. Randomized Efficacy Study of Tirofiban for Outcomes and Restenosis. *J Am Coll Cardiol* 1999; 34:1061–1066.
120. Weintraub WS, Culler SD, Kosinski A, et al. Economics, health-related quality of life, and cost-effectiveness methods for the TACTICS (Treat Angina with Aggrastat [tirofiban] and Determine Cost of Therapy with Invasive or Conservative Strategy): TIMI 18 trial. *Am J Cardiol* 1999; 83:317–322.

121. Braunwald E, McCabe CH, Cannon CP, et al. Effects of tissue plasminogen activator and a comparison of early invasive and conservative strategies in unstable angina and non-Q-wave myocardial infarction: Results of the TIMI IIIB trial. *Circulation* 1994; 89:1545–1556.
122. Boden WE, O'Rourke RA, Crawford MH, et al. Outcomes in patients with acute non-Q-wave myocardial infarction randomly assigned to an invasive as compared with a conservative management strategy. *N Engl J Med* 1998; 338:1785–1792.
123. Ragmin F, Wallentin L, Swahn E, et al. Invasive compared with non-invasive treatment in unstable coronary-artery disease: FRISC II prospective randomised multicentre study. *Lancet* 1999; 354:708–715.
124. Cannon CP, Weintraub WS, Demopoulos LA, et al. Invasive versus Conservative Strategies in Unstable Angina and Non-Q Wave Myocardial Infarction Following Treatment with Tirofiban: Rationale and study design of the International TACTICS-TIMI 18 trial. *Am J Cardiol* 1998; 82:731–736.
125. Yusuf S, Peto R, Lewis J, et al. Beta blockade during and after myocardial infarction: An overview of the randomized trials. *Prog Cardiovasc Dis* 1985; 27:335–371.
126. Goldman L, Sia ST, Cook EF, et al. Costs and effectiveness of routine therapy with long-term beta-adrenergic antagonists after acute myocardial infarction. *N Engl J Med* 1988; 319:152–157.
127. Brown NJ, Vaughan DE. Angiotensin-converting enzyme inhibitors. *Circulation* 1998; 97:1411–1420.
128. Tsevat J, Duke D, Goldman L, et al. Cost-effectiveness of captopril therapy after myocardial infarction. *J Am Coll Cardiol* 1995; 26:914–919.
129. McMurray JJ, McGuire A, Davie AP, et al. Cost-effectiveness of different ACE inhibitor treatment scenarios post-myocardial infarction. *Eur Heart J* 1997; 18:1411–1415.
130. Ades PA. Pashkow FJ. Nestor JR. Cost-effectiveness of cardiac rehabilitation after myocardial infarction. *J Cardpulm Rehabil* 1997; 17:222–231.
131. Weintraub WS, Ghazzal ZMB, Douglas JS Jr, et al. Trends in outcome and costs of coronary intervention in the 1990s. *Circulation* 1997; 96:I-456.
132. Cowper PA, DeLong ER, Peterson ED, et al. Geographic variation in resource use for coronary artery bypass surgery. IHD Port Investigators. *Med Care* 1997; 35:320–333.
133. Peterson ED, Cowper PA, Zidar JP, et al. In-hospital costs of coronary stenting (with or without Coumadin) compared to angioplasty. *Circulation* 1996; 94:1891A.
134. Cohen DJ, Krumholz HM, Sukin CA, et al. In-hospital and one-year economic outcomes after coronary stenting or balloon angioplasty: Results from a randomized clinical trial. *Circulation* 1995; 92:2480–2487.
135. Mark DB, Talley JD, Topol EJ, et al. Economic assessment of platelet glycoprotein IIb/IIIa inhibition for prevention of ischemic complications of high-risk coronary angioplasty: EPIC Investigators. *Circulation* 1996; 94:629–635.
136. Weintraub WS, Culler S, Boccuzzi SJ, et al. Economic impact of GPIIB/IIIA blockade after high-risk angioplasty: Results from the RESTORE trial. *J Am Coll Cardiol* 1999; 34:1061–1066.
137. Weintraub WS, Boccuzzi SJ, Shen Y, et al. Targeting patients for thrombus inhibition after angioplasty: Clinical and economic implications. *J Am Coll Cardiol* 1997; 29:500A.
138. Weintraub WS. Evaluating the cost of therapy for restenosis: Considerations for brachytherapy. *Int J Radiat Oncol Biol Phys* 1996; 36:949–958.
139. Wong JB, Sonnenberg FA, Salem DN, et al. Myocardial revascularization for chronic stable angina: Analysis of the role of percutaneous transluminal coronary angioplasty based on data available in 1989. *Ann Intern Med* 1990; 113:852–871.
140. Detre KM, Guo P, Holubkov R, et al. Coronary revascularization in diabetic patients: A comparison of the randomized and observational components of the bypass angioplasty revascularization investigation (BARI). *Circulation* 1999; 99:633–640.
141. Rodriguez A, Palacios IF, Navia J, et al. Argentine Randomized Study: Coronary angioplasty with stenting versus coronary artery bypass surgery in patients with multiple vessel disease (ERACI II): 30-day and long-term follow-up results. *Circulation* 1999; 100:I-234.
142. Parisi AF, Folland ED, Hartigan P, on behalf of the Veterans Affairs ACME Investigators. Comparison of angioplasty with medical therapy in the treatment of single-vessel coronary artery disease. *N Engl J Med* 1992; 326:10–16.
143. Pitt B, Waters D, Brown WV, et al. Aggressive lipid-lowering therapy compared with angioplasty in stable coronary artery disease. *N Engl J Med* 1999; 341:70–76.
144. Chamberlain DH, Fox KAA, Henderson RA, et al. Coronary angioplasty versus medical therapy for angina: The second randomised intervention treatment of angina (RITA-2) trial. *Lancet* 1997; 350:461–468.
145. Kinlay S, Leitch JW, Neil A, et al. Cardiac event recorders yield more diagnoses and are more cost-effective than 48-hour Holter monitoring in patients with palpitations: A controlled clinical trial. *Ann Intern Med* 1996; 124(1 pt 1):16–20.
146. Kupersmith J, Hogan A, Guerrero P, et al. Evaluating and improving the cost-effectiveness of the implantable cardioverter-defibrillator. *Am Heart J* 1995; 130(3 pt 1):507–515.
147. Levine JH, Mellits ED, Baumgardner RA, et al. Predictors of first discharge and subsequent survival in patients with automatic implantable cardioverter defibrillators. *Circulation* 1991; 84: 558–566.
148. Owens DK, Sanders GD, Harris RA, et al. Cost-effectiveness of implantable cardioverter defibrillators relative to amiodarone for prevention of sudden cardiac death. *Ann Intern Med* 1997; 126: 1–12.
149. Larsen GC, Manolis AS, Sonnenberg FA, et al. Cost-effectiveness of the implantable cardioverter-defibrillator: Effect of improved battery life and comparison with amiodarone therapy. *J Am Coll Cardiol* 1992; 19:1323–1334.
150. Kuppermann M, Luce BR, McGovern B, et al. An analysis of the cost effectiveness of the implantable defibrillator. *Circulation* 1990; 81:91–100.
151. Wever EF, Hauer RN, Schrijvers G, et al. Cost-effectiveness of implantable defibrillator as first-choice therapy versus electrophysiologically guided, tiered strategy in postinfarct sudden death survivors. *Circulation* 1996; 93:489–496.
152. Mushlin AI, Hall WJ, Zwanziger J, et al. The cost-effectiveness of automatic implantable cardiac defibrillators: Results from MADIT. Multicenter Automatic Defibrillator Implantation Trial. *Circulation* 1998; 97:2129–2135.
153. Mitchell JB, Surge RT, Lee AJ, et al. *Per Case Prospective Payment for Episodes of Hospital Care* (final report prepared for the Health Care Financing Administration under contract no 500-92-0020). Waltham, MA: Health Economics Research; 1995.
154. Kalbfleisch SJ, Calkins H, Langberg JJ, et al. Comparison of the cost of radiofrequency catheter modification of the atrioventricular node and medical therapy for drug-refractory atrioventricular node reentrant tachycardia. *J Am Coll Cardiol* 1992; 19:1583–1587.
155. Kertes PJ, Kalman JM, Tonkin AM. Cost effectiveness of radiofrequency catheter ablation in the treatment of symptomatic supraventricular tachyarrhythmias. *Aust NZ J Med* 1993; 23: 433–436.
156. Weerasooriya HR, Murdock CJ, Harris AH, et al. The cost-effectiveness of treatment of supraventricular arrhythmias related to an accessory atrioventricular pathway: Comparison of catheter ablation, surgical division and medical treatment. *Aust NZ J Med* 1994; 24:161–167.
157. Hogenhuis W, Stevens SK, Wang P, et al. Cost-effectiveness of

radiofrequency ablation compared with other strategies in Wolff-Parkinson-White syndrome. *Circulation* 1993; 88(suppl II):II-437–II-446.
158. Stamato NJ, O'Toole MF, Enger EL. Permanent pacemaker implantation in the cardiac catheterization laboratory versus the operating room: An analysis of hospital charges and complications. *Pacing Clin Electrophysiol* 1992; 15:2236–2239.
159. Sutton R, Bourgeois I. Cost benefit analysis of single and dual chamber pacing for sick sinus syndrome and atrioventricular block: An economic sensitivity analysis of the literature. *Eur Heart J* 1996; 17:574–582.
160. Falk RH. Impact of prospective peer review on pacemaker implantation rates in Massachusetts. *J Am Coll Cardiol* 1990; 15:1087–1092.
161. Parsonnet V. Role of peer review of pacemaker implantations. *J Am Coll Cardiol* 1990; 15:1093–1094.
162. Dreifus LS, Fisch C, Griffin JC, et al. Guidelines for implantation of cardiac pacemakers and antiarrhythmia devices. *Circulation* 1991; 84:455–467.
163. Ray SG, Griffith MJ, Jamieson S, et al. Impact of the recommendations of the British Pacing and Electrophysiology Group on pacemaker prescription and on the immediate costs of pacing in the Northern Region. *Br Heart J* 1992; 68:531–534.
164. Gage BF, Cardinalli AB, Albers GW, et al. Cost-effectiveness of warfarin and aspirin for prophylaxis of stroke in patients with nonvalvular atrial fibrillation. *JAMA* 1995; 274:1839–1845.
165. Barnett HJM, Eliasziw M, Meldrum HE. Drugs and surgery in the prevention of ischemic stroke. *N Engl J Med* 1995; 332:238–248.
166. Laupacis A, Boysen G, Connolly S, et al. Risk factors for stroke and efficacy of antithrombotic therapy in atrial fibrillation: Analysis of pooled data from five randomized controlled trials. *Arch Intern Med* 1994; 154:1449–1457.
167. Gustafsson C, Asplund K, Britton M, et al. Cost-effectiveness of primary stroke prevention in atrial fibrillation: Swedish national perspective. *Br Med J* 1992; 305:1457–1460.
168. Lightowlers S, McGuire A. Cost-effectiveness of anticoagulation in nonrheumatic atrial fibrillation in the primary prevention of ischemic stroke. *Stroke* 1998; 29:1827–1832.
169. Eckman MH, Falk RH, Pauker SG. Cost-effectiveness of therapies for patients with nonvalvular atrial fibrillation. *Arch Intern Med* 1998; 158:1669–1677.
170. Catherwood E, Fitzpatrick WD, Greenberg ML, et al. Cost-effectiveness of cardioversion and antiarrhythmic therapy in nonvalvular atrial fibrillation. *Ann Intern Med* 1999; 130:625–636.
171. Seto TB, Taira DA, Tsevat J, et al. Cost-effectiveness of transesophageal echocardiographic-guided cardioversion: A decision analytic model for patients admitted to the hospital with atrial fibrillation. *J Am Coll Cardiol* 1997; 29:122–130.
172. Ward RE, Gheorghiade M, Young JB, et al. Economic outcomes of withdrawal of digoxin therapy in adult patients with stable congestive heart failure. *J Am Coll Cardiol* 1995; 26:93–101.
173. Uretsky BF, Young JB, Shahidi FE, et al. Randomized study assessing the effect of digoxin withdrawal in patients with mild to moderate chronic congestive heart failure: Results of the PROVED trial. *J Am Coll Cardiol* 1993; 22:955–962.
174. Packer M, Gheorghiade M, Young JB, et al. Withdrawal of digoxin from patients with chronic heart failure treated with angiotensin-converting-enzyme inhibitors. *N Engl J Med* 1993; 329:1–7.
175. Garg R, Gorlin R, Smith T, et al. The effect of digoxin on mortality and morbidity in patients with heart failure. *N Engl J Med* 1997; 336:525–533.
176. Mark, DB. Medical economics in cardiovascular medicine. In: Topol EJ, ed. *Cardiovascular Medicine*. Philadelphia: Lippincott-Williams & Wilkins; 1997:1193.
177. Garg R, Yusuf S, for the Collaborative Group on ACE Inhibitor Trials. Overview of randomized trials of angiotensin-converting-enzyme inhibitors on mortality and morbidity in patients with heart failure. *JAMA* 1995; 273:1450–1456.
178. The SOLVD Investigators. Effect of enalapril on survival in patients with reduced left ventricular ejection fractions and congestive heart failure. *N Engl J Med* 1991; 325:293–302.
179. Glick H, Cook J, Kinosian B, et al. Costs and effects of enalapril therapy in patients with symptomatic heart failure: An economic analysis of the Studies of Left Ventricular Dysfunction (SOLVD) treatment trial. *J Cardiac Failure* 1995; 1:371–379.
180. Boyko WL Jr, Glick HA, Schulman KA. Economics and cost-effectiveness in evaluating the value of cardiovascular therapies. ACE inhibitors in the management of congestive heart failure: Comparative economic data. *Am Heart J* 1999; 137:S115–S119.
181. Paul SD, Kuntz KM, Eagle KA, et al. Costs and effectiveness of angiotensin converting enzyme inhibition in patients with congestive heart failure. *Arch Intern Med* 1994; 154:1143–1149.
182. Kleber FX. Socioeconomic aspects of ACE inhibition in the secondary prevention in cardiovascular disease. *Am J Hypertens* 1994; 7:112S–116S.
183. Van Hout BA, Wielink G, Bonsel GJ, et al. Effects of ACE inhibitors on heart failure in the Netherlands: A pharmacoeconomic model. *Pharmacoeconomics* 1993; 3:387–397.
184. Hart W, Rhodes G, McMurray J. The cost effectiveness of enalapril in the treatment of chronic heart failure. *Br J Med Econ* 1993; 6:91–98.
185. Packer M, Bristol MR, Cohn JN, et al. The effect of carvedilol on morbidity and mortality in patients with chronic heart failure. *N Engl J Med* 1996; 334:1349–1355.
186. Delea TE, Vera-Llonch M, Richner RE, et al. Cost effectiveness of carvedilol for heart failure. *Am J Cardiol* 1999; 83:890–896.
187. Rich MW, Beckham V, Wittenberg C, et al. A multidisciplinary intervention to prevent the readmission of elderly patients with congestive heart failure. *N Engl J Med* 1995; 333:1190.
188. Weinberger M, Oddone EZ, Henderson WG. Does increased access to primary care reduce hospital readmissions? Veterans Affairs Cooperative Study Group on Primary Care and Hospital Readmission. *N Engl J Med* 1996; 334:1441–1447.
189. West JA, Miller NH, Parker KM, et al. A comprehensive management system for heart failure improves clinical outcomes and reduces medical resource utilization. *Am J Cardiol* 1997; 79: 58–63.
190. Kornowski R, Zeeli D, Averbuch M, et al. Intensive home-care surveillance prevents hospitalization and improves morbidity rates among elderly patients with severe congestive heart failure. *Am Heart J* 1995; 129:762–766.
191. Rich MW. Heart failure disease management: A critical review. *J Cardiac Failure* 1999; 5:64–75.
192. Philbin EF. Comprehensive multidisciplinary programs for the management of patients with congestive heart failure. *J Gen Intern Med* 1999; 14:130–135.
193. Evans RW. Cost-effectiveness analysis of transplantation. *Surg Clin North Am* 1986; 66:603–616.
194. Garber AM, Solomon NA. Cost-effectiveness of alternative test strategies for the diagnosis of coronary artery disease. *Ann Intern Med* 1999; 130:719–728.
195. Kim C, Kwok YS, Saha S, et al. Diagnosis of suspected coronary artery disease in women: A cost-effectiveness analysis. *Am Heart J* 1999; 137:1019–1027.
196. Kuntz KM, Fleischmann KE, Hunink MG, et al. Cost-effectiveness of diagnostic strategies for patients with chest pain. *Ann Intern Med* 1999; 130:709–718.
197. Dittus RS, Roberts SD, Adolph RJ. Cost-effectiveness analysis of patient management alternatives after uncomplicated myocardial infarction: A model. *JAMA* 1987; 10:869–878.
198. Kuntz KM, Tsevat J, Goldman L, et al. Cost-effectiveness of routine coronary angiography after acute myocardial infarction. *Circulation* 1996; 94:957–965.

CHAPTER 95

INSURANCE ISSUES IN PATIENTS WITH HEART DISEASE

Michael B. Clark / William T. Friedewald

INSURANCE MEDICINE AND CARDIOLOGY

The purpose of insurance is to provide for financial relief in the event of significant economic loss. Insurance usually takes the form of a contract—a legal agreement between insurer and insured—specifying those losses that are to be covered and the insurance benefit agreed upon. Under specific conditions, including definable losses that occur by chance within large populations at risk, the laws of probability can be applied, using actuarial methods to predict the total amount of loss for a group of individuals over some defined period of time.[1] For life and health insurance, an evaluation process described as *insurance underwriting* serves to identify the potential risk of loss for each individual. When a premium proportional to that risk is assessed, the result is an insurance system that allows for economic risk to be spread over large groups of people, with contributions from each insured proportional to the risk assumed by the insurer for that individual.

These concepts of insurance and insurance underwriting are not new; insurance for commercial ventures existed in some form by the Middle Ages, and life insurance had appeared by the seventeenth century. Private medical insurance, usually for catastrophic illnesses, was available in the 1800s.[2] Within the past 100 years, there has been an explosion in the amount of life and health insurance available and in the diversity of insurance products. This includes group employee-sponsored health and life insurance, insurance options offered by health maintenance and managed care organizations, and government-sponsored health insurance plans for indigent, disabled, and elderly populations. Within the medical community, the impact of this changing insurance climate has been enormous.[3,4] Nevertheless, as medical care providers and as consultants, cardiologists continue to play an important role in insurance underwriting evaluation.

MEDICAL UNDERWRITING FOR LIFE INSURANCE

Medical Risk Assessment

As a first step in the risk assessment process for an insurance applicant with a cardiac impairment, the patient's physician submits medical information to the insurance company in the form of the Attending Physician Statement (APS). This may include an outline of recent medical history and will often contain office and hospital records for review. Clinical problems identified in the APS are analyzed for severity of disease, extent of clinical evaluation, and thoroughness of clinical follow-up to provide data for risk assessment.

After the development of any additional information provided by authorized query to one of the national insurance company data-base exchanges, the next step in the medical underwriting evaluation involves, in most cases, the insurance medical examination. Comprehensive history taking and physical examination are routine in these examinations. Noninvasive cardiac testing may also be required by the insurance company, particularly if large amounts of insurance are requested or if additional information is required to permit a proper assessment of cardiac risk. A cardiology consultant may serve as a member of the medical underwriting team itself at this stage, reviewing all of the cardiac information obtained as part of the evaluation, including electrocardiograms and stress test tracings.

To complete the risk assessment process, each medical condition identified during the medical underwriting evaluation must be correlated with long-term survival data relevant to that disease process. From these data, a mortality ratio is derived (observed deaths in a population of individuals affected by the condition divided by the expected deaths for a comparable standard population).[5,6] This quantitative prognostic index serves as a standard, which is useful for comparing mortality projections among the various medical conditions. In general, the higher the mortality ratio calculated for a particular impairment, the greater the mortality and, thus, the greater the relative risk assumed by the company to provide insurance for individuals affected by that impairment. The mortality ratios calculated for various medical conditions are integrated into a table of risk classes or "ratings"; applicants within a rating class are grouped together to be assessed similar insurance premiums. The relationship of risk class to premium is complex and often varies by company and by insurance product, but the final result is coverage for financial loss, with the contribution to the total insurance pool proportional to the medical risk assumed by the insurance company. This equitable arrangement has the additional benefit of making insurance coverage possible for many people with cardiac disease who would otherwise be uninsurable.[7,8]

Published data relevant to mortality assessment derive from several sources. Excellent long-term follow-up data are available for insured populations based on medical conditions, demographic characteristics, and personal habits identified at the time of original insurance application (Table 95-1). Results are usually expressed as mortality ratios to address directly the prognostic, as opposed to diagnostic, significance of examination and laboratory abnormalities, such as "heart murmur on exam" or "low serum albumin." This information, while particularly relevant to insurance underwriting, may not be directly comparable to standard mortality data derived from the general population, as the insured population data more precisely relate to large groups of *selected* individuals (those people willing and able to purchase life insurance). A further limitation of such data is that they typically involve follow-up intervals as long as 20 to 30 years. Significant medical advances, as well as changes in demographics or personal lifestyles that occur during the period of study, may significantly limit the applicability of the information developed.

Long-term clinical and epidemiologic studies published in the medical literature are also useful for mortality assessment and are generally readily available for most medical impairments. In such studies, the survival data as reported can be extrapolated to provide actuarial information useful to the calculation of mortality risk. A common shortcoming in such clinical studies, however, is the single reporting of the observed mortality for the population recruited into the study without sufficient information to allow one to extrapolate the findings to the larger population from which they were selected.[9] This actuarial problem for many of the studies reported in the clinical literature was recently identified in a review[10] of a reported study of survivors of asymptomatic myocardial infarction.[11] "Good long-term prognosis" was the conclusion of the clinical investigation, which followed 48 patients with a mean age of 36 years for approximately 6 years; the observed mortality in this population was 10 percent for the entire period. However, reference to the U.S. Standard Life Tables (1979–1981) reveals a much lower expected mortality (approximately 1.46 percent) at this age for the same length of follow-up. The estimated mortality ratio of 685 percent (10 percent/1.46 percent × 100) represents a high substandard risk level for life insurance purposes, even though it may represent good clinical results in young patients with severe cardiac disease.

TABLE 95-1 Mortality Ratios in Cardiac Impairments: Selected Data

Medical Finding or Condition	Age Interval, Years	Number of Patients	Mortality Ratio, Percent
ECG findings in males	40–64	21,415	
Axis deviation (symptomatic)			225
Axis deviation (asymptomatic)			139
ST depression (symptomatic)			420
ST depression (asymptomatic)			220
Heart murmurs	50–59	21,295	
Apical systolic (not transmitted to neck; presumed functional)			114
Apical systolic (transmitted)			178
Basal systolic			276
Acute myocardial infarction	30–59	1,608	145
Coronary bypass reoperation	50–59	1,608	145

SOURCE: Adapted from Refs. 14, 33, 36, and 37.

CORONARY HEART DISEASE: ANGINA PECTORIS AND MYOCARDIAL INFARCTION

One long-term follow-up study in the insured population[12] has shown initial and short-term mortality following the diagnosis of coronary disease to be relatively high (estimated at up to 1150 percent of standard mortality depending on the presenting manifestations of disease) and quite variable for clinical subpopulations. This initial period of unstable risk is followed by a plateau phase during which the mortality rate (found to be close to 390 percent of standard) is relatively stable and thus more predictable. Other studies in insured individuals have confirmed this pattern,[13,14] which has led to the common practice of postponing consideration for life insurance for periods of up to 1 year following the initial presentation of coronary heart disease (CHD). Over the next several years, the excess *short-term* mortality demonstrated for this disease is reflected in a series of short-term extra premium charges. Upon reaching the more predictable plateau phase, a permanent, somewhat substandard rating is usually applied to correspond to the more stable but still greater than expected mortality rate seen in individuals with CHD.

To facilitate appropriate risk assessment, special attention is directed to the presence of known CHD risk factors, such as high blood pressure, diabetes mellitus, hyperlipidemia, smoking history, and obesity. In addition, a strong family history of cardiovascular disease has been confirmed in studies in insured as well as in other broader-based epidemiologic populations to be an independent risk factor for coronary heart disease, with mortality ratios in insureds of 189 and 121 percent for men and women, respectively.[14]

Long-term prognosis in patients with CHD may be influenced by intercurrent clinical interventions, such as the use of thrombolytic drugs or the performance of coronary angioplasty and coronary bypass surgery.[36,37] Commonly, life insurance consideration for patients having undergone these procedures is initially postponed to allow for review of the clinical course soon after the intervention. Underwriting risk assessment after this initial period is quite similar to that for the coronary syndromes, as described above, with particular consideration given to the status of left ventricular function before and after intervention, the number and extent of coronary artery lesions seen on coronary angiography, and the results of electrocardiographic, echocardiographic, and radionuclide stress testing. In addition, the presence or absence of coronary artery risk factors, in particular smoking, will influence the level of the final medical rating. The frequency and thoroughness of follow-up care may also influence the medical underwriter in otherwise borderline cases.

Mortality risk assessment is considerably more difficult when only limited information is available. For example, the record from the patient's physician may include, in its assessment of an individual presenting with chest pain, a simple statement such as "possible angina, trial of nitroglycerin initiated" with no further cardiac testing indicated at the time of insurance review. For purposes of risk assessment, this information would commonly be rated as "definite angina" until further clinical follow-up or noninvasive cardiac testing results were made available. Exercise electrocardiograms are, in general, routinely required for applicants requesting large amounts of insurance, although some insurance companies have recently discontinued this requirement. Even for such companies, however, these tests continue to be ordered when indicated by the presence of strong risk factors for CHD or by suggestive clinical presentations documented in the attending physician's medical summary forwarded to the insurance company. An abnormal stress test will, in most cases, result in a recommendation for a less than standard insurance rating. These judgments can be revised, however, based on supplementary evidence provided by the applicant's personal physician, including the results of stress testing with cardiac imaging or the findings on coronary angiography.

HIGH BLOOD PRESSURE

Since 1925, the life insurance industry has published several major comprehensive studies demonstrating increased mortality among insured populations with high blood pressure.[15–17] All of these show a direct, nearly linear relation between systolic and diastolic blood pressure and mortality. The 1979 Blood Pressure Study[17] dealt in the main with the mortality experience between 1954 and 1972 of 4,350,000 men and women aged 15 to 60. An estimated 530,000 of these men and women had borderline or definite high blood pressure, obviously an unusually large population of people with this diagnosis. During this study's follow-up phase, the first effective (and later routinely) used treatment for high blood pressure was introduced in the United States, and thus the 1979 study, unlike previous studies, was influenced by the increasing use of antihypertensive medication. Mortality ratios for mildly or moderately hypertensive individuals were approximately 20 percent lower than for those with more severe elevations of blood pressure. In a subgroup of applicants who were taking antihypertensive medication at the time of entry and whose blood pressure was well controlled, mortality was closer to normal (mortality ratio in males under 50 years of age at the time of insurance review, 175 percent; in males over 50 years old, 95 percent). More recently, the Multiple Medical Impairment Study underscored the necessity for adequate blood pressure control. Identification of elevated blood pressure as part of the insurance risk assessment examination was found to impact negatively on the mortality experience of most of the other medical impairments studied.[18] It follows, then, that consideration of less than standard or declined insurance applications would generally apply only to patients with untreated hypertension, for noncompliance with prescribed medical regimens, or with hypertension complicated by end-organ damage (ventricular hypertrophy or cerebrovascular or renal disease). Although such developments are often identified in the clinical record, at times additional testing is performed by the insurance company and may include electrocardiography and qualitative urinary protein measurement. On rare occasions, echocardiography may be ordered to assess the degree of cardiac impairment as a result of long-standing hypertension where other clues are ambiguous or contradictory.

VALVULAR HEART DISEASE

The Medical Impairment Study of 1983 provided long-term survival data in the insured population with heart murmurs.[14] Information extracted from that study has been used to provide mortality projections in people with valvular heart disease (Table 95-1). Advances in cardiac diagnostic technology since publication of that study, particularly the development of echocardiographic and Doppler imaging systems, have allowed better definition of valvular pathology. With these and other advances in medical and surgical intervention, it has become more difficult to accumulate data concerning the natural history of unoperated cardiac valvular impairments.[19,20]

Mitral Valve Prolapse

This is, at present, the most common valve condition reported to insurance companies. Although most such patients are offered standard insurance rates, a small subset of patients with frequent chest pain, cardiac arrhythmias, and significant mitral regurgitation may be rated below standard.[21]

Congenital Valvular Heart Disease

Most companies postpone consideration of life insurance for an infant with known or suspected congenital heart disease until the child reaches 1 or 2 years of age. Even then, the history must include a definitively proven diagnosis as well as successful repair of all surgically correctable lesions before the applicant can be considered for life insurance. After successful restoration of normal cardiac hemodynamics, most applicants with congenital defects—including those with atrial and ventricular septal defects, corrected pulmonic stenosis, patent ductus, or coarctation of the aorta (once blood pressure has returned to normal)—can be considered as standard risks.[22] Uninsurable applicants would include most cases of transposition of the great vessels, Ebstein's anomaly, anomalous venous return, and Eisenmenger's syndrome.

Congenital bicuspid aortic valve remains a difficult clinical and underwriting problem.[8] Estimation of prognosis in this impairment when applicants present in the second and third decades of life is often problematic. In the absence of associated echocardiographic evidence of left ventricular enlargement, most companies are willing to assess this risk as only mildly substandard. Left ventricular dilatation or hypertrophy seen on echocardiography, or the presence by Doppler analysis of any significant degree of aortic stenosis or regurgitation, will usually require a more substantial rating assessment.

Acquired Valvular Heart Disease

To perform risk assessment in applicants known to have acquired valvular disease, the underwriter will usually first consider the clinical and electrocardiographic findings on the insurance examination. The degree of cardiac enlargement and severity of left ventricular dysfunction will also be considered and will commonly be outlined in the APS. The medical underwriter will also give consideration to the attendant risk of anticipated surgical valve repair or replacement as well as to the risk of lifelong anticoagulation following such surgery. Applicants with valvular disease who show evidence of marked cardiomegaly, especially with prior history or physical examination findings consistent with left-sided or right-sided heart failure, cannot usually be offered life insurance. Other significant complications, such as new-onset atrial fibrillation or systemic embolization, will usually result in a postponement for up to 1 year prior to reconsideration. In most other cases, life insurance can be offered, albeit at rates significantly below standard.[8,20,23] Early follow-up studies of patients undergoing surgical procedures that preserve the native cardiac valve have demonstrated an improvement in perioperative and short-term postoperative survival.[21] As more complete long-term data in patients undergoing these procedures become available, further liberalization of risk penalties may be possible.

OTHER CARDIAC DISEASES OR ABNORMAL LABORATORY FINDINGS

Cardiomyopathy

Insurance risk assessment of the applicant with cardiomyopathy is based on the initial clinical presentation of the patient and the subsequent clinical and physiologic evaluation. Life insurance cannot usually be offered to those diagnosed with dilated (congestive) cardiomyopathy or amyloid heart disease. Systemic diseases with cardiac involvement, such as scleroderma and sarcoidosis, are most often assessed on the basis of overall disease activity and response to therapy. Insurance, however, may be available to many in this latter group of patients, albeit at rates below standard.[8]

Evaluation of the asymptomatic individual with a strong family history of inheritable heart disease or in whom a heart murmur has been discovered may at times produce findings consistent with the obstructive or nonobstructive cardiomyopathies. Complete information concerning the natural history of these impairments is not yet available, particularly in the mild, asymptomatic cases.[24] In the past, many clinical reports were of severe and fatal outcomes, leading many insurance companies to decline or rate highly any applicant with an established diagnosis of hypertrophic cardiomyopathy.[8] More recent experience in defining mortality outcomes in hypertrophic cardiomyopathy has been much more favorable[25,26] and may allow for more favorable mortality risk assessment in the future.[27]

Arrhythmias

Most insurance companies will consider applicants who give a history of paroxysmal or chronic atrial arrhythmias in the context of the presence and severity of coexisting cardiac disease. One series in an insured population with paroxysmal atrial tachycardia noted mortality rates quite similar to those of the standard population; the mortality ratio for this condition was estimated to be 73 percent.[14] This can be contrasted with mortality ratios of 700 percent or greater in the presence of atrial fibrillation.[28] In the apparently asymptomatic young individual with new-onset atrial arrhythmias, particular attention is paid to social history and habits such as smoking or excessive alcohol use. In the middle-aged or older applicant, the possibility of asymptomatic coronary heart disease must also be assessed.

Ventricular arrhythmias have remained a difficult risk-assessment problem. In many cases, isolated ventricular ectopy can be rated in the context of the underlying cardiac impairment, such as coronary artery or valvular heart disease. Particular attention is directed during the review of the medical record to the results of clinical cardiac evaluation, including stress testing and noninvasive analysis of cardiac function.[29] Survivors of sudden death will, in most cases, be declined—a situation that may change as long-term data on the benefits of automatic implantable defibrillator (AID) become available. This change would probably apply to those patients in whom AID implantation has been performed as prophylaxis in the setting of high clinical risk for sudden death[30] (see also Chap. 33).

Heart Transplantation

Heart transplantation techniques and immunosuppressive strategies have continued to evolve and have been associated with significant improvement in 5- to 10-year survival (see also Chap. 22). Most insurance companies would continue to decline such patients, however, until additional long-term survival data became available.

Insurance Laboratory Evaluation Abnormalities

Life insurance underwriting protocols generally include a clinical laboratory panel with a full lipid profile and a resting electrocardiogram. Depending on the age of the applicant and the amount of life insurance requested, additional testing, including stress testing and echocardiography, may be required. In most cases, abnormalities revealed during this laboratory evaluation are fully consistent with the clinical history as reported in the APS. In a minority of applicants, however, medical history is scanty or medical records are unavailable. In such patients, medical underwriting risk assessment is then based primarily on the findings from the insurance physical and laboratory examination. Studies in insured as well as in general populations provide the necessary mortality projections for underwriting risk assessment using these parameters (Table 95-1). The Medical Impairment Study (1983), for example, confirmed the benign prognosis of incidental bradycardia found on insurance examination, with mortality ratios of 73 to 80 percent reported.[14] On the other hand, a relative mortality of 250 percent was found for the finding of tachycardia.[14] Additional information is available to perform risk assessment for findings such as overweight and underweight,[12,31] low serum albumin,[32] and an abnormal electrocardiogram.[33,34]

HEALTH AND DISABILITY INSURANCE

Health insurance continues to evolve in terms of overall cost, quality, and availability within the current environment of health care reform. Further, the delivery of health care under managed care plans by both governmental and employer insurance plans has begun to redefine many aspects of the traditional patient–doctor, doctor–doctor, and doctor–insurer relationships.[3,4]

Within this environment, cardiologists remain vitally important, functioning both as clinical consultants to primary care providers as well as professional consultants to managed care organizations and indemnity insurance plans. This latter role deserves special emphasis. Cardiologists will often be called upon to provide the expertise essential to the determination of the medical necessity and appropriateness of care for health insurance case management and claim review. Assessment of new technology in its evolution from experimental procedure to accepted standard of care is a particularly important responsibility of the insurance consultant in the managed care environment.[35]

The role of the physician in disability determination is more complex, often requiring legal interpretation of disability based on the results of medical data available. The expertise of medical specialists—including physiatrists, physical and occupational therapists, and social workers—may be required for complete evaluation and recommendations. In general, thorough analysis coupled with appropriate goal-directed therapy often allows for return to work in a supportive environment accommodated to individual needs.

For practical purposes, the patient with known heart disease of any kind is going to have difficulty in obtaining standard individual health or disability insurance. As in patients with high blood pressure, however, effective subclassification of patients and effective new therapies may allow insurance to become available to more and more patients who were considered unacceptable insurance risks in the past.

ACKNOWLEDGMENTS

We gratefully acknowledge the work of Dr. M. Irene Ferrer and Dr. Joseph A. Wilber in previous editions of this textbook, from which we drew for this current chapter.

References

1. Morton GA. *Principles of Life and Health Insurance.* Atlanta: Life Office Management Association; 1984.
2. Brackenridge RDC, Brown AE. A historical survey of the development of life assurance. In: Brackenridge RDC, Elder WJ, eds. *Medical Selection of Life Risks,* 3rd ed. New York: Stockton Press; 1992:3–17.
3. Billi JE, Wise CG, Bills EA, Mitchell RL. Potential effects of managed care on specialty practice at a university medical center. *N Engl J Med* 1995; 333:979–983.
4. Weisbuch JB, Roberts NK. Without the denominator, where is the quality improvement paradigm in the nation's health care reform? *J Ins Med* 1995; 27:12–14.
5. Pokorski RJ. Mortality methodology and analysis seminar test. *J Ins Med* 1995; 20:20–45.
6. Seltzer F. Choosing a standard for adjusted mortality rates. *Stat Bull* 1996; 77:13–19.
7. Cumming GR, Croxson R. Cardiovascular disorders: Part I. Coronary heart disease. In: Brackenridge RDC, Elder WJ, eds. *Medical Selection of Life Risks,* 3rd ed. New York: Stockton Press; 1992:251–323.
8. Croxson RS. Cardiovascular disorders: Part II. Other cardiovascular disorders. In: Brackenridge RDC, Elder WJ, eds. *Medical Selection of Life Risks,* 3rd ed. New York: Stockton Press; 1992:324–431.
9. Singer RB. Pitfalls of inferring annual mortality from inspection of published survival curves. *J Ins Med* 1994; 26:333–338.
10. Iacovino JR. A "quick hit" method to assess insurance mortality from a clinical article. *J Ins Med* 1994; 26:317–318.
11. Negus BH. Coronary anatomy and prognosis of young, asymptomatic survivors of myocardial infarction. *Am J Med* 1994; 96:354–358.
12. Clarke RD. Mortality of impaired lives 1964–73 (abstr). *J Inst Act* 1979; 100 (part 1). In: Lew EA, Gajewski J, eds. *Medical Risks: Trends in Mortality by Age and Time Elapsed.* New York: Praeger; 1990:7–120.
13. Jarvis HJ. Development of the diabetic, coronary, and blood pressure pools (abstr). *Cooperation internationale pour les assurances des risques aggraves,* 1986. In: Lew EA, Gajewski J, eds. *Medical Risks: Trends in Mortality by Age and Time Elapsed.* New York: Praeger; 1990:7–122.
14. Medical Impairment Study 1983 (abstr) I. Boston: Society of Actuaries and Association of Life Insurance Medical Directors of America, 1986. In: Lew EA, Gajewski J, eds. *Medical Risks: Trends in Mortality by Age and Time Elapsed.* New York: Praeger; 1990:6–78.
15. *Build and Blood Pressure Study 1959.* Chicago: Society of Actuaries; 1959.
16. *Mortality Investigation of Declined Lives in Japan.* Tokyo: The Life Insurance Association of Japan; 1979.
17. *Blood Pressure Study 1979.* Boston: Society of Actuaries and Association of Life Insurance Medical Directors of America; 1980.
18. *Multiple Medical Impairment Study.* Westwood, MA: Center for Medico-Actuarial Statistics of MIB, Inc.; 1998.
19. Borer JS, Kligfield P. Aortic regurgitation: Making management decisions. *ACC Curr J Rev* 1995; 4:30–32.
20. MacKenzie BR. Long-term mortality and complications of Bjork-Shiley spherical-disc valves—A life table analysis. *J Ins Med* 1992; 24:128–132.
21. Jeresaty RM. Mitral valve prolapse: An update. In: Arnold CB, ed. *Transactions of The American Academy of Insurance Medicine: One Hundred and First Annual Meeting.* Tampa, FL: Klay Printing; 1993:24–33.
22. Singer RB, Gajewski J. Cardiovascular diseases I. In: Lew EA, Gajewski J, eds. *Medical Risks: Trends in Mortality by Age and Time Elapsed, 1.* New York: Praeger; 1990:6-30–6-38.
23. Cumming GR. Survival after valve replacement. In: Arnold CB, ed. *Transactions of The America Academy of Insurance Medicine: One Hundred and First Annual Meeting.* Tampa, FL: Klay Printing; 1993:40–55.

24. Elliott PM, Saumarez RC, McKenna WJ. Recent clinical advances in hypertrophic cardiomyopathy. *Heart Failure* 1995; 11:15–25.
25. Cannan CR, Reeder GS, Bailey KR, et al. Natural history of hypertrophic cardiomyopathy: A population-based study, 1976 through 1990. *Circulation* 1995; 92:2488–2495.
26. Ten Cate FJ. Prognosis of hypertrophic cardiomyopathy. *J Ins Med* 1996; 28:42–45.
27. Iacovino JR. The nonmortality of hypertrophic cardiomyopathy in an unselected, community diagnosed and treated population. *J Ins Med* 1996; 28:51–54.
28. Gajewski J, Singer RB. Mortality in an insured population with atrial fibrillation. *JAMA* 1981; 245:1540–1544.
29. Chait L. Electrocardiography. In: Brackenridge RDC, Elder WJ, eds. *Medical Selection of Life Risks,* 3rd ed. New York: Stockton Press; 1992:433–472.
30. Gorlin R. Cost-effectiveness of ICD therapy for ventricular arrhythmias. *Prim Cardiol* 1995; 21:32–38.
31. *Build Study 1979*. Boston: Society of Actuaries and Association of Life Insurance Medical Directors of America; 1980.
32. Segel L. Serum albumin: "Phoenix" of the blood profile. *On the Risk* 1995; 11:81–83.
33. Rose G, Baxter PJ, Reid DD, McCartney P. Prevalence and prognosis of electrocardiographic findings in middle-aged men (abstr). *Br Heart J* 1978; 40:636–643. In: Lew EA, Gajewski J, eds. *Medical Risks: Trends in Mortality by Age and Time Elapsed*. New York: Praeger; 1990.
34. Ferrer MI. A survey of 19,734 electrocardiograms obtained in insurance applicants. *J Ins Med* 1985; 16:6–13.
35. Privette M, ed. Court overrules HCFA 1986 investigational devices payment policy. *Cardiology* 1996; 25:4.
36. Singer RB. Comparative mortality by sex and age in residents of Rochester, Minnesota, with acute myocardial infarction during 1960–1979 (sudden deaths included). *J Ins Med* 1995–1996; 27:235–240.
37. Hutchinson R. Additional follow-up of patients with coronary bypass reoperation at Cleveland Clinic. *J Ins Med* 1994; 26: 324–328.

CHAPTER 96

CARDIAC EVALUATIONS FOR LEGAL PURPOSES

Elliot L. Sagall* / Ira S. Nash

INTRODUCTION

This chapter describes for the physician the scope of the legal areas where issues concerning heart disorder are key elements of the litigation. The following topics will be discussed: (a) the essential components of a medicolegal cardiac evaluation; (b) the legal and medical concepts, definitions, and criteria for determinations of diagnosis and the time of occurrence of specific cardiac lesions, causality, disability, medical malpractice, prognosis, life expectancy, and other medicolegal assessments; and (c) the formulation of a report of the physician's findings and opinions that will be meaningful and helpful to the legal forum assigned to resolve the disputed medical problems of the case in hand.

The socioeconomic ramifications of heart disease have long been a source of vexing legal as well as medical problems with no easy resolution as yet forthcoming. Nationwide, claims instituted by heart patients and/or their beneficiaries alleging heart disorder, disability, and cardiac death as a workplace or accidental injury or as due to the negligent action of a health care provider are burgeoning in number and scope. The existence of a heart disorder may also be the key issue in the legal determination of an individual's physical capacity to participate as a defendant or witness in a legal proceeding, to drive a motor vehicle, to pilot an airplane, to engage in "substantial" gainful activity, to write a legally valid will or contract, to enable an insurer to recover some of the moneys paid to a worker as compensation for a work-related injury, or to invalidate a life insurance policy. It may be the basis for suit by a disabled employee against the employer for illegal job discrimination.

The rapidly expanding interrelationships of heart disorders and the law necessarily will involve physicians who examine and treat cardiac patients more and more frequently in one or combinations of several roles, as follows: (a) as a factual witness called upon to present the history personally received and the findings of physical and other examinations performed and treatment rendered; (b) as an expert witness called by one side or the other in a legal dispute to present opinions on the issues under consideration; (c) as an impartial witness called by the presiding judicial arbiter for opinion testimony; or (d) as a defendant in a suit for medical malpractice.

The question of a cardiac patient's eligibility for certain statutory or common law benefits is basically a legal rather than a medical issue. Accordingly, the ultimate determination is assigned to a court, jury, administrative agency, commissioner, referee, or some other duly appointed person or persons referred to as a *fact finder.* The legal resolution of disputed issues of a medical nature, however, almost invariably necessitates consideration of expert medical opinion testimony. Crucial areas such as diagnosis, extent, degree, and causation of disability, the existence and time frame of "conscious" pain and suffering, the necessity and reasonableness of past and projected medical and surgical treatment, the charges rendered, the role of preexisting conditions, losses of bodily functions, scarring and disfigurement, reduction of life expectancy, prognosis, whether an "end result" has been reached, and the many other items that determine damages to be awarded to the victim of a cardiac injury or benefits available under covering workers' compensation or other legislative acts, and the causal relationship of each to the alleged injury, generally require medical substantiation or refutation.

LEGAL ACTIONS REQUIRING CARDIAC MEDICAL EVALUATIONS

The spectrum of legal actions where medical evaluations relating to cardiology become key issues is vast, varied, and limited only by the ingenuity and imagination of the claimants' attorneys.[1-3] The most common areas include the following:

1. Claims brought under various state workers' compensation statutes and similar federal legislation (e.g., the Federal Longshoremen's and Harbor Workers' Compensation Act and the Federal Employees' Compensation Act), where cardiac disorder disability, treatment, or death is alleged

* This chapter is dedicated to the memory of Dr. Elliot L. Sagall.

a consequence of a work-related heart "injury" or an "occupational disease."

2. Tort claims under common law seeking damages for alleged cardiac "injury" due to negligence on the part of another person or persons, including suits for medical malpractice.
3. Claims against insurers, including the Social Security Disability Insurance program, for pensions, covered medical expenses, losses of income, or accidental death benefits resulting from heart disease.
4. Questions as to the fitness of a person with a heart disorder to return to a specific job, to drive a motor vehicle, to operate machinery or other equipment, to pilot an airplane, to participate in a legal proceeding, to serve a prison sentence, or to prepare a will.
5. Claims instituted by insurers alleging preexistent heart disease as a basis for qualifying under "second injury funds" for reimbursement of workers' compensation benefits, the voiding of an insurance contract by reason of the applicant's fraudulent concealment of a preexisting heart disorder, or the nonpayment of special benefits provided in the insurance contract for death or injury due to an accident because of the contribution of a preexistent cardiac disorder.
6. Claims under the Americans with Disabilities Act.

Of these, the most commonly encountered are claims that a cardiac disorder is a workplace injury covered by the applicable workers' compensation statute.

Although individual state and federal workers' compensation acts differ somewhat in requirements for eligibility and benefits provided to injured workers and their dependents,[4] the fundamental social principle common to all compensation statutes is that the financial costs of work-related injuries should be assumed to a large extent by the employer as an expense of production and not by the injured worker or by public funds. Without exception, all compensation acts embrace the basic concept that the right to compensation for work-incurred injury is provided to the injured employee without regard to fault or to demonstrable negligence of the employer. Legal defenses available under common law to employers to avoid or to mitigate liability such as assumption of the risk of the job by the employee's acceptance of the employment or contributory negligence by the employee or fellow employees are specifically excluded from workers' compensation. In turn, the benefits potentially accruing to an injured employee are generally limited to a portion of the lost wages plus allowances for dependents and reasonable and necessary medical expenses. Items such as pain and suffering and loss of consortium, which may play a large role in the determination of an award to an injured person in actions for tort (negligence) under common law, are excluded. In workers' compensation, legal liability attaches to the employer (or insurance carrier) for the consequences of an injury, including heart disorder, disability, or death,[1,4–8] demonstrated to have occurred during "the course of" and to have arisen "out of" employment—a formula that has aptly been characterized as "deceptively simple and litigiously prolific."

Under some compensation statutes, the basic formula of compensable injury has been modified by specific legislative restrictive definitions that require that the alleged work injury be suffered "by accident" or be due to "unusual stress" or to "stress greater than normal nonwork life" or to have been contributed "substantially" to by the work. In most jurisdictions, an identified time and place of injury must be demonstrated for coverage to apply. And in one compensation act (Wyoming's), further restriction has been placed for legal acceptance of an alleged work-related cardiac injury in that no more than 4 h must elapse between the claimed time of injury and the first clinical manifestations of same.[9]

The imposition of these restrictions indicates a legislative attempt to distinguish alleged work-related heart injuries from those that occur as a result of the natural progression of the underlying disease—an effort not often successful. Along these lines, one state (Nevada) even went so far as to exclude "coronary thrombosis, coronary occlusion, or any other ailment or disorder of the heart, and any death or disability ensuing therefrom" as an injury by accident arising out of and in the course of employment, except under certain circumstances for firefighters, police officers, prison guards, and several other favored categories of public employees.[10]

In many states the concept of "accidental disability"* for purposes of workers' compensation or retirement has been extended for certain named occupational groups, particularly uniformed police and firefighters, by legislative inclusion in the covering statutes of a presumption of job causation for disabling heart disease or hypertension. Although theoretically rebuttable, such presumptions, from a practical viewpoint, generally cannot be overcome, particularly if the worker has no clear risk factors for heart disease. The result is that applicants under these laws (commonly referred to as "Heart Laws") often need only establish the existence of a disabling heart disorder or hypertension and not the causal connection to the employment, although in some jurisdictions, (e.g., Massachusetts) the existence of significant nonemployment risk factors such as tobacco abuse may overcome the presumption of job-related causation. The Massachusetts statute 11 is a typical example:

> Notwithstanding the provisions of any general or special law to the contrary . . . any condition of impairment of health caused by hypertension and heart disease resulting in total or partial disability or death to a uniformed member of a paid fire department or permanent member of a police department . . . shall, if he successfully passed a physical examination on entry into such service which examination failed to reveal any evidence of such condition, be presumed to have been suffered in line of duty, unless the contrary be shown by competent evidence.[11]

The first step in the process of determining eligibility of an applicant for the benefits provided under this statute usually is an examination by a medical panel appointed for the purpose of determining the existence of heart disease or hypertension, the resulting job disability, and job causation. The medical

* Accidental disability retirement applies to a permanent work incapacity as a result of a work-related injury or a hazard experienced in the performance of job duties. Ordinary disability retirement applies to permanent work incapacity due to sickness or injury that is not job-related. Since the financial benefits of an accidental disability retirement generally are significantly greater than those of an ordinary disability retirement in that the awards usually are free from federal and state income tax, applicants for disability understandably seek the greater "take-home" pay of an "accidental disability."

panel's findings, however, are only advisory and are not binding on the designated retirement board. Since the etiology of most forms of heart disease and hypertension is not currently known, the medical panel, most often, cannot provide "competent evidence" to offset the legislative presumption of job causation embodied in the covering statute. An accidental disability can then be awarded if the medical panel has found the existence of a disabling cardiac or hypertensive condition. The applicant's task under many of these statutes is further eased by the definition of *job disability* as an incapability of the applicant to perform the full range or "all" of the duties, including response to emergency situations inherent in the course of police or firefighting activities. The legal dependents of retirees under the Heart Law do not automatically receive death benefits. They usually have the burden of establishing by medical evidence that the death was causally related to the condition for which retirement was awarded. Thus, a statement on a death certificate that the immediate cause of death was "cardiac arrest" is not sufficient to establish legal causation, since cardiac arrest is frequently only a terminal event, not necessarily related to a condition of preexistent heart disease or hypertension. However, medical opinion that the death was hastened to some degree (even by as short a period as seconds to minutes) by reason of reduced cardiac reserve related to the underlying heart disorder may be sufficient to satisfy the legal issue of causality.

Particularly important in adjudication of claims for cardiac injury, disability, or death under workers' compensation and in actions in tort for injury due to negligence is the universal legal acceptance of the common law precept that prior infirmity is no bar to benefits even though the injured person would not have suffered injury, as is the case in most cardiac claims, had there not been underlying heart disease. Legally, the injured person may be entitled to benefits if it can be shown that the employment or an act of negligence in some way aggravated a preexisting condition to lead to injury, disability, or death sooner than would otherwise have been expected during the natural history of the underlying disorder. Under many state compensation acts, the burden of proving job causation generally assigned to the claimant is eliminated when the worker is found deceased or otherwise medically unable to testify at the place of employment. By the statutory adoption of presumption of work relationship in such situations, the burden of disproving causation is placed upon the employer. Under the Federal Longshoremen's and Harbor Workers' Compensation Act, a set of presumptions effectively requires that the employer establish noncausation to the job for almost all medical conditions that may render an employee permanently or partially disabled from work.[12]

Under actions in tort in common law, recovery of "damages" may be obtained when the plaintiff or those claiming through the plaintiff can show that the disorder and its consequences arose from or were aggravated by the negligent activity of another (commonly referred to as a *tortfeasor*). Unlike the doctrine of workers' compensation, liability in actions of tort is predicated on fault. To be awarded "damages," the injured party must show (1) that the defendant owed the plaintiff a duty, i.e., the duty to adhere to an accepted standard of medical care and the duty to refrain from negligence; (2) that the defendant's conduct breached that duty; (3) that the plaintiff suffered injuries or "harms"; (4) that the defendant's negligent conduct was the proximate cause of the damage (harms) allegedly suffered by the plaintiff; and (5) that the victim's own negligence did not contribute to his or her harms (the *doctrine of contributory negligence*). Again, susceptibility to injury by reason of preexisting infirmity does not bar recovery.

Actions in tort alleging cardiac injury most commonly arise from motor vehicle accidents where it is claimed that a myocardial contusion, an acute coronary artery occlusion, an acute myocardial infarction, a cardiac death, or some other acute cardiac episode resulted from, or was hastened by, physical trauma or the psychological consequences of the accident. Most difficult in both medical determinations and legal handling are those situations where it is alleged that a preexisting condition of stable angina pectoris has been aggravated, as evidenced by a change in a preexisting symptom complex, but with no objective evidence to support the claimed aggravation. Another commonly encountered vexing medicolegal problem is whether a fatal cardiac episode was "the result of" or "the cause of" an accident—a determination also of importance when insurance contracts provide double indemnity or other specified benefits for "accidental" death or injury. Other frequently encountered actions in tort involving cardiac patients are those in which it is alleged that heart problems have stemmed from trauma or stress subsequent to negligent conduct, such as from falling objects, slipping, and other accidentally induced falls; from exposure to food poisonings; from toxic fumes; from menacing animals; and from long-term psychological "stress." In addition, the Americans with Disabilities Act, initially phased in on July 26, 1992, promises new areas of litigation by prohibiting employment discrimination against an employee "who meets the skill, experience, education and other job-related requirements of a position held or desired, and who, with or without reasonable accommodation, can perform the essential functions of a job."[13]

Medical malpractice suits fall within the province of actions in tort and are subject to the same legal considerations affecting all claims for "damages" due to "negligence." In malpractice cases, as with other actions in tort, the aggrieved patient or those acting for the plaintiff have the burden of demonstrating (1) that the defendant breached a standard of care owed, and (2) that this breach caused the plaintiff "harm." In evidentiary proof, the plaintiff must define by expert medical opinion the standard of care alleged to have been breached. The plaintiff must further establish the existence of alleged "harms" or "damage" and also must then show, again by expert medical opinion, that the alleged deviation from the acceptable standard of care was the cause of the claimed "damages." Finally, in many jurisdictions it must further be demonstrated that the plaintiff's conduct did not negligently contribute to the claimed harms. Unless all these criteria are satisfied, a directed verdict for the defendant may be ordered by the judge.

In some legal actions, the known existence of a prior cardiac disorder is of importance in the assessment of financial awards. Under the Second Injury Funds of the Federal Longshoremen's and Harbor Workers' Compensation Act and of many state workers' compensation acts, some financial relief is afforded the employer or insurer for disability payments to an injured worker if it can be demonstrated that the work incapacity following an accepted or assigned work injury was made substantially greater than would otherwise have been the case because of a known preexistent medical condition or that death would not have occurred without the preexisting physical impairment.

In other instances, the demonstration of a heart disorder may be of key importance in a legal decision as to whether a worker can return to a prior job that an employer claims involves physical or psychological stress potentially harmful to a person with known heart disease or where the operation of machinery by a person subject to sudden incapacity, as from an acute cardiac dysrhythmia, would endanger others; whether a person should be rejected from driving a motor vehicle, particularly one used in public transportation, or from piloting an airplane; whether a heart patient can participate in a court trial as a defendant or witness or serve a prison term, write a valid will, or be forced to pay alimony or other financial assessment; whether certain items claimed as income-tax–deductible medical expenses are medically justified as treatment; whether an insurance contract can be voided because of the applicant's fraudulent concealment of a known cardiac disorder in the original application for the policy; and in other situations where the question of preexistent heart disorder may be of importance for legal and insurance determinations of eligibility for "accidental death" benefits.

A large area of litigation involving heart disorder concerns the many applicants for disability benefits under the Social Security Disability Insurance Program, public welfare programs, the Veterans Administration service- and non-service-related pensions, and privately purchased disability, accident, and health insurance contracts. In most of these situations, the legal issue to be decided is the work capacity of the individual, as defined in the covering statute or insurance contract, based on a demonstrated medical condition, not the question of causation. Miscellaneous legal actions that may require expert medical opinions on heart disorders and their consequences include determination of the existence and extent of "conscious pain and suffering" as an element of tort "damages," losses of bodily functions under certain workers' compensation statutes, reduction of life and/or work-year expectancy due to a cardiac disorder or worsening thereof, projected reasonable medical expenses of future treatment in a cardiac patient, relation of coronary artery bypass grafting or other treatments to a compensable myocardial infarction, prognosis, projected life span, and other medicolegal issues.

THE CARDIOLOGIST IN THE COURTROOM

It is in the role of an expert witness that cardiologists most often find themselves involved with the legal profession. Any duly licensed physician, however, whether a general practitioner or a specialist, is considered legally qualified to present opinion testimony when the medical issues in hand are not a matter of common knowledge. The appropriateness of a particular physician's competency to testify as an expert, however, can be raised by either side of the dispute and put before the court for its evaluation on the basis of the physician's training, experience, and demonstrated bias. Once a physician has been accepted as an expert witness, the weight to be attached to the medical conclusions presented is determined by a legally appointed fact-finding body. Since the current state of scientific knowledge in cardiology often does not provide clear-cut answers to many of the courtroom medical questions, there is often a difference between the conclusions reached by the expert witnesses called by the two sides in a case. In such instances, the legal fact finder can adopt the opinion believed most likely to conform to the facts and reach a decision on that basis. In some legal actions the fact finder may elect to call on an outside court-appointed physician for an "impartial" opinion. Thus, almost every legal decision in medical matters has to be supported by the testimony of a physician "expert witness." It is imperative, therefore, that legal decisions should be in accord with the main current of medical thinking and the testimony of the "experts" should be within the boundaries of presently acceptable scientific beliefs and concepts.

The physician who testifies as an expert witness need not have personally examined the claimant or even have any personal knowledge of the claimant's medical condition prior to or following an alleged incident. The medical expert may reach conclusions solely from a review of the medical records and other factual data that have been admitted into evidence. Alternatively, the expert may be presented by either counsel with a hypothetical question that contains a set of facts to be utilized for the conclusions reached and the opinions expressed. The law, however, does require that those facts put forth in hypothetical questions be supported by the evidence presented in the case. Thus, the fact finder cannot adopt the opinion expressed by an expert in answer to a hypothetical question unless the evidence on hand is sufficient to establish the truth of the supposition. When the factual evidence is conflicting, as is frequently the case, it is within the province of the fact finder to determine which evidence is to be believed and adopted as "factual."

The hypothetical question posed to a medical expert in courtroom proceedings need not include all the evidence previously presented in the case. It may be limited to a partisan recital of that evidence most favorable to the proponent's side. The adversary party, in cross-examination of the expert, however, can propose a counterhypothetical recital of alleged facts to provide data omitted or now added to the original question. The medical expert can then be asked whether the newly assumed facts alter the opinions previously expressed. In this manner, both parties in the legal dispute have full opportunity to pose to medical experts respective versions of what they believe is factual. Again, however, the ultimate determination of medical issues for legal purposes rests with the duly appointed fact finder, not with the medical experts.

Generally, it is not sufficient for an expert witness to present conclusions alone without supporting reasoning. The basis on which the opinion rendered rests also may be subject to attack in cross-examination so that the testimony presented can be weighed by the fact finder. In formulating an opinion, the medical expert must appreciate the degree of certainty required in reaching medical conclusions in a legal forum. The legal system recognizes the current inability of medical science to answer definitively and with absolute certainty many of the medical questions raised in individual cases. Yet the legal body responsible for final legal resolution must answer as best it can all the issues raised at the time of trial. Legal proof cannot be equated with scientific proof. In civil cases, decisions are based primarily upon standards such as a preponderance of the evidence and clear and convincing evidence. In criminal matters, the requirements are more stringent, usually beyond a reasonable doubt. The law generally requires that answers to medical questions be expressed in terms of reasonable medical certainty or probability rather than mere possibility. In essence, this means that the conclusions reached by an expert are believed to be more likely than not true even though the level of certainty would not be acceptable to a body of scientists. In accord with this legal philosophy, reasonable medical certainty generally means reasonable legal certainty—a far less exacting criterion of proof than that required for medical scientific certainty.

In cases involving cardiac claims, as in most civil cases, the burden of proof generally is placed on the claimant, who must show by a preponderance of supporting evidence, including expert opinion when necessary, that the allegations are true. For example, in a claim alleging a cardiac disorder and its consequences as a workplace injury, the claimant must provide the fact finder with sufficient supporting medical expert testimony attesting not only to the existence of a cardiac disorder but also to its causal relationship to some element of the employment. A claimant's burden of proof generally is not met when a medical expert merely acknowledges the possibility of the truth of the allegations rather than asserting their probability. Phraseology frequently employed by physicians in medical reports and testimony such as *may, could,* or *might have* serves no useful purpose in the courtroom. Additionally, the burden of proof is not met, nor is it sustained, when the medical supportive conclusions are shown to be based on speculation, rather than on reasonable medical certainty, or when the medical expert admits that acceptance and denial of the allegations are equal possibilities that cannot be differentiated.

As pointed out earlier in this chapter, under many workers' compensation acts, when a worker is found dead or unable to testify at the place of employment, the burden of disproving causation by the job is placed on the employer. The Federal Longshoremen's and Harbor Workers' Compensation Act even goes a step further by stating, "In any proceeding for the enforcement of a claim for compensation under this Act it shall be presumed, in the absence of substantial evidence to the contrary. . . . That the claim comes within the provisions of this Act. . . ."[12] In actions for medical malpractice the burden of proof of lack of causation by negligence may be shifted to the defendant health care provider when the doctrines of *res ipsa loquitur* ("the thing speaks for itself") and the *captain of the ship,* i.e., the operating room surgeon, become applicable. When expert medical opinions presented by the respective litigants contradict or conflict, the fact finder must choose between them. The choice is subject to reversal on appeal to a higher court only when contrary to the weight of the evidence or the result of an error in legal procedure. Since the legal fact finder often lacks an adequate scientific background, legal decisions may appear contrary to medical thinking.

THE MEDICOLEGAL CARDIAC EVALUATION

Medical examinations and evaluations performed specifically for legal and insurance reasons necessarily emphasize aspects of the medical situation not customarily addressed by physicians, since the primary purpose of such evaluations is the answering of legal questions and not the providing of medical care.

The scope of potential medicolegal questions where heart disorder is germane to the litigation is too broad to be reviewed completely here. Certain inquiries, however, are fundamental to most claims alleging cardiac injury, dysfunction, or death. These are (1) the cardiac diagnosis accepted legally as established in a given claimant; (2) the time of onset of each specific cardiac lesion; (3) the causal relation, if any, between the factor or factors under legal examination and the cardiac disorder found; (4) the medical determination of the impairment based on the claimant's overall cardiovascular status; and (5) the medical considerations in allegations of professional negligence. Additionally, in some legal actions arising under workers' compensation and some insurance policies, questions as to the role of preexisting disease or infirmity in contributing to the covered impairment or death may be of paramount importance in determining eligibility for benefits as well as the amount of benefits to be paid by the employer or insurer.

Defining the Cardiac Diagnosis

From the medical viewpoint, the diagnosis is the foundation on which the treatment of the patient is constructed. From the legal viewpoint, the diagnosis is the foundation upon which many decisions and rulings concerning issues of causation, eligibility for disability and retirement pensions, awards for damages, and many other matters arising in the litigation on hand are made. Although the diagnosis has to be made by a physician based upon medical data, legally it is considered only one of the various factual determinations in the case. The diagnosis reached by a physician after the gathering, reviewing, and studying of the medical data is, in essence, merely an opinion based on the individual examiner's specialized training, study, experience, and interpretation of the medical findings. As such, it is open to question both medically and legally as to reasonableness, accuracy, and completeness. Since different examiners may make different diagnoses, opinions expressed in court are subject to interrogation by counsel during cross-examination. The cardiac diagnosis should be established in each instance as fully as possible in terms of (1) an etiologic diagnosis that describes the underlying disease processes; (2) an anatomic diagnosis that describes the specific structural abnormalities (lesions) found in the cardiovascular examination; and (3) a physiologic diagnosis that describes the resulting disturbances of cardiovascular action and function. These should be delineated in generally accepted terminology, such as recommended by the Criteria Committee of the New York Heart Association in that committee's publication, "Nomenclature and Criteria for Diagnosis of the Heart and Great Vessels."[14] Because of varying connotations and implications, nonspecific terms, such as heart attack, coronary, mild or massive heart attack, and heart disease, without adequate qualification as to specific meaning, should not be employed in the cardiac evaluator's written report or testimony. Similarly, umbrella terms, such as *unstable angina, preinfarction angina, acute coronary deficiency,* and *acute coronary insufficiency,* should be avoided unless they are precisely defined.

The etiologic diagnosis should be reached after consideration of both the structural and functional disturbances found. If two or more etiologic bases for a person's heart disorder are present, each should be listed. Legally, the identification of the etiologic basis of a cardiac disorder or disorders becomes important in a causality assessment where worsening of a preexistent cardiac condition is claimed as a "personal injury" (and must be differentiated from the expected natural progression) and in legal actions where an estimation of life expectancy is of importance in determining awards for "damages" or in settlement proceedings.

The anatomic diagnosis comprises that component of the total cardiac diagnosis that describes the specific structural lesions present in the heart and great vessels. A complete description of the anatomic alterations often constitutes an important aspect of the legal determinations of a cardiac "personal injury" and of disability. Thus, for example, there may be considerable differences in the benefits or awards available legally for the sustaining of an episode of prolonged ischemic cardiac pain when diagnosed as an intermediate coronary syndrome with no documented new myocardial damage or when diagnosed as acute myocardial necrosis with resulting permanent new or added heart damage.

Anatomic lesions of the heart and great vessels frequently can be delineated clinically on the basis of the history, the findings of physical examination, and the results of specialized cardiac diagnostic studies. Certain anatomic lesions, e.g., a coronary artery thrombotic occlusion, however, cannot be diagnosed with reasonable certainty unless established by coronary angiography or other reliable objective means. Thus, diagnoses of *coronary thrombosis* and *microscopic myocardial necrosis,* terms not infrequently encountered in cardiac medicolegal reports and expert testimony, should usually be reserved for the radiologist or pathologist. When more than one anatomic abnormality is found, each should be included in the final diagnosis.

The physiologic diagnosis specifies the alterations in cardiovascular dynamics and function that have resulted from the cardiac pathology. The physiologic diagnosis may include a description of the cardiac rhythm; disturbances in cardiac impulse conduction; disturbances in supravalvular, valvular, or subvalvular function; malfunctions of prostheses, homografts, and cardiac pacemakers; disturbances in myocardial pump action; disturbances in intravascular pressures; abnormal communications (shunts) in the heart or great vessels; and the anginal syndromes. A cardiac diagnosis presented in the courtroom should be supported, wherever possible, by objective measures of cardiac structure and function, where indicated and within limitations of practicality and risk. A diagnosis based solely on a claimant's history, although in many cases the only diagnostic tool available to the medical expert, is not on secure grounds and, accordingly, is subject to strong attack on cross-examination. Many symptoms common to cardiac disorders, such as chest pain, shortness of breath on exertion, palpitations, and fatigue, are not pathognomonic for heart disorder. Symptoms alone are difficult to evaluate, since they may be exaggerated for self-serving purposes. Symptoms, per se, also defy quantifying. In contrast, the severity of symptoms in cardiac patients often does not correlate with the degree and severity of the found impairment of heart structure and function, and some cardiac disorders may result in no, minimal, or nonspecific symptoms.

The physician performing a cardiac evaluation for legal purposes must determine whether the patient-claimant had heart disease prior to the alleged potentially harmful exposure under legal consideration and, if so, whether there was a change in the preexistent cardiac status after the exposure. If a change is found, the physician must then define its nature and extent and whether it is permanent or temporary. It is also important to distinguish between a demonstrated structural change in a preexisting heart disorder and an alleged hastening of an expected consequence.

Diagnoses, as with other medical opinions, presented to a legal forum must be established in terms of reasonable medical certainty. Possible, potential, or suspected heart disorder has no place in the courtroom or in other legal determinations.

Timing the Onset of Cardiac Lesions

Determining the time of onset of specific cardiac pathology is an essential part of many cardiac medicolegal evaluations. It is often the crux of causation or of eligibility for the benefits of an insurance contract. Because of the variability of clinical presentations, individual differences in response to and manifestations of illness, and the frequent initial "silent" development of many cardiac pathologies, it may be impossible to time the onset of cardiac conditions within the precise framework sought by the law. Yet, the time of onset of cardiac lesions and dysfunction must be defined by the cardiac examiner as best as it can be with reasonable medical certainty and probability.

Determining the time of onset of a myocardial infarction may be difficult because of variable clinical presentations. The classic textbook presentation of sudden crushing anterior chest pain associated with profuse diaphoresis, dyspnea, and weakness is a generally acceptable index of the occurrence at that time of significant discrete acute myocardial tissue necrosis, although the possibility that some degree of myocardial necrosis has occurred previously (silently or with atypical manifestations) cannot be excluded. In some patients, an acute myocardial infarction, although evident at a later date on an electrocardiogram or at postmortem examination, is clinically silent. In other patients, the clinical picture is one of waxing and waning ischemic symptoms or signs over the course of 1 or more days with or without a bout of classic, prolonged chest discomfort. In patients with previous angina pectoris, an acute myocardial infarction may be manifested by an anginal attack of greater severity and duration or of radiation and location different from that previously experienced.

Unless otherwise determinable, the time of onset of a cardiac arrhythmia generally is accepted as the time of occurrence of identifying symptoms such as palpitations or a sudden collapse, as with a cardiac arrest due to ventricular tachycardia or fibrillation. The time of onset of coronary atherosclerotic, valvular, hypertensive, and most other heart disorders generally cannot be determined medically with any greater accuracy other than that the underlying etiologic condition must have been present for some time (usually only measurable in months or years) prior to the initial clinical manifestations. The occurrence of sudden collapse, acute pulmonary edema, cardiogenic shock, or severe pain provides an index of the time of rupture of an aortic aneurysm of a cardiac valve, papillary muscle, or of chordae tendineae, or infarcted myocardium. However, the commencement of the pathophysiologic processes underlying such rupture cannot be pinpointed with accuracy because of subtle or absent manifestations for a variable period of time preceding the catastrophic event.

Assessment of Causality

The determination of causation is vital to legal actions in which a heart disorder or its consequences is claimed as a compensable "work injury," as an injury due to "negligence," or as an "accident" under an insurance contract in which benefits are specifically provided for injury, disability, or death due to an "accident" rather than "illness." In general, legal claims of cardiac injury or sudden cardiac death generally allege as *a* or *the* cause of (1) an isolated, specifically identified incident, event, accident, trauma, or exposure; (2) a complication of medical or surgical treatment or other alleged so-called triggers[5,6] or (as in a malpractice action) a negligent treatment or negligent failure to institute indicated treatment; (3) a set of repetitive, cumulative factors[7] that, although subliminal individually, have combined in additive effect to produce cardiovascular harm (e.g., repeated subthreshold inhalation of carbon monoxide); (4) a long-term "overall" job or situational physical or psychological "stress"; or (5) a combination of one or more of the preceding.[6,7] In such actions, the claimant must first establish the existence of a cardiac disorder that can be accepted as an "injury" and then establish a causal connection between such injury and the alleged harmful consequences (disability, medical and surgical treatment and diagnostic expenses, pain and suffering, death, and other items of "harms") for which benefits are claimed. The claimant usually has the further burden of disproving any contributions to the alleged harms from intervening causes or from personal negligence if such charges are raised by the defendant.

In disputed issues involving causality questions in medical disorders, the legal fact finder must rely on the evidence put forth by the respective litigants, particularly expert medical opinion testimony. Physicians presenting such testimony in cause-and-effect assessments must appreciate the different weights assigned by the legal profession to the various elements that comprise a legal causality determination from those assigned by the medical profession to a pure medical assessment of causality (see Table 96-1). Causation often means one thing to a physician and quite another to an attorney, judge, or administrative hearing official. On occasions, medical opinion testimony based on traditional medical concepts of causality differs dramatically from answers based primarily on legal concepts utilized by a fact finder in reaching courtroom decisions.

TABLE 96-1 Medical Versus Legal Emphasis in Causality Assessment

Medical Emphasis	Legal Emphasis
The etiologic bases of a disease or disorder	The proximate ("triggering") cause of an injury, disability, or death
The causes of disease	A cause of injury, disability, or death
The producing cause of the entire disorder	An aggravation of a preexisting condition
The key role of preexisting disease	"The victim is taken as found," not as a normal, healthy person, but subject to whatever existing medical disorders were present at the time of exposure
The end result was inevitable because of the expected progression of the preexisting disease	A determination of whether the end result was hastened, not the time amount of hastening
The degree of aggravation was small in the light of the entire clinical picture	The crux is aggravation, not degree
The alleged causative element(s) not unique or unusual	The key element is the causative element(s), not the characteristics
The multiplicity of causes and their interrelationships	The key is the causative element(s) under legal scrutiny, independent of other coexisting or interrelating causes
Scientific proof of causation required	Establishment of causation generally is defined in terms of reasonable medical certainty, i.e., probable vs. possible, more likely than not, a 50.1% chance of relationship
Equally consistent theories of causation acceptable in differential diagnosis and choice of therapies	Equally consistent theories of causation do not satisfy standards for legal proof
The ultimate answer to causations can be deferred, pending new scientific advances	The issue of causation must be decided legally when presented
In assessment of damages (harms), there should be an apportionment of the role of each causative element	Generally, a total responsibility is assigned for the end result, if such is deemed due to a legally indicated exposure

SOURCE: Adapted from Sagall and Reed,[3] Sagall,[18] and Danner and Sagall.[19]

There are many differences between the medical and legal approaches to solving causality problems.[15-20] The physician, for example, in viewing a patient's medical problems, instinctively searches for the basic cause or causes underlying the overall disorder, whereas legal and judiciary professionals generally limit their concern to the one or more items under legal scrutiny as an "injury," independent of other causes. The physician generally defines cause as the production of a new condition or a new pathology or dysfunction, whereas the law in its definition accepts the aggravation of an underlying disorder by the worsening, hastening, or acceleration of its progression. The law thus includes in its framework of causation not only the production of a de novo condition but also the "triggering" or "proximate precipitation" of a new stage of pathology or of a new dysfunction in an underlying disorder and the worsening of an ongoing pathologic process. Physicians are reluctant to assign causal responsibility when the degree of aggravation of a preexisting condition is small in relation to the extent of the underlying abnormality or when the degree of hastening of an inevitable end result is minor. The law, in comparison, emphasizes the fact of hastening or aggravation, not the quantitative aspects. The crux of legal causation thus is the occurrence of an aggravation of an underlying disorder, not the degree to which it was aggravated, or the hastening of an end result, not the extent to which it was hastened.

Physicians are usually impressed that the alleged injury would not have occurred in the absence of a preexisting disorder that rendered the patient susceptible to harm from the alleged exposure. Legal fact finders, however, see it as immaterial that the event in question would not have caused injurious consequences had the victim been in good or average health. In all personal injury legal actions, the victim is "taken as he is found." Preexisting infirmity does not bar legal recovery, nor is it an acceptable excuse to relieve a defendant from legal responsibility or to mitigate the damages to be assessed. An illustration is the case of the proverbial "straw that broke the camel's back." To the physician, the proverb emphasizes the obvious predisposition to break down because of existing overload. The physician thus assigns the cause of the camel's collapse to the prior strain on his back, not to the added straw. The law, in comparison, asserts that although loaded to the breaking point, the back had held up without breaking. Accordingly, the added straw must be viewed as the cause of the collapse and the person who placed the straw on that loaded back as legally responsible for the consequences. Most often, the assignment of legal liability in such situations is made without attempt to apportion a percentage of harm between the triggering straw and the preexisting load. Unfortunately, the many current deficiencies in medical knowledge concerning the etiology and pathogenesis of most cardiac disorders and the limitations of presently available cardiac diagnostic testing procedures often prevent defining precisely the complete cardiac diagnosis, the nature and extent of the underlying pathology, the pathophysiologic mechanisms that have led to the end result, the sequence in which pathologic lesions have developed, the time of onset of certain lesions, and the answers to the many medical questions that may be of key importance in the legal matter on hand. The medical determination of causation is further made difficult because the very nature of most cardiac disorders categorized legally as personal injuries does not, in contrast to lesions such as burns or lacerations, present clinical or pathologic features pathognomonic of trauma or of an external cause. Thus, the question of whether some identified external element or stress played a contributory or precipitating role in their development or whether the disorder found stemmed from the natural, expected progression of an underlying cardiac disease unrelated to and unaffected by the item under legal scrutiny quite frequently is not amenable to clear-cut answers.

Similarly, differences in the provisions of the individual state and territorial workers' compensation acts under which most cardiac claims arise, differences in legal philosophy among the many persons assigned fact-finding roles in disputed litigation, subtle differences in claims that are seemingly identical, and the often diametrically opposed medical conclusions presented in a given case by equally competent medical experts preclude the formulation of legal standards of causality that can be applied uniformly to cover all instances. Accordingly, each case must be decided, both medically and legally, on its own set of facts and medical testimony. Certain precepts, however, should govern medical assessments of causality in cardiac claims. For an alleged causal connection to be accepted in a cardiac case as probable or with reasonable medical certainty, the following criteria should be satisfied:

- The cardiac diagnosis should be delineated completely and established, as far as reasonably possible, by objective means, and those portions of the cardiac condition under consideration as potential "injuries" specified.
- The alleged causative element presented for legal consideration should be one that is currently recognized medically and scientifically as capable, under appropriate circumstances, of producing the heart disorder or injury found.
- Conversely, the cardiac condition or dysfunction diagnosed must be one generally recognized medically as a possible result of the alleged harmful exposure.
- The time interval elapsing between the alleged noxious exposure and the medically manifest evidence of heart damage or dysfunction must be consistent with currently accepted scientific concepts of pathogenesis.
- The proposed cause-and-effect relation, although not always fully explainable in terms of present-day scientific knowledge, must still be consistent with current scientific concepts.

As an aid to medical assessment of causality in coronary artery heart disease and its ischemic sequelae, the reader is referred to the "Report of the American Heart Association's Committee on Stress, Strain, and Heart Disease."[20] Although originally published in 1977, the conclusions of this committee, supported by more recent studies,[21–32] are currently valid with only minor modification, have not been supplanted by any other formal set of medical causality guidelines, and are generally accepted by the medical profession. The conclusions currently pertinent to a medical assessment of causality in cardiac claims are subsequently summarized:

- Long-term repetitive physical effort, such as is inherent in many occupations, cannot currently be regarded medically as a causative element in the development of atherosclerotic coronary heart disease. Such activity, if playing any role in this disease process, is believed beneficial by preventing or slowing the rate of atherosclerotic progression.[20]
- Long-term repeated physical effort of work and/or nonwork activities in persons with underlying heart disease theoretically may hasten the development of congestive heart failure by reason of the additional workload imposed upon an already weakened heart. It is not possible within the present state of medical knowledge, however, to determine in any given heart patient when congestive heart failure would have occurred as the result of the expected natural progression of the underlying cardiac disorder in the absence of such exertional efforts; hence in these situations a causative or aggravating role to such stress most often cannot be assigned with "reasonable medical certainty."[20]
- Continued, psychological emotional stress and job demands to which an individual may have been subjected over a protracted period of time, though commonly accepted by the public and many physicians, have not been established scientifically as a causative or worsening agent in the genesis or acceleration of atherosclerotic disease,[20–36] although the possibility of some contribution cannot be excluded in individual cases.
- A single, isolated, identified physical or emotional stress in individuals rendered susceptible by reason of preexistent heart disease, is capable of eliciting adverse cardiac responses that, in turn, can "trigger" or hasten certain cardiac lesions and dysfunctions such as an attack of angina pectoris, a myocardial infarction, a sudden cardiac dysrhythmia, sudden

cardiac death, rupture of a diseased cardiac structure, coronary artery vasospasm, and flash pulmonary edema.[20–32]

- The shorter the time interval between the exposure of an individual to a potentially noxious stimulus and the appearance of clinical or pathologic evidence of new heart disease or dysfunction, the more likely there is a causal relation between the two. Conversely, the farther apart in time, the less likely is a cause-and-effect relation.[20]
- The exposure of a person with underlying heart disease to a stimulus potentially capable of eliciting harmful cardiovascular responses does not necessarily mean that such will be elicited, even when the exposure would be advised against medically because of the possibility of ensuing harm.[20]

The elements most often accepted by workers' compensation adjudicators in cardiac cases as work-related competent-producing causes of injury, disability, or death are identified incidents of physical work effort (usual, unusual, or of a degree greater than accustomed nonwork exertion, depending on the covering compensation act requirements); adverse work environments, (e.g., excessive heat or cold); and acute psychological trauma such as a heated argument or a sudden fright; an accidental electric shock; a severe nonpenetrating blow or other mechanical injury to the chest; and adverse cardiac reactions to medical, surgical, corrective, and rehabilitative therapy of an industrial injury not originally involving the cardiovascular system.

Nationwide, burgeoning claims under workers' compensation alleging illnesses such as coronary heart disease, hypertension, stroke, gastrointestinal disorders, and neuropsychiatric states as initiated or worsened by overall job-related "stress" are straining the workers' compensation system.[36] Frequently cited as "harmful" to the cardiovascular system are adverse mental reactions stemming from harassment by superiors, frustration from dealing with the public, tension created by imposed deadlines and quotas, boredom or excessive responsibility in job duties, threats of job termination or changes, insufficient vacations and time off, changing work shifts, long work hours, and ongoing business financial problems. In the cardiac "stress" cases that have reached state supreme court levels on appeals, the decisions have been mixed and have not established uniform case law precedents. For example, note the following cases:

- In New Hampshire, medical opinion that the continuing "stress" of a failing business over a 2-year period did not cause the fatal myocardial infarction suffered by the owner on a Sunday morning at home was upheld and compensation to his widow denied.[37]
- In contrast, a Rhode Island trial commissioner's denial of compensation to the widow of a newspaper sports editor who suffered a fatal cerebral hemorrhage at home was reversed. The court concluded that medical testimony that the deceased was suffering from high blood pressure of the type that would rise whenever he was under stress plus evidence that the decedent attended a professional football game earlier in the day of his death that placed him "under pressure" to meet a reporting deadline were sufficient to support the claim that his death that night was due to a cerebral hemorrhage resulting from aggravation of his preexisting hypertension. [38]
- In Colorado, the denial of compensation by the Industrial Commission to the widow of a fire department lieutenant with preexisting mitral valve prolapse and hypertension who died at home on the tenth day of a vacation absence from work was vacated. As grounds for the reversal and for an award of compensation, the court concluded that uncontroverted testimony from the fire chief, coworkers, and widow that the decedent had suffered a great deal of cumulative tension and frustration relating to his being overlooked in favor of junior firefighters for promotion and to his differing from superiors in department training and communication policies qualified this "stress" as an injury or occupational disease arising out of and in the course of employment. On this basis, the court remanded the claim to the referee to make specific findings whether the job-related stress was the proximate cause of the death. The decedent's doctor testified that the likely cause of death was an irregular heart rhythm that, when combined with a preexisting mitral valve prolapse and job-related stress, resulted in a fatal arrhythmia. The doctor further testified that the imminence of the decedent's return to work may have exacerbated his stress level, and was a contributory cause of his death.[39]
- In Connecticut, the court affirmed a commissioner's decision that unjust criticism of a bank employee on a number of occasions by superiors so aggravated her condition of obstructive coronary disease as to lead to a continued work disability from angina pectoris. This despite the presence of multiple coronary atherosclerosis risk factors including extensive cigarette smoking, obesity, and a positive family history of premature coronary disease.[40]

Major risk factors for coronary heart disease, such as cigarette smoking, elevated blood cholesterol, diabetes mellitus, hypertension, and positive family history of coronary disease, are often put forth by defense counsels as mitigating elements arguing against the claim's validity in questions of causality in coronary heart disease. Conversely, in a New Hampshire Supreme Court decision, the absence of identified risk factors in a firefighter with catheter-documented coronary atherosclerotic disease was deemed to support the *prima facie* presumption in the state's Workers' Compensation Act that heart disease in firefighters is occupationally related.[41]

In evaluating the role of risk factors in cardiac claims, it should be recognized that risk factors are of importance primarily in epidemiologic studies applicable to groups, not to an individual. For any given person, the presence or absence of medical background risk factors does not necessarily indicate the premature development of this condition. Thus, although statistically related to the presence of coronary heart disease, generally accepted risk factors for coronary atherosclerosis cannot be viewed medically as legally causative elements in the production of the disease.

Not all cardiac claims require legal causality determinations. For example, in claims instituted under the Social Security Disability Insurance Program, the primary issue is whether the applicant is unable to engage in substantial gainful employment as defined in the covering statute, not the medical or legal relationship of the disability to a particular causative element. Similarly, eligibility for benefits in most privately acquired insurance contracts is based on the fact of disability, generally independent of cause.

Evaluation of Disability

Evaluation of disability for legal and insurance purposes is a complex process necessarily involving more than one professional discipline. The evaluation generally requires interrelating the fields of medicine, law, insurance, judiciary, vocational counseling, and rehabilitation. As a minimum, a cardiac disability evaluation is twofold: first, a medical assessment must be made both in terms of what the patient cannot do and what the patient should not do by reason of the cardiac disorder and, second, there must be a legal translation of the medically determined impairment into the specific definition of disability in the applicable statute or insurance contract. The latter often involves questions concerning disability being total versus partial, permanent, house-confining, and other qualifying or restrictive adjectives that may affect benefits. As with most medicolegal evaluations, contested claims for disability benefits are decided by legal or administrative fact finders, with the physician's role limited to providing the fact finder with medical data and opinion testimony that can be utilized in reaching a conclusion. As a minimum, the physician examining a patient-claimant for disability evaluation purposes should attempt to determine the following issues:

- The full cardiac diagnosis, including etiology when known, and all anatomic and functional derangements found, together with the supporting clinical evidence.
- The clinical manifestations of the disorder revealed by the medical examination, including all subjective complaints and, more important, all objective confirmatory findings that support the presence of a heart disease or disorder medically recognized as capable of producing the symptoms alleged as the basis for disability.
- The impairment in the patient's physical activities and mental capacity in terms of limitations of walking, stair climbing, standing, sitting, reaching, lifting, bending, pushing, pulling, gripping, running, work hours, work pace, ability to concentrate, and capacity to work under conditions of tension, heat, cold, etc.
- The restrictions of nonwork and work activities medically imposed to prevent an aggravation of the underlying heart disorder or to prevent further heart damage, such as advice to post-myocardial infarction patients not to subject themselves to sudden bursts of strenuous physical effort. In those instances where the law requires that causation be apportioned between the parties (e.g., work-related versus non-work-related disabilities), the physician may be asked to furnish an opinion as to the causation of each of the impairments found. For example, in claims based on myocardial infarction, the physician may be asked what aspects of the impairments found are related to the underlying coronary atherosclerotic disease for which there may not be legal liability and what are related to the myocardial infarction itself for which there may exist legal responsibility.

In those situations where a patient-claimant has impairments coexisting from cardiac as well as noncardiac disorders, the physician may be asked to separate the impairments due to each disorder and, in assessing the overall combined impairments, whether noncardiac impairments magnify those attributable to the heart disorder. Where workers' compensation acts provide second injury funds, the examining or treating physician may be asked whether the disability from a cardiac injury in an employee with a known physical impairment from a congenital or acquired heart condition was made substantially greater by the combined effects of such impairment and subsequent personal injury.

In reaching the conclusions expressed in the medical assessment of disability, all currently available objective means of diagnosis and measurement of cardiac function should be used within practical limits of risk to the patient, cost of the testing, and value of the information to be obtained. Wherever feasible, medical evaluations of disability should be based on objective findings to obviate depending only on subjective complaints, which are often unreliable because they are self-serving. Medical assessments of cardiac impairment are significantly hampered by the following items:

1. Reliance on subjective complaints.
2. Individual variations in symptoms, motivation, adjustment, and return-to-work desires among persons with similar cardiac abnormalities.
3. Limitations of currently available means for quantitative measurement of cardiac functional reserves.
4. Frequent discrepancy between objective findings and subjective complaints.
5. Difficulties in transferring the results of objective test measurements, such as those of exercise stress testing, into the variable environment of the workplace or other real-life settings.
6. Susceptibility of most cardiac impairments to sudden change so that an impairment assessment or disability evaluation at a given date may be invalid for a later time.

The definition of disability from cardiovascular and/or other conditions for adults to qualify for benefits under the Social Security Insurance program requires an "inability to engage in any substantial gainful employment by reason of any medically determinable physical or mental impairment which can be expected to result in death or has lasted or is expected to last for a continuous period of not less than 12 months." The listing of impairment for each major body system, the applicable medical criteria, and the key concepts of medical evaluations are outlined and defined in the agency's handbook, *Disability Evaluation under Social Security,* [42] and on its web site on the Internet. [43]

In workers' compensation, for both cardiac and noncardiac conditions, administrators in more and more states have turned to the American Medical Association's *Guides to the Evaluation of Permanent Impairment*[44] for determinations of qualifying disability, as well as for rating the impairment in terms of percentage degree of functional loss that may qualify the injured worker for additional benefits in addition to lost wages. The New York Heart Association's[14] grading system of cardiac functional capacity provides an easily understood, readily applicable guide to the medical description of cardiovascular impairment:

Class I. Patients with cardiac disease, but without resulting limitation of physical activity. Ordinary physical activity does not cause undue fatigue, palpitation, dyspnea, or anginal pain.

Class II. Patients with cardiac disease resulting in slight limitations of physical activity. They are comfortable at rest. Ordinary physical activity results in fatigue, palpitation, dyspnea, or anginal pain.

Class III. Patients with marked limitation of physical activity.

They are comfortable at rest. Less than ordinary physical activity causes fatigue, palpitation, dyspnea, or anginal pain.

Class IV. Patients with cardiac disease resulting in inability to carry on any physical activity without discomfort. Symptoms of heart failure or of the anginal syndrome may be present even at rest. If any physical activity is undertaken, discomfort is increased.

For further discussion of medical evaluations and legal definitions of disability under a variety of situations plus extensive legal and medical references to disability assessments the reader is referred to the *Disability Handbook* of Balsam and Zabin[45] and its updated supplements.[46] The legal aspects of commonly sought medical assessments of physical impairment by third-party physicians and the legal relationship of the third-party physician and the person being examined are discussed by Rothstein.[47]

As with causality assessments, medical and legal assessments of disability may vary considerably because of the difference in emphasis necessarily placed by each profession on individual aspects of the impairment in the disability rating process. Although a physician might consider a patient not disabled and, therefore, employable, the fact finder may declare the same person disabled from work activity under the terms of the applicable law or insurance contract. Here the physician must appreciate that in reaching the legal decision as to work capacity, the fact finder frequently has to include nonmedical elements such as age, sex, educational background, motivation, and prior work training and experience. Additionally, the fact finder's decision may be influenced by the availability of certain types of employment in the local or national labor market, the problems imposed by transportation to and from work sites, language or other communication problems, and other factors that, as a practical matter, so restrict a given person's opportunity for gainful employment as to make that individual practically disabled from gainful employment although medically cleared for work.

It is also important to recognize that because of differing statutory and contractual definitions, a person declared disabled and awarded benefits under one disability program may not be deemed eligible for benefits under another program. Thus, an award for disability by one agency or insurer does not, by itself, bind another agency or insurer. Each insurance contract or other disability benefit program or statute must be considered individually and separately for each claim raised, although the claim in each instance is based on the same medical disorders and impairments.

Prognosis and Life Expectancy Assessments

When considering a lump sum settlement of a disputed cardiac claim or when setting up a dollar reserve to cover future benefits, defendant attorneys and insurers often ask their cardiology expert for an opinion as to a claimant's future course, anticipated future treatment, and/or life expectancy. Estimates of the number of years a claimant with heart disease can reasonably be expected to live not only are utilized legally to establish economic and other losses in the consideration of awards for "damages" in tort cases of cardiac injury, but also may be significant in limiting potential "damages" by reason of the heart condition's expected reduction of life span in cases where the legal liability is for a noncardiac injury.[48] Prognostic and life expectancy determinations realistically have to be based to a large extent upon statistical considerations and parameters in reported series involving large numbers of patients. While statistical conclusions do not necessarily apply to a given individual patient, a medical assessment of a cardiac patient's expected need for and extent of future treatment and of life expectancy, formulated after thorough medical examination and based on valid scientific guidelines, can be relatively accurate within certain ranges and, of practical usefulness to the legal resolution of cardiac claims of persons with heart disease.

Determination of Malpractice

The risk of a physician being sued for professional negligence is an inescapable fact of today's professional life. Choosing cardiology as a specialty increases this risk[49] because of a variety of reasons, particularly (1) the ever-present threat of sudden, unpredicted death due to the nature of heart diseases; (2) the inherent hazards and complications of invasive procedures and cardiac surgery; (3) the often-encountered lack of clear-cut diagnostic evidence or an atypical clinical presentation in the early stages of an acute myocardial infarction; (4) the unavoidable mortality and morbidity associated with heroic medical and surgical treatment of desperately ill patients in the end stages of heart disease; and (5) the many problems involved in obtaining informed consent for procedures beyond the understanding of most lay persons, particularly when frightened by the threats of a cardiac illness.

In medical malpractice cases, those instituting the claim have the legal burden of demonstrating by factual and opinion evidence (1) that the defendant doctor or other health care provider owed a duty to the plaintiff as is legally and morally implied in the physician-patient relationship; (2) that the defendant violated that duty by breaching the standard of care; (3) that the patient suffered injury or harm; (4) that the physician or other health care provider's negligence was the proximate cause of that harm; and (5) in some jurisdictions, that the patient's conduct did not negligently contribute to the alleged harm (the doctrine of contributory negligence). Unless all these elements are established in the courtroom by the plaintiff, the legal action will fail.

The evidentiary proof required of the plaintiff in establishing the bases of his or her action generally necessitates that expert medical opinion be provided that (1) defines the standard of care due the plaintiff by the defendants; (2) establishes the breach or failure to conform to that standard of care; (3) defines the injuries or "harms" claimed; and (4) causally relates the harms found to the claimed negligent action or failure to act on the part of the defendants. Should a patient suffer harm during the course of medical diagnosis and treatment, the physician and/or other health care providers may be liable, separately or additionally, to two other legal actions. The first constitutes charges that the patient was not given sufficient information by the responsible professional persons to allow a legally valid "informed" consent to be made to a medically prescribed diagnostic test or treatment that resulted in injury. Therefore, performance of the procedure or treatment was legally an "assault," subject to evidentiary requirements less stringent than those required in actions in tort as well as protected by a different statute of limitations. The second possible legal action is one based on alleged breach of contract should a particular result or cure allegedly promised not be achieved. In both of these actions, supportive expert medical opinions may not be necessary to substantiate the claim, since the legal issue in dispute often hinges on the factual determination of whether the defendant physician did or did not say what the patient alleges and not a separate demonstration of professional negligence.

Medical evaluation of a malpractice claim requires a careful review of all the claimant's medical records with particular attention, first, to whether the defendant's professional actions were in accord with generally accepted and proper standards of professional conduct and, second, to whether the alleged "harms" were causally related to the defendant's professional actions or failure to act.

As discussed in detail in Chap. 97, clinical practice guidelines are intended to help improve medical practice by providing clear and well-documented statements regarding appropriate medical services for particular medical conditions. Such guidelines can therefore, at least in theory, act as objective references for the standard of care in medical malpractice suits. Indeed, one of the factors that has promoted the development of practice guidelines has been the belief that physicians could model their practices on the guideline recommendations and avoid the tendency to practice "defensive medicine"—a pattern of excessive diagnostic testing and interventions designed to avoid legal liability.[50] The actual impact of practice guidelines on medical malpractice has been more complex.

First, practice guidelines have not uniformly been accepted as admissible evidence by the courts.[50] In some cases, courts have held that the guidelines are "hearsay" and could not be admitted into evidence unless the experts who developed them testified directly and were subject to cross-examination. In other cases, the courts have allowed the use of guidelines at trial, but have not automatically granted them status as a valid statement of the standard of practice. Most observers now believe that guidelines will be routinely admissible into evidence and granted appropriate weight as long as there is expert testimony offered to attest to the guideline's validity and authority.[51]

It is also the case that guidelines may be used as both a "sword" and "shield"[52] in particular cases of malpractice. That is, physicians may be sued for their failure to meet published guidelines, even as many had hoped that guidelines would protect physicians from frivolous suits. The most extensive examination of this issue[53] found that in a review of 259 cases of medical malpractice, clinical practice guidelines were cited in 17. Of those, guidelines were used to build a case against the physician (inculpatory) in 12 cases and to provide a defense for the physician (exculpatory) in 4 cases. The authors acknowledge that their study was biased, in that the presence of exculpatory guidelines may have prevented plaintiffs from pursuing a malpractice claim. Nevertheless, a survey of malpractice attorneys reported in the same paper found that guidelines were more than twice as likely to be used as inculpatory rather than exculpatory once a suit was filed.[53]

In a medical evaluation of alleged professional negligence, the fact that a patient suffered injurious effects during or after a prescribed treatment or procedure does not by itself raise a legal presumption of negligence as a causative factor. A physician is not legally responsible for a poor patient outcome unless it is proved that it followed from lack of professional care and diligence ordinarily possessed by others in the profession.

THE MEDICOLEGAL CARDIAC EXAMINATION

The techniques employed in medicolegal cardiac examinations are essentially the same as in medical examinations performed for treatment purposes. Generally, the basic components of history taking, physical examination, resting electrocardiogram, and chest roentgenogram plus review and study of the available medical records suffice. In claims where the patient-claimant is not available for examination, the evaluation may have to be made entirely on the basis of medical records. Rarely do the legal questions require the employment of more advanced diagnostic testing. In such cases, the recommending physician must keep in mind the information it can be expected to provide, the limitations of results, the pitfalls in interpretation, the availability and cost of the procedure, and the inherent risks and hazards to the patient. All must be weighed carefully against the legal need for the information to be obtained.

When cardiac disorders have legal consequences, the content of the medical history ultimately accepted by the legal arbiter frequently makes or breaks the action instituted by the plaintiff-claimant. For example, in many workers' compensation cases there is often no dispute concerning insurance coverage and the presence of a disabling cardiac disorder for which benefits might be available under the law; rather, the key issue is whether a work-connected factor played a role in precipitating, triggering, hastening, aggravating, or otherwise "causing" the disorder. The crucial element in such causality assessments frequently is the medical history ultimately accepted by the fact finder as depicting the sequence of events and circumstances surrounding the occurrence of cardiac symptoms. In those situations where it is alleged or where it can be anticipated that it will later be alleged that the patient's heart disorder arose in some part out of employment, thereby entitling the person to workers' compensation benefits for disability, the examining physician should inquire about and include in the written history the sequence of events preceding and leading to the onset of symptoms for which the patient sought medical attention. Inquiry should also be made as to the specific work activities engaged in before, during, and after an alleged cardiac incident; whether these were customary and usual for the employee; and whether there were associated environmental conditions that could have intensified the potential physiologic demands. Similarly, in situations where mechanical trauma is alleged to be a cause of heart injury, as in tort cases involving motor vehicle accidents, inquiry should be directed to the exact type of mechanical forces involved, particularly the point or points of bodily contact; the effect on the patient's body; the development and objective evidence of trauma such as cuts, external bleeding, and ecchymoses; and the precise time and sequence of occurrence of symptoms and signs consistent with cardiac injury. The list of potential questions that may be pertinent in the medicolegal history thus is virtually endless. In each case, therefore, the examiner's questioning must be tailored to provide the information needed to reach a reasonable medical conclusion for the facts on hand. Hospital records generally contain more than one written history. Significant historic facts, often of key legal significance, may be found in the admitting histories and progress notes of attending physicians, interns, residents, nurses, and medical students and in reports of consultants and occupational and physical therapists as well as in less obvious places, such as in requests for x-rays, laboratory determinations, and various diagnostic tests and reports. Accordingly, the physician asked to make a medical evaluation for legal purposes should request the complete hospital records rather than only the discharge summary.

Because the medical history is derived by an interview between a physician and a patient and simultaneously or later transposed into a written record, it is subject to many limitations of content, distortion, and error that may affect its legal value. Many of these limitations stem from a failure of the interviewer to ask pertinent questions, a failure of the interviewed patient to understand the questions asked or to respond appropriately, a bias of the interviewer, and self-serving motives of the patient. Typically, histories contained in hospital records are devoid of those items that later are of key importance in legal resolution of the claim. This is quite common in the history recorded at the time the patient is first seen with an actual or suspected acute myocardial infarction. In such situations, brevity in history taking is essential because of the urgent need to establish a diagnosis and institute lifesaving therapy rapidly. Characteristically, such histories make no mention of details relevant to causation that are crucial in later legal actions. In many instances, the attending physician, not aware of the potential legal actions that may stem from the patient's cardiac disorder, fails to record the detailed history necessary to resolve the legal aspects of the patient's illness, making it necessary to obtain a detailed history at a later date when the patient has become less reliable because of elements of financial or other gain associated with the institution of a claim for benefits.

THE MEDICOLEGAL REPORT

The report prepared by the physician of the cardiac evaluation is an important document with far-reaching practical consequences.[54] For the attorney or insurer to whom it is addressed, the report forms the basis for determining the pretrial acceptance or denial of the claim, the consideration of settlement negotiations, the pretrial preparation, and the courtroom presentation of the medical aspects of the case. For the physician, the time put forth in compiling a comprehensive medical report of the examination findings, summary of medical records, and conclusions drawn therefrom will later provide a useful refresher of the pertinent medical findings and the bases for the conclusions reached should the matter come to trial at some later date. Carelessly composed, poorly prepared, or obviously biased medical reports frequently prove damaging and embarrassing to the physician called upon to testify at trial.

The composition of a medical report for legal and insurance purposes differs from that of the usual medical report in that it often requires inclusion of information not directly related to the treatment of a patient but essential for answering the various medical questions posed by the impending litigation. In most situations, the medicolegal report of a cardiac examination and findings is best presented in narrative form. As a minimum such a report should cover the following topics, preferably in the order listed:

- A recounting of the history personally related to the examining physician by the patient-claimant or outlined in the medical records reviewed, with particular emphasis on the sequence of events leading to the seeking of medical attention. In a workers' compensation claim, adequate facts must be recorded in the medical history as to the overall job duties and requirements, including consideration of possible noxious occupational exposures and psychological "stress." There should also be detailed recounting of the work activity before, during, and after an alleged cardiac event. In an automobile accident or other situation where trauma is alleged as a cause of a cardiac "injury," there should be a description of the mechanical aspects of the contact or psychological sequelae. The significant past medical history should be detailed, with particular reference to recognized background medical risk factors favoring premature development of atherosclerotic coronary heart disease and the existence of prior heart disorder or of other conditions that might affect the patient's susceptibility to cardiac injury and/or current medical status.
- A chronologic listing, with summary of the contents deemed important, of the various hospital and medical reports and other data reviewed by the physician and utilized in the formulation of the opinions reached. If death has occurred, the pertinent findings of autopsy should be included.
- A detailing of the physical examination findings with description of all the abnormalities detected as well as the important negatives.
- The results of the various diagnostic studies performed or utilized by the examining physician in reaching conclusions of the evaluation.
- A statement of the complete cardiac diagnosis with substantiating reasons.
- The examiner's opinion concerning each of the various medicolegal questions posed in the individual case with substantiating reasons that support the conclusions expressed.

The medicolegal report should conclude with the physician's signature in black ink for photocopy purposes and a certification—a simple maneuver that in many cases suffices for the report to be accepted into evidence without need for the personal appearance of the author to verify its authenticity. The following is an example that has been successfully employed:

> CERTIFICATION: I hereby swear that I am a physician duly licensed in the state of __________ and further state that this written report of __________ pages dated __________ represents my report concerning __________ and is signed under the pains and penalties of perjury pursuant to the laws of this state, as cited in Chapter ______, Section ______.
> Signed ______________________________
> Board-certified in Internal Medicine and Cardiovascular Diseases

Finally, it is imperative that the physician submitting a medicolegal report recognize that the report, in most cases, will be made available to opposing counsel in sufficient time for detailed close study and conference with his or her medical expert in preparation for a potential intensive cross-examination.

References

1. McNiece HF. *Heart Disease and the Law*. Englewood Cliffs, NJ: Prentice-Hall; 1961.
2. Sagall EL, Reed BC. *The Heart and the Law—A Practical Guide to Medicolegal Cardiology*. New York: Macmillan; 1968.

3. Sagall EL, Reed BC. *The Law and Clinical Medicine*. Philadelphia: Lippincott; 1970.
4. "Analysis of Workers' Compensation Laws," prepared and published annually by the Chamber of Commerce of the United States, 1615 H Street, NW, Washington, DC 20062; 1999.
5. Sagall EL. Heart disease, workmen's compensation and the practicing physician. *N Engl J Med* 1961; 264:699–705.
6. Sagall EL. Compensable heart disease. *Trial* 1969; 5:29–31.
7. LaDou J, Mulryan LE, McCarthy KJ. Cumulative injury or disease claims: An attempt to define employers' liability for workers' compensation. *Am J Law Med* 1980; 6:1–28.
8. Sullivan RT. Heart injuries under workers' compensation: Medical and legal considerations. *Suffolk Univ Law Rev* 1980; 14:1365–1401.
9. Wyo Stat §27-12-603(b) (1977).
10. (a) Nev Rev Stat Ann, Title 53, Ch 616.110 (1985). (b) Nev Rev Stat Ann, Title 53, Ch 617.457 (1973).
11. Mass. Gen. Laws Ch 32 §94 (1956).
12. Longshoremen's and Harbor Workers' Compensation Act, Amendments of 1972, Sec. 20.
13. The Americans with Disabilities Act 42 U.S.C. 12101, et seq.
14. Criteria Committee of the New York Heart Association. *Nomenclature and Criteria for Diagnosis of Diseases of the Heart and Great Vessels*, 9th ed. Boston: Little, Brown; 1994.
15. Small B. Gaffing at a thing called cause: Medico-legal conflicts in the concept of causation. *Texas Law Rev* 1953; 31:630–659.
16. Sagall EL. Heart disease and the law—medico-legal considerations of causality. *Tenn Law Rev* 1963; 30:517–535.
17. Sagall EL, Reed BC. The legal assessment of causality. *Med Sci* 1967; 18(July):51–54.
18. Sagall EL. Causality assessment—Medical vs. legal. *Trial* 1969; 5(June/July):59–60.
19. Danner D, Sagall EL. Medicolegal causation: A source of professional misunderstanding. *Am J Law Med* 1977; 3:303–308.
20. American Heart Association. Report of the Committee on Stress, Strain, and Heart Disease. *Circulation* 1977; 55:825A–835A.
21. Muller JE, Toffler GH, Stone PH. Circadian variation and triggers of onset of acute cardiovascular disease. *Circulation* 1989; 79:733–743.
22. Brodsky MA, Allen BJ. Stress, cardiac arrhythmias, and sudden cardiac death. *Pract Cardiol* 1989; 15:49A–55A.
23. Muller JE, Toffler GH, eds. A symposium: Triggering and circadian variation of acute cardiovascular disease. *Am J Cardiol* 1990; 66:1G–70G.
24. Johnson RJ. Sudden death during exercise. A cruel turn of events. *Postgrad Med* 1992; 92:195–206.
25. Mittleman MA, Maclure M, Toffler GH, et al. Triggering of acute myocardial infarction by heavy physical exertion. Protection against triggering by regular exertion. *N Engl J Med* 1993; 329:1677–1690.
26. Muller JE, Abela GS, Nesto RW, Toffler GH. Triggers, acute risk factors and vulnerable plaques: The lexicon of a new frontier. *J Am Coll Cardiol* 1994; 23:809–813.
27. Taylor CB. Anger, angina, and ischemia. *J Myocard Ischem* 1994; 6:11–17.
28. Gottdiener JS, Krantz DS, Howell RH, et al. Induction of silent myocardial ischemia with mental stress testing: Relation to triggers of ischemia during daily life activities and to ischemic functional severity. *J Am Coll Cardiol* 1994; 24:1645–1651.
29. Maron BJ, Poliac LC, Kaplan JA, Myeller FO. Blunt impact to the chest leading to sudden death from cardiac arrest during sports activities. *N Engl J Med* 1995; 333:337–342.
30. Mittleman MA, Maclure M, Sherwood JB, et al. Triggering of acute myocardial onset by episodes of anger. *Circulation* 1995; 92:1720–1725.
31. Gabbay FH, Krantz DS, Kop WJ, et al. Triggers of myocardial ischemia during daily life in patients with coronary artery disease: Physical and mental activities, anger and smoking. *J Am Coll Cardiol* 1996; 27:585–592.
32. Krantz DS, Kop WJ, Gabbay FH, et al. Circadian variation of ambulatory myocardial ischemia. Triggering by daily activities and evidence of an endogenous circadian component. *Circulation* 1996; 93:1364–1371.
33. Sagall EL, Reed BC. Heart disorder due to emotional stress: Medical and legal aspects. *Med Counterpoint* 1969; 1(April): 15–43.
34. *Proceedings of the Conference on Stress, Strain, Heart Disease and the Law*, Boston, Jan. 26–28, 1978. US Government Printing Office, Publication 790-281-412/107, 1979.
35. *Stress in the Workplace: Costs, Liability and Prevention*. Rockville, MD: The Bureau of National Affairs; 1987.
36. Hlatky MA, Lam LC, Lee KL, et al. Job strain and the prevalence and outcome of coronary artery disease. *Circulation* 1995; 92:327–333.
37. *New Hampshire Supply Company, Inc. et al. v. Edith Steinberg et al.* 121 N.H. 506, 433 A.2d 1247 (1981).
38. *Helen F. Mulcahey v. New England Newspapers, Inc.* 488 A.2d 681 (R.I. 1985).
39. *City of Boulder v. Barbara E. Streeb et al.* 706 P.2d 786 (Colo. 1985).
40. *Rosalie McDonough v. Connecticut Bank and Trust Company et al.* 204 Conn. 104 527 A.2d 664 (1987).
41. *Cunningham v. City of Manchester Fire Department*. 129 N.H. 232.
42. *Disability Evaluation under Social Security*. DHEW Publication No. 05-10089, Washington, DC, US Government Printing Office, February 1986.
43. http://www.ohsu.edu/disability/adult.html.
44. Committee on Rating of Mental and Physical Impairment, American Medical Association. *Guides to the Evaluation of Permanent Impairment*, 4th ed. Chicago: American Medical Association; 1993.
45. Balsam A, Zabin AP. *Disability Handbook*. Colorado Springs: Shepard's/McGraw-Hill; 1990.
46. Balsam A, Zabin AP. *Disability Handbook. 1995 cumulative supplement*. Current through December, 1994. Colorado Springs: Shepard's/McGraw-Hill; 1995.
47. Rothstein MA. Legal issues in the medical assessment of physical impairment by third-party physicians. *J Leg Med* 1984; 5:503–548.
48. Sagall EL. Life expectancy determination. *Trial* 1969; 5(Aug/Sep):59–62.
49. Sagall EL, Lucas I, eds. *Malpractice Hazards in Cardiology* (proceedings, symposium, Boston, May 12, 1971). Boston: Massachusetts Heart Association; 1973.
50. Eagle KA, Lee TH, Brennan TA, et al. Task force 2: Guideline implementation. *J Am Coll Cardiol* 1997; 29:1141–1147.
51. Jacobson PD. Legal and policy considerations in using clinical practice guidelines. *Am J Cardiol* 1997; 80:74H–79H.
52. Pelly JE, Newby L, Tito F, et al. Clinical practice guidelines before the law: Sword or shield? *Med J Aust* 1998; 169:330–333.
53. Hyams AL, Brandenburg JA, Lipsitz SR, et al. Practice guidelines and malpractice litigation: A two-way street. *Ann Intern Med* 1995; 122:450–455.
54. Sagall EL. Physician's medical report. *Trial* 1972; 8(Jan/Feb):59–62.

CHAPTER 97

PRACTICE GUIDELINES IN CARDIOVASCULAR CARE

Ira S. Nash

INTRODUCTION

The delivery of medical care in the United States is an enormous enterprise which now accounts for approximately 14 percent of the entire economic activity of the nation and for which about $1 trillion changes hands each year.[1] The rapid growth of medical expenditures throughout the 1970s and 1980s—and, in particular, the burden of those expenditures borne by businesses through their provision of employee health insurance benefits—fostered an intense and unprecedented scrutiny of the practice of medicine. This scrutiny, which has continued to grow, is actually just a single component of a broader transformation in the delivery of medical care, which has been termed the "industrialization" of medicine. Kleinke describes this as a movement to "rationalize health care delivery, measure the costs and benefits of treatments, and compare the outcomes of different providers."[2] He goes on to say that "the compulsion to identify, measure and emulate 'best practices' is the essence of true industrialization." Others have referred to this being nothing less than a "revolution" in medical care.[3]

Physicians, long accustomed to the autonomous, small-scale practice of medicine, are understandably often bewildered by this transformation and are, as a rule, unschooled in the techniques required to understand and lead it.[4] This chapter deals with one of the new tools—clinical practice guidelines—which have the potential to keep physicians in the forefront of medicine's transformation and simultaneously to facilitate the transformation itself.

We first address the context in which practice guidelines have achieved their current prominence. Next, the nature of guidelines is presented, including the criteria by which the value of particular guidelines may be judged and how specific guidelines are and ought to be developed. Following the general discussion of guidelines, we present the key provisions of the most important practice guidelines in cardiovascular medicine. Finally, the success of practice guidelines in improving cardiovascular medicine is examined.

QUALITY OF CARE

Practice Variation

One of the most striking aspects of the delivery of medical care in the United States is its enormous inhomogeneity.[5–7] Much of the evidence of this practice variation comes from the examination of treatments for cardiovascular illnesses. Substantial differences in the way cardiology is practiced—what diagnostic tests are performed, what interventions are undertaken, how specific diseases or syndromes are approached—have been well documented across an array of patient and provider characteristics. African Americans are offered coronary angiography and revascularization less frequently than whites with similar disease severity.[8,9] Rates of rehospitalization after acute infarction differ markedly among different cities, in the absence of clinical differences among the populations.[10] Following a myocardial infarction, one is much more likely to undergo catheterization in Texas than New York,[11] or in the South compared with New England.[12] As the cost, complexity, and potential benefit of medical care (and cardiac care in particular) have grown, so too has the importance of addressing this variation. Which of the different approaches to care is "right"? Which leads to the greatest benefit for patients? Could similar benefits be achieved at a lower cost? How could one tell? Addressing these and related questions is the essence of evaluating the quality of medical care. Evaluating the quality of care is a necessary prerequisite for improving it.

Defining Quality

Many different definitions of quality have been proposed. Leaders in the field have suggested that this multiplicity of definitions may make sense, given the complexity of medical care and the wide range of specific, local goals associated with assessing its quality.[13] The Institute of Medicine put forth a definition of the quality of medical care which has been widely adopted: "the degree to which health services for individuals and populations increase the likelihood of desired health outcomes and are consistent with current professional knowledge."[14] Simply put, good medical practice is necessarily based on sound medical knowledge, and if done right, benefits patients. Note that even under the best of circumstances, quality medical care improves the *likelihood* of good outcomes but cannot guarantee them. A patient with cardiogenic shock on the basis of an extensive myocardial infarction is at high risk of dying even with the best medical care. Likewise, many patients will recover without incident after an infarction even if they do not receive effective therapies such as thrombolysis or postinfarction beta blockade. It is therefore inappropriate to examine only patient outcomes (such as mortality following an infarction) to judge the quality of care they received.

Measuring Quality: Structure, Process, and Outcome

A more complete assessment of the quality of care depends on considering three fundamental components of medical practice, which, taken together, paint a more complete picture: the structure, process, and outcome of care.[15] The structure of care is a characterization of the environment in which care is delivered. The process of care encompasses the myriad steps in the actual delivery of services, and the outcome of care is some result of interest to patients or providers. Consider, as an example, the assessment of the quality of care provided by a cardiac catheterization laboratory.

The structure of care provided by the lab includes the physical attributes of the facility, such as the modernity of the fluoroscopic equipment and the sophistication of the patient hemodynamic monitor. Perhaps less obviously, it also encompasses the staffing levels of the laboratory (e.g., nurse/patient ratios, nurse/technologist ratios), the level of training of the personnel (e.g., advanced cardiac life support certification, or "cross-training" of nursing and technical staff), and the maintenance of the equipment (e.g., the frequency of radiation safety inspections and film processor calibration). The structure of the laboratory also extends beyond its own physical boundaries. Is the laboratory a free-standing facility? Is it in a community hospital, where it may be used for general vascular radiology as well as coronary angiography? Is there a cardiac surgical program at the same institution?

The process of care addresses what providers do and how they do it. For the catheterization laboratory, this runs the gamut from how patients are scheduled for their procedure (indeed, how they are identified as candidates for a procedure) through the steps that are taken to prepare them for the catheterization (including patient education and the solicitation of informed consent) and all the details of the procedure and postprocedure care. Clearly, this includes an enormous number of potential points of quality assessment. How are patients prepared for the catheterization? Do cardiology trainees perform part (or all) of the procedure under supervision? How are patients monitored after their procedure? Are there dedicated personnel who remove the arterial introducing sheaths? How much heparin is used? How long are patients required to stay in bed? The list goes on.

Finally, an assessment of the quality of the laboratory may rightfully include an examination of the outcomes of the patients who were treated. This may include traditional outcomes such as complications and mortality, but can also be construed more broadly to include "patient-centered outcomes" such as patients' satisfaction with the care they received[16,17] or the functional capacity of patients who have undergone percutaneous interventions.[18]

Quality Assessment and Improvement

With the dimensions of quality more broadly drawn, the assessment and improvement of care can be specified more precisely with reference to the definition of quality offered by the Institute of Medicine. This assessment may then, in turn, form the basis for quality improvement or for comparisons among providers. Some component of the structure, process, or outcome of a particular aspect of medical care must be selected, defined, and measured. In order for the quality assessment to be meaningful (and, ultimately useful as a vehicle for improving care), certain criteria must be met.[19,20]

First, the focus of the assessment must be something under the control of the providers of care. There may be particular health outcomes which are of interest to patients and providers; but if they remain outside the ability of medical care to influence them, then measuring them would neither inform a judgment about the quality of care delivered nor form the basis for improving it. For example, the frequency with which patients with hypertrophic cardiomyopathy experience potentially life-threatening arrhythmias is of great interest to affected patients and their physicians. Yet tracking such events in a given population says little about the quality of medical care they received, since there are no therapies currently available that can reliably influence the outcome.

A measurable outcome of care must therefore be linked with a controllable structure or process of care. The mortality associated with coronary artery bypass graft (CABG) surgery is arguably the most intensively tracked outcome in all of medicine and has drawn the attention of a large number of investigators[21–24] as well as government agencies.[25,26] One critical factor in making this outcome a useful quality measure is that it can be influenced by changing the environment and processes of care.[27] Mortality following CABG depends, in part, on how well patients are treated. Tracking outcomes can therefore stimulate examination of, and changes in, the way care is delivered which can then result in improved outcomes.[28]

A measurable process of care can also be the focus of quality assessment and improvement activities as long as it is closely linked to an important health outcome. The National Cooperative Cardiovascular Project (CCP), sponsored by the Health Care Finance Administration (HCFA), is an excellent example of a large-scale quality assessment and improvement project predicated on this principle.[29] Drawing on a large body of randomized controlled clinical trials of therapies for patients with acute myocardial infarction, investigators developed a series of quality indicators. These indicators were measures of specific processes of care; that is, they specified which patients received which therapy. Based on the evidence from clinical trials, the investigators also specified which patients *should* get which therapy. They determined in this way the percentage of candidates for a given therapy who actually received it. Since the clinical trials established, for example, the connection between early aspirin administration and improved survival,[30] measuring the extent to which patients actually did receive aspirin serves as a measure of the quality of the care delivered. In situations such as this, where process and outcome are so well linked by clinical evidence, measuring some specific step in the delivery of care instead of the final outcome offers several important advantages. First, it provides an important efficiency. Since every patient treated for a particular condition such as myocardial infarction is exposed to a system of care but only a small percentage of patients (regardless of the care they receive) is likely to experience a particular outcome such as death, many more patients must be studied if the quality of care they receive is to be judged solely on the outcomes they experience.

Mant and Hicks[31] estimated the relative numbers of patients required to detect differences in the quality of care provided to patients with acute myocardial infarction based on process versus outcome measures. After applying estimates of the efficacy of a variety of medical therapies for myocardial infarction derived from randomized trials, they constructed a model for calculating the sample size needed to detect a given difference in mortality between two hospitals treating populations with the same risk of dying. For example, detecting a reduction in mortality from 30 percent (the assumed baseline mortality in the absence of any effective therapies) to 25 percent (achievable with the adoption of 31 percent of effective interventions) with a power of 80 percent and a significance level of 5 percent, would require the examination of records from nearly 1300 patients with myocardial infarction. To detect the difference in frequency of use of effective therapeutic interventions that could lead to a reduction in mortality of the same magnitude (the process instead of the outcome of care), they derived a minimum sample size of only 27 patients. Clearly, tremendous economy of effort could be achieved by focusing on process instead of outcome.

In addition, if only the outcomes of care are tracked, then any efforts directed at improving outcomes must still ultimately identify and improve those aspects of the delivery of care which drive the outcome. So, for example, if hospitals tracked only infarction mortality without measuring the extent to which their patients receive aspirin, then the discovery of high mortality rates would necessarily lead to an investigation of care, including critical steps such as the use of aspirin. Following aspirin utilization directly focuses attention where it must eventually be paid.[32]

Another criterion that any useful quality measure must fulfill rests on the fact that resources devoted to assessing one aspect of care are necessarily unavailable for a similar examination of some other aspect of care.[33] Maximizing the impact of quality assessment and improvement activities therefore requires prioritization in favor of high-cost, prevalent conditions. One of the most important reasons why cardiovascular medicine has come under so much scrutiny is the large economic impact of cardiovascular disease and its treatment.[34]

Finally, a range of practical issues must be considered in choosing a useful measure of the structure, process, or outcome of care. The collection of necessary data must be feasible within the constraints of time and resources. Quality measures must also be reliable (measurable in a consistent way over time), valid (a true measure of what one hopes to measure), and sensitive to change over time and differences among systems of care.

Ultimately, regardless of which type of quality measure is selected, its interpretation often rests on comparing local findings or practices against an objective standard. Such standards serve to link the desired health outcomes, which are the centerpiece of the definition of quality, with the elements of care that providers can control. They specify the setting and conditions or particular processes of care which, if adhered to, maximize the likelihood of good patient outcomes. These compilations of standards are clinical practice guidelines.

CLINICAL PRACTICE GUIDELINES

Definition

In 1989, a new federal agency, The Agency for Health Care Policy and Research (AHCPR) was created with the charge to "enhance the quality, appropriateness, and effectiveness of health care services, through the establishment of a broad base of scientific research and through the promotion of improvements in clinical practice and in the organization, financing and delivery of health care services."[35] Specifically included in the legislation was the charge that the agency put forth "clinically relevant guidelines that may be used by physicians, educators, and health care practitioners to assist in determining how diseases, disorders, and other health conditions can most effectively and appropriately be prevented, diagnosed, treated and managed clinically."[36] In order to assist the newly formed agency in fulfilling its mandate, the Institute of Medicine convened an advisory committee, which issued its report in 1990.[37] That report defined practice guidelines as "systematically developed statements to assist practitioner and patient decisions about appropriate health care for specific clinical circumstances."[38] The intended utility of practice guidelines was expressed in a follow-up report by the Institute of Medicine in 1992[39]: "Scientific evidence and clinical judgement can be systematically combined to produce clinically valid, operational recommendations for appropriate care that can and will be used to persuade clinicians, patients, and others to change their practices in ways that lead to better health outcomes and lower health care costs." While the report acknowledged the existence of substantial barriers to the realization of this ideal, it remains a concise statement of the potential utility of practice guidelines.

Other Aids to Clinical Practice

As the perceived need to improve the quality of care has grown, so too has the range of tools available to practitioners. Many of these share some characteristics of practice guidelines. Unfortunately, there is no universal agreement about the names used to describe them, which has led to some confusion. *Medical review criteria* are "systematically developed statements that can be used to assess the appropriateness of specific health care decisions, services, and outcomes."[40] These are generally derived from clinical practice guidelines and allow for their application in assessing and improving care. They may be "restatements of specific guideline recommendations into forms suitable for . . . review of clinical practice."[41] For example, the AHCPR guideline for the management of congestive heart failure states that patients with a reduced ejection fraction (EF) should be treated with an angiotensin converting enzyme (ACE) inhibitor.[42] The medical review criterion derived from that recommendation states that "patients with EF ≤35 percent should be receiving an ACE inhibitor at appropriate doses unless hyperkalemic, documented intolerance, patient hypotensive."[41] The standards by which care was judged in the CCP were also medical review criteria.

Another quality improvement tool closely related to practice guidelines is a *critical pathway.* A critical pathway may also be referred to as a critical path, a clinical pathway, a clinical plan, a care map, or a care plan[43] (although others have drawn distinctions among these[44]). These are usually locally developed, highly detailed accounts of how the process of care should unfold for a focused episode of care. They typically deal with the direction and coordination of inpatient services for a particular diagnosis or procedure. For instance, a CABG critical pathway may specify what each of several different providers of care should do during each day of a patient's stay. This would include items such as nursing instruction in the use of incentive spirometry on postoperative day 1, the removal of chest tubes by the surgeon on day 3, climbing stairs with the physical therapist on day 5, and so on. Developing explicit statements of this sort forces groups of providers to examine their practices and achieve local consensus about how care should be delivered, and the final products serve as real-time references to those caring for patients.

For critical pathways, clinical practice guidelines or other statements regarding the quality of medical care to achieve their intended effect, the tools themselves must be of high quality, and they must be used in an effective way.

Guideline Attributes

Several observers have suggested lists of attributes which good practice guidelines should have. The Institute of Medicine report lists eight important qualities[45] (Table 97-1). *Validity* implies that the guidelines, if adopted, will actually lead to the anticipated improvements in health outcomes and/or cost of care. *Reliability or reproducibility* is achieved if another group of guideline developers would create equivalent guidelines, if they relied on the same evidence, and if the guidelines are "interpreted and applied consistently by practitioners."[45] Good

TABLE 97-1 Desirable Attributes of Clinical Practice Guidelines Identified by the Institute of Medicine

Validity	Clarity
Reliability	Multidisciplinary development
Clinical applicability	Scheduled review
Flexibility	Documentation

SOURCE: From Field and Lohr,[45] with permission.

guidelines should also have clear *clinical applicability,* so that they pertain to a broad, well-defined, and explicitly stated population. Guidelines must also allow for some *flexibility* of medical practice and acknowledge the appropriate role of clinical judgment and possible exceptions to broad dictates. *Clarity* of recommendations is another important attribute and should be promoted through the use of precise definitions of terms, unambiguous recommendations, and a variety of presentation techniques. Ideally, guidelines should be developed through *a multidisciplinary process,* which elicits the input of a broad range of stakeholders in the field. Given the rapid pace of medical research and the attendant changes in clinical practice over time, good guidelines should include a provision for *scheduled revision* or an "expiration date." Finally, the institute report suggests that good guidelines should be *well documented,* so that users will know the "procedures followed in developing guidelines, the participants involved, the evidence used, the assumptions and rationales accepted, and the analytic methods employed."[45]

The Evidence-Based Medicine Working Group has put forth its own criteria for judging the quality of practice guidelines. They posed a series of questions, the affirmative answers to which indicate a good guideline[46]:

- Were all important options and outcomes clearly specified?
- Was an explicit and sensible process used to identify, select, and combine evidence?
- Was an explicit and sensible process used to consider the relative value of different outcomes?
- Is the guideline likely to account for important recent developments?
- Has the guideline been subject to peer review and testing?
- Are practical, clinically important recommendations made?
- How strong are the recommendations?

They conclude: "A good guideline, based on solid scientific evidence and an explicit process for judging the value of alternative practices, allows you to review, at one sitting, links between multiple options and outcomes."[47]

Weingarten endorsed this same series of questions to assess the quality of practice guidelines,[48] but Selker offered a slightly different set of criteria.[49] He proposed that guidelines must have the following attributes to warrant adoption:

- Face validity: they must appear "reasonable and appropriate to relevant experts in the field."
- Content validity: they must be based on sound medical evidence.
- Clinical practicality: they must balance specificity with flexibility.
- Consensus validity: they must reflect the achievement of consensus by affected parties.
- Demonstrated safety and effectiveness: they should be tested and proved useful in clinical trials.
- Transportability: they must be useful across a range of practice settings.
- Timeliness: they should be up to date, reflecting current medical knowledge.

Achieving each of these goals is a challenging task for guideline developers, as the promulgators of the standards have themselves acknowledged. It is also not a trivial process even to determine whether these quality criteria are met.

That is why The American Medical Association (AMA), which compiles a list of practice guidelines,[50] has included guidelines based on how they were developed rather than on their content.

How Do Guidelines Measure Up?

There are now a huge number of practice guidelines put forth by a large number of organizations and dealing with a broad array of clinical issues. The AMA directory lists nearly 2000 guidelines by roughly 80 organizations dealing with issues from allergy testing to wound care.[50] The National Guideline Clearinghouse, a collaborative effort of the AHCPR, the AMA, and the American Association of Health Plans, has more restrictive criteria for inclusion than the AMA directory and still lists over 550 practice guidelines on its web site.[51] With such a large number of guidelines in the published literature, a number of investigators have attempted to assess how well they fulfill the criteria discussed above.

Shaneyfelt and colleagues explicitly judged a total of 279 clinical practice guidelines published between 1985 and 1997.[52] They first devised an evaluation tool that consisted of 25 specific standards that guidelines should ideally fulfill. These criteria were separated into standards of development and format, standards of evidence identification and summary, and standards on the formulation of recommendations. No attempt was made to prioritize the standards, and the authors acknowledge that it is extremely unlikely that any guideline would fulfill all of them. Nevertheless, they reported that the guidelines met a mean of only 43.1 percent of the quality standards and concluded that most guidelines "do not adhere well to established methodologic standards," especially in regard to how the underlying medical evidence is gathered and critically combined.[52] Cook and Giacomini, in an accompanying editorial, commented that the findings revealed "the diversity of guideline methodologies . . . and [are a] call for greater transparency of guideline reporting and more rigorous peer review."[53] Parmley, in a critique[54] of an abbreviated version[55] of the AHCPR guidelines for congestive heart failure,[42] made similar observations regarding the importance (and practical difficulty) of peer review of clinical practice guidelines. In order to create guidelines of the highest quality, their development should follow an organized process.

Guideline Development

Although some of the desirable attributes of guidelines discussed previously—such as multidisciplinary input—speak to how guidelines should be developed, some groups have approached the process of guideline development more explicitly. Task Force 1 of the 28th Bethesda Conference of the American College of Cardiology detailed eight phases of successful clinical practice guideline development.[56] Within each of these phases, they outlined specific tasks to be accomplished (Table 97-2).

Perhaps no other step in guideline development is as critical as systematically evaluating the strength of the evidence upon which recommendations are based. Unless, as is rarely the case, all of the available evidence supports a particular clinical approach, guideline developers must weigh one bit of evidence against another. Even in the less problematic circumstance of general concordance of the available data, the quality of the data may have important implications for the confidence the guideline drafters have in one or more of their recommendations.

Some research findings (or other pieces of evidence) reported in the medical literature are more reliable than others. That is, some reported findings are likely to be a true effect, while others may be only an artifact of a study design flaw or a statistical quirk. There is a generally accepted hierarchy of study design, based on the premise that the systematic minimization of potential bias improves the reliability of research results.[57] The most reliable research results come from randomized controlled trials (RCTs),[58] and among RCTs, those that re-

TABLE 97-2 Phases of Guideline Development and Associated Tasks Identified by the 28th Bethesda Conference

Phase 1. Administrative oversight
- Task 1. Identify specific goals
- Task 2. Prioritize possible guideline topics
- Task 3. Review the literature to define task, costs, and time line

Phase 2. Select expert panel
- Task 1. Members must bring expertise, diversity, enthusiasm, and commitment
- Task 2. Convene panel electronically (videoconference, e-mail) to begin plans
- Task 3. Confirm outline, map patient care algorithm

Phase 3. Literature search and evidence review
- Task 1. Computerized literature search
- Task 2. Match literature to guideline outline, rate evidence
- Task 3. Create evidence tables for each topic
- Task 4. Base wording of recommendations on strength of relevant evidence

Phase 4. Consensus process
- Task 1. Converge on recommendations by an explicit process

Phase 5. Computerize guideline documents in format for clinical use
- Task 1. Link recommendations with related evidence
- Task 2. Create preformatted documents to capture data and facilitate care
- Task 3. Create database to store information regarding guideline compliance

Phase 6. Test and revise guideline
- Task 1. Expert panel tests computerized guideline in actual patient care
- Task 2. Final revision of guidelines based on testing

Phase 7. Disseminate guideline
- Task 1. Publish printed version, disseminate computerized version
- Task 2. Encourage local customization

Phase 8. Revise and refine guideline
- Task 1. Maintain ongoing literature review
- Task 2. Refine management strategies based on patient outcomes associated with guideline use

SOURCE: From Jones et al.,[56] with permission.

cruited larger cohorts of patients are generally more reliable than smaller studies.[57] In descending order of reliability (ascending vulnerability to bias), the remaining sources of data are cohort studies, case-control studies, case series and registries, and case reports and expert opinion.[57] The AHCPR guideline developers have divided the different levels of available evidence into three classes. A-level evidence is derived from RCTs (both large and small), meta-analyses of RCTs, well-conducted cohort studies, and metanalyses of well-conducted cohort studies. B-level evidence is drawn from studies with other kinds of designs. C-level evidence is based on expert opinion only.[57] Other guideline developers have adopted a similar method of ranking the evidence upon which their recommendations rest.[59]

Although evidence of consistently high quality may form the basis for strong guideline recommendations, it must be noted that there are legitimate circumstances where this concordance is violated. If several large RCTs provide conflicting conclusions, then the quality of the available evidence may be high but the recommendation necessarily weak. On the other hand, if there is such universal agreement that a particular element of care is so essential that no RCT is ever likely to be done (e.g., the necessity of examining a patient[56]), then a strong recommendation may be appropriate in the absence of rigorous evidence. Guideline developers have therefore developed separate systems for indicating the strength of their recommendations.

A very good system for classifying recommendations is used by the Joint Task Force on Practice Guidelines of the American College of Cardiology (ACC) and the American Heart Association (AHA). They use the classification scheme in Table 97-3 to summarize the indications for a particular treatment or therapy. This classification has been slightly modified in some of the joint ACC/AHA guidelines. For example, in the guideline for the treatment of myocardial infarction,[59] class I indications are those which are "beneficial, useful, and effective." In the guidelines on assessing cardiac risk in patients undergoing noncardiac surgery,[60] class I indications are defined as those where the treatment is "of benefit." The preoperative evaluation guidelines also do not distinguish between classes IIa and IIb. The myocardial infarction guidelines have a more forceful description of class III indications than the preoperative evaluation guidelines, stating that the procedure or treatment "may be harmful," while the other guidelines state that class III procedures and treatments are just "not necessary." Despite these minor variations, the broad classes remain uniform in basic meaning across all of the ACC/AHA guidelines.

TABLE 97-3 American College of Cardiology/American Heart Association Classification of Guideline Recommendations

Class I: Conditions for which there is evidence and/or general agreement that a given procedure or treatment is of benefit

Class II: Conditions for which there is conflicting evidence and/or a divergence of opinion about the usefulness or efficacy of a procedure or treatment

- Class IIa: weight of evidence in favor or usefulness or efficacy
- Class IIb: usefulness or efficacy is less well established

Class III: Conditions for which there is evidence and/or general agreement that the procedure/treatment is not useful/effective and in some cases may be harmful

Guideline Implementation

Clinical practice guidelines are a tool for improving patient care. Much of that potential can be realized only by changing physician behavior, since physicians are ultimately responsible for directing care. Even a well-crafted guideline, then, will not benefit patients unless and until it actually changes how doctors act under particular circumstances.

Multiple studies have demonstrated that just making information available to physicians is generally insufficient to change their practice.[61] Successful implementation of clinical practice guidelines must therefore go beyond making the guidelines themselves accessible through publication in the medical literature or by electronic means. The extent to which cardiovascular clinical practice guidelines have been successful in improving care is reviewed later in this chapter. Here, we review some of the barriers to guideline implementation and the strategies for overcoming them.

Perhaps the greatest barrier to guideline implementation is the complexity of the health care delivery system itself. Medical care is provided in a broad range of settings, from private physicians' offices to large academic medical centers and by a host of practitioners with different levels of interest and expertise in particular clinical conditions. Given the financial pressure present in many medical delivery systems, guideline implementation may well be seen as another burden or expense rather than as an aid to clinical practice. Even if guideline adoption is seen as desirable, limitations of physician time and practice resources may hinder efforts to move forward. Where physician time and practice resources do not constrain efforts at guideline adoption, the complexity and diversity of clinical encounters still make routine application of uniform standards of practice difficult. The inadequacy of many clinical information systems, which under ideal circumstances could identify patients who meet guideline criteria and remind providers of current recommendation, is another important institutional barrier to successful guideline implementation.[62]

Skepticism among clinicians about the value of guidelines is also a significant barrier to their implementation. This skepticism, in turn, may be a result of a general mistrust of "cookbook"[54] approaches to clinical practice, a rejection of national (in favor of local) standards of practice,[63] concerns regarding malpractice liability,[64] or differences in physician training and experience.[65] Certainly, deficiencies in the guidelines themselves—including conflicting recommendations among different guidelines addressing the same conditions, lack of clarity of recommendations, or any other failure of the guidelines to achieve the high standards discussed previously—contribute to physician skepticism and decrease the likelihood of successful guideline implementation.[66]

Just as the barriers to guideline implementation are diverse, there is no single proven strategy for successful guideline adoption. For guideline developers, close attention to the principles of rigorous data synthesis and the straightforward presentation of well-documented recommendations is essential. Explicit discussion of potential conflicts with other guidelines and the reasons for different recommendations should be included. Guideline writers should include clear statements regarding the limitations of their own guidelines with respect to the patients or conditions to which they apply. Guideline developers should also recognize that guidelines are not "self-implementing."[67]

Those who are charged with implementing practice guidelines must be prepared to address the barriers discussed above. Clear demonstration of the value of guideline adoption, through the feedback of local data demonstrating improvements in patient outcomes, is often part of a successful strategy. Simultaneous development of the infrastructure to support clinical practice guidelines, including modifying the incentives of clinicians and investing in clinical information systems, is also helpful.

CARDIOVASCULAR CLINICAL PRACTICE GUIDELINES

Finding Practice Guidelines

Clinical practice guidelines in cardiovascular medicine have been developed by many different organizations on a wide array of topics. New guidelines are constantly being produced in order to cover new subjects and to incorporate new data about previously addressed conditions. Just keeping track of the guidelines themselves has become challenging for clinicians and policymakers. Fortunately, there are several ways to find relevant guidelines.

Most clinical practice guidelines are published in peer-reviewed medical journals. Often, the journals are the official publication of the same parent organization that produced the guideline. So, for example, the guidelines compiled by the American College of Physicians/American Society of Internal Medicine are published in the *Annals of Internal Medicine;* those of the American College of Chest Physicians appear in *Chest,* and the guidelines of the joint efforts of the ACC/AHA are published in both the *Journal of the American College of Cardiology* and *Circulation*. Guidelines by lesser-known groups are also generally published in mainstream journals. Even government agencies, which have their own publishing capabilities, often seek to have part or all of their guidelines published in journals as well. As a consequence, a computer search of the MEDLINE database of peer-reviewed journals can produce a list of many of the sought guidelines. This process is far from perfect, however, in part because of the wide variety of key terms used to index published guidelines.

The National Library of Medicine periodically publishes the results of its own electronic searches of the medical literature as part of its series *Current Bibliographies in Medicine*. One such search for practice guidelines, prepared in 1992, utilized a total of 39 search terms to obtain a comprehensive list.[68] Such a search strategy is not only daunting for even the most facile users of computerized medical database search engines but also inevitably yields a large number of references of minimal relevance, which must then be manually culled from the bibliography in a rather laborious fashion.

Guidelines have been compiled by other parties as well. The American Medical Association annually publishes its *Clinical Practice Guideline Directory*.[50] Although the guidelines themselves are not included in the directory, there are listings of guidelines by subject and sponsoring organization as well as sections on guidelines in development, contact information for all the sponsoring groups, bibliographic references for published guidelines, and a listing of withdrawn (obsolete or superseded) guidelines.

The electronic compendium of guidelines maintained by the National Guideline Clearinghouse[51] is very useful. This searchable web site allows the user to specify the subject and/or sponsor of guidelines. The interface is user-friendly, and the list generated by the search contains links to the specified guideline. So, for example, if one specifies *cardiovascular disease,* a total of 55 listed guidelines is presented, along with suggested search terms ("*heart disease,* "*vascular disease,* etc., and the number of guidelines fitting those search criteria). The links allow a user to go directly from the list to a brief summary of the guideline prepared by the National Guideline Clearinghouse as well as to the full text of a particular guideline, often at the web site of the sponsoring organization.

Categorizing Cardiovascular Clinical Practice Guidelines

The large number of cardiovascular clinical practice guidelines, as well as their detail and rapid evolution, makes it impossible to present a comprehensive discussion of all of their provisions here. For example, the 1996 ACC/AHA guidelines for the management of patients with acute myocardial infarction[59] are 100 pages long and cover every aspect of myocardial infarction care, from the prophylactic use of antiarrhythmic agents to the indications for temporary transvenous pacing. An even more focused guideline, such as the physician monograph from the National Cholesterol Education Program (NCEP) on cholesterol management in patients with established coronary heart disease,[69] is over 25 pages long and contains information and detailed recommendations about dietary management as well as dosing information about specific lipid-lowering medications.

Instead of trying to present all cardiovascular guidelines, the most prominent guidelines are presented here and several of their key findings and recommendations are discussed. These guidelines generally follow the criteria previously outlined. The guidelines are divided into five broad categories, which are discussed in turn. The first group are those dealing with the assessment and treatment of risk factors for cardiovascular disease. The second group includes the guidelines for screening asymptomatic populations for the presence of specific cardiovascular diseases. Next, we review the guidelines that pertain to the diagnosis and treatment of established cardiovascular conditions. The fourth group of guidelines speaks to the application of various technologies for diagnosis and treatment. The final group covers specific interventions and/or treatments.

Assessment and Treatment of Risk Factors for Cardiovascular Disease

Because cardiovascular and, in particular, coronary disease may present in sudden and catastrophic fashion, attention has long been paid to identifying those factors that may predict the development of overt disease. More recently, the accumulation of compelling data demonstrating the efficacy of risk-factor interventions in improving clinical outcomes[70,71] has reinforced the value of risk-factor modification. In addition, the identification of previously unrecognized risk factors continues[72,73] to focus attention on the prevention of cardiovascular illness.

HYPERTENSION

The most comprehensive and definitive guideline on hypertension is the Sixth Report of the Joint National Committee on Prevention, Detection, Evaluation and Treatment of High Blood Pressure, commonly referred to as JNC VI.[74] The JNC report is divided into four sections. The first provides introductory information, including data on the prevalence of hypertension and its clinical consequences. It also includes a discussion of the workings of the JNC, such as the methodology they used to evaluate the quality and reliability of available scientific evidence for each of their recommendations. The second section addresses blood pressure measurement and the clinical evaluation of hypertensive patients. Section 3 covers the prevention and treatment of high blood pressure, and the final section deals with special populations and situations.

Section 1 of JNC VI concludes that:

- "Hypertension awareness, treatment, and control rates have increased during the last 3 decades."[74]
- Age-adjusted mortality rates for stroke and coronary heart disease (CHD) declined during the same period of time.
- End-stage renal disease and congestive heart failure (important consequences of uncontrolled hypertension) are increasing.
- RCTs are the best source of information, but they have some limitations.
- Prevention and treatment of hypertension and target-organ damage should remain public health priorities.

Section 2 defines normal and elevated blood pressure (Table 97-4). It also proposes that blood pressure be evaluated as part of a more comprehensive cardiovascular risk assessment, so that a patient with other risk factors would have his blood pressure controlled more vigorously than someone without other risk factors (Table 97-5). Similarly, hypertensive damage to another organ system should trigger more intensive antihypertensive efforts (Table 97-6). This approach, of recommending intensified treatment of a particular risk factor—in this case, hypertension—based on both the degree to which that risk factor is present and the presence of other risk factors or overt cardiovascular disease, is a general model of most guidelines for risk-factor modification. It implicitly recognizes that risk factors do not operate independently of one another[75] and that a particular patient's overall cardiovascular risk reflects the integration of many different factors.[76,77]

Section 3 details the myriad treatment options open to clinicians for the control of hypertension. The major conclusions are as follows:

- Lifestyle modification can lower blood pressure and prevent cardiovascular disease.
- Diuretics and beta blockers should be chosen as initial therapy in the absence of specific indications for other agents.

Details are also provided concerning the treatment of hypertensive emergencies and strategies that may be employed to improve patient compliance with antihypertensive regimens.

HYPERLIPIDEMIA

There are several important guidelines that address the assessment and management of hyperlipidemia as a risk factor for cardiovascular disease. The oldest, and still most influential from a national policy perspective, is the second report of the adult treatment panel of the NCEP.[78] The NCEP subsequently published a physician monograph (and accompanying patient education materials) addressing cholesterol management in patients with established coronary heart disease.[69] The American College of Physicians issued a clinical guideline on screening asymptomatic adults for the presence of hyperlipidemia in

TABLE 97-4 Blood Pressure Classification from JNC VI[a]

Category	Systolic Blood Pressure, mmHg		Diastolic Blood Pressure, mmHg
Optimal	<120	and	<80
Normal	<130	and	<85
High normal	130–139	or	85–89
Stage 1 hypertension	140–159	or	90–99
Stage 2 hypertension	160–179	or	100–109
Stage 3 hypertension	≥180	or	≥110

[a]When systolic and diastolic pressures fall into different categories, the patient is assigned on the basis of the higher of the two categories. Elevated readings should be based on the average of two or more readings, taken at each of two more visits after initial screening.

SOURCE: From JNC VI,[74] with permission.

TABLE 97-5 Cardiovascular Risk Stratification in Patients with Hypertension

- Major risk factors
  - Smoking
  - Dyslipidemia
  - Diabetes mellitus
  - Age >60 years
  - Sex (men and postmenopausal women)
  - Family history of cardiovascular disease (women <65 years or men <55 years)
- Target organ damage/clinical cardiovascular disease
  - Heart diseases
    - Left ventricular hypertrophy
    - Angina or prior myocardial infarction
    - Prior coronary revascularization
    - Heart failure
  - Stroke or transient ischemic attack
  - Nephropathy
  - Peripheral arterial disease
  - Retinopathy

SOURCE: From JNC VI,[74] with permission.

1996,[79] which proved to be quite controversial.[80,81] Finally, the AHA has issued several related scientific statements regarding cholesterol assessment and management as a primary preventive measure for individuals without CHD[82] or as a secondary measure for those who do have CHD.[83,84] The AHA guidelines are in close agreement with those of the NCEP, and the key recommendations of the latter are presented.

As with the hypertension guidelines discussed previously, the NCEP recommends a comprehensive assessment of overall cardiovascular risk as the basis for clinical decision making. The risk factors to be assessed are shown in Table 97-7 and are slightly different from the risk factors listed in Table 97-5, though the broad overlap between the two lists is apparent. Note that a high level of high-density lipoprotein (HDL) cholesterol is considered a "negative risk factor." That is, an individual with an HDL cholesterol above 60 mg/dL may be treated as if he or she had one fewer other risk factors.

The key treatment recommendations of the NCEP are summarized in Table 97-8. Note that treatment is to be based on the level of low-density lipoprotein (LDL) cholesterol rather than on the total cholesterol. For patients at greatest risk for future morbid events—those with established CHD—the goal of treatment is the achievement of an LDL cholesterol of ≤100 mg/dL through a combination of dietary and drug therapy. For those without established CHD but with two or more risk factors (Table 97-7), the LDL goal is <130 mg/dL. For individuals at low risk, the LDL goal is <160 mg/dL. Differential thresholds for the initiation of drug and dietary therapy are recommended. This approach is echoed in the AHA statements.

The dietary therapy recommended by the NCEP is summarized by the Step I and Step II Diets.[78] The Step I Diet, recommended by the AHA for the general population, is characterized by a total dietary fat intake of <30 percent of total calories, with <10 percent of total calories derived from saturated fat. Dietary cholesterol should be limited to <300 mg per day. The Step II Diet calls for a reduction in total calories derived from saturated fat to <8 percent and a reduction in dietary cholesterol to <200 mg per day.

The NCEP guidelines were issued prior to the availability of clinical trials evidence demonstrating the efficacy of HMG-CoA reductase inhibitors (statins) in reducing mortality and morbidity from CHD.[70] These data were the basis for the recommendations in the AHA statements that statin drugs are the first choice for lowering LDL cholesterol in those individuals identified as candidates for drug treatment provided that they have no specific contraindications to the medications and their tryglyceride levels are below 400 mg/dL.[84]

DIABETES MELLITUS

The assessment and management of this complex disease is beyond the scope of this chapter. However, insofar as diabetes is a major risk factor for the development of cardiovascular disease, the recommendations of the AHA for diabetes management as a means of both primary[82] and secondary[84] prevention of CHD are quite simple. Both documents call for "appropriate hypoglycemic therapy to achieve near normal fasting plasma glucose as indicated by HbA1c" and "treatment of other risk factors" in accord with other guidelines.

Addressing a related issue, the ACC and the American Diabetes Association have issued a joint statement of recommendations for diagnosing CHD in patients with diabetes.[85]

CIGARETTE SMOKING

The link between cigarette smoking and cardiovascular disease is firmly established. Smoking cessation is therefore an important component of risk-factor modification for the prevention of cardiovascular disease. The definitive guideline on smoking cessation was produced by the AHCPR.[86] This provides extensive background information and a careful review of the efficacy of available methods of promoting smoking cessation. A much more concise document, in the form of a science advisory from

TABLE 97-6 Risk Stratification and Treatment of High Blood Pressure

	Risk Group		
Blood Pressure Stage	A	B	C
High-normal	Lifestyle modification	Lifestyle modification	Drug therapy[a]
1	Lifestyle modification (up to 12 months)	Lifestyle modification (up to 6 months)[b]	Drug therapy
2	Drug therapy	Drug therapy	Drug therapy

Risk group A: No risk factors; no target-organ damage or clinical cadiovascular disease.
Risk group B: At least one risk factor not including diabetes mellitus; no target-organ damage or clinical cardiovascular disease.
Risk group C: Target-organ damage or clinical cardiovascular disease and/or diabetes mellitus, with or without other risk factors.
[a]Consider drug therapy as initial therapy if multiple risk factors present.
[b]For those with heart failure, renal insufficiency, or diabete mellitus.
SOURCE: From JNC VI,[74] with permission.

TABLE 97-7 Non-LDL-Cholesterol Risk Factors for CHD Identified by the National Cholesterol Education Program

Positive risk factors
- Age: male ≥45 years; female ≥55 (or premature menopause without hormone replacement)
- Family history: premature (<55 years in men, <65 years in women) CHD in first-order relative
- Current cigarette smoking
- Hypertension: blood pressure ≥140/90 or use of antihypertensive medication
- Low HDL cholesterol: <35 mg/dL
- Diabetes mellitus

Negative risk factor
- High HDL cholesterol: ≥60 mg/dL

SOURCE: From the Expert Panel on Detection, Evaluation, and Treatment of High Blood Cholesterol in Adults,[78] with permission.

TABLE 97-8 Treatment Recommendations of the National Cholesterol Education Program

Patient Category	LDL Level at Which to Initiate Treatment mg/dL		
	Dietary Treatment	Drug Treatment	LDL Goal, mg/dL
No CHD and fewer than two risk factors	≥160	≥190	<160
No CHD and two or more risk factors	≥130	≥160	<130
Established CHD	>100	≥130[a]	≤100

[a]Drug therapy should be considered if the LDL cholesterol is between 100 and 129 mg/dL.

SOURCE: From the Expert Panel on Detection, Evaluation, and Treatment of High Blood Cholesterol in Adults,[78] with permission.

the AHA,[87] is a useful reference for most physicians. Although science advisories are not labeled as "practice guidelines" by the AHA, they fulfill the definition of a practice guideline offered earlier in this chapter and so are considered here. The AHA advisory recommends the following smoking cessation steps:

- Every smoker should be counseled to quit on every physician office visit; maintenance should be discussed with all ex-smokers.
- Every patient should be asked about tobacco use.
- Clinicians should receive training in smoking cessation counseling.
- Office systems to facilitate cessation programs should be established.

The "minimal intervention" to promote smoking cessation should include the following elements:

- Asking about smoking
- Recommending cessation
- Helping those who want to quit through the provision of educational materials, referral to specialists, or other community resources
- Scheduling a quit date
- Arranging for follow-up

Although the authors acknowledge the barriers to successful smoking cessation, they review a large body of evidence supporting the efficacy of the recommended interventions.

OBESITY

Obesity is defined by the National Heart Lung and Blood Institute of the National Institutes of Health (NIH) as a body mass index—BMI = [weight (kg)/height (m)^2]—of 30 kg/m^2 or more; overweight is defined as a BMI of 25 to 29.9 kg/m^2.[88] Although traditionally considered to increase the risk of CHD only through its influence on other risk factors such as hypertension, hyperlipidemia, and diabetes, obesity is now recognized as a risk factor for CHD in its own right.[89] In addition to the NIH guidelines, the American Association of Clinical Endocrinologists (AACE) and the American College of Endocrinology (ACE) have jointly issued a position statement on obesity.[90] The NIH guidelines are summarized here. The principal recommendations are:

- The use of the BMI as a tool to assess overweight and obesity
- Comprehensive assessment of other cardiovascular risk factors
- The establishment of clear goals for weight loss, with an initial goal of a 10 percent reduction in body weight, followed by additional weight loss as needed and an ongoing weight maintenance program
- Weight loss should be achieved primarily through the reduction of dietary calories
- Physical activity should be part of a comprehensive weight reduction program
- Drug therapy with FDA-approved agents should be considered for those individuals with a BMI ≥30
- Weight loss surgery should be considered for individuals with severe obesity, defined as a BMI >40, or a BMI >35 in the presence of other significant comorbidities

PHYSICAL INACTIVITY

As is the case with obesity, physical inactivity is an independent risk factor for coronary artery disease.[91] Two important guidelines have formulated recommendations for increasing the general level of physical activity among the general population. The Consensus Statement of the NIH, while not presented as a formal guideline, reports as its intent "to advance understanding of the . . . issue in question and to be useful to health professionals and the public"[92] and so fulfills the definition of a generic guideline. The Statement on Exercise of the AHA[91] is a conceptually similar document.

The NIH document states that "All Americans should engage in regular physical activity at a level appropriate to their capacity, needs and interest. Children and adults alike should set a goal of accumulating at least 30 minutes of moderate-intensity physical activity on most, and preferably, all days of the week."[92]

The AHA recommendations are very similar: ". . . dynamic exercise of the large muscles for extended periods of time (30–60 minutes, three to six times weekly) is recommended. This may include short periods of moderate intensity . . . that total 30 minutes on most days."[91]

Screening for Cardiovascular Diseases

There are few nationally recognized clinical practice guidelines that primarily address the issue of screening for cardiovascular disease in the asymptomatic population. The use of specific technologies that are sometimes used as screening tools is discussed later in this chapter. This section addresses the recommendations for screening per se. All of the guidelines in this section are part of the *Guide to Clinical Preventive Services,* a comprehensive document dealing with the detection and prevention of a broad range of conditions, which was developed by the U.S. Preventive Services Task Force.[93]

CORONARY ARTERY DISEASE

Screening for coronary disease among asymptomatic individuals was not recommended. The guideline states:

> There is insufficient evidence to recommend for or against screening middle-aged and older men and women for asymptomatic coronary artery disease. . . . Recommendations against routine screening can be made on other grounds for individuals who are not at high risk of developing clinical heart disease. Routine screening is not recommended as part of the periodic health visit or preparticipation sports examination for children, adolescents, or young adults.[93]

The guideline left open the question of the utility of screening individuals at high risk, stating that such screening would be justified if the results would influence treatment. The task force also found that screening individuals in certain occupations (e.g., airline pilots) may be justified on public health grounds.

CAROTID ARTERY STENOSIS

The U.S. Preventive Services Task Force recommendations regarding screening for asymptomatic carotid artery stenosis are very similar to those regarding screening for coronary artery disease.[94] The guidelines state that there is insufficient evidence to recommend for or against general screening, whether by ultrasound or other techniques. Rather, they recommend discussing the potential value of screening with patients who may be at high risk. Even that recommendation is qualified, in that it applies only if high-quality vascular surgery (defined as surgical mortality and morbidity from carotid endarterectomy of less than 3 percent) is available.

ABDOMINAL AORTIC ANEURYSM

Screening for abdominal aortic aneurysm is the third and final cardiovascular condition addressed by the screening guidelines of the U.S. Preventive Services Task Force.[95] Here again, they report that there is insufficient evidence to recommend for or against routine screening. While stating that there is no evidence, even in high-risk populations, that screening leads to lower morbidity and mortality, the guidelines concede that clinicians may wish to screen selected high-risk patients because of the significant prevalence of the disease and the efficacy of surgical repair. Screening is recommended only for patients who are candidates for abdominal surgery, regardless of their risk.

Established Cardiovascular Conditions

There are five broad cardiovascular conditions for which well-formulated clinical practice guidelines have been written. These are atrial fibrillation, chronic stable angina, heart failure, myocardial infarction, and valvular heart disease. The AHCPR also issued clinical practice guidelines for unstable angina,[96] but these were published in 1994, and the approach to unstable angina has progressed very rapidly since that time. As a result, those guidelines are not included here.

ATRIAL FIBRILLATION

The best guidelines available for the approach to patients with atrial fibrillation are those that were prepared by a committee sponsored by the AHA.[97] Although the document produced was not formally labeled a practice guideline, it contains specific evidence-based recommendations intended to guide clinical practice.

The guideline establishes three therapeutic goals for each patient with atrial fibrillation: rate control, maintenance of sinus rhythm, and the prevention of thromboembolism. The first goal should be achieved for all patients, whereas the approach to the other two requires a careful weighing of individualized risks and benefits. The recommendations for achieving each of these goals are presented below.

Rate Control Control of the ventricular response to atrial fibrillation avoids a tachycardia-induced myopathy and reduces patients' symptoms.[97] It can be achieved by pharmacologic or nonpharmacologic means. The guidelines recommend the intravenous use of verapamil, diltiazem, or a beta blocker for acute rate control and the same drugs in oral formulations for chronic use. They state that digoxin is less effective and should be considered a front-line agent only in patients who also have congestive heart failure and also that some patients will require combination therapy. Nonpharmacologic rate control can be achieved with catheter ablation or modification of the AV node.

Maintanence of Sinus Rhythm Sinus rhythm preserves atrioventricular synchrony, maintains cardiac output, and reduces symptoms associated with an irregular rhythm. Restoration of sinus rhythm may also reduce the risk of future thromoboembolic events. Despite these important goals, there are few data to guide rational clinical decision making regarding overall strategies of cardioversion and antiarrhythmic drug therapy. The document states that the "selection of an antiarrhythmic agent should be individualized and will depend in part on renal and hepatic function, concomitant illnesses and drugs, and cardiovascular function."[97]

Preventing Thromboembolism The guidelines recommend identifying patients with atrial fibrillation who are at high risk for stroke based on the presence of one or more "high-risk variables." These are age >65 years, hypertension, prior stroke or transient ischemic attack (TIA), diabetes, or recent heart failure. Individuals at high risk should be treated with warfarin titrated to an International Normalized Ratio (INR) of 2.0 to 3.0. Low-risk patients may be treated with 325 mg of aspirin daily. For all individuals who are undergoing elective cardioversion by electrical or pharmacologic means, anticoagulants should be administered for at least 3 weeks prior and 4 weeks after.

CHRONIC STABLE ANGINA

Definitive guidelines for the management of patients with chronic stable angina were recently published.[98] These are particularly valuable because they represent the collaborative effort not just of the ACC and the AHA but also of the American College of Physicians—American Society of Internal Medicine (ACP-ASIM).

The guidelines clearly specify a rational, evidence-based approach to the patient with angina, beginning with establishing the diagnosis. A useful classification of chest pain is presented to aid the clinician in determining the risk of ischemic heart disease. Chest pain should be considered (definite) angina if it:

1. Is substernal in location, with a characteristic quality and duration
2. Is provoked by exertion or emotional stress
3. Is relieved by rest or nitroglycerin

Chest pain that fulfills two of the preceding criteria is considered probable or atypical angina and chest pain that meets one or fewer of the criteria is considered noncardiac chest pain, not angina.

The assessment of patients presenting with chest pain is outlined in a flow diagram (Fig. 97-1). The key elements of the assessment algorithm are the risk stratification of the patient on clinical grounds; the exclusion of other, related conditions such as unstable angina or acute myocardial infarction; and the evaluation of possible precipitating factors, such as anemia and hyperthyroidism. Those patients who, after such an assessment, are thought to have a high probability of coronary artery disease are then candidates for the treatment algorithms specifying the approach to stress testing and angiography (Fig. 97-2) and treatment (Fig. 97-3).

The guidelines recommend (class I) cardiac catheterization and coronary angiography for a particular subset of patients with chronic stable angina. They include patients with

- Disabling chronic stable angina (Canadian Cardiovascular Society classes III and IV) despite medical therapy
- High-risk criteria on noninvasive testing regardless of anginal severity
- Angina who have survived sudden cardiac death or have serious ventricular arrhythmias
- Angina and symptoms and signs of congestive heart failure
- Clinical characteristics that indicate a high likelihood of severe coronary artery disease

Pharmacologic treatment of patients with angina (Fig. 97-3) should be directed at reducing symptoms as well as lowering the risk of future ischemic events. The key elements of the treatment include:

- Aspirin unless specifically contraindicated
- Beta blockers unless specifically contraindicated
- Calcium antagonists and/or long-acting nitrates when beta blockers are contraindicated, fail to control symptoms, or are associated with intolerable side effects
- Sublingual nitroglycerin or nitroglycerin spray for the immediate relief of angina
- Lipid-lowering therapy for appropriate patients (see guidelines for hyperlipidemia, above)

In addition to the medications specified above, the guidelines urge a comprehensive treatment plan according to the following mnemonic:

A. Aspirin and antianginals
B. Beta blockers and blood pressure control
C. Cigarette smoking cessation and cholesterol reduction
D. Diet and diabetes control
E. Education and exercise

Intensive efforts at risk factor identification and modification are considered essential elements of the treatment of all patients with chronic angina, and the spe-

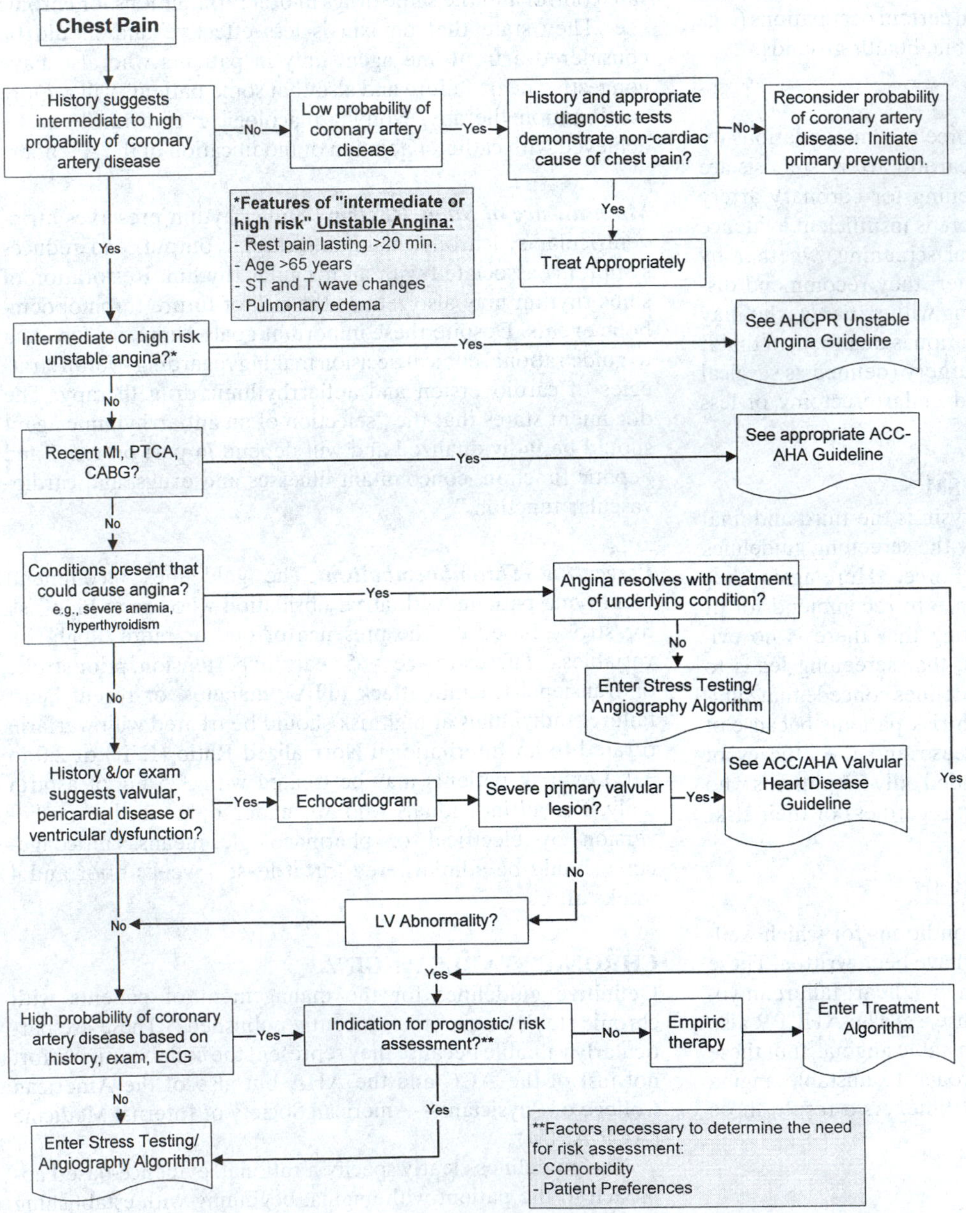

FIGURE 97-1 Algorithm for the clinical assessment of patients with chest pain. (From Gibbons et al.,[98] with permission.)

cific recommendations follow the guidelines for risk factor modification discussed earlier in this chapter.

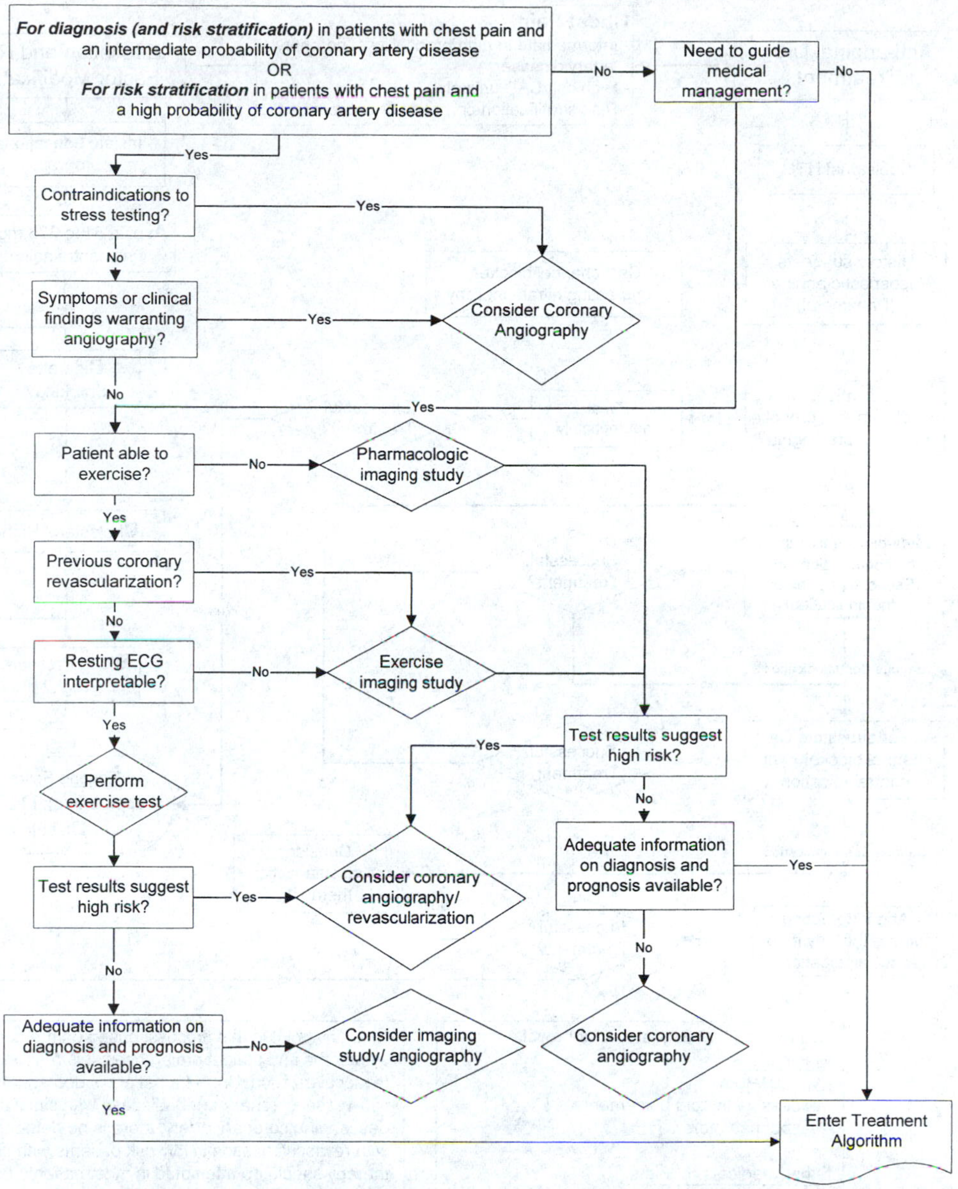

FIGURE 97-2 Algorithm for the use of stress testing and angiography in patients with angina. (From Gibbons et al.,[98] with permission.)

HEART FAILURE

Two major guidelines exist to help the clinician in the care of patients with congestive heart failure and/or depressed left ventricular function. The AHCPR published its guidelines in 1994.[42] The ACC and AHA published their joint guidelines in 1995.[99] Both documents address the role of diagnostic testing in heart failure and make recommendations about appropriate pharmacologic therapy.

Diagnostic Testing For patients with chronic or stabilized heart failure, the ACC/AHA guidelines identify the following elements of the diagnostic workup as class I:

- Complete blood count and urinalysis
- Blood serum: electrolytes, blood urea nitrogen, creatinine, glucose, phosphorus, magnesium, calcium, and albumin levels
- Thyroid-stimulating hormone levels
- Chest radiograph and electrocardiogram
- Transthoracic echocardiogram
- Noninvasive stress testing to detect ischemia in patients who would be candidates for revascularization
- Coronary arteriography in patients with a previous infarction who would be candidates for revascularization
- Cardiac catheterization and coronary arteriography in patients with angina, those with large areas of ischemia on noninvasive testing and those at risk for CHD who are undergoing surgical correction of noncoronary cardiac lesions

The AHCPR guidelines are generally consistent with these recommendations. Among the diagnostic tests and procedures that are not *routinely* recommended by either guidelines (although allowances are made for exceptions) are:

- Endomyocardial biopsy
- Multiple echocardiograms or radionuclide ventriculograms as a means of routine follow-up
- Holter monitoring or signal-averaged electrocardiography

Pharmacologic Treatment The two major guidelines are also very similar in their recommendations regarding drug treatment for heart failure. The class I recommendations of the ACC/AHA are:

- Angiotensin converting enzyme (ACE) inhibitors for all patients with reduced left ventricular ejection fraction unless contraindicated
- Hydralazine and isosorbide dinitrate in patients who cannot take ACE inhibitors
- Digoxin in patients with heart failure due to systolic dysfunction not adequately responsive to ACE inhibitors and diuretic drugs
- Digoxin in patients with atrial fibrillation and rapid ventricular rates
- Diuretic drugs for patients with fluid overload

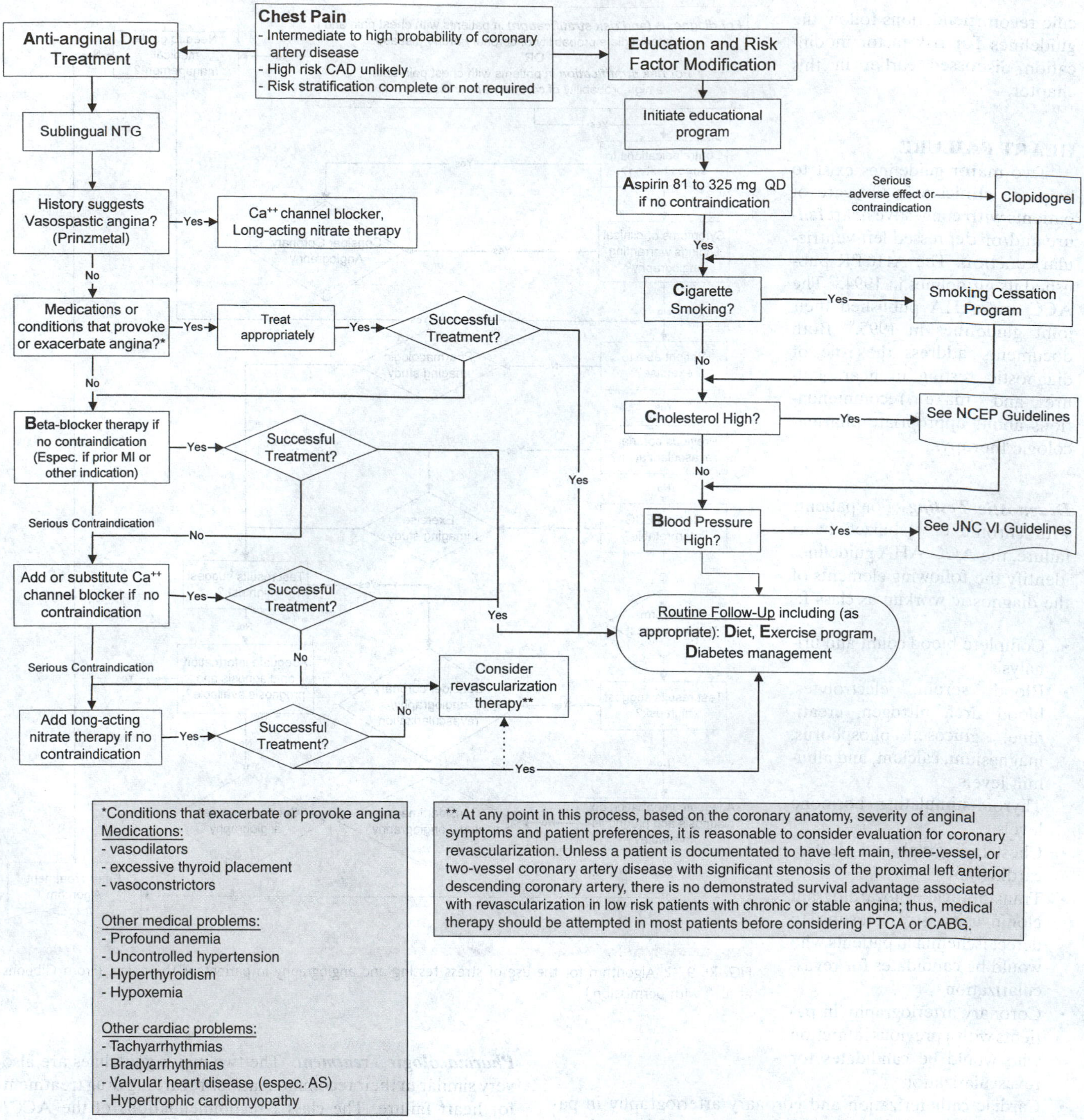

FIGURE 97-3 Algorithm for the treatment of chronic stable angina. (From Gibbons et al.,[98] with permission.)

- Anticoagulation in patients with atrial fibrillation or a previous history of systemic or pulmonary embolism
- Beta blockers for high risk patients after an acute myocardial infarction

Note that the routine use of beta blockers was not recommended in these guidelines. Newer evidence in support of the use of these agents is reviewed in Chap. 21. Among the treatments that are not recommended by the ACC/AHA (class III) are:

- Drugs with positive inotropic effect in the absence of systolic dysfunction
- Treatment of asymptomatic arrhythmias

The AHCPR guidelines also indicate that routine anticoagulation of heart failure patients is not indicated.

MYOCARDIAL INFARCTION

The ACC/AHA guidelines for the care of acute myocardial infarction are the most definitive and up to date. These were originally published in 1990,[100] revised in 1996,[59] and updated again in 1999.[101] The most important class I recommendations from the 1999 guideline update are presented.

With regard to prehospital and initial emergency department management, the following are class I recommendations:

- Availability of 911 emergency access
- Availability of emergency medical services with the capability of defibrillating patients in the field
- Emergency department standards to assure clinical evaluation of patients at risk for myocardial infarction (MI) within 10 min of hospital arrival and thrombolysis (if indicated) within 30 min
- Oxygen for all patients with pulmonary congestion or demonstrated arterial desaturation
- Aspirin for all patients without clear contraindication
- Intravenous nitroglycerin for the first 24 to 48 h in patients with CHF, large anterior infarcts, persistent ischemia, or hypertension

Strategies for early coronary revascularization are also highlighted. Pharmacologic thrombolysis and direct coronary angioplasty are considered alternative therapies, based on locally available resources and expertise. Class I indications for thrombolysis include:

- ST elevation >0.1 mV in two or more contiguous leads, time to therapy 12 h or less, and age less than 75 years
- Bundle branch block that obscures ST analysis and clinical history suggestive of acute infarction

Class I indications for primary angioplasty are:

- As an alternative to thrombolysis in patients who meet the same electrocardiographic criteria, in whom the procedure can be performed within 90 min (time to balloon inflation) of presentation, by operators who perform ≥75 procedures per year in centers that perform ≥200 procedures per year and have cardiac surgical programs
- In patients who are within 36 h of infarction and develop cardiogenic shock and in whom revascularization can be accomplished within 18 h of the development of shock

The class I indications for emergent or urgent coronary artery bypass graft surgery are:

- Failed angioplasty with persistent pain or hemodynamic instability, given suitable coronary anatomy
- Persistent or refractory ischemia in patients who are not suitable candidates for percutaneous intervention
- Coincident CABG at the time of surgical repair of postinfarction ventricular septal defect (VSD) or mitral regurgitation

Key pharmacologic therapy (class I) for patients with acute infarction, beyond the use of thrombolytics are:

- Heparin in all patients undergoing percutaneous or surgical revascularization
- Early (intravenous) beta blockers for patients without contraindications who can be treated within 12 h, or who have continuing or recurrent ischemia or tachyarrhythmias
- ACE inhibitors within 24 h in patients with anterior infarctions, clinical heart failure, or demonstrated left ventricular systolic dysfunction (ejection fraction <40 percent)

Of note, there are no class I indications for calcium channel blockers or magnesium, so that these agents should not be considered part of the routine management of MI patients. Secondary prevention—the long-term, postdischarge management of MI patients—is also addressed by the guidelines. The critical class I indications for secondary prevention include:

- Management of lipids, through the initiation of the Step II Diet in all patients, and the use of lipid-lowering agents in patients with an LDL cholesterol of >125 mg/dL
- Long-term use of beta blockers in all but low-risk patients
- Long-term use of aspirin in all patients
- Long-term anticoagulation in patients unable to take aspirin and in those with atrial fibrillation or left ventricular thrombus

The guidelines also address the indications for coronary angiography and revascularization in patients who did not undergo primary angioplasty. Such a strategy is not recommended as a routine procedure after successful thrombolysis but is indicated in the presence of:

- Spontaneous or easily provoked ischemia early after infarction
- Hemodynamic instability
- A planned repair of a mechanical complication of infarction (VSD, mitral regurgitation)

VALVULAR HEART DISEASE

There are few areas of clinical decision making in cardiology as complex as the assessment and management of patients with valvular heart disease. The reader is referred to Chaps. 55 through 58 for a comprehensive discussion of the approach to particular valvular lesions, since the complexity of their management precludes a complete discussion here. This section briefly presents some of the key elements of the ACC/AHA guideline pertaining to valvular heart disease.[102]

Class I indications for the assessment of patients with known or suspected valvular heart disease include the following:

- Echocardiography for diastolic, continuous, holosystolic, or loud systolic murmurs, or in patients with murmurs and signs or symptoms of heart failure, ischemia or endocarditis
- Catheterization prior to valve replacement surgery

Specific indications for the use of percutaneous balloon valvotomy for aortic stenosis and mitral stenosis are presented. There are no class I indications for balloon aortic valvotomy, and it should not be considered a satisfactory alternative to surgery for aortic valve replacement. Mitral valvotomy is indicated (class I) in symptomatic patients with a mitral valve area of <1.5 cm^2 and valvular morphology favorable to balloon valvotomy as long as there is no atrial thrombus present and no significant mitral regurgitation.

The guidelines present useful flow diagrams to aid the clinician in dealing with particularly challenging circumstances, such as determining the appropriate timing for valve repair or replacement in patients with chronic mitral regurgitation (Fig. 97-4) and chronic aortic regurgitation (Fig. 97-5).

The use of anticoagulants in patients with prosthetic heart valves is also discussed. Class I indications for the use of warfarin include:

- All patients for the first 3 months following valve replacement surgery (INR 2.5 to 3.5)
- Mechanical aortic or mitral prosthesis

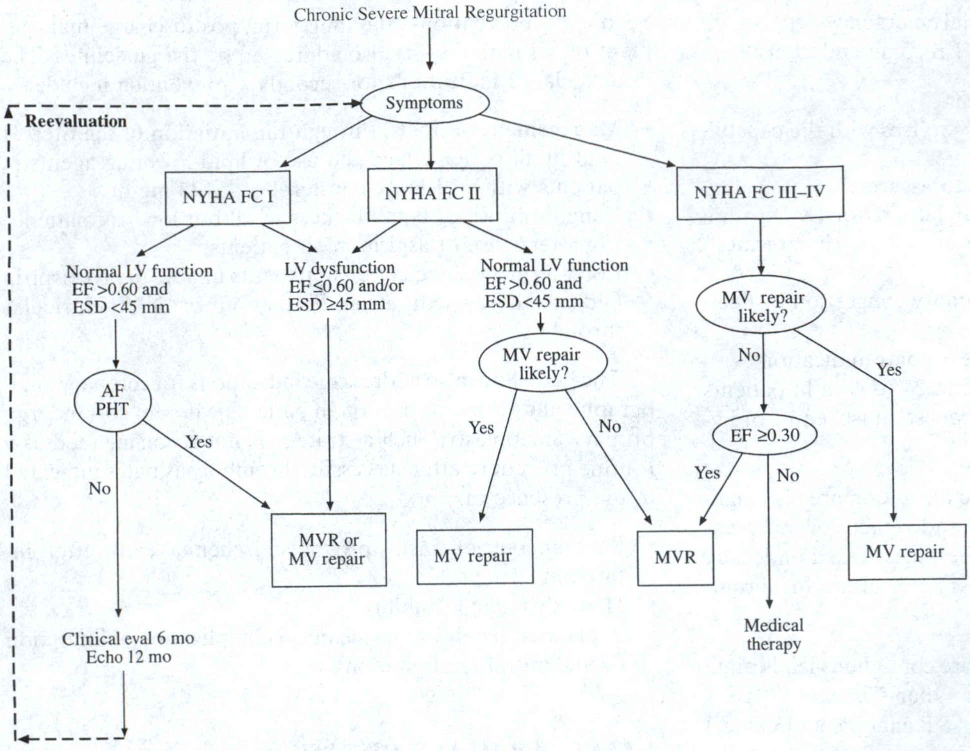

FIGURE 97-4 Algorithm for the management of patients with chronic severe mitral regurgitation. AF, atrial fibrillation; EF, ejection fraction; ESD, end-systolic diameter; FC, functional class; MV, mitral valve; NYHA, New York Heart Association; PHT, pulmonary hypertension. (From Bonow et al.,[102] with permission.)

- Bioprosthetic aortic or mitral valve in the presence of atrial fibrillation, left ventricular dysfunction, previous thromboembolism, or hypercoagulable state

Use of Cardiovascular Technology

Cardiovascular medicine is extremely technology-intensive and is becoming more so with the continuous development of new and highly sophisticated techniques for patient assessment and treatment. This section presents the highlights of clinical practice guidelines that have been developed to aid physicians in the rational use of this technology. There are national guidelines on exercise testing, echocardiography, coronary angiography, and electrophysiologic testing. We also present recommendations for risk-stratifying patients with known or suspected cardiac disease prior to noncardiac surgery, since this risk assessment often depends on the use of the other technologies discussed.

EXERCISE TESTING

The most authoritative practice guidelines for exercise testing are a product of the ACC/AHA Task Force on Practice Guidelines.[103] Those guidelines describe the following class I indications:

- As a diagnostic tool in patients with an intermediate pretest probability of coronary artery disease (CAD) and an electrocardiogram with less than 1 mm of resting ST-segment depression
- As a means of risk assessment in patients with known or suspected CAD
- Before discharge following myocardial infarction, for prognosis, assessment of medical therapy, or activity prescription
- Evaluation of exercise capacity in patients with heart failure
- Demonstration of ischemia prior to planned coronary revascularization or reassessment of symptoms following revascularization
- Identification of appropriate programmable parameters for patients with rate-adaptive pacemakers

The ACC/AHA Task Force has also produced guidelines for the use of radionuclide imaging in both with and without exercise testing,[104] as has the Society of Nuclear Medicine.[105]

ECHOCARDIOGRAPHY

There is considerable overlap between the previously discussed ACC/AHA guideline on valvular heart disease[102] and the ACC/AHA guideline devoted specifically to the use of echocardiography.[106] Once again, key class I indications for the use of echocardiography are presented:

- Evaluation of heart murmurs in symptomatic patients or in patients whose murmur has a moderate probability of reflecting structural heart disease
- Assessment of hemodynamic severity of known valvular lesions
- Evaluation of the patient with known or suspected endocarditis in order to assess the degree of hemodynamic compromise or to detect and characterize vegetations
- Evaluation of patients with known valvular lesions (or prosthetic valves) who have a change in functional status
- Evaluation of left ventricular function in ischemic heart disease, heart failure, or symptoms suggestive of either
- Evaluation of suspected pericardial disease, including trauma, constriction, pericarditis, or pericardial tamponade
- Evaluation of possible cardiac masses
- Evaluation of possible aortic dissection, aneurysm, or rupture (may be best accomplished via transesophageal techniques)
- Evaluation of pulmonary hypertension and/or suspected pulmonary embolism
- Search for a cardiac source of systemic or cerebral embolism
- Evaluation of possible underlying structural heart disease in patients with arrhythmias or syncope

Additional class I indications are listed for the evaluation of critically ill or hemodynamically unstable patients as well as patients with congenital heart disease.

CORONARY ANGIOGRAPHY

Cardiac catheterization is performed more than a million times per year in the United States, and the frequency of its use continues to grow.[107] The ACC/AHA guidelines on coronary angiography[107] seek to provide a framework for the appropriate use of this technique. The class I indications for coronary angiography include:

- Canadian Cardiovascular Society class III or IV angina despite medical therapy
- High-risk criteria on noninvasive testing, including depressed left ventricular function, a large stress-induced (especially anterior) perfusion defect, or a strongly positive treadmill exercise test
- Resuscitation following an episode of sudden cardiac death
- Unstable angina (in high- or intermediate-risk patients) that has not fully responded to medical therapy
- Recurrent symptoms within 9 months of prior percutaneous coronary intervention
- As an alternative to thrombolytic therapy for acute MI (if done with an intent to perform percutaneous transluminal coronary angioplasty)
- Spontaneous or easily provoked ischemia in the immediate postinfarction period or as a precursor to the surgical repair of a mechanical complication of acute infarction
- Hemodynamic instability in the peri- or immediate postinfarction period
- Prior to valve surgery or balloon valvotomy in patients with ischemic symptoms or at high risk for CAD
- Prior to surgical correction of congenital heart disease in patients at high risk for CAD on the basis of symptoms, risk factors, or particular congenital lesions
- Heart failure due to systolic dysfunction with noninvasive evidence of underlying CAD

The preceding list is not exhaustive, either in its presentation of indications considered by the guidelines or in terms of other settings when coronary angiography may be appropriate. As the guidelines themselves state: "This report is not intended to provide strict indications and contraindications for coronary angiography because, in the individual patient, multiple other considerations may be relevant, including the family setting, occupational needs, and individual lifestyle preferences."[107]

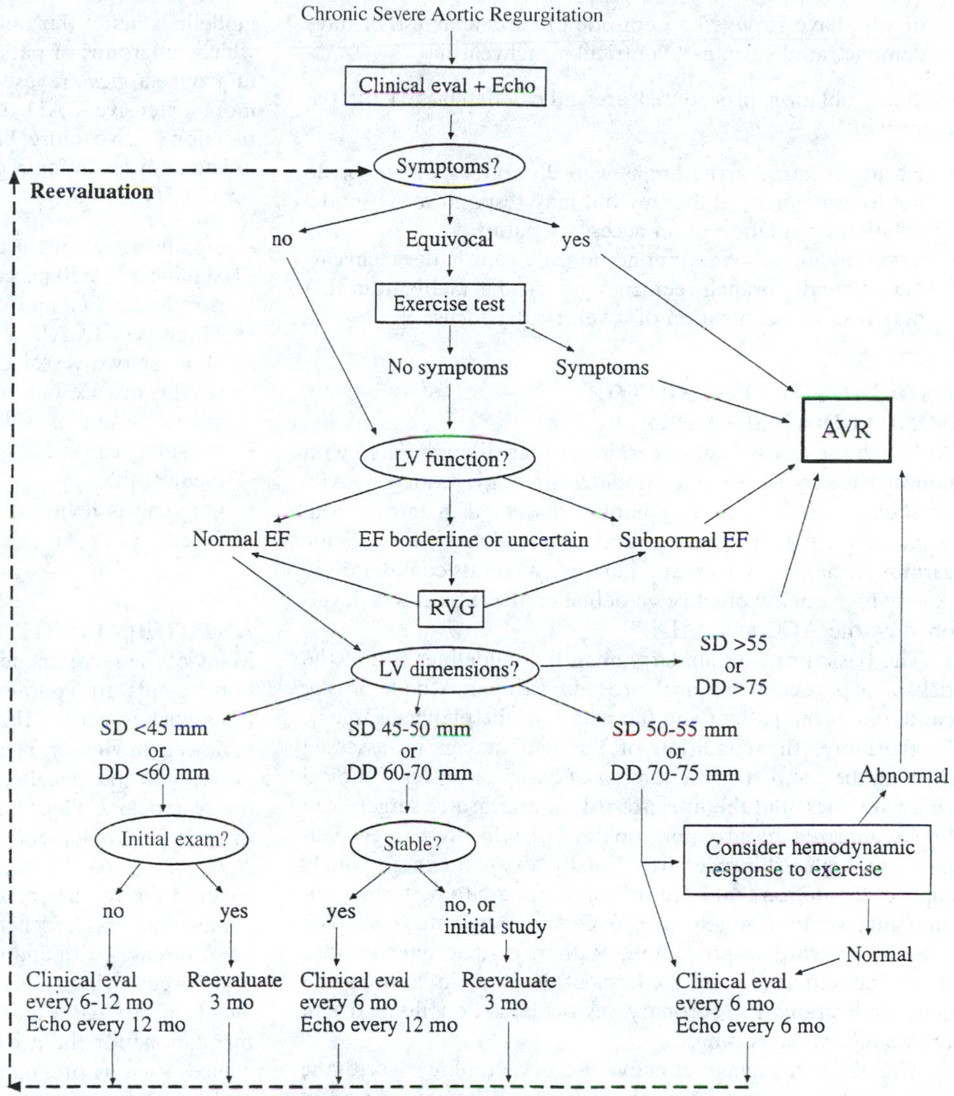

FIGURE 97-5 Algorithm for the management of patients with chronic severe aortic regurgitation. DD, end-diastolic dimension; RVG, radionuclide ventriculography; SD, end-systolic dimension. (From Bonow et al.,[102] with permission.)

ELECTROPHYSIOLOGIC TESTING

The North American Society of Pacing and Electrophysiology, the American College of Cardiology, and the AHA collaborated to produce guidelines for invasive electrophysiologic testing and catheter ablation procedures, which were published in 1995.[108] Class I indications for electrophysiologic testing identified by the guidelines include patients with

- Sinus node dysfunction as the suspected cause of symptoms
- Second- or third-degree AV block who remain symptomatic following pacemaker insertion and in whom another arrhythmia is suspected as the cause of symptoms
- Narrow QRS complex tachycardias who do not respond to or do not tolerate medical therapy
- The Wolff-Parkinson-White syndrome who have survived an episode of cardiac arrest, have unexplained syncope, or are candidates for ablation of an accessory pathway
- Suspected structural heart disease with unexplained syncope,

or who have survived an episode of cardiac arrest, or have demonstrated sustained ventricular tachycardia

Catheter ablation procedures are indicated (class I) for patients with

- Recurrent atrial arrhythmias who do not respond to or do not tolerate medical therapy but may respond to AV nodal ablation or ablation of an accessory pathway
- Symptomatic sustained monomorphic ventricular tachycardia or bundle branch reentrant ventricular tachycardia that may respond to ablation of a ventricular focus

CARDIAC EVALUATION FOR NONCARDIAC SURGERY

Although the assessment of cardiovascular risk associated with noncardiac surgery is not a specific technology, it draws heavily on the use of the other techniques discussed in this section. In addition, it is a major clinical responsibility of practicing cardiovascular specialists and therefore warrants consideration. A very high quality practice guideline on the subject was developed by the ACC and AHA.[60]

The basic principle underpinning the guidelines is that the risk of a particular surgical procedure depends both on the condition of the patient and the nature of the planned surgery. Furthermore, the condition of the patient can be assessed through the use of a small number of easily ascertained clinical characteristics, and the intrinsic risk of noncardiac surgery can be summarized by grouping operations into low-, intermediate-, and high-risk procedures. Finally, the guidelines strongly support the notion that it is rarely appropriate to perform coronary interventions solely to reduce the anticipated risk of a planned noncardiac procedure. Rather, cardiac interventions should be undertaken on the basis of the same indications and contraindications for coronary revascularization that exist in the nonoperative setting.

The guidelines make effective use of a graphic, algorithmic approach to risk assessment that has also been reproduced in pocket form as a quick reference. The principal algorithm is reproduced as Fig. 97-6. High-risk surgical procedures include emergent major operations, aortic and major vascular procedures, and those anticipated to involve large shifts of fluids or prolonged time under anesthesia. Intermediate-risk procedures include carotid endarterectomy as well as orthopedic and prostate operations. Low-risk surgeries include cataract extractions, breast procedures, and endoscopies.

Specific Interventions and Treatments

The range of specific cardiovascular interventions and therapies for which specific guidelines exist is broad. The following four areas were chosen to illustrate this range: CABG, the use of antithrombotic therapies, the implantation of cardiac pacemakers and antiarrhythmia devices, and the use of cardiac rehabilitation programs.

CORONARY ARTERY BYPASS GRAFT SURGERY

As the ACC/AHA guidelines on the subject state, "CABG surgery is among the most common operations performed in the world and accounts for more resources expended in cardiovascular medicine than any other single procedure."[109] The guidelines detail the randomized trial evidence that identifies which subgroups of patients with CAD derive the most benefit from surgical revascularization. In general, patients with more extensive CAD and depressed left ventricular systolic function derive more benefit than similar patients with less ischemia or less impaired ventricles. Specific class I indications for CABG include:

- Significant left main coronary artery stenosis
- Significant (≥70 percent) stenosis of the proximal left anterior descending and proximal left circumflex arteries
- Three-vessel CAD
- One- or two-vessel CAD without left anterior descending (LAD) disease but with a large area of viable myocardium at risk on noninvasive testing
- Disabling chronic angina or ongoing unstable angina despite medical therapy
- Ongoing ischemia or hemodynamic instability following a failed PTCA

ANTITHROMBOTIC THERAPY

Many of the recommendations regarding the use of antithrombotic agents are contained in guidelines for particular conditions, such as acute MI and atrial fibrillation, which have been reviewed previously. They are mentioned here primarily to draw attention to the excellent compilation of recommendations by the American College of Chest Physicians. These were detailed in a special supplement to *Chest*[110] and summarized in the *Quick Reference Guide for Clinicians* in 1999.[111] Among the subjects covered are the use of antithrombotic agents in the following conditions: CAD, ischemic stroke, atrial fibrillation, valvular heart disease (with and without prosthetic valves), and peripheral vascular disease. In addition, the role of antithrombotic agents after CABG and PTCA is reviewed, along with recommendations for the use of these agents under special circumstances such as pregnancy, and the management of excessive anticoagulation.

PACEMAKERS AND ANTIARRHYTHMIC DEVICES

The guidelines for the use of these devices come from the ACC and the AHA.[112] Class I indications for the implantation of a permanent pacemaker generally depend on the presence of a bradycardic rhythm and an established connection between the rhythm and symptoms. These include:

- Third-degree AV block associated with:
  —Symptomatic bradycardia, or the need for drugs (for other conditions) that induce symptomatic bradycardia
  —Periods of asystole ≥3 s or an escape rate <40 beats per minute (even in the absence of symptoms)
  —Postoperative AV block not expected to resolve
  —Neuromuscular disorders with associated AV block
- Second-degree AV block with associated symptomatic bradycardia
- Intermittent third-degree AV block or type II second-degree AV block with chronic bifascicular or trifascicular block
- Persistent and symptomatic second- and third-degree AV block following MI
- Transient second- or third-degree infranodal AV block with associated bundle branch block

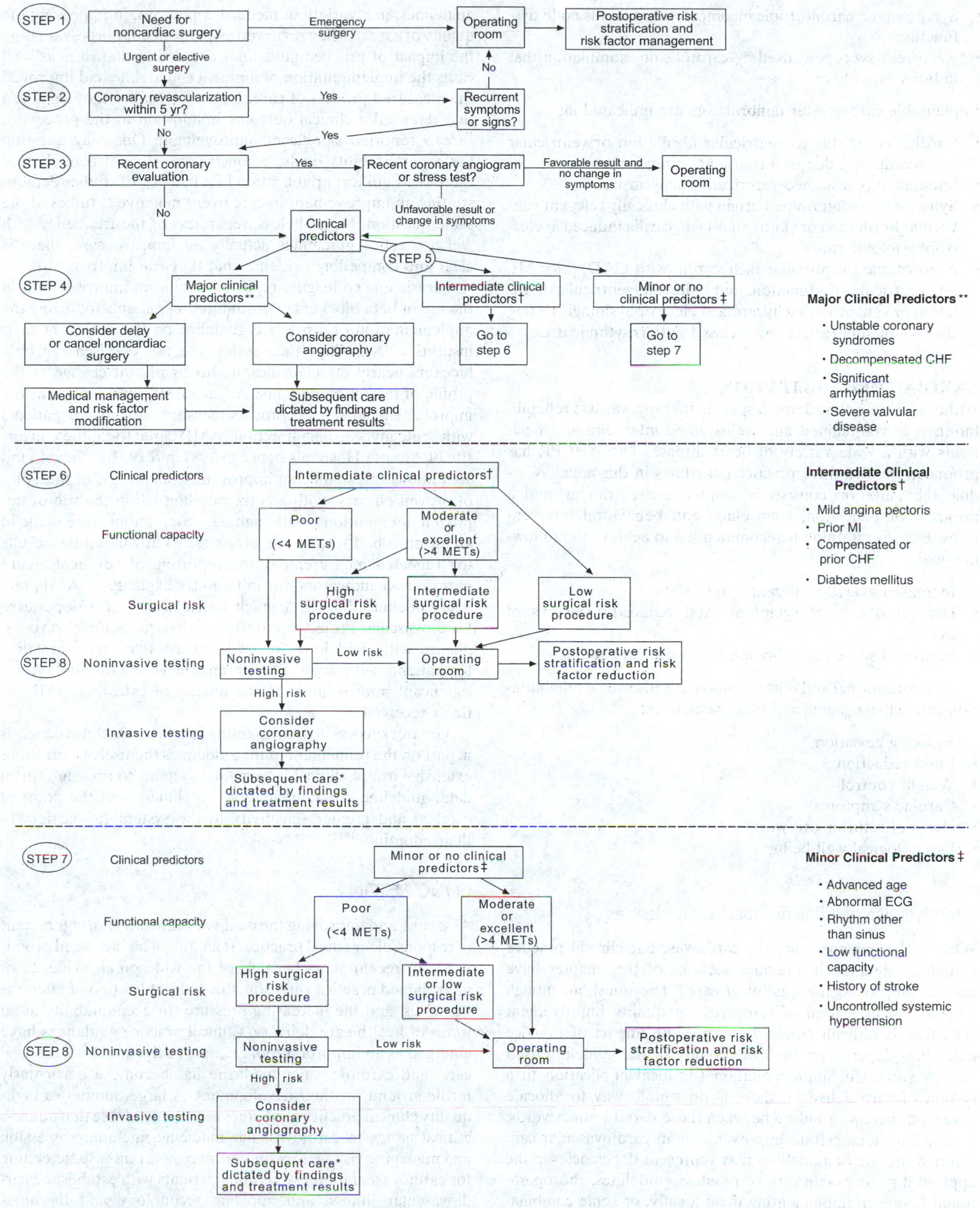

FIGURE 97-6 Algorithm for the preoperative assessment of cardiac risk. (From Eagle et al.,[60] with permission.)

- Symptomatic chronotropic incompetence or sinus node dysfunction
- Recurrent syncope caused by carotid sinus stimulation that induces asystole of >3 s

Implantable cardioverter defibrillators are indicated in:

- Cardiac arrest due to ventricular fibrillation or ventricular tachycardia not due to a transient or reversible cause
- Spontaneous sustained ventricular tachycardia
- Syncope of undetermined origin with clinically relevant ventricular fibrillation or ventricular tachycardia induced at electrophysiologic study
- Nonsustained ventricular tachycardia with CAD, prior MI, left ventricular dysfunction, and inducible ventricular fibrillation or ventricular tachycardia at electrophysiologic testing that is not suppressible by a class I antiarrhythmic drug

CARDIAC REHABILITATION

Although rarely considered a specific therapy, cardiac rehabilitation is a well-defined and well-studied intervention for patients with a wide variety of heart disease. The AHCPR has produced the definitive practice guidelines in this area.[113] Cardiac rehabilitation consists of both exercise training and a program of education, counseling, and behavioral interventions. Exercise training is recommended to achieve the following goals:

- Increased exercise tolerance and habits
- Decreased anginal symptoms and reduced measures of ischemia
- Improved sense of well-being and social functioning

The educational and other components of cardiac rehabilitation can achieve significant improvement in:

- Smoking cessation
- Lipid reduction
- Weight control
- Cardiac symptoms
- Rates of returning to work
- Psychological well-being

Effectiveness of Clinical Practice Guidelines

What is the evidence that the cardiovascular clinical practice guidelines detailed in previous sections of this chapter have actually improved the quality of care? The question, though vital to the allocation of resources for quality improvement activities, is difficult to answer. Since the impact of practice guidelines depends on both the quality of the guideline itself and its successful implementation (its local application to a system of care delivery), there is no simple way to allocate observed success or failure between these two. In other words, a failure to demonstrate improvements in cardiovascular care through the use of guidelines may represent deficiencies in the applicability or practicality of practice guidelines, the operational failure of implementing them locally, or some combination of both. In addition, it is challenging to perform randomized trials of guideline use. Fortunately, there are data to suggest that guidelines can improve care. Grimshaw and Russell compiled the most rigorous assessment of the success of practice guidelines, in a variety of medical conditions, in improving the quality of care.[114] They reviewed 59 published reports evaluating the impact of practice guidelines and found that in nearly all cases the implementation of a practice guideline had improved the measured process of care. Of the 11 studies they reviewed that reported a clinical outcome in addition to the process of care, 9 reported significant improvement. One may question the generalizability of these conclusions, since it is likely that there is a significant publication bias in favor of studies demonstrating an improvement in care over "negative" studies of the same question. Nevertheless, regardless of the frequency with which practice guidelines actually *do* improve care, there is clear and compelling evidence that they *can* improve care.

Sarasin and colleagues reported significant improvements in the use of beta blockers in postinfarction patients following the implementation of a practice guideline on the subject at their institution.[115] In their time series, the use of discharge beta blockers nearly doubled, despite no significant change in the profile of infarction patients. A Canadian group looked at the improvement in several process measures of care for patients with acute myocardial infarction (AMI) cared for at the University of Alberta Hospitals between 1987 and 1993.[116] They found continuous and significant improvement in the use of therapies of proven efficacy, with a corresponding fall in the use of unproven interventions. Although the observations were made in an uncontrolled setting, the investigators attributed the results to "repeated measurement and reporting of key health care performance indicators, and initiation of explicit . . . AMI practice guidelines."[116] On a much larger scale, the Cooperative Cardiovascular Project demonstrated that the feedback on compliance with guidelines for critical process of care measures for patients with myocardial infarction was associated with a significant improvement in the quality of care that AMI patients received.[117]

Greater success in implementing practice guidelines depends in part on the refinement of the guidelines themselves, the more extensive use of clinical information systems to present critical data, guideline recommendations to clinicians at the point of care, [118] and greater sensitivity to the systematic barriers to their adoption.[119,120]

CONCLUSION

Assessing and improving the quality of care is a vital component of responsible medical practice. It has taken on increased prominence in recent years because of the widespread evidence of unexplained practice variation, the underutilization of effective therapies, and the increasing pressure for accountability at all levels of health care delivery. Clinical practice guidelines have emerged as an important tool to improve the quality of medical care, and cardiovascular medicine has become a particularly fertile ground for their development. A large number of high-quality clinical practice guidelines are now available that address critical issues in cardiovascular medicine, including assessing and managing risk factors for coronary heart disease, screening for cardiovascular illness, treating patients with established cardiovascular illness, and applying technology and therapies appropriately. When they are based on dependable, rigorous evidence, written in clear language, and implemented with sensitivity to the myriad local issues that can thwart their success, clinical practice guidelines can help improve patient care.

References

1. Health Care Financing Administration, 1999. ⟨http://www.hcfa.gov/stats/nhe-oact⟩
2. Kleinke JD. Medicine's industrial revolution. *Wall Street Journal,* August 21, 1995, p A7.
3. Relman AS. Assessment and accountability: The third revolution in medical care. *N Engl J Med* 1988; 319:1220–1222.
4. Berwick DM, Nolan TW. Physicians as leaders in improving health care: A new series in Annals of Internal Medicine. *Ann Intern Med* 1998; 128:289–292.
5. Wennberg JE, Gittelsohn AM. Small area variations in health care delivery. *Science* 1973; 321:1168–1173.
6. Chassin MR, Kosecoff J, Park RE, et al. Variations in the use of medical and surgical services by the Medicare population. *N Engl J Med* 1986; 314:285–290.
7. Gornick ME, Eggers PW, Reilly TW, et al. Effects of race and income on mortality and use of services among Medicare beneficiaries. *N Engl J Med* 1996; 335:791–799.
8. Ayanian JZ, Udvarhelyi S, Gatsonis CA, et al. Racial differences in the use of revascularization procedures after coronary angiography. *JAMA* 1993; 269:2642–2646.
9. Peterson ED, Wright SM, Daley J, et al. Racial variation in cardiac procedure use and survival following acute myocardial infarction in the Department of Veteran Affairs. *JAMA* 1994; 271:1175–1180.
10. Fisher ES, Wennberg JE, Stukel TA, et al. Hospital readmission rates for cohorts of Medicare beneficiaries in Boston and New Haven. *N Engl J Med* 1994; 331:989–995.
11. Guadagnoli E, Hauptman PJ, Ayanian JZ, et al. Variation in the use of cardiac procedures after acute myocardial infarction. *N Engl J Med* 1995; 333:573–578.
12. Pilote L, Califf RM, Sapp S, et al. Regional variation across the United States in the management of acute myocardial infarction. *N Engl J Med* 1995; 333:565–572.
13. Blumenthal D. Quality of care—What is it? *N Engl J Med* 1996; 335:891–894.
14. Institute of Medicine. *Medicare: A Strategy for Quality Assurance.* Washington, DC: National Academy Press; 1990.
15. Donabedian A. *Explorations in Quality Assessment and Monitoring: Vol 1. The Definition of Quality and Approaches to Its Assessment.* Ann Arbor, MI: Health Administration Press; 1980.
16. Nash IS. Improving outcomes of percutaneous coronary intervention. *Am Heart J* 1999; 137:979–982.
17. Cleary P, Edgman-Levitan S. Health care quality: Incorporating consumer perspectives. *JAMA* 1997; 278:1608–1612.
18. Nash IS, Curtis LH, Rubin H. Predictors of patient reported physical and mental health six months after percutaneous coronary revascularization. *Am Heart J* 1999; 138:422–429.
19. Hammermeister KE, Shroyer AL, Sethi GK, Grover FL. Why it is important to demonstrate linkages between outcomes of care and processes and structures of care. *Med Care* 1995; 33(10 suppl):OS5–OS16.
20. Siu A. personal communication.
21. Williams SV, Nash DB, Goldfarb. Differences in mortality from coronary bypass graft surgery at five teaching hospitals. *JAMA* 1991; 266:810–815.
22. O'Connor GT, Plume SK, Olmstead EM, et al. Multivariate prediction of in-hospital mortality associated with coronary artery bypass graft surgery: Northern New England Cardiovascular Disease Study Group. *Circulation* 1992; 85:2110–2118.
23. Luft HS, Romano PS. Chance, continuity, and change in hospital mortality rates: Coronary artery bypass graft patients in California hospitals, 1983–1989. *JAMA* 1993; 270:331–337.
24. Hannan EL, Kilburn H, Bernard H, et al. Coronary artery bypass surgery: The relationship between in-hospital mortality rate and surgical volume after controlling for clinical risk factors. *Med Care* 1991; 29:1094–1107.
25. New York State Department of Health. *Coronary Artery Bypass Surgery in New York State, 1994–1996.* Albany, NY: New York State Department of Health; 1998.
26. Pennsylvania Health Care Cost Containment Council. *Pennsylvania's Guide to Coronary Artery Bypass Graft Surgery 1994–1995.* Harrisburg, PA: Pennsylvania Health Care Cost Containment Council; 1998.
27. Kasper JF, Plume SK, O'Connor GT. A methodology for QI in the coronary artery bypass grafting procedure involving comparative process analysis. *QRB Quality Rev Bull* 1992; 18(4):129–133.
28. Dziuban SW, McIlduff JB, Miller SJ, Dal Col RH. How a New York cardiac surgery program uses outcomes data. *Ann Thorac Surg* 1994; 58:1871–1876.
29. Ellerbeck EF, Jencks SF, Radford MJ, et al. Quality of care for Medicare patients with acute myocardial infarction. *JAMA* 1995; 273:1509–1514.
30. ISIS-2 (Second International Study of Infarct Survival) Collaborative Group. Randomised trial of intravenous streptokinase, oral aspirin, both, or neither among 17,187 cases of suspected acute myocardial infarction: ISIS-2. *Lancet* 1988; 2:349–360.
31. Mant J, Hicks N. Detecting differences in quality of care: The sensitivity of measures of process and outcome in treating acute myocardial infarction. *Br Med J* 1995; 311:793–796.
32. Saketkhou BB, Conte FJ, Noris M, et al. Emergency department use of aspirin in patients with possible acute myocardial infarction. *Ann Intern Med* 1997; 127:126–129.
33. Casalino LP. The unintended consequences of measuring quality on the quality of medical care. *N Engl J Med* 1999; 341:1147–1150.
34. Topol EJ, Califf RM. Scorecard cardiovascular medicine: Its impact and future directions. *Ann Intern Med* 1994; 120:65–70.
35. Public Law 101-239, the Omnibus Budget Reconciliation Act of 1989, section 901.
36. Public Law 101-239, the Omnibus Budget Reconciliation Act of 1989, section 912.
37. Field MJ, Lohr KN, eds. *Clinical Practice Guidelines: Directions for a New Program.* Washington, DC: National Academy Press; 1990.
38. Field MJ, Lohr KN, eds. *Clinical Practice Guidelines: Directions for a New Program.* Washington, DC: National Academy Press; 1990:8.
39. Field MJ, Lohr KN, *Guidelines for Clinical Practice: From Development to Use.* Washington, DC: National Academy Press; 1992:4.
40. Field MJ, Lohr KN, eds. *Clinical Practice Guidelines: Directions for a New Program.* Washington, DC: National Academy Press; 1990:50.
41. Hadorn DC, Baker DW, Kamberg CJ, Brook RH. Phase II of the AHCPR-sponsored heart failure guideline: Translating practice recommendations into review criteria. *Jt Comm J Qual Improv* 1996; 22:265–276.
42. Konstam MA, Dracup K, Baker DW, et al. *Heart Failure: Evaluation and Care of Patients with Left Ventricular Systolic Dysfunction. Clinical Practice Guideline No. 11.* Rockville, MD: US Department of Health and Human Services, Agency for Health Care Policy and Research; 1994.
43. Pearson SD, Goulart-Fisher D, Lee TH. Critical pathways as a strategy for improving care: Problems and potential. *Ann Intern Med* 1995; 123:941–948.
44. Ritchie JL, Forrester JS, Jones RH, et al. 28th Bethesda conference: Practice guidelines and the quality of care. *J Am Coll Cardiol* 1997; 29:1125–1179.
45. Field MJ, Lohr KN, eds. *Clinical Practice Guidelines: Directions for a New Program.* Washington, DC: National Academy Press; 1990:59.
46. Hayward RSA, Wilson MC, Tunis SR, et al. User's guide to the medical literature: VIII. How to use clinical practice guide-

lines. A: Are the recommendations valid? *JAMA* 1995; 274: 570–574.

47. Wilson MC, Hayward RAS, Tunis SR, et al. User's guide to the medical literature: VIII. How to use clinical practice guidelines. B: What are the recommendations and will they help you in caring for your patients? *JAMA* 1999; 274:1630–1632.
48. Weingarten S. Using practice guidelines compendiums to provide better preventive care. *Ann Intern Med* 1999; 130:454–458.
49. Selker HP. Criteria for adoption of medical practice guidelines. *Am J Cardiol* 1993; 71:339–341.
50. American Medical Association. *Clinical Practice Guidelines Directory 1999*. Chicago: American Medical Association; 1999.
51. http://www.guidelines.gov/index.asp
52. Shaneyfelt TM, Mayo-Smith MF, Rothwangle J. Are guidelines following guidelines? The methodological quality of clinical practice guidelines in the peer-reviewed medical literature. *JAMA* 1999; 281:1900–1905.
53. Cook D, Giacomini M. The trials and tribulations of clinical practice guidelines. *JAMA* 1999; 281:1950–1951.
54. Parmley WW. Clinical practice guidelines: Does the cookbook have enough recipes? *JAMA* 1994; 272:1374–1375.
55. Baker DW, Konstam MA, Bottorff M, Pitt B. Management of heart failure, I: Pharmacologic treatment. *JAMA* 1994; 272: 1361–1366.
56. Jones RH, Ritchie JL, Fleming BB, et al. Task Force 1: Clinical practice guideline development, dissemination and computerization. *J Am Coll Cardiol* 1997; 29:1133–1141.
57. Hadorn DC, Baker D, Hodges JS, et al. Rating the quality of evidence for clinical practice guidelines. *J Clin Epidemiol* 1996; 49:749–754.
58. U.S. Preventive Services Task Force. *Guide to Clinical Preventive Services*. Baltimore, MD: Williams & Wilkins; 1989.
59. Ryan TJ, Anderson JL, Antman EM, et al. ACC/AHA guidelines for the management of patients with acute myocardial infarction: A report of the American College of Cardiology/American Heart Association Task Force on Practice Guidelines (Committee on Management of Acute Myocardial Infarction). *J Am Coll Cardiol* 1996; 28:1328–1428.
60. Eagle KA, Brundage BH, Chiatman BR, et al. ACC/AHA guidelines for perioperative cardiovascular evaluation for noncardiac surgery: A report of the American College of Cardiology/American Heart Association Task Force on Practice Guidelines (Committee on Perioperative Cardiovascular Evaluation for Noncardiac Surgery). *J Am Coll Cardiol* 1996; 27:910–948.
61. Lee TH, Pearson SD, Johnson PA, et al. Failure of information as an intervention to modify clinical management: A time-series trial in patients with acute chest pain. *Ann Intern Med* 1995; 122:434–437.
62. Field MJ, Lohr KN, eds. *Clinical Practice Guidelines: Directions for a New Program*. Washington, DC: National Academy Press; 1990:12.
63. Grimshaw JM, Russell IT. Achieving health gain through clinical guidelines: II. Ensuring guidelines change medical practice. *Quality Health Care* 1994; 3:45–51.
64. Pelly JE, Newby L, Tito F, et al. Clinical practice guidelines before the law: Sword or shield? *Med J Aust* 1998; 169:330–333.
65. Chodoff P, Crowley K. Clinical practice guidelines: Roadblocks to their acceptance and implementation. *J Outcomes Mgt* 1995; 2(2):5–10.
66. Grol R, Dalhuijsen J, Thomas S, et al. Attributes of clinical guidelines that influence use of guidelines in general practice: Observational study. *Br Med J* 1998; 317:858–861.
67. Field MJ, Lohr KN, eds. *Clinical Practice Guidelines: Directions for a New Program*. Washington, DC: National Academy Press; 1990:78.
68. Scannell KM, Miller N, Glock M. *Current Biographies in Medicine 92-14: Practice Guidelines*. Washington, DC: National Library of Medicine; 1992.
69. National Cholesterol Education Program. *Cholesterol Lowering in the Patient with Coronary Heart Disease: Physician Monograph*. National Institutes of Health Publication 97-3794. Bethesda, MD: National Institutes of Health; 1997.
70. Scandinavian Simvastatin Survival Study Group. Randomised trial of cholesterol lowering in 4444 patients with coronary heart disease: The Scandinavian Simvastatin Survival Study (4S). *Lancet* 1994; 344:1001–1009.
71. Sacks FM, Pfeffer MA, Moye LA, et al. The effect of pravastatin on coronary events after myocardial infarction in patients with average cholesterol levels. *N Engl J Med* 1996; 335:1001–1009.
72. Ridker PM. Are associations between infection and coronary disease causal or due to confounding? *Am J Med* 1999; 106:376–377.
73. Bostom AG, Selhub J. Homocysteine and arteriosclerosis: Subclinical and clinical disease associations. *Circulation* 1999; 99:2361–2363.
74. Joint National Committee on Prevention, Detection, Evaluation and Treatment of High Blood Pressure. The sixth report of the Joint National Committee on Prevention, Detection, Evaluation and Treatment of High Blood Pressure. *Arch Intern Med* 1997; 157:2413–2446.
75. Pasternak RC, Grundy SM, Levy D, et al. Spectrum of risk factors for coronary heart disease. *J Am Coll Cardiol* 1996; 27:978–990.
76. Swan HJC, Gersh BJ, Grayboys TB, et al. Evaluation and management of risk factors for the individual patient (case management). *J Am Coll Cardiol* 1996; 27:1030–1039.
77. Grundy SM, Paternak R, Greenland P, et al. Assessment of cardiovascular risk by use of multiple-risk-factor assessment equations: A statement for healthcare professionals from the American Heart Association and the American College of Cardiology. *Circulation* 1999; 100:1481–1492.
78. Expert Panel on Detection, Evaluation, and Treatment of High Blood Cholesterol in Adults. Summary of the second report of the National Cholesterol Education Program (NCEP) Expert Panel on Detection, Evaluation, and Treatment of High Blood Cholesterol in Adults (Adult Treatment Panel II). *JAMA* 1993; 269:3015–3023.
79. Garber AM, Browner WS, Hulley SB. Clinical guideline, part 2: Cholesterol screening in asymptomatic adults, revisited. *Ann Intern Med* 1996; 124:518–531.
80. Task Force on Risk Reduction, American Heart Association. Cholesterol screening in asymptomatic adults: No cause to change. *Circulation* 1996; 93:1067–1068.
81. Garber AM, Browner WS. Cholesterol screening guidelines: Consensus, evidence, and common sense. *Circulation* 1997; 95:1642–1645.
82. Consensus Panel Statement. Guide to primary prevention of cardiovascular diseases. *Circulation* 1997; 95:2330.
83. Grundy SM, Balady GJ, Criqui MH, et al. When to start cholesterol-lowering therapy in patients with coronary heart disease: A statement for healthcare professionals from the American Heart Association Task Force on Risk Reduction. *Circulation* 1997; 95:1683–1685.
84. Consensus Panel Statement. Preventing heart attack and death in patients with coronary disease. *Circulation* 1995; 92:2–4.
85. Summary report from the Consensus Development Conference on Diagnosis of Coronary Heart Disease in People with Diabetes. (http://www.acc.org)
86. Fiore MC, Bailey WC, Cohen SJ, et al. *Smoking Cessation: Clinical Practice Guideline No 18*. Rockville, MD: U.S. Department of Health and Human Services, Public Health Service, Agency for Health Care Policy and Research; 1996.
87. Ockene IS, Houston-Miller, N. Cigarette smoking, cardiovascular disease, and stroke: A statement for healthcare professionals

from the American Heart Association. *Circulation* 1997; 96:3243–3247.

88. *Obesity Education Initiative: Clinical Guidelines on the Identification, Evaluation, and Treatment of Overweight and Obesity in Adults*. Bethesda, MD: National Institutes of Health, National Heart, Lung, and Blood Institute; 1998.
89. Eckel RH, for the Nutrition Committee. Obesity and heart disease: A statement for healthcare professionals from the Nutrition Committee, American Heart Association. *Circulation* 1997; 96:3248–3250.
90. AACE/ACE Obesity Task Force. AACE/ACE position statement on the prevention, diagnosis, and treatment of obesity. *Endocrinol Pract* 1997; 3:162–208.
91. Fletcher GF, Balady G, Blair SN, et al. Statement on exercise: Benefits and recommendations for physical activity programs for all Americans: A statement for health professionals by the Committee on Exercise and Cardiac Rehabilitation of the Council on Clinical Cardiology, American Heart Association. *Circulation* 1996; 94:857–862.
92. *Physical Activity and Cardiovascular Health: National Institutes of Health Consensus Statement*. Bethesda, MD: National Institutes of Health; 1995; 13(3):1–33.
93. *Guide to Clinical Preventive Services,* 2d ed. Baltimore, MD: Williams & Wilkins; 1996:3–14.
94. *Guide to Clinical Preventive Services,* 2d ed. Baltimore, MD: Williams & Wilkins; 1996:53–61.
95. *Guide to Clinical Preventive Services*, 2d ed. Baltimore, MD: Williams & Wilkins; 1996:67–72.
96. Braunwald E, Mark DB, Jones RH, et al. *Unstable Angina: Diagnosis and Management. Clinical Practice Guideline No. 10*. AHCPR Publication no. 94-0602. Rockville, MD: Agency for Health Care Policy and Research and the National Heart, Lung, and Blood Institute, Public Health Service, U.S. Department of Health and Human Services; March 1994.
97. Prystowsky EN, Benson DW, Fuster V, et al. Management of patients with atrial fibrillation: A statement for healthcare professionals from the Subcommittee on Electrocardiography and Electrophysiology, American Heart Association. *Circulation* 1996; 93:1262–1277.
98. Gibbons RJ, Chatterjee K, Daley J, et al. ACC/AHA/ACP-ISM guidelines for the management of patients with chronic stable angina: A report of the American College of Cardiology/American Heart Association Task Force on Practice Guidelines (Committee on Management of Patients with Chronic Stable Angina). *Circulation* 1999; 99:2829–2848.
99. Ritchie JL, Cheitlin MD, Eagle KA, et al. Guidelines for the evaluation and management of heart failure: A report of the American College of Cardiology/American Heart Association Task Force on Practice Guidelines (Committee on Evaluation and Management of Heart Failure). *J Am Coll Cardiol* 1995; 26:1376–1398.
100. Gunnar RM, Bourdillon PDV, Dixon DW, et al. Guidelines for the early management of patients with acute myocardial infarction: A report of the American College of Cardiology/American Heart Association Task Force on Assessment of Diagnostic and Therapeutic Cardiovascular Procedures (Subcommittee to Develop Guidelines for the Early Management of Patients with Acute Myocardial Infarction). *J Am Coll Cardiol* 1990; 16:249–292.
101. Ryan TJ, Antman EM, Brooks NH, et al. 1999 update: ACC/AHA guidelines for the management of patients with acute myocardial infarction: Executive summary and recommendations: A report of the American College of Cardiology/American Heart Association Task Force on Practice Guidelines (Committee on Management of Acute Myocardial Infarction). *Circulation* 1999; 100:1016–1030.
102. Bonow RO, Carabello B, deLeon AC Jr, et al. ACC/AHA guidelines for the management of patients with valvular heart disease: A report of the American College of Cardiology/American Heart Association Task Force on Practice Guidelines (Committee on Management of Patients with Valvular Heart Disease). *J Am Coll Cardiol* 1998; 32:1486–1588.
103. Gibbons RJ, Balady GJ, Beasley JW, et al. ACC/AHA guidelines for exercise testing: A report of the American College of Cardiology/American Heart Association Task Force on Practice Guidelines (Committee on Exercise Testing). *J Am Coll Cardiol* 1997; 30:260–311.
104. Ritchie JL, Bateman TM, Bonow RO, et al. ACC/AHA guidelines for clinical use of cardiac radionuclide imaging: A report of the American College of Cardiology/American Heart Association Task Force on Practice Guidelines (Committee on Radionuclide Imaging). *J Am Coll Cardiol* 1995; 25:521–547.
105. Strauss HW, Miller DD, Wittry MD, et al. *Procedure Guideline for Myocardial Perfusion Imaging*. Reston, VA: Society of Nuclear Medicine; 1999.
106. Cheitlan MD, Alpert JS. ACC/AHA guidelines for the clinical application of echocardiography: A report of the American College of Cardiology/American Heart Association Task Force on Practice Guidelines (Committee on Clinical Application of Echocardiography). *Circulation* 1997; 95:1686–1744.
107. Scanlon PJ, Faxon DP, Audet AM, et al. ACC/AHA guidelines for coronary angiography: A report of the American College of Cardiology/American Heart Association Task Force on Practice Guidelines (Committee on Coronary Angiography), developed in collaboration with the Society for Cardiac Angiography and Interventions. *J Am Coll Cardiol* 1999; 33:1756–1816.
108. Zipes DP, DiMarco JP, Gillette PC, et al. ACC/AHA guidelines for clinical intracardiac electrophysiological and catheter ablation procedures: A report of the American College of Cardiology/American Heart Association Task Force on Practice Guidelines (Committee on Clinical Intracardiac Electrophysiologic and Catheter Ablation Procedures), developed in collaboration with the North American Society of Pacing and Electrophysiology. *Circulation* 1995; 92:673–691.
109. Eagle KA, Guyton RA, Davidoff R, et al. ACC/AHA guidelines for coronary artery bypass graft surgery: A report of the American College of Cardiology/American Heart Association Task Force on Practice Guidelines (Committee to Revise the 1991 Guidelines for Coronary Artery Bypass Graft Surgery). *J Am Coll Cardiol* 1999; 34:1262–1347.
110. American College of Chest Physicians. *Fifth ACCP Consensus Conference on Antithrombotic Therapy. Chest* 1998; 144 (suppl):439S–769S.
111. Dalen JE, Hirsh J, for the American College of Chest Physicians. *Fifth ACCP Consensus Conference on Antithrombotic Therapy (1998): Summary Recommendations*. Northbrook, IL: American College of Chest Physicians; 1999.
112. Gregoratos G, Cheitlin MD, Conill A, et al. ACC/AHA guidelines for implantation of cardiac pacemakers and antiarrhythmia devices: A report of the American College of Cardiology/American Heart Association Task Force on Practice Guidelines (Committee on Pacemaker Implementation). *J Am Coll Cardiol* 1998; 31:1175–1209.
113. USDHHS. *Cardiac Rehabilitation: Clinical Practice Guideline No. 16*. Rockville, MD: U.S. Department of Health and Human Services, Agency for Health Care Policy and Research, 1995.
114. Grimshaw JM, Russell IT, Effect of clinical guidelines on medical practice: A systematic review of rigorous evaluations. *Lancet* 1993; 342:1317–1322.
115. Sarasin FP, Maschiangelo ML, Schaller MD, et al. Successful implementation of guidelines for encouraging the use of beta blockers in patients after acute myocardial infarction. *Am J Med* 1999; 106:499–505.

116. Montague T, Taylor L, Martin S, et al. Can practice patterns and outcomes be successfully altered? Examples from cardiovascular medicine. *Can J Cardiol* 1995; 11:487–492.
117. Marciniak TA, Ellerbeck EF, Radford MJ, et al. Improving the quality of care for Medicare patients with acute myocardial infarction: Results from the Cooperative Cardiovascular Project. *JAMA* 1998; 279:1351–1357.
118. Tierney WM, Overhage JM, Takesue BY, et al. Computerizing guidelines to improve care and patient outcomes: The example of heart failure. *JAMA* 1995; 2:316–322.
119. Cabana MD, Rand CS, Powe NR, et al. Why don't physicians follow clinical practice guidelines? A framework for improvement. *JAMA* 1999; 282:1458–1465.
120. James PA, Cowan TM, Graham RP. Patient-centered clinical decisions and their impact on physician adherence to clinical guidelines. *J Fam Pract* 1998; 46:311–318.

CHAPTER 98

BEHAVIORAL MEDICINE IN THE TREATMENT OF HEART DISEASE

Thomas G. Pickering / Karina Davidson / William Gerin

In an assessment of the causes of death in the United States in 1993, McGinnis and Foege[1] estimated that approximately 50 percent of deaths (the majority of which were due to heart disease) were attributable to behavioral or lifestyle factors, including tobacco use, poor diet, physical inactivity, and alcohol consumption. Although genetic factors undoubtedly contribute to individual susceptibility to these factors, a prime ingredient is individual behavior. The costs of treating heart disease are escalating at an alarming rate because of the widespread use of sophisticated and increasingly expensive treatments such as coronary artery stents and gene therapy. Most efforts to contain the rise in health care costs have focused on limiting supply (a largely unfulfilled promise of managed care) and imposing some sort of rationing. However, in 1993, Fries and associates[2] pointed out that restricting demand could achieve the same objective. They identified six factors, including four that are relevant to this chapter:

1. Much disease is preventable.
2. Risky behavior costs money. Lifetime medical costs, which averaged $225,000 per person, are clearly related to health behavior habits; for example, those costs are approximately one-third higher in smokers than in nonsmokers.
3. Self-management can result in savings. Several studies have shown that providing medical consumers with information about and guidelines for self-management can lower the use of medical services 10 percent or more.
4. Health behavior promotion at work has reduced medical costs. This has been documented in numerous studies.

This chapter focuses on the major behavioral and psychological factors that influence the course of heart disease and discusses how they can be treated. The behavioral factors are smoking, obesity, and physical inactivity, and the psychological factors are hostility, depression, and anxiety.

A dramatic example of the effects of environmental and psychosocial factors on cardiovascular disease is provided by a recent analysis of changing mortality rates in Russia.[3] Over a 4-year period after the breakup of the Soviet Union, life expectancy declined 5 years, most of which could be attributed to increased mortality in men age 25 to 64 resulting from accidents and cardiovascular disease. Factors that might have contributed to those changes include economic instability, stress, depression, and increased intake of alcohol and tobacco. An equally dramatic example of the influence of lifestyle factors comes from the Honolulu Heart Program, in which it was found that retired men who walked less than 1 mile a day were nearly twice as likely to die over a 12-year period than were men who walked more than 2 miles daily.[4]

Psychosocial factors can influence the course of chronic disease by two main pathways: by inducing behavioral or lifestyle patterns, such as smoking, that are injurious and through a direct effect of social and environmental factors such as socioeconomic status and stress on the disease process. Individual characteristics interact with both pathways, influencing how people choose their lifestyles and how they react to stress. An example of the multiplicity of pathways linking psychosocial factors and disease is provided by hostility, a personality characteristic that has been shown to be a risk factor for coronary heart disease. It has been hypothesized that hostile persons show an exaggerated cardiovascular reactivity to stress, which contributes to the development of atherosclerosis or may trigger an acute event (see below). Hostile persons are also more likely to smoke and less likely to quit.[5]

Although it is widely accepted that behavioral and lifestyle factors may play an important role in the development of coronary heart disease, most practicing cardiologists are not involved in the primary prevention of disease as much as they are in the treatment of existent disease. One factor that is not widely appreciated is how important lifestyle and psychological factors can be in influencing the progression of established coronary heart disease. For example, a study at the Mayo Clinic evaluated a cohort of 381 patients referred to a cardiac rehabilitation unit after hospitalization for an acute coronary event [unstable angina, myocardial infarction (MI), bypass surgery, or angioplasty]. In addition to the traditional risk factors, patients were evaluated for psychological distress (a term that includes depression and vital exhaustion). Over a 6-month follow-up period, it was found that persons high in psychological distress were three times more likely to be hospitalized for recurrent coronary events [i.e., an odds ratio (OR) of 3.05]; other less powerful predictive factors included no previous bypass procedure (OR = 2.73), diabetes (OR = 2.65), and ejection fraction <40 percent (OR = 1.98). Interestingly, smoking and the use of beta blockers did not predict relapse. A second example comes from a study of patients undergoing coronary angioplasty, after which new cardiac events occur in 20 to 30 percent of patients within 1 year. The study found that after controlling for standard risk factors, men who scored high on anger had a threefold increase in the rate of recurrent events compared with men with lower scores.[6]

BASIC PRINCIPLES OF BEHAVIORAL MEDICINE

It has long been recognized that knowledge alone does not provide sufficient motivation to change behavior.[7] A fundamental problem is that intervention studies commonly produce improvements in the behavior being manipulated that last a few weeks or months, but by 1 year there is almost always a relapse. An example is the Trials of Hypertension Prevention, in which patients were asked to reduce their weight or salt intake (Fig. 98-1).

Some of the basic principles that may be employed to obtain sustained behavioral change can be illustrated by the example of dietary intervention, but the same principles apply to modalities such as smoking cessation and exercise.

TABLE 98-1 Stages of Change

1. Precontemplation. Patient is not yet thinking about changing behavior
2. Contemplation. Patient is considering but is not yet ready to engage in behavior change
3. Preparation. Patient intends to take action in the next month
4. Action. Patient begins actual process of behavior change
5. Maintenance. Patient develops strategies to prevent relapse

As with other types of behavioral intervention, many studies of dietary intervention have reported disappointing or at best modest lipid-lowering results even when trained dietitians and knowledgeable health professionals were involved in the intervention process.[8–10] One reason for these disappointing results is suggested by recent behavioral studies that indicate that the method used to deliver dietary interventions may be less than optimal. Earlier intervention studies typically applied a didactic, informative approach with little attention paid to what now are recognized as important differences in learning styles or levels of motivation to change behavior.[11] More recent behavioral models identify psychosocial factors that influence food choices and delineate the process of motivating changes in behavior.[12] Several behavioral models have evolved, and these models are potentially additive. The social learning theory model incorporates behavior modification methods that include cognitive, interpersonal, and environmental influences on behavior.[13] The basic components of this approach include self-monitoring and analysis of behavior; self-management, including stimulus control of external cues; the replacement of less desirable (i.e., high-fat foods) behaviors with more desirable behaviors; and the reinforcement of desirable behaviors.[7] Strongly related is the construct of "self-efficacy,"[14] which refers to a person's degree of confidence that she or he has the ability to gain control over specific behaviors, such as eating and dieting. Increased self-efficacy has been found to be a critical element in motivation to engage in healthy behaviors.[14]

Over the last decade, research on the stages of change model has yielded valuable insights regarding how, why, and when persons will change behavior.[15] This model suggests that behavior change is achieved through a series of stages: precontemplation, contemplation, preparation, action, and maintenance[16] (Table 98-1).

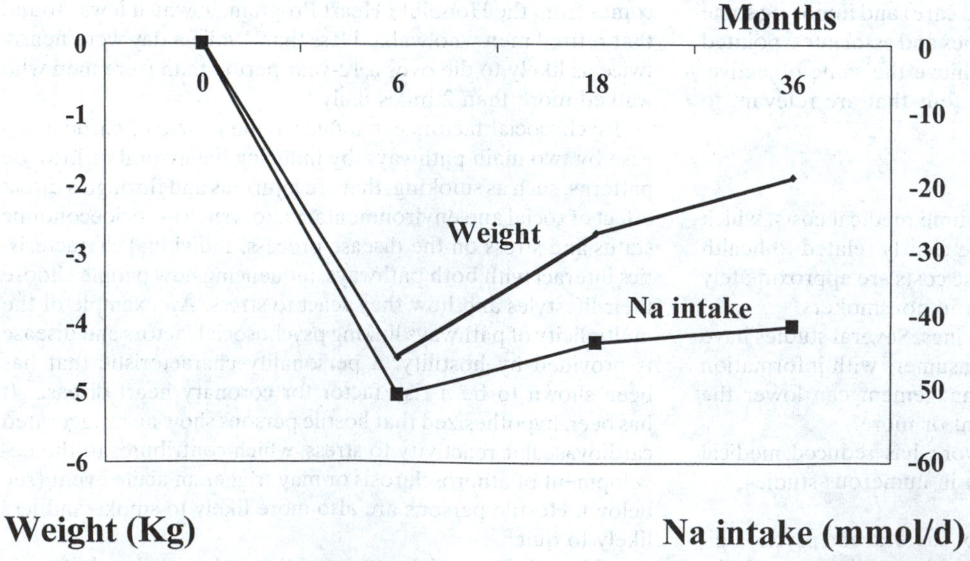

FIGURE 98-1 The trials of hypertension prevention.

Since most dietary intervention studies have applied approaches suitable for the action stage, it is not surprising that adherence has been disappointing. It is likely that many participants were overwhelmed, uncommitted, or simply not ready to adopt the recommended eating pattern.

Barriers to Behavioral Intervention and the Role of Collaborative Management of Patients with Heart Disease

A basic issue in the treatment of behavioral and lifestyle factors is the concept of collaborative management. Heart disease is usually chronic, and its successful management requires active collaboration between the patient and the health care providers. There is a large gap between the care that is prescribed and what is actually achieved. A classic example is control of hypertension, in which despite the availability of numerous powerful medications, blood pressure is adequately controlled in fewer than one-third of patients.[17] Some of the barriers to the more successful implementation of recommended lifestyle and other changes are summarized in Table 98-2. These barriers can be categorized as relating to the patient, the physician, or the health care system.

Patients often lack the knowledge and motivation to make behavior changes, and the training of cardiologists rarely includes behavior and behavioral intervention. Physicians generally have a low opinion of the effectiveness of behavioral interventions and little incentive to implement them, let alone the time. Because neither patients nor physicians have pressured the health care system to recognize the importance of making these changes, behavioral interventions rarely are reimbursed.

Despite these limitations, health care providers can and should use behavioral techniques to improve self-care in patients with chronic illnesses such as heart disease. These techniques include contracting with the patient to reach specific goals, evaluating the patient's readiness for self-care, breaking self-care tasks into small manageable steps, providing personalized feedback to the patient, self-monitoring of health-related behaviors, enlisting social support, and checking the patient's commitment to key tasks. One of the first steps is to define problems clearly. Physicians usually are concerned with items such as poor compliance and unhealthy behavior, while patients are more concerned with symptoms and emotional distress. Few physicians ask patients to identify the biggest problems they face in managing illness.

In light of the lack of training in behavioral techniques and the severe time limitations of cardiologists, the solution to this dilemma ideally should be a team approach. Behavioral interventions tend to require relatively large amounts of time, but a lot can be achieved by persons whose training and time is less costly than those of the physician. These persons include nurses, psychologists, dietitians, and social workers.

At the end of this chapter specific strategies are discussed that can be used easily by the physician to help patients make the necessary changes in their behavior.

TABLE 98-2 Barriers to Implementation of Behavioral Changes

Patient
Lack of knowledge
Lack of motivation
Low self-efficacy (confidence in the ability to effect changes)
Unreadiness to commit to behavior change
Lack of access to care
Social and cultural factors
Physician
Time constraints
Problem-based focus
Perceived ineffectiveness of interventions
Lack of behavioral skills
Lack of incentives
Health care system
Focus on acute care
Failure to provide team approach
Failure to provide reimbursement
Lack of policies and standards

SMOKING CESSATION

Smoking kills more than 400,000 Americans every year, and more than half of these deaths are due to cardiovascular disease and stroke. Smoking has been recognized for many years as one of the "big three" risk factors for cardiovascular disease (the others being hypertension and hyperlipidemia) and is responsible for about 30 percent of cardiovascular morbidity and mortality.[18] Smoking more than doubles the incidence of coronary artery disease and increases mortality 70 percent.[19] The economic cost of tobacco smoking has been estimated to be over $50 billion a year. The risks associated with smoking are almost completely reversible after quitting,[20,21] and smoking cessation has been shown to be one of the most cost-effective interventions in the field of medicine.[22] However, smoking cessation programs rarely are reimbursed by health insurance programs.

AHCPR Guidelines

The science and effectiveness of smoking cessation programs have been reviewed extensively by the Agency for Health Care Policy (AHCPR), which issued its guidelines in 1996.[18] The guidelines stress that health care clinics such as cardiology practices are ideal settings for the promotion of smoking cessation treatments. More than 70 percent of smokers report that they see a physician at least once a year.[23] The guidelines emphasize that a variety of effective strategies can be adopted, some very simple and others more complex. The recommended steps are summarized below.

- Clearly, step 1 is to identify smokers. Although this seems obvious, data show that only about 50 percent of smokers report ever having been asked by a physician if they smoked.[24]
- Step 2 is advising a smoker to quit, an intervention that takes 3 min at most. Although this may seem trivial, an analysis of several studies has shown that the quit rate will increase from 7.9 percent to 10.2 percent, an increment that may seem insubstantial except that each smoker who quits will add up to 15 years to his or her life expectancy.[18] Moreover, this

number will increase with each succeeding examination in which the physician advises the patient to quit.

- Step 3 is the assessment of a smoker's willingness to quit. The mnemonic STOP is advocated: *s*upport from the physician in the quit attempt; *t*ry, acknowledging that the patient is making a commitment to try, not necessarily to quit; *o*ptions, reviewing the various treatment options open to the patient; and *p*icking a quit day.
- Step 4 deals with a smoker who is unwilling to attempt to quit. This involves promoting the patient's readiness to quit, and emphasizes the four Rs: personal *r*elevance to the patient's medical and social situation, the *r*isks associated with smoking, the *r*ewards of quitting, and the *r*epetition of a stop-smoking message. A good way to assess a patient's readiness to quit is to use the stages of change model described above.[25] The important message here is that all smokers should be given advice about smoking, but the advice should differ according to the patient's stage of change.
- Step 5 deals with the strategy that is chosen for a patient who is willing to quit. A general rule is that "more is better," or that the quit rate is proportional to the amount of effort that is put into it. The options, which are not mutually exclusive, include counseling, which has two basic components: providing social support and boosting skills in problem solving. Other components include the use of nicotine replacement therapy, which can be delivered in a variety of ways, including gum, skin patches, and nasal sprays. A number of clinical trials have shown that the nicotine patches can double quit rates.[26] Finally, the use of the antidepressant drug bupropion (Zyban) has been found to be very effective. A study published after the AHCPR guidelines were published found that bupropion approximately doubled the quit rate[27] and that the best results were obtained with a combination of counseling, nicotine patches, and bupropion treatment.

Nicotine Gum and Patch

Since 1995, nicotine gum (Nicorette) and nicotine skin patches (Nicoderm, Nicotrol) have been approved as over-the-counter drugs. The gum is available in 2- or 4-mg doses, and it is recommended that one to two pieces be chewed per hour. The lower dose is for persons who smoke fewer than 25 cigarettes daily, and the higher dose is for those who smoke more. The regular dose is used for 6 weeks, followed by 6 weeks of tapering.

The Nicotrol patch label instructs patients to use the patch for 16 h a day for 6 weeks, with no tapering period. The Nicoderm CQ patch is used for 16 h a day at a high dose (21 mg/day) for 6 weeks, followed by 14 mg/day for 2 weeks and then 7 mg/day for 2 weeks. Both the gum and the patch have been subjected to several placebo-controlled clinical trials that have shown that the use of either one leads to an approximate doubling of the quit rate.[28]

Nicotine Nasal Spray and Inhaler

The spray is available as a prescription drug (Nicotrol nasal spray) that is designed to deliver the nicotine more rapidly than does the gum or patch. It is administered once or twice per hour for up to 3 months. Its use doubles the quit rate; side effects include sore throat and rhinitis, both of which are usually transient.[28] Another prescription formulation is the Nicotrol inhaler, which has pharmacokinetics similar to those of the nicotine gum. Its effectiveness is comparable to that of the other nicotine replacement therapies.[28]

Bupropion

Bupropion originally was developed as an antidepressant, for which it is not very effective. As an antismoking adjuvant, it is available in a long-acting form as Zyban, which has been found to lead to a doubling of the quit rate. The recommended dose is 300 mg/day, which is started 1 week before the quit date and continued for 7 to 12 weeks. It has been found to work equally well whether or not the smoker is depressed, suggesting that its antidepressant activity is not its primary mode of action.[29] Side effects include dry mouth and insomnia.

Reimbursement Issues

One of the reasons why so little attention is given to smoking cessation programs is that those programs rarely are reimbursed by insurance companies. A survey of managed care companies found that only 9 percent reimbursed physicians for implementing the AHCPR recommendations fully, while another 39 percent reimbursed partially and 53 percent did not reimburse at all.[30] Approximately half the companies surveyed were not aware of the existence of the guidelines. Whereas 54 percent of managed care organizations (MCOs) offered some self-help materials for smokers, only 17.6 percent provided reimbursement for bupropion use.

The almost total lack of reimbursement for smoking cessation programs stands in stark contrast to the reimbursement for the treatment of the other two major risk factors for heart disease: hypertension and hyperlipidemia. Smoking cessation has been labeled "the gold standard of health care cost-effectiveness"[22] and is dramatically more cost-effective in terms of life-years saved (LYS) than is treatment for hypertension or hyperlipidemia with medications (Table 98-3).

One commonly given reason why smoking cessation is not reimbursed more often is that the benefits are delayed for about 5 to 10 years, which may be longer than the life span of many

TABLE 98-3 Cost-effectiveness of Treatment of the Big Three Cardiovascular Risk Factors

Intervention	Cost per Life-Year Saved, $
Smoking cessation[a]	
Brief advice from doctor	1000–3000
High intensity	6000–15,000
Treatment of hypertension[b]	11,000–72,000
Treatment of hyperlipidemia[c]	9000–297,000

SOURCE: [a]From Warner.[22] [b]From Edelson JT, Weinstein MC, Tosteson AN, et al. Long-term cost-effectiveness of various initial monotherapies for mild to moderate hypertension [see comments]. *JAMA* 1990; 266:407. [c]From Hay JW, Wittels EH, Gotto AMJ. An economic evaluation of lovastatin for cholesterol lowering and coronary artery disease reduction [see comments]. *Am J Cardiol* 1991; 67:789.

MCOs; hence, no net cost savings for the MCO will result from the program. However, this is a double standard: Coronary bypass surgery and angioplasty are reimbursed routinely, and no one ever questions whether they reduce health care costs for an MCO, which clearly they do not.

In light of these numbers, why do so few physicians pay attention to smoking cessation? There are several reasons: First, physicians are not trained in behavioral techniques such as counseling even though this is an activity to which they devote substantial time. They believe that their patients already know that smoking is harmful and that counseling is unlikely to have a significant effect. Second, the fact that it is not reimbursed automatically gives counseling a low priority. Thus, it has been established that brief (3 mins or so) counseling from a physician can double the spontaneous quit rate of smokers, which is about 2.5 percent per year. If a physician counsels 100 patients per year, 95 percent will continue to smoke, a dispiritingly large number for the physician. However, of the 2.5 smokers who quit as a result of physician counseling—in addition to the other 2.5 smokers who will quit spontaneously—one ex-smoker will avoid a premature smoking-related death and another will gain up to 15 years of life expectancy. The cost of this benefit will have been 3 h and 20 min of the physician's time.

DIETARY INTERVENTIONS

Dietary factors have a substantial impact on the development of cardiovascular disease (CVD). Many studies show that saturated fat and lipid intake is associated with rates of CVD-related death and all-cause mortality.[31,32] On the basis of epidemiologic and observational studies in men, women, African-Americans, and elderly persons as well as postmortem angiographic studies in young persons, the National Institutes of Health and the European Atherosclerosis Society have concluded that the level of serum lipids is a causal factor in coronary artery disease.[32–34]

Low-density lipoprotein cholesterol (LDL-C) and other components of the lipid profile are affected by dietary interventions.[35] This has led to strong recommendations by the National Cholesterol Education Program that dietary counseling should form the basis of lipid-regulating regimens for both the prevention and the clinical management of CVD.[36] Reductions in lipid levels are readily achievable through careful adherence to dietary changes.

Compared with pharmacologic intervention, dietary intervention has produced less net reduction in total cholesterol (TC) and LDL-C levels in randomized trials.[37] However, two secondary intervention trials—one with medication (Scandinavian Simvastatin Survival Study) and one with a Mediterranean, alpha-linolenic-rich diet (Lyon Diet Heart Study)—reported remarkably similar reductions in cardiac deaths over 5 years.[8–10,38]

Comprehensive reviews of dietary intervention studies[11,32,39] lead to the conclusion that aggressive treatment with a diet low in total and saturated fat produces lowered serum lipid levels and positive angiographic changes as well as potentially helping improve angina and other non-lipid-related symptoms. However, achieving and maintaining dietary adherence on a long-term basis remains a major challenge.

On the basis of the cumulative scientific evidence from epidemiologic and controlled clinical trials, the National Cholesterol Education Program (NCEP) advocated diet as the cornerstone of treatment in its reports of the Adult Treatment Panel as well as in its Population Based Panel and Pediatric Panel reports.[36,40] In 1989, both NCEP and the American Heart Association (AHA) announced populationwide recommendations for step I and step II diets as primary strategies for the prevention and treatment of high blood lipids.[36,41]

The last two decades have seen improvement in some aspects of the U.S. diet and corresponding declines in blood lipid levels.[11,39] Although the vast majority of U.S. adults still eat more than the recommended 30 percent of total calories as fat, the country as a whole has had a major downward shift in total fat intake.

Obesity and weight are increasing at epidemic rates, however, especially among young women and children.[34] This is due to other factors, such as levels of inactivity, and other aspects of the diet such as energy sources. For example, a potential contributor is the low intake of total dietary fiber. The AHA recommends 25 to 30 g of dietary fiber a day from whole grains, vegetables, and fruits. Because the population eats on average less than half the recommended daily minimum of five servings of fruits and vegetables, the intake of more energy-dense but nutrient-poor foods is the likely consequence.[34] It has been estimated that 52 million Americans are candidates for diet therapy to reduce high blood lipids; however, according to several surveys, fewer than 10 percent have been prescribed such diets.[42,43]

Other Nutrients, Antioxidants, and Homocysteine

Other nutrients have been explored in regard to their impact on blood lipids. The antioxidant vitamins E and C and beta-carotene delay and reduce the oxidation of LDL-C in vitro and may be especially important among smokers.[44–47] Observational studies in female nurses and male health professionals have reported favorable reductions in coronary heart disease (CHD) risk among those who take vitamin E supplements, but no intervention trials have been completed.[46] The use of vitamin E supplements was associated with a 35 percent reduction in CHD after adjustment for other risk factors, multiple vitamins, beta-carotene, and vitamin C.[45,46] Conversely, iron has been suggested to serve as a prooxidant in the arterial wall, potentially contributing to LDL-C oxidation, endothelial injury, and myocardial injury.[48] Studies on iron and the risk of CHD have been inconclusive.

Elevated levels of homocysteine damage endothelial cells and promote arterial occlusion.[49] Homocysteine is produced by the demethylation of methionine, an amino acid found mainly in animal protein foods. This conversion is dependent on folic acid, with vitamins B_6- and B_{12}-dependent enzymes playing a role as well. If these factors are reduced or inactivated, elevations in homocysteine can result. Diets rich in dark green and yellow fruits and vegetables and whole grains that provide an optimal amount of 400 mg/day of folate are adequate to produce serum folate levels of 15 μmol/L.

OBESITY

Independent of the qualitative objectives of dietary adherence, obesity directly and indirectly plays a major causal role in CHD and stroke.[50] It contributes to dyslipidemia, diabetes, and hypertension, and its strong association with reduced physical activity further exacerbates cardiovascular disease.[51–53] The national prevalence of obesity is currently estimated at 30 percent among adults and children.[54,55]

Excess body weight has been causally linked with deleterious changes in the lipoprotein profile.[51] Several studies have documented the fact that lipoprotein abnormalities are induced with weight gain and reversed with weight loss.[56,57] Particularly in obese children, even small degrees of weight loss can result in dramatic normalization of the lipid profile.[57]

In summary, the research strongly suggests that a diet reduced in total and saturated fat, lipids, trans-fatty acids, homocysteine, sodium, and excess calories and increased in dietary fiber (especially soluble fiber), antioxidants, folate, vitamin B_6, and n-3 fatty acids will lower cardiovascular risk for most persons. The resulting diet is rich in fruits and vegetables, whole grains and cereals, low-fat and skim dairy products, and fish, lean meats, and/or soy protein foods. Foods should be cooked without added saturated fat or cooked in a small amount of liquid vegetable oil, preferably olive oil, canola oil, or another monounsaturated nonhydrogenated liquid oil. Egg yolks should be limited to fewer than two per week.

Prevention and Treatment of Obesity

A recent National Institutes of Health (NIH) conference on voluntary methods for weight loss and control concluded that most existing adult obesity interventions are ineffective, with one-third to two-thirds of the lost weight being regained in 1 year and almost all the weight being regained within 5 years.[55] Training and calorie restrictions and the use of packaged diet food are not effective in the long term. The greatest success in treating the obese adult has occurred with combined dietary fat restriction, behavioral skill development, and regular exercise.[58,59] Other effective strategies include family-oriented interventions and booster sessions.[60] Pharmacologic appetite suppressants and gene therapy may offer promising options in the future for some patients, but inevitably diet and energy balance must be addressed.

Practical Steps toward Achieving Dietary Adherence

In a review of 30 studies reporting changes in fat intake, Barnard and coworkers[61] summarized the factors that were commonly associated with increased adherence. Those factors include the following:

- Stricter limits on fat intake. The lower the limit, the closer the average level of adherence.
- Frequent monitoring. At least monthly monitoring is recommended.
- Vegetarian diets. The use of a vegetarian diet more often achieved recommended fat intake than did nonvegetarian approaches.
- Initial residential components. These components provide intensive training, monitoring, provision of food, and group support in the short term, resulting in better adherence to self-selected diets in the long term. However, these components may be impractical in many cases.
- Family involvement. Involvement by family members results in improved adherence.
- Group support. This is not mandatory but can be helpful.
- Providing food. Entire meals are not required, but some provision of acceptable products is important.
- Symptomatic patients. These patients appear to be more motivated to comply with dietary regimens; healthy, high-risk patients appear to be less motivated.

Relevant sources of total and saturated fat and lipids should be identified before one attempts to prescribe a new dietary pattern for any patient. Two large-scale controlled clinical trials reported that meats, fats and oils, dairy foods, and baked goods contributed more total and saturated fat to the diets of adults than did any other food groups.[62,63] Fortunately, there are now many acceptable alternatives to these high-fat foods. Substitution of lower-fat or fat-free versions for high-fat foods (e.g., skim milk for whole milk, fat-free salad dressing for full-fat salad dressing) and the addition of more servings of fruits, vegetables, and grains to compensate for fewer servings of high-fat meats, dairy products, and baked goods are essential components. The food industry has responded aggressively to the request for lower-fat and no-fat products. The greater challenge lies in achieving the desired shift to a higher intake of foods with complex carbohydrates.

Changing Dietary Behavior One Patient at a Time

On the basis of these behavioral principles and the accumulated knowledge about diet and risk reduction, Van Horn and Kavey[34] have made the following suggestions, which can help promote successful dietary adherence:

- Start with dietary assessment and then individualize the dietary intervention. Assessing baseline intake is the only way to identify the foods that are contributing the most saturated fat and lipids to a patient's diet. In adults, this is often meats, fats, and sweets. In children, it is often whole-milk dairy products. In children who consume the recommended four servings of dairy foods per day, it may be possible to achieve adherence to the step I diet (≤10% saturated fat acids) by switching to skim milk and low-fat dairy products at school and at home.
- Provide clear, identifiable goals for each person. For example, current food labels make it possible to establish a fixed "fat gram goal" rather than following the less precise recommendations to get less than 30 percent of calories from total fat. This provides each person with an objective target he or she can self-monitor. Similarly, establishing the goal number of servings of fruits, vegetables, and grains can further help an individual achieve increased fiber, folate, and antioxidant intake.
- Assess the current state of change and determine the person's level of confidence (self-efficacy) in achieving a self-determined adherence goal. Reassess the person's status at each subsequent visit.
- Encourage self-monitoring through the use of food records and/or other simplified fat and fiber goal-counting records. Also, encourage the use of nonfood self-rewards when goals are met.
- Promote the benefit of adopting other health-oriented behaviors, including exercise, relaxation techniques, and stress reduction.
- Prevent relapse through ongoing follow-up, reassessment, and the establishment of new goals as needed.

- Patients who are referred to registered dietitians or other trained nutrition counselors may require relatively few follow-up sessions. Comprehensive feedback on dietary adherence can be provided to the referring physician by these other health professionals for consideration in determining future treatment plans.

EXERCISE

Physical inactivity is widely recognized as a major risk factor for cardiovascular disease, and numerous studies have shown that even mild exercise can reduce the probability of morbid events and even improve longevity. Only 22 percent of adults engage in 30 min or more of light to moderate exercise five or more times a week, the recommended amount for cardiovascular benefit.[64] Despite the fact that patients with cardiac disease are seen regularly by both cardiologists and primary care physicians, most physicians do not counsel their patients about physical activity.[65,66] One of the goals of the national Health Promotion Objectives for the year 2000 is to increase to at least 50 percent the number of primary care physicians who assess and advise their patients about exercise.

Two studies have investigated the efficacy of exercise counseling by physicians. Both used the stages of change model described above. One study, the Physician-based Assessment and Counseling for Exercise (PACE),[67] gave patients a brief questionnaire in the waiting room to assess their readiness for change: precontemplation, not intending to exercise; contemplation, willing to consider becoming more active; and active, already exercising. Physicians were given a manual describing the intervention and spent about 5 min describing it to the patients. There was also a 10-min follow-up call from a health educator. This simple intervention resulted in an approximate doubling in the number of minutes of walking per week in the intervention group (an average increase of 37 min) without any significant change in the controls. However, the participants in this study were followed for only 6 weeks. A second trial, Physically Active for Life (PAL),[68] used a similar design and demonstrated a marginally significant positive effect at 6 weeks, but the effect disappeared when assessed at 8 months. One reason for the more disappointing results in PAL might have been that the participants were older (average age, 65).

Whereas it is often recommended that exercise should occur in bouts of 30 min or so, there is evidence that shorter bouts can be equally effective in improving cardiovascular fitness. One study[69] compared the effects of a single 30-min bout, three 10-min bouts, and bouts of 5 min or more totaling 30 min and found that all three produced roughly the same degree of improvement in blood pressure and body fat.

As with any form of behavioral intervention, a number of methods help improve adherence to exercise regimens. The first is to educate and motivate patients about the benefits of exercise (moving them from precontemplation to contemplation). The second is to set reasonable goals that can be increased gradually over time. It may be helpful for the patient and the interventionist to agree on a "behavioral contract" with a date set for achieving a particular goal. Self-monitoring is also helpful (keeping a log of daily activities, for example), and feedback and reinforcement should be provided regularly to the participant. It is also important to identify barriers that may hinder progress and find ways to overcome them. For example, if a patient has no easy means of getting to a gym, a home exercise program can be recommended.

PSYCHOSOCIAL RISK FACTORS

Stress, depression, anger and hostility, the type A behavior pattern, and anxiety have been proposed as possible cardiovascular disease risk factors. Unfortunately, the supporting or contradictory evidence for each construct is often considered interchangeable in the evaluation of its role in the development and manifestation of cardiovascular disease. Each construct, however, is theoretically and operationally distinct from the others, and the empirical support for each one as a cardiovascular disease risk factor varies. Further, recent technology and animal experiments suggest that some of these psychosocial factors contribute to the pathogenesis of cardiovascular disease whereas others do not.[70]

Stress

Stress is listed as one of the major factors causing heart disease when patients and lay persons are asked and is listed more frequently than high blood pressure and high lipids by those persons.[71] However, the investigation of stress as a cardiovascular disease risk factor has been vexed by definitional difficulties. Stress to the layperson typically encompasses, among other issues, work and family stress, social isolation, and the occurrence of recent acute and chronic life events. Work stress, which is defined as having low control over the way in which work is done but high work demands, has been implicated as a reliable and consistent predictor of the progression of hypertension,[72] carotid atherosclerosis,[73] and cardiac events and death.[74-76] Other theorists have argued that work stress is better assessed as low job control, and this index of work stress also has been found to predict future cardiac events.[77] Family stress rarely has been studied in regard to its relation to cardiovascular disease recurrence and mortality. However, it has been hypothesized that women with dual roles—both family and work stress—would have increased cardiovascular disease incidence, but in fact these women seem to have lower cardiovascular disease risk.[78]

Social isolation (few friends, family members, or close others) and perceived lack of social support consistently have been found to predict acute MI and cardiac death. As has been noted by Rozanski and colleagues,[70] the relative risks in the most recent 15 studies indicate a threefold mortality risk for cardiovascular disease patients who are socially isolated and/or perceive poor social support.

Acute mental stress such as the sudden loss of a loved one or an earthquake consistently has been shown to provoke silent myocardial ischemia and predict increased cardiovascular disease incidence and death in epidemiologic studies.[79]

Depression

Depressive symptoms and depressive disorders predict cardiac recurrence and mortality with a relative risk ranging from 2.6 to 7.8 in cardiac patients.[80-83] These risk ratios remain when all other known predictors of MI recurrence are controlled for, and depressive symptoms predict MI recurrence in a gradient fashion. Thus, there is considerable evidence that a cardiac patient who is depressed is at substantially higher risk for a future event. As is reviewed in Chap. 79, many studies have examined the mechanisms that may underlie this relationship as well as some interventions that may reduce this excess risk.

Anxiety

There have been fewer investigations of the relation of anxiety to cardiac disease and recurrence.[81,82,84,85] Most studies of anxiety disorders have examined the increased occurrence of cardiovascular disease mortality in psychiatric patients known to have some type of anxiety disorder,[86–88] although some small studies have found a relation between anxiety and sudden cardiac death in cardiovascular disease patients.[70] However, anxiety symptoms were not associated with MI recurrence in these studies. Rozanski and associates, among others,[70,89,90] have hypothesized that anxiety disorders and the associated symptoms may cause an alteration in cardiac autonomic tone through impaired vagal control, reduced heart rate variability, or both to cause an increased risk of sudden cardiac death in cardiac patients. A further discussion of the role of anxiety and related disorders can be found in Chap. 79.

Type A Behavior Pattern

Friedman and Rosenman[91] first proposed that a constellation of competitive, hostile, time-pressured behaviors constitutes a personality trait ("type A") that predisposes patients to cardiovascular disease. Although the Western Collaborative Group study found a twofold risk for cardiovascular disease and a fivefold MI recurrence risk in those in the type A-B categorization, several later studies failed to find that difference.[92] Many theorists have suggested that hostility, or the tendency to view others with suspicion and skepticism, may be the toxic component of the type A behavioral pattern and that this component should be evaluated independently for its prediction of increased risk in cardiac patients. Four small studies of cardiovascular disease patients found that the presence of a high level of hostility is associated with more rapid progression of atherosclerosis, more ischemia, a faster rate of restenosis after angioplasty, and a higher probability of recurrent MI.[6,93–96]

Psychosocial Interventions

In light of the emphasis cardiovascular disease patients place on stress and psychosocial factors as contributors to their disease and some of the recent evidence suggesting that psychosocial factors predict cardiovascular disease recurrence and death, offering psychosocial interventions for cardiovascular disease patients seems reasonable. However, there are many different types of interventions that are aimed at different psychosocial factors and different outcomes.

Linden and associates[97] conducted a meta-analysis of 23 controlled psychosocial intervention studies. All the patients were receiving standard medical and surgical care, and most additionally were receiving standard cardiac rehabilitation interventions. For follow-up periods of less than 2 years, there was a 41 percent reduction in mortality and a 46 percent reduction in MI recurrence as a result of psychosocial interventions. There were also significant and clinically meaningful reductions in measures of psychosocial distress such as depression and anxiety and in cardiovascular risk factors such as blood pressure and lipid levels. Only three randomized trials reported results for more than 2 years of follow-up, and in none of them did the effects of psychosocial intervention on mortality or MI recurrence remain significant.

Two large studies of psychosocial interventions merit special comment. In 1989, Frasure-Smith and coinvestigators reported favorable survival results for post-MI patients ($n = 229$) who received a home- and telephone-based stress-monitoring nursing intervention. As a result of this outcome, a larger randomized trial of a similar intervention was conducted ($n = 1376$). In this trial, there was no overall survival impact of the program, and in elderly women, there was increased cardiac and all-cause mortality.[98] In the second study, Jones and West[99] conducted a randomized controlled psychological intervention trial in 2328 post-MI patients and also found no difference in cardiac event recurrence and mortality at 12 months of follow-up. Two important features of these studies may explain their negative results. First, neither one actually achieved the objective of significantly reducing stress when this is operationalized as decreased scores on standardized depression and anxiety scales. Second, neither study screened patients to determine whether they in fact exhibited any symptoms of stress or of the psychological factor that was targeted by the intervention. Frasure-Smith[100] conducted a reanalysis of her original nursing intervention and reported that only patients who reported distress during hospitalization benefited from the psychosocial intervention; this is consistent with the author's speculation that those not at risk for psychosocial difficulties will not benefit from a psychosocial intervention. However, firm conclusions about the efficacy of psychosocial interventions in cardiac patients awaits larger randomized trials that target those at risk. A trial of this sort has recently been funded by NIH, to examine the efficacy of cognitive-behavioral interventions on cardiac, psychosocial, and cardiovascular disease risk factor outcomes in lonely and/or depressed post-MI patients.

Clinical Implications

Because of the dearth of large, randomly assigned psychosocial interventions, there is not yet sufficient evidence to recommend or caution against psychosocial interventions for altering cardiac outcomes in patients with CHD. There is, however, ample evidence that improvement in psychosocial functioning can be obtained through the use of standardized, empirically supported therapy protocols administered by mental health professionals to patients who are at psychosocial risk. Improving the quality of life and decreasing the psychological distress of cardiac patients also may have other benefits. First, many of the mechanisms proposed to account for the association between psychosocial factors and cardiovascular disease are behavioral. Thus, decreasing depressive symptoms is hypothesized to decrease smoking rates, increase engagement in physical activity, and improve dietary habits.[101] Second, decreasing psychosocial distress is thought to increase patient compliance with physicians' recommendations, but testing these behavioral mechanisms, as well as the pathophysiologic mechanisms addressed elsewhere, awaits larger, controlled trials.

Cardiologists should be aware of psychosocial risk factors present in their patients. Asking about social support and recent symptoms of depression will identify patients at increased risk of event recurrence or death. Referring such patients to mental health specialists for further diagnostic and intervention investigations may improve patients' quality of life and their behavioral risk factor profile, if not their cardiac outcome.

Cost Implications

Thorough cost-effectiveness and cost-offset analyses are being conducted in some of the recent psychosocial trials. For example, the average cost of adding a behavioral intervention to the treatment of a cardiac patient in one study was $790.[102] The longest and most comprehensive psychosocial intervention (for reducing type A behavior), the Recurrent Coronary Care Project in California, showed MI recurrence decreases for the intervention patients, but treatment required an average of 58 hours per patient. This amount of therapy, when delivered in a group format, as occurred in this trial, would cost on average $1200 per patient.

COMPLIANCE: THE KEY TO SUCCESSFUL INTERVENTIONS

The evidence for the intervention strategies reviewed in this chapter points to the inescapable conclusion that changing lifestyle habits can significantly reduce the risk for cardiovascular disease. No matter how efficacious the intervention strategy is, however, it is doomed to failure unless the patient complies with the requirements of the intervention. Nonadherence crosses treatment regimens, age and gender groups, and socioeconomic strata and, moreover, varies across the treatment course.[1,2] Thus, persons are asked to change their diets, eat less, exercise more, quit smoking, reduce the amount of stress they experience, and change the ways in which they express anger. These changes are difficult. Knowledge of the risks is clearly insufficient to produce changes; most persons know by now that smoking is bad for them, that their diet could be improved, and so on. These behaviors, however, are reinforcing in their own right. Smoking is pleasurable, as is the avoidance of nicotine withdrawal; high-fat foods taste good; and exercise is time-consuming and may be boring and even painful for many persons. Coping with stress and anger means having to examine one's life in ways that may be unpleasant and even traumatic. Thus, poor health habits that may have been reinforced over the course of a lifetime are very resistant to change. Clearly, it is vitally important to begin establishing healthy behavior habits early in life; however, parents and teachers may provide poor models for these behaviors, having been enculturated in a time during which such concerns were virtually nonexistent.

Much of the adherence problem occurs early in treatment. It has been estimated that 50 percent of persons discontinue participation in cardiac rehabilitation programs within the first year.[3] The smoking cessation literature reports a 79 percent relapse rate in the first 6 months.[4] Not only are early adherence problems likely, early adherence rates are predictive of longer-term adherence.[5-7]

The primary care physician and the cardiologist can play a major role in helping persons alter poor health habits and establish healthy behaviors. A physician is regarded by many patients as a source of authority and can have a large impact on behavior change.[103] In addition, a physician can refer patients to other health professionals, such as nutrition and exercise counselors and stress- and anger-reduction therapists. This often does not occur, however, for a number of reasons. First, while most physicians are undoubtedly aware of the importance of healthy behaviors, they may be convinced that patients will not engage in them or may not know how to suggest such changes or to whom to refer these patients. Second, given the current reimbursement climate, many physicians have only a very few minutes to spend with each patient.

The fact is that a great deal is now known about how to maximize the likelihood that patients will adhere to health behavior regimens. One review provides a great amount of detail concerning these regimens[104]; a brief summary is provided below that briefly describes strategies that have been demonstrated to be successful in improving compliance to cardiovascular disease behavioral intervention strategies.

- Signed agreements. A written contract is drawn up between the patient and the physician or other health professional in which a specific set of behaviors to be followed by the patient is agreed on. These behaviors should be as specific as possible (e.g., number of calories per day, number of servings of fruits and vegetables per day, number of minutes of cardiovascular-strengthening exercise, number of hours of stress-reduction therapy). Behavioral logs should be maintained by the patient.
- Behavioral skill training. Patients can attend classes that teach healthy cooking, proper stretching techniques before and after exercise, and how to respond to an anger-provoking situation. Patients may want to engage in healthy behaviors, but without the skills, they tend to fall back on old behaviors.
- Self-monitoring. Many patients are truly unaware of the extent to which they engage in certain unhealthy behaviors. It is useful to have them monitor the number of cigarettes they smoke, their daily intake of fat (current packaging requirements make this relatively easy), and so on. The first step in changing behavior is to establish a baseline so that the patient can see improvement.
- Self-efficacy enhancement. Patients' confidence in their ability to engage in a particular behavior, such as eating in more healthy ways or exercising with a specified frequency, has been shown to be an important factor in their motivation to engage in these behaviors. Self-monitoring (discussed above) provides a baseline level and can document improvement. Even small changes will increase a patient's self-efficacy for a given behavior, so that he or she is motivated to continue. This will produce additional positive change, which then enhances self-efficacy even more, and so on. The physician or other health professional can focus on such improvement as a means of further enhancing the patient's self-efficacy for behavior change.
- Telephone and/or mail contact. Such reminders have been shown to have a positive effect on compliance.
- Spouse and/or social support. A great deal of research has shown that others in the patient's social environment can have a dramatic impact on compliance. When a physician discusses behavior change with the patient, it is helpful for such a support person to be present as well. If an exercise and/or diet regimen is agreed on, possibly using a contract, as was described above, having a support person participate will significantly enhance the likelihood that the patient will

stay with the program. Having an immediate other, such as a spouse, continue in her or his own unhealthy behavior patterns, conversely, such as continuing to smoke or to express anger in an abusive or unhealthy manner, will hinder the possibility for change on the part of the patient.

- Stages of change. Earlier in this chapter, it was noted that different persons may be in different stages of readiness to change behavior.[16] Thus, one patient may be ready only to begin discussing the need to stop smoking, while another may be ready to begin the actual quitting. Research shows that it is helpful to tailor advice to the patient's current stage of readiness. The techniques described above are clearly additive; more than one may be combined usefully to help the patient comply. It is also clear that in trying, many patients will fail. However, it is worth noting that a patient cannot quit smoking until she or he first *tries* to quit, and so efforts to produce this behavior are a good investment of the physician's time.
- The authors strongly recommend that primary care physicians develop a network of health care professionals who can support their efforts and to whom patients can be referred for help with specific intervention strategies.
- Physicians are a long way from eliminating the need for medication and surgical intervention for cardiovascular disease. However, the situation is better than it was only a relatively short time ago. If physicians advocate such strategies, prescribe them, discuss them with patients, and refer patients to other health professionals, a substantial proportion of the need for more traditional interventions can be eliminated.

CONCLUSIONS

The potential applications of behavioral techniques in cardiology are enormous and largely unrealized. In principle, they can help prevent the onset of disease, treat it once it is established, and be used in conjunction with virtually any other kind of treatment. In practice, few cardiologists have the time or interest to pay much attention to them despite the demonstrated efficacy of many programs. Future success depends on better education of physicians, the incorporation of a team approach, and recognition of the value of behavioral interventions by third-party payers.

References

1. McGinnis JM, Foege WH. Actual causes of death in the United States. *JAMA* 1993; 270:2207.
2. Fries JF, Koop CE, Beadle CE, et al. Reducing health care costs by reducing the need and demand for medical services: The Health Project Consortium. *N Engl J Med* 1993; 329:321.
3. Notzon FC, Komarov YM, Ermakov SP, et al. Causes of declining life expectancy in Russia. *JAMA* 1998; 279:793.
4. Hakim AA, Petrovitch H, Burchfiel CM, et al. Effects of walking on mortality among nonsmoking retired men. *N Engl J Med* 1998; 338:94.
5. Lipkus IM, Barefoot JC, Williams RB, et al. Personality measures as predictors of smoking initiation and cessation in the UNC Alumni Heart Study. *Health Psychol* 1994; 13:149.
6. De Leon CFM, Kop WJ, de Swart HB, et al. Psychosocial characteristics and recurrent events after percutaneous transluminal coronary angioplasty. *Am J Cardiol* 1996; 77:252.
7. Glanz K. Nutrition education for risk factor reduction and patient education: A review. *Prev Med* 1999; 14:721.
8. De Lorgeril M, Renaud S, Mamelle N, et al. Mediterranean alpha-linolenic acid-rich diet in secondary prevention of coronary heart disease. *Lancet* 1994; 343:1454.
9. Randomized trial of cholesterol lowering in 4,444 patients with coronary heart disease: Scandinavian Simvastatin Survival Study (4S). *Lancet* 1994; 344:1383.
10. Walden CE, Retzlaff BM, Buck BL, et al. Lipoprotein lipid response to the National Cholesterol Education Program Step II diet by hypercholesterolic and combined hyperlipidemic women and men. *Arterioscler Thromb Vasc Biol* 1997; 17:375.
11. Buefel RR. Assessment of the U.S diet in national nutrition surveys: National collaborative efforts and NHANES. *Am J Clin Nutr* 1994; 59(suppl):1645.
12. Glanz K, Eriksen MP. Individual and community models for dietary behavior change. *J Nutr Educ* 1993; 25:80.
13. Bandura A. *Social Foundations of Thought and Action: A Social Cognitive Theory.* Englewood Cliffs, NJ: Prentice-Hall; 1986.
14. Bandura A. *Self-Efficacy: The Exercise of Control.* New York: Freeman; 1997.
15. Prochaska JO, DiClemente CC. Transtheoretical therapy: Toward a more integrative model of change. *Psycho Ther Res Pract* 1982; 19:276.
16. Prochaska JO, DiClemente CC, Norcross JC. In search of how people change: Applications to addictive behaviors. *Am Psychol* 1992; 47:1102.
17. The sixth report of the Joint National Committee on prevention, detection, evaluation, and treatment of high blood pressure. *Arch Intern Med* 1997; 157:2413.
18. Fiore MC, Jorenby DE, Baker TB. Smoking cessation: Principles and practice based upon the AHCPR Guideline, 1996: Agency for Health Care Policy and Research. *Ann Behav Med* 1997; 19:213.
19. Weintraub WS, Klein LW, Seelaus PA, et al. Importance of total life consumption of cigarettes as a risk factor for coronary artery disease. *Am J Cardiol* 1985; 55:669.
20. Rosenberg L, Kaufman DW, Helmrich SP, et al. The risk of myocardial infarction after quitting smoking in men under 55 years of age. *N Engl J Med* 1985; 313:1511.
21. Gordon T, Kannel WB, McGee D, et al. Death and coronary attacks in men after giving up cigarette smoking: A report from the Framingham study. *Lancet* 1974; 2:1345.
22. Warner KE. Smoking out the incentives for tobacco control in managed care settings. *Tob Control* 1998; 7(suppl):S50.
23. Tomar SL, Husten CG, Manley MW. Do dentists and physicians advise tobacco users to quit? *J Am Dent Assoc* 1996; 127:259.
24. Anda RF, Remington PL, Sienko DG, et al. Are physicians advising smokers to quit? The patient's perspective. *JAMA* 1987; 257:1916.
25. Prochaska JO, Di Clemente CC, Velicer WF, et al. Standardized, individualized, interactive, and personalized self-help programs for smoking cessation. *Health Psychol* 1993; 12:399.
26. Silagy C, Mant D, Fowler G, et al. Meta-analysis on efficacy of nicotine replacement therapies in smoking cessation. *Lancet* 1994; 343:139.
27. Jorenby DE, Leischow SJ, Nides MA, et al. A controlled trial of sustained-release bupropion, a nicotine patch, or both for smoking cessation. *N Engl J Med* 1999; 340:685.
28. Hughes JR, Goldstein MG, Hurt RD, et al. Recent advances in the pharmacotherapy of smoking. *JAMA* 1999; 281:72.
29. Hayford KE, Patten CA, Rummans TA, et al. Efficacy of bupropion for smoking cessation in smokers with a former history of major depression or alcoholism. *Br J Psychiatry* 1999; 174:173.
30. McPhillips-Tangum C. Results from the first annual survey on addressing tobacco in managed care. *Tob Control* 1998; 7(suppl): S11.
31. Keys A. *Seven Countries: A Multivariate Analysis of Death and*

Coronary Heart Disease. Cambridge, MA: Harvard University Press; 1980.

32. Levine G, Keaney J, Vita J. Cholesterol reduction in cardiovascular disease. *N Engl J Med* 1995; 332:512.
33. Lipid Research Clinics Program. The Lipid Research Clinics Coronary Primary Prevention Trial results: I. Reduction in incidence of coronary heart disease. *JAMA* 1984; 251:351.
34. Van Horn L, Kavey RE. Diet and cardiovascular disease prevention: What works? *Ann Behav Med* 1997; 19:197–212.
35. Greenland P, Hayman L. Making cardiovascular disease prevention a reality. *Ann Behav Med* 1997; 19:193.
36. National Cholesterol Education Program: *Report of the Expert Panel on Population Strategies for Blood Cholesterol Reduction*. DHHS Publication No. (NIH) 90-30-46. Bethesda, MD: U.S. Department of Health and Human Services, Public Health Service, National Institutes of Health, National Heart, Lung and Blood Institute; 1990.
37. Holme I. An analysis of randomized trials evaluating the effect of cholesterol reduction on total mortality and coronary heart disease incidence. *Circulation* 1990; 82:1916.
38. Renaud S, de Lorgeril M, Delaye J, et al. Cretan Mediterranean diet for prevention of coronary heart disease. *Am J Clin Nutr* 1995; 61(suppl):1360S.
39. *Nationwide Food Consumption Survey, Continuing Survey of Food Intake by Individuals: Women 19–50 Years and Children 1–5 Years, 4 Days*. Washington, DC: U.S. Department of Agriculture, Human Nutrition Information Service; 1996.
40. Expert Panel on Detection Evaluation and Treatment of High Blood Cholesterol in Adults. Summary of the Second Report of the National Cholesterol Education Program (NCEP) Expert Panel on Detection, Evaluation, and Treatment of High Blood Cholesterol in Adults (Adult Treatment Panel II). *JAMA* 1993; 269:3015.
41. LaRosa JC, Hunninghake D, Bush D, et al. The cholesterol facts: A summary of the evidence relating dietary facts, serum cholesterol, and coronary heart disease: A joint statement by the American Heart Association and the National Heart, Lung, and Blood Institute. *Circulation* 1990; 81:1721.
42. Sempos C, Cleeman J, Carroll M, et al. Prevalence of high blood cholesterol among U.S. adults. *JAMA* 1993; 269:3009.
43. Schucker B, Wittes JT, Santanello NC, et al. Change in cholesterol awareness and action: Results from national physician and public surveys. *Arch Intern Med* 1991; 151:666.
44. Stone NJ. Diet, blood cholesterol levels, and coronary heart disease. *Coron Artery Dis* 1993; 4:871.
45. Princen HM, Van Poppel G, Vogelezang C, et al. Supplementation with vitamin E but not beta-carotene in vivo protects low density lipoprotein from lipid peroxidation in vitro: Effect of cigarette smoking. *Arterioscler Thromb* 1992; 12:554.
46. Stamler MJ, Hennekens CH, Manson JE, et al. Vitamin E consumption and the risk of coronary disease in women. *N Engl J Med* 1993; 328:1444.
47. Steinberg D, Parthasarathy S, Carew TE, et al. Beyond cholesterol: Modifications of low-density lipoprotein that increase its atherogenicity. *N Engl J Med* 1989; 320:915.
48. Hoffman RM, Garewal HS. Antioxidants and the prevention of coronary heart disease. *Arch Intern Med* 1995; 155:241.
49. Boushey CJ, Beresford SAA, Omenn GS, et al. A quantitative assessment of plasma homocysteine as a risk factor for vascular disease: Probable benefits of increasing folic acid intakes. *JAMA* 1995; 274:1049.
50. Hubert HB, Feinleib M, McNamara PM, et al. Obesity as an independent risk factor for cardiovascular disease: A 26-year follow-up of participants in the Framingham Heart Study. *Circulation* 1983; 67:968.
51. Denke MA, Sempos CT, Grundy SM. Excess body weight: An underrecognized contributor to high blood cholesterol levels. *Arch Intern Med* 1993; 153:1093.
52. Medalie JH, Papier CM, Goldbourt U, et al. Major factors in the development of diabetes mellitus in 10,000 men. *Arch Intern Med* 1975; 135:811.
53. Tobian L. Hypertension and obesity. *N Engl J Med* 1978; 298:46.
54. McCarron D. Calcium metabolism in hypertension. *Keio J Med* 1995; 44:105.
55. Health implications of obesity: National Institutes of Health Consensus Development Conference Statement. *Ann Inter Med* 1985; 103:1073.
56. Wood PD, Stefanick ML, Williams PT, et al. The effects on plasma lipoprotein of a prudent weight-reducing diet, with or without exercise, in overweight men and women. *N Engl J Med* 1988; 319:1173.
57. Becque MD, Katch VL, Rocchini AP, et al. Coronary risk incidence of obese adolescents: Reduction by exercise plus diet intervention. *Pediatrics* 1988; 81:605.
58. O'Leary KD, Wilson GT. *Behavior Therapy: Application and Outcome*. Englewood Cliffs, NJ: Prentice-Hall; 1975.
59. Brownell KD, Heckerman C, Westlake R. The behavior control: A descriptive analysis of a large scale program. *J Clin Psychol* 1979; 35:864.
60. Garner D, Wooley S. Confronting the failure of behavior and dietary treatments for obesity. *Clin Psychol Rev* 1991; 11:729.
61. Barnard N, Akhtar A, Nicholson A. Factors that facilitate compliance to lower fat intake. *Arch Fam Med* 1995; 4:153.
62. Tinker L, Burrows E, Henry H, et al. The Women's Health Initiative: Overview of the nutrition components. In: Krummel D, Kris-Etherton P, eds. *Nutrition in Women's Health*. Garthersberg, MD: Aspen; 1996:510.
63. Dolecek TA, Milas NC, Van Horn LV, et al. A long-term nutrition intervention experience: Lipid responses and dietary adherence patterns in the Multiple Risk Factor Intervention Trial (MRFIT). *J Am Diet Assoc* 1986; 86:752.
64. U.S. Department of Health and Human Services. *Healthy People 2000: National Health Promotion and Disease Prevention Objectives*. DHHS Publication No. (PHS) 91-50212. Washington, DC: U.S. Department of Health and Human Services; 1990.
65. Wells KB, Lewis CE, Leake B, et al. The practices of general and subspecialty internists in counseling about smoking and exercise. *Am J Public Health* 1986; 76:1009.
66. Orleans CT, George LK, Houpt JL, et al. Health promotion in primary care: A survey of U.S. family practitioners. *Prev Med* 1985; 14:636.
67. Calfas KJ, Long BJ, Sallis JF, et al. A controlled trial of physician counseling to promote the adoption of physical activity. *Prev Med* 1996; 25:225.
68. Goldstein MG, Pinto BM, Lynn H, et al. Physician-based physical activity counseling for middle-aged and older adults: A randomized trial. *Ann Behav Med* 1999; 21:40.
69. Coleman KJ, Raynor HR, Mueller DM, et al. Providing sedentary adults with choices for meeting their walking goals. *Prev Med* 1999; 28:510.
70. Rozanski A, Blumenthal JA, Kaplan J. Impact of psychological factors on the pathogenesis of cardiovascular disease and implications for therapy. *Circulation* 1999; 99:2192.
71. Kirkland SA, MacLean DR, Langille DB, et al. Knowledge and awareness of risk factors for cardiovascular disease among Canadians 55 to 74 years of age: Results from the Canadian Heart Health Surveys, 1986–1992. *Can Med Assoc J* 1999; 161(suppl 8):S10.
72. Schnall PL, Schwartz JE, Landsbergis PA, et al. A longitudinal study of job strain and ambulatory blood pressure: Results from a three year follow up. *Psychosom Med* 1999; 60:697.
73. Lynch J, Krause N, Kaplan GA, et al. Work place demands,

economic reward, and progression of carotid atherosclerosis. *Circulation* 1997; 96:302.

74. Karasek RA, Baker D, Marxer F, et al. Job decision latitude, job demands, and cardiovascular disease: A prospective study of Swedish men. *Am J Public Health* 1981; 75:694.
75. Karasek RA, Theorell T, Schwartz JE, et al. Job characteristics in relation to the prevalence of myocardial infarction in the U.S. Health Examination Survey (HESS) and the Health and Nutrition Examination Survey (HAINES). *Am J Public Health* 1988; 78:910.
76. Theorell T, Tsutsumi A, Hallqist J, et al. Decision latitude, job strain, and myocardial infarction: A study of working men in Stockholm. *Am J Public Health* 1998; 88:382.
77. Johnson JV, Stewart W, Hall EM, et al. Long-term psychosocial work environment and cardiovascular mortality among Swedish men. *Am J Public Health* 1996; 86:324.
78. Gove WR. Gender differences in mental and physical illness: The effects of fixed roles and nurturant roles. *Soc Sci Med* 1984; 19(2):77.
79. Gabbay FH, Krantz DS, Kop WJ, et al. Triggers of myocardial ischemia during daily life in patients with coronary artery disease: Physical and mental activities, anger and smoking. *J Am Coll Cardiol* 1996; 27:585.
80. Frasure-Smith N, Lesperance F, Juneau M, et al. Gender, depression, and one-year prognosis after myocardial infarction. *Psychosom Med* 1999; 61:26.
81. Denollet J, Brutsaert DL. Personality, disease severity, and the risk of long-term cardiac events in patients with a decreased ejection fraction after myocardial infarction. *Circulation* 1998; 97:167.
82. Hermann C, Brand-Driehorst S, Kaminsky B, et al. Diagnosis groups and depressed mood as predictors of 22-month mortality in medical patients. *Psychosom Med* 1998; 60:570.
83. Frasure-Smith N, Lesperance F, Talajic M. Depression and 18-month prognosis after myocardial infarction. *Circulation* 1995; 91:999.
84. Frasure-Smith N, Lesperance F, Talajic M. The impact of negative emotions on prognosis following myocardial infarction: Is it more than depression? *Health Psychol* 1995; 14:388.
85. Moser DK, Dracup K. Is anxiety early after myocardial infarction associated with subsequent ischemic and arrhythmic events? *Psychosom Med* 1996; 58:395.
86. Haines AP, Imeson JD, Meade TW. Phobic anxiety and ischemic heart disease. *Br Med J* 1987; 295:297.
87. Kawachi I, Colditz GA, Ascherio A, et al. Prospective study of phobic anxiety and risk of coronary heart disease in men. *Circulation* 1994; 89:1992.
88. Kawachi I, Sparrow D, Vokonas PS, et al. Symptoms of anxiety and risk of coronary heart disease: The Normative Aging Study. *Circulation* 1994; 90:2225.
89. Kawachi I, Sparrow D, Vokonas PS, et al. Decreased heart rate variability in men with phobic anxiety (data from the Normative Aging Study). *Am J Cardiol* 1995; 75:882.
90. Watkins LL, Grossman P, Krishnan R, et al. Anxiety and vagal control of heart risk. *Psychosom Med* 1998; 60:498.
91. Friedman M, Rosenman RH. Association of specific overt behavior pattern with blood and cardiovascular findings: Blood cholesterol level, blood clotting time, incidence of arcus senilis, and clinical coronary artery disease. *JAMA* 1959; 169:1286.
92. Miller TQ, Turner CW, Tindale RS, et al. Reasons for the trend toward null findings in research on Type A behavior. *Psychol Bull* 1991; 110:469.
93. Koskenvuo M, Kaprio J, Rose RJ, et al. Hostility as a risk factor for mortality and ischemic heart disease in men. *Psychosom Med* 1988; 50:330.
94. Hecker MHL, Chesney MA, Blacks GW, et al. Coronary-prone behaviors in the Western Collaborative Group Study. *Psychosom Med* 1988; 50:153.
95. Dembroski TM, MacDougall JM, Costa PT, et al. Components of hostility as predictors of sudden death and myocardial infarction in the Multiple Risk Factor Intervention Trial. *Psychosom Med* 1989; 51:514.
96. Lau J, Antman EM, Jimenez-Silva J, et al. Cumulative meta-analysis of therapeutic trials for myocardial infarction. *N Engl J Med* 1992; 327:248.
97. Linden W, Stossel C, Maurice J. Psychosocial interventions for patients with coronary artery disease: A meta-analysis. *Arch Intern Med* 1996; 156:745.
98. Frasure-Smith N, Lesperance F, Prince RH, et al. Randomized trial of home-based psychosocial nursing intervention for patients recovering from myocardial infarction. *Lancet* 1997; 350:473.
99. Jones DA, West RR. Psychological rehabilitation after myocardial infarction: Multicentre randomized controlled trial. *Br Med J* 1996; 313:1517.
100. Frasure-Smith N. In-hospital symptoms of psychological stress as predictors of long-term outcome after acute myocardial infarction in men. *Am J Cardiol* 1991; 67:121.
101. Davidson K, Jonas B, Dixon K, et al. Do depression symptoms predict early hypertension incidence in young adults from the CARDIA study? *Arch Intern Med* 2000; 160:1495.
102. Oldridge N, Furlong W, Feeny D, et al. Economic evaluation of cardiac rehabilitation soon after acute myocardial infarction. *Am J Cardiol* 1993; 72:154.
103. Caggiula A, Watson J, Kuller L, et al. Cholesterol-lowering intervention program: Effect of the Step I diet in community office practices. *Arch Intern Med* 1996; 156:1205.
104. Ammerman A, Caggiula A, Elmer PJ, et al. Putting medical practice guidelines into practice: The cholesterol model. *Am J Prev Med* 1994; 10:209.

INDEX

NOTE: Boldface numbers indicate the start of the main discussion of the topic; numbers followed by an *f* or a *t* refer to figures and tables, respectively.

C

D

F

J

K

M

O

Q

R

T

ISBN 0-07-135694-0
90000
9 780071 356947
FUSTER/HURST'S THE HEART
10E